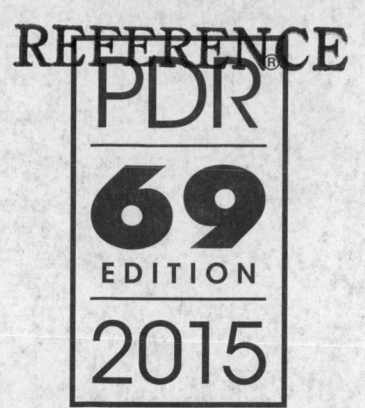

REFERENCE

PDR

69 EDITION

2015

PHYSICIANS' DESK REFERENCE®

TOURO COLLEGE LIBRARY

Kings Hwy

Chief Executive Officer: Mark Heinold
Chief Medical Officer: Salvatore Volpe, MD, FAAP, FACP, CHCQM

Executive Vice President and Chief Financial Officer: Gary Lubin
Chief Technology Officer: David Cheng
Senior Vice President, Marketing, Business Analytics & Pharmacy Discount Program: Barbara Senich, BSN, MBA, MPH
Senior Vice President, Digital Products: Eugene Lee
Senior Vice President, Strategy & Innovation: Stephen Buck

Vice President, Sales: Dennis McCormack
Director, Customer Services & Sales Operations: Karen Fass
Directors, Strategic Accounts: Mike Baczynski, Nick Clark, Robert Davison, Chris McCarthy, William Springgate, Dan Stokes

Vice President, Clinical & Regulatory Solutions: Mukesh Mehta, DPh, MBA, RPh

Associate Director, Clinical Operations: Anila Patel, PharmD
Associate Manager, Clinical Content Development: Demyana Farag, PharmD

Associate Manager, Clinical Operations: Pauline Lee, PharmD
Senior Drug Information Specialist: Kristine Mecca, PharmD
Drug Information Specialists: Vanessa Azevedo, PharmD; Autri Sajedeen, PharmD
Managing Clinical Editor: Julia Tonelli, MD
Medical Editor: Christa Mary Kronick, MA

Senior Director, Marketing: Kim Marich
Manager, Corporate Communications: Thomas W. Eck
Manager, Art Department: Livio Udina

Associate Vice President, Operations: Jeffrey D. Schaefer
Director, Manufacturing & Distribution: Thomas Westburgh
Associate Director, Operations: Noel Deloughery
Senior Content Operations Specialist: Allison O'Hare
Senior Production Coordinator: Yasmin Hernández
Production Coordinator: Eric Udina
Associate Manager, Fulfillment: Gary Lew
Senior Client Services Manager: Jennifer Park
Customer Service Supervisor: Ricardo Plaisir

Copyright ©2014 PDR Network, LLC. Published by PDR Network, LLC at Montvale, NJ 07645-1725. All rights reserved. None of the content of this publication may be reproduced, stored in a retrieval system, resold, redistributed, or transmitted in any form or by any means (electronic, mechanical, photocopying, recording, or otherwise) without the prior written permission of PDR Network, LLC. Physicians' Desk Reference®, PDR Network®, PDR.net®, *mobile*PDR®, and PDR® are registered trademarks of PDR Network, LLC. PDR® for Nonprescription Drugs; PDR® Pharmacopoeia; PDR® BRIEF, PDR®+, PDR® Search, and PDR®3D are trademarks of PDR Network, LLC.

WITHDRAWN

D0845631

KH

REFERENCE
PDR
69
EDITION
2015

PHYSICIANS

ISBN: 978-1-56363-830-5

8/10/15

FOREWORD TO THE 69th EDITION

About PDR Network, LLC

PDR Network, LLC (PDR Network) is committed to ensuring that prescribers have access to the right drug labeling, safety, and other clinically relevant information at the point of prescribing. PDR Network distributes this information through the PDR® suite of digital and print services, which includes: (1) the *Physicians' Desk Reference® (PDR®)*, the most highly trusted drug information reference available in the U.S., now available in multiple formats; (2) PDR interactive drug information services for prescribers embedded in their Electronic Health Record (EHR) systems; (3) PDR.net®, the Internet home of the *PDR*; (4) *mobile*PDR®; and (5) PDR Drug Alerts, the only specialty-specific service that provides electronic delivery of U.S. Food and Drug Administration (FDA)-approved Drug Alerts to physicians and other healthcare professionals.

By improving the communication of important medication information and FDA-approved Drug Alerts, PDR Network's unique services enhance patient safety and may help to reduce prescribers' medical liability. For more information or to sign up for electronic PDR Drug Alerts, visit PDR.net.

About the *Physicians' Desk Reference (PDR)*

The *PDR* book and related products are produced by PDR Network in cooperation with participating manufacturers, and contains FDA-approved product labeling. In accordance with current FDA policies, *PDR* also includes prescribing information provided by manufacturers for products marketed without FDA approval, as well as information on some dietary supplements and other products. PDR Network makes this information available in multiple formats, including both the classic print edition and the new digital eBook version.

For ease of use, *PDR* includes color-coded indices (designated with white, pink, or blue pages at the front of the book), and a Generic/Brand Cross-Reference Table in Section 2. This table can help prescribers quickly locate the brand names associated with specific active ingredients as well as their product indications. In addition, manufacturer-supplied information on dietary supplements is listed separately in Section 6.

Each full-length product information entry in *PDR* provides you with an exact, formatted copy of the product's FDA-approved or other manufacturer-supplied labeling. Under the Federal Food, Drug, and Cosmetic (FD&C) Act, a drug approved for marketing may be labeled, promoted, and advertised by the manufacturer for only those uses for which the drug's safety and effectiveness have been established. The Code of Federal Regulations [Title 21 Section 201.100(d)(1)] pertaining to labeling for prescription products requires that for *PDR* content "indications, effects, dosages, routes, methods, and frequency and duration of administration, and any relevant warnings, hazards, contraindications, side effects, and precautions" must be the "*same in language and emphasis*" as the approved labeling for the products. The FDA regards the words *same in language and emphasis* as requiring VERBATIM use of the approved labeling when providing such information. Furthermore, information that is emphasized in the FDA-approved labeling by the use of type set in a box, or in capitals, boldface, or italics, must be given the same emphasis in *PDR*.

The FDA has acknowledged that the FD&C Act does not limit the manner in which a physician may use an approved drug. Once a product has been approved for marketing, a physician may choose to prescribe it for uses, treatment regimens, or patient populations that are not included in the approved labeling. The FDA also observed that accepted medical practice includes drug use that is not reflected in approved drug labeling. In addition, the dietary supplements listed in Section 6 are marketed under the Dietary Supplement Health and Education Act of 1994 (DSHEA). Products marketed under the DSHEA do not receive formal evaluation or approval from the FDA. The following disclaimer applies to all product information listed in Section 6, as mandated by the federal government: *These statements have not been evaluated by the Food and Drug Administration. This product is not intended to diagnose, treat, cure, or prevent any disease.*

The function of PDR Network is the compilation, organization, and distribution of this information. All product information appearing in *PDR* is made possible through the courtesy of the manufacturers whose products appear in it. The information concerning each product has been provided by its manufacturer and in each instance fully approved by such manufacturer prior to publication by PDR Network. In organizing and presenting the material in *PDR*, PDR Network does not warrant or guarantee any of the products described, or perform any independent analysis in connection with any of the product information contained herein. PDR Network does not assume, and expressly disclaims, any obligation to obtain and include any information other than that provided to it by the manufacturers. It should be understood that by making this material available, PDR Network is not advocating the use of any product described herein, nor is PDR Network responsible for the use of a product, or the use and/or misuse of a product due to typographical error. Additional information on any product may be obtained from the manufacturer.

Updates to *PDR*

The book edition of *PDR* contains the latest information available when the edition closes for new material. As new drugs are released and new research data, clinical findings, and safety information emerge throughout the year, it is the responsibility of the manufacturer to provide that information to the medical community and revise that information accordingly in PDR's database. These revisions are distributed in *PDR Updates*, on PDR.net, *mobile*PDR, and within EHR systems and other healthcare IT systems where integrated. To be certain that prescribers have the most current data, they should always consult the *PDR Updates*, PDR.net, *mobile*PDR, and the eDrug Updates or the applicable *PDR* modules in their EHR before prescribing or administering any product described in the following pages.

Electronic PDR Resources

PDR.net

PDR.net, a web portal designed specifically for prescribers, provides trusted, professional drug information, including full FDA-approved labeling as well as concise point-of-care drug information. **PDR.net** provides prescribers with online access to the authoritative drug information they need to support their treatment decisions.

mobilePDR

mobilePDR provides the only source for FDA-approved full product labeling and concise point-of-care drug information from the PDR database directly on a mobile device. Prescribing information on more than 2,500 drugs, full-color product images, and frequent updates provide up-to-date drug information. **mobilePDR** is free for U.S.-based MDs, DOs, NPs, and PAs in full-time patient practice and can be downloaded for all major mobile platforms from PDR.net. A new version of **mobilePDR** is currently in development and scheduled to be released this spring. Visit PDR.net for more information on the new mobile product, including the launch announcement and directions for downloading (when available).

PDR Drug Alerts

FDA-approved Drug Alerts are delivered electronically to physicians and other prescribers who register to receive them at PDR.net, through participating medical societies, or by returning the verification form distributed with complimentary copies of *PDR*.

Electronic Health Records

PDR Network's services for EHRs offer prescribers a comprehensive suite of free, interactive EHR tools—including drug labeling information, boxed warnings, drug safety alerts, and patient education and financial support programs that deliver critical drug information to help prescribers provide optimal patient care.

PDR Network's services for EHRs are convenient and readily accessible for prescribers within their workflow at no cost to prescribers or their patients. Many medical societies and medical insurance and malpractice carriers have endorsed the use of such services to their prescribing members and clients. To request PDR Network's services in their EHR, prescribers should contact their EHR vendor. PDR Network services for EHRs include:

PDR® BRIEF

PDR BRIEF offers an intuitive dashboard of full labeling information and provider resources delivered within the prescriber's EHR system to support their treatment decisions within their workflow. **PDR BRIEF** surfaces when a medication is selected, to ensure prescribers have the most current full prescribing information, label updates, boxed warnings, patient education, financial support, adherence, and other clinically relevant resources available.

PDR®+ *for Patients*

PDR+ *for Patients* drug education guides are designed to help patients understand the drugs prescribed by their physicians. Available in the EHR workflow, the guides are easy to print and hand out during an office visit or automatically send to the Patient Portal. By addressing potential concerns early on and sharing **PDR+ *for Patients***, physicians can help their patients start and stay on therapy.

PDR® Search

PDR Search delivers an unparalleled interactive and searchable drug database of drug labeling and safety and product support information. **PDR Search** supplies full drug prescribing information and prescribing summaries with access to FDA and PDR Drug Alerts, as well as patient education, financial support, adherence and other clinically relevant resources, directly through their EHR application.

Patient Financial Support

PDR® Pharmacy Discount Card

This free program provides patients with access to medications at discounted prices, helping them save up to 75% and an average of 38% on their prescriptions at more than 60,000 pharmacies nationwide. PDR Network distributes this program via healthcare provider offices, allowing them to share the program with their patients directly. The program is offered at no cost to participating providers or their patients. If prescribers are not already enrolled, they can call 800-232-7379 or visit PDR.net/PharmacyDiscountCard.

For more information on these or any other PDR Network products, please call toll-free 800-232-7379; fax 201-722-2680; or visit PDRNetwork.com. To order a PDR Network publication, visit PDRBooks.com.

Any portion of PDR Network's products that is reproduced, duplicated, copied, downloaded, sold, resold, or otherwise exploited for any commercial purpose without the express written consent of PDR Network, is prohibited. Any use of trademarks, logos, or other proprietary information (including images, text, page layout, and form) of PDR Network's products and/or its affiliates without the express written consent of PDR Network is also prohibited. For more information about licensing PDR Network content, please contact Gary Lubin at (201) 358-7161 or Gary.Lubin@PDR.net.

CONTENTS

CONTENTS

SECTION 1

MANUFACTURERS' INDEX

Listed in this index are all manufacturers participating in the *Physicians' Desk Reference®*. It is through their courtesy that the *PDR®* is brought to the medical profession.

Each company's entry may include the address, phone, and fax number of its headquarters and regional offices, as well as email address, website, and contacts for inquiries, orders, and medical emergency information. Products with entries in the Product Information section are listed with their page numbers. Other products available from the manufacturer are listed following the described products.

If an entry in the index lists multiple page numbers, the first one shown refers to images of the product; the last one refers to its prescribing information.

- **Bold page numbers** indicate full prescribing information.

- *Italic page numbers* signify partial information.

- The ◆ symbol marks drugs shown in the Product Identification Guide.

◆ **Shown in Product Identification Guide**

Italic Page Number **Indicates Brief Listing**

MANUFACTURERS' INDEX

NSE PRODUCTS, INC.   **2457**
(PHARMANEX)
75 West Center Street
Provo, UT 84601

For Information and Product Support:
1-(800) 487-1000
Website: www.nuskin.com

Products Described:
ageLOC R² Day Capsules.........2457
ageLOC R² Night Capsules.......2457
ageLOC TR90 Control Capsules....2457
ageLOC TR90 Fit Capsules......2457
ageLOC TR90 JumpStart
  Powder......................2457
ageLOC TR90 TrimShake
  Powder......................2457
CordyMax Cs-4 Capsules.........2457
LifePak Capsules...............2457
MarineOmega Softgel Capsules....2458
ReishiMax GLp Capsules.........2458
Tegreen 97 Capsules............2458

ONYX   **311, 2071**
PHARMACEUTICALS,
INC.
249 E. Grand Avenue
South San Francisco, CA 94080

Direct Inquiries to:
Phone: 877-ONYX-121 (669-9121)
Fax: 877-ONX-PHRM (669-7476)
Email: medinfo@onyx.com

Products Described:
◆Kyprolis for Injection.........311, 2071

OTSUKA AMERICA   **311, 2075**
PHARMACEUTICAL,
INC.
2440 Research Boulevard
Rockville, MD 20850

Direct Medical Inquiries to:
Medical Affairs
Otsuka America Pharmaceutical, Inc.
(800) 441-6763
Fax: (301) 212-8634

To Request Routine or Emergency Medical Information, or to Report an Adverse Experience:
(800) 438-9927

Products Described:
◆Abilify Maintena
  Extended-Release Injectable
  Suspension.................311, 2075
◆Samsca Tablets................311, 2441

PERQUE INTEGRATIVE   **2458**
HEALTH
44621 Guilford Drive, Suite 150
Ashburn, VA 20147

Direct Inquiries to:
(800) 525-7372

Products Described:
Perque Life Guard Tabsules........2458
Perque Potent C Guard Powder....2459
Perque Repair Guard Tabsules......2459
Perque Vessel Health Guard
  Lozenges....................2459
Perque Whey Guard Repair
  Powder......................2459

PFIZER INC.   **2084**
235 East 42nd Street
New York, NY 10017-5755

For updates to the product information listed below, please check the Pfizer Web site http://www.pfizerpro.com or call (800) 438-1985.

For Medical Information, Contact:
(800) 438-1985
24 hours a day, 7 days a week

Distribution:
1855 Shelby Oaks Drive North
Memphis, TN 38134
(901) 387-5200

Customer Service:
(800) 533-4535

Pfizer Companies Include:
Agouron Pharmaceuticals
King Pharmaceuticals, Inc.
Parke-Davis
Pharmacia & Upjohn
G.D. Searle & Co.
Wyeth Pharmaceuticals

◆ **Shown in Product Identification Guide**

Products Described:
Viagra Tablets.................2084
Xeljanz Tablets................2091

Other Products Available:
Accupril Tablets
Accuretic Tablets
Aldactazide Tablets
Alsuma Injection
Altace Capsules
Aromasin Tablets
Arthrotec Tablets
Atgam Sterile Solution
Avinza Capsules
Azulfidine Tablets, EN-Tabs
Bicillin L-A Injection
Bosulif Tablets
Caduet Tablets
Calan Tablets, SR Caplets
Camptosar for Injection
Cardura Tablets, XL Tablets
Caverject
Celebrex Capsules
Celontin Capsules
Chantix Tablets
Cleocin HCl Capsules
Cleocin Pediatric for Oral Solution, USP
Cleocin Phosphate Sterile Solution
Cleocin T Topical Gel, Lotion, Solution
Cleocin Vaginal Cream, Ovules
Colestid Tablets, Oral Suspension
Colestid/Flavored Colestid for Oral
  Suspension
Cortef Tablets
Daypro Caplets
Depo-Estradiol Injectable Solution
Depo-Medrol Injectable Suspension
Depo-Provera
depo-subQ provera Injectable Suspension
Depo-Testosterone Injection
Detrol Tablets
Detrol LA Capsules
Didrex Tablets
Diflucan
Dilantin
Elelyso Injection
Ellence Injection
Embeda Extended Release Capsules
Emcyt Capsules
Eraxis for Injection
Estring Vaginal Ring
Feldene Capsules
Flagyl
Flector Patch
Gelfilm Sterile Film
Gelfoam Sterile Powder, Sponge
Genotropin Lyophilized Powder
Geodon
Glucotrol Tablets, XL Tablets
Glynase PresTab Tablets
Glyset Tablets
Halcion Tablets
Hemabate Sterile Solution (Sales
  restricted to hospitals only)
Idamycin
Inlyta Tablets
Inspra Tablets
Levoxyl Tablets
Lincocin Sterile Solution
Lipitor Tablets
Lomotil Tablets
Lopid Tablets
Lyrica Capsules, Oral Solution
Medrol Tablets and Dosepak
Mycobutin Capsules
Nardil Tablets
Neurontin Capsules, Tablets, Oral
  Solution
Nitrostat Tablets
Norpace
Norvasc Tablets
Oxecta Tablets
Pfizerpen for Injection
Prepidil Gel
Procardia Capsules, XL Tablets
Prostin E2 Vaginal Suppository
Prostin VR Pediatric Sterile Solution
Provera Tablets
Relpax Tablets
Revatio Injection, Tablets
R-Gene 10 for Intravenous Use
Skelaxin Tablets
Solu-Cortef Injection
Solu-Medrol Injection
Somavert for Injection
Sutent Capsules
Tikosyn Capsules
Toviaz Extended-Release Tablets
Unasyn
VFEND
Vibramycin
Xalatan Sterile Ophthalmic Solution
Xalkori Capsules
Xanax Tablets, XR Tablets
Zithromax
Zmax for Oral Suspension
Zoloft
Zyvox

PIVOTAL   **311, 2098**
THERAPEUTICS INC.
81 Zenway Blvd.
Unit #10
Woodbridge, Ontario L4H 0S5
Canada
Telephone: 1-905-856-9797

Direct Inquiries to:
Pivotal Therapeutics (US), Inc.
3651 FAU Blvd., Suite 400
Boca Raton, FL 33431
United States
Telephone: 1-888-358-2080
Telephone: 1-561-288-5231
Email: info@pivotaltherapeutics.us
Website: www.pivotaltherapeutics.us

Products Described:
◆Vascazen......................311, 2098

PURDUE PHARMA L.P.   **312, 2101**
One Stamford Forum
Stamford, CT 06901-3431

For Medical Inquiries:
(888) 726-7535

Adverse Drug Experiences:
(888) 726-7535

Customer Service:
(800) 877-5666
FAX: (800) 877-3210

Products Described:
◆Butrans Transdermal
  System....................312, 2101
◆Dilaudid Injection............312, 2112
◆Dilaudid Oral Liquid.........312, 2110
◆Dilaudid Tablets.............312, 2110
◆Dilaudid-HP Injection........312, 2112
◆Dilaudid-HP Lyophilized
  Powder 250 mg............312, 2112
◆Intermezzo Sublingual
  Tablet...................312, 2117
◆OxyContin Tablets............312, 2122

RANBAXY   **312, 2129**
LABORATORIES INC.
9431 Florida Mining Boulevard East
Jacksonville, Florida 32257

Direct Inquiries to:
(609) 720-9200

Products Described:
◆Absorica Capsules............312, 2129

RECORDATI RARE   **312, 2136**
DISEASES, INC.
100 Corporate Drive
Lebanon, NJ 08833

Direct Inquiries to:
(908) 236-0888

Products Described:
◆Chemet Capsules.............312, 2136
NeoProfen Injection...............2138
◆Panhematin for Injection......313, 2140

RLC LABS, INC.   **312, 2141**
Cave Creek, AZ 85331

For Product Information:
(877) 797-7997
sales@rlclabs.com

For Customer Service & Ordering Information:
(877) 797-7997
FAX: (623) 879-8683
customerservice@rlclabs.com
www.rlclabs.com

Products Described:
◆Nature-Throid Tablets.........312, 2141
◆WP Thyroid Tablets...........312, 2143

SALIX   **313, 2145**
PHARMACEUTICALS,
INC.
8510 Colonnade Center Drive
Raleigh, NC 27615

Direct Inquiries to:
(866) 669-7597 Phone
(919) 862-1817 Fax
www.salix.com

For adverse events, product quality complaints and patient information requests:
Product Information Center
(800) 508-0024 Phone
(510) 595-8183 Fax
E-mail: customerservice@salix.com

Products Described:
◆Apriso Extended-Release
  Capsules..................313, 2145
◆Cycloset Tablets.............313, 2147
◆Fulyzaq Delayed-Release
  Tablets...................313, 2152
◆MoviPrep Powder for Oral
  Solution..................313, 2154
◆Relistor Subcutaneous
  Injection.................313, 2157
◆Uceris Extended-Release
  Tablets...................313, 2165
◆Xifaxan Tablets..............313, 2168

Other Products Available:
Anusol-HC Cream 2.5%
Anusol-HC Suppository 25 mg
Azasan Tablets
Deflux
Diuril Oral Suspension
Fenoglide Tablets
Giazo Tablets
Glumetza Extended-Release Tablets
Metozolv Orally Disintegrating Tablets
OsmoPrep Tablets
Pepcid Oral Suspension
Proctocort Cream 1%
Proctocort Suppository 30 mg
Ruconest C1 Esterase Inhibitor
  (Recombinant)
Solesta Syringes
Zegerid Capsules
Zegerid Powder for Oral Suspension

SCHERING CORP.
(See MERCK)

SMITH & NEPHEW, INC.   **313, 2172**
3909 Hulen Street
Fort Worth, TX 76107

Direct Inquiries to:
(800) 441-8227

Products Described:
◆Collagenase Santyl
  Ointment..................313, 2172

STIEFEL   **2173**
LABORATORIES, INC.
20 T. W. Alexander Drive
Research Triangle Park
North Carolina 27709

Direct Inquiries to:
GSK Response Center
1-888-825-5249
www.gsk.com

Products Described:
Altabax Ointment..................2173
Bactroban Cream..................2176
Bactroban Nasal..................2177
Bactroban Ointment...............2178
Duac Gel........................2178
Fabior Foam.....................2181
Soriatane Capsules................2184
Sorilux Foam, 0.005%............2192
Veltin Gel......................2194

SUNOVION   **313, 2197**
PHARMACEUTICALS
INC.
84 Waterford Drive
Marlborough, MA 01752
(508) 481-6700

For Medical Information Inquiries:
Medical Information
(800) 739-0565
minfo@sunovion.com
www.SunovionMedical.com
For Adverse Event Reporting:
(877) 737-7226
For Customer Service:
(888) 394-7377
CAC@sunovion.com

Products Described:
◆Aptiom Tablets...............313, 2197
◆Brovana Inhalation Solution...313, 2203
◆Latuda Tablets...............313, 2209

Italic Page Number **Indicates Brief Listing**

MANUFACTURERS' INDEX

◆ **Shown in Product Identification Guide**   *Italic Page Number* **Indicates Brief Listing**

BRAND AND GENERIC NAME INDEX

This index includes all entries in the Product Information section. Products are listed alphabetically by both brand and generic name. Generic names are underlined; brand names are not. Under each generic name, you will find a list of the brand names that are associated with the generic product. This enables you to find a product by either of its names. For example, the brand Amerge appears once in the A's, and again under its generic name, naratriptan hydrochloride.

Each time a brand name appears, it is followed by the manufacturer's name and the page number to consult for further information. If multiple page numbers appear, the first one refers to images of the product; the last one refers to its prescribing information. Under a generic heading, all fully described brands are listed first, followed by those with only partial information.

- **Bold page numbers** indicate full prescribing information.

- *Italic page numbers* signify partial information.

- The ◆ symbol marks drugs shown in the Product Identification Guide.

BRAND AND GENERIC NAME INDEX

BRAND AND GENERIC NAME INDEX

BRAND AND GENERIC NAME INDEX

BRAND AND GENERIC NAME INDEX

◆ Shown in Product Identification Guide   Underline Denotes Generic Name   *Italic Page Number* Indicates Brief Listing

BRAND AND GENERIC NAME INDEX

BRAND AND GENERIC NAME INDEX

BRAND AND GENERIC NAME INDEX

BRAND AND GENERIC NAME INDEX

◆ **Shown in Product Identification Guide**   <u>Underline</u> **Denotes Generic Name**   *Italic Page Number* **Indicates Brief Listing**

GENERIC/BRAND CROSS-REFERENCE TABLE

This table includes a list of more than 200 of the top prescribed products dispensed in the pharmacy setting, identified by generic name. For ease of use, products are listed alphabetically with reference to the corresponding brand name(s) available on the market. Additionally, the table contains indications for each product; if indications differ either by the way the drug is supplied (ie, injection, cream, etc.) or by specific brand, it is noted.

Products with full prescribing information listed in the *PDR®* are in **boldface** in the Brand(s) column. Please go to PDR.net® to view prescribing information on a particular product.

GENERIC	BRAND(S)	INDICATION(S)
Abatacept	**Orencia**	arthritis; arthritis, juvenile idiopathic; arthritis, rheumatoid
Abiraterone	Zytiga	cancer, prostate
Acellular Pertussis/ Reduced Diphtheria Toxoid/ Tetanus Toxoid	**Boostrix**	vaccine
Acetaminophen/Hydrocodone	Anexsia, Lorcet, Lortab, Maxidone, Norco, **Vicodin**, **Vicodin ES**, Zydone	pain
Adalimumab	**Humira**	ankylosing spondylitis; arthritis, psoriatic; arthritis, rheumatoid; colitis, ulcerative; Crohn's disease; psoriasis
Adapalene/Benzoyl Peroxide	Epiduo	acne
Albuterol Sulfate	Albuterol Tabs/Syrup (generic), **ProAir HFA**, **Proventil HFA**, **Ventolin HFA**	asthma, bronchospasm
Albuterol Sulfate/Ipratropium Bromide	Combivent, Combivent Respimat, Duoneb	bronchospasm, COPD
Aliskiren	**Tekturna**	hypertension
Amlodipine Besylate/ Hydrochlorothiazide/Olmesartan	Tribenzor	hypertension
Amlodipine Besylate/ Hydrochlorothiazide/Valsartan	**Exforge HCT**	hypertension
Amlodipine Besylate/ Olmesartan Medoxomil	Azor	hypertension
Amlodipine Besylate/Valsartan	**Exforge**	hypertension
Amphetamine/ Dextroamphetamine	Adderall, Adderall XR	Adderall: narcolepsy Adderall, Adderall XR: ADHD
Apixaban	**Eliquis**	deep vein thrombosis; pulmonary embolism; stroke, reduce risk; surgical adjunct/aid; thrombosis prevention
Aripiprazole	Abilify	autistic disorder, irritability; bipolar disorder; depression; major depressive disorder; mania; psychosis; schizophrenia
Armodafinil	Nuvigil	narcolepsy, shift work disorder
Ascorbic Acid/Polyethylene Glycol 3350/Potassium Chloride/ Sodium Ascorbate/Sodium Chloride/Sodium Sulfate	**MoviPrep**	bowel cleansing, diagnostic aid

Please go to **PDR.net** to view Prescribing Information for these and other products.

Aspirin/Dipyridamole	Aggrenox	stroke; stroke, reduce risk
Atazanavir	**Reyataz**	AIDS, HIV
Atomoxetine	Strattera	ADHD
Atorvastatin Calcium	Lipitor	angina, reduce risk; hypercholesterolemia; hyperlipidemia; myocardial infarction, reduce risk; revascularization, reduce risk; stroke, reduce risk
Azelaic Acid	Azelex, Finacea	Azelex: acne Finacea: rosacea
Azelastine HCl	Astelin, Astepro	allergy, rhinitis
Azelastine/Fluticasone Propionate	Dymista	allergy, rhinitis
Beclomethasone Dipropionate	Qvar	asthma
Bendamustine	Treanda	leukemia, non-Hodgkin's lymphoma
Besifloxacin	Besivance	conjunctivitis; infections, bacterial/ophthalmic
Bevacizumab	Avastin	cancer, cervical; cancer, colorectal; cancer, lung; cancer, renal; glioblastoma
Bimatoprost	Latisse, Lumigan	Latisse: hypotrichosis Lumigan: glaucoma/IOP
Bortezomib	Velcade	lymphoma, multiple myeloma
Brimonidine Tartrate	Alphagan P	glaucoma/IOP
Brimonidine Tartrate/ Timolol Maleate	Combigan	glaucoma/IOP
Brinzolamide	Azopt	glaucoma/IOP
Budesonide	Pulmicort Flexhaler	asthma
Budesonide/Formoterol Fumarate Dihydrate	Symbicort	asthma, COPD
Buprenorphine HCl	Buprenex, **Butrans**	pain
Buprenorphine HCl/Naloxone	Suboxone, Zubsolv	opioid dependence
Canagliflozin	Invokana	diabetes
Capecitabine	Xeloda	cancer, breast; cancer, colon; cancer, colorectal
Carvedilol	**Coreg, Coreg CR**	congestive heart failure; hypertension; myocardial infarction, postmanagement
Celecoxib	Celebrex	ankylosing spondylitis; arthritis, osteo; arthritis, rheumatoid; dysmenorrhea; pain
Cinacalcet	Sensipar	hypercalcemia of malignancy, hyperparathyroidism
Ciprofloxacin HCl/ Dexamethasone	Ciprodex	infections, otic; inflammation, otic; otitis externa; otitis media
Cobicistat/Elvitegravir/ Emtricitabine/Tenofovir Disoproxil Fumarate	**Stribild**	AIDS, HIV
Colchicine	**Colcrys**	Familial Mediterranean fever, gout
Colesevelam HCl	WelChol	diabetes, hypercholesterolemia, hyperlipidemia

GENERIC/BRAND CROSS-REFERENCE TABLE

Please go to **PDR.net** to view Prescribing Information for these and other products.

Conjugated Estrogens	Cenestin, Enjuvia, Premarin Tablets, Premarin Vaginal	Cenestin, Enjuvia: menopause; vaginitis, atrophic Premarin Tablets: cancer, breast; cancer, prostate; hypoestrogenism; menopause; osteoporosis; vaginitis, atrophic Premarin Vaginal: vaginitis, atrophic
Conjugated Estrogens/ Medroxyprogesterone	Prempro	menopause; osteoporosis; vaginitis, atrophic
Cyclosporine Ophthalmic	Restasis	inflammation, ophthalmic; keratoconjunctivitis sicca
Dabigatran Etexilate Mesylate	Pradaxa	deep vein thrombosis; pulmonary embolism; stroke, reduce risk; thrombosis prevention
Dapsone Topical	Aczone	acne
Daptomycin	Cubicin	bacteremia; endocarditis; infections, bacterial/skin; infections, bacterial/systemic
Darbepoetin Alfa	Aranesp	anemia, chemotherapy adjunct
Darunavir	Prezista	AIDS, HIV
Denosumab	Xgeva	bone metastases; cancer, bone
Desvenlafaxine	Pristiq	depression, major depressive disorder
Dexlansoprazole	**Dexilant**	erosive esophagitis, GERD, heartburn
Dexmethylphenidate HCl	Focalin, **Focalin XR**	ADHD
Diclofenac Sodium	Pennsaid, Solaraze, Voltaren Gel, Voltaren Ophthalmic, Voltaren-XR	Pennsaid: arthritis, osteo; pain Solaraze: keratosis Voltaren Gel: osteoarthritis Voltaren Ophthalmic: inflammation, ophthalmic; pain, ophthalmic; surgical adjunct/aid Voltaren-XR: arthritis, osteo; arthritis, rheumatoid
Difluprednate	Durezol	inflammation, ophthalmic; pain, ophthalmic; uveitis
Dimethyl Fumarate	Tecfidera	multiple sclerosis
Divalproex Sodium	Depakote, **Depakote ER**, Depakote Sprinkle	bipolar disorder, mania; migraine, tension headache; seizures
Doxycycline	Oracea	rosacea
Dronedarone	Multaq	arrhythmia
Drospirenone/Ethinyl Estradiol/ Levomefolate	Beyaz, Safyral	Beyaz: acne, contraception, premenstrual dysphoric disorder Safyral: contraception
Duloxetine HCl	Cymbalta	anxiety; depression; fibromyalgia; major depressive disorder; pain; pain, neuropathic
Dutasteride	**Avodart**	benign prostatic hypertrophy
Efavirenz/Emtricitabine/Tenofovir Disoproxil Fumarate	**Atripla**	AIDS, HIV
Eletriptan Hydrobromide	Relpax	migraine
Emtricitabine/Rilpivirine/ Tenofovir Disoproxil Fumarate	**Complera**	AIDS, HIV

GENERIC/BRAND CROSS-REFERENCE TABLE

Please go to **PDR.net** to view Prescribing Information for these and other products.

GENERIC/BRAND CROSS-REFERENCE TABLE

Emtricitabine/Tenofovir Disoproxil Fumarate	**Truvada**	AIDS, HIV
Epinephrine	Adrenaclick, Auvi-Q, EpiPen, EpiPen Jr	allergy, anaphylaxis
Epoetin Alfa	Epogen, Procrit	AIDS adjunct, anemia; chemotherapy adjunct; surgical adjunct/aid
Erlotinib	Tarceva	cancer, lung; cancer, pancreas
Escitalopram Oxalate	Lexapro	anxiety, depression, major depressive disorder
Esomeprazole Magnesium	Nexium	erosive esophagitis; GERD; *Helicobacter pylori* eradication; heartburn; hypersecretory conditions; ulcer, gastrointestinal; Zollinger-Ellison syndrome
Estradiol Oral	Estrace, Estradiol Tablets	cancer, breast; cancer, prostate; hypoestrogenism; menopause; osteoporosis; vaginitis, atrophic
Estradiol Transdermal	Alora, Climara, Menostar, Minivelle, Vivelle-Dot	Alora, Climara, Vivelle-Dot: hypoestrogenism; menopause; osteoporosis; vaginitis, atrophic Menostar: osteoporosis Minivelle: menopause
Estradiol Vaginal	Estring, Vagifem	Estring: atrophic vaginitis Vagifem: menopause; vaginitis, atrophic
Eszopiclone	Lunesta	insomnia
Etanercept	Enbrel	ankylosing spondylitis; arthritis; arthritis, psoriatic; arthritis, rheumatoid; psoriasis
Ethinyl Estradiol/Etonogestrel	**NuvaRing**	contraception
Ethinyl Estradiol/ Ferrous Fumarate/ Norethindrone Acetate	Generess Fe, Gildess Fe, Junel Fe, Loestrin Fe, Lo Loestrin Fe, Microgestin Fe, Minastrin 24 Fe	contraception
Ethinyl Estradiol/Norelgestromin	Ortho Evra	contraception
Ethinyl Estradiol/Norgestimate	MonoNessa, Ortho-Cyclen, Ortho Tri-Cyclen, Ortho Tri-Cyclen Lo, Sprintec	Ortho Tri-Cyclen: acne, contraception MonoNessa, Ortho-Cyclen, Ortho Tri-Cyclen Lo, Sprintec: contraception
Everolimus	**Afinitor**, **Afinitor Disperz**, **Zortress**	Afinitor: cancer, brain; cancer, breast; cancer, pancreas; cancer, renal Afinitor Disperz: cancer, brain Zortress: organ and transplant rejection
Exenatide	Bydureon, Byetta	diabetes
Ezetimibe	**Zetia**	elevated sitosterolemia, hypercholesterolemia, hyperlipidemia
Ezetimibe/Simvastatin	**Vytorin**	hypercholesterolemia, hyperlipidemia
Febuxostat	**Uloric**	gout, hyperuricemia
Fenofibrate	Antara, Fenoglide, Lipofen, Lofibra, **Tricor**, Triglide,	hypercholesterolemia, hyperlipidemia, hypertriglyceridemia
Fenofibric Acid	Fibricor, **Trilipix**	hypercholesterolemia, hyperlipidemia, hypertriglyceridemia
Fentanyl	Abstral, Actiq, Duragesic, Fentanyl Injection, Lazanda, Onsolis, Subsys	pain; pain, cancer Fentanyl Injection: anesthesia

Please go to **PDR.net** to view Prescribing Information for these and other products.

Fesoterodine Fumarate	Toviaz	bladder, overactive; urinary incontinence
Filgrastim	Neupogen	bone marrow transplant; chemotherapy adjunct; febrile neutropenia; neutropenia, severe/chronic; peripheral blood progenitor cell collection and therapy
Fingolimod	**Gilenya**	multiple sclerosis
Fluticasone Furoate	**Veramyst**	allergy, rhinitis
Fluticasone Propionate	**Flovent Diskus**, **Flovent HFA**	asthma
Fluticasone Propionate/ Salmeterol	**Advair Diskus**, **Advair HFA**	Advair Diskus: asthma, bronchitis, COPD, emphysema Advair HFA: asthma
Formoterol Fumarate Dihydrate/ Mometasone Furoate	**Dulera**	asthma
Glatiramer	Copaxone	multiple sclerosis
Guanfacine	Intuniv, Tenex	Intuniv: ADHD Tenex: hypertension
Human Papillomavirus Recombination	**Gardasil**	vaccine
Hydrochlorothiazide/ Olmesartan Medoxomil	Benicar HCT	hypertension
Hydrochlorothiazide/Telmisartan	Micardis HCT	hypertension
Hydrochlorothiazide/Valsartan	**Diovan HCT**	hypertension
Imatinib	**Gleevec**	cancer, gastrointestinal; dermatofibrosarcoma protuberans; hypereosinophilic syndrome; leukemia; mastocytosis; myelodysplastic syndrome
Infliximab	Remicade	ankylosing spondylitis; arthritis, psoriatic; arthritis, rheumatoid; colitis, ulcerative; Crohn's disease; psoriasis
Influenza Virus Vaccine	Afluria, **Fluarix Quadrivalent**, Flucelvax, **Flulaval**, Fluvirin, Fluzone, Fluzone HD, Fluzone Intradermal	influenza vaccine
Insulin Aspart	**NovoLog**, **NovoLog FlexPen**	diabetes
Insulin Aspart Protamine/ Insulin Aspart	NovoLog Mix 50/50, **NovoLog Mix 70/30**	diabetes
Insulin Detemir	**Levemir**, **Levemir FlexPen**	diabetes
Insulin Glargine	Lantus, Lantus Solostar	diabetes
Insulin Lispro	Humalog, Humalog KwikPen	diabetes
Insulin Lispro Protamine/ Insulin Lispro	Humalog Mix50/50, Humalog Mix75/25, Humalog Mix75/25 KwikPen	diabetes
Interferon beta-1a	Rebif	multiple sclerosis
Interferon beta-1b	Betaseron	multiple sclerosis
Ipratropium Bromide	Atrovent HFA, Atrovent Nasal	Atrovent HFA: bronchitis, bronchospasm, COPD, emphysema Atrovent Nasal: allergy, rhinitis
Lacosamide	Vimpat	seizures

Please go to **PDR.net** to view Prescribing Information for these and other products.

GENERIC/BRAND CROSS-REFERENCE TABLE

Lansoprazole	Prevacid, Prevacid SoluTab	erosive esophagitis; GERD; heartburn; *Helicobacter pylori* eradication; hypersecretory conditions; ulcer, gastrointestinal; Zollinger-Ellison syndrome
Levalbuterol Tartrate	Xopenex HFA	asthma, bronchospasm
Levothyroxine Sodium	Levothroid, Levoxyl, **Synthroid**, Unithroid	cancer, thyroid; goiter; hypothyroidism; surgical adjunct/aid; TSH suppression
Lidocaine	Lidoderm Patch	pain; pain, neuropathic; postherpetic neuralgia
Linaclotide	Linzess	constipation, irritable bowel syndrome
Linagliptin	Tradjenta	diabetes
Linezolid	Zyvox	infections, bacterial/respiratory tract; infections, bacterial/skin; infections, bacterial/systemic; pneumonia, bacterial
Liraglutide	**Victoza**	diabetes
Lisdexamfetamine Dimesylate	Vyvanse	ADHD
Loteprednol Etabonate	Lotemax Gel, Lotemax Ointment, Lotemax Suspension	Lotemax Gel, Lotemax Ointment: inflammation, ophthalmic; pain, ophthalmic; surgical adjunct/aid Lotemax Suspension: conjunctivitis; inflammation, ophthalmic
Lubiprostone	**Amitiza**	constipation, irritable bowel syndrome
Lurasidone HCl	**Latuda**	bipolar disorder, schizophrenia
Magnesium Sulfate/ Potassium Sulfate/ Sodium Sulfate	Suprep Bowel Prep	bowel cleansing, diagnostic aid
Memantine HCl	Namenda, Namenda XR	Alzheimer's disease
Mesalamine	Asacol HD, Delzicol, Lialda	colitis, ulcerative
Metformin HCl/Saxagliptin	Kombiglyze XR	diabetes
Metformin HCl/Sitagliptin	**Janumet, Janumet XR**	diabetes
Methylphenidate	Concerta, Daytrana, Metadate CD, Metadate ER, Methylin, Quillivant XR, Ritalin, Ritalin LA, Ritalin-SR	Metadate ER, Methylin, Ritalin, Ritalin-SR: ADHD, narcolepsy Concerta, Daytrana, Metadate CD, Quillivant XR, Ritalin LA: ADHD
Metoprolol Succinate	Toprol-XL	angina, heart failure, hypertension
Milnacipran HCl	Savella	fibromyalgia
Mirabegron	Myrbetriq	bladder, overactive; urinary incontinence
Modafinil	Provigil	narcolepsy
Mometasone Furoate	**Asmanex, Elocon Cream, Elocon Lotion, Elocon Ointment**	Asmanex: asthma Elocon Cream, Elocon Lotion, Elocon Ointment: dermatitis; inflammation, topical; pruritus, topical
Mometasone Furoate Monohydrate	**Nasonex**	allergy, nasal polyps, rhinitis
Montelukast Sodium	Singulair	allergy, asthma, rhinitis, exercise-induced bronchoconstriction
Moxifloxacin HCl Ophthalmic	Moxeza, Vigamox	conjunctivitis; infections, bacterial/ophthalmic

Please go to **PDR.net** to view Prescribing Information for these and other products.

Moxifloxacin HCl Oral	**Avelox**	bronchitis; infections, bacterial/respiratory tract; infections, bacterial/skin; infections, intra-abdominal; pneumonia, bacterial; sinusitis
Nebivolol	Bystolic	hypertension
Nepafenac	Ilevro, Nevanac	inflammation, ophthalmic; pain, ophthalmic; surgical adjunct/aid
Niacin	**Niaspan**	coronary artery disease; hypercholesterolemia; hyperlipidemia; hypertriglyceridemia; myocardial infarction, reduce risk
Nitroglycerin	Minitran, Nitro-Bid, **Nitro-Dur**, Nitrolingual, Nitromist, Nitrostat, Transderm Nitro	angina
Octreotide	**Sandostatin LAR**	acromegaly, diarrhea
Olmesartan Medoxomil	Benicar	hypertension
Olopatadine HCl Nasal	Patanase	allergy, rhinitis
Olopatadine HCl Ophthalmic	Pataday, Patanol	allergy, conjunctivitis
Omalizumab	**Xolair**	asthma, urticaria
Omega-3-Acid Ethyl Esters	**Lovaza**	hypertriglyceridemia
Omeprazole	Prilosec, Prilosec OTC	erosive esophagitis; GERD; heartburn; *Helicobacter pylori* eradication; hypersecretory conditions; mastocytosis; ulcer, gastrointestinal; Zollinger-Ellison syndrome
Oseltamivir Phosphate	Tamiflu	infections, viral/systemic; influenza
Oxycodone HCl	Oxecta, **Oxycontin**, Roxicodone	pain
Oxymorphone HCl	Opana, Opana ER	pain
Paliperidone	Invega Sustenna	schizophrenia
Palivizumab	Synagis	respiratory syncytial virus
Pancrelipase	**Creon**	cystic fibrosis, enzyme deficiency, pancreatitis
Pegfilgrastim	Neulasta	chemotherapy adjunct, neutropenia
Pemetrexed	Alimta	lung cancer, mesothelioma
Phenytoin	Dilantin, Dilantin Infatabs, Dilantin-125, Phenytek	seizures
Pitavastatin	**Livalo**	hypercholesterolemia, hyperlipidemia, hypertriglyceridemia
Pneumococcal 13 Valent Conjugated	Prevnar 13	vaccine
Pneumococcal Vaccine Polyvalent	**Pneumovax 23**	vaccine
Prasugrel	Effient	angina; coronary syndrome; myocardial infarction, postmanagement; percutaneous coronary intervention; thrombosis prevention
Pregabalin	Lyrica	fibromyalgia; pain; pain, neuropathic; postherpetic neuralgia; seizures

Please go to **PDR.net** to view Prescribing Information for these and other products.

Quetiapine Fumarate	Seroquel, Seroquel XR	Seroquel: bipolar disorder, mania, schizophrenia Seroquel XR: bipolar disorder, depression, major depressive disorder, mania, schizophrenia
Rabeprazole Sodium	Aciphex, Aciphex Sprinkles	GERD; heartburn; *Helicobacter pylori* eradication; hypersecretory conditions; ulcer, gastrointestinal; Zollinger-Ellison syndrome
Raloxifene HCl	Evista	cancer, breast; osteoporosis
Raltegravir	**Isentress**	AIDS, HIV
Ranolazine	**Ranexa**	angina
Rifaximin	**Xifaxan**	hepatic encephalopathy; travelers' diarrhea
Risedronate Sodium	Actonel, Atelvia	Actonel: osteoporosis, Paget's disease Atelvia: osteoporosis
Ritonavir	**Norvir**	AIDS, HIV
Rituximab	Rituxan	arthritis, rheumatoid; leukemia; non-Hodgkin's lymphoma; vasculitis
Rivaroxaban	Xarelto	deep vein thrombosis; pulmonary embolism; stroke, reduce risk; surgical adjunct/aid; thrombosis prevention
Rivastigmine	**Exelon Patch**, Exelon Capsules and Oral Solution	Alzheimer's disease, Parkinson's disease
Roflumilast	Daliresp	bronchitis, COPD
Rosuvastatin Calcium	Crestor	coronary artery disease; hypercholesterolemia; hyperlipidemia; myocardial infarction, reduce risk; revascularization, reduce risk; stroke, reduce risk
Saxagliptin	Onglyza	diabetes
Scopolamine	Transderm Scop	anesthesia, adjunct; motion sickness; nausea; vomiting
Sevelamer Carbonate	Renvela	hyperphosphatemia
Sildenafil Citrate	**Viagra**	erectile dysfunction
Silodosin	Rapaflo	benign prostatic hypertrophy
Sitagliptin	**Januvia**	diabetes
Sodium Fluoride	Denta 5000 Plus, PreviDent 5000, PreviDent 5000 Plus	dental caries
Solifenacin Succinate	Vesicare	bladder, overactive; urinary incontinence
Sucralfate	Carafate	gastrointestinal ulcer
Tadalafil	Cialis	benign prostatic hypertrophy, erectile dysfunction
Tapentadol	**Nucynta**, **Nucynta ER**	Nucynta: pain Nucynta ER: pain; pain, neuropathic
Telaprevir	Incivek	Hepatitis
Telmisartan	Micardis	hypertension; myocardial infarction, reduce risk; stroke, reduce risk
Tenofovir Disoproxil Fumarate	**Viread**	AIDS, HIV, hepatitis

GENERIC/BRAND CROSS-REFERENCE TABLE

Please go to **PDR.net** to view Prescribing Information for these and other products.

Testosterone Topical	Androderm, **Androgel**, **Androgel Pump**, Axiron, Fortesta, Testim, Testoderm, Testoderm TTS, Striant, Vogelxo	hypogonadism, testosterone replacement
Thyroid	Armour Thyroid, **Nature-Throid**, Westhroid, **WP Thyroid**	Armour Thyroid: cancer, thyroid; goiter; hypothyroidism; TSH suppression Nature-Throid, Westhroid, WP Thyroid: cancer, thyroid; diagnostic aid; goiter; hypothyroidism; TSH suppression
Ticagrelor	Brilinta	angina; coronary syndrome; myocardial infarction; myocardial infarction, reduce risk; stroke, reduce risk; thrombosis prevention
Tiotropium Bromide	Spiriva Handihaler	bronchitis, bronchospasm, COPD, emphysema
Tolterodine Tartrate	Detrol, Detrol LA	overactive bladder
Trastuzumab	Herceptin	cancer, breast; cancer, gastric - chronic
Travoprost	Travatan Z	glaucoma/IOP
Valsartan	**Diovan**	heart failure; hypertension; myocardial infarction, postmanagement
Vardenafil HCl	Levitra	erectile dysfunction
Varenicline	Chantix, Chantix Continuing Month Pak, Chantix Starting Month Pak	smoking cessation
Vilazodone HCl	Viibryd	depression, major depressive disorder
Warfarin Sodium	**Coumadin**, Jantoven	myocardial infarction, postmanagement; myocardial infarction, reduce risk; pulmonary embolism; stroke, reduce risk; thrombosis prevention
Zostavax Vaccine Live	**Zostavax**	shingles, vaccine

GENERIC/BRAND CROSS-REFERENCE TABLE

Please go to **PDR.net** to view Prescribing Information for these and other products.

PRODUCT CATEGORY INDEX

This index lists products by prescribing category, allowing you to quickly and easily identify all agents with a given therapeutic use or mechanism of action. Categories are based on the latest medical terminology and are comprehensively cross-referenced. All fully described products in the Product Information section of the *PDR®* are included here.

If an entry in the index lists multiple page numbers, the first one shown refers to images of the product; the last one refers to its prescribing information.

PRODUCT CATEGORY INDEX

PRODUCT CATEGORY INDEX

PRODUCT CATEGORY INDEX

Key to Controlled Substances Schedule

Products listed with the symbols shown below are subject to the Controlled Substances Act of 1970. These drugs are categorized according to their potential for abuse. The greater the potential, the more severe the limitations on their prescription.

SCHEDULE	INTERPRETATION
C II	**HIGH POTENTIAL FOR ABUSE.** Use may lead to severe physical or psychological dependence.
C III	**POTENTIAL FOR ABUSE LESS THAN THE DRUGS OR OTHER SUBSTANCES IN C-II.** Use may lead to low-to-moderate physical dependence or high psychological dependence.
C IV	**LOW POTENTIAL FOR ABUSE RELATIVE TO DRUGS OR OTHER SUBSTANCES IN C-III.** Use may lead to limited physical or psychological dependence relative to the drugs or other substances in C-III.
C V	**LOW POTENTIAL FOR ABUSE RELATIVE TO DRUGS OR OTHER SUBSTANCES IN C-IV.** Use may lead to limited physical or psychological dependence relative to the drugs or other substances in C-IV.

Key to FDA Use-in-Pregnancy Ratings

The FDA use-in-pregnancy rating system weighs the degree to which available information has ruled out risk to the fetus against the drug's potential benefit to the patient. The ratings, and their interpretations, are as follows:

SCHEDULE	INTERPRETATION
A	**CONTROLLED STUDIES SHOW NO RISK.** Adequate, well-controlled studies in pregnant women have failed to demonstrate a risk to the fetus in the first trimester of pregnancy (and there is no evidence of a risk in later trimesters).
B	**NO EVIDENCE OF RISK IN HUMANS.** Adequate, well-controlled studies in pregnant women are lacking, and animal studies have not shown increased risk of fetal abnormalities. The chance of fetal harm is remote, but remains a possibility.
C	**RISK CANNOT BE RULED OUT.** Adequate, well-controlled human studies in pregnant women are lacking, and animal studies have shown a risk to the fetus. There is a chance of fetal harm if the drug is administered during pregnancy, but the potential benefits may outweigh the potential risk.
D	**POSITIVE EVIDENCE OF RISK.** Studies in humans, or investigational or postmarketing data, have demonstrated fetal risk. Nevertheless, potential benefits from the use of the drug may outweigh the potential risk. For example, the drug may be acceptable if needed in a life-threatening situation or serious disease for which safer drugs cannot be used or are ineffective.
X	**CONTRAINDICATED IN PREGNANCY.** Studies in animals or humans have demonstrated fetal abnormalities or if there is positive evidence of fetal risk based on adverse reaction reports from investigational or marketing experience, or both, and risk of use clearly outweighs any possible benefit.

U.S. FOOD AND DRUG ADMINISTRATION

Medical Product Reporting Programs

MedWatch (24-hour service).. 800-332-1088
Reporting of adverse events related to drugs, biologics (except vaccines), devices, combination products, special nutritional products, cosmetics, or foods/beverages.

Vaccine Adverse Event Reporting System (24-hour service)................................. 800-822-7967
Reporting of vaccine-related adverse events.

Mandatory Medical Device Reporting... 301-796-6670
Reporting required from device user facilities regarding medical device-related deaths and serious injuries.

Veterinary Adverse Drug Reaction Program 888-332-8387
Reporting of adverse drug experiences in animals.

Information for Health Professionals

Center for Drug Evaluation and Research 855-543-3784
Information on human drugs, including hormones.

Center for Biologics Evaluation and Research 800-835-4709
Information on biological products, including vaccines and blood.

Center for Devices and Radiological Health... 800-638-2041
Automated request for information on medical devices and radiation-emitting products.

Office of Prescription Drug Promotion 301-796-1200
Inquiries from health professionals regarding product promotion.

Emergency Operations... 866-300-4374
Emergencies involving food, drugs, medical devices, dietary supplements, or cosmetics.

Office of Orphan Products Development 301-796-8660
Information on products for rare diseases.

General Information

General Consumer Inquiries 888-463-6332
Consumer information on regulated products/issues.

Division of Freedom of Information 301-796-3900
Requests for publicly available FDA documents.

Office of Media Affairs.. 301-796-4540
Interviews/press inquiries on FDA activities.

Center for Food Safety and Applied Nutrition... 888-723-3366
Information on food and cosmetics safety.

Consumer Information Service, Center for Devices and Radiological Health... 800-638-2041
Information on medical devices, mammography facilities, and radiation-emitting products.

POISON ANTIDOTES

This information has been assembled by the Illinois Poison Center, as a resource for the uses and suggested minimum stock quantities for poison antidotes for Illinois hospitals with emergency departments. Requirements and special circumstances in other areas of the U.S. may justify different stocking quantities or products (eg, antivenoms for other varieties of snakes, scorpions, spiders). Contact your nearest regional PCC via the nationwide Poison Help Line at **1-800-222-1222** (available 24 hours a day) for treatment information regarding any exposure, including indications for use of antidote therapy.

ANTIDOTE	POISON/DRUG/TOXIN	SUGGESTED MINIMUM STOCK QUANTITY	RATIONALE/COMMENTS
N-Acetylcysteine (Mucomyst, Acetadote)	Acetaminophen Carbon tetrachloride Other hepatotoxins	IV: 300 mL (60 g) Acetadote PO: 750 mL (150 mg) of 20% NAC	Acetaminophen is the most common drug involved in intentional and unintentional poisonings. 750 mL (150 g) of the oral product provides enough to treat three 100 kg adults for 24 h. Several vials may be stocked in the ED to provide a loading dose, and the remaining vials stocked in the pharmacy. 300 mL (60 g) of IV product will treat two 100 kg adult patients for the entire 21-h IV protocol.
Antivenin, *Crotalidae* Polyvalent Immune Fab – Ovine (CroFab)	Pit viper envenomation (eg, rattlesnakes, cottonmouths, and copperheads)	12-18 vials	Advised in geographic areas in Illinois with endemic populations of copperhead, water moccasin, eastern massasauga, or timber rattlesnake. In low-risk areas, know nearest alternate source of antivenin. This product has a lower risk of hypersensitivity reaction than previously marketed equine product. 12 vials will cover 8 h of treatment, while 18 vials will cover 24 h of treatment. Stock in pharmacy. Store in refrigerator. Equine product was discontinued March 31, 2007 and is no longer available for purchase.
Antivenin, *Latrodectus mactans* (Black widow spider)	Black widow spider envenomation	0 to 1 vial	Serious *Latrodectus* envenomations are rare in Illinois. This product is only used for severe envenomations. Antivenin must be given in a critical care setting since it is an equine-derived product that may cause anaphylaxis. Stock in pharmacy. Product must be refrigerated at all times. Know the nearest source of antidote.

(Continued)

©Illinois Poison Center March, 2014. PDR has secured written permission to reprint the Antidote Chart for the sole purpose of providing an additional educational reference within this publication. Reproduction or resale of this list without the written authorization from the Illinois Poison Center is strictly prohibited.

ANTIDOTE	POISON/DRUG/TOXIN	SUGGESTED MINIMUM STOCK QUANTITY	RATIONALE/COMMENTS
Atropine sulfate	Alpha$_2$ agonists (eg, clonidine, guanabenz and guanfacine) Alzheimer drugs (eg, donepezil, galantamine, rivastigmine, tacrine) Antimyasthenic agents (eg, pyridostigmine) Bradyarrhythmia-producing agents (eg, beta blockers, calcium channel blockers and digitalis glycosides)	175 mg or greater Available in various formulations: 0.4 mg/mL (1 mL, 0.4 mg vial); 0.4 mg/mL (20 mL, 8 mg vial); 0.1 mg/mL (10 mL; 1 mg vial) Atropine Sulfate military-style auto-injectors: (Atropen): 2 mg/0.7 mL, 1 mg/0.7 mL, 0.5 mg/0.7 mL, 0.25 mg/0.3 mL Atropine Sulfate 2.1 mg/0.7 mL with Pralidoxime chloride 600 mg/2 mL (DuoDote)	The product should be immediately available in the ED. Some also may be stored in the pharmacy or other hospital sites, but should be easily mobilized if a severely poisoned patient needs treatment. Note: Product is necessary to be adequately prepared for WMD incidents; the suggested amount may not be sufficient for mass casualty events. Auto-injectors are available from Bound Tree Medical, Inc (800-533-0523). Drug stocked in chempack containers is intended only for use in mass casualty events.
Atropine sulfate *(Continued)*	Cholinergic agonists (eg, bethanechol) Muscarine-containing mushrooms (eg, *Clitocybe* and *Inocybe*) Nerve agents (eg, sarin, soman, tabun, and VX) Organophosphate and carbamate insecticides		
Botulinum antitoxin As of March 13, 2010, the only botulinum antitoxin available is HBAT (heptavalent types A-G). This product replaces bivalent antitoxins type AB and antitoxin type E. Baby Botulism Immune Globulin (BIG)	Food-borne botulism Wound botulism Botulism as a biological weapon Note: Heptavalent antitoxin not currently recommended for infant botulism	None. Product is stored at 9 CDC regional centers (including the Chicago Quarantine). To obtain antitoxin, hospitals must call their Local or State Department of Public Health, which will contact the CDC in Atlanta. The CDC emergency operation center can be reached at 770-488-7100.	Antitoxin must be given in a critical care setting since it is an equine-derived product. Note: Product must be refrigerated at all times. Heptavalent antitoxin is stored in the CDC SNS. BabyBIG is available for infant botulism types A and B, through the Infant Botulism Treatment and Prevention Program, sponsored by the California Department of Public Health, telephone: 510-231-7600, www.infantbotulism.org/physician/obtain.php.
Calcium disodium EDTA (Versenate)	Lead Zinc salts (eg, zinc chloride)	2x 5 mL vials (200 mg/mL)	One vial provides 1 day of therapy for a child. 2 to 4 g per 24 h may be necessary in adult patients. Stock in pharmacy. Important note: Edetate disodium (Endrate) is not the same as calcium disodium EDTA, and is used primarily as an IV chelator for emergent treatment of hypercalcemia.

©Illinois Poison Center March, 2014. PDR has secured written permission to reprint the Antidote Chart for the sole purpose of providing an additional educational reference within this publication. Reproduction or resale of this list without the written authorization from the Illinois Poison Center is strictly prohibited.

ANTIDOTE	POISON/DRUG/TOXIN	SUGGESTED MINIMUM STOCK QUANTITY	RATIONALE/COMMENTS
Calcium chloride and Calcium gluconate	Fluoride salts (eg, NaF) Hydrofluoric acid (HF) Hyperkalemia (not digoxin-induced) Hypermagnesemia	10% calcium chloride: 10x 10 mL vials 10% calcium gluconate: 30x 10 mL vials	Many vials of calcium chloride may be necessary in life-threatening HF poisoning. Stock in ED. More may be stocked in pharmacy. The chloride salt provides 3x more calcium than the gluconate salt. Calcium chloride is very irritating and administration through a central line is preferable. Topical calcium gluconate or carbonate gels may be extemporaneously prepared by the pharmacy. Calgonate (calcium gluconate 2.5% gel) is not FDA approved but is manufactured in an FDA-GMP approved facility and is distributed by Calgonate Corp in Port St. Lucie, Florida.
Centruroides Immune F(ab)$_2$ – Equine (Anascorp)	Scorpion envenomation	None	This product is manufactured in Mexico by the Instituto Bioclon. In the U.S., it is marketed by Rare Disease Therapeutics, Inc. in Nashville, Tennessee. It was approved by the FDA in 2011 and can be stored at room temperature. Usual dose: 1 to 3 vials.
Cyanide Antidote: Sodium nitrite and sodium thiosulfate (Nithiodote)	Acetonitrile Acrylonitrile Bromates (thiosulfate only) Chlorates (thiosulfate only) Cyanide (eg, HCN, KCN, and NaCN) Cyanogen chloride Cyanogenic glycoside natural sources (eg, apricot pits and peach pits) Hydrogen sulfide (nitrites only) Laetrile Mustard agents (thiosulfate only) Nitroprusside (thiosulfate only) Smoke inhalation (combustion of synthetic materials)	2-4 kits Each kit contains: 1 vial (10 mL) sodium nitrite (300 mg); 1 vial (50 mL) sodium thiosulfate (12.5 g) Stocking this kit may be unnecessary if an adequate supply of hydroxocobalamin HCl is available.	Stock 2 kits in the ED. Consider also stocking 2 kits in the pharmacy. Note: This kit has a short shelf life of 24 months. Significant adverse reactions include methemoglobinemia and hypotension. For smoke inhalation victims, thiosulfate without the use of nitrites may be considered. In 2012, the cyanide kit containing 12 amyl nitrite pearls, two 10 mL sodium nitrite vials, and two 50 mL sodium thiosulfate vials was discontinued by the manufacturer and is no longer available in the U.S. Amyl nitrite ampules may be ordered separately.
Deferoxamine mesylate (Desferal)	Iron Deferoxamine has also been used for chronic aluminum toxicity in chronic kidney disease patients.	12-36 g (Available in 500 mg and 2 g vials)	Quantity recommended supplies 8 to 24 h of therapy for a 100 kg adult. Per package insert, the maximum daily dose is 6 g (12 vials). However, this dose may be exceeded in serious acute iron poisonings. Stock in pharmacy.

(Continued)

©Illinois Poison Center March, 2014. PDR has secured written permission to reprint the Antidote Chart for the sole purpose of providing an additional educational reference within this publication. Reproduction or resale of this list without the written authorization from the Illinois Poison Center is strictly prohibited.

ANTIDOTE	POISON/DRUG/TOXIN	SUGGESTED MINIMUM STOCK QUANTITY	RATIONALE/COMMENTS
Digoxin immune Fab (Digibind, Digifab)	Cardiac glycoside-containing plants (eg, foxglove and oleander) Digitoxin Digoxin	15 vials Each vial (38 mg) neutralizes 0.5 mg of digoxin	An initial dose of 2-3 vials for chronic poisoning or 10 vials for acute poisoning may be given to a digoxin-poisoned patient in whom the digoxin level is unknown. More may be necessary in severe intoxications. 15 vials would effectively neutralize a steady-state digoxin level of 15 ng/mL in a 100 kg patient. Know nearest source of additional supply. Stock in ED or pharmacy.
Dimercaprol (BAL in oil)	Arsenic Copper Gold Lead Lewisite Mercury	4x 3 mL vials (100 mg/mL)	This amount provides 3 doses of 3 to 5 mg/kg/dose given q 4 h to treat 1 seriously poisoned adult (up to 100 kg) or provides enough to treat a 15 kg child for more than 24 h. Stock in pharmacy.
Ethanol	Ethylene glycol Methanol	Ethanol is unnecessary if adequate amounts of fomepizole are stocked. Consider stocking 180-360 g in the form of 95% ethanol or equivalents (10% ethanol can be prepared from dehydrated alcohol and D5W for IV use).	180 g provides loading and maintenance doses for a 100 kg adult for 8-24 h. More alcohol or fomepizole will be needed during dialysis or prolonged treatment. 95% or 40% alcohol diluted in juice may be given PO if IV alcohol is unavailable. Stock in pharmacy. Note: See also fomepizole in this chart. Ethanol may cause hypotension or metabolic abnormalities (eg, hypoglycemia) especially in pediatric patients. Since ethanol treatment for toxic alcohol poisoning is not FDA approved and fomepizole offers greater efficacy and safety, fomepizole is the preferred alcohol dehydrogenase inhibitor.
Fat emulsion (Intralipid, Liposyn II, Liposyn III)	Local anesthetics and possibly other cardiac toxins (eg, bupropion, calcium channel blockers, cocaine, beta blockers, tricyclic antidepressants)	Quantity determined by institution. Available in 100 mL of 20% emulsion.	Fat emulsion is an experimental therapy showing promise in the reverse of cardiac toxicity induced by local anesthetics and other cardiac toxins. The evidence for the efficacy of fat emulsion therapy is based on animal studies and human case reports, and its safety has not yet been established. Consultation with a regional PCC toxicologist is advised. Initial dose: 1.5 mL/kg IV over 1 minute. Follow with infusion of 0.25 mL/kg/min over 30 minutes. Loading dose may be repeated once. Rate may be increased to 0.5 mL/kg/min for 60 minutes if blood pressure drops. Maximum total dose is 8 mL/kg. Consider storage in pharmacy, ED, and possibly surgical units.

©Illinois Poison Center March, 2014. PDR has secured written permission to reprint the Antidote Chart for the sole purpose of providing an additional educational reference within this publication. Reproduction or resale of this list without the written authorization from the Illinois Poison Center is strictly prohibited.

ANTIDOTE	POISON/DRUG/TOXIN	SUGGESTED MINIMUM STOCK QUANTITY	RATIONALE/COMMENTS
Flumazenil (Romazicon)	Benzodiazepines	Total 6-12 mg Available in 5 and 10 mL vials (0.1 mg/mL)	Due to risk of seizures, use with extreme caution, if at all, in poisoned patients. More may be stocked in the pharmacy for use in reversal of conscious sedation. Stock in ED, pharmacy, and any unit where procedural sedation is performed.
Folic acid and Folinic acid (Leucovorin)	Formaldehyde/Formic acid Methanol Methotrexate, Trimetrexate Pyrimethamine Trimethoprim	Folic acid: 3x 50 mg vials Folinic acid: 1x 50 mg vial	For adjunctive treatment of methanol-poisoned patients with an acidosis, give 50 mg folinic acid initially, then 50 mg of folic acid q 4 h for 6 doses. For methotrexate-poisoned patients, administer folinic acid only; consult PCC for dosing information. Stock in pharmacy.
Fomepizole (Antizol) 4-methylpyrazole (4-MP)	Ethylene glycol Methanol	1 to 2x 1.5 g vials Note: Available in a kit of 4x 1.5 g vials	One 1.5 g vial provides an initial dose of 15 mg/kg/12 h to an adult weighing up to 100 kg. Hospitals with critical care and hemodialysis capabilities should consider stocking 1 kit of 4 vials or more. More frequent dosing (ie, every 4 h) is required if the patient is dialyzed. Ethanol is unnecessary if adequate supply of fomepizole is stocked. Fomepizole is preferred to ethanol because of ease of use, fewer adverse effects, simplicity of dosing, and less need for close monitoring. Stock in pharmacy. Know where nearest alternate supply is located.
Glucagon HCl	Beta blockers	50 to 90x 1 mg vials	This quantity provides 4 to 8 h of maximum dosing, ie, a 10 mg IV bolus dose followed by 10 mg/h. More may be necessary. Know where nearest alternate supply is located. Stock 30 mg in ED and remainder in pharmacy.
Hydroxocobalamin HCl (Cyanokit)	Acetonitrile Acrylonitrile Cyanide (eg, HCN, KCN, and NaCN) Cyanogen chloride Cyanogenic glycoside natural sources (eg, apricot pits and peach pits) Laetrile Nitroprusside Smoke inhalation (combustion of synthetic materials)	2 to 4 kits Each kit contains one 5 g vial. Note: Diluent is not included in the kit.	Seriously poisoned cyanide patients may require 5 to 10 g (1 to 2 kits). Stock 2 kits in ED. Consider also stocking 2 kits in the pharmacy. The product has a shelf life of 30 months post-manufacture.

(Continued)

©Illinois Poison Center March, 2014. PDR has secured written permission to reprint the Antidote Chart for the sole purpose of providing an additional educational reference within this publication. Reproduction or resale of this list without the written authorization from the Illinois Poison Center is strictly prohibited.

ANTIDOTE	POISON/DRUG/TOXIN	SUGGESTED MINIMUM STOCK QUANTITY	RATIONALE/COMMENTS
Hyperbaric oxygen (HBO)	Carbon monoxide and possibly the following: Carbon tetrachloride Cyanide Hydrogen sulfide Methemoglobinemia	Post the location and phone number of nearest HBO chamber in the ED.	Consult PCC to determine if HBO treatment is indicated.
Insulin and dextrose	Calcium channel blockers (diltiazem, nifedipine, verapamil)	Quantity determined by institution. Humulin R is available as 100 units/mL in a 1.5 mL cartridge and 10 mL bottle. Dextrose 50% in water is available in 50 mL ampules and syringes. Dextrose 25% is available in 10 mL vials and syringes for pediatric use.	High dose insulin and dextrose therapy can reverse cardiovascular toxicity associated with calcium channel blocker overdose. IV Bolus: Recommended starting dose of 1 unit/kg regular insulin (with 1 amp D_{50}); The lowest maintenance dose is 0.5-1 units/kg/h. Higher doses may be considered under consultation with medical toxicologist. Stock in ED and pharmacy.
Methylene blue	Methemoglobin-inducing agents including: Aniline dyes Dapsone Dinitrophenol Local anesthetics (eg, benzocaine) Metoclopramide Monomethylhydrazine-containing mushrooms (eg, *Gyromitra*) Naphthalene Nitrates and nitrites Nitrobenzene Phenazopyridine	6x 10 mL vials (10 mg/mL)	The usual dose is 1 to 2 mg/kg IV (0.1 to 0.2 mL/kg). A second dose may be given in 1 h. More may be necessary. 6 vials provide 3 doses of 2 mg/kg for a 100 kg adult. Stock in pharmacy.
Naloxone (Narcan)	Alpha$_2$ agonists (eg, clonidine, guanabenz, and guanfacine) Unknown poisoning with mental status depression Opioids (eg, codeine, diphenoxylate, fentanyl, heroin, meperidine, morphine, and propoxyphene)	Naloxone: total of 40 mg, any combination of 0.4 mg and 2 mg vials	Stock 20 mg naloxone in the ED and 20 mg elsewhere in the institution.
Octreotide acetate (Sandostatin)	Sulfonylurea hypoglycemic agents (eg, glipizide, glyburide)	225 mcg Available in 1 mL vials (0.05 mg/mL, 0.1 mg/mL, and 0.5 mg/mL) and 5 mL multidose vials (0.2 mg/mL and 1 mg/mL)	Octreotide acetate blocks the release of insulin from pancreatic beta cells that, along with IV dextrose, can reverse sulfonylurea-induced hypoglycemia. The usual adult dose is 50 to 100 mcg IV or SC q 6 to 12 h. The usual pediatric dose is 1 to 1.5 mcg/kg IV or SC q 6 to 12 h. 225 mcg provides 4x 75 mcg adult doses. Stock in pharmacy.

©Illinois Poison Center March, 2014. PDR has secured written permission to reprint the Antidote Chart for the sole purpose of providing an additional educational reference within this publication. Reproduction or resale of this list without the written authorization from the Illinois Poison Center is strictly prohibited.

ANTIDOTE	POISON/DRUG/TOXIN	SUGGESTED MINIMUM STOCK QUANTITY	RATIONALE/COMMENTS
D-Penicillamine (Cuprimine)	Arsenic Copper Lead Mercury	None required as an antidote. Available in bottles of 100 (250 mg capsules)	D-Penicillamine is no longer considered the drug of choice for heavy metal poisonings. It may be stocked in the pharmacy for other indications such as Wilson's disease or rheumatoid arthritis.
Physostigmine salicylate (Antilirium)	Anticholinergic alkaloid-containing plants (eg, deadly nightshade and jimson weed) Antihistamines Atropine and other anticholinergic agents	2x 2 mL vials (1 mg/mL)	Usual adult dose is 1 to 2 mg slow IV push. Note: Duration of effect is 30 to 60 minutes. Stock in ED or pharmacy.
Phytonadione (Vitamin K$_1$) (Aquamephyton, Mephyton)	Indandione derivatives Long-acting anticoagulant rodenticides (eg, brodifacoum and bromadiolone) Warfarin	100 mg injectable; 100 mg oral Available as: 0.5 mL vials (2 mg/mL) and 1 mL vials (10 mg/mL) 5 mg tablets in packages of 10, 12, and 100	Patients who are poisoned by long-acting anticoagulant rodenticides may require 50 to 100 mg/day or more for weeks to months to maintain normal INRs. An oral suspension for pediatric patients may be extemporaneously prepared by the pharmacy. Stock in pharmacy.
Pralidoxime chloride (2-PAM) (Protopam)	OPIs Nerve agents (eg, sarin, soman, tabun, and VX) And possibly: Antimyasthenic agents (eg, pyridostigmine) Tacrine	18x 1 g vials. Also available as: Pralidoxime chloride military-style auto-injectors: 600 mg/2 mL Atropine Sulfate 2.1 mg/0.7 mL with Pralidoxime chloride 600 mg/2 mL (DuoDote)	18 g provides an adult dose of 750 mg/h for 24 h. More may be needed in severe poisoning. Healthcare facilities located in agricultural areas where OPIs are used should maintain adequate supplies. Product is necessary to be adequately prepared for WMD incidents; the suggested amount may not be sufficient for mass casualty events. Auto-injectors are available from Bound Tree Medical, Inc (800-533-0523). The drugs stocked in chempack containers are intended for use in mass casualty events only. Stock in ED or pharmacy.
Protamine sulfate	Heparin Low molecular weight heparins (eg, enoxaparin, dalteparin, tinzaparin)	Variable, consider recommendation of hospital Pharmacy and Therapeutics Committee Available as 5 mL vials (10 mg/mL) and 25 mL vials (250 mg/25 mL)	The usual dose is 1 to 1.5 mg for each 100 units of heparin. Stock in pharmacy in refrigerator. Preservative-free formulation does not require refrigeration.
Pyridoxine HCl (Vitamin B$_6$)	Acrylamide Ethylene glycol Hydrazine Hydrazine MAOIs (isocarboxazid, phenelzine) Isoniazid (INH) Monomethylhydrazine-containing mushrooms (eg, Gyromitra)	10 g (100 vials) Available as 1 mL vials (100 mg/mL)	Usual dose is 1 g pyridoxine HCl for each g of INH ingested. If amount ingested is unknown, give 5 g of pyridoxine. Repeat 5 g dose if seizures are uncontrolled. More may be necessary. Know nearest source of additional supply. For ethylene glycol, a dose of 100 mg/day may enhance the clearance of toxic metabolite. Stock in ED or pharmacy.

(Continued)

©Illinois Poison Center March, 2014. PDR has secured written permission to reprint the Antidote Chart for the sole purpose of providing an additional educational reference within this publication. Reproduction or resale of this list without the written authorization from the Illinois Poison Center is strictly prohibited.

ANTIDOTE	POISON/DRUG/TOXIN	SUGGESTED MINIMUM STOCK QUANTITY	RATIONALE/COMMENTS
Silibinin (Legalon-SIL)	Cyclopeptide-containing mushrooms (eg, Amanita phalloides, Amanita verna, Amanita virosa, Galerina autumnalis, Lepiota josserandi, and others)	None 350 mg/vial	Silibinin is a water-soluble preparation of silymarin; a flavolignone extracted from the milk thistle plant. It inhibits uptake of cyclopeptides in hepatocytes. These hepatotoxins are responsible for high morbidity and mortality following ingestion of these mushrooms. Silibinin is manufactured by Madaus, Inc. in Germany, and has been widely used in Europe since 1984. The initial adult loading dose consists of a 1 h infusion of 5 mg/kg followed by the recommended daily dosage of 20 mg/kg via continuous IV infusion. Product is now available in the U.S. under an open-treatment investigational new drug application. Physicians can obtain the product free-of-charge by contacting the primary investigator at 866-520-4412.
Sodium bicarbonate	Chlorine gas Hyperkalemia Serum Alkalinization: Agents producing a quinidine-like effect as noted by widened QRS complex on EKG (eg, amantadine, carbamazepine, chloroquine, cocaine, diphenhydramine, flecainide, propafenone, propoxyphene, tricyclic antidepressants, quinidine, and related agents) Urine Alkalinization: Weakly acidic agents (eg, chlorophenoxy herbicides, chlorpropamide, methotrexate, phenobarbital, and salicylates)	20 to 25x 50 mL vials of either 8.4% (50 mEq/50 mL) or 7.5% (44 mEq/50 mL) Consider stocking 4.2% (5 mEq/10 mL) for pediatric patients.	Stock 20 vials in ED and remainder in pharmacy. Nebulized 2.5-5% sodium bicarbonate has been demonstrated in anecdotal case reports to provide symptomatic relief for chlorine gas inhalation.
Succimer (Chemet) Dimercaptosuccinic acid (DMSA)	Arsenic Lead Lewisite Mercury	0 to 10 capsules Available in bottles of 100 capsules (100 mg/capsule)	Initial treatment of severely symptomatic heavy metal poisoning consists of parenterally administered chelators, eg, BAL or calcium disodium EDTA. Patients who markedly improve may eventually be started on oral DMSA. Asymptomatic or minimally symptomatic patients do not require parenteral therapy and are often treated as outpatients with an oral chelator. FDA approved only for pediatric lead poisoning, however it has shown efficacy for other heavy metal poisonings. 10 capsules represent an initial dose of 10 mg/kg in a 100 kg adult. Stock in pharmacy.

©Illinois Poison Center March, 2014. PDR has secured written permission to reprint the Antidote Chart for the sole purpose of providing an additional educational reference within this publication. Reproduction or resale of this list without the written authorization from the Illinois Poison Center is strictly prohibited.

ADJUNCTIVE AGENTS

ADJUNCTIVE AGENT	POISON/DRUG/TOXIN	SUGGESTED MINIMUM STOCK QUANTITY	RATIONALE/COMMENTS
Benztropine mesylate (Cogentin)	Medications causing a dystonic reaction or other EPS	Quantity determined by institution. Available in tablets of 0.5 mg, 1 mg, 2 mg (bottles of 100 or 1,000) and in 1 mg/mL injectable (2 mL vial) form.	Maximum daily adult dose is 6 mg/d. Stock some in ED and some in pharmacy. See also diphenhydramine.
L-Carnitine (Carnitor)	Valproic acid	Quantity determined by institution. Available as 330 mg and 500 mg tablets, 250 mg capsules, 200 mg/mL IV solution, and 100 mg/mL PO solution.	L-Carnitine may be considered in valproate intoxication associated with elevated serum ammonia levels and/or hepatotoxicity. Doses of 100 mg/kg/d up to 2 g a day PO divided into 3 doses, or 150-500 mg/kg/d IV (maximum 3 g daily) in 3 or 4 divided doses are recommended for a period of 3 to 4 days or until clinical improvement. Stock in pharmacy.
Cyproheptadine HCl (Periactin)	Medications causing serotonin syndrome	Quantity determined by institution. Available in 4 mg tablets (bottles of 100, 250, 500, and 1,000) and 2 mg/5 mL PO solution.	Cyproheptadine HCl is a nonspecific 5-HT antagonist that has been used in the treatment of serotonin syndrome. Adult dose is 12 mg PO initially, followed by 2 mg every 2 h if symptoms persist. Maintenance dose is 8 mg every 6 h. Maximum of 32 mg/day. Pediatric dose is 0.25 mg/kg/day divided every 6 h, with a max dose of 12 mg/day. Stock in pharmacy.
Dantrolene sodium (Dantrium)	Medications causing NMS Medications causing malignant hyperthermia	Quantity determined by institution. Available in 25, 50, and 100 mg capsules (bottles of 100 or 500) and injectable 20 mg/vial form.	The recommended dose for NMS is 1 mg/kg IV; may repeat as needed every 5 to 10 minutes for a maximum of 10 mg/kg. Dantrolene sodium inhibits calcium release from the sarcoplasmic reticulum of skeletal muscle and thereby reduces rigidity. Stock in pharmacy. Any hospital using inhalational anesthetics should strongly consider stocking dantrolene for treatment of malignant hyperthermia.

(Continued)

©Illinois Poison Center March, 2014. PDR has secured written permission to reprint the Antidote Chart for the sole purpose of providing an additional educational reference within this publication. Reproduction or resale of this list without the written authorization from the Illinois Poison Center is strictly prohibited.

ADJUNCTIVE AGENTS *(Continued)*

ADJUNCTIVE AGENT	POISON/DRUG/TOXIN	SUGGESTED MINIMUM STOCK QUANTITY	RATIONALE/COMMENTS
Diazepam (Valium)	Chloroquine and related antimalarial drugs NMS Serotonin syndrome Severe agitation from any toxic exposure/overdose (eg, cocaine, PCP, methamphetamine)	Quantity determined by institution. Available as 5 mg/mL injectables in 2 mL ampules, 2 mL disposable syringes, and 10 mL multidose vials. Diazepam military-style auto-injectors for nerve agent-induced seizures: 10 mg/2 mL.	Diazepam and other benzodiazepines are also used in poisoned and nonpoisoned patients as an anticonvulsant, muscle relaxant, and antianxiety agent. They are usually the first-line therapy for drug-induced agitation, tachycardia, and hypertension. Benzodiazepines are a mainstay in the treatment of NMS and serotonin syndrome. Stock in ED and pharmacy. Adequate supply is necessary to be prepared for WMD incidents. Auto-injectors are available from Bound Tree Medical, Inc (800-533-0523). Diazepam is used in conjunction with epinephrine for patients with chloroquine/hydroxychloroquine toxicity (seizures, dysrhythmias, hypotension) or if the amount ingested is more than 5 g. Intravenous loading dose 2 mg/kg over 30 minutes. Maintenance dose of 1 to 2 mg/kg per day for 2 to 4 days.
Diphenhydramine HCL (Benadryl)	Medications causing a dystonic reaction or other EPS	Quantity determined by institution. Available in 25 and 50 mg capsules (bottles of 30, 100, or 1,000). Also in oral liquid formulation of 12.5 mg/5 mL (4 ounce bottle) and 50 mg/mL injectable syringes.	In addition to its use as an anticholinergic agent, diphenhydramine is a widely used antihistamine in the management of minor or severe allergic reactions. Stock in ED and pharmacy.
Glycopyrrolate bromide (Robinul)	OPIs Nerve agents	Quantity determined by institution. Available as 0.2 mg/mL in vials of 1 mL, 2 mL, 5 mL, and 20 mL.	The dose of glycopyrrolate for OPI poisoning is 0.01 to 0.02 mg/kg IV. Glycopyrrolate is a quaternary ammonium antimuscarinic agent that may assist in the control of hypersecretions caused by acetylcholinesterase inhibition. This agent produces less tachycardia and CNS effects than atropine. Stock in ED and pharmacy.
Phentolamine mesylate (Regitine)	Catecholamine extravasation Intradigital epinephrine injection	Quantity determined by institution. Available as a 5 mg/vial powder with 1 mL diluent.	Phentolamine is an alpha-adrenergic antagonist that will reverse vasoconstriction and peripheral ischemia associated with extravasation of adrenergic agents. When phentolamine is not available, consider using subcutaneous terbutaline sulfate (Brethine). Phentolamine also offers an additional option in the management of drug-induced hypertension. Stock in ED and pharmacy.

©Illinois Poison Center March, 2014. PDR has secured written permission to reprint the Antidote Chart for the sole purpose of providing an additional educational reference within this publication. Reproduction or resale of this list without the written authorization from the Illinois Poison Center is strictly prohibited.

ADJUNCTIVE AGENTS (Continued)

ADJUNCTIVE AGENT	POISON/DRUG/TOXIN	SUGGESTED MINIMUM STOCK QUANTITY	RATIONALE/COMMENTS
Sodium nitrite	Hydrogen sulfide (H_2S)	0 to 1 vial. Available as 3% sodium nitrite in 10 mL vials.	Nitrite therapy for H_2S poisoning is controversial. Seriously poisoned patients should receive nitrites within 1 h of exposure. Sodium thiosulfate is not administered in H_2S poisoning. The product is available from Hope Pharmaceuticals in Scottsdale, Arizona. If the amyl nitrite/sodium nitrite/sodium thiosulfate cyanide antidote kits are stocked, additional sodium nitrite vials may not be necessary. Stock in pharmacy.
Sodium thiosulfate	Bromates Chlorates Mustard agents Nitroprusside Smoke inhalation	Quantity determined by institution. Available in 100 mg/mL, 10 mL vials and 250 mg/mL, 50 mL vials.	Sodium thiosulfate (without nitrites) has been advocated in the treatment of smoke inhalation related to cyanide exposure; however, it is not necessary if hydroxocobalamin is available. Sodium thiosulfate may be used in conjunction with cisplatin to reduce toxicity of this chemotherapy agent. Sodium thiosulfate is found in the amyl nitrite/sodium nitrite/sodium thiosulfate cyanide antidote kits; however, additional vials may be stocked. Stock in pharmacy.
Thiamine	Ethanol Ethylene glycol	Quantity determined by institution. Available as 100 mg/mL in 2 mL vials.	Parenteral thiamine precedes IV dextrose in patients with chronic ethanol abuse. Thiamine 100 mg every 6 h enhances clearance of toxic metabolites of ethylene glycol. Stock in ED and pharmacy.

AGENTS FOR RADIOLOGICAL EXPOSURES

AGENT	POISON/DRUG/TOXIN	SUGGESTED MINIMUM STOCK QUANTITY	RATIONALE/COMMENTS
Calcium-diethylenetriamine pentaacetic acid (Ca-DTPA; Pentetate calcium trisodium injection) Zinc-diethylenetriamine pentaacetic acid (Zn-DTPA; Pentetate zinc trisodium injection)	Internal contamination with transuranium elements: americium, curium, plutonium	Quantity determined by institution. Supplied as 200 mg/mL, 5 mL ampules for IV or inhalation administration. The product is sponsored through Hameln Pharmaceuticals, GmbH, of Hameln, Germany. Distributed in the U.S. by Akorn, Inc.	1 ampule provides the usual adult dose of 1 g q 24 h. More would be necessary in a mass casualty event. Ca-DTPA and Zn-DTPA are available through the SNS and REAC/TS, Oak Ridge, Tennessee at 865-576-3131 (business hours) or 865-576-1005 (after hours).

(Continued)

©Illinois Poison Center March, 2014. PDR has secured written permission to reprint the Antidote Chart for the sole purpose of providing an additional educational reference within this publication. Reproduction or resale of this list without the written authorization from the Illinois Poison Center is strictly prohibited.

AGENTS FOR RADIOLOGICAL EXPOSURES *(Continued)*

AGENT	POISON/DRUG/TOXIN	SUGGESTED MINIMUM STOCK QUANTITY	RATIONALE/COMMENTS
Potassium iodide, KI tablets (Iosat, Thyrosafe) KI liquid (Thyroshield, SSKI)	Prevents thyroid uptake of radioactive iodine (I-131)	Quantity determined by institution. Available in 130 mg and 65 mg tablets, and PO solutions: 65 mg/mL (30 mL bottle) and 1 g/mL (30 mL and 240 mL bottle).	One 130 mg tablet represents the initial daily adult dose. More would be necessary in a mass casualty event. KI tablets and oral solution are OTC. The Illinois Emergency Management Association makes KI tablets available to healthcare facilities and the general public located near nuclear reactors.
Prussian blue, ferric hexacyanoferrate (Radiogardase)	Radioactive cesium (Cs-137), radioactive thallium (Tl-201), and non-radioactive thallium	None recommended at the present time. Available in bottles of 30 capsules (500 mg/capsule).	The usual oral adult dose is 3 g, 3 times a day. The product is manufactured by Haupt Pharma Berlin GmbH for distribution by HEYL Chemisch-pharmazeutische Fabrik GmbH & Co. KG, Berlin, Germany, and is available in the U.S. from Heyltex Corporation. Prussian Blue is also available through the SNS and REAC/TS, Oak Ridge, Tennessee at 865-576-3131 (business hours) or 865-576-1005 (after hours).

Abbreviations: BAL = British anti-Lewisite; CDC = Centers for Disease Control and Prevention; ED = emergency department; EPS = extrapyramidal symptom; NMS = neuroleptic malignant syndrome; OPI = organophosphate insecticide; PCC = poison control center; REAC/TS = radiation emergency assistance center/training site; SNS = Strategic National Stockpile; WMD = weapons of mass destruction.

©Illinois Poison Center March, 2014. PDR has secured written permission to reprint the Antidote Chart for the sole purpose of providing an additional educational reference within this publication. Reproduction or resale of this list without the written authorization from the Illinois Poison Center is strictly prohibited.

DRUGS EXCRETED IN BREAST MILK

The following list is not comprehensive; generic forms and alternate brands of some products may be available. When recommending drugs to pregnant or nursing patients, always check labeling for specific precautions.

Abstral
Accolate
Accupril
Accuretic
Acetaminophen/Codeine
Aclovate
Actiq
Activella
Acyclovir
Adalat CC
Adderall XR
Advicor
Aggrenox
Aldactazide
Aldactone
Allegra-D
Aloprim
Alora
Altace
Ambien
Ambien CR
Amcinonide
Amiloride/HCTZ
Amitriptyline
Amoxapine
Amoxicillin
Ampicillin
Amturnide
Anafranil
Analpram-HC
Angeliq
Ansaid
Anusol-HC Cream
Aplenzin
Apriso
Armour Thyroid
Arthrotec
Asacol
Astramorph PF
Atacand HCT
ATryn
Atuss DS
Augmentin
Augmentin ES-600
Augmentin XR

Avalide
AVC
Avelox
Aviane
Avinza
Aygestin
Azactam
Azasan
Azulfidine
Azulfidine EN
Bactrim
Banzel
Benicar HCT
Bentyl
BenzaClin
Benzamycin
Betamethasone Dipropionate
Betamethasone Valerate
Betapace
Betapace AF
Beyaz
Bicillin C-R
Bicillin L-A
Biltricide
Buprenex
Butisol
Butorphanol
Butrans
Calan
Calan SR
Capex
Carbatrol
Cardene IV
Cardizem
Cardizem CD
Catapres
Cayston
Cefaclor ER
Cefazolin
Cefotetan
Cefoxitin
Cefpodoxime
Cefprozil
Ceftin

Ceftriaxone
Celebrex
Celestone
Celexa
Cenestin
Cephadyn
Cephalexin
Ceredase
Chloral Hydrate
Chlorothiazide
Chlorpromazine
Chlorthalidone
Cipro
Cipro XR
Cisplatin
Claforan
Clarinex
Clarinex-D
Clenia
Cleocin
Cleocin T
Climara
Climara Pro
Clindagel
Clindamax
Clobex
Cloderm
Co-Gesic
Colcrys
CombiPatch
Combivir
Compro
Cordarone
Cordran
Corgard
Cortifoam
Cortisporin
Corzide
Cosopt
Covera-HS
Crinone
Cutivate
Cyclessa
Cyklokapron
Cymbalta

Cytomel
Cytotec
Dantrium IV
Dapsone
Daraprim
Delestrogen
Demeclocycline HCl
Demerol
Depacon
Depakote
Depakote ER
DepoDur
Depo-Estradiol
Depo-Provera
depo-subQ provera 104
Derma-Smoothe/FS
Dermatop
DermOtic Oil
Desonate
Dexamethasone
Dexedrine Spansules
Dexferrum
Dextroamphetamine Sulfate
Diabinese
Diclegis
Dicloxacillin
Didrex
Diethylpropion
Diflorasone
Diflucan
Diflunisal
Dilacor XR
Dilantin
Dilaudid
Diltiazem
Diovan HCT
Dipentum
Diprivan
Diprolene
Dipyridamole
Divigel
Dolophine
Doral
Doryx
Doxorubicin HCl

(Continued)

Droxia	Femring	Isoniazid	Marcaine Spinal
Duac	Femtrace	Isoptin SR	Marinol
Duexis	Fentora	Jenloga	Maxipime
Duragesic	Fioricet	Jentadueto	Maxitrol Ointment
Duramorph	Fioricet w/Codeine	Kadian	Maxzide
Dyazide	Fiorinal	Kapvay ER	MDP-25
Dynacin	Fiorinal w/Codeine	Kenalog	Meclofenamate
E.E.S.	Flagyl	Keppra	Mefloquine
Edarbyclor	Flagyl ER	Keppra XR	Menest
Effexor XR	Flagyl IV	Ketoconazole	Menostar
Elestrin	Fleet Enema	Ketorolac	Meperidine
Elixophyllin	Flo-Pred	Korlym	Meprobamate
Elocon	Fludrocortisone	Labetalol	Meruvax II
Embeda	Fluocinolone Acetonide	Lamictal	Methadone
EMLA	Fluocinonide	Lamictal XR	Methadose
Enalapril/HCTZ	Fluorescite	Lamisil	Methotrexate
Enalaprilat	Fluoxetine	Lanoxin	Methyclothiazide
Endometrin	Fluvoxamine	Lazanda	Methyldopa
Enjuvia	Folic Acid	Levaquin	Methyldopa/HCTZ
Epifoam	Forfivo XL	Levbid	Methyldopate
Epivir	Fortaz	Levoxyl	Metoclopramide
Epivir-HBV	Fosamax Plus D	Levsin	Metoprolol/HCTZ
Epzicom	Fosinopril/HCTZ	Lexapro	Metozolv ODT
Equetro	Fragmin	Lialda	MetroGel-Vaginal
Ergomar	Furosemide	Lidocaine Cream	Mexiletine
ERYC	Gablofen	Lidoderm Patch	Micardis HCT
EryPed	Gadavist	Lindane	Microzide
Ery-Tab	Gengraf Capsules	Lioresal	Midazolam
Erythrocin	Gleevec	Lipitor	Minipress
Erythrocin Lactobionate	Glyset	Lithium	Minoxidil
Erythromycin	Gralise	Lithium ER	Mircette
Erythromycin Ethylsuccinate	Guanidine HCl	Lo Loestrin Fe	Mirena
and Sulfisoxazole Acetyl	Haldol Decanoate	Lo/Ovral	M-M-R II
Esgic	Halog	Locoid	Modicon
Esgic-Plus	Haloperidol	Loestrin 21	Monodox
Estrace	Helidac	Loestrin 24 Fe	Monopril
Estraderm	Hydrea	Loestrin Fe	Morphine
Estradiol	Hydrochlorothiazide	Lopressor	Moxeza
Estrasorb	Hyzaar	Lorcet	MS Contin
Estring	Ifex	Lortab	Myambutol
EstroGel	Imitrex	Loseasonique	Myochrysine
Estropipate	Implanon	Lotensin	Mysoline
Estrostep Fe	Imuran	Lotensin HCT	Nafcillin Sodium
Evamist	Inderal LA	Lotrel	Nalbuphine
Evoclin	Indomethacin	Lusedra	Naprelan
Exalgo	INFeD	Luvox CR	Naprosyn
Exforge HCT	Infumorph	Luxiq	Natazia
Exparel	InnoPran XL	Lysteda	Nature-Throid
Famotidine	Intermezzo	Magnevist	Necon 10/11
Felbatol	Invanz	Makena	Nembutal Sodium Solution
Feldene	Invega	Maprotiline	Neomycin/Polymyxin B/
femhrt	Invega Sustenna	Marcaine	Dexamethasone

Neoral
Neurontin
Nexiclon XR
Nexplanon
Nexterone
Niaspan
Nicotrol Nasal Spray
Niravam
Nizatidine
Norco
Nordette-28
Norinyl 1/50
Noritate
Nor-QD
Novacort
Novantrone
NuvaRing
Ofirmev
Ofloxacin
Olux-E
Onfi
Onsolis
Oracea
Orapred
Oraqix
Ortho Evra
Ortho Micronor
Ortho Tri-Cyclen
Ortho Tri-Cyclen Lo
Ortho-Cept
Ortho-Cyclen
Ortho-Novum 1/35
Ortho-Novum 7/7/7
Ovcon-35
Oxecta
Oxistat
Oxycodone IR
OxyContin
Pandel
Paxil
Paxil CR
PCE
Pediapred
Peganone
Penicillin G Potassium
Penicillin G Procaine
Pentasa
Percocet
Percodan
Periostat

Persantine
Pexeva
Pfizerpen
Phenobarbital
Phoslyra
Phrenilin Forte
Plexion
Poly-Pred
Ponstel
Pramosone
Pravachol
Prefest
Premarin
Premphase
Prevpac
Prilosec
Primsol
Prinzide
Pristiq
Proctocort Cream
ProctoFoam-HC
Progesterone
Prograf
Promethazine w/Codeine
Promethazine VC w/Codeine
Prometrium
Propranolol
Propranolol/HCTZ
Propylthiouracil
Proquin XR
Prosed EC
Protonix
Protopic
Provera
Prozac
Pulmicort
Pylera
Pyrazinamide
Qsymia
Qualaquin
Quinidine Gluconate
Quinidine Sulfate
Quixin
Qvar
Rayos
Reserpine
Restasis
Retrovir
Rezira

Rhinocort Aqua
Rifater
Risperdal
Risperdal Consta
Robaxin
Rocaltrol
Rosac
Roxicet
Roxicodone
Rybix ODT
Rythmol SR
Sabril
Safyral
Salsalate
Sandimmune
Sarafem
Seasonale
Seconal Sodium
Sectral
Semprex-D
Sensorcaine-MPF
Septra
Seromycin
Seroquel
Seroquel XR
Silenor
Simcor
Sinemet CR
Solodyn
Solu-Cortef
Solu-Medrol
Soma
Soma Compound
Soma Compound w/Codeine
Soriatane
Spectracef
Sporanox
Sprix
SSKi
St. Joseph 81 mg Aspirin
Stavzor
Stelara
Streptomycin
Stribild
Stromectol
Suboxone Sublingual Film
Subsys
Sumycin
Symbyax

Synthroid
Taclonex
Tambocor
Tapazole
Tarka
Tazicef
Tegretol
Tekturna HCT
Tenoretic
Tenormin
Teveten HCT
Theo-24
Theophylline
Thyrolar
Tiazac
Tilia Fe
Timoptic
Tindamax
Topamax
Toprol-XL
Transderm Scop
Tranxene T-Tab
Trental
Treximet
Triamcinolone
Tribenzor
Trileptal
Tri-Luma
Trimethoprim
Triphasil
Trisenox
Trivora
Trizivir
Tysabri
Tudorza Pressair
Ultane
Ultracet
Ultravate
Unasyn
Uniretic
Unithroid
Urex
Urogesic Blue
UTA
Utira-C
Vagifem
Valium
Valtrex
Vandazole

(Continued)

Vanos	Viread	Xyzal	Zinacef
Vascepa	Visudyne	Yasmin	Zolpimist
Vasotec	Vivelle-Dot	YAZ	Zonalon
Venlafaxine	Vivitrol	Zanaflex	Zonegran
Verapamil	Vyvanse	Zantac	Zosyn
Verdeso	Wellbutrin SR	Zarah	Zovia
Verelan	Wellbutrin XL	Zarontin	Zovirax Oral
Verelan PM	Westcort	Zebutal	Zubsolv
Vibramycin	Westhroid	Zegerid	Zyban
Vicodin	Xanax	Zestoretic	Zydone
Vigamox	Xanax XR	Zevalin	Zyprexa
Vimovo	Ximino	Ziac	Zyprexa Relprevv
Viramune	Xylocaine Jelly	Ziana	

Abbreviation: HCTZ = hydrochlorothiazide

PRODUCT IDENTIFICATION GUIDE

To aid in quick identification, this section provides full-color, actual-sized images of tablets and capsules. A variety of other dosage forms and packages are shown at less than actual size.

Products in this section are arranged alphabetically by manufacturer. Some exceptions, however, have been made based on space available in this section. Late submissions appear alphabetically by manufacturer at the end of the section. In some instances, not all dosage forms and sizes are pictured. If others are available, a † symbol precedes the product's name. Letters or numbers representing the manufacturer's identification code are followed by a * symbol.

For more information on any of the products in this section, please turn to the Product Information section, or check directly with the manufacturer. The page number of each product's text entry appears with its images.

While every effort has been made to guarantee faithful reproduction of the images in this section, changes in size, color, and design are always a possibility. Be sure to confirm a product's identity with the manufacturer or a pharmacist.

INDEX BY MANUFACTURER

This section is made possible through the courtesy of the manufacturers whose products appear on the following pages.

4LIFE

DS   4LIFE   P. 2448

4Life Transfer Factor®
Tri-Factor® Formula

While every effort has been made to reproduce products faithfully, this section is to be considered a quick reference identification aid. In cases of suspected overdosing, etc., chemical analysis should be done.

A&Z PHARMACEUTICAL

OTC   A&Z PHARMACEUTICAL   P. 2449

Calcium 300 mg

60 Chewable Tablets

D-Cal®
(calcium carbonate/vitamin D₃)

OTC   A&Z PHARMACEUTICAL   P. 2449

Calcium 300 mg
10 pouches

Granules

D-Cal® Kids
(calcium carbonate)

Products in this section are arranged alphabetically by manufacturer. In some instances, not all dosage forms and/or sizes are pictured. If others are available, a † symbol precedes the product's name. Letters or numbers representing the manufacturer's identification code are followed by a * symbol.

ABBVIE INC.

For description of Abbo-Code Identifications, see Abbo-Code index at the beginning of the AbbVie Information Section.

RX   AbbVie Inc.   P. 402

502
500 mg/20 mg

752
750 mg/20 mg

1002
1000 mg/20 mg

1004
1000 mg/40 mg

Advicor®
(niacin extended-release/lovastatin tablets)

C-III   AbbVie Inc.   P. 409

AndroGel® 1%
(testosterone gel)

C-III   AbbVie Inc.   P. 414

AndroGel® 1.62%
(testosterone gel)

RX   AbbVie Inc.   P. 420

KJ* 500 mg

Biaxin® XL Filmtab®
(clarithromycin extended-release tablets)

RX   AbbVie Inc.   P. 420

KT* 250 mg

KL* 500 mg

Biaxin® Filmtab®
(clarithromycin tablets, USP)

RX   AbbVie Inc.   P. 420

250 mg/5 mL

†Biaxin® Granules
(clarithromycin for oral suspension, USP)

RX   AbbVie Inc.   P. 431

Creon®
(pancrelipase)
Delayed-Release Capsules

RX   AbbVie Inc.   P. 435

250 mg

†Depakene®
(valproic acid)
Capsules and Oral Solution

RX   AbbVie Inc.   P. 435

NT* 125 mg

NR* 250 mg

NS* 500 mg

Depakote®
(divalproex sodium)
Tablets for Oral Use

RX   AbbVie Inc.   P. 435

125 mg

Depakote® Sprinkle Capsules
(divalproex sodium delayed release capsules)

RX   AbbVie Inc.   P. 435

HF* 250 mg

HC* 500 mg

Depakote® ER
(divalproex sodium)
Tablets, Extended-Release for Oral Use

RX   AbbVie Inc.   P. 445

OR* 25 mg

OT* 100 mg

Gengraf® Capsules
(cyclosporine capsules USP [MODIFIED])

RX   AbbVie Inc.   P. 455

prefilled syringe

40 mg/0.8 mL
pen

†HUMIRA®
(adalimumab)

RX   AbbVie Inc.   P. 469

80 mg-20 mg/mL
160 mL bottle

Kaletra®
(lopinavir/ritonavir)
Solution for Oral Use

RX   AbbVie Inc.   P. 469

100 mg/25 mg

Kaletra®
(lopinavir/ritonavir)
Tablet Film-Coated for Oral Use

RX   AbbVie Inc.   P. 469

200 mg/50 mg

Kaletra®
(lopinavir/ritonavir)
Tablet Film-Coated for Oral Use

RX   AbbVie Inc.   P. 484, 491

1-Month 3.75 mg/5 mg

3-Month 11.25 mg/5 mg

Lupaneta Pack®
(leuprolide acetate for depot suspension and norethindrone acetate tablets)

RX   AbbVie Inc.   P. 497, 504

1-Month 3.75 mg

3-Month 11.25 mg

Lupron Depot® GYN
(leuprolide acetate for depot suspension)

RX   AbbVie Inc.   P. 514

1-Month 7.5 mg

11.25 mg

1-Month 15 mg

Lupron Depot–PED®
(leuprolide acetate for depot suspension)

The pictured forms shown in this section may not necessarily be the only dosage forms and/or sizes available. Where a product name is preceded by a † symbol, refer to the description in the Product Information Section for other dosage forms and/or sizes.

*AbbVie Abbo-Code identification letters. Filmtab® Film-sealed tablets, AbbVie.

†Additional dosage forms and sizes available.

RX AbbVie Inc. P. 502, 509	

1-Month 7.5 mg

3-Month 22.5 mg

4-Month 30 mg

Lupron Depot® URO
(leuprolide acetate for depot suspension)

RX   AbbVie Inc.   P. 519

FT* 1 mg

FX* 2 mg

FZ* 4 mg

Mavik®
(trandolapril tablets)

RX   AbbVie Inc.   P. 522

200 mg

400 mg

600 mg

Moderiba™
(ribavirin, USP) Tablets

Help your patients save on prescription medications with the PDR® Pharmacy Discount Card. For more, visit PDR.net/PharmacyDiscountCard.

RX   AbbVie Inc.   P. 529

500 mg

750 mg

1000 mg

Niaspan® Tablets
(niacin extended-release)
Tablet, Film-Coated, Extended-Release
for Oral Use

RX   AbbVie Inc.   P. 536

10 mg/5 mL
(2 mg/mL)

20 mg/10 mL
(2 mg/mL)

200 mg/20 mL
(10 mg/mL)

Nimbex®
(cisatracurium besylate) Injection

RX   AbbVie Inc.   P. 542

DS* 100 mg

Norvir®
(ritonavir)
Capsules, Soft Gelatin for Oral Use

RX   AbbVie Inc.   P. 552

80 mg/mL
240 mL bottle

Norvir®
(ritonavir oral solution)

RX   AbbVie Inc.   P. 552

100 mg

Norvir®
(ritonavir) Tablet for Oral Use

RX   AbbVie Inc.   P. 568

500-20

500 mg/20 mg

750-20

750 mg/20 mg

1000-20

1000 mg/20 mg

500-40

500 mg/40 mg

1000-40

1000 mg/40 mg

Simcor®
(niacin extended-release/
simvastatin) Tablets

RX   AbbVie Inc.   P. 575

4 mL

8 mL

Survanta®
(beractant)
Intratracheal Suspension

RX   AbbVie Inc.   P. 578

25 mcg   **50 mcg**   **75 mcg**

88 mcg   **100 mcg**   **112 mcg**

125 mcg   **137 mcg**   **150 mcg**

175 mcg   **200 mcg**   **300 mcg**

Synthroid®
(levothyroxine sodium tablets, USP)

RX   AbbVie Inc.   P. 582

182

2 mg/180 mg

241

1 mg/240 mg

242

2 mg/240 mg

244

4 mg/240 mg

Tarka®
(trandolapril/verapamil
hydrochloride ER tablets)

RX   AbbVie Inc.   P. 587

FI* 48 mg

FO* 145 mg

Tricor®
(fenofibrate) Tablet for Oral Use

RX   AbbVie Inc.   P. 592

45

45 mg

135

135 mg

Trilipix®
(fenofibric acid) Capsule,
Delayed-Release for Oral Use

RX   AbbVie Inc.   P. 598

250 mL

Ultane®
(sevoflurane)
Volatile Liquid for Inhalation

C-III   AbbVie Inc.   P. 605

VICODIN

5 mg/500 mg

Vicodin®
(hydrocodone bitartrate and
acetaminophen tablets, USP)

C-III   AbbVie Inc.   P. 607

VICODIN ES

7.5 mg/750 mg

Vicodin ES®
(hydrocodone bitartrate and
acetaminophen tablets, USP)

C-III   AbbVie Inc.   P. 609

VICODIN HP

10 mg/660 mg

Vicodin HP®
(hydrocodone bitartrate and
acetaminophen tablets, USP)

---

*Manufacturer's Identification Code

The trusted *Physicians' Desk Reference*® is now available digitally. Visit <u>PDR.net</u> to download your free *PDR*® eBook today.

RX   AbbVie Inc.   P. 614

1 mcg   2 mcg

Zemplar® Capsules
(paricalcitol)

ALTO
DS   ALTO PHARMACEUTICALS, INC. P. 2449

220 mg
Zinc-220®
(zinc sulfate, USP)

Register at <u>PDR.net</u> today to receive free PDR® Drug Alerts, monthly eDrug Updates, and FDA-required Drug Safety Alerts via email.

AMGEN INC.
RX   AMGEN INC.   P. 621

60 mg/1 mL
Prolia®
(denosumab)

ANDORRA LIFE
DS   ANDORRA LIFE   P. 2449

Advanced Blood Sugar Control

C-III   AbbVie Inc.   P. 604

5 mg/300 mg

Vicodin®
(hydrocodone bitartrate and acetaminophen tablets, USP)

C-III   AbbVie Inc.   P. 604

7.5 mg/300 mg

Vicodin ES®
(hydrocodone bitartrate and acetaminophen tablets, USP)

C-iii   AbbVie Inc.   P. 604

10 mg/300 mg

Vicodin HP®
(hydrocodone bitartrate and acetaminophen tablets, USP)

C-III   AbbVie Inc.   P. 610

VP* 7.5 mg/200 mg

Vicoprofen®
(hydrocodone bitartrate and ibuprofen tablets)

*Manufacturer's Identification Code

DS   ANDORRA LIFE   P. 2450

Advanced Lung Cleanse

DS   ANDORRA LIFE   P. 2451

CholesteRight

DS   ANDORRA LIFE   P. 2452

OPC Supreme

ARIIX
DS   ARIIX   P. 2453

Optimal-M™

Optimal-V™

Optimal

AWARENESSLIFE/ PURETRIM
DS   AWARENESSLIFE/PURETRIM   P. 2454

Experience®

DS   AWARENESSLIFE/PURETRIM   P. 2454

30 fl. oz./886 mL

Liquid Daily Complete®

DS   AWARENESSLIFE/PURETRIM   P. 2454

LiverMaster®

DS   AWARENESSLIFE/PURETRIM   P. 2454

PureTrim Mediterranean Truffles®

Look for PDR® services in your EHR with PDR® BRIEF and PDR®+ *for Patients*.

DS   AWARENESSLIFE/PURETRIM   P. 2454

PureTrim® Mediterranean Wellness Shake™

BAYER HEALTHCARE LLC
RX   BAYER HEALTHCARE LLC   P. 627

200 mg

Nexavar®
(sorafenib) tablets

RX   BAYER HEALTHCARE LLC   P. 635

40 mg

Stivarga®
(regorafenib) tablets

RX   BAYER HEALTHCARE LLC   P. 641

1000 kBq/mL

Xofigo™
(radium Ra 223 dichloride) injection

BRISTOL-MYERS SQUIBB COMPANY

RX   BRISTOL-MYERS SQUIBB COMPANY   P. 645
& GILEAD SCIENCES, LLC

600 mg/200 mg/300 mg

ATRIPLA®
(efavirenz/emtricitabine/tenofovir
disoproxil fumarate)

RX   BRISTOL-MYERS SQUIBB COMPANY   P. 658

0.5 mg

1.0 mg

Also available as 0.05 mg/mL oral solution

Baraclude®
(entecavir) tablets

RX   BRISTOL-MYERS SQUIBB COMPANY   P. 666

1 mg   2 mg   2½ mg

3 mg   4 mg   5 mg

6 mg   7½ mg   10 mg

Also available as 5 mg vial for
intravenous use

Coumadin® Tablets
(warfarin sodium tablets, USP) crystalline

RX   BRISTOL-MYERS SQUIBB COMPANY   P. 672

2.5 mg

5 mg

Eliquis®
(apixaban) tablets

RX   BRISTOL-MYERS SQUIBB COMPANY   P. 681

100 mg/50 mL

200 mg/100 mL

ERBITUX®
(cetuximab) injection

RX   BRISTOL-MYERS SQUIBB COMPANY   P. 688

15 mg/vial for injection and
8 mL DILUENT for IXEMPRA/vial

45 mg/vial for injection and
23.5 mL DILUENT for IXEMPRA/vial

IXEMPRA® Kit
(ixabepilone) for injection

RX   BRISTOL-MYERS SQUIBB COMPANY   P. 694

250 mg/vial

Nulojix®
(belatacept) for injection

RX   BRISTOL-MYERS SQUIBB COMPANY   P. 702

125 mg/mL Prefilled Syringe with
UltraSafe Passive® Needle Guard

250 mg/vial for intravenous use

Orencia®
(abatacept)

RX   BRISTOL-MYERS SQUIBB COMPANY   P. 712

150 mg

200 mg

300 mg

Reyataz®
(atazanavir) capsules

RX   BRISTOL-MYERS SQUIBB COMPANY   P. 732

20 mg   50 mg

70 mg   80 mg

100 mg   140 mg

Sprycel®
(dasatinib) tablets

RX   BRISTOL-MYERS SQUIBB COMPANY   P. 739

50 mg

200 mg

600 mg

SUSTIVA®
(efavirenz) capsules and tablets

While every effort has been
made to reproduce products
faithfully, this section is to be
considered a quick reference
identification aid. In cases of
suspected overdosing, etc.,
chemical analysis should
be done.

RX   BRISTOL-MYERS SQUIBB COMPANY   P. 752

50 mg/10 mL

Yervoy®
(ipilimumab) Injection

200 mg/40 mL

Yervoy®
(ipilimumab) injection for intravenous
infusion

Products in this section are
arranged alphabetically by
manufacturer. In some instances,
not all dosage forms and/or
sizes are pictured. If others are
available, a † symbol precedes
the product's name. Letters or
numbers representing the
manufacturer's identification code
are followed by a * symbol.

CONCORDIA PHARMACEUTICALS INC.

RX   CONCORDIA   P. 2417
PHARMACEUTICALS INC.

0.1037 mg/0.0194 mg/
0.0065 mg/16.2 mg

Donnatal®
(hyoscyamine sulfate/atropine sulfate/
scopolamine HBr/phenobarbital) tablets

EDGEMONT PHARMACEUTICALS

RX   EDGEMONT PHARMACEUTICALS P. 2417

60 mg

Fluoxetine Tablets, USP

RX   EDGEMONT PHARMACEUTICALS P. 2428

450 mg

Forfivo XL
(bupropion hydrochloride
extended-release tablets)

ESSENTIA WATER, LLC.

DS   ESSENTIA WATER, LLC.   P. 2454

Essentia® Water

GILEAD

RX   BRISTOL-MYERS SQUIBB &   P. 774
GILEAD SCIENCES, LLC

600 mg/200 mg/300 mg

ATRIPLA®
(efavirenz/emtricitabine/tenofovir
disoproxil fumarate)

RX   GILEAD SCIENCES, INC.   P. 774

75 mg/vial

CAYSTON®
(aztreonam for inhalation solution)

RX   GILEAD SCIENCES, INC.   P. 777

200 mg/25 mg/300 mg

COMPLERA®
(emtricitabine/rilpivirine/
tenofovir disoproxil fumarate)

The pictured forms shown in this
section may not necessarily be
the only dosage forms and/or
sizes available. Where a product
name is preceded by a †
symbol, refer to the description
in the Product Information
Section for other dosage forms
and/or sizes.

RX   GILEAD SCIENCES, INC.   P. 788

GSI | 5

5 mg

GSI | 10

10 mg

LETAIRIS®
(ambrisentan)

RX   GILEAD SCIENCES, INC.   P. 793

GSI 500

500 mg

GSI 1000

1000 mg

RANEXA®
(ranolazine) extended-release tablets

RX   GILEAD SCIENCES, INC.   P. 797

GSI

7977

400 mg

SOVALDI®
(sofosbuvir)

RX   GILEAD SCIENCES, INC.   P. 804

GSI

1

150 mg/150 mg/200 mg/300 mg

STRIBILD®
(elvitegravir/cobicistat/emtricitabine/
tenofovir disoproxil fumarate)

RX   GILEAD SCIENCES, INC.   P. 815

GILEAD

701

200 mg/300 mg

TRUVADA®
(emtricitabine/tenofovir
disoproxil fumarate)

RX   GILEAD SCIENCES, INC.   P. 825

GSI | 150

150 mg

GSI | 200

200 mg

GSI | 250

250 mg

GILEAD
4331 | 300

300 mg

VIREAD®
(tenofovir disoproxil fumarate)

40 mg/scoop

RX   GILEAD SCIENCES, INC.   P. 837

GSI | 100

100 mg

GSI | 150

150 mg

ZYDELIG®
(idelalisib)

GLENWOOD

RX   GLENWOOD   P. 1275

POTABA 51 | POTABA 51

500 mg

Potaba®
(aminobenzoate potassium, USP)

Help your patients save on
prescription medications
with the PDR® Pharmacy
Discount Card. For more, visit
PDR.net/PharmacyDiscountCard.

GORDON LABORATORIES

RX   GORDON LABORATORIES   P. 1276

FORMADON

10%
Available in 60 mL and 120 mL

Formadon
(formaldehyde solution)

OTC   GORDON LABORATORIES   P. 1276

Gordochom

25%
30 mL

Gordochom
(undecylenic acid)

**HALOZYME
THERAPEUTICS, INC.**

RX   HALOZYME THERAPEUTICS, INC. P. 1276

Hylenex 4 x 1 mL

150 USP units/mL
4 x 1 mL single dose vials

Hylenex® recombinant
(hyaluronidase human injection)

HEEL INC.

RX   HEEL INC.   P. 1278

Traumeel

2.2 mL

Traumeel®
Injection Solution

RX   HEEL INC.   P. 1279

Zeel

2 mL

Zeel®
Injection Solution

HIGH CHEMICAL

RX   HIGH CHEMICAL   P. 1281

SARAPIN | SARAPIN

50 mL Multiple Dose Vial

SARAPIN®
(sarraceniaceae)

**JANSSEN
PHARMACEUTICALS, INC.**

C-II   JANSSEN
PHARMACEUTICALS, INC.   P. 1290

50 | O-M

NUCYNTA | NUCYNTA

50 mg

75 | O-M

NUCYNTA | NUCYNTA

75 mg

100 | O-M

NUCYNTA | NUCYNTA

100 mg

NUCYNTA®
(tapentadol)
Immediate-Release Tablets

C-II   JANSSEN
PHARMACEUTICALS, INC.   P. 1295

OMJ 50

50 mg

OMJ 100

100 mg

OMJ 150

150 mg

OMJ 200

200 mg

OMJ 250

250 mg

NUCYNTA® ER
(tapentadol)
Extended-Release Tablets

**KOWA PHARMACEUTICALS
AMERICA, INC.**

RX   KOWA PHARMACEUTICALS,   P. 1309
AMERICA INC.

1

1 mg

2

2 mg

4

4 mg

Livalo®
(pitavastatin) Tablets

The trusted *Physicians' Desk
Reference®* is now available
digitally. Visit PDR.net to
download your free *PDR®*
eBook today.

**LIFEPHARM GLOBAL
NETWORK**

DS   LIFEPHARM GLOBAL NETWORK P. 2455

Laminine

Laminine

Laminine®

MANNKIND CORPORATION

RX   MANNKIND CORPORATION   P. 1314

4 U and 8 U
single-use cartridges

Afrezza®
(insulin human) Inhalation Powder

Register at PDR.net today to
receive free PDR® Drug Alerts,
monthly eDrug Updates, and
FDA-required Drug Safety Alerts
via email.

MERCK

RX   MERCK   P. 1329

400 mg

Avelox®
(moxifloxacin HCI)

RX   MERCK   P. 1339

50 mg

70 mg

Cancidas®
(caspofungin acetate) for Injection

RX   MERCK   P. 1351

5 mg
Also available in 0.5 mg/1 mL oral solution

Clarinex®
(desloratadine)

RX   MERCK   P. 1356

2.5 mg/120 mg

Clarinex-D® 12 Hour
(desloratadine/pseudoephedrine sulfate)

RX   MERCK   P. 1364

2%/0.5%
0.2 mL

Cosopt® PF
(dorzolamide HCI - timolol maleate
ophthalmic solution)

Look for PDR® services in your
EHR with PDR® BRIEF and
PDR®+ *for Patients.*

RX   MERCK   P. 1368

200 mg

400 mg

Crixivan®
(indinavir sulfate)

RX   MERCK   P. 1380

100 mcg/5 mcg   200 mcg/5 mcg

Dulera®
(mometasone furoate and formoterol
fumarate dihydrate) Inhalation Aerosol

RX   MERCK   P. 1395

464* 40 mg

461* 80 mg

462* 125 mg

†Emend®
(aprepitant)

RX   MERCK   P. 1426

Foradil® Aerolizer®
(formoterol fumarate inhalation powder)

12 mcg per capsule

Foradil® Aerolizer®
(formoterol fumarate inhalation powder)

RX   MERCK   P. 1442

710* 70 mg/2800 IU

270* 70 mg/5600 IU

Fosamax® Plus D
(alendronate sodium/cholecalciferol)

RX   MERCK   P. 1434

31* 70 mg

Fosamax®
(alendronate sodium)

RX   MERCK   P. 1463

2800 BAU

Grastek®
(timothy grass pollen allergen extract)
Tablet for Sublingual Use

RX   MERCK   P. 1467

68 mg

IMPLANON®
(etonogestrel implant)

RX   MERCK   P. 1474

0.75 mg/mL   2 mg/mL

Integrilin®
(eptifibatide) injection

RX   MERCK   P. 1478

10 MIU/0.2 mL
Available in 3, 5, and 10 million IU
Multidose Pens

5 MIU/0.5 mL
Available in 18 and 25 million IU
Multidose Vials

INTRON® A
(interferon alfa-2b, recombinant)
solution for injection

RX   MERCK   P. 1502

473* 25 mg

477* 100 mg

227* 400 mg

ISENTRESS®
(raltegravir) tablets

While every effort has been
made to reproduce products
faithfully, this section is to be
considered a quick reference
identification aid. In cases of
suspected overdosing, etc.,
chemical analysis should
be done.

RX   MERCK   P. 1512

575* 50 mg/500 mg

577* 50 mg/1000 mg

Janumet®
(sitagliptin/metformin HCI) tablets

RX   MERCK   P. 1522

78* 50 mg/500 mg

80* 50 mg/1000 mg

81* 100 mg/1000 mg

Janumet® XR
(sitagliptin/metformin HCI
extended-release) tablets

RX   MERCK   P. 1533

221* 25 mg

112* 50 mg

277* 100 mg

Januvia®
(sitagliptin)

RX   MERCK   P. 1544

10 mg/10 mg

10 mg/20 mg

10 mg/40 mg

10 mg/80 mg

Liptruzet™
(ezetimibe and atorvastatin) tablets

RX   MERCK   P. 1558

50 mcg/actuation
17 g, 120 metered sprays

Nasonex®
(mometasone furoate monohydrate)

RX   MERCK   P. 1571

0.4
mg/hr
(20 cm²)

0.4 mg/hr
Also available in 0.1 mg/hr, 0.2 mg/hr,
0.3 mg/hr, 0.6 mg/hr, and 0.8 mg/hr

Nitro-Dur®
(nitroglycerin)
Transdermal Infusion System

RX   MERCK   P. 1586

delivers 0.120 mg/0.015 mg per day

NuvaRing®
(etonogestrel/ethinyl estradiol
vaginal ring)

---

*Manufacturer's Identification Code   †Additional dosage forms and sizes available

RX   MERCK   P. 1596

50 mcg/0.5 mL

Also available in 80 mcg/0.5 mL, 120 mcg/0.5 mL, and 150 mcg/0.5 mL

PegIntron®
(peginterferon alfa-2b)

RX   MERCK   P. 1621

19* 5 mg

106* 10 mg

207* 20 mg

PRINIVIL®
(lisinopril) tablets

RX   MERCK   P. 1626

1 mg

Propecia®
(finasteride)

RX   MERCK   P. 1640

72* 5 mg

Proscar®
(finasteride)

Products in this section are arranged alphabetically by manufacturer. In some instances, not all dosage forms and/or sizes are pictured. If others are available, a † symbol precedes the product's name. Letters or numbers representing the manufacturer's identification code are followed by a * symbol.

RX   MERCK   P. 1649

12 Amb a 1-U

Ragwitek™
(short ragweed pollen allergen extract)
Tablet for Sublingual Use

RX   MERCK   P. 1652

200 mg
Capsules

40 mg/mL
Oral Solution

Rebetol®
(ribavirin, USP)

RX   MERCK   P. 1667

15 mg

30 mg   45 mg

REMERON®
(mirtazapine) Tablets

RX   MERCK   P. 1673

15 mg

30 mg

45 mg
Orally Disintegrating Tablets

REMERONSolTab®
(mirtazapine)

RX   MERCK   P. 1684

5 mg

10 mg

Saphris®
(asenapine) sublingual tablets

RX   MERCK   P. 1697

32* 3 mg

Stromectol®
(ivermectin)

RX   MERCK   P. 1705

5 mg

20 mg

100 mg

140 mg

250 mg
Also available as 180 mg capsules and 100 mg vials for injection

Temodar®
(temozolomide)

RX   MERCK   P. 1726

200 mg

VICTRELIS®
(boceprevir) Capsules

RX   MERCK   P. 1739

311* 10/10 mg   **312*** 10/20 mg

313* 10/40 mg   **315*** 10/80 mg

Vytorin®
(ezetimibe/simvastatin)

RX   MERCK   P. 1750

10 x 5 mL multiple dose vials

Zemuron® Injection
(rocuronium bromide)

RX   MERCK   P. 1756

414* 10 mg

Zetia®
(ezetimibe)

RX   MERCK   P. 1762

0.0015%
0.3 mL

ZIOPTAN™
(tafluprost ophthalmic solution)

RX   MERCK   P. 1765

726* 5 mg

735* 10 mg

740* 20 mg

749* 40 mg

543* 80 mg

Zocor®
(simvastatin)

RX   MERCK   P. 1772

100 mg

Zolinza®
(vorinostat)

RX   MERCK   P. 1776

2.08 mg

Zontivity™
(vorapaxar) Tablets

The pictured forms shown in this section may not necessarily be the only dosage forms and/or sizes available. Where a product name is preceded by a † symbol, refer to the description in the Product Information Section for other dosage forms and/or sizes.

NOVARTIS PHARMACEUTICALS CORPORATION

RX   NOVARTIS PHARMACEUTICALS   P. 1801
CORPORATION

5 mg
Other side: imprinted "NVR"

10 mg
Other side: imprinted "NVR"
Also available in 2.5 mg and 7.5 mg

Afinitor®
(everolimus) Tablets

Also available in tablets for oral suspension as Afinitor Disperz in 2 mg, 3 mg, and 5 mg

RX   NOVARTIS PHARMACEUTICALS   P. 1816
CORPORATION

150 mg/5 mg/12.5 mg

300 mg/5 mg/12.5 mg

300 mg/5 mg/25 mg

300 mg/10 mg/12.5 mg

300 mg/10 mg/25 mg

Amturnide™
(aliskiren/amlodipine/hydrochlorothiazide) Tablets

RX   NOVARTIS PHARMACEUTICALS   P. 1824
CORPORATION

75 mcg

arcapta™ neohaler™
(indacaterol inhalation powder)

RX   NOVARTIS PHARMACEUTICALS   P. 1838
CORPORATION

20 mg/120 mg

Coartem®
(artemether/lumefantrine) Tablets

*Manufacturer's Identification Code

RX　NOVARTIS PHARMACEUTICALS P. 1844
CORPORATION

40 mg　80 mg

160 mg

320 mg
Other Side: debossed with "NVR"

Diovan®
(valsartan)

RX　NOVARTIS PHARMACEUTICALS P. 1850
CORPORATION

HGH* 80 mg/12.5 mg
Other side: debossed with "CG"

HHH* 160 mg/12.5 mg
Other side: debossed with "CG"

HXH* 160 mg/25 mg
Other side: debossed with "NVR"

HIL* 320 mg/12.5 mg
Other side: debossed with "NVR"

CTI* 320 mg/25 mg
Other side: debossed with "NVR"

Diovan HCT®
(valsartan/hydrochlorothiazide)

RX　NOVARTIS PHARMACEUTICALS P. 1856
CORPORATION

4.6 mg/24 hours

9.5 mg/24 hours

13.3 mg/24 hours
Patches not actual size
Exelon® Patch
(rivastigmine transdermal system)

Help your patients save on
prescription medications
with the PDR® Pharmacy
Discount Card. For more, visit
PDR.net/PharmacyDiscountCard.

The trusted *Physicians' Desk
Reference®* is now available
digitally. Visit PDR.net to
download your free *PDR®*
eBook today.

RX　NOVARTIS PHARMACEUTICALS P. 1863
CORPORATION

ECE
5 mg/160 mg

UIC
10 mg/160 mg

CSF
5 mg/320 mg

LUF
10 mg/320 mg

Exforge®
(amlodipine/valsartan) Tablets

RX　NOVARTIS PHARMACEUTICALS P. 1870
CORPORATION

VCL
5 mg/160 mg/12.5 mg

VDL
10 mg/160 mg/12.5 mg

VEL
5 mg/160 mg/25 mg

VHL
10 mg/160 mg/25 mg

VFL
10 mg/320 mg/25 mg

Exforge HCT®
(amlodipine/valsartan/hydrochlorothiazide)
Tablets

RX　NOVARTIS PHARMACEUTICALS P. 1877
CORPORATION

J
125
125 mg

J
250
250 mg

J
500
500 mg

Exjade®
(deferasirox)
Tablets for Oral Suspension

RX　NOVARTIS PHARMACEUTICALS P. 1882
CORPORATION

1 mg

2 mg

4 mg

6 mg

8 mg

10 mg

12 mg

DOSAGE INSTRUCTIONS:

Titration Pack

Fanapt®
(iloperidone) Tablets

Register at PDR.net today to
receive free PDR® Drug Alerts,
monthly eDrug Updates, and
FDA-required Drug Safety Alerts
via email.

RX　NOVARTIS PHARMACEUTICALS P. 1888
CORPORATION

FV* 2.5 mg
Other side: imprinted "CG"
Femara®
(letrozole)

While every effort has been
made to reproduce products
faithfully, this section is to be
considered a quick reference
identification aid. In cases of
suspected overdosing, etc.,
chemical analysis should
be done.

Look for PDR® services in your
EHR with PDR® BRIEF and
PDR®+ *for Patients*.

C-II　NOVARTIS PHARMACEUTICALS P. 1895
CORPORATION

NVR D5
5 mg

NVR D10
10 mg

NVR D15
15 mg

NVR D20
20 mg

NVR D25
25 mg

NVR D30
30 mg

NVR D35
35 mg

NVR D40
40 mg

Extended-Release Capsules

Focalin® XR
(dexmethylphenidate HCl)

RX　NOVARTIS PHARMACEUTICALS P. 1901
CORPORATION

GILENYA
(fingolimod)
capsules
0.5 mg

0.5 mg

Gilenya™
(fingolimod) Capsules

RX　NOVARTIS PHARMACEUTICALS P. 1907
CORPORATION

NVR
100 mg

400 mg

Gleevec®
(imatinib mesylate)

RX　NOVARTIS PHARMACEUTICALS P. 1932
CORPORATION

ILARIS
(canakinumab)
For Injection
180 mg sterile powder for reconstitution/vial
For Subcutaneous Use

180 mg

Ilaris®
(canakinumab)

RX　NOVARTIS PHARMACEUTICALS P. 1936
CORPORATION

C
180 mg

CT
360 mg

Myfortic®
(mycophenolic acid*)
delayed-release tablets
*as mycophenolate sodium

RX　NOVARTIS PHARMACEUTICALS P. 1944
CORPORATION

NEORAL Oral
Solution
100 mg/mL
50 mL

100 mg/mL
50 mL

NEORAL® Oral Solution
(cyclosporine oral solution, USP) MODIFIED

RX　NOVARTIS PHARMACEUTICALS P. 1944
CORPORATION

NEORAL
25mg
25 mg

NEORAL
100mg
100 mg

**NEORAL® Soft Gelatin
Capsules**
(cyclosporine capsules, USP) MODIFIED

RX　NOVARTIS PHARMACEUTICALS P. 1953
CORPORATION

Reclast
(zoledronic acid) injection
5 mg/100 mL
Solution for Intravenous Infusion

5 mg/100 mL

Reclast®
(zoledronic acid) Injection

RX NOVARTIS PHARMACEUTICALS P. 1966 CORPORATION

50 mcg/mL   100 mcg/mL   500 mcg/mL
1 mL ampuls

Products in this section are arranged alphabetically by manufacturer. In some instances, not all dosage forms and/or sizes are pictured. If others are available, a † symbol precedes the product's name. Letters or numbers representing the manufacturer's identification code are followed by a * symbol.

200 mcg/mL   1000 mcg/mL
5 mL multi-dose vials

Sandostatin®
(octreotide acetate injection)

RX NOVARTIS PHARMACEUTICALS P. 1968 CORPORATION

10 mg/vial

20 mg/vial

30 mg/vial

Sandostatin® LAR Depot
(octreotide acetate for injectable suspension)

Help your patients save on prescription medications with the PDR® Pharmacy Discount Card. For more, visit PDR.net/PharmacyDiscountCard.

RX NOVARTIS PHARMACEUTICALS P. 1973 CORPORATION

20 mg/vial
Also available in 10 mg vial

Simulect® for Injection
(basiliximab)

RX NOVARTIS PHARMACEUTICALS P. 1976 CORPORATION

NVR   BCR

150 mg

NVR   TKI

200 mg

Tasigna®
(nilotinib) Capsules

RX NOVARTIS PHARMACEUTICALS P. 1984 CORPORATION

T2
150 mg/5 mg

T11
300 mg/5 mg

T7
150 mg/10 mg

T12
300 mg/10 mg

Tekamlo™
(aliskiren/amlodipine) Tablets

RX NOVARTIS PHARMACEUTICALS P. 1990 CORPORATION

IL
150 mg

IU
300 mg

Tekturna®
(aliskiren) Tablets

RX NOVARTIS PHARMACEUTICALS P. 1996 CORPORATION

CVI
300 mg/12.5 mg

CVV
300 mg/25 mg

LCT   CLL
150 mg/12.5 mg   150 mg/25 mg

Tekturna HCT®
(aliskiren/hydrochlorothiazide) Tablets

RX NOVARTIS PHARMACEUTICALS P. 2003 CORPORATION

TOBI

300 mg/5 mL ampules

TOBI®
(tobramycin inhalation solution)

RX NOVARTIS PHARMACEUTICALS P. 2006 CORPORATION

28 mg per capsule
112 mg per dose

TOBI® Podhaler™
(tobramycin inhalation powder)

RX NOVARTIS PHARMACEUTICALS P. 2435 CORPORATION/GENENTECH

Xolair
Omalizumab

150 mg/5 mL single-use vial

XOLAIR®
(omalizumab) Injection

The trusted *Physicians' Desk Reference®* is now available digitally. Visit PDR.net to download your free *PDR®* eBook today.

RX NOVARTIS PHARMACEUTICALS P. 2011 CORPORATION

4 mg/5 mL single-use vial of concentrate

4 mg/100 mL single-use ready-to-use bottle

ZOMETA®
(zoledronic acid) Injection

RX NOVARTIS PHARMACEUTICALS P. 2018 CORPORATION

C
0.25 mg

CH
0.5 mg

CL
0.75 mg

Zortress®
(everolimus) Tablets

RX NOVARTIS PHARMACEUTICALS P. 2028 CORPORATION

NVR   LDK 150M

150 mg

Zykadia™
(ceritinib) Capsules

Register at PDR.net today to receive free PDR® Drug Alerts, monthly eDrug Updates, and FDA-required Drug Safety Alerts via email.

NOVO NORDISK

RX NOVO NORDISK P. 2033

Levemir FlexTouch

100 units/mL

Levemir® FlexTouch®
(insulin detemir [rDNA origin] injection)

RX NOVO NORDISK P. 2060

Victoza

6 mg/mL

Victoza®
(liraglutide [rDNA origin] injection)

ONYX PHARMACEUTICALS, INC.

RX ONYX PHARMACEUTICALS, INC. P. 2071

Kyprolis
60 mg/vial

60 mg/vial

Kyprolis™
(carfilzomib) for Injection

OTSUKA AMERICA PHARMACEUTICAL, INC.

RX OTSUKA AMERICA PHARMACEUTICAL, INC. P. 2075

300 mg

400 mg

Extended-Release

Abilify Maintena®
(aripiprazole) injectable suspension, for intramuscular use

RX OTSUKA AMERICA P. 2441 PHARMACEUTICAL, INC.

15 mg

30 mg

SAMSCA®
(tolvaptan) tablets

Look for PDR® services in your EHR with PDR® BRIEF and PDR®+ *for Patients.*

PIVOTAL THERAPEUTICS INC.

RX PIVOTAL THERAPEUTICS INC. P. 2098

VASCAZEN

VASCAZEN®
(omega-3-acid ethyl esters) capsules

While every effort has been made to reproduce products faithfully, this section is to be considered a quick reference identification aid. In cases of suspected overdosing, etc., chemical analysis should be done.

PURDUE PHARMA L.P.

C-III　　PURDUE PHARMA L.P.　　P. 2101

5 mcg/hour

7.5 mcg/hour

10 mcg/hour

15 mcg/hour

20 mcg/hour

Butrans®
(buprenorphine) Transdermal System

C-II　　PURDUE PHARMA L.P.　　P. 2110

1 mg/1 mL

Dilaudid® Oral Liquid
(hydromorphone HCl)

C-II　　PURDUE PHARMA L.P.　　P. 2110

2 mg

4 mg

8 mg

Dilaudid® Tablets
(hydromorphone HCl)

C-II　　PURDUE PHARMA L.P.　　P. 2112

1 mg/mL

2 mg/mL

4 mg/mL

Dilaudid® Injection
(hydromorphone HCl)

C-II　　PURDUE PHARMA L.P.　　P. 2112

10 mg/mL

50 mg/5 mL

250 mg

500 mg/50 mL

Dilaudid-HP® Injection
(hydromorphone HCl)

C-IV　　PURDUE PHARMA L.P.　　P. 2117

1.75 mg

3.5 mg

Intermezzo®
(zolpidem tartrate) sublingual tablet

Products in this section are arranged alphabetically by manufacturer. In some instances, not all dosage forms and/or sizes are pictured. If others are available, a † symbol precedes the product's name. Letters or numbers representing the manufacturer's identification code are followed by a * symbol.

C-II　　PURDUE PHARMA L.P.　　P. 2122

10 mg

15 mg

20 mg

30 mg

40 mg

60 mg

80 mg

Extended-Release Tablets

OxyContin®
(oxycodone HCl extended-release tablets)

Help your patients save on prescription medications with the PDR® Pharmacy Discount Card. For more, visit PDR.net/PharmacyDiscountCard.

RANBAXY LABORATORIES INC.

RX　　RANBAXY LABORATORIES INC. P. 2129

G 240　10

10 mg

20 mg

G 342　25

25 mg

G 242　30

30 mg

G 343　35

35 mg

G 325　40

40 mg

ABSORICA®
(isotretinoin) capsules

The pictured forms shown in this section may not necessarily be the only dosage forms and/or sizes available. Where a product name is preceded by a † symbol, refer to the description in the Product Information Section for other dosage forms and/or sizes.

RLC LABS, INC.

RX　　RLC LABS, INC.　　P. 2141

16.25 mg (1/4 gr.)

32.5 mg (1/2 gr.)

48.75 mg (3/4 gr.)

65 mg (1 gr.)

81.25 mg (1.25 gr.)

97.5 mg (1.5 gr.)

113.75 mg (1.75 gr.)

130 mg (2 gr.)

146.25 mg (2.25 gr.)

162.5 mg (2.5 gr.)

195 mg (3 gr.)

260 mg (4 gr.)

325 mg (5 gr.)

Nature-Throid®
(Thyroid USP) tablets

RX　　RLC LABS, INC.　　P. 2143

16.25 mg (1/4 gr.)

32.5 mg (1/2 gr.)

48.75 mg (3/4 gr.)

65 mg (1 gr.)

81.25 mg (1.25 gr.)

97.5 mg (1.5 gr.)

113.75 mg (1.75 gr.)

130 mg (2 gr.)

146.25 mg (2.25 gr.)

162.5 mg (2.5 gr.)

195 mg (3 gr.)

WP Thyroid®
(Thyroid USP) tablets

The trusted *Physicians' Desk Reference®* is now available digitally. Visit PDR.net to download your free *PDR®* eBook today.

RECORDATI RARE DISEASES INC.

RX　　RECORDATI RARE DISEASES INC. P. 2136

100 mg

Chemet®
(succimer) capsules

RX RECORDATI RARE DISEASES INC. P. 2140

313 mg
Hemin per Vial

Panhematin®
(hemin for injection)

Register at <u>PDR.net</u> today to
receive free PDR® Drug Alerts,
monthly eDrug Updates, and
FDA-required Drug Safety Alerts
via email.

SALIX PHARMACEUTICALS, INC.

RX SALIX PHARMACEUTICALS, INC. P. 2145

0.375 g

Apriso™
(mesalamine)
Extended-Release Capsules

RX SALIX PHARMACEUTICALS, INC. P. 2147

0.8 mg

Cycloset®
(bromocriptine mesylate) Tablets

RX SALIX PHARMACEUTICALS, INC. P. 2145

125SLXP

125 mg

Fulyzaq®
(crofelemer)
Delayed-Release Tablets

RX SALIX PHARMACEUTICALS, INC. P. 2154

MoviPrep®
(PEG-3350, sodium sulfate,
sodium chloride, potassium chloride,
sodium ascorbate, and ascorbic acid
for oral solution)

Look for PDR® services in your
EHR with PDR® BRIEF and
PDR®+ for Patients.

RX SALIX PHARMACEUTICALS, INC. P. 2157

12 mg/0.6 mL per syringe
Also available in 8 mg/0.4 mL per syringe

12 mg/0.6 mL per vial

Relistor®
(methylnaltrexone bromide)
Subcutaneous Injection

While every effort has been
made to reproduce products
faithfully, this section is to be
considered a quick reference
identification aid. In cases of
suspected overdosing, etc.,
chemical analysis should
be done.

RX SALIX PHARMACEUTICALS, INC. P. 2165

MX9

9 mg

Uceris®
(budesonide)
Extended-Release Tablets

RX SALIX PHARMACEUTICALS, INC. P. 2168

200 mg

RfX

550 mg

Xifaxan®
(rifaximin) Tablets

Products in this section are
arranged alphabetically by
manufacturer. In some instances,
not all dosage forms and/or
sizes are pictured. If others are
available, a † symbol precedes
the product's name. Letters or
numbers representing the
manufacturer's identification code
are followed by a * symbol.

SMITH & NEPHEW

RX SMITH & NEPHEW P. 2172

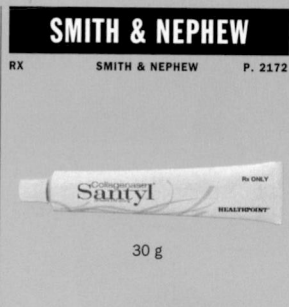

30 g

SANTYL® Ointment
(collagenase)

Help your patients save on
prescription medications
with the PDR® Pharmacy
Discount Card. For more, visit
<u>PDR.net/PharmacyDiscountCard</u>.

SUNOVION PHARMACEUTICALS INC.

RX SUNOVION PHARMACEUTICALS INC. P. 2197

ESL200	SL400
200 mg	400 mg

ESL600	ESL800
600 mg	800 mg

Aptiom®
(eslicarbazepine acetate) Tablets

RX SUNOVION PHARMACEUTICALS INC. P. 2203

Brovana®
(arformoterol tartrate)
Inhalation Solution

15 mcg/2 mL

Brovana®
(arformoterol tartrate)
Inhalation Solution

RX SUNOVION PHARMACEUTICALS INC. P. 2209

L 20	L 40
20 mg	40 mg

L 60	L 80
60 mg	80 mg

L 120

120 mg

Latuda®
(lurasidone HCl)

SUPERNUS PHARMACEUTICALS

RX SUPERNUS PHARMACEUTICALS P. 2221

150

150 mg

300

300 mg

600

600 mg
Extended-Release Tablets

Oxtellar XR™
(oxcarbazepine)

RX SUPERNUS PHARMACEUTICALS P. 2228

SPN 25

25 mg

SPN 50

50 mg

SPN 100

100 mg

SPN 200

200 mg
Extended-Release Capsules

Trokendi XR™
(topiramate)

SYNERGY WORLDWIDE, INC.

DS SYNERGY WORLDWIDE, INC. P. 2460

ProArgi-9+
(l-arginine complexer)

TAKEDA PHARMACEUTICALS

RX TAKEDA PHARMACEUTICALS P. 2242

SPI

8 mcg

SPI

24 mcg

Amitiza®
(lubiprostone)

RX TAKEDA PHARMACEUTICALS P. 2246

S	TL
5 mg	

10	TL
10 mg	

20	TL
20 mg	

Also available as 15 mg tablet

Brintellix®
(vortioxetine)

RX TAKEDA PHARMACEUTICALS P. 2253

AB37x

0.6 mg

Colcrys®
(colchicine, USP) tablets

RX TAKEDA PHARMACEUTICALS P. 2260

NB-890

8 mg/90 mg
Extended-Release Tablets

Contrave®
(naltrexone HCl and bupropion HCl)

RX TAKEDA PHARMACEUTICALS P. 2271

30 mg

DEXILANT
dexlansoprazole
delayed release
capsules

60 mg
Delayed-Release Capsules

DEXILANT™
(dexlansoprazole)

The pictured forms shown in this
section may not necessarily be
the only dosage forms and/or
sizes available. Where a product
name is preceded by a †
symbol, refer to the description
in the Product Information
Section for other dosage forms
and/or sizes.

RX   TAKEDA PHARMACEUTICALS   P. 2276

12.5 mg/500 mg

12.5 mg/1000 mg

Kazano®
(alogliptin and metformin hydrochloride)
tablets

RX   TAKEDA PHARMACEUTICALS   P. 2284

6.25 mg

12.5 mg

25 mg

Nesina®
(alogliptin) tablets

RX   TAKEDA PHARMACEUTICALS   P. 2292

12.5 mg/15 mg

12.5 mg/30 mg

12.5 mg/45 mg

25 mg/15 mg

25 mg/30 mg

25 mg/45 mg

Oseni®
(alogliptin and pioglitazone) tablets

RX   TAKEDA PHARMACEUTICALS   P. 2303

40 mg   80 mg

Uloric®
(febuxostat)

TEVA RESPIRATORY, LLC

RX   TEVA RESPIRATORY, LLC   P. 2307

90 mcg/inh
8.5 g canister
200 actuations

ProAir® HFA
(albuterol sulfate)

TEVA SELECT BRANDS

RX   TEVA SELECT BRANDS   P. 2313

ADASUVE®
(loxapine) inhalation powder 10 mg

RX   TEVA SELECT BRANDS   P. 2318

5 mg (15 IU)

Tev-Tropin®
[somatropin (rDNA origin)] for Injection

THE MEDICINES COMPANY

RX   THE MEDICINES COMPANY   P. 2321

400 mg/vial

Orbactiv™
(oritavancin) for injection

TRIVITA, INC.

DS   TRIVITA, INC.   P. 2460

32 fl. oz.

nopalea™

UNICITY INTERNATIONAL, INC.

DS   UNICITY INTERNATIONAL, INC.   P. 2461

Dietary Supplement

Bios Life® Cardio

DS   UNICITY INTERNATIONAL, INC.   P. 2462

Dietary Supplement

CM Plex®

DS   UNICITY INTERNATIONAL, INC.   P. 2463

Dietary Supplement

Unicity Balance™

DS   UNICITY INTERNATIONAL, INC.   P. 2463

Dietary Supplement

Joint Mobility™

VANDA PHARMACEUTICALS

RX   VANDA PHARMACEUTICALS   P. 2326

20 mg

Hetlioz™
(tasimelteon) Capsules

![PDR Network logo] PDR Network®

Today's Physicians' Desk Reference®

Innovation to Meet Healthcare Providers' Needs

PDR® is committed to prescribers, pioneering new ways to deliver our trusted prescribing and patient safety information. We understand that today's prescribers face greater challenges and that the demands on their time are higher than ever before. With increasing responsibilities, prescribers require tools that offer support throughout the day – both inside and outside of the office. These tools must support workflow, increase efficiency, and save time for what's most important – the patient.

Our latest digital innovations deliver critical information within workflow to efficiently offer the tools needed to provide optimal patient care. Developed with today's prescribers in mind, these offerings ensure access to the right information at the right time to support prescribing decisions. Whether online, via email, mobile, our eBook, or through the EHR, PDR provides the resources that prescribers rely on and trust.

©2014 PDR Network, LLC. All Rights Reserved. *Physicians' Desk Reference, PDR, PDR.net, mobilePDR,* and *PDR Network* are registered trademarks of PDR Network, LLC.

Innovative Products, Trusted Content

While new technology continues to change the way medicine is practiced, the need for critical drug reference information remains. PDR® delivers that critical drug information in multiple ways to suit each provider's preference and fit their respective workflow. Whether you access PDR online, via email, mobile, or through your EHR system, PDR puts trusted information at your fingertips.

EHR Innovations

PDR® BRIEF
- An intuitive dashboard of full labeling information and provider resources surfacing within EHR workflow to support prescribing decisions.

PDR®+ *for Patients*
- Patient-focused prescribing information to help patients better understand their treatment, accessible when prescribing to print for your patients or send to the patient portal.

PDR® Search
- An integrated database providing access to detailed drug information on-demand directly through the EHR.

Digital Properties

Physicians' Desk Reference® eBook
- Trusted FDA-approved full prescribing information, available in a convenient eBook format for all desktop and tablet platforms.

mobilePDR®
- The single, go-to source for trusted drug information available anywhere, anytime via mobile devices, available across platforms.

PDR.net®
- A web portal designed specifically for providers, offering trusted drug information quickly and easily online.

Communications Services

eDrug Updates
- Monthly updates of FDA-approved labeling information delivered via email.

Drug Alerts
- Critical, time-sensitive updates on prescription drugs, delivered via email as information becomes available.

Dear HCP Letters
- Important notifications from bio/pharmaceutical manufacturers detailing new information about their products.

REMS Communications
- Detailed Risk Evaluation and Mitigation Strategy (REMS) plans to support patient safety when prescribing designated medications.

Recalls, Withdrawals, and Other Notifications
- Timely communications to keep up-to-date on changing prescribing information, product availability, and other key issues that may impact prescribing decisions.

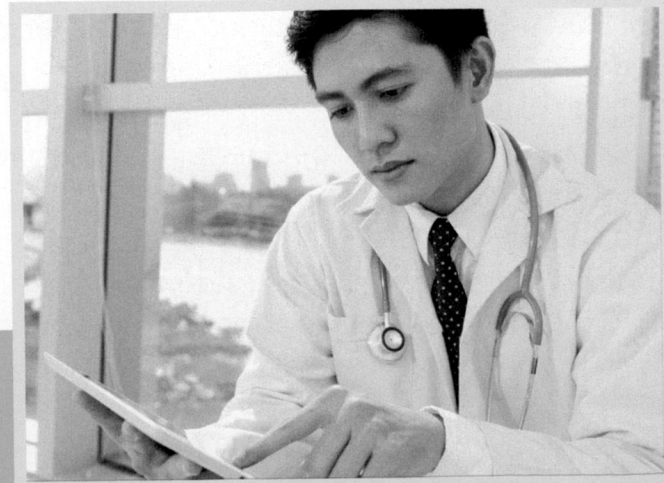

Feedback
As a member of the PDR Network, we welcome any feedback that you may have to shape our products. Please feel free to share your suggestions with us via email at ProviderFeedback@PDR.net.

Critical drug information and patient support resources right within EHR workflow. No more searching multiple resources outside of workflow, and no more wondering if the drug information you rely upon is complete and current.

PDR Drug Information at Your Fingertips

> Current prescribing and drug safety information

> Boxed Warnings, Drug Alerts, & REMS

Melavin
(melavinus)

☏ @ ✕

❗ Recent Major Change: Aug 2014
Full Prescribing Information

Patient Drug Info

Updated Aug 2014
Boxed WARNING

Alerts

REMS

Melavin – new 5mg dose available

Important Safety Information

Patient coupon available:
Eligible patients pay no more than $15

Important Safety Information

Terms of Service

✓ PDR® BRIEF

> Printable PDR+ patient drug education guides to improve medication adherence

> Provider & patient support resources

With PDR BRIEF, key drug and safety information, as well as pertinent patient resources, are delivered on-screen when you select a medication.

Don't have PDR in your EHR? Tell us at EHR@PDR.net.

©2014 PDR Network, LLC. All Rights Reserved. *PDR* and *PDR Network* are registered trademarks of PDR Network, LLC.

PDR®+ *for Patients*

Free Patient Education from PDR

PDR+ helps educate your patients about their prescriptions from the moment that you write the prescription. Available through your EHR or online, PDR+ helps patients start and stay on their medications.

▶ **Easy to Read**
- Clearly written drug names and simple Q&A format

▶ **Easy to Understand**
- Patient-friendly prescription information

▶ **Easy to Help Patients Save**
- Includes a PDR® Pharmacy Discount Card

▶ **Easy to Access**
- Available through your EHR to print or send via the patient portal
- Also available online at PDR.net

For illustrative purposes only.

✔PDR+
Trusted by Doctors and Patients

Melavin
Generic name: (melavinus)

Other Brands: ranbavinus, tevavinus, mylavinus
Last Revised: 08/2013

⚠ Dr. Smith has prescribed Melavin for you. It is important that you fill your prescription and use this medication as prescribed. It is also important for you to read this information carefully, as it includes key facts you should know about your medicine.

℞ **What is this medication and its most common uses?**

Melavin is a medicine known as an angiotensin receptor blocker (ARB), used alone or in combination with other medications to treat high blood pressure. Melavin is also used to treat heart failure, or to lower the risk of death from heart problems in people who have had a heart attack.

What should I know when beginning and continuing on this medication?

How does this medication work?

Melavin lowers high blood pressure by blocking a chemical in your body that causes blood vessels to narrow. By blocking this chemical, Melavin relaxes and widens your blood vessels, allowing your blood to flow through with less resistance.

What are the beneficial effects of this medication and when should I begin to have results?

What: High Blood Pressure: By lowering your blood pressure, Melavin may lower your risk of a stroke or heart attack.

Heart Failure: Melavin is proven to lower the need for hospitalization from heart failure.

After a Heart Attack: Melavin is proven to reduce the chance of death after a heart attack in people who have certain types of heart problems.

When: Melavin may start lowering your blood pressure within 2 weeks. Though you may not feel an improvement or change in the way you feel, it is very important to keep taking your medicine as prescribed to keep your condition under control.

How do I know it is working?

Check your blood pressure regularly. Your healthcare provider will also check your blood pressure at every visit. Following an appropriate diet and exercise plan will also affect your blood pressure results.

What are the possible side effects of this medication?

The following is not a full list of side effects. Side effects cannot be anticipated. If any develop or change in intensity, tell your healthcare provider as soon as possible. Only your healthcare provider can determine if it is safe for you to continue taking this medication.

Page 1 of 4

☀Melavin
(melavinus)   ☎ ✕

! **Recent Major Change: Dec 2014**   Patient
! Full Prescribing Information   Drug Info

Updated Apr 2014   Alerts   REMS
Boxed WARNING

Melavin – new 5mg dose available
                              Important Safety Information

Patient coupon available:
Eligible patients pay no more than $15
                              Important Safety Information

Terms of Service   ✔**PDR® BRIEF**

✂ Cut here

✔PDR®
Physicians' Desk Reference®

Pharmacy Discount Card
Save up to 75% on your medications.
Includes more than 50,000 drugs at over 60,000 pharmacies in the U.S., Puerto Rico, Guam, and the U.S.V.I.

This card is not insurance.   BioScrip PBM Services

MEMBER INSTRUCTIONS
1. Carry this card in your wallet and present it to the pharmacist every time you or a family member fills a prescription.
2. Make sure the pharmacist enters your account information into their system. Ask for your PDR Discount every time!

For more information or questions regarding your card, please visit www.pdr.net/DiscountCard or call 1-855-737-1737.
By using this card, the holder agrees to the terms and conditions under which it was issued.

PHARMACIST INSTRUCTIONS
Covered prescriptions may be filled at participating pharmacies. For information regarding claims transmission or becoming a participating pharmacy, please call the Pharmacy Service at 1-855-737-1737.

✔PDR

This discount plan is NOT insurance or a Medicare prescription drug plan. The plan is not

---

Patients prefer PDR+.

"PDR+ would make me feel more comfortable about my medicine."

"If I'm not afraid of my medication I will stay on it."

"...if the doctor tells me everything I need to know about my medication, it shows he really cares about me and my health."

70% of patients have never received printed drug information from their physician, but two out of three said they wish they had.

Source: PDR Patient Research, July 2013.

©2014 PDR Network, LLC. All Rights Reserved. *PDR* and *PDR Network* are registered trademarks of PDR Network, LLC.

Look for PDR in Your EHR

No reason to leave workflow to get critical drug and patient support information.

PDR® BRIEF

Key drug and safety information, as well as pertinent patient and provider resources, delivered on-screen. PDR BRIEF is activated when a medication is selected, to ensure access to the most current information available.

- Full prescribing information, including label updates and boxed warnings
- Education, financial support, and adherence resources for patients
- Provider resources including dosing guides, new indications, new research, and more

Melavin (melavinus)

Recent Major Change: Aug 2014
Full Prescribing Information — Patient Drug Info

Updated Aug 2014
Boxed WARNING — Alerts — REMS

Melavin — new 5mg dose available

Important Safety Information

Patient coupon available:
Eligible patients pay no more than $15

Important Safety Information

Terms of Service — PDR® BRIEF

PDR® + for Patients

Medication-specific patient drug education guides you can print and give to your patient. Written in patient-friendly language, PDR+ guides go beyond the information typically given out by the pharmacy.

- Helps patients better understand their medications
- Conveniently accessed via PDR BRIEF to be printed or sent to the patient portal
- Available to patients on PDR.net

PDR+

For illustrative purposes only.

Melavin
Generic name: (melavinus)

Other Brands: ranbavinus, tevavinus, mylavinus
Last Revised: 08/2013

Dr. Smith has prescribed Melavin for you. It is important that you fill your prescription and use this medication as prescribed. It is also important for you to read this information carefully, as it includes key facts you should know about your medicine.

What is this medication and its most common uses?
Melavin is a medicine known as an angiotensin receptor blocker (ARB), used alone or in combination with other medications to treat high blood pressure. Melavin is also used to treat heart failure, or to lower the risk of death from heart problems in people who have had a heart attack.

What should I know when beginning and continuing on this medication?
How does this medication work?
Melavin lowers high blood pressure by blocking a chemical in your body that causes blood vessels to narrow. By blocking this chemical, Melavin relaxes and widens your blood vessels, allowing your blood to flow through with less resistance.

What are the beneficial effects of this medication and when should I begin to have results?
What: High Blood Pressure: By lowering your blood pressure, Melavin may lower your risk of a stroke or heart attack.

Heart Failure: Melavin is proven to lower the need for hospitalization from heart failure.

After a Heart Attack: Melavin is proven to reduce the chance of death after a heart attack in people who have certain types of heart problems.

When: Melavin may start lowering your blood pressure within 2 weeks. Though you may not feel an improvement or change in the way you feel, it is very important to keep taking your medicine as prescribed to keep your condition under control.

How do I know it is working?
Check your blood pressure regularly. Your healthcare provider will also check your blood pressure at every visit. Following an appropriate diet and exercise plan will also affect your blood pressure results.

What are the possible side effects of this medication?
The following is not a full list of side effects. Side effects cannot be anticipated. If any develop or change in intensity, tell your healthcare provider as soon as possible. Only your healthcare provider can determine if it is safe for you to continue taking this medication.

Page 1 of 4

PDR® Search

Interactive and searchable drug label and safety database.

- Full FDA-approved prescribing information and prescribing summaries
- FDA and PDR Drug Safety Alerts

PDR Search — Type medication name here

Don't have PDR in your EHR? Tell us at EHR@PDR.net.

©2014 PDR Network, LLC. All Rights Reserved. *PDR, Physicians' Desk Reference,* and *PDR Network* are registered trademarks of PDR Network, LLC.

PDR Network®

PDR.net®: Your Online Home of the PDR®
Trusted Drug Information Online

A web portal designed specifically for prescribers, providing trusted, professional drug information, including full FDA-approved labeling as well as concise point-of-care prescribing information. PDR.net offers online access to authoritative drug information to support treatment decisions.

©2014 PDR Network, LLC. All Rights Reserved. *PDR*, *PDR.net*, and *PDR Network* are registered trademarks of PDR Network, LLC.

Coming Soon: Updated & Expanded
mobilePDR®

*mobile*PDR has always been the source for FDA-approved full product labeling and concise point-of-care drug information from PDR for your mobile device. This spring, PDR Network will release a new version of *mobile*PDR. Developed with the prescriber in mind, this new platform will deliver more robust drug information to your mobile device than ever before.

Coming this Spring!

Reserve Now
Visit PDR.net/GetMobile for more information and to pre-register

*mobile***PDR** is free for U.S.-based MDs, DOs, NPs, and PAs in full-time patient practice and can be downloaded for all major mobile platforms.

©2014 PDR Network, LLC. All Rights Reserved. *PDR*, *PDR.net*, *mobilePDR*, and *PDR Network* are registered trademarks of PDR Network, LLC.

Pharmacy Discount Card
Save up to 75% on your medications.
Includes more than 50,000 drugs at over 60,000 pharmacies in the U.S., Puerto Rico, Guam, and the U.S.V.I.
This card is not insurance.
BIN 900020
PCN CLAIMNE
GRP 0000000
Member ID PDR0000000
BioScrip PBM Services

Helping your patients save money on medications is just a few steps away.

Step 1: Enroll in this FREE program

Step 2: Receive your complete program kit

Step 3: Encourage your patients to use their preactivated PDR® Pharmacy Discount Cards on a regular basis for maximum savings

Enrolling is easy.
Call: **800-232-7379**
Visit: **PDR.net/PharmacyDiscountCard**

Benefits of the PDR® Pharmacy Discount Card Program:

- Anyone paying cash prices for a prescription is eligible

- Patients save up to 75% on brand & generic drugs

- Includes over 50,000 drugs at 60,000 pharmacies nationwide

- Kits available in English or Spanish

In a recent survey,
94% of physicians
indicated they prefer a
pharmacy discount card
from PDR®

DOCTORS' CHOICE

(PDR Research: Feb 2013; N= 1,772)

This discount plan is NOT insurance or a Medicare prescription drug plan. The plan is not intended as a substitute for insurance and does not meet creditable coverage requirements under state or federal law. The plan provides discounts at participating pharmacies on certain pharmaceutical supplies, prescription drugs, or medical equipment and supplies. The range of discounts will vary depending on the products received. Members are obligated to pay the pharmacy the entire amount of the discounted rate for such products at the point of sale. The plan does not pay pharmacies for products provided to members. No enrollment or periodic fees apply. The pharmacy may pay the plan a fee from amounts the pharmacy collects from the member. The discount plan organization is BioScrip PBM Services, LLC, 100 Clearbrook Road, Elmsford, NY 10523, 1-888-299-5383. Customer service is provided by PDR Network, LLC, 5 Paragon Drive, Montvale, NJ 07645, 1-800-232-7379, PDR.net/PharmacyDiscountCard, CustomerService@PDR.net.

©2014 PDR Network, LLC. All Rights Reserved. PDR, Physicians' Desk Reference, and PDR Network are registered trademarks of PDR Network, LLC.

PRODUCT INFORMATION

This edition of the *PDR®* contains the latest full label product information available when the book went to press. Listings are arranged alphabetically by manufacturer; late submissions appear alphabetically by manufacturer at the end of this section. As new drugs are released, and new research data, clinical findings, and safety information emerge throughout the year, it is the responsibility of the manufacturer to provide that information to the medical community and to revise that information in the PDR database.

Revisions are published six times annually in the *PDR Updates*, more frequently on PDR.net® and *mobile*PDR®, as well as emailed via the *PDR® eDrug Update* and *PDR® Drug Alerts*. These updates can also be found in the Electronic Health Record (EHR) of PDR's growing network of EHR partners. To be certain that you have the most current information, always consult PDR.net, *mobile*PDR, *PDR eDrug Update*, *PDR Updates*, or PDR drug information within your EHR before prescribing or administering any product described in the following pages.

AbbVie Inc.
1 North Waukegan Road
North Chicago, IL 60064

Direct Inquiries to:
Customer Service:
(800) 255-5162
Patient Access Program:
(800) 441-4987
For Medical Services Department:
(800) 633-9110 or www.abbviemedinfo.com
Adverse experiences or side effects
(for all AbbVie drug products):
(800) 633-9110 or www.abbviemedinfo.com
Sales and Ordering:
(800) 255-5162

ABBO–CODE™ INDEX

The Abbo-Code identification system provides positive identification of a drug and dosage strength. The following AbbVie products are imprinted or debossed with an Abbo-Code designation:

ADVICOR®   ℞

[ăd-vĭ-kŏr]

(niacin extended-release/lovastatin tablets)

DESCRIPTION

ADVICOR® (niacin extended-release and lovastatin) is intended to facilitate the daily administration of its individual components, Niaspan® and lovastatin, when used together for the intended patient population (see INDICATIONS AND USAGE and DOSAGE AND ADMINISTRATION).
ADVICOR contains niacin extended-release and lovastatin in combination. Lovastatin, an inhibitor of 3-hydroxy-3-methylglutaryl-coenzyme A (HMG-CoA) reductase, and niacin are both lipid-altering agents.
Niacin is nicotinic acid, or 3-pyridinecarboxylic acid. Niacin is a white, nonhygroscopic crystalline powder that is very soluble in water, boiling ethanol and propylene glycol. It is insoluble in ethyl ether. The empirical formula of niacin is $C_6H_5NO_2$ and its molecular weight is 123.11. Niacin has the following structural formula:

Lovastatin is [1S -[1(alpha)(R *), 3(alpha), 7(beta), 8(beta)(2S *, 4S *), 8a(beta)]]-1,2,3, 7,8,8a-hexahydro-3,7-dimethyl-8-[2-(tetrahydro-4-hydroxy-6-oxo-2H-pyran-2-yl) ethyl]-1-naphthalenyl 2-methylbutanoate. Lovastatin is a white, nonhygroscopic crystalline powder that is insoluble in water and sparingly soluble in ethanol, methanol, and acetonitrile. The empirical formula of lovastatin is $C_{24}H_{36}O_5$ and its molecular weight is 404.55. Lovastatin has the following structural formula:

ADVICOR tablets contain the labeled amount of niacin and lovastatin and have the following inactive ingredients: hypromellose, povidone, stearic acid, polyethylene glycol, titanium dioxide, polysorbate 80.
The individual tablet strengths (expressed in terms of mg niacin/mg lovastatin) contain the following coloring agents:
ADVICOR 500 mg/20 mg - Iron Oxide Yellow, Iron Oxide Red.
ADVICOR 750 mg/20 mg - FD&C Yellow #6/Sunset Yellow FCF Aluminum Lake.
ADVICOR 1000 mg/20 mg - Iron Oxide Red, Iron Oxide Yellow, Iron Oxide Black.
ADVICOR 1000 mg/40 mg - Iron Oxide Red.

CLINICAL PHARMACOLOGY

A variety of clinical studies have demonstrated that elevated levels of total cholesterol (TC), low-density lipoprotein cholesterol (LDL-C), and apolipoprotein B-100 (Apo B) promote human atherosclerosis. Similarly, decreased levels of high-density lipoprotein cholesterol (HDL-C) are associated with the development of atherosclerosis. Epidemiological investigations have established that cardiovascular morbidity and mortality vary directly with the level of TC and LDL-C, and inversely with the level of HDL-C.
Cholesterol-enriched triglyceride-rich lipoproteins, including very low-density lipoproteins (VLDL), intermediate-density lipoproteins (IDL), and their remnants, can also promote atherosclerosis. Elevated plasma triglycerides (TG) are frequently found in a triad with low HDL-C levels and small LDL particles, as well as in association with non-lipid metabolic risk factors for coronary heart disease (CHD). As such, total plasma TG have not consistently been shown to be an independent risk factor for CHD.
As an adjunct to diet, the efficacy of niacin and lovastatin in improving lipid profiles (either individually, or in combination with each other, or niacin in combination with other statins) for the treatment of dyslipidemia has been well documented. The effect of combined therapy with niacin and lovastatin on cardiovascular morbidity and mortality has not been determined.

Effects on lipids
ADVICOR
ADVICOR reduces LDL-C, TC, and TG, and increases HDL-C due to the individual actions of niacin and lovastatin. The magnitude of individual lipid and lipoprotein responses may be influenced by the severity and type of underlying lipid abnormality.
Niacin
Niacin functions in the body after conversion to nicotinamide adenine dinucleotide (NAD) in the NAD coenzyme system. Niacin (but not nicotinamide) in gram doses reduces LDL-C, Apo B, Lp(a), TG, and TC, and increases HDL-C. The increase in HDL-C is associated with an increase in apolipoprotein A-I (Apo A-I) and a shift in the distribution of HDL subfractions. These shifts include an increase in the $HDL_2:HDL_3$ ratio, and an elevation in lipoprotein A-I (Lp A-I, an HDL-C particle containing only Apo A-I). In addition, preliminary reports suggest that niacin causes favorable LDL particle size transformations, although the clinical relevance of this effect is not yet clear.
Lovastatin
Lovastatin has been shown to reduce both normal and elevated LDL-C concentrations. Apo B also falls substantially during treatment with lovastatin. Since each LDL-C particle contains one molecule of Apo B, and since little Apo B is found in other lipoproteins, this strongly suggests that lovastatin does not merely cause cholesterol to be lost from LDL-C, but also reduces the concentration of circulating LDL particles. In addition, lovastatin can produce increases of variable magnitude in HDL-C, and modestly reduces VLDL-C and plasma TG. The effects of lovastatin on Lp(a),

fibrinogen, and certain other independent biochemical risk markers for coronary heart disease are not well characterized.

Mechanism of Action

Niacin

The mechanism by which niacin alters lipid profiles is not completely understood and may involve several actions, including partial inhibition of release of free fatty acids from adipose tissue, and increased lipoprotein lipase activity (which may increase the rate of chylomicron triglyceride removal from plasma). Niacin decreases the rate of hepatic synthesis of VLDL-C and LDL-C, and does not appear to affect fecal excretion of fats, sterols, or bile acids.

Lovastatin

Lovastatin is a specific inhibitor of 3-hydroxy-3-methylglutaryl-coenzyme A (HMG-CoA) reductase, the enzyme that catalyzes the conversion of HMG-CoA to mevalonate. The conversion of HMG-CoA to mevalonate is an early step in the biosynthetic pathway for cholesterol. Lovastatin is a prodrug and has little, if any, activity until hydrolyzed to its active beta-hydroxyacid form, lovastatin acid. The mechanism of the LDL-lowering effect of lovastatin may involve both reduction of VLDL-C concentration and induction of the LDL receptor, leading to reduced production and/or increased catabolism of LDL-C.

Pharmacokinetics

Absorption and Bioavailability

ADVICOR

In single-dose studies of ADVICOR, rate and extent of niacin and lovastatin absorption were bioequivalent under fed conditions to that from NIASPAN® (niacin extended-release tablets) and Mevacor® (lovastatin) tablets, respectively. After administration of two ADVICOR 1000 mg/20 mg tablets, peak niacin concentrations averaged about 18 mcg/mL and occurred about 5 hours after dosing; about 72% of the niacin dose was absorbed according to the urinary excretion data. Peak lovastatin concentrations averaged about 11 ng/mL and occurred about 2 hours after dosing.

The extent of niacin absorption from ADVICOR was increased by administration with food. The administration of two ADVICOR 1000 mg/20 mg tablets under low-fat or high-fat conditions resulted in a 22 to 30% increase in niacin bioavailability relative to dosing under fasting conditions. Lovastatin bioavailability is affected by food. Lovastatin C_{max} was increased 48% and 21% after a high- and a low-fat meal, respectively, but the lovastatin AUC was decreased 26% and 24% after a high- and a low-fat meal, respectively, compared to those under fasting conditions.

A relative bioavailability study results indicated that ADVICOR tablet strengths (i.e., two tablets of 500 mg/20 mg and one tablet of 1000 mg/40 mg) are not interchangeable.

Niacin

Due to extensive and saturable first-pass metabolism, niacin concentrations in the general circulation are dose dependent and highly variable. Peak steady-state niacin concentrations were 0.6, 4.9, and 15.5 mcg/mL after doses of 1000, 1500, and 2000 mg NIASPAN once daily (given as two 500 mg, two 750 mg, and two 1000 mg tablets, respectively).

Lovastatin

Lovastatin appears to be incompletely absorbed after oral administration. Because of extensive hepatic extraction, the amount of lovastatin reaching the systemic circulation as active inhibitors after oral administration is low (<5%) and shows considerable inter-individual variation. Peak concentrations of active and total inhibitors occur within 2 to 4 hours after Mevacor® administration.

Lovastatin absorption appears to be increased by at least 30% by grapefruit juice; however, the effect is dependent on the amount of grapefruit juice consumed and the interval between grapefruit juice and lovastatin ingestion. With a once-a-day dosing regimen, plasma concentrations of total inhibitors over a dosing interval achieved a steady-state between the second and third days of therapy and were about 1.5 times those following a single dose of Mevacor®.

Although the mechanism is not fully understood, cyclosporine has been shown to increase the AUC of HMG-CoA reductase inhibitors. The increase in AUC for lovastatin and lovastatin acid is presumably due, in part, to inhibition of CYP3A4.

Distribution

Niacin

Niacin is less than 20% bound to human serum proteins and distributes into milk. Studies using radiolabeled niacin in mice show that niacin and its metabolites concentrate in the liver, kidney, and adipose tissue.

Lovastatin

Both lovastatin and its beta-hydroxyacid metabolite are highly bound (>95%) to human plasma proteins. Distribution of lovastatin or its metabolites into human milk is unknown; however, lovastatin distributes into milk in rats. In animal studies, lovastatin concentrated in the liver, and crossed the blood-brain and placental barriers.

Metabolism

Niacin

Niacin undergoes rapid and extensive first-pass metabolism that is dose-rate specific and, at the doses used to treat dyslipidemia, saturable. In humans, one pathway is through a simple conjugation step with glycine to form nicotinuric acid (NUA). NUA is then excreted, although there may be a small amount of reversible metabolism back to niacin. The other pathway results in the formation of NAD. It is unclear whether nicotinamide is formed as a precursor to, or following the synthesis of, NAD. Nicotinamide is further metabolized to at least N-methylnicotinamide (MNA) and nicotinamide-N-oxide (NNO). MNA is further metabolized to two other compounds, N-methyl-2-pyridone-5-carboxamide (2PY) and N-methyl-4-pyridone-5-carboxamide (4PY). The formation of 2PY appears to predominate over 4PY in humans.

Lovastatin

Lovastatin undergoes extensive first-pass extraction and metabolism by cytochrome P450 3A4 in the liver, its primary site of action. The major active metabolites present in human plasma are the beta-hydroxyacid of lovastatin (lovastatin acid), its 6′-hydroxy derivative, and two additional metabolites.

Elimination

ADVICOR

Niacin is primarily excreted in urine mainly as metabolites. After a single dose of ADVICOR, at least 60% of the niacin dose was recovered in urine as unchanged niacin and its metabolites. The plasma half-life for lovastatin was about 4.5 hours in single-dose studies.

Niacin

The plasma half-life for niacin is about 20 to 48 minutes after oral administration and dependent on dose administered. Following multiple oral doses of NIASPAN, up to 12% of the dose was recovered in urine as unchanged niacin depending on dose administered. The ratio of metabolites recovered in the urine was also dependent on the dose administered.

Lovastatin

Lovastatin is excreted in urine and bile, based on studies of Mevacor®. Following an oral dose of radiolabeled lovastatin in man, 10% of the dose was excreted in urine and 83% in feces. The latter represents absorbed drug equivalents excreted in bile, as well as any unabsorbed drug.

Special Populations

Hepatic

No pharmacokinetic studies have been conducted in patients with hepatic insufficiency for either niacin or lovastatin (see WARNINGS, Liver Dysfunction).

Renal

No information is available on the pharmacokinetics of niacin in patients with renal insufficiency.

In a study of patients with severe renal insufficiency (creatinine clearance 10 to 30 mL/min), the plasma concentra-

---

Table 1. Mean percent change from baseline at endpoint for LDL-C, HDL-C and TG by gender

	ADVICOR 2000 mg/40 mg		NIASPAN 2000 mg		Lovastatin 40 mg	
	Women (n=22)	Men (n=30)	Women (n=28)	Men (n=28)	Women (n=21)	Men (n=38)
LDL-C	-47%	-34%	-12%	-9%	-31%	-31%
HDL-C	+33%	+24%	+22%	+15%	+3%	+7%
TG	-48%	-35%	-25%	-15%	-15%	-23%

Table 2. The Effects of Other Drugs on Lovastatin Exposure When Both Were Co-administered

Drug	N	Dose of Co-administered Drug or Grapefruit Juice	Dosing of Lovastatin	AUC Ratio* (with / without co-administered drug)	
				Lovastatin	Lovastatin Acid
Gemfibrozil	11	600 mg BID for 3 days	40 mg	0.96	2.80
Itraconazole‡	12	200 mg QD for 4 days	40 mg on Day 4	> 36§	22
	10	100 mg QD for 4 days	40 mg on Day 4	> 14.8§	15.4
Grapefruit Juice¶ (high dose)	10	200 mL of double-strength TID#	80 mg single dose	15.3	5.0
Grapefruit Juice¶ (low dose)	16	8 oz (about 250 mL) of single-strengthᵇ for 4 days	40 mg single dose	1.94	1.57
Cyclosporine	16	Not describedᵝ	10 mg QD for 10 days	5- to 8-fold	NDᵃ

	Number of Subjects	Dosing of Coadministered Drug or Grapefruit Juice	Dosing of Lovastatin	AUC Ratio* (with / without co-administered drug) No Effect = 1.00
				Total Lovastatin Acid ᵉ
Diltiazem	10	120 mg BID for 14 days	20 mg	3.57ᵉ

* Results based on a chemical assay.
† Lovastatin acid refers to the β-hydroxyacid of lovastatin.
‡ The mean total AUC of lovastatin without itraconazole phase could not be determined accurately. Results could be representative of strong CYP3A4 inhibitors such as ketoconazole, posaconazole, clarithromycin, telithromycin, HIV protease inhibitors, and nefazodone.
§ Estimated minimum change.
¶ The effect of amounts of grapefruit juice between those used in these two studies on lovastatin pharmacokinetics has not been studied.
# Double-strength: one can of frozen concentrate diluted with one can of water. Grapefruit juice was administered TID for 2 days, and 200 mL together with single dose lovastatin and 30 and 90 minutes following single dose lovastatin on Day 3.
ᵇ Single-strength: one can of frozen concentrate diluted with 3 cans of water. Grapefruit juice was administered with breakfast for 3 days, and lovastatin was administered in the evening on Day 3.
ᵝ Cyclosporine-treated patients with psoriasis or post kidney or heart transplant patients with stable graft function, transplanted at least 9 months prior to study.
ᵃ ND = Analyte not determined.
ᵉ Lactone converted to acid by hydrolysis prior to analysis. Figure represents total unmetabolized acid and lactone.

Information on the AbbVie, Inc. products listed on these pages is from the prescribing information in use as of July 31, 2014. For more information, please visit rxabbvie.com or call 1-800-633-9110.

Table 3. LDL-C mean percent change from baseline

Week	ADVICOR			NIASPAN			Lovastatin		
	n*	Dose (mg/mg)	LDL	n*	Dose (mg)	LDL	n*	Dose (mg)	LDL
Baseline	57	-	190.9 mg/dL	61	-	189.7 mg/dL	61	-	185.6 mg/dL
12	47	1000/20	-30%	46	1000	-3%	56	20	-29%
16	45	1000/40	-36%	44	1000	-6%	56	40	-31%
20	42	1500/40	-37%	43	1500	-12%	54	40	-34%
28	42	2000/40	-42%	41	2000	-14%	53	40	-32%

*n = number of patients remaining in the trial at each timepoint

Table 4. HDL-C mean percent change from baseline

Week	ADVICOR			NIASPAN			Lovastatin		
	n*	Dose (mg/mg)	HDL	n*	Dose (mg)	HDL	n*	Dose (mg)	HDL
Baseline	57	-	45 mg/dL	61	-	47 mg/dL	61	-	43 mg/dL
12	47	1000/20	+20%	46	1000	+14%	56	20	+3%
16	45	1000/40	+20%	44	1000	+15%	56	40	+5%
20	42	1500/40	+27%	43	1500	+22%	54	40	+6%
28	42	2000/40	+30%	41	2000	+24%	53	40	+6%

*n = number of patients remaining in the trial at each timepoint

Table 5. TG median percent change from baseline

Week	ADVICOR			NIASPAN			Lovastatin		
	n*	Dose (mg/mg)	TG	n*	Dose (mg)	TG	n*	Dose (mg)	TG
Baseline	57	-	174 mg/dL	61	-	186 mg/dL	61	-	171 mg/dL
12	47	1000/20	-32%	46	1000	-22%	56	20	-20%
16	45	1000/40	-39%	44	1000	-23%	56	40	-17%
20	42	1500/40	-44%	43	1500	-31%	54	40	-21%
28	42	2000/40	-44%	41	2000	-31%	53	40	-20%

*n = number of patients remaining in the trial at each timepoint

Table 6. Lp(a) median percent change from baseline

Week	ADVICOR			NIASPAN			Lovastatin		
	n*	Dose (mg/mg)	Lp(a)	n*	Dose (mg)	Lp(a)	n*	Dose (mg)	Lp(a)
Baseline	57	-	34 mg/dL	61	-	41 mg/dL	60	-	42 mg/dL
12	47	1000/20	-9%	46	1000	-8%	55	20	+8%
16	45	1000/40	-9%	44	1000	-12%	55	40	+8%
20	42	1500/40	-17%	43	1500	-22%	53	40	+6%
28	42	2000/40	-22%	41	2000	-32%	52	40	0%

*n = number of patients remaining in the trial at each timepoint

tions of total inhibitors after a single dose of lovastatin were approximately two-fold higher than those in healthy volunteers.

ADVICOR should be used with caution in patients with renal disease.

Gender

Plasma concentrations of niacin and metabolites after single- or multiple-dose administration of niacin are generally higher in women than in men, with the magnitude of the difference varying with dose and metabolite. Recovery of niacin and metabolites in urine, however, is generally similar for men and women, indicating similar absorption for both genders. The gender differences observed in plasma niacin and metabolite levels may be due to gender-specific differences in metabolic rate or volume of distribution. Data from clinical trials suggest that women have a greater hypolipidemic response than men at equivalent doses of NIASPAN and ADVICOR.

In a multiple-dose study, plasma concentrations of active and total HMG-CoA reductase inhibitors were 20 to 50% higher in women than in men. In two single-dose studies with ADVICOR, lovastatin concentrations were about 30% higher in women than men, and total HMG-CoA reductase inhibitor concentrations were about 20 to 25% greater in women.

In a multi-center, randomized, double-blind, active-comparator study in patients with Type IIa and IIb hyperlipidemia, ADVICOR was compared to single-agent treatment (NIASPAN and lovastatin). The treatment effects of ADVICOR compared to lovastatin and NIASPAN differed for males and females with a significantly larger treatment effect seen for females. The mean percent change from baseline at endpoint for LDL-C, TG, and HDL-C by gender are as follows (Table 1):
[See table 1 at top of previous page]

Drug-drug Interactions
[See table 2 at top of previous page]

Clinical Studies
In a multi-center, randomized, double-blind, parallel, 28-week, active-comparator study in patients with Type IIa and IIb hyperlipidemia, ADVICOR was compared to each of its components (NIASPAN and lovastatin). Using a forced dose-escalation study design, patients received each dose for at least 4 weeks. Patients randomized to treatment with ADVICOR initially received 500 mg/20 mg. The dose was increased at 4-week intervals to a maximum of 1000 mg/20 mg in one-half of the patients and 2000 mg/40 mg in the other half. The NIASPAN monotherapy group underwent a similar titration from 500 mg to 2000 mg. The patients randomized to lovastatin monotherapy received 20 mg for 12 weeks titrated to 40 mg for up to 16 weeks. Up to a third of the patients randomized to ADVICOR or NIASPAN discontinued prior to Week 28. In this study, ADVICOR decreased LDL-C, TG and Lp(a), and increased HDL-C in a dose-dependent fashion (Tables 3, 4, 5 and 6 below). Results from this study for LDL-C mean percent change from baseline (the primary efficacy variable) showed that:

1. LDL-lowering with ADVICOR was significantly greater than that achieved with lovastatin 40 mg only after 28 weeks of titration to a dose of 2000 mg/40 mg ($p<.0001$)
2. ADVICOR at doses of 1000 mg/20 mg or higher achieved greater LDL-lowering than NIASPAN ($p<.0001$) The LDL-C results are summarized in Table 3.

[See table 3 above]

ADVICOR achieved significantly greater HDL-raising compared to lovastatin and NIASPAN monotherapy at all doses (Table 4).
[See table 4 above]

In addition, ADVICOR achieved significantly greater TG-lowering at doses of 1000 mg/20 mg or greater compared to lovastatin and NIASPAN monotherapy (Table 5).
[See table 5 above]

The Lp(a) lowering effects of ADVICOR and NIASPAN were similar, and both were superior to lovastatin (Table 6). The independent effect of lowering Lp(a) with NIASPAN or ADVICOR on the risk of coronary and cardiovascular morbidity and mortality has not been determined.
[See table 6 above]

ADVICOR Long-Term Study
A total of 814 patients were enrolled in a long-term (52-week), open-label, single-arm study of ADVICOR. Patients were force dose-titrated to 2000 mg/40 mg over 16 weeks. After titration, patients were maintained on the maximum tolerated dose of ADVICOR for a total of 52 weeks. Five hundred-fifty (550) patients (68%) completed the study, and fifty-six percent (56%) of all patients were able to maintain a dose of 2000 mg/40 mg for the 52 weeks of treatment. The lipid-altering effects of ADVICOR peaked after 4 weeks on the maximum tolerated dose, and were maintained for the duration of treatment. These effects were comparable to what was observed in the double-blind study of ADVICOR (Tables 3-5).

INDICATIONS AND USAGE

Therapy with lipid-altering agents should be only one component of multiple risk-factor intervention in individuals at significantly increased risk for atherosclerotic vascular disease due to hypercholesterolemia. Drug therapy is indicated as an adjunct to diet when the response to a diet restricted in saturated fat and cholesterol and other nonpharmacologic measures alone has been inadequate (see also Table 8 and the NCEP treatment guidelines[1]).

ADVICOR
ADVICOR (niacin extended-release and lovastatin) is indicated for use when treatment with both NIASPAN and lovastatin is appropriate. As described in the labeling for Niaspan and lovastatin below, the components of ADVICOR are both indicated for the treatment of hypercholesterolemia. Patients receiving treatment with ADVICOR should be on a standard cholesterol-lowering diet and should continue on this diet during treatment.

NIASPAN (niacin extended-release)
Hypercholesterolemia
NIASPAN is indicated as an adjunct to diet for reduction of elevated TC, LDL-C, Apo B and TG levels, and to increase HDL-C in patients with primary hypercholesterolemia (heterozygous familial and nonfamilial) and mixed dyslipidemia (Table 7), when the response to an appropriate diet has been inadequate.

Secondary Prevention of Cardiovascular Events
In patients with a history of myocardial infarction and hypercholesterolemia, niacin is indicated to reduce the risk of recurrent nonfatal myocardial infarction.

Hypertriglyceridemia
Niacin is also indicated as adjunctive therapy for treatment of adult patients with very high serum triglyceride levels (Table 7) who present a risk of pancreatitis and who do not respond adequately to a determined dietary effort to control them. Such patients typically have serum TG levels over 2000 mg/dL and have elevations of VLDL-C as well as fasting chylomicrons (Table 7). Patients who consistently have total serum or plasma TG below 1000 mg/dL are unlikely to develop pancreatitis. Therapy with niacin may be considered for those patients with TG elevations between 1000 and 2000 mg/dL who have a history of pancreatitis or of recurrent abdominal pain typical of pancreatitis. Some patients with TG under 1000 mg/dL may, through dietary or alcohol indiscretion, convert to a pattern with massive TG elevations accompanying fasting chylomicronemia, but the influence of niacin therapy on risk of pancreatitis in such situations has not been adequately studied. Drug therapy is not indicated for patients with hyperlipoproteinemia, who have elevations of chylomicrons and plasma TG, but who have normal levels of VLDL-C.

Lovastatin
Hypercholesterolemia
Lovastatin is indicated as an adjunct to diet for the reduction of elevated TC and LDL-C levels in patients with primary hypercholesterolemia (Table 7), when the response to diet restricted in saturated fat and cholesterol and to other nonpharmacological measures alone has been inadequate.

Primary Prevention of Cardiovascular Events

In individuals without symptomatic cardiovascular disease, average to moderately elevated TC and LDL-C, and below average HDL-C, lovastatin is indicated to reduce the risk of:
- Myocardial infarction
- Unstable angina
- Coronary revascularization procedures

Secondary Prevention of Cardiovascular Events

Lovastatin is also indicated to slow the progression of coronary atherosclerosis in patients with coronary heart disease as part of a treatment strategy to lower TC and LDL-C to target levels.

The National Cholesterol Education Program (NCEP) Treatment Guidelines are summarized below:

Table 7. Classification of Hyperlipoproteinemias

Type	Lipoproteins Elevated	Lipid Elevations	
		Major	Minor
I (rare)	Chylomicrons	TG	↑→TC
IIa	LDL	TG	↑→TC
IIb	LDL,VLDL	TC	-
III (rare)	IDL	TC	TG
IV	VLDL	TC/TG	-
V (rare)	Chylomicrons, VLDL	TG	↑→TC

TC = total cholesterol; TG = triglycerides; LDL = low-density lipoprotein; VLDL = very low-density lipoprotein; IDL = intermediate-density lipoprotein ↑→ = increased or no change

General Recommendations

Prior to initiating therapy with a lipid-lowering agent, secondary causes for hypercholesterolemia (e.g., poorly controlled diabetes mellitus, hypothyroidism, nephrotic syndrome, dysproteinemias, obstructive liver disease, other drug therapy, alcoholism) should be excluded, and a lipid profile performed to measure TC, HDL-C, and TG. For patients with TG < 400 mg/dL, LDL-C can be estimated using the following equation:

$$LDL\text{-}C = TC - [(0.20 \times TG) + HDL\text{-}C]$$

For TG levels > 400 mg/dL, this equation is less accurate and LDL-C concentrations should be determined by ultracentrifugation. Lipid determinations should be performed at intervals of no less than 4 weeks and dosage adjusted according to the patient's response to therapy. The NCEP Treatment Guidelines are summarized in Table 8.

[See table 8 above]

After the LDL-C goal has been achieved, if the TG is still ≥200 mg/dL, non-HDL-C (TC minus HDL-C) becomes a secondary target of therapy. Non-HDL-C goals are set 30 mg/dL higher than LDL-C goals for each risk category.

CONTRAINDICATIONS

ADVICOR is contraindicated in patients with a known hypersensitivity to niacin, lovastatin or any component of this medication, active liver disease or unexplained persistent elevations in serum transaminases (see WARNINGS), active peptic ulcer disease, or arterial bleeding.

Concomitant administration with strong CYP3A4 inhibitors (e.g., itraconazole, ketoconazole, posaconazole, HIV protease inhibitors, boceprevir, telaprevir, erythromycin, clarithromycin, telithromycin and nefazodone) (see WARNINGS, Myopathy/Rhabdomyolysis).

Pregnancy and lactation - Atherosclerosis is a chronic process and the discontinuation of lipid-lowering drugs during pregnancy should have little impact on the outcome of long-term therapy of primary hypercholesterolemia. Moreover, cholesterol and other products of the cholesterol biosynthesis pathway are essential components for fetal development, including synthesis of steroids and cell membranes. Because of the ability of inhibitors of HMG-CoA reductase, such as lovastatin, to decrease the synthesis of cholesterol and possibly other products of the cholesterol biosynthesis pathway, ADVICOR is contraindicated in women who are pregnant and in lactating mothers. ADVICOR may cause fetal harm when administered to pregnant women. **ADVICOR should be administered to women of childbearing age only when such patients are highly unlikely to conceive.** If the patient becomes pregnant while taking this drug, ADVICOR should be discontinued immediately and the patient should be apprised of the potential hazard to the fetus (see PRECAUTIONS, Pregnancy).

Table 8. NCEP Treatment Guidelines: LDL-C Goals and Cutpoints for Therapeutic Lifestyle Changes and Drug Therapy in Different Risk Categories

Risk Category	LDL Goal (mg/dL)	LDL Level at Which to Initiate Therapeutic Lifestyle Changes (mg/dL)	LDL Level at Which to Consider Drug Therapy (mg/dL)
CHD[†] or CHD risk equivalents (10-year risk >20%)	<100	≥ 100	≥ 130 (100-129:drug optional) [††]
2+ Risk factors (10-year risk ≤20%)	<130	≥ 130	10-year risk 10%-20%: ≥ 130 10-year risk <10%: ≥ 160
0-1 Risk factor [†††]	<160	≥ 160	≥ 190 (160-189:LDL-lowering drug optional)

[†] CHD, coronary heart disease

[††] Some authorities recommend use of LDL-lowering drugs in this category if an LDL-C level of <100 mg/dL cannot be achieved by therapeutic lifestyle changes. Others prefer use of drugs that primarily modify triglycerides and HDL-C, e.g., nicotinic acid or fibrate. Clinical judgement also may call for deferring drug therapy in this subcategory.

[†††] Almost all people with 0-1 risk factor have 10-year risk <10%; thus, 10-year risk assessment in people with 0-1 risk factor is not necessary.

WARNINGS

ADVICOR should not be substituted for equivalent doses of immediate-release (crystalline) niacin. For patients switching from immediate-release niacin to NIASPAN, therapy with NIASPAN should be initiated with low doses (i.e., 500 mg once daily at bedtime) and the NIASPAN dose should then be titrated to the desired therapeutic response (see DOSAGE AND ADMINISTRATION).

Liver Dysfunction

Cases of severe hepatic toxicity, including fulminant hepatic necrosis, have occurred in patients who have substituted sustained-release (modified-release, timed-release) niacin products for immediate-release (crystalline) niacin at equivalent doses.

ADVICOR should be used with caution in patients who consume substantial quantities of alcohol and/or have a past history of liver disease. Active liver disease or unexplained transaminase elevations are contraindications to the use of ADVICOR.

Niacin preparations and lovastatin preparations have been associated with abnormal liver tests. In studies using NIASPAN alone, 0.8% of patients were discontinued for transaminase elevations. In studies using lovastatin alone, 0.2% of patients were discontinued for transaminase elevations.[2] In three safety and efficacy studies involving titration to final daily ADVICOR doses ranging from 500 mg/10 mg to 2500 mg/40 mg, ten of 1028 patients (1.0%) experienced reversible elevations in AST/ALT to more than 3 times the upper limit of normal (ULN). Three of ten elevations occurred at doses outside the recommended dosing limit of 2000 mg/40 mg; no patient receiving 1000 mg/20 mg had 3-fold elevations in AST/ALT.

In clinical studies with ADVICOR, elevations in transaminases did not appear to be related to treatment duration; elevations in AST and ALT levels did appear to be dose related. Transaminase elevations were reversible upon discontinuation of ADVICOR.

It is recommended that liver enzyme tests be obtained prior to initiating therapy with ADVICOR and repeated as clinically indicated.

There have been rare postmarketing reports of fatal and non-fatal hepatic failure in patients taking statins, including lovastatin. If serious liver injury with clinical symptoms and/or hyperbilirubinemia or jaundice occurs during treatment with ADVICOR, promptly interrupt therapy. If an alternate etiology is not found do not restart ADVICOR.

Myopathy/Rhabdomyolysis

Lovastatin and other inhibitors of HMG-CoA reductase occasionally cause myopathy, which is manifested as muscle pain or weakness associated with grossly elevated creatine kinase (> 10 times ULN). **Rhabdomyolysis, with or without acute renal failure secondary to myoglobinuria, has been reported rarely and can occur at any time.** In a large, long-term, clinical safety and efficacy study (the EXCEL study)[3,4] with lovastatin, myopathy occurred in up to 0.2% of patients treated with lovastatin 20 to 80 mg for up to 2 years. When drug treatment was interrupted or discontinued in these patients, muscle symptoms and creatine kinase (CK) increases promptly resolved. The risk of myopathy is increased by concomitant therapy with certain drugs, some of which were excluded by the EXCEL study design.

The risk of myopathy/rhabdomyolysis is increased by concomitant use of lovastatin with the following:

Strong inhibitors of CYP3A4: The risk of myopathy appears to be increased by high levels of HMG-CoA reductase inhibitory activity in plasma. Lovastatin is metabolized by the cytochrome P450 isoform 3A4. Certain drugs which share this metabolic pathway can raise the plasma levels of lovastatin and may increase the risk of myopathy. These include itraconazole, ketoconazole, and posaconazole, the macrolide antibiotics erythromycin and clarithromycin, the ketolide antibiotic telithromycin, HIV protease inhibitors, boceprevir, telaprevir, the antidepressant nefazodone, or large quantities of grapefruit juice (>1 quart daily). Combination of these drugs with lovastatin is contraindicated. If treatment with itraconazole, ketoconazole, erythromycin, clarithromycin or telithromycin is unavoidable, therapy with lovastatin should be suspended during the course of treatment.

Although not studied clinically, voriconazole has been shown to inhibit lovastatin metabolism *in vitro* (human liver microsomes). Therefore, voriconazole is likely to increase the plasma concentration of lovastatin. It is recommended that dose adjustment of lovastatin be considered during coadministration. Increased lovastatin concentration in plasma has been associated with an increased risk of myopathy/rhabdomyolysis.

Gemfibrozil: The combined use of lovastatin with gemfibrozil should be avoided.

Other fibrates: Caution should be used when prescribing other fibrates with lovastatin, as these agents can cause myopathy when given alone. **The benefit of further alterations in lipid levels by the combined use of lovastatin with other fibrates should be carefully weighed against the potential risks of this combination.**

Cyclosporine: The use of lovastatin with cyclosporine should be avoided.

Danazol, diltiazem or verapamil with higher doses of lovastatin: In patients taking concomitant danazol, diltiazem or verapamil, the dose of lovastatin should not exceed 20 mg (see DOSAGE AND ADMINISTRATION), as the risk of myopathy increases at higher doses. The benefits of the use of lovastatin in patients receiving danazol, diltiazem, or verapamil should be carefully weighed against the risks of these combinations.

Amiodarone: In patients taking concomitant amiodarone, the dose of lovastatin should not exceed 40 mg (see DOSAGE AND ADMINISTRATION), as the risk of myopathy increases at higher doses.

Colchicine: Cases of myopathy, including rhabdomyolysis, have been reported with lovastatin coadministered with colchicine, and caution should be exercised when prescribing lovastatin with colchicine.

Ranolazine: The risk of myopathy, including rhabdomyolysis, may be increased by concomitant administration of ranolazine. Dose adjustment of lovastatin may be considered during co-administration with ranolazine.

Prescribing recommendations for interacting agents are summarized in Table 9.

Information on the AbbVie, Inc. products listed on these pages is from the prescribing information in use as of July 31, 2014. For more information, please visit rxabbvie.com or call 1-800-633-9110.

**Table 9.
Drug Interactions Associated with Increased
Risk of Myopathy/Rhabdomyolysis**

Interacting Agents	Prescribing Recommendations
Strong CYP3A4 inhibitors, e.g.: Ketoconazole Itraconazole Posaconazole Erythromycin Clarithromycin Telithromycin HIV protease inhibitors Boceprevir Telaprevir Nefazodone	Contraindicated with lovastatin
Gemfibrozil Cyclosporine	Avoid with lovastatin
Danazol Diltiazem Verapamil	Do not exceed 20 mg lovastatin daily
Amiodarone	Do not exceed 40 mg lovastatin daily
Grapefruit juice	Avoid large quantities of grapefruit juice (>1 quart daily)

ADVICOR

Myopathy and/or rhabdomyolysis have been reported when lovastatin is used in combination with lipid-altering doses (≥1g/day) of niacin. Physicians contemplating the use of ADVICOR, a combination of lovastatin and niacin, should weigh the potential benefits and risks, and should carefully monitor patients for any signs and symptoms of muscle pain, tenderness, or weakness, particularly during the initial month of treatment or during any period of upward dosage titration of either drug. Periodic CK determinations may be considered in such situations, but there is no assurance that such monitoring will prevent myopathy. In clinical studies, no cases of rhabdomyolysis and one suspected case of myopathy have been reported in 1079 patients who were treated with ADVICOR at doses up to 2000 mg/40 mg for periods up to 2 years.

There have been rare reports of immune-mediated necrotizing myopathy (IMNM), an autoimmune myopathy, associated with statin use. IMNM is characterized by: proximal muscle weakness and elevated serum creatine kinase, which persist despite discontinuation of statin treatment; muscle biopsy showing necotizing myopathy without significant inflammation; improvement with immunosuppressive agents.

All patients starting therapy with ADVICOR, or whose dose of ADVICOR is being increased, should be advised of the risk of myopathy, and told to report promptly unexplained muscle pain, tenderness, or weakness particularly if accompanied by malaise or fever or if muscle signs and symptoms persist after discontinuing ADVICOR. A CK level above 10 times ULN in a patient with unexplained muscle symptoms indicates myopathy. ADVICOR therapy should be discontinued immediately if myopathy is diagnosed or suspected.

In patients with complicated medical histories predisposing to rhabdomyolysis, such as preexisting renal insufficiency, dose escalation requires caution. ADVICOR therapy should be discontinued if markedly elevated CPK levels occur or myopathy is diagnosed or suspected. ADVICOR therapy should also be temporarily withheld in any patient experiencing an acute or serious condition predisposing to the development of renal failure secondary to rhabdomyolysis, e.g., sepsis; hypotension; major surgery; trauma; severe metabolic, endocrine, or electrolyte disorders; or uncontrolled epilepsy.

PRECAUTIONS
General
Before instituting therapy with a lipid-altering medication, an attempt should be made to control dyslipidemia with appropriate diet, exercise, and weight reduction in obese patients, and to treat other underlying medical problems (see INDICATIONS AND USAGE).

Patients with a past history of jaundice, hepatobiliary disease, or peptic ulcer should be observed closely during ADVICOR therapy. Frequent monitoring of liver function tests and blood glucose should be performed to ascertain that the drug is producing no adverse effects on these organ systems.

Diabetic patients may experience a dose-related rise in fasting blood sugar (FBS). In three clinical studies, which included 1028 patients exposed to ADVICOR (6 to 22% of whom had diabetes type II at baseline), increases in FBS above normal occurred in 46 to 65% of patients at any time during study treatment with ADVICOR. Fourteen patients (1.4%) were discontinued from study treatment: 3 patients for worsening diabetes, 10 patients for hyperglycemia and 1 patient for a new diagnosis of diabetes. In the studies in which lovastatin and NIASPAN were used as active controls, 24 to 41% of patients receiving lovastatin and 43 to 58% of patients receiving NIASPAN also had increases in FBS above normal. One patient (1.1%) receiving lovastatin was discontinued for hyperglycemia. Diabetic or potentially diabetic patients should be observed closely during treatment with ADVICOR, and adjustment of diet and/or hypoglycemic therapy may be necessary.

In one long-term study of 106 patients treated with ADVICOR, elevations in prothrombin time (PT) >3 times ULN occurred in 2 patients (2%) during study drug treatment. In a long-term study of 814 patients treated with ADVICOR, 7 patients were noted to have platelet counts <100,000 during study drug treatment. Four of these patients were discontinued, and one patient with a platelet count <100,000 had prolonged bleeding after a tooth extraction. Prior studies have shown that NIASPAN can be associated with dose-related reductions in platelet count (mean of -11% with 2000 mg) and increases of PT (mean of approximately +4%). Accordingly, patients undergoing surgery should be carefully evaluated. In controlled studies, ADVICOR has been associated with small but statistically significant dose-related reductions in phosphorus levels (mean of -10% with 2000 mg/40 mg). Phosphorus levels should be monitored periodically in patients at risk for hypophosphatemia. In clinical studies with ADVICOR, hypophosphatemia was more common in males than in females. The clinical relevance of hypophosphatemia in this population is not known.

Niacin
Caution should also be used when ADVICOR is used in patients with unstable angina or in the acute phase of MI, particularly when such patients are also receiving vasoactive drugs such as nitrates, calcium channel blockers, or adrenergic blocking agents.

Elevated uric acid levels have occurred with niacin therapy; therefore, in patients predisposed to gout, niacin therapy should be used with caution. Niacin is rapidly metabolized by the liver, and excreted through the kidneys. ADVICOR is contraindicated in patients with significant or unexplained hepatic dysfunction (see CONTRAINDICATIONS and WARNINGS) and should be used with caution in patients with renal dysfunction.

Lovastatin
Lovastatin may elevate creatine phosphokinase and transaminase levels (see WARNINGS and ADVERSE REACTIONS). This should be considered in the differential diagnosis of chest pain in a patient on therapy with lovastatin.

Endocrine function - Increases in HbA1c and fasting serum glucose levels have been reported with HMG-CoA reductase inhibitors, including lovastatin.

HMG-CoA reductase inhibitors interfere with cholesterol synthesis and as such might theoretically blunt adrenal and/or gonadal steroid production. Results of clinical studies with drugs in this class have been inconsistent with regard to drug effects on basal and reserve steroid levels. However, clinical studies have shown that lovastatin does not reduce basal plasma cortisol concentration or impair adrenal reserve, and does not reduce basal plasma testosterone concentration. Another HMG-CoA reductase inhibitor has been shown to reduce the plasma testosterone response to human chorionic gonadotropin (HCG). In the same study, the mean testosterone response to HCG was slightly but not significantly reduced after treatment with lovastatin 40 mg daily for 16 weeks in 21 men. The effects of HMG-CoA reductase inhibitors on male fertility have not been studied in adequate numbers of male patients. The effects, if any, on the pituitary-gonadal axis in premenopausal women are unknown. Patients treated with lovastatin who develop clinical evidence of endocrine dysfunction should be evaluated appropriately. Caution should also be exercised if an HMG-CoA reductase inhibitor or other agent used to lower cholesterol levels is administered to patients also receiving other drugs (e.g., spironolactone, cimetidine) that may decrease the levels or activity of endogenous steroid hormones.

CNS toxicity - Lovastatin produced optic nerve degeneration (Wallerian degeneration of retinogeniculate fibers) in clinically normal dogs in a dose-dependent fashion starting at 60 mg/kg/day, a dose that produced mean plasma drug levels about 30 times higher than the mean drug level in humans taking the highest recommended dose (as measured by total enzyme inhibitory activity). Vestibulocochlear Wallerian-like degeneration and retinal ganglion cell chromatolysis were also seen in dogs treated for 14 weeks at

180 mg/kg/day, a dose which resulted in a mean plasma drug level (C_{max}) similar to that seen with the 60 mg/kg/day dose.

CNS vascular lesions, characterized by perivascular hemorrhage and edema, mononuclear cell infiltration of perivascular spaces, perivascular fibrin deposits and necrosis of small vessels, were seen in dogs treated with lovastatin at a dose of 180 mg/kg/day, a dose which produced plasma drug levels (C_{max}) which were about 30 times higher than the mean values in humans taking 80 mg/day.

Similar optic nerve and CNS vascular lesions have been observed with other drugs of this class.

Cataracts were seen in dogs treated with lovastatin for 11 and 28 weeks at 180 mg/kg/day and 1 year at 60 mg/kg/day.

Information for Patients
Patients should be advised of the following:
• to report promptly unexplained muscle pain, tenderness, or weakness particularly if accompanied by malaise or fever or if muscle signs and symptoms persist after discontinuing ADVICOR (see WARNINGS, Myopathy/Rhabdomyolysis);
• to report promptly any symptoms that may indicate liver injury, including fatigue, anorexia, right upper abdominal discomfort, dark urine or jaundice (see WARNINGS, Liver Dysfunction);
• to take ADVICOR at bedtime, with a low-fat snack. Administration on an empty stomach is not recommended;
• to carefully follow the prescribed dosing regimen (see DOSAGE AND ADMINISTRATION);
• that flushing is a common side effect of niacin therapy that usually subsides after several weeks of consistent niacin use. Flushing may last for several hours after dosing, may vary in severity, and will, by taking ADVICOR at bedtime, most likely occur during sleep. If awakened by flushing, especially if taking antihypertensives, rise slowly to minimize the potential for dizziness and/or syncope;
• that taking aspirin (up to approximately 30 minutes before taking ADVICOR) may minimize flushing;
• to avoid ingestion of alcohol, hot beverages and spicy foods around the time of ADVICOR administration, to minimize flushing;
• should not be administered with grapefruit juice;
• that if ADVICOR therapy is discontinued for an extended length of time, their physician should be contacted prior to re-starting therapy; re-titration is recommended (see DOSAGE AND ADMINISTRATION);
• to notify their physician if they are taking vitamins or other nutritional supplements containing niacin or related compounds such as nicotinamide (see Drug Interactions);
• to notify their physician if symptoms of dizziness occur;
• if diabetic, to notify their physician of changes in blood glucose;
• that ADVICOR tablets should not be broken, crushed, or chewed, but should be swallowed whole.

Drug Interactions
Niacin
Antihypertensive Therapy - Niacin may potentiate the effects of ganglionic blocking agents and vasoactive drugs resulting in postural hypotension.

Aspirin - Concomitant aspirin may decrease the metabolic clearance of niacin. The clinical relevance of this finding is unclear.

Bile Acid Sequestrants - An *in vitro* study was carried out investigating the niacin-binding capacity of colestipol and cholestyramine. About 98% of available niacin was bound to colestipol, with 10 to 30% binding to cholestyramine. These results suggest that 4 to 6 hours, or as great an interval as possible, should elapse between the ingestion of bile acid-binding resins and the administration of ADVICOR.

Other - Concomitant alcohol or hot drinks may increase the side effects of flushing and pruritus and should be avoided around the time of ADVICOR ingestion. Vitamins or other nutritional supplements containing large doses of niacin or related compounds such as nicotinamide may potentiate the adverse effects of ADVICOR.

Lovastatin
Lovastatin is metabolized by CYP3A4 but has no CYP3A4 inhibitory activity; therefore it is not expected to affect the plasma concentrations of other drugs metabolized by CYP3A4. Strong inhibitors of CYP3A4 (e.g., itraconazole, ketoconazole, posaconazole, clarithromycin, telithromycin, HIV protease inhibitors, boceprevir, telaprevir, nefazodone, and erythromycin), and large quantities of grapefruit juice (>1 quart daily) increase the risk of myopathy by reducing the elimination of lovastatin (see WARNINGS, Myopathy/Rhabdomyolysis).

In vitro studies have demonstrated that voriconazole inhibits the metabolism of lovastatin. Adjustment of the lovastatin dose may be needed to reduce the risk of myopathy, including rhabdomyolysis, if voriconazole must be used concomitantly with lovastatin.

Interactions With Lipid-Lowering Drugs That Can Cause Myopathy When Given Alone

The risk of myopathy is also increased by the following lipid-lowering drugs that are not strong CYP3A4 inhibitors, but which can cause myopathy when given alone (see WARNINGS, Myopathy/Rhabdomyolysis).

Gemfibrozil

Other fibrates

Other Drug Interactions

Cyclosporine: The risk of myopathy/rhabdomyolysis is increased by concomitant administration of cyclosporine (see WARNINGS, Myopathy/Rhabdomyolysis).

Danazol, Diltiazem, or Verapamil: The risk of myopathy/rhabdomyolysis is increased by concomitant administration of danazol, diltiazem, or verapamil particularly with higher doses of lovastatin (see WARNINGS, Myopathy/Rhabdomyolysis and CLINICAL PHARMACOLOGY, Pharmacokinetics).

Amiodarone: The risk of myopathy/rhabdomyolysis is increased when amiodarone is used concomitantly with a closely related member of the HMGCoA reductase inhibitor class (see WARNINGS, Myopathy/Rhabdomyolysis).

Coumarin Anticoagulants - In a small clinical study in which lovastatin was administered to warfarin-treated patients, no effect on PT was detected. However, another HMG-CoA reductase inhibitor has been found to produce a less than two seconds increase in PT in healthy volunteers receiving low doses of warfarin. Also, bleeding and/or increased PT have been reported in a few patients taking coumarin anticoagulants concomitantly with lovastatin. It is recommended that in patients taking anticoagulants, PT be determined before starting ADVICOR and frequently enough during early therapy to insure that no significant alteration of PT occurs. Once a stable PT has been documented, PT can be monitored at the intervals usually recommended for patients on coumarin anticoagulants. If the dose of ADVICOR is changed, the same procedure should be repeated.

Colchicine - Cases of myopathy, including rhabdomyolysis, have been reported with lovastatin coadministered with colchicine.

Ranolazine - The risk of myopathy, including rhabdomyolysis, may be increased by concomitant administration of ranolazine.

Propranolol - In normal volunteers, there was no clinically significant pharmacokinetic or pharmacodynamic interaction with concomitant administration of single doses of lovastatin and propranolol.

Digoxin - In patients with hypercholesterolemia, concomitant administration of lovastatin and digoxin resulted in no effect on digoxin plasma concentrations.

Oral Hypoglycemic Agents - In pharmacokinetic studies of lovastatin in hypercholesterolemic, non-insulin dependent diabetic patients, there was no drug interaction with glipizide or with chlorpropamide.

Drug/Laboratory Test Interactions

Niacin may produce false elevations in some fluorometric determinations of plasma or urinary catecholamines. Niacin may also give false-positive reactions with cupric sulfate solution (Benedict's reagent) in urine glucose tests.

Carcinogenesis, Mutagenesis, Impairment of Fertility

No studies have been conducted with ADVICOR regarding carcinogenesis, mutagenesis, or impairment of fertility.

Niacin

Niacin, administered to mice for a lifetime as a 1% solution in drinking water, was not carcinogenic. The mice in this study received approximately 6 to 8 times a human dose of 3000 mg/day as determined on a mg/m² basis. Niacin was negative for mutagenicity in the Ames test. No studies on impairment of fertility have been performed.

Lovastatin

In a 21-month carcinogenic study in mice, there was a statistically significant increase in the incidence of hepatocellular carcinomas and adenomas in both males and females at 500 mg/kg/day. This dose produced a total plasma drug exposure 3 to 4 times that of humans given the highest recommended dose of lovastatin (drug exposure was measured as total HMG-CoA reductase inhibitory activity in extracted plasma). Tumor increases were not seen at 20 and 100 mg/kg/day, doses that produced drug exposures of 0.3 to 2 times that of humans at the 80 mg/day dose. A statistically significant increase in pulmonary adenomas was seen in female mice at approximately 4 times the human drug exposure. (Although mice were given 300 times the human dose on a mg/kg body weight basis, plasma levels of total inhibitory activity were only 4 times higher in mice than in humans given 80 mg of lovastatin.)

There was an increase in incidence of papilloma in the nonglandular mucosa of the stomach of mice beginning at exposures of 1 to 2 times that of humans. The glandular mucosa was not affected. The human stomach contains only glandular mucosa.

In a 24-month carcinogenicity study in rats, there was a positive dose-response relationship for hepatocellular carcinogenicity in males at drug exposures between 2 to 7 times that of human exposure at 80 mg/day (doses in rats were 5, 30, and 180 mg/kg/day).

An increased incidence of thyroid neoplasms in rats appears to be a response that has been seen with other HMG-CoA reductase inhibitors.

A drug in this class chemically similar to lovastatin was administered to mice for 72 weeks at 25, 100, and 400 mg/kg body weight, which resulted in mean serum drug levels approximately 3, 15, and 33 times higher than the mean human serum drug concentration (as total inhibitory activity) after a 40 mg oral dose. Liver carcinomas were significantly increased in high-dose females and mid- and high-dose males, with a maximum incidence of 90% in males. The incidence of adenomas of the liver was significantly increased in mid- and high-dose females. Drug treatment also significantly increased the incidence of lung adenomas in mid- and high-dose males and females. Adenomas of the Harderian gland (a gland of the eye of rodents) were significantly higher in high-dose mice than in controls.

No evidence of mutagenicity was observed in a microbial mutagen test using mutant strains of *Salmonella typhimurium* with or without rat or mouse liver metabolic activation. In addition, no evidence of damage to genetic material was noted in an *in vitro* alkaline elution assay using rat or mouse hepatocytes, a V-79 mammalian cell forward mutation study, an *in vitro* chromosome aberration study in CHO cells, or an *in vivo* chromosomal aberration assay in mouse bone marrow.

Drug-related testicular atrophy, decreased spermatogenesis, spermatocytic degeneration and giant cell formation were seen in dogs starting at 20 mg/kg/day. Similar findings were seen with another drug in this class. No drug-related effects on fertility were found in studies with lovastatin in rats. However, in studies with a similar drug in this class, there was decreased fertility in male rats treated for 34 weeks at 25 mg/kg body weight, although this effect was not observed in a subsequent fertility study when this same dose was administered for 11 weeks (the entire cycle of spermatogenesis, including epididymal maturation). In rats treated with this same reductase inhibitor at 180 mg/kg/day, seminiferous tubule degeneration (necrosis and loss of spermatogenic epithelium) was observed. No microscopic changes were observed in the testes from rats of either study. The clinical significance of these findings is unclear.

Pregnancy

Pregnancy Category X — See CONTRAINDICATIONS.

ADVICOR should be administered to women of childbearing potential only when such patients are highly unlikely to conceive and have been informed of the potential hazard. Safety in pregnant women has not been established and there is no apparent benefit to therapy with ADVICOR during pregnancy (see CONTRAINDICATIONS). Treatment should be immediately discontinued as soon as pregnancy is recognized.

Niacin

Animal reproduction studies have not been conducted with niacin or with ADVICOR. It is also not known whether niacin at doses typically used for lipid disorders can cause fetal harm when administered to pregnant women or whether it can affect reproductive capacity. If a woman receiving niacin or ADVICOR for primary hypercholesterolemia becomes pregnant, the drug should be discontinued.

Lovastatin

Rare reports of congenital anomalies have been received following intrauterine exposure to HMG-CoA reductase inhibitors. In a review[5] of approximately 100 prospectively followed pregnancies in women exposed to lovastatin or another structurally related HMG-CoA reductase inhibitor, the incidences of congenital anomalies, spontaneous abortions and fetal deaths/stillbirths did not exceed what would be expected in the general population. The number of cases is adequate only to exclude a 3- to 4-fold increase in congenital anomalies over the background incidence. In 89% of the prospectively followed pregnancies, drug treatment was initiated prior to pregnancy and was discontinued at some point in the first trimester when pregnancy was identified. Lovastatin has been shown to produce skeletal malformations at plasma levels 40 times the human exposure (for mouse fetus) and 80 times the human exposure (for rat fetus) based on mg/m² surface area (doses were 800 mg/kg/day). No drug-induced changes were seen in either species at multiples of 8 times (rat) or 4 times (mouse) based on surface area. No evidence of malformations was noted in rabbits at exposures up to 3 times the human exposure (dose of 15 mg/kg/day, highest tolerated dose).

Labor and Delivery

No studies have been conducted on the effect of ADVICOR, niacin or lovastatin on the mother or the fetus during labor or delivery, on the duration of labor or delivery, or on the growth, development, and functional maturation of the child.

Nursing Mothers

No studies have been conducted with ADVICOR in nursing mothers.

Because of the potential for serious adverse reactions in nursing infants from lipid-altering doses of niacin and lovastatin (see CONTRAINDICATIONS), ADVICOR should not be taken while a woman is breastfeeding.

Niacin has been reported to be excreted in human milk. It is not known whether lovastatin is excreted in human milk. A small amount of another drug in this class is excreted in human breast milk.

Pediatric Use

No studies in patients under 18 years-of-age have been conducted with ADVICOR. Because pediatric patients are not likely to benefit from cholesterol lowering for at least a decade and because experience with this drug or its active ingredients is limited, treatment of pediatric patients with ADVICOR is not recommended at this time.

Geriatric Use

Of the 214 patients who received ADVICOR in double-blind clinical studies, 37.4% were 65 years-of-age and older, and of the 814 patients who received ADVICOR in open-label clinical studies, 36.2% were 65 years-of-age and older. Responses in LDL-C, HDL-C, and TG were similar in geriatric patients. No overall differences in the percentage of patients with adverse events were observed between older and younger patients. No overall differences were observed in selected chemistry values between the two groups except for amylase which was higher in older patients.

ADVERSE REACTIONS

Overview

In controlled clinical studies, 40/214 (19%) of patients randomized to ADVICOR discontinued therapy prior to study completion. Of the 214 patients enrolled 18 (8%) discontinued due to flushing. In the same controlled studies, 9/94 (10%) of patients randomized to lovastatin and 19/92 (21%) of patients randomized to NIASPAN also discontinued treatment prior to study completion secondary to adverse events. Flushing episodes (i.e., warmth, redness, itching and/or tingling) were the most common treatment-emergent adverse events, and occurred in 53% to 83% of patients treated with ADVICOR. Spontaneous reports with NIASPAN and clinical studies with ADVICOR suggest that flushing may also be accompanied by symptoms of dizziness or syncope, tachycardia, palpitations, shortness of breath, sweating, burning sensation/skin burning sensation, chills, and/or edema.

Adverse Reactions Information

Because clinical studies are conducted under widely varying conditions, adverse reaction rates observed in clinical studies of a drug cannot be directly compared to rates in the clinical studies of another drug and may not reflect the rates observed in clinical practice. The adverse reaction information from clinical studies does, however provide a basis for identifying the adverse events that appear to be related to drug use and for approximating rates.

The data described in this section reflect the exposure to ADVICOR in two double-blind, controlled clinical studies of 400 patients. The population was 28 to 86 years-of-age, 54% male, 85% Caucasian, 9% Black, and 7% Other, and had mixed dyslipidemia.

In addition to flushing, other adverse events occurring in 5% or greater of patients treated with ADVICOR are shown in Table 10 below.

Table 10. Treatment-Emergent Adverse Events in ≥ 5% of Patients (Events Irrespective of Causality; Data from Controlled, Double-Blind Studies)

Adverse Event	ADVICOR	NIASPAN	Lovastatin
Total Number of Patients	214	92	94
Cardiovascular	**163 (76%)**	**66 (72%)**	**24 (26%)**
Flushing	152 (71%)	60 (65%)	17 (18%)
Body as a Whole	**104 (49%)**	**50 (54%)**	**42 (45%)**
Asthenia	10 (5%)	6 (7%)	5 (5%)
Flu Syndrome	12 (6%)	7 (8%)	4 (4%)
Headache	20 (9%)	12 (13%)	5 (5%)
Infection	43 (20%)	14 (15%)	19 (20%)
Pain	18 (8%)	3 (3%)	9 (10%)
Pain, Abdominal	9 (4%)	1 (1%)	6 (6%)
Pain, Back	10 (5%)	5 (5%)	5 (5%)

Information on the AbbVie, Inc. products listed on these pages is from the prescribing information in use as of July 31, 2014. For more information, please visit rxabbvie.com or call 1-800-633-9110.

Digestive System	51 (24%)	26 (28%)	16 (17%)
Diarrhea	13 (6%)	8 (9%)	2 (2%)
Dyspepsia	6 (3%)	5 (5%)	4 (4%)
Nausea	14 (7%)	11 (12%)	2 (2%)
Vomiting	7 (3%)	5 (5%)	0
Metabolic and Nutrit. System	37 (17%)	18 (20%)	13 (14%)
Hyperglycemia	8 (4%)	6 (7%)	6 (6%)
Musculoskeletal System	19 (9%)	9 (10%)	17 (18%)
Myalgia	6 (3%)	5 (5%)	8 (9%)
Skin and Appendages	38 (18%)	19 (21%)	11 (12%)
Pruritus	14 (7%)	7 (8%)	3 (3%)
Rash	11 (5%)	11 (12%)	3 (3%)

Note: Percentages are calculated from the total number of patients in each column.

See also the full prescribing information for niacin extended release (Niaspan) and lovastatin products.

The following adverse events have also been reported with niacin, lovastatin, and/or other HMG-CoA reductase inhibitors, but not necessarily with ADVICOR, either during clinical studies or in routine patient management.

Body as a Whole:	chest pain; abdominal pain; edema; chills; malaise
Cardiovascular:	atrial fibrillation; tachycardia; palpitations, and other cardiac arrhythmias; postural hypotension, orthostasis; hypotension; syncope
Eye:	toxic amblyopia; cystoid macular edema; ophthalmoplegia; eye irritation, blurred vision, progression of cataracts
Gastrointestinal:	activation of peptic ulcers and peptic ulceration; dyspepsia; vomiting; anorexia; constipation; flatulence, pancreatitis; hepatitis; fatty change in liver; jaundice; and rarely, cirrhosis, fulminant hepatic necrosis, and hepatoma, eructation, fatal and non-fatal hepatic failure
Metabolic:	gout, decreased glucose tolerance
Musculoskeletal:	muscle cramps; myopathy; rhabdomyolysis; arthralgia, myalgia. There have been rare reports of immune-mediated necrotizing myopathy with statin use (see WARNINGS).
Nervous:	dizziness; insomnia; dry mouth; paresthesia; anxiety; tremor; vertigo; peripheral neuropathy; psychic disturbances; dysfunction of certain cranial nerves, nervousness, burning sensation/skin burning sensation, peripheral nerve palsy
Psychiatric	depression
Skin:	hyper-pigmentation; acanthosis nigricans; urticaria; alopecia; dry skin; sweating; and a variety of skin changes (e.g., nodules, discoloration, dryness of mucous membranes, changes to hair/nails), vesiculobullous rash, maculopapular rash
Respiratory:	dyspnea; rhinitis
Urogenital:	gynecomastia; loss of libido; erectile dysfunction

Hypersensitivity reactions:	An apparent hypersensitivity syndrome has been reported rarely, which has included one or more of the following features: anaphylaxis, angioedema, tongue edema, larynx edema, face edema, peripheral edema, laryngismus, lupus erythematous-like syndrome, polymyalgia rheumatica, vasculitis, purpura, thrombocytopenia, leukopenia, hemolytic anemia, positive ANA, ESR increase, eosinophilia, arthritis, arthralgia, urticaria, asthenia, photosensitivity, fever, chills, flushing, malaise, dyspnea, toxic epidermal necrolysis, erythema multiforme, including Stevens-Johnson syndrome, dermatomyositis
Other:	migraine

There have been rare postmarketing reports of cognitive impairment (e.g., memory loss, forgetfulness, amnesia, memory impairment, confusion) associated with statin use. These cognitive issues have been reported for all statins. The reports are generally nonserious, and reversible upon statin discontinuation, with variable times to symptom onset (1 day to years) and symptom resolution (median of 3 weeks).

Clinical Laboratory Abnormalities
Chemistry
Elevations in serum transaminases (see WARNINGS - Liver Dysfunction), CPK and fasting glucose, and reductions in phosphorus. Niacin extended-release tablets have been associated with slight elevations in LDH, uric acid, total bilirubin, amylase and creatine kinase. Lovastatin and/or HMG-CoA reductase inhibitors have been associated with elevations in alkaline phosphatase, γ-glutamyl transpeptidase and bilirubin, and thyroid function abnormalities.
Hematology
Niacin extended-release tablets have been associated with slight reductions in platelet counts and prolongation in PT (see WARNINGS).

DRUG ABUSE AND DEPENDENCE
Neither niacin nor lovastatin is a narcotic drug. ADVICOR has no known addiction potential in humans.

OVERDOSAGE
Information on acute overdose with ADVICOR in humans is limited. Until further experience is obtained, no specific treatment of overdose with ADVICOR can be recommended. The patient should be carefully observed and given supportive treatment.
Niacin
The s.c. LD50 of niacin is 5 g/kg in rats.
The signs and symptoms of an acute overdose of niacin can be anticipated to be those of excessive pharmacologic effect: severe flushing, nausea/vomiting, diarrhea, dyspepsia, dizziness, syncope, hypotension, possibly cardiac arrhythmias and clinical laboratory abnormalities. Insufficient information is available on the potential for the dialyzability of niacin.
Lovastatin
After oral administration of lovastatin to mice the median lethal dose observed was >15 g/m².
Five healthy human volunteers have received up to 200 mg of lovastatin as a single dose without clinically significant adverse experiences. A few cases of accidental overdose have been reported; no patients had any specific symptoms, and all patients recovered without sequelae. The maximum dose taken was 5 or 6 g. The dialyzability of lovastatin and its metabolites in man is not known at present.

DOSAGE AND ADMINISTRATION
The patient should be placed on a standard cholesterol-lowering diet before receiving ADVICOR or its individual active components and should continue on this diet during treatment with lipid-altering therapy (see NCEP Treatment Guidelines for details on dietary therapy).
ADVICOR
ADVICOR should be taken at bedtime, with a low-fat snack. ADVICOR tablets should be taken whole and should not be broken, crushed, or chewed before swallowing. Patients not currently on NIASPAN must start ADVICOR at the lowest initial ADVICOR dose, a single 500 mg/20 mg tablet once daily at bedtime. The dose of ADVICOR should not be increased by more than 500 mg daily (based on the NIASPAN component) every 4 weeks. The dose of ADVICOR should be individualized based on targeted goals for cholesterol and triglycerides, and on patient response. Doses of ADVICOR greater than 2000 mg/40 mg daily are not recommended. **If ADVICOR therapy is discontinued for an extended period (>7 days), reinstitution of therapy should begin with the lowest dose of ADVICOR.**

Flushing of the skin (see ADVERSE REACTIONS) may be reduced in frequency or severity by pretreatment with aspirin up to the recommended dose of 325 mg (taken up to approximately 30 minutes prior to ADVICOR dose). Flushing, pruritus, and gastrointestinal distress are also greatly reduced by slowly increasing the dose of niacin and avoiding administration on an empty stomach.
Equivalent doses of ADVICOR may be substituted for equivalent doses of NIASPAN but should not be substituted for other modified-release (sustained-release or time-release) niacin preparations or immediate-release (crystalline) niacin preparations (see WARNINGS). Patients previously receiving niacin products other than NIASPAN should be started on NIASPAN with the recommended NIASPAN titration schedule, and the dose should subsequently be individualized based on patient response. A relative bioavailability study results indicated that ADVICOR tablet strengths (i.e. two tablets of 500 mg/20 mg and one tablet of 1000 mg/40 mg) are not interchangeable.
NIASPAN
NIASPAN should be taken at bedtime, after a low-fat snack, and doses should be individualized according to patient response. Therapy with NIASPAN must be initiated at 500 mg at bedtime in order to reduce the incidence and severity of side effects which may occur during early therapy. NIASPAN must be titrated and the dose should not be increased by more than 500 mg every 4 weeks up to a maximum dose of 2000 mg a day. The recommended dose escalation is shown in Table 11 below. Patients already receiving a stable dose of NIASPAN may be switched directly to a niacin-equivalent dose of ADVICOR.

Table 11. Recommended Dosing

	Week(s)	Daily dose	NIASPAN Dosage
INITIAL TITRATION SCHEDULE	1 to 4	500 mg	1 NIASPAN 500 mg tablet at bedtime
	5 to 8	1000 mg	2 NIASPAN 500 mg tablets at bedtime
	*	1500 mg	2 NIASPAN 750 mg tablets or 3 NIASPAN 500 mg tablets at bedtime
	*	2000 mg	2 NIASPAN 1000 mg tablets or 4 NIASPAN 500 mg tablets at bedtime

* After Week 8, titrate to patient response and tolerance. If response to 1000 mg daily is inadequate, increase dose to 1500 mg daily; may subsequently increase dose to 2000 mg daily. Daily dose should not be increased more than 500 mg in a 4-week period, and doses above 2000 mg daily are not recommended. Women may respond at lower doses than men.

Maintenance Dose:
The daily dosage of NIASPAN should not be increased by more than 500 mg in any 4-week period. The recommended maintenance dose is 1000 mg (two 500 mg tablets) to 2000 mg (two 1000 mg tablets or four 500 mg tablets) once daily at bedtime. Doses greater than 2000 mg daily are not recommended. Women may respond at lower NIASPAN doses than men.
Flushing of the skin (see ADVERSE REACTIONS) may be reduced in frequency or severity by pretreatment with aspirin up to the recommended dose of 325 mg (taken 30 minutes prior to NIASPAN dose). Tolerance to this flushing develops rapidly over the course of several weeks. Flushing, pruritus, and gastrointestinal distress are also greatly reduced by slowly increasing the dose of niacin and avoiding administration on an empty stomach. Concomitant alcoholic, hot drinks or spicy foods may increase the side effects of flushing and pruritus and should be avoided around the time of ADVICOR ingestion.
Equivalent doses of NIASPAN should **not** be substituted for sustained-release (modified-release, timed-release) niacin preparations or immediate-release (crystalline) niacin (see WARNINGS). Patients previously receiving other niacin products should be started with the recommended NIASPAN titration schedule (see Table 11), and the dose should subsequently be individualized based on patient response. Single-dose bioavailability studies have demonstrated that NIASPAN tablet strengths are not interchangeable.
If NIASPAN therapy is discontinued for an extended period, reinstitution of therapy should include a titration phase (see Table 11).
NIASPAN tablets should be taken whole and should not be broken, crushed or chewed before swallowing.
Concomitant Therapy
Concomitant Therapy with Lovastatin
Patients already receiving a stable dose of lovastatin who require further TG-lowering or HDL-raising (e.g., to achieve NCEP non-HDL-C goals), may receive concomitant dosage titration with NIASPAN per NIASPAN recommended initial titration schedule (see Table 10, DOSAGE AND ADMINISTRATION section). For patients already receiving a stable dose of NIASPAN who require further LDL-lowering (e.g., to achieve NCEP LDL-C goals; Table 8), the usual recom-

mended starting dose of lovastatin is 20 mg once a day. Dose adjustments should be made at intervals of 4 weeks or more. Combination therapy with NIASPAN and lovastatin should not exceed doses of 2000 mg and 40 mg daily, respectively.

Dosage in Patients with Renal or Hepatic Insufficiency

Use of NIASPAN in patients with renal or hepatic insufficiency has not been studied. NIASPAN is contraindicated in patients with significant or unexplained hepatic dysfunction (see WARNINGS, PRECAUTIONS). NIASPAN should be used with caution in patients with renal insufficiency (see CLINICAL PHARMACOLOGY).

Lovastatin

The usual recommended starting dose is 20 mg once a day given with the evening meal. The recommended dosing range is 10-80 mg/day in single or two divided doses; the maximum recommended dose is 80 mg/day. Doses should be individualized according to the recommended goal of therapy (see NCEP Guidelines and CLINICAL PHARMACOLOGY). Patients requiring reductions in LDL cholesterol of 20% or more to achieve their goal (see INDICATIONS AND USAGE) should be started on 20 mg/day of lovastatin. A starting dose of 10 mg may be considered for patients requiring smaller reductions. Adjustments should be made at intervals of 4 weeks or more.

Cholesterol levels should be monitored periodically and consideration should be given to reducing the dosage of lovastatin if cholesterol levels fall significantly below the targeted range.

Dosage in Patients taking Danazol, Diltiazem or Verapamil

In patients taking danazol, diltiazem, or verapamil concomitantly with lovastatin (see WARNINGS, Myopathy/Rhabdomyolysis), therapy should begin with 10 mg of lovastatin and should not exceed 20 mg/day.

Dosage in Patients taking Amiodarone

In patients taking amiodarone concomitantly with lovastatin, the dose should not exceed 40 mg/day (see WARNINGS, Myopathy/Rhabdomyolysis and PRECAUTIONS, Drug Interactions, Other drug interactions).

Concomitant Lipid-Lowering Therapy

Use of lovastatin with gemfibrozil should be avoided. Caution should be used when prescribing other fibrates with lovastatin, as fibrates can cause myopathy when given alone.

Dosage in Patients with Renal Insufficiency

In patients with severe renal insufficiency (creatinine clearance <30 mL/min), dosage increases above 20 mg/day should be carefully considered and, if deemed necessary, implemented cautiously (see CLINICAL PHARMACOLOGY and WARNINGS, Myopathy/Rhabdomyolysis).

HOW SUPPLIED

ADVICOR is an unscored capsule-shaped tablet containing either 500, 750, or 1000 mg of extended-release niacin, and 20 mg of immediate-release lovastatin (ADVICOR 500 mg/20 mg, 750 mg/20 mg, 1000 mg/20 mg), or 1000 mg of extended-release niacin and 40 mg of immediate-release lovastatin (ADVICOR 1000 mg/40 mg). Tablets are color-coated and printed with the "a" logo and a code number specific to the tablet strength on the same side. ADVICOR 500 mg/20 mg tablets are light yellow, code "502". ADVICOR 750 mg/20 mg tablets are light orange, code "752". ADVICOR 1000 mg/20 mg tablets are dark pink/light purple, code "1002". ADVICOR 1000 mg/40 mg tablets are reddish brown, code "1004." Tablets are supplied in bottles of 90 tablets as shown below.

500 mg/20 mg tablets: bottles of 90 - NDC# 0074-3005-90
750 mg/20 mg tablets: bottles of 90 - NDC# 0074-3072-90
1000 mg/20 mg tablets: bottles of 90 - NDC# 0074-3007-90
1000 mg/40 mg tablets: bottles of 90 - NDC# 0074-3010-90
Store at room temperature (20° to 25°C or 68° to 77°F).
NIASPAN is a registered trademark of AbbVie Inc., and Mevacor is a registered trademark of Merck & Co., Inc.

REFERENCES

1. Executive Summary of the Third Report of the National Cholesterol Education Program (NCEP) Expert Panel on Detection, Evaluation, and Treatment of High Blood Cholesterol in Adults (Adult Treatment Panel III). *JAMA* 2001; 285:2486-2497.
2. Downs JR, et al. *JAMA* 1998; 279:1615-1622.
3. Bradford RH, et al. *Arch Intern Med* 1991;151:43-49.
4. Bradford RH, et al. *Am J Cardiol* 1994; 74:667-673.
5. Manson JM, et al. *Reprod Toxicol* 1996; 10(6): 439-446.

Manufactured by AbbVie LTD, Barceloneta, PR 00617 for AbbVie Inc., North Chicago, IL 60064, U.S.A.
© 2013 AbbVie Inc.
Ref: 03-A745-R8-Revised February, 2013
Shown in Product Identification Guide, page 303

ANDROGEL® 1%
[ăn drō-jĕl]
(testosterone gel) for topical use   ℞ CIII

HIGHLIGHTS OF PRESCRIBING INFORMATION

These highlights do not include all the information needed to use AndroGel 1% safely and effectively. See full prescribing information for AndroGel 1%.
AndroGel® (testosterone gel) 1% for topical use CIII
Initial U.S. Approval: 1953

WARNING: SECONDARY EXPOSURE TO TESTOSTERONE

See full prescribing information for complete boxed warning.

- Virilization has been reported in children who were secondarily exposed to testosterone gel. (5.2, 6.2)
- Children should avoid contact with unwashed or unclothed application sites in men using testosterone gel. (2.2, 5.2)
- Healthcare providers should advise patients to strictly adhere to recommended instructions for use. (2.2, 5.2, 17)

———RECENT MAJOR CHANGES———
Indications and Usage. (1) 09/2012

———INDICATIONS AND USAGE———
AndroGel 1% is an androgen indicated for replacement therapy in males for conditions associated with a deficiency or absence of endogenous testosterone:
- Primary hypogonadism (congenital or acquired). (1)
- Hypogonadotropic hypogonadism (congenital or acquired). (1)

Important limitations of use:
- Safety and efficacy of AndroGel 1% in males less than 18 years old have not been established. (8.4)
- Topical testosterone products may have different doses, strengths or application instructions that may result in different systemic exposure. (1, 12.3)

———DOSAGE AND ADMINISTRATION———
- Dosage and Administration for AndroGel 1% differs from AndroGel 1.62 %. For dosage and administration of AndroGel 1.62% refer to its full prescribing information. (2)
- Starting dose of AndroGel 1% is 50 mg of testosterone (4 pump actuations, two 25 mg packets, or one 50 mg packet), applied once daily in the morning. (2.1)
- Apply to clean, dry, intact skin of shoulders and upper arms and/or abdomen. Do NOT apply AndroGel 1% to any other parts of the body including the genitals, chest or back. (2.2)
- Dose adjustment: AndroGel 1% can be dose adjusted using 50 mg, 75 mg, or 100 mg of testosterone on the basis of total serum testosterone concentration. The dose should be titrated based on the serum testosterone concentration. Additionally, serum testosterone concentration should be assessed periodically. (2.1)
- Patients should wash hands immediately with soap and water after applying AndroGel 1% and cover the application site(s) with clothing after the gel has dried. Wash the application site thoroughly with soap and water prior to any situation where skin-to-skin contact of the application site with another person is anticipated. (2.2)

———DOSAGE FORMS AND STRENGTHS———
AndroGel (testosterone gel) 1% for topical use is available as follows:
- Metered-dose pump that delivers 12.5 mg of testosterone per actuation. (3)
- Packets containing 25 mg of testosterone. (3)
- Packets containing 50 mg of testosterone. (3)

———CONTRAINDICATIONS———
- Men with carcinoma of the breast or known or suspected prostate cancer. (4, 5.1)
- Pregnant or breastfeeding women. Testosterone may cause fetal harm. (4, 8.1, 8.3)

———WARNINGS AND PRECAUTIONS———
- Monitor patients with benign prostatic hyperplasia (BPH) for worsening of signs and symptoms of BPH. (5.1)
- Avoid unintentional exposure of women or children to AndroGel 1%. Secondary exposure to testosterone can produce signs of virilization. AndroGel 1% should be discontinued until the cause of virilization is identified. (5.2)
- Exogenous administration of androgens may lead to azoospermia. (5.5)
- Edema, with or without congestive heart failure (CHF), may be a complication in patients with preexisting cardiac, renal, or hepatic disease. (5.7, 6.2)
- Sleep apnea may occur in those with risk factors. (5.9)
- Monitor serum testosterone, prostate specific antigen (PSA), hemoglobin, hematocrit, liver function tests, and lipid concentrations periodically. (5.1, 5.3, 5.6, 5.10)
- AndroGel 1% is flammable until dry. (5.13)

———ADVERSE REACTIONS———
Most common adverse reactions (incidence ≥ 5%) are acne, application site reaction, abnormal lab tests, and prostatic disorders. (6.1)

To report SUSPECTED ADVERSE REACTIONS, contact AbbVie Inc. at 1-800-633-9110 or FDA at 1-800-FDA-1088 or www.fda.gov/medwatch.

———DRUG INTERACTIONS———
- Androgens may decrease blood glucose and therefore may decrease insulin requirements in diabetic patients. (7.1)
- Changes in anticoagulant activity may be seen with androgens. More frequent monitoring of INR and prothrombin time is recommended. (7.2)
- Use of testosterone with adrenocorticotrophic hormone (ACTH) or corticosteroids may result in increased fluid retention. Use with caution, particularly in patients with cardiac, renal, or hepatic disease. (7.3)

———USE IN SPECIFIC POPULATIONS———
- There are insufficient long-term safety data in geriatric patients using AndroGel 1% to assess the potential risks of cardiovascular disease and prostate cancer. (8.5)

See 17 for PATIENT COUNSELING INFORMATION and Medication Guide

Revised: 05/2013

FULL PRESCRIBING INFORMATION: CONTENTS*

Information on the AbbVie, Inc. products listed on these pages is from the prescribing information in use as of July 31, 2014. For more information, please visit rxabbvie.com or call 1-800-633-9110.

* Sections or subsections omitted from the full prescribing information are not listed

FULL PRESCRIBING INFORMATION

> **WARNING: SECONDARY EXPOSURE TO TESTOSTERONE**
> - Virilization has been reported in children who were secondarily exposed to testosterone gel *[see Warnings and Precautions (5.2) and Adverse Reactions (6.2)]*.
> - Children should avoid contact with unwashed or unclothed application sites in men using testosterone gel *[see Dosage and Administration (2.2) and Warnings and Precautions (5.2)]*.
> - Healthcare providers should advise patients to strictly adhere to recommended instructions for use *[see Dosage and Administration (2.2), Warnings and Precautions (5.2) and Patient Counseling Information (17)]*.

---

1   INDICATIONS AND USAGE

AndroGel 1% is an androgen indicated for replacement therapy in adult males for conditions associated with a deficiency or absence of endogenous testosterone:

- Primary hypogonadism (congenital or acquired): testicular failure due to conditions such as cryptorchidism, bilateral torsion, orchitis, vanishing testis syndrome, orchiectomy, Klinefelter's syndrome, chemotherapy, or toxic damage from alcohol or heavy metals. These men usually have low serum testosterone concentrations and gonadotropins (follicle-stimulating hormone [FSH], luteinizing hormone [LH]) above the normal range.
- Hypogonadotropic hypogonadism (congenital or acquired): idiopathic gonadotropin or luteinizing hormone-releasing hormone (LHRH) deficiency or pituitary-hypothalamic injury from tumors, trauma, or radiation. These men have low testosterone serum concentrations, but have gonadotropins in the normal or low range.

Important limitations of use:

- Safety and efficacy of AndroGel 1% in males less than 18 years old have not been established *[see Use in Specific Populations (8.4)]*.
- Topical testosterone products may have different doses, strengths or application instructions that may result in different systemic exposure (1, 12.3).

2   DOSAGE AND ADMINISTRATION

Dosage and Administration for AndroGel 1% differs from AndroGel 1.62%. For dosage and administration of AndroGel 1.62% refer to its full prescribing information. (2)

2.1   Dosing and Dose Adjustment

The recommended starting dose of AndroGel 1% is 50 mg of testosterone (4 pump actuations, two 25 mg packets, or one 50 mg packet), applied topically once daily in the morning to the shoulders and upper arms and/or abdomen area (preferably at the same time every day).

Dose Adjustment

To ensure proper dosing, serum testosterone concentrations should be measured at intervals. If the serum testosterone concentration is below the normal range, the daily AndroGel 1% dose may be increased from 50 mg to 75 mg and from 75 mg to 100 mg for adult males as instructed by the physician (see Table 1, Dosing Information for AndroGel 1%). If the serum testosterone concentration exceeds the normal range, the daily AndroGel 1% dose may be decreased. If the serum testosterone concentration consistently exceeds the normal range at a daily dose of 50 mg, AndroGel 1% therapy should be discontinued. In addition, serum testosterone concentrations should be assessed periodically.

The application site and dose of AndroGel 1% are not interchangeable with other topical testosterone products.

2.2   Administration Instructions

AndroGel 1% should be applied to clean, dry, healthy, intact skin of the right and left upper arms/shoulders and/or right and left abdomen. Area of application should be limited to the area that will be covered by the patient's short sleeve T-shirt. Do not apply AndroGel 1% to any other part of the body including the genitals, chest or back. AndroGel 1% should be evenly distributed between the right and left upper arms/shoulders or both sides of the abdomen.

The prescribed daily dose of AndroGel 1% should be applied to the right and left upper arms/shoulders and/or right/left abdomen as shown in the shaded areas in the figure below.

[See figure at top of next column]

After applying the gel, the application site should be allowed to dry prior to dressing. Hands should be washed thoroughly with soap and water after application. Avoid fire, flames or smoking until the gel has dried since alcohol based products, including AndroGel 1%, are flammable.

The patient should be advised to avoid swimming or showering for at least 5 hours after the application of AndroGel 1%.

Multi-Dose Pump

To obtain a full first dose, it is necessary to prime the canister pump. To do so, with the canister in the upright position, slowly and fully depress the actuator three times. Safely discard the gel from the first three actuations. It is only necessary to prime the pump before the first dose. After the priming procedure, patients should completely depress the pump one time actuation for every 12.5 mg of testosterone required to achieve the daily prescribed dosage. The product should be delivered directly into the palm of the hand and then applied to the desired application sites. Alternatively, AndroGel 1% can be applied directly to the application sites. Table 1 provides dosing information for adult males.

Table 1: Dosing Information for AndroGel 1%

Amount of Testosterone	Number of Pump Actuations
50 mg	4 (once daily)
75 mg	6 (once daily)
100 mg	8 (once daily)

Packets

The entire contents should be squeezed into the palm of the hand and immediately applied to the application sites. Alternately, patients may squeeze a portion of the gel from the packet into the palm of the hand and apply to application sites. Repeat until entire contents have been applied.

Strict adherence to the following precautions is advised in order to minimize the potential for secondary exposure to testosterone from AndroGel 1%-treated skin:

- Children and women should avoid contact with unwashed or unclothed application site(s) of men using AndroGel 1%.
- Patients should wash hands with soap and water immediately after application of AndroGel 1%.
- Patients should cover the application site(s) with clothing (e.g., a T-shirt) after the gel has dried.
- Prior to situation in which direct skin-to-skin contact is anticipated, patients should wash the application site thoroughly with soap and water to remove any testosterone residue.
- In the event that unwashed or unclothed skin to which AndroGel 1% has been applied comes in direct contact with the skin of another person, the general area of contact on the other person should be washed with soap and water as soon as possible.

3   DOSAGE FORMS AND STRENGTHS

AndroGel (testosterone gel) 1% for topical use is available as follows:

- A metered-dose pump. Each pump actuation delivers 12.5 mg of testosterone in 1.25 g of gel.
- A unit dose packet containing 25 mg of testosterone provided in 2.5 g of gel.
- A unit dose packet containing 50 mg of testosterone provided in 5 g of gel.

4   CONTRAINDICATIONS

- AndroGel 1% is contraindicated in men with carcinoma of the breast or known or suspected carcinoma of the prostate *[see Warnings and Precautions (5.1), Adverse Reactions (6.1), and Nonclinical Toxicology (13.1)]*.
- AndroGel 1% is contraindicated in women who are or may become pregnant, or who are breastfeeding. AndroGel 1% may cause fetal harm when administered to a pregnant

woman. AndroGel 1% may cause serious adverse reactions in nursing infants. Exposure of a female fetus or nursing infant to androgens may result in varying degrees of virilization. Pregnant women or those who may become pregnant need to be aware of the potential for transfer of testosterone from men treated with AndroGel 1%. If a pregnant woman is exposed to AndroGel 1%, she should be apprised of the potential hazard to the fetus *[see Warnings and Precautions (5.2) and Use in Specific Populations (8.1, 8.3)]*.

5   WARNINGS AND PRECAUTIONS

5.1   Worsening of Benign Prostatic Hyperplasia (BPH) and Potential Risk of Prostate Cancer

- Patients with BPH treated with androgens are at an increased risk for worsening of signs and symptoms of BPH. Monitor patients with BPH for worsening signs and symptoms.
- Patients treated with androgens may be at increased risk for prostate cancer. Evaluate patients for prostate cancer prior to initiating and during treatment with androgens *[see Contraindications (4), Adverse Reactions (6.1) and Nonclinical Toxicology (13.1)]*.

5.2   Potential for Secondary Exposure to Testosterone

Cases of secondary exposure resulting in virilization of children have been reported in postmarketing surveillance. Signs and symptoms have included enlargement of the penis or clitoris, development of pubic hair, increased erections and libido, aggressive behavior, and advanced bone age. In most cases, these signs and symptoms regressed with removal of the exposure to testosterone gel. In a few cases, however, enlarged genitalia did not fully return to age-appropriate normal size, and bone age remained modestly greater than chronological age. The risk of transfer was increased in some of these cases by not adhering to precautions for the appropriate use of the topical testosterone product. Children and women should avoid contact with unwashed or unclothed application sites in men using AndroGel 1% *[see Dosage and Administration (2.2), Use in Specific Populations (8.1) and Clinical Pharmacology (12.3)]*.

Inappropriate changes in genital size or development of pubic hair or libido in children, or changes in body hair distribution, significant increase in acne, or other signs of virilization in adult women should be brought to the attention of a physician and the possibility of secondary exposure to testosterone gel should also be brought to the attention of a physician. Testosterone gel should be promptly discontinued until the cause of virilization has been identified.

5.3   Polycythemia

Increases in hematocrit, reflective of increases in red blood cell mass, may require lowering or discontinuation of testosterone. Check hematocrit prior to initiating treatment. It would also be appropriate to re-evaluate the hematocrit 3 to 6 months after starting treatment, and then annually. If hematocrit becomes elevated, stop therapy until hematocrit decreases to an acceptable concentration. An increase in red blood cell mass may increase the risk of thromboembolic events.

5.4   Use in Women

Due to lack of controlled evaluations in women and potential virilizing effects, AndroGel 1% is not indicated for use in women *[see Contraindications (4) and Use in Specific Populations (8.1, 8.3)]*.

5.5   Potential for Adverse Effects on Spermatogenesis

With large doses of exogenous androgens, including AndroGel 1%, spermatogenesis may be suppressed through feedback inhibition of pituitary follicle-stimulating hormone (FSH) which could possibly lead to adverse effects on semen parameters including sperm count.

5.6   Hepatic Adverse Effects

Prolonged use of high doses of orally active 17-alpha-alkyl androgens (e.g., methyltestosterone) has been associated with serious hepatic adverse effects (peliosis hepatis, hepatic neoplasms, cholestatic hepatitis, and jaundice). Peliosis hepatis can be a life-threatening or fatal complication. Long-term therapy with intramuscular testosterone enanthate has produced multiple hepatic adenomas. AndroGel 1% is not known to cause these adverse effects.

5.7   Edema

Androgens, including AndroGel 1%, may promote retention of sodium and water. Edema, with or without congestive heart failure, may be a serious complication in patients with preexisting cardiac, renal, or hepatic disease *[see Adverse Reactions (6.2)]*.

5.8   Gynecomastia

Gynecomastia may develop and persist in patients being treated with androgens, including AndroGel 1%, for hypogonadism.

5.9   Sleep Apnea

The treatment of hypogonadal men with testosterone may potentiate sleep apnea in some patients, especially those with risk factors such as obesity or chronic lung diseases *[see Adverse Reactions (6.2)]*.

5.10   Lipids

Changes in serum lipid profile may require dose adjustment or discontinuation of testosterone therapy.

5.11   Hypercalcemia

Androgens, including AndroGel 1%, should be used with caution in cancer patients at risk of hypercalcemia (and associated hypercalciuria). Regular monitoring of serum calcium concentrations is recommended in these patients.

5.12   Decreased Thyroxine-binding Globulin

Androgens, including AndroGel 1%, may decrease concentrations of thyroxin-binding globulins, resulting in decreased total T4 serum concentrations and increased resin uptake of T3 and T4. Free thyroid hormone concentrations remain unchanged, however, and there is no clinical evidence of thyroid dysfunction.

5.13   Flammability

Alcohol based products, including AndroGel 1%, are flammable; therefore, patients should be advised to avoid fire, flame or smoking until the AndroGel 1% has dried.

6   ADVERSE REACTIONS

6.1   Clinical Trial Experience

Because clinical trials are conducted under widely varying conditions, adverse reaction rates observed in the clinical trials of a drug cannot be directly compared to rates in the clinical trials of another drug and may not reflect the rates observed in practice.

Clinical Trials in Hypogonadal Men

Table 2 shows the incidence of all adverse events judged by the investigator to be at least possibly related to treatment with AndroGel 1% and reported by >1% of patients in a 180 Day, Phase 3 study.

Table 2: Adverse Events Possibly, Probably or Definitely Related to Use of AndroGel 1% in the 180-Day Controlled Clinical Trial

Adverse Event	Dose of AndroGel 1%		
	50 mg	75 mg	100 mg
	N = 77	N = 40	N = 78
Acne	1%	3%	8%
Alopecia	1%	0%	1%
Application Site Reaction	5%	3%	4%
Asthenia	0%	3%	1%
Depression	1%	0%	1%
Emotional Lability	0%	3%	3%
Gynecomastia	1%	0%	3%
Headache	4%	3%	3%
Hypertension	3%	0%	3%
Lab Test Abnormal*	6%	5%	3%
Libido Decreased	0%	3%	1%
Nervousness	0%	3%	1%
Pain Breast	1%	3%	1%
Prostate Disorder**	3%	3%	5%
Testis Disorder***	3%	0%	0%

Lab test abnormal occurred in nine patients with one or more of the following events reported: elevated hemoglobin or hematocrit, hyperlipidemia, elevated triglycerides, hypokalemia, decreased HDL, elevated glucose, elevated creatinine, elevated total bilirubin.

**Prostate disorders* included five patients with enlarged prostate, one with BPH, and one with elevated PSA results.

***Testis disorders* were reported in two patients: one with left varicocele and one with slight sensitivity of left testis.

Other less common adverse reactions, reported in fewer than 1% of patients included: amnesia, anxiety, discolored hair, dizziness, dry skin, hirsutism, hostility, impaired urination, paresthesia, penis disorder, peripheral edema, sweating, and vasodilation.

In this 180 day clinical trial, skin reactions at the site of application were reported with AndroGel 1%, but none was severe enough to require treatment or discontinuation of drug.

Six patients (4%) in this trial had adverse events that led to discontinuation of AndroGel 1%. These events included: cerebral hemorrhage, convulsion (neither of which were considered related to AndroGel 1% administration), depression, sadness, memory loss, elevated prostate specific antigen, and hypertension. No AndroGel 1% patient discontinued due to skin reactions.

In a separate uncontrolled pharmacokinetic study of 10 patients, two had adverse events associated with AndroGel 1%; these were asthenia and depression in one patient and increased libido and hyperkinesia in the other.

In a 3 year, flexible dose, extension study, the incidence of all adverse events judged by the investigator to be at least possibly related to treatment with AndroGel 1% and reported by > 1% of patients is shown in Table 3.

Table 3: Adverse Events Possibly, Probably or Definitely Related to Use of AndroGel 1% in the 3 Year, Flexible Dose, Extension Study

Adverse Event	Percent of Subjects
	(N = 162)
Lab Test Abnormal+	9.3
Skin dry	1.9
Application Site Reaction	5.6
Acne	3.1
Pruritus	1.9
Enlarged Prostate	11.7
Carcinoma of Prostate	1.2
Urinary Symptoms*	3.7
Testis Disorder**	1.9
Gynecomastia	2.5
Anemia	2.5

+*Lab test abnormal* occurred in 15 patients with one or more of the following events reported: elevated AST, elevated ALT, elevated testosterone, elevated hemoglobin or hematocrit, elevated cholesterol, elevated cholesterol/LDL ratio, elevated triglycerides, elevated HDL, elevated serum creatinine.

Urinary symptoms included nocturia, urinary hesitancy, urinary incontinence, urinary retention, urinary urgency and weak urinary stream.

**Testis disorders* included three patients. There were two with a non-palpable testis and one with slight right testicular tenderness.

Two patients reported serious adverse events considered possibly related to treatment: deep vein thrombosis (DVT) and prostate disorder requiring a transurethral resection of the prostate (TURP).

Discontinuation for adverse events in this study included: two patients with application site reactions, one with kidney failure, and five with prostate disorders (including increase in serum PSA in 4 patients, and increase in PSA with prostate enlargement in a fifth patient).

Increases in Serum PSA Observed in Clinical Trials of Hypogonadal Men

During the initial 6-month study, the mean change in PSA values had a statistically significant increase of 0.26 ng/mL. Serum PSA was measured every 6 months thereafter in the 162 hypogonadal men on AndroGel 1% in the 3-year extension study. There was no additional statistically significant increase observed in mean PSA from 6 months through 36 months. However, there were increases in serum PSA observed in approximately 18% of individual patients. The overall mean change from baseline in serum PSA values for the entire group from month 6 to 36 was 0.11 ng/mL.

Twenty-nine patients (18%) met the per-protocol criterion for increase in serum PSA, defined as >2X the baseline or any single serum PSA >6 ng/mL. Most of these (25/29) met this criterion by at least doubling of their PSA from baseline. In most cases where PSA at least doubled (22/25), the maximum serum PSA value was still <2 ng/mL. The first occurrence of a pre-specified, post-baseline increase in serum PSA was seen at or prior to Month 12 in most of the patients who met this criterion (23 of 29; 79%).

Four patients met this criterion by having a serum PSA >6 ng/mL and in these, maximum serum PSA values were 6.2 ng/mL, 6.6 ng/mL, 6.7 ng/mL, and 10.7 ng/mL. In two of these patients, prostate cancer was detected on biopsy. The first patient's PSA levels were 4.7 ng/mL and 6.2 ng/mL at baseline and at Month 6/Final, respectively. The second patient's PSA levels were 4.2 ng/mL, 5.2 ng/mL, 5.8 ng/mL, and 6.6 ng/mL at baseline, Month 6, Month 12, and Final, respectively.

6.2   Postmarketing Experience

The following adverse reactions have been identified during post approval use of AndroGel 1%. Because the reactions are reported voluntarily from a population of uncertain size, it is not always possible to reliably estimate their frequency or establish a causal relationship to drug exposure (Table 4).

Table 4: Adverse Drug Reactions from Postmarketing Experience of AndroGel 1% by MedDRA System Organ Class

Blood and the lymphatic system disorders:	Elevated Hgb, Hct (polycythemia)
Endocrine disorders:	Hirsutism
Gastrointestinal disorders:	Nausea
General disorders and administration site reactions:	Asthenia, edema, malaise
Genitourinary disorders:	Impaired urination
Hepatobiliary disorders:	Abnormal liver function tests (e.g. transaminases, elevated GGTP, bilirubin)
Investigations:	Elevated PSA, electrolyte changes (nitrogen, calcium, potassium, phosphorus, sodium), changes in serum lipids (hyperlipidemia, elevated triglycerides, decreased HDL), impaired glucose tolerance, fluctuating testosterone concentrations, weight increase
Neoplasms benign, malignant and unspecified (cysts and polyps):	Prostate cancer
Nervous system:	Headache, dizziness, sleep apnea, insomnia
Psychiatric disorders:	Depression, emotional lability, decreased libido, nervousness, hostility, amnesia, anxiety
Reproductive system and breast disorders:	Gynecomastia, mastodynia, prostatic enlargement, testicular atrophy, oligospermia, priapism (frequent or prolonged erections)
Respiratory disorders:	Dyspnea
Skin and subcutaneous tissue disorders:	Acne, alopecia, application site reaction (pruritus, dry skin, erythema, rash, discolored hair, paresthesia), sweating
Vascular disorders:	Hypertension, vasodilation (hot flushes)

Secondary Exposure to Testosterone in Children

Cases of secondary exposure to testosterone resulting in virilization of children have been reported in postmarket surveillance. Signs and symptoms of these reported cases have included enlargement of the clitoris (with surgical intervention) or the penis, development of pubic hair, increased erections and libido, aggressive behavior, and advanced bone age. In most cases with a reported outcome, these signs and symptoms were reported to have regressed with removal of the testosterone gel exposure. In a few cases, however, enlarged genitalia did not fully return to age appropriate normal size, and bone age remained modestly greater than chronological age. In some of the cases, direct contact with the sites of application on the skin of men using testosterone gel was reported. In at least one reported case, the reporter considered the possibility of secondary exposure from items such as the testosterone gel user's shirts and/or other fabric, such as towels and sheets *[see Warnings and Precautions (5.2)].*

7   DRUG INTERACTIONS

7.1   Insulin

Changes in insulin sensitivity or glycemic control may occur in patients treated with androgens. In diabetic patients, the metabolic effects of androgens may decrease blood glucose and, therefore, may decrease insulin requirements.

7.2   Oral Anticoagulants

Changes in anticoagulant activity may be seen with androgens, therefore more frequent monitoring of international normalized ratio (INR) and prothrombin time are recommended in patients taking anticoagulants, especially at the initiation and termination of androgen therapy.

7.3   Corticosteroids

The concurrent use of testosterone with adrenocorticotropic hormone (ACTH) or corticosteroids may result in increased fluid retention and requires careful monitoring particularly in patients with cardiac, renal or hepatic disease.

8   USE IN SPECIFIC POPULATIONS

8.1   Pregnancy

Pregnancy Category X *[see Contraindications (4)]*: AndroGel 1% is contraindicated during pregnancy or in

Information on the AbbVie, Inc. products listed on these pages is from the prescribing information in use as of July 31, 2014. For more information, please visit rxabbvie.com or call 1-800-633-9110.

women who may become pregnant. Testosterone is teratogenic and may cause fetal harm. Exposure of a female fetus to androgens may result in varying degrees of virilization. If this drug is used during pregnancy, or if the patient becomes pregnant while taking this drug, the patient should be apprised of the potential hazard to a fetus.

8.3 Nursing Mothers
Although it is not known how much testosterone transfers into human milk, AndroGel 1% is contraindicated in nursing women because of the potential for serious adverse reactions in nursing infants. Testosterone and other androgens may adversely affect lactation [see Contraindications (4)].

8.4 Pediatric Use
The safety and efficacy of AndroGel 1% in pediatric patients less than 18 years old has not been established. Improper use may result in acceleration of bone age and premature closure of epiphyses.

8.5 Geriatric Use
There have not been sufficient numbers of geriatric patients involved in controlled clinical studies utilizing AndroGel 1% to determine whether efficacy in those over 65 years of age differs from younger subjects. Additionally, there is insufficient long-term safety data in geriatric patients to assess the potential risks of cardiovascular disease and prostate cancer.
Geriatric patients treated with androgens may also be at risk for worsening of signs and symptoms of BPH.

8.6 Renal Impairment
No studies were conducted in patients with renal impairment.

8.7 Hepatic Impairment
No studies were conducted in patients with hepatic impairment.

9 DRUG ABUSE AND DEPENDENCE
9.1 Controlled Substance
AndroGel 1% contains testosterone, a Schedule III controlled substance in the Controlled Substances Act.

9.2 Abuse
Anabolic steroids, such as testosterone, are abused. Abuse is often associated with adverse physical and psychological effects.

9.3 Dependence
Although drug dependence is not documented in individuals using therapeutic doses of anabolic steroids for approved indications, dependence is observed in some individuals abusing high doses of anabolic steroids. In general, anabolic steroid dependence is characterized by any three of the following:
- Taking more drug than intended
- Continued drug use despite medical and social problems
- Significant time spent in obtaining adequate amounts of drug
- Desire for anabolic steroids when supplies of the drugs are interrupted
- Difficulty in discontinuing use of the drug despite desires and attempts to do so
- Experience of a withdrawal syndrome upon discontinuation of anabolic steroid use

10 OVERDOSAGE
There is one report of acute overdosage with use of an approved injectable testosterone product: this subject had serum testosterone concentrations of up to 11,400 ng/dL with a cerebrovascular accident.
Treatment of overdosage would consist of discontinuation of AndroGel 1%, washing the application site with soap and water, and appropriate symptomatic and supportive care.

11 DESCRIPTION
AndroGel (testosterone gel) 1% is a clear, colorless hydroalcoholic gel containing testosterone.
The active pharmacological ingredient in AndroGel 1% is testosterone, an androgen. Testosterone USP is a white to practically white crystalline powder chemically described as 17-beta hydroxyandrost-4-en-3-one. The structural formula is:

Testosterone

$C_{19}H_{28}O_2$ MW 288.42

Pharmacologically inactive ingredients in AndroGel 1% are carbomer 980, ethanol 67.0%, isopropyl myristate, purified water, and sodium hydroxide. These ingredients are not pharmacologically active.

12 CLINICAL PHARMACOLOGY
12.1 Mechanism of Action
Endogenous androgens, including testosterone and dihydrotestosterone (DHT), are responsible for the normal growth and development of the male sex organs and for maintenance of secondary sex characteristics. These effects include the growth and maturation of prostate, seminal vesicles, penis and scrotum; the development of male hair distribution, such as facial, pubic, chest and axillary hair; laryngeal enlargement, vocal chord thickening, alterations in body musculature and fat distribution. Testosterone and DHT are necessary for the normal development of secondary sex characteristics. Male hypogonadism results from insufficient secretion of testosterone and is characterized by low serum testosterone concentrations. Signs/symptoms associated with male hypogonadism include erectile dysfunction and decreased sexual desire, fatigue and loss of energy, mood depression, regression of secondary sexual characteristics and osteoporosis.
Male hypogonadism can present as primary hypogonadism caused by defects of the gonads, such as Klinefelter's Syndrome or Leydig cell aplasia while secondary hypogonadism is the failure of the hypothalamus or pituitary to produce sufficient gonadotropins (FSH, LH).

12.2 Pharmacodynamics
No specific pharmacodynamic studies were conducted using AndroGel 1%.

12.3 Pharmacokinetics
Absorption
AndroGel 1% delivers physiologic amounts of testosterone, producing circulating testosterone concentrations that approximate normal concentrations (298 - 1043 ng/dL) seen in healthy men. AndroGel 1% provides continuous transdermal delivery of testosterone for 24 hours following a single application to intact, clean, dry skin of the shoulders, upper arms and/or abdomen.
AndroGel 1% is a hydroalcoholic formulation that dries quickly when applied to the skin surface. The skin serves as a reservoir for the sustained release of testosterone into the systemic circulation. Approximately 10% of the testosterone dose applied on the skin surface from AndroGel is absorbed into systemic circulation. In a study with AndroGel 1% 100 mg , all patients showed an increase in serum testosterone within 30 minutes, and eight of nine patients had a serum testosterone concentration within normal range by 4 hours after the initial application. Absorption of testosterone into the blood continues for the entire 24-hour dosing interval. Serum concentrations approximate the steady-state concentration by the end of the first 24 hours and are at steady state by the second or third day of dosing. With single daily applications of AndroGel 1%, follow-up measurements 30, 90 and 180 days after starting treatment have confirmed that serum testosterone concentrations are generally maintained within the eugonadal range. Figure 1 summarizes the 24-hour pharmacokinetic profiles of testosterone for hypogonadal men (less than 300 ng/dL) maintained on AndroGel 1% 50 mg or 100 mg for 30 days. The average (± SD) daily testosterone concentration produced by AndroGel 1% 100 mg on Day 30 was 792 (± 294) ng/dL and by AndroGel 1% 50 mg 566 (± 262) ng/dL.

Figure 1: Mean (± SD) Steady-State Serum Testosterone Concentrations on Day 30 in Patients Applying AndroGel 1% Once Daily

Distribution
Circulating testosterone is primarily bound in the serum to sex hormone-binding globulin (SHBG) and albumin. Approximately 40% of testosterone in plasma is bound to SHBG, 2% remains unbound (free) and the rest is bound to albumin and other proteins.

Metabolism
Testosterone is metabolized to various 17-keto steroids through two different pathways. The major active metabolites of testosterone are estradiol and dihydrotestosterone (DHT).
DHT concentrations increased in parallel with testosterone concentrations during AndroGel 1% treatment. The mean steady-state DHT/T ratio during 180 days of AndroGel

treatment ranged from 0.23 to 0.29 (50 mg of AndroGel 1%/day) and from 0.27 to 0.33 (100 mg of AndroGel 1%/day).

Excretion
There is considerable variation in the half-life of testosterone concentration as reported in the literature, ranging from 10 to 100 minutes. About 90% of a dose of testosterone given intramuscularly is excreted in the urine as glucuronic and sulfuric acid conjugates of testosterone and its metabolites. About 6% of a dose is excreted in the feces, mostly in the unconjugated form. Inactivation of testosterone occurs primarily in the liver.
When AndroGel 1% treatment is discontinued after achieving steady state, serum testosterone concentrations remain in the normal range for 24 to 48 hours but return to their pretreatment concentrations by the fifth day after the last application.

Testosterone Transfer from Male Patients to Female Partners
The potential for dermal testosterone transfer following AndroGel 1% use was evaluated in a clinical study between males dosed with AndroGel 1% and their untreated female partners. Two (2) to 12 hours after application of 100 mg of testosterone administered as AndroGel 1% by the male subjects, the couples (N = 38 couples) engaged in daily, 15-minute sessions of vigorous skin-to-skin contact so that the female partners gained maximum exposure to the AndroGel 1% application sites. Under these study conditions, all unprotected female partners had a serum testosterone concentration >2 times the baseline value at some time during the study. When a shirt covered the application site(s), the transfer of testosterone from the males to the female partners was completely prevented.

13 NONCLINICAL TOXICOLOGY
13.1 Carcinogenesis, Mutagenesis, Impairment of Fertility
Testosterone has been tested by subcutaneous injection and implantation in mice and rats. In mice, the implant induced cervical-uterine tumors which metastasized in some cases. There is suggestive evidence that injection of testosterone into some strains of female mice increases their susceptibility to hepatoma. Testosterone is also known to increase the number of tumors and decrease the degree of differentiation of chemically induced carcinomas of the liver in rats. Testosterone was negative in the *in vitro* Ames and in the *in vivo* mouse micronucleus assays. The administration of exogenous testosterone has been reported to suppress spermatogenesis in the rat, dog and non-human primates, which was reversible on cessation of the treatment.

14 CLINICAL STUDIES
14.1 Clinical Trials in Adult Hypogonadal Males
AndroGel 1% was evaluated in a multi-center, randomized, parallel-group, active-controlled, 180-day trial in 227 hypogonadal men. The study was conducted in 2 phases. During the Initial Treatment Period (Days 1-90), 73 patients were randomized to AndroGel 1% 50 mg daily, 78 patients to AndroGel 1% 100 mg daily, and 76 patients to a non-scrotal testosterone transdermal system. The study was double-blind for dose of AndroGel 1% but open-label for active control. Patients who were originally randomized to AndroGel 1% and who had single-sample serum testosterone concentrations above or below the normal range on Day 60 were titrated to 75 mg daily on Day 91. During the Extended Treatment Period (Days 91-180), 51 patients continued on AndroGel 1% 50 mg daily, 52 patients continued on AndroGel 1% 100 mg daily, 41 patients continued on a non-scrotal testosterone transdermal system (5 mg daily), and 40 patients received AndroGel 1% 75 mg daily. Upon completion of the initial study, 163 enrolled and 162 patients received treatment in an open-label extension study of AndroGel 1% for an additional period of up to 3 years.
Mean peak, trough and average serum testosterone concentrations within the normal range (298-1043 ng/dL) were achieved on the first day of treatment with doses of 50 mg and 100 mg of AndroGel 1%. In patients continuing on AndroGel 1% 50 mg and 100 mg, these mean testosterone concentrations were maintained within the normal range for the 180-day duration of the original study. Figure 2 summarizes the 24-hour pharmacokinetic profiles of testosterone administered as AndroGel 1% for 30, 90 and 180 days. Testosterone concentrations were maintained as long as the patient continued to properly apply the prescribed AndroGel 1% treatment.
[See figure 2 at top of next column]
Table 5 summarizes the mean testosterone concentrations on Treatment Day 180 for patients receiving 50 mg, 75 mg, or 100 mg of AndroGel 1%. The 75 mg dose produced mean concentrations intermediate to those produced by 50 mg and 100 mg of AndroGel 1%.

Figure 2: Mean Steady-State Testosterone Concentrations in Patients with Once-Daily AndroGel 1% Therapy

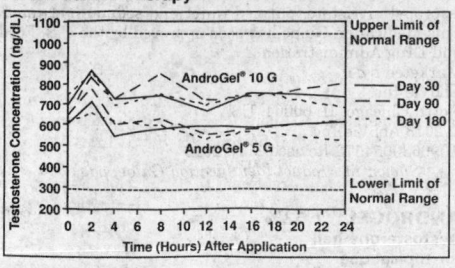

Table 5: Mean (± SD) Steady-State Serum Testosterone Concentrations During Therapy (Day 180)

	50 mg N = 44	75 mg N = 37	100 mg N = 48
C_{avg}	555 ± 225	601 ± 309	713 ± 209
C_{max}	830 ± 347	901 ± 471	1083 ± 434
C_{min}	371 ± 165	406 ± 220	485 ± 156

Of 129 hypogonadal men who were appropriately titrated with AndroGel 1% and who had sufficient data for analysis, 87% achieved an average serum testosterone concentration within the normal range on Treatment Day 180.

In patients treated with AndroGel 1%, there were no observed differences in the average daily serum testosterone concentrations at steady-state based on age, cause of hypogonadism, or body mass index.

AndroGel 1% 50 mg/day and 100 mg/day resulted in significant increases over time in total body mass and total body lean mass, while total body fat mass and the percent body fat decreased significantly. These changes were maintained for 180 days of treatment during the original study. Changes in the 75 mg dose group were similar. Bone mineral density in both hip and spine increased significantly from Baseline to Day 180 with AndroGel 1% 100 mg.

AndroGel 1% treatment at 50 mg/day and 100 mg/day for 90 days produced significant improvement in libido (measured by sexual motivation, sexual activity and enjoyment of sexual activity as assessed by patient responses to a questionnaire). The degree of penile erection as subjectively estimated by the patients, increased with AndroGel 1% treatment, as did the subjective score for "satisfactory duration of erection." AndroGel 1% treatment at 50 mg/day and 100 mg/day produced positive effects on mood and fatigue. Similar changes were seen after 180 days of treatment and in the group treated with the 75 mg dose. DHT concentrations increased in parallel with testosterone concentrations at AndroGel 1% doses of 50 mg/day and 100 mg/day, but the DHT/T ratio stayed within the normal range, indicating enhanced availability of the major physiologically active androgen. Serum estradiol (E2) concentrations increased significantly within 30 days of starting treatment with AndroGel 1% 50 or 100 mg/day and remained elevated throughout the treatment period but remained within the normal range for eugonadal men. Serum levels of SHBG decreased very slightly (1 to 11%) during AndroGel 1% treatment. In men with hypergonadotropic hypogonadism, serum levels of LH and FSH fell in a dose- and time-dependent manner during treatment with AndroGel 1%.

14.2   Phototoxicity in Humans
The phototoxic potential of AndroGel 1% was evaluated in a double-blind, single-dose study in 27 subjects with photosensitive skin types. The Minimal Erythema Dose (MED) of ultraviolet radiation was determined for each subject. A single 24 (+1) hour application of duplicate patches containing test articles (placebo gel, testosterone gel, or saline) was made to naive skin sites on Day 1. On Day 2, each subject received five exposure times of ultraviolet radiation, each exposure being 25% greater than the previous one. Skin evaluations were made on Days 2 to 5. Exposure of test and control article application sites to ultraviolet light did not produce increased inflammation relative to non-irradiated sites, indicating no phototoxic effect.

16   HOW SUPPLIED/STORAGE AND HANDLING
AndroGel 1% is supplied in non-aerosol, metered-dose pumps that deliver 12.5 mg of testosterone per complete pump actuation. The pumps are composed of plastic and stainless steel and an LDPE/aluminum foil inner liner encased in rigid plastic with a polypropylene cap. Each 88 g metered-dose pump is capable of dispensing 75 g of gel or 60-metered pump actuations; each pump actuation dispenses 1.25 g of gel.

AndroGel 1% is also supplied in unit-dose aluminum foil packets in cartons of 30. Each packet of 2.5 g or 5 g gel contains 25 mg or 50 mg testosterone, respectively.

NDC Number	Package Size
0051-8488-88	2 × 75 g pump (each pump dispenses 60 metered pump actuations with each pump actuation containing 12.5 mg of testosterone in 1.25 g of gel)
0051-8425-30	30 packets (a unit dose packet containing 25 mg of testosterone provided in 2.5 g of gel)
0051-8450-30	30 packets (a unit dose packet containing 50 mg of testosterone provided in 5 g of gel)

Storage
Store at 25°C (77°F); excursions permitted to 15° to 30°C (59° to 86°F) [see USP Controlled Room Temperature].
Disposal
Used AndroGel 1% pumps or used AndroGel 1% packets should be discarded in household trash in a manner that prevents accidental application or ingestion by children or pets.

17   PATIENT COUNSELING INFORMATION
See FDA-Approved Patient Labeling (Medication Guide)
Patients should be informed of the following:
17.1   Use in Men with Known or Suspected Prostate or Breast Cancer
Men with known or suspected prostate or breast cancer should not use AndroGel 1% [see Contraindications (4) and Warnings and Precautions (5.1)].

17.2   Potential for Secondary Exposure to Testosterone and Steps to Prevent Secondary Exposure
Secondary exposure to testosterone in children and women can occur with the use of testosterone gel in men. Cases of secondary exposure to testosterone have been reported in children.

Physicians should advise patients of the reported signs and symptoms of secondary exposure which may include the following:
• In children; unexpected sexual development including inappropriate enlargement of the penis or clitoris, premature development of pubic hair, increased erections, and aggressive behavior
• In women; changes in hair distribution, increase in acne, or other signs of testosterone effects
• The possibility of secondary exposure to testosterone gel should be brought to the attention of a healthcare provider
• AndroGel 1% should be promptly discontinued until the cause of virilization is identified

Strict adherence to the following precautions is advised to minimize the potential for secondary exposure to testosterone from testosterone gel in men [see Medication Guide]:
• **Children and women should avoid contact with unwashed or unclothed application site(s)** of men using testosterone gel
• Patients using AndroGel 1% should apply the product as directed and strictly adhere to the following:
  ◦ **Wash hands** with soap and water after application
  ◦ **Cover the application site(s)** with clothing after the gel has dried
  ◦ **Wash the application site(s) thoroughly** with soap and water prior to any situation where skin-to-skin contact of the application site with another person is anticipated
  • In the event that unwashed or unclothed skin to which AndroGel 1% has been applied comes in contact with the skin of another person, the general area of contact on the other person should be washed with soap and water as soon as possible [see Dosage and Administration (2.2), Warnings and Precautions (5.2) and Clinical Pharmacology (12.3)].

17.3   Potential Adverse Reactions with Androgens
Patients should be informed that treatment with androgens may lead to adverse reactions which include:
• Changes in urinary habits such as increased urination at night, trouble starting your urine stream, passing urine many times during the day, having an urge that you have to go to the bathroom right away, having a urine accident, being unable to pass urine and weak urine flow.
• Breathing disturbances, including those associated with sleep, or excessive daytime sleepiness.
• Too frequent or persistent erections of the penis.
• Nausea, vomiting, changes in skin color, or ankle swelling.

17.4   Patients Should Be Advised of the Following Instructions for Use:
• **Read the Medication Guide before starting AndroGel 1% therapy and to reread it each time the prescription is renewed**
• **AndroGel 1% should be applied and used appropriately to maximize the benefits and to minimize the risk of secondary exposure in children and women**
• **Keep AndroGel 1% out of the reach of children**

• **AndroGel 1% is an alcohol based product and is flammable; therefore avoid fire, flame or smoking until the gel has dried**
• **It is important to adhere to all recommended monitoring**
• **Report any changes in their state of health, such as changes in urinary habits, breathing, sleep, and mood**
• AndroGel 1% is prescribed to meet the patient's specific needs; therefore, the patient should never share AndroGel 1% with anyone.
• Wait 5 hours before swimming or washing following application of AndroGel 1%. This will ensure that the greatest amount of AndroGel 1% is absorbed into their system.

Medication Guide
ANDROGEL® (AN DROW JEL) (III)
(testosterone gel) 1%
Read this Medication Guide that comes with ANDROGEL 1% before you start taking it and each time you get a refill. There may be new information. This Medication Guide does not take the place of talking to your healthcare provider about your medical condition or your treatment.
What is the most important information I should know about ANDROGEL 1%?
1. **Early signs and symptoms of puberty have happened in young children who were accidentally exposed to testosterone through contact with men using ANDROGEL 1%.**
   Signs and symptoms of early puberty in a child may include:
   • enlarged penis or clitoris
   • early development of pubic hair
   • increased erections or sex drive
   • aggressive behavior
   ANDROGEL 1% can transfer from your body to others.
2. **Women and children should avoid contact with unwashed or unclothed area where ANDROGEL 1% has been applied to your skin.**
   Stop using ANDROGEL 1% and call your healthcare provider right away if you see any signs and symptoms in a child or a woman that may have occurred through accidental exposure to ANDROGEL 1%.
   Signs and symptoms of exposure to ANDROGEL 1% in children may include:
   • enlarged penis or clitoris
   • early development of pubic hair
   • increased erections or sex drive
   • aggressive behavior
   Signs and symptoms of exposure to ANDROGEL 1% in women may include:
   • changes in body hair
   • a large increase in acne
• **To lower the risk of transfer of ANDROGEL 1% from your body to others, you should follow these important instructions:**
   ◦ Apply ANDROGEL 1% only to areas that will be covered by a short sleeve T-shirt. These areas are your shoulders and upper arms, or stomach area (abdomen), or shoulders, upper arms and stomach area.
   ◦ Wash your hands **right away** with soap and water after applying ANDROGEL 1%.
   ◦ After the gel has dried, **cover the application area with clothing.** Keep the area covered until you have washed the application area well or have showered.
   ◦ If you expect to have skin-to-skin contact with another person, first wash the application area well with soap and water.
   ◦ If a woman or child makes contact with the ANDROGEL 1% application area, that area on the woman or child should be washed well with soap and water right away.
What is ANDROGEL 1%?
ANDROGEL 1% is a prescription medicine that contains testosterone. ANDROGEL 1% is used to treat adult males who have low or no testosterone.
Your healthcare provider will test your blood before you start and while you are taking ANDROGEL 1%.
It is not known if ANDROGEL 1% is safe or effective in children younger than 18 years old. Improper use of ANDROGEL 1% may affect bone growth in children.
ANDROGEL 1% is a controlled substance (CIII) because it contains testosterone that can be a target for people who abuse prescription medicines. Keep your ANDROGEL 1% in a safe place to protect it. Never give your ANDROGEL 1% to anyone else, even if they have the same symptoms you have. Selling or giving away this medicine may harm others and is against the law.
ANDROGEL 1% is not meant for use in women.

Information on the AbbVie, Inc. products listed on these pages is from the prescribing information in use as of July 31, 2014. For more information, please visit rxabbvie.com or call 1-800-633-9110.

Who should not use ANDROGEL 1%?
Do not use ANDROGEL 1% if you:
• have breast cancer
• have or might have prostate cancer
• are pregnant or may become pregnant or breast-feeding. ANDROGEL 1% may harm your unborn or breast-feeding baby.
  Women who are pregnant or who may become pregnant should avoid contact with the area of skin where ANDROGEL 1% has been applied.
Talk to your healthcare provider before taking this medicine if you have any of the above conditions.
What should I tell my healthcare provider before using ANDROGEL 1%?
Before you use ANDROGEL 1%, tell your healthcare provider if you:
• have breast cancer
• have or might have prostate cancer
• have urinary problems due to an enlarged prostate
• have heart problems
• have liver or kidney problems
• have problems breathing while you sleep (sleep apnea)
• have any other medical conditions
Tell your healthcare provider about all the medicines you take, including prescription and non-prescription medicines, vitamins, and herbal supplements.
Using ANDROGEL 1% with certain other medicines can affect each other.
Especially, tell your healthcare provider if you take:
• insulin
• corticosteroids
• medicines that decrease blood clotting
Know the medicines you take. Ask your healthcare provider or pharmacist for a list of these medicines, if you are not sure. Keep a list of them and show it to your healthcare provider and pharmacist when you get a new medicine.
How should I use ANDROGEL 1%?
• It is important that you apply ANDROGEL 1% exactly as your healthcare provider tells you to.
• Your healthcare provider will tell you how much ANDROGEL 1% to apply and when to apply it.
• Your healthcare provider may change your ANDROGEL 1% dose. **Do not** change your ANDROGEL 1% dose without talking to your healthcare provider.
• **ANDROGEL 1% is to be applied to the area of your shoulders, upper arms, or abdomen that will be covered by a short sleeve t-shirt. Do not** apply ANDROGEL 1% to any other parts of your body such as your penis, scrotum, chest, or back.
• Apply AndroGel 1% at the same time each morning. ANDROGEL 1% should be applied after showering or bathing.
• **Wash your hands right away** with soap and water after applying ANDROGEL 1%.
• Avoid showering, swimming, or bathing for at least 5 hours after you apply ANDROGEL 1%.
• ANDROGEL 1% is flammable until dry. Let ANDROGEL 1% dry before smoking or going near an open flame.
• Let the application areas dry completely before putting on a t-shirt.
Applying ANDROGEL 1%:
ANDROGEL 1% comes in a pump or in packets.
• **Before applying ANDROGEL 1%, make sure that your shoulders, upper arms, and abdomen are clean, dry, and there is no broken skin.**
• The application sites for ANDROGEL 1% are the shoulders, upper arms, or abdomen that will be covered by a short sleeve t-shirt (See Figure A).

(Figure A)

If you are using the ANDROGEL 1% pump:
• Before using a new bottle of ANDROGEL 1% for the first time, you will need to prime the pump. To prime the ANDROGEL 1% pump, slowly push the pump all the way down 3 times. **Do not** use any ANDROGEL 1% that came out while priming. Wash it down the sink to avoid accidental exposure to others. Your ANDROGEL 1% pump is ready to use.
• Remove the cap from the pump. Then, position the nozzle over the palm of your hand and slowly push the pump all the way down. Apply ANDROGEL 1% to the application site. You may also apply ANDROGEL 1% directly to the application site.
• **Wash your hands with soap and water right away.**
• Your healthcare provider will tell you the number of times to press the pump for each dose.
If you are using ANDROGEL 1% packets:
• Tear open the packet completely at the dotted line. Squeeze from the bottom of the packet to the top.
• Squeeze all of the ANDROGEL 1% out of the packet into the palm of your hand. Apply ANDROGEL 1% to the application site. You may also apply ANDROGEL 1% from the packet directly to the application site.
• ANDROGEL 1% should be applied right away.
• **Wash your hands with soap and water right away.**
What are the possible side effects of ANDROGEL 1%?
See "What is the most important information I should know about ANDROGEL 1%?"
ANDROGEL 1% can cause serious side effects including:
• **If you already have enlargement of your prostate gland your signs and symptoms can get worse while using ANDROGEL 1%.** This can include:
  ○ increased urination at night
  ○ trouble starting your urine stream
  ○ having to pass urine many times during the day
  ○ having an urge that you have to go to the bathroom right away
  ○ having a urine accident
  ○ being unable to pass urine or weak urine flow
• **Possible increased risk of prostate cancer.** Your healthcare provider should check you for prostate cancer or any other prostate problems before you start and while you use ANDROGEL 1%.
• **In large doses ANDROGEL 1% may lower your sperm count.**
• **Swelling of your ankles, feet, or body, with or without heart failure.**
• **Enlarged or painful breasts.**
• **Have problems breathing while you sleep (sleep apnea).**
• **Blood clots in the legs.** This can include pain, swelling or redness of your legs.
Call your healthcare provider right away if you have any of the serious side effects listed above.
The most common side effects of ANDROGEL 1% include:
• acne
• skin irritation where ANDROGEL 1% is applied
• lab test changes
• increased prostate specific antigen (a test used to screen for prostate cancer)
Other side effects include more erections than are normal for you or erections that last a long time.
Tell your healthcare provider if you have any side effect that bothers you or that does not go away.
These are not all the possible side effects of ANDROGEL 1%. For more information, ask your healthcare provider or pharmacist.
Call your doctor for medical advice about side effects. You may report side effects to FDA at 1-800-FDA-1088.
How should I store ANDROGEL 1%?
• Store ANDROGEL 1% between 59°F to 86°F (15°C to 30°C).
• Safely throw away used ANDROGEL 1% in household trash. Be careful to prevent accidental exposure of children or pets.
• Keep ANDROGEL 1% away from fire.
Keep ANDROGEL 1% and all medicines out of the reach of children.
General information about the safe and effective use of ANDROGEL 1%
Medicines are sometimes prescribed for purposes other than those listed in a Medication Guide. Do not use ANDROGEL 1% for a condition for which it was not prescribed. Do not give ANDROGEL 1% to other people, even if they have the same symptoms you have. It may harm them.
This Medication Guide summarizes the most important information about ANDROGEL 1%. If you would like more information, talk to your healthcare provider. You can ask your pharmacist or healthcare provider for information about ANDROGEL 1% that is written for health professionals.
For more information, go to www.ANDROGEL.com or call 1-800-633-9110.

What are the ingredients in ANDROGEL 1%?
Active ingredient: testosterone
Inactive ingredients: carbomer 980, ethyl alcohol 67.0%, isopropyl myristate, purified water and sodium hydroxide. This Medication Guide has been approved by the U.S. Food and Drug Administration.
Marketed by:
AbbVie Inc.
North Chicago, IL 60064, USA
© 2013 AbbVie Inc.
A090630054573 Revised May, 2013
Shown in Product Identification Guide, page 303

ANDROGEL® 1.62%   ℂⅢℝ
(testosterone gel)
for topical use

HIGHLIGHTS OF PRESCRIBING INFORMATION
These highlights do not include all the information needed to use ANDROGEL 1.62% safely and effectively. See full prescribing information for ANDROGEL 1.62%.
AndroGel® (testosterone gel) 1.62% for topical use CIII
Initial U.S. Approval: 1953

> **WARNING: SECONDARY EXPOSURE TO TESTOSTERONE**
> *See full prescribing information for complete boxed warning.*
> • Virilization has been reported in children who were secondarily exposed to testosterone gel (5.2, 6.2).
> • Children should avoid contact with unwashed or unclothed application sites in men using testosterone gel (2.2, 5.2).
> • Healthcare providers should advise patients to strictly adhere to recommended instructions for use (2.2, 5.2, 17).

————RECENT MAJOR CHANGES————
Indications and Usage. (1) 09/2012
————INDICATIONS AND USAGE————
AndroGel 1.62% is an androgen indicated for replacement therapy in males for conditions associated with a deficiency or absence of endogenous testosterone:
• Primary hypogonadism (congenital or acquired) (1)
• Hypogonadotropic hypogonadism (congenital or acquired) (1)
Important limitations of use:
• Safety and efficacy of AndroGel 1.62% in males less than 18 years old have not been established. (1, 8.4)
• Topical testosterone products may have different doses, strengths, or application instructions that may result in different systemic exposure. (1, 12.3)
————DOSAGE AND ADMINISTRATION————
• **Dosage and Administration for AndroGel 1.62% differs from AndroGel 1%. For dosage and administration of AndroGel 1% refer to its full prescribing information. (2)**
• Starting dose of AndroGel 1.62% is 40.5 mg of testosterone (2 pump actuations or a single 40.5 mg packet), applied topically once daily in the morning. (2.1)
• Apply to clean, dry, intact skin of the shoulders and upper arms. Do not apply AndroGel 1.62% to any other parts of the body including the abdomen or genitals. (2.2, 12.3)
• Dose adjustment: AndroGel 1.62% can be dose adjusted between a minimum of 20.25 mg of testosterone (1 pump actuation or a single 20.25 mg packet) and a maximum of 81 mg of testosterone (4 pump actuations or two 40.5 mg packets). The dose should be titrated based on the pre-dose morning serum testosterone concentration at approximately 14 days and 28 days after starting treatment or following dose adjustment. Additionally, serum testosterone concentration should be assessed periodically thereafter. (2.1)
• Patients should wash hands immediately with soap and water after applying AndroGel 1.62% and cover the application site(s) with clothing after the gel has dried. Wash the application site thoroughly with soap and water prior to any situation where skin-to-skin contact of the application site with another person is anticipated. (2.2)
————DOSAGE FORMS AND STRENGTHS————
AndroGel (testosterone gel) 1.62% for topical use is available as follows:
• a metered-dose pump that delivers 20.25 mg testosterone per actuation. (3)
• packets containing 20.25 mg testosterone. (3)
• packets containing 40.5 mg testosterone. (3)
————CONTRAINDICATIONS————
• Men with carcinoma of the breast or known or suspected prostate cancer (4, 5.1)
• Pregnant or breast-feeding women. Testosterone may cause fetal harm (4, 8.1, 8.3)
————WARNINGS AND PRECAUTIONS————
• Monitor patients with benign prostatic hyperplasia (BPH) for worsening of signs and symptoms of BPH (5.1)

- Avoid unintentional exposure of women or children to AndroGel 1.62%. Secondary exposure to testosterone can produce signs of virilization. AndroGel 1.62% should be discontinued until the cause of virilization is identified (5.2)
- Exogenous administration of androgens may lead to azoospermia (5.5)
- Edema with or without congestive heart failure (CHF) may be a complication in patients with preexisting cardiac, renal, or hepatic disease (5.7)
- Sleep apnea may occur in those with risk factors (5.9)
- Monitor serum testosterone, prostate specific antigen (PSA), hemoglobin, hematocrit, liver function tests and lipid concentrations periodically (5.1, 5.3, 5.6, 5.10)
- AndroGel 1.62% is flammable until dry (5.13)

────────ADVERSE REACTIONS────────

The most common adverse reaction (incidence ≥ 5%) is an increase in prostate specific antigen (PSA). (6.1)

To report SUSPECTED ADVERSE REACTIONS, contact AbbVie Inc. at 1-800-633-9110 or FDA at 1-800-FDA-1088 or www.fda.gov/medwatch.

────────DRUG INTERACTIONS────────

- Androgens may decrease blood glucose and therefore may decrease insulin requirements in diabetic patients (7.1)
- Changes in anticoagulant activity may be seen with androgens. More frequent monitoring of International Normalized Ratio (INR) and prothrombin time is recommended (7.2)
- Use of testosterone with adrenocorticotrophic hormone (ACTH) or corticosteroids may result in increased fluid retention. Use with caution, particularly in patients with cardiac, renal, or hepatic disease (7.3)

────USE IN SPECIFIC POPULATIONS────

There are insufficient long-term safety data in geriatric patients using AndroGel 1.62% to assess the potential risks of cardiovascular disease and prostate cancer. (8.5)

See 17 for PATIENT COUNSELING INFORMATION and Medication Guide

Revised: 05/2013

FULL PRESCRIBING INFORMATION: CONTENTS*

FULL PRESCRIBING INFORMATION

WARNING: SECONDARY EXPOSURE TO TESTOSTERONE
- **Virilization has been reported in children who were secondarily exposed to testosterone gel *[see Warnings and Precautions (5.2) and Adverse Reactions (6.2)]*.**
- **Children should avoid contact with unwashed or unclothed application sites in men using testosterone gel *[see Dosage and Administration (2.2) and Warnings and Precautions (5.2)]*.**
- **Healthcare providers should advise patients to strictly adhere to recommended instructions for use *[see Dosage and Administration (2.2), Warnings and Precautions (5.2) and Patient Counseling Information (17)]*.**

---

1   INDICATIONS AND USAGE

AndroGel 1.62% is an androgen indicated for replacement therapy in adult males for conditions associated with a deficiency or absence of endogenous testosterone:
- Primary hypogonadism (congenital or acquired): testicular failure due to conditions such as cryptorchidism, bilateral torsion, orchitis, vanishing testis syndrome, orchiectomy, Klinefelter's syndrome, chemotherapy, or toxic damage from alcohol or heavy metals. These men usually have low serum testosterone concentrations and gonadotropins (follicle-stimulating hormone [FSH], luteinizing hormone [LH]) above the normal range.
- Hypogonadotropic hypogonadism (congenital or acquired): idiopathic gonadotropin or luteinizing hormone-releasing hormone (LHRH) deficiency or pituitary-hypothalamic injury from tumors, trauma, or radiation. These men have low testosterone serum concentrations, but have gonadotropins in the normal or low range.

Important limitations of use:
- Safety and efficacy of AndroGel 1.62% in males less than 18 years old have not been established *[see Use in Specific Populations (8.4)]*.
- Topical testosterone products may have different doses, strengths, or application instructions that may result in different systemic exposure *[see Indications and Usage (1), and Clinical Pharmacology (12.3)]*.

2   DOSAGE AND ADMINISTRATION

Dosage and Administration for AndroGel 1.62% differs from AndroGel 1%. For dosage and administration of AndroGel 1% refer to its full prescribing information. (2)

2.1   Dosing and Dose Adjustment

The recommended starting dose of AndroGel 1.62% is 40.5 mg of testosterone (2 pump actuations or a single 40.5 mg packet) applied topically once daily in the morning to the shoulders and upper arms.

The dose can be adjusted between a minimum of 20.25 mg of testosterone (1 pump actuation or a single 20.25 mg packet) and a maximum of 81 mg of testosterone (4 pump actuations or two 40.5 mg packets). To ensure proper dosing, the dose should be titrated based on the pre-dose morning serum testosterone concentration from a single blood draw at approximately 14 days and 28 days after starting treatment or following dose adjustment. In addition, serum testosterone concentration should be assessed periodically thereafter. Table 1 describes the dose adjustments required at each titration step.

Table 1: Dose Adjustment Criteria

Pre-Dose Morning Total Serum Testosterone Concentration	Dose Titration
Greater than 750 ng/dL	Decrease daily dose by 20.25 mg (1 pump actuation or the equivalent of one 20.25 mg packet)
Equal to or greater than 350 and equal to or less than 750 ng/dL	No change: continue on current dose
Less than 350 ng/dL	Increase daily dose by 20.25 mg (1 pump actuation or the equivalent of one 20.25 mg packet)

The application site and dose of AndroGel 1.62% are not interchangeable with other topical testosterone products.

2.2   Administration Instructions

AndroGel 1.62% should be applied to clean, dry, intact skin of the upper arms and shoulders. Do not apply AndroGel 1.62% to any other parts of the body, including the abdomen or genitals *[see Clinical Pharmacology (12.3)]*. Area of application should be limited to the area that will be covered by the patient's short sleeve t-shirt. Patients should be instructed to use the palm of the hand to apply AndroGel 1.62% and spread across the maximum surface area as directed in Table 2 (for pump) and Table 3 (for packets) and in Figure 1.

Table 2: Application Sites for AndroGel 1.62%, Pump

Total Dose of Testosterone	Total Pump Actuations	Pump Actuations Per Upper Arm and Shoulder	
		Upper Arm and Shoulder #1	Upper Arm and Shoulder #2
20.25 mg	1	1	0
40.5 mg	2	1	1
60.75 mg	3	2	1
81 mg	4	2	2

Table 3: Application Sites for AndroGel 1.62%, Packets

Total Dose of Testosterone	Total packets	Gel Applications Per Upper Arm and Shoulder	
		Upper Arm and Shoulder #1	Upper Arm and Shoulder #2
20.25 mg	One 20.25 mg packet	One 20.25 mg packet	0
40.5 mg	One 40.5 mg packet	Half of contents of One 40.5 mg packet	Half of contents of One 40.5 mg packet
60.75 mg	One 20.25 mg packet AND One 40.5 mg packet	One 40.5 mg packet	One 20.25 mg packet
81 mg	Two 40.5 mg packets	One 40.5 mg packet	One 40.5 mg packet

The prescribed daily dose of AndroGel 1.62% should be applied to the right and left upper arms and shoulders as shown in the shaded areas in Figure 1.

Figure 1. Application Sites for AndroGel 1.62%

Once the application site is dry, the site should be covered with clothing *[see Clinical Pharmacology (12.3)]*. Wash hands thoroughly with soap and water. Avoid fire, flames or smoking until the gel has dried since alcohol based products, including AndroGel 1.62%, are flammable.

Information on the AbbVie, Inc. products listed on these pages is from the prescribing information in use as of July 31, 2014. For more information, please visit rxabbvie.com or call 1-800-633-9110.

The patient should avoid swimming or showering or washing the administration site for a minimum of 2 hours after application [see Clinical Pharmacology (12.3)].

To obtain a full first dose, it is necessary to prime the canister pump. To do so, with the canister in the upright position, slowly and fully depress the actuator three times. Safely discard the gel from the first three actuations. It is only necessary to prime the pump before the first dose.

After the priming procedure, fully depress the actuator once for every 20.25 mg of AndroGel 1.62%. AndroGel 1.62% should be delivered directly into the palm of the hand and then applied to the application sites.

When using packets, the entire contents should be squeezed into the palm of the hand and immediately applied to the application sites. When 40.5 mg packets need to be split between the left and right shoulder, patients may squeeze a portion of the gel from the packet into the palm of the hand and apply to application sites. Repeat until entire contents have been applied. Alternatively, AndroGel 1.62% can be applied directly to the application sites from the pump or packets.

Strict adherence to the following precautions is advised in order to minimize the potential for secondary exposure to testosterone from AndroGel 1.62%-treated skin:

• Children and women should avoid contact with unwashed or unclothed application site(s) of men using AndroGel 1.62%.

• AndroGel 1.62% should only be applied to the upper arms and shoulders. The area of application should be limited to the area that will be covered by a short sleeve t-shirt.

• Patients should wash their hands with soap and water immediately after applying AndroGel 1.62%.

• Patients should cover the application site(s) with clothing (e.g., a t-shirt) after the gel has dried.

• Prior to situations in which direct skin-to-skin contact is anticipated, patients should wash the application site(s) thoroughly with soap and water to remove any testosterone residue.

• In the event that unwashed or unclothed skin to which AndroGel 1.62% has been applied comes in direct contact with the skin of another person, the general area of contact on the other person should be washed with soap and water as soon as possible.

3 DOSAGE FORMS AND STRENGTHS

AndroGel (testosterone gel) 1.62% for topical use only, is available as follows:

• A metered-dose pump. Each pump actuation delivers 20.25 mg of testosterone in 1.25 g of gel.

• A unit dose packet containing 20.25 mg of testosterone in 1.25 g of gel.

• A unit dose packet containing 40.5 mg of testosterone in 2.5 g of gel.

4 CONTRAINDICATIONS

• AndroGel 1.62% is contraindicated in men with carcinoma of the breast or known or suspected carcinoma of the prostate [see Warnings and Precautions (5.1) and Adverse Reactions (6.1)].

• AndroGel 1.62% is contraindicated in women who are or may become pregnant, or who are breastfeeding. AndroGel 1.62% may cause fetal harm when administered to a pregnant woman. AndroGel 1.62% may cause serious adverse reactions in nursing infants. Exposure of a fetus or nursing infant to androgens may result in varying degrees of virilization. Pregnant women or those who may become pregnant need to be aware of the potential for transfer of testosterone from men treated with AndroGel 1.62%. If a pregnant woman is exposed to AndroGel 1.62%, she should be apprised of the potential hazard to the fetus [see Warnings and Precautions (5.2) and Use in Specific Populations (8.1, 8.3)].

5 WARNINGS AND PRECAUTIONS

5.1 Worsening of Benign Prostatic Hyperplasia (BPH) and Potential Risk of Prostate Cancer

• Patients with BPH treated with androgens are at an increased risk for worsening of signs and symptoms of BPH. Monitor patients with BPH for worsening signs and symptoms.

• Patients treated with androgens may be at increased risk for prostate cancer. Evaluation of patients for prostate cancer prior to initiating and during treatment with androgens is appropriate [see Contraindications (4)].

5.2 Potential for Secondary Exposure to Testosterone

Cases of secondary exposure resulting in virilization of children have been reported in postmarketing surveillance of testosterone gel products. Signs and symptoms have included enlargement of the penis or clitoris, development of pubic hair, increased erections and libido, aggressive behavior, and advanced bone age. In most cases, these signs and symptoms regressed with removal of the exposure to testosterone gel. In a few cases, however, enlarged genitalia did not fully return to age-appropriate normal size, and bone age remained modestly greater than chronological age.

The risk of transfer was increased in some of these cases by not adhering to precautions for the appropriate use of the topical testosterone product. Children and women should avoid contact with unwashed or unclothed application sites in men using AndroGel 1.62% [see Dosage and Administration (2.2), Use in Specific Populations (8.1) and Clinical Pharmacology (12.3)].

Inappropriate changes in genital size or development of pubic hair or libido in children, or changes in body hair distribution, significant increase in acne, or other signs of virilization in adult women should be brought to the attention of a physician and the possibility of secondary exposure to testosterone gel should also be brought to the attention of a physician. Testosterone gel should be promptly discontinued until the signs of virilization has been identified.

5.3 Polycythemia

Increases in hematocrit, reflective of increases in red blood cell mass, may require lowering or discontinuation of testosterone. Check hematocrit prior to initiating treatment. It would also be appropriate to re-evaluate the hematocrit 3 to 6 months after starting treatment, and then annually. If hematocrit becomes elevated, stop therapy until hematocrit decreases to an acceptable concentration. An increase in red blood cell mass may increase the risk of thromboembolic events.

5.4 Use in Women

Due to the lack of controlled evaluations in women and potential virilizing effects, AndroGel 1.62% is not indicated for use in women [see Contraindications (4) and Use in Specific Populations (8.1, 8.3)].

5.5 Potential for Adverse Effects on Spermatogenesis

With large doses of exogenous androgens, including AndroGel 1.62%, spermatogenesis may be suppressed through feedback inhibition of pituitary FSH possibly leading to adverse effects on semen parameters including sperm count.

5.6 Hepatic Adverse Effects

Prolonged use of high doses of orally active 17-alpha-alkyl androgens (e.g., methyltestosterone) has been associated with serious hepatic adverse effects (peliosis hepatis, hepatic neoplasms, cholestatic hepatitis, and jaundice). Peliosis hepatis can be a life-threatening or fatal complication. Long-term therapy with intramuscular testosterone enanthate has produced multiple hepatic adenomas. AndroGel 1.62% is not known to cause these adverse effects.

5.7 Edema

Androgens, including AndroGel 1.62%, may promote retention of sodium and water. Edema, with or without congestive heart failure, may be a serious complication in patients with preexisting cardiac, renal, or hepatic disease [see Adverse Reactions (6.2)].

5.8 Gynecomastia

Gynecomastia may develop and persist in patients being treated with androgens, including AndroGel 1.62%, for hypogonadism.

5.9 Sleep Apnea

The treatment of hypogonadal men with testosterone may potentiate sleep apnea in some patients, especially those with risk factors such as obesity or chronic lung diseases.

5.10 Lipids

Changes in serum lipid profile may require dose adjustment or discontinuation of testosterone therapy.

5.11 Hypercalcemia

Androgens, including AndroGel 1.62 %, should be used with caution in cancer patients at risk of hypercalcemia (and associated hypercalciuria). Regular monitoring of serum calcium concentrations is recommended in these patients.

5.12 Decreased Thyroxine-binding Globulin

Androgens, including AndroGel 1.62%, may decrease concentrations of thyroxin-binding globulins, resulting in decreased total T4 serum concentrations and increased resin uptake of T3 and T4. Free thyroid hormone concentrations remain unchanged, however, and there is no clinical evidence of thyroid dysfunction.

5.13 Flammability

Alcohol based products, including AndroGel 1.62%, are flammable; therefore, patients should be advised to avoid fire, flame or smoking until the AndroGel 1.62% has dried.

6 ADVERSE REACTIONS

6.1 Clinical Trial Experience

Because clinical trials are conducted under widely varying conditions, adverse reaction rates observed in the clinical trials of a drug cannot be directly compared to rates in the clinical trials of another drug and may not reflect the rates observed in practice.

AndroGel 1.62% was evaluated in a two-phase, 364-day, controlled clinical study. The first phase was a multi-center, randomized, double-blind, parallel-group, placebo-controlled period of 182 days, in which 234 hypogonadal men were treated with AndroGel 1.62% and 40 received placebo. Patients could continue in an open-label, non-comparative, maintenance period for an additional 182 days [see Clinical Studies (14.1)].

The most common adverse reaction reported in the double-blind period was increased prostate specific antigen (PSA) reported in 26 AndroGel 1.62%-treated patients (11.1%). In 17 patients, increased PSA was considered an adverse event by meeting one of the two pre-specified criteria for abnormal PSA values, defined as (1) average serum PSA >4 ng/mL based on two separate determinations, or (2) an average change from baseline in serum PSA of greater than 0.75 ng/mL on two determinations.

During the 182-day, double-blind period of the clinical trial, the mean change in serum PSA value was 0.14 ng/mL for patients receiving AndroGel 1.62% and -0.12 ng/mL for the patients in the placebo group. During the double-blind period, seven patients had a PSA value >4.0 ng/mL, four of these seven patients had PSA less than or equal to 4.0 ng/mL upon repeat testing. The other three patients did not undergo repeat PSA testing.

During the 182-day, open-label period of the study, the mean change in serum PSA values was 0.10 ng/mL for both patients continuing on active therapy and patients transitioning onto active from placebo. During the open-label period, three patients had a serum PSA value > 4.0 ng/mL, two of whom had a serum PSA less than or equal to 4.0 ng/mL upon repeated testing. The other patient did not undergo repeat PSA testing. Among previous placebo patients, 3 of 28 (10.7%), had increased PSA as an adverse event in the open-label period.

Table 4 shows adverse reactions reported by >2% of patients in the 182-day, double-blind period of the AndroGel 1.62% clinical trial and more frequent in the AndroGel 1.62% treated group versus placebo.

Table 4: Adverse Reactions Reported in >2% of Patients in the 182-Day, Double-Blind Period of AndroGel 1.62% Clinical Trial

Adverse Reaction	Number (%) of Patients	
	AndroGel 1.62% N=234	Placebo N= 40
PSA increased*	26 (11.1%)	0%
Emotional lability**	6 (2.6%)	0%
Hypertension	5 (2.1%)	0%
Hematocrit or hemoglobin increased	5 (2.1%)	0%
Contact dermatitis***	5 (2.1%)	0%

*__PSA increased__ includes: PSA values that met pre-specified criteria for abnormal PSA values (an average change from baseline > 0.75 ng/mL and/or an average PSA value >4.0 ng/mL based on two measurements) as well as those reported as adverse events.

**__Emotional lability__ includes: mood swings, affective disorder, impatience, anger, and aggression.

***__Contact dermatitis__ includes: 4 patients with dermatitis at non-application sites.

Other adverse reactions occurring in less than or equal to 2% of AndroGel 1.62%-treated patients and more frequently than placebo included: frequent urination, and hyperlipidemia.

In the open-label period of the study (N=191), the most commonly reported adverse reaction (experienced by greater than 2% of patients) was increased PSA (n=13; 6.2%) and sinusitis. Other adverse reactions reported by less than or equal to 2% of patients included increased hemoglobin or hematocrit, hypertension, acne, libido decreased, insomnia, and benign prostatic hypertrophy.

During the 182-day, double-blind period of the clinical trial, 25 AndroGel 1.62%-treated patients (10.7%) discontinued treatment because of adverse reactions. These adverse reactions included 17 patients with PSA increased and 1 report each of: hematocrit increased, blood pressure increased, frequent urination, diarrhea, fatigue, pituitary tumor, dizziness, skin erythema and skin nodule (same patient – neither at application site), vasovagal syncope, and diabetes mellitus. During the 182-day, open-label period, 9 patients discontinued treatment because of adverse reactions. These adverse reactions included 6 reports of PSA increased, 2 of hematocrit increased, and 1 each of triglycerides increased and prostate cancer.

Application Site Reactions

In the 182-day double-blind period of the study, application site reactions were reported in two (2/234; 0.9%) patients receiving AndroGel 1.62%, both of which resolved. Neither of these patients discontinued the study due to application site adverse reactions. In the open-label period of the study, application site reactions were reported in three (3/219; 1.4%) additional patients that were treated with AndroGel 1.62%. None of these subjects were discontinued from the study due to application site reactions.

6.2 Postmarketing Experience

The following adverse reactions have been identified during post approval use of AndroGel 1%. Because the reactions are reported voluntarily from a population of uncertain size, it is not always possible to reliably estimate their frequency or establish a causal relationship to drug exposure (Table 5).

Table 5: Adverse Reactions from Post Approval Experience of AndroGel 1% by System Organ Class

System Organ Class	Adverse Reaction
Blood and lymphatic system disorders:	Elevated hemoglobin or hematocrit, polycythemia, anemia
Endocrine disorders:	Hirsutism
Gastrointestinal disorders:	Nausea
General disorders:	Asthenia, edema, malaise
Genitourinary disorders:	Impaired urination*
Hepatobiliary disorders:	Abnormal liver function tests
Investigations:	Lab test abnormal**, elevated PSA, electrolyte changes (nitrogen, calcium, potassium [includes hypokalemia], phosphorus, sodium), impaired glucose tolerance, hyperlipidemia, HDL, fluctuating testosterone levels, weight increase
Neoplasms:	Prostate cancer
Nervous system disorders:	Dizziness, headache, insomnia, sleep apnea
Psychiatric disorders:	Amnesia, anxiety, depression, hostility, emotional lability, decreased libido, nervousness
Reproductive system and breast disorders:	Gynecomastia, mastodynia, oligospermia, priapism (frequent or prolonged erections), prostate enlargement, BPH, testis disorder***
Respiratory disorders:	Dyspnea
Skin and subcutaneous tissue disorders:	Acne, alopecia, application site reaction (discolored hair, dry skin, erythema, paresthesia, pruritus, rash), skin dry, pruritus, sweating
Vascular disorders:	Hypertension, vasodilation (hot flushes)

* *Impaired urination* includes nocturia, urinary hesitancy, urinary incontinence, urinary retention, urinary urgency and weak urinary stream

***Lab test abnormal* includes elevated AST, elevated ALT, elevated testosterone, elevated hemoglobin or hematocrit, elevated cholesterol, elevated cholesterol/LDL ratio, elevated triglycerides, or elevated serum creatinine

***Testis disorder includes atrophy or non-palpable testis, varicocele, testis sensitivity or tenderness

Secondary Exposure to Testosterone in Children
Cases of secondary exposure to testosterone resulting in virilization of children have been reported in postmarketing surveillance of testosterone gel products. Signs and symptoms of these reported cases have included enlargement of the clitoris (with surgical intervention) or the penis, development of pubic hair, increased erections and libido, aggressive behavior, and advanced bone age. In most cases with a reported outcome, these signs and symptoms were reported to have regressed with removal of the testosterone gel exposure. In a few cases, however, enlarged genitalia did not fully return to age appropriate normal size, and bone age remained modestly greater than chronological age. In some of the cases, direct contact with the sites of application on the skin of men using testosterone gel was reported. In at least one reported case, the reporter considered the possibility of secondary exposure from items such as the testosterone gel user's shirts and/or other fabric, such as towels and sheets [see Warnings and Precautions (5.2)].

7 DRUG INTERACTIONS

7.1 Insulin

Changes in insulin sensitivity or glycemic control may occur in patients treated with androgens. In diabetic patients, the metabolic effects of androgens may decrease blood glucose and, therefore, may decrease insulin requirements.

7.2 Oral Anticoagulants

Changes in anticoagulant activity may be seen with androgens, therefore more frequent monitoring of international normalized ratio (INR) and prothrombin time are recommended in patients taking anticoagulants, especially at the initiation and termination of androgen therapy.

7.3 Corticosteroids

The concurrent use of testosterone with adrenocorticotropic hormone (ACTH) or corticosteroids may result in increased fluid retention and requires careful monitoring particularly in patients with cardiac, renal or hepatic disease.

8 USE IN SPECIFIC POPULATIONS

8.1 Pregnancy

Pregnancy Category X [see Contraindications (4)]: AndroGel 1.62% is contraindicated during pregnancy or in women who may become pregnant. Testosterone is teratogenic and may cause fetal harm. Exposure of a fetus to androgens may result in varying degrees of virilization. If this drug is used during pregnancy, or if the patient becomes pregnant while taking this drug, the patient should be made aware of the potential hazard to the fetus.

8.3 Nursing Mothers

Although it is not known how much testosterone transfers into human milk, AndroGel 1.62% is contraindicated in nursing women because of the potential for serious adverse reactions in nursing infants. Testosterone and other androgens may adversely affect lactation [see Contraindications (4)].

8.4 Pediatric Use

The safety and effectiveness of AndroGel 1.62% in pediatric patients less than 18 years old has not been established. Improper use may result in acceleration of bone age and premature closure of epiphyses.

8.5 Geriatric Use

There have not been sufficient numbers of geriatric patients involved in controlled clinical studies utilizing AndroGel 1.62% to determine whether efficacy in those over 65 years of age differs from younger subjects. Of the 234 patients enrolled in the clinical trial utilizing AndroGel 1.62%, 21 were over 65 years of age. Additionally, there is insufficient long-term safety data in geriatric patients to assess the potentially increased risks of cardiovascular disease and prostate cancer.

Geriatric patients treated with androgens may also be at risk for worsening of signs and symptoms of BPH.

8.6 Renal Impairment

No studies were conducted involving patients with renal impairment.

8.7 Hepatic Impairment

No studies were conducted in patients with hepatic impairment.

9 DRUG ABUSE AND DEPENDENCE

9.1 Controlled Substance

AndroGel 1.62% contains testosterone, a Schedule III controlled substance in the Controlled Substances Act.

9.2 Abuse

Anabolic steroids, such as testosterone, are abused. Abuse is often associated with adverse physical and psychological effects.

9.3 Dependence

Although drug dependence is not documented in individuals using therapeutic doses of anabolic steroids for approved indications, dependence is observed in some individuals abusing high doses of anabolic steroids. In general, anabolic steroid dependence is characterized by any three of the following:
- Taking more drug than intended
- Continued drug use despite medical and social problems
- Significant time spent in obtaining adequate amounts of drug
- Desire for anabolic steroids when supplies of the drugs are interrupted
- Difficulty in discontinuing use of the drug despite desires and attempts to do so
- Experience of a withdrawal syndrome upon discontinuation of anabolic steroid use

10 OVERDOSAGE

There is a single report of acute overdosage after parenteral administration of an approved testosterone product in the literature. This subject had serum testosterone concentrations of up to 11,400 ng/dL, which were implicated in a cerebrovascular accident. There were no reports of overdosage in the AndroGel 1.62% clinical trial.

Treatment of overdosage would consist of discontinuation of AndroGel 1.62%, washing the application site with soap and water, and appropriate symptomatic and supportive care.

11 DESCRIPTION

AndroGel 1.62% for topical use is a clear, colorless gel containing testosterone. Testosterone is an androgen. AndroGel 1.62% is available in a metered-dose pump or unit dose packets.

The active pharmacologic ingredient in AndroGel 1.62% is testosterone. Testosterone USP is a white to almost white powder chemically described as 17-beta hydroxyandrost-4-en-3-one. The structural formula is:

Testosterone

$C_{19}H_{28}O_2$ MW 288.42

The inactive ingredients in AndroGel 1.62% are: carbopol 980, ethyl alcohol, isopropyl myristate, purified water, and sodium hydroxide.

12 CLINICAL PHARMACOLOGY

12.1 Mechanism of Action

Endogenous androgens, including testosterone and dihydrotestosterone (DHT), are responsible for the normal growth and development of the male sex organs and for maintenance of secondary sex characteristics. These effects include the growth and maturation of prostate, seminal vesicles, penis and scrotum; the development of male hair distribution, such as facial, pubic, chest and axillary hair; laryngeal enlargement; vocal chord thickening; and alterations in body musculature and fat distribution. Testosterone and DHT are necessary for the normal development of secondary sex characteristics. Male hypogonadism results from insufficient secretion of testosterone and is characterized by low serum testosterone concentrations. Signs/symptoms associated with male hypogonadism include erectile dysfunction and decreased sexual desire, fatigue and loss of energy, mood depression, regression of secondary sexual characteristics and osteoporosis.

Male hypogonadism can present as primary hypogonadism caused by defects of the gonads, such as Klinefelter's Syndrome or Leydig cell aplasia while secondary hypogonadism is the failure of the hypothalamus or pituitary to produce sufficient gonadotropins (FSH, LH).

12.2 Pharmacodynamics

No specific pharmacodynamic studies were conducted using AndroGel 1.62%.

12.3 Pharmacokinetics

Absorption

AndroGel 1.62% delivers physiologic amounts of testosterone, producing circulating testosterone concentrations that approximate normal levels (300 – 1000 ng/dL) seen in healthy men. AndroGel 1.62% provides continuous transdermal delivery of testosterone for 24 hours following once daily application to clean, dry, intact skin of the shoulders and upper arms. Average serum testosterone concentrations over 24 hours (C_{avg}) observed when AndroGel 1.62% was applied to the upper arms/shoulders were comparable to average serum testosterone concentrations (C_{avg}) when AndroGel 1.62% was applied using a rotation method utilizing the abdomen and upper arms/shoulders. The rotation of abdomen and upper arms/shoulders was a method used in the pivotal clinical trial [see Clinical Studies (14.1)].

Figure 2: Mean (±SD) Serum Total Testosterone Concentrations on Day 7 in Patients Following AndroGel 1.62% Once-Daily Application of 81 mg of Testosterone (N=33) for 7 Days

Information on the AbbVie, Inc. products listed on these pages is from the prescribing information in use as of July 31, 2014. For more information, please visit rxabbvie.com or call 1-800-633-9110.

Table 6: Mean (SD) Testosterone Concentrations (C_{avg} and C_{max}) by final dose on Days 112 and 364

Parameter	Final Dose on Day 112					
	Placebo (n=27)	20.25 mg (n=12)	40.5 mg (n=34)	60.75 mg (n=54)	81 mg (n=79)	All Active (n=179)
C_{avg} (ng/dL)	303 (135)	457 (275)	524 (228)	643 (285)	537 (240)	561 (259)
C_{max} (ng/dL)	450 (349)	663 (473)	798 (439)	958 (497)	813 (479)	845 (480)
	Final Dose on Day 364					
		20.25 mg (n=7)	40.5 mg (n=26)	60.75 mg (n=29)	81 mg (n=74)	Continuing Active (n=136)
C_{avg} (ng/dL)		386 (130)	474 (176)	513 (222)	432 (186)	455 (192)
C_{max} (ng/dL)		562 (187)	715 (306)	839 (568)	649 (329)	697 (389)

Distribution

Circulating testosterone is primarily bound in the serum to sex hormone-binding globulin (SHBG) and albumin. Approximately 40% of testosterone in plasma is bound to SHBG, 2% remains unbound (free) and the rest is loosely bound to albumin and other proteins.

Metabolism

Testosterone is metabolized to various 17-keto steroids through two different pathways. The major active metabolites of testosterone are estradiol and DHT.

Excretion

There is considerable variation in the half-life of testosterone concentration as reported in the literature, ranging from 10 to 100 minutes. About 90% of a dose of testosterone given intramuscularly is excreted in the urine as glucuronic acid and sulfuric acid conjugates of testosterone and its metabolites. About 6% of a dose is excreted in the feces, mostly in the unconjugated form. Inactivation of testosterone occurs primarily in the liver.
When AndroGel 1.62% treatment is discontinued, serum testosterone concentrations return to approximately baseline concentrations within 48-72 hours after administration of the last dose.

Potential for testosterone transfer

The potential for testosterone transfer following administration of AndroGel 1.62% when it was applied only to upper arms/shoulders was evaluated in two clinical studies of males dosed with AndroGel 1.62% and their untreated female partners. In one study, 8 male subjects applied a single dose of AndroGel 1.62% 81 mg to their shoulders and upper arms. Two (2) hours after application, female subjects rubbed their hands, wrists, arms, and shoulders to the application site of the male subjects for 15 minutes. Serum concentrations of testosterone were monitored in female subjects for 24 hours after contact occurred. After direct skin-to-skin contact with the site of application, mean testosterone C_{avg} and C_{max} in female subjects increased by 280% and 267%, respectively, compared to mean baseline testosterone concentrations. In a second study evaluating transfer of testosterone, 12 male subjects applied a single dose of AndroGel 1.62% 81 mg to their shoulders and upper arms. Two (2) hours after application, female subjects rubbed their hands, wrists, arms, and shoulders to the application site of the male subjects for 15 minutes while the site of application was covered by a t-shirt. When a t-shirt was used to cover the site of application, mean testosterone C_{avg} and C_{max} in female subjects increased by 6% and 11%, respectively, compared to mean baseline testosterone concentrations.
A separate study was conducted to evaluate the potential for testosterone transfer from 16 males dosed with AndroGel 1.62% 81 mg when it was applied to abdomen only for 7 days, a site of application not approved for AndroGel 1.62%. Two (2) hours after application to the males on each day, the female subjects rubbed their abdomens for 15 minutes to the abdomen of the males. The males had covered the application area with a T-shirt. The mean testosterone C_{avg} and C_{max} in female subjects on day 1 increased by 43% and 47%, respectively, compared to mean baseline testosterone concentrations. The mean testosterone C_{avg} and C_{max} in female subjects on day 7 increased by 60% and 58%, respectively, compared to mean baseline testosterone concentrations.

Effect of showering

In a randomized, 3-way (3 treatment periods without washout period) crossover study in 24 hypogonadal men, the effect of showering on testosterone exposure was assessed after once daily application of AndroGel 1.62% 81 mg to upper arms/shoulders for 7 days in each treatment period. On the 7th day of each treatment period, hypogonadal men took a shower with soap and water at either 2, 6, or 10 hours after drug application. The effect of showering at 2 or 6 hours

post-dose on Day 7 resulted in 13% and 12% decreases in mean C_{avg}, respectively, compared to Day 6 when no shower was taken after drug application. Showering at 10 hours after drug application had no effect on bioavailability. The amount of testosterone remaining in the outer layers of the skin at the application site on the 7th day was assessed using a tape stripping procedure and was reduced by at least 80% after showering 2-10 hours post-dose compared to on the 6th day when no shower was taken after drug application.

Effect of sunscreen or moisturizing lotion on absorption of testosterone

In a randomized, 3-way (3 treatment periods without washout period) crossover study in 18 hypogonadal males, the effect of applying a moisturizing lotion or a sunscreen on the absorption of testosterone was evaluated with the upper arms/shoulders as application sites. For 7 days, moisturizing lotion or sunscreen (SPF 50) was applied daily to the AndroGel 1.62% application site 1 hour after the application of AndroGel 1.62% 40.5 mg. Application of moisturizing lotion increased mean testosterone C_{avg} and C_{max} by 14% and 17%, respectively, compared to AndroGel 1.62% administered alone. Application of sunscreen increased mean testosterone C_{avg} and C_{max} by 8% and 13%, respectively, compared to AndroGel 1.62% applied alone.

13 NONCLINICAL TOXICOLOGY

13.1 Carcinogenesis, Mutagenesis, Impairment of Fertility

Testosterone has been tested by subcutaneous injection and implantation in mice and rats. In mice, the implant induced cervical-uterine tumors which metastasized in some cases. There is suggestive evidence that injection of testosterone into some strains of female mice increases their susceptibility to hepatoma. Testosterone is also known to increase the number of tumors and decrease the degree of differentiation of chemically induced carcinomas of the liver in rats. Testosterone was negative in the *in vitro* Ames and in the *in vivo* mouse micronucleus assays. The administration of exogenous testosterone has been reported to suppress spermatogenesis in the rat, dog and non-human primates, which was reversible on cessation of the treatment.

14 CLINICAL STUDIES

14.1 Clinical Trials in Hypogonadal Males

AndroGel 1.62% was evaluated in a multi-center, randomized, double-blind, parallel-group, placebo-controlled study (182-day double-blind period) in 274 hypogonadal men with body mass index (BMI) 18-40 kg/m² and 18-80 years of age (mean age 53.8 years). The patients had an average serum testosterone concentration of <300 ng/dL, as determined by two morning samples collected on the same visit. Patients were Caucasian 83%, Black 13%, Asian or Native American 4%. 7.5% of patients were Hispanic.
Patients were randomized to receive active treatment or placebo using a rotation method utilizing the abdomen and upper arms/shoulders for 182 days. All patients were started at a daily dose of 40.5 mg (two pump actuations) AndroGel 1.62% or matching placebo on Day 1 of the study. Patients returned to the clinic on Day 14, Day 28, and Day 42 for predose serum total testosterone assessments. The patient's daily dose was titrated up or down in 20.25 mg increments if the predose serum testosterone value was outside the range of 350-750 ng/dL. The study included four active AndroGel 1.62% doses: 20.25 mg, 40.5 mg, 60.75 mg, and 81 mg daily.
The primary endpoint was the percentage of patients with C_{avg} within the normal range of 300-1000 ng/dL on Day 112. In patients treated with AndroGel 1.62%, 81.6% (146/179) had C_{avg} within the normal range at Day 112. The secondary endpoint was the percentage of patients, with C_{max} above three pre-determined limits. The percentages of patients with C_{max} greater than 1500 ng/dL, and between 1800

and 2499 ng/dL on Day 112 were 11.2% and 5.5%, respectively. Two patients had a C_{max} >2500 ng/dL on Day 112 (2510 ng/dL and 2550 ng/dL, respectively); neither of these 2 patients demonstrated an abnormal C_{max} on prior or subsequent assessments at the same dose.
Patients could agree to continue in an open-label, active treatment maintenance period of the study for an additional 182 days.
Dose titrations on Days 14, 28, and 42 resulted in final doses of 20.25 mg – 81 mg on Day 112 as shown in Table 6. [See table 6 above]
Figure 3 summarizes the pharmacokinetic profile of total testosterone in patients completing 112 days of AndroGel 1.62% treatment administered as a starting dose of 40.5 mg of testosterone (2 pump actuations) for the initial 14 days followed by possible titration according to the follow-up testosterone measurements.

Figure 3: Mean (±SD) Steady-State Serum Total Testosterone Concentrations on Day 112

Efficacy was maintained in the group of men that received AndroGel 1.62% for one full year. In that group, 78% (106/136) had average serum testosterone concentrations in the normal range at Day 364. Figure 4 summarizes the mean total testosterone profile for these patients on Day 364.

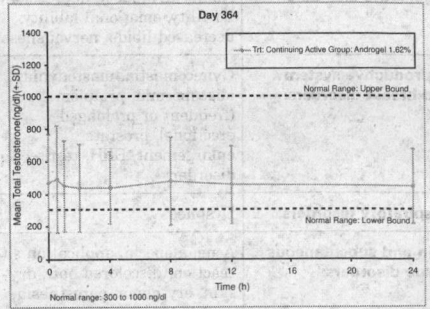

Figure 4: Mean (±SD) Steady-State Serum Total Testosterone Concentrations on Day 364

The mean estradiol and DHT concentration profiles paralleled the changes observed in testosterone. The levels of LH and FSH decreased with testosterone treatment. The decreases in levels of LH and FSH are consistent with reports published in the literature of long-term treatment with testosterone.

16 HOW SUPPLIED/STORAGE AND HANDLING

AndroGel 1.62% is supplied in non-aerosol, metered-dose pumps that deliver 20.25 mg of testosterone per complete pump actuation. The pumps are composed of plastic and stainless steel and an LDPE/aluminum foil inner liner encased in rigid plastic with a polypropylene cap. Each 88 g metered-dose pump is capable of dispensing 75 g of gel or 60-metered pump actuations; each pump actuation dispenses 1.25 g of gel.
AndroGel 1.62% is also supplied in unit-dose aluminum foil packets in cartons of 30. Each packet of 1.25 g or 2.5 g gel contains 20.25 mg or 40.5 mg testosterone, respectively.

NDC Number	Package Size
0051-8462-33	88 g pump (each pump dispenses 60 metered pump actuations with each pump actuation containing 20.25 mg of testosterone in 1.25 g of gel)
0051-8462-12	Each unit dose packet contains 20.25 mg of testosterone provided in 1.25 g of gel
0051-8462-31	30 packets (each unit dose packet contains 20.25 mg of testosterone provided in 1.25 g of gel)
0051-8462-01	Each unit dose packet contains 40.5 mg of testosterone provided in 2.5 g of gel

0051-8462-30   30 packets (each unit dose packet contains 40.5 mg of testosterone provided in 2.5 g of gel)

Store at controlled room temperature 20°-25°C (68°-77°F); excursions permitted to 15°- 30°C (59°- 86°F) [see USP Controlled Room Temperature].
Used AndroGel 1.62% pumps or used AndroGel 1.62% packets should be discarded in household trash in a manner that prevents accidental application or ingestion by children or pets.

17   PATIENT COUNSELING INFORMATION
See FDA-Approved Medication Guide
Patients should be informed of the following:
17.1   Use in Men with Known or Suspected Prostate or Breast Cancer
Men with known or suspected prostate or breast cancer should not use AndroGel 1.62% [see Contraindications (4) and Warnings and Precautions (5.1)].
17.2   Potential for Secondary Exposure to Testosterone and Steps to Prevent Secondary Exposure
Secondary exposure to testosterone in children and women can occur with the use of testosterone gel in men. Cases of secondary exposure to testosterone have been reported in children.
Physicians should advise patients of the reported signs and symptoms of secondary exposure, which may include the following:
- In children: unexpected sexual development including inappropriate enlargement of the penis or clitoris, premature development of pubic hair, increased erections, and aggressive behavior.
- In women: changes in hair distribution, increase in acne, or other signs of testosterone effects.
- The possibility of secondary exposure to testosterone gel should be brought to the attention of a healthcare provider.
- AndroGel 1.62% should be promptly discontinued until the cause of virilization is identified.

Strict adherence to the following precautions is advised to minimize the potential for secondary exposure to testosterone from AndroGel 1.62% in men [see Medication Guide]:
- **Children and women should avoid contact with unwashed or unclothed application site(s)** of men using AndroGel 1.62%.
- Patients using AndroGel 1.62% should apply the product as directed and strictly adhere to the following:
  - **Wash hands** with soap and water immediately after application.
  - **Cover the application site(s)** with clothing after the gel has dried.
  - **Wash the application site(s) thoroughly** with soap and water prior to any situation where skin-to-skin contact of the application site with another person is anticipated.
- In the event that unwashed or unclothed skin to which AndroGel 1.62% has been applied comes in contact with the skin of another person, the general area of contact on the other person should be washed with soap and water as soon as possible [see Dosage and Administration (2.2), Warnings and Precautions (5.2) and Clinical Pharmacology (12.3)].

17.3   Potential Adverse Reactions with Androgens
Patients should be informed that treatment with androgens may lead to adverse reactions which include:
- Changes in urinary habits such as increased urination at night, trouble starting the urine stream, passing urine many times during the day, having an urge to go to the bathroom right away, having a urine accident, being unable to pass urine and weak urine flow.
- Breathing disturbances, including those associated with sleep, or excessive daytime sleepiness.
- Too frequent or persistent erections of the penis.
- Nausea, vomiting, changes in skin color, or ankle swelling.

17.4   Patients Should Be Advised of the Following Instructions for Use
- **Read the Medication Guide** before starting AndroGel 1.62% therapy and to reread it each time the prescription is renewed.
- AndroGel 1.62% should be applied and used appropriately to maximize the benefits and to minimize the risk of secondary exposure in children and women.
- Keep AndroGel 1.62% out of the reach of children.
- **AndroGel 1.62% is an alcohol based product and is flammable; therefore avoid fire, flame or smoking until the gel has dried.**
- It is important to adhere to all recommended monitoring.
- Report any changes in their state of health, such as changes in urinary habits, breathing, sleep, and mood.
- AndroGel 1.62% is prescribed to meet the patient's specific needs; therefore, the patient should never share AndroGel 1.62% with anyone.

Find Your Dose as Prescribed by Your Healthcare Provider		Application Method
1 PUMP DEPRESSION	20.25 mg	Apply 1 pump depression of ANDROGEL 1.62% to 1 upper arm and shoulder.
2 PUMP DEPRESSIONS	40.5 mg	Apply 1 pump depression of ANDROGEL 1.62% to 1 upper arm and shoulder and then apply 1 pump depression of ANDROGEL 1.62% to the opposite upper arm and shoulder.
3 PUMP DEPRESSIONS	60.75 mg	Apply 2 pump depressions of ANDROGEL 1.62% to 1 upper arm and shoulder and then apply 1 pump depression of ANDROGEL 1.62% to the opposite upper arm and shoulder.
4 PUMP DEPRESSIONS	81 mg	Apply 2 pump depressions of ANDROGEL 1.62% to 1 upper arm and shoulder and then apply 2 pump depressions of ANDROGEL 1.62% to the opposite upper arm and shoulder.

Find Your Dose as Prescribed by Your Healthcare Provider		Application Method
One 20.25 mg packet	20.25 mg	Apply 1 packet of ANDROGEL 1.62% to 1 upper arm and shoulder.
One 40.5 mg packet	40.5 mg	Apply half of the 40.5 mg packet of ANDROGEL 1.62% to 1 upper arm and shoulder and then apply the remaining packet contents to the opposite upper arm and shoulder.
One 40.5 mg packet and one 20.25 mg packet	60.75 mg	Apply one 40.5 mg packet of ANDROGEL 1.62% to 1 upper arm and shoulder and then apply one 20.25 mg packet of ANDROGEL 1.62% to the opposite upper arm and shoulder.
Two 40.5 mg packets	81 mg	Apply one 40.5 mg packet of ANDROGEL 1.62% to 1 upper arm and shoulder and then apply one 40.5 mg packet of ANDROGEL 1.62% to the opposite upper arm and shoulder.

- Wait 2 hours before swimming or washing following application of AndroGel 1.62%. This will ensure that the greatest amount of AndroGel 1.62% is absorbed into their system.

Medication Guide
ANDROGEL® (AN DROW JEL) ℂⅢ
(testosterone gel) 1.62%
Read this Medication Guide before you start using ANDROGEL 1.62% and each time you get a refill. There may be new information. This information does not take the place of talking with your healthcare provider about your medical condition or treatment.
What is the most important information I should know about ANDROGEL 1.62%?
1. **Early signs and symptoms of puberty have happened in young children who were accidentally exposed to testosterone through contact with men using ANDROGEL 1.62%.**
   Signs and symptoms of early puberty in a child may include:
   - enlarged penis or clitoris
   - early development of pubic hair
   - increased erections or sex drive
   - aggressive behavior
   ANDROGEL 1.62% can transfer from your body to others.
2. **Women and children should avoid contact with the unwashed or unclothed area where ANDROGEL 1.62% has been applied to your skin.**
   Stop using ANDROGEL 1.62% and call your healthcare provider right away if you see any signs and symptoms in a child or a woman that may have occurred through accidental exposure to ANDROGEL 1.62%.
   Signs and symptoms of exposure to ANDROGEL 1.62% in children may include:
   - enlarged penis or clitoris
   - early development of pubic hair
   - increased erections or sex drive
   - aggressive behavior
   Signs and symptoms of exposure to ANDROGEL 1.62% in women may include:
   - changes in body hair
   - a large increase in acne
- **To lower the risk of transfer of ANDROGEL 1.62% from your body to others, you should follow these important instructions:**
  - Apply ANDROGEL 1.62% **only** to your shoulders and upper arms that will be covered by a short sleeve t-shirt.
  - Wash your hands **right away** with soap and water after applying ANDROGEL 1.62%.
  - After the gel has dried, **cover the application area with clothing.** Keep the area covered until you have washed the application area or have showered.

- **If you expect to have skin-to-skin contact with another person, first wash the application area well with soap and water.**
- **If a woman or child makes contact with the ANDROGEL 1.62% application area, that area on the woman or child should be washed well with soap and water right away.**
What is ANDROGEL 1.62%?
ANDROGEL 1.62% is a prescription medicine that contains testosterone. ANDROGEL 1.62% is used to treat adult males who have low or no testosterone.
Your healthcare provider will test your blood before you start and while you are taking ANDROGEL 1.62%.
It is not known if ANDROGEL 1.62% is safe or effective in children younger than 18 years old. Improper use of ANDROGEL 1.62% may affect bone growth in children.
ANDROGEL 1.62% is a controlled substance (CIII) because it contains testosterone that can be a target for people who abuse prescription medicines. Keep your ANDROGEL 1.62% in a safe place to protect it. Never give your ANDROGEL 1.62% to anyone else, even if they have the same symptoms you have. Selling or giving away this medicine may harm others and is against the law.
ANDROGEL 1.62% is not meant for use in women.
Who should not use ANDROGEL 1.62%?
Do not use ANDROGEL 1.62% if you:
- have breast cancer
- have or might have prostate cancer
- are pregnant or may become pregnant or are breast-feeding. ANDROGEL 1.62% may harm your unborn or breast-feeding baby.
  Women who are pregnant or who may become pregnant should avoid contact with the area of skin where ANDROGEL 1.62% has been applied.
Talk to your healthcare provider before taking this medicine if you have any of the above conditions.
What should I tell my healthcare provider before using ANDROGEL 1.62%?
Before you use ANDROGEL 1.62%, tell your healthcare provider if you:
- have breast cancer
- have or might have prostate cancer
- have urinary problems due to an enlarged prostate
- have heart problems
- have kidney or liver problems
- have problems breathing while you sleep (sleep apnea)
- have any other medical conditions

Information on the AbbVie, Inc. products listed on these pages is from the prescribing information in use as of July 31, 2014. For more information, please visit rxabbvie.com or call 1-800-633-9110.

Tell your healthcare provider about all the medicines you take, including prescription and non-prescription medicines, vitamins, and herbal supplements.

Using ANDROGEL 1.62% with certain other medicines can affect each other.

Especially, tell your healthcare provider if you take:
• insulin
• medicines that decrease blood clotting
• corticosteroids

Know the medicines you take. Ask your healthcare provider or pharmacist for a list of all of your medicines, if you are not sure. Keep a list of them and show it to your healthcare provider and pharmacist when you get a new medicine.

How should I use ANDROGEL 1.62%?
• It is important that you apply ANDROGEL 1.62% exactly as your healthcare provider tells you to.
• Your healthcare provider will tell you how much ANDROGEL 1.62% to apply and when to apply it.
• Your healthcare provider may change your ANDROGEL 1.62% dose. **Do not** change your ANDROGEL 1.62% dose without talking to your healthcare provider.
• **ANDROGEL 1.62% is to be applied to the area of your shoulders and upper arms that will be covered by a short sleeve t-shirt.** Do not apply ANDROGEL 1.62% to any other parts of your body such as your stomach area (abdomen), penis, or scrotum.
• Apply ANDROGEL 1.62% at the same time each morning. ANDROGEL 1.62% should be applied after showering or bathing.
• **Wash your hands right away** with soap and water after applying ANDROGEL 1.62%.
• Avoid showering, swimming or bathing for at least 2 hours after you apply ANDROGEL 1.62%.
• ANDROGEL 1.62% is flammable until dry. Let ANDROGEL 1.62% dry before smoking or going near an open flame.
• Let the application site dry completely before putting on a t-shirt.

Applying ANDROGEL 1.62%:
ANDROGEL 1.62% comes in a pump or in packets.
• **Before applying ANDROGEL 1.62% make sure that your shoulders and upper arms are clean, dry, and that there is no broken skin.**
• The application sites for ANDROGEL 1.62% are the upper arms and shoulders that will be covered by a short sleeve t-shirt (See Figure A).

(Figure A)

If you are using ANDROGEL 1.62% pump:
• Before using a new bottle of ANDROGEL 1.62 % for the first time, you will need to prime the pump. To prime the ANDROGEL 1.62% pump, slowly push the pump all the way down 3 times. **Do not** use any ANDROGEL 1.62% that came out while priming. Wash it down the sink to avoid accidental exposure to others. Your ANDROGEL 1.62% pump is now ready to use.
• Remove the cap from the pump. Then, position the nozzle over the palm of your hand and slowly push the pump all the way down. Apply ANDROGEL 1.62% to the application site. You may also apply ANDROGEL 1.62% directly to the application site.
• **Wash your hands with soap and water right away.**
[See first table at top of previous page]
If you are using ANDROGEL 1.62% packets:
• Tear open the packet completely at the dotted line. Squeeze from the bottom of the packet to the top.
• Squeeze all of the ANDROGEL 1.62% out of the packet into the palm of your hand. Apply ANDROGEL 1.62% to the application site. You may also apply ANDROGEL 1.62% directly to the application site.
• ANDROGEL 1.62% should be applied right away.
• **Wash your hands with soap and water right away.**
[See second table at top of previous page]

What are the possible side effects of ANDROGEL 1.62%?
See "What is the most important information I should know about ANDROGEL 1.62%?"
ANDROGEL 1.62% can cause serious side effects including:
• **If you already have enlargement of your prostate gland your signs and symptoms can get worse while using ANDROGEL 1.62%.** This can include:
  ○ increased urination at night
  ○ trouble starting your urine stream
  ○ having to pass urine many times during the day
  ○ having an urge that you have to go to the bathroom right away
  ○ having a urine accident
  ○ being unable to pass urine or weak urine flow
• **Possible increased risk of prostate cancer.** Your healthcare provider should check you for prostate cancer or any other prostate problems before you start and while you use ANDROGEL 1.62%.
• **In large doses ANDROGEL 1.62% may lower your sperm count.**
• **Swelling of your ankles, feet, or body, with or without heart failure.**
• **Enlarged or painful breasts.**
• **Have problems breathing while you sleep (sleep apnea).**
• **Blood clots in the legs.** This can include pain, swelling, or redness of your legs.
Call your healthcare provider right away if you have any of the serious side effects listed above.
The most common side effects of ANDROGEL 1.62% include:
• increased prostate specific antigen (a test used to screen for prostate cancer)
• mood swings
• hypertension
• increased red blood cell count
• skin irritation where ANDROGEL 1.62% is applied
Other side effects include more erections than are normal for you or erections that last a long time.
Tell your healthcare provider if you have any side effect that bothers you or that does not go away.
These are not all the possible side effects of ANDROGEL 1.62%. For more information, ask your healthcare provider or pharmacist.
Call your doctor for medical advice about side effects. You may report side effects to FDA at 1-800-FDA-1088.
How should I store ANDROGEL 1.62%?
• Store ANDROGEL 1.62% at 59°F to 86°F (15°C to 30°C).
• When it is time to throw away the pump or packets, safely throw away used ANDROGEL 1.62% in household trash. Be careful to prevent accidental exposure of children or pets.
• Keep ANDROGEL 1.62% away from fire.
Keep ANDROGEL 1.62% and all medicines out of the reach of children.
General information about the safe and effective use of ANDROGEL 1.62%
Medicines are sometimes prescribed for purposes other than those listed in a Medication Guide. Do not use ANDROGEL 1.62% for a condition for which it was not prescribed. Do not give ANDROGEL 1.62% to other people, even if they have the same symptoms you have. It may harm them.
This Medication Guide summarizes the most important information about ANDROGEL 1.62%. If you would like more information, talk to your healthcare provider. You can ask your pharmacist or healthcare provider for information about ANDROGEL 1.62% that is written for health professionals.
For more information, go to www.androgel.com or call 1-800-633-9110.
What are the ingredients in ANDROGEL 1.62%?
Active ingredient: testosterone
Inactive ingredients: carbopol 980, ethyl alcohol, isopropyl myristate, purified water and sodium hydroxide.
This Medication Guide has been approved by the U.S. Food and Drug Administration.
Marketed by:
AbbVie Inc.
North Chicago, IL 60064, USA
© 2013 AbbVie Inc.
A090630054574 Revised May, 2013
Shown in Product Identification Guide, page 303

BIAXIN® FILMTAB®
[bi ax ən]
(clarithromycin tablets, USP)

BIAXIN® XL FILMTAB®
(clarithromycin extended-release tablets)

BIAXIN® GRANULES
(clarithromycin for oral suspension, USP)

To reduce the development of drug-resistant bacteria and maintain the effectiveness of BIAXIN and other antibacte-rial drugs, BIAXIN should be used only to treat or prevent infections that are proven or strongly suspected to be caused by bacteria.

DESCRIPTION
Clarithromycin is a semi-synthetic macrolide antibiotic. Chemically, it is 6-0-methylerythromycin. The molecular formula is $C_{38}H_{69}NO_{13}$, and the molecular weight is 747.96. The structural formula is:

Clarithromycin is a white to off-white crystalline powder. It is soluble in acetone, slightly soluble in methanol, ethanol, and acetonitrile, and practically insoluble in water.
BIAXIN is available as immediate-release tablets, extended-release tablets, and granules for oral suspension. Each yellow oval film-coated immediate-release BIAXIN tablet (clarithromycin tablets, USP) contains 250 mg or 500 mg of clarithromycin and the following inactive ingredients:
250 mg tablets: hypromellose, hydroxypropyl cellulose, croscarmellose sodium, D&C Yellow No. 10, FD&C Blue No. 1, magnesium stearate, microcrystalline cellulose, povidone, pregelatinized starch, propylene glycol, silicon dioxide, sorbic acid, sorbitan monooleate, stearic acid, talc, titanium dioxide, and vanillin.
500 mg tablets: hypromellose, hydroxypropyl cellulose, colloidal silicon dioxide, croscarmellose sodium, D&C Yellow No. 10, magnesium stearate, microcrystalline cellulose, povidone, propylene glycol, sorbic acid, sorbitan monooleate, titanium dioxide, and vanillin.
Each yellow oval film-coated BIAXIN XL tablet (clarithromycin extended-release tablets) contains 500 mg of clarithromycin and the following inactive ingredients: cellulosic polymers, D&C Yellow No. 10, lactose monohydrate, magnesium stearate, propylene glycol, sorbic acid, sorbitan monooleate, talc, titanium dioxide, and vanillin.
After constitution, each 5 mL of BIAXIN suspension (clarithromycin for oral suspension, USP) contains 125 mg or 250 mg of clarithromycin. Each bottle of BIAXIN granules contains 1250 mg (50 mL size), 2500 mg (50 and 100 mL sizes) or 5000 mg (100 mL size) of clarithromycin and the following inactive ingredients: carbomer, castor oil, citric acid, hypromellose phthalate, maltodextrin, potassium sorbate, povidone, silicon dioxide, sucrose, xanthan gum, titanium dioxide and fruit punch flavor.

CLINICAL PHARMACOLOGY
Pharmacokinetics
Clarithromycin is rapidly absorbed from the gastrointestinal tract after oral administration. The absolute bioavailability of 250 mg clarithromycin tablets was approximately 50%. For a single 500 mg dose of clarithromycin, food slightly delays the onset of clarithromycin absorption, increasing the peak time from approximately 2 to 2.5 hours. Food also increases the clarithromycin peak plasma concentration by about 24%, but does not affect the extent of clarithromycin bioavailability. Food does not affect the onset of formation of the antimicrobially active metabolite, 14-OH clarithromycin or its peak plasma concentration but does slightly decrease the extent of metabolite formation, indicated by an 11% decrease in area under the plasma concentration-time curve (AUC). Therefore, BIAXIN tablets may be given without regard to food.
In nonfasting healthy human subjects (males and females), peak plasma concentrations were attained within 2 to 3 hours after oral dosing. Steady-state peak plasma clarithromycin concentrations were attained within 3 days and were approximately 1 to 2 mcg/mL with a 250 mg dose administered every 12 hours and 3 to 4 mcg/mL with a 500 mg dose administered every 8 to 12 hours. The elimination half-life of clarithromycin was about 3 to 4 hours with 250 mg administered every 12 hours but increased to 5 to 7 hours with 500 mg administered every 8 to 12 hours. The nonlinearity of clarithromycin pharmacokinetics is slight at the recommended doses of 250 mg and 500 mg administered every 8 to 12 hours. With a 250 mg every 12 hours dosing, the principal metabolite, 14-OH clarithromycin, attains a peak steady-state concentration of about 0.6 mcg/mL and has an elimination half-life of 5 to 6 hours. With a 500 mg

every 8 to 12 hours dosing, the peak steady-state concentration of 14-OH clarithromycin is slightly higher (up to 1 mcg/mL), and its elimination half-life is about 7 to 9 hours. With any of these dosing regimens, the steady-state concentration of this metabolite is generally attained within 3 to 4 days.

After a 250 mg tablet every 12 hours, approximately 20% of the dose is excreted in the urine as clarithromycin, while after a 500 mg tablet every 12 hours, the urinary excretion of clarithromycin is somewhat greater, approximately 30%. In comparison, after an oral dose of 250 mg (125 mg/5 mL) suspension every 12 hours, approximately 40% is excreted in urine as clarithromycin. The renal clearance of clarithromycin is, however, relatively independent of the dose size and approximates the normal glomerular filtration rate. The major metabolite found in urine is 14-OH clarithromycin, which accounts for an additional 10% to 15% of the dose with either a 250 mg or a 500 mg tablet administered every 12 hours.

Steady-state concentrations of clarithromycin and 14-OH clarithromycin observed following administration of 500 mg doses of clarithromycin every 12 hours to adult patients with HIV infection were similar to those observed in healthy volunteers. In adult HIV-infected patients taking 500- or 1000-mg doses of clarithromycin every 12 hours, steady-state clarithromycin C_{max} values ranged from 2 to 4 mcg/mL and 5 to 10 mcg/mL, respectively.

The steady-state concentrations of clarithromycin in subjects with impaired hepatic function did not differ from those in normal subjects; however, the 14-OH clarithromycin concentrations were lower in the hepatically impaired subjects. The decreased formation of 14-OH clarithromycin was at least partially offset by an increase in renal clearance of clarithromycin in the subjects with impaired hepatic function when compared to healthy subjects. The pharmacokinetics of clarithromycin was also altered in subjects with impaired renal function (see **PRECAUTIONS** and **DOSAGE AND ADMINISTRATION**).

Clarithromycin and the 14-OH clarithromycin metabolite distribute readily into body tissues and fluids. There are no data available on cerebrospinal fluid penetration. Because of high intracellular concentrations, tissue concentrations are higher than serum concentrations. Examples of tissue and serum concentrations are presented below.

CONCENTRATION (after 250 mg q12h)

Tissue Type	Tissue (mcg/g)	Serum (mcg/mL)
Tonsil	1.6	0.8
Lung	8.8	1.7

Clarithromycin extended-release tablets provide extended absorption of clarithromycin from the gastrointestinal tract after oral administration. Relative to an equal total daily dose of immediate-release clarithromycin tablets, clarithromycin extended-release tablets provide lower and later steady-state peak plasma concentrations but equivalent 24-hour AUC's for both clarithromycin and its microbiologically-active metabolite, 14-OH clarithromycin. While the extent of formation of 14-OH clarithromycin following administration of BIAXIN XL tablets (2 × 500 mg once daily) is not affected by food, administration under fasting conditions is associated with approximately 30% lower clarithromycin AUC relative to administration with food. Therefore, BIAXIN XL tablets should be taken with food.

Steady-State Clarithromycin Plasma Concentration-Time Profiles

In healthy human subjects, steady-state peak plasma clarithromycin concentrations of approximately 2 to

Clarithromycin Tissue Concentrations 2 hours after Dose (mcg/mL)/(mcg/g)

Treatment	N	antrum	fundus	N	mucus
Clarithromycin	5	10.48 ± 2.01	20.81 ± 7.64	4	4.15 ± 7.74
Clarithromycin + Omeprazole	5	19.96 ± 4.71	24.25 ± 6.37	4	39.29 ± 32.79

3 mcg/mL were achieved about 5 to 8 hours after oral administration of 2 × 500 mg BIAXIN XL tablets once daily; for 14-OH clarithromycin, steady-state peak plasma concentrations of approximately 0.8 mcg/mL were attained about 6 to 9 hours after dosing. Steady-state peak plasma clarithromycin concentrations of approximately 1 to 2 mcg/mL were achieved about 5 to 6 hours after oral administration of a single 500 mg BIAXIN XL tablet once daily; for 14-OH clarithromycin, steady-state peak plasma concentrations of approximately 0.6 mcg/mL were attained about 6 hours after dosing.

When 250 mg doses of clarithromycin as BIAXIN suspension were administered to fasting healthy adult subjects, peak plasma concentrations were attained around 3 hours after dosing. Steady-state peak plasma concentrations were attained in 2 to 3 days and were approximately 2 mcg/mL for clarithromycin and 0.7 mcg/mL for 14-OH clarithromycin when 250-mg doses of the clarithromycin suspension were administered every 12 hours. Elimination half-life of clarithromycin (3 to 4 hours) and that of 14-OH clarithromycin (5 to 7 hours) were similar to those observed at steady state following administration of equivalent doses of BIAXIN tablets.

For adult patients, the bioavailability of 10 mL of the 125 mg/5 mL suspension or 10 mL of the 250 mg/5 mL suspension is similar to a 250 mg or 500 mg tablet, respectively.

In children requiring antibiotic therapy, administration of 7.5 mg/kg q12h doses of clarithromycin as the suspension generally resulted in steady-state peak plasma concentrations of 3 to 7 mcg/mL for clarithromycin and 1 to 2 mcg/mL for 14-OH clarithromycin.

In HIV-infected children taking 15 mg/kg every 12 hours, steady-state clarithromycin peak concentrations generally ranged from 6 to 15 mcg/mL.

Clarithromycin penetrates into the middle ear fluid of children with secretory otitis media.

CONCENTRATION (after 7.5 mg/kg q12h for 5 doses)

Analyte	Middle Ear Fluid (mcg/mL)	Serum (mcg/mL)
Clarithromycin	2.5	1.7
14-OH Clarithromycin	1.3	0.8

In adults given 250 mg clarithromycin as suspension (n = 22), food appeared to decrease mean peak plasma clarithromycin concentrations from 1.2 (± 0.4) mcg/mL to 1.0 (± 0.4) mcg/mL and the extent of absorption from 7.2 (± 2.5) hr•mcg/mL to 6.5 (± 3.7) hr•mcg/mL.

When children (n = 10) were administered a single oral dose of 7.5 mg/kg suspension, food increased mean peak plasma clarithromycin concentrations from 3.6 (± 1.5) mcg/mL to 4.6 (± 2.8) mcg/mL and the extent of absorption from 10.0 (± 5.5) hr•mcg/mL to 14.2 (± 9.4) hr•mcg/mL.

Clarithromycin 500 mg every 8 hours was given in combination with omeprazole 40 mg daily to healthy adult males. The plasma levels of clarithromycin and 14-hydroxy-clarithromycin were increased by the concomitant administration of omeprazole. For clarithromycin, the mean C_{max} was 10% greater, the mean C_{min} was 27% greater, and the mean AUC_{0-8} was 15% greater when clarithromycin was administered with omeprazole than when clarithromycin was administered alone. Similar results were seen for 14-hydroxy-clarithromycin, the mean C_{max} was 45% greater, the mean C_{min} was 57% greater, and the mean AUC_{0-8} was 45% greater. Clarithromycin concentrations in the gastric tissue and mucus were also increased by concomitant administration of omeprazole.

[See table above]

For information about other drugs indicated in combination with BIAXIN, refer to the **CLINICAL PHARMACOLOGY** section of their package inserts.

Microbiology

Clarithromycin exerts its antibacterial action by binding to the 50S ribosomal subunit of susceptible bacteria resulting in inhibition of protein synthesis.

Clarithromycin is active *in vitro* against a variety of aerobic and anaerobic Gram-positive and Gram-negative bacteria as well as most *Mycobacterium avium* complex (MAC) bacteria.

Additionally, the 14-OH clarithromycin metabolite also has clinically significant antimicrobial activity. The 14-OH clarithromycin is twice as active against *Haemophilus influenzae* microorganisms as the parent compound. However,

for *Mycobacterium avium* complex (MAC) isolates the 14-OH metabolite is 4 to 7 times less active than clarithromycin. The clinical significance of this activity against *Mycobacterium avium* complex is unknown.

Clarithromycin has been shown to be active against most strains of the following microorganisms both *in vitro* and in clinical infections as described in the **INDICATIONS AND USAGE** section:

Gram-Positive Microorganisms
Staphylococcus aureus
Streptococcus pneumoniae
Streptococcus pyogenes
Gram-Negative Microorganisms
Haemophilus influenzae
Haemophilus parainfluenzae
Moraxella catarrhalis
Other Microorganisms
Mycoplasma pneumoniae
Chlamydophila pneumoniae (TWAR) [previously *Chlamydia pneumoniae*]
Mycobacteria
Mycobacterium avium complex (MAC) consisting of:
Mycobacterium avium
Mycobacterium intracellulare

Beta-lactamase production should have no effect on clarithromycin activity.

NOTE: Most isolates of methicillin-resistant and oxacillin-resistant staphylococci are resistant to clarithromycin.

Omeprazole/clarithromycin dual therapy; ranitidine bismuth citrate/clarithromycin dual therapy; omeprazole/clarithromycin/amoxicillin triple therapy; and lansoprazole/clarithromycin/amoxicillin triple therapy have been shown to be active against most strains of *Helicobacter pylori in vitro* and in clinical infections as described in the **INDICATIONS AND USAGE** section.

Helicobacter
Helicobacter pylori
Pretreatment Resistance

Clarithromycin pretreatment resistance rates were 3.5% (4/113) in the omeprazole/clarithromycin dual therapy studies (M93-067, M93-100) and 9.3% (41/439) in the omeprazole/clarithromycin/amoxicillin triple therapy studies (126, 127, M96-446). Clarithromycin pretreatment resistance was 12.6% (44/348) in the ranitidine bismuth citrate/clarithromycin b.i.d. versus t.i.d. clinical study (H2BA3001). Clarithromycin pretreatment resistance rates were 9.5% (91/960) by E-test and 11.3% (12/106) by agar dilution in the lansoprazole/clarithromycin/amoxicillin triple therapy clinical trials (M93-125, M93-130, M93-131, M95-392, and M95-399).

Amoxicillin pretreatment susceptible isolates (< 0.25 mcg/mL) were found in 99.3% (436/439) of the patients in the omeprazole/clarithromycin/amoxicillin clinical studies (126, 127, M96-446). Amoxicillin pretreatment minimum inhibitory concentrations (MICs) > 0.25 mcg/mL occurred in 0.7% (3/439) of the patients, all of whom were in the clarithromycin/amoxicillin study arm. Amoxicillin pretreatment susceptible isolates (< 0.25 mcg/mL) occurred in 97.8% (936/957) and 98.0% (98/100) of the patients in the lansoprazole/clarithromycin/amoxicillin triple-therapy clinical trials by E-test and agar dilution, respectively. Twenty-one of the 957 patients (2.2%) by E-test and 2 of 100 patients (2.0%) by agar dilution had amoxicillin pretreatment MICs of > 0.25 mcg/mL. Two patients had an unconfirmed pretreatment amoxicillin minimum inhibitory concentration (MIC) of > 256 mcg/mL by E-test.

[See table at top of next page]

Patients not eradicated of *H. pylori* following omeprazole/clarithromycin, ranitidine bismuth citrate/clarithromycin, omeprazole/clarithromycin/amoxicillin, or lansoprazole/clarithromycin/amoxicillin therapy would likely have clarithromycin resistant *H. pylori* isolates. Therefore, for patients who fail therapy, clarithromycin susceptibility testing should be done, if possible. Patients with clarithromycin resistant *H. pylori* should not be treated with any of the following: omeprazole/clarithromycin dual therapy; ranitidine bismuth citrate/clarithromycin dual therapy; omeprazole/clarithromycin/amoxicillin triple therapy; lansoprazole/

Information on the AbbVie, Inc. products listed on these pages is from the prescribing information in use as of July 31, 2014. For more information, please visit rxabbvie.com or call 1-800-633-9110.

Clarithromycin Susceptibility Test Results and Clinical/Bacteriological Outcomes[a]

Clarithromycin Pretreatment Results	Clarithromycin Post-treatment Results					
	H. pylori negative - eradicated	H. pylori positive - not eradicated Post-treatment susceptibility results				
		S[b]	I[b]	R[b]	No MIC	
Omeprazole 40 mg q.d./clarithromycin 500 mg t.i.d. for 14 days followed by omeprazole 20 mg q.d. for another 14 days (M93-067, M93-100)						
Susceptible[b]	108	72	1	26	9	
Intermediate[b]	1		1			
Resistant[b]	4			4		
Ranitidine bismuth citrate 400 mg b.i.d./clarithromycin 500 mg t.i.d. for 14 days followed by ranitidine bismuth citrate 400 mg b.i.d. for another 14 days (H2BA3001)						
Susceptible[b]	124	98	4	14	8	
Intermediate[b]	3	2			1	
Resistant[b]	17	1		15	1	
Ranitidine bismuth citrate 400 mg b.i.d./clarithromycin 500 mg b.i.d. for 14 days followed by ranitidine bismuth citrate 400 mg b.i.d. for another 14 days (H2BA3001)						
Susceptible[b]	125	106	1	1	12	5
Intermediate[b]	2		1			
Resistant[b]	20	1			19	
Omeprazole 20 mg b.i.d./clarithromycin 500 mg b.i.d./amoxicillin 1 g b.i.d. for 10 days (126, 127, M96-446)						
Susceptible[b]	171	153	7		3	8
Intermediate[b]						
Resistant[b]	14	4	1		6	3
Lansoprazole 30 mg b.i.d./clarithromycin 500 mg b.i.d./amoxicillin 1 g b.i.d. for 14 days (M95-399, M93-131, M95-392)						
Susceptible[b]	112	105				7
Intermediate[b]	3	3				
Resistant[b]	17	6			7	4
Lansoprazole 30 mg b.i.d./clarithromycin 500 mg b.i.d./amoxicillin 1 g b.i.d. for 10 days (M95-399)						
Susceptible[b]	42	40	1		1	
Intermediate[b]						
Resistant[b]	4	1			3	

a Includes only patients with pretreatment clarithromycin susceptibility tests

b Breakpoints for antimicrobial susceptibility testing at the time of studies were: Susceptible (S) MIC < 0.25 mcg/mL, Intermediate (I) MIC 0.5-1.0 mcg/mL, Resistant (R) MIC > 2 mcg/mL. For current antimicrobial susceptibility testing guidelines see reference 4. For current susceptibility test interpretive criteria, see Susceptibility Test for *Helicobacter pylori* below.

clarithromycin/amoxicillin triple therapy; or other regimens which include clarithromycin as the sole antimicrobial agent.

Amoxicillin Susceptibility Test Results and Clinical/Bacteriological Outcomes

In the omeprazole/clarithromycin/amoxicillin triple-therapy clinical trials, 84.9% (157/185) of the patients who had pretreatment amoxicillin susceptible MICs (< 0.25 mcg/mL) were eradicated of *H. pylori* and 15.1% (28/185) failed therapy. Of the 28 patients who failed triple therapy, 11 had no post-treatment susceptibility test results, and 17 had post-treatment *H. pylori* isolates with amoxicillin susceptible MICs. Eleven of the patients who failed triple therapy also had post-treatment *H. pylori* isolates with clarithromycin resistant MICs.

In the lansoprazole/clarithromycin/amoxicillin triple-therapy clinical trials, 82.6% (195/236) of the patients that had pretreatment amoxicillin susceptible MICs (< 0.25 mcg/mL) were eradicated of *H. pylori*. Of those with pretreatment amoxicillin MICs of > 0.25 mcg/mL, three of six had the *H. pylori* eradicated. A total of 12.8% (22/172) of the patients failed the 10- and 14-day triple-therapy regimens. Post-treatment susceptibility results were not obtained on 11 of the patients who failed therapy. Nine of the 11 patients with amoxicillin post-treatment MICs that failed the triple-therapy regimen also had clarithromycin resistant *H. pylori* isolates.

The following *in vitro* data are available, **but their clinical significance is unknown**. Clarithromycin exhibits *in vitro* activity against most isolates of the following bacteria; however, the safety and effectiveness of clarithromycin in treating clinical infections due to these bacteria have not been established in adequate and well-controlled clinical trials.

Gram-Positive Bacteria
Streptococcus agalactiae
Streptococci (Groups C, F, G)
Viridans group streptococci
Gram-Negative Bacteria
Bordetella pertussis
Legionella pneumophila
Pasteurella multocida
Gram-Positive Bacteria
Clostridium perfringens
Peptococcus niger
Propionibacterium acnes
Gram-Negative Anaerobic Bacteria
Prevotella melaninogenica (formerly *Bacteriodes melaninogenicus*)

Susceptibility Testing Methods (Excluding Mycobacteria and Helicobacter)
Dilution Techniques
Quantitative methods are used to determine antimicrobial minimum inhibitory concentrations (MICs). These MICs provide estimates of the susceptibility of bacteria to antimicrobial compounds. The MICs should be determined using a standardized procedure. Standardized procedures are based on a dilution method[1] (broth or agar) or equivalent with standardized inoculum concentrations and standardized concentrations of clarithromycin powder. The MIC values should be interpreted according to the following criteria[2]:

Susceptibility Test Interpretive Criteria for *Staphylococcus aureus*

MIC (mcg/mL)	Interpretation
≤ 2.0	Susceptible (S)
4.0	Intermediate (I)
≥ 8.0	Resistant (R)

Susceptibility Test Interpretive Criteria for *Streptococcus pyogenes* and *Streptococcus pneumoniae*[a]

MIC (mcg/mL)	Interpretation
≤ 0.25	Susceptible (S)
0.5	Intermediate (I)
≥ 1.0	Resistant (R)

a These interpretive standards are applicable only to broth microdilution susceptibility tests using cation-adjusted Mueller-Hinton broth with 2-5% lysed horse blood.

For testing *Haemophilus* spp.[b]

MIC (mcg/mL)	Interpretation
≤ 8.0	Susceptible (S)
16.0	Intermediate (I)
≥ 32.0	Resistant (R)

b These interpretive standards are applicable only to broth microdilution susceptibility tests with *Haemophilus* spp. using Haemophilus Testing Medium (HTM).[1]

Note: When testing *Streptococcus pyogenes* and *Streptococcus pneumoniae*, susceptibility and resistance to clarithromycin can be predicted using erythromycin.

A report of "Susceptible" indicates that the pathogen is likely to be inhibited if the antimicrobial compound in the blood reaches the concentrations usually achievable. A report of "Intermediate" indicates that the result should be considered equivocal, and, if the microorganism is not fully susceptible to alternative, clinically feasible drugs, the test should be repeated. This category implies possible clinical applicability in body sites where the drug is physiologically concentrated or in situations where high dosage of drug can be used. This category also provides a buffer zone which prevents small uncontrolled technical factors from causing major discrepancies in interpretation. A report of "Resistant" indicates that the pathogen is not likely to be inhibited if the antimicrobial compound in the blood reaches the concentrations usually achievable; other therapy should be selected.

Quality Control
Standardized susceptibility test procedures require the use of laboratory control bacteria to monitor and ensure the accuracy and precision of supplies and reagents in the assay, and the techniques of the individual performing the test.[1,2] Standard clarithromycin powder should provide the following MIC ranges.

QC Strain		MIC (mcg/mL)
S. aureus	ATCC® 29213[c]	0.12 to 0.5
S. pneumoniae[d]	ATCC 49619	0.03 to 0.12
Haemophilus influenzae[e]	ATCC 49247	4 to 16

c ATCC is a registered trademark of the American Type Culture Collection.
d This quality control range is applicable only to *S. pneumoniae* ATCC 49619 tested by a microdilution procedure using cation-adjusted Mueller-Hinton broth with 2-5% lysed horse blood.
e This quality control range is applicable only to *H. influenzae* ATCC 49247 tested by a microdilution procedure using HTM[1].

Diffusion Techniques
Quantitative methods that require measurement of zone diameters also provide reproducible estimates of the susceptibility of bacteria to antimicrobial compounds. The zone size provides an estimate of the susceptibility of bacteria to antimicrobial compounds. The zone size should be determined using a standardized method.[2,3] The procedure uses paper disks impregnated with 15 mcg of clarithromycin to test the susceptibility of bacteria. The disk diffusion interpretive criteria are provided below.

Susceptibility Test Interpretive Criteria for *Staphylococcus aureus*

Zone diameter (mm)	Interpretation
≥ 18	Susceptible (S)
14 to 17	Intermediate (I)
≤ 13	Resistant (R)

Susceptibility Test Interpretive Criteria for *Streptococcus pyogenes* and *Streptococcus pneumoniae*[f]

Zone diameter (mm)	Interpretation
≥ 21	Susceptible (S)
17 to 20	Intermediate (I)
≤ 16	Resistant (R)

f These zone diameter standards only apply to tests performed using Mueller-Hinton agar supplemented with 5% sheep blood incubated in 5% CO_2.

For testing *Haemophilus* spp.[g]

Zone diameter (mm)	Interpretation
≥ 13	Susceptible (S)
11 to 12	Intermediate (I)
≤ 10	Resistant (R)

g These zone diameter standards are applicable only to tests with *Haemophilus* spp. using HTM[2].

Note: When testing *Streptococcus pyogenes* and *Streptococcus pneumoniae*, susceptibility and resistance to clarithromycin can be predicted using erythromycin.

Quality Control

Standardized susceptibility test procedures require the use of laboratory control bacteria to monitor and ensure the accuracy and precision of supplies and reagents in the assay, and the techniques of the individual performing the test.[2,3] For the diffusion technique using the 15 mcg disk, the criteria in the following table should be achieved.

Acceptable Quality Control Ranges for Clarithromycin

QC Strain		Zone diameter (mm)
S. aureus	ATCC 25923	26 to 32
S. pneumoniae[h]	ATCC 49619	25 to 31
Haemophilus influenzae[i]	ATCC 49247	11 to 17

h This quality control range is applicable only to tests performed by disk diffusion using Mueller-Hinton agar supplemented with 5% defibrinated sheep blood.
i This quality control limit applies to tests conducted with *Haemophilus influenzae* ATCC 49247 using HTM[2].

In vitro Activity of Clarithromycin against Mycobacteria
Clarithromycin has demonstrated *in vitro* activity against *Mycobacterium avium* complex (MAC) microorganisms isolated from both AIDS and non-AIDS patients. While gene probe techniques may be used to distinguish *M. avium* species from *M. intracellulare*, many studies only reported results on *M. avium* complex (MAC) isolates.
Various *in vitro* methodologies employing broth or solid media at different pH's, with and without oleic acid-albumin-dextrose-catalase (OADC), have been used to determine clarithromycin MIC values for mycobacterial species. In general, MIC values decrease more than 16-fold as the pH of Middlebrook 7H12 broth media increases from 5.0 to 7.4. At pH 7.4, MIC values determined with Mueller-Hinton agar were 4- to 8-fold higher than those observed with Middlebrook 7H12 media. Utilization of oleic acid-albumin-dextrose-catalase (OADC) in these assays has been shown to further alter MIC values.
Clarithromycin activity against 80 MAC isolates from AIDS patients and 211 MAC isolates from non-AIDS patients was evaluated using a microdilution method with Middlebrook 7H9 broth. Results showed an MIC value of ≤ 4.0 mcg/mL in 81% and 89% of the AIDS and non-AIDS MAC isolates, respectively. Twelve percent of the non-AIDS isolates had an MIC value ≤ 0.5 mcg/mL. Clarithromycin was also shown to be active against phagocytized *M. avium* complex (MAC) in mouse and human macrophage cell cultures as well as in the beige mouse infection model.
Clarithromycin activity was evaluated against *Mycobacterium tuberculosis* microorganisms. In one study utilizing the agar dilution method with Middlebrook 7H10 media, 3 of 30 clinical isolates had an MIC of 2.5 mcg/mL. Clarithromycin inhibited all isolates at > 10.0 mcg/mL.
Susceptibility Testing for *Mycobacterium avium* Complex (MAC)
The disk diffusion and dilution techniques for susceptibility testing against gram-positive and gram-negative bacteria should not be used for determining clarithromycin MIC values against mycobacteria. *In vitro* susceptibility testing methods and diagnostic products currently available for determining minimum inhibitory concentration (MIC) values against *Mycobacterium avium* complex (MAC) organisms have not been standardized or validated. Clarithromycin MIC values will vary depending on the susceptibility testing method employed, composition and pH of the media, and the utilization of nutritional supplements. Breakpoints to determine whether clinical isolates of *M. avium* or *M. intracellulare* are susceptible or resistant to clarithromycin have not been established.
Susceptibility Test for *Helicobacter pylori*
The reference methodology for susceptibility testing of *H. pylori* is agar dilution MICs.[4] One to three microliters of an inoculum equivalent to a No. 2 McFarland standard (1×10^7-1×10^8 CFU/mL for *H. pylori*) are inoculated directly onto freshly prepared antimicrobial containing Mueller-Hinton agar plates with 5% aged defibrinated sheep blood (> 2-weeks old). The agar dilution plates are incubated at 35°C in a microaerobic environment produced by a gas generating system suitable for *Campylobacter* species. After 3 days of incubation, the MICs are recorded as the lowest concentration of antimicrobial agent required to inhibit growth of the organism. The clarithromycin and amoxicillin MIC values should be interpreted according to the following criteria:

Susceptibility Test Interpretive Criteria for *H. pylori*

Clarithromycin MIC (mcg/mL)[j]	Interpretation
≤ 0.25	Susceptible (S)
0.5	Intermediate (I)
≥ 1.0	Resistant (R)

Susceptibility Test Interpretive Criteria for *H. pylori*

Amoxicillin MIC (mcg/mL)[j,k]	Interpretation
< 0.25	Susceptible (S)

j These are tentative breakpoints for the agar dilution methodology, and should not be used to interpret results obtained using alternative methods.
k There were not enough organisms with MICs > 0.25 mcg/mL to determine a resistance breakpoint.

Standardized susceptibility test procedures require the use of laboratory control bacteria to monitor and ensure the accuracy and precision of supplies and reagents in the assay, and the techniques of the individual performing the test. Standard clarithromycin or amoxicillin powder should provide the following MIC ranges.

Acceptable Quality Control Ranges		Antimicrobial Agent	MIC (mcg/mL)[l]
H. pylori	ATCC 43504	Clarithromycin	0.015-0.12 mcg/mL
H. pylori	ATCC 43504	Amoxicillin	0.015-0.12 mcg/mL

l These are quality control ranges for the agar dilution methodology and should not be used to control test results obtained using alternative methods.

INDICATIONS AND USAGE

BIAXIN Filmtab (clarithromycin tablets, USP) and BIAXIN Granules (clarithromycin for oral suspension, USP) are indicated for the treatment of mild to moderate infections caused by susceptible isolates of the designated bacteria in the conditions as listed below:
Adults (BIAXIN Filmtab Tablets and Granules for Oral Suspension)
Pharyngitis/Tonsillitis due to *Streptococcus pyogenes* (The usual drug of choice in the treatment and prevention of streptococcal infections and the prophylaxis of rheumatic fever is penicillin administered by either the intramuscular or the oral route. Clarithromycin is generally effective in the eradication of *S. pyogenes* from the nasopharynx; however, data establishing the efficacy of clarithromycin in the subsequent prevention of rheumatic fever are not available at present).
Acute maxillary sinusitis due to *Haemophilus influenzae*, *Moraxella catarrhalis*, or *Streptococcus pneumoniae*.
Acute bacterial exacerbation of chronic bronchitis due to *Haemophilus influenzae*, *Haemophilus parainfluenzae*, *Moraxella catarrhalis*, or *Streptococcus pneumoniae*.
Community-Acquired Pneumonia due to *Haemophilus influenzae*, *Mycoplasma pneumoniae*, *Streptococcus pneumoniae*, or *Chlamydophila pneumoniae* (TWAR).
Uncomplicated skin and skin structure infections due to *Staphylococcus aureus*, or *Streptococcus pyogenes* (Abscesses usually require surgical drainage).
Disseminated mycobacterial infections due to *Mycobacterium avium*, or *Mycobacterium intracellulare*
BIAXIN (clarithromycin) Filmtab tablets in combination with amoxicillin and PREVACID (lansoprazole) or PRILOSEC (omeprazole) Delayed-Release Capsules, as triple therapy, are indicated for the treatment of patients with *Helicobacter pylori* infection and duodenal ulcer disease (active or five-year history of duodenal ulcer) to eradicate *H. pylori*.
BIAXIN Filmtab tablets in combination with PRILOSEC (omeprazole) capsules or TRITEC (ranitidine bismuth citrate) tablets are also indicated for the treatment of patients with an active duodenal ulcer associated with *H. pylori* infection. However, regimens which contain clarithromycin as the single antimicrobial agent are more likely to be associated with the development of clarithromycin resistance among patients who fail therapy. Clarithromycin-containing regimens should not be used in patients with known or suspected clarithromycin resistant isolates because the efficacy of treatment is reduced in this setting.
In patients who fail therapy, susceptibility testing should be done if possible. If resistance to clarithromycin is demonstrated, a non-clarithromycin-containing therapy is recommended. (For information on development of resistance see **Microbiology** section.) The eradication of *H. pylori* has been demonstrated to reduce the risk of duodenal ulcer recurrence.
Children (BIAXIN Filmtab Tablets and Granules for Oral Suspension)
Pharyngitis/Tonsillitis due to *Streptococcus pyogenes*.
Community-Acquired Pneumonia due to *Mycoplasma pneumoniae*, *Streptococcus pneumoniae*, or *Chlamydophila pneumoniae* (TWAR)
Acute maxillary sinusitis due to *Haemophilus influenzae*, *Moraxella catarrhalis*, or *Streptococcus pneumoniae*
Acute otitis media due to *Haemophilus influenzae*, *Moraxella catarrhalis*, or *Streptococcus pneumoniae*
NOTE: For information on otitis media, see **CLINICAL STUDIES - Otitis Media.**
Uncomplicated skin and skin structure infections due to *Staphylococcus aureus*, or *Streptococcus pyogenes* (Abscesses usually require surgical drainage.)
Disseminated mycobacterial infections due to *Mycobacterium avium*, or *Mycobacterium intracellulare*
Adults (BIAXIN XL Filmtab Tablets)
BIAXIN XL Filmtab (clarithromycin extended-release tablets) are indicated for the treatment of adults with mild to moderate infection caused by susceptible strains of the designated microorganisms in the conditions listed below:
Acute maxillary sinusitis due to *Haemophilus influenzae*, *Moraxella catarrhalis*, or *Streptococcus pneumoniae*
Acute bacterial exacerbation of chronic bronchitis due to *Haemophilus influenzae*, *Haemophilus parainfluenzae*, *Moraxella catarrhalis*, or *Streptococcus pneumoniae*
Community-Acquired Pneumonia due to *Haemophilus influenzae*, *Haemophilus parainfluenzae*, *Moraxella catarrhalis*, *Streptococcus pneumoniae*, *Chlamydophila pneumoniae* (TWAR), or *Mycoplasma pneumoniae*
THE EFFICACY AND SAFETY OF BIAXIN XL IN TREATING OTHER INFECTIONS FOR WHICH OTHER FORMULATIONS OF BIAXIN ARE APPROVED HAVE NOT BEEN ESTABLISHED.
Prophylaxis
BIAXIN Filmtab tablets and BIAXIN Granules for oral suspension are indicated for the prevention of disseminated *Mycobacterium avium* complex (MAC) disease in patients with advanced HIV infection.
To reduce the development of drug-resistant bacteria and maintain the effectiveness of BIAXIN and other antibacterial drugs, BIAXIN should be used only to treat or prevent infections that are proven or strongly suspected to be caused by susceptible bacteria. When culture and susceptibility information are available, they should be considered in selecting or modifying antibacterial therapy. In the absence of such data, local epidemiology and susceptibility patterns may contribute to the empiric selection of therapy.

CONTRAINDICATIONS

Clarithromycin is contraindicated in patients with a known hypersensitivity to clarithromycin or any of its excipients, erythromycin, or any of the macrolide antibiotics.
Clarithromycin is contraindicated in patients with a history of cholestatic jaundice/hepatic dysfunction associated with prior use of clarithromycin.
Concomitant administration of clarithromycin and any of the following drugs is contraindicated: cisapride, pimozide, astemizole, terfenadine, and ergotamine or dihydroergotamine (see **Drug Interactions**). There have been postmarketing reports of drug interactions when clarithromycin and/or erythromycin are coadministered with cisapride, pimozide, astemizole, or terfenadine resulting in cardiac arrhythmias (QT prolongation, ventricular tachycardia, ventricular fibrillation, and torsades de pointes) most likely due to inhibition of metabolism of these drugs by erythromycin and clarithromycin. Fatalities have been reported.
Concomitant administration of clarithromycin and colchicine is contraindicated in patients with renal or hepatic impairment.
Clarithromycin should not be given to patients with history of QT prolongation or ventricular cardiac arrhythmia, including *torsades de pointes*.
Clarithromycin should not be used concomitantly with HMG-CoA reductase inhibitors (statins) that are extensively metabolized by CYP3A4 (lovastatin or simvastatin), due to the increased risk of myopathy, including rhabdomyolysis (see **WARNINGS**).
For information about contraindications of other drugs indicated in combination with BIAXIN, refer to the **CONTRAINDICATIONS** section of their package inserts.

Information on the AbbVie, Inc. products listed on these pages is from the prescribing information in use as of July 31, 2014. For more information, please visit rxabbvie.com or call 1-800-633-9110.

WARNINGS

Use In Pregnancy

CLARITHROMYCIN SHOULD NOT BE USED IN PREGNANT WOMEN EXCEPT IN CLINICAL CIRCUMSTANCES WHERE NO ALTERNATIVE THERAPY IS APPROPRIATE. IF PREGNANCY OCCURS WHILE TAKING THIS DRUG, THE PATIENT SHOULD BE APPRISED OF THE POTENTIAL HAZARD TO THE FETUS. CLARITHROMYCIN HAS DEMONSTRATED ADVERSE EFFECTS OF PREGNANCY OUTCOME AND/OR EMBRYO-FETAL DEVELOPMENT IN MONKEYS, RATS, MICE, AND RABBITS AT DOSES THAT PRODUCED PLASMA LEVELS 2 TO 17 TIMES THE SERUM LEVELS ACHIEVED IN HUMANS TREATED AT THE MAXIMUM RECOMMENDED HUMAN DOSES (see PRECAUTIONS - Pregnancy).

Hepatotoxicity

Hepatic dysfunction, including increased liver enzymes, and hepatocellular and/or cholestatic hepatitis, with or without jaundice, has been reported with clarithromycin. This hepatic dysfunction may be severe and is usually reversible. In some instances, hepatic failure with fatal outcome has been reported and generally has been associated with serious underlying diseases and/or concomitant medications. Symptoms of hepatitis can include anorexia, jaundice, dark urine, pruritus, or tender abdomen. Discontinue clarithromycin immediately if signs and symptoms of hepatitis occur.

QT Prolongation

Clarithromycin has been associated with prolongation of the QT interval and infrequent cases of arrhythmia. Cases of *torsades de pointes* have been spontaneously reported during postmarketing surveillance in patients receiving clarithromycin. Fatalities have been reported. Clarithromycin should be avoided in patients with ongoing proarrhythmic conditions such as uncorrected hypokalemia or hypomagnesemia, clinically significant bradycardia (see CONTRAINDICATIONS) and in patients receiving Class IA (quinidine, procainamide) or Class III (dofetilide, amiodarone, sotalol) antiarrhythmic agents. Elderly patients may be more susceptible to drug-associated effects on the QT interval.

Drug Interactions

Serious adverse reactions have been reported in patients taking clarithromycin concomitantly with CYP3A4 substrates. These include colchicine toxicity with colchicine; rhabdomyolysis with simvastatin, lovastatin, and atorvastatin; and hypotension with calcium channel blockers metabolized by CYP3A4 (e.g., verapamil, amlodipine, diltiazem) (see CONTRAINDICATIONS and PRECAUTIONS - Drug Interactions). Clarithromycin should be used with caution when administered concurrently with medications that induce the cytochrome CYP3A4 enzyme (see PRECAUTIONS - Drug Interactions).

Colchicine

Life-threatening and fatal drug interactions have been reported in patients treated with clarithromycin and colchicine. Clarithromycin is a strong CYP3A4 inhibitor and this interaction may occur while using both drugs at their recommended doses. If co-administration of clarithromycin and colchicine is necessary in patients with normal renal and hepatic function, the dose of colchicine should be reduced. Patients should be monitored for clinical symptoms of colchicine toxicity. Concomitant administration of clarithromycin and colchicine is contraindicated in patients with renal or hepatic impairment (see CONTRAINDICATIONS and PRECAUTIONS - Drug Interactions).

Benzodiazepines

Increased sedation and prolongation of sedation have been reported with concomitant administration of clarithromycin and triazolobenzodiazepines, such as triazolam, and midazolam.

Oral Hypoglycemic Agents/Insulin

The concomitant use of clarithromycin and oral hypoglycemic agents and/or insulin can result in significant hypoglycemia. With certain hypoglycemic drugs such as nateglinide, pioglitazone, repaglinide and rosiglitazone, inhibition of CYP3A enzyme by clarithromycin may be involved and could cause hypoglycemia when used concomitantly. Careful monitoring of glucose is recommended.

Oral Anticoagulants

There is a risk of serious hemorrhage and significant elevations in INR and prothrombin time when clarithromycin is co-administered with warfarin. INR and prothrombin times should be frequently monitored while patients are receiving clarithromycin and oral anticoagulants concurrently.

HMG-CoA Reductase Inhibitors (statins)

Concomitant use of clarithromycin with lovastatin or simvastatin is contraindicated (see CONTRAINDICATIONS) as these statins are extensively metabolized by CYP3A4, and concomitant treatment with clarithromycin increases their plasma concentration, which increases the risk of myopathy, including rhabdomyolysis. Cases of rhabdomyolysis have been reported in patients taking clarithromycin concomitantly with these statins. If treatment with clarithromycin cannot be avoided, therapy with lovastatin or simvastatin must be suspended during the course of treatment.

Caution should be exercised when prescribing clarithromycin with statins. In situations where the concomitant use of clarithromycin with atorvastatin or pravastatin cannot be avoided, atorvastatin dose should not exceed 20 mg daily and pravastatin dose should not exceed 40 mg daily. Use of a statin that is not dependent on CYP3A metabolism (e.g. fluvastatin) can be considered. It is recommended to prescribe the lowest registered dose if concomitant use cannot be avoided.

Clostridium difficile Associated Diarrhea

Clostridium difficile associated diarrhea (CDAD) has been reported with use of nearly all antibacterial agents, including BIAXIN, and may range in severity from mild diarrhea to fatal colitis. Treatment with antibacterial agents alters the normal flora of the colon leading to overgrowth of *C. difficile*.

C. difficile produces toxins A and B which contribute to the development of CDAD. Hypertoxin producing strains of *C. difficile* cause increased morbidity and mortality, as these infections can be refractory to antimicrobial therapy and may require colectomy. CDAD must be considered in all patients who present with diarrhea following antibiotic use. Careful medical history is necessary since CDAD has been reported to occur over two months after the administration of antibacterial agents.

If CDAD is suspected or confirmed, ongoing antibiotic use not directed against *C. difficile* may need to be discontinued. Appropriate fluid and electrolyte management, protein supplementation, antibiotic treatment of *C. difficile*, and surgical evaluation should be instituted as clinically indicated.

Acute Hypersensitivity Reactions

In the event of severe acute hypersensitivity reactions, such as anaphylaxis, Stevens-Johnson Syndrome, toxic epidermal necrolysis, drug rash with eosinophilia and systemic symptoms (DRESS), and Henoch-Schonlein purpura clarithromycin therapy should be discontinued immediately and appropriate treatment should be urgently initiated.

Combination Therapy with Other Drugs

For information about warnings of other drugs indicated in combination with BIAXIN, refer to the WARNINGS section of their package inserts.

PRECAUTIONS

General

Prescribing BIAXIN in the absence of a proven or strongly suspected bacterial infection or a prophylactic indication is unlikely to provide benefit to the patient and increases the risk of the development of drug-resistant bacteria.

Clarithromycin is principally excreted via the liver and kidney. Clarithromycin may be administered without dosage adjustment to patients with hepatic impairment and normal renal function. However, in the presence of severe renal impairment with or without coexisting hepatic impairment, decreased dosage or prolonged dosing intervals may be appropriate.

Clarithromycin in combination with ranitidine bismuth citrate therapy is not recommended in patients with creatinine clearance less than 25 mL/min (see DOSAGE AND ADMINISTRATION).

Clarithromycin in combination with ranitidine bismuth citrate should not be used in patients with a history of acute porphyria.

Exacerbation of symptoms of myasthenia gravis and new onset of symptoms of myasthenic syndrome has been reported in patients receiving clarithromycin therapy.

For information about precautions of other drugs indicated in combination with BIAXIN, refer to the PRECAUTIONS section of their package inserts.

Information to Patients

Patients should be counseled that antibacterial drugs including BIAXIN should only be used to treat bacterial infections. They do not treat viral infections (e.g., the common cold). When BIAXIN is prescribed to treat a bacterial infection, patients should be told that although it is common to feel better early in the course of therapy, the medication should be taken exactly as directed. Skipping doses or not completing the full course of therapy may (1) decrease the effectiveness of the immediate treatment and (2) increase the likelihood that bacteria will develop resistance and will not be treatable by BIAXIN or other antibacterial drugs in the future.

Diarrhea is a common problem caused by antibiotics which usually ends when the antibiotic is discontinued. Sometimes after starting treatment with antibiotics, patients can develop watery and bloody stools (with or without stomach cramps and fever) even as late as two or more months after having taken the last dose of the antibiotic. If this occurs, patients should contact their physician as soon as possible. BIAXIN may interact with some drugs; therefore patients should be advised to report to their doctor the use of any other medications.

BIAXIN tablets and oral suspension can be taken with or without food and can be taken with milk; however, BIAXIN XL tablets should be taken with food. Do NOT refrigerate the suspension.

Drug Interactions

Clarithromycin use in patients who are receiving theophylline may be associated with an increase of serum theophylline concentrations. Monitoring of serum theophylline concentrations should be considered for patients receiving high doses of theophylline or with baseline concentrations in the upper therapeutic range. In two studies in which theophylline was administered with clarithromycin (a theophylline sustained-release formulation was dosed at either 6.5 mg/kg or 12 mg/kg together with 250 or 500 mg q12h clarithromycin), the steady-state levels of C_{max}, C_{min}, and the area under the serum concentration time curve (AUC) of theophylline increased about 20%.

Hypotension, bradyarrhythmias, and lactic acidosis have been observed in patients receiving concurrent verapamil, belonging to the calcium channel blockers drug class.

Concomitant administration of single doses of clarithromycin and carbamazepine has been shown to result in increased plasma concentrations of carbamazepine. Blood level monitoring of carbamazepine may be considered.

When clarithromycin and terfenadine were coadministered, plasma concentrations of the active acid metabolite of terfenadine were threefold higher, on average, than the values observed when terfenadine was administered alone. The pharmacokinetics of clarithromycin and the 14-OH-clarithromycin were not significantly affected by coadministration of terfenadine once clarithromycin reached steady-state conditions. Concomitant administration of clarithromycin with terfenadine is contraindicated (see CONTRAINDICATIONS).

Clarithromycin 500 mg every 8 hours was given in combination with omeprazole 40 mg daily to healthy adult subjects. The steady-state plasma concentrations of omeprazole were increased (C_{max}, AUC_{0-24}, and $t_{1/2}$ increases of 30%, 89%, and 34%, respectively), by the concomitant administration of clarithromycin. The mean 24-hour gastric pH value was 5.2 when omeprazole was administered alone and 5.7 when coadministered with clarithromycin.

Coadministration of clarithromycin with ranitidine bismuth citrate resulted in increased plasma ranitidine concentrations (57%), increased plasma bismuth trough concentrations (48%), and increased 14-hydroxy-clarithromycin plasma concentrations (31%). These effects are clinically insignificant.

Simultaneous oral administration of BIAXIN tablets and zidovudine to HIV-infected adult patients may result in decreased steady-state zidovudine concentrations. Following administration of clarithromycin 500 mg tablets twice daily with zidovudine 100 mg every 4 hours, the steady-state zidovudine AUC decreased 12% compared to administration of zidovudine alone (n=4). Individual values ranged from a decrease of 34% to an increase of 14%. When clarithromycin tablets were administered two to four hours prior to zidovudine, the steady-state zidovudine C_{max} increased 100% whereas the AUC was unaffected (n=24). Administration of clarithromycin and zidovudine should be separated by at least two hours. The impact of co-administration of clarithromycin extended-release tablets and zidovudine has not been evaluated.

Simultaneous administration of BIAXIN tablets and didanosine to 12 HIV-infected adult patients resulted in no statistically significant change in didanosine pharmacokinetics.

Following administration of fluconazole 200 mg daily and clarithromycin 500 mg twice daily to 21 healthy volunteers, the steady-state clarithromycin C_{min} and AUC increased 33% and 18%, respectively. Steady-state concentrations of 14-OH clarithromycin were not significantly affected by concomitant administration of fluconazole. No dosage adjustment of clarithromycin is necessary when co-administered with fluconazole.

Ritonavir

Concomitant administration of clarithromycin and ritonavir (n = 22) resulted in a 77% increase in clarithromycin AUC and a 100% decrease in the AUC of 14-OH clarithromycin. Clarithromycin may be administered without dosage adjustment to patients with normal renal function taking ritonavir. Since concentrations of 14-OH clarithromycin are significantly reduced when clarithromycin is co-administered with ritonavir, alternative antibacterial therapy should be considered for indications other than infections due to *Mycobacterium avium* complex (see PRECAUTIONS - Drug Interactions). Doses of clarithromycin greater than 1000 mg per day should not be co-administered with protease inhibitors.

Spontaneous reports in the post-marketing period suggest that concomitant administration of clarithromycin and oral anticoagulants may potentiate the effects of the oral anticoagulants. Prothrombin times should be carefully monitored while patients are receiving clarithromycin and oral anticoagulants simultaneously.

Digoxin is a substrate for P-glycoprotein (Pgp) and clarithromycin is known to inhibit Pgp. When clarithromycin and digoxin are co-administered, inhibition of Pgp by clarithromycin may lead to increased exposure of digoxin. Elevated digoxin serum concentrations in patients receiving clarithromycin and digoxin concomitantly have been reported in post-marketing surveillance. Some patients have shown clinical signs consistent with digoxin toxicity, including potentially fatal arrhythmias. Monitoring of serum digoxin concentrations should be considered, especially for patients with digoxin concentrations in the upper therapeutic range.

Co-administration of clarithromycin, known to inhibit CYP3A, and a drug primarily metabolized by CYP3A may be associated with elevations in drug concentrations that could increase or prolong both therapeutic and adverse effects of the concomitant drug.

Clarithromycin should be used with caution in patients receiving treatment with other drugs known to be CYP3A enzyme substrates, especially if the CYP3A substrate has a narrow safety margin (e.g., carbamazepine) and/or the substrate is extensively metabolized by this enzyme. Dosage adjustments may be considered, and when possible, serum concentrations of drugs primarily metabolized by CYP3A should be monitored closely in patients concurrently receiving clarithromycin.

The following are examples of some clinically significant CYP3A based drug interactions. Interactions with other drugs metabolized by the CYP3A isoform are also possible.

Carbamazepine and Terfenadine
Increased serum concentrations of carbamazepine and the active acid metabolite of terfenadine were observed in clinical trials with clarithromycin.

Colchicine
Colchicine is a substrate for both CYP3A and the efflux transporter, P-glycoprotein (Pgp). Clarithromycin and other macrolides are known to inhibit CYP3A and Pgp. When a single dose of colchicine 0.6 mg was administered with clarithromycin 250 mg BID for 7 days, the colchicine C_{max} increased 197% and the $AUC_{0-\infty}$ increased 239% compared to administration of colchicine alone. The dose of colchicine should be reduced when co-administered with clarithromycin in patients with normal renal and hepatic function. Concomitant use of clarithromycin and colchicine is contraindicated in patients with renal or hepatic impairment (see **WARNINGS**).

Efavirenz, Nevirapine, Rifampicin, Rifabutin, and Rifapentine
Inducers of CYP3A enzymes, such as efavirenz, nevirapine, rifampicin, rifabutin, and rifapentine will increase the metabolism of clarithromycin, thus decreasing plasma concentrations of clarithromycin, while increasing those of 14-OH-clarithromycin. Since the microbiological activities of clarithromycin and 14-OH-clarithromycin are different for different bacteria, the intended therapeutic effect could be impaired during concomitant administration of clarithromycin and enzyme inducers. Alternative antibacterial treatment should be considered when treating patients receiving inducers of CYP3A. Concomitant administration of rifabutin and clarithromycin resulted in an increase in rifabutin, and decrease in clarithromycin serum levels together with an increased risk of uveitis.

Etravirine
Clarithromycin exposure was decreased by etravirine; however, concentrations of the active metabolite, 14-OH-clarithromycin, were increased. Because 14-OH-clarithromycin has reduced activity against *Mycobacterium avium* complex (MAC), overall activity against this pathogen may be altered; therefore alternatives to clarithromycin should be considered for the treatment of MAC.

Sildenafil, Tadalafil, and Vardenafil
Each of these phosphodiesterase inhibitors is primarily metabolized by CYP3A, and CYP3A will be inhibited by concomitant administration of clarithromycin. Co-administration of clarithromycin with sildenafil, tadalafil, or vardenafil will result in increased exposure of these phosphodiesterase inhibitors. Co-administration of these phosphodiesterase inhibitors with clarithromycin is not recommended.

Tolterodine
The primary route of metabolism for tolterodine is via CYP2D6. However, in a subset of the population devoid of CYP2D6, the identified pathway of metabolism is via CYP3A. In this population subset, inhibition of CYP3A results in significantly higher serum concentrations of tolterodine. Tolterodine 1 mg twice daily is recommended in patients deficient in CYP2D6 activity (poor metabolizers) when co-administered with clarithromycin.

Triazolobenzodiazepines (e.g., alprazolam, midazolam, triazolam)
When a single dose of midazolam was co-administered with clarithromycin tablets (500 mg twice daily for 7 days), midazolam AUC increased 174% after intravenous administration of midazolam and 600% after oral administration.

When oral midazolam is co-administered with clarithromycin, dose adjustments may be necessary and possible prolongation and intensity of effect should be anticipated. Caution and appropriate dose adjustments should be considered when triazolam or alprazolam is co-administered with clarithromycin. For benzodiazepines which are not metabolized by CYP3A (e.g., temazepam, nitrazepam, lorazepam), a clinically important interaction with clarithromycin is unlikely.

There have been post-marketing reports of drug interactions and central nervous system (CNS) effects (e.g., somnolence and confusion) with the concomitant use of clarithromycin and triazolam. Monitoring the patient for increased CNS pharmacological effects is suggested.

Atazanavir
Both clarithromycin and atazanavir are substrates and inhibitors of CYP3A, and there is evidence of a bi-directional drug interaction. Following administration of clarithromycin (500 mg twice daily) with atazanavir (400 mg once daily), the clarithromycin AUC increased 94%, the 14-OH clarithromycin AUC decreased 70% and the atazanavir AUC increased 28%. When clarithromycin is co-administered with atazanavir, the dose of clarithromycin should be decreased by 50%. Since concentrations of 14-OH clarithromycin are significantly reduced when clarithromycin is co-administered with atazanavir, alternative antibacterial therapy should be considered for indications other than infections due to *Mycobacterium avium* complex (see **PRECAUTIONS - Drug Interactions**). Doses of clarithromycin greater than 1000 mg per day should not be co-administered with protease inhibitors.

Itraconazole
Both clarithromycin and itraconazole are substrates and inhibitors of CYP3A, potentially leading to a bi-directional drug interaction when administered concomitantly. Clarithromycin may increase the plasma concentrations of itraconazole, while itraconazole may increase the plasma concentrations of clarithromycin. Patients taking itraconazole and clarithromycin concomitantly should be monitored closely for signs or symptoms of increased or prolonged adverse reactions.

Saquinavir
Both clarithromycin and saquinavir are substrates and inhibitors of CYP3A and there is evidence of a bi-directional drug interaction. Following administration of clarithromycin (500 mg bid) and saquinavir (soft gelatin capsules, 1200 mg tid) to 12 healthy volunteers, the steady-state saquinavir AUC and C_{max} increased 177% and 187% respectively compared to administration of saquinavir alone. Clarithromycin AUC and C_{max} increased 45% and 39% respectively, whereas the 14–OH clarithromycin AUC and C_{max} decreased 24% and 34% respectively, compared to administration with clarithromycin alone. No dose adjustment of clarithromycin is necessary when clarithromycin is co-administered with saquinavir in patients with normal renal function. When saquinavir is co-administered with ritonavir, consideration should be given to the potential effects of ritonavir on clarithromycin (refer to interaction between clarithromycin and ritonavir) (see **PRECAUTIONS - Drug Interactions**).

The following CYP3A based drug interactions have been observed with erythromycin products and/or with clarithromycin in post-marketing experience:

Antiarrhythmics
There have been post-marketing reports of torsades de pointes occurring with concurrent use of clarithromycin and quinidine or disopyramide. Electrocardiograms should be monitored for QTc prolongation during coadministration of clarithromycin with these drugs. Serum concentrations of these medications should also be monitored.

Ergotamine/Dihydroergotamine
Post-marketing reports indicate that coadministration of clarithromycin with ergotamine or dihydroergotamine has been associated with acute ergot toxicity characterized by vasospasm and ischemia of the extremities and other tissues including the central nervous system. Concomitant administration of clarithromycin with ergotamine or dihydroergotamine is contraindicated (see **CONTRAINDICATIONS**).

Triazolobenzodiazepines (Such as Triazolam and Alprazolam) and Related Benzodiazepines (Such as Midazolam)
Erythromycin has been reported to decrease the clearance of triazolam and midazolam, and thus, may increase the pharmacologic effect of these benzodiazepines. There have been post-marketing reports of drug interactions and CNS effects (e.g., somnolence and confusion) with the concomitant use of clarithromycin and triazolam.

Sildenafil (Viagra)
Erythromycin has been reported to increase the systemic exposure (AUC) of sildenafil. A similar interaction may occur with clarithromycin; reduction of sildenafil dosage should be considered. (See Viagra package insert.)

There have been spontaneous or published reports of CYP3A based interactions of erythromycin and/or clarithromycin with cyclosporine, carbamazepine, tacrolimus, alfentanil, disopyramide, rifabutin, quinidine, methylprednisolone, cilostazol, bromocriptine, vinblastine, phenobarbital and St. John's Wort.

Concomitant administration of clarithromycin with cisapride, pimozide, astemizole, or terfenadine is contraindicated (see **CONTRAINDICATIONS**).

In addition, there have been reports of interactions of erythromycin or clarithromycin with drugs not thought to be metabolized by CYP3A, including hexobarbital, phenytoin, and valproate.

Carcinogenesis, Mutagenesis, Impairment of Fertility
The following *in vitro* mutagenicity tests have been conducted with clarithromycin:
Salmonella/Mammalian Microsomes Test
Bacterial Induced Mutation Frequency Test
In Vitro Chromosome Aberration Test
Rat Hepatocyte DNA Synthesis Assay
Mouse Lymphoma Assay
Mouse Dominant Lethal Study
Mouse Micronucleus Test

All tests had negative results except the *In Vitro* Chromosome Aberration Test which was weakly positive in one test and negative in another.

In addition, a Bacterial Reverse-Mutation Test (Ames Test) has been performed on clarithromycin metabolites with negative results.

Fertility and reproduction studies have shown that daily doses of up to 160 mg/kg/day (1.3 times the recommended maximum human dose based on mg/m^2) to male and female rats caused no adverse effects on the estrous cycle, fertility, parturition, or number and viability of offspring. Plasma levels in rats after 150 mg/kg/day were 2 times the human serum levels.

In the 150 mg/kg/day monkey studies, plasma levels were 3 times the human serum levels. When given orally at 150 mg/kg/day (2.4 times the recommended maximum human dose based on mg/m^2), clarithromycin was shown to produce embryonic loss in monkeys. This effect has been attributed to marked maternal toxicity of the drug at this high dose.

In rabbits, *in utero* fetal loss occurred at an intravenous dose of 33 mg/m^2, which is 17 times less than the maximum proposed human oral daily dose of 618 mg/m^2.

Long-term studies in animals have not been performed to evaluate the carcinogenic potential of clarithromycin.

Pregnancy
Teratogenic Effects
Pregnancy Category C
Four teratogenicity studies in rats (three with oral doses and one with intravenous doses up to 160 mg/kg/day administered during the period of major organogenesis) and two in rabbits at oral doses up to 125 mg/kg/day (approximately 2 times the recommended maximum human dose based on mg/m^2) or intravenous doses of 30 mg/kg/day administered during gestation days 6 to 18 failed to demonstrate any teratogenicity from clarithromycin. Two additional oral studies in a different rat strain at similar doses and similar conditions demonstrated a low incidence of cardiovascular anomalies at doses of 150 mg/kg/day administered during gestation days 6 to 15. Plasma levels after 150 mg/kg/day were 2 times the human serum levels. Four studies in mice revealed a variable incidence of cleft palate following oral doses of 1000 mg/kg/day (2 and 4 times the recommended maximum human dose based on mg/m^2, respectively) during gestation days 6 to 15. Cleft palate was also seen at 500 mg/kg/day. The 1000 mg/kg/day exposure resulted in plasma levels 17 times the human serum levels. In monkeys, an oral dose of 70 mg/kg/day (an approximate equidose of the recommended maximum human dose based on mg/m^2) produced fetal growth retardation at plasma levels that were 2 times the human serum levels.

There are no adequate and well-controlled studies in pregnant women. Clarithromycin should be used during pregnancy only if the potential benefit justifies the potential risk to the fetus (see **WARNINGS**).

Nursing Mothers
Clarithromycin and its active metabolite 14-hydroxy clarithromycin are excreted in human milk. Serum and milk samples were obtained after 3 days of treatment, at steady state, from one published study of 12 lactating women who were taking clarithromycin 250 mg orally twice daily. Based on the limited data from this study, and assuming milk consumption of 150 mL/kg/day, an exclusively human milk fed infant would receive an estimated average of

Information on the AbbVie, Inc. products listed on these pages is from the prescribing information in use as of July 31, 2014. For more information, please visit rxabbvie.com or call 1-800-633-9110.

ADULT DOSAGE GUIDELINES

Infection	BIAXIN Tablets Dosage (q12h)	Duration (days)	BIAXIN XL Tablets Dosage (q24h)	Duration (days)
Pharyngitis/Tonsillitis due to				
S. pyogenes	250 mg	10	-	-
Acute maxillary sinusitis due to	500 mg	14	2 × 500 mg	14
H. influenzae				
M. catarrhalis				
S. pneumoniae				
Acute exacerbation of chronic bronchitis due to				
H. influenzae	500 mg	7-14	2 × 500 mg	7
H. parainfluenzae	500 mg	7	2 × 500 mg	7
M. catarrhalis	250 mg	7-14	2 × 500 mg	7
S. pneumoniae	250 mg	7-14	2 × 500 mg	7
Community-Acquired Pneumonia due to				
H. influenzae	250 mg	7	2 × 500 mg	7
H. parainfluenzae	-	-	2 × 500 mg	7
M. catarrhalis	-	-	2 × 500 mg	7
S. pneumoniae	250 mg	7-14	2 × 500 mg	7
C. pneumoniae	250 mg	7-14	2 × 500 mg	7
M. pneumoniae	250 mg	7-14	2 × 500 mg	7
Uncomplicated skin and skin structure	250 mg	7-14	-	-
S. aureus				
S. pyogenes				

136 mcg/kg/day of clarithromycin and its active metabolite, with this maternal dosage regimen. This is less than 2% of the maternal weight-adjusted dose (7.8 mg/kg/day, based on the average maternal weight of 64 kg), and less than 1% of the pediatric dose (15 mg/kg/day) for children greater than 6 months of age.

A prospective observational study of 55 breastfed infants of mothers taking a macrolide antibiotic (6 were exposed to clarithromycin) were compared to 36 breastfed infants of mothers taking amoxicillin. Adverse reactions were comparable in both groups. Adverse reactions occurred in 12.7% of infants exposed to macrolides and included rash, diarrhea, loss of appetite, and somnolence.

Caution should be exercised when clarithromycin is administered to nursing women. The development and health benefits of human milk feeding should be considered along with the mother's clinical need for Biaxin and any potential adverse effects on the human milk fed child from the drug or from the underlying maternal condition.

Pediatric Use

Safety and effectiveness of clarithromycin in pediatric patients under 6 months of age have not been established. The safety of clarithromycin has not been studied in MAC patients under the age of 20 months. Neonatal and juvenile animals tolerated clarithromycin in a manner similar to adult animals. Young animals were slightly more intolerant to acute overdosage and to subtle reductions in erythrocytes, platelets and leukocytes but were less sensitive to toxicity in the liver, kidney, thymus, and genitalia.

Geriatric Use

In a steady-state study in which healthy elderly subjects (age 65 to 81 years old) were given 500 mg every 12 hours, the maximum serum concentrations and area under the curves of clarithromycin and 14-OH clarithromycin were increased compared to those achieved in healthy young adults. These changes in pharmacokinetics parallel known age-related decreases in renal function. In clinical trials, elderly patients did not have an increased incidence of adverse events when compared to younger patients. Dosage adjustment should be considered in elderly patients with severe renal impairment. Elderly patients may be more susceptible to development of *torsades de pointes* arrhythmias than younger patients (see **WARNINGS** and **PRECAUTIONS**).

ADVERSE REACTIONS

The most frequent and common adverse reactions related to clarithromycin therapy for both adult and pediatric populations are abdominal pain, diarrhea, nausea, vomiting and dysgeusia. These adverse reactions are consistent with the known safety profile of macrolide antibiotics.

There was no significant difference in the incidence of these gastrointestinal adverse reactions during clinical trials between the patient population with or without preexisting mycobacterial infections.

Adverse Reactions Observed During Clinical Trials of Clarithromycin

The following adverse reactions were observed in clinical trials with clarithromycin at a rate greater than or equal to 1%:

Gastrointestinal Disorders

Diarrhea, vomiting, dyspepsia, nausea, abdominal pain

Hepatobiliary Disorders

Liver function test abnormal

Immune System Disorders

Anaphylactoid reaction

Infection and Infestations

Candidiasis

Nervous System Disorders

Dysgeusia, headache

Psychiatric Disorders

Insomnia

Skin and Subcutaneous Tissue Disorders

Rash

Other Adverse Reactions Observed During Clinical Trials of Clarithromycin

The following adverse reactions were observed in clinical trials with clarithromycin at a rate less than 1%:

Blood and Lymphatic System Disorders

Leukopenia, neutropenia, thrombocythemia, eosinophilia

Cardiac Disorders

Electrocardiogram QT prolonged, cardiac arrest, atrial fibrillation, extrasystoles, palpitations

Ear and Labyrinth Disorders

Vertigo, tinnitus, hearing impaired

Gastrointestinal Disorders

Stomatitis, glossitis, esophagitis, gastrooesophageal reflux disease, gastritis, proctalgia, abdominal distension, constipation, dry mouth, eructation, flatulence

General Disorders and Administration Site Conditions

Malaise, pyrexia, asthenia, chest pain, chills, fatigue

Hepatobiliary Disorders

Cholestasis, hepatitis

Immune System Disorders

Hypersensitivity

Infections and Infestations

Cellulitis, gastroenteritis, infection, vaginal infection

Investigations

Blood bilirubin increased, blood alkaline phosphatase increased, blood lactate dehydrogenase increased, albumin globulin ratio abnormal

Metabolism and Nutrition Disorders

Anorexia, decreased appetite

Musculoskeletal and Connective Tissue Disorders

Myalgia, muscle spasms, nuchal rigidity

Nervous System Disorders

Dizziness, tremor, loss of consciousness, dyskinesia, somnolence

Psychiatric Disorders

Anxiety, nervousness

Renal and Urinary Disorders

Blood creatinine increased, blood urea increased

Respiratory, Thoracic and Mediastinal Disorders

Asthma, epistaxis, pulmonary embolism

Skin and Subcutaneous Tissue Disorders

Urticaria, dermatitis bullous, pruritus, hyperhidrosis, rash maculo-papular

In the acute exacerbation of chronic bronchitis and acute maxillary sinusitis studies overall gastrointestinal adverse events were reported by a similar proportion of patients taking either BIAXIN tablets or BIAXIN XL tablets; however, patients taking BIAXIN XL tablets reported significantly less severe gastrointestinal symptoms compared to patients taking BIAXIN tablets. In addition, patients taking BIAXIN XL tablets had significantly fewer premature discontinuations for drug-related gastrointestinal or abnormal taste adverse events compared to BIAXIN tablets.

In community-acquired pneumonia studies conducted in adults comparing clarithromycin to erythromycin base or erythromycin stearate, there were fewer adverse events involving the digestive system in clarithromycin-treated patients compared to erythromycin-treated patients (13% vs 32%; p < 0.01). Twenty percent of erythromycin-treated patients discontinued therapy due to adverse events compared to 4% of clarithromycin-treated patients.

In two U.S. studies of acute otitis media comparing clarithromycin to amoxicillin/potassium clavulanate in pediatric patients, there were fewer adverse events involving the digestive system in clarithromycin-treated patients compared to amoxicillin/potassium clavulanate-treated patients (21% vs. 40%, p < 0.001). One-third as many clarithromycin-treated patients reported diarrhea as did amoxicillin/potassium clavulanate-treated patients.

Post-Marketing Experience

The following adverse reactions have been identified during post approval use of clarithromycin. Because these reactions are reported voluntarily from a population of uncertain size, it is not always possible to reliably estimate their frequency or establish a causal relationship to drug exposure.

Blood and Lymphatic System Disorders

Thrombocytopenia, agranulocytosis

Cardiac Disorders

Torsades de pointes, ventricular tachycardia, ventricular arrhythmia

Ear and Labyrinth Disorders

Deafness was reported chiefly in elderly women and was usually reversible.

Gastrointestinal Disorders

Pancreatitis acute, tongue discoloration, tooth discoloration was reported and was usually reversible with professional cleaning upon discontinuation of the drug. There have been reports of BIAXIN XL tablets in the stool, many of which have occurred in patients with anatomic (including ileostomy or colostomy) or functional gastrointestinal disorders with shortened GI transit times. In several reports, tablet residues have occurred in the context of diarrhea. It is recommended that patients who experience tablet residue in the stool and no improvement in their condition should be switched to a different clarithromycin formulation (e.g. suspension) or another antibacterial drug.

Hepatobiliary Disorders

Hepatic failure, jaundice hepatocellular. Adverse reactions related to hepatic dysfunction have been reported with clarithromycin (see **WARNINGS - Hepatotoxicity**).

Immune System Disorders

Anaphylactic reaction

Infections and Infestations

Pseudomembranous colitis

Investigations

Prothrombin time prolonged, white blood cell count decreased, international normalized ratio increased. Abnormal urine color has been reported, associated with hepatic failure.

Metabolism and Nutrition Disorders

Hypoglycemia has been reported in patients taking oral hypoglycemic agents or insulin.

Musculoskeletal and Connective Tissue Disorders

Myopathy, rhabdomyolysis was reported and in some of the reports, clarithromycin was administered concomitantly with statins, fibrates, colchicine or allopurinol (see **CONTRAINDICATIONS** and **WARNINGS**).

Nervous System Disorders

Convulsion, ageusia, parosmia, anosmia, paraesthesia

Psychiatric Disorders

Psychotic disorder, confusional state, depersonalization, depression, disorientation, manic behavior, hallucination, abnormal behavior, abnormal dreams. These disorders usually resolve upon discontinuation of the drug.

There are no data on the effect of clarithromycin on the ability to drive or use machines. The potential for dizziness, vertigo, confusion and disorientation, which may occur with the medication, should be taken into account before patients drive or use machines.

Renal and Urinary Disorders

Nephritis interstitial, renal failure

Skin and Subcutaneous Tissue Disorders

Stevens-Johnson syndrome, toxic epidermal necrolysis, drug rash with eosinophilia and systemic symptoms (DRESS), Henoch-Schonlein purpura, acne

Vascular Disorders

Hemorrhage

There have been reports of colchicine toxicity with concomitant use of clarithromycin and colchicine, especially in the elderly, some of which occurred in patients with renal insufficiency. Deaths have been reported in some such patients (see **WARNINGS** and **PRECAUTIONS**).

OVERDOSAGE

Overdosage of clarithromycin can cause gastrointestinal symptoms such as abdominal pain, vomiting, nausea, and diarrhea.

Adverse reactions accompanying overdosage should be treated by the prompt elimination of unabsorbed drug and supportive measures. As with other macrolides, clarithromycin serum concentrations are not expected to be appreciably affected by hemodialysis or peritoneal dialysis.

DOSAGE AND ADMINISTRATION

BIAXIN® Filmtab (clarithromycin tablets, USP) and BIAXIN® Granules (clarithromycin for oral suspension, USP) may be given with or without food. BIAXIN® XL Filmtab® (clarithromycin extended-release tablets) should be taken with food. BIAXIN XL tablets should be swallowed whole and not chewed, broken or crushed.

Clarithromycin may be administered without dosage adjustment in the presence of hepatic impairment if there is normal renal function. In patients with severe renal impairment ($CL_{CR} < 30$ mL/min), the dose of clarithromycin should be reduced by 50%. However, when patients with moderate or severe renal impairment are taking clarithromycin concomitantly with atazanavir or ritonavir, the dose of clarithromycin should be reduced by 50% or 75% for patients with CL_{CR} of 30 to 60 mL/min or < 30 mL/min, respectively.

[See table at top of previous page]

H. pylori Eradication to Reduce the Risk of Duodenal Ulcer Recurrence

Triple therapy: BIAXIN/lansoprazole/amoxicillin
The recommended adult dose is 500 mg BIAXIN, 30 mg lansoprazole, and 1 gram amoxicillin, all given twice daily (q12h) for 10 or 14 days (see **INDICATIONS AND USAGE** and **CLINICAL STUDIES** sections).

Triple therapy: BIAXIN/omeprazole/amoxicillin
The recommended adult dose is 500 mg BIAXIN, 20 mg omeprazole, and 1 gram amoxicillin, all given twice daily (q12h) for 10 days (see **INDICATIONS AND USAGE** and **CLINICAL STUDIES** sections). In patients with an ulcer present at the time of initiation of therapy, an additional 18 days of omeprazole 20 mg once daily is recommended for ulcer healing and symptom relief.

Dual therapy: BIAXIN/omeprazole
The recommended adult dose is 500 mg BIAXIN given three times daily (q8h) and 40 mg omeprazole given once daily (qAM) for 14 days (see **INDICATIONS AND USAGE** and **CLINICAL STUDIES** sections). An additional 14 days of omeprazole 20 mg once daily is recommended for ulcer healing and symptom relief.

Dual therapy: BIAXIN/ranitidine bismuth citrate
The recommended adult dose is 500 mg BIAXIN given twice daily (q12h) or three times daily (q8h) and 400 mg ranitidine bismuth citrate given twice daily (q12h) for 14 days. An additional 14 days of 400 mg twice daily is recommended for ulcer healing and symptom relief. BIAXIN and ranitidine bismuth citrate combination therapy is not recommended in patients with creatinine clearance less than 25 mL/min (see **INDICATIONS AND USAGE** and **CLINICAL STUDIES** sections).

Children
The usual recommended daily dosage is 15 mg/kg/day divided q12h for 10 days.

PEDIATRIC DOSAGE GUIDELINES

Weight		Dose (q12h)	Based on Body Weight Dosing Calculated on 7.5 mg/kg q12h	
Kg	lbs		125 mg/5 mL	250 mg/5 mL
9	20	62.5 mg	2.5 mL q12h	1.25 mL q12h
17	37	125 mg	5 mL q12h	2.5 mL q12h
25	55	187.5 mg	7.5 mL q12h	3.75 mL q12h
33	73	250 mg	10 mL q12h	5 mL q12h

Mycobacterial Infections
Prophylaxis
The recommended dose of BIAXIN for the prevention of disseminated *Mycobacterium avium* disease is 500 mg b.i.d. In children, the recommended dose is 7.5 mg/kg b.i.d. up to 500 mg b.i.d. No studies of clarithromycin for MAC prophylaxis have been performed in pediatric populations and the doses recommended for prophylaxis are derived from MAC treatment studies in children. Dosing recommendations for children are in the table above.
Treatment
Clarithromycin is recommended as the primary agent for the treatment of disseminated infection due to *Mycobacterium avium* complex. Clarithromycin should be used in combination with other antimycobacterial drugs that have shown *in vitro* activity against MAC or clinical benefit in MAC treatment (see **CLINICAL STUDIES**). The recommended dose for mycobacterial infections in adults is 500 mg b.i.d. In children, the recommended dose is 7.5 mg/kg b.i.d. up to 500 mg b.i.d. Dosing recommendations for children are in the table above.
Clarithromycin therapy should continue if clinical response is observed. Clarithromycin can be discontinued when the patient is considered at low risk of disseminated infection.

Total Volume After Constitution	Clarithromycin Concentration After Constitution	Clarithromycin Contents Per Bottle	NDC
50 mL	125 mg/5 mL	1250 mg	0074-3163-50
100 mL	125 mg/5 mL	2500 mg	0074-3163-13
50 mL	250 mg/5 mL	2500 mg	0074-3188-50
100 mL	250 mg/5 mL	5000 mg	0074-3188-13

Constituting Instructions
The table below indicates the volume of water to be added when constituting:

Total Volume After Constitution	Clarithromycin Concentration After Constitution	Amount of Water to be Added*
50 mL	125 mg/5 mL	27 mL
100 mL	125 mg/5 mL	55 mL
50 mL	250 mg/5 mL	27 mL
100 mL	250 mg/5 mL	55 mL

* see instructions below.

Add half the volume of water to the bottle and shake vigorously. Add the remainder of water to the bottle and shake. Shake well before each use. Oversize bottle provides shake space. Keep tightly closed. Do not refrigerate. After mixing, store below 25°C (77°F) and use within 14 days.

HOW SUPPLIED
BIAXIN® Filmtab® (clarithromycin tablets, USP) are supplied as yellow oval film-coated tablets in the following packaging sizes:
250 mg tablets: (imprinted in blue with the "a" logo and code KT)
Bottles of 60 (**NDC** 0074-3368-60) and unit dose strip packages of 100 (**NDC** 0074-3368-11).
Store BIAXIN 250 mg tablets at controlled room temperature 15° to 30°C (59° to 86°F) in a well-closed container. Protect from light.
500 mg tablets: (debossed with the "a" logo on one side and code KL on the opposite side)
Bottles of 60 (**NDC** 0074-2586-60) and unit dose strip packages of 100 (**NDC** 0074-2586-11).
Store BIAXIN 500 mg tablets at controlled room temperature 20° to 25°C (68° to 77°F) in a well-closed container.
BIAXIN® XL Filmtab® (clarithromycin extended-release tablets) are supplied as yellow oval film-coated 500 mg tablets debossed (on one side) with the "a" logo and a two-letter code designation, KJ in the following packaging sizes:
500 mg tablets:
Bottles of 60 (**NDC** 0074-3165-60), unit dose strip packages of 100 (**NDC** 0074-3165-11), and BIAXIN® XL PAC carton of 4 blister packages 14 tablets each (**NDC** 0074-3165-41).
Store BIAXIN XL tablets at 20° to 25°C (68° to 77°F). Excursions permitted to 15° to 30°C (59° to 86°F). [See USP Controlled Room Temperature.]
BIAXIN® Granules (clarithromycin for oral suspension, USP) is supplied in the following strengths and sizes:
[See table above]
Store BIAXIN granules for oral suspension below 25°C (77°F) in a well-closed container. Do not refrigerate BIAXIN suspension.

CLINICAL STUDIES
Mycobacterial Infections
Prophylaxis
A randomized, double-blind study (561) compared clarithromycin 500 mg b.i.d. to placebo in patients with CDC-defined AIDS and CD_4 counts < 100 cells/µL. This study accrued 682 patients from November 1992 to January 1994, with a median CD_4 cell count at study entry of 30 cells/µL. Median duration of clarithromycin was 10.6 months vs. 8.2 months for placebo. More patients in the placebo arm than the clarithromycin arm discontinued prematurely from the study (75.6% and 67.4%, respectively). However, if premature discontinuations due to MAC or death are excluded, approximately equal percentages of patients on each arm (54.8% on clarithromycin and 52.5% on placebo) discontinued study drug early for other reasons. The study was designed to evaluate the following endpoints:
1. MAC bacteremia, defined as at least one positive culture for *M. avium* complex bacteria from blood or another normally sterile site.
2. Survival.
3. Clinically significant disseminated MAC disease, defined as MAC bacteremia accompanied by signs or symptoms of serious MAC infection, including fever, night sweats, weight loss, anemia, or elevations in liver function tests.
MAC Bacteremia
In patients randomized to clarithromycin, the risk of MAC bacteremia was reduced by 69% compared to placebo. The

difference between groups was statistically significant (p < 0.001). On an intent-to-treat basis, the one-year cumulative incidence of MAC bacteremia was 5.0% for patients randomized to clarithromycin and 19.4% for patients randomized to placebo. While only 19 of the 341 patients randomized to clarithromycin developed MAC, 11 of these cases were resistant to clarithromycin. The patients with resistant MAC bacteremia had a median baseline CD_4 count of 10 cells/mm³ (range 2 to 25 cells/mm³). Information regarding the clinical course and response to treatment of the patients with resistant MAC bacteremia is limited. The 8 patients who received clarithromycin and developed susceptible MAC bacteremia had a median baseline CD_4 count of 25 cells/mm³ (range 10 to 80 cells/mm³). Comparatively, 53 of the 341 placebo patients developed MAC; none of these isolates were resistant to clarithromycin. The median baseline CD_4 count was 15 cells/mm³ (range 2 to 130 cells/mm³) for placebo patients that developed MAC.
Survival
A statistically significant survival benefit was observed.

Survival All Randomized Patients

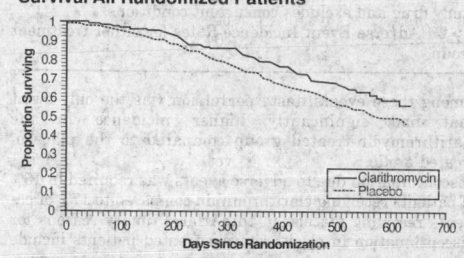

		Mortality	Reduction in Mortality on Clarithromycin
	Placebo	Clarithromycin	
6 month	9.4%	6.5%	31%
12 month	29.7%	20.5%	31%
18 month	46.4%	37.5%	20%

Since the analysis at 18 months includes patients no longer receiving prophylaxis the survival benefit of clarithromycin may be underestimated.
Clinically Significant Disseminated MAC Disease
In association with the decreased incidence of bacteremia, patients in the group randomized to clarithromycin showed reductions in the signs and symptoms of disseminated MAC disease, including fever, night sweats, weight loss, and anemia.
Safety
In AIDS patients treated with clarithromycin over long periods of time for prophylaxis against *M. avium*, it was often difficult to distinguish adverse events possibly associated with clarithromycin administration from underlying HIV disease or intercurrent illness. Median duration of treatment was 10.6 months for the clarithromycin group and 8.2 months for the placebo group.

Treatment-related* Adverse Event Incidence Rates (%) in Immunocompromised Adult Patients Receiving Prophylaxis Against *M. avium* Complex

Body System‡ Adverse Event	Clarithromycin (n = 339) %	Placebo (n = 339) %
Body as a Whole		
Abdominal pain	5.0%	3.5%
Headache	2.7%	0.9%
Digestive		
Diarrhea	7.7%	4.1%
Dyspepsia	3.8%	2.7%

Information on the AbbVie, Inc. products listed on these pages is from the prescribing information in use as of July 31, 2014. For more information, please visit rxabbvie.com or call 1-800-633-9110.

b.i.d. dose (mg)	Resolution of Fever		
	% ever afebrile	% afebrile ≥ 6 weeks	
500	67%	23%	
1000	67%	12%	
2000	62%	22%	

b.i.d. dose (mg)	Resolution of Night Sweats	
	% ever resolving	% resolving ≥ 6 weeks
500	85%	42%
1000	70%	33%
2000	72%	36%

b.i.d. dose (mg)	Weight Gain > 3%	
	% ever gaining	% gaining ≥ 6 weeks
500	33%	14%
1000	26%	17%
2000	26%	12%

b.i.d. dose (mg)	Hemoglobin Increase > 1 gm	
	% ever increasing	% increasing ≥ 6 weeks
500	58%	26%
1000	37%	6%
2000	62%	18%

Flatulence	2.4%	0.9%
Nausea	11.2%	7.1%
Vomiting	5.9%	3.2%
Skin & Appendages		
Rash	3.2%	3.5%
Special Senses		
Taste Perversion	8.0%	0.3%

* Includes those events possibly or probably related to study drug and excludes concurrent conditions.
‡ > 2% Adverse Event Incidence Rates for either treatment group.

Among these events, taste perversion was the only event that had significantly higher incidence in the clarithromycin-treated group compared to the placebo-treated group.

Discontinuation due to adverse events was required in 18% of patients receiving clarithromycin compared to 17% of patients receiving placebo in this trial. Primary reasons for discontinuation in clarithromycin treated patients include headache, nausea, vomiting, depression and taste perversion.

Changes in Laboratory Values of Potential Clinical Importance
In immunocompromised patients receiving prophylaxis against *M. avium*, evaluations of laboratory values were made by analyzing those values outside the seriously abnormal value (i.e., the extreme high or low limit) for the specified test.

Percentage of Patients[a] Exceeding Extreme Laboratory Value in Patients Receiving Prophylaxis Against *M. avium* Complex

		Clarithromycin 500 mg b.i.d.	Placebo
Hemoglobin	< 8 g/dL	4/118 3%	5/103 5%
Platelet Count	< 50 × 10⁹/L	11/249 4%	12/250 5%
WBC Count	< 1 × 10⁹/L	2/103 4%	0/95 0%
SGOT	> 5 × ULN[b]	7/196 4%	5/208 2%
SGPT	> 5 × ULN[b]	6/217 3%	4/232 2%
Alk. Phos.	> 5 × ULN[b]	5/220 2%	5/218 2%

(a) Includes only patients with baseline values within the normal range or borderline high (hematology variables) and within the normal range or borderline low (chemistry variables).
(b) ULN = Upper Limit of Normal

Treatment
Three randomized studies (500, 577, and 521) compared different dosages of clarithromycin in patients with CDC-defined AIDS and CD₄ counts < 100 cells/µL. These studies accrued patients from May 1991 to March 1992. Study 500 was randomized, double-blind; Study 577 was open-label compassionate use. Both studies used 500 and 1000 mg b.i.d. doses; Study 500 also had a 2000 mg b.i.d. group. Study 521 was a pediatric study at 3.75, 7.5, and 15 mg/kg b.i.d. Study 500 enrolled 154 adult patients, Study 577 enrolled 469 adult patients, and Study 521 enrolled 25 patients between the ages of 1 to 20. The majority of patients had CD₄ cell counts < 50/µL at study entry. The studies were designed to evaluate the following end points:
1. Change in MAC bacteremia or blood cultures negative for *M. avium*.
2. Change in clinical signs and symptoms of MAC infection including one or more of the following: fever, night sweats, weight loss, diarrhea, splenomegaly, and hepatomegaly.

The results for the 500 study are described below. The 577 study results were similar to the results of the 500 study. Results with the 7.5 mg/kg b.i.d. dose in the pediatric study were comparable to those for the 500 mg b.i.d. regimen in the adult studies.

Study 069 compared the safety and efficacy of clarithromycin in combination with ethambutol versus clarithromycin in combination with ethambutol and clofazimine for the treatment of disseminated MAC (dMAC) infection.[4,5] This 24-week study enrolled 106 patients with AIDS and dMAC, with 55 patients randomized to receive clarithromycin and ethambutol, and 51 patients randomized to receive clarithromycin, ethambutol, and clofazimine. Baseline characteristics between study arms were similar with the exception of median CFU counts being at least 1 log higher in the clarithromycin, ethambutol, and clofazimine arm.

Compared to prior experience with clarithromycin monotherapy, the two-drug regimen of clarithromycin and ethambutol was well tolerated and extended the time to microbiologic relapse, largely through suppressing the emergence of clarithromycin resistant strains. However, the addition of clofazimine to the regimen added no additional microbiologic or clinical benefit. Tolerability of both multidrug regimens was comparable with the most common adverse events being gastrointestinal in nature. Patients receiving the clofazimine-containing regimen had reduced survival rates; however, their baseline mycobacterial colony counts were higher. The results of this trial support the addition of ethambutol to clarithromycin for the treatment of initial dMAC infections but do not support adding clofazimine as a third agent.

MAC Bacteremia
Decreases in MAC bacteremia or negative blood cultures were seen in the majority of patients in all dose groups. Mean reductions in colony forming units (CFU) are shown below. Included in the table are results from a separate study with a four drug regimen[6] (ciprofloxacin, ethambutol, rifampicin, and clofazimine). Since patient populations and study procedures may vary between these two studies, comparisons between the clarithromycin results and the combination therapy results should be interpreted cautiously.

Mean Reductions in Log CFU from Baseline (After 4 Weeks of Therapy)

500 mg b.i.d. (N = 35)	1000 mg b.i.d. (N = 32)	2000 mg b.i.d. (N = 26)	Four Drug Regimen (N = 24)
1.5	2.3	2.3	1.4

Although the 1000 mg and 2000 mg b.i.d. doses showed significantly better control of bacteremia during the first four weeks of therapy, no significant differences were seen beyond that point. The percent of patients whose blood was sterilized as shown by one or more negative cultures at any time during acute therapy was 61% (30/49) for the 500 mg b.i.d. group and 59% (29/49) and 52% (25/48) for the 1000 and 2000 mg b.i.d. groups, respectively. The percent of patients who had 2 or more negative cultures during acute therapy that were sustained through study Day 84 was 25% (12/49) in both the 500 and 1000 mg b.i.d. groups and 8% (4/48) for the 2000 mg b.i.d. group. By Day 84, 23% (11/49), 37% (18/49), and 56% (27/48) of patients had died or discontinued from the study, and 14% (7/49), 12% (6/49), and 13% (6/48) of patients had relapsed in the 500, 1000, and 2000 mg b.i.d. dose groups, respectively. All of the isolates had an MIC < 8 mcg/mL at pre-treatment. Relapse was almost always accompanied by an increase in MIC. The median time to first negative culture was 54, 41, and 29 days for the 500, 1000, and 2000 mg b.i.d. groups, respectively.

The time to first decrease of at least 1 log in CFU count was significantly shorter with the 1000 and 2000 mg b.i.d. doses (median equal to 16 and 15 days, respectively) in comparison to the 500 mg b.i.d. group (median equal to 29 days). The median time to first positive culture or study discontinuation following the first negative culture was 43, 59 and 43 days for the 500, 1000, and 2000 mg b.i.d. groups, respectively.
Clinically Significant Disseminated MAC Disease
Among patients experiencing night sweats prior to therapy, 84% showed resolution or improvement at some point during the 12 weeks of clarithromycin at 500 to 2000 mg b.i.d. doses. Similarly, 77% of patients reported resolution or improvement in fevers at some point. Response rates for clinical signs of MAC are given below:
[See first table above]
[See second table above]
The median duration of response, defined as improvement or resolution of clinical signs and symptoms, was 2 to 6 weeks.
Since the study was not designed to determine the benefit of monotherapy beyond 12 weeks, the duration of response may be underestimated for the 25 to 33% of patients who continued to show clinical response after 12 weeks.
Survival
Median survival time from study entry (Study 500) was 249 days at the 500 mg b.i.d. dose compared to 215 days with the 1000 mg b.i.d. dose. However, during the first 12 weeks of therapy, there were 2 deaths in 53 patients in the 500 mg b.i.d. group versus 13 deaths in 51 patients in the 1000 mg b.i.d. group. The reason for this apparent mortality difference is not known. Survival in the two groups was similar beyond 12 weeks. The median survival times for these dosages were similar to recent historical controls with MAC when treated with combination therapies.[6]
Median survival time from study entry in Study 577 was 199 days for the 500 mg b.i.d. dose and 179 days for the 1000 mg b.i.d. dose. During the first four weeks of therapy, while patients were maintained on their originally assigned dose, there were 11 deaths in 255 patients taking 500 mg b.i.d. and 18 deaths in 214 patients taking 1000 mg b.i.d.
Safety
The adverse event profiles showed that both the 500 and 1000 mg b.i.d. doses were well tolerated. The 2000 mg b.i.d. dose was poorly tolerated and resulted in a higher proportion of premature discontinuations.
In AIDS patients and other immunocompromised patients treated with the higher doses of clarithromycin over long periods of time for mycobacterial infections, it was often difficult to distinguish adverse events possibly associated with clarithromycin administration from underlying signs of HIV disease or intercurrent illness.
The following analyses summarize experience during the first 12 weeks of therapy with clarithromycin. Data are reported separately for Study 500 (randomized, double-blind) and Study 577 (open-label, compassionate use) and also combined. Adverse events were reported less frequently in Study 577, which may be due in part to differences in monitoring between the two studies. In adult patients receiving clarithromycin 500 mg b.i.d., the most frequently reported adverse events, considered possibly or probably related to study drug, with an incidence of 5% or greater, are listed below. Most of these events were mild to moderate in severity, although 5% (Study 500: 8%; Study 577: 4%) of patients receiving 500 mg b.i.d. and 5% (Study 500: 4%; Study 577: 6%) of patients receiving 1000 mg b.i.d. reported severe adverse events. Excluding those patients who discontinued therapy or died due to complications of their underlying non-mycobacterial disease, approximately 8% (Study 500: 15%; Study 577: 7%) of the patients who received 500 mg b.i.d. and 12% (Study 500: 14%; Study 577: 12%) of the patients who received 1000 mg b.i.d. discontinued therapy due to drug-related events during the first 12 weeks of therapy. Overall, the 500 and 1000 mg b.i.d. doses had similar adverse event profiles.

Treatment-related* Adverse Event Incidence Rates (%) in Immunocompromised Adult Patients During the First 12 Weeks of Therapy with 500 mg b.i.d. Clarithromycin Dose

Adverse Event	Study 500 (n = 53)	Study 577 (n = 255)	Combined (n = 308)
Abdominal Pain	7.5	2.4	3.2
Diarrhea	9.4	1.6	2.9
Flatulence	7.5	0.0	1.3
Headache	7.5	0.4	1.6
Nausea	28.3	9.0	12.3
Rash	9.4	2.0	3.2
Taste Perversion	18.9	0.4	3.6
Vomiting	24.5	3.9	7.5

* Includes those events possibly or probably related to study drug and excludes concurrent conditions.

Per-Protocol and Intent-to-Treat H. pylori Eradication Rates % of Patients Cured [95% Confidence Interval]

| | Clarithromycin + omeprazole + amoxicillin | | Clarithromycin + amoxicillin | |
	Per-Protocol [†]	Intent-to-Treat [‡]	Per-Protocol [†]	Intent-to-Treat [‡]
Study 126	*77 [64, 86] (n = 64)	69 [57, 79] (n = 80)	43 [31, 56] (n = 67)	37 [27, 48] (n = 84)
Study 127	*78 [67, 88] (n = 65)	73 [61, 82] (n = 77)	41 [29, 54] (n = 68)	36 [26, 47] (n = 84)
Study M96-446	*90 [80, 96] (n = 69)	83 [74, 91] (n = 84)	33 [24, 44] (n = 93)	32 [23, 42] (n = 99)

[†] Patients were included in the analysis if they had confirmed duodenal ulcer disease (active ulcer studies 126 and 127; history of ulcer within 5 years, study M96-446) and H. pylori infection at baseline defined as at least two of three positive endoscopic tests from CLOtest®, histology, and/or culture. Patients were included in the analysis if they completed the study. Additionally, if patients dropped out of the study due to an adverse event related to the study drug, they were included in the analysis as failures of therapy. The impact of eradication on ulcer recurrence has not been assessed in patients with a past history of ulcer.

[‡] Patients were included in the analysis if they had documented H. pylori infection at baseline and had confirmed duodenal ulcer disease. All dropouts were included as failures of therapy.

* p < 0.05 versus clarithromycin plus amoxicillin.

A limited number of pediatric AIDS patients have been treated with clarithromycin suspension for mycobacterial infections. The most frequently reported adverse events, excluding those due to the patient's concurrent condition, were consistent with those observed in adult patients.

Changes in Laboratory Values
In immunocompromised patients treated with clarithromycin for mycobacterial infections, evaluations of laboratory values were made by analyzing those values outside the seriously abnormal level (i.e., the extreme high or low limit) for the specified test.

Percentage of Patients[(a)] Exceeding Extreme Laboratory Value Limits During First 12 Weeks of Treatment 500 mg b.i.d. Dose[(b)]

		Study 500	Study 577	Combined
BUN	> 50 mg/dL	0%	< 1%	< 1%
Platelet Count	< 50 × 10⁹/L	0%	< 1%	< 1%
SGOT	> 5 × ULN[(c)]	0%	3%	2%
SGPT	> 5 × ULN[(c)]	0%	2%	1%
WBC	< 1 × 10⁹/L	0%	1%	1%

(a) Includes only patients with baseline values within the normal range or borderline high (hematology variables) and within the normal range or borderline low (chemistry variables)
(b) Includes all values within the first 12 weeks for patients who start on 500 mg b.i.d.
(c) ULN = Upper Limit of Normal

Otitis Media
In a controlled clinical study of acute otitis media performed in the United States, where significant rates of beta-lactamase producing organisms were found, clarithromycin was compared to an oral cephalosporin. In this study, very strict evaluability criteria were used to determine clinical response. For the 223 patients who were evaluated for clinical efficacy, the clinical success rate (i.e., cure plus improvement) at the post-therapy visit was 88% for clarithromycin and 91% for the cephalosporin.
In a smaller number of patients, microbiologic determinations were made at the pre-treatment visit. The following presumptive bacterial eradication/clinical cure outcomes (i.e., clinical success) were obtained:

U.S. Acute Otitis Media Study Clarithromycin vs. Oral Cephalosporin EFFICACY RESULTS

PATHOGEN	OUTCOME
S. pneumoniae	clarithromycin success rate, 13/15 (87%), control 4/5
H. influenzae*	clarithromycin success rate, 10/14 (71%), control 3/4
M. catarrhalis	clarithromycin success rate, 4/5, control 1/1
S. pyogenes	clarithromycin success rate, 3/3, control 0/1
Overall	clarithromycin success rate, 30/37 (81%), control 8/11 (73%)

* None of the H. influenzae isolated pre-treatment was resistant to clarithromycin; 6% were resistant to the control agent.

Safety
The incidence of adverse events in all patients treated, primarily diarrhea and vomiting, did not differ clinically or statistically for the two agents.

In two other controlled clinical trials of acute otitis media performed in the United States, where significant rates of beta-lactamase producing organisms were found, clarithromycin was compared to an oral antimicrobial agent that contained a specific beta-lactamase inhibitor. In these studies, very strict evaluability criteria were used to determine the clinical responses. In the 233 patients who were evaluated for clinical efficacy, the combined clinical success rate (i.e., cure and improvement) at the post-therapy visit was 91% for both clarithromycin and the control.
For the patients who had microbiologic determinations at the pre-treatment visit, the following presumptive bacterial eradication/clinical cure outcomes (i.e., clinical success) were obtained:

Two U.S. Acute Otitis Media Studies Clarithromycin vs. Antimicrobial/Beta-lactamase Inhibitor EFFICACY RESULTS

PATHOGEN	OUTCOME
S. pneumoniae	clarithromycin success rate, 43/51 (84%), control 55/56 (98%)
H. influenzae*	clarithromycin success rate, 36/45 (80%), control 31/33 (94%)
M. catarrhalis	clarithromycin success rate, 9/10 (90%), control 6/6
S. pyogenes	clarithromycin success rate, 3/3, control 5/5
Overall	clarithromycin success rate, 91/109 (83%), control 97/100 (97%)

* Of the H. influenzae isolated pre-treatment, 3% were resistant to clarithromycin and 10% were resistant to the control agent.

Safety
The incidence of adverse events in all patients treated, primarily diarrhea (15% vs. 38%) and diaper rash (3% vs. 11%) in young children, was clinically and statistically lower in the clarithromycin arm versus the control arm.

Duodenal Ulcer Associated with H. pylori Infection
Clarithromycin + Lansoprazole and Amoxicillin
H. pylori Eradication for Reducing the Risk of Duodenal Ulcer Recurrence
Two U.S. randomized, double-blind clinical studies in patients with H. pylori and duodenal ulcer disease (defined as an active ulcer or history of an active ulcer within one year) evaluated the efficacy of clarithromycin in combination with lansoprazole and amoxicillin capsules as triple 14-day therapy for eradication of H. pylori. Based on the results of these studies, the safety and efficacy of the following eradication regimen were established:
Triple therapy: BIAXIN (clarithromycin) 500 mg b.i.d. + lansoprazole 30 mg b.i.d. + amoxicillin 1 gm b.i.d.
Treatment was for 14 days. H. pylori eradication was defined as two negative tests (culture and histology) at 4 to 6 weeks following the end of treatment.
The combination of BIAXIN plus lansoprazole and amoxicillin as triple therapy was effective in eradicating H. pylori. Eradication of H. pylori has been shown to reduce the risk of duodenal ulcer recurrence.
A randomized, double-blind clinical study performed in the U.S. in patients with H. pylori and duodenal ulcer disease (defined as an active ulcer or history of an ulcer within one year) compared the efficacy of clarithromycin in combination with lansoprazole and amoxicillin as triple therapy for 10 and 14 days. This study established that the 10-day triple therapy was equivalent to the 14-day triple therapy in eradicating H. pylori.

H. pylori Eradication Rates-Triple Therapy (BIAXIN/lansoprazole/amoxicillin) Percent of Patients Cured [95% Confidence Interval] (number of patients)

Study	Duration	Triple Therapy Evaluable Analysis*	Triple Therapy Intent-to-Treat Analysis#
M93-131	14 days	92[†] [80.0-97.7] (n = 48)	86[†] [73.3-93.5] (n = 55)
M95-392	14 days	86[‡] [75.7-93.6] (n = 66)	83[‡] [72.0-90.8] (n = 70)
M95-399¶	14 days	85 [77.0-91.0] (N = 113)	82 [73.9-88.1] (N = 126)
	10 days	84 [76.0-89.8] (N = 123)	81 [73.9-87.6] (N = 135)

* Based on evaluable patients with confirmed duodenal ulcer (active or within one year) and H. pylori infection at baseline defined as at least two of three positive endoscopic tests from CLOtest (Delta West LTD., Bentley, Australia), histology, and/or culture. Patients were included in the analysis if they completed the study. Additionally, if patients were dropped out of the study due to an adverse event related to the study drug, they were included in the analysis as evaluable failures of therapy.
# Patients were included in the analysis if they had documented H. pylori infection at baseline as defined above and had a confirmed duodenal ulcer (active or within one year). All dropouts were included as failures of therapy.
[†] (p < 0.05) versus BIAXIN/lansoprazole and lansoprazole/amoxicillin dual therapy.
[‡] (p < 0.05) versus BIAXIN/amoxicillin dual therapy.
¶ The 95% confidence interval for the difference in eradication rates, 10-day minus 14-day, is (-10.5, 8.1) in the evaluable analysis and (-9.7, 9.1) in the intent-to-treat analysis.

Clarithromycin + Omeprazole and Amoxicillin Therapy
H. pylori Eradication for Reducing the Risk of Duodenal Ulcer Recurrence
Three U.S., randomized, double-blind clinical studies in patients with H. pylori infection and duodenal ulcer disease (n = 558) compared clarithromycin plus omeprazole and amoxicillin to clarithromycin plus amoxicillin. Two studies (Studies 126 and 127) were conducted in patients with an active duodenal ulcer, and the third study (Study 446) was conducted in patients with a duodenal ulcer in the past 5 years, but without an ulcer present at the time of enrollment. The dosage regimen in the studies was clarithromycin 500 mg b.i.d. plus omeprazole 20 mg b.i.d. plus amoxicillin 1 gram b.i.d. for 10 days. In Studies 126 and 127, patients who took the omeprazole regimen also received an additional 18 days of omeprazole 20 mg q.d. Endpoints studied were eradication of H. pylori and duodenal ulcer healing (studies 126 and 127 only). H. pylori status was determined by CLOtest®, histology, and culture in all three studies. For a given patient, H. pylori was considered eradicated if at least two of these tests were negative, and none was positive. The combination of clarithromycin plus omeprazole and amoxicillin was effective in eradicating H. pylori.
[See table above]
Safety
In clinical trials using combination therapy with clarithromycin plus omeprazole and amoxicillin, no adverse reactions peculiar to the combination of these drugs have been observed. Adverse reactions that have occurred have been limited to those that have been previously reported with clarithromycin, omeprazole, or amoxicillin.
The most frequent adverse experiences observed in clinical trials using combination therapy with clarithromycin plus omeprazole and amoxicillin (n = 274) were diarrhea (14%), taste perversion (10%), and headache (7%).
For information about adverse reactions with omeprazole or amoxicillin, refer to the **ADVERSE REACTIONS** section of their package inserts.
Clarithromycin + Omeprazole Therapy
Four randomized, double-blind, multi-center studies (067, 100, 812b, and 058) evaluated clarithromycin 500 mg t.i.d. plus omeprazole 40 mg q.d. for 14 days, followed by omeprazole 20 mg q.d. (067, 100, and 058) or by omeprazole 40 mg q.d. (812b) for an additional 14 days in patients with active duodenal ulcer associated with H. pylori. Studies 067 and 100 were conducted in the U.S. and Canada and enrolled

Information on the AbbVie, Inc. products listed on these pages is from the prescribing information in use as of July 31, 2014. For more information, please visit rxabbvie.com or call 1-800-633-9110.

H. pylori Eradication Rates in Study H2BA-3001

Analysis	RBC 400 mg + Clarithromycin 500 mg b.i.d.	RBC 400 mg + Clarithromycin 500 mg t.i.d.	95% CI Rate Difference
ITT	65% (122/188) [58%, 72%]	63% (122/195) [55%, 69%]	(-8%, 12%)
Per-Protocol	72% (117/162) [65%, 79%]	71% (120/170) [63%, 77%]	(-9%, 12%)

242 and 256 patients, respectively. H. pylori infection and duodenal ulcer were confirmed in 219 patients in Study 067 and 228 patients in Study 100. These studies compared the combination regimen to omeprazole and clarithromycin monotherapies. Studies 812b and 058 were conducted in Europe and enrolled 154 and 215 patients, respectively. H. pylori infection and duodenal ulcer were confirmed in 148 patients in Study 812b and 208 patients in Study 058. These studies compared the combination regimen to omeprazole monotherapy. The results for the efficacy analyses for these studies are described below.

Duodenal Ulcer Healing

The combination of clarithromycin and omeprazole was as effective as omeprazole alone for healing duodenal ulcer.

End-of-Treatment Ulcer Healing Rates Percent of Patients Healed (n/N)

Study	Clarithromycin + Omeprazole	Omeprazole	Clarithromycin
U.S. Studies			
Study 100	94% (58/62)[†]	88% (60/68)	71% (49/69)
Study 067	88% (56/64)[†]	85% (55/65)	64% (44/69)
Non-U.S. Studies			
Study 058	99% (84/85)	95% (82/86)	N/A
Study 812b[1]	100% (64/64)	99% (71/72)	N/A

[†] p < 0.05 for clarithromycin + omeprazole versus clarithromycin monotherapy.

[1] In Study 812b patients received omeprazole 40 mg daily for days 15 to 28.

Eradication of H. pylori Associated with Duodenal Ulcer
The combination of clarithromycin and omeprazole was effective in eradicating H. pylori.

H. pylori Eradication Rates (Per-Protocol Analysis) at 4 to 6 weeks Percent of Patients Cured (n/N)

Study	Clarithromycin + Omeprazole	Omeprazole	Clarithromycin
U.S. Studies			
Study 100	64% (39/61)[†‡]	0% (0/59)	39% (17/44)
Study 067	74% (39/53)[†‡]	0% (0/54)	31% (13/42)
Non-U.S. Studies			
Study 058	74% (64/86)[‡]	1% (1/90)	N/A
Study 812b	83% (50/60)[‡]	1% (1/74)	N/A

[†] Statistically significantly higher than clarithromycin monotherapy (p < 0.05).
[‡] Statistically significantly higher than omeprazole monotherapy (p < 0.05).

H. pylori eradication was defined as no positive test (culture or histology) at 4 weeks following the end of treatment, and two negative tests were required to be considered eradicated. In the per-protocol analysis, the following patients were excluded: dropouts, patients with major protocol violations, patients with missing H. pylori tests post-treatment, and patients that were not assessed for H. pylori eradication at 4 weeks after the end of treatment because they were found to have an unhealed ulcer at the end of treatment. Ulcer recurrence at 6-months following the end of treatment was assessed for patients in whom ulcers were healed post-treatment.

Ulcer Recurrence at 6 months by H. pylori Status at 4-6 Weeks

	H. pylori Negative	H. pylori Positive
U.S. Studies		
Study 100		
Clarithromycin + Omeprazole	6% (2/34)	56% (9/16)
Omeprazole	- (0/0)	71% (35/49)
Clarithromycin	12% (2/17)	32% (7/22)
Study 067		
Clarithromycin + Omeprazole	38% (11/29)	50% (6/12)
Omeprazole	- (0/0)	67% (31/46)
Clarithromycin	18% (2/11)	52% (14/27)
Non-U.S. Studies		
Study 058		
Clarithromycin + Omeprazole	6% (3/53)	24% (4/17)
Omeprazole	0% (0/3)	55% (39/71)
Study 812b*		
Clarithromycin + Omeprazole	5% (2/42)	0% (0/7)
Omeprazole	0% (0/1)	54% (32/59)
***12-month recurrence rates:**		
Clarithromycin + Omeprazole	3% (1/40)	0% (0/6)
Omeprazole	0% (0/1)	67% (29/43)

Thus, in patients with duodenal ulcer associated with H. pylori infection, eradication of H. pylori reduced ulcer recurrence.

Safety

The adverse event profiles for the four studies showed that the combination of clarithromycin 500 mg t.i.d. and omeprazole 40 mg q.d. for 14 days, followed by omeprazole 20 mg q.d. (067, 100, and 058) or 40 mg q.d. (812b) for an additional 14 days was well tolerated. Of the 346 patients who received the combination, 12 (3.5%) patients discontinued study drug due to adverse events.

Adverse Events with an Incidence of 3% or Greater

Adverse Event	Clarithromycin + Omeprazole (N = 346) % of Patients	Omeprazole (N = 355) % of Patients	Clarithromycin (N = 166) % of Patients*
Taste Perversion	15%	1%	16%
Nausea	5%	1%	3%
Headache	5%	6%	9%
Diarrhea	4%	3%	7%
Vomiting	4%	< 1%	1%
Abdominal Pain	3%	2%	1%
Infection	3%	4%	2%

* Studies 067 and 100, only.

Most of these events were mild to moderate in severity.
Changes in Laboratory Values

Changes in laboratory values with possible clinical significance in patients taking clarithromycin and omeprazole were as follows:

Hepatic - elevated direct bilirubin < 1%; GGT < 1%; SGOT (AST) < 1%; SGPT (ALT) < 1%.

Renal - elevated serum creatinine < 1%.

For information on omeprazole, refer to the **ADVERSE REACTIONS** section of the PRILOSEC package insert.
Clarithromycin + Ranitidine Bismuth Citrate Therapy
In a U.S. double-blind, randomized, multicenter, dose-comparison trial, ranitidine bismuth citrate 400 mg b.i.d. for 4 weeks plus clarithromycin 500 mg b.i.d. for the first 2 weeks was found to have an equivalent H. pylori eradication rate (based on culture and histology) when compared to ranitidine bismuth citrate 400 mg b.i.d. for 4 weeks plus clarithromycin 500 mg t.i.d. for the first 2 weeks. The intent-to-treat H. pylori eradication rates are shown below: [See table above]

H. pylori eradication was defined as no positive test at 4 weeks following the end of treatment. Patients must have had two tests performed, and these must have been negative to be considered eradicated of H. pylori. The following

patients were excluded from the per-protocol analysis: patients not infected with H. pylori prestudy, dropouts, patients with major protocol violations, patients with missing H. pylori tests. Patients excluded from the intent-to-treat analysis included those not infected with H. pylori prestudy and those with missing H. pylori tests prestudy. Patients were assessed for H. pylori eradication (4 weeks following treatment) regardless of their healing status (at the end of treatment).

The relationship between H. pylori eradication and duodenal ulcer recurrence was assessed in a combined analysis of six U.S. randomized, double-blind, multicenter, placebo-controlled trials using ranitidine bismuth citrate with or without antibiotics. The results from approximately 650 U.S. patients showed that the risk of ulcer recurrence within 6 months of completing treatment was two times less likely in patients whose H. pylori infection was eradicated compared to patients in whom H. pylori infection was not eradicated.

Safety

In clinical trials using combination therapy with clarithromycin plus ranitidine bismuth citrate, no adverse reactions peculiar to the combination of these drugs (using clarithromycin twice daily or three times a day) were observed. Adverse reactions that have occurred have been limited to those reported with clarithromycin or ranitidine bismuth citrate. (See **ADVERSE REACTIONS** section of the Tritec package insert.) The most frequent adverse experiences observed in clinical trials using combination therapy with clarithromycin (500 mg three times a day) with ranitidine bismuth citrate (n = 329) were taste disturbance (11%), diarrhea (5%), nausea and vomiting (3%). The most frequent adverse experiences observed in clinical trials using combination therapy with clarithromycin (500 mg twice daily) with ranitidine bismuth citrate (n = 196) were taste disturbance (8%), nausea and vomiting (5%), and diarrhea (4%).

ANIMAL PHARMACOLOGY AND TOXICOLOGY

Clarithromycin is rapidly and well-absorbed with dose-linear kinetics, low protein binding, and a high volume of distribution. Plasma half-life ranged from 1 to 6 hours and was species dependent. High tissue concentrations were achieved, but negligible accumulation was observed. Fecal clearance predominated. Hepatotoxicity occurred in all species tested (i.e., in rats and monkeys at doses 2 times greater than and in dogs at doses comparable to the maximum human daily dose, based on mg/m^2). Renal tubular degeneration (calculated on a mg/m^2 basis) occurred in rats at doses 2 times, in monkeys at doses 8 times, and in dogs at doses 12 times greater than the maximum human daily dose. Testicular atrophy (on a mg/m^2 basis) occurred in rats at doses 7 times, in dogs at doses 3 times, and in monkeys at doses 8 times greater than the maximum human daily dose. Corneal opacity (on a mg/m^2 basis) occurred in dogs at doses 12 times and in monkeys at doses 8 times greater than the maximum human daily dose. Lymphoid depletion (on a mg/m^2 basis) occurred in dogs at doses 3 times greater than and in monkeys at doses 2 times greater than the maximum human daily dose. These adverse events were absent during clinical trials.

REFERENCES

1. Clinical and Laboratory Standards Institute (CLSI). Methods for Dilution Antimicrobial Susceptibility Tests for Bacteria that Grow Aerobically - 9th edition. Approved Standard. CLSI Document M07-A9, CLSI. 950 West Valley Rd, Suite 2500, Wayne, PA 19087, 2012.
2. CLSI. Performance Standards for Antimicrobial Susceptibility Testing, 23rd Informational Supplement, CLSI Document M100-S23, 2013.
3. CLSI. Performance Standards for Antimicrobial Disk Susceptibility Tests, 11th edition. Approved Standard CLSI Document M02-A11, 2012.
4. CLSI. Methods for Antimicrobial Dilution and Disk Diffusion Susceptibility Testing of Infrequently Isolated or Fastidious Bacteria - 2nd edition. CLSI document M45-A2, 2010.
5. Chaisson RE, et al. Clarithromycin and Ethambutol with or without Clofazimine for the Treatment of Bacteremic Mycobacterium avium Complex Disease in Patients with HIV Infection. AIDS. 1997;11:317-317.
6. Kemper CA, et al. Treatment of Mycobacterium avium Complex Bacteremia in AIDS with a Four-Drug Oral Regimen. Ann Intern Med. 1992;116:466-472.

Filmtab® - Film-sealed tablets, AbbVie Inc.

Biaxin Filmtab 250 mg and 500 mg and Biaxin XL 500 mg Mfd. by AbbVie LTD, Barceloneta, PR 00617

Biaxin Granules for Oral Suspension, 125 mg/5 mL and 250 mg/5 mL

Mfd. by AbbVie Inc., North Chicago, IL 60064
For AbbVie Inc., North Chicago, IL 60064, U.S.A.
03-A897 October, 2013

Shown in Product Identification Guide, page 303

CREON®
[krē′ŏn]
(pancrelipase)
delayed-release capsules for oral use

HIGHLIGHTS OF PRESCRIBING INFORMATION
These highlights do not include all the information needed to use CREON safely and effectively. See full prescribing information for CREON.
CREON (pancrelipase) delayed-release capsules for oral use
Initial U.S. Approval: 2009

―――――INDICATIONS AND USAGE―――――
CREON is a combination of porcine-derived lipases, proteases, and amylases indicated for the treatment of exocrine pancreatic insufficiency due to cystic fibrosis, chronic pancreatitis, pancreatectomy, or other conditions. (1)

―――――DOSAGE AND ADMINISTRATION―――――
CREON is not interchangeable with any other pancrelipase product. (2.1)
Do not crush or chew capsules and capsule contents. For infants or patients unable to swallow intact capsules, the contents may be sprinkled on soft acidic food, e.g., applesauce. (2.1) Dosing should not exceed the recommended maximum dosage set forth by the Cystic Fibrosis Foundation Consensus Conferences Guidelines. (2.2)

Infants (up to 12 months)
• Prior to each feeding, infants may be given 3,000 lipase units (one capsule) per 120 mL of formula or per breast-feeding. (2.1)
• Do not mix CREON capsule contents directly into formula or breast milk prior to administration. (2.1)

Children Older than 12 Months and Younger than 4 Years
• Begin with 1,000 lipase units/kg of body weight per meal for children less than age 4 years to a maximum of 2,500 lipase units/kg of body weight per meal (or less than or equal to 10,000 lipase units/kg of body weight per day), or less than 4,000 lipase units/g fat ingested per day. (2.2)

Children 4 Years and Older and Adults
• Begin with 500 lipase units/kg of body weight per meal for those older than age 4 years to a maximum of 2,500 lipase units/kg of body weight per meal (or less than or equal to 10,000 lipase units/kg of body weight per day), or less than 4,000 lipase units/g fat ingested per day. (2.2)

Adults with Exocrine Pancreatic Insufficiency Due to Chronic Pancreatitis or Pancreatectomy
• Individualize dosage based on clinical symptoms, the degree of steatorrhea present and the fat content of the diet. (2.2)

―――――DOSAGE FORMS AND STRENGTHS―――――
• Delayed-Release Capsules: 3,000 USP units of lipase; 9,500 USP units of protease; 15,000 USP units of amylase (3)
• Delayed-Release Capsules: 6,000 USP units of lipase; 19,000 USP units of protease; 30,000 USP units of amylase (3)
• Delayed-Release Capsules: 12,000 USP units of lipase; 38,000 USP units of protease; 60,000 USP units of amylase (3)
• Delayed-Release Capsules: 24,000 USP units of lipase; 76,000 USP units of protease; 120,000 USP units of amylase (3)
• Delayed-Release Capsules: 36,000 USP units of lipase; 114,000 USP units of protease; 180,000 USP units of amylase (3)

―――――CONTRAINDICATIONS―――――
None (4)

―――――WARNINGS AND PRECAUTIONS―――――
• Fibrosing colonopathy is associated with high-dose use of pancreatic enzyme replacement in the treatment of cystic fibrosis patients. Exercise caution when doses of CREON exceed 2,500 lipase units/kg of body weight per meal (or greater than 10,000 lipase units/kg of body weight per day). (5.1)
• To avoid irritation of oral mucosa, do not chew CREON or retain in the mouth. (5.2)
• Exercise caution when prescribing CREON to patients with gout, renal impairment, or hyperuricemia. (5.3)
• There is theoretical risk of viral transmission with all pancreatic enzyme products including CREON. (5.4)
• Exercise caution when administering pancrelipase to a patient with a known allergy to proteins of porcine origin. (5.5)

―――――ADVERSE REACTIONS―――――
• Adverse reactions occurring in at least 2 cystic fibrosis patients (greater than or equal to 4%) receiving CREON are vomiting, dizziness, and cough. (6.1)
• Adverse reactions that occurred in at least 1 chronic pancreatitis or pancreatectomy patient (greater than or equal to 4%) receiving CREON are hyperglycemia, hypoglycemia, abdominal pain, abnormal feces, flatulence, frequent bowel movements, and nasopharyngitis. (6.1)

To report SUSPECTED ADVERSE REACTIONS, contact AbbVie Inc. at 1-800-633-9110 or FDA at 1-800-FDA-1088 or www.fda.gov/medwatch.

See 17 for PATIENT COUNSELING INFORMATION and Medication Guide
Revised: 03/2013

―――――――――――――――――――――

FULL PRESCRIBING INFORMATION: CONTENTS*
WARNING:
* Sections or subsections omitted from the full prescribing information are not listed

―――――――――――――――――――――

FULL PRESCRIBING INFORMATION

1   INDICATIONS AND USAGE

CREON® (pancrelipase) is indicated for the treatment of exocrine pancreatic insufficiency due to cystic fibrosis, chronic pancreatitis, pancreatectomy, or other conditions.

2   DOSAGE AND ADMINISTRATION

CREON is not interchangeable with other pancrelipase products.
CREON is orally administered. Therapy should be initiated at the lowest recommended dose and gradually increased. The dosage of CREON should be individualized based on clinical symptoms, the degree of steatorrhea present, and the fat content of the diet as described in the Limitations on Dosing below [see Dosage and Administration (2.2) and Warnings and Precautions (5.1)].

2.1   Administration
Infants (up to 12 months)
CREON should be administered to infants immediately prior to each feeding, using a dosage of 3,000 lipase units per 120 mL of formula or prior to breast-feeding. Contents of the capsule may be administered directly to the mouth or with a small amount of applesauce. Administration should be followed by breast milk or formula. Contents of the capsule should not be mixed directly into formula or breast milk as this may diminish efficacy. Care should be taken to ensure that CREON is not crushed or chewed or retained in the mouth, to avoid irritation of the oral mucosa.

Children and Adults
CREON should be taken during meals or snacks, with sufficient fluid. CREON capsules and capsule contents should not be crushed or chewed. Capsules should be swallowed whole.
For patients who are unable to swallow intact capsules, the capsules may be carefully opened and the contents added to a small amount of acidic soft food with a pH of 4.5 or less, such as applesauce, at room temperature. The CREON-soft food mixture should be swallowed immediately without crushing or chewing, and followed with water or juice to ensure complete ingestion. Care should be taken to ensure that no drug is retained in the mouth.

2.2   Dosage
Dosage recommendations for pancreatic enzyme replacement therapy were published following the Cystic Fibrosis Foundation Consensus Conferences.[1, 2, 3] CREON should be

administered in a manner consistent with the recommendations of the Cystic Fibrosis Foundation Consensus Conferences (also known as Conferences) provided in the following paragraphs, except for infants. Although the Conferences recommend doses of 2,000 to 4,000 lipase units in infants up to 12 months, CREON is available in a 3,000 lipase unit capsule. Therefore, the recommended dose of CREON in infants up to 12 months is 3,000 lipase units per 120 mL of formula or per breast-feeding. Patients may be dosed on a fat ingestion-based or actual body weight-based dosing scheme.
Additional recommendations for pancreatic enzyme therapy in patients with exocrine pancreatic insufficiency due to chronic pancreatitis or pancreatectomy are based on a clinical trial conducted in these populations.

Infants (up to 12 months)
CREON is available in the strength of 3,000 USP units of lipase thus infants may be given 3,000 lipase units (one capsule) per 120 mL of formula or per breast-feeding. Do not mix CREON capsule contents directly into formula or breast milk prior to administration [see Administration (2.1)].

Children Older than 12 Months and Younger than 4 Years
Enzyme dosing should begin with 1,000 lipase units/kg of body weight per meal for children less than age 4 years to a maximum of 2,500 lipase units/kg of body weight per meal (or less than or equal to 10,000 lipase units/kg of body weight per day), or less than 4,000 lipase units/g fat ingested per day.

Children 4 Years and Older and Adults
Enzyme dosing should begin with 500 lipase units/kg of body weight per meal for those older than age 4 years to a maximum of 2,500 lipase units/kg of body weight per meal (or less than or equal to 10,000 lipase units/kg of body weight per day), or less than 4,000 lipase units/g fat ingested per day.
Usually, half of the prescribed CREON dose for an individualized full meal should be given with each snack. The total daily dose should reflect approximately three meals plus two or three snacks per day.
Enzyme doses expressed as lipase units/kg of body weight per meal should be decreased in older patients because they weigh more but tend to ingest less fat per kilogram of body weight.

Adults with Exocrine Pancreatic Insufficiency Due to Chronic Pancreatitis or Pancreatectomy
The initial starting dose and increases in the dose per meal should be individualized based on clinical symptoms, the degree of steatorrhea present, and the fat content of the diet.
In one clinical trial, patients received CREON at a dose of 72,000 lipase units per meal while consuming at least 100 g of fat per day [see Clinical Studies (14.2)]. Lower starting doses recommended in the literature are consistent with the 500 lipase units/kg of body weight per meal lowest starting dose recommended for adults in the Cystic Fibrosis Foundation Consensus Conferences Guidelines.[1, 2, 3, 4] Usually, half of the prescribed CREON dose for an individualized full meal should be given with each snack.

Limitations on Dosing
Dosing should not exceed the recommended maximum dosage set forth by the Cystic Fibrosis Foundation Consensus Conferences Guidelines.[1, 2, 3] If symptoms and signs of steatorrhea persist, the dosage may be increased by the healthcare professional. Patients should be instructed not to increase the dosage on their own. There is great interindividual variation in response to enzymes; thus, a range of doses is recommended. Changes in dosage may require an adjustment period of several days. If doses are to exceed 2,500 lipase units/kg of body weight per meal, further investigation is warranted. Doses greater than 2,500 lipase units/kg of body weight per meal (or greater than 10,000 lipase units/kg of body weight per day) should be used with caution and only if they are documented to be effective by 3-day fecal fat measures that indicate a significantly improved coefficient of fat absorption. Doses greater than 6,000 lipase units/kg of body weight per meal have been associated with colonic stricture, indicative of fibrosing colonopathy, in children less than 12 years of age [see Warnings and Precautions (5.1)]. Patients currently receiving higher doses than 6,000 lipase units/kg of body weight per meal should be examined and the dosage either immediately decreased or titrated downward to a lower range.

3   DOSAGE FORMS AND STRENGTHS

The active ingredient in CREON evaluated in clinical trials is lipase. CREON is dosed by lipase units.

―――――――――――――――――――――

Information on the AbbVie, Inc. products listed on these pages is from the prescribing information in use as of July 31, 2014. For more information, please visit rxabbvie.com or call 1-800-633-9110.

Other active ingredients include protease and amylase. Each CREON delayed-release capsule strength contains the specified amounts of lipase, protease, and amylase as follows:

- 3,000 USP units of lipase; 9,500 USP units of protease; 15,000 USP units of amylase delayed-release capsules have a white opaque cap with imprint "CREON 1203" and a white opaque body.
- 6,000 USP units of lipase; 19,000 USP units of protease; 30,000 USP units of amylase delayed-release capsules have an orange opaque cap with imprint "CREON 1206" and a blue opaque body.
- 12,000 USP units of lipase; 38,000 USP units of protease; 60,000 USP units of amylase delayed-release capsules have a brown opaque cap with imprint "CREON 1212" and a colorless transparent body.
- 24,000 USP units of lipase; 76,000 USP units of protease; 120,000 USP units of amylase delayed-release capsules have an orange opaque cap with imprint "CREON 1224" and a colorless transparent body.
- 36,000 USP units of lipase; 114,000 USP units of protease; 180,000 USP units of amylase delayed-release capsules have a blue opaque cap with imprint "CREON 1236" and a colorless transparent body.

4 CONTRAINDICATIONS
None.

5 WARNINGS AND PRECAUTIONS
5.1 Fibrosing Colonopathy
Fibrosing colonopathy has been reported following treatment with different pancreatic enzyme products.[5, 6] Fibrosing colonopathy is a rare, serious adverse reaction initially described in association with high-dose pancreatic enzyme use, usually over a prolonged period of time and most commonly reported in pediatric patients with cystic fibrosis. The underlying mechanism of fibrosing colonopathy remains unknown. Doses of pancreatic enzyme products exceeding 6,000 lipase units/kg of body weight per meal have been associated with colonic stricture in children less than 12 years of age.[1] Patients with fibrosing colonopathy should be closely monitored because some patients may be at risk of progressing to stricture formation. It is uncertain whether regression of fibrosing colonopathy occurs.[1] It is generally recommended, unless clinically indicated, that enzyme doses should be less than 2,500 lipase units/kg of body weight per meal (or less than 10,000 lipase units/kg of body weight per day) or less than 4,000 lipase units/g fat ingested per day [see Dosage and Administration (2.1)].
Doses greater than 2,500 lipase units/kg of body weight per meal (or greater than 10,000 lipase units/kg of body weight per day) should be used with caution and only if they are documented to be effective by 3-day fecal fat measures that indicate a significantly improved coefficient of fat absorption. Patients receiving higher doses than 6,000 lipase units/kg of body weight per meal should be examined and the dosage either immediately decreased or titrated downward to a lower range.

5.2 Potential for Irritation to Oral Mucosa
Care should be taken to ensure that no drug is retained in the mouth. CREON should not be crushed or chewed or mixed in foods having a pH greater than 4.5. These actions can disrupt the protective enteric coating resulting in early release of enzymes, irritation of oral mucosa, and/or loss of enzyme activity [see Dosage and Administration (2.2) and Patient Counseling Information (17.1)]. For patients who are unable to swallow intact capsules, the capsules may be carefully opened and the contents added to a small amount of acidic soft food with a pH of 4.5 or less, such as applesauce, at room temperature. The CREON-soft food mixture should be swallowed immediately and followed with water or juice to ensure complete ingestion.

5.3 Potential for Risk of Hyperuricemia
Caution should be exercised when prescribing CREON to patients with gout, renal impairment, or hyperuricemia. Porcine-derived pancreatic enzyme products contain purines that may increase blood uric acid levels.

5.4 Potential Viral Exposure from the Product Source
CREON is sourced from pancreatic tissue from swine used for food consumption. Although the risk that CREON will transmit an infectious agent to humans has been reduced by testing for certain viruses during manufacturing and by inactivating certain viruses during manufacturing, there is a theoretical risk for transmission of viral disease, including diseases caused by novel or unidentified viruses. Thus, the presence of porcine viruses that might infect humans cannot be definitely excluded. However, no cases of transmission of an infectious illness associated with the use of porcine pancreatic extracts have been reported.

5.5 Allergic Reactions
Caution should be exercised when administering pancrelipase to a patient with a known allergy to proteins of porcine origin. Rarely, severe allergic reactions including anaphylaxis, asthma, hives, and pruritus, have been re-

ported with other pancreatic enzyme products with different formulations of the same active ingredient (pancrelipase). The risks and benefits of continued CREON treatment in patients with severe allergy should be taken into consideration with the overall clinical needs of the patient.

6 ADVERSE REACTIONS
The most serious adverse reactions reported with different pancreatic enzyme products of the same active ingredient (pancrelipase) that are described elsewhere in the label include fibrosing colonopathy, hyperuricemia and allergic reactions [see Warnings and Precautions (5)].
6.1 Clinical Trials Experience
Because clinical trials are conducted under widely varying conditions, adverse reaction rates observed in the clinical trials of a drug cannot be directly compared to the rates in the clinical trials of another drug and may not reflect the rates observed in practice.
The short-term safety of CREON was assessed in clinical trials conducted in 121 patients with exocrine pancreatic insufficiency (EPI): 67 patients with EPI due to cystic fibrosis (CF) and 25 patients with EPI due to chronic pancreatitis or pancreatectomy were treated with CREON.
Cystic Fibrosis
Studies 1 and 2 were randomized, double-blind, placebo-controlled, crossover studies of 49 patients, ages 7 to 43 years, with EPI due to CF. Study 1 included 32 patients ages 12 to 43 years and Study 2 included 17 patients ages 7 to 11 years. In these studies, patients were randomized to receive CREON at a dose of 4,000 lipase units/g fat ingested per day or matching placebo for 5 to 6 days of treatment, followed by crossover to the alternate treatment for an additional 5 to 6 days. The mean exposure to CREON during these studies was 5 days.
In Study 1, one patient experienced duodenitis and gastritis of moderate severity 16 days after completing treatment with CREON. Transient neutropenia without clinical sequelae was observed as an abnormal laboratory finding in one patient receiving CREON and a macrolide antibiotic.
In Study 2, adverse reactions that occurred in at least 2 patients (greater than or equal to 12%) treated with CREON were vomiting and headache. Vomiting occurred in 2 patients treated with CREON and did not occur in patients treated with placebo; headache occurred in 2 patients treated with CREON and did not occur in patients treated with placebo.
The most common adverse reactions (greater than or equal to 4%) in Studies 1 and 2 were vomiting, dizziness, and cough. Table 1 enumerates adverse reactions that occurred in at least 2 patients (greater than or equal to 4%) treated with CREON at a higher rate than with placebo in Studies 1 and 2.

Table 1: Adverse Reactions Occurring in at Least 2 Patients (greater than or equal to 4%) in Cystic Fibrosis (Studies 1 and 2)

Adverse Reaction	CREON Capsules n = 49 (%)	Placebo n = 47 (%)
Vomiting	3 (6)	1 (2)
Dizziness	2 (4)	1 (2)
Cough	2 (4)	0

An additional open-label, single-arm study assessed the short-term safety and tolerability of CREON in 18 infants and children, ages 4 months to 6 years, with EPI due to cystic fibrosis. Patients received their usual pancreatic enzyme replacement therapy (mean dose of 7,000 lipase units/kg/day for a mean duration of 18.2 days) followed by CREON (mean dose of 7,500 lipase units/kg/day for a mean duration of 12.6 days). There were no serious adverse reactions. Adverse reactions that occurred in patients during treatment with CREON were vomiting, irritability, and decreased appetite, each occurring in 6% of patients.
Chronic Pancreatitis or Pancreatectomy
A randomized, double-blind, placebo-controlled, parallel group study was conducted in 54 adult patients, ages 32 to 75 years, with EPI due to chronic pancreatitis or pancreatectomy. Patients received single-blind placebo treatment during a 5-day run-in period followed by an intervening period of up to 16 days of investigator-directed treatment with no restrictions on pancreatic enzyme replacement therapy. Patients were then randomized to receive CREON or matching placebo for 7 days. The CREON dose was 72,000 lipase units per main meal (3 main meals) and 36,000 lipase units per snack (2 snacks). The mean exposure to CREON during this study was 6.8 days in the 25 patients that received CREON.
The most common adverse reactions reported during the study were related to glycemic control and were reported more commonly during CREON treatment than during placebo treatment.

Table 2 enumerates adverse reactions that occurred in at least 1 patient (greater than or equal to 4%) treated with CREON at a higher rate than with placebo.

Table 2: Adverse Reactions in at Least 1 Patient (greater than or equal to 4%) in the Chronic Pancreatitis or Pancreatectomy Trial

Adverse Reaction	CREON Capsules n = 25 (%)	Placebo n = 29 (%)
Hyperglycemia	2 (8)	2 (7)
Hypoglycemia	1 (4)	1 (3)
Abdominal Pain	1 (4)	1 (3)
Abnormal Feces	1 (4)	0
Flatulence	1 (4)	0
Frequent Bowel Movements	1 (4)	0
Nasopharyngitis	1 (4)	0

6.2 Postmarketing Experience
Postmarketing data from this formulation of CREON have been available since 2009. The following adverse reactions have been identified during post approval use of this formulation of CREON. Because these reactions are reported voluntarily from a population of uncertain size, it is not always possible to reliably estimate their frequency or establish a causal relationship to drug exposure.
Gastrointestinal disorders (including abdominal pain, diarrhea, flatulence, constipation and nausea), skin disorders (including pruritus, urticaria and rash), blurred vision, myalgia, muscle spasm, and asymptomatic elevations of liver enzymes have been reported with this formulation of CREON.
Delayed- and immediate-release pancreatic enzyme products with different formulations of the same active ingredient (pancrelipase) have been used for the treatment of patients with exocrine pancreatic insufficiency due to cystic fibrosis and other conditions, such as chronic pancreatitis. The long-term safety profile of these products has been described in the medical literature. The most serious adverse reactions included fibrosing colonopathy, distal intestinal obstruction syndrome (DIOS), recurrence of pre-existing carcinoma, and severe allergic reactions including anaphylaxis, asthma, hives, and pruritus.

7 DRUG INTERACTIONS
No drug interactions have been identified. No formal interaction studies have been conducted.

8 USE IN SPECIFIC POPULATIONS
8.1 Pregnancy
Teratogenic effects
Pregnancy Category C: Animal reproduction studies have not been conducted with pancrelipase. It is also not known whether pancrelipase can cause fetal harm when administered to a pregnant woman or can affect reproduction capacity. CREON should be given to a pregnant woman only if clearly needed. The risk and benefit of pancrelipase should be considered in the context of the need to provide adequate nutritional support to a pregnant woman with exocrine pancreatic insufficiency. Adequate caloric intake during pregnancy is important for normal maternal weight gain and fetal growth. Reduced maternal weight gain and malnutrition can be associated with adverse pregnancy outcomes.
8.3 Nursing Mothers
It is not known whether this drug is excreted in human milk. Because many drugs are excreted in human milk, caution should be exercised when CREON is administered to a nursing woman. The risk and benefit of pancrelipase should be considered in the context of the need to provide adequate nutritional support to a nursing mother with exocrine pancreatic insufficiency.
8.4 Pediatric Use
The short-term safety and effectiveness of CREON were assessed in two randomized, double-blind, placebo-controlled, crossover studies of 49 patients with EPI due to cystic fibrosis, 25 of whom were pediatric patients. Study 1 included 8 adolescents between 12 and 17 years of age. Study 2 included 17 children between 7 and 11 years of age. The safety and efficacy in pediatric patients in these studies were similar to adult patients [see Adverse Reactions (6.1) and Clinical Studies (14)].
An open-label, single-arm, short-term study of CREON was conducted in 18 infants and children, ages 4 months to six years of age, with EPI due to cystic fibrosis. Patients received their usual pancreatic enzyme replacement therapy (mean dose of 7,000 lipase units/kg/day for a mean duration of 18.2 days) followed by CREON (mean dose of 7,500 lipase

units/kg/day for a mean duration of 12.6 days). The mean daily fat intake was 48 grams during treatment with usual pancreatic enzyme replacement therapy and 47 grams during treatment with CREON. When patients were switched from their usual pancreatic enzyme replacement therapy to CREON, they demonstrated similar spot fecal fat testing results; the clinical relevance of spot fecal fat testing has not been demonstrated. Adverse reactions that occurred in patients during treatment with CREON were vomiting, irritability, and decreased appetite *[see Adverse Reactions (6.1)].*
The safety and efficacy of pancreatic enzyme products with different formulations of pancrelipase consisting of the same active ingredient (lipases, proteases, and amylases) for treatment of children with exocrine pancreatic insufficiency due to cystic fibrosis have been described in the medical literature and through clinical experience.
Dosing of pediatric patients should be in accordance with recommended guidance from the Cystic Fibrosis Foundation Consensus Conferences *[see Dosage and Administration (2.1)].* Doses of other pancreatic enzyme products exceeding 6,000 lipase units/kg of body weight per meal have been associated with fibrosing colonopathy and colonic strictures in children less than 12 years of age *[see Warnings and Precautions (5.1)].*

8.5 Geriatric Use

Clinical studies of CREON did not include sufficient numbers of subjects aged 65 and over to determine whether they respond differently from younger subjects. Other reported clinical experience has not identified differences in responses between the elderly and younger patients.

10 OVERDOSAGE

There have been no reports of overdose in clinical trials or postmarketing surveillance with this formulation of CREON. Chronic high doses of pancreatic enzyme products have been associated with fibrosing colonopathy and colonic strictures *[see Dosage and Administration (2.2) and Warnings and Precautions (5.1)].* High doses of pancreatic enzyme products have been associated with hyperuricosuria and hyperuricemia, and should be used with caution in patients with a history of hyperuricemia, gout, or renal impairment *[see Warnings and Precautions (5.3)].*

11 DESCRIPTION

CREON is a pancreatic enzyme preparation consisting of pancrelipase, an extract derived from porcine pancreatic glands. Pancrelipase contains multiple enzyme classes, including porcine-derived lipases, proteases, and amylases.
Pancrelipase is a beige-white amorphous powder. It is miscible in water and practically insoluble or insoluble in alcohol and ether.
Each delayed-release capsule for oral administration contains enteric-coated spheres (0.71–1.60 mm in diameter).
The active ingredient evaluated in clinical trials is lipase. CREON is dosed by lipase units.
Other active ingredients include protease and amylase.
CREON contains the following inactive ingredients: cetyl alcohol, dimethicone, hypromellose phthalate, polyethylene glycol, and triethyl citrate.
3,000 USP units of lipase; 9,500 USP units of protease; 15,000 USP units of amylase delayed-release capsules have a white opaque cap with imprint "CREON 1203" and a white opaque body. The shells contain titanium dioxide and hypromellose.
6,000 USP units of lipase; 19,000 USP units of protease; 30,000 USP units of amylase delayed-release capsules have a Swedish-orange opaque cap with imprint "CREON 1206" and a blue opaque body. The shells contain FD&C Blue No. 2, gelatin, red iron oxide, sodium lauryl sulfate, titanium dioxide, and yellow iron oxide.
12,000 USP units of lipase; 38,000 USP units of protease; 60,000 USP units of amylase delayed-release capsules have a brown opaque cap with imprint "CREON 1212" and a colorless transparent body. The shells contain black iron oxide, gelatin, red iron oxide, sodium lauryl sulfate, titanium dioxide, and yellow iron oxide.
24,000 USP units of lipase; 76,000 USP units of protease; 120,000 USP units of amylase delayed-release capsules have a Swedish-orange opaque cap with imprint "CREON 1224" and a colorless transparent body. The shells contain gelatin, red iron oxide, sodium lauryl sulfate, titanium dioxide, and yellow iron oxide.
36,000 USP units of lipase; 114,000 USP units of protease; 180,000 USP units of amylase delayed-release capsules have a blue opaque cap with imprint "CREON 1236" and a colorless transparent body. The shells contain gelatin, titanium dioxide, FD&C Blue No. 2 and sodium lauryl sulfate.

12 CLINICAL PHARMACOLOGY

12.1 Mechanism of Action

The pancreatic enzymes in CREON® (pancrelipase) catalyze the hydrolysis of fats to monoglyceride, glycerol and free fatty acids, proteins into peptides and amino acids, and starches into dextrins and short chain sugars such as malt-

ose and maltriose in the duodenum and proximal small intestine, thereby acting like digestive enzymes physiologically secreted by the pancreas.

12.3 Pharmacokinetics

The pancreatic enzymes in CREON are enteric-coated to minimize destruction or inactivation in gastric acid. CREON is designed to release most of the enzymes *in vivo* at an approximate pH of 5.5 or greater. Pancreatic enzymes are not absorbed from the gastrointestinal tract in appreciable amounts.

13 NONCLINICAL TOXICOLOGY

13.1 Carcinogenesis, Mutagenesis, Impairment of Fertility

Carcinogenicity, genetic toxicology, and animal fertility studies have not been performed with pancrelipase.

14 CLINICAL STUDIES

The short-term efficacy of CREON was evaluated in three studies conducted in 103 patients with exocrine pancreatic insufficiency (EPI). Two studies were conducted in 49 patients with EPI due to cystic fibrosis (CF); one study was conducted in 54 patients with EPI due to chronic pancreatitis or pancreatectomy.

14.1 Cystic Fibrosis

Studies 1 and 2 were randomized, double-blind, placebo-controlled, crossover studies in 49 patients, ages 7 to 43 years, with exocrine pancreatic insufficiency due to cystic fibrosis. Study 1 included patients aged 12 to 43 years (n = 32). The final analysis population was limited to 29 patients; 3 patients were excluded due to protocol deviations. Study 2 included patients aged 7 to 11 years (n = 17). The final analysis population was limited to 16 patients; 1 patient withdrew consent prior to stool collection during treatment with CREON. In each study, patients were randomized to receive CREON at a dose of 4,000 lipase units/g fat ingested per day or matching placebo for 5 to 6 days of treatment, followed by crossover to the alternate treatment for an additional 5 to 6 days. All patients consumed a high-fat diet (greater than or equal to 90 grams of fat per day, 40% of daily calories derived from fat) during the treatment periods.
The coefficient of fat absorption (CFA) was determined by a 72-hour stool collection during both treatments, when both fat excretion and fat ingestion were measured. Each patient's CFA during placebo treatment was used as their no-treatment CFA value.
In Study 1, mean CFA was 89% with CREON treatment compared to 49% with placebo treatment. The mean difference in CFA was 41 percentage points in favor of CREON treatment with 95% CI: (34, 47) and p<0.001.
In Study 2, mean CFA was 83% with CREON treatment compared to 47% with placebo treatment. The mean difference in CFA was 35 percentage points in favor of CREON treatment with 95% CI: (27, 44) and p<0.001.
Subgroup analyses of the CFA results in Studies 1 and 2 showed that mean change in CFA with CREON treatment was greater in patients with lower no-treatment (placebo) CFA values than in patients with higher no-treatment (placebo) CFA values. There were no differences in response to CREON by age or gender, with similar responses to CREON observed in male and female patients, and in younger (under 18 years of age) and older patients.
The coefficient of nitrogen absorption (CNA) was determined by a 72-hour stool collection during both treatments, when nitrogen excretion was measured and nitrogen ingestion from a controlled diet was estimated (based on the assumption that proteins contain 16% nitrogen). Each patient's CNA during placebo treatment was used as their no-treatment CNA value.
In Study 1, mean CNA was 86% with CREON treatment compared to 49% with placebo treatment. The mean difference in CNA was 37 percentage points in favor of CREON treatment with 95% CI: (31, 42) and p<0.001.
In Study 2, mean CNA was 80% with CREON treatment compared to 45% with placebo treatment. The mean difference in CNA was 35 percentage points in favor of CREON treatment with 95% CI: (26, 45) and p<0.001.

14.2 Chronic Pancreatitis or Pancreatectomy

A randomized, double-blind, placebo-controlled, parallel group study was conducted in 54 adult patients, ages 32 to 75 years, with EPI due to chronic pancreatitis or pancreatectomy. The final analysis population was limited to 52 patients; 2 patients were excluded due to protocol violations. Ten patients had a history of pancreatectomy (7 were treated with CREON). In this study, patients received placebo for 5 days (run-in period), followed by pancreatic enzyme replacement therapy as directed by the investigator for 16 days; this was followed by randomization to CREON or matching placebo for 7 days of treatment (double-blind period). Only patients with CFA less than 80% in the run-in period were randomized to the double-blind period. The dose of CREON during the double-blind period was 72,000 lipase units per main meal (3 main meals) and 36,000 lipase

units per snack (2 snacks). All patients consumed a high-fat diet (greater than or equal to 100 grams of fat per day) during the treatment period.
The CFA was determined by a 72-hour stool collection during the run-in and double-blind treatment periods, when both fat excretion and fat ingestion were measured. The mean change in CFA from the run-in period to the end of the double-blind period in the CREON and Placebo groups is shown in Table 3.

Table 3: Change in CFA in the Chronic Pancreatitis and Pancreatectomy Trial (Run-in Period to End of Double-Blind Period)

	CREON n = 24	Placebo n = 28
CFA [%]		
Run-in Period (Mean, SD)	54 (19)	57 (21)
End of Double-Blind Period (Mean, SD)	86 (6)	66 (20)
Change in CFA * [%]		
Run-in Period to End of Double-Blind Period (Mean, SD)	32 (18)	9 (13)
Treatment Difference (95% CI)	21 (14, 28)	

*p<0.0001

Subgroup analyses of the CFA results showed that mean change in CFA was greater in patients with lower run-in period CFA values than in patients with higher run-in period CFA values. Only 1 of the patients with a history of total pancreatectomy was treated with CREON in the study. That patient had a CFA of 26% during the run-in period and a CFA of 73% at the end of the double-blind period. The remaining 6 patients with a history of partial pancreatectomy treated with CREON on the study had a mean CFA of 42% during the run-in period and a mean CFA of 84% at the end of the double-blind period.

15 REFERENCES

[1] Borowitz DS, Grand RJ, Durie PR, et al. Use of pancreatic enzyme supplements for patients with cystic fibrosis in the context of fibrosing colonopathy. *Journal of Pediatrics.* 1995; 127: 681-684.
[2] Borowitz DS, Baker RD, Stallings V. Consensus report on nutrition for pediatric patients with cystic fibrosis. *Journal of Pediatric Gastroenterology Nutrition.* 2002 Sep; 35: 246-259.
[3] Stallings VA, Stark LJ, Robinson KA, et al. Evidence-based practice recommendations for nutrition-related management of children and adults with cystic fibrosis and pancreatic insufficiency: results of a systematic review. *Journal of the American Dietetic Association.* 2008; 108: 832-839.
[4] Dominguez-Munoz JE. Pancreatic enzyme therapy for pancreatic exocrine insufficiency. *Current Gastroenterology Reports.* 2007; 9: 116-122.
[5] Smyth RL, Ashby D, O'Hea U, et al. Fibrosing colonopathy in cystic fibrosis: results of a case-control study. *Lancet.* 1995; 346: 1247-1251.
[6] FitzSimmons SC, Burkhart GA, Borowitz DS, et al. High-dose pancreatic-enzyme supplements and fibrosing colonopathy in children with cystic fibrosis. *New England Journal of Medicine.* 1997; 336: 1283-1289.

16 HOW SUPPLIED/STORAGE AND HANDLING

CREON® (pancrelipase) Delayed-Release Capsules
3,000 USP units of lipase; 9,500 USP units of protease; 15,000 USP units of amylase
Each CREON capsule is available as a two piece hypromellose capsule with a white opaque cap with imprint "CREON 1203" and a white opaque body that contains tan colored, delayed-release pancrelipase supplied in bottles of:
• 70 capsules (NDC 0032-1203-70)
CREON (pancrelipase) Delayed-Release Capsules
6,000 USP units of lipase; 19,000 USP units of protease; 30,000 USP units of amylase
Each CREON capsule is available as a two-piece gelatin capsule with orange opaque cap with imprint "CREON 1206" and a blue opaque body that contains tan-colored, delayed-release pancrelipase supplied in bottles of:
• 100 capsules (NDC 0032-1206-01)
• 250 capsules (NDC 0032-1206-07)

Information on the AbbVie, Inc. products listed on these pages is from the prescribing information in use as of July 31, 2014. For more information, please visit rxabbvie.com or call 1-800-633-9110.

CREON (pancrelipase) Delayed-Release Capsules

12,000 USP units of lipase; 38,000 USP units of protease; 60,000 USP units of amylase

Each CREON capsule is available as a two-piece gelatin capsule with a brown opaque cap with imprint "CREON 1212" and a colorless transparent body that contains tan-colored, delayed-release pancrelipase supplied in bottles of:

• 100 capsules (NDC 0032-1212-01)
• 250 capsules (NDC 0032-1212-07)

CREON (pancrelipase) Delayed-Release Capsules

24,000 USP units of lipase; 76,000 USP units of protease; 120,000 USP units of amylase

Each CREON capsule is available as a two-piece gelatin capsule with orange opaque cap with imprint "CREON 1224" and a colorless transparent body that contains tan-colored, delayed-release pancrelipase supplied in bottles of:

• 100 capsules (NDC 0032-1224-01)
• 250 capsules (NDC 0032-1224-07)

CREON (pancrelipase) Delayed-Release Capsules

36,000 USP units of lipase; 114,000 USP units of protease; 180,000 USP units of amylase

Each CREON capsule is available as a two-piece gelatin capsule with blue opaque cap with imprint "CREON 1236" and a colorless transparent body that contains tan-colored, delayed-release pancrelipase supplied in bottles of:

• 100 capsules (NDC 0032-3016-13)
• 250 capsules (NDC 0032-3016-28)

Storage and Handling

CREON must be stored at room temperature up to 25°C (77°F) and protected from moisture. Temperature excursions are permitted between 25°C to 40°C (77°F and 104°F) for up to 30 days. Product should be discarded if exposed to higher temperature and moisture conditions higher than 70%. After opening, keep bottle tightly closed between uses to protect from moisture.

Bottles of CREON 3,000 USP units of lipase must be stored and dispensed in the original container.

Do not crush CREON delayed-release capsules or the capsule contents.

17 PATIENT COUNSELING INFORMATION

See FDA-approved patient labeling (Medication Guide)

17.1 Dosing and Administration

• Instruct patients and caregivers that CREON should only be taken as directed by their healthcare professional. Patients should be advised that the total daily dose should not exceed 10,000 lipase units/kg body weight/day unless clinically indicated. This needs to be especially emphasized for patients eating multiple snacks and meals per day. Patients should be informed that if a dose is missed, the next dose should be taken with the next meal or snack as directed. Doses should not be doubled [see Dosage and Administration (2)].

• Instruct patients and caregivers that CREON should always be taken with food. Patients should be advised that CREON delayed-release capsules and the capsule contents must not be crushed or chewed as doing so could cause early release of enzymes and/or loss of enzymatic activity. Patients should swallow the intact capsules with adequate amounts of liquid at mealtimes. If necessary, the capsule contents can also be sprinkled on soft acidic foods [see Dosage and Administration (2)].

17.2 Fibrosing Colonopathy

Advise patients and caregivers to follow dosing instructions carefully, as doses of pancreatic enzyme products exceeding 6,000 lipase units/kg of body weight per meal have been associated with colonic strictures in children below the age of 12 years [see Dosage and Administration (2)].

17.3 Allergic Reactions

Advise patients and caregivers to contact their healthcare professional immediately if allergic reactions to CREON develop [see Warnings and Precautions (5.5)].

17.4 Pregnancy and Breast Feeding

• Instruct patients to notify their healthcare professional if they are pregnant or are thinking of becoming pregnant during treatment with CREON [see Use in Specific Populations (8.1)].

• Instruct patients to notify their healthcare professional if they are breast feeding or are thinking of breast feeding during treatment with CREON [see Use in Specific Populations (8.3)].

Manufactured by:
Abbott Laboratories GmbH
Hannover, Germany
Marketed by:
AbbVie Inc.
North Chicago, IL 60064, U.S.A.
© 2012 AbbVie Inc.
1083531 March, 2013

MEDICATION GUIDE
CREON® (krē ´ŏn)
(pancrelipase)
Delayed-Release Capsules

Read this Medication Guide before you start taking CREON and each time you get a refill. There may be new information. This information does not take the place of talking to your doctor about your medical condition or treatment.

What is the most important information I should know about CREON?

CREON may increase your chance of having a rare bowel disorder called fibrosing colonopathy. This condition is serious and may require surgery. The risk of having this condition may be reduced by following the dosing instructions that your doctor gave you. Call your doctor right away if you have any unusual or severe:

• stomach area (abdominal) pain
• bloating
• trouble passing stool (having bowel movements)
• nausea, vomiting, or diarrhea

Take CREON exactly as prescribed. Do not take more or less CREON than directed by your doctor.

What is CREON?

CREON is a prescription medicine used to treat people who cannot digest food normally because their pancreas does not make enough enzymes due to cystic fibrosis, swelling of the pancreas that lasts a long time (chronic pancreatitis), removal of some or all of the pancreas (pancreatectomy), or other conditions. CREON may help your body use fats, proteins, and sugars from food.

CREON contains a mixture of digestive enzymes including lipases, proteases, and amylases from pig pancreas.

What should I tell my doctor before taking CREON?

Before taking CREON, tell your doctor about all your medical conditions, including if you:

• are allergic to pork (pig) products
• have a history of intestinal blockage of your intestines, or scarring or thickening of your bowel wall (fibrosing colonopathy)
• have gout, kidney disease, or high blood uric acid (hyperuricemia)
• have trouble swallowing capsules
• have any other medical condition
• are pregnant or plan to become pregnant. It is not known if CREON will harm your unborn baby.
• are breast-feeding or plan to breast-feed. It is not known if CREON passes into your breast milk.

Tell your doctor about all the medicines you take, including prescription and nonprescription medicines, vitamins, and herbal supplements.

Know the medicines you take. Keep a list of them and show it to your doctor and pharmacist when you get a new medicine.

How should I take CREON?

• **Take CREON exactly as your doctor tells you.**

• You should not switch CREON with any other pancreatic enzyme product without first talking to your doctor.

• Do not take more capsules in a day than the number your doctor tells you to take (total daily dose).

• Always take CREON with a meal or snack and enough liquid to swallow CREON completely. If you eat a lot of meals or snacks in a day, be careful not to go over your total daily dose.

• Your doctor may change your dose based on the amount of fatty foods you eat or based on your weight.

• **Do not crush or chew CREON capsules or its contents, and do not hold the capsule or capsule contents in your mouth.** Crushing, chewing or holding the CREON capsules in your mouth may cause irritation in your mouth or change the way CREON works in your body.

Giving CREON to infants (children up to 12 months)

1. Give CREON right before each feeding of formula or breast milk.

2. Do not mix CREON capsule contents directly into formula or breast milk.

3. Open the capsules and sprinkle the contents directly into your infant's mouth or mix the contents in a small amount of room temperature acidic soft food such as applesauce. These foods should be the kind found in baby food jars that you buy at the store, or other food recommended by your doctor.

4. If you sprinkle the CREON on food, give the CREON and food mixture to your child right away. Do not store CREON that is mixed with food.

5. Give your child enough liquid to completely swallow the CREON contents or the CREON and food mixture.

6. Look in your child's mouth to make sure that all of the medicine has been swallowed.

Giving CREON to children and adults

1. Swallow CREON capsules whole and take them with enough liquid to swallow them right away.

2. If you have trouble swallowing capsules, open the capsules and sprinkle the contents on a small amount of room temperature acidic food such as applesauce. Ask your doctor about other foods you can mix with CREON.

3. If you sprinkle CREON on food, swallow it right after you mix it and drink enough water or juice to make sure the medicine is swallowed completely. Do not store CREON that is mixed with food.

4. If you forget to take CREON, call your doctor or wait until your next meal and take your usual number of capsules. Take your next dose at your usual time. **Do not make up for missed doses.**

What are the possible side effects of CREON?

CREON may cause serious side effects, including:

• See " What is the most important information I should know about CREON? "

• **Irritation of the inside of your mouth.** This can happen if CREON is not swallowed completely.

• **Increase in blood uric acid levels.** This may cause worsening of swollen, painful joints (gout) caused by an increase in your blood uric acid levels.

• **Allergic reactions, including trouble with breathing, skin rashes, or swollen lips.**

Call your doctor right away if you have any of these symptoms.

The most common side effects of CREON include:

• Blood sugar increase (hyperglycemia) or decrease (hypoglycemia)
• Pain in your stomach (abdominal area)
• Frequent or abnormal bowel movements
• Gas
• Vomiting
• Dizziness
• Sore throat and cough

Other Possible Side Effects:

CREON and other pancreatic enzyme products are made from the pancreas of pigs, the same pigs people eat as pork. These pigs may carry viruses. Although it has never been reported, it may be possible for a person to get a viral infection from taking pancreatic enzyme products that come from pigs.

Tell your doctor if you have any side effect that bothers you or that does not go away.

These are not all the side effects of CREON. For more information, ask your doctor or pharmacist.

Call your doctor for medical advice about side effects. You may report side effects to the FDA at 1-800-FDA-1088.

You may also report side effects to AbbVie Inc. at 1-800-633-9110.

How should I store CREON?

• Store CREON® (pancrelipase) at room temperature below 77°F (25°C). Avoid heat.

• You may store CREON at a temperature between 77°F to 104°F (25°C to 40°C) for up to 30 days. Throw away any CREON stored at these temperatures for more than 30 days.

• Keep CREON in a dry place and in the original container.

• After opening the bottle, keep it closed tightly between uses to protect from moisture.

Keep CREON and all medicines out of the reach of children.

General information about CREON

Medicines are sometimes prescribed for purposes other than those listed in a Medication Guide. Do not use CREON for a condition for which it was not prescribed. Do not give CREON to other people to take, even if they have the same symptoms you have. It may harm them.

This Medication Guide summarizes the most important information about CREON. If you would like more information, talk to your doctor. You can ask your doctor or pharmacist for information about CREON that is written for healthcare professionals. For more information, go to www.creon-us.com or call toll-free [1-800-633-9110].

What are the ingredients in CREON?

Active Ingredient: lipase, protease, amylase

Inactive Ingredients: cetyl alcohol, dimethicone, hypromellose phthalate, polyethylene glycol, and triethyl citrate.

The shells of the CREON 6,000 USP units of lipase, 12,000 USP units of lipase, and 24,000 USP units of lipase strengths contain: gelatin, red iron oxide, sodium lauryl sulfate, titanium dioxide, and yellow iron oxide.

In addition:

The shells for the CREON 3,000 USP units of lipase strength capsules contain titanium dioxide and hypromellose.

The shells of the CREON 6,000 USP units of lipase strength capsules contain FD&C Blue No. 2.

The shells of the CREON 12,000 USP units of lipase strength capsules contain black iron oxide.

The shells of the CREON 36,000 USP units of lipase strength capsules contain gelatin, titanium dioxide, sodium lauryl sulfate and FD&C Blue No. 2.

This Medication Guide has been approved by the U.S. Food and Drug Administration.

Manufactured for:
AbbVie Inc.
North Chicago, IL 60064, U.S.A.
© 2012 AbbVie Inc.
1083531 March, 2013

Shown in Product Identification Guide, page 303

DEPAKOTE® ER   ℞
[dĕp'ă-kōte]
(divalproex sodium)
Extended Release Tablet for Oral Use

HIGHLIGHTS OF PRESCRIBING INFORMATION
These highlights do not include all the information needed
to use Depakote ER safely and effectively. See full prescribing information for Depakote ER.
Depakote ER (divalproex sodium) Tablet, Extended Release
for Oral use
Initial U.S. Approval: 2000

**WARNING: LIFE THREATENING ADVERSE REAC-
TIONS**
*See full prescribing information for complete boxed
warning.*
- **Hepatotoxicity, including fatalities, usually during
first 6 months of treatment. Children under the age
of two years and patients with mitochondrial disorders are at higher risk. Monitor patients closely, and
perform serum liver testing prior to therapy and at
frequent intervals thereafter (5.1)**
- **Fetal Risk, particularly neural tube defects, other
major malformations, and decreased IQ (5.2, 5.3,
5.4)**
- **Pancreatitis, including fatal hemorrhagic cases (5.5)**

———————RECENT MAJOR CHANGES———————
Boxed Warning, Hepatotoxicity 07/2013
Boxed Warning, Fetal Risk 06/2013
Indications and Usage, Important Limitations (1.4)
06/2013
Contraindications, Known or Suspected Mitochondrial Dis-
orders (4) 07/2013
Contraindications, Prophylaxis of Migraines in Pregnancy
(4) 06/2013
Warnings and Precautions, Hepatotoxicity (5.1) 07/2013
Warnings and Precautions, Birth Defects (5.2) 06/2013
Warnings and Precautions, Decreased IQ (5.3) 06/2013
Warnings and Precautions, Use in Women of Childbearing
Potential (5.4) 06/2013
Warnings and Precautions, Brain Atrophy (5.7) 05/2013

———————INDICATIONS AND USAGE———————
Depakote ER is an anti-epileptic drug indicated for:
- Acute treatment of manic or mixed episodes associated
with bipolar disorder, with or without psychotic features
(1.1)
- Monotherapy and adjunctive therapy of complex partial
seizures and simple and complex absence seizures; adjunctive therapy in patients with multiple seizure types that
include absence seizures (1.2)
- Prophylaxis of migraine headaches (1.3)

———————DOSAGE AND ADMINISTRATION———————
- Depakote ER is intended for once-a-day oral administration. Depakote ER should be swallowed whole and should
not be crushed or chewed (2.1, 2.2).
- Mania: Initial dose is 25 mg/kg/day, increasing as rapidly as possible to achieve therapeutic response or desired
plasma level (2.1). The maximum recommended dosage is
60 mg/kg/day (2.1, 2.2).
- Complex Partial Seizures: Start at 10 to 15 mg/kg/day,
increasing at 1 week intervals by 5 to 10 mg/kg/day to
achieve optimal clinical response; if response is not satisfactory, check valproate plasma level; see full prescribing
information for conversion to monotherapy (2.2). The
maximum recommended dose is 60 mg/kg/day (2.1, 2.2).
- Absence Seizures: Start at 15 mg/kg/day, increasing at 1
week intervals by 5 to 10 mg/kg/day until seizure control
or limiting side effects (2.2). The maximum recommended
dosage is 60 mg/kg/day (2.1, 2.2).
- Migraine: The recommended starting dose is 500 mg/day
for 1 week, thereafter increasing to 1000 mg/day (2.3).

———————DOSAGE FORMS AND STRENGTHS———————
Tablets: 250 mg and 500 mg (3)

———————CONTRAINDICATIONS———————
- Hepatic disease or significant hepatic dysfunction (4, 5.1)
- Known mitochondrial disorders caused by mutations in
mitochondrial DNA polymerase γ (POLG) (4, 5.1)
- Suspected POLG-related disorder in children under two
years of age (4, 5.1)
- Known hypersensitivity to the drug (4, 5.13)
- Urea cycle disorders (4, 5.6)
- Pregnant patients treated for prophylaxis of migraine
headaches (4, 8.1)

———————WARNINGS AND PRECAUTIONS———————
- Hepatotoxicity; evaluate high risk populations and monitor serum liver tests (5.1)
- Birth defects and decreased IQ following *in utero* exposure; only use to treat pregnant women with epilepsy or
bipolar disorder if other medications are unacceptable;
should not be administered to a woman of childbearing potential unless essential (5.2, 5.3, 5.4)

- Pancreatitis; Depakote ER should ordinarily be discontinued (5.5)
- Brain Atrophy; evaluate for continued use in the presence
of suspected or apparent signs of reversible or irreversible
cerebral and cerebellar atrophy (5.7)
- Suicidal behavior or ideation; Antiepileptic drugs, including Depakote ER, increase the risk of suicidal thoughts or
behavior (5.8)
- Thrombocytopenia; monitor platelet counts and coagulation tests (5.9)
- Hyperammonemia and hyperammonemic encephalopathy;
measure ammonia level if unexplained lethargy and vomiting or changes in mental status, and also with concomitant topiramate use; consider discontinuation of valproate
therapy (5.6, 5.10, 5.11)
- Hypothermia; Hypothermia has been reported during valproate therapy with or without associated hyperammonemia. This adverse reaction can also occur in patients using
concomitant topiramate (5.12)
- Multi-organ hypersensitivity reaction; discontinue
Depakote ER (5.13)
- Somnolence in the elderly can occur. Depakote ER dosage
should be increased slowly and with regular monitoring
for fluid and nutritional intake (5.15)

———————ADVERSE REACTIONS———————
- Most common adverse reactions (reported >5%) reported
in adult studies are nausea, somnolence, dizziness, vomiting, asthenia, abdominal pain, dyspepsia, rash, diarrhea,
increased appetite, tremor, weight gain, back pain, alopecia, headache, fever, anorexia, constipation, diplopia, am-
blyopia/blurred, ataxia, nystagmus, emotional lability,
thinking abnormal, amnesia, flu syndrome, infection,
bronchitis, rhinitis, ecchymosis, peripheral edema, insomnia, nervousness, depression, pharyngitis, dyspnea, tinnitus (6.1, 6.2, 6.3, 6.4).
- The safety and tolerability of valproate in pediatric patients were shown to be comparable to those in adults
(8.4).

**To report SUSPECTED ADVERSE REACTIONS, contact
AbbVie Inc. at 1-800-633-9110 or FDA at 1-800-FDA-1088 or
www.fda.gov/medwatch**

———————DRUG INTERACTIONS———————
- Hepatic enzyme-inducing drugs (e.g., phenytoin, carbamazepine, primidone, phenobarbital, rifampin) can increase valproate clearance, while enzyme inhibitors (e.g.,
felbamate) can decrease valproate clearance. Therefore increased monitoring of valproate and concomitant drug
concentrations and dose adjustment is indicated whenever
enzyme-inducing or inhibiting drugs are introduced or
withdrawn (7.1)
- Aspirin, carbapenem antibiotics: Monitoring of valproate concentrations are recommended (7.1)
- Co-administration of valproate can affect the pharmacokinetics of other drugs (e.g. diazepam, ethosuximide, lamotrigine, phenytoin) by inhibiting their metabolism or protein binding displacement (7.2)
- Dosage adjustment of amitryptyline/nortriptyline, warfarin, and zidovudine may be necessary if used concomitantly with Depakote ER (7.2)
- Topiramate: Hyperammonemia and encephalopathy (5.10,
7.3)

———————USE IN SPECIFIC POPULATIONS———————
- Pregnancy: Depakote ER can cause congenital malformations including neural tube defects and decreased IQ.
(5.2, 5.3, 8.1)
- Pediatric: Children under the age of two years are at
considerably higher risk of fatal hepatotoxicity (5.1, 8.4)
- Geriatric: Reduce starting dose; increase dosage more
slowly; monitor fluid and nutritional intake, and somnolence (5.15, 8.5)

**See 17 for PATIENT COUNSELING INFORMATION
and Medication Guide.**

Revised: 04/2014

FULL PRESCRIBING INFORMATION: CONTENTS*
WARNING: LIFE THREATENING ADVERSE REAC-
TIONS

*Sections or subsections omitted from the full prescribing
information are not listed.

FULL PRESCRIBING INFORMATION

**WARNING: LIFE THREATENING ADVERSE
REACTIONS**

Hepatotoxicity

General Population: Hepatic failure resulting in fatalities has occurred in patients receiving valproate
and its derivatives. These incidents usually have
occurred during the first six months of treatment. Serious or fatal hepatotoxicity may be preceded by nonspecific symptoms such as malaise, weakness, lethargy, facial edema, anorexia, and vomiting. In
patients with epilepsy, a loss of seizure control may
also occur. Patients should be monitored closely for
appearance of these symptoms. Serum liver tests
should be performed prior to therapy and at frequent
intervals thereafter, especially during the first six
months *[see Warnings and Precautions (5.1)]*.

Children under the age of two years are at a considerably increased risk of developing fatal hepatotoxicity, especially those on multiple anticonvulsants,
those with congenital metabolic disorders, those
with severe seizure disorders accompanied by mental
retardation, and those with organic brain disease.
When Depakote ER is used in this patient group, it
should be used with extreme caution and as a sole

Information on the AbbVie, Inc. products listed on these
pages is from the prescribing information in use as
of July 31, 2014. For more information, please visit
rxabbvie.com or call 1-800-633-9110.

agent. The benefits of therapy should be weighed against the risks. The incidence of fatal hepatotoxicity decreases considerably in progressively older patient groups.

Patients with Mitochondrial Disease: There is an increased risk of valproate-induced acute liver failure and resultant deaths in patients with hereditary neurometabolic syndromes caused by DNA mutations of the mitochondrial DNA Polymerase γ (POLG) gene (e.g. Alpers Huttenlocher Syndrome). Depakote ER is contraindicated in patients known to have mitochondrial disorders caused by POLG mutations and children under two years of age who are clinically suspected of having a mitochondrial disorder *[see Contraindications (4)]*. In patients over two years of age who are clinically suspected of having a hereditary mitochondrial disease, Depakote ER should only be used after other anticonvulsants have failed. This older group of patients should be closely monitored during treatment with Depakote ER for the development of acute liver injury with regular clinical assessments and serum liver testing. POLG mutation screening should be performed in accordance with current clinical practice *[see Warnings and Precautions (5.1)]*.

Fetal Risk
Valproate can cause major congenital malformations, particularly neural tube defects (e.g., spina bifida). In addition, valproate can cause decreased IQ scores following *in utero* exposure.

Valproate is therefore contraindicated in pregnant women treated for prophylaxis of migraine *[see Contraindications (4)]*. Valproate should only be used to treat pregnant women with epilepsy or bipolar disorder if other medications have failed to control their symptoms or are otherwise unacceptable.

Valproate should not be administered to a woman of childbearing potential unless the drug is essential to the management of her medical condition. This is especially important when valproate use is considered for a condition not usually associated with permanent injury or death (e.g., migraine). Women should use effective contraception while using valproate *[see Warnings and Precautions (5.2, 5.3, 5.4)]*.

A Medication Guide describing the risks of valproate is available for patients *[see Patient Counseling Information (17)]*.

Pancreatitis
Cases of life-threatening pancreatitis have been reported in both children and adults receiving valproate. Some of the cases have been described as hemorrhagic with a rapid progression from initial symptoms to death. Cases have been reported shortly after initial use as well as after several years of use. Patients and guardians should be warned that abdominal pain, nausea, vomiting and/or anorexia can be symptoms of pancreatitis that require prompt medical evaluation. If pancreatitis is diagnosed, valproate should ordinarily be discontinued. Alternative treatment for the underlying medical condition should be initiated as clinically indicated *[see Warnings and Precautions (5.5)]*.

1 INDICATIONS AND USAGE
1.1 Mania
Depakote ER is a valproate and is indicated for the treatment of acute manic or mixed episodes associated with bipolar disorder, with or without psychotic features. A manic episode is a distinct period of abnormally and persistently elevated, expansive, or irritable mood. Typical symptoms of mania include pressure of speech, motor hyperactivity, reduced need for sleep, flight of ideas, grandiosity, poor judgment, aggressiveness, and possible hostility. A mixed episode is characterized by the criteria for a manic episode in conjunction with those for a major depressive episode (depressed mood, loss of interest or pleasure in nearly all activities).

The efficacy of Depakote ER is based in part on studies of Depakote (divalproex sodium delayed release tablets) in this indication, and was confirmed in a 3-week trial with patients meeting DSM-IV TR criteria for bipolar I disorder, manic or mixed type, who were hospitalized for acute mania *[see Clinical Studies (14.1)]*.

The effectiveness of valproate for long-term use in mania, i.e., more than 3 weeks, has not been demonstrated in controlled clinical trials. Therefore, healthcare providers who elect to use Depakote ER for extended periods should continually reevaluate the long-term risk-benefits of the drug for the individual patient.

1.2 Epilepsy
Depakote ER is indicated as monotherapy and adjunctive therapy in the treatment of adult patients and pediatric patients down to the age of 10 years with complex partial seizures that occur either in isolation or in association with other types of seizures. Depakote ER is also indicated for use as sole and adjunctive therapy in the treatment of simple and complex absence seizures in adults and children 10 years of age or older, and adjunctively in adults and children 10 years of age or older with multiple seizure types that include absence seizures.

Simple absence is defined as very brief clouding of the sensorium or loss of consciousness accompanied by certain generalized epileptic discharges without other detectable clinical signs. Complex absence is the term used when other signs are also present.

1.3 Migraine
Depakote ER is indicated for prophylaxis of migraine headaches. There is no evidence that Depakote ER is useful in the acute treatment of migraine headaches.

1.4 Important Limitations
Because of the risk to the fetus of decreased IQ, neural tube defects, and other major congenital malformations, which may occur very early in pregnancy, valproate should not be administered to a woman of childbearing potential unless the drug is essential to the management of her medical condition *[see Warnings and Precautions (5.2, 5.3, 5.4), Use in Specific Populations (8.1), and Patient Counseling Information (17.3)]*.

Depakote ER is contraindicated for prophylaxis of migraine headaches in women who are pregnant.

2 DOSAGE AND ADMINISTRATION
Depakote ER is an extended-release product intended for once-a-day oral administration. Depakote ER tablets should be swallowed whole and should not be crushed or chewed.

2.1 Mania
Depakote ER tablets are administered orally. The recommended initial dose is 25 mg/kg/day given once daily. The dose should be increased as rapidly as possible to achieve the lowest therapeutic dose which produces the desired clinical effect or the desired range of plasma concentrations. In a placebo-controlled clinical trial of acute mania or mixed type, patients were dosed to a clinical response with a trough plasma concentration between 85 and 125 mcg/mL. The maximum recommended dosage is 60 mg/kg/day.

There is no body of evidence available from controlled trials to guide a clinician in the longer term management of a patient who improves during Depakote ER treatment of an acute manic episode. While it is generally agreed that pharmacological treatment beyond an acute response in mania is desirable, both for maintenance of the initial response and for prevention of new manic episodes, there are no data to support the benefits of Depakote ER in such longer-term treatment (i.e., beyond 3 weeks).

2.2 Epilepsy
Depakote ER (divalproex sodium) extended release tablets are administered orally, and must be swallowed whole. As Depakote ER dosage is titrated upward, concentrations of clonazepam, diazepam, ethosuximide, lamotrigine, tolbutamide, phenobarbital, carbamazepine, and/or phenytoin may be affected *[see Drug Interactions (7.2)]*.

Complex Partial Seizures
For adults and children 10 years of age or older.

Monotherapy (Initial Therapy)
Depakote ER has not been systematically studied as initial therapy. Patients should initiate therapy at 10 to 15 mg/kg/day. The dosage should be increased by 5 to 10 mg/kg/week to achieve optimal clinical response. Ordinarily, optimal clinical response is achieved at daily doses below 60 mg/kg/day. If satisfactory clinical response has not been achieved, plasma levels should be measured to determine whether or not they are in the usually accepted therapeutic range (50 to 100 mcg/mL). No recommendation regarding the safety of valproate for use at doses above 60 mg/kg/day can be made. The probability of thrombocytopenia increases significantly at total trough valproate plasma concentrations above 110 mcg/mL in females and 135 mcg/mL in males. The benefit of improved seizure control with higher doses should be weighed against the possibility of a greater incidence of adverse reactions.

Conversion to Monotherapy
Patients should initiate therapy at 10 to 15 mg/kg/day. The dosage should be increased by 5 to 10 mg/kg/week to achieve optimal clinical response. Ordinarily, optimal clinical response is achieved at daily doses below 60 mg/kg/day. If satisfactory clinical response has not been achieved, plasma levels should be measured to determine whether or not they are in the usually accepted therapeutic range (50 - 100 mcg/mL). No recommendation regarding the safety of valproate for use at doses above 60 mg/kg/day can be made.

Concomitant antiepilepsy drug (AED) dosage can ordinarily be reduced by approximately 25% every 2 weeks. This reduction may be started at initiation of Depakote ER therapy, or delayed by 1 to 2 weeks if there is a concern that seizures are likely to occur with a reduction. The speed and duration of withdrawal of the concomitant AED can be highly variable, and patients should be monitored closely during this period for increased seizure frequency.

Adjunctive Therapy
Depakote ER may be added to the patient's regimen at a dosage of 10 to 15 mg/kg/day. The dosage may be increased by 5 to 10 mg/kg/week to achieve optimal clinical response. Ordinarily, optimal clinical response is achieved at daily doses below 60 mg/kg/day. If satisfactory clinical response has not been achieved, plasma levels should be measured to determine whether or not they are in the usually accepted therapeutic range (50 to 100 mcg/mL). No recommendation regarding the safety of valproate for use at doses above 60 mg/kg/day can be made.

In a study of adjunctive therapy for complex partial seizures in which patients were receiving either carbamazepine or phenytoin in addition to valproate, no adjustment of carbamazepine or phenytoin dosage was needed *[see Clinical Studies (14.2)]*. However, since valproate may interact with these or other concurrently administered AEDs as well as other drugs, periodic plasma concentration determinations of concomitant AEDs are recommended during the early course of therapy *[see Drug Interactions (7)]*.

Simple and Complex Absence Seizures
The recommended initial dose is 15 mg/kg/day, increasing at one week intervals by 5 to 10 mg/kg/day until seizures are controlled or side effects preclude further increases. The maximum recommended dosage is 60 mg/kg/day.

A good correlation has not been established between daily dose, serum concentrations, and therapeutic effect. However, therapeutic valproate serum concentration for most patients with absence seizures is considered to range from 50 to 100 mcg/mL. Some patients may be controlled with lower or higher serum concentrations *[see Clinical Pharmacology (12.3)]*.

As Depakote ER dosage is titrated upward, blood concentrations of phenobarbital and/or phenytoin may be affected *[see Drug Interactions (7.2)]*.

Antiepilepsy drugs should not be abruptly discontinued in patients in whom the drug is administered to prevent major seizures because of the strong possibility of precipitating status epilepticus with attendant hypoxia and threat to life.

2.3 Migraine
Depakote ER is indicated for prophylaxis of migraine headaches in adults.

The recommended starting dose is 500 mg once daily for 1 week, thereafter increasing to 1000 mg once daily. Although doses other than 1000 mg once daily of Depakote ER have not been evaluated in patients with migraine, the effective dose range of Depakote (divalproex sodium delayed-release tablets) in these patients is 500-1000 mg/day. As with other valproate products, doses of Depakote ER should be individualized and dose adjustment may be necessary. If a patient requires smaller dose adjustments than that available with Depakote ER, Depakote should be used instead.

2.4 Conversion from Depakote to Depakote ER
In adult patients and pediatric patients 10 years of age or older with epilepsy previously receiving Depakote, Depakote ER should be administered once-daily using a dose 8 to 20% higher than the total daily dose of Depakote (Table 1). For patients whose Depakote total daily dose cannot be directly converted to Depakote ER, consideration may be given at the clinician's discretion to increase the patient's Depakote total daily dose to the next higher dosage before converting to the appropriate total daily dose of Depakote ER.

Table 1. Dose Conversion

Depakote Total Daily Dose (mg)	Depakote ER (mg)
500* - 625	750
750* - 875	1000
1000*-1125	1250
1250-1375	1500
1500-1625	1750
1750	2000
1875-2000	2250
2125-2250	2500
2375	2750
2500-2750	3000
2875	3250
3000-3125	3500

* These total daily doses of Depakote cannot be directly converted to an 8 to 20% higher total daily dose of Depakote ER because the required dosing strengths of Depakote ER are not available. Consideration may be given at the clinician's discretion to increase the patient's Depakote total daily dose to the next higher dosage before converting to the appropriate total daily dose of Depakote ER.

There is insufficient data to allow a conversion factor recommendation for patients with DEPAKOTE doses above 3125 mg/day. Plasma valproate C_{min} concentrations for DEPAKOTE ER on average are equivalent to DEPAKOTE, but may vary across patients after conversion. If satisfactory clinical response has not been achieved, plasma levels should be measured to determine whether or not they are in the usually accepted therapeutic range (50 to 100 mcg/mL) *[see Clinical Pharmacology (12.2)]*.

2.5 General Dosing Advice

Dosing in Elderly Patients

Due to a decrease in unbound clearance of valproate and possibly a greater sensitivity to somnolence in the elderly, the starting dose should be reduced in these patients. Starting doses in the elderly lower than 250 mg can only be achieved by the use of Depakote. Dosage should be increased more slowly and with regular monitoring for fluid and nutritional intake, dehydration, somnolence, and other adverse reactions. Dose reductions or discontinuation of valproate should be considered in patients with decreased food or fluid intake and in patients with excessive somnolence. The ultimate therapeutic dose should be achieved on the basis of both tolerability and clinical response *[see Warnings and Precautions (5.15), Use in Specific Populations (8.5) and Clinical Pharmacology (12.3)]*.

Dose-Related Adverse Reactions

The frequency of adverse effects (particularly elevated liver enzymes and thrombocytopenia) may be dose-related. The probability of thrombocytopenia appears to increase significantly at total valproate concentrations of ≥ 110 mcg/mL (females) or ≥ 135 mcg/mL (males) *[see Warnings and Precautions (5.9)]*. The benefit of improved therapeutic effect with higher doses should be weighed against the possibility of a greater incidence of adverse reactions.

G.I. Irritation

Patients who experience G.I. irritation may benefit from administration of the drug with food or by slowly building up the dose from an initial low level.

Compliance

Patients should be informed to take Depakote ER every day as prescribed. If a dose is missed it should be taken as soon as possible, unless it is almost time for the next dose. If a dose is skipped, the patient should not double the next dose.

3 DOSAGE FORMS AND STRENGTHS

Depakote ER 250 mg is available as white ovaloid tablets with the "a" logo and the code (HF). Each Depakote ER tablet contains divalproex sodium equivalent to 250 mg of valproic acid.

Depakote ER 500 mg is available as gray ovaloid tablets with the "a" logo and the code HC. Each Depakote ER tablet contains divalproex sodium equivalent to 500 mg of valproic acid.

4 CONTRAINDICATIONS

- Depakote ER should not be administered to patients with hepatic disease or significant hepatic dysfunction *[see Warnings and Precautions (5.1)]*.
- Depakote ER is contraindicated in patients known to have mitochondrial disorders caused by mutations in mitochondrial DNA polymerase γ (POLG; e.g., Alpers-Huttenlocher Syndrome) and children under two years of age who are suspected of having a POLG-related disorder *[see Warnings and Precautions (5.1)]*.
- Depakote ER is contraindicated in patients with known hypersensitivity to the drug *[see Warnings and Precautions (5.13)]*.
- Depakote ER is contraindicated in patients with known urea cycle disorders *[see Warnings and Precautions (5.6)]*.
- Depakote ER is contraindicated for use in prophylaxis of migraine headaches in pregnant women *[see Warnings and Precautions (5.3) and Use in Specific Populations (8.1)]*.

5 WARNINGS AND PRECAUTIONS

5.1 Hepatotoxicity

General Information on Hepatotoxicity

Hepatic failure resulting in fatalities has occurred in patients receiving valproate. These incidents usually have occurred during the first six months of treatment. Serious or fatal hepatotoxicity may be preceded by non-specific symptoms such as malaise, weakness, lethargy, facial edema, anorexia, and vomiting. In patients with epilepsy, a loss of seizure control may also occur. Patients should be monitored closely for appearance of these symptoms. Serum liver tests should be performed prior to therapy and at frequent intervals thereafter, especially during the first six months. However, healthcare providers should not rely totally on serum biochemistry since these tests may not be abnormal in all instances, but should also consider the results of careful interim medical history and physical examination.

Caution should be observed when administering valproate products to patients with a prior history of hepatic disease. Patients on multiple anticonvulsants, children, those with congenital metabolic disorders, those with severe seizure disorders accompanied by mental retardation, and those with organic brain disease may be at particular risk. See below, "Patients with Known or Suspected Mitochondrial Disease."

Experience has indicated that children under the age of two years are at a considerably increased risk of developing fatal hepatotoxicity, especially those with the aforementioned conditions. When Depakote ER is used in this patient group, it should be used with extreme caution and as a sole agent. The benefits of therapy should be weighed against the risks. In progressively older patient groups experience in epilepsy has indicated that the incidence of fatal hepatotoxicity decreases considerably.

Patients with Known or Suspected Mitochondrial Disease

Depakote ER is contraindicated in patients known to have mitochondrial disorders caused by POLG mutations and children under two years of age who are clinically suspected of having a mitochondrial disorder *[see Contraindications (4)]*. Valproate-induced acute liver failure and liver-related deaths have been reported in patients with hereditary neurometabolic syndromes caused by mutations in the gene for mitochondrial DNA polymerase γ (POLG) (e.g., Alpers-Huttenlocher Syndrome) at a higher rate than those without these syndromes. Most of the reported cases of liver failure is in patients with these syndromes have been identified in children and adolescents.

POLG-related disorders should be suspected in patients with a family history or suggestive symptoms of a POLG-related disorder, including but not limited to unexplained encephalopathy, refractory epilepsy (focal, myoclonic), status epilepticus at presentation, developmental delays, psychomotor regression, axonal sensorimotor neuropathy, myopathy cerebellar ataxia, opthalmoplegia, or complicated migraine with occipital aura. POLG mutation testing should be performed in accordance with current clinical practice for the diagnostic evaluation of such disorders. The A467T and W748S mutations are present in approximately 2/3 of patients with autosomal recessive POLG-related disorders.

In patients over two years of age who are clinically suspected of having a hereditary mitochondrial disease, Depakote ER should only be used after other anticonvulsants have failed. This older group of patients should be closely monitored during treatment with Depakote ER for the development of acute liver injury with regular clinical assessments and serum liver test monitoring.

The drug should be discontinued immediately in the presence of significant hepatic dysfunction, suspected or apparent. In some cases, hepatic dysfunction has progressed in spite of discontinuation of drug *[see Boxed Warning and Contraindications (4)]*.

5.2 Birth Defects

Valproate can cause fetal harm when administered to a pregnant woman. Pregnancy registry data show that maternal valproate use can cause neural tube defects and other structural abnormalities (e.g., craniofacial defects, cardiovascular malformations and malformations involving various body systems). The rate of congenital malformations among babies born to mothers using valproate is about four times higher than the rate among babies born to epileptic mothers using other anti-seizure monotherapies. Evidence suggests that folic acid supplementation prior to conception and during the first trimester of pregnancy decreases the risk for congenital neural tube defects in the general population.

5.3 Decreased IQ Following *in utero* Exposure

Valproate can cause decreased IQ scores following *in utero* exposure. Published epidemiological studies have indicated that children exposed to valproate *in utero* have lower cognitive test scores than children exposed *in utero* to either another antiepileptic drug or to no antiepileptic drugs. The largest of these studies[1] is a prospective cohort study conducted in the United States and United Kingdom that found that children with prenatal exposure to valproate (n=62) had lower IQ scores at age 6 (97 [95% C.I. 94-101]) than children with prenatal exposure to the other antiepileptic drug monotherapy treatments evaluated: lamotrigine (108 [95% C.I. 105–110]), carbamazepine (105 [95% C.I. 102–108]), and phenytoin (108 [95% C.I. 104–112]). It is not known when during pregnancy cognitive effects in valproate-exposed children occur. Because the women in this study were exposed to antiepileptic drugs throughout pregnancy, whether the risk for decreased IQ was related to a particular time period during pregnancy could not be assessed.

Although all of the available studies have methodological limitations, the weight of the evidence supports the conclusion that valproate exposure *in utero* can cause decreased IQ in children.

In animal studies, offspring with prenatal exposure to valproate had malformations similar to those seen in humans and demonstrated neurobehavioral deficits *[see Use in Specific Populations (8.1)]*.

Valproate use is contraindicated during pregnancy in women being treated for prophylaxis of migraine headaches. Women with epilepsy or bipolar disorder who are pregnant or who plan to become pregnant should not be treated with valproate unless other treatments have failed to provide adequate symptom control or are otherwise unacceptable. In such women, the benefits of treatment with valproate during pregnancy may still outweigh the risks.

5.4 Use in Women of Childbearing Potential

Because of the risk to the fetus of decreased IQ and major congenital malformations (including neural tube defects), which may occur very early in pregnancy, valproate should not be administered to a woman of childbearing potential unless the drug is essential to the management of her medical condition. This is especially important when valproate use is considered for a condition not usually associated with permanent injury or death (e.g., migraine). Women should use effective contraception while using valproate. Women who are planning a pregnancy should be counseled regarding the relative risks and benefits of valproate use during pregnancy, and alternative therapeutic options should be considered for these patients *[see Boxed Warning and Use in Specific Populations (8.1)]*.

To prevent major seizures, valproate should not be discontinued abruptly, as this can precipitate status epilepticus with resulting maternal and fetal hypoxia and threat to life. Evidence suggests that folic acid supplementation prior to conception and during the first trimester of pregnancy decreases the risk for congenital neural tube defects in the general population. It is not known whether the risk of neural tube defects or decreased IQ in the offspring of women receiving valproate is reduced by folic acid supplementation. Dietary folic acid supplementation both prior to conception and during pregnancy should be routinely recommended for patients using valproate.

5.5 Pancreatitis

Cases of life-threatening pancreatitis have been reported in both children and adults receiving valproate. Some of the cases have been described as hemorrhagic with rapid progression from initial symptoms to death. Some cases have occurred shortly after initial use as well as after several years of use. The rate based upon the reported cases exceeds that expected in the general population and there have been cases in which pancreatitis recurred after rechallenge with valproate. In clinical trials, there were 2 cases of pancreatitis without alternative etiology in 2416 patients, representing 1044 patient-years experience. Patients and guardians should be warned that abdominal pain, nausea, vomiting, and/or anorexia can be symptoms of pancreatitis that require prompt medical evaluation. If pancreatitis is diagnosed, Depakote ER should ordinarily be discontinued. Alternative treatment for the underlying medical condition should be initiated as clinically indicated *[see Boxed Warning]*.

5.6 Urea Cycle Disorders

Depakote ER is contraindicated in patients with known urea cycle disorders (UCD). Hyperammonemic encephalopathy, sometimes fatal, has been reported following initiation of valproate therapy in patients with urea cycle disorders, a group of uncommon genetic abnormalities, particularly ornithine transcarbamylase deficiency. Prior to the initiation of Depakote ER therapy, evaluation for UCD should be considered in the following patients: 1) those with a history of unexplained encephalopathy or coma, encephalopathy associated with a protein load, pregnancy-related or postpartum encephalopathy, unexplained mental retardation, or history of elevated plasma ammonia or glutamine; 2) those with cyclical vomiting and lethargy, episodic extreme irritability, ataxia, low BUN, or protein avoidance; 3) those with a family history of UCD or a family history of unexplained infant deaths (particularly males); 4) those with other signs or symptoms of UCD. Patients who develop symptoms of unexplained hyperammonemic encephalopathy while receiving valproate therapy should receive prompt treatment (including discontinuation of valproate therapy) and be evaluated for underlying urea cycle disorders *[see Contraindications (4) and Warnings and Precautions (5.11)]*.

5.7 Brain Atrophy

There have been postmarketing reports of reversible and irreversible cerebral and cerebellar atrophy temporally associated with the use of valproate products; in some cases, patients recovered with permanent sequelae *[see Adverse Reactions (6.4)]*. The motor and cognitive functions of patients on valproate should be routinely monitored and drug should be evaluated for continued use in the presence of suspected or apparent signs of brain atrophy.

Reports of cerebral atrophy have also been reported in children who were exposed *in utero* to valproate products *[see Use in Specific Populations (8.1)]*.

Information on the AbbVie, Inc. products listed on these pages is from the prescribing information in use as of July 31, 2014. For more information, please visit rxabbvie.com or call 1-800-633-9110.

Table 2. Risk by indication for antiepileptic drugs in the pooled analysis

Indication	Placebo Patients with Events Per 1000 Patients	Drug Patients with Events Per 1000 Patients	Relative Risk: Incidence of Events in Drug Patients/ Incidence in Placebo Patients	Risk Difference: Additional Drug Patients with Events Per 1000 Patients
Epilepsy	1.0	3.4	3.5	2.4
Psychiatric	5.7	8.5	1.5	2.9
Other	1.0	1.8	1.9	0.9
Total	2.4	4.3	1.8	1.9

5.8   Suicidal Behavior and Ideation
Antiepileptic drugs (AEDs), including Depakote ER, increase the risk of suicidal thoughts or behavior in patients taking these drugs for any indication. Patients treated with any AED for any indication should be monitored for the emergence or worsening of depression, suicidal thoughts or behavior, and/or any unusual changes in mood or behavior. Pooled analyses of 199 placebo-controlled clinical trials (mono- and adjunctive therapy) of 11 different AEDs showed that patients randomized to one of the AEDs had approximately twice the risk (adjusted Relative Risk 1.8, 95% CI:1.2, 2.7) of suicidal thinking or behavior compared to patients randomized to placebo. In these trials, which had a median treatment duration of 12 weeks, the estimated incidence rate of suicidal behavior or ideation among 27,863 AED-treated patients was 0.43%, compared to 0.24% among 16,029 placebo-treated patients, representing an increase of approximately one case of suicidal thinking or behavior for every 530 patients treated. There were four suicides in drug-treated patients in the trials and none in placebo-treated patients, but the number is too small to allow any conclusion about drug effect on suicide.
The increased risk of suicidal thoughts or behavior with AEDs was observed as early as one week after starting drug treatment with AEDs and persisted for the duration of treatment assessed. Because most trials included in the analysis did not extend beyond 24 weeks, the risk of suicidal thoughts or behavior beyond 24 weeks could not be assessed.
The risk of suicidal thoughts or behavior was generally consistent among drugs in the data analyzed. The finding of increased risk with AEDs of varying mechanisms of action and across a range of indications suggests that the risk applies to all AEDs used for any indication. The risk did not vary substantially by age (5-100 years) in the clinical trials analyzed.
Table 2 shows absolute and relative risk by indication for all evaluated AEDs.
[See table 2 above]
The relative risk for suicidal thoughts or behavior was higher in clinical trials for epilepsy than in clinical trials for psychiatric or other conditions, but the absolute risk differences were similar for the epilepsy and psychiatric indications.
Anyone considering prescribing Depakote ER or any other AED must balance the risk of suicidal thoughts or behavior with the risk of untreated illness. Epilepsy and many other illnesses for which AEDs are prescribed are themselves associated with morbidity and mortality and an increased risk of suicidal thoughts and behavior. Should suicidal thoughts and behavior emerge during treatment, the prescriber needs to consider whether the emergence of these symptoms in any given patient may be related to the illness being treated.
Patients, their caregivers, and families should be informed that AEDs increase the risk of suicidal thoughts and behavior and should be advised of the need to be alert for the emergence or worsening of the signs and symptoms of depression, any unusual changes in mood or behavior, or the emergence of suicidal thoughts, behavior, or thoughts about self-harm. Behaviors of concern should be reported immediately to healthcare providers.

5.9   Thrombocytopenia
The frequency of adverse effects (particularly elevated liver enzymes and thrombocytopenia) may be dose-related. In a clinical trial of valproate as monotherapy in patients with epilepsy, 34/126 patients (27%) receiving approximately 50 mg/kg/day on average, had at least one value of platelets ≤ 75 × 10⁹/L. Approximately half of these patients had treatment discontinued, with return of platelet counts to normal. In the remaining patients, platelet counts normalized with continued treatment. In this study, the probability of thrombocytopenia appeared to increase significantly at total valproate concentrations of ≥ 110 mcg/mL (females) or ≥ 135 mcg/mL (males). The therapeutic benefit which may accompany the higher doses should therefore be weighed against the possibility of a greater incidence of adverse effects.

Because of reports of thrombocytopenia, inhibition of the secondary phase of platelet aggregation, and abnormal coagulation parameters, (e.g., low fibrinogen), platelet counts and coagulation tests are recommended before initiating therapy and at periodic intervals. It is recommended that patients receiving Depakote ER be monitored for platelet count and coagulation parameters prior to planned surgery. Evidence of hemorrhage, bruising, or a disorder of hemostasis/coagulation is an indication for reduction of the dosage or withdrawal of therapy.

5.10   Hyperammonemia
Hyperammonemia has been reported in association with valproate therapy and may be present despite normal liver function tests. In patients who develop unexplained lethargy and vomiting or changes in mental status, hyperammonemic encephalopathy should be considered and an ammonia level should be measured. Hyperammonemia should also be considered in patients who present with hypothermia [see Warnings and Precautions (5.12)]. If ammonia is increased, valproate therapy should be discontinued. Appropriate interventions for treatment of hyperammonemia should be initiated, and such patients should undergo investigation for underlying urea cycle disorders [see Contraindications (4) and Warnings and Precautions (5.6, 5.10, 5.11)]. During the placebo controlled pediatric mania trial, one (1) in twenty (20) adolescents (5%) treated with valproate developed increased plasma ammonia levels compared to no (0) patients treated with placebo.
Asymptomatic elevations of ammonia are more common and when present, require close monitoring of plasma ammonia levels. If the elevation persists, discontinuation of valproate therapy should be considered.

5.11   Hyperammonemia and Encephalopathy associated with Concomitant Topiramate Use
Concomitant administration of topiramate and valproate has been associated with hyperammonemia with or without encephalopathy in patients who have tolerated either drug alone. Clinical symptoms of hyperammonemic encephalopathy often include acute alterations in level of consciousness and/or cognitive function with lethargy or vomiting. Hypothermia can also be a manifestation of hyperammonemia [see Warnings and Precautions (5.12)]. In most cases, symptoms and signs abated with discontinuation of either drug. This adverse event is not due to a pharmacokinetic interaction. It is not known if topiramate monotherapy is associated with hyperammonemia. Patients with inborn errors of metabolism or reduced hepatic mitochondrial activity may be at an increased risk for hyperammonemia with or without encephalopathy. Although not studied, an interaction of topiramate and valproate may exacerbate existing defects or unmask deficiencies in susceptible persons. In patients who develop unexplained lethargy, vomiting, or changes in mental status, hyperammonemic encephalopathy should be considered and an ammonia level should be measured [see Contraindications (4) and Warnings and Precautions (5.6, 5.10)].

5.12   Hypothermia
Hypothermia, defined as an unintentional drop in body core temperature to < 35°C (95°F), has been reported in association with valproate therapy both in conjunction with and in the absence of hyperammonemia. This adverse reaction can also occur in patients using concomitant topiramate with valproate after starting topiramate treatment or after increasing the daily dose of topiramate [see Drug Interactions (7.3)]. Consideration should be given to stopping valproate in patients who develop hypothermia, which may be manifested by a variety of clinical abnormalities including lethargy, confusion, coma, and significant alterations in other major organ systems such as the cardiovascular and respiratory systems. Clinical management and assessment should include examination of blood ammonia levels.

5.13   Multi-Organ Hypersensitivity Reactions
Multi-organ hypersensitivity reactions have been rarely reported in close temporal association to the initiation of valproate therapy in adult and pediatric patients (median time to detection 21 days: range 1 to 40 days). Although there have been a limited number of reports, many of these cases resulted in hospitalization and at least one death has been

reported. Signs and symptoms of this disorder were diverse; however, patients typically, although not exclusively, presented with fever and rash associated with other organ system involvement. Other associated manifestations may include lymphadenopathy, hepatitis, liver function test abnormalities, hematological abnormalities (e.g., eosinophilia, thrombocytopenia, neutropenia), pruritus, nephritis, oliguria, hepato-renal syndrome, arthralgia, and asthenia. Because the disorder is variable in its expression, other organ system symptoms and signs, not noted here, may occur. If this reaction is suspected, valproate should be discontinued and an alternative treatment started. Although the existence of cross sensitivity with other drugs that produce this syndrome is unclear, the experience amongst drugs associated with multi-organ hypersensitivity would indicate this to be a possibility.

5.14   Interaction with Carbapenem Antibiotics
Carbapenem antibiotics (for example, ertapenem, imipenem, meropenem; this is not a complete list) may reduce serum valproate concentrations to subtherapeutic levels, resulting in loss of seizure control. Serum valproate concentrations should be monitored frequently after initiating carbapenem therapy. Alternative antibacterial or anticonvulsant therapy should be considered if serum valproate concentrations drop significantly or seizure control deteriorates [see Drug Interactions (7.1)].

5.15   Somnolence in the Elderly
In a double-blind, multicenter trial of valproate in elderly patients with dementia (mean age = 83 years), doses were increased by 125 mg/day to a target dose of 20 mg/kg/day. A significantly higher proportion of valproate patients had somnolence compared to placebo, and although not statistically significant, there was a higher proportion of patients with dehydration. Discontinuations for somnolence were also significantly higher than with placebo. In some patients with somnolence (approximately one-half), there was associated reduced nutritional intake and weight loss. There was a trend for the patients who experienced these events to have a lower baseline albumin concentration, lower valproate clearance, and a higher BUN. In elderly patients, dosage should be increased more slowly and with regular monitoring for fluid and nutritional intake, dehydration, somnolence, and other adverse reactions. Dose reductions or discontinuation of valproate should be considered in patients with decreased food or fluid intake and in patients with excessive somnolence [see Dosage and Administration (2.4)].

5.16   Monitoring: Drug Plasma Concentration
Since valproate may interact with concurrently administered drugs which are capable of enzyme induction, periodic plasma concentration determinations of valproate and concomitant drugs are recommended during the early course of therapy [see Drug Interactions (7)].

5.17   Effect on Ketone and Thyroid Function Tests
Valproate is partially eliminated in the urine as a ketometabolite which may lead to a false interpretation of the urine ketone test.
There have been reports of altered thyroid function tests associated with valproate. The clinical significance of these is unknown.

5.18   Effect on HIV and CMV Viruses Replication
There are in vitro studies that suggest valproate stimulates the replication of the HIV and CMV viruses under certain experimental conditions. The clinical consequence, if any, is not known. Additionally, the relevance of these in vitro findings is uncertain for patients receiving maximally suppressive antiretroviral therapy. Nevertheless, these data should be borne in mind when interpreting the results from regular monitoring of the viral load in HIV infected patients receiving valproate or when following CMV infected patients clinically.

5.19   Medication Residue in the Stool
There have been rare reports of medication residue in the stool. Some patients have had anatomic (including ileostomy or colostomy) or functional gastrointestinal disorders with shortened GI transit times. In some reports, medication residues have occurred in the context of diarrhea. It is recommended that plasma valproate levels be checked in patients who experience medication residue in the stool, and patients' clinical condition should be monitored. If clinically indicated, alternative treatment may be considered.

6   ADVERSE REACTIONS

The following adverse reactions are discussed in greater detail in other sections of the labeling:
Hepatic failure (5.1)
Birth defects (5.2)
Decreased IQ following in utero exposure (5.3)
Pancreatitis (5.5)
Thrombocytopenia (5.9)
Hyperammonemic encephalopathy (5.6, 5.10, 5.11)
Multi-organ hypersensitivity reactions (5.13)
Somnolence in the elderly (5.15)

Because clinical studies are conducted under widely varying conditions, adverse reaction rates observed in the clinical studies of a drug cannot be directly compared to rates in the clinical studies of another drug and may not reflect the rates observed in practice.

Information on pediatric adverse reactions is presented in section 8.

6.1 Mania

The incidence of treatment-emergent events has been ascertained based on combined data from two three week placebo-controlled clinical trials of Depakote ER in the treatment of manic episodes associated with bipolar disorder.

Table 3 summarizes those adverse reactions reported for patients in these trials where the incidence rate in the Depakote ER-treated group was greater than 5% and greater than the placebo incidence.

Table 3. Adverse Reactions Reported by > 5% of Depakote-Treated Patients During Placebo-Controlled Trials of Acute Mania[1]

Adverse Event	Depakote ER (n=338)	Placebo (n=263)
Somnolence	26%	14%
Dyspepsia	23%	11%
Nausea	19%	13%
Vomiting	13%	5%
Diarrhea	12%	8%
Dizziness	12%	7%
Pain	11%	10%
Abdominal pain	10%	5%
Accidental injury	6%	5%
Asthenia	6%	5%
Pharyngitis	6%	5%

1. The following adverse reactions/event occurred at an equal or greater incidence for placebo than for Depakote ER: headache

The following additional adverse reactions were reported by greater than 1% but not more than 5% of the Depakote ER-treated patients in controlled clinical trials:

Body as a Whole: Back Pain, Flu Syndrome, Infection, Infection Fungal
Cardiovascular System: Hypertension
Digestive System: Constipation, Dry Mouth, Flatulence
Hemic and Lymphatic System: Ecchymosis
Metabolic and Nutritional Disorders: Peripheral Edema
Musculoskeletal System: Myalgia
Nervous System: Abnormal Gait, Hypertonia, Tremor
Respiratory System: Rhinitis
Skin and Appendages: Pruritus, Rash
Special Senses: Conjunctivitis
Urogenital System: Urinary Tract Infection, Vaginitis

6.2 Epilepsy

Based on a placebo-controlled trial of adjunctive therapy for treatment of complex partial seizures, Depakote was generally well tolerated with most adverse reactions rated as mild to moderate in severity. Intolerance was the primary reason for discontinuation in the Depakote-treated patients (6%), compared to 1% of placebo-treated patients.

Table 4 lists treatment-emergent adverse reactions which were reported by ≥ 5% of Depakote-treated patients and for which the incidence was greater than in the placebo group, in the placebo-controlled trial of adjunctive therapy for treatment of complex partial seizures. Since patients were also treated with other antiepilepsy drugs, it is not possible, in most cases, to determine whether the following adverse reactions can be ascribed to Depakote alone, or the combination of Depakote and other antiepilepsy drugs.

Table 4. Adverse Reactions Reported by ≥ 5% of Patients Treated with Valproate During Placebo-Controlled Trial of Adjunctive Therapy for Complex Partial Seizures

Body System/Event	Depakote (%) (N=77)	Placebo (%) (N=70)
Body as a Whole		
Headache	31	21
Asthenia	27	7
Fever	6	4
Gastrointestinal System		
Nausea	48	14
Vomiting	27	7
Abdominal pain	23	6
Diarrhea	13	6
Anorexia	12	0
Dyspepsia	8	4
Constipation	5	1
Nervous System		
Somnolence	27	11
Tremor	25	6
Dizziness	25	13
Diplopia	16	9
Amblyopia/Blurred Vision	12	9
Ataxia	8	1
Nystagmus	8	1
Emotional Lability	6	4
Thinking Abnormal	6	0
Amnesia	5	1
Respiratory System		
Flu Syndrome	12	9
Infection	12	6
Bronchitis	5	1
Rhinitis	5	4
Other		
Alopecia	6	1
Weight Loss	6	0

Table 5 lists treatment-emergent adverse reactions which were reported by ≥ 5% of patients in the high dose valproate group, and for which the incidence was greater than in the low dose group, in a controlled trial of Depakote monotherapy treatment of complex partial seizures. Since patients were being titrated off another antiepilepsy drug during the first portion of the trial, it is not possible, in many cases, to determine whether the following adverse reactions can be ascribed to Depakote alone, or the combination of valproate and other antiepilepsy drugs.

Table 5. Adverse Reactions Reported by ≥ 5% of Patients in the High Dose Group in the Controlled Trial of Valproate Monotherapy for Complex Partial Seizures[1]

Body System/Event	High Dose (%) (n=131)	Low Dose (%) (n=134)
Body as a Whole		
Asthenia	21	10
Digestive System		
Nausea	34	26
Diarrhea	23	19
Vomiting	23	15
Abdominal pain	12	9
Anorexia	11	4
Dyspepsia	11	10
Hemic/Lymphatic System		
Thrombocytopenia	24	1
Ecchymosis	5	4
Metabolic/Nutritional		
Weight Gain	9	4
Peripheral Edema	8	3
Nervous System		
Tremor	57	19
Somnolence	30	18
Dizziness	18	13
Insomnia	15	9
Nervousness	11	7
Amnesia	7	4
Nystagmus	7	1
Depression	5	4
Respiratory System		
Infection	20	13
Pharyngitis	8	2
Dyspnea	5	1
Skin and Appendages		
Alopecia	24	13
Special Senses		
Amblyopia/Blurred Vision	8	4
Tinnitus	7	1

1. Headache was the only adverse event that occurred in ≥5% of patients in the high dose group and at an equal or greater incidence in the low dose group.

The following additional adverse reactions were reported by greater than 1% but less than 5% of the 358 patients treated with valproate in the controlled trials of complex partial seizures:

Body as a Whole: Back pain, chest pain, malaise.

Cardiovascular System: Tachycardia, hypertension, palpitation.
Digestive System: Increased appetite, flatulence, hematemesis, eructation, pancreatitis, periodontal abscess.
Hemic and Lymphatic System: Petechia.
Metabolic and Nutritional Disorders: SGOT increased, SGPT increased.
Musculoskeletal System: Myalgia, twitching, arthralgia, leg cramps, myasthenia.
Nervous System: Anxiety, confusion, abnormal gait, paresthesia, hypertonia, incoordination, abnormal dreams, personality disorder.
Respiratory System: Sinusitis, cough increased, pneumonia, epistaxis.
Skin and Appendages: Rash, pruritus, dry skin.
Special Senses: Taste perversion, abnormal vision, deafness, otitis media.
Urogenital System: Urinary incontinence, vaginitis, dysmenorrhea, amenorrhea, urinary frequency.

6.3 Migraine

Based on two placebo-controlled clinical trials and their long term extension, valproate was generally well tolerated with most adverse reactions rated as mild to moderate in severity. Of the 202 patients exposed to valproate in the placebo-controlled trials, 17% discontinued for intolerance. This is compared to a rate of 5% for the 81 placebo patients. Including the long term extension study, the adverse reactions reported as the primary reason for discontinuation by ≥ 1% of 248 valproate-treated patients were alopecia (6%), nausea and/or vomiting (5%), weight gain (2%), tremor (2%), somnolence (1%), elevated SGOT and/or SGPT (1%), and depression (1%).

Table 6 includes those adverse reactions reported for patients in the placebo-controlled trial where the incidence rate in the Depakote ER-treated group was greater than 5% and was greater than that for placebo patients.

Table 6. Adverse Reactions Reported by >5% of Depakote ER-Treated Patients During the Migraine Placebo-Controlled Trial with a Greater Incidence than Patients Taking Placebo[1]

Body System Event	Depakote ER (n=122)	Placebo (n=115)
Gastrointestinal System		
Nausea	15%	9%
Dyspepsia	7%	4%
Diarrhea	7%	3%
Vomiting	7%	2%
Abdominal Pain	7%	5%
Nervous System		
Somnolence	7%	2%
Other		
Infection	15%	14%

1. The following adverse reactions occurred in greater than 5% of Depakote ER-treated patients and at a greater incidence for placebo than for Depakote ER: asthenia and flu syndrome.

The following additional adverse reactions were reported by greater than 1% but not more than 5% of Depakote ER-treated patients and with a greater incidence than placebo in the placebo-controlled clinical trial for migraine prophylaxis:

Body as a Whole: Accidental injury, viral infection.
Digestive System: Increased appetite, tooth disorder.
Metabolic and Nutritional Disorders: Edema, weight gain.
Nervous System: Abnormal gait, dizziness, hypertonia, insomnia, nervousness, tremor, vertigo.
Respiratory System: Pharyngitis, rhinitis.
Skin and Appendages: Rash.
Special Senses: Tinnitus.

Table 7 includes those adverse reactions reported for patients in the placebo-controlled trials where the incidence rate in the valproate-treated group was greater than 5% and was greater than that for placebo patients.

Information on the AbbVie, Inc. products listed on these pages is from the prescribing information in use as of July 31, 2014. For more information, please visit rxabbvie.com or call 1-800-633-9110.

Table 7. Adverse Reactions Reported by > 5% of Valproate-Treated Patients During Migraine Placebo-Controlled Trials with a Greater Incidence than Patients Taking Placebo[1]

Body System Reaction	Depakote (n=202)	Placebo (n=81)
Gastrointestinal System		
Nausea	31%	10%
Dyspepsia	13%	9%
Diarrhea	12%	7%
Vomiting	11%	1%
Abdominal pain	9%	4%
Increased appetite	6%	4%
Nervous System		
Asthenia	20%	9%
Somnolence	17%	5%
Dizziness	12%	6%
Tremor	9%	0%
Other		
Weight gain	8%	2%
Back pain	8%	6%
Alopecia	7%	1%

1. The following adverse reactions occurred in greater than 5% of Depakote-treated patients and at a greater incidence for placebo than for Depakote: flu syndrome and pharyngitis.

The following additional adverse reactions were reported by greater than 1% but not more than 5% of the 202 valproate-treated patients in the controlled clinical trials:
Body as a Whole: Chest pain.
Cardiovascular System: Vasodilatation.
Digestive System: Constipation, dry mouth, flatulence, and stomatitis.
Hemic and Lymphatic System: Ecchymosis.
Metabolic and Nutritional Disorders: Peripheral edema.
Musculoskeletal System: Leg cramps.
Nervous System: Abnormal dreams, confusion, paresthesia, speech disorder, and thinking abnormalities.
Respiratory System: Dyspnea, and sinusitis.
Skin and Appendages: Pruritus.
Urogenital System: Metrorrhagia.

6.4 Other Patient Populations
Mania
The following adverse reactions not listed previously were reported by greater than 1% of Depakote-treated patients and with a greater incidence than placebo in placebo-controlled trials of manic episodes associated with bipolar disorder:
Body as a Whole: Chills, chills and fever, drug level increased, neck rigidity.
Cardiovascular System: Arrhythmia, hypotension, postural hypotension.
Digestive System: Dysphagia, fecal incontinence, gastroenteritis, glossitis, gum hemorrhage, mouth ulceration.
Hemic and Lymphatic System: Anemia, bleeding time increased, leucopenia.
Metabolic and Nutritional Disorders: Hypoproteinemia.
Musculoskeletal System: Arthrosis.
Nervous System: Agitation, catatonic reaction, dysarthria, hallucinations, hypokinesia, psychosis, reflexes increased, sleep disorder, tardive dyskinesia.
Respiratory System: Hiccup.
Skin and Appendages: Discoid lupus erythematosus, erythema nodosum, furunculosis, maculopapular rash, seborrhea, sweating, vesiculobullous rash.
Special Senses: Conjunctivitis, dry eyes, eye disorder, eye pain, photophobia, taste perversion.
Urogenital System: Cystitis, menstrual disorder.

Epilepsy
Adverse reactions that have been reported with all dosage forms of valproate from epilepsy trials, spontaneous reports, and other sources are listed below by body system.
Gastrointestinal
The most commonly reported side effects at the initiation of therapy are nausea, vomiting, and indigestion. These effects are usually transient and rarely require discontinuation of therapy. Diarrhea, abdominal cramps, and constipation have been reported. Both anorexia with some weight loss and increased appetite with weight gain have also been reported. The administration of delayed-release divalproex sodium may result in reduction of gastrointestinal side effects in some patients.
CNS Effects
Sedative effects have occurred in patients receiving valproate alone but occur most often in patients receiving combination therapy. Sedation usually abates upon reduction of other antiepileptic medication. Tremor (may be dose-related), hallucinations, ataxia, headache, nystagmus, di-

plopia, asterixis, "spots before eyes", dysarthria, dizziness, confusion, hypesthesia, vertigo, incoordination, and parkinsonism have been reported with the use of valproate. Rare cases of coma have occurred in patients receiving valproate alone or in conjunction with phenobarbital. In rare instances encephalopathy with or without fever has developed shortly after the introduction of valproate monotherapy without evidence of hepatic dysfunction or inappropriately high plasma valproate levels. Although recovery has been described following drug withdrawal, there have been fatalities in patients with hyperammonemic encephalopathy, particularly in patients with underlying urea cycle disorders [see Warnings and Precautions (5.6)].
There have been postmarketing reports of reversible and irreversible cerebral and cerebellar atrophy temporally associated with the use of valproate products. In some cases the patients recovered with permanent sequelae [see Warnings and Precautions (5.7)]. Cerebral atrophy has been reported in children exposed to valproate in utero [see Use in Specific Populations (8.1)].
Dermatologic
Transient hair loss, skin rash, photosensitivity, generalized pruritus, erythema multiforme, and Stevens-Johnson syndrome. Rare cases of toxic epidermal necrolysis have been reported including a fatal case in a 6 month old infant taking valproate and several other concomitant medications. An additional case of toxic epidermal necrosis resulting in death was reported in a 35 year old patient with AIDS taking several concomitant medications and with a history of multiple cutaneous drug reactions. Serious skin reactions have been reported with concomitant administration of lamotrigine and valproate [see Drug Interactions (7.2)].
Psychiatric
Emotional upset, depression, psychosis, aggression, hyperactivity, hostility, and behavioral deterioration.
Musculoskeletal
Weakness.
Hematologic
Thrombocytopenia and inhibition of the secondary phase of platelet aggregation may be reflected in altered bleeding time, petechiae, bruising, hematoma formation, epistaxis, and frank hemorrhage [see Warnings and Precautions (5.9) and Drug Interactions (7)]. Relative lymphocytosis, macrocytosis, hypofibrinogenemia, leukopenia, eosinophilia, anemia including macrocytic with or without folate deficiency, bone marrow suppression, pancytopenia, aplastic anemia, agranulocytosis, and acute intermittent porphyria.
Hepatic
Minor elevations of transaminases (e.g., SGOT and SGPT) and LDH are frequent and appear to be dose-related. Occasionally, laboratory test results include increases in serum bilirubin and abnormal changes in other liver function tests. These results may reflect potentially serious hepatotoxicity [see Warnings and Precautions (5.1)].
Endocrine
Irregular menses, secondary amenorrhea, breast enlargement, galactorrhea, and parotid gland swelling. Abnormal thyroid function tests [see Warnings and Precautions (5.17)]. There have been rare spontaneous reports of polycystic ovary disease. A cause and effect relationship has not been established.
Pancreatic
Acute pancreatitis including fatalities [see Warnings and Precautions (5.5)].
Metabolic
Hyperammonemia [see Warnings and Precautions (5.10, 5.11)], hyponatremia, and inappropriate ADH secretion.
There have been rare reports of Fanconi's syndrome occurring chiefly in children.
Decreased carnitine concentrations have been reported although the clinical relevance is undetermined.
Hyperglycinemia has occurred and was associated with a fatal outcome in a patient with preexistent nonketotic hyperglycinemia.
Genitourinary
Enuresis and urinary tract infection.
Special Senses
Hearing loss, either reversible or irreversible, has been reported; however, a cause and effect relationship has not been established. Ear pain has also been reported.
Other
Allergic reaction, anaphylaxis, edema of the extremities, lupus erythematosus, bone pain, cough increased, pneumonia, otitis media, bradycardia, cutaneous vasculitis, fever, and hypothermia [see Warnings and Precautions (5.12)].
There have been reports of developmental delay, autism and/or autism spectrum disorder in the offspring of women exposed to valproate during pregnancy.

7 DRUG INTERACTIONS
7.1 Effects of Co-Administered Drugs on Valproate Clearance
Drugs that affect the level of expression of hepatic enzymes, particularly those that elevate levels of glucuronosyltrans-

ferases, may increase the clearance of valproate. For example, phenytoin, carbamazepine, and phenobarbital (or primidone) can double the clearance of valproate. Thus, patients on monotherapy will generally have longer half-lives and higher concentrations than patients receiving polytherapy with antiepilepsy drugs.
In contrast, drugs that are inhibitors of cytochrome P450 isozymes, e.g., antidepressants, may be expected to have little effect on valproate clearance because cytochrome P450 microsomal mediated oxidation is a relatively minor secondary metabolic pathway compared to glucuronidation and beta-oxidation.
Because of these changes in valproate clearance, monitoring of valproate and concomitant drug concentrations should be increased whenever enzyme inducing drugs are introduced or withdrawn.
The following list provides information about the potential for an influence of several commonly prescribed medications on valproate pharmacokinetics. The list is not exhaustive nor could it be, since new interactions are continuously being reported.
Drugs for which a potentially important interaction has been observed
Aspirin
A study involving the co-administration of aspirin at antipyretic doses (11 to 16 mg/kg) with valproate to pediatric patients (n=6) revealed a decrease in protein binding and an inhibition of metabolism of valproate. Valproate free fraction was increased 4-fold in the presence of aspirin compared to valproate alone. The β-oxidation pathway consisting of 2-E-valproic acid, 3-OH-valproic acid, and 3-keto valproic acid was decreased from 25% of total metabolites excreted on valproate alone to 8.3% in the presence of aspirin. Whether or not the interaction observed in this study applies to adults is unknown, but caution should be observed if valproate and aspirin are to be co-administered.
Carbapenem Antibiotics
A clinically significant reduction in serum valproic acid concentration has been reported in patients receiving carbapenem antibiotics (for example, ertapenem, imipenem, meropenem; this is not a complete list) and may result in loss of seizure control. The mechanism of this interaction in not well understood. Serum valproic acid concentrations should be monitored frequently after initiating carbapenem therapy. Alternative antibacterial or anticonvulsant therapy should be considered if serum valproic acid concentrations drop significantly or seizure control deteriorates [see Warnings and Precautions (5.14)].
Felbamate
A study involving the co-administration of 1200 mg/day of felbamate with valproate to patients with epilepsy (n=10) revealed an increase in mean valproate peak concentration by 35% (from 86 to 115 mcg/mL) compared to valproate alone. Increasing the felbamate dose to 2400 mg/day increased the mean valproate peak concentration to 133 mcg/mL (another 16% increase). A decrease in valproate dosage may be necessary when felbamate therapy is initiated.
Rifampin
A study involving the administration of a single dose of valproate (7 mg/kg) 36 hours after 5 nights of daily dosing with rifampin (600 mg) revealed a 40% increase in the oral clearance of valproate. Valproate dosage adjustment may be necessary when it is co-administered with rifampin.
Drugs for which either no interaction or a likely clinically unimportant interaction has been observed
Antacids
A study involving the co-administration of valproate 500 mg with commonly administered antacids (Maalox, Trisogel, and Titralac - 160 mEq doses) did not reveal any effect on the extent of absorption of valproate.
Chlorpromazine
A study involving the administration of 100 to 300 mg/day of chlorpromazine to schizophrenic patients already receiving valproate (200 mg BID) revealed a 15% increase in trough plasma levels of valproate.
Haloperidol
A study involving the administration of 6 to 10 mg/day of haloperidol to schizophrenic patients already receiving valproate (200 mg BID) revealed no significant changes in valproate trough plasma levels.
Cimetidine and Ranitidine
Cimetidine and ranitidine do not affect the clearance of valproate.
7.2 Effects of Valproate on Other Drugs
Valproate has been found to be a weak inhibitor of some P450 isozymes, epoxide hydrase, and glucuronosyltransferases.
The following list provides information about the potential for an influence of valproate co-administration on the pharmacokinetics or pharmacodynamics of several commonly prescribed medications. The list is not exhaustive, since new interactions are continuously being reported.

Drugs for which a potentially important valproate interaction has been observed

Amitriptyline/Nortriptyline
Administration of a single oral 50 mg dose of amitriptyline to 15 normal volunteers (10 males and 5 females) who received valproate (500 mg BID) resulted in a 21% decrease in plasma clearance of amitriptyline and a 34% decrease in the net clearance of nortriptyline. Rare postmarketing reports of concurrent use of valproate and amitriptyline resulting in an increased amitriptyline level have been received. Concurrent use of valproate and amitriptyline has rarely been associated with toxicity. Monitoring of amitriptyline levels should be considered for patients taking valproate concomitantly with amitriptyline. Consideration should be given to lowering the dose of amitriptyline/nortriptyline in the presence of valproate.

Carbamazepine/carbamazepine-10,11-Epoxide
Serum levels of carbamazepine (CBZ) decreased 17% while that of carbamazepine-10,11-epoxide (CBZ-E) increased by 45% upon co-administration of valproate and CBZ to epileptic patients.

Clonazepam
The concomitant use of valproate and clonazepam may induce absence status in patients with a history of absence type seizures.

Diazepam
Valproate displaces diazepam from its plasma albumin binding sites and inhibits its metabolism. Co-administration of valproate (1500 mg daily) increased the free fraction of diazepam (10 mg) by 90% in healthy volunteers (n=6). Plasma clearance and volume of distribution for free diazepam were reduced by 25% and 20%, respectively, in the presence of valproate. The elimination half-life of diazepam remained unchanged upon addition of valproate.

Ethosuximide
Valproate inhibits the metabolism of ethosuximide. Administration of a single ethosuximide dose of 500 mg with valproate (800 to 1600 mg/day) to healthy volunteers (n=6) was accompanied by a 25% increase in elimination half-life of ethosuximide and a 15% decrease in its total clearance as compared to ethosuximide alone. Patients receiving valproate and ethosuximide, especially along with other anticonvulsants, should be monitored for alterations in serum concentrations of both drugs.

Lamotrigine
In a steady-state study involving 10 healthy volunteers, the elimination half-life of lamotrigine increased from 26 to 70 hours with valproate co-administration (a 165% increase). The dose of lamotrigine should be reduced when co-administered with valproate. Serious skin reactions (such as Stevens-Johnson syndrome and toxic epidermal necrolysis) have been reported with concomitant lamotrigine and valproate administration. See lamotrigine package insert for details on lamotrigine dosing with concomitant valproate administration.

Phenobarbital
Valproate was found to inhibit the metabolism of phenobarbital. Co-administration of valproate (250 mg BID for 14 days) with phenobarbital to normal subjects (n=6) resulted in a 50% increase in half-life and a 30% decrease in plasma clearance of phenobarbital (60 mg single-dose). The fraction of phenobarbital dose excreted unchanged increased by 50% in presence of valproate.
There is evidence for severe CNS depression, with or without significant elevations of barbiturate or valproate serum concentrations. All patients receiving concomitant barbiturate therapy should be closely monitored for neurological toxicity. Serum barbiturate concentrations should be obtained, if possible, and the barbiturate dosage decreased, if appropriate.
Primidone, which is metabolized to a barbiturate, may be involved in a similar interaction with valproate.

Phenytoin
Valproate displaces phenytoin from its plasma albumin binding sites and inhibits its hepatic metabolism. Co-administration of valproate (400 mg TID) with phenytoin (250 mg) in normal volunteers (n=7) was associated with a 60% increase in the free fraction of phenytoin. Total plasma clearance and apparent volume of distribution of phenytoin increased 30% in the presence of valproate. Both the clearance and apparent volume of distribution of free phenytoin were reduced by 25%.
In patients with epilepsy, there have been reports of breakthrough seizures occurring with the combination of valproate and phenytoin. The dosage of phenytoin should be adjusted as required by the clinical situation.

Tolbutamide
From in vitro experiments, the unbound fraction of tolbutamide was increased from 20% to 50% when added to plasma samples taken from patients treated with valproate. The clinical relevance of this displacement is unknown.

Warfarin
In an in vitro study, valproate increased the unbound fraction of warfarin by up to 32.6%. The therapeutic relevance of this is unknown; however, coagulation tests should be monitored if valproate therapy is instituted in patients taking anticoagulants.

Zidovudine
In six patients who were seropositive for HIV, the clearance of zidovudine (100 mg q8h) was decreased by 38% after administration of valproate (250 or 500 mg q8h); the half-life of zidovudine was unaffected.

Drugs for which either no interaction or a likely clinically unimportant interaction has been observed

Acetaminophen
Valproate had no effect on any of the pharmacokinetic parameters of acetaminophen when it was concurrently administered to three epileptic patients.

Clozapine
In psychotic patients (n=11), no interaction was observed when valproate was co-administered with clozapine.

Lithium
Co-administration of valproate (500 mg BID) and lithium carbonate (300 mg TID) to normal male volunteers (n=16) had no effect on the steady-state kinetics of lithium.

Lorazepam
Concomitant administration of valproate (500 mg BID) and lorazepam (1 mg BID) in normal male volunteers (n=9) was accompanied by a 17% decrease in the plasma clearance of lorazepam.

Olanzapine
No dose adjustment for olanzapine is necessary when olanzapine is administered concomitantly with valproate. Co-administration of valproate (500 mg BID) and Olanzapine (5 mg) to healthy adults (n=10) caused 15% reduction in C_{max} and 35% reduction in AUC of olanzapine.

Oral Contraceptive Steroids
Administration of a single-dose of ethinyloestradiol (50 mcg)/levonorgestrel (250 mcg) to 6 women on valproate (200 mg BID) therapy for 2 months did not reveal any pharmacokinetic interaction.

7.3 Topiramate
Concomitant administration of valproate and topiramate has been associated with hyperammonemia with and without encephalopathy [see Contraindications (4) and Warnings and Precautions (5.10, 5.11)]. Concomitant administration of topiramate with valproate has also been associated with hypothermia in patients who have tolerated either drug alone. It may be prudent to examine blood ammonia levels in patients in whom the onset of hypothermia has been reported [see Warnings and Precautions (5.10, 5.12)].

8 USE IN SPECIFIC POPULATIONS
8.1 Pregnancy
Pregnancy Category D for epilepsy and for manic episodes associated with bipolar disorder [see Warnings and Precautions (5.2, 5.3)].
Pregnancy Category X for prophylaxis of migraine headaches [see Contraindications (4)].

Pregnancy Registry
To collect information on the effects of in utero exposure to Depakote, physicians should encourage pregnant patients taking Depakote to enroll in the North American Antiepileptic Drug (NAAED) Pregnancy Registry. This can be done by calling toll free 1-888-233-2334, and must be done by the patients themselves. Information on the registry can be found at the website, http://www.aedpregnancyregistry.org/.

Fetal Risk Summary
All pregnancies have a background risk of birth defects (about 3%), pregnancy loss (about 15%), or other adverse outcomes regardless of drug exposure. Maternal valproate use during pregnancy for any indication increases the risk of congenital malformations, particularly neural tube defects, but also malformations involving other body systems (e.g., craniofacial defects, cardiovascular malformations). The risk of major structural abnormalities is greatest during the first trimester; however, other serious developmental effects can occur with valproate use throughout pregnancy. The rate of congenital malformations among babies born to epileptic mothers who used valproate during pregnancy has been shown to be about four times higher than the rate among babies born to epileptic mothers who used other anti-seizure monotherapies [see Warnings and Precautions (5.3)].
Exposure in utero to valproate products has been associated with cerebral atrophy [see Warnings and Precautions (5.7) and Adverse Reactions (6.4)].
Several published epidemiological studies have indicated that children exposed to valproate in utero have lower IQ scores than children exposed to either another antiepileptic drug in utero or to no antiepileptic drugs in utero [see Warnings and Precautions (5.3)].
In animal studies, offspring with prenatal exposure to valproate had structural malformations similar to those seen in humans and demonstrated neurobehavioral deficits.

Clinical Considerations
• Neural tube defects are the congenital malformation most strongly associated with maternal valproate use. The risk of spina bifida following in utero valproate exposure is generally estimated as 1-2%, compared to an estimated general population risk for spina bifida of about 0.06 to 0.07% (6 to 7 in 10,000 births).
• Valproate can cause decreased IQ scores in children whose mothers were treated with valproate during pregnancy.
• Because of the risks of decreased IQ, neural tube defects, and other fetal adverse events, which may occur very early in pregnancy:
  • Valproate should not be administered to a woman of childbearing potential unless the drug is essential to the management of her medical condition. This is especially important when valproate use is considered for a condition not usually associated with permanent injury or death (e.g., migraine).
  • Valproate is contraindicated during pregnancy in women being treated for prophylaxis of migraine headaches.
  • Valproate should not be used to treat women with epilepsy or bipolar disorder who are pregnant or who plan to become pregnant unless other treatments have failed to provide adequate symptom control or are otherwise unacceptable. In such women, the benefits of treatment with valproate during pregnancy may still outweigh the risks. When treating a pregnant woman or a woman of childbearing potential, carefully consider both the potential risks and benefits of treatment and provide appropriate counseling.
• To prevent major seizures, women with epilepsy should not discontinue valproate abruptly, as this can precipitate status epilepticus with resulting maternal and fetal hypoxia and threat to life. Even minor seizures may pose some hazard to the developing embryo or fetus. However, discontinuation of the drug may be considered prior to and during pregnancy in individual cases if the seizure disorder severity and frequency do not pose a serious threat to the patient.
• Available prenatal diagnostic testing to detect neural tube and other defects should be offered to pregnant women using valproate.
• Evidence suggests that folic acid supplementation prior to conception and during the first trimester of pregnancy decreases the risk for congenital neural tube defects in the general population. It is not known whether the risk of neural tube defects or decreased IQ in the offspring of women receiving valproate is reduced by folic acid supplementation. Dietary folic acid supplementation both prior to conception and during pregnancy should be routinely recommended for patients using valproate.
• Patients taking valproate may develop clotting abnormalities [see Warnings and Precautions (5.9)]. A patient who had low fibrinogen when taking multiple anticonvulsants including valproate gave birth to an infant with afibrinogenemia who subsequently died of hemorrhage. If valproate is used in pregnancy, the clotting parameters should be monitored carefully.
• Patients taking valproate may develop hepatic failure [see Boxed Warning and Warnings and Precautions (5.1)]. Fatal cases of hepatic failure in infants exposed to valproate in utero have also been reported following maternal use of valproate during pregnancy.

Data
Human
There is an extensive body of evidence demonstrating that exposure to valproate in utero increases the risk of neural tube defects and other structural abnormalities. Based on published data from the CDC's National Birth Defects Prevention Network, the risk of spina bifida in the general population is about 0.06 to 0.07%. The risk of spina bifida following in utero valproate exposure has been estimated to be approximately 1 to 2%.
In one study using NAAED Pregnancy Registry data, 16 cases of major malformations following prenatal valproate exposure were reported among offspring of 149 enrolled women who used valproate during pregnancy. Three of the 16 cases were neural tube defects; the remaining cases included craniofacial defects, cardiovascular malformations and malformations of varying severity involving other body systems. The NAAED Pregnancy Registry has reported a major malformation rate of 10.7% (95% C.I. 6.3% – 16.9%) in the offspring of women exposed to an average of 1,000 mg/day of valproate monotherapy during pregnancy (dose range 500 – 2000 mg/day). The major malformation rate among the internal comparison group of 1,048 epileptic women who received any other antiepileptic drug monotherapy during pregnancy was 2.9% (95% CI 2.0% to 4.1%). These data show a four-fold increased risk for any major malformation (Odds Ratio 4.0; 95% CI 2.1 to 7.4) following

Information on the AbbVie, Inc. products listed on these pages is from the prescribing information in use as of July 31, 2014. For more information, please visit rxabbvie.com or call 1-800-633-9110.

Table 9. Bioavailability of Depakote ER Tablets Relative to Depakote When Depakote ER Dose is 8 to 20% Higher

Study Population	Regimens	Relative Bioavailability		
	Depakote ER vs. Depakote	AUC_{24}	C_{max}	C_{min}
Healthy Volunteers (N=35)	1000 & 1500 mg Depakote ER vs. 875 & 1250 mg Depakote	1.059	0.882	1.173
Patients with epilepsy on concomitant enzyme-inducing antiepilepsy drugs (N = 64)	1000 to 5000 mg Depakote ER vs. 875 to 4250 mg Depakote	1.008	0.899	1.022

valproate exposure *in utero* compared to the risk following exposure *in utero* to any other antiepileptic drug monotherapy.

Published epidemiological studies have indicated that children exposed to valproate *in utero* have lower IQ scores than children exposed to either another antiepileptic drug *in utero* or to no antiepileptic drugs *in utero*. The largest of these studies is a prospective cohort study conducted in the United States and United Kingdom that found that children with prenatal exposure to valproate (n=62) had lower IQ scores at age 6 (97 [95% C.I. 94-101]) than children with prenatal exposure to the other anti-epileptic drug monotherapy treatments evaluated: lamotrigine (108 [95% C.I. 105–110]), carbamazepine (105 [95% C.I. 102–108]) and phenytoin (108 [95% C.I. 104–112]). It is not known when during pregnancy cognitive effects in valproate-exposed children occur. Because the women in this study were exposed to antiepileptic drugs throughout pregnancy, whether the risk for decreased IQ was related to a particular time period during pregnancy could not be assessed.

Although all of the available studies have methodological limitations, the weight of the evidence supports a causal association between valproate exposure *in utero* and subsequent adverse effects on cognitive development.

There are published case reports of fatal hepatic failure in offspring of women who used valproate during pregnancy.

Animal

In developmental toxicity studies conducted in mice, rats, rabbits, and monkeys, increased rates of fetal structural abnormalities, intrauterine growth retardation, and embryo-fetal death occurred following treatment of pregnant animals with valproate during organogenesis at clinically relevant doses (calculated on a body surface area basis). Valproate induced malformations of multiple organ systems, including skeletal, cardiac, and urogenital defects. In mice, in addition to other malformations, fetal neural tube defects have been reported following valproate administration during critical periods of organogenesis, and the teratogenic response correlated with peak maternal drug levels. Behavioral abnormalities (including cognitive, locomotor, and social interaction deficits) and brain histopathological changes have also been reported in mice and rat offspring exposed prenatally to clinically relevant doses of valproate.

8.3   Nursing Mothers

Valproate is excreted in human milk. Caution should be exercised when valproate is administered to a nursing woman.

8.4   Pediatric Use

Experience has indicated that pediatric patients under the age of two years are at a considerably increased risk of developing fatal hepatotoxicity, especially those with the aforementioned conditions *[see Boxed Warning and Warnings and Precautions (5.1)]*. When valproate is used in this patient group, it should be used with extreme caution and as a sole agent. The benefits of therapy should be weighed against the risks. Above the age of 2 years, experience in epilepsy has indicated that the incidence of fatal hepatotoxicity decreases considerably in progressively older patient groups.

Younger children, especially those receiving enzyme inducing drugs, will require larger maintenance doses to attain targeted total and unbound valproate concentrations. Pediatric patients (i.e., between 3 months and 10 years) have 50% higher clearances expressed on weight (i.e., mL/min/kg) than do adults. Over the age of 10 years, children have pharmacokinetic parameters that approximate those of adults.

The variability in free fraction limits the clinical usefulness of monitoring total serum valproic acid concentration. Interpretation of valproic acid concentrations in children should include consideration of factors that affect hepatic metabolism and protein binding.

Pediatric Clinical Trials

Depakote was studied in seven pediatric clinical trials.

Two of the pediatric studies were double-blinded placebo-controlled trials to evaluate the efficacy of Depakote ER for the indications of mania (150 patients aged 10 to 17 years, 76 of whom were on Depakote ER) and migraine (304 patients aged 12 to 17 years, 231 of whom were on Depakote

ER). Efficacy was not established for either the treatment of migraine or the treatment of mania. The most common drug-related adverse reactions (reported >5% and twice the rate of placebo) reported in the controlled pediatric mania study were nausea, upper abdominal pain, somnolence, increased ammonia, gastritis and rash.

The remaining five trials were long term safety studies. Two six-month pediatric studies were conducted to evaluate the long-term safety of Depakote ER for the indication of mania (292 patients aged 10 to 17 years). Two twelve-month pediatric studies were conducted to evaluate the long-term safety of Depakote ER for the indication of migraine (353 patients aged 12 to 17 years). One twelve-month study was conducted to evaluate the safety of Depakote Sprinkle Capsules in the indication of partial seizures (169 patients aged 3 to 10 years).

In these seven clinical trials, the safety and tolerability of Depakote in pediatric patients were shown to be comparable to those in adults *[see Adverse Reactions (6)]*.

Juvenile Animal Toxicology

In studies of valproate in immature animals, toxic effects not observed in adult animals included retinal dysplasia in rats treated during the neonatal period (from postnatal day 4) and nephrotoxicity in rats treated during the neonatal and juvenile (from postnatal day 14) periods. The no-effect dose for these findings was less than the maximum recommended human dose on a mg/m² basis.

8.5   Geriatric Use

No patients above the age of 65 years were enrolled in double-blind prospective clinical trials of mania associated with bipolar illness. In a case review study of 583 patients, 72 patients (12%) were greater than 65 years of age. A higher percentage of patients above 65 years of age reported accidental injury, infection, pain, somnolence, and tremor. Discontinuation of valproate was occasionally associated with the latter two events. It is not clear whether these events indicate additional risk or whether they result from preexisting medical illness and concomitant medication use among these patients.

A study of elderly patients with dementia revealed drug related somnolence and discontinuation for somnolence *[see Warnings and Precautions (5.15)]*. The starting dose should be reduced in these patients, and dosage reductions or discontinuation should be considered in patients with excessive somnolence *[see Dosage and Administration (2.5)]*.

There is insufficient information available to discern the safety and effectiveness of valproate for the prophylaxis of migraines in patients over 65.

The capacity of elderly patients (age range: 68 to 89 years) to eliminate valproate has been shown to be reduced compared to younger adults (age range: 22 to 26 years) *[see Clinical Pharmacology (12.3)]*.

8.6   Effect of Disease

Liver Disease

[(See Boxed Warning, Contraindications (4), Warnings and Precautions (5), and Clinical Pharmacology (12.3)]. Liver disease impairs the capacity to eliminate valproate.

10   OVERDOSAGE

Over dosage with valproate may result in somnolence, heart block, and deep coma. Fatalities have been reported; however patients have recovered from valproate levels as high as 2120 mcg/mL.

In overdose situations, the fraction of drug not bound to protein is high and hemodialysis or tandem hemodialysis plus hemoperfusion may result in significant removal of drug. The benefit of gastric lavage or emesis will vary with the time since ingestion. General supportive measures should be applied with particular attention to the maintenance of adequate urinary output.

Naloxone has been reported to reverse the CNS depressant effects of valproate over dosage. Because naloxone could theoretically also reverse the antiepileptic effects of valproate, it should be used with caution in patients with epilepsy.

11   DESCRIPTION

Divalproex sodium is a stable co-ordination compound comprised of sodium valproate and valproic acid in a 1:1 molar

relationship and formed during the partial neutralization of valproic acid with 0.5 equivalent of sodium hydroxide. Chemically it is designated as sodium hydrogen bis(2-propylpentanoate). Divalproex sodium has the following structure:

Divalproex sodium occurs as a white powder with a characteristic odor.

Depakote ER 250 and 500 mg tablets are for oral administration. Depakote ER tablets contain divalproex sodium in a once-a-day extended-release formulation equivalent to 250 and 500 mg of valproic acid.

Inactive Ingredients

Depakote ER 250 and 500 mg tablets: FD&C Blue No. 1, hypromellose, lactose, microcrystalline cellulose, polyethylene glycol, potassium sorbate, propylene glycol, silicon dioxide, titanium dioxide, and triacetin.

In addition, 500 mg tablets contain iron oxide and polydextrose.

12   CLINICAL PHARMACOLOGY

12.1   Mechanism of Action

Divalproex sodium dissociates to the valproate ion in the gastrointestinal tract. The mechanisms by which valproate exerts its therapeutic effects have not been established. It has been suggested that its activity in epilepsy is related to increased brain concentrations of gamma-aminobutyric acid (GABA).

12.2   Pharmacodynamics

The relationship between plasma concentration and clinical response is not well documented. One contributing factor is the nonlinear, concentration dependent protein binding of valproate which affects the clearance of the drug. Thus, monitoring of total serum valproate may not provide a reliable index of the bioactive valproate species.

For example, because the plasma protein binding of valproate is concentration dependent, the free fraction increases from approximately 10% at 40 mcg/mL to 18.5% at 130 mcg/mL. Higher than expected free fractions occur in the elderly, in hyperlipidemic patients, and in patients with hepatic and renal diseases.

Epilepsy

The therapeutic range in epilepsy is commonly considered to be 50 to 100 mcg/mL of total valproate, although some patients may be controlled with lower or higher plasma concentrations.

Mania

In placebo-controlled clinical trials of acute mania, patients were dosed to clinical response with trough plasma concentrations between 85 and 125 mcg/mL *[see Dosage and Administration (2.1)]*.

12.3   Pharmacokinetics

Absorption/Bioavailability

The absolute bioavailability of Depakote ER tablets administered as a single dose after a meal was approximately 90% relative to intravenous infusion.

When given in equal total daily doses, the bioavailability of Depakote ER is less than that of Depakote (divalproex sodium delayed-release tablets). In five multiple-dose studies in healthy subjects (N=82) and in subjects with epilepsy (N=86), when administered under fasting and nonfasting conditions, Depakote ER given once daily produced an average bioavailability of 89% relative to an equal total daily dose of Depakote given BID, TID, or QID. The median time to maximum plasma valproate concentrations (C_{max}) after Depakote ER administration ranged from 4 to 17 hours. After multiple once-daily dosing of Depakote ER, the peak-to-trough fluctuation in plasma valproate concentrations was 10-20% lower than that of regular Depakote given BID, TID, or QID.

Conversion from Depakote to Depakote ER

When Depakote ER is given in doses 8 to 20% higher than the total daily dose of Depakote, the two formulations are bioequivalent. In two randomized, crossover studies, multiple daily doses of Depakote were compared to 8 to 20% higher once-daily doses of Depakote ER. In these two studies, Depakote ER and Depakote regimens were equivalent with respect to area under the curve (AUC; a measure of the extent of bioavailability). Additionally, valproate C_{max} was lower, and C_{min} was either higher or not different, for Depakote ER relative to Depakote regimens (see Table 9). [See table 9 above]

Concomitant antiepilepsy drugs (topiramate, phenobarbital, carbamazepine, phenytoin, and lamotrigine were evaluated) that induce the cytochrome P450 isozyme system did not significantly alter valproate bioavailability when converting between Depakote and Depakote ER.

Distribution
Protein Binding

The plasma protein binding of valproate is concentration dependent and the free fraction increases from approximately 10% at 40 mcg/mL to 18.5% at 130 mcg/mL. Protein binding of valproate is reduced in the elderly, in patients with chronic hepatic diseases, in patients with renal impairment, and in the presence of other drugs (e.g., aspirin). Conversely, valproate may displace certain protein-bound drugs (e.g., phenytoin, carbamazepine, warfarin, and tolbutamide) [see Drug Interactions (7.2) for more detailed information on the pharmacokinetic interactions of valproate with other drugs].

CNS Distribution

Valproate concentrations in cerebrospinal fluid (CSF) approximate unbound concentrations in plasma (about 10% of total concentration).

Metabolism

Valproate is metabolized almost entirely by the liver. In adult patients on monotherapy, 30-50% of an administered dose appears in urine as a glucuronide conjugate. Mitochondrial β-oxidation is the other major metabolic pathway, typically accounting for over 40% of the dose. Usually, less than 15-20% of the dose is eliminated by other oxidative mechanisms. Less than 3% of an administered dose is excreted unchanged in urine.

The relationship between dose and total valproate concentration is nonlinear; concentration does not increase proportionally with the dose, but rather, increases to a lesser extent due to saturable plasma protein binding. The kinetics of unbound drug are linear.

Elimination

Mean plasma clearance and volume of distribution for total valproate are 0.56 L/hr/1.73 m^2 and 11 L/1.73 m^2, respectively. Mean plasma clearance and volume of distribution for free valproate are 4.6 L/hr/1.73 m^2 and 92 L/1.73 m^2. Mean terminal half-life for valproate monotherapy ranged from 9 to 16 hours following oral dosing regimens of 250 to 1000 mg.

The estimates cited apply primarily to patients who are not taking drugs that affect hepatic metabolizing enzyme systems. For example, patients taking enzyme-inducing antiepileptic drugs (carbamazepine, phenytoin, and phenobarbital) will clear valproate more rapidly. Because of these changes in valproate clearance, monitoring of antiepileptic concentrations should be intensified whenever concomitant antiepileptics are introduced or withdrawn.

Special Populations
Effect of Age
Pediatric

The valproate pharmacokinetic profile following administration of Depakote ER was characterized in a multiple-dose, non-fasting, open label, multi-center study in children and adolescents. Depakote ER once daily doses ranged from 250-1750 mg. Once daily administration of Depakote ER in pediatric patients (10-17 years) produced plasma VPA concentration-time profiles similar to those that have been observed in adults.

Elderly

The capacity of elderly patients (age range: 68 to 89 years) to eliminate valproate has been shown to be reduced compared to younger adults (age range: 22 to 26). Intrinsic clearance is reduced by 39%; the free fraction is increased by 44%. Accordingly, the initial dosage should be reduced in the elderly [see Dosage and Administration (2.4)].

Effect of Sex

There are no differences in the body surface area adjusted unbound clearance between males and females (4.8±0.17 and 4.7±0.07 L/hr per 1.73 m^2, respectively).

Effect of Race

The effects of race on the kinetics of valproate have not been studied.

Effect of Disease
Liver Disease

Liver disease impairs the capacity to eliminate valproate. In one study, the clearance of free valproate was decreased by 50% in 7 patients with cirrhosis and by 16% in 4 patients with acute hepatitis, compared with 6 healthy subjects. In that study, the half-life of valproate was increased from 12 to 18 hours. Liver disease is also associated with decreased albumin concentrations and larger unbound fractions (2 to 2.6 fold increase) of valproate. Accordingly, monitoring of total concentrations may be misleading since free concentrations may be substantially elevated in patients with hepatic disease whereas total concentrations may appear to be normal [see Boxed Warning, Contraindications (4), and Warnings and Precautions (5.1)].

Renal Disease

A slight reduction (27%) in the unbound clearance of valproate has been reported in patients with renal failure (creatinine clearance < 10 mL/minute); however, hemodialysis typically reduces valproate concentrations by about 20%. Therefore, no dosage adjustment appears to be necessary in patients with renal failure. Protein binding in these patients is substantially reduced; thus, monitoring total concentrations may be misleading.

13 NONCLINICAL TOXICOLOGY
13.1 Carcinogenesis, Mutagenesis, and Impairment of Fertility
Carcinogenesis

Valproate was administered orally to rats and mice at doses of 80 and 170 mg/kg/day (less than the maximum recommended human dose on a mg/m^2 basis) for two years. The primary findings were an increase in the incidence of subcutaneous fibrosarcomas in high-dose male rats receiving valproate and a dose-related trend for benign pulmonary adenomas in male mice receiving valproate. The significance of these findings for humans is unknown.

Mutagenesis

Valproate was not mutagenic in an in vitro bacterial assay (Ames test), did not produce dominant lethal effects in mice, and did not increase chromosome aberration frequency in an in vivo cytogenetic study in rats. Increased frequencies of sister chromatid exchange (SCE) have been reported in a study of epileptic children taking valproate, but this association was not observed in another study conducted in adults. There is some evidence that increased SCE frequencies may be associated with epilepsy. The biological significance of an increase in SCE frequency is not known.

Fertility

Chronic toxicity studies of valproate in juvenile and adult rats and dogs demonstrated reduced spermatogenesis and testicular atrophy at oral doses of 400 mg/kg/day or greater in rats (approximately equivalent to or greater than the maximum recommended human dose (MRHD) on a mg/m^2 basis) and 150 mg/kg/day or greater in dogs (approximately 1.4 times the MRHD or greater on a mg/m^2 basis). Fertility studies in rats have shown no effect on fertility at oral doses of valproate up to 350 mg/kg/day (approximately equal to the MRHD on a mg/m^2 basis) for 60 days. The effect of valproate on testicular development and on sperm production and fertility in humans is unknown.

14 CLINICAL STUDIES
14.1 Mania

The effectiveness of Depakote ER for the treatment of acute mania is based in part on studies establishing the effectiveness of Depakote (divalproex sodium delayed release tablets) for this indication. Depakote ER's effectiveness was confirmed in a randomized, double-blind, placebo-controlled, parallel group, 3-week, multicenter study. The study was designed to evaluate the safety and efficacy of Depakote ER in the treatment of bipolar I disorder, manic or mixed type, in adults. Adult male and female patients who had a current DSM-IV TR primary diagnosis of bipolar I disorder, manic or mixed type, and who were hospitalized for acute mania, were enrolled into this study. Depakote ER was initiated at a dose of 25 mg/kg/day given once daily, increased by 500 mg/day on Day 3, then adjusted to achieve plasma valproate concentrations in the range of 85-125 mcg/mL. Mean daily Depakote ER doses for observed cases were 2362 mg (range: 500-4000), 2874 mg (range: 1500-4500), 2993 mg (range: 1500-4500), 3181 mg (range: 1500-5000), and 3353 mg (range: 1500-5500) at Days 1, 5, 10, 15, and 21, respectively. Mean valproate concentrations were 96.5 mcg/mL, 102.1 mcg/mL, 98.5 mcg/mL, 89.5 mcg/mL at Days 5, 10, 15 and 21, respectively. Patients were assessed on the Mania Rating Scale (MRS; score ranges from 0-52).

Depakote ER was significantly more effective than placebo in reduction of the MRS total score.

14.2 Epilepsy

The efficacy of valproate in reducing the incidence of complex partial seizures (CPS) that occur in isolation or in association with other seizure types was established in two controlled trials.

In one, multi-clinic, placebo controlled study employing an add-on design, (adjunctive therapy) 144 patients who continued to suffer eight or more CPS per 8 weeks during an 8 week period of monotherapy with doses of either carbamazepine or phenytoin sufficient to assure plasma concentrations within the "therapeutic range" were randomized to receive, in addition to their original antiepilepsy drug (AED), either Depakote or placebo. Randomized patients were to be followed for a total of 16 weeks. The following Table presents the findings.

Table 10. Adjunctive Therapy Study Median Incidence of CPS per 8 Weeks

Add-on Treatment	Number of Patients	Baseline Incidence	Experimental Incidence
Depakote	75	16.0	8.9*
Placebo	69	14.5	11.5

* Reduction from baseline statistically significantly greater for valproate than placebo at p ≤ 0.05 level.

Figure 1 presents the proportion of patients (X axis) whose percentage reduction from baseline in complex partial seizure rates was at least as great as that indicated on the Y axis in the adjunctive therapy study. A positive percent reduction indicates an improvement (i.e., a decrease in seizure frequency), while a negative percent reduction indicates worsening. Thus, in a display of this type, the curve for an effective treatment is shifted to the left of the curve for placebo. This Figure shows that the proportion of patients achieving any particular level of improvement was consistently higher for valproate than for placebo. For example, 45% of patients treated with valproate had a ≥ 50% reduction in complex partial seizure rate compared to 23% of patients treated with placebo.

Figure 1

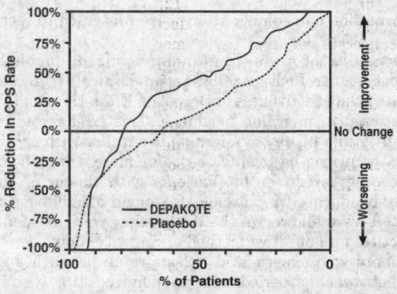

The second study assessed the capacity of valproate to reduce the incidence of CPS when administered as the sole AED. The study compared the incidence of CPS among patients randomized to either a high or low dose treatment arm. Patients qualified for entry into the randomized comparison phase of this study only if 1) they continued to experience 2 or more CPS per 4 weeks during an 8 to 12 week long period of monotherapy with adequate doses of an AED (i.e., phenytoin, carbamazepine, phenobarbital, or primidone) and 2) they made a successful transition over a two week interval to valproate. Patients entering the randomized phase were then brought to their assigned target dose, gradually tapered off their concomitant AED and followed for an interval as long as 22 weeks. Less than 50% of the patients randomized, however, completed the study. In patients converted to Depakote monotherapy, the mean total valproate concentrations during monotherapy were 71 and 123 mcg/mL in the low dose and high dose groups, respectively.

The following Table presents the findings for all patients randomized who had at least one post-randomization assessment.

Table 11. Monotherapy Study Median Incidence of CPS per 8 Weeks

Treatment	Number of Patients	Baseline Incidence	Randomized Phase Incidence
High dose Valproate	131	13.2	10.7*
Low dose Valproate	134	14.2	13.8

* Reduction from baseline statistically significantly greater for high dose than low dose at p ≤ 0.05 level.

Figure 2 presents the proportion of patients (X axis) whose percentage reduction from baseline in complex partial seizure rates was at least as great as that indicated on the Y

Information on the AbbVie, Inc. products listed on these pages is from the prescribing information in use as of July 31, 2014. For more information, please visit rxabbvie.com or call 1-800-633-9110.

axis in the monotherapy study. A positive percent reduction indicates an improvement (i.e., a decrease in seizure frequency), while a negative percent reduction indicates worsening. Thus, in a display of this type, the curve for a more effective treatment is shifted to the left of the curve for a less effective treatment. This Figure shows that the proportion of patients achieving any particular level of reduction was consistently higher for high dose valproate than for low dose valproate. For example, when switching from carbamazepine, phenytoin, phenobarbital or primidone monotherapy to high dose valproate monotherapy, 63% of patients experienced no change or a reduction in complex partial seizure rates compared to 54% of patients receiving low dose valproate.

Figure 2

Information on pediatric studies are presented in section 8.

14.3   Migraine
The results of a multicenter, randomized, double-blind, placebo-controlled, parallel-group clinical trial demonstrated the effectiveness of Depakote ER in the prophylactic treatment of migraine headache. This trial recruited patients with a history of migraine headaches with or without aura occurring on average twice or more a month for the preceding three months. Patients with cluster or chronic daily headaches were excluded. Women of childbearing potential were allowed in the trial if they were deemed to be practicing an effective method of contraception.

Patients who experienced ≥ 2 migraine headaches in the 4-week baseline period were randomized in a 1:1 ratio to Depakote ER or placebo and treated for 12 weeks. Patients initiated treatment on 500 mg once daily for one week, and were then increased to 1000 mg once daily with an option to permanently decrease the dose back to 500 mg once daily during the second week of treatment if intolerance occurred. Ninety-eight of 114 Depakote ER-treated patients (86%) and 100 of 110 placebo-treated patients (91%) treated at least two weeks maintained the 1000 mg once daily dose for the duration of their treatment periods. Treatment outcome was assessed on the basis of reduction in 4-week migraine headache rate in the treatment period compared to the baseline period.

Patients (50 male, 187 female) ranging in age from 16 to 69 were treated with Depakote ER (N=122) or placebo (N=115). Four patients were below the age of 18 and 3 were above the age of 65. Two hundred and two patients (101 in each treatment group) completed the treatment period. The mean reduction in 4-week migraine headache rate was 1.2 from a baseline mean of 4.4 in the Depakote ER group, versus 0.6 from a baseline mean of 4.2 in the placebo group. The treatment difference was statistically significant (see Figure 3).

Figure 3 Mean Reduction In 4-Week Migraine Headache Rates

* p=0.006

15   REFERENCES
1. Meador KJ, Baker GA, Browning N, et al. Fetal antiepileptic drug exposure and cognitive outcomes at age 6 years (NEAD study): a prospective observational study. Lancet Neurology 2013; 12 (3):244-252.

16   HOW SUPPLIED/STORAGE AND HANDLING
Depakote ER 250 mg is available as white ovaloid tablets with the "a" logo and the code (HF). Each Depakote ER tablet contains divalproex sodium equivalent to 250 mg of valproic acid in the following package sizes:

Bottles of 60 ....(NDC 0074-3826-60).
Bottles of 100 ....(NDC 0074-3826-13).
Bottles of 500 ....(NDC 0074-3826-53).
Unit Dose Packages of 100.................(NDC 0074-3826-11).
Depakote ER 500 mg is available as gray ovaloid tablets with the "a" logo and the code HC. Each Depakote ER tablet contains divalproex sodium equivalent to 500 mg of valproic acid in the following packaging sizes:
Bottles of 100 ....(NDC 0074-7126-13).
Bottles of 500 ....(NDC 0074-7126-53).
Unit Dose Packages of 100.................(NDC 0074-7126-11).
Recommended Storage
Store tablets at 25°C (77°F); excursions permitted to 15-30°C (59-86°F) [see USP Controlled Room Temperature].

17   PATIENT COUNSELING INFORMATION
See FDA-Approved Medication Guide
17.1   Hepatotoxicity
Warn patients and guardians that nausea, vomiting, abdominal pain, anorexia, diarrhea, asthenia, and/or jaundice can be symptoms of hepatotoxicity and, therefore, require further medical evaluation promptly [see Warnings and Precautions (5.1)].
17.2   Pancreatitis
Warn patients and guardians that abdominal pain, nausea, vomiting, and/or anorexia can be symptoms of pancreatitis and, therefore, require further medical evaluation promptly [see Warnings and Precautions (5.5)].
17.3   Birth Defects and Decreased IQ
Inform pregnant women and women of childbearing potential that use of valproate during pregnancy increases the risk of birth defects and decreased IQ in children who were exposed. Advise women to use effective contraception while using valproate. When appropriate, counsel these patients about alternative therapeutic options. This is particularly important when valproate use is considered for a condition not usually associated with permanent injury or death. Advise patients to read the Medication Guide, which appears as the last section of the labeling [see Warnings and Precautions (5.2, 5.3, 5.4) and Use in Specific Populations (8.1)]. Advise women of childbearing potential to discuss pregnancy planning with their doctor and to contact their doctor immediately if they think they are pregnant.
Encourage patients to enroll in the NAAED Pregnancy Registry if they become pregnant. This registry is collecting information about the safety of antiepileptic drugs during pregnancy. To enroll, patients can call the toll free number 1-888-233-2334 [see Use in Specific Populations (8.1)].
17.4   Suicidal Thinking and Behavior
Counsel patients, their caregivers, and families that AEDs, including Depakote ER, may increase the risk of suicidal thoughts and behavior and should be advised of the need to be alert for the emergence or worsening of symptoms of depression, any unusual changes in mood or behavior, or the emergence of suicidal thoughts, behavior, or thoughts about self-harm. Instruct patients, caregivers, and families to report behaviors of concern immediately to the healthcare providers [see Warnings and Precautions (5.8)].
17.5   Hyperammonemia
Inform patients of the signs and symptoms associated with hyperammonemic encephalopathy and be told to inform the prescriber if any of these symptoms occur [see Warnings and Precautions (5.10, 5.11)].
17.6   CNS Depression
Since valproate products may produce CNS depression, especially when combined with another CNS depressant (e.g., alcohol), advise patients not to engage in hazardous activities, such as driving an automobile or operating dangerous machinery, until it is known that they do not become drowsy from the drug.
17.7   Multi-organ Hypersensitivity Reaction
Instruct patients that a fever associated with other organ system involvement (rash, lymphadenopathy, etc.) may be drug-related and should be reported to the physician immediately [see Warnings and Precautions (5.13)].
17.8   Medication Residue in the Stool
Instruct patients to notify their healthcare provider if they notice a medication residue in the stool [see Warnings and Precautions (5.19)].
250 mg is Mfd. by AbbVie LTD, Barceloneta, PR 00617
500 mg is Mfd. by AbbVie Inc., North Chicago, IL 60064 U.S.A. or
AbbVie LTD, Barceloneta, PR 00617
For AbbVie Inc., North Chicago, IL 60064 U.S.A.

MEDICATION GUIDE
DEPAKOTE ER (dep-a-kOte)
(divalproex sodium)
Extended Release Tablets
DEPAKOTE (dep-a-kOte)
(divalproex sodium)
Tablets
DEPAKOTE (dep-a-kOte)
(divalproex sodium)

Sprinkle Capsules
DEPAKENE (dep-a-keen)
(valproic acid)
Capsules and Oral Solution
Read this Medication Guide before you start taking Depakote or Depakene and each time you get a refill. There may be new information. This information does not take the place of talking to your healthcare provider about your medical condition or treatment.
What is the most important information I should know about Depakote and Depakene?
Do not stop taking Depakote or Depakene without first talking to your healthcare provider.
Stopping Depakote or Depakene suddenly can cause serious problems.
Depakote and Depakene can cause serious side effects, including:
1. **Serious liver damage that can cause death, especially in children younger than 2 years old.** The risk of getting this serious liver damage is more likely to happen within the first 6 months of treatment.
   Call your healthcare provider right away if you get any of the following symptoms:
   ○ nausea or vomiting that does not go away
   ○ loss of appetite
   ○ pain on the right side of your stomach (abdomen)
   ○ dark urine
   ○ swelling of your face
   ○ yellowing of your skin or the whites of your eyes
   In some cases, liver damage may continue despite stopping the drug.
2. **Depakote or Depakene may harm your unborn baby.**
   • If you take Depakote or Depakene during pregnancy for any medical condition, your baby is at risk for serious birth defects. The most common birth defects with Depakote or Depakene affect the brain and spinal cord and are called spina bifida or neural tube defects. These defects occur in 1 to 2 out of every 100 babies born to mothers who use this medicine during pregnancy. These defects can begin in the first month, even before you know you are pregnant. Other birth defects can happen.
   • Birth defects may occur even in children born to women who are not taking any medicines and do not have other risk factors.
   • Taking folic acid supplements before getting pregnant and during early pregnancy can lower the chance of having a baby with a neural tube defect.
   • If you take Depakote or Depakene during pregnancy for any medical condition, your child is at risk for having a lower IQ.
   • There may be other medicines to treat your condition that have a lower chance of causing birth defects and decreased IQ in your child.
   • Women who are pregnant must not take Depakote or Depakene to prevent migraine headaches.
   • **All women of child-bearing age should talk to their healthcare provider about using other possible treatments instead of Depakote or Depakene. If the decision is made to use Depakote or Depakene, you should use effective birth control (contraception).**
   • Tell your healthcare provider right away if you become pregnant while taking Depakote or Depakene. You and your healthcare provider should decide if you will continue to take Depakote or Depakene while you are pregnant.
   Pregnancy Registry: If you become pregnant while taking Depakote or Depakene, talk to your healthcare provider about registering with the North American Antiepileptic Drug Pregnancy Registry. You can enroll in this registry by calling 1-888-233-2334. The purpose of this registry is to collect information about the safety of antiepileptic drugs during pregnancy.
3. **Inflammation of your pancreas that can cause death.**
   Call your healthcare provider right away if you have any of these symptoms:
   • severe stomach pain that you may also feel in your back
   • nausea or vomiting that does not go away
4. **Like other antiepileptic drugs, Depakote or Depakene may cause suicidal thoughts or actions in a very small number of people, about 1 in 500.**
   Call a healthcare provider right away if you have any of these symptoms, especially if they are new, worse, or worry you:
   ○ thoughts about suicide or dying
   ○ attempts to commit suicide
   ○ new or worse depression
   ○ new or worse anxiety
   ○ feeling agitated or restless
   ○ panic attacks
   ○ trouble sleeping (insomnia)
   ○ new or worse irritability
   ○ acting aggressive, being angry, or violent
   ○ acting on dangerous impulses
   ○ an extreme increase in activity and talking (mania)

○ other unusual changes in behavior or mood

How can I watch for early symptoms of suicidal thoughts and actions?

○ Pay attention to any changes, especially sudden changes in mood, behaviors, thoughts, or feelings.

○ Keep all follow-up visits with your healthcare provider as scheduled.

Call your healthcare provider between visits as needed, especially if you are worried about symptoms.

Do not stop Depakote or Depakene without first talking to a healthcare provider. Stopping Depakote or Depakene suddenly can cause serious problems. Stopping a seizure medicine suddenly in a patient who has epilepsy can cause seizures that do not stop (status epilepticus).

Suicidal thoughts or actions can be caused by things other than medicines. If you have suicidal thoughts or actions, your healthcare provider may check for other causes.

What are Depakote and Depakene?

Depakote and Depakene come in different dosage forms with different usages.

Depakote Tablets and Depakote Extended Release Tablets are prescription medicines used:
• to treat manic episodes associated with bipolar disorder.
• alone or with other medicines to treat:
  ○ complex partial seizures in adults and children 10 years of age and older
  ○ simple and complex absence seizures, with or without other seizure types
• to prevent migraine headaches

Depakene (solution and liquid capsules) and Depakote Sprinkles are prescription medicines used alone or with other medicines, to treat:
• complex partial seizures in adults and children 10 years of age and older
• simple and complex absence seizures, with or without other seizure types

Who should not take Depakote or Depakene?

Do not take Depakote or Depakene if you:
• have liver problems
• have or think you have a genetic liver problem caused by a mitochondrial disorder (e.g. Alpers-Huttenlocher syndrome)
• are allergic to divalproex sodium, valproic acid, sodium valproate, or any of the ingredients in Depakote or Depakene. See the end of this leaflet for a complete list of ingredients in Depakote and Depakene.
• have a genetic problem called urea cycle disorder
• are pregnant for the prevention of migraine headaches

What should I tell my healthcare provider before taking Depakote or Depakene?

Before you take Depakote or Depakene, tell your healthcare provider if you:
• have a genetic liver problem caused by a mitochondrial disorder (e.g. Alpers-Huttenlocher syndrome)
• drink alcohol
• are pregnant or breastfeeding. Depakote or Depakene can pass into breast milk. Talk to your healthcare provider about the best way to feed your baby if you take Depakote or Depakene.
• have or have had depression, mood problems, or suicidal thoughts or behavior
• have any other medical conditions

Tell your healthcare provider about all the medicines you take, including prescription and non-prescription medicines, vitamins, herbal supplements and medicines that you take for a short period of time.

Taking Depakote or Depakene with certain other medicines can cause side effects or affect how well they work. Do not start or stop other medicines without talking to your healthcare provider.

Know the medicines you take. Keep a list of them and show it to your healthcare provider and pharmacist each time you get a new medicine.

How should I take Depakote or Depakene?

• Take Depakote or Depakene exactly as your healthcare provider tells you. Your healthcare provider will tell you how much Depakote or Depakene to take and when to take it.
• Your healthcare provider may change your dose.
• Do not change your dose of Depakote or Depakene without talking to your healthcare provider.
• **Do not stop taking Depakote or Depakene without first talking to your healthcare provider.** Stopping Depakote or Depakene suddenly can cause serious problems.
• Swallow Depakote tablets, Depakote ER tablets or Depakene capsules whole. Do not crush or chew Depakote tablets, Depakote ER tablets, or Depakene capsules. Tell your healthcare provider if you cannot swallow Depakote or Depakene whole. You may need a different medicine.
• Depakote Sprinkle Capsules may be swallowed whole, or they may be opened and the contents may be sprinkled on a small amount of soft food, such as applesauce or pud-

ding. See the Patient Instructions for Use at the end of this Medication Guide for detailed instructions on how to use Depakote Sprinkle Capsules.
• If you take too much Depakote or Depakene, call your healthcare provider or local Poison Control Center right away.

What should I avoid while taking Depakote or Depakene?

• Depakote and Depakene can cause drowsiness and dizziness. Do not drink alcohol or take other medicines that make you sleepy or dizzy while taking Depakote or Depakene, until you talk with your doctor. Taking Depakote or Depakene with alcohol or drugs that cause sleepiness or dizziness may make your sleepiness or dizziness worse.
• Do not drive a car or operate dangerous machinery until you know how Depakote or Depakene affect you. Depakote and Depakene can slow your thinking and motor skills.

What are the possible side effects of Depakote or Depakene?

• See "What is the most important information I should know about Depakote or Depakene?"

Depakote or Depakene may cause other serious side effects including:

• **Low blood count:** red or purple spots on your skin, bruising, bleeding from your mouth, teeth or nose.
• **High ammonia levels in your blood:** feeling tired, vomiting, changes in mental status.
• **Low body temperature (hypothermia):** drop in your body temperature to less than 95°F, feeling tired, confusion, coma.
• **Allergic (hypersensitivity) reactions:** fever, skin rash, hives, sores in your mouth, blistering and peeling of your skin, swelling of your lymph nodes, swelling of your face, eyes, lips, tongue, or throat, trouble swallowing or breathing.
• **Drowsiness or sleepiness in the elderly.** This extreme drowsiness may cause you to eat or drink less than you normally would. Tell your doctor if you are not able to eat or drink as you normally do. Your doctor may start you at a lower dose of Depakote or Depakene.

Call your healthcare provider right away, if you have any of the symptoms listed above.

The common side effects of Depakote and Depakene include:
• nausea
• headache
• sleepiness
• vomiting
• weakness
• tremor
• dizziness
• stomach pain
• blurry vision
• double vision
• diarrhea
• increased appetite
• weight gain
• hair loss
• loss of appetite
• problems with walking or coordination

These are not all of the possible side effects of **Depakote or Depakene.** For more information, ask your healthcare provider or pharmacist.

Tell your healthcare provider if you have any side effect that bothers you or that does not go away.

Call your doctor for medical advice about side effects. You may report side effects to FDA at 1-800-FDA-1088.

How should I store Depakote or Depakene?

• Store Depakote Extended Release Tablets between 59°F to 86°F (15°C to 30°C).
• Store Depakote Delayed Release Tablets below 86°F (30°C).
• Store Depakote Sprinkle Capsules below 77°F (25°C).
• Store Depakene Capsules at 59°F to 77°F (15°C to 25°C).
• Store Depakene Oral Solution below 86°F (30°C).

Keep Depakote or Depakene and all medicines out of the reach of children.

General information about the safe and effective use of Depakote or Depakene

Medicines are sometimes prescribed for purposes other than those listed in a Medication Guide. Do not use Depakote or Depakene for a condition for which it was not prescribed. Do not give Depakote or Depakene to other people, even if they have the same symptoms that you have. It may harm them.

This Medication Guide summarizes the most important information about Depakote or Depakene. If you would like more information, talk with your healthcare provider. You can ask your pharmacist or healthcare provider for information about Depakote or Depakene that is written for health professionals.

For more information, go to www.rxabbvie.com or call 1-800-633-9110.

What are the ingredients in Depakote or Depakene?

Depakote:

Active ingredient: divalproex sodium

Inactive ingredients:
• **Depakote Extended Release Tablets:** FD&C Blue No. 1, hypromellose, lactose, microcrystalline cellulose, polyethylene glycol, potassium sorbate, propylene glycol, silicon dioxide, titanium dioxide, and triacetin. The 500 mg tablets also contain iron oxide and polydextrose.
• **Depakote Tablets:** cellulosic polymers, diacetylated monoglycerides, povidone, pregelatinized starch (contains corn starch), silica gel, talc, titanium dioxide, and vanillin. Individual tablets also contain:
125 mg tablets: FD&C Blue No. 1 and FD&C Red No. 40,
250 mg tablets: FD&C Yellow No. 6 and iron oxide,
500 mg tablets: D&C Red No. 30, FD&C Blue No. 2, and iron oxide.
• **Depakote Sprinkle Capsules:** cellulosic polymers, D&C Red No. 28, FD&C Blue No. 1 gelatin, iron oxide, magnesium stearate, silica gel, titanium dioxide, and triethyl citrate.

Depakene:

Active ingredient: valproic acid

Inactive ingredients:
• **Depakene Capsules:** corn oil, FD&C Yellow No. 6, gelatin, glycerin, iron oxide, methylparaben, propylparaben, and titanium dioxide.
• **Depakene Oral Solution:** FD&C Red No. 40, glycerin, methylparaben, propylparaben, sorbitol, sucrose, water, and natural and artificial flavors.

Depakote ER:
250 mg is Mfd. by AbbVie LTD, Barceloneta, PR 00617
500 mg is Mfd. by AbbVie Inc., North Chicago, IL 60064 U.S.A. or
AbbVie LTD, Barceloneta, PR 00617
For AbbVie Inc., North Chicago, IL 60064 U.S.A.
Depakote Tablets:
Mfd. by AbbVie LTD, Barceloneta, PR 00617
For AbbVie Inc., North Chicago, IL 60064, U.S.A.
Depakote Sprinkle Capsules:
AbbVie Inc., North Chicago, IL 60064, U.S.A.
Depakene Capsules:
Mfd. by Banner Pharmacaps, Inc., High Point, NC 27265 U.S.A.
For AbbVie Inc., North Chicago, IL 60064, U.S.A.
Depakene Oral solution:
Mfd. by AbbVie Inc., North Chicago, IL 60064, U.S.A.
OR by DPT Laboratories, Ltd., San Antonio, TX 78215, U.S.A.
For AbbVie Inc., North Chicago, IL 60064, U.S.A.
This Medication Guide has been approved by the U.S. Food and Drug Administration.
©2014 AbbVie Inc.
Ref: 03-A916-R17-Revised March, 2014

Shown in Product Identification Guide, page 303

GENGRAF® CAPSULES ℞
[jen-graf]
(cyclosporine capsules USP [MODIFIED])

WARNING

Only physicians experienced in the management of systemic immunosuppressive therapy for the indicated disease should prescribe Gengraf® Capsules (cyclosporine capsules, USP [**MODIFIED**]). At doses used in solid organ transplantation, only physicians experienced in immunosuppressive therapy and management of organ transplant recipients should prescribe Gengraf®. Patients receiving the drug should be managed in facilities equipped and staffed with adequate laboratory and supportive medical resources. The physician responsible for maintenance therapy should have complete information requisite for the follow-up of the patient.

Gengraf®, a systemic immunosuppressant, may increase the susceptibility to infection and the development of neoplasia. In kidney, liver, and heart transplant patients Gengraf® may be administered with other immunosuppressive agents. Increased susceptibility to infection and the possible development of lymphoma and other neoplasms may result from the increase in the degree of immunosuppression in transplant patients.

Gengraf® Capsules (cyclosporine capsules, USP [**MODIFIED**]) has increased bioavailability in compari-

---

Information on the AbbVie, Inc. products listed on these pages is from the prescribing information in use as of July 31, 2014. For more information, please visit rxabbvie.com or call 1-800-633-9110.

Pharmacokinetic Parameters (mean± SD)

Patient Population	Dose/day[1] (mg/d)	Dose/ weight (mg/kg/d)	AUC[2] (ng·hr/mL)	C_{max} (ng/mL)	Trough[3] (ng/mL)	CL/F (mL/min)	CL/F (mL/min/kg)
De novo renal transplant[4] Week 4 (N = 37)	597 ± 174	7.95 ± 2.81	8772 ± 2089	1802 ± 428	361 ± 129	593 ± 204	7.8 ± 2.9
Stable renal transplant[4] (N = 55)	344 ± 122	4.10 ± 1.58	6035 ± 2194	1333 ± 469	251 ± 116	492 ± 140	5.9 ± 2.1
De novo liver transplant[5] Week 4 (N = 18)	458 ± 190	6.89 ± 3.68	7187 ± 2816	1555 ± 740	268 ± 101	577 ± 309	8.6 ± 5.7
De novo rheumatoid arthritis[6] (N = 23)	182 ± 55.6	2.37 ± 0.36	2641 ± 877	728 ± 263	96.4 ± 37.7	613 ± 196	8.3 ± 2.8
De novo psoriasis[6] Week 4 (N = 18)	189 ± 69.8	2.48 ± 0.65	2324 ± 1048	655 ± 186	74.9 ± 46.7	723 ± 186	10.2 ± 3.9

[1] Total daily dose was divided into two doses administered every 12 hours.
[2] AUC was measured over one dosing interval.
[3] Trough concentration was measured just prior to the morning cyclosporine (**MODIFIED**) dose, approximately 12 hours after the previous dose.
[4] Assay: TDx specific monoclonal fluorescence polarization immunoassay.
[5] Assay: Cyclo-trac specific monoclonal radioimmunoassay.
[6] Assay: INCSTAR specific monoclonal radioimmunoassay.

Pediatric Pharmacokinetic Parameters (mean ± SD)

Patient Population	Dose/ day (mg/d)	Dose/ weight (mg/kg/d)	AUC[1] (ng·hr/mL)	C_{max} (ng/mL)	CL/F (mL/min)	CL/F (mL/min/kg)
Stable liver transplant [2]						
Age 2-8, Dosed TID (N = 9)	101 ± 25	5.95 ± 1.32	2163 ± 801	629 ± 219	285 ± 94	16.6 ± 4.3
Age 8-15, Dosed BID (N = 8)	188 ± 55	4.96 ± 2.09	4272 ± 1462	975 ± 281	378 ± 80	10.2 ± 4.0
Stable liver transplant [3]						
Age 3, Dosed BID (N = 1)	120	8.33	5832	1050	171	11.9
Age 8-15, Dosed BID (N = 5)	158 ± 55	5.51 ± 1.91	4452 ± 2475	1013 ± 635	328 ± 121	11.0 ± 1.9
Stable renal transplant [3]						
Age 7-15, Dosed BID (N = 5)	328 ± 83	7.37 ± 4.11	6922 ± 1988	1827 ± 487	418 ± 143	8.7 ± 2.9

[1] AUC was measured over one dosing interval.
[2] Assay: Cyclo-trac specific monoclonal radioimmunoassay.
[3] Assay: TDx specific monoclonal fluorescence polarization immunoassay.

son to Sandimmune® Soft Gelatin Capsules (cyclosporine capsules, USP). Gengraf® and Sandimmune® are not bioequivalent and cannot be used interchangeably without physician supervision. For a given trough concentration, cyclosporine exposure will be greater with Gengraf® than with Sandimmune®. If a patient who is receiving exceptionally high doses of Sandimmune® is converted to Gengraf®, particular caution should be exercised. Cyclosporine blood concentrations should be monitored in transplant and rheumatoid arthritis patients taking Gengraf® to avoid toxicity due to high concentrations. Dose adjustments should be made in transplant patients to minimize possible organ rejection due to low concentrations. Comparison of blood concentrations in the published literature with blood concentrations obtained using current assays must be done with detailed knowledge of the assay methods employed.

For Psoriasis Patients (see also Boxed WARNINGS above)

Psoriasis patients previously treated with PUVA and to a lesser extent, methotrexate or other immunosuppressive agents, UVB, coal tar, or radiation therapy, are at an increased risk of developing skin malignancies when taking Gengraf® Capsules (cyclosporine capsules, USP [**MODIFIED**]).

Cyclosporine, the active ingredient in Gengraf®, in recommended dosages, can cause systemic hypertension and nephrotoxicity. The risk increases with increasing dose and duration of cyclosporine therapy. Renal dysfunction, including structural kidney damage, is a potential consequence of cyclosporine; and therefore, renal function must be monitored during therapy.

DESCRIPTION

Gengraf® Capsules (cyclosporine capsules, USP [**MODIFIED**]) is a modified oral formulation of cyclosporine that forms an aqueous dispersion in an aqueous environment.

Cyclosporine, the active principle in Gengraf®, is a cyclic polypeptide immunosuppressant agent consisting of 11 amino acids. It is produced as a metabolite by the fungus species *Aphanocladium album*.

Chemically, cyclosporine is designated as [R-[R*,R*-(E)]]-cyclic-(L-alanyl-D-alanyl-N-methyl-L-leucyl-N -methyl-L-leucyl-N-methyl-L-valyl-3-hydroxy-N,4-dimethyl- L-2-amino-6-octenoyl-L-α-amino-butyryl-N-methylglycyl-N -methyl-L-leucyl-L-valyl-N-methyl-L-leucyl).

Gengraf® Capsules (cyclosporine capsules, USP [**MODIFIED**]) are available in 25 mg and 100 mg strengths.

Each 25 mg capsule contains
cyclosporine, 25 mg, alcohol, USP, absolute, 12.8% v/v (10.1% wt/vol.).

Each 100 mg capsule contains
cyclosporine, 100 mg, alcohol, USP, absolute, 12.8% v/v (10.1% wt/vol.).

Inactive Ingredients
FD&C Blue No. 2, gelatin NF, polyethylene glycol NF, polyoxyl 35 castor oil NF, polysorbate 80 NF, propylene glycol USP, sorbitan monooleate NF, titanium dioxide.

The chemical structure for cyclosporine USP is:
[See chemical structure at top of next column]

CLINICAL PHARMACOLOGY

Cyclosporine is a potent immunosuppressive agent that in animals prolongs survival of allogeneic transplants involving skin, kidney, liver, heart, pancreas, bone marrow, small intestine, and lung. Cyclosporine has been demonstrated to suppress some humoral immunity and to a greater extent,

$C_{62}H_{111}N_{11}O_{12}$ Mol. Wt. 1202.61

cell-mediated immune reactions such as allograft rejection, delayed hypersensitivity, experimental allergic encephalomyelitis, Freund's adjuvant arthritis, and graft vs. host disease in many animal species for a variety of organs.

The effectiveness of cyclosporine results from specific and reversible inhibition of immunocompetent lymphocytes in the G_0- and G_1-phase of the cell cycle. T-lymphocytes are preferentially inhibited. The T-helper cell is the main target, although the T-suppressor cell may also be suppressed. Cyclosporine also inhibits lymphokine production and release including interleukin-2.

No effects on phagocytic function (changes in enzyme secretions, chemotactic migration of granulocytes, macrophage migration, carbon clearance *in vivo*) have been detected in animals. Cyclosporine does not cause bone marrow suppression in animal models or man.

Pharmacokinetics

The immunosuppressive activity of cyclosporine is primarily due to parent drug. Following oral administration, absorption of cyclosporine is incomplete. The extent of absorption of cyclosporine is dependent on the individual patient, the patient population, and the formulation. Elimination of cyclosporine is primarily biliary with only 6% of the dose (parent drug and metabolites) excreted in urine. The disposition of cyclosporine from blood is generally biphasic, with a terminal half-life of approximately 8.4 hours (range 5 to 18 hours). Following intravenous administration, the blood clearance of cyclosporine (assay: HPLC) is approximately 5 to 7 mL/min/kg in adult recipients of renal or liver allografts. Blood cyclosporine clearance appears to be slightly slower in cardiac transplant patients.

The Gengraf® Capsules (cyclosporine capsules, USP [**MODIFIED**]) and Gengraf® Oral Solution (cyclosporine oral solution, USP [**MODIFIED**]) are bioequivalent.

The relationship between administered dose and exposure (area under the concentration versus time curve, AUC) is linear within the therapeutic dose range. The intersubject variability (total, % CV) of cyclosporine exposure (AUC) when cyclosporine (**MODIFIED**) or Sandimmune® is administered ranges from approximately 20% to 50% in renal transplant patients. This intersubject variability contributes to the need for individualization of the dosing regimen for optimal therapy (see **DOSAGE AND ADMINISTRATION**). Intrasubject variability of AUC in renal transplant recipients (% CV) was 9% to 21% for cyclosporine (**MODIFIED**) and 19% to 26% for Sandimmune®. In the same studies, intrasubject variability of trough concentrations (% CV) was 17% to 30% for cyclosporine (**MODIFIED**) and 16% to 38% for Sandimmune®.

Absorption

Cyclosporine (**MODIFIED**) has increased bioavailability compared to Sandimmune®. The absolute bioavailability of cyclosporine administered as Sandimmune® is dependent on the patient population, estimated to be less than 10% in liver transplant patients and as great as 89% in some renal transplant patients. The absolute bioavailability of cyclosporine administered as cyclosporine (**MODIFIED**) has not been determined in adults. In studies of renal transplant, rheumatoid arthritis and psoriasis patients, the mean cyclosporine AUC was approximately 20% to 50% greater and the peak blood cyclosporine concentration (C_{max}) was approximately 40% to 106% greater following administration of cyclosporine (**MODIFIED**) compared to following administration of Sandimmune®. The dose normalized AUC in *de novo* liver transplant patients administered cyclosporine (**MODIFIED**) 28 days after transplantation was 50% greater and C_{max} was 90% greater than in those patients administered Sandimmune®. AUC and C_{max} are also increased (cyclosporine [**MODIFIED**] relative to Sandimmune®) in heart transplant patients, but data are very limited. Although the AUC and C_{max} values are higher on cyclosporine (**MODIFIED**) relative to Sandimmune®, the pre-dose trough concentrations (dose-normalized) are similar for the two formulations.

Following oral administration of cyclosporine (**MODIFIED**), the time to peak blood cyclosporine concentrations (T_{max}) ranged from 1.5 to 2.0 hours. The administration of food with cyclosporine (**MODIFIED**) decreases the cyclosporine AUC and C_{max}. A high fat meal (669 kcal, 45 grams fat) consumed within one-half hour before cyclosporine (**MODIFIED**) administration decreased the AUC by 13% and C_{max} by 33%. The effects of a low fat meal (667 kcal, 15 grams fat) were similar.

The effect of T-tube diversion of bile on the absorption of cyclosporine from cyclosporine (**MODIFIED**) was investigated in eleven *de novo* liver transplant patients. When the patients were administered cyclosporine (**MODIFIED**) with and without T-tube diversion of bile, very little difference in absorption was observed, as measured by the change in maximal cyclosporine blood concentrations from pre-dose values with the T-tube closed relative to when it was open: $6.9 \pm 41\%$ (range -55% to 68%).

[See first table at top of previous page]

Distribution

Cyclosporine

Cyclosporine is distributed largely outside the blood volume. The steady state volume of distribution during intravenous dosing has been reported as 3 to 5 L/kg in solid organ transplant recipients. In blood, the distribution is concentration dependent. Approximately 33% to 47% is in plasma, 4% to 9% in lymphocytes, 5% to 12% in granulocytes, and 41% to 58% in erythrocytes. At high concentrations, the binding capacity of leukocytes and erythrocytes becomes saturated. In plasma, approximately 90% is bound to proteins, primarily lipoproteins. Cyclosporine is excreted in human milk (see **PRECAUTIONS - Nursing Mothers**).

Metabolism

Cyclosporine is extensively metabolized by the cytochrome P-450 III-A enzyme system in the liver, and to a lesser degree in the gastrointestinal tract, and the kidney. The metabolism of cyclosporine can be altered by the coadministration of a variety of agents (see **PRECAUTIONS - Drug Interactions**). At least 25 metabolites have been identified from human bile, feces, blood, and urine. The biological activity of the metabolites and their contributions to toxicity are considerably less than those of the parent compound. The major metabolites (M1, M9, and M4N) result from oxidation at the 1-beta, 9-gamma, and 4-N-demethylated positions, respectively. At steady state following the oral administration of Sandimmune®, the mean AUCs for blood concentrations of M1, M9 and M4N are about 70%, 21%, and 7.5% of the AUC for blood cyclosporine concentrations, respectively. Based on blood concentration data from stable renal transplant patients (13 patients administered cyclosporine [**MODIFIED**] and Sandimmune® in a crossover study), and bile concentration data from *de novo* liver transplant patients (4 administered cyclosporine [**MODIFIED**], 3 administered Sandimmune®), the percentage of dose present as M1, M9, and M4N metabolites is similar when either cyclosporine (**MODIFIED**) or Sandimmune® is administered.

Excretion

Only 0.1% of a cyclosporine dose is excreted unchanged in the urine. Elimination is primarily biliary with only 6% of the dose (parent drug and metabolites) excreted in the urine. Neither dialysis nor renal failure alter cyclosporine clearance significantly.

Drug Interactions

(See **PRECAUTIONS - Drug Interactions**). When diclofenac or methotrexate was coadministered with cyclosporine in rheumatoid arthritis patients, the AUC of diclofenac and methotrexate, each was significantly increased (see **PRECAUTIONS - Drug Interactions**). No clinically significant pharmacokinetic interactions occurred between cyclosporine and aspirin, ketoprofen, piroxicam, or indomethacin.

Specific Populations

Renal Impairment

In a study performed in 4 subjects with end-stage renal disease (creatinine clearance <5 mL/min), an intravenous infusion of 3.5 mg/kg of cyclosporine over 4 hours administered at the end of a hemodialysis session resulted in a mean volume of distribution (Vdss) of 3.49 L/kg and systemic clearance (CL) of 0.369 L/hr/kg. This systemic CL (0.369 L/hr/kg) was approximately two thirds of the mean systemic CL (0.56 L/hr/kg) of cyclosporine in historical control subjects with normal renal function. In 5 liver transplant patients, the mean clearance of cyclosporine on and off hemodialysis was 463 mL/min and 398 mL/min, respectively. Less than 1% of the dose of cyclosporine was recovered in the dialysate.

Hepatic Impairment

Cyclosporine is extensively metabolized by the liver. Since severe hepatic impairment may result in significantly increased cyclosporine exposures, the dosage of cyclosporine may need to be reduced in these patients.

Pediatric Population

Pharmacokinetic data from pediatric patients administered cyclosporine (**MODIFIED**) or Sandimmune® are very limited. In 15 renal transplant patients aged 3 to 16 years, cyclosporine whole blood clearance after IV administration of Sandimmune® was 10.6 ± 3.7 mL/min/kg (assay: Cyclotrac specific RIA). In a study of 7 renal transplant patients aged 2 to 16, the cyclosporine clearance ranged from 9.8 to 15.5 mL/min/kg. In 9 liver transplant patients aged 0.6 to 5.6 years, clearance was 9.3 ± 5.4 mL/min/kg (assay: HPLC).

In the pediatric population, cyclosporine (**MODIFIED**) also demonstrates an increased bioavailability as compared to Sandimmune®. In 7 liver *de novo* transplant patients aged 1.4 to 10 years, the absolute bioavailability of cyclosporine (**MODIFIED**) was 43% (range 30% to 68%) and for Sandimmune® in the same individuals absolute bioavailability was 28% (range 17% to 42%).

[See second table at top of previous page]

Geriatric Population

Comparison of single dose data from both normal elderly volunteers (N = 18, mean age 69 years) and elderly rheumatoid arthritis patients (N = 16, mean age 68 years) to single dose data in young adult volunteers (N = 16, mean age 26 years) showed no significant difference in the pharmacokinetic parameters.

CLINICAL TRIALS

Rheumatoid Arthritis

The effectiveness of Sandimmune® and cyclosporine (**MODIFIED**) in the treatment of severe rheumatoid arthritis was evaluated in five clinical studies involving a total of 728 cyclosporine treated patients and 273 placebo treated patients.

A summary of the results is presented for the "responder" rates per treatment group, with a responder being defined as a patient having *completed* the trial with a 20% improvement in the tender and the swollen joint count and a 20% improvement in 2 of 4 of investigator global, patient global, disability, and erythrocyte sedimentation rates (ESR) for the Studies 651 and 652 and 3 of 5 of investigator global, patient global, disability, visual analog pain, and ESR for Studies 2008, 654, and 302.

Study 651 enrolled 264 patients with active rheumatoid arthritis with at least 20 involved joints, who had failed at least one major RA drug, using a 3:3:2 randomization to one of the following three groups: (1) cyclosporine dosed at 2.5 to 5 mg/kg/day, (2) methotrexate at 7.5 to 15 mg/week, or (3) placebo. Treatment duration was 24 weeks. The mean cyclosporine dose at the last visit was 3.1 mg/kg/day. See Graph below.

Study 652 enrolled 250 patients with active RA with > 6 active painful or tender joints who had failed at least one major RA drug. Patients were randomized using a 3:3:2 randomization to 1 of 3 treatment arms: (1) 1.5 to 5 mg/kg/day of cyclosporine, (2) 2.5 to 5 mg/kg/day of cyclosporine, and (3) placebo. Treatment duration was 16 weeks. The mean cyclosporine dose for group 2 at the last visit was 2.92 mg/kg/day. See Graph below.

Study 2008 enrolled 144 patients with active RA and > 6 active joints who had unsuccessful treatment courses of aspirin and gold or Penicillamine. Patients were randomized to one of two treatment groups: (1) cyclosporine 2.5 to 5 mg/kg/day with adjustments after the first month to achieve a target trough level and (2) placebo. Treatment duration was 24 weeks. The mean cyclosporine dose at the last visit was 3.63 mg/kg/day. See Graph below.

Study 654 enrolled 148 patients who remained with active joint counts of 6 or more despite treatment with maximally tolerated methotrexate doses for at least three months. Patients continued to take their current dose of methotrexate and were randomized to receive, in addition, one of the following medications: (1) cyclosporine 2.5 mg/kg/day with dose increases of 0.5 mg/kg/day at Weeks 2 and 4 if there was no evidence of toxicity and further increases of 0.5 mg/kg/day at Weeks 8 and 16 if a < 30% decrease in active joint count occurred without any significant toxicity; dose decreases could be made at any time for toxicity or (2) placebo. Treatment duration was 24 weeks. The mean cyclosporine dose at the last visit was 2.8 mg/kg/day (range: 1.3 to 4.1). See Graph below.

Study 302 enrolled 299 patients with severe active RA, 99% of whom were unresponsive or intolerant to at least one prior major RA drug. Patients were randomized to 1 of 2 treatment groups (1) cyclosporine (**MODIFIED**) and (2) Sandimmune® both of which were started at 2.5 mg/kg/day and increased after 4 weeks for inefficacy in increments of 0.5 mg/kg/day to a maximum of 5 mg/kg/day and decreased at any time for toxicity. Treatment duration was 24 weeks. The mean cyclosporine dose at the last visit was 2.91 mg/kg/day (range: 0.72 to 5.17) for cyclosporine (**MODIFIED**) and 3.27 mg/kg/day (range: 0.73 to 5.68) for Sandimmune®. See Graph below.

Numbers on columns are p-values vs. placebo, unless indicated otherwise

ACR Responders Randomized

INDICATIONS AND USAGE

Kidney, Liver and Heart Transplantation

Gengraf® Capsules (cyclosporine capsules, USP [**MODIFIED**]) is indicated for the prophylaxis of organ rejection in kidney, liver, and heart allogeneic transplants. Cyclosporine (**MODIFIED**) has been used in combination with azathioprine and corticosteroids.

Rheumatoid Arthritis

Gengraf® Capsules (cyclosporine capsules, USP [**MODIFIED**]) is indicated for the treatment of patients with severe active, rheumatoid arthritis where the disease has not adequately responded to methotrexate. Gengraf® can be used in combination with methotrexate in rheumatoid arthritis patients who do not respond adequately to methotrexate alone.

Psoriasis

Gengraf® Capsules (cyclosporine capsules, USP [**MODIFIED**]) is indicated for the treatment of *adult, nonimmunocompromised* patients with severe (i.e., extensive and/or disabling), recalcitrant, plaque psoriasis who have failed to respond to at least one systemic therapy (e.g., PUVA, retinoids, or methotrexate) or in patients for whom other systemic therapies are contraindicated, or cannot be tolerated.

While rebound rarely occurs, most patients will experience relapse with Gengraf® as with other therapies upon cessation of treatment.

CONTRAINDICATIONS

General

Gengraf® Capsules (cyclosporine capsules, USP [**MODIFIED**]) is contraindicated in patients with a hypersensitivity to cyclosporine or to any of the ingredients of the formulation.

Rheumatoid Arthritis

Rheumatoid arthritis patients with abnormal renal function, uncontrolled hypertension or malignancies should not receive Gengraf® Capsules (cyclosporine capsules, USP [**MODIFIED**]).

Psoriasis

Psoriasis patients who are treated with Gengraf® Capsules (cyclosporine capsules, USP [**MODIFIED**]) should not receive concomitant PUVA or UVB therapy, methotrexate or other immunosuppressive agents, coal tar or radiation therapy. Psoriasis patients with abnormal renal function, uncontrolled hypertension, or malignancies should not receive Gengraf®.

WARNINGS

(See also **Boxed WARNINGS**).

All Patients

Cyclosporine, the active ingredient of Gengraf® Capsules (cyclosporine capsules, USP [**MODIFIED**]), can cause nephrotoxicity and hepatotoxicity. The risk increases with increasing doses of cyclosporine. Renal dysfunction including structural kidney damage is a potential consequence of Gengraf® and therefore renal function must be monitored during therapy. **Care should be taken in using cyclosporine with nephrotoxic drugs (see PRECAUTIONS).**

Patients receiving Gengraf® require frequent monitoring of serum creatinine (see Special Monitoring under **DOSAGE AND ADMINISTRATION**). Elderly patients should be monitored with particular care, since decreases in renal function also occur with age. If patients are not properly monitored and doses are not properly adjusted, cyclosporine therapy can be associated with the occurrence of structural kidney damage and persistent renal dysfunction.

An increase in serum creatinine and BUN may occur during Gengraf® therapy and reflect a reduction in the glomerular filtration rate. Impaired renal function at any time requires close monitoring, and frequent dosage adjustment may be indicated. The frequency and severity of serum creatinine elevations increase with dose and duration of cyclosporine therapy. These elevations are likely to become more pronounced without dose reduction or discontinuation.

Because Gengraf® Capsules (cyclosporine capsules, USP [MODIFIED]) is not bioequivalent to Sandimmune® Soft Gelatin Capsules (cyclosporine capsules, USP), conversion from Gengraf® to Sandimmune® using a 1:1 ratio (mg/kg/day) may result in lower cyclosporine blood concentrations. Conversion from Gengraf® to Sandimmune® should be made with increased monitoring to avoid the potential of underdosing.

Kidney, Liver, and Heart Transplant

Nephrotoxicity

Cyclosporine, the active ingredient of Gengraf® Capsules (cyclosporine capsules, USP [**MODIFIED**]), can cause nephrotoxicity and hepatotoxicity when used in high doses. It is

Information on the AbbVie, Inc. products listed on these pages is from the prescribing information in use as of July 31, 2014. For more information, please visit rxabbvie.com or call 1-800-633-9110.

Parameter	Nephrotoxicity vs. Rejection	
	Nephrotoxicity	Rejection
History	Donor > 50 years old or hypotensive Prolonged kidney preservation Prolonged anastomosis time Concomitant nephrotoxic drugs	Anti-donor immune response Retransplant patient
Clinical	Often > 6 weeks postop[b] Prolonged initial nonfunction (acute tubular necrosis)	Often < 4 weeks postop[b] Fever > 37.5°C Weight gain > 0.5 kg Graft swelling and tenderness Decrease in daily urine volume > 500 mL (or 50%)
Laboratory	CyA serum trough level > 200 ng/mL Gradual rise in Cr (< 0.15 mg/dL/day)[a] Cr plateau < 25% above baseline BUN/Cr ≥ 20	CyA serum trough level < 150 ng/mL Rapid rise in Cr (> 0.3 mg/dL/day)[a] Cr > 25% above baseline BUN/Cr < 20
Biopsy	Arteriolopathy (medial hypertrophy[a], hyalinosis, nodular deposits, intimal thickening, endothelial vacuolization, progressive scarring) Tubular atrophy, isometric vacuolization, isolated calcifications Minimal edema Mild focal infiltrates[c] Diffuse interstitial fibrosis, often striped form	Endovasculitis[c] (proliferation[a], intimal arteritis[b], necrosis, sclerosis) Tubulitis with RBC[b] and WBC[b] casts, some irregular vacuolization Interstitial edema[c] and hemorrhage[b] Diffuse moderate to severe mononuclear infiltrates[d] Glomerulitis (mononuclear cells)[c]
Aspiration Cytology	CyA deposits in tubular and endothelial cells Fine isometric vacuolization of tubular cells	Inflammatory infiltrate with mononuclear phagocytes, macrophages, lymphoblastoid cells, and activated T-cells These strongly express HLA-DR antigens
Urine Cytology	Tubular cells with vacuolization and granularization	Degenerative tubular cells, plasma cells, and lymphocyturia > 20% of sediment
Manometry Ultrasonography	Intracapsular pressure < 40 mm Hg[b] Unchanged graft cross sectional area	Intracapsular pressure > 40 mm Hg[b] Increase in graft cross sectional area AP diameter ≥ Transverse diameter
Magnetic Resonance Imagery	Normal appearance	Loss of distinct corticomedullary junction, swelling image intensity of parachyma approaching that of psoas, loss of hilar fat
Radionuclide Scan	Normal or generally decreased perfusion Decrease in tubular function (^{131} I-hippuran) > decrease in perfusion (^{99m} Tc DTPA)	Patchy arterial flow Decrease in perfusion > decrease in tubular function Increased uptake of Indium 111 labeled platelets or Tc-99m in colloid
Therapy	Responds to decreased cyclosporine	Responds to increased steroids or antilymphocyte globulin

[a] p < 0.05, [b] p < 0.01, [c] p < 0.001, [d] p < 0.0001

not unusual for serum creatinine and BUN levels to be elevated during cyclosporine therapy. These elevations in renal transplant patients do not necessarily indicate rejection, and each patient must be fully evaluated before dosage adjustment is initiated.

Based on the historical Sandimmune® experience with oral solution, nephrotoxicity associated with cyclosporine had been noted in 25% of cases of renal transplantation, 38% of cases of cardiac transplantation, and 37% of cases of liver transplantation. Mild nephrotoxicity was generally noted 2 to 3 months after renal transplant and consisted of an arrest in the fall of the pre-operative elevations of BUN and creatinine at a range of 35 to 45 mg/dL and 2.0 to 2.5 mg/dL respectively. These elevations were often responsive to cyclosporine dosage reduction.

More overt nephrotoxicity was seen early after transplantation and was characterized by a rapidly rising BUN and creatinine. Since these events are similar to renal rejection episodes, care must be taken to differentiate between them. This form of nephrotoxicity is usually responsive to cyclosporine dosage reduction.

Although specific diagnostic criteria which reliably differentiate renal graft rejection from drug toxicity have not been found, a number of parameters have been significantly associated with one or the other. It should be noted however, that up to 20% of patients may have simultaneous nephrotoxicity and rejection.

[See table above]

A form of a cyclosporine-associated nephropathy is characterized by serial deterioration in renal function and morphologic changes in the kidneys. From 5% to 15% of transplant recipients who have received cyclosporine will fail to show a reduction in rising serum creatinine despite a decrease or discontinuation of cyclosporine therapy. Renal biopsies from these patients will demonstrate one or several of the following alterations: tubular vacuolization, tubular microcalcifications, peritubular capillary congestion, arteri-

olopathy, and a striped form of interstitial fibrosis with tubular atrophy. Though none of these morphologic changes is entirely specific, a diagnosis of cyclosporine-associated structural nephrotoxicity requires evidence of these findings.

When considering the development of cyclosporine-associated nephropathy, it is noteworthy that several authors have reported an association between the appearance of interstitial fibrosis and higher cumulative doses or persistently high circulating trough concentrations of cyclosporine. This is particularly true during the first 6 post-transplant months when the dosage tends to be highest and when, in kidney recipients, the organ appears to be most vulnerable to the toxic effects of cyclosporine. Among other contributing factors to the development of interstitial fibrosis in these patients are prolonged perfusion time, warm ischemia time, as well as episodes of acute toxicity, and acute and chronic rejection. The reversibility of interstitial fibrosis and its correlation to renal function have not yet been determined. Reversibility of arteriolopathy has been reported after stopping cyclosporine or lowering the dosage.

Impaired renal function at any time requires close monitoring, and frequent dosage adjustment may be indicated.

In the event of severe and unremitting rejection, when rescue therapy with pulse steroids and monoclonal antibodies fail to reverse the rejection episode, it may be preferable to switch to alternative immunosuppressive therapy rather than increase the Gengraf® dose to excessive blood concentrations.

Due to the potential for additive or synergistic impairment of renal function, caution should be exercised when coadministering Gengraf® with other drugs that may impair renal function (see PRECAUTIONS - Drug Interactions).

Thrombotic Microangiopathy

Occasionally patients have developed a syndrome of thrombocytopenia and microangiopathic hemolytic anemia which

may result in graft failure. The vasculopathy can occur in the absence of rejection and is accompanied by avid platelet consumption within the graft as demonstrated by Indium 111 labeled platelet studies. Neither the pathogenesis nor the management of this syndrome is clear. Though resolution has occurred after reduction or discontinuation of cyclosporine and 1) administration of streptokinase and heparin or 2) plasmapheresis, this appears to depend upon early detection with Indium 111 labeled platelet scans (see ADVERSE REACTIONS).

Hyperkalemia

Significant hyperkalemia (sometimes associated with hyperchloremic metabolic acidosis) and hyperuricemia have been seen occasionally in individual patients.

Hepatotoxicity

Cases of hepatotoxicity and liver injury including cholestasis, jaundice, hepatitis and liver failure have been reported in patients treated with cyclosporine. Most reports included patients with significant co-morbidities, underlying conditions and other confounding factors including infectious complications and comedications with hepatotoxic potential. In some cases, mainly in transplant patients, fatal outcomes have been reported (see ADVERSE REACTIONS, Postmarketing Experience, Kidney, Liver and Heart Transplantation).

Hepatotoxicity usually manifested by elevations of hepatic enzymes and bilirubin, was reported in patients treated with cyclosporine in clinical trials: 4% in renal transplantation, 7% in cardiac transplantation, and 4% in liver transplantation. This was usually noted during the first month of therapy when high doses of cyclosporine were used. The chemistry elevations usually decreased with a reduction in dosage.

Malignancies

As in patients receiving other immunosuppressants, those patients receiving cyclosporine are at increased risk for development of lymphomas and other malignancies, particularly those of the skin. Patients taking cyclosporine should be warned to avoid excess ultraviolet light exposure. The increased risk appears related to the intensity and duration of immunosuppression rather than to the use of specific agents. Because of the danger of oversuppression of the immune system resulting in increased risk of infection or malignancy, a treatment regimen containing multiple immunosuppressants should be used with caution. Some malignancies may be fatal. Transplant patients receiving cyclosporine are at increased risk for serious infection with fatal outcome.

Serious Infections

Patients receiving immunosuppressants, including Gengraf®, are at increased risk of developing bacterial, viral, fungal, and protozoal infections, including opportunistic infections. These infections may lead to serious, including fatal, outcomes (see Boxed WARNING and ADVERSE REACTIONS).

Polyoma Virus Infections

Patients receiving immunosuppressants including Gengraf® are at increased risk for opportunistic infections, including polyoma virus infections. Polyoma virus infections in transplant patients may have serious, and sometimes, fatal outcomes. These include cases of JC virus-associated progressive multifocal leukoencephalopathy (PML) and polyoma virus-associated nephropathy (PVAN) especially due to BK virus infection which have been observed in patients receiving cyclosporine. PVAN is associated with serious outcomes, including deteriorating renal function and renal graft loss, (see ADVERSE REACTIONS/Postmarketing Experience, Kidney, Liver and Heart Transplantation). Patient monitoring may help detect patients at risk for PVAN.

Cases of PML have been reported in patients treated with Gengraf®. PML, which is sometimes fatal, commonly presents with hemiparesis, apathy, confusion, cognitive deficiencies and ataxia. Risk factors for PML include treatment with immunosuppressant therapies and impairment of immune function. In immunosuppressed patients, physicians should consider PML in the differential diagnosis in patients reporting neurological symptoms and consultation with a neurologist should be considered as clinically indicated.

Consideration should be given to reducing the total immunosuppression in transplant patients who develop PML or PVAN. However, reduced immunosuppression may place the graft at risk.

Neurotoxicity

There have been reports of convulsions in adult and pediatric patients receiving cyclosporine, particularly in combination with high dose methylprednisolone.

Encephalopathy, including Posterior Reversible Encephalopathy Syndrome (PRES), has been described both in postmarketing reports and in the literature. Manifestations include impaired consciousness, convulsions, visual disturbances (including blindness), loss of motor function, movement disorders and psychiatric disturbances. In many cases, changes in the white matter have been detected using imaging techniques and pathologic specimens. Predisposing factors such as hypertension, hypomagnesemia, hypocholesterolemia, high-dose corticosteroids, high cyclosporine blood concentrations, and graft-versus-host disease have been noted in many but not all of the reported cases. The changes in most cases have been reversible upon discontinuation of cyclosporine, and in some cases improvement was noted after reduction of dose. It appears that patients receiving liver transplant are more susceptible to encephalopathy than those receiving kidney transplant. Another rare manifestation of cyclosporine-induced neurotoxicity, occurring in transplant patients more frequently than in other indications, is optic disc edema including papilloedema, with possible visual impairment, secondary to benign intracranial hypertension.

Care should be taken in using cyclosporine with nephrotoxic drugs (see **PRECAUTIONS**).

Rheumatoid Arthritis

Cyclosporine nephropathy was detected in renal biopsies of six out of 60 (10%) rheumatoid arthritis patients after the average treatment duration of 19 months. Only one patient, out of these 6 patients, was treated with a dose ≤ 4 mg/kg/day. Serum creatinine improved in all but one patient after discontinuation of cyclosporine. The "maximal creatinine increase" appears to be a factor in predicting cyclosporine nephropathy.

There is a potential, as with other immunosuppressive agents, for an increase in the occurrence of malignant lymphomas with cyclosporine. It is not clear whether the risk with cyclosporine is greater than that in rheumatoid arthritis patients or in rheumatoid arthritis patients on cytotoxic treatment for this indication. Five cases of lymphoma were detected: four in a survey of approximately 2,300 patients treated with cyclosporine for rheumatoid arthritis, and another case of lymphoma was reported in a clinical trial. Although other tumors (12 skin cancers, 24 solid tumors of diverse types, and 1 multiple myeloma) were also reported in this survey, epidemiologic analyses did not support a relationship to cyclosporine other than for malignant lymphomas.

Patients should be thoroughly evaluated before and during Gengraf® Capsules (cyclosporine capsules, USP [MODIFIED]) treatment for the development of malignancies. Moreover, use of Gengraf® therapy with other immunosuppressive agents may induce an excessive immunosuppression which is known to increase the risk of malignancy.

Psoriasis

(See also **Boxed WARNINGS** for Psoriasis)

Since cyclosporine is a potent immunosuppressive agent with a number of potentially serious side effects, the risks and benefits of using Gengraf® Capsules (cyclosporine capsules, USP [MODIFIED]) should be considered before treatment of patients with psoriasis. Cyclosporine, the active ingredient in Gengraf®, can cause nephrotoxicity and hypertension (see **PRECAUTIONS**) and the risk increases with increasing dose and duration of therapy. Patients who may be at increased risk such as those with abnormal renal function, uncontrolled hypertension or malignancies, should not receive Gengraf®.

Renal dysfunction is a potential consequence of Gengraf®, therefore renal function must be monitored during therapy. Patients receiving Gengraf® require frequent monitoring of serum creatinine (see Special Monitoring under **DOSAGE AND ADMINISTRATION**). Elderly patients should be monitored with particular care, since decreases in renal function also occur with age. If patients are not properly monitored and doses are not properly adjusted, cyclosporine therapy can cause structural kidney damage and persistent renal dysfunction.

An increase in serum creatinine and BUN may occur during Gengraf® therapy and reflects a reduction in the glomerular filtration rate.

Kidney biopsies from 86 psoriasis patients treated for a mean duration of 23 months with 1.2 to 7.6 mg/kg/day of cyclosporine showed evidence of cyclosporine nephropathy in 18/86 (21%) of the patients. The pathology consisted of renal tubular atrophy and interstitial fibrosis. On repeat biopsy of 13 of these patients maintained on various dosages of cyclosporine for a mean of 2 additional years, the number with cyclosporine induced nephropathy rose to 26/86 (30%). The majority of patients (19/26) were on a dose of ≥ 5 mg/kg/day (the highest recommended dose is 4 mg/kg/day). The patients were also on cyclosporine for greater than 15 months (18/26) and/or had a clinically significant increase in serum creatinine for greater than 1 month (21/26). Creatinine levels returned to normal range in 7 of 11 patients in whom cyclosporine therapy was discontinued.

There is an increased risk for the development of skin and lymphoproliferative malignancies in cyclosporine-treated psoriasis patients. The relative risk of malignancies is comparable to that observed in psoriasis patients treated with other immunosuppressive agents.

Drugs That May Potentiate Renal Dysfunction

Antibiotics	Antineoplastics	Anti-inflammatory Drugs	Gastrointestinal Agents
ciprofloxacin	melphalan	azapropazon	cimetidine
gentamicin		colchicine	ranitidine
tobramycin	**Antifungals**	diclofenac	
vancomycin	amphotericin B	naproxen	**Immunosuppressives**
trimethoprim with	ketoconazole	sulindac	tacrolimus
sulfamethoxazole			
			Other Drugs
			fibric acid derivatives (e.g., bezafibrate, fenofibrate)
			methotrexate

1. Drugs That Increase Cyclosporine Concentrations

Calcium Channel Blockers	Antifungals	Antibiotics	Glucocorticoids	Other Drugs
diltiazem	fluconazole	azithromycin	methylprednisolone	allopurinol
nicardipine	itraconazole	clarithromycin		amiodarone
verapamil	ketoconazole	erythromycin		bromocriptine
	voriconazole	quinupristin/ dalfopristin		colchicine
				danazol
				imatinib
				metoclopramide
				nefazodone
				oral contraceptives

Tumors were reported in 32 (2.2%) of 1439 psoriasis patients treated with cyclosporine worldwide from clinical trials. Additional tumors have been reported in 7 patients in cyclosporine postmarketing experience. Skin malignancies were reported in 16 (1.1%) of these patients; all but 2 of them had previously received PUVA therapy. Methotrexate was received by 7 patients. UVB and coal tar had been used by 2 and 3 patients, respectively. Seven patients had either a history of previous skin cancer or a potentially predisposing lesion was present prior to cyclosporine exposure. Of the 16 patients with skin cancer, 11 patients had 18 squamous cell carcinomas and 7 patients had 10 basal cell carcinomas. There were two lymphoproliferative malignancies; one case of non-Hodgkin's lymphoma which required chemotherapy, and one case of mycosis fungoides which regressed spontaneously upon discontinuation of cyclosporine. There were four cases of benign lymphocytic infiltration: 3 regressed spontaneously upon discontinuation of cyclosporine, while the fourth regressed despite continuation of the drug. The remainder of the malignancies, 13 cases (0.9%), involved various organs.

Patients should not be treated concurrently with cyclosporine and PUVA or UVB, other radiation therapy, or other immunosuppressive agents, because of the possibility of excessive immunosuppression and the subsequent risk of malignancies (see CONTRAINDICATIONS). Patients should also be warned to protect themselves appropriately when in the sun, and to avoid excessive sun exposure. Patients should be thoroughly evaluated before and during treatment for the presence of malignancies remembering that malignant lesions may be hidden by psoriatic plaques. Skin lesions not typical of psoriasis should be biopsied before starting treatment. Patients should be treated with Gengraf® Capsules (cyclosporine capsules, USP [MODIFIED]) only after complete resolution of suspicious lesions, and only if there are no other treatment options (see Special Monitoring for Psoriasis Patients).

Special Excipients

Alcohol (ethanol)

The alcohol content (see **DESCRIPTION**) of Gengraf® should be taken into account when given to patients in whom alcohol intake should be avoided or minimized, e.g., pregnant or breastfeeding women, in patients presenting with liver disease or epilepsy, in alcoholic patients, or pediatric patients. For an adult weighing 70 kg, the maximum daily oral dose would deliver about 1 gram of alcohol which is approximately 6% of the amount of alcohol contained in a standard drink.

PRECAUTIONS

General

Hypertension

Cyclosporine is the active ingredient of Gengraf® Capsules (cyclosporine capsules, USP [MODIFIED]). Hypertension is a common side effect of cyclosporine therapy which may persist (see **ADVERSE REACTIONS** and **DOSAGE AND ADMINISTRATION** for monitoring recommendations). Mild or moderate hypertension is encountered more frequently than severe hypertension and the incidence decreases over time. In recipients of kidney, liver, and heart allografts treated with cyclosporine, antihypertensive therapy may be required (see **Special Monitoring of Rheumatoid Arthritis and Psoriasis Patients**). However, since cyclosporine may cause hyperkalemia, potassium-sparing diuretics should not be used. While calcium antagonists can

be effective agents in treating cyclosporine-associated hypertension, they can interfere with cyclosporine metabolism (see **PRECAUTIONS - Drug Interactions**).

Vaccination

During treatment with cyclosporine, vaccination may be less effective; and the use of live attenuated vaccines should be avoided.

Special Monitoring of Rheumatoid Arthritis Patients

Before initiating treatment, a careful physical examination, including blood pressure measurements (on at least two occasions) and two creatinine levels to estimate baseline should be performed. Blood pressure and serum creatinine should be evaluated every 2 weeks during the initial 3 months and then monthly if the patient is stable. It is advisable to monitor serum creatinine and blood pressure always after an increase of the dose of nonsteroidal anti-inflammatory drugs and after initiation of new nonsteroidal anti-inflammatory drug therapy during Gengraf® Capsules (cyclosporine capsules, USP [MODIFIED]) treatment. If co-administered with methotrexate, CBC and liver function tests are recommended to be monitored monthly (see also **PRECAUTIONS - General, Hypertension**).

In patients who are receiving cyclosporine, the dose of Gengraf® should be decreased by 25% to 50% if hypertension occurs. If hypertension persists, the dose of Gengraf® should be further reduced or blood pressure should be controlled with antihypertensive agents. In most cases, blood pressure has returned to baseline when cyclosporine was discontinued.

In placebo-controlled trials of rheumatoid arthritis patients, systolic hypertension (defined as an occurrence of two systolic blood pressure readings > 140 mmHg) and diastolic hypertension (defined as two diastolic blood pressure readings > 90 mmHg) occurred in 33% and 19% of patients treated with cyclosporine, respectively. The corresponding placebo rates were 22% and 8%.

Special Monitoring for Psoriasis Patients

Before initiating treatment, a careful dermatological and physical examination, including blood pressure measurements (on at least two occasions) should be performed. Since Gengraf® (cyclosporine capsules, USP [MODIFIED]) is an immunosuppressive agent, patients should be evaluated for the presence of occult infection on their first physical examination and for the presence of tumors initially, and throughout treatment with Gengraf®. Skin lesions not typical for psoriasis should be biopsied before starting Gengraf®. Patients with malignant or premalignant changes of the skin should be treated with Gengraf® only after appropriate treatment of such lesions and if no other treatment option exists.

Baseline laboratories should include serum creatinine (on two occasions), BUN, CBC, serum magnesium, potassium, uric acid, and lipids.

The risk of cyclosporine nephropathy is reduced when the starting dose is low (2.5 mg/kg/day), the maximum dose does not exceed 4 mg/kg/day, serum creatinine is monitored regularly while cyclosporine is administered, and the dose

Information on the AbbVie, Inc. products listed on these pages is from the prescribing information in use as of July 31, 2014. For more information, please visit rxabbvie.com or call 1-800-633-9110.

of Gengraf® is decreased when the rise in creatinine is greater than or equal to 25% above the patients pretreatment level. The increase in creatinine is generally reversible upon timely decrease of the dose of Gengraf® or its discontinuation.

Serum creatinine and BUN should be evaluated every 2 weeks during the initial 3 months of therapy and then monthly if the patient is stable. If the serum creatinine is greater than or equal to 25% above the patient's pretreatment level, serum creatinine should be repeated within two weeks. If the change in serum creatinine remains greater than or equal to 25% above baseline, Gengraf® should be reduced by 25% to 50%. If at **any time** the serum creatinine increases by greater than or equal to 50% above pretreatment level, Gengraf® should be reduced by 25% to 50%. Gengraf® should be discontinued if reversibility (within 25% of baseline) of serum creatinine is not achievable after two dosage modifications. It is advisable to monitor serum creatinine after an increase of the dose of nonsteroidal anti-inflammatory drug and after initiation of new nonsteroidal anti-inflammatory therapy during Gengraf® treatment.

Blood pressure should be evaluated every 2 weeks during the initial 3 months of therapy and then monthly if the patient is stable, or more frequently when dosage adjustments are made. Patients without a history of previous hypertension before initiation of treatment with Gengraf®, should have the drug reduced by 25% to 50% if found to have sustained hypertension. If the patient continues to be hypertensive despite multiple reductions of Gengraf®, then Gengraf® should be discontinued. For patients with treated hypertension, before the initiation of Gengraf® therapy, their medication should be adjusted to control hypertension while on Gengraf®. Gengraf® should be discontinued if a change in hypertension management is not effective or tolerable.

CBC, uric acid, potassium, lipids, and magnesium should also be monitored every 2 weeks for the first 3 months of therapy, and then monthly if the patient is stable or more frequently when dosage adjustments are made. Gengraf® dosage should be reduced by 25% to 50% for any abnormality of clinical concern.

In controlled trials of cyclosporine in psoriasis patients, cyclosporine blood concentrations did not correlate well with either improvement or with side effects such as renal dysfunction.

Information for Patients

Patients should be advised that any change of cyclosporine formulation should be made cautiously and only under physician supervision because it may result in the need for a change in dosage.

Patients should be informed of the necessity of repeated laboratory tests while they are receiving cyclosporine. Patients should be advised of the potential risks during pregnancy and informed of the increased risk of neoplasia. Patients should also be informed of the risk of hypertension and renal dysfunction.

Patients should be advised that during treatment with cyclosporine, vaccination may be less effective and the use of live attenuated vaccines should be avoided.

Patients should be advised to take Gengraf® on a consistent schedule with regard to time of day and relation to meals. Grapefruit and grapefruit juice affect metabolism, increasing blood concentration of cyclosporine, thus should be avoided.

Laboratory Tests

In all patients treated with cyclosporine, renal and liver functions should be assessed repeatedly by measurement of serum creatinine, BUN, serum bilirubin, and liver enzymes. Serum lipids, magnesium, and potassium should also be monitored. Cyclosporine blood concentrations should be routinely monitored in transplant patients (see **DOSAGE AND ADMINISTRATION - Blood Concentration Monitoring in Transplant Patients**), and periodically monitored in rheumatoid arthritis patients.

Drug Interactions

A. Effect of Drugs and Other Agents on Cyclosporine Pharmacokinetics and/or Safety

All of the individual drugs cited below are well substantiated to interact with cyclosporine. In addition, concomitant use of non-steroidal anti-inflammatory drugs with cyclosporine, particularly in the setting of dehydration, may potentiate renal dysfunction. Caution should be exercised when using other drugs which are known to impair renal function (see **WARNINGS - Nephrotoxicity**).

[See first table at top of previous page]

During the concomitant use of a drug that may exhibit additive or synergistic renal impairment with cyclosporine, close monitoring of renal function (in particular serum creatinine) should be performed. If a significant impairment of renal function occurs, the dosage of the coadministered drug should be reduced or an alternative treatment considered.

Cyclosporine is extensively metabolized by CYP 3A isoenzymes, in particular CYP3A4, and is a substrate of the multidrug efflux transporter P-glycoprotein. Various agents are known to either increase or decrease plasma or whole blood concentrations of cyclosporine usually by inhibition or induction of CYP3A4 or P-glycoprotein transporter or both. Compounds that decrease cyclosporine absorption such as orlistat should be avoided. Appropriate Gengraf® dosage adjustment to achieve the desired cyclosporine concentrations is essential when drugs that significantly alter cyclosporine concentrations are used concomitantly (see **DOSAGE AND ADMINISTRATION - Blood Concentration Monitoring**).

[See second table at top of previous page]

HIV protease inhibitors

The HIV protease inhibitors (e.g., indinavir, nelfinavir, ritonavir, and saquinavir) are known to inhibit cytochrome P-450 III-A and thus could potentially increase the concentrations of cyclosporine, however no formal studies of the interaction are available. Care should be exercised when these drugs are administered concomitantly.

Grapefruit Juice

Grapefruit and grapefruit juice affect metabolism, increasing blood concentrations of cyclosporine, thus should be avoided.

---

2. Drugs/Dietary Supplements That Decrease Cyclosporine Concentrations

Antibiotics	Anticonvulsants	Other Drugs/Dietary Supplements
nafcillin	carbamazepine	
rifampin	oxcarbazepine	
	phenobarbital	bosentan
	phenytoin	octreotide
		orlistat
		sulfinpyrazone
		St. John's Wort
		terbinafine
		ticlopidine

Bosentan

Coadministration of bosentan (250-1000 mg every 12 hours based on tolerability) and cyclosporine (300 mg every 12 hours for 2 days then dosing to achieve a C_{min} of 200-250 ng/mL) for 7 days in healthy subjects resulted in decreases in the cyclosporine mean dose-normalized AUC, C_{max}, and trough concentration of approximately 50%, 30%, and 60%, respectively, compared to when cyclosporine was given alone (see also *Effect of Cyclosporine on the Pharmacokinetics and/or Safety of Other Drugs or Agents*).

Boceprevir

Coadministration of boceprevir (800 mg three times daily for 7 days) and cyclosporine (100 mg single dose) in healthy subjects resulted in increases in the mean AUC and C_{max} of cyclosporine approximately 2.7-fold and 2-fold, respectively, compared to when cyclosporine was given alone.

Telaprevir

Coadministration of telaprevir (750 mg every 8 hours for 11 days) with cyclosporine (10 mg on day 8) in healthy subjects resulted in increases in the mean dose-normalized AUC and C_{max} of cyclosporine approximately 4.5-fold and 1.3-fold, respectively, compared to when cyclosporine (100 mg single dose) was given alone.

St. John's Wort

There have been reports of a serious drug interaction between cyclosporine and the herbal dietary supplement, St. John's Wort. This interaction has been reported to produce a marked reduction in the blood concentrations of cyclosporine, resulting in subtherapeutic levels, rejection of transplanted organs, and graft loss.

Rifabutin

Rifabutin is known to increase the metabolism of other drugs metabolized by the cytochrome P-450 system. The interaction between rifabutin and cyclosporine has not been studied. Care should be exercised when these two drugs are administered concomitantly.

B. Effect of Cyclosporine on the Pharmacokinetics and/or Safety of Other Drugs or Agents

Cyclosporine is an inhibitor of CYP3A4 and of the multidrug efflux transporter P-glycoprotein and may increase plasma concentrations of comedications that are substrates of CYP3A4 or P-glycoprotein or both.

Cyclosporine may reduce the clearance of digoxin, colchicine, prednisolone, and HMG-CoA reductase inhibitors (statins) and, aliskiren, repaglinide, NSAIDs, sirolimus, etoposide, and other drugs. See the full prescribing information of the other drug for further information and specific recommendations. The decision on co-administration of cyclosporine with other drugs or agents should be made by the physician following the careful assessment of benefits and risks.

Digoxin

Severe digitalis toxicity has been seen within days of starting cyclosporine in several patients taking digoxin. If digoxin is used concurrently with cyclosporine, serum digoxin concentrations should be monitored.

Colchicine

There are reports on the potential of cyclosporine to enhance the toxic effects of colchicine such as myopathy and neuropathy, especially in patients with renal dysfunction. Concomitant administration of cyclosporine and colchicine results in significant increases in colchicine plasma concentrations. If colchicine is used concurrently with cyclosporine, a reduction in the dosage of colchicine is recommended.

HMG-CoA reductase inhibitors (statins)

Literature and postmarketing cases of myotoxicity, including muscle pain and weakness, myositis, and rhabdomyolysis, have been reported with concomitant administration of cyclosporine with lovastatin, simvastatin, atorvastatin, pravastatin, and, rarely, fluvastatin. When concurrently administered with cyclosporine, the dosage of these statins should be reduced according to label recommendations. Statin therapy needs to be temporarily withheld or discontinued in patients with signs and symptoms of myopathy or those with risk factors predisposing to severe renal injury, including renal failure, secondary to rhabdomyolysis.

Repaglinide

Cyclosporine may increase the plasma concentrations of repaglinide and thereby increase the risk of hypoglycemia. In 12 healthy male subjects who received two doses of 100 mg cyclosporine capsule orally 12 hours apart with a single dose of 0.25 mg repaglinide tablet (one half of a 0.5 mg tablet) orally 13 hours after the cyclosporine initial dose, the repaglinide mean C_{max} and AUC were increased 1.8 fold (range: 0.6 to 3.7 fold) and 2.4 fold (range 1.2 to 5.3 fold), respectively. Close monitoring of blood glucose level is advisable for a patient taking cyclosporine and repaglinide concomitantly.

Ambrisentan

Coadministration of ambrisentan (5 mg daily) and cyclosporine (100-150 mg twice daily initially, then dosing to achieve C_{min} 150-200 ng/mL) for 8 days in healthy subjects resulted in mean increases in ambrisentan AUC and C_{max} of approximately 2-fold and 1.5-fold, respectively, compared to ambrisentan alone.

Anthracycline antibiotics

High doses of cyclosporine (e.g., at starting intravenous dose of 16 mg/kg/day) may increase the exposure to anthracycline antibiotics (e.g., doxorubicin, mitoxantrone, daunorubicin) in cancer patients.

Aliskiren

Cyclosporine alters the pharmacokinetics of aliskiren, a substrate of P-glycoprotein and CYP3A4. In 14 healthy subjects who received concomitantly single doses of cyclosporine (200 mg) and reduced dose aliskiren (75 mg), the mean C_{max} of aliskiren was increased by approximately 2.5 fold (90% CI: 1.96 to 3.17) and the mean AUC by approximately 4.3 fold (90% CI: 3.52 to 5.21), compared to when these subjects received aliskiren alone. The concomitant administration of aliskiren with cyclosporine prolonged the median aliskiren elimination half-life (26 hours versus 43 to 45 hours) and the T_{max} (0.5 hours versus 1.5 to 2.0 hours). The mean AUC and C_{max} of cyclosporine were comparable to reported literature values. Co-administration of cyclosporine and aliskiren in these subjects also resulted in an increase in the number and/or intensity of adverse events, mainly headache, hot flush, nausea, vomiting, and somnolence. The co-administration of cyclosporine with aliskiren is not recommended.

Bosentan

In healthy subjects, coadministration of bosentan and cyclosporine resulted in mean increases in dose-normalized bosentan trough concentrations on day 1 and day 8 of approximately 21-fold and 2-fold , respectively, compared to when bosentan was given alone as a single dose on day 1 (see also *Effect of Drugs and Other Agents on Cyclosporine Pharmacokinetics and/or Safety*).

Potassium-Sparing Diuretics

Cyclosporine should not be used with potassium sparing diuretics because hyperkalemia can occur. Caution is also required when cyclosporine is coadministered with potassium sparing drugs (e.g. angiotensin converting enzyme inhibitors, angiotensin II receptor antagonists), potassium containing drugs as well as in patients on a potassium rich diet. Control of potassium levels in these situations is advisable.

Nonsteroidal Anti-Inflammatory Drugs (NSAIDs)

Clinical status and serum creatinine should be closely monitored when cyclosporine is used with nonsteroidal anti-inflammatory agents in rheumatoid arthritis patients (see **WARNINGS**).

Pharmacodynamic interactions have been reported to occur between cyclosporine and both naproxen and sulindac, in that concomitant use is associated with additive decreases in renal function, as determined by ^{99m}Tc-diethylenetriaminepentaacetic acid (DTPA) and (*p*-aminohippuric acid) PAH clearances. Although concomitant administration of diclofenac does not affect blood concentrations of cyclosporine, it has been associated with approximate doubling of diclofenac blood concentrations and occa-

Body System / Adverse Reactions	Randomized Kidney Patients		Cyclosporine Patients (Sandimmune®)		
	Sandimmune® (N = 227) %	Azathioprine (N = 228) %	Kidney (N = 705) %	Heart (N = 112) %	Liver (N = 75) %
Genitourinary					
Renal Dysfunction	32	6	25	38	37
Cardiovascular					
Hypertension	26	18	13	53	27
Cramps	4	< 1	2	< 1	0
Skin					
Hirsutism	21	< 1	21	28	45
Acne	6	8	2	2	1
Central Nervous System					
Tremor	12	0	21	31	55
Convulsions	3	1	1	4	5
Headache	2	<1	2	15	4
Gastrointestinal					
Gum Hyperplasia	4	0	9	5	16
Diarrhea	3	< 1	3	4	8
Nausea/Vomiting	2	< 1	4	10	4
Hepatotoxicity	< 1	< 1	4	7	4
Abdominal Discomfort	< 1	0	<1	7	0
Autonomic Nervous System					
Paresthesia	3	0	1	2	1
Flushing	< 1	0	4	1	4
Hematopoietic					
Leukopenia	2	19	< 1	6	0
Lymphoma	< 1	0	1	6	1
Respiratory					
Sinusitis	< 1	0	4	3	7
Miscellaneous					
Gynecomastia	< 1	0	< 1	4	3

sional reports of reversible decreases in renal function. Consequently, the dose of diclofenac should be in the lower end of the therapeutic range.

Methotrexate Interaction

Preliminary data indicate that when methotrexate and cyclosporine were co-administered to rheumatoid arthritis patients (N=20), methotrexate concentrations (AUCs) were increased approximately 30% and the concentrations (AUCs) of its metabolite, 7-hydroxy methotrexate, were decreased by approximately 80%. The clinical significance of this interaction is not known. Cyclosporine concentrations do not appear to have been altered (N=6).

Sirolimus

Elevations in serum creatinine were observed in studies using sirolimus in combination with full-dose cyclosporine. This effect is often reversible with cyclosporine dose reduction. Simultaneous coadministration of cyclosporine significantly increases blood levels of sirolimus. To minimize increases in sirolimus blood concentrations, it is recommended that sirolimus be given 4 hours after cyclosporine administration.

Nifedipine

Frequent gingival hyperplasia when nifedipine is given concurrently with cyclosporine have been reported. The concomitant use of nifedipine should be avoided in patients in whom gingival hyperplasia develops as a side effect of cyclosporine.

Methyprednisolone

Convulsions when high dose methylprednisolone is given concomitantly with cyclosporine have been reported.

Other Immunosuppressive Drugs and Agents

Psoriasis patients receiving other immunosuppressive agents or radiation therapy (including PUVA and UVB) should not receive concurrent cyclosporine because of the possibility of excessive immunosuppression.

C. Effect of Cyclosporine on the Efficacy of Live Vaccines

During treatment with cyclosporine, vaccination may be less effective. The use of live vaccines should be avoided. For additional information on Cyclosporine Drug Interactions please contact AbbVie Inc. Medical Information Department at 1-800-633-9110.

Carcinogenesis, Mutagenesis, and Impairment of Fertility

Carcinogenicity studies were carried out in male and female rats and mice. In the 78-week mouse study, evidence of a statistically significant trend was found for lymphocytic lymphomas in females, and the incidence of hepatocellular carcinomas in mid-dose males significantly exceeded the control value. In the 24-month rat study, pancreatic islet cell adenomas significantly exceeded the control rate in the low dose level. Doses used in the mouse and rat studies were 0.01 to 0.16 times the clinical maintenance dose (6 mg/kg). The hepatocellular carcinomas and pancreatic islet cell adenomas were not dose related. Published reports indicate the co-treatment of hairless mice with UV irradia-

tion and cyclosporine or other immunosuppressive agents shorten the time to skin tumor formation compared to UV irradiation alone.

Cyclosporine was not mutagenic in appropriate test systems. Cyclosporine has not been found to be mutagenic/genotoxic in the Ames Test, the V79-HGPRT Test, the micronucleus test in mice and Chinese hamsters, the chromosome-aberration tests in Chinese hamster bone-marrow, the mouse dominant lethal assay, and the DNA-repair test in sperm from treated mice. A recent study analyzing sister chromatid exchange (SCE) induction by cyclosporine using human lymphocytes *in vitro* gave indication of a positive effect (i.e., induction of SCE), at high concentrations in this system. In two published research studies, rabbits exposed to cyclosporine *in utero* (10 mg/kg/day subcutaneously) demonstrated reduced numbers of nephrons, renal hypertrophy, systemic hypertension and progressive renal insufficiency up to 35 weeks of age. Pregnant rats which received 12 mg/kg/day of cyclosporine intravenously (twice the recommended human intravenous dose) had fetuses with an increased incidence of ventricular septal defect. These findings have not been demonstrated in other species and their relevance for humans is unknown. No impairment in fertility was demonstrated in studies in male and female rats.

Widely distributed papillomatosis of the skin was observed after chronic treatment of dogs with cyclosporine at 9 times the human initial psoriasis treatment dose of 2.5 mg/kg, where doses are expressed on a body surface area basis. This papillomatosis showed a spontaneous regression upon discontinuation of cyclosporine.

An increased incidence of malignancy is a recognized complication of immunosuppression in recipients of organ transplants and patients with rheumatoid arthritis and psoriasis. The most common forms of neoplasms are non-Hodgkin's lymphoma and carcinomas of the skin. The risk of malignancies in cyclosporine recipients is higher than in the normal, healthy population but similar to that in patients receiving other immunosuppressive therapies. Reduction or discontinuance of immunosuppression may cause the lesions to regress.

In psoriasis patients on cyclosporine, development of malignancies, especially those of the skin has been reported (see **WARNINGS**). Skin lesions not typical for psoriasis should be biopsied before starting cyclosporine treatment. Patients with malignant or premalignant changes of the skin should be treated with cyclosporine only after appropriate treatment of such lesions and if no other treatment option exists.

Pregnancy

Pregnancy Category C

Animal studies have shown reproductive toxicity in rats and rabbits. Cyclosporine gave no evidence of mutagenic or teratogenic effects in the standard test systems with oral application (rats up to 17 mg/kg and rabbits up to 30 mg/kg per day orally). Only at dose levels toxic to dams, were ad-

verse effects seen in reproduction studies in rats. Cyclosporine has been shown to be embryo- and fetotoxic in rats and rabbits following oral administration at maternally toxic doses. Fetal toxicity was noted in rats at 0.8 and rabbits at 5.4 times the transplant doses in humans of 6 mg/kg, where dose corrections are based on body surface area. Cyclosporine was embryo- and fetotoxic as indicated by increased pre- and postnatal mortality and reduced fetal weight together with related skeletal retardation.

There are no adequate and well-controlled studies in pregnant women and, therefore, Gengraf® Capsules (cyclosporine capsules, USP [MODIFIED]) should not be used during pregnancy unless the potential benefit to the mother justifies the potential risk to the fetus.

In pregnant transplant recipients who are being treated with immunosuppressants the risk of premature births is increased. The following data represent the reported outcomes of 116 pregnancies in women receiving cyclosporine during pregnancy, 90% of whom were transplant patients, and most of whom received cyclosporine throughout the entire gestational period. The only consistent patterns of abnormality were premature birth (gestational period of 28 to 36 weeks) and low birth weight for gestational age. Sixteen fetal losses occurred. Most of the pregnancies (85 of 100) were complicated by disorders; including, pre-eclampsia, eclampsia, premature labor, abruptio placentae, oligohydramnios, Rh incompatibility and fetoplacental dysfunction. Pre-term delivery occurred in 47%. Seven malformations were reported in 5 viable infants and in 2 cases of fetal loss. Twenty-eight percent of the infants were small for gestational age. Neonatal complications occurred in 27%. Therefore, the risks and benefits of using Gengraf® during pregnancy should be carefully weighed.

A limited number of observations in children exposed to cyclosporine *in utero* is available, up to an age of approximately 7 years. Renal function and blood pressure in these children were normal.

Because of the possible disruption of maternal-fetal interaction, the risk/benefit ratio of using Gengraf® in psoriasis patients during pregnancy should carefully be weighed with serious consideration for discontinuation of Gengraf®.

The alcohol content of the Gengraf® formulations should also be taken into account in pregnant women (see **WARNINGS - Special Excipients**).

Nursing Mothers

Cyclosporine is present in breast milk. Because of the potential for serious adverse drug reactions in nursing infants from Gengraf®, a decision should be made whether to discontinue nursing or to discontinue the drug, taking into account the importance of the drug to the mother. Gengraf® contains ethanol. Ethanol will be present in human milk at levels similar to that found in maternal serum and if present in breast milk will be orally absorbed by a nursing infant (see **WARNINGS**).

Pediatric Use

Although no adequate and well-controlled studies have been completed in children, transplant recipients as young as one year of age have received cyclosporine (MODIFIED) with no unusual adverse effects. The safety and efficacy of cyclosporine (MODIFIED) treatment in children with juvenile rheumatoid arthritis or psoriasis below the age of 18 have not been established.

Geriatric Use

In rheumatoid arthritis clinical trials with cyclosporine, 17.5% of patients were age 65 or older. These patients were more likely to develop systolic hypertension on therapy, and more likely to show serum creatinine rises ≥ 50% above the baseline after 3 to 4 months of therapy.

Clinical studies of cyclosporine oral solution (modified) in transplant and psoriasis patients did not include a sufficient number of subjects aged 65 and over to determine whether they respond differently from younger subjects. Other reported clinical experiences have not identified differences in response between the elderly and younger patients. In general, dose selection for an elderly patient should be cautious, usually starting at the low end of the dosing range, reflecting the greater frequency of decreased hepatic, renal, or cardiac function, and of concomitant disease or other drug therapy.

ADVERSE REACTIONS

Kidney, Liver, and Heart Transplantation

The principal adverse reactions of cyclosporine therapy are renal dysfunction, tremor, hirsutism, hypertension, and gum hyperplasia.

Hypertension

Hypertension, which is usually mild to moderate, may occur in approximately 50% of patients following renal transplantation and in most cardiac transplant patients.

Information on the AbbVie, Inc. products listed on these pages is from the prescribing information in use as of July 31, 2014. For more information, please visit rxabbvie.com or call 1-800-633-9110.

Cyclosporine (MODIFIED)/Sandimmune® Rheumatoid Arthritis Percentage of Patients with Adverse Events ≥ 3% in any Cyclosporine Treated Group

Body System	Preferred Term	Studies 651+652+2008 Sandimmune®† (N = 269)	Study 302 Sandimmune® (N = 155)	Study 654 Methotrexate & Sandimmune® (N = 74)	Study 654 Methotrexate & Placebo (N = 73)	Study 302 Cyclosporine (MODIFIED) (N = 143)	Studies 651+652 +2008 Placebo (N = 201)
Autonomic Nervous System Disorders							
	Flushing	2%	2%	3%	0%	5%	2%
Body As A Whole - General Disorders							
	Accidental Trauma	0%	1%	10%	4%	4%	0%
	Edema NOS*	5%	14%	12%	4%	10%	< 1%
	Fatigue	6%	3%	8%	12%	3%	7%
	Fever	2%	3%	0%	0%	2%	4%
	Influenza-like symptoms	< 1%	6%	1%	0%	3%	2%
	Pain	6%	9%	10%	15%	13%	4%
	Rigors	1%	1%	4%	0%	3%	1%
Cardiovascular Disorders							
	Arrhythmia	2%	5%	5%	6%	2%	1%
	Chest Pain	4%	5%	1%	1%	6%	1%
	Hypertension	8%	26%	16%	12%	25%	2%
Central and Peripheral Nervous System Disorders							
	Dizziness	8%	6%	7%	3%	8%	3%
	Headache	17%	23%	22%	11%	25%	9%
	Migraine	2%	3%	0%	0%	3%	1%
	Paresthesia	8%	7%	8%	4%	11%	1%
	Tremor	8%	7%	7%	3%	13%	4%
Gastrointestinal System Disorders							
	Abdominal Pain	15%	15%	15%	7%	15%	10%
	Anorexia	3%	3%	1%	0%	3%	3%
	Diarrhea	12%	12%	18%	15%	13%	8%
	Dyspepsia	12%	12%	10%	8%	8%	4%
	Flatulence	5%	5%	5%	4%	4%	1%
	Gastrointestinal Disorder NOS*	0%	2%	1%	4%	4%	0%
	Gingivitis	4%	3%	0%	0%	0%	1%
	Gum Hyperplasia	2%	4%	1%	3%	4%	1%
	Nausea	23%	14%	24%	15%	18%	14%
	Rectal Hemorrhage	0%	3%	0%	0%	1%	1%
	Stomatitis	7%	5%	16%	12%	6%	8%
	Vomiting	9%	8%	14%	7%	6%	5%
Hearing and Vestibular Disorders							
	Ear Disorders NOS*	0%	5%	0%	0%	1%	0%
Metabolic and Nutritional Disorders							
	Hypomagnesemia	0%	4%	0%	0%	6%	0%
Musculoskeletal System Disorders							
	Arthropathy	0%	5%	0%	1%	4%	0%
	Leg Cramps/ Involuntary Muscle Contractions	2%	11%	11%	3%	12%	1%
Psychiatric Disorders							
	Depression	3%	6%	3%	1%	1%	2%
	Insomnia	4%	1%	1%	0%	3%	2%
Renal							
	Creatinine elevations ≥ 30%	43%	39%	55%	19%	48%	13%
	Creatinine elevations ≥ 50%	24%	18%	26%	8%	18%	3%
Reproductive Disorders, Female							
	Leukorrhea	1%	0%	4%	0%	1%	0%
	Menstrual Disorder	3%	2%	1%	0%	1%	1%
Respiratory System Disorders							
	Bronchitis	1%	3%	1%	0%	1%	3%
	Coughing	5%	3%	5%	7%	4%	4%
	Dyspnea	5%	1%	3%	3%	1%	2%
	Infection NOS*	9%	5%	0%	7%	3%	10%
	Pharyngitis	3%	5%	5%	6%	4%	4%
	Pneumonia	1%	0%	4%	0%	1%	1%
	Rhinitis	0%	3%	11%	10%	1%	0%
	Sinusitis	4%	4%	8%	4%	3%	3%
	Upper Respiratory Tract	0%	14%	23%	15%	13%	0%
Skin and Appendages Disorders							
	Alopecia	3%	0%	1%	1%	4%	4%
	Bullous Eruption	1%	0%	4%	1%	1%	1%
	Hypertrichosis	19%	17%	12%	0%	15%	3%
	Rash	7%	12%	10%	7%	8%	10%
	Skin Ulceration	1%	1%	3%	4%	0%	2%
Urinary System Disorders							
	Dysuria	0%	0%	11%	3%	1%	2%
	Micturition Frequency	2%	4%	3%	1%	2%	2%
	NPN, Increased	0%	19%	12%	0%	18%	0%
	Urinary Tract Infection	0%	3%	5%	4%	3%	0%
Vascular (Extracardiac) Disorders							
	Purpura	3%	4%	1%	1%	2%	0%

† Includes patients in 2.5 mg/kg/day dose group only.
* NOS = Not Otherwise Specified.

Glomerular Capillary Thrombosis

Glomerular capillary thrombosis has been found in patients treated with cyclosporine and may progress to graft failure. The pathologic changes resembled those seen in the hemolytic-uremic syndrome and include thrombosis of the renal microvasculature, with platelet-fibrin thrombi occluding glomerular capillaries and afferent arterioles, microangiopathic hemolytic anemia, thrombocytopenia, and decreased renal function. Similar findings have been observed when other immunosuppressives have been employed post-transplantation.

Hypomagnesemia

Hypomagnesemia has been reported in some, but not all, patients exhibiting convulsions while on cyclosporine therapy. Although magnesium-depletion studies in normal subjects suggest that hypomagnesemia is associated with neurologic disorders, multiple factors, including hypertension, high dose methylprednisolone, hypocholesterolemia, and nephrotoxicity associated with high plasma concentrations of cyclosporine appear to be related to the neurological manifestations of cyclosporine toxicity.

Clinical Studies

In controlled studies, the nature, severity and incidence of the adverse events that were observed in 493 transplanted patients treated with cyclosporine (MODIFIED) were comparable with those observed in 208 transplanted patients who received Sandimmune® Soft Gelatin Capsules (cyclosporine capsules, USP) in these same studies when the dosage of the two drugs was adjusted to achieve the same cyclosporine blood trough concentrations.

Based on the historical experience with Sandimmune®, the following reactions occurred in 3% or greater of 892 patients involved in clinical trials of kidney, heart, and liver transplants.

[See table at top of page 451]

Among 705 kidney transplant patients treated with cyclosporine oral solution (Sandimmune®) in clinical trials, the reason for treatment discontinuation was renal toxicity in 5.4%, infection in 0.9%, lack of efficacy in 1.4%, acute tubular necrosis in 1.0%, lymphoproliferative disorders in 0.3%, hypertension in 0.3%, and other reasons in 0.7% of the patients.

The following reactions occurred in 2% or less of cyclosporine-treated patients: allergic reactions, anemia, anorexia, confusion, conjunctivitis, edema, fever, brittle fingernails, gastritis, hearing loss, hiccups, hyperglycemia, migraine (Gengraf®), muscle pain, peptic ulcer, thrombocytopenia, tinnitus.

The following reactions occurred rarely: anxiety, chest pain, constipation, depression, hair breaking, hematuria, joint pain, lethargy, mouth sores, myocardial infarction, night sweats, pancreatitis, pruritus, swallowing difficulty, tingling, upper GI bleeding, visual disturbance, weakness, weight loss.

Patients receiving immunosuppressive therapies, including cyclosporine and cyclosporine-containing regimens, are at increased risk of infections (viral, bacterial, fungal, parasitic). Both generalized and localized infections can occur. Pre-existing infections may also be aggravated. Fatal outcomes have been reported (see **WARNINGS**).

Infectious Complications in Historical Randomized Studies in Renal Transplant Patients Using Sandimmune®

Complication	Cyclosporine Treatment (N = 227) % of Complications	Azathioprine with Steroids* (N = 228) % of Complications
Septicemia	5.3	4.8
Abscesses	4.4	5.3
Systemic Fungal Infection	2.2	3.9
Local Fungal Infection	7.5	9.6
Cytomegalovirus	4.8	12.3
Other Viral Infections	15.9	18.4
Urinary Tract Infections	21.1	20.2
Wound and Skin Infections	7.0	10.1
Pneumonia	6.2	9.2

* Some patients also received ALG.

Postmarketing Experience, Kidney, Liver and Heart Transplantation

Hepatotoxicity

Cases of hepatotoxicity and liver injury including cholestasis, jaundice, hepatitis and liver failure; serious and/or fatal outcomes have been reported. [See **WARNINGS, Hepatotoxicity**]

Adverse Events Occurring in 3% or More of Psoriasis Patients in Controlled Clinical Trials

Body System*	Preferred Term	Cyclosporine (MODIFIED) (N = 182)	Sandimmune® (N = 185)
Infection or Potential Infection		24.7%	24.3%
	Influenza-like Symptoms	9.9%	8.1%
	Upper Respiratory Tract Infections	7.7%	11.3%
Cardiovascular System		28.0%	25.4%
	Hypertension**	27.5%	25.4%
Urinary System		24.2%	16.2%
	Increased Creatinine	19.8%	15.7%
Central and Peripheral Nervous System		26.4%	20.5%
	Headache	15.9%	14.0%
	Paresthesia	7.1%	4.8%
Musculoskeletal System		13.2%	8.7%
	Arthralgia	6.0%	1.1%
Body As a Whole – General		29.1%	22.2%
	Pain	4.4%	3.2%
Metabolic and Nutritional		9.3%	9.7%
Reproductive, Female		8.5% (4 of 47 females)	11.5% (6 of 52 females)
Resistance Mechanism		18.7%	21.1%
Skin and Appendages		17.6%	15.1%
	Hypertrichosis	6.6%	5.4%
Respiratory System		5.0%	6.5%
	Bronchospasm, Coughing, Dyspnea, Rhinitis	5.0%	4.9%
Psychiatric		5.0%	3.8%
Gastrointestinal System		19.8%	28.7%
	Abdominal Pain	2.7%	6.0%
	Diarrhea	5.0%	5.9%
	Dyspepsia	2.2%	3.2%
	Gum Hyperplasia	3.8%	6.0%
	Nausea	5.5%	5.9%
White cell and RES		4.4%	2.7%

* Total percentage of events within the system.
** Newly occurring hypertension = SBP ≥160 mm Hg and/or DBP ≥90 mm Hg.

Increased Risk of Infections

Cases of JC virus-associated progressive multifocal leukoencephalopathy (PML), sometimes fatal; and polyoma virus-associated nephropathy (PVAN), especially BK virus resulting in graft loss have been reported. [See **WARNINGS, Polyoma Virus Infection**]

Headache, including Migraine

Cases of migraine have been reported. In some cases, patients have been unable to continue cyclosporine, however the final decision on treatment discontinuation should be made by the treating physician following the careful assessment of benefits versus risks.

Rheumatoid Arthritis

The principal adverse reactions associated with the use of cyclosporine in rheumatoid arthritis are renal dysfunction (see **WARNINGS**), hypertension (see **PRECAUTIONS**), headache, gastrointestinal disturbances and hirsutism/hypertrichosis.

In rheumatoid arthritis patients treated in clinical trials within the recommended dose range, cyclosporine therapy was discontinued in 5.3% of the patients because of hypertension and in 7% of the patients because of increased creatinine. These changes are usually reversible with timely dose decrease or drug discontinuation. The frequency and severity of serum creatinine elevations increase with dose and duration of cyclosporine therapy. These elevations are likely to become more pronounced without dose reduction or discontinuation.

The following adverse events occurred in controlled clinical trials

[See table on previous page]

In addition, the following adverse events have been reported in 1% to < 3% of the rheumatoid arthritis patients in the cyclosporine treatment group in controlled clinical trials.

Autonomic Nervous System
dry mouth, increased sweating
Body as a Whole
allergy, asthenia, hot flushes, malaise, overdose, procedure NOS*, tumor NOS*, weight decrease, weight increase
Cardiovascular
abnormal heart sounds, cardiac failure, myocardial infarction, peripheral ischemia
Central and Peripheral Nervous System
hypoesthesia, neuropathy, vertigo
Endocrine
goiter
Gastrointestinal
constipation, dysphagia, enanthema, eructation, esophagitis, gastric ulcer, gastritis, gastroenteritis, gingival bleeding, glossitis, peptic ulcer, salivary gland enlargement, tongue disorder, tooth disorder
Infection
abscess, bacterial infection, cellulitis, folliculitis, fungal infection, herpes simplex, herpes zoster, renal abscess, moniliasis, tonsillitis, viral infection
Hematologic
anemia, epistaxis, leukopenia, lymphadenopathy
Liver and Biliary System
bilirubinemia
Metabolic and Nutritional
diabetes mellitus, hyperkalemia, hyperuricemia, hypoglycemia
Musculoskeletal System
arthralgia, bone fracture, bursitis, joint dislocation, myalgia, stiffness, synovial cyst, tendon disorder
Neoplasms
breast fibroadenosis, carcinoma
Psychiatric
anxiety, confusion, decreased libido, emotional lability, impaired concentration, increased libido, nervousness, paroniria, somnolence
Reproductive (Female)
breast pain, uterine hemorrhage
Respiratory System
abnormal chest sounds, bronchospasm
Skin and Appendages
abnormal pigmentation, angioedema, dermatitis, dry skin, eczema, nail disorder, pruritus, skin disorder, urticaria
Special Senses
abnormal vision, cataract, conjunctivitis, deafness, eye pain, taste perversion, tinnitus, vestibular disorder
Urinary System
abnormal urine, hematuria, increased BUN, micturition urgency, nocturia, polyuria, pyelonephritis, urinary incontinence

* NOS = Not Otherwise Specified.

Information on the AbbVie, Inc. products listed on these pages is from the prescribing information in use as of July 31, 2014. For more information, please visit rxabbvie.com or call 1-800-633-9110.

Psoriasis

The principal adverse reactions associated with the use of cyclosporine in patients with psoriasis are renal dysfunction, headache, hypertension, hypertriglyceridemia, hirsutism/hypertrichosis, paresthesia or hyperesthesia, influenza-like symptoms, nausea/vomiting, diarrhea, abdominal discomfort, lethargy, and musculoskeletal or joint pain.

In psoriasis patients treated in U.S. controlled clinical studies within the recommended dose range, cyclosporine therapy was discontinued in 1.0% of the patients because of hypertension and in 5.4% of the patients because of increased creatinine. In the majority of cases, these changes were reversible after dose reduction or discontinuation of cyclosporine.

There has been one reported death associated with the use of cyclosporine in psoriasis. A 27 year old male developed renal deterioration and was continued on cyclosporine. He had progressive renal failure leading to death.

Frequency and severity of serum creatinine increases with dose and duration of cyclosporine therapy. These elevations are likely to become more pronounced and may result in irreversible renal damage without dose reduction or discontinuation.

[See table at top of previous page]

The following events occurred in 1% to less than 3% of psoriasis patients treated with cyclosporine:

Body as a Whole
fever, flushes, hot flushes
Cardiovascular
chest pain
Central and Peripheral Nervous System
appetite increased, insomnia, dizziness, nervousness, vertigo
Gastrointestinal
abdominal distention, constipation, gingival bleeding
Liver and Biliary System
hyperbilirubinemia
Neoplasms
skin malignancies [squamous cell (0.9%) and basal cell (0.4%) carcinomas]
Reticuloendothelial
platelet, bleeding, and clotting disorders, red blood cell disorder
Respiratory
infection, viral and other infection
Skin and Appendages
acne, folliculitis, keratosis, pruritus, rash, dry skin
Urinary System
micturition frequency
Vision
abnormal vision.

Mild hypomagnesemia and hyperkalemia may occur but are asymptomatic. Increases in uric acid may occur and attacks of gout have been rarely reported. A minor and dose related hyperbilirubinemia has been observed in the absence of hepatocellular damage. Cyclosporine therapy may be associated with a modest increase of serum triglycerides or cholesterol. Elevations of triglycerides (> 750 mg/dL) occur in about 15% of psoriasis patients; elevations of cholesterol (> 300 mg/dL) are observed in less than 3% of psoriasis patients. Generally these laboratory abnormalities are reversible upon dose reduction or discontinuation of cyclosporine.

Postmarketing Experience, Psoriasis

Cases of transformation to erythrodermic psoriasis or generalized pustular psoriasis upon either withdrawal or reduction of cyclosporine in patients with chronic plaque psoriasis have been reported.

OVERDOSAGE

There is a minimal experience with cyclosporine overdosage. Forced emesis and gastric lavage can be of value up to 2 hours after administration of Gengraf® Capsules (cyclosporine capsules, USP [MODIFIED]). Transient hepatotoxicity and nephrotoxicity may occur which should resolve following drug withdrawal. Oral doses of cyclosporine up to 10 g (about 150 mg/kg) have been tolerated with relatively minor clinical consequences, such as vomiting, drowsiness, headache, tachycardia and, in a few patients, moderately severe, reversible impairment of renal function. However, serious symptoms of intoxication have been reported following accidental parenteral overdosage with cyclosporine in premature neonates. General supportive measures and symptomatic treatment should be followed in all cases of overdosage. Cyclosporine is not dialyzable to any great extent, nor is it cleared well by charcoal hemoperfusion. The oral dosage at which half of experimental animals are estimated to die is 31 times, 39 times and > 54 times the human maintenance dose for transplant patients (6 mg/kg; corrections based on body surface area) in mice, rats, and rabbits.

DOSAGE AND ADMINISTRATION

Gengraf® Capsules (cyclosporine capsules, USP [MODIFIED]) has increased bioavailability in comparison to Sandimmune® Soft Gelatin Capsules (cyclosporine capsules, USP). Gengraf® and Sandimmune® are not bioequivalent and cannot be used interchangeably without physician supervision.

The daily dose of Gengraf® Capsules (cyclosporine capsules, USP [MODIFIED]) should always be given in two divided doses (BID). It is recommended that Gengraf® be administered on a consistent schedule with regard to time of day and relation to meals. Grapefruit and grapefruit juice affect metabolism, increasing blood concentration of cyclosporine, thus should be avoided.

Specific Populations

Renal Impairment in Kidney, Liver, and Heart Transplantation

Cyclosporine undergoes minimal renal elimination and its pharmacokinetics do not appear to be significantly altered in patients with end-stage renal disease who receive routine hemodialysis treatments (see CLINICAL PHARMACOLOGY). However, due to its nephrotoxic potential (see WARNINGS), careful monitoring of renal function is recommended; cyclosporine dosage should be reduced if indicated (see WARNINGS and PRECAUTIONS).

Renal Impairment in Rheumatoid Arthritis and Psoriasis

Patients with impaired renal function should not receive cyclosporine (see CONTRAINDICATIONS, WARNINGS and PRECAUTIONS).

Hepatic Impairment

The clearance of cyclosporine may be significantly reduced in severe liver disease patients (see CLINICAL PHARMACOLOGY). Dose reduction may be necessary in patients with severe liver impairment to maintain blood concentrations within the recommended target range (see WARNINGS and PRECAUTIONS).

Newly Transplanted Patients

The initial oral dose of Gengraf® Capsules (cyclosporine capsules, USP [MODIFIED]) can be given 4 to 12 hours prior to transplantation or be given postoperatively. The initial dose of Gengraf® varies depending on the transplanted organ and the other immunosuppressive agents included in the immunosuppressive protocol. In newly transplanted patients, the initial oral dose of Gengraf® is the same as the initial oral dose of Sandimmune®. Suggested initial doses are available from the results of a 1994 survey of the use of Sandimmune® in U.S. transplant centers. The mean ± SD initial doses were 9 ± 3 mg/kg/day for renal transplant patients (75 centers), 8 ± 4 mg/kg/day for liver transplant patients (30 centers), and 7 ± 3 mg/kg/day for heart transplant patients (24 centers). Total daily doses were divided into two equal daily doses. The Gengraf® dose is subsequently adjusted to achieve a pre-defined cyclosporine blood concentration (see DOSAGE AND ADMINISTRATION - Blood Concentration Monitoring in Transplant Patients, below). If cyclosporine trough blood concentrations are used, the target range is the same for Gengraf® as for Sandimmune®. Using the same trough concentration target range for Gengraf® as for Sandimmune® results in greater cyclosporine exposure when Gengraf® is administered (see CLINICAL PHARMACOLOGY - Pharmacokinetics, Absorption). Dosing should be titrated based on clinical assessments of rejection and tolerability. Lower Gengraf® doses may be sufficient as maintenance therapy.

Adjunct therapy with adrenal corticosteroids is recommended initially. Different tapering dosage schedules of prednisone appear to achieve similar results. A representative dosage schedule based on the patient's weight started with 2 mg/kg/day for the first 4 days tapered to 1 mg/kg/day by 1 week, 0.6 mg/kg/day by 2 weeks, 0.3 mg/kg/day by 1 month, and 0.15 mg/kg/day by 2 months and thereafter as a maintenance dose. Steroid doses may be further tapered on an individualized basis depending on status of patient and function of graft. Adjustments in dosage of prednisone must be made according to the clinical situation.

Conversion from Sandimmune® (Cyclosporine) to Gengraf® Capsules (Cyclosporine Capsules, USP [MODIFIED]) in Transplant Patients

In transplanted patients who are considered for conversion to Gengraf® from Sandimmune® (cyclosporine), Gengraf® should be started with the same daily dose as was previously used with Sandimmune® (cyclosporine) (1:1 dose conversion). The Gengraf® dose should subsequently be adjusted to attain the pre-conversion cyclosporine blood trough concentration. Using the same trough concentration target range for Gengraf® as for Sandimmune® (cyclosporine) results in greater cyclosporine exposure when Gengraf® is administered (see CLINICAL PHARMACOLOGY - Pharmacokinetics, Absorption). Patients with suspected poor absorption of Sandimmune® (cyclosporine) require different dosing strategies (see DOSAGE AND ADMINISTRATION - Transplant Patients with Poor Absorption of Sandimmune® (cyclosporine), below). In some patients, the increase in blood trough concentration is more pronounced and may be of clinical significance.

Until the blood trough concentration attains the pre-conversion value, it is strongly recommended that the cyclosporine blood trough concentration be monitored every 4 to 7 days after conversion to Gengraf®. In addition, clinical safety parameters such as serum creatinine and blood pressure should be monitored every two weeks during the first two months after conversion. If the blood trough concentrations are outside the desired range and/or if the clinical safety parameters worsen, the dosage of Gengraf® must be adjusted accordingly.

Transplant Patients with Poor Absorption of Sandimmune® (Cyclosporine)

Patients with lower than expected cyclosporine blood trough concentrations in relation to the oral dose of Sandimmune® (cyclosporine) may have poor or inconsistent absorption of cyclosporine from Sandimmune® (cyclosporine). After conversion to Gengraf® Capsules (cyclosporine capsules, USP [MODIFIED]), patients tend to have higher cyclosporine concentrations. Due to the increase in bioavailability of cyclosporine following conversion to Gengraf®, the cyclosporine blood trough concentration may exceed the target range. Particular caution should be exercised when converting patients to Gengraf® at doses greater than 10 mg/kg/day. The dose of Gengraf® should be titrated individually based on cyclosporine trough concentrations, tolerability, and clinical response. In this population the cyclosporine blood trough concentration should be measured more frequently, at least twice a week (daily, if initial dose exceeds 10 mg/kg/day) until the concentration stabilizes within the desired range.

Rheumatoid Arthritis

The initial dose of Gengraf® Capsules (cyclosporine capsules, USP [MODIFIED]) is 2.5 mg/kg/day, taken twice daily as a divided (BID) oral dose. Salicylates, nonsteroidal anti-inflammatory agents, and oral corticosteroids may be continued (see WARNINGS and PRECAUTIONS - Drug Interactions). Onset of action generally occurs between 4 and 8 weeks. If insufficient clinical benefit is seen and tolerability is good (including serum creatinine less than 30% above baseline), the dose may be increased by 0.5 to 0.75 mg/kg/day after 8 weeks and again after 12 weeks to a maximum of 4 mg/kg/day. If no benefit is seen by 16 weeks of therapy, Gengraf® therapy should be discontinued.

Dose decreases by 25% to 50% should be made at any time to control adverse events, e.g., hypertension elevations in serum creatinine (30% above patient's pretreatment level) or clinically significant laboratory abnormalities (see WARNINGS and PRECAUTIONS).

If dose reduction is not effective in controlling abnormalities or if the adverse event or abnormality is severe, Gengraf® should be discontinued. The same initial dose and dosage range should be used if Gengraf® is combined with the recommended dose of methotrexate. Most patients can be treated with Gengraf® doses of 3 mg/kg/day or below when combined with methotrexate doses of up to 15 mg/week (see CLINICAL PHARMACOLOGY - Clinical Trials).

There is limited long-term treatment data. Recurrence of rheumatoid arthritis disease activity is generally apparent within four weeks after stopping cyclosporine.

Psoriasis

The initial dose of Gengraf® Capsules (cyclosporine capsules, USP [MODIFIED]) should be 2.5 mg/kg/day. Gengraf® should be taken twice daily, as a divided (1.25 mg/kg BID) oral dose. Patients should be kept at that dose for at least 4 weeks, barring adverse events. If significant clinical improvement has not occurred in patients by that time, the patient's dosage should be increased at 2 week intervals. Based on patient response, dose increases of approximately 0.5 mg/kg/day should be made to a maximum of 4 mg/kg/day.

Dose decreases by 25% to 50% should be made at any time to control adverse events, e.g., hypertension, elevations in serum creatinine (≥ 25% above the patient's pretreatment level), or clinically significant laboratory abnormalities.

If dose reduction is not effective in controlling abnormalities, or if the adverse event or abnormality is severe, Gengraf® should be discontinued (see PRECAUTIONS - Special Monitoring of Psoriasis Patients).

Patients generally show some improvement in the clinical manifestations of psoriasis in 2 weeks. Satisfactory control and stabilization of the disease may take 12 to 16 weeks to achieve. Results of a dose-titration clinical trial with Gengraf® indicate that an improvement of psoriasis by 75% or more (based on PASI) was achieved in 51% of the patients after 8 weeks and in 79% of the patients after 16 weeks. Treatment should be discontinued if satisfactory response cannot be achieved after 6 weeks at 4 mg/kg/day or the patient's maximum tolerated dose. Once a patient is adequately controlled and appears stable the dose of Gengraf® should be lowered, and the patient treated with the lowest dose that maintains an adequate response (this should not necessarily be total clearing of the patient). In clinical trials, cyclosporine doses at the lower end of the recommended dosage range were effective in maintaining a satisfactory response in 60% of the patients. Doses below 2.5 mg/kg/day may also be equally effective.

Upon stopping treatment with cyclosporine, relapse will occur in approximately six weeks (50% of the patients) to 16 weeks (75% of the patients). In the majority of patients rebound does not occur after cessation of treatment with cyclosporine. Thirteen cases of transformation of chronic plaque psoriasis to more severe forms of psoriasis have been reported. There were 9 cases of pustular and 4 cases of erythrodermic psoriasis. Long term experience with Gengraf® in psoriasis patients is limited and continuous treatment for extended periods greater than one year is not recommended. Alternation with other forms of treatment should be considered in the long term management of patients with this life long disease.

Blood Concentration Monitoring in Transplant Patients
Transplant centers have found blood concentration monitoring of cyclosporine to be an essential component of patient management. Of importance to blood concentration analysis are the type of assay used, the transplanted organ, and other immunosuppressant agents being administered. While no fixed relationship has been established, blood concentration monitoring may assist in the clinical evaluation of rejection and toxicity, dose adjustments, and the assessment of compliance.

Various assays have been used to measure blood concentrations of cyclosporine. Older studies using a non-specific assay often cited concentrations that were roughly twice those of the specific assays. Therefore, comparison between concentrations in the published literature and an individual patient concentration using current assays must be made with detailed knowledge of the assay methods employed. Current assay results are also not interchangeable and their use should be guided by their approved labeling. A discussion of the different assay methods is contained in Annals of Clinical Biochemistry 1994;31:420-446. While several assays and assay matrices are available, there is a consensus that parent-compound-specific assays correlate best with clinical events. Of these, HPLC is the standard reference, but the monoclonal antibody RIAs and the monoclonal antibody FPIA offer sensitivity, reproducibility, and convenience. Most clinicians base their monitoring on trough cyclosporine concentrations. Applied Pharmacokinetics, Principles of Therapeutic Drug Monitoring (1992) contains a broad discussion of cyclosporine pharmacokinetics and drug monitoring techniques. Blood concentration monitoring is not a replacement for renal function monitoring or tissue biopsies.

HOW SUPPLIED
Gengraf® Capsules (Cyclosporine Capsules, USP [MODIFIED])
25 mg
Oval, white imprinted in blue, the "a" logo, 25 mg, and the code OR. Packages of 30 unit-dose blisters. (**NDC** 0074-6463-32).
100 mg
Oval, white, with two blue stripes, imprinted in blue, the "a" logo, 100 mg, and the code OT. Packages of 30 unit-dose blisters. (**NDC** 0074-6479-32).
Store and Dispense
In the original unit-dose container at controlled room temperature
68°-77°F (20°-25°C). (See USP Controlled Room Temperature).
Sandimmune® is a registered trademark of Novartis Pharmaceuticals Corporation.
© AbbVie Inc. 2013
AbbVie Inc., North Chicago, IL 60064, U.S.A.
03-A831-R15-Revised July, 2013
Shown in Product Identification Guide, page 303

HUMIRA®   ℞
[hu-mare-ah]
(adalimumab)
injection, for subcutaneous use

HIGHLIGHTS OF PRESCRIBING INFORMATION
These highlights do not include all the information needed to use HUMIRA safely and effectively. See full prescribing information for HUMIRA.
HUMIRA (adalimumab) injection, for subcutaneous use
Initial U.S. Approval: 2002

> **WARNING: SERIOUS INFECTIONS AND MALIGNANCY**
> *See full prescribing information for complete boxed warning.*
> **SERIOUS INFECTIONS (5.1, 6.1):**
> - Increased risk of serious infections leading to hospitalization or death, including tuberculosis (TB), bacterial sepsis, invasive fungal infections (such as histoplasmosis), and infections due to other opportunistic pathogens.
> - Discontinue HUMIRA if a patient develops a serious infection or sepsis during treatment.

> - Perform test for latent TB; if positive, start treatment for TB prior to starting HUMIRA.
> - Monitor all patients for active TB during treatment, even if initial latent TB test is negative.
> **MALIGNANCY (5.2):**
> - Lymphoma and other malignancies, some fatal, have been reported in children and adolescent patients treated with TNF blockers including HUMIRA.
> - Post-marketing cases of hepatosplenic T-cell lymphoma (HSTCL), a rare type of T-cell lymphoma, have occurred in adolescent and young adults with inflammatory bowel disease treated with TNF blockers including HUMIRA.

————RECENT MAJOR CHANGES————
Warnings and Precautions, Serious Infections (5.1)	5/2013
Warnings and Precautions, Malignancies (5.2)	5/2013
Warnings and Precautions, Hypersensitivity Reactions (5.3)	5/2013

————INDICATIONS AND USAGE————
HUMIRA is a tumor necrosis factor (TNF) blocker indicated for treatment of:
- **Rheumatoid Arthritis (RA) (1.1):** Reducing signs and symptoms, inducing major clinical response, inhibiting the progression of structural damage, and improving physical function in adult patients with moderately to severely active RA.
- **Juvenile Idiopathic Arthritis (JIA) (1.2):** Reducing signs and symptoms of moderately to severely active polyarticular JIA in pediatric patients 4 years of age and older.
- **Psoriatic Arthritis (PsA) (1.3):** Reducing signs and symptoms, inhibiting the progression of structural damage, and improving physical function in adult patients with active PsA.
- **Ankylosing Spondylitis (AS) (1.4):** Reducing signs and symptoms in adult patients with active AS.
- **Crohn's Disease (CD) (1.5):** Reducing signs and symptoms and inducing and maintaining clinical remission in adult patients with moderately to severely active Crohn's disease who have had an inadequate response to conventional therapy. Reducing signs and symptoms and inducing clinical remission in these patients if they have also lost response to or are intolerant to infliximab.
- **Ulcerative Colitis (UC) (1.6):** Inducing and sustaining clinical remission in adult patients with moderately to severely active ulcerative colitis who have had an inadequate response to immunosuppressants such as corticosteroids, azathioprine or 6-mercaptopurine (6-MP). The effectiveness of HUMIRA has not been established in patients who have lost response to or were intolerant to TNF blockers.
- **Plaque Psoriasis (Ps) (1.7):** The treatment of adult patients with moderate to severe chronic plaque psoriasis who are candidates for systemic therapy or phototherapy, and when other systemic therapies are medically less appropriate.

————DOSAGE AND ADMINISTRATION————
- Administered by subcutaneous injection (2)
Rheumatoid Arthritis, Psoriatic Arthritis, Ankylosing Spondylitis (2.1):
- 40 mg every other week.
- Some patients with RA not receiving methotrexate may benefit from increasing the frequency to 40 mg every week.
Juvenile Idiopathic Arthritis (2.2):
- *15 kg (33 lbs) to < 30 kg (66 lbs):* 20 mg every other week
- *≥30 kg (66 lbs):* 40 mg every other week
Crohn's Disease and Ulcerative Colitis (2.3, 2.4):
- Initial dose (Day 1): 160 mg (four 40 mg injections in one day or two 40 mg injections per day for two consecutive days)
- Second dose two weeks later (Day 15): 80 mg
  - Two weeks later (Day 29): Begin a maintenance dose of 40 mg every other week.
- For patients with Ulcerative Colitis only: Only continue HUMIRA in patients who have shown evidence of clinical remission by eight weeks (Day 57) of therapy.
Plaque Psoriasis (2.5):
- 80 mg initial dose, followed by 40 mg every other week starting one week after initial dose.

————DOSAGE FORMS AND STRENGTHS————
- Injection: 40 mg/0.8 mL in a single-use prefilled pen (HUMIRA Pen) (3)
- Injection: 40 mg/0.8 mL in a single-use prefilled glass syringe (3)
- Injection: 20 mg/0.4 mL in a single-use prefilled glass syringe (3)
- Injection: 40 mg/0.8 mL in a single-use glass vial for institutional use only (3)

————CONTRAINDICATIONS————
None (4)

————WARNINGS AND PRECAUTIONS————
- *Serious infections:* Do not start HUMIRA during an active infection. If an infection develops, monitor carefully, and stop HUMIRA if infection becomes serious (5.1)
- *Invasive fungal infections:* For patients who develop a systemic illness on HUMIRA, consider empiric antifungal therapy for those who reside or travel to regions where mycoses are endemic (5.1)
- *Malignancies:* Incidence of malignancies was greater in HUMIRA-treated patients than in controls (5.2)
- *Anaphylaxis or serious allergic reactions* may occur (5.3)
- *Hepatitis B virus reactivation:* Monitor HBV carriers during and several months after therapy. If reactivation occurs, stop HUMIRA and begin anti-viral therapy (5.4)
- *Demyelinating disease:* Exacerbation or new onset, may occur (5.5)
- *Cytopenias, pancytopenia:* Advise patients to seek immediate medical attention if symptoms develop, and consider stopping HUMIRA (5.6)
- *Heart failure:* Worsening or new onset, may occur (5.8)
- *Lupus-like syndrome:* Stop HUMIRA if syndrome develops (5.9)

————ADVERSE REACTIONS————
Most common adverse reactions (incidence >10%): infections (e.g. upper respiratory, sinusitis), injection site reactions, headache and rash (6.1)
To report SUSPECTED ADVERSE REACTIONS, contact AbbVie Inc. at 1-800-633-9110 or FDA at 1-800-FDA-1088 or www.fda.gov/medwatch

————DRUG INTERACTIONS————
- *Abatacept:* Increased risk of serious infection (5.1, 5.11, 7.2)
- *Anakinra:* Increased risk of serious infection (5.1, 5.7, 7.2)
- *Live vaccines:* Avoid use with HUMIRA (5.10, 7.3)
See 17 for PATIENT COUNSELING INFORMATION and Medication Guide.

Revised: 05/2014

FULL PRESCRIBING INFORMATION: CONTENTS*
WARNING: SERIOUS INFECTIONS AND MALIGNANCY
1 INDICATIONS AND USAGE
    1.1 Rheumatoid Arthritis
    1.2 Juvenile Idiopathic Arthritis
    1.3 Psoriatic Arthritis
    1.4 Ankylosing Spondylitis
    1.5 Crohn's Disease
    1.6 Ulcerative Colitis
    1.7 Plaque Psoriasis
2 DOSAGE AND ADMINISTRATION
    2.1 Rheumatoid Arthritis, Psoriatic Arthritis, and Ankylosing Spondylitis
    2.2 Juvenile Idiopathic Arthritis
    2.3 Crohn's Disease
    2.4 Ulcerative Colitis
    2.5 Plaque Psoriasis
    2.6 Monitoring to Assess Safety
    2.7 General Considerations for Administration
3 DOSAGE FORMS AND STRENGTHS
4 CONTRAINDICATIONS
5 WARNINGS AND PRECAUTIONS
    5.1 Serious Infections
    5.2 Malignancies
    5.3 Hypersensitivity Reactions
    5.4 Hepatitis B Virus Reactivation
    5.5 Neurologic Reactions
    5.6 Hematological Reactions
    5.7 Use with Anakinra
    5.8 Heart Failure
    5.9 Autoimmunity
    5.10 Immunizations
    5.11 Use with Abatacept
6 ADVERSE REACTIONS
    6.1 Clinical Trials Experience
    6.2 Postmarketing Experience
7 DRUG INTERACTIONS
    7.1 Methotrexate
    7.2 Biological Products
    7.3 Live Vaccines
    7.4 Cytochrome P450 Substrates
8 USE IN SPECIFIC POPULATIONS
    8.1 Pregnancy
    8.3 Nursing Mothers
    8.4 Pediatric Use
    8.5 Geriatric Use
10 OVERDOSAGE

Information on the AbbVie, Inc. products listed on these pages is from the prescribing information in use as of July 31, 2014. For more information, please visit rxabbvie.com or call 1-800-633-9110.

FULL PRESCRIBING INFORMATION

WARNING: SERIOUS INFECTIONS AND MALIGNANCY

SERIOUS INFECTIONS

Patients treated with HUMIRA are at increased risk for developing serious infections that may lead to hospitalization or death [see Warnings and Precautions (5.1)]. Most patients who developed these infections were taking concomitant immunosuppressants such as methotrexate or corticosteroids.

Discontinue HUMIRA if a patient develops a serious infection or sepsis.

Reported infections include:

• Active tuberculosis (TB), including reactivation of latent TB. Patients with TB have frequently presented with disseminated or extrapulmonary disease. Test patients for latent TB before HUMIRA use and during therapy. Initiate treatment for latent TB prior to HUMIRA use.

• Invasive fungal infections, including histoplasmosis, coccidioidomycosis, candidiasis, aspergillosis, blastomycosis, and pneumocystosis. Patients with histoplasmosis or other invasive fungal infections may present with disseminated, rather than localized, disease. Antigen and antibody testing for histoplasmosis may be negative in some patients with active infection. Consider empiric anti-fungal therapy in patients at risk for invasive fungal infections who develop severe systemic illness.

• Bacterial, viral and other infections due to opportunistic pathogens, including Legionella and Listeria.

Carefully consider the risks and benefits of treatment with HUMIRA prior to initiating therapy in patients with chronic or recurrent infection.

Monitor patients closely for the development of signs and symptoms of infection during and after treatment with HUMIRA, including the possible development of TB in patients who tested negative for latent TB infection prior to initiating therapy [see Warnings and Precautions (5.1) and Adverse Reactions (6.1)].

MALIGNANCY

Lymphoma and other malignancies, some fatal, have been reported in children and adolescent patients treated with TNF blockers including HUMIRA [see Warnings and Precautions (5.2)]. Post-marketing cases of hepatosplenic T-cell lymphoma (HSTCL), a rare type of T-cell lymphoma, have been reported in patients treated with TNF blockers including HUMIRA. These cases have had a very aggressive disease course and have been fatal. The majority of reported TNF blocker cases have occurred in patients with Crohn's disease or ulcerative colitis and the majority were in adolescent and young adult males. Almost all these patients had received treatment with azathioprine or 6-mercaptopurine (6-MP) concomitantly with a TNF blocker at or prior to diagnosis. It is uncertain whether the occurrence of HSTCL is related to use of a TNF blocker or a TNF blocker in combination with these other immunosuppressants [see Warnings and Precautions (5.2)].

---

1 INDICATIONS AND USAGE

1.1 Rheumatoid Arthritis

HUMIRA is indicated for reducing signs and symptoms, inducing major clinical response, inhibiting the progression of structural damage, and improving physical function in adult patients with moderately to severely active rheumatoid arthritis. HUMIRA can be used alone or in combination with methotrexate or other non-biologic disease-modifying anti-rheumatic drugs (DMARDs).

1.2 Juvenile Idiopathic Arthritis

HUMIRA is indicated for reducing signs and symptoms of moderately to severely active polyarticular juvenile idiopathic arthritis in pediatric patients 4 years of age and older. HUMIRA can be used alone or in combination with methotrexate.

1.3 Psoriatic Arthritis

HUMIRA is indicated for reducing signs and symptoms, inhibiting the progression of structural damage, and improving physical function in adult patients with active psoriatic arthritis. HUMIRA can be used alone or in combination with non-biologic DMARDs.

1.4 Ankylosing Spondylitis

HUMIRA is indicated for reducing signs and symptoms in adult patients with active ankylosing spondylitis.

1.5 Crohn's Disease

HUMIRA is indicated for reducing signs and symptoms and inducing and maintaining clinical remission in adult patients with moderately to severely active Crohn's disease who have had an inadequate response to conventional therapy. HUMIRA is indicated for reducing signs and symptoms and inducing clinical remission in these patients if they have also lost response to or are intolerant to infliximab.

1.6 Ulcerative Colitis

HUMIRA is indicated for inducing and sustaining clinical remission in adult patients with moderately to severely active ulcerative colitis who have had an inadequate response to immunosuppressants such as corticosteroids, azathioprine or 6-mercaptopurine (6-MP). The effectiveness of HUMIRA has not been established in patients who have lost response to or were intolerant to TNF blockers [see Clinical Studies (14.6)].

1.7 Plaque Psoriasis

HUMIRA is indicated for the treatment of adult patients with moderate to severe chronic plaque psoriasis who are candidates for systemic therapy or phototherapy, and when other systemic therapies are medically less appropriate. HUMIRA should only be administered to patients who will be closely monitored and have regular follow-up visits with a physician [see Boxed Warning and Warnings and Precautions (5)].

2 DOSAGE AND ADMINISTRATION

HUMIRA is administered by subcutaneous injection.

2.1 Rheumatoid Arthritis, Psoriatic Arthritis, and Ankylosing Spondylitis

The recommended dose of HUMIRA for adult patients with rheumatoid arthritis (RA), psoriatic arthritis (PsA), or ankylosing spondylitis (AS) is 40 mg administered every other week. Methotrexate (MTX), other non-biologic DMARDS, glucocorticoids, nonsteroidal anti-inflammatory drugs (NSAIDs), and/or analgesics may be continued during treatment with HUMIRA. In the treatment of RA, some patients not taking concomitant MTX may derive additional benefit from increasing the dosing frequency of HUMIRA to 40 mg every week.

2.2 Juvenile Idiopathic Arthritis

The recommended dose of HUMIRA for pediatric patients 4 to 17 years of age with polyarticular juvenile idiopathic arthritis (JIA) is based on weight as shown below. MTX, glucocorticoids, NSAIDs, and/or analgesics may be continued during treatment with HUMIRA.

Pediatric Patients (4 to 17 years)	Dose
15 kg (33 lbs) to <30 kg (66 lbs)	20 mg every other week (20 mg Prefilled Syringe)
≥30 kg (66 lbs)	40 mg every other week (HUMIRA Pen or 40 mg Prefilled Syringe)

Limited data are available for HUMIRA treatment in pediatric patients with a weight below 15 kg.

2.3 Crohn's Disease

The recommended HUMIRA dose regimen for adult patients with Crohn's disease (CD) is 160 mg initially on Day 1 (given as four 40 mg injections in one day or as two 40 mg injections per day for two consecutive days), followed by 80 mg two weeks later (Day 15). Two weeks later (Day 29) begin a maintenance dose of 40 mg every other week. Aminosalicylates and/or corticosteroids may be continued during treatment with HUMIRA. Azathioprine, 6-mercaptopurine (6-MP) [see Warnings and Precautions (5.2)] or MTX may be continued during treatment with HUMIRA if necessary. The use of HUMIRA in CD beyond one year has not been evaluated in controlled clinical studies.

2.4 Ulcerative Colitis

The recommended HUMIRA dose regimen for adult patients with ulcerative colitis (UC) is 160 mg initially on Day 1 (given as four 40 mg injections in one day or as two 40 mg injections per day for two consecutive days), followed by 80 mg two weeks later (Day 15). Two weeks later (Day 29) continue with a dose of 40 mg every other week.

Only continue HUMIRA in patients who have shown evidence of clinical remission by eight weeks (Day 57) of therapy. Aminosalicylates and/or corticosteroids may be continued during treatment with HUMIRA. Azathioprine and 6-mercaptopurine (6-MP) [see Warnings and Precautions (5.2)] may be continued during treatment with HUMIRA if necessary.

2.5 Plaque Psoriasis

The recommended dose of HUMIRA for adult patients with plaque psoriasis (Ps) is an initial dose of 80 mg, followed by 40 mg given every other week starting one week after the initial dose. The use of HUMIRA in moderate to severe chronic Ps beyond one year has not been evaluated in controlled clinical studies.

2.6 Monitoring to Assess Safety

Prior to initiating HUMIRA and periodically during therapy, evaluate patients for active tuberculosis and test for latent infection [see Warnings and Precautions (5.1)].

2.7 General Considerations for Administration

HUMIRA is intended for use under the guidance and supervision of a physician. A patient may self-inject HUMIRA if a physician determines that it is appropriate, and with medical follow-up, as necessary, after proper training in subcutaneous injection technique.

Carefully inspect the solution in the HUMIRA Pen or prefilled syringe for particulate matter and discoloration prior to subcutaneous administration. If particulates and discolorations are noted, do not use the product. HUMIRA does not contain preservatives; therefore, discard unused portions of drug remaining from the syringe. NOTE: Instruct patients sensitive to latex not to handle the needle cover of the syringe because it contains dry rubber (latex).

Instruct patients using the HUMIRA Pen or prefilled syringe to inject the full amount in the syringe (0.8 mL), which provides 40 mg of HUMIRA, according to the directions provided in the Instructions for Use [see Instructions for Use].

Instruct patients (15 kg to <30 kg) using the pediatric prefilled syringe, or their caregivers, to inject the full amount in the syringe (0.4 mL), which provides 20 mg of HUMIRA, according to the directions provided in the Instructions for Use.

Rotate injection sites and do not give injections into areas where the skin is tender, bruised, red or hard.

The HUMIRA institutional use vial is for use and administration within an institutional setting only, such as a hospital, physician's office or clinic. Withdraw the dose using a sterile needle and syringe and administer promptly by a healthcare provider within an institutional setting. Only administer one dose per vial. The vial does not contain preservatives; therefore, discard unused portions.

3 DOSAGE FORMS AND STRENGTHS

• Pen

Injection: A single-use pen (HUMIRA Pen), containing a 1 mL prefilled glass syringe with a fixed 27 gauge ½ inch needle, providing 40 mg (0.8 mL) of HUMIRA.

• Prefilled Syringe

Injection: A single-use, 1 mL prefilled glass syringe with a fixed 27 gauge ½ inch needle, providing 40 mg (0.8 mL) of HUMIRA.

Injection: A single-use, 1 mL prefilled glass syringe with a fixed 27 gauge ½ inch needle, providing 20 mg (0.4 mL) of HUMIRA.

• Institutional Use Vial

Injection: A single-use, glass vial, providing 40 mg (0.8 mL) of HUMIRA for institutional use only.

4 CONTRAINDICATIONS

None.

5 WARNINGS AND PRECAUTIONS

5.1 Serious Infections

Patients treated with HUMIRA are at increased risk for developing serious infections involving various organ systems and sites that may lead to hospitalization or death [see Boxed Warning]. Opportunistic infections due to bacterial, mycobacterial, invasive fungal, viral, parasitic, or other opportunistic pathogens including aspergillosis, blastomycosis, candidiasis, coccidioidomycosis, histoplasmosis, legionellosis, listeriosis, pneumocystosis and tuberculosis have been reported with TNF blockers. Patients have frequently presented with disseminated rather than localized disease. The concomitant use of a TNF blocker and abatacept or anakinra was associated with a higher risk of serious infections in patients with rheumatoid arthritis (RA); therefore, the concomitant use of HUMIRA and these biologic products is not recommended in the treatment of patients with RA [see Warnings and Precautions (5.7, 5.11) and Drug Interactions (7.2)].

Treatment with HUMIRA should not be initiated in patients with an active infection, including localized infections. Patients greater than 65 years of age, patients with co-morbid conditions and/or patients taking concomitant immunosuppressants (such as corticosteroids or methotrexate), may be at greater risk of infection. Consider the risks and benefits of treatment prior to initiating therapy in patients:

• with chronic or recurrent infection;
• who have been exposed to tuberculosis;
• with a history of an opportunistic infection;
• who have resided or traveled in areas of endemic tuberculosis or endemic mycoses, such as histoplasmosis, coccidioidomycosis, or blastomycosis; or
• with underlying conditions that may predispose them to infection.

Tuberculosis

Cases of reactivation of tuberculosis and new onset tuberculosis infections have been reported in patients receiving HUMIRA, including patients who have previously received treatment for latent or active tuberculosis. Reports included cases of pulmonary and extrapulmonary (i.e., disseminated) tuberculosis. Evaluate patients for tuberculosis risk factors and test for latent infection prior to initiating HUMIRA and periodically during therapy.

Treatment of latent tuberculosis infection prior to therapy with TNF blocking agents has been shown to reduce the risk of tuberculosis reactivation during therapy. Prior to initiating HUMIRA, assess if treatment for latent tuberculosis is needed; and consider an induration of ≥ 5 mm a positive tuberculin skin test result, even for patients previously vaccinated with Bacille Calmette-Guerin (BCG).

Consider anti-tuberculosis therapy prior to initiation of HUMIRA in patients with a past history of latent or active tuberculosis in whom an adequate course of treatment cannot be confirmed, and for patients with a negative test for latent tuberculosis but having risk factors for tuberculosis infection. Despite prophylactic treatment for tuberculosis, cases of reactivated tuberculosis have occurred in patients treated with HUMIRA. Consultation with a physician with expertise in the treatment of tuberculosis is recommended to aid in the decision whether initiating anti-tuberculosis therapy is appropriate for an individual patient.

Strongly consider tuberculosis in the differential diagnosis in patients who develop a new infection during HUMIRA treatment, especially in patients who have previously or recently traveled to countries with a high prevalence of tuberculosis, or who have had close contact with a person with active tuberculosis.

Monitoring

Closely monitor patients for the development of signs and symptoms of infection during and after treatment with HUMIRA, including the development of tuberculosis in patients who tested negative for latent tuberculosis infection prior to initiating therapy. Tests for latent tuberculosis infection may also be falsely negative while on therapy with HUMIRA.

Discontinue HUMIRA if a patient develops a serious infection or sepsis. For a patient who develops a new infection during treatment with HUMIRA, closely monitor them, perform a prompt and complete diagnostic workup appropriate for an immunocompromised patient, and initiate appropriate antimicrobial therapy.

Invasive Fungal Infections

If patients develop a serious systemic illness and they reside or travel in regions where mycoses are endemic, consider invasive fungal infection in the differential diagnosis. Antigen and antibody testing for histoplasmosis may be negative in some patients with active infection. Consider appropriate empiric antifungal therapy, taking into account both the risk for severe fungal infection and the risks of antifungal therapy, while a diagnostic workup is being performed. To aid in the management of such patients, consider consultation with a physician with expertise in the diagnosis and treatment of invasive fungal infections.

5.2   Malignancies

Consider the risks and benefits of TNF-blocker treatment including HUMIRA prior to initiating therapy in patients with a known malignancy other than a successfully treated non-melanoma skin cancer (NMSC) or when considering continuing a TNF blocker in patients who develop a malignancy.

Malignancies in Adults

In the controlled portions of clinical trials of some TNF-blockers, including HUMIRA, more cases of malignancies have been observed among TNF-blocker-treated adult patients compared to control-treated adult patients. During the controlled portions of 34 global HUMIRA clinical trials in adult patients with rheumatoid arthritis (RA), psoriatic arthritis (PsA), ankylosing spondylitis (AS), Crohn's disease (CD), ulcerative colitis (UC) and plaque psoriasis (Ps), malignancies, other than non-melanoma (basal cell and squamous cell) skin cancer, were observed at a rate (95% confidence interval) of 0.6 (0.38, 0.91) per 100 patient-years among 7304 HUMIRA-treated patients versus a rate of 0.6

(0.30, 1.03) per 100 patient-years among 4232 control-treated patients (median duration of treatment of 4 months for HUMIRA-treated patients and 4 months for control-treated patients). In 47 global controlled and uncontrolled clinical trials of HUMIRA in adult patients with RA, PsA, AS, CD, UC, and Ps, the most frequently observed malignancies, other than lymphoma and NMSC, were breast, colon, prostate, lung, and melanoma. The malignancies in HUMIRA-treated patients in the controlled and uncontrolled portions of the studies were similar in type and number to what would be expected in the general U.S. population according to the SEER database (adjusted for age, gender, and race).[1]

In controlled trials of other TNF blockers in adult patients at higher risk for malignancies (i.e., patients with COPD with a significant smoking history and cyclophosphamide-treated patients with Wegener's granulomatosis), a greater portion of malignancies occurred in the TNF blocker group compared to the control group.

Non-Melanoma Skin Cancer

During the controlled portions of 34 global HUMIRA clinical trials in adult patients with RA, PsA, AS, CD, UC, and Ps, the rate (95% confidence interval) of NMSC was 0.7 (0.49, 1.08) per 100 patient-years among HUMIRA-treated patients and 0.2 (0.08, 0.59) per 100 patient-years among control-treated patients. Examine all patients, and in particular patients with a medical history of prior prolonged immunosuppressant therapy or psoriasis patients with a history of PUVA treatment for the presence of NMSC prior to and during treatment with HUMIRA.

Lymphoma and Leukemia

In the controlled portions of clinical trials of all the TNF-blockers in adults, more cases of lymphoma have been observed among TNF-blocker-treated patients compared to control-treated patients. In the controlled portions of 34 global HUMIRA clinical trials in adult patients with RA, PsA, AS, CD, UC and Ps, 3 lymphomas occurred among 7304 HUMIRA-treated patients versus 1 among 4232 control-treated patients. In 47 global controlled and uncontrolled clinical trials of HUMIRA in adult patients with RA, PsA, AS, CD, UC and Ps with a median duration of approximately 0.6 years, including 23,036 patients and over 34,000 patient-years of HUMIRA, the observed rate of lymphomas was approximately 0.11 per 100 patient-years. This is approximately 3-fold higher than expected in the general U.S. population according to the SEER database (adjusted for age, gender, and race).[1] Rates of lymphoma in clinical trials of HUMIRA cannot be compared to rates of lymphoma in clinical trials of other TNF blockers and may not predict the rates observed in a broader patient population. Patients with RA and other chronic inflammatory diseases, particularly those with highly active disease and/or chronic exposure to immunosuppressant therapies, may be at a higher risk (up to several fold) than the general population for the development of lymphoma, even in the absence of TNF blockers. Post-marketing cases of acute and chronic leukemia have been reported in association with TNF-blocker use in RA and other indications. Even in the absence of TNF-blocker therapy, patients with RA may be at a higher risk (approximately 2-fold) than the general population for the development of leukemia.

Malignancies in Pediatric Patients and Young Adults

Malignancies, some fatal, have been reported among children, adolescents, and young adults who received treatment with TNF-blockers (initiation of therapy ≤ 18 years of age), of which HUMIRA is a member *[see Boxed Warning]*. Approximately half the cases were lymphomas, including Hodgkin's and non-Hodgkin's lymphoma. The other cases represented a variety of different malignancies and included rare malignancies usually associated with immunosuppression and malignancies that are not usually observed in children and adolescents. The malignancies occurred after a median of 30 months of therapy (range 1 to 84 months). Most of the patients were receiving concomitant immunosuppressants. These cases were reported post-marketing and are derived from a variety of sources including registries and spontaneous postmarketing reports.

Postmarketing cases of hepatosplenic T-cell lymphoma (HSTCL), a rare type of T-cell lymphoma, have been reported in patients treated with TNF blockers including HUMIRA *[see Boxed Warning]*. These cases have had a very aggressive disease course and have been fatal. The majority of reported TNF blocker cases have occurred in patients with Crohn's disease or ulcerative colitis and the majority were in adolescent and young adult males. Almost all of these patients had received treatment with the immunosuppressants azathioprine or 6-mercaptopurine (6–MP) concomitantly with a TNF blocker at or prior to diagnosis. It is uncertain whether the occurrence of HSTCL is related to use of a TNF blocker or a TNF blocker in combination with these other immunosuppressants. The potential risk with the combination of azathioprine or 6-mercaptopurine and HUMIRA should be carefully considered.

5.3   Hypersensitivity Reactions

Anaphylaxis and angioneurotic edema have been reported following HUMIRA administration. If an anaphylactic or other serious allergic reaction occurs, immediately discontinue administration of HUMIRA and institute appropriate therapy. In clinical trials of HUMIRA in adults, allergic reactions (e.g., allergic rash, anaphylactoid reaction, fixed drug reaction, non-specified drug reaction, urticaria) have been observed.

5.4   Hepatitis B Virus Reactivation

Use of TNF blockers, including HUMIRA, may increase the risk of reactivation of hepatitis B virus (HBV) in patients who are chronic carriers of this virus. In some instances, HBV reactivation occurring in conjunction with TNF blocker therapy has been fatal. The majority of these reports have occurred in patients concomitantly receiving other medications that suppress the immune system, which may also contribute to HBV reactivation. Evaluate patients at risk for HBV infection for prior evidence of HBV infection before initiating TNF blocker therapy. Exercise caution in prescribing TNF blockers for patients identified as carriers of HBV. Adequate data are not available on the safety or efficacy of treating patients who are carriers of HBV with anti-viral therapy in conjunction with TNF blocker therapy to prevent HBV reactivation. For patients who are carriers of HBV and require treatment with TNF blockers, closely monitor such patients for clinical and laboratory signs of active HBV infection throughout therapy and for several months following termination of therapy. In patients who develop HBV reactivation, stop HUMIRA and initiate effective anti-viral therapy with appropriate supportive treatment. The safety of resuming TNF blocker therapy after HBV reactivation is controlled is not known. Therefore, exercise caution when considering resumption of HUMIRA therapy in this situation and monitor patients closely.

5.5   Neurologic Reactions

Use of TNF blocking agents, including HUMIRA, has been associated with rare cases of new onset or exacerbation of clinical symptoms and/or radiographic evidence of central nervous system demyelinating disease, including multiple sclerosis (MS) and optic neuritis, and peripheral demyelinating disease, including Guillain-Barré syndrome. Exercise caution in considering the use of HUMIRA in patients with preexisting or recent-onset central or peripheral nervous system demyelinating disorders.

5.6   Hematological Reactions

Rare reports of pancytopenia including aplastic anemia have been reported with TNF blocking agents. Adverse reactions of the hematologic system, including medically significant cytopenia (e.g., thrombocytopenia, leukopenia) have been infrequently reported with HUMIRA. The causal relationship of these reports to HUMIRA remains unclear. Advise all patients to seek immediate medical attention if they develop signs and symptoms suggestive of blood dyscrasias or infection (e.g., persistent fever, bruising, bleeding, pallor) while on HUMIRA. Consider discontinuation of HUMIRA therapy in patients with confirmed significant hematologic abnormalities.

5.7   Use with Anakinra

Concurrent use of anakinra (an interleukin-1 antagonist) and another TNF-blocker, was associated with a greater proportion of serious infections and neutropenia and no added benefit compared with the TNF-blocker alone in patients with RA. Therefore, the combination of HUMIRA and anakinra is not recommended *[see Drug Interactions (7.2)]*.

5.8   Heart Failure

Cases of worsening congestive heart failure (CHF) and new onset CHF have been reported with TNF blockers. Cases of worsening CHF have also been observed with HUMIRA. HUMIRA has not been formally studied in patients with CHF; however, in clinical trials of another TNF blocker, a higher rate of serious CHF-related adverse reactions was observed. Exercise caution when using HUMIRA in patients who have heart failure and monitor them carefully.

5.9   Autoimmunity

Treatment with HUMIRA may result in the formation of autoantibodies and, rarely, in the development of a lupus-like syndrome. If a patient develops symptoms suggestive of a lupus-like syndrome following treatment with HUMIRA, discontinue treatment *[see Adverse Reactions (6.1)]*.

5.10   Immunizations

In a placebo-controlled clinical trial of patients with RA, no difference was detected in anti-pneumococcal antibody response between HUMIRA and placebo treatment groups when the pneumococcal polysaccharide vaccine and influenza vaccine were administered concurrently with HUMIRA. Similar proportions of patients developed protec-

Information on the AbbVie, Inc. products listed on these pages is from the prescribing information in use as of July 31, 2014. For more information, please visit rxabbvie.com or call 1-800-633-9110.

tive levels of anti-influenza antibodies between HUMIRA and placebo treatment groups; however, titers in aggregate to influenza antigens were moderately lower in patients receiving HUMIRA. The clinical significance of this is unknown. Patients on HUMIRA may receive concurrent vaccinations, except for live vaccines. No data are available on the secondary transmission of infection by live vaccines in patients receiving HUMIRA.

It is recommended that JIA patients, if possible, be brought up to date with all immunizations in agreement with current immunization guidelines prior to initiating HUMIRA therapy. Patients on HUMIRA may receive concurrent vaccinations, except for live vaccines.

5.11 Use with Abatacept

In controlled trials, the concurrent administration of TNF-blockers and abatacept was associated with a greater proportion of serious infections than the use of a TNF-blocker alone; the combination therapy, compared to the use of a TNF-blocker alone, has not demonstrated improved clinical benefit in the treatment of RA. Therefore, the combination of abatacept with TNF-blockers including HUMIRA is not recommended [see Drug Interactions (7.2)].

6 ADVERSE REACTIONS

The most serious adverse reactions described elsewhere in the labeling include the following:
- Serious Infections [see Warnings and Precautions (5.1)]
- Malignancies [see Warnings and Precautions (5.2)]

6.1 Clinical Trials Experience

Because clinical trials are conducted under widely varying and controlled conditions, adverse reaction rates observed in clinical trials of a drug cannot be directly compared to rates in the clinical trials of another drug and may not predict the rates observed in a broader patient population in clinical practice.

The most common adverse reaction with HUMIRA was injection site reactions. In placebo-controlled trials, 20% of patients treated with HUMIRA developed injection site reactions (erythema and/or itching, hemorrhage, pain or swelling), compared to 14% of patients receiving placebo. Most injection site reactions were described as mild and generally did not necessitate drug discontinuation.

The proportion of patients who discontinued treatment due to adverse reactions during the double-blind, placebo-controlled portion of studies in patients with RA (i.e., Studies RA-I, RA-II, RA-III and RA-IV) was 7% for patients taking HUMIRA and 4% for placebo-treated patients. The most common adverse reactions leading to discontinuation of HUMIRA in these RA studies were clinical flare reaction (0.7%), rash (0.3%) and pneumonia (0.3%).

Infections

In the controlled portions of the 34 global HUMIRA clinical trials in adult patients with RA, PsA, AS, CD, UC and Ps, the rate of serious infections was 4.6 per 100 patient-years in 7304 HUMIRA-treated patients versus a rate of 3.1 per 100 patient-years in 4232 control-treated patients. Serious infections observed included pneumonia, septic arthritis, prosthetic and post-surgical infections, erysipelas, cellulitis, diverticulitis, and pyelonephritis [see Warnings and Precautions (5.1)].

Tuberculosis and Opportunistic Infections

In 47 global controlled and uncontrolled clinical trials in RA, PsA, AS, CD, UC and Ps that included 23,036 HUMIRA-treated patients, the rate of reported active tuberculosis was 0.22 per 100 patient-years and the rate of positive PPD conversion was 0.08 per 100 patient-years. In a subgroup of 9396 U.S. and Canadian HUMIRA-treated patients, the rate of reported active TB was 0.07 per 100 patient-years and the rate of positive PPD conversion was 0.08 per 100 patient-years. These trials included reports of miliary, lymphatic, peritoneal, and pulmonary TB. Most of the TB cases occurred within the first eight months after initiation of therapy and may reflect recrudescence of latent disease. In these global clinical trials, cases of serious opportunistic infections have been reported at an overall rate of 0.08 per 100 patient-years. Some cases of serious opportunistic infections and TB have been fatal [see Warnings and Precautions (5.1)].

Autoantibodies

In the rheumatoid arthritis controlled trials, 12% of patients treated with HUMIRA and 7% of placebo-treated patients that had negative baseline ANA titers developed positive titers at week 24. Two patients out of 3046 treated with HUMIRA developed clinical signs suggestive of new-onset lupus-like syndrome. The patients improved following discontinuation of therapy. No patients developed lupus nephritis or central nervous system symptoms. The impact of long-term treatment with HUMIRA on the development of autoimmune diseases is unknown.

Liver Enzyme Elevations

There have been reports of severe hepatic reactions including acute liver failure in patients receiving TNF-blockers. In controlled Phase 3 trials of HUMIRA (40 mg SC every other week) in patients with RA, PsA, and AS with control period

duration ranging from 4 to 104 weeks, ALT elevations $\geq 3 \times$ ULN occurred in 3.5% of HUMIRA-treated patients and 1.5% of control-treated patients. Since many of these patients in these trials were also taking medications that cause liver enzyme elevations (e.g., NSAIDS, MTX), the relationship between HUMIRA and the liver enzyme elevations is not clear. In controlled Phase 3 trials of HUMIRA (initial doses of 160 mg and 80 mg, or 80 mg and 40 mg on Days 1 and 15, respectively, followed by 40 mg every other week) in patients with CD with control period duration ranging from 4 to 52 weeks, ALT elevations $\geq 3 \times$ ULN occurred in 0.9% of HUMIRA-treated patients and 0.9% of control-treated patients. In controlled Phase 3 trials of HUMIRA (initial doses of 160 mg and 80 mg on Days 1 and 15 respectively, followed by 40 mg every other week) in patients with UC with control period duration ranging from 1 to 52 weeks, ALT elevations $\geq 3 \times$ ULN occurred in 1.5% of HUMIRA-treated patients and 1.0% of control-treated patients. In controlled Phase 3 trials of HUMIRA (initial dose of 80 mg then 40 mg every other week) in patients with Ps with control period duration ranging from 12 to 24 weeks, ALT elevations $\geq 3 \times$ ULN occurred in 1.8% of HUMIRA-treated patients and 1.8% of control-treated patients.

Immunogenicity

Patients in Studies RA-I, RA-II, and RA-III were tested at multiple time points for antibodies to adalimumab during the 6- to 12-month period. Approximately 5% (58 of 1062) of adult RA patients receiving HUMIRA developed low-titer antibodies to adalimumab at least once during treatment, which were neutralizing *in vitro*. Patients treated with concomitant methotrexate (MTX) had a lower rate of antibody development than patients on HUMIRA monotherapy (1% versus 12%). No apparent correlation of antibody development to adverse reactions was observed. With monotherapy, patients receiving every other week dosing may develop antibodies more frequently than those receiving weekly dosing. In patients receiving the recommended dosage of 40 mg every other week as monotherapy, the ACR 20 response was lower among antibody-positive patients than among antibody-negative patients. The long-term immunogenicity of HUMIRA is unknown.

In patients with JIA, adalimumab antibodies were identified in 16% of HUMIRA-treated patients. In patients receiving concomitant MTX, the incidence was 6% compared to 26% with HUMIRA monotherapy.

In patients with AS, the rate of development of antibodies to adalimumab in HUMIRA-treated patients was comparable to patients with RA.

In patients with PsA, the rate of antibody development in patients receiving HUMIRA monotherapy was comparable to patients with RA; however, in patients receiving concomitant MTX the rate was 7% compared to 1% in RA.

In patients with CD, the rate of antibody development was 3%.

In patients with moderately to severely active UC, the rate of antibody development in patients receiving HUMIRA was 5%. However, due to the limitation of the assay conditions, antibodies to adalimumab could be detected only when serum adalimumab levels were < 2 ug/ml. Among the patients whose serum adalimumab levels were < 2 ug/ml (approximately 25% of total patients studied), the immunogenicity rate was 20.7%.

In patients with Ps, the rate of antibody development with HUMIRA monotherapy was 8%. However, due to the limitation of the assay conditions, antibodies to adalimumab could be detected only when serum adalimumab levels were < 2 ug/ml. Among the patients whose serum adalimumab levels were < 2 ug/ml (approximately 40% of total patients studied), the immunogenicity rate was 20.7%. In Ps patients who were on HUMIRA monotherapy and subsequently withdrawn from the treatment, the rate of antibodies to adalimumab after retreatment was similar to the rate observed prior to withdrawal.

The data reflect the percentage of patients whose test results were considered positive for antibodies to adalimumab in an ELISA assay, and are highly dependent on the sensitivity and specificity of the assay. The observed incidence of antibody (including neutralizing antibody) positivity in an assay is highly dependent on several factors including assay sensitivity and specificity, assay methodology, sample handling, timing of sample collection, concomitant medications, and underlying disease. For these reasons, comparison of the incidence of antibodies to adalimumab with the incidence of antibodies to other products may be misleading.

Other Adverse Reactions

Rheumatoid Arthritis Clinical Studies

The data described below reflect exposure to HUMIRA in 2468 patients, including 2073 exposed for 6 months, 1497 exposed for greater than one year and 1380 in adequate and well-controlled studies (Studies RA-I, RA-II, RA-III, and RA-IV). HUMIRA was studied primarily in placebo-controlled trials and in long-term follow up studies for up to 36 months duration. The population had a mean age of 54

years, 77% were female, 91% were Caucasian and had moderately to severely active rheumatoid arthritis. Most patients received 40 mg HUMIRA every other week.

Table 1 summarizes reactions reported at a rate of at least 5% in patients treated with HUMIRA 40 mg every other week compared to placebo and with an incidence higher than placebo. In Study RA-III, the types and frequencies of adverse reactions in the second year open-label extension were similar to those observed in the one-year double-blind portion.

Table 1. Adverse Reactions Reported by ≥5% of Patients Treated with HUMIRA During Placebo-Controlled Period of Pooled RA Studies (Studies RA-I, RA-II, RA-III, and RA-IV)

Adverse Reaction (Preferred Term)	HUMIRA 40 mg subcutaneous Every Other Week (N=705)	Placebo (N=690)
Respiratory		
Upper respiratory infection	17%	13%
Sinusitis	11%	9%
Flu syndrome	7%	6%
Gastrointestinal		
Nausea	9%	8%
Abdominal pain	7%	4%
Laboratory Tests*		
Laboratory test abnormal	8%	7%
Hypercholesterolemia	6%	4%
Hyperlipidemia	7%	5%
Hematuria	5%	4%
Alkaline phosphatase increased	5%	3%
Other		
Headache	12%	8%
Rash	12%	6%
Accidental injury	10%	8%
Injection site reaction **	8%	1%
Back pain	6%	4%
Urinary tract infection	8%	5%
Hypertension	5%	3%

* Laboratory test abnormalities were reported as adverse reactions in European trials

** Does not include injection site erythema, itching, hemorrhage, pain or swelling

Less Common Adverse Reactions in Rheumatoid Arthritis Clinical Studies

Other infrequent serious adverse reactions that do not appear in the Warnings and Precautions or Adverse Reaction sections that occurred at an incidence of less than 5% in HUMIRA-treated patients in RA studies were:

Body As A Whole: Pain in extremity, pelvic pain, surgery, thorax pain

Cardiovascular System: Arrhythmia, atrial fibrillation, chest pain, coronary artery disorder, heart arrest, hypertensive encephalopathy, myocardial infarct, palpitation, pericardial effusion, pericarditis, syncope, tachycardia

Digestive System: Cholecystitis, cholelithiasis, esophagitis, gastroenteritis, gastrointestinal hemorrhage, hepatic necrosis, vomiting

Endocrine System: Parathyroid disorder

Hemic And Lymphatic System: Agranulocytosis, polycythemia

Metabolic And Nutritional Disorders: Dehydration, healing abnormal, ketosis, paraproteinemia, peripheral edema

Musculo-Skeletal System: Arthritis, bone disorder, bone fracture (not spontaneous), bone necrosis, joint disorder, muscle cramps, myasthenia, pyogenic arthritis, synovitis, tendon disorder

Neoplasia: Adenoma

Nervous System: Confusion, paresthesia, subdural hematoma, tremor

Respiratory System: Asthma, bronchospasm, dyspnea, lung function decreased, pleural effusion

Special Senses: Cataract

Thrombosis: Thrombosis leg

Urogenital System: Cystitis, kidney calculus, menstrual disorder

Juvenile Idiopathic Arthritis Clinical Studies

In general, the adverse reactions in the HUMIRA-treated pediatric patients in the juvenile idiopathic arthritis (JIA) trial were similar in frequency and type to those seen in adult patients [see Warnings and Precautions (5), Adverse Reactions (6)]. Important findings and differences from adults are discussed in the following paragraphs.

HUMIRA was studied in 171 pediatric patients, 4 to 17 years of age, with polyarticular JIA. Severe adverse reactions reported in the study included neutropenia, streptococcal pharyngitis, increased aminotransferases, herpes zoster, myositis, metrorrhagia, appendicitis. Serious infections were observed in 4% of patients within approximately 2 years of initiation of treatment with HUMIRA and included cases of herpes simplex, pneumonia, urinary tract infection, pharyngitis, and herpes zoster.

A total of 45% of children experienced an infection while receiving HUMIRA with or without concomitant MTX in the first 16 weeks of treatment. The types of infections reported in HUMIRA-treated patients were generally similar to those commonly seen in JIA patients who are not treated with TNF blockers. Upon initiation of treatment, the most common adverse reactions occurring in the pediatric population treated with HUMIRA were injection site pain and injection site reaction (19% and 16%, respectively). A less commonly reported adverse event in children receiving HUMIRA was granuloma annulare which did not lead to discontinuation of HUMIRA treatment.

In the first 48 weeks of treatment, non-serious hypersensitivity reactions were seen in approximately 6% of children and included primarily localized allergic hypersensitivity reactions and allergic rash.

Isolated mild to moderate elevations of liver aminotransferases (ALT more common than AST) were observed in children with JIA exposed to HUMIRA alone; liver enzyme test elevations were more frequent among those treated with the combination of HUMIRA and MTX than those treated with HUMIRA alone. In general, these elevations did not lead to discontinuation of HUMIRA treatment.

In the JIA trial, 10% of patients treated with HUMIRA who had negative baseline anti-dsDNA antibodies developed positive titers after 48 weeks of treatment. No patient developed clinical signs of autoimmunity during the clinical trial.

Approximately 15% of children treated with HUMIRA developed mild-to-moderate elevations of creatine phosphokinase (CPK). Elevations exceeding 5 times the upper limit of normal were observed in several patients. CPK levels decreased or returned to normal in all patients. Most patients were able to continue HUMIRA without interruption.

Psoriatic Arthritis and Ankylosing Spondylitis Clinical Studies
HUMIRA has been studied in 395 patients with psoriatic arthritis (PsA) in two placebo-controlled trials and in an open label study and 393 patients with ankylosing spondylitis (AS) in two placebo-controlled studies. The safety profile for patients with PsA and AS treated with HUMIRA 40 mg every other week was similar to the safety profile seen in patients with RA, HUMIRA Studies RA-I through IV.

Crohn's Disease Clinical Studies
HUMIRA has been studied in 1478 patients with Crohn's disease (CD) in four placebo-controlled and two open-label extension studies. The safety profile for patients with CD treated with HUMIRA was similar to the safety profile seen in patients with RA.

Ulcerative Colitis Clinical Studies
HUMIRA has been studied in 1010 patients with ulcerative colitis (UC) in two placebo-controlled studies and one open-label extension study. The safety profile for patients with UC treated with HUMIRA was similar to the safety profile seen in patients with RA.

Plaque Psoriasis Clinical Studies
HUMIRA has been studied in 1696 patients with plaque psoriasis (Ps) in placebo-controlled and open-label extension studies. The safety profile for patients with Ps treated with HUMIRA was similar to the safety profile seen in patients with RA with the following exceptions. In the placebo-controlled portions of the clinical trials in Ps patients, HUMIRA-treated patients had a higher incidence of arthralgia when compared to controls (3% *vs.* 1%).

6.2   Postmarketing Experience
The following adverse reactions have been identified during post-approval use of HUMIRA. Because these reactions are reported voluntarily from a population of uncertain size, it is not always possible to reliably estimate their frequency or establish a causal relationship to HUMIRA exposure.
Gastrointestinal disorders: Diverticulitis, large bowel perforations including perforations associated with diverticulitis and appendiceal perforations associated with appendicitis, pancreatitis
General disorders and administration site conditions: Pyrexia
Hepato-biliary disorders: Liver failure, hepatitis
Immune system disorders: Sarcoidosis
Neoplasms benign, malignant and unspecified (incl cysts and polyps):   Merkel Cell Carcinoma (neuroendocrine carcinoma of the skin)
Nervous system disorders: Demyelinating disorders (e.g., optic neuritis, Guillain-Barré syndrome), cerebrovascular accident

Respiratory disorders: Interstitial lung disease, including pulmonary fibrosis, pulmonary embolism
Skin reactions: Stevens Johnson Syndrome, cutaneous vasculitis, erythema multiforme, new or worsening psoriasis (all sub-types including pustular and palmoplantar), alopecia
Vascular disorders: Systemic vasculitis, deep vein thrombosis

7   DRUG INTERACTIONS
7.1   Methotrexate
HUMIRA has been studied in rheumatoid arthritis (RA) patients taking concomitant methotrexate (MTX). Although MTX reduced the apparent adalimumab clearance, the data do not suggest the need for dose adjustment of either HUMIRA or MTX [see Clinical Pharmacology (12.3)].
7.2   Biological Products
In clinical studies in patients with RA, an increased risk of serious infections has been seen with the combination of TNF blockers with anakinra or abatacept, with no added benefit; therefore, use of HUMIRA with abatacept or anakinra is not recommended in patients with RA [see Warnings and Precautions (5.7 and 5.11)]. A higher rate of serious infections has also been observed in patients with RA treated with rituximab who received subsequent treatment with a TNF blocker. There is insufficient information regarding the concomitant use of HUMIRA and other biologic products for the treatment of RA, PsA, AS, CD, UC, and Ps. Concomitant administration of HUMIRA with other biologic DMARDS (e.g., anakinra and abatacept) or other TNF blockers is not recommended based upon the possible increased risk for infections and other potential pharmacological interactions.
7.3   Live Vaccines
Avoid the use of live vaccines with HUMIRA [see Warnings and Precautions (5.10)].
7.4   Cytochrome P450 Substrates
The formation of CYP450 enzymes may be suppressed by increased levels of cytokines (e.g., TNFα, IL-6) during chronic inflammation. It is possible for a molecule that antagonizes cytokine activity, such as adalimumab, to influence the formation of CYP450 enzymes. Upon initiation or discontinuation of HUMIRA in patients being treated with CYP450 substrates with a narrow therapeutic index, monitoring of the effect (e.g., warfarin) or drug concentration (e.g., cyclosporine or theophylline) is recommended and the individual dose of the drug product may be adjusted as needed.

8   USE IN SPECIFIC POPULATIONS
8.1   Pregnancy
Pregnancy Category B
Risk Summary
Adequate and well controlled studies with HUMIRA have not been conducted in pregnant women. Adalimumab is an IgG1 monoclonal antibody and IgG1 is actively transferred across the placenta during the third trimester of pregnancy. Adalimumab serum levels were obtained from ten women treated with HUMIRA during pregnancy and eight newborn infants suggest active placental transfer of adalimumab. No fetal harm was observed in reproductive studies performed in cynomolgus monkeys. Because animal reproductive studies are not always predictive of human response, this drug should be used during pregnancy only if clearly needed.
Clinical Considerations
In general, monoclonal antibodies are transported across the placenta in a linear fashion as pregnancy progresses, with the largest amount transferred during the third trimester.
Human Data
In an independent clinical study conducted in ten pregnant women with inflammatory bowel disease treated with HUMIRA, adalimumab concentrations were measured in maternal blood as well as in cord (n=10) and infant blood (n=8) on the day of birth. The last dose of HUMIRA was given between 1 and 56 days prior to delivery. Adalimumab concentrations were 0.16-19.7 µg/mL in cord blood, 4.28-17.7 µg/mL in infant blood, and 0-16.1 µg/mL in maternal blood. In all but one case, the cord blood level of adalimumab was higher than the maternal level, suggesting adalimumab actively crosses the placenta. In addition, one infant had levels at each of the following: 6 weeks (1.94 µg/mL), 7 weeks (1.31 µg/mL), 8 weeks (0.93 µg/mL), and 11 weeks (0.53 µg/mL), suggesting adalimumab can be detected in the serum of infants exposed in utero for at least 3 months from birth.
Animal Data
An embryo-fetal perinatal developmental toxicity study has been performed in cynomolgus monkeys at dosages up to 100 mg/kg (266 times human AUC when given 40 mg subcutaneously with methotrexate every week or 373 times human AUC when given 40 mg subcutaneously without methotrexate) and has revealed no evidence of harm to the fetuses due to adalimumab.

8.3   Nursing Mothers
Limited data from published literature indicate that adalimumab is present in low levels in human milk and is

not likely to be absorbed by a breastfed infant. However, no data is available on the absorption of adalimumab from breastmilk in newborn or preterm infants. Caution should be exercised when HUMIRA is administered to a nursing woman.

8.4   Pediatric Use
Safety and efficacy of HUMIRA in pediatric patients for uses other than juvenile idiopathic arthritis (JIA) have not been established. Due to its inhibition of TNFα, HUMIRA administered during pregnancy could affect immune response in the in utero-exposed newborn and infant. Data from eight infants exposed to HUMIRA in utero, suggest adalimumab crosses the placenta [see Use in Specific Populations (8.1)]. The clinical significance of elevated adalimumab levels in infants is unknown. The safety of administering live or live-attenuated vaccines in exposed infants is unknown. Risks and benefits should be considered prior to vaccinating (live or live-attenuated) exposed infants.
Post-marketing cases of lymphoma, including hepatosplenic T-cell lymphoma and other malignancies, some fatal, have been reported among children, adolescents, and young adults who received treatment with TNF-blockers including HUMIRA [see Boxed Warning and Warnings and Precautions (5.2)].
Juvenile Idiopathic Arthritis
In the JIA trial, HUMIRA was shown to reduce signs and symptoms of active polyarticular JIA in patients 4 to 17 years of age [see Clinical Studies (14.2)]. HUMIRA has not been studied in children less than 4 years of age, and there are limited data on HUMIRA treatment in children with weight <15 kg.
The safety of HUMIRA in pediatric patients in the JIA trial was generally similar to that observed in adults with certain exceptions [see Adverse Reactions (6.1)].
8.5   Geriatric Use
A total of 519 RA patients 65 years of age and older, including 107 patients 75 years of age and older, received HUMIRA in clinical studies RA-I through IV. No overall difference in effectiveness was observed between these patients and younger patients. The frequency of serious infection and malignancy among HUMIRA treated patients over 65 years of age was higher than for those under 65 years of age. Because there is a higher incidence of infections and malignancies in the elderly population, use caution when treating the elderly.

10   OVERDOSAGE
Doses up to 10 mg/kg have been administered to patients in clinical trials without evidence of dose-limiting toxicities. Incase of overdosage, it is recommended that the patient be monitored for any signs or symptoms of adverse reactions or effects and appropriate symptomatic treatment instituted immediately.

11   DESCRIPTION
HUMIRA (adalimumab) is a recombinant human IgG1 monoclonal antibody specific for human tumor necrosis factor (TNF). HUMIRA was created using phage display technology resulting in an antibody with human derived heavy and light chain variable regions and human IgG1:k constant regions. Adalimumab is produced by recombinant DNA technology in a mammalian cell expression system and is purified by a process that includes specific viral inactivation and removal steps. It consists of 1330 amino acids and has a molecular weight of approximately 148 kilodaltons.
HUMIRA is supplied as a sterile, preservative-free solution of adalimumab for subcutaneous administration. The drug product is supplied as either a single-use, prefilled pen (HUMIRA Pen) or as a single-use, 1 mL prefilled glass syringe. Enclosed within the pen is a single-use, 1 mL prefilled glass syringe. The solution of HUMIRA is clear and colorless, with a pH of about 5.2.
Each prefilled syringe delivers 0.8 mL (40 mg) of drug product. Each 0.8 mL of HUMIRA contains 40 mg adalimumab, 4.93 mg sodium chloride, 0.69 mg monobasic sodium phosphate dihydrate, 1.22 mg dibasic sodium phosphate dihydrate, 0.24 mg sodium citrate, 1.04 mg citric acid monohydrate, 9.6 mg mannitol, 0.8 mg polysorbate 80, and Water for Injection, USP. Sodium hydroxide added as necessary to adjust pH.
Each pediatric prefilled syringe delivers 0.4 mL (20 mg) of drug product. Each 0.4 mL of HUMIRA contains 20 mg adalimumab, 2.47 mg sodium chloride, 0.34 mg monobasic sodium phosphate dihydrate, 0.61 mg dibasic sodium phosphate dihydrate, 0.12 mg sodium citrate, 0.52 mg citric acid monohydrate, 4.8 mg mannitol, 0.4 mg polysorbate 80, and Water for Injection, USP. Sodium hydroxide added as necessary to adjust pH.

Information on the AbbVie, Inc. products listed on these pages is from the prescribing information in use as of July 31, 2014. For more information, please visit rxabbvie.com or call 1-800-633-9110.

Table 2. ACR Responses in Studies RA-II and RA-III (Percent of Patients)

Response	Study RA-II Monotherapy (26 weeks)			Study RA-III Methotrexate Combination (24 and 52 weeks)	
	Placebo	HUMIRA 40 mg every other week	HUMIRA 40 mg weekly	Placebo/MTX	HUMIRA/MTX 40 mg every other week
	N=110	N=113	N=103	N=200	N=207
ACR20					
Month 6	19%	46%*	53%*	30%	63%*
Month 12	NA	NA	NA	24%	59%*
ACR50					
Month 6	8%	22%*	35%*	10%	39%*
Month 12	NA	NA	NA	10%	42%*
ACR70					
Month 6	2%	12%*	18%*	3%	21%*
Month 12	NA	NA	NA	5%	23%*

* p<0.01, HUMIRA *vs.* placebo

12 CLINICAL PHARMACOLOGY

12.1 Mechanism of Action

Adalimumab binds specifically to TNF-alpha and blocks its interaction with the p55 and p75 cell surface TNF receptors. Adalimumab also lyses surface TNF expressing cells *in vitro* in the presence of complement. Adalimumab does not bind or inactivate lymphotoxin (TNF-beta). TNF is a naturally occurring cytokine that is involved in normal inflammatory and immune responses. Elevated levels of TNF are found in the synovial fluid of patients with RA, JIA, PsA, and AS and play an important role in both the pathologic inflammation and the joint destruction that are hallmarks of these diseases. Increased levels of TNF are also found in psoriasis plaques. In Ps, treatment with HUMIRA may reduce the epidermal thickness and infiltration of inflammatory cells. The relationship between these pharmacodynamic activities and the mechanism(s) by which HUMIRA exerts its clinical effects is unknown.

Adalimumab also modulates biological responses that are induced or regulated by TNF, including changes in the levels of adhesion molecules responsible for leukocyte migration (ELAM-1, VCAM-1, and ICAM-1 with an IC_{50} of $1-2 \times 10^{-10}$M).

12.2 Pharmacodynamics

After treatment with HUMIRA, a decrease in levels of acute phase reactants of inflammation (C-reactive protein [CRP] and erythrocyte sedimentation rate [ESR]) and serum cytokines (IL-6) was observed compared to baseline in patients with rheumatoid arthritis. A decrease in CRP levels was also observed in patients with Crohn's disease and ulcerative colitis. Serum levels of matrix metalloproteinases (MMP-1 and MMP-3) that produce tissue remodeling responsible for cartilage destruction were also decreased after HUMIRA administration.

12.3 Pharmacokinetics

The maximum serum concentration (C_{max}) and the time to reach the maximum concentration (T_{max}) were 4.7 ± 1.6 μg/mL and 131 ± 56 hours respectively, following a single 40 mg subcutaneous administration of HUMIRA to healthy adult subjects. The average absolute bioavailability of adalimumab estimated from three studies following a single 40 mg subcutaneous dose was 64%. The pharmacokinetics of adalimumab were linear over the dose range of 0.5 to 10.0 mg/kg following a single intravenous dose.

The single dose pharmacokinetics of adalimumab in RA patients were determined in several studies with intravenous doses ranging from 0.25 to 10 mg/kg. The distribution volume (V_{ss}) ranged from 4.7 to 6.0 L. The systemic clearance of adalimumab is approximately 12 mL/hr. The mean terminal half-life was approximately 2 weeks, ranging from 10 to 20 days across studies. Adalimumab concentrations in the synovial fluid from five rheumatoid arthritis patients ranged from 31 to 96% of those in serum.

In RA patients receiving 40 mg HUMIRA every other week, adalimumab mean steady-state trough concentrations of approximately 5 μg/mL and 8 to 9 μg/mL, were observed without and with methotrexate (MTX), respectively. MTX reduced adalimumab apparent clearance after single and multiple dosing by 29% and 44% respectively, in patients with RA. Mean serum adalimumab trough levels at steady state increased approximately proportionally with dose following 20, 40, and 80 mg every other week and every week subcutaneous dosing. In long-term studies with dosing more than two years, there was no evidence of changes in clearance over time.

Adalimumab mean steady-state trough concentrations were slightly higher in psoriatic arthritis patients treated with 40 mg HUMIRA every other week (6 to 10 μg/mL and 8.5 to 12 μg/mL, without and with MTX, respectively) compared to the concentrations in RA patients treated with the same dose.

The pharmacokinetics of adalimumab in patients with AS were similar to those in patients with RA.

In patients with CD, the loading dose of 160 mg HUMIRA on Week 0 followed by 80 mg HUMIRA on Week 2 achieves mean serum adalimumab trough levels of approximately 12 μg/mL at Week 2 and Week 4. Mean steady-state trough levels of approximately 7 μg/mL were observed at Week 24 and Week 56 in CD patients after receiving a maintenance dose of 40 mg HUMIRA every other week.

In patients with UC, the loading dose of 160 mg HUMIRA on Week 0 followed by 80 mg HUMIRA on Week 2 achieves mean serum adalimumab trough levels of approximately 12 μg/mL at Week 2 and Week 4. Mean steady-state trough level of approximately 8 μg/mL was observed at Week 52 in UC patients after receiving a dose of 40 mg HUMIRA every other week, and approximately 15 μg/mL at Week 52 in UC patients who increased to a dose of 40 mg HUMIRA every week.

In patients with Ps, the mean steady-state trough concentration was approximately 5 to 6 μg/mL during HUMIRA 40 mg every other week monotherapy treatment.

Population pharmacokinetic analyses in patients with RA revealed that there was a trend toward higher apparent clearance of adalimumab in the presence of anti-adalimumab antibodies, and lower clearance with increasing age in patients aged 40 to >75 years.

Minor increases in apparent clearance were also predicted in RA patients receiving doses lower than the recommended dose and in RA patients with high rheumatoid factor or CRP concentrations. These increases are not likely to be clinically important.

No gender-related pharmacokinetic differences were observed after correction for a patient's body weight. Healthy volunteers and patients with rheumatoid arthritis displayed similar adalimumab pharmacokinetics.

No pharmacokinetic data are available in patients with hepatic or renal impairment.

In subjects with JIA (4 to 17 years of age), the mean steady-state trough serum adalimumab concentrations for subjects weighing <30 kg receiving 20 mg HUMIRA subcutaneously every other week as monotherapy or with concomitant methotrexate were 6.8 μg/mL and 10.9 μg/mL, respectively. The mean steady-state trough serum adalimumab concentrations for subjects weighing ≥30 kg receiving 40 mg HUMIRA subcutaneously every other week as monotherapy or with concomitant methotrexate were 6.6 μg/mL and 8.1 μg/mL, respectively.

13 NONCLINICAL TOXICOLOGY

13.1 Carcinogenesis, Mutagenesis, Impairment of Fertility

Long-term animal studies of HUMIRA have not been conducted to evaluate the carcinogenic potential or its effect on fertility. No clastogenic or mutagenic effects of HUMIRA were observed in the *in vivo* mouse micronucleus test or the *Salmonella-Escherichia coli* (Ames) assay, respectively.

14 CLINICAL STUDIES

14.1 Rheumatoid Arthritis

The efficacy and safety of HUMIRA were assessed in five randomized, double-blind studies in patients ≥18 years of age with active rheumatoid arthritis (RA) diagnosed according to American College of Rheumatology (ACR) criteria. Patients had at least 6 swollen and 9 tender joints. HUMIRA was administered subcutaneously in combination with methotrexate (MTX) (12.5 to 25 mg, Studies RA-I,

RA-III and RA-V) or as monotherapy (Studies RA-II and RA-V) or with other disease-modifying anti-rheumatic drugs (DMARDs) (Study RA-IV).

Study RA-I evaluated 271 patients who had failed therapy with at least one but no more than four DMARDs and had inadequate response to MTX. Doses of 20, 40 or 80 mg of HUMIRA or placebo were given every other week for 24 weeks.

Study RA-II evaluated 544 patients who had failed therapy with at least one DMARD. Doses of placebo, 20 or 40 mg of HUMIRA were given as monotherapy every other week or weekly for 26 weeks.

Study RA-III evaluated 619 patients who had an inadequate response to MTX. Patients received placebo, 40 mg of HUMIRA every other week with placebo injections on alternate weeks, or 20 mg of HUMIRA weekly for up to 52 weeks. Study RA-III had an additional primary endpoint at 52 weeks of inhibition of disease progression (as detected by X-ray results). Upon completion of the first 52 weeks, 457 patients enrolled in an open-label extension phase in which 40 mg of HUMIRA was administered every other week for up to 5 years.

Study RA-IV assessed safety in 636 patients who were either DMARD-naive or were permitted to remain on their pre-existing rheumatologic therapy provided that therapy was stable for a minimum of 28 days. Patients were randomized to 40 mg of HUMIRA or placebo every other week for 24 weeks.

Study RA-V evaluated 799 patients with moderately to severely active RA of less than 3 years duration who were ≥18 years old and MTX naïve. Patients were randomized to receive either MTX (optimized to 20 mg/week by week 8), HUMIRA 40 mg every other week or HUMIRA/MTX combination therapy for 104 weeks. Patients were evaluated for signs and symptoms, and for radiographic progression of joint damage. The median disease duration among patients enrolled in the study was 5 months. The median MTX dose achieved was 20 mg.

Clinical Response

The percent of HUMIRA treated patients achieving ACR 20, 50 and 70 responses in Studies RA-II and III are shown in Table 2.

[See table 2 above]

The results of Study RA-I were similar to Study RA-III; patients receiving HUMIRA 40 mg every other week in Study RA-I also achieved ACR 20, 50 and 70 response rates of 65%, 52% and 24%, respectively, compared to placebo responses of 13%, 7% and 3% respectively, at 6 months (p<0.01).

The results of the components of the ACR response criteria for Studies RA-II and RA-III are shown in Table 3. ACR response rates and improvement in all components of ACR response were maintained to week 104. Over the 2 years in Study RA-III, 20% of HUMIRA patients receiving 40 mg every other week (EOW) achieved a major clinical response, defined as maintenance of an ACR 70 response over a 6-month period. ACR responses were maintained in similar proportions of patients for up to 5 years with continuous HUMIRA treatment in the open-label portion of Study RA-III.

[See table 3 at top of next page]

The time course of ACR 20 response for Study RA-III is shown in Figure 1.

In Study RA-III, 85% of patients with ACR 20 responses at week 24 maintained the response at 52 weeks. The time course of ACR 20 response for Study RA-I and Study RA-II were similar.

Figure 1. Study RA-III ACR 20 Responses over 52 Weeks

In Study RA-IV, 53% of patients treated with HUMIRA 40 mg every other week plus standard of care had an ACR 20 response at week 24 compared to 35% on placebo plus

standard of care (p<0.001). No unique adverse reactions related to the combination of HUMIRA (adalimumab) and other DMARDs were observed.

In Study RA-V with MTX naïve patients with recent onset RA, the combination treatment with HUMIRA plus MTX led to greater percentages of patients achieving ACR responses than either MTX monotherapy or HUMIRA monotherapy at Week 52 and responses were sustained at Week 104 (see Table 4).

[See table 4 above]

At Week 52, all individual components of the ACR response criteria for Study RA-V improved in the HUMIRA/MTX group and improvements were maintained to Week 104.

Radiographic Response

In Study RA-III, structural joint damage was assessed radiographically and expressed as change in Total Sharp Score (TSS) and its components, the erosion score and Joint Space Narrowing (JSN) score, at month 12 compared to baseline. At baseline, the median TSS was approximately 55 in the placebo and 40 mg every other week groups. The results are shown in Table 5. HUMIRA/MTX treated patients demonstrated less radiographic progression than patients receiving MTX alone at 52 weeks.

[See table 5 above]

In the open-label extension of Study RA-III, 77% of the original patients treated with any dose of HUMIRA were evaluated radiographically at 2 years. Patients maintained inhibition of structural damage, as measured by the TSS. Fifty-four percent had no progression of structural damage as defined by a change in the TSS of zero or less. Fifty-five percent (55%) of patients originally treated with 40 mg HUMIRA every other week have been evaluated radiographically at 5 years. Patients had continued inhibition of structural damage with 50% showing no progression of structural damage defined by a change in the TSS of zero or less.

In Study RA-V, structural joint damage was assessed as in Study RA-III. Greater inhibition of radiographic progression, as assessed by changes in TSS, erosion score and JSN was observed in the HUMIRA/MTX combination group as compared to either the MTX or HUMIRA monotherapy group at Week 52 as well as at Week 104 (see Table 6).

[See table 6 above]

Physical Function Response

In studies RA-I through IV, HUMIRA showed significantly greater improvement than placebo in the disability index of Health Assessment Questionnaire (HAQ-DI) from baseline to the end of study, and significantly greater improvement than placebo in the health-outcomes as assessed by The Short Form Health Survey (SF 36). Improvement was seen in both the Physical Component Summary (PCS) and the Mental Component Summary (MCS).

In Study RA-III, the mean (95% CI) improvement in HAQ-DI from baseline at week 52 was 0.60 (0.55, 0.65) for the HUMIRA patients and 0.25 (0.17, 0.33) for placebo/MTX (p<0.001) patients. Sixty-three percent of HUMIRA-treated patients achieved a 0.5 or greater improvement in HAQ-DI at week 52 in the double-blind portion of the study. Eighty-two percent of these patients maintained that improvement through week 104 and a similar proportion of patients maintained this response through week 260 (5 years) of open-label treatment. Mean improvement in the SF-36 was maintained through the end of measurement at week 156 (3 years).

In Study RA-V, the HAQ-DI and the physical component of the SF-36 showed greater improvement (p<0.001) for the HUMIRA/MTX combination therapy group versus either the MTX monotherapy or the HUMIRA monotherapy group at Week 52, which was maintained through Week 104.

14.2   Juvenile Idiopathic Arthritis

The safety and efficacy of HUMIRA were assessed in a multicenter, randomized, withdrawal, double-blind, parallel-group study in 171 children (4 to 17 years of age) with polyarticular juvenile idiopathic arthritis (JIA). In the study, the patients were stratified into two groups: MTX-treated or non-MTX-treated. All subjects had to show signs of active moderate or severe disease despite previous treatment with NSAIDs, analgesics, corticosteroids, or DMARDS. Subjects who received prior treatment with any biologic DMARDS were excluded from the study.

The study included four phases: an open-label lead in phase (OL-LI; 16 weeks), a double-blind randomized withdrawal phase (DB; 32 weeks), an open-label extension phase (OLE-BSA; up to 136 weeks), and an open-label fixed dose phase (OLE-FD; 16 weeks). In the first three phases of the study, HUMIRA was administered based on body surface area at a dose of 24 mg/m² up to a maximum total body dose of 40 mg subcutaneously (SC) every other week. In the OLE-FD phase, the patients were treated with 20 mg of HUMIRA SC every other week if their weight was less than 30 kg and with 40 mg of HUMIRA SC every other week if their weight was 30 kg or greater. Patients remained on stable doses of NSAIDs and or prednisone (≤0.2 mg/kg/day or 10 mg/day maximum).

Patients demonstrating a Pediatric ACR 30 response at the end of OL-LI phase were randomized into the double blind (DB) phase of the study and received either HUMIRA or placebo every other week for 32 weeks or until disease flare. Disease flare was defined as a worsening of ≥30% from baseline in ≥3 of 6 Pediatric ACR core criteria, ≥2 active joints, and improvement of >30% in no more than 1 of the 6 criteria. After 32 weeks or at the time of disease flare during the DB phase, patients were treated in the open-label extension phase based on the BSA regimen (OLE-BSA), before converting to a fixed dose regimen based on body weight (OLE-FD phase).

Clinical Response

At the end of the 16-week OL-LI phase, 94% of the patients in the MTX stratum and 74% of the patients in the non-MTX stratum were Pediatric ACR 30 responders. In the DB phase significantly fewer patients who received HUMIRA

experienced disease flare compared to placebo, both without MTX (43% vs. 71%) and with MTX (37% vs. 65%). More patients treated with HUMIRA continued to show pediatric ACR 30/50/70 responses at Week 48 compared to patients treated with placebo. Pediatric ACR responses were maintained for up to two years in the OLE phase in patients who received HUMIRA throughout the study.

14.3   Psoriatic Arthritis

The safety and efficacy of HUMIRA was assessed in two randomized, double-blind, placebo controlled studies in 413 patients with psoriatic arthritis (PsA). Upon completion of

---

Table 3. Components of ACR Response in Studies RA-II and RA-III

Parameter (median)	Study RA-II				Study RA-III			
	Placebo N=110		HUMIRA[a] N=113		Placebo/MTX N=200		HUMIRA[a]/MTX N=207	
	Baseline	Wk 26	Baseline	Wk 26	Baseline	Wk 24	Baseline	Wk 24
Number of tender joints (0-68)	35	26	31	16*	26	15	24	8*
Number of swollen joints (0-66)	19	16	18	10*	17	11	18	5*
Physician global assessment[b]	7.0	6.1	6.6	3.7*	6.3	3.5	6.5	2.0*
Patient global assessment[b]	7.5	6.3	7.5	4.5*	5.4	3.9	5.2	2.0*
Pain[b]	7.3	6.1	7.3	4.1*	6.0	3.8	5.8	2.1*
Disability index (HAQ)[c]	2.0	1.9	1.9	1.5*	1.5	1.3	1.5	0.8*
CRP (mg/dL)	3.9	4.3	4.6	1.8*	1.0	0.9	1.0	0.4*

[a] 40 mg HUMIRA administered every other week
[b] Visual analogue scale; 0 = best, 10 = worst
[c] Disability Index of the Health Assessment Questionnaire; 0 = best, 3 = worst, measures the patient's ability to perform the following: dress/groom, arise, eat, walk, reach, grip, maintain hygiene, and maintain daily activity
* p<0.001, HUMIRA vs. placebo, based on mean change from baseline

---

Table 4. ACR Response in Study RA-V (Percent of Patients)

Response	MTX[b] N=257	HUMIRA[c] N=274	HUMIRA/MTX N=268
ACR20			
Week 52	63%	54%	73%
Week 104	56%	49%	69%
ACR50			
Week 52	46%	41%	62%
Week 104	43%	37%	59%
ACR70			
Week 52	27%	26%	46%
Week 104	28%	28%	47%
Major Clinical Response[a]	28%	25%	49%

[a] Major clinical response is defined as achieving an ACR70 response for a continuous six month period
[b] p<0.05, HUMIRA/MTX vs. MTX for ACR 20
p<0.001, HUMIRA/MTX vs. MTX for ACR 50 and 70, and Major Clinical Response
[c] p<0.001, HUMIRA/MTX vs. HUMIRA

Table 5. Radiographic Mean Changes Over 12 Months in Study RA-III

	Placebo/MTX	HUMIRA/MTX 40 mg every other week	Placebo/MTX- HUMIRA/MTX (95% Confidence Interval*)	P-value**
Total Sharp score	2.7	0.1	2.6 (1.4, 3.8)	<0.001
Erosion score	1.6	0.0	1.6 (0.9, 2.2)	<0.001
JSN score	1.0	0.1	0.9 (0.3, 1.4)	0.002

*95% confidence intervals for the differences in change scores between MTX and HUMIRA.
**Based on rank analysis

Table 6. Radiographic Mean Change* in Study RA-V

		MTX[a] N=257	HUMIRA[a,b] N=274	HUMIRA/MTX N=268
52 Weeks	Total Sharp score	5.7 (4.2, 7.3)	3.0 (1.7, 4.3)	1.3 (0.5, 2.1)
	Erosion score	3.7 (2.7, 4.8)	1.7 (1.0, 2.4)	0.8 (0.4, 1.2)
	JSN score	2.0 (1.2, 2.8)	1.3 (0.5, 2.1)	0.5 (0.0, 1.0)
104 Weeks	Total Sharp score	10.4 (7.7, 13.2)	5.5 (3.6, 7.4)	1.9 (0.9, 2.9)
	Erosion score	6.4 (4.6, 8.2)	3.0 (2.0, 4.0)	1.0 (0.4, 1.6)
	JSN score	4.1 (2.7, 5.4)	2.6 (1.5, 3.7)	0.9 (0.3, 1.5)

* mean (95% confidence interval)
[a] p<0.001, HUMIRA/MTX vs. MTX at 52 and 104 weeks and for HUMIRA/MTX vs. HUMIRA at 104 weeks
[b] p<0.01, for HUMIRA/MTX vs. HUMIRA at 52 weeks

Information on the AbbVie, Inc. products listed on these pages is from the prescribing information in use as of July 31, 2014. For more information, please visit rxabbvie.com or call 1-800-633-9110.

both studies, 383 patients enrolled in an open-label extension study, in which 40 mg HUMIRA was administered every other week.

Study PsA-I enrolled 313 adult patients with moderately to severely active PsA (>3 swollen and >3 tender joints) who had an inadequate response to NSAID therapy in one of the following forms: (1) distal interphalangeal (DIP) involvement (N=23); (2) polyarticular arthritis (absence of rheumatoid nodules and presence of plaque psoriasis) (N=210); (3) arthritis mutilans (N=1); (4) asymmetric PsA (N=77); or (5) AS-like (N=2). Patients on MTX therapy (158 of 313 patients) at enrollment (stable dose of ≤30 mg/week for >1 month) could continue MTX at the same dose. Doses of HUMIRA 40 mg or placebo every other week were administered during the 24-week double-blind period of the study. Compared to placebo, treatment with HUMIRA resulted in improvements in the measures of disease activity (see Tables 7 and 8). Among patients with PsA who received HUMIRA, the clinical responses were apparent in some patients at the time of the first visit (two weeks) and were maintained up to 88 weeks in the ongoing open-label study. Similar responses were seen in patients with each of the subtypes of psoriatic arthritis, although few patients were enrolled with the arthritis mutilans and ankylosing spondylitis-like subtypes. Responses were similar in patients who were or were not receiving concomitant MTX therapy at baseline.

Patients with psoriatic involvement of at least three percent body surface area (BSA) were evaluated for Psoriatic Area and Severity Index (PASI) responses. At 24 weeks, the proportions of patients achieving a 75% or 90% improvement in the PASI were 59% and 42% respectively, in the HUMIRA group (N=69), compared to 1% and 0% respectively, in the placebo group (N=69) (p<0.001). PASI responses were apparent in some patients at the time of the first visit (two weeks). Responses were similar in patients who were or were not receiving concomitant MTX therapy at baseline.

Table 7. ACR Response in Study PsA-I (Percent of Patients)

	Placebo N=162	HUMIRA* N=151
ACR20		
Week 12	14%	58%
Week 24	15%	57%
ACR50		
Week 12	4%	36%
Week 24	6%	39%
ACR70		
Week 12	1%	20%
Week 24	1%	23%

* p<0.001 for all comparisons between HUMIRA and placebo

[See table 8 above]

Similar results were seen in an additional, 12-week study in 100 patients with moderate to severe psoriatic arthritis who had suboptimal response to DMARD therapy as manifested by ≥3 tender joints and ≥3 swollen joints at enrollment.

Radiographic Response

Radiographic changes were assessed in the PsA studies. Radiographs of hands, wrists, and feet were obtained at baseline and Week 24 during the double-blind period when patients were on HUMIRA or placebo and at Week 48 when all patients were on open-label HUMIRA. A modified Total Sharp Score (mTSS), which included distal interphalangeal joints (i.e., not identical to the TSS used for rheumatoid arthritis), was used by readers blinded to treatment group to assess the radiographs.

HUMIRA-treated patients demonstrated greater inhibition of radiographic progression compared to placebo-treated patients and this effect was maintained at 48 weeks (see Table 9).

Table 9. Change in Modified Total Sharp Score in Psoriatic Arthritis

	Placebo N=141	HUMIRA N=133	
	Week 24	Week 24	Week 48
Baseline mean	22.1	23.4	23.4
Mean Change ± SD	0.9 ± 3.1	-0.1 ± 1.7	-0.2 ± 4.9*

* <0.001 for the difference between HUMIRA, Week 48 and Placebo, Week 24 (primary analysis)

Physical Function Response

In Study PsA-I, physical function and disability were assessed using the HAQ Disability Index (HAQ-DI) and the SF-36 Health Survey. Patients treated with 40 mg of HUMIRA every other week showed greater improvement from baseline in the HAQ-DI score (mean decreases of 47%

Table 8. Components of Disease Activity in Study PsA-I

Parameter: median	Placebo N=162 Baseline	24 weeks	HUMIRA* N=151 Baseline	24 weeks
Number of tender joints[a]	23.0	17.0	20.0	5.0
Number of swollen joints[b]	11.0	9.0	11.0	3.0
Physician global assessment[c]	53.0	49.0	55.0	16.0
Patient global assessment[c]	49.5	49.0	48.0	20.0
Pain[c]	49.0	49.0	54.0	20.0
Disability index (HAQ)[d]	1.0	0.9	1.0	0.4
CRP (mg/dL)[e]	0.8	0.7	0.8	0.2

* p<0.001 for HUMIRA *vs.* placebo comparisons based on median changes
[a] Scale 0-78
[b] Scale 0-76
[c] Visual analog scale; 0=best, 100=worst
[d] Disability Index of the Health Assessment Questionnaire; 0=best, 3=worst; measures the patient's ability to perform the following: dress/groom, arise, eat, walk, reach, grip, maintain hygiene, and maintain daily activity.
[e] Normal range: 0-0.287 mg/dL

Table 10. Components of Ankylosing Spondylitis Disease Activity

	Placebo N=107 Baseline mean	Week 24 mean	HUMIRA N=208 Baseline mean	Week 24 mean
ASAS 20 Response Criteria*				
Patient's Global Assessment of Disease Activity[a]*	65	60	63	38
Total back pain*	67	58	65	37
Inflammation[b]*	6.7	5.6	6.7	3.6
BASFI[c]*	56	51	52	34
BASDAI[d] score*	6.3	5.5	6.3	3.7
BASMI[e] score*	4.2	4.1	3.8	3.3
Tragus to wall (cm)	15.9	15.8	15.8	15.4
Lumbar flexion (cm)	4.1	4.0	4.2	4.4
Cervical rotation (degrees)	42.2	42.1	48.4	51.6
Lumbar side flexion (cm)	8.9	9.0	9.7	11.7
Intermalleolar distance (cm)	92.9	94.0	93.5	100.8
CRP[f]*	2.2	2.0	1.8	0.6

[a] Percent of subjects with at least a 20% and 10-unit improvement measured on a Visual Analog Scale (VAS) with 0 = "none" and 100 = "severe"
[b] mean of questions 5 and 6 of BASDAI (defined in 'd')
[c] Bath Ankylosing Spondylitis Functional Index
[d] Bath Ankylosing Spondylitis Disease Activity Index
[e] Bath Ankylosing Spondylitis Metrology Index
[f] C-Reactive Protein (mg/dL)
* statistically significant for comparisons between HUMIRA and placebo at Week 24

and 49% at Weeks 12 and 24 respectively) in comparison to placebo (mean decreases of 1% and 3% at Weeks 12 and 24 respectively). At Weeks 12 and 24, patients treated with HUMIRA showed greater improvement from baseline in the SF-36 Physical Component Summary score compared to patients treated with placebo, and no worsening in the SF-36 Mental Component Summary score. Improvement in physical function based on the HAQ-DI was maintained for up to 84 weeks through the open-label portion of the study.

14.4 Ankylosing Spondylitis

The safety and efficacy of HUMIRA 40 mg every other week was assessed in 315 adult patients in a randomized, 24 week double-blind, placebo-controlled study in patients with active ankylosing spondylitis (AS) who had an inadequate response to glucocorticoids, NSAIDs, analgesics, methotrexate or sulfasalazine. Active AS was defined as patients who fulfilled at least two of the following three criteria: (1) a Bath AS disease activity index (BASDAI) score ≥4 cm, (2) a visual analog score (VAS) for total back pain ≥ 40 mm, and (3) morning stiffness ≥ 1 hour. The blinded period was followed by an open-label period during which patients received HUMIRA 40 mg every other week subcutaneously for up to an additional 28 weeks.

Improvement in measures of disease activity was first observed at Week 2 and maintained through 24 weeks as shown in Figure 2 and Table 10.

Responses of patients with total spinal ankylosis (n=11) were similar to those without total ankylosis.

[See figure 2 at top of next column]

At 12 weeks, the ASAS 20/50/70 responses were achieved by 58%, 38%, and 23%, respectively, of patients receiving HUMIRA, compared to 21%, 10%, and 5% respectively, of patients receiving placebo (p <0.001). Similar responses were seen at Week 24 and were sustained in patients receiving open-label HUMIRA for up to 52 weeks.

A greater proportion of patients treated with HUMIRA (22%) achieved a low level of disease activity at 24 weeks (defined as a value <20 [on a scale of 0 to 100 mm] in each of the four ASAS response parameters) compared to patients treated with placebo (6%).

Figure 2. ASAS 20 Response By Visit, Study AS-I

[See table 10 above]

A second randomized, multicenter, double-blind, placebo-controlled study of 82 patients with ankylosing spondylitis showed similar results.

Patients treated with HUMIRA achieved improvement from baseline in the Ankylosing Spondylitis Quality of Life Questionnaire (ASQoL) score (-3.6 *vs.* -1.1) and in the Short Form Health Survey (SF-36) Physical Component Summary (PCS) score (7.4 *vs.* 1.9) compared to placebo-treated patients at Week 24.

14.5 Crohn's Disease

The safety and efficacy of multiple doses of HUMIRA were assessed in adult patients with moderately to severely active Crohn's disease, CD, (Crohn's Disease Activity Index (CDAI) ≥ 220 and ≤ 450) in randomized, double-blind, placebo-controlled studies. Concomitant stable doses of aminosalicylates, corticosteroids, and/or immunomodulatory agents were permitted, and 79% of patients continued to receive at least one of these medications.

Induction of clinical remission (defined as CDAI < 150) was evaluated in two studies. In Study CD-I, 299 TNF-blocker naïve patients were randomized to one of four treatment groups: the placebo group received placebo at Weeks 0 and 2, the 160/80 group received 160 mg HUMIRA at Week 0 and 80 mg at Week 2, the 80/40 group received 80 mg at Week 0 and 40 mg at Week 2, and the 40/20 group received 40 mg at Week 0 and 20 mg at Week 2. Clinical results were assessed at Week 4.

In the second induction study, Study CD-II, 325 patients who had lost response to, or were intolerant to, previous infliximab therapy were randomized to receive either 160 mg HUMIRA at Week 0 and 80 mg at Week 2, or placebo at Weeks 0 and 2. Clinical results were assessed at Week 4. Maintenance of clinical remission was evaluated in Study CD-III. In this study, 854 patients with active disease received open-label HUMIRA, 80 mg at week 0 and 40 mg at Week 2. Patients were then randomized at Week 4 to 40 mg HUMIRA every other week, 40 mg HUMIRA every week, or placebo. The total study duration was 56 weeks. Patients in clinical response (decrease in CDAI ≥70) at Week 4 were stratified and analyzed separately from those not in clinical response at Week 4.

Induction of Clinical Remission
A greater percentage of the patients treated with 160/80 mg HUMIRA achieved induction of clinical remission versus placebo at Week 4 regardless of whether the patients were TNF blocker naïve (CD-I), or had lost response to or were intolerant to infliximab (CD-II) (see Table 11).
[See table 11 above]

Maintenance of Clinical Remission
In Study CD-III at Week 4, 58% (499/854) of patients were in clinical response and were assessed in the primary analysis. At Weeks 26 and 56, greater proportions of patients who were in clinical response at Week 4 achieved clinical remission in the HUMIRA 40 mg every other week maintenance group compared to patients in the placebo maintenance group (see Table 12). The group that received HUMIRA therapy every week did not demonstrate significantly higher remission rates compared to the group that received HUMIRA every other week.

Table 12. Maintenance of Clinical Remission in CD-III (Percent of Patients)

	Placebo N=170	40 mg HUMIRA every other week N=172
Week 26		
Clinical remission	17%	40%*
Clinical response	28%	54%*
Week 56		
Clinical remission	12%	36%*
Clinical response	18%	43%*

Clinical remission is CDAI score < 150; clinical response is decrease in CDAI of at least 70 points.

*p<0.001 for HUMIRA vs. placebo pairwise comparisons of proportions

Of those in response at Week 4 who attained remission during the study, patients in the HUMIRA every other week group maintained remission for a longer time than patients in the placebo maintenance group. Among patients who were not in response by Week 12, therapy continued beyond 12 weeks did not result in significantly more responses.

14.6 Ulcerative Colitis
The safety and efficacy of HUMIRA were assessed in adult patients with moderately to severely active ulcerative colitis (Mayo score 6 to 12 on a 12 point scale, with an endoscopy subscore of 2 to 3 on a scale of 0 to 3) despite concurrent or prior treatment with immunosuppressants such as corticosteroids, azathioprine, or 6-MP in two randomized, double-blind, placebo-controlled clinical studies (Studies UC-I and UC-II). Both studies enrolled TNF-blocker naïve patients, but Study UC-II also allowed entry of patients who lost response to or were intolerant to TNF-blockers. Forty percent (40%) of patients enrolled in Study UC-II had previously used another TNF-blocker.
Concomitant stable doses of aminosalicylates and immunosuppressants were permitted. In Studies UC-I and II, patients were receiving aminosalicylates (69%), corticosteroids (59%) and/or azathioprine or 6-MP (37%) at baseline. In both studies, 92% of patients received at least one of these medications.
Induction of clinical remission (defined as Mayo score ≤ 2 with no individual subscores > 1) at Week 8 was evaluated in both studies. Clinical remission at Week 52 and sustained clinical remission (defined as clinical remission at both Weeks 8 and 52) were evaluated in Study UC-II.
In Study UC-I, 390 TNF-blocker naïve patients were randomized to one of three treatment groups for the primary efficacy analysis. The placebo group received placebo at Weeks 0, 2, 4 and 6. The 160/80 group received 160 mg

Table 11. Induction of Clinical Remission in Studies CD-I and CD-II (Percent of Patients)

	CD-I		CD-II	
	Placebo N=74	HUMIRA 160/80 mg N=76	Placebo N=166	HUMIRA 160/80 mg N=159
Week 4				
Clinical remission	12%	36%*	7%	21%*
Clinical response	34%	58%**	34%	52%**

Clinical remission is CDAI score < 150; clinical response is decrease in CDAI of at least 70 points.
* p<0.001 for HUMIRA vs. placebo pairwise comparison of proportions
** p<0.01 for HUMIRA vs. placebo pairwise comparison of proportions

Table 13. Induction of Clinical Remission in Studies UC-I and UC-II and Sustained Clinical Remission in Study UC-II (Percent of Patients)

	Study UC-I			Study UC-II		
	Placebo N=130	HUMIRA 160/80 mg N=130	Treatment Difference (95% CI)	Placebo N=246	HUMIRA 160/80 mg N=248	Treatment Difference (95% CI)
Induction of Clinical Remission (Clinical Remission at Week 8)	9.2%	18.5%	9.3%* (0.9%, 17.6%)	9.3%	16.5%	7.2%* (1.2%, 12.9%)
Sustained Clinical Remission (Clinical Remission at both Weeks 8 and 52)	N/A	N/A	N/A	4.1%	8.5%	4.4%* (0.1%, 8.6%)

Clinical remission is defined as Mayo score ≤ 2 with no individual subscores > 1.
CI=Confidence interval
* p<0.05 for HUMIRA vs. placebo pairwise comparison of proportions

HUMIRA at Week 0 and 80 mg at Week 2, and the 80/40 group received 80 mg HUMIRA at Week 0 and 40 mg at Week 2. After Week 2, patients in both HUMIRA treatment groups received 40 mg every other week (eow).
In Study UC-II, 518 patients were randomized to receive either HUMIRA 160 mg at Week 0, 80 mg at Week 2, and 40 mg eow starting at Week 4 through Week 50, or placebo starting at Week 0 and eow through Week 50. Corticosteroid taper was permitted starting at Week 8.
In both Studies UC-I and UC-II, a greater percentage of the patients treated with 160/80 mg of HUMIRA compared to patients treated with placebo achieved induction of clinical remission. In Study UC-II, a greater percentage of the patients treated with 160/80 mg of HUMIRA compared to patients treated with placebo achieved sustained clinical remission (clinical remission at both Weeks 8 and 52) (Table 13).
[See table 13 above]
In Study UC-I, there was no statistically significant difference in clinical remission observed between the HUMIRA 80/40 mg group and the placebo group at Week 8.
In Study UC-II, 17.3% (43/248) in the HUMIRA group were in clinical remission at Week 52 compared to 8.5% (21/246) in the placebo group (treatment difference: 8.8%; 95% confidence interval (CI): [2.8%, 14.5%]; p<0.05).
In the subgroup of patients in Study UC-II with prior TNF-blocker use, the treatment difference for induction of clinical remission appeared to be lower than that seen in the whole study population, and the treatment differences for sustained clinical remission and clinical remission at Week 52 appeared to be similar to those seen in the whole study population. The subgroup of patients with prior TNF-blocker use achieved induction of clinical remission at 9% (9/98) in the HUMIRA group versus 7% (7/101) in the placebo group, and sustained clinical remission at 5% (5/98) in the HUMIRA group versus 1% (1/101) in the placebo group. In the subgroup of patients with prior TNF-blocker use, 10% (10/98) were in clinical remission at Week 52 in the HUMIRA group versus 3% (3/101) in the placebo group.

14.7 Plaque Psoriasis
The safety and efficacy of HUMIRA were assessed in randomized, double-blind, placebo-controlled studies in 1696 adult patients with moderate to severe chronic plaque psoriasis (Ps) who were candidates for systemic therapy or phototherapy.
Study Ps-I evaluated 1212 patients with chronic Ps with ≥10% body surface area (BSA) involvement, Physician's Global Assessment (PGA) of at least moderate disease severity, and Psoriasis Area and Severity Index (PASI) ≥12 within three treatment periods. In period A, patients received placebo or HUMIRA at an initial dose of 80 mg at Week 0 followed by a dose of 40 mg every other week starting at Week 1. After 16 weeks of therapy, patients who achieved at least a PASI 75 response at Week 16, defined as

a PASI score improvement of at least 75% relative to baseline, entered period B and received open-label 40 mg HUMIRA every other week. After 17 weeks of open label therapy, patients who maintained at least a PASI 75 response at Week 33 and were originally randomized to active therapy in period A were re-randomized in period C to receive 40 mg HUMIRA every other week or placebo for an additional 19 weeks. Across all treatment groups the mean baseline PASI score was 19 and the baseline Physician's Global Assessment score ranged from "moderate" (53%) to "severe" (41%) to "very severe" (6%).
Study Ps-II evaluated 99 patients randomized to HUMIRA and 48 patients randomized to placebo with chronic plaque psoriasis with ≥10% BSA involvement and PASI ≥12. Patients received placebo, or an initial dose of 80 mg HUMIRA at Week 0 followed by 40 mg every other week starting at Week 1 for 16 weeks. Across all treatment groups the mean baseline PASI score was 21 and the baseline PGA score ranged from "moderate" (41%) to "severe" (51%) to "very severe" (8%).
Studies Ps-I and II evaluated the proportion of patients who achieved "clear" or "minimal" disease on the 6-point PGA scale and the proportion of patients who achieved a reduction in PASI score of at least 75% (PASI 75) from baseline at Week 16 (see Table 14 and 15).
Additionally, Study Ps-I evaluated the proportion of subjects who maintained a PGA of "clear" or "minimal" disease or a PASI 75 response after Week 33 and on or before Week 52.

Table 14. Efficacy Results at 16 Weeks in Study Ps-I Number of Patients (%)

	HUMIRA 40 mg every other week N = 814	Placebo N = 398
PGA: Clear or minimal*	506 (62%)	17 (4%)
PASI 75	578 (71%)	26 (7%)

* Clear = no plaque elevation, no scale, plus or minus hyperpigmentation or diffuse pink or red coloration
Minimal = possible but difficult to ascertain whether there is slight elevation of plaque above normal skin, plus or minus surface dryness with some white coloration, plus or minus up to red coloration

Information on the AbbVie, Inc. products listed on these pages is from the prescribing information in use as of July 31, 2014. For more information, please visit rxabbvie.com or call 1-800-633-9110.

Table 15. Efficacy Results at 16 Weeks in Study Ps-II Number of Patients (%)

	HUMIRA 40 mg every other week N = 99	Placebo N = 48
PGA: Clear or minimal*	70 (71%)	5 (10%)
PASI 75	77 (78%)	9 (19%)

* Clear = no plaque elevation, no scale, plus or minus hyperpigmentation or diffuse pink or red coloration
Minimal = possible but difficult to ascertain whether there is slight elevation of plaque above normal skin, plus or minus surface dryness with some white coloration, plus or minus up to red coloration

Additionally, in Study Ps-I, subjects on HUMIRA who maintained a PASI 75 were re-randomized to HUMIRA (N = 250) or placebo (N = 240) at Week 33. After 52 weeks of treatment with HUMIRA, more patients on HUMIRA maintained efficacy when compared to subjects who were re-randomized to placebo based on maintenance of PGA of "clear" or "minimal" disease (68% *vs.* 28%) or a PASI 75 (79% *vs.* 43%).

A total of 347 stable responders participated in a withdrawal and retreatment evaluation in an open-label extension study. Median time to relapse (decline to PGA "moderate" or worse) was approximately 5 months. During the withdrawal period, no subject experienced transformation to either pustular or erythrodermic psoriasis. A total of 178 subjects who relapsed re-initiated treatment with 80 mg of HUMIRA, then 40 mg eow beginning at week 1. At week 16, 69% (123/178) of subjects had a response of PGA "clear" or "minimal".

15 REFERENCES

1. National Cancer Institute. Surveillance, Epidemiology, and End Results Database (SEER) Program. SEER Incidence Crude Rates, 11 Registries, 1993-2001.

16 HOW SUPPLIED/STORAGE AND HANDLING

HUMIRA® (adalimumab) is supplied as a preservative-free, sterile solution for subcutaneous administration. The following packaging configurations are available.

• HUMIRA Pen Carton
HUMIRA is dispensed in a carton containing two alcohol preps and two dose trays. Each dose tray consists of a single-use pen, containing a 1 mL prefilled glass syringe with a fixed 27 gauge ½ inch needle, providing 40 mg (0.8 mL) of HUMIRA. The NDC number is 0074-4339-02.

• HUMIRA Pen – Crohn's Disease/Ulcerative Colitis Starter Package
HUMIRA is dispensed in a carton containing 6 alcohol preps and 6 dose trays (Crohn's Disease/Ulcerative Colitis Starter Package). Each dose tray consists of a single-use pen, containing a 1 mL prefilled glass syringe with a fixed 27 gauge ½ inch needle, providing 40 mg (0.8 mL) of HUMIRA. The NDC number is 0074-4339-06.

• HUMIRA Pen – Psoriasis Starter Package
HUMIRA is dispensed in a carton containing 4 alcohol preps and 4 dose trays (Psoriasis Starter Package). Each dose tray consists of a single-use pen, containing a 1 mL prefilled glass syringe with a fixed 27 gauge ½ inch needle, providing 40 mg (0.8 mL) of HUMIRA. The NDC number is 0074-4339-07.

• Prefilled Syringe Carton – 40 mg
HUMIRA is dispensed in a carton containing two alcohol preps and two dose trays. Each dose tray consists of a single-use, 1 mL prefilled glass syringe with a fixed 27 gauge ½ inch needle, providing 40 mg (0.8 mL) of HUMIRA. The NDC number is 0074-3799-02.

• Pediatric Prefilled Syringe Carton – 20 mg
HUMIRA is supplied for pediatric use only in a carton containing two alcohol preps and two dose trays. Each dose tray consists of a single-use, 1 mL pre-filled glass syringe with a fixed 27 gauge ½ inch needle, providing 20 mg (0.4 mL) of HUMIRA. The NDC number is 0074-9374-02.

• Institutional Use Vial Carton – 40 mg
HUMIRA is supplied for institutional use only in a carton containing a single-use, glass vial, providing 40 mg (0.8 mL) of HUMIRA. The NDC number is 0074-3797-01.

Storage and Stability
Do not use beyond the expiration date on the container. HUMIRA must be refrigerated at 36°F to 46°F (2°C to 8°C). DO NOT FREEZE. Do not use if frozen even if it has been thawed. When traveling, store HUMIRA in a cool carrier with an ice pack. Protect the prefilled syringe from exposure to light. Store in original carton until time of administration.

17 PATIENT COUNSELING INFORMATION

See FDA-approved patient labeling (Medication Guide and Instructions for Use).

17.1 Patient Counseling

Provide the HUMIRA "Medication Guide" to patients or their caregivers, and provide them an opportunity to read it and ask questions prior to initiation of therapy and prior to each time the prescription is renewed. If patients develop signs and symptoms of infection, instruct them to seek medical evaluation immediately.
Advise patients of the potential benefits and risks of HUMIRA.

• Infections
Inform patients that HUMIRA may lower the ability of their immune system to fight infections. Instruct patients of the importance of contacting their doctor if they develop any symptoms of infection, including tuberculosis, invasive fungal infections, and reactivation of hepatitis B virus infections.

• Malignancies
Counsel patients about the risk of malignancies while receiving HUMIRA.

• Allergic Reactions
Advise patients to seek immediate medical attention if they experience any symptoms of severe allergic reactions. Advise latex-sensitive patients that the needle cap of the prefilled syringe contains latex.

• Other Medical Conditions
Advise patients to report any signs of new or worsening medical conditions such as congestive heart failure, neurological disease, autoimmune disorders, or cytopenias. Advise patients to report any symptoms suggestive of a cytopenia such as bruising, bleeding, or persistent fever.

17.2 Instruction on Injection Technique

Inform patients that the first injection is to be performed under the supervision of a qualified health care professional. If a patient or caregiver is to administer HUMIRA, instruct them in injection techniques and assess their ability to inject subcutaneously to ensure the proper administration of HUMIRA *[see Instructions for Use]*.
For patients who will use the HUMIRA Pen, tell them that they:

• Will hear a **loud 'click'** when the plum-colored activator button is pressed. The loud click means the **start** of the injection.
• Must keep holding the HUMIRA Pen against their squeezed, raised skin until all of the medicine is injected. This can take up to 10 seconds.
• Will know that the injection has finished when the yellow marker fully appears in the window view and stops moving.

Instruct patients to dispose of their used needles and syringes or used Pen in a FDA-cleared sharps disposal container immediately after use. **Instruct patients not to dispose of loose needles and syringes or Pen in their household trash.**
Instruct patients that if they do not have a FDA-cleared sharps disposal container, they may use a household container that is made of a heavy-duty plastic, can be closed with a tight-fitting and puncture-resistant lid without sharps being able to come out, upright and stable during use, leak-resistant, and properly labeled to warn of hazardous waste inside the container.
Instruct patients that when their sharps disposal container is almost full, they will need to follow their community guidelines for the correct way to dispose of their sharps disposal container. Instruct patients that there may be state or local laws regarding disposal of used needles and syringes. Refer patients to the FDA's website at http://www.fda.gov/safesharpsdisposal for more information about safe sharps disposal, and for specific information about sharps disposal in the state that they live in.
Instruct patients not to dispose of their used sharps disposal container in their household trash unless their community guidelines permit this. Instruct patients not to recycle their used sharps disposal container.
AbbVie Inc.
North Chicago, IL 60064, U.S.A.
03-A985 May 2014
MEDICATION GUIDE
HUMIRA® (Hu-MARE-ah)
(adalimumab)
injection
Read the Medication Guide that comes with HUMIRA before you start taking it and each time you get a refill. There may be new information. This Medication Guide does not take the place of talking with your doctor about your medical condition or treatment.
What is the most important information I should know about HUMIRA?
HUMIRA is a medicine that affects your immune system. HUMIRA can lower the ability of your immune system to fight infections. **Serious infections have happened in people taking HUMIRA. These serious infections include tuberculosis (TB) and infections caused by viruses, fungi or bacteria that have spread throughout the body. Some people have died from these infections.**

• Your doctor should test you for TB before starting HUMIRA.
• Your doctor should check you closely for signs and symptoms of TB during treatment with HUMIRA.
You should not start taking HUMIRA if you have any kind of infection unless your doctor says it is okay.
Before starting HUMIRA, tell your doctor if you:
• think you have an infection or have symptoms of infection such as:

• fever, sweats, or chills	• warm, red, or painful skin or sores on your body
• muscle aches	
• cough	• diarrhea or stomach pain
• shortness of breath	• burning when you urinate or urinate more often than normal
• blood in phlegm	
• weight loss	• feel very tired

• are being treated for an infection
• get a lot of infections or have infections that keep coming back
• have diabetes
• have TB, or have been in close contact with someone with TB
• were born in, lived in, or traveled to countries where there is more risk for getting TB. Ask your doctor if you are not sure.
• live or have lived in certain parts of the country (such as the Ohio and Mississippi River valleys) where there is an increased risk for getting certain kinds of fungal infections (histoplasmosis, coccidioidomycosis, or blastomycosis). These infections may happen or become more severe if you use HUMIRA. Ask your doctor if you do not know if you have lived in an area where these infections are common.
• have or have had hepatitis B
• use the medicine ORENCIA® (abatacept), KINERET® (anakinra), RITUXAN® (rituximab), IMURAN® (azathioprine), or PURINETHOL® (6-mercaptopurine, 6-MP).
• are scheduled to have major surgery
After starting HUMIRA, call your doctor right away if you have an infection, or any sign of an infection.
HUMIRA can make you more likely to get infections or make any infection that you may have worse.
Cancer
• For children and adults taking TNF-blockers, including HUMIRA, the chances of getting cancer may increase.
• There have been cases of unusual cancers in children, teenagers, and young adults using TNF-blockers.
• People with RA, especially more serious RA, may have a higher chance for getting a kind of cancer called lymphoma.
• If you use TNF blockers including HUMIRA your chance of getting two types of skin cancer may increase (basal cell cancer and squamous cell cancer of the skin). These types of cancer are generally not life-threatening if treated. Tell your doctor if you have a bump or open sore that doesn't heal.
• Some people receiving TNF blockers including HUMIRA developed a rare type of cancer called hepatosplenic T-cell lymphoma. This type of cancer often results in death. Most of these people were male teenagers or young men. Also, most people were being treated for Crohn's disease or ulcerative colitis with another medicine called IMURAN® (azathioprine) or PURINETHOL® (6-mercaptopurine, 6-MP).
See the "What are the possible side effects of HUMIRA?" section.
What is HUMIRA?
HUMIRA is a medicine called a Tumor Necrosis Factor (TNF) blocker. HUMIRA is used:
• To reduce the signs and symptoms of:
   • **moderate to severe rheumatoid arthritis (RA) in adults.** HUMIRA can be used alone, with methotrexate, or with certain other medicines.
   • **moderate to severe polyarticular juvenile idiopathic arthritis (JIA) in children** 4 years and older. HUMIRA can be used alone, with methotrexate, or with certain other medicines.
   • **psoriatic arthritis (PsA) in adults.** HUMIRA can be used alone or with certain other medicines.
   • **ankylosing spondylitis (AS) in adults.**
   • **moderate to severe Crohn's disease (CD) in adults** when other treatments have not worked well enough.
• In adults, to help get **moderate to severe ulcerative colitis (UC)** under control (induce remission) and keep it under control (sustain remission) when certain other medicines have not worked well enough. It is not known if HUMIRA is effective in people who stopped responding to or could not tolerate TNF-blocker medicines.
• To treat **moderate to severe chronic (lasting a long time) plaque psoriasis (Ps) in adults** who have the condition in many areas of their body and who may benefit from taking injections or pills (systemic therapy) or phototherapy (treatment using ultraviolet light alone or with pills).
What should I tell my doctor before taking HUMIRA?
HUMIRA may not be right for you. Before starting HUMIRA, tell your doctor about all of your health conditions, including if you:

- have an infection. See "**What is the most important information I should know about HUMIRA?**"
- have or have had cancer.
- have any numbness or tingling or have a disease that affects your nervous system such as multiple sclerosis or Guillain-Barré syndrome.
- have or had heart failure.
- have recently received or are scheduled to receive a vaccine. You may receive vaccines, except for live vaccines while using HUMIRA. Children with juvenile idiopathic arthritis should be brought up to date with all vaccines before starting HUMIRA.
- are allergic to rubber or latex. The needle cover on the pre-filled syringe contains dry natural rubber. Tell your doctor if you have any allergies to rubber or latex.
- are allergic to HUMIRA or to any of its ingredients. See the end of this Medication Guide for a list of ingredients in HUMIRA.
- are pregnant or planning to become pregnant. It is not known if HUMIRA will harm your unborn baby. HUMIRA should only be used during a pregnancy if needed.
- breastfeeding or plan to breastfeed. You and your doctor should decide if you will breastfeed or use HUMIRA. You should not do both.

Tell your doctor about all the medicines you take, including prescription and non-prescription medicines, vitamins, and herbal supplements.

Especially tell your doctor if you use:
- ORENCIA® (abatacept), KINERET® (anakinra), REMICADE® (infliximab), ENBREL® (etanercept), CIMZIA® (certolizumab pegol) or SIMPONI® (golimumab), because you should not use HUMIRA while you are also taking one of these medicines.
- RITUXAN® (rituximab). Your doctor may not want to give you HUMIRA if you have received RITUXAN® (rituximab) recently.
- IMURAN® (azathioprine) or PURINETHOL® (6–mercaptopurine, 6-MP).

Keep a list of your medicines with you to show your doctor and pharmacist each time you get a new medicine.

How should I take HUMIRA?
- HUMIRA is given by an injection under the skin. Your doctor will tell you how often to take an injection of HUMIRA. This is based on your condition to be treated. **Do not inject HUMIRA more often than you were prescribed.**
- See the **Instructions for Use** inside the carton for complete instructions for the right way to prepare and inject HUMIRA.
- Make sure you have been shown how to inject HUMIRA before you do it yourself. You can call your doctor or 1-800-4HUMIRA (1-800-448-6472) if you have any questions about giving yourself an injection. Someone you know can also help you with your injection after he/she has been shown how to prepare and inject HUMIRA.
- **Do not** try to inject HUMIRA yourself until you have been shown the right way to give the injections. If your doctor decides that you or a caregiver may be able to give your injections of HUMIRA at home, you should receive training on the right way to prepare and inject HUMIRA.
- Do not miss any doses of HUMIRA unless your doctor says it is okay. If you forget to take HUMIRA, inject a dose as soon as you remember. Then, take your next dose at your regular scheduled time. This will put you back on schedule. In case you are not sure when to inject HUMIRA, call your doctor or pharmacist.
- If you take more HUMIRA than you were told to take, call your doctor.

What are the possible side effects of HUMIRA?
HUMIRA can cause serious side effects, including:
See "**What is the most important information I should know about HUMIRA?**"
- **Serious Infections.**
  Your doctor will examine you for TB and perform a test to see if you have TB. If your doctor feels that you are at risk for TB, you may be treated with medicine for TB before you begin treatment with HUMIRA and during treatment with HUMIRA. Even if your TB test is negative your doctor should carefully monitor you for TB infections while you are taking HUMIRA. People who had a negative TB skin test before receiving HUMIRA have developed active TB. Tell your doctor if you have any of the following symptoms while taking or after taking HUMIRA:
  - cough that does not go away
  - low grade fever
  - weight loss
  - loss of body fat and muscle (wasting)
- **Hepatitis B infection in people who carry the virus in their blood.**
  If you are a carrier of the hepatitis B virus (a virus that affects the liver), the virus can become active while you use HUMIRA. Your doctor should do blood tests before you start treatment, while you are using HUMIRA, and for several months after you stop treatment with HUMIRA. Tell your doctor if you have any of the following symptoms of a possible hepatitis B infection:

- muscle aches
- feel very tired
- dark urine
- skin or eyes look yellow
- little or no appetite
- vomiting
- clay-colored bowel movements
- fever
- chills
- stomach discomfort
- skin rash

- **Allergic reactions.** Allergic reactions can happen in people who use HUMIRA. Call your doctor or get medical help right away if you have any of these symptoms of a serious allergic reaction:
  - hives
  - swelling of your face, eyes, lips or mouth
  - trouble breathing
- **Nervous system problems.** Signs and symptoms of a nervous system problem include: numbness or tingling, problems with your vision, weakness in your arms or legs, and dizziness.
- **Blood problems.** Your body may not make enough of the blood cells that help fight infections or help to stop bleeding. Symptoms include a fever that does not go away, bruising or bleeding very easily, or looking very pale.
- **New heart failure or worsening of heart failure you already have. Call your doctor right away** if you get new worsening symptoms of heart failure while taking HUMIRA, including:
  - shortness of breath
  - swelling of your ankles or feet
  - sudden weight gain.
- **Immune reactions including a lupus-like syndrome.** Symptoms include chest discomfort or pain that does not go away, shortness of breath, joint pain, or a rash on your cheeks or arms that gets worse in the sun. Symptoms may improve when you stop HUMIRA.
- **Liver Problems.** Liver problems can happen in people who use TNF-blocker medicines. These problems can lead to liver failure and death. Call your doctor right away if you have any of these symptoms:
  - feel very tired
  - skin or eyes look yellow
  - poor appetite or vomiting
  - pain on the right side of your stomach (abdomen)
- **Psoriasis.** Some people using HUMIRA had new psoriasis or worsening of psoriasis they already had. Tell your doctor if you develop red scaly patches or raised bumps that are filled with pus. Your doctor may decide to stop your treatment with HUMIRA.

Call your doctor or get medical care right away if you develop any of the above symptoms. Your treatment with HUMIRA may be stopped.
Common side effects with HUMIRA include:
- injection site reactions: redness, rash, swelling, itching, or bruising. These symptoms usually will go away within a few days. Call your doctor right away if you have pain, redness or swelling around the injection site that does not go away within a few days or gets worse.
- upper respiratory infections (including sinus infections)
- headaches
- rash
- nausea

These are not all the possible side effects with HUMIRA. Tell your doctor if you have any side effect that bothers you or that does not go away. Ask your doctor or pharmacist for more information.

Call your doctor for medical advice about side effects. You may report side effects to the FDA at 1-800-FDA-1088.

How should I store HUMIRA?
- Store HUMIRA in a refrigerator at 36°F to 46°F (2°C to 8°C) in the original container until it is used. Protect from light.
- When traveling, HUMIRA should be stored in a cool carrier with an ice pack.
- **Do not freeze HUMIRA.** Do not use HUMIRA if frozen, even if it has been thawed.
- Refrigerated HUMIRA may be used until the expiration date printed on the HUMIRA carton, dose tray, Pen or pre-filled syringe.
- Do not use a Pen or prefilled syringe if the liquid is cloudy, discolored, or has flakes or particles in it.
- Do not drop or crush HUMIRA. The prefilled syringe is glass.
- **Keep HUMIRA, injection supplies, and all other medicines out of the reach of children.**

General information about HUMIRA
Medicines are sometimes prescribed for purposes other than those listed in a Medication Guide. Do not use HUMIRA for a condition for which it was not prescribed. Do not give HUMIRA to other people, even if they have the same condition. It may harm them.
This Medication Guide summarizes the most important information about HUMIRA. If you would like more informa-

tion, talk with your doctor. You can ask your doctor or pharmacist for information about HUMIRA that was written for healthcare professionals.
For more information go to www.HUMIRA.com or you can enroll in a patient support program by calling 1-800-4HUMIRA (1-800-448-6472).

What are the ingredients in HUMIRA?
Active ingredient: adalimumab
Inactive ingredients: sodium chloride, monobasic sodium phosphate dihydrate, dibasic sodium phosphate dihydrate, sodium citrate, citric acid monohydrate, mannitol, polysorbate 80, and Water for Injection. Sodium hydroxide is added as necessary to adjust pH.
This Medication Guide has been approved by the U.S. Food and Drug Administration.
AbbVie Inc.
North Chicago, IL 60064, U.S.A.
03-A830-R7
Content revised 05/2013

INSTRUCTIONS FOR USE
HUMIRA® (Hu-MARE-ah)
(adalimumab)
SINGLE-USE PEN
Do not try to inject HUMIRA yourself until you have been shown the right way to give the injections. If your doctor decides that you or a caregiver may be able to give your injections of HUMIRA at home, you should receive training on the right way to prepare and inject HUMIRA. It is important that you read, understand, and follow these instructions so that you inject HUMIRA the right way. Call your healthcare provider if you or your caregiver has any questions about the right way to inject HUMIRA.
IMPORTANT:
- Do not use HUMIRA if frozen, even if it has been thawed.
- The HUMIRA Pen contains glass. Do not drop or crush the Pen because the glass inside may break.
- Do not remove the gray cap or the plum-colored cap until right before your injection.
- When the plum-colored button on the HUMIRA Pen is pressed to give your dose of HUMIRA, you will hear a loud "click" sound.
  - You must practice injecting HUMIRA with your doctor or nurse so that you are not startled by this click when you start giving yourself the injections at home.
  - The loud click sound means the start of the injection.
  - You will know that the injection has finished when the yellow marker appears fully in the window view and stops moving.

See the section below called "**Prepare the HUMIRA Pen**".
How should I store HUMIRA?
- Store HUMIRA in a refrigerator at 36°F to 46°F (2°C to 8°C) in the original container until it is used. Protect from light.
- When traveling, HUMIRA should be stored in a cool carrier with an ice pack.
- **Do not freeze HUMIRA.** Do not use HUMIRA if frozen, even if it has been thawed.
- Refrigerated HUMIRA may be used until the expiration date printed on the HUMIRA carton, dose tray, and Pen.
- Do not use a Pen if the liquid is cloudy, discolored, or has flakes or particles in it.
- Do not drop or crush HUMIRA.
- **Keep HUMIRA, injection supplies, and all other medicines out of the reach of children.**

Gather the Supplies for Your Injection
- You will need the following supplies for your injection of HUMIRA.
  Find a clean, flat surface to place the supplies on.
  - 1 alcohol swab
  - 1 cotton ball or gauze pad (not included in your HUMIRA carton)
  - 1 HUMIRA Pen (See Figure A)
  - 1 FDA-cleared sharps disposal container for HUMIRA Pen disposal (not included in your HUMIRA carton)

If you do not have all of the supplies you need to give yourself an injection, go to a pharmacy or call your pharmacist. The diagram below shows what the HUMIRA Pen looks like. See Figure A.
[See figure A at top of next column]
Check the carton, dose tray, and HUMIRA Pen.
1. Make sure the name HUMIRA appears on the carton, dose tray, and HUMIRA Pen label.
2. **Do not** use and call your doctor or pharmacist if:
- you drop or crush your HUMIRA Pen.
- the seals on the top or bottom of the carton are broken or missing.

Information on the AbbVie, Inc. products listed on these pages is from the prescribing information in use as of July 31, 2014. For more information, please visit rxabbvie.com or call 1-800-633-9110.

Figure A

Plum-colored Cap (Cap #2)

Plum-colored Activator Button

Window

White Needle Sleeve

Gray Cap (Cap #1)

- the expiration date on the carton, dose tray, and Pen has passed.
- the HUMIRA Pen has been frozen or left in direct sunlight. See the section: **"How should I store HUMIRA?"** at the beginning of these Instructions For Use.

3. Hold the Pen with the gray cap (Cap # 1) pointed down.

4. Make sure the amount of liquid in the Pen is at the fill line or close to the fill line seen through the window. This is the full dose of HUMIRA that you will inject. See Figure B.

5. If the Pen does not have the full amount of liquid, **do not use that Pen**. Call your pharmacist.

Figure B

Fill Line

6. Turn the Pen over and hold the Pen with the gray cap (Cap # 1) pointed up. See Figure C.

7. Check the solution through the windows on the side of the Pen to make sure the liquid is clear and colorless. **Do not use** your HUMIRA Pen if the liquid is cloudy, discolored, or if it has flakes or particles in it. Call your pharmacist. It is normal to see one or more bubbles in the window.

Figure C

Choose the Injection Site

8. Wash and dry your hands well.

9. Choose an injection site on:
- the front of your thighs or
- your lower abdomen (belly). If you choose your abdomen, do not use the area 2 inches around your belly button (navel). See Figure D.

[See figure D at top of next column]

- Choose a different site each time you give yourself an injection. Each new injection should be given at least one inch from a site you used before.
- **Do not** inject HUMIRA into skin that is:
  - sore (tender)

Figure D

Injectable Areas

- bruised
- red
- hard
- scarred or where you have stretch marks
- If you have psoriasis, **do not** inject directly into any raised, thick, red or scaly skin patches or lesions on your skin.
- Do not inject through your clothes.

Prepare the Injection Site

10. Wipe the injection site with an alcohol prep (swab) using a circular motion.

- **Do not** touch this area again before giving the injection. Allow the skin to dry before injecting. **Do not** fan or blow on the clean area.

Preparing the HUMIRA Pen

11. **Do not remove the gray cap (Cap # 1) or the plum-colored cap (Cap # 2) until right before your injection.**

12. Hold the middle of the Pen (gray body) with one hand so that you are not touching the gray cap (Cap # 1) or the plum-colored cap (Cap # 2). Turn the Pen so that the gray cap (Cap # 1) is pointing up. See Figure E.

Figure E

13. With your other hand, pull the gray cap (Cap # 1) straight off (do not twist the cap). Make sure the small gray needle cover of the syringe has come off with the gray cap (Cap # 1). See Figure F.

14. Throw away the gray cap (Cap # 1).

Figure F

- **Do not** put the gray cap (Cap # 1) back on the Pen. Putting the gray cap (Cap # 1) back on may damage the needle.
- The white needle sleeve, which covers the needle, can now be seen.

- **Do not** touch the needle with your fingers or let the needle touch anything.
- You may see a few drops of liquid come out of the needle. This is normal.

15. Remove the plum-colored cap (Cap # 2) from the bottom of the Pen by pulling it straight off (do not twist the cap). The Pen is now activated. Throw away the plum-colored cap.

- Do not put the plum-colored cap (Cap # 2) back on the Pen because it could cause medicine to come out of the syringe.

The plum-colored activator button:

- Turn the Pen so the plum-colored activator button is pointed up. See Figure G.

Figure G

- **Do not** press the plum-colored activator button until you are ready to inject HUMIRA. Pressing the plum-colored activator button will release the medicine from the Pen.
- Hold the Pen so that you can see the window. See Figure H. It is normal to see one or more bubbles in the window.

Figure H

Position the Pen and Inject HUMIRA

16. **Position the Pen:**

- Gently squeeze the area of the cleaned skin and hold it firmly. See Figure I. You will inject into this raised area of skin.

Figure I

17. Place the white end of the Pen straight (at a 90° angle) and flat against the raised area of your skin that you are squeezing. Place the Pen so that it will not inject the needle into your fingers that are holding the raised skin. See Figure J.

Figure J

18. Inject HUMIRA
• With your index finger or your thumb, press the plum-colored activator button to begin the injection. Try not to cover the window. See Figure K.

Figure K

((click))

• You will hear a loud "click" when you press the plum-colored activator button. The loud click means the start of the injection.
• Keep pressing the plum-colored activator button and continue to hold the Pen against your squeezed, raised skin until all of the medicine is injected. This can take up to 10 seconds, so count slowly to ten. Keep holding the Pen against the squeezed, raised skin of your injection site for the whole time so you get the full dose of medicine.
• You will know that the injection has finished when the yellow marker fully appears in the window view and stops moving. See Figure L.

Figure L

Yellow Indicator

19. When the injection is finished, slowly pull the Pen from your skin. The white needle sleeve will move to cover the needle tip. See Figure M.
• Do not touch the needle. The white needle sleeve is there to prevent you from touching the needle.
[See figure M at top of next column]
• Press a cotton ball or gauze pad over the injection site and hold it for 10 seconds. Do **not** rub the injection site. You may have slight bleeding. This is normal.
20. Dispose of your used HUMIRA Pen. See the section "How should I dispose of the used HUMIRA Pen?"
21. Keep a record of the dates and location of your injection sites. To help you remember when to take HUMIRA, you can mark your calendar ahead of time.

Figure M

White Needle Sleeve

Yellow Window Marker

How should I dispose of the used HUMIRA Pen?
• Put your Pen in a FDA-cleared sharps disposal container right away after use. See Figure N. **Do not throw away (dispose of) the Pen in your household trash.**
• Do not try to touch the needle. The white needle sleeve is there to prevent you from touching the needle.

Figure N

• If you do not have a FDA-cleared sharps disposal container, you may use a household container that is:
  ○ made of a heavy-duty plastic,
  ○ can be closed with a tight-fitting, puncture-resistant lid, without sharps being able to come out,
  ○ upright and stable during use,
  ○ leak-resistant, and
  ○ properly labeled to warn of hazardous waste inside the container.
• When your sharps disposal container is almost full, you will need to follow your community guidelines for the right way to dispose of your sharps disposal container. There may be state or local laws about how you should throw away used needles and syringes. For more information about safe sharps disposal, and for specific information about sharps disposal in the state that you live in, go to the FDA's website at: http://www.fda.gov/safesharpsdisposal.
• For the safety and health of you and others, never re-use your HUMIRA Pens.
• The used alcohol pads, cotton balls, dose trays and packaging may be placed in your household trash.
• **Do not dispose of your used sharps disposal container in your household trash unless your community guidelines permit this. Do not recycle your used sharps disposal container.**
• **Always keep the sharps container out of the reach of children.**

This Instructions for Use has been approved by the U.S. Food and Drug Administration.
AbbVie Inc.
North Chicago, IL 60064, U.S.A.
03-A857-R7
Content revised 07/2013
INSTRUCTIONS FOR USE
HUMIRA® (Hu-MARE-ah)
(adalimumab)
SINGLE-USE PREFILLED SYRINGE
Do not try to inject HUMIRA yourself until you have been shown the right way to give the injections. If your doctor decides that you or a caregiver may be able to give your injections of HUMIRA at home, you should receive training on the right way to prepare and inject HUMIRA. It is important that you read, understand, and follow these instruc-

tions so that you inject HUMIRA the right way. Call your healthcare provider if you or your caregiver has any questions about the right way to inject HUMIRA.
How should I store HUMIRA?
• Store HUMIRA in a refrigerator at 36°F to 46°F (2°C to 8°C) in the original container until it is used. Protect from light.
• When traveling, HUMIRA should be stored in a cool carrier with an ice pack.
• **Do not freeze HUMIRA.** Do not use HUMIRA if frozen, even if it has been thawed.
• Refrigerated HUMIRA may be used until the expiration date printed on the HUMIRA carton, dose tray and prefilled syringe.
• Do not use a prefilled syringe if the liquid is cloudy, discolored, or has flakes or particles in it.
• Do not drop or crush HUMIRA. The prefilled syringe is glass.
• **Keep HUMIRA, injection supplies, and all other medicines out of the reach of children.**
Gather the Supplies for Your Injection
• You will need the following supplies for your injection of HUMIRA.
  Find a clean, flat surface to place the supplies on.
  • 1 alcohol swab
  • 1 cotton ball or gauze pad (not included in your HUMIRA carton)
  • 1 HUMIRA prefilled syringe (See Figure A)
  • 1 FDA-cleared sharps disposal container for HUMIRA prefilled syringe disposal (not included in your HUMIRA carton)
If you do not have all of the supplies you need to give yourself an injection, go to a pharmacy or call your pharmacist. The diagram below shows what a prefilled syringe looks like. See Figure A.

Figure A

Plunger Rod

Finger Grip

Needle Cover

Check the carton, dose tray, and prefilled syringe
1. Make sure the name HUMIRA appears on the dose tray and prefilled syringe label.
2. **Do not use** and call your doctor or pharmacist if:
• the seals on top and bottom of the carton are broken or missing.
• the HUMIRA labeling has an expired date. Check the expiration date on your HUMIRA carton and do not use if the date has passed.
• the prefilled syringe that has been frozen or left in direct sunlight. See the section: **"How should I store HUMIRA?"** at the beginning of these Instructions for Use.
• the liquid in the prefilled syringe is cloudy, discolored or has flakes or particles in it. Make sure the liquid is clear and colorless.
Choose the Injection Site
3. Wash and dry your hands well.
4. Choose an injection site on:
• the front of your thighs or
• your lower abdomen (belly). If you choose your abdomen, do not use the area 2 inches around your belly button (navel). See Figure B.
[See figure B at top of next column]
• Choose a different site each time you give yourself an injection. Each new injection should be given at least one inch from a site you used before.
• **Do not** inject into skin that is:
• sore (tender)
• bruised
• red
• hard

Information on the AbbVie, Inc. products listed on these pages is from the prescribing information in use as of July 31, 2014. For more information, please visit rxabbvie.com or call 1-800-633-9110.

Figure B

Injectable Areas

• scarred or where you have stretch marks
• If you have psoriasis, do not inject directly into any raised, thick, red or scaly skin patches or lesions on your skin.
• Do not inject through your clothes.

Prepare the Injection Site

5. Wipe the injection site with an alcohol prep (swab) using a circular motion.

6. Do **not** touch this area again before giving the injection. Allow the skin to dry before injecting. Do not fan or blow on the clean area.

Prepare the Syringe and Needle

7. Check the fluid level in the syringe:
• Always hold the prefilled syringe by the body of the syringe. Hold the syringe with the covered needle pointing down. See Figure C.

Figure C

• Hold the syringe at eye level. Look closely to make sure that the amount of liquid in the syringe is the same or close to the:
  • 0.8 mL line for the 40 mg prefilled syringe
  • 0.4 mL line for the 20 mg pediatric prefilled syringe. See Figure D.
[See figure D at top of next column]

8. The top of the liquid may be curved. If the syringe does not have the correct amount of liquid, **do not use that syringe**. Call your pharmacist.

9. Remove the needle cover:
• Hold the syringe in one hand. With the other hand gently remove the needle cover. See Figure E.
• Throw away the needle cover.
[See figure E at top of next column]
• Do not touch the needle with your fingers or let the needle touch anything.

10. Turn the syringe so the needle is facing up and hold the syringe at eye level with one hand so you can see the air in the syringe. Using your other hand, slowly push the plunger in to push the air out through the needle. See Figure F.
[See figure F at top of next column]
• You may see a drop of liquid at the end of the needle. This is normal.

Figure D

0.8 mL ➤   ◄ 0.4 mL

0.8 mL Prefilled Syringe   0.4 mL Pediatric Prefilled Syringe

Figure E

Figure F

Position the Prefilled Syringe and Inject HUMIRA

Position the Syringe

11. Hold the body of the prefilled syringe in one hand between the thumb and index finger. Hold the syringe in your hand like a pencil. See Figure G.
[See figure G at top of next column]
• **Do not** pull back on the plunger at any time.
• With your other hand, gently squeeze the area of the cleaned skin and hold it firmly. See Figure H.
[See figure H at top of next column]

Inject HUMIRA

12. Using a quick, dart-like motion, insert the needle into the squeezed skin at about a **45-degree angle**. See Figure I.
[See figure I at top of next column]
• After the needle is in, let go of the skin. Pull back gently on the plunger.

If blood appears in the syringe:
• It means that you have entered a blood vessel.
• **Do not** inject HUMIRA.

Figure G

Figure H

Figure I

45°

• Pull the needle out of the skin while keeping the syringe at the same angle.
• Press a cotton ball or gauze pad over the injection site and hold it for 10 seconds. See Figure J.
[See figure J at top of next column]
• **Do not** use the same syringe and needle again. Throw away the needle and syringe in your special sharps container.
• **Do not** rub the injection site. You may have slight bleeding. This is normal.
• Repeat Steps 1 through 12 with a new prefilled syringe.

If no blood appears in the syringe:
• Slowly push the plunger all the way in until all of the liquid is injected and the syringe is empty.
• Pull the needle out of the skin while keeping the syringe at the same angle.
• Press a cotton ball or gauze pad over the injection site and hold it for 10 seconds. Do **not** rub the injection site. You may have slight bleeding. This is normal.

Figure J

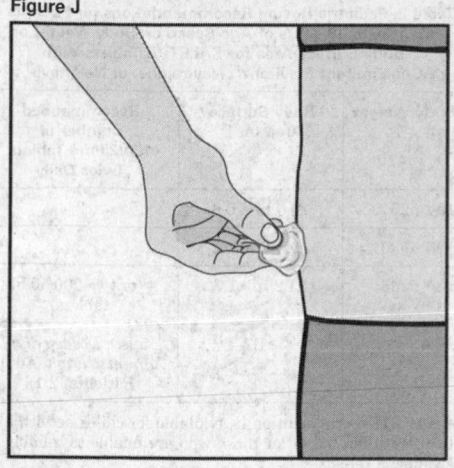

13. Throw away the used prefilled syringe and needle. See **"How should I dispose of used prefilled syringes and needles?"**

14. Keep a record of the dates and location of your injection sites. To help you remember when to take HUMIRA, you can mark your calendar ahead of time.

How should I dispose of used prefilled syringes and needles?

- Put your used needles and syringes in a FDA-cleared sharps disposal container right away after use. See Figure K. **Do not throw away (dispose of) loose needles and syringes in your household trash.**
- Do not try to touch the needle.

Figure K

- If you do not have a FDA-cleared sharps disposal container, you may use a household container that is:
  ∘ made of a heavy-duty plastic,
  ∘ can be closed with a tight-fitting, puncture-resistant lid, without sharps being able to come out,
  ∘ upright and stable during use,
  ∘ leak-resistant, and
  ∘ properly labeled to warn of hazardous waste inside the container.
- When your sharps disposal container is almost full, you will need to follow your community guidelines for the right way to dispose of your sharps disposal container. There may be state or local laws about how you should throw away used needles and syringes. For more information about safe sharps disposal, and for specific information about sharps disposal in the state that you live in, go to the FDA's website at: http://www.fda.gov/safesharpsdisposal.
- For the safety and health of you and others, needles and used syringes **must never** be re-used.
- The used alcohol pads, cotton balls, dose trays and packaging may be placed in your household trash.
- **Do not dispose of your used sharps disposal container in your household trash unless your community guidelines permit this. Do not recycle your used sharps disposal container.**
- **Always keep the sharps container out of the reach of children.**

This Instructions for Use has been approved by the U.S. Food and Drug Administration.

AbbVie Inc.
North Chicago, IL 60064, U.S.A.
03-A763-R6
Content revised 01/2013
Shown in Product Identification Guide, page 303

KALETRA® ℞
[*kuh-LEE-tra*]
(lopinavir/ritonavir)
tablet, film coated for oral use
Rx only
KALETRA
(lopinavir/ritonavir)
solution for oral use
Rx only

HIGHLIGHTS OF PRESCRIBING INFORMATION
These highlights do not include all the information needed to use KALETRA safely and effectively. See full prescribing information for KALETRA.
KALETRA (lopinavir/ritonavir) tablet, film coated for oral use
KALETRA (lopinavir/ritonavir) solution for oral use
Initial U.S. Approval: 2000

———**RECENT MAJOR CHANGES**———
Indications and Usage. (1)   01/2013

———**INDICATIONS AND USAGE**———
KALETRA is an HIV-1 protease inhibitor indicated in combination with other antiretroviral agents for the treatment of HIV-1 infection in adults and pediatric patients (14 days and older). (1)

———**DOSAGE AND ADMINISTRATION**———
Tablets: May be taken with or without food, swallowed whole and not chewed, broken, or crushed. (2)
Oral solution: must be taken with food. (2)
Do not use once daily administration of KALETRA in:
- HIV-1 infected patients with three or more of the following lopinavir resistance-associated substitutions: L10F/I/R/V, K20M/N/R, L24I, L33F, M36I, I47V, G48V, I54L/T/V, V82A/C/F/S/T, and I84V. (2.1)
- Combination with efavirenz, nevirapine, nelfinavir, carbamazepine, phenobarbital, or phenytoin. (2.1, 7.3)
- Pediatric patients. (2.2)
Adult Patients:
- 400/100 mg (two 200/50 mg tablets or 5 mL oral solution) twice daily.
  or
- 800/200 mg (four 200/50 mg tablets or 10 mL oral solution) once daily in patients with less than three lopinavir resistance-associated substitutions. (2.1)
Pediatric Patients (14 days and older):
- Twice daily dose is based on body weight or body surface area. (2.2)
Concomitant Therapy in Adults and Pediatric Patients:
- Dose adjustments of KALETRA may be needed when co-administering with efavirenz, nevirapine, or nelfinavir. (2.1, 2.2, 7.3)
KALETRA oral solution should not be administered to neonates before a postmenstrual age (first day of the mother's last menstrual period to birth plus the time elapsed after birth) of 42 weeks and a postnatal age of at least 14 days has been attained (2.2, 5.2)

———**DOSAGE FORMS AND STRENGTHS**———
- Film-coated tablets: 200 mg lopinavir and 50 mg ritonavir (3)
- Film-coated tablets: 100 mg lopinavir and 25 mg ritonavir (3)
- Oral solution: 80 mg lopinavir and 20 mg ritonavir per milliliter (3)

———**CONTRAINDICATIONS**———
Hypersensitivity to KALETRA (e.g., toxic epidermal necrolysis, Stevens-Johnson syndrome, erythema multiforme, urticaria, angioedema) or any of its ingredients, including ritonavir. (4)
Co-administration with:
- drugs highly dependent on CYP3A for clearance and for which elevated plasma levels may result in serious and/or life-threatening events. (4)
- potent CYP3A inducers where significantly reduced lopinavir plasma concentrations may be associated with the potential for loss of virologic response and possible resistance and cross resistance. (4)

———**WARNINGS AND PRECAUTIONS**———
The following have been observed in patients receiving KALETRA:
- Drug Interactions: Higher plasma concentrations of concomitant medications may occur; consider drug-drug interaction potential to reduce risk of serious or life-threatening adverse reactions. (5.1)
- Toxicity in preterm neonates: KALETRA oral solution should not be used in preterm neonates in the immediate postnatal period because of possible toxicities. A safe and effective dose of KALETRA oral solution in this patient population has not been established. (2.2, 5.2).

- Pancreatitis: Fatalities have occurred; suspend therapy as clinically appropriate. (5.3)
- Hepatotoxicity: Fatalities have occurred. Monitor liver function before and during therapy, especially in patients with underlying hepatic disease, including hepatitis B and hepatitis C, or marked transaminase elevations. (5.4, 8.6)
- QT interval prolongation and isolated cases of torsade de pointes have been reported although causality could not be established. Avoid use in patients with congenital long QT syndrome, those with hypokalemia, and with other drugs that prolong the QT interval. (5.1, 5.5, 12.3)
- PR interval prolongation may occur in some patients. Cases of second and third degree heart block have been reported. Use with caution in patients with pre-existing conduction system disease, ischemic heart disease, cardiomyopathy, underlying structural heart disease or when administering with other drugs that may prolong the PR interval. (5.1, 5.6, 12.3)
- Patients may develop new onset or exacerbations of diabetes mellitus, hyperglycemia (5.7), immune reconstitution syndrome (5.8), redistribution/accumulation of body fat. (5.10)
- Total cholesterol and triglycerides elevations. Monitor prior to therapy and periodically thereafter. (5.9)
- Hemophilia: Spontaneous bleeding may occur, and additional factor VIII may be required. (5.11)

———**ADVERSE REACTIONS**———
Commonly reported adverse reactions to KALETRA included diarrhea, nausea, vomiting, hypertriglyceridemia and hypercholesterolemia. (6.1, 6.2)

To report SUSPECTED ADVERSE REACTIONS, contact AbbVie Inc. at 1-800-633-9110 or FDA at 1-800-FDA-1088 or www.fda.gov/medwatch
———**DRUG INTERACTIONS**———
Co-administration of KALETRA can alter the plasma concentrations of other drugs and other drugs may alter the plasma concentrations of lopinavir. The potential for drug-drug interactions must be considered prior to and during therapy. (4, 5.1, 7, 12.3)

See 17 for PATIENT COUNSELING INFORMATION and Medication Guide

Revised: 11/2013

———————————————————
FULL PRESCRIBING INFORMATION: CONTENTS*

———————————————————
Information on the AbbVie, Inc. products listed on these pages is from the prescribing information in use as of July 31, 2014. For more information, please visit rxabbvie.com or call 1-800-633-9110.

13 NONCLINICAL TOXICOLOGY
  13.1 Carcinogenesis, Mutagenesis, Impairment of Fertility

14 CLINICAL STUDIES
  14.1 Adult Patients without Prior Antiretroviral Therapy
  14.2 Adult Patients with Prior Antiretroviral Therapy
  14.3 Other Studies Supporting Approval in Adult Patients
  14.4 Pediatric Studies

16 HOW SUPPLIED/STORAGE AND HANDLING
  16.1 KALETRA Tablets, 200 mg lopinavir/50 mg ritonavir
  16.2 KALETRA Tablets, 100 mg lopinavir/25 mg ritonavir
  16.3 KALETRA Oral Solution

17 PATIENT COUNSELING INFORMATION
* Sections or subsections omitted from the full prescribing information are not listed

FULL PRESCRIBING INFORMATION

1   INDICATIONS AND USAGE
KALETRA is indicated in combination with other antiretroviral agents for the treatment of HIV-1 infection in adults and pediatric patients (14 days and older).
The following points should be considered when initiating therapy with KALETRA:
• The use of other active agents with KALETRA is associated with a greater likelihood of treatment response [see Microbiology (12.4) and Clinical Studies (14)].
• Genotypic or phenotypic testing and/or treatment history should guide the use of KALETRA [see Microbiology (12.4)]. The number of baseline lopinavir resistance-associated substitutions affects the virologic response to KALETRA [see Microbiology (12.4)].

2   DOSAGE AND ADMINISTRATION
KALETRA tablets may be taken with or without food. The tablets should be swallowed whole and not chewed, broken, or crushed.
KALETRA oral solution must be taken with food.

2.1   Adult Patients
• KALETRA tablets 400/100 mg (given as two 200/50 mg tablets) twice daily.
• KALETRA oral solution 400/100 mg (5 mL) twice daily.
• KALETRA tablets 800/200 mg (given as four 200/50 mg tablets) once daily in patients with less than three lopinavir resistance-associated substitutions.
• KALETRA oral solution 800/200 mg (10 mL) once daily in patients with less than three lopinavir resistance-associated substitutions.
Once daily administration of KALETRA is not recommended for adult patients with three or more of the following lopinavir resistance-associated substitutions: L10F/I/R/V, K20M/N/R, L24I, L33F, M36I, I47V, G48V, I54L/T/V, V82A/C/F/S/T, and I84V [see Microbiology (12.4)].
KALETRA should not be administered once daily in combination with carbamazepine, phenobarbital, or phenytoin [see Drug Interactions (7)].
Concomitant Therapy: Efavirenz, Nevirapine, or Nelfinavir
[see Clinical Pharmacology (12.3) and Drug Interactions (7.3)]
KALETRA tablets and oral solution should not be administered as a once daily regimen in combination with efavirenz, nevirapine, or nelfinavir.
• A dose increase is recommended for all patients who use KALETRA tablets. The recommended dose of KALETRA tablets is 500/125 mg (such as two 200/50 tablets and one 100/25 mg tablet) twice daily in combination with efavirenz, nevirapine, or nelfinavir.
• A dose increase is recommended for all patients who use KALETRA oral solution. The recommended dose of KALETRA oral solution is 533/133 mg (6.5 mL) twice daily when used in combination with efavirenz, nevirapine, or nelfinavir.

2.2   Pediatric Patients
KALETRA tablets and oral solution should not be administered once daily in pediatric patients < 18 years of age.
KALETRA oral solution should not be administered to neonates before a postmenstrual age (first day of the mother's last menstrual period to birth plus the time elapsed after birth) of 42 weeks and a postnatal age of at least 14 days has been attained [see Warnings and Precautions (5.2)].
KALETRA oral solution contains 42.4% (v/v) alcohol and 15.3% (w/v) propylene glycol. Special attention should be given to accurate calculation of the dose of KALETRA, transcription of the medication order, dispensing information and dosing instructions to minimize the risk for medication errors, and overdose. This is especially important for infants and young children. Total amounts of alcohol and propylene glycol from all medicines that are to be given to pediatric patients 14 days to 6 months of age should be taken

into account in order to avoid toxicity from these excipients [see Warnings and Precautions (5.2) and Overdosage (10)]. Prescribers should calculate the appropriate dose of KALETRA for each individual child based on body weight (kg) or body surface area (BSA) to avoid underdosing or exceeding the recommended adult dose.
Body surface area (BSA) can be calculated as follows:

$$\text{BSA (m}^2) = \sqrt{\frac{\text{Ht (Cm)} \times \text{Wt (kg)}}{3600}}$$

The KALETRA dose can be calculated based on weight or BSA:
Based on Weight:
Patient Weight (kg) × Prescribed lopinavir dose (mg/kg) = Administered lopinavir dose (mg)
Based on BSA:
Patient BSA (m²) × Prescribed lopinavir dose (mg/m²) = Administered lopinavir dose (mg)
If KALETRA oral solution is used, the volume (mL) of KALETRA solution can be determined as follows:
Volume of KALETRA solution (mL) = Administered lopinavir dose (mg) ÷ 80 (mg/mL)
The dose of the oral solution should be administered using a calibrated dosing syringe.
Before prescribing KALETRA 100/25 mg tablets, children should be assessed for the ability to swallow intact tablets. If a child is unable to reliably swallow a KALETRA tablet, the KALETRA oral solution formulation should be prescribed.
14 Days to 6 Months:
In pediatric patients 14 days to 6 months of age, the recommended dosage of lopinavir/ritonavir using KALETRA oral solution is 16/4 mg/kg or 300/75 mg/m² twice daily. Prescribers should calculate the appropriate dose based on body weight or body surface area.
Because no data exists for dosage when administered with efavirenz, nevirapine, or nelfinavir, it is recommended that KALETRA not be administered in combination with these drugs in patients < 6 months of age.
6 Months to 18 Years:
Without Concomitant Efavirenz, Nevirapine, or Nelfinavir
Dosing recommendations using oral solution
In children 6 months to 18 years of age, the recommended dosage of lopinavir/ritonavir using KALETRA oral solution without concomitant efavirenz, nevirapine, or nelfinavir is 230/57.5 mg/m² given twice daily, not to exceed the recommended adult dose (400/100 mg [5 mL] twice daily). If weight-based dosing is preferred, the recommended dosage of lopinavir/ritonavir for patients < 15 kg is 12/3 mg/kg given twice daily and the dosage for patients ≥ 15 kg to 40 kg is 10/2.5 mg/kg given twice daily.
Dosing recommendations using tablets
Table 1 provides the dosing recommendations for pediatric patients 6 months to 18 years of age based on body weight or body surface area for KALETRA tablets.

Table 1. Pediatric Dosing Recommendations for Patients 6 Months to 18 Years of Age Based on Body Weight or Body Surface Area for KALETRA Tablets Without Concomitant Efavirenz, Nevirapine, or Nelfinavir

Body Weight (kg)	Body Surface Area (m²)*	Recommended number of 100/25 mg Tablets Twice Daily
15 to 25	≥0.6 to < 0.9	2
>25 to 35	≥0.9 to < 1.4	3
>35	≥1.4	4 (or two 200/50 mg tablets)

* KALETRA oral solution is available for children with a BSA less than 0.6 m² or those who are unable to reliably swallow a tablet.

Concomitant Therapy: Efavirenz, Nevirapine, or Nelfinavir
Dosing recommendations using oral solution
A dose increase of KALETRA to 300/75 mg/m² using KALETRA oral solution is needed when co-administered with efavirenz, nevirapine, or nelfinavir in children (both treatment-naïve and treatment-experienced) 6 months to 18 years of age, not to exceed the recommended adult dose (533/133 mg [6.5 mL] twice daily). If weight-based dosing is preferred, the recommended dosage for patients <15 kg is 13/3.25 mg/kg given twice daily and the dosage for patients >15 kg to 45 kg is 11/2.75 mg/kg given twice daily.
Dosing recommendations using tablets
Table 2 provides the dosing recommendations for pediatric patients 6 months to 18 years of age based on body weight or body surface area for KALETRA tablets when given in combination with efavirenz, nevirapine, or nelfinavir.

Table 2. Pediatric Dosing Recommendations for Patients 6 Months to 18 Years of Age Based on Body Weight or Body Surface Area for KALETRA Tablets With Concomitant Efavirenz[†], Nevirapine, or Nelfinavir[†]

Body Weight (kg)	Body Surface Area (m²)*	Recommended number of 100/25 mg Tablets Twice Daily
15 to 20	≥0.6 to < 0.8	2
>20 to 30	≥0.8 to < 1.2	3
>30 to 45	≥1.2 to <1.7	4 (or two 200/50 mg tablets)
>45	≥1.7	5 [see Dosage and Administration, Adult Patients (2.1)]

* KALETRA oral solution is available for children with a BSA less than 0.6 m² or those who are unable to reliably swallow a tablet.
† Please refer to the individual product labels for appropriate dosing in children.

3   DOSAGE FORMS AND STRENGTHS
• **KALETRA Tablets, 200 mg lopinavir/50 mg ritonavir**
Yellow, film-coated, ovaloid tablets debossed with the "a" logo and the code KA providing 200 mg lopinavir/50 mg ritonavir.
• **KALETRA Tablets, 100 mg lopinavir/25 mg ritonavir**
Pale yellow, film-coated, ovaloid tablets debossed with the "a" logo and the code KC providing 100 mg lopinavir/25 mg ritonavir.
• **KALETRA Oral Solution**
Light yellow to orange colored liquid containing 400 mg lopinavir/100 mg ritonavir per 5 mL (80 mg lopinavir/20 mg ritonavir per mL).

4   CONTRAINDICATIONS
• KALETRA is contraindicated in patients with previously demonstrated clinically significant hypersensitivity (e.g., toxic epidermal necrolysis, Stevens-Johnson syndrome, erythema multiforme, urticaria, angioedema) to any of its ingredients, including ritonavir.
• Co-administration of KALETRA is contraindicated with drugs that are highly dependent on CYP3A for clearance and for which elevated plasma concentrations are associated with serious and/or life-threatening reactions.
• Co-administration of KALETRA is contraindicated with potent CYP3A inducers where significantly reduced lopinavir plasma concentrations may be associated with the potential for loss of virologic response and possible resistance and cross-resistance. These drugs are listed in Table 3.
[See table 3 at top of next page]

5   WARNINGS AND PRECAUTIONS
5.1   Drug Interactions - CYP3A Enzyme Inhibition
KALETRA is a CYP3A inhibitor. Initiating treatment with KALETRA in patients receiving medications metabolized by CYP3A or initiating medications metabolized by CYP3A in patients already maintained on KALETRA may result in increased plasma concentrations of concomitant medications. Higher plasma concentrations of concomitant medications can result in increased or prolonged therapeutic or adverse effects, potentially leading to severe, life-threatening or fatal events. The potential for drug-drug interactions must be considered prior to and during therapy with KALETRA. Review of other medications taken by patients and monitoring of patients for adverse effects is recommended during therapy with KALETRA.
See Tables 3 and 9 for listing of drugs that are contraindicated for use with KALETRA due to potentially life-threatening adverse events, significant drug interactions, or loss of virologic activity [see Contraindications (4) and Drug Interactions (7)].
5.2   Toxicity in Preterm Neonates
KALETRA oral solution contains the excipients alcohol (42.4% v/v) and propylene glycol (15.3% w/v). When administered concomitantly with propylene glycol, ethanol competitively inhibits the metabolism of propylene glycol, which may lead to elevated concentrations. Preterm neonates may be at increased risk of propylene glycol-associated adverse events due to diminished ability to metabolize propylene glycol, thereby leading to accumulation and potential adverse events. Postmarketing life-threatening cases of cardiac toxicity (including complete AV block, bradycardia, and cardiomyopathy), lactic acidosis, acute renal failure, CNS

Table 3. Drugs That are Contraindicated with KALETRA

Drug Class	Drugs Within Class That are Contraindicated with KALETRA	Clinical Comments
Alpha 1- Adrenoreceptor Antagonist	Alfuzosin	Potentially increased alfuzosin concentrations can result in hypotension.
Antimycobacterial	Rifampin	May lead to loss of virologic response and possible resistance to KALETRA or to the class of protease inhibitors or other co-administered antiretroviral agents [see Drug Interactions (7)].
Ergot Derivatives	Dihydroergotamine, ergotamine, methylergonovine	Potential for acute ergot toxicity characterized by peripheral vasospasm and ischemia of the extremities and other tissues.
GI Motility Agent	Cisapride	Potential for cardiac arrhythmias.
Herbal Products	St. John's Wort (hypericum perforatum)	May lead to loss of virologic response and possible resistance to KALETRA or to the class of protease inhibitors.
HMG-CoA Reductase Inhibitors	Lovastatin, simvastatin	Potential for myopathy including rhabdomyolysis.
PDE5 Enzyme Inhibitor	Sildenafil[a] (Revatio®) when used for the treatment of pulmonary arterial hypertension	A safe and effective dose has not been established when used with KALETRA. There is an increased potential for sildenafil-associated adverse events, including visual abnormalities, hypotension, prolonged erection, and syncope [see Drug Interactions (7)].
Neuroleptic	Pimozide	Potential for cardiac arrhythmias.
Sedative/Hypnotics	Triazolam; orally administered midazolam[b]	Prolonged or increased sedation or respiratory depression.

[a] see Drug Interactions (7), *Table 8* for co-administration of sildenafil in patients with erectile dysfunction.
[b] see Drug Interactions (7), *Table 8* for parenterally administered midazolam.

depression and respiratory complications leading to death have been reported, predominantly in preterm neonates receiving KALETRA oral solution.

KALETRA oral solution should not be used in preterm neonates in the immediate postnatal period because of possible toxicities. A safe and effective dose of KALETRA oral solution in this patient population has not been established. However, if the benefit of using KALETRA oral solution to treat HIV infection in infants immediately after birth outweighs the potential risks, infants should be monitored closely for increases in serum osmolality and serum creatinine, and for toxicity related to KALETRA oral solution including: hyperosmolality, with or without lactic acidosis, renal toxicity, CNS depression (including stupor, coma, and apnea), seizures, hypotonia, cardiac arrhythmias and ECG changes, and hemolysis. Total amounts of alcohol and propylene glycol from all medicines that are to be given to infants should be taken into account in order to avoid toxicity from these excipients [see Dosage and Administration (2.2) and Overdosage (10)].

5.3 Pancreatitis
Pancreatitis has been observed in patients receiving KALETRA therapy, including those who developed marked triglyceride elevations. In some cases, fatalities have been observed. Although a causal relationship to KALETRA has not been established, marked triglyceride elevations are a risk factor for development of pancreatitis [see Warnings and Precautions (5.9)]. Patients with advanced HIV-1 disease may be at increased risk of elevated triglycerides and pancreatitis, and patients with a history of pancreatitis may be at increased risk for recurrence during KALETRA therapy.

Pancreatitis should be considered if clinical symptoms (nausea, vomiting, abdominal pain) or abnormalities in laboratory values (such as increased serum lipase or amylase values) suggestive of pancreatitis occur. Patients who exhibit these signs or symptoms should be evaluated and KALETRA and/or other antiretroviral therapy should be suspended as clinically appropriate.

5.4 Hepatotoxicity
Patients with underlying hepatitis B or C or marked elevations in transaminase prior to treatment may be at increased risk for developing or worsening of transaminase elevations or hepatic decompensation with use of KALETRA. There have been postmarketing reports of hepatic dysfunction, including some fatalities. These have generally occurred in patients with advanced HIV-1 disease taking multiple concomitant medications in the setting of underlying chronic hepatitis or cirrhosis. A causal relationship with KALETRA therapy has not been established.

Elevated transaminases with or without elevated bilirubin levels have been reported in HIV-1 mono-infected and uninfected patients as early as 7 days after the initiation of KALETRA in conjunction with other antiretroviral agents. In some cases, the hepatic dysfunction was serious; however, a definitive causal relationship with KALETRA therapy has not been established.

Appropriate laboratory testing should be conducted prior to initiating therapy with KALETRA and patients should be monitored closely during treatment. Increased AST/ALT monitoring should be considered in the patients with underlying chronic hepatitis or cirrhosis, especially during the first several months of KALETRA treatment [see Use in Specific Populations (8.6)].

5.5 QT Interval Prolongation
Postmarketing cases of QT interval prolongation and torsade de pointes have been reported although causality of KALETRA could not be established. Avoid use in patients with congenital long QT syndrome, those with hypokalemia, and with other drugs that prolong the QT interval [see Clinical Pharmacology (12.3)].

5.6 PR Interval Prolongation
Lopinavir/ritonavir prolongs the PR interval in some patients. Cases of second or third degree atrioventricular block have been reported. KALETRA should be used with caution in patients with underlying structural heart disease, pre-existing conduction system abnormalities, ischemic heart disease or cardiomyopathies, as these patients may be at increased risk for developing cardiac conduction abnormalities.

The impact on the PR interval of co-administration of KALETRA with other drugs that prolong the PR interval (including calcium channel blockers, beta-adrenergic blockers, digoxin and atazanavir) has not been evaluated. As a result, co-administration of KALETRA with these drugs should be undertaken with caution, particularly with those drugs metabolized by CYP3A. Clinical monitoring is recommended [see Clinical Pharmacology (12.3)].

5.7 Diabetes Mellitus/Hyperglycemia
New onset diabetes mellitus, exacerbation of pre-existing diabetes mellitus, and hyperglycemia have been reported during post-marketing surveillance in HIV-1 infected patients receiving protease inhibitor therapy. Some patients required either initiation or dose adjustments of insulin or oral hypoglycemic agents for treatment of these events. In some cases, diabetic ketoacidosis has occurred. In those patients who discontinued protease inhibitor therapy, hyperglycemia persisted in some cases. Because these events have been reported voluntarily during clinical practice, estimates of frequency cannot be made and a causal relationship between protease inhibitor therapy and these events has not been established.

5.8 Immune Reconstitution Syndrome
Immune reconstitution syndrome has been reported in patients treated with combination antiretroviral therapy, in-

cluding KALETRA. During the initial phase of combination antiretroviral treatment, patients whose immune system responds may develop an inflammatory response to indolent or residual opportunistic infections (such as *Mycobacterium avium* infection, cytomegalovirus, *Pneumocystis jirovecii* pneumonia [PCP], or tuberculosis) which may necessitate further evaluation and treatment.

Autoimmune disorders (such as Graves' disease, polymyositis, and Guillain-Barré syndrome) have also been reported to occur in the setting of immune reconstitution, however, the time to onset is more variable, and can occur many months after initiation of treatment.

5.9 Lipid Elevations
Treatment with KALETRA has resulted in large increases in the concentration of total cholesterol and triglycerides [see Adverse Reactions (6.1)]. Triglyceride and cholesterol testing should be performed prior to initiating KALETRA therapy and at periodic intervals during therapy. Lipid disorders should be managed as clinically appropriate, taking into account any potential drug-drug interactions with KALETRA and HMG-CoA reductase inhibitors [see Contraindications (4) and Drug Interactions (7.3)].

5.10 Fat Redistribution
Redistribution/accumulation of body fat including central obesity, dorsocervical fat enlargement (buffalo hump), peripheral wasting, facial wasting, breast enlargement, and "cushingoid appearance" have been observed in patients receiving antiretroviral therapy. The mechanism and long-term consequences of these events are currently unknown. A causal relationship has not been established.

5.11 Patients with Hemophilia
Increased bleeding, including spontaneous skin hematomas and hemarthrosis have been reported in patients with hemophilia type A and B treated with protease inhibitors. In some patients additional factor VIII was given. In more than half of the reported cases, treatment with protease inhibitors was continued or reintroduced. A causal relationship between protease inhibitor therapy and these events has not been established.

5.12 Resistance/Cross-resistance
Because the potential for HIV cross-resistance among protease inhibitors has not been fully explored in KALETRA-treated patients, it is unknown what effect therapy with KALETRA will have on the activity of subsequently administered protease inhibitors [see Microbiology (12.4)].

6 ADVERSE REACTIONS
The following adverse reactions are discussed in greater detail in other sections of the labeling.
- QT Interval Prolongation, PR Interval Prolongation [see Warnings and Precautions (5.5, 5.6)]
- Drug Interactions [see Warnings and Precautions (5.1)]
- Pancreatitis [see Warnings and Precautions (5.3)]
- Hepatotoxicity [see Warnings and Precautions (5.4)]

Because clinical trials are conducted under widely varying conditions, adverse reactions rates observed in the clinical trials of a drug cannot be directly compared to rates in the clinical trials of another drug and may not reflect the rates observed in clinical practice.

6.1 Adult Clinical Trial Experience
Treatment-Emergent Adverse Reactions
The safety of KALETRA has been investigated in about 2,600 patients in Phase II-IV clinical trials, of which about 700 have received a dose of 800/200 mg (6 capsules or 4 tablets) once daily. Along with nucleoside reverse transcriptase inhibitors (NRTIs), in some studies, KALETRA was used in combination with efavirenz or nevirapine.

In clinical studies the incidence of diarrhea in patients treated with either KALETRA capsules or tablets was greater in those patients treated once daily than in those patients treated twice daily. Any grade of diarrhea was reported by at least half of patients taking once daily Kaletra capsules or tablets. At the time of treatment discontinuation, 4.2-6.3% of patients taking once daily Kaletra and 1.8-3.7% of those taking twice daily Kaletra reported ongoing diarrhea.

Commonly reported adverse reactions to KALETRA included diarrhea, nausea, vomiting, hypertriglyceridemia and hypercholesterolemia. Diarrhea, nausea and vomiting may occur at the beginning of the treatment while hypertriglyceridemia and hypercholesterolemia may occur later. The following have been identified as adverse reactions of moderate or severe intensity (Table 4):

Information on the AbbVie, Inc. products listed on these pages is from the prescribing information in use as of July 31, 2014. For more information, please visit rxabbvie.com or call 1-800-633-9110.

Table 4. Treatment-Emergent Adverse Reactions of Moderate or Severe Intensity Occurring in at Least 0.1% of Adult Patients Receiving KALETRA in Combined Phase II/IV Studies (N=2,612)

System Organ Class (SOC) and Adverse Reaction	n	%
BLOOD AND LYMPHATIC SYSTEM DISORDERS		
anemia*	54	2.1
leukopenia and neutropenia*	44	1.7
lymphadenopathy*	35	1.3
CARDIAC DISORDERS		
atherosclerosis such as myocardial infarction*	10	0.4
atrioventricular block*	3	0.1
tricuspid valve incompetence*	3	0.1
EAR AND LABYRINTH DISORDERS		
vertigo*	7	0.3
tinnitus	6	0.2
ENDOCRINE DISORDERS		
hypogonadism*	16	0.8[1]
EYE DISORDERS		
visual impairment*	8	0.3
GASTROINTESTINAL DISORDERS		
diarrhea*	510	19.5
nausea	269	10.3
vomiting*	177	6.8
abdominal pain (upper and lower)*	160	6.1
gastroenteritis and colitis*	66	2.5
dyspepsia	53	2.0
pancreatitis*	45	1.7
Gastroesophageal Reflux Disease (GERD)*	40	1.5
hemorrhoids	39	1.5
flatulence	36	1.4
abdominal distension	34	1.3
constipation*	26	1.0
stomatitis and oral ulcers*	24	0.9
duodenitis and gastritis*	20	0.8
gastrointestinal hemorrhage including rectal hemorrhage*	13	0.5
dry mouth	9	0.3
gastrointestinal ulcer*	6	0.2
fecal incontinence	5	0.2
GENERAL DISORDERS AND ADMINISTRATION SITE CONDITIONS		
fatigue including asthenia*	198	7.6
HEPATOBILIARY DISORDERS		
hepatitis including AST, ALT, and GGT increases*	91	3.5
hepatomegaly	5	0.2
cholangitis	3	0.1

System Organ Class (SOC) and Adverse Reaction	n	%
hepatic steatosis	3	0.1
IMMUNE SYSTEM DISORDERS		
hypersensitivity including urticaria and angioedema*	70	2.7
immune reconstitution syndrome	3	0.1
INFECTIONS AND INFESTATIONS		
upper respiratory tract infection*	363	13.9
lower respiratory tract infection*	202	7.7
skin infections including cellulitis, folliculitis, and furuncle*	86	3.3
METABOLISM AND NUTRITION DISORDERS		
hypercholesterolemia*	192	7.4
hypertriglyceridemia*	161	6.2
weight decreased*	61	2.3
decreased appetite	52	2.0
blood glucose disorders including diabetes mellitus*	30	1.1
weight increased*	20	0.8
lactic acidosis*	11	0.4
increased appetite	5	0.2
MUSCULOSKELETAL AND CONNECTIVE TISSUE DISORDERS		
musculoskeletal pain including arthralgia and back pain*	166	6.4
myalgia*	46	1.8
muscle disorders such as weakness and spasms*	34	1.3
rhabdomyolysis*	18	0.7
osteonecrosis	3	0.1
NERVOUS SYSTEM DISORDERS		
headache including migraine*	165	6.3
insomnia*	99	3.8
neuropathy and peripheral neuropathy*	51	2.0
dizziness*	45	1.7
ageusia*	19	0.7
convulsion*	9	0.3
tremor*	9	0.3
cerebral vascular event*	6	0.2
PSYCHIATRIC DISORDERS		
anxiety*	101	3.9
abnormal dreams*	19	0.7
libido decreased	19	0.7
RENAL AND URINARY DISORDERS		
renal failure*	31	1.2
hematuria*	20	0.8
nephritis*	3	0.1
REPRODUCTIVE SYSTEM AND BREAST DISORDERS		
erectile dysfunction*	34	1.7[1]
menstrual disorders - amenorrhea, menorrhagia*	10	1.7[2]

System Organ Class (SOC) and Adverse Reaction	n	%
SKIN AND SUBCUTANEOUS TISSUE DISORDERS		
rash including maculopapular rash*	99	3.8
lipodystrophy acquired including facial wasting*	58	2.2
dermatitis/rash including eczema and seborrheic dermatitis*	50	1.9
night sweats*	42	1.6
pruritus*	29	1.1
alopecia	10	0.4
capillaritis and vasculitis*	3	0.1
VASCULAR DISORDERS		
hypertension*	47	1.8
deep vein thrombosis*	17	0.7

*Represents a medical concept including several similar MedDRA PTs
[1]. Percentage of male population (N=2,038)
[2]. Percentage of female population (N=574)

Laboratory Abnormalities
The percentages of adult patients treated with combination therapy with Grade 3-4 laboratory abnormalities are presented in Table 5 (treatment-naïve patients) and Table 6 (treatment-experienced patients).
[See table 5 at top of next page]
[See table 6 at top of page 474]

6.2   Pediatric Clinical Trial Experience
KALETRA oral solution dosed up to 300/75 mg/m^2 has been studied in 100 pediatric patients 6 months to 12 years of age. The adverse reaction profile seen during Study 940 was similar to that for adult patients.

Dysgeusia (22%), vomiting (21%), and diarrhea (12%) were the most common adverse reactions of any severity reported in pediatric patients treated with combination therapy for up to 48 weeks in Study 940. A total of 8 patients experienced adverse reactions of moderate to severe intensity. The adverse reactions meeting these criteria and reported for the 8 subjects include: hypersensitivity (characterized by fever, rash and jaundice), pyrexia, viral infection, constipation, hepatomegaly, pancreatitis, vomiting, alanine aminotransferase increased, dry skin, rash, and dysgeusia. Rash was the only event of those listed that occurred in 2 or more subjects (N = 3).

KALETRA oral solution dosed at 300/75 mg/m^2 has been studied in 31 pediatric patients 14 days to 6 months of age. The adverse reaction profile in Study 1030 was similar to that observed in older children and adults. No adverse reaction was reported in greater than 10% of subjects. Adverse drug reactions of moderate to severe intensity occurring in 2 or more subjects included decreased neutrophil count (N=3), anemia (N=2), high potassium (N=2), and low sodium (N=2).

KALETRA oral solution and soft gelatin capsules dosed at higher than recommended doses including 400/100 mg/m^2 (without concomitant NNRTI) and 480/120 mg/m^2 (with concomitant NNRTI) have been studied in 26 pediatric patients 7 to 18 years of age in Study 1038. Patients also had saquinavir mesylate added to their regimen at Week 4. Rash (12%), blood cholesterol abnormal (12%) and blood triglycerides abnormal (12%) were the only adverse reactions reported in greater than 10% of subjects. Adverse drug reactions of moderate to severe intensity occurring in 2 or more subjects included rash (N=3), blood triglycerides abnormal (N=3), and electrocardiogram QT prolonged (N=2). Both subjects with QT prolongation had additional predisposing conditions such as electrolyte abnormalities, concomitant medications, or pre-existing cardiac abnormalities.

Laboratory Abnormalities
The percentages of pediatric patients treated with combination therapy including KALETRA with Grade 3-4 laboratory abnormalities are presented in Table 7.

Table 7. Grade 3-4 Laboratory Abnormalities Reported in ≥ 2% Pediatric Patients in Study 940

Variable	Limit[1]	KALETRA Twice Daily + RTIs (N = 100)
Chemistry	**High**	
Sodium	> 149 mEq/L	3%
Total Bilirubin	≥ 3.0 × ULN	3%

SGOT/AST	> 180 U/L	8%
SGPT/ALT	> 215 U/L	7%
Total Cholesterol	> 300 mg/dL	3%
Amylase	> 2.5 × ULN	7%[2]
Chemistry	**Low**	
Sodium	< 130 mEq/L	3%
Hematology	**Low**	
Platelet Count	< 50 × 10⁹/L	4%
Neutrophils	< 0.40 × 10⁹/L	2%

[1] ULN = upper limit of the normal range.
[2] Subjects with Grade 3-4 amylase confirmed by elevations in pancreatic amylase.

6.3 Postmarketing Experience

The following adverse reactions have been reported during postmarketing use of KALETRA. Because these reactions are reported voluntarily from a population of unknown size, it is not possible to reliably estimate their frequency or establish a causal relationship to KALETRA exposure.

Body as a Whole
Redistribution/accumulation of body fat has been reported *[see Warnings and Precautions (5.10)]*.

Cardiovascular
Bradyarrhythmias. First-degree AV block, second-degree AV block, third-degree AV block, QTc interval prolongation, torsades (torsade) de pointes *[see Warnings and Precautions (5.5, 5.6)]*.

Skin and Appendages
Toxic epidermal necrolysis (TEN), Stevens-Johnson syndrome and erythema multiforme.

7 DRUG INTERACTIONS

See also Contraindications (4), Warnings and Precautions (5.1), Clinical Pharmacology (12.3)

7.1 Potential for KALETRA to Affect Other Drugs

Lopinavir/ritonavir is an inhibitor of CYP3A and may increase plasma concentrations of agents that are primarily metabolized by CYP3A. Agents that are extensively metabolized by CYP3A and have high first pass metabolism appear to be the most susceptible to large increases in AUC (> 3-fold) when co-administered with KALETRA. Thus, co-administration of KALETRA with drugs highly dependent on CYP3A for clearance and for which elevated plasma concentrations are associated with serious and/or life-threatening events is contraindicated. Co-administration with other CYP3A substrates may require a dose adjustment or additional monitoring as shown in Table 8.
Additionally, KALETRA induces glucuronidation.

7.2 Potential for Other Drugs to Affect Lopinavir

Lopinavir/ritonavir is a CYP3A substrate; therefore, drugs that induce CYP3A may decrease lopinavir plasma concentrations and reduce KALETRA's therapeutic effect. Although not observed in the KALETRA/ketoconazole drug interaction study, co-administration of KALETRA and other drugs that inhibit CYP3A may increase lopinavir plasma concentrations.

7.3 Established and Other Potentially Significant Drug Interactions

Table 8 provides a listing of established or potentially clinically significant drug interactions. Alteration in dose or regimen may be recommended based on drug interaction studies or predicted interaction *[see Clinical Pharmacology (12.3) for magnitude of interaction]*.
[See table 8 on pages 475 through 479]

7.4 Drugs with No Observed or Predicted Interactions with KALETRA

Drug interaction or clinical studies reveal no clinically significant interaction between KALETRA and desipramine (CYP2D6 probe), pitavastatin, pravastatin, stavudine, lamivudine, omeprazole, raltegravir, or ranitidine.
Based on known metabolic profiles, clinically significant drug interactions are not expected between KALETRA and dapsone, trimethoprim/sulfamethoxazole, azithromycin, erythromycin, or fluconazole.

8 USE IN SPECIFIC POPULATIONS

8.1 Pregnancy

Pregnancy Category C.
Antiretroviral Pregnancy Registry: To monitor maternal-fetal outcomes of pregnant women exposed to KALETRA, an Antiretroviral Pregnancy Registry has been established. Physicians are encouraged to register patients by calling 1-800-258-4263.

Table 5. Grade 3-4 Laboratory Abnormalities Reported in ≥ 2% of Adult Antiretroviral-Naïve Patients

Variable	Limit[1]	Study 863 (48 Weeks) KALETRA 400/100 mg Twice Daily + d4T +3TC (N = 326)	Study 863 (48 Weeks) Nelfinavir 750 mg Three Times Daily + d4T + 3TC (N = 327)	Study 720 (360 Weeks) KALETRA Twice Daily + d4T + 3TC (N = 100)	Study 730 (48 Weeks) KALETRA Once Daily + TDF +FTC (N=333)	Study 730 (48 Weeks) KALETRA Twice Daily + TDF +FTC (N=331)
Chemistry	**High**					
Glucose	> 250 mg/dL	2%	2%	4%	0%	<1%
Uric Acid	> 12 mg/dL	2%	2%	5%	<1%	1%
SGOT/AST[2]	> 180 U/L	2%	4%	10%	1%	2%
SGPT/ALT[2]	>215 U/L	4%	4%	11%	1%	1%
GGT	>300 U/L	N/A	N/A	10%	N/A	N/A
Total Cholesterol	>300 mg/dL	9%	5%	27%	4%	3%
Triglycerides	>750 mg/dL	9%	1%	29%	3%	6%
Amylase	>2 × ULN	3%	2%	4%	N/A	N/A
Lipase	>2 × ULN	N/A	N/A	N/A	3%	5%
Chemistry	**Low**					
Calculated Creatinine Clearance	<50 mL/min	N/A	N/A	N/A	2%	2%
Hematology	**Low**					
Neutrophils	<0.75 × 10⁹/L	1%	3%	5%	2%	1%

[1] ULN = upper limit of the normal range; N/A = Not Applicable.
[2] Criterion for Study 730 was >5x ULN (AST/ALT).

Human Data

There are no adequate and well-controlled studies in pregnant women. KALETRA should be used during pregnancy only if the potential benefit justifies the potential risk to the fetus.

Antiretroviral Pregnancy Registry

As of January 2011, the Antiretroviral Pregnancy Registry (APR) has received prospective reports of 2458 exposures to lopinavir containing regimens (738 exposed in the first trimester and 1720 exposed in the second and third trimester). Birth defects occurred in 16 of the 738 (2.2%) live births (first trimester exposure) and 41 of the 1720 (2.4%) live births (second/third trimester exposure). Among pregnant women in the U.S. reference population, the background rate of birth defects is 2.7%. There was no association between lopinavir and overall birth defects observed in the APR.

Animal Data

No treatment-related malformations were observed when lopinavir in combination with ritonavir was administered to pregnant rats or rabbits. Embryonic and fetal developmental toxicities (early resorption, decreased fetal viability, decreased fetal body weight, increased incidence of skeletal variations and skeletal ossification delays) occurred in rats at a maternally toxic dosage. Based on AUC measurements, the drug exposures in rats at the toxic doses were approximately 0.7-fold for lopinavir and 1.8-fold for ritonavir for males and females that of the exposures in humans at the recommended therapeutic dose (400/100 mg twice daily). In a peri- and postnatal study in rats, a developmental toxicity (a decrease in survival in pups between birth and postnatal Day 21) occurred.
No embryonic and fetal developmental toxicities were observed in rabbits at a maternally toxic dosage. Based on AUC measurements, the drug exposures in rabbits at the toxic doses were approximately 0.6-fold for lopinavir and 1.0-fold for ritonavir that of the exposures in humans at the recommended therapeutic dose (400/100 mg twice daily).

8.3 Nursing Mothers

The Centers for Disease Control and Prevention recommend that HIV-1 infected mothers not breastfeed their infants to avoid risking postnatal transmission of HIV-1. Studies in rats have demonstrated that lopinavir is secreted in milk. It is not known whether lopinavir is secreted in human milk. Because of both the potential for HIV-1 transmission and the potential for serious adverse reactions in nursing infants, mothers should be instructed not to breastfeed if they are receiving KALETRA.

8.4 Pediatric Use

The safety, efficacy, and pharmacokinetic profiles of KALETRA in pediatric patients below the age of 14 days have not been established. KALETRA once daily has not been evaluated in pediatric patients.
An open-label, multi-center, dose-finding trial was performed to evaluate the pharmacokinetic profile, tolerability, safety and efficacy of KALETRA oral solution containing lopinavir 80 mg/mL and ritonavir 20 mg/mL at a dose of 300/75 mg/m² twice daily plus two NRTIs in HIV-infected infants ≥14 days and < 6 months of age. Results revealed that infants younger than 6 months of age generally had lower lopinavir AUC₁₂ than older children (6 months to 12 years of age), however, despite the lower lopinavir drug exposure observed, antiviral activity was demonstrated as reflected in the proportion of subjects who achieved HIV-1 RNA <400 copies/mL at Week 24 *[see Adverse Reactions (6.2), Clinical Pharmacology (12.3), Clinical Studies (14.4)]*. Safety and efficacy in pediatric patients > 6 months of age was demonstrated in a clinical trial in 100 patients. The clinical trial was an open-label, multicenter trial evaluating the pharmacokinetic profile, tolerability, safety, and efficacy of KALETRA oral solution containing lopinavir 80 mg/mL and ritonavir 20 mg/mL in 100 antiretroviral naïve and experienced pediatric patients ages 6 months to 12 years. Dose selection for patients 6 months to 12 years of age was based on the following results. The 230/57.5 mg/m² oral solution twice daily regimen without nevirapine and the 300/75 mg/m² oral solution twice daily regimen with nevirapine provided lopinavir plasma concentrations similar to those obtained in adult patients receiving the 400/100 mg twice daily regimen (without nevirapine) *[see Adverse Reactions (6.2), Clinical Pharmacology (12.3), Clinical Studies (14.4)]*.
A prospective multicenter, open-label trial evaluated the pharmacokinetic profile, tolerability, safety and efficacy of

Information on the AbbVie, Inc. products listed on these pages is from the prescribing information in use as of July 31, 2014. For more information, please visit rxabbvie.com or call 1-800-633-9110.

Table 6. Grade 3-4 Laboratory Abnormalities Reported in ≥ 2% of Adult Protease Inhibitor-Experienced Patients

| Variable | Limit[1] | Study 888 (48 Weeks) | | Study 957[2] and Study 765[3] (84-144 Weeks) | Study 802 (48 Weeks) | |
		KALETRA 400/100 mg Twice Daily + NVP + NRTIs (N = 148)	Investigator-Selected Protease Inhibitor(s) + NVP + NRTIs (N = 140)	KALETRA Twice Daily + NNRTI + NRTIs (N = 127)	KALETRA 800/200 mg Once Daily +NRTIs (N=300)	KALETRA 400/100 mg Twice Daily +NRTIs (N=299)
Chemistry	**High**					
Glucose	>250 mg/dL	1%	2%	5%	2%	2%
Total Bilirubin	>3.48 mg/dL	1%	3%	1%	1%	1%
SGOT/AST[4]	>180 U/L	5%	11%	8%	3%	2%
SGPT/ALT[4]	>215 U/L	6%	13%	10%	2%	2%
GGT	>300 U/L	N/A	N/A	29%	N/A	N/A
Total Cholesterol	>300 mg/dL	20%	21%	39%	6%	7%
Triglycerides	>750 mg/dL	25%	21%	36%	5%	6%
Amylase	>2 × ULN	4%	8%	8%	4%	4%
Lipase	>2 × ULN	N/A	N/A	N/A	4%	1%
Creatine Phosphokinase	>4 × ULN	N/A	N/A	N/A	4%	5%
Chemistry	**Low**					
Calculated Creatinine Clearance	<50 mL/min	N/A	N/A	N/A	3%	3%
Inorganic Phosphorus	<1.5 mg/dL	1%	0%	2%	1%	<1%
Hematology	**Low**					
Neutrophils	$<0.75 \times 10^9$/L	1%	2%	4%	3%	4%
Hemoglobin	<80 g/L	1%	1%	1%	1%	2%

[1] ULN = upper limit of the normal range; N/A = Not Applicable.
[2] Includes clinical laboratory data from patients receiving 400/100 mg twice daily (n = 29) or 533/133 mg twice daily (n = 28) for 84 weeks. Patients received KALETRA in combination with NRTIs and efavirenz.
[3] Includes clinical laboratory data from patients receiving 400/100 mg twice daily (n = 36) or 400/200 mg twice daily (n = 34) for 144 weeks. Patients received KALETRA in combination with NRTIs and nevirapine.
[4] Criterion for Study 802 was >5x ULN (AST/ALT).

high-dose KALETRA with or without concurrent NNRTI therapy (Group 1: 400/100 mg/m[2] twice daily + ≥ 2 NRTIs; Group 2: 480/120 mg/m[2] twice daily + ≥ 1 NRTI + 1 NNRTI) in 26 children and adolescents ≥ 2 years to < 18 years of age who had failed prior therapy. Patients also had saquinavir mesylate added to their regimen. This strategy was intended to assess whether higher than approved doses of KALETRA could overcome protease inhibitor cross-resistance. High doses of KALETRA exhibited a safety profile similar to those observed in previous trials; changes in HIV-1 RNA were less than anticipated; three patients had HIV-1 RNA <400 copies/mL at Week 48. CD4+ cell count increases were noted in the eight patients who remained on treatment for 48 weeks [see Adverse Reactions (6.2), Clinical Pharmacology (12.3)].

8.5 Geriatric Use
Clinical studies of KALETRA did not include sufficient numbers of subjects aged 65 and over to determine whether they respond differently from younger subjects. In general, appropriate caution should be exercised in the administration and monitoring of KALETRA in elderly patients reflecting the greater frequency of decreased hepatic, renal, or cardiac function, and of concomitant disease or other drug therapy.

8.6 Hepatic Impairment
KALETRA is principally metabolized by the liver; therefore, caution should be exercised when administering this drug to patients with hepatic impairment, because lopinavir concentrations may be increased [see Warnings and Precautions (5.4) and Clinical Pharmacology (12.3)].

10 OVERDOSAGE
Overdoses with KALETRA oral solution have been reported. One of these reports described fatal cardiogenic shock in a 2.1 kg infant who received a single dose of 6.5 mL of KALETRA oral solution (520 mg lopinavir, approximately 10-fold above the recommended lopinavir dose) nine days prior. The following events have been reported in association with unintended overdoses in preterm neonates: complete AV block, cardiomyopathy, lactic acidosis, and acute renal failure [see Warnings and Precautions (5.2)]. Healthcare professionals should be aware that KALETRA oral solution is highly concentrated and therefore, should pay special attention to accurate calculation of the dose of KALETRA, transcription of the medication order, dispensing information and dosing instructions to minimize the risk for medication errors and overdose. This is especially important for infants and young children.

KALETRA oral solution contains 42.4% alcohol (v/v) and 15.3% propylene glycol (w/v). Ingestion of the product over the recommended dose by an infant or a young child could result in significant toxicity and could potentially be lethal. Human experience of acute overdosage with KALETRA is limited. Treatment of overdose with KALETRA should consist of general supportive measures including monitoring of vital signs and observation of the clinical status of the patient. There is no specific antidote for overdose with KALETRA. If indicated, elimination of unabsorbed drug should be achieved by gastric lavage. Administration of activated charcoal may also be used to aid in removal of unabsorbed drug. Since lopinavir is highly protein bound, dialysis is unlikely to be beneficial in significant removal of the drug. However, dialysis can remove both alcohol and propylene glycol in the case of overdose with KALETRA oral solution.

11 DESCRIPTION
KALETRA (lopinavir/ritonavir) is a co-formulation of lopinavir and ritonavir. Lopinavir is an inhibitor of the HIV-1 protease. As co-formulated in KALETRA, ritonavir inhibits the CYP3A-mediated metabolism of lopinavir, thereby providing increased plasma levels of lopinavir. Lopinavir is chemically designated as [1S-[1R*,(R*), 3R*, 4R*]]-N-[4-[[(2,6-dimethylphenoxy)acetyl]amino]-3-hydroxy-5-phenyl-1-(phenylmethyl)pentyl]tetrahydro-alpha-(1-methylethyl)-2-oxo-1(2H)-pyrimidineacetamide. Its molecular formula is $C_{37}H_{48}N_4O_5$, and its molecular weight is 628.80. Lopinavir is a white to light tan powder. It is freely soluble in methanol and ethanol, soluble in isopropanol and practically insoluble in water. Lopinavir has the following structural formula:

Ritonavir is chemically designated as 10-hydroxy-2-methyl-5-(1-methylethyl)-1- [2-(1-methylethyl)-4-thiazolyl]-3,6-dioxo-8,11-bis(phenylmethyl)-2,4,7,12-tetraazatridecan-13-oic acid, 5-thiazolylmethyl ester, [5S-(5R*,8R*,10R*,11R*)]. Its molecular formula is $C_{37}H_{48}N_6O_5S_2$, and its molecular weight is 720.95. Ritonavir is a white to light tan powder. It is freely soluble in methanol and ethanol, soluble in isopropanol and practically insoluble in water. Ritonavir has the following structural formula:

KALETRA film-coated tablets are available for oral administration in two strengths:
• Yellow tablets containing 200 mg of lopinavir and 50 mg of ritonavir
• Pale yellow tablets containing 100 mg of lopinavir and 25 mg of ritonavir

The yellow, 200 mg lopinavir/50 mg ritonavir, tablets contain the following inactive ingredients: copovidone, sorbitan monolaurate, colloidal silicon dioxide, and sodium stearyl fumarate. The following are the ingredients in the film coating: hypromellose, titanium dioxide, polyethylene glycol 400, hydroxypropyl cellulose, talc, colloidal silicon dioxide, polyethylene glycol 3350, yellow ferric oxide E172, and polysorbate 80.

The pale yellow, 100 mg lopinavir/25 mg ritonavir, tablets contain the following inactive ingredients: copovidone, sorbitan monolaurate, colloidal silicon dioxide, and sodium stearyl fumarate. The following are the ingredients in the film coating: polyvinyl alcohol, titanium dioxide, talc, polyethylene glycol 3350, and yellow ferric oxide E172.

KALETRA oral solution is available for oral administration as 80 mg lopinavir and 20 mg ritonavir per milliliter with the following inactive ingredients: acesulfame potassium, alcohol, artificial cotton candy flavor, citric acid, glycerin, high fructose corn syrup, Magnasweet-110 flavor, menthol, natural & artificial vanilla flavor, peppermint oil, polyoxyl 40 hydrogenated castor oil, povidone, propylene glycol, saccharin sodium, sodium chloride, sodium citrate, and water. KALETRA oral solution contains 42.4% alcohol (v/v).

12 CLINICAL PHARMACOLOGY
12.1 Mechanism of Action
Lopinavir is an antiviral drug [see Microbiology (12.4)]. As co-formulated in KALETRA, ritonavir inhibits the CYP3A-mediated metabolism of lopinavir, thereby providing increased plasma levels of lopinavir.

12.3 Pharmacokinetics
The pharmacokinetic properties of lopinavir co-administered with ritonavir have been evaluated in healthy adult volunteers and in HIV-1 infected patients; no substantial differences were observed between the two groups. Lopinavir is essentially completely metabolized by CYP3A. Ritonavir inhibits the metabolism of lopinavir, thereby increasing the plasma levels of lopinavir. Across studies, administration of KALETRA 400/100 mg twice daily yields mean steady-state lopinavir plasma concentrations 15- to 20-fold higher than those of ritonavir in HIV-1 infected patients. The plasma levels of ritonavir are less than 7% of those obtained after the ritonavir dose of 600 mg twice daily. The in vitro antiviral EC_{50} of lopinavir is approximately 10-fold lower than that of ritonavir. Therefore, the antiviral activity of KALETRA is due to lopinavir.

Table 8. Established and Other Potentially Significant Drug Interactions

Concomitant Drug Class: Drug Name	Effect on Concentration of Lopinavir or Concomitant Drug	Clinical Comments
HIV-1 Antiviral Agents		
HIV-1 Protease Inhibitor: fosamprenavir/ritonavir	↓ amprenavir ↓ lopinavir	An increased rate of adverse reactions has been observed with co-administration of these medications. Appropriate doses of the combinations with respect to safety and efficacy have not been established.
HIV-1 Protease Inhibitor: indinavir*	↑ indinavir	Decrease indinavir dose to 600 mg twice daily, when co-administered with KALETRA 400/100 mg twice daily [see *Clinical Pharmacology (12.3)*]. KALETRA once daily has not been studied in combination with indinavir.
HIV-1 Protease Inhibitor: nelfinavir*	↑ nelfinavir ↑ M8 metabolite of nelfinavir ↓ lopinavir	KALETRA should not be administered once daily in combination with nelfinavir [see *Dosage and Administration (2.1)* and *Clinical Pharmacology (12.3)*].
HIV-1 Protease Inhibitor: ritonavir*	↑ lopinavir	Appropriate doses of additional ritonavir in combination with KALETRA with respect to safety and efficacy have not been established.
HIV-1 Protease Inhibitor: saquinavir*	↑ saquinavir	The saquinavir dose is 1000 mg twice daily, when co-administered with KALETRA 400/100 mg twice daily. KALETRA once daily has not been studied in combination with saquinavir.
HIV-1 Protease Inhibitor: tipranavir	↓ lopinavir AUC and C_{min}	KALETRA should not be administered with tipranavir (500 mg twice daily) co-administered with ritonavir (200 mg twice daily).
HIV CCR5 – Antagonist: maraviroc	↑ maraviroc	Concurrent administration of maraviroc with KALETRA will increase plasma levels of maraviroc. When co-administered, patients should receive 150 mg twice daily of maraviroc. For further details see complete prescribing information for Selzentry® (maraviroc).
Non-nucleoside Reverse Transcriptase Inhibitors: efavirenz*, nevirapine*	↓ lopinavir	KALETRA dose increase is recommended in all patients [see *Dosage and Administration (2.1)* and *Clinical Pharmacology (12.3)*]. Increasing the dose of KALETRA tablets to 500/125 mg (given as two 200/50 mg tablets and one 100/25 mg tablet) twice daily co-administered with efavirenz resulted in similar lopinavir concentrations compared to KALETRA tablets 400/100 mg (given as two 200/50 mg tablets) twice daily without efavirenz. Increasing the dose of KALETRA tablets to 600/150 mg (given as three 200/50 mg tablets) twice daily co-administered with efavirenz resulted in significantly higher lopinavir plasma concentrations compared to KALETRA tablets 400/100 mg twice daily without efavirenz. KALETRA should not be administered once daily in combination with efavirenz or nevirapine [see *Dosage and Administration (2.1)* and *Clinical Pharmacology (12.3)*].
Non-nucleoside Reverse Transcriptase Inhibitor: delavirdine	↑ lopinavir	Appropriate doses of the combination with respect to safety and efficacy have not been established.
Nucleoside Reverse Transcriptase Inhibitor: didanosine		KALETRA tablets can be administered simultaneously with didanosine without food. For KALETRA oral solution, it is recommended that didanosine be administered on an empty stomach; therefore, didanosine should be given one hour before or two hours after KALETRA oral solution (given with food).
Nucleoside Reverse Transcriptase Inhibitor: tenofovir	↑ tenofovir	KALETRA increases tenofovir concentrations. The mechanism of this interaction is unknown. Patients receiving KALETRA and tenofovir should be monitored for adverse reactions associated with tenofovir.
Nucleoside Reverse Transcriptase Inhibitors: abacavir zidovudine	↓ abacavir ↓ zidovudine	KALETRA induces glucuronidation; therefore, KALETRA has the potential to reduce zidovudine and abacavir plasma concentrations. The clinical significance of this potential interaction is unknown.
Other Agents		
Antiarrhythmics e.g.: amiodarone, bepridil, lidocaine (systemic), quinidine	↑ antiarrhythmics	Caution is warranted and therapeutic concentration monitoring (if available) is recommended for antiarrhythmics when co-administered with KALETRA.

(Table continued on next page)

Figure 1 displays the mean steady-state plasma concentrations of lopinavir and ritonavir after KALETRA 400/100 mg twice daily with food for 3 weeks from a pharmacokinetic study in HIV-1 infected adult subjects (n = 19).

Figure 1. Mean Steady-State Plasma Concentrations with 95% Confidence Intervals (CI) for HIV-1 Infected Adult Subjects (N = 19)

Absorption

In a pharmacokinetic study in HIV-1 positive subjects (n = 19), multiple dosing with 400/100 mg KALETRA twice daily with food for 3 weeks produced a mean ± SD lopinavir peak plasma concentration (C_{max}) of 9.8 ± 3.7 µg/mL, occurring approximately 4 hours after administration. The mean steady-state trough concentration prior to the morning dose was 7.1 ± 2.9 µg/mL and minimum concentration within a dosing interval was 5.5 ± 2.7 µg/mL. Lopinavir AUC over a 12 hour dosing interval averaged 92.6 ± 36.7 µg·h/mL. The absolute bioavailability of lopinavir co-formulated with ritonavir in humans has not been established. Under non-fasting conditions (500 kcal, 25% from fat), lopinavir concentrations were similar following administration of KALETRA co-formulated capsules and oral solution. When administered under fasting conditions, both the mean AUC and C_{max} of lopinavir were 22% lower for the KALETRA oral solution relative to the capsule formulation.

Plasma concentrations of lopinavir and ritonavir after administration of two 200/50 mg KALETRA tablets are similar to three 133.3/33.3 mg KALETRA capsules under fed conditions with less pharmacokinetic variability.

Effects of Food on Oral Absorption

KALETRA Tablets

No clinically significant changes in C_{max} and AUC were observed following administration of KALETRA tablets under fed conditions compared to fasted conditions. Relative to fasting, administration of KALETRA tablets with a moderate fat meal (500 - 682 Kcal, 23 to 25% calories from fat) increased lopinavir AUC and C_{max} by 26.9% and 17.6%, respectively. Relative to fasting, administration of KALETRA tablets with a high fat meal (872 Kcal, 56% from fat) increased lopinavir AUC by 18.9% but not C_{max}. Therefore, KALETRA tablets may be taken with or without food.

KALETRA Oral Solution

Relative to fasting, administration of KALETRA oral solution with a moderate fat meal (500 - 682 Kcal, 23 to 25% calories from fat) increased lopinavir AUC and C_{max} by 80 and 54%, respectively. Relative to fasting, administration of KALETRA oral solution with a high fat meal (872 Kcal, 56% from fat) increased lopinavir AUC and C_{max} by 130% and 56%, respectively. To enhance bioavailability and minimize pharmacokinetic variability KALETRA oral solution should be taken with food.

Distribution

At steady state, lopinavir is approximately 98-99% bound to plasma proteins. Lopinavir binds to both alpha-1-acid glycoprotein (AAG) and albumin; however, it has a higher affinity for AAG. At steady state, lopinavir protein binding remains constant over the range of observed concentrations after 400/100 mg KALETRA twice daily, and is similar between healthy volunteers and HIV-1 positive patients.

Metabolism

In vitro experiments with human hepatic microsomes indicate that lopinavir primarily undergoes oxidative metabolism. Lopinavir is extensively metabolized by the hepatic cytochrome P450 system, almost exclusively by the CYP3A isozyme. Ritonavir is a potent CYP3A inhibitor which inhibits the metabolism of lopinavir, and therefore increases plasma levels of lopinavir. A ^{14}C-lopinavir study in humans showed that 89% of the plasma radioactivity after a single 400/100 mg KALETRA dose was due to parent drug. At

Information on the AbbVie, Inc. products listed on these pages is from the prescribing information in use as of July 31, 2014. For more information, please visit rxabbvie.com or call 1-800-633-9110.

Help Patients Save on Rx Drugs: PDR.net/PharmacyDiscountCard

Table 8 *(cont.).* **Established and Other Potentially Significant Drug Interactions**

Concomitant Drug Class: Drug Name	Effect on Concentration of Lopinavir or Concomitant Drug	Clinical Comments
	Other Agents (cont.)	
Anticancer Agents: vincristine, vinblastine, dasatinib, nilotinib	↑ anticancer agents	Concentrations of these drugs may be increased when co-administered with KALETRA resulting in the potential for increased adverse events usually associated with these anticancer agents. For vincristine and vinblastine, consideration should be given to temporarily withholding the ritonavir-containing antiretroviral regimen in patients who develop significant hematologic or gastrointestinal side effects when KALETRA is administered concurrently with vincristine or vinblastine. If the antiretroviral regimen must be withheld for a prolonged period, consideration should be given to initiating a revised regimen that does not include a CYP3A or P-gp inhibitor. A decrease in the dosage or an adjustment of the dosing interval of nilotinib and dasatinib may be necessary for patients requiring co-administration with strong CYP3A inhibitors such as KALETRA. Please refer to the nilotinib and dasatinib prescribing information for dosing instructions.
Anticoagulants: warfarin, rivaroxaban	↑ rivaroxaban	Concentrations of warfarin may be affected. It is recommended that INR (international normalized ratio) be monitored. Avoid concomitant use of rivaroxaban and KALETRA. Co-administration of KALETRA and rivaroxaban is expected to result in increased exposure of rivaroxaban which may lead to risk of increased bleeding.
Anticonvulsants: carbamazepine, phenobarbital, phenytoin	↓ lopinavir ↓ phenytoin	KALETRA may be less effective due to decreased lopinavir plasma concentrations in patients taking these agents concomitantly and should be used with caution. KALETRA should not be administered once daily in combination with carbamazepine, phenobarbital, or phenytoin. In addition, co-administration of phenytoin and KALETRA may cause decreases in steady-state phenytoin concentrations. Phenytoin levels should be monitored when co-administering with KALETRA.
Anticonvulsants: lamotrigine, valproate	↓ lamotrigine ↓ or ↔ valproate	Co-administration of KALETRA and lamotrigine or valproate may decrease the exposure of lamotrigine or valproate. A dose increase of lamotrigine or valproate may be needed when co-administered with KALETRA and therapeutic concentration monitoring for lamotrigine may be indicated; particularly during dosage adjustments.
Antidepressant: bupropion	↓ bupropion ↓ active metabolite, hydroxybupropion	Concurrent administration of bupropion with KALETRA may decrease plasma levels of both bupropion and its active metabolite (hydroxybupropion). Patients receiving KALETRA and bupropion concurrently should be monitored for an adequate clinical response to bupropion.
Antidepressant: trazodone	↑ trazodone	Concomitant use of trazodone and KALETRA may increase concentrations of trazodone. Adverse reactions of nausea, dizziness, hypotension and syncope have been observed following co-administration of trazodone and ritonavir. If trazodone is used with a CYP3A4 inhibitor such as ritonavir, the combination should be used with caution and a lower dose of trazodone should be considered.
Anti-infective: clarithromycin	↑ clarithromycin	For patients with renal impairment, the following dosage adjustments should be considered: • For patients with CL_{CR} 30 to 60 mL/min the dose of clarithromycin should be reduced by 50%. • For patients with CL_{CR} < 30 mL/min the dose of clarithromycin should be decreased by 75%. No dose adjustment for patients with normal renal function is necessary.
Antifungals: ketoconazole*, itraconazole, voriconazole	↑ ketoconazole ↑ itraconazole ↓ voriconazole	High doses of ketoconazole (>200 mg/day) or itraconazole (> 200 mg/day) are not recommended. Co-administration of voriconazole with KALETRA has not been studied. However, a study has been shown that administration of voriconazole with ritonavir 100 mg every 12 hours decreased voriconazole steady-state AUC by an average of 39%; therefore, co-administration of KALETRA and voriconazole may result in decreased voriconazole concentrations and the potential for decreased voriconazole effectiveness and should be avoided, unless an assessment of the benefit/risk to the patient justifies the use of voriconazole. Otherwise, alternative antifungal therapies should be considered in these patients.

(Table continued on next page)

least 13 lopinavir oxidative metabolites have been identified in man. Ritonavir has been shown to induce metabolic enzymes, resulting in the induction of its own metabolism. Pre-dose lopinavir concentrations decline with time during multiple dosing, stabilizing after approximately 10 to 16 days.

Elimination

Following a 400/100 mg ^{14}C-lopinavir/ritonavir dose, approximately 10.4 ± 2.3% and 82.6 ± 2.5% of an administered dose of ^{14}C-lopinavir can be accounted for in urine and feces, respectively, after 8 days. Unchanged lopinavir accounted for approximately 2.2 and 19.8% of the administered dose in urine and feces, respectively. After multiple dosing, less than 3% of the lopinavir dose is excreted unchanged in the urine. The apparent oral clearance (CL/F) of lopinavir is 5.98 ± 5.75 L/hr (mean ± SD, n = 19).

Once Daily Dosing

The pharmacokinetics of once daily KALETRA have been evaluated in HIV-1 infected subjects naïve to antiretroviral treatment. KALETRA 800/200 mg was administered in combination with emtricitabine 200 mg and tenofovir DF 300 mg as part of a once daily regimen. Multiple dosing of 800/200 mg KALETRA once daily for 4 weeks with food (n = 24) produced a mean ± SD lopinavir peak plasma concentration (C_{max}) of 11.8 ± 3.7 µg/mL, occurring approximately 6 hours after administration. The mean steady-state lopinavir trough concentration prior to the morning dose was 3.2 ± 2.1 µg/mL and minimum concentration within a dosing interval was 1.7 ± 1.6 µg/mL. Lopinavir AUC over a 24 hour dosing interval averaged 154.1 ± 61.4 µg• h/mL. The pharmacokinetics of once daily KALETRA has also been evaluated in treatment experienced HIV-1 infected subjects. Lopinavir exposure (C_{max}, $AUC_{[0-24h]}$, C_{trough}) with once daily KALETRA administration in treatment experienced subjects is comparable to the once daily lopinavir exposure in treatment naïve subjects.

Effects on Electrocardiogram

QTcF interval was evaluated in a randomized, placebo and active (moxifloxacin 400 mg once daily) controlled crossover study in 39 healthy adults, with 10 measurements over 12 hours on Day 3. The maximum mean time-matched (95% upper confidence bound) differences in QTcF interval from placebo after baseline-correction were 5.3 (8.1) and 15.2 (18.0) mseconds (msec) for 400/100 mg twice daily and supratherapeutic 800/200 mg twice daily KALETRA, respectively. KALETRA 800/200 mg twice daily resulted in a Day 3 mean C_{max} approximately 2-fold higher than the mean C_{max} observed with the approved once daily and twice daily KALETRA doses at steady state.

PR interval prolongation was also noted in subjects receiving KALETRA in the same study on Day 3. The maximum mean (95% upper confidence bound) difference from placebo in the PR interval after baseline-correction were 24.9 (21.5, 28.3) and 31.9 (28.5, 35.3) msec for 400/100 mg twice daily and supratherapeutic 800/200 mg twice daily KALETRA, respectively *[see Warnings and Precautions (5.5, 5.6)]*.

Special Populations

Gender, Race and Age

No gender related pharmacokinetic differences have been observed in adult patients. No clinically important pharmacokinetic differences due to race have been identified. Lopinavir pharmacokinetics have not been studied in elderly patients.

Pediatric Patients

The pharmacokinetics of KALETRA oral solution 300/75 mg/m² twice daily and 230/57.5 mg/m² twice daily have been studied in a total of 53 pediatric patients in Study 940, ranging in age from 6 months to 12 years *[see Clinical Studies (14.4)]*. The 230/57.5 mg/m² twice daily regimen without nevirapine and the 300/75 mg/m² twice daily regimen with nevirapine provided lopinavir plasma concentrations similar to those obtained in adult patients receiving the 400/100 mg twice daily regimen (without nevirapine). The mean steady-state lopinavir AUC, C_{max}, and C_{min} were 72.6 ± 31.1 µg•h/mL, 8.2 ± 2.9 and 3.4 ± 2.1 µg/mL, respectively after KALETRA oral solution 230/57.5 mg/m² twice daily without nevirapine (n = 12), and were 85.8 ± 36.9 µg• h/mL, 10.0 ± 3.3 and 3.6 ± 3.5 µg/mL, respectively, after 300/75 mg/m² twice daily with nevirapine (n = 12). The nevirapine regimen was 7 mg/kg twice daily (6 months to 8 years) or 4 mg/kg twice daily (> 8 years).

The pharmacokinetics of KALETRA oral solution at approximately 300/75 mg/m² twice daily have also been evaluated in infants at approximately 6 weeks of age (n = 9) and between 6 weeks and 6 months of age (n = 18) in Study 1030. The mean steady-state lopinavir AUC_{12}, C_{max}, and C_{12} were 43.4 ± 14.8 µg• h/mL, 5.2 ± 1.8 µg/mL and 1.9 ± 1.1 µg/mL, respectively, in infants at approximately 6 weeks of age, and 74.5 ± 37.9 µg• h/mL, 9.4 ± 4.9 and 3.1 ± 1.8 µg/mL, respectively, in infants between 6 weeks and 6 months of age after KALETRA oral solution was administered at approximately 300/75 mg/m² twice daily without concomitant NNRTI therapy.

Table 8 (cont.). Established and Other Potentially Significant Drug Interactions

Concomitant Drug Class: Drug Name	Effect on Concentration of Lopinavir or Concomitant Drug	Clinical Comments
Other Agents (cont.)		
Anti-gout: colchicine	↑ colchicine	Patients with renal or hepatic impairment should not be given colchicine with KALETRA. Treatment of gout flares-co-administration of colchicine in patients on KALETRA: 0.6 mg (1 tablet) × 1 dose, followed by 0.3 mg (half tablet) 1 hour later. Dose to be repeated no earlier than 3 days. Prophylaxis of gout flares-co-administration of colchicine in patients on KALETRA: If the original colchicine regimen was 0.6 mg twice a day, the regimen should be adjusted to 0.3 mg once a day. If the original colchicine regimen was 0.6 mg once a day, the regimen should be adjusted to 0.3 mg once every other day. Treatment of familial Mediterranean fever (FMF)-co-administration of colchicine in patients on KALETRA: Maximum daily dose of 0.6 mg (may be given as 0.3 mg twice a day).
Antimycobacterial: rifabutin*	↑ rifabutin and rifabutin metabolite	Dosage reduction of rifabutin by at least 75% of the usual dose of 300 mg/day is recommended (i.e., a maximum dose of 150 mg every other day or three times per week). Increased monitoring for adverse reactions is warranted in patients receiving the combination. Further dosage reduction of rifabutin may be necessary.
Antimycobacterial: rifampin	↓ lopinavir	May lead to loss of virologic response and possible resistance to KALETRA or to the class of protease inhibitors or other co-administered antiretroviral agents. A study evaluated combination of rifampin 600 mg once daily, with KALETRA 800/200 mg twice daily or KALETRA 400/100 mg + ritonavir 300 mg twice daily. Pharmacokinetic and safety results from this study do not allow for a dose recommendation. Nine subjects (28%) experienced a ≥ grade 2 increase in ALT/AST, of which seven (21%) prematurely discontinued study per protocol. Based on the study design, it is not possible to determine whether the frequency or magnitude of the ALT/AST elevations observed is higher than what would be seen with rifampin alone [see Clinical Pharmacology (12.3) for magnitude of interaction].
Antiparasitic: atovaquone	↓ atovaquone	Clinical significance is unknown; however, increase in atovaquone doses may be needed.
Benzodiazepines: parenterally administered midazolam	↑ midazolam	Midazolam is extensively metabolized by CYP3A4. Increases in the concentration of midazolam are expected to be significantly higher with oral than with parenteral administration. Therefore, KALETRA should not be given with orally administered midazolam [see Contraindications (4)]. If KALETRA is co-administered with parenteral midazolam, close clinical monitoring for respiratory depression and/or prolonged sedation should be exercised and dosage adjustment should be considered.
Contraceptive: ethinyl estradiol*	↓ ethinyl estradiol	Because contraceptive steroid concentrations may be altered when KALETRA is co-administered with oral contraceptives or with the contraceptive patch, alternative methods of nonhormonal contraception are recommended.
Corticosteroids (systemic): e.g. budesonide, dexamethasone, prednisone	↓ lopinavir ↑ glucocorticoids	Use with caution. KALETRA may be less effective due to decreased lopinavir plasma concentrations in patients taking these agents concomitantly. Concomitant use may result in increased steroid concentrations and reduced serum cortisol concentrations. Concomitant use of glucocorticoids that are metabolized by CYP3A, particularly for long-term use, should consider the potential benefit of treatment versus the risk of systemic corticosteroid effects. Concomitant use may increase the risk for development of systemic corticosteroid effects including Cushing's syndrome and adrenal suppression.
Dihydropyridine Calcium Channel Blockers: e.g. felodipine, nifedipine, nicardipine	↑ dihydropyridine calcium channel blockers	Caution is warranted and clinical monitoring of patients is recommended.
Disulfiram/metronidazole		KALETRA oral solution contains alcohol, which can produce disulfiram-like reactions when co-administered with disulfiram or other drugs that produce this reaction (e.g., metronidazole).

(Table continued on next page)

The pharmacokinetics of KALETRA soft gelatin capsule and oral solution (Group 1: 400/100 mg/m² twice daily + 2 NRTIs; Group 2: 480/120 mg/m² twice daily + ≥ 1 NRTI + 1 NNRTI) have been evaluated in children and adolescents age ≥ 2 years to < 18 years of age who had failed prior therapy (n=26) in Study 1038. KALETRA doses of 400/100 and 480/120 mg/m² resulted in high lopinavir exposure, as almost all subjects had lopinavir AUC₁₂ above 100 μg•h/mL. Both groups of subjects also achieved relatively high average minimum lopinavir concentrations.

KALETRA once daily has not been evaluated in pediatric patients.

Renal Impairment

Lopinavir pharmacokinetics have not been studied in patients with renal impairment; however, since the renal clearance of lopinavir is negligible, a decrease in total body clearance is not expected in patients with renal impairment.

Hepatic Impairment

Lopinavir is principally metabolized and eliminated by the liver. Multiple dosing of KALETRA 400/100 mg twice daily to HIV-1 and HCV co-infected patients with mild to moderate hepatic impairment (n = 12) resulted in a 30% increase in lopinavir AUC and 20% increase in C_{max} compared to HIV-1 infected subjects with normal hepatic function (n = 12). Additionally, the plasma protein binding of lopinavir was statistically significantly lower in both mild and moderate hepatic impairment compared to controls (99.09 vs. 99.31%, respectively). Caution should be exercised when administering KALETRA to subjects with hepatic impairment. KALETRA has not been studied in patients with severe hepatic impairment [see Warnings and Precautions (5.4) and Use in Specific Populations (8.6)].

Drug Interactions

KALETRA is an inhibitor of the P450 isoform CYP3A *in vitro*. Co-administration of KALETRA and drugs primarily metabolized by CYP3A may result in increased plasma concentrations of the other drug, which could increase or prolong its therapeutic and adverse effects [see Contraindications (4) and Drug Interactions (7)].

KALETRA does not inhibit CYP2D6, CYP2C9, CYP2C19, CYP2E1, CYP2B6 or CYP1A2 at clinically relevant concentrations.

KALETRA has been shown *in vivo* to induce its own metabolism and to increase the biotransformation of some drugs metabolized by cytochrome P450 enzymes and by glucuronidation.

KALETRA is metabolized by CYP3A. Drugs that induce CYP3A activity would be expected to increase the clearance of lopinavir, resulting in lowered plasma concentrations of lopinavir. Although not noted with concurrent ketoconazole, co-administration of KALETRA and other drugs that inhibit CYP3A may increase lopinavir plasma concentrations.

Drug interaction studies were performed with KALETRA and other drugs likely to be co-administered and some drugs commonly used as probes for pharmacokinetic interactions. The effects of co-administration of KALETRA on the AUC, C_{max} and C_{min} are summarized in Table 9 (effect of other drugs on lopinavir) and Table 10 (effect of KALETRA on other drugs). The effects of other drugs on ritonavir are not shown since they generally correlate with those observed with lopinavir (if lopinavir concentrations are decreased, ritonavir concentrations are decreased) unless otherwise indicated in the table footnotes. For information regarding clinical recommendations, see Table 8 in *Drug Interactions (7)*.

[See table 9 on pages 480 and 481]
[See table 10 on pages 482 and 483]

12.4   Microbiology
Mechanism of Action
Lopinavir, an inhibitor of the HIV-1 protease, prevents cleavage of the Gag-Pol polyprotein, resulting in the production of immature, non-infectious viral particles.

Antiviral Activity
The antiviral activity of lopinavir against laboratory HIV strains and clinical HIV-1 isolates was evaluated in acutely infected lymphoblastic cell lines and peripheral blood lymphocytes, respectively. In the absence of human serum, the mean 50% effective concentration (EC₅₀) values of lopinavir against five different HIV-1 subtype B laboratory strains ranged from 10-27 nM (0.006-0.017 μg/mL, 1 μg/mL = .6 μM) and ranged from 4-11 nM (0.003-0.007 μg/mL) against several HIV-1 subtype B clinical isolates (n = 6). In the presence of 50% human serum, the mean EC₅₀ values of lopinavir against these five HIV-1 laboratory strains ranged from 65-289 nM (0.04-0.18 μg/mL), representing a 7 to 11-fold attenuation. Combination antiviral drug activity studies with lopinavir in cell cultures demonstrated additive to antagonistic activity with nelfinavir and additive to synergistic activity with amprenavir, atazanavir, indinavir, saquinavir and tipranavir. The EC₅₀ values of lopinavir against three different HIV-2 strains ranged from 12-180 nM (0.008-113 μg/mL).

Information on the AbbVie, Inc. products listed on these pages is from the prescribing information in use as of July 31, 2014. For more information, please visit rxabbvie.com or call 1-800-633-9110.

Table 8 (cont.). Established and Other Potentially Significant Drug Interactions

Concomitant Drug Class: Drug Name	Effect on Concentration of Lopinavir or Concomitant Drug	Clinical Comments
	Other Agents (cont.)	
Endothelin Receptor Antagonists: bosentan	↑ bosentan	Co-administration of bosentan in patients on KALETRA: In patients who have been receiving KALETRA for at least 10 days, start bosentan at 62.5 mg once daily or every other day based upon individual tolerability. Co-administration of KALETRA in patients on bosentan: Discontinue use of bosentan at least 36 hours prior to initiation of KALETRA. After at least 10 days following the initiation of KALETRA, resume bosentan at 62.5 mg once daily or every other day based upon individual tolerability.
HCV-Protease Inhibitor: boceprevir	↓ lopinavir ↓ boceprevir ↓ ritonavir	It is not recommended to co-administer KALETRA and boceprevir. Concomitant administration of KALETRA and boceprevir reduced boceprevir, lopinavir and ritonavir steady-state exposures [see Clinical Pharmacology (12.3)].
HCV-Protease Inhibitor: telaprevir	↓ telaprevir ↔ lopinavir	It is not recommended to co-administer KALETRA and telaprevir. Concomitant administration of KALETRA and telaprevir reduced steady-state telaprevir exposure, while the steady-state lopinavir exposure was not affected [see Clinical Pharmacology (12.3)].
HMG-CoA Reductase Inhibitors: atorvastatin rosuvastatin	↑ atorvastatin ↑ rosuvastatin	Use atorvastatin with caution and at the lowest necessary dose. Titrate rosuvastatin dose carefully and use the lowest necessary dose; do not exceed rosuvastatin 10 mg/day. See Drugs with No Observed or Predicted Interactions with KALETRA (7.4) and Clinical Pharmacology (12.3) for drug interaction data with other HMG-CoA reductase inhibitors.
Immunosuppressants: e.g. cyclosporine, tacrolimus, sirolimus	↑ immunosuppressants	Therapeutic concentration monitoring is recommended for immunosuppressant agents when co-administered with KALETRA.
Inhaled or Intranasal Steroids e.g.: fluticasone, budesonide	↑ glucocorticoids	Concomitant use of KALETRA and fluticasone or other glucocorticoids that are metabolized by CYP3A is not recommended unless the potential benefit of treatment outweighs the risk of systemic corticosteroid effects. Concomitant use may result in increased steroid concentrations and reduce serum cortisol concentrations. Systemic corticosteroid effects including Cushing's syndrome and adrenal suppression have been reported during postmarketing use in patients when certain ritonavir-containing products have been co-administered with fluticasone propionate or budesonide.
Long-acting beta-adrenoceptor Agonist: salmeterol	↑ salmeterol	Concurrent administration of salmeterol and KALETRA is not recommended. The combination may result in increased risk of cardiovascular adverse events associated with salmeterol, including QT prolongation, palpitations and sinus tachycardia.
Narcotic Analgesics: methadone,* fentanyl	↓ methadone ↑ fentanyl	Dosage of methadone may need to be increased when co-administered with KALETRA. Concentrations of fentanyl are expected to increase. Careful monitoring of therapeutic and adverse effects (including potentially fatal respiratory depression) is recommended when fentanyl is concomitantly administered with KALETRA.

(Table continued on next page)

Resistance

HIV-1 isolates with reduced susceptibility to lopinavir have been selected in cell culture. The presence of ritonavir does not appear to influence the selection of lopinavir-resistant viruses in cell culture.

The selection of resistance to KALETRA in antiretroviral treatment naïve patients has not yet been characterized. In a study of 653 antiretroviral treatment naïve patients (Study 863), plasma viral isolates from each patient on treatment with plasma HIV-1 RNA > 400 copies/mL at Week 24, 32, 40 and/or 48 were analyzed. No evidence of resistance to KALETRA was observed in 37 evaluable KALETRA-treated patients (0%). Evidence of genotypic resistance to nelfinavir, defined as the presence of the D30N and/or L90M substitution in HIV-1 protease, was observed in 25/76 (33%) of evaluable nelfinavir-treated patients. The selection of resistance to KALETRA in antiretroviral treatment naïve pediatric patients (Study 940) appears to be consistent with that seen in adult patients (Study 863). Resistance to KALETRA has been noted to emerge in patients treated with other protease inhibitors prior to KALETRA therapy. In studies of 227 antiretroviral treatment naïve and protease inhibitor experienced patients, iso-

lates from 4 of 23 patients with quantifiable (> 400 copies/mL) viral RNA following treatment with KALETRA for 12 to 100 weeks displayed significantly reduced susceptibility to lopinavir compared to the corresponding baseline viral isolates. Three of these patients had previously received treatment with a single protease inhibitor (indinavir, nelfinavir, or saquinavir) and one patient had received treatment with multiple protease inhibitors (indinavir, ritonavir, and saquinavir). All four of these patients had at least 4 substitutions associated with protease inhibitor resistance immediately prior to KALETRA therapy. Following viral rebound, isolates from these patients all contained additional substitutions, some of which are recognized to be associated with protease inhibitor resistance. However, there are insufficient data at this time to identify patterns of lopinavir resistance-associated substitutions in isolates from patients on KALETRA therapy. The assessment of these patterns is under study.

Cross-resistance - Preclinical Studies

Varying degrees of cross-resistance have been observed among HIV-1 protease inhibitors. Little information is available on the cross-resistance of viruses that developed decreased susceptibility to lopinavir during KALETRA therapy.

The antiviral activity in cell culture of lopinavir against clinical isolates from patients previously treated with a single protease inhibitor was determined. Isolates that displayed > 4-fold reduced susceptibility to nelfinavir (n = 13) and saquinavir (n = 4), displayed < 4-fold reduced susceptibility to lopinavir. Isolates with > 4-fold reduced susceptibility to indinavir (n = 16) and ritonavir (n = 3) displayed a mean of 5.7- and 8.3-fold reduced susceptibility to lopinavir, respectively. Isolates from patients previously treated with two or more protease inhibitors showed greater reductions in susceptibility to lopinavir, as described in the following paragraph.

Clinical Studies - Antiviral Activity of KALETRA in Patients with Previous Protease Inhibitor Therapies

The clinical relevance of reduced susceptibility in cell culture to lopinavir has been examined by assessing the virologic response to KALETRA therapy in treatment-experienced patients, with respect to baseline viral genotype in three studies and baseline viral phenotype in one study.

Virologic response to KALETRA has been shown to be affected by the presence of three or more of the following amino acid substitutions in protease at baseline: L10F/I/R/V, K20M/N/R, L24I, L33F, M36I, I47V, G48V, I54L/T/V, V82A/C/F/S/T, and I84V. Table 11 shows the 48-week virologic response (HIV-1 RNA <400 copies/mL) according to the number of the above protease inhibitor resistance-associated substitutions at baseline in studies 888 and 765 [see Clinical Studies (14.2) and (14.3)] and study 957 (see below). Once daily administration of KALETRA for adult patients with three or more of the above substitutions is not recommended.

[See table 11 on page 483]

Virologic response to KALETRA therapy with respect to phenotypic susceptibility to lopinavir at baseline was examined in Study 957. In this study 56 NNRTI-naïve patients with HIV-1 RNA >1,000 copies/mL despite previous therapy with at least two protease inhibitors selected from indinavir, nelfinavir, ritonavir, and saquinavir were randomized to receive one of two doses of KALETRA in combination with efavirenz and nucleoside reverse transcriptase inhibitors (NRTIs). The EC_{50} values of lopinavir against the 56 baseline viral isolates ranged from 0.5- to 96-fold the wild-type EC_{50} value. Fifty-five percent (31/56) of these baseline isolates displayed >4-fold reduced susceptibility to lopinavir. These 31 isolates had a median reduction in lopinavir susceptibility of 18-fold. Response to therapy by baseline lopinavir susceptibility is shown in Table 12.

Table 12. HIV-1 RNA Response at Week 48 by Baseline Lopinavir Susceptibility[1]

Lopinavir susceptibility[2] at baseline	HIV-1 RNA <400 copies/mL (%)	HIV-1 RNA <50 copies/mL (%)
< 10 fold	25/27 (93%)	22/27 (81%)
> 10 and < 40 fold	11/15 (73%)	9/15 (60%)
≥ 40 fold	2/8 (25%)	2/8 (25%)

[1] Lopinavir susceptibility was determined by recombinant phenotypic technology performed by Virologic.
[2] Fold change in susceptibility from wild type.

13   NONCLINICAL TOXICOLOGY

13.1   Carcinogenesis, Mutagenesis, Impairment of Fertility

Carcinogenesis

Lopinavir/ritonavir combination was evaluated for carcinogenic potential by oral gavage administration to mice and rats for up to 104 weeks. Results showed an increase in the incidence of benign hepatocellular adenomas and an increase in the combined incidence of hepatocellular adenomas plus carcinoma in both males and females in mice and males in rats at doses that produced approximately 1.6-2.2 times (mice) and 0.5 times (rats) the human exposure (based on AUC_{0-24hr} measurement) at the recommended dose of 400/100 mg KALETRA twice daily. Administration of lopinavir/ritonavir did not cause a statistically significant increase in the incidence of any other benign or malignant neoplasm in mice or rats.

Carcinogenicity studies in mice and rats have been carried out on ritonavir. In male mice, there was a dose dependent increase in the incidence of both adenomas and combined adenomas and carcinomas in the liver. Based on AUC measurements, the exposure at the high dose was approximately 4-fold for males that of the exposure in humans with the recommended therapeutic dose (400/100 mg KALETRA twice daily). There were no carcinogenic effects seen in females at the dosages tested. The exposure at the high dose was approximately 9-fold for the females that of the exposure in humans. There were no carcinogenic effects in rats. In this study, the exposure at the high dose was approximately 0.7-fold that of the exposure in humans with the

400/100 mg KALETRA twice daily regimen. Based on the exposures achieved in the animal studies, the significance of the observed effects is not known.

Mutagenesis

Neither lopinavir nor ritonavir was found to be mutagenic or clastogenic in a battery of *in vitro* and *in vivo* assays including the Ames bacterial reverse mutation assay using *S. typhimurium* and *E. coli*, the mouse lymphoma assay, the mouse micronucleus test and chromosomal aberration assays in human lymphocytes.

Impairment of Fertility

Lopinavir in combination with ritonavir at a 2:1 ratio produced no effects on fertility in male and female rats at levels of 10/5, 30/15 or 100/50 mg/kg/day. Based on AUC measurements, the exposures in rats at the high doses were approximately 0.7-fold for lopinavir and 1.8-fold for ritonavir of the exposures in humans at the recommended therapeutic dose (400/100 mg twice daily).

14 CLINICAL STUDIES

14.1 Adult Patients without Prior Antiretroviral Therapy

Study 863: KALETRA Capsules twice daily + stavudine + lamivudine compared to nelfinavir three times daily + stavudine + lamivudine

Study 863 was a randomized, double-blind, multicenter trial comparing treatment with KALETRA capsules (400/100 mg twice daily) plus stavudine and lamivudine versus nelfinavir (750 mg three times daily) plus stavudine and lamivudine in 653 antiretroviral treatment naïve patients. Patients had a mean age of 38 years (range: 19 to 84), 57% were Caucasian, and 80% were male. Mean baseline CD4+ cell count was 259 cells/mm^3 (range: 2 to 949 cells/mm^3) and mean baseline plasma HIV-1 RNA was 4.9 log$_{10}$ copies/mL (range: 2.6 to 6.8 log$_{10}$ copies/mL). Treatment response and outcomes of randomized treatment are presented in Table 13.

Table 13. Outcomes of Randomized Treatment Through Week 48 (Study 863)

Outcome	KALETRA+ d4T+3TC (N = 326)	Nelfinavir+ d4T+3TC (N = 327)
Responder[1]	75%	62%
Virologic failure[2]	9%	25%
Rebound	7%	15%
Never suppressed through Week 48	2%	9%
Death	2%	1%
Discontinued due to adverse events	4%	4%
Discontinued for other reasons[3]	10%	8%

[1] Patients achieved and maintained confirmed HIV-1 RNA < 400 copies/mL through Week 48.
[2] Includes confirmed viral rebound and failure to achieve confirmed < 400 copies/mL through Week 48.
[3] Includes lost to follow-up, patient's withdrawal, non-compliance, protocol violation and other reasons.

Overall discontinuation through Week 48, including patients who discontinued subsequent to virologic failure, was 17% in the KALETRA arm and 24% in the nelfinavir arm.

Through 48 weeks of therapy, there was a statistically significantly higher proportion of patients in the KALETRA arm compared to the nelfinavir arm with HIV-1 RNA < 400 copies/mL (75% vs. 62%, respectively) and HIV-1 RNA < 50 copies/mL (67% vs. 52%, respectively). Treatment response by baseline HIV-1 RNA level subgroups is presented in Table 14.

[See table 14 at bottom of page 483]

Through 48 weeks of therapy, the mean increase from baseline in CD4+ cell count was 207 cells/mm^3 for the KALETRA arm and 195 cells/mm^3 for the nelfinavir arm.

Study 730: KALETRA Tablets once daily + tenofovir DF + emtricitabine compared to KALETRA Tablets twice daily + tenofovir DF + emtricitabine

Study 730 was a randomized, open-label, multicenter trial comparing treatment with KALETRA 800/200 mg once daily plus tenofovir DF and emtricitabine versus KALETRA 400/100 mg twice daily plus tenofovir DF and emtricitabine in 664 antiretroviral treatment-naïve patients. Patients were randomized in a 1:1 ratio to receive either KALETRA 800/200 mg once daily (n = 333) or KALETRA 400/100 mg twice daily (n = 331). Further stratification within each group was 1:1 (tablet vs. capsule). Patients administered the capsule were switched to the tablet formulation at Week 8 and maintained on their randomized dosing schedule. Pa-

Table 8 (cont.). Established and Other Potentially Significant Drug Interactions

Concomitant Drug Class: Drug Name	Effect on Concentration of Lopinavir or Concomitant Drug	Clinical Comments
Other Agents (cont.)		
PDE5 inhibitors: avanafil, sildenafil, tadalafil, vardenafil	↑ avanafil ↑ sildenafil ↑ tadalafil ↑ vardenafil	Do not use KALETRA with avanafil because a safe and effective avanafil dosage regimen has not been established. Particular caution should be used when prescribing sildenafil, tadalafil, or vardenafil in patients receiving KALETRA. Co-administration of KALETRA with these drugs is expected to substantially increase their concentrations and may result in an increase in PDE5 inhibitor associated adverse reactions including hypotension, syncope, visual changes and prolonged erection. Use of PDE5 inhibitors for pulmonary arterial hypertension (PAH): Sildenafil (Revatio®) is contraindicated when used for the treatment of pulmonary arterial hypertension (PAH) because a safe and effective dose has not been established when used with KALETRA [see Contraindications (4)]. The following dose adjustments are recommended for use of tadalafil (Adcirca®) with KALETRA: Co-administration of ADCIRCA in patients on KALETRA: In patients receiving KALETRA for at least one week, start ADCIRCA at 20 mg once daily. Increase to 40 mg once daily based upon individual tolerability. Co-administration of KALETRA in patients on ADCIRCA: Avoid use of ADCIRCA during the initiation of KALETRA. Stop ADCIRCA at least 24 hours prior to starting KALETRA. After at least one week following the initiation of KALETRA, resume ADCIRCA at 20 mg once daily. Increase to 40 mg once daily based upon individual tolerability. Use of PDE5 inhibitors for erectile dysfunction: It is recommended not to exceed the following doses: • Sildenafil: 25 mg every 48 hours • Tadalafil: 10 mg every 72 hours • Vardenafil: 2.5 mg every 72 hours Use with increased monitoring for adverse events.

* see Clinical Pharmacology (12.3) for magnitude of interaction.

tients were administered emtricitabine 200 mg once daily and tenofovir DF 300 mg once daily. Mean age of patients enrolled was 39 years (range: 19 to 71); 75% were Caucasian, and 78% were male. Mean baseline CD4+ cell count was 216 cells/mm^3 (range: 20 to 775 cells/mm^3) and mean baseline plasma HIV-1 RNA was 5.0 log$_{10}$ copies/mL (range: 1.7 to 7.0 log$_{10}$ copies/mL).
Treatment response and outcomes of randomized treatment through Week 48 are presented in Table 15.

Table 15. Outcomes of Randomized Treatment Through Week 48 (Study 730)

Outcome	KALETRA Once Daily + TDF + FTC (n = 333)	KALETRA Twice Daily + TDF + FTC (n = 331)
Responder[1]	78%	77%
Virologic failure[2]	10%	8%
Rebound	5%	5%
Never suppressed through Week 48	5%	3%
Death	1%	<1%
Discontinued due to adverse events	4%	3%
Discontinued for other reasons[3]	8%	11%

[1] Patients achieved and maintained confirmed HIV-1 RNA < 50 copies/mL through Week 48.
[2] Includes confirmed viral rebound and failure to achieve confirmed < 50 copies/mL through Week 48.
[3] Includes lost to follow-up, patient's withdrawal, non-compliance, protocol violation and other reasons.

Through 48 weeks of therapy, 78% in the KALETRA once daily arm and 77% in the KALETRA twice daily arm achieved and maintained HIV-1 RNA < 50 copies/mL (95% confidence interval for the difference, -5.9% to 6.8%). Mean CD4+ cell count increases at Week 48 were 186 cells/mm^3 for the KALETRA once daily arm and 198 cells/mm^3 for the KALETRA twice daily arm.

14.2 Adult Patients with Prior Antiretroviral Therapy

Study 888: KALETRA Capsules twice daily + nevirapine + NRTIs compared to investigator-selected protease inhibitor(s) + nevirapine + NRTIs

Study 888 was a randomized, open-label, multicenter trial comparing treatment with KALETRA capsules (400/100 mg twice daily) plus nevirapine and nucleoside reverse transcriptase inhibitors versus investigator-selected protease inhibitor(s) plus nevirapine and nucleoside reverse transcriptase inhibitors in 288 single protease inhibitor-experienced, non-nucleoside reverse transcriptase inhibitor (NNRTI)-naïve patients. Patients had a mean age of 40 years (range: 18 to 74), 68% were Caucasian, and 86% were male. Mean baseline CD4+ cell count was 322 cells/mm^3 (range: 10 to 1059 cells/mm^3) and mean baseline plasma HIV-1 RNA was 4.1 log$_{10}$ copies/mL (range: 2.6 to 6.0 log$_{10}$ copies/mL). Treatment response and outcomes of randomized treatment through Week 48 are presented in Table 16.

Table 16. Outcomes of Randomized Treatment Through Week 48 (Study 888)

Outcome	KALETRA + nevirapine + NRTIs (n = 148)	Investigator-Selected Protease Inhibitor(s) + nevirapine + NRTIs (n = 140)
Responder[1]	57%	33%
Virologic failure[2]	24%	41%
Rebound	11%	19%
Never suppressed through Week 48	13%	23%
Death	1%	2%
Discontinued due to adverse events	5%	11%

Information on the AbbVie, Inc. products listed on these pages is from the prescribing information in use as of July 31, 2014. For more information, please visit rxabbvie.com or call 1-800-633-9110.

Discontinued for other reasons[3]	14%	13%	

[1] Patients achieved and maintained confirmed HIV-1 RNA < 400 copies/mL through Week 48.
[2] Includes confirmed viral rebound and failure to achieve confirmed < 400 copies/mL through Week 48.
[3] Includes lost to follow-up, patient's withdrawal, non-compliance, protocol violation and other reasons.

Through 48 weeks of therapy, there was a statistically significantly higher proportion of patients in the KALETRA arm compared to the investigator-selected protease inhibitor(s) arm with HIV-1 RNA < 400 copies/mL (57% vs. 33%, respectively).
Through 48 weeks of therapy, the mean increase from baseline in CD4+ cell count was 111 cells/mm[3] for the KALETRA arm and 112 cells/mm[3] for the investigator-selected protease inhibitor(s) arm.
Study 802: KALETRA Tablets 800/200 mg Once Daily Versus 400/100 mg Twice Daily when Co-administered with Nucleoside/Nucleotide Reverse Transcriptase Inhibitors in Antiretroviral-Experienced, HIV-1 Infected Subjects
M06-802 was a randomized open-label study comparing the safety, tolerability, and antiviral activity of once daily and twice daily dosing of KALETRA tablets in 599 subjects with detectable viral loads while receiving their current antiviral therapy. Of the enrolled subjects, 55% on both treatment arms had not been previously treated with a protease inhibitor and 81 – 88% had received prior NNRTIs as part of their anti-HIV treatment regimen. Patients were randomized in a 1:1 ratio to receive either KALETRA 800/200 mg once daily (n = 300) or KALETRA 400/100 mg twice daily (n = 299). Patients were administered at least two nucleoside/nucleotide reverse transcriptase inhibitors selected by the investigator. Mean age of patients enrolled was 41 years (range: 21 to 73); 51% were Caucasian, and 66% were male. Mean baseline CD4+ cell count was 254 cells/mm[3] (range: 4 to 952 cells/mm[3]) and mean baseline plasma HIV-1 RNA was 4.3 $\log_{10}$ copies/mL (range: 1.7 to 6.6 $\log_{10}$ copies/mL). Treatment response and outcomes of randomized treatment through Week 48 are presented in Table 17.

Table 17. Outcomes of Randomized Treatment Through Week 48 (Study 802)

Outcome	KALETRA Once Daily + NRTIs (n = 300)	KALETRA Twice Daily + NRTIs (n = 299)
Virologic Success (HIV-1 RNA <50 copies/mL)	57%	54%
Virologic failure[1]	22%	24%
No virologic data in Week 48 window		
Discontinued study due to adverse event or death[2]	5%	7%
Discontinued study for other reasons[3]	13%	12%
Missing data during window but on study	3%	3%

[1] Includes patients who discontinued prior to Week 48 for lack or loss of efficacy and patients with HIV-1 RNA ≥ 50 copies/mL at Week 48.
[2] Includes patients who discontinued due to adverse events or death at any time from Day 1 through Week 48 if this resulted in no virologic data on treatment at Week 48.
[3] Includes withdrawal of consent, loss to follow-up, non-compliance, protocol violation and other reasons.

Through 48 weeks of treatment, the mean change from baseline for CD4+ cell count was 135 cells/mm[3] for the once daily group and 122 cells/mm[3] for the twice daily group.
14.3   Other Studies Supporting Approval in Adult Patients
Study 720: KALETRA twice daily + stavudine + lamivudine
Study 765: KALETRA twice daily + nevirapine + NRTIs
Study 720 (patients without prior antiretroviral therapy) and study 765 (patients with prior protease inhibitor therapy) were randomized, blinded, multi-center trials evaluating treatment with KALETRA at up to three dose levels (200/100 mg twice daily [720 only], 400/100 mg twice daily, and 400/200 mg twice daily). In Study 720, all patients

Table 9. Drug Interactions: Pharmacokinetic Parameters for Lopinavir in the Presence of the Co-administered Drug for Recommended Alterations in Dose or Regimen

Co-administered Drug	Dose of Co-administered Drug (mg)	Dose of KALETRA (mg)	n	Ratio (in combination with Co-administered drug/alone) of Lopinavir Pharmacokinetic Parameters (90% CI); No Effect = 1.00		
				C_{max}	AUC	C_{min}
Boceprevir	800 q8h, 6 d	400/100 tablet twice daily, 22 d	13	0.70 (0.65, 0.77)	0.66[12] (0.60, 0.72)	0.57 (0.49, 0.65)
Efavirenz[1,2]	600 at bedtime, 9 d	400/100 capsule twice daily, 9 d	11, 7*	0.97 (0.78, 1.22)	0.81 (0.64, 1.03)	0.61 (0.38, 0.97)
	600 at bedtime, 9 d	500/125 tablet twice daily, 10 d	19	1.12 (1.02, 1.23)	1.06 (0.96, 1.17)	0.90 (0.78, 1.04)
	600 at bedtime, 9 d	600/150 tablet twice daily, 10 d	23	1.36 (1.28, 1.44)	1.36 (1.28, 1.44)	1.32 (1.21, 1.44)
Fosamprenavir[3]	700 twice daily plus ritonavir 100 twice daily, 14 d	400/100 capsule twice daily, 14 d	18	1.30 (0.85, 1.47)	1.37 (0.80, 1.55)	1.52 (0.72, 1.82)
Ketoconazole	200 single dose	400/100 capsule twice daily, 16 d	12	0.89 (0.80, 0.99)	0.87 (0.75, 1.00)	0.75 (0.55, 1.00)
Nelfinavir	1000 twice daily, 10 d	400/100 capsule twice daily, 21 d	13	0.79 (0.70, 0.89)	0.73 (0.63, 0.85)	0.62 (0.49, 0.78)
Nevirapine	200 twice daily, steady-state (> 1 yr)[4#]	400/100 capsule twice daily, steady-state	22, 19*	0.81 (0.62, 1.05)	0.73 (0.53, 0.98)	0.49 (0.28, 0.74)
	7 mg/kg or 4 mg/kg once daily, 2 wk; twice daily 1 wk[5]	(> 1 yr) 300/75 mg/m[2] oral solution twice daily, 3 wk	12, 15*	0.86 (0.64, 1.16)	0.78 (0.56, 1.09)	0.45 (0.25, 0.81)
Omeprazole	40 once daily, 5 d	400/100 tablet twice daily, 10 d	12	1.08 (0.99, 1.17)	1.07 (0.99, 1.15)	1.03 (0.90, 1.18)
	40 once daily, 5 d	800/200 tablet once daily, 10 d	12	0.94 (0.88, 1.00)	0.92 (0.86, 0.99)	0.71 (0.57, 0.89)
Pitavastatin[6]	4 mg once daily, 5 d	400/100 tablet twice daily, 16 d	23	0.93 (0.88-0.98)	0.91 (0.86-0.97)	NA
Pravastatin	20 once daily, 4 d	400/100 capsule twice daily, 14 d	12	0.98 (0.89, 1.08)	0.95 (0.85, 1.05)	0.88 (0.77, 1.02)
Rifabutin	150 once daily, 10 d	400/100 capsule twice daily, 20 d	14	1.08 (0.97, 1.19)	1.17 (1.04, 1.31)	1.20 (0.96, 1.65)
Ranitidine	150 single dose	400/100 tablet twice daily, 10 d	12	0.99 (0.95, 1.03)	0.97 (0.93, 1.01)	0.90 (0.85, 0.95)
	150 single dose	800/200 tablet once daily, 10 d	10	0.97 (0.95, 1.00)	0.95 (0.91, 0.99)	0.82 (0.74, 0.91)
Rifampin	600 once daily, 10 d	400/100 capsule twice daily, 20 d	22	0.45 (0.40, 0.51)	0.25 (0.21, 0.29)	0.01 (0.01, 0.02)
	600 once daily, 14 d	800/200 capsule twice daily, 9 d[7]	10	1.02 (0.85, 1.23)	0.84 (0.64, 1.10)	0.43 (0.19, 0.96)
	600 once daily, 14 d	400/400 capsule twice daily, 9 d[8]	9	0.93 (0.81, 1.07)	0.98 (0.81, 1.17)	1.03 (0.68, 1.56)

(Table continued on next page)

switched to 400/100 mg twice daily between Weeks 48-72. Patients in study 720 had a mean age of 35 years, 70% were Caucasian, and 96% were male, while patients in study 765 had a mean age of 40 years, 73% were Caucasian, and 90% were male. Mean (range) baseline CD4+ cell counts for patients in study 720 and study 765 were 338 (3-918) and 372 (72-807) cells/mm[3], respectively. Mean (range) baseline plasma HIV-1 RNA levels for patients in study 720 and study 765 were 4.9 (3.3 to 6.3) and 4.0 (2.9 to 5.8) $\log_{10}$ copies/mL, respectively.
Through 360 weeks of treatment in study 720, the proportion of patients with HIV-1 RNA < 400 (< 50) copies/mL was 61% (59%) [n = 100]. Among patients completing 360 weeks of treatment with CD4+ cell count measurements [n=60], the mean (median) increase in CD4+ cell count was 501 (457) cells/mm[3]. Thirty-nine patients (39%) discontinued the study, including 13 (13%) discontinuations due to adverse reactions and 1 (1%) death.
Through 144 weeks of treatment in study 765, the proportion of patients with HIV-1 RNA < 400 (< 50) copies/mL was 54% (50%) [n = 70], and the corresponding mean increase in

CD4+ cell count was 212 cells/mm[3]. Twenty-seven patients (39%) discontinued the study, including 5 (7%) discontinuations secondary to adverse reactions and 2 (3%) deaths.
14.4   Pediatric Studies
Study 1030 was an open-label, multicenter, dose-finding trial evaluating the pharmacokinetic profile, tolerability, safety and efficacy of KALETRA oral solution containing lopinavir 80 mg/mL and ritonavir 20 mg/mL at a dose of 300/75 mg/m[2] twice daily plus 2 NRTIs in HIV-1 infected infants ≥14 days and <6 months of age.
Ten infants, ≥14 days and <6 wks of age, were enrolled at a median (range) age of 5.7 (3.6-6.0) weeks and all completed 24 weeks. At entry, median (range) HIV-1 RNA was 6.0 (4.7-7.2) $\log_{10}$ copies/mL. Seven of 10 infants had HIV-1 RNA <400 copies/mL at Week 24. At entry, median (range) CD4+ percentage was 41 (16-59) with a median decrease of 1% (95% CI: -10, 18) from baseline to week 24 in 6 infants with available data.
Twenty-one infants, between 6 weeks and 6 months of age, were enrolled at a median (range) age of 14.7 (6.9-25.7) weeks and 19 of 21 infants completed 24 weeks. At entry,

median (range) HIV RNA level was 5.8 (3.7-6.9) $\log_{10}$ copies/mL. Ten of 21 infants had HIV RNA <400 copies/mL at Week 24. At entry, the median (range) CD4+ percentage was 32 (11-54) with a median increase of 4% (95% CI: -1, 9) from baseline to week 24 in 19 infants with available data. *See Clinical Pharmacology (12.3) for pharmacokinetic results.*

Study 940 was an open-label, multicenter trial evaluating the pharmacokinetic profile, tolerability, safety and efficacy of KALETRA oral solution containing lopinavir 80 mg/mL and ritonavir 20 mg/mL in 100 antiretroviral naïve (44%) and experienced (56%) pediatric patients. All patients were non-nucleoside reverse transcriptase inhibitor naïve. Patients were randomized to either 230 mg lopinavir/57.5 mg ritonavir per m^2 or 300 mg lopinavir/75 mg ritonavir per m^2. Naïve patients also received lamivudine and stavudine. Experienced patients received nevirapine plus up to two nucleoside reverse transcriptase inhibitors.

Safety, efficacy and pharmacokinetic profiles of the two dose regimens were assessed after three weeks of therapy in each patient. After analysis of these data, all patients were continued on the 300 mg lopinavir/75 mg ritonavir per m^2 dose. Patients had a mean age of 5 years (range 6 months to 12 years) with 14% less than 2 years. Mean baseline CD4+ cell count was 838 cells/mm³ and mean baseline plasma HIV-1 RNA was 4.7 $\log_{10}$ copies/mL.

Through 48 weeks of therapy, the proportion of patients who achieved and sustained an HIV-1 RNA < 400 copies/mL was 80% for antiretroviral naïve patients and 71% for antiretroviral experienced patients. The mean increase from baseline in CD4+ cell count was 404 cells/mm³ for antiretroviral naïve and 284 cells/mm³ for antiretroviral experienced patients treated through 48 weeks. At 48 weeks, two patients (2%) had prematurely discontinued the study. One antiretroviral naïve patient prematurely discontinued secondary to an adverse reaction, while one antiretroviral experienced patient prematurely discontinued secondary to an HIV-1 related event.

Dose selection in pediatric patients was based on the following:

• Among patients 14 days to 6 months of age receiving 300/75 mg/m² twice daily without nevirapine, plasma concentrations were lower than those observed in adults or in older children. This dose resulted in HIV-1 RNA < 400 copies/mL in 55% of patients (70% in those initiating treatment at <6 weeks of age).

• Among patients 6 months to 12 years of age, the 230/57.5 mg/m² oral solution twice daily regimen without nevirapine and the 300/75 mg/m² oral solution twice daily regimen with nevirapine provided lopinavir plasma concentrations similar to those obtained in adult patients receiving the 400/100 mg twice daily regimen (without nevirapine). These doses resulted in treatment benefit (proportion of patients with HIV-1 RNA < 400 copies/mL) similar to that seen in the adult clinical trials.

• Among patients 12 to 18 years of age receiving 400/100 mg/m² or 480/120 mg/m² (with efavirenz) twice daily, plasma concentrations were 60-100% higher than among 6 to 12 year old patients receiving 230/57.5 mg/m². Mean apparent clearance was similar to that observed in adult patients receiving standard dose and in patients 6 to 12 years of age. Although changes in HIV-1 RNA in patients with prior treatment failure were less than anticipated, the pharmacokinetic data supports use of similar dosing as in patients 6 to 12 years of age, not to exceed the recommended adult dose.

• For all age groups, the body surface area dosing was converted to body weight dosing using the patient's prescribed lopinavir dose.

16 HOW SUPPLIED/STORAGE AND HANDLING

KALETRA® (lopinavir/ritonavir) Film-Coated tablets and Oral Solution are available in the following strengths and package sizes:

16.1 KALETRA Tablets, 200 mg lopinavir/50 mg ritonavir

Yellow film-coated ovaloid tablets debossed with the "a" logo and the code KA:

Bottles of 120 tablets.............................(NDC 0074-6799-22)
Recommended Storage
Store KALETRA film-coated tablets at 20°-25°C (68°-77°F); excursions permitted to 15°-30°C (59° to 86°F)[see USP controlled room temperature]. Dispense in original container or USP equivalent tight container (250 mL or less). For patient use: exposure of this product to high humidity outside the original container or USP equivalent tight container (250 mL or less) for longer than 2 weeks is not recommended.

16.2 KALETRA Tablets, 100 mg lopinavir/25 mg ritonavir

Pale yellow film-coated ovaloid tablets debossed with the "a" logo and the code KC:

Bottles of 60 tablets.............................(NDC 0074-0522-60)

Table 9 (cont.). Drug Interactions: Pharmacokinetic Parameters for Lopinavir in the Presence of the Co-administered Drug for Recommended Alterations in Dose or Regimen

Co-administered Drug	Dose of Co-administered Drug (mg)	Dose of KALETRA (mg)	n	Ratio (in combination with Co-administered drug/ alone) of Lopinavir Pharmacokinetic Parameters (90% CI); No Effect = 1.00		
				C_{max}	AUC	C_{min}
Ritonavir[4]	100 twice daily, 3-4 wk[#]	400/100 capsule twice daily, 3-4 wk	8, 21*	1.28 (0.94, 1.76)	1.46 (1.04, 2.06)	2.16 (1.29, 3.62)
Telaprevir	750 q8h, 10 days	400/100 tablet twice daily, 20 days	12[13]	0.96 (0.87, 1.05)	1.06 (0.96, 1.17)	1.14 (0.96, 1.36)
Tenofovir[9]	300 mg once daily, 14 d	400/100 capsule twice daily, 14 d	24	NC†	NC†	NC†
Tipranavir/ ritonavir[4]	500/200 mg twice daily (28 doses)[#]	400/100 capsule twice daily (27 doses)	21 69	0.53 (0.40, 0.69)[10]	0.45 (0.32, 0.63)[10]	0.30 (0.17, 0.51)[10] 0.48 (0.40, 0.58)[11]

All interaction studies conducted in healthy, HIV-1 negative subjects unless otherwise indicated.
[1] The pharmacokinetics of ritonavir are unaffected by concurrent efavirenz.
[2] Reference for comparison is lopinavir/ritonavir 400/100 mg twice daily without efavirenz.
[3] Data extracted from the fosamprenavir package insert.
[4] Study conducted in HIV-1 positive adult subjects.
[5] Study conducted in HIV-1 positive pediatric subjects ranging in age from 6 months to 12 years.
[6] Data extracted from the pitavastatin package insert and results presented at the 2011 International AIDS Society Conference on HIV Pathogenesis, Treatment and Prevention (Morgan, et al, poster #MOPE170).
[7] Titrated to 800/200 twice daily as 533/133 twice daily × 1 d, 667/167 twice daily × 1 d, then 800/200 twice daily × 7 d, compared to 400/100 twice daily × 10 days alone.
[8] Titrated to 400/400 twice daily as 400/200 twice daily × 1 d, 400/300 twice daily × 1 d, then 400/400 twice daily × 7 d, compared to 400/100 twice daily × 10 days alone.
[9] Data extracted from the tenofovir package insert.
[10] Intensive PK analysis.
[11] Drug levels obtained at 8-16 hrs post-dose.
[12] AUC parameter is AUC$_{(0-last)}$.
[13] N=12 for test arm, 19 for reference arm
* Parallel group design; n for KALETRA + co-administered drug, n for KALETRA alone.
† NC = No change.
# For the nevirapine 200 mg twice daily study, ritonavir, and tipranavir/ritonavir studies, KALETRA was administered with or without food. For all other studies, KALETRA was administered with food.

Recommended Storage
Store KALETRA film-coated tablets at 20°-25°C (68°-77°F); excursions permitted to 15°-30°C (59° to 86°F)[see USP controlled room temperature]. Dispense in original container or USP equivalent tight container (100 mL or less). For patient use: exposure of this product to high humidity outside the original container or USP equivalent tight container (100 mL or less) for longer than 2 weeks is not recommended.

16.3 KALETRA Oral Solution

KALETRA (lopinavir/ritonavir) oral solution is a light yellow to orange colored liquid supplied in amber-colored multiple-dose bottles containing 400 mg lopinavir/100 mg ritonavir per 5 mL (80 mg lopinavir/20 mg ritonavir per mL) packaged with a marked dosing cup in the following size:

160 mL bottle ....(NDC 0074-3956-46)
Recommended Storage
Store KALETRA oral solution at 2°-8°C (36°-46°F) until dispensed. Avoid exposure to excessive heat. For patient use, refrigerated KALETRA oral solution remains stable until the expiration date printed on the label. If stored at room temperature up to 25°C (77°F), oral solution should be used within 2 months.

17 PATIENT COUNSELING INFORMATION

See FDA-approved patient labeling (Medication Guide)
Information For Patients
Patients or parents of patients should be informed that:
General Information
☐ They should pay special attention to accurate administration of their dose to minimize the risk of accidental overdose or underdose of KALETRA.
☐ They should inform their healthcare provider if their children's weight changes in order to make sure that the child's KALETRA dose is the correct one.
☐ They should take the prescribed dose of KALETRA as directed and to set up a daily routine in order to do so.
☐ KALETRA tablets may be taken with or without food. KALETRA oral solution should be taken with food to enhance absorption.
☐ Sustained decreases in plasma HIV-1 RNA have been associated with a reduced risk of progression to AIDS and death. Patients should remain under the care of a physician while using KALETRA. Patients should be advised to take KALETRA and other concomitant antiretroviral therapy every day as prescribed. KALETRA must always be used in combination with other antiretroviral drugs. Patients should not alter the dose or discontinue therapy without consulting with their doctor. If a dose of KALETRA is missed patients should take the dose as soon as possible and then return to their normal schedule. However, if a dose is skipped the patient should not double the next dose. The amount of HIV-1 virus in their blood may increase if the medicine is stopped for even a short time. The virus may become resistant to KALETRA and become harder to treat.
☐ KALETRA is not a cure for HIV-1 infection and patients may continue to experience illnesses associated with HIV-1 infection, including opportunistic infections. Patients should remain under the care of a physician when using KALETRA.
Patients should be advised to avoid doing things that can spread HIV-1 infection to others.
• **Do not share needles or other injection equipment.**
• **Do not share personal items that can have blood or body fluids on them, like toothbrushes and razor blades.**
• **Do not have any kind of sex without protection.** Always practice safe sex by using a latex or polyurethane condom to lower the chance of sexual contact with semen, vaginal secretions, or blood.
• **Do not breastfeed.** We do not know if KALETRA can be passed to the baby through breast milk and whether it could harm the baby. Also, mothers with HIV-1 should not breastfeed because HIV-1 can be passed to the baby in the breast milk.
Drug Interactions
☐ KALETRA may interact with some drugs; therefore, patients should be advised to report to their doctor the use of any other prescription, non-prescription medication or herbal products, particularly St. John's Wort.
☐ KALETRA tablets can be taken at the same time as didanosine without food. Patients taking didanosine should take didanosine one hour before or two hours after KALETRA oral solution.
☐ If they are receiving avanafil, sildenafil, tadalafil, or vardenafil for the treatment of erectile dysfunction, there

Information on the AbbVie, Inc. products listed on these pages is from the prescribing information in use as of July 31, 2014. For more information, please visit rxabbvie.com or call 1-800-633-9110.

Table 10. Drug Interactions: Pharmacokinetic Parameters for Co-administered Drug in the Presence of KALETRA for Recommended Alterations in Dose or Regimen

Co-administered Drug	Dose of Co-administered Drug (mg)	Dose of KALETRA (mg)	n	Ratio (in combination with KALETRA/alone) of Co-administered Drug Pharmacokinetic Parameters (90% CI); No Effect = 1.00		
				C_{max}	AUC	C_{min}
Boceprevir	800 q8h, 6 d	400/100 tablet twice daily, 22 d	13[8]	0.50 (0.45, 0.55)	0.55 (0.49, 0.61)	0.43 (0.36, 0.53)
Desipramine[2]	100 single dose	400/100 capsule twice daily, 10 d	15	0.91 (0.84, 0.97)	1.05 (0.96, 1.16)	N/A
Efavirenz	600 at bedtime, 9 d	400/100 capsule twice daily, 9 d	11, 12*	0.91 (0.72, 1.15)	0.84 (0.62, 1.15)	0.84 (0.58, 1.20)
Ethinyl Estradiol	35 µg once daily, 21 d (Ortho Novum®)	400/100 capsule twice daily, 14 d	12	0.59 (0.52, 0.66)	0.58 (0.54, 0.62)	0.42 (0.36, 0.49)
Fosamprenavir[3]	700 twice daily plus ritonavir 100 twice daily, 14 d	400/100 capsule twice daily, 14 d	18	0.42 (0.30, 0.58)	0.37 (0.28, 0.49)	0.35 (0.27, 0.46)
Indinavir[1]	600 twice daily, 10 d combo nonfasting vs. 800 three times daily, 5 d alone fasting	400/100 capsule twice daily, 15 d	13	0.71 (0.63, 0.81)	0.91 (0.75, 1.10)	3.47 (2.60, 4.64)
Ketoconazole	200 single dose	400/100 capsule twice daily, 16 d	12	1.13 (0.91, 1.40)	3.04 (2.44, 3.79)	N/A
Methadone	5 single dose	400/100 capsule twice daily, 10 d	11	0.55 (0.48, 0.64)	0.47 (0.42, 0.53)	N/A
Nelfinavir[1]	1000 twice daily, 10 d combo vs. 1250 twice daily 14 d alone	400/100 capsule twice daily, 21 d	13	0.93 (0.82, 1.05)	1.07 (0.95, 1.19)	1.86 (1.57, 2.22)
M8 metabolite				2.36 (1.91, 2.91)	3.46 (2.78, 4.31)	7.49 (5.85, 9.58)
Nevirapine	200 once daily, 14 d; twice daily, 6 d	400/100 capsule twice daily, 20 d	5, 6*	1.05 (0.72, 1.52)	1.08 (0.72, 1.64)	1.15 (0.71, 1.86)
Norethindrone	1 once daily, 21 d (Ortho Novum®)	400/100 capsule twice daily, 14 d	12	0.84 (0.75, 0.94)	0.83 (0.73, 0.94)	0.68 (0.54, 0.85)
Pitavastatin[4]	4 mg once daily, 5 d	400/100 tablet twice daily, 16 d	23	0.96 (0.84-1.10)	0.80 (0.73-0.87)	N/A
Pravastatin	20 once daily, 4 d	400/100 capsule twice daily, 14 d	12	1.26 (0.87, 1.83)	1.33 (0.91, 1.94)	N/A
Rifabutin	150 once daily, 10 d; combo vs. 300 once daily, 10 d; alone	400/100 capsule twice daily, 10 d	12	2.12 (1.89, 2.38)	3.03 (2.79, 3.30)	4.90 (3.18, 5.76)

(Table continued on next page)

may be an increased risk of associated adverse reactions including hypotension, visual changes, and sustained erection, and should promptly report any symptoms to their doctor. If they are currently using or planning to use avanafil or tadalafil (for the treatment of pulmonary arterial hypertension) they should ask their doctor about potential adverse reactions these medications may cause when taken with KALETRA. The doctor may choose not to keep them on avanafil, or may adjust the dose of tadalafil while initiating treatment with KALETRA.

☐ If they are receiving estrogen-based hormonal contraceptives, additional or alternate contraceptive measures should be used during therapy with KALETRA.

☐ If they are taking or before they begin using Serevent® (salmeterol) and KALETRA, they should talk to their doctor about problems these two medications may cause when taken together. The doctor may choose not to keep someone on Serevent® (salmeterol).

☐ If they are taking or before they begin taking Advair® (salmeterol in combination with fluticasone propionate) and KALETRA, they should talk to their doctor about problems these two medications may cause when taken together. The doctor may choose not to keep someone on Advair® (salmeterol in combination with fluticasone propionate).

Potential Adverse Effects

☐ Skin rashes ranging in severity from mild to toxic epidermal necrolysis (TEN), Stevens-Johnson syndrome, erythema multiforme, urticaria, and angioedema have been reported in patients receiving KALETRA or its components lopinavir and/or ritonavir. Patients should be advised to contact their healthcare provider if they develop a rash while taking KALETRA. The healthcare provider will determine if treatment should be continued or an alternative antiretroviral regimen used.

☐ Patients should be advised that appropriate liver function testing will be conducted prior to initiating and during therapy with KALETRA. Pre-existing liver disease including Hepatitis B or C can worsen with use of KALETRA. This can be seen as worsening of transaminase elevations or hepatic decompensation. Patients should be advised that their liver function tests will need to be monitored closely especially during the first several months of KALETRA treat-

ment and that they should notify their healthcare provider if they develop the signs and symptoms of worsening liver disease including loss of appetite, abdominal pain, jaundice, and itchy skin.

☐ New onset of diabetes or exacerbation of pre-existing diabetes mellitus, and hyperglycemia have been reported during KALETRA use. Patients should be advised to notify their healthcare provider if they develop the signs and symptoms of diabetes mellitus including frequent urination, excessive thirst, extreme hunger or unusual weight loss and/or an increased blood sugar while on KALETRA as they may require a change in their diabetes treatment or new treatment.

☐ KALETRA might produce changes in the electrocardiogram (e.g., PR and/or QT prolongation). Patients should consult their physician if they experience symptoms such as dizziness, lightheadedness, abnormal heart rhythm or loss of consciousness.

☐ They should seek medical assistance immediately if they develop a sustained penile erection lasting more than 4 hours while taking KALETRA and a PDE 5 Inhibitor such as Viagra, Cialis or Levitra.

☐ Redistribution or accumulation of body fat may occur in patients receiving antiretroviral therapy and that the cause and long term health effects of these conditions are not known at this time.

☐ Patients should be informed that there may be a greater chance of developing diarrhea with the once daily regimen as compared with the twice daily regimen.

MEDICATION GUIDE
KALETRA® (kuh-LEE-tra)
(lopinavir/ritonavir)
Tablets
KALETRA® (kuh-LEE-tra)
(lopinavir/ritonavir)
Oral Solution

Read this Medication Guide before you start taking KALETRA and each time you get a refill. There may be new information. This information does not take the place of talking with your doctor about your medical condition or treatment. You and your doctor should talk about your treatment with KALETRA before you start taking it and at regular check-ups. You should stay under your doctor's care when taking KALETRA.

What is the most important information I should know about KALETRA?

KALETRA may cause serious side effects, including:

• **Interactions with other medicines. It is important to know the medicines that should not be taken with KALETRA.** For more information, see "Who should not take KALETRA?"

• **Changes in your heart rhythm and the electrical activity of your heart.** These changes may be seen on an EKG (electrocardiogram) and can lead to serious heart problems. Your risk for these problems may be higher if you:
 ◦ already have a history of abnormal heart rhythm or other types of heart disease.
 ◦ take other medicines that can affect your heart rhythm while you take KALETRA.

Tell your doctor right away if you have any of these symptoms while taking KALETRA:

• dizziness
• lightheadedness
• fainting
• sensation of abnormal heartbeats

See "What are the possible side effects of KALETRA?" for more information about serious side effects.

What is KALETRA?

KALETRA is a prescription HIV-1 medicine that is used with other HIV medicines to treat HIV-1 (Human Immunodeficiency Virus) infection in adults and children 14 days of age and older. HIV is the virus that causes AIDS (Acquired Immune Deficiency Syndrome). KALETRA is a type of HIV medicine called a protease inhibitor. KALETRA contains two medicines: lopinavir and ritonavir.

When used with other HIV medicines, KALETRA may help to reduce the amount of HIV in your blood (called "viral load"). KALETRA may also help to increase the number of white blood cells called CD4 (T) cell which help fight off other infections. Reducing the amount of HIV and increasing the CD4 (T) cell count may improve your immune system. This may reduce your risk of death or infections that can happen when your immune system is weak (opportunistic infections).

It is not known if KALETRA is safe and effective in children under 14 days old.

KALETRA does not cure HIV infection or AIDS. People taking KALETRA may develop infections or other conditions associated with HIV infection, including opportunistic infections (for example, pneumonia and herpes virus infections). Avoid doing things that can spread HIV-1 infection to others:

• **Do not share needles or other injection equipment.**

- **Do not share personal items** that can have blood or body fluids on them, like toothbrushes and razor blades.
- **Do not have any kind of sex without protection.** Always practice safe sex by using a latex or polyurethane condom to lower the chance of sexual contact with semen, vaginal secretions, or blood.

Ask your doctor if you have any questions on how to prevent passing HIV to other people.

Who should not take KALETRA?

Do not take KALETRA if you take any of the following medicines:

- alfuzosin (Uroxatral®)
- cisapride (Propulsid®, Quicksolv®)
- ergot containing medicines including
  - ◦ ergotamine tartrate (Cafergot®, Migergot®, Ergomar®, Ergostat®, Medihaler®, Ergotamine, Wigraine®, Wigrettes®)
  - ◦ dihydroergotamine mesylate (D.H.E. 45®, Migranal®)
  - ◦ methylergonovine (Methergine®)
- lovastatin (Advicor®, Altoprev®, Mevacor®)
- midazolam oral syrup
- pimozide (Orap®)
- rifampin (Rifadin®, Rifamate®, Rifater®, Rimactane®)
- sildenafil (Revatio®), when used for the treatment of pulmonary arterial hypertension
- simvastatin (Zocor®, Vytorin®, Simcor®)
- St. John's Wort (Hypericum perforatum)
- triazolam (Halcion®)

Serious problems can happen if you or your child take any of the medicines listed above with KALETRA.

- **Do not take KALETRA if you are allergic** to lopinavir, ritonavir or any of the ingredients in KALETRA. See the end of this Medication Guide for a complete list of ingredients in KALETRA.

What should I tell my doctor before taking KALETRA?

KALETRA may not be right for you. Tell your doctor about all your medical conditions, including if you:

- have any heart problems, including if you have a condition called Congenital Long QT Syndrome.
- have or had pancreas problems.
- have liver problems, including Hepatitis B or Hepatitis C.
- have diabetes.
- have hemophilia. People who take KALETRA may have increased bleeding.
- have low potassium in your blood.
- are pregnant or plan to become pregnant. It is not known if KALETRA will harm your unborn baby.

Pregnancy Registry. There is a pregnancy registry for women who take antiretroviral medicines during pregnancy. The purpose of the pregnancy registry is to collect information about the health of you and your baby. Talk to your doctor about how you can take part in this registry.

- **Do not breastfeed.** We do not know if KALETRA can be passed to the baby through your breast milk and whether it could harm your baby. Also, mothers with HIV-1 should not breastfeed because HIV-1 can be passed to the baby in the breast milk.

Tell your doctor about all the medicines you take, including prescription and non-prescription medicines, vitamins, and herbal supplements. Many medicines interact with KALETRA. Do not start taking a new medicine without telling your doctor or pharmacist. Your doctor can tell you if it is safe to take KALETRA with other medicines. Your doctor may need to change the dose of other medicines while you take KALETRA.

Especially tell your doctor if you take:

- medicine to treat HIV
- estrogen-based contraceptives (birth control pills and patches). KALETRA may reduce the effectiveness of estrogen-based contraceptives. During treatment with KALETRA, you should use a different type or an extra form of birth control. Talk to your doctor about what types of birth control you can use to prevent pregnancy while taking KALETRA.
- medicines to prevent organ transplant rejection
- medicines to treat cancer
- amiodarone (Cordarone®, Pacerone®)
- atorvastatin (Lipitor®)
- atovaquone (Marlarone®, Mepron®)
- avanafil (Stendra®), sildenafil (Viagra®), tadalafil (Cialis®), or vardenafil (Levitra®) for the treatment of erectile dysfunction (ED). If you get dizzy or faint (low blood pressure), have vision changes or have an erection that last longer than 4 hours, call your doctor or get medical help right away
- bepridil (Bepadin®, Vascor®)
- boceprevir (Victrelis®)
- bosentan (Tracleer®)
- budesonide (Rhinocort®, Symbicort®, Pulmicort®, Entocort EC®)
- bupropion (Aplenzin®, Forfivo XL®, Wellbutrin®, Zyban®)
- carbamazepine (Carbatrol®, Epitol®, Equetro®, Tegretol®)
- clarithromycin (Biaxin®, Prevpac®)
- colchicine (Colcrys®)

- dexamethasone (Maxidex®, Ozurdex®)
- disulfiram
- felodipine
- fentanyl (Abstral®, Actiq®, Duragesic®, Fentora®, Lazanda®, Onsolis®, Subsys®)
- fluticasone (Cutivate®, Flonase®, Flovent®, Flovent Diskus®, Flovent HFA®, Veramyst®)
- itraconazole (Onmel®, Sporanox®)
- ketoconazole (Extina®, Ketozole®, Nizoral®, Xolegel®)
- lamotrigine (Lamictal®)
- lidocaine

- methadone hydrochloride (Dolphine hydrochloride, Methadose®)
- metronidazole
- nicardipine (Cardene®)
- nifedipine (Adalat CC®, Afeditab CR®, Procardia®)

Information on the AbbVie, Inc. products listed on these pages is from the prescribing information in use as of July 31, 2014. For more information, please visit rxabbvie.com or call 1-800-633-9110.

Table 10 (cont.). Drug Interactions: Pharmacokinetic Parameters for Co-administered Drug in the Presence of KALETRA for Recommended Alterations in Dose or Regimen

Co-administered Drug	Dose of Co-administered Drug (mg)	Dose of KALETRA (mg)	n	Ratio (in combination with KALETRA/alone) of Co-administered Drug Pharmacokinetic Parameters (90% CI); No Effect = 1.00		
				C_{max}	AUC	C_{min}
25-O-desacetyl rifabutin				23.6 (13.7, 25.3)	47.5 (29.3, 51.8)	94.9 (74.0, 122)
Rifabutin + 25-O-desacetyl rifabutin[5]				3.46 (3.07, 3.91)	5.73 (5.08, 6.46)	9.53 (7.56, 12.01)
Rosuvastatin[6]	20 mg once daily, 7 d	400/100 tablet twice daily, 7 d	15	4.66 (3.4, 6.4)	2.08 (1.66, 2.6)	1.04 (0.9, 1.2)
Telaprevir	750 q8h, 10 days	400/100 tablet twice daily, 20 days	12[9]	0.47 (0.41, 0.52)	0.46 (0.41, 0.52)	0.48 (0.40, 0.56)
Tenofovir[7]	300 mg once daily, 14 d	400/100 capsule twice daily, 14 d	24	NC[†]	1.32 (1.26, 1.38)	1.51 (1.32, 1.66)

All interaction studies conducted in healthy, HIV-1 negative subjects unless otherwise indicated.
[1] Ratio of parameters for indinavir, and nelfinavir, are not normalized for dose.
[2] Desipramine is a probe substrate for assessing effects on CYP2D6-mediated metabolism.
[3] Data extracted from the fosamprenavir package insert.
[4] Data extracted from the pitavastatin package insert and results presented at the 2011 International AIDS Society Conference on HIV Pathogenesis, Treatment and Prevention (Morgan, *et al*, poster #MOPE170).
[5] Effect on the dose-normalized sum of rifabutin parent and 25-O-desacetyl rifabutin active metabolite.
[6] Kiser, et al. J Acquir Immune Defic Syndr. 2008 Apr 15;47(5):570-8.
[7] Data extracted from the tenofovir package insert.
[8] N=12 for C_{min} (test arm)
[9] N=12 for the test arm, 14 for reference arm
* Parallel group design; n for KALETRA + co-administered drug, n for co-administered drug alone.
N/A = Not available.
† NC = No change.

Table 11. Virologic Response (HIV-1 RNA <400 copies/mL) at Week 48 by Baseline KALETRA Susceptibility and by Number of Protease Substitutions Associated with Reduced Response to KALETRA[1]

Number of protease inhibitor substitutions at baseline[1]	Study 888 (Single protease inhibitor-experienced[2], NNRTI-naïve) n=130	Study 765 (Single protease inhibitor-experienced[3], NNRTI-naïve) n=56	Study 957 (Multiple protease inhibitor-experienced[4], NNRTI-naïve) n=50
0-2	76/103 (74%)	34/45 (76%)	19/20 (95%)
3-5	13/26 (50%)	8/11 (73%)	18/26 (69%)
6 or more	0/1 (0%)	N/A	1/4 (25%)

[1] Substitutions considered in the analysis included L10F/I/R/V, K20M/N/R, L24I, L33F, M36I, I47V, G48V, I54L/T/V, V82A/C/F/S/T, and I84V.
[2] 43% indinavir, 42% nelfinavir, 10% ritonavir, 15% saquinavir.
[3] 41% indinavir, 38% nelfinavir, 4% ritonavir, 16% saquinavir.
[4] 86% indinavir, 54% nelfinavir, 80% ritonavir, 70% saquinavir.

Table 14. Proportion of Responders Through Week 48 by Baseline Viral Load (Study 863)

Baseline Viral Load (HIV-1 RNA copies/mL)	KALETRA +d4T+3TC			Nelfinavir +d4T+3TC		
	<400 copies/mL[1]	<50 copies/mL[2]	n	<400 copies/mL[1]	<50 copies/mL[2]	n
< 30,000	74%	71%	82	79%	72%	87
≥ 30,000 to < 100,000	81%	73%	79	67%	54%	79
≥ 100,000 to < 250,000	75%	64%	83	60%	47%	72
≥ 250,000	72%	60%	82	44%	33%	89

[1] Patients achieved and maintained confirmed HIV-1 RNA < 400 copies/mL through Week 48.
[2] Patients achieved HIV-1 RNA < 50 copies/mL at Week 48.

- phenobarbital
- phenytoin (Dilantin®, Phenytek®)
- prednisone
- quinidine (Quinidex®)
- rifabutin (Mycobutin®)
- rivaroxaban (Xarelto®)
- rosuvastatin (Crestor®)
- salmeterol (Serevent®) or salmeterol when taken in combination with fluticasone (Advair Diskus®, Advair HFA®)
- tadalafil (Adcirca®) for the treatment of pulmonary arterial hypertension
- telaprevir (Incivek®)
- trazodone (Oleptro®)
- valproate (Depakote®, Depakene®, Depacon®)
- voriconazole (Vfend®)
- warfarin (Coumadin®, Jantoven®)

KALETRA should not be administered once daily in combination with carbamazepine (Carbatrol®, Epitol®, Equetro®, Tegretol®), phenobarbital, or phenytoin (Dilantin®, Phenytek®)

Ask your doctor or pharmacist if you are not sure if your medicine is one that is listed above.

Know all the medicines that you take. Keep a list of them with you to show doctors and pharmacists when you get a new medicine.

If you are not sure if you are taking a medicine above, ask your doctor.

How should I take KALETRA?

- Take KALETRA every day exactly as prescribed by your doctor.
- It is very important to set up a dosing schedule and follow it every day.
- Do not change your treatment or stop treatment without first talking with your doctor.
- Swallow KALETRA tablets whole. Do not chew, break, or crush KALETRA tablets.
- KALETRA tablets can be taken with or without food.
- If you are taking both didanosine (Videx®) and KALETRA:
  ○ didanosine can be taken at the same time as KALETRA tablets, without food.
  ○ take didanosine either one hour before or two hours after taking KALETRA oral solution.
- Do not miss a dose of KALETRA. This could make the virus harder to treat. If you forget to take KALETRA, take the missed dose right away. If it is almost time for your next dose, do not take the missed dose. Instead, follow your regular dosing schedule by taking your next dose at its regular time. Do not take more than one dose of KALETRA at one time.
- If you take more than the prescribed dose of KALETRA, call your doctor or go to the nearest emergency room right away.
- Take KALETRA oral solution with food to help it work better.
- If your child is prescribed KALETRA, tell your doctor if your child's weight changes.
- KALETRA **should not** be given one time each day in children. When giving KALETRA to your child, give KALETRA exactly as prescribed.
- KALETRA oral solution contains propylene glycol and a large amount of alcohol. KALETRA oral solution **should not** be given to babies younger than 14 days of age unless your doctor thinks it is right for your baby.
  ○ If a young child drinks more than the recommended dose, it could make them sick. Contact your local poison control center or emergency room right away.
  ○ Talk with your doctor if you take or plan to take metronidazole or disulfiram. You can have severe nausea and vomiting if you take these medicines with KALETRA.
- When your KALETRA supply starts to run low, get more from your doctor or pharmacy. It is important not to run out of KALETRA. The amount of HIV-1 virus in your blood may increase if the medicine is stopped for even a short time. The virus may become resistant to KALETRA and become harder to treat.

What are the possible side effects of KALETRA?

KALETRA can cause serious side effects, including:

- See "What is the most important information I should know about KALETRA?"
- **Inflammation of the pancreas (pancreatitis)**. Some people who take KALETRA get inflammation of the pancreas which may be serious and cause death. You have a higher chance of getting pancreatitis if you have had it before. Tell your doctor if you have nausea, vomiting, or abdominal pain while taking KALETRA. These may be signs of pancreatitis.
- **Liver problems.** Liver problems, including death, can happen in people who take KALETRA. Your doctor should do blood tests before and during your treatment with KALETRA to check your liver function. Some people with liver disease such as Hepatitis B and Hepatitis C who take KALETRA may have worsening liver disease. Tell your doctor right away if you have any of these signs and symptoms of liver problems:

  ○ loss of appetite
  ○ yellow skin and whites of eyes (jaundice)
  ○ dark-colored urine
  ○ pale colored stools
  ○ itchy skin
  ○ stomach area (abdominal) pain.
- **Diabetes and high blood sugar (hyperglycemia).** Some people who take protease inhibitors including KALETRA get new or more serious diabetes, or high blood sugar. Tell your doctor if you notice an increase in thirst or urinate often while taking KALETRA.
- **Changes in your immune system (Immune Reconstitution Syndrome)** can happen when you start taking HIV medicines. Your immune system may get stronger and begin to fight infections that have been hidden in your body for a long time. Call your doctor right away if you start having new symptoms after starting your HIV medicine.
- **Increases in certain fat (triglycerides and cholesterol) levels in your blood.** Large increases of triglycerides and cholesterol can be seen in blood test results of some people who take KALETRA. Your doctor should do blood tests to check your cholesterol and triglyceride levels before you start taking KALETRA and during your treatment.
- **Changes in body fat.** Changes in body fat in some people who take antiretroviral therapy. These changes may include increased amount of fat in the upper back and neck ("buffalo hump"), breast, and around the trunk. Loss of fat from the legs, arms and face may also happen. The cause and long-term health effects of these conditions are not known at this time.
- **Increased bleeding for hemophiliacs.** Some people with hemophilia have increased bleeding with protease inhibitors including KALETRA.
- **Allergic reactions.** Skin rashes, some of them severe, can occur in people who take KALETRA. Tell your healthcare provider if you had a rash when you took another medicine for your HIV-1 infection or if you notice any skin rash when you take KALETRA.
- **Babies taking KALETRA oral solution may have side effects.** KALETRA oral solution contains alcohol and propylene glycol. Call your doctor right away if your baby appears too sleepy or their breathing has changed.

Common side effects of KALETRA include:

- diarrhea
- nausea
- increased fats in blood (triglycerides or cholesterol)
- vomiting

Tell your doctor about any side effect that bothers you or that does not go away.

These are not all of the possible side effects of KALETRA. For more information, ask your doctor or pharmacist.

Call your doctor for medical advice about side effects. You may report side effects to FDA at 1-800-FDA-1088.

How should I store KALETRA?

KALETRA tablets:

- Store KALETRA tablets at room temperature, between 59°F to 86°F (15°C to 30°C).
- Do not keep KALETRA tablets out of the container it comes in for longer than 2 weeks, especially in areas where there is a lot of humidity. Keep the container closed tightly.

KALETRA oral solution:

- Store KALETRA oral solution in a refrigerator, between 36°F to 46°F (2°C to 8°C). KALETRA oral solution that is kept refrigerated may be used until the expiration date printed on the label.
- KALETRA oral solution that is stored at room temperature (less than 77°F or 25°C) should be used within 2 months.
- Keep KALETRA away from high heat.

Throw away any medicine that is out of date or that you no longer need.

Keep KALETRA and all medicines out of the reach of children.

General information about KALETRA

Medicines are sometimes prescribed for purposes other than those listed in a Medication Guide. Do not use KALETRA for a condition for which it was not prescribed. Do not give KALETRA to other people, even if they have the same condition you have. It may harm them.

This Medication Guide summarizes the most important information about KALETRA. If you would like more information, talk with your doctor. You can ask your pharmacist or doctor for information about KALETRA that is written for health professionals. For more information about KALETRA call 1-800-633-9110 or go to www.KALETRA.com.

What are the ingredients in KALETRA?

Active ingredients: lopinavir and ritonavir

Inactive ingredients:

KALETRA 200 mg lopinavir and 50 mg ritonavir tablets: copovidone, sorbitan monolaurate, colloidal silicon dioxide, and sodium stearyl fumarate. The film coating contains: hypromellose, titanium dioxide, polyethylene glycol 400, hydroxypropyl cellulose, talc, colloidal silicon dioxide, polyethylene glycol 3350, yellow ferric oxide 172, and polysorbate 80.

KALETRA 100 mg lopinavir and 25 mg ritonavir tablets: copovidone, sorbitan monolaurate, colloidal silicon dioxide, and sodium stearyl fumarate. The film coating contains: polyvinyl alcohol, titanium dioxide, talc, polytheylene glycol 3350, and yellow ferric oxide E172.

KALETRA oral solution: acesulfame potassium, alcohol, artificial cotton candy flavor, citric acid, glycerin, high fructose corn syrup, Magnasweet-110 flavor, menthol, natural and artificial vanilla flavor, peppermint oil, polyoxyl 40 hydrogenated castor oil, povidone, propylene glycol, saccharin sodium, sodium chloride, sodium citrate, and water.

KALETRA oral solution contains 42.4% alcohol (v/v). "See How should I take KALETRA?".

This Medication Guide has been approved by the U.S. Food and Drug Administration.

2013, ALL RIGHTS RESERVED

* The brands listed are trademarks of their respective owners and are not trademarks of AbbVie Inc. The makers of these brands are not affiliated with and do not endorse AbbVie Inc. or its products.

KALETRA Tablets, 200 mg lopinavir/50 mg ritonavir Manufactured by AbbVie LTD, Barceloneta, PR 00617 for AbbVie Inc., North Chicago, IL 60064 USA

KALETRA Tablets, 100 mg lopinavir/25 mg ritonavir and KALETRA Oral Solution

AbbVie Inc., North Chicago, IL 60064 USA

Ref. 03-A841-R17-Rev. November, 2013

Shown in Product Identification Guide, page 303

LUPANETA PACK™ ℞
Leuprolide Acetate for Depot Suspension
3.75 mg for intramuscular injection
only and Norethindrone Acetate
tablets, 5 mg for oral administration

HIGHLIGHTS OF PRESCRIBING INFORMATION

These highlights do not include all the information needed to use LUPANETA PACK safely and effectively. See full prescribing information for LUPANETA PACK.

LUPANETA PACK (leuprolide acetate for depot suspension; norethindrone acetate tablets), co-packaged for intramuscular use and for oral use, respectively

Initial U.S. Approval: 2012

————INDICATIONS AND USAGE————

LUPANETA PACK contains leuprolide acetate, a gonadotropin-releasing hormone (GnRH) agonist and norethindrone acetate, a progestin, indicated for

- Initial management of the painful symptoms of endometriosis (1)
- Management of recurrence of symptoms (1)

Limitations of Use: Initial treatment course is limited to 6 months and use is not recommended longer than a total of 12 months due to concerns about adverse impact on bone mineral density. (1, 2.1, 5.1)

————DOSAGE AND ADMINISTRATION————

- Leuprolide acetate for depot suspension 3.75 mg given by a healthcare provider as a single intramuscular injection every month for up to six injections (6 months of therapy) (2.1)
- Norethindrone acetate 5 mg tablets taken orally by the patient once per day for up to 6 months (2.1)
- If endometriosis symptoms recur after initial course of therapy, consider retreatment for up to another six months (2.1)
- Assess bone density before retreatment begins (2.1, 5.1)
- Reconstitute leuprolide acetate prior to use, see important administration instructions (2.3)

————DOSAGE FORMS AND STRENGTHS————

- Leuprolide acetate for depot suspension 3.75 mg syringe (3)
- Norethindrone acetate 5 mg tablets; 30 count bottle (3)

————CONTRAINDICATIONS————

- Hypersensitivity to GnRH, GnRH agonist or any of the excipients in leuprolide acetate for depot suspension or norethindrone acetate (4)
- Undiagnosed abnormal uterine bleeding (4)
- Pregnancy or suspected pregnancy (4, 8.1)
- Women who are breast-feeding (4)
- Known, suspected or history of breast or other hormone-sensitive cancer (4)
- Thrombotic or thromboembolic disorders (4)
- Liver tumors or liver disease (4)

————WARNINGS AND PRECAUTIONS————

- Loss of bone mineral density: do not use for more than two six-month treatment courses. (1, 2.1, 5.1)
- Exclude pregnancy before starting treatment and discontinue use if pregnancy occurs; use non-hormonal methods of contraception only. (5.2)
- Discontinue in case of sudden loss of vision or onset of proptosis, diplopia or migraine. (5.3)

- Carefully observe patients with history of depression and discontinue the drug if the depression recurs to a serious degree. (5.4)
- Assess and manage risk factors for cardiovascular disease before starting LUPANETA PACK. (5.6)

ADVERSE REACTIONS

Leuprolide acetate for depot suspension: Most common related adverse reactions (>10%) were hot flashes/sweats, headache/migraine, depression/emotional lability, nausea/vomiting, nervousness/anxiety, insomnia, pain, acne, asthenia, vaginitis, weight gain, constipation/diarrhea (6.1)
Progestins: breakthrough bleeding, spotting (6.1)
To report SUSPECTED ADVERSE REACTIONS, contact AbbVie Inc. at 1-800-633-9110 or FDA at 1-800-FDA-1088 or www.fda.gov/medwatch

USE IN SPECIFIC POPULATIONS

Pediatric: Safety and effectiveness of LUPANETA PACK has not been established in pediatric patients. (8.4)
Geriatric: LUPANETA PACK has not been studied in women over 65 years of age and is not indicated in this population. (8.5)
See 17 for PATIENT COUNSELING INFORMATION and FDA-approved patient labeling

Revised: 03/2013

FULL PRESCRIBING INFORMATION: CONTENTS*

FULL PRESCRIBING INFORMATION

1 INDICATIONS AND USAGE

LUPANETA PACK (leuprolide acetate for depot suspension and norethindrone acetate tablets) is indicated for initial management of the painful symptoms of endometriosis and for management of recurrence of symptoms.
Limitation of Use: Duration of use is limited due to concerns about adverse impact on bone mineral density [see Warnings and Precautions (5.1)]. The initial treatment course of LUPANETA PACK is limited to six months. A single retreatment course of not more than six months may be administered after the initial course of treatment if symptoms recur. Use of LUPANETA PACK for longer than a total of 12 months is not recommended.

2 DOSAGE AND ADMINISTRATION

2.1 Dosing Information

LUPANETA PACK is a co-packaging of leuprolide acetate for depot suspension for intramuscular use and norethindrone acetate tablets for oral use. Administer as follows:

- 3.75 mg of leuprolide acetate by intramuscular injection once a month for up to six injections (6 months of therapy); to be administered by a healthcare provider

Figure 1:

Plunger — End Stopper — Middle Stoppers — Barrel — Front Stopper — Needle and Cap — Finger Grip — Diluent — Blue Line — LuproLoc® Safety Device — Leuprolide Acetate Microsphere Powder

- 5 mg of norethindrone acetate orally once daily for up to 6 months of therapy

The initial course of treatment with leuprolide acetate for depot suspension 3.75 mg in combination with norethindrone acetate 5 mg daily is not to exceed six months.
If the symptoms of endometriosis recur after the initial course of therapy, consider retreatment with LUPANETA PACK for up to another six months. It is recommended that bone density be assessed before retreatment begins [see Warnings and Precautions (5.1)].
Treatment beyond two six-month courses has not been studied and is not recommended due to concerns about adverse impact on bone mineral density.

2.2 Different Formulations of Leuprolide Acetate

Due to the specific release characteristics of the 1-month depot formulation, HCPs should not administer 3 doses of the 3.75 mg 1-month formulation simultaneously to mimic the pharmacological profile of the 11.25 mg 3-month formulation.

2.3 Reconstitution and Administration for Injection of Leuprolide Acetate

- Reconstitute and administer the lyophilized microspheres as a single intramuscular injection.
- Inject the suspension immediately or discard if not used within two hours, because leuprolide acetate for depot suspension does not contain a preservative.
1. Visually inspect the leuprolide acetate for depot suspension powder. DO NOT USE the syringe if clumping or caking is evident. A thin layer of powder on the wall of the syringe is considered normal prior to mixing with the diluent. The diluent should appear clear.
2. To prepare for injection, screw the white plunger into the end stopper until the stopper begins to turn (see Figure 1 and Figure 2).

[See figure 1 above]

Figure 2:

3. Hold the syringe UPRIGHT. Release the diluent by SLOWLY PUSHING (6 to 8 seconds) the plunger until the first middle stopper is at the blue line in the middle of the barrel (see Figure 3).

Figure 3:

← blue line

4. Keep the syringe UPRIGHT. Mix the microspheres (powder) thoroughly by gently shaking the syringe until the powder forms a uniform suspension. The suspension will appear milky. If the powder adheres to the stopper or caking/clumping is present, tap the syringe with your finger to disperse. DO NOT USE if any of the powder has not gone into suspension (see Figure 4).

Figure 4:

5. Keep the syringe UPRIGHT. With the opposite hand pull the needle cap upward without twisting.
6. Keep the syringe UPRIGHT. Advance the plunger to expel the air from the syringe. Now the syringe is ready for injection.
7. After cleaning the injection site with an alcohol swab, administer the intramuscular injection by inserting the needle at a 90 degree angle into the gluteal area, anterior thigh, or deltoid (see Figure 5). Alternate injection sites.

Figure 5:

NOTE: If a blood vessel is accidentally penetrated, aspirated blood will be visible just below the luer lock (see Figure 6) and can be seen through the transparent LuproLoc safety device. If blood is present, remove the needle immediately. Do not inject the medication.

Figure 6:

If a blood vessel is injured, blood will be visible in this section of the syringe.

8. Inject the entire contents of the syringe intramuscularly.
9. Withdraw the needle. Once the syringe has been withdrawn, immediately activate the LuproLoc® safety device by pushing the arrow on the lock upward towards the

Information on the AbbVie, Inc. products listed on these pages is from the prescribing information in use as of July 31, 2014. For more information, please visit rxabbvie.com or call 1-800-633-9110.

Table 1. Adverse Reactions Occurring in the First Six Months of Treatment in ≥ 5% of Patients with Endometriosis

	Controlled Study				Open Label Study	
	LA-Only*		LA/N†		LA/N†	
	N=51		N=55		N=136	
Adverse Reactions	N	%	N	%	N	%
Any Adverse Reaction	50	98	53	96	126	93
Body as a Whole						
Asthenia		18		18		11
Headache/Migraine		65		51		46
Injection Site Reaction		2		9		3
Pain		24		29		21
Cardiovascular System						
Hot flashes/Sweats		98		87		57
Digestive System						
Altered Bowel Function (constipation, diarrhea)		14		15		10
Changes in Appetite		4		0		6
GI Disturbance (dyspepsia, flatulence)		4		7		4
Nausea/Vomiting		25		29		13
Metabolic and Nutritional Disorders						
Edema		0		9		7
Weight Gain		12		13		4
Nervous System						
Depression/Emotional Lability		31		27		34
Dizziness/Vertigo		16		11		7
Insomnia/Sleep Disorder		31		13		15
Decreased Libido		10		4		7
Memory Disorder		6		2		4
Nervousness/Anxiety		8		4		11
Neuromuscular Disorder (leg cramps, paresthesia)		2		9		3
Skin and Appendages						
Androgen-Like Effects (acne, alopecia)		4		5		18
Skin/Mucous Membrane Reaction		4		9		11
Urogenital System						
Breast Changes/Pain/Tenderness		6		13		8
Menstrual Disorders		2		0		5
Vaginitis		20		15		8

* LA-Only = leuprolide acetate 3.75 mg
† LA/N = leuprolide acetate 3.75 mg plus norethindrone acetate 5 mg

needle tip with the thumb or finger, as illustrated, until the needle cover of the safety device over the needle is fully extended and a CLICK is heard or felt (see Figure 7).

Figure 7:

CLICK

10. Dispose of the syringe according to local regulations/procedures [see References (15)].

3 DOSAGE FORMS AND STRENGTHS
LUPANETA PACK 1-month copackaged kit contains two separate components:
- Leuprolide acetate for depot suspension 3.75 mg for 1-month administration: Leuprolide acetate lyophilized powder for reconstitution with supplied diluent in a pre-filled dual chamber syringe
- Norethindrone acetate 5 mg tablets: White to off-white oval, flat-faced beveled edged, uncoated debossed with 'G with breakline' on one side and 304 on other side

4 CONTRAINDICATIONS
LUPANETA PACK is contraindicated in women with the following:
- Hypersensitivity to gonadotropin-releasing hormone (GnRH), GnRH agonist analogs, any of the excipients in leuprolide acetate for depot suspension, or norethindrone acetate
- Undiagnosed abnormal uterine bleeding
- Known, suspected or planned pregnancy during the course of therapy [see Use in Specific Populations (8.1)]
- Lactating women [see Use in Specific Populations (8.3)]
- Known, suspected or history of breast cancer or other hormone-sensitive cancer
- Current or history of thrombotic or thromboembolic disorder
- Liver tumors or liver disease

5 WARNINGS AND PRECAUTIONS
5.1 Loss of Bone Mineral Density
Leuprolide acetate for depot suspension induces a hypoestrogenic state that results in loss of bone mineral density (BMD), some of which may not be reversible. Concurrent use of norethindrone acetate is effective in reducing the loss of BMD that occurs with leuprolide acetate [see Clinical Studies (14)]. Nonetheless, duration of use of LUPANETA PACK is limited to two six-month courses of treatment due to concerns about the adverse impact on BMD. It is recommended that BMD be assessed before retreatment. Retreatment with leuprolide acetate for depot suspension alone is not recommended.
In women with major risk factors for decreased BMD such as chronic alcohol (> 3 units per day) or tobacco use, strong family history of osteoporosis, or chronic use of drugs that can decrease BMD, such as anticonvulsants or corticosteroids, use of LUPANETA PACK may pose an additional risk, and the risks and benefits should be weighed carefully.
5.2 Pregnancy Risk
Leuprolide acetate for depot suspension may cause fetal harm if administered to a pregnant woman. Exclude pregnancy before initiating treatment with LUPANETA PACK. When used at the recommended dose and dosing interval, leuprolide acetate for depot suspension usually inhibits ovulation and stops menstruation. Contraception, however, is not ensured by taking leuprolide acetate for depot suspension. Therefore, patients should use nonhormonal methods of contraception. Advise patients to notify their healthcare provider if they believe they may be pregnant. Discontinue LUPANETA PACK if a patient becomes pregnant during treatment and inform the patient of potential risk to the fetus [see Contraindications (4) and Use in Specific Populations (8.1)].
5.3 Visual Abnormalities
Discontinue norethindrone acetate tablets in the LUPANETA PACK pending examination if there is a sudden partial or complete loss of vision or if there is sudden onset of proptosis, diplopia, or migraine. Discontinue LUPANETA PACK if examination reveals papilledema or retinal vascular lesions.
5.4 Clinical Depression
Depression may occur or worsen during treatment with LUPANETA PACK. Carefully observe patients with a history of clinical depression and discontinue LUPANETA PACK if the depression recurs to a serious degree.
5.5 Serious Allergic Reactions
In clinical trials of LUPANETA PACK, adverse events of asthma were reported in women with pre-existing histories of asthma, sinusitis and environmental or drug allergies. Symptoms consistent with an anaphylactoid or asthmatic process have been reported postmarketing.
5.6 Cardiovascular and Metabolic Disorders
Assess and manage risk factors for cardiovascular disease before starting LUPANETA PACK. Closely monitor women on norethindrone acetate who have risk factors for arterial vascular disease (e.g., hypertension, diabetes mellitus, tobacco use, hypercholesterolemia, and obesity) and/or venous thromboembolism (e.g., family history of VTE, obesity, and smoking) when using LUPANETA PACK. [see Contraindications (4)].
5.7 Initial Flare of Symptoms
Following the first dose of leuprolide acetate, sex steroids temporarily rise above baseline because of the physiologic effect of the drug. Therefore, an increase in symptoms associated with endometriosis may be observed during the initial days of therapy, but these should dissipate with continued therapy.
5.8 Fluid Retention
Because norethindrone acetate may cause some degree of fluid retention, carefully observe women with conditions that might be influenced by this effect, such as epilepsy, migraine, cardiac or renal dysfunctions.

6 ADVERSE REACTIONS
6.1 Clinical Trials Experience
Because clinical trials are conducted under widely varying conditions, adverse reaction rates observed in the clinical trials of a drug cannot be directly compared to rates in the clinical trials of another drug and may not reflect the rates observed in clinical practice.
The safety of co-administering leuprolide acetate for depot suspension and norethindrone acetate was evaluated in two clinical studies in which a total of 242 women were treated for up to one year. Women were treated with monthly IM injections of leuprolide acetate 3.75 mg (13 injections) alone

or monthly IM injections of leuprolide acetate 3.75 mg (13 injections) and 5 mg norethindrone acetate daily. The population age range was 17-43 years old. The majority of patients were Caucasian (87%).

One study was a controlled clinical trial in which 106 women were randomized to one year of treatment with leuprolide acetate for depot suspension alone or with leuprolide acetate for depot suspension and norethindrone acetate. The other study was an open-label single arm clinical study in 136 women of one year of treatment with leuprolide acetate for depot suspension and norethindrone acetate, with follow-up for up to 12 months after completing treatment.

Adverse Reactions (>1%) Leading to Study Discontinuation: In the controlled study, 18% of patients treated monthly with leuprolide acetate and 18% of patients treated monthly with leuprolide acetate plus norethindrone acetate discontinued therapy due to adverse reactions, most commonly hot flashes (6%) and insomnia (4%) in the leuprolide acetate alone group and hot flashes and emotional lability (4% each) in the leuprolide acetate and norethindrone group.

In the open label study, 13% of patients treated monthly with leuprolide acetate plus norethindrone acetate discontinued therapy due to adverse reactions, most commonly depression (4%) and acne (2%).

Common Adverse Reactions:

Table 1 lists the adverse reactions observed in at least 5% of patients in any treatment group, during the first 6 months of treatment in the add-back clinical studies, in which patients were treated with monthly leuprolide acetate for depot suspension 3.75 mg with or without norethindrone acetate co-treatment. The most frequently-occurring adverse reactions observed in these studies were hot flashes and headaches.

[See table 1 at top of previous page]

In the controlled clinical trial, 50 of 51 (98%) patients in the leuprolide acetate alone group and 48 of 55 (87%) patients in the leuprolide acetate and norethindrone group reported experiencing hot flashes on one or more occasions during treatment. Table 2 presents hot flash data in the last month of treatment.

[See table 2 above]

Serious Adverse Reactions:

Urinary tract infection, renal calculus, depression

Changes in Laboratory Values during Treatment:

Liver Enzymes

In the two clinical trials of women with endometriosis, 4 of 191 patients receiving leuprolide acetate and norethindrone acetate for up to 12 months developed an elevated (at least twice the upper limit of normal) SGPT and 2 of 136 developed an elevated GGT. Five of the 6 increases were observed beyond 6 months of treatment. None was associated with an elevated bilirubin concentration.

Lipids

Percent changes from baseline for serum lipids and percentages of patients with serum lipid values outside of the normal range in the two studies of leuprolide acetate and norethindrone acetate are summarized in the tables below. The major impact of adding norethindrone acetate to treatment with leuprolide acetate for depot suspension was a decrease in serum HDL cholesterol and an increase in the LDL/HDL ratio.

[See table 3 above]

Changes from baseline tended to be greater at Week 52. After treatment, mean serum lipid levels from patients with follow up data (105 of 158 patients) returned to pretreatment values.

[See table 4 above]

6.2 Postmarketing Experience

The following adverse reactions have been identified during postapproval use of leuprolide acetate for depot suspension or norethindrone acetate. Because these reactions are reported voluntarily from a population of uncertain size, it is not always possible to reliably estimate their frequency or establish a causal relationship to drug exposure.

Leuprolide Acetate for Depot Suspension

During postmarketing surveillance with other dosage forms and in the same or different populations, the following adverse reactions were reported:

• Allergic reactions (anaphylactic, rash, urticaria, and photosensitivity reactions)
• Mood swings, including depression
• Suicidal ideation and attempt
• Symptoms consistent with an anaphylactoid or asthmatic process
• Localized reactions including induration and abscess at the site of injection
• Symptoms consistent with fibromyalgia (e.g., joint and muscle pain, headaches, sleep disorders, gastrointestinal distress, and shortness of breath), individually and collectively

Other adverse reactions reported are:

Hepato-biliary disorder - Serious liver injury

Injury, poisoning and procedural complications - Spinal fracture

Investigations - Decreased white blood count

Musculoskeletal and connective tissue disorder - Tenosynovitis-like symptoms

Nervous System disorder - Convulsion, peripheral neuropathy, paralysis

Vascular disorder - Hypotension, Hypertension

Serious venous and arterial thrombotic and thromboembolic events, including deep vein thrombosis, pulmonary embolism, myocardial infarction, stroke, and transient ischemic attack

Pituitary apoplexy

During post-marketing surveillance, cases of pituitary apoplexy (a clinical syndrome secondary to infarction of the pituitary gland) have been reported after the administration of leuprolide acetate and other GnRH agonists. In a majority of these cases, a pituitary adenoma was diagnosed, with a majority of pituitary apoplexy cases occurring within 2 weeks of the first dose, and some within the first hour. In these cases, pituitary apoplexy has presented as sudden headache, vomiting, visual changes, ophthalmoplegia, altered mental status, and sometimes cardiovascular collapse. Immediate medical attention has been required.

7 DRUG INTERACTIONS

7.1 Drug-Drug Interactions

Leuprolide Acetate for Depot Suspension

No pharmacokinetic-based drug-drug interaction studies have been conducted with leuprolide acetate for depot suspension. However, drug interactions associated with cytochrome P-450 enzymes or protein binding would not be expected to occur *[see Clinical Pharmacology (12.3)].*

Norethindrone Acetate

No pharmacokinetic drug interaction studies investigating any drug-drug interactions with norethindrone acetate have been conducted. Drugs or herbal products that induce or inhibit certain enzymes, including CYP3A4, may decrease or increase the serum concentrations of norethindrone.

Information on the AbbVie, Inc. products listed on these pages is from the prescribing information in use as of July 31, 2014. For more information, please visit rxabbvie.com or call 1-800-633-9110.

Table 2. Hot Flashes in the Month Prior to the Assessment Visit (Controlled Study)

Assessment Visit	Treatment Group	Number of Patients Reporting Hot Flashes		Number of Days with Hot Flashes		Maximum Number of Hot Flashes in 24 Hours	
		N	(%)	N[2]	Mean	N[2]	Mean
Week 24	LA-Only*	32/37	86	37	19	36	5.8
	LA/N†	22/38	58[1]	38	7[1]	38	1.9[1]

* LA-Only = leuprolide acetate 3.75 mg
† LA/N = leuprolide acetate 3.75 mg plus norethindrone acetate 5 mg
[1] Statistically significantly less than the LA-Only group (p<0.01)
[2] Number of patients assessed.

Table 3. Serum Lipids: Mean Percent Changes from Baseline Values at Treatment Week 24

	leuprolide acetate 3.75 mg		leuprolide acetate for depot suspension 3.75 mg plus norethindrone acetate 5 mg daily			
	Controlled Study (n=39)		Controlled Study (n=41)		Open Label Study (n=117)	
	Baseline Value*	Wk 24% Change	Baseline Value*	Wk 24% Change	Baseline Value*	Wk 24% Change
Total Cholesterol	170.5	9.2%	179.3	0.2%	181.2	2.8%
HDL Cholesterol	52.4	7.4%	51.8	-18.8%	51.0	-14.6%
LDL Cholesterol	96.6	10.9%	101.5	14.1%	109.1	13.1%
LDL/HDL Ratio	2.0†	5.0%	2.1†	43.4%	2.3†	39.4%
Triglycerides	107.8	17.5%	130.2	9.5%	105.4	13.8%

* mg/dL
† ratio

Table 4. Percent of Patients with Serum Lipid Values Outside of the Normal Range

	leuprolide acetate for depot suspension 3.75 mg plus norethindrone acetate 5 mg daily			
	Controlled Study (n=41)		Open Label Study (n=117)	
	Baseline	Wk 24*	Baseline	Wk 24*
Total Cholesterol (>240 mg/dL)	15%	20%	6%	7%
HDL Cholesterol (<40 mg/dL)	15%	44%	15%	41%
LDL Cholesterol (>160 mg/dL)	5%	7%	9%	11%
LDL/HDL Ratio (>4.0)	2%	15%	7%	21%
Triglycerides (>200 mg/dL)	12%	10%	5%	9%

* Includes all patients regardless of baseline value.

Figure 8. Mean Norethindrone Plasma Concentration Profile after a Single Dose of 5 mg Norethindrone Acetate Administered to 29 Healthy Female Volunteers under Fasting Conditions

7.2 Drug/Laboratory Test Interactions
Leuprolide Acetate for Depot Suspension

Administration of leuprolide acetate for depot suspension in therapeutic doses results in suppression of the pituitary-gonadal system. Normal function is usually restored within three months after treatment is discontinued. Therefore, diagnostic tests of pituitary gonadotropic and gonadal functions conducted during treatment and for up to three months after discontinuation of leuprolide acetate for depot suspension may be affected.

8   USE IN SPECIFIC POPULATIONS
8.1   Pregnancy
Pregnancy Category X – *[See Contraindications (4)]*
Teratogenic Effects

LUPANETA PACK is contraindicated in women who are or may become pregnant while receiving the drug *[see Contraindications (4)]*. Before starting and during treatment with leuprolide acetate for depot suspension, establish whether the patient is pregnant. Leuprolide acetate for depot suspension is not a contraceptive. In reproductively capable women, a non-hormonal method of contraception should be used *[see Warnings and Precautions (5.4)]*.

Leuprolide acetate for depot suspension may cause fetal harm when administered to a pregnant woman.

When administered on day 6 of pregnancy at test dosages of 0.00024, 0.0024, and 0.024 mg/kg (1/300 to 1/3 of the human dose) to rabbits, leuprolide acetate for depot suspension produced a dose-related increase in major fetal abnormalities. Similar studies in rats failed to demonstrate an increase in fetal malformations. There was increased fetal mortality and decreased fetal weights with the two higher doses of leuprolide acetate for depot suspension in rabbits and with the highest dose (0.024 mg/kg) in rats.

8.3   Nursing Mothers
Do not use LUPANETA PACK in nursing mothers because the effects of leuprolide acetate for depot suspension on lactation and/or the breast-fed child have not been determined. It is not known whether leuprolide acetate for depot suspension is excreted in human milk.

Detectable amounts of progestins have been identified in the milk of mothers receiving them *[see Contraindications (4)]*.

8.4   Pediatric Use
LUPANETA PACK is not indicated in premenarcheal adolescents. Safety and effectiveness of LUPANETA PACK have not been established in pediatric patients. Experience with LUPANETA PACK for treatment of endometriosis has been limited to women 18 years of age and older.

8.5   Geriatric Use
LUPANETA PACK is not indicated in postmenopausal women and has not been studied in women over 65 years of age.

11   DESCRIPTION
LUPANETA PACK (leuprolide acetate for depot suspension; norethindrone acetate tablets) 1-month contains one dual chamber syringe with leuprolide acetate for depot suspension 3.75 mg and norethindrone acetate tablets USP: 5 mg (bottle of 30 tablets).

Leuprolide Acetate for Depot Suspension

Leuprolide acetate for depot suspension is a synthetic nonapeptide analog of gonadotropin-releasing hormone (GnRH or LH-RH), a GnRH agonist. The chemical name is 5- oxo-L-prolyl-L-histidyl-L-tryptophyl-L-seryl-L-tyrosyl-D-leucyl-L-leucyl-L-arginyl-N-ethyl-L-prolinamide acetate (salt) with the following structural formula:
[See chemical structure above]

Leuprolide acetate for depot suspension 3.75 mg is available in a prefilled dual-chamber syringe containing sterile lyophilized microspheres which, when mixed with diluent, become a suspension intended as an intramuscular injection. The front chamber of leuprolide acetate for depot suspension 3.75 mg prefilled dual-chamber syringe contains leuprolide acetate for depot suspension (3.75 mg), purified gelatin (0.65 mg), DL-lactic and glycolic acids copolymer (33.1 mg), and D-mannitol (6.6 mg). The second chamber of diluent contains carboxymethylcellulose sodium (5 mg), D-mannitol (50 mg), polysorbate 80 (1 mg), water for injection, USP, and glacial acetic acid, USP to control pH. During the manufacture of leuprolide acetate for depot suspension, acetic acid is lost, leaving the peptide.

Norethindrone Acetate

Norethindrone acetate tablets USP - 5 mg oral tablets.

Norethindrone acetate USP, (17-hydroxy-19-nor-17α-pregn-4-en-20-yn-3-one acetate), a synthetic, orally active progestin, is the acetic acid ester of norethindrone. It is a white, or creamy white, crystalline powder.

Norethindrone acetate tablets USP, 5 mg contain the following inactive ingredients: colloidal silicon dioxide, lactose monohydrate, magnesium stearate, microcrystalline cellulose and talc.

12   CLINICAL PHARMACOLOGY
12.1   Mechanism of Action
Leuprolide Acetate for Depot Suspension

Leuprolide acetate for depot suspension is a long-acting GnRH analog. A single injection of leuprolide acetate for depot suspension results in an initial elevation followed by a prolonged suppression of pituitary gonadotropins. Repeated dosing at quarterly intervals results in decreased secretion of gonadal steroids; consequently, tissues and functions that depend on gonadal steroids for their maintenance become quiescent. This effect is reversible on discontinuation of drug therapy.

Leuprolide acetate is not active when given orally.

Norethindrone Acetate

Norethindrone acetate induces secretory changes in an estrogen-primed endometrium.

12.2   Pharmacodynamics
In a pharmacokinetic/pharmacodynamic study of leuprolide acetate 11.25 mg for 3-month administration in healthy female subjects (N=20), the onset of estradiol suppression was observed for individual subjects between day 4 and week 4 after dosing. By the third week following the injection, the mean estradiol concentration (8 pg/mL) was in the menopausal range. Throughout the remainder of the dosing period, mean serum estradiol levels ranged from the menopausal to the early follicular range.

Serum estradiol was suppressed to ≤20 pg/mL in all subjects within four weeks and remained suppressed (≤40 pg/mL) in 80% of subjects until the end of the 12-week dosing interval, at which time two of these subjects had a value between 40 and 50 pg/mL. Four additional subjects had at least two consecutive elevations of estradiol (range 43-240 pg/mL) levels during the 12-week dosing interval, but there was no indication of luteal function for any of the subjects during this period.

12.3   Pharmacokinetics
Absorption
Leuprolide Acetate for Depot Suspension

Following a single injection of the three month formulation of leuprolide acetate for depot suspension (11.25 mg) in female subjects, a mean plasma leuprolide concentration of 36.3 ng/mL was observed at 4 hours. Leuprolide appeared to be released at a constant rate following the onset of steady-state levels during the third week after dosing and mean levels then declined gradually to near the lower limit of detection by 12 weeks. The mean (± standard deviation) leuprolide concentration from 3 to 12 weeks was 0.23 ± 0.09 ng/mL. However, intact leuprolide and an inactive major metabolite could not be distinguished by the assay which was employed in the study. The initial burst, followed by the rapid decline to a steady-state level, was similar to the release pattern seen with the monthly formulation.

Norethindrone Acetate

Norethindrone acetate is deacetylated to norethindrone after oral administration, and the disposition of norethindrone acetate is indistinguishable from that of orally administered norethindrone. Norethindrone acetate is absorbed from norethindrone acetate tablets, with maximum plasma concentration of norethindrone generally occurring at about 2 hours post-dose (see Figure 8). The pharmacokinetic parameters of norethindrone following single oral administration of 5 mg norethindrone acetate under fasting conditions in 29 healthy female volunteers are summarized in Table 5.

Table 5. Pharmacokinetic Parameters after a Single Dose of Norethindrone Acetate in Healthy Women

Norethindrone Acetate (n=29) Arithmetic Mean ± SD	
Norethindrone	
AUC (0-inf) (ng/ml*h)	166.90 ± 56.28
C_{max} (ng/ml)	26.19 ± 6.19
t_{max} (h)	1.83 ± 0.58
$t_{1/2}$ (h)	8.51 ± 2.19

AUC = area under the curve,
C_{max} = maximum plasma concentration,
t_{max} = time at maximum plasma concentration,
$t_{1/2}$ = half-life,
SD = standard deviation

[See figure 8 above]
Effect of Food:
The effect of food administration on the pharmacokinetics of norethindrone acetate has not been studied.

Distribution
Leuprolide Acetate for Depot Suspension

The mean steady-state volume of distribution of leuprolide following intravenous bolus administration to healthy male volunteers was 27 L. *In vitro* binding to human plasma proteins ranged from 43% to 49%.

Norethindrone Acetate

Norethindrone is 36% bound to sex hormone-binding globulin (SHBG) and 61% bound to albumin. Volume of distribution of norethindrone is about 4 L/kg.

Metabolism
Leuprolide Acetate for Depot Suspension

In healthy male volunteers, a 1 mg bolus of leuprolide administered intravenously revealed that the mean systemic clearance was 7.6 L/h, with a terminal elimination half-life of approximately 3 hours based on a two compartment model.

In rats and dogs, administration of ^{14}C-labeled leuprolide was shown to be metabolized to smaller inactive peptides, a pentapeptide (Metabolite I), tripeptides (Metabolites II and III) and a dipeptide (Metabolite IV). These fragments may be further catabolized.

In a pharmacokinetic/pharmacodynamic study of endometriosis patients, intramuscular 11.25 mg leuprolide acetate for depot suspension (n=19) every 12 weeks or intramuscular 3.75 mg leuprolide acetate for depot suspension (n=15) every 4 weeks was administered for 24 weeks. There was no statistically significant difference in changes of serum estradiol concentration from baseline between the 2 treatment groups.

M-I plasma concentrations measured in 5 prostate cancer patients reached maximum concentration 2 to 6 hours after dosing and were approximately 6% of the peak parent drug concentration. One week after dosing, mean plasma M-I concentrations were approximately 20% of mean leuprolide concentrations.

Norethindrone Acetate
Norethindrone undergoes extensive biotransformation, primarily via reduction, followed by sulfate and glucuronide conjugation. The majority of metabolites in the circulation are sulfates, with glucuronides accounting for most of the urinary metabolites.

Excretion
Leuprolide Acetate for Depot Suspension
Following administration of leuprolide acetate for depot suspension 3.75 mg for 1-month administration to 3 patients, less than 5% of the dose was recovered as parent and M-I metabolite in the urine.

Norethindrone Acetate
Plasma clearance value for norethindrone is approximately 0.4 L/hr/kg. Norethindrone is excreted in both urine and feces, primarily as metabolites. The mean terminal elimination half-life of norethindrone following a single dose administration of norethindrone acetate is approximately 9 hours.

Specific Populations
Hepatic Impairment
The effect of hepatic disease on the disposition of norethindrone after norethindrone acetate administration has not been evaluated. However, norethindrone acetate is contraindicated in markedly impaired liver function or liver disease [see Contraindications (4)].
The pharmacokinetics of the leuprolide acetate for depot suspension in hepatically impaired patients has not been determined.

Renal Impairment
The effect of renal disease on the disposition of norethindrone after norethindrone acetate administration has not been evaluated. In pre-menopausal women with chronic renal failure undergoing peritoneal dialysis who received multiple doses of an oral contraceptive containing ethinyl estradiol and norethindrone, plasma norethindrone concentration was unchanged compared to concentrations in pre-menopausal women with normal renal function.
The pharmacokinetics of the leuprolide acetate for depot suspension in renally impaired patients has not been determined.

Race
The effect of race on the disposition of norethindrone after norethindrone acetate administration has not been evaluated.

Drug Interactions
Leuprolide Acetate for Depot Suspension
Leuprolide acetate for depot suspension is a peptide that is primarily degraded by peptidase and not by cytochrome P-450 enzymes as noted in specific studies, and the drug is only about 46% bound to plasma proteins, drug interactions would not be expected to occur.

13 NONCLINICAL TOXICOLOGY
13.1 Carcinogenesis, Mutagenesis, Impairment of Fertility
Leuprolide Acetate for Depot Suspension
A two-year carcinogenicity study was conducted in rats and mice. In rats, a dose-related increase of benign pituitary hyperplasia and benign pituitary adenomas was noted at 24 months when the drug was administered subcutaneously at high daily doses (0.6 to 4 mg/kg). There was a significant but not dose-related increase of pancreatic islet-cell adenomas in females and of testicular interstitial cell adenomas in males (highest incidence in the low dose group). In mice, no leuprolide acetate-induced tumors or pituitary abnormalities were observed at a dose as high as 60 mg/kg for two years. Patients have been treated with leuprolide acetate for up to three years with doses as high as 10 mg/day and for two years with doses as high as 20 mg/day without demonstrable pituitary abnormalities.
Mutagenicity studies have been performed with leuprolide acetate using bacterial and mammalian systems. These studies provided no evidence of a mutagenic potential.
Clinical and pharmacologic studies in adults (>18 years) with leuprolide acetate and similar analogs have shown reversibility of fertility suppression when the drug is discontinued after continuous administration for periods of up to 24 weeks. Although no clinical studies have been completed in children to assess the full reversibility of fertility suppression, animal studies (prepubertal and adult rats and monkeys) with leuprolide acetate and other GnRH analogs have shown functional recovery.

14 CLINICAL STUDIES
Leuprolide Acetate for Depot Suspension
Initial endometriosis efficacy data for leuprolide acetate for depot suspension were based on the 3.75 mg dose administered once monthly.
A pharmacokinetic/pharmacodynamic study in 41 women that included both the 3.75 mg dose administered once monthly and the 11.25 mg dose administered once every three months did not reveal clinically significant differences in terms of efficacy in reducing painful symptoms of endometriosis or magnitude of the decrease in bone mineral density (BMD) associated with use of leuprolide acetate.

Leuprolide Acetate for Depot Suspension Plus Norethindrone Acetate
Two clinical studies with treatment duration of 12 months were conducted to evaluate the effect of coadministration of leuprolide acetate for depot suspension and norethindrone acetate on the loss of bone mineral density (BMD) associated with leuprolide acetate for depot suspension and on the efficacy of leuprolide acetate for depot suspension in relieving symptoms of endometriosis. (All patients in these studies received calcium supplementation with 1000 mg elemental calcium). A total of 242 women were treated with monthly administration of leuprolide acetate 3.75 mg (13 injections) and with 5 mg norethindrone acetate taken daily. The population age range was 17-43 years old. The majority of patients were Caucasian (87%).
One coadministration study was a controlled, randomized and double-blind study included 51 women treated monthly with leuprolide acetate for depot suspension alone and 55 women treated monthly with leuprolide acetate for depot suspension plus norethindrone acetate daily. Women in this trial were followed for up to 24 months after completing one year of treatment. The other study was an open-label single arm clinical study in 136 women of one year of treatment with leuprolide acetate for depot suspension and norethindrone acetate, with follow-up for up to 12 months after completing treatment.
The second study was an open label, single arm study in which 136 women were treated monthly with leuprolide acetate for depot suspension plus norethindrone acetate daily, with follow-up for up to 12 months after completing treatment.
The assessment of efficacy was based on the investigator's or the patient's monthly assessment of five signs or symptoms of endometriosis (dysmenorrhea, pelvic pain, deep dyspareunia, pelvic tenderness and pelvic induration).
Table 6 below provides detailed efficacy data regarding relief of symptoms of endometriosis based on the two studies of coadministration of leuprolide acetate and norethindrone acetate.
[See table 6 above]
Suppression of menses (menses was defined as three or more consecutive days of menstrual bleeding) was maintained throughout treatment in 84% and 73% of patients receiving leuprolide acetate and norethindrone acetate, in the controlled study and open label study, respectively. The median time for menses resumption after treatment with leuprolide acetate and norethindrone acetate was 8 weeks.

Changes in Bone Density
The effect of leuprolide acetate for depot suspension and norethindrone acetate on bone mineral density was evaluated by dual energy x-ray absorptiometry (DXA) scan in the two clinical trials. For the open-label study, success in mitigating BMD loss was defined as the lower bound of the 95% confidence interval around the change from baseline at one year of treatment not to exceed –2.2%. The bone mineral density data of the lumbar spine from these two studies are presented in Table 7.

Table 6. Percentages of Patients with Symptoms of Endometriosis and Mean Clinical Severity Scores

Variable	Study	Group	Percent of Patients with Symptom — Baseline N[1]	Baseline (%)[2]	Final (%)	Clinical Pain Severity Score — Baseline N[1]	Baseline Value[3]	Final Change
Dysmenorrhea	Controlled Study	LA*	51	(100)	(4)	50	3.2	-2.0
		LA/N†	55	(100)	(4)	54	3.1	-2.0
	Open Label Study	LA/N	136	(99)	(9)	134	3.3	-2.1
Pelvic Pain	Controlled Study	LA	51	(100)	(66)	50	2.9	-1.1
		LA/N	55	(96)	(56)	54	3.1	-1.1
	Open Label Study	LA/N	136	(99)	(63)	134	3.2	-1.2
Deep Dyspareunia	Controlled Study	LA	42	(83)	(37)	25	2.4	-1.0
		LA/N	43	(84)	(45)	30	2.7	-0.8
	Open Label Study	LA/N	102	(91)	(53)	94	2.7	-1.0
Pelvic Tenderness	Controlled Study	LA	51	(94)	(34)	50	2.5	-1.0
		LA/N	54	(91)	(34)	52	2.6	-0.9
	Open Label Study	LA/N	136	(99)	(39)	134	2.9	-1.4
Pelvic Induration	Controlled Study	LA	51	(51)	(12)	50	1.9	-0.4
		LA/N	54	(46)	(17)	52	1.6	-0.4
	Open Label Study	LA/N	136	(75)	(21)	134	2.2	-0.9

* LA = leuprolide acetate 3.75 mg
† LA/N = leuprolide acetate 3.75 mg plus norethindrone acetate 5 mg
[1] Number of patients that were included in the assessment
[2] Percentage of patients with the symptom/sign
[3] Value description: 1=none; 2= mild; 3= moderate; 4= severe

Information on the AbbVie, Inc. products listed on these pages is from the prescribing information in use as of July 31, 2014. For more information, please visit rxabbvie.com or call 1-800-633-9110.

Table 7. Mean Percent Change from Baseline in BMD of Lumbar Spine

| | leuprolide acetate for depot suspension 3.75 mg | | leuprolide acetate for depot suspension 3.75 mg plus norethindrone acetate 5 mg daily | | | |
| | Controlled Study | | Controlled Study | | Open Label Study | |
	N	Change (Mean, 95% CI)#	N	Change (Mean, 95% CI)#	N	Change (Mean, 95% CI)#
Week 24*	41	-3.2% (-3.8, -2.6)	42	-0.3% (-0.8, 0.3)	115	-0.2% (-0.6, 0.2)
Week 52†	29	-6.3% (-7.1, -5.4)	32	-1.0% (-1.9, -0.1)	84	-1.1% (-1.6, -0.5)

* Includes on-treatment measurements that fell within 2-252 days after the first day of treatment.
† Includes on-treatment measurements >252 days after the first day of treatment.
# 95% CI: 95% Confidence Interval

Table 8. Mean Percent Change from Baseline in BMD of Lumbar Spine in Post-Treatment Follow-up Period

| Post Treatment Measurement | Controlled Study | | | | | | Open Label Study | | |
| | LA-Only | | | LA/N | | | LA/N | | |
	N	Mean % Change	95% CI (%)	N	Mean % Change	95% CI (%)	N	Mean % Change	95% CI (%)[2]
Month 8	19	-3.3	(-4.9, -1.8)	23	-0.9	(-2.1, 0.4)	89	-0.6	(-1.2, 0.0)
Month 12	16	-2.2	(-3.3, -1.1)	12	-0.7	(-2.1, 0.6)	65	0.1	(-0.6, 0.7)

[1] Patients with post treatment measurements
[2] 95% CI (2-sided) of percent change in BMD values from baseline

[See table 7 above]
The change in BMD following discontinuation of treatment is shown in Table 8.
[See table 8 above]
These clinical studies demonstrated that coadministration of leuprolide acetate and norethindrone acetate 5 mg daily is effective in significantly reducing the loss of bone mineral density that occurs with leuprolide acetate for depot suspension treatment, and in relieving symptoms of endometriosis.

15   REFERENCES

Leuprolide Acetate for Depot Suspension
1. NIOSH Alert: Preventing occupational exposures to antineoplastic and other hazardous drugs in healthcare settings. 2004. U.S. Department of Health and Human Services, Public Health Service, Centers for Disease Control and Prevention, National Institute for Occupational Safety and Health, DHHS (NIOSH) Publication No. 2004-165.
2. OSHA Technical Manual, TED 1-0.15A, Section VI: Chapter 2. Controlling Occupational Exposure to Hazardous Drugs. OSHA, 1999. http://www.osha.gov/dts/osta/otm/otm_vi/otm_vi_2.html
3. American Society of Health-System Pharmacists. ASHP guidelines on handling hazardous drugs. *Am J Health-Syst Pharm.* 2006; 63; 1172-1193.
4. Polovich, M., White, J.M., & Kelleher, L.O. (eds.) 2005. Chemotherapy and biotherapy guidelines and recommendations for practice (2nd. Ed.) Pittsburgh, PA: Oncology Nursing Society.

16   HOW SUPPLIED/STORAGE AND HANDLING

LUPANETA PACK for 1-month copackaged kit (NDC 0074-1052-05) is available in
cartons containing: leuprolide acetate for depot suspension 3.75 mg for 1-month
administration Kit (NDC 0074-3641-04)
norethindrone acetate 5 mg tablets; 30 count bottle (NDC 0074-1049-02)
1. Leuprolide acetate for depot suspension 3.75 mg for 1-month administration kit contains:
   • one prefilled dual-chamber syringe
   • one plunger
   • two alcohol swab
   Each syringe contains sterile lyophilized microspheres of leuprolide acetate incorporated in a biodegradable copolymer of lactic and glycolic acids. When mixed with diluent, leuprolide acetate for depot suspension 3.75 mg for 1-month administration is administered as a single intramuscular injection.
2. Norethindrone acetate 5 mg 30 count bottle
   White to off-white oval, flat faced beveled edged, uncoated tablets debossed with 'G with breakline' on one side and 304 on other side.
Store at 25°C (77°F); excursions permitted to 15 to 30°C (59 to 86°F) [See USP Controlled Room Temperature]

17   PATIENT COUNSELING INFORMATION

See FDA-approved patient labeling (Patient Information)
Counsel patients about the Warnings and Precautions for LUPANETA PACK, including:
• Do not use this drug if they have experienced an allergic reaction to GnRH agonists or progestins
• Do not use this drug if they are pregnant or planning a pregnancy, suspect they may be pregnant, or are breast-feeding
• Risk of loss of bone mineral density and limitation of treatment to two six-month courses of treatment
• Risk to an exposed fetus and need to use nonhormonal contraception
• Discontinue norethindrone if they develop sudden loss of vision, double vision or sudden migraine
• The possibility of development or worsening of depression during treatment with leuprolide acetate for depot suspension
• Need for close monitoring if they have cardiovascular risk factors, or conditions like epilepsy, migraine or renal dysfunction
• Notify their healthcare provider if they develop new or worsened symptoms after beginning treatment

PATIENT INFORMATION
LUPANETA PACK™ (loo-pan-e-tə pæk)
(leuprolide acetate for depot suspension and norethindrone acetate tablets)
Read this Patient Information before you start taking LUPANETA PACK and each time you get a refill. There may be new information. This information does not take the place of talking with your doctor about your medical condition or your treatment.

What is LUPANETA PACK?
LUPANETA PACK contains 2 different prescription medicines:
• **leuprolide acetate for depot suspension** is a medicine injected into your muscle and used to treat pain due to endometriosis.
• **norethindrone acetate tablets** is a medicine taken by mouth and used to help lower the side effect of bone thinning that is caused by leuprolide acetate for depot suspension.
LUPANETA PACK should not be used longer than 6 months at a time after you first start treatment for your endometriosis symptoms. LUPANETA PACK should not be used for more than a total of 12 months during your treatment.
It is not known if LUPANETA PACK is safe and effective in children under 18 years of age.
Who should not take LUPANETA PACK?
Do not take LUPANETA PACK if you:
• have had an allergic reaction to medicines like leuprolide acetate for depot suspension or norethindrone acetate tablets. See the end of this leaflet for a complete list of ingredients in LUPANETA PACK.
• have uterine bleeding for which a cause has not been found.

• are pregnant or may be pregnant. LUPANETA PACK may harm your unborn baby.
• are breast-feeding or plan to breast-feed. It is not known if LUPANETA PACK passes into your breast milk.
• had or have breast cancer or other cancers that are sensitive to hormones.
• have problems with blood clots, a stroke or a heart attack.
• have liver problems.
What should I tell my doctor before taking LUPANETA PACK?
Before you take LUPANETA PACK, tell your doctor if you:

• drink alcohol
• have a family history of bone loss (osteoporosis)
• have high cholesterol
• have migraine headaches
• have epilepsy
• smoke
• have depression
• have had blood clots, a stroke or a heart attack
• have diabetes
• have kidney problems

Tell your doctor about all the medicines you take, including prescription and non-prescription medicines, vitamins, and herbal supplements.
Especially tell your doctor if you take anticonvulsant (seizure) or corticosteroid medicines.
Ask your doctor for a list of these medicines if you are not sure.
Know the medicines you take. Keep a list of them to show your doctor and pharmacist when you get a new medicine.
How should I take LUPANETA PACK?
• **Leuprolide acetate for depot suspension** for 1 month administration is injected into your muscle 1 time every month by a healthcare professional in your doctor's office.
• **Take norethindrone acetate tablets** exactly as your doctor tells you to take them. Take 1 norethindrone acetate tablet by mouth every day for 1 month after you receive your injection.
• Talk to your doctor about the birth control method that is right for you before you start taking LUPANETA PACK. You will need to use a form of birth control that does not contain hormones, such as:
  ○ a diaphragm with spermicide
  ○ condoms with spermicide
  ○ a copper IUD
• If you become pregnant while taking LUPANETA PACK, stop taking the norethindrone acetate tablets and call your doctor right away.
How well does LUPANETA PACK work?
LUPANETA PACK is used to treat pain due to endometriosis. The pain from endometriosis can happen when you have your period, during times of the month, or during intercourse (sex). Most women feel some relief from their endometriosis pain after taking both drugs in LUPANETA PACK.
The tablets in LUPANETA PACK help lower the side effect of bone thinning that is caused by leuprolide acetate for depot suspension. Women taking both drugs in LUPANETA PACK lost an average of 1% of their bone density after about 1 year of treatment. Women regained some of their bone density about 1 year after they stopped treatment with LUPANETA PACK.
What are the possible side effects of LUPANETA PACK?
LUPANETA PACK may cause serious side effects, including:
• **bone thinning** (decreased bone mineral density)
• **harm to your unborn baby**
• **vision problems.** Call your doctor right away if you have sudden loss of vision, double vision, bulging eyes, or migraine headaches.
• **depression or worsening depression**
• **allergic reactions.** Get medical help right away if you have any of these symptoms of a serious allergic reaction:
  ○ swelling of your face, lips, mouth, or tongue
  ○ trouble breathing
  ○ wheezing
  ○ severe itching
  ○ skin rash, redness, or swelling
  ○ dizziness or fainting
  ○ fast heartbeat or pounding in your chest (tachycardia)
  ○ sweating
• **worsening endometriosis symptoms when you start taking LUPANETA PACK**
• **swelling (fluid retention)**
The most common side effects of LUPANETA PACK include:
• hot flashes and sweats
• headaches or migraine headaches
• depression and mood swings
• nausea and vomiting
• problems sleeping
• nervousness or feeling anxious
• pain
• acne
• weakness
• vaginal infection or inflammation
• weight gain
• constipation or diarrhea
Tell your doctor if you have any side effect that bothers you or that does not go away.

These are not all the possible side effects of LUPANETA PACK. For more information, ask your doctor or pharmacist.

Call your doctor for medical advice about side effects. You may report side effects to FDA at 1-800-FDA-1088.

How should I store norethindrone acetate tablets in the LUPANETA PACK?

• Store norethindrone acetate tablets at room temperature between 68°F to 77°F (20°C to 25°C).

Keep LUPANETA PACK and all medicines out of the reach of children.

General information about the safe and effective use of LUPANETA PACK.

Medicines are sometimes prescribed for purposes other than those listed in a Patient Information leaflet. Do not use LUPANETA PACK for a condition for which it was not prescribed. Do not give LUPANETA PACK to other people, even if they have the same symptoms that you have. It may harm them.

This Patient Information leaflet summarizes the most important information about LUPANETA PACK. If you would like more information, talk with your doctor. You can ask your pharmacist or doctor for information about LUPANETA PACK that is written for health professionals. For more information, go to www.lupanetapack.com or call 1-800-633-9110.

What are the ingredients in LUPANETA PACK?

leuprolide acetate for depot suspension:

Active Ingredients: leuprolide acetate for depot suspension

Inactive Ingredients: purified gelatin, DL-lactic and glycolic acids copolymer, D-mannitol, carboxymethylcellulose sodium, polysorbate 80, water for injection, USP, and glacial acetic acid, USP to control pH.

norethindrone acetate tablets:

Active Ingredients: norethindrone acetate USP

Inactive Ingredients: colloidal silicon dioxide, lactose monohydrate, magnesium stearate, microcrystalline cellulose and talc.

This Patient Information has been approved by the U.S. Food and Drug Administration.

Leuprolide Acetate for Depot Suspension:

Manufactured for
AbbVie Inc.
North Chicago, IL 60064
By Takeda Pharmaceutical Company Limited
Osaka, Japan 540-8645

Norethindrone Acetate:

Manufactured for
AbbVie Inc.
North Chicago, IL 60064
By Glenmark Generics Ltd.
Colvale-Bardez, Goa
403 513, India

LUPANETA PACK
Packaged by:
AbbVie Inc.
North Chicago, IL 60064

™ - Trademark
® - Registered Trademark
©AbbVie Inc. 2013
03-A586 March, 2013
Shown in Product Identification Guide, page 303

LUPANETA PACK™   ℞
**Leuprolide Acetate for Depot Suspension,
11.25 mg for intramuscular injection only
and Norethindrone Acetate tablets, 5 mg
for oral administration**

HIGHLIGHTS OF PRESCRIBING INFORMATION
These highlights do not include all the information needed to use LUPANETA PACK safely and effectively. See full prescribing information for LUPANETA PACK.
LUPANETA PACK (leuprolide acetate for depot suspension; norethindrone acetate tablets), co-packaged for intramuscular use and for oral use, respectively
Initial U.S. Approval: 2012

———INDICATIONS AND USAGE———
LUPANETA PACK contains leuprolide acetate, a gonadotropin-releasing hormone (GnRH) agonist and norethindrone acetate, a progestin, indicated for
• Initial management of the painful symptoms of endometriosis (1)
• Management of recurrence of symptoms (1)
Limitations of Use: Initial treatment course is limited to 6 months and use is not recommended longer than a total of 12 months due to concerns about adverse impact on bone mineral density. (1, 2.1, 5.1)

———DOSAGE AND ADMINISTRATION———
• Leuprolide acetate for depot suspension 11.25 mg given by a healthcare provider as a single intramuscular injection every 3 months for up to two injections (6 months of therapy) (2.1)
• Norethindrone acetate 5 mg tablets taken orally by the patient once per day for up to 6 months (2.1)
• If endometriosis symptoms recur after initial course of therapy, consider retreatment for up to another six months (2.1)
• Assess bone density before retreatment begins (2.1, 5.1)
• Reconstitute leuprolide acetate prior to use, see important administration instructions (2.3)

———DOSAGE FORMS AND STRENGTHS———
• Leuprolide acetate for depot suspension 11.25 mg syringe (3)
• Norethindrone acetate 5 mg tablets; 90 count bottle (3)

———CONTRAINDICATIONS———
• Hypersensitivity to GnRH, GnRH agonist or any of the excipients in leuprolide acetate for depot suspension or norethindrone acetate (4)
• Undiagnosed abnormal uterine bleeding (4)
• Pregnancy or suspected pregnancy (4, 8.1)
• Women who are breast-feeding (4)
• Known, suspected or history of breast or other hormone-sensitive cancer (4)
• Thrombotic or thromboembolic disorders (4)
• Liver tumors or liver disease (4)

———WARNINGS AND PRECAUTIONS———
• Loss of bone mineral density: do not use for more than two six-month treatment courses. (1, 2.1, 5.1)
• Exclude pregnancy before starting treatment and discontinue use if pregnancy occurs; use non-hormonal methods of contraception only. (5.2)
• Discontinue in case of sudden loss of vision or onset of proptosis, diplopia or migraine. (5.3)
• Carefully observe patients with history of depression and discontinue the drug if the depression recurs to a serious degree. (5.4)
• Assess and manage risk factors for cardiovascular disease before starting LUPANETA PACK. (5.6)

———ADVERSE REACTIONS———
Leuprolide acetate for depot suspension: Most common related adverse reactions (>10%) were hot flashes/sweats, headache/migraine, depression/emotional lability, nausea/vomiting, nervousness/anxiety, insomnia, pain, acne, asthenia, vaginitis, weight gain, constipation/diarrhea (6.1)
Progestins: breakthrough bleeding, spotting (6.1)
To report SUSPECTED ADVERSE REACTIONS, contact AbbVie Inc. at 1-800-633-9110 or FDA at 1-800-FDA-1088 or www.fda.gov/medwatch

———USE IN SPECIFIC POPULATIONS———
Pediatric: Safety and effectiveness of LUPANETA PACK has not been established in pediatric patients. (8.4)
Geriatric: LUPANETA PACK has not been studied in women over 65 years of age and is not indicated in this population. (8.5)

See 17 for PATIENT COUNSELING INFORMATION and FDA-approved patient labeling

Revised: 03/2013

FULL PRESCRIBING INFORMATION

1 INDICATIONS AND USAGE

LUPANETA PACK (leuprolide acetate for depot suspension and norethindrone acetate tablets) is indicated for initial management of the painful symptoms of endometriosis and for management of recurrence of symptoms.
Limitation of Use: Duration of use is limited due to concerns about adverse impact on bone mineral density *[see Warnings and Precautions (5.1)]*. The initial treatment course of LUPANETA PACK is limited to six months. A single retreatment course of not more than six months may be administered after the initial course of treatment if symptoms recur. Use of LUPANETA PACK for longer than a total of 12 months is not recommended.

2 DOSAGE AND ADMINISTRATION
2.1 Dosing Information
LUPANETA PACK is a co-packaging of leuprolide acetate for depot suspension for intramuscular use and norethindrone acetate tablets for oral use. Administer as follows:
• 11.25 mg of leuprolide acetate by intramuscular injection once every three months for up to two injections (6 months of therapy); to be administered by a healthcare provider
• 5 mg of norethindrone acetate orally once daily for up to 6 months of therapy
The initial course of treatment with leuprolide acetate for depot suspension 11.25 mg in combination with norethindrone acetate 5 mg daily is not to exceed six months.
If the symptoms of endometriosis recur after the initial course of therapy, consider retreatment with LUPANETA PACK for up to another six months. It is recommended that bone density be assessed before retreatment begins *[see Warnings and Precautions (5.1)]*.
Treatment beyond two six-month courses has not been studied and is not recommended due to concerns about adverse impact on bone mineral density.
2.2 Different Formulations of Leuprolide Acetate
Due to different release characteristics, a fractional dose of the leuprolide acetate for depot suspension 3-month depot formulation is not equivalent to the same dose of the monthly formulation and should not be given.
2.3 Reconstitution and Administration for Injection of Leuprolide Acetate
• Reconstitute and administer the lyophilized microspheres as a single intramuscular injection.
• Inject the suspension immediately or discard if not used within two hours, because leuprolide acetate for depot suspension does not contain a preservative.
  1. Visually inspect the leuprolide acetate for depot suspension powder. DO NOT USE the syringe if clumping or caking is evident. A thin layer of powder on the wall of the syringe is considered normal prior to mixing with the diluent. The diluent should appear clear.
  2. To prepare for injection, screw the white plunger into the end stopper until the stopper begins to turn (see Figure 1 and Figure 2).
[See figures 1 and 2 at top of next page]
  3. Hold the syringe UPRIGHT. Release the diluent by SLOWLY PUSHING (6 to 8 seconds) the plunger until the first middle stopper is at the blue line in the middle of the barrel (see Figure 3).
[See figure 3 at top of next column]
  4. Keep the syringe UPRIGHT. Mix the microspheres (powder) thoroughly by gently shaking the syringe until the powder forms a uniform suspension. The suspension will appear milky. If the powder adheres to the stopper or caking/clumping is present, tap the syringe with your finger to disperse. DO NOT USE if any of the powder has not gone into suspension (see Figure 4).
[See figure 4 at top of next column]
  5. Keep the syringe UPRIGHT. With the opposite hand pull the needle cap upward without twisting.

Information on the AbbVie, Inc. products listed on these pages is from the prescribing information in use as of July 31, 2014. For more information, please visit rxabbvie.com or call 1-800-633-9110.

Figure 1:

10. Dispose of the syringe according to local regulations/procedures [see References (15)].

Figure 2:

Figure 3:

← blue line

Figure 4:

6. Keep the syringe UPRIGHT. Advance the plunger to expel the air from the syringe. Now the syringe is ready for injection.
7. After cleaning the injection site with an alcohol swab, administer the intramuscular injection by inserting the needle at a 90 degree angle into the gluteal area, anterior thigh, or deltoid (see Figure 5).

Figure 5:

NOTE: If a blood vessel is accidentally penetrated, aspirated blood will be visible just below the luer lock (see Figure 6) and can be seen through the transparent

LuproLoc safety device. If blood is present, remove the needle immediately. Do not inject the medication.

Figure 6:

If a blood vessel is injured, blood will be visible in this section of the syringe.

8. Inject the entire contents of the syringe intramuscularly.
9. Withdraw the needle. Once the syringe has been withdrawn, immediately activate the LuproLoc® safety device by pushing the arrow on the lock upward towards the needle tip with the thumb or finger, as illustrated, until the needle cover of the safety device over the needle is fully extended and a CLICK is heard or felt (see Figure 7).

Figure 7:

CLICK

10. Dispose of the syringe according to local regulations/procedures [see References (15)].

3   DOSAGE FORMS AND STRENGTHS

LUPANETA PACK 3-month copackaged kit contains two separate components:
- Leuprolide acetate for depot suspension 11.25 mg for 3-month administration: Leuprolide acetate lyophilized powder for reconstitution with supplied diluent in a prefilled dual chamber syringe
- Norethindrone acetate 5 mg tablets: White to off-white oval, flat-faced beveled edged, uncoated debossed with 'G with breakline' on one side and 304 on other side

4   CONTRAINDICATIONS

LUPANETA PACK is contraindicated in women with the following:
- Hypersensitivity to gonadotropin-releasing hormone (GnRH), GnRH agonist analogs, any of the excipients in leuprolide acetate for depot suspension, or norethindrone acetate
- Undiagnosed abnormal uterine bleeding
- Known, suspected or planned pregnancy during the course of therapy [see Use in Specific Populations (8.1)]
- Lactating women [see Use in Specific Populations (8.3)]
- Known, suspected or history of breast cancer or other hormone-sensitive cancer
- Current or history of thrombotic or thromboembolic disorder
- Liver tumors or liver disease

5   WARNINGS AND PRECAUTIONS
5.1   Loss of Bone Mineral Density

Leuprolide acetate for depot suspension induces a hypoestrogenic state that results in loss of bone mineral density (BMD), some of which may not be reversible. Concurrent use of norethindrone acetate is effective in reducing the loss of BMD that occurs with leuprolide acetate [see Clinical Studies (14)]. Nonetheless, duration of use of LUPANETA

PACK is limited to two six-month courses of treatment due to concerns about the adverse impact on BMD. It is recommended that BMD be assessed before retreatment. Retreatment with leuprolide acetate for depot suspension alone is not recommended.

In women with major risk factors for decreased BMD such as chronic alcohol (> 3 units per day) or tobacco use, strong family history of osteoporosis, or chronic use of drugs that can decrease BMD, such as anticonvulsants or corticosteroids, use of LUPANETA PACK may pose an additional risk, and the risks and benefits should be weighed carefully.

5.2   Pregnancy Risk

Leuprolide acetate for depot suspension may cause fetal harm if administered to a pregnant woman. Exclude pregnancy before initiating treatment with LUPANETA PACK. When used at the recommended dose and dosing interval, leuprolide acetate for depot suspension usually inhibits ovulation and stops menstruation. Contraception, however, is not ensured by taking leuprolide acetate for depot suspension. Therefore, patients should use nonhormonal methods of contraception. Advise patients to notify their healthcare provider if they believe they may be pregnant. Discontinue LUPANETA PACK if a patient becomes pregnant during treatment and inform the patient of potential risk to the fetus [see Contraindications (4) and Use in Specific Populations (8.1)].

5.3   Visual Abnormalities

Discontinue norethindrone acetate tablets in the LUPANETA PACK pending examination if there is a sudden partial or complete loss of vision or if there is sudden onset of proptosis, diplopia, or migraine. Discontinue LUPANETA PACK if examination reveals papilledema or retinal vascular lesions.

5.4   Clinical Depression

Depression may occur or worsen during treatment with LUPANETA PACK. Carefully observe patients with a history of clinical depression and discontinue LUPANETA PACK if the depression recurs to a serious degree.

5.5   Serious Allergic Reactions

In clinical trials of LUPANETA PACK, adverse events of asthma were reported in women with pre-existing histories of asthma, sinusitis and environmental or drug allergies. Symptoms consistent with an anaphylactoid or asthmatic process have been reported postmarketing.

5.6   Cardiovascular and Metabolic Disorders

Assess and manage risk factors for cardiovascular disease before starting LUPANETA PACK. Closely monitor women on norethindrone acetate who have risk factors for arterial vascular disease (e.g., hypertension, diabetes mellitus, tobacco use, hypercholesterolemia, and obesity) and/or venous thromboembolism (e.g., family history of VTE, obesity, and smoking) when using LUPANETA PACK [see Contraindications (4)].

5.7   Initial Flare of Symptoms

Following the first dose of leuprolide acetate, sex steroids temporarily rise above baseline because of the physiologic effect of the drug. Therefore, an increase in symptoms associated with endometriosis may be observed during the initial days of therapy, but these should dissipate with continued therapy.

5.8   Fluid Retention

Because norethindrone acetate may cause some degree of fluid retention, carefully observe women with conditions that might be influenced by this effect, such as epilepsy, migraine, cardiac or renal dysfunctions.

6   ADVERSE REACTIONS
6.1   Clinical Trials Experience

Because clinical trials are conducted under widely varying conditions, adverse reaction rates observed in the clinical trials of a drug cannot be directly compared to rates in the clinical trials of another drug and may not reflect the rates observed in clinical practice.

The safety of co-administering leuprolide acetate for depot suspension and norethindrone acetate was evaluated in two clinical studies in which a total of 242 women were treated for up to one year. Women were treated with monthly IM injections of leuprolide acetate 3.75 mg (13 injections) alone or monthly IM injections of leuprolide acetate 3.75 mg (13 injections) and 5 mg norethindrone acetate daily. The population age range was 17-43 years old. The majority of patients were Caucasian (87%).

One study was a controlled clinical trial in which 106 women were randomized to one year of treatment with leuprolide acetate for depot suspension alone or with leuprolide acetate for depot suspension and norethindrone acetate. The other study was an open-label single arm clinical study in 136 women of one year of treatment with leuprolide acetate for depot suspension and norethindrone acetate, with follow-up for up to 12 months after completing treatment.

Adverse Reactions (>1%) Leading to Study Discontinuation: In the controlled study, 18% of patients treated monthly with leuprolide acetate and 18% of patients treated monthly with leuprolide acetate plus norethindrone acetate discontinued therapy due to adverse reactions, most commonly hot flashes (6%) and insomnia (4%) in the leuprolide acetate alone group and hot flashes and emotional lability (4% each) in the leuprolide acetate and norethindrone group.

Table 1. Adverse Reactions Occurring in the First Six Months of Treatment in ≥ 5% of Patients with Endometriosis

Adverse Reactions	Controlled Study LA-Only* N=51		Controlled Study LA/N† N=55		Open Label Study LA/N† N=136	
	N	%	N	%	N	%
Any Adverse Reaction	50	98	53	96	126	93
Body as a Whole						
Asthenia		18		18		11
Headache/Migraine		65		51		46
Injection Site Reaction		2		9		3
Pain		24		29		21
Cardiovascular System						
Hot flashes/Sweats		98		87		57
Digestive System						
Altered Bowel Function (constipation, diarrhea)		14		15		10
Changes in Appetite		4		0		6
GI Disturbance (dyspepsia, flatulence)		4		7		4
Nausea/Vomiting		25		29		13
Metabolic and Nutritional Disorders						
Edema		0		9		7
Weight Gain		12		13		4
Nervous System						
Depression/Emotional Lability		31		27		34
Dizziness/Vertigo		16		11		7
Insomnia/Sleep Disorder		31		13		15
Decreased Libido		10		4		7
Memory Disorder		6		2		4
Nervousness/Anxiety		8		4		11
Neuromuscular Disorder (leg cramps, paresthesia)		2		9		3
Skin and Appendages						
Androgen-Like Effects (acne, alopecia)		4		5		18
Skin/Mucous Membrane Reaction		4		9		11
Urogenital System						
Breast Changes/Pain/Tenderness		6		13		8
Menstrual Disorders		2		0		5
Vaginitis		20		15		8

* LA-Only = leuprolide acetate 3.75 mg
† LA/N = leuprolide acetate 3.75 mg plus norethindrone acetate 5 mg

Table 2. Hot Flashes in the Month Prior to the Assessment Visit (Controlled Study)

Assessment Visit	Treatment Group	Number of Patients Reporting Hot Flashes		Number of Days with Hot Flashes		Maximum Number Hot Flashes in 24 Hours	
		N	(%)	N²	Mean	N²	Mean
Week 24	LA-Only*	32/37	86	37	19	36	5.8
	LA/N†	22/38	58¹	38	7¹	38	1.9¹

* LA-Only = leuprolide acetate 3.75 mg
† LA/N = leuprolide acetate 3.75 mg plus norethindrone acetate 5 mg
[1] Statistically significantly less than the LA-Only group (p<0.01)
[2] Number of patients assessed.

Table 3. Serum Lipids: Mean Percent Changes from Baseline Values at Treatment Week 24

	leuprolide acetate 3.75 mg Controlled Study (n=39)		leuprolide acetate for depot suspension 3.75 mg plus norethindrone acetate 5 mg daily Controlled Study (n=41)		Open Label Study (n=117)	
	Baseline Value*	Wk 24 % Change	Baseline Value*	Wk 24 % Change	Baseline Value*	Wk 24 % Change
Total Cholesterol	170.5	9.2%	179.3	0.2%	181.2	2.8%
HDL Cholesterol	52.4	7.4%	51.8	-18.8%	51.0	-14.6%
LDL Cholesterol	96.6	10.9%	101.5	14.1%	109.1	13.1%
LDL/HDL Ratio	2.0†	5.0%	2.1†	43.4%	2.3†	39.4%
Triglycerides	107.8	17.5%	130.2	9.5%	105.4	13.8%

* mg/dL
† ratio

In the open label study, 13% of patients treated monthly with leuprolide acetate plus norethindrone acetate discontinued therapy due to adverse reactions, most commonly depression (4%) and acne (2%).
Common Adverse Reactions:
Table 1 lists the adverse reactions observed in at least 5% of patients in any treatment group, during the first 6 months of treatment in the add-back clinical studies, in which patients were treated with monthly leuprolide acetate for depot suspension 3.75 mg with or without norethindrone acetate co-treatment. The most frequently-occurring adverse reactions observed in these studies were hot flashes and headaches.
[See table 1 above]
In the controlled clinical trial, 50 of 51 (98%) patients in the leuprolide acetate alone group and 48 of 55 (87%) patients in the leuprolide acetate and norethindrone group reported experiencing hot flashes on one or more occasions during treatment. Table 2 presents hot flash data in the last month of treatment.
[See table 2 above]
Serious Adverse Reactions:
Urinary tract infection, renal calculus, depression
Changes in Laboratory Values during Treatment:
Liver Enzymes
In the two clinical trials of women with endometriosis, 4 of 191 patients receiving leuprolide acetate and norethindrone acetate for up to 12 months developed an elevated (at least twice the upper limit of normal) SGPT and 2 of 136 developed an elevated GGT. Five of the 6 increases were observed beyond 6 months of treatment. None was associated with an elevated bilirubin concentration.
Lipids
Percent changes from baseline for serum lipids and percentages of patients with serum lipid values outside of the normal range in the two studies of leuprolide acetate and norethindrone acetate are summarized in the tables below. The major impact of adding norethindrone acetate to treatment with leuprolide acetate for depot suspension was a decrease in serum HDL cholesterol and an increase in the LDL/HDL ratio.
[See table 3 above]
Changes from baseline tended to be greater at Week 52. After treatment, mean serum lipid levels from patients with follow up data (105 of 158 patients) returned to pretreatment values.

Table 4. Percent of Patients with Serum Lipid Values Outside of the Normal Range

	leuprolide acetate for depot suspension 3.75 mg plus norethindrone acetate 5 mg daily			
	Controlled Study (n=41)		Open Label Study (n=117)	
	Baseline	Wk 24*	Baseline	Wk 24*
Total Cholesterol (>240 mg/dL)	15%	20%	6%	7%
HDL Cholesterol (<40 mg/dL)	15%	44%	15%	41%
LDL Cholesterol (>160 mg/dL)	5%	7%	9%	11%
LDL/HDL Ratio (>4.0)	2%	15%	7%	21%
Triglycerides (>200 mg/dL)	12%	10%	5%	9%

* Includes all patients regardless of baseline value.

6.2 Postmarketing Experience
The following adverse reactions have been identified during postapproval use of leuprolide acetate for depot suspension or norethindrone acetate. Because these reactions are reported voluntarily from a population of uncertain size, it is not always possible to reliably estimate their frequency or establish a causal relationship to drug exposure.
Leuprolide Acetate for Depot Suspension
During postmarketing surveillance with other dosage forms and in the same or different populations, the following adverse reactions were reported:
• Allergic reactions (anaphylactic, rash, urticaria, and photosensitivity reactions)
• Mood swings, including depression
• Suicidal ideation and attempt
• Symptoms consistent with an anaphylactoid or asthmatic process
• Localized reactions including induration and abscess at the site of injection
• Symptoms consistent with fibromyalgia (e.g., joint and muscle pain, headaches, sleep disorders, gastrointestinal distress, and shortness of breath), individually and collectively

Other adverse reactions reported are:
Hepato-biliary disorder - Serious liver injury
Injury, poisoning and procedural complications - Spinal fracture

Information on the AbbVie, Inc. products listed on these pages is from the prescribing information in use as of July 31, 2014. For more information, please visit rxabbvie.com or call 1-800-633-9110.

Investigations - Decreased white blood count
Musculoskeletal and connective tissue disorder - Tenosynovitis-like symptoms
Nervous System disorder - Convulsion, peripheral neuropathy, paralysis
Vascular disorder - Hypotension, Hypertension
Serious venous and arterial thrombotic and thromboembolic events, including deep vein thrombosis, pulmonary embolism, myocardial infarction, stroke, and transient ischemic attack

Pituitary apoplexy
During post-marketing surveillance, cases of pituitary apoplexy (a clinical syndrome secondary to infarction of the pituitary gland) have been reported after the administration of leuprolide acetate and other GnRH agonists. In a majority of these cases, a pituitary adenoma was diagnosed, with a majority of pituitary apoplexy cases occurring within 2 weeks of the first dose, and some within the first hour. In these cases, pituitary apoplexy has presented as sudden headache, vomiting, visual changes, ophthalmoplegia, altered mental status, and sometimes cardiovascular collapse. Immediate medical attention has been required.

7 DRUG INTERACTIONS
7.1 Drug-Drug Interactions
Leuprolide Acetate for Depot Suspension
No pharmacokinetic-based drug-drug interaction studies have been conducted with leuprolide acetate for depot suspension. However, drug interactions associated with cytochrome P-450 enzymes or protein binding would not be expected to occur *[see Clinical Pharmacology (12.3)]*.
Norethindrone Acetate
No pharmacokinetic drug interaction studies investigating any drug-drug interactions with norethindrone acetate have been conducted. Drugs or herbal products that induce or inhibit certain enzymes, including CYP3A4, may decrease or increase the serum concentrations of norethindrone.
7.2 Drug/Laboratory Test Interactions
Leuprolide Acetate for Depot Suspension
Administration of leuprolide acetate for depot suspension in therapeutic doses results in suppression of the pituitary-gonadal system. Normal function is usually restored within three months after treatment is discontinued. Therefore, diagnostic tests of pituitary gonadotropic and gonadal functions conducted during treatment and for up to three months after discontinuation of leuprolide acetate for depot suspension may be affected.

8 USE IN SPECIFIC POPULATIONS
8.1 Pregnancy
Pregnancy Category X – *[See Contraindications (4)]*
Teratogenic Effects
LUPANETA PACK is contraindicated in women who are or may become pregnant while receiving the drug *[see Contraindications (4)]*. Before starting and during treatment with leuprolide acetate for depot suspension, establish whether the patient is pregnant. Leuprolide acetate for depot suspension is not a contraceptive. In reproductively capable women, a non-hormonal method of contraception should be used *[see Warnings and Precautions (5.4)]*.
Leuprolide acetate for depot suspension may cause fetal harm when administered to a pregnant woman.
When administered on day 6 of pregnancy at test dosages of 0.00024, 0.0024, and 0.024 mg/kg (1/300 to 1/3 of the human dose) to rabbits, leuprolide acetate for depot suspension produced a dose-related increase in major fetal abnormalities. Similar studies in rats failed to demonstrate an increase in fetal malformations. There was increased fetal mortality and decreased fetal weights with the two higher doses of leuprolide acetate for depot suspension in rabbits and with the highest dose (0.024 mg/kg) in rats.
8.3 Nursing Mothers
Do not use LUPANETA PACK in nursing mothers because the effects of leuprolide acetate for depot suspension on lactation and/or the breast-fed child have not been determined. It is not known whether leuprolide acetate for depot suspension is excreted in human milk.
Detectable amounts of progestins have been identified in the milk of mothers receiving them *[see Contraindications (4)]*.

8.4 Pediatric Use
LUPANETA PACK is not indicated in premenarcheal adolescents. Safety and effectiveness of LUPANETA PACK have not been established in pediatric patients. Experience with LUPANETA PACK for treatment of endometriosis has been limited to women 18 years of age and older.
8.5 Geriatric Use
LUPANETA PACK is not indicated in postmenopausal women and has not been studied in women over 65 years of age.

11 DESCRIPTION
LUPANETA PACK (leuprolide acetate for depot suspension; norethindrone acetate tablets) 3-month contains one dual chamber syringe with leuprolide acetate for depot suspension 11.25 mg and norethindrone acetate tablets USP: 5 mg (bottle of 90 tablets).
Leuprolide Acetate for Depot Suspension
Leuprolide acetate for depot suspension is a synthetic nonapeptide analog of gonadotropin-releasing hormone (GnRH or LH-RH), a GnRH agonist. The chemical name is 5- oxo-L-prolyl-L-histidyl-L-tryptophyl-L-seryl-L-tyrosyl-D-leucyl-L-leucyl-L-arginyl-N-ethyl-L-prolinamide acetate (salt) with the following structural formula:
[See chemical structure above]
Leuprolide acetate for depot suspension 11.25 mg is available in a prefilled dual-chamber syringe containing sterile lyophilized microspheres which, when mixed with diluent, become a suspension intended as an intramuscular injection.
The front chamber of leuprolide acetate for depot suspension 11.25 mg for 3-month administration prefilled dual-chamber syringe contains leuprolide acetate for depot suspension (11.25 mg), polylactic acid (99.3 mg) and D-mannitol (19.45 mg). The second chamber of diluent contains carboxymethylcellulose sodium (7.5 mg), D-mannitol (75 mg), polysorbate 80 (1.5 mg), water for injection, USP, and glacial acetic acid, USP to control pH.
During the manufacture of leuprolide acetate for depot suspension, acetic acid is lost, leaving the peptide.
Norethindrone Acetate
Norethindrone acetate tablets USP - 5 mg oral tablets. Norethindrone acetate USP, (17-hydroxy-19-nor-17α-pregn-4-en-20-yn-3-one acetate), a synthetic, orally active progestin, is the acetic acid ester of norethindrone. It is a white, or creamy white, crystalline powder.

Norethindrone acetate tablets USP, 5 mg contain the following inactive ingredients: colloidal silicon dioxide, lactose monohydrate, magnesium stearate, microcrystalline cellulose and talc.

12 CLINICAL PHARMACOLOGY
12.1 Mechanism of Action
Leuprolide Acetate for Depot Suspension
Leuprolide acetate for depot suspension is a long-acting GnRH analog. A single injection of leuprolide acetate for depot suspension results in an initial elevation followed by a prolonged suppression of pituitary gonadotropins. Repeated dosing at quarterly intervals results in decreased secretion of gonadal steroids; consequently, tissues and functions that depend on gonadal steroids for their maintenance become quiescent. This effect is reversible on discontinuation of drug therapy.
Leuprolide acetate is not active when given orally.

Norethindrone Acetate
Norethindrone acetate induces secretory changes in an estrogen-primed endometrium.
12.2 Pharmacodynamics
In a pharmacokinetic/pharmacodynamic study of leuprolide acetate 11.25 mg for 3-month administration in healthy female subjects (N=20), the onset of estradiol suppression was observed for individual subjects between day 4 and week 4 after dosing. By the third week following the injection, the mean estradiol concentration (8 pg/mL) was in the menopausal range. Throughout the remainder of the dosing period, mean serum estradiol levels ranged from the menopausal to the early follicular range.
Serum estradiol was suppressed to ≤20 pg/mL in all subjects within four weeks and remained suppressed (≤40 pg/mL) in 80% of subjects until the end of the 12-week dosing interval, at which time two of these subjects had a value between 40 and 50 pg/mL. Four additional subjects had at least two consecutive elevations of estradiol (range 43-240 pg/mL) levels during the 12-week dosing interval, but there was no indication of luteal function for any of the subjects during this period.
12.3 Pharmacokinetics
Absorption
Leuprolide Acetate for Depot Suspension
Following a single injection of the three month formulation of leuprolide acetate for depot suspension (11.25 mg) in female subjects, a mean plasma leuprolide concentration of 36.3 ng/mL was observed at 4 hours. Leuprolide appeared to be released at a constant rate following the onset of steady-state levels during the third week after dosing and mean levels then declined gradually to near the lower limit of detection by 12 weeks. The mean (± standard deviation) leuprolide concentration from 3 to 12 weeks was 0.23 ± 0.09 ng/mL. However, intact leuprolide and an inactive major metabolite could not be distinguished by the assay which was employed in the study. The initial burst, followed by the rapid decline to a steady-state level, was similar to the release pattern seen with the monthly formulation.

Norethindrone Acetate
Norethindrone acetate is deacetylated to norethindrone after oral administration, and the disposition of norethindrone acetate is indistinguishable from that of orally administered norethindrone. Norethindrone acetate is absorbed from norethindrone acetate tablets, with maximum plasma concentration of norethindrone generally occurring at about 2 hours post-dose (see Figure 8). The pharmacokinetic parameters of norethindrone following single oral administration of 5 mg norethindrone acetate under fasting conditions in 29 healthy female volunteers are summarized in Table 5.

Table 5. Pharmacokinetic Parameters after a Single Dose of Norethindrone Acetate in Healthy Women

Norethindrone Acetate (n=29)	Arithmetic Mean ± SD
Norethindrone	
AUC (0-inf) (ng/ml*h)	166.90 ± 56.28
C_{max} (ng/ml)	26.19 ± 6.19
t_{max} (h)	1.83 ± 0.58
$t_{1/2}$ (h)	8.51 ± 2.19

AUC = area under the curve,
C_{max} = maximum plasma concentration,
t_{max} = time at maximum plasma concentration,
$t_{1/2}$ = half-life,
SD = standard deviation

[See figure 8 at top of next page]
Effect of Food:
The effect of food administration on the pharmacokinetics of norethindrone acetate has not been studied.
Distribution
Leuprolide Acetate for Depot Suspension
The mean steady-state volume of distribution of leuprolide following intravenous bolus administration to healthy male volunteers was 27 L. *In vitro* binding to human plasma proteins ranged from 43% to 49%.
Norethindrone Acetate
Norethindrone is 36% bound to sex hormone-binding globulin (SHBG) and 61% bound to albumin. Volume of distribution of norethindrone is about 4 L/kg.
Metabolism
Leuprolide Acetate for Depot Suspension
In healthy male volunteers, a 1 mg bolus of leuprolide administered intravenously revealed that the mean systemic

Figure 8. Mean Norethindrone Plasma Concentration Profile after a Single Dose of 5 mg Norethindrone Acetate Administered to 29 Healthy Female Volunteers under Fasting Conditions

Table 6. Percentages of Patients with Symptoms of Endometriosis and Mean Clinical Severity Scores

Variable	Study	Group	Percent of Patients with Symptom			Clinical Pain Severity Score		
			Baseline		Final	Baseline		Final
			N[1]	(%)[2]	(%)	N[1]	Value[3]	Change
Dysmenorrhea	Controlled Study	LA*	51	(100)	(4)	50	3.2	-2.0
		LA/N†	55	(100)	(4)	54	3.1	-2.0
	Open Label Study	LA/N	136	(99)	(9)	134	3.3	-2.1
Pelvic Pain	Controlled Study	LA	51	(100)	(66)	50	2.9	-1.1
		LA/N	55	(96)	(56)	54	3.1	-1.1
	Open Label Study	LA/N	136	(99)	(63)	134	3.2	-1.2
Deep Dyspareunia	Controlled Study	LA	42	(83)	(37)	25	2.4	-1.0
		LA/N	43	(84)	(45)	30	2.7	-0.8
	Open Label Study	LA/N	102	(91)	(53)	94	2.7	-1.0
Pelvic Tenderness	Controlled Study	LA	51	(94)	(34)	50	2.5	-1.0
		LA/N	54	(91)	(34)	52	2.6	-0.9
	Open Label Study	LA/N	136	(99)	(39)	134	2.9	-1.4
Pelvic Induration	Controlled Study	LA	51	(51)	(12)	50	1.9	-0.4
		LA/N	54	(46)	(17)	52	1.6	-0.4
	Open Label Study	LA/N	136	(75)	(21)	134	2.2	-0.9

* LA = leuprolide acetate 3.75 mg assessment
† LA/N = leuprolide acetate 3.75 mg plus norethindrone acetate 5 mg
[1] Number of patients that were included in the assessment
[2] Percentage of patients with the symptom/sign
[3] Value description: 1=none; 2= mild; 3= moderate; 4= severe

clearance was 7.6 L/h, with a terminal elimination half-life of approximately 3 hours based on a two compartment model.

In rats and dogs, administration of ^{14}C-labeled leuprolide was shown to be metabolized to smaller inactive peptides, a pentapeptide (Metabolite I), tripeptides (Metabolites II and III) and a dipeptide (Metabolite IV). These fragments may be further catabolized.

In a pharmacokinetic/pharmacodynamic study of endometriosis patients, intramuscular 11.25 mg leuprolide acetate for depot suspension (n=19) every 12 weeks or intramuscular 3.75 mg leuprolide acetate for depot suspension (n=15) every 4 weeks was administered for 24 weeks. There was no statistically significant difference in changes of serum estradiol concentration from baseline between the 2 treatment groups.

M-I plasma concentrations measured in 5 prostate cancer patients reached maximum concentration 2 to 6 hours after dosing and were approximately 6% of the peak parent drug concentration. One week after dosing, mean plasma M-I concentrations were approximately 20% of mean leuprolide concentrations.

Norethindrone Acetate
Norethindrone undergoes extensive biotransformation, primarily via reduction, followed by sulfate and glucuronide conjugation. The majority of metabolites in the circulation are sulfates, with glucuronides accounting for most of the urinary metabolites.

Excretion
Leuprolide Acetate for Depot Suspension
Following administration of leuprolide acetate for depot suspension 3.75 mg for 1-month administration to 3 patients, less than 5% of the dose was recovered as parent and M-I metabolite in the urine.

Norethindrone Acetate
Plasma clearance value for norethindrone is approximately 0.4 L/hr/kg. Norethindrone is excreted in both urine and feces, primarily as metabolites. The mean terminal elimina-

tion half-life of norethindrone following a single dose administration of norethindrone acetate is approximately 9 hours.

Specific Populations
Hepatic Impairment
The effect of hepatic disease on the disposition of norethindrone after norethindrone acetate administration has not been evaluated. However, norethindrone acetate is contraindicated in markedly impaired liver function or liver disease [see Contraindications (4)].

The pharmacokinetics of the leuprolide acetate for depot suspension in hepatically impaired patients has not been determined.

Renal Impairment
The effect of renal disease on the disposition of norethindrone after norethindrone acetate administration has not been evaluated. In pre-menopausal women with chronic renal failure undergoing peritoneal dialysis who received multiple doses of an oral contraceptive containing ethinyl estradiol and norethindrone, plasma norethindrone concentration was unchanged compared to concentrations in pre-menopausal women with normal renal function.

The pharmacokinetics of the leuprolide acetate for depot suspension in renally impaired patients has not been determined.

Race
The effect of race on the disposition of norethindrone after norethindrone acetate administration has not been evaluated.

Drug Interactions
Leuprolide Acetate for Depot Suspension
Leuprolide acetate for depot suspension is a peptide that is primarily degraded by peptidase and not by cytochrome P-450 enzymes as noted in specific studies, and the drug is only about 46% bound to plasma proteins, drug interactions would not be expected to occur.

13 NONCLINICAL TOXICOLOGY
13.1 Carcinogenesis, Mutagenesis, Impairment of Fertility
Leuprolide Acetate for Depot Suspension
A two-year carcinogenicity study was conducted in rats and mice. In rats, a dose-related increase of benign pituitary hyperplasia and benign pituitary adenomas was noted at 24 months when the drug was administered subcutaneously at high daily doses (0.6 to 4 mg/kg). There was a significant but not dose-related increase of pancreatic islet-cell adenomas in females and of testicular interstitial cell adenomas in males (highest incidence in the low dose group). In mice, no leuprolide acetate-induced tumors or pituitary abnormalities were observed at a dose as high as 60 mg/kg for two years. Patients have been treated with leuprolide acetate for up to three years with doses as high as 10 mg/day and for two years with doses as high as 20 mg/day without demonstrable pituitary abnormalities.

Mutagenicity studies have been performed with leuprolide acetate using bacterial and mammalian systems. These studies provided no evidence of a mutagenic potential.

Clinical and pharmacologic studies in adults (> 18 years) with leuprolide acetate and similar analogs have shown reversibility of fertility suppression when the drug is discontinued after continuous administration for periods of up to 24 weeks. Although no clinical studies have been completed in children to assess the full reversibility of fertility suppression, animal studies (prepubertal and adult rats and monkeys) with leuprolide acetate and other GnRH analogs have shown functional recovery.

14 CLINICAL STUDIES
Leuprolide Acetate for Depot Suspension
Initial endometriosis efficacy data for leuprolide acetate for depot suspension were based on the 3.75 mg dose administered once monthly.

A pharmacokinetic/pharmacodynamic study in 41 women that included both the 3.75 mg dose administered once monthly and the 11.25 mg dose administered once every three months did not reveal clinically significant differences in terms of efficacy in reducing painful symptoms of endometriosis or magnitude of the decrease in bone mineral density (BMD) associated with use of leuprolide acetate.

Leuprolide Acetate for Depot Suspension Plus Norethindrone Acetate
Two clinical studies with treatment duration of 12 months were conducted to evaluate the effect of coadministration of leuprolide acetate for depot suspension and norethindrone acetate on the loss of bone mineral density (BMD) associated with leuprolide acetate for depot suspension and on the efficacy of leuprolide acetate for depot suspension in reliev-

Information on the AbbVie, Inc. products listed on these pages is from the prescribing information in use as of July 31, 2014. For more information, please visit rxabbvie.com or call 1-800-633-9110.

Table 7. Mean Percent Change from Baseline In BMD of Lumbar Spine

	leuprolide acetate for depot suspension 3.75 mg		leuprolide acetate for depot suspension 3.75 mg plus norethindrone acetate 5 mg daily				
	Controlled Study		Controlled Study		Open Label Study		
	N	Change (Mean, 95% CI)#	N	Change (Mean, 95% CI)#	N	Change (Mean, 95% CI)#	
Week 24*	41	-3.2% (-3.8, -2.6)	42	-0.3% (-0.8, 0.3)	115	-0.2% (-0.6, 0.2)	
Week 52†	29	-6.3% (-7.1, -5.4)	32	-1.0% (-1.9, -0.1)	84	-1.1% (-1.6, -0.5)	

* Includes on-treatment measurements that fell within 2-252 days after the first day of treatment.
† Includes on-treatment measurements >252 days after the first day of treatment.
# 95% CI: 95% Confidence Interval

Table 8. Mean Percent Change from Baseline in BMD of Lumbar Spine in Post-Treatment Follow-up Period

Post Treatment Measurement	Controlled Study						Open Label Study		
	LA-Only			LA/N			LA/N		
	N	Mean % Change	95% CI (%)	N	Mean % Change	95% CI (%)	N	Mean % Change	95% CI (%)²
Month 8	19	-3.3	(-4.9, -1.8)	23	-0.9	(-2.1, 0.4)	89	-0.6	(-1.2, 0.0)
Month 12	16	-2.2	(-3.3, -1.1)	12	-0.7	(-2.1, 0.6)	65	0.1	(-0.6, 0.7)

¹ Patients with post treatment measurements
² 95% CI (2-sided) of percent change in BMD values from baseline

ing symptoms of endometriosis. (All patients in these studies received calcium supplementation with 1000 mg elemental calcium). A total of 242 women were treated with monthly administration of leuprolide acetate 3.75 mg (13 injections) and with 5 mg norethindrone acetate taken daily. The population age range was 17-43 years old. The majority of patients were Caucasian (87%).

One coadministration study was a controlled, randomized and double-blind study included 51 women treated monthly with leuprolide acetate for depot suspension alone and 55 women treated monthly with leuprolide acetate for depot suspension plus norethindrone acetate daily. Women in this trial were followed for up to 24 months after completing one year of treatment. The other study was an open-label single arm clinical study in 136 women of one year of treatment with leuprolide acetate for depot suspension and norethindrone acetate, with follow-up for up to 12 months after completing treatment.

The second study was an open label, single arm study in which 136 women were treated monthly with leuprolide acetate for depot suspension plus norethindrone acetate daily, with follow-up for up to 12 months after completing treatment.

The assessment of efficacy was based on the investigator's or the patient's monthly assessment of five signs or symptoms of endometriosis (dysmenorrhea, pelvic pain, deep dyspareunia, pelvic tenderness and pelvic induration).

Table 6 below provides detailed efficacy data regarding relief of symptoms of endometriosis based on the two studies of coadministration of leuprolide acetate and norethindrone acetate.

[See table 6 at top of previous page]

Suppression of menses (menses was defined as three or more consecutive days of menstrual bleeding) was maintained throughout treatment in 84% and 73% of patients receiving leuprolide acetate and norethindrone acetate, in the controlled study and open label study, respectively. The median time for menses resumption after treatment with leuprolide acetate and norethindrone acetate was 8 weeks.

Changes in Bone Density
The effect of leuprolide acetate for depot suspension and norethindrone acetate on bone mineral density was evaluated by dual energy x-ray absorptiometry (DXA) scan in the two clinical trials. For the open-label study, success in mitigating BMD loss was defined as the lower bound of the 95% confidence interval around the change from baseline at one year of treatment not to exceed -2.2%. The bone mineral density data of the lumbar spine from these two studies are presented in Table 7.

[See table 7 above]

The change in BMD following discontinuation of treatment is shown in Table 8.

[See table 8 above]

These clinical studies demonstrated that coadministration of leuprolide acetate and norethindrone acetate 5 mg daily is effective in significantly reducing the loss of bone mineral density that occurs with leuprolide acetate for depot suspension treatment, and in relieving symptoms of endometriosis.

15 REFERENCES

Leuprolide Acetate for Depot Suspension
1. NIOSH Alert: Preventing occupational exposures to antineoplastic and other hazardous drugs in healthcare settings. 2004. U.S. Department of Health and Human Services, Public Health Service, Centers for Disease Control and Prevention, National Institute for Occupational Safety and Health, DHHS (NIOSH) Publication No. 2004-165.
2. OSHA Technical Manual, TED 1-0.15A, Section VI: Chapter 2. Controlling Occupational Exposure to Hazardous Drugs. OSHA, 1999. http://www.osha.gov/dts/osta/otm/otm_vi/otm_vi_2.html
3. American Society of Health-System Pharmacists. ASHP guidelines on handling hazardous drugs. *Am J Health-Syst Pharm.* 2006; 63; 1172-1193.
4. Polovich, M., White, J.M., & Kelleher, L.O. (eds.) 2005. Chemotherapy and biotherapy guidelines and recommendations for practice (2nd. Ed.) Pittsburgh, PA: Oncology Nursing Society.

16 HOW SUPPLIED/STORAGE AND HANDLING

LUPANETA PACK for 3-month copackaged kit (NDC 0074-1053-05) is available in cartons containing:
leuprolide acetate for depot suspension 11.25 mg for 3-month administration Kit (NDC 0074-3663-04)
norethindrone acetate 5 mg tablets; 90 count bottle (NDC 0074-1049-04)
1. Leuprolide acetate for depot suspension 11.25 mg for 3-month administration kit contains:
   • one prefilled dual-chamber syringe
   • one plunger
   • two alcohol swabs
   Each syringe contains sterile lyophilized microspheres of leuprolide acetate incorporated in a biodegradable polymer of polylactic acid. When mixed with 1.5 mL of the diluent, leuprolide acetate for depot suspension 11.25 mg for 3-month administration is administered as a single intramuscular injection.
2. Norethindrone acetate 5 mg 90 count bottle
   White to off-white oval, flat faced beveled edged, uncoated tablets debossed with 'G with breakline' on one side and 304 on other side.
   Store at 25°C (77°F); excursions permitted to 15 to 30°C (59 to 86°F) [See USP Controlled Room Temperature]

17 PATIENT COUNSELING INFORMATION

See FDA-approved patient labeling (Patient Information)
Counsel patients about the Warnings and Precautions for LUPANETA PACK, including:
• Do not use this drug if they have experienced an allergic reaction to GnRH agonists or progestins
• Do not use this drug if they are pregnant or planning a pregnancy, suspect they may be pregnant, or are breastfeeding
• Risk of loss of bone mineral density and limitation of treatment to two six-month courses of treatment
• Risk to an exposed fetus and need to use nonhormonal contraception
• Discontinue norethindrone if they develop sudden loss of vision, double vision or sudden migraine
• The possibility of development or worsening of depression during treatment with leuprolide acetate for depot suspension
• Need for close monitoring if they have cardiovascular risk factors, or conditions like epilepsy, migraine or renal dysfunction
• Notify their healthcare provider if they develop new or worsened symptoms after beginning treatment

PATIENT INFORMATION
LUPANETA PACK™ (loo-pan-e-tə pæk)
(leuprolide acetate for depot suspension and norethindrone acetate tablets)
Read this Patient Information before you start taking LUPANETA PACK and each time you get a refill. There may be new information. This information does not take the place of talking with your doctor about your medical condition or your treatment.

What is LUPANETA PACK?
LUPANETA PACK contains 2 different prescription medicines:
• **leuprolide acetate for depot suspension** is a medicine injected into your muscle and used to treat pain due to endometriosis.
• **norethindrone acetate tablets** is a medicine taken by mouth and used to help lower the side effect of bone thinning that is caused by leuprolide acetate for depot suspension.

LUPANETA PACK should not be used longer than 6 months at a time after you first start treatment for your endometriosis symptoms. LUPANETA PACK should not be used for more than a total of 12 months during your treatment.
It is not known if LUPANETA PACK is safe and effective in children under 18 years of age.

Who should not take LUPANETA PACK?
Do not take LUPANETA PACK if you:
• have had an allergic reaction to medicines like leuprolide acetate for depot suspension or norethindrone acetate tablets. See the end of this leaflet for a complete list of ingredients in LUPANETA PACK.
• have uterine bleeding for which a cause has not been found
• are pregnant or may be pregnant. LUPANETA PACK may harm your unborn baby.
• are breastfeeding or plan to breastfeed. It is not known if LUPANETA PACK passes into your breast milk.
• had or have breast cancer or other cancers that are sensitive to hormones
• have problems with blood clots, a stroke or a heart attack
• have liver problems

What should I tell my doctor before taking LUPANETA PACK?
Before you take LUPANETA PACK, tell your doctor if you:

• drink alcohol	• smoke
• have a family history of bone loss (osteoporosis)	• have depression
• have high cholesterol	• have had blood clots, a stroke or a heart attack
• have migraine headaches	• have diabetes
• have epilepsy	• have kidney problems

Tell your doctor about all the medicines you take, including prescription and non-prescription medicines, vitamins, and herbal supplements.
Especially tell your doctor if you take anticonvulsant (seizure) or corticosteroid medicines.
Ask your doctor for a list of these medicines if you are not sure.
Know the medicines you take. Keep a list of them to show your doctor and pharmacist when you get a new medicine.
How should I take LUPANETA PACK?
• **Leuprolide acetate for depot suspension** for 3-month administration is injected into your muscle 1 time every 3 months by a healthcare professional in your doctor's office.
• **Take norethindrone acetate tablets** exactly as your doctor tells you to take them. Take 1 norethindrone acetate tablet by mouth every day for 3 months after you receive your injection.
• Talk to your doctor about the birth control method that is right for you before you start taking LUPANETA PACK. You will need to use a form of birth control that does not contain hormones, such as:
  ◦ a diaphragm with spermicide
  ◦ condoms with spermicide
  ◦ a copper IUD
• If you become pregnant while taking LUPANETA PACK, stop taking the norethindrone acetate tablets and call your doctor right away.

How well does LUPANETA PACK work?

LUPANETA PACK is used to treat pain due to endometriosis. The pain from endometriosis can happen when you have your period, during other times of the month, or during intercourse (sex). Most women feel some relief from their endometriosis pain after taking both drugs in LUPANETA PACK.

The tablets in LUPANETA PACK help lower the side effect of bone thinning that is caused by leuprolide acetate for depot suspension. Women taking both drugs in LUPANETA PACK lost an average of 1% of their bone density after about 1 year of treatment. Women regained some of their bone density about 1 year after they stopped treatment with LUPANETA PACK.

What are the possible side effects of LUPANETA PACK?
LUPANETA PACK may cause serious side effects, including:
• **bone thinning (decreased bone mineral density)**
• **harm to your unborn baby**
• **vision problems.** Call your doctor right away if you have sudden loss of vision, double vision, bulging eyes, or migraine headaches.
• **depression or worsening depression**
• **allergic reactions.** Get medical help right away if you have any of these symptoms of a serious allergic reaction:
  ○ swelling of your face, lips, mouth, or tongue
  ○ trouble breathing
  ○ wheezing
  ○ severe itching
  ○ skin rash, redness, or swelling
  ○ dizziness or fainting
  ○ fast heartbeat or pounding in your chest (tachycardia)
  ○ sweating
• **worsening endometriosis symptoms when you start taking LUPANETA PACK**
• **swelling (fluid retention)**

The most common side effects of LUPANETA PACK include:
• hot flashes and sweats
• headaches or migraine headaches
• depression and mood swings
• nausea and vomiting
• problems sleeping
• nervousness or feeling anxious
• pain
• acne
• weakness
• vaginal infection or inflammation
• weight gain
• constipation or diarrhea
Tell your doctor if you have any side effect that bothers you or that does not go away.

These are not all the possible side effects of LUPANETA PACK. For more information, ask your doctor or pharmacist.
Call your doctor for medical advice about side effects. You may report side effects to FDA at 1-800-FDA-1088.
How should I store norethindrone acetate tablets in the LUPANETA PACK?
• Store norethindrone acetate tablets at room temperature between 68°F to 77°F (20°C to 25°C).
Keep LUPANETA PACK and all medicines out of the reach of children.
General information about the safe and effective use of LUPANETA PACK.
Medicines are sometimes prescribed for purposes other than those listed in a Patient Information leaflet. Do not use LUPANETA PACK for a condition for which it was not prescribed. Do not give LUPANETA PACK to other people, even if they have the same symptoms that you have. It may harm them.
This Patient Information leaflet summarizes the most important information about LUPANETA PACK. If you would like more information, talk with your doctor. You can ask your pharmacist or doctor for information about LUPANETA PACK that is written for health professionals. For more information, go to www.lupanetapack.com or call 1-800-633-9110.
What are the ingredients in LUPANETA PACK?
leuprolide acetate for depot suspension:
Active Ingredients: leuprolide acetate for depot suspension
Inactive Ingredients: polylactic acid, D-mannitol, carboxymethylcellulose sodium, polysorbate 80, water for injection, USP, and glacial acetic acid, USP
norethindrone acetate tablets:
Active Ingredients: norethindrone acetate USP
Inactive Ingredients: colloidal silicon dioxide, lactose monohydrate, magnesium stearate, microcrystalline cellulose and talc.
This Patient Information has been approved by the U.S. Food and Drug Administration.
Leuprolide Acetate for Depot Suspension:
Manufactured for
AbbVie Inc.
North Chicago, IL 60064

By Takeda Pharmaceutical Company Limited
Osaka, Japan 540-8645
Norethindrone Acetate:
Manufactured for
AbbVie Inc.
North Chicago, IL 60064
By Glenmark Generics Ltd.
Colvale-Bardez, Goa
403 513, India
LUPANETA PACK
Packaged by:
AbbVie Inc.
North Chicago, IL 60064
™ - Trademark
® - Registered Trademark
©2013 AbbVie Inc.
03-A587 March, 2013
Shown in Product Identification Guide, page 303

LUPRON DEPOT® 3.75 mg   ℞
[lew-prŏn]
(leuprolide acetate for depot suspension)
Rx only

This is combined labeling. Examples of different fonts and colors appear below.
• General information
• Information on endometriosis
• Information on uterine fibroids

DESCRIPTION

Leuprolide acetate is a synthetic nonapeptide analog of naturally occurring gonadotropin-releasing hormone (GnRH or LH-RH). The analog possesses greater potency than the natural hormone. The chemical name is 5-oxo-L-prolyl-L-histidyl-L-tryptophyl-L-seryl-L-tyrosyl-D-leucyl-L-leucyl-L-arginyl-N-ethyl-L-prolinamide acetate (salt) with the following structural formula:
[See chemical structure at top of next page]
LUPRON DEPOT is available in a prefilled dual-chamber syringe containing sterile lyophilized microspheres which, when mixed with diluent, become a suspension intended as a monthly intramuscular injection.
The front chamber of LUPRON DEPOT 3.75 mg prefilled dual-chamber syringe contains leuprolide acetate (3.75 mg), purified gelatin (0.65 mg), DL-lactic and glycolic acids copolymer (33.1 mg), and D-mannitol (6.6 mg). The second chamber of diluent contains carboxymethylcellulose sodium (5 mg), D-mannitol (50 mg), polysorbate 80 (1 mg), water for injection, USP, and glacial acetic acid, USP to control pH. During the manufacture of LUPRON DEPOT 3.75 mg, acetic acid is lost, leaving the peptide.

CLINICAL PHARMACOLOGY

Leuprolide acetate is a long-acting GnRH analog. A single monthly injection of LUPRON DEPOT 3.75 mg results in an initial stimulation followed by a prolonged suppression of pituitary gonadotropins.
Repeated dosing at monthly intervals results in decreased secretion of gonadal steroids; consequently, tissues and functions that depend on gonadal steroids for their maintenance become quiescent. This effect is reversible on discontinuation of drug therapy.
Leuprolide acetate is not active when given orally. Intramuscular injection of the depot formulation provides plasma concentrations of leuprolide over a period of one month.
Pharmacokinetics
Absorption
A single dose of LUPRON DEPOT 3.75 mg was administered by intramuscular injection to healthy female volunteers. The absorption of leuprolide was characterized by an initial increase in plasma concentration, with peak concentration ranging from 4.6 to 10.2 ng/mL at four hours postdosing. However, intact leuprolide and an inactive metabolite could not be distinguished by the assay used in the study. Following the initial rise, leuprolide concentrations started to plateau within two days after dosing and remained relatively stable for about four to five weeks with plasma concentrations of about 0.30 ng/mL.
Distribution
The mean steady-state volume of distribution of leuprolide following intravenous bolus administration to healthy male volunteers was 27 L. *In vitro* binding to human plasma proteins ranged from 43% to 49%.
Metabolism
In healthy male volunteers, a 1 mg bolus of leuprolide administered intravenously revealed that the mean systemic clearance was 7.6 L/h, with a terminal elimination half-life of approximately 3 hours based on a two compartment model.
In rats and dogs, administration of ^{14}C-labeled leuprolide was shown to be metabolized to smaller inactive peptides, a

pentapeptide (Metabolite I), tripeptides (Metabolites II and III) and a dipeptide (Metabolite IV). These fragments may be further catabolized.
The major metabolite (M-I) plasma concentrations measured in 5 prostate cancer patients reached maximum concentration 2 to 6 hours after dosing and were approximately 6% of the peak parent drug concentration. One week after dosing, mean plasma M-I concentrations were approximately 20% of mean leuprolide concentrations.
Excretion
Following administration of LUPRON DEPOT 3.75 mg to 3 patients, less than 5% of the dose was recovered as parent and M-I metabolite in the urine.
Special Populations
The pharmacokinetics of the drug in hepatically and renally impaired patients have not been determined.
Drug Interactions
No pharmacokinetic-based drug-drug interaction studies have been conducted with LUPRON DEPOT. However, because leuprolide acetate is a peptide that is primarily degraded by peptidase and not by cytochrome P-450 enzymes as noted in specific studies, and the drug is only about 46% bound to plasma proteins, drug interactions would not be expected to occur.

CLINICAL STUDIES
Endometriosis
In controlled clinical studies, LUPRON DEPOT 3.75 mg monthly for six months was shown to be comparable to danazol 800 mg/day in relieving the clinical sign/symptoms of endometriosis (pelvic pain, dysmenorrhea, dyspareunia, pelvic tenderness, and induration) and in reducing the size of endometrial implants as evidenced by laparoscopy. The clinical significance of a decrease in endometriotic lesions is not known at this time, and in addition laparoscopic staging of endometriosis does not necessarily correlate with the severity of symptoms.
LUPRON DEPOT 3.75 mg monthly induced amenorrhea in 74% and 98% of the patients after the first and second treatment months respectively. Most of the remaining patients reported episodes of only light bleeding or spotting. In the first, second and third post-treatment months, normal menstrual cycles resumed in 7%, 71% and 95% of patients, respectively, excluding those who became pregnant.
Figure 1 illustrates the percent of patients with symptoms at baseline, final treatment visit and sustained relief at 6 and 12 months following discontinuation of treatment for the various symptoms evaluated during two controlled clinical studies. This included all patients at end of treatment and those who elected to participate in the follow-up period. This might provide a slight bias in the results at follow-up as 75% of the original patients entered the follow-up study, and 36% were evaluated at 6 months and 26% at 12 months.
[See figure 1 at top of next page]
Hormonal replacement therapy
Two clinical studies with a treatment duration of 12 months indicate that concurrent hormonal therapy (norethindrone acetate 5 mg daily) is effective in significantly reducing the loss of bone mineral density associated with LUPRON, without compromising the efficacy of LUPRON in relieving symptoms of endometriosis. (All patients in these studies received calcium supplementation with 1000 mg elemental calcium.) One controlled, randomized and double-blind study included 51 women treated with LUPRON DEPOT alone and 55 women treated with LUPRON plus norethindrone acetate 5 mg daily. The second study was an open label study in which 136 women were treated with LUPRON plus norethindrone acetate 5 mg daily. This study confirmed the reduction in loss of bone mineral density that was observed in the controlled study. Suppression of menses was maintained throughout treatment in 84% and 73% of patients receiving LD/N in the controlled study and open label study, respectively. The median time for menses resumption after treatment with LD/N was 8 weeks.
Figure 2 illustrates the mean pain scores for the LD/N group from the controlled study.
[See figure 2 at top of next page]
Uterine Leiomyomata (Fibroids)
In controlled clinical trials, administration of LUPRON DEPOT 3.75 mg for a period of three or six months was shown to decrease uterine and fibroid volume, thus allowing for relief of clinical symptoms (abdominal bloating, pelvic pain, and pressure). Excessive vaginal bleeding (menorrhagia and menometrorrhagia) decreased, resulting in improvement in hematologic parameters.
In three clinical trials, enrollment was not based on hematologic status. Mean uterine volume decreased by 41% and myoma volume decreased by 37% at final visit as evidenced by ultrasound or MRI. These patients also experienced a decrease in symptoms including excessive vaginal bleeding and pelvic discomfort. Benefit occurred by three months of therapy,

---

Information on the AbbVie, Inc. products listed on these pages is from the prescribing information in use as of July 31, 2014. For more information, please visit rxabbvie.com or call 1-800-633-9110.

FIGURE 1–PERCENT OF PATIENTS WITH SIGN/SYMPTOMS AT BASELINE, FINAL TREATMENT VISIT, AND AFTER 6 AND 12 MONTHS OF FOLLOW-UP

B = BASELINE
F = FINAL TREATMENT VISIT
6 = 6 MO. FOLLOW-UP (36%)*
12 = 12 MO. FOLLOW-UP (26%)*

* % refers to % of original patients who elected to participate in the follow-up study. Only 75% of the original patients enrolled in the follow-up study.

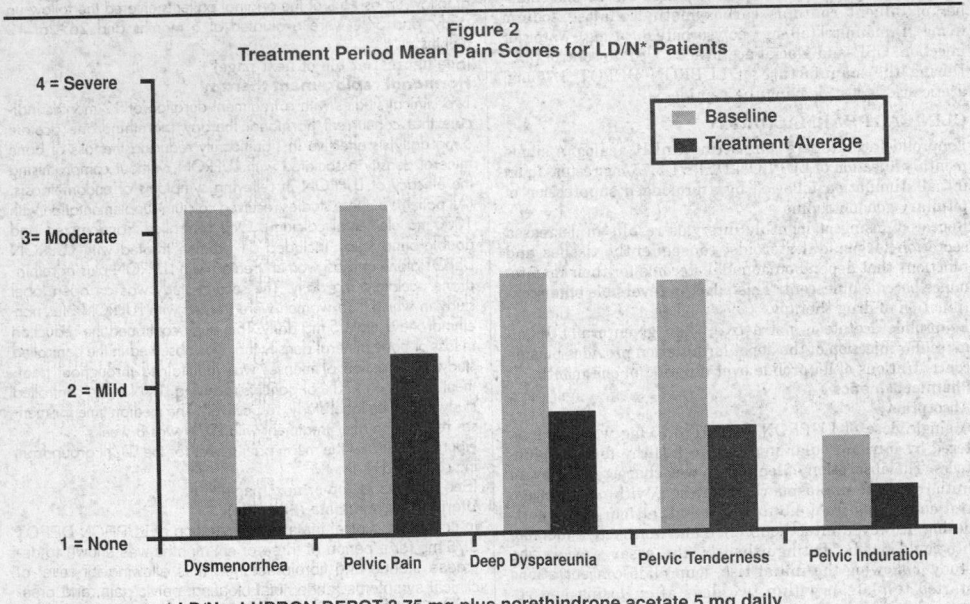

Figure 2
Treatment Period Mean Pain Scores for LD/N* Patients

Baseline
Treatment Average

* LD/N = LUPRON DEPOT 3.75 mg plus norethindrone acetate 5 mg daily

but additional gain was observed with an additional three months of LUPRON DEPOT 3.75 mg. Ninety-five percent of these patients became amenorrheic with 61%, 25%, and 4% experiencing amenorrhea during the first, second, and third treatment months respectively.

Post-treatment follow-up was carried out for a small percentage of LUPRON DEPOT 3.75 mg patients among the 77% who demonstrated a ≥ 25% decrease in uterine volume while on therapy. Menses usually returned within two months of cessation of therapy. Mean time to return to pretreatment uterine size was 8.3 months. Regrowth did not appear to be related to pretreatment uterine volume.

In another controlled clinical study, enrollment was based on hematocrit ≤ 30% and/or hemoglobin ≤ 10.2 g/dL. Administration of LUPRON DEPOT 3.75 mg, concomitantly with iron, produced an increase of ≥ 6% hematocrit and ≥ 2 g/dL hemoglo-

bin in 77% of patients at three months of therapy. The mean change in hematocrit was 10.1% and the mean change in hemoglobin was 4.2 g/dL. Clinical response was judged to be a hematocrit of ≥ 36% and hemoglobin of ≥ 12 g/dL, thus allowing for autologous blood donation prior to surgery. At three months, 75% of patients met this criterion.

At three months, 80% of patients experienced relief from either menorrhagia or menometrorrhagia. As with the previous studies, episodes of spotting and menstrual-like bleeding were noted in some patients.

In this same study, a decrease of ≥ 25% was seen in uterine and myoma volumes in 60% and 54% of patients respectively. LUPRON DEPOT 3.75 mg was found to relieve symptoms of bloating, pelvic pain, and pressure.

There is no evidence that pregnancy rates are enhanced or adversely affected by the use of LUPRON DEPOT 3.75 mg.

INDICATIONS AND USAGE

Endometriosis

LUPRON DEPOT 3.75 mg is indicated for management of endometriosis, including pain relief and reduction of endometriotic lesions. LUPRON DEPOT monthly with norethindrone acetate 5 mg daily is also indicated for initial management of endometriosis and for management of recurrence of symptoms. (Refer also to norethindrone acetate prescribing information for WARNINGS, PRECAUTIONS, CONTRAINDICATIONS and ADVERSE REACTIONS associated with norethindrone acetate). Duration of initial treatment or retreatment should be limited to 6 months.

Uterine Leiomyomata (Fibroids)

LUPRON DEPOT 3.75 mg concomitantly with iron therapy is indicated for the preoperative hematologic improvement of patients with anemia caused by uterine leiomyomata. The clinician may wish to consider a one-month trial period on iron alone inasmuch as some of the patients will respond to iron alone. (See **Table 1**.) LUPRON may be added if the response to iron alone is considered inadequate. Recommended duration of therapy with LUPRON DEPOT 3.75 mg is **up to three** months.

Experience with LUPRON DEPOT in females has been limited to women 18 years of age and older.

Table 1 PERCENT OF PATIENTS ACHIEVING HEMOGLOBIN ≥ 12 GM/DL

Treatment Group	Week 4	Week 8	Week 12
LUPRON DEPOT 3.75 mg with Iron	41*	71†	79*
Iron Alone	17	40	56

* P-Value < 0.01
† P-Value < 0.001

CONTRAINDICATIONS

1. Hypersensitivity to GnRH, GnRH agonist analogs or any of the excipients in LUPRON DEPOT.
2. Undiagnosed abnormal vaginal bleeding.
3. LUPRON DEPOT is contraindicated in women who are or may become pregnant while receiving the drug. LUPRON DEPOT may cause fetal harm when administered to a pregnant woman. Major fetal abnormalities were observed in rabbits but not in rats after administration of LUPRON DEPOT throughout gestation. There was increased fetal mortality and decreased fetal weights in rats and rabbits. (See **Pregnancy** section.) The effects on fetal mortality are expected consequences of the alterations in hormonal levels brought about by the drug. If this drug is used during pregnancy, or if the patient becomes pregnant while taking this drug, the patient should be apprised of the potential hazard to the fetus.
4. Use in women who are breast-feeding. (See **Nursing Mothers** section.)
5. Norethindrone acetate is contraindicated in women with the following conditions:
   ○ Thrombophlebitis, thromboembolic disorders, cerebral apoplexy, or a past history of these conditions
   ○ Markedly impaired liver function or liver disease
   ○ Known or suspected carcinoma of the breast

WARNINGS

Safe use of leuprolide acetate or norethindrone acetate in pregnancy has not been established clinically. Before starting treatment with LUPRON DEPOT, pregnancy must be excluded.

When used monthly at the recommended dose, LUPRON DEPOT usually inhibits ovulation and stops menstruation. Contraception is not insured, however, by taking LUPRON DEPOT. Therefore, patients should use non-hormonal methods of contraception.

Patients should be advised to see their physician if they believe they may be pregnant. If a patient becomes pregnant during treatment, the drug must be discontinued and the patient must be apprised of the potential risk to the fetus. During the early phase of therapy, sex steroids temporarily rise above baseline because of the physiologic effect of the drug. Therefore, an increase in clinical signs and symptoms may be observed during the initial days of therapy, but these will dissipate with continued therapy.

Symptoms consistent with an anaphylactoid or asthmatic process have been rarely reported post-marketing.

The following applies to co-treatment with LUPRON and norethindrone acetate:

Norethindrone acetate treatment should be discontinued if there is a sudden partial or complete loss of vision or if there is sudden onset of proptosis, diplopia, or migraine. If examination reveals papilledema or retinal vascular lesions, medication should be withdrawn.

Because of the occasional occurrence of thrombophlebitis and pulmonary embolism in patients taking progestogens, the physician should be alert to the earliest manifestations of the disease in women taking norethindrone acetate.

Assessment and management of risk factors for cardiovascular disease is recommended prior to initiation of add-back therapy with norethindrone acetate. Norethindrone acetate should be used with caution in women with risk factors, including lipid abnormalities or cigarette smoking.

PRECAUTIONS

Information for Patients

Patients should be aware of the following information:

1. Since menstruation usually stops with effective doses of LUPRON DEPOT, the patient should notify her physician if regular menstruation persists. Patients missing successive doses of LUPRON DEPOT may experience breakthrough bleeding.

2. Patients should not use LUPRON DEPOT if they are pregnant, breast feeding, have undiagnosed abnormal vaginal bleeding, or are allergic to any of the ingredients in LUPRON DEPOT.

3. Safe use of the drug in pregnancy has not been established clinically. Therefore, a non-hormonal method of contraception should be used during treatment. Patients should be advised that if they miss successive doses of LUPRON DEPOT, breakthrough bleeding or ovulation may occur with the potential for conception. If a patient becomes pregnant during treatment, she should discontinue treatment and consult her physician.

4. Adverse events occurring in clinical studies with LUPRON DEPOT that are associated with hypoestrogenism include: hot flashes, headaches, emotional lability, decreased libido, acne, myalgia, reduction in breast size, and vaginal dryness. Estrogen levels returned to normal after treatment was discontinued.

5. Patients should be counseled on the possibility of the development or worsening of depression and the occurrence of memory disorders.

6. The induced hypoestrogenic state **also** results in a loss in bone density over the course of treatment, some of which may not be reversible. Clinical studies show that concurrent hormonal therapy with norethindrone acetate 5 mg daily is effective in reducing loss of bone mineral density that occurs with LUPRON. (All patients received calcium supplementation with 1000 mg elemental calcium.) (See *Changes in Bone Density* section.)

7. If the symptoms of endometriosis recur after a course of therapy, retreatment with a six-month course of LUPRON DEPOT and norethindrone acetate 5 mg daily may be considered. Retreatment beyond this one six month course cannot be recommended. It is recommended that bone density be assessed before retreatment begins to ensure that values are within normal limits. Retreatment with LUPRON DEPOT alone is not recommended.

8. In patients with major risk factors for decreased bone mineral content such as chronic alcohol and/or tobacco use, strong family history of osteoporosis, or chronic use of drugs that can reduce bone mass such as anticonvulsants or corticosteroids, LUPRON DEPOT therapy may pose an additional risk. In these patients, the risks and benefits must be weighed carefully before therapy with LUPRON DEPOT alone is instituted, and concomitant treatment with norethindrone acetate 5 mg daily should be considered. Retreatment with gonadotropin-releasing hormone analogs, including LUPRON is not advisable in patients with major risk factors for loss of bone mineral content.

9. Because norethindrone acetate may cause some degree of fluid retention, conditions which might be influenced by this factor, such as epilepsy, migraine, asthma, cardiac or renal dysfunctions require careful observation during norethindrone acetate add-back therapy.

10. Patients who have a history of depression should be carefully observed during treatment with norethindrone acetate and norethindrone acetate should be discontinued if severe depression occurs.

Convulsions

There have been postmarketing reports of convulsions in patients on leuprolide acetate therapy. These included patients with and without concurrent medications and comorbid conditions.

Table 2 ADVERSE EVENTS REPORTED TO BE CAUSALLY RELATED TO DRUG IN ≥ 5% OF PATIENTS

| | Endometriosis (2 Studies) | | | | | | Uterine Fibroids (4 Studies) | | | |
| | LUPRON DEPOT 3.75 mg N=166 | | Danazol N=136 | | Placebo N=31 | | LUPRON DEPOT 3.75 mg N=166 | | Placebo N=163 | |
	N	(%)	N	(%)	N	(%)	N	(%)	N	(%)
Body as a Whole										
Asthenia	5	(3)	9	(7)	0	(0)	14	(8.4)	8	(4.9)
General pain	31	(19)	22	(16)	1	(3)	14	(8.4)	10	(6.1)
Headache*	53	(32)	30	(22)	2	(6)	43	(25.9)	29	(17.8)
Cardiovascular System										
Hot flashes/sweats*	139	(84)	77	(57)	9	(29)	121	(72.9)	29	(17.8)
Gastrointestinal System										
Nausea/vomiting	21	(13)	17	(13)	1	(3)	8	(4.8)	6	(3.7)
GI disturbances*	11	(7)	8	(6)	1	(3)	5	(3.0)	2	(1.2)
Metabolic and Nutritional Disorders										
Edema	12	(7)	17	(13)	1	(3)	9	(5.4)	2	(1.2)
Weight gain/loss	22	(13)	36	(26)	0	(0)	5	(3.0)	2	(1.2)
Endocrine System										
Acne	17	(10)	27	(20)	0	(0)	0	(0)	0	(0)
Hirsutism	2	(1)	9	(7)	1	(3)	1	(0.6)	0	(0)
Musculoskeletal System										
Joint disorder*	14	(8)	11	(8)	0	(0)	13	(7.8)	5	(3.1)
Myalgia*	1	(1)	7	(5)	0	(0)	1	(0.6)	0	(0)
Nervous System										
Decreased libido*	19	(11)	6	(4)	0	(0)	3	(1.8)	0	(0)
Depression/emotional lability*	36	(22)	27	(20)	1	(3)	18	(10.8)	7	(4.3)
Dizziness	19	(11)	4	(3)	0	(0)	3	(1.8)	6	(3.7)
Nervousness*	8	(5)	11	(8)	0	(0)	8	(4.8)	1	(0.6)
Neuromuscular disorders*	11	(7)	17	(13)	0	(0)	3	(1.8)	0	(0)
Paresthesias	12	(7)	11	(8)	0	(0)	2	(1.2)	1	(0.6)
Skin and Appendages										
Skin reactions	17	(10)	20	(15)	1	(3)	5	(3.0)	2	(1.2)
Urogenital System										
Breast changes/tenderness/pain*	10	(6)	12	(9)	0	(0)	3	(1.8)	7	(4.3)
Vaginitis*	46	(28)	23	(17)	0	(0)	19	(11.4)	3	(1.8)

In these same studies, symptoms reported in <5% of patients included: *Body as a Whole* - Body odor, Flu syndrome, Injection site reactions; *Cardiovascular System* - Palpitations, Syncope, Tachycardia; *Digestive System* - Appetite changes, Dry mouth, Thirst; *Endocrine System* - Androgen-like effects; *Hemic and Lymphatic System* - Ecchymosis, Lymphadenopathy; *Nervous System* – Anxiety*, Insomnia/Sleep disorders*, Delusions, Memory disorder, Personality disorder; *Respiratory System* - Rhinitis; *Skin and Appendages* - Alopecia, Hair disorder, Nail disorder; *Special Senses* - Conjunctivitis, Ophthalmologic disorders*, Taste perversion; *Urogenital System* - Dysuria*, Lactation, Menstrual disorders.

* = Possible effect of decreased estrogen.

Laboratory Tests

See **ADVERSE REACTIONS** section.

Drug Interactions

See **CLINICAL PHARMACOLOGY, Pharmacokinetics**.

Drug/Laboratory Test interactions

Administration of LUPRON DEPOT in therapeutic doses results in suppression of the pituitary-gonadal system. Normal function is usually restored within three months after treatment is discontinued. Therefore, diagnostic tests of pituitary gonadotropic and gonadal functions conducted during treatment and for up to three months after discontinuation of LUPRON DEPOT may be misleading.

Carcinogenesis, Mutagenesis, Impairment of Fertility

A two-year carcinogenicity study was conducted in rats and mice. In rats, a dose-related increase of benign pituitary hyperplasia and benign pituitary adenomas was noted at 24 months when the drug was administered subcutaneously at high daily doses (0.6 to 4 mg/kg). There was a significant but not dose-related increase of pancreatic islet-cell adenomas in females and of testicular interstitial cell adenomas in males (highest incidence in the low dose group). In mice, no leuprolide acetate-induced tumors or pituitary abnormalities were observed at a dose as high as 60 mg/kg for two years. Patients have been treated with leuprolide acetate for up to three years with doses as high as 10 mg/day and for two years with doses as high as 20 mg/day without demonstrable pituitary abnormalities.

Mutagenicity studies have been performed with leuprolide acetate using bacterial and mammalian systems. These studies provided no evidence of a mutagenic potential.

Clinical and pharmacologic studies in adults (>18 years) with leuprolide acetate and similar analogs have shown reversibility of fertility suppression when the drug is discontinued after continuous administration for periods of up to 24 weeks. Although no clinical studies have been completed in children to assess the full reversibility of fertility suppression, animal studies (prepubertal and adult rats and monkeys) with leuprolide acetate and other GnRH analogs have shown functional recovery.

Pregnancy

Teratogenic Effects

Pregnancy Category X (see **CONTRAINDICATIONS** section). When administered on day 6 of pregnancy at test dosages of 0.00024, 0.0024, and 0.024 mg/kg (1/300 to 1/3 of the human dose) to rabbits, LUPRON DEPOT produced a dose-related increase in major fetal abnormalities. Similar studies in rats failed to demonstrate an increase in fetal malformations. There was increased fetal mortality and decreased fetal weights with the two higher doses of LUPRON DEPOT in rabbits and with the highest dose (0.024 mg/kg) in rats.

Nursing Mothers

It is not known whether LUPRON DEPOT is excreted in human milk. Because many drugs are excreted in human milk, and because the effects of LUPRON DEPOT on lactation and/or the breast-fed child have not been determined, LUPRON DEPOT should not be used by nursing mothers.

Pediatric Use

Experience with LUPRON DEPOT 3.75 mg for treatment of endometriosis has been limited to women 18 years of age and older. See LUPRON DEPOT-PED® (leuprolide acetate for depot suspension) labeling for the safety and effectiveness in children with central precocious puberty.

Geriatric Use

This product has not been studied in women over 65 years of age and is not indicated in this population.

ADVERSE REACTIONS

Clinical Trials

Estradiol levels may increase during the first weeks following the initial injection of LUPRON, but then decline to menopausal levels. This transient increase in estradiol can be associated with a temporary worsening of signs and symptoms (see **WARNINGS** section).

As would be expected with a drug that lowers serum estradiol levels, the most frequently reported adverse reactions were those related to hypoestrogenism.

The **monthly formulation of LUPRON DEPOT 3.75 mg** was utilized in controlled clinical trials that studied the drug in 166 endometriosis and 166 uterine fibroids patients. Ad-

Information on the AbbVie, Inc. products listed on these pages is from the prescribing information in use as of July 31, 2014. For more information, please visit rxabbvie.com or call 1-800-633-9110.

Table 3 TREATMENT-RELATED ADVERSE EVENTS OCCURRING IN ≥5% OF PATIENTS

| | Controlled Study | | | | Open Label Study | |
| | LD - Only* N=51 | | LD/N† N=55 | | LD/N† N=136 | |
Adverse Events	N	(%)	N	(%)	N	(%)
Any Adverse Event	50	(98)	53	(96)	126	(93)
Body as a Whole						
Asthenia	9	(18)	10	(18)	15	(11)
Headache/Migraine	33	(65)	28	(51)	63	(46)
Injection Site Reaction	1	(2)	5	(9)	4	(3)
Pain	12	(24)	16	(29)	29	(21)
Cardiovascular System						
Hot flashes/sweats	50	(98)	48	(87)	78	(57)
Digestive System						
Altered Bowel Function	7	(14)	8	(15)	14	(10)
Changes in Appetite	2	(4)	0	(0)	8	(6)
GI Disturbance	2	(4)	4	(7)	6	(4)
Nausea/Vomiting	13	(25)	16	(29)	17	(13)
Metabolic and Nutritional Disorders						
Edema	0	(0)	5	(9)	9	(7)
Weight Changes	6	(12)	7	(13)	6	(4)
Nervous System						
Anxiety	3	(6)	0	(0)	11	(8)
Depression/Emotional Lability	16	(31)	15	(27)	46	(34)
Dizziness/Vertigo	8	(16)	6	(11)	10	(7)
Insomnia/Sleep Disorder	16	(31)	7	(13)	20	(15)
Libido Changes	5	(10)	2	(4)	10	(7)
Memory Disorder	3	(6)	1	(2)	6	(4)
Nervousness	4	(8)	2	(4)	15	(11)
Neuromuscular Disorder	1	(2)	5	(9)	4	(3)
Skin and Appendages						
Alopecia	0	(0)	5	(9)	4	(3)
Androgen-Like Effects	2	(4)	3	(5)	24	(18)
Skin/Mucous Membrane Reaction	2	(4)	5	(9)	15	(11)
Urogenital System						
Breast Changes/Pain/Tenderness	3	(6)	7	(13)	11	(8)
Menstrual Disorders	1	(2)	0	(0)	7	(5)
Vaginitis	10	(20)	8	(15)	11	(8)

* LD-Only = LUPRON DEPOT 3.75 mg
† LD/N = LUPRON DEPOT 3.75 mg plus norethindrone acetate 5 mg

Table 4 MEAN PERCENT CHANGE FROM BASELINE IN BONE MINERAL DENSITY OF LUMBAR SPINE

| | LUPRON DEPOT 3.75 mg Controlled Study | | LUPRON DEPOT 3.75 mg plus norethindrone acetate 5 mg daily | | | |
| | | | Controlled Study | | Open Label Study | |
	N	Change (Mean, 95% CI)#	N	Change (Mean, 95% CI)#	N	Change (Mean, 95% CI)#
Week 24*	41	-3.2% (-3.8, -2.6)	42	-0.3% (-0.8, 0.3)	115	-0.2% (-0.6, 0.2)
Week 52†	29	-6.3% (-7.1, -5.4)	32	-1.0% (-1.9, -0.1)	84	-1.1% (-1.6, -0.5)

* Includes on-treatment measurements that fell within 2–252 days after the first day of treatment.
† Includes on-treatment measurements >252 days after the first day of treatment.
\# 95% CI: 95% Confidence Interval

verse events reported in ≥5% of patients in either of these populations and thought to be potentially related to drug are noted in the following table.
[See table 2 at top of previous page]
In one controlled clinical trial utilizing the monthly formulation of LUPRON DEPOT, patients diagnosed with uterine fibroids received a higher dose (7.5 mg) of LUPRON DEPOT. Events seen with this dose that were thought to be potentially related to drug and were not seen at the lower dose included glossitis, hypesthesia, lactation, pyelonephritis, and urinary disorders. Generally, a higher incidence of hypoestrogenic effects was observed at the higher dose.
Table 3 lists the potentially drug-related adverse events observed in at least 5% of patients in any treatment group during the first 6 months of treatment in the add-back clinical studies.
In the controlled clinical trial, 50 of 51 (98%) patients in the LD group and 48 of 55 (87%) patients in the LD/N group reported experiencing hot flashes on one or more occasions during treatment. During Month 6 of treatment, 32 of 37 (86%) patients in the LD group and 22 of 38 (58%) patients in the LD/N group reported having experienced hot flashes. The mean number of days on which hot flashes were reported during this month of treatment was 19 and 7 in the LD and LD/N treatment groups, respectively. The mean maximum number of hot flashes in a day during this month of treatment was 5.8 and 1.9 in the LD and LD/N treatment groups, respectively.
[See table 3 above]
Changes in Bone Density
In controlled clinical studies, patients with endometriosis (six months of therapy) or uterine fibroids (three months of therapy) were treated with LUPRON DEPOT 3.75 mg. In endometriosis patients, vertebral bone density as measured by dual energy x-ray absorptiometry (DEXA) decreased by an average of 3.2% at six months compared with the pretreatment value. Clinical studies demonstrate that concurrent hormonal therapy (norethindrone acetate 5 mg daily) and calcium supplementation is effective in significantly reducing the loss of bone mineral density that occurs with LUPRON treatment, without compromising the efficacy of LUPRON in relieving symptoms of endometriosis.
LUPRON DEPOT 3.75 mg plus norethindrone acetate 5 mg daily was evaluated in two clinical trials. The results from this regimen were similar in both studies. LUPRON DEPOT 3.75 mg was used as a control group in one study. The bone mineral density data of the lumbar spine from these two studies are presented in Table 4.
[See table 4 above]
When LUPRON DEPOT 3.75 mg was administered for three months in uterine fibroid patients, vertebral trabecular bone mineral density as assessed by quantitative digital radiography (QDR) revealed a mean decrease of 2.7% compared with baseline. Six months after discontinuation of therapy, a trend toward recovery was observed. Use of LUPRON DEPOT for longer than three months (uterine fibroids) or six months (endometriosis) or in the presence of other known risk factors for decreased bone mineral content may cause additional bone loss **and is not recommended**.
Changes in Laboratory Values During Treatment
Plasma Enzymes
Endometriosis
During early clinical trials with LUPRON DEPOT 3.75 mg, regular laboratory monitoring revealed that AST levels were more than twice the upper limit of normal in only one patient. There was no clinical or other laboratory evidence of abnormal liver function.

In two other clinical trials, 6 of 191 patients receiving LUPRON DEPOT 3.75 mg plus norethindrone acetate 5 mg daily for up to 12 months developed an elevated (at least twice the upper limit of normal) SGPT or GGT. Five of the 6 increases were observed beyond 6 months of treatment. None were associated with elevated bilirubin concentration.
Uterine Leiomyomata (Fibroids)
In clinical trials with LUPRON DEPOT 3.75 mg, five (3%) patients had a post-treatment transaminase value that was at least twice the baseline value and above the upper limit of the normal range. None of the laboratory increases were associated with clinical symptoms.
Lipids
Endometriosis
In earlier clinical studies, 4% of the LUPRON DEPOT 3.75 mg patients and 1% of the danazol patients had total cholesterol values above the normal range at enrollment. These patients also had cholesterol values above the normal range at the end of treatment. Of those patients whose pretreatment cholesterol values were in the normal range, 7% of the LUPRON DEPOT 3.75 mg patients and 9% of the danazol patients had post-treatment values above the normal range.
The mean (±SEM) pretreatment values for total cholesterol from all patients were 178.8 (2.9) mg/dL in the LUPRON DEPOT 3.75 mg groups and 175.3 (3.0) mg/dL in the danazol group. At the end of treatment, the mean values for total cholesterol from all patients were 193.3 mg/dL in the LUPRON DEPOT 3.75 mg group and 194.4 mg/dL in the danazol group. These increases from the pretreatment values were statistically significant (p<0.03) in both groups.
Triglycerides were increased above the upper limit of normal in 12% of the patients who received LUPRON DEPOT 3.75 mg and in 6% of the patients who received danazol.
At the end of treatment, HDL cholesterol fractions decreased below the lower limit of the normal range in 2% of the LUPRON DEPOT 3.75 mg patients compared with 54% of those receiving danazol. LDL cholesterol fractions increased above the upper limit of the normal range in 6% of the patients receiving LUPRON DEPOT 3.75 mg compared with 23% of those receiving danazol. There was no increase in the LDL/HDL ratio in patients receiving LUPRON DEPOT 3.75 mg but there was approximately a two-fold increase in the LDL/HDL ratio in patients receiving danazol.
In two other clinical trials, LUPRON DEPOT 3.75 mg plus norethindrone acetate 5 mg daily was evaluated for 12 months of treatment. LUPRON DEPOT 3.75 mg was used as a control group in one study. Percent changes from baseline for serum lipids and percentages of patients with serum lipid values outside of the normal range in the two studies are summarized in the tables below.
[See table 5 at top of next page]
Changes from baseline tended to be greater at Week 52. After treatment, mean serum lipid levels from patients with follow up data returned to pretreatment values.
[See table 6 at top of next page]
Low HDL-cholesterol (<40 mg/dL) and elevated LDL-cholesterol (>160 mg/dL) are recognized risk factors for cardiovascular disease. The long-term significance of the observed treatment-related changes in serum lipids in women with endometriosis is unknown. Therefore assessment of cardiovascular risk factors should be considered prior to initiation of concurrent treatment with LUPRON and norethindrone acetate.
Uterine Leiomyomata (Fibroids)
In patients receiving LUPRON DEPOT 3.75 mg, mean changes in cholesterol (+11 mg/dL to +29 mg/dL), LDL cholesterol (+8 mg/dL to +22 mg/dL), HDL cholesterol (0 to +6 mg/dL), and the LDL/HDL ratio (-0.1 to +0.5) were observed across studies. In the one study in which triglycerides were determined, the mean increase from baseline was 32 mg/dL.
Other Changes
Endometriosis
The following changes were seen in approximately 5% to 8% of patients. In the earlier comparative studies, LUPRON DEPOT 3.75 mg was associated with elevations of LDH and phosphorus, and decreases in WBC counts. Danazol therapy was associated with increases in hematocrit, platelet count, and LDH. In the hormonal add-back studies LUPRON DEPOT in combination with norethindrone acetate was associated with elevations of GGT and SGPT.
Uterine Leiomyomata (Fibroids)
Hematology: (see **CLINICAL STUDIES** section) In LUPRON DEPOT 3.75 mg treated patients, although there were statistically significant mean decreases in platelet counts from baseline to final visit, the last mean platelet counts were within the normal range. Decreases in total WBC count and neutrophils were observed, but were not clinically significant.
Chemistry: Slight to moderate mean increases were noted for glucose, uric acid, BUN, creatinine, total protein, albumin, bilirubin, alkaline phosphatase, LDH, calcium, and phosphorus. None of these increases were clinically significant.
Postmarketing
The following adverse reactions have been identified during postapproval use of LUPRON DEPOT. Because these reactions are reported voluntarily from a population of uncer-

tain size, it is not always possible to reliably estimate their frequency or establish a causal relationship to drug exposure.

During postmarketing surveillance, the following adverse events were reported. Like other drugs in this class, mood swings, including depression, have been reported. There have been rare reports of suicidal ideation and attempt. Many, but not all, of these patients had a history of depression or other psychiatric illness. Patients should be counseled on the possibility of development or worsening of depression during treatment with LUPRON.

Symptoms consistent with an anaphylactoid or asthmatic process have been rarely reported. Rash, urticaria, and photosensitivity reactions have also been reported.

Localized reactions including induration and abscess have been reported at the site of injection. Symptoms consistent with fibromyalgia (eg: joint and muscle pain, headaches, sleep disorder, gastrointestinal distress, and shortness of breath) have been reported individually and collectively. Other events reported are:

Hepato-biliary disorder: Rarely reported serious liver injury

Injury, poisoning and procedural complications: Spinal fracture

Investigations: Decreased WBC

Musculoskeletal and Connective tissue disorder: Tenosynovitis-like symptoms

Nervous System Disorder: Convulsion, peripheral neuropathy, paralysis

Vascular Disorder: Hypotension

Cases of serious venous and arterial thromboembolism have been reported, including deep vein thrombosis, pulmonary embolism, myocardial infarction, stroke, and transient ischemic attack. Although a temporal relationship was reported in some cases, most cases were confounded by risk factors or concomitant medication use. It is unknown if there is a causal association between the use of GnRH analogs and these events.

Pituitary apoplexy

During post-marketing surveillance, rare cases of pituitary apoplexy (a clinical syndrome secondary to infarction of the pituitary gland) have been reported after the administration of gonadotropin-releasing hormone agonists. In a majority of these cases, a pituitary adenoma was diagnosed, with a majority of pituitary apoplexy cases occurring within 2 weeks of the first dose, and some within the first hour. In these cases, pituitary apoplexy has presented as sudden headache, vomiting, visual changes, ophthalmoplegia, altered mental status, and sometimes cardiovascular collapse. Immediate medical attention has been required.

See other LUPRON DEPOT and LUPRON Injection package inserts for other events reported in different patient populations.

OVERDOSAGE

In rats subcutaneous administration of 250 to 500 times the recommended human dose, expressed on a per body weight basis, resulted in dyspnea, decreased activity, and local irritation at the injection site. There is no evidence that there is a clinical counterpart of this phenomenon. In early clinical trials using daily subcutaneous leuprolide acetate in patients with prostate cancer, doses as high as 20 mg/day for up to two years caused no adverse effects differing from those observed with the 1 mg/day dose.

DOSAGE AND ADMINISTRATION

LUPRON DEPOT Must Be Administered Under The Supervision Of A Physician.

Endometriosis

The recommended duration of treatment with LUPRON DEPOT 3.75 mg alone or in combination with norethindrone acetate is six months. The choice of LUPRON DEPOT alone or LUPRON DEPOT plus norethindrone acetate therapy for initial management of the symptoms and signs of endometriosis should be made by the health care professional in consultation with the patient and should take into consideration the risks and benefits of the addition of norethindrone to LUPRON DEPOT alone.

If the symptoms of endometriosis recur after a course of therapy, retreatment with a six-month course of LUPRON DEPOT administered monthly and norethindrone acetate 5 mg daily may be considered. Retreatment beyond this one six-month course cannot be recommended. It is recommended that bone density be assessed before retreatment begins to ensure that values are within normal limits. LUPRON DEPOT alone is not recommended for retreatment. If norethindrone acetate is contraindicated for the individual patient, then retreatment is not recommended.

An assessment of cardiovascular risk and management of risk factors such as cigarette smoking is recommended before beginning treatment with LUPRON DEPOT and norethindrone acetate.

Uterine Leiomyomata (Fibroids)

Recommended duration of therapy with *LUPRON DEPOT 3.75 mg is* **up to 3 months.** *The symptoms associated with uterine leiomyomata will recur following discontinuation of therapy. If additional treatment with LUPRON DEPOT 3.75 mg is*

Table 5 SERUM LIPIDS: MEAN PERCENT CHANGES FROM BASELINE VALUES AT TREATMENT WEEK 24

| | LUPRON Controlled Study (n=39) | | LUPRON plus norethindrone acetate 5 mg daily | | | |
| | | | Controlled Study (n=41) | | Open Label Study (n=117) | |
	Baseline Value*	Wk 24 % Change	Baseline Value*	Wk 24 % Change	Baseline Value*	Wk 24 % Change
Total Cholesterol	170.5	9.2%	179.3	0.2%	181.2	2.8%
HDL Cholesterol	52.4	7.4%	51.8	-18.8%	51.0	-14.6%
LDL Cholesterol	96.6	10.9%	101.5	14.1%	109.1	13.1%
LDL/HDL Ratio	2.0†	5.0%	2.1†	43.4%	2.3†	39.4%
Triglycerides	107.8	17.5%	130.2	9.5%	105.4	13.8%

* mg/dL
† ratio

Table 6 PERCENTAGE OF PATIENTS WITH SERUM LIPID VALUES OUTSIDE OF THE NORMAL RANGE

| | LUPRON Controlled Study (n=39) | | LUPRON plus norethindrone acetate 5 mg daily | | | |
| | | | Controlled Study (n=41) | | Open Label Study (n=117) | |
	Wk 0	Wk 24*	Wk 0	Wk 24*	Wk 0	Wk 24*
Total Cholesterol (>240 mg/dL)	15%	23%	15%	20%	6%	7%
HDL Cholesterol (<40 mg/dL)	15%	10%	15%	44%	15%	41%
LDL Cholesterol (>160 mg/dL)	0%	8%	5%	7%	9%	11%
LDL/HDL Ratio (>4.0)	0%	3%	2%	15%	7%	21%
Triglycerides (>200 mg/dL)	13%	13%	12%	10%	5%	9%

* Includes all patients regardless of baseline value.

contemplated, bone density should be assessed prior to initiation of therapy to ensure that values are within normal limits. The recommended dose of LUPRON DEPOT is 3.75 mg, incorporated in a depot formulation.

For optimal performance of the prefilled dual chamber syringe (PDS), read and follow the following instructions:

Reconstitution and Administration Instructions

- The lyophilized microspheres are to be reconstituted and administered as a single intramuscular injection.
- Since LUPRON DEPOT does not contain a preservative, the suspension should be injected immediately or discarded if not used within two hours.
- As with other drugs administered by injection, the injection site should be varied periodically.

1. The LUPRON DEPOT powder should be visually inspected and the syringe should NOT BE USED if clumping or caking is evident. A thin layer of powder on the wall of the syringe is considered normal prior to mixing with the diluent. The diluent should appear clear.

2. To prepare for injection, screw the white plunger into the end stopper until the stopper begins to turn.

3. Hold the syringe UPRIGHT. Release the diluent by SLOWLY PUSHING (6 to 8 seconds) the plunger until the first stopper is at the blue line in the middle of the barrel.

← blue line

4. Keep the syringe UPRIGHT. Mix the microspheres (powder) thoroughly by gently shaking the syringe until the

powder forms a uniform suspension. The suspension will appear milky. If the powder adheres to the stopper or caking/clumping is present, tap the syringe with your finger to disperse. DO NOT USE if any of the powder has not gone into suspension.

5. Hold the syringe UPRIGHT. With the opposite hand pull the needle cap upward without twisting.

6. Keep the syringe UPRIGHT. Advance the plunger to expel the air from the syringe. Now the syringe is ready for injection.

7. After cleaning the injection site with an alcohol swab, the intramuscular injection should be performed by inserting the needle at a 90 degree angle into the gluteal area, anterior thigh, or deltoid; injection sites should be alternated.

NOTE: Aspirated blood would be visible just below the luer lock connection if a blood vessel is accidentally penetrated. If present, blood can be seen through the transparent LuproLoc® safety device. If blood is present remove the needle immediately. Do not inject the medication.

[See figure at top of next column]

8. Inject the entire contents of the syringe intramuscularly at the time of reconstitution. The suspension settles very quickly following reconstitution; therefore, LUPRON DEPOT should be mixed and used immediately.

AFTER INJECTION

9. Withdraw the needle. Once the syringe has been withdrawn, activate immediately the LuproLoc® safety device by pushing the arrow on the lock upward towards the

Information on the AbbVie, Inc. products listed on these pages is from the prescribing information in use as of July 31, 2014. For more information, please visit rxabbvie.com or call 1-800-633-9110.

CLICK

needle tip with the thumb or finger, as illustrated, until the needle cover of the safety device over the needle is fully extended and a CLICK is heard or felt.

ADDITIONAL INFORMATION
- Dispose of the syringe according to local regulations/procedures.

HOW SUPPLIED
Each LUPRON DEPOT 3.75 mg kit (NDC 0074-3641-03) contains:
- one prefilled dual-chamber syringe
- one plunger
- two alcohol swabs
- a complete prescribing information enclosure

Each syringe contains sterile lyophilized microspheres, which is leuprolide incorporated in a biodegradable copolymer of lactic and glycolic acids. When mixed with diluent, LUPRON DEPOT 3.75 mg is administered as a single monthly IM injection.

Store at 25°C (77°F); excursions permitted to 15-30°C (59-86°F) [See USP Controlled Room Temperature]

REFERENCES
1. NIOSH Alert: Preventing occupational exposures to antineoplastic and other hazardous drugs in healthcare settings. 2004. U.S. Department of Health and Human Services, Public Health Service, Centers for Disease Control and Prevention, National Institute for Occupational Safety and Health, DHHS (NIOSH) Publication No. 2004-165.
2. OSHA Technical Manual, TED 1-0.15A, Section VI: Chapter 2. Controlling Occupational Exposure to Hazardous Drugs. OSHA, 1999. http://www.osha.gov/dts/osta/otm/otm_vi/otm_vi_2.html
3. American Society of Health-System Pharmacists. ASHP guidelines on handling hazardous drugs. *Am J Health-Syst Pharm.* 2006; 63; 1172-1193.
4. Polovich, M., White, J.M., & Kelleher, L.O. (eds.) 2005. Chemotherapy and biotherapy guidelines and recommendations for practice (2nd. Ed.) Pittsburgh, PA: Oncology Nursing Society.

Manufactured for
AbbVie Inc.
North Chicago, IL 60064
by Takeda Pharmaceutical Company Limited
Osaka, Japan 540-8645
™ - Trademark
® - Registered Trademark
(No. 3641)
Ref: 03-A891-Revised October, 2013
© 2013 AbbVie Inc.
Shown in Product Identification Guide, page 303

LUPRON DEPOT® 7.5 mg for 1-month administration
[*lew-prŏn*]
(leuprolide acetate for depot suspension)   ℞

Rx only

DESCRIPTION
Leuprolide acetate is a synthetic nonapeptide analog of naturally occurring gonadotropin-releasing hormone (GnRH or LH-RH). The analog possesses greater potency than the natural hormone. The chemical name is 5-oxo-L-prolyl-L-histidyl-L-tryptophyl-L-seryl-L-tyrosyl-D-leucyl-L-leucyl-L-arginyl-N-ethyl-L-prolinamide acetate (salt) with the following structural formula:
[See chemical structure above]
LUPRON DEPOT is available in a prefilled dual-chamber syringe containing sterile lyophilized microspheres which, when mixed with diluent, becomes a suspension intended as a monthly intramuscular injection.

The front chamber of LUPRON DEPOT 7.5 mg for 1-month administration prefilled dual-chamber syringe contains leuprolide acetate (7.5 mg), purified gelatin (1.3 mg), DL-lactic and glycolic acids copolymer (66.2 mg), and D-mannitol (13.2 mg). The second chamber of diluent contains carboxymethylcellulose sodium (5 mg), D-mannitol (50 mg), polysorbate 80 (1 mg), water for injection, USP, and glacial acetic acid, USP to control pH.
During the manufacture of LUPRON DEPOT 7.5 mg for 1-month administration, acetic acid is lost, leaving the peptide.

CLINICAL PHARMACOLOGY
Mechanism of Action
Leuprolide acetate, a GnRH agonist, acts as a potent inhibitor of gonadotropin secretion. Animal studies indicate that following an initial stimulation, chronic administration of leuprolide acetate results in suppression of ovarian and testicular steroidogenesis. This effect is reversible upon discontinuation of drug therapy.
Administration of leuprolide acetate has resulted in inhibition of the growth of certain hormone dependent tumors (prostatic tumors in Noble and Dunning male rats and DMBA-induced mammary tumors in female rats) as well as atrophy of the reproductive organs.

Pharmacodynamics
In humans, administration of leuprolide acetate results in an initial increase in circulating levels of luteinizing hormone (LH) and follicle stimulating hormone (FSH), leading to a transient increase in levels of the gonadal steroids (testosterone and dihydrotestosterone in males, and estrone and estradiol in premenopausal females). However, continuous administration of leuprolide acetate results in decreased levels of LH and FSH. In males, testosterone is reduced to castrate levels. In premenopausal females, estrogens are reduced to postmenopausal levels. These decreases occur within two to four weeks after initiation of treatment, and castrate levels of testosterone in prostatic cancer patients have been demonstrated for more than five years.
Leuprolide acetate is not active when given orally.

Pharmacokinetics
Absorption
Following a single injection of LUPRON DEPOT 7.5 mg for 1-month administration to patients, mean plasma leuprolide concentration was almost 20 ng/mL at 4 hours and 0.36 ng/mL at 4 weeks. However, intact leuprolide and an inactive major metabolite could not be distinguished by the assay which was employed in the study. Nondetectable leuprolide plasma concentrations have been observed during chronic LUPRON DEPOT 7.5 mg administration, but testosterone levels appear to be maintained at castrate levels.

Distribution
The mean steady-state volume of distribution of leuprolide following intravenous bolus administration to healthy male volunteers was 27 L. *In vitro* binding to human plasma proteins ranged from 43% to 49%.

Metabolism
In healthy male volunteers, a 1 mg bolus of leuprolide administered intravenously revealed that the mean systemic clearance was 7.6 L/h, with a terminal elimination half-life of approximately 3 hours based on a two compartment model.
In rats and dogs, administration of ^{14}C-labeled leuprolide was shown to be metabolized to smaller inactive peptides, a pentapeptide (Metabolite I), tripeptides (Metabolites II and III) and a dipeptide (Metabolite IV). These fragments may be further catabolized.
The major metabolite (M-I) plasma concentrations measured in 5 prostate cancer patients reached maximum concentration 2 to 6 hours after dosing and were approximately 6% of the peak parent drug concentration. One week after dosing, mean plasma M-I concentrations were approximately 20% of mean leuprolide concentrations.

Excretion
Following administration of LUPRON DEPOT 3.75 mg to 3 patients, less than 5% of the dose was recovered as parent and M-I metabolite in the urine.

Special Populations
The pharmacokinetics of the drug in hepatically and renally impaired patients have not been determined.

CLINICAL STUDIES
In an open-label, non-comparative, multicenter clinical study of LUPRON DEPOT 7.5 mg for 1-month administration, 56 patients with stage D_2 prostatic adenocarcinoma and no prior systemic treatment were enrolled. The objectives were to determine if a 7.5 mg depot formulation of leuprolide injected once every 4 weeks would reduce and maintain serum testosterone to castrate range (≤50 ng/dL), to evaluate objective clinical response, and to assess the safety of the formulation. During the initial 24 weeks, serum testosterone was measured weekly, biweekly, or every four weeks and objective tumor response assessments were performed at Weeks 12 and 24. Once the patient completed the initial 24-week treatment phase, treatment continued at the investigator's discretion. Data from the initial 24-week treatment phase are summarized in this section.
In the majority of patients, serum testosterone increased by 50% or more above baseline during the first week of treatment. Serum testosterone suppressed to the castrate range within 30 days of the initial depot injection in 94% (51/54) of patients for whom testosterone suppression was achieved (2 patients withdrew prior to onset of suppression) and within 66 days in all 54 patients. Mean serum testosterone suppressed to castrate level by Week 3. The median dosing interval between injections was 28 days. One escape from suppression (2 consecutive testosterone values greater than 50 ng/dL after achieving castrate level) was noted at Week 18, associated with a substantial dosing delay. In this patient, serum testosterone returned to the castrate range at the next monthly measurement. Serum testosterone was minimally above the castrate range on a single occasion for 4 other patients. No clinical significance was attributed to these rises in testosterone.

Lupron Depot 7.5 mg
Mean Serum Testosterone Concentrations

[Graph: y-axis "Serum Testosterone (ng/dL)" from 0 to 700; x-axis "Weeks" from 0 to 24. Injection arrows labeled Inj. #1 through Inj. #6. Dashed line "50 ng/dL = castrate level".]

Secondary efficacy endpoints evaluated included objective tumor response, assessed by clinical evaluations of tumor burden (complete response, partial response, objectively stable, and progression), as well as changes in local disease status, assessed by digital rectal examination, and changes in prostatic acid phosphatase (PAP). These evaluations were performed at Weeks 12 and 24. The objective tumor response analysis showed a "no progression" (ie. complete or partial response, or stable disease) in 77% (40/52) of patients at Week 12, and in 84% (42/50) of patients at Week 24. Local disease improved or remained stable in all (42) patients evaluated at Week 12 and in 98% (41/42) of patients elevated at Week 24. PAP normalized or decreased at Week 12 and/or 24 in the majority of patients with elevated baseline PAP.
Periodic monitoring of serum testosterone and PSA levels is recommended, especially if the anticipated clinical or biochemical response to treatment has not been achieved. It should be noted that results of testosterone determinations are dependent on assay methodology. It is advisable to be aware of the type and precision of the assay methodology to make appropriate clinical and therapeutic decisions.

INDICATIONS AND USAGE
LUPRON DEPOT 7.5 mg for 1-month administration is indicated in the palliative treatment of advanced prostatic cancer.

CONTRAINDICATIONS

1. LUPRON DEPOT is contraindicated in individuals with known hypersensitivity to GnRH agonists or any of the excipients in LUPRON DEPOT. Reports of anaphylactic reactions to GnRH agonist analogs have been reported in the medical literature.
2. LUPRON DEPOT may cause fetal harm when administered to a pregnant woman. Expected hormonal changes that occur with LUPRON DEPOT increase the risk for pregnancy loss and fetal harm when administered to a pregnant woman (see **Pregnancy Category X**). LUPRON DEPOT is contraindicated in women who are or may become pregnant. If this drug is used during pregnancy, or if the patient becomes pregnant while taking this drug, the patient should be apprised of the potential hazard to the fetus.

WARNINGS

Tumor Flare

Initially, LUPRON DEPOT, like other GnRH agonists, causes increases in serum levels of testosterone to approximately 50% above baseline during the first week of treatment. Isolated cases of ureteral obstruction and spinal cord compression have been observed, which may contribute to paralysis with or without fatal complications. Transient worsening of symptoms may develop. A small number of patients may experience a temporary increase in bone pain, which can be managed symptomatically.

PRECAUTIONS

Information for Patients

- If they experience an allergic reaction to other drugs like LUPRON DEPOT, they should not use this drug.
- The most common side effects associated with LUPRON DEPOT are hot flashes, pain (especially joint pain and back pain), injection site pain and fatigue.
- LUPRON DEPOT may cause impotence.
- The increase in testosterone that occurs during the first weeks of therapy can cause an increase in urinary symptoms or pain.
- If they have metastatic cancer to the spine or urinary tract, they need close medical attention during the first weeks of therapy.
- They should notify their doctor if they develop new or worsened symptoms after beginning LUPRON DEPOT treatment.

General

Patients with metastatic vertebral lesions and/or with urinary tract obstruction should be closely observed during the first few weeks of therapy (see **WARNINGS** section).

Hyperglycemia and Diabetes

Hyperglycemia and an increased risk of developing diabetes have been reported in men receiving GnRH agonists. Hyperglycemia may represent development of diabetes mellitus or worsening of glycemic control in patients with diabetes. Monitor blood glucose and/or glycosylated hemoglobin (HbA1c) periodically in patients receiving a GnRH agonist and manage with current practice for treatment of hyperglycemia or diabetes.

Cardiovascular Diseases

Increased risk of developing myocardial infarction, sudden cardiac death and stroke has been reported in association with use of GnRH agonists in men. The risk appears low based on the reported odds ratios, and should be evaluated carefully along with cardiovascular risk factors when determining a treatment for patients with prostate cancer. Patients receiving a GnRH agonist should be monitored for symptoms and signs suggestive of development of cardiovascular disease and be managed according to current clinical practice.

Effect on QT/QTc Interval

Long-term androgen deprivation therapy prolongs the QT interval. Physicians should consider whether the benefits of androgen deprivation therapy outweigh the potential risks in patients with congenital long QT syndrome, electrolyte abnormalities, or congestive heart failure and in patients taking class IA (e.g., quinidine, procainamide) or Class III (e.g., amiodarone, sotalol) antiarrhythmic medications.

Convulsions

Postmarketing reports of convulsions have been observed in patients on leuprolide acetate therapy. These included patients with a history of seizures, epilepsy, cerebrovascular disorders, central nervous system anomalies or tumors, and in patients on concomitant medications that have been associated with convulsions such as bupropion and SSRIs. Convulsions have also been reported in patients in the absence of any of the conditions mentioned above. Patients receiving a GnRH agonist who experience convulsions should be managed according to current clinical practice.

Laboratory Tests

Response to LUPRON DEPOT 7.5 mg for 1-month administration should be monitored by measuring serum levels of testosterone. In the majority of patients, testosterone levels increased above baseline, declining thereafter to castration levels (<50 ng/dL) within four weeks (see **CLINICAL STUDIES** section).

Drug Interactions

No pharmacokinetic-based drug-drug interaction studies have been conducted with LUPRON DEPOT. However, because leuprolide acetate is a peptide that is primarily degraded by peptidase and not by Cytochrome P-450 enzymes as noted in specific studies, and the drug is only about 46% bound to plasma proteins, drug interactions would not be expected to occur (see **Pharmacokinetics**).

Drug/Laboratory Test Interactions

Administration of LUPRON DEPOT in therapeutic doses results in suppression of the pituitary-gonadal system. Normal function is usually restored within three months after treatment is discontinued. Due to the suppression of the pituitary-gonadal system by LUPRON DEPOT, diagnostic tests of pituitary gonadotropic and gonadal functions conducted during treatment and for up to three months after discontinuation of LUPRON DEPOT may be affected.

Carcinogenesis, Mutagenesis, Impairment of Fertility

Two-year carcinogenicity studies were conducted in rats and mice. In rats, a dose-related increase of benign pituitary hyperplasia and benign pituitary adenomas was noted at 24 months when the drug was administered subcutaneously at high daily doses (0.6 to 4 mg/kg). There was a significant but not dose-related increase of pancreatic islet-cell adenomas in females and of testicular interstitial cell adenomas in males (highest incidence in the low dose group). In mice, no leuprolide acetate-induced tumors or pituitary abnormalities were observed at a dose as high as 60 mg/kg for two years. Patients have been treated with leuprolide acetate for up to three years with doses as high as 10 mg/day and for two years with doses as high as 20 mg/day without demonstrable pituitary abnormalities.

Genotoxicity studies were conducted with leuprolide acetate using bacterial and mammalian systems. These studies provided no evidence of a mutagenic potential or chromosomal aberrations.

Leuprolide may reduce male and female fertility. Administration of leuprolide acetate to male and female rats at dose of 0.024, 0.24, and 2.4 mg/kg as monthly depot formulation for up to 3 months (approximately as low as 1/30 of the human dose based on body surface area using an estimated daily dose in animals and humans) caused atrophy of the reproductive organs, and suppression of reproductive function. These changes were reversible upon cessation of treatment. Clinical and pharmacologic studies in adults (≥ 18 years) with leuprolide acetate and similar analogs have shown reversibility of fertility suppression when the drug is discontinued after continuous administration for periods of up to 24 weeks.

Clinical and pharmacologic studies in adults (≥ 18 years) with leuprolide acetate and similar analogs have shown reversibility of fertility suppression when the drug is discontinued after continuous administration for periods of up to 24 weeks.

Pregnancy Category X

See **CONTRAINDICATIONS** section.

LUPRON DEPOT is contraindicated in women who are or may become pregnant while receiving the drug. Expected hormonal changes that occur with LUPRON DEPOT treatment increase the risk for pregnancy loss and fetal harm when administered to a pregnant woman. If this drug is used during pregnancy, or if the patient becomes pregnant while taking this drug, the patient should be apprised of the potential hazard to the fetus.

Major fetal abnormalities were observed in rabbits after a single administration of the monthly formulation of LUPRON DEPOT on day 6 of pregnancy at doses of 0.00024, 0.0024, and 0.024 mg/kg (approximately 1/1600 to 1/16 the human dose based on body surface area using an estimated daily dose in animals and humans). Since a depot formulation was utilized in the study, a sustained exposure to leuprolide was expected throughout the period of organogenesis and to the end of gestation. Similar studies in rats did not demonstrate an increase in fetal malformations, however, there was increased fetal mortality and decreased fetal weights with the two higher doses of the monthly formulation of LUPRON DEPOT in rabbits and with the highest dose (0.024 mg/kg) in rats.

Nursing Mothers

LUPRON DEPOT is not indicated for women (see **INDICATIONS AND USAGE** section). It is not known whether leuprolide is excreted in human milk. Because many drugs are excreted in human milk and because of the potential for serious adverse reactions in nursing infants from LUPRON DEPOT, a decision should be made to discontinue nursing or discontinue the drug taking into account the importance of the drug to the mother.

Pediatric Use

See LUPRON DEPOT-PED® (leuprolide acetate for depot suspension) labeling for the safety and effectiveness in children with central precocious puberty.

Geriatric Use

In the clinical trials for LUPRON DEPOT in prostate cancer, the majority (80%) of the subjects studied were at least 65 years of age. Therefore, the labeling reflects the pharmacokinetics, efficacy and safety of LUPRON DEPOT in this population.

ADVERSE REACTIONS

Clinical Trials

In the majority of patients testosterone levels increased above baseline during the first week, declining thereafter to baseline levels or below by the end of the second week of treatment.

Potential exacerbations of signs and symptoms during the first few weeks of treatment is a concern in patients with vertebral metastases and/or urinary obstruction or hematuria which, if aggravated, may lead to neurological problems such as temporary weakness and/or paresthesia of the lower limbs or worsening of urinary symptoms (see **WARNINGS** section).

In a clinical trial of LUPRON DEPOT 7.5 mg for 1-month administration, the following adverse reactions were reported in 5% or more of the patients during the initial 24-week treatment period regardless of causality.

LUPRON DEPOT 7.5 mg for 1-Month Administration (N=56)

	N	(%)
Body as a Whole		
General pain	13	(23.2)
Infection	3	(5.4)
Cardiovascular System		
Hot flashes/sweats*	32	(57.1)
Digestive System		
GI disorders	8	(14.3)
Metabolic and Nutritional Disorders		
Edema	8	(14.3)
Nervous System		
Libido decreased*	3	(5.4)
Respiratory System		
Respiratory disorder	6	(10.7)
Urogenital System		
Urinary disorder	7	(12.5)
Impotence*	3	(5.4)
Testicular atrophy*	3	(5.4)

* Due to the expected physiologic effect of decreased testosterone levels.

In this same study, the following adverse reactions were reported in less than 5% of the patients on LUPRON DEPOT 7.5 mg for 1-month administration.
Body as a Whole - Asthenia, Cellulitis, Fever, Headache, Injection site reaction, Neoplasm; *Cardiovascular System* - Angina, Congestive heart failure; *Digestive System* - Anorexia, Dysphagia, Eructation, Peptic ulcer; *Hemic and Lymphatic System* - Ecchymosis; *Musculoskeletal System* - Myalgia; *Nervous System* - Agitation, Insomnia/sleep disorders, Neuromuscular disorders; *Respiratory System* - Emphysema, Hemoptysis, Lung edema, Sputum increased; *Skin and Appendages* - Hair disorder, Skin reaction; *Urogenital System* - Balanitis, Breast enlargement, Urinary tract infection.

Laboratory: Abnormalities of certain parameters were observed, but their relationship to drug treatment are difficult to assess in this population. The following were recorded in ≥5% of patients at final visit: Decreased albumin, decreased hemoglobin/hematocrit, decreased prostatic acid phosphatase, decreased total protein, decreased urine specific gravity, hyperglycemia, hyperuricemia, increased BUN, increased creatinine, increased liver function tests (AST, LDH), increased phosphorus, increased platelets, increased prostatic acid phosphatase, increased total cholesterol, increased urine specific gravity, leukopenia.

Postmarketing

The following adverse reactions have been identified during postapproval use of LUPRON DEPOT. Because these reactions are reported voluntarily from a population of uncertain size, it is not always possible to reliably estimate their frequency or establish a causal relationship to drug exposure.

During postmarketing surveillance, which includes other dosage forms and other patient populations, the following adverse events were reported.

Like other drugs in this class, mood swings, including depression, have been reported. There have been very rare reports of suicidal ideation and attempt. Many, but not all, of these patients had a history of depression or other psychi-

Information on the AbbVie, Inc. products listed on these pages is from the prescribing information in use as of July 31, 2014. For more information, please visit rxabbvie.com or call 1-800-633-9110.

atric illness. Patients should be counseled on the possibility of development or worsening of depression during treatment with LUPRON.

Symptoms consistent with an anaphylactoid or asthmatic process have been rarely (incidence rate of about 0.002%) reported. Rash, urticaria, and photosensitivity reactions have also been reported.

Changes in Bone Density: Decreased bone density has been reported in the medical literature in men who have had orchiectomy or who have been treated with an LH-RH agonist analog. In a clinical trial, 25 men with prostate cancer, 12 of whom had been treated previously with leuprolide acetate for at least six months, underwent bone density studies as a result of pain. The leuprolide-treated group had lower bone density scores than the nontreated control group. It can be anticipated that long periods of medical castration in men will have effects on bone density.

Pituitary apoplexy: During post-marketing surveillance, rare cases of pituitary apoplexy (a clinical syndrome secondary to infarction of the pituitary gland) have been reported after the administration of gonadotropin-releasing hormone agonists. In a majority of these cases, a pituitary adenoma was diagnosed, with a majority of pituitary apoplexy cases occurring within 2 weeks of the first dose, and some within the first hour. In these cases, pituitary apoplexy has presented as sudden headache, vomiting, visual changes, ophthalmoplegia, altered mental status, and sometimes cardiovascular collapse. Immediate medical attention has been required.

Localized reactions including induration and abscess have been reported at the site of injection.

Symptoms consistent with fibromyalgia (eg, joint and muscle pain, headaches, sleep disorders, gastrointestinal distress, and shortness of breath) have been reported individually and collectively.

Cardiovascular System – Hypotension, Myocardial infarction, Pulmonary embolism;

Respiratory, thoracic and mediastinal disorder – Interstitial lung disease;

Hepato-biliary disorder: Serious drug-induced liver injury

Hemic and Lymphatic System – Decreased WBC;

Central/Peripheral Nervous System – Convulsion, Peripheral neuropathy, Spinal fracture/paralysis;

Endocrine System – Diabetes;

Musculoskeletal System – Tenosynovitis-like symptoms;

Urogenital System – Prostate pain.

See other LUPRON DEPOT and LUPRON Injection package inserts for other events reported in women and pediatric populations.

OVERDOSAGE

There is no experience of overdosage in clinical trials. In rats, a single subcutaneous dose of 100 mg/kg (approximately 4,000 times the estimated daily human dose based on body surface area), resulted in dyspnea, decreased activity, and excessive scratching. In early clinical trials with daily subcutaneous leuprolide acetate, doses as high as 20 mg/day for up to two years caused no adverse effects differing from those observed with the 1 mg/day dose.

DOSAGE AND ADMINISTRATION

LUPRON DEPOT must be administered under the supervision of a physician.

The recommended dose of LUPRON DEPOT is 7.5 mg for 1-month administration, incorporated in a depot formulation. Due to different release characteristics, a fractional dose, or a combination of doses of this depot formulation is not equivalent to the same dose of the monthly formulation and should not be given.

Incorporated in a depot formulation, the lyophilized microspheres are to be reconstituted and administered every 4 weeks as a single intramuscular injection.

For optimal performance of the prefilled dual chamber syringe (PDS), read and follow the following instructions:

- The lyophilized microspheres are to be reconstituted and administered as a single intramuscular injection.
- Since LUPRON DEPOT does not contain a preservative, the suspension should be injected immediately or discarded if not used within two hours.
- As with other drugs administered by injection, the injection site should be varied periodically.

1. The LUPRON DEPOT powder should be visually inspected and the syringe should NOT BE USED if clumping or caking is evident. A thin layer of powder on the wall of the syringe is considered normal prior to mixing with the diluent. The diluent should appear clear.
2. To prepare for injection, screw the white plunger into the end stopper until the stopper begins to turn. [See first figure at top of next column]
3. Hold the syringe UPRIGHT. Release the diluent by SLOWLY PUSHING (6 to 8 seconds) the plunger until the first stopper is at the blue line in the middle of the barrel. [See second figure at top of next column]
4. Keep the syringe UPRIGHT. Gently mix the microspheres (powder) thoroughly to form a uniform

← blue line

suspension. The suspension will appear milky. If the powder adheres to the stopper or caking/clumping is present, tap the syringe with your finger to disperse. DO NOT USE if any of the powder has not gone into suspension.

5. Hold the syringe UPRIGHT. With the opposite hand pull the needle cap upward without twisting.
6. Keep the syringe UPRIGHT. Advance the plunger to expel the air from the syringe.
7. After cleaning the injection site with an alcohol swab, insert the needle completely at a 90 degree angle.

NOTE: Aspirated blood would be visible just below the luer lock connection if a blood vessel is accidentally penetrated. If present, blood can be seen through the transparent LuproLoc® safety device. If blood is present remove the needle immediately. Do not inject the medication.

8. Inject the entire contents of the syringe intramuscularly at the time of reconstitution. The suspension settles very quickly following reconstitution; therefore, LUPRON DEPOT should be mixed and used immediately.
AFTER INJECTION
9. Withdraw the needle. Immediately activate the LuproLoc® safety device by pushing the arrow forward with the thumb or finger, as illustrated, until the device is fully extended and a CLICK is heard or felt.

CLICK

HOW SUPPLIED

Each LUPRON DEPOT 7.5 mg for 1-month administration kit (NDC 0074-3642-03) contains:
- one prefilled dual-chamber syringe containing needle with LuproLoc® safety device
- one plunger
- two alcohol swabs
- a complete prescribing information enclosure

The prefilled dual-chamber syringe contains sterile lyophilized microspheres of leuprolide acetate incorporated in a biodegradable lactic acid/glycolic acid copolymer. When mixed with 1 mL of accompanying diluent, LUPRON DEPOT 7.5 mg for 1-month administration is administered as a single monthly intramuscular injection.

Store at 25°C (77°F); excursions permitted to 15–30°C (59–86°F) [See USP Controlled Room Temperature]

REFERENCES

1. NIOSH Alert: Preventing occupational exposures to antineoplastic and other hazardous drugs in healthcare settings. 2004. U.S. Department of Health and Human Services, Public Health Service, Centers for Disease Control and Prevention, National Institute for Occupational Safety and Health, DHHS (NIOSH) Publication No. 2004-165.
2. OSHA Technical Manual, TED 1-0.15A, Section VI: Chapter 2. Controlling Occupational Exposure to Hazardous Drugs. OSHA, 1999. http://www.osha.gov/dts/osta/otm/otm_vi/otm_vi_2.html
3. American Society of Health-System Pharmacists. ASHP guidelines on handling hazardous drugs. Am J Health-Syst Pharm. 2006; 63; 1172-1193.
4. Polovich, M., White, J.M., & Kelleher, L.O. (eds.) 2005. Chemotherapy and biotherapy guidelines and recommendations for practice (2nd Ed.) Pittsburgh, PA: Oncology Nursing Society.

Manufactured for
AbbVie Inc.
North Chicago, IL 60064
by Takeda Pharmaceutical Company Limited
Osaka, Japan 540-8645
™ - Trademark
® - Registered Trademark
(No. 3642)
03-A852 July, 2013
©2013 AbbVie Inc.
Shown in Product Identification Guide, page 304

LUPRON DEPOT® -3 MONTH 11.25 MG   ℞
[lew-prŏn]
(leuprolide acetate for depot suspension)
3-MONTH FORMULATION

Rx only
This is combined labeling. Examples of different fonts and colors appear below.
- General information
- Information on endometriosis
- Information on uterine fibroids

DESCRIPTION

Leuprolide acetate is a synthetic nonapeptide analog of naturally occurring gonadotropin-releasing hormone (GnRH or LH-RH). The analog possesses greater potency than the natural hormone. The chemical name is 5-oxo-L-prolyl-L-histidyl-L-tryptophyl-L-seryl-L-tyrosyl-D-leucyl-L-leucyl-L-arginyl-N-ethyl-L-prolinamide acetate (salt) with the following structural formula:
[See chemical structure at top of next page]
LUPRON DEPOT–3 Month 11.25 mg is available in a prefilled dual-chamber syringe containing sterile lyophilized microspheres which, when mixed with diluent, become a suspension intended as an intramuscular injection to be given **ONCE EVERY THREE MONTHS**.
The front chamber of LUPRON DEPOT–3 Month 11.25 mg prefilled dual-chamber syringe contains leuprolide acetate

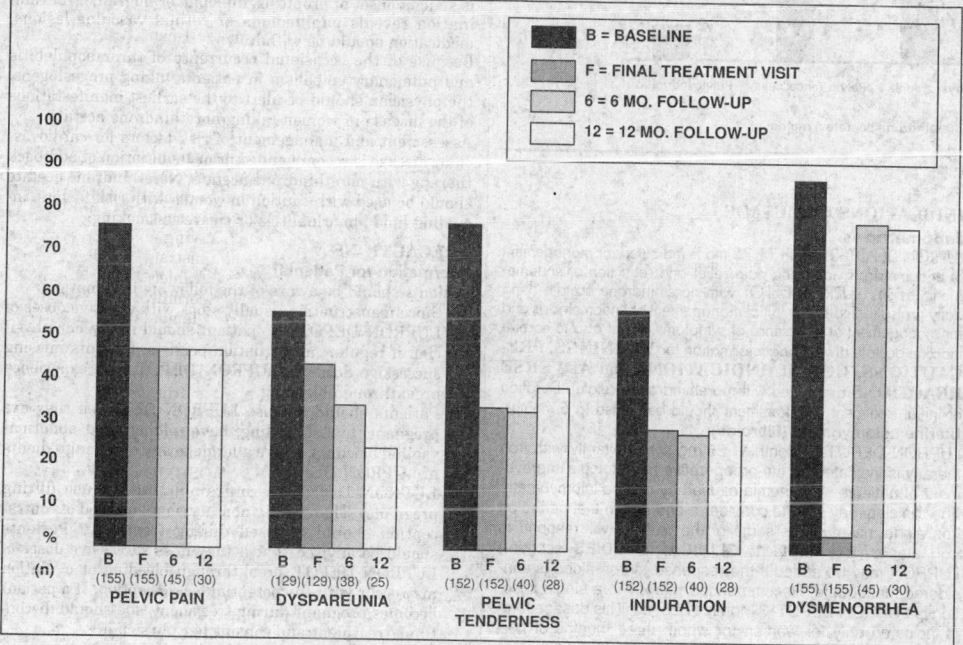

FIGURE 1 – PERCENT OF PATIENTS WITH SIGN/SYMPTOMS OF ENDOMETRIOSIS AT BASELINE, FINAL TREATMENT VISIT, AND AFTER 6 AND 12 MONTHS OF FOLLOW-UP

B = BASELINE
F = FINAL TREATMENT VISIT
6 = 6 MO. FOLLOW-UP
12 = 12 MO. FOLLOW-UP

(Chart categories: PELVIC PAIN, DYSPAREUNIA, PELVIC TENDERNESS, INDURATION, DYSMENORRHEA)

PELVIC PAIN: B (155) F (155) 6 (45) 12 (30)
DYSPAREUNIA: B (129) F (129) 6 (38) 12 (25)
PELVIC TENDERNESS: B (152) F (152) 6 (40) 12 (28)
INDURATION: B (152) F (152) 6 (40) 12 (28)
DYSMENORRHEA: B (155) F (155) 6 (45) 12 (30)

was observed for individual subjects between day 4 and week 4 after dosing. By the third week following the injection, the mean estradiol concentration (8 pg/mL) was in the menopausal range. Throughout the remainder of the dosing period, mean serum estradiol levels ranged from the menopausal to the early follicular range.

Serum estradiol was suppressed to ≤20 pg/mL in all subjects within four weeks and remained suppressed (≤40 pg/mL) in 80% of subjects until the end of the 12-week dosing interval, at which time two of these subjects had a value between 40 and 50 pg/mL. Four additional subjects had at least two consecutive elevations of estradiol (range 43-240 pg/mL) levels during the 12-week dosing interval, but there was no indication of luteal function for any of the subjects during this period.

LUPRON DEPOT–3 Month 11.25 mg induced amenorrhea in 85% (N=17) of subjects during the initial month and 100% during the second month following the injection. All subjects remained amenorrheic through the remainder of the 12-week dosing interval. Episodes of light bleeding and spotting were reported by a majority of subjects during the first month after the injection and in a few subjects at later time-points. Menses resumed on average 12 weeks (range 2.9 to 20.4 weeks) following the end of the 12-week dosing interval.

LUPRON DEPOT–3 Month 11.25 mg produced similar pharmacodynamic effects in terms of hormonal and menstrual suppression to those achieved with monthly injections of LUPRON DEPOT 3.75 mg during the controlled clinical trials for the management of endometriosis and the anemia caused by uterine fibroids.

Endometriosis

In a Phase IV pharmacokinetic/pharmacodynamic study of patients, LUPRON DEPOT–3 Month 11.25 mg (N=21) was shown to be comparable to monthly LUPRON DEPOT 3.75 mg (N=20) in relieving the clinical signs/symptoms of endometriosis (dysmenorrhea, non-menstrual pelvic pain, pelvic tenderness and pelvic induration). In both treatment groups, suppression of menses was achieved in 100% of the patients who remained in the study for at least 60 days. Suppression is defined as no new menses for at least 60 consecutive days.

In controlled clinical studies, LUPRON DEPOT 3.75 mg monthly for six months was shown to be comparable to danazol 800 mg/day in relieving the clinical sign/symptoms of endometriosis (pelvic pain, dysmenorrhea, dyspareunia, pelvic tenderness, and induration) and in reducing the size of endometrial implants as evidenced by laparoscopy.

The clinical significance of a decrease in endometriotic lesions is not known at this time, and in addition laparoscopic staging of endometriosis does not necessarily correlate with the severity of symptoms.

LUPRON DEPOT 3.75 mg monthly induced amenorrhea in 74% and 98% of the patients after the first and second treatment months respectively. Most of the remaining patients reported episodes of only light bleeding or spotting. In the first, second and third post-treatment months, normal menstrual cycles resumed in 7%, 71% and 95% of patients, respectively, excluding those who became pregnant.

Figure 1 illustrates the percent of patients with symptoms at baseline, final treatment visit and sustained relief at 6 and 12 months following discontinuation of treatment for the various symptoms evaluated during the two controlled clinical studies. A total of 166 patients received LUPRON DEPOT 3.75 mg. Seventy-five percent (N=125) of these patients elected to participate in the follow-up period. Of these patients, 36% and 24% are included in the 6 month and 12 month follow-up analysis, respectively. All the patients who had a pain evaluation at baseline and at a minimum of one treatment visit, are included in the Baseline (B) and final treatment visit (F) analysis.

[See figure 1 above]

Hormonal add-back therapy

Two clinical studies with a treatment duration of 12 months indicate that concurrent hormonal therapy (norethindrone acetate 5 mg daily) is effective in significantly reducing the loss of bone mineral density associated with LUPRON, without compromising the efficacy of LUPRON in relieving symptoms of endometriosis. (All patients in these studies received calcium supplementation with 1000 mg elemental calcium). One controlled, randomized and double-blind study included 51 women treated with LUPRON DEPOT 3.75 mg alone and 55 women treated with LUPRON DEPOT 3.75 mg plus norethindrone acetate 5 mg (LD/N) daily. The second study was an open label study in which 136 women were treated with monthly LUPRON DEPOT 3.75 mg plus norethindrone acetate 5 mg daily. This study confirmed the reduction in loss of bone mineral density that was observed in the controlled study. Suppression of menses was maintained throughout treat-

(11.25 mg), polylactic acid (99.3 mg) and D-mannitol (19.45 mg). The second chamber of diluent contains carboxymethylcellulose sodium (7.5 mg), D-mannitol (75.0 mg), polysorbate 80 (1.5 mg), water for injection, USP, and glacial acetic acid, USP to control pH.

During the manufacture of LUPRON DEPOT–3 Month 11.25 mg, acetic acid is lost, leaving the peptide.

CLINICAL PHARMACOLOGY

Leuprolide acetate is a long-acting GnRH analog. A single injection of LUPRON DEPOT–3 Month 11.25 mg will result in an initial stimulation followed by a prolonged suppression of pituitary gonadotropins. Repeated dosing at quarterly (LUPRON DEPOT–3 Month 11.25 mg) intervals results in decreased secretion of gonadal steroids; consequently, tissues and functions that depend on gonadal steroids for their maintenance become quiescent. This effect is reversible on discontinuation of drug therapy.

Leuprolide acetate is not active when given orally.

Pharmacokinetics

Absorption

Following a single injection of the three month formulation of LUPRON DEPOT–3 Month 11.25 mg in female subjects, a mean plasma leuprolide concentration of 36.3 ng/mL was observed at 4 hours. Leuprolide appeared to be released at a constant rate following the onset of steady-state levels during the third week after dosing and mean levels then declined gradually to near the lower limit of detection by 12 weeks. The mean (± standard deviation) leuprolide concentration from 3 to 12 weeks was 0.23 ± 0.09 ng/mL. However, intact leuprolide and an inactive major metabolite could not be distinguished by the assay which was employed in the study. The initial burst, followed by the rapid decline to a steady-state level, was similar to the release pattern seen with the monthly formulation.

Distribution

The mean steady-state volume of distribution of leuprolide following intravenous bolus administration to healthy male volunteers was 27 L. In vitro binding to human plasma proteins ranged from 43% to 49%.

Metabolism

In healthy male volunteers, a 1 mg bolus of leuprolide administered intravenously revealed that the mean systemic clearance was 7.6 L/h, with a terminal elimination half-life of approximately 3 hours based on a two compartment model.

In rats and dogs, administration of ^{14}C-labeled leuprolide was shown to be metabolized to smaller inactive peptides, a pentapeptide (Metabolite I), tripeptides (Metabolites II and III) and a dipeptide (Metabolite IV). These fragments may be further catabolized.

In a pharmacokinetic/pharmacodynamic study of endometriosis patients, intramuscular 11.25 mg LUPRON DEPOT (n=19) every 12 weeks or intramuscular 3.75 mg LUPRON DEPOT (n=15) every 4 weeks was administered for 24 weeks. There was no statistically significant difference in changes of serum estradiol concentration from baseline between the 2 treatment groups.

M-I plasma concentrations measured in 5 prostate cancer patients reached maximum concentration 2 to 6 hours after dosing and were approximately 6% of the peak parent drug concentration. One week after dosing, mean plasma M-I concentrations were approximately 20% of mean leuprolide concentrations.

Excretion

Following administration of LUPRON DEPOT 3.75 mg to 3 patients, less than 5% of the dose was recovered as parent and M-I metabolite in the urine.

Special Populations

The pharmacokinetics of the drug in hepatically and renally impaired patients have not been determined.

Drug Interactions

No pharmacokinetic-based drug-drug interaction studies have been conducted with LUPRON DEPOT. However, because leuprolide acetate is a peptide that is primarily degraded by peptidase and not by cytochrome P-450 enzymes as noted in specific studies, and the drug is only about 46% bound to plasma proteins, drug interactions would not be expected to occur.

CLINICAL STUDIES

In a pharmacokinetic/pharmacodynamic study of healthy female subjects (N=20), the onset of estradiol suppression

Information on the AbbVie, Inc. products listed on these pages is from the prescribing information in use as of July 31, 2014. For more information, please visit rxabbvie.com or call 1-800-633-9110.

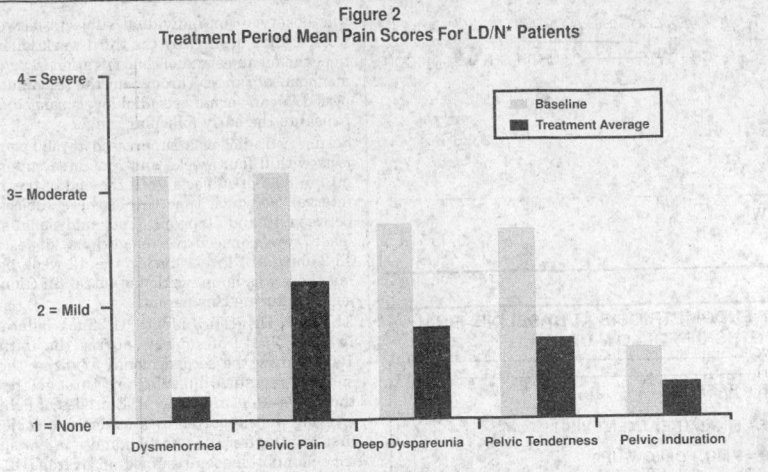

Figure 2
Treatment Period Mean Pain Scores For LD/N* Patients

* LD/N = LUPRON DEPOT 3.75 mg plus norethindrone acetate 5 mg daily

ment in 84% and 73% of patients receiving LD/N, in the controlled study and open label study, respectively. The median time for menses resumption after treatment with LD/N was 8 weeks.
Figure 2 illustrates the mean pain scores for the LD/N group from the controlled study.
[See figure 2 above]

Uterine Leiomyomata (Fibroids)
LUPRON DEPOT 3.75 mg for a period of three to six months was studied in four controlled clinical trials.
In one of these clinical studies, enrollment was based on hematocrit ≤ 30% and/or hemoglobin ≤ 10.2 g/dL. Administration of LUPRON DEPOT 3.75 mg, concomitantly with iron, produced an increase of ≥ 6% hematocrit and ≥ 2 g/dL hemoglobin in 77% of patients at three months of therapy. The mean change in hematocrit was 10.1% and the mean change in hemoglobin was 4.2 g/dL. Clinical response was judged to be a hematocrit of ≥ 36% and hemoglobin of ≥ 12 g/dL, thus allowing for autologous blood donation prior to surgery. At two and three months respectively, 71% and 75% of patients met this criterion (Table 1). These data suggest however, that some patients may benefit from iron alone or 1 to 2 months of LUPRON DEPOT 3.75 mg.

Table 1 PERCENT OF PATIENTS ACHIEVING HEMATOCRIT ≥ 36% AND HEMOGLOBIN ≥ 12 GM/DL

Treatment Group	Week 4	Week 8	Week 12
LUPRON DEPOT 3.75 mg with Iron (N=104)	40*	71†	75*
Iron Alone (N=98)	17	39	49

* P-Value < 0.01
† P-Value < 0.001

Excessive vaginal bleeding (menorrhagia or menometrorrhagia) decreased in 80% of patients at three months. Episodes of spotting and menstrual-like bleeding were noted in 16% of patients at final visit.
In this same study, a decrease of ≥ 25% was seen in uterine and myoma volumes in 60% and 54% of patients respectively. The mean fibroid diameter was 6.3 cm at pretreatment and decreased to 5.6 cm at the end of treatment. LUPRON DEPOT 3.75 mg was found to relieve symptoms of bloating, pelvic pain, and pressure.
In three other controlled clinical trials, enrollment was not based on hematologic status. Mean uterine volume decreased by 41% and myoma volume decreased by 37% at final visit as evidenced by ultrasound or MRI. The mean fibroid diameter was 5.6 cm at pretreatment and decreased to 4.7 cm at the end of treatment. These patients also experienced a decrease in symptoms including excessive vaginal bleeding and pelvic discomfort. Ninety-five percent of these patients became amenorrheic with 61%, 25%, and 4% experiencing amenorrhea during the first, second, and third treatment months respectively.
In addition, posttreatment follow-up was carried out in one clinical trial for a small percentage of LUPRON DEPOT 3.75 mg patients (N=46) among the 77% who demonstrated a ≥ 25% decrease in uterine volume while on therapy. Menses usually returned within two months of cessation of therapy. Mean time to return to pretreatment uterine size was 8.3 months. Regrowth did not appear to be related to pretreatment uterine volume.
There is no evidence that pregnancy rates are enhanced or adversely affected by the use of LUPRON DEPOT.

INDICATIONS AND USAGE

Endometriosis
LUPRON DEPOT–3 Month 11.25 mg is indicated for management of endometriosis, including pain relief and reduction of endometriotic lesions. LUPRON DEPOT with norethindrone acetate 5 mg daily is also indicated for initial management of endometriosis and for management of recurrence of symptoms. (Refer also to norethindrone acetate prescribing information for **WARNINGS, PRECAUTIONS, CONTRAINDICATIONS** and **ADVERSE REACTIONS** associated with norethindrone acetate). Duration of initial treatment or retreatment should be limited to 6 months.

Uterine Leiomyomata (Fibroids)
LUPRON DEPOT–3 Month 11.25 mg concomitantly with iron therapy is indicated for the preoperative hematologic improvement of patients with anemia caused by uterine leiomyomata. The clinician may wish to consider a one-month trial period on iron alone inasmuch as some of the patients will respond to iron alone. (See **Table 1, CLINICAL STUDIES** section.) LUPRON may be added if the response to iron alone is considered inadequate. Recommended therapy is a single injection of LUPRON DEPOT–3 Month 11.25 mg. This dosage form is indicated only for women for whom three months of hormonal suppression is deemed necessary.
Experience with LUPRON DEPOT–3 Month 11.25 mg in females has been limited to women 18 years of age and older treated for no more than 6 months.

CONTRAINDICATIONS

1. Hypersensitivity to GnRH, GnRH agonist analogs or any of the excipients in LUPRON DEPOT.
2. Undiagnosed abnormal vaginal bleeding.
3. LUPRON DEPOT is contraindicated in women who are or may become pregnant while receiving the drug. LUPRON DEPOT may cause fetal harm when administered to a pregnant woman. Major fetal abnormalities were observed in rabbits but not in rats after administration of LUPRON DEPOT throughout gestation. There was increased fetal mortality and decreased fetal weights in rats and rabbits. (See **Pregnancy** section.) The effects on fetal mortality are expected consequences of the alterations in hormonal levels brought about by the drug. If this drug is used during pregnancy or if the patient becomes pregnant while taking this drug, the patient should be apprised of the potential hazard to the fetus.
4. Use in women who are breast-feeding. (See **Nursing Mothers** section.)
5. Norethindrone acetate is contraindicated in women with the following conditions:
   ◦ Thrombophlebitis, thromboembolic disorders, cerebral apoplexy, or a past history of these conditions
   ◦ Markedly impaired liver function or liver disease
   ◦ Known or suspected carcinoma of the breast

WARNINGS

1. As the effects of LUPRON DEPOT–3 Month 11.25 mg are present throughout the course of therapy, the drug should only be used in patients who require hormonal suppression for at least three months.
2. Experience with LUPRON DEPOT–3 Month 11.25 mg in females has been limited to six months; therefore, exposure should be limited to six months of therapy.
3. Safe use of leuprolide acetate or norethindrone acetate in pregnancy has not been established clinically. Before starting treatment with LUPRON DEPOT pregnancy must be excluded.
4. When used at the recommended dose and dosing interval, LUPRON DEPOT usually inhibits ovulation and stops

menstruation. Contraception is not insured, however, by taking LUPRON DEPOT. Therefore, patients should use non-hormonal methods of contraception. Patients should be advised to see their physician if they believe they may be pregnant. If a patient becomes pregnant during treatment, the drug must be discontinued and the patient must be apprised of the potential risk to the fetus. (See **CONTRAINDICATIONS** section.)
5. During the early phase of therapy, sex steroids temporarily rise above baseline because of the physiologic effect of the drug. Therefore, an increase in clinical signs and symptoms may be observed during the initial days of therapy, but these will dissipate with continued therapy.
6. Symptoms consistent with an anaphylactoid or asthmatic process have been rarely reported post-marketing.
7. The following applies to co-treatment with LUPRON and norethindrone acetate:
Norethindrone acetate treatment should be discontinued if there is a sudden partial or complete loss of vision or if there is sudden onset of proptosis, diplopia, or migraine. If examination reveals papilledema or retinal vascular lesions, medication should be withdrawn.
Because of the occasional occurrence of thrombophlebitis and pulmonary embolism in patients taking progestogens, the physician should be alert to the earliest manifestations of the disease in women taking norethindrone acetate. Assessment and management of risk factors for cardiovascular disease is recommended prior to initiation of add-back therapy with norethindrone acetate. Norethindrone acetate should be used with caution in women with risk factors, including lipid abnormalities or cigarette smoking.

PRECAUTIONS

Information for Patients
Patients should be aware of the following information:
1. Since menstruation usually stops with effective doses of LUPRON DEPOT, the patient should notify her physician if regular menstruation persists. Patients missing successive doses of LUPRON DEPOT may experience breakthrough bleeding.
2. Patients should not use LUPRON DEPOT if they are pregnant, breast feeding, have undiagnosed abnormal vaginal bleeding, or are allergic to any of the ingredients in LUPRON DEPOT.
3. LUPRON DEPOT is contraindicated for use during pregnancy. Therefore, a non-hormonal method of contraception should be used during treatment. Patients should be advised that if they miss successive doses of LUPRON DEPOT, breakthrough bleeding or ovulation may occur with the potential for conception. If a patient becomes pregnant during treatment, she should discontinue treatment and consult her physician.
4. Adverse events occurring in clinical studies with LUPRON DEPOT that are associated with hypoestrogenism include: hot flashes, headaches, emotional lability, decreased libido, acne, myalgia, reduction in breast size, and vaginal dryness. Estrogen levels returned to normal after treatment was discontinued.
5. Patients should be counseled on the possibility of the development or worsening of depression and the occurrence of memory disorders.
6. The induced hypoestrogenic state **also** results in a loss in bone density over the course of treatment, some of which may not be reversible. Clinical studies show that concurrent hormonal therapy with norethindrone acetate 5 mg daily is effective in reducing loss of bone mineral density that occurs with LUPRON. (All patients received calcium supplementation with 1000 mg elemental calcium.) (See **Changes in Bone Density** section).
7. If the symptoms of endometriosis recur after a course of therapy, retreatment with a six-month course of LUPRON DEPOT and norethindrone acetate 5 mg daily may be considered. Retreatment beyond this one six-month course cannot be recommended. It is recommended that bone density be assessed before retreatment begins to ensure that values are within normal limits. Retreatment with LUPRON DEPOT alone is not recommended.
8. In patients with major risk factors for decreased bone mineral content such as chronic alcohol and/or tobacco use, strong family history of osteoporosis, or chronic use of drugs that can reduce bone mass such as anticonvulsants or corticosteroids, LUPRON DEPOT therapy may pose an additional risk. In these patients, the risks and benefits must be weighed carefully before therapy with LUPRON DEPOT alone is instituted, and concomitant treatment with norethindrone acetate 5 mg daily should be considered. Retreatment with gonadotropin-releasing hormone analogs, including LUPRON is not advisable in patients with major risk factors for loss of bone mineral content.
9. Because norethindrone acetate may cause some degree of fluid retention, conditions which might be influenced by this factor, such as epilepsy, migraine, asthma, cardiac or renal dysfunctions require careful observation during norethindrone acetate add-back therapy.

10. Patients who have a history of depression should be carefully observed during treatment with norethindrone acetate and norethindrone acetate should be discontinued if severe depression occurs.

Convulsions

There have been postmarketing reports of convulsions in patients on leuprolide acetate therapy. These included patients with and without concurrent medications and comorbid conditions.

Laboratory Tests

See **ADVERSE REACTIONS** section.

Drug Interactions

See **CLINICAL PHARMACOLOGY, Pharmacokinetics.**

Drug/Laboratory Test Interactions

Administration of LUPRON DEPOT in therapeutic doses results in suppression of the pituitary-gonadal system. Normal function is usually restored within three months after treatment is discontinued. Therefore, diagnostic tests of pituitary gonadotropic and gonadal functions conducted during treatment and for up to three months after discontinuation of LUPRON DEPOT may be misleading.

Carcinogenesis, Mutagenesis, Impairment of Fertility

A two-year carcinogenicity study was conducted in rats and mice. In rats, a dose-related increase of benign pituitary hyperplasia and benign pituitary adenomas was noted at 24 months when the drug was administered subcutaneously at high daily doses (0.6 to 4 mg/kg). There was a significant but not dose-related increase of pancreatic islet-cell adenomas in females and of testicular interstitial cell adenomas in males (highest incidence in the low dose group). In mice, no leuprolide acetate-induced tumors or pituitary abnormalities were observed at a dose as high as 60 mg/kg for two years. Patients have been treated with leuprolide acetate for up to three years with doses as high as 10 mg/day and for two years with doses as high as 20 mg/day without demonstrable pituitary abnormalities.

Mutagenicity studies have been performed with leuprolide acetate using bacterial and mammalian systems. These studies provided no evidence of a mutagenic potential.

Clinical and pharmacologic studies in adults (> 18 years) with leuprolide acetate and similar analogs have shown reversibility of fertility suppression when the drug is discontinued after continuous administration for periods of up to 24 weeks. Although no clinical studies have been completed in children to assess the full reversibility of fertility suppression, animal studies (prepubertal and adult rats and monkeys) with leuprolide acetate and other GnRH analogs have shown functional recovery.

Pregnancy

Teratogenic Effects

Pregnancy Category X (See **CONTRAINDICATIONS** section). When administered on day 6 of pregnancy at test dosages of 0.00024, 0.0024, and 0.024 mg/kg (1/300 to 1/3 of the human dose) to rabbits, LUPRON DEPOT produced a dose-related increase in major fetal abnormalities. Similar studies in rats failed to demonstrate an increase in fetal malformations. There was increased fetal mortality and decreased fetal weights with the two higher doses of LUPRON DEPOT in rabbits and with the highest dose (0.024 mg/kg) in rats.

Nursing Mothers

It is not known whether LUPRON DEPOT is excreted in human milk. Because many drugs are excreted in human milk, and because the effects of LUPRON DEPOT on lactation and/or the breast-fed child have not been determined, LUPRON DEPOT should not be used by nursing mothers.

Pediatric Use

Safety and effectiveness of LUPRON DEPOT–3 Month 11.25 mg have not been established in pediatric patients. Experience with LUPRON DEPOT for treatment of endometriosis has been limited to women 18 years of age and older. See LUPRON DEPOT-PED® (leuprolide acetate for depot suspension) labeling for the safety and effectiveness in children with central precocious puberty.

Geriatric Use

This product has not been studied in women over 65 years of age and is not indicated in this population.

ADVERSE REACTIONS

Clinical Trials

The **monthly formulation of LUPRON DEPOT 3.75 mg** was utilized in controlled clinical trials that studied the drug in 166 endometriosis and 166 uterine fibroids patients. Adverse events reported in ≥ 5% of patients in either of these populations and thought to be potentially related to drug are noted in the following table.

[See table 2 above]

In one controlled clinical trial utilizing the monthly formulation of LUPRON DEPOT, patients diagnosed with uterine fibroids received a higher dose (7.5 mg) of LUPRON DEPOT. Events seen with this dose that were thought to be potentially related to drug and were not seen at the lower dose included glossitis, hypesthesia, lactation, pyelonephritis, and urinary disorders. Generally, a higher incidence of hypoestrogenic effects was observed at the higher dose.

Table 2 ADVERSE EVENTS REPORTED TO BE CAUSALLY RELATED TO DRUG IN ≥ 5% OF PATIENTS

	Endometriosis (2 Studies)						Uterine Fibroids (4 Studies)			
	LUPRON DEPOT 3.75 mg N=166		Danazol N=136		Placebo N=31		LUPRON DEPOT 3.75 mg N=166		Placebo N=163	
	N	(%)	N	(%)	N	(%)	N	(%)	N	(%)
Body as a Whole										
Asthenia	5	(3)	9	(7)	0	(0)	14	(8.4)	8	(4.9)
General pain	31	(19)	22	(16)	1	(3)	14	(8.4)	10	(6.1)
Headache*	53	(32)	30	(22)	2	(6)	43	(25.9)	29	(17.8)
Cardiovascular System										
Hot flashes/sweats*	139	(84)	77	(57)	9	(29)	121	(72.9)	29	(17.8)
Gastrointestinal System										
Nausea/vomiting	21	(13)	17	(13)	1	(3)	8	(4.8)	6	(3.7)
GI disturbances*	11	(7)	8	(6)	1	(3)	5	(3.0)	2	(1.2)
Metabolic and Nutritional Disorders										
Edema	12	(7)	17	(13)	1	(3)	9	(5.4)	2	(1.2)
Weight gain/loss	22	(13)	36	(26)	0	(0)	5	(3.0)	2	(1.2)
Endocrine System										
Acne	17	(10)	27	(20)	0	(0)	0	(0)	0	(0)
Hirsutism	2	(1)	9	(7)	1	(3)	1	(0.6)	0	(0)
Musculoskeletal System										
Joint disorder*	14	(8)	11	(8)	0	(0)	13	(7.8)	5	(3.1)
Myalgia*	1	(1)	7	(5)	0	(0)	1	(0.6)	0	(0)
Nervous System										
Decreased libido*	19	(11)	6	(4)	0	(0)	3	(1.8)	0	(0)
Depression/emotional lability*	36	(22)	27	(20)	1	(3)	18	(10.8)	7	(4.3)
Dizziness	19	(11)	4	(3)	0	(0)	3	(1.8)	6	(3.7)
Nervousness*	8	(5)	11	(8)	0	(0)	8	(4.8)	1	(0.6)
Neuromuscular disorders*	11	(7)	17	(13)	0	(0)	3	(1.8)	0	(0)
Paresthesias	12	(7)	11	(8)	0	(0)	2	(1.2)	1	(0.6)
Skin and Appendages										
Skin reactions	17	(10)	20	(15)	1	(3)	5	(3.0)	2	(1.2)
Urogenital System										
Breast changes/tenderness/pain*	10	(6)	12	(9)	0	(0)	3	(1.8)	7	(4.3)
Vaginitis*	46	(28)	23	(17)	0	(0)	19	(11.4)	3	(1.8)

In these same studies, symptoms reported in < 5% of patients included: *Body as a Whole* - Body odor, Flu syndrome, Injection site reactions; *Cardiovascular System* - Palpitations, Syncope, Tachycardia; *Digestive System* - Appetite changes, Dry mouth, Thirst; *Endocrine System* - Androgen-like effects; *Hemic and Lymphatic System* - Ecchymosis, Lymphadenopathy; *Nervous System* - Anxiety*, Insomnia/Sleep disorders*, Delusions, Memory disorder, Personality disorder; *Respiratory System* - Rhinitis; *Skin and Appendages* - Alopecia, Hair disorder, Nail disorder; *Special Senses* - Conjunctivitis, Ophthalmologic disorders*, Taste perversion; *Urogenital System* - Dysuria*, Lactation, Menstrual disorders.

* = Possible effect of decreased estrogen.

In a pharmacokinetic trial involving 20 healthy female subjects receiving LUPRON DEPOT–3 Month 11.25 mg, a few adverse events were reported with this formulation that were not reported previously. These included face edema, agitation, laryngitis, and ear pain.

In a Phase IV study involving endometriosis patients receiving LUPRON DEPOT 3.75 mg (N=20) or LUPRON DEPOT–3 Month 11.25 mg (N=21), similar adverse events were reported by the two groups of patients. In general the safety profiles of the two formulations were comparable in this study.

Table 3 lists the potentially drug-related adverse events observed in at least 5% of patients in any treatment group, during the first 6 months of treatment in the add-back clinical studies, in which patients were treated with monthly LUPRON DEPOT 3.75 mg with or without norethindrone acetate co-treatment.

[See table 3 at top of next page]

In the controlled clinical trial, 50 of 51 (98%) patients in the LD group (LUPRON DEPOT 3.75 mg) and 48 of 55 (87%) patients in the LD/N group (LUPRON DEPOT 3.75 mg plus norethindrone acetate 5 mg daily) reported experiencing hot flashes on one or more occasions during treatment. During Month 6 of treatment, 32 of 37 (86%) patients in the LD group and 22 of 38 (58%) patients in the LD/N group reported having experienced hot flashes. The mean number of days on which hot flashes were reported during this month of treatment was 19 and 7 in the LD and LD/N treatment groups, respectively. The mean maximum number of hot flashes in a day during this month of treatment was 5.8 and 1.9 in the LD and LD/N treatment groups, respectively.

Changes in Bone Density

In controlled clinical studies, patients with endometriosis (six months of therapy) or uterine fibroids (three months of therapy) were treated with LUPRON DEPOT 3.75 mg. In endometriosis patients, vertebral bone density as measured by dual energy x-ray absorptiometry (DEXA) decreased by an average of 3.2% at six months compared with the pre-treatment value. Clinical studies demonstrate that concurrent hormonal therapy (norethindrone acetate 5 mg daily) and calcium supplementation is effective in significantly reducing the loss of bone mineral density that occurs with LUPRON treatment, without compromising the efficacy of LUPRON in relieving symptoms of endometriosis. LUPRON DEPOT 3.75 mg plus norethindrone acetate 5 mg daily was evaluated in two clinical trials. The results from this regimen were similar in both studies. LUPRON DEPOT 3.75 mg was used as a control group in one study. The bone mineral density data of the lumbar spine from these two studies are presented in Table 4.

[See table 4 at top of next page]

In the Phase IV, six-month pharmacokinetic/pharmacodynamic study in endometriosis patients who were treated with LUPRON DEPOT 3.75 mg or LUPRON DEPOT–3 Month 11.25 mg (N=21), vertebral bone density measured by DEXA decreased compared with baseline by an average of 3.0% and 2.8% at six months for the two groups, respectively.

When LUPRON DEPOT 3.75 mg was administered for three months in uterine fibroid patients, vertebral trabecular bone mineral density as assessed by quantitative digital radiography (QDR) revealed a mean decrease of 2.7% compared with baseline. Six months after discontinuation of therapy, a trend toward recovery was observed. Use of LUPRON DEPOT for longer than three months (uterine fibroids) or six months (endometriosis) or in the presence of other known risk factors for decreased bone mineral content may cause additional bone loss **and is not recommended.**

Changes in Laboratory Values During Treatment

Liver Enzymes

Three percent of uterine fibroid patients treated with LUPRON DEPOT 3.75 mg, manifested posttreatment transaminase values that were at least twice the baseline value and above the upper limit of the normal range. None of the laboratory increases were associated with clinical symptoms.

In two other clinical trials, 6 of 191 patients receiving LUPRON DEPOT 3.75 mg plus norethindrone acetate 5 mg daily for up to 12 months developed an elevated (at least twice the upper limit of normal) SGPT or GGT. Five of the 6 increases were observed beyond 6 months of treatment. None were associated with an elevated bilirubin concentration.

Information on the AbbVie, Inc. products listed on these pages is from the prescribing information in use as of July 31, 2014. For more information, please visit rxabbvie.com or call 1-800-633-9110.

Table 3 TREATMENT-RELATED ADVERSE EVENTS OCCURRING IN ≥ 5% OF PATIENTS

	Controlled Study				Open Label Study	
	LD - Only* N=51		LD/N† N=55		LD/N† N=136	
Adverse Events	N	(%)	N	(%)	N	(%)
Any Adverse Event	50	(98)	53	(96)	126	(93)
Body as a Whole						
Asthenia	9	(18)	10	(18)	15	(11)
Headache/Migraine	33	(65)	28	(51)	63	(46)
Injection Site Reaction	1	(2)	5	(9)	4	(3)
Pain	12	(24)	16	(29)	29	(21)
Cardiovascular System						
Hot flashes/Sweats	50	(98)	48	(87)	78	(57)
Digestive System						
Altered Bowel Function	7	(14)	8	(15)	14	(10)
Changes in Appetite	2	(4)	0	(0)	8	(6)
GI Disturbance	2	(4)	4	(7)	6	(4)
Nausea/Vomiting	13	(25)	16	(29)	17	(13)
Metabolic and Nutritional Disorders						
Edema	0	(0)	5	(9)	9	(7)
Weight Changes	6	(12)	7	(13)	6	(4)
Nervous System						
Anxiety	3	(6)	0	(0)	11	(8)
Depression/Emotional Lability	16	(31)	15	(27)	46	(34)
Dizziness/Vertigo	8	(16)	6	(11)	10	(7)
Insomnia/Sleep Disorder	16	(31)	7	(13)	20	(15)
Libido Changes	5	(10)	2	(4)	10	(7)
Memory Disorder	3	(6)	1	(2)	6	(4)
Nervousness	4	(8)	2	(4)	15	(11)
Neuromuscular Disorder	1	(2)	5	(9)	4	(3)
Skin and Appendages						
Alopecia	0	(0)	5	(9)	4	(3)
Androgen-Like Effects	2	(4)	3	(5)	24	(18)
Skin/Mucous Membrane Reaction	2	(4)	5	(9)	15	(11)
Urogenital System						
Breast Changes/Pain/Tenderness	3	(6)	7	(13)	11	(8)
Menstrual Disorders	1	(2)	0	(0)	7	(5)
Vaginitis	10	(20)	8	(15)	11	(8)

* LD-Only = LUPRON DEPOT 3.75 mg
† LD/N = LUPRON DEPOT 3.75 mg plus norethindrone acetate 5 mg

Table 4 MEAN PERCENT CHANGE FROM BASELINE IN BONE MINERAL DENSITY OF LUMBAR SPINE

	LUPRON DEPOT 3.75 mg		LUPRON DEPOT 3.75 mg plus norethindrone acetate 5 mg daily			
	Controlled Study		Controlled Study		Open Label Study	
	N	Change (Mean, 95% CI)#	N	Change (Mean, 95% CI)#	N	Change (Mean, 95% CI)#
Week 24*	41	-3.2% (-3.8, -2.6)	42	-0.3% (-0.8, 0.3)	115	-0.2% (-0.6, 0.2)
Week 52†	29	-6.3% (-7.1, -5.4)	32	-1.0% (-1.9, -0.1)	84	-1.1% (-1.6, -0.5)

* Includes on-treatment measurements that fell within 2-252 days after the first day of treatment.
† Includes on-treatment measurements >252 days after the first day of treatment.
\# 95% CI: 95% Confidence Interval

Table 5 SERUM LIPIDS: MEAN PERCENT CHANGES FROM BASELINE VALUES AT TREATMENT WEEK 24

	LUPRON DEPOT 3.75 mg		LUPRON DEPOT 3.75 mg plus norethindrone acetate 5 mg daily			
	Controlled Study (n=39)		Controlled Study (n=41)		Open Label Study (n=117)	
	Baseline Value*	Wk 24 % Change	Baseline Value*	Wk 24 % Change	Baseline Value*	Wk 24 % Change
Total Cholesterol	170.5	9.2%	179.3	0.2%	181.2	2.8%
HDL Cholesterol	52.4	7.4%	51.8	-18.8%	51.0	-14.6%
LDL Cholesterol	96.6	10.9%	101.5	14.1%	109.1	13.1%
LDL/HDL Ratio	2.0†	5.0%	2.1†	43.4%	2.3†	39.4%
Triglycerides	107.8	17.5%	130.2	9.5%	105.4	13.8%

* mg/dL
† ratio

Lipids
Triglycerides were increased above the upper limit of normal in 12% of the endometriosis patients who received LUPRON DEPOT 3.75 mg and in 32% of the subjects receiving LUPRON DEPOT–3 Month 11.25 mg.
Of those endometriosis and uterine fibroid patients whose pretreatment cholesterol values were in the normal range, mean change following therapy was +16 mg/dL to +17 mg/dL in endometriosis patients and +11 mg/dL to +29 mg/dL in uterine fibroid patients. In the endometriosis treated patients, increases from the pretreatment values were statistically significant (p<0.03). There was essentially no increase in the LDL/HDL ratio in patients from either population receiving LUPRON DEPOT 3.75 mg.
In two other clinical trials, LUPRON DEPOT 3.75 mg plus norethindrone acetate 5 mg daily were evaluated for 12 months of treatment. LUPRON DEPOT 3.75 mg was used as a control group in one study. Percent changes from base-

line for serum lipids and percentages of patients with serum lipid values outside of the normal range in the two studies are summarized in the tables below.
[See table 5 above]
Changes from baseline tended to be greater at Week 52. After treatment, mean serum lipid levels from patients with follow up data returned to pretreatment values.
[See table 6 at top of next page]
Low HDL-cholesterol (<40 mg/dL) and elevated LDL-cholesterol (>160 mg/dL) are recognized risk factors for cardiovascular disease. The long-term significance of the observed treatment-related changes in serum lipids in women with endometriosis is unknown. Therefore assessment of cardiovascular risk factors should be considered prior to initiation of concurrent treatment with LUPRON and norethindrone acetate.

Chemistry
Slight to moderate mean increases were noted for glucose, uric acid, BUN, creatinine, total protein, albumin, bilirubin, alkaline phosphatase, LDH, calcium, and phosphorus. None of these increases were clinically significant. In the hormonal add-back studies LUPRON DEPOT in combination with norethindrone acetate was associated with elevations of GGT and SGPT in 6% to 7% of patients.

Postmarketing
The following adverse reactions have been identified during postapproval use of LUPRON DEPOT. Because these reactions are reported voluntarily from a population of uncertain size, it is not always possible to reliably estimate their frequency or establish a causal relationship to drug exposure.
During postmarketing surveillance with other dosage forms and in the same and/or different populations, the following adverse events were reported. Like other drugs in this class, mood swings, including depression, have been reported. There have been rare reports of suicidal ideation and attempt. Many, but not all, of these patients had a history of depression or other psychiatric illness. Patients should be counseled on the possibility of development or worsening of depression during treatment with LUPRON.
Symptoms consistent with an anaphylactoid or asthmatic process have been rarely reported. Rash, urticaria, and photosensitivity reactions have also been reported.
Localized reactions including induration and abscess have been reported at the site of injection.
Symptoms consistent with fibromyalgia (eg: joint and muscle pain, headaches, sleep disorders, gastrointestinal distress, and shortness of breath) have been reported individually and collectively.
Other events reported are:
Hepato-biliary disorder: Rarely reported serious liver injury
Injury, poisoning and procedural complications: Spinal fracture
Investigations: Decreased WBC
Musculoskeletal and Connective tissue disorder: Tenosynovitis-like symptoms
Nervous System Disorder: Convulsion, peripheral neuropathy, paralysis
Vascular Disorder: Hypotension
Cases of serious venous and arterial thromboembolism have been reported, including deep vein thrombosis, pulmonary embolism, myocardial infarction, stroke, and transient ischemic attack. Although a temporal relationship was reported in some cases, most cases were confounded by risk factors or concomitant medication use. It is unknown if there is a causal association between the use of GnRH analogs and these events.
Pituitary apoplexy
During post-marketing surveillance, rare cases of pituitary apoplexy (a clinical syndrome secondary to infarction of the pituitary gland) have been reported after the administration of gonadotropin-releasing hormone agonists. In a majority of these cases, a pituitary adenoma was diagnosed, with a majority of pituitary apoplexy cases occurring within 2 weeks of the first dose, and some within the first hour. In these cases, pituitary apoplexy has presented as sudden headache, vomiting, visual changes, ophthalmoplegia, altered mental status, and sometimes cardiovascular collapse. Immediate medical attention has been required.
See other LUPRON DEPOT and LUPRON Injection package inserts for other events reported in the same and different patient populations.

OVERDOSAGE
In clinical trials using daily subcutaneous leuprolide acetate in patients with prostate cancer, doses as high as 20 mg/day for up to two years caused no adverse effects differing from those observed with the 1 mg/day dose.

DOSAGE AND ADMINISTRATION
LUPRON DEPOT Must Be Administered Under the Supervision of a Physician.
Endometriosis
The recommended duration of treatment with LUPRON DEPOT–3 Month 11.25 mg alone or in combination with norethindrone

acetate is six months. The choice of LUPRON DEPOT alone or LUPRON DEPOT plus norethindrone acetate therapy for initial management of the symptoms and signs of endometriosis should be made by the health care professional in consultation with the patient and should take into consideration the risks and benefits of the addition of norethindrone to LUPRON DEPOT alone.

If the symptoms of endometriosis recur after a course of therapy, retreatment with a six-month course of LUPRON DEPOT-3 Month 11.25 mg administered every three months and norethindrone acetate 5 mg daily may be considered. Retreatment beyond this one six-month course cannot be recommended. It is recommended that bone density be assessed before retreatment begins to ensure that values are within normal limits. LUPRON DEPOT alone is not recommended for retreatment. If norethindrone acetate is contraindicated for the individual patient, then retreatment is not recommended.

An assessment of cardiovascular risk and management of risk factors such as cigarette smoking is recommended before beginning treatment with LUPRON DEPOT and norethindrone acetate.

Uterine Leiomyomata (Fibroids)

The recommended dose of LUPRON DEPOT-3 Month 11.25 mg is one injection. The symptoms associated with uterine leiomyomata will recur following discontinuation of therapy. If additional treatment with LUPRON DEPOT-3 Month 11.25 mg is contemplated, bone density should be assessed prior to initiation of therapy to ensure that values are within normal limits

Due to different release characteristics, a fractional dose of the 3-month depot formulation is not equivalent to the same dose of the monthly formulation and should not be given.

For optimal performance of the prefilled dual chamber syringe (PDS), read and follow the following instructions:
Reconstitution and Administration Instructions

- The lyophilized microspheres are to be reconstituted and administered as a single intramuscular injection.
- Since LUPRON DEPOT does not contain a preservative, the suspension should be injected immediately or discarded if not used within two hours.
- As with other drugs administered by injection, the injection site should be varied periodically.

1. The LUPRON DEPOT powder should be visually inspected and the syringe should NOT BE USED if clumping or caking is evident. A thin layer of powder on the wall of the syringe is considered normal prior to mixing with the diluent. The diluent should appear clear.
2. To prepare for injection, screw the white plunger into the end stopper until the stopper begins to turn.

3. Hold the syringe UPRIGHT. Release the diluent by SLOWLY PUSHING (6 to 8 seconds) the plunger until the first stopper is <u>at the blue line</u> in the middle of the barrel.

← blue line

4. Keep the syringe UPRIGHT. Mix the microspheres (powder) thoroughly by gently shaking the syringe until the powder forms a uniform suspension. The suspension will appear milky. If the powder adheres to the stopper or caking/clumping is present, tap the syringe with your finger to disperse. DO NOT USE if any of the powder has not gone into suspension.

Table 6 PERCENTAGE OF PATIENTS WITH SERUM LIPID VALUES OUTSIDE OF THE NORMAL RANGE

| | LUPRON DEPOT 3.75 mg | | LUPRON DEPOT 3.75 mg plus norethindrone acetate 5 mg daily | | | |
| | Controlled Study (n=39) | | Controlled Study (n=41) | | Open Label Study (n=117) | |
	Wk 0	Wk 24*	Wk 0	Wk 24*	Wk 0	Wk 24*
Total Cholesterol (>240 mg/dL)	15%	23%	15%	20%	6%	7%
HDL Cholesterol (<40 mg/dL)	15%	10%	15%	44%	15%	41%
LDL Cholesterol (>160 mg/dL)	0%	8%	5%	7%	9%	11%
LDL/HDL Ratio (>4.0)	0%	3%	2%	15%	7%	21%
Triglycerides (>200 mg/dL)	13%	13%	12%	10%	5%	9%

* Includes all patients regardless of baseline value.

5. Hold the syringe UPRIGHT. With the opposite hand pull the needle cap upward without twisting.
6. Keep the syringe UPRIGHT. Advance the plunger to expel the air from the syringe. Now the syringe is ready for injection.
7. After cleaning the injection site with an alcohol swab, the intramuscular injection should be performed by inserting the needle at a 90 degree angle into the gluteal area, anterior thigh, or deltoid; injection sites should be alternated.

NOTE: Aspirated blood would be visible just below the luer lock connection if a blood vessel is accidentally penetrated. If present, blood can be seen through the transparent LuproLoc® safety device. If blood is present remove the needle immediately. Do not inject the medication.

8. Inject the entire contents of the syringe intramuscularly at the time of reconstitution. The suspension settles very quickly following reconstitution; therefore, LUPRON DEPOT should be mixed and used immediately.

AFTER INJECTION

9. Withdraw the needle. Once the syringe has been withdrawn, activate immediately the LuproLoc® safety device by pushing the arrow on the lock upward towards the needle tip with the thumb or finger, as illustrated, until the needle cover of the safety device over the needle is fully extended and a CLICK is heard or felt.

CLICK

ADDITIONAL INFORMATION

- Dispose of the syringe according to local regulations/procedures.

HOW SUPPLIED

Each LUPRON DEPOT – 3 Month 11.25 mg kit (NDC 0074-3663-03) contains:
- one prefilled dual-chamber syringe
- one plunger
- two alcohol swabs
- a complete prescribing information enclosure

Each syringe contains sterile lyophilized microspheres which are leuprolide acetate incorporated in a biodegradable polymer of polylactic acid. When mixed with 1.5 mL of the diluent, LUPRON DEPOT–3 Month 11.25 mg is administered as a single IM injection **EVERY THREE MONTHS.** Store at 25°C (77°F); excursions permitted to 15-30°C (59-86°F) [See USP Controlled Room Temperature]

REFERENCES

1. NIOSH Alert: Preventing occupational exposures to antineoplastic and other hazardous drugs in healthcare settings. 2004. U.S. Department of Health and Human Services, Public Health Service, Centers for Disease Control and Prevention, National Institute for Occupational Safety and Health, DHHS (NIOSH) Publication No. 2004-165.
2. OSHA Technical Manual, TED 1-0.15A, Section VI: Chapter 2. Controlling Occupational Exposure to Hazardous Drugs. OSHA, 1999. http://www.osha.gov/dts/osta/otm/otm_vi/otm_vi_2.html
3. American Society of Health-System Pharmacists. ASHP guidelines on handling hazardous drugs. *Am J Health-Syst Pharm.* 2006; 63; 1172-1193.
4. Polovich, M., White, J.M., & Kelleher, L.O. (eds.) 2005. Chemotherapy and biotherapy guidelines and recommendations for practice (2nd. Ed.) Pittsburgh, PA: Oncology Nursing Society.

Manufactured for
AbbVie Inc.
North Chicago, IL 60064
by Takeda Pharmaceutical Company Limited
Osaka, Japan 540-8645
™ - Trademark
® - Registered Trademark
(No. 3663)
Ref: 03-A892 - Revised October, 2013
© 2013, AbbVie Inc.
Shown in Product Identification Guide, page 303

LUPRON DEPOT ℞

[lū-prŏn]
(leuprolide acetate for depot suspension)
22.5 mg for 3-Month Administration
30 mg for 4-Month Administration
45 mg for 6-Month Administration

HIGHLIGHTS OF PRESCRIBING INFORMATION

These highlights do not include all the information needed to use Lupron Depot safely and effectively. See full prescribing information for Lupron Depot.
Lupron Depot (leuprolide acetate for depot suspension)
Initial U.S. Approval: 1995

-----RECENT MAJOR CHANGES-----

Warnings and Precautions, Convulsions (5.5) 7/2013

-----INDICATIONS AND USAGE-----

LUPRON DEPOT is a gonadotropin releasing hormone (GnRH) agonist indicated for:
- palliative treatment of advanced prostatic cancer (1)

Information on the AbbVie, Inc. products listed on these pages is from the prescribing information in use as of July 31, 2014. For more information, please visit rxabbvie.com or call 1-800-633-9110.

Help Patients Save on Rx Drugs: PDR.net/PharmacyDiscountCard

DOSAGE AND ADMINISTRATION

LUPRON DEPOT must be administered under the supervision of a physician. Due to different release characteristics, the dosage strengths are not additive and must be selected based upon the desired dosing schedule. (2)

- LUPRON DEPOT 22.5 mg for 3–month administration, given as a single intramuscular injection every 12 weeks (2.1)
- LUPRON DEPOT 30 mg for 4–month administration, given as a single intramuscular injection every 16 weeks (2.2)
- LUPRON DEPOT 45 mg for 6–month administration, given as a single intramuscular injection every 24 weeks (2.3)

DOSAGE FORMS AND STRENGTHS

22.5 mg, 30 mg, and 45 mg injections in a kit with prefilled dual chamber syringe (3)

CONTRAINDICATIONS

- Hypersensitivity to GnRH, GnRH agonist or any of the excipients in LUPRON DEPOT (4.1)
- Pregnancy (4.2, 8.1)

WARNINGS AND PRECAUTIONS

- Increased serum testosterone (~ 50% above baseline) during first week of treatment; monitor serum testosterone and PSA (5.1, 5.6)
  - Isolated cases of transient worsening of symptoms, or additional signs and symptoms of prostate cancer during the first few weeks of treatment. (5.1)
  - A small number of patients may experience a temporary increase in bone pain which can be managed symptomatically. (5.1)
  - Isolated cases of ureteral obstruction and spinal cord compression have been reported with GnRH agonists, which may contribute to paralysis with or without fatal complications. (5.1)
- Hyperglycemia and Diabetes: Hyperglycemia and an increased risk of developing diabetes have been reported in men receiving GnRH analogs. Monitor blood glucose level and manage according to current clinical practice. (5.2)
- Cardiovascular Diseases: Increased risk of myocardial infarction, sudden cardiac death and stroke has been reported in association with use of GnRH analogs in men. Monitor for cardiovascular disease and manage according to current clinical practice. (5.3)
- Long-term androgen deprivation therapy prolongs the QT interval. Consider risks and benefits. (5.4)
- Convulsions have been observed in patients with or without a history of predisposing factors. Manage convulsions according to the current clinical practice. (5.5)

ADVERSE REACTIONS

- LUPRON DEPOT 22.5 mg for 3–month administration: The most common related adverse reactions (>10%) were general pain, injection site reaction, hot flashes/sweats, GI disorders, joint disorders, testicular atrophy, urinary disorders. (6.1)
- LUPRON DEPOT 30 mg for 4–month administration: The most common adverse reactions (>10%) were asthenia, flu syndrome, general pain, headache, injection site reaction, hot flashes/sweats, GI disorders, edema, skin reaction, urinary disorders. (6.2)
- LUPRON DEPOT 45 mg for 6–month administration: The most common adverse reactions (>10%) were hot flush, injection site pain, upper respiratory infection, and fatigue. (6.3)

In postmarketing experience, mood swings, depression, rare reports of suicidal ideation and attempt, rare reports of pituitary apoplexy, and rare reports of serious drug-induced liver injury have been reported. (6.4)

To report SUSPECTED ADVERSE REACTIONS, contact AbbVie Inc. at 1-800-633-9110 or FDA at 1-800-FDA-1088 or www.fda.gov/medwatch

DRUG INTERACTIONS

- No interactions with LUPRON DEPOT are expected. (7)

USE IN SPECIFIC POPULATIONS

- Pediatric: These LUPRON DEPOT formulations are not indicated for use in children. See the LUPRON DEPOT PED® package insert for the use of leuprolide acetate in children with central precocious puberty.
- Geriatric: This label reflects clinical trials for LUPRON DEPOT in prostate cancer in which the majority of the subjects studied were at least 65 years of age.

See 17 for PATIENT COUNSELING INFORMATION

Revised: 07/2013

FULL PRESCRIBING INFORMATION: CONTENTS*

FULL PRESCRIBING INFORMATION

1 INDICATIONS AND USAGE

LUPRON DEPOT 22.5 mg for 3–month administration, 30 mg for 4–month administration, and 45 mg for 6–month administration (leuprolide acetate) are indicated in the palliative treatment of advanced prostatic cancer.

LUPRON DEPOT is a gonadotropin releasing hormone (GnRH) agonist.

2 DOSAGE AND ADMINISTRATION

LUPRON DEPOT must be administered under the supervision of a physician.

[See table 1 above]

2.1 LUPRON DEPOT 22.5 mg for 3-Month Administration

The recommended dose of LUPRON DEPOT 22.5 mg for 3-month administration is one injection every 12 weeks. Due to different release characteristics, a fractional dose, or a combination of doses of this depot formulation is not equivalent to the same dose of the monthly formulation and should not be given.

Incorporated in a depot formulation, the lyophilized microspheres are to be reconstituted and administered every 12 weeks as a single intramuscular injection.

For optimal performance of the prefilled dual chamber syringe (PDS), read and follow the instructions in Section 2.4.

2.2 LUPRON DEPOT 30 mg for 4-Month Administration

The recommended dose of LUPRON DEPOT 30 mg for 4-month administration is one injection every 16 weeks. Due to different release characteristics, a fractional dose, or a combination of doses of this depot formulation is not equivalent to the same dose of the monthly formulation and should not be given.

Incorporated in a depot formulation, the lyophilized microspheres are to be reconstituted and administered every 16 weeks as a single intramuscular injection.

For optimal performance of the prefilled dual chamber syringe (PDS), read and follow the instructions in Section 2.4.

2.3 LUPRON DEPOT 45 mg for 6-Month Administration

The recommended dose of LUPRON DEPOT 45 mg for 6-month administration is one injection every 24 weeks. Due to different release characteristics, a fractional dose, or a combination of doses of this depot formulation is not equivalent to the same dose of the monthly formulation and should not be given.

Incorporated in a depot formulation, the lyophilized microspheres are to be reconstituted and administered every 24 weeks as a single intramuscular injection.

For optimal performance of the prefilled dual chamber syringe (PDS), read and follow the instructions in Section 2.4.

2.4 Administration of Injection

- The lyophilized microspheres are to be reconstituted and administered as a single intramuscular injection.
- Since LUPRON DEPOT does not contain a preservative, the suspension should be injected immediately or discarded if not used within two hours.
- As with other drugs administered by injection, the injection site should be varied periodically.

1. The LUPRON DEPOT powder should be visually inspected and the syringe should NOT BE USED if clumping or caking is evident. A thin layer of powder on the wall of the syringe is considered normal prior to mixing with the diluent. The diluent should appear clear.
2. To prepare for injection, screw the white plunger into the end stopper until the stopper begins to turn.

3. Hold the syringe UPRIGHT. Release the diluent by SLOWLY PUSHING (6 to 8 seconds) the plunger until the first stopper is <u>at the blue line</u> in the middle of the barrel.

← blue line

4. Keep the syringe UPRIGHT. Gently mix the microspheres (powder) thoroughly to form a uniform suspension. The suspension will appear milky. If the powder adheres to the stopper or caking/clumping is present, tap the syringe with your finger to disperse. DO NOT USE if any of the powder has not gone into suspension. [See figure at top of next column]
5. Hold the syringe UPRIGHT. With the opposite hand pull the needle cap upward without twisting.
6. Keep the syringe UPRIGHT. Advance the plunger to expel the air from the syringe.

Table 1 LUPRON DEPOT Recommended Dosing

Dosage	22.5 mg for 3-Month Administration	30 mg for 4-Month Administration	45 mg for 6-Month Administration
Recommended dose	1 injection every 12 weeks	1 injection every 16 weeks	1 injection every 24 weeks

7. After cleaning the injection site with an alcohol swab, insert the needle completely at a 90 degree angle.

NOTE: Aspirated blood would be visible just below the luer lock connection if a blood vessel is accidentally penetrated. If present, blood can be seen through the transparent LuproLoc® safety device. If blood is present remove the needle immediately. Do not inject the medication

8. Inject the entire contents of the syringe intramuscularly at the time of reconstitution. The suspension settles very quickly following reconstitution; therefore, LUPRON DEPOT should be mixed and used immediately.

AFTER INJECTION

9. Withdraw the needle. Immediately activate the Lupro-Loc® safety device by pushing the arrow forward with the thumb or finger, as illustrated, until the device is fully extended and a CLICK is heard or felt.

CLICK

ADDITIONAL INFORMATION

- Please see the handling information in the Reference Section 15.0.
- Dispose of the syringe according to local regulations/procedures.

3 DOSAGE FORMS AND STRENGTHS

LUPRON DEPOT 22.5 mg for 3-month administration, 30 mg for 4-month administration, and 45 mg for 6-month administration are each supplied as a kit with prefilled dual chamber syringe.

4 CONTRAINDICATIONS

4.1 Hypersensitivity

LUPRON DEPOT is contraindicated in individuals with known hypersensitivity to GnRH agonists or any of the excipients in LUPRON DEPOT. Reports of anaphylactic reactions to GnRH agonists have been reported in the medical literature.

4.2 Pregnancy

LUPRON DEPOT may cause fetal harm when administered to a pregnant woman. Expected hormonal changes that occur with LUPRON DEPOT treatment increase the risk for pregnancy loss and fetal harm when administered to a pregnant woman [see Use in Specific Populations (8.1)]. LUPRON DEPOT is contraindicated in women who are or may become pregnant. If this drug is used during pregnancy, or if the patient becomes pregnant while taking this drug, the patient should be apprised of the potential hazard to the fetus.

5 WARNINGS AND PRECAUTIONS

5.1 Tumor Flare

Initially, LUPRON DEPOT, like other GnRH agonists, causes increases in serum levels of testosterone to approximately 50% above baseline during the first weeks of treatment. Isolated cases of ureteral obstruction and spinal cord compression have been observed, which may contribute to paralysis with or without fatal complications. Transient worsening of symptoms may develop. A small number of patients may experience a temporary increase in bone pain, which can be managed symptomatically.

Patients with metastatic vertebral lesions and/or with urinary tract obstruction should be closely observed during the first few weeks of therapy.

5.2 Hyperglycemia and Diabetes

Hyperglycemia and an increased risk of developing diabetes have been reported in men receiving GnRH agonists. Hyperglycemia may represent development of diabetes mellitus or worsening of glycemic control in patients with diabetes. Monitor blood glucose and/or glycosylated hemoglobin (HbA1c) periodically in patients receiving a GnRH agonist and manage with current practice for treatment of hyperglycemia or diabetes.

5.3 Cardiovascular Diseases

Increased risk of developing myocardial infarction, sudden cardiac death and stroke has been reported in association with use of GnRH agonists in men. The risk appears low based on the reported odds ratios, and should be evaluated carefully along with cardiovascular risk factors when determining a treatment for patients with prostate cancer. Patients receiving a GnRH agonist should be monitored for symptoms and signs suggestive of development of cardiovascular disease and be managed according to current clinical practice.

5.4 Effect on QT/QTc Interval

Long-term androgen deprivation therapy prolongs the QT interval. Physicians should consider whether the benefits of androgen deprivation therapy outweigh the potential risks in patients with congenital long QT syndrome, electrolyte abnormalities, or congestive heart failure and in patients taking class IA (e.g., quinidine, procainamide) or Class III (e.g., amiodarone, sotalol) antiarrhythmic medications.

5.5 Convulsions

Postmarketing reports of convulsions have been observed in patients on leuprolide acetate therapy. These included patients with a history of seizures, epilepsy, cerebrovascular disorders, central nervous system anomalies or tumors, and in patients on concomitant medications that have been associated with convulsions such as bupropion and SSRIs. Convulsions have also been reported in patients in the absence of any of the conditions mentioned above. Patients receiving a GnRH agonist who experience convulsion should be managed according to current clinical practice.

5.6 Laboratory Tests

Response to LUPRON DEPOT 22.5 mg for 3-month administration, 30 mg for 4-month administration, and 45 mg for 6-month administration should be monitored by measuring serum levels of testosterone. In the majority of patients, testosterone levels increased above baseline, declining thereafter to castrate levels (< 50 ng/dL) within four weeks. [see Clinical Studies (14) and Adverse Reactions (6)].

6 ADVERSE REACTIONS

Because clinical studies are conducted under widely varying conditions, adverse reaction rates observed in the clinical studies of a drug cannot be directly compared to rates in the clinical studies of another drug and may not reflect the rates observed in practice.

6.1 LUPRON DEPOT 22.5 mg for 3-Month Administration

Clinical Trials

In two clinical trials of LUPRON DEPOT 22.5 mg for 3-month administration, the following adverse reactions were reported to have a possible or probable relationship to drug as ascribed by the treating physician in 5% or more of the patients receiving the drug. **Often, causality is difficult to assess in patients with metastatic prostate cancer.** Reactions considered not drug-related are excluded.

Table 2. Adverse Reactions Reported in ≥ 5% of Patients

LUPRON DEPOT 22.5 mg for 3-Month Administration		
Body System/Reaction	**N=94**	**(%)**
Body As A Whole		
Asthenia	7	(7.4)
General Pain	25	(26.6)
Headache	6	(6.4)
Injection Site Reaction	13	(13.8)
Cardiovascular System		
Hot flashes/Sweats	55	(58.5)
Digestive System		
GI Disorders	15	(16.0)
Musculoskeletal System		
Joint Disorders	11	(11.7)
Central/Peripheral Nervous System		
Dizziness/Vertigo	6	(6.4)
Insomnia/Sleep Disorders	8	(8.5)
Neuromuscular Disorders	9	(9.6)
Respiratory System		
Respiratory Disorders	6	(6.4)
Skin and Appendages		
Skin Reaction	8	(8.5)
Urogenital System		
Testicular Atrophy	19	(20.2)
Urinary Disorders	14	(14.9)

In these same studies, the following adverse reactions were reported in less than 5% of the patients on LUPRON DEPOT 22.5 mg for 3-month administration.

Body As A Whole - Enlarged abdomen, Fever

Cardiovascular System - Arrhythmia, Bradycardia, Heart failure, Hypertension, Hypotension, Varicose vein

Digestive System - Anorexia, Duodenal ulcer, Increased appetite, Thirst/dry mouth

Hemic and Lymphatic System - Anemia, Lymphedema

Metabolic and Nutritional Disorders - Dehydration, Edema

Central/Peripheral Nervous System - Anxiety, Delusions, Depression, Hypesthesia, Libido decreased*, Nervousness, Paresthesia

Respiratory System - Epistaxis, Pharyngitis, Pleural effusion, Pneumonia

Special Senses - Abnormal vision, Amblyopia, Dry eyes, Tinnitus

Urogenital System - Gynecomastia, Impotence*, Penis disorders, Testis disorders.

* Physiologic effect of decreased testosterone.

Laboratory

Abnormalities of certain parameters were observed, but are difficult to assess in this population. The following were recorded in ≥5% of patients: Increased BUN, Hyperglycemia, Hyperlipidemia (total cholesterol, LDL-cholesterol, triglycerides), Hyperphosphatemia, Abnormal liver function tests, Increased PT, Increased PTT. Additional laboratory abnormalities reported were: Decreased platelets, Decreased potassium and Increased WBC.

6.2 LUPRON DEPOT 30 mg for 4-Month Administration Clinical Trials

The 4-month formulation of LUPRON DEPOT 30 mg was utilized in clinical trials that studied the drug in 49 non-orchiectomized prostate cancer patients for 32 weeks or longer and in 24 orchiectomized prostate cancer patients for 20 weeks.

In the above described clinical trials, the following adverse reactions were reported in ≥ 5% of the patients during the treatment period regardless of causality.

[See table 3 at top of next page]

In these same studies, the following adverse reactions were reported in less than 5% of the patients on LUPRON DEPOT 30 mg for 4-month administration.

Body As a Whole - Abscess, Accidental injury, Allergic reaction, Cyst, Fever, Generalized edema, Hernia, Neck pain, Neoplasm

Cardiovascular System - Atrial fibrillation, Deep thrombophlebitis, Hypertension

Digestive System - Anorexia, Eructation, Gastrointestinal hemorrhage, Gingivitis, Gum hemorrhage, Hepatomegaly, Increased appetite, Intestinal obstruction, Periodontal abscess

Hemic and Lymphatic System - Lymphadenopathy

Metabolic and Nutritional Disorders - Healing abnormal, Hypoxia, Weight loss

Musculoskeletal System - Leg cramps, Pathological fracture, Ptosis

Nervous System - Abnormal thinking, Amnesia, Confusion, Convulsion, Dementia, Depression, Insomnia/sleep disorders, Libido decreased*, Neuropathy, Paralysis

Respiratory System - Asthma, Bronchitis, Hiccup, Lung disorder, Sinusitis, Voice alteration

Skin and Appendages - Herpes zoster, Melanosis

Urogenital System - Bladder carcinoma, Epididymitis, Impotence*, Prostate disorder, Testicular atrophy*, Urinary incontinence, Urinary tract infection.

* Physiologic effect of decreased testosterone.

Information on the AbbVie, Inc. products listed on these pages is from the prescribing information in use as of July 31, 2014. For more information, please visit rxabbvie.com or call 1-800-633-9110.

Table 3. Adverse Events Regardless of Causality Reported in ≥ 5% of Patients

LUPRON DEPOT 30 mg for 4-Month Administration

Body System/Events	Nonorchiectomized Study 013 N=49	(%)	Orchiectomized Study 012 N=24	(%)
Body As a Whole				
Asthenia	6	(12.2)	1	(4.2)
Flu Syndrome	6	(12.2)	0	(0.0)
General Pain	16	(32.7)	1	(4.2)
Headache	5	(10.2)	1	(4.2)
Injection Site Reaction	4	(8.2)	9	(37.5)
Cardiovascular System				
Hot flashes/Sweats	23	(46.9)	2	(8.3)
Digestive System				
GI Disorders	5	(10.2)	3	(12.5)
Metabolic and Nutritional Disorders				
Dehydration	4	(8.2)	0	(0.0)
Edema	4	(8.2)	5	(20.8)
Musculoskeletal System				
Joint Disorder	8	(16.3)	1	(4.2)
Myalgia	4	(8.2)	0	(0.0)
Nervous System				
Dizziness/Vertigo	3	(6.1)	2	(8.3)
Neuromuscular Disorders	3	(6.1)	1	(4.2)
Paresthesia	4	(8.2)	1	(4.2)
Respiratory System				
Respiratory Disorder	4	(8.2)	1	(4.2)
Skin and Appendages				
Skin Reaction	6	(12.2)	0	(0.0)
Urogenital System				
Urinary Disorders	5	(10.2)	4	(16.7)

Table 4. Adverse Events in ≥ 5% of Patients

LUPRON DEPOT 45 mg for 6-Month Administration

Adverse Event	Treatment Emergent N = 151	(%)	Treatment Related N = 151	(%)
Hot Flush/Flushing	89	58.9	88	58.3
Injection Site Pain/Discomfort	29	19.2	16	10.6
Upper Respiratory Tract Infection/Influenza-like Illness[1]	32	21.2	0	0
Fatigue/Lethargy	20	13.2	18	11.9
Constipation	15	9.9	5	3.3
Arthralgia	14	9.3	2	1.3
Insomnia/Sleep Disorder	13	8.6	5	3.3
Headache/Sinus Headache	12	7.9	3	2.0
Musculoskeletal Pain/ Myalgia	12	7.9	3	2.0
Second Primary Neoplasm[2]	11	7.3	0	0
Cough	10	6.6	2	1.3
Hematuria/Hemorrhagic Cystitis	10	6.6	0	0
Hypertension/BP Increased	10	6.6	3	2.0
Rash	9	6.0	3	2.0
Dysuria	9	6.0	1	0.7
Urinary Tract Infection/Cystitis	9	6.0	0	0
Anemia/Hemoglobin Decreased	10	6.6	2	1.3
Back Pain	8	5.3	0	0
COPD	8	5.3	0	0
Dizziness	8	5.3	3	2.0
Dyspnea/Dyspnea on Exertion	8	5.3	2	1.3
Nocturia	8	5.3	2	1.3
Peripheral/Pitting Edema	8	5.3	2	1.3
Coronary Artery Disease/Angina	8	5.3	1	0.7

[1]Includes influenza, nasal congestion, nasopharyngitis, rhinorrhea, upper respiratory tract infection, and viral upper respiratory tract infection
[2]Includes basal cell carcinoma, bladder transitional cell carcinoma, lung neoplasm, malignant melanoma, non-Hodgkin's lymphoma, and squamous cell carcinoma

Laboratory

Abnormalities of certain parameters were observed, but their relationship to drug treatment is difficult to assess in this population. The following were recorded in ≥ 5% of patients: Decreased bicarbonate, Decreased hemoglobin/hematocrit/RBC, Hyperlipidemia (total cholesterol, LDL-cholesterol, triglycerides), Decreased HDL-cholesterol, Eosinophilia, Increased glucose, Increased liver function tests (ALT, AST, GGTP, LDH), Increased phosphorus. Additional laboratory abnormalities were reported: Increased BUN and PT, Leukopenia, Thrombocytopenia, Uricaciduria.

6.3 LUPRON DEPOT 45 mg for 6-Month Administration Clinical Trials

One open label, multicenter study was conducted with LUPRON DEPOT 45 mg for 6-month administration in 151 prostate cancer patients. Patients were treated for 48 weeks, with 139/151 receiving two injections 24 weeks apart.

In the above described clinical trial, the following adverse events were reported in ≥ 5% of the patients during the treatment period. The Table 4 includes all adverse events reported in ≥ 5% of patients as well as the incidences of these adverse events that were considered, by the treating physician, to have a definite or possible relationship to LUPRON.

[See table 4 above]

The following adverse events led to discontinuation; fatigue, hot flush, second primary neoplasm, asthenia, coronary artery disease, constipation, hyperkalemia, and sleep disorder. Serious adverse events in ≥ 2% of patients, regardless of causality, included chronic obstructive pulmonary disease, coronary artery disease/angina, cerebrovascular accident/transient ischemic attack, pneumonia, and second primary neoplasms.

Laboratory

At baseline, 13.9% of patients had a CTCAE v4.0 grade 1 or 2 decreased hemoglobin. During the study, 42.4% of subjects had grade 1 decreased hemoglobin (10 - <12·5 g/dL), 2.0% had grade 2 (8 - <10 g/dL) and 1.3% of subjects had grade 3 or 4 (<8 g/dL). Likewise, 28.5% of patients had a grade 1 or 2 increased cholesterol at baseline while 55.0% had grade 1 increased cholesterol (>199- 300 mg/dL), 3.3% had a grade 2 increase (>300-400 mg/dL), and 0.7% of subjects had grade 3 (>400 mg/dL) during the study.

6.4 Postmarketing

The following adverse reactions have been identified during postapproval use of LUPRON DEPOT. Because these reactions are reported voluntarily from a population of uncertain size, it is not always possible to reliably estimate their frequency or establish a causal relationship to drug exposure.

During postmarketing surveillance, which includes other dosage forms and other patient populations, the following adverse reactions were reported.

Like other drugs in this class, mood swings, including depression, have been reported. There have been very rare reports of suicidal ideation and attempt. Many, but not all, of these patients had a history of depression or other psychiatric illness. Patients should be counseled on the possibility of development or worsening of depression during treatment with LUPRON.

Symptoms consistent with an anaphylactoid or asthmatic process have been rarely (incidence rate of about 0.002%) reported. Rash, urticaria, and photosensitivity reactions have also been reported.

Changes in Bone Density - Decreased bone density has been reported in the medical literature in men who have had orchiectomy or who have been treated with a GnRH agonist analog. In a clinical trial, 25 men with prostate cancer, 12 of whom had been treated previously with leuprolide acetate for at least six months, underwent bone density studies as a result of pain. The leuprolide-treated group had lower bone density scores than the nontreated control group. It can be anticipated that long periods of medical castration in men will have effects on bone density.

Pituitary apoplexy - During post-marketing surveillance, rare cases of pituitary apoplexy (a clinical syndrome secondary to infarction of the pituitary gland) have been reported after the administration of gonadotropin-releasing hormone agonists. In a majority of these cases, a pituitary adenoma was diagnosed, with a majority of pituitary apoplexy cases occurring within 2 weeks of the first dose, and some within the first hour. In these cases, pituitary apoplexy has presented as sudden headache, vomiting, visual changes, ophthalmoplegia, altered mental status, and sometimes cardiovascular collapse. Immediate medical attention has been required.

Localized reactions including induration and abscess have been reported at the site of injection.

Symptoms consistent with fibromyalgia (e.g., joint and muscle pain, headaches, sleep disorders, gastrointestinal distress, and shortness of breath) have been reported individually and collectively.

Cardiovascular System – Hypotension, Myocardial infarction, Pulmonary embolism
Respiratory, thoracic and mediastinal disorder – Interstitial lung disease
Hepato-biliary disorder: Serious drug-induced liver injury
Hemic and Lymphatic System - Decreased WBC
Central/Peripheral Nervous System - Convulsion, Peripheral neuropathy, Spinal fracture/paralysis
Endocrine System – Diabetes
Musculoskeletal System - Tenosynovitis-like symptoms
Urogenital System - Prostate pain

See other LUPRON DEPOT and LUPRON Injection package inserts for other reactions reported in women and pediatric populations.

7 DRUG INTERACTIONS

No pharmacokinetic-based drug-drug interaction studies have been conducted with LUPRON DEPOT. However, because leuprolide acetate is a peptide that is primarily degraded by peptidase and not by Cytochrome P-450 enzymes as noted in specific studies, and the drug is only about 46% bound to plasma proteins, drug interactions would not be expected to occur.

See Clinical Pharmacology (12.3).

7.1 Drug/Laboratory Test Interactions

Administration of LUPRON DEPOT in therapeutic doses results in suppression of the pituitary-gonadal system. Normal function is usually restored within three months after treatment is discontinued. Due to the suppression of the pituitary-gonadal system by LUPRON DEPOT, diagnostic tests of pituitary gonadotropic and gonadal functions conducted during treatment and up to three months after discontinuation of LUPRON DEPOT may be affected.

8 USE IN SPECIFIC POPULATIONS

8.1 Pregnancy

Pregnancy Category X *[see Contraindications (4.2)]*.

LUPRON DEPOT is contraindicated in women who are or may become pregnant while receiving the drug. Expected hormonal changes that occur with LUPRON DEPOT treatment increase the risk for pregnancy loss and fetal harm when administered to a pregnant woman. If this drug is used during pregnancy, or if the patient becomes pregnant while taking this drug, the patient should be apprised of the potential hazard to the fetus.

Major fetal abnormalities were observed in rabbits after a single administration of the monthly formulation of LUPRON DEPOT on day 6 of pregnancy at doses of 0.00024, 0.0024, and 0.024 mg/kg (approximately 1/1600 to 1/16 the human dose based on body surface area using an estimated daily dose in animals and humans). Since a depot formulation was utilized in the study, a sustained exposure to leuprolide was expected throughout the period of organogenesis and to the end of gestation. Similar studies in rats did not demonstrate an increase in fetal malformations, however, there was increased fetal mortality and decreased fetal weights with the two higher doses of the monthly formulation of LUPRON DEPOT in rabbits and with the highest dose (0.024 mg/kg) in rats.

8.3 Nursing Mothers

LUPRON DEPOT is not indicated for women [see Indications and Usage (1)]. It is not known whether leuprolide is excreted in human milk. Because many drugs are excreted in human milk and because of the potential for serious adverse reactions in nursing infants from LUPRON DEPOT, a decision should be made to discontinue nursing or discontinue the drug taking into account the importance of the drug to the mother.

8.4 Pediatric Use

See LUPRON DEPOT-PED® (leuprolide acetate for depot suspension) labeling for the safety and effectiveness in children with central precocious puberty.

8.5 Geriatric Use

In the clinical trials for LUPRON DEPOT in prostate cancer, the majority (approximately 80%) of the subjects studied were at least 65 years of age. Therefore, the labeling reflects the pharmacokinetics, efficacy and safety of LUPRON DEPOT in this population.

10 OVERDOSAGE

There is no experience of overdosage in clinical trials. In rats, a single subcutaneous dose of 100 mg/kg (approximately 4,000 times the estimated daily human dose based on body surface area), resulted in dyspnea, decreased activity, and excessive scratching. In early clinical trials with daily subcutaneous leuprolide acetate, doses as high as 20 mg/day for up to two years caused no adverse effects differing from those observed with the 1 mg/day dose.

11 DESCRIPTION

Leuprolide acetate is a synthetic nonapeptide analog of naturally occurring gonadotropin-releasing hormone (GnRH). The analog possesses greater potency than the natural hormone. The chemical name is 5-oxo-L-prolyl-L-histidyl-L-tryptophyl-L-seryl-L-tyrosyl-D-leucyl-L-leucyl-L-arginyl-N-ethyl-L-prolinamide acetate (salt) with the following structural formula:

[See chemical structure above]

LUPRON DEPOT 22.5 mg for 3-month administration is available in a prefilled dual-chamber syringe containing sterile lyophilized microspheres which, when mixed with diluent, become a suspension intended as an intramuscular injection to be given **ONCE EVERY 12 WEEKS.**

The front chamber of LUPRON DEPOT 22.5 mg for 3-month administration prefilled dual-chamber syringe contains leuprolide acetate (22.5 mg), polylactic acid (198.6 mg) and D-mannitol (38.9 mg). The second chamber of diluent contains carboxymethylcellulose sodium (7.5 mg), D-mannitol (75.0 mg), polysorbate 80 (1.5 mg), water for injection, USP, and glacial acetic acid, USP to control pH.

LUPRON DEPOT 30 mg for 4-month administration is available in a prefilled dual-chamber syringe containing sterile lyophilized microspheres which, when mixed with diluent, become a suspension intended as an intramuscular injection to be given **ONCE EVERY 16 WEEKS.**

The front chamber of LUPRON DEPOT 30 mg for 4-month administration prefilled dual-chamber syringe contains leuprolide acetate (30 mg), polylactic acid (264.8 mg) and D-mannitol (51.9 mg). The second chamber of diluent contains carboxymethylcellulose sodium (7.5 mg), D-mannitol (75.0 mg), polysorbate 80 (1.5 mg), water for injection, USP, and glacial acetic acid, USP to control pH.

LUPRON DEPOT 45 mg for 6-month administration is available in a prefilled dual-chamber syringe containing sterile lyophilized microspheres which, when mixed with diluent, become a suspension intended as an intramuscular injection to be given **ONCE EVERY 24 WEEKS.**

The front chamber of LUPRON DEPOT 45 mg for 6-month administration prefilled dual-chamber syringe contains leuprolide acetate (45 mg), polylactic acid (169.9 mg), D-mannitol (39.7 mg), and stearic acid (10.1 mg). The second chamber of diluent contains carboxymethylcellulose sodium (7.5 mg), D-mannitol (75.0 mg), polysorbate 80 (1.5 mg), water for injection, USP, and glacial acetic acid, USP to control pH.

During the manufacture of LUPRON DEPOT 22.5 mg for 3-month administration, 30 mg for 4-month administration, and 45 mg for 6-month administration, acetic acid is lost, leaving the peptide.

12 CLINICAL PHARMACOLOGY

12.1 Mechanism of Action

Leuprolide acetate, a GnRH agonist, acts as an inhibitor of gonadotropin secretion. Animal studies indicate that following an initial stimulation, continuous administration of leuprolide acetate results in suppression of ovarian and testicular steroidogenesis. This effect was reversible upon discontinuation of drug therapy.

Administration of leuprolide acetate has resulted in inhibition of the growth of certain hormone dependent tumors (prostatic tumors in Noble and Dunning male rats and DMBA-induced mammary tumors in female rats) as well as atrophy of the reproductive organs.

12.2 Pharmacodynamics

In humans, administration of leuprolide acetate results in an initial increase in circulating levels of luteinizing hormone (LH) and follicle stimulating hormone (FSH), leading to a transient increase in levels of the gonadal steroids (testosterone and dihydrotestosterone in males, and estrone and estradiol in premenopausal females). However, continuous administration of leuprolide acetate results in decreased levels of LH and FSH. In males, testosterone is reduced to castrate levels. In premenopausal females, estrogens are reduced to postmenopausal levels. These decreases occur within two to four weeks after initiation of treatment, and castrate levels of testosterone in prostatic cancer patients have been demonstrated for more than five years.

Leuprolide acetate is not active when given orally.

12.3 Pharmacokinetics

Absorption

LUPRON DEPOT 22.5 mg for 3-Month Administration

Following a single injection of LUPRON DEPOT 22.5 mg for 3-month administration in patients, mean peak plasma leuprolide concentration of 48.9 ng/mL was observed at 4 hours and then declined to 0.67 ng/mL at 12 weeks. Leuprolide appeared to be released at a constant rate following the onset of steady-state levels during the third week after dosing, providing steady plasma concentrations through the 12-week dosing interval. However, intact leuprolide and an inactive major metabolite could not be distinguished by the assay which was employed in the study. Detectable levels of leuprolide were present at all measurement points in all patients. The initial burst, followed by the rapid decline to a steady-state level, was similar to the release pattern seen with the monthly formulation.

LUPRON DEPOT 30 mg for 4-Month Administration

Following a single injection of LUPRON DEPOT 30 mg for 4-month administration in sixteen orchiectomized prostate cancer patients, mean peak plasma leuprolide concentration of 59.3 ng/mL was observed at 4 hours and the mean concentration then declined to 0.30 ng/mL at 16 weeks. The mean plasma concentration of leuprolide from weeks 3.5 to 16 was 0.44 ± 0.20 ng/mL (range: 0.20-1.06). Leuprolide appeared to be released at a constant rate following the onset of steady-state levels during the fourth week after dosing, providing steady plasma concentrations throughout the 16-week dosing interval. However, intact leuprolide and an inactive major metabolite could not be distinguished by the assay which was employed in the study. The initial burst, followed by the rapid decline to a steady-state level, was similar to the release pattern seen with the other depot formulations.

LUPRON DEPOT 45 mg for 6-Month Administration

Following a single injection of LUPRON DEPOT 45 mg for 6-month administration in 26 prostate cancer patients, mean peak plasma leuprolide concentration of 6.7 ng/mL was observed at 2 hours and the mean concentration then declined to 0.07 ng/mL at 24 weeks. Leuprolide appeared to be released continuously following the onset of steady-state levels during the third week after dosing providing steady plasma concentrations through the 24-week dosing interval. The initial burst, followed by the rapid decline to a steady-state level, was similar to the release pattern seen with the other depot formulations. In this study, mean leuprolide plasma concentration-time profiles were similar after the first and second dose.

Distribution

The mean steady-state volume of distribution of leuprolide following intravenous bolus administration to healthy male volunteers was 27 L. In vitro binding to human plasma proteins ranged from 43% to 49%.

Metabolism

In healthy male volunteers, a 1 mg bolus of leuprolide administered intravenously revealed that the mean systemic clearance was 7.6 L/h, with a terminal elimination half-life of approximately 3 hours based on a two compartment model.

In rats and dogs, administration of ^{14}C-labeled leuprolide was shown to be metabolized to smaller inactive peptides, a pentapeptide (Metabolite I), tripeptides (Metabolites II and III) and a dipeptide (Metabolite IV). These fragments may be further catabolized.

The major metabolite (M-I) plasma concentrations measured in 5 prostate cancer patients reached maximum concentration 2 to 6 hours after dosing and were approximately 6% of the peak parent drug concentration. One week after dosing, mean plasma M-I concentrations were approximately 20% of mean leuprolide concentrations.

Excretion

Following administration of LUPRON DEPOT 3.75 mg to 3 patients, less than 5% of the dose was recovered as parent and M-I metabolite in the urine.

Special Populations

The pharmacokinetics of the drug in hepatically and renally impaired patients have not been determined.

13 NONCLINICAL TOXICOLOGY

13.1 Carcinogenesis, Mutagenesis, Impairment of Fertility

Two-year carcinogenicity studies were conducted in rats and mice. In rats, a dose-related increase of benign pituitary hyperplasia and benign pituitary adenomas was noted at 24 months when the drug was administered subcutaneously at daily doses (0.6 to 4 mg/kg). There was a significant but not dose-related increase of pancreatic islet-cell adenomas in females and of testicular interstitial cell adenomas in males (highest incidence in the low dose group). In mice, no pituitary abnormalities were observed at a dose as high as 60 mg/kg for two years. Patients have been treated with leuprolide acetate for up to three years with doses as high as 10 mg/day and for two years with doses as high as 20 mg/day without demonstrable pituitary abnormalities.

Genotoxicity studies were conducted with leuprolide acetate using bacterial and mammalian systems. These studies provided no evidence of mutagenic effects or chromosomal aberrations.

Leuprolide may reduce male and female fertility. Administration of leuprolide acetate to male and female rats at dose of 0.024, 0.24, and 2.4 mg/kg as monthly depot formulation for up to 3 months (approximately as low as 1/30 of the human dose based on body surface area using an estimated daily dose in animals and humans) caused atrophy of the reproductive organs, and suppression of reproductive function. These changes were reversible upon cessation of treatment. Clinical and pharmacologic studies in adults (≥ 18 years) with leuprolide acetate and similar analogs have shown reversibility of fertility suppression when the drug is discontinued after continuous administration for periods of up to 24 weeks.

Clinical and pharmacologic studies in adults (≥ 18 years) with leuprolide acetate and similar analogs have shown reversibility of fertility suppression when the drug is discontinued after continuous administration for periods of up to 24 weeks.

14 CLINICAL STUDIES

14.1 LUPRON DEPOT 22.5 mg for 3-Month Administration

In clinical studies, serum testosterone was suppressed to castrate within 30 days in 87 of 92 (95%) patients and within an additional two weeks in three patients. Two patients did not suppress for 15 and 28 weeks, respectively. Suppression was maintained in all of these patients with the exception of transient minimal testosterone elevations in one of them, and in another an increase in serum testosterone to above the castrate range was recorded during the 12 hour observation period after a subsequent injection. This represents stimulation of gonadotropin secretion.

Information on the AbbVie, Inc. products listed on these pages is from the prescribing information in use as of July 31, 2014. For more information, please visit rxabbvie.com or call 1-800-633-9110.

Figure 1. LUPRON DEPOT 22.5 mg for 3-Month Administration Mean Serum Testosterone Concentrations

Note: Measurements were taken in a subset of patients from one study at Weeks 10.5, 11.5, 12.5, 22.5 and 23.5

Figure 3. LUPRON DEPOT 45 mg for 6-Month Administration Serum Testosterone Concentrations (Mean + SE)

An 85% rate of "no progression" was achieved during the initial 24 weeks of treatment. A decrease from baseline in serum PSA of ≥90% was reported in 71% of the patients and a change to within the normal range (≤3.99 ng/mL) in 63% of the patients.

Periodic monitoring of serum testosterone and PSA levels is recommended, especially if the anticipated clinical or biochemical response to treatment has not been achieved. It should be noted that results of testosterone determinations are dependent on assay methodology. It is advisable to be aware of the type and precision of the assay methodology to make appropriate clinical and therapeutic decisions.

14.2   LUPRON DEPOT 30 mg for 4-Month Administration

In an open-label, noncomparative, multicenter clinical study of LUPRON DEPOT 30 mg for 4-month administration, 49 patients with stage D2 prostatic adenocarcinoma (with no prior treatment) were enrolled. The objectives were to determine whether a 30 mg depot formulation of leuprolide injected once every 16 weeks would reduce and maintain serum testosterone levels at castrate levels (≤ 50 ng/dL), and to assess the safety of the formulation. The study was divided into an initial 32-week treatment phase and a long-term treatment phase. Serum testosterone levels were determined biweekly or weekly during the first 32 weeks of treatment. Once the patient completed the initial 32-week treatment period, treatment continued at the investigator's discretion with serum testosterone levels being done every 4 months prior to the injection.

In the majority of patients, testosterone levels increased 50% or more above the baseline during the first week of treatment. Mean serum testosterone subsequently suppressed to castrate levels within 30 days of the first injection in 94% of patients and within 43 days in all 49 patients during the initial 32-week treatment period. The median dosing interval between injections was 112 days. One escape from suppression (two consecutive testosterone values greater than 50 ng/dL after castrate levels achieved) was noted at Week 16. In this patient, serum testosterone increased to above the castrate range following the second depot injection (Week 16) but returned to the castrate level by Week 18. No adverse reactions were associated with this rise in serum testosterone. A second patient had a rise in testosterone at Week 17, then returned to the castrate level by Week 18 and remained there through Week 32. In the long-term treatment phase two patients experienced testosterone elevations, both at Week 48. Testosterone for one patient returned to the castrate range at Week 52, and one patient discontinued the study at Week 48 due to disease progression.

Secondary efficacy endpoints evaluated in the study were the objective tumor response as assessed by clinical evaluations of tumor burden (complete response, partial response, objectively stable and progression) and evaluations of changes in prostatic involvement and prostate-specific antigen (PSA). These evaluations were performed at Weeks 16 and 32 of the treatment phase. The long-term treatment phase monitored PSA at each visit (every 16 weeks). The objective tumor response analysis showed "no progression" (i.e. complete or partial response, or stable disease) in 86% (37/43) of patients at Week 16, and in 77% (37/48) of patients at Week 32. Local disease improved or remained stable in all patients evaluated at Week 16 and/or 32. For patients with elevated baseline PSA, 50% (23/46) had a normal PSA (less than 4.0 ng/mL) at Week 16, and 51% (19/37) had a normal PSA at Week 32.

Periodic monitoring of serum testosterone and PSA levels is recommended, especially if the anticipated clinical or biochemical response to treatment has not been achieved. It should be noted that results of testosterone determinations are dependent on assay methodology. It is advisable to be aware of the type and precision of the assay methodology to make appropriate clinical and therapeutic decisions. Using historical comparisons, the safety and efficacy of LUPRON DEPOT 30 mg for 4-month administration appear similar to the other LUPRON DEPOT formulations.

Figure 2. LUPRON DEPOT 30 mg for 4-Month Administration Mean Serum Testosterone Concentrations

Note: Measurements were taken in a subset of patients from one study at Weeks 14.5, 15.5 16.5, 30.5, 31 and 31.5

14.3   LUPRON DEPOT 45 mg for 6-Month Administration

An open-label, non-comparative, multicenter clinical study of LUPRON DEPOT 45 mg for 6-month administration enrolled 151 patients with prostate cancer. The study drug was administered as two intramuscular injections of LUPRON DEPOT 45 mg at 24 week intervals (139/151 received 2 injections), and patients were followed for a total of 48 weeks.

Among 148 patients who had testosterone value at Week 4, serum testosterone was suppressed to castrate levels (< 50 ng/dL) from Week 4 through Week 48 in an estimated 93.4% (two-sided 95% CI: 89.2%, 97.6%) of patients. One patient failed to achieve testosterone suppression by Week 4, and eight patients had escapes from suppression (any testosterone value > 50 ng/dL after castrate levels were achieved). Mean testosterone levels increased to 608 ng/dL from a baseline of 435 ng/dL during the first week of treatment. By Week 4, the mean testosterone concentration had decreased to below castrate levels (16 ng/dL).

Periodic monitoring of serum testosterone levels is recommended, especially if the anticipated clinical or biochemical response to treatment has not been achieved. Testosterone determinations are dependent on assay methodology and it is advisable to be aware of the type and precision of the assay methodology to make appropriate clinical and therapeutic decisions.

Figure 3 below shows the mean testosterone concentration at various time points.
[See figure 3 above]

15   REFERENCES

1. NIOSH Alert: Preventing occupational exposures to antineoplastic and other hazardous drugs in healthcare settings. 2004. U.S. Department of Health and Human Services, Public Health Service, Centers for Disease Control and Prevention, National Institute for Occupational Safety and Health, DHHS (NIOSH) Publication No. 2004-165.
2. OSHA Technical Manual, TED 1-0.15A, Section VI: Chapter 2. Controlling Occupational Exposure to Hazardous Drugs. OSHA, 1999. http://www.osha.gov/dts/osta/otm/otm_vi/otm_vi_2.html
3. American Society of Health-System Pharmacists. ASHP guidelines on handling hazardous drugs. *Am J Health-Syst Pharm.* 2006; 63; 1172-1193.
4. Polovich, M., White, J.M., & Kelleher, L.O. (eds.) 2005. Chemotherapy and biotherapy guidelines and recommendations for practice (2nd Ed.) Pittsburgh, PA: Oncology Nursing Society.

16   HOW SUPPLIED/STORAGE AND HANDLING

Each LUPRON DEPOT 22.5 mg for 3-month administration (NDC 0074-3346-03), 30 mg for 4-month administration (NDC 0074-3683-03), 45 mg for 6-month administration (NDC 0074-3473-03) contains:
• one prefilled dual-chamber syringe containing needle with LuproLoc® safety device
• one plunger
• two alcohol swabs
• a complete prescribing information enclosure

The prefilled dual-chamber syringe contains sterile lyophilized microspheres of leuprolide acetate incorporated in a biodegradable lactic acid polymer.

When mixed with 1.5 mL of accompanying diluent, LUPRON DEPOT 22.5 mg for 3-month administration is administered as a single intramuscular injection **EVERY 12 WEEKS**.

When mixed with 1.5 mL of accompanying diluent, LUPRON DEPOT 30 mg for 4-month administration is administered as a single intramuscular injection **EVERY 16 WEEKS**.

When mixed with 1.5 mL of accompanying diluent, LUPRON DEPOT 45 mg for 6-month administration is administered as a single intramuscular injection **EVERY 24 WEEKS**.

Store at 25°C (77°F); excursions permitted to 15–30°C (59–86°F) [See USP Controlled Room Temperature].

17   PATIENT COUNSELING INFORMATION

Information for Patients
Patients should be informed that:
• If they experience an allergic reaction to other drugs like LUPRON DEPOT, they should not use this drug.
• The most common side effects associated with LUPRON DEPOT are hot flashes, pain (especially joint pain and back pain), injection site pain and fatigue.
• LUPRON DEPOT may cause impotence.
• The increase in testosterone that occurs during the first weeks of therapy can cause an increase in urinary symptoms or pain.
• If they have metastatic cancer to the spine or urinary tract, they need close medical attention during the first weeks of therapy.
• They should notify their doctor if they develop new or worsened symptoms after beginning LUPRON DEPOT treatment.

Manufactured for
AbbVie Inc.
North Chicago, IL 60064
by Takeda Pharmaceutical Company Limited
Osaka, Japan 540-8645
™-Trademark
®-Registered Trademark
(No. 3346) (No. 3683) (No. 3473)
03-A853-R5 July, 2013
©2013 AbbVie Inc.
Shown in Product Identification Guide, page 304

LUPRON DEPOT-PED®   ℞
(leuprolide acetate for depot suspension)
7.5 mg, 11.25 mg, 15 mg, and 30 mg

HIGHLIGHTS OF PRESCRIBING INFORMATION
These highlights do not include all the information needed to use LUPRON DEPOT-PED safely and effectively. See full prescribing information for LUPRON DEPOT-PED.
LUPRON DEPOT-PED (leuprolide acetate for depot suspension) Injection, Powder, Lyophilized, For Suspension
Initial U.S. Approval: 1993

INDICATIONS AND USAGE

LUPRON DEPOT-PED is a gonadotropin releasing hormone (GnRH) agonist indicated in the treatment of children with central precocious puberty. (1)

DOSAGE AND ADMINISTRATION

- LUPRON DEPOT-PED is administered as a single intramuscular injection. The starting dose 7.5 mg, 11.25 mg, or 15 mg for 1-month administration is based on the child's weight. (2)
- LUPRON DEPOT-PED is administered as a single intramuscular injection. The doses are either 11.25 mg or 30 mg for 3-month administration.(2)
- Hormonal and clinical parameters should be monitored during treatment to ensure adequate suppression. (2)
- The injection site should be varied periodically. (2)

DOSAGE FORMS AND STRENGTHS

LUPRON DEPOT-PED 7.5 mg, 11.25 mg, or 15 mg for 1-month administration and LUPRON DEPOT-PED 11.25 mg or 30 mg for 3-month administration are provided in a prefilled dual chamber syringe for intramuscular injection. (3)

CONTRAINDICATIONS

- Hypersensitivity reactions. (4)
- Pregnancy. (4,8.1)

WARNINGS AND PRECAUTIONS

- An increase in clinical signs and symptoms of puberty may be observed during the first 2-4 weeks of therapy since gonadotropins and sex steroids rise above baseline because of the initial stimulatory effect of the drug before being suppressed. (5.1)
- Convulsions have been observed in patients with or without a history of seizures, epilepsy, cerebrovascular disorders, central nervous system anomalies or tumors, and in patients on concomitant medications that have been associated with convulsions. (5.2)

ADVERSE REACTIONS

- Adverse events related to suppression of endogenous sex steroid secretion may occur with LUPRON DEPOT-PED 7.5 mg, 11.25 mg, or 15 mg for 1-month administration. (6.1, 6.3)
- In clinical studies for LUPRON DEPOT-PED 11.25 mg or 30 mg for 3-month administration, the most frequent (≥ 2 patients) adverse reactions were: injection site pain, weight increased, headache, mood altered, and injection site swelling. (6.2)

To report SUSPECTED ADVERSE REACTIONS, contact AbbVie Inc. at 1-800-633-9110 or FDA at 1-800-FDA-1088 or www.fda.gov/medwatch

USE IN SPECIFIC POPULATIONS

- The use of LUPRON DEPOT-PED in children under 2 years is not recommended. (8.4)

See 17 for PATIENT COUNSELING INFORMATION

Revised: 06/2013

FULL PRESCRIBING INFORMATION: CONTENTS*

FULL PRESCRIBING INFORMATION

1 INDICATIONS AND USAGE

LUPRON DEPOT-PED is indicated in the treatment of children with central precocious puberty (CPP).

CPP is defined as early onset of secondary sexual characteristics (generally earlier than 8 years of age in girls and 9 years of age in boys) associated with pubertal pituitary gonadotropin activation. It may show a significantly advanced bone age that can result in diminished adult height.

Prior to initiation of treatment a clinical diagnosis of CPP should be confirmed by measurement of blood concentrations of luteinizing hormone (LH) (basal or stimulated with a GnRH analog), sex steroids, and assessment of bone age versus chronological age. Baseline evaluations should include height and weight measurements, diagnostic imaging of the brain (to rule out intracranial tumor), pelvic/testicular/adrenal ultrasound (to rule out steroid secreting tumors), human chorionic gonadotropin levels (to rule out a chorionic gonadotropin secreting tumor), and adrenal steroid measurements to exclude congenital adrenal hyperplasia.

2 DOSAGE AND ADMINISTRATION

2.1 Dose and Principles of Dosing 7.5 mg, 11.25 mg, or 15 mg for 1-month administration

LUPRON DEPOT-PED must be administered under the supervision of a physician.

LUPRON DEPOT-PED is administered as a single intramuscular injection once a month. The starting dose will be dictated by the child's weight, as indicated in the table below.

Table 1. Dosing Recommendations Based on Body Weight for LUPRON DEPOT-PED 1-month Formulations

Body Weight	Recommended Dose
≤ 25 kg	7.5 mg
> 25-37.5 kg	11.25 mg
> 37.5 kg	15 mg

The dose of LUPRON DEPOT-PED must be individualized for each child. If adequate hormonal and clinical suppression is not achieved with the starting dose, it should be increased to the next available higher dose (e.g. 11.25 mg or 15 mg at the next monthly injection). Similarly, the dose may be adjusted with changes in body weight. The injection site should be varied periodically.

The goal of therapy is to suppress pituitary gonadotropins and peripheral sex steroids, and to arrest progression of secondary sexual characteristics. Hormonal and clinical parameters should be monitored after 1–2 months of initiating therapy and with each dose change to ensure adequate pituitary gonadotropin suppression. Once a dose that results in adequate hormonal suppression is found, it can often be maintained for the duration of therapy in most children. It is recommended, however, that adequate hormonal suppression be verified in such patients as weight can increase significantly while on therapy.

Each LUPRON DEPOT-PED strength and formulation has different release characteristics. Do not use partial syringes or a combination of syringes to achieve a particular dose.

LUPRON DEPOT-PED should be discontinued at the appropriate age of onset of puberty at the discretion of the physician.

For optimal performance of the prefilled dual chamber syringe (PDS), read and follow the instructions in Section 2.3.

2.2 Dose and Principles of Dosing 11.25 mg or 30 mg for 3-month administration

LUPRON DEPOT-PED 11.25 mg or 30 mg for 3-month administration must be administered under the supervision of a physician.

LUPRON DEPOT-PED 11.25 mg or 30 mg for 3-month administration should be administered once every three months (12 weeks) as a single intramuscular injection. Regardless of the dose chosen, the goal of therapy is to suppress pituitary gonadotropins and peripheral sex steroids, and to arrest progression of secondary sexual characteris-

tics. Hormonal and clinical parameters should be monitored during treatment, for instance at month 2-3, month 6 and further as judged clinically appropriate, to ensure adequate suppression. In case of inadequate suppression, other available GnRH agonists indicated for the treatment of CPP should be considered.

Each LUPRON DEPOT-PED 11.25 mg or 30 mg for 3-month administration strength and formulation has different release characteristics. Do not use partial syringes or a combination of syringes to achieve a particular dose.

LUPRON DEPOT-PED 11.25 mg or 30 mg for 3-month administration treatment should be discontinued at the appropriate age of onset of puberty at the discretion of the physician.

For optimal performance of the prefilled dual chamber syringe (PDS), read and follow the instructions in Section 2.3.

2.3 Reconstitution and Administration Instructions

- The lyophilized microspheres are to be reconstituted and administered as a single intramuscular injection.
- Since LUPRON DEPOT-PED does not contain a preservative, the suspension should be injected immediately or discarded if not used within two hours.
- As with other drugs administered by injection, the injection site should be varied periodically.

1. The LUPRON DEPOT-PED powder should be visually inspected and the syringe should NOT BE USED if clumping or caking is evident. A thin layer of powder on the wall of the syringe is considered normal prior to mixing with the diluent. The diluent should appear clear.
2. To prepare for injection, screw the white plunger into the end stopper until the stopper begins to turn.

3. Hold the syringe UPRIGHT. Release the diluent by SLOWLY PUSHING (6 to 8 seconds) the plunger until the first stopper is at the blue line in the middle of the barrel.

← blue line

4. Keep the syringe UPRIGHT. Mix the microspheres (powder) thoroughly by gently shaking the syringe until the powder forms a uniform suspension. The suspension will appear milky. If the powder adheres to the stopper or caking/clumping is present, tap the syringe with your finger to disperse. DO NOT USE if any of the powder has not gone into suspension.

[See figure at top of next column]

5. Hold the syringe UPRIGHT. With the opposite hand pull the needle cap upward without twisting.
6. Keep the syringe UPRIGHT. Advance the plunger to expel the air from the syringe.
Now the syringe is ready for injection.

Information on the AbbVie, Inc. products listed on these pages is from the prescribing information in use as of July 31, 2014. For more information, please visit rxabbvie.com or call 1-800-633-9110.

7. After cleaning the injection site with an alcohol swab, the intramuscular injection should be performed by inserting the needle at a 90 degree angle into the gluteal area, anterior thigh, or shoulder; injection sites should be alternated.

NOTE: Aspirated blood would be visible just below the luer lock connection if a blood vessel is accidentally penetrated. If present, blood can be seen through the transparent LuproLoc® safety device. If blood is present remove the needle immediately. Do not inject the medication.

8. Inject the entire contents of the syringe intramuscularly at the time of reconstitution. The suspension settles very quickly following reconstitution; therefore, LUPRON DEPOT-PED should be mixed and used immediately.

AFTER INJECTION

9. Withdraw the needle. Once the syringe has been withdrawn, activate immediately the LuproLoc® safety device by pushing the arrow on the lock upward towards the needle tip with the thumb or finger, as illustrated, until the needle cover of the safety device is fully extended over the needle and a CLICK is heard or felt.

ADDITIONAL INFORMATION

• Dispose of the syringe according to local regulations/procedures.

---

3 DOSAGE FORMS AND STRENGTHS

LUPRON DEPOT-PED 7.5 mg, 11.25 mg, or 15 mg for 1-month administration and LUPRON DEPOT-PED 11.25 mg or 30 mg for 3-month administration is provided in a prefilled dual chamber syringe for intramuscular injection.

4 CONTRAINDICATIONS

• Hypersensitivity to GnRH, GnRH agonists or any of the excipients in LUPRON DEPOT-PED. Reports of anaphylactic reactions to GnRH agonists have been reported in the medical literature.
• All formulations of LUPRON DEPOT may cause fetal harm if administered to a pregnant woman. When LUPRON DEPOT was administered subcutaneously to rabbits it produced a dose related increase in major fetal abnormalities, and fetal mortality. The possibility exists that spontaneous abortion may occur if the drug is administered during pregnancy. LUPRON DEPOT-PED is contraindicated in women who are or may become pregnant. If this drug is inadvertently used during pregnancy, or if the patient becomes pregnant while taking this drug, the patient should be apprised of the potential hazard to the fetus.

5 WARNINGS AND PRECAUTIONS

5.1 Initial Rise of Gonadotropins and Sex Steroid Levels
During the early phase of therapy, gonadotropins and sex steroids rise above baseline because of the initial stimulatory effect of the drug. Therefore, an increase in clinical signs and symptoms of puberty may be observed [see Clinical Pharmacology (12.3)].

5.2 Convulsions
Postmarketing reports of convulsions have been observed in patients on leuprolide acetate therapy. These included patients with a history of seizures, epilepsy, cerebrovascular disorders, central nervous system anomalies or tumors, and patients on concomitant medications that have been associated with convulsions such as bupropion and SSRIs. Convulsions have also been reported in patients in the absence of any of the conditions mentioned above.

5.3 Monitoring and Laboratory Tests
Response to LUPRON DEPOT-PED 7.5 mg, 11.25 mg, or 15 mg for 1-month administration should be monitored with a GnRHa stimulation test, basal LH or serum concentration of sex steroid levels beginning 1-2 months following initiation of therapy, with changing doses, or potentially during therapy in order to confirm maintenance of efficacy. Measurement of bone age for advancement should be done every 6-12 months.

Response to LUPRON DEPOT-PED 11.25 mg or 30 mg for 3-month administration should be monitored with a GnRHa stimulation test, basal LH or serum concentration of sex steroid levels at months 2-3, month 6 and further as judged clinically appropriate, to ensure adequate suppression. Additionally, height (for calculation of growth rate) and bone age should be assessed every 6-12 months.

Once a therapeutic dose has been established, gonadotropin and sex steroid levels will decline to prepubertal levels. Gonadotropins and/or sex steroids may increase or rise above prepubertal levels if the dose is inadequate. Noncompliance with drug regimen or inadequate dosing may result in inadequate control of the pubertal process with gonadotropins and/or sex steroids increasing above prepubertal levels [see Clinical Studies (14) and Adverse Reactions (6)].

6 ADVERSE REACTIONS

The most common adverse reactions with GnRH agonists including LUPRON DEPOT-PED 7.5 mg, 11.25 mg, or 15 mg for 1-month administration and LUPRON DEPOT-PED 11.25 mg or 30 mg for 3-month administration are injection site reactions/pain including abscess, general pain, headache, emotional lability and hot flushes/sweating.

During the early phase of therapy, gonadotropins and sex steroids rise above baseline because of the initial stimulatory effect of the drug (hormonal flare effect). Therefore, an increase in clinical signs and symptoms of puberty may be observed [see Warnings and Precautions (5.1)].

6.1 LUPRON DEPOT-PED 7.5 mg, 11.25 mg, or 15 mg for 1-month administration - Clinical Trials Experience
Because clinical studies are conducted under widely varying conditions, adverse reaction rates observed in the clinical studies of a drug cannot be directly compared to rates in the clinical studies of another drug and may not reflect the rates observed in practice.

In two studies of children with central precocious puberty, in 2% or more of the patients receiving the drug, the following adverse reactions were reported to have a possible or probable relationship to drug as ascribed by the treating physician. Reactions which are not considered drug-related are excluded.

Table 2. Percentage of Patients with Treatment-Emergent Adverse Reactions Occurring in ≥ 2% of Pediatric Patients Receiving LUPRON DEPOT-PED 1-month

	Number of Patients (N = 421)	
	N	(%)
Body as a Whole		
Injection Site Reactions Including Abscess*	37	(9)
General Pain	12	(3)
Headache	11	(3)
Cardiovascular System		
Vasodilation	9	(2)
Integumentary System (Skin and Appendages)		
Acne/Seborrhea	13	(3)
Rash Including Erythema Multiforme	12	(3)
Nervous System		
Emotional Lability	19	(5)
Urogenital System		
Vaginitis/Vaginal Bleeding/ Vaginal Discharge	13	(3)

* Most events were mild or moderate in severity.

Less Common Adverse Reactions
The following treatment-emergent adverse reactions were reported in less than 2% of the patients and are listed below by body system.
Body as a Whole – aggravation of preexisting tumor and decreased vision, allergic reaction, body odor, fever, flu syndrome, hypertrophy, infection; Cardiovascular System – bradycardia, hypertension, peripheral vascular disorder, syncope; Digestive System – constipation, dyspepsia, dysphagia, gingivitis, increased appetite, nausea/vomiting; Endocrine System – accelerated sexual maturity, feminization, goiter; Hemic and Lymphatic System – purpura; Metabolic and Nutritional Disorders – growth retarded, peripheral edema, weight gain; Musculoskeletal System – arthralgia, joint disorder, myalgia, myopathy; Nervous System – depression, hyperkinesia, nervousness, somnolence; Respiratory System – asthma, epistaxis, pharyngitis, rhinitis, sinusitis; Integumentary System (Skin and Appendages) – alopecia, hair disorder, hirsutism, leukoderma, nail disorder, skin hypertrophy; Urogenital System – cervix disorder/neoplasm, dysmenorrhea, gynecomastia/breast disorders, menstrual disorder, urinary incontinence.
Laboratory: The following laboratory events were reported as adverse reactions: antinuclear antibody present and increased sedimentation rate.

6.2 LUPRON DEPOT-PED 11.25 mg or 30 mg for 3-month administration - Clinical Trials Experience
Because clinical studies are conducted under widely varying conditions, adverse reaction rates observed in the clinical studies of a drug cannot be directly compared to rates in the clinical studies of another drug and may not reflect the rates observed in practice.
[See table 3 at top of next page]
Less Common Adverse Reactions
The following treatment-emergent adverse reactions were reported in one patient and are listed below by system organ class:
Gastrointestinal Disorders – abdominal pain, nausea; General Disorders and Administration Site Conditions – asthenia, gait disturbance, injection site abscess sterile, injection site hematoma, injection site induration, injection site warmth, irritability; Metabolic and Nutritional Disorders – decreased appetite, obesity; Musculoskeletal and Connective Tissue Disorders - musculoskeletal pain, pain in extremity; Nervous System Disorders – crying, dizziness; Psychiatric Disorders – tearfulness; Respiratory, Thoracic and Mediastinal Disorders – cough; Skin and Subcutaneous Tissue Disorders – hyperhidrosis; Vascular Disorders – pallor.

6.3 Postmarketing
The following adverse events have been observed with this or other formulations of leuprolide acetate injection. As leuprolide has multiple indications, and therefore patient populations, some of these adverse events may not be applicable to every patient.

Allergic reactions (anaphylactic, rash, urticaria, and photo-sensitivity reactions) have also been reported.

Gastrointestinal Disorders: nausea, abdominal pain, vomiting;

General Disorders and Administration Site Conditions: chest pain, injection site reactions including induration and abscess have been reported;

Investigations: decreased WBC, weight increased;

Metabolism and Nutrition Disorders: diabetes mellitus;

Musculoskeletal and Connective Tissue Disorders: tenosynovitis-like symptoms;

Nervous System Disorders: neuropathy peripheral, convulsion, spinal fracture/paralysis;

Skin and Subcutaneous Tissue Disorders: hot flush, flushing, hyperhidrosis;

Reproductive System and Breast Disorders: prostate pain;

Vascular Disorders: hypertension, hypotension.

Pituitary apoplexy: During post-marketing surveillance, rare cases of pituitary apoplexy (a clinical syndrome secondary to infarction of the pituitary gland) have been reported after the administration of gonadotropin-releasing hormone agonists. In a majority of these cases, a pituitary adenoma was diagnosed, with a majority of pituitary apoplexy cases occurring within 2 weeks of the first dose, and some within the first hour. In these cases, pituitary apoplexy has presented as sudden headache, vomiting, visual changes, ophthalmoplegia, altered mental status, and sometimes cardiovascular collapse. Immediate medical attention has been required.

See other LUPRON DEPOT and LUPRON Injection package inserts for other events reported in different patient populations.

7 DRUG INTERACTIONS

No pharmacokinetic-based drug-drug interaction studies have been conducted; however, drug interactions are not expected to occur [see Clinical Pharmacology (12.3)].

7.1 Drug/Laboratory Test Interactions

Administration of LUPRON DEPOT-PED in therapeutic doses results in suppression of the pituitary-gonadal system. Therefore, diagnostic tests of pituitary gonadotropic and gonadal functions conducted during treatment and up to six months after discontinuation of LUPRON DEPOT-PED may be affected. Normal pituitary-gonadal function is usually restored within six months after treatment with LUPRON DEPOT-PED is discontinued.

8 USE IN SPECIFIC POPULATIONS

8.1 Pregnancy

Pregnancy Category X

LUPRON DEPOT-PED is contraindicated in women who are or may become pregnant while receiving the drug [see Contraindications (4)].

Safe use of leuprolide acetate in pregnancy has not been established in clinical studies. Before starting and during treatment with leuprolide acetate, it is advisable to establish whether the patient is pregnant. Leuprolide acetate is not a contraceptive. If contraception is required, a non-hormonal method of contraception should be used.

When LUPRON DEPOT was administered subcutaneously to groups of rabbits as one time dosing on day 6 of pregnancy at test dosages of 0.00024, 0.0024, and 0.024 mg/kg (1/1900 to 1/19 of the human pediatric dose) it produced a dose-related increase in major fetal abnormalities. Similar studies in rats failed to demonstrate an increase in fetal malformations. There was increased fetal mortality and decreased fetal weights with the two higher doses of LUPRON DEPOT in rabbits and with the highest dose in rats. No fetal malformations but increase in fetal resorptions and mortality were observed in rat and rabbit when the daily injection formulation of leuprolide acetate was dosed subcutaneously once daily at lower doses (0.1-1 mcg/kg/day in rabbit; 10 mcg/kg/day in rat) during the period of organogenesis. The effects on fetal mortality are logical consequences of the alterations in hormonal levels brought about by this drug. Therefore, the possibility exists that spontaneous abortion may occur if the drug is administered during pregnancy.

8.3 Nursing Mothers

It is not known whether leuprolide acetate is excreted in human milk. LUPRON DEPOT-PED should not be used by nursing mothers.

8.4 Pediatric Use

Safety and effectiveness in pediatric patients below the age of 2 years have not been established. The use of LUPRON DEPOT-PED in children under 2 years is not recommended.

8.5 Geriatric Use

LUPRON DEPOT 1-month 7.5 mg and 4-month 30 mg are indicated for the palliative treatment of advanced prostate cancer. For LUPRON DEPOT-PED 11.25 mg or 15 mg for 1-month administration and LUPRON DEPOT-PED 11.25 mg or 30 mg for 3-month administration, no clinical information is available for persons aged 65 and over.

Table 3. Percentage of Patients with Treatment-Emergent Adverse Reactions Occurring in ≥ 2 Pediatric Patients Receiving LUPRON DEPOT-PED 11.25 mg or 30 mg for 3-month administration.

	11.25 mg every 3 Months N=42		30 mg every 3 Months N=42		Overall N = 84	
	N	%	N	%	N	%
Injection site pain	8	(19)	9	(21)	17	(20)
Weight increased	3	(7)	3	(7)	6	(7)
Headache	1	(2)	3	(7)	4	(5)
Mood altered	2	(5)	2	(5)	4	(5)
Injection site swelling	1	(2)	1	(2)	2	(2)

10 OVERDOSAGE

In early clinical trials using leuprolide acetate in adult patients, doses as high as 20 mg/day for up to two years caused no adverse effects differing from those observed with the 1 mg/day dose.

In rats, subcutaneous administration of leuprolide acetate as a single dose 225 times the recommended human pediatric dose, expressed on a per body weight basis, resulted in dyspnea, decreased activity, and local irritation at the injection site. There is no evidence at present that there is a clinical counterpart of this phenomenon.

In cases of overdosage, standard of care monitoring and management principles should be followed.

11 DESCRIPTION

Leuprolide acetate is a synthetic nonapeptide analog of naturally occurring gonadotropin-releasing hormone (GnRH or LH-RH). The analog possesses greater potency than the natural hormone. The chemical name is 5-oxo-L-prolyl-L-histidyl-L-tryptophyl-L-seryl-L-tyrosyl-D-leucyl-L-leucyl-L-arginyl-N-ethyl-L-prolinamide acetate (salt) with the following structural formula:

[See chemical structure above]

LUPRON DEPOT-PED 7.5 mg, 11.25 mg, or 15 mg for 1-month administration

LUPRON DEPOT-PED is available in a prefilled dual-chamber syringe containing sterile lyophilized microspheres which, when mixed with diluent, become a suspension intended as a single intramuscular injection.

The front chamber of LUPRON DEPOT-PED 7.5 mg, 11.25 mg, and 15 mg prefilled dual-chamber syringe contains leuprolide acetate (7.5/11.25/15 mg), purified gelatin (1.3/1.95/2.6 mg), DL-lactic and glycolic acids copolymer (66.2/99.3/132.4 mg), and D-mannitol (13.2/19.8/26.4 mg). The second chamber of diluent contains carboxymethylcellulose sodium (5 mg), D-mannitol (50 mg), polysorbate 80 (1 mg), water for injection, USP, and glacial acetic acid, USP to control pH.

LUPRON DEPOT-PED 11.25 mg or 30 mg for 3-month administration

LUPRON DEPOT-PED 11.25 mg or 30 mg for 3-month administration is available in a prefilled dual-chamber syringe containing sterile lyophilized microspheres which, when mixed with diluent, become a suspension intended as an intramuscular injection to be given **ONCE EVERY THREE MONTHS**.

The front chamber of LUPRON DEPOT-PED 11.25 mg for 3-month administration prefilled dual-chamber syringe contains leuprolide acetate (11.25 mg), polylactic acid (99.3 mg) and D-mannitol (19.45 mg). The second chamber of diluent contains carboxymethylcellulose sodium (7.5 mg), D-mannitol (75.0 mg), polysorbate 80 (1.5 mg), water for injection, USP, and glacial acetic acid, USP to control pH.

The front chamber of LUPRON DEPOT-PED 30 mg for 3-month administration prefilled dual-chamber syringe contains leuprolide acetate (30 mg), polylactic acid (264.8 mg) and D-mannitol (51.9 mg). The second chamber of diluent contains carboxymethylcellulose sodium (7.5 mg), D-mannitol (75.0 mg), polysorbate 80 (1.5 mg), water for injection, USP, and glacial acetic acid, USP to control pH.

12 CLINICAL PHARMACOLOGY

12.1 Mechanism of Action

Leuprolide acetate, a GnRH agonist, acts as a potent inhibitor of gonadotropin secretion when given continuously and in therapeutic doses. Human studies indicate that following an initial stimulation of gonadotropins, chronic stimulation with leuprolide acetate results in suppression or "downregulation" of these hormones and consequent suppression of ovarian and testicular steroidogenesis. These effects are reversible on discontinuation of drug therapy.

Leuprolide acetate is not active when given orally.

12.3 Pharmacokinetics

Absorption

LUPRON DEPOT-PED 7.5 mg, 11.25 mg, or 15 mg for 1-month administration

Following a single LUPRON DEPOT-PED 7.5 mg for 1-month administration to adult patients, mean peak leuprolide plasma concentration was almost 20 ng/mL at 4 hours and then declined to 0.36 ng/mL at 4 weeks. However, intact leuprolide and an inactive major metabolite could not be distinguished by the assay which was employed in the study. Nondetectable leuprolide plasma concentrations have been observed during chronic LUPRON DEPOT-PED 7.5 mg administration, but testosterone levels appear to be maintained at castrate levels.

In a study of 55 children with central precocious puberty, doses of 7.5 mg, 11.25 mg and 15.0 mg of LUPRON DEPOT-PED were given every 4 weeks and in a subset of 22 children, trough leuprolide plasma levels were determined according to weight categories as summarized below:

Patient Weight Range (kg)	Group Weight Average (kg)	Dose (mg)	Trough Plasma Leuprolide Level Mean ±SD (ng/mL)*
20.2 - 27.0	22.7	7.5	0.77±0.033
28.4 - 36.8	32.5	11.25	1.25±1.06
39.3 - 57.5	44.2	15.0	1.59±0.65

* Group average values determined at Week 4 immediately prior to leuprolide injection. Drug levels at 12 and 24 weeks were similar to respective 4 week levels.

LUPRON DEPOT-PED 11.25 mg or 30 mg for 3-month administration

Following a single LUPRON DEPOT-PED 11.25 mg or 30 mg for 3-month administration to children with CPP, leuprolide concentrations increased with increasing dose with mean peak leuprolide plasma concentration of 19.1

Information on the AbbVie, Inc. products listed on these pages is from the prescribing information in use as of July 31, 2014. For more information, please visit rxabbvie.com or call 1-800-633-9110.

Table 5. Suppression of Peak-Stimulated LH from Month 2 Through Month 6

Parameter	LUPRON DEPOT-PED 11.25 mg every 3 Months			LUPRON DEPOT-PED 30 mg every 3 Months		
	Naïve N = 21	Prev Trt[a] N = 21	Total N = 42	Naïve N = 21	Prev Trt[a] N = 21	Total N = 42
Percent with Suppression	76.2	81.0	78.6	90.5	100	95.2
2-sided 95% CI	52.8, 91.8	58.1, 94.6	63.2, 89.7	69.6, 98.8	83.9, 100	83.8, 99.4

a. Previously treated with GnRHa for at least 6 months prior to enrollment in pivotal Study L-CP07-167.

and 52.5 ng/mL at 1 hour for the 11.25 and 30 mg dose levels, respectively. The concentrations then declined to 0.08 and 0.25 ng/mL at 2 weeks after dosing for the 11.25 and 30 mg dose levels. Mean leuprolide plasma concentration remained constant from month 1 to month 3 for both 11.25 and 30 mg doses. The mean leuprolide concentrations 3 months after the first and second injections were similar indicating no accumulation of leuprolide from repeated administration.

Distribution

The mean steady-state volume of distribution of leuprolide following intravenous bolus administration to healthy male volunteers was 27 L. *In vitro* binding to human plasma proteins ranged from 43% to 49%.

Metabolism

In healthy male volunteers, a 1 mg bolus of leuprolide administered intravenously revealed that the mean systemic clearance was 7.6 L/h, with a terminal elimination half-life of approximately 3 hours based on a two compartment model.

In rats and dogs, administration of ^{14}C-labeled leuprolide was shown to be metabolized to smaller inactive peptides; a pentapeptide (Metabolite I), tripeptides (Metabolites II and III) and a dipeptide (Metabolite IV). These fragments may be further catabolized.

The major metabolite (M-I) plasma concentrations measured in 5 prostate cancer patients reached maximum concentration 2 to 6 hours after dosing and were approximately 6% of the peak parent drug concentration. One week after dosing, mean plasma M-I concentrations were approximately 20% of mean leuprolide concentrations.

Excretion

Following administration of LUPRON DEPOT 3.75 mg to 3 patients, less than 5% of the dose was recovered as parent and M-I metabolite in the urine.

Specific Populations

The pharmacokinetics of LUPRON DEPOT-PED has not been determined in patients with hepatic or renal impairment.

Drug-Drug Interactions

No pharmacokinetic-based drug-drug interaction studies have been conducted with LUPRON DEPOT-PED. However, because leuprolide acetate is a peptide that is primarily degraded by peptidase and not by cytochrome P-450 enzymes as noted in specific studies, and the drug is only about 46% bound to plasma proteins, drug interactions are not expected to occur.

13 NONCLINICAL TOXICOLOGY

13.1 Carcinogenesis, Mutagenesis, Impairment of Fertility

A two-year carcinogenicity study was conducted in rats and mice. In rats, a dose-related increase of benign pituitary hyperplasia and benign pituitary adenomas was noted at 24 months when the drug was administered subcutaneously at high daily doses (0.6 to 4 mg/kg). There was a significant but not dose-related increase of pancreatic islet-cell adenomas in females and of testicular interstitial cell adenomas in males (highest incidence in the low dose group). In mice, no leuprolide acetate-induced tumors or pituitary abnormalities were observed at a dose as high as 60 mg/kg for two years. Adult patients have been treated with leuprolide acetate for up to three years with doses as high as 10 mg/day and for two years with doses as high as 20 mg/day without demonstrable pituitary abnormalities.

Following subcutaneous administration of LUPRON DEPOT to male and female rats before mating there was atrophy of the reproductive organs and suppression of reproductive performance.

Following a study with leuprolide acetate, immature male rats demonstrated tubular degeneration in the testes even after a recovery period. In spite of the failure to recover histologically, the treated males proved to be as fertile as the controls. Also, no histologic changes were observed in the female rats following the same protocol. In both sexes, the offspring of the treated animals appeared normal. The effect of the treatment of the parents on the reproductive performance of the F1 generation has been evaluated using LUPRON DEPOT formulation to groups of rats as one-time subcutaneous dose of 0.024 mg/kg (1/19 of the pediatric

dose) on Day 15 of gestation or dosing on parturition day at doses up to 8 mg/kg (18 fold of the pediatric dose). There was no effect on growth, morphological development and reproductive performance of F1 generation.

14 CLINICAL STUDIES

14.1 LUPRON DEPOT-PED 7.5 mg, 11.25 mg, or 15 mg for 1-month administration

In children with central precocious puberty (CPP), therapeutic doses of LUPRON DEPOT-PED reduce stimulated and basal gonadotropins to prepubertal levels. Testosterone and estradiol are also reduced to prepubertal levels in males and females respectively. Reduction of gonadotropins and sex steroids allow a return to age-appropriate physical and psychological growth and development. The following effects have been noted with the chronic administration of leuprolide: cessation of menses (in girls), normalization and stabilization of linear growth and bone age advancement, stabilization of clinical signs and symptoms of puberty.

55 CPP subjects (49 females and 6 males, naïve to previous GnRHa treatment), were treated with LUPRON DEPOT-PED 1-month formulations until age appropriate for entry into puberty (see treatment period data below) and a subset of 40 subjects were then followed post-treatment (see follow-up period data below).

Treatment Period Data:

During the treatment period, LUPRON DEPOT-PED suppressed gonadotropins and sex steroids to prepubertal levels. Suppression of peak stimulated LH concentrations to < 1.75 mIU/mL was achieved in 96% of subjects by month 1. Five subjects required increased doses of study drug to achieve or retain LH suppression. The number and percentage of subjects with suppression of peak stimulated LH < 1.75 mIU/mL and mean ± SD peak stimulated LH over time is shown in Table 4. The mean ± SD age at the start of treatment was 7 ± 2 years and the duration of treatment was 4 ± 2 years. Six months after the treatment period was finished, the mean peak stimulated LH was 20.6 ± SD 13.7 mIU/mL (n=30).

Table 4. The number and percentage of patients with peak stimulated LH < 1.75 mIU/mL and Mean (SD) peak LH at each clinic visit

Weeks on Study	n with peak stimulated LH < 1.75 mIU/mL/N with a LH measurement for that week		Mean (SD) peak LH
	n/N	%	
Baseline	0/55	0%	35.0 (21.32)
Week 4	53/55	96.4%	0.8 (0.57)
Week 12	48/54	88.9%	1.1 (1.77)
Week 24	48/53	90.6%	0.8 (0.79)
Week 36	51/54	94.4%	0.6 (0.43)
Week 48	51/54	94.4%	0.6 (0.47)
Week 72	52/52	100%	0.5 (0.30)
Week 96	46/46	100%	0.4 (0.33)
Week 120	40/40	100%	0.4 (0.27)
Week 144	36/36	100%	0.4 (0.24)
Week 168	27/28	96.4%	1.2 (4.58)
Week 216	18/19	94.7%	0.5 (0.90)
Week 240	16/17	94.1%	0.4 (0.62)
Week 264	14/15	95.3%	0.4 (0.41)
Week 288	11/11	100%	0.3 (0.22)
Week 312	9/9	100%	0.4 (0.20)
Week 336	6/6	100%	0.3 (0.10)
Week 360	6/6	100%	0.3 (0.13)
Week 384	5/5	100%	0.2 (0.10)
Week 408	3/3	100%	0.2 (0.09)
Week 432	2/2	100%	0.3 (0.04)
Week 456	2/2	100%	0.2 (0.04)
Week 480	1/1	100%	0.2 (NA)
Week 504	1/1	100%	0.2 (NA)

Suppression (defined as regression or no change) of the clinical/physical signs of puberty was achieved in most patients. In females, suppression of breast development ranged from 66.7 to 90.6% of subjects during the first 5 years of treatment. The mean stimulated estradiol was 15.1 pg/mL at baseline, decreased to the lower level of detection (5.0 pg/mL) by Week 4 and was maintained there during the first 5 years of treatment. In males, suppression of genitalia development ranged from 60% to 100% of subjects during the first 5 years of treatment. The mean stimulated testosterone was 347.7 ng/dL at baseline and was maintained at levels no greater than 25.3 ng/dL during the first 5 years of treatment.

A "flare effect" of transient bleeding or spotting during the first 4 weeks of treatment was observed in 19.4% (7/36) females who had not reached menarche at baseline. After the first 4 weeks for the remainder of the treatment period, no subject reported menstrual-like bleeding, and only rare spotting was noted.

In many subjects, growth rate decreased on treatment, as did bone age: chronological age ratio. Through year 5, the mean growth rate ranged between 3.4 and 5.6 cm/yr. The mean ratio of bone age to chronological age decreased from 1.5 at baseline to 1.1 by end of treatment. The mean height standard deviation score changed from 1.6 at baseline to 0.7 at the end of the treatment phase.

Follow-up Period Data:

35 females and 5 males participated in a post-treatment follow-up period to assess reproductive function (in females) and final height. At 6 months post-treatment, most subjects reverted to pubertal levels of LH (87.9%) and clinical signs of resumption of pubertal progression were evident with increase in breast development in girls (66.7%) and increase in genitalia development in boys (80%).

Of the 40 patients evaluated in the follow-up, 33 were observed until they reached final or near-final adult height. These patients had a mean increase in final adult height compared to baseline predicted adult height. The mean final adult height standard deviation score was -0.2.

After stopping treatment, regular menses were reported for all female subjects who reached 12 years of age during follow-up; mean time to menses was approximately 1.5 years; mean age of onset of menstruation after stopping treatment was 12.9 years. Data to assess reproductive function was collected in a post-study survey of 20 girls who reached adulthood (ages 18-26): menstrual cycles were reported to be normal in 80% of women; 12 pregnancies were reported for a total of 7 of the 20 subjects, including multiple pregnancies for 4 subjects.

14.2 LUPRON DEPOT-PED 11.25 mg or 30 mg for 3-month administration

In a randomized, open-label clinical study of LUPRON DEPOT-PED 3-Month formulations, 84 subjects (76 female, 8 male) between 1 and 11 years of age received the LUPRON DEPOT-PED 11.25 mg or 30 mg for 3-month administration formulation. Each dose group had an equal number of treatment-naïve patients who had pubertal LH levels and patients previously treated with GnRHa therapies who had prepubertal LH levels at the time of study entry. The percentage of subjects with suppression of peak-stimulated LH to < 4.0 mIU/mL, as determined by assessments at months 2, 3 and 6 is 78.6% in the 11.25 mg dose and 95.2% in the 30 mg dose as shown in Table 5.

[See table 5 above]

The mean peak stimulated LH levels for all visits are shown by dose and subgroup (naïve vs. previously treated subjects) in Figures 1 and 2.

[See figure 1 at top of next page]

[See figure 2 at top of next page]

For the LUPRON DEPOT-PED 11.25 mg dose for 3-month administration, 93% (39/42) of subjects and for LUPRON DEPOT-PED 30 mg dose for 3-month administration 100% (42/42) of subjects had sex steroid (estradiol or testosterone) suppressed to prepubertal levels at all visits. Clinical suppression of puberty in female patients was observed in 29 of 32 (90.6%) and 28 of 34 (82.4%) of patients in the 11.25 mg and 30 mg groups, respectively, at month 6. Clinical suppression of puberty in males was observed in 1 of 2 (50.0%)

Figure 1. Mean Peak Stimulated LH for LUPRON DEPOT-PED 11.25 mg for 3-month administration

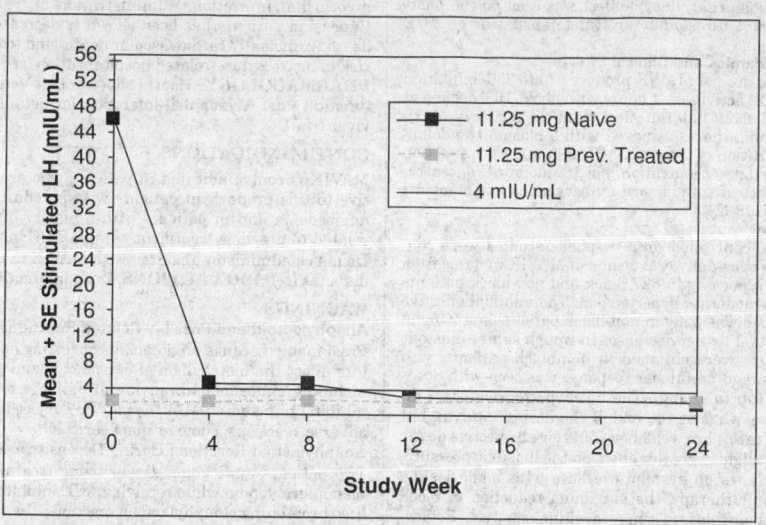

- During the first weeks of treatment, signs of puberty, e.g., vaginal bleeding, may occur. This is a common initial effect of the drug. If these symptoms continue beyond the second month of treatment, the physician should be notified.
- The most common side effects related to treatment with LUPRON DEPOT-PED for 1-month or 3-month administration in clinical studies are: pain, acne/seborrhea, injection site reactions including pain, swelling and abscess, rash including erythema multiforme, vaginitis/bleeding/discharge, increased weight, headache, and altered mood.
- After injection, some pain and irritation is expected; however if more severe symptoms occur, the physician should be contacted. Any unusual signs or symptoms should be reported to the physician.
- The parents should notify the physician if new or worsened symptoms develop after beginning treatment.

Manufactured for
AbbVie Inc.
North Chicago, IL 60064
by Takeda Pharmaceutical Company Limited
Osaka, Japan 540-8645
™ - Trademark
® - Registered Trademark
Ref: 03-A822-R23-Revised: June, 2013
©2013 AbbVie Inc.
Shown in Product Identification Guide, page 303

Figure 2. Mean Peak Stimulated LH for LUPRON DEPOT-PED 30 mg for 3-month administration

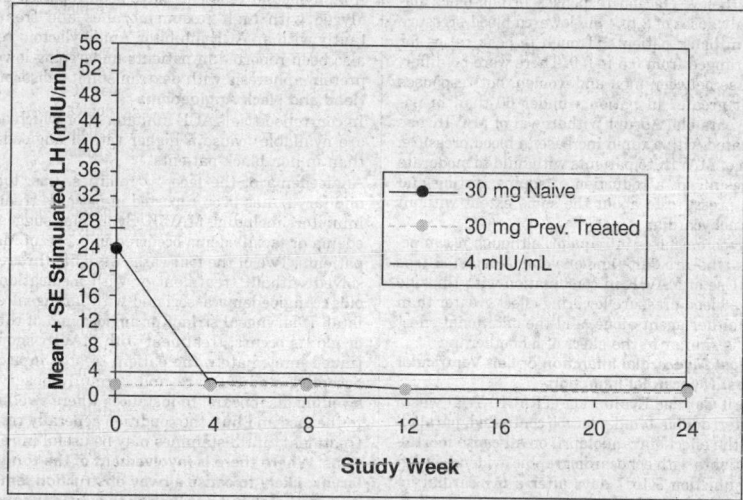

MAVIK® ℞
[*MAH-vic*]
(trandolapril tablets)

> **WARNING: FETAL TOXICITY**
> - When pregnancy is detected, discontinue MAVIK as soon as possible.
> - Drugs that act directly on the renin-angiotensin system can cause injury and death to the developing fetus (See **WARNINGS: Fetal Toxicity**).

DESCRIPTION
Trandolapril is the ethyl ester prodrug of a nonsulfhydryl angiotensin converting enzyme (ACE) inhibitor, trandolaprilat. Trandolapril is chemically described as (2S, 3aR, 7aS)-1-[(S)-N-[(S)-1-Carboxy-3-phenylpropyl]alanyl] hexahydro-2-indolinecarboxylic acid, 1-ethyl ester. Its empirical formula is $C_{24}H_{34}N_2O_5$ and its structural formula is

M.W. = 430.54
Melting Point = 125°C
Trandolapril is a white or almost white powder that is soluble (> 100 mg/mL) in chloroform, dichloromethane, and methanol. MAVIK tablets contain 1 mg, 2 mg, or 4 mg of trandolapril for oral administration. Each tablet also contains corn starch, croscarmellose sodium, hypromellose, iron oxide, lactose monohydrate, povidone, sodium stearyl fumarate.

CLINICAL PHARMACOLOGY
Mechanism of Action
Trandolapril is deesterified to the diacid metabolite, trandolaprilat, which is approximately eight times more active as an inhibitor of ACE activity. ACE is a peptidyl dipeptidase that catalyzes the conversion of angiotensin I to the vasoconstrictor, angiotensin II. Angiotensin II is a potent peripheral vasoconstrictor that also stimulates secretion of aldosterone by the adrenal cortex and provides negative feedback for renin secretion. The effect of trandolapril in hypertension appears to result primarily from the inhibition of circulating and tissue ACE activity thereby reducing angiotensin II formation, decreasing vasoconstriction, decreasing aldosterone secretion, and increasing plasma renin. Decreased aldosterone secretion leads to diuresis, natriuresis, and a small increase in serum potassium. In controlled clin-

and 2 of 5 (40.0%) patients in the 11.25 mg and 30 mg groups, respectively, at month 6. In subjects with complete data for bone age, 29 of 33 (87.9 %) in the 11.25 mg group and 30 of 40 in the 30 mg group (75.0%) had a decrease in the ratio of bone age to chronological age at month 6 compared to screening.

16 HOW SUPPLIED/STORAGE AND HANDLING

LUPRON DEPOT-PED 7.5 mg, 11.25 mg, or 15 mg for 1-month administration is packaged as follows:

1-month Kit with prefilled dual-chamber syringe	7.5 mg	NDC 0074-2108-03
1-month Kit with prefilled dual-chamber syringe	11.25 mg	NDC 0074-2282-03
1-month Kit with prefilled dual-chamber syringe	15 mg	NDC 0074-2440-03

LUPRON DEPOT-PED 11.25 mg or 30 mg for 3-month administration is packaged as follows:

3-month Kit with prefilled dual-chamber syringe	11.25 mg	NDC 0074-3779-03
3-month Kit with prefilled dual-chamber syringe	30 mg	NDC 0074-9694-03

LUPRON DEPOT-PED prefilled syringe for 1-month administration contains sterile lyophilized microspheres of leuprolide acetate incorporated in a biodegradable lactic acid/glycolic acid copolymer.

LUPRON DEPOT-PED prefilled syringe for 3-month administration contains sterile lyophilized microspheres of leuprolide acetate incorporated in a biodegradable lactic acid polymer.
When mixed with 1 milliliter of accompanying diluent, LUPRON DEPOT-PED for 1-month administration is administered as a single intramuscular injection. When mixed with 1.5 milliliter of accompanying diluent, LUPRON DEPOT-PED for 3-month administration is administered as a single intramuscular injection.
Each kit contains:
- one prefilled dual-chamber syringe containing 1½ inch needle with LuproLoc® safety device
- one plunger
- two alcohol swabs
- population, dose and frequency confirmation insert
- a complete prescribing information enclosure
Store at 25°C (77°F); excursions permitted to 15-30°C (59-86°F) [See USP Controlled Room Temperature]

17 PATIENT COUNSELING INFORMATION
Information for Parents
Prior to starting therapy with LUPRON DEPOT-PED, patients should be informed that:
- All formulations are contraindicated in women who are or may become pregnant. If this drug is used during pregnancy, or if the patient becomes pregnant while taking the drug, the patient should be informed of the potential risk to the fetus.
- Continuous therapy is important and that adherence to the recommended drug administration schedule (monthly for LUPRON DEPOT-PED for 1-month administration and every three months for LUPRON DEPOT-PED for 3-month administration) must be accepted if therapy is to be successful. If the injection schedule is not followed, pubertal development may begin again.

Information on the AbbVie, Inc. products listed on these pages is from the prescribing information in use as of July 31, 2014. For more information, please visit rxabbvie.com or call 1-800-633-9110.

ical trials, treatment with MAVIK alone resulted in mean increases in potassium of 0.1 mEq/L (see **PRECAUTIONS.**)

ACE is identical to kininase II, an enzyme that degrades bradykinin, a potent peptide vasodilator; whether increased levels of bradykinin play a role in the therapeutic effect of trandolapril remains to be elucidated.

While the principal mechanism of antihypertensive effect is thought to be through the renin-angiotensin-aldosterone system, trandolapril exerts antihypertensive actions even in patients with low-renin hypertension. MAVIK was an effective antihypertensive in all races studied. Both black patients (usually a predominantly low-renin group) and non-black patients responded to 2 to 4 mg of MAVIK.

Pharmacokinetics and Metabolism
Pharmacokinetics

Trandolapril's ACE-inhibiting activity is primarily due to its diacid metabolite, trandolaprilat. Cleavage of the ester group of trandolapril, primarily in the liver, is responsible for conversion. Absolute bioavailability after oral administration of trandolapril is about 10% as trandolapril and 70% as trandolaprilat. After oral trandolapril under fasting conditions, peak trandolapril levels occur at about one hour and peak trandolaprilat levels occur between 4 and 10 hours. The elimination half-life of trandolapril is about 6 hours. At steady state, the effective half-life of trandolaprilat is 22.5 hours. Like all ACE inhibitors, trandolaprilat also has a prolonged terminal elimination phase, involving a small fraction of administered drug, probably representing binding to plasma and tissue ACE. During multiple dosing of trandolapril, there is no significant accumulation of trandolaprilat. Food slows absorption of trandolapril, but does not affect AUC or C_{max} of trandolaprilat or C_{max} of trandolapril.

Metabolism and Excretion

After oral administration of trandolapril, about 33% of parent drug and metabolites are recovered in urine, mostly as trandolaprilat, with about 66% in feces. The extent of the absorbed dose which is biliary excreted has not been determined. Plasma concentrations (C_{max} and AUC of trandolapril and C_{max} of trandolaprilat) are dose proportional over the 1-4 mg range, but the AUC of trandolaprilat is somewhat less than dose proportional. In addition to trandolaprilat, at least 7 other metabolites have been found, principally glucuronides or deesterification products.

Serum protein binding of trandolapril is about 80%, and is independent of concentration. Binding of trandolaprilat is concentration-dependent, varying from 65% at 1000 ng/mL to 94% at 0.1 ng/mL, indicating saturation of binding with increasing concentration.

The volume of distribution of trandolapril is about 18 liters. Total plasma clearances of trandolapril and trandolaprilat after approximately 2 mg IV doses are about 52 liters/hour and 7 liters/hour respectively. Renal clearance of trandolaprilat varies from 1-4 liters/hour, depending on dose.

Special Populations
Pediatric

Trandolapril pharmacokinetics have not been evaluated in patients < 18 years of age.

Geriatric and Gender

Trandolapril pharmacokinetics have been investigated in the elderly (> 65 years) and in both genders. The plasma concentration of trandolapril is increased in elderly hypertensive patients, but the plasma concentration of trandolaprilat and inhibition of ACE activity are similar in elderly and young hypertensive patients. The pharmacokinetics of trandolapril and trandolaprilat and inhibition of ACE activity are similar in male and female elderly hypertensive patients.

Race

Pharmacokinetic differences have not been evaluated in different races.

Renal Insufficiency

Compared to normal subjects, the plasma concentrations of trandolapril and trandolaprilat are approximately 2-fold greater and renal clearance is reduced by about 85% in patients with creatinine clearance below 30 ml/min and in patients on hemodialysis. Dosage adjustment is recommended in renally impaired patients (see **DOSAGE AND ADMINISTRATION**).

Hepatic Insufficiency

Following oral administration in patients with mild to moderate alcoholic cirrhosis, plasma concentrations of trandolapril and trandolaprilat were, respectively, 9-fold and 2-fold greater than in normal subjects, but inhibition of ACE activity was not affected. Lower doses should be considered in patients with hepatic insufficiency (see **DOSAGE AND ADMINISTRATION**).

Drug Interactions

Trandolapril did not affect the plasma concentration (predose and 2 hours post-dose) of oral digoxin (0.25 mg). Coadministration of trandolapril and cimetidine led to an increase of about 44% in C_{max} for trandolapril, but no difference in the pharmacokinetics of trandolaprilat or in

ACE inhibition. Coadministration of trandolapril and furosemide led to an increase of about 25% in the renal clearance of trandolaprilat, but no effect was seen on the pharmacokinetics of furosemide or trandolaprilat or on ACE inhibition.

Pharmacodynamics and Clinical Effects
A single 2-mg dose of MAVIK produces 70 to 85% inhibition of plasma ACE activity at 4 hours with about 10% decline at 24 hours and about half the effect manifest at 8 days. Maximum ACE inhibition is achieved with a plasma trandolaprilat concentration of 2 ng/mL. ACE inhibition is a function of trandolaprilat concentration, not trandolapril concentration. The effect of trandolapril on exogenous angiotensin I was not measured.

Hypertension

Four placebo-controlled dose response studies were conducted using once-daily oral dosing of MAVIK in doses from 0.25 to 16 mg per day in 827 black and non-black patients with mild to moderate hypertension. The minimal effective once-daily dose was 1 mg in non-black patients and 2 mg in black patients. Further decreases in trough supine diastolic blood pressure were obtained in non-black patients with higher doses, and no further response was seen with doses above 4 mg (up to 16 mg). The antihypertensive effect diminished somewhat at the end of the dosing interval, but trough/peak ratios are well above 50% for all effective doses. There was a slightly greater effect on the diastolic pressure, but no difference on systolic pressure with b.i.d. dosing. During chronic therapy, the maximum reduction in blood pressure with any dose is achieved within one week. Following 6 weeks of monotherapy in placebo-controlled trials in patients with mild to moderate hypertension, once-daily doses of 2 to 4 mg lowered supine or standing systolic/diastolic blood pressure 24 hours after dosing by an average 7-10/4-5 mmHg below placebo responses in non-black patients. Once-daily doses of 2 to 4 mg lowered blood pressure 4-6/3-4 mmHg in black patients. Trough to peak ratios for effective doses ranged from 0.5 to 0.9. There were no differences in response between men and women, but responses were somewhat greater in patients under 60 than in patients over 60 years old. Abrupt withdrawal of MAVIK has not been associated with a rapid increase in blood pressure. Administration of MAVIK to patients with mild to moderate hypertension results in a reduction of supine, sitting and standing blood pressure to about the same extent without compensatory tachycardia.

Symptomatic hypotension is infrequent, although it can occur in patients who are salt- and/or volume-depleted (see **WARNINGS**). Use of MAVIK in combination with thiazide diuretics gives a blood pressure lowering effect greater than that seen with either agent alone, and the additional effect of trandolapril is similar to the effect of monotherapy.

Heart Failure Post Myocardial Infarction or Left Ventricular Dysfunction Post Myocardial Infarction
The Trandolapril Cardiac Evaluation (TRACE) Trial was a Danish, 27-center, double-blind, placebo controlled, parallel-group study of the effect of trandolapril on all-cause mortality in stable patients with echocardiographic evidence of left ventricular dysfunction 3 to 7 days after a myocardial infarction. Subjects with residual ischemia or overt heart failure were included. Patients tolerant of a test dose of 1 mg trandolapril were randomized to placebo (n=873) or trandolapril (n=876) and followed for 24 months. Among patients randomized to trandolapril, who began treatment on 1 mg, 62% were successfully titrated to a target dose of 4 mg once daily over a period of weeks. The use of trandolapril was associated with a 16% reduction in the risk of all-cause mortality (p=0.042), largely cardiovascular mortality. Trandolapril was also associated with a 20% reduction in the risk of progression of heart failure (p=0.047), defined by a time-to-first-event analysis of death attributed to heart failure, hospitalization for heart failure, or requirement for open-label ACE inhibitor for the treatment of heart failure. There was no significant effect of treatment on other endpoints: subsequent hospitalization, incidence of recurrent myocardial infarction, exercise tolerance, ventricular function, ventricular dimensions, or NYHA class.

The population in TRACE was entirely Caucasian and had less usage than would be typical in a U.S. population of other post-infarction interventions: 42% thrombolysis, 16% beta-adrenergic blockade, and 6.7% PTCA or CABG during the entire period of follow-up. Blood pressure control, especially in the placebo group, was poor: 47 to 53% of patients randomized to placebo and 32 to 40% of patients randomized to trandolapril had blood pressures > 140/95 at 90-day follow-up visits.

INDICATIONS AND USAGE
Hypertension

MAVIK is indicated for the treatment of hypertension. It may be used alone or in combination with other antihypertensive medication such as hydrochlorothiazide.

Heart Failure Post Myocardial Infarction or Left-Ventricular Dysfunction Post Myocardial Infarction
MAVIK is indicated in stable patients who have evidence of left-ventricular systolic dysfunction (identified by wall mo-

tion abnormalities) or who are symptomatic from congestive heart failure within the first few days after sustaining acute myocardial infarction. Administration of trandolapril to Caucasian patients has been shown to decrease the risk of death (principally cardiovascular death) and to decrease the risk of heart failure-related hospitalization (see **CLINICAL PHARMACOLOGY - Heart Failure or Left-Ventricular Dysfunction Post Myocardial Infarction** for details of the survival trial).

CONTRAINDICATIONS
MAVIK is contraindicated in patients who are hypersensitive to this product, in patients with hereditary/idiopathic angioedema and in patients with a history of angioedema related to previous treatment with an ACE inhibitor.

Do not co-administer aliskiren with MAVIK in patients with diabetes (see **PRECAUTIONS, Drug Interactions**).

WARNINGS
Anaphylactoid and Possibly Related Reactions

Presumably because angiotensin converting enzyme inhibitors affect the metabolism of eicosanoids and polypeptides, including endogenous bradykinin, patients receiving ACE inhibitors, including MAVIK, may be subject to a variety of adverse reactions, some of them serious.

Anaphylactoid Reactions During Desensitization

Two patients undergoing desensitizing treatment with hymenoptera venom while receiving ACE inhibitors sustained life-threatening anaphylactoid reactions. In the same patients, these reactions did not occur when ACE inhibitors were temporarily withheld, but they reappeared when the ACE inhibitors were inadvertently readministered.

Anaphylactoid Reactions During Membrane Exposure

Anaphylactoid reactions have been reported in patients dialyzed with high-flux membranes and treated concomitantly with an ACE inhibitor. Anaphylactoid reactions have also been reported in patients undergoing low-density lipoprotein apheresis with dextran sulfate absorption.

Head and Neck Angioedema

In controlled trials ACE inhibitors (for which adequate data are available) cause a higher rate of angioedema in black than in non-black patients.

Angioedema of the face, extremities, lips, tongue, glottis, and larynx has been reported in patients treated with ACE inhibitors, including MAVIK. Symptoms suggestive of angioedema or facial edema occurred in 0.13% of MAVIK-treated patients. Two of the four cases were life-threatening and resolved without treatment or with medication (corticosteroids). Angioedema associated with laryngeal edema can be fatal. If laryngeal stridor or angioedema of the face, tongue or glottis occurs, treatment with MAVIK should be discontinued immediately, the patient treated in accordance with accepted medical care and carefully observed until the swelling disappears. In instances where swelling is confined to the face and lips, the condition generally resolves without treatment; antihistamines may be useful in relieving symptoms. **Where there is involvement of the tongue, glottis, or larynx, likely to cause airway obstruction, emergency therapy, including but not limited to subcutaneous epinephrine solution 1:1,000 (0.3 to 0.5 mL) should be promptly administered** (see **PRECAUTIONS - Information for Patients** and **ADVERSE REACTIONS**).

Intestinal Angioedema

Intestinal angioedema has been reported in patients treated with ACE inhibitors. These patients presented with abdominal pain (with or without nausea or vomiting); in some cases there was no prior history of facial angioedema and C-1 esterase levels were normal. The angioedema was diagnosed by procedures including abdominal CT scan or ultrasound, or at surgery, and symptoms resolved after stopping the ACE inhibitor. Intestinal angioedema should be included in the differential diagnosis of patients on ACE inhibitors presenting with abdominal pain.

Hypotension

MAVIK can cause symptomatic hypotension. Like other ACE inhibitors, MAVIK has only rarely been associated with symptomatic hypotension in uncomplicated hypertensive patients. Symptomatic hypotension is most likely to occur in patients who have been salt- or volume-depleted as a result of prolonged treatment with diuretics, dietary salt restriction, dialysis, diarrhea, or vomiting. Volume and/or salt depletion should be corrected before initiating treatment with MAVIK (see **PRECAUTIONS - Drug Interactions** and **ADVERSE REACTIONS**). In controlled and uncontrolled studies, hypotension was reported as an adverse event in 0.6% of patients and led to discontinuations in 0.1% of patients.

In patients with concomitant congestive heart failure, with or without associated renal insufficiency, ACE inhibitor therapy may cause excessive hypotension, which may be associated with oliguria or azotemia, and rarely, with acute renal failure and death. In such patients, MAVIK therapy should be started at the recommended dose under close medical supervision. These patients should be followed closely during the first 2 weeks of treatment and, thereafter, whenever the dosage of MAVIK or diuretic is increased (see **DOSAGE AND ADMINISTRATION**). Care in avoiding hypotension should also be taken in patients with ischemic heart disease, aortic stenosis, or cerebrovascular disease.

If symptomatic hypotension occurs, the patient should be placed in the supine position and, if necessary, normal saline may be administered intravenously. A transient hypotensive response is not a contraindication to further doses; however, lower doses of MAVIK or reduced concomitant diuretic therapy should be considered.

Neutropenia/Agranulocytosis

Another ACE inhibitor, captopril, has been shown to cause agranulocytosis and bone marrow depression rarely in patients with uncomplicated hypertension, but more frequently in patients with renal impairment, especially if they also have a collagen-vascular disease such as systemic lupus erythematosus or scleroderma. Available data from clinical trials of trandolapril is insufficient to show that trandolapril does not cause agranulocytosis at similar rates. As with other ACE inhibitors, periodic monitoring of white blood cell counts in patients with collagen-vascular disease and/or renal disease should be considered.

Hepatic Failure

ACE inhibitors rarely have been associated with a syndrome of cholestatic jaundice, fulminant hepatic necrosis, and death. The mechanism of this syndrome is not understood. Patients receiving ACE inhibitors who develop jaundice should discontinue the ACE inhibitor and receive appropriate medical follow-up.

Fetal Toxicity

Pregnancy Category D

Use of drugs that act on the renin-angiotensin system during the second and third trimesters of pregnancy reduces fetal renal function and increases fetal and neonatal morbidity and death. Resulting oligohydramnios can be associated with fetal lung hypoplasia and skeletal deformations. Potential neonatal adverse effects include skull hypoplasia, anuria, hypotension, renal failure, and death. When pregnancy is detected, discontinue MAVIK as soon as possible. These adverse outcomes are usually associated with use of these drugs in the second and third trimester of pregnancy. Most epidemiologic studies examining fetal abnormalities after exposure to antihypertensive use in the first trimester have not distinguished drugs affecting the renin-angiotensin system from other antihypertensive agents. Appropriate management of maternal hypertension during pregnancy is important to optimize outcomes for both mother and fetus.

In the unusual case that there is no appropriate alternative to therapy with drugs affecting the renin-angiotensin system for a particular patient, apprise the mother of the potential risk to the fetus. Perform serial ultrasound examinations to assess the intra-amniotic environment. If oligohydramnios is observed, discontinue MAVIK, unless it is considered lifesaving for the mother. Fetal testing may be appropriate, based on the week of pregnancy. Patients and physicians should be aware, however, that oligohydramnios may not appear until after the fetus has sustained irreversible injury. Closely observe infants with histories of in utero exposure to MAVIK for hypotension, oliguria, and hyperkalemia (See **PRECAUTIONS, Pediatric Use**).

Doses of 0.8 mg/kg/day (9.4 mg/m^2/day) in rabbits, 1000 mg/kg/day (7000 mg/m^2/day) in rats, and 25 mg/kg/day (295 mg/m^2/day) in cynomolgus monkeys did not produce teratogenic effects. These doses represent 10 and 3 times (rabbits), 1250 and 2564 times (rats), and 312 and 108 times (monkeys) the maximum projected human dose of 4 mg based on body-weight and body-surface-area, respectively assuming a 50 kg woman.

PRECAUTIONS

General

Impaired Renal Function

As a consequence of inhibiting the renin-angiotensin-aldosterone system, changes in renal function may be anticipated in susceptible individuals. In patients with severe heart failure whose renal function may depend on the activity of the renin-angiotensin-aldosterone system, treatment with ACE inhibitors, including MAVIK® (trandolapril), may be associated with oliguria and/or progressive azotemia and rarely with acute renal failure and/or death.

In hypertensive patients with unilateral or bilateral renal artery stenosis, increases in blood urea nitrogen and serum creatinine have been observed in some patients following ACE inhibitor therapy. These increases were almost always reversible upon discontinuation of the ACE inhibitor and/or diuretic therapy. In such patients, renal function should be monitored during the first few weeks of therapy.

Some hypertensive patients with no apparent preexisting renal vascular disease have developed increases in blood urea and serum creatinine, usually minor and transient, especially when ACE inhibitors have been given concomitantly with a diuretic. This is more likely to occur in pa-

tients with preexisting renal impairment. Dosage reduction and/or discontinuation of any diuretic and/or the ACE inhibitor may be required. **Evaluation of hypertensive patients should always include assessment of renal function** (see **DOSAGE AND ADMINISTRATION**).

Hyperkalemia and Potassium-sparing Diuretics

In clinical trials, hyperkalemia (serum potassium > 6.00 mEq/L) occurred in approximately 0.4% of hypertensive patients receiving MAVIK. In most cases, elevated serum potassium levels were isolated values, which resolved despite continued therapy. None of these patients were discontinued from the trials because of hyperkalemia. Risk factors for the development of hyperkalemia include renal insufficiency, diabetes mellitus, and the concomitant use of potassium-sparing diuretics, potassium supplements, and/or potassium-containing salt substitutes, which should be used cautiously, if at all, with MAVIK (see **PRECAUTIONS - Drug Interactions**).

Cough

Presumably due to the inhibition of the degradation of endogenous bradykinin, persistent nonproductive cough has been reported with all ACE inhibitors, always resolving after discontinuation of therapy. ACE inhibitor-induced cough should be considered in the differential diagnosis of cough. In controlled trials of trandolapril, cough was present in 2% of trandolapril patients and 0% of patients given placebo. There was no evidence of a relationship to dose.

Surgery/Anesthesia

In patients undergoing major surgery or during anesthesia with agents that produce hypotension, MAVIK will block angiotensin II formation secondary to compensatory renin release. If hypotension occurs and is considered to be due to this mechanism, it can be corrected by volume expansion.

Information for Patients

Angioedema

Angioedema, including laryngeal edema, may occur at any time during treatment with ACE inhibitors, including MAVIK. Patients should be so advised and told to report immediately any signs or symptoms suggesting angioedema (swelling of face, extremities, eyes, lips, tongue, difficulty in swallowing or breathing) and to stop taking the drug until they have consulted with their physician (see **WARNINGS** and **ADVERSE REACTIONS**).

Symptomatic Hypotension

Patients should be cautioned that light-headedness can occur, especially during the first days of MAVIK therapy, and should be reported to a physician. If actual syncope occurs, patients should be told to stop taking the drug until they have consulted with their physician (see **WARNINGS**).

All patients should be cautioned that inadequate fluid intake, excessive perspiration, diarrhea, or vomiting, resulting in reduced fluid volume, may precipitate an excessive fall in blood pressure with the same consequences of light-headedness and possible syncope.

Patients planning to undergo any surgery and/or anesthesia should be told to inform their physician that they are taking an ACE inhibitor that has a long duration of action.

Hyperkalemia

Patients should be told not to use potassium supplements or salt substitutes containing potassium without consulting their physician (see **PRECAUTIONS**).

Neutropenia

Patients should be told to report promptly any indication of infection (e.g., sore throat, fever) which could be a sign of neutropenia.

Pregnancy

Female patients of childbearing age should be told about the consequences of exposure to MAVIK during pregnancy. Discuss treatment options with women planning to become pregnant. Patients should be asked to report pregnancies to their physicians as soon as possible.

NOTE: As with many other drugs, certain advice to patients being treated with MAVIK is warranted. This information is intended to aid in the safe and effective use of this medication. It is not a disclosure of all possible adverse or intended effects.

Drug Interactions

Dual Blockade of the Renin-Angiotensin System (RAS)

Dual blockade of the RAS with angiotensin receptor blockers, ACE inhibitors, or aliskiren is associated with increased risks of hypotension, hyperkalemia, and changes in renal function (including acute renal failure) compared to monotherapy. Closely monitor blood pressure, renal function and electrolytes in patients on MAVIK and other agents that affect the RAS.

Do not co-administer aliskiren with MAVIK in patients with diabetes. Avoid use of aliskiren with MAVIK in patients with renal impairment (GFR <60 ml/min).

Concomitant Diuretic Therapy

As with other ACE inhibitors, patients on diuretics, especially those on recently instituted diuretic therapy, may experience an excessive reduction of blood pressure after initiation of therapy with MAVIK. The possibility of exacerbation of hypotensive effects with MAVIK may be

minimized by either discontinuing the diuretic or cautiously increasing salt intake prior to initiation of treatment with MAVIK. If it is not possible to discontinue the diuretic, the starting dose of trandolapril should be reduced (see **DOSAGE AND ADMINISTRATION**).

Agents Increasing Serum Potassium

Trandolapril can attenuate potassium loss caused by thiazide diuretics and increase serum potassium when used alone. Use of potassium-sparing diuretics (spironolactone, triamterene, or amiloride), potassium supplements, or potassium-containing salt substitutes concomitantly with ACE inhibitors can increase the risk of hyperkalemia. If concomitant use of such agents is indicated, they should be used with caution and with appropriate monitoring of serum potassium (see **PRECAUTIONS**).

Antidiabetic Agents

Concomitant use of ACE inhibitors and antidiabetic medicines (insulin or oral hypoglycemic agents) may cause an increased blood glucose lowering effect with greater risk of hypoglycemia.

Lithium

Increased serum lithium levels and symptoms of lithium toxicity have been reported in patients receiving concomitant lithium and ACE inhibitor therapy. These drugs should be coadministered with caution, and frequent monitoring of serum lithium levels is recommended. If a diuretic is also used, the risk of lithium toxicity may be increased.

Non-Steroidal Anti-Inflammatory Agents including Selective Cyclooxygenase-2 Inhibitors (COX-2 Inhibitors)

In patients who are elderly, volume-depleted (including those on diuretic therapy), or with compromised renal function, co-administration of NSAIDs, including selective COX-2 inhibitors, with ACE inhibitors, including trandolapril, may result in deterioration of renal function, including possible acute renal failure. These effects are usually reversible. Monitor renal function periodically in patients receiving trandolapril and NSAID therapy.

The antihypertensive effect of ACE inhibitors, including trandolapril may be attenuated by NSAIDs.

Gold

Nitritoid reactions (symptoms include facial flushing, nausea, vomiting and hypotension) have been reported rarely in patients on therapy with injectable gold (sodium aurothiomalate) and concomitant ACE inhibitor therapy including MAVIK.

Other

No clinically significant pharmacokinetic interaction has been found between trandolaprilat and food, cimetidine, digoxin, or furosemide.

The anticoagulant effect of warfarin was not significantly changed by trandolapril.

The hypotensive effect of certain inhalation anesthetics may be enhanced by ACE inhibitors including trandolapril (see **PRECAUTIONS-Surgery/Anesthesia**).

Carcinogenesis, Mutagenesis, Impairment of Fertility

Long-term studies were conducted with oral trandolapril administered by gavage to mice (78 weeks) and rats (104 and 106 weeks). No evidence of carcinogenic potential was seen in mice dosed up to 25 mg/kg/day (85 mg/m^2/day) or rats dosed up to 8 mg/kg/day (60 mg/m^2/day). These doses are 313 and 32 times (mice), and 100 and 23 times (rats) the maximum recommended human daily dose (MRHDD) of 4 mg based on body-weight and body-surface-area, respectively assuming a 50 kg individual. The genotoxic potential of trandolapril was evaluated in the microbial mutagenicity (Ames) test, the point mutation and chromosome aberration assays in Chinese hamster V79 cells, and the micronucleus test in mice. There was no evidence of mutagenic or clastogenic potential in these in vitro and in vivo assays.

Reproduction studies in rats did not show any impairment of fertility at doses up to 100 mg/kg/day (710 mg/m^2/day) of trandolapril, or 1250 and 260 times the MRHDD on the basis of body-weight and body-surface-area, respectively.

Nursing Mothers

Radiolabeled trandolapril or its metabolites are secreted in rat milk. MAVIK should not be administered to nursing mothers.

Geriatric Use

In placebo-controlled studies of MAVIK, 31.1% of patients were 60 years and older, 20.1% were 65 years and older, and 2.3% were 75 years and older. No overall differences in effectiveness or safety were observed between these patients and younger patients. (Greater sensitivity of some older individual patients cannot be ruled out).

Pediatric Use

Neonates with a history of in utero exposure to MAVIK: If oliguria or hypotension occurs, direct attention toward support of blood pressure and renal perfusion. Exchange

---

Information on the AbbVie, Inc. products listed on these pages is from the prescribing information in use as of July 31, 2014. For more information, please visit rxabbvie.com or call 1-800-633-9110.

TOURO COLLEGE LIBRARY

transfusions or dialysis may be required as a means of reversing hypotension and/or substituting for disordered renal function.

The safety and effectiveness of MAVIK in pediatric patients have not been established.

ADVERSE REACTIONS

The safety experience in U.S. placebo-controlled trials included 1069 hypertensive patients, of whom 832 received MAVIK. Nearly 200 hypertensive patients received MAVIK for over one year in open-label trials. In controlled trials, withdrawals for adverse events were 2.1% on placebo and 1.4% on MAVIK. Adverse events considered at least possibly related to treatment occurring in 1% of MAVIK-treated patients and more common on MAVIK than placebo, pooled for all doses, are shown below, together with the frequency of discontinuation of treatment because of these events.

ADVERSE EVENTS IN PLACEBO-CONTROLLED HYPERTENSION TRIALS

	Occurring at 1% or greater	
	MAVIK (N=832) % Incidence (% Discontinuance)	PLACEBO (N=237) % Incidence (% Discontinuance)
Cough	1.9 (0.1)	0.4 (0.4)
Dizziness	1.3 (0.2)	0.4 (0.4)
Diarrhea	1.0 (0.0)	0.4 (0.0)

Headache and fatigue were all seen in more than 1% of MAVIK-treated patients but were more frequently seen on placebo. Adverse events were not usually persistent or difficult to manage.

Left Ventricular Dysfunction Post Myocardial Infarction

Adverse reactions related to MAVIK occurring at a rate greater than that observed in placebo-treated patients with left ventricular dysfunction, are shown below. The incidences represent the experiences from the TRACE study. The follow-up time was between 24 and 50 months for this study.

Percentage of Patients with Adverse Events Greater Than Placebo

Adverse Event	Placebo-Controlled (TRACE) Mortality Study	
	Trandolapril N=876	Placebo N=873
Cough	35	22
Dizziness	23	17
Hypotension	11	6.8
Elevated serum uric acid	15	13
Elevated BUN	9.0	7.6
PICA or CABG	7.3	6.1
Dyspepsia	6.4	6.0
Syncope	5.9	3.3
Hyperkalemia	5.3	2.8
Bradycardia	4.7	4.4
Hypocalcemia	4.7	3.9
Myalgia	4.7	3.1
Elevated creatinine	4.7	2.4
Gastritis	4.2	3.6
Cardiogenic shock	3.8	< 2
Intermittent claudication	3.8	< 2
Stroke	3.3	3.2
Asthenia	3.3	2.6

Clinical adverse experiences possibly or probably related or of uncertain relationship to therapy occurring in 0.3% to 1.0% (except as noted) of the patients treated with MAVIK (with or without concomitant calcium ion antagonist or diuretic) in controlled or uncontrolled trials (N=1134) and less frequent, clinically significant events seen in clinical trials or post-marketing experience include (listed by body system):
General Body Function
Chest pain.
Cardiovascular
AV first degree block, bradycardia, edema, flushing, and palpitations.
Central Nervous System
Drowsiness, insomnia, paresthesia, vertigo.
Dermatologic
Pruritus, rash, pemphigus.
Eye, Ear, Nose, Throat
Epistaxis, throat inflammation, upper respiratory tract infection.

Emotional, Mental, Sexual States
Anxiety, impotence, decreased libido.
Gastrointestinal
Abdominal distention, abdominal pain/cramps, constipation, dyspepsia, diarrhea, vomiting, nausea.
Hemopoietic
Decreased leukocytes, decreased neutrophils.
Metabolism and Endocrine
Increased liver enzymes including SGPT (ALT).
Musculoskeletal System
Extremity pain, muscle cramps, gout.
Pulmonary
Dyspnea.

Postmarketing

The following adverse reactions were identified during post approval use of MAVIK. Because these reactions are reported voluntarily from a population of uncertain size, it is not always possible to reliably estimate their frequency or establish a causal relationship to drug exposure.
General Body Function
Malaise, fever.
Cardiovascular
Myocardial infarction, myocardial ischemia, angina pectoris, cardiac failure, ventricular tachycardia, tachycardia, transient ischemic attack, arrhythmia.
Central Nervous System
Cerebral hemorrhage.
Dermatologic
Alopecia, sweating, Stevens-Johnson syndrome and toxic epidermal necrolysis.
Emotional, Mental, Sexual States
Hallucination, depression.
Gastrointestinal
Dry mouth, pancreatitis, jaundice and hepatitis.
Hemopoietic
Agranulocytosis, pancytopenia.
Metabolism and Endocrine
Increased SGOT (AST).
Pulmonary
Bronchitis.
Renal and Urinary
Renal failure.
Clinical Laboratory Test Findings
Hematology
Thrombocytopenia.
Serum Electrolytes
Hyponatremia.
Creatinine and Blood Urea Nitrogen
Increases in creatinine levels occurred in 1.1% of patients receiving MAVIK alone and 7.3% of patients treated with MAVIK, a calcium ion antagonist and a diuretic. Increases in blood urea nitrogen levels occurred in 0.6% of patients receiving MAVIK alone and 1.4% of patients receiving MAVIK, a calcium ion antagonist, and a diuretic. None of these increases required discontinuation of treatment. Increases in these laboratory values are more likely to occur in patients with renal insufficiency or those pretreated with a diuretic and, based on experience with other ACE inhibitors, would be expected to be especially likely in patients with renal artery stenosis (see **PRECAUTIONS** and **WARNINGS**).
Liver Function Tests
Occasional elevation of transaminases at the rate of 3X upper normals occurred in 0.8% of patients and persistent increase in bilirubin occurred in 0.2% of patients. Discontinuation for elevated liver enzymes occurred in 0.2% of patients.

Other

Another potentially important adverse experience, eosinophilic pneumonitis, has been attributed to other ACE inhibitors.

OVERDOSAGE

No data are available with respect to overdosage in humans. The oral LD_{50} of trandolapril in mice was 4875 mg/Kg in males and 3990 mg/Kg in females. In rats, an oral dose of 5000 mg/Kg caused low mortality (1 male out of 5; 0 females). In dogs, an oral dose of 1000 mg/Kg did not cause mortality and abnormal clinical signs were not observed. In humans, the most likely clinical manifestation would be symptoms attributable to severe hypotension. Symptoms also expected with ACE inhibitors are hypotension, hyperkalemia, and renal failure.
Laboratory determinations of serum levels of trandolapril and its metabolites are not widely available, and such determinations have, in any event, no established role in the management of trandolapril overdose. No data are available to suggest that physiological maneuvers (e.g., maneuvers to change the pH of the urine) might accelerate elimination of trandolapril and its metabolites. Trandolaprilat is removed by hemodialysis. Angiotensin II could presumably serve as a specific antagonist antidote in the setting of trandolapril overdose, but angiotensin II is essentially unavailable outside of scattered research facilities. Because the hypoten-

sive effect of trandolapril is achieved through vasodilation and effective hypovolemia, it is reasonable to treat trandolapril overdose by infusion of normal saline solution.

DOSAGE AND ADMINISTRATION

Hypertension

The recommended initial dosage of MAVIK for patients not receiving a diuretic is 1 mg once daily in non-black patients and 2 mg in black patients. Dosage should be adjusted according to the blood pressure response. Generally, dosage adjustments should be made at intervals of at least 1 week. Most patients have required dosages of 2 to 4 mg once daily. There is little clinical experience with doses above 8 mg. Patients inadequately treated with once-daily dosing at 4 mg may be treated with twice-daily dosing. If blood pressure is not adequately controlled with MAVIK monotherapy, a diuretic may be added.

In patients who are currently being treated with a diuretic, symptomatic hypotension occasionally can occur following the initial dose of MAVIK. To reduce the likelihood of hypotension, the diuretic should, if possible, be discontinued two to three days prior to beginning therapy with MAVIK (see **WARNINGS**). Then, if blood pressure is not controlled with MAVIK alone, diuretic therapy should be resumed. If the diuretic cannot be discontinued, an initial dose of 0.5 mg MAVIK should be used with careful medical supervision for several hours until blood pressure has stabilized. The dosage should subsequently be titrated (as described above) to the optimal response (see **WARNINGS, PRECAUTIONS,** and **DRUG INTERACTIONS**).

Concomitant administration of MAVIK with potassium supplements, potassium salt substitutes, or potassium sparing diuretics can lead to increases of serum potassium (see **PRECAUTIONS**).

Heart Failure Post Myocardial Infarction or Left-Ventricular Dysfunction Post Myocardial Infarction

The recommended starting dose is 1 mg, once daily. Following the initial dose, all patients should be titrated (as tolerated) toward a target dose of 4 mg, once daily. If a 4 mg dose is not tolerated, patients can continue therapy with the greatest tolerated dose.

Dosage Adjustment in Renal Impairment or Hepatic Cirrhosis

For patients with a creatinine clearance < 30 mL/min. or with hepatic cirrhosis, the recommended starting dose, based on clinical and pharmacokinetic data, is 0.5 mg daily. Patients should subsequently have their dosage titrated (as described above) to the optimal response.

HOW SUPPLIED

MAVIK® (trandolapril tablets) are supplied as follows:
1 mg tablet - Salmon colored, round shaped, scored, compressed tablets, with the "a" logo on one side and code identification letters FT on the other side. NDC 0074-2278-13 - bottles of 100 NDC 0074-2278-11 - unit dose packs of 100
2 mg tablet - Yellow colored, round shaped, compressed tablets, with the "a" logo on one side and code identification letters FX on the other side. NDC 0074-2279-13 - bottles of 100 NDC 0074-2279-11 - unit dose packs of 100
4 mg tablet - Rose colored, round shaped, compressed tablets, with the "a" logo on one side and code identification letters FZ on the other side. NDC 0074-2280-13 - bottles of 100 NDC 0074-2280-11 - unit dose packs of 100
Dispense in well-closed container with safety closure.

Storage

Store at controlled room temperature: 20-25°C (68-77°F) see USP.

Manufactured by
Halo Pharmaceutical Inc.
Whippany, N.J. 07981, U.S.A.
for
AbbVie Inc.
North Chicago, IL 60064, U.S.A.
03-A670 December 2012
Shown in Product Identification Guide, page 304

MODERIBA™

[mah-duh-RYE-bah]
[ribavirin, USP]
tablet, film coated

R

HIGHLIGHTS OF PRESCRIBING INFORMATION

These highlights do not include all the information needed to use Moderiba (ribavirin, USP) safely and effectively. See full prescribing information for Moderiba (ribavirin, USP).
Moderiba™ (ribavirin, USP) Tablets
Initial U.S. Approval: 2002

> **WARNING: RISK OF SERIOUS DISORDERS AND RIBAVIRIN-ASSOCIATED EFFECTS**
> *See full prescribing information for complete boxed warning*
> • Ribavirin monotherapy, including Moderiba (ribavirin, USP), is not effective for the treatment of chronic hepatitis C virus infection (Boxed Warning).

- The hemolytic anemia associated with ribavirin therapy may result in worsening of cardiac disease and lead to fatal and nonfatal myocardial infarctions. Patients with a history of significant or unstable cardiac disease should not be treated with Moderiba (ribavirin, USP) (2.3, 5.2, 6.1).
- Significant teratogenic and embryocidal effects have been demonstrated in all animal species exposed to ribavirin. Therefore, Moderiba (ribavirin, USP) is contraindicated in women who are pregnant and in the male partners of women who are pregnant. Extreme care must be taken to avoid pregnancy during therapy and for 6 months after completion of treatment in both female patients and in female partners of male patients who are taking Moderiba (ribavirin, USP) therapy (4, 5.1, 8.1).

INDICATIONS AND USAGE

Moderiba (ribavirin, USP) is a nucleoside analogue indicated for the treatment of chronic hepatitis C (CHC) virus infection in combination with peginterferon alfa-2a in adults with compensated liver disease not previously treated with interferon alpha, and in CHC patients coinfected with HIV (1)

DOSAGE AND ADMINISTRATION

- CHC: Moderiba (ribavirin, USP) is administered according to body weight and genotype (2.1)
- CHC with HIV coinfection: 800 mg by mouth daily for a total of 48 weeks, regardless of genotype (2.2)
- Dose reduction or discontinuation is recommended in patients experiencing certain adverse reactions or renal impairment (2.4, 2.5)

DOSAGE FORMS AND STRENGTHS

- Moderiba (ribavirin, USP) tablets 200 mg (3)
- Moderiba (ribavirin, USP) tablets 400 mg (3)
- Moderiba (ribavirin, USP) tablets 600 mg (3)

CONTRAINDICATIONS

- Pregnant women and men whose female partners are pregnant (4, 5.1, 8.1)
- Hemoglobinopathies (4)
- Coadministration with didanosine (4, 7.1)

Moderiba (ribavirin, USP) in combination with peginterferon alfa-2a is contraindicated in patients with:

- Autoimmune hepatitis (4)
- Hepatic decompensation in cirrhotic patients (4, 5.3)

WARNINGS AND PRECAUTIONS

- Birth defects and fetal death with ribavirin: Do not use in pregnancy and for 6 months after treatment. Patients must have a negative pregnancy test prior to therapy, use at least 2 forms of contraception and undergo monthly pregnancy tests (4, 5.1, 8.1)

Peginterferon alfa-2a/Moderiba (ribavirin, USP): Patients exhibiting the following conditions should be closely monitored and may require dose reduction or discontinuation of therapy:

- Hemolytic anemia may occur with a significant initial drop in hemoglobin. This may result in worsening cardiac disease leading to fatal or nonfatal myocardial infarctions (5.2, 6.1)
- Risk of hepatic failure and death: Monitor hepatic function during treatment and discontinue treatment for hepatic decompensation (5.3)
- Severe hypersensitivity reactions including urticaria, angioedema, bronchoconstriction, and anaphylaxis, and serious skin reactions such as Stevens-Johnson Syndrome (5.4)
- Pulmonary disorders, including pulmonary function impairment and pneumonitis, including fatal cases of pneumonia (5.6)
- Severe depression and suicidal ideation, autoimmune and infectious disorders, suppression of bone marrow function, pancreatitis, and diabetes (5)
- Bone marrow suppression with azathioprine coadministration (5.7)

ADVERSE REACTIONS

The most common adverse reactions (frequency > 40%) in adults receiving combination therapy are fatigue/asthenia, pyrexia, myalgia, and headache (6.1)

To report SUSPECTED ADVERSE REACTIONS, contact AbbVie Inc. at 1-800-633-9110 or FDA at 1-800-FDA-1088 or www.fda.gov/medwatch

DRUG INTERACTIONS

- Nucleoside analogues: Closely monitor for toxicities. Discontinue nucleoside reverse transcriptase inhibitors or reduce dose or discontinue interferon, ribavirin or both with worsening toxicities (7.1)

- Azathioprine: Concomitant use of azathioprine with ribavirin has been reported to induce severe pancytopenia and may increase the risk of azathioprine-related myelotoxicity (7.3)

USE IN SPECIFIC POPULATIONS

- Ribavirin Pregnancy Registry: 1-800-593-2214
- Pediatrics: Safety and efficacy in patients < 18 years old have not been established (8.4)
- Renal Impairment: Do not use in patients with GFR < 50 mL/min (8.7)
- Organ transplant: Safety and efficacy have not been studied (8.10)

See 17 for PATIENT COUNSELING INFORMATION and Medication Guide

Revised: 11/2013

FULL PRESCRIBING INFORMATION: CONTENTS*
WARNING: RISK OF SERIOUS DISORDERS AND RIBAVIRIN-ASSOCIATED EFFECTS
*Sections or subsections omitted from the full prescribing information are not listed

FULL PRESCRIBING INFORMATION

WARNING: RISK OF SERIOUS DISORDERS AND RIBAVIRIN-ASSOCIATED EFFECTS

Moderiba (ribavirin, USP) monotherapy is not effective for the treatment of chronic hepatitis C virus infection and should not be used alone for this indication.

The primary clinical toxicity of ribavirin is hemolytic anemia. The anemia associated with ribavirin therapy may result in worsening of cardiac disease and lead to fatal and nonfatal myocardial infarctions. Patients with a history of significant or unstable cardiac disease should not be treated with Moderiba (ribavirin, USP) [see Warnings and Precautions (5.2), Adverse Reactions (6.1), and Dosage and Administration (2.3)].

Significant teratogenic and/or embryocidal effects have been demonstrated in all animal species exposed to ribavirin. In addition, ribavirin has a multiple dose half-life of 12 days, and it may persist in nonplasma compartments for as long as 6 months. Therefore, ribavirin, including Moderiba (ribavirin, USP), is contraindicated in women who are pregnant and in the male partners of women who are pregnant. Extreme care must be taken to avoid pregnancy during therapy and for 6 months after completion of therapy in both female patients and in female partners of male patients who are taking ribavirin therapy. At least two reliable forms of effective contraception must be utilized during treatment and during the 6-month post treatment follow-up period [see Contraindications (4), Warnings and Precautions (5.1), and Use in Specific Populations (8.1)].

1   INDICATIONS AND USAGE

Moderiba (ribavirin, USP) in combination with peginterferon alfa-2a is indicated for the treatment of adults with chronic hepatitis C (CHC) virus infection who have compensated liver disease and have not been previously treated with interferon alpha.

The following points should be considered when initiating Moderiba (ribavirin, USP) combination therapy with peginterferon alfa-2a:

- This indication is based on clinical trials of combination therapy in patients with CHC and compensated liver disease, some of whom had histological evidence of cirrhosis (Child-Pugh class A), and in patients with clinically stable HIV disease and CD4 count > 100 cells/mm^3.
- This indication is based on achieving undetectable HCV-RNA after treatment for 24 or 48 weeks, based on HCV genotype, and maintaining a Sustained Virologic Response (SVR) 24 weeks after the last dose.
- Safety and efficacy data are not available for treatment longer than 48 weeks.
- The safety and efficacy of ribavirin and peginterferon alfa-2a therapy have not been established in liver or other organ transplant recipients, patients with decompensated liver disease, or previous non-responders to interferon therapy.
- The safety and efficacy of ribavirin therapy for the treatment of adenovirus, RSV, parainfluenza or influenza infections have not been established. Moderiba (ribavirin, USP) should not be used for these indications. Ribavirin for inhalation has a separate package insert, which should be consulted if ribavirin inhalation therapy is being considered.

2   DOSAGE AND ADMINISTRATION

2.1   Chronic Hepatitis C Monoinfection

The recommended dose of Moderiba (ribavirin, USP) tablets is provided in **Table 1**. The recommended duration of treatment for patients previously untreated with ribavirin and interferon is 24 to 48 weeks.

The daily dose of Moderiba (ribavirin, USP) is 800 mg to 1200 mg administered orally in two divided doses. The dose should be individualized to the patient depending on baseline disease characteristics (e.g., genotype), response to therapy, and tolerability of the regimen (see **Table 1**). Moderiba (ribavirin, USP) should be taken with food.

Table 1 Peginterferon alfa-2a and Moderiba (ribavirin, USP) Dosing Recommendations

Hepatitis C Virus (HCV) Genotype	Peginterferon alfa-2a Dose*	Moderiba (ribavirin, USP) Dose	Duration
Genotypes 1, 4	180 mcg	<75 kg = 1000 mg	48 weeks
		≥75 kg = 1200 mg	48 weeks
Genotypes 2, 3	180 mcg	800 mg	24 weeks

Genotypes 2 and 3 showed no increased response to treatment beyond 24 weeks (see **Table 6**).
Data on genotypes 5 and 6 are insufficient for dosing recommendations.
*See peginterferon alfa-2a Package Insert for further details on peginterferon alfa-2a dosing and administration.

2.2   Chronic Hepatitis C with HIV Coinfection

The recommended dose for treatment of chronic hepatitis C in patients coinfected with HIV is peginterferon alfa-2a

Information on the AbbVie, Inc. products listed on these pages is from the prescribing information in use as of July 31, 2014. For more information, please visit rxabbvie.com or call 1-800-633-9110.

180 mcg subcutaneous once weekly and Moderiba (ribavirin, USP) 800 mg by mouth daily for a total duration of 48 weeks, regardless of HCV genotype.

Moderiba™ (ribavirin, USP) should be taken with food.

2.3 Dose Modifications

If severe adverse reactions or laboratory abnormalities develop during combination Moderiba (ribavirin, USP)/peginterferon alfa-2a therapy, the dose should be modified or discontinued, if appropriate, until the adverse reactions abate or decrease in severity. If intolerance persists after dose adjustment, Moderiba (ribavirin, USP)/peginterferon alfa-2a therapy should be discontinued. **Table 2** provides guidelines for dose modifications and discontinuation based on the patient's hemoglobin concentration and cardiac status.

Moderiba (ribavirin, USP) should be administered with caution to patients with pre-existing cardiac disease. Patients should be assessed before commencement of therapy and should be appropriately monitored during therapy. If there is any deterioration of cardiovascular status, therapy should be stopped [see Warnings and Precautions (5.2)].

Table 2 Moderiba (ribavirin, USP) Dosage Modification Guidelines

Laboratory Values	Reduce Only Moderiba (ribavirin, USP) Dose to 600 mg/day* if:	Discontinue Moderiba (ribavirin, USP) if:
Hemoglobin in patients with no cardiac disease	<10 g/dL	<8.5 g/dL
Hemoglobin in patients with history of stable cardiac disease	≥2 g/dL decrease in hemoglobin during any 4 week period treatment	<12 g/dL despite 4 weeks at reduced dose

*One 200 mg tablet in the morning and either two 200 mg tablets or one 400 mg tablet in the evening.

Once Moderiba (ribavirin, USP) has been withheld due to either a laboratory abnormality or clinical manifestation, an attempt may be made to restart Moderiba (ribavirin, USP) at 600 mg daily and further increase the dose to 800 mg daily. However, it is not recommended that Moderiba (ribavirin, USP) be increased to its original assigned dose (1000 mg to 1200 mg).

See Peginterferon alfa-2a full prescribing information for recommendations on peginterferon alfa-2a dose modification.

2.4 Discontinuation of Dosing

Discontinuation of peginterferon alfa-2a/ Moderiba (ribavirin, USP) therapy should be considered if the patient has failed to demonstrate at least a 2 log₁₀ reduction from baseline in HCV RNA by 12 weeks of therapy, or undetectable HCV RNA levels after 24 weeks of therapy.

Peginterferon alfa-2a/ Moderiba (ribavirin, USP) therapy should be discontinued in patients who develop hepatic decompensation during treatment [see Warnings and Precautions (5.3)].

2.5 Renal Impairment

Moderiba (ribavirin, USP) should not be used in patients with creatinine clearance <50 mL/min [see Use in Specific Populations (8.7)].

3 DOSAGE FORMS AND STRENGTHS

Moderiba (ribavirin, USP) is available as tablets for oral administration.

Each Moderiba (ribavirin, USP) 200-mg tablet contains 200 mg of ribavirin and is a capsule-shaped, light blue colored, film-coated tablet, debossed with "200" on one side and the logo "3RP" on the other side.

Each Moderiba (ribavirin, USP) 400-mg tablet contains 400 mg of ribavirin and is a capsule-shaped, medium blue colored, film-coated tablet, debossed with "400" on one side and the logo "3RP" on the other side.

Each Moderiba (ribavirin, USP) 600-mg tablet contains 600 mg of ribavirin and is a capsule-shaped, dark blue colored, film-coated tablet, debossed with "600" on one side and the logo "3RP" on the other side.

4 CONTRAINDICATIONS

Moderiba (ribavirin, USP) is contraindicated in:

• Women who are pregnant. Moderiba (ribavirin, USP) may cause fetal harm when administered to a pregnant woman. Moderiba (ribavirin, USP) is contraindicated in women who are or may become pregnant. If this drug is used during pregnancy, or if the patient becomes pregnant while taking this drug, the patient should be apprised of the potential hazard to the fetus [see Warnings and Precautions (5.1), Use in Specific Populations (8.1), and Patient Counseling Information (17)].

• Men whose female partners are pregnant.

• Patients with hemoglobinopathies (e.g., thalassemia major or sickle-cell anemia).

• In combination with didanosine. Reports of fatal hepatic failure, as well as peripheral neuropathy, pancreatitis, and symptomatic hyperlactatemia/lactic acidosis have been reported in clinical trials [see Drug Interactions (7.1)].

Moderiba (ribavirin, USP) and peginterferon alfa-2a combination therapy is contraindicated in patients with:

• Autoimmune hepatitis.

• Hepatic decompensation (Child-Pugh score greater than 6; class B and C) in cirrhotic CHC monoinfected patients before treatment [see Warnings and Precautions (5.3)].

• Hepatic decompensation (Child-Pugh score greater than or equal to 6) in cirrhotic CHC patients coinfected with HIV before treatment [see Warnings and Precautions (5.3)].

5 WARNINGS AND PRECAUTIONS

Significant adverse reactions associated with Moderiba (ribavirin, USP)/peginterferon alfa-2a combination therapy include severe depression and suicidal ideation, hemolytic anemia, suppression of bone marrow function, autoimmune and infectious disorders, ophthalmologic disorders, cerebrovascular disorders, pulmonary dysfunction, colitis, pancreatitis, and diabetes.

The Peginterferon alfa-2a Package Insert should be reviewed in its entirety for additional safety information prior to initiation of combination treatment.

5.1 Pregnancy

Moderiba (ribavirin, USP) may cause birth defects and/or death of the exposed fetus. Ribavirin has demonstrated significant teratogenic and/or embryocidal effects in all animal species in which adequate studies have been conducted. These effects occurred at doses as low as one twentieth of the recommended human dose of ribavirin.

Moderiba (ribavirin, USP) therapy should not be started unless a report of a negative pregnancy test has been obtained immediately prior to planned initiation of therapy. Extreme care must be taken to avoid pregnancy in female patients and in female partners of male patients. Patients should be instructed to use at least two forms of effective contraception during treatment and for 6 months after treatment has been stopped. Pregnancy testing should occur monthly during Moderiba (ribavirin, USP) therapy and for 6 months after therapy has stopped [see Boxed Warning, Contraindications (4), Use in Specific Populations (8.1), and Patient Counseling Information (17)].

5.2 Anemia

The primary toxicity of ribavirin is hemolytic anemia, which was observed in approximately 13% of all ribavirin/peginterferon alfa-2a- treated subjects in clinical trials. Anemia associated with ribavirin occurs within 1 to 2 weeks of initiation of therapy. Because the initial drop in hemoglobin may be significant, it is advised that hemoglobin or hematocrit be obtained pretreatment and at week 2 and week 4 of therapy or more frequently if clinically indicated. Patients should then be followed as clinically appropriate. Caution should be exercised in initiating treatment in any patient with baseline risk of severe anemia (e.g., spherocytosis, history of gastrointestinal bleeding) [see Dosage and Administration (2.3)].

Fatal and nonfatal myocardial infarctions have been reported in patients with anemia caused by ribavirin. Patients should be assessed for underlying cardiac disease before initiation of ribavirin therapy. Patients with pre-existing cardiac disease should have electrocardiograms administered before treatment, and should be appropriately monitored during therapy. If there is any deterioration of cardiovascular status, therapy should be suspended or discontinued [see Dosage and Administration (2.3)]. Because cardiac disease may be worsened by drug-induced anemia, patients with a history of significant or unstable cardiac disease should not use Moderiba (ribavirin, USP) [see Boxed Warning, and Dosage and Administration (2.3)].

5.3 Hepatic Failure

Chronic hepatitis C (CHC) patients with cirrhosis may be at risk of hepatic decompensation and death when treated with alpha interferons, including peginterferon alfa-2a. Cirrhotic CHC patients coinfected with HIV receiving highly active antiretroviral therapy (HAART) and interferon alfa-2a with or without ribavirin appear to be at increased risk for the development of hepatic decompensation compared to patients not receiving HAART. In Study NR15961 [see Clinical Studies (14.3)], among 129 CHC/HIV cirrhotic patients receiving HAART, 14 (11%) of these patients across all treatment arms developed hepatic decompensation resulting in 6 deaths. All 14 patients were on NRTIs, including stavudine, didanosine, abacavir, zidovudine, and lamivudine. These small numbers of patients do not permit discrimination between specific NRTIs or the associated risk. During treatment, patients' clinical status and hepatic function should be closely monitored for signs and symptoms of hepatic decompensation. Treatment with peginter-

feron alfa-2a/Moderiba (ribavirin, USP) should be discontinued immediately in patients with hepatic decompensation [see Contraindications (4)].

5.4 Hypersensitivity

Severe acute hypersensitivity reactions (e.g., urticaria, angioedema, bronchoconstriction, and anaphylaxis) have been observed during alpha interferon and ribavirin therapy. If such a reaction occurs, therapy with peginterferon alfa-2a and Moderiba (ribavirin, USP) should be discontinued immediately and appropriate medical therapy instituted. Serious skin reactions including vesiculobullous eruptions, reactions in the spectrum of Stevens-Johnson Syndrome (erythema multiforme major) with varying degrees of skin and mucosal involvement and exfoliative dermatitis (erythroderma) have been reported in patients receiving peginterferon alfa-2a with and without ribavirin. Patients developing signs or symptoms of severe skin reactions must discontinue therapy [see Adverse Reactions (6.2)].

5.5 Renal Impairment

Moderiba (ribavirin, USP) should not be used in patients with creatinine clearance <50 mL/min [see Use in Specific Populations (8.7)].

5.6 Pulmonary Disorders

Dyspnea, pulmonary infiltrates, pneumonitis, pulmonary hypertension, and pneumonia have been reported during therapy with ribavirin and interferon. Occasional cases of fatal pneumonia have occurred. In addition, sarcoidosis or the exacerbation of sarcoidosis has been reported. If there is evidence of pulmonary infiltrates or pulmonary function impairment, patients should be closely monitored and, if appropriate, combination Moderiba (ribavirin, USP)/Peginterferon alfa-2a treatment should be discontinued.

5.7 Bone Marrow Suppression

Pancytopenia (marked decreases in RBCs, neutrophils and platelets) and bone marrow suppression have been reported in the literature to occur within 3 to 7 weeks after the concomitant administration of pegylated interferon/ribavirin and azathioprine. In this limited number of patients (n=8), myelotoxicity was reversible within 4 to 6 weeks upon withdrawal of both HCV antiviral therapy and concomitant azathioprine and did not recur upon reintroduction of either treatment alone. Peginterferon alfa-2a, Moderiba (ribavirin, USP), and azathioprine should be discontinued for pancytopenia, and pegylated interferon/ribavirin should not be reintroduced with concomitant azathioprine [see Drug Interactions (7.3)].

5.8 Pancreatitis

Moderiba (ribavirin, USP) and peginterferon alfa-2a therapy should be suspended in patients with signs and symptoms of pancreatitis, and discontinued in patients with confirmed pancreatitis.

5.9 Laboratory Tests

Before beginning peginterferon alfa-2a/Moderiba (ribavirin, USP) combination therapy, standard hematological and biochemical laboratory tests are recommended for all patients. Pregnancy screening for women of childbearing potential must be performed. Patients who have pre-existing cardiac abnormalities should have electrocardiograms administered before treatment with peginterferon alfa-2a/Moderiba (ribavirin, USP).

After initiation of therapy, hematological tests should be performed at 2 weeks and 4 weeks and biochemical tests should be performed at 4 weeks. Additional testing should be performed periodically during therapy. In the clinical studies, the CBC (including hemoglobin level and white blood cell and platelet counts) and chemistries (including liver function tests and uric acid) were measured at 1, 2, 4, 6, and 8 weeks, and then every 4 to 6 weeks or more frequently if abnormalities were found. Thyroid stimulating hormone (TSH) was measured every 12 weeks. Monthly pregnancy testing should be performed during combination therapy and for 6 months after discontinuing therapy.

The entrance criteria used for the clinical studies of ribavirin and peginterferon alfa-2a may be considered as a guideline to acceptable baseline values for initiation of treatment:

• Platelet count ≥ 90,000 cells/mm³ (as low as 75,000 cells/mm³ in HCV patients with cirrhosis or 70,000 cells/mm³ in patients with CHC and HIV)

• Absolute neutrophil count (ANC) ≥ 1500 cells/mm³

• TSH and T₄ within normal limits or adequately controlled thyroid function

• CD4+ cell count ≥ 200 cells/mcL or CD4+ cell count ≥ 100 cells/mcL but < 200 cells/mcL and HIV-1 RNA <5000 copies/mL in patients coinfected with HIV

• Hemoglobin ≥ 12 g/dL for women and ≥ 13 g/dL for men in CHC monoinfected patients

• Hemoglobin ≥ 11 g/dL for women and ≥ 12 g/dL for men in patients with CHC and HIV

6 ADVERSE REACTIONS

Peginterferon alfa-2a in combination with ribavirin causes a broad variety of serious adverse reactions [see Boxed Warning and Warnings and Precautions (5)]. The most common serious or life-threatening adverse reactions induced or aggravated by ribavirin/peginterferon alfa-2a include depression, suicide, relapse of drug abuse/overdose, and bacterial infections each occurring at a frequency of < 1%. Hepatic decompensation occurred in 2% (10/574) CHC/HIV patients [see Warnings and Precautions (5.3)].

6.1 Clinical Studies Experience

Because clinical trials are conducted under widely varying conditions, adverse reaction rates observed in the clinical trials of a drug cannot be directly compared to rates in the clinical trials of another drug and may not reflect the rates observed in clinical practice.

In the pivotal registration trials NV15801 and NV15942, 886 patients received ribavirin for 48 weeks at doses of 1000/1200 mg based on body weight. In these trials, one or more serious adverse reactions occurred in 10% of CHC monoinfected subjects and in 19% of CHC/HIV subjects receiving peginterferon alfa-2a alone or in combination with ribavirin. The most common serious adverse event (3% in CHC and 5% in CHC/HIV) was bacterial infection (e.g., sepsis, osteomyelitis, endocarditis, pyelonephritis, pneumonia). Other serious adverse reactions occurred at a frequency of <1% and included: suicide, suicidal ideation, psychosis, aggression, anxiety, drug abuse and drug overdose, angina, hepatic dysfunction, fatty liver, cholangitis, arrhythmia, diabetes mellitus, autoimmune phenomena (e.g., hyperthyroidism, hypothyroidism, sarcoidosis, systemic lupus erythematosus, rheumatoid arthritis), peripheral neuropathy, aplastic anemia, peptic ulcer, gastrointestinal bleeding, pancreatitis, colitis, corneal ulcer, pulmonary embolism, coma, myositis, cerebral hemorrhage, thrombotic thrombocytopenic purpura, psychotic disorder, and hallucination.

The percentage of patients in clinical trials who experienced one or more adverse events was 98%. The most commonly reported adverse reactions were psychiatric reactions, including depression, insomnia, irritability, anxiety, and flu-like symptoms such as fatigue, pyrexia, myalgia, headache and rigors. Other common reactions were anorexia, nausea and vomiting, diarrhea, arthralgias, injection site reactions, alopecia, and pruritus. **Table 3** shows rates of adverse events occurring in ≥5% subjects receiving pegylated interferon and ribavirin combination therapy in the CHC Clinical Trial, NV15801.

Ten percent of CHC monoinfected patients receiving 48 weeks of therapy with peginterferon alfa-2a in combination with ribavirin discontinued therapy; 16% of CHC/HIV coinfected patients discontinued therapy. The most common reasons for discontinuation of therapy were psychiatric, flu-like syndrome (e.g., lethargy, fatigue, headache), dermatologic and gastrointestinal disorders and laboratory abnormalities (thrombocytopenia, neutropenia, and anemia).

Overall 39% of patients with CHC or CHC/HIV required modification of peginterferon alfa-2a and/or ribavirin therapy. The most common reason for dose modification of peginterferon alfa-2a in CHC and CHC/HIV patients was for laboratory abnormalities; neutropenia (20% and 27%, respectively) and thrombocytopenia (4% and 6%, respectively). The most common reason for dose modification of ribavirin in CHC and CHC/HIV patients was anemia (22% and 16%, respectively).

Peginteferon alfa-2a dose was reduced in 12% of patients receiving 1000 mg to 1200 mg ribavirin for 48 weeks and in 7% of patients receiving 800 mg ribavirin for 24 weeks. Ribavirin dose was reduced in 21% of patients receiving 1000 mg to 1200 mg ribavirin for 48 weeks and in 12% of patients receiving 800 mg ribavirin for 24 weeks.

Chronic hepatitis C monoinfected patients treated for 24 weeks with peginterferon alfa-2a and 800 mg ribavirin were observed to have lower incidence of serious adverse events (3% vs. 10%), hemoglobin <10g/dL (3% vs. 15%), dose modification of peginterferon alfa-2a (30% vs. 36%) and ribavirin (19% vs. 38%), and of withdrawal from treatment (5% vs. 15%) compared to patients treated for 48 weeks with peginterferon alfa-2a and 1000 mg or 1200 mg ribavirin. On the other hand, the overall incidence of adverse events appeared to be similar in the two treatment groups.

Table 3 Adverse Reactions Occurring in ≥5% of Patients in Chronic Hepatitis C Clinical Trials (Study NV15801)

Body System	CHC Combination Therapy Study NV15801	
	peginterferon alfa-2a 180 mcg + 1000 mg or 1200 mg ribavirin tablets 48 weeks N=451 %	interferon alfa-2b + 1000 mg or 1200 mg ribavirin capsules 48 weeks N=443 %
Application Site Disorders		
Injection site reaction	23	16
Endocrine Disorders		
Hypothyroidism	4	5
Flu-like Symptoms and Signs		
Fatigue/Asthenia	65	68
Pyrexia	41	55
Rigors	25	37
Pain	10	9
Gastrointestinal		
Nausea/Vomiting	25	29
Diarrhea	11	10
Abdominal pain	8	9
Dry mouth	4	7
Dyspepsia	6	5
Hematologic*		
Lymphopenia	14	12
Anemia	11	11
Neutropenia	27	8
Thrombocytopenia	5	<1
Metabolic and Nutritional		
Anorexia	24	26
Weight decrease	10	10
Musculoskeletal, Connective Tissue and Bone		
Myalgia	40	49
Arthralgia	22	23
Back pain	5	5
Neurological		
Headache	43	49
Dizziness (excluding vertigo)	14	14
Memory impairment	6	5
Psychiatric		
Irritability/Anxiety/Nervousness	33	38
Insomnia	30	37
Depression	20	28
Concentration impairment	10	13
Mood alteration	5	6
Resistance Mechanism Disorders		
Overall	12	10
Respiratory, Thoracic and Mediastinal		
Dyspnea	13	14
Cough	10	7
Dyspnea exertional	4	7
Skin and Subcutaneous Tissue		
Alopecia	28	33
Pruritus	19	18
Dermatitis	16	13
Dry skin	10	13
Rash	8	5
Sweating increased	6	5
Eczema	5	4
Visual Disorders		
Vision blurred	5	2

* Severe hematologic abnormalities (lymphocyte <0.5 × 10^9/L; hemoglobin <10 g/dL; neutrophil <0.75 × 10^9/L; platelet <50 × 10^9/L).

Common Adverse Reactions in CHC with HIV Coinfection

The adverse event profile of coinfected patients treated with peginterferon alfa-2a/ribavirin in Study NR15961 was generally similar to that shown for monoinfected patients in Study NV15801 (**Table 3**). Events occurring more frequently in coinfected patients were neutropenia (40%), anemia (14%), thrombocytopenia (8%), weight decrease (16%), and mood alteration (9%).

Laboratory Test Abnormalities

Anemia due to hemolysis is the most significant toxicity of ribavirin therapy. Anemia (hemoglobin <10 g/dL) was observed in 13% of all ribavirin and peginterferon alfa-2a combination-treated patients in clinical trials. The maximum drop in hemoglobin occurred during the first 8 weeks of initiation of ribavirin therapy [see Dosage and Administration (2.3)].

Table 4 Selected Laboratory Abnormalities During Treatment With Ribavirin in Combination With Either Peginterferon alfa-2a or Interferon alfa-2b

Laboratory Parameter	Peginterferon alfa-2a + Ribavirin 1000/1200 mg 48 wks (N=887)	Interferon alfa-2b + Ribavirin 1000/1200 mg 48 wks (N=443)
Neutrophils (×10^9/L)		
1.0 – 1.49	34%	38%
0.5 – 0.99	49%	21%
< 0.5	5%	1%
Platelets (×10^9/L)		
50 – 74.9	11%	4%
20 – 49.9	5%	< 1%
< 20	0	0
Hemoglobin (g/dL)		
8.5 – 9.9	11%	11%
< 8.5	2%	< 1%

6.2 Postmarketing Experience

The following adverse reactions have been identified and reported during post-approval use of peginterferon alfa-2a/ribavirin combination therapy. Because these reactions are reported voluntarily from a population of uncertain size, it is not always possible to reliably estimate their frequency or establish a causal relationship to drug exposure.

Blood and Lymphatic System disorders
Pure red cell aplasia
Ear and Labyrinth disorders
Hearing impairment, hearing loss
Eye disorders
Serous retinal detachment
Immune disorders
Liver and renal graft rejection
Metabolism and Nutrition disorders
Dehydration
Skin and Subcutaneous Tissue disorders
Stevens-Johnson Syndrome (SJS)
Toxic epidermal necrolysis (TEN)

7 DRUG INTERACTIONS

Results from a pharmacokinetic sub-study demonstrated no pharmacokinetic interaction between peginterferon alfa-2a and ribavirin.

7.1 Nucleoside Reverse Transcriptase Inhibitors (NRTIs)

In vitro data indicate ribavirin reduces phosphorylation of lamivudine, stavudine, and zidovudine. However, no pharmacokinetic (e.g., plasma concentrations or intracellular triphosphorylated active metabolite concentrations) or pharmacodynamic (e.g., loss of HIV/HCV virologic suppression) interaction was observed when ribavirin and lamivudine (n=18), stavudine (n=10), or zidovudine (n=6) were co-administered as part of a multi-drug regimen to HCV/HIV coinfected patients.

In Study NR15961 among the CHC/HIV coinfected cirrhotic patients receiving NRTIs cases of hepatic decompensation (some fatal) were observed [see Warnings and Precautions (5.3)].

Patients receiving peginterferon alfa-2a/Moderiba™ (ribavirin, USP) and NRTIs should be closely monitored for treatment associated toxicities. Physicians should refer to prescribing information for the respective NRTIs for guidance regarding toxicity management. In addition, dose reduction or discontinuation of peginterferon alfa-2a, Moderiba (ribavirin, USP) or both should also be considered if worsening toxicities are observed, including hepatic decompensation (e.g., Child-Pugh ≥6) [see Warnings and Precautions (5.3) and Dosage and Administration (2.3)].

Didanosine
Co-administration of Moderiba (ribavirin, USP) and didanosine is contraindicated. Didanosine or its active metabolite (dideoxyadenosine 5'-triphosphate) concentrations are increased when didanosine is co-administered with ribavirin, which could cause or worsen clinical toxicities. Reports of fatal hepatic failure, as well as peripheral neuropathy, pancreatitis, and symptomatic hyperlactatemia/lactic acidosis have been reported in clinical trials [see Contraindications (4)].

Zidovudine
In Study NR15961, patients who were administered zidovudine in combination with peginterferon alfa-2a/ribavirin developed severe neutropenia (ANC <500) and severe anemia (hemoglobin <8 g/dL) more frequently than similar patients

Information on the AbbVie, Inc. products listed on these pages is from the prescribing information in use as of July 31, 2014. For more information, please visit rxabbvie.com or call 1-800-633-9110.

not receiving zidovudine (neutropenia 15% vs. 9%) (anemia 5% vs. 1%). Discontinuation of zidovudine should be considered as medically appropriate.

7.2 Drugs Metabolized by Cytochrome P450
In vitro studies indicate that ribavirin does not inhibit CYP 2C9, CYP 2C19, CYP 2D6 or CYP 3A4.

7.3 Azathioprine
The use of ribavirin to treat chronic hepatitis C in patients receiving azathioprine has been reported to induce severe pancytopenia and may increase the risk of azathioprine-related myelotoxicity. Inosine monophosphate dehydrogenase (IMDH) is required for one of the metabolic pathways of azathioprine. Ribavirin is known to inhibit IMDH, thereby leading to accumulation of an azathioprine metabolite, 6-methylthioinosine monophosphate (6-MTITP), which is associated with myelotoxicity (neutropenia, thrombocytopenia, and anemia). Patients receiving azathioprine with ribavirin should have complete blood counts, including platelet counts, monitored weekly for the first month, twice monthly for the second and third months of treatment, then monthly or more frequently if dosage or other therapy changes are necessary *[see Warnings and Precautions (5.7)]*.

8 USE IN SPECIFIC POPULATIONS

8.1 Pregnancy
Pregnancy: Category X *[see Contraindications (4)]*.
Ribavirin produced significant embryocidal and/or teratogenic effects in all animal species in which adequate studies have been conducted. Malformations of the skull, palate, eye, jaw, limbs, skeleton, and gastrointestinal tract were noted. The incidence and severity of teratogenic effects increased with escalation of the drug dose. Survival of fetuses and offspring was reduced *[see Contraindications (4), Warnings and Precautions (5.1)]*.
In conventional embryotoxicity/teratogenicity studies in rats and rabbits, observed no-effect dose levels were well below those for proposed clinical use (0.3 mg/kg/day for both the rat and rabbit; approximately 0.06 times the recommended daily human dose of ribavirin). No maternal toxicity or effects on offspring were observed in a peri/postnatal toxicity study in rats dosed orally at up to 1 mg/kg/day (approximately 0.01 times the maximum recommended daily human dose of ribavirin).

Treatment and Post treatment: Potential Risk to the Fetus
Ribavirin is known to accumulate in intracellular components from where it is cleared very slowly. It is not known whether ribavirin is contained in sperm, and if so, will exert a potential teratogenic effect upon fertilization of the ova. However, because of the potential human teratogenic effects of ribavirin, male patients should be advised to take every precaution to avoid risk of pregnancy for their female partners.
Moderiba (ribavirin, USP) should not be used by pregnant women or by men whose female partners are pregnant. Female patients of childbearing potential and male patients with female partners of childbearing potential should not receive Moderiba (ribavirin, USP) unless the patient and his/her partner are using effective contraception (two reliable forms) during therapy and for 6 months post therapy *[see Contraindications (4)]*.

Ribavirin Pregnancy Registry
A Ribavirin Pregnancy Registry has been established to monitor maternal-fetal outcomes of pregnancies of female patients and female partners of male patients exposed to ribavirin during treatment and for 6 months following cessation of treatment. Healthcare providers and patients are encouraged to report such cases by calling 1-800-593-2214.

8.3 Nursing Mothers
It is not known whether ribavirin is excreted in human milk. Because many drugs are excreted in human milk and to avoid any potential for serious adverse reactions in nursing infants from ribavirin, a decision should be made either to discontinue nursing or therapy with Moderiba (ribavirin, USP), based on the importance of the therapy to the mother.

8.4 Pediatric Use
Pharmacokinetic evaluations in pediatric patients have not been performed.
Safety and effectiveness of Moderiba (ribavirin, USP) tablets have not been established in patients below the age of 18.

8.5 Geriatric Use
Clinical studies of ribavirin and peginterferon alfa-2a did not include sufficient numbers of subjects aged 65 or over to determine whether they respond differently from younger subjects. Specific pharmacokinetic evaluations for ribavirin in the elderly have not been performed. The risk of toxic reactions to this drug may be greater in patients with impaired renal function. Moderiba (ribavirin, USP) should not be administered to patients with creatinine clearance <50 mL/min.

8.6 Race
A pharmacokinetic study in 42 subjects demonstrated there is no clinically significant difference in ribavirin pharmacokinetics among Black (n=14), Hispanic (n=13) and Caucasian (n=15) subjects.

8.7 Renal Impairment
The pharmacokinetics of ribavirin following administration of ribavirin have not been studied in patients with renal impairment and there are limited data from clinical trials on administration of ribavirin in patients with creatinine clearance <50 mL/min. Therefore, patients with creatinine clearance <50 mL/min should not be treated with ribavirin *[see Warnings and Precautions (5.5) and Dosage and Administration (2.5)]*.

8.8 Hepatic Impairment
The effect of hepatic impairment on the pharmacokinetics of ribavirin following administration of ribavirin has not been evaluated. The clinical trials of ribavirin were restricted to patients with Child-Pugh class A disease.

8.9 Gender
No clinically significant differences in the pharmacokinetics of ribavirin were observed between male and female subjects.
Ribavirin pharmacokinetics, when corrected for weight, are similar in male and female patients.

8.10 Organ Transplant Recipients
The safety and efficacy of peginterferon alfa-2a and ribavirin treatment have not been established in patients with liver and other transplantations. As with other alpha interferons, liver and renal graft rejections have been reported on peginterferon alfa-2a, alone or in combination with ribavirin *[see Adverse Reactions (6.2)]*.

10 OVERDOSAGE

No cases of overdose with ribavirin have been reported in clinical trials. Hypocalcemia and hypomagnesemia have been observed in persons administered greater than the recommended dosage of ribavirin. In most of these cases, ribavirin was administered intravenously at dosages up to and in some cases exceeding four times the recommended maximum oral daily dose.

11 DESCRIPTION

Moderiba (ribavirin, USP) is a nucleoside analogue with antiviral activity. The chemical name of ribavirin is 1-β-D-ribofuranosyl-1*H*-1,2,4-triazole-3-carboxamide and has the following structural formula:

The molecular formula of ribavirin is $C_8H_{12}N_4O_5$ and the molecular weight is 244.2. Ribavirin is a white to off-white powder. It is freely soluble in water and slightly soluble in anhydrous alcohol.
Moderiba (ribavirin, USP) is available as a blue-colored (shade depending on strength), capsule-shaped, film-coated tablet for oral administration. Each tablet contains 200 mg, 400 mg, or 600 mg of ribavirin and the following inactive ingredients: microcrystalline cellulose, lactose monohydrate, croscarmellose sodium, povidone K27-33, magnesium stearate, and purified water. The coating of the 200 mg tablet contains partially hydrolyzed polyvinyl alcohol, titanium dioxide, polyethylene glycol 3350, talc, FD&C blue #2 [indigo carmine aluminum lake], and carnauba wax. The coating of the 400 mg and 600 mg tablet contains partially hydrolyzed polyvinyl alcohol, titanium dioxide, polyethylene glycol 3350, talc, FD&C blue #1 [brilliant blue FCF aluminum lake], and carnauba wax.

12 CLINICAL PHARMACOLOGY

12.1 Mechanism of Action
Ribavirin is an antiviral drug *[see Clinical Pharmacology (12.4)]*.

12.3 Pharmacokinetics
Multiple dose ribavirin pharmacokinetic data are available for HCV patients who received ribavirin in combination with peginterferon alfa-2a. Following administration of 1200 mg/day with food for 12 weeks mean±SD (n=39; body weight >75 kg) AUC_{0-12hr} was 25,361±7110 ng•hr/mL and C_{max} was 2748±818 ng/mL. The average time to reach C_{max} was 2 hours. Trough ribavirin plasma concentrations following 12 weeks of dosing with food were 1662±545 ng/mL in HCV infected patients who received 800 mg/day (n=89), and 2112±810 ng/mL in patients who received 1200 mg/day (n=75; body weight >75 kg).
The terminal half-life of ribavirin following administration of a single oral dose of ribavirin is about 120 to 170 hours. The total apparent clearance following administration of a single oral dose of ribavirin is about 26 L/h. There is extensive accumulation of ribavirin after multiple dosing (twice daily) such that the C_{max} at steady state was four-fold higher than that of a single dose.

Effect of Food on Absorption of Ribavirin
Bioavailability of a single oral dose of ribavirin was increased by co-administration with a high-fat meal. The absorption was slowed (T_{max} was doubled) and the AUC_{0-192h} and C_{max} increased by 42% and 66%, respectively, when ribavirin was taken with a high-fat meal compared with fasting conditions *[see Dosage and Administration (2.1) and Patient Counseling Information (17)]*.

Elimination and Metabolism
The contribution of renal and hepatic pathways to ribavirin elimination after administration of ribavirin is not known. *In vitro* studies indicate that ribavirin is not a substrate of CYP450 enzymes.

12.4 Microbiology
Mechanism of Action
The mechanism by which ribavirin contributes to its antiviral efficacy in the clinic is not fully understood. Ribavirin has direct antiviral activity in tissue culture against many RNA viruses. Ribavirin increases the mutation frequency in the genomes of several RNA viruses and ribavirin triphosphate inhibits HCV polymerase in a biochemical reaction.

Antiviral Activity in Cell Culture
In the stable HCV cell culture model system (HCV replicon), ribavirin inhibited autonomous HCV RNA replication with a 50% effective concentration (EC_{50}) value of 11-21 mcM. In the same model, PEG-IFN α-2a also inhibited HCV RNA replication, with an EC_{50} value of 0.1-3 ng/mL. The combination of PEG-IFN α-2a and ribavirin was more effective at inhibiting HCV RNA replication than either agent alone.

Resistance
Different HCV genotypes display considerable clinical variability in their response to PEG-IFN-α and ribavirin therapy. Viral genetic determinants associated with the variable response have not been definitively identified.

Cross-resistance
Cross-resistance between IFN α and ribavirin has not been observed.

13 NONCLINICAL TOXICOLOGY

13.1 Carcinogenesis, Mutagenesis, Impairment of Fertility
Carcinogenesis
In a p53 (+/-) mouse carcinogenicity study up to the maximum tolerated dose of 100 mg/kg/day, ribavirin was not oncogenic. Ribavirin was also not oncogenic in a rat 2-year carcinogenicity study at doses up to the maximum tolerated dose of 60 mg/kg/day. On a body surface area basis, these doses are approximately 0.5 and 0.6 times the maximum recommended daily human dose of ribavirin, respectively.

Mutagenesis
Ribavirin demonstrated mutagenic activity in the *in vitro* mouse lymphoma assay. No clastogenic activity was observed in an *in vivo* mouse micronucleus assay at doses up to 2000 mg/kg. However, results from studies published in the literature show clastogenic activity in the *in vivo* mouse micronucleus assay at oral doses up to 2000 mg/kg. A dominant lethal assay in rats was negative, indicating that if mutations occurred in rats they were not transmitted through male gametes. However, potential carcinogenic risk to humans cannot be excluded.

Impairment of Fertility
In a fertility study in rats, ribavirin showed a marginal reduction in sperm counts at the dose of 100 mg/kg/day with no effect on fertility. Upon cessation of treatment, total recovery occurred after 1 spermatogenesis cycle. Abnormalities in sperm were observed in studies in mice designed to evaluate the time course and reversibility of ribavirin-induced testicular degeneration at doses of 15 to 150 mg/kg/day (approximately 0.1 to 0.8 times the maximum recommended daily human dose of ribavirin) administered for 3 to 6 months. Upon cessation of treatment, essentially total recovery from ribavirin-induced testicular toxicity was apparent within 1 or 2 spermatogenic cycles.
Female patients of childbearing potential and male patients with female partners of childbearing potential should not receive Moderiba™ (ribavirin, USP) unless the patient and his/her partner are using effective contraception (two reliable forms). Based on a multiple dose half-life ($t_{1/2}$) of ribavirin of 12 days, effective contraception must be utilized for 6 months post therapy (i.e., 15 half-lives of clearance for ribavirin).
No reproductive toxicology studies have been performed using peginterferon alfa-2a in combination with ribavirin. However, peginterferon alfa-2a and ribavirin when administered separately, each has adverse effects on reproduction. It should be assumed that the effects produced by either agent alone would also be caused by the combination of the two agents.

13.2 Animal Toxicology and/or Pharmacology
In a study in rats, it was concluded that dominant lethality was not induced by ribavirin at doses up to 200 mg/kg for 5 days (up to 1.7 times the maximum recommended human dose of ribavirin).
Long-term studies in the mouse and rat (18 to 24 months; dose 20 to 75, and 10 to 40 mg/kg/day, respectively, approx-

imately 0.1 to 0.4 times the maximum daily human dose of ribavirin) have demonstrated a relationship between chronic ribavirin exposure and an increased incidence of vascular lesions (microscopic hemorrhages) in mice. In rats, retinal degeneration occurred in controls, but the incidence was increased in ribavirin-treated rats.

14 CLINICAL STUDIES

14.1 Chronic Hepatitis C Patients

The safety and effectiveness of peginterferon alfa-2a in combination with ribavirin for the treatment of hepatitis C virus infection were assessed in two randomized controlled clinical trials. All patients were adults, had compensated liver disease, detectable hepatitis C virus, liver biopsy diagnosis of chronic hepatitis, and were previously untreated with interferon. Approximately 20% of patients in both studies had compensated cirrhosis (Child-Pugh class A). Patients coinfected with HIV were excluded from these studies.

In Study NV15801, patients were randomized to receive either peginterferon alfa-2a 180 mcg subcutaneous once weekly with an oral placebo, peginterferon alfa-2a 180 mcg once weekly with ribavirin 1000 mg by mouth (body weight <75 kg) or 1200 mg by mouth (body weight ≥75 kg) or interferon alfa-2b 3 MIU subcutaneous three times a week plus ribavirin 1000 mg or 1200 mg by mouth. All patients received 48 weeks of therapy followed by 24 weeks of treatment-free follow-up. Ribavirin or placebo treatment assignment was blinded. Sustained virological response was defined as undetectable (<50 IU/mL) HCV RNA on or after study week 68. Peginterferon alfa-2a in combination with ribavirin resulted in a higher SVR compared to peginterferon alfa-2a alone or interferon alfa-2b and ribavirin (**Table 5**). In all treatment arms, patients with viral genotype 1, regardless of viral load, had a lower response rate to peginterferon alfa-2a in combination with ribavirin compared to patients with other viral genotypes.

[See table 5 above]

In Study NV15942, all patients received peginterferon alfa-2a 180 mcg subcutaneous once weekly and were randomized to treatment for either 24 or 48 weeks and to a ribavirin dose of either 800 mg or 1000 mg/1200 mg (for body weight <75 kg/≥75 kg). Assignment to the four treatment arms was stratified by viral genotype and baseline HCV viral titer. Patients with genotype 1 and high viral titer (defined as >2 × 10^6 HCV RNA copies/mL serum) were preferentially assigned to treatment for 48 weeks.

Sustained Virologic Response (SVR) and HCV Genotype

HCV 1 and 4- Irrespective of baseline viral titer, treatment for 48 weeks with peginterferon alfa-2a and 1000 mg or 1200 mg of ribavirin resulted in higher SVR (defined as undetectable HCV RNA at the end of the 24-week treatment-free follow-up period) compared to shorter treatment (24 weeks) and/or 800 mg ribavirin.

HCV 2 and 3- Irrespective of baseline viral titer, treatment for 24 weeks with peginterferon alfa-2a and 800 mg of ribavirin resulted in a similar SVR compared to longer treatment (48 weeks) and/or 1000 mg or 1200 mg of ribavirin (see **Table 6**).

The numbers of patients with genotype 5 and 6 were too few to allow for meaningful assessment.

[See table 6 above]

14.2 Other Treatment Response Predictors

Treatment response rates are lower in patients with poor prognostic factors receiving pegylated interferon alpha therapy. In studies NV15801 and NV15942, treatment response rates were lower in patients older than 40 years (50% vs. 66%), in patients with cirrhosis (47% vs. 59%), in patients weighing over 85 kg (49% vs. 60%), and in patients with genotype 1 with high vs. low viral load (43% vs. 56%). African-American patients had lower response rates compared to Caucasians.

In studies NV15801 and NV15942, lack of early virologic response by 12 weeks (defined as HCV RNA undetectable or >2 log$_{10}$ lower than baseline) was grounds for discontinuation of treatment. Of patients who lacked an early viral response by 12 weeks and completed a recommended course of therapy despite a protocol-defined option to discontinue therapy, 5/39 (13%) achieved an SVR. Of patients who lacked an early viral response by 24 weeks, 19 completed a full course of therapy and none achieved an SVR.

14.3 Chronic Hepatitis C/HIV Coinfected Patients

In Study NR15961, patients with CHC/HIV were randomized to receive either peginterferon alfa-2a 180 mcg subcutaneous once weekly plus an oral placebo, peginterferon alfa-2a 180 mcg once weekly plus ribavirin 800 mg by mouth daily or interferon alfa-2a, 3 MIU subcutaneous three times a week plus ribavirin 800 mg by mouth daily. All patients received 48 weeks of therapy and sustained virologic response (SVR) was assessed at 24 weeks of treatment-free follow-up. Ribavirin or placebo treatment assignment was blinded in the peginterferon alfa-2a treatment arms. All patients were adults, had compensated liver disease, detectable hepatitis C virus, liver biopsy diagnosis

of chronic hepatitis C, and were previously untreated with interferon. Patients also had CD4+ cell count ≥200 cells/mcL or CD4+ cell count ≥100 cells/mcL but <200 cells/mcL and HIV-1 RNA <5000 copies/mL, and stable status of HIV. Approximately 15% of patients in the study had cirrhosis. Results are shown in **Table 7**.

[See table 7 above]

Treatment response rates were lower in CHC/HIV patients with poor prognostic factors (including HCV genotype 1, HCV RNA >800,000 IU/mL, and cirrhosis) receiving pegylated interferon alpha therapy.

Of the patients who did not demonstrate either undetectable HCV RNA or at least a 2 log$_{10}$ reduction from baseline in HCV RNA titer by 12 weeks of peginterferon alfa-2a and ribavirin combination therapy, 2% (2/85) achieved an SVR. In CHC patients with HIV coinfection who received 48 weeks of peginterferon alfa-2a alone or in combination with ribavirin treatment, mean and median HIV RNA titers did not increase above baseline during treatment or 24 weeks post treatment.

16 HOW SUPPLIED/STORAGE AND HANDLING

Moderiba (ribavirin, USP) is available as tablets for oral administration.

Each Moderiba (ribavirin, USP) 200-mg tablet contains 200 mg of ribavirin and is a capsule-shaped, light blue colored, film-coated tablet, debossed with "200" on one side and the logo "3RP" on the other side.

Each Moderiba (ribavirin, USP) 400-mg tablet contains 400 mg of ribavirin and is a capsule-shaped, medium blue colored, film-coated tablet, debossed with "400" on one side and the logo "3RP" on the other side.

Each Moderiba (ribavirin, USP) 600-mg tablet contains 600 mg of ribavirin and is a capsule-shaped, dark blue colored, film-coated tablet, debossed with "600" on one side and the logo "3RP" on the other side.

They are packaged as follows:

200 mg   Bottles of 168   NDC 0074-3197-16

Moderiba™ is also available in blister packs as follows:

Moderiba™ 600 Dose Pack Carton contains a total of 28 - 200 mg Moderiba (ribavirin, USP) tablets and 28 - 400 mg Moderiba (ribavirin, USP) tablets. Each carton contains 4 individual Moderiba™ 600 Dose Packs. Each individual Moderiba™ 600 Dose Pack contains 7 (seven) - 200 mg Moderiba (ribavirin, USP) tablets and 7 (seven) - 400 mg Moderiba (ribavirin, USP) tablets.

Each 200 mg Moderiba (ribavirin, USP) tablet contains 200 mg of ribavirin and is a capsule-shaped, light blue colored, film-coated tablet, debossed with "200" on one side and the logo "3RP" on the other side. Each 400 mg Moderiba (ribavirin, USP) tablet contains 400 mg of ribavirin and is a capsule-shaped, medium blue colored, film-coated tablet, debossed with "400" on one side and the logo "3RP" on the other side.

Moderiba™ 600 Dose Pack Carton
NDC: 0074-3224-56
Moderiba™ 600 Dose Pack
NDC: 0074-3224-14
Moderiba™ 800 Dose Pack Carton contains a total of 56 - 400 mg Moderiba (ribavirin, USP) tablets. Each carton contains 4 individual Moderiba 800 Dose Packs. Each individual Moderiba 800 Dose Pack contains 14 (fourteen) - 400 mg Moderiba (ribavirin, USP) tablets.

Each 400 mg Moderiba (ribavirin, USP) tablet contains 400 mg of ribavirin and is a capsule-shaped, medium blue colored, film-coated tablet, debossed with "400" on one side and the logo "3RP" on the other side.

Moderiba™ 800 Dose Pack Carton
NDC: 0074-3239-56
Moderiba™ 800 Dose Pack
NDC: 0074-3239-14
Moderiba™ 1000 Dose Pack Carton contains a total of 28 - 400 mg Moderiba (ribavirin, USP) tablets and 28 - 600 mg Moderiba (ribavirin, USP) tablets. Each carton contains 4 individual Moderiba 1000 Dose Packs. Each individual Moderiba 1000 Dose Pack contains 7 (seven) - 400 mg Moderiba (ribavirin, USP) tablets and 7 (seven) - 600 mg Moderiba (ribavirin, USP) tablets. Each 400 mg Moderiba (ribavirin, USP) tablet contains 400 mg of ribavirin and is a capsule-shaped, medium blue colored, film-coated tablet, debossed with "400" on one side and the logo "3RP" on the other side. Each 600 mg Moderiba (ribavirin, USP) tablet contains 600 mg of ribavirin and is a capsule-shaped, dark blue colored, film-coated tablet, debossed with "600" on one side and the logo "3RP" on the other side.

Moderiba™ 1000 Dose Pack Carton
NDC: 0074-3271-56
Moderiba™ 1000 Dose Pack
NDC: 0074-3271-14
Moderiba™ 1200 Dose Pack Carton contains a total of 56 - 600 mg Moderiba (ribavirin, USP) tablets. Each carton contains 4 individual Moderiba 1200 Dose Packs. Each individual Moderiba 1200 Dose Pack contains 14 (fourteen) - 600 mg Moderiba (ribavirin, USP) tablets.

Each 600 mg Moderiba (ribavirin, USP) tablet contains 600 mg of ribavirin and is a capsule-shaped, dark blue colored, film-coated tablet, debossed with "600" on one side and the logo "3RP" on the other side.

Moderiba™ 1200 Dose Pack Carton
NDC: 0074-3282-56
Moderiba™ 1200 mg Dose Pack
NDC: 0074-3282-14

Information on the AbbVie, Inc. products listed on these pages is from the prescribing information in use as of July 31, 2014. For more information, please visit rxabbvie.com or call 1-800-633-9110.

Table 5 Sustained Virologic Response (SVR) to Combination Therapy (Study NV15801)

	Interferon alfa-2b + Ribavirin 1000 mg or 1200 mg	Peginterferon alfa-2a + placebo	Peginterferon alfa-2a + Ribavirin Tablets 1000 mg or 1200 mg
All Patients	197/444 (44%)	65/224 (29%)	241/453 (53%)
Genotype 1	103/285 (36%)	29/145 (20%)	132/298 (44%)
Genotypes 2–6	94/159 (59%)	36/79 (46%)	109/155 (70%)

Difference in overall treatment response (Peginterferon alfa-2a /ribavirin – Interferon alfa-2b/ribavirin) was 9% (95% CI 2.3, 15.3).

Table 6 Sustained Virologic Response as a Function of Genotype (Study NV15942)

	24 Weeks Treatment		48 Weeks Treatment	
	Peginterferon alfa-2a + Ribavirin 800 mg (N=207)	Peginterferon alfa-2a + Ribavirin 1000 mg or 1200 mg* (N=280)	Peginterferon alfa-2a + Ribavirin 800 mg (N=361)	Peginterferon alfa-2a + Ribavirin 1000 mg or 1200 mg* (N=436)
Genotype 1	29/101 (29%)	48/118 (41%)	99/250 (40%)	138/271 (51%)
Genotypes 2,3	79/96 (82%)	116/144 (81%)	75/99 (76%)	117/153 (76%)
Genotype 4	0/5 (0%)	7/12 (58%)	5/8 (63%)	9/11 (82%)

*1000 mg for body weight <75 kg; 1200 mg for body weight ≥75 kg.

Table 7 Sustained Virologic Response in Patients With Chronic Hepatitis C Coinfected With HIV (Study NR15961)

	Interferon alfa-2a + Ribavirin 800 mg (N=289)	peginterferon alfa-2a + Placebo (N=289)	peginterferon alfa-2a + Ribavirin 800 mg (N=290)
All patients	33 (11%)	58 (20%)	116 (40%)
Genotype 1	12/171 (7%)	24/175 (14%)	51/176 (29%)
Genotypes 2, 3	18/89 (20%)	32/90 (36%)	59/95 (62%)

Storage and Handling

Store the Moderiba™ Tablets bottle at 25°C (77°F); excursions are permitted between 15°C and 30°C (59°F and 86°F) [see USP Controlled Room Temperature]. Keep bottle tightly closed.

17   PATIENT COUNSELING INFORMATION

See FDA-approved Medication Guide

Pregnancy

Patients must be informed that ribavirin may cause birth defects and/or death of the exposed fetus. Moderiba (ribavirin, USP) therapy must not be used by women who are pregnant or by men whose female partners are pregnant. Extreme care must be taken to avoid pregnancy in female patients and in female partners of male patients taking Moderiba (ribavirin, USP) therapy and for 6 months post therapy. Moderiba (ribavirin, USP) therapy should not be initiated until a report of a negative pregnancy test has been obtained immediately prior to initiation of therapy. Patients must perform a pregnancy test monthly during therapy and for 6 months post therapy.

Female patients of childbearing potential and male patients with female partners of childbearing potential must be advised of the teratogenic/embryocidal risks and must be instructed to practice effective contraception during Moderiba (ribavirin, USP) therapy and for 6 months post therapy. Patients should be advised to notify the healthcare provider immediately in the event of a pregnancy [see Contraindications (4) and Warnings and Precautions (5.1)].

Anemia

The most common adverse event associated with ribavirin is anemia, which may be severe [see Boxed Warning, Warnings and Precautions (5.2) and Adverse Reactions (6.1)]. Patients should be advised that laboratory evaluations are required prior to starting Moderiba (ribavirin, USP) therapy and periodically thereafter [see Warnings and Precautions (5.9)]. It is advised that patients be well hydrated, especially during the initial stages of treatment.

Patients who develop dizziness, confusion, somnolence, and fatigue should be cautioned to avoid driving or operating machinery.

Patients should be advised to take Moderiba (ribavirin, USP) with food.

Patients should be questioned about prior history of drug abuse before initiating Moderiba (ribavirin, USP)/peginterferon alfa-2a, as relapse of drug addiction and drug overdoses have been reported in patients treated with interferons.

Patients should be advised not to drink alcohol, as alcohol may exacerbate chronic hepatitis C infection.

Patient should be informed about what to do in the event they miss a dose of Moderiba (ribavirin, USP). The missed doses should be taken as soon as possible during the same day. Patients should not double the next dose. Patients should be advised to call their healthcare provider if they have questions.

Patients should be informed that the effect of peginterferon alfa-2a/Moderiba (ribavirin, USP) treatment of hepatitis C infection on transmission is not known, and that appropriate precautions to prevent transmission of hepatitis C virus should be taken.

Patients should be informed regarding the potential benefits and risks attendant to the use of Moderiba (ribavirin, USP). Instructions on appropriate use should be given, including review of the contents of the enclosed MEDICATION GUIDE, which is not a disclosure of all or possible adverse effects.

U.S. Patent No. 7,723,310
C139.00011 v. 1.0
70009910

MEDICATION GUIDE

FDA-approved Medication Guide
Moderiba™ (Mah-duh-RYE-bah)
(ribavirin, USP)
Tablets

Read this Medication Guide carefully before you start taking Moderiba™ (ribavirin, USP) and read the Medication Guide each time you get more Moderiba (ribavirin, USP). There may be new information. This information does not take the place of talking to your healthcare provider about your medical condition or your treatment.

Also read the Medication Guide for PEGASYS[1] (peginterferon alfa-2a).

What is the most important information I should know about Moderiba (ribavirin, USP)?

1. **You should not take Moderiba (ribavirin, USP) alone to treat chronic hepatitis C infection.** Moderiba (ribavirin, USP) should be used with peginterferon alfa-2a to treat chronic hepatitis C infection.

2. **Moderiba (ribavirin, USP) may cause you to have a blood problem (hemolytic anemia) that can worsen any heart problems you have, and cause you to have a heart attack or die.** Tell your healthcare provider if you have ever had

any heart problems. Moderiba (ribavirin, USP) may not be right for you. If you have chest pain while you take Moderiba (ribavirin, USP), get emergency medical attention right away.

3. **Moderiba (ribavirin, USP) may cause birth defects or death of your unborn baby.** If you are pregnant or your sexual partner is pregnant, do not take Moderiba (ribavirin, USP). You or your sexual partner should not become pregnant while you take Moderiba (ribavirin, USP) and for 6 months after treatment is over. You must use two forms of birth control when you take Moderiba (ribavirin, USP) and for the 6 months after treatment.

• Females must have a pregnancy test before starting Moderiba (ribavirin, USP), every month while treated with Moderiba (ribavirin, USP), and every month for the 6 months after treatment with Moderiba (ribavirin, USP).

• **If you or your female sexual partner becomes pregnant** while taking Moderiba (ribavirin, USP) or within 6 months after you stop taking Moderiba (ribavirin, USP), tell your healthcare provider right away. You or your healthcare provider should contact the **Ribavirin Pregnancy Registry** by calling **1-800-593-2214**. The Ribavirin Pregnancy Registry collects information about what happens to mothers and their babies if the mother takes Moderiba (ribavirin, USP) while she is pregnant.

What is Moderiba (ribavirin, USP)?

Moderiba (ribavirin, USP) is a medicine used with another medicine called peginterferon alfa-2a to treat chronic (lasting a long time) hepatitis C infection in people whose liver still works normally, and who have not been treated before with a medicine called an interferon alpha. It is not known if Moderiba (ribavirin, USP) is safe and will work in children under 18 years of age.

Who should not take Moderiba (ribavirin, USP)?

See "What is the most important information I should know about Moderiba (ribavirin, USP)?"

Do not take Moderiba (ribavirin, USP) if you:

• **have certain types of hepatitis** caused by your immune system attacking your liver (autoimmune hepatitis)

• **have certain blood disorders, such as thalassemia major or sickle-cell anemia (hemoglobinopathies)**

• **have severe kidney disease**

• **take didanosine** (Videx or Videx EC)

Talk to your healthcare provider before starting treatment with Moderiba (ribavirin, USP) if you have any of these medical conditions.

What should I tell my healthcare provider before taking Moderiba (ribavirin, USP)?

Before you take Moderiba (ribavirin, USP), tell your healthcare provider if you have or have had:

• **treatment for hepatitis C that did not work for you**

• **serious allergic reactions to Moderiba (ribavirin, USP) or to any of the ingredients in Moderiba (ribavirin, USP).** See the end of this Medication Guide for a list of ingredients.

• **breathing problems.** Moderiba (ribavirin, USP) may cause or worsen your breathing problems you already have.

• **vision problems.** Moderiba (ribavirin, USP) may cause eye problems or worsen eye problems you already have. You should have an eye exam before you start treatment with Moderiba (ribavirin, USP).

• **certain blood disorders such as anemia**

• **high blood pressure, heart problems or have had a heart attack.** Your healthcare provider should test your blood and heart before you start treatment with Moderiba (ribavirin, USP).

• **thyroid problems**

• **diabetes.** Moderiba (ribavirin, USP) and peginterferon alfa-2a combination therapy may make your diabetes worse or harder to treat.

• **liver problems** other than hepatitis C virus infection

• **human immunodeficiency virus (HIV) or other immunity problems**

• **mental health problems,** including depression or thoughts of suicide

• **kidney problems**

• **an organ transplant**

• **drug addiction or abuse**

• **infection with hepatitis B virus**

• **any other medical condition**

• **are breast-feeding.** It is not known if Moderiba (ribavirin, USP) passes into your breast milk. You and your healthcare provider should decide if you will take Moderiba (ribavirin, USP) or breast-feed.

Tell your healthcare provider about all the medicines you take, including prescription and non-prescription medicines, vitamins and herbal supplements. Some medicines can cause serious side effects if taken while you also take Moderiba (ribavirin, USP). Some medicines may affect how Moderiba (ribavirin, USP) works or Moderiba (ribavirin, USP) may affect how your other medicines work.

Especially tell your healthcare provider if you take any medicines to treat HIV, including didanosine (Videx or Videx EC), or if you take azathioprine (Imuran®[2] or Azasan).

Know the medicines you take. Keep a list of them to show your healthcare provider or pharmacist when you get a new medicine.

How should I take Moderiba (ribavirin, USP)?

• Take Moderiba (ribavirin, USP) exactly as your healthcare provider tells you. Your healthcare provider will tell you how much Moderiba (ribavirin, USP) to take and when to take it.

• Take Moderiba (ribavirin, USP) with food.

• If you miss a dose of Moderiba (ribavirin, USP), take the missed dose as soon as possible during the same day. Do not double the next dose. If you have questions about what to do, call your healthcare provider.

• If you take too much Moderiba (ribavirin, USP), call your healthcare provider or local Poison Control Center right away, or go to the nearest hospital emergency room right away.

• Your healthcare provider should do blood tests before you start treatment with Moderiba (ribavirin, USP), at weeks 2 and 4 of treatment, and then as needed to see how well you are tolerating treatment and to check for side effects. Your healthcare provider may change your dose of Moderiba (ribavirin, USP) based on blood test results or side effects you may have.

• If you have heart problems, your healthcare provider should check your heart by doing an electrocardiogram before you start treatment with Moderiba (ribavirin, USP), and if needed during treatment.

What should I avoid while taking Moderiba (ribavirin, USP)?

• **Moderiba (ribavirin, USP) can make you feel tired, dizzy, or confused. You should not drive or operate machinery if you have any of these symptoms.**

• **Do not drink alcohol,** including beer, wine, and liquor. This may make your liver disease worse.

What are the possible side effects of Moderiba (ribavirin, USP)?

Moderiba (ribavirin, USP) may cause serious side effects including:

See "What is the most important information I should know about Moderiba (ribavirin, USP)?"

• **Swelling and irritation of your pancreas (pancreatitis).** You may have stomach pain, nausea, vomiting or diarrhea.

• **Severe allergic reactions.** Symptoms may include hives, wheezing, trouble breathing, chest pain, swelling of your mouth, tongue, or lips, or severe rash.

• **Serious breathing problems.** Difficulty breathing may be a sign of a serious lung infection (pneumonia) that can lead to death.

• **Serious eye problems** that may lead to vision loss or blindness.

• **Liver problems.** Some people may get worsening of liver function. Tell your healthcare provider right away if you have any of these symptoms: stomach bloating, confusion, brown urine, and yellow eyes.

• **Severe depression**

• **Suicidal thoughts and attempts**

Call your healthcare provider or get medical help right away if you have any of the symptoms listed above. These may be signs of serious side effects of Moderiba (ribavirin, USP) treatment.

Common side effects of Moderiba (ribavirin, USP) taken with peginterferon alfa-2a include:

• flu-like symptoms-feeling tired, headache, shaking along with high temperature (fever), and muscle or joint aches

• mood changes, feeling irritable, anxiety, and difficulty sleeping

• loss of appetite, nausea, vomiting, and diarrhea

• hair loss

• itching

Tell your healthcare provider about any side effect that bothers you or that does not go away.

These are not all the possible side effects of Moderiba™ (ribavirin, USP) treatment. For more information, ask your healthcare provider or pharmacist.

Call your doctor for medical advice about side effects. You may report side effects to FDA at 1-800-FDA-1088.

You may also report side effects to AbbVie Inc. at 1-800-633-9110.

How should I store Moderiba (ribavirin, USP)?

• Store Moderiba (ribavirin, USP) tablets between 59°F and 86°F (15°C and 30°C).

• Keep the bottle tightly closed.

Keep Moderiba (ribavirin, USP) and all medicines out of the reach of children.

General information about the safe and effective use of Moderiba (ribavirin, USP)

It is not known if treatment with Moderiba (ribavirin, USP) can cure hepatitis C or if it can prevent liver damage (cirrhosis), liver failure or liver cancer that is caused by hepatitis C virus infections. It is not known if treatment with Moderiba (ribavirin, USP) will prevent an infected person from spreading the hepatitis C virus to another person.

Medicines are sometimes prescribed for purposes other than those listed in a Medication Guide. Do not use Moderiba (ribavirin, USP) for a condition for which it was not prescribed. Do not give Moderiba (ribavirin, USP) to other people, even if they have the same symptoms that you have. It may harm them.

This Medication Guide summarizes the most important information about Moderiba (ribavirin, USP). If you would like more information, talk with your healthcare provider. You can ask your healthcare provider or pharmacist for information about Moderiba (ribavirin, USP) that is written for healthcare professionals.

What are the ingredients in Moderiba (ribavirin, USP)?
Active Ingredient: ribavirin
Inactive Ingredients: microcrystalline cellulose, lactose monohydrate, croscarmellose sodium, povidone K27-33, magnesium stearate, and purified water. The tablet is coated with partially hydrolyzed polyvinyl alcohol, polyethylene glycol 3350, talc, titanium dioxide, FD&C blue #2 [indigo carmine aluminum lake] (200 mg tablet only), FD&C blue #1 [brilliant blue FCF aluminum lake] (400 mg and 600 mg tablets only), and carnauba wax.
This Medication Guide has been approved by the U.S. Food and Drug Administration.

[1]PEGASYS is a trademark of Hoffmann-La Roche Inc.
[2]Imuran is a registered trademark of Prometheus Laboratories, Inc.
Distributed by
AbbVie Inc.
North Chicago, IL 60064 USA
C139.00002 v. 1.0
70009911
Printed in USA
U.S. Patent No. 7,723,310
Copyright © 2013 by Kadmon Pharmaceuticals, LLC. All rights reserved.
Ref. C139.00011 - Rev. November, 2013
Shown in Product Identification Guide, page 304

NIASPAN® TABLETS   ℞
[ny-a-span]
(niacin extended-release)
tablet, film coated, extended release for oral use.

HIGHLIGHTS OF PRESCRIBING INFORMATION
These highlights do not include all the information needed to use NIASPAN® safely and effectively. See full prescribing information for NIASPAN.
NIASPAN (niacin extended-release) tablet, film coated, extended release for oral use.
Initial U.S. Approval: 1997

——————RECENT MAJOR CHANGES——————
Indications and Usage: Limitations of Use (1)	02/2013
Warnings and Precautions, Mortality and Coronary Heart Disease Morbidity (5.1)	02/2013

——————INDICATIONS AND USAGE——————
NIASPAN contains extended-release niacin (nicotinic acid), and is indicated:
• To reduce elevated TC, LDL-C, Apo B and TG, and to increase HDL-C in patients with primary hyperlipidemia and mixed dyslipidemia. (1)
• In combination with simvastatin or lovastatin: to treat primary hyperlipidemia and mixed dyslipidemia when treatment with NIASPAN, simvastatin, or lovastatin monotherapy is considered inadequate. (1)
• To reduce the risk of recurrent nonfatal myocardial infarction in patients with a history of myocardial infarction and hyperlipidemia. (1)
• In combination with a bile acid binding resin:
  ◦ Slows progression or promotes regression of atherosclerotic disease in patients with a history of coronary artery disease (CAD) and hyperlipidemia. (1)
  ◦ As an adjunct to diet to reduce elevated TC and LDL-C in adult patients with primary hyperlipidemia. (1)
• To reduce TG in adult patients with severe hypertriglyceridemia. (1)
Limitations of use:
No incremental benefit of NIASPAN coadministered with simvastatin or lovastatin on cardiovascular morbidity and mortality over and above that demonstrated for niacin, simvastatin and lovastatin monotherapy, has been established. NIASPAN, at doses of 1,500-2,000 mg/day, in combination with simvastatin, did not reduce the incidence of cardiovascular events more than simvastatin in a randomized controlled trial of patients with cardiovascular disease and mean baseline LDL-C levels of 74 mg per deciliter (5.1).

——————DOSAGE AND ADMINISTRATION——————
• NIASPAN should be taken at bedtime with a low-fat snack. (2)
• Dose range: 500 mg to 2000 mg once daily. (2)
• Therapy with NIASPAN must be initiated at 500 mg at bedtime in order to reduce the incidence and severity of side effects which may occur during early therapy and should not be increased by more than 500 mg in any four week period. (2)
• Maintenance dose: 1000 to 2000 mg once daily. (2)
• Doses greater than 2000 mg daily are not recommended. (2)
• Concomitant therapy with lovastatin: Initial dose of lovastatin is 20 mg once a day; combination therapy with NIASPAN and lovastatin should not exceed doses of 2000 mg and 40 mg daily, respectively. (2)
• Concomitant therapy with simvastatin: Initial dose of simvastatin is 20 mg once a day; combination therapy with NIASPAN and simvastatin should not exceed doses of 2000 mg and 40 mg daily, respectively. (2)

——————DOSAGE FORMS AND STRENGTHS——————
Unscored film-coated tablets for oral administration: 500, 750 and 1000 mg niacin extended-release. (3)

——————CONTRAINDICATIONS——————
• Active liver disease, which may include unexplained persistent elevations in hepatic transaminase levels. (4, 5.3)
• Active peptic ulcer disease. (4)
• Arterial bleeding. (4)
• Known hypersensitivity to product components. (4, 6.1)

——————WARNINGS AND PRECAUTIONS——————
• Severe hepatic toxicity has occurred in patients substituting sustained-release niacin for immediate-release niacin at equivalent doses. (5.3)
• Myopathy has been reported in patients taking NIASPAN. The risk for myopathy and rhabdomyolysis are increased when lovastatin or simvastatin are coadministered with NIASPAN, particularly in elderly patients and patients with diabetes, renal failure, or uncontrolled hypothyroidism. (5.2)
• Liver enzyme abnormalities and monitoring: Persistent elevations in hepatic transaminase can occur. Monitor liver enzymes before and during treatment. (5.3)
• Use with caution in patients with unstable angina or in the acute phase of an MI. (5)
• NIASPAN can increase serum glucose levels. Glucose levels should be closely monitored in diabetic or potentially diabetic patients particularly during the first few months of use or dose adjustment. (5.4)

——————ADVERSE REACTIONS——————
Most common adverse reactions (incidence >5% and greater than placebo) are flushing, diarrhea, nausea, vomiting, increased cough, and pruritus. (6.1)
Flushing of the skin may be reduced in frequency or severity by pretreatment with aspirin (up to the recommended dose of 325 mg taken 30 minutes prior to NIASPAN dose). (2)
To report SUSPECTED ADVERSE REACTIONS, contact AbbVie Inc. at 1-800-633-9110 or FDA at 1-800-FDA-1088 or www.fda.gov/medwatch.

——————DRUG INTERACTIONS——————
• Statins: Caution should be used when prescribing niacin with statins as these agents can increase risk of myopathy/rhabdomyolysis. (5.2, 7.1)
• Bile Acid Sequestrants: Bile acid sequestrants have a high niacin-binding capacity and should be taken at least 4 - 6 hours before NIASPAN administration. (7.2)

——————USE IN SPECIFIC POPULATIONS——————
• Renal impairment: NIASPAN should be used with caution in patients with renal impairment. (5, 8.6)
• Hepatic impairment: NIASPAN is contraindicated in active liver disease or significant or unexplained hepatic dysfunction or unexplained elevations of serum transaminases. (4,5, 5.3, 8.7)
See 17 for PATIENT COUNSELING INFORMATION and FDA-approved patient labeling

Revised: 03/2013

——————FULL PRESCRIBING INFORMATION: CONTENTS*——————

FULL PRESCRIBING INFORMATION

1 INDICATIONS AND USAGE

Therapy with lipid-altering agents should be only one component of multiple risk factor intervention in individuals at significantly increased risk for atherosclerotic vascular disease due to hyperlipidemia. Niacin therapy is indicated as an adjunct to diet when the response to a diet restricted in saturated fat and cholesterol and other nonpharmacologic measures alone has been inadequate.

1. NIASPAN is indicated to reduce elevated TC, LDL-C, Apo B and TG levels, and to increase HDL-C in patients with primary hyperlipidemia and mixed dyslipidemia.
2. NIASPAN in combination with simvastatin or lovastatin is indicated for the treatment of primary hyperlipidemia and mixed dyslipidemia when treatment with NIASPAN, simvastatin, or lovastatin monotherapy is considered inadequate.
3. In patients with a history of myocardial infarction and hyperlipidemia, niacin is indicated to reduce the risk of recurrent nonfatal myocardial infarction.
4. In patients with a history of coronary artery disease (CAD) and hyperlipidemia, niacin, in combination with a bile acid binding resin, is indicated to slow progression or promote regression of atherosclerotic disease.
5. NIASPAN in combination with a bile acid binding resin is indicated to reduce elevated TC and LDL-C levels in adult patients with primary hyperlipidemia.
6. Niacin is also indicated as adjunctive therapy for treatment of adult patients with severe hypertriglyceridemia who present a risk of pancreatitis and who do not respond adequately to a determined dietary effort to control them.

Limitations of Use
No incremental benefit of NIASPAN coadministered with simvastatin or lovastatin on cardiovascular morbidity and mortality over and above that demonstrated for niacin, simvastatin, or lovastatin monotherapy has been established.
NIASPAN, at doses of 1,500-2,000 mg/day, in combination with simvastatin, did not reduce the incidence of cardiovascular events more than simvastatin in a randomized controlled trial of patients with cardiovascular disease and mean baseline LDL-C levels of 74 mg per deciliter *[see Warnings and Precautions (5.1)]*.

2 DOSAGE AND ADMINISTRATION

NIASPAN should be taken at bedtime, after a low-fat snack, and doses should be individualized according to patient response. Therapy with NIASPAN must be initiated at 500 mg at bedtime in order to reduce the incidence and severity of side effects which may occur during early therapy. The recommended dose escalation is shown in Table 1 below.
[See table 1 at top of next page]
Maintenance Dose
The daily dosage of NIASPAN should not be increased by more than 500 mg in any 4-week period. The recommended maintenance dose is 1000 mg (two 500 mg tablets or one 1000 mg tablet) to 2000 mg (two 1000 mg tablets or four 500 mg tablets) once daily at bedtime. Doses greater than 2000 mg daily are not recommended. Women may respond at lower NIASPAN doses than men *[see Clinical Studies (14.2)]*.

Information on the AbbVie, Inc. products listed on these pages is from the prescribing information in use as of July 31, 2014. For more information, please visit rxabbvie.com or call 1-800-633-9110.

Table 1. Recommended Dosing

	Week(s)	Daily dose	NIASPAN Dosage
INITIAL TITRATION SCHEDULE	1 to 4	500 mg	1 NIASPAN 500 mg tablet at bedtime
	5 to 8	1000 mg	1 NIASPAN 1000 mg tablet or 2 NIASPAN 500 mg tablets at bedtime
	*	1500 mg	2 NIASPAN 750 mg tablets or 3 NIASPAN 500 mg tablets at bedtime
	*	2000 mg	2 NIASPAN 1000 mg tablets or 4 NIASPAN 500 mg tablets at bedtime

* After Week 8, titrate to patient response and tolerance. If response to 1000 mg daily is inadequate, increase dose to 1500 mg daily; may subsequently increase dose to 2000 mg daily. Daily dose should not be increased more than 500 mg in a 4-week period, and doses above 2000 mg daily are not recommended. Women may respond at lower doses than men.

Single-dose bioavailability studies have demonstrated that two of the 500 mg and one of the 1000 mg tablet strengths are interchangeable but three of the 500 mg and two of the 750 mg tablet strengths are not interchangeable.

If lipid response to NIASPAN alone is insufficient or if higher doses of NIASPAN are not well tolerated, some patients may benefit from combination therapy with a bile acid binding resin or statin *[see Drug Interactions (7.3), Concomitant Therapy below and Clinical Studies (14.3, 14.4)]*.

Flushing of the skin *[see Adverse Reactions (6.1)]* may be reduced in frequency or severity by pretreatment with aspirin (up to the recommended dose of 325 mg taken 30 minutes prior to NIASPAN dose). Tolerance to this flushing develops rapidly over the course of several weeks. Flushing, pruritus, and gastrointestinal distress are also greatly reduced by slowly increasing the dose of niacin and avoiding administration on an empty stomach. Concomitant alcoholic, hot drinks or spicy foods may increase the side effects of flushing and pruritus and should be avoided around the time of NIASPAN ingestion.

Equivalent doses of NIASPAN should not be substituted for sustained-release (modified-release, timed-release) niacin preparations or immediate-release (crystalline) niacin *[see Warnings and Precautions (5)]*. Patients previously receiving other niacin products should be started with the recommended NIASPAN titration schedule (see Table 1), and the dose should subsequently be individualized based on patient response.

If NIASPAN therapy is discontinued for an extended period, reinstitution of therapy should include a titration phase (see Table 1).

NIASPAN tablets should be taken whole and should not be broken, crushed or chewed before swallowing.

Concomitant Therapy
Concomitant Therapy with Lovastatin or Simvastatin
Patients already receiving a stable dose of lovastatin or simvastatin who require further TG-lowering or HDL-raising (e.g., to achieve NCEP non-HDL-C goals), may receive concomitant dosage titration with NIASPAN per NIASPAN recommended initial titration schedule *[see Dosage and Administration (2)]*. For patients already receiving a stable dose of NIASPAN who require further LDL-lowering (e.g., to achieve NCEP LDL-C goals), the usual recommended starting dose of lovastatin and simvastatin is 20 mg once a day. Dose adjustments should be made at intervals of 4 weeks or more. Combination therapy with NIASPAN and lovastatin or NIASPAN and simvastatin should not exceed doses of 2000 mg NIASPAN and 40 mg lovastatin or simvastatin daily.

Dosage in Patients with Renal or Hepatic Impairment
Use of NIASPAN in patients with renal or hepatic impairment has not been studied. NIASPAN is contraindicated in patients with significant or unexplained hepatic dysfunction. NIASPAN should be used with caution in patients with renal impairment *[see Warnings and Precautions (5)]*.

3   DOSAGE FORMS AND STRENGTHS
- 500 mg unscored, medium-orange, film-coated, capsule-shaped tablets
- 750 mg unscored, medium-orange, film-coated, capsule-shaped tablets
- 1000 mg unscored, medium-orange, film-coated, capsule-shaped tablets

4   CONTRAINDICATIONS
NIASPAN is contraindicated in the following conditions:
- Active liver disease or unexplained persistent elevations in hepatic transaminases *[see Warnings and Precautions (5.3)]*
- Patients with active peptic ulcer disease
- Patients with arterial bleeding
- Hypersensitivity to niacin or any component of this medication *[see Adverse Reactions (6.1)]*

5   WARNINGS AND PRECAUTIONS
NIASPAN preparations should not be substituted for equivalent doses of immediate-release (crystalline) niacin. For patients switching from immediate-release niacin to NIASPAN, therapy with NIASPAN should be initiated with low doses (i.e., 500 mg at bedtime) and the NIASPAN dose should then be titrated to the desired therapeutic response *[see Dosage and Administration (2)]*.
Caution should also be used when NIASPAN is used in patients with unstable angina or in the acute phase of an MI, particularly when such patients are also receiving vasoactive drugs such as nitrates, calcium channel blockers, or adrenergic blocking agents.
Niacin is rapidly metabolized by the liver, and excreted through the kidneys. NIASPAN is contraindicated in patients with significant or unexplained hepatic impairment *[see Contraindications (4) and Warnings and Precautions (5.3)]* and should be used with caution in patients with renal impairment. Patients with a past history of jaundice, hepatobiliary disease, or peptic ulcer should be observed closely during NIASPAN therapy.

5.1   Mortality and Coronary Heart Disease Morbidity
The Atherothrombosis Intervention in Metabolic Syndrome with Low HDL/High Triglycerides: Impact on Global Health Outcomes (AIM-HIGH) trial was a randomized placebo-controlled trial of 3414 patients with stable, previously diagnosed cardiovascular disease. Mean baseline lipid levels were LDL-C 74 mg/dL, HDL-C 35 mg/dL, non-HDL-C 111 mg/dL and median triglyceride level of 163-177 mg/dL. Ninety-four percent of patients were on background statin therapy prior to entering the trial. All participants received simvastatin, 40 to 80 mg per day, plus ezetimibe 10 mg per day if needed, to maintain an LDL-C level of 40-80 mg/dL, and were randomized to receive NIASPAN 1500-2000 mg/day (n=1718) or matching placebo (IR Niacin, 100-150 mg, n=1696). On-treatment lipid changes at two years for LDL-C were -12.0% for the simvastatin plus NIASPAN group and -5.5% for the simvastatin plus placebo group. HDL-C increased by 25.0% to 42 mg/dL in the simvastatin plus NIASPAN group and by 9.8% to 38 mg/dL in the simvastatin plus placebo group (P<0.001). Triglyceride levels decreased by 28.6% in the simvastatin plus NIASPAN group and by 8.1% in the simvastatin plus placebo group. The primary outcome was an ITT composite of the first study occurrence of coronary heart disease death, nonfatal myocardial infarction, ischemic stroke, hospitalization for acute coronary syndrome or symptom-driven coronary or cerebral revascularization procedures. The trial was stopped after a mean follow-up period of 3 years owing to a lack of efficacy. The primary outcome occurred in 282 patients in the simvastatin plus NIASPAN group (16.4%) and in 274 patients in the simvastatin plus placebo group (16.2%) (HR 1.02 [95% CI, 0.87-1.21], P=0.79. In an ITT analysis, there were 42 cases of first occurrence of ischemic stroke reported, 27 (1.6%) in the simvastatin plus NIASPAN group and 15 (0.9%) in the simvastatin plus placebo group, a non-statistically significant result (HR 1.79, [95%CI = 0.95-3.36], p=0.071). The on-treatment ischemic stroke events were 19 for the simvastatin plus NIASPAN group and 15 for the simvastatin plus placebo group *[see Adverse Reactions (6.1)]*.

5.2   Skeletal Muscle
Cases of rhabdomyolysis have been associated with concomitant administration of lipid-altering doses (≥1 g/day) of niacin and statins. Physicians contemplating combined therapy with statins and NIASPAN should carefully weigh the potential benefits and risks and should carefully monitor patients for any signs and symptoms of muscle pain, tenderness, or weakness, particularly during the initial months of therapy and during any periods of upward dosage titration of either drug. Periodic serum creatine phosphokinase (CPK) and potassium determinations should be considered in such situations, but there is no assurance that such monitoring will prevent the occurrence of severe myopathy.

The risk for myopathy and rhabdomyolysis are increased when lovastatin or simvastatin are coadministered with NIASPAN, particularly in elderly patients and patients with diabetes, renal failure, or uncontrolled hypothyroidism.

5.3   Liver Dysfunction
Cases of severe hepatic toxicity, including fulminant hepatic necrosis, have occurred in patients who have substituted sustained-release (modified-release, timed-release) niacin products for immediate-release (crystalline) niacin at equivalent doses.
NIASPAN should be used with caution in patients who consume substantial quantities of alcohol and/or have a past history of liver disease. Active liver diseases or unexplained transaminase elevations are contraindications to the use of NIASPAN.
Niacin preparations have been associated with abnormal liver tests. In three placebo-controlled clinical trials involving titration to final daily NIASPAN doses ranging from 500 to 3000 mg, 245 patients received NIASPAN for a mean duration of 17 weeks. No patient with normal serum transaminase levels (AST, ALT) at baseline experienced elevations to more than 3 times the upper limit of normal (ULN) during treatment with NIASPAN. In these studies, fewer than 1% (2/245) of NIASPAN patients discontinued due to transaminase elevations greater than 2 times the ULN.
In three safety and efficacy studies with a combination tablet of NIASPAN and lovastatin involving titration to final daily doses (expressed as mg of niacin/ mg of lovastatin) 500 mg/10 mg to 2500 mg/40 mg, ten of 1028 patients (1.0%) experienced reversible elevations in AST/ALT to more than 3 times the ULN. Three of ten elevations occurred at doses outside the recommended dosing limit of 2000 mg/40 mg; no patient receiving 1000 mg/20 mg had 3-fold elevations in AST/ALT.
Niacin extended-release and simvastatin can cause abnormal liver tests. In a simvastatin-controlled, 24 week study with a fixed dose combination of NIASPAN and simvastatin in 641 patients, there were no persistent increases (more than 3× the ULN) in serum transaminases. In three placebo-controlled clinical studies of extended-release niacin there were no patients with normal serum transaminase levels at baseline who experienced elevations to more than 3× the ULN. Persistent increases (more than 3× the ULN) in serum transaminases have occurred in approximately 1% of patients who received simvastatin in clinical studies. When drug treatment was interrupted or discontinued in these patients, the transaminases levels usually fell slowly to pretreatment levels. The increases were not associated with jaundice or other clinical signs or symptoms. There was no evidence of hypersensitivity.
In the placebo-controlled clinical trials and the long-term extension study, elevations in transaminases did not appear to be related to treatment duration; elevations in AST levels did appear to be dose related. Transaminase elevations were reversible upon discontinuation of NIASPAN.
Liver function tests should be performed on all patients during therapy with NIASPAN. Serum transaminase levels, including AST and ALT (SGOT and SGPT), should be monitored before treatment begins, every 6 to 12 weeks for the first year, and periodically thereafter (e.g., at approximately 6-month intervals). Special attention should be paid to patients who develop elevated serum transaminase levels, and in these patients, measurements should be repeated promptly and then performed more frequently. If the transaminase levels show evidence of progression, particularly if they rise to 3 times ULN and are persistent, or if they are associated with symptoms of nausea, fever, and/or malaise, the drug should be discontinued.

5.4   Laboratory Abnormalities
Increase in Blood Glucose: Niacin treatment can increase fasting blood glucose. Frequent monitoring of blood glucose should be performed to ascertain that the drug is producing no adverse effects. Diabetic patients may experience a dose-related increase in glucose intolerance. Diabetic or potentially diabetic patients should be observed closely during treatment with NIASPAN, particularly during the first few months of use or dose adjustment; adjustment of diet and/or hypoglycemic therapy may be necessary.
Reduction in platelet count: NIASPAN has been associated with small but statistically significant dose-related reductions in platelet count (mean of -11% with 2000 mg). Caution should be observed when NIASPAN is administered concomitantly with anticoagulants; platelet counts should be monitored closely in such patients.
Increase in Prothrombin Time (PT):   NIASPAN has been associated with small but statistically significant increases in prothrombin time (mean of approximately +4%); accordingly, patients undergoing surgery should be carefully evaluated. Caution should be observed when NIASPAN is administered concomitantly with anticoagulants; prothrombin time should be monitored closely in such patients.
Increase in Uric Acid: Elevated uric acid levels have occurred with niacin therapy, therefore use with caution in patients predisposed to gout.

Decrease in Phosphorus: In placebo-controlled trials, NIASPAN has been associated with small but statistically significant, dose-related reductions in phosphorus levels (mean of -13% with 2000 mg). Although these reductions were transient, phosphorus levels should be monitored periodically in patients at risk for hypophosphatemia.

6 ADVERSE REACTIONS

Because clinical studies are conducted under widely varying conditions, adverse reaction rates observed in the clinical studies of a drug cannot be directly compared to rates in the clinical studies of another drug and may not reflect the rates observed in practice.

6.1 Clinical Studies Experience

In the placebo-controlled clinical trials database of 402 patients (age range 21-75 years, 33% women, 89% Caucasians, 7% Blacks, 3% Hispanics, 1% Asians) with a median treatment duration of 16 weeks, 16% of patients on NIASPAN and 4% of patients on placebo discontinued due to adverse reactions. The most common adverse reactions in the group of patients treated with NIASPAN that led to treatment discontinuation and occurred at a rate greater than placebo were flushing (6% vs. 0%), rash (2% vs. 0%), diarrhea (2% vs. 0%), nausea (1% vs. 0%), and vomiting (1% vs. 0%). The most commonly reported adverse reactions (incidence >5% and greater than placebo) in the NIASPAN controlled clinical trial database of 402 patients were flushing, diarrhea, nausea, vomiting, increased cough and pruritus.

In the placebo-controlled clinical trials, flushing episodes (i.e., warmth, redness, itching and/or tingling) were the most common treatment-emergent adverse reactions (reported by as many as 88% of patients) for NIASPAN. Spontaneous reports suggest that flushing may also be accompanied by symptoms of dizziness, tachycardia, palpitations, shortness of breath, sweating, burning sensation/skin burning sensation, chills, and/or edema, which in rare cases may lead to syncope. In pivotal studies, 6% (14/245) of NIASPAN patients discontinued due to flushing. In comparisons of immediate-release (IR) niacin and NIASPAN, although the proportion of patients who flushed was similar, fewer flushing episodes were reported by patients who received NIASPAN. Following 4 weeks of maintenance therapy at daily doses of 1500 mg, the incidence of flushing over the 4-week period averaged 8.6 events per patient for IR niacin versus 1.9 following NIASPAN.

Other adverse reactions occurring in ≥5% of patients treated with NIASPAN and at an incidence greater than placebo are shown in Table 2 below.

[See table 2 above]

In general, the incidence of adverse events was higher in women compared to men.

Atherothrombosis Intervention in Metabolic Syndrome with Low HDL/ High Triglycerides: Impact on Global Health Outcomes (AIM-HIGH)

In AIM-HIGH involving 3414 patients (mean age of 64 years, 15% women, 92% Caucasians, 34% with diabetes mellitus) with stable, previously diagnosed cardiovascular disease, all patients received simvastatin, 40 to 80 mg per day, plus ezetimibe 10 mg per day if needed, to maintain an LDL-C level of 40-80 mg/dL, and were randomized to receive NIASPAN 1500-2000 mg/day (n=1718) or matching placebo (IR Niacin, 100-150 mg, n=1696). The incidence of the adverse reactions of "blood glucose increased" (6.4% vs. 4.5%) and "diabetes mellitus" (3.6% vs. 2.2%) was significantly higher in the simvastatin plus NIASPAN group as compared to the simvastatin plus placebo group. There were 5 cases of rhabdomyolysis reported, 4 (0.2%) in the simvastatin plus NIASPAN group and one (<0.1%) in the simvastatin plus placebo group [see Warnings and Precautions (5.1)].

6.2 Postmarketing Experience

Because the below reactions are reported voluntarily from a population of uncertain size, it is generally not possible to reliably estimate their frequency or establish a causal relationship to drug exposure.

The following additional adverse reactions have been identified during post-approval use of NIASPAN:

Hypersensitivity reactions, including anaphylaxis, angioedema, urticaria, flushing, dyspnea, tongue edema, larynx edema, face edema, peripheral edema, laryngismus, and vesiculobullous rash; maculopapular rash; dry skin; tachycardia; palpitations; atrial fibrillation; other cardiac arrhythmias; syncope; hypotension; postural hypotension; blurred vision; macular edema; peptic ulcers; eructation; flatulence; hepatitis; jaundice; decreased glucose tolerance; gout; myalgia; myopathy; dizziness; insomnia; asthenia; nervousness; paresthesia; dyspnea; sweating; burning sensation/skin burning sensation; skin discoloration, and migraine.

Clinical Laboratory Abnormalities

Chemistry: Elevations in serum transaminases [see Warnings and Precautions (5.3)], LDH, fasting glucose, uric acid, total bilirubin, amylase and creatine kinase, and reduction in phosphorus.

Table 2. Treatment-Emergent Adverse Reactions by Dose Level in ≥ 5% of Patients and at an Incidence Greater than Placebo; Regardless of Causality Assessment in Placebo-Controlled Clinical Trials

	Placebo-Controlled Studies NIASPAN Treatment[@]				
				Recommended Daily Maintenance Doses [†]	
	Placebo (n = 157) %	500 mg[‡] (n = 87) %	1000 mg (n = 110) %	1500 mg (n = 136) %	2000 mg (n = 95) %
Gastrointestinal Disorders					
Diarrhea	13	7	10	10	14
Nausea	7	5	6	4	11
Vomiting	4	0	2	4	9
Respiratory					
Cough, Increased	6	3	2	< 2	8
Skin and Subcutaneous Tissue Disorders					
Pruritus	2	8	0	3	0
Rash	0	5	5	5	0
Vascular Disorders					
Flushing[&]	19	68	69	63	55

Note: Percentages are calculated from the total number of patients in each column.
[†] Adverse reactions are reported at the initial dose where they occur.
[@] Pooled results from placebo-controlled studies; for NIASPAN, n = 245 and median treatment duration = 16 weeks.
Number of NIASPAN patients (n) are not additive across doses.
[‡] The 500 mg/day dose is outside the recommended daily maintenance dosing range [see Dosage and Administration (2)].
[&] 10 patients discontinued before receiving 500 mg, therefore they were not included.

Hematology: Slight reductions in platelet counts and prolongation in prothrombin time [see Warnings and Precautions (5.4)].

7 DRUG INTERACTIONS

7.1 Statins

Caution should be used when prescribing niacin (≥1 gm/day) with statins as these drugs can increase risk of myopathy/rhabdomyolysis. Combination therapy with NIASPAN and lovastatin or NIASPAN and simvastatin should not exceed doses of 2000 mg NIASPAN and 40 mg lovastatin or simvastatin daily. [see Warnings and Precautions (5) and Clinical Pharmacology (12.3)].

7.2 Bile Acid Sequestrants

An *in vitro* study results suggest that the bile acid-binding resins have high niacin binding capacity. Therefore, 4 to 6 hours, or as great an interval as possible, should elapse between the ingestion of bile acid-binding resins and the administration of NIASPAN [see Clinical Pharmacology (12.3)].

7.3 Aspirin

Concomitant aspirin may decrease the metabolic clearance of nicotinic acid. The clinical relevance of this finding is unclear.

7.4 Antihypertensive Therapy

Niacin may potentiate the effects of ganglionic blocking agents and vasoactive drugs resulting in postural hypotension.

7.5 Other

Vitamins or other nutritional supplements containing large doses of niacin or related compounds such as nicotinamide may potentiate the adverse effects of NIASPAN.

7.6 Laboratory Test Interactions

Niacin may produce false elevations in some fluorometric determinations of plasma or urinary catecholamines. Niacin may also give false-positive reactions with cupric sulfate solution (Benedict's reagent) in urine glucose tests.

8 USE IN SPECIFIC POPULATIONS

8.1 Pregnancy

Pregnancy Category C.

Animal reproduction studies have not been conducted with niacin or with NIASPAN. It is also not known whether niacin at doses typically used for lipid disorders can cause fetal harm when administered to pregnant women or whether it can affect reproductive capacity. If a woman receiving niacin for primary hyperlipidemia becomes pregnant, the drug should be discontinued. If a woman being treated with niacin for hypertriglyceridemia conceives, the benefits and risks of continued therapy should be assessed on an individual basis.

All statins are contraindicated in pregnant and nursing women. When NIASPAN is administered with a statin in a woman of childbearing potential, refer to the pregnancy category and product labeling for the statin.

8.3 Nursing Mothers

Niacin is excreted into human milk but the actual infant dose or infant dose as a percent of the maternal dose is not known. Because of the potential for serious adverse reactions in nursing infants from lipid-altering doses of nicotinic acid, a decision should be made whether to discontinue nursing or to discontinue the drug, taking into account the importance of the drug to the mother. No studies have been conducted with NIASPAN in nursing mothers.

8.4 Pediatric Use

Safety and effectiveness of niacin therapy in pediatric patients (≤16 years) have not been established.

8.5 Geriatric Use

Of 979 patients in clinical studies of NIASPAN, 21% of the patients were age 65 and over. No overall differences in safety and effectiveness were observed between these patients and younger patients, and other reported clinical experience has not identified differences in responses between the elderly and younger patients, but greater sensitivity of some older individuals cannot be ruled out.

8.6 Renal Impairment

No studies have been performed in this population. NIASPAN should be used with caution in patients with renal impairment [see Warnings and Precautions (5)].

8.7 Hepatic Impairment

No studies have been performed in this population. NIASPAN should be used with caution in patients with a past history of liver disease and/or who consume substantial quantities of alcohol. Active liver disease, unexplained transaminase elevations and significant or unexplained hepatic dysfunction are contraindications to the use of NIASPAN [see Contraindications (4.0) and Warnings and Precautions (5.3)].

8.8 Gender

Data from the clinical trials suggest that women have a greater hypolipidemic response than men at equivalent doses of NIASPAN.

10 OVERDOSAGE

Supportive measures should be undertaken in the event of an overdose.

11 DESCRIPTION

NIASPAN (niacin tablet, film-coated extended-release), contains niacin, which at therapeutic doses is an antihyperlipidemic agent. Niacin (nicotinic acid, or 3-pyridinecarboxylic acid) is a white, crystalline powder, very soluble in water, with the following structural formula:

$C_6H_5NO_2$ M.W.: 123.11

NIASPAN is an unscored, medium-orange, film-coated tablet for oral administration and is available in three tablet strengths containing 500, 750, and 1000 mg niacin. NIASPAN tablets also contain the inactive ingredients hypromellose, povidone, stearic acid, and polyethylene glycol, and the following coloring agents: FD&C yellow #6/sunset yellow FCF Aluminum Lake, synthetic red and yellow iron oxides, and titanium dioxide.

Information on the AbbVie, Inc. products listed on these pages is from the prescribing information in use as of July 31, 2014. For more information, please visit rxabbvie.com or call 1-800-633-9110.

12 CLINICAL PHARMACOLOGY

12.1 Mechanism of Action

The mechanism by which niacin alters lipid profiles has not been well defined. It may involve several actions including partial inhibition of release of free fatty acids from adipose tissue, and increased lipoprotein lipase activity, which may increase the rate of chylomicron triglyceride removal from plasma. Niacin decreases the rate of hepatic synthesis of VLDL and LDL, and does not appear to affect fecal excretion of fats, sterols, or bile acids.

12.2 Pharmacodynamics

Niacin functions in the body after conversion to nicotinamide adenine dinucleotide (NAD) in the NAD coenzyme system. Niacin (but not nicotinamide) in gram doses reduces total cholesterol (TC), low density lipoprotein cholesterol (LDL-C), and triglycerides (TG), and increases high-density lipoprotein cholesterol (HDL-C). The magnitude of individual lipid and lipoprotein responses may be influenced by the severity and type of underlying lipid abnormality. The increase in HDL-C is associated with an increase in apolipoprotein A-I (Apo A-I) and a shift in the distribution of HDL subfractions. These shifts include an increase in the $HDL_2:HDL_3$ ratio, and an elevation in lipoprotein A-I (Lp A-I, an HDL-C particle containing only Apo A-I). Niacin treatment also decreases serum levels of apolipoprotein B-100 (Apo B), the major protein component of the very low-density lipoprotein (VLDL) and LDL fractions, and of Lp(a), a variant form of LDL independently associated with coronary risk. In addition, preliminary reports suggest that niacin causes favorable LDL particle size transformations, although the clinical relevance of this effect requires further investigation. The effect of niacin-induced changes in lipids/proteins on cardiovascular morbidity or mortality in individuals without preexisting coronary disease has not been established.

A variety of clinical studies have demonstrated that elevated levels of TC, LDL-C, and Apo B promote human atherosclerosis. Similarly, decreased levels of HDL-C are associated with the development of atherosclerosis. Epidemiological investigations have established that cardiovascular morbidity and mortality vary directly with the level of Total-C and LDL-C, and inversely with the level of HDL-C.

Like LDL, cholesterol-enriched triglyceride-rich lipoproteins, including VLDL, intermediate-density lipoprotein (IDL), and their remnants, can also promote atherosclerosis. Elevated plasma TG are frequently found in a triad with low HDL-C levels and small LDL particles, as well as in association with non-lipid metabolic risk factors for coronary heart disease (CHD). As such, total plasma TG has not consistently been shown to be an independent risk factor for CHD. Furthermore, the independent effect of raising HDL-C or lowering TG on the risk of coronary and cardiovascular morbidity and mortality has not been determined.

12.3 Pharmacokinetics

Absorption

Due to extensive and saturable first-pass metabolism, niacin concentrations in the general circulation are dose dependent and highly variable. Time to reach the maximum niacin plasma concentrations was about 5 hours following NIASPAN. To reduce the risk of gastrointestinal (GI) upset, administration of NIASPAN with a low-fat meal or snack is recommended.

Single-dose bioavailability studies have demonstrated that the 500 mg and 1000 mg tablet strengths are dosage form equivalent but the 500 mg and 750 mg tablet strengths are not dosage form equivalent.

Metabolism

The pharmacokinetic profile of niacin is complicated due to extensive first-pass metabolism that is dose-rate specific and, at the doses used to treat dyslipidemia, saturable. In humans, one pathway is through a simple conjugation step with glycine to form nicotinuric acid (NUA). NUA is then excreted in the urine, although there may be a small amount of reversible metabolism back to niacin. The other pathway results in the formation of nicotinamide adenine dinucleotide (NAD). It is unclear whether nicotinamide is formed as a precursor to, or following the synthesis of, NAD. Nicotinamide is further metabolized to at least N-methylnicotinamide (MNA) and nicotinamide-N-oxide (NNO). MNA is further metabolized to two other compounds, N-methyl-2-pyridone-5-carboxamide (2PY) and N-methyl-4-pyridone-5-carboxamide (4PY). The formation of 2PY appears to predominate over 4PY in humans. At the doses used to treat hyperlipidemia, these metabolic pathways are saturable, which explains the nonlinear relationship between niacin dose and plasma concentrations following multiple-dose NIASPAN administration.

Nicotinamide does not have hypolipidemic activity; the activity of the other metabolites is unknown.

Elimination

Following single and multiple doses, approximately 60 to 76% of the niacin dose administered as NIASPAN was recovered in urine as niacin and metabolites; up to 12% was recovered as unchanged niacin after multiple dosing. The ratio of metabolites recovered in the urine was dependent on the dose administered.

Pediatric Use

No pharmacokinetic studies have been performed in this population (≤16 years) [see Use in Specific Populations (8.4)].

Geriatric Use

No pharmacokinetic studies have been performed in this population (> 65 years) [see Use in Specific Populations (8.5)].

Renal Impairment

No pharmacokinetic studies have been performed in this population. NIASPAN should be used with caution in patients with renal disease [see Warnings and Precautions (5)].

Hepatic Impairment

No pharmacokinetic studies have been performed in this population. Active liver disease, unexplained transaminase elevations and significant or unexplained hepatic dysfunction are contraindications to the use of NIASPAN [see Contraindications (4) and Warnings and Precautions (5.3)].

Gender

Steady-state plasma concentrations of niacin and metabolites after administration of NIASPAN are generally higher in women than in men, with the magnitude of the difference varying with dose and metabolite. This gender differences observed in plasma levels of niacin and its metabolites may be due to gender-specific differences in metabolic rate or volume of distribution. Recovery of niacin and metabolites in urine, however, is generally similar for men and women, indicating that absorption is similar for both genders [see Gender (8.8)].

Drug interactions

Fluvastatin

Niacin did not affect fluvastatin pharmacokinetics [see Drug Interactions (7.1)].

Lovastatin

When NIASPAN 2000 mg and lovastatin 40 mg were co-administered, NIASPAN increased lovastatin C_{max} and AUC by 2% and 14%, respectively, and decreased lovastatin acid C_{max} and AUC by 22% and 2%, respectively. Lovastatin reduced NIASPAN bioavailability by 2-3% [see Drug Interactions (7.1)].

Simvastatin

When NIASPAN 2000 mg and simvastatin 40 mg were co-administered, NIASPAN increased simvastatin C_{max} and AUC by 1% and 9%, respectively, and simvastatin acid C_{max} and AUC by 2% and 18%, respectively. Simvastatin reduced NIASPAN bioavailability by 2% [see Drug Interactions (7.1)].

Bile Acid Sequestrants

An in vitro study was carried out investigating the niacin-binding capacity of colestipol and cholestyramine. About 98% of available niacin was bound to colestipol, with 10 to 30% binding to cholestyramine [see Drug Interactions (7.2)].

13 NONCLINICAL TOXICOLOGY

13.1 Carcinogenesis and Mutagenesis and Impairment of Fertility

Niacin administered to mice for a lifetime as a 1% solution in drinking water was not carcinogenic. The mice in this study received approximately 6 to 8 times a human dose of 3000 mg/day as determined on a mg/m^2 basis. Niacin was negative for mutagenicity in the Ames test. No studies on impairment of fertility have been performed. No studies have been conducted with NIASPAN regarding carcinogenesis, mutagenesis, or impairment of fertility.

14 CLINICAL STUDIES

14.1 Niacin Clinical Studies

The role of LDL-C in atherogenesis is supported by pathological observations, clinical studies, and many animal experiments. Observational epidemiological studies have clearly established that high TC or LDL-C and low HDL-C are risk factors for CHD. Additionally, elevated levels of Lp(a) have been shown to be independently associated with CHD risk.

Niacin's ability to reduce mortality and the risk of definite, nonfatal myocardial infarction (MI) has been assessed in long-term studies. The Coronary Drug Project, completed in 1975, was designed to assess the safety and efficacy of niacin and other lipid-altering drugs in men 30 to 64 years old with a history of MI. Over an observation period of 5 years, niacin treatment was associated with a statistically significant reduction in nonfatal, recurrent MI. The incidence of definite, nonfatal MI was 8.9% for the 1,119 patients randomized to nicotinic acid versus 12.2% for the 2,789 patients who received placebo (p<0.004). Total mortality was similar in the two groups at 5 years (24.4% with nicotinic acid versus 25.4% with placebo; p=N.S.). At the time of a 15-year follow-up, there were 11% (69) fewer deaths in the niacin group compared to the placebo cohort (52.0% versus 58.2%; p=0.0004). However, mortality at 15 years was not an original endpoint of the Coronary Drug Project. In addition, patients had not received niacin for approximately 9 years, and confounding variables such as concomitant medication use and medical or surgical treatments were not controlled.

The Cholesterol-Lowering Atherosclerosis Study (CLAS) was a randomized, placebo-controlled, angiographic trial testing combined colestipol and niacin therapy in 162 non-smoking males with previous coronary bypass surgery. The primary, per-subject cardiac endpoint was global coronary artery change score. After 2 years, 61% of patients in the placebo cohort showed disease progression by global change score (n=82), compared with only 38.8% of drug-treated subjects (n=80), when both native arteries and grafts were con-

Table 3. Lipid Response to NIASPAN Therapy

Treatment	n	TC	LDL-C	HDL-C	TC/HDL-C	TG	Lp(a)	Apo B	Apo A-I
				Mean Percent Change from Baseline to Week 16*					
NIASPAN 1000 mg at bedtime	41	-3	-5	+18	-17	-21	-13	-6	+9
NIASPAN 2000 mg at bedtime	41	-10	-14	+22	-25	-28	-27	-16	+8
Placebo	40	0	-1	+4	-3	0	0	+1	+3
NIASPAN 1500 mg at bedtime	76	-8	-12	+20	-20	-13	-15	-12	+8
Placebo	73	+2	+1	+2	+1	+12	+2	+1	+2

n = number of patients at baseline;
* Mean percent change from baseline for all NIASPAN doses was significantly different (p < 0.05) from placebo for all lipid parameters shown except Apo A-I at 2000 mg.

Table 4. Lipid Response in Dose-Escalation Study

Treatment	n	TC	LDL-C	HDL-C	TC/HDL-C	TG	Lp(a)	Apo B	Apo A-I
				Mean Percent Change from Baseline*					
Placebo‡	44	-2	-1	+5	-7	-6	-5	-2	+4
NIASPAN	87								
500 mg at bedtime		-2	-3	+10	-10	-5	-3	-2	+5
1000 mg at bedtime		-5	-9	+15	-17	-11	-12	-7	+8
1500 mg at bedtime		-11	-14	+22	-26	-28	-20	-15	+10
2000 mg at bedtime		-12	-17	+26	-29	-35	-24	-16	+12

n = number of patients enrolled;
‡ Placebo data shown are after 24 weeks of placebo treatment.
* For all NIASPAN doses except 500 mg, mean percent change from baseline was significantly different (p < 0.05) from placebo for all lipid parameters shown except Lp(a) and Apo A-I which were significantly different from placebo starting with 1500 mg and 2000 mg, respectively.

sidered (p<0.005); disease regression also occurred more frequently in the drug-treated group (16.2% versus 2.4%; p=0.002). In a follow-up to this trial in a subgroup of 103 patients treated for 4 years, again, significantly fewer patients in the drug-treated group demonstrated progression than in the placebo cohort (48% versus 85%, respectively; p<0.0001).

The Familial Atherosclerosis Treatment Study (FATS) in 146 men ages 62 and younger with Apo B levels ≥125 mg/dL, established coronary artery disease, and family histories of vascular disease, assessed change in severity of disease in the proximal coronary arteries by quantitative arteriography. Patients were given dietary counseling and randomized to treatment with either conventional therapy with double placebo (or placebo plus colestipol if the LDL-C was elevated); lovastatin plus colestipol; or niacin plus colestipol. In the conventional therapy group, 46% of patients had disease progression (and no regression) in at least one of nine proximal coronary segments; regression was the only change in 11%. In contrast, progression (as the only change) was seen in only 25% in the niacin plus colestipol group, while regression was observed in 39%. Though not an original endpoint of the trial, clinical events (death, MI, or revascularization for worsening angina) occurred in 10 of 52 patients who received conventional therapy, compared with 2 of 48 who received niacin plus colestipol.

The Harvard Atherosclerosis Reversibility Project (HARP) was a randomized placebo-controlled, 2.5-year study of the effect of a stepped-care antihyperlipidemic drug regimen on 91 patients (80 men and 11 women) with CHD and average baseline TC levels less than 250 mg/dL and ratios of TC to HDL-C greater than 4.0. Drug treatment consisted of an HMG-CoA reductase inhibitor administered alone as initial therapy followed by addition of varying dosages of either a slow-release nicotinic acid, cholestyramine, or gemfibrozil. Addition of nicotinic acid to the HMG-CoA reductase inhibitor resulted in further statistically significant mean reductions in TC, LDL-C, and TG, as well as a further increase in HDL-C in a majority of patients (40 of 44 patients). The ratios of TC to HDL-C and LDL-C to HDL-C were also significantly reduced by this combination drug regimen [see Warnings and Precautions (5.2)].

14.2 NIASPAN Clinical Studies

Placebo-Controlled Clinical Studies in Patients with Primary Hyperlipidemia and Mixed Dyslipidemia: In two randomized, double-blind, parallel, multi-center, placebo-controlled trials, NIASPAN dosed at 1000, 1500 or 2000 mg daily at bedtime with a low-fat snack for 16 weeks (including 4 weeks of dose escalation) favorably altered lipid profiles compared to placebo (Table 3). Women appeared to have a greater response than men at each NIASPAN dose level (see *Gender Effect,* below).

[See table 3 at top of previous page]

In a double-blind, multi-center, forced dose-escalation study, monthly 500 mg increases in NIASPAN dose resulted in incremental reductions of approximately 5% in LDL-C and Apo B levels in the daily dose range of 500 mg through 2000 mg (Table 4). Women again tended to have a greater response to NIASPAN than men (see *Gender Effect,* below).

[See table 4 at top of previous page]

Pooled results for major lipids from these three placebo-controlled studies are shown below (Table 5).

[See table 5 above]

Gender Effect: Combined data from the three placebo-controlled NIASPAN studies in patients with primary hyperlipidemia and mixed dyslipidemia suggest that, at each NIASPAN dose level studied, changes in lipid concentrations are greater for women than for men (Table 6).

[See table 6 above]

Other Patient Populations: In a double-blind, multi-center, 19-week study the lipid-altering effects of NIASPAN (forced titration to 2000 mg at bedtime) were compared to baseline in patients whose primary lipid abnormality was a low level of HDL-C (HDL-C ≤40 mg/dL, TG ≤400 mg/dL, and LDL-C ≤160, or <130 mg/dL in the presence of CHD). Results are shown below (Table 7).

[See table 7 above]

At NIASPAN 2000 mg/day, median changes from baseline (25th, 75th percentiles) for LDL-C, HDL-C, and TG were -3% (-14, +12%), +27% (+13, +38%), and -33% (-50, -19%), respectively.

14.3 NIASPAN and Lovastatin Clinical Studies

Combination NIASPAN and Lovastatin Study: In a multi-center, randomized, double-blind, parallel, 28-week study, a combination tablet of NIASPAN and lovastatin was compared to each individual component in patients with Type IIa and IIb hyperlipidemia. Using a forced dose-escalation study design, patients received each dose for at least 4 weeks. Patients randomized to treatment with the combination tablet of NIASPAN and lovastatin initially received 500 mg/20 mg (expressed as mg of niacin/mg of lovastatin) once daily before bedtime. The dose was increased by 500 mg at 4-week intervals (based on the NIASPAN component) to a maximum dose of 1000 mg/20 mg in one-half of

the patients and 2000 mg/40 mg in the other half. The NIASPAN monotherapy group underwent a similar titration from 500 mg to 2000 mg. The patients randomized to lovastatin monotherapy received 20 mg for 12 weeks titrated to 40 mg for up to 16 weeks. Up to a third of the patients randomized to the combination tablet of NIASPAN and lovastatin or NIASPAN monotherapy discontinued prior to Week 28. Results from this study showed that combination therapy decreased LDL-C, TG and Lp(a), and increased HDL-C in a dose-dependent fashion (Tables 8, 9, 10, and 11). Results from this study for LDL-C mean percent change from baseline (the primary efficacy variable) showed that:

1. LDL-lowering with the combination tablet of NIASPAN and lovastatin was significantly greater than that achieved with lovastatin 40 mg only after 28 weeks of titration to a dose of 2000 mg/40 mg (p<0.0001)
2. The combination tablet of NIASPAN and lovastatin at doses of 1000 mg/20 mg or higher achieved greater LDL-lowering than NIASPAN (p<0.0001)

The LDL-C results are summarized in Table 8.

[See table 8 above]

Combination therapy achieved significantly greater HDL-raising compared to lovastatin and NIASPAN monotherapy at all doses (Table 9).

[See table 9 at top of next page]

In addition, combination therapy achieved significantly greater TG lowering at doses of 1000 mg/20 mg or greater compared to lovastatin and NIASPAN monotherapy (Table 10).

[See table 10 at top of next page]

The Lp(a)-lowering effects of combination therapy and NIASPAN monotherapy were similar, and both were superior to lovastatin (Table 11). The independent effect of low-

Information on the AbbVie, Inc. products listed on these pages is from the prescribing information in use as of July 31, 2014. For more information, please visit rxabbvie.com or call 1-800-633-9110.

Table 5. Selected Lipid Response to NIASPAN in Placebo-Controlled Clinical Studies*

Mean Baseline and Median Percent Change from Baseline (25th, 75th Percentiles)

NIASPAN Dose	n	LDL-C	HDL-C	TG
1000 mg at bedtime	104			
Baseline (mg/dL)		218	45	172
Percent Change		-7 (-15, 0)	+14 (+7, +23)	-16 (-34, +3)
1500 mg at bedtime	120			
Baseline (mg/dL)		212	46	171
Percent Change		-13 (-21, -4)	+19 (+9, +31)	-25 (-45, -2)
2000 mg at bedtime	85			
Baseline (mg/dL)		220	44	160
Percent Change		-16 (-26, -7)	+22 (+15, +34)	-38 (-52, -14)

* Represents pooled analyses of results; minimum duration on therapy at each dose was 4 weeks.

Table 6. Effect of Gender on NIASPAN Dose Response

Mean Percent Change from Baseline

NIASPAN	n	LDL-C		HDL-C		TG		Apo B	
Dose	(M/F)	M	F	M	F	M	F	M	F
500 mg at bedtime	50/37	-2	-5	+11	+8	-3	-9	-1	-5
1000 mg at bedtime	76/52	-6*	-11*	+14	+20	-10	-20	-5*	-10*
1500 mg at bedtime	104/59	-12	-16	+19	+24	-17	-28	-13	-15
2000 mg at bedtime	75/53	-15	-18	+23	+26	-30	-36	-16	-16

n = number of male/female patients enrolled.
* Percent change significantly different between genders (p < 0.05).

Table 7. Lipid Response to NIASPAN in Patients with Low HDL-C

Mean Baseline and Mean Percent Change from Baseline*

	n	TC	LDL-C	HDL-C	TC/HDL-C	TG	Lp(a)†	Apo B†	Apo A-I†	Lp A-I††
Baseline (mg/dL)	88	190	120	31	6	194	8	106	105	32
Week 19 (% Change)	71	-3	0	+26	-22	-30	-20	-9	+11	+20

n = number of patients
* Mean percent change from baseline was significantly different (p < 0.05) for all lipid parameters shown except LDL-C.
† n = 72 at baseline and 69 at week 19.
†† n = 30 at baseline and week 19.

Table 8. LDL-C mean percent change from baseline

Week	Combination Tablet of NIASPAN and Lovastatin			NIASPAN			Lovastatin		
	n*	Dose (mg/mg)	LDL	n*	Dose (mg)	LDL	n*	Dose (mg)	LDL
Baseline	57	–	190.9 mg/dL	61	–	189.7 mg/dL	61	–	185.6 mg/dL
12	47	1000/20	-30%	46	1000	-3%	56	20	-29%
16	45	1000/40	-36%	44	1000	-6%	56	40	-31%
20	42	1500/40	-37%	43	1500	-12%	54	40	-34%
28	42	2000/40	-42%	41	2000	-14%	53	40	-32%

* n = number of patients remaining in trial at each time point

Table 9. HDL-C mean percent change from baseline

Week	Combination Tablet of NIASPAN and Lovastatin			NIASPAN			Lovastatin		
	n*	Dose (mg/mg)	HDL	n*	Dose (mg)	HDL	n*	Dose (mg)	HDL
Baseline	57	–	45 mg/dL	61	–	47 mg/dL	61	–	43 mg/dL
12	47	1000/20	+20%	46	1000	+14%	56	20	+3%
16	45	1000/40	+20%	44	1000	+15%	56	40	+5%
20	42	1500/40	+27%	43	1500	+22%	54	40	+6%
28	42	2000/40	+30%	41	2000	+24%	53	40	+6%

* n = number of patients remaining in trial at each time point

Table 10. TG median percent change from baseline

Week	Combination Tablet of NIASPAN and Lovastatin			NIASPAN			Lovastatin		
	n*	Dose (mg/mg)	TG	n*	Dose (mg)	TG	n*	Dose (mg)	TG
Baseline	57	–	174 mg/dL	61	–	186 mg/dL	61	–	171 mg/dL
12	47	1000/20	-32%	46	1000	-22%	56	20	-20%
16	45	1000/40	-39%	44	1000	-23%	56	40	-17%
20	42	1500/40	-44%	43	1500	-31%	54	40	-21%
28	42	2000/40	-44%	41	2000	-31%	53	40	-20%

* n = number of patients remaining in trial at each time point

Table 11. Lp(a) median percent change from baseline

Week	Combination Tablet of NIASPAN and Lovastatin			NIASPAN			Lovastatin		
	n*	Dose (mg/mg)	Lp(a)	n*	Dose (mg)	Lp(a)	n*	Dose (mg)	Lp(a)
Baseline	57	–	34 mg/dL	61	–	41 mg/dL	60	–	42 mg/dL
12	47	1000/20	-9%	46	1000	-8%	55	20	+8%
16	45	1000/40	-9%	44	1000	-12%	55	40	+8%
20	42	1500/40	-17%	43	1500	-22%	53	40	+6%
28	42	2000/40	-22%	41	2000	-32%	52	40	0%

* n = number of patients remaining in trial at each time point

Table 12. Non-HDL Treatment Response Following 24-Week Treatment Mean Percent Change from Simvastatin 20-mg Treated Baseline

Group A								
	Combination Tablet of NIASPAN and Simvastatin 2000/20			Combination Tablet of NIASPAN and Simvastatin 1000/20			Simvastatin 20		
Week	n[a]	Dose (mg/mg)	Non-HDL[b]	n[a]	Dose (mg/mg)	Non-HDL[b]	n[a]	Dose (mg/mg)	Non-HDL[b]
Baseline	56	–	163.1 mg/dL	108	–	164.8 mg/dL	102	–	163.7 mg/dL
4	52	500/20	-12.9%	86	500/20	-12.8%	91	20	-8.3%
8	46	1000/20	-17.5%	91	1000/20	-15.5%	95	20	-8.3%
12	46	1500/20	-18.9%	90	1000/20	-14.8%	96	20	-6.4%
24	40	2000/20	-19.5%[†]	78	1000/20	-13.6%[†]	90	20	-5.0%
Dropouts by week 24:	28.6%			27.8%			11.8%		

[a] n=number of subjects with values in the analysis window at each timepoint
[b] The percent change from baseline is the model-based mean from a repeated measures mixed model with no imputation for missing data from study dropouts.
[†] significant vs. simvastatin 20 mg at the primary endpoint (Week 24), p<0.05

ering Lp(a) with NIASPAN or combination therapy on the risk of coronary and cardiovascular morbidity and mortality has not been determined.
[See table 11 above]

14.4 NIASPAN and Simvastatin Clinical Studies
In a double-blind, randomized, multicenter, multi-national, active-controlled, 24-week study, the lipid effects of a combination tablet of NIASPAN and simvastatin were compared to simvastatin 20 mg and 80 mg in 641 patients with type II hyperlipidemia or mixed dyslipidemia. Following a lipid qualification phase, patients were eligible to enter one of two treatment groups. In Group A, patients on simvastatin 20 mg monotherapy, with elevated non-HDL levels and LDL-C levels at goal per the NCEP guidelines, were randomized to one of three treatment arms: combination tablet of NIASPAN and simvastatin 1000/20 mg, combination tablet of NIASPAN and simvastatin 2000/20 mg, or simvastatin 20 mg. In Group B, patients on simvastatin 40 mg monotherapy, with elevated non-HDL levels per the NCEP guidelines regardless of attainment of LDL-C goals, were randomized to one of three treatment arms: combination tablet of NIASPAN and simvastatin 1000/40 mg, combination tablet of NIASPAN and simvastatin 2000/40 mg, or simvastatin 80 mg. Therapy was initiated at the 500 mg dose of combination tablet of NIASPAN and simvastatin and increased by 500 mg every four weeks. Thus patients were titrated to the 1000 mg dose of combination tablet of NIASPAN and simvastatin after four weeks and to the 2000 mg dose of combination tablet of NIASPAN and simvastatin after 12 weeks. All patients randomized to simvastatin monotherapy received 50 mg immediate-release niacin daily in an attempt to keep the study from becoming unblinded due to flushing in the combination tablet of NIASPAN and simvastatin groups. Patients were instructed to take one 325 mg aspirin or 200 mg ibuprofen 30 minutes prior to taking the double-blind medication to help minimize flushing effects.

In Group A, the primary efficacy analysis was a comparison of the mean percent change in non-HDL levels between the combination tablet of NIASPAN and simvastatin 2000/20 mg and simvastatin 20 mg groups, and if statistically significant, then a comparison was conducted between the combination tablet of NIASPAN and simvastatin 1000/20 mg and simvastatin 20 mg groups. In Group B, the primary efficacy analysis was a determination of whether the mean percent change in non-HDL in the combination tablet of NIASPAN and simvastatin 2000/40 mg group was non-inferior to the mean percent change in the simvastatin 80 mg group, and if so, whether the mean percent change in non-HDL in the combination tablet of NIASPAN and simvastatin 1000/40 mg group was non-inferior to the mean percent change in the simvastatin 80 mg group.
In Group A, the non-HDL-C lowering with combination tablet of NIASPAN and simvastatin 2000/20 and combination tablet of NIASPAN and simvastatin 1000/20 was statistically significantly greater than that achieved with simvastatin 20 mg after 24 weeks (p<0.05; Table 12). The completion rate after 24 weeks was 72% for the combination tablet of NIASPAN and simvastatin arms and 88% for the simvastatin 20 mg arm. In Group B, the non-HDL-C lowering with combination tablet of NIASPAN and simvastatin 2000/40 and combination tablet of NIASPAN and simvastatin 1000/40 was non-inferior to that achieved with simvastatin 80 mg after 24 weeks (Table 13). The completion rate after 24 weeks was 78% for the combination tablet of NIASPAN and simvastatin arms and 80% for the simvastatin 80 mg arm.
The combination tablet of NIASPAN and simvastatin was not superior to simvastatin in lowering LDL-C in either Group A or Group B. However, the combination tablet of NIASPAN and simvastatin was superior to simvastatin in both groups in lowering TG and raising HDL (Tables 14 and 15).
[See table 12 above]
[See table 13 at top of next page]
[See table 14 at top of next page]
[See table 15 at top of next page]

16 HOW SUPPLIED/STORAGE AND HANDLING
NIASPAN tablets are supplied as unscored, medium-orange, film-coated, capsule-shaped (containing 500 or 750 mg of niacin) or oval shaped (containing 1000 mg of niacin) tablets, in an extended-release formulation. Tablets are printed with the "a" logo and the tablet strength (500, 750 or 1000). Tablets are supplied in bottles of 30 and 90 as shown below.
500 mg tablets: bottles of 30 - NDC# 0074–3074–30
500 mg tablets: bottles of 90 - NDC# 0074–3074–90
750 mg tablets: bottles of 30 - NDC# 0074–3079–30
750 mg tablets: bottles of 90 - NDC# 0074–3079–90
1000 mg tablets: bottles of 30 - NDC# 0074–3080–30
1000 mg tablets: bottles of 90 - NDC# 0074–3080–90
Storage: Store at room temperature 20° to 25°C (68° to 77°F).

17 PATIENT COUNSELING INFORMATION
17.1 Patient Counseling
Patients should be advised to adhere to their National Cholesterol Education Program (NCEP) recommended diet, a regular exercise program, and periodic testing of a fasting lipid panel.
Patients should be advised to inform other healthcare professionals prescribing a new medication that they are taking NIASPAN.
The patient should be informed of the following:
Dosing Time
NIASPAN tablets should be taken at bedtime, after a low-fat snack. Administration on an empty stomach is not recommended.
Tablet Integrity
NIASPAN tablets should not be broken, crushed or chewed, but should be swallowed whole.
Dosing Interruption
If dosing is interrupted for any length of time, their physician should be contacted prior to restarting therapy; re-titration is recommended.
Muscle Pain
Notify their physician of any unexplained muscle pain, tenderness, or weakness promptly. They should discuss all medication, both prescription and over the counter, with their physician.
Flushing
Flushing (warmth, redness, itching and/or tingling of the skin) is a common side effect of niacin therapy that may subside after several weeks of consistent NIASPAN use. Flushing may vary in severity and is more likely to occur with initiation of therapy, or during dose increases. By dosing at bedtime, flushing will most likely occur during sleep. However, if awakened by flushing at night, the patient should get up slowly, especially if feeling dizzy, feeling faint, or taking blood pressure medications. Advise patients of the symptoms of flushing and how they differ from the symptoms of a myocardial infarction.

Use of Aspirin Medication

Taking aspirin (up to the recommended dose of 325 mg) approximately 30 minutes before dosing can minimize flushing.

Diet

Avoid ingestion of alcohol, hot beverages and spicy foods around the time of taking NIASPAN to minimize flushing.

Supplements

Notify their physician if they are taking vitamins or other nutritional supplements containing niacin or nicotinamide.

Dizziness

Notify their physician if symptoms of dizziness occur.

Diabetics

If diabetic, to notify their physician of changes in blood glucose.

Pregnancy

Discuss future pregnancy plans with your patients, and discuss when to stop NIASPAN if they are trying to conceive. Patients should be advised that if they become pregnant, they should stop taking NIASPAN and call their healthcare professional.

Breastfeeding

Women who are breastfeeding should be advised to not use NIASPAN. Patients, who have a lipid disorder and are breastfeeding, should be advised to discuss the options with their healthcare professional.

© AbbVie Inc. 2013

Manufactured for AbbVie Inc., North Chicago, IL 60064, U.S.A.

500 mg tablets

by Norwich Pharmaceuticals, Inc., Norwich, NY 13815

or

500 mg, 750 mg and 1000 mg tablets

by AbbVie LTD, Barceloneta, PR 00617

Ref. 03-A751-R8-Revised March, 2013

PATIENT INFORMATION

NIASPAN® (ny-a-span)

(niacin extended-release) tablets

Read this information carefully before you start taking NIASPAN and each time you get a refill. There may be new information. This information does not take the place of talking with your doctor about your medical condition or your treatment.

What is NIASPAN?

NIASPAN is a prescription medicine used with diet and exercise to increase the good cholesterol (HDL) and lower the bad cholesterol (LDL) and fats (triglycerides) in your blood.

• NIASPAN can be used by itself or with other cholesterol-lowering medicines.

• NIASPAN is also used to lower the risk of heart attack in people who have had a heart attack and have high cholesterol.

• In people with coronary artery disease and high cholesterol, NIASPAN, when used with a bile acid-binding resin (another cholesterol medicine) can slow down or lessen the build-up of plaque (fatty deposits) in your arteries.

• In people with heart problems and well-controlled cholesterol, taking NIASPAN with another cholesterol-lowering medicine (simvastatin) has not been shown to reduce heart attacks or strokes more than taking simvastatin alone.

It is not known if NIASPAN is safe and effective in children 16 years of age and under.

Who should not take NIASPAN?

Do not take NIASPAN if you have:

• liver problems

• a stomach ulcer

• bleeding problems

• an allergy to niacin or any of the ingredients in NIASPAN. See the end of this leaflet for a complete list of ingredients in NIASPAN.

What should I tell my doctor before taking NIASPAN?

Before you take NIASPAN, tell your doctor, if you:

• have diabetes. Tell your doctor if your blood sugar levels change after you take NIASPAN.

• have gout

• have kidney problems

• are pregnant or plan to become pregnant. It is not known if NIASPAN will harm your unborn baby. Talk to your doctor if you are pregnant or plan to become pregnant while taking NIASPAN.

• are breastfeeding or plan to breastfeed. NIASPAN can pass into your breast milk. You and your doctor should decide if you will take NIASPAN or breastfeed. You should not do both. Talk to your doctor about the best way to feed your baby if you take NIASPAN.

Tell your doctor about all the medicines you take, including prescription and non-prescription medicines, vitamins, herbal supplements or other nutritional supplements containing niacin or nicotinamide. NIASPAN and other medicines may affect each other causing side effects. NIASPAN may affect the way other medicines work, and other medicines may affect how NIASPAN works.

Table 13. Non-HDL Treatment Response Following 24-Week Treatment Mean Percent Change from Simvastatin 40-mg Treated Baseline

Group B

Week	n[a]	Dose (mg/mg)	Non-HDL[b]	n[a]	Dose (mg/mg)	Non-HDL[b]	n[a]	Dose (mg/mg)	Non-HDL[b]
	Combination Tablet of NIASPAN and Simvastatin 2000/40			Combination Tablet of NIASPAN and Simvastatin 1000/40			Simvastatin 80		
Baseline	98	–	144.4 mg/dL	111	–	141.2 mg/dL	113	–	134.5 mg/dL
4	96	500/40	-6.0%	108	500/40	-5.9%	110	80	-11.3%
8	93	1000/40	-15.5%	100	1000/40	-16.2%	104	80	-13.7%
12	90	1500/40	-18.4%	97	1000/40	-12.6%	100	80	-9.5%
24	80	2000/40	-7.6%[c]	82	1000/40	-6.7%[d]	90	80	-6.0%
Dropouts by week 24:	18.4%			26.1%			20.4%		

[a] n=number of subjects with values in the analysis window at each timepoint

[b] The percent change from baseline is the model-based mean from a repeated measures mixed model with no imputation for missing data from study dropouts

[c] non-inferior to simvastatin 80 arm; 95% confidence interval of mean difference in non-HDL for the combination tablet of NIASPAN and simvastatin 2000/40 vs. simvastatin 80 is (-7.7%, 4.5%)

[d] non-inferior to simvastatin 80 arm; 95% confidence interval of mean difference in non-HDL for combination tablet of NIASPAN and simvastatin 1000/40 vs. combination tablet of NIASPAN and simvastatin 80 is (-6.6%, 5.3%)

Table 14. Mean Percent Change from Baseline to Week 24 in Lipoprotein Lipid Levels

Treatment Group A

TREATMENT	N	LDL-C	Total-C	HDL-C	TG[a]	Apo B
Baseline (mg/dL)*	266	120	207	43	209	102
Simvastatin 20 mg	102	-6.7%	-4.5%	7.8%	-15.3%	-5.6%
Combination Tablet of NIASPAN and Simvastatin 1000/20	108	-11.9%	-8.8%	20.7%	-26.5%	-13.2%
Combination Tablet of NIASPAN and Simvastatin 2000/20	56	-14.3%	-11.1%	29.0%	-38.0%	-18.5%

* either treatment naïve or after receiving simvastatin 20 mg

[a] medians are reported for TG

Table 15. Mean Percent Change from Baseline to Week 24 in Lipoprotein Lipid Levels

Treatment Group B

TREATMENT	N	LDL-C	Total-C	HDL-C	TG[a]	Apo B
Baseline (mg/dL)*	322	108	187	47	145	93
Simvastatin 80 mg	113	-11.4%	-6.2%	0.1%	0.3%	-7.5%
Combination Tablet of NIASPAN and Simvastatin 1000/40	111	-7.1%	-3.1%	15.4%	-22.8%	-7.7%
Combination Tablet of NIASPAN and Simvastatin 2000/40	98	-5.1	-1.6%	24.4%	-31.8%	-10.5%

* after receiving simvastatin 40 mg

[a] medians are reported for TG

Especially tell your doctor if you take:

• other medicines to lower cholesterol or triglycerides

• aspirin

• blood pressure medicines

• blood thinner medicines

• large amounts of alcohol

Know the medicines you take. Keep a list of them to show your doctor and pharmacist when you get a new medicine.

How should I take NIASPAN?

• Take NIASPAN exactly as your doctor tells you to take it.

• Take NIASPAN tablets whole. Do not break, crush or chew NIASPAN tablets before swallowing.

• Take NIASPAN 1 time a day at bedtime after a low-fat snack. NIASPAN should not be taken on an empty stomach.

• All forms of niacin are not the same as NIASPAN. Do not switch between forms of niacin without first talking to your doctor as severe liver damage can occur.

• Do not change your dose or stop taking NIASPAN unless your doctor tells you to.

• If you need to stop taking NIASPAN, call your doctor before you start taking NIASPAN again. Your doctor may need to lower your dose of NIASPAN.

• If you forget to take a dose of NIASPAN, take it as soon as you remember.

• If you take too much NIASPAN, call your doctor right away.

• Medicines used to lower your cholesterol called bile acid resins, such as colestipol and cholestyramine, should not be taken at the same time of day as NIASPAN. You should take NIASPAN and the bile acid resin medicine at least 4 to 6 hours apart.

• Your doctor may do blood tests before you start taking NIASPAN and during your treatment. You should see your doctor regularly to check your cholesterol and triglyceride levels and to check for side effects.

What are the possible side effects of NIASPAN?

NIASPAN may cause serious side effects, including:

• **severe liver problems. Signs of liver problems include:**

  ○ increased tiredness

  ○ dark colored urine (tea-colored)

  ○ loss of appetite

  ○ light colored stools

  ○ nausea

  ○ right upper stomach (abdomen) pain

  ○ yellowing of your skin or whites of your eye

  ○ itchy skin

• **unexplained muscle pain, tenderness or weakness**

• **high blood sugar level (glucose)**

Call your doctor right away if you have any of the side effects listed above.

The most common side effects of NIASPAN include:

• flushing

• diarrhea

• nausea

• vomiting

• increased cough

• rash

Flushing is the most common side effect of NIASPAN.

Flushing happens when tiny blood vessels near the surface of the skin (especially on the face, neck, chest and/or back) open wider. Symptoms of flushing may include any or all of the following:

• warmth

• redness

• itching

• tingling of the skin

Flushing does not always happen. If it does, it is usually within 2 to 4 hours after taking a dose of NIASPAN. Flushing may last for a few hours. Flushing is more likely to happen when you first start taking NIASPAN or when your dose of NIASPAN is increased. Flushing may get better after several weeks.

Information on the AbbVie, Inc. products listed on these pages is from the prescribing information in use as of July 31, 2014. For more information, please visit rxabbvie.com or call 1-800-633-9110.

If you wake up at night because of flushing, get up slowly, especially if you:

- feel dizzy or faint
- take blood pressure medicines

To lower your chance of flushing:

- Ask your doctor if you can take aspirin to help lower the flushing side effect from NIASPAN. You can take aspirin (up to the recommended dose of 325 mg) about 30 minutes before you take NIASPAN to help lower the flushing side effect.
- Do not drink hot beverages (including coffee), alcohol, or eat spicy foods around the time you take NIASPAN.
- Take NIASPAN with a low-fat snack to lessen upset stomach.

People with high cholesterol and heart disease are at risk for a heart attack. Symptoms of a heart attack may be different from a flushing reaction from NIASPAN. **The following may be symptoms of a heart attack due to heart disease and not a flushing reaction:**

- chest pain
- pain in other areas of your upper body such as one or both arms, back, neck, jaw or stomach
- shortness of breath
- sweating
- nausea
- lightheadedness

The chest pain you have with a heart attack may feel like uncomfortable pressure, squeezing, fullness or pain that lasts more than a few minutes, or that goes away and comes back. Heart attacks may be sudden and intense, but often start slowly, with mild pain or discomfort.

Call your doctor right away if you have any symptoms of a heart attack.

Tell your doctor if you have any side effect that bothers you or does not go away.

These are not all the possible side effects of NIASPAN. For more information, ask your doctor or pharmacist.

Call your doctor for medical advice about side effects. You may report side effects to FDA at 1-800-FDA-1088.

How should I store NIASPAN?

- Store NIASPAN at 68°F to 77°F (20°C to 25°C).

Keep NIASPAN and all medicines out of the reach of children.

General information about the safe and effective use of NIASPAN.

Medicines are sometimes prescribed for purposes other than those listed in a Patient Information leaflet. Do not use NIASPAN for a condition for which it was not prescribed. Do not give NIASPAN to other people, even if they have the same symptoms that you have. It may harm them.

This leaflet summarizes the most important information about NIASPAN. If you would like more information, talk with your doctor. You can ask your pharmacist or doctor for information about NIASPAN that is written for health professionals.

For more information, go to www.NIASPAN.com or call AbbVie Inc. Medical Information at 1-800-633-9110.

What are the ingredients in NIASPAN?

Active ingredient: niacin

Inactive Ingredients: hypromellose, povidone, stearic acid, and polyethylene glycol, and the following coloring agents: FD&C yellow #6/sunset yellow FCF Aluminum Lake, synthetic red and yellow iron oxides, and titanium dioxide.

This Patient Information has been approved by the U.S. Food and Drug Administration.

Manufactured for AbbVie Inc., North Chicago, IL 60064, U.S.A.

500 mg tablets by Norwich Pharmaceuticals, Inc., Norwich, NY 13815

or 500 mg, 750 mg and 1000 mg tablets by AbbVie LTD, Barceloneta, PR 00617

Ref. 03-A751-R8-Revised March, 2013

Shown in Product Identification Guide, page 304

NIMBEX®
[nǐm-běks]
(cisatracurium besylate)
Injection

℞

This drug should be administered only by adequately trained individuals familiar with its actions, characteristics, and hazards.

NOT FOR USE IN NEONATES
CONTAINS BENZYL ALCOHOL

DESCRIPTION

NIMBEX® (cisatracurium besylate) is a nondepolarizing skeletal muscle relaxant for intravenous administration. Compared to other neuromuscular blocking agents, it is intermediate in its onset and duration of action. Cisatracurium besylate is one of 10 isomers of atracurium besylate and constitutes approximately 15% of that mixture. Cisatracurium besylate is [1R-[1α,2α(1′R*,2′R*)]]-2,2′- [1,5-pentanediylbis[oxy(3-oxo-3,1-propanediyl)]]bis[1-

[(3,4-dimethoxyphenyl)methyl]-1,2,3,4-tetrahydro-6,7-dimethoxy-2-methylisoquinolinium] dibenzenesulfonate. The molecular formula of the cisatracurium parent bis-cation is $C_{53}H_{72}N_2O_{12}$ and the molecular weight is 929.2. The molecular formula of cisatracurium as the besylate salt is $C_{65}H_{82}N_2O_{18}S_2$ and the molecular weight is 1243.50. The structural formula of cisatracurium besylate is:

The log of the partition coefficient of cisatracurium besylate is -2.12 in a 1-octanol/distilled water system at 25°C.

NIMBEX Injection is a sterile, non-pyrogenic aqueous solution provided in 5 mL, 10 mL, and 20 mL vials. The pH is adjusted to 3.25 to 3.65 with benzenesulfonic acid. The 5 mL and 10 mL vials each contain cisatracurium besylate, equivalent to 2 mg/mL cisatracurium. The 20 mL vial, **intended for ICU use only**, contains cisatracurium besylate, equivalent to 10 mg/mL cisatracurium. The 10 mL vial, intended for multiple-dose use, contains 0.9% benzyl alcohol as a preservative. The 5 mL and 20 mL vials are single-use vials and do not contain benzyl alcohol.

Cisatracurium besylate slowly loses potency with time at a rate of approximately 5% per year under refrigeration (5°C). NIMBEX should be refrigerated at 2° to 8°C (36° to 46°F) in the carton to preserve potency. The rate of loss in potency increases to approximately 5% per *month* at 25°C (77°F). Upon removal from refrigeration to room temperature storage conditions (25°C/77°F), use NIMBEX within 21 days, even if rerefrigerated.

CLINICAL PHARMACOLOGY

NIMBEX binds competitively to cholinergic receptors on the motor end-plate to antagonize the action of acetylcholine, resulting in block of neuromuscular transmission. This action is antagonized by acetylcholinesterase inhibitors such as neostigmine.

Pharmacodynamics

The neuromuscular blocking potency of NIMBEX is approximately threefold that of atracurium besylate. The time to maximum block is up to 2 minutes longer for equipotent doses of NIMBEX compared to atracurium besylate. The clinically effective duration of action and rate of spontaneous recovery from equipotent doses of NIMBEX and atracurium besylate are similar.

The average ED_{95} (dose required to produce 95% suppression of the adductor pollicis muscle twitch response to ulnar nerve stimulation) of cisatracurium is 0.05 mg/kg (range: 0.048 to 0.053) in adults receiving opioid/nitrous oxide/oxygen anesthesia. For comparison, the average ED_{95} for atracurium when also expressed as the parent bis-cation is 0.17 mg/kg under similar anesthetic conditions.

The pharmacodynamics of $2 \times ED_{95}$ to $8 \times ED_{95}$ doses of cisatracurium administered over 5 to 10 seconds during opioid/nitrous oxide/oxygen anesthesia are summarized in Table 1. When the dose is doubled, the clinically effective duration of block increases by approximately 25 minutes. Once recovery begins, the rate of recovery is independent of dose. Isoflurane or enflurane administered with nitrous oxide/oxygen to achieve 1.25 MAC [Minimum Alveolar Concentration] may prolong the clinically effective duration of action of initial and maintenance doses, and decrease the average infusion rate requirement of NIMBEX. The magnitude of these effects may depend on the duration of administration of the volatile agents. Fifteen to 30 minutes of exposure to 1.25 MAC isoflurane or enflurane had minimal effects on the duration of action of initial doses of NIMBEX and therefore, no adjustment to the initial dose should be necessary when NIMBEX is administered shortly after initiation of volatile agents. In long surgical procedures during enflurane or isoflurane anesthesia, less frequent maintenance dosing, lower maintenance doses, or reduced infusion rates of NIMBEX may be necessary. The average infusion rate requirement may be decreased by as much as 30% to 40%.

The onset, duration of action, and recovery profiles of NIMBEX during propofol/oxygen or propofol/nitrous oxide/oxygen anesthesia are similar to those during opioid/nitrous oxide/oxygen anesthesia.

[See table 1 above]

When administered during the induction of adequate anesthesia using propofol, nitrous oxide/oxygen, and co-induction agents (e.g., fentanyl and midazolam), GOOD or EXCELLENT conditions for tracheal intubation occurred in 96/102 (94%) patients in 1.5 to 2.0 minutes following 0.15 mg/kg cisatracurium and in 97/110 (88%) patients in 1.5 minutes following 0.2 mg/kg cisatracurium.

In one intubation study during thiopental anesthesia in which fentanyl and midazolam were administered two min-

Table 1. Pharmacodynamic Dose Response* of NIMBEX During Opioid/Nitrous Oxide/Oxygen Anesthesia

Initial Dose of NIMBEX (mg/kg)	Time to 90% Block (min)	Time to Maximum Block (min)	5% Recovery (min)	Time to Spontaneous Recovery			T_4:T_1 Ratio‡≥70% (min)	25%-75% Recovery Index (min)
				25% Recovery† (min)	95% Recovery (min)			
Adults								
0.1 (2 × ED_{95}) (n§=98)	3.3 (1.0-8.7)	5.0 (1.2-17.2)	33 (15-51)	42 (22-63)	64 (25-93)		64 (32-91)	13 (5-30)
0.15 (3 × ED_{95}) (n=39)	2.6 (1.0-4.4)	3.5 (1.6-6.8)	46 (28-65)	55 (44-74)	76 (60-103)		75 (63-98)	13 (11-16)
0.2 (4 × ED_{95}) (n=30)	2.4 (1.5-4.5)	2.9 (1.9-5.2)	59 (31-103)	65 (43-103)	81 (53-114)		85 (55-114)	12 (2-30)
0.25 (5 × ED_{95}) (n=15)	1.6 (0.8-3.3)	2.0 (1.2-3.7)	70 (58-85)	78 (66-86)	91 (76-109)		97 (82-113)	8 (5-12)
0.4 (8 × ED_{95}) (n=15)	1.5 (1.3-1.8)	1.9 (1.4-2.3)	83 (37-103)	91 (59-107)	121 (110-134)		126 (115-137)	14 (10-18)
Infants (1-23 mos.)								
0.15** (n=18-26)	1.5 (0.7-3.2)	2.0 (1.3-4.3)	36 (28-50)	43 (34-58)	64 (54-84)		59 (49-76)	11.3 (7.3-18.3)
Children (2-12 yr)								
0.08¶ (2 × ED_{95}) (n=60)	2.2 (1.2-6.8)	3.3 (1.7-9.7)	22 (11-38)	29 (20-46)	52 (37-64)		50 (37-62)	11 (7-15)
0.1 (n=16)	1.7 (1.3-2.7)	2.8 (1.8-6.7)	21 (13-31)	28 (21-38)	46 (37-58)		44 (36-58)	10 (7-12)
0.15** (n=23-24)	2.1 (1.3-2.8)	3.0 (1.5-8.0)	29 (19-38)	36 (29-46)	55 (45-72)		54 (44-66)	10.6 (8.5-17.7)

* Values shown are medians of means from individual studies. Values in parentheses are ranges of individual patient values.
† Clinically effective duration of block.
‡ Train-of-four ratio.
§ n=the number of patients with Time to Maximum Block data.
‖ Propofol anesthesia.
¶ Halothane anesthesia.
** Thiopentone, alfentanil, N_2O/O_2 anesthesia

utes prior to induction, intubation conditions were assessed at 120 seconds. Table 2 displays these results in this study of 51 patients.

Table 2. Study of Tracheal Intubation Comparing Two Doses of Cisatracurium (Thiopental Anesthesia)

Intubating Conditions at 120 seconds	$3 \times ED_{95}$ 0.15 mg/kg n = 26	$4 \times ED_{95}$ 0.20 mg/kg n = 25
Excellent and Good		
Proportion	23/26	24/25
Percent	88%	96%
95% CI	76,100	88,100
Excellent		
Proportion	8/26	15/26
Percent	31%	60%
Good		
Proportion	15/26	9/25
Percent	58%	36%

While GOOD or EXCELLENT intubation conditions were achieved in the majority of patients in this setting, EXCELLENT intubation conditions were more frequently achieved with the 0.2 mg/kg dose (60%) than the 0.15 mg/kg dose (31%) when intubation was attempted 2.0 minutes following cisatracurium.

A second study evaluated intubation conditions after 3 and $4 \times ED_{95}$ (0.15 mg/kg and 0.20 mg/kg) following induction with fentanyl and midazolam and either thiopental or propofol anesthesia. This study compared intubation conditions produced by these doses of cisatracurium after 1.5 minutes. Table 3 displays these results.

[See table 3 above]

EXCELLENT intubation conditions were more frequently observed with the 0.2 mg/kg dose when intubation was attempted 1.5 minutes following cisatracurium.

A third study in pediatric patients (ages 1 month to 12 years) evaluated intubation conditions at 120 seconds after 0.15 mg/kg NIMBEX following induction with either halothane (with halothane/nitrous oxide/oxygen maintenance) or thiopentone and fentanyl (with thiopentone/fentanyl nitrous oxide/oxygen maintenance). The results are summarized in Table 4.

[See table 4 above]

EXCELLENT or GOOD intubating conditions were produced 120 seconds following 0.15 mg/kg NIMBEX in 88/90 (98%) of patients induced with halothane and in 85/90 (94%) of patients induced with thiopentone and fentanyl. There were no patients for whom intubation was not possible, but there were 7/120 patients ages 1-12 years for whom intubating conditions were described as poor.

Repeated administration of maintenance doses or a continuous infusion of NIMBEX for up to 3 hours is not associated with development of tachyphylaxis or cumulative neuromuscular blocking effects. The time needed to recover from successive maintenance doses does not change with the number of doses administered as long as partial recovery is allowed to occur between doses. Maintenance doses can therefore be administered at relatively regular intervals with predictable results. The rate of spontaneous recovery of neuromuscular function after infusion is independent of the duration of infusion and comparable to the rate of recovery following initial doses (Table 1).

Long-term infusion (up to 6 days) of NIMBEX during mechanical ventilation in the ICU has been evaluated in two studies. In a randomized, double-blind study using presence of a single twitch during train-of-four (TOF) monitoring to regulate dosage, patients treated with NIMBEX (n = 19) recovered neuromuscular function ($T_4:T_1$ ratio ≥ 70%) following termination of infusion in approximately 55 minutes (range: 20 to 270) whereas those treated with vecuronium (n = 12) recovered in 178 minutes (range: 40 minutes to 33 hours). In another study comparing NIMBEX and atracurium, patients recovered neuromuscular function in approximately 50 minutes for both NIMBEX (range: 20 to 175; n = 34) and atracurium (range: 35 to 85; n = 15).

The neuromuscular block produced by NIMBEX is readily antagonized by anticholinesterase agents once recovery has started. As with other nondepolarizing neuromuscular blocking agents, the more profound the neuromuscular block at the time of reversal, the longer the time required for recovery of neuromuscular function.

In children (2 to 12 years) cisatracurium has a lower ED_{95} than in adults (0.04 mg/kg, halothane/nitrous oxide/oxygen anesthesia). At 0.1 mg/kg during opioid anesthesia, cisatracurium had a faster onset and shorter duration of action in children than in adults (Table 1). Recovery following reversal is faster in children than in adults.

At 0.15 mg/kg during opioid anesthesia, cisatracurium had a faster onset and longer clinically effective duration of action in infants aged 1-23 months compared to children aged 2-12 years (Table 1).

Table 3. Study of Tracheal Intubation Comparing Three Doses of Cisatracurium (Thiopental or Propofol Anesthesia)

Intubating Conditions at 90 seconds	$3 \times ED_{95}$ 0.15 mg/kg Propofol n = 31	$3 \times ED_{95}$ 0.15 mg/kg Thiopental n = 31	$4 \times ED_{95}$ 0.20 mg/kg Propofol n = 30	$4 \times ED_{95}$ 0.20 mg/kg Thiopental n = 28
Excellent and Good				
Proportion	29/31	28/31	28/30	27/28
Percent	94%	90%	93%	96%
95% CI	85,100	80,100	84,100	90,100
Excellent				
Proportion	18/31	17/31	22/30	16/28
Percent	58%	55%	70%	57%
Good				
Proportion	11/31	11/31	6/30	11/28
Percent	35%	35%	20%	39%

Table 4. Study of Tracheal Intubation for Pediatrics Stratified by Age Group (0.15 mg/kg NIMBEX with Halothane or Thiopentone/Fentanyl Anesthesia)

Intubating Conditions at 120 seconds**	NIMBEX 0.15 mg/kg 1-11 mo. n = 30 Halothane Anesthesia	NIMBEX 0.15 mg/kg 1-11 mo. n = 30 Thiopentone/ Fentanyl Anesthesia	NIMBEX 0.15 mg/kg 1-4 years n = 31 Halothane Anesthesia	NIMBEX 0.15 mg/kg 1-4 years n = 31 Thiopentone/ Fentanyl Anesthesia	NIMBEX 0.15 mg/kg 5-12 years n = 30 Halothane Anesthesia	NIMBEX 0.15 mg/kg 5-12 years n = 30 Thiopentone/ Fentanyl Anesthesia
Excellent and Good						
Proportion	30/30	30/30	29/30	26/30	29/30	29/30
Percent	100%	100%	97%	87%	97%	97%
Excellent						
Proportion	30/30	25/30	27/30	19/30	22/30	21/30
Percent	100%	83%	90%	63%	73%	70%
Good						
Proportion	0	5/30	2/30	7/30	7/30	8/30
Percent	0%	17%	7%	23%	23%	27%
Poor						
Proportion	0/30	0/30	1/30	4/30	1/30	1/30
Percent	0%	0%	3%	13%	3%	3%

** **Excellent:** Easy passage of the tube without coughing. Vocal cords relaxed and abducted.
Good: Passage of tube with slight coughing and/or bucking. Vocal cords relaxed and abducted.
Poor: Passage of tube with moderate coughing and/or bucking. Vocal cords moderately adducted. Response of patient requires adjustment of ventilation pressure and/or rate.

Studies were conducted during both opioid-based and halothane-based anesthesia in children aged 1-11 months, 1-4 years, and 5-12 years. Cisatracurium had a faster onset and longer duration of action in infants 1-11 months compared to children 1-4 years, who in turn have a faster onset and longer duration of action for cisatracurium compared to children 5-12 years.

The mean time to onset of maximum T_1 suppression was generally faster for pediatric patients induced with halothane compared to thiopentone/fentanyl and the clinically effective duration (time to 25% recovery) was longer (by up to 15%) for pediatric patients under halothane anesthesia.

Hemodynamics Profile

The cardiovascular profile of NIMBEX allows it to be administered by rapid bolus at higher multiples of the ED_{95} than atracurium. NIMBEX has no dose-related effects on mean arterial blood pressure (MAP) or heart rate (HR) following doses ranging from 2 to $8 \times ED_{95}$ (> 0.1 to > 0.4 mg/kg), administered over 5 to 10 seconds, in healthy adult patients (Figure 1) or in patients with serious cardiovascular disease (Figure 2).

A total of 141 patients undergoing coronary artery bypass grafting (CABG) have been administered NIMBEX in three active controlled clinical trials and have received doses ranging from 2 to $8 \times ED_{95}$. While the hemodynamic profile was comparable in both the NIMBEX and active control groups, data for doses above 0.3 mg/kg in this population are limited.

Unlike atracurium, NIMBEX® (cisatracurium besylate), at therapeutic doses of $2 \times ED_{95}$ to $8 \times ED_{95}$ (0.1 to 0.4 mg/kg), administered over 5 to 10 seconds, does not cause dose-related elevations in mean plasma histamine concentration.

[See figure 1 at top of next column]
[See figure 2 at top of next page]

No clinically significant changes in MAP or HR were observed following administration of doses up to 0.1 mg/kg NIMBEX over 5 to 10 seconds in 2- to 12-year-old children receiving either halothane/nitrous oxide/oxygen or opioid/nitrous oxide/oxygen anesthesia. Doses of 0.15 mg/kg NIMBEX administered over 5 seconds were not consistently associated with changes in HR and MAP in pediatric patients aged 1 month to 12 years receiving opioid/nitrous oxide/oxygen or halothane/nitrous oxide/oxygen anesthesia.

[See figure 3 at top of next page]
[See figure 4 at top of next page]

Figure 1. Maximum Percent Change from Preinjection in Heart Rate (HR) and Mean Arterial Pressure (MAP) During First 5 Minutes after Initial 4 x ED_{95} to 8 x ED_{95} Doses of NIMBEX in Healthy Adult Patients Receiving Opioid/Nitrous Oxide/Oxygen Anesthesia (n = 44)

Pharmacokinetics

General

The neuromuscular blocking activity of NIMBEX is due to parent drug. Cisatracurium plasma concentration-time data following IV bolus administration are best described by a two-compartment open model (with elimination from both compartments) with an elimination half-life ($t_{1/2}\beta$) of 22 minutes, a plasma clearance (CL) of 4.57 mL/min/kg, and a volume of distribution at steady state (V_{ss}) of 145 mL/kg. Cisatracurium undergoes organ-independent Hofmann elimination (a chemical process dependent on pH and temperature) to form the monoquaternary acrylate metabolite and laudanosine, neither of which has any neuromuscular blocking activity (see **Pharmacokinetics** -Metabolism sec-

Information on the AbbVie, Inc. products listed on these pages is from the prescribing information in use as of July 31, 2014. For more information, please visit rxabbvie.com or call 1-800-633-9110.

Figure 2. Percent Change from Preinjection in Heart Rate (HR) and Mean Arterial Pressure (MAP) 10 Minutes After an Initial 4 x ED95 to 8 x ED95 Dose of NIMBEX in Patients Undergoing CABG Surgery Receiving Oxygen/Fentanyl/Midazolam/ Anesthesia (n = 54)

Figure 3. Heart Rate and MAP Change at 1 Minute After the Initial Dose, By Age Group Treatment Group: NIMBEX 0:3 x ED95 Opioid Intubation at 120 Sec.

1-11 Months

1-5 Years

5-13 Years

Figure 4. Heart Rate and MAP Change at 1 Minute After the Initial Dose, By Age Group Treatment Group: NIMBEX H:3 x ED95 Halothane Intubation at 120 Sec.

1-11 Months

1-5 Years

5-13 Years

curium) has been noted to cause transient hypotension and, in higher doses, cerebral excitatory effects when administered to several animal species. The relationship between CNS excitation and laudanosine concentrations in humans has not been established (see **PRECAUTIONS - Long-term Use in the Intensive Care Unit**). Because cisatracurium is three times more potent than atracurium and lower doses are required, the corresponding laudanosine concentrations following cisatracurium are one third of those that would be expected following an equipotent dose of atracurium (see **Pharmacokinetics** - Special Populations -*Intensive Care Unit Patients*).

Results from population pharmacokinetic/pharmacodynamic (PK/PD) analyses from 241 healthy surgical patients are summarized in Table 5.

Table 5. Key Population PK/PD Parameter Estimates for Cisatracurium in Healthy Surgical Patients* Following 0.1 (2 × ED95) to 0.4 mg/kg (8 × ED95) NIMBEX

Parameter	Estimate[†]	Magnitude of Interpatient Variability (CV)[‡]
CL (mL/min/kg)	4.57	16%
V_{ss} (mL/kg)[§]	145	27%
k_{eo} (min-1)[∥]	0.0575	61%
EC_{50} (ng/mL)[¶]	141	52%

* Healthy male non-obese patients 19-64 years of age with creatinine clearance values greater than 70 mL/min who received cisatracurium during opioid anesthesia and had venous samples collected.
† The percent standard error of the mean (%SEM) ranged from 3% to 12% indicating good precision for the PK/PD estimates.
‡ Expressed as a coefficient of variation; the %SEM ranged from 20% to 35% indicating adequate precision for the estimates of interpatient variability.
§ V_{ss} is the volume of distribution at steady state estimated using a two-compartment model with elimination from both compartments. V_{ss} is equal to the sum of the volume in the central compartment (V_c) and the volume in the peripheral compartment (Vp); interpatient variability could only be estimated for V_c.
∥ Rate constant describing the equilibration between plasma concentrations and neuromuscular block.
¶ Concentration required to produce 50% T_1 suppression; an index of patient sensitivity.

The magnitude of interpatient variability in CL was low (16%), as expected based on the importance of Hofmann elimination (see **Pharmacokinetics** -Elimination). The magnitudes of interpatient variability in CL and volume of distribution were low in comparison to those for k_{eo} and EC_{50}. This suggests that any alterations in the time course of cisatracurium-induced block are more likely to be due to variability in the pharmacodynamic parameters than in the pharmacokinetic parameters. Parameter estimates from the population pharmacokinetic analyses were supported by noncompartmental pharmacokinetic analyses on data from healthy patients and from special patient populations. Conventional pharmacokinetic analyses have shown that the pharmacokinetics of cisatracurium are proportional to dose between 0.1 (2 × ED95) and 0.2 (4 × ED95) mg/kg cisatracurium. In addition, population pharmacokinetic analyses revealed no statistically significant effect of initial dose on CL for doses between 0.1 (2 × ED95) and 0.4 (8 × ED95) mg/kg cisatracurium.

Distribution
The volume of distribution of cisatracurium is limited by its large molecular weight and high polarity. The V_{ss} was equal to 145 mL/kg (Table 4) in healthy 19- to 64-year-old surgical patients receiving opioid anesthesia. The V_{ss} was 21% larger in similar patients receiving inhalation anesthesia (see **Pharmacokinetics** - Special Populations -*Other Patient Factors*).

Protein Binding
The binding of cisatracurium to plasma proteins has not been successfully studied due to its rapid degradation at physiologic pH. Inhibition of degradation requires nonphysiological conditions of temperature and pH which are associated with changes in protein binding.

Metabolism
The degradation of cisatracurium is largely independent of liver metabolism. Results from *in vitro* experiments suggest that cisatracurium undergoes Hofmann elimination (a pH and temperature-dependent chemical process) to form laudanosine (see **PRECAUTIONS - Long-term Use in the Intensive Care Unit**) and the monoquaternary acrylate metabolite. The monoquaternary acrylate undergoes hydrolysis by non-specific plasma esterases to form the monoquaternary alcohol (MQA) metabolite. The MQA metabolite can also undergo Hofmann elimination but at a much slower rate than cisatracurium. Laudanosine is further metabolized to desmethyl metabolites which are conjugated with glucuronic acid and excreted in the urine.

Organ-independent Hofmann elimination is the predominant pathway for the elimination of cisatracurium. The liver and kidney play a minor role in the elimination of cisatracurium but are primary pathways for the elimination of metabolites. Therefore, the $t_{1/2}\beta$ values of metabolites (including laudanosine) are longer in patients with kidney or liver dysfunction and metabolite concentrations may be higher after long-term administration (see **PRECAUTIONS - Long-term Use in the Intensive Care Unit**). Most importantly, C_{max} values of laudanosine are significantly lower in healthy surgical patients receiving infusions of NIMBEX than in patients receiving infusions of atracurium (mean ± SD C_{max}: 60 ± 52 and 342 ± 93 ng/mL, respectively).

Elimination
Clearance and Half-life
Mean CL values for cisatracurium ranged from 4.5 to 5.7 mL/min/kg in studies of healthy surgical patients. Compartmental pharmacokinetic modeling suggests that approximately 80% of the CL is accounted for by Hofmann elimination and the remaining 20% by renal and hepatic elimination. These findings are consistent with the low magnitude of interpatient variability in CL (16%) estimated as part of the population PK/PD analyses and with the recovery of parent and metabolites in urine. Following ^{14}C-cisatracurium administration to 6 healthy male patients,

tion). Following administration of radiolabeled cisatracurium, 95% of the dose was recovered in the urine; less than 10% of the dose was excreted as unchanged parent drug. Laudanosine, a metabolite of cisatracurium (and atra-

95% of the dose was recovered in the urine (mostly as conjugated metabolites) and 4% in the feces; less than 10% of the dose was excreted as unchanged parent drug in the urine. In 12 healthy surgical patients receiving nonradiolabeled cisatracurium who had Foley catheters placed for surgical management, approximately 15% of the dose was excreted unchanged in the urine.

In studies of healthy surgical patients, mean $t_{1/2}\beta$ values of cisatracurium ranged from 22 to 29 minutes and were consistent with the $t_{1/2}\beta$ of cisatracurium in vitro (29 minutes). The mean ± SD $t_{1/2}\beta$ values of laudanosine were 3.1 ± 0.4 and 3.3 ± 2.1 hours in healthy surgical patients receiving NIMBEX (n = 10) or atracurium (n = 10), respectively. During IV infusions of NIMBEX, peak plasma concentrations (C_{max}) of laudanosine and the MQA metabolite are approximately 6% and 11% of the parent compound, respectively.

Special Populations
Geriatric Patients (≥ 65 years)
The results of conventional pharmacokinetic analysis from a study of 12 healthy elderly patients and 12 healthy young adult patients receiving a single IV dose of 0.1 mg/kg NIMBEX are summarized in Table 6. Plasma clearances of cisatracurium were not affected by age; however, the volumes of distribution were slightly larger in elderly patients than in young patients resulting in slightly longer $t_{1/2}\beta$ values for cisatracurium. The rate of equilibration between plasma cisatracurium concentrations and neuromuscular block was slower in elderly patients than in young patients (mean ± SD k_{eo}: 0.071 ± 0.036 and 0.105 ± 0.021 minutes^{-1}, respectively); there was no difference in the patient sensitivity to cisatracurium-induced block, as indicated by EC_{50} values (mean ± SD EC_{50}: 91 ± 22 and 89 ± 23 ng/mL, respectively). These changes were consistent with the 1-minute slower times to maximum block in elderly patients receiving 0.1 mg/kg NIMBEX, when compared to young patients receiving the same dose. The minor differences in PK/PD parameters of cisatracurium between elderly patients and young patients were not associated with clinically significant differences in the recovery profile of NIMBEX® (cisatracurium besylate).

Table 6. Pharmacokinetic Parameters* of Cisatracurium in Healthy Elderly and Young Adult Patients Following 0.1 mg/kg (2 × ED$_{95}$) NIMBEX (Isoflurane/Nitrous Oxide/Oxygen Anesthesia)

Parameter	Healthy Elderly Patients	Healthy Young Adult Patients
Elimination Half-Life ($t_{1/2}\beta$, min)	25.8 ± 3.6†	22.1 ± 2.5
Volume of Distribution at Steady State‡ (mL/kg)	156 ± 17†	133 ± 15
Plasma Clearance (mL/min/kg)	5.7 ± 1.0	5.3 ± 0.9

* Values presented are mean ± SD.
† P < 0.05 for comparisons between healthy elderly and healthy young adult patients.
‡ Volume of distribution is underestimated because elimination from the peripheral compartment is ignored.

Patients with Hepatic Disease
Table 7 summarizes the conventional pharmacokinetic analysis from a study of NIMBEX in 13 patients with end-stage liver disease undergoing liver transplantation and 11 healthy adult patients undergoing elective surgery. The slightly larger volumes of distribution in liver transplant patients were associated with slightly higher plasma clearances of cisatracurium. The parallel changes in these parameters resulted in no difference in $t_{1/2}\beta$ values. There were no differences in k_{eo} or EC_{50} between patient groups. The times to maximum block were approximately one minute faster in liver transplant patients than in healthy adult patients receiving 0.1 mg/kg NIMBEX. These minor differences in pharmacokinetics were not associated with clinically significant differences in the recovery profile of NIMBEX.

The $t_{1/2}\beta$ values of metabolites are longer in patients with hepatic disease and concentrations may be higher after long-term administration (see Pharmacokinetics - Special Populations - Intensive Care Unit Patients).

Table 7. Pharmacokinetic Parameters* of Cisatracurium in Healthy Adult Patients and in Patients Undergoing Liver Transplantation Following 0.1 mg/kg (2 × ED$_{95}$) NIMBEX (Isoflurane/Nitrous Oxide/Oxygen Anesthesia)

Parameter	Liver Transplant Patients	Healthy Adult Patients
Elimination Half-Life ($t_{1/2}\beta$, min)	24.4 ± 2.9	23.5 ± 3.5

Table 9. Parameter Estimates* for Cisatracurium, Atracurium, and Metabolites in ICU Patients After Long-Term (24-48 Hour) Administration of NIMBEX or Atracurium Besylate

	Parameter	Cisatracurium (n = 6)	Atracurium (n = 6)
Parent Compound	CL (mL/min/kg)	7.45 ± 1.02	7.49 ± 0.66†
	$t_{1/2}\beta$ (min)	26.8 ± 11.1	16.5 ± 6.0†
	Vβ (mL/kg)‡	280 ± 103	178 ± 71†
Laudanosine	C_{max} (ng/mL)	707 ± 360	2318 ± 1498
	$t_{1/2}\beta$ (hrs)	6.6 ± 4.1	8.4 ± 7.3
MQA metabolite	C_{max} (ng/mL)	152-181§	943 ± 333‖
	$t_{1/2}\beta$ (min)	26-31§	21-58§

* Presented as mean ± standard deviation.
† n = 5.
‡ Volume of distribution during the terminal elimination phase, an underestimate because elimination from the peripheral compartment is ignored.
§ n = 2, range presented.
‖ n = 3.

Volume of Distribution at Steady State‡ (mL/kg)	195 ± 38†	161 ± 23
Plasma Clearance (mL/min/kg)	6.6 ± 1.1†	5.7 ± 0.8

* Values presented are mean ± SD.
† P < 0.05 for comparisons between liver transplant patients and healthy adult patients.
‡ Volume of distribution is underestimated because elimination from the peripheral compartment is ignored.

Patients with Renal Dysfunction
Results from a conventional pharmacokinetic study of NIMBEX in 13 healthy adult patients and 15 patients with end-stage renal disease (ESRD) undergoing elective surgery are summarized in Table 8. The PK/PD parameters of cisatracurium were similar in healthy adult patients and ESRD patients. The times to 90% block were approximately one minute slower in ESRD patients following 0.1 mg/kg NIMBEX. There were no differences in the durations or rates of recovery of NIMBEX between ESRD and healthy adult patients.

The $t_{1/2}\beta$ values of metabolites are longer in patients with renal failure and concentrations may be higher after long-term administration (see Pharmacokinetics - Special Populations - Intensive Care Unit Patients).

Table 8. Pharmacokinetic Parameters* for Cisatracurium in Healthy Adult Patients and in Patients With End-Stage Renal Disease (ESRD) Receiving 0.1 mg/kg (2 × ED$_{95}$) NIMBEX (Opioid/Nitrous Oxide/Oxygen Anesthesia)

Parameter	Healthy Adult Patients	ESRD Patients
Elimination Half-Life ($t_{1/2}\beta$, min)	29.4 ± 4.1	32.3 ± 6.3
Volume of Distribution at Steady State† (mL/kg)	149 ± 35	160 ± 32
Plasma Clearance (mL/min/kg)	4.66 ± 0.86	4.26 ± 0.62

* Values presented are mean ± SD.
† Volume of distribution is underestimated because elimination from the peripheral compartment is ignored.

Population pharmacokinetic analyses revealed that patients with creatinine clearances ≤ 70 mL/min had a slower rate of equilibration between plasma concentrations and neuromuscular block than patients with normal renal function; this change was associated with a slightly slower (~ 40 seconds) predicted time to 90% T_1 suppression in patients with renal dysfunction following 0.1 mg/kg NIMBEX. There was no clinically significant alteration in the recovery profile of NIMBEX in patients with renal dysfunction. The recovery profile of NIMBEX is unchanged in the presence of renal or hepatic failure, which is consistent with predominantly organ-independent elimination.

Intensive Care Unit (ICU) Patients
The pharmacokinetics of cisatracurium, atracurium, and their metabolites were determined in six ICU patients receiving NIMBEX and in six ICU patients receiving atracurium and are presented in Table 9. The plasma clearances of cisatracurium and atracurium are similar. The volume of distribution was larger and the $t_{1/2}\beta$ was longer for cisatracurium than for atracurium. The relationships between plasma cisatracurium or atracurium concentrations and neuromuscular block have not been evaluated in ICU patients. The minor differences in pharmacokinetics were not associated with any differences in the recovery profiles of NIMBEX and atracurium in ICU patients.
[See table 9 above]

Plasma metabolite pharmacokinetics are listed in Table 9. Limited pharmacokinetic data are available for patients with liver/kidney dysfunction receiving NIMBEX. Data from studies of atracurium demonstrate that renal/hepatic failure in ICU patients produces little to no effect on its pharmacokinetics, but decreases the biotransformation and elimination of the metabolites. Following atracurium, $t_{1/2}\beta$ values for laudanosine are longer in ICU patients with renal failure than in ICU patients with normal renal function (15 and 6 hours, respectively). The $t_{1/2}\beta$ values of laudanosine were 39 ± 14 hours in ICU patients with liver failure receiving atracurium after an unsuccessful liver transplantation and 5 ± 2 hours in similar ICU patients after successful liver transplantation. Therefore, relative to ICU patients with normal renal and hepatic function receiving NIMBEX, metabolite concentrations (plasma and tissues) may be higher in ICU patients with renal or hepatic failure (see Precautions - Long-term Use in the Intensive Care Unit). Consistent with the decreased infusion rate requirements for NIMBEX, metabolite concentrations were lower in patients receiving NIMBEX than in patients receiving atracurium besylate.

Pediatric Patients
The population PK/PD of cisatracurium were described in 20 healthy pediatric patients during halothane anesthesia, using the same model developed for healthy adult patients. The CL was higher in healthy pediatric patients (5.89 mL/min/kg) than in healthy adult patients (4.57 mL/min/kg) during opioid anesthesia. The rate of equilibration between plasma concentrations and neuromuscular block, as indicated by k_{eo}, was faster in healthy pediatric patients receiving halothane anesthesia (0.1330 minutes^{-1}) than in healthy adult patients receiving opioid anesthesia (0.0575 minutes^{-1}). The EC_{50} in healthy pediatric patients (125 ng/mL) was similar to the value in healthy adult patients (141 ng/mL) during opioid anesthesia. The minor differences in the PK/PD parameters of cisatracurium were associated with a faster time to onset and a shorter duration of cisatracurium-induced neuromuscular block in pediatric patients.

Other Patient Factors
Population PK/PD analyses revealed that gender and obesity were associated with statistically significant effects on the pharmacokinetics and/or pharmacodynamics of cisatracurium; these factors were not associated with clinically significant alterations in the predicted onset or recovery profile of NIMBEX. The use of inhalation agents was associated with a 21% larger V_{ss}, a 78% larger k_{eo}, and a 15% lower EC_{50} for cisatracurium. These changes resulted in a slightly faster (~45 seconds) predicted time to 90% T_1 suppression in patients receiving 0.1 mg/kg cisatracurium during inhalation anesthesia than in patients receiving the same dose of cisatracurium during opioid anesthesia; however, there were no clinically significant differences in the predicted recovery profile of NIMBEX between patient groups.

Individualization of Dosages
DOSES OF NIMBEX SHOULD BE INDIVIDUALIZED AND A PERIPHERAL NERVE STIMULATOR SHOULD BE USED TO MEASURE NEUROMUSCULAR FUNCTION DURING ADMINISTRATION OF NIMBEX IN ORDER TO MONITOR DRUG EFFECT, TO DETERMINE THE NEED FOR ADDITIONAL DOSES, AND TO CONFIRM RECOVERY FROM NEUROMUSCULAR BLOCK.

Based on the known action of NIMBEX and other neuromuscular blocking agents, the following factors should be considered when administering NIMBEX.

Information on the AbbVie, Inc. products listed on these pages is from the prescribing information in use as of July 31, 2014. For more information, please visit rxabbvie.com or call 1-800-633-9110.

Renal and Hepatic Disease
See **PRECAUTIONS** section.

Long-Term Use in the Intensive Care Unit (ICU)
The long-term infusion (up to 6 days) of NIMBEX during mechanical ventilation in the ICU has been evaluated in two studies. Average infusion rates of approximately 3 mcg/kg/min (range: 0.5 to 10.2) were required to achieve adequate neuromuscular block. As with other neuromuscular blocking agents, these data indicate the presence of wide interpatient variability in dosage requirements. In addition, dosage requirements may increase or decrease with time (see **PRECAUTIONS**). Use of NIMBEX in the ICU for longer than 6 days has not been studied.

Drugs or Conditions Causing Potentiation of or Resistance to Neuromuscular Block
Persons with certain pre-existing conditions or receiving certain drugs may require individualization of dosing (see **PRECAUTIONS**).

Burns
Patients with burns have been shown to develop resistance to nondepolarizing neuromuscular blocking agents, and may require individualization of dosing (see **PRECAUTIONS**).

INDICATIONS AND USAGE
NIMBEX is an intermediate-onset/intermediate-duration neuromuscular blocking agent indicated for inpatients and outpatients as an adjunct to general anesthesia, to facilitate tracheal intubation, and to provide skeletal muscle relaxation during surgery or mechanical ventilation in the ICU.

CONTRAINDICATIONS
NIMBEX is contraindicated in patients with known hypersensitivity to the product and its components. The 10 mL multiple-dose vials of Nimbex is contraindicated for use in premature infants because the formulation contains benzyl alcohol. (See **WARNINGS** and **PRECAUTIONS – Pediatric Use**).

WARNINGS
Anaphylaxis
Severe anaphylactic reactions to neuromuscular blocking agents, including NIMBEX, have been reported. These reactions have in some cases been life-threatening and fatal. Due to the potential severity of these reactions, the necessary precautions, such as the immediate availability of appropriate emergency treatment, should be taken. Precautions should also be taken in those individuals who have had previous anaphylactic reactions to other neuromuscular blocking agents since cross-reactivity between neuromuscular blocking agents, both depolarizing and non-depolarizing, has been reported in this class of drugs.

Administration
NIMBEX SHOULD BE ADMINISTERED IN CAREFULLY ADJUSTED DOSAGE BY OR UNDER THE SUPERVISION OF EXPERIENCED CLINICIANS WHO ARE FAMILIAR WITH THE DRUG'S ACTIONS AND THE POSSIBLE COMPLICATIONS OF ITS USE. THE DRUG SHOULD NOT BE ADMINISTERED UNLESS PERSONNEL AND FACILITIES FOR RESUSCITATION AND LIFE SUPPORT (TRACHEAL INTUBATION, ARTIFICIAL VENTILATION, OXYGEN THERAPY), AND AN ANTAGONIST OF NIMBEX ARE IMMEDIATELY AVAILABLE. IT IS RECOMMENDED THAT A PERIPHERAL NERVE STIMULATOR BE USED TO MEASURE NEUROMUSCULAR FUNCTION DURING THE ADMINISTRATION OF NIMBEX IN ORDER TO MONITOR DRUG EFFECT, DETERMINE THE NEED FOR ADDITIONAL DOSES, AND CONFIRM RECOVERY FROM NEUROMUSCULAR BLOCK.

NIMBEX HAS NO KNOWN EFFECT ON CONSCIOUSNESS, PAIN THRESHOLD, OR CEREBRATION. TO AVOID DISTRESS TO THE PATIENT, NEUROMUSCULAR BLOCK SHOULD NOT BE INDUCED BEFORE UNCONSCIOUSNESS.

NIMBEX Injection is acidic (pH 3.25 to 3.65) and may not be compatible with alkaline solutions having a pH greater than 8.5 (e.g., barbiturate solutions).

The 10 mL multiple-dose vials of NIMBEX contain benzyl alcohol, which is potentially toxic when administered locally to neural tissue. Exposure to excessive amounts of benzyl alcohol has been associated with toxicity (hypotension, metabolic acidosis), particularly in neonates, and an increased incidence of kernicterus, particularly in small preterm infants. There have been rare reports of deaths, primarily in preterm infants, associated with exposure to excessive amounts of benzyl alcohol. The amount of benzyl alcohol from medications is usually considered negligible compared to that received in flush solution containing benzyl alcohol. Administration of high dosages of medications containing this preservative must take into account the total amount of benzyl alcohol administered. The amount of benzyl alcohol at which toxicity may occur is not known. If the patient requires more than the recommended dosages or other medications containing this preservative, the practitioner must

consider the daily metabolic load of benzyl alcohol from these combined sources. Single-use vials (5 mL and 20 mL) of NIMBEX do not contain benzyl alcohol (see **WARNINGS** and **PRECAUTIONS - Pediatric Use**).

PRECAUTIONS
Because of its intermediate onset of action, NIMBEX is not recommended for rapid sequence endotracheal intubation. Recommended doses of NIMBEX® (cisatracurium besylate) have no clinically significant effects on heart rate; therefore, NIMBEX will not counteract the bradycardia produced by many anesthetic agents or by vagal stimulation.

Neuromuscular blocking agents may have a profound effect in patients with neuromuscular diseases (e.g., myasthenia gravis and the myasthenic syndrome). In these and other conditions in which prolonged neuromuscular block is a possibility (e.g., carcinomatosis), the use of a peripheral nerve stimulator and a dose of not more than 0.02 mg/kg NIMBEX is recommended to assess the level of neuromuscular block and to monitor dosage requirements.

Patients with burns have been shown to develop resistance to nondepolarizing neuromuscular blocking agents, including atracurium. The extent of altered response depends upon the size of the burn and the time elapsed since the burn injury. NIMBEX has not been studied in patients with burns; however, based on its structural similarity to atracurium, the possibility of increased dosing requirements and shortened duration of action must be considered if NIMBEX is administered to burn patients.

Patients with hemiparesis or paraparesis also may demonstrate resistance to nondepolarizing muscle relaxants in the affected limbs. To avoid inaccurate dosing, neuromuscular monitoring should be performed on a non-paretic limb.

Acid-base and/or serum electrolyte abnormalities may potentiate or antagonize the action of neuromuscular blocking agents. No data are available to support the use of NIMBEX by intramuscular injection.

Allergic Reactions
Since allergic cross-reactivity has been reported in this class, request information from your patients about previous anaphylactic reactions to other neuromuscular blocking agents. In addition, inform your patients that severe anaphylactic reactions to neuromuscular blocking agents, including NIMBEX have been reported (see **CONTRAINDICATIONS**).

Renal and Hepatic Disease
No clinically significant alterations in the recovery profile were observed in patients with renal dysfunction or in patients with end-stage liver disease following a 0.1 mg/kg dose of cisatracurium. The onset time was approximately 1 minute faster in patients with end-stage liver disease and approximately 1 minute slower in patients with renal dysfunction than in healthy adult control patients.

Malignant Hyperthermia (MH)
In a study of MH-susceptible pigs, cisatracurium besylate (highest dose 2000 mcg/kg equivalent to $3 \times ED_{95}$ in pigs and $40 \times ED_{95}$ in humans) did not trigger MH. Cisatracurium besylate has not been studied in MH-susceptible patients. Because MH can develop in the absence of established triggering agents, the clinician should be prepared to recognize and treat MH in any patient undergoing general anesthesia.

Long-Term Use in the Intensive Care Unit (ICU)
Long-term infusion (up to 6 days) of NIMBEX during mechanical ventilation in the ICU has been safely used in two studies. Dosage requirements may increase or decrease with time (see **CLINICAL PHARMACOLOGY - Individualization of Doses**).

Little information is available on the plasma levels and clinical consequences of cisatracurium metabolites that may accumulate during days to weeks of cisatracurium administration in ICU patients. Laudanosine, a major, biologically active metabolite of atracurium and cisatracurium without neuromuscular blocking activity, produces transient hypotension and, in higher doses, cerebral excitatory effects (generalized muscle twitching and seizures) when administered to several species of animals. There have been rare spontaneous reports of seizures in ICU patients who have received atracurium or other agents. These patients usually had predisposing causes (such as cranial trauma, cerebral edema, hypoxic encephalopathy, viral encephalitis, uremia). There are insufficient data to determine whether or not laudanosine contributes to seizures in ICU patients. Consistent with the decreased infusion rate requirements for NIMBEX, laudanosine concentrations were lower in patients receiving NIMBEX than in patients receiving atracurium for up to 48 hours (see **Pharmacokinetics -Special Populations - Intensive Care Unit Patients**).

In a randomized, double-blind study using train-of-four nerve stimulator monitoring to maintain at least one visible twitch, evaluable patients treated with NIMBEX (n = 19) recovered neuromuscular function (T_4:T_1 ratio $\geq 70\%$) following termination of infusion in approximately 55 minutes (range: 20 to 270) whereas evaluable vecuronium-treated

patients (n = 12) recovered in 178 minutes (range: 40 minutes to 33 hours). In another study comparing NIMBEX and atracurium, patients recovered neuromuscular function in approximately 50 minutes for both NIMBEX (range: 20 to 175; n = 34) and atracurium (range: 35 to 85; n = 15).

WHENEVER THE USE OF NIMBEX OR ANY OTHER NEUROMUSCULAR BLOCKING AGENT IN THE ICU IS CONTEMPLATED, IT IS RECOMMENDED THAT NEUROMUSCULAR FUNCTION BE MONITORED DURING ADMINISTRATION WITH A NERVE STIMULATOR. ADDITIONAL DOSES OF NIMBEX OR ANY OTHER NEUROMUSCULAR BLOCKING AGENT SHOULD NOT BE GIVEN BEFORE THERE IS A DEFINITE RESPONSE TO NERVE STIMULATION. IF NO RESPONSE IS ELICITED, INFUSION ADMINISTRATION SHOULD BE DISCONTINUED UNTIL A RESPONSE RETURNS.

The effects of hemofiltration, hemodialysis, and hemoperfusion on plasma levels of NIMBEX and its metabolites are unknown.

Drug Interactions
NIMBEX has been used safely following varying degrees of recovery from succinylcholine-induced neuromuscular block. Administration of 0.1 mg/kg ($2 \times ED_{95}$) NIMBEX at 10% or 95% recovery following an intubating dose of succinylcholine (1 mg/kg) produced $\geq 95\%$ neuromuscular block. The time to onset of maximum block following NIMBEX is approximately 2 minutes faster with prior administration of succinylcholine. Prior administration of succinylcholine had no effect on the duration of neuromuscular block following initial or maintenance bolus doses of NIMBEX. Infusion requirements of NIMBEX in patients administered succinylcholine prior to infusions of NIMBEX were comparable to or slightly greater than when succinylcholine was not administered.

The use of NIMBEX before succinylcholine to attenuate some of the side effects of succinylcholine has not been studied.

Although not studied systematically in clinical trials, no drug interactions were observed when vecuronium, pancuronium, or atracurium were administered following varying degrees of recovery from single doses or infusions of NIMBEX.

Isoflurane or enflurane administered with nitrous oxide/oxygen to achieve 1.25 MAC [Minimum Alveolar Concentration] may prolong the clinically effective duration of action of initial and maintenance doses of NIMBEX and decrease the required infusion rate of NIMBEX. The magnitude of these effects may depend on the duration of administration of the volatile agents. Fifteen to 30 minutes of exposure to 1.25 MAC isoflurane or enflurane had minimal effects on the duration of action of initial doses of NIMBEX and therefore, no adjustment to the initial dose should be necessary when NIMBEX is administered shortly after initiation of volatile agents. In long surgical procedures during enflurane or isoflurane anesthesia, less frequent maintenance dosing, lower maintenance doses, or reduced infusion rates of NIMBEX may be necessary. The average infusion rate requirement may be decreased by as much as 30% to 40%.

In clinical studies propofol had no effect on the duration of action or dosing requirements for NIMBEX.

Other drugs which may enhance the neuromuscular blocking action of nondepolarizing agents such as NIMBEX include certain antibiotics (e.g., aminoglycosides, tetracyclines, bacitracin, polymyxins, lincomycin, clindamycin, colistin, and sodium colistemethate); magnesium salts, lithium, local anesthetics, procainamide, and quinidine.

Resistance to the neuromuscular blocking action of nondepolarizing neuromuscular blocking agents has been demonstrated in patients chronically administered phenytoin or carbamazepine. While the effects of chronic phenytoin or carbamazepine therapy on the action of NIMBEX are unknown, slightly shorter durations of neuromuscular block may be anticipated and infusion rate requirements may be higher.

Drug/Laboratory Test Interactions
None known.

Carcinogenesis, Mutagenesis, Impairment of Fertility
Carcinogenesis and fertility studies have not been performed. Cisatracurium besylate was evaluated in a battery of four short-term mutagenicity tests. It was non-mutagenic in the Ames Salmonella assay, a rat bone marrow cytogenetic assay, and an *in vitro* human lymphocyte cytogenetics assay. As was the case with atracurium, the mouse lymphoma assay was positive both in the presence and absence of exogenous metabolic activation (rat liver S-9). In the absence of S-9, cisatracurium besylate was positive at *in vitro* cisatracurium concentrations of 40 mcg/mL and higher. The highest non-mutagenic concentration (30 mcg/mL) and incubation time (4 hours) resulted in an AUC approximately 120 times that noted in clinical studies and approximately 8.5 times the mean peak clinical concentration noted. In the presence of S-9, cisatracurium besylate was positive at a cisatracurium concentration of 300 mcg/mL but not at lower or higher concentrations.

Pregnancy
Teratogenic Effects
Pregnancy Category B
Teratology testing in nonventilated pregnant rats treated subcutaneously with maximum subparalyzing doses (4 mg/kg daily; equivalent to 8 × the human ED_{95} following a bolus dose of 0.2 mg/kg IV) and in ventilated rats treated intravenously with paralyzing doses of NIMBEX at 0.5 and 1.0 mg/kg; equivalent to 10 × and 20 × the human ED_{95} dose, respectively, revealed no maternal or fetal toxicity or teratogenic effects. There are no adequate and well-controlled studies of NIMBEX in pregnant women. Because animal studies are not always predictive of human response, NIMBEX should be used during pregnancy only if clearly needed.

Labor and Delivery
The use of NIMBEX during labor, vaginal delivery, or cesarean section has not been studied in humans and it is not known whether NIMBEX administered to the mother has effects on the fetus. Doses of 0.2 or 0.4 mg/kg cisatracurium given to female beagles undergoing cesarean section resulted in negligible levels of cisatracurium in umbilical vessel blood of neonates and no deleterious effects on the puppies. The action of neuromuscular blocking agents may be enhanced by magnesium salts administered for the management of toxemia of pregnancy.

Nursing Mothers
It is not known whether cisatracurium besylate is excreted in human milk. Because many drugs are excreted in human milk, caution should be exercised following administration of NIMBEX to a nursing woman.

Pediatric Use
NIMBEX has not been studied in pediatric patients below the age of 1 month (see CLINICAL PHARMACOLOGY and DOSAGE AND ADMINISTRATION for clinical experience and recommendations for use in children 1 month to 12 years of age). Intubation of the trachea in patients 1-4 years old was facilitated more reliably when NIMBEX was used in combination with Halothane than when opioids and nitrous oxide were used for induction of anesthesia.

The 10 mL multiple-dose vials of NIMBEX contain benzyl alcohol as a preservative. Benzyl alcohol, a component of this product, has been associated with serious adverse events and death, particularly in pediatric patients. The "gasping syndrome", (characterized by central nervous system depression, metabolic acidosis, gasping respirations, and high levels of benzyl alcohol and its metabolites found in the blood and urine) has been associated with benzyl alcohol dosages >99 mg/kg/day in neonates and low-birth-weight neonates. Additional symptoms may include gradual neurological deterioration, seizures, intracranial hemorrhage, hematologic abnormalities, skin breakdown, hepatic and renal failure, hypotension, bradycardia, and cardiovascular collapse. Although normal therapeutic doses of this product deliver amounts of benzyl alcohol that are substantially lower than those reported in association with the "gasping syndrome", the minimum amount of benzyl alcohol at which toxicity may occur is not known. Premature and low-birth-weight infants, as well as patients receiving high dosages, may be more likely to develop toxicity. Practitioners administering this and other medications containing benzyl alcohol should consider the combined daily metabolic load of benzyl alcohol from all sources.

Geriatric Use
Of the total number of subjects in clinical studies of NIMBEX, 57 were 65 and over, 63 were 70 and over, and 15 were 80 and over. The geriatric population included a subset of patients with significant cardiovascular disease (see CLINICAL PHARMACOLOGY - Hemodynamics Profile and Special Populations - Geriatric Patients subsections). No overall differences in safety or effectiveness were observed between these subjects and younger subjects, and other reported clinical experience has not identified differences in responses between elderly and younger subjects, but greater sensitivity of some older individuals to NIMBEX cannot be ruled out.

Minor differences in the pharmacokinetics of cisatracurium between elderly and young adult patients are not associated with clinically significant differences in the recovery profile of NIMBEX following a single 0.1 mg/kg dose; the time to maximum block is approximately 1 minute slower in elderly patients (see CLINICAL PHARMACOLOGY - Pharmacokinetics).

ADVERSE REACTIONS
Observed in Clinical Trials of Surgical Patients
Adverse experiences were uncommon among the 945 surgical patients who received NIMBEX in conjunction with other drugs in US and European clinical studies in the course of a wide variety of procedures in patients receiving opioid, propofol, or inhalation anesthesia. The following adverse experiences were judged by investigators during the clinical trials to have a possible causal relationship to administration of NIMBEX:
Incidence Greater than 1%
None.
Incidence Less than 1%

Cardiovascular
bradycardia (0.4%)
hypotension (0.2%)
flushing (0.2%).
Respiratory
bronchospasm (0.2%).
Dermatological
rash (0.1%).

Observed in Clinical Trials of Intensive Care Unit Patients
Adverse experiences were uncommon among the 68 ICU patients who received NIMBEX in conjunction with other drugs in US and European clinical studies. One patient experienced bronchospasm. In one of the two ICU studies, a randomized and double-blind study of ICU patients using TOF neuromuscular monitoring, there were two reports of prolonged recovery (167 and 270 minutes) among 28 patients administered NIMBEX and 13 reports of prolonged recovery (range: 90 minutes to 33 hours) among 30 patients administered vecuronium.

Observed During Clinical Practice
In addition to adverse events reported from clinical trials, the following events have been identified during post-approval use of cisatracurium besylate in conjunction with one or more anesthetic agents in clinical practice. Because they are reported voluntarily from a population of unknown size, estimates of frequency cannot be made. These events have been chosen for inclusion due to a combination of their seriousness, frequency of reporting, or potential causal connection to cisatracurium besylate.
General
Histamine release, hypersensitivity reactions including anaphylactic or anaphylactoid reactions which in some cases have been life threatening and fatal. Because these reactions were reported voluntarily from a population of uncertain size, it is not possible to reliably estimate their frequency (see WARNINGS and PRECAUTIONS). There are rare reports of wheezing, laryngospasm, bronchospasm, rash and itching following administration of NIMBEX in children. These reported adverse events were not serious and their etiology could not be established with certainty.
Musculoskeletal
Prolonged neuromuscular block, inadequate neuromuscular block, muscle weakness, and myopathy.

OVERDOSAGE
Overdosage with neuromuscular blocking agents may result in neuromuscular block beyond the time needed for surgery and anesthesia. The primary treatment is maintenance of a patent airway and controlled ventilation until recovery of normal neuromuscular function is assured. Once recovery from neuromuscular block begins, further recovery may be facilitated by administration of an anticholinesterase agent (e.g., neostigmine, edrophonium) in conjunction with an appropriate anticholinergic agent (see Antagonism of Neuromuscular Block below).

Antagonism of Neuromuscular Block
ANTAGONISTS (SUCH AS NEOSTIGMINE AND EDROPHONIUM) SHOULD NOT BE ADMINISTERED WHEN COMPLETE NEUROMUSCULAR BLOCK IS EVIDENT OR SUSPECTED. THE USE OF A PERIPHERAL NERVE STIMULATOR TO EVALUATE RECOVERY AND ANTAGONISM OF NEUROMUSCULAR BLOCK IS RECOMMENDED.
Administration of 0.04 to 0.07 mg/kg neostigmine at approximately 10% recovery from neuromuscular block (range: 0 to 15%) produced 95% recovery of the muscle twitch response and a T_4:T_1 ratio ≥ 70% in an average of 9 to 10 minutes. The times from 25% recovery of the muscle twitch response to a T_4:T_1 ratio ≥ 70% following these doses of neostigmine averaged 7 minutes. The mean 25% to 75% recovery index following reversal was 3 to 4 minutes.
Administration of 1.0 mg/kg edrophonium at approximately 25% recovery from neuromuscular block (range: 16% to 30%) produced 95% recovery and a T_4:T_1 ratio ≥ 70% in an average of 3 to 5 minutes.
Patients administered antagonists should be evaluated for evidence of adequate clinical recovery (e.g., 5-second head lift and grip strength). Ventilation must be supported until no longer required.
The onset of antagonism may be delayed in the presence of debilitation, cachexia, carcinomatosis, and the concomitant use of certain broad spectrum antibiotics, or anesthetic agents and other drugs which enhance neuromuscular block or separately cause respiratory depression (see PRECAUTIONS - Drug Interactions). Under such circumstances the management is the same as that of prolonged neuromuscular block (see OVERDOSAGE).

DOSAGE AND ADMINISTRATION
NOTE: CONTAINS BENZYL ALCOHOL (see WARNINGS and PRECAUTIONS – Pediatric Use)
NIMBEX SHOULD ONLY BE ADMINISTERED INTRAVENOUSLY.
The dosage information provided below is intended as a guide only. Doses of NIMBEX should be individualized (see

CLINICAL PHARMACOLOGY - Individualization of Dosages).
The use of a peripheral nerve stimulator will permit the most advantageous use of NIMBEX, minimize the possibility of overdosage or underdosage, and assist in the evaluation of recovery.
Adults
Initial Doses
One of two intubating doses of NIMBEX may be chosen, based on the desired time to tracheal intubation and the anticipated length of surgery. In addition to the dose of neuromuscular blocking agent, the presence of co-induction agents (e.g., fentanyl and midazolam) and the depth of anesthesia are factors that can influence intubation conditions. Doses of 0.15 (3 × ED_{95}) and 0.20 (4 × ED_{95}) mg/kg NIMBEX, as components of a propofol/nitrous oxide/oxygen induction-intubation technique, may produce generally GOOD or EXCELLENT conditions for intubation in 2.0 and 1.5 minutes, respectively. Similar intubation conditions may be expected when these doses of NIMBEX are administered as components of a thiopental/nitrous oxide/oxygen induction-intubation technique. In two intubation studies using thiopental or propofol and midazolam and fentanyl as co-induction agents, EXCELLENT intubation conditions were most frequently achieved with the 0.2 mg/kg compared to 0.15 mg/kg dose of cisatracurium. The clinically effective durations of action for 0.15 and 0.20 mg/kg NIMBEX during propofol anesthesia are 55 minutes (range: 44 to 74 minutes) and 61 minutes (range: 41 to 81 minutes), respectively. Lower doses may result in a longer time for the development of satisfactory intubation conditions. Doses up to 8 × ED_{95} NIMBEX have been safely administered to healthy adult patients and patients with serious cardiovascular disease. These larger doses are associated with longer clinically effective durations of action (see CLINICAL PHARMACOLOGY).
Because slower times to onset of complete neuromuscular block were observed in elderly patients and patients with renal dysfunction, extending the interval between administration of NIMBEX and the intubation attempt for these patients may be required to achieve adequate intubation conditions.
A dose of 0.03 mg/kg NIMBEX is recommended for maintenance of neuromuscular block during prolonged surgical procedures. Maintenance doses of 0.03 mg/kg each sustain neuromuscular block for approximately 20 minutes. Maintenance dosing is generally required 40 to 50 minutes following an initial dose of 0.15 mg/kg NIMBEX and 50 to 60 minutes following an initial dose of 0.20 mg/kg NIMBEX, but the need for maintenance doses should be determined by clinical criteria. For shorter or longer durations of action, smaller or larger maintenance doses may be administered. Isoflurane or enflurane administered with nitrous oxide/oxygen to achieve 1.25 MAC (Minimum Alveolar Concentration) may prolong the clinically effective duration of action of initial and maintenance doses. The magnitude of these effects may depend on the duration of administration of the volatile agents. Fifteen to 30 minutes of exposure to 1.25 MAC isoflurane or enflurane had minimal effects on the duration of action of initial doses of NIMBEX and therefore, no adjustment to the initial dose should be necessary when NIMBEX is administered shortly after initiation of volatile agents. In long surgical procedures during enflurane or isoflurane anesthesia, less frequent maintenance dosing or lower maintenance doses of NIMBEX may be necessary. No adjustments to the initial dose of NIMBEX are required when used in patients receiving propofol anesthesia.
Children
Initial Doses
The recommended dose of NIMBEX for children 2 to 12 years of age is 0.10-0.15 mg/kg administered over 5 to 10 seconds during either halothane or opioid anesthesia. When administered during stable opioid/nitrous oxide/oxygen anesthesia, 0.10 mg/kg NIMBEX produces maximum neuromuscular block in an average of 2.8 minutes (range: 1.8 to 6.7 minutes) and clinically effective block for 28 minutes (range: 21 to 38 minutes). When administered during stable opioid/nitrous oxide/oxygen anesthesia, 0.15 mg/kg NIMBEX produces maximum neuromuscular block in about 3.0 minutes (range: 1.5 to 8.0 minutes) and clinically effective block (time to 25% recovery) for 36 minutes (range: 29 to 46 minutes).
Infants
Initial Doses
The recommended dose of NIMBEX for intubation of infants 1 month to 23 months is 0.15 mg/kg administered over 5 to 10 seconds during either halothane or opioid anesthesia. When administered during stable opioid/nitrous oxide/oxygen anesthesia, 0.15 mg/kg NIMBEX produces maximum neuromuscular block in about 2.0 minutes (range: 1.3 to 3.4

Information on the AbbVie, Inc. products listed on these pages is from the prescribing information in use as of July 31, 2014. For more information, please visit rxabbvie.com or call 1-800-633-9110.

minutes) and clinically effective block (time to 25% recovery) for about 43 minutes (range: 34 to 58 minutes).

Use by Continuous Infusion
Infusion in the Operating Room (OR)
After administration of an initial bolus dose of NIMBEX, a diluted solution of NIMBEX can be administered by continuous infusion to adults and children aged 2 or more years for maintenance of neuromuscular block during extended surgical procedures. Infusion of NIMBEX should be individualized for each patient. The rate of administration should be adjusted according to the patient's response as determined by peripheral nerve stimulation. Accurate dosing is best achieved using a precision infusion device.

Infusion of NIMBEX should be initiated only after early evidence of spontaneous recovery from the initial bolus dose. An initial infusion rate of 3 mcg/kg/min may be required to rapidly counteract the spontaneous recovery of neuromuscular function. Thereafter, a rate of 1 to 2 mcg/kg/min should be adequate to maintain continuous neuromuscular block in the range of 89% to 99% in most pediatric and adult patients under opioid/nitrous oxide/oxygen anesthesia.

Reduction of the infusion rate by up to 30% to 40% should be considered when NIMBEX is administered during stable isoflurane or enflurane anesthesia (administered with nitrous oxide/oxygen at the 1.25 MAC level). Greater reductions in the infusion rate of NIMBEX may be required with longer durations of administration of isoflurane or enflurane.

The rate of infusion of atracurium required to maintain adequate surgical relaxation in patients undergoing coronary artery bypass surgery with induced hypothermia (25° to 28°C) is approximately half the rate required during normothermia. Based on the structural similarity between NIMBEX and atracurium, a similar effect on the infusion rate of NIMBEX may be expected.

Spontaneous recovery from neuromuscular block following discontinuation of infusion of NIMBEX may be expected to proceed at a rate comparable to that following administration of a single bolus dose.

Infusion in the Intensive Care Unit (ICU)
The principles for infusion of NIMBEX in the OR are also applicable to use in the ICU. An infusion rate of approximately 3 mcg/kg/min (range: 0.5 to 10.2 mcg/kg/min) should provide adequate neuromuscular block in adult patients in the ICU. There may be wide interpatient variability in dosage requirements and these may increase or decrease with time (see **PRECAUTIONS - Long-Term Use in the Intensive Care Unit [ICU]**). Following recovery from neuromuscular block, readministration of a bolus dose may be necessary to quickly re-establish neuromuscular block prior to reinstitution of the infusion.

Infusion Rate Tables
The amount of infusion solution required per minute will depend upon the concentration of NIMBEX in the infusion solution, the desired dose of NIMBEX, and the patient's weight. The contribution of the infusion solution to the fluid requirements of the patient also must be considered. Tables 10 and 11 provide guidelines for delivery, in mL/hr (equivalent to microdrops/minute when 60 microdrops = 1 mL), of NIMBEX solutions in concentrations of 0.1 mg/mL (10 mg/100 mL) or 0.4 mg/mL (40 mg/100 mL).

Table 10. Infusion Rates of NIMBEX for Maintenance of Neuromuscular Block During Opioid/Nitrous Oxide/Oxygen Anesthesia for a Concentration of 0.1 mg/mL

	Drug Delivery Rate (mcg/kg/min)				
	1.0	1.5	2.0	3.0	5.0
Patient Weight (kg)	Infusion Delivery Rate (mL/hr)				
10	6	9	12	18	30
45	27	41	54	81	135
70	42	63	84	126	210
100	60	90	120	180	300

Table 11. Infusion Rates of NIMBEX for Maintenance of Neuromuscular Block During Opioid/Nitrous Oxide/Oxygen Anesthesia for a Concentration of 0.4 mg/mL

	Drug Delivery Rate (mcg/kg/min)				
	1.0	1.5	2.0	3.0	5.0
Patient Weight (kg)	Infusion Delivery Rate (mL/hr)				
10	1.5	2.3	3.0	4.5	7.5
45	6.8	10.1	13.5	20.3	33.8
70	10.5	15.8	21.0	31.5	52.5
100	15.0	22.5	30.0	45.0	75.0

NIMBEX Injection Compatibility and Admixtures
Y-site Administration
NIMBEX Injection is acidic (pH = 3.25 to 3.65) and may not be compatible with alkaline solution having a pH greater than 8.5 (e.g., barbiturate solutions).

Studies have shown that NIMBEX Injection is compatible with:
- 5% Dextrose Injection, USP
- 0.9% Sodium Chloride Injection, USP
- 5% Dextrose and 0.9% Sodium Chloride Injection, USP
- SUFENTA® (sufentanil citrate) Injection, diluted as directed
- ALFENTA® (alfentanil hydrochloride) Injection, diluted as directed
- SUBLIMAZE® (fentanyl citrate) Injection, diluted as directed
- VERSED® (midazolam hydrochloride) Injection, diluted as directed
- Droperidol Injection, diluted as directed

NIMBEX Injection is not compatible with DIPRIVAN® (propofol) Injection or TORADOL® (ketorolac) Injection for Y-site administration. Studies of other parenteral products have not been conducted.

Dilution Stability
NIMBEX Injection diluted in 5% Dextrose Injection, USP; 0.9% Sodium Chloride Injection, USP; or 5% Dextrose and 0.9% Sodium Chloride Injection, USP to 0.1 mg/mL may be stored either under refrigeration or at room temperature for 24 hours without significant loss of potency. Dilutions to 0.1 mg/mL or 0.2 mg/mL in 5% Dextrose and Lactated Ringer's Injection may be stored under refrigeration for 24 hours.

NIMBEX Injection should not be diluted in Lactated Ringer's Injection, USP due to chemical instability.

NOTE: Parenteral drug products should be inspected visually for particulate matter and discoloration prior to administration whenever solution and container permit. Solutions which are not clear, or contain visible particulates, should not be used. NIMBEX Injection is a colorless to slightly yellow or greenish-yellow solution.

HOW SUPPLIED
NIMBEX Injection, 2 mg cisatracurium per mL, is supplied in the following:

List No.	Container	Size
4378	Single-dose Vial	5 mL
4380	Multiple-dose Vial	10 mL

NOTE: 10 mL Multiple-dose Vials contain 0.9% w/v benzyl alcohol as a preservative (see **WARNINGS** concerning newborn infants).

NIMBEX Injection, 10 mg cisatracurium per mL is supplied in the following:

4382	Single-dose Vial	20 mL

Intended only for use in the ICU.
STORAGE
NIMBEX Injection should be refrigerated at 2° to 8°C (36° to 46°F) in the carton to preserve potency. Protect from light. DO NOT FREEZE. Upon removal from refrigeration to room temperature storage conditions (25°C/77°F), use NIMBEX Injection within 21 days even if rerefrigerated.

Nimbex® is a registered trademark of GlaxoSmithKline, licensed for use by AbbVie Inc.
©2013 AbbVie Inc.
Mfd By: Hospira, Inc.
Lake Forest, IL 60045 USA
For: AbbVie Inc.
North Chicago, IL 60064 USA
EN-3172 Revised January, 2013
Shown in Product Identification Guide, page 304

NORVIR®   ℞
[nor - veer]
(ritonavir)
Capsules, Soft Gelatin for Oral use

HIGHLIGHTS OF PRESCRIBING INFORMATION
These highlights do not include all the information needed to use NORVIR safely and effectively. See full prescribing information for NORVIR.

NORVIR (ritonavir) capsules, soft gelatin for oral use
Initial U.S. Approval: 1996

WARNING: DRUG-DRUG INTERACTIONS LEADING TO POTENTIALLY SERIOUS AND/OR LIFE THREATENING REACTIONS
See full prescribing information for complete boxed warning
- Co-administration of NORVIR with several classes of drugs including sedative hypnotics, antiarrhythmics, or ergot alkaloid preparations may result in potentially serious and/or life-threatening adverse events

due to possible effects of NORVIR on the hepatic metabolism of certain drugs. Review medications taken by patients prior to prescribing NORVIR or when prescribing other medications to patients already taking NORVIR [see Contraindications (4), Warnings and Precautions (5.1), Drug Interactions (7), and Clinical Pharmacology (12.3)].

—INDICATIONS AND USAGE—
NORVIR is an HIV protease inhibitor indicated in combination with other antiretroviral agents for the treatment of HIV-1 infection. (1)

—DOSAGE AND ADMINISTRATION—
- Dose modification for NORVIR is necessary when used with other protease inhibitors. (2)
- Adult patients: 600 mg twice-daily with meals if possible. (2.1)
- Pediatrics patients: The recommended twice daily dose for children greater than one month of age is based on body surface area and should not exceed 600 mg twice daily with meals if possible. (2.2)

—DOSAGE FORMS AND STRENGTHS—
- Capsule, Soft Gelatin: 100 mg. (3)

—CONTRAINDICATIONS—
- NORVIR is contraindicated in patients with known hypersensitivity to ritonavir (e.g., toxic epidermal necrolysis, Stevens-Johnson syndrome) or any of its ingredients. (4)
- Co-administration with drugs highly dependent on CYP3A for clearance and for which elevated plasma concentrations may be associated with serious and/or life-threatening events. (4)
- Co-administration with drugs that significantly reduce ritonavir. (4)

—WARNINGS AND PRECAUTIONS—
The following have been observed in patients receiving NORVIR:
- Drug Interactions: Consider drug-drug interaction potential to reduce risk of serious or life-threatening adverse reactions. (5.1)
- Hepatic Reactions: Fatalities have occurred. Monitor liver function before and during therapy, especially in patients with underlying hepatic disease, including hepatitis B and hepatitis C, or marked transaminase elevations. (5.2, 8.6)
- Pancreatitis: Fatalities have occurred; suspend therapy as clinically appropriate. (5.3)
- Allergic Reactions/Hypersensitivity: Allergic reactions have been reported and include anaphylaxis, toxic epidermal necrolysis, Stevens-Johnson syndrome, bronchospasm and angioedema. Discontinue treatment if severe reactions develop. (5.4, 6.3)
- PR interval prolongation may occur in some patients. Cases of second and third degree heart block have been reported. Use with caution with patients with preexisting conduction system disease, ischemic heart disease, cardiomyopathy, underlying structural heart disease or when administering with other drugs that may prolong the PR interval. (5.5, 12.3)
- Total cholesterol and triglycerides elevations: Monitor prior to therapy and periodically thereafter. (5.6)
- Patients may develop new onset or exacerbations of diabetes mellitus, hyperglycemia. (5.7)
- Patients may develop immune reconstitution syndrome. (5.8)
- Patients may develop redistribution/accumulation of body fat. (5.9)
- Hemophilia: Spontaneous bleeding may occur, and additional factor VIII may be required. (5.10)

—ADVERSE REACTIONS—
The most frequently reported adverse drug reactions among patients receiving NORVIR alone or in combination with other antiretroviral drugs were gastrointestinal (including diarrhea, nausea, vomiting, abdominal pain (upper and lower)), neurological disturbances (including paresthesia and oral paresthesia), rash, and fatigue/asthenia (6.1)

To report SUSPECTED ADVERSE REACTIONS, contact AbbVie Inc. at 1-800-633-9110 or FDA at 1-800-FDA-1088 or www.fda.gov/medwatch

—DRUG INTERACTIONS—
- Co-administration of NORVIR can alter the concentrations of other drugs. The potential for drug-drug interactions must be considered prior to and during therapy. (4, 5.1, 7, 12.3)

—USE IN SPECIFIC POPULATIONS—
- Nursing Mothers: Because of both the potential for HIV transmission and the potential for serious adverse reactions in nursing infants, mothers should be instructed not to breastfeed if they are receiving NORVIR. (8.3)

See 17 for PATIENT COUNSELING INFORMATION and FDA-approved patient labeling

Revised: 11/2013

FULL PRESCRIBING INFORMATION: CONTENTS*

FULL PRESCRIBING INFORMATION

> **WARNING: DRUG-DRUG INTERACTIONS LEADING TO POTENTIALLY SERIOUS AND/OR LIFE THREATENING REACTIONS**
>
> **Co-administration of NORVIR with several classes of drugs including sedative hypnotics, antiarrhythmics, or ergot alkaloid preparations may result in potentially serious and/or life-threatening adverse events due to possible effects of NORVIR on the hepatic metabolism of certain drugs. Review medications taken by patients prior to prescribing NORVIR or when prescribing other medications to patients already taking NORVIR [see Contraindications (4), Warnings and Precautions (5.1), Drug Interactions (7), and Clinical Pharmacology (12.3)].**

1   INDICATIONS AND USAGE

NORVIR is indicated in combination with other antiretroviral agents for the treatment of HIV-1 infection.

2   DOSAGE AND ADMINISTRATION

NORVIR is administered orally in combination with other antiretroviral agents. It is recommended that NORVIR be taken with meals if possible.

General Dosing Guidelines
Patients should be aware that frequently observed adverse events, such as mild to moderate gastrointestinal disturbances and paraesthesias, may diminish as therapy is continued.

Dose modification for NORVIR
Dose reduction of NORVIR is necessary when used with other protease inhibitors: atazanavir, darunavir, fosamprenavir, saquinavir, and tipranavir.

Prescribers should consult the full prescribing information and clinical study information of these protease inhibitors if they are co-administered with a reduced dose of ritonavir [see Warnings and Precautions (5), and Drug Interactions (7)].

2.1   Adult Patients

Recommended Dosage for treatment of HIV-1
The recommended dosage of ritonavir is 600 mg twice daily by mouth. Use of a dose titration schedule may help to reduce treatment-emergent adverse events while maintaining appropriate ritonavir plasma levels. Ritonavir should be started at no less than 300 mg twice daily and increased at 2 to 3 day intervals by 100 mg twice daily. The maximum dose of 600 mg twice daily should not be exceeded upon completion of the titration.

2.2   Pediatric Patients

The recommended dosage of ritonavir in children greater than 1 month is 350 to 400 mg per m^2 twice daily by mouth and should not exceed 600 mg twice daily. Ritonavir should be started at 250 mg per m^2 twice daily and increased at 2 to 3 day intervals by 50 mg per m^2 twice daily. If patients do not tolerate 400 mg per m^2 twice daily due to adverse events, the highest tolerated dose may be used for maintenance therapy in combination with other antiretroviral agents, however, alternative therapy should be considered. The use of NORVIR oral solution is recommended for children greater than 1 month who cannot swallow capsules. Please refer to the NORVIR oral solution full prescribing information for pediatric dosage and administration.

Table 1. Drugs that are Contraindicated with NORVIR

Drug Class	Drugs Within Class That Are Contraindicated With NORVIR**	Clinical Comments
Alpha₁-adrenoreceptor antagonist	Alfuzosin HCL	Potential for hypotension.
Antiarrhythmics	Amiodarone, flecainide, propafenone, quinidine	Potential for cardiac arrhythmias.
Antifungal	Voriconazole	Co-administration of voriconazole with ritonavir 400 mg every 12 hours significantly decreases voriconazole plasma concentrations and may lead to loss of antifungal response. Voriconazole is contraindicated with ritonavir doses of 400 mg every 12 hours or greater [see Drug Interactions (7.2)].
Ergot Derivatives	Dihydroergotamine, ergonovine, ergotamine, methylergonovine	Potential for acute ergot toxicity characterized by vasospasm and ischemia of the extremities and other tissues including the central nervous system.
GI Motility Agent	Cisapride	Potential for cardiac arrhythmias.
Herbal Products	St. John's Wort (hypericum perforatum)	Co-administration of NORVIR with St. John's Wort may result in decreased ritonavir plasma concentrations and may lead to loss of virologic response and possible resistance to NORVIR or to the class of protease inhibitors.
HMG-CoA Reductase Inhibitors	Lovastatin, simvastatin	Potential for myopathy including rhabdomyolysis.
Neuroleptic	Pimozide	Potential for cardiac arrhythmias.
PDE5 enzyme inhibitor	Sildenafil* (Revatio®) only when used for the treatment of pulmonary arterial hypertension (PAH)	A safe and effective dose has not been established when used with ritonavir. There is an increased potential for sildenafil-associated adverse events, including visual abnormalities, hypotension, prolonged erection, and syncope [see Drug Interactions (7)].
Sedative/hypnotics	Oral midazolam, triazolam	Prolonged or increased sedation or respiratory depression [see Drug Interactions (7.2)].

*see Drug Interactions (7) for co-administration of sildenafil in patients with erectile dysfunction.
** For additional information for these contraindicated drugs, see also Drug Interactions (7).

3   DOSAGE FORMS AND STRENGTHS

• NORVIR (ritonavir) capsules, soft gelatin
White soft gelatin capsules imprinted with the "a" logo, 100 and the code DS, providing 100 mg of ritonavir.

4   CONTRAINDICATIONS

• When co-administering NORVIR with other protease inhibitors, see the full prescribing information for that protease inhibitor including contraindication information.
• NORVIR is contraindicated in patients with known hypersensitivity (e.g., toxic epidermal necrolysis (TEN) or Stevens-Johnson syndrome) to ritonavir or any of its ingredients.
• Co-administration of NORVIR with several classes of drugs (including sedative hypnotics, antiarrhythmics, or ergot alkaloid preparations) is contraindicated and may result in potentially serious and/or life-threatening adverse events due to possible effects of NORVIR on the hepatic metabolism of these drugs (see Table 1). Voriconazole and St. John's Wort are exceptions in that co-administration of NORVIR and voriconazole results in a significant decrease in plasma concentrations of voriconazole, and co-administration of NORVIR with St. John's Wort may result in decreased ritonavir plasma concentrations.

[See table 1 above]

Information on the AbbVie, Inc. products listed on these pages is from the prescribing information in use as of July 31, 2014. For more information, please visit rxabbvie.com or call 1-800-633-9110.

5   WARNINGS AND PRECAUTIONS

When co-administering NORVIR with other protease inhibitors, see the full prescribing information for that protease inhibitor including Warnings and Precautions.

5.1   Drug Interactions

NORVIR is a CYP3A inhibitor. Initiating treatment with NORVIR in patients receiving medications metabolized by CYP3A or initiating medications metabolized by CYP3A in patients already maintained on NORVIR may result in increased plasma concentrations of concomitant medications. Higher plasma concentrations of concomitant medications can result in increased or prolonged therapeutic or adverse effects, potentially leading to severe, life-threatening or fatal events. The potential for drug-drug interactions must be considered prior to and during therapy with NORVIR. Review of other medications taken by patients and monitoring of patients for adverse effects is recommended during therapy with NORVIR.

See Table 1 for a listing of drugs that are contraindicated with NORVIR due to potentially life-threatening adverse events, significant drug interactions, or loss of virologic activity. Also, see Table 4 for a listing of drugs with established and other significant drug interactions [see Contraindications (4), Drug Interactions (7), and Clinical Pharmacology (12.3)].

5.2   Hepatic Reactions

Hepatic transaminase elevations exceeding 5 times the upper limit of normal, clinical hepatitis, and jaundice have occurred in patients receiving NORVIR alone or in combination with other antiretroviral drugs (see Table 3). There may be an increased risk for transaminase elevations in patients with underlying hepatitis B or C. Therefore, caution should be exercised when administering NORVIR to patients with pre-existing liver diseases, liver enzyme abnormalities, or hepatitis. Increased AST/ALT monitoring should be considered in these patients, especially during the first three months of NORVIR treatment [see Use In Specific Populations (8.6)].

There have been postmarketing reports of hepatic dysfunction, including some fatalities. These have generally occurred in patients taking multiple concomitant medications and/or with advanced AIDS.

5.3   Pancreatitis

Pancreatitis has been observed in patients receiving NORVIR therapy, including those who developed hypertriglyceridemia. In some cases fatalities have been observed. Patients with advanced HIV-1 disease may be at increased risk of elevated triglycerides and pancreatitis [see Warnings and Precautions (5.8)]. Pancreatitis should be considered if clinical symptoms (nausea, vomiting, abdominal pain) or abnormalities in laboratory values (such as increased serum lipase or amylase values) suggestive of pancreatitis should occur. Patients who exhibit these signs or symptoms should be evaluated and NORVIR therapy should be discontinued if a diagnosis of pancreatitis is made.

5.4   Allergic Reactions/Hypersensitivity

Allergic reactions including urticaria, mild skin eruptions, bronchospasm, and angioedema have been reported. Cases of anaphylaxis, toxic epidermal necrolysis (TEN), and Stevens-Johnson syndrome have also been reported. Discontinue treatment if severe reactions develop.

5.5   PR Interval Prolongation

Ritonavir prolongs the PR interval in some patients. Post marketing cases of second or third degree atrioventricular block have been reported in patients.

NORVIR should be used with caution in patients with underlying structural heart disease, preexisting conduction system abnormalities, ischemic heart disease, cardiomyopathies, as these patients may be at increased risk for developing cardiac conduction abnormalities.

The impact on the PR interval of co-administration of ritonavir with other drugs that prolong the PR interval (including calcium channel blockers, beta-adrenergic blockers, digoxin and atazanavir) has not been evaluated. As a result, co-administration of ritonavir with these drugs should be undertaken with caution, particularly with those drugs metabolized by CYP3A. Clinical monitoring is recommended [see Drug Interactions (7), and Clinical Pharmacology (12.3)].

5.6   Lipid Disorders

Treatment with NORVIR therapy alone or in combination with saquinavir has resulted in substantial increases in the concentration of total cholesterol and triglycerides [see Adverse Reactions (6.1)]. Triglyceride and cholesterol testing should be performed prior to initiating NORVIR therapy and at periodic intervals during therapy. Lipid disorders

should be managed as clinically appropriate, taking into account any potential drug-drug interactions with NORVIR and HMG CoA reductase inhibitors [see Contraindications (4), and Drug Interactions (7)].

5.7   Diabetes Mellitus/Hyperglycemia

New onset diabetes mellitus, exacerbation of pre-existing diabetes mellitus, and hyperglycemia have been reported during postmarketing surveillance in HIV-1 infected patients receiving protease inhibitor therapy. Some patients required either initiation or dose adjustments of insulin or oral hypoglycemic agents for treatment of these events. In some cases, diabetic ketoacidosis has occurred. In those patients who discontinued protease inhibitor therapy, hyperglycemia persisted in some cases. Because these events have been reported voluntarily during clinical practice, estimates of frequency cannot be made and a causal relationship between protease inhibitor therapy and these events has not been established.

5.8   Immune Reconstitution Syndrome

Immune reconstitution syndrome has been reported in HIV-1 infected patients treated with combination antiretroviral therapy, including NORVIR. During the initial phase of combination antiretroviral treatment, patients whose immune system responds may develop an inflammatory response to indolent or residual opportunistic infections (such as Mycobacterium avium infection, cytomegalovirus, Pneumocystis jiroveci pneumonia (PCP), or tuberculosis), which may necessitate further evaluation and treatment.

Autoimmune disorders (such as Graves' disease, polymyositis, and Guillain-Barré syndrome) have also been reported to occur in the setting of immune reconstitution, however, the time to onset is more variable, and can occur many months after initiation of treatment.

5.9   Fat Redistribution

Redistribution/accumulation of body fat including central obesity, dorsocervical fat enlargement (buffalo hump), peripheral wasting, facial wasting, breast enlargement, and "cushingoid appearance" have been observed in patients receiving antiretroviral therapy. The mechanism and long-term consequences of these events are currently unknown. A causal relationship has not been established.

5.10   Patients with Hemophilia

There have been reports of increased bleeding, including spontaneous skin hematomas and hemarthrosis, in patients with hemophilia type A and B treated with protease inhibitors. In some patients additional factor VIII was given. In more than half of the reported cases, treatment with protease inhibitors was continued or reintroduced. A causal relationship between protease inhibitor therapy and these events has not been established.

5.11   Resistance/Cross-resistance

Varying degrees of cross-resistance among protease inhibitors have been observed. Continued administration of ritonavir 600 mg twice daily following loss of viral suppression may increase the likelihood of cross-resistance to other protease inhibitors [see Microbiology (12.4)].

5.12   Laboratory Tests

Ritonavir has been shown to increase triglycerides, cholesterol, SGOT (AST), SGPT (ALT), GGT, CPK, and uric acid. Appropriate laboratory testing should be performed prior to initiating NORVIR therapy and at periodic intervals or if any clinical signs or symptoms occur during therapy.

6   ADVERSE REACTIONS

The following adverse reactions are discussed in greater detail in other sections of the labeling.
• Drug Interactions [see Warnings and Precautions (5.1)]
• Hepatotoxicity [see Warnings and Precautions (5.2)]
• Pancreatitis [see Warnings and Precautions (5.3)]
• Allergic Reactions/Hypersensitivity [see Warnings and Precautions (5.4)]

When co-administering NORVIR with other protease inhibitors, see the full prescribing information for that protease inhibitor including adverse reactions.

6.1   Adult Clinical Trial Experience

Because clinical trials are conducted under widely varying conditions, adverse reaction rates observed in the clinical trials of a drug cannot be directly compared to rates in the clinical trials of another drug and may not reflect the rates observed in clinical practice.

The safety of NORVIR alone and in combination with other antiretroviral agents was studied in 1,755 adult patients. Table 2 lists treatment-emergent Adverse Reactions (with possible or probable relationship to study drug) occurring in greater than or equal to 1% of adult patients receiving NORVIR in combined Phase II/IV studies.

The most frequently reported adverse drug reactions among patients receiving NORVIR alone or in combination with other antiretroviral drugs were gastrointestinal (including diarrhea, nausea, vomiting, abdominal pain (upper and lower)), neurological disturbances (including paresthesia and oral paresthesia), rash, and fatigue/asthenia.

Table 2. Treatment-Emergent Adverse Reactions (With Possible or Probable Relationship to Study Drug) Occurring in greater than or equal to 1% of Adult Patients Receiving NORVIR in Combined Phase II/IV Studies (N = 1,755)

Adverse Reactions	n	%
Eye disorders		
Blurred vision	113	6.4
Gastrointestinal disorders		
Abdominal Pain (upper and lower)*	464	26.4
Diarrhea including severe with electrolyte imbalance*	1,192	67.9
Dyspepsia	201	11.5
Flatulence	142	8.1
Gastrointestinal hemorrhage*	41	2.3
Gastroesophageal reflux disease (GERD)	19	1.1
Nausea	1,007	57.4
Vomiting*	559	31.9
General disorders and administration site conditions		
Fatigue including asthenia*	811	46.2
Hepatobiliary disorders		
Blood bilirubin increased (including jaundice)*	25	1.4
Hepatitis (including increased AST, ALT, GGT)*	153	8.7
Immune system disorders		
Hypersensivity including urticatria and face edema*	114	8.2
Metabolism and nutrition disorders		
Edema and peripheral edema*	110	6.3
Gout*	24	1.4
Hypercholesterolemia*	52	3.0
Hypertriglyceridemia*	158	9.0
Lipodystrophy acquired*	51	2.9
Musculoskeletal and connective tissue disorders		
Arthralgia and back pain*	326	18.6
Myopathy/creatine phosphokinase increased*	66	3.8
Myalgia	156	8.9
Nervous system disorders		
Dizziness*	274	15.6
Dysgeusia*	285	16.2
Paresthesia (including oral paresthesia)*	889	50.7
Peripheral neuropathy	178	10.1
Syncope*	58	3.3
Psychiatric disorders		
Confusion*	52	3.0
Disturbance in attention	44	2.5
Renal and urinary disorders		
Increased urination*	74	4.2

Respiratory, thoracic and mediastinal disorders

Coughing*	380	21.7
Oropharyngeal Pain*	279	15.9

Skin and subcutaneous tissue disorders

Acne*	67	3.8
Pruritus*	214	12.2
Rash (includes erythematous and maculopapular)*	475	27.1

Vascular disorders

Flushing, feeling hot*	232	13.2
Hypertension*	58	3.3
Hypotension including orthostatic hypotension*	30	1.7
Peripheral coldness*	21	1.2

* Represents a medical concept including several similar MedDRA PTs

Laboratory Abnormalities
Table 3 shows the percentage of adult patients who developed marked laboratory abnormalities.
[See table 3 above]

6.2 Pediatric Clinical Trial Experience
NORVIR has been studied in 265 pediatric patients greater than 1 month to 21 years of age. The adverse event profile observed during pediatric clinical trials was similar to that for adult patients.
Vomiting, diarrhea, and skin rash/allergy were the only drug-related clinical adverse events of moderate to severe intensity observed in greater than or equal to 2% of pediatric patients enrolled in NORVIR clinical trials.
Laboratory Abnormalities
The following Grade 3-4 laboratory abnormalities occurred in greater than 3% of pediatric patients who received treatment with NORVIR either alone or in combination with reverse transcriptase inhibitors: neutropenia (9%), hyperamylasemia (7%), thrombocytopenia (5%), anemia (4%), and elevated AST (3%).

6.3 Postmarketing Experience
The following adverse events have been reported during post-marketing use of NORVIR. Because these reactions are reported voluntarily from a population of unknown size, it is not possible to reliably estimate their frequency or establish a causal relationship to NORVIR exposure.
Body as a Whole
Dehydration, usually associated with gastrointestinal symptoms, and sometimes resulting in hypotension, syncope, or renal insufficiency has been reported. Syncope, orthostatic hypotension, and renal insufficiency have also been reported without known dehydration.
Co-administration of ritonavir with ergotamine or dihydroergotamine has been associated with acute ergot toxicity characterized by vasospasm and ischemia of the extremities and other tissues including the central nervous system.
Cardiovascular System
First-degree AV block, second-degree AV block, third-degree AV block, right bundle branch block have been reported [see Warnings and Precautions (5.5)].
Cardiac and neurologic events have been reported when ritonavir has been co-administered with disopyramide, mexiletine, nefazodone, fluoxetine, and beta blockers. The possibility of drug interaction cannot be excluded.
Endocrine System
Cushing's syndrome and adrenal suppression have been reported when ritonavir has been co-administered with fluticasone propionate or budesonide.
Nervous System
There have been postmarketing reports of seizure. Also, see Cardiovascular System.
Skin and subcutaneous tissue disorders
Toxic epidermal necrolysis (TEN) has been reported.

7 DRUG INTERACTIONS
See also Contraindications (4), Warnings and Precautions (5.1), and Clinical Pharmacology (12.3)
When co-administering NORVIR with other protease inhibitors (atazanavir, darunavir, fosamprenavir, saquinavir, and tipranavir), see the full prescribing information for that protease inhibitor including important information for drug interactions.

7.1 Potential for NORVIR to Affect Other Drugs
Ritonavir has been found to be an inhibitor of cytochrome P450 3A (CYP3A) and may increase plasma concentrations of agents that are primarily metabolized by CYP3A. Agents that are extensively metabolized by CYP3A and have high first pass metabolism appear to be the most susceptible to large increases in AUC (greater than 3-fold) when co-administered with ritonavir. Thus, co-administration of NORVIR with drugs highly dependent on CYP3A for clearance and for which elevated plasma concentrations are associated with serious and/or life-threatening events is contraindicated. Co-administration with other CYP3A substrates may require a dose adjustment or additional monitoring as shown in Table 4.
Ritonavir also inhibits CYP2D6 to a lesser extent. Co-administration of substrates of CYP2D6 with ritonavir could result in increases (up to 2-fold) in the AUC of the other agent, possibly requiring a proportional dosage reduction. Ritonavir also appears to induce CYP3A, CYP1A2, CYP2C9, CYP2C19, and CYP2B6 as well as other enzymes, including glucuronosyl transferase.

7.2 Established and Other Potentially Significant Drug Interactions
Table 4 provides a list of established or potentially clinically significant drug interactions. Alteration in dose or regimen may be recommended based on drug interaction studies or predicted interaction [see Clinical Pharmacology (12.3) for magnitude of interaction].
[See table 4 on pages 547 through 550]

8 USE IN SPECIFIC POPULATIONS
When co-administering NORVIR with other protease inhibitors, see the full prescribing information for the co-administered protease inhibitor including important information for use in special populations.

8.1 Pregnancy
Pregnancy Category B
Antiretroviral Pregnancy Registry: To monitor maternal-fetal outcomes of pregnant women exposed to NORVIR, an Antiretroviral Pregnancy Registry has been established. Physicians are encouraged to register patients by calling 1-800-258-4263.
Human Data
There are no adequate and well-controlled studies in pregnant women. NORVIR should be used during pregnancy only if the potential benefit justifies the potential risk to the fetus.
Antiretroviral Pregnancy Registry:
As of January 2012, the Antiretroviral Pregnancy Registry (APR) has received prospective reports of 3860 exposures to ritonavir containing regimens (1567 exposed in the first trimester and 2293 exposed in the second and third trimester). Birth defects occurred in 35 of the 1567 (2.2%) live births (first trimester exposure) and 59 of the 2293 (2.6%) live births (second/third trimester exposure).
Among pregnant women in the U.S. reference population, the background rate of birth defects is 2.7%. There was no association between ritonavir and overall birth defects observed in the APR.
Animal Data
No treatment related malformations were observed when ritonavir was administered to pregnant rats or rabbits. Developmental toxicity observed in rats (early resorptions, decreased fetal body weight and ossification delays and developmental variations) occurred at a maternally toxic dosage at an exposure equivalent to approximately 30% of that achieved with the proposed therapeutic dose. A slight increase in the incidence of cryptorchidism was also noted in rats at an exposure approximately 22% of that achieved with the proposed therapeutic dose.
Developmental toxicity observed in rabbits (resorptions, decreased litter size and decreased fetal weights) also occurred at a maternally toxic dosage equivalent to 1.8 times the proposed therapeutic dose based on a body surface area conversion factor.

8.3 Nursing Mothers
The Centers for Disease Control and Prevention recommend that HIV-infected mothers not breastfeed their infants to avoid risking postnatal transmission of HIV. It is not known whether ritonavir is secreted in human milk. Because of both the potential for HIV transmission and the potential for serious adverse reactions in nursing infants, mothers should be instructed not to breastfeed if they are receiving NORVIR.

8.4 Pediatric Use
In HIV-1 infected patients age greater than 1 month to 21 years, the antiviral activity and adverse event profile seen during clinical trials and through postmarketing experience were similar to that for adult patients.

8.5 Geriatric Use
Clinical studies of NORVIR did not include sufficient numbers of subjects aged 65 and over to determine whether they respond differently from younger subjects. In general, dose selection for an elderly patient should be cautious, usually starting at the low end of the dosing range, reflecting the greater frequency of decreased hepatic, renal or cardiac function, and of concomitant disease or other drug therapy.

Information on the AbbVie, Inc. products listed on these pages is from the prescribing information in use as of July 31, 2014. For more information, please visit rxabbvie.com or call 1-800-633-9110.

Table 3. Percentage of Adult Patients, by Study and Treatment Group, with Chemistry and Hematology Abnormalities Occurring in greater than 3% of Patients Receiving NORVIR

Variable	Limit	Study 245 Naive Patients			Study 247 Advanced Patients		Study 462 PI-Naive Patients
		NORVIR plus ZDV	NORVIR	ZDV	NORVIR	Placebo	NORVIR plus Saquinavir
Chemistry	**High**						
Cholesterol	> 240 mg/dL	30.7	44.8	9.3	36.5	8.0	65.2
CPK	> 1000 IU/L	9.6	12.1	11.0	9.1	6.3	9.9
GGT	> 300 IU/L	1.8	5.2	1.7	19.6	11.3	9.2
SGOT (AST)	> 180 IU/L	5.3	9.5	2.5	6.4	7.0	7.8
SGPT (ALT)	> 215 IU/L	5.3	7.8	3.4	8.5	4.4	9.2
Triglycerides	> 800 mg/dL	9.6	17.2	3.4	33.6	9.4	23.4
Triglycerides	> 1500 mg/dL	1.8	2.6	-	12.6	0.4	11.3
Triglycerides Fasting	> 1500 mg/dL	1.5	1.3	-	9.9	0.3	-
Uric Acid	> 12 mg/dL	-	-	-	3.8	0.2	1.4
Hematology	**Low**						
Hematocrit	< 30%	2.6	-	0.8	17.3	22.0	0.7
Hemoglobin	< 8.0 g/dL	0.9	-	-	3.8	3.9	-
Neutrophils	≤ 0.5 × 10⁹/L	-	-	-	6.0	8.3	-
RBC	< 3.0 × 10¹²/L	1.8	-	5.9	18.6	24.4	-
WBC	< 2.5 × 10⁹/L	-	0.9	6.8	36.9	59.4	3.5

- Indicates no events reported.

Table 4. Established and Other Potentially Significant Drug Interactions

Concomitant Drug Class: Drug Name	Effect on Concentration of Ritonavir or Concomitant Drug	Clinical Comments
	HIV-Antiviral Agents	
HIV-1 Protease Inhibitor: atazanavir	When co-administered with reduced doses of atazanavir and ritonavir ↑ atazanavir (↑ AUC, ↑ C_{max}, ↑ C_{min})	Atazanavir plasma concentrations achieved with atazanavir 300 mg once daily and ritonavir 100 mg once daily are higher than those achieved with atazanavir 400 mg once daily. See the complete prescribing information for Reyataz® (atazanavir) for details on co-administration of atazanavir 300 mg once daily with ritonavir 100 mg once daily.
HIV-1 Protease Inhibitor: darunavir	When co-administered with reduced doses of ritonavir ↑ darunavir (↑ AUC, ↑ C_{max}, ↑ C_{min})	See the complete prescribing information for Prezista® (darunavir) for details on co-administration of darunavir 600 mg twice daily with ritonavir 100 mg twice daily or darunavir 800 mg once daily with ritonavir 100 mg once daily.
HIV-1 Protease Inhibitor: fosamprenavir	When co-administered with reduced doses of ritonavir ↑ amprenavir (↑ AUC, ↑ C_{max}, ↑ C_{min})	See the complete prescribing information for Lexiva® (fosamprenavir) for details on co-administration of fosamprenavir 700 mg twice daily with ritonavir 100 mg twice daily, fosamprenavir 1400 mg once daily with ritonavir 200 mg once daily or fosamprenavir 1400 mg once daily with ritonavir 100 mg once daily.
HIV-1 Protease Inhibitor: indinavir	When co-administered with reduced doses of indinavir and ritonavir ↑ indinavir (↔ AUC, ↓ C_{max}, ↑ C_{min})	Alterations in concentrations are noted when reduced doses of indinavir are co-administered with NORVIR. Appropriate doses for this combination, with respect to efficacy and safety, have not been established.
HIV-1 Protease Inhibitor: saquinavir	When co-administered with reduced doses of ritonavir ↑ saquinavir (↑ AUC, ↑ C_{max}, ↑ C_{min})	See the complete prescribing information for Invirase® (saquinavir) for details on co-administration of saquinavir 1000 mg twice daily with ritonavir 100 mg twice daily. Saquinavir/ritonavir should not be given together with rifampin, due to the risk of severe hepatotoxicity (presenting as increased hepatic transaminases) if the three drugs are given together.
HIV-1 Protease Inhibitor: tipranavir	When co-administered with reduced doses of ritonavir ↑ tipranavir (↑ AUC, ↑ C_{max}, ↑ C_{min})	See the complete prescribing information for Aptivus® (tipranavir) for details on co-administration of tipranavir 500 mg twice daily with ritonavir 200 mg twice daily. There have been reports of clinical hepatitis and hepatic decompensation including some fatalities. All patients should be followed closely with clinical and laboratory monitoring, especially those with chronic hepatitis B or C co-infection, as these patients have an increased risk of hepatotoxicity. Liver function tests should be performed prior to initiating therapy with tipranavir/ritonavir, and frequently throughout the duration of treatment.
Non-Nucleoside Reverse Transcriptase Inhibitor: delavirdine	↑ ritonavir (↑AUC, ↑C_{max}, ↑ C_{min})	Appropriate doses of this combination with respect to safety and efficacy have not been established.
HIV-1 CCR5 – antagonist: maraviroc	↑ maraviroc	Concurrent administration of maraviroc with ritonavir will increase plasma levels of maraviroc. For specific dosage adjustment recommendations, please refer to the complete prescribing information for Selzentry® (maraviroc).
Integrase Inhibitor: Raltegravir	↓ raltegravir	The effects of ritonavir on raltegravir with ritonavir dosage regimens greater than 100 mg twice daily have not been evaluated, however raltegravir concentrations may be decreased with ritonavir coadministration.
	Other Agents	
Analgesics, Narcotic: tramadol, propoxyphene		A dose decrease may be needed for these drugs when co-administered with ritonavir.
Anesthetic: meperidine	↓ meperidine/ ↑ normeperidine (metabolite)	Dosage increase and long-term use of meperidine with ritonavir are not recommended due to the increased concentrations of the metabolite normeperidine which has both analgesic activity and CNS stimulant activity (e.g., seizures).
Antialcoholics: disulfiram/ metronidazole		Ritonavir formulations contain alcohol, which can produce disulfiram-like reactions when co-administered with disulfiram or other drugs that produce this reaction (e.g., metronidazole).
Antiarrhythmics: disopyramide, lidocaine, mexiletine	↑ antiarrhythmics	Caution is warranted and therapeutic concentration monitoring is recommended for antiarrhythmics when co-administered with ritonavir, if available.

(Table continued on next page)

8.6   Hepatic Impairment

No dose adjustment of ritonavir is necessary for patients with either mild (Child-Pugh Class A) or moderate (Child-Pugh Class B) hepatic impairment. No pharmacokinetic or safety data are available regarding the use of ritonavir in subjects with severe hepatic impairment (Child-Pugh Class C), therefore, ritonavir is not recommended for use in patients with severe hepatic impairment [see *Warnings and Precautions (5.2)*, and *Clinical Pharmacology (12.3)*].

10   OVERDOSAGE

10.1   Acute Overdosage - Human Overdose Experience

Human experience of acute overdose with NORVIR is limited. One patient in clinical trials took NORVIR 1500 mg per day for two days. The patient reported paresthesias which resolved after the dose was decreased. A post-marketing case of renal failure with eosinophilia has been reported with ritonavir overdose.

The approximate lethal dose was found to be greater than 20 times the related human dose in rats and 10 times the related human dose in mice.

10.2   Management of Overdosage

Treatment of overdose with NORVIR consists of general supportive measures including monitoring of vital signs and observation of the clinical status of the patient. There is no specific antidote for overdose with NORVIR. If indicated, elimination of unabsorbed drug should be achieved by emesis or gastric lavage; usual precautions should be observed to maintain the airway. Administration of activated charcoal may also be used to aid in removal of unabsorbed drug. Since ritonavir is extensively metabolized by the liver and is highly protein bound, dialysis is unlikely to be beneficial in significant removal of the drug. A Certified Poison Control Center should be consulted for up-to-date information on the management of overdose with NORVIR.

11   DESCRIPTION

NORVIR (ritonavir) is an inhibitor of HIV-1 protease with activity against the Human Immunodeficiency Virus (HIV) type 1.

Ritonavir is chemically designated as 10-Hydroxy-2-methyl-5-(1-methylethyl)-1-[2-(1-methylethyl)-4-thiazolyl]-3,6-di-oxo-8,11-bis(phenylmethyl)-2,4,7,12- tetraazatridecan-13-oic acid, 5-thiazolylmethyl ester, [5S-(5R*,8R*,10R*,11R*)]. Its molecular formula is $C_{37}H_{48}N_6O_5S_2$, and its molecular weight is 720.95. Ritonavir has the following structural formula:

Ritonavir is a white-to-light-tan powder. Ritonavir has a bitter metallic taste. It is freely soluble in methanol and ethanol, soluble in isopropanol and practically insoluble in water.

NORVIR soft gelatin capsules are available for oral administration in a strength of 100 mg ritonavir with the following inactive ingredients: Butylated hydroxytoluene, ethanol, gelatin, iron oxide, oleic acid, polyoxyl 35 castor oil, and titanium dioxide.

12   CLINICAL PHARMACOLOGY

12.1   Mechanism of Action

Ritonavir is an antiviral drug [see *Microbiology (12.4)*].

12.3   Pharmacokinetics

The pharmacokinetics of ritonavir have been studied in healthy volunteers and HIV-1 infected patients (CD_4 greater than or equal to 50 cells per μL). See Table 5 for ritonavir pharmacokinetic characteristics.

Absorption

The absolute bioavailability of ritonavir has not been determined.

Effect of Food on Oral Absorption

After a single 600 mg dose under non-fasting conditions, in two separate studies, the soft gelatin capsule (n = 57) formulation yielded a mean ± SD area under the plasma concentration-time curve (AUC) of 121.7 ± 53.8. Relative to fasting conditions, the extent of absorption of ritonavir from the soft gelatin capsule formulation was 13% higher when administered with a meal (615 KCal; 14.5% fat, 9% protein, and 76% carbohydrate).

Metabolism

Nearly all of the plasma radioactivity after a single oral 600 mg dose of ^{14}C-ritonavir oral solution (n = 5) was attributed to unchanged ritonavir. Five ritonavir metabolites have been identified in human urine and feces. The isopropylthiazole oxidation metabolite (M-2) is the major metabolite and has antiviral activity similar to that of parent drug; however, the concentrations of this metabolite in plasma are low. *In vitro* studies utilizing human liver microsomes have demonstrated that cytochrome P450 3A (CYP3A) is the major isoform involved in ritonavir metabolism, although CYP2D6 also contributes to the formation of M-2.

Elimination

In a study of five subjects receiving a 600 mg dose of ^{14}C-ritonavir oral solution, 11.3 ± 2.8% of the dose was excreted into the urine, with 3.5 ± 1.8% of the dose excreted as unchanged parent drug. In that study, 86.4 ± 2.9% of the dose was excreted in the feces with 33.8 ± 10.8% of the dose excreted as unchanged parent drug. Upon multiple dosing, ritonavir accumulation is less than predicted from a single dose possibly due to a time and dose-related increase in clearance.

Table 5. Ritonavir Pharmacokinetic Characteristics

Parameter	n	Values (Mean ± SD)
$V_\beta/F^\ddagger$	91	0.41 ± 0.25 L/kg
$t_{1/2}$		3 - 5 h
CL/F SS[†]	10	8.8 ± 3.2 L/h
CL/F[‡]	91	4.6 ± 1.6 L/h
CL_R	62	< 0.1 L/h
RBC/Plasma Ratio		0.14
Percent Bound*		98 to 99%

† SS = steady state; patients taking ritonavir 600 mg q12h.
‡ Single ritonavir 600 mg dose.
* Primarily bound to human serum albumin and alpha-1 acid glycoprotein over the ritonavir concentration range of 0.01 to 30 µg/mL.

Effects on Electrocardiogram
QTcF interval was evaluated in a randomized, placebo and active (moxifloxacin 400 mg once-daily) controlled crossover study in 45 healthy adults, with 10 measurements over 12 hours on Day 3. The maximum mean (95% upper confidence bound) time-matched difference in QTcF from placebo after baseline correction was 5.5 (7.6) milliseconds (msec) for 400 mg twice-daily ritonavir. Ritonavir 400 mg twice daily resulted in Day 3 ritonavir exposure that was approximately 1.5 fold higher than observed with ritonavir 600 mg twice-daily dose at steady state.
PR interval prolongation was also noted in subjects receiving ritonavir in the same study on Day 3. The maximum mean (95% confidence interval) difference from placebo in the PR interval after baseline correction was 22 (25) msec for 400 mg twice-daily ritonavir [see Warnings and Precautions (5.5)].

Special Populations
Gender, Race and Age
No age-related pharmacokinetic differences have been observed in adult patients (18 to 63 years). Ritonavir pharmacokinetics have not been studied in older patients.
A study of ritonavir pharmacokinetics in healthy males and females showed no statistically significant differences in the pharmacokinetics of ritonavir. Pharmacokinetic differences due to race have not been identified.

Pediatric Patients
Steady-state pharmacokinetics were evaluated in 37 HIV-1 infected patients ages 2 to 14 years receiving doses ranging from 250 mg per m^2 twice-daily to 400 mg per m^2 twice-daily in PACTG Study 310, and in 41 HIV-1 infected patients ages 1 month to 2 years at doses of 350 and 450 mg per m^2 twice-daily in PACTG Study 345. Across dose groups, ritonavir steady-state oral clearance (CL per F per m^2) was approximately 1.5 to 1.7 times faster in pediatric patients than in adult subjects. Ritonavir concentrations obtained after 350 to 400 mg per m^2 twice-daily in pediatric patients greater than 2 years were comparable to those obtained in adults receiving 600 mg (approximately 330 mg per m^2) twice-daily. The following observations were seen regarding ritonavir concentrations after administration with 350 or 450 mg per m^2 twice-daily in children less than 2 years of age. Higher ritonavir exposures were not evident with 450 mg per m^2 twice-daily compared to the 350 mg per m^2 twice-daily. Ritonavir trough concentrations were somewhat lower than those obtained in adults receiving 600 mg twice-daily. The area under the ritonavir plasma concentration-time curve and trough concentrations obtained after administration with 350 or 450 mg per m^2 twice-daily in children less than 2 years were approximately 16% and 60% lower, respectively, than that obtained in adults receiving 600 mg twice-daily.

Renal Impairment
Ritonavir pharmacokinetics have not been studied in patients with renal impairment, however, since renal clearance is negligible, a decrease in total body clearance is not expected in patients with renal impairment.

Hepatic Impairment
Dose-normalized steady-state ritonavir concentrations in subjects with mild hepatic impairment (400 mg twice-daily, n = 6) were similar to those in control subjects dosed with 500 mg twice-daily. Dose-normalized steady-state ritonavir exposures in subjects with moderate hepatic impairment (400 mg twice-daily, n= 6) were about 40% lower than those in subjects with normal hepatic function (500 mg twice-daily, n = 6). Protein binding of ritonavir was not statistically significantly affected by mild or moderately impaired hepatic function. No dose adjustment is recommended in patients with mild or moderate hepatic impairment. However, health care providers should be aware of the potential for lower ritonavir concentrations in patients with moderate hepatic impairment and should monitor patient response carefully. Ritonavir has not been studied in patients with severe hepatic impairment.

Table 4 (cont.). Established and Other Potentially Significant Drug Interactions

Concomitant Drug Class: Drug Name	Effect on Concentration of Ritonavir or Concomitant Drug	Clinical Comments
Other Agents (cont.)		
Anticancer Agents: dasatinib, nilotinib, vincristine, vinblastine	↑ anticancer agents	Concentrations of these drugs may be increased when co-administered with ritonavir resulting in the potential for increased adverse events usually associated with these anticancer agents. For vincristine and vinblastine, consideration should be given to temporarily withholding the ritonavir containing antiretroviral regimen in patients who develop significant hematologic or gastrointestinal side effects when ritonavir is administered concurrently with vincristine or vinblastine. Clinicians should be aware that if the ritonavir containing regimen is withheld for a prolonged period, consideration should be given to altering the regimen to not include a CYP3A or P-gp inhibitor in order to control HIV-1 viral load. A decrease in the dosage or an adjustment of the dosing interval of nilotinib and dasatinib may be necessary for patients requiring co-administration with strong CYP3A inhibitors such as NORVIR. Please refer to the nilotinib and dasatinib prescribing information for dosing instructions.
Anticoagulant: warfarin	↓ R-warfarin ↓↑ S-warfarin	Initial frequent monitoring of the INR during ritonavir and warfarin co-administration is indicated.
Anticoagulant: rivaroxaban	↑ rivaroxaban	Avoid concomitant use of rivaroxaban and ritonavir. Co-administration of ritonavir and rivaroxaban is expected to result in increased exposure of rivaroxaban which may lead to risk of increased bleeding.
Anticonvulsants: carbamazepine, clonazepam, ethosuximide	↑ anticonvulsants	Use with caution. A dose decrease may be needed for these drugs when co-administered with ritonavir and therapeutic concentration monitoring is recommended for these anticonvulsants, if available.
Anticonvulsants: divalproex, lamotrigine, phenytoin	↓ anticonvulsants	Use with caution. A dose increase may be needed for these drugs when co-administered with ritonavir and therapeutic concentration monitoring is recommended for these anticonvulsants, if available.
Antidepressants: nefazodone, selective serotonin reuptake inhibitors (SSRIs): e.g. fluoxetine, paroxetine, tricyclics: e.g. amitriptyline, nortriptyline	↑ antidepressants	A dose decrease may be needed for these drugs when co-administered with ritonavir.
Antidepressant: bupropion	↓ bupropion ↓ active metabolite, hydroxybupropion	Concurrent administration of bupropion with ritonavir may decrease plasma levels of both bupropion and its active metabolite (hydroxybupropion). Patients receiving ritonavir and bupropion concurrently should be monitored for an adequate clinical response to bupropion.
Antidepressant: desipramine	↑ desipramine	Dosage reduction and concentration monitoring of desipramine is recommended.
Antidepressant: trazodone	↑ trazodone	Concomitant use of trazodone and NORVIR increases plasma concentrations of trazodone. Adverse events of nausea, dizziness, hypotension and syncope have been observed following co-administration of trazodone and NORVIR. If trazodone is used with a CYP3A4 inhibitor such as ritonavir, the combination should be used with caution and a lower dose of trazodone should be considered.
Antiemetic: dronabinol	↑ dronabinol	A dose decrease of dronabinol may be needed when co-administered with ritonavir.
Antifungal: ketoconazole itraconazole voriconazole	↑ ketoconazole ↑ itraconazole ↓ voriconazole	High doses of ketoconazole or itraconazole (greater than 200 mg per day) are not recommended. Co-administration of voriconazole and ritonavir doses of 400 mg every 12 hours or greater is contraindicated. Co-administration of voriconazole and ritonavir 100 mg should be avoided, unless an assessment of the benefit/risk to the patient justifies the use of voriconazole.

(Table continued on next page)

Information on the AbbVie, Inc. products listed on these pages is from the prescribing information in use as of July 31, 2014. For more information, please visit rxabbvie.com or call 1-800-633-9110.

Table 4 (cont.). Established and Other Potentially Significant Drug Interactions

Concomitant Drug Class: Drug Name	Effect on Concentration of Ritonavir or Concomitant Drug	Clinical Comments
	Other Agents (cont.)	
Anti-gout: colchicine	↑ colchicine	Patients with renal or hepatic impairment should not be given colchicine with ritonavir. Treatment of gout flares-co-administration of colchicine in patients on ritonavir: 0.6 mg (one tablet) for one dose, followed by 0.3 mg (half tablet) one hour later. Dose to be repeated no earlier than three days. Prophylaxis of gout flares-co-administration of colchicine in patients on ritonavir: If the original colchicine regimen was 0.6 mg twice a day, the regimen should be adjusted to 0.3 mg once a day. If the original colchicine regimen was 0.6 mg once a day, the regimen should be adjusted to 0.3 mg once every other day. Treatment of familial Mediterranean fever (FMF)-co-administration of colchicine in patients on ritonavir: Maximum daily dose of 0.6 mg (may be given as 0.3 mg twice a day).
Anti-infective: clarithromycin	↑ clarithromycin	For patients with renal impairment the following dosage adjustments should be considered: • For patients with CL_{CR} 30 to 60 mL per min the dose of clarithromycin should be reduced by 50%. • For patients with CL_{CR} less than 30 mL per min the dose of clarithromycin should be decreased by 75%. No dose adjustment for patients with normal renal function is necessary.
Antimycobacterial: rifabutin	↑ rifabutin and rifabutin metabolite	Dosage reduction of rifabutin by at least three-quarters of the usual dose of 300 mg per day is recommended (e.g., 150 mg every other day or three times a week). Further dosage reduction may be necessary.
Antimycobacterial: rifampin	↓ ritonavir	May lead to loss of virologic response. Alternate antimycobacterial agents such as rifabutin should be considered (see Antimycobacterial: rifabutin, for dose reduction recommendations).
Antiparasitic: atovaquone	↓ atovaquone	Clinical significance is unknown; however, increase in atovaquone dose may be needed.
Antiparasitic: quinine	↑ quinine	A dose decrease of quinine may be needed when co-administered with ritonavir.
β-Blockers: metoprolol, timolol	↑ Beta-Blockers	Caution is warranted and clinical monitoring of patients is recommended. A dose decrease may be needed for these drugs when co-administered with ritonavir.
Bronchodilator: theophylline	↓ theophylline	Increased dosage of theophylline may be required; therapeutic monitoring should be considered.
Calcium channel blockers: diltiazem, nifedipine, verapamil	↑ calcium channel blockers	Caution is warranted and clinical monitoring of patients is recommended. A dose decrease may be needed for these drugs when co-administered with ritonavir.
Digoxin	↑ digoxin	Concomitant administration of ritonavir with digoxin may increase digoxin levels. Caution should be exercised when co-administering ritonavir with digoxin, with appropriate monitoring of serum digoxin levels.
Endothelin receptor antagonists: bosentan	↑ bosentan	Co-administration of bosentan in patients on ritonavir: In patients who have been receiving ritonavir for at least 10 days, start bosentan at 62.5 mg once daily or every other day based upon individual tolerability. Co-administration of ritonavir in patients on bosentan: Discontinue use of bosentan at least 36 hours prior to initiation of ritonavir. After at least 10 days following the initiation of ritonavir, resume bosentan at 62.5 mg once daily or every other day based upon individual tolerability.
HMG-CoA Reductase Inhibitor: atorvastatin rosuvastatin	↑ atorvastatin ↑ rosuvastatin	Titrate atorvastatin and rosuvastatin dose carefully and use the lowest necessary dose. If NORVIR is used with another protease inhibitor, see the complete prescribing information for the concomitant protease inhibitor for details on co-administration with atorvastatin and rosuvastatin.
Immunosuppressants: cyclosporine, tacrolimus, sirolimus (rapamycin)	↑ immunosuppressants	Therapeutic concentration monitoring is recommended for immunosuppressant agents when co-administered with ritonavir.

(Table continued on next page)

Drug Interactions
[see also Contraindications (4), Warnings and Precautions (5.1), and Drug Interactions (7)]

Table 6 and Table 7 summarize the effects on AUC and C_{max}, with 95% confidence intervals (95% CI), of co-administration of ritonavir with a variety of drugs. For in-formation about clinical recommendations see Table 4 in *Drug Interactions (7)*.
[See table 6 at top of page 550]
[See table 7 on pages 551 and 552]

12.4   Microbiology
Mechanism of Action
Ritonavir is a peptidomimetic inhibitor of the HIV-1 protease. Inhibition of HIV protease renders the enzyme incapable of processing the *gag-pol* polyprotein precursor which leads to production of non-infectious immature HIV-1 particles.

Antiviral Activity in Cell Culture
The activity of ritonavir was assessed in acutely infected lymphoblastoid cell lines and in peripheral blood lymphocytes. The concentration of drug that inhibits 50% (EC_{50}) value of viral replication ranged from 3.8 to 153 nM depending upon the HIV-1 isolate and the cells employed. The average EC_{50} for low passage clinical isolates was 22 nM (n = 13). In MT_4 cells, ritonavir demonstrated additive effects against HIV-1 in combination with either didanosine (ddI) or zidovudine (ZDV). Studies which measured cytotoxicity of ritonavir on several cell lines showed that greater than 20 µM was required to inhibit cellular growth by 50% resulting in a cell culture therapeutic index of at least 1,000.

Resistance
HIV-1 isolates with reduced susceptibility to ritonavir have been selected in cell culture. Genotypic analysis of these isolates showed mutations in the HIV-1 protease gene encoding at amino acid substitutions I84V, V82F, A71V, and M46I. Phenotypic (n = 18) and genotypic (n = 48) changes in HIV-1 isolates from selected patients treated with ritonavir were monitored in phase I/II trials over a period of 3 to 32 weeks. Substitutions associated with the HIV-1 viral protease in isolates obtained from 43 patients appeared to occur in a stepwise and ordered fashion; in sequence, these substitutions were position V82A/F/T/S, I54V, A71V/T, and I36L, followed by combinations of substitutions at an additional 5 specific amino acid positions (M46I/L, K20R, I84V, L33F and L90M). Of 18 patients for whom both phenotypic and genotypic analysis were performed on free virus isolated from plasma, 12 showed reduced susceptibility to ritonavir in cell culture. All 18 patients possessed one or more substitutions in the viral protease gene. The V82A/F substitution appeared to be necessary but not sufficient to confer phenotypic resistance. Phenotypic resistance was defined as a greater than or equal to 5-fold decrease in viral sensitivity in cell culture from baseline.

Cross-Resistance to Other Antiretrovirals
Among protease inhibitors variable cross-resistance has been recognized. Serial HIV-1 isolates obtained from six patients during ritonavir therapy showed a decrease in ritonavir susceptibility in cell culture but did not demonstrate a concordant decrease in susceptibility to saquinavir in cell culture when compared to matched baseline isolates. However, isolates from two of these patients demonstrated decreased susceptibility to indinavir in cell culture (8-fold). Isolates from 5 patients were also tested for cross-resistance to amprenavir and nelfinavir; isolates from 3 patients had a decrease in susceptibility to nelfinavir (6- to 14-fold), and none to amprenavir. Cross-resistance between ritonavir and reverse transcriptase inhibitors is unlikely because of the different enzyme targets involved. One ZDV-resistant HIV-1 isolate tested in cell culture retained full susceptibility to ritonavir.

13   NONCLINICAL TOXICOLOGY
13.1   Carcinogenesis, Mutagenesis, Impairment of Fertility
Carcinogenesis
Carcinogenicity studies in mice and rats have been carried out on ritonavir. In male mice, at levels of 50, 100 or 200 mg per kg per day, there was a dose dependent increase in the incidence of both adenomas and combined adenomas and carcinomas in the liver. Based on AUC measurements, the exposure at the high dose was approximately 0.3-fold for males that of the exposure in humans with the recommended therapeutic dose (600 mg twice-daily). There were no carcinogenic effects seen in females at the dosages tested. The exposure at the high dose was approximately 0.6-fold for the females that of the exposure in humans. In rats dosed at levels of 7, 15 or 30 mg per kg per day there were no carcinogenic effects. In this study, the exposure at the high dose was approximately 6% that of the exposure in humans with the recommended therapeutic dose. Based on the exposures achieved in the animal studies, the significance of the observed effects is not known.

Mutagenesis
Ritonavir was found to be negative for mutagenic or clastogenic activity in a battery of *in vitro* and *in vivo* assays including the Ames bacterial reverse mutation assay using *S. typhimurium* and *E. coli*, the mouse lymphoma assay, the mouse micronucleus test and chromosomal aberration assays in human lymphocytes.

Table 4 (cont.). Established and Other Potentially Significant Drug Interactions

Concomitant Drug Class: Drug Name	Effect on Concentration of Ritonavir or Concomitant Drug	Clinical Comments
		Other Agents (cont.)
Inhaled or Intranasal Steroid: e.g. fluticasone budesonide	↑ glucocorticoids	Concomitant use of ritonavir and fluticasone or other glucocorticoids that are metabolized by CYP3A is not recommended unless the potential benefit of treatment outweighs the risk of systemic corticosteroid effects. Concomitant use may result in increased steroid concentrations and reduced serum cortisol concentrations. Systemic corticosteroid effects including Cushing's syndrome and adrenal suppression have been reported during postmarketing use in patients when ritonavir has been coadministered with fluticasone propionate or budesonide.
Long-acting beta-adrenoceptor agonist: salmeterol	↑ salmeterol	Concurrent administration of salmeterol and ritonavir is not recommended. The combination may result in increased risk of cardiovascular adverse events associated with salmeterol, including QT prolongation, palpitations and sinus tachycardia.
Narcotic Analgesic: methadone fentanyl	↓ methadone ↑ fentanyl	Dosage increase of methadone may be considered. Concentrations of fentanyl are expected to increase. Careful monitoring of therapeutic and adverse effects (including potentially fatal respiratory depression) is recommended when fentanyl is concomitantly administered with NORVIR.
Neuroleptics: perphenazine, risperidone, thioridazine	↑ neuroleptics	A dose decrease may be needed for these drugs when co-administered with ritonavir.
Oral Contraceptives or Patch Contraceptives: ethinyl estradiol	↓ ethinyl estradiol	Alternate methods of contraception should be considered.
PDE5 Inhibitors: avanafil sildenafil, tadalafil, vardenafil	↑ avanafil ↑ sildenafil ↑ tadalafil ↑ vardenafil	Do not use ritonavir with avanafil because a safe and effective avanafil dosage regimen has not been established. Particular caution should be used when prescribing sildenafil, tadalafil or vardenafil in patients receiving ritonavir. Co-administration of ritonavir with these drugs is expected to substantially increase their concentrations and may result in an increase in PDE5 inhibitor associated adverse events, including hypotension, syncope, visual changes, and prolonged erection. Use of PDE5 inhibitors for pulmonary arterial hypertension (PAH): Sildenafil (Revatio®) is contraindicated when used for the treatment of pulmonary arterial hypertension (PAH) because a safe and effective dose has not been established when used with ritonavir [see Contraindications (4)]. The following dose adjustments are recommended for use of tadalafil (Adcirca™) with ritonavir: Co-administration of ADCIRCA in patients on ritonavir: In patients receiving ritonavir for at least one week, start ADCIRCA at 20 mg once daily. Increase to 40 mg once daily based upon individual tolerability. Co-administration of ritonavir in patients on ADCIRCA: Avoid use of ADCIRCA during the initiation of ritonavir. Stop ADCIRCA at least 24 hours prior to starting ritonavir. After at least one week following the initiation of ritonavir, resume ADCIRCA at 20 mg once daily. Increase to 40 mg once daily based upon individual tolerability. Use of PDE5 inhibitors for the treatment of erectile dysfunction: It is recommended not to exceed the following doses: • Sildenafil: 25 mg every 48 hours • Tadalafil: 10 mg every 72 hours • Vardenafil: 2.5 mg every 72 hours Use with increased monitoring for adverse events.
Sedative/hypnotics: buspirone, clorazepate, diazepam, estazolam, flurazepam, zolpidem	↑ sedative/hypnotics	A dose decrease may be needed for these drugs when co-administered with ritonavir.
Sedative/hypnotics: Parenteral midazolam	↑ midazolam	Co-administration of oral midazolam with NORVIR is CONTRAINDICATED. Concomitant use of parenteral midazolam with NORVIR may increase plasma concentrations of midazolam. Co-administration should be done in a setting which ensures close clinical monitoring and appropriate medical management in case of respiratory depression and/or prolonged sedation. Dosage reduction for midazolam should be considered, especially if more than a single dose of midazolam is administered.

(Table continued on next page)

Impairment of Fertility

Ritonavir produced no effects on fertility in rats at drug exposures approximately 40% (male) and 60% (female) of that achieved with the proposed therapeutic dose. Higher dosages were not feasible due to hepatic toxicity.

14 CLINICAL STUDIES

The activity of NORVIR as monotherapy or in combination with nucleoside reverse transcriptase inhibitors has been evaluated in 1446 patients enrolled in two double-blind, randomized trials.

14.1 Advanced Patients with Prior Antiretroviral Therapy

Study 247 was a randomized, double-blind trial (with open-label follow-up) conducted in HIV-1 infected patients with at least nine months of prior antiretroviral therapy and baseline CD_4 cell counts less than or equal to 100 cells per μL. NORVIR 600 mg twice-daily or placebo was added to each patient's baseline antiretroviral therapy regimen, which could have consisted of up to two approved antiretroviral agents. The study accrued 1090 patients, with mean baseline CD_4 cell count at study entry of 32 cells per μL. After the clinical benefit of NORVIR therapy was demonstrated, all patients were eligible to switch to open-label NORVIR for the duration of the follow-up period. Median duration of double-blind therapy with NORVIR and placebo was 6 months. The median duration of follow-up through the end of the open-label phase was 13.5 months for patients randomized to NORVIR and 14 months for patients randomized to placebo.

The cumulative incidence of clinical disease progression or death during the double-blind phase of Study 247 was 26% (140/543) for patients initially randomized to NORVIR compared to 42% (229/547) for patients initially randomized to placebo. This difference in rates was statistically significant.

Cumulative mortality through the end of the open-label follow-up phase for patients enrolled in Study 247 was 18% (99/543) for patients initially randomized to NORVIR compared to 26% (142/547) for patients initially randomized to placebo. This difference in rates was statistically significant. However, since the analysis at the end of the open-label phase includes patients in the placebo arm who were switched from placebo to NORVIR therapy, the survival benefit of NORVIR cannot be precisely estimated.

During the double-blind phase of Study 247, CD_4 cell counts increases from baseline for patients randomized to NORVIR at Week 2 and Week 4 were observed. From Week 4 and through Week 24, mean CD_4 cell counts for patients randomized to NORVIR appeared to plateau. In contrast, there was no apparent change in mean CD_4 cell counts for patients randomized to placebo at any visit between baseline and Week 24 of the double-blind phase of Study 247.

14.2 Patients Without Prior Antiretroviral Therapy

In Study 245, 356 antiretroviral-naive HIV-1 infected patients (mean baseline of CD_4 = 364 cells/μL) were randomized to receive either NORVIR 600 mg twice-daily, zidovudine 200 mg three-times-daily, or a combination of these drugs. During the double-blind phase of study 245, greater mean CD_4 cell count increases were observed from baseline to Week 12 in the NORVIR-containing arms compared to the zidovudine arms. Mean CD_4 cell count changes subsequently appeared to plateau through Week 24 in the NORVIR arm, whereas mean CD_4 cell counts gradually diminished through Week 24 in the zidovudine and NORVIR plus zidovudine arms.

Greater mean reductions in plasma HIV-1 RNA levels were observed from baseline to Week 2 for the NORVIR-containing arms compared to the zidovudine arm. After Week 2 and through Week 24, mean plasma HIV-1 RNA levels either remained stable in the NORVIR and zidovudine arms or gradually rebounded toward baseline in the NORVIR plus zidovudine arm.

15 REFERENCES

1. Sewester CS. Calculations. In: Drug Facts and Comparisons. St. Louis, MO: J.B. Lippincott Co; January, 1997:xix.

16 HOW SUPPLIED/STORAGE AND HANDLING

NORVIR (ritonavir) soft gelatin capsules are white capsules imprinted with the "a" logo, 100 and the code DS, available in the following package size:
Bottles of 120 capsules each (**NDC** 0074-6633-22).
Bottles of 30 capsules each (**NDC** 0074-6633-30).
Recommended Storage
Store NORVIR soft gelatin capsules in the refrigerator between 2°-8°C (36°-46°F) until dispensed. Refrigeration of NORVIR soft gelatin capsules by the patient is recommended, but not required if used within 30 days and stored below 25°C (77°F). Protect from light. Avoid exposure to excessive heat.
Product should be stored and dispensed in the original container.
Keep cap tightly closed.

Information on the AbbVie, Inc. products listed on these pages is from the prescribing information in use as of July 31, 2014. For more information, please visit rxabbvie.com or call 1-800-633-9110.

17 PATIENT COUNSELING INFORMATION

See FDA-approved patient labeling (Patient Information)

Information For Patients

Patients or parents of patients should be informed that:

Underline: General Information

☐ They should pay special attention to accurate administration of their dose to minimize the risk of accidental overdose or underdose of NORVIR.

☐ They should inform their healthcare provider if their children's weight changes in order to make sure that the child's NORVIR dose is the correct one.

☐ Take NORVIR with meals.

☐ For adult patients taking NORVIR capsules, the maximum dose of 600 mg twice daily by mouth with meals should not be exceeded.

☐ Patients should remain under the care of a physician while using NORVIR. Patients should be advised to take NORVIR and other concomitant antiretroviral therapy every day as prescribed. NORVIR must always be used in combination with other antiretroviral drugs. Patients should not alter the dose or discontinue therapy without consulting with their doctor. If a dose of NORVIR is missed patients should take the dose as soon as possible and then return to their normal schedule. However, if a dose is skipped the patient should not double the next dose.

☐ NORVIR is not a cure for HIV-1 infection and patients may continue to experience illnesses associated with HIV-1 infection, including opportunistic infections. Patients should remain under the care of a physician when using NORVIR.

Patients should be advised to avoid doing things that can spread HIV-1 infection to others.

• **Do not share needles or other injection equipment.**
• **Do not share personal items that can have blood or body fluids on them, like toothbrushes and razor blades.**
• **Do not have any kind of sex without protection.** Always practice safe sex by using a latex or polyurethane condom to lower the chance of sexual contact with semen, vaginal secretions, or blood.
• **Do not breastfeed.** We do not know if NORVIR can be passed to the baby through breast milk and whether it could harm the baby. Also, mothers with HIV-1 should not breastfeed because HIV-1 can be passed to the baby in the breast milk.

☐ Sustained decreases in plasma HIV-1 RNA have been associated with a reduced risk of progression to AIDS and death.

Underline: Drug Interactions

☐ NORVIR may interact with some drugs; therefore, patients should be advised to report to their doctor the use of any other prescription, non-prescription medication or herbal products, particularly St. John's Wort.

☐ If they are receiving estrogen-based hormonal contraceptives, additional or alternate contraceptive measures should be used during therapy with NORVIR.

Underline: Potential Adverse Effects

☐ Pre-existing liver disease including Hepatitis B or C can worsen with use of NORVIR. This can be seen as worsening of transaminase elevations or hepatic decompensation. Patients should be advised that their liver function tests will need to be monitored closely especially during the first several months of NORVIR treatment and that they should notify their healthcare provider if they develop the signs and symptoms of worsening liver disease including loss of appetite, abdominal pain, jaundice, and itchy skin.

☐ Pancreatitis, including some fatalities, has been observed in patients receiving NORVIR therapy. Your patients should let you know of signs and symptoms (nausea, vomiting, and abdominal pain) that might be suggestive of pancreatitis.

☐ Skin rashes ranging in severity from mild to Stevens-Johnson syndrome have been reported in patients receiving NORVIR. Patients should be advised to contact their healthcare provider if they develop a rash while taking NORVIR. The healthcare provider will determine if treatment should be continued or an alternative antiretroviral regimen used.

☐ NORVIR may produce changes in the electrocardiogram (e.g., PR prolongation). Patients should consult their physician if they experience symptoms such as dizziness, lightheadedness, abnormal heart rhythm or loss of consciousness.

☐ Treatment with NORVIR therapy can result in substantial increases in the concentration of total cholesterol and triglycerides.

☐ New onset of diabetes mellitus, and exacerbation of pre-existing diabetes mellitus, and hyperglycemia have been reported. Patients should be advised to notify their healthcare provider if they develop the signs and symptoms of diabetes mellitus including frequent urination, excessive thirst, extreme hunger or unusual weight loss and/or an increased blood sugar while on NORVIR as they may require a change in their diabetes treatment or new treatment.

☐ Immune reconstitution syndrome has been reported in HIV-1 infected patients treated with combination antiretroviral therapy, including NORVIR.

☐ Redistribution or accumulation of body fat may occur in patients receiving antiretroviral therapy and that the cause and long term health effects of these conditions are not known at this time.

☐ Patients with hemophilia may experience increased bleeding when treated with protease inhibitors such as NORVIR.

☐ If they are receiving avanafil, sildenafil, tadalafil, or vardenafil for the treatment of erectile dysfunction, they may be at an increased risk of associated adverse reactions including hypotension, visual changes, and sustained erection, and should promptly report any symptoms to their doctor. They should seek medical assistance immediately if they develop a sustained penile erection lasting more than 4 hours while taking NORVIR and a PDE5 Inhibitor such as Stendra®, Viagra®, Cialis® or Levitra®. If they are currently using or planning to use avanafil or tadalafil (for the treatment of pulmonary arterial hypertension) they should ask their doctor about potential adverse reactions these medications may cause when taken with NORVIR. The doctor may choose not to keep them on avanafil, or may adjust the dose of tadalafil while initiating treatment with NORVIR. Concomitant use of Revatio® (sildenafil) with NORVIR is contraindicated in patients with pulmonary arterial hypertension (PAH).

☐ Continued NORVIR therapy at a dose of 600 mg twice daily following loss of viral suppression may increase the likelihood of cross-resistance to other protease inhibitors.

NORVIR 100 mg soft gelatin capsules are manufactured for:
AbbVie Inc.
North Chicago, IL 60064 USA

Patient Information

NORVIR® (NOR-VEER)

(ritonavir)

capsules Soft Gelatin

Read this Patient Information before you start taking NORVIR and each time you get a refill. There may be new information. This information does not take the place of talking to your doctor about your medical condition or your treatment.

Table 4 (cont.). Established and Other Potentially Significant Drug Interactions

Concomitant Drug Class: Drug Name	Effect on Concentration of Ritonavir or Concomitant Drug	Clinical Comments
Other Agents (cont.)		
Steroids (systemic): e.g. budesonide, dexamethasone, prednisone	↑ glucocorticoids	Concomitant use of glucocorticoids that are metabolized by CYP3A is not recommended unless the potential benefit of treatment outweighs the risk of systemic corticosteroid effects. Concomitant use may result in increased steroid concentrations and reduced serum cortisol concentrations. This may increase the risk for development of systemic corticosteroid effects including Cushing's syndrome and adrenal suppression.
Stimulant: methamphetamine	↑ methamphetamine	Use with caution. A dose decrease of methamphetamine may be needed when co-administered with ritonavir.

Table 6. Drug Interactions - Pharmacokinetic Parameters for Ritonavir in the Presence of the Co-administered Drug

Co-administered Drug	Dose of Co-administered Drug (mg)	Dose of NORVIR (mg)	n	AUC % (95% CI)	C_{max} (95% CI)	C_{min} (95% CI)
Clarithromycin	500 q12h, 4 d	200 q8h, 4 d	22	↑ 12% (2, 23%)	↑ 15% (2, 28%)	↑ 14% (-3, 36%)
Didanosine	200 q12h, 4 d	600 q12h, 4 d	12	↔	↔	↔
Fluconazole	400 single dose, day 1; 200 daily, 4 d	200 q6h, 4 d	8	↑ 12% (5, 20%)	↑ 15% (7, 22%)	↑ 14% (0, 26%)
Fluoxetine	30 q12h, 8 d	600 single dose, 1 d	16	↑ 19% (7, 34%)	↔	ND
Ketoconazole	200 daily, 7 d	500 q12h, 10 d	12	↑ 18% (-3, 52%)	↑ 10% (-11, 36%)	ND
Rifampin	600 or 300 daily, 10 d	500 q12h, 20 d	7, 9*	↓ 35% (7, 55%)	↓ 25% (-5, 46%)	↓ 49% (-14, 91%)
Voriconazole	400 q12h, 1 d; then 200 q12h, 8 d	400 q12h, 9 d		↔	↔	ND
Zidovudine	200 q8h, 4 d	300 q6h, 4 d	10	↔	↔	↔

What is the most important information I should know about NORVIR?

• NORVIR can interact with other medicines and cause serious side effects. It is important to know the medicines that should not be taken with NORVIR. **See the section "Who should not take NORVIR?"**

What is NORVIR?

NORVIR is a prescription anti-HIV medicine used with other anti-HIV medicines to treat people with human immunodeficiency virus (HIV) infection. NORVIR is a type of anti-HIV medicine called a protease inhibitor. HIV is the virus that causes AIDS (Acquired Immune Deficiency Syndrome).

When used with other HIV medicines, NORVIR may reduce the amount of HIV in your blood (called "viral load"). NORVIR may also help to increase the number of CD_4 (T) cells in your blood which help fight off other infections. Reducing the amount of HIV and increasing the CD_4 (T) cell count may improve your immune system. This may reduce your risk of death or infections that can happen when your immune system is weak (opportunistic infections).

NORVIR does not cure HIV infection or AIDS and you may continue to experience illnesses associated with HIV-1 infection, including opportunistic infections. You should remain under the care of a doctor when using NORVIR.

Avoid doing things that can spread HIV-1 infection:

• Do not share needles or other injection equipment.
• Do not share personal items that can have blood or body fluids on them, like toothbrushes and razor blades.
• Do not have any kind of sex without protection. Always practice safe sex by using a latex or polyurethane condom to lower the chance of sexual contact with semen, vaginal secretions, or blood.

Who should not take NORVIR?

Do not take NORVIR if you are allergic to ritonavir or any of the ingredients in NORVIR. See the end of this leaflet for a complete list of ingredients in NORVIR.

Do not take NORVIR with any of the following medicines:

• alfuzosin (Uroxatral)
• amiodarone (Cordarone, Nexterone, Pacerone), flecainide (Tambocor), propafenone (Rhythmol) or quinidine (Nuedext, Quinaglute, Cardioquin, Quinidex, and others)
• voriconazole (VFend) if NORVIR dose is 400 mg every 12 hours or greater

- dihydroergotamine (D.H.E. 45, Embolex, Migranal), ergonovine, ergotamine (Cafergot, Ergomar) methylergonovine (Methergine)
- cisapride (Propulsid)
- St. John's Wort (Hypericum perforatum)
- the cholesterol lowering medicines lovastatin (Mevacor, Altoprev, Advicor) or simvastatin (Zocor, Simcor, Vytorin)
- pimozide (Orap)
- sildenafil (Revatio) only when used for the treatment of pulmonary arterial hypertension
- oral midazolam or triazolam (Halcion)

Serious problems can happen if you or your child takes any of these medicines with NORVIR.

What should I tell my doctor before taking NORVIR?

Before taking NORVIR, tell your doctor if you:

- have liver problems, including Hepatitis B or Hepatitis C.
- have heart problems.
- have high blood sugar (diabetes).
- have bleeding problems or hemophilia.
- are pregnant or plan to become pregnant. It is not known if NORVIR can harm your unborn baby.
  Pregnancy Registry: There is a pregnancy registry for women who take antiviral medicines during pregnancy. The purpose of the registry is to collect information about the health of you and your baby. Talk to your doctor about how you can take part in this registry.
- are breastfeed. **Do not breastfeed if you take NORVIR.**
  - You should not breastfeed if you have HIV-1 because of the risk of passing HIV-1 to your baby.
  - It is not known if NORVIR passes into your breast milk
  - Talk to your doctor about the best way to feed your baby.

Tell your doctor about all the medicines you take including prescription and nonprescription medicines, vitamins, and herbal supplements. Taking NORVIR and certain other medicines may affect each other causing serious side effects. NORVIR may affect the way other medicines work and other medicines may affect how NORVIR works.

Especially tell your doctor if you take:
- medicine to treat HIV
- estrogen-based contraceptives (birth control). NORVIR might reduce the effectiveness of estrogen-based contraceptives. You must take additional precautions for birth control such as a condom.
- medicine for pain such as tramadol (Ryzolt, Ultracet, Conzip, Ultram), propoxyphene, or meperidine (Demerol)
- medicine to treat alcohol abuse such as disulfiram (Antabuse)
- medicine for your heart such as disopyramide (Norpace), lidocaine (Xylocaine Viscous), mexiletine, digoxin (Lanoxin), nifedipine (Procardia, Adalat, Afeditab CR), diltiazem (Cardizem, Dilacor, Cartia, Diltzac, Dilt, Taztia, Tiazac) or verapamil (Calan, Covera, Isoptin, Tarka, Verelan)
- medicines for panic disorder or anxiety such as buspirone, clorazepate, diazepam, estazolam, flurazepam, and zolpidem
- medicine for cancer such as dasatinib (Sprycel), nilotinib (Tasigna) vincristine, or vinblastine
- warfarin (Coumadin, Jantoven), rivaroxaban (Xarelto)
- medicine for seizures such as carbamazepine (Carbatrol, Equetro, Tegretol, Epitol), clonazepam (Klonopin), ethosuximide (Zarontin, Ethosuximide), divalproex (Depakote, Divalproex Sodium), lamotrigine (Lamictal) or phenytoin (Dilantin, Phenytek)
- medicine for depression such as nefazodone, bupropion (Wellbutrin, Aplenzin, Zyban), desipramine (Norpramin) or trazodone, fluoxetine (Prozac), paroxetine (Paxil), amitriptyline, or nortriptyline
- medicine for nausea and vomiting such as dronabinol (Marinol) or perphenazine
- medicine for fungal infections such as ketoconazole (Nizoral), itraconazole (Sporanox, Onmel) or voriconazole (VFend)
- colchicine (Colcrys, Col-Probenecid, Probenecid and Colchine)
- medicine for infections such as clarithromycin (Prevpac, Biaxin), rifabutin (Mycobutin), rifampin (Rimactane, Rifadin, Rifater, Rifamate), atovaquone (Mepron, Malarone), quinine (Qualaquin) or metronidazole (Flagyl, Helidac, Metrocream)
- medicine used to treat blood pressure, a heart attack, heart failure, or to lower pressure in the eye such as metoprolol (Lopressor, Toprol-XL), timolol (Cosopt, Betimol, Timoptic, Isatolol, Combigan)
- medicine for lung disease such as theophylline and salmeterol (Serevent)
- bosentan (Tracleer)
- medicine to prevent organ transplant failure such as cyclosporine (Gengraf, Sandimmune, Neoral), tacrolimus (Prograf,) sirolimus (Rapamune)
- steroids such as dexamethasone, fluticasone (Advair Diskus, Veramyst, Flovent, Flonase), budesonide (Entocort EC, Pulmicort, Rhinocort), or prednisone
- a narcotic medicine such as methadone (Methadose, Dolophine Hydrochloride) or fentanyl (Abstral, Actiq, Fentora, Lazanda, Onsolis, Duragesic)

Table 7. Drug Interactions - Pharmacokinetic Parameters for Co-administered Drug in the Presence of NORVIR

Co-administered Drug	Dose of Co-administered Drug (mg)	Dose of NORVIR (mg)	n	AUC % (95% CI)	C_{max} (95% CI)	C_{min} (95% CI)
Alprazolam	1, single dose	500 q12h, 10 d	12	↓ 12% (-5, 30%)	↓ 16% (5, 27%)	ND
Avanafil	50, single dose	600 q12h	14[6]	↑ 13-fold	↑ 2.4-fold	ND
Clarithromycin	500 q12h, 4 d	200 q8h, 4 d	22	↑ 77% (56, 103%)	↑ 31% (15, 51%)	↑ 2.8-fold (2.4, 3.3×)
14-OH clarithromycin metabolite				↓ 100%	↓ 99%	↓ 100%
Desipramine	100, single dose	500 q12h, 12 d	14	↑ 145% (103, 211%)-	↑ 22% (12, 35%)	ND
2-OH desipramine metabolite				↓ 15% (3, 26%)	↓ 67% (62, 72%)	ND
Didanosine	200 q12h, 4 d	600 q12h, 4 d	12	↓ 13% (0, 23%)	↓ 16% (5, 26%)	↔
Ethinyl estradiol	50 µg single dose	500 q12h, 16 d	23	↓ 40% (31, 49%)	↓ 32% (24, 39%)	ND
Fluticasone propionate aqueous nasal spray	200 mcg qd, 7 d	100 mg q12h, 7 d	18	↑ approximately 350-fold[5]	↑ approximately 25-fold[5]	
Indinavir[1] Day 14 Day 15	400 q12h, 15 d	400 q12h, 15 d	10	↑ 6% (-14, 29%) ↓ 7% (-22, 28%)	↓ 51% (40, 61%) ↓ 62% (52, 70%)	↑ 4-fold (2.8, 6.8×) ↑ 4-fold (2.5, 6.5×)
Ketoconazole	200 daily, 7 d	500 q12h, 10 d	12	↑ 3.4-fold (2.8, 4.3×)	↑ 55% (40, 72%)	ND
Meperidine Normeperidine metabolite	50 oral single dose	500 q12h, 10 d	8 6	↓ 62% (59, 65%) ↑ 47% (-24, 345%)	↓ 59% (42, 72%) ↑ 87% (42, 147%)	ND ND
Methadone[2]	5, single dose	500 q12h, 15 d	11	↓ 36% (16, 52%)	↓ 38% (28, 46%)	ND
Raltegravir	400, single dose	100 q12h, 16 d	10	↓ 16% (-30, 1%)	↓ 24% (-45, 4%)	↓ 1% (-30, 40%)
Rivaroxaban	10, single dose (days 0 and 7)	600 q12h (days 2 to 7)	12	↑ 150% (130-170%)[7]	↑ 60% (40-70%)[7]	ND
Rifabutin 25-O-desacetyl rifabutin metabolite	150 daily, 16 d	500 q12h, 10 d	5, 11*	↑ 4-fold (2.8, 6.1×) ↑ 38-fold (28, 56×)	↑ 2.5-fold (1.9, 3.4×) ↑ 16-fold (13, 20×)	↑ 6-fold (3.5, 18.3×) ↑ 181-fold (ND)
Sildenafil	100, single dose	500 twice daily, 8 d	28	↑ 11-fold	↑ 4-fold	ND
Sulfamethoxazole[3]	800, single dose	500 q12h, 12 d	15	↓ 20% (16, 23%)	↔	ND
Tadalafil	20 mg, single dose	200 mg q12h		↑ 124%	↔	ND
Theophylline	3 mg/kg q8h, 15 d	500 q12h, 10 d	13, 11*	↓ 43% (42, 45%)	↓ 32% (29, 34%)	↓ 57% (55, 59%)
Trazodone	50 mg, single dose	200 mg q12h, 4 doses	10	↑ 2.4-fold	↑ 34%	
Trimethoprim[3]	160, single dose	500 q12h, 12 d	15	↑ 20% (3, 43%)	↔	ND

(Table continued on next page)

- medicine to treat schizophrenia such as risperidone (Risperdal) or thioridazine
- medicine to treat erectile dysfunction or pulmonary hypertension such as avanafil (Stendra), sildenafil (Viagra, Revatio), vardenafil (Levitra, Staxyn), tadalafil (Cialis, Adcirca). If you are taking avanafil (Stendra), your doctor may need to change it to a different medicine.
- midazolam by injection
- methamphetamine (Desoxyn)
- cholesterol lowering medicine such as atorvastatin (Lipitor) or rosuvastatin (Crestor)

This is not a complete list of medicines that you should tell your doctor that you are taking. Ask your doctor, provider or pharmacist if you are not sure if your medicine is one that is listed above.

Know the medicines you take. Keep a list of them to show your doctor or pharmacist when you get a new medicine. Do not start any new medicines while you are taking NORVIR without first talking with your doctor.

How should I take NORVIR?
- Take NORVIR exactly as prescribed by your doctor.
- You should stay under a doctor's care when taking NORVIR. Do not change your dose of NORVIR or stop treatment without talking with your doctor first.
- If your child is taking NORVIR, your child's doctor will decide the right dose based on your child's height and weight. Tell your doctor if your child's weight changes. Your child should take NORVIR with food.
- Take NORVIR with food if possible.
- Do not run out of NORVIR. Get your NORVIR prescription refilled from you doctor or pharmacy before you run out.

Information on the AbbVie, Inc. products listed on these pages is from the prescribing information in use as of July 31, 2014. For more information, please visit rxabbvie.com or call 1-800-633-9110.

Table 7 (cont.). Drug Interactions - Pharmacokinetic Parameters for Co-administered Drug in the Presence of NORVIR

Co-administered Drug	Dose of Co-administered Drug (mg)	Dose of NORVIR (mg)	n	AUC % (95% CI)	Cmax (95% CI)	Cmin (95% CI)
Vardenafil	5 mg	600 q12h		↑ 49-fold	↑ 13-fold	ND
Voriconazole	400 q12h, 1 d; then 200 q12h, 8 d	400 q12h, 9 d		↓ 82%	↓ 66%	
	400 q12h, 1 d; then 200 q12h, 8 d	100 q12h, 9 d		↓ 39%	↓ 24%	
Warfarin S-Warfarin R-Warfarin	5, single dose	400 q12h, 12d	12	↑ 9% (-17, 44%)[4] ↓ 33% (-38, -27%)[4]	↓ 9% (-16, -2%)[4] ↔	ND ND
Zidovudine	200 q8h, 4 d	300 q6h, 4 d	9	↓ 25% (15, 34%)	↓ 27% (4, 45%)	ND

1 Ritonavir and indinavir were co-administered for 15 days; Day 14 doses were administered after a 15%-fat breakfast (757 Kcal) and 9%-fat evening snack (236 Kcal), and Day 15 doses were administered after a 15%-fat breakfast (757 Kcal) and 32%-fat dinner (815 Kcal). Indinavir C_{min} was also increased 4-fold. Effects were assessed relative to an indinavir 800 mg q8h regimen under fasting conditions.
2 Effects were assessed on a dose-normalized comparison to a methadone 20 mg single dose.
3 Sulfamethoxazole and trimethoprim taken as single combination tablet.
4 90% CI presented for R- and S-warfarin AUC and C_{max} ratios.
5 This significant increase in plasma fluticasone propionate exposure resulted in a significant decrease (86%) in plasma cortisol AUC.
6 For the reference arm: N=14 for C_{max} and $AUC_{(0-inf)}$ and for the test arm: N=13 for C_{max} and N=4 for $AUC_{(0-inf)}$.
7 90% CI presented for rivaroxaban
↑ Indicates increase.
↓ Indicates decrease.
↔ Indicates no change.
* Parallel group design; entries are subjects receiving combination and control regimens, respectively.

- If you miss a dose of NORVIR, take it as soon as possible and then take your next scheduled dose at its regular time. If it is almost time for your next dose, wait and take the next dose at the regular time. Do not double the next dose.
- If you take too much NORVIR, call your local poison control center or go to the nearest hospital emergency room right away.

What are the possible side effects of NORVIR?
NORVIR can cause serious side effects including:
- **See "What is the most important information I should know about NORVIR?"**
- **Liver disease.** Some people taking NORVIR in combination with other anti-HIV medicines have developed liver problems which may be life-threatening. Your doctor should do regular blood tests during your combination treatment with NORVIR. If you have chronic hepatitis B or C infection, your doctor should check your blood tests more often because you have an increased chance of developing liver problems. Tell your doctor if you have any of the below signs and symptoms of liver problems:
  - loss of appetite
  - pain or tenderness on your right side below your ribs
  - yellowing of your skin or whites of your eyes
  - itchy skin
- **Swelling of your pancreas (Pancreatitis).** NORVIR can cause serious pancreas problems, which may lead to death. Tell your doctor right away if you have signs or symptoms of pancreatitis such as:
  - nausea
  - vomiting
  - stomach (abdomen) pain
- **Allergic Reactions.** Sometimes these allergic reactions can become severe and require treatment in a hospital. You should call your doctor right away if you develop a rash. Stop taking NORVIR and get medical help right away if you have any of the following symptoms of a severe allergic reaction:
  - trouble breathing
  - wheezing
  - dizziness or fainting
  - throat tightness or hoarseness
  - fast heartbeat or pounding in your chest (tachycardia)
  - sweating
  - swelling of your face, lips or tongue
  - muscle or joint pain
  - blisters or skin lesions
  - mouth sores or ulcers
- **Changes in the electrical activity of your heart called PR prolongation. PR prolongation can cause irregular heartbeats.** Tell your doctor right away if you have symptoms such as:
  - dizziness
  - lightheadedness

- feeling faint or passing out
- abnormal heart beat
- **Increase in some fats (cholesterol and triglyceride levels) in your blood.** Treatment with NORVIR may increase your blood levels of cholesterol and triglycerides. Your doctor should do blood tests before you start your treatment with NORVIR and regularly to check for an increase in your cholesterol and triglycerides levels.
- **Diabetes and high blood sugar (hyperglycemia).** Some people who take protease inhibitors including NORVIR can get high blood sugar, develop diabetes, or their diabetes can get worse. Tell your doctor if you notice an increase in thirst or urinate often while taking NORVIR.
- **Changes in your immune system (Immune reconstitution syndrome)** can happen when you start taking HIV medicines. Your immune system may get stronger and begin to fight infections that have been hidden in your body for a long time. Call your doctor right away if you start having new symptoms after starting your HIV medicine.
- **Change in body fat.** These changes can happen in people who take antiretroviral therapy. The changes may include an increase amount of fat in the upper back and neck ("buffalo hump"), breast, and around the back and stomach area. Loss of fat from the legs, arms, and face may also happen. The exact cause and long-term health effects of these conditions are not known.
- **Increased bleeding for hemophiliacs.** Some people with hemophilia have increased bleeding with protease inhibitors including NORVIR.

The most common side effects of NORVIR include:
- diarrhea
- nausea
- vomiting
- upper and lower stomach (abdomen) pain
- tingling feeling or numbness in hands or feet or around the lips
- rash
- feeling weak or tired

Tell your doctor if you have any side effect that bothers you or that does not go away.
These are not all of the possible side effects of NORVIR. For more information, ask your doctor or pharmacist.
Call your doctor for medical advice about side effects. You may report side effects to FDA at 1-800-FDA-1088.

How do I Store NORVIR?
Store NORVIR soft gelatin capsules in the refrigerator between 36°F to 46°F (2°C to 8°C) NORVIR soft gelatin capsules may be stored below 77°F (25°C) if used within 30 days.
- Protect NORVIR soft gelatin capsules from light.
- Keep NORVIR soft gelatin capsules away from heat.
- Store NORVIR soft gelatin capsules tightly closed in the original container.
- Use NORVIR soft gelatin capsules by the expiration date on the bottle.

Keep NORVIR and all medicines out of the reach of children.

General information about NORVIR
Medicines are sometimes prescribed for purposes other than those listed in a Patient Information Leaflet. Do not use this medicine for a condition for which it was not prescribed. Do not share this medicine with other people.
This leaflet summarizes the most important information about NORVIR. If you would like more information, talk to your doctor. You can ask your doctor or pharmacist for information about NORVIR that is written for healthcare professionals.
For more information, call 1-800-633-9110.

What are the ingredients in NORVIR?
Active ingredient: ritonavir
Inactive ingredients:
NORVIR soft gelatin capsules: butylated hydroxytoluene, ethanol, gelatin, iron oxide, oleic acid, polyoxyl 35 castor oil, and titanium dioxide
This Patient Information has been approved by the U.S. Food and Drug Administration.
NORVIR 100 mg soft gelatin capsules are manufactured for:
AbbVie Inc.
North Chicago, IL 60064 USA
* The brands listed are trademarks of their respective owners and are not trademarks of AbbVie Inc. The makers of these brands are not affiliated with and do not endorse AbbVie Inc. or its products.
Ref. 03 - A843-R34-Rev. November, 2013
Shown in Product Identification Guide, page 304

NORVIR® ℞
[NOR-VEER]
(ritonavir)
tablet for oral use

NORVIR®
(ritonavir)
solution for oral use

HIGHLIGHTS OF PRESCRIBING INFORMATION
These highlights do not include all the information needed to use NORVIR safely and effectively. See full prescribing information for NORVIR.
NORVIR (ritonavir) tablet for oral use
NORVIR (ritonavir) solution for oral use
Initial U.S. Approval: 1996

WARNING: DRUG-DRUG INTERACTIONS LEADING TO POTENTIALLY SERIOUS AND/OR LIFE THREATENING REACTIONS
See full prescribing information for complete boxed warning
Co-administration of NORVIR with several classes of drugs including sedative hypnotics, antiarrhythmics, or ergot alkaloid preparations may result in potentially serious and/or life-threatening adverse events due to possible effects of NORVIR on the hepatic metabolism of certain drugs. Review medications taken by patients prior to prescribing NORVIR or when prescribing other medications to patients already taking NORVIR *[see Contraindications (4), Warnings and Precautions (5.1), Drug Interactions (7), and Clinical Pharmacology (12.3)].*

————INDICATIONS AND USAGE————
NORVIR is an HIV protease inhibitor indicated in combination with other antiretroviral agents for the treatment of HIV-1 infection (1)

————DOSAGE AND ADMINISTRATION————
- Dose modification for NORVIR is necessary when used with other protease inhibitors (2)
- Adult patients: 600 mg twice-day with meals (2.1)
- Pediatrics patients: The recommended twice daily dose for children greater than one month of age is based on body surface area and should not exceed 600 mg twice daily with meals (2.2)
- NORVIR oral solution should not be administered to neonates before a postmenstrual age (first day of the mother's last menstrual period to birth plus the time elapsed after birth) of 44 weeks has been attained (2.2, 5.2)

————DOSAGE FORMS AND STRENGTHS————
- Tablet: 100 mg ritonavir (3)
- Oral solution: 80 mg ritonavir per milliliter (3)

CONTRAINDICATIONS

- NORVIR is contraindicated in patients with known hypersensitivity to ritonavir (e.g., toxic epidermal necrolysis, Stevens-Johnson syndrome) or any of its ingredients (4)
- Co-administration with drugs highly dependent on CYP3A for clearance and for which elevated plasma concentrations may be associated with serious and/or life-threatening events (4)
- Co-administration with drugs that significantly reduce ritonavir (4)

WARNINGS AND PRECAUTIONS

The following have been observed in patients receiving NORVIR:

- Drug Interactions: Consider drug-drug interaction potential to reduce risk of serious or life-threatening adverse reactions (5.1)
- Toxicity in preterm neonates: NORVIR oral solution should not be used in preterm neonates in the immediate postnatal period because of possible toxicities. A safe and effective dose of NORVIR oral solution in this patient population has not been established (2.2, 5.2)
- Hepatic Reactions: Fatalities have occurred. Monitor liver function before and during therapy, especially in patients with underlying hepatic disease, including hepatitis B and hepatitis C, or marked transaminase elevations (5.3, 8.6)
- Pancreatitis: Fatalities have occurred; suspend therapy as clinically appropriate (5.4)
- Allergic Reactions/Hypersensitivity: Allergic reactions have been reported and include anaphylaxis, toxic epidermal necrolysis, Stevens-Johnson syndrome, bronchospasm and angioedema. Discontinue treatment if severe reactions develop (5.5, 6.3)
- PR interval prolongation may occur in some patients. Cases of second and third degree heart block have been reported. Use with caution with patients with preexisting conduction system disease, ischemic heart disease, cardiomyopathy, underlying structural heart disease or when administering with other drugs that may prolong the PR interval (5.6, 12.3)
- Total cholesterol and triglycerides elevations: Monitor prior to therapy and periodically thereafter (5.7)
- Patients may develop new onset or exacerbations of diabetes mellitus, hyperglycemia (5.8)
- Patients may develop immune reconstitution syndrome (5.9)
- Patients may develop redistribution/accumulation of body fat (5.10)
- Hemophilia: Spontaneous bleeding may occur, and additional factor VIII may be required (5.11)

ADVERSE REACTIONS

The most frequently reported adverse drug reactions among patients receiving NORVIR alone or in combination with other antiretroviral drugs were gastrointestinal (including diarrhea, nausea, vomiting, abdominal pain (upper and lower)), neurological disturbances (including paresthesia and oral paresthesia), rash, and fatigue/asthenia (6.1)

To report SUSPECTED ADVERSE REACTIONS, contact AbbVie Inc. at 1-800-633-9110 or FDA at 1-800-FDA-1088 or www.fda.gov/medwatch.

DRUG INTERACTIONS

- Co-administration of NORVIR can alter the concentrations of other drugs. The potential for drug-drug interactions must be considered prior to and during therapy (4, 5.1, 7, 12.3)

USE IN SPECIFIC POPULATIONS

- Nursing Mothers: Because of both the potential for HIV transmission and the potential for serious adverse reactions in nursing infants, mothers should be instructed not to breastfeed if they are receiving NORVIR (8.3)

See 17 for PATIENT COUNSELING INFORMATION and the FDA-approved patient labeling

Revised: 11/2013

FULL PRESCRIBING INFORMATION: CONTENTS*

FULL PRESCRIBING INFORMATION

> **WARNING: DRUG-DRUG INTERACTIONS LEADING TO POTENTIALLY SERIOUS AND/OR LIFE THREATENING REACTIONS**
>
> Co-administration of NORVIR with several classes of drugs including sedative hypnotics, antiarrhythmics, or ergot alkaloid preparations may result in potentially serious and/or life-threatening adverse events due to possible effects of NORVIR on the hepatic metabolism of certain drugs. Review medications taken by patients prior to prescribing NORVIR or when prescribing other medications to patients already taking NORVIR [see Contraindications (4), Warnings and Precautions (5.1), Drug Interactions (7), and Clinical Pharmacology (12.3)].

1   INDICATIONS AND USAGE

NORVIR is indicated in combination with other antiretroviral agents for the treatment of HIV-1 infection.

2   DOSAGE AND ADMINISTRATION

NORVIR is administered orally. NORVIR tablets should be swallowed whole, and not chewed, broken or crushed. Take NORVIR with meals. Patients may improve the taste of NORVIR oral solution by mixing with chocolate milk, Ensure®, or Advera® within one hour of dosing.

General Dosing Guidelines

Patients who take the 600 mg twice daily soft gel capsule NORVIR dose may experience more gastrointestinal side effects such as nausea, vomiting, abdominal pain or diarrhea when switching from the soft gel capsule to the tablet formulation because of greater maximum plasma concentration (C_{max}) achieved with the tablet formulation relative to the soft gel capsule [see Clinical Pharmacology (12.3)]. Patients should also be aware that these adverse events (gastrointestinal or paresthesias) may diminish as therapy is continued.

Dose Modification for NORVIR

Dose reduction of NORVIR is necessary when used with other protease inhibitors: atazanavir, darunavir, fosamprenavir, saquinavir, and tipranavir.

Prescribers should consult the full prescribing information and clinical study information of these protease inhibitors if they are co-administered with a reduced dose of ritonavir [see Warnings and Precautions (5), and Drug Interactions (7)].

2.1   Adult Patients

Recommended Dosage for Treatment of HIV-1:

The recommended dosage of ritonavir is 600 mg twice daily by mouth to be taken with meals. Use of a dose titration schedule may help to reduce treatment-emergent adverse events while maintaining appropriate ritonavir plasma levels. Ritonavir should be started at no less than 300 mg twice daily and increased at 2 to 3 day intervals by 100 mg twice daily. The maximum dose of 600 mg twice daily should not be exceeded upon completion of the titration.

2.2   Pediatric Patients

Ritonavir should be used in combination with other antiretroviral agents [see Dosage and Administration (2)]. The recommended dosage of ritonavir in children greater than 1 month is 350 to 400 mg per m^2 twice daily by mouth to be taken with meals and should not exceed 600 mg twice daily. Ritonavir should be started at 250 mg per m^2 twice daily and increased at 2 to 3 day intervals by 50 mg per m^2 twice daily. If patients do not tolerate 400 mg per m^2 twice daily due to adverse events, the highest tolerated dose may be used for maintenance therapy in combination with other antiretroviral agents, however, alternative therapy should be considered. When possible, dose should be administered using a calibrated dosing syringe.

NORVIR oral solution should not be administered to neonates before a postmenstrual age (first day of the mother's last menstrual period to birth plus the time elapsed after birth) of 44 weeks has been attained [see Warnings and Precautions (5.2)].

NORVIR oral solution contains 43.2% (v/v) alcohol and 26.57% (w/v) propylene glycol. Special attention should be given to accurate calculation of the dose of NORVIR, transcription of the medication order, dispensing information and dosing instructions to minimize the risk for medication errors, and overdose. This is especially important for young children. Total amounts of alcohol and propylene glycol from all medicines that are to be given to pediatric patients 1 to 6 months of age should be taken into account in order to avoid toxicity from these excipients [see Warnings and Precautions (5.2) and Overdosage (10)].

[See table 1 above]

Body surface area (BSA) can be calculated as follows[1]:

$$BSA\ (m^2) = \sqrt{\frac{Ht\ (Cm) \times Wt\ (kg)}{3600}}$$

3   DOSAGE FORMS AND STRENGTHS

- NORVIR Tablets

White film-coated ovaloid tablets debossed with the "a" logo and the code NK providing 100 mg ritonavir.

Table 1. Pediatric Dosage Guidelines

Body Surface Area (m²)	Twice Daily Dose 250 mg per m²	Twice Daily Dose 300 mg per m²	Twice Daily Dose 350 mg per m²	Twice Daily Dose 400 mg per m²
0.20	0.6 mL (50 mg)	0.75 mL (60 mg)	0.9 mL (70 mg)	1.0 mL (80 mg)
0.25	0.8 mL (62.5 mg)	0.9 mL (75 mg)	1.1 mL (87.5 mg)	1.25 mL (100 mg)
0.50	1.6 mL (125 mg)	1.9 mL (150 mg)	2.2 mL (175 mg)	2.5 mL (200 mg)
0.75	2.3 mL (187.5 mg)	2.8 mL (225 mg)	3.3 mL (262.5 mg)	3.75 mL (300 mg)
1.00	3.1 mL (250 mg)	3.75 mL (300 mg)	4.4 mL (350 mg)	5 mL (400 mg)
1.25	3.9 mL (312.5 mg)	4.7 mL (375 mg)	5.5 mL (437.5 mg)	6.25 mL (500 mg)
1.50	4.7 mL (375 mg)	5.6 mL (450 mg)	6.6 mL (525 mg)	7.5 mL (600 mg)

Information on the AbbVie, Inc. products listed on these pages is from the prescribing information in use as of July 31, 2014. For more information, please visit rxabbvie.com or call 1-800-633-9110.

Table 2. Drugs that are Contraindicated with NORVIR

Drug Class	Drugs Within Class That Are Contraindicated With NORVIR**	Clinical Comments
Alpha$_1$-adrenoreceptor antagonist	Alfuzosin HCL	Potential for hypotension.
Antiarrhythmics	Amiodarone, flecainide, propafenone, quinidine	Potential for cardiac arrhythmias.
Antifungal	Voriconazole	Co-administration of voriconazole with ritonavir 400 mg every 12 hours significantly decreases voriconazole plasma concentrations and may lead to loss of antifungal response. Voriconazole is contraindicated with ritonavir doses of 400 mg every 12 hours or greater [see Drug Interactions (7.2)].
Ergot Derivatives	Dihydroergotamine, ergonovine, ergotamine, methylergonovine	Potential for acute ergot toxicity characterized by vasospasm and ischemia of the extremities and other tissues including the central nervous system.
GI Motility Agent	Cisapride	Potential for cardiac arrhythmias.
Herbal Products	St. John's Wort (hypericum perforatum)	Co-administration of NORVIR with St. John's Wort may result in decreased ritonavir plasma concentrations and may lead to loss of virologic response and possible resistance to NORVIR or to the class of protease inhibitors.
HMG-CoA Reductase Inhibitors:	Lovastatin, simvastatin	Potential for myopathy including rhabdomyolysis.
Neuroleptic	Pimozide	Potential for cardiac arrhythmias.
PDE5 enzyme inhibitor	Sildenafil* (Revatio®) only when used for the treatment of pulmonary arterial hypertension (PAH)	A safe and effective dose has not been established when used with ritonavir. There is an increased potential for sildenafil-associated adverse events, including visual abnormalities, hypotension, prolonged erection, and syncope [see Drug Interactions (7.2)].
Sedative/hypnotics	Oral midazolam, triazolam	Prolonged or increased sedation or respiratory depression [see Drug Interactions (7.2)].

*see Drug Interactions (7) for co-administration of sildenafil in patients with erectile dysfunction.
** For additional information for these contraindicated drugs, see also Drug Interactions (7).

• NORVIR Oral Solution
Orange-colored liquid containing 600 mg ritonavir per 7.5 mL marked dosage cup (80 mg per mL).

4   CONTRAINDICATIONS

• When co-administering NORVIR with other protease inhibitors, see the full prescribing information for that protease inhibitor including contraindication information.
• NORVIR is contraindicated in patients with known hypersensitivity (e.g., toxic epidermal necrolysis (TEN) or Stevens-Johnson syndrome) to ritonavir or any of its ingredients.
• Co-administration of NORVIR with several classes of drugs (including sedative hypnotics, antiarrhythmics, or ergot alkaloid preparations) is contraindicated and may result in potentially serious and/or life-threatening adverse events due to possible effects of NORVIR on the hepatic metabolism of these drugs (see Table 2). Voriconazole and St. John's Wort are exceptions in that co-administration of NORVIR and voriconazole results in a significant decrease in plasma concentrations of voriconazole, and co-administration of NORVIR with St. John's Wort may result in decreased ritonavir plasma concentrations.
[See table 2 above]

5   WARNINGS AND PRECAUTIONS

When co-administering NORVIR with other protease inhibitors, see the full prescribing information for that protease inhibitor including important Warnings and Precautions.

5.1   Drug Interactions

NORVIR is a CYP3A inhibitor. Initiating treatment with NORVIR in patients receiving medications metabolized by CYP3A or initiating medications metabolized by CYP3A in patients already maintained on NORVIR may result in increased plasma concentrations of concomitant medications. Higher plasma concentrations of concomitant medications can result in increased or prolonged therapeutic or adverse effects, potentially leading to severe, life-threatening or fatal events. The potential for drug-drug interactions must be considered prior to and during therapy with NORVIR. Review of other medications taken by patients and monitoring of patients for adverse effects is recommended during therapy with NORVIR.
See Table 2 for a listing of drugs that are contraindicated with NORVIR due to potentially life-threatening adverse events, significant drug interactions, or loss of virologic ac-

tivity. Also, see Table 5 for a listing of drugs with established and other significant drug interactions [see Contraindications (4), Drug Interactions (7), and Clinical Pharmacology (12.3)].

5.2   Toxicity in Preterm Neonates

NORVIR oral solution contains the excipients alcohol (43.2% v/v) and propylene glycol (26.57% w/v). When administered concomitantly with propylene glycol, ethanol competitively inhibits the metabolism of propylene glycol, which may lead to elevated concentrations. Preterm neonates may be at an increased risk of propylene glycol-associated adverse events due to diminished ability to metabolize propylene glycol, thereby leading to accumulation and potential adverse events. Postmarketing life-threatening cases of cardiac toxicity (including complete AV block, bradycardia, and cardiomyopathy), lactic acidosis, acute renal failure, CNS depression and respiratory complications leading to death have been reported, predominantly in preterm neonates receiving lopinavir/ritonavir oral solution which also contains the excipients alcohol and propylene glycol.
NORVIR oral solution should not be used in preterm neonates in the immediate postnatal period because of possible toxicities. However, if the benefit of using NORVIR oral solution to treat HIV infection in infants immediately after birth outweighs the potential risks, infants should be monitored closely for increases in serum osmolality and serum creatinine, and for toxicity related to NORVIR oral solution including: hyperosmolality, with or without lactic acidosis, renal toxicity, CNS depression (including stupor, coma, and apnea), seizures, hypotonia, cardiac arrhythmias and ECG changes, and hemolysis. Total amounts of alcohol and propylene glycol from all medicines that are to be given to infants should be taken into account in order to avoid toxicity from these excipients [see Dosage and Administration (2.2) and Overdosage (10)].

5.3   Hepatic Reactions

Hepatic transaminase elevations exceeding 5 times the upper limit of normal, clinical hepatitis, and jaundice have occurred in patients receiving NORVIR alone or in combination with other antiretroviral drugs (see Table 4). There may be an increased risk for transaminase elevations in patients with underlying hepatitis B or C. Therefore, caution should be exercised when administering NORVIR to patients with pre-existing liver diseases, liver enzyme abnormalities, or hepatitis. Increased AST/ALT monitoring should be considered in these patients, especially during the first three months of NORVIR treatment [see Use in Specific Populations (8.6)].

There have been postmarketing reports of hepatic dysfunction, including some fatalities. These have generally occurred in patients taking multiple concomitant medications and/or with advanced AIDS.

5.4   Pancreatitis

Pancreatitis has been observed in patients receiving NORVIR therapy, including those who developed hypertriglyceridemia. In some cases fatalities have been observed. Patients with advanced HIV disease may be at increased risk of elevated triglycerides and pancreatitis [see Warnings and Precautions (5.7)]. Pancreatitis should be considered if clinical symptoms (nausea, vomiting, abdominal pain) or abnormalities in laboratory values (such as increased serum lipase or amylase values) suggestive of pancreatitis should occur. Patients who exhibit these signs or symptoms should be evaluated and NORVIR therapy should be discontinued if a diagnosis of pancreatitis is made.

5.5   Allergic Reactions/Hypersensitivity

Allergic reactions including urticaria, mild skin eruptions, bronchospasm, and angioedema have been reported. Cases of anaphylaxis, toxic epidermal necrolysis (TEN), and Stevens-Johnson syndrome have also been reported. Discontinue treatment if severe reactions develop.

5.6   PR Interval Prolongation

Ritonavir prolongs the PR interval in some patients. Post marketing cases of second or third degree atrioventricular block have been reported in patients.
NORVIR should be used with caution in patients with underlying structural heart disease, preexisting conduction system abnormalities, ischemic heart disease, cardiomyopathies, as these patients may be at increased risk for developing cardiac conduction abnormalities.
The impact on the PR interval of co-administration of ritonavir with other drugs that prolong the PR interval (including calcium channel blockers, beta-adrenergic blockers, digoxin and atazanavir) has not been evaluated. As a result, co-administration of ritonavir with these drugs should be undertaken with caution, particularly with those drugs metabolized by CYP3A. Clinical monitoring is recommended [see Drug Interactions (7), and Clinical Pharmacology (12.3)].

5.7   Lipid Disorders

Treatment with NORVIR therapy alone or in combination with saquinavir has resulted in substantial increases in the concentration of total cholesterol and triglycerides [see Adverse Reactions (6.1)]. Triglyceride and cholesterol testing should be performed prior to initiating NORVIR therapy and at periodic intervals during therapy. Lipid disorders should be managed as clinically appropriate, taking into account any potential drug-drug interactions with NORVIR and HMG CoA reductase inhibitors [see Contraindications (4) and Drug Interactions (7)].

5.8   Diabetes Mellitus/Hyperglycemia

New onset diabetes mellitus, exacerbation of pre-existing diabetes mellitus, and hyperglycemia have been reported during postmarketing surveillance in HIV-infected patients receiving protease inhibitor therapy. Some patients required either initiation or dose adjustments of insulin or oral hypoglycemic agents for treatment of these events. In some cases, diabetic ketoacidosis has occurred. In those patients who discontinued protease inhibitor therapy, hyperglycemia persisted in some cases. Because these events have been reported voluntarily during clinical practice, estimates of frequency cannot be made and a causal relationship between protease inhibitor therapy and these events has not been established.

5.9   Immune Reconstitution Syndrome

Immune reconstitution syndrome has been reported in HIV-infected patients treated with combination antiretroviral therapy, including NORVIR. During the initial phase of combination antiretroviral treatment, patients whose immune system responds may develop an inflammatory response to indolent or residual opportunistic infections (such as Mycobacterium avium infection, cytomegalovirus, Pneumocystis jiroveci pneumonia, or tuberculosis), which may necessitate further evaluation and treatment.
Autoimmune disorders (such as Graves' disease, polymyositis, and Guillain-Barré syndrome) have also been reported to occur in the setting of immune reconstitution, however, the time to onset is more variable, and can occur many months after initiation of treatment.

5.10   Fat Redistribution

Redistribution/accumulation of body fat including central obesity, dorsocervical fat enlargement (buffalo hump), peripheral wasting, facial wasting, breast enlargement, and "cushingoid appearance" have been observed in patients receiving antiretroviral therapy. The mechanism and long-term consequences of these events are currently unknown. A causal relationship has not been established.

5.11   Patients with Hemophilia

There have been reports of increased bleeding, including spontaneous skin hematomas and hemarthrosis, in patients with hemophilia type A and B treated with protease inhibitors. In some patients additional factor VIII was given. In more than half of the reported cases, treatment with protease inhibitors was continued or reintroduced. A causal relationship between protease inhibitor therapy and these events has not been established.

5.12 Resistance/Cross-resistance
Varying degrees of cross-resistance among protease inhibitors have been observed. Continued administration of ritonavir 600 mg twice daily following loss of viral suppression may increase the likelihood of cross-resistance to other protease inhibitors *[see Microbiology (12.4)].*

5.13 Laboratory Tests
Ritonavir has been shown to increase triglycerides, cholesterol, SGOT (AST), SGPT (ALT), GGT, CPK, and uric acid. Appropriate laboratory testing should be performed prior to initiating NORVIR therapy and at periodic intervals or if any clinical signs or symptoms occur during therapy.

6 ADVERSE REACTIONS
The following adverse reactions are discussed in greater detail in other sections of the labeling.
- Drug Interactions *[see Warnings and Precautions (5.1)]*
- Hepatotoxicity *[see Warnings and Precautions (5.3)]*
- Pancreatitis *[see Warnings and Precautions (5.4)]*
- Allergic Reactions/Hypersensitivity *[see Warnings and Precautions (5.5)]*

When co-administering NORVIR with other protease inhibitors, see the full prescribing information for that protease inhibitor including adverse reactions.

6.1 Adult Clinical Trial Experience
Because clinical trials are conducted under widely varying conditions, adverse reactions rates observed in the clinical trials of a drug cannot be directly compared to rates in the clinical trials of another drug and may not reflect the rates observed in practice.

The safety of NORVIR alone and in combination with other antiretroviral agents was studied in 1,755 adult patients. Table 3 lists treatment-emergent Adverse Reactions (with possible or probable relationship to study drug) occurring in greater than or equal to 1% of adult patients receiving NORVIR in combined Phase II/IV studies.

The most frequently reported adverse drug reactions among patients receiving NORVIR alone or in combination with other antiretroviral drugs were gastrointestinal (including diarrhea, nausea, vomiting, abdominal pain (upper and lower)), neurological disturbances (including paresthesia and oral paresthesia), rash, and fatigue/asthenia.

Table 3. Treatment-Emergent Adverse Reactions (With Possible or Probable Relationship to Study Drug) Occurring in greater than or equal to 1% of Adult Patients Receiving NORVIR in Combined Phase II/IV Studies (N = 1,755)

Adverse Reactions	n	%
Eye disorders		
Blurred vision	113	6.4
Gastrointestinal disorders		
Abdominal Pain (upper and lower)*	464	26.4
Diarrhea including severe with electrolyte imbalance*	1,192	67.9
Dyspepsia	201	11.5
Flatulence	142	8.1
Gastrointestinal hemorrhage*	41	2.3
Gastroesophageal reflux disease (GERD)	19	1.1
Nausea	1,007	57.4
Vomiting*	559	31.9
General disorders and administration site conditions		
Fatigue including asthenia*	811	46.2
Hepatobiliary disorders		
Blood bilirubin increased (including jaundice)*	25	1.4
Hepatitis (including increased AST, ALT, GGT)*	153	8.7
Immune system disorders		
Hypersensivity including urticatria and face edema*	114	8.2

Table 4. Percentage of Adult Patients, by Study and Treatment Group, with Chemistry and Hematology Abnormalities Occurring in greater than 3% of Patients Receiving NORVIR

Variable	Limit	Study 245 Naive Patients			Study 247 Advanced Patients		Study 462 PI-Naive Patients
		NORVIR plus ZDV	NORVIR	ZDV	NORVIR	Placebo	NORVIR plus Saquinavir
Chemistry	**High**						
Cholesterol	> 240 mg/dL	30.7	44.8	9.3	36.5	8.0	65.2
CPK	> 1000 IU/L	9.6	12.1	11.0	9.1	6.3	9.9
GGT	> 300 IU/L	1.8	5.2	1.7	19.6	11.3	9.2
SGOT (AST)	> 180 IU/L	5.3	9.5	2.5	6.4	7.0	7.8
SGPT (ALT)	> 215 IU/L	5.3	7.8	3.4	8.5	4.4	9.2
Triglycerides	> 800 mg/dL	9.6	17.2	3.4	33.6	9.4	23.4
Triglycerides	> 1500 mg/dL	1.8	2.6	-	12.6	0.4	11.3
Triglycerides Fasting	> 1500 mg/dL	1.5	1.3	-	9.9	0.3	-
Uric Acid	> 12 mg/dL	-	-	-	3.8	0.2	1.4
Hematology	**Low**						
Hematocrit	< 30%	2.6	-	0.8	17.3	22.0	0.7
Hemoglobin	< 8.0 g/dL	0.9	-	-	3.8	3.9	-
Neutrophils	≤ 0.5 × 10⁹/L	-	-	-	6.0	8.3	-
RBC	< 3.0 × 10¹²/L	1.8	-	5.9	18.6	24.4	-
WBC	< 2.5 × 10⁹/L	-	0.9	6.8	36.9	59.4	3.5

- Indicates no events reported.

Metabolism and nutrition disorders		
Edema and peripheral edema*	110	6.3
Gout*	24	1.4
Hypercholesterolemia*	52	3.0
Hypertriglyceridemia*	158	9.0
Lipodystrophy acquired*	51	2.9
Musculoskeletal and connective tissue disorders		
Arthralgia and back pain*	326	18.6
Myopathy/creatine phosphokinase increased*	66	3.8
Myalgia	156	8.9
Nervous system disorders		
Dizziness*	274	15.6
Dysgeusia*	285	16.2
Paresthesia (including oral paresthesia)*	889	50.7
Peripheral neuropathy	178	10.1
Syncope*	58	3.3
Psychiatric disorders		
Confusion*	52	3.0
Disturbance in attention	44	2.5
Renal and urinary disorders		
Increased urination*	74	4.2
Respiratory, thoracic and mediastinal disorders		
Coughing*	380	21.7
Oropharyngeal Pain*	279	15.9

Skin and subcutaneous tissue disorders		
Acne*	67	3.8
Pruritus*	214	12.2
Rash (includes erythematous and maculopapular)*	475	27.1
Vascular disorders		
Flushing, feeling hot*	232	13.2
Hypertension*	58	3.3
Hypotension including orthostatic hypotension*	30	1.7
Peripheral coldness*	21	1.2

* Represents a medical concept including several similar MedDRA PTs

Laboratory Abnormalities
Table 4 shows the percentage of adult patients who developed marked laboratory abnormalities.
[See table 4 above]

6.2 Pediatric Clinical Trial Experience
NORVIR has been studied in 265 pediatric patients greater than 1 month to 21 years of age. The adverse event profile observed during pediatric clinical trials was similar to that for adult patients.

Vomiting, diarrhea, and skin rash/allergy were the only drug-related clinical adverse events of moderate to severe intensity observed in greater than or equal to 2% of pediatric patients enrolled in NORVIR clinical trials.

Laboratory Abnormalities
The following Grade 3-4 laboratory abnormalities occurred in greater than 3% of pediatric patients who received treatment with NORVIR either alone or in combination with re-

Information on the AbbVie, Inc. products listed on these pages is from the prescribing information in use as of July 31, 2014. For more information, please visit rxabbvie.com or call 1-800-633-9110.

Table 5. Established and Other Potentially Significant Drug Interactions

Concomitant Drug Class: Drug Name	Effect on Concentration of Ritonavir or Concomitant Drug	Clinical Comment
	HIV-Antiviral Agents	
HIV-1 Protease Inhibitor: atazanavir	When co-administered with reduced doses of atazanavir and ritonavir ↑ atazanavir (↑ AUC, ↑ C_{max}, ↑ C_{min})	Atazanavir plasma concentrations achieved with atazanavir 300 mg once daily and ritonavir 100 mg once daily are higher than those achieved with atazanavir 400 mg once daily. See the complete prescribing information for Reyataz® (atazanavir) for details on co-administration of atazanavir 300 mg once daily with ritonavir 100 mg once daily.
HIV-1 Protease Inhibitor: darunavir	When co-administered with reduced doses of ritonavir ↑ darunavir (↑ AUC, ↑ C_{max}, ↑ C_{min})	See the complete prescribing information for Prezista® (darunavir) for details on co-administration of darunavir 600 mg twice daily with ritonavir 100 mg twice daily or darunavir 800 mg once daily with ritonavir 100 mg once daily.
HIV-1 Protease Inhibitor: fosamprenavir	When co-administered with reduced doses of ritonavir ↑ amprenavir (↑ AUC, ↑ C_{max}, ↑ C_{min})	See the complete prescribing information for Lexiva® (fosamprenavir) for details on co-administration of fosamprenavir 700 mg twice daily with ritonavir 100 mg twice daily, fosamprenavir 1400 mg once daily with ritonavir 200 mg once daily or fosamprenavir 1400 mg once daily with ritonavir 100 mg once daily.
HIV-1 Protease Inhibitor: indinavir	When co-administered with reduced doses of indinavir and ritonavir ↑ indinavir (↔ AUC, ↓ C_{max}, ↑ C_{min})	Alterations in concentrations are noted when reduced doses of indinavir are co-administered with NORVIR. Appropriate doses for this combination, with respect to efficacy and safety, have not been established.
HIV-1 Protease Inhibitor: saquinavir	When co-administered with reduced doses of ritonavir ↑ saquinavir (↑ AUC, ↑ C_{max}, ↑ C_{min})	See the complete prescribing information for Invirase® (saquinavir) for details on co-administration of saquinavir 1000 mg twice daily with ritonavir 100 mg twice daily. Saquinavir/ritonavir should not be given together with rifampin, due to the risk of severe hepatotoxicity (presenting as increased hepatic transaminases) if the three drugs are given together.
HIV-1 Protease Inhibitor: tipranavir	When co-administered with reduced doses of ritonavir ↑ tipranavir (↑ AUC, ↑ C_{max}, ↑ C_{min})	See the complete prescribing information for Aptivus® (tipranavir) for details on co-administration of tipranavir 500 mg twice daily with ritonavir 200 mg twice daily. There have been reports of clinical hepatitis and hepatic decompensation including some fatalities. All patients should be followed closely with clinical and laboratory monitoring, especially those with chronic hepatitis B or C co-infection, as these patients have an increased risk of hepatotoxicity. Liver function tests should be performed prior to initiating therapy with tipranavir/ritonavir, and frequently throughout the duration of treatment.
Non-Nucleoside Reverse Transcriptase Inhibitor: delavirdine	↑ ritonavir (↑AUC, ↑C_{max}, ↑ C_{min})	Appropriate doses of this combination with respect to safety and efficacy have not been established.
HIV-1 CCR5 – antagonist: maraviroc	↑ maraviroc	Concurrent administration of maraviroc with ritonavir will increase plasma levels of maraviroc. For specific dosage adjustment recommendations, please refer to the complete prescribing information for Selzentry® (maraviroc).
Integrase Inhibitor: Raltegravir	↓ raltegravir	The effects of ritonavir on raltegravir with ritonavir dosage regimens greater than 100 mg twice daily have not been evaluated, however raltegravir concentrations may be decreased with ritonavir coadministration.
	Other Agents	
Analgesics, Narcotic: tramadol, propoxyphene		A dose decrease may be needed for these drugs when co-administered with ritonavir.
Anesthetic: meperidine	↓ meperidine/ ↑ normeperidine (metabolite)	Dosage increase and long-term use of meperidine with ritonavir are not recommended due to the increased concentrations of the metabolite normeperidine which has both analgesic activity and CNS stimulant activity (e.g., seizures).
Antialcoholics: disulfiram/ metronidazole		Ritonavir formulations contain alcohol, which can produce disulfiram-like reactions when co-administered with disulfiram or other drugs that produce this reaction (e.g., metronidazole).
Antiarrhythmics: disopyramide, lidocaine, mexiletine	↑ antiarrhythmics	Caution is warranted and therapeutic concentration monitoring is recommended for antiarrhythmics when co-administered with ritonavir, if available.

(Table continued on next page)

verse transcriptase inhibitors: neutropenia (9%), hyperamylasemia (7%), thrombocytopenia (5%), anemia (4%), and elevated AST (3%).

6.3 Postmarketing Experience
The following adverse events (not previously mentioned in the labeling) have been reported during post-marketing use of NORVIR. Because these reactions are reported voluntarily from a population of unknown size, it is not possible to reliably estimate their frequency or establish a causal relationship to NORVIR exposure.
Body as a Whole
Dehydration, usually associated with gastrointestinal symptoms, and sometimes resulting in hypotension, syncope, or renal insufficiency has been reported. Syncope, or-

thostatic hypotension, and renal insufficiency have also been reported without known dehydration.

Co-administration of ritonavir with ergotamine or dihydroergotamine has been associated with acute ergot toxicity characterized by vasospasm and ischemia of the extremities and other tissues including the central nervous system.
Cardiovascular System
First-degree AV block, second-degree AV block, third-degree AV block, right bundle branch block have been reported *[see Warnings and Precautions (5.6)]*.
Cardiac and neurologic events have been reported when ritonavir has been co-administered with disopyramide, mexiletine, nefazodone, fluoxetine, and beta blockers. The possibility of drug interaction cannot be excluded.
Endocrine System
Cushing's syndrome and adrenal suppression have been reported when ritonavir has been co-administered with fluticasone propionate or budesonide.
Nervous System
There have been postmarketing reports of seizure. Also, see Cardiovascular System.
Skin and subcutaneous tissue disorders
Toxic epidermal necrolysis (TEN) has been reported.

7   DRUG INTERACTIONS
See also Contraindications (4), Warnings and Precautions (5.1), and Clinical Pharmacology (12.3)
When co-administering NORVIR with other protease inhibitors (atazanavir, darunavir, fosamprenavir, saquinavir, and tipranavir), see the full prescribing information for that protease inhibitor including important information for drug interactions.
7.1   Potential for NORVIR to Affect Other Drugs
Ritonavir has been found to be an inhibitor of cytochrome P450 3A (CYP3A) and may increase plasma concentrations of agents that are primarily metabolized by CYP3A. Agents that are extensively metabolized by CYP3A and have high first pass metabolism appear to be the most susceptible to large increases in AUC (greater than 3-fold) when co-administered with ritonavir. Thus, co-administration of NORVIR with drugs highly dependent on CYP3A for clearance and for which elevated plasma concentrations are associated with serious and/or life-threatening events is contraindicated. Co-administration with other CYP3A substrates may require a dose adjustment or additional monitoring as shown in Table 5.
Ritonavir also inhibits CYP2D6 to a lesser extent. Co-administration of substrates of CYP2D6 with ritonavir could result in increases (up to 2-fold) in the AUC of the other agent, possibly requiring a proportional dosage reduction. Ritonavir also appears to induce CYP3A, CYP1A2, CYP2C9, CYP2C19, and CYP2B6 as well as other enzymes, including glucuronosyl transferase.
7.2   Established and Other Potentially Significant Drug Interactions
Table 5 provides a list of established or potentially clinically significant drug interactions. Alteration in dose or regimen may be recommended based on drug interaction studies or predicted interaction *[see Clinical Pharmacology (12.3) for magnitude of interaction]*.
[See table 5 on pages 556 through 560]

8   USE IN SPECIFIC POPULATIONS
When co-administering NORVIR with other protease inhibitors, see the full prescribing information for the co-administered protease inhibitor including important information for use in special populations.
8.1   Pregnancy
Pregnancy Category B
Antiretroviral Pregnancy Registry: To monitor maternal-fetal outcomes of pregnant women exposed to NORVIR, an Antiretroviral Pregnancy Registry has been established. Physicians are encouraged to register patients by calling 1–800–258–4263.
Human Data:
There are no adequate and well-controlled studies in pregnant women. NORVIR should be used during pregnancy only if the potential benefit justifies the potential risk to the fetus.
Antiretroviral Pregnancy Registry:
As of January 2012, the Antiretroviral Pregnancy Registry (APR) has received prospective reports of 3860 exposures to ritonavir containing regimens (1567 exposed in the first trimester and 2293 exposed in the second and third trimester). Birth defects occurred in 35 of the 1567 (2.2%) live births (first trimester exposure) and 59 of the 2293 (2.6%) live births (second/third trimester exposure).
Among pregnant women in the U.S. reference population, the background rate of birth defects is 2.7%. There was no association between ritonavir and overall birth defects observed in the APR.

Table 5 (cont.). Established and Other Potentially Significant Drug Interactions

Concomitant Drug Class: Drug Name	Effect on Concentration of Ritonavir or Concomitant Drug	Clinical Comment
	Other Agents (cont.)	
Anticancer Agents: dasatinib, nilotinib, vincristine, vinblastine	↑ anticancer agents	Concentrations of these drugs may be increased when co-administered with ritonavir resulting in the potential for increased adverse events usually associated with these anticancer agents. For vincristine and vinblastine, consideration should be given to temporarily withholding the ritonavir containing antiretroviral regimen in patients who develop significant hematologic or gastrointestinal side effects when ritonavir is administered concurrently with vincristine or vinblastine. Clinicians should be aware that if the ritonavir containing regimen is withheld for a prolonged period, consideration should be given to altering the regimen to not include a CYP3A or P-gp inhibitor in order to control HIV-1 viral load. A decrease in the dosage or an adjustment of the dosing interval of nilotinib and dasatinib may be necessary for patients requiring co-administration with strong CYP3A inhibitors such as NORVIR. Please refer to the nilotinib and dasatinib prescribing information for dosing instructions.
Anticoagulant: warfarin	↓ R-warfarin ↓↑ S-warfarin	Initial frequent monitoring of the INR during ritonavir and warfarin co-administration is indicated.
Anticoagulant: rivaroxaban	↑ rivaroxaban	Avoid concomitant use of rivaroxaban and ritonavir. Co-administration of ritonavir and rivaroxaban is expected to result in increased exposure of rivaroxaban which may lead to risk of increased bleeding.
Anticonvulsants: carbamazepine, clonazepam, ethosuximide	↑ anticonvulsants	Use with caution. A dose decrease may be needed for these drugs when co-administered with ritonavir and therapeutic concentration monitoring is recommended for these anticonvulsants, if available.
Anticonvulsants: divalproex, lamotrigine, phenytoin	↓ anticonvulsants	Use with caution. A dose increase may be needed for these drugs when co-administered with ritonavir and therapeutic concentration monitoring is recommended for these anticonvulsants, if available.
Antidepressants: nefazodone, selective serotonin reuptake inhibitors (SSRIs): e.g. fluoxetine, paroxetine, tricyclics: e.g. amitriptyline, nortriptyline	↑ antidepressants	A dose decrease may be needed for these drugs when co-administered with ritonavir.
Antidepressant: bupropion	↓ bupropion ↓ active metabolite, hydroxybupropion	Concurrent administration of bupropion with ritonavir may decrease plasma levels of both bupropion and its active metabolite (hydroxybupropion). Patients receiving ritonavir and bupropion concurrently should be monitored for an adequate clinical response to bupropion.
Antidepressant: desipramine	↑ desipramine	Dosage reduction and concentration monitoring of desipramine is recommended.
Antidepressant: trazodone	↑ trazodone	Concomitant use of trazodone and NORVIR increases plasma concentrations of trazodone. Adverse events of nausea, dizziness, hypotension and syncope have been observed following co-administration of trazodone and NORVIR. If trazodone is used with a CYP3A4 inhibitor such as ritonavir, the combination should be used with caution and a lower dose of trazodone should be considered.
Antiemetic: dronabinol	↑ dronabinol	A dose decrease of dronabinol may be needed when co-administered with ritonavir.
Antifungal: ketoconazole itraconazole voriconazole	↑ ketoconazole ↑ itraconazole ↓ voriconazole	High doses of ketoconazole or itraconazole (greater than 200 mg per day) are not recommended. Co-administration of voriconazole and ritonavir doses of 400 mg every 12 hours or greater is contraindicated. Co-administration of voriconazole and ritonavir 100 mg should be avoided, unless an assessment of the benefit/risk to the patient justifies the use of voriconazole.

(Table continued on next page)

Animal Data

No treatment related malformations were observed when ritonavir was administered to pregnant rats or rabbits. Developmental toxicity observed in rats (early resorptions, decreased fetal body weight and ossification delays and developmental variations) occurred at a maternally toxic dosage at an exposure equivalent to approximately 30% of that achieved with the proposed therapeutic dose. A slight increase in the incidence of cryptorchidism was also noted in rats at an exposure approximately 22% of that achieved with the proposed therapeutic dose.

Developmental toxicity observed in rabbits (resorptions, decreased litter size and decreased fetal weights) also occurred at a maternally toxic dosage equivalent to 1.8 times the proposed therapeutic dose based on a body surface area conversion factor.

8.3   Nursing Mothers

The Centers for Disease Control and Prevention recommend that HIV-infected mothers not breastfeed their infants to avoid risking postnatal transmission of HIV. It is not known whether ritonavir is secreted in human milk. Because of both the potential for HIV transmission and the potential for serious adverse reactions in nursing infants, mothers should be instructed not to breastfeed if they are receiving NORVIR.

8.4   Pediatric Use

In HIV-infected patients age greater than 1 month to 21 years, the antiviral activity and adverse event profile seen during clinical trials and through postmarketing experience were similar to that for adult patients.

8.5   Geriatric Use

Clinical studies of NORVIR did not include sufficient numbers of subjects aged 65 and over to determine whether they respond differently from younger subjects. In general, dose selection for an elderly patient should be cautious, usually starting at the low end of the dosing range, reflecting the greater frequency of decreased hepatic, renal or cardiac function, and of concomitant disease or other drug therapy.

8.6   Hepatic Impairment

No dose adjustment of ritonavir is necessary for patients with either mild (Child-Pugh Class A) or moderate (Child-Pugh Class B) hepatic impairment. No pharmacokinetic or safety data are available regarding the use of ritonavir in subjects with severe hepatic impairment (Child-Pugh Class C), therefore, ritonavir is not recommended for use in patients with severe hepatic impairment *[see Warnings and Precautions (5.3), Clinical Pharmacology (12.3)]*.

10   OVERDOSAGE

10.1   Acute Overdosage - Human Overdose Experience

Human experience of acute overdose with NORVIR is limited. One patient in clinical trials took NORVIR 1500 mg per day for two days. The patient reported paresthesias which resolved after the dose was decreased. A postmarketing case of renal failure with eosinophilia has been reported with ritonavir overdose.

The approximate lethal dose was found to be greater than 20 times the related human dose in rats and 10 times the related human dose in mice.

10.2   Management of Overdosage

NORVIR oral solution contains 43.2% (v/v) alcohol and 26.57% (w/v) propylene glycol. Ingestion of the product over the recommended dose by a young child could result in significant toxicity and could potentially be lethal.

Treatment of overdose with NORVIR consists of general supportive measures including monitoring of vital signs and observation of the clinical status of the patient. There is no specific antidote for overdose with NORVIR. If indicated, elimination of unabsorbed drug should be achieved by gastric lavage; usual precautions should be observed to maintain the airway. Administration of activated charcoal may also be used to aid in removal of unabsorbed drug. Since ritonavir is extensively metabolized by the liver and is highly protein bound, dialysis is unlikely to be beneficial in significant removal of the drug. However, dialysis can remove both alcohol and propylene glycol in the case of overdose with ritonavir oral solution. A Certified Poison Control Center should be consulted for up-to-date information on the management of overdose with NORVIR.

11   DESCRIPTION

NORVIR (ritonavir) is an inhibitor of HIV protease with activity against the Human Immunodeficiency Virus (HIV).

Ritonavir is chemically designated as 10-Hydroxy-2-methyl-5-(1-methylethyl)-1-[2-(1-methylethyl)-4-thiazolyl]-3,6-dioxo-8,11-bis(phenylmethyl)-2,4,7,12- tetraazatridecan-13-oic acid, 5-thiazolylmethyl ester, [5S-(5R*,8R*,10R*,11R*)]. Its molecular formula is $C_{37}H_{48}N_6O_5S_2$, and its molecular weight is 720.95. Ritonavir has the following structural formula:

Information on the AbbVie, Inc. products listed on these pages is from the prescribing information in use as of July 31, 2014. For more information, please visit rxabbvie.com or call 1-800-633-9110.

Table 5 (cont.). Established and Other Potentially Significant Drug Interactions

Concomitant Drug Class: Drug Name	Effect on Concentration of Ritonavir or Concomitant Drug	Clinical Comment
Other Agents (cont.)		
Anti-gout: colchicine	↑ colchicine	Patients with renal or hepatic impairment should not be given colchicine with ritonavir. Treatment of gout flares-co-administration of colchicine in patients on ritonavir: 0.6 mg (one tablet) for one dose, followed by 0.3 mg (half tablet) one hour later. Dose to be repeated no earlier than three days. Prophylaxis of gout flares-co-administration of colchicine in patients on ritonavir: If the original colchicine regimen was 0.6 mg twice a day, the regimen should be adjusted to 0.3 mg once a day. If the original colchicine regimen was 0.6 mg once a day, the regimen should be adjusted to 0.3 mg once every other day. Treatment of familial Mediterranean fever (FMF)-co-administration of colchicine in patients on ritonavir: Maximum daily dose of 0.6 mg (may be given as 0.3 mg twice a day).
Anti-infective: clarithromycin	↑ clarithromycin	For patients with renal impairment the following dosage adjustments should be considered: • For patients with CL_{CR} 30 to 60 mL per min the dose of clarithromycin should be reduced by 50%. • For patients with CL_{CR} less than 30 mL per min the dose of clarithromycin should be decreased by 75%. No dose adjustment for patients with normal renal function is necessary.
Antimycobacterial: rifabutin	↑ rifabutin and rifabutin metabolite	Dosage reduction of rifabutin by at least three-quarters of the usual dose of 300 mg per day is recommended (e.g., 150 mg every other day or three times a week). Further dosage reduction may be necessary.
Antimycobacterial: rifampin	↓ ritonavir	May lead to loss of virologic response. Alternate antimycobacterial agents such as rifabutin should be considered (see Antimycobacterial: rifabutin, for dose reduction recommendations).
Antiparasitic: atovaquone	↓ atovaquone	Clinical significance is unknown; however, increase in atovaquone dose may be needed.
Antiparasitic: quinine	↑ quinine	A dose decrease of quinine may be needed when co-administered with ritonavir.
β-Blockers: metoprolol, timolol	↑ Beta-Blockers	Caution is warranted and clinical monitoring of patients is recommended. A dose decrease may be needed for these drugs when co-administered with ritonavir.
Bronchodilator: theophylline	↓ theophylline	Increased dosage of theophylline may be required; therapeutic monitoring should be considered.
Calcium channel blockers: diltiazem, nifedipine, verapamil	↑ calcium channel blockers	Caution is warranted and clinical monitoring of patients is recommended. A dose decrease may be needed for these drugs when co-administered with ritonavir.
Digoxin	↑ digoxin	Concomitant administration of ritonavir with digoxin may increase digoxin levels. Caution should be exercised when co-administering ritonavir with digoxin, with appropriate monitoring of serum digoxin levels.
Endothelin receptor antagonists: bosentan	↑ bosentan	Co-administration of bosentan in patients on ritonavir: In patients who have been receiving ritonavir for at least 10 days, start bosentan at 62.5 mg once daily or every other day based upon individual tolerability. Co-administration of ritonavir in patients on bosentan: Discontinue use of bosentan at least 36 hours prior to initiation of ritonavir. After at least 10 days following the initiation of ritonavir, resume bosentan at 62.5 mg once daily or every other day based upon individual tolerability.
HMG-CoA Reductase Inhibitor: atorvastatin rosuvastatin	↑ atorvastatin ↑ rosuvastatin	Titrate atorvastatin and rosuvastatin dose carefully and use the lowest necessary dose. If NORVIR is used with another protease inhibitor, see the complete prescribing information for the concomitant protease inhibitor for details on co-administration with atorvastatin and rosuvastatin.
Immunosuppressants: cyclosporine, tacrolimus, sirolimus (rapamycin)	↑ immunosuppressants	Therapeutic concentration monitoring is recommended for immunosuppressant agents when co-administered with ritonavir.

(Table continued on next page)

Ritonavir is a white-to-light-tan powder. Ritonavir has a bitter metallic taste. It is freely soluble in methanol and ethanol, soluble in isopropanol and practically insoluble in water.

NORVIR tablets are available for oral administration in a strength of 100 mg ritonavir with the following inactive ingredients: copovidone, anhydrous dibasic calcium phosphate, sorbitan monolaurate, colloidal silicon dioxide, and sodium stearyl fumarate. The following are the ingredients in the film coating: hypromellose, titanium dioxide, polyethylene glycol 400, hydroxypropyl cellulose, talc, polyethylene glycol 3350, colloidal silicon dioxide, and polysorbate 80.

NORVIR oral solution is available for oral administration as 80 mg per mL of ritonavir in a peppermint and caramel flavored vehicle. Each 8-ounce bottle contains 19.2 grams of ritonavir. NORVIR oral solution also contains ethanol, water, polyoxyl 35 castor oil, propylene glycol, anhydrous citric acid to adjust pH, saccharin sodium, peppermint oil, creamy caramel flavoring, and FD&C Yellow No. 6.

12 CLINICAL PHARMACOLOGY

12.1 Mechanism of Action

Ritonavir is an antiviral drug *[see Microbiology (12.4)]*.

12.3 Pharmacokinetics

The pharmacokinetics of ritonavir have been studied in healthy volunteers and HIV-infected patients (CD_4 greater than or equal to 50 cells per μL). See Table 6 for ritonavir pharmacokinetic characteristics.

Absorption

The absolute bioavailability of ritonavir has not been determined. After a 600 mg dose of oral solution, peak concentrations of ritonavir were achieved approximately 2 hours and 4 hours after dosing under fasting and non-fasting (514 KCal; 9% fat, 12% protein, and 79% carbohydrate) conditions, respectively.

NORVIR tablets are not bioequivalent to NORVIR capsules. Under moderate fat conditions (857 kcal; 31% fat, 13% protein, 56% carbohydrates), when a single 100 mg NORVIR dose was administered as a tablet compared with a capsule, $AUC_{(0-\infty)}$ met equivalence criteria but mean C_{max} was increased by 26% (92.8% confidence intervals: ↑15 - ↑39%).

No information is available comparing NORVIR tablets to NORVIR capsules under fasting conditions.

Effect of Food on Oral Absorption

When the oral solution was given under non-fasting conditions, peak ritonavir concentrations decreased 23% and the extent of absorption decreased 7% relative to fasting conditions. Dilution of the oral solution, within one hour of administration, with 240 mL of chocolate milk, Advera® or Ensure® did not significantly affect the extent and rate of ritonavir absorption. Administration of a single 600 mg dose oral solution under non-fasting conditions yielded mean ± SD areas under the plasma concentration-time curve (AUCs) of 129.0 ± 39.3 mg•h per mL.

A food effect is observed for NORVIR tablets. Food decreased the bioavailability of the ritonavir tablets when a single 100 mg dose of NORVIR was administered. Under high fat conditions (907 kcal; 52% fat, 15% protein, 33% carbohydrates), a 23% decrease in mean $AUC_{(0-\infty)}$ [90% confidence intervals: ↓30%-↓15%], and a 23% decrease in mean C_{max} [90% confidence intervals: ↓34%-↓11%]) was observed relative to fasting conditions. Under moderate fat conditions, a 21% decrease in mean $AUC_{(0-\infty)}$ [90% confidence intervals: ↓28%-↓13%], and a 22% decrease in mean C_{max} [90% confidence intervals: ↓33%-↓9%]) was observed relative to fasting conditions.

However, the type of meal administered did not change ritonavir tablet bioavailability when high fat was compared to moderate fat meals.

Metabolism

Nearly all of the plasma radioactivity after a single oral 600 mg dose of ^{14}C-ritonavir oral solution (n = 5) was attributed to unchanged ritonavir. Five ritonavir metabolites have been identified in human urine and feces. The isopropylthiazole oxidation metabolite (M-2) is the major metabolite and has antiviral activity similar to that of parent drug; however, the concentrations of this metabolite in plasma are low. *In vitro* studies utilizing human liver microsomes have demonstrated that cytochrome P450 3A (CYP3A) is the major isoform involved in ritonavir metabolism, although CYP2D6 also contributes to the formation of M–2.

Elimination

In a study of five subjects receiving a 600 mg dose of ^{14}C-ritonavir oral solution, 11.3 ± 2.8% of the dose was excreted into the urine, with 3.5 ± 1.8% of the dose excreted as unchanged parent drug. In that study, 86.4 ± 2.9% of the dose was excreted in the feces with 33.8 ± 10.8% of the dose excreted as unchanged parent drug. Upon multiple dosing, ritonavir accumulation is less than predicted from a single dose possibly due to a time and dose-related increase in clearance.

Table 6. Ritonavir Pharmacokinetic Characteristics

Parameter	N	Values (Mean ± SD)
$V_\beta/F^\ddagger$	91	0.41 ± 0.25 L/kg
$t_{1/2}$		3 - 5 h
CL/F SS†	10	8.8 ± 3.2 L/h
CL/F‡	91	4.6 ± 1.6 L/h
CL_R	62	< 0.1 L/h
RBC/Plasma Ratio		0.14
Percent Bound*		98 to 99%

† SS = steady state; patients taking ritonavir 600 mg q12h.
‡ Single ritonavir 600 mg dose.
* Primarily bound to human serum albumin and alpha-1 acid glycoprotein over the ritonavir concentration range of 0.01 to 30 µg/mL.

Effects on Electrocardiogram
QTcF interval was evaluated in a randomized, placebo and active (moxifloxacin 400 mg once-daily) controlled crossover study in 45 healthy adults, with 10 measurements over 12 hours on Day 3. The maximum mean (95% upper confidence bound) time-matched difference in QTcF from placebo after baseline correction was 5.5 (7.6) milliseconds (msec) for 400 mg twice-daily ritonavir. Ritonavir 400 mg twice daily resulted in Day 3 ritonavir exposure that was approximately 1.5 fold higher than observed with ritonavir 600 mg twice-daily dose at steady state.
PR interval prolongation was also noted in subjects receiving ritonavir in the same study on Day 3. The maximum mean (95% confidence interval) difference from placebo in the PR interval after baseline correction was 22 (25) msec for 400 mg twice-daily ritonavir [see Warnings and Precautions (5.6)].
Special Populations
Gender, Race and Age
No age-related pharmacokinetic differences have been observed in adult patients (18 to 63 years). Ritonavir pharmacokinetics have not been studied in older patients.
A study of ritonavir pharmacokinetics in healthy males and females showed no statistically significant differences in the pharmacokinetics of ritonavir. Pharmacokinetic differences due to race have not been identified.
Pediatric Patients
Steady-state pharmacokinetics were evaluated in 37 HIV-infected patients ages 2 to 14 years receiving doses ranging from 250 mg per m^2 twice-daily to 400 mg per m^2 twice-daily in PACTG Study 310, and in 41 HIV-infected patients ages 1 month to 2 years at doses of 350 and 450 mg per m^2 twice-daily in PACTG Study 345. Across dose groups, ritonavir steady-state oral clearance (CL/F/m^2) was approximately 1.5 to 1.7 times faster in pediatric patients than in adult subjects. Ritonavir concentrations obtained after 350 to 400 mg per m^2 twice-daily in pediatric patients greater than 2 years were comparable to those obtained in adults receiving 600 mg (approximately 330 mg per m^2) twice-daily. The following observations were seen regarding ritonavir concentrations after administration with 350 or 450 mg per m^2 twice-daily in children less than 2 years of age. Higher ritonavir exposures were not evident with 450 mg per m^2 twice-daily compared to the 350 mg per m^2 twice-daily. Ritonavir trough concentrations were somewhat lower than those obtained in adults receiving 600 mg twice-daily. The area under the ritonavir plasma concentration time curve and trough concentrations obtained after administration with 350 or 450 mg per m^2 twice-daily in children less than 2 years were approximately 16% and 60% lower, respectively, than that obtained in adults receiving 600 mg twice daily.
Renal Impairment
Ritonavir pharmacokinetics have not been studied in patients with renal impairment, however, since renal clearance is negligible, a decrease in total body clearance is not expected in patients with renal impairment.
Hepatic Impairment
Dose-normalized steady-state ritonavir concentrations in subjects with mild hepatic impairment (400 mg twice-daily, n = 6) were similar to those in control subjects dosed with 500 mg twice-daily. Dose-normalized steady-state ritonavir exposures in subjects with moderate hepatic impairment (400 mg twice-daily, n= 6) were about 40% lower than those in subjects with normal hepatic function (500 mg twice-daily, n = 6). Protein binding of ritonavir was not statistically significantly affected by mild or moderately impaired hepatic function. No dose adjustment is recommended in patients with mild or moderate hepatic impairment. How-

ever, health care providers should be aware of the potential for lower ritonavir concentrations in patients with moderate hepatic impairment and should monitor patient response carefully. Ritonavir has not been studied in patients with severe hepatic impairment.
Drug Interactions
[see also Contraindications (4), Warnings and Precautions (5.1), and Drug Interactions (7)]
Table 7 and Table 8 summarize the effects on AUC and C_{max}, with 95% confidence intervals (95% CI), of co-administration of ritonavir with a variety of drugs. For information about clinical recommendations see Table 5 in *Drug Interactions (7)*.

Table 5 (cont.). Established and Other Potentially Significant Drug Interactions

Concomitant Drug Class: Drug Name	Effect on Concentration of Ritonavir or Concomitant Drug	Clinical Comment
Other Agents (cont.)		
Inhaled or Intranasal Steroid: e.g. fluticasone budesonide	↑ glucocorticoids	Concomitant use of ritonavir and fluticasone or other glucocorticoids that are metabolized by CYP3A is not recommended unless the potential benefit of treatment outweighs the risk of systemic corticosteroid effects. Concomitant use may result in increased steroid concentrations and reduced serum cortisol concentrations. Systemic corticosteroid effects including Cushing's syndrome and adrenal suppression have been reported during postmarketing use in patients when ritonavir has been coadministered with fluticasone propionate or budesonide.
Long-acting beta-adrenoceptor agonist: salmeterol	↑ salmeterol	Concurrent administration of salmeterol and ritonavir is not recommended. The combination may result in increased risk of cardiovascular adverse events associated with salmeterol, including QT prolongation, palpitations and sinus tachycardia.
Narcotic Analgesic: methadone fentanyl	↓ methadone ↑ fentanyl	Dosage increase of methadone may be considered. Concentrations of fentanyl are expected to increase. Careful monitoring of therapeutic and adverse effects (including potentially fatal respiratory depression) is recommended when fentanyl is concomitantly administered with NORVIR.
Neuroleptics: perphenazine, risperidone, thioridazine	↑ neuroleptics	A dose decrease may be needed for these drugs when co-administered with ritonavir.
Oral Contraceptives or Patch Contraceptives: ethinyl estradiol	↓ ethinyl estradiol	Alternate methods of contraception should be considered.
PDE5 Inhibitors: avanafil sildenafil, tadalafil, vardenafil	↑ avanafil ↑ sildenafil ↑ tadalafil ↑ vardenafil	Do not use ritonavir with avanafil because a safe and effective avanafil dosage regimen has not been established. Particular caution should be used when prescribing sildenafil, tadalafil or vardenafil in patients receiving ritonavir. Co-administration of ritonavir with these drugs is expected to substantially increase their concentrations and may result in an increase in PDE5 inhibitor associated adverse events, including hypotension, syncope, visual changes, and prolonged erection. Use of PDE5 inhibitors for pulmonary arterial hypertension (PAH): Sildenafil (Revatio®) is contraindicated when used for the treatment of pulmonary arterial hypertension (PAH) because a safe and effective dose has not been established when used with ritonavir [see Contraindications (4)]. The following dose adjustments are recommended for use of tadalafil (Adcirca™) with ritonavir: Co-administration of ADCIRCA in patients on ritonavir: In patients receiving ritonavir for at least one week, start ADCIRCA at 20 mg once daily. Increase to 40 mg once daily based upon individual tolerability. Co-administration of ritonavir in patients on ADCIRCA: Avoid use of ADCIRCA during the initiation of ritonavir. Stop ADCIRCA at least 24 hours prior to starting ritonavir. After at least one week following the initiation of ritonavir, resume ADCIRCA at 20 mg once daily. Increase to 40 mg once daily based upon individual tolerability. Use of PDE5 inhibitors for the treatment of erectile dysfunction: It is recommended not to exceed the following doses: • Sildenafil: 25 mg every 48 hours • Tadalafil: 10 mg every 72 hours • Vardenafil: 2.5 mg every 72 hours Use with increased monitoring for adverse events.
Sedative/hypnotics: buspirone, clorazepate, diazepam, estazolam, flurazepam, zolpidem	↑ sedative/hypnotics	A dose decrease may be needed for these drugs when co-administered with ritonavir.

(Table continued on next page)

[See table 7 at top of next page]
[See table 8 on pages 561 and 562]
12.4   Microbiology
Mechanism of Action
Ritonavir is a peptidomimetic inhibitor of the HIV-1 protease. Inhibition of HIV protease renders the enzyme incapa-

Information on the AbbVie, Inc. products listed on these pages is from the prescribing information in use as of July 31, 2014. For more information, please visit rxabbvie.com or call 1-800-633-9110.

Table 5 *(cont.)*. Established and Other Potentially Significant Drug Interactions

Concomitant Drug Class: Drug Name	Effect on Concentration of Ritonavir or Concomitant Drug	Clinical Comment
Other Agents (cont.)		
Sedative/hypnotics: Parenteral midazolam	↑ midazolam	Co-administration of oral midazolam with NORVIR is CONTRAINDICATED. Concomitant use of parenteral midazolam with NORVIR may increase plasma concentrations of midazolam. Co-administration should be done in a setting which ensures close clinical monitoring and appropriate medical management in case of respiratory depression and/or prolonged sedation. Dosage reduction for midazolam should be considered, especially if more than a single dose of midazolam is administered.
Steroids (systemic): e.g. budesonide, dexamethasone, prednisone	↑ glucocorticoids	Concomitant use of glucocorticoids that are metabolized by CYP3A is not recommended unless the potential benefit of treatment outweighs the risk of systemic corticosteroid effects. Concomitant use may result in increased steroid concentrations and reduced serum cortisol concentrations. This may increase the risk for development of systemic corticosteroid effects including Cushing's syndrome and adrenal suppression.
Stimulant: methamphetamine	↑ methamphetamine	Use with caution. A dose decrease of methamphetamine may be needed when co-administered with ritonavir.

Table 7. Drug Interactions - Pharmacokinetic Parameters for Ritonavir in the Presence of the Co-administered Drug

Co-administered Drug	Dose of Co-administered Drug (mg)	Dose of NORVIR (mg)	N	AUC % (95% CI)	C_{max} (95% CI)	C_{min} (95% CI)
Clarithromycin	500 q12h, 4 d	200 q8h, 4 d	22	↑ 12% (2, 23%)	↑ 15% (2, 28%)	↑ 14% (-3, 36%)
Didanosine	200 q12h, 4 d	600 q12h, 4 d	12	↔	↔	↔
Fluconazole	400 single dose, day 1; 200 daily, 4 d	200 q6h, 4 d	8	↑ 12% (5, 20%)	↑ 15% (7, 22%)	↑ 14% (0, 26%)
Fluoxetine	30 q12h, 8 d	600 single dose, 1 d	16	↑ 19% (7, 34%)	↔	ND
Ketoconazole	200 daily, 7 d	500 q12h, 10 d	12	↑ 18% (-3, 52%)	↑ 10% (-11, 36%)	ND
Rifampin	600 or 300 daily, 10 d	500 q12h, 20 d	7, 9*	↓ 35% (7, 55%)	↓ 25% (-5, 46%)	↓ 49% (-14, 91%)
Voriconazole	400 q12h, 1 d; then 200 q12h, 8 d	400 q12h, 9 d				ND
Zidovudine	200 q8h, 4 d	300 q6h, 4 d	10	↔	↔	↔

ble of processing the *gag-pol* polyprotein precursor which leads to production of non-infectious immature HIV particles.

Antiviral Activity in Cell Culture
The activity of ritonavir was assessed in acutely infected lymphoblastoid cell lines and in peripheral blood lymphocytes. The concentration of drug that inhibits 50% (EC_{50}) value of viral replication ranged from 3.8 to 153 nM depending upon the HIV-1 isolate and the cells employed. The average EC_{50} value for low passage clinical isolates was 22 nM (n = 13). In MT_4 cells, ritonavir demonstrated additive effects against HIV-1 in combination with either didanosine (ddI) or zidovudine (ZDV). Studies which measured cytotoxicity of ritonavir on several cell lines showed that greater than 20 μM was required to inhibit cellular growth by 50% resulting in a cell culture therapeutic index of at least 1000.
Resistance
HIV-1 isolates with reduced susceptibility to ritonavir have been selected in cell culture. Genotypic analysis of these isolates showed mutations in the HIV-1 protease gene leading to amino acid substitutions I84V, V82F, A71V, and M46I. Phenotypic (n = 18) and genotypic (n = 48) changes in HIV-1 isolates from selected patients treated with ritonavir were monitored in phase I/II trials over a period of 3 to 32 weeks. Substitutions associated with the HIV-1 viral protease in isolates obtained from 43 patients appeared to occur in a stepwise and ordered fashion at positions V82A/F/T/S, I54V, A71V/T, and I36L, followed by combinations of substitutions at an additional 5 specific amino acid positions (M46I/L, K20R, I84V, L33F and L90M). Of 18 patients for whom both phenotypic and genotypic analysis were performed on free virus isolated from plasma, 12 showed reduced susceptibility to ritonavir in cell culture. All 18 patients possessed one or more substitutions in the viral protease gene. The V82A/F substitution appeared to be necessary but not suf-

ficient to confer phenotypic resistance. Phenotypic resistance was defined as a greater than or equal to 5-fold decrease in viral sensitivity in cell culture from baseline.

Cross-Resistance to Other Antiretrovirals
Among protease inhibitors variable cross-resistance has been recognized. Serial HIV-1 isolates obtained from six patients during ritonavir therapy showed a decrease in ritonavir susceptibility in cell culture but did not demonstrate a concordant decrease in susceptibility to saquinavir in cell culture when compared to matched baseline isolates. However, isolates from two of these patients demonstrated decreased susceptibility to indinavir in cell culture (8-fold). Isolates from 5 patients were also tested for cross-resistance to amprenavir and nelfinavir; isolates from 3 patients had a decrease in susceptibility to nelfinavir (6- to 14-fold), and none to amprenavir. Cross-resistance between ritonavir and reverse transcriptase inhibitors is unlikely because of the different enzyme targets involved. One ZDV-resistant HIV-1 isolate tested in cell culture retained full susceptibility to ritonavir.

13　NONCLINICAL TOXICOLOGY
13.1　Carcinogenesis, Mutagenesis, Impairment of Fertility
Carcinogenesis
Carcinogenicity studies in mice and rats have been carried out on ritonavir. In male mice, at levels of 50, 100 or 200 mg per kg per day, there was a dose dependent increase in the incidence of both adenomas and combined adenomas and carcinomas in the liver. Based on AUC measurements, the exposure at the high dose was approximately 0.3-fold for males that of the exposure in humans with the recommended therapeutic dose (600 mg twice-daily). There were no carcinogenic effects seen in females at the dosages tested. The exposure at the high dose was approximately

0.6-fold for the females that of the exposure in humans. In rats dosed at levels of 7, 15 or 30 mg per kg per day there were no carcinogenic effects. In this study, the exposure at the high dose was approximately 6% that of the exposure in humans with the recommended therapeutic dose. Based on the exposures achieved in the animal studies, the significance of the observed effects is not known.
Mutagenesis
However, ritonavir was found to be negative for mutagenic or clastogenic activity in a battery of in *in vitro* and *in vivo* assays including the Ames bacterial reverse mutation assay using *S. typhimurium* and *E. coli*, the mouse lymphoma assay, the mouse micronucleus test and chromosomal aberration assays in human lymphocytes.
Impairment of Fertility
Ritonavir produced no effects on fertility in rats at drug exposures approximately 40% (male) and 60% (female) of that achieved with the proposed therapeutic dose. Higher dosages were not feasible due to hepatic toxicity.

14　CLINICAL STUDIES
The activity of NORVIR as monotherapy or in combination with nucleoside reverse transcriptase inhibitors has been evaluated in 1446 patients enrolled in two double-blind, randomized trials.
14.1　Advanced Patients with Prior Antiretroviral Therapy
Study 247 was a randomized, double-blind trial (with open-label follow-up) conducted in HIV-infected patients with at least nine months of prior antiretroviral therapy and baseline CD_4 cell counts less than or equal to 100 cells per μL. NORVIR 600 mg twice-daily or placebo was added to each patient's baseline antiretroviral therapy regimen, which could have consisted of up to two approved antiretroviral agents. The study accrued 1,090 patients, with mean baseline CD_4 cell count at study entry of 32 cells per μL. After the clinical benefit of NORVIR therapy was demonstrated, all patients were eligible to switch to open-label NORVIR for the duration of the follow-up period. Median duration of double-blind therapy with NORVIR and placebo was 6 months. The median duration of follow-up through the end of the open-label phase was 13.5 months for patients randomized to NORVIR and 14 months for patients randomized to placebo.
The cumulative incidence of clinical disease progression or death during the double-blind phase of Study 247 was 26% for patients initially randomized to NORVIR compared to 42% for patients initially randomized to placebo. This difference in rates was statistically significant.
Cumulative mortality through the end of the open-label follow-up phase for patients enrolled in Study 247 was 18% (99/543) for patients initially randomized to NORVIR compared to 26% (142/547) for patients initially randomized to placebo. This difference in rates was statistically significant. However, since the analysis at the end of the open-label phase includes patients in the placebo arm who were switched from placebo to NORVIR therapy, the survival benefit of NORVIR cannot be precisely estimated.
During the double-blind phase of Study 247, CD_4 cell counts increases from baseline for patients randomized to NORVIR at Week 2 and Week 4 were observed. From Week 4 and through Week 24, mean CD_4 cell counts for patients randomized to NORVIR appeared to plateau. In contrast, there was no apparent change in mean CD_4 cell counts for patients randomized to placebo at any visit between baseline and Week 24 of the double-blind phase of Study 247.
14.2　Patients without Prior Antiretroviral Therapy
In Study 245, 356 antiretroviral-naive HIV-infected patients (mean baseline CD_4 = 364 cells per μL) were randomized to receive either NORVIR 600 mg twice-daily, zidovudine 200 mg three-times-daily, or a combination of these drugs.
During the double-blind phase of study 245, greater mean CD_4 cell count increases were observed from baseline to Week 12 in the NORVIR-containing arms compared to the zidovudine arms. Mean CD_4 cell count changes subsequently appeared to plateau through Week 24 in the NORVIR arm, whereas mean CD_4 cell counts gradually diminished through Week 24 in the zidovudine and NORVIR plus zidovudine arms.
Greater mean reductions in plasma HIV-1 RNA levels were observed from baseline to Week 2 for the NORVIR-containing arms compared to the zidovudine arm. After Week 2 and through Week 24, mean plasma HIV-1 RNA levels either remained stable in the NORVIR and zidovudine arms or gradually rebounded toward baseline in the NORVIR plus zidovudine arm.

15　REFERENCES
1. Sewester CS. Calculations. In: Drug Facts and Comparisons. St. Louis, MO: J.B. Lippincott Co; January, 1997:xix.

16　HOW SUPPLIED/STORAGE AND HANDLING
NORVIR (ritonavir) tablets and NORVIR (ritonavir) oral solution are available in the following strengths and package sizes:

16.1   NORVIR Tablets, 100 mg Ritonavir

NORVIR (ritonavir) tablets are white film-coated ovaloid tablets debossed with the "a" logo and the code NK. Bottles of 30 tablets each (**NDC** 0074-3333-30).

Recommended Storage

Store at or below 30°C (86°F). Exposure to temperatures up to 50°C (122°F) for seven days permitted. Dispense in original container or USP equivalent tight container (60 mL or less). For patient use: exposure of this product to high humidity outside the original or USP equivalent tight container (60 mL or less) for longer than 2 weeks is not recommended.

16.2   NORVIR Oral Solution, 80 mg per mL Ritonavir

NORVIR (ritonavir) oral solution is an orange-colored liquid, supplied in amber-colored, multi-dose bottles containing 600 mg ritonavir per 7.5 mL marked dosage cup (80 mg per mL).

240 mL bottles (**NDC** 0074-1940-63).

Recommended Storage

Store NORVIR oral solution at room temperature 20°-25°C (68°-77°F). Do not refrigerate. Shake well before each use. Use by product expiration date.

Product should be stored and dispensed in the original container.

Avoid exposure to excessive heat. Keep cap tightly closed.

17   PATIENT COUNSELING INFORMATION

See FDA-approved patient labeling (Patient Information)

Information For Patients

Patients or parents of patients should be informed that:

General Information

☐ They should pay special attention to accurate administration of their dose to minimize the risk of accidental overdose or underdose of NORVIR.

☐ They should inform their healthcare provider if their children's weight changes in order to make sure that the child's NORVIR dose is the correct one.

☐ Take NORVIR with meals.

☐ For adult patients taking NORVIR tablets, the maximum dose of 600 mg twice daily by mouth with meals should not be exceeded.

☐ Patients should remain under the care of a physician while using NORVIR. Patients should be advised to take NORVIR and other concomitant antiretroviral therapy every day as prescribed. NORVIR must always be used in combination with other antiretroviral drugs. Patients should not alter the dose or discontinue therapy without consulting with their doctor. If a dose of NORVIR is missed patients should take the dose as soon as possible and then return to their normal schedule. However, if a dose is skipped the patient should not double the next dose.

☐ NORVIR is not a cure for HIV-1 infection and patients may continue to experience illnesses associated with HIV-1 infection, including opportunistic infections. Patients should remain under the care of a physician when using NORVIR.

Patients should be advised to avoid doing things that can spread HIV-1 infection to others.

• **Do not share needles or other injection equipment.**

• **Do not share personal items that can have blood or body fluids on them, like toothbrushes and razor blades.**

• **Do not have any kind of sex without protection.** Always practice safe sex by using a latex or polyurethane condom to lower the chance of sexual contact with semen, vaginal secretions, or blood.

• **Do not breastfeed.** We do not know if NORVIR can be passed to the baby through breast milk and whether it could harm the baby. Also, mothers with HIV-1 should not breastfeed because HIV-1 can be passed to the baby in the breast milk.

☐ Sustained decreases in plasma HIV-1 RNA have been associated with a reduced risk of progression to AIDS and death.

Drug Interactions

☐ NORVIR may interact with some drugs; therefore, patients should be advised to report to their doctor the use of any other prescription, non-prescription medication or herbal products, particularly St. John's Wort.

☐ If they are receiving estrogen-based hormonal contraceptives, additional or alternate contraceptive measures should be used during therapy with NORVIR.

Potential Adverse Effects

☐ Pre-existing liver disease including Hepatitis B or C can worsen with use of NORVIR. This can be seen as worsening of transaminase elevations or hepatic decompensation. Patients should be advised that their liver function tests will need to be monitored closely especially during the first several months of NORVIR treatment and that they should notify their healthcare provider if they develop the signs and symptoms of worsening liver disease including loss of appetite, abdominal pain, jaundice, and itchy skin.

☐ Pancreatitis, including some fatalities, has been observed in patients receiving NORVIR therapy. Your patients should let you know of signs and symptoms (nausea, vomiting, and abdominal pain) that might be suggestive of pancreatitis.

☐ Skin rashes ranging in severity from mild to Stevens-Johnson syndrome have been reported in patients receiving NORVIR. Patients should be advised to contact their healthcare provider if they develop a rash while taking NORVIR. The healthcare provider will determine if treatment should be continued or an alternative antiretroviral regimen used.

☐ NORVIR may produce changes in the electrocardiogram (e.g., PR prolongation). Patients should consult their physician if they experience symptoms such as dizziness, lightheadedness, abnormal heart rhythm or loss of consciousness.

☐ Treatment with NORVIR therapy can result in substantial increases in the concentration of total cholesterol and triglycerides.

☐ New onset of diabetes or exacerbation of pre-existing diabetes mellitus, and hyperglycemia have been reported. Patients should be advised to notify their healthcare provider if they develop the signs and symptoms of diabetes mellitus including frequent urination, excessive thirst, extreme hunger or unusual weight loss and/or an increased blood sugar while on NORVIR as they may require a change in their diabetes treatment or new treatment.

☐ Immune reconstitution syndrome has been reported in HIV-infected patients treated with combination antiretroviral therapy, including NORVIR.

☐ Redistribution or accumulation of body fat may occur in patients receiving antiretroviral therapy and that the cause and long term health effects of these conditions are not known at this time.

☐ Patients with hemophilia may experience increased bleeding when treated with protease inhibitors such as NORVIR.

☐ If they are receiving avanafil, sildenafil, tadalafil, or vardenafil for the treatment of erectile dysfunction, they may be at an increased risk of associated adverse reactions

Table 8. Drug Interactions - Pharmacokinetic Parameters for Co-administered Drug in the Presence of NORVIR

Co-administered Drug	Dose of Co-administered Drug (mg)	Dose of NORVIR (mg)	N	AUC % (95% CI)	C_{max} (95% CI)	C_{min} (95% CI)
Alprazolam	1, single dose	500 q12h, 10 d	12	↓ 12% (-5, 30%)	↓ 16% (5, 27%)	ND
Avanafil	50, single dose	600 q12h	14[6]	↑ 13-fold	↑ 2.4-fold	ND
Clarithromycin	500 q12h, 4 d	200 q8h, 4 d	22	↑ 77% (56, 103%)	↑ 31% (15, 51%)	↑ 2.8-fold (2.4, 3.3×)
14-OH clarithromycin metabolite				↓ 100%	↓ 99%	↓ 100%
Desipramine	100, single dose	500 q12h, 12 d	14	↑ 145% (103, 211%)	↑ 22% (12, 35%)	ND
2-OH desipramine metabolite				↓ 15% (3, 26%)	↓ 67% (62, 72%)	ND
Didanosine	200 q12h, 4 d	600 q12h, 4 d	12	↓ 13% (0, 23%)	↓ 16% (5, 26%)	↔
Ethinyl estradiol	50 µg single dose	500 q12h, 16 d	23	↓ 40% (31, 49%)	↓ 32% (24, 39%)	ND
Fluticasone propionate aqueous nasal spray	200 mcg qd, 7 d	100 mg q12h, 7 d	18	↑ approximately 350-fold[5]	↑ approximately 25-fold[5]	
Indinavir[1] Day 14 Day 15	400 q12h, 15 d	400 q12h, 15 d	10	↑ 6% (-14, 29%) ↓ 7% (-22, 28%)	↓ 51% (40, 61%) ↓ 62% (52, 70%)	↑ 4-fold (2.8, 6.8×) ↑ 4-fold (2.5, 6.5×)
Ketoconazole	200 daily, 7 d	500 q12h, 10 d	12	↑ 3.4-fold (2.8, 4.3×)	↑ 55% (40, 72%)	ND
Meperidine Normeperidine metabolite	50 oral single dose	500 q12h, 10 d	8 6	↓ 62% (59, 65%) ↑ 47% (-24, 345%)	↓ 59% (42, 72%) ↑ 87% (42, 147%)	ND ND
Methadone[2]	5, single dose	500 q12h, 15 d	11	↓ 36% (16, 52%)	↓ 38% (28, 46%)	ND
Raltegravir	400, single dose	100 q12h, 16 d	10	↓ 16% (-30, 1%)	↓ 24% (-45, 4%)	↓ 1% (-30, 40%)
Rivaroxaban	10, single dose (days 0 and 7)	600 q12h (days 2 to 7)	12	↑ 150% (130-170%)[7]	↑ 60% (40-70%)[7]	ND
Rifabutin 25-O-desacetyl rifabutin metabolite	150 daily, 16 d	500 q12h, 10 d	5, 11*	↑ 4-fold (2.8, 6.1×) ↑ 38-fold (28, 56×)	↑ 2.5-fold (1.9, 3.4×) ↑ 16-fold (13, 20×)	↑ 6-fold (3.5, 18.3×) ↑ 181-fold (ND)
Sildenafil	100, single dose	500 twice daily, 8 d	28	↑ 11-fold	↑ 4-fold	ND
Sulfamethoxazole[3]	800, single dose	500 q12h, 12 d	15	↓ 20% (16, 23%)	↔	ND
Tadalafil	20 mg, single dose	200 mg q12h		↑ 124%	↔	ND
Theophylline	3 mg/kg q8h, 15 d	500 q12h, 10 d	13, 11*	↓ 43% (42, 45%)	↓ 32% (29, 34%)	↓ 57% (55, 59%)
Trazodone	50 mg, single dose	200 mg q12h, 4 doses	10	↑ 2.4-fold	↑ 34%	
Trimethoprim[3]	160, single dose	500 q12h, 12 d	15	↑ 20% (3, 43%)	↔	ND

(Table continued on next page)

Information on the AbbVie, Inc. products listed on these pages is from the prescribing information in use as of July 31, 2014. For more information, please visit rxabbvie.com or call 1-800-633-9110.

Table 8 (cont.). Drug Interactions - Pharmacokinetic Parameters for Co-administered Drug in the Presence of NORVIR

Co-administered Drug	Dose of Co-administered Drug (mg)	Dose of NORVIR (mg)	N	AUC % (95% CI)	C_{max} (95% CI)	C_{min} (95% CI)
Vardenafil	5 mg	600 q12h		↑ 49-fold	↑ 13-fold	ND
Voriconazole	400 q12h, 1 d; then 200 q12h, 8 d	400 q12h, 9 d		↓ 82%	↓ 66%	
	400 q12h, 1 d; then 200 q12h, 8 d	100 q12h, 9 d		↓ 39%	↓ 24%	
Warfarin S-Warfarin R-Warfarin	5, single dose	400 q12h, 12d	12	↑ 9% (-17, 44%)[4] ↓ 33% (-38, -27%)[4]	↓ 9% (-16, -2%)[4] ↔	ND ND
Zidovudine	200 q8h, 4 d	300 q6h, 4 d	9	↓ 25% (15, 34%)	↓ 27% (4, 45%)	ND

1 Ritonavir and indinavir were co-administered for 15 days; Day 14 doses were administered after a 15%-fat breakfast (757 Kcal) and 9%-fat evening snack (236 Kcal), and Day 15 doses were administered after a 15%-fat breakfast (757 Kcal) and 32%-fat dinner (815 Kcal). Indinavir C_{min} was also increased 4-fold. Effects were assessed relative to an indinavir 800 mg q8h regimen under fasting conditions.

2 Effects were assessed on a dose-normalized comparison to a methadone 20 mg single dose.

3 Sulfamethoxazole and trimethoprim taken as single combination tablet.

4 90% CI presented for R- and S-warfarin AUC and C_{max} ratios.

5 This significant increase in plasma fluticasone propionate exposure resulted in a significant decrease (86%) in plasma cortisol AUC.

6 For the reference arm: N=14 for C_{max} and $AUC_{(0-inf)}$, and for the test arm: N=13 for C_{max} and N=4 for $AUC_{(0-inf)}$.

7 90% CI presented for rivaroxaban

↑ Indicates increase.

↓ Indicates decrease.

↔ Indicates no change.

* Parallel group design; entries are subjects receiving combination and control regimens, respectively.

---

including hypotension, visual changes, and sustained erection, and should promptly report any symptoms to their doctor. They should seek medical assistance immediately if they develop a sustained penile erection lasting more than 4 hours while taking NORVIR and a PDE 5 Inhibitor such as Stendra®, Viagra®, Cialis® or Levitra®. If they are currently using or planning to use avanafil or tadalafil (for the treatment of pulmonary arterial hypertension) they should ask their doctor about potential adverse reactions these medications may cause when taken with NORVIR. The doctor may choose not to keep them on avanafil, or may adjust the dose of tadalafil while initiating treatment with NORVIR. Concomitant use of Revatio® (sildenafil) with NORVIR is contraindicated in patients with pulmonary arterial hypertension (PAH).

☐ Continued NORVIR therapy at a dose of 600 mg twice daily following loss of viral suppression may increase the likelihood of cross-resistance to other protease inhibitors.

Patient Information

NORVIR® (NOR-VEER)

(ritonavir) Tablet

(ritonavir) Oral Solution

Read this Patient Information before you start taking NORVIR and each time you get a refill. There may be new information. This information does not take the place of talking to your doctor about your medical condition or your treatment.

What is the most important information I should know about NORVIR?

• NORVIR can interact with other medicines and cause serious side effects. It is important to know the medicines that should not be taken with NORVIR. See the section "Who should not take NORVIR?"

What is NORVIR?

NORVIR is a prescription anti-HIV medicine used with other anti-HIV medicines to treat people with human immunodeficiency virus (HIV) infection. NORVIR is a type of anti-HIV medicine called a protease inhibitor. HIV is the virus that causes AIDS (Acquired Immune Deficiency Syndrome).

When used with other HIV medicines, NORVIR may reduce the amount of HIV in your blood (called "viral load"). NORVIR may also help to increase the number of CD_4 (T) cells in your blood which help fight off other infections. Reducing the amount of HIV and increasing the CD_4 (T) cell count may improve your immune system. This may reduce your risk of death or infections that can happen when your immune system is weak (opportunistic infections). Patients who took NORVIR in clinical studies had significant reductions in both death and AIDS defining diseases; however NORVIR may not have these effects in all patients.

NORVIR does not cure HIV infection or AIDS and you may continue to experience illnesses associated with HIV-1 infection, including opportunistic infections. You should remain under the care of a doctor when using NORVIR.

Avoid doing things that can spread HIV-1 infection.

• **Do not share needles or other injection equipment.**

• **Do not share personal items that can have blood or body fluids on them, like toothbrushes and razor blades.**

• **Do not have any kind of sex without protection.** Always practice safe sex by using a latex or polyurethane condom to lower the chance of sexual contact with semen, vaginal secretions, or blood.

Who should not take NORVIR?

Do not take NORVIR if you are allergic to ritonavir or any of the ingredients in NORVIR. See the end of this leaflet for a complete list of ingredients in NORVIR.

Do not take NORVIR with any of the following medicines:

• alfuzosin (Uroxatral)

• amiodarone (Cordarone, Nexterone, Pacerone), flecainide (Tambocor), propafenone (Rhythmol) or quinidine (Nuedext, Quinaglute, Cardioquin, Quinidex, and others)

• voriconazole (VFend) if NORVIR dose is 400 mg every 12 hours or greater

• dihydroergotamine (D.H.E. 45, Embolex, Migranal), ergonovine, ergotamine (Cafergot, Ergomar) methylergonovine (Methergine)

• cisapride (Propulsid)

• St. John's Wort (Hypericum perforatum)

• the cholesterol lowering medicines lovastatin (Mevacor, Altoprev, Advicor) or simvastatin (Zocor, Simcor, Vytorin)

• pimozide (Orap)

• sildenafil (Revatio) only when used for the treatment of pulmonary arterial hypertension

• oral midazolam or triazolam (Halcion)

Serious problems can happen if you or your child takes any of these medicines with NORVIR.

What should I tell my doctor before taking NORVIR?

Before taking NORVIR, tell your doctor if you:

• have liver problems, including Hepatitis B or Hepatitis C.

• have heart problems.

• have high blood sugar (diabetes).

• have bleeding problems or hemophilia.

• are pregnant or plan to become pregnant. It is not known if NORVIR can harm your unborn baby. **Pregnancy Registry:** There is a pregnancy registry for women who take antiviral medicines during pregnancy. The purpose of the registry is to collect information about the health of you and your baby. Talk to your doctor about how you can take part in this registry.

• are breastfeeding. **Do not breastfeed if you take NORVIR**

• You should not breastfeed if you have HIV-1 because of the risk of passing HIV-1 to your baby.

• It is not known if NORVIR passes into your breast milk.

• Talk to your doctor about the best way to feed your baby.

Tell your doctor about all the medicines you take including prescription and nonprescription medicines, vitamins, and herbal supplements. Taking NORVIR and certain other medicines may affect each other causing serious side effects. NORVIR may affect the way other medicines work and other medicines may affect how NORVIR works.

Especially tell your doctor if you take:

• medicine to treat HIV

• estrogen-based contraceptives (birth control). NORVIR might reduce the effectiveness of estrogen-based contraceptives. You must take additional precautions for birth control such as a condom.

• medicine for pain such as tramadol (Ryzolt, Ultracet, Conzip, Ultram), propoxyphene, or meperidine (Demerol)

• medicine to treat alcohol abuse such as disulfiram (Antabuse)

• medicine for your heart such as disopyramide (Norpace), lidocaine (Xylocaine Viscous), mexiletine, digoxin (Lanoxin), nifedipine (Procardia, Adalat, Afeditab CR), diltiazem (Cardizem, Dilacor, Cartia, Diltzac, Dilt, Taztia, Tiazac) or verapamil (Calan, Covera, Isoptin, Tarka, Verelan)

• medicines for panic disorder or anxiety such as buspirone, clorazepate, diazepam, estazolam, flurazepam, and zolpidem

• medicine for cancer such as dasatinib (Sprycel), nilotinib (Tasigna) vincristine, or vinblastine

• warfarin (Coumadin, Jantoven), rivaroxaban (Xarelto)

• medicine for seizures such as carbamazepine (Carbatrol, Equetro, Tegretol, Epitol), clonazepam (Klonopin), ethosuximide (Zarontin, Ethosuximide), divalproex (Depakote, Divalproex Sodium), lamotrigine (Lamictal) or phenytoin (Dilantin, Phenytek)

• medicine for depression such as nefazodone, bupropion (Wellbutrin, Aplenzin, Zyban), desipramine (Norpramin) or trazodone, fluoxetine (Prozac), paroxetine (Paxil), amitriptyline, or nortriptyline

• medicine for nausea and vomiting such as dronabinol (Marinol) or perphenazine

• medicine for fungal infections such as ketoconazole (Nizoral), itraconazole (Sporanox, Onmel) or voriconazole (VFend)

• colchicine (Colcrys, Col-Probenecid, Probenecid and Colchine)

• medicine for infections such as clarithromycin (Prevpac, Biaxin), rifabutin (Mycobutin), rifampin (Rimactane, Rifadin, Rifater, Rifamate), atovaquone (Mepron, Malarone), quinine (Qualaquin) or metronidazole (Flagyl, Helidac, Metrocream)

• medicine used to treat blood pressure, a heart attack, heart failure, or to lower pressure in the eye such as metoprolol (Lopressor, Toprol-XL), timolol (Cosopt, Betimol, Timoptic, Isatolol, Combigan)

• medicine for lung disease such as theophylline and salmeterol (Serevent)

• bosentan (Tracleer)

• medicine to prevent organ transplant failure such as cyclosporine (Gengraf, Sandimmune, Neoral), tacrolimus (Prograf), sirolimus (Rapamune)

• steroids such as dexamethasone, fluticasone (Advair Diskus, Veramyst, Flovent, Flonase), budesonide (Entocort EC, Pulmicort, Rhinocort), or prednisone

• a narcotic medicine such as methadone (Methadose, Dolophine Hydrochloride) or fentanyl (Abstral, Actiq, Fentora, Lazanda, Onsolis, Duragesic)

• medicine to treat schizophrenia such as risperidone (Risperdal) or thioridazine

• medicine to treat erectile dysfunction or pulmonary hypertension such as avanafil (Stendra), sildenafil (Viagra, Revatio), vardenafil (Levitra, Staxyn), tadalafil (Cialis, Adcirca). If you are taking avanafil (Stendra), your doctor may need to change it to a different medicine.

• midazolam by injection

• methamphetamine (Desoxyn)

• cholesterol lowering medicine such as atorvastatin (Lipitor) or rosuvasatin (Crestor)

This is not a complete list of medicines that you should tell your doctor that you are taking. Ask your doctor, provider or pharmacist if you are not sure if your medicine is one that is listed above.

Know the medicines you take. Keep a list of them to show your doctor or pharmacist when you get a new medicine. Do not start any new medicines while you are taking NORVIR without first talking with your doctor.

How should I take NORVIR?

• Take NORVIR exactly as prescribed by your doctor.

• You should stay under a doctor's care when taking NORVIR. Do not change your dose of NORVIR or stop your treatment without talking with your doctor.

• If your child is taking NORVIR, your child's doctor will decide the right dose based on your child's height and weight. Tell your doctor if your child's weight changes.

Your child should take NORVIR with food. If your child does not tolerate NORVIR Oral Solution, ask your child's doctor for advice.

- Swallow NORVIR tablets whole. Do not chew, break, or crush tablets before swallowing. If you cannot swallow NORVIR tablets whole, tell your doctor. You may need a different medicine.
- Take NORVIR with meals.
- NORVIR Oral Solution is peppermint or caramel flavored. You can take it alone, or may improve the taste by mixing it with 8 ounces of chocolate milk, Ensure®, or Advera®. NORVIR Oral Solution should be taken within 1 hour if mixed with these fluids. Ask your doctor, nurse or pharmacist about other ways to improve the taste of NORVIR Oral Solution.
- Do not run out of NORVIR. Get your NORVIR prescription refilled from you doctor or pharmacy before you run out.
- If you miss a dose of NORVIR, take it as soon as possible and then take your next scheduled dose at its regular time. If it is almost time for your next dose, wait and take the next dose at the regular time. Do not double the next dose.
- If you take too much NORVIR, call your local poison control center or go to the nearest hospital emergency room right away.

What are the possible side effects of NORVIR?
NORVIR can cause serious side effects including:
- See "What is the most important information I should know about NORVIR?"
- **Liver disease.** Some people taking NORVIR in combination with other anti-HIV medicines have developed liver problems which may be life-threatening. Your doctor should do regular blood tests during your combination treatment with NORVIR. If you have chronic hepatitis B or C infection, your doctor should check your blood tests more often because you have an increased chance of developing liver problems. Tell your doctor if you have any of the below signs and symptoms of liver problems:
  - loss of appetite
  - pain or tenderness on your right side below your ribs
  - yellowing of your skin or whites of your eyes
  - itchy skin
- **Swelling of your pancreas (Pancreatitis).** NORVIR can cause serious pancreas problems, which may lead to death. Tell your doctor right away if you have signs or symptoms of pancreatitis such as:
  - nausea
  - vomiting
  - stomach (abdomen) pain
- **Allergic Reactions.** Sometimes these allergic reactions can become severe and require treatment in a hospital. You should call your doctor right away if you develop a rash. Stop taking NORVIR and get medical help right away if you have any of the following symptoms of a severe allergic reaction:
  - trouble breathing
  - wheezing
  - dizziness or fainting
  - throat tightness or hoarseness
  - fast heartbeat or pounding in your chest (tachycardia)
  - sweating
  - swelling of your face, lips or tongue
  - muscle or joint pain
  - blisters or skin lesions
  - mouth sores or ulcers
- **Changes in the electrical activity of your heart called PR prolongation.** PR prolongation can cause irregular heartbeats. Tell your doctor right away if you have symptoms such as:
  - dizziness
  - lightheadedness
  - feel faint or pass out
  - abnormal heart beat
- **Increase in cholesterol and triglyceride levels.** Treatment with NORVIR may increase your blood levels of cholesterol and triglycerides. Your doctor should do blood tests before you start your treatment with NORVIR and regularly to check for an increase in your cholesterol and triglycerides levels.
- **Diabetes and high blood sugar (hyperglycemia).** Some people who take protease inhibitors including NORVIR can get high blood sugar, develop diabetes, or your diabetes can get worse. Tell your doctor if you notice an increase in thirst or urinate often while taking NORVIR.
- **Changes in your immune system (Immune reconstitution syndrome)** can happen when you start taking HIV medicines. Your immune system may get stronger and begin to fight infections that have been hidden in your body for a long time. Call your doctor right away if you start having new symptoms after starting your HIV medicine.
- **Change in body fat.** These changes can happen in people who take antiretroviral therapy. The changes may include an increase amount of fat in the upper back and neck ("buffalo hump"), breast, and around the back and stom-

ach area. Loss of fat from the legs, arms, and face may also happen. The exact cause and long-term health effects of these conditions are not known.
- **Increased bleeding for hemophiliacs.** Some people with hemophilia have increased bleeding with protease inhibitors including NORVIR.

The most common side effects of NORVIR include:
- diarrhea
- nausea
- vomiting
- upper and lower stomach (abdomen) pain
- tingling feeling or numbness in hands or feet or around the lips
- rash
- feeling weak or tired

NORVIR liquid contains a large amount of alcohol. If a toddler or young child accidentally drinks more than the recommended dose of NORVIR, it could make him/her sick from too much alcohol. Contact your local poison control center or emergency room immediately if this happens.
Tell your doctor if you have any side effect that bothers you or that does not go away.
These are not all of the possible side effects of NORVIR. For more information, ask your doctor or pharmacist.
Call your doctor for medical advice about side effects. You may report side effects to FDA at 1-800-FDA-1088.

How should I store NORVIR?
- Store NORVIR Oral Solution at room temperature between 68°F to 77°F (20°C to 25°C).
- Store NORVIR tablets below 30°C (86°F). Exposure to temperatures up to 50°C (122°F) for seven days permitted.
- Do not refrigerate NORVIR Oral Solution.
- Shake NORVIR Oral Solution well before each use.
- Keep NORVIR Oral Solution away from heat.
- Store NORVIR tablets and NORVIR oral solution in the original container given to you by the pharmacist.
- Exposure of NORVIR tablets to high humidity outside the original container for longer than 2 weeks is not recommended.
- Use NORVIR tablets and NORVIR Oral Solution by the expiration date on the bottle.

Keep NORVIR and all medicines out of the reach of children.

General information about NORVIR
Medicines are sometimes prescribed for purposes other than those listed in a Patient Information Leaflet. Do not use this medicine for a condition for which it was not prescribed. Do not share this medicine with other people.
This leaflet summarizes the most important information about NORVIR. If you would like more information, talk to your doctor. You can ask your doctor or pharmacist for information about NORVIR that is written for healthcare professionals.
For more information, call 1-800-633-9110.

What are the ingredients in NORVIR?
Active ingredient: ritonavir
Inactive ingredients:
NORVIR Tablet: copovidone, anhydrous dibasic calcium phosphate, sorbitan monolaurate, colloidal silicon dioxide, and sodium stearyl fumarate. The film coating contains: hypromellose, titanium dioxide, polyethylene glycol 400, hydroxypropyl cellulose, talc, polyethylene glycol 3350, colloidal silicon dioxide, and polysorbate 80.
NORVIR Oral Solution: ethanol, water, polyoxyl 35 castor oil, propylene glycol, anhydrous citric acid to adjust pH, saccharin sodium, peppermint oil, creamy caramel flavoring, and FD&C Yellow No. 6.
This Patient Information has been approved by the U.S. Food and Drug Administration.
* The brands listed are trademarks of their respective owners and are not trademarks of AbbVie Inc. The makers of these brands are not affiliated with and do not endorse AbbVie Inc. or its products.
NORVIR tablets and oral solution are manufactured by: AbbVie Inc.
North Chicago, IL 60064 USA
Ref: 03-A842-R9-Rev. November, 2013
Shown in Product Identification Guide, page 304

PROMETRIUM® ℞
[pro-mē-trē-um]
(progesterone, USP)
Capsules 100 mg
Capsules 200 mg

> **WARNING: CARDIOVASCULAR DISORDERS, BREAST CANCER AND PROBABLE DEMENTIA FOR ESTROGEN PLUS PROGESTIN THERAPY**
> **Cardiovascular Disorders and Probable Dementia**
> Estrogens plus progestin therapy should not be used for the prevention of cardiovascular disease or dementia. (See **CLINICAL STUDIES** and **WARNINGS, Cardiovascular disorders** and **Probable dementia**.)

The Women's Health Initiative (WHI) estrogen plus progestin substudy reported increased risks of deep vein thrombosis, pulmonary embolism, stroke and myocardial infarction in postmenopausal women (50 to 79 years of age) during 5.6 years of treatment with daily oral conjugated estrogens (CE) [0.625 mg] combined with medroxyprogesterone acetate (MPA) [2.5 mg], relative to placebo. (See **CLINICAL STUDIES** and **WARNINGS, Cardiovascular disorders**.)
The WHI Memory Study (WHIMS) estrogen plus progestin ancillary study of the WHI reported an increased risk of developing probable dementia in postmenopausal women 65 years of age or older during 4 years of treatment with daily CE (0.625 mg) combined with MPA (2.5 mg), relative to placebo. It is unknown whether this finding applies to younger postmenopausal women. (See **CLINICAL STUDIES** and **WARNINGS, Probable dementia** and **PRECAUTIONS, Geriatric Use**.)
Breast Cancer
The WHI estrogen plus progestin substudy also demonstrated an increased risk of invasive breast cancer. (See **CLINICAL STUDIES** and **WARNINGS, Malignant neoplasms, *Breast Cancer*.**)
In the absence of comparable data, these risks should be assumed to be similar for other doses of CE and MPA, and other combinations and dosage forms of estrogens and progestins.
Progestins with estrogens should be prescribed at the lowest effective doses and for the shortest duration consistent with treatment goals and risks for the individual woman.

DESCRIPTION
PROMETRIUM® (progesterone, USP) Capsules contain micronized progesterone for oral administration. Progesterone has a molecular weight of 314.47 and a molecular formula of $C_{21}H_{30}O_2$. Progesterone (pregn-4-ene-3, 20-dione) is a white or creamy white, odorless, crystalline powder practically insoluble in water, soluble in alcohol, acetone and dioxane and sparingly soluble in vegetable oils, stable in air, melting between 126° and 131°C. The structural formula is:

Progesterone is synthesized from a starting material from a plant source and is chemically identical to progesterone of human ovarian origin. PROMETRIUM Capsules are available in multiple strengths to afford dosage flexibility for optimum management. PROMETRIUM Capsules contain 100 mg or 200 mg micronized progesterone.
The inactive ingredients for PROMETRIUM Capsules 100 mg include: peanut oil NF, gelatin NF, glycerin USP, lecithin NF, titanium dioxide USP, FD&C Red No. 40, and D&C Yellow No. 10.
The inactive ingredients for PROMETRIUM Capsules 200 mg include: peanut oil NF, gelatin NF, glycerin USP, lecithin NF, titanium dioxide USP, D&C Yellow No. 10, and FD&C Yellow No. 6.

CLINICAL PHARMACOLOGY
PROMETRIUM Capsules are an oral dosage form of micronized progesterone which is chemically identical to progesterone of ovarian origin. The oral bioavailability of progesterone is increased through micronization.
Pharmacokinetics
A. Absorption
After oral administration of progesterone as a micronized soft-gelatin capsule formulation, maximum serum concentrations were attained within 3 hours. The absolute bioavailability of micronized progesterone is not known. Table 1 summarizes the mean pharmacokinetic parameters in postmenopausal women after five oral daily doses of PROMETRIUM Capsules 100 mg as a micronized soft-gelatin capsule formulation.

Information on the AbbVie, Inc. products listed on these pages is from the prescribing information in use as of July 31, 2014. For more information, please visit rxabbvie.com or call 1-800-633-9110.

TABLE 1. Pharmacokinetic Parameters of PROMETRIUM Capsules

Parameter	PROMETRIUM Capsules Daily Dose		
	100 mg	200 mg	300 mg
C_{max} (ng/mL)	17.3 ± 21.9[a]	38.1 ± 37.8	60.6 ± 72.5
T_{max} (hr)	1.5 ± 0.8	2.3 ± 1.4	1.7 ± 0.6
$AUC_{(0-10)}$ (ng × hr/mL)	43.3 ± 30.8	101.2 ± 66.0	175.7 ± 170.3

[a] Mean ± S.D.

Serum progesterone concentrations appeared linear and dose proportional following multiple dose administration of PROMETRIUM® (progesterone, USP) Capsules 100 mg over the dose range 100 mg per day to 300 mg per day in postmenopausal women. Although doses greater than 300 mg per day were not studied in females, serum concentrations from a study in male volunteers appeared linear and dose proportional between 100 mg per day and 400 mg per day. The pharmacokinetic parameters in male volunteers were generally consistent with those seen in postmenopausal women.

B. Distribution
Progesterone is approximately 96 percent to 99 percent bound to serum proteins, primarily to serum albumin (50 to 54 percent) and transcortin (43 to 48 percent).

C. Metabolism
Progesterone is metabolized primarily by the liver largely to pregnanediols and pregnanolones. Pregnanediols and pregnanolones are conjugated in the liver to glucuronide and sulfate metabolites. Progesterone metabolites which are excreted in the bile may be deconjugated and may be further metabolized in the intestine via reduction, dehydroxylation, and epimerization.

D. Excretion
The glucuronide and sulfate conjugates of pregnanediol and pregnanolone are excreted in the bile and urine. Progesterone metabolites are eliminated mainly by the kidneys. Progesterone metabolites which are excreted in the bile may undergo enterohepatic recycling or may be excreted in the feces.

E. Special Populations
The pharmacokinetics of PROMETRIUM Capsules have not been assessed in low body weight or obese patients.
Hepatic Insufficiency: The effect of hepatic impairment on the pharmacokinetics of PROMETRIUM Capsules has not been studied.
Renal Insufficiency: The effect of renal impairment on the pharmacokinetics of PROMETRIUM Capsules has not been studied.

F. Food–Drug Interaction
Concomitant food ingestion increased the bioavailability of PROMETRIUM Capsules relative to a fasting state when administered to postmenopausal women at a dose of 200 mg.

G. Drug Interactions
The metabolism of progesterone by human liver microsomes was inhibited by ketoconazole ($IC_{50} < 0.1$ μM). Ketoconazole is a known inhibitor of cytochrome P450 3A4, hence these data suggest that ketoconazole or other known inhibitors of this enzyme may increase the bioavailability of progesterone. The clinical relevance of the *in vitro* findings is unknown.
Coadministration of conjugated estrogens and PROMETRIUM Capsules to 29 postmenopausal women over a 12-day period resulted in an increase in total estrone concentrations (C_{max} 3.68 ng/mL to 4.93 ng/mL) and total equilin concentrations (C_{max} 2.27 ng/mL to 3.22 ng/mL) and a decrease in circulating 17β estradiol concentrations (C_{max} 0.037 ng/mL to 0.030 ng/mL). The half-life of the conjugated estrogens was similar with coadministration of PROMETRIUM Capsules. Table 2 summarizes the pharmacokinetic parameters.
[See table 2 above]

CLINICAL STUDIES
Effects on the endometrium
In a randomized, double-blind clinical trial, 358 postmenopausal women, each with an intact uterus, received treatment for up to 36 months. The treatment groups were: PROMETRIUM® (progesterone, USP) Capsules at the dose of 200 mg per day for 12 days per 28-day cycle in combination with conjugated estrogens 0.625 mg per day (n=120); conjugated estrogens 0.625 mg per day only (n=119); or placebo (n=119). The subjects in all three treatment groups were primarily Caucasian women (87 percent or more of each group). The results for the incidence of endometrial hyperplasia in women receiving up to 3 years of treatment are shown in Table 3. A comparison of the PROMETRIUM Cap-

TABLE 2. Mean (± S.D.) Pharmacokinetic Parameters for Estradiol, Estrone, and Equilin Following Coadministration of Conjugated Estrogens 0.625 mg and PROMETRIUM Capsules 200 mg for 12 Days to Postmenopausal Women

Drug	Conjugated Estrogens			Conjugated Estrogens plus PROMETRIUM Capsules		
	C_{max} (ng/mL)	T_{max} (hr)	$AUC_{(0-24h)}$ (ng × h/mL)	C_{max} (ng/mL)	T_{max} (hr)	$AUC_{(0-24h)}$ (ng × h/mL)
Estradiol	0.037 ± 0.048	12.7 ± 9.1	0.676 ± 0.737	0.030 ± 0.032	17.32 ± 1.21	0.561 ± 0.572
Estrone Total[a]	3.68 ± 1.55	10.6 ± 6.8	61.3 ± 26.36	4.93 ± 2.07	7.5 ± 3.8	85.9 ± 41.2
Equilin Total[a]	2.27 ± 0.95	6.0 ± 4.0	28.8 ± 13.0	3.22 ± 1.13	5.3 ± 2.6	38.1 ± 20.2

[a] Total estrogens is the sum of conjugated and unconjugated estrogen.

TABLE 3. Incidence of Endometrial Hyperplasia in Women Receiving 3 Years of Treatment

Endometrial Diagnosis	Treatment Group					
	Conjugated Estrogens 0.625 mg + PROMETRIUM Capsules 200 mg (cyclical)		Conjugated Estrogens 0.625 mg (alone)		Placebo	
	Number of patients	% of patients	Number of patients	% of patients	Number of patients	% of patients
	n=117		n=115		n=116	
HYPERPLASIA [a]	7	6	74	64	3	3
Adenocarcinoma	0	0	0	0	1	1
Atypical hyperplasia	1	1	14	12	0	0
Complex hyperplasia	0	0	27	23	1	1
Simple hyperplasia	6	5	33	29	1	1

[a] Most advanced result to least advanced result:
Adenocarcinoma > atypical hyperplasia > complex hyperplasia > simple hyperplasia

sules plus conjugated estrogens treatment group to the conjugated estrogens only group showed a significantly lower rate of hyperplasia (6 percent combination product versus 64 percent estrogen alone) in the PROMETRIUM Capsules plus conjugated estrogens treatment group throughout 36 months of treatment.
[See table 3 above]
The times to diagnosis of endometrial hyperplasia over 36 months of treatment are shown in Figure 1. This figure illustrates graphically that the proportion of patients with hyperplasia was significantly greater for the conjugated estrogens group (64 percent) compared to the conjugated estrogens plus PROMETRIUM Capsules group (6 percent).

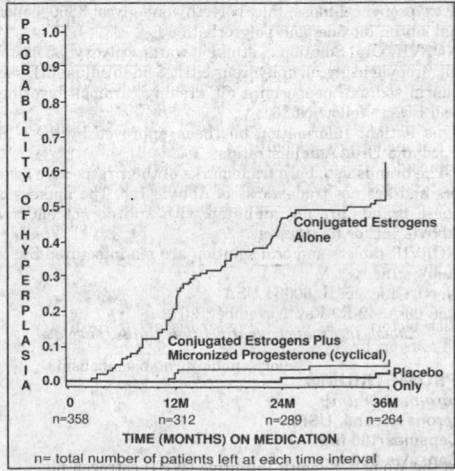

n= total number of patients left at each time interval

Figure 1. Time to Hyperplasia in Women Receiving up to 36 Months of Treatment

The discontinuation rates due to hyperplasia over the 36 months of treatment are as shown in Table 4. For any degree of hyperplasia, the discontinuation rate for patients who received conjugated estrogens plus PROMETRIUM Capsules was similar to that of the placebo only group, while the discontinuation rate for patients who received

conjugated estrogens alone was significantly higher. Women who permanently discontinued treatment due to hyperplasia were similar in demographics to the overall study population.
[See table 4 at top of next page]

Effects on secondary amenorrhea
In a single-center, randomized, double-blind clinical study that included premenopausal women with secondary amenorrhea for at least 90 days, administration of 10 days of PROMETRIUM® (progesterone, USP) Capsules therapy resulted in 80 percent of women experiencing withdrawal bleeding within 7 days of the last dose of PROMETRIUM Capsules, 300 mg per day (n=20), compared to 10 percent of women experiencing withdrawal bleeding in the placebo group (n=21).
In a multicenter, parallel-group, open label, postmarketing dosing study that included premenopausal women with secondary amenorrhea for at least 90 days, administration of 10 days of PROMETRIUM Capsules during two 28-day treatment cycles, 300 mg per day (n=107) or 400 mg per day (n=99), resulted in 73.8 percent and 76.8 percent of women, respectively, experiencing withdrawal bleeding.
The rate of secretory transformation was evaluated in a multicenter, randomized, double-blind clinical study in estrogen-primed postmenopausal women. PROMETRIUM Capsules administered orally for 10 days at 400 mg per day (n=22) induced complete secretory changes in the endometrium in 45 percent of women compared to 0 percent in the placebo group (n=23).
A second multicenter, parallel-group, open label postmarketing dosing study in premenopausal women with secondary amenorrhea for at least 90 days also evaluated the rate of secretory transformation. All subjects received daily oral conjugated estrogens over 3 consecutive 28-day treatment cycles and PROMETRIUM Capsules, 300 mg per day (n=107) or 400 mg per day (n=99) for 10 days of each treatment cycle. The rate of complete secretory transformation was 21.5 percent and 28.3 percent, respectively.

Women's Health Initiative Studies
The Women's Health Initiative (WHI) enrolled approximately 27,000 predominantly healthy postmenopausal women in two substudies to assess the risks and benefits of daily oral conjugated estrogens (CE) [0.625 mg]-alone or in combination with medroxyprogesterone acetate (MPA) [2.5 mg] compared to placebo in the prevention of certain chronic diseases. The primary endpoint was the incidence of

coronary heart disease [(CHD) defined as nonfatal myocardial infarction (MI), silent MI and CHD death], with invasive breast cancer as the primary adverse outcome. A "global index" included the earliest occurrence of CHD, invasive breast cancer, stroke, pulmonary embolism (PE), endometrial cancer (only in the CE plus MPA substudy), colorectal cancer, hip fracture, or death due to other cause. These sub studies did not evaluate the effects of CE–alone or CE plus MPA on menopausal symptoms.

WHI Estrogen Plus Progestin Substudy
The WHI estrogen plus progestin substudy was stopped early. According to the predefined stopping rule, after an average follow-up of 5.6 years of treatment, the increased risk of breast cancer and cardiovascular events exceeded the specified benefits included in the "global index." The absolute excess risk of events in the "global index" was 19 per 10,000 women-years.

For those outcomes included in the WHI "global index" that reached statistical significance after 5.6 years of follow-up, the absolute excess risks per 10,000 women-years in the group treated with CE plus MPA were 7 more CHD events, 8 more strokes, 10 more PEs, and 8 more invasive breast cancers, while the absolute risk reductions per 10,000 women-years were 6 fewer colorectal cancers and 5 fewer hip fractures.

Results of the estrogen plus progestin substudy, which included 16,608 women (average 63 years of age, range 50 to 79; 83.9 percent White, 6.8 percent Black, 5.4 percent Hispanic, 3.9 percent Other) are presented in Table 5. These results reflect centrally adjudicated data after an average follow-up of 5.6 years.

[See table 5 above]

Timing of the initiation of estrogen plus progestin therapy relative to the start of menopause may affect the overall risk benefit profile. The WHI estrogen plus progestin substudy stratified for age showed in women 50 to 59 years of age a non-significant trend toward reducing risk of overall mortality [hazard ratio (HR) 0.69 (95 percent CI, 0.44-1.07)].

Women's Health Initiative Memory Study
The estrogen plus progestin Women's Health Initiative Memory Study (WHIMS), an ancillary study of WHI, enrolled 4,532 predominantly healthy postmenopausal women 65 years of age and older (47 percent were 65 to 69 years of age; 35 percent were 70 to 74 years of age; and 18 percent were 75 years of age and older) to evaluate the effects of daily CE (0.625 mg) plus MPA (2.5 mg) on the incidence of probable dementia (primary outcome) compared to placebo. After an average follow-up of 4 years, the relative risk of probable dementia for CE plus MPA versus placebo was 2.05 (95 percent CI, 1.21 – 3.48). The absolute risk of probable dementia for CE plus MPA versus placebo was 45 versus 22 per 10,000 women-years. Probable dementia as defined in this study included Alzheimer's disease (AD), vascular dementia (VaD) and mixed type (having features of both AD and VaD). The most common classification of probable dementia in the treatment group and the placebo group was AD. Since the ancillary study was conducted in women 65 to 79 years of age, it is unknown whether these findings apply to younger postmenopausal women. (See **WARNINGS, Probable dementia** and **PRECAUTIONS, Geriatric Use**.)

INDICATIONS AND USAGE
PROMETRIUM® (progesterone, USP) Capsules are indicated for use in the prevention of endometrial hyperplasia in nonhysterectomized postmenopausal women who are receiving conjugated estrogens tablets. They are also indicated for use in secondary amenorrhea.

CONTRAINDICATIONS
PROMETRIUM Capsules should not be used in women with any of the following conditions:
1. **PROMETRIUM Capsules should not be used in patients with known hypersensitivity to its ingredients. PROMETRIUM Capsules contain peanut oil and should never be used by patients allergic to peanuts.**
2. Undiagnosed abnormal genital bleeding.
3. Known, suspected, or history of breast cancer.
4. Active deep vein thrombosis, pulmonary embolism or history of these conditions.
5. Active arterial thromboembolic disease (for example, stroke and myocardial infarction), or a history of these conditions.
6. Known liver dysfunction or disease.
7. Known or suspected pregnancy.

WARNINGS
See **BOXED WARNING.**
1. Cardiovascular disorders
An increased risk of pulmonary embolism, deep vein thrombosis (DVT), stroke, and myocardial infarction has been reported with estrogen plus progestin therapy. Should any of these occur or be suspected, estrogen with progestin therapy should be discontinued immediately.

TABLE 4. Discontinuation Rate Due to Hyperplasia Over 36 Months of Treatment

Most Advanced Biopsy Result Through 36 Months of Treatment	Treatment Group					
	Conjugated Estrogens + PROMETRIUM Capsules (cyclical)		Conjugated Estrogens (alone)		Placebo	
	n=120		n=119		n=119	
	Number of patients	% of patients	Number of patients	% of patients	Number of patients	% of patients
Adenocarcinoma	0	0	0	0	1	1
Atypical hyperplasia	1	1	10	8	0	0
Complex hyperplasia	0	0	21	18	1	1
Simple hyperplasia	1	1	13	11	0	0

TABLE 5. Relative and Absolute Risk Seen in the Estrogen Plus Progestin Substudy of WHI at an Average of 5.6 Years[a, b]

Event	Relative Risk CE/MPA versus Placebo (95% nCI [c])	CE/MPA n = 8,506	Placebo n = 8,102
		Absolute Risk per 10,000 Women-Years	
CHD events	1.23 (0.99-1.53)	41	34
Non-fatal MI	*1.28 (1.00-1.63)*	*31*	*25*
CHD death	*1.10 (0.70-1.75)*	*8*	*8*
All stroke	1.31 (1.03-1.88)	33	25
Ischemic Stroke	*1.44 (1.09-1.90)*	*26*	*18*
Deep vein thrombosis [d]	1.95 (1.43-2.67)	26	13
Pulmonary embolism	2.13 (1.45-3.11)	18	8
Invasive breast cancer [e]	1.24 (1.01-1.54)	41	33
Colorectal cancer	0.61 (0.42-0.87)	10	16
Endometrial cancer [d]	0.81 (0.48-1.36)	6	7
Cervical cancer [d]	1.44 (0.47-4.42)	2	1
Hip fracture	0.67 (0.47-0.96)	11	16
Vertebral fractures [d]	0.65 (0.46-0.92)	11	17
Lower arm/wrist fractures [d]	0.71 (0.59-0.85)	44	62
Total fractures [d]	0.76 (0.69-0.83)	152	199
Overall mortality [f]	1.00 (0.83-1.19)	52	52
Global Index [g]	1.13 (1.02-1.25)	184	165

[a] Adapted from numerous WHI publications. WHI publications can be viewed at www.nhlbi.nih.gov/whi.
[b] Results are based on centrally adjudicated data.
[c] Nominal confidence intervals unadjusted for multiple looks and multiple comparisons.
[d] Not included in Global Index.
[e] Includes metastatic and non-metastatic breast cancer with the exception of *in situ* breast cancer.
[f] All deaths, except from breast or colorectal cancer, definite or probable CHD, PE or cerebrovascular disease.
[g] A subset of the events was combined in a "global index" defined as the earliest occurrence of CHD events, invasive breast cancer, stroke, pulmonary embolism, endometrial cancer, colorectal cancer, hip fracture, or death due to other causes.

Risk factors for arterial vascular disease (for example, hypertension, diabetes mellitus, tobacco use, hypercholesterolemia, and obesity) and/or venous thromboembolism (for example, personal history or family history of venous thromboembolism [VTE], obesity, and systemic lupus erythematosus) should be managed appropriately.

a. Stroke
In the Women's Health Initiative (WHI) estrogen plus progestin substudy, a statistically significant increased risk of stroke was reported in women 50 to 79 years of age receiving daily CE (0.625 mg) plus MPA (2.5 mg) compared to women in the same age group receiving placebo (33 versus 25 per 10,000 women-years). The increase in risk was demonstrated after the first year and persisted. (See **CLINICAL STUDIES.**) Should a stroke occur or be suspected, estrogen plus progestin therapy should be discontinued immediately.

b. Coronary Heart Disease
In the WHI estrogen plus progestin substudy, there was a statistically non-significant increased risk of coronary heart disease (CHD) events (defined as nonfatal myocardial infarction [MI], silent MI, or CHD death) reported in women receiving daily CE (0.625 mg) plus MPA (2.5 mg) compared to women receiving placebo (41 versus 34 per 10,000 women-years). An increase in relative risk was demonstrated in year 1 and a trend toward decreasing relative risk was reported in years 2 through 5. (See **CLINICAL STUDIES.**)

Information on the AbbVie, Inc. products listed on these pages is from the prescribing information in use as of July 31, 2014. For more information, please visit rxabbvie.com or call 1-800-633-9110.

In postmenopausal women with documented heart disease (n = 2,763, average age 66.7 years), in a controlled clinical trial of secondary prevention of cardiovascular disease (Heart and Estrogen/Progestin Replacement Study [HERS]), treatment with daily CE (0.625 mg) plus MPA (2.5 mg) demonstrated no cardiovascular benefit. During an average follow-up of 4.1 years, treatment with CE plus MPA did not reduce the overall rate of CHD events in postmenopausal women with established coronary heart disease. There were more CHD events in the CE plus MPA-treated group than in the placebo group in year 1, but not during the subsequent years. Two thousand, three hundred and twenty-one (2,321) women from the original HERS trial agreed to participate in an open-label extension of HERS, HERS II. Average follow-up in HERS II was an additional 2.7 years, for a total of 6.8 years overall. Rates of CHD events were comparable among women in the CE plus MPA group and the placebo group in HERS, HERS II, and overall.

c. Venous Thromboembolism
In the WHI estrogen plus progestin substudy, a statistically significant 2-fold greater rate of VTE (DVT and pulmonary embolism [PE]) was reported in women receiving daily CE (0.625 mg) plus MPA (2.5 mg) compared to women receiving placebo (35 versus 17 per 10,000 women-years). Statistically significant increases in risk for both DVT (26 versus 13 per 10,000 women-years) and PE (18 versus 8 per 10,000 women-years) were also demonstrated. The increase in VTE risk was demonstrated during the first year and persisted. (See **CLINICAL STUDIES**.) Should a VTE occur or be suspected, estrogen plus progestin therapy should be discontinued immediately.

If feasible, estrogens with progestins should be discontinued at least 4 to 6 weeks before surgery of the type associated with an increased risk of thromboembolism, or during periods of prolonged immobilization.

2. Malignant neoplasms
a. Breast Cancer
The most important randomized clinical trial providing information about breast cancer in estrogen plus progestin users is the Women's Health Initiative (WHI) substudy of daily CE (0.625 mg) plus MPA (2.5 mg). After a mean follow-up of 5.6 years, the estrogen plus progestin substudy reported an increased risk of invasive breast cancer in women who took daily CE plus MPA. In this substudy, prior use of estrogen-alone or estrogen plus progestin therapy was reported by 26 percent of the women. The relative risk of invasive breast cancer was 1.24 (95 percent nCI, 1.01-1.54), and the absolute risk was 41 versus 33 cases per 10,000 women-years, for CE plus MPA compared with placebo.

Among women who reported prior use of hormone therapy, the relative risk of invasive breast cancer was 1.86, and the absolute risk was 46 versus 25 cases per 10,000 women-years, for estrogen plus progestin compared with placebo. Among women who reported no prior use of hormone therapy, the relative risk of invasive breast cancer was 1.09, and the absolute risk was 40 versus 36 cases per 10,000 women-years for CE plus MPA compared with placebo. In the same substudy, invasive breast cancers were larger, were more likely to be node positive, and were diagnosed at a more advanced stage in the CE (0.625 mg) plus MPA (2.5 mg) group compared with the placebo group. Metastatic disease was rare, with no apparent difference between the two groups. Other prognostic factors such as histologic subtype, grade and hormone receptor status did not differ between the groups. (See **CLINICAL STUDIES**.)

Consistent with the WHI clinical trials, observational studies have also reported an increased risk of breast cancer for estrogen plus progestin therapy, and a smaller increased risk for estrogen-alone therapy, after several years of use. The risk increased with duration of use, and appeared to return to baseline over about 5 years after stopping treatment (only the observational studies have substantial data on risk after stopping). Observational studies also suggest that the risk of breast cancer was greater, and became apparent earlier, with estrogen plus progestin therapy as compared to estrogen-alone therapy. However, these studies have not generally found significant variation in the risk of breast cancer among different estrogen plus progestin combinations, doses, or routes of administration.

The use of estrogen plus progestin has been reported to result in an increase in abnormal mammograms requiring further evaluation. All women should receive yearly breast examinations by a healthcare provider and perform monthly breast self-examinations. In addition, mammography examinations should be scheduled based on patient age, risk factors, and prior mammogram results.

b. Endometrial Cancer
An increased risk of endometrial cancer has been reported with the use of unopposed estrogen therapy in a woman with a uterus. The reported endometrial cancer risk among unopposed estrogen users is about 2 to 12 times greater than in non-users, and appears dependent on duration of treatment and on estrogen dose. Most studies show no significant increased risk associated with the use of estrogens for less than 1 year. The greatest risk appears associated with prolonged use, with increased risks of 15- to 24-fold for 5 to 10 years or more and this risk has been shown to persist for at least 8 to 15 years after estrogen therapy is discontinued.

Clinical surveillance of all women using estrogen plus progestin therapy is important. Adequate diagnostic measures, including directed or random endometrial sampling when indicated, should be undertaken to rule out malignancy in all cases of undiagnosed persistent or recurring abnormal genital bleeding. There is no evidence that the use of natural estrogens results in a different endometrial risk profile than synthetic estrogens of equivalent estrogen dose. Adding a progestin to estrogen therapy in postmenopausal women has been shown to reduce the risk of endometrial hyperplasia, which may be a precursor to endometrial cancer.

c. Ovarian Cancer
The WHI estrogen plus progestin substudy reported a statistically non-significant increased risk of ovarian cancer. After an average follow-up of 5.6 years, the relative risk for ovarian cancer for CE plus MPA versus placebo was 1.58 (95 percent nCI, 0.77 – 3.24). The absolute risk for CE plus MPA versus placebo was 4 versus 3 cases per 10,000 women-years. In some epidemiologic studies, the use of estrogen plus progestin and estrogen-only products, in particular for 5 or more years, has been associated with an increased risk of ovarian cancer. However, the duration of exposure associated with increased risk is not consistent across all epidemiologic studies and some report no association.

3. Probable dementia
In the estrogen plus progestin Women's Health Initiative Memory Study (WHIMS), an ancillary study of WHI, a population of 4,532 postmenopausal women 65 to 79 years of age was randomized to daily CE (0.625 mg) plus MPA (2.5 mg) or placebo.

In the WHIMS estrogen plus progestin ancillary study, after an average follow-up of 4 years, 40 women in the CE plus MPA group and 21 women in the placebo group were diagnosed with probable dementia. The relative risk of probable dementia for estrogen plus progestin versus placebo was 2.05 (95 percent CI, 1.21-3.48). The absolute risk of probable dementia for CE plus MPA versus placebo was 45 versus 22 cases per 10,000 women-years. It is unknown whether these findings apply to younger postmenopausal women. (See **CLINICAL STUDIES** and **PRECAUTIONS, Geriatric Use**.)

4. Vision abnormalities
Retinal vascular thrombosis has been reported in patients receiving estrogen. Discontinue estrogen plus progestin therapy pending examination if there is sudden partial or complete loss of vision, or if there is a sudden onset of proptosis, diplopia or migraine. If examination reveals papilledema or retinal vascular lesions, estrogen plus progestin therapy should be permanently discontinued.

PRECAUTIONS
A. General
1. Addition of a progestin when a woman has not had a hysterectomy
Studies of the addition of a progestin for 10 or more days of a cycle of estrogen administration, or daily with estrogen in a continuous regimen, have reported a lowered incidence of endometrial hyperplasia than would be induced by estrogen treatment alone. Endometrial hyperplasia may be a precursor to endometrial cancer.

There are, however, possible risks that may be associated with the use of progestins with estrogens compared with estrogen-alone regimens. These include an increased risk of breast cancer.

2. Fluid Retention
Progesterone may cause some degree of fluid retention. Women with conditions that might be influenced by this factor, such as cardiac or renal dysfunction, warrant careful observation.

3. Dizziness and Drowsiness
PROMETRIUM® (progesterone, USP) Capsules may cause transient dizziness and drowsiness and should be used with caution when driving a motor vehicle or operating machinery. PROMETRIUM Capsules should be taken as a single daily dose at bedtime.

B. Patient Information
General: This product contains peanut oil and should not be used if you are allergic to peanuts.
Physicians are advised to discuss the contents of the Patient Information leaflet with patients for whom they prescribe PROMETRIUM Capsules.

C. Drug-Laboratory Test Interactions
The following laboratory results may be altered by the use of estrogen plus progestin therapy:
- Increased sulfobromophthalein retention and other hepatic function tests.
- Coagulation tests: increase in prothrombin factors VII, VIII, IX and X.
- Pregnanediol determination.
- Thyroid function: increase in PBI, and butanol extractable protein bound iodine and decrease in T3 uptake values.

D. Carcinogenesis, Mutagenesis, Impairment of Fertility
Progesterone has not been tested for carcinogenicity in animals by the oral route of administration. When implanted into female mice, progesterone produced mammary carcinomas, ovarian granulosa cell tumors and endometrial stromal sarcomas. In dogs, long-term intramuscular injections produced nodular hyperplasia and benign and malignant mammary tumors. Subcutaneous or intramuscular injections of progesterone decreased the latency period and increased the incidence of mammary tumors in rats previously treated with a chemical carcinogen.

Progesterone did not show evidence of genotoxicity in *in vitro* studies for point mutations or for chromosomal damage. *In vivo* studies for chromosome damage have yielded positive results in mice at oral doses of 1000 mg/kg and 2000 mg/kg. Exogenously administered progesterone has been shown to inhibit ovulation in a number of species and it is expected that high doses given for an extended duration would impair fertility until the cessation of treatment.

E. Pregnancy
PROMETRIUM Capsules should not be used during pregnancy. (See **CONTRAINDICATIONS**).
Pregnancy Category B: Reproductive studies have been performed in mice at doses up to 9 times the human oral dose, in rats at doses up to 44 times the human oral dose, in rabbits at a dose of 10 mcg/day delivered locally within the uterus by an implanted device, in guinea pigs at doses of approximately one-half the human oral dose and in rhesus monkeys at doses approximately the human dose, all based on body surface area, and have revealed little or no evidence of impaired fertility or harm to the fetus due to progesterone.

F. Nursing Women
Detectable amounts of progestin have been identified in the milk of nursing women receiving progestins. Caution should be exercised when PROMETRIUM Capsules are administered to a nursing woman.

G. Pediatric Use
PROMETRIUM Capsules are not indicated in children. Clinical studies have not been conducted in the pediatric population.

H. Geriatric Use
There have not been sufficient numbers of geriatric women involved in clinical studies utilizing PROMETRIUM Capsules to determine whether those over 65 years of age differ from younger subjects in their response to PROMETRIUM Capsules.
The Women's Health Initiative Study
In the Women's Health Initiative (WHI) estrogen plus progestin substudy (daily CE [0.625 mg] plus MPA [2.5 mg] versus placebo), there was a higher relative risk of nonfatal stroke and invasive breast cancer in women greater than 65 years of age. (See **CLINICAL STUDIES** and **WARNINGS, Cardiovascular disorders** and **Malignant neoplasms**.)
The Women's Health Initiative Memory Study
In the Women's Health Initiative Memory Study (WHIMS) of postmenopausal women 65 to 79 years of age, there was an increased risk of developing probable dementia in the estrogen plus progestin ancillary study when compared to placebo. (See **CLINICAL STUDIES** and **WARNINGS, Probable dementia**.)

ADVERSE REACTIONS
See **BOXED WARNING**, **WARNINGS** and **PRECAUTIONS**.

Because clinical trials are conducted under widely varying conditions, adverse reaction rates observed in the clinical trials of a drug cannot be directly compared to rates in the clinical trials of another drug and may not reflect the rates observed in practice.

In a multicenter, randomized, double-blind, placebo-controlled clinical trial, the effects of PROMETRIUM Capsules on the endometrium was studied in a total of 875 postmenopausal women. Table 6 lists adverse reactions greater than or equal to 2 percent of women who received cyclic

PROMETRIUM Capsules 200 mg daily (12 days per calendar month cycle) with 0.625 mg conjugated estrogens or placebo.

TABLE 6. Adverse Reactions (≥ 2%) Reported in an 875 Patient Placebo-Controlled Trial in Postmenopausal Women Over a 3-Year Period [Percentage (%) of Patients Reporting]

	PROMETRIUM Capsules 200 mg with Conjugated Estrogens 0.625 mg	Placebo
	(n=178)	(n=174)
Headache	31	27
Breast Tenderness	27	6
Joint Pain	20	29
Depression	19	12
Dizziness	15	9
Abdominal Bloating	12	5
Hot Flashes	11	35
Urinary Problems	11	9
Abdominal Pain	10	10
Vaginal Discharge	10	3
Nausea / Vomiting	8	7
Worry	8	4
Chest Pain	7	5
Diarrhea	7	4
Night Sweats	7	17
Breast Pain	6	2
Swelling of Hands and Feet	6	9
Vaginal Dryness	6	10
Constipation	3	2
Breast Carcinoma	2	<1
Breast Excisional Biopsy	2	<1
Cholecystectomy	2	<1

Effects on Secondary Amenorrhea

In a multicenter, randomized, double-blind, placebo-controlled clinical trial, the effects of PROMETRIUM® (progesterone, USP) Capsules on secondary amenorrhea was studied in 49 estrogen-primed postmenopausal women. Table 7 lists adverse reactions greater than or equal to 5 percent of women who received PROMETRIUM Capsules or placebo.

TABLE 7. Adverse Reactions (≥ 5%) Reported in Patients Using 400 mg/day in a Placebo-Controlled Trial in Estrogen-Primed Postmenopausal Women

Adverse Experience	PROMETRIUM Capsules 400 mg	Placebo
	n=25	n=24
	Percentage (%) of Patients	
Fatigue	8	4
Headache	16	8
Dizziness	24	4
Abdominal Distention (Bloating)	8	8
Abdominal Pain (Cramping)	20	13
Diarrhea	8	4
Nausea	8	0
Back Pain	8	8
Musculoskeletal Pain	12	4
Irritability	8	4
Breast Pain	16	8
Infection Viral	12	0
Coughing	8	0

In a multicenter, parallel-group, open label postmarketing dosing study consisting of three consecutive 28-day treatment cycles, 220 premenopausal women with secondary amenorrhea were randomized to receive daily conjugated estrogens therapy (0.625 mg conjugated estrogens) and PROMETRIUM Capsules, 300 mg per day (n=113) or PROMETRIUM Capsules, 400 mg per /day (n=107) for 10 days of each treatment cycle. Overall, the most frequently reported treatment-emergent adverse reactions, reported in greater than or equal to 5 percent of subjects, were nausea, fatigue, vaginal mycosis, nasopharyngitis, upper respiratory tract infection, headache, dizziness, breast tenderness, abdominal distension, acne, dysmenorrhea, mood swing, and urinary tract infection.

Postmarketing Experience:
The following additional adverse reactions have been reported with PROMETRIUM Capsules. Because these reactions are reported voluntarily from a population of uncertain size, it is not always possible to reliably estimate the frequency or establish a causal relationship to drug exposure.
Genitourinary System: endometrial carcinoma, hypospadia, intra-uterine death, menorrhagia, menstrual disorder, metrorrhagia, ovarian cyst, spontaneous abortion.
Cardiovascular: circulatory collapse, congenital heart disease (including ventricular septal defect and patent ductus arteriosus), hypertension, hypotension, tachycardia.
Gastrointestinal: acute pancreatitis, cholestasis, cholestatic hepatitis, dysphagia, hepatic failure, hepatic necrosis, hepatitis, increased liver function tests (including alanine aminotransferase increased, aspartate aminotransferase increased, gamma-glutamyl transferase increased), jaundice, swollen tongue.
Skin: alopecia, pruritus, urticaria.
Eyes: blurred vision, diplopia, visual disturbance.
Central Nervous System: aggression, convulsion, depersonalization, depressed consciousness, disorientation, dysarthria, loss of consciousness, paresthesia, sedation, stupor, syncope (with and without hypotension), transient ischemic attack, suicidal ideation.
During initial therapy, a few women have experienced a constellation of many or all of the following symptoms: extreme dizziness and/or drowsiness, blurred vision, slurred speech, difficulty walking, loss of consciousness, vertigo, confusion, disorientation, feeling drunk, and shortness of breath.
Miscellaneous: abnormal gait, anaphylactic reaction, arthralgia, blood glucose increased, choking, cleft lip, cleft palate, difficulty walking, dyspnea, face edema, feeling abnormal, feeling drunk, hypersensitivity, asthma, muscle cramp, throat tightness, tinnitus, vertigo, weight decreased, weight increased.

OVERDOSAGE

No studies on overdosage have been conducted in humans. In the case of overdosage, PROMETRIUM® (progesterone, USP) Capsules should be discontinued and the patient should be treated symptomatically.

DOSAGE AND ADMINISTRATION
Prevention of Endometrial Hyperplasia
PROMETRIUM Capsules should be given as a single daily dose at bedtime, 200 mg orally for 12 days sequentially per 28-day cycle, to a postmenopausal woman with a uterus who is receiving daily conjugated estrogens tablets.
Treatment of Secondary Amenorrhea
PROMETRIUM Capsules may be given as a single daily dose of 400 mg at bedtime for 10 days.
Some women may experience difficulty swallowing PROMETRIUM Capsules. For these women, PROMETRIUM Capsules should be taken with a glass of water while in the standing position.

HOW SUPPLIED
PROMETRIUM (progesterone, USP) Capsules 100 mg are round, peach-colored capsules branded with black imprint "SV."
NDC 0032-1708-01 (Bottle of 100)
PROMETRIUM (progesterone, USP) Capsules 200 mg are oval, pale yellow-colored capsules branded with black imprint "SV2."
NDC 0032-1711-01 (Bottle of 100)

Store at 25°C (77°F); excursions permitted to 15° to 30°C (59° to 86°F) [See USP Controlled Room Temperature].
Protect from excessive moisture.
Dispense in tight, light-resistant container as defined in USP/NF, accompanied by a Patient Insert.
Keep out of reach of children.
Manufactured by:
Catalent Pharma Solutions
St. Petersburg, FL 33716
Marketed by:
AbbVie Inc.
North Chicago, IL 60064, USA
© AbbVie Inc. 2013
Ref: 500032 Rev 09/13 - Revised: September, 2013

PATIENT INFORMATION
PROMETRIUM® (progesterone, USP)
Capsules 100 mg
Capsules 200 mg
Read this PATIENT INFORMATION before you start taking PROMETRIUM® (progesterone, USP) Capsules and read what you get each time you refill your PROMETRIUM Capsules prescription. There may be new information. This information does not take the place of talking to your healthcare provider about your medical condition or your treatment.

> **WHAT IS THE MOST IMPORTANT INFORMATION I SHOULD KNOW ABOUT PROMETRIUM CAPSULES (A Progesterone Hormone)?**
> - Progestins with estrogens should not be used to prevent heart disease, heart attacks, strokes, or dementia.
> - Using progestins with estrogens may increase your chance of getting heart attacks, strokes, breast cancer, and blood clots.
> - Using progestins with estrogens may increase your chance of getting dementia, based on a study of women age 65 and older.
> - You and your healthcare provider should talk regularly about whether you still need treatment with PROMETRIUM Capsules.

THIS PRODUCT CONTAINS PEANUT OIL AND SHOULD NOT BE USED IF YOU ARE ALLERGIC TO PEANUTS.
What is PROMETRIUM Capsules?
PROMETRIUM Capsules contain the female hormone called progesterone.
What is PROMETRIUM Capsules used for?
Treatment of Menstrual Irregularities
PROMETRIUM Capsules are used for the treatment of secondary amenorrhea (absence of menstrual periods in women who have previously had a menstrual period) due to a decrease in progesterone. When you do not produce enough progesterone, menstrual irregularities can occur. If your healthcare provider has determined your body does not produce enough progesterone on its own, PROMETRIUM Capsules may be prescribed to provide the progesterone you need.
Protection of the Endometrium (Lining of the Uterus)
PROMETRIUM Capsules are used in combination with estrogen-containing medications in a postmenopausal woman with a uterus (womb). Taking estrogen-alone increases the chance of developing a condition called endometrial hyperplasia that may lead to cancer of the lining of the uterus (womb). The addition of a progestin is generally recommended for a woman with a uterus to reduce the chance of getting cancer of the uterus (womb).
Who should not take PROMETRIUM Capsules?
Do not start taking PROMETRIUM Capsules if you:
- Are allergic to peanuts
- Have unusual vaginal bleeding
- Currently have or have had certain cancers
  Estrogen plus progestin treatment may increase the chance of getting certain types of cancers, including cancer of the breast or uterus. If you have or have had cancer, talk with your healthcare provider about whether you should take PROMETRIUM Capsules.
- Had a stroke or heart attack
- Currently have or have had blood clots
- Currently have or have had liver problems
- Are allergic to PROMETRIUM Capsules or any of its ingredients
  See the list of ingredients in PROMETRIUM Capsules at the end of this leaflet.
- Think you may be pregnant

Information on the AbbVie, Inc. products listed on these pages is from the prescribing information in use as of July 31, 2014. For more information, please visit rxabbvie.com or call 1-800-633-9110.

Tell your healthcare provider:
- **If you are breastfeeding.** The hormone in PROMETRIUM Capsules can pass into your breast milk.
- **About all of your medical problems.** Your healthcare provider may need to check you more carefully if you have certain conditions, such as asthma (wheezing), epilepsy (seizures), diabetes, migraine, endometriosis, lupus, problems with your heart, liver, thyroid, or kidneys, or have high calcium levels in your blood.
- **About all the medicines you take.** This includes prescription and nonprescription medicines, vitamins, and herbal supplements. Some medicines may affect how PROMETRIUM Capsules work. PROMETRIUM Capsules may also affect how your other medicines work.

How should I take PROMETRIUM Capsules?
1. Prevention of Endometrial Hyperplasia: A postmenopausal woman with a uterus who is taking estrogens should take a single daily dose of 200 mg PROMETRIUM Capsules at bedtime for 12 continuous days per 28-day cycle.
2. Secondary Amenorrhea: PROMETRIUM Capsules may be given as a single daily dose of 400 mg at bedtime for 10 days.
3. **PROMETRIUM Capsules are to be taken at bedtime as some women become very drowsy and/or dizzy after taking PROMETRIUM Capsules. In a few cases, symptoms may include blurred vision, difficulty speaking, difficulty with walking, and feeling abnormal. If you experience these symptoms, discuss them with your healthcare provider right away.**
4. If you experience difficulty in swallowing PROMETRIUM Capsules, it is recommended that you take your daily dose at bedtime with a glass of water while in the standing position.

What are the possible side effects of PROMETRIUM Capsules?
Side effects are grouped by how serious they are and how often they happen when you are treated:
Serious, but less common side effects include:
- *Risk to the Fetus:* Cases of cleft palate, cleft lip, hypospadias, ventricular septal defect, patent ductus arteriosus, and other congenital heart defects.
- *Abnormal Blood Clotting:* Stroke, heart attack, pulmonary embolus, visual loss or blindness.

Some of the warning signs of serious side effects include:
- Changes in vision or speech
- Sudden new severe headaches
- Severe pains in your chest or legs with or without shortness of breath, weakness and fatigue
- Dizziness and faintness
- Vomiting

Call your healthcare provider right away if you get any of these warning signs, or any other unusual symptoms that concern you.

Less serious, but common side effects include:
- Headaches
- Breast pain
- Irregular vaginal bleeding or spotting
- Stomach or abdominal cramps, bloating
- Nausea and vomiting
- Hair loss
- Fluid retention
- Vaginal yeast infection

These are not all the possible side effects of PROMETRIUM Capsules. For more information, ask your healthcare provider or pharmacist for advice about side effects. You may report side effects to AbbVie Inc. at 1-800-633-9110 or to FDA at 1-800-FDA-1088.

What can I do to lower my chances of getting a serious side effect with PROMETRIUM Capsules?
- Talk with your healthcare provider regularly about whether you should continue taking PROMETRIUM Capsules.
- See your healthcare provider right away if you get unusual vaginal bleeding while taking PROMETRIUM Capsules.
- Have a pelvic exam, breast exam, and mammogram (breast X-ray) every year unless your healthcare provider tells you something else. If members of your family have had breast cancer or if you have ever had breast lumps or an abnormal mammogram, you may need to have breast exams more often.
- If you have high blood pressure, high cholesterol (fat in the blood), diabetes, are overweight, or if you use tobacco, you may have higher chances for getting heart disease. Ask your healthcare provider for ways to lower your chances for getting heart disease.

General information about safe and effective use of PROMETRIUM Capsules
- Medicines are sometimes prescribed for conditions that are not mentioned in patient information leaflets. Do not take PROMETRIUM Capsules for conditions for which it was not prescribed.

- Your healthcare provider has prescribed this drug for you and you alone. Do not give PROMETRIUM Capsules to other people, even if they have the same symptoms you have. It may harm them.
- PROMETRIUM Capsules should be taken as a single daily dose at bedtime. Some women may experience extreme dizziness and/or drowsiness during initial therapy. In a few cases, symptoms may include blurred vision, difficulty speaking, difficulty with walking, and feeling abnormal. If you experience these symptoms, discuss them with your healthcare provider right away.
- Use caution when driving a motor vehicle or operating machinery as dizziness or drowsiness may occur.

Keep PROMETRIUM Capsules out of the reach of children.
This leaflet provides a summary of the most important information about PROMETRIUM Capsules. If you would like more information, talk with your healthcare provider or pharmacist. You can ask for information about PROMETRIUM Capsules that is written for health professionals. You can get more information by calling the toll free number 1-800-633-9110.

What are the ingredients in PROMETRIUM Capsules?
Active ingredient: 100 mg or 200 mg micronized progesterone
The inactive ingredients for PROMETRIUM Capsules 100 mg include: peanut oil NF, gelatin NF, glycerin USP, lecithin NF, titanium dioxide USP, FD&C Red No. 40, and D&C Yellow No. 10.
The inactive ingredients for PROMETRIUM Capsules 200 mg include: peanut oil NF, gelatin NF, glycerin USP, lecithin NF, titanium dioxide USP, D&C Yellow No. 10, and FD&C Yellow No. 6.

HOW SUPPLIED
PROMETRIUM Capsules 100 mg are round, peach-colored capsules branded with black imprint "SV."
PROMETRIUM Capsules 200 mg are oval, pale yellow-colored capsules branded with black imprint "SV2."
Store at 25°C (77°F); excursions permitted to 15° to 30°C (59° to 86°F) [See USP Controlled Room Temperature].
Protect from excessive moisture.
Manufactured by:
Catalent Pharma Solutions
St. Petersburg, FL 33716
Marketed by:
AbbVie Inc.
North Chicago, IL 60064, USA
© AbbVie Inc. 2013
Ref: 500033 Rev 09/13 - Revised: September, 2013

SIMCOR®
[sĭm-kŏr]
(niacin extended-release/simvastatin)
tablets

Rx

HIGHLIGHTS OF PRESCRIBING INFORMATION
These highlights do not include all the information needed to use SIMCOR® safely and effectively. See full prescribing information for SIMCOR.
SIMCOR (niacin extended-release/simvastatin) tablet, film coated for oral use.
Initial U.S. Approval: 2008

RECENT MAJOR CHANGES

Warnings and Precautions, Myopathy/Rhabdomyolysis (5.2)	10/2012
Adverse Reactions, Postmarketing Experience (6.2)	10/2012
Indications and Usage, Limitations of Use (1.1)	02/2013
Warnings and Precautions, Mortality and Coronary Heart Disease Morbidity (5.1)	02/2013
Adverse Reactions, Clinical Studies Experience (6.1)	02/2013

INDICATIONS AND USAGE

SIMCOR is a combination of simvastatin, an HMG-Co-A reductase inhibitor, and niacin extended-release (NIASPAN), nicotinic acid. SIMCOR is indicated to:
- Reduce elevated Total-C, LDL-C, Apo B, non-HDL-C, TG, or to increase HDL-C in patients with primary hypercholesterolemia and mixed dyslipidemia when treatment with simvastatin monotherapy or niacin extended-release monotherapy is considered inadequate. (1.1)
- Reduce TG in patients with hypertriglyceridemia when treatment with simvastatin monotherapy or niacin extended-release monotherapy is considered inadequate. (1.1)

Limitations of use:
No incremental benefit of SIMCOR on cardiovascular morbidity and mortality over and above that demonstrated for simvastatin monotherapy and niacin monotherapy has been established. (1.1)
Niacin extended-release, one of the components of SIMCOR, at doses of 1,500 – 2,000 mg/day, in combination with simvastatin, did not reduce the incidence of cardiovascular

events more than simvastatin in a randomized controlled trial of patients with cardiovascular disease and mean baseline LDL-C levels of 74 mg per deciliter (5.1).

DOSAGE AND ADMINISTRATION

- SIMCOR should be taken at bedtime with a low-fat snack. (2)
- Dose range: 500/20 mg to 2000/40 mg once daily. (2)
- Initial dose for patients naïve to or switching from immediate-release niacin: 500/20 mg once daily. (2)
- The initial dose for patients already receiving niacin extended-release should not exceed 2000/40 mg once daily. (2)
- Maintenance dose: 1000/20 mg to 2000/40 mg once daily. (2)
- Doses greater than 2000/40 mg daily are not recommended. (2)

DOSAGE FORMS AND STRENGTHS

- Unscored film-coated tablets:
  500 mg niacin extended-release/20 mg simvastatin (3)
  500 mg niacin extended-release/40 mg simvastatin (3)
  750 mg niacin extended-release/20 mg simvastatin (3)
  1000 mg niacin extended-release/20 mg simvastatin (3)
  1000 mg niacin extended-release/40 mg simvastatin (3)

CONTRAINDICATIONS

- Active liver disease, which may include unexplained persistent elevations in hepatic transaminase levels (4, 5.3)
- Active peptic ulcer disease (4)
- Arterial bleeding (4)
- Concomitant administration of strong CYP3A4 inhibitors (4, 5.2)
- Concomitant administration of gemfibrozil, cyclosporine, or danazol (4, 5.2)
- Concomitant administration of verapamil or diltiazem (4, 5.2)
- Women who are pregnant or may become pregnant (4, 8.1)
- Nursing mothers (4, 8.3)
- Known hypersensitivity to product components (4, 6.1)

WARNINGS AND PRECAUTIONS

- Skeletal muscle effects (e.g., myopathy and rhabdomyolysis): Risks increase with higher doses and concomitant use of certain medicines. Predisposing factors include advanced age (≥ 65), female gender, uncontrolled hypothyroidism, and renal impairment. Patients should be advised to report promptly any unexplained and/or persistent muscle pain, tenderness, or weakness. SIMCOR therapy should be discontinued immediately if myopathy is diagnosed or suspected. (4, 5.2, 8.5, 8.7)
- Liver enzyme abnormalities: Persistent elevations in hepatic transaminases can occur. Check liver enzyme tests before initiating therapy and as clinically indicated thereafter. (5.3)
- Severe hepatic toxicity has occurred in patients substituting sustained-release niacin for immediate-release niacin at equivalent doses. If switching from niacin preparations other than niacin extended-release (NIASPAN), initiate with lowest SIMCOR dose; niacin extended-release can be converted at equivalent doses. (5.3)
- Niacin extended-release can increase serum glucose levels. Glucose levels should be closely monitored in diabetic or potentially diabetic patients particularly during the first few months of use. (5.4)

ADVERSE REACTIONS

The most common (incidence > 3%) adverse reactions with SIMCOR are flushing, headache, back pain, diarrhea, nausea, and pruritus. (6.1)

To report SUSPECTED ADVERSE REACTIONS, contact AbbVie Inc. at 1-800-633-9110 or FDA at 1-800-FDA-1088 or www.fda.gov/medwatch.

DRUG INTERACTIONS

Drug Interactions Associated with Increased Risk of Myopathy/Rhabdomyolysis (2.2, 4, 5.2, 7.1, 7.2, 7.3, 7.4, 12.3)

Interacting Agents	Prescribing Recommendations
Strong CYP3A4 inhibitors (e.g., itraconazole, ketoconazole, posaconazole, erythromycin, clarithromycin, telithromycin, HIV protease inhibitors, boceprevir, telaprevir, nefazodone), gemfibrozil, cyclosporine, danazol, verapamil, diltiazem	Contraindicated with SIMCOR

| Amiodarone, amlodipine, ranolazine | Do not exceed 1000/20 mg SIMCOR daily |
| Grapefruit juice | Avoid large quantities of grapefruit juice (>1 quart daily) |

- Fenofibrate: Combination with SIMCOR increases the risk of adverse skeletal muscle effects and should be avoided. (7.3)
- Coumarin anticoagulants: Combination prolongs INR. Achieve stable INR prior to starting SIMCOR. Monitor INR frequently until stable upon initiation or alteration of SIMCOR therapy. (7.7)

——————USE IN SPECIFIC POPULATIONS——————

- Severe renal impairment (not on dialysis): SIMCOR should be used with extreme caution. (8.7)

See 17 for PATIENT COUNSELING INFORMATION

Revised: 03/2013

FULL PRESCRIBING INFORMATION: CONTENTS*

Table 2. SIMCOR Tablet Strengths

	500mg/20mg	500mg/40mg	750mg/20mg	1000mg/20mg	1000mg/40mg
Niacin extended-release equivalent (mg)	500	500	750	1000	1000
simvastatin equivalent (mg)	20	40	20	20	40

FULL PRESCRIBING INFORMATION

1 INDICATIONS AND USAGE

Therapy with lipid-altering agents should be only one component of multiple risk factor intervention in individuals at significantly increased risk for atherosclerotic vascular disease due to hypercholesterolemia. Drug therapy is indicated as an adjunct to diet when the response to a diet restricted in saturated fat and cholesterol and other nonpharmacologic measures alone has been inadequate.

1.1 Patients with Hypercholesterolemia Requiring Modifications of Lipid Profiles

SIMCOR

SIMCOR is indicated to reduce Total-C, LDL-C, Apo B, non-HDL-C, TG, or to increase HDL-C in patients with primary hypercholesterolemia and mixed dyslipidemia when treatment with simvastatin monotherapy or niacin extended-release monotherapy is considered inadequate.

SIMCOR is indicated to reduce TG in patients with hypertriglyceridemia when treatment with simvastatin monotherapy or niacin extended-release monotherapy is considered inadequate.

Limitations of use

No incremental benefit of SIMCOR on cardiovascular morbidity and mortality over and above that demonstrated for simvastatin monotherapy and niacin monotherapy has been established.

Niacin extended-release, one of the components of SIMCOR, at doses of 1,500 – 2,000 mg/day, in combination with simvastatin, did not reduce the incidence of cardiovascular events more than simvastatin in a randomized controlled trial of patients with cardiovascular disease and mean baseline LDL-C levels of 74 mg per deciliter [see Warnings and Precautions (5.1)].

2 DOSAGE AND ADMINISTRATION

2.1 Recommended Dosing

SIMCOR should be taken as a single daily dose at bedtime, with a low fat snack. Patients not currently on niacin extended-release and patients currently on niacin products other than niacin extended-release should start SIMCOR at a single 500/20 mg tablet daily at bedtime. Patients already taking simvastatin 20 to 40 mg who need additional management of their lipid levels may be started on a SIMCOR dose of 500/40 mg once daily at bedtime [see Warnings and Precautions (5.3)]. The dose of niacin extended-release should not be increased by more than 500 mg daily every 4 weeks - see Table 1.

Table 1. Recommended niacin extended-release dosing

	Week(s)	Daily dose of niacin extended-release
Initial Titration Schedule	1 to 4	500 mg
	5 to 8	1000 mg
	*	1500 mg
	*	2000 mg

* After Week 8, titrate to patient response and tolerance. If response to 1000 mg daily is inadequate, increase dose to 1500 mg daily; may subsequently increase dose to 2000 mg daily. Daily dose should not be increased more than 500 mg in a 4-week period, and doses above 2000 mg daily are not recommended.

The recommended maintenance dose for SIMCOR is 1000/20 mg to 2000/40 mg (two 1000/20 mg tablets) once daily depending on patient tolerability and lipid levels. **The efficacy and safety of doses of SIMCOR greater than 2000/40 mg daily have not been studied and are therefore not recommended.**

If SIMCOR therapy is discontinued for an extended period of time (> 7 days), re-titration as tolerated is recommended. SIMCOR tablets should be taken whole and should not be broken, crushed, or chewed before swallowing.

Due to the increased risk of hepatotoxicity with other modified-release (sustained-release or time-release) niacin preparations or immediate-release (crystalline) niacin, SIMCOR should only be substituted for equivalent doses of niacin extended-release (NIASPAN).

Flushing [see Adverse Reactions (6.1)] may be reduced in frequency or severity by pretreatment with aspirin up to the recommended dose of 325 mg (taken approximately 30 minutes prior to SIMCOR dose). Flushing, pruritus, and gastrointestinal distress are also reduced by gradually increasing the dose of niacin (refer to Table 1) and avoiding administration on an empty stomach. Concomitant alcoholic, hot drinks or spicy foods may increase the side effects of flushing and pruritus and should be avoided around the time of SIMCOR ingestion.

2.2 Coadministration with Other Drugs

Patients taking Amiodarone, Amlodipine or Ranolazine

- The dose of SIMCOR should not exceed 1000/20 mg/day [see Warnings and Precautions (5.2), Drug Interactions (7.4), and Clinical Pharmacology (12.3)].

2.3 Chinese Patients Taking SIMCOR

Because of an increased risk for myopathy in Chinese patients taking simvastatin 40 mg coadministered with lipid-modifying doses (≥1 g/day niacin) of niacin-containing products, caution should be used when prescribing SIMCOR in doses that exceed 1000/20 mg/day to Chinese patients. The cause of the increased risk of myopathy is not known. It is also unknown if the risk for myopathy with coadministration of simvastatin with lipid-modifying doses of niacin-containing products observed in Chinese patients applies to other Asian patients [see Warnings and Precautions (5.2)].

3 DOSAGE FORMS AND STRENGTHS

SIMCOR tablets are formulated for oral administration in the following strength combinations:
[See table 2 above]

4 CONTRAINDICATIONS

SIMCOR is contraindicated in the following conditions:
- Active liver disease, which may include unexplained persistent elevations in hepatic transaminase levels [see Warnings and Precautions (5.3)]
- Patients with active peptic ulcer disease
- Patients with arterial bleeding
- Concomitant administration of strong CYP3A4 inhibitors (e.g. itraconazole, ketoconazole, posaconazole, HIV protease inhibitors, boceprevir, telaprevir, erythromycin, clarithromycin, telithromycin and nefazodone) [see Warnings and Precautions (5.2)]
- Concomitant administration of gemfibrozil, cyclosporine, or danazol [see Warnings and Precautions (5.2)]
- Concomitant administration of verapamil or diltiazem [see Warnings and Precautions (5.2)]
- Women who are pregnant or may become pregnant. SIMCOR may cause fetal harm when administered to a pregnant woman. Serum cholesterol and triglycerides increase during normal pregnancy, and cholesterol or cholesterol derivatives are essential for fetal development. Atherosclerosis is a chronic process and discontinuation of lipid-lowering drugs during pregnancy should have little impact on long-term outcomes of primary hypercholesterolemia therapy. There are no adequate and well-controlled studies of SIMCOR use during pregnancy; however in rare reports congenital anomalies were observed following intrauterine exposure to HMG-CoA reductase inhibitors. If SIMCOR is used during pregnancy or if the patient becomes pregnant while taking this drug, the patient should be apprised of the potential hazard to the fetus [see Use In Specific Populations (8.1)]. In rat and rabbit animal reproduction studies, simvastatin revealed no evidence of teratogenicity. There are no animal reproductive studies conducted with niacin.
- Nursing mothers. SIMCOR contains simvastatin and nicotinic acid. Nicotinic acid is excreted into human milk and it is not known whether simvastatin is excreted in human milk; however a small amount of another drug in this class does pass into breast milk. Because of the potential for serious adverse reactions in nursing infants, women who require SIMCOR treatment should not breastfeed their infants [see Use In Specific Populations (8.3)].
- Patients with a known hypersensitivity to any component of this product. Hypersensitivity reactions including one or more of the following adverse reactions have been reported for simvastatin and/or niacin extended-release: anaphylaxis, angioedema, urticaria, fever, dyspnea,

Information on the AbbVie, Inc. products listed on these pages is from the prescribing information in use as of July 31, 2014. For more information, please visit rxabbvie.com or call 1-800-633-9110.

tongue edema, larynx edema, face edema, peripheral edema, laryngismus, and flushing [see Adverse Reactions (6.1)].

5 WARNINGS AND PRECAUTIONS

SIMCOR should not be substituted for equivalent doses of immediate-release (crystalline) niacin. For patients switching from immediate-release niacin to SIMCOR, therapy with SIMCOR should be initiated at 500/20 mg and appropriately titrated to the desired therapeutic response. Patients already taking simvastatin 20-40 mg who need additional management of their lipid levels may be started on a SIMCOR dose of 500/40 mg once daily at bedtime. Doses of SIMCOR greater than 2000/40 mg are not recommended.

5.1 Mortality and Coronary Heart Disease Morbidity

The Atherothrombosis Intervention in Metabolic Syndrome with Low HDL/High Triglycerides: Impact on Global Health Outcomes (AIM-HIGH) trial was a randomized placebo-controlled trial of 3414 patients with stable, previously diagnosed cardiovascular disease. Mean baseline lipid levels were LDL-C 74 mg/dL, HDL-C 35 mg/dL, non-HDL-C 111 mg/dL and median triglyceride level of 163-177 mg/dL. Ninety-four percent of patients were on background statin therapy prior to entering the trial. All participants received simvastatin, 40 to 80 mg per day, plus ezetimibe 10 mg per day if needed, to maintain an LDL-C level of 40-80 mg/dL, and were randomized to receive niacin extended-release tablets 1500-2000 mg/day (n=1718) or matching placebo (niacin immediate-release tablets, 100-150 mg, n=1696). On-treatment lipid changes at two years for LDL-C were -12.0% for the simvastatin plus niacin extended-release group and -5.5% for the simvastatin plus placebo group. HDL-C increased by 25.0% to 42 mg/dL in the simvastatin plus niacin extended-release group and by 9.8% to 38 mg/dL in the simvastatin plus placebo group (P<0.001). Triglyceride levels decreased by 28.6% in the simvastatin plus niacin extended-release group and by 8.1% in the simvastatin plus placebo group.

The primary outcome was an ITT composite of the first study occurrence of coronary heart disease death, nonfatal myocardial infarction, ischemic stroke, hospitalization for acute coronary syndrome or symptom-driven coronary or cerebral revascularization procedures. The trial was stopped after a mean follow-up period of 3 years owing to a lack of efficacy. The primary outcome occurred in 282 patients in the simvastatin plus niacin extended-release group (16.4%) and in 274 patients in the simvastatin plus placebo group (16.2%) (HR 1.02 [95% CI, 0.87-1.21], P=0.79.

In an ITT analysis, there were 42 cases of first occurrence of ischemic stroke reported, 27 (1.6%) in the simvastatin plus niacin extended-release group and 15 (0.9%) in the simvastatin plus placebo group, a non-statistically significant result (HR 1.79, [95%CI = 0.95-3.36], p=0.071). The on-treatment ischemic stroke events were 19 for the simvastatin plus niacin extended-release group and 15 for the simvastatin plus placebo group [see Adverse Reactions (6.1)].

5.2 Myopathy/Rhabdomyolysis

Simvastatin

Simvastatin occasionally causes myopathy manifested as muscle pain, tenderness or weakness with creatine kinase (CK) above ten times the upper limit of normal (ULN). Myopathy sometimes takes the form of rhabdomyolysis with or without acute renal failure secondary to myoglobinuria, and rare fatalities have occurred. The risk of myopathy is increased by high levels of HMG-CoA reductase inhibitory activity in plasma. Predisposing factors for myopathy include advanced age (≥65 years), female gender, uncontrolled hypothyroidism, and renal impairment.

The risk of myopathy/rhabdomyolysis is dose related. In a clinical trial database in which 41,413 patients were treated with simvastatin with 24,747 (approximately 60%) of whom were enrolled in studies with a median follow-up of at least 4 years, the incidence of myopathy was approximately 0.03% and 0.08% at 20 and 40 mg/day, respectively. The incidence of myopathy with 80 mg (0.61%) was disproportionately higher than that observed at the lower doses. In these trials, patients were carefully monitored and some interacting medicinal products were excluded.

In a clinical trial in which 12,064 patients with a history of myocardial infarction were treated with ZOCOR (mean follow-up 6.7 years), the incidence of myopathy (defined as unexplained muscle weakness or pain with a serum creatine kinase [CK] >10 times upper limit of normal [ULN]) in patients on 80 mg/day was approximately 0.9% compared with 0.02% for patients on 20 mg/day; the incidence of rhabdomyolysis (defined as myopathy with a CK >40 times ULN) was approximately 0.4% in patients on 80 mg/day compared with 0% for patients on 20 mg/day. The incidence of myopathy, including rhabdomyolysis, was highest during the first year and then notably decreased during the subsequent years of treatment. In this trial, patients were carefully monitored and some interacting medicinal products were excluded.

There have been rare reports of immune-mediated necrotizing myopathy (IMNM), an autoimmune myopathy, associated with statin use. IMNM is characterized by: proximal muscle weakness and elevated serum creatine kinase, which persist despite discontinuation of statin treatment; muscle biopsy showing necrotizing myopathy without significant inflammation; improvement with immunosuppressive agents.

All patients starting therapy with SIMCOR, or whose dose of SIMCOR is being increased, should be advised of the risk of myopathy, including rhabdomyolysis, and told to report promptly any unexplained muscle pain, tenderness or weakness particularly if accompanied by malaise or fever or if muscle signs and symptoms persist after discontinuing SIMCOR. SIMCOR therapy should be discontinued immediately if myopathy is diagnosed or suspected. In most cases, muscle symptoms and CK increases resolved when treatment was promptly discontinued. Periodic CK determinations may be considered in patients starting therapy with SIMCOR or whose dose is being increased, but there is no assurance that such monitoring will prevent myopathy. Many of the patients who have developed rhabdomyolysis on therapy with simvastatin have had complicated medical histories, including renal insufficiency usually as a consequence of long-standing diabetes mellitus. Such patients merit closer monitoring. SIMCOR therapy should be discontinued if markedly elevated CPK levels occur or myopathy is diagnosed or suspected. SIMCOR therapy should also be temporarily withheld in any patient experiencing an acute or serious condition predisposing to the development of renal failure secondary to rhabdomyolysis, e.g., sepsis; hypotension; major surgery; trauma; severe metabolic, endocrine, or electrolyte disorders; or uncontrolled epilepsy.

Drug Interactions

The risk of myopathy and rhabdomyolysis is increased by high levels of statin activity in plasma. Simvastatin is metabolized by the cytochrome P450 isoform 3A4. Certain drugs which inhibit this metabolic pathway can raise the plasma levels of simvastatin and may increase the risk of myopathy. These include itraconazole, ketoconazole, and posaconazole, the macrolide antibiotics erythromycin and clarithromycin, and the ketolide antibiotic telithromycin, HIV protease inhibitors, boceprevir, telaprevir, the antidepressant nefazodone, or large quantities of grapefruit juice (>1 quart daily), and combination of these drugs with SIMCOR is contraindicated. If treatment with itraconazole, ketoconazole, posaconazole, erythromycin, clarithromycin or telithromycin is unavoidable, therapy with SIMCOR must be suspended during the course of treatment [see Contraindications (4) and Drug Interactions (7.1)]. In vitro studies have demonstrated a potential for voriconazole to inhibit the metabolism of simvastatin. Adjustment of the SIMCOR dose may be needed to reduce the risk of myopathy/rhabdomyolysis if voriconazole must be used concomitantly with simvastatin [see Drug Interactions (7.1)].

The combined use of SIMCOR with gemfibrozil, cyclosporine, or danazol is contraindicated [see Contraindications (4) and Drug Interactions (7.1)].

The combined use of SIMCOR with verapamil or diltiazem is contraindicated, because dosages of simvastatin are not to exceed 10 mg when these drugs are co-administered and all doses of SIMCOR contain simvastatin in excess of 10 mg [see Contraindications (4) and Drug Interactions (7.2)].

The combined use of SIMCOR with drugs that cause myopathy/rhabdomyolysis when given alone, such as fibrates, should be avoided [see Drug Interactions (7.3)].

Cases of myopathy, including rhabdomyolysis, have been reported with simvastatin coadministered with colchicine, and caution should be exercised when prescribing SIMCOR with colchicine [see Drug Interactions (7.8)].

The benefits of the combined use of SIMCOR with amlodipine or ranolazine should be carefully weighed against the potential risks of combination [see Drug Interactions (7.4)]. Periodic CK determinations may be considered in patients starting therapy with or increasing the dose of these agents, but there is no assurance that such monitoring will prevent myopathy.

Cases of myopathy, including rhabdomyolysis, have been observed with simvastatin coadministered with lipid-modifying doses (≥1 g/day niacin) of niacin-containing products. In an ongoing, double-blind, randomized cardiovascular outcomes trial, an independent safety monitoring committee identified that the incidence of myopathy is higher in Chinese compared with non-Chinese patients taking simvastatin 40 mg coadministered with lipid modifying doses of a niacin-containing product. Caution should be used when prescribing SIMCOR in doses that exceed 1000/20 mg/day to Chinese patients. It is unknown if the risk for myopathy with coadministration of simvastatin with lipid modifying doses of niacin-containing products observed in Chinese patients applies to other Asian patients [see Dosage and Administration (2.3)].

Prescribing recommendations for interacting agents are summarized in Table 3 [see also Dosage and Administration (2.2), Contraindications (4), Drug Interactions (7), Clinical Pharmacology (12.3)].

Table 3.
Drug Interactions Associated with Increased Risk of Myopathy/Rhabdomyolysis

Interacting Agents	Prescribing Recommendations
Strong CYP3A4 inhibitors, e.g., Itraconazole Ketoconazole Posaconazole Erythromycin Clarithromycin Telithromycin HIV protease inhibitors Boceprevir Telaprevir Nefazodone Gemfibrozil Cyclosporine Danazol Verapamil Diltiazem	Contraindicated with SIMCOR
Amiodarone Amlodipine Ranolazine	Do not exceed 1000/20 mg SIMCOR daily
Grapefruit juice	Avoid large quantities of grapefruit juice (>1 quart daily)

SIMCOR

Myopathy and/or rhabdomyolysis have been reported when simvastatin is used in combination with lipid-altering doses (≥ 1 gram/day) of niacin. Physicians contemplating the use of SIMCOR, a combination of simvastatin and niacin extended-release (NIASPAN), should weigh the potential benefits and risks, and should carefully monitor for any signs and symptoms of muscle pain, tenderness, or weakness, particularly during the initial month of treatment or during any period of upward dosage titration of either drug. Periodic determination of serum creatine kinase (CK) determinations may be considered in such situations, but there is no assurance that such monitoring will prevent myopathy. Patients starting therapy with SIMCOR should be advised of the risk of myopathy, and told to report promptly unexplained muscle pain, tenderness, or weakness. A CK level above ten times the upper limit of normal (ULN) in a patient with unexplained muscle symptoms indicates myopathy. SIMCOR therapy should be discontinued if myopathy is diagnosed or suspected.

In patients with complicated medical histories predisposing to rhabdomyolysis, such as renal insufficiency, dose escalation requires caution. Also, as there are no known adverse consequences of brief interruption of therapy, treatment with SIMCOR should be stopped for a few days before elective major surgery and when any major acute medical or surgical condition supervenes (e.g., sepsis, hypotension, dehydration, major surgery, trauma, severe metabolic, endocrine, and electrolyte disorders, or uncontrolled seizures).

5.3 Liver Dysfunction

Cases of severe hepatic toxicity, including fulminant hepatic necrosis, have occurred in patients who have substituted sustained-release (modified-release, timed-release) niacin products for immediate-release (crystalline) niacin at equivalent doses. Patients previously receiving niacin products other than niacin extended-release (NIASPAN) should be started on SIMCOR at the lowest recommended starting dose [see Dosage and Administration (2)].

SIMCOR should be used with caution in patients who consume substantial quantities of alcohol and/or have a past history of liver disease. Active liver disease or unexplained transaminase elevations are contraindications to the use of SIMCOR [see Contraindications (4)].

Niacin extended-release (NIASPAN) and simvastatin can cause abnormal liver tests. In a simvastatin-controlled, 24 week study with SIMCOR in 641 patients, there were no persistent increases (to more than 3× the ULN) in serum transaminases. In three placebo-controlled clinical studies of niacin extended-release, patients with normal serum transaminases levels at baseline did not experience any transaminase elevations greater than 3× the ULN. Persistent increases (to more than 3× the ULN) in serum transaminases have occurred in approximately 1% of patients who received simvastatin in clinical studies. When drug treatment was interrupted or discontinued in these patients, the transaminases levels usually fell slowly to pretreatment levels. The increases were not associated with jaundice or other clinical signs or symptoms. There was no evidence of hypersensitivity.

It is recommended that liver enzyme tests be obtained prior to initiating therapy with SIMCOR and repeated as clinically indicated. There have been rare postmarketing reports of fatal and non-fatal hepatic failure in patients taking statins, including simvastatin. If serious liver injury with clinical symptoms and/or hyperbilirubinemia or jaundice occurs during treatment with SIMCOR, promptly interrupt therapy. If an alternate etiology is not found do not restart SIMCOR. Note that ALT may emanate from muscle, therefore ALT rising with CK may indicate myopathy [see Warnings and Precautions (5.2)].

5.4 Laboratory Abnormalities

Increase in Blood Glucose: Niacin treatment can increase fasting blood glucose. In a simvastatin-controlled, 24-week study with SIMCOR the change from baseline in glycosylated hemoglobin levels was 0.2% for SIMCOR-treated patients and 0.2% for simvastatin-treated patients. Diabetic or potentially diabetic patients should be observed closely during treatment with SIMCOR, particularly during the first few months of therapy. Adjustment of diet and/or hypoglycemic therapy or discontinuation of SIMCOR may be necessary.

Reduction in platelet count: Niacin can reduce platelet count. In a simvastatin-controlled, 24-week study with SIMCOR the mean percent change from baseline for patients treated with 2000/40 mg daily was -5.6%.

Increase in ProthrombinTime (PT): Niacin can cause small increases in PT. In a simvastatin-controlled, 24-week study with SIMCOR this effect was not seen.

Increase in Uric Acid: Elevated uric acid levels have occurred with niacin therapy. In a simvastatin-controlled, 24-week study with SIMCOR this effect was not seen. Nevertheless, in patients predisposed to gout, SIMCOR therapy should be used with caution.

Decrease in Phosphorus: Small dose-related reductions in phosphorous levels were seen in clinical studies with niacin. In a simvastatin-controlled, 24-week study with SIMCOR this effect was not seen.

5.5 Endocrine Function

Increases in HbA1c and fasting serum glucose levels have been reported with HMG-CoA reductase inhibitors, including simvastatin.

6 ADVERSE REACTIONS

Overview

In a controlled clinical study, 14% of patients randomized to SIMCOR discontinued therapy due to an adverse event. Flushing episodes (i.e., warmth, redness, itching and/or tingling) were the most common treatment-emergent adverse reactions, occurring in up to 59% of patients treated with SIMCOR. Spontaneous reports with niacin extended-release and clinical studies of SIMCOR suggest that flushing may be accompanied by symptoms of dizziness or syncope, tachycardia, palpitations, shortness of breath, sweating, burning sensation/skin burning sensation, chills, and/or edema.

6.1 Clinical Studies Experience

SIMCOR

Because clinical studies are conducted under widely varying conditions, adverse reaction rates observed in the clinical studies of a drug cannot be directly compared to rates in the clinical studies of another drug and may not reflect the rates observed in practice.

The safety data described below reflect exposure to SIMCOR in 403 patients in a controlled study for a period of 6 months.

Flushing: Flushing (warmth, redness, itching and/or tingling) occurred in up to 59% of patients treated with SIMCOR. Flushing resulted in study discontinuation for 6.0% of patients.

More Common Adverse Reactions: In addition to flushing, adverse reactions occurring in ≥ 3% of patients (irrespective of investigator causality) treated with SIMCOR are shown in Table 4 below:

Table 4. Adverse Reactions Occurring in ≥ 3% of Patients in a Controlled Clinical Trial

Adverse Event	SIMCOR overall *	Simvastatin overall **
Total Number of Patients	N=403	N=238
Headache	18 (4.5%)	11 (4.6%)
Pruritus	13 (3.2%)	0 (0.0%)
Nausea	13 (3.2%)	10 (4.2%)
Back Pain	13 (3.2%)	5 (2.1%)
Diarrhea	12 (3.0%)	7 (2.9%)

* SIMCOR overall included all doses from 500/20 mg to 2000/40 mg
** Simvastatin overall included 20 mg, 40 mg, and 80 mg doses

Atherothrombosis Intervention in Metabolic Syndrome with Low HDL/High Triglycerides: Impact on Global Health Outcomes (AIM-HIGH)

In AIM-HIGH involving 3414 patients (mean age of 64 years, 15% women, 92% Caucasians, 34% with diabetes

mellitus) with stable, previously diagnosed cardiovascular disease, all patients received simvastatin, 40 to 80 mg per day, plus ezetimibe 10 mg per day if needed, to maintain an LDL-C level of 40-80 mg/dL, and were randomized to receive NIASPAN 1500-2000 mg/day (n=1718) or matching placebo (IR Niacin, 100-150 mg, n=1696). The incidence of the adverse reactions of "blood glucose increased" (6.4% vs. 4.5%) and "diabetes mellitus" (3.6% vs. 2.2%) was significantly higher in the simvastatin plus NIASPAN group as compared to the simvastatin plus placebo group. There were 5 cases of rhabdomyolysis reported, 4 (0.2%) in the simvastatin plus NIASPAN group and one (<0.1%) in the simvastatin plus placebo group [see Warnings and Precautions (5.1)].

Simvastatin

In pre-marketing controlled clinical studies and their open extensions (2,423 patients with mean duration of follow-up of approximately 18 months) 1.4% of patients discontinued due to adverse reactions. The most commonly reported adverse reactions (incidence > 1%) in simvastatin controlled clinical trials were: headache (3.5%), abdominal pain (3.5%), constipation (2.3%), upper respiratory infection (2.1%), diarrhea (1.9%), and flatulence (1.9%).

Other Clinical Studies

In a clinical trial in which 12,064 patients with a history of myocardial infarction were treated with simvastatin (mean follow-up 6.7 years), the incidence of myopathy (defined as unexplained muscle weakness or pain with a serum creatine kinase [CK] >10 times upper limit of normal [ULN]) in patients on 80 mg/day was approximately 0.9% compared with 0.02% for patients on 20 mg/day. The incidence of rhabdomyolysis (defined as myopathy with a CK >40 times ULN) in patients on 80 mg/day was approximately 0.4% compared with 0% for patients on 20 mg/day. The incidence of myopathy, including rhabdomyolysis, was highest during the first year and then notably decreased during the subsequent years of treatment.

Niacin Extended-Release

In placebo-controlled clinical trials (n=245), flushing episodes were the most common treatment-emergent adverse events (up to 88% of patients) for niacin extended-release. Other adverse events occurring in 5% or greater of patients treated with niacin extended-release are headache (9%), diarrhea (7%), nausea (5%), rhinitis (5%), and dyspepsia (4%) at a maintenance dose of 1000mg daily.

Clinical Laboratory Abnormalities:

SIMCOR

Chemistry

Elevations in serum transaminases [see Warnings and Precautions (5.3)], CK, fasting glucose, uric acid, alkaline phosphatase, LDH, amylase, γ-glutamyl transpeptidase, bilirubin, and reductions in phosphorus, and abnormal thyroid function tests.

Hematology

Reductions in platelet counts and prolongation of PT [see Warnings and Precautions (5.4)].

6.2 Postmarketing Experience

See also the full prescribing information for niacin extended release (Niaspan) and simvastatin products.

Because the below reactions are reported voluntarily from a population of uncertain size, it is generally not possible to reliably estimate their frequency or establish a causal relationship to drug exposure.

Simvastatin

The following additional adverse reactions have been identified during postapproval use of simvastatin. Hypersensitivity reaction including one or more of the following features: anaphylaxis, angioedema, lupus erythematous-like syndrome, vasculitis, purpura, thrombocytopenia, leucopenia, hemolytic anemia, positive ANA, ESR increase, eosinophilia, arthritis, photosensitivity, chills, toxic epidermal necrolysis, erythema multiforme, Stevens-Johnson syndrome, urticaria, fever, dyspnea, and arthralgia; pancreatitis, hepatitis, fatal and non-fatal hepatic failure, pruritus, cataracts, polymyositis, dermatomyositis, polymyalgia rheumatica, tendon rupture, peripheral neuropathy, erectile dysfunction, depression, interstitial lung disease, alopecia, a variety of skin changes (e.g., nodules, discoloration, dryness of skin/mucous membranes, changes to hair/nails), muscle cramps, vomiting, malaise.

There have been rare reports of immune-mediated necrotizing myopathy with statin use [see Warnings and Precautions (5.2)].

There have been rare postmarketing reports of cognitive impairment (e.g., memory loss, forgetfulness, amnesia, memory impairment, confusion) associated with statin use. These cognitive issues have been reported for all statins. The reports are generally nonserious, and reversible upon statin discontinuation, with variable times to symptom onset (1 day to years) and symptom resolution (median of 3 weeks).

NIASPAN

The following additional adverse reactions have been identified during post-approval use of NIASPAN. Hypersensitiv-

ity reaction including one or more of the following features: anaphylaxis, dyspnea, angioedema, tongue edema, larynx edema, face edema, laryngismus; tachycardia, atrial fibrillation, other cardiac arrhythmias, palpitations, hypotension, postural hypotension, dizziness, syncope, flushing, burning sensation/skin burning sensation, paresthesia, urticaria, vesiculobullous rash, maculopapular rash, sweating, dry skin, skin discoloration, blurred vision, macular edema, myalgia, myopathy, peptic ulcers, eructation, flatulence, hepatitis, jaundice, peripheral edema, asthenia, nervousness, insomnia, migraine, gout, and decreased glucose tolerance.

7 DRUG INTERACTIONS

No drug interaction studies were conducted with SIMCOR. However, the following interactions have been noted with the individual components of SIMCOR:

Simvastatin

7.1 Strong CYP3A4 Inhibitors, Cyclosporine, or Danazol

Strong CYP3A4 inhibitors: Simvastatin, like several other inhibitors of HMG-CoA reductase, is a substrate of CYP3A4. Simvastatin is metabolized by CYP3A4 but has no CYP3A4 inhibitory activity; therefore it is not expected to affect the plasma concentrations of other drugs metabolized by CYP3A4.

Elevated plasma levels of HMG-CoA reductase inhibitory activity increases the risk of myopathy and rhabdomyolysis, particularly with higher doses of SIMCOR [see Warnings and Precautions (5.2) and Clinical Pharmacology (12.3)]. Concomitant use of drugs labeled as having a strong inhibitory effect on CYP3A4 is contraindicated [see Contraindications (4)]. If treatment with itraconazole, ketoconazole, posaconazole, erythromycin, clarithromycin or telithromycin is unavoidable, therapy with SIMCOR must be suspended during the course of treatment.

Although not studied clinically, voriconazole has been shown to inhibit lovastatin metabolism *in vitro* (human liver microsomes). Therefore, voriconazole is likely to increase the plasma concentration of simvastatin. It is recommended that dose adjustment of SIMCOR be considered during concomitant use of voriconazole and SIMCOR to reduce the risk of myopathy, including rhabdomyolysis [see Warnings and Precautions (5.2)].

Cyclosporine or Danazol: The risk of myopathy, including rhabdomyolysis is increased by concomitant administration of cyclosporine or danazol. Therefore, concomitant use of these drugs is contraindicated [see Contraindications (4), Warnings and Precautions (5.2) and Clinical Pharmacology (12.3)].

7.2 Verapamil or Diltiazem

The risk of myopathy, including rhabdomyolysis is increased by concomitant administration of verapamil or diltiazem with doses of simvastatin exceeding 10 mg. Because all doses of SIMCOR contain simvastatin in excess of 10 mg, concomitant use of these drugs is contraindicated [see Contraindications (4), Warnings and Precautions (5.2) and Clinical Pharmacology (12.3)].

7.3 Lipid-Lowering Drugs That Can Cause Myopathy When Given Alone

Gemfibrozil: Contraindicated with SIMCOR [see Contraindications (4) and Warnings and Precautions (5.2)]. Other fibrates: Combined use with SIMCOR should be avoided [see Warnings and Precautions (5.2)].

7.4 Amlodipine or Ranolazine

The risk of myopathy, including rhabdomyolysis, is increased by concomitant administration of amlodipine or ranolazine [see Dosage and Administration (2.2) and Warnings and Precautions (5.2) and Table 5 in Clinical Pharmacology (12.3)].

7.5 Propranolol

In healthy male volunteers there was a significant decrease in mean C_{max}, but no change in AUC, for simvastatin total and active inhibitors with concomitant administration of single doses of simvastatin and propranolol. The clinical relevance of this finding is unclear. The pharmacokinetics of the enantiomers of propranolol were not affected.

7.6 Digoxin

Concomitant administration of a single dose of digoxin in healthy male volunteers receiving simvastatin resulted in a slight elevation (less than 0.3 ng/mL) in digoxin concentrations in plasma (as measured by a radioimmunoassay) compared to concomitant administration of placebo and digoxin. Patients taking digoxin should be monitored appropriately when SIMCOR is initiated.

7.7 Coumarin Anticoagulants

In normal volunteers and hypercholesterolemic patients, simvastatin 20-40 mg/day modestly potentiated the effect of

Information on the AbbVie, Inc. products listed on these pages is from the prescribing information in use as of July 31, 2014. For more information, please visit rxabbvie.com or call 1-800-633-9110.

coumarin anticoagulants since the prothrombin time, reported as International Normalized Ratio (INR), increased from a baseline of 1.7 to 1.8 and from 2.6 to 3.4 in the volunteers and patients, respectively. With other reductase inhibitors, clinically evident bleeding and/or increased prothrombin time has been reported in a few patients taking coumarin anticoagulants concomitantly. In such patients, prothrombin time should be determined before starting SIMCOR and frequently enough during early therapy to ensure that no significant alteration of prothrombin time occurs. Once a stable prothrombin time has been documented, prothrombin times can be monitored at the intervals usually recommended for patients on coumarin anticoagulants. If the dose of SIMCOR is changed or discontinued, the same procedure should be repeated.

7.8 Colchicine
Cases of myopathy, including rhabdomyolysis, have been reported with simvastatin coadministered with colchicine, and caution should be exercised when prescribing SIMCOR with colchicine [see Warnings and Precautions (5.2)].

Niacin
7.9 Aspirin
Concomitant use of aspirin may decrease the metabolic clearance of niacin. The clinical relevance of this finding is unclear.

7.10 Antihypertensive Therapy
Niacin may potentiate the effects of ganglionic blocking agents and vasoactive drugs resulting in postural hypotension.

7.11 Bile Acid Sequestrants
An in vitro study was carried out investigating the niacin-binding capacity of colestipol and cholestyramine. About 98% of available niacin was bound to colestipol, with 10 to 30% binding to cholestyramine. These results suggest that 4 to 6 hours, or as great an interval as possible, should elapse between the ingestion of bile acid-binding resins and the administration of SIMCOR.

7.12 Other
Nutritional supplements containing large doses of niacin or related compounds may potentiate the adverse effects of SIMCOR.

8 USE IN SPECIFIC POPULATIONS
8.1 Pregnancy
Pregnancy Category X – [see Contraindications (4)]
SIMCOR is contraindicated in women who are or may become pregnant. Lipid lowering drugs offer no benefit during pregnancy, because cholesterol and cholesterol derivatives are needed for normal fetal development. Serum cholesterol and triglycerides increase during normal pregnancy. Atherosclerosis is a chronic process, and discontinuation of lipid-lowering drugs during pregnancy should have little impact on long-term outcomes of primary hypercholesterolemia therapy. There are no adequate and well-controlled studies of SIMCOR use during pregnancy; however, there are rare reports of congenital anomalies in infants exposed to HMG-CoA reductase inhibitors in utero. Animal reproduction studies of simvastatin in rats and rabbits showed no evidence of teratogenicity. SIMCOR may cause fetal harm when administered to a pregnant woman. If SIMCOR is used during pregnancy or if the patient becomes pregnant while taking this drug, the patient should be apprised of the potential hazard to the fetus.
SIMCOR contains simvastatin (a HMG-CoA reductase inhibitor) and niacin (nicotinic acid). There are rare reports of congenital anomalies following intrauterine exposure to HMG-CoA reductase inhibitors. In a review of approximately 100 prospectively followed pregnancies in women exposed to simvastatin or another structurally related HMG-CoA reductase inhibitor, the incidences of congenital anomalies, spontaneous abortions, and fetal deaths/stillbirths did not exceed those expected in the general population. However, the study was only able to exclude a 3- to 4-fold increased risk of congenital anomalies over the background rate. In 89% of these cases, drug treatment was initiated prior to pregnancy and was discontinued during the first trimester when pregnancy was identified. It is not known whether niacin at doses used for lipid disorders can cause fetal harm when administered to a pregnant woman. Simvastatin was not teratogenic in rats or rabbits at doses that resulted in 3 times the human exposure based on mg/m^2 surface area. However, in studies with another structurally-related HMG-CoA reductase inhibitor, skeletal malformations were observed in rats and mice. Animal reproduction studies have not been conducted with niacin.
Women of childbearing potential, who require SIMCOR treatment for a lipid disorder, should use effective contraception. Patients trying to conceive should contact their prescriber to discuss stopping SIMCOR treatment. If pregnancy occurs, SIMCOR should be immediately discontinued.

8.3 Nursing Mothers
It is not known whether simvastatin is excreted into human milk; however, a small amount of another drug in this class does pass into breast milk. Niacin is excreted into human milk but the actual infant dose or infant dose as a percent of the maternal dose is not known. Because of the potential for serious adverse reactions in nursing infants, nursing mothers who require SIMCOR treatment should not breastfeed their infants. A decision should be made whether to discontinue nursing or discontinue drug, taking into account the importance of the drug to the mother [see Contraindications (4)].

8.4 Pediatric Use
The safety and effectiveness of SIMCOR in pediatric patients have not been established.

8.5 Geriatric Use
There were 281 (30.8%) patients aged 65 years and older treated with SIMCOR in Phase III clinical studies. No overall differences in safety and effectiveness were observed between these patients and younger patients, but greater sensitivity of some older individuals cannot be ruled out. A pharmacokinetic study with simvastatin showed the mean plasma level of HMG-CoA reductase inhibitory activity to be approximately 45% higher in elderly patients between 70-78 years of age compared with patients between 18-30 years of age.
Because advanced age (≥65 years) is a predisposing factor for myopathy, including rhabdomyolysis, SIMCOR should be prescribed with caution in the elderly. In a clinical trial of patients treated with simvastatin 80 mg/day, patients ≥65 years of age had an increased risk of myopathy, including rhabdomyolysis, compared to patients <65 years of age [see Warnings and Precautions (5.2) and Clinical Pharmacology (12.3)].

8.6 Gender
Data from the clinical trials suggest that women have a greater hypolipidemic response than men at equivalent doses of niacin extended-release. No consistent gender differences in efficacy and safety were observed in SIMCOR studies.

8.7 Renal Impairment
No pharmacokinetic studies have been conducted in patients with renal impairment for SIMCOR. Caution should be exercised when SIMCOR is administered to patients with renal disease. For patients with severe renal insufficiency, SIMCOR should not be started unless the patient has already tolerated treatment with simvastatin at a dose of 10 mg or higher. Caution should be exercised when SIMCOR is administered to these patients and they should be closely monitored.

8.8 Hepatic Impairment
No pharmacokinetic studies have been conducted in patients with hepatic insufficiency for SIMCOR [see Warnings and Precautions (5.3)].

10 OVERDOSAGE
Supportive measures should be taken in the event of an overdose. The dialyzability of niacin, or of simvastatin and its metabolites, is not known.
A few cases of overdosage with simvastatin have been reported; the maximum dose taken was 3.6 g. All patients recovered without sequelae.

11 DESCRIPTION
SIMCOR tablets contain niacin extended-release (NIASPAN) and simvastatin in combination. Simvastatin, an inhibitor of HMG-CoA reductase, and niacin are both lipid-altering agents.

Niacin Extended-Release
Niacin is nicotinic acid, or 3-pyridinecarboxylic acid. Niacin is a white, nonhygroscopic crystalline powder that is very soluble in water, boiling ethanol, and propylene glycol. It is insoluble in ethyl ether. The empirical formula of niacin is $C_6H_5NO_2$ and its molecular weight is 123.11. Niacin has the following structural formula:

Simvastatin
Simvastatin is butanoic acid, 2,2-dimethyl-,1,2,3,7,8,8a-hexahydro-3-7-dimethyl-8-[2-(tetrahydro-4-hydroxy-6-oxo-2H-pyran-2-yl)-ethyl]-1-naphthalenyl ester, [1S-[1α,3α,7β,8β(2S*4S*),-8aβ]]. Simvastatin is a white to off-white, nonhygroscopic, crystalline powder that is practically insoluble in water and freely soluble in chloroform, methanol, and ethanol. The empirical formula of simvastatin is $C_{25}H_{38}O_5$ and its molecular weight is 418.57. Simvastatin has the following structural formula:
[See chemical structure above]
SIMCOR is available for oral administration as tablets containing 500 mg of niacin extended-release (NIASPAN) and 20 mg simvastatin (SIMCOR 500/20 mg), 500 mg of niacin extended-release (NIASPAN) and 40 mg simvastatin (SIMCOR 500/40 mg), 750 mg of niacin extended-release (NIASPAN) and 20 mg simvastatin (SIMCOR 750/20 mg), 1000 mg of niacin extended-release (NIASPAN) and 20 mg simvastatin (SIMCOR 1000/20 mg) and 1000 mg of niacin extended-release (NIASPAN) and 40 mg simvastatin (SIMCOR 1000/40 mg). Each tablet contains the following inactive ingredients: hypromellose, povidone, stearic acid, polyethylene glycol, butylated hydroxyanisole, FD&C Blue #2, lactose monohydrate, titanium dioxide, triacetin. SIMCOR 500/20 mg, SIMCOR 750/20 mg, and SIMCOR 1000/20 mg also contain iron oxide.

12 CLINICAL PHARMACOLOGY
12.1 Mechanism of Action
Niacin
Niacin functions in the body after conversion to nicotinamide adenine dinucleotide (NAD) in the NAD coenzyme system. The mechanism by which niacin alters lipid profiles is not completely understood and may involve several actions, including partial inhibition of release of free fatty acids from adipose tissue, and increased lipoprotein lipase activity (which may increase the rate of chylomicron triglyceride removal from plasma). Niacin decreases the rate of hepatic synthesis of VLDL-C and LDL-C, and does not appear to affect fecal excretion of fats, sterols, or bile acids.

Simvastatin
Simvastatin is a prodrug and is hydrolyzed to its active β-hydroxyacid form, simvastatin acid, after administration. Simvastatin is a specific inhibitor of 3-hydroxy-3-methylglutaryl-coenzyme A (HMG-CoA) reductase, the enzyme that catalyzes the conversion of HMG-CoA to mevalonate, an early and rate-limiting step in the biosynthetic pathway for cholesterol. In addition, simvastatin reduces VLDL and TG and increases HDL-C.

12.2 Pharmacodynamics
A variety of clinical studies have demonstrated that elevated levels of Total-C, LDL-C, and Apo B promote human atherosclerosis. Similarly, decreased levels of HDL-C are associated with the development of atherosclerosis. Epidemiological investigations have established that cardiovascular morbidity and mortality vary directly with the level of Total-C and LDL-C, and inversely with the level of HDL-C. Like LDL, cholesterol-enriched triglyceride-rich lipoproteins, including VLDL, intermediate-density lipoprotein (IDL), and their remnants, can also promote atherosclerosis. Elevated plasma TG are frequently found in a triad with low HDL-C levels and small LDL particles, as well as in association with non-lipid metabolic risk factors for coronary heart disease (CHD). As such, total plasma TG has not consistently been shown to be an independent risk factor for CHD. Furthermore, the independent effect of raising HDL-C or lowering TG on the risk of coronary and cardiovascular morbidity and mortality has not been determined.

SIMCOR
SIMCOR reduces Total-C, LDL-C, non-HDL-C, Apo B, TG, and Lp(a) levels and increases HDL-C in patients with primary hyperlipidemia, mixed dyslipidemia, or hypertriglyceridemia.

Niacin
Niacin (but not nicotinamide) in gram doses reduces LDL-C, Apo B, Lp(a), TG, and Total-C, and increases HDL-C. The magnitude of individual lipid and lipoprotein responses may be influenced by the severity and type of underlying lipid abnormality. The increase in HDL-C is associated with an increase in apolipoprotein A-I (Apo A-I) and a shift in the distribution of HDL subfractions. These shifts include an increase in the HDL2:HDL3 ratio, and an elevation in lipoprotein A-I (Lp A-I, an HDL-C particle containing only Apo A-I). Niacin treatment also decreases serum levels of apolipoprotein B-100 (Apo B), the major protein component of the very low-density lipoprotein (VLDL) and LDL fractions, and of Lp(a), a variant form of LDL independently associated with coronary risk. In addition, preliminary reports suggest that niacin causes favorable LDL particle size transformations, although the clinical relevance of this effect requires further investigation.

Simvastatin
Simvastatin reduces elevated Total-C, LDL-C, Apo B, and TG, and increases HDL-C in patients with primary heterozygous familial and nonfamilial hypercholesterolemia and mixed dyslipidemia. Simvastatin reduces Total-C and LDL-C in patients with homozygous familial hypercholesterolemia. Simvastatin decreases VLDL, Total-C/HDL-C ratio, and LDL-C/HDL-C ratio.

Table 5.
Effect of Coadministered Drugs or Grapefruit Juice on Simvastatin Systemic Exposure

Coadministered Drug or Grapefruit Juice	Dosing of Coadministered Drug or Grapefruit Juice	Dosing of Simvastatin		Geometric Mean Ratio (Ratio* with / without coadministered drug) No Effect = 1.00	
				AUC	C_{max}
Contraindicated with simvastatin *[see Contraindications (4) and Warnings and Precautions (5.2)]*					
Telithromycin[†]	200 mg QD for 4 days	80 mg	simvastatin acid[‡]	12	15
			simvastatin	8.9	5.3
Nelfinavir[†]	1250 mg BID for 14 days	20 mg QD for 28 days	simvastatin acid[‡]	6	6.2
			simvastatin		
Itraconazole[†]	200 mg QD for 4 days	80 mg	simvastatin acid[‡]		13.1
			simvastatin		13.1
Posaconazole	100 mg (oral suspension) QD for 13 days	40 mg	simvastatin acid	7.3	9.2
			simvastatin	10.3	9.4
	200 mg (oral suspension) QD for 13 days	40 mg	simvastatin acid	8.5	9.5
			simvastatin	10.6	11.4
Gemfibrozil	600 mg BID for 3 days	40 mg	simvastatin acid	2.85	2.18
			simvastatin	1.35	0.91
Avoid >1 quart of grapefruit juice with simvastatin *[see Warnings and Precautions (5.2)]*					
Grapefruit Juice[§] (high dose)	200 mL of double-strength TID[¶]	60 mg single dose	simvastatin acid	7	
			simvastatin	16	
Grapefruit Juice[§] (low dose)	8 oz (about 237 mL) of single-strength[#]	20 mg single dose	simvastatin acid	1.3	
			simvastatin	1.9	
Avoid taking with >10 mg simvastatin, based on clinical and/or post-marketing experience *[see Warnings and Precautions (5.2)]*					
Verapamil SR	240 mg QD Days 1-7 then 240 mg BID on Days 8-10	80 mg on Day 10	simvastatin acid	2.3	2.4
			simvastatin	2.5	2.1
Diltiazem	120 mg BID for 10 days	80 mg on Day 10	simvastatin acid	2.69	2.69
			simvastatin	3.10	2.88
Diltiazem	120 mg BID for 14 days	20 mg on Day 14	simvastatin	4.6	3.6
Avoid taking with >20 mg simvastatin, based on clinical and/or post-marketing experience *[see Warnings and Precautions (5.2)]*					
Amiodarone	400 mg QD for 3 days	40 mg on Day 3	simvastatin acid	1.75	1.72
			simvastatin	1.76	1.79
Amlodipine	10 mg QD for 10 days	80 mg on Day 10	simvastatin acid	1.58	1.56
			simvastatin	1.77	1.47
Ranolazine SR	1000 mg BID for 7 days	80 mg on Day 1, and Day 6-9	simvastatin acid	2.26	2.28
			simvastatin	1.86	1.75
No dosing adjustments required for the following:					
Fenofibrate	160 mg QD for 14 days	80 mg QD on Days 8-14	simvastatin acid	0.64	0.89
			simvastatin	0.89	0.83
Niacin extended-release[Þ]	2 g single dose	20 mg single dose	simvastatin acid	1.6	1.84
			simvastatin	1.4	1.08
Propranolol	80 mg single dose	80 mg single dose	total inhibitor	0.79	↓ from 33.6 to 21.1 ng●eq/mL
			active inhibitor	0.79	↓ from 7.0 to 4.7 ng●eq/mL

* Results based on a chemical assay except results with propranolol as indicated.
[†] Results could be representative of the following CYP3A4 inhibitors: ketoconazole, erythromycin, clarithromycin, HIV protease inhibitors, and nefazodone.
[‡] Simvastatin acid refers to the β-hydroxyacid of simvastatin.
[§] The effect of amounts of grapefruit juice between those used in these two studies on simvastatin pharmacokinetics has not been studied.

[¶] Double-strength: one can of frozen concentrate diluted with one can of water. Grapefruit juice was administered TID for 2 days, and 200 mL together with single dose simvastatin and 30 and 90 minutes following single dose simvastatin on Day 3.
[#] Single-strength: one can of frozen concentrate diluted with 3 cans of water. Grapefruit juice was administered with breakfast for 3 days, and simvastatin was administered in the evening on Day 3.

[Þ] Because Chinese patients have an increased risk for myopathy with simvastatin coadministered with lipid-modifying doses (≥1 gram/day niacin) of niacin-containing products, and the risk is dose-related, Chinese patients should not receive simvastatin 80 mg coadministered with lipid-modifying doses of niacin-containing products *[see Warnings and Precautions (5.2)]*.

12.3   Pharmacokinetics
Absorption and Bioavailability
SIMCOR
The relative bioavailability of niacin (Nicotinuric acid, NUA, C_{max} and total urinary excretion as the surrogate), simvastatin, and simvastatin acid was evaluated under a light snack conditions in healthy volunteers (n=42), following administration of two 1000/20 mg SIMCOR tablets. Niacin exposure (C_{max} and AUC) after SIMCOR was similar to that of a niacin extended-release formulation. However, simvastatin and simvastatin acid AUC after SIMCOR increased by 23% and 41%, respectively, compared to those of a simvastatin immediate release formulation. The mean time to C_{max} (T_{max}) for niacin ranged from 4.6 to 4.9 hours and simvastatin from 1.9 to 2.0 hours. Following administration of $2 \times 1000/20$ mg SIMCOR, the mean C_{max}, T_{max} and $AUC_{(0-t)}$ for simvastatin acid, active metabolite of simvastatin, were 3.29 ng/mL, 6.56 hours and 30.81 ng●hr/mL respectively.

Bioequivalence has not been evaluated among different SIMCOR dosage strengths except between 1000/40 and 500/20 mg. SIMCOR tablets 1000/40 mg and 500/20 mg were bioequivalent following a single dose of 2000/80 mg. Therefore, dosage strengths of SIMCOR should not be considered exchangeable except between these two strengths.

Niacin
Due to extensive and saturable first-pass metabolism, niacin concentrations in the general circulation are dose dependent and highly variable. Peak steady-state niacin concentrations were 0.6, 4.9, and 15.5 mcg/mL after doses of 1000, 1500, and 2000 mg NIASPAN once daily (given as two 500 mg, two 750 mg, and two 1000 mg tablets, respectively). To reduce the risk of gastrointestinal upset, administration of niacin extended-release with a low-fat meal or snack is recommended.

Simvastatin
Since simvastatin undergoes extensive first-pass extraction in the liver, the availability of the drug to the general circulation is low (<5%). Peak plasma concentrations of both active and total inhibitors were attained within 1.3 to 2.4 hours postdose. Following an oral dose of ^{14}C-labeled simvastatin in man, plasma concentration of total radioactivity (simvastatin plus ^{14}C-metabolites) peaked at 4 hours and declined rapidly to about 10% of peak by 12 hours postdose. Relative to the fasting state, the plasma profile of inhibitors was not affected when simvastatin was administered immediately before an American Heart Association recommended low-fat meal.

Metabolism
SIMCOR
Following administration of SIMCOR, niacin and simvastatin undergo rapid and extensive first-pass metabolism as described in the following niacin and simvastatin sections. Following administration of $2 \times 1000/20$ mg SIMCOR in healthy volunteers, 10.2%, 10.7%, and 29.5% of the administered niacin dose was recovered in urine as niacin metabolites, NUA, N-methylnicotinamide (MNA), and N-methyl-2-pyridone-5-carboxamide (2PY), respectively. Following administration of $2 \times 1000/20$ mg SIMCOR, the mean C_{max}, T_{max}, and $AUC_{(0-t)}$ for the simvastatin metabolite, simvastatin acid were 3.29 ng/mL, 6.56 hours, and 30.81 ng●hr/mL respectively.

Niacin
Niacin undergoes rapid and extensive first-pass metabolism that is dose-rate specific and, at the doses used to treat dyslipidemia, saturable. In humans, one pathway is through a simple conjugation step with glycine to form NUA. NUA is then excreted, although there may be a small amount of reversible metabolism back to niacin. The other pathway results in the formation of nicotinamide adenine dinucleotide (NAD). It is unclear whether nicotinamide is formed as a precursor to, or following the synthesis of, NAD. Nicotinamide is further metabolized to at least MNA and nicotinamide-N-oxide NNO. MNA is further metabolized to two other compounds, 2PY and N-methyl-4-pyridone-5-carboxamide (4PY). The formation of 2PY appears to predominate over 4PY in humans.

Simvastatin
Simvastatin is a substrate of CYP3A4. Simvastatin is a lactone that is readily hydrolyzed *in vivo* to the corresponding β-hydroxyacid, a potent inhibitor of HMG-CoA reductase. The major active metabolites of simvastatin present in human plasma are the β-hydroxyacid of simvastatin and its 6'-hydroxy, 6'-hydroxymethyl, and 6'-exomethylene derivatives.

Information on the AbbVie, Inc. products listed on these pages is from the prescribing information in use as of July 31, 2014. For more information, please visit rxabbvie.com or call 1-800-633-9110.

Table 6. Non-HDL Treatment Response Following 24-Week Treatment Mean Percent Change from Simvastatin 20-mg Treated Baseline

Group A

Week	n[a]	SIMCOR 2000/20 dose (mg/mg)	non-HDL[b]	n[a]	SIMCOR 1000/20 Dose (mg/mg)	non-HDL[b]	n[a]	Simvastatin 20 Dose (mg/mg)	non-HDL[b]
Baseline	56	---	163.1 mg/dL	108	---	164.8 mg/dL	102	---	163.7 mg/dL
4	52	500/20	-12.9%	86	500/20	-12.8%	91	20	-8.3%
8	46	1000/20	-17.5%	91	1000/20	-15.5%	95	20	-8.3%
12	46	1500/20	-18.9%	90	1000/20	-14.8%	96	20	-6.4%
24	40	2000/20	-19.5%[†]	78	1000/20	-13.6%[†]	90	20	-5.0%
Dropouts by week 24:	28.6%			27.8%			11.8%		

[a] n=number of subjects with values in the analysis window at each timepoint
[b] The percent change from baseline is the model-based mean from a repeated measures mixed model with no imputation for missing data from study dropouts.
[†] significant vs. simvastatin 20 mg at the primary endpoint (Week 24), p<0.05

Table 7. Non-HDL Treatment Response Following 24-Week Treatment Mean Percent Change from Simvastatin 40-mg Treated Baseline

Group B

Week	n[a]	SIMCOR 2000/40 dose (mg/mg)	non-HDL[b]	n[a]	SIMCOR 1000/40 Dose (mg/mg)	non-HDL[b]	n[a]	Simvastatin 80 Dose (mg/mg)	non-HDL[b]
Baseline	98	---	144.4 mg/dL	111	---	141.2 mg/dL	113	---	134.5 mg/dL
4	96	500/40	-6.0%	108	500/40	-5.9%	110	80	-11.3%
8	93	1000/40	-15.5%	100	1000/40	-16.2%	104	80	-13.7%
12	90	1500/40	-18.4%	97	1000/40	-12.6%	100	80	-9.5%
24	80	2000/40	-7.6%[c]	82	1000/40	-6.7%[d]	90	80	-6.0%
Dropouts by week 24:	18.4%			26.1%			20.4%		

[a] n=number of subjects with values in the analysis window at each timepoint
[b] The percent change from baseline is the model-based mean from a repeated measures mixed model with no imputation for missing data from study dropouts.
[c] non-inferior to Simvastatin 80 arm; 95% confidence interval of mean difference in non-HDL for SIMCOR 2000/40 vs. Simvastatin 80 is (-7.7%, 4.5%)
[d] non-inferior to Simvastatin 80 arm; 95% confidence interval of mean difference in non-HDL for SIMCOR 1000/40 vs. SIMCOR 80 is (-6.6%, 5.3%)

Elimination

SIMCOR

Following 2 × 1000/20 mg SIMCOR administration, approximately 54% of the niacin dose administered was recovered in urine in 96 hours as niacin and metabolites of which 3.6% was recovered as niacin.

After SIMCOR administration, the mean terminal plasma half-life for simvastatin was 4.2 to 4.9 hours and for simvastatin acid was 4.6 to 5.0 hours.

Niacin

Niacin and its metabolites are rapidly eliminated in the urine. Following single and multiple doses of 1500 to 2000 mg niacin, approximately 53 to 77% of the niacin dose administered as NIASPAN was recovered in urine as niacin and metabolites; up to 7.7% of the dose was recovered in urine as unchanged niacin after multiple dosing with 2 × 1000 mg NIASPAN. The ratio of metabolites recovered in the urine was dependent on the dose administered.

Simvastatin

Simvastatin is excreted in urine, based on studies in humans. Following an oral dose of ^{14}C-labeled simvastatin in man, 13% of the dose was excreted in urine and 60% in feces.

Special Populations

A pharmacokinetic study with simvastatin showed the mean plasma level of HMG-CoA reductase inhibitory activity to be approximately 45% higher in elderly patients between 70-78 years of age compared with patients between 18-30 years of age.

Steady-state plasma concentrations of niacin and metabolites after administration of niacin extended-release are generally higher in women than in men, with the magnitude of the difference varying with dose and metabolite. Recovery of niacin and metabolites in urine, however, is generally similar for men and women, indicating that absorption is similar for both genders. The gender differences observed in plasma levels of niacin and its metabolites may be due to gender-specific differences in metabolic rate or volume of distribution.

Pharmacokinetic studies with a statin having a similar principal route of elimination to that of simvastatin have suggested that for a given dose level, higher systemic exposure may be achieved in patients with severe renal insufficiency (as measured by creatinine clearance).

Drug Interaction

Effect of other drugs on simvastatin:

[See table on previous page]

Simvastatin effect on other drugs:

In a study of 12 healthy volunteers, simvastatin at the 80-mg dose had no effect on the metabolism of the probe cytochrome P450 isoform 3A4 (CYP3A4) substrates midazolam and erythromycin. This indicates that simvastatin is not an inhibitor of CYP3A4, and, therefore, is not expected to affect the plasma levels of other drugs metabolized by CYP3A4.

Coadministration of simvastatin (40 mg QD for 10 days) resulted in an increase in the maximum mean levels of cardioactive digoxin (given as a single 0.4 mg dose on day 10) by approximately 0.3 ng/mL.

Niacin effect on other drugs:

Niacin did not affect fluvastatin pharmacokinetics.

When NIASPAN 2000 mg and lovastatin 40 mg were coadministered, NIASPAN increased lovastatin C_{max} and AUC by 2% and 14%, respectively, and decreased lovastatin acid C_{max} and AUC by 22% and 2%, respectively. Lovastatin reduced NIASPAN bioavailability by 2-3%.

13   NONCLINICAL TOXICOLOGY

13.1   Carcinogenesis, Mutagenesis, Impairment of Fertility

No studies have been conducted with SIMCOR regarding carcinogenesis, mutagenesis, or impairment of fertility.

Niacin

Niacin, administered to mice for a lifetime as a 1% solution in drinking water, was not carcinogenic. The mice in this study received approximately 6 to 8 times a human dose of 3000 mg/day as determined on a mg/m^2 basis. Niacin was negative for mutagenicity in the Ames test. No studies on impairment of fertility have been performed.

Simvastatin

In a 72-week carcinogenicity study, mice were administered daily doses of simvastatin of 25, 100, and 400 mg/kg body weight, which resulted in mean plasma drug levels approximately 1, 4, and 8 times higher than the mean human plasma drug level, respectively (as total inhibitory activity based on AUC) after an 80-mg oral dose. Liver carcinomas were significantly increased in high-dose females and mid- and high-dose males with a maximum incidence of 90% in males. The incidence of adenomas of the liver was significantly increased in mid- and high-dose females. Drug treatment also significantly increased the incidence of lung adenomas in mid- and high-dose males and females. Adenomas of the Harderian gland (a gland of the eye of rodents) were significantly higher in high-dose mice than in controls. No evidence of a tumorigenic effect was observed at 25 mg/kg/day.

In a separate 92-week carcinogenicity study in mice at doses up to 25 mg/kg/day, no evidence of a tumorigenic effect was observed (mean plasma drug levels were 1 times higher than humans given 80 mg simvastatin as measured by AUC). In a two-year study in rats at 25 mg/kg/day, there was a statistically significant increase in the incidence of thyroid follicular adenomas in female rats exposed to approximately 11 times higher levels of simvastatin than in humans given 80 mg simvastatin (as measured by AUC). A second two-year rat carcinogenicity study with doses of 50 and 100 mg/kg/day produced hepatocellular adenomas and carcinomas (in female rats at both doses and in males at 100 mg/kg/day). Thyroid follicular cell adenomas were increased in males and females at both doses; thyroid follicular cell carcinomas were increased in females at 100 mg/kg/day. The increased incidence of thyroid neoplasms appears to be consistent with findings from other HMG-CoA reductase inhibitors. These treatment levels represented plasma drug levels (AUC) of approximately 7 and 15 times (males) and 22 and 25 times (females) the mean human plasma drug exposure after an 80 milligram daily dose. No evidence of mutagenicity was observed in a microbial mutagenicity (Ames) test with or without rat or mouse liver metabolic activation. In addition, no evidence of damage to genetic material was noted in an in vitro alkaline elution assay using rat hepatocytes, a V-79 mammalian cell forward mutation study, an in vitro chromosome aberration study in CHO cells, or an in vivo chromosomal aberration assay in mouse bone marrow. There was decreased fertility in male rats treated with simvastatin for 34 weeks at 25 mg/kg body weight (4 times the maximum human exposure level, based on AUC, in patients receiving 80 mg/day); however, this effect was not observed during a subsequent fertility study in which simvastatin was administered at this same dose level to male rats for 11 weeks (the entire cycle of spermatogenesis including epididymal maturation). No microscopic changes were observed in the testes of rats from either study. At 180 mg/kg/day, (which produces exposure levels 22 times higher than those in humans taking 80 mg/day based on surface area, mg/m^2), seminiferous tubule degeneration (necrosis and loss of spermatogenic epithelium) was observed. In dogs, there was drug-related testicular atrophy, decreased spermatogenesis, spermatocytic degeneration and giant cell formation at 10 mg/kg/day, (approximately 2 times the human exposure, based on AUC, at 80 mg/day). The clinical significance of these findings is unclear.

13.2   Animal Toxicology and/or Pharmacology

SIMCOR

No animal toxicology or pharmacology studies were done with SIMCOR.

Niacin

No animal toxicology or pharmacology studies were done with niacin extended-release.

Simvastatin

Optic nerve degeneration was seen in clinically normal dogs treated with simvastatin for 14 weeks at 180 mg/kg/day, a dose that produced mean plasma drug levels about 12 times higher than the mean plasma drug level in humans taking 80 mg/day. A chemically similar drug in this class also produced optic nerve degeneration (Wallerian degeneration of retinogeniculate fibers) in clinically normal dogs in a dose-dependent fashion starting at 60 mg/kg/day, a dose that produced mean plasma drug levels about 30 times higher than the mean plasma drug level in humans taking the highest recommended dose (as measured by total enzyme inhibitory activity). This same drug also produced vestibulocochlear Wallerian-like degeneration and retinal ganglion cell chromatolysis in dogs treated for 14 weeks at 180 mg/kg/day, a dose that resulted in a mean plasma drug level similar to that seen with the 60 mg/kg/day dose.

Central Nervous System (CNS) vascular lesions, characterized by perivascular hemorrhage and edema, mononuclear cell infiltration of perivascular spaces, perivascular fibrin deposits and necrosis of small vessels were seen in dogs treated with simvastatin at a dose of 360 mg/kg/day, a dose that produced mean plasma drug levels that were about 14 times higher than the mean plasma drug levels in humans taking 80 mg/day. Similar CNS vascular lesions have been observed with several other drugs of this class.

There were cataracts in female rats after two years of simvastatin treatment with 50 and 100 mg/kg/day (22 and 25 times the human AUC at 80 mg/day, respectively) and in dogs after three months at 90 mg/kg/day (19 times) and at two years at 50 mg/kg/day (5 times).

Reproductive Toxicology Studies

Simvastatin was not teratogenic in rats at doses of 25 mg/kg/day or in rabbits at doses up to 10 mg/kg/day. These doses resulted in 3 times (rat) or 3 times (rabbit) the human exposure based on mg/m^2 surface area. However, in studies with another structurally-related HMG-CoA reductase inhibitor, skeletal malformations were observed in rats and mice.

14 CLINICAL STUDIES

14.1 Modifications of Lipid Profiles

SIMCOR

In a double-blind, randomized, multicenter, multi-national, active-controlled, 24-week study, the lipid effects of SIMCOR were compared to simvastatin 20 mg and 80 mg in 641 patients with type II hyperlipidemia or mixed dyslipidemia. Following a lipid qualification phase, patients were eligible to enter one of two treatment groups. In Group A, patients on simvastatin 20 mg monotherapy with elevated non-HDL levels and LDL-C levels at goal, per the NCEP guidelines, were randomized to one of three treatment arms: SIMCOR 1000/20 mg, SIMCOR 2000/20 mg, or simvastatin 20 mg. In Group B, patients on simvastatin 40 mg monotherapy, with elevated non-HDL levels per the NCEP guidelines regardless of attainment of LDL-C goals, were randomized to one of three treatment arms: SIMCOR 1000/40 mg, SIMCOR 2000/40 mg, or simvastatin 80 mg. Therapy was initiated at the 500 mg dose of SIMCOR and increased by 500 mg every four weeks. Thus patients were titrated to the 1000 mg dose of SIMCOR after four weeks and to the 2000 mg dose of SIMCOR after 12 weeks. All patients randomized to simvastatin monotherapy received 50 mg immediate-release niacin daily in an attempt to keep the study from becoming unblinded due to flushing in the SIMCOR groups. Patients were instructed to take one 325 mg aspirin 30 minutes prior to taking the double-blind medication to help minimize flushing effects.

In Group A, the primary efficacy analysis was a comparison of the mean percent change in non-HDL levels between the SIMCOR 2000/20 mg and simvastatin 20 mg groups, and if statistically significant, then a comparison was conducted between the SIMCOR 1000/20 mg and simvastatin 20 mg groups. In Group B, the primary efficacy analysis was a determination of whether the mean percent change in non-HDL in the SIMCOR 2000/40 mg group was non-inferior to the mean percent change in the simvastatin 80 mg group, and if so, whether the mean percent change in non-HDL in the SIMCOR 1000/40 mg group was non-inferior to the mean percent change in the simvastatin 80 mg group.

In Group A, the non-HDL-C lowering with SIMCOR 2000/20 and SIMCOR 1000/20 was statistically significantly greater than that achieved with simvastatin 20 mg after 24 weeks (p<0.05; Table 6). The completion rate after 24 weeks was 72% for the SIMCOR arms and 88% for the simvastatin 20 mg arm. In Group B, the non-HDL-C lowering with SIMCOR 2000/40 and SIMCOR 1000/40 was non-inferior to that achieved with simvastatin 80 mg after 24 weeks (Table 7). The completion rate after 24 weeks was 78% for the SIMCOR arms and 80% for the simvastatin 80 mg arm.

SIMCOR was not superior to simvastatin in lowering LDL-C in either Group A or Group B. However, SIMCOR was superior to simvastatin in both groups in lowering TG and raising HDL (Tables 8 and 9).

[See table 6 at top of previous page]
[See table 7 at top of previous page]
[See table 8 above]
[See table 9 above]

16 HOW SUPPLIED/STORAGE AND HANDLING

SIMCOR 500 mg/20 mg, 750 mg/20 mg and 1000 mg/20 mg tablets are available as blue, unscored, tablets, printed with black ink and packaged in bottles of 90 tablets. SIMCOR 500 mg/40 mg and 1000 mg/40 mg tablets are available as dark blue, unscored, tablets, printed with white ink and packaged in bottles of 90 tablets. Each tablet is printed on one side with the "a" logo and a code number specific to the tablet strength. Please see the table below:

SIMCOR Tablet Strength	Printed ID	NDC Number
500 mg/20 mg	a 500-20	0074-3312-90
500 mg/40 mg	a 500-40	0074-3459-90
750 mg/20 mg	a 750-20	0074-3315-90
1000 mg/20 mg	a 1000-20	0074-3455-90
1000 mg/40 mg	a 1000-40	0074-3457-90

Storage: Store at controlled room temperature 20°-25°C (68°-77°F).

Table 8. Mean Percent Change from Baseline to Week 24 in Lipoprotein Lipid Levels

TREATMENT	N	Treatment Group A				
		LDL-C	Total-C	HDL-C	TG[a]	Apo B
Baseline (mg/dL)*	266	120	207	43	209	102
Simvastatin 20 mg	102	-6.7%	-4.5%	7.8%	-15.3%	-5.6%
SIMCOR 1000/20	108	-11.9%	-8.8%	20.7%	-26.5%	-13.2%
SIMCOR 2000/20	56	-14.3%	-11.1%	29.0%	-38.0%	-18.5%

* either treatment naïve or after receiving simvastatin 20 mg
[a] medians are reported for TG

Table 9. Mean Percent Change from Baseline to Week 24 in Lipoprotein Lipid Levels

TREATMENT	N	Treatment Group B				
		LDL-C	Total-C	HDL-C	TG[a]	Apo B
Baseline (mg/dL)*	322	108	187	47	145	93
Simvastatin 80 mg	113	-11.4%	-6.2%	0.1%	0.3%	-7.5%
SIMCOR 1000/40	111	-7.1%	-3.1%	15.4%	-22.8%	-7.7%
SIMCOR 2000/40	98	-5.1%	-1.6%	24.4%	-31.8%	-10.5%

* after receiving simvastatin 40 mg
[a] medians are reported for TG

17 PATIENT COUNSELING INFORMATION

Patients should be advised to adhere to their National Cholesterol Education Program (NCEP)-recommended diet, a regular exercise program, and periodic testing of a fasting lipid panel.

Patients should be advised about substances they should not take concomitantly with simvastatin [see Contraindications (4) and Warnings and Precautions (5.2)]. Patients should also be advised to inform other healthcare professionals prescribing a new medication or increasing the dose of an existing medication that they are taking SIMCOR.

17.1 Muscle Pain

All patients starting therapy with SIMCOR should be advised of the risk of myopathy, including rhabdomyolysis, and told to report promptly any unexplained muscle pain, tenderness or weakness particularly if accompanied by malaise or fever or if these muscle signs or symptoms persist after discontinuing SIMCOR. The risk of myopathy, including rhabdomyolysis, occurring with the use of SIMCOR is increased when taking certain types of medication or consuming larger quantities of grapefruit juice. Patients should discuss all medication, both prescription and over the counter, with their healthcare professional.

17.2 Liver Enzymes

It is recommended that liver enzyme tests be performed before the initiation of SIMCOR, and if signs or symptoms of liver injury occur. All patients treated with SIMCOR should be advised to report promptly any symptoms that may indicate liver injury, including fatigue, anorexia, right upper abdominal discomfort, dark urine or jaundice.

17.3 Dosing Time

SIMCOR tablets should be taken at bedtime, after a low-fat snack. Administration on an empty stomach is not recommended.

17.4 Tablet Integrity

SIMCOR tablets should not be broken, crushed or chewed, but should be swallowed whole.

17.5 Dosing Interruption

If dosing is interrupted for any length of time, their physician should be contacted prior to re-starting therapy; retitration is recommended.

17.6 Flushing

Flushing is a common side effect of niacin therapy that may subside after several weeks of consistent SIMCOR use. Flushing may vary in severity and is more likely to occur with initiation of therapy, or during dose increases. By dosing at bedtime, flushing will most likely occur during sleep. However, if awakened by flushing at night, the patient should get up slowly, especially if feeling dizzy, feeling faint, or taking blood pressure medications.

17.7 Use of Aspirin

Taking aspirin approximately 30 minutes before dosing can minimize flushing.

17.8 Diet

To avoid ingestion of alcohol, hot beverages and spicy foods around the time of taking SIMCOR to minimize flushing.

17.9 Supplements

To notify their physician if they are taking vitamins or other nutritional supplements containing niacin or nicotinamide.

17.10 Dizziness

To notify their physician if symptoms of dizziness occur.

17.11 Diabetics

If diabetic, to notify their physician of changes in blood glucose.

17.12 Pregnancy

Women of childbearing age should use an effective method of birth control to prevent pregnancy while using SIMCOR. Discuss future pregnancy plans with your healthcare professional, and discuss when to stop SIMCOR if you are trying to conceive. If you are pregnant, stop SIMCOR and call your healthcare professional.

17.13 Breastfeeding

Women who are breastfeeding should not use SIMCOR. If you have a lipid disorder and are breastfeeding, speak with your healthcare professionals about your lipid disorder and whether or not you should breastfeed your infant.

Manufactured by AbbVie LTD, Barceloneta, PR 00617 for AbbVie Inc., North Chicago, IL 60064, U.S.A.

Ref: 03-A744-R10-Revised March, 2013

Shown in Product Identification Guide, page 304

SURVANTA® ℞

(beractant)

intratracheal suspension

Sterile Suspension

For Intratracheal Administration Only

DESCRIPTION

SURVANTA® (beractant) Intratracheal Suspension is a sterile, non-pyrogenic pulmonary surfactant intended for intratracheal use only. It is a natural bovine lung extract containing phospholipids, neutral lipids, fatty acids, and surfactant-associated proteins to which colfosceril palmitate (dipalmitoylphosphatidylcholine), palmitic acid, and tripalmitin are added to standardize the composition and to mimic surface-tension lowering properties of natural lung surfactant. The resulting composition provides 25 mg/mL phospholipids (including 11.0-15.5 mg/mL disaturated phosphatidylcholine), 0.5-1.75 mg/mL triglycerides, 1.4-3.5 mg/mL free fatty acids, and less than 1.0 mg/mL protein. It is suspended in 0.9% sodium chloride solution, and heat-sterilized. SURVANTA contains no preservatives. Its protein content consists of two hydrophobic, low molecular weight, surfactant-associated proteins commonly known as SP-B and SP-C. It does not contain the hydrophilic, large molecular weight surfactant-associated protein known as SP-A.

Information on the AbbVie, Inc. products listed on these pages is from the prescribing information in use as of July 31, 2014. For more information, please visit rxabbvie.com or call 1-800-633-9110.

Each mL of SURVANTA contains 25 mg of phospholipids. It is an off-white to light brown liquid supplied in single-use glass vials containing 4 mL (100 mg phospholipids) or 8 mL (200 mg phospholipids).

CLINICAL PHARMACOLOGY

Endogenous pulmonary surfactant lowers surface tension on alveolar surfaces during respiration and stabilizes the alveoli against collapse at resting transpulmonary pressures. Deficiency of pulmonary surfactant causes Respiratory Distress Syndrome (RDS) in premature infants. SURVANTA replenishes surfactant and restores surface activity to the lungs of these infants.

Activity

In vitro, SURVANTA reproducibly lowers minimum surface tension to less than 8 dynes/cm as measured by the pulsating bubble surfactometer and Wilhelmy Surface Balance. *In situ*, SURVANTA restores pulmonary compliance to excised rat lungs artificially made surfactant-deficient. *In vivo*, single SURVANTA doses improve lung pressure-volume measurements, lung compliance, and oxygenation in premature rabbits and sheep.

Animal Metabolism

SURVANTA is administered directly to the target organ, the lungs, where biophysical effects occur at the alveolar surface. In surfactant-deficient premature rabbits and lambs, alveolar clearance of radio-labelled lipid components of SURVANTA is rapid. Most of the dose becomes lung-associated within hours of administration, and the lipids enter endogenous surfactant pathways of reutilization and recycling. In surfactant-sufficient adult animals, SURVANTA clearance is more rapid than in premature and young animals. There is less reutilization and recycling of surfactant in adult animals.

Limited animal experiments have not found effects of SURVANTA on endogenous surfactant metabolism. Precursor incorporation and subsequent secretion of saturated phosphatidylcholine in premature sheep are not changed by SURVANTA treatments.

No information is available about the metabolic fate of the surfactant-associated proteins in SURVANTA. The metabolic disposition in humans has not been studied.

Clinical Studies

Clinical effects of SURVANTA were demonstrated in six single-dose and four multiple-dose randomized, multi-center, controlled clinical trials involving approximately 1700 infants. Three open trials, including a Treatment IND, involved more than 8500 infants. Each dose of SURVANTA in all studies was 100 mg phospholipids/kg birth weight and was based on published experience with Surfactant TA, a lyophilized powder dosage form of SURVANTA having the same composition.

Prevention Studies

Infants of 600-1250 g birth weight and 23 to 29 weeks estimated gestational age were enrolled in two *multiple-dose* studies. A dose of SURVANTA was given within 15 minutes of birth to prevent the development of RDS. Up to three additional doses in the first 48 hours, as often as every 6 hours, were given if RDS subsequently developed and infants required mechanical ventilation with an $FiO_2 \geq 0.30$. Results of the studies at 28 days of age are shown in Table 1.

TABLE 1

Study 1

	SURVANTA	Control	P-Value
Number infants studied	119	124	
Incidence of RDS (%)	27.6	63.5	< 0.001
Death due to RDS (%)	2.5	19.5	< 0.001
Death or BPD due to RDS (%)	48.7	52.8	0.536
Death due to any cause (%)	7.6	22.8	0.001
Air Leaks[a] (%)	5.9	21.7	0.001
Pulmonary interstitial emphysema (%)	20.8	40.0	0.001

Study 2[b]

	SURVANTA	Control	P-Value
Number infants studied	91	96	
Incidence of RDS (%)	28.6	48.3	0.007
Death due to RDS (%)	1.1	10.5	0.006
Death or BPD due to RDS (%)	27.5	44.2	0.018
Death due to any cause [c] (%)	16.5	13.7	0.633
Air Leaks [a] (%)	14.5	19.6	0.374

Pulmonary interstitial emphysema (%)	26.5	33.2	0.298

[a]Pneumothorax or pneumopericardium
[b]Study discontinued when Treatment IND initiated
[c]No cause of death in the SURVANTA group was significantly increased; the higher number of deaths in this group was due to the sum of all causes.

Rescue Studies

Infants of 600-1750 g birth weight with RDS requiring mechanical ventilation and an $FiO_2 \geq 0.40$ were enrolled in two *multiple-dose* rescue studies. The initial dose of SURVANTA was given after RDS developed and before 8 hours of age. Infants could receive up to three additional doses in the first 48 hours, as often as every 6 hours, if they required mechanical ventilation and an $FiO_2 \geq 0.30$. Results of the studies at 28 days of age are shown in Table 2.

TABLE 2

Study 3[a]

	SURVANTA	Control	P-Value
Number infants studied	198	193	
Death due to RDS (%)	11.6	18.1	0.071
Death or BPD due to RDS (%)	59.1	66.8	0.102
Death due to any cause (%)	21.7	26.4	0.285
Air Leaks[b] (%)	11.8	29.5	<0.001
Pulmonary interstitial emphysema (%)	16.3	34.0	<0.001

Study 4

	SURVANTA	Control	P-Value
Number infants studied	204	203	
Death due to RDS (%)	6.4	22.3	< 0.001
Death or BPD due to RDS (%)	43.6	63.4	< 0.001
Death due to any cause (%)	15.2	28.2	0.001
Air Leaks[b] (%)	11.2	22.2	0.005
Pulmonary interstitial emphysema (%)	20.8	44.4	< 0.001

[a]Study discontinued when Treatment IND initiated
[b]Pneumothorax or pneumopericardium

Acute Clinical Effects

Marked improvements in oxygenation may occur within minutes of administration of SURVANTA.

All controlled clinical studies with SURVANTA provided information regarding the acute effects of SURVANTA on the arterial-alveolar oxygen ratio (a/APO$_2$), FiO_2, and mean airway pressure (MAP) during the first 48 to 72 hours of life. Significant improvements in these variables were sustained for 48-72 hours in SURVANTA-treated infants in four single-dose and two multiple-dose rescue studies and in two multiple-dose prevention studies. In the single-dose prevention studies, the FiO_2 improved significantly.

Indications and Usage

SURVANTA is indicated for prevention and treatment ("rescue") of Respiratory Distress Syndrome (RDS) (hyaline membrane disease) in premature infants. SURVANTA significantly reduces the incidence of RDS, mortality due to RDS and air leak complications.

Prevention

In premature infants less than 1250 g birth weight or with evidence of surfactant deficiency, give SURVANTA as soon as possible, preferably within 15 minutes of birth.

Rescue

To treat infants with RDS confirmed by x-ray and requiring mechanical ventilation, give SURVANTA as soon as possible, preferably by 8 hours of age.

Contraindications

None known.

Warnings

SURVANTA is intended for intratracheal use only.
SURVANTA CAN RAPIDLY AFFECT OXYGENATION AND LUNG COMPLIANCE. Therefore, its use should be restricted to a highly supervised clinical setting with immediate availability of clinicians experienced with intubation, ventilator management, and general care of premature infants. Infants receiving SURVANTA should be frequently monitored with arterial or transcutaneous measurement of systemic oxygen and carbon dioxide.
DURING THE DOSING PROCEDURE, TRANSIENT EPISODES OF BRADYCARDIA AND DECREASED OXYGEN

SATURATION HAVE BEEN REPORTED. If these occur, stop the dosing procedure and initiate appropriate measures to alleviate the condition. After stabilization, resume the dosing procedure.

Precautions

General

Rales and moist breath sounds can occur transiently after administration. Endotracheal suctioning or other remedial action is not necessary unless clear-cut signs of airway obstruction are present.

Increased probability of post-treatment nosocomial sepsis in SURVANTA-treated infants was observed in the controlled clinical trials (Table 3). The increased risk for sepsis among SURVANTA-treated infants was not associated with increased mortality among these infants. The causative organisms were similar in treated and control infants. There was no significant difference between groups in the rate of post-treatment infections other than sepsis.

Use of SURVANTA in infants less than 600 g birth weight or greater than 1750 g birth weight has not been evaluated in controlled trials. There is no controlled experience with use of SURVANTA in conjunction with experimental therapies for RDS (eg, high-frequency ventilation or extracorporeal membrane oxygenation).

No information is available on the effects of doses other than 100 mg phospholipids/kg, more than four doses, dosing more frequently than every 6 hours, or administration after 48 hours of age.

Carcinogenesis, Mutagenesis, Impairment of Fertility

Carcinogenicity studies have not been performed with SURVANTA. SURVANTA was negative when tested in the Ames test for mutagenicity. Using the maximum feasible dose volume, SURVANTA up to 500 mg phospholipids/kg/day (approximately one-third the premature infant dose based on mg/m^2/day) was administered subcutaneously to newborn rats for 5 days. The rats reproduced normally and there were no observable adverse effects in their offspring.

Adverse Reactions

The most commonly reported adverse experiences were associated with the dosing procedure. In the multiple-dose controlled clinical trials, each dose of SURVANTA was divided into four quarter-doses which were instilled through a catheter inserted into the endotracheal tube by briefly disconnecting the endotracheal tube from the ventilator. Transient bradycardia occurred in 11.9% of *doses*. Oxygen desaturation occurred with 9.8% of *doses*.

Other reactions during the dosing procedure occurred with fewer than 1% of doses and included endotracheal tube reflux, pallor, vasoconstriction, hypotension, endotracheal tube blockage, hypertension, hypocarbia, hypercarbia, and apnea. No deaths occurred during the dosing procedure, and all reactions resolved with symptomatic treatment.

The occurrence of concurrent illnesses common in premature infants was evaluated in the controlled trials. The rates in all controlled studies are in Table 3.

TABLE 3

	All Controlled Studies		
Concurrent Event	SURVANTA (%)	Control (%)	P-Value[a]
Patent ductus arteriosus	46.9	47.1	0.814
Intracranial hemorrhage	48.1	45.2	0.241
Severe intracranial hemorrhage	24.1	23.3	0.693
Pulmonary air leaks	10.9	24.7	< 0.001
Pulmonary interstitial emphysema	20.2	38.4	< 0.001
Necrotizing enterocolitis	6.1	5.3	0.427
Apnea	65.4	59.6	0.283
Severe apnea	46.1	42.5	0.114
Post-treatment sepsis	20.7	16.1	0.019
Post-treatment infection	10.2	9.1	0.345
Pulmonary hemorrhage	7.2	5.3	0.166

[a]P-value comparing groups in controlled studies

When all controlled studies were pooled, there was no difference in intracranial hemorrhage. However, in one of the single-dose rescue studies and one of the multiple-dose prevention studies, the rate of intracranial hemorrhage was significantly higher in SURVANTA patients than control patients (63.3% v 30.8%, P = 0.001; and 48.8% v 34.2%, P = 0.047, respectively). The rate in a Treatment IND involving approximately 8100 infants was lower than in the controlled trials.

In the controlled clinical trials, there was no effect of SURVANTA on results of common laboratory tests: white blood cell count and serum sodium, potassium, bilirubin, and creatinine.

More than 4300 pretreatment and post-treatment serum samples from approximately 1500 patients were tested by Western Blot Immunoassay for antibodies to surfactant-associated proteins SP-B and SP-C. No IgG or IgM antibodies were detected.

Several other complications are known to occur in premature infants. The following conditions were reported in the controlled clinical studies. The rates of the complications were not different in treated and control infants, and none of the complications were attributed to SURVANTA.

Respiratory
lung consolidation, blood from the endotracheal tube, deterioration after weaning, respiratory decompensation, subglottic stenosis, paralyzed diaphragm, respiratory failure.

Cardiovascular
hypotension, hypertension, tachycardia, ventricular tachycardia, aortic thrombosis, cardiac failure, cardio-respiratory arrest, increased apical pulse, persistent fetal circulation, air embolism, total anomalous pulmonary venous return.

Gastrointestinal
abdominal distention, hemorrhage, intestinal perforations, volvulus, bowel infarct, feeding intolerance, hepatic failure, stress ulcer.

Renal
renal failure, hematuria.

Hematologic
coagulopathy, thrombocytopenia, disseminated intravascular coagulation.

Central Nervous System
seizures.

Endocrine/Metabolic
adrenal hemorrhage, inappropriate ADH secretion, hyperphosphatemia.

Musculoskeletal
inguinal hernia.

Systemic
fever, deterioration.

Follow-Up Evaluations
To date, no long-term complications or sequelae of SURVANTA therapy have been found.

Single-Dose Studies
Six-month adjusted-age follow-up evaluations of 232 infants (115 treated) demonstrated no clinically important differences between treatment groups in pulmonary and neurologic sequelae, incidence or severity of retinopathy of prematurity, rehospitalizations, growth, or allergic manifestations.

Multiple-Dose Studies
Six-month adjusted age follow-up evaluations have been completed in 631 (345 treated) of 916 surviving infants. There were significantly less cerebral palsy and need for supplemental oxygen in SURVANTA infants than controls. Wheezing at the time of examination was significantly more frequent among SURVANTA infants, although there was no difference in bronchodilator therapy.

Final twelve-month follow-up data from the multiple-dose studies are available from 521 (272 treated) of 909 surviving infants. There was significantly less wheezing in SURVANTA infants than controls, in contrast to the six-month results. There was no difference in the incidence of cerebral palsy at twelve months.

Twenty-four month adjusted age evaluations were completed in 429 (226 treated) of 906 surviving infants. There were significantly fewer SURVANTA infants with rhonchi, wheezing, and tachypnea at the time of examination. No other differences were found.

Overdosage
Overdosage with SURVANTA has not been reported. Based on animal data, overdosage might result in acute airway obstruction. Treatment should be symptomatic and supportive.

Rales and moist breath sounds can transiently occur after SURVANTA is given, and do not indicate overdosage. Endotracheal suctioning or other remedial action is not required unless clear-cut signs of airway obstruction are present.

Dosage and Administration
FOR INTRATRACHEAL ADMINISTRATION ONLY.
SURVANTA should be administered by or under the supervision of clinicians experienced in intubation, ventilator management, and general care of premature infants.

Marked improvements in oxygenation may occur within minutes of administration of SURVANTA. Therefore, frequent and careful clinical observation and monitoring of systemic oxygenation are essential to avoid hyperoxia.

Review of audiovisual instructional materials describing dosage and administration procedures is recommended before using SURVANTA. Materials are available upon request from AbbVie Inc.

Dosage
Each dose of SURVANTA is 100 mg of phospholipids/kg birth weight (4 mL/kg). The SURVANTA DOSING CHART shows the total dosage for a range of birth weights.

SURVANTA DOSING CHART			
Weight (grams)	Total Dose (mL)	Weight (grams)	Total Dose (mL)
600-650	2.6	1301-1350	5.4
651-700	2.8	1351-1400	5.6
701-750	3.0	1401-1450	5.8
751-800	3.2	1451-1500	6.0
801-850	3.4	1501-1550	6.2
851-900	3.6	1551-1600	6.4
901-950	3.8	1601-1650	6.6
951-1000	4.0	1651-1700	6.8
1001-1050	4.2	1701-1750	7.0
1051-1100	4.4	1751-1800	7.2
1101-1150	4.6	1801-1850	7.4
1151-1200	4.8	1851-1900	7.6
1201-1250	5.0	1901-1950	7.8
1251-1300	5.2	1951-2000	8.0

Four doses of SURVANTA can be administered in the first 48 hours of life. Doses should be given no more frequently than every 6 hours.

Directions for Use
SURVANTA should be inspected visually for discoloration prior to administration. The color of SURVANTA is off-white to light brown. If settling occurs during storage, swirl the vial gently (DO NOT SHAKE) to redisperse. Some foaming at the surface may occur during handling and is inherent in the nature of the product.

SURVANTA is stored refrigerated (2-8°C). Date and time need to be recorded in the box on front of the carton or vial, whenever SURVANTA is removed from the refrigerator. Before administration, SURVANTA should be warmed by standing at room temperature for at least 20 minutes or warmed in the hand for at least 8 minutes. ARTIFICIAL WARMING METHODS SHOULD NOT BE USED. If a prevention dose is to be given, preparation of SURVANTA should begin before the infant's birth.

Unopened, unused vials of SURVANTA that have been warmed to room temperature may be returned to the refrigerator within 24 hours of warming, and stored for future use. SURVANTA SHOULD NOT BE REMOVED FROM THE REFRIGERATOR FOR MORE THAN 24 HOURS. SURVANTA SHOULD NOT BE WARMED AND RETURNED TO THE REFRIGERATOR MORE THAN ONCE. Each single-use vial of SURVANTA should be entered only once. Used vials with residual drug should be discarded. SURVANTA DOES NOT REQUIRE RECONSTITUTION OR SONICATION BEFORE USE.

Dosing Procedures
General
SURVANTA is administered intratracheally by instillation through a 5 French end-hole catheter. The catheter can be inserted into the infant's endotracheal tube without interrupting ventilation by passing the catheter through a neonatal suction valve attached to the endotracheal tube. Alternatively, SURVANTA can be instilled through the catheter by briefly disconnecting the endotracheal tube from the ventilator.

The neonatal suction valve used for administering SURVANTA should be a type that allows entry of the catheter into the endotracheal tube without interrupting ventilation and also maintains a closed airway circuit system by sealing the valve around the catheter.

If the neonatal suction valve is used, the catheter should be rigid enough to pass easily into the endotracheal tube. A very soft and pliable catheter may twist or curl within the neonatal suction valve. The length of the catheter should be shortened so that the tip of the catheter protrudes just beyond the end of the endotracheal tube above the infant's carina. SURVANTA should not be instilled into a mainstem bronchus.

To ensure homogenous distribution of SURVANTA throughout the lungs, each dose is divided into *four quarter-doses*. Each quarter-dose is administered with the infant in a different position. The recommended positions are:
• Head and body inclined 5-10° down, head turned to the right
• Head and body inclined 5-10° down, head turned to the left
• Head and body inclined 5-10° up, head turned to the right
• Head and body inclined 5-10° up, head turned to the left
The dosing procedure is facilitated if one person administers the dose while another person positions and monitors the infant.

First Dose
Determine the total dose of SURVANTA from the SURVANTA DOSING CHART based on the infant's birth weight. Slowly withdraw the entire contents of the vial into a plastic syringe through a large-gauge needle (eg, at least 20 gauge). DO NOT FILTER SURVANTA AND AVOID SHAKING.

Attach the premeasured 5 French end-hole catheter to the syringe. Fill the catheter with SURVANTA. Discard excess SURVANTA through the catheter so that only the total dose to be given remains in the syringe.

BEFORE ADMINISTERING SURVANTA, assure proper placement and patency of the endotracheal tube. At the discretion of the clinician, the endotracheal tube may be suctioned before administering SURVANTA. The infant should be allowed to stabilize before proceeding with dosing.

In the prevention strategy, weigh, intubate and stabilize the infant. Administer the dose as soon as possible after birth, preferably within 15 minutes. Position the infant appropriately and gently inject the first quarter-dose through the catheter over 2-3 seconds.

After administration of the first quarter-dose, remove the catheter from the endotracheal tube. Manually ventilate with a hand-bag with sufficient oxygen to prevent cyanosis, at a rate of 60 breaths/minute, and sufficient positive pressure to provide adequate air exchange and chest wall excursion.

In the rescue strategy, the first dose should be given as soon as possible after the infant is placed on a ventilator for management of RDS. In the clinical trials, immediately before instilling the first quarter-dose, the infant's ventilator settings were changed to rate 60/minute, inspiratory time 0.5 second, and FiO$_2$ 1.0.

Position the infant appropriately and gently inject the first quarter-dose through the catheter over 2-3 seconds. After administration of the first quarter-dose, remove the catheter from the endotracheal tube and continue mechanical ventilation.

In both strategies, ventilate the infant for at least 30 seconds or until stable. Reposition the infant for instillation of the next quarter-dose.

Instill the remaining quarter-doses using the same procedures. After instillation of each quarter-dose, remove the catheter and ventilate for at least 30 seconds or until the infant is stabilized. After instillation of the final quarter-dose, remove the catheter without flushing it. Do not suction the infant for 1 hour after dosing unless signs of significant airway obstruction occur.

AFTER COMPLETION OF THE DOSING PROCEDURE, RESUME USUAL VENTILATOR MANAGEMENT AND CLINICAL CARE.

Repeat Doses
The dosage of SURVANTA for repeat doses is also 100 mg phospholipids/kg and is based on the infant's birth weight. The infant should not be reweighed for determination of the SURVANTA dosage. Use the SURVANTA DOSING CHART to determine the total dosage.

The need for additional doses of SURVANTA is determined by evidence of continuing respiratory distress. Using the following criteria for redosing, significant reductions in mortality due to RDS were observed in the multiple-dose clinical trials with SURVANTA.

Dose no sooner than 6 hours after the preceding dose if the infant remains intubated and requires at least 30% inspired oxygen to maintain a PaO$_2$ less than or equal to 80 torr.

Radiographic confirmation of RDS should be obtained before administering additional doses to those who received a prevention dose.

Prepare SURVANTA and position the infant for administration of each quarter-dose as previously described. After instillation of each quarter-dose, remove the dosing catheter from the endotracheal tube and ventilate the infant for at least 30 seconds or until stable.

In the clinical studies, ventilator settings used to administer repeat doses were different than those used for the first dose. For repeat doses, the FiO$_2$ was increased by 0.20 or an amount sufficient to prevent cyanosis. The ventilator delivered a rate of 30/minute with an inspiratory time less than 1.0 second. If the infant's pretreatment rate was 30 or greater, it was left unchanged during SURVANTA instillation.

Manual hand-bag ventilation should not be used to administer repeat doses. DURING THE DOSING PROCEDURE, VENTILATOR SETTINGS MAY BE ADJUSTED AT THE DISCRETION OF THE CLINICIAN TO MAINTAIN APPROPRIATE OXYGENATION AND VENTILATION.

AFTER COMPLETION OF THE DOSING PROCEDURE, RESUME USUAL VENTILATOR MANAGEMENT AND CLINICAL CARE.

Dosing Precautions
If an infant experiences bradycardia or oxygen desaturation during the dosing procedure, stop the dosing procedure and

Information on the AbbVie, Inc. products listed on these pages is from the prescribing information in use as of July 31, 2014. For more information, please visit rxabbvie.com or call 1-800-633-9110.

initiate appropriate measures to alleviate the condition. After the infant has stabilized, resume the dosing procedure. Rales and moist breath sounds can occur transiently after administration of SURVANTA. Endotracheal suctioning or other remedial action is unnecessary unless clear-cut signs of airway obstruction are present.

How Supplied

SURVANTA (beractant) Intratracheal Suspension is supplied in single-use glass vials containing 4 mL (NDC 0074-1040-04) or 8 mL of SURVANTA (NDC 0074-1040-08). Each milliliter contains 25 mg of phospholipids suspended in 0.9% sodium chloride solution. The color is off-white to light brown.

Store unopened vials at refrigeration temperature (2-8°C). Protect from light. Store vials in carton until ready for use. Vials are for single use only. Upon opening, discard unused drug.

LITHO IN USA

AbbVie Inc.

North Chicago, IL 60064, U.S.A.

03-A683 December, 2012

Shown in Product Identification Guide, page 304

SYNTHROID® ℞

[sĭn-thrŏĭd]

(levothyroxine sodium tablets, USP)

DESCRIPTION

SYNTHROID (levothyroxine sodium tablets, USP) contain synthetic crystalline L-3,3',5,5'-tetraiodothyronine sodium salt [levothyroxine (T_4) sodium]. Synthetic T_4 is identical to that produced in the human thyroid gland. Levothyroxine (T_4) sodium has an empirical formula of $C_{15}H_{10}I_4N\ NaO_4 \cdot H_2O$, molecular weight of 798.86 g/mol (anhydrous), and structural formula as shown:

Inactive Ingredients

Acacia, confectioner's sugar (contains corn starch), lactose monohydrate, magnesium stearate, povidone, and talc. The following are the color additives by tablet strength:

Strength (mcg)	Color additive(s)
25	FD&C Yellow No. 6 Aluminum Lake*
50	None
75	FD&C Red No. 40 Aluminum Lake, FD&C Blue No. 2 Aluminum Lake
88	FD&C Blue No. 1 Aluminum Lake, FD&C Yellow No. 6 Aluminum Lake*, D&C Yellow No. 10 Aluminum Lake
100	D&C Yellow No. 10 Aluminum Lake, FD&C Yellow No. 6 Aluminum Lake*
112	D&C Red No. 27 & 30 Aluminum Lake
125	FD&C Yellow No. 6 Aluminum Lake*, FD&C Red No. 40 Aluminum Lake, FD&C Blue No. 1 Aluminum Lake
137	FD&C Blue No. 1 Aluminum Lake
150	FD&C Blue No. 2 Aluminum Lake
175	FD&C Blue No. 1 Aluminum Lake, D&C Red No. 27 & 30 Aluminum Lake
200	FD&C Red No. 40 Aluminum Lake
300	D&C Yellow No. 10 Aluminum Lake, FD&C Yellow No. 6 Aluminum Lake*, FD&C Blue No. 1 Aluminum Lake

*Note – FD&C Yellow No. 6 is orange in color.
Meets USP Dissolution Test 3

CLINICAL PHARMACOLOGY

Thyroid hormone synthesis and secretion is regulated by the hypothalamic-pituitary-thyroid axis. Thyrotropin-releasing hormone (TRH) released from the hypothalamus stimulates secretion of thyrotropin-stimulating hormone, TSH, from the anterior pituitary. TSH, in turn, is the physiologic stimulus for the synthesis and secretion of thyroid hormones, L-thyroxine (T_4) and L-triiodothyronine (T_3), by the thyroid gland. Circulating serum T_3 and T_4 levels exert a feedback effect on both TRH and TSH secretion. When serum T_3 and T_4 levels increase, TRH and TSH secretion decrease. When thyroid hormone levels decrease, TRH and TSH secretion increase.

The mechanisms by which thyroid hormones exert their physiologic actions are not completely understood, but it is thought that their principal effects are exerted through con-

Table 1. Pharmacokinetic Parameters of Thyroid Hormones in Euthyroid Patients

Hormone	Ratio in Thyroglobulin	Biologic Potency	$t_{1/2}$ (days)	Protein Binding (%)[2]
Levothyroxine (T_4)	10 - 20	1	6-7[1]	99.96
Liothyronine (T_3)	1	4	≤ 2	99.5

[1] 3 to 4 days in hyperthyroidism, 9 to 10 days in hypothyroidism
[2] Includes TBG, TBPA, and TBA

---

trol of DNA transcription and protein synthesis. T_3 and T_4 diffuse into the cell nucleus and bind to thyroid receptor proteins attached to DNA. This hormone nuclear receptor complex activates gene transcription and synthesis of messenger RNA and cytoplasmic proteins.

Thyroid hormones regulate multiple metabolic processes and play an essential role in normal growth and development, and normal maturation of the central nervous system and bone. The metabolic actions of thyroid hormones include augmentation of cellular respiration and thermogenesis, as well as metabolism of proteins, carbohydrates and lipids. The protein anabolic effects of thyroid hormones are essential to normal growth and development.

The physiological actions of thyroid hormones are produced predominantly by T_3, the majority of which (approximately 80%) is derived from T_4 by deiodination in peripheral tissues.

Levothyroxine, at doses individualized according to patient response, is effective as replacement or supplemental therapy in hypothyroidism of any etiology, except transient hypothyroidism during the recovery phase of subacute thyroiditis.

Levothyroxine is also effective in the suppression of pituitary TSH secretion in the treatment or prevention of various types of euthyroid goiters, including thyroid nodules, Hashimoto's thyroiditis, multinodular goiter and, as adjunctive therapy in the management of thyrotropin-dependent well-differentiated thyroid cancer (see **INDICATIONS AND USAGE**, **PRECAUTIONS**, and **DOSAGE AND ADMINISTRATION**).

Pharmacokinetics

Absorption

Absorption of orally administered T_4 from the gastrointestinal (GI) tract ranges from 40% to 80%. The majority of the levothyroxine dose is absorbed from the jejunum and upper ileum. The relative bioavailability of SYNTHROID tablets, compared to an equal nominal dose of oral levothyroxine sodium solution, is approximately 93%. T_4 absorption is increased by fasting, and decreased in malabsorption syndromes and by certain foods such as soybean infant formula. Dietary fiber decreases bioavailability of T_4. Absorption may also decrease with age. In addition, many drugs and foods affect T_4 absorption (see **PRECAUTIONS - Drug Interactions** and **Drug-Food Interactions**).

Distribution

Circulating thyroid hormones are greater than 99% bound to plasma proteins, including thyroxine-binding globulin (TBG), thyroxine-binding prealbumin (TBPA), and albumin (TBA), whose capacities and affinities vary for each hormone. The higher affinity of both TBG and TBPA for T_4 partially explains the higher serum levels, slower metabolic clearance, and longer half-life of T_4 compared to T_3. Protein-bound thyroid hormones exist in reverse equilibrium with small amounts of free hormone. Only unbound hormone is metabolically active. Many drugs and physiologic conditions affect the binding of thyroid hormones to serum proteins (see **PRECAUTIONS - Drug Interactions** and **Drug-Laboratory Test Interactions**). Thyroid hormones do not readily cross the placental barrier (see **PRECAUTIONS - Pregnancy**).

Metabolism

T_4 is slowly eliminated (see **Table 1**). The major pathway of thyroid hormone metabolism is through sequential deiodination. Approximately eighty-percent of circulating T_3 is derived from peripheral T_4 by monodeiodination. The liver is the major site of degradation for both T_4 and T_3, with T_4 deiodination also occurring at a number of additional sites, including the kidney and other tissues. Approximately 80% of the daily dose of T_4 is deiodinated to yield equal amounts of T_3 and reverse T_3 (rT_3). T_3 and rT_3 are further deiodinated to diiodothyronine. Thyroid hormones are also metabolized via conjugation with glucuronides and sulfates and excreted directly into the bile and gut where they undergo enterohepatic recirculation.

Elimination

Thyroid hormones are primarily eliminated by the kidneys. A portion of the conjugated hormone reaches the colon unchanged and is eliminated in the feces. Approximately 20% of T_4 is eliminated in the stool. Urinary excretion of T_4 decreases with age.

[See table 1 above]

INDICATIONS AND USAGE

Levothyroxine sodium is used for the following indications:

Hypothyroidism

As replacement or supplemental therapy in congenital or acquired hypothyroidism of any etiology, except transient hypothyroidism during the recovery phase of subacute thyroiditis. Specific indications include: primary (thyroidal), secondary (pituitary), and tertiary (hypothalamic) hypothyroidism and subclinical hypothyroidism. Primary hypothyroidism may result from functional deficiency, primary atrophy, partial or total congenital absence of the thyroid gland, or from the effects of surgery, radiation, or drugs, with or without the presence of goiter.

Pituitary TSH Suppression

In the treatment or prevention of various types of euthyroid goiters (see **WARNINGS** and **PRECAUTIONS**), including thyroid nodules (see **WARNINGS** and **PRECAUTIONS**), subacute or chronic lymphocytic thyroiditis (Hashimoto's thyroiditis), multinodular goiter (see **WARNINGS** and **PRECAUTIONS**) and, as an adjunct to surgery and radioiodine therapy in the management of thyrotropin-dependent well-differentiated thyroid cancer.

CONTRAINDICATIONS

Levothyroxine is contraindicated in patients with untreated subclinical (suppressed serum TSH level with normal T_3 and T_4 levels) or overt thyrotoxicosis of any etiology and in patients with acute myocardial infarction. Levothyroxine is contraindicated in patients with uncorrected adrenal insufficiency since thyroid hormones may precipitate an acute adrenal crisis by increasing the metabolic clearance of glucocorticoids (see **PRECAUTIONS**). SYNTHROID is contraindicated in patients with hypersensitivity to any of the inactive ingredients in SYNTHROID tablets (See **DESCRIPTION - Inactive Ingredients**).

WARNINGS

> **Boxed Warning**
> **WARNING: Thyroid hormones, including SYNTHROID, either alone or with other therapeutic agents, should not be used for the treatment of obesity or for weight loss. In euthyroid patients, doses within the range of daily hormonal requirements are ineffective for weight reduction. Larger doses may produce serious or even life threatening manifestations of toxicity, particularly when given in association with sympathomimetic amines such as those used for their anorectic effects.**

Levothyroxine sodium should not be used in the treatment of male or female infertility unless this condition is associated with hypothyroidism.

In patients with nontoxic diffuse goiter or nodular thyroid disease, particularly the elderly or those with underlying cardiovascular disease, levothyroxine sodium therapy is contraindicated if the serum TSH level is already suppressed due to the risk of precipitating overt thyrotoxicosis (see **CONTRAINDICATIONS**). If the serum TSH level is not suppressed, SYNTHROID should be used with caution in conjunction with careful monitoring of thyroid function for evidence of hyperthyroidism and clinical monitoring for potential associated adverse cardiovascular signs and symptoms of hyperthyroidism.

PRECAUTIONS

General

Levothyroxine has a narrow therapeutic index. Regardless of the indication for use, careful dosage titration is necessary to avoid the consequences of over- or under-treatment. These consequences include, among others, effects on growth and development, cardiovascular function, bone metabolism, reproductive function, cognitive function, emotional state, gastrointestinal function, and on glucose and lipid metabolism. Many drugs interact with levothyroxine sodium necessitating adjustments in dosing to maintain therapeutic response (see **Drug Interactions**).

Effects on Bone Mineral Density

In women, long-term levothyroxine sodium therapy has been associated with increased bone resorption, thereby decreasing bone mineral density, especially in postmenopausal women on greater than replacement doses or in women who are receiving suppressive doses of levothyroxine sodium. The increased bone resorption may be associated with increased serum levels and urinary excretion of calcium and phosphorous, elevations in bone alkaline phosphatase and suppressed serum parathyroid hormone levels. Therefore, it is recommended that patients receiving levothyroxine sodium be given the minimum dose necessary to achieve the desired clinical and biochemical response.

Patients with Underlying Cardiovascular Disease

Exercise caution when administering levothyroxine to patients with cardiovascular disorders and to the elderly in whom there is an increased risk of occult cardiac disease. In these patients, levothyroxine therapy should be initiated at lower doses than those recommended in younger individuals or in patients without cardiac disease (see **WARNINGS, PRECAUTIONS - Geriatric Use,** and **DOSAGE AND ADMINISTRATION**). If cardiac symptoms develop or worsen, the levothyroxine dose should be reduced or withheld for one week and then cautiously restarted at a lower dose. Overtreatment with levothyroxine sodium may have adverse cardiovascular effects such as an increase in heart rate, cardiac wall thickness, and cardiac contractility and may precipitate angina or arrhythmias. Patients with coronary artery disease who are receiving levothyroxine therapy should be monitored closely during surgical procedures, since the possibility of precipitating cardiac arrhythmias may be greater in those treated with levothyroxine. Concomitant administration of levothyroxine and sympathomimetic agents to patients with coronary artery disease may precipitate coronary insufficiency.

Patients with Nontoxic Diffuse Goiter or Nodular Thyroid Disease

Exercise caution when administering levothyroxine to patients with nontoxic diffuse goiter or nodular thyroid disease in order to prevent precipitation of thyrotoxicosis (see **WARNINGS**). If the serum TSH is already suppressed, levothyroxine sodium should not be administered (see **CONTRAINDICATIONS**).

Associated Endocrine Disorders

Hypothalamic/pituitary hormone deficiencies

In patients with secondary or tertiary hypothyroidism, additional hypothalamic/pituitary hormone deficiencies should be considered, and, if diagnosed, treated (see **PRECAUTIONS - Autoimmune polyglandular syndrome** for adrenal insufficiency).

Autoimmune polyglandular syndrome

Occasionally, chronic autoimmune thyroiditis may occur in association with other autoimmune disorders such as adrenal insufficiency, pernicious anemia, and insulin-dependent diabetes mellitus. Patients with concomitant adrenal insufficiency should be treated with replacement glucocorticoids prior to initiation of treatment with levothyroxine sodium. Failure to do so may precipitate an acute adrenal crisis when thyroid hormone therapy is initiated, due to increased metabolic clearance of glucocorticoids by thyroid hormone. Patients with diabetes mellitus may require upward adjustments of their antidiabetic therapeutic regimens when treated with levothyroxine (see **PRECAUTIONS - Drug Interactions**).

Other associated medical conditions

Infants with congenital hypothyroidism appear to be at increased risk for other congenital anomalies, with cardiovascular anomalies (pulmonary stenosis, atrial septal defect, and ventricular septal defect) being the most common association.

Information for Patients

Patients should be informed of the following information to aid in the safe and effective use of SYNTHROID:

1. Notify your physician if you are allergic to any foods or medicines, are pregnant or intend to become pregnant, are breast-feeding or are taking any other medications, including prescription and over-the-counter preparations.
2. Notify your physician of any other medical conditions you may have, particularly heart disease, diabetes, clotting disorders, and adrenal or pituitary gland problems. Your dose of medications used to control these other conditions may need to be adjusted while you are taking SYNTHROID. If you have diabetes, monitor your blood and/or urinary glucose levels as directed by your physician and immediately report any changes to your physician. If you are taking anticoagulants (blood thinners), your clotting status should be checked frequently.
3. Use SYNTHROID only as prescribed by your physician. Do not discontinue or change the amount you take or how often you take it, unless directed to do so by your physician.
4. The levothyroxine in SYNTHROID is intended to replace a hormone that is normally produced by your thyroid gland. Generally, replacement therapy is to be taken for life, except in cases of transient hypothyroidism, which is usually associated with an inflammation of the thyroid gland (thyroiditis).
5. Take SYNTHROID as a single dose, preferably on an empty stomach, one-half to one hour before breakfast. Levothyroxine absorption is increased on an empty stomach.

6. It may take several weeks before you notice an improvement in your symptoms.
7. Notify your physician if you experience any of the following symptoms: rapid or irregular heartbeat, chest pain, shortness of breath, leg cramps, headache, nervousness, irritability, sleeplessness, tremors, change in appetite, weight gain or loss, vomiting, diarrhea, excessive sweating, heat intolerance, fever, changes in menstrual periods, hives or skin rash, or any other unusual medical event.
8. Notify your physician if you become pregnant while taking SYNTHROID. It is likely that your dose of SYNTHROID will need to be increased while you are pregnant.
9. Notify your physician or dentist that you are taking SYNTHROID prior to any surgery.
10. Partial hair loss may occur rarely during the first few months of SYNTHROID therapy, but this is usually temporary.
11. SYNTHROID should not be used as a primary or adjunctive therapy in a weight control program.
12. Keep SYNTHROID out of the reach of children. Store SYNTHROID away from heat, moisture, and light.
13. Agents such as iron and calcium supplements and antacids can decrease the absorption of levothyroxine sodium tablets. Therefore, levothyroxine sodium tablets should not be administered within 4 hours of these agents.

Laboratory Tests

General

The diagnosis of hypothyroidism is confirmed by measuring TSH levels using a sensitive assay (second generation assay sensitivity ≤ 0.1 mIU/L or third generation assay sensitivity ≤ 0.01 mIU/L) and measurement of free-T_4.

The adequacy of therapy is determined by periodic assessment of appropriate laboratory tests and clinical evaluation. The choice of laboratory tests depends on various factors including the etiology of the underlying thyroid disease, the presence of concomitant medical conditions, including pregnancy, and the use of concomitant medications (see **PRECAUTIONS - Drug Interactions** and **Drug-Laboratory Test Interactions**). Persistent clinical and laboratory evidence of hypothyroidism despite an apparent adequate replacement dose of SYNTHROID may be evidence of inadequate absorption, poor compliance, drug interactions, or decreased T_4 potency of the drug product.

Adults

In adult patients with primary (thyroidal) hypothyroidism, serum TSH levels (using a sensitive assay) alone may be used to monitor therapy. The frequency of TSH monitoring during levothyroxine dose titration depends on the clinical situation but it is generally recommended at 6-8 week intervals until normalization. For patients who have recently initiated levothyroxine therapy and whose serum TSH has normalized or in patients who have had their dosage or brand of levothyroxine changed, the serum TSH concentration should be measured after 8-12 weeks. When the optimum replacement dose has been attained, clinical (physical examination) and biochemical monitoring may be performed every 6-12 months, depending on the clinical situation, and whenever there is a change in the patient's status. It is recommended that a physical examination and a serum TSH measurement be performed at least annually in patients receiving SYNTHROID (see **WARNINGS, PRECAUTIONS,** and **DOSAGE AND ADMINISTRATION**).

Pediatrics

In patients with congenital hypothyroidism, the adequacy of replacement therapy should be assessed by measuring both serum TSH (using a sensitive assay) and total- or free- T_4. During the first three years of life, the serum total- or free-T_4 should be maintained at all times in the upper half of the normal range. While the aim of therapy is to also normalize the serum TSH level, this is not always possible in a small percentage of patients, particularly in the first few months of therapy. TSH may not normalize due to a resetting of the pituitary-thyroid feedback threshold as a result of *in utero* hypothyroidism. Failure of the serum T_4 to increase into the upper half of the normal range within 2 weeks of initiation of SYNTHROID therapy and/or of the serum TSH to decrease below 20 mU/L within 4 weeks should alert the physician to the possibility that the child is not receiving adequate therapy. Careful inquiry should then be made regarding compliance, dose of medication administered, and method of administration prior to raising the dose of SYNTHROID.

The recommended frequency of monitoring of TSH and total or free T_4 in children is as follows: at 2 and 4 weeks after the initiation of treatment; every 1-2 months during the first year of life; every 2-3 months between 1 and 3 years of age; and every 3 to 12 months thereafter until growth is completed. More frequent intervals of monitoring may be necessary if poor compliance is suspected or abnormal values are obtained. It is recommended that TSH and T_4 levels, and a physical examination, if indicated, be performed 2

weeks after any change in SYNTHROID dosage. Routine clinical examination, including assessment of mental and physical growth and development, and bone maturation, should be performed at regular intervals (see **PRECAUTIONS - Pediatric Use** and **DOSAGE AND ADMINISTRATION**).

Secondary (Pituitary) and Tertiary (Hypothalamic) Hypothyroidism

Adequacy of therapy should be assessed by measuring serum free-T_4 levels, which should be maintained in the upper half of the normal range in these patients.

Drug Interactions

Many drugs affect thyroid hormone pharmacokinetics and metabolism (e.g., absorption, synthesis, secretion, catabolism, protein binding, and target tissue response) and may alter the therapeutic response to SYNTHROID. In addition, thyroid hormones and thyroid status have varied effects on the pharmacokinetics and actions of other drugs. A listing of drug-thyroidal axis interactions is contained in Table 2.

The list of drug-thyroidal axis interactions in Table 2 may not be comprehensive due to the introduction of new drugs that interact with the thyroidal axis or the discovery of previously unknown interactions. The prescriber should be aware of this fact and should consult appropriate reference sources (e.g., package inserts of newly approved drugs, medical literature) for additional information if a drug-drug interaction with levothyroxine is suspected.

[See table 2 on pages 580 through 582]

Oral anticoagulants

Levothyroxine increases the response to oral anticoagulant therapy. Therefore, a decrease in the dose of anticoagulant may be warranted with correction of the hypothyroid state or when the SYNTHROID dose is increased. Prothrombin time should be closely monitored to permit appropriate and timely dosage adjustments (see **Table 2**).

Digitalis glycosides

The therapeutic effects of digitalis glycosides may be reduced by levothyroxine. Serum digitalis glycoside levels may be decreased when a hypothyroid patient becomes euthyroid, necessitating an increase in the dose of digitalis glycosides (see **Table 2**).

Drug-Food Interactions

Consumption of certain foods may affect levothyroxine absorption thereby necessitating adjustments in dosing. Soybean flour (infant formula), cotton seed meal, walnuts, and dietary fiber may bind and decrease the absorption of levothyroxine sodium from the GI tract.

Drug-Laboratory Test Interactions

Changes in TBG concentration must be considered when interpreting T_4 and T_3 values, which necessitates measurement and evaluation of unbound (free) hormone and/or determination of the free T_4 index (FT_4I). Pregnancy, infectious hepatitis, estrogens, estrogen-containing oral contraceptives, and acute intermittent porphyria increase TBG concentrations. Decreases in TBG concentrations are observed in nephrosis, severe hypoproteinemia, severe liver disease, acromegaly, and after androgen or corticosteroid therapy (see also **Table 2**). Familial hyper- or hypothyroxine binding globulinemias have been described, with the incidence of TBG deficiency approximating 1 in 9000.

Carcinogenesis, Mutagenesis, and Impairment of Fertility

Animal studies have not been performed to evaluate the carcinogenic potential, mutagenic potential or effects on fertility of levothyroxine. The synthetic T_4 in SYNTHROID is identical to that produced naturally by the human thyroid gland. Although there has been a reported association between prolonged thyroid hormone therapy and breast cancer, this has not been confirmed. Patients receiving SYNTHROID for appropriate clinical indications should be titrated to the lowest effective replacement dose.

Pregnancy

Category A

Studies in women taking levothyroxine sodium during pregnancy have not shown an increased risk of congenital abnormalities. Therefore, the possibility of fetal harm appears remote. SYNTHROID should not be discontinued during pregnancy and hypothyroidism diagnosed during pregnancy should be promptly treated.

Hypothyroidism during pregnancy is associated with a higher rate of complications, including spontaneous abortion, pre-eclampsia, stillbirth and premature delivery. Maternal hypothyroidism may have an adverse effect on fetal and childhood growth and development. During pregnancy, serum T_4 levels may decrease and serum TSH levels increase to values outside the normal range. Since elevations in serum TSH may occur as early as 4 weeks gestation, pregnant women taking SYNTHROID should have their

Information on the AbbVie, Inc. products listed on these pages is from the prescribing information in use as of July 31, 2014. For more information, please visit rxabbvie.com or call 1-800-633-9110.

TSH measured during each trimester. An elevated serum TSH level should be corrected by an increase in the dose of SYNTHROID. Since postpartum TSH levels are similar to preconception values, the SYNTHROID dosage should return to the pre-pregnancy dose immediately after delivery. A serum TSH level should be obtained 6-8 weeks postpartum.

Thyroid hormones cross the placental barrier to some extent as evidenced by levels in cord blood of athyreotic fetuses being approximately one-third maternal levels. Transfer of thyroid hormone from the mother to the fetus, however, may not be adequate to prevent *in utero* hypothyroidism.

Nursing Mothers
Although thyroid hormones are excreted only minimally in human milk, caution should be exercised when SYNTHROID is administered to a nursing woman. However, adequate replacement doses of levothyroxine are generally needed to maintain normal lactation.

Pediatric Use
General
The goal of treatment in pediatric patients with hypothyroidism is to achieve and maintain normal intellectual and physical growth and development.

The initial dose of levothyroxine varies with age and body weight (see **DOSAGE AND ADMINISTRATION - Table 3**). Dosing adjustments are based on an assessment of the individual patient's clinical and laboratory parameters (see **PRECAUTIONS - Laboratory Tests**).

In children in whom a diagnosis of permanent hypothyroidism has not been established, it is recommended that levothyroxine administration be discontinued for a 30-day trial period, but only after the child is at least 3 years of age. Serum T_4 and TSH levels should then be obtained. If the T_4 is low and the TSH high, the diagnosis of permanent hypothyroidism is established, and levothyroxine therapy should be reinstituted. If the T_4 and TSH levels are normal, euthyroidism may be assumed and, therefore, the hypothyroidism can be considered to have been transient. In this instance, however, the physician should carefully monitor the child and repeat the thyroid function tests if any signs or symptoms of hypothyroidism develop. In this setting, the clinician should have a high index of suspicion of relapse. If the results of the levothyroxine withdrawal test are inconclusive, careful follow-up and subsequent testing will be necessary.

Since some more severely affected children may become clinically hypothyroid when treatment is discontinued for 30 days, an alternate approach is to reduce the replacement dose of levothyroxine by half during the 30-day trial period. If, after 30 days, the serum TSH is elevated above 20 mU/L, the diagnosis of permanent hypothyroidism is confirmed, and full replacement therapy should be resumed. However, if the serum TSH has not risen to greater than 20 mU/L, levothyroxine treatment should be discontinued for another 30-day trial period followed by repeat serum T_4 and TSH testing.

The presence of concomitant medical conditions should be considered in certain clinical circumstances and, if present, appropriately treated (see **PRECAUTIONS**).

Congenital Hypothyroidism
(see **PRECAUTIONS - Laboratory Tests** and **DOSAGE AND ADMINISTRATION**)
Rapid restoration of normal serum T_4 concentrations is essential for preventing the adverse effects of congenital hypothyroidism on intellectual development as well as on overall physical growth and maturation. Therefore, SYNTHROID therapy should be initiated immediately upon diagnosis and is generally continued for life.

During the first 2 weeks of SYNTHROID therapy, infants should be closely monitored for cardiac overload, arrhythmias, and aspiration from avid suckling.

The patient should be monitored closely to avoid undertreatment or overtreatment. Undertreatment may have deleterious effects on intellectual development and linear growth. Overtreatment has been associated with craniosynostosis in infants, and may adversely affect the tempo of brain maturation and accelerate the bone age with resultant premature closure of the epiphyses and compromised adult stature.

Acquired Hypothyroidism in Pediatric Patients
The patient should be monitored closely to avoid undertreatment and overtreatment. Undertreatment may result in poor school performance due to impaired concentration and slowed mentation and in reduced adult height. Overtreatment may accelerate the bone age and result in premature epiphyseal closure and compromised adult stature.

Treated children may manifest a period of catch-up growth, which may be adequate in some cases to normalize adult height. In children with severe or prolonged hypothyroidism, catch-up growth may not be adequate to normalize adult height.

Geriatric Use
Because of the increased prevalence of cardiovascular disease among the elderly, levothyroxine therapy should not be

initiated at the full replacement dose (see **WARNINGS, PRECAUTIONS**, and **DOSAGE AND ADMINISTRATION**).

ADVERSE REACTIONS
Adverse reactions associated with levothyroxine therapy are primarily those of hyperthyroidism due to therapeutic overdosage (see **PRECAUTIONS** and **OVERDOSAGE**). They include the following:

General
fatigue, increased appetite, weight loss, heat intolerance, fever, excessive sweating;
Central nervous system
headache, hyperactivity, nervousness, anxiety, irritability, emotional lability, insomnia;
Musculoskeletal
tremors, muscle weakness;

Table 2. Drug-Thyroidal Axis Interactions

Drug or Drug Class	Effect
Drugs that may reduce TSH secretion – the reduction is not sustained; therefore, hypothyroidism does not occur	
Dopamine/Dopamine Agonists Glucocorticoids Octreotide	Use of these agents may result in a transient reduction in TSH secretion when administered at the following doses: Dopamine (≥ 1 mcg/kg/min); Glucocorticoids (hydrocortisone ≥ 100 mg/day or equivalent); Octreotide (> 100 mcg/day).
Drugs that alter thyroid hormone secretion	
Drugs that may decrease thyroid hormone secretion, which may result in hypothyroidism	
Aminoglutethimide Amiodarone Iodide (including iodine-containing radiographic contrast agents) Lithium Methimazole Propylthiouracil (PTU) Sulfonamides Tolbutamide	Long-term lithium therapy can result in goiter in up to 50% of patients, and either subclinical or overt hypothyroidism, each in up to 20% of patients. The fetus, neonate, elderly and euthyroid patients with underlying thyroid disease (e.g., Hashimoto's thyroiditis or with Grave's disease previously treated with radioiodine or surgery) are among those individuals who are particularly susceptible to iodine-induced hypothyroidism. Oral cholecystographic agents and amiodarone are slowly excreted, producing more prolonged hypothyroidism than parenterally administered iodinated contrast agents. Long-term aminoglutethimide therapy may minimally decrease T_4 and T_3 levels and increase TSH, although all values remain within normal limits in most patients.
Drugs that may increase thyroid hormone secretion, which may result in hyperthyroidism	
Amiodarone Iodide (including iodine-containing radiographic contrast agents)	Iodide and drugs that contain pharmacologic amounts of iodide may cause hyperthyroidism in euthyroid patients with Grave's disease previously treated with antithyroid drugs or in euthyroid patients with thyroid autonomy (e.g., multinodular goiter or hyperfunctioning thyroid adenoma). Hyperthyroidism may develop over several weeks and may persist for several months after therapy discontinuation. Amiodarone may induce hyperthyroidism by causing thyroiditis.
Drugs that may decrease T_4 absorption, which may result in hypothyroidism	
Antacids - Aluminum & Magnesium Hydroxides - Simethicone Bile Acid Sequestrants - Cholestyramine - Colestipol Calcium Carbonate Cation Exchange Resins - Kayexalate Ferrous Sulfate Orlistat Sucralfate	Concurrent use may reduce the efficacy of levothyroxine by binding and delaying or preventing absorption, potentially resulting in hypothyroidism. Calcium carbonate may form an insoluble chelate with levothyroxine, and ferrous sulfate likely forms a ferric-thyroxine complex. Administer levothyroxine at least 4 hours apart from these agents. Patients treated concomitantly with orlistat and levothyroxine should be monitored for changes in thyroid function.

Drugs that may alter T_4 and T_3 serum transport - but FT_4 concentration remains normal; and therefore, the patient remains euthyroid

Drugs that may increase serum TBG concentration	Drugs that may decrease serum TBG concentration
Clofibrate Estrogen-containing oral contraceptives Estrogens (oral) Heroin / Methadone 5-Fluorouracil Mitotane Tamoxifen	Androgens / Anabolic Steroids Asparaginase Glucocorticoids Slow-Release Nicotinic Acid

Drugs that may cause protein-binding site displacement	
Furosemide (> 80 mg IV) Heparin Hydantoins Non Steroidal Anti-Inflammatory Drugs - Fenamates - Phenylbutazone Salicylates (> 2 g/day)	Administration of these agents with levothyroxine results in an initial transient increase in FT_4. Continued administration results in a decrease in serum T_4 and normal FT_4 and TSH concentrations and, therefore, patients are clinically euthyroid. Salicylates inhibit binding of T_4 and T_3 to TBG and transthyretin. An initial increase in serum FT_4 is followed by return of FT_4 to normal levels with sustained therapeutic serum salicylate concentrations, although total-T_4 levels may decrease by as much as 30%.

(Table continued on next page)

Table 2 (cont.). Drug-Thyroidal Axis Interactions

Drug or Drug Class	Effect
Drugs that may alter T_4 and T_3 metabolism	
Drugs that may increase hepatic metabolism, which may result in hypothyroidism	
Carbamazepine Hydantoins Phenobarbital Rifampin	Stimulation of hepatic microsomal drug-metabolizing enzyme activity may cause increased hepatic degradation of levothyroxine, resulting in increased levothyroxine requirements. Phenytoin and carbamazepine reduce serum protein binding of levothyroxine, and total- and free- T_4 may be reduced by 20% to 40%, but most patients have normal serum TSH levels and are clinically euthyroid.
Drugs that may decrease T_4 5'-deiodinase activity	
Amiodarone Beta-adrenergic antagonists - (e.g., Propranolol > 160 mg/day) Glucocorticoids - (e.g., Dexamethasone ≥ 4 mg/day) Propylthiouracil (PTU)	Administration of these enzyme inhibitors decreases the peripheral conversion of T_4 to T_3, leading to decreased T_3 levels. However, serum T_4 levels are usually normal but may occasionally be slightly increased. In patients treated with large doses of propranolol (> 160 mg/day), T_3 and T_4 levels change slightly, TSH levels remain normal, and patients are clinically euthyroid. It should be noted that actions of particular beta-adrenergic antagonists may be impaired when the hypothyroid patient is converted to the euthyroid state. Short-term administration of large doses of glucocorticoids may decrease serum T_3 concentrations by 30% with minimal change in serum T_4 levels. However, long-term glucocorticoid therapy may result in slightly decreased T_3 and T_4 levels due to decreased TBG production (see above).
Miscellaneous	
Anticoagulants (oral) - Coumarin Derivatives - Indandione Derivatives	Thyroid hormones appear to increase the catabolism of vitamin K-dependent clotting factors, thereby increasing the anticoagulant activity of oral anticoagulants. Concomitant use of these agents impairs the compensatory increases in clotting factor synthesis. Prothrombin time should be carefully monitored in patients taking levothyroxine and oral anticoagulants and the dose of anticoagulant therapy adjusted accordingly.
Antidepressants - Tricyclics (e.g., Amitriptyline) - Tetracyclics (e.g., Maprotiline) - Selective Serotonin Reuptake Inhibitors (SSRIs; e.g., Sertraline)	Concurrent use of tri/tetracyclic antidepressants and levothyroxine may increase the therapeutic and toxic effects of both drugs, possibly due to increased receptor sensitivity to catecholamines. Toxic effects may include increased risk of cardiac arrhythmias and CNS stimulation; onset of action of tricyclics may be accelerated. Administration of sertraline in patients stabilized on levothyroxine may result in increased levothyroxine requirements.
Antidiabetic Agents - Biguanides - Meglitinides - Sulfonylureas - Thiazolidinediones - Insulin	Addition of levothyroxine to antidiabetic or insulin therapy may result in increased antidiabetic agent or insulin requirements. Careful monitoring of diabetic control is recommended, especially when thyroid therapy is started, changed, or discontinued.
Cardiac Glycosides	Serum digitalis glycoside levels may be reduced in hyperthyroidism or when the hypothyroid patient is converted to the euthyroid state. Therapeutic effect of digitalis glycosides may be reduced.
Cytokines - Interferon-α - Interleukin-2	Therapy with interferon-α has been associated with the development of antithyroid microsomal antibodies in 20% of patients and some have transient hypothyroidism, hyperthyroidism, or both. Patients who have antithyroid antibodies before treatment are at higher risk for thyroid dysfunction during treatment. Interleukin-2 has been associated with transient painless thyroiditis in 20% of patients. Interferon-β and -γ have not been reported to cause thyroid dysfunction.
Growth Hormones - Somatrem - Somatropin	Excessive use of thyroid hormones with growth hormones may accelerate epiphyseal closure. However, untreated hypothyroidism may interfere with growth response to growth hormone.
Ketamine	Concurrent use may produce marked hypertension and tachycardia; cautious administration to patients receiving thyroid hormone therapy is recommended.
Methylxanthine Bronchodilators - (e.g., Theophylline)	Decreased theophylline clearance may occur in hypothyroid patients; clearance returns to normal when the euthyroid state is achieved.

(Table continued on next page)

Cardiovascular
palpitations, tachycardia, arrhythmias, increased pulse and blood pressure, heart failure, angina, myocardial infarction, cardiac arrest;
Respiratory
dyspnea;
Gastrointestinal
diarrhea, vomiting, abdominal cramps and elevations in liver function tests;
Dermatologic
hair loss, flushing;
Endocrine
decreased bone mineral density;
Reproductive
menstrual irregularities, impaired fertility.
Pseudotumor cerebri and slipped capital femoral epiphysis have been reported in children receiving levothyroxine therapy. Overtreatment may result in craniosynostosis in infants and premature closure of the epiphyses in children with resultant compromised adult height.
Seizures have been reported rarely with the institution of levothyroxine therapy.
Inadequate levothyroxine dosage will produce or fail to ameliorate the signs and symptoms of hypothyroidism.
Hypersensitivity reactions to inactive ingredients have occurred in patients treated with thyroid hormone products. These include urticaria, pruritus, skin rash, flushing, angioedema, various GI symptoms (abdominal pain, nausea, vomiting and diarrhea), fever, arthralgia, serum sickness and wheezing. Hypersensitivity to levothyroxine itself is not known to occur.

Overdosage
The signs and symptoms of overdosage are those of hyperthyroidism (see **PRECAUTIONS** and **ADVERSE REACTIONS**). In addition, confusion and disorientation may occur. Cerebral embolism, shock, coma, and death have been reported. Seizures have occurred in a child ingesting 18 mg of levothyroxine. Symptoms may not necessarily be evident or may not appear until several days after ingestion of levothyroxine sodium.
Treatment of Overdosage
Levothyroxine sodium should be reduced in dose or temporarily discontinued if signs or symptoms of overdosage occur.
Acute Massive Overdosage
This may be a life-threatening emergency, therefore, symptomatic and supportive therapy should be instituted immediately. If not contraindicated (e.g., by seizures, coma, or loss of the gag reflex), the stomach should be emptied by emesis or gastric lavage to decrease gastrointestinal absorption. Activated charcoal or cholestyramine may also be used to decrease absorption. Central and peripheral increased sympathetic activity may be treated by administering β-receptor antagonists, e.g., propranolol, provided there are no medical contraindications to their use. Provide respiratory support as needed; control congestive heart failure and arrhythmia; control fever, hypoglycemia, and fluid loss as necessary. Large doses of antithyroid drugs (e.g., methimazole or propylthiouracil) followed in one to two hours by large doses of iodine may be given to inhibit synthesis and release of thyroid hormones. Glucocorticoids may be given to inhibit the conversion of T_4 to T_3. Plasmapheresis, charcoal hemoperfusion and exchange transfusion have been reserved for cases in which continued clinical deterioration occurs despite conventional therapy. Because T_4 is highly protein bound, very little drug will be removed by dialysis.

DOSAGE AND ADMINISTRATION
General Principles
The goal of replacement therapy is to achieve and maintain a clinical and biochemical euthyroid state. The goal of suppressive therapy is to inhibit growth and/or function of abnormal thyroid tissue. The dose of SYNTHROID that is adequate to achieve these goals depends on a variety of factors including the patient's age, body weight, cardiovascular status, concomitant medical conditions, including pregnancy, concomitant medications, and the specific nature of the condition being treated (see **WARNINGS** and **PRECAUTIONS**). Hence, the following recommendations serve only as dosing guidelines. Dosing must be individualized and adjustments made based on periodic assessment of the patient's clinical response and laboratory parameters (see **PRECAUTIONS - Laboratory Tests**).
SYNTHROID is administered as a single daily dose, preferably one-half to one-hour before breakfast. SYNTHROID should be taken at least 4 hours apart from drugs that are known to interfere with its absorption (see **PRECAUTIONS - Drug Interactions**).

Information on the AbbVie, Inc. products listed on these pages is from the prescribing information in use as of July 31, 2014. For more information, please visit rxabbvie.com or call 1-800-633-9110.

Table 2 (cont.). Drug-Thyroidal Axis Interactions

Drug or Drug Class	Effect
Radiographic Agents	Thyroid hormones may reduce the uptake of ^{123}I, ^{131}I, and ^{99m}Tc.
Sympathomimetics	Concurrent use may increase the effects of sympathomimetics or thyroid hormone. Thyroid hormones may increase the risk of coronary insufficiency when sympathomimetic agents are administered to patients with coronary artery disease.
Chloral Hydrate Diazepam Ethionamide Lovastatin Metoclopramide 6-Mercaptopurine Nitroprusside Para-aminosalicylate sodium Perphenazine Resorcinol (excessive topical use) Thiazide Diuretics	These agents have been associated with thyroid hormone and/or TSH level alterations by various mechanisms.

Strength (mcg)	Color	NDC# for bottles of 90	NDC # for bottles of 100	NDC # for bottles of 1000	NDC # for unit dose cartons of 100
25	orange	0074-4341-90	0074-4341-13	0074-4341-19	--
50	white	0074-4552-90	0074-4552-13	0074-4552-19	0074-4552-11
75	violet	0074-5182-90	0074-5182-13	0074-5182-19	0074-5182-11
88	olive	0074-6594-90	0074-6594-13	0074-6594-19	--
100	yellow	0074-6624-90	0074-6624-13	0074-6624-19	0074-6624-11
112	rose	0074-9296-90	0074-9296-13	0074-9296-19	--
125	brown	0074-7068-90	0074-7068-13	0074-7068-19	0074-7068-11
137	turquoise	0074-3727-90	0074-3727-13	0074-3727-19	--
150	blue	0074-7069-90	0074-7069-13	0074-7069-19	0074-7069-11
175	lilac	0074-7070-90	0074-7070-13	0074-7070-19	--
200	pink	0074-7148-90	0074-7148-13	0074-7148-19	0074-7148-11
300	green	0074-7149-90	0074-7149-13	0074-7149-19	--

Due to the long half-life of levothyroxine, the peak therapeutic effect at a given dose of levothyroxine sodium may not be attained for 4-6 weeks.

Caution should be exercised when administering SYNTHROID to patients with underlying cardiovascular disease, to the elderly, and to those with concomitant adrenal insufficiency (see **PRECAUTIONS**).

Specific Patient Populations
Hypothyroidism in Adults and in Children in Whom Growth and Puberty are Complete
(see **WARNINGS** and **PRECAUTIONS - Laboratory Tests**)
Therapy may begin at full replacement doses in otherwise healthy individuals less than 50 years old and in those older than 50 years who have been recently treated for hyperthyroidism or who have been hypothyroid for only a short time (such as a few months). The average full replacement dose of levothyroxine sodium is approximately 1.7 mcg/kg/day (e.g., **100-125 mcg/day** for a 70 kg adult). Older patients may require less than 1 mcg/kg/day. Levothyroxine sodium doses greater than 200 mcg/day are seldom required. An inadequate response to daily doses ≥ 300 mcg/day is rare and may indicate poor compliance, malabsorption, and/or drug interactions.

For most patients older than 50 years or for patients under 50 years of age with underlying cardiac disease, an initial starting dose of **25-50 mcg/day** of levothyroxine sodium is recommended, with gradual increments in dose at 6-8 week intervals, as needed. The recommended starting dose of levothyroxine sodium in elderly patients with cardiac disease is **12.5-25 mcg/day**, with gradual dose increments at 4-6 week intervals. The levothyroxine sodium dose is generally adjusted in 12.5-25 mcg increments until the patient with primary hypothyroidism is clinically euthyroid and the serum TSH has normalized.

In patients with severe hypothyroidism, the recommended initial levothyroxine sodium dose is **12.5-25 mcg/day** with increases of 25 mcg every 2-4 weeks, accompanied by clinical and laboratory assessment, until the TSH level is normalized.

In patients with secondary (pituitary) or tertiary (hypothalamic) hypothyroidism, the levothyroxine sodium dose should be titrated until the patient is clinically euthyroid and the serum free- T_4 level is restored to the upper half of the normal range.

Pediatric Dosage - Congenital or Acquired Hypothyroidism
(see **PRECAUTIONS - Laboratory Tests**)
General Principles
In general, levothyroxine therapy should be instituted at full replacement doses as soon as possible. Delays in diagnosis and institution of therapy may have deleterious effects on the child's intellectual and physical growth and development.

Undertreatment and overtreatment should be avoided (see **PRECAUTIONS - Pediatric Use**). SYNTHROID may be administered to infants and children who cannot swallow intact tablets by crushing the tablet and suspending the freshly crushed tablet in a small amount (5-10 mL or 1-2 teaspoons) of water. This suspension can be administered by spoon or by dropper. **DO NOT STORE THE SUSPENSION.** Foods that decrease absorption of levothyroxine, such as soybean infant formula, should not be used for administering levothyroxine sodium tablets (see **PRECAUTIONS - Drug-Food Interactions**).

Newborns
The recommended starting dose of levothyroxine sodium in newborn infants is **10-15 mcg/kg/day** . A lower starting dose (e.g., 25 mcg/day) should be considered in infants at risk for cardiac failure, and the dose should be increased in 4-6 weeks as needed based on clinical and laboratory response to treatment. In infants with very low (< 5 mcg/dL) or undetectable serum T_4 concentrations, the initial starting dose is **50 mcg/day** of levothyroxine sodium.

Infants and Children
Levothyroxine therapy is usually initiated at full replacement doses, with the recommended dose per body weight decreasing with age (see **Table 3**). However, in children with chronic or severe hypothyroidism, an initial dose of **25 mcg/day** of levothyroxine sodium is recommended with increments of 25 mcg every 2-4 weeks until the desired effect is achieved.

Hyperactivity in an older child can be minimized if the starting dose is one-fourth of the recommended full replacement dose, and the dose is then increased on a weekly basis by an amount equal to one-fourth the full-recommended replacement dose until the full recommended replacement dose is reached.

Table 3. Levothyroxine Sodium Dosing Guidelines for Pediatric Hypothyroidism

AGE	Daily Dose Per Kg Body Weight[a]
0-3 months	10-15 mcg/kg/day
3-6 months	8-10 mcg/kg/day
6-12 months	6-8 mcg/kg/day
1-5 years	5-6 mcg/kg/day
6-12 years	4-5 mcg/kg/day
> 12 years but growth and puberty incomplete	2-3 mcg/kg/day
Growth and puberty complete	1.7 mcg/kg/day

[a] The dose should be adjusted based on clinical response and laboratory parameters (see **PRECAUTIONS - Laboratory Tests and Pediatric Use**).

Pregnancy
Pregnancy may increase levothyroxine requirements (see **PREGNANCY**).
Subclinical Hypothyroidism
If this condition is treated, a lower levothyroxine sodium dose (e.g., **1 mcg/kg/day**) than that used for full replacement may be adequate to normalize the serum TSH level. Patients who are not treated should be monitored yearly for changes in clinical status and thyroid laboratory parameters.
TSH Suppression in Well-differentiated Thyroid Cancer and Thyroid Nodules
The target level for TSH suppression in these conditions has not been established with controlled studies. In addition, the efficacy of TSH suppression for benign nodular disease is controversial. Therefore, the dose of SYNTHROID used for TSH suppression should be individualized based on the specific disease and the patient being treated.
In the treatment of well-differentiated (papillary and follicular) thyroid cancer, levothyroxine is used as an adjunct to surgery and radioiodine therapy. Generally, TSH is suppressed to < 0.1 mU/L, and this usually requires a levothyroxine sodium dose of **greater than 2 mcg/kg/day**. However, in patients with high-risk tumors, the target level for TSH suppression may be < 0.01 mU/L.
In the treatment of benign nodules and nontoxic multinodular goiter, TSH is generally suppressed to a higher target (e.g., 0.1 to either 0.5 or 1.0 mU/L) than that used for the treatment of thyroid cancer. Levothyroxine sodium is contraindicated if the serum TSH is already suppressed due to the risk of precipitating overt thyrotoxicosis (see **CONTRAINDICATIONS, WARNINGS** and **PRECAUTIONS**).
Myxedema Coma
Myxedema coma is a life-threatening emergency characterized by poor circulation and hypometabolism, and may result in unpredictable absorption of levothyroxine sodium from the gastrointestinal tract. Therefore, oral thyroid hormone drug products are not recommended to treat this condition. Thyroid hormone products formulated for intravenous administration should be administered.

HOW SUPPLIED

SYNTHROID® **(levothyroxine sodium tablets, USP)** are round, color coded, scored and debossed with "SYNTHROID" on one side and potency on the other side. They are supplied as follows:
[See second table above]
Storage Conditions
Store at 25°C (77°F); excursions permitted to 15-30°C (59-86°F) [see USP Controlled Room Temperature]. SYNTHROID tablets should be protected from light and moisture.
(Nos. 4341, 4552, 5182, 6594, 9296, 7068, 3727, 7069, 7070, 7148, 7149)
03-A663-R7-Rev. September, 2012
AbbVie Inc.
North Chicago, IL 60064, U.S.A.
Shown in Product Identification Guide, page 304

TARKA®
(trandolapril/verapamil hydrochloride ER tablets) ℞

> **WARNING: FETAL TOXICITY**
> • When pregnancy is detected, discontinue TARKA as soon as possible.
> • Drugs that act directly on the renin-angiotensin system can cause injury and death to the developing fetus (see **WARNINGS: Fetal Toxicity**).

DESCRIPTION

TARKA® (trandolapril/verapamil hydrochloride ER) combines a slow release formulation of a calcium channel blocker, verapamil hydrochloride, and an immediate release formulation of an angiotensin converting enzyme inhibitor, trandolapril.
Verapamil Component
Verapamil hydrochloride is chemically described as benzeneacetonitrile, $\alpha[3-[[2-(3,4-dimethoxyphenyl)ethyl]methylamino]propyl]-3$, $4-dimethoxy-\alpha-(1-methylethyl)$ hydrochloride. Its empirical formula is $C_{27}H_{38}N_2O_4 \cdot HCl$ and its structural formula is:

Verapamil hydrochloride is an almost white crystalline powder, with a molecular weight of 491.08. It is soluble in water, chloroform, and methanol. It is practically free of odor, with a bitter taste.

Trandolapril Component

Trandolapril is the ethyl ester prodrug of a nonsulfhydryl angiotensin converting enzyme (ACE) inhibitor, trandolaprilat. It is chemically described as (2S,3aR,7aS)-1-[(S)-N-[(S)-1-Carboxy-3-phenylpropyl]alanyl] hexahydro-2-indolinecarboxylic acid, 1-ethyl ester. Its empirical formula is $C_{24}H_{34}N_2O_5$ and its structural formula is:

Trandolapril is a white or almost white powder with a molecular weight of 430.54. It is soluble (>100 mg/mL) in chloroform, dichloromethane, and methanol.

TARKA tablets are formulated for oral administration, containing verapamil hydrochloride as a controlled release formulation and trandolapril as an immediate release formulation. The tablet strengths are trandolapril 2 mg/verapamil hydrochloride ER 180 mg, trandolapril 1 mg/verapamil hydrochloride ER 240 mg, trandolapril 2 mg/verapamil hydrochloride ER 240 mg, and trandolapril 4 mg/verapamil hydrochloride ER 240 mg. The tablets also contain the following ingredients: corn starch, dioctyl sodium sulfosuccinate, ethanol, hydroxypropyl cellulose, hypromellose, lactose monohydrate, magnesium stearate, microcrystalline cellulose, polyethylene glycol, povidone, purified water, silicon dioxide, sodium alginate, sodium stearyl fumarate, synthetic iron oxides, talc, and titanium dioxide.

CLINICAL PHARMACOLOGY

Verapamil hydrochloride and trandolapril have been used individually and in combination for the treatment of hypertension. For the four dosing strengths, the antihypertensive effect of the combination is approximately additive to the individual components.

Verapamil Component

Verapamil is a calcium channel blocker that exerts its pharmacologic effects by modulating the influx of ionic calcium across the cell membrane of the arterial smooth muscle as well as in conductile and contractile myocardial cells. Verapamil exerts antihypertensive effects by decreasing systemic vascular resistance, usually without orthostatic decreases in blood pressure or reflex tachycardia. During isometric or dynamic exercise, verapamil does not alter systolic cardiac function in patients with normal ventricular function. Verapamil does not alter total serum calcium levels.

Trandolapril Component

Trandolapril is de-esterified to its diacid metabolite, trandolaprilat. Both inhibit angiotensin-converting enzyme (ACE) in human subjects and in animals. Trandolaprilat is about 8 times more potent than trandolapril. ACE is a peptidyl dipeptidase that catalyzes the conversion of angiotensin I to the vasoconstrictor, angiotensin II. Angiotensin II also stimulates aldosterone secretion by the adrenal cortex. Inhibition of ACE results in decreased plasma angiotensin II, which leads to decreased vasopressor activity and to decreased aldosterone secretion. The latter decrease may result in a small increase of serum potassium. In controlled clinical trials, treatment with TARKA resulted in mean increases in potassium of 0.1 mEq/L (see **PRECAUTIONS**). Removal of angiotensin II negative feedback on renin secretion leads to increased plasma renin activity (PRA).

ACE is identical to kininase II, an enzyme that degrades bradykinin. Whether increased levels of bradykinin, a potent vasodepressor peptide, play a role in the therapeutic effect of TARKA remains to be elucidated.

While the mechanism through which trandolapril lowers blood pressure is believed to be primarily suppression of the renin-angiotensin-aldosterone system, trandolapril has an antihypertensive effect even in patients with low renin hypertension. Trandolapril is an effective antihypertensive in all races studied. Both black patients (usually a predominantly low renin group) and non-black patients respond to 2 to 4 mg of trandolapril.

Pharmacokinetics and Metabolism

TARKA

Following a single oral dose of TARKA in healthy subjects, peak plasma concentrations are reached within 0.5-2 hours for trandolapril and within 4-15 hours for verapamil. Peak plasma concentrations of the active desmethyl metabolite of verapamil, norverapamil, are reached within 5-15 hours.

Cleavage of the ester group converts trandolapril to its active diacid metabolite, trandolaprilat, which reaches peak plasma concentrations within 2-12 hours. The pharmacokinetics of trandolapril and trandolaprilat are not altered when trandolapril is administered in combination with verapamil, compared to monotherapy.

The AUC and C_{max} for both verapamil and norverapamil are increased when 240 mg of controlled release verapamil is administered concomitantly with 4 mg trandolapril. The increase in C_{max} is 54 and 30% and the AUC is increased by 65 and 32% for verapamil and norverapamil, respectively. Administration of TARKA 4/240 (4 mg trandolapril and 240 mg verapamil hydrochloride ER) with a high-fat meal does not alter the bioavailability of trandolapril whereas verapamil peak concentrations and area under the curve (AUC) decrease 37% and 28%, respectively. Food thus decreases verapamil bioavailability and the time to peak plasma concentration for both verapamil and norverapamil are delayed by approximately 7 hours. Both optical isomers of verapamil are similarly affected.

The elimination half life of trandolapril is about 6 hours. At steady state, the effective half-life of trandolaprilat is 22.5 hours. Like all ACE inhibitors, trandolaprilat also has a prolonged terminal elimination phase, involving a small fraction of administered drug, probably representing binding to plasma and tissue ACE.

The terminal half-life of verapamil is 6-11 hours. Steady-state plasma concentrations of the two components are achieved after about a week of once-daily dosing of TARKA. At steady-state, plasma concentrations of verapamil and trandolaprilat are up to two-fold higher than those observed after a single oral TARKA dose.

The pharmacokinetics of verapamil and trandolaprilat are significantly different in the elderly (≥65 years) than in younger subjects. The bioavailability of verapamil and norverapamil are increased by 87% and 77%, respectively, and that of trandolapril by approximately 35% in the elderly. AUCs are approximately 80% and 35% higher, respectively.

Verapamil Component

With the immediate release formulation, more than 90% of the orally administered dose is absorbed with peak plasma concentrations of verapamil observed 1 to 2 hours after dosing. A delayed rate but similar extent of absorption is observed for the sustained release formulation when compared to the immediate release formulation. Because of the rapid biotransformation of verapamil during its first pass through the portal circulation, absolute bioavailability ranges from 20% to 35%. A nonlinear correlation exists between verapamil dose and plasma concentrations.

In early dose titration with verapamil, a relationship exists between plasma concentrations of verapamil and prolongation of the PR interval. However, during chronic administration, this relationship may disappear. No relationship has been established between the plasma concentration of verapamil and reduction in blood pressure.

In healthy subjects, orally administered verapamil undergoes extensive metabolism in the liver. Twelve metabolites have been identified in plasma; all except norverapamil are present in trace amounts only. Approximately 70% of an administered dose is excreted as metabolites in the urine and 16% or more in the feces within 5 days. Urinary excretion of unchanged drug is about 3% to 4% of the dose. Verapamil is approximately 90% bound to plasma proteins.

In patients with hepatic insufficiency, verapamil clearance is decreased about 30% and the elimination half-life is prolonged up to 14 to 16 hours (see **PRECAUTIONS**). In patients with liver dysfunction, a dosage adjustment may be required. In the elderly (≥65 years), verapamil clearance is reduced resulting in increases in elimination half-life.

Trandolapril Component

Following oral administration of trandolapril, the absolute bioavailability of trandolapril is approximately 10% as trandolapril and 70% as trandolaprilat. Plasma concentrations of trandolaprilat but not trandolapril increase in proportion with dose. Plasma concentrations of trandolaprilat decline in a triphasic manner. The more prolonged terminal elimination phase probably represents a small fraction of dose saturably bound to ACE.

After an oral radiolabeled dose of trandolapril, excretion of trandolapril and metabolites account for 33% of the dose in the urine and about 66% in the feces. Less than 1% of the dose is excreted in the urine as unchanged drug. Serum protein binding of trandolapril is about 80%, and is independent of concentration. Binding of trandolaprilat is concentration-dependent, varying from 65% at 1000 ng/mL to 94% at 0.1 ng/mL, indicating saturation of binding with increasing concentration.

Compared to normal subjects, the plasma concentrations of trandolapril and trandolaprilat are approximately 2-fold greater and renal clearance is reduced by about 85% in patients with creatinine clearance below 30 mL/min and in patients on hemodialysis. Dosage adjustment is recommended in renally impaired patients (see **DOSAGE AND ADMINISTRATION**).

Following oral administration in patients with mild to moderate alcoholic cirrhosis, plasma concentrations of trandolapril and trandolaprilat were, respectively, 9-fold and 2-fold greater than in normal subjects, but inhibition of ACE activity was not affected. Lower doses should be considered in patients with hepatic insufficiency (see **DOSAGE AND ADMINISTRATION**).

Pharmacodynamics

TARKA

Verapamil does not interfere with ACE inhibition by trandolapril. Trandolapril does not alter the effect of verapamil on intra-cardiac conduction.

Verapamil Component

Verapamil dilates the main coronary arteries and coronary arterioles, both in normal and ischemic regions, and is a potent inhibitor of coronary artery spasm. This property increases myocardial oxygen delivery in patients with coronary artery spasm, and is responsible for the effectiveness of verapamil in vasospastic (Prinzmetal's or variant) as well as unstable angina at rest.

Verapamil regularly reduces the total systemic resistance (afterload) by dilating peripheral arterioles. By decreasing the influx of calcium, verapamil prolongs the effective refractory period within the AV node and slows AV conduction in a rate-related manner.

Normal sinus rhythm is usually not affected, but in patients with sick sinus syndrome, verapamil may interfere with sinus node impulse generation and may induce sinus arrest or sinoatrial block. Atrioventricular block can occur in patients without preexisting conduction defects (see **WARNINGS**).

Verapamil does not alter the normal atrial action potential or intraventricular conduction time, but depresses amplitude, velocity of depolarization and conduction in depressed atrial fibers. Verapamil may shorten the antegrade effective refractory period of accessory bypass tracts. Acceleration of ventricular rate and/or ventricular fibrillation has been reported in patients with atrial flutter or atrial fibrillation and a coexisting accessory AV pathway following administration of verapamil (see **WARNINGS**).

Hemodynamics and Myocardial Metabolism: Verapamil reduces afterload and myocardial contractility. Improved left ventricular diastolic function in patients with idiopathic hypertrophic subaortic stenosis (IHSS) and those with coronary heart disease has also been observed with verapamil therapy. In most patients, including those with organic cardiac disease, the negative inotropic action of verapamil is countered by a reduction of afterload and cardiac index is usually not reduced. However, in patients with severe left ventricular dysfunction (e.g., pulmonary wedge pressure about 20 mmHg or ejection fraction less than 30%), or in patients taking beta-adrenergic blocking agents or other cardio-depressant drugs, deterioration of ventricular function may occur (see **PRECAUTIONS - Drug Interactions**).

Pulmonary Function: Verapamil does not induce bronchoconstriction and hence, does not impair ventilatory function.

Trandolapril Component

After a single 2 mg dose of trandolapril, inhibition of ACE activity reaches a maximum (70-85%) at 4 hours with about 10% decline at 24 hours. Eight days after dosing, ACE inhibition is still 40%.

Four placebo-controlled dose response studies were conducted using once daily oral dosing of trandolapril in doses from 0.25 to 16 mg per day in 827 black and non-black patients with mild to moderate hypertension. The minimal effective once daily dose was 1.0 mg in non-black patients and 2.0 mg in black patients. Further decreases in trough supine diastolic blood pressure were obtained in non-black patients with higher doses, and no further response was seen with doses above 4 mg (up to 16 mg). The antihypertensive effect diminished somewhat at the end of the dosing interval.

During chronic therapy, the maximum reduction in blood pressure with any dose is achieved within one week. Following 6 weeks of monotherapy in placebo-controlled trials in patients with mild to moderate hypertension, once daily doses of 2 to 4 mg lowered supine or standing systolic/diastolic blood pressure 24 hours after dosing by an average 7-10/4-5 mmHg below placebo responses in non-black patients. Once daily doses of 2 to 4 mg lowered blood pressures 4-6/3-4 mmHg below placebo responses in black patients.

CLINICAL STUDIES

In controlled clinical trials, once daily doses of TARKA, trandolapril 4 mg/verapamil HCl ER 240 mg or trandolapril 2 mg/verapamil HCl ER 180 mg, decreased placebo-corrected seated pressure (systolic/diastolic) 24 hours after

Information on the AbbVie, Inc. products listed on these pages is from the prescribing information in use as of July 31, 2014. For more information, please visit rxabbvie.com or call 1-800-633-9110.

dosing by about 7-12/6-8 mmHg. Each of the components of TARKA added to the antihypertensive effect. Treatment effects were consistent across age groups (<65, ≥65 years), and gender (male, female).

Blood pressure reductions were significantly greater for the TARKA 4/240 combination than for either of the components used alone.

The antihypertensive effects of TARKA have continued during therapy for at least 1 year.

INDICATIONS AND USAGE

TARKA is indicated for the treatment of hypertension.

This fixed combination drug is not indicated for the initial therapy of hypertension (see DOSAGE AND ADMINISTRATION).

In using TARKA, consideration should be given to the fact that an angiotensin converting enzyme inhibitor, captopril, has caused agranulocytosis, particularly in patients with renal impairment or collagen vascular disease, and that available data are insufficient to show that trandolapril does not have similar risk (see **WARNINGS - Neutropenia/Agranulocytosis**).

CONTRAINDICATIONS

TARKA is contraindicated in patients who are hypersensitive to any ACE inhibitor or verapamil.

Because of the verapamil component, TARKA is contraindicated in:

1. Severe left ventricular dysfunction (see **WARNINGS**).
2. Hypotension (systolic pressure less than 90 mmHg) or cardiogenic shock.
3. Sick sinus syndrome (except in patients with a functioning artificial ventricular pacemaker).
4. Second- or third-degree AV block (except in patients with a functioning artificial ventricular pacemaker).
5. Patients with atrial flutter or atrial fibrillation and an accessory bypass tract (e.g. Wolff-Parkinson-White, Lown-Ganong-Levine syndromes) (see **WARNINGS**).

Because of the trandolapril component, TARKA is contraindicated in patients with a history of angioedema related to previous treatment with an angiotensin converting enzyme (ACE) inhibitor.

Do not co-administer aliskiren with TARKA in patients with diabetes (see **PRECAUTIONS, Drug Interactions**).

WARNINGS

Heart Failure
Verapamil Component
Verapamil has a negative inotropic effect which, in most patients, is compensated by its afterload reduction (decreased systemic vascular resistance) properties without a net impairment of ventricular performance. In clinical experience with 4,954 patients, 87 (1.8%) developed congestive heart failure or pulmonary edema. Verapamil should be avoided in patients with severe left ventricular dysfunction (e.g., ejection fraction less than 30%, pulmonary wedge pressure above 20 mmHg, or severe symptoms of cardiac failure) and in patients with any degree of ventricular dysfunction if they are receiving a beta adrenergic blocker (see **PRECAUTIONS - Drug Interactions**). Patients with milder ventricular dysfunction should, if possible, be controlled with optimum doses of digitalis and/or diuretics before verapamil treatment (Note interactions with digoxin under: **PRECAUTIONS**).

Trandolapril Component
Trandolapril, as an ACE inhibitor, may cause excessive hypotension in patients with congestive heart failure (see **WARNINGS - Hypotension**).

Hypotension
Verapamil Component
Occasionally, the pharmacologic action of verapamil may produce a decrease in blood pressure below normal levels which may result in dizziness or symptomatic hypotension.

Trandolapril Component
Trandolapril can cause symptomatic hypotension. Like other ACE inhibitors, trandolapril has only rarely been associated with symptomatic hypotension in uncomplicated hypertensive patients. Symptomatic hypotension is most likely to occur in patients who are salt- or volume-depleted as a result of prolonged treatment with diuretics, dietary salt restriction, dialysis, diarrhea, or vomiting. Volume and/or salt depletion should be corrected before initiating treatment with trandolapril (see **PRECAUTIONS - Drug Interactions and ADVERSE REACTIONS**).

In controlled studies, hypotension was observed in 0.6% of patients receiving any combination of trandolapril and verapamil HCl ER.

In patients with concomitant congestive heart failure, with or without associated renal insufficiency, ACE inhibitor therapy may cause excessive hypotension, which may be associated with oliguria or azotemia and, rarely, with acute renal failure and death (see **DOSAGE AND ADMINISTRATION**).

If symptomatic hypotension occurs, the patient should be placed in the supine position and, if necessary, normal sa-

line may be administered intravenously. A transient hypotensive response is not a contraindication to further doses; however, lower doses of verapamil HCl ER and/or trandolapril or reduced concomitant diuretic therapy should be considered.

Elevated Liver Enzymes/Hepatic Failure
Verapamil Component
Elevations of transaminases with and without concomitant elevations in alkaline phosphatase and bilirubin have been reported. Such elevations have sometimes been transient and may disappear even in the face of continued verapamil treatment. Several cases of hepatocellular injury related to verapamil have been proven by rechallenge; half of these had clinical symptoms (malaise, fever, and/or right upper quadrant pain) in addition to elevations of SGOT, SGPT, and alkaline phosphatase.

Trandolapril Component
ACE inhibitors rarely have been associated with a syndrome of cholestatic jaundice, fulminant hepatic necrosis, and death. The mechanism of this syndrome is not understood. Patients receiving ACE inhibitors who develop jaundice should discontinue the ACE inhibitor and receive appropriate medical follow-up.

Liver abnormalities were noted in 3.2% of patients taking any of several combinations of trandolapril/verapamil doses. Periodic monitoring of liver function in patients taking TARKA is therefore prudent.

Accessory Bypass Tract (Wolff-Parkinson-White or Lown-Ganong-Levine Syndromes)
Verapamil Component
Some patients with paroxysmal and/or chronic atrial fibrillation or atrial flutter and a coexisting accessory AV pathway have developed increased antegrade conduction across the accessory pathway bypassing the AV node, producing a very rapid ventricular response or ventricular fibrillation after receiving intravenous verapamil (or digitalis). Although a risk of this occurring with oral verapamil has not been established, such patients receiving oral verapamil may be at risk and its use in these patients is contraindicated (see **CONTRAINDICATIONS**).

Treatment is usually DC-cardioversion. Cardioversion has been used safely and effectively after oral verapamil.

Atrioventricular Block
Verapamil Component
The effect of verapamil on AV conduction and the SA node may lead to asymptomatic first-degree AV block and transient bradycardia, sometimes accompanied by nodal escape rhythms. PR interval prolongation is correlated with verapamil plasma concentrations, especially during the early titration phases of therapy. Higher degrees of AV block, however, were infrequently (0.8%) observed. Marked first-degree block or progressive development to second- or third-degree AV block requires a reduction in dosage or, in rare instances, discontinuation of verapamil HCl and institution of appropriate therapy depending upon the clinical situation.

Patients with Hypertrophic Cardiomyopathy (IHSS)
Verapamil Component
In 120 patients with hypertrophic cardiomyopathy (most of them refractory or intolerant to propranolol) who received therapy with verapamil at doses up to 720 mg/day, a variety of serious adverse effects were seen. Three patients died in pulmonary edema; all had severe left ventricular outflow obstruction and a past history of left ventricular dysfunction. Eight other patients had pulmonary edema and/or severe hypotension; abnormally high (over 20 mmHg) capillary wedge pressure and a marked left ventricular outflow obstruction were present in most of these patients. Sinus bradycardia occurred in 11% of the patients, second-degree AV block in 4% and sinus arrest in 2%. It must be appreciated that this group of patients had a serious disease with a high mortality rate. Most adverse effects responded well to dose reduction and only rarely did verapamil have to be discontinued.

Anaphylactoid and Possibly Related Reactions
Presumably because angiotensin-converting enzyme inhibitors affect the metabolism of eicosanoids and polypeptides, including endogenous bradykinin, patients receiving ACE inhibitors, including trandolapril may be subject to a variety of adverse reactions, some of them serious.

Angioedema
Angioedema of the face, extremities, lips, tongue, glottis, and larynx has been reported in patients treated with ACE inhibitors including trandolapril. Symptoms suggestive of angioedema or facial edema occurred in 0.13% of trandolapril-treated patients. Two of the four cases were life-threatening and resolved without treatment or with medication (corticosteroids). Angioedema associated with laryngeal edema can be fatal. If laryngeal stridor or angioedema of the face, tongue or glottis occurs, treatment with TARKA should be discontinued immediately, the patient treated in accordance with accepted medical care and carefully observed until the swelling disappears. In instances where swelling is confined to the face and lips, the condition

generally resolves without treatment; antihistamines may be useful in relieving symptoms. **Where there is involvement of the tongue, glottis, or larynx, likely to cause airway obstruction, emergency therapy, including but not limited to subcutaneous epinephrine solution 1:1,000 (0.3 to 0.5 mL) should be promptly administered (see PRECAUTIONS and ADVERSE REACTIONS).**

Anaphylactoid Reactions During Desensitization
Two patients undergoing desensitizing treatment with hymenoptera venom while receiving ACE inhibitors sustained life-threatening anaphylactoid reactions. In the same patients, these reactions did not occur when ACE inhibitors were temporarily withheld, but they reappeared when the ACE inhibitors were inadvertently readministered.

Anaphylactoid Reactions During Membrane Exposure
Anaphylactoid reactions have been reported in patients dialyzed with high-flux membranes and treated concomitantly with an ACE inhibitor. Anaphylactoid reactions have also been reported in patients undergoing low-density lipoprotein apheresis with dextran sulfate absorption.

Neutropenia/Agranulocytosis
Trandolapril Component
Another ACE inhibitor, captopril, has been shown to cause agranulocytosis and bone marrow depression rarely in patients with uncomplicated hypertension, but more frequently in patients with renal impairment, especially if they also have a collagen-vascular disease such as systemic lupus erythematosus or scleroderma. Available data from clinical trials of trandolapril or TARKA are insufficient to show that trandolapril does not cause agranulocytosis at similar rates. As with other ACE inhibitors, periodic monitoring of white blood cell counts in patients with collagen-vascular disease and/or renal disease should be considered.

Fetal Toxicity
Pregnancy Category D
Trandolapril Component
Use of drugs that act on the renin-angiotensin system during the second and third trimesters of pregnancy reduces fetal renal function and increases fetal and neonatal morbidity and death. Resulting oligohydramnios can be associated with fetal lung hypoplasia and skeletal deformations. Potential neonatal adverse effects include skull hypoplasia, anuria, hypotension, renal failure, and death. When pregnancy is detected, discontinue TARKA as soon as possible. These adverse outcomes are usually associated with use of these drugs in the second and third trimester of pregnancy. Most epidemiologic studies examining fetal abnormalities after exposure to antihypertensive use in the first trimester have not distinguished drugs affecting the renin-angiotensin system from other antihypertensive agents. Appropriate management of maternal hypertension during pregnancy is important to optimize outcomes for both mother and fetus.

In the unusual case that there is no appropriate alternative to therapy with drugs affecting the renin-angiotensin system for a particular patient, apprise the mother of the potential risk to the fetus. Perform serial ultrasound examinations to assess the intra-amniotic environment. If oligohydramnios is observed, discontinue TARKA, unless it is considered lifesaving for the mother. Fetal testing may be appropriate, based on the week of pregnancy. Patients and physicians should be aware, however, that oligohydramnios may not appear until after the fetus has sustained irreversible injury. Closely observe infants with histories of *in utero* exposure to TARKA for hypotension, oliguria, and hyperkalemia (see **PRECAUTIONS - Pediatric Use**).

Doses of 0.8 mg/kg/day (9.4 mg/m2/day) in rabbits, 1000 mg/kg/day (7000 mg/m2/day) in rats, and 25 mg/kg/day (295 mg/m2/day) in cynomolgus monkeys did not produce teratogenic effects. These doses represent 10 and 3 times (rabbits), 1250 and 2564 times (rats), and 312 and 108 times (monkeys) the maximum projected human dose of 4 mg based on body-weight and body-surface-area, respectively assuming a 50 kg woman.

Trandolapril in doses of 0.8 mg/kg/day in rabbits, 100.0 mg/kg/day in rats, and 25 mg/kg/day in cynomolgus monkeys (10, 1250, and 312 times the maximum projected human dose, respectively, assuming a 50 kg woman) did not produce teratogenic effects.

PRECAUTIONS
Use in Patients with Impaired Hepatic Function
TARKA has not been evaluated in subjects with impaired hepatic function.

Verapamil Component
Since verapamil is highly metabolized by the liver, it should be administered cautiously to patients with impaired hepatic function. Severe liver dysfunction prolongs the elimination half-life of immediate release verapamil to about 14 to 16 hours; hence, approximately 30% of the dose given to patients with normal liver function should be administered to these patients.

Careful monitoring for abnormal prolongation of the PR interval or other signs of excessive pharmacologic effects (see **OVERDOSAGE**) should be carried out.

Trandolapril Component
Trandolapril and trandolaprilat concentrations increase in patients with impaired liver function.

Use in Patients with Impaired Renal Function
TARKA has not been evaluated in patients with impaired renal function.

Verapamil Component
About 70% of an administered dose of verapamil is excreted as metabolites in the urine. Verapamil is not removed by hemodialysis. Until further data are available, verapamil should be administered cautiously to patients with impaired renal function. These patients should be carefully monitored for abnormal prolongation of the PR interval or other signs of overdosage (see **OVERDOSAGE**).

Trandolapril Component
As a consequence of inhibiting the renin-angiotensin-aldosterone system, changes in renal function may be anticipated in susceptible individuals. In patients with severe heart failure whose renal function may depend on the activity of the renin-angiotensin-aldosterone system, treatment with ACE inhibitors, including trandolapril, may be associated with oliguria and/or progressive azotemia and rarely with acute renal failure and/or death.

In hypertensive patients with unilateral or bilateral renal artery stenosis, increases in blood urea nitrogen and serum creatinine have been observed in some patients following ACE inhibitor therapy. These increases were almost always reversible upon discontinuation of the ACE inhibitor and/or diuretic therapy. In such patients, renal function should be monitored during the first few weeks of therapy.

Some hypertensive patients with no apparent pre-existing renal vascular disease have developed increases in blood urea and serum creatinine, usually minor and transient, especially when ACE inhibitors have been given concomitantly with a diuretic. This is more likely to occur in patients with pre-existing renal impairment. Dosage reduction and/or discontinuation of any diuretic and/or the ACE inhibitor may be required.

Evaluation of hypertensive patients should always include assessment of renal function (see **DOSAGE AND ADMINISTRATION**).

Use in Patients with Attenuated (Decreased) Neuromuscular Transmission
Verapamil Component
It has been reported that verapamil decreases neuromuscular transmission in patients with Duchenne's muscular dystrophy, and that verapamil prolongs recovery from the neuromuscular blocking agent vecuronium. It may be necessary to decrease the dosage of verapamil when it is administered to patients with attenuated neuromuscular transmission (see **PRECAUTIONS - Surgery/Anesthesia**).

Hyperkalemia and Potassium-sparing Diuretics
Trandolapril Component
In clinical trials, hyperkalemia (serum potassium > 6.00 mEq/L) occurred in approximately 0.4 percent of hypertensive patients receiving trandolapril and in 0.8% of patients receiving a dose of trandolapril (0.5-8 mg) in combination with a dose of verapamil SR (120-240 mg). In most cases, elevated serum potassium levels were isolated values, which resolved despite continued therapy. None of these patients were discontinued from the trials because of hyperkalemia. Risk factors for the development of hyperkalemia include renal insufficiency, diabetes mellitus, and the concomitant use of potassium-sparing diuretics, potassium supplements, and/or potassium-containing salt substitutes, which should be used cautiously, if at all, with trandolapril (see **PRECAUTIONS - Drug Interactions**).

Cough
Presumably due to the inhibition of the degradation of endogenous bradykinin, persistent nonproductive cough has been reported with all ACE inhibitors, always resolving after discontinuation of therapy. ACE inhibitor-induced cough should be considered in the differential diagnosis of cough. In controlled trials of trandolapril, cough was present in 2% of trandolapril patients and 0% of patients given placebo. There was no evidence of a relationship to dose.

Surgery/anesthesia
Trandolapril Component
In patients undergoing major surgery or during anesthesia with agents that produce hypotension, trandolapril will block angiotensin II formation secondary to compensatory renin release. If hypotension occurs and is considered to be due to this mechanism, it can be corrected by volume expansion (see **PRECAUTIONS - Use in Patients with Attenuated (Decreased) Neuromuscular Transmission**).

Drug Interactions
In vitro metabolic studies indicate that verapamil is metabolized by cytochrome P450 including CYP3A4, CYP1A2, CYP2C8, CYP2C9 and CYP2C18. Verapamil has been shown to be an inhibitor of CYP3A4 enzymes and P-glycoprotein (P-gp).
Clinically significant interactions have been reported with inhibitors of CYP3A4 (e.g. erythromycin, ritonavir) causing elevation of plasma levels of verapamil while inducers of CYP3A4 (e.g. rifampin) have caused a lowering of plasma levels of verapamil. Therefore, patients receiving inhibitors or inducers of the cytochrome P450 system should be monitored for drug interactions.

Digitalis
Clinical use of verapamil in digitalized patients has shown the combination to be well tolerated if digoxin doses are properly adjusted. Chronic verapamil treatment can increase serum digoxin levels by 50 to 75% during the first week of therapy, and this can result in digoxin toxicity. In patients with hepatic cirrhosis, the influence of verapamil on digoxin kinetics is magnified. Verapamil may reduce total body clearance and extrarenal clearance of digitoxin by 27% and 29%, respectively. Maintenance digoxin doses should be reduced when verapamil is administered, and the patient should be carefully monitored to avoid over- or under-digitalization. Whenever overdigitalization is suspected, the daily dose of digoxin should be reduced or temporarily discontinued. Upon discontinuation of any verapamil-containing regime including TARKA® (trandolapril/verapamil hydrochloride ER), the patient should be reassessed to avoid underdigitalization. No clinically significant pharmacokinetic interaction has been found between trandolapril (or its metabolites) and digoxin.

Lithium
Verapamil Component
Increased sensitivity to the effects of lithium (neurotoxicity) has been reported during concomitant verapamil-lithium therapy with either no change or an increase in serum lithium levels. Increased serum lithium levels and symptoms of lithium toxicity have been reported in patients receiving concomitant lithium and ACE inhibitor therapy. TARKA and lithium should be coadministered with caution, and frequent monitoring of serum lithium levels is recommended. If a diuretic is also used, the risk of lithium toxicity may be increased.

Clarithromycin
Hypotension, bradyarrhythmias, and lactic acidosis have been observed in patients receiving concurrent clarithromycin.

Erythromycin
Hypotension, bradyarrhythmias, and lactic acidosis have been observed in patients receiving concurrent erythromycin ethylsuccinate.

Cimetidine
The interaction between cimetidine and chronically administered verapamil has not been studied. Variable results on clearance have been obtained in acute studies of healthy volunteers; clearance of verapamil was either reduced or unchanged. No clinically significant pharmacokinetic interaction has been found between trandolapril (or its metabolites) and cimetidine.

Antiarrhythmic Agents
Verapamil Component
Disopyramide Phosphate
Data on possible interactions between verapamil and disopyramide phosphate are not available. Therefore, disopyramide should not be administered within 48 hours before or 24 hours after verapamil administration.

Flecainide
A study of healthy volunteers showed that the concomitant administration of flecainide and verapamil may have additive effects on myocardial contractility, AV conduction, and repolarization. Concomitant therapy with flecainide and verapamil may result in additive negative inotropic effect and prolongation of atrioventricular conduction.

Quinidine
In a small number of patients with hypertrophic cardiomyopathy (IHSS), concomitant use of verapamil and quinidine resulted in significant hypotension. Until further data are obtained, combined therapy of verapamil and quinidine in patients with hypertrophic cardiomyopathy should probably be avoided.
The electrophysiological effects of quinidine and verapamil on AV conduction were studied in 8 patients. Verapamil significantly counteracted the effects of quinidine on AV conduction. There has been a report of increased quinidine levels during verapamil therapy.

Antihypertensive Agents
Concomitant use of TARKA with other antihypertensive agents including diuretics, vasodilators, beta-adrenergic blockers, and alpha-antagonists may result in additive hypotensive effects. There are reports that verapamil may result in higher concentrations of the alpha-agonists prazosin and terazosin.

Dual Blockade of the Renin-Angiotensin System (RAS)
Trandolapril Component
Dual blockade of the RAS with angiotensin receptor blockers, ACE inhibitors, or aliskiren is associated with increased risks of hypotension, hyperkalemia, and changes in renal function (including acute renal failure) compared to monotherapy. Closely monitor blood pressure, renal function and electrolytes in patients on TARKA and other agents that affect the RAS.

Do not co-administer aliskiren with TARKA in patients with diabetes. Avoid use of aliskiren with TARKA in patients with renal impairment (GFR <60 ml/min).

Beta Blockers
Verapamil Component
Concomitant therapy with beta-adrenergic blockers and verapamil may result in additive negative effects on heart rate, atrioventricular conduction, and/or cardiac contractility. Drug interaction studies have indicated that the maximum concentrations of metoprolol and propanolol are increased after the administration of verapamil. The use of verapamil in combination with a beta-adrenergic blocker should be used only with caution, and close monitoring. Asymptomatic bradycardia (36 beats/min) with a wandering atrial pacemaker has been observed in a patient receiving concomitant timolol (a beta-adrenergic blocker) eyedrops and oral verapamil.

Concomitant Diuretic Therapy
Trandolapril Component
As with other ACE inhibitors, patients on diuretics, especially those on recently instituted diuretic therapy, may occasionally experience an excessive reduction of blood pressure after initiation of therapy with TARKA. The possibility of exacerbation of hypotensive effects with TARKA may be minimized by either discontinuing the diuretic or cautiously increasing salt intake prior to initiation of treatment with TARKA. If it is not possible to discontinue the diuretic, the starting dose of TARKA should be reduced (see **DOSAGE AND ADMINISTRATION**). No clinically significant pharmacokinetic interaction has been found between trandolapril (or its metabolites) and furosemide.

Agents Increasing Serum Potassium
Trandolapril Component
Trandolapril can attenuate potassium loss caused by thiazide diuretics and increase serum potassium when used alone. Use of potassium-sparing diuretics (spironolactone, triamterene, or amiloride), potassium supplements, or potassium-containing salt substitutes concomitantly with ACE inhibitors can increase the risk of hyperkalemia. If concomitant use of such agents is indicated, they should be used with caution and with appropriate monitoring of serum potassium (see **PRECAUTIONS**).

HMG-CoA Reductase Inhibitors ("Statins")
Verapamil component
The use of HMG-CoA reductase inhibitors that are CYP3A4 substrates in combination with verapamil has been associated with reports of myopathy/rhabdomyolysis.
Co-administration of multiple doses of 10 mg of verapamil with 80 mg simvastatin resulted in exposure to simvastatin 2.5-fold that following simvastatin alone. Limit the dose of simvastatin in patients on verapamil to 10 mg daily. Limit the daily dose of lovastatin to 40 mg. Lower starting and maintenance doses of other CYP3A4 substrates (e.g., atorvastatin) may be required as verapamil may increase the plasma concentration of these drugs.

Non-Steroidal Anti-Inflammatory Agents including Selective Cyclooxygenase-2 Inhibitors (COX-2 Inhibitors)
Trandolapril component
In patients who are elderly, volume-depleted (including those on diuretic therapy), or with compromised renal function, co-administration of NSAIDs, including selective COX-2 inhibitors, with ACE inhibitors, including trandolapril, may result in deterioration of renal function, including possible acute renal failure. These effects are usually reversible. Monitor renal function periodically in patients receiving trandolapril and NSAID therapy.
The antihypertensive effect of ACE inhibitors, including trandolapril may be attenuated by NSAIDs.

Other (Verapamil Component)
Nitrates
Verapamil has been given concomitantly with short- and long-acting nitrates without any undesirable drug interactions. The pharmacologic profile of both drugs and the clinical experience suggest beneficial interactions.

Carbamazepine
Verapamil may increase carbamazepine concentrations during combined therapy. This may produce carbamazepine side effects such as diplopia, headache, ataxia, or dizziness.

Anti-infective Agents
Therapy with rifampin may markedly reduce oral verapamil bioavailability. There have been reports that erythromycin and telithromycin may increase concentrations of verapamil.

Barbiturates
Phenobarbital therapy may increase verapamil clearance.

Immunosuppressive Agents

Information on the AbbVie, Inc. products listed on these pages is from the prescribing information in use as of July 31, 2014. For more information, please visit rxabbvie.com or call 1-800-633-9110.

ADVERSE EVENTS OCCURRING in ≥ 1% of TARKA PATIENTS IN U.S. PLACEBO-CONTROLLED TRIALS

	TARKA (N = 541) % Incidence (% Discontinuance)	PLACEBO (N = 206) % Incidence (% Discontinuance)
AV Block First Degree	3.9 (0.2)	0.5 (0.0)
Bradycardia	1.8 (0.0)	0.0 (0.0)
Bronchitis	1.5 (0.0)	0.5 (0.0)
Chest Pain	2.2 (0.0)	1.0 (0.0)
Constipation	3.3 (0.0)	1.0 (0.0)
Cough	4.6 (0.0)	2.4 (0.0)
Diarrhea	1.5 (0.2)	1.0 (0.0)
Dizziness	3.1 (0.0)	1.9 (0.5)
Dyspnea	1.3 (0.4)	0.0 (0.0)
Edema	1.3 (0.0)	2.4 (0.0)
Fatigue	2.8 (0.4)	2.4 (0.0)
Headache(s)+	8.9 (0.0)	9.7 (0.5)
Increased Liver Enzymes*	2.8 (0.2)	1.0 (0.0)
Nausea	1.5 (0.2)	0.5 (0.0)
Pain Extremity(ies)	1.1 (0.2)	0.5 (0.0)
Pain Back+	2.2 (0.0)	2.4 (0.0)
Pain Joint(s)	1.7 (0.0)	1.0 (0.0)
Upper Respiratory Tract Infection(s)+	5.4 (0.0)	7.8 (0.0)
Upper Respiratory Tract Congestion+	2.4 (0.0)	3.4 (0.0)

* Also includes increase in SGPT, SGOT, Alkaline Phosphatase
+ Incidence of adverse events is higher in Placebo group than TARKA patients

Verapamil therapy may increase serum levels of cyclosporin, sirolimus and tacrolimus.

Theophylline
Verapamil therapy may inhibit the clearance and increase the plasma levels of theophylline.

Tranquilizers/ Anti-depressants
Due to metabolism via the CYP enzyme system, there have been reports that verapamil may increase the concentrations of buspirone, midazolam, almotriptan and imipramine.

Colchicine
Colchicine is a substrate for both CYP3A and the efflux transporter, P-gp. Verapamil is known to inhibit CYP3A and P-gp. When verapamil and colchicine are administered together, the potential inhibition of P-gp and/or CYP3A by verapamil may lead to increased exposure to colchicine (see **PRECAUTIONS - Drug Interactions**).

Other
Concentrations of verapamil may be increased by the concomitant administration of protease inhibitors such as ritonavir, and reduced by the concomitant administration of sulfinpyrazone, or St John's Wort.
Concentrations of doxorubicin may be increased by the administration of verapamil.
There have been reports that verapamil may elevate the concentrations of the oral anti-diabetic glyburide.

Inhalation Anesthetics
Animal experiments have shown that inhalation anesthetics depress cardiovascular activity by decreasing the inward movement of calcium ions. When used concomitantly, inhalation anesthetics and calcium antagonists, such as verapamil, should be titrated carefully to avoid excessive cardiovascular depression.

Neuromuscular Blocking Agents
Clinical data and animal studies suggest that verapamil may potentiate the activity of neuromuscular blocking agents (curare-like and depolarizing). It may be necessary to decrease the dose of verapamil and/or the dose of the neuromuscular blocking agent when the drugs are used concomitantly.

Gold
Nitritoid reactions (symptoms include facial flushing, nausea, vomiting and hypotension) have been reported rarely in patients on therapy with injectable gold (sodium aurothiomalate) and concomitant ACE inhibitor therapy including TARKA.

Other (Trandolapril Component)
No clinically significant pharmacokinetic interaction has been found between trandolapril (or its metabolites) and nifedipine.
The anticoagulant effect of warfarin was not significantly changed by trandolapril.

Anti-diabetic Agents
The concomitant use of ACE inhibitors such as trandolapril with antidiabetic medications (insulin or oral hypoglycemic agents) may result in increased blood glucose lowering effects.

Carcinogenesis, Mutagenesis, Impairment of Fertility
Verapamil Component
An 18-month toxicity study in rats, at a low multiple (6 fold) of the maximum recommended human dose, and not the maximum tolerated dose, did not suggest a tumorigenic potential. There was no evidence of a carcinogenic potential of verapamil administered in the diet of rats for two years at doses of 10, 35, and 120 mg/kg per day or approximately 1×, 3.5×, and 12×, respectively, the maximum recommended human daily dose (480 mg per day or 9.6 mg/kg/day).
Verapamil was not mutagenic in the Ames test in 5 test strains at 3 mg per plate, with or without metabolic activation.
Studies in female rats at daily dietary doses up to 5.5 times (55 mg/kg/day) the maximum recommended human dose did not show impaired fertility. Effects on male fertility have not been determined.
Long-term studies were conducted with oral trandolapril administered by gavage to mice (78 weeks) and rats (104 and 106 weeks). No evidence of carcinogenic potential was seen in mice dosed up to 25 mg/kg/day (85 mg/m²/day) or rats dosed up to 8 mg/kg/day (60 mg/m²/day). These doses are 313 and 32 times (mice), and 100 and 23 times (rats) the maximum recommended human daily dose (MRHDD) of 4 mg based on body-weight and body-surface-area, respectively assuming a 50 kg individual. The genotoxic potential of trandolapril was evaluated in the microbial mutagenicity (Ames) test, the point mutation and chromosome aberration assays in Chinese hamster V79 cells, and the micronucleus test in mice. There was no evidence of mutagenic or clastogenic potential in these *in vitro* and *in vivo* assays.
Reproduction studies in rats did not show any impairment of fertility at doses up to 100 mg/kg/day (710 mg/m²/day) of trandolapril, or 1250 and 260 times the MRHDD on the basis of body-weight and body-surface-area, respectively.

Pregnancy
Female patients of childbearing age should be told about the consequences of exposure to TARKA during pregnancy. Discuss treatment options with women planning to become pregnant. Patients should be asked to report pregnancies to their physicians as soon as possible.

Nursing Mothers
Verapamil is excreted in human milk. Radiolabeled trandolapril or its metabolites are secreted in rat milk. TARKA should not be administered to nursing mothers.

Geriatric Use
In placebo-controlled studies, where 23% of patients receiving TARKA were 65 years and older, and 2.4% were 75 years and older, no overall differences in effectiveness or safety were observed between these patients and younger patients. However, greater sensitivity of some older individual patients cannot be ruled out.

Pediatric Use
Neonates with a history of *in utero* exposure to TARKA:
If oliguria or hypotension occurs, direct attention toward support of blood pressure and renal perfusion. Exchange transfusions or dialysis may be required as a means of reversing hypotension and/or substituting for disordered renal function.
The safety and effectiveness of TARKA in children below the age of 18 have not been established.

Animal Pharmacology and/or Animal Toxicology
In chronic animal toxicology studies, verapamil caused lenticular and/or suture line changes at 30 mg/kg/day or greater and frank cataracts at 62.5 mg/kg/day or greater in the beagle dog but not the rat. Development of cataracts due to verapamil has not been reported in man.

ADVERSE REACTIONS

TARKA has been evaluated in over 1,957 subjects and patients. Of these, 541 patients, including 23% elderly patients, participated in U.S. controlled clinical trials, and 251 were studied in foreign controlled clinical trials. In clinical trials with TARKA, no adverse experiences peculiar to this combination drug have been observed. Adverse experiences that have occurred have been limited to those that have been previously reported with verapamil or trandolapril. TARKA has been evaluated for long-term safety in 272 patients treated for 1 year or more. Adverse experiences were usually mild and transient.
Discontinuation of therapy because of adverse events in U.S. placebo-controlled hypertension studies was required in 2.6% and 1.9% of patients treated with TARKA and placebo, respectively.
Adverse experiences occurring in 1% or more of the 541 patients in placebo-controlled hypertension trials who were treated with a range of trandolapril (0.5-8 mg) and verapamil (120-240 mg) combinations are shown below. [See table above]
Other clinical adverse experiences possibly, probably, or definitely related to drug treatment occurring in 0.3% or more of patients treated with trandolapril/verapamil combinations with or without concomitant diuretic in controlled or uncontrolled trials (N = 990) and less frequent, clinically significant events (in italics) include the following:

Cardiovascular
Angina, AV block second degree, bundle branch block, edema, flushing, hypotension, myocardial infarction , palpitations, premature ventricular contractions, nonspecific ST-T changes, near syncope, tachycardia.

Central Nervous System
Drowsiness, hypesthesia, insomnia, loss of balance, paresthesia, vertigo.

Dermatologic
Pruritus, rash.

Emotional, Mental, Sexual States
Anxiety, impotence, abnormal mentation.

Eye, Ear, Nose, Throat
Epistaxis, tinnitus, upper respiratory tract infection, blurred vision.

Gastrointestinal
Diarrhea, dyspepsia, dry mouth, nausea.

General Body Function
Chest pain, malaise, weakness.

Genitourinary
Endometriosis, hematuria, nocturia, polyuria, proteinuria.

Hemopoietic
Decreased leukocytes, decreased neutrophils.

Musculoskeletal System
Arthralgias/myalgias, gout (increased uric acid).

Pulmonary
Dyspnea.

Angioedema
Angioedema has been reported in 3 (0.15%) patients receiving TARKA in U.S. and foreign studies (N = 1,957). Angioedema associated with laryngeal edema may be fatal. If angioedema of the face, extremities, lips, tongue, glottis, and/or larynx occurs, treatment with TARKA should be discontinued and appropriate therapy instituted immediately (see **WARNINGS**).

Hypotension
(See **WARNINGS**). In hypertensive patients, hypotension occurred in 0.6% and near syncope occurred in 0.1%. Hypotension or syncope was a cause for discontinuation of therapy in 0.4% of hypertensive patients.

Treatment of Acute Cardiovascular Adverse Reactions
The frequency of cardiovascular adverse reactions which require therapy is rare, hence, experience with their treatment is limited. Whenever severe hypotension or complete AV block occur following oral administration of TARKA (verapamil component), the appropriate emergency measures should be applied immediately, e.g., intravenously administered isoproterenol HCl, levarterenol bitartrate, atropine (all in the usual doses), or calcium gluconate (10% solution). In patients with hypertrophic cardiomyopathy (IHSS), alpha-adrenergic agents (phenylephrine, metaraminol bitartrate or methoxamine) should be used to maintain blood pressure, and isoproterenol and levarterenol should be avoided. If further support is necessary, inotropic agents (dopamine or dobutamine) may be administered. Actual treatment and dosage should depend on the severity and the clinical situation and the judgment and experience of the treating physician.
Other adverse experiences (in addition to those in table and listed above) that have been reported with the individual components are listed below.
Verapamil Component
Cardiovascular
(See **WARNINGS**). CHF/pulmonary edema, AV block 3°, atrioventricular dissociation, claudication, purpura (vasculitis), syncope.
Digestive System
Gingival hyperplasia. Reversible, (upon discontinuation of verapamil) nonobstructive, paralytic ileus has been infrequently reported in association with the use of verapamil.

Hemic and Lymphatic
Ecchymosis or bruising.
Nervous System
Cerebrovascular accident, confusion, psychotic symptoms, shakiness, somnolence.
Skin
Exanthema, hair loss, hyperkeratosis, maculae, sweating, urticaria, Stevens-Johnson syndrome, erythema multiforme.
Urogenital
Gynecomastia, galactorrhea/hyperprolactinemia, increased urination, spotty menstruation.
Trandolapril Component
Emotional, Mental, Sexual States
Decreased libido.
Gastrointestinal
Pancreatitis.

Clinical Laboratory Test Findings
Hematology
(See **WARNINGS**). Low white blood cells, low neutrophils, low lymphocytes, low platelets.
Serum Electrolytes
Hyperkalemia (see **PRECAUTIONS**), hyponatremia.
Renal Function Tests
Increases in creatinine and blood urea nitrogen levels occurred in 1.1 percent and 0.3 percent, respectively, of patients receiving TARKA with or without hydrochlorothiazide therapy. None of these increases required discontinuation of treatment. Increases in these laboratory values are more likely to occur in patients with renal insufficiency or those pretreated with a diuretic and, based on experience with other ACE inhibitors, would be expected to be especially likely in patients with renal artery stenosis (see **PRECAUTIONS** and **WARNINGS**).
Liver Function Tests
Elevations of liver enzymes (SGOT, SGPT, LDH, and alkaline phosphatase) and/or serum bilirubin occurred. Discontinuation for elevated liver enzymes occurred in 0.9 percent of patients (see **WARNINGS**).
Post Marketing Experience
There has been a single postmarketing report of paralysis (tetraparesis) associated with the combined use of verapamil and colchicine. This may have been caused by colchicine crossing the blood-brain barrier due to CYP3A4 and P-gp inhibition by verapamil. Combined use of verapamil and colchicine is not recommended (see **PRECAUTIONS - Drug Interactions**).

OVERDOSAGE

No specific information is available on the treatment of overdosage with TARKA.
Verapamil Component
Overdose with verapamil may lead to pronounced hypotension, bradycardia, and conduction system abnormalities (e.g., junctional rhythm with AV dissociation and high degree AV block, including asystole). Other symptoms secondary to hypoperfusion (e.g., metabolic acidosis, hyperglycemia, hyperkalemia, renal dysfunction, and convulsions) may be evident.
Treat all verapamil overdoses as serious and maintain observation for at least 48 hours, preferably under continuous hospital care. Delayed pharmacodynamic consequences may occur with the sustained release formulation. Verapamil is known to decrease gastrointestinal transit time. In cases of overdose, tablets of ISOPTIN SR have occasionally been reported to form concretions within the stomach or intestines. These concretions have not been visible on plain radiographs of the abdomen, and no medical means of gastrointestinal emptying is of proven efficacy in removing them. Endoscopy might reasonably be considered in cases of overdose when symptoms are unusually prolonged. Verapamil cannot be removed by hemodialysis.
Treatment of overdosage should be supportive. Beta adrenergic stimulation or parenteral administration of calcium solutions may increase calcium ion flux across the slow channel, and have been used effectively in treatment of deliberate overdosage with verapamil. The following measures may be considered:
Bradycardia and Conduction System Abnormalities
Atropine, isoproterenol, and cardiac pacing.
Hypotension
Intravenous fluids, vasopressors (e.g., dopamine, dobutamine), calcium solutions (e.g., 10% calcium chloride solution).
Cardiac Failures
Inotropic agents (e.g., isoproterenol, dopamine, dobutamine), diuretics. Asystole should be handled by the usual measures including cardiopulmonary resuscitation.
Trandolapril Component
The oral LD_{50} of trandolapril in mice was 4875 mg/kg in males and 3990 mg/kg in females. In rats, an oral dose of 5000 mg/kg caused low mortality (1 male out of 5; 0 females). In dogs, an oral dose of 1000 mg/kg did not cause mortality and abnormal clinical signs were not observed.

In humans, the most likely clinical manifestation would be symptoms attributable to severe hypotension. Laboratory determinations of serum levels of trandolapril and its metabolites are not widely available, and such determinations have, in any event, no established role in the management of trandolapril overdose. No data are available to suggest that physiological maneuvers (e.g., maneuvers to change pH of the urine) might accelerate elimination of trandolapril and its metabolites. It is not known if trandolapril or trandolaprilat can be usefully removed from the body by hemodialysis.
Angiotensin II could presumably serve as a specific antagonist antidote in the setting of trandolapril overdose, but angiotensin II is essentially unavailable outside of scattered research facilities. Because the hypotensive effect of trandolapril is achieved through vasodilation and effective hypovolemia, it is reasonable to treat trandolapril overdose by infusion of normal saline solution.

DOSAGE AND ADMINISTRATION

The recommended usual dosage range of trandolapril for hypertension is 1 to 4 mg per day administered in a single dose or two divided doses. The recommended usual dosage range of Isoptin-SR for hypertension is 120 to 480 mg per day administered in a single dose or two divided doses.
The hazards (see **WARNINGS**) of trandolapril are generally independent of dose; those of verapamil are a mixture of dose-dependent phenomena (primarily dizziness, AV block, constipation) and dose-independent phenomena, the former much more common than the latter. Therapy with any combination of trandolapril and verapamil will thus be associated with both sets of dose-independent hazards. The dose-dependent side effects of verapamil have not been shown to be decreased by the addition of trandolapril nor vice versa. Rarely, the dose-independent hazards of trandolapril are serious. To minimize dose-independent hazards, it is usually appropriate to begin therapy with TARKA only after a patient has either (a) failed to achieve the desired antihypertensive effect with one or the other monotherapy at its respective maximally recommended dose and shortest dosing interval, or (b) the dose of one or the other monotherapy cannot be increased further because of dose-limiting side effects.
Clinical trials with TARKA have explored only once-a-day doses. The antihypertensive effect and or adverse effects of adding 4 mg of trandolapril once-a-day to a dose of 240 mg Isoptin-SR administered twice-a-day has not been studied, nor have the effects of adding as little of 180 mg Isoptin-SR to 2 mg trandolapril administered twice-a-day been evaluated. Over the dose range of Isoptin-SR 120 to 240 mg once-a-day and trandolapril 0.5 to 8 mg once-a-day, the effects of the combination increase with increasing doses of either component.

Replacement Therapy
For convenience, patients receiving trandolapril (up to 8 mg) and verapamil (up to 240 mg) in separate tablets, administered once-a-day, may instead wish to receive tablets of TARKA containing the same component doses.
TARKA should be administered with food.

HOW SUPPLIED

TARKA 2/180 mg tablets are supplied as pink, oval, film-coated tablets containing 2 mg trandolapril in an immediate release form and 180 mg verapamil hydrochloride in a sustained release form. The tablet is debossed with a triangle and 182 on one side and plain on the other side.
NDC 0074-3287-13 - bottles of 100
TARKA 1/240 mg tablets are supplied as white, oval, film-coated tablets containing 1 mg trandolapril in an immediate release form and 240 mg verapamil hydrochloride in a sustained release form. The tablet is debossed with a triangle and 241 on one side and plain on the other side.
NDC 0074-3288-13 - bottles of 100
TARKA 2/240 mg tablets are supplied as gold, oval, film-coated tablets containing 2 mg trandolapril in an immediate release form and 240 mg verapamil hydrochloride in a sustained release form. The tablet is debossed with a triangle and 242 on one side and plain on the other side.
NDC 0074-3289-13 - bottles of 100
TARKA 4/240 mg tablets are supplied as reddish-brown, oval, film-coated tablets containing 4 mg trandolapril in an immediate release form and 240 mg verapamil hydrochloride in a sustained release form. The tablet is debossed with a triangle and 244 on one side and plain on the other side.
NDC 0074-3290-13 - bottles of 100
Dispense in well-closed container with safety closure.
Storage
Store at 15°-25°C (59°-77°F) see USP.
AbbVie Inc.
North Chicago, IL 60064, U.S.A.
03-A778 February, 2013
Shown in Product Identification Guide, page 304

TRICOR®
[*tri cŏr*]
(fenofibrate)
Tablet for oral use

HIGHLIGHTS OF PRESCRIBING INFORMATION
These highlights do not include all the information needed to use TRICOR safely and effectively. See full prescribing information for TRICOR.
TRICOR (fenofibrate) Tablet for oral use
Initial U.S. Approval: 1993

——————**INDICATIONS AND USAGE**——————
TRICOR is a peroxisome proliferator receptor alpha (PPARα) activator indicated as an adjunct to diet:
• To reduce elevated LDL-C, Total-C, TG and Apo B, and to increase HDL-C in adult patients with primary hypercholesterolemia or mixed dyslipidemia (1.1).
• For treatment of adult patients with severe hypertriglyceridemia (1.2).
Important Limitations of Use: Fenofibrate was not shown to reduce coronary heart disease morbidity and mortality in patients with type 2 diabetes mellitus (5.1).

——————**DOSAGE AND ADMINISTRATION**——————
• Primary hypercholesterolemia or mixed dyslipidemia: Initial dose of 145 mg once daily (2.2).
• Severe hypertriglyceridemia: Initial dose of 48 to 145 mg once daily. Maximum dose is 145 mg (2.3).
• Renally impaired patients: Initial dose of 48 mg once daily (2.4).
• Geriatric patients: Select the dose on the basis of renal function (2.5).
• Maybe taken without regard to meals (2.1).

——————**DOSAGE FORMS AND STRENGTHS**——————
Oral Tablets: 48 mg and 145 mg (3).

——————**CONTRAINDICATIONS**——————
• Severe renal dysfunction, including patients receiving dialysis (4, 8.6, 12.3).
• Active liver disease (4, 5.3).
• Gallbladder disease (4, 5.5).
• Known hypersensitivity to fenofibrate (4).
• Nursing mothers (4, 8.3).

——————**WARNINGS AND PRECAUTIONS**——————
• Myopathy and rhabdomyolysis have been reported in patients taking fenofibrate. The risks for myopathy and rhabdomyolysis are increased when fibrates are co-administered with a statin (with a significantly higher rate observed for gemfibrozil), particularly in elderly patients and patients with diabetes, renal failure, or hypothyroidism (5.2).
• TRICOR can increase serum transaminases. Monitor liver tests, including ALT, periodically during therapy (5.3).
• TRICOR can reversibly increase serum creatinine levels (5.4). Monitor renal function periodically in patients with renal impairment (8.6).
• TRICOR increases cholesterol excretion into the bile, leading to risk of cholelithiasis. If cholelithiasis is suspected, gallbladder studies are indicated (5.5).
• Exercise caution in concomitant treatment with oral coumarin anticoagulants. Adjust the dosage of coumarin anticoagulant to maintain the prothrombin time/INR at the desired level to prevent bleeding complications (5.6).

——————**ADVERSE REACTIONS**——————
The most common adverse reactions (> 2% and at least 1% greater than placebo) are abnormal liver tests, increased AST, increased ALT, increased CPK, and rhinitis (6).

To report SUSPECTED ADVERSE REACTIONS, contact AbbVie Inc. at 1-800-633-9110 or FDA at 1-800-FDA-1088 or www.fda.gov/medwatch.

——————**DRUG INTERACTIONS**——————
• Coumarin anticoagulants: (7.1).
• Immunosuppressants: (7.2).
• Bile acid resins: (7.3).

——————**USE IN SPECIFIC POPULATIONS**——————
• Geriatric Use: Determine dose selection based on renal function (8.5).
• Renal Impairment: Avoid use in patients with severe renal impairment. Dose reduction is required in patients with mild to moderate renal impairment (8.6).
See 17 for PATIENT COUNSELING INFORMATION
Revised: 02/2013

FULL PRESCRIBING INFORMATION: CONTENTS*
1   INDICATIONS AND USAGE

Information on the AbbVie, Inc. products listed on these pages is from the prescribing information in use as of July 31, 2014. For more information, please visit rxabbvie.com or call 1-800-633-9110.

2 **DOSAGE AND ADMINISTRATION**
  2.1 General Considerations
  2.2 Primary Hypercholesterolemia or Mixed Dyslipidemia
  2.3 Severe Hypertriglyceridemia
  2.4 Impaired Renal Function
  2.5 Geriatric Patients
3 **DOSAGE FORMS AND STRENGTHS**
4 **CONTRAINDICATIONS**
5 **WARNINGS AND PRECAUTIONS**
  5.1 Mortality and Coronary Heart Disease Morbidity
  5.2 Skeletal Muscle
  5.3 Liver Function
  5.4 Serum Creatinine
  5.5 Cholelithiasis
  5.6 Coumarin Anticoagulants
  5.7 Pancreatitis
  5.8 Hematologic Changes
  5.9 Hypersensitivity Reactions
  5.10 Venothromboembolic Disease
  5.11 Paradoxical Decreases in HDL Cholesterol Levels
6 **ADVERSE REACTIONS**
  6.1 Clinical Trials Experience
  6.2 Postmarketing Experience
7 **DRUG INTERACTIONS**
  7.1 Coumarin Anticoagulants
  7.2 Immunosuppressants
  7.3 Bile Acid Binding Resins
  7.4 Colchicine
8 **USE IN SPECIFIC POPULATIONS**
  8.1 Pregnancy
  8.3 Nursing Mothers
  8.4 Pediatric Use
  8.5 Geriatric Use
  8.6 Renal Impairment
  8.7 Hepatic Impairment
10 **OVERDOSAGE**
11 **DESCRIPTION**
12 **CLINICAL PHARMACOLOGY**
  12.1 Mechanism of Action
  12.2 Pharmacodynamics
  12.3 Pharmacokinetics
13 **NONCLINICAL TOXICOLOGY**
  13.1 Carcinogenesis and Mutagenesis and Impairment of Fertility
14 **CLINICAL STUDIES**
  14.1 Primary Hypercholesterolemia (Heterozygous Familial and Nonfamilial) and Mixed Dyslipidemia
  14.2 Severe Hypertriglyceridemia
16 **HOW SUPPLIED/STORAGE AND HANDLING**
17 **PATIENT COUNSELING INFORMATION**
* Sections or subsections omitted from the full prescribing information are not listed

---

FULL PRESCRIBING INFORMATION

1 **INDICATIONS AND USAGE**
1.1 Primary Hypercholesterolemia or Mixed Dyslipidemia
TRICOR is indicated as adjunctive therapy to diet to reduce elevated low-density lipoprotein cholesterol (LDL-C), total cholesterol (Total-C), Triglycerides and apolipoprotein B (Apo B), and to increase high-density lipoprotein cholesterol (HDL-C) in adult patients with primary hypercholesterolemia or mixed dyslipidemia.
1.2 Severe Hypertriglyceridemia
TRICOR is also indicated as adjunctive therapy to diet for treatment of adult patients with severe hypertriglyceridemia. Improving glycemic control in diabetic patients showing fasting chylomicronemia will usually obviate the need for pharmacologic intervention.
Markedly elevated levels of serum triglycerides (e.g. > 2,000 mg/dL) may increase the risk of developing pancreatitis. The effect of fenofibrate therapy on reducing this risk has not been adequately studied.
1.3 Important Limitations of Use
Fenofibrate at a dose equivalent to 145 mg of TRICOR was not shown to reduce coronary heart disease morbidity and mortality in a large, randomized controlled trial of patients with type 2 diabetes mellitus [see Warnings and Precautions (5.1)].

2 **DOSAGE AND ADMINISTRATION**
2.1 General Considerations
Patients should be placed on an appropriate lipid-lowering diet before receiving TRICOR, and should continue this diet during treatment with TRICOR. TRICOR tablets can be given without regard to meals.
The initial treatment for dyslipidemia is dietary therapy specific for the type of lipoprotein abnormality. Excess body weight and excess alcoholic intake may be important factors in hypertriglyceridemia and should be addressed prior to any drug therapy. Physical exercise can be an important ancillary measure. Diseases contributory to hyperlipidemia,

such as hypothyroidism or diabetes mellitus should be looked for and adequately treated. Estrogen therapy, thiazide diuretics and beta-blockers, are sometimes associated with massive rises in plasma triglycerides, especially in subjects with familial hypertriglyceridemia. In such cases, discontinuation of the specific etiologic agent may obviate the need for specific drug therapy of hypertriglyceridemia. Lipid levels should be monitored periodically and consideration should be given to reducing the dosage of TRICOR if lipid levels fall significantly below the targeted range.
Therapy should be withdrawn in patients who do not have an adequate response after two months of treatment with the maximum recommended dose of 145 mg once daily.
2.2 Primary Hypercholesterolemia or Mixed Dyslipidemia
The initial dose of TRICOR is 145 mg once daily.
2.3 Severe Hypertriglyceridemia
The initial dose is 48 to 145 mg per day. Dosage should be individualized according to patient response, and should be adjusted if necessary following repeat lipid determinations at 4 to 8 week intervals. The maximum dose is 145 mg once daily.
2.4 Impaired Renal Function
Treatment with TRICOR should be initiated at a dose of 48 mg per day in patients having mild to moderately impaired renal function, and increased only after evaluation of the effects on renal function and lipid levels at this dose. The use of TRICOR should be avoided in patients with severe renal impairment [see Use in Specific Populations (8.6) and Clinical Pharmacology (12.3)].
2.5 Geriatric Patients
Dose selection for the elderly should be made on the basis of renal function [see Use in Specific Populations (8.5)].

3 **DOSAGE FORMS AND STRENGTHS**
• 48 mg yellow tablets, imprinted with the "a" logo and code identification letters "FI".
• 145 mg white tablets, imprinted with the "a" logo and code identification letters "FO".

4 **CONTRAINDICATIONS**
TRICOR is contraindicated in:
• patients with severe renal impairment, including those receiving dialysis [see Clinical Pharmacology (12.3)].
• patients with active liver disease, including those with primary biliary cirrhosis and unexplained persistent liver function abnormalities [see Warnings and Precautions (5.3)].
• patients with preexisting gallbladder disease [see Warnings and Precautions (5.5)].
• nursing mothers [see Use in Specific Populations (8.3)].
• patients with known hypersensitivity to fenofibrate or fenofibric acid [see Warnings and Precautions (5.9)].

5 **WARNINGS AND PRECAUTIONS**
5.1 Mortality and Coronary Heart Disease Morbidity
The effect of TRICOR on coronary heart disease morbidity and mortality and non-cardiovascular mortality has not been established.
The Action to Control Cardiovascular Risk in Diabetes Lipid (ACCORD Lipid) trial was a randomized placebo-controlled study of 5518 patients with type 2 diabetes mellitus on background statin therapy treated with fenofibrate. The mean duration of follow-up was 4.7 years. Fenofibrate plus statin combination therapy showed a non-significant 8% relative risk reduction in the primary outcome of major adverse cardiovascular events (MACE), a composite of non-fatal myocardial infarction, non-fatal stroke, and cardiovascular disease death (hazard ratio [HR] 0.92, 95% CI 0.79-1.08) (p=0.32) as compared to statin monotherapy. In a gender subgroup analysis, the hazard ratio for MACE in men receiving combination therapy versus statin monotherapy was 0.82 (95% CI 0.69-0.99), and the hazard ratio for MACE in women receiving combination therapy versus statin monotherapy was 1.38 (95% CI 0.98-1.94) (interaction p=0.01). The clinical significance of this subgroup finding is unclear.
The Fenofibrate Intervention and Event Lowering in Diabetes (FIELD) study was a 5-year randomized, placebo-controlled study of 9795 patients with type 2 diabetes mellitus treated with fenofibrate. Fenofibrate demonstrated a non-significant 11% relative reduction in the primary outcome of coronary heart disease events (hazard ratio [HR] 0.89, 95% CI 0.75-1.05, p=0.16) and a significant 11% reduction in the secondary outcome of total cardiovascular disease events (HR 0.89 [0.80-0.99], p=0.04). There was a non-significant 11% (HR 1.11 [0.95, 1.29], p=0.18) and 19% (HR 1.19 [0.90, 1.57], p=0.22) increase in total and coronary heart disease mortality, respectively, with fenofibrate as compared to placebo.
Because of chemical, pharmacological, and clinical similarities between TRICOR (fenofibrate tablets), clofibrate, and gemfibrozil, the adverse findings in 4 large randomized, placebo-controlled clinical studies with these other fibrate drugs may also apply to TRICOR.

In the Coronary Drug Project, a large study of post myocardial infarction of patients treated for 5 years with clofibrate, there was no difference in mortality seen between the clofibrate group and the placebo group. There was however, a difference in the rate of cholelithiasis and cholecystitis requiring surgery between the two groups (3.0% vs. 1.8%).
In a study conducted by the World Health Organization (WHO), 5000 subjects without known coronary artery disease were treated with placebo or clofibrate for 5 years and followed for an additional one year. There was a statistically significant, higher age - adjusted all-cause mortality in the clofibrate group compared with the placebo group (5.70% vs. 3.96%, p = < 0.01). Excess mortality was due to a 33% increase in non-cardiovascular causes, including malignancy, post-cholecystectomy complications, and pancreatitis. This appeared to confirm the higher risk of gallbladder disease seen in clofibrate-treated patients studied in the Coronary Drug Project.
The Helsinki Heart Study was a large (n=4081) study of middle-aged men without a history of coronary artery disease. Subjects received either placebo or gemfibrozil for 5 years, with a 3.5 year open extension afterward. Total mortality was numerically higher in the gemfibrozil randomization group but did not achieve statistical significance (p = 0.19, 95% confidence interval for relative risk G:P = .91-1.64). Although cancer deaths trended higher in the gemfibrozil group (p = 0.11), cancers (excluding basal cell carcinoma) were diagnosed with equal frequency in both study groups. Due to the limited size of the study, the relative risk of death from any cause was not shown to be different than that seen in the 9 year follow-up data from World Health Organization study (RR=1.29).
A secondary prevention component of the Helsinki Heart Study enrolled middle-aged men excluded from the primary prevention study because of known or suspected coronary heart disease. Subjects received gemfibrozil or placebo for 5 years. Although cardiac deaths trended higher in the gemfibrozil group, this was not statistically significant (hazard ratio 2.2, 95% confidence interval: 0.94-5.05). The rate of gallbladder surgery was not statistically significant between study groups, but did trend higher in the gemfibrozil group, (1.9% vs. 0.3%, p = 0.07).
5.2 Skeletal Muscle
Fibrates increase the risk for myopathy and have been associated with rhabdomyolysis. The risk for serious muscle toxicity appears to be increased in elderly patients and in patients with diabetes, renal insufficiency, or hypothyroidism.
Myopathy should be considered in any patient with diffuse myalgias, muscle tenderness or weakness, and/or marked elevations of creatine phosphokinase (CPK) levels.
Patients should be advised to report promptly unexplained muscle pain, tenderness or weakness, particularly if accompanied by malaise or fever. CPK levels should be assessed in patients reporting these symptoms, and TRICOR therapy should be discontinued if markedly elevated CPK levels occur or myopathy/myositis is suspected or diagnosed.
Data from observational studies indicate that the risk for rhabdomyolysis is increased when fibrates, in particular gemfibrozil, are co-administered with an HMG-CoA reductase inhibitor (statin). The combination should be avoided unless the benefit of further alterations in lipid levels is likely to outweigh the increased risk of this drug combination [see Clinical Pharmacology (12.3)].
Cases of myopathy, including rhabdomyolysis, have been reported with fenofibrates co-administered with colchicine, and caution should be exercised when prescribing fenofibrate with colchicine [see Drug Interactions (7.4)].
5.3 Liver Function
Fenofibrate at doses equivalent to 96 mg to 145 mg TRICOR per day has been associated with increases in serum transaminases [AST (SGOT) or ALT (SGPT)]. In a pooled analysis of 10 placebo-controlled trials, increases to > 3 times the upper limit of normal occurred in 5.3% of patients taking fenofibrate versus 1.1% of patients treated with placebo.
When transaminase determinations were followed either after discontinuation of treatment or during continued treatment, a return to normal limits was usually observed. The incidence of increases in transaminases related to fenofibrate therapy appear to be dose related. In an 8-week dose-ranging study, the incidence of ALT or AST elevations to at least three times the upper limit of normal was 13% in patients receiving dosages equivalent to 96 mg to 145 mg TRICOR per day and was 0% in those receiving dosages equivalent to 48 mg or less TRICOR per day, or placebo. Hepatocellular, chronic active and cholestatic hepatitis associated with fenofibrate therapy have been reported after exposures of weeks to several years. In extremely rare cases, cirrhosis has been reported in association with chronic active hepatitis.
Baseline and regular periodic monitoring of liver function, including serum ALT (SGPT) should be performed for the duration of therapy with TRICOR, and therapy discontinued if enzyme levels persist above three times the normal limit.

5.4 Serum Creatinine

Elevations in serum creatinine have been reported in patients on fenofibrate. These elevations tend to return to baseline following discontinuation of fenofibrate. The clinical significance of these observations is unknown. Monitor renal function in patients with renal impairment taking TRICOR. Renal monitoring should also be considered for patients taking TRICOR at risk for renal insufficiency such as the elderly and patients with diabetes.

5.5 Cholelithiasis

Fenofibrate, like clofibrate and gemfibrozil, may increase cholesterol excretion into the bile, leading to cholelithiasis. If cholelithiasis is suspected, gallbladder studies are indicated. TRICOR therapy should be discontinued if gallstones are found.

5.6 Coumarin Anticoagulants

Caution should be exercised when coumarin anticoagulants are given in conjunction with TRICOR because of the potentiation of coumarin-type anticoagulant effects in prolonging the Prothrombin Time/International Normalized Ratio (PT/INR). To prevent bleeding complications, frequent monitoring of PT/INR and dose adjustment of the anticoagulant are recommended until PT/INR has stabilized *[see Drug Interactions (7.1)]*.

5.7 Pancreatitis

Pancreatitis has been reported in patients taking fenofibrate, gemfibrozil, and clofibrate. This occurrence may represent a failure of efficacy in patients with severe hypertriglyceridemia, a direct drug effect, or a secondary phenomenon mediated through biliary tract stone or sludge formation with obstruction of the common bile duct.

5.8 Hematologic Changes

Mild to moderate hemoglobin, hematocrit, and white blood cell decreases have been observed in patients following initiation of fenofibrate therapy. However, these levels stabilize during long-term administration. Thrombocytopenia and agranulocytosis have been reported in individuals treated with fenofibrate. Periodic monitoring of red and white blood cell counts are recommended during the first 12 months of TRICOR administration.

5.9 Hypersensitivity Reactions

Acute hypersensitivity reactions such as Stevens-Johnson syndrome and toxic epidermal necrolysis requiring patient hospitalization and treatment with steroids have been reported in individuals treated with fenofibrates. Urticaria was seen in 1.1 vs. 0%, and rash in 1.4 vs. 0.8% of fenofibrate and placebo patients respectively in controlled trials.

5.10 Venothromboembolic Disease

In the FIELD trial, pulmonary embolus (PE) and deep vein thrombosis (DVT) were observed at higher rates in the fenofibrate- than the placebo-treated group. Of 9,795 patients enrolled in FIELD, there were 4,900 in the placebo group and 4,895 in the fenofibrate group. For DVT, there were 48 events (1%) in the placebo group and 67 (1%) in the fenofibrate group (p = 0.074); and for PE, there were 32 (0.7%) events in the placebo group and 53 (1%) in the fenofibrate group (p = 0.022).

In the Coronary Drug Project, a higher proportion of the clofibrate group experienced definite or suspected fatal or nonfatal pulmonary embolism or thrombophlebitis than the placebo group (5.2% vs. 3.3% at five years; p < 0.01).

5.11 Paradoxical Decreases in HDL Cholesterol Levels

There have been postmarketing and clinical trial reports of severe decreases in HDL cholesterol levels (as low as 2 mg/dL) occurring in diabetic and non-diabetic patients initiated on fibrate therapy. The decrease in HDL-C is mirrored by a decrease in apolipoprotein A1. This decrease has been reported to occur within 2 weeks to years after initiation of fibrate therapy. The HDL-C levels remain depressed until fibrate therapy has been withdrawn; the response to withdrawal of fibrate therapy is rapid and sustained. The clinical significance of this decrease in HDL-C is unknown. It is recommended that HDL-C levels be checked within the first few months after initiation of fibrate therapy. If a severely depressed HDL-C level is detected, fibrate therapy should be withdrawn, and the HDL-C level monitored until it has returned to baseline, and fibrate therapy should not be re-initiated.

6 ADVERSE REACTIONS

6.1 Clinical Trials Experience

Because clinical studies are conducted under widely varying conditions, adverse reaction rates observed in the clinical studies of a drug cannot be directly compared to rates in the clinical studies of another drug and may not reflect the rates observed in practice.

Adverse events reported by 2% or more of patients treated with fenofibrate (and greater than placebo) during the double-blind, placebo-controlled trials, regardless of causality, are listed in Table 1 below. Adverse events led to discontinuation of treatment in 5.0% of patients treated with fenofibrate and in 3.0% treated with placebo. Increases in liver function tests were the most frequent events, causing discontinuation of fenofibrate treatment in 1.6% of patients in double-blind trials.

Table 1. Adverse Reactions Reported by 2% or More of Patients Treated with Fenofibrate and Greater than Placebo During the Double-Blind, Placebo-Controlled Trials

BODY SYSTEM	Fenofibrate*	Placebo
Adverse Reaction	(N=439)	(N=365)
BODY AS A WHOLE		
Abdominal Pain	4.6%	4.4%
Back Pain	3.4%	2.5%
Headache	3.2%	2.7%
DIGESTIVE		
Nausea	2.3%	1.9%
Constipation	2.1%	1.4%
METABOLIC AND NUTRITIONAL DISORDERS		
Abnormal Liver Function Tests	7.5%**	1.4%
Increased ALT	3.0%	1.6%
Increased CPK	3.0%	1.4%
Increased AST	3.4%**	0.5%
RESPIRATORY		
Respiratory Disorder	6.2%	5.5%
Rhinitis	2.3%	1.1%

* Dosage equivalent to 145 mg TRICOR.
** Significantly different from Placebo.

6.2 Postmarketing Experience

The following adverse reactions have been identified during postapproval use of fenofibrate: myalgia, rhabdomyolysis, pancreatitis, acute renal failure, muscle spasm, hepatitis, cirrhosis, anemia, arthralgia, decreases in hemoglobin, decreases in hematocrit, white blood cell decreases, asthenia, and severely depressed HDL-cholesterol levels. Because these reactions are reported voluntarily from a population of uncertain size, it is not always possible to reliably estimate their frequency or establish a causal relationship to drug exposure.

7 DRUG INTERACTIONS

7.1 Coumarin Anticoagulants

Potentiation of coumarin-type anticoagulant effects has been observed with prolongation of the PT/INR.

Caution should be exercised when coumarin anticoagulants are given in conjunction with TRICOR. The dosage of the anticoagulants should be reduced to maintain the PT/INR at the desired level to prevent bleeding complications. Frequent PT/INR determinations are advisable until it has been definitely determined that the PT/INR has stabilized *[see Warnings and Precautions (5.6)]*.

7.2 Immunosuppressants

Immunosuppressants such as cyclosporine and tacrolimus can produce nephrotoxicity with decreases in creatinine clearance and rises in serum creatinine, and because renal excretion is the primary elimination route of fibrate drugs including TRICOR, there is a risk that an interaction will lead to deterioration of renal function. The benefits and risks of using TRICOR (fenofibrate tablets) with immunosuppressants and other potentially nephrotoxic agents should be carefully considered, and the lowest effective dose employed and renal function monitored.

7.3 Bile Acid Binding Resins

Since bile acid binding resins may bind other drugs given concurrently, patients should take TRICOR at least 1 hour before or 4 to 6 hours after a bile acid binding resin to avoid impeding its absorption.

7.4 Colchicine

Cases of myopathy, including rhabdomyolysis, have been reported with fenofibrates co-administered with colchicine, and caution should be exercised when prescribing fenofibrate with colchicine.

8 USE IN SPECIFIC POPULATIONS

8.1 Pregnancy

Pregnancy Category C

Safety in pregnant women has not been established. There are no adequate and well controlled studies of fenofibrate in pregnant women. Fenofibrate should be used during pregnancy only if the potential benefit justifies the potential risk to the fetus.

In female rats given oral dietary doses of 15, 75, and 300 mg/kg/day of fenofibrate from 15 days prior to mating through weaning, maternal toxicity was observed at 0.3 times the MRHD, based on body surface area comparisons; mg/m^2.

In pregnant rats given oral dietary doses of 14, 127, and 361 mg/kg/day from gestation day 6-15 during the period of organogenesis, adverse developmental findings were not observed at 14 mg/kg/day (less than 1 times the MRHD, based on body surface area comparisons; mg/m^2). At higher multiples of human doses evidence of maternal toxicity was observed.

In pregnant rabbits given oral gavage doses of 15, 150, and 300 mg/kg/day from gestation day 6-18 during the period of organogenesis and allowed to deliver, aborted litters were observed at 150 mg/kg/day (10 times the MRHD, based on body surface area comparisons: mg/m^2). No developmental findings were observed at 15 mg/kg/day (at less than 1 times the MRHD, based on body surface area comparisons; mg/m^2).

In pregnant rats given oral dietary doses of 15, 75, and 300 mg/kg/day from gestation day 15 through lactation day 21 (weaning), maternal toxicity was observed at less than 1 times the maximum recommended human dose (MRHD), based on body surface area comparisons; mg/m^2.

8.3 Nursing Mothers

Fenofibrate should not be used in nursing mothers. A decision should be made whether to discontinue nursing or to discontinue the drug, taking into account the importance of the drug to the mother.

8.4 Pediatric Use

Safety and effectiveness have not been established in pediatric patients.

8.5 Geriatric Use

Fenofibric acid is known to be substantially excreted by the kidney, and the risk of adverse reactions to this drug may be greater in patients with impaired renal function. Fenofibric acid exposure is not influenced by age. Since elderly patients have a higher incidence of renal impairment, dose selection for the elderly should be made on the basis of renal function *[see Dosage and Administration (2.5) and Clinical Pharmacology (12.3)]*. Elderly patients with normal renal function should require no dose modifications. Consider monitoring renal function in elderly patients taking TRICOR.

8.6 Renal Impairment

The use of TRICOR should be avoided in patients who have severe renal impairment *[see Contraindications (4)]*. Dose reduction is required in patients with mild to moderate renal impairment *[see Dosage and Administration (2.4) and Clinical Pharmacology (12.3)]*. Monitoring renal function in patients with renal impairment is recommended.

8.7 Hepatic Impairment

The use of TRICOR has not been evaluated in subjects with hepatic impairment *[see Contraindications (4) and Clinical Pharmacology (12.3)]*.

10 OVERDOSAGE

There is no specific treatment for overdose with TRICOR. General supportive care of the patient is indicated, including monitoring of vital signs and observation of clinical status, should an overdose occur. If indicated, elimination of unabsorbed drug should be achieved by emesis or gastric lavage; usual precautions should be observed to maintain the airway. Because fenofibric acid is highly bound to plasma proteins, hemodialysis should not be considered.

11 DESCRIPTION

TRICOR (fenofibrate tablets), is a lipid regulating agent available as tablets for oral administration. Each tablet contains 48 mg or 145 mg of fenofibrate. The chemical name for fenofibrate is 2-[4-(4-chlorobenzoyl) phenoxyl-2-methylpropanoic acid, 1-methylethyl ester with the following structural formula:

The empirical formula is $C_{20}H_{21}O_4Cl$ and the molecular weight is 360.83; fenofibrate is insoluble in water. The melting point is 79-82°C. Fenofibrate is a white solid which is stable under ordinary conditions.

Inactive Ingredients

Each tablet contains hypromellose 2910 (3 cps), docusate sodium, sucrose, sodium lauryl sulfate, lactose monohydrate, silicified microcrystalline cellulose, crospovidone, and magnesium stearate.

Information on the AbbVie, Inc. products listed on these pages is from the prescribing information in use as of July 31, 2014. For more information, please visit rxabbvie.com or call 1-800-633-9110.

Table 2. Effects of Co-Administered Drugs on Fenofibric Acid Systemic Exposure from Fenofibrate Administration

Co-Administered Drug	Dosage Regimen of Co-Administered Drug	Dosage Regimen of Fenofibrate	Changes in Fenofibric Acid Exposure	
			AUC	C_{max}
Lipid-lowering agents				
Atorvastatin	20 mg once daily for 10 days	Fenofibrate 160 mg[1] once daily for 10 days	↓2%	↓4%
Pravastatin	40 mg as a single dose	Fenofibrate 3×67 mg[2] as a single dose	↓1%	↓2%
Fluvastatin	40 mg as a single dose	Fenofibrate 160 mg[1] as a single dose	↓2%	↓10%
Anti-diabetic agents				
Glimepiride	1 mg as a single dose	Fenofibrate 145 mg[1] once daily for 10 days	↑1%	↓1%
Metformin	850 mg three times daily for 10 days	Fenofibrate 54 mg[1] three times daily for 10 days	↓9%	↓6%
Rosiglitazone	8 mg once daily for 5 days	Fenofibrate 145 mg[1] once daily for 14 days	↑10%	↑3%

[1] TriCor (fenofibrate) oral tablet
[2] TriCor (fenofibrate) oral micronized capsule

Table 3. Effects of Fenofibrate Co-Administration on Systemic Exposure of Other Drugs

Dosage Regimen of Fenofibrate	Dosage Regimen of Co-Administered Drug	Change in Co-Administered Drug Exposure		
		Analyte	AUC	C_{max}
Lipid-lowering agents				
Fenofibrate 160 mg[1] once daily for 10 days	Atorvastatin, 20 mg once daily for 10 days	Atorvastatin	↓17%	0%
Fenofibrate 3×67 mg[2] as a single dose	Pravastatin, 40 mg as a single dose	Pravastatin	↑13%	↑13%
		3α-Hydroxyl-iso-pravastatin	↑26%	↑29%
Fenofibrate 160 mg[1] as a single dose	Fluvastatin, 40 mg as a single dose	(+)-3R, 5S-Fluvastatin	↑15%	↑16%
Anti-diabetic agents				
Fenofibrate 145 mg[1] once daily for 10 days	Glimepiride, 1 mg as a single dose	Glimepiride	↑35%	↑18%
Fenofibrate 54 mg[1] three times daily for 10 days	Metformin, 850 mg three times daily for 10 days	Metformin	↑3%	↑6%
Fenofibrate 145 mg[1] once daily for 14 days	Rosiglitazone, 8 mg once daily for 5 days	Rosiglitazone	↑6%	↓1%

[1] TriCor (fenofibrate) oral tablet
[2] TriCor (fenofibrate) oral micronized capsule

In addition, individual tablets contain:
48 mg tablets
polyvinyl alcohol, titanium dioxide, talc, soybean lecithin, xanthan gum, D&C Yellow #10 aluminum lake, FD&C Yellow #6 /sunset yellow FCF aluminum lake, FD&C Blue #2 /indigo carmine aluminum lake.
145 mg tablets
polyvinyl alcohol, titanium dioxide, talc, soybean lecithin, xanthan gum.

12   CLINICAL PHARMACOLOGY
12.1   Mechanism of Action
The active moiety of TRICOR is fenofibric acid. The pharmacological effects of fenofibric acid in both animals and humans have been extensively studied through oral administration of fenofibrate.

The lipid-modifying effects of fenofibric acid seen in clinical practice have been explained *in vivo* in transgenic mice and *in vitro* in human hepatocyte cultures by the activation of peroxisome proliferator activated receptor α (PPARα). Through this mechanism, fenofibrate increases lipolysis and elimination of triglyceride-rich particles from plasma by activating lipoprotein lipase and reducing production of apoprotein C-III (an inhibitor of lipoprotein lipase activity).
The resulting decrease in TG produces an alteration in the size and composition of LDL from small, dense particles (which are thought to be atherogenic due to their suscepti-

bility to oxidation), to large buoyant particles. These larger particles have a greater affinity for cholesterol receptors and are catabolized rapidly. Activation of PPARα also induces an increase in the synthesis of apolipoproteins AI, A-II and HDL-cholesterol.
Fenofibrate also reduces serum uric acid levels in hyperuricemic and normal individuals by increasing the urinary excretion of uric acid.
12.2   Pharmacodynamics
A variety of clinical studies have demonstrated that elevated levels of total-C, LDL-C, and apo B, an LDL membrane complex, are associated with human atherosclerosis. Similarly, decreased levels of HDL-C and its transport complex, apolipoprotein A (apo AI and apo AII) are associated with the development of atherosclerosis. Epidemiologic investigations have established that cardiovascular morbidity and mortality vary directly with the level of total-C, LDL-C, and TG, and inversely with the level of HDL-C. The independent effect of raising HDL-C or lowering triglycerides (TG) on the risk of cardiovascular morbidity and mortality has not been determined.
Fenofibric acid, the active metabolite of fenofibrate, produces reductions in total cholesterol, LDL cholesterol, apolipoprotein B, total triglycerides and triglyceride rich lipoprotein (VLDL) in treated patients. In addition, treatment with fenofibrate results in increases in high density lipoprotein (HDL) and apolipoproteins apoAI and apoAII.

12.3   Pharmacokinetics
Plasma concentrations of fenofibric acid after administration of three 48 mg or one 145 mg tablets are equivalent under fed conditions to one 200 mg micronized fenofibrate capsule.
Fenofibrate is a pro-drug of the active chemical moiety fenofibric acid. Fenofibrate is converted by ester hydrolysis in the body to fenofibric acid which is the active constituent measurable in the circulation.
Absorption
The absolute bioavailability of fenofibrate cannot be determined as the compound is virtually insoluble in aqueous media suitable for injection. However, fenofibrate is well absorbed from the gastrointestinal tract. Following oral administration in healthy volunteers, approximately 60% of a single dose of radiolabelled fenofibrate appeared in urine, primarily as fenofibric acid and its glucuronate conjugate, and 25% was excreted in the feces. Peak plasma levels of fenofibric acid occur within 6 to 8 hours after administration.
Exposure to fenofibric acid in plasma, as measured by C_{max} and AUC, is not significantly different when a single 145 mg dose of fenofibrate is administered under fasting or nonfasting conditions.
Distribution
Upon multiple dosing of fenofibrate, fenofibric acid steady state is achieved within 9 days. Plasma concentrations of fenofibric acid at steady state are approximately double of those following a single dose. Serum protein binding was approximately 99% in normal and hyperlipidemic subjects.
Metabolism
Following oral administration, fenofibrate is rapidly hydrolyzed by esterases to the active metabolite, fenofibric acid; no unchanged fenofibrate is detected in plasma.
Fenofibric acid is primarily conjugated with glucuronic acid and then excreted in urine. A small amount of fenofibric acid is reduced at the carbonyl moiety to a benzhydrol metabolite which is, in turn, conjugated with glucuronic acid and excreted in urine.
In vivo metabolism data indicate that neither fenofibrate nor fenofibric acid undergo oxidative metabolism (e.g., cytochrome P450) to a significant extent.
Elimination
After absorption, fenofibrate is mainly excreted in the urine in the form of metabolites, primarily fenofibric acid and fenofibric acid glucuronide. After administration of radiolabelled fenofibrate, approximately 60% of the dose appeared in the urine and 25% was excreted in the feces.
Fenofibric acid is eliminated with a half-life of 20 hours, allowing once daily dosing.
Special Populations
Geriatrics
In elderly volunteers 77 to 87 years of age, the oral clearance of fenofibric acid following a single oral dose of fenofibrate was 1.2 L/h, which compares to 1.1 L/h in young adults. This indicates that a similar dosage regimen can be used in elderly with normal renal function, without increasing accumulation of the drug or metabolites *[see Dosage and Administration (2.5) and Use in Specific Populations (8.5)]*.
Pediatrics
The pharmacokinetics of TRICOR has not been studied in pediatric populations.
Gender
No pharmacokinetic difference between males and females has been observed for fenofibrate.
Race
The influence of race on the pharmacokinetics of fenofibrate has not been studied, however fenofibrate is not metabolized by enzymes known for exhibiting inter-ethnic variability.
Renal Impairment
The pharmacokinetics of fenofibric acid was examined in patients with mild, moderate, and severe renal impairment. Patients with severe renal impairment (estimated glomerular filtration rate [eGFR] < 30 mL/min/1.73m^2) showed 2.7-fold increase in exposure for fenofibric acid and increased accumulation of fenofibric acid during chronic dosing compared to that of healthy subjects. Patients with mild to moderate renal impairment (eGFR 30-59 mL/min/1.73m^2) had similar exposure but an increase in the half-life for fenofibric acid compared to that of healthy subjects. Based on these findings, the use of TRICOR should be avoided in patients who have severe renal impairment and dose reduction is required in patients having mild to moderate renal impairment *[see Dosage and Administration (2.4)]*.
Hepatic Impairment
No pharmacokinetic studies have been conducted in patients with hepatic impairment.
Drug-drug Interactions
In vitro studies using human liver microsomes indicate that fenofibrate and fenofibric acid are not inhibitors of cytochrome (CYP) P450 isoforms CYP3A4, CYP2D6, CYP2E1,

Table 4. Mean Percent Change in Lipid Parameters at End of Treatment[†]

Treatment Group	Total-C	LDL-C	HDL-C	TG
Pooled Cohort				
Mean baseline lipid values (n=646)	306.9 mg/dL	213.8 mg/dL	52.3 mg/dL	191.0 mg/dL
All FEN (n=361)	-18.7%*	-20.6%*	+11.0%*	-28.9%*
Placebo (n=285)	-0.4%	-2.2%	+0.7%	+7.7%
Baseline LDL-C > 160 mg/dL and TG < 150 mg/dL				
Mean baseline lipid values (n=334)	307.7 mg/dL	227.7 mg/dL	58.1 mg/dL	101.7 mg/dL
All FEN (n=193)	-22.4%*	-31.4%*	+9.8%*	-23.5%*
Placebo (n=141)	+0.2%	-2.2%	+2.6%	+11.7%
Baseline LDL-C >160 mg/dL and TG ≥ 150 mg/dL				
Mean baseline lipid values (n=242)	312.8 mg/dL	219.8 mg/dL	46.7 mg/dL	231.9 mg/dL
All FEN (n=126)	-16.8%*	-20.1%*	+14.6%*	-35.9%*
Placebo (n=116)	-3.0%	-6.6%	+2.3%	+0.9%

† Duration of study treatment was 3 to 6 months.
* p = < 0.05 vs. Placebo

Table 5. Effects of TRICOR in Patients With Severe Hypertriglyceridemia

Study 1		Placebo				TRICOR		
Baseline TG levels 350 to 499 mg/dL	N	Baseline (Mean)	Endpoint (Mean)	% Change (Mean)	N	Baseline (Mean)	Endpoint (Mean)	% Change (Mean)
Triglycerides	28	449	450	-0.5	27	432	223	-46.2*
VLDL Triglycerides	19	367	350	2.7	19	350	178	-44.1*
Total Cholesterol	28	255	261	2.8	27	252	227	-9.1*
HDL Cholesterol	28	35	36	4	27	34	40	19.6*
LDL Cholesterol	28	120	129	12	27	128	137	14.5
VLDL Cholesterol	27	99	99	5.8	27	92	46	-44.7*
Study 2		**Placebo**				**TRICOR**		
Baseline TG levels 500 to 1500 mg/dL	N	Baseline (Mean)	Endpoint (Mean)	% Change (Mean)	N	Baseline (Mean)	Endpoint (Mean)	% Change (Mean)
Triglycerides	44	710	750	7.2	48	726	308	-54.5*
VLDL Triglycerides	29	537	571	18.7	33	543	205	-50.6*
Total Cholesterol	44	272	271	0.4	48	261	223	-13.8*
HDL Cholesterol	44	27	28	5.0	48	30	36	22.9*
LDL Cholesterol	42	100	90	-4.2	45	103	131	45.0*
VLDL Cholesterol	42	137	142	11.0	45	126	54	-49.4*

* =p < 0.05 vs. Placebo

or CYP1A2. They are weak inhibitors of CYP2C8, CYP2C19 and CYP2A6, and mild-to-moderate inhibitors of CYP2C9 at therapeutic concentrations.
Table 2 describes the effects of co-administered drugs on fenofibric acid systemic exposure. Table 3 describes the effects of coadministered fenofibrate or fenofibric acid on other drugs.
[See table 2 at top of previous page]
[See table 3 at top of previous page]

13   NONCLINICAL TOXICOLOGY
13.1   Carcinogenesis and Mutagenesis and Impairment of Fertility
Two dietary carcinogenicity studies have been conducted in rats with fenofibrate. In the first 24-month study, Wistar rats were dosed with fenofibrate at 10, 45, and 200 mg/kg/day, approximately 0.3, 1, and 6 times the maximum recommended human dose (MRHD), based on body surface area comparisons (mg/m^2). At a dose of 200 mg/kg/day (at 6 times the MRHD), the incidence of liver carcinomas was significantly increased in both sexes. A statistically significant increase in pancreatic carcinomas was observed in males at 1 and 6 times the MRHD; an increase in pancreatic adenomas

and benign testicular interstitial cell tumors was observed at 6 times the MRHD in males. In a second 24-month rat carcinogenicity study in a different strain of rats (Sprague-Dawley), doses of 10 and 60 mg/kg/day (0.3 and 2 times the MRHD) produced significant increases in the incidence of pancreatic acinar adenomas in both sexes and increases in testicular interstitial cell tumors in males at 2 times the MRHD.
A 117-week carcinogenicity study was conducted in rats comparing three drugs: fenofibrate 10 and 60 mg/kg/day (0.3 and 2 times the MRHD), clofibrate (400 mg/kg/day; 2 times the human dose), and gemfibrozil (250 mg/kg/day; 2 times the human dose, based on mg/m^2 surface area). Fenofibrate increased pancreatic acinar adenomas in both sexes. Clofibrate increased hepatocellular carcinoma and pancreatic acinar adenomas in males and hepatic neoplastic nodules in females. Gemfibrozil increased hepatic neoplastic nodules in males and females, while all three drugs increased testicular interstitial cell tumors in males.
In a 21-month study in CF-1 mice, fenofibrate 10, 45, and 200 mg/kg/day (approximately 0.2, 1, and 3 times the MRHD on the basis of mg/m^2 surface area) significantly increased the liver carcinomas in both sexes at 3 times the

MRHD. In a second 18-month study at 10, 60, and 200 mg/kg/day, fenofibrate significantly increased the liver carcinomas in male mice and liver adenomas in female mice at 3 times the MRHD.
Electron microscopy studies have demonstrated peroxisomal proliferation following fenofibrate administration to the rat. An adequate test for peroxisome proliferation in humans has not been done, but changes in peroxisome morphology and numbers have been observed in humans after treatment with other members of the fibrate class when liver biopsies were compared before and after treatment in the same individual.
Mutagenesis: Fenofibrate has been demonstrated to be devoid of mutagenic potential in the following tests: Ames, mouse lymphoma, chromosomal aberration and unscheduled DNA synthesis in primary rat hepatocytes.
Impairment of Fertility: In fertility studies rats were given oral dietary doses of fenofibrate, males received 61 days prior to mating and females 15 days prior to mating through weaning which resulted in no adverse effect on fertility at doses up to 300 mg/kg/day (~10 times the MRHD, based on mg/m^2 surface area comparisons).

14   CLINICAL STUDIES
14.1   Primary Hypercholesterolemia (Heterozygous Familial and Nonfamilial) and Mixed Dyslipidemia
The effects of fenofibrate at a dose equivalent to 145 mg TRICOR (fenofibrate tablets) per day were assessed from four randomized, placebo-controlled, double-blind, parallel-group studies including patients with the following mean baseline lipid values: total-C 306.9 mg/dL; LDL-C 213.8 mg/dL; HDL-C 52.3 mg/dL; and triglycerides 191.0 mg/dL. TRICOR therapy lowered LDL-C, Total-C, and the LDL-C/HDL-C ratio. TRICOR therapy also lowered triglycerides and raised HDL-C (see Table 4).
[See table 4 above]
In a subset of the subjects, measurements of apo B were conducted. TRICOR treatment significantly reduced apo B from baseline to endpoint as compared with placebo (-25.1% vs. 2.4%, p < 0.0001, n=213 and 143 respectively).
14.2   Severe Hypertriglyceridemia
The effects of fenofibrate on serum triglycerides were studied in two randomized, double-blind, placebo-controlled clinical trials of 147 hypertriglyceridemic patients. Patients were treated for eight weeks under protocols that differed only in that one entered patients with baseline TG levels of 500 to 1500 mg/dL, and the other TG levels of 350 to 500 mg/dL. In patients with hypertriglyceridemia and normal cholesterolemia with or without hyperchylomicronemia, treatment with fenofibrate at dosages equivalent to TRICOR 145 mg per day decreased primarily very low density lipoprotein (VLDL) triglycerides and VLDL cholesterol. Treatment of patients with elevated triglycerides often results in an increase of LDL-C (see Table 5).
[See table 5 above]
The effect of TRICOR on cardiovascular morbidity and mortality has not been determined.

16   HOW SUPPLIED/STORAGE AND HANDLING
TRICOR® (fenofibrate tablets) is available in two strengths:
48 mg yellow tablets, imprinted with the "a" logo and code identification letters "FI", available in bottles of 90 (NDC 0074-6122-90).
145 mg white tablets, imprinted with the "a" logo and code identification letters "FO", available in bottles of 90 (NDC 0074-6123-90).
Storage
Store at 25°C (77°F); excursions permitted to 15-30°C (59-86°F).
[See USP Controlled Room Temperature]. Keep out of the reach of children. Protect from moisture.

17   PATIENT COUNSELING INFORMATION
Patients should be advised:
• of the potential benefits and risks of TRICOR.
• not to use TRICOR if there is a known hypersensitivity to fenofibrate or fenofibric acid.
• of medications that should not be taken in combination with TRICOR.
• that if they are taking coumarin anticoagulants, TRICOR may increase their anti-coagulant effect, and increased monitoring may be necessary.
• to continue to follow an appropriate lipid-modifying diet while taking TRICOR.
• to take TRICOR once daily, without regard to food, at the prescribed dose, swallowing each tablet whole.
• to return for routine monitoring.

Information on the AbbVie, Inc. products listed on these pages is from the prescribing information in use as of July 31, 2014. For more information, please visit rxabbvie.com or call 1-800-633-9110.

- to inform their physician of all medications, supplements, and herbal preparations they are taking and any change to their medical condition. Patients should also be advised to inform their physicians prescribing a new medication that they are taking TRICOR.
- to inform their physician of any muscle pain, tenderness, or weakness; onset of abdominal pain; or any other new symptoms.

Manufactured for AbbVie Inc., North Chicago, IL 60064, U.S.A.

by Fournier Laboratories Ireland Limited, Anngrove, Carrigtwohill Co. Cork, Ireland.

03-A774-R8, Revised: February, 2013

Shown in Product Identification Guide, page 304

TRILIPIX® ℞
[try-lip-iks]
(fenofibric acid)
capsule, delayed release for oral use

HIGHLIGHTS OF PRESCRIBING INFORMATION
These highlights do not include all the information needed to use TRILIPIX safely and effectively. See full prescribing information for TRILIPIX.

TRILIPIX (fenofibric acid) capsule, delayed release for oral use

Initial U.S. Approval: 2008

——————RECENT MAJOR CHANGES——————
Warnings and Precautions, Skeletal Muscle (5.2) 09/2012
Warnings and Precautions, Paradoxical Decreased in HDL Cholesterol Levels (5.11) 09/2012

——————INDICATIONS AND USAGE——————
Trilipix is a peroxisome proliferator receptor alpha (PPARα) activator indicated:
- In combination with a statin to reduce TG and increase HDL-C in patients with mixed dyslipidemia and CHD or a CHD risk equivalent who are on optimal statin therapy to achieve their LDL-C goal (1.1).
- As monotherapy to reduce TG in patients with severe hypertriglyceridemia (1.2).
- As monotherapy to reduce elevated LDL-C, Total-C, TG and Apo B, and to increase HDL-C in patients with primary hyperlipidemia or mixed dyslipidemia (1.3).

Important Limitations of Use: No incremental benefit of Trilipix on cardiovascular morbidity and mortality over and above that demonstrated for statin monotherapy has been established. Fenofibrate at a dose equivalent to 135 mg of Trilipix was not shown to reduce coronary heart disease morbidity and mortality in patients with type 2 diabetes mellitus.

——————DOSAGE AND ADMINISTRATION——————
- Mixed dyslipidemia: 135 mg once daily (2.2).
- Hypertriglyceridemia: 45 to 135 mg once daily (2.3).
- Renally impaired patients: 45 mg once daily (2.5).
- Maximum dose: 135 mg once daily (2.1).
- May be taken without regard to food (2.1).
- May be taken at the same time as a statin (2.2).
- Co-administration with the maximum dose of a statin has not been evaluated in clinical studies and should be avoided unless the benefits are expected to outweigh the risks (2.2).

——————DOSAGE FORMS AND STRENGTHS——————
Oral Delayed Release Capsules: 45 mg and 135 mg (3).

——————CONTRAINDICATIONS——————
- Severe renal dysfunction, including patients receiving dialysis (4, 12.3).
- Active liver disease (4, 5.3).
- Gallbladder disease (4, 5.4).
- Nursing mothers (4, 8.3).
- Known hypersensitivity to fenofibric acid or fenofibrate (4, 5.9).

——————WARNINGS AND PRECAUTIONS——————
- Myopathy and rhabdomyolysis have been reported in patients taking fenofibrate. The risks for myopathy and rhabdomyolysis are increased when fibrates are co-administered with a statin (with a significantly higher rate observed for gemfibrozil), particularly in elderly patients and patients with diabetes, renal failure, or hypothyroidism (5.1).
- Trilipix can increase serum transaminases. Liver tests should be monitored periodically (5.3).
- Trilipix can reversibly increase serum creatinine levels (5.2). Renal function should be monitored periodically in patients with renal insufficiency (8.6).
- Trilipix increases cholesterol excretion into the bile, leading to risk of cholelithiasis. If cholelithiasis is suspected, gallbladder studies are indicated (5.4).
- Exercise caution in concomitant treatment with oral coumarin anticoagulants. Adjust the dosage of coumarin anticoagulant to maintain the prothrombin time/INR at the desired level to prevent bleeding complications (5.5).

——————ADVERSE REACTIONS——————
The most common adverse events (≥ 3% of patients receiving Trilipix or Trilipix co-administered with statins) are headache, back pain, nasopharyngitis, nausea, myalgia, diarrhea, and upper respiratory tract infection (6.1).

To report SUSPECTED ADVERSE REACTIONS, contact AbbVie Inc. at 1-800-633-9110 or FDA at 1-800-FDA-1088 or www.fda.gov/medwatch

——————DRUG INTERACTIONS——————
- Coumarin Anticoagulants: (7.1).
- Bile Acid Binding Resins: (7.2).
- Immunosuppressants: (7.3).

——————USE IN SPECIFIC POPULATIONS——————
- Geriatric Use: Dose selection for the elderly should be made on the basis of renal function (8.5).
- Renal Impairment: Trilipix should be avoided in patients with severe renal impairment. Dose adjustment is required in patients with mild to moderate renal impairment (8.6).

See 17 for PATIENT COUNSELING INFORMATION and Medication Guide

Revised: 03/2013

FULL PRESCRIBING INFORMATION

1 INDICATIONS AND USAGE

1.1 Co-administration Therapy with Statins for the Treatment of Mixed Dyslipidemia
Trilipix is indicated as an adjunct to diet in combination with a statin to reduce TG and increase HDL-C in patients with mixed dyslipidemia and CHD or a CHD risk equivalent who are on optimal statin therapy to achieve their LDL-C goal.
CHD risk equivalents comprise:
- Other clinical forms of atherosclerotic disease (peripheral arterial disease, abdominal aortic aneurysm, and symptomatic carotid artery disease);
- Diabetes;
- Multiple risk factors that confer a 10-year risk for CHD > 20%

1.2 Treatment of Severe Hypertriglyceridemia
Trilipix is indicated as adjunctive therapy to diet to reduce TG in patients with severe hypertriglyceridemia. Improving glycemic control in diabetic patients showing fasting chylomicronemia will usually obviate the need for pharmacological intervention. Markedly elevated levels of serum triglycerides (e.g. > 2,000 mg/dL) may increase the risk of developing pancreatitis. The effect of Trilipix therapy on reducing this risk has not been adequately studied.

1.3 Treatment of Primary Hypercholesterolemia or Mixed Dyslipidemia
Trilipix is indicated as adjunctive therapy to diet to reduce elevated low-density lipoprotein cholesterol (LDL-C), total cholesterol (Total-C), triglycerides (TG), and apolipoprotein B (Apo B), and to increase high-density lipoprotein cholesterol (HDL-C) in patients with primary hypercholesterolemia or mixed dyslipidemia.

1.4 Important Limitations of Use
No incremental benefit of Trilipix on cardiovascular morbidity and mortality over and above that demonstrated for statin monotherapy has been established. Fenofibrate at a dose equivalent to 135 mg of Trilipix was not shown to reduce coronary heart disease morbidity and mortality in 2 large, randomized controlled trials of patients with type 2 diabetes mellitus.

1.5 General Considerations for Treatment
Laboratory studies should be performed to establish that lipid levels are abnormal before instituting Trilipix therapy. Every reasonable attempt should be made to control serum lipids with non-drug methods including appropriate diet, exercise, weight loss in obese patients, and control of any medical problems such as diabetes mellitus and hypothyroidism that may be contributing to the lipid abnormalities. Medications known to exacerbate hypertriglyceridemia (beta-blockers, thiazides, estrogens) should be discontinued or changed if possible, and excessive alcohol intake should be addressed before triglyceride-lowering drug therapy is considered. If the decision is made to use lipid-altering drugs, the patient should be instructed that this does not reduce the importance of adhering to diet.
Drug therapy is not indicated for patients who have elevations of chylomicrons and plasma triglycerides, but who have normal levels of VLDL.

2 DOSAGE AND ADMINISTRATION

2.1 General Considerations
Patients should be placed on an appropriate lipid-lowering diet before receiving Trilipix as monotherapy or co-administered with a statin, and should continue this diet during treatment. Trilipix delayed release capsules can be taken without regard to meals. Patients should be advised to swallow Trilipix capsules whole. Do not open, crush, dissolve, or chew capsules. Serum lipids should be monitored periodically.

2.2 Co-administration Therapy with Statins for the Treatment of Mixed Dyslipidemia
Trilipix 135 mg may be co-administered with an HMG-CoA reductase inhibitor (statin) in patients with mixed dyslipidemia. For convenience, the daily dose of Trilipix may be taken at the same time as a statin, according to the dosing recommendations for each medication. Co-administration with the maximum dose of a statin has not been evaluated in clinical studies and should be avoided unless the benefits are expected to outweigh the risks.

2.3 Severe Hypertriglyceridemia
The initial dose of Trilipix is 45 to 135 mg once daily. Dosage should be individualized according to patient response, and should be adjusted if necessary following repeat lipid determinations at 4 to 8 week intervals. The maximum dose is 135 mg once daily.

2.4 Primary Hypercholesterolemia or Mixed Dyslipidemia
The dose of Trilipix is 135 mg once daily.

2.5 Impaired Renal Function
Treatment with Trilipix should be initiated at a dose of 45 mg once daily in patients with mild to moderate renal impairment and should only be increased after evaluation of the effects on renal function and lipid levels at this dose.

The use of Trilipix should be avoided in patients with severely impaired renal function [see Use in Specific Populations (8.6) and Clinical Pharmacology (12.3)].

2.6   Geriatric Patients
Dose selection for the elderly should be made on the basis of renal function [see Use in Specific Populations (8.5)].

3   DOSAGE FORMS AND STRENGTHS

- 45 mg capsules with a reddish-brown cap imprinted in white ink the "a" logo and a yellow body imprinted in black ink the number "45".
- 135 mg capsules with a blue cap imprinted in white ink the "a" logo and a yellow body imprinted in black ink the number "135".

4   CONTRAINDICATIONS

Trilipix is contraindicated in:

- patients with severe renal impairment, including those receiving dialysis [see Clinical Pharmacology (12.3)].
- patients with active liver disease, including those with primary biliary cirrhosis and unexplained persistent liver function abnormalities [see Warnings and Precautions (5.3)].
- patients with preexisting gallbladder disease [see Warnings and Precautions (5.5)].
- nursing mothers [see Use in Specific Populations (8.3)].
- patients with hypersensitivity to fenofibric acid or fenofibrate [see Warnings and Precautions (5.9)].

When Trilipix is co-administered with a statin, refer to the Contraindications section of the respective statin labeling.

5   WARNINGS AND PRECAUTIONS

5.1   Mortality and Coronary Heart Disease Morbidity
The effect of Trilipix on coronary heart disease morbidity and mortality and non-cardiovascular mortality has not been established. Because of similarities between Trilipix and fenofibrate, clofibrate, and gemfibrozil, the findings in the following large randomized, placebo-controlled clinical studies with these fibrate drugs may also apply to Trilipix. The Action to Control Cardiovascular Risk in Diabetes Lipid (ACCORD Lipid) trial was a randomized placebo-controlled study of 5518 patients with type 2 diabetes mellitus on background statin therapy treated with fenofibrate. The mean duration of follow-up was 4.7 years. Fenofibrate plus statin combination therapy showed a non-significant 8% relative risk reduction in the primary outcome of major adverse cardiovascular events (MACE), a composite of non-fatal myocardial infarction, non-fatal stroke, and cardiovascular disease death (hazard ratio [HR] 0.92, 95% CI 0.79-1.08) (p=0.32) as compared to statin monotherapy. In a gender subgroup analysis, the hazard ratio for MACE in men receiving combination therapy versus statin monotherapy was 0.82 (95% CI 0.69-0.99), and the hazard ratio for MACE in women receiving combination therapy versus statin monotherapy was 1.38 (95% CI 0.98-1.94) (interaction p=0.01). The clinical significance of this subgroup finding is unclear.

The Fenofibrate Intervention and Event Lowering in Diabetes (FIELD) study was a 5-year randomized, placebo-controlled study of 9795 patients with type 2 diabetes mellitus treated with fenofibrate. Fenofibrate demonstrated a non-significant 11% relative reduction in the primary outcome of coronary heart disease events (hazard ratio [HR] 0.89, 95% CI 0.75-1.05, p = 0.16) and a significant 11% reduction in the secondary outcome of total cardiovascular disease events (HR 0.89 [0.80-0.99], p = 0.04). There was a non-significant 11% (HR 1.11 [0.95, 1.29], p = 0.18) and 19% (HR 1.19 [0.90, 1.57], p = 0.22) increase in total and coronary heart disease mortality, respectively, with fenofibrate as compared to placebo.

In the Coronary Drug Project, a large study of post-myocardial infarction patients treated for 5 years with clofibrate, there was no difference in mortality seen between the clofibrate group and the placebo group. There was, however, a difference in the rate of cholelithiasis and cholecystitis requiring surgery between the two groups (3.0% vs. 1.8%).

In a study conducted by the World Health Organization (WHO), 5000 subjects without known coronary artery disease were treated with placebo or clofibrate for 5 years and followed for an additional one year. There was a statistically significant, higher age-adjusted all-cause mortality in the clofibrate group compared with the placebo group (5.70% vs. 3.96%, p = < 0.01). Excess mortality was due to a 33% increase in non-cardiovascular causes, including malignancy, post-cholecystectomy complications, and pancreatitis. This appeared to confirm the higher risk of gallbladder disease seen in clofibrate-treated patients studied in the Coronary Drug Project.

The Helsinki Heart Study was a large (N = 4081) study of middle-aged men without a history of coronary artery disease. Subjects received either placebo or gemfibrozil for 5 years, with a 3.5 year open extension afterward. Total mortality was numerically higher in the gemfibrozil randomization group but did not achieve statistical significance (p = 0.19, 95% confidence interval for relative risk G:P = 0.91-1.64). Although cancer deaths trended higher in the gemfibrozil group (p = 0.11), cancers (excluding basal cell carcinoma) were diagnosed with equal frequency in both study groups. Due to the limited size of the study, the relative risk of death from any cause was not shown to be different than that seen in the 9 year follow-up data from WHO study (RR = 1.29). A secondary prevention component of the Helsinki Heart Study enrolled middle-aged men excluded from the primary prevention study because of known or suspected coronary heart disease. Subjects received gemfibrozil or placebo for 5 years. Although cardiac deaths trended higher in the gemfibrozil group, this was not statistically significant (hazard ratio 2.2, 95% confidence interval: 0.94-5.05).

5.2   Skeletal Muscle
Fibrate and statin monotherapy increase the risk of myositis or myopathy, and have been associated with rhabdomyolysis. Data from observational studies suggest that the risk for rhabdomyolysis is increased when fibrates are co-administered with a statin (with a numerically higher rate observed with gemfibrozil/statin combination use compared to fenofibrate/statin combination use). Refer to the respective statin labeling for important drug-drug interactions that increase statin levels and could increase this risk. The risk for serious muscle toxicity appears to be increased in elderly patients and in patients with diabetes, renal failure, or hypothyroidism.

In phase 3 clinical trials with Trilipix, myalgia was reported in 3.3% of patients treated with Trilipix monotherapy and 3.1% to 3.5% of patients treated with Trilipix co-administered with statins compared to 4.7% to 6.1% of patients treated with statin monotherapy. Increases in creatine phosphokinase (CPK) to > 5 times upper limit of normal occurred in no patients treated with Trilipix monotherapy and 0.2% to 1.2% of patients treated with Trilipix co-administered with statins compared to 0.4% to 1.3% of patients treated with statin monotherapy.

Myopathy should be considered in any patient with diffuse myalgias, muscle tenderness or weakness, and/or marked elevations of CPK levels. Patients should promptly report unexplained muscle pain, tenderness or weakness, particularly if accompanied by malaise or fever. CPK levels should be assessed in patients reporting these symptoms, and Trilipix and statin therapy should be discontinued if markedly elevated CPK levels occur or myopathy or myositis is suspected or diagnosed.

Cases of myopathy, including rhabdomyolysis, have been reported with fenofibrates co-administered with colchicine, and caution should be exercised when prescribing fenofibrate with colchicine [see Drug Interactions (7.4)].

5.3   Liver Function
Trilipix at a dose of 135 mg once daily administered as monotherapy or co-administered with low to moderate doses of statins has been associated with increases in serum transaminases [AST (SGOT) or ALT (SGPT)]. In a pooled analysis of three double-blind controlled studies of Trilipix administered as monotherapy or in combination with statins, increases to > 3 times the upper limit of normal on two consecutive occasions in ALT and AST occurred in 1.9% and 0.2%, respectively, of patients receiving Trilipix monotherapy and in 1.3% and 0.4%, respectively, of patients receiving Trilipix co-administered with statins. Increases to > 3 times the upper limit of normal in ALT and AST occurred in no patients receiving low- to moderate-dose statin monotherapy. Increases to > 3 times the upper limit of normal in ALT and AST occurred in 0.8% and 0.4%, respectively, in patients receiving high-dose statin monotherapy. In a long-term study of Trilipix co-administered with statins for up to 52 weeks, increases of > 3 times the upper limit of normal on two consecutive occasions of ALT and AST occurred in 1.2% and 0.5% of patients, respectively. When transaminase determinations were followed either after discontinuation of treatment or during continued treatment, a return to normal limits was usually observed. Increases in ALT and/or AST were not accompanied by increases in bilirubin or clinically significant increases in alkaline phosphatase.

In a pooled analysis of 10 placebo-controlled trials of fenofibrate, increases to > 3 times the upper limit of normal in ALT occurred in 5.3% of patients taking fenofibrate versus 1.1% of patients treated with placebo. The incidence of increases in transaminases observed with fenofibrate therapy may be dose related. In an 8-week dose-ranging study of fenofibrate in hypertriglyceridemia, the incidence of ALT or AST elevations ≥ 3 times the upper limit of normal was 13% in patients receiving dosages equivalent to 90 mg to 135 mg Trilipix once daily and was 0% in those receiving dosages equivalent to 45 mg Trilipix once daily or less, or placebo. Hepatocellular, chronic active, and cholestatic hepatitis observed with fenofibrate therapy have been reported after exposures of weeks to several years. In extremely rare cases, cirrhosis has been reported in association with chronic active hepatitis.

Baseline and regular monitoring of liver function, including serum ALT (SGPT) should be performed for the duration of therapy with Trilipix, and therapy discontinued if enzyme levels persist above 3 times the upper limit of normal.

5.4   Serum Creatinine
Reversible elevations in serum creatinine have been reported in patients receiving Trilipix as monotherapy or co-administered with statins as well as patients receiving fenofibrate. In the pooled analysis of three double-blind controlled studies of Trilipix administered as monotherapy or in combination with statins, increases in creatinine to > 2 mg/dL occurred in 0.8% of patients treated with Trilipix monotherapy and 1.1% to 1.3% of patients treated with Trilipix co-administered with statins compared to 0% to 0.4% of patients treated with statin monotherapy. Elevations in serum creatinine were generally stable over time with no evidence for continued increases in serum creatinine with long-term therapy and tended to return to baseline following discontinuation of treatment. The clinical significance of these observations is unknown. Monitoring renal function in patients with renal impairment taking Trilipix is suggested. Renal monitoring should be considered for patients at risk for renal insufficiency, such as the elderly and those with diabetes.

5.5   Cholelithiasis
Trilipix, like fenofibrate, clofibrate, and gemfibrozil, may increase cholesterol excretion into the bile, potentially leading to cholelithiasis. If cholelithiasis is suspected, gallbladder studies are indicated. Trilipix therapy should be discontinued if gallstones are found.

5.6   Coumarin Anticoagulants
Caution should be exercised when Trilipix is given in conjunction with oral coumarin anticoagulants. Trilipix may potentiate the anticoagulant effects of these agents resulting in prolongation of the prothrombin time/International Normalized Ratio (PT/INR). Frequent monitoring of PT/INR and dose adjustment of the oral anticoagulant are recommended until the PT/INR has stabilized in order to prevent bleeding complications [see Drug Interactions (7.1)].

5.7   Pancreatitis
Pancreatitis has been reported in patients taking drugs of the fibrate class, including Trilipix. This occurrence may represent a failure of efficacy in patients with severe hypertriglyceridemia, a direct drug effect, or a secondary phenomenon mediated through biliary tract stone or sludge formation with obstruction of the common bile duct.

5.8   Hematological Changes
Mild to moderate hemoglobin, hematocrit, and white blood cell decreases have been observed in patients following initiation of Trilipix and fenofibrate therapy. However, these levels stabilize during long-term administration. Thrombocytopenia and agranulocytosis have been reported in individuals treated with fenofibrates. Periodic monitoring of red and white blood cell counts are recommended during the first 12 months of Trilipix administration.

5.9   Hypersensitivity Reactions
Acute hypersensitivity reactions such as Stevens-Johnson syndrome and toxic necrolysis requiring patient hospitalization and treatment with steroids have been reported in individuals treated with fenofibrates.

5.10   Venothromboembolic Disease
In the FIELD trial, pulmonary embolus (PE) and deep vein thrombosis (DVT) were observed at higher rates in the fenofibrate- than the placebo-treated group. Of 9,795 patients enrolled in FIELD, there were 4,900 in the placebo group and 4,895 in the fenofibrate group. For DVT, there were 48 events (1%) in the placebo group and 67 (1%) in the fenofibrate group (p = 0.074); and for PE, there were 32 (0.7%) events in the placebo group and 53 (1%) in the fenofibrate group (p = 0.022).

In the Coronary Drug Project, a higher proportion of the clofibrate group experienced definite or suspected fatal or nonfatal PE or thrombophlebitis than the placebo group (5.2% vs. 3.3% at five years; p < 0.01).

5.11   Paradoxical Decreases in HDL Cholesterol Levels
There have been postmarketing and clinical trial reports of severe decreases in HDL cholesterol levels (as low as 2 mg/dL) occurring in diabetic and non-diabetic patients initiated on fibrate therapy. The decrease in HDL-C is mirrored by a decrease in apolipoprotein A1. This decrease has been reported to occur within 2 weeks to years after initiation of fibrate therapy. The HDL-C levels remain depressed until fibrate therapy has been withdrawn; the response to withdrawal of fibrate therapy is rapid and sustained. The clinical significance of this decrease in HDL-C is unknown. It is recommended that HDL-C levels be checked within the first few months after initiation of fibrate therapy. If a se-

Information on the AbbVie, Inc. products listed on these pages is from the prescribing information in use as of July 31, 2014. For more information, please visit rxabbvie.com or call 1-800-633-9110.

Table 1. Treatment-Emergent Adverse Events Reported in ≥ 3% of Patients Receiving Trilipix or Trilipix Co-Administered with a Statin During Double-Blind Controlled Studies [Number (%)]

Adverse Event	Trilipix (N = 490)	Low-Dose Statin (N = 493)	Trilipix + Low-Dose Statin (N = 490)	Moderate-Dose Statin (N = 491)	Trilipix + Moderate-Dose Statin (N = 489)	High-Dose Statin (N = 245)
Gastrointestinal Disorders						
Constipation	16 (3.3)	11 (2.2)	16 (3.3)	13 (2.6)	15 (3.1)	6 (2.4)
Diarrhea	19 (3.9)	16 (3.2)	15 (3.1)	24 (4.9)	18 (3.7)	17 (6.9)
Dyspepsia	18 (3.7)	13 (2.6)	13 (2.7)	17 (3.5)	23 (4.7)	6 (2.4)
Nausea	21 (4.3)	18 (3.7)	17 (3.5)	22 (4.5)	27 (5.5)	10 (4.1)
General Disorders and Administration Site Conditions						
Fatigue	10 (2.0)	13 (2.6)	13 (2.7)	13 (2.6)	16 (3.3)	5 (2.0)
Pain	17 (3.5)	9 (1.8)	16 (3.3)	8 (1.6)	7 (1.4)	8 (3.3)
Infections and Infestations						
Nasopharyngitis	17 (3.5)	29 (5.9)	23 (4.7)	16 (3.3)	21 (4.3)	9 (3.7)
Sinusitis	16 (3.3)	4 (0.8)	14 (2.9)	8 (1.6)	17 (3.5)	4 (1.6)
Upper Respiratory Tract Infection	26 (5.3)	13 (2.6)	18 (3.7)	23 (4.7)	23 (4.7)	7 (2.9)
Investigations						
ALT Increased	6 (1.2)	2 (0.4)	15 (3.1)	2 (0.4)	12 (2.5)	4 (1.6)
Musculoskeletal and Connective Tissue Disorders						
Arthralgia	19 (3.9)	22 (4.5)	21 (4.3)	21 (4.3)	17 (3.5)	12 (4.9)
Back Pain	31 (6.3)	31 (6.3)	30 (6.1)	32 (6.5)	20 (4.1)	8 (3.3)
Muscle Spasms	8 (1.6)	18 (3.7)	12 (2.4)	24 (4.9)	15 (3.1)	6 (2.4)
Myalgia	16 (3.3)	24 (4.9)	17 (3.5)	23 (4.7)	15 (3.1)	15 (6.1)
Pain in Extremity	22 (4.5)	24 (4.9)	14 (2.9)	21 (4.3)	13 (2.7)	9 (3.7)
Nervous System Disorders						
Dizziness	20 (4.1)	8 (1.6)	19 (3.9)	11 (2.2)	16 (3.3)	2 (0.8)
Headache	62 (12.7)	64 (13.0)	64 (13.1)	82 (16.7)	58 (11.9)	32 (13.1)

Low-dose statin = rosuvastatin 10 mg, simvastatin 20 mg, or atorvastatin 20 mg
Moderate-dose statin = rosuvastatin 20 mg, simvastatin 40 mg, or atorvastatin 40 mg
High-dose statin = rosuvastatin 40 mg, simvastatin 80 mg, or atorvastatin 80 mg

verely depressed HDL-C level is detected, fibrate therapy should be withdrawn, and the HDL-C level monitored until it has returned to baseline, and fibrate therapy should not be re-initiated.

6 ADVERSE REACTIONS
6.1 Clinical Trials Experience
Because clinical studies are conducted under widely varying conditions, adverse event rates observed in the clinical studies of a drug cannot be directly compared to rates in the clinical studies of another drug.
Trilipix (fenofibric acid)
Monotherapy
Treatment-emergent adverse events reported in 3% or more of patients treated with Trilipix during the randomized controlled trials are listed in Table 1 below.
Co-Administration Therapy with Statins (Double-blind Controlled Trials)
Treatment-emergent adverse events reported in 3% or more of patients treated with Trilipix co-administered with statins during the randomized controlled trials are listed in Table 1 below.
[See table 1 above]
Co-Administration Therapy with Statins (Long-Term Exposure for up to 64 Weeks)
Patients successfully completing any one of the three double-blind, controlled studies were eligible to participate in a 52-week long-term extension study where they received Trilipix co-administered with the moderate dose statin. A total of 2201 patients received at least one dose of Trilipix co-administered with a statin in the double-blind controlled study or the long-term extension study for up to a total of 64 weeks of treatment. Additional treatment-emergent adverse events (not listed in Table 1 above) reported in 3% or more of patients receiving Trilipix co-administered with a statin in either the double-blind controlled studies or the long-term extension study are provided below.
Infections and Infestations
Bronchitis, influenza, and urinary tract infection.
Investigations
AST increased, blood CPK increased, and hepatic enzyme increased.
Musculoskeletal and Connective Tissue Disorders
Musculoskeletal pain.
Psychiatric Disorders
Insomnia.
Respiratory, Thoracic, and Mediastinal Disorders
Cough and pharyngolaryngeal pain.
Vascular Disorders
Hypertension.
Fenofibrate
Fenofibric acid is the active metabolite of fenofibrate. Adverse events reported by 2% or more of patients treated with fenofibrate and greater than placebo during double-

blind, placebo-controlled trials are listed in Table 2. Adverse events led to discontinuation of treatment in 5.0% of patients treated with fenofibrate and in 3.0% treated with placebo. Increases in liver tests were the most frequent events, causing discontinuation of fenofibrate treatment in 1.6% of patients in double-blind trials.

Table 2. Adverse Events Reported by 2% or More of Patients Treated with Fenofibrate and Greater than Placebo During the Double-Blind, Placebo-Controlled Trials

BODY SYSTEM Adverse Event	Fenofibrate* (N = 439)	Placebo (N = 365)
BODY AS A WHOLE		
Abdominal Pain	4.6%	4.4%
Back Pain	3.4%	2.5%
Headache	3.2%	2.7%
DIGESTIVE		
Nausea	2.3%	1.9%
Constipation	2.1%	1.4%
INVESTIGATIONS		
Abnormal Liver Tests	7.5%	1.4%
Increased AST	3.4%	0.5%
Increased ALT	3.0%	1.6%
Increased Creatine Phosphokinase	3.0%	1.4%
RESPIRATORY		
Respiratory Disorder	6.2%	5.5%
Rhinitis	2.3%	1.1%

* Dosage equivalent to 135 mg Trilipix

6.2 Postmarketing Experience
The following adverse events have been identified during postapproval use of fenofibrate: myalgia, rhabdomyolysis, pancreatitis, renal failure, muscle spasms, acute renal failure, hepatitis, cirrhosis, anemia, arthralgia, asthenia, and severely depressed HDL-cholesterol levels.
Because these events are reported voluntarily from a population of uncertain size, it is not always possible to reliably estimate their frequency or establish a casual relationship to drug exposure.

7 DRUG INTERACTIONS
7.1 Coumarin Anticoagulants
Potentiation of coumarin-type anticoagulant effect has been observed with prolongation of the PT/INR.
Caution should be exercised when oral coumarin anticoagulants are given in conjunction with Trilipix. The dosage of the anticoagulant should be reduced to maintain the PT/INR at the desired level to prevent bleeding complications.

Frequent PT/INR determinations are advisable until it has been definitely determined that the PT/INR has stabilized [see Warnings and Precautions (5.6)].
7.2 Bile Acid Binding Resins
Since bile acid binding resins may bind other drugs given concurrently, patients should take Trilipix at least 1 hour before or 4 to 6 hours after a bile acid resin to avoid impeding its absorption.
7.3 Immunosuppressants
Immunosuppressants such as cyclosporine and tacrolimus can produce nephrotoxicity with decreases in creatinine clearance and rises in serum creatinine, and because renal excretion is the primary elimination route of drugs of the fibrate class including Trilipix, there is a risk that an interaction will lead to deterioration of renal function. The benefits and risks of using Trilipix with immunosuppressants and other potentially nephrotoxic agents should be carefully considered, and the lowest effective dose employed.
7.4 Colchicine
Cases of myopathy, including rhabdomyolysis, have been reported with fenofibrates co-administered with colchicine, and caution should be exercised when prescribing fenofibrate with colchicine.

8 USE IN SPECIFIC POPULATIONS
8.1 Pregnancy
Pregnancy Category: C
The safety of Trilipix in pregnant women has not been established. There are no adequate and well controlled studies of Trilipix in pregnant women. Trilipix should be used during pregnancy only if the potential benefit justifies the potential risk to the fetus.
When Trilipix is administered with a statin in a woman of childbearing potential, refer to pregnancy category and product labeling for the statin. All statins are contraindicated in pregnant women.
In pregnant rats given oral dietary doses of 14, 127, and 361 mg/kg/day from gestation day 6-15 during the period of organogenesis, adverse developmental findings were not observed at 14 mg/kg/day (less than 1 times the maximum recommended human dose [MRHD], based on body surface area comparisons; mg/m^2). At higher multiples of human doses evidence of maternal toxicity was observed.
In pregnant rabbits given oral gavage doses of 15, 150, and 300 mg/kg/day from gestation day 6-18 during the period of organogenesis and allowed to deliver, aborted litters were observed at 150 mg/kg/day (10 times the MRHD, based on body surface area comparisons; mg/m^2). No developmental findings were observed at 15 mg/kg/day (at less than 1 times the MRHD, based on body surface area comparisons; mg/m^2).
In pregnant rats given oral dietary doses of 15, 75, and 300 mg/kg/day from gestation day 15 through lactation day 21 (weaning), maternal toxicity was observed at less than 1 times the MRHD, based on body surface area comparisons; mg/m^2.
8.3 Nursing Mothers
Trilipix should not be used in nursing mothers. A decision should be made whether to discontinue nursing or to discontinue the drug taking into account the importance of the drug to the mother.
8.4 Pediatric Use
The safety and effectiveness of Trilipix monotherapy or co-administration with a statin in pediatric patients have not been established.
8.5 Geriatric Use
Trilipix is substantially excreted by the kidney as fenofibric acid and fenofibric acid glucuronide, and the risk of adverse reactions to this drug may be greater in patients with impaired renal function. Fenofibric acid exposure is not influenced by age. Since elderly patients have a higher incidence of renal impairment, dose selection for the elderly should be made on the basis of renal function [see Dosage and Administration (2.6) and Clinical Pharmacology (12.3)]. Elderly patients with normal renal function should require no dose modifications. Consider monitoring renal function in elderly patients taking Trilipix.
8.6 Renal Impairment
The use of Trilipix should be avoided in patients who have severe renal impairment [see Contraindications (4)]. Dose reduction is required in patients with mild to moderate renal impairment [see Dosage and Administration (2.5) and Clinical Pharmacology (12.3)]. Monitoring renal function in patients with renal impairment is recommended.
8.7 Hepatic Impairment
The use of Trilipix has not been evaluated in subjects with hepatic impairment [see Contraindications (4) and Clinical Pharmacology (12.3)].

10 OVERDOSAGE
There is no specific treatment for overdose with Trilipix. General supportive care of the patient is indicated, including monitoring of vital signs and observation of clinical status, should an overdose occur. If indicated, elimination of

unabsorbed drug should be achieved by emesis or gastric lavage; usual precautions should be observed to maintain the airway. Because Trilipix is highly bound to plasma proteins, hemodialysis should not be considered.

11 DESCRIPTION

Trilipix (fenofibric acid) is a lipid regulating agent available as delayed release capsules for oral administration. Each delayed release capsule contains choline fenofibrate, equivalent to 45 mg or 135 mg of fenofibric acid. The chemical name for choline fenofibrate is ethanaminium, 2-hydroxy-N,N,N-trimethyl, 2-[4-(4-chlorobenzoyl)phenoxy]-2-methylpropanoate (1:1) with the following structural formula:

The empirical formula is $C_{22}H_{28}ClNO_5$ and the molecular weight is 421.91. Choline fenofibrate is freely soluble in water. The melting point is approximately 210°C. Choline fenofibrate is a white to yellow powder, which is stable under ordinary conditions.

Each delayed release capsule contains enteric coated minitablets comprised of choline fenofibrate and the following inactive ingredients: hypromellose, povidone, water, hydroxylpropyl cellulose, colloidal silicon dioxide, sodium stearyl fumarate, methacrylic acid copolymer, talc, triethyl citrate. The capsule shell of the 45 mg capsule contains the following inactive ingredients: gelatin, titanium dioxide, yellow iron oxide, black iron oxide, and red iron oxide. The capsule shell of the 135 mg capsule contains the following inactive ingredients: gelatin, titanium dioxide, yellow iron oxide, and FD&C Blue #2.

12 CLINICAL PHARMACOLOGY

12.1 Mechanism of Action

The active moiety of Trilipix is fenofibric acid. The pharmacological effects of fenofibric acid in both animals and humans have been extensively studied through oral administration of fenofibrate.

The lipid-modifying effects of fenofibric acid seen in clinical practice have been explained *in vivo* in transgenic mice and *in vitro* in human hepatocyte cultures by the activation of peroxisome proliferator activated receptor α (PPARα). Through this mechanism, fenofibric acid increases lipolysis and elimination of triglyceride-rich particles from plasma by activating lipoprotein lipase and reducing production of Apo CIII (an inhibitor of lipoprotein lipase activity).

The resulting decrease in TG produces an alteration in the size and composition of LDL from small, dense particles (which are thought to be atherogenic due to their susceptibility to oxidation), to large buoyant particles. These larger particles have a greater affinity for cholesterol receptors and are catabolized rapidly. Activation of PPARα also induces an increase in the synthesis of HDL-C and Apo AI and AII.

12.2 Pharmacodynamics

Elevated levels of Total-C, LDL-C, and Apo B, and decreased levels of HDL-C and its transport complex, Apo AI and Apo AII, are risk factors for human atherosclerosis. Epidemiologic studies have established that cardiovascular morbidity and mortality vary directly with the levels of Total-C, LDL-C, and TG, and inversely with the level of HDL-C. The independent effect of raising HDL-C or lowering TG on the risk of cardiovascular morbidity and mortality has not been determined.

Fenofibric acid, the active metabolite of fenofibrate, produces reductions in TC, LDL-C, Apo B, TG, and triglyceride-rich lipoprotein (VLDL) in treated patients. In addition, treatment with fenofibric acid results in increases in HDL-C and Apo AI and Apo AII.

12.3 Pharmacokinetics

Trilipix contains fenofibric acid, which is the only circulating pharmacologically active moiety in plasma after oral administration of Trilipix. Fenofibric acid is also the circulating pharmacologically active moiety in plasma after oral administration of fenofibrate, the ester of fenofibric acid. Plasma concentrations of fenofibric acid after administration of one 135 mg Trilipix delayed release capsule are equivalent to those after one 200 mg capsule of micronized fenofibrate administered under fed conditions.

Absorption

Fenofibric acid is well absorbed throughout the gastrointestinal tract. The absolute bioavailability of fenofibric acid is approximately 81%.

Peak plasma levels of fenofibric acid occur within 4 to 5 hours after a single dose administration of Trilipix capsule under fasting conditions.

Table 3. Effects of Co-Administered Drugs on Fenofibric Acid Systemic Exposure from Trilipix or Fenofibrate Administration

Co-Administered Drug	Dosage Regimen of Co-Administered Drug	Dosage Regimen of Trilipix or Fenofibrate	Changes in Fenofibric Acid Exposure	
			AUC	C_{max}
Lipid-lowering agents				
Rosuvastatin	40 mg once daily for 10 days	Trilipix 135 mg once daily for 10 days	↓2%	↓2%
Atorvastatin	20 mg once daily for 10 days	Fenofibrate 160 mg[1] once daily for 10 days	↓2%	↓4%
Atorvastatin + ezetimibe	Atorvastatin, 80 mg once daily and ezetimibe, 10 mg once daily for 10 days	Trilipix 135 mg once daily for 10 days	↑5%	↑5%
Pravastatin	40 mg as a single dose	Fenofibrate 3 × 67 mg[2] as a single dose	↓1%	↓2%
Fluvastatin	40 mg as a single dose	Fenofibrate 160 mg[1] as a single dose	↓2%	↓10%
Simvastatin	80 mg once daily for 7 days	Fenofibrate 160 mg[1] once daily for 7 days	↓5%	↓11%
Anti-diabetic agents				
Glimepiride	1 mg as a single dose	Fenofibrate 145 mg[1] once daily for 10 days	↑1%	↓1%
Metformin	850 mg 3 times daily for 10 days	Fenofibrate 54 mg[1] 3 times daily for 10 days	↓9%	↓6%
Rosiglitazone	8 mg once daily for 5 days	Fenofibrate 145 mg[1] once daily for 14 days	↑10%	↑3%
Gastrointestinal agents				
Omeprazole	40 mg once daily for 5 days	Trilipix 135 mg as a single dose fasting	↑6%	↑17%
Omeprazole	40 mg once daily for 5 days	Trilipix 135 mg as a single dose with food	↑4%	↓2%

[1] TriCor (fenofibrate) oral tablet
[2] TriCor (fenofibrate) oral micronized capsule

Fenofibric acid exposure in plasma, as measured by C_{max} and AUC, is not significantly different when a single 135 mg dose of Trilipix is administered under fasting or nonfasting conditions.

Distribution

Upon multiple dosing of Trilipix, fenofibric acid levels reach steady state within 8 days. Plasma concentrations of fenofibric acid at steady state are approximately slightly more than double those following a single dose. Serum protein binding is approximately 99% in normal and dyslipidemic subjects.

Metabolism

Fenofibric acid is primarily conjugated with glucuronic acid and then excreted in urine. A small amount of fenofibric acid is reduced at the carbonyl moiety to a benzhydrol metabolite which is, in turn, conjugated with glucuronic acid and excreted in urine.

In vivo metabolism data after fenofibrate administration indicate that fenofibric acid does not undergo oxidative metabolism (e.g., cytochrome P450) to a significant extent.

Elimination

After absorption, Trilipix is primarily excreted in the urine in the form of fenofibric acid and fenofibric acid glucuronide. Fenofibric acid is eliminated with a half-life of approximately 20 hours, allowing once daily administration of Trilipix.

Specific Populations

Geriatrics

In five elderly volunteers 77 to 87 years of age, the oral clearance of fenofibric acid following a single oral dose of fenofibrate was 1.2 L/h, which compares to 1.1 L/h in young adults. This indicates that an equivalent dose of Trilipix can be used in elderly subjects with normal renal function, without increasing accumulation of the drug or metabolites *[see Use in Specific Populations (8.5)]*.

Pediatrics

The pharmacokinetics of Trilipix has not been studied in pediatric populations.

Gender

No pharmacokinetic difference between males and females has been observed for Trilipix.

Race

The influence of race on the pharmacokinetics of Trilipix has not been studied; however, fenofibric acid is not metabolized by enzymes known for exhibiting inter-ethnic variability.

Renal Impairment

The pharmacokinetics of fenofibric acid was examined in patients with mild, moderate, and severe renal impairment. Patients with severe renal impairment (estimated glomerular filtration rate [eGFR] <30 mL/min/1.73m²) showed a 2.7-fold increase in exposure for fenofibric acid and increased accumulation of fenofibric acid during chronic dosing compared to that of healthy subjects. Patients with mild to moderate renal impairment (eGFR 30-59 mL/min/1.73m²) had similar exposure but an increase in the half-life of fenofibric acid compared to that of healthy subjects. Based on these findings, the use of Trilipix should be avoided in patients who have severe renal impairment and dose reduction is required in patients having mild to moderate renal impairment *[see Dosage and Administration (2.5)]*.

Hepatic Impairment

No pharmacokinetic studies have been conducted in patients with hepatic impairment.

Drug-drug Interactions

In vitro studies using human liver microsomes indicate that fenofibric acid is not an inhibitor of cytochrome (CYP) P450 isoforms CYP3A4, CYP2D6, CYP2E1, or CYP1A2. It is a weak inhibitor of CYP2C8, CYP2C19, and CYP2A6, and mild-to-moderate inhibitor of CYP2C9 at therapeutic concentrations.

Comparison of atorvastatin exposures when atorvastatin (80 mg once daily for 10 days) is given in combination with fenofibric acid (Trilipix 135 mg once daily for 10 days) and ezetimibe (10 mg once daily for 10 days) versus when atorvastatin is given in combination with ezetimibe only (ezetimibe 10 mg once daily and atorvastatin, 80 mg once daily for 10 days): The C_{max} decreased by 1% for atorvastatin and ortho-hydroxy-atorvastatin and increased by 2% for parahydroxy-atorvastatin. The AUC decreased 6% and 9% for atorvastatin and orthohydroxy-atorvastatin, respectively, and did not change for para-hydroxy-atorvastatin.

Comparison of ezetimibe exposures when ezetimibe (10 mg once daily for 10 days) is given in combination with fenofibric acid (Trilipix 135 mg once daily for 10 days) and atorvastatin (80 mg once daily for 10 days) versus when ezetimibe is given in combination with atorvastatin only (ezetimibe 10 mg once daily and atorvastatin, 80 mg once daily for 10 days): The C_{max} increased by 26% and 7% for total and free ezetimibe, respectively. The AUC increased by 27% and 12% for total and free ezetimibe, respectively.

Table 3 describes the effects of co-administered drugs on fenofibric acid systemic exposure. Table 4 describes the effects of co-administered fenofibric acid on other drugs.

[See table 3 above]
[See table 4 at top of next page]

13 NONCLINICAL TOXICOLOGY

13.1 Carcinogenesis, Mutagenesis, Impairment of Fertility

Trilipix (fenofibric acid)

No carcinogenicity and fertility studies have been conducted with choline fenofibrate or fenofibric acid. However, because fenofibrate is rapidly converted to its active metabolite, fenofibric acid, either during or immediately following absorption both in animals and humans, studies conducted with fenofibrate are relevant for the assessment of the tox-

Information on the AbbVie, Inc. products listed on these pages is from the prescribing information in use as of July 31, 2014. For more information, please visit rxabbvie.com or call 1-800-633-9110.

Table 4. Effects of Trilipix or Fenofibrate Co-Administration on Systemic Exposure of Other Drugs

Dosage Regimen of Trilipix or Fenofibrate	Dosage Regimen of Co-Administered Drug	Change in Co-Administered Drug Exposure		
		Analyte	AUC	C_{max}
Lipid-lowering agents				
Trilipix 135 mg once daily for 10 days	Rosuvastatin, 40 mg once daily for 10 days	Rosuvastatin	↑6%	↑20%
Fenofibrate 160 mg[1] once daily for 10 days	Atorvastatin, 20 mg once daily for 10 days	Atorvastatin	↓17%	0%
Fenofibrate 3 × 67 mg[2] as a single dose	Pravastatin, 40 mg as a single dose	Pravastatin	↑13%	↑13%
		3α-Hydroxyl-iso-pravastatin	↑26%	↑29%
Fenofibrate 160 mg[1] as a single dose	Fluvastatin, 40 mg as a single dose	(+)-3R, 5S-Fluvastatin	↑15%	↑16%
Fenofibrate 160 mg[1] once daily for 7 days	Simvastatin, 80 mg once daily for 7 days	Simvastatin acid	↓36%	↓11%
		Simvastatin Active	↓11%	↓17%
		HMG-CoA Inhibitors	↓12%	↓1%
		Total HMG-CoA Inhibitors	↓8%	↓10%
Anti-diabetic agents				
Fenofibrate 145 mg[1] once daily for 10 days	Glimepiride, 1 mg as a single dose	Glimepiride	↑35%	↑18%
Fenofibrate 54 mg[1] 3 times daily for 10 days	Metformin, 850 mg 3 times daily for 10 days	Metformin	↑3%	↑6%
Fenofibrate 145 mg[1] once daily for 14 days	Rosiglitazone, 8 mg once daily for 5 days	Rosiglitazone	↑6%	↓1%

[1] TriCor (fenofibrate) oral tablet
[2] TriCor (fenofibrate) oral micronized capsule

Table 5. Mean Percent Change from Baseline to the Final Value in HDL-C, TG, and LDL-C (Pooled Double-Blind, Controlled Studies)

	Trilipix	Low-Dose Statin	Trilipix + Low-Dose Statin	Between-group Δ (p-value)	Moderate-Dose Statin	Trilipix + Moderate-Dose Statin	Between-group Δ (p-value)	High-Dose Statin
HDL-C (mg/dL)	(N = 420)	(N = 455)	(N = 423)		(N = 430)	(N = 422)		(N = 217)
BL mean	38.4	38.4	38.2		38.4	38.1		38.0
Mean % Δ	16.3%	7.4%	18.1%	10.7%[a] (< 0.001)	8.7%	17.5%	8.8%[a] (< 0.001)	7.9%
TG (mg/dL)	(N = 459)	(N = 477)	(N = 470)		(N = 472)	(N = 462)		(N = 235)
BL mean	280.7	286.1	282.1		287.9	286.1		282.5
Mean % Δ	-31.0%	-16.8%	-43.9%	-27.2%[a] (< 0.001)	-23.7%	-42.0%	-18.3%[a] (< 0.001)	-28.1%
LDL-C (mg/dL)	(N = 427)	(N = 463)	(N = 436)		(N = 439)	(N = 434)		(N = 225)
BL mean	158.4	153.8	155.7		158.0	156.4		156.1
Mean % Δ	-5.1%	-33.9%	-33.1%	-28.0%[b] (< 0.001)	-40.6%	-34.6%	-29.5%[b] (< 0.001)	-47.1%

[a] Combination therapy vs. corresponding statin monotherapy
[b] Combination therapy vs. Trilipix monotherapy
Low-dose statin = rosuvastatin 10 mg, simvastatin 20 mg, or atorvastatin 20 mg
Moderate-dose statin = rosuvastatin 20 mg, simvastatin 40 mg, or atorvastatin 40 mg
High-dose statin = rosuvastatin 40 mg, simvastatin 80 mg, or atorvastatin 80 mg
BL = Baseline
% Δ = Percent change from baseline to final value

icity profile of fenofibric acid. A similar toxicity spectrum is expected after treatment with either Trilipix or fenofibrate.
Fenofibrate
Two dietary carcinogenicity studies have been conducted in rats with fenofibrate. In the first 24-month study, Wistar rats were dosed with fenofibrate at 10, 45, and 200 mg/kg/day, approximately 0.3, 1, and 6 times the maximum recommended human dose (MRHD), based on body surface area comparisons (mg/m²). At a dose of 200 mg/kg/day (6 times the MRHD), the incidence of liver carcinomas was significantly increased in both sexes. A statistically significant increase in pancreatic carcinomas was observed in males at 1 and 6 times the MRHD; an increase in pancreatic adenomas and benign testicular interstitial cell tumors was observed at 6 times the MRHD in males. In a second 24-month rat carcinogenicity study in a different strain of rats (Sprague-Dawley), (doses of 10 and 60 mg/kg/day (0.3 and 2 times the MRHD), produced significant increases in the incidence of pancreatic acinar adenomas in both sexes and increases in interstitial cell tumors of the testes at 2 times the MRHD.
A 117-week carcinogenicity study was conducted in rats comparing three drugs: fenofibrate 10 and 60 mg/kg/day (0.3 and 2 times the MRHD), clofibrate (400 mg/kg/day; 2 times the human dose), and gemfibrozil (250 mg/kg/day; 2

times the MRHD). Fenofibrate increased pancreatic acinar adenomas in both sexes. Clofibrate increased hepatocellular carcinoma and pancreatic acinar adenomas in males and hepatic neoplastic nodules in females. Gemfibrozil increased hepatic neoplastic nodules in males and females, while all three drugs increased testicular interstitial cell tumors in males.
In a 21-month study in CF-1 mice, fenofibrate 10, 45, and 200 mg/kg/day (approximately 0.2, 1, and 3 times the MRHD on the basis of mg/m² surface area) significantly increased the liver carcinomas in both sexes at 3 times the MRHD. In a second 18-month study at 10, 60, and 200 mg/kg/day, fenofibrate significantly increased the liver carcinomas in male and female mice at 3 times the MRHD. Electron microscopy studies have demonstrated peroxisomal proliferation following fenofibrate administration to the rat. An adequate study to test for peroxisome proliferation in humans has not been done, but changes in peroxisome morphology and numbers have been observed in humans after treatment with other members of the fibrate class when liver biopsies were compared before and after treatment in the same individual.
Mutagenesis: Fenofibrate has been demonstrated to be devoid of mutagenic potential in the following tests: Ames, and micronucleus *in vivo*/rat. In addition, fenofibric acid,

has been demonstrated to be devoid of mutagenic potential in the following tests: Ames, mouse lymphoma, chromosomal aberration and sister chromatid exchange in human lymphocytes, and unscheduled DNA synthesis in primary rat hepatocytes.
Impairment of Fertility: In a fertility study, rats were given oral dietary doses of fenofibrate. Males received doses for 61 days prior to mating and females for 15 days prior to mating through weaning, which resulted in no adverse effect on fertility at doses up to 300 mg/kg/day (~10 times the MRHD, based on mg/m² surface area comparisons).

14   CLINICAL STUDIES
14.1   Co-Administration Therapy with Statins
Efficacy and safety of Trilipix co-administered with statins were assessed in three 12-week, double-blind, controlled Phase 3 studies and one 52-week, long-term, open-label extension study in 2698 patients with mixed dyslipidemia. Patients were required to meet the following fasting lipid entry criteria: TG ≥ 150 mg/dL, and HDL-C < 40 mg/dL (males) and < 50 mg/dL (females), and LDL-C ≥ 130 mg/dL. The three multicenter, randomized, double-blind, controlled studies had similar designs, differing primarily in the statin used for combination therapy/monotherapy. Each study compared the effects of 135 mg Trilipix co-administered with either a low dose or a moderate dose of statin with Trilipix monotherapy and statin monotherapy at the corresponding dose on CHD lipid risk factors. A smaller group of patients received a high dose of statin monotherapy. In study 1, patients received Trilipix co-administered with 10 mg or 20 mg rosuvastatin. In study 2, patients received Trilipix co-administered with 20 mg or 40 mg simvastatin. In study 3, patients received Trilipix co-administered with 20 mg or 40 mg atorvastatin.
Patients were enrolled for a total of approximately 22 weeks, consisting of a 6-week diet run-in/washout period, a 12-week treatment period, and a 30-day safety follow up period. Patients who completed the 12-week treatment period were eligible to participate in the 52-week long-term extension study. Of the 2698 randomized and treated subjects in the controlled studies, 51.6% were female and 48.4% were male; 92.6% of all subjects were White, 4.7% were Black, and 2.8% were of other races. Hispanics comprised 9.9% of the study population. Mean age was 54.9 years.
The primary efficacy endpoints for all three studies were mean percent changes from baseline to final value in HDL-C, TG, and LDL-C. For each statin dose co-administered with Trilipix, there were three primary comparisons. For HDL-C and TG, Trilipix co-administered with each statin dose was compared with statin monotherapy at the corresponding dose. For LDL-C, Trilipix co-administered with each statin dose was compared with Trilipix monotherapy. In order to declare combination therapy successful for a particular statin dose, all three primary comparisons were required to demonstrate superiority of the combination therapy over the corresponding monotherapy. The primary efficacy results were consistent in the three studies and were confirmed by the pooled analysis of the three studies. The results from the individual studies and the pooled analysis demonstrated that Trilipix co-administered with low-dose statins and moderate-dose statins was superior to the corresponding monotherapy. Statistically significant differences were observed for all three primary efficacy comparisons for both doses of combination therapy in all three double-blind, controlled studies as well as the pooled analysis.
In the pooled analysis, Trilipix co-administered with both low-dose statins and moderate-dose statins resulted in mean percent increases (18.1% and 17.5%) in HDL-C and mean percent decreases (-43.9% and -42.0%) in TG that were significantly greater than the corresponding dose of statin monotherapy (7.4% and 8.7% for HDL-C; -16.8% and -23.7% for TG). In addition, both doses of combination therapy resulted in mean percent decreases (-33.1% and -34.6%) in LDL-C that were significantly greater than Trilipix monotherapy (-5.1%). The results of the pooled analysis are described in Table 5.
[See table 5 above]
Secondary efficacy endpoints in all three double-blind, controlled studies were percent changes in non-HDL-C (Trilipix co-administered with statin compared to Trilipix monotherapy and corresponding statin monotherapy), and percent changes in VLDL-C, Total-C, and Apo B (Trilipix co-administered with statin compared to corresponding statin monotherapy). Co-administration of Trilipix with statins resulted in the following changes in secondary parameters (Table 6).
[See table 6 at top of next page]
A total of 1895 patients who completed 12 weeks of treatment in the double-blind, controlled studies were treated in the 52-week, long-term extension study. Patients received Trilipix co-administered with the moderate-dose of the statin that had been used in the double-blind, controlled study in which they were enrolled. Whether combination therapy was initiated during the double-blind, controlled studies or introduced during the long-term extension study,

the treatment effect of combination therapy was observed within four weeks, and was sustained over the duration of treatment in the long-term study. A total of 568 patients completed 52 weeks of treatment with Trilipix co-administered with statins. Mean 52-week values and mean percent change from baseline (at time of enrollment in randomized controlled trials) were 91.7 mg/dL (-38.2%) for LDL-C, 47.3 mg/dL (+24.0%) for HDL-C, 135.5 mg/dL (-47.6%) for TG, 117.9 mg/dL (-45.7%) for non-HDL-C, 26.2 mg/dL (-53.1%) for VLDL-C, 165.2 mg/dL (-35.4%) for Total-C, and 81.4 mg/dL (-43.6%) for Apo B.

14.2 Severe Hypertriglyceridemia

The effects of fenofibrate on serum triglycerides were studied in two randomized, double-blind, placebo-controlled clinical trials of 147 hypertriglyceridemic patients. Patients were treated for eight weeks under protocols that differed only in that one entered patients with baseline TG levels of 500 to 1500 mg/dL, and the other TG levels of 350 to 500 mg/dL. In patients with hypertriglyceridemia and normal cholesterolemia with or without hyperchylomicronemia, treatment with fenofibrate at dosages equivalent to 135 mg once daily of Trilipix decreased primarily VLDL-TG and VLDL-C. Treatment of patients with elevated TG often results in an increase of LDL-C (Table 7).
[See table 7 above]

14.3 Primary Hypercholesterolemia (Heterozygous Familial and Nonfamilial) and Mixed Dyslipidemia

The effects of fenofibrate at a dose equivalent to Trilipix 135 mg once daily were assessed from four randomized, placebo-controlled, double-blind, parallel-group studies including patients with the following mean baseline lipid values: Total-C 306.9 mg/dL; LDL-C 213.8 mg/dL; HDL-C 52.3 mg/dL; and triglycerides 191.0 mg/dL. Fenofibrate therapy lowered LDL-C, Total-C, and the LDL-C/HDL-C ratio. Fenofibrate therapy also lowered triglycerides and raised HDL-C (Table 8).
[See table 8 at top of next page]
In a subset of the subjects, measurements of Apo B were conducted. Fenofibrate treatment significantly reduced Apo B from baseline to endpoint as compared with placebo (-25.1% vs. 2.4%, p < 0.0001, n = 213 and 143, respectively).

16 HOW SUPPLIED/STORAGE AND HANDLING

Trilipix (fenofibric acid) delayed release capsules 45 mg have a reddish-brown cap imprinted in white ink the "a" logo and a yellow body imprinted in black ink the number "45".
Cartons of 30 (NDC 0074-9642-10) and bottles of 90 (NDC 0074-9642-90).
Trilipix (fenofibric acid) delayed release capsules 135 mg have a blue cap imprinted in white ink the "a" logo and a yellow body imprinted in black ink the number "135".
Cartons of 30 (NDC 0074-9189-10) and bottles of 90 (NDC 0074-9189-90).
Store at 25°C (77°F); excursions permitted to 15°-30°C (59° to 86°F) [See USP controlled room temperature]. Keep out of the reach of children. Protect from moisture.

17 PATIENT COUNSELING INFORMATION

See Medication Guide

17.1 Patient Counseling

Patients should be advised:
- of the potential benefits and risks of Trilipix.
- to read the Medication Guide before starting Trilipix therapy and to reread it each time the prescription is renewed.
- of medications that should not be taken in combination with Trilipix.
- to continue to follow an appropriate lipid-modifying diet while taking Trilipix.
- to take Trilipix once daily, without regard to food, at the prescribed dose, swallowing each capsule whole. If Trilipix is co-administered with a statin, they may be taken together.
- to return for routine monitoring.
- to inform their physician of all medications, supplements, and herbal preparations they are taking and any change to their medical condition. Patients should also be advised to inform their physicians prescribing a new medication that they are taking Trilipix.
- to inform their physician of any muscle pain, tenderness, or weakness; onset of abdominal pain; or any other new symptoms.

© AbbVie Inc, 2013
Manufactured for AbbVie Inc., North Chicago, IL 60064, U.S.A. by Fournier Laboratories Ireland Limited, Anngrove, Carrigtwohill Co. Cork, Ireland, or AbbVie LTD, Barceloneta, PR 00617.
03-A785 March, 2013

MEDICATION GUIDE

Trilipix®
(try-lip-iks)
(fenofibric acid, delayed release capsules)
Read this Medication Guide before you start taking Trilipix and each time you get a refill. There may be new informa-

---

Table 6. Percent Change from Baseline to the Final Value in Non-HDL-C, VLDL-C, Total-C, and Apo B (Pooled Double-Blind, Controlled Studies)

Secondary Endpoints	Trilipix	Low-Dose Statin	Trilipix + Low-Dose Statin	Between-group Δ	Moderate-Dose Statin	Trilipix + Moderate-Dose Statin	Between-group Δ	High-Dose Statin
Non HDL-C (mg/dL)	(N = 420)	(N = 454)	(N = 422)		(N = 431)	(N = 420)		(N = 217)
BL mean	222.5	217.6	219.9		222.4	218.9		220.2
Mean % Δ	-17.3%	-34.9%	-40.4%	-23.1%ᵃ / -5.5%ᵇ	-42.4%	-42.0%	-24.8%ᵃ / 0.4%ᵇ	-47.3%
VLDL-C (mg/dL)	(N = 449)	(N = 463)	(N = 455)		(N = 458)	(N = 449)		(N = 232)
BL mean	65.0	66.0	65.5		67.8	64.5		66.1
Mean % Δ	-34.2%	-32.1%	-50.0%	-18.0%ᵇ	-38.9%	-51.2%	-12.3%ᵇ	-42.1%
Total-C (mg/dL)	(N = 459)	(N = 477)	(N = 469)		(N = 472)	(N = 462)		(N = 235)
BL mean	260.9	257.0	258.6		261.3	257.3		258.8
Mean % Δ	-12.4%	-28.7%	-31.5%	-2.8%ᵇ	-34.7%	-33.3%	1.4%ᵇ	-39.5%
Apo B (mg/dL)	(N = 455)	(N = 470)	(N = 465)		(N = 468)	(N = 455)		(N = 229)
BL mean	146.2	145.0	146.1		147.1	145.0		146.0
Mean % Δ	-15.6%	-31.1%	-36.3%	-5.2%ᵇ	-36.9%	-36.7%	0.2%ᵇ	-42.4%

ᵃ Trilipix + statin vs. Trilipix monotherapy
ᵇ Trilipix + statin vs. corresponding statin monotherapy
Low-dose statin = rosuvastatin 10 mg, simvastatin 20 mg, or atorvastatin 20 mg
Moderate-dose statin = rosuvastatin 20 mg, simvastatin 40 mg, or atorvastatin 40 mg
High-dose statin = rosuvastatin 40 mg, simvastatin 80 mg, or atorvastatin 80 mg
BL = Baseline
% Δ = Percent change from baseline to final value

Table 7. Effects of Fenofibrate in Patients With Severe Hypertriglyceridemia

Study 1 Baseline TG levels 350 to 499 mg/dL	Placebo N	Baseline Mean (mg/dL)	Endpoint Mean (mg/dL)	Mean % Change	Fenofibrate N	Baseline Mean (mg/dL)	Endpoint Mean (mg/dL)	Mean % Change
Triglycerides	28	449	450	-0.5	27	432	223	-46.2*
VLDL Triglycerides	19	367	350	2.7	19	350	178	-44.1*
Total Cholesterol	28	255	261	2.8	27	252	227	-9.1*
HDL Cholesterol	28	35	36	4	27	34	40	19.6*
LDL Cholesterol	28	120	129	12	27	128	137	14.5
VLDL Cholesterol	27	99	99	5.8	27	92	46	-44.7*
Study 2 Baseline TG levels 500 to 1500 mg/dL	**Placebo N**	Baseline Mean (mg/dL)	Endpoint Mean (mg/dL)	Mean % Change	**Fenofibrate N**	Baseline Mean (mg/dL)	Endpoint Mean (mg/dL)	Mean % Change
Triglycerides	44	710	750	7.2	48	726	308	-54.5*
VLDL Triglycerides	29	537	571	18.7	33	543	205	-50.6*
Total Cholesterol	44	272	271	0.4	48	261	223	-13.8*
HDL Cholesterol	44	27	28	5.0	48	30	36	22.9*
LDL Cholesterol	42	100	90	-4.2	45	103	131	45.0*
VLDL Cholesterol	42	137	142	11.0	45	126	54	-49.4*

* = p < 0.05 vs. Placebo

---

tion. This information does not take the place of talking to your healthcare provider about your medical condition or your treatment.

What is the most important information I should know about Trilipix?
Trilipix can be used with other cholesterol-lowering medicines called statins. Statins include:
- atorvastatin (Lipitor, Caduet)
- fluvastatin (Lescol, Lescol XL)
- lovastatin (Altoprev, Mevacor, Advicor)
- pitavastatin (Livalo)
- pravastatin (Pravachol)
- rosuvastatin (Crestor)
- simvastatin (Zocor, Simcor, Vytorin)

Statins can cause muscle pain, tenderness or weakness, which may be symptoms of a rare but serious muscle condition called rhabdomyolysis. In some cases rhabdomyolysis can cause kidney damage and death. The risk of rhabdomyolysis may be higher when Trilipix is given with statins. If you take a statin, tell your healthcare provider.

Other medicines or large amounts of grapefruit juice (more than a quart) may raise the levels of statins in your body, and could then raise the risk of muscle problems. Tell your healthcare provider if you are taking any medicines listed below.
- Heart medicine
- Stomach medicine
- Antibiotic
- Anti-fungal
- Cholesterol-lowering medicine
- Hormones
- HIV/AIDS medicine
- Antidepressant
- Immunosuppressant
- Anti-seizure medicine

Ask your healthcare provider or pharmacist for a list of these medicines, if you are not sure.
Tell your healthcare provider if you drink grapefruit juice.

What is Trilipix?
Trilipix is a prescription medicine used to treat cholesterol in the blood by lowering the total amount of triglycerides and LDL (bad) cholesterol, and increasing the HDL (good) cholesterol. **Trilipix has not been shown to lower your risk of having heart problems or a stroke.** You should be on a low fat and low cholesterol diet while you take Trilipix.
The safety and effectiveness of Trilipix in children is not known.

Who should not take Trilipix?
Do not take Trilipix if you:
- are allergic to fenofibric acid, or any of the ingredients in Trilipix. See the end of this Medication Guide for a list of all the ingredients in Trilipix.
- have severe kidney disease.
- have liver disease.
- have gallbladder disease.
- are a nursing mother.

Talk to your healthcare provider before you take Trilipix if you have any of these conditions.

Information on the AbbVie, Inc. products listed on these pages is from the prescribing information in use as of July 31, 2014. For more information, please visit rxabbvie.com or call 1-800-633-9110.

Table 8. Mean Percent Change in Lipid Parameters at End of Treatment[†]

Treatment Group	Total-C (mg/dL)	LDL-C (mg/dL)	HDL-C (mg/dL)	TG (mg/dL)
Pooled Cohort				
Mean baseline lipid values (n = 646)	306.9	213.8	52.3	191.0
All Fenofibrate (n = 361)	-18.7%*	-20.6%*	+11.0%*	-28.9%*
Placebo (n = 285)	-0.4%	-2.2%	+0.7%	+7.7%
Baseline LDL-C > 160 mg/dL and TG < 150 mg/dL				
Mean baseline lipid values (n = 334)	307.7	227.7	58.1	101.7
All Fenofibrate (n = 193)	-22.4%*	-31.4%*	+9.8%*	-23.5%*
Placebo (n = 141)	+0.2%	-2.2%	+2.6%	+11.7%
Baseline LDL-C > 160 mg/dL and TG ≥ 150 mg/dL				
Mean baseline lipid values (n = 242)	312.8	219.8	46.7	231.9
All Fenofibrate (n = 126)	-16.8%*	-20.1%*	+14.6%*	-35.9%*
Placebo (n = 116)	-3.0%	-6.6%	+2.3%	+0.9%

[†] Duration of study treatment was 3 to 6 months
* $p = < 0.05$ vs. Placebo

What should I tell my healthcare provider before taking Trilipix?

Before taking Trilipix, tell your healthcare provider about all your medical conditions, including if you:

- are allergic to any medicines.
- have ever had kidney problems.
- have ever had liver problems.
- have ever had gallbladder problems.
- are pregnant or if you plan to become pregnant. It is not known if Trilipix will harm your unborn baby.
- are breastfeeding or plan to breastfeed. It is not known if Trilipix passes into your breast milk. You and your health-care provider should decide if you will take Trilipix or breastfeed. You should not do both.

Tell your healthcare provider about all the medicines you take, including prescription and non-prescription medicines, vitamins and herbal supplements.

Using Trilipix with certain other medicines can affect the way these medicines work and other medicines may affect how Trilipix works. In some cases, using Trilipix with other medicines can cause serious side effects.

Know all the medicines you take. Keep a list of them and show it to your healthcare provider when you get a new medicine.

It is especially important to tell your healthcare provider if you take any of the medicines mentioned in, "What is the most important information I should know about Trilipix?" or any of the medicines listed below:

- **anticoagulants,** also known as blood thinners (warfarin, Coumadin)
- **bile acid resins**
- **cyclosporine**

Ask your healthcare provider if you are not sure if your medicine is one of these.

How should I take Trilipix?

- You should be on a low fat and low cholesterol diet while you take Trilipix.
- Take Trilipix one time each day as prescribed by your healthcare provider.
- Take Trilipix with or without food.
- Swallow Trilipix capsules whole. Do not break, crush, dissolve, or chew Trilipix capsules before swallowing. If you cannot swallow Trilipix capsules whole, tell your health-care provider, you may need a different medicine.
- If you take a medicine called a statin, you can take Trilipix and your statin at the same time of day.
- If you miss a dose of Trilipix, take it as soon as you remember. If it is almost time for your next dose, just skip the missed dose. Take the next dose at your regular time. If you are not sure about your dosing, call your healthcare provider. **Do not take more than one dose of Trilipix a day unless your healthcare provider tells you to.**
- If you take too much Trilipix, contact your healthcare provider or your local emergency department.
- Do not change your dose or stop Trilipix unless your healthcare provider tells you to.
- Your healthcare provider may do blood tests before you start taking Trilipix and during treatment. See your healthcare provider regularly to check your cholesterol and triglyceride levels and to check for side effects.

What are the possible side effects with Trilipix?

Trilipix may cause serious side effects, including:

- **muscle pain, tenderness, or weakness.** See "What is the most important information that I should know about Trilipix?"
- **tiredness and fever.**
- **abdominal pain, nausea, or vomiting.** These may be signs of inflammation (swelling) of the gallbladder or pancreas.

Call your healthcare provider right away if you have any of these serious side effects.

The most common side effects with Trilipix include:

- headache
- heartburn (indigestion)
- nausea
- muscle aches
- increases in muscle or liver enzymes that are measured by blood tests

Tell your healthcare provider if you have any side effect that bothers you or that does not go away. These are not all the possible side effects of Trilipix. For more information, ask your healthcare provider or pharmacist.

Call your doctor for medical advice about side effects. You may report side effects to FDA at 1-800-FDA-1088.

How do I store Trilipix?

- Store Trilipix between 59° to 86° F (15° to 30° C).
- Protect Trilipix from moisture.

Keep Trilipix and all medicines out of the reach of children.

General information about the safe and effective use of Trilipix

Medicines are sometimes prescribed for conditions that are not mentioned in the Medication Guide. Do not use Trilipix for a condition for which it was not prescribed. Do not give Trilipix to other people, even if they have the same condition you have. It may harm them.

This Medication Guide summarizes the most important information about Trilipix. If you would like more information, talk to your healthcare provider. You can also ask your pharmacist or healthcare provider for information that is written for health professionals.

For more information go to www.Trilipix.com or call 1-800-633-9110.

What are the ingredients in Trilipix?

Active Ingredient: Fenofibric acid

Inactive Ingredients: Hypromellose, povidone, water, hydroxylpropyl cellulose, colloidal silicon dioxide, sodium stearyl fumarate, methacrylic acid copolymer, talc, triethyl citrate, gelatin, titanium dioxide, and yellow iron oxide. Additionally, the 45 mg capsule shell contains black iron oxide and red iron oxide, and the 135 mg capsule shell contains FD&C Blue #2.

© AbbVie Inc. 2013

Manufactured for AbbVie Inc., North Chicago, IL 60064, U.S.A. by Fournier Laboratories Ireland Limited, Anngrove, Carrigtwohill Co. Cork, Ireland, or AbbVie LTD, Barceloneta, PR 00617.

Ref: 03-A785 March, 2013

This Medication Guide has been approved by the U.S. Food and Drug Administration.

Shown in Product Identification Guide, page 304

ULTANE®

[ul-tān]

(sevoflurane)

volatile liquid for inhalation

℞

DESCRIPTION

ULTANE (sevoflurane), volatile liquid for inhalation, a nonflammable and nonexplosive liquid administered by vaporization, is a halogenated general inhalation anesthetic drug. Sevoflurane is fluoromethyl 2,2,2,-trifluoro-1-(trifluoromethyl) ethyl ether and its structural formula is:

Sevoflurane, Physical Constants are:

Molecular weight	200.05
Boiling point at 760 mm Hg	58.6°C
Specific gravity at 20°C	1.520 - 1.525
Vapor pressure in mm Hg	157 mm Hg at 20°C
	197 mm Hg at 25°C
	317 mm Hg at 36°C

Distribution Partition Coefficients at 37°C:

Blood/Gas	0.63 - 0.69
Water/Gas	0.36
Olive Oil/Gas	47 - 54
Brain/Gas	1.15

Mean Component/Gas Partition Coefficients at 25°C for Polymers Used Commonly in Medical Applications:

Conductive rubber	14.0
Butyl rubber	7.7
Polyvinylchloride	17.4
Polyethylene	1.3

Sevoflurane is nonflammable and nonexplosive as defined by the requirements of International Electrotechnical Commission 601-2-13.

Sevoflurane is a clear, colorless, liquid containing no additives. Sevoflurane is not corrosive to stainless steel, brass, aluminum, nickel-plated brass, chrome-plated brass or copper beryllium. Sevoflurane is nonpungent. It is miscible with ethanol, ether, chloroform, and benzene, and it is slightly soluble in water. Sevoflurane is stable when stored under normal room lighting conditions according to instructions. No discernible degradation of sevoflurane occurs in the presence of strong acids or heat. When in contact with alkaline CO_2 absorbents (e.g Baralyme® and to a lesser extent soda lime) within the anesthesia machine, sevoflurane can undergo degradation under certain conditions. Degradation of sevoflurane is minimal, and degradants are either undetectable or present in non-toxic amounts when used as directed with fresh absorbents. Sevoflurane degradation and subsequent degradant formation are enhanced by increasing absorbent temperature increased sevoflurane concentration, decreased fresh gas flow and desiccated CO_2 absorbents (especially with potassium hydroxide containing absorbents e.g. Baralyme).

Sevoflurane alkaline degradation occurs by two pathways. The first results from the loss of hydrogen fluoride with the formation of pentafluoroisopropenyl fluoromethyl ether, (PIFE, $C_4H_2F_6O$), also known as Compound A, and trace amounts of pentafluoromethoxy isopropyl fluoromethyl ether, (PMFE, $C_5H_6F_6O$), also known as Compound B. The second pathway for degradation of sevoflurane, which occurs primarily in the presence of desiccated CO_2 absorbents, is discussed later.

In the first pathway, the defluorination pathway, the production of degradants in the anesthesia circuit results from the extraction of the acidic proton in the presence of a strong base (KOH and/or NaOH) forming an alkene (Compound A) from sevoflurane similar to formation of 2-bromo-2-chloro-1,1-difluoro ethylene (BCDFE) from halothane. Laboratory simulations have shown that the concentration of these degradants is inversely correlated with the fresh gas flow rate (See Figure 1).

Figure 1. Fresh Gas Flow Rate versus Compound A Levels in a Circle Absorber System

Since the reaction of carbon dioxide with absorbents is exothermic, the temperature increase will be determined by quantities of CO_2 absorbed, which in turn will depend on fresh gas flow in the anesthesia circle system, metabolic status of the patient, and ventilation. The relationship of temperature produced by varying levels of CO_2 and

Compound A production is illustrated in the following *in vitro* simulation where CO_2 was added to a circle absorber system.

Figure 2. Carbon Dioxide Flow versus Compound A and Maximum Temperature

Compound A concentration in a circle absorber system increases as a function of increasing CO_2 absorbent temperature and composition (Baralyme producing higher levels than soda lime), increased body temperature, and increased minute ventilation, and decreasing fresh gas flow rates. It has been reported that the concentration of Compound A increases significantly with prolonged dehydration of Baralyme. Compound A exposure in patients also has been shown to rise with increased sevoflurane concentrations and duration of anesthesia. In a clinical study in which sevoflurane was administered to patients under low flow conditions for ≥ 2 hours at flow rates of 1 Liter/minute, Compound A levels were measured in an effort to determine the relationship between MAC hours and Compound A levels produced. The relationship between Compound A levels and sevoflurane exposure are shown in Figure 2a.

Figure 2a. ppm-hr versus MAC-hr at Flow Rate of 1 L/min

Compound A has been shown to be nephrotoxic in rats after exposures that have varied in duration from one to three hours. No histopathologic change was seen at a concentration of up to 270 ppm for one hour. Sporadic single cell necrosis of proximal tubule cells has been reported at a concentration of 114 ppm after a 3-hour exposure to Compound A in rats. The LC_{50} reported at 1 hour is 1050-1090 ppm (male-female) and, at 3 hours, 350-490 ppm (male-female).

An experiment was performed comparing sevoflurane plus 75 or 100 ppm Compound A with an active control to evaluate the potential nephrotoxicity of Compound A in non-human primates. A single 8-hour exposure of Sevoflurane in the presence of Compound A produced single-cell renal tubular degeneration and single-cell necrosis in cynomolgus monkeys. These changes are consistent with the increased urinary protein, glucose level and enzymic activity noted on days one and three on the clinical pathology evaluation. This nephrotoxicity produced by Compound A is dose and duration of exposure dependent.

At a fresh gas flow rate of 1 L/min, mean maximum concentrations of Compound A in the anesthesia circuit in clinical settings are approximately 20 ppm (0.002%) with soda lime and 30 ppm (0.003%) with Baralyme in adult patients; mean maximum concentrations in pediatric patients with soda lime are about half those found in adults. The highest concentration observed in a single patient with Baralyme was 61 ppm (0.0061%) and 32 ppm (0.0032%) with soda lime. The levels of Compound A at which toxicity occurs in humans is not known.

The second pathway for degradation of sevoflurane occurs primarily in the presence of desiccated CO_2 absorbents and leads to the dissociation of sevoflurane into hexafluoroisopropanol (HFIP) and formaldehyde. HFIP is inactive, non-genotoxic, rapidly glucuronidated and cleared by the liver. Formaldehyde is present during normal metabolic processes. Upon exposure to a highly desiccated absorbent, formaldehyde can further degrade into methanol and formate. Formate can contribute to the formation of carbon monoxide in the presence of high temperature that can be associated with desiccated Baralyme®. Methanol can react with Compound A to form the methoxy addition product Compound B. Compound B can undergo further HF elimination to form Compounds C, D, and E.

Sevoflurane degradants were observed in the respiratory circuit of an experimental anesthesia machine using desiccated CO_2 absorbents and maximum sevoflurane concentrations (8%) for extended periods of time (> 2 hours). Concentrations of formaldehyde observed with desiccated soda lime in this experimental anesthesia respiratory circuit were consistent with levels that could potentially result in respiratory irritation. Although KOH containing CO_2 absorbents are no longer commercially available, in the laboratory experiments, exposure of sevoflurane to the desiccated KOH containing CO_2 absorbent, Baralyme, resulted in the detection of substantially greater degradant levels.

CLINICAL PHARMACOLOGY

Sevoflurane is an inhalational anesthetic agent for use in induction and maintenance of general anesthesia. Minimum alveolar concentration (MAC) of sevoflurane in oxygen for a 40-year-old adult is 2.1%. The MAC of sevoflurane decreases with age (see **DOSAGE AND ADMINISTRATION** for details).

Pharmacokinetics

Uptake and Distribution

Solubility

Because of the low solubility of sevoflurane in blood (blood/gas partition coefficient @ 37°C = 0.63-0.69), a minimal amount of sevoflurane is required to be dissolved in the blood before the alveolar partial pressure is in equilibrium with the arterial partial pressure. Therefore there is a rapid rate of increase in the alveolar (end-tidal) concentration (F_A) toward the inspired concentration (F_I) during induction.

Induction of Anesthesia

In a study in which seven healthy male volunteers were administered 70% N_2O/30%O_2 for 30 minutes followed by 1.0% sevoflurane and 0.6% isoflurane for another 30 minutes the F_A/F_I ratio was greater for sevoflurane than isoflurane at all time points. The time for the concentration in the alveoli to reach 50% of the inspired concentration was 4-8 minutes for isoflurane and approximately 1 minute for sevoflurane. F_A/F_I data from this study were compared with F_A/F_I data of other halogenated anesthetic agents from another study. When all data were normalized to isoflurane, the uptake and distribution of sevoflurane was shown to be faster than isoflurane and halothane, but slower than desflurane. The results are depicted in Figure 3.

Recovery from Anesthesia

The low solubility of sevoflurane facilitates rapid elimination via the lungs. The rate of elimination is quantified as the rate of change of the alveolar (end-tidal) concentration following termination of anesthesia (F_A), relative to the last alveolar concentration (Fa_0) measured immediately before discontinuance of the anesthetic. In the healthy volunteer study described above, rate of elimination of sevoflurane was similar compared with desflurane, but faster compared with either halothane or isoflurane. These results are depicted in Figure 4.

Figure 3. Ratio of Concentration of Anesthetic in Alveolar Gas to Inspired Gas

[See figure 4 at top of next column]

Yasuda N, Lockhart S, Eger EI II, et al: Comparison of kinetics of sevoflurane and isoflurane in humans. Anesth Analg 72:316, 1991.

Protein Binding

The effects of sevoflurane on the displacement of drugs from serum and tissue proteins have not been investigated. Other fluorinated volatile anesthetics have been shown to displace drugs from serum and tissue proteins *in vitro*. The clinical significance of this is unknown. Clinical studies have shown no untoward effects when sevoflurane is administered to patients taking drugs that are highly bound and have a small volume of distribution (e.g., phenytoin).

Metabolism

Sevoflurane is metabolized by cytochrome P450 2E1, to hexafluoroisopropanol (HFIP) with release of inorganic fluoride and CO_2. Once formed HFIP is rapidly conjugated with glucuronic acid and eliminated as a urinary metabolite. No other metabolic pathways for sevoflurane have been identified. *In vivo* metabolism studies suggest that approximately 5% of the sevoflurane dose may be metabolized. Cytochrome P450 2E1 is the principal isoform identified for sevoflurane metabolism and this may be induced by chronic exposure to isoniazid and ethanol. This is similar to the metabolism of isoflurane and enflurane and is distinct from that of methoxyflurane which is metabolized via a variety of cytochrome P450 isoforms. The metabolism of sevoflurane is not inducible by barbiturates. As shown in Figure 5, inorganic fluoride concentrations peak within 2 hours of the end of sevoflurane anesthesia and return to baseline concentrations within 48 hours post-anesthesia in the majority of cases (67%). The rapid and extensive pulmonary elimination of sevoflurane minimizes the amount of anesthetic available for metabolism.

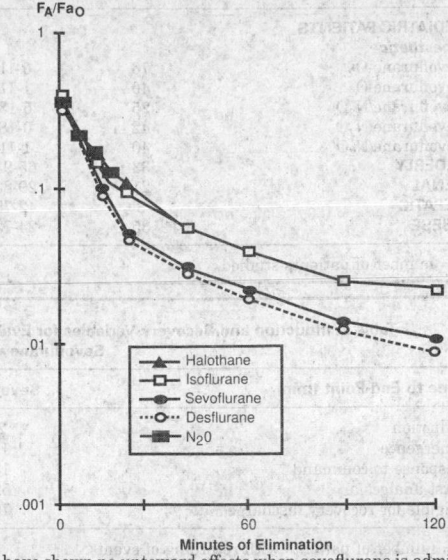

Figure 4. Concentration of Anesthetic in Alveolar Gas Following Termination of Anesthesia

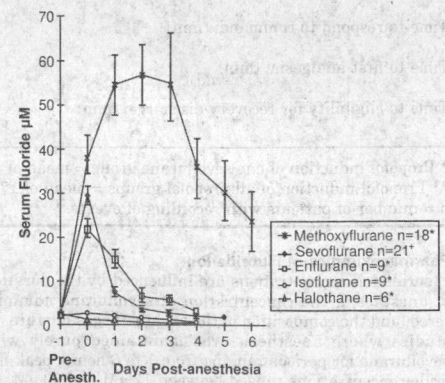

Figure 5. Serum Inorganic Fluoride Concentrations for Sevoflurane and Other Volatile Anesthetics

Cousins M.J., Greenstein L.R., Hitt B.A., et al: Metabolism and renal effects of enflurane in man. Anesthesiology 44:44; 1976* and Sevo-93-044+.
Legend:
Pre-Anesth. = Pre-anesthesia

Elimination

Up to 3.5% of the sevoflurane dose appears in the urine as inorganic fluoride. Studies on fluoride indicate that up to 50% of fluoride clearance is nonrenal (via fluoride being taken up into bone).

Information on the AbbVie, Inc. products listed on these pages is from the prescribing information in use as of July 31, 2014. For more information, please visit rxabbvie.com or call 1-800-633-9110.

Table 1. Fluoride Ion Estimates in Special Populations Following Administration of Sevoflurane

	n	Age (yr)	Duration (hr)	Dose (MAC·hr)	C_{max} (µM)
PEDIATRIC PATIENTS					
Anesthetic					
Sevoflurane-O_2	76	0-11	0.8	1.1	12.6
Sevoflurane-O_2	40	1-11	2.2	3.0	16.0
Sevoflurane/N_2O	25	5-13	1.9	2.4	21.3
Sevoflurane/N_2O	42	0-18	2.4	2.2	18.4
Sevoflurane/N_2O	40	1-11	2.0	2.6	15.5
ELDERLY	33	65-93	2.6	1.4	25.6
RENAL	21	29-83	2.5	1.0	26.1
HEPATIC	8	42-79	3.6	2.2	30.6
OBESE	35	24-73	3.0	1.7	38.0

n = number of patients studied.

Table 2. Induction and Recovery Variables for Evaluable Pediatric Patients in Two Comparative Studies: Sevoflurane versus Halothane

Time to End-Point (min)	Sevoflurane Mean ± SEM	Halothane Mean ± SEM
Induction	2.0 ± 0.2 (n=294)	2.7 ± 0.2 (n=252)
Emergence	11.3 ± 0.7 (n=293)	15.8 ± 0.8 (n=252)
Response to command	13.7 ± 1.0 (n=271)	19.3 ± 1.1 (n=230)
First analgesia	52.2 ± 8.5 (n=216)	67.6 ± 10.6 (n=150)
Eligible for recovery discharge	76.5 ± 2.0 (n=292)	81.1 ± 1.9 (n=246)

n = number of patients with recording of events.

Table 3. Recovery Variables for Evaluable Adult Patients in Two Comparative Studies: Sevoflurane versus Isoflurane

Time to Parameter: (min)	Sevoflurane Mean ± SEM	Isoflurane Mean ± SEM
Emergence	7.7 ± 0.3 (n = 395)	9.1 ± 0.3 (n = 348)
Response to command	8.1 ± 0.3 (n = 395)	9.7 ± 0.3 (n = 345)
First analgesia	42.7 ± 3.0 (n = 269)	52.9 ± 4.2 (n = 228)
Eligible for recovery discharge	87.6 ± 5.3 (n = 244)	79.1 ± 5.2 (n = 252)

n = number of patients with recording of recovery events.

Table 4. Meta-Analyses for Induction and Emergence Variables for Evaluable Adult Patients in Comparative Studies: Sevoflurane versus Propofol

Parameter	No. of Studies	Sevoflurane Mean ± SEM	Propofol Mean ± SEM
Mean maintenance anesthesia exposure	3	1.0 MAC·hr. ± 0.8 (n=259)	7.2 mg/kg/hr ± 2.6 (n=258)
Time to induction: (min)	1	3.1 ± 0.18* (n=93)	2.2 ± 0.18** (n=93)
Time to emergence: (min)	3	8.6 ± 0.57 (n=255)	11.0 ± 0.57 (n=260)
Time to respond to command: (min)	3	9.9 ± 0.60 (n=257)	12.1 ± 0.60 (n=260)
Time to first analgesia: (min)	3	43.8 ± 3.79 (n=177)	57.9 ± 3.68 (n=179)
Time to eligibility for recovery discharge: (min)	3	116.0 ± 4.15 (n=257)	115.6 ± 3.98 (n=261)

* Propofol induction of one sevoflurane group = mean of 178.8 mg ±72.5 SD (n=165)
** Propofol induction of all propofol groups = mean of 170.2 mg ±60.6 SD (n=245)
n = number of patients with recording of events.

Pharmacokinetics of Fluoride Ion

Fluoride ion concentrations are influenced by the duration of anesthesia, the concentration of sevoflurane administered, and the composition of the anesthetic gas mixture. In studies where anesthesia was maintained purely with sevoflurane for periods ranging from 1 to 6 hours, peak fluoride concentrations ranged between 12 µM and 90 µM. As shown in Figure 6, peak concentrations occur within 2 hours of the end of anesthesia and are less than 25 µM (475 ng/mL) for the majority of the population after 10 hours. The half-life is in the range of 15-23 hours.

It has been reported that following administration of methoxyflurane, serum inorganic fluoride concentrations >50 µM were correlated with the development of vasopressin-resistant, polyuric, renal failure. In clinical trials with sevoflurane, there were no reports of toxicity associated with elevated fluoride ion levels.
[See figure 6 at top of next column]

Fluoride Concentrations After Repeat Exposure and in Special Populations

Fluoride concentrations have been measured after single, extended, and repeat exposure to sevoflurane in normal surgical and special patient populations, and pharmacokinetic parameters were determined.

Figure 6. Fluoride Ion Concentrations Following Administration of Sevoflurane (mean MAC = 1.27, mean duration = 2.06 hr) Mean Fluoride Ion Concentrations (n = 48)

— mean concentration
— mean conc + 1 sd
--- mean conc + 2 sd
--- mean conc + 3 sd

Compared with healthy individuals, the fluoride ion half-life was prolonged in patients with renal impairment, but not in the elderly. A study in 8 patients with hepatic impairment suggests a slight prolongation of the half-life. The mean half-life in patients with renal impairment averaged approximately 33 hours (range 21-61 hours) as compared to a mean of approximately 21 hours (range 10-48 hours) in normal healthy individuals. The mean half-life in the el-

derly (greater than 65 years) approximated 24 hours (range 18-72 hours). The mean half-life in individuals with hepatic impairment was 23 hours (range 16-47 hours). Mean maximal fluoride values (C_{max}) determined in individual studies of special populations are displayed below.
[See table 1 above]

Pharmacodynamics

Changes in the depth of sevoflurane anesthesia rapidly follow changes in the inspired concentration.

In the sevoflurane clinical program, the following recovery variables were evaluated:

1. **Time to events measured from the end of study drug:**
   - Time to removal of the endotracheal tube (extubation time)
   - Time required for the patient to open his/her eyes on verbal command (emergence time)
   - Time to respond to simple command (e.g., squeeze my hand) or demonstrates purposeful movement (response to command time, orientation time)

2. **Recovery of cognitive function and motor coordination was evaluated based on:**
   - psychomotor performance tests (Digit Symbol Substitution Test [DSST], Treiger Dot Test)
   - the results of subjective (Visual Analog Scale [VAS]) and objective (objective pain-discomfort scale [OPDS]) measurements
   - time to administration of the first post-anesthesia analgesic medication
   - assessments of post-anesthesia patient status

3. **Other recovery times were:**
   - time to achieve an Aldrete Score of ≥ 8
   - time required for the patient to be eligible for discharge from the recovery area, per standard criteria at site
   - time when the patient was eligible for discharge from the hospital
   - time when the patient was able to sit up or stand without dizziness

Some of these variables are summarized as follows:
[See table 2 above]
[See table 3 above]
[See table 4 above]

Cardiovascular Effects

Sevoflurane was studied in 14 healthy volunteers (18-35 years old) comparing sevoflurane-O_2 (Sevo/O_2) to sevoflurane-N_2O/O_2 (Sevo/N_2O/O_2) during 7 hours of anesthesia. During controlled ventilation, hemodynamic parameters measured are shown in Figures 7-10:

Figure 7. Heart Rate

Figure 8. Mean Arterial Pressure

Figure 9. Systemic Vascular Resistance

Figure 10. Cardiac Index

Sevoflurane is a dose-related cardiac depressant. Sevoflurane does not produce increases in heart rate at doses less than 2 MAC.

A study investigating the epinephrine induced arrhythmogenic effect of sevoflurane versus isoflurane in adult patients undergoing transsphenoidal hypophysectomy demonstrated that the threshold dose of epinephrine (i.e., the dose at which the first sign of arrhythmia was observed) producing multiple ventricular arrhythmias was 5 mcg/kg with both sevoflurane and isoflurane. Consequently, the interaction of sevoflurane with epinephrine appears to be equal to that seen with isoflurane.

Clinical Trials

Sevoflurane was administered to a total of 3185 patients prior to sevoflurane NDA submission. The types of patients are summarized as follows:

Table 5. Patients Receiving Sevoflurane in Clinical Trials

Type of Patients	Number Studied
ADULT	2223
Cesarean Delivery	29
Cardiovascular and patients at risk of myocardial ischemia	246
Neurosurgical	22
Hepatic impairment	8
Renal impairment	35
PEDIATRIC	962

Clinical experience with these patients is described below.

Adult Anesthesia

The efficacy of sevoflurane in comparison to isoflurane, enflurane, and propofol was investigated in 3 outpatient and 25 inpatient studies involving 3591 adult patients. Sevoflurane was found to be comparable to isoflurane, enflurane, and propofol for the maintenance of anesthesia in adult patients. Patients administered sevoflurane showed shorter times (statistically significant) to some recovery events (extubation, response to command, and orientation) than patients who received isoflurane or propofol.

Mask Induction

Sevoflurane has a nonpungent odor and does not cause respiratory irritability. Sevoflurane is suitable for mask induction in adults. In 196 patients, mask induction was smooth and rapid, with complications occurring with the following frequencies: cough, 6%; breathholding, 6%; agitation, 6%; laryngospasm, 5%.

Ambulatory Surgery

Sevoflurane was compared to isoflurane and propofol for maintenance of anesthesia supplemented with N_2O in two studies involving 786 adult (18-84 years of age) ASA Class I, II, or III patients. Shorter times to emergence and response to commands (statistically significant) were observed with sevoflurane compared to isoflurane and propofol.

[See table 6 above]

Inpatient Surgery

Sevoflurane was compared to isoflurane and propofol for maintenance of anesthesia supplemented with N_2O in two multicenter studies involving 741 adult ASA Class I, II, or III (18-92 years of age) patients. Shorter times to emergence, command response, and first post-anesthesia analgesia (statistically significant) were observed with sevoflurane compared to isoflurane and propofol.

[See table 7 above]

Pediatric Anesthesia

The concentration of sevoflurane required for maintenance of general anesthesia is age-dependent (see **DOSAGE AND ADMINISTRATION**). Sevoflurane or halothane was used to anesthetize 1620 pediatric patients aged 1 day to 18 years, and ASA physical status I or II (948 sevoflurane, 672 halothane). In one study involving 90 infants and children, there were no clinically significant decreases in heart rate compared to awake values at 1 MAC. Systolic blood pressure decreased 15-20% in comparison to awake values following administration of 1 MAC sevoflurane; however, clinically significant hypotension requiring immediate intervention did not occur. Overall incidences of bradycardia [more than 20 beats/min lower than normal (80 beats/

Table 6. Recovery Parameters in Two Outpatient Surgery Studies: Least Squares Mean ± SEM

	Sevoflurane/N$_2$O	Isoflurane/N$_2$O	Sevoflurane/N$_2$O	Propofol/N$_2$O
Mean Maintenance Anesthesia Exposure ± SD	0.64 ± 0.03 MAC•hr. (n=245)	0.66 ± 0.03 MAC•hr. (n=249)	0.8 ± 0.5 MAC•hr. (n=166)	7.3 ± 2.3 mg/kg/hr. (n=166)
Time to Emergence (min)	8.2 ± 0.4 (n=246)	9.3 ± 0.3 (n=251)	8.3 ± 0.7 (n=137)	10.4 ± 0.7 (n=142)
Time to Respond to Commands (min)	8.5 ± 0.4 (n=246)	9.8 ± 0.4 (n=248)	9.1 ± 0.7 (n=139)	11.5 ± 0.7 (n=143)
Time to First Analgesia (min)	45.9 ± 4.7 (n=160)	59.1 ± 6.0 (n=252)	46.1 ± 5.4 (n=83)	60.0 ± 4.7 (n=88)
Time to Eligibility for Discharge from Recovery Area (min)	87.6 ± 5.3 (n=244)	79.1 ± 5.2 (n=252)	103.1 ± 3.8 (n=139)	105.1 ± 3.7 (n=143)

n = number of patients with recording of recovery events.

Table 7. Recovery Parameters in Two Inpatient Surgery Studies: Least Squares Mean ± SEM

	Sevoflurane/N$_2$O	Isoflurane/N$_2$O	Sevoflurane/N$_2$O	Propofol/N$_2$O
Mean Maintenance Anesthesia Exposure ± SD	1.27 MAC•hr. ± 0.05 (n=271)	1.58 MAC•hr. ± 0.06 (n=282)	1.43 MAC•hr. ± 0.94 (n=93)	7.0 mg/kg/hr ± 2.9 (n=92)
Time to Emergence (min)	11.0 ± 0.6 (n=270)	16.4 ± 0.6 (n=281)	8.8 ± 1.2 (n=92)	13.2 ± 1.2 (n=92)
Time to Respond to Commands (min)	12.8 ± 0.7 (n=270)	18.4 ± 0.7 (n=281)	11.0 ± 1.20 (n=92)	14.4 ± 1.21 (n=91)
Time to First Analgesia (min)	46.1 ± 3.0 (n=233)	55.4 ± 3.2 (n=242)	37.8 ± 3.3 (n=82)	49.2 ± 3.3 (n=79)
Time to Eligibility for Discharge from Recovery Area (min)	139.2 ± 15.6 (n=268)	165.9 ± 16.3 (n=282)	148.4 ± 8.9 (n=92)	141.4 ± 8.9 (n=92)

n = number of patients with recording of recovery events.

min)] in comparative studies was 3% for sevoflurane and 7% for halothane. Patients who received sevoflurane had slightly faster emergence times (12 vs. 19 minutes), and a higher incidence of post-anesthesia agitation (14% vs. 10%). Sevoflurane (n=91) was compared to halothane (n=89) in a single-center study for elective repair or palliation of congenital heart disease. The patients ranged in age from 9 days to 11.8 years with an ASA physical status of II, III, and IV (18%, 68%, and 13% respectively). No significant differences were demonstrated between treatment groups with respect to the primary outcome measures: cardiovascular decompensation and severe arterial desaturation. Adverse event data was limited to the study outcome variables collected during surgery and before institution of cardiopulmonary bypass.

Mask Induction

Sevoflurane has a nonpungent odor and is suitable for mask induction in pediatric patients. In controlled pediatric studies in which mask induction was performed, the incidence of induction events is shown below (see **ADVERSE REACTIONS**).

Table 8. Incidence of Pediatric Induction Events

	Sevoflurane (n=836)	Halothane (n=660)
Agitation	14%	11%
Cough	6%	10%
Breathholding	5%	6%
Secretions	3%	3%
Laryngospasm	2%	2%
Bronchospasm	<1%	0%

n = number of patients.

Ambulatory Surgery

Sevoflurane (n=518) was compared to halothane (n=382) for the maintenance of anesthesia in pediatric outpatients. All patients received N_2O and many received fentanyl, midazolam, bupivacaine, or lidocaine. The time to eligibility for discharge from post-anesthesia care units was similar between agents (see **CLINICAL PHARMACOLOGY** and **ADVERSE REACTIONS**).

Cardiovascular Surgery

Coronary Artery Bypass Graft (CABG) Surgery

Sevoflurane was compared to isoflurane as an adjunct with opioids in a multicenter study of 273 patients undergoing CABG surgery. Anesthesia was induced with midazolam (0.1-0.3 mg/kg); vecuronium (0.1-0.2 mg/kg), and fentanyl (5-15 mcg/kg). Both isoflurane and sevoflurane were administered at loss of consciousness in doses of 1.0 MAC and titrated until the beginning of cardiopulmonary bypass to a maximum of 2.0 MAC. The total dose of fentanyl did not exceed 25 mcg/kg. The average MAC dose was 0.49 for sevoflurane and 0.53 for isoflurane. There were no significant differences in hemodynamics, cardioactive drug use, or

ischemia incidence between the two groups. Outcome was also equivalent. In this small multicenter study, sevoflurane appears to be as effective and as safe as isoflurane for supplementation of opioid anesthesia for coronary bypass grafting.

Non-Cardiac Surgery Patients at Risk for Myocardial Ischemia

Sevoflurane-N_2O was compared to isoflurane-N_2O for maintenance of anesthesia in a multicenter study in 214 patients, age 40-87 years who were at mild-to-moderate risk for myocardial ischemia and were undergoing elective noncardiac surgery. Forty-six percent (46%) of the operations were cardiovascular, with the remainder evenly divided between gastrointestinal and musculoskeletal and small numbers of other surgical procedures. The average duration of surgery was less than 2 hours. Anesthesia induction usually was performed with thiopental (2-5 mg/kg) and fentanyl (1-5 mcg/kg). Vecuronium (0.1-0.2 mg/kg) was also administered to facilitate intubation, muscle relaxation or immobility during surgery. The average MAC dose was 0.49 for both anesthetics. There was no significant difference between the anesthetic regimens for intraoperative hemodynamics, cardioactive drug use, or ischemic incidents, although only 83 patients in the sevoflurane group and 85 patients in the isoflurane group were successfully monitored for ischemia. The outcome was also equivalent in terms of adverse events, death, and postoperative myocardial infarction. Within the limits of this small multicenter study in patients at mild-to-moderate risk for myocardial ischemia, sevoflurane was a satisfactory equivalent to isoflurane in providing supplemental inhalation anesthesia to intravenous drugs.

Cesarean Section

Sevoflurane (n=29) was compared to isoflurane (n=27) in ASA Class I or II patients for the maintenance of anesthesia during cesarean section. Newborn evaluations and recovery events were recorded. With both anesthetics, Apgar scores averaged 8 and 9 at 1 and 5 minutes, respectively.

Use of sevoflurane as part of general anesthesia for elective cesarean section produced no untoward effects in mother or neonate. Sevoflurane and isoflurane demonstrated equivalent recovery characteristics. There was no difference between sevoflurane and isoflurane with regard to the effect on the newborn, as assessed by Apgar Score and Neurological and Adaptive Capacity Score (average=29.5). The safety of sevoflurane in labor and vaginal delivery has not been evaluated.

Neurosurgery

Three studies compared sevoflurane to isoflurane for maintenance of anesthesia during neurosurgical procedures. In a study of 20 patients, there was no difference between

Information on the AbbVie, Inc. products listed on these pages is from the prescribing information in use as of July 31, 2014. For more information, please visit rxabbvie.com or call 1-800-633-9110.

sevoflurane and isoflurane with regard to recovery from anesthesia. In 2 studies, a total of 22 patients with intracranial pressure (ICP) monitors received either sevoflurane or isoflurane. There was no difference between sevoflurane and isoflurane with regard to ICP response to inhalation of 0.5, 1.0, and 1.5 MAC inspired concentrations of volatile agent during N_2O-O_2-fentanyl anesthesia. During progressive hyperventilation from $PaCO_2$ = 40 to $PaCO_2$ = 30, ICP response to hypocarbia was preserved with sevoflurane at both 0.5 and 1.0 MAC concentrations. In patients at risk for elevations of ICP, sevoflurane should be administered cautiously in conjunction with ICP-reducing maneuvers such as hyperventilation.

Hepatic Impairment
A multicenter study (2 sites) compared the safety of sevoflurane and isoflurane in 16 patients with mild-to-moderate hepatic impairment utilizing the lidocaine MEGX assay for assessment of hepatocellular function. All patients received intravenous propofol (1-3 mg/kg) or thiopental (2-7 mg/kg) for induction and succinylcholine, vecuronium, or atracurium for intubation. Sevoflurane or isoflurane was administered in either 100% O_2 or up to 70% N_2O/O_2. Neither drug adversely affected hepatic function. No serum inorganic fluoride level exceeded 45 μM/L, but sevoflurane patients had prolonged terminal disposition of fluoride, as evidenced by longer inorganic fluoride half-life than patients with normal hepatic function (23 hours vs. 10-48 hours).

Renal Impairment
Sevoflurane was evaluated in renally impaired patients with baseline serum creatinine >1.5 mg/dL. Fourteen patients who received sevoflurane were compared with 12 patients who received isoflurane. In another study, 21 patients who received sevoflurane were compared with 20 patients who received enflurane. Creatinine levels increased in 7% of patients who received sevoflurane, 8% of patients who received isoflurane, and 10% of patients who received enflurane. Because of the small number of patients with renal insufficiency (baseline serum creatinine greater than 1.5 mg/dL) studied, the safety of sevoflurane administration in this group has not yet been fully established. Therefore, sevoflurane should be used with caution in patients with renal insufficiency (see **WARNINGS**).

INDICATIONS AND USAGE
Sevoflurane is indicated for induction and maintenance of general anesthesia in adult and pediatric patients for inpatient and outpatient surgery.

Sevoflurane should be administered only by persons trained in the administration of general anesthesia. Facilities for maintenance of a patent airway, artificial ventilation, oxygen enrichment, and circulatory resuscitation must be immediately available. Since level of anesthesia may be altered rapidly, only vaporizers producing predictable concentrations of sevoflurane should be used.

CONTRAINDICATIONS
Sevoflurane can cause malignant hyperthermia. It should not be used in patients with known sensitivity to sevoflurane or to other halogenated agents nor in patients with known or suspected susceptibility to malignant hyperthermia.

WARNINGS
Although data from controlled clinical studies at low flow rates are limited, findings taken from patient and animal studies suggest that there is a potential for renal injury which is presumed due to Compound A. Animal and human studies demonstrate that sevoflurane administered for more than 2 MAC•hours and at fresh gas flow rates of <2 L/min may be associated with proteinuria and glycosuria.

While a level of Compound A exposure at which clinical nephrotoxicity might be expected to occur has not been established, it is prudent to consider all of the factors leading to Compound A exposure in humans, especially duration of exposure, fresh gas flow rate, and concentration of sevoflurane. During sevoflurane anesthesia the clinician should adjust inspired concentration and fresh gas flow rate to minimize exposure to Compound A. To minimize exposure to Compound A, sevoflurane exposure should not exceed 2 MAC•hours at flow rates of 1 to <2 L/min. Fresh gas flow rates <1 L/min are not recommended.

Because clinical experience in administering sevoflurane to patients with renal insufficiency (creatinine >1.5 mg/dL) is limited, its safety in these patients has not been established.

Sevoflurane may be associated with glycosuria and proteinuria when used for long procedures at low flow rates. The safety of low flow sevoflurane on renal function was evaluated in patients with normal preoperative renal function. One study compared sevoflurane (N=98) to an active control (N=90) administered for ≥ 2 hours at a fresh gas flow rate of ≤1 Liter/minute. Per study defined criteria (Hou et al.) one patient in the sevoflurane group developed elevations of creatinine, in addition to glycosuria and proteinuria. This pa-

tient received sevoflurane at fresh gas flow rates of ≤800 mL/minute. Using these same criteria, there were no patients in the active control group who developed treatment emergent elevations in serum creatinine.

Sevoflurane may present an increased risk in patients with known sensitivity to volatile halogenated anesthetic agents. KOH containing CO_2 absorbents are not recommended for use with sevoflurane.

Reports of QT prolongation, associated with torsade de pointes (in exceptional cases, fatal), have been received. Caution should be exercised when administering sevoflurane to susceptible patients (e.g. patients with congenital Long QT Syndrome or patients taking drugs that can prolong the QT interval).

Malignant Hyperthermia
In susceptible individuals, potent inhalation anesthetic agents, including sevoflurane, may trigger a skeletal muscle hypermetabolic state leading to high oxygen demand and the clinical syndrome known as malignant hyperthermia. Sevoflurane can induce malignant hyperthermia in genetically susceptible individuals, such as those with certain inherited ryanodine receptor mutations. The clinical syndrome is signaled by hypercapnia, and may include muscle rigidity, tachycardia, tachypnea, cyanosis, arrhythmias, and/or unstable blood pressure. Some of these nonspecific signs may also appear during light anesthesia, acute hypoxia, hypercapnia, and hypovolemia.

In clinical trials, one case of malignant hyperthermia was reported. In addition, there have been postmarketing reports of malignant hyperthermia. Some of these cases have been fatal.

Treatment of malignant hyperthermia includes discontinuation of triggering agents (e.g., sevoflurane), administration of intravenous dantrolene sodium (consult prescribing information for intravenous dantrolene sodium for additional information on patient management), and application of supportive therapy. Supportive therapy may include efforts to restore body temperature, respiratory and circulatory support as indicated, and management of electrolyte-fluid-acid-base abnormalities. Renal failure may appear later, and urine flow should be monitored and sustained if possible.

Perioperative Hyperkalemia
Use of inhaled anesthetic agents has been associated with rare increases in serum potassium levels that have resulted in cardiac arrhythmias and death in pediatric patients during the postoperative period. Patients with latent as well as overt neuromuscular disease, particularly Duchenne muscular dystrophy, appear to be most vulnerable. Concomitant use of succinylcholine has been associated with most, but not all, of these cases. These patients also experienced significant elevations in serum creatine kinase levels and, in some cases, changes in urine consistent with myoglobinuria. Despite the similarity in presentation to malignant hyperthermia, none of these patients exhibited signs or symptoms of muscle rigidity or hypermetabolic state. Early and aggressive intervention to treat the hyperkalemia and resistant arrhythmias is recommended; as is subsequent evaluation for latent neuromuscular disease.

PRECAUTIONS
During the maintenance of anesthesia, increasing the concentration of sevoflurane produces dose-dependent decreases in blood pressure. Due to sevoflurane's insolubility in blood, these hemodynamic changes may occur more rapidly than with other volatile anesthetics. Excessive decreases in blood pressure or respiratory depression may be related to depth of anesthesia and may be corrected by decreasing the inspired concentration of sevoflurane.

Rare cases of seizures have been reported in association with sevoflurane use (see **PRECAUTIONS – Pediatric Use** and **ADVERSE REACTIONS**).

The recovery from general anesthesia should be assessed carefully before a patient is discharged from the post-anesthesia care unit.

Drug Interactions
In clinical trials, no significant adverse reactions occurred with other drugs commonly used in the perioperative period, including: central nervous system depressants, autonomic drugs, skeletal muscle relaxants, anti-infective agents, hormones and synthetic substitutes, blood derivatives, and cardiovascular drugs.

Intravenous Anesthetics
Sevoflurane administration is compatible with barbiturates, propofol, and other commonly used intravenous anesthetics.

Benzodiazepines and Opioids
Benzodiazepines and opioids would be expected to decrease the MAC of sevoflurane in the same manner as with other inhalational anesthetics. Sevoflurane administration is compatible with benzodiazepines and opioids as commonly used in surgical practice.

Nitrous Oxide
As with other halogenated volatile anesthetics, the anesthetic requirement for sevoflurane is decreased when administered in combination with nitrous oxide. Using 50%

N_2O, the MAC equivalent dose requirement is reduced approximately 50% in adults, and approximately 25% in pediatric patients (see **DOSAGE AND ADMINISTRATION**).

Neuromuscular Blocking Agents
As is the case with other volatile anesthetics, sevoflurane increases both the intensity and duration of neuromuscular blockade induced by nondepolarizing muscle relaxants. When used to supplement alfentanil-N_2O anesthesia, sevoflurane and isoflurane equally potentiate neuromuscular block induced with pancuronium, vecuronium or atracurium. Therefore, during sevoflurane anesthesia, the dosage adjustments for these muscle relaxants are similar to those required with isoflurane.

Potentiation of neuromuscular blocking agents requires equilibration of muscle with delivered partial pressure of sevoflurane. Reduced doses of neuromuscular blocking agents during induction of anesthesia may result in delayed onset of conditions suitable for endotracheal intubation or inadequate muscle relaxation.

Among available nondepolarizing agents, only vecuronium, pancuronium and atracurium interactions have been studied during sevoflurane anesthesia. In the absence of specific guidelines:
1. For endotracheal intubation, do not reduce the dose of nondepolarizing muscle relaxants.
2. During maintenance of anesthesia, the required dose of nondepolarizing muscle relaxants is likely to be reduced compared to that during N_2O/opioid anesthesia. Administration of supplemental doses of muscle relaxants should be guided by the response to nerve stimulation.

The effect of sevoflurane on the duration of depolarizing neuromuscular blockade induced by succinylcholine has not been studied.

Hepatic Function
Results of evaluations of laboratory parameters (e.g., ALT, AST, alkaline phosphatase, and total bilirubin, etc.), as well as investigator-reported incidence of adverse events relating to liver function, demonstrate that sevoflurane can be administered to patients with normal or mild-to-moderately impaired hepatic function. However, patients with severe hepatic dysfunction were not investigated.

Occasional cases of transient changes in postoperative hepatic function tests were reported with both sevoflurane and reference agents. Sevoflurane was found to be comparable to isoflurane with regard to these changes in hepatic function.

Very rare cases of mild, moderate and severe post-operative hepatic dysfunction or hepatitis with or without jaundice have been reported from postmarketing experiences. Clinical judgement should be exercised when sevoflurane is used in patients with underlying hepatic conditions or under treatment with drugs known to cause hepatic dysfunction (see **ADVERSE REACTIONS**).

It has been reported that previous exposure to halogenated hydrocarbon anesthetics may increase the potential for hepatic injury.

Desiccated CO_2 Absorbents
An exothermic reaction occurs when sevoflurane is exposed to CO_2 absorbents. This reaction is increased when the CO_2 absorbent becomes desiccated, such as after an extended period of dry gas flow through the CO_2 absorbent canisters. Rare cases of extreme heat, smoke, and/or spontaneous fire in the anesthesia breathing circuit have been reported during sevoflurane use in conjunction with the use of desiccated CO_2 absorbent, specifically those containing potassium hydroxide (e.g. Baralyme). KOH containing CO_2 absorbents are not recommended for use with sevoflurane. An unusually delayed rise or unexpected decline of inspired sevoflurane concentration compared to the vaporizer setting may be associated with excessive heating of the CO_2 absorbent and chemical breakdown of sevoflurane.

As with other inhalational anesthetics, degradation and production of degradation products can occur when sevoflurane is exposed to desiccated absorbents. When a clinician suspects that the CO_2 absorbent may be desiccated, it should be replaced. The color indicator of most CO_2 absorbents may not change upon desiccation. Therefore, the lack of significant color change should not be taken as an assurance of adequate hydration. CO_2 absorbents should be replaced routinely regardless of the state of the color indicator.

Carcinogenesis, Mutagenesis, Impairment of Fertility
Studies on carcinogenesis have not been performed for either sevoflurane or Compound A. No mutagenic effect of sevoflurane was noted in the Ames test, mouse micronucleus test, mouse lymphoma mutagenicity assay, human lymphocyte culture assay, mammalian cell transformation assay, ^{32}P DNA adduct assay, and no chromosomal aberrations were induced in cultured mammalian cells.

Similarly, no mutagenic effect of Compound A was noted in the Ames test, the Chinese hamster chromosomal aberration assay and the *in vivo* mouse micronucleus assay. However, positive responses were observed in the human lymphocyte chromosome aberration assay. These responses were seen only at high concentrations and in the absence of metabolic activation (human S-9).

Pregnancy Category B
Reproduction studies have been performed in rats and rabbits at doses up to 1 MAC (minimum alveolar concentration) without CO_2 absorbent and have revealed no evidence of impaired fertility or harm to the fetus due to sevoflurane at 0.3 MAC, the highest nontoxic dose. Developmental and reproductive toxicity studies of sevoflurane in animals in the presence of strong alkalies (i.e., degradation of sevoflurane and production of Compound A) have not been conducted. There are no adequate and well-controlled studies in pregnant women. Because animal reproduction studies are not always predictive of human response, sevoflurane should be used during pregnancy only if clearly needed.

Labor and Delivery
Sevoflurane has been used as part of general anesthesia for elective cesarean section in 29 women. There were no untoward effects in mother or neonate (see **PHARMACODYNAMICS - Clinical Trials**). The safety of sevoflurane in labor and delivery has not been demonstrated.

Nursing Mothers
The concentrations of sevoflurane in milk are probably of no clinical importance 24 hours after anesthesia. Because of rapid washout, sevoflurane concentrations in milk are predicted to be below those found with many other volatile anesthetics.

Geriatric Use
MAC decreases with increasing age. The average concentration of sevoflurane to achieve MAC in an 80 year old is approximately 50% of that required in a 20 year old.

Pediatric Use
Induction and maintenance of general anesthesia with sevoflurane have been established in controlled clinical trials in pediatric patients aged 1 to 18 years (see **PHARMACODYNAMICS - Clinical Trials** and **ADVERSE REACTIONS**). Sevoflurane has a nonpungent odor and is suitable for mask induction in pediatric patients.

The concentration of sevoflurane required for maintenance of general anesthesia is age dependent. When used in combination with nitrous oxide, the MAC equivalent dose of sevoflurane should be reduced in pediatric patients. MAC in premature infants has not been determined (see **PRECAUTIONS - Drug Interactions** and **DOSAGE AND ADMINISTRATION** for recommendations in pediatric patients 1 day of age and older).

The use of sevoflurane has been associated with seizures (see **PRECAUTIONS** and **ADVERSE REACTIONS**). The majority of these have occurred in children and young adults starting from 2 months of age, most of whom had no predisposing risk factors. Clinical judgement should be exercised when using sevoflurane in patients who may be at risk for seizures.

ADVERSE REACTIONS
Adverse events are derived from controlled clinical trials conducted in the United States, Canada, and Europe. The reference drugs were isoflurane, enflurane, and propofol in adults and halothane in pediatric patients. The studies were conducted using a variety of premedications, other anesthetics, and surgical procedures of varying length. Most adverse events reported were mild and transient, and may reflect the surgical procedures, patient characteristics (including disease) and/or medications administered.

Of the 5182 patients enrolled in the clinical trials, 2906 were exposed to sevoflurane, including 118 adults and 507 pediatric patients who underwent mask induction. Each patient was counted once for each type of adverse event. Adverse events reported in clinical trials and considered to be possibly or probably related to sevoflurane are presented within each body system in order of decreasing frequency in the following listings. One case of malignant hyperthermia was reported in pre-registration clinical trials.

Adverse Events During the Induction Period (from Onset of Anesthesia by Mask Induction to Surgical Incision) Incidence >1%
Adult Patients (N = 118)
Cardiovascular
Bradycardia 5%, Hypotension 4%, Tachycardia 2%
Nervous System
Agitation 7%
Respiratory System
Laryngospasm 8%, Airway obstruction 8%, Breathholding 5%, Cough Increased 5%
Pediatric Patients (N = 507)
Cardiovascular
Tachycardia 6%, Hypotension 4%
Nervous System
Agitation 15%
Respiratory System
Breathholding 5%, Cough Increased 5%, Laryngospasm 3%, Apnea 2%

Digestive System
Increased salivation 2%
Adverse Events During Maintenance and Emergence Periods, Incidence >1% (N = 2906)
Body as a whole
Fever 1%, Shivering 6%, Hypothermia 1%, Movement 1%, Headache 1%
Cardiovascular
Hypotension 11%, Hypertension 2%, Bradycardia 5%, Tachycardia 2%
Nervous System
Somnolence 9%, Agitation 9%, Dizziness 4%, Increased salivation 4%
Digestive System
Nausea 25%, Vomiting 18%
Respiratory System
Cough increased 11%, Breathholding 2%, Laryngospasm 2%
Adverse Events, All Patients in Clinical Trials (N = 2906), All Anesthetic Periods, Incidence <1% (Reported in 3 or More Patients)
Body as a whole
Asthenia, Pain
Cardiovascular
Arrhythmia, Ventricular Extrasystoles, Supraventricular Extrasystoles, Complete AV Block, Bigeminy, Hemorrhage, Inverted T Wave, Atrial Fibrillation, Atrial Arrhythmia, Second Degree AV Block, Syncope, S-T Depressed
Nervous System
Crying, Nervousness, Confusion, Hypertonia, Dry Mouth, Insomnia
Respiratory System
Sputum Increased, Apnea, Hypoxia, Wheezing, Bronchospasm, Hyperventilation, Pharyngitis, Hiccup, Hypoventilation, Dyspnea, Stridor
Metabolism and Nutrition
Increases in LDH, AST, ALT, BUN, Alkaline Phosphatase, Creatinine, Bilirubinemia, Glycosuria, Fluorosis, Albuminuria, Hypophosphatemia, Acidosis, Hyperglycemia
Hemic and Lymphatic System
Leucocytosis, Thrombocytopenia
Skin and Special Senses
Amblyopia, Pruritus, Taste Perversion, Rash, Conjunctivitis
Urogenital
Urination Impaired, Urine Abnormality, Urinary Retention, Oliguria
See **WARNINGS** for information regarding malignant hyperthermia.

Post-Marketing Adverse Events
The following adverse events have been identified during post-approval use of Ultane (sevoflurane USP). Due to the spontaneous nature of these reports, the actual incidence and relationship of Ultane to these events cannot be established with certainty.
CNS
Seizures - Post-marketing reports indicate that sevoflurane use has been associated with seizures. The majority of cases were in children and young adults, most of whom had no medical history of seizures. Several cases reported no concomitant medications, and at least one case was confirmed by EEG. Although many cases were single seizures that resolved spontaneously or after treatment, cases of multiple seizures have also been reported. Seizures have occurred during, or soon after sevoflurane induction, during emergence, and during post-operative recovery up to a day following anesthesia.
Cardiac
Cardiac arrest
Hepatic
• Cases of mild, moderate and severe post-operative hepatic dysfunction or hepatitis with or without jaundice have been reported. Histological evidence was not provided for any of the reported hepatitis cases. In most of these cases, patients had underlying hepatic conditions or were under treatment with drugs known to cause hepatic dysfunction. Most of the reported events were transient and resolved spontaneously (see **PRECAUTIONS**).
• Hepatic necrosis
• Hepatic failure
Other
• Malignant hyperthermia (see **CONTRAINDICATIONS** and **WARNINGS**)
• Allergic reactions, such as rash, urticaria, pruritus, bronchospasm, anaphylactic or anaphylactoid reactions (see **CONTRAINDICATIONS**)
• Reports of hypersensitivity (including contact dermatitis, rash, dyspnea, wheezing, chest discomfort, swelling face, or anaphylactic reaction) have been received, particularly in association with long-term occupational exposure to inhaled anesthetic agents, including sevoflurane (see **OCCUPATIONAL CAUTION**).
Laboratory Findings
• Transient elevations in glucose, liver function tests, and white blood cell count may occur as with use of other anesthetic agents.

OVERDOSAGE
In the event of overdosage, or what may appear to be overdosage, the following action should be taken: discontinue administration of sevoflurane, maintain a patent airway, initiate assisted or controlled ventilation with oxygen, and maintain adequate cardiovascular function.

DOSAGE AND ADMINISTRATION
The concentration of sevoflurane being delivered from a vaporizer during anesthesia should be known. This may be accomplished by using a vaporizer calibrated specifically for sevoflurane. The administration of general anesthesia must be individualized based on the patient's response.

Replacement of Desiccated CO_2 Absorbents
When a clinician suspects that the CO_2 absorbent may be desiccated, it should be replaced. The exothermic reaction that occurs with sevoflurane and CO_2 absorbents is increased when the CO_2 absorbent becomes desiccated, such as after an extended period of dry gas flow through the CO_2 absorbent canisters (see **PRECAUTIONS**).

Pre-anesthetic Medication
No specific premedication is either indicated or contraindicated with sevoflurane. The decision as to whether or not to premedicate and the choice of premedication is left to the discretion of the anesthesiologist.

Induction
Sevoflurane has a nonpungent odor and does not cause respiratory irritability; it is suitable for mask induction in pediatrics and adults.

Maintenance
Surgical levels of anesthesia can usually be achieved with concentrations of 0.5 - 3% sevoflurane with or without the concomitant use of nitrous oxide. Sevoflurane can be administered with any type of anesthesia circuit.

Table 9. MAC Values for Adults and Pediatric Patients According to Age

Age of Patient (years)	Sevoflurane in Oxygen	Sevoflurane in 65% N_2O/35% O_2
0 - 1 months #	3.3%	
1 - < 6 months	3.0%	
6 months - < 3 years	2.8%	2.0%[@]
3 - 12	2.5%	
25	2.6%	1.4%
40	2.1%	1.1%
60	1.7%	0.9%
80	1.4%	0.7%

Neonates are full-term gestational age. MAC in premature infants has not been determined.
[@] In 1 - < 3 year old pediatric patients, 60% N_2O/40% O_2 was used.

HOW SUPPLIED
ULTANE (sevoflurane), Volatile Liquid for Inhalation, is packaged in amber colored bottles containing 250 mL sevoflurane, List 4456, NDC # 0074-4456-04 (plastic).
SAFETY AND HANDLING
Occupational Caution
There is no specific work exposure limit established for sevoflurane. However, the National Institute for Occupational Safety and Health has recommended an 8 hour time-weighted average limit of 2 ppm for halogenated anesthetic agents in general (0.5 ppm when coupled with exposure to N_2O) (see **ADVERSE REACTIONS**).
Storage
Store at controlled room temperature, 15° - 30°C (59° - 86°F). See USP.

Product of Japan

Product inquiries should be directed to AbbVie Inc., North Chicago, IL 60064, USA
Manufactured by:
AbbVie Inc., North Chicago, IL 60064, USA under license from Maruishi Pharmaceutical Company LTD. 2-3-5, Fushimi-machi, Chuo-Ku, Osaka, Japan.
©AbbVie Inc. 2014
Ref. 03-A903-R7-Rev. March, 2014
Shown in Product Identification Guide, page 304

Information on the AbbVie, Inc. products listed on these pages is from the prescribing information in use as of July 31, 2014. For more information, please visit rxabbvie.com or call 1-800-633-9110.

VICODIN®
VICODIN ES®
VICODIN HP®

(hydrocodone bitartrate and acetaminophen)
Tablets, USP

Ⅲ Ŗ

WARNING

> **HEPATOTOXICITY**
> ACETAMINOPHEN HAS BEEN ASSOCIATED WITH CASES OF ACUTE LIVER FAILURE, AT TIMES RESULTING IN LIVER TRANSPLANT AND DEATH. MOST OF THE CASES OF LIVER INJURY ARE ASSOCIATED WITH THE USE OF ACETAMINOPHEN AT DOSES THAT EXCEED 4000 MILLIGRAMS PER DAY, AND OFTEN INVOLVE MORE THAN ONE ACETAMINOPHEN-CONTAINING PRODUCT.

DESCRIPTION

Hydrocodone bitartrate and acetaminophen is supplied in tablet form for oral administration.

WARNING: May be habit-forming (see **PRECAUTIONS, Information for Patients/Caregivers,** and **DRUG ABUSE AND DEPENDENCE**).

Hydrocodone bitartrate is an opioid analgesic and antitussive and occurs as fine, white crystals or as a crystalline powder. It is affected by light. The chemical name is $4,5\alpha$-epoxy-3-methoxy-17-methylmorphinan-6-one tartrate (1:1) hydrate (2:5). It has the following structural formula:

$C_{18}H_{21}NO_3 \cdot C_4H_6O_6 \cdot 2\frac{1}{2}H_2O$ M.W. = 494.490

Acetaminophen, 4'-hydroxyacetanilide, a slightly bitter, white, odorless, crystalline powder, is a non-opiate, non-salicylate analgesic and antipyretic. It has the following structural formula:

$C_8H_9NO_2$ M.W. = 151.16

Hydrocodone Bitartrate and Acetaminophen Tablets, USP is available in the following strengths:

VICODIN®: Hydrocodone Bitartrate............. 5 mg
WARNING: May be habit-forming.
Acetaminophen................................ 300 mg
VICODIN ES®: Hydrocodone Bitartrate....... 7.5 mg
WARNING: May be habit-forming.
Acetaminophen................................ 300 mg
VICODIN HP®: Hydrocodone Bitartrate...... 10 mg
WARNING: May be habit-forming.
Acetaminophen................................ 300 mg

In addition each tablet contains the following inactive ingredients: colloidal silicon dioxide, crospovidone, magnesium stearate, microcrystalline cellulose, povidone, pregelatinized starch, and stearic acid.

This product complies with USP dissolution test 2.

CLINICAL PHARMACOLOGY

Hydrocodone is a semisynthetic narcotic analgesic and antitussive with multiple actions qualitatively similar to those of codeine. Most of these involve the central nervous system and smooth muscle. The precise mechanism of action of hydrocodone and other opiates is not known, although it is believed to relate to the existence of opiate receptors in the central nervous system. In addition to analgesia, narcotics may produce drowsiness, changes in mood and mental clouding.

The analgesic action of acetaminophen involves peripheral influences, but the specific mechanism is as yet undetermined. Antipyretic activity is mediated through hypothalamic heat regulating centers. Acetaminophen inhibits prostaglandin synthetase. Therapeutic doses of acetaminophen have negligible effects on the cardiovascular or respiratory systems; however, toxic doses may cause circulatory failure and rapid, shallow breathing.

Pharmacokinetics

The behavior of the individual components is described below.

Hydrocodone

Following a 10 mg oral dose of hydrocodone administered to five adult male subjects, the mean peak concentration was 23.6 ± 5.2 ng/mL. Maximum serum levels were achieved at 1.3 ± 0.3 hours and the half-life was determined to be 3.8 ± 0.3 hours. Hydrocodone exhibits a complex pattern of metabolism including O-demethylation, N-demethylation and 6-keto reduction to the corresponding 6-α- and 6-β-hydroxy- metabolites. See **OVERDOSAGE** for toxicity information.

Acetaminophen

Acetaminophen is rapidly absorbed from the gastrointestinal tract and is distributed throughout most body tissues. The plasma half-life is 1.25 to 3 hours, but may be increased by liver damage and following overdosage. Elimination of acetaminophen is principally by liver metabolism (conjugation) and subsequent renal excretion of metabolites. Approximately 85% of an oral dose appears in the urine within 24 hours of administration, most as the glucuronide conjugate, with small amounts of other conjugates and unchanged drug. See **OVERDOSAGE** for toxicity information.

INDICATIONS AND USAGE

Hydrocodone bitartrate and acetaminophen tablets are indicated for the relief of moderate to moderately severe pain.

CONTRAINDICATIONS

This product should not be administered to patients who have previously exhibited hypersensitivity to hydrocodone or acetaminophen.

Patients known to be hypersensitive to other opioids may exhibit cross sensitivity to hydrocodone.

WARNINGS

Hepatotoxicity

Acetaminophen has been associated with cases of acute liver failure, at times resulting in liver transplant and death. Most of the cases of liver injury are associated with the use of acetaminophen at doses that exceed 4000 milligrams per day, and often involve more than one acetaminophen-containing product. The excessive intake of acetaminophen may be intentional to cause self-harm or unintentional as patients attempt to obtain more pain relief or unknowingly take other acetaminophen-containing products.

The risk of acute liver failure is higher in individuals with underlying liver disease and in individuals who ingest alcohol while taking acetaminophen.

Instruct patients to look for acetaminophen or APAP on package labels and not to use more than one product that contains acetaminophen. Instruct patients to seek medical attention immediately upon ingestion of more than 4000 milligrams of acetaminophen per day, even if they feel well.

Serious skin reactions

Rarely, acetaminophen may cause serious skin reactions such as acute generalized exanthematous pustulosis (AGEP), Stevens-Johnson Syndrome (SJS), and toxic epidermal necrolysis (TEN), which can be fatal. Patients should be informed about the signs of serious skin reactions, and use of the drug should be discontinued at the first appearance of skin rash or any other sign of hypersensitivity.

Hypersensitivity/anaphylaxis

There have been post-marketing reports of hypersensitivity and anaphylaxis associated with use of acetaminophen. Clinical signs included swelling of the face, mouth and throat, respiratory distress, urticaria, rash, pruritus, and vomiting. There were infrequent reports of life-threatening anaphylaxis requiring emergency medical attention. Instruct patients to discontinue hydrocodone bitartrate and acetaminophen tablets immediately and seek medical care if they experience these symptoms. Do not prescribe hydrocodone bitartrate and acetaminophen tablets for patients with acetaminophen allergy.

Respiratory Depression

At high doses or in sensitive patients, hydrocodone may produce dose-related respiratory depression by acting directly on the brain stem respiratory center. Hydrocodone also affects the center that controls respiratory rhythm, and may produce irregular and periodic breathing.

Head Injury and Increased Intracranial Pressure

The respiratory depressant effects of narcotics and their capacity to elevate cerebrospinal fluid pressure may be markedly exaggerated in the presence of head injury, other intracranial lesions or a preexisting increase in intracranial pressure. Furthermore, narcotics produce adverse reactions which may obscure the clinical course of patients with head injuries.

Acute Abdominal Conditions

The administration of narcotics may obscure the diagnosis or clinical course of patients with acute abdominal conditions.

PRECAUTIONS

General

Special Risk Patients

As with any narcotic analgesic agent, hydrocodone bitartrate and acetaminophen tablets should be used with caution in elderly or debilitated patients and those with severe impairment of hepatic or renal function, hypothyroidism, Addison's disease, prostatic hypertrophy or urethral stricture. The usual precautions should be observed and the possibility of respiratory depression should be kept in mind.

Cough Reflex

Hydrocodone suppresses the cough reflex; as with all narcotics, caution should be exercised when hydrocodone bitartrate and acetaminophen tablets are used postoperatively and in patients with pulmonary disease.

Information for Patients/Caregivers

• Do not take hydrocodone bitartrate and acetaminophen tablets if you are allergic to any of its ingredients.

• If you develop signs of allergy such as a rash or difficulty breathing stop taking hydrocodone bitartrate and acetaminophen tablets and contact your healthcare provider immediately.

• Do not take more than 4000 milligrams of acetaminophen per day. Call your doctor if you took more than the recommended dose.

Hydrocodone, like all narcotics, may impair the mental and/or physical abilities required for the performance of potentially hazardous tasks such as driving a car or operating machinery; patients should be cautioned accordingly.

Alcohol and other CNS depressants may produce an additive CNS depression, when taken with this combination product, and should be avoided.

Hydrocodone may be habit forming. Patients should take the drug only for as long as it is prescribed, in the amounts prescribed, and no more frequently than prescribed.

Laboratory Tests

In patients with severe hepatic or renal disease, effects of therapy should be monitored with serial liver and/or renal function tests.

Drug Interactions

Patients receiving other narcotics, antihistamines, antipsychotics, antianxiety agents, or other CNS depressants (including alcohol) concomitantly with hydrocodone bitartrate and acetaminophen tablets may exhibit an additive CNS depression. When combined therapy is contemplated, the dose of one or both agents should be reduced.

The use of MAO inhibitors or tricyclic antidepressants with hydrocodone preparations may increase the effect of either the antidepressant or hydrocodone.

Drug/Laboratory Test Interactions

Acetaminophen may produce false-positive test results for urinary 5-hydroxyindoleacetic acid.

Carcinogenesis, Mutagenesis, Impairment of Fertility

No adequate studies have been conducted in animals to determine whether hydrocodone or acetaminophen have a potential for carcinogenesis, mutagenesis, or impairment of fertility.

Pregnancy

Teratogenic Effects

Pregnancy Category C

There are no adequate and well-controlled studies in pregnant women. Hydrocodone bitartrate and acetaminophen tablets should be used during pregnancy only if the potential benefit justifies the potential risk to the fetus.

Nonteratogenic Effects

Babies born to mothers who have been taking opioids regularly prior to delivery will be physically dependent. The withdrawal signs include irritability and excessive crying, tremors, hyperactive reflexes, increased respiratory rate, increased stools, sneezing, yawning, vomiting, and fever. The intensity of the syndrome does not always correlate with the duration of maternal opioid use or dose. There is no consensus on the best method of managing withdrawal.

Labor and Delivery

As with all narcotics, administration of this product to the mother shortly before delivery may result in some degree of respiratory depression in the newborn, especially if higher doses are used.

Nursing Mothers

Acetaminophen is excreted in breast milk in small amounts, but the significance of its effects on nursing infants is not known. It is not known whether hydrocodone is excreted in human milk. Because many drugs are excreted in human milk and because of the potential for serious adverse reactions in nursing infants from hydrocodone and acetaminophen, a decision should be made whether to discontinue nursing or to discontinue the drug, taking into account the importance of the drug to the mother.

Pediatric Use

Safety and effectiveness in pediatric patients have not been established.

Geriatric Use

Clinical studies of hydrocodone bitartrate and acetaminophen tablets did not include sufficient numbers of subjects aged 65 and over to determine whether they respond differently from younger subjects. Other reported clinical experience has not identified differences in responses between the elderly and younger patients. In general, dose selection for an elderly patient should be cautious, usually starting at the low end of the dosing range, reflecting the greater frequency of decreased hepatic, renal, or cardiac function, and of concomitant disease or other drug therapy.

Hydrocodone and the major metabolites of acetaminophen are known to be substantially excreted by the kidney. Thus the risk of toxic reactions may be greater in patients with impaired renal function due to accumulation of the parent compound and/or metabolites in the plasma. Because elderly patients are more likely to have decreased renal function, care should be taken in dose selection, and it may be useful to monitor renal function.

Hydrocodone may cause confusion and over-sedation in the elderly; elderly patients generally should be started on low doses of hydrocodone bitartrate and acetaminophen tablets and observed closely.

ADVERSE REACTIONS

The most frequently reported adverse reactions are lightheadedness, dizziness, sedation, nausea and vomiting. These effects seem to be more prominent in ambulatory than in nonambulatory patients, and some of these adverse reactions may be alleviated if the patient lies down.
Other adverse reactions include:

Central Nervous System
Drowsiness, mental clouding, lethargy, impairment of mental and physical performance, anxiety, fear, dysphoria, psychic dependence, mood changes.

Gastrointestinal System
Prolonged administration of hydrocodone bitartrate and acetaminophen tablets may produce constipation.

Genitourinary System
Ureteral spasm, spasm of vesical sphincters and urinary retention have been reported with opiates.

Respiratory Depression
Hydrocodone bitartrate may produce dose-related respiratory depression by acting directly on the brain stem respiratory centers (see **OVERDOSAGE**).

Special Senses
Cases of hearing impairment or permanent loss have been reported predominantly in patients with chronic overdose.

Dermatological
Skin rash, pruritus.
The following adverse drug events may be borne in mind as potential effects of acetaminophen: allergic reactions, rash, thrombocytopenia, agranulocytosis, Stevens-Johnson syndrome, toxic epidermal necrolysis.
Potential effects of high dosage are listed in the **OVERDOSAGE** section.

DRUG ABUSE AND DEPENDENCE

Controlled Substance
Hydrocone bitartrate and acetaminophen tablets is classified as a Schedule III controlled substance.

Abuse and Dependence
Psychic dependence, physical dependence, and tolerance may develop upon repeated administration of narcotics; therefore, this product should be prescribed and administered with caution. However, psychic dependence is unlikely to develop when hydrocodone bitartrate and acetaminophen tablets are used for a short time for the treatment of pain. Physical dependence, the condition in which continued administration of the drug is required to prevent the appearance of a withdrawal syndrome, assumes clinically significant proportions only after several weeks of continued narcotic use, although some mild degree of physical dependence may develop after a few days of narcotic therapy. Tolerance, in which increasingly large doses are required in order to produce the same degree of analgesia, is manifested initially by a shortened duration of analgesic effect, and subsequently by decreases in the intensity of analgesia. The rate of development of tolerance varies among patients.

OVERDOSAGE

Following an acute overdosage, toxicity may result from hydrocodone or acetaminophen.

Signs and Symptoms
Hydrocodone: Serious overdose with hydrocodone is characterized by respiratory depression (a decrease in respiratory rate and/or tidal volume, Cheyne-Stokes respiration, cyanosis), extreme somnolence progressing to stupor or coma, skeletal muscle flaccidity, cold and clammy skin, and sometimes bradycardia and hypotension. In severe overdosage, apnea, circulatory collapse, cardiac arrest and death may occur.

Acetaminophen: In acetaminophen overdosage: dose-dependent, potentially fatal hepatic necrosis is the most serious adverse effect. Renal tubular necrosis, hypoglycemic coma, and coagulation defects may also occur.
Early symptoms following a potentially hepatotoxic overdose may include: nausea, vomiting, diaphoresis and general malaise. Clinical and laboratory evidence of hepatic toxicity may not be apparent until 48 to 72 hours post-ingestion.

Treatment
A single or multiple drug overdose with hydrocodone and acetaminophen is a potentially lethal polydrug overdose, and consultation with a regional poison control center is recommended.

Immediate treatment includes support of cardiorespiratory function and measures to reduce drug absorption.
Oxygen, intravenous fluids, vasopressors, and other supportive measures should be employed as indicated. Assisted or controlled ventilation should also be considered.

For hydrocodone overdose, primary attention should be given to the reestablishment of adequate respiratory exchange through provision of a patent airway and the institution of assisted or controlled ventilation. The narcotic antagonist naloxone hydrochloride is a specific antidote against respiratory depression which may result from overdosage or unusual sensitivity to narcotics, including hydrocodone. Since the duration of action of hydrocodone may exceed that of the antagonist, the patient should be kept under continued surveillance, and repeated doses of the antagonist should be administered as needed to maintain adequate respiration. A narcotic antagonist should not be administered in the absence of clinically significant respiratory or cardiovascular depression.

Gastric decontamination with activated charcoal should be administered just prior to N-acetylcysteine (NAC) to decrease systemic absorption if acetaminophen ingestion is known or suspected to have occurred within a few hours of presentation. Serum acetaminophen levels should be obtained immediately if the patient presents 4 hours or more after ingestion to assess potential risk of hepatotoxicity; acetaminophen levels drawn less than 4 hours post-ingestion may be misleading. To obtain the best possible outcome, NAC should be administered as soon as possible where impending or evolving liver injury is suspected. Intravenous NAC may be administered when circumstances preclude oral administration.

Vigorous supportive therapy is required in severe intoxication. Procedures to limit the continuing absorption of the drug must be readily performed since the hepatic injury is dose dependent and occurs early in the course of intoxication.

DOSAGE AND ADMINISTRATION

Dosage should be adjusted according to the severity of the pain and the response of the patient. However, it should be kept in mind that tolerance to hydrocodone can develop with continued use and that the incidence of untoward effects is dose related.

VICODIN® (Hydrocodone Bitartrate and Acetaminophen Tablets, USP 5 mg/300 mg): The usual adult dosage is one or two tablets every four to six hours as needed for pain. The total daily dosage should not exceed 8 tablets.

VICODIN ES® (Hydrocodone Bitartrate and Acetaminophen Tablets, USP 7.5 mg/300 mg): The usual adult dosage is one tablet every four to six hours as needed for pain. The total daily dosage should not exceed 6 tablets.

VICODIN HP® (Hydrocodone Bitartrate and Acetaminophen Tablets, USP 10 mg/300 mg): The usual adult dosage is one tablet every four to six hours as needed for pain. The total daily dosage should not exceed 6 tablets.

HOW SUPPLIED

VICODIN®, VICODIN ES® and VICODIN HP® (Hydrocodone Bitartrate and Acetaminophen) Tablets, USP are supplied as follows:

VICODIN® 5 mg/300 mg
White, capsule-shaped, bisected tablets, debossed "5" score "300"on one side and "VICODIN" on the other side in bottles of 100 and 500 tablets:
Bottles of 100 - NDC 0074-3041-13
Bottles of 500 - NDC 0074-3041-53

VICODIN ES® 7.5 mg/300 mg
White, capsule-shaped, bisected tablets, debossed "7.5" score "300" on one side and "VICODIN ES" on the other side in bottles of 100 and 500 tablets:
Bottles of 100 - NDC 0074-3043-13
Bottles of 500 - NDC 0074-3043-53

VICODIN HP® 10 mg/300 mg
White, capsule-shaped, bisected tablets, debossed "10" score "300" on one side and "VICODIN HP" on the other side in bottles of 100 and 500 tablets:
Bottles of 100 - NDC 0074-3054-13
Bottles of 500 - NDC 0074-3054-53

STORAGE

Store at 20° to 25°C (68° to 77°F). [See USP Controlled Room Temperature].
PHARMACIST: Dispense in a tight, light-resistant container with a child-resistant closure.
A Schedule III Narcotic
© AbbVie Inc. 2013
Manufactured for
AbbVie Inc.
North Chicago, IL 60064 U.S.A.

Manufactured by:
Mikart, Inc.
Atlanta, GA 30318
Ref. 1122F00 Rev.10/13 - Rev. October, 2013
Shown in Product Identification Guide, page 305

VICODIN® ℞
(hydrocodone bitartrate and acetaminophen tablets, USP)
5 mg/500 mg

BOXED WARNING

Hepatotoxicity
Acetaminophen has been associated with cases of acute liver failure, at times resulting in liver transplant and death. Most of the cases of liver injury are associated with the use of acetaminophen at doses that exceed 4000 milligrams per day, and often involve more than one acetaminophen-containing product.

DESCRIPTION

Hydrocodone bitartrate and acetaminophen is supplied in tablet form for oral administration.
Hydrocodone bitartrate is an opioid analgesic and antitussive and occurs as fine, white crystals or as a crystalline powder. It is affected by light. The chemical name is: 4,5α-epoxy-3-methoxy-17-methylmorphinan-6-one tartrate (1:1) hydrate (2:5). It has the following structural formula:

$C_{18}H_{21}NO_3 \cdot C_4H_6O_6 \cdot 2\frac{1}{2}H_2O$ M.W. 494.50

Acetaminophen, 4'-hydroxyacetanilide, a slightly bitter, white, odorless, crystalline powder, is a non-opiate, non-salicylate analgesic and antipyretic. It has the following structural formula:

$C_8H_9NO_2$ M.W. 151.16

Each VICODIN tablet contains:
Hydrocodone Bitartrate 5 mg
Acetaminophen 500 mg
In addition each tablet contains the following inactive ingredients: colloidal silicon dioxide, starch, croscarmellose sodium, dibasic calcium phosphate, magnesium stearate, microcrystalline cellulose, povidone, and stearic acid.
Meets USP Dissolution Test 2.

CLINICAL PHARMACOLOGY

Hydrocodone is a semisynthetic narcotic analgesic and antitussive with multiple actions qualitatively similar to those of codeine. Most of these involve the central nervous system and smooth muscle. The precise mechanism of action of hydrocodone and other opiates is not known, although it is believed to relate to the existence of opiate receptors in the central nervous system. In addition to analgesia, narcotics may produce drowsiness, changes in mood and mental clouding.

The analgesic action of acetaminophen involves peripheral influences, but the specific mechanism is as yet undetermined. Antipyretic activity is mediated through hypothalamic heat regulating centers. Acetaminophen inhibits prostaglandin synthetase. Therapeutic doses of acetaminophen have negligible effects on the cardiovascular or respiratory systems; however, toxic doses may cause circulatory failure and rapid, shallow breathing.

Pharmacokinetics
The behavior of the individual components is described below.
Hydrocodone
Following a 10 mg oral dose of hydrocodone administered to five adult male subjects, the mean peak concentration was

Information on the AbbVie, Inc. products listed on these pages is from the prescribing information in use as of July 31, 2014. For more information, please visit rxabbvie.com or call 1-800-633-9110.

23.6 ± 5.2 ng/mL. Maximum serum levels were achieved at 1.3 ± 0.3 hours and the half-life was determined to be 3.8 ± 0.3 hours. Hydrocodone exhibits a complex pattern of metabolism including O-demethylation, N-demethylation and 6-keto reduction to the corresponding 6-α- and 6-β-hydroxymetabolites. See **OVERDOSAGE** for toxicity information.

Acetaminophen

Acetaminophen is rapidly absorbed from the gastrointestinal tract and is distributed throughout most body tissues. The plasma half-life is 1.25 to 3 hours, but may be increased by liver damage and following overdosage. Elimination of acetaminophen is principally by liver metabolism (conjugation) and subsequent renal excretion of metabolites. Approximately 85% of an oral dose appears in the urine within 24 hours of administration, most as the glucuronide conjugate, with small amounts of other conjugates and unchanged drug. See OVERDOSAGE for toxicity information.

INDICATIONS AND USAGE

VICODIN tablets are indicated for the relief of moderate to moderately severe pain.

CONTRAINDICATIONS

This product should not be administered to patients who have previously exhibited hypersensitivity to hydrocodone or acetaminophen.

Patients known to be hypersensitive to other opioids may exhibit cross-sensitivity to hydrocodone.

WARNINGS
Hepatotoxicity

Acetaminophen has been associated with cases of acute liver failure, at times resulting in liver transplant and death. Most of the cases of liver injury are associated with the use of acetaminophen at doses that exceed 4000 milligrams per day, and often involve more than one acetaminophen-containing product. The excessive intake of acetaminophen may be intentional to cause self-harm or unintentional as patients attempt to obtain more pain relief or unknowingly take other acetaminophen-containing products.

The risk of acute liver failure is higher in individuals with underlying liver disease and in individuals who ingest alcohol while taking acetaminophen.

Instruct patients to look for acetaminophen or APAP on package labels and not to use more than one product that contains acetaminophen. Instruct patients to seek medical attention immediately upon ingestion of more than 4000 milligrams of acetaminophen per day, even if they feel well.

Serious skin reactions

Rarely, acetaminophen may cause serious skin reactions such as acute generalized exanthematous pustulosis (AGEP), Stevens-Johnson Syndrome (SJS), and toxic epidermal necrolysis (TEN), which can be fatal. Patients should be informed about the signs of serious skin reactions, and use of the drug should be discontinued at the first appearance of skin rash or any other sign of hypersensitivity.

Hypersensitivity/anaphylaxis

There have been post-marketing reports of hypersensitivity and anaphylaxis associated with use of acetaminophen. Clinical signs included swelling of the face, mouth, and throat, respiratory distress, urticaria, rash, pruritis, and vomiting. There were infrequent reports of life-threatening anaphylaxis requiring emergency medical attention. Instruct patients to discontinue VICODIN Tablets immediately and seek medical care if they experience these symptoms. Do not prescribe VICODIN Tablets for patients with acetaminophen allergy.

Respiratory Depression

At high doses or in sensitive patients, hydrocodone may produce dose-related respiratory depression by acting directly on the brain stem respiratory center. Hydrocodone also affects the center that controls respiratory rhythm, and may produce irregular and periodic breathing.

Head Injury and Increased Intracranial Pressure

The respiratory depressant effects of narcotics and their capacity to elevate cerebrospinal fluid pressure may be markedly exaggerated in the presence of head injury, other intracranial lesions or a preexisting increase in intracranial pressure. Furthermore, narcotics produce adverse reactions which may obscure the clinical course of patients with head injuries.

Acute Abdominal Conditions

The administration of narcotics may obscure the diagnosis or clinical course of patients with acute abdominal conditions.

Misuse, Abuse, and Diversion of Opioids

VICODIN tablets contains hydrocodone an opioid agonist, and is a Schedule III controlled substance. Opioid agonists have the potential for being abused and are sought by abusers and people with addiction disorders, and are subject to diversion.

VICODIN tablets can be abused in a manner similar to other opioid agonists, legal or illicit. This should be consid-

ered when prescribing or dispensing VICODIN tablets in situations where the physician or pharmacist is concerned about an increased risk of misuse, abuse or diversion (see **DRUG ABUSE AND DEPENDENCE**).

PRECAUTIONS
General
Special Risk Patients

As with any narcotic analgesic agent, VICODIN Tablets should be used with caution in elderly or debilitated patients and those with severe impairment of hepatic or renal function, hypothyroidism, Addison's disease, prostatic hypertrophy or urethral stricture. The usual precautions should be observed and the possibility of respiratory depression should be kept in mind.

Cough Reflex

Hydrocodone suppresses the cough reflex; as with all narcotics, caution should be exercised when VICODIN Tablets are used postoperatively and in patients with pulmonary disease.

Information for Patients/Caregivers

• Do not take VICODIN Tablets if you are allergic to any of its ingredients.

• If you develop signs of allergy such as a rash or difficulty breathing stop taking VICODIN Tablets and contact your healthcare provider immediately.

• Do not take more than 4000 milligrams of acetaminophen per day. Call your doctor if you took more than the recommended dose.

Hydrocodone, like all narcotics, may impair the mental and/or physical abilities required for the performance of potentially hazardous tasks such as driving a car or operating machinery; patients should be cautioned accordingly. Alcohol and other CNS depressants may produce an additive CNS depression, when taken with this combination product, and should be avoided.

Hydrocodone may be habit forming. Patients should take the drug only for as long as it is prescribed, in the amounts prescribed, and no more frequently than prescribed.

Laboratory Tests

In patients with severe hepatic or renal disease, effects of therapy should be monitored with serial liver and/or renal function tests.

Drug Interactions

Patients receiving other narcotic analgesics, antihistamines, antipsychotics, antianxiety agents, or other CNS depressants (including alcohol) concomitantly with VICODIN Tablets may exhibit an additive CNS depression. When combined therapy is contemplated, the dose of one or both agents should be reduced.

The use of MAO inhibitors or tricyclic antidepressants with hydrocodone preparations may increase the effect of either the antidepressant or hydrocodone.

Drug/Laboratory Test Interactions

Acetaminophen may produce false-positive test results for urinary 5-hydroxyindoleacetic acid.

Carcinogenesis, Mutagenesis, Impairment of Fertility

No adequate studies have been conducted in animals to determine whether hydrocodone or acetaminophen have a potential for carcinogenesis, mutagenesis, or impairment of fertility.

Pregnancy
Teratogenic Effects
Pregnancy Category C

There are no adequate and well-controlled studies in pregnant women. VICODIN Tablets should be used during pregnancy only if the potential benefit justifies the potential risk to the fetus.

Nonteratogenic Effects

Babies born to mothers who have been taking opioids regularly prior to delivery will be physically dependent. The withdrawal signs include irritability and excessive crying, tremors, hyperactive reflexes, increased respiratory rate, increased stools, sneezing, yawning, vomiting, and fever. The intensity of the syndrome does not always correlate with the duration of maternal opioid use or dose. There is no consensus on the best method of managing withdrawal.

Labor and Delivery

As with all narcotics, administration of VICODIN Tablets to the mother shortly before delivery may result in some degree of respiratory depression in the newborn, especially if higher doses are used.

Nursing Mothers

Acetaminophen is excreted in breast milk in small amounts, but the significance of its effects on nursing infants is not known. It is not known whether hydrocodone is excreted in human milk. Because many drugs are excreted in human milk and because of the potential for serious adverse reactions in nursing infants from hydrocodone and acetaminophen, a decision should be made whether to discontinue nursing or to discontinue the drug, taking into account the importance of the drug to the mother.

Pediatric Use

Safety and effectiveness in the pediatric population have not been established.

Geriatric Use

Clinical studies of VICODIN (hydrocodone bitartrate 5 mg and acetaminophen 500 mg) did not include sufficient numbers of subjects aged 65 and over to determine whether they respond differently from younger subjects. Other reported clinical experience has not identified differences in responses between the elderly and younger patients. In general, dose selection for an elderly patient should be cautious, usually starting at the low end of the dosing range, reflecting the greater frequency of decreased hepatic, renal, or cardiac function, and of concomitant disease or other drug therapy.

Hydrocodone and the major metabolites of acetaminophen are known to be substantially excreted by the kidney. Thus the risk of toxic reactions may be greater in patients with impaired renal function due to accumulation of the parent compound and/or metabolites in the plasma. Because elderly patients are more likely to have decreased renal function, care should be taken in dose selection, and it may be useful to monitor renal function.

Hydrocodone may cause confusion and over-sedation in the elderly; elderly patients generally should be started on low doses of hydrocodone bitartrate and acetaminophen tablets and observed closely.

ADVERSE REACTIONS

The most frequently reported adverse reactions include: lightheadedness, dizziness, sedation, nausea and vomiting. These effects seem to be more prominent in ambulatory than in nonambulatory patients and some of these adverse reactions may be alleviated if the patient lies down.

Other adverse reactions include:

Central Nervous System

Drowsiness, mental clouding, lethargy, impairment of mental and physical performance, anxiety, fear, dysphoria, psychic dependence, mood changes.

Gastrointestinal System

Prolonged administration of VICODIN Tablets may produce constipation.

Genitourinary System

Ureteral spasm, spasm of vesical sphincters and urinary retention have been reported with opiates.

Respiratory Depression

Hydrocodone bitartrate may produce dose-related respiratory depression by acting directly on the brain stem respiratory center. (see **OVERDOSAGE**).

Special Senses

Cases of hearing impairment or permanent loss have been reported predominantly in patients with chronic overdose.

Dermatological

Skin rash, pruritus.

The following adverse drug events may be borne in mind as potential effects of acetaminophen: allergic reactions, rash, thrombocytopenia, agranulocytosis, Stevens-Johnson syndrome, toxic epidermal necrolysis.

Potential effects of high dosage are listed in the **OVERDOSAGE** section.

DRUG ABUSE AND DEPENDENCE
Misuse, Abuse, and Diversion of Opioids

VICODIN contains hydrocodone, an opioid agonist, and is a Schedule III controlled substance. VICODIN, and other opioids used in analgesia can be abused and are subject to criminal diversion.

Addiction is a primary, chronic, neurobiologic disease, with genetic, psychosocial, and environmental factors influencing its development and manifestations. It is characterized by behaviors that include one or more of the following: impaired control over drug use, compulsive use, continued use despite harm, and craving. Drug addiction is a treatable disease utilizing a multidisciplinary approach, but relapse is common.

"Drug seeking" behavior is very common in addicts and drug abusers. Drug-seeking tactics include emergency calls or visits near the end of office hours, refusal to undergo appropriate examination, testing or referral, repeated "loss" of prescriptions, tampering with prescriptions and reluctance to provide prior medical records or contact information for other treating physician(s). "Doctor shopping" to obtain additional prescriptions is common among drug abusers and people suffering from untreated addiction.

Abuse and addiction are separate and distinct from physical dependence and tolerance. Physical dependence usually assumes clinically significant dimensions only after several weeks of continued opioid use, although a mild degree of physical dependence may develop after a few days of opioid therapy. Tolerance, in which increasingly large doses are required in order to produce the same degree of analgesia, is manifested initially by a shortened duration of analgesic effect, and subsequently by decreases in the intensity of analgesia. The rate of development of tolerance varies among patients. Physicians should be aware that abuse of opioids can occur in the absence of true addiction and is characterized by misuse for non-medical purposes, often in combination with other psychoactive substances. VICODIN, like other opioids, may be diverted for non-medical use. Record-keeping of prescribing information, including quantity, frequency, and renewal requests is strongly advised.

Proper assessment of the patient, proper prescribing practices, periodic re-evaluation of therapy, and proper dispensing and storage are appropriate measures that help to limit abuse of opioid drugs.

OVERDOSAGE

Following an acute overdosage, toxicity may result from hydrocodone or acetaminophen.

Signs and Symptoms

Hydrocodone: Serious overdose with hydrocodone is characterized by respiratory depression (a decrease in respiratory rate and/or tidal volume, Cheyne-Stokes respiration, cyanosis), extreme somnolence progressing to stupor or coma, skeletal muscle flaccidity, cold and clammy skin, and sometimes bradycardia and hypotension. In severe overdosage, apnea, circulatory collapse, cardiac arrest and death may occur.

Acetaminophen: In acetaminophen overdosage: dose-dependent, potentially fatal hepatic necrosis is the most serious adverse effect. Renal tubular necrosis, hypoglycemic coma, and coagulation defects may also occur.

Early symptoms following a potentially hepatotoxic overdose may include: nausea, vomiting, diaphoresis and general malaise. Clinical and laboratory evidence of hepatic toxicity may not be apparent until 48 to 72 hours post-ingestion.

Treatment

A single or multiple drug overdose with hydrocodone and acetaminophen is a potentially lethal polydrug overdose, and consultation with a regional poison control center is recommended.

Immediate treatment includes support of cardiorespiratory function and measures to reduce drug absorption. Oxygen, intravenous fluids, vasopressors, and other supportive measures should be employed as indicated. Assisted or controlled ventilation should also be considered.

For hydrocodone overdose, primary attention should be given to the reestablishment of adequate respiratory exchange through provision of a patent airway and the institution of assisted or controlled ventilation. The narcotic antagonist naloxone hydrochloride is a specific antidote against respiratory depression which may result from overdosage or unusual sensitivity to narcotics, including hydrocodone. Since the duration of action of hydrocodone may exceed that of the antagonist, the patient should be kept under continued surveillance, and repeated doses of the antagonist should be administered as needed to maintain adequate respiration. A narcotic antagonist should not be administered in the absence of clinically significant respiratory or cardiovascular depression.

Gastric decontamination with activated charcoal should be administered just prior to N-acetylcysteine (NAC) to decrease systemic absorption if acetaminophen ingestion is known or suspected to have occurred within a few hours of presentation. Serum acetaminophen levels should be obtained immediately if the patient presents 4 hours or more after ingestion to assess potential risk of hepatotoxicity; acetaminophen levels drawn less than 4 hours post-ingestion may be misleading. To obtain the best possible outcome, NAC should be administered as soon as possible where impending or evolving liver injury is suspected. Intravenous NAC may be administered when circumstances preclude oral administration.

Vigorous supportive therapy is required in severe intoxication. Procedures to limit the continuing absorption of the drug must be readily performed since the hepatic injury is dose dependent and occurs early in the course of intoxication.

DOSAGE AND ADMINISTRATION

Dosage should be adjusted according to the severity of the pain and the response of the patient. However, it should be kept in mind that tolerance to hydrocodone can develop with continued use and that the incidence of untoward effects is dose related.

The usual adult dosage is one or two tablets every four to six hours as needed for pain. The total daily dosage should not exceed 8 tablets.

HOW SUPPLIED

VICODIN is supplied as white, capsule-shaped tablets containing 5 mg hydrocodone bitartrate and 500 mg acetaminophen, bisected on one side and debossed with "VICODIN" on the other.

Bottles of 100-NDC 0074-1949-14.
Bottles of 500-NDC 0074-1949-54.
Hospital Unit Dose Package-100 tablets (4 × 25 tablets)-NDC 0074-1949-12.

Storage

Store at 25°C (77°F); excursions permitted to 15°-30°C (59°-86°F). [See USP Controlled Room Temperature].

Dispense in a tight, light-resistant container as defined in the USP.

A Schedule ℃ controlled drug substance.
©AbbVie Inc. 2013
Manufactured for
AbbVie Inc.
North Chicago, IL 60064 U.S.A.
by Halo Pharmaceutical Inc.
Whippany, NJ 07981 U.S.A.
Ref. DN2846V2 - Rev. October, 2013
Shown in Product Identification Guide, page 304

VICODIN ES® ℃ ℞
(hydrocodone bitartrate and acetaminophen tablets, USP)
7.5 mg/750 mg

BOXED WARNING

Hepatotoxicity

Acetaminophen has been associated with cases of acute liver failure, at times resulting in liver transplant and death. Most of the cases of liver injury are associated with the use of acetaminophen at doses that exceed 4000 milligrams per day, and often involve more than one acetaminophen-containing product.

DESCRIPTION

Hydrocodone bitartrate and acetaminophen is supplied in tablet form for oral administration.

Hydrocodone bitartrate is an opioid analgesic and antitussive and occurs as fine, white crystals or as a crystalline powder. It is affected by light. The chemical name is: 4,5α-epoxy-3-methoxy-17-methylmorphinan-6-one tartrate (1:1) hydrate (2:5). It has the following structural formula:

$C_{18}H_{21}NO_3 \cdot C_4H_6O_6 \cdot 2\frac{1}{2}H_2O$ M.W. = 494.50

Acetaminophen, 4'-hydroxyacetanilide, a slightly bitter, white, odorless, crystalline powder, is a non-opiate, non-salicylate analgesic and antipyretic. It has the following structural formula:

$C_8H_9NO_2$ M.W.151.16

Each VICODIN ES Tablet contains:
Hydrocodone Bitartrate 7.5 mg
Acetaminophen 750 mg
In addition each tablet contains the following inactive ingredients: Colloidal silicon dioxide, pregelatinized starch, magnesium stearate, croscarmellose sodium povidone, and stearic acid.
Meets USP Dissolution Test 2.

CLINICAL PHARMACOLOGY

Hydrocodone is a semisynthetic narcotic analgesic and antitussive with multiple actions qualitatively similar to those of codeine. Most of these involve the central nervous system and smooth muscle. The precise mechanism of action of hydrocodone and other opiates is not known, although it is believed to relate to the existence of opiate receptors in the central nervous system. In addition to analgesia, narcotics may produce drowsiness, changes in mood and mental clouding.

The analgesic action of acetaminophen involves peripheral influences, but the specific mechanism is as yet undetermined. Antipyretic activity is mediated through hypothalamic heat regulating centers. Acetaminophen inhibits prostaglandin synthetase. Therapeutic doses of acetaminophen have negligible effects on the cardiovascular or respiratory systems; however, toxic doses may cause circulatory failure and rapid, shallow breathing.

Pharmacokinetics

The behavior of the individual components is described below.

Hydrocodone

Following a 10 mg oral dose of hydrocodone administered to five adult male subjects, the mean peak concentration was

23.6 ± 5.2 ng/mL. Maximum serum levels were achieved at 1.3 ± 0.3 hours and the half-life was determined to be 3.8 ± 0.3 hours. Hydrocodone exhibits a complex pattern of metabolism including O-demethylation, N-demethylation and 6-keto reduction to the corresponding 6-α and 6-β- hydroxy-metabolites. See **OVERDOSAGE** for toxicity information.

Acetaminophen

Acetaminophen is rapidly absorbed from the gastrointestinal tract and is distributed throughout most body tissues. The plasma half-life is 1.25 to 3 hours, but may be increased by liver damage and following hepatic necrosis. Elimination of acetaminophen is principally by liver metabolism (conjugation) and subsequent renal excretion of metabolites. Approximately 85% of an oral dose appears in the urine within 24 hours of administration, most as the glucuronide conjugate, with small amounts of other conjugates and unchanged drug. See **OVERDOSAGE** for toxicity information.

INDICATIONS AND USAGE

VICODIN ES Tablets are indicated for the relief of moderate to moderately severe pain.

CONTRAINDICATIONS

This product should not be administered to patients who have previously exhibited hypersensitivity to hydrocodone or acetaminophen.

Patients known to be hypersensitive to other opioids may exhibit cross-sensitivity to hydrocodone.

WARNINGS

Hepatotoxicity

Acetaminophen has been associated with cases of acute liver failure, at times resulting in liver transplant and death. Most of the cases of liver injury are associated with the use of acetaminophen at doses that exceed 4000 milligrams per day, and often involve more than one acetaminophen-containing product. The excessive intake of acetaminophen may be intentional to cause self-harm or unintentional as patients attempt to obtain more pain relief or unknowingly take other acetaminophen-containing products.

The risk of acute liver failure is higher in individuals with underlying liver disease and in individuals who ingest alcohol while taking acetaminophen.

Instruct patients to look for acetaminophen or APAP on package labels and not to use more than one product that contains acetaminophen. Instruct patients to seek medical attention immediately upon ingestion of more than 4000 milligrams of acetaminophen per day, even if they feel well.

Serious skin reactions

Rarely, acetaminophen may cause serious skin reactions such as acute generalized exanthematous pustulosis (AGEP), Stevens-Johnson Syndrome (SJS), and toxic epidermal necrolysis (TEN), which can be fatal. Patients should be informed about the signs of serious skin reactions, and use of the drug should be discontinued at the first appearance of skin rash or any other sign of hypersensitivity.

Hypersensitivity/anaphylaxis

There have been post-marketing reports of hypersensitivity and anaphylaxis associated with use of acetaminophen. Clinical signs included swelling of the face, mouth, and throat, respiratory distress, urticaria, rash, pruritis, and vomiting. There were infrequent reports of life-threatening anaphylaxis requiring emergency medical attention. Instruct patients to discontinue VICODIN ES Tablets immediately and seek medical care if they experience these symptoms. Do not prescribe VICODIN ES Tablets for patients with acetaminophen allergy.

Respiratory Depression

At high doses or in sensitive patients, hydrocodone may produce dose-related respiratory depression by acting directly on the brain stem respiratory center. Hydrocodone also affects the center that controls respiratory rhythm, and may produce irregular and periodic breathing.

Head Injury and Increased Intracranial Pressure

The respiratory depressant effects of narcotics and their capacity to elevate cerebrospinal fluid pressure may be markedly exaggerated in the presence of head injury, other intracranial lesions or a preexisting increase in intracranial pressure. Furthermore, narcotics produce adverse reactions, which may obscure the clinical course of patients with head injuries.

Acute Abdominal Conditions

The administration of narcotics may obscure the diagnosis or clinical course of patients with acute abdominal conditions.

Information on the AbbVie, Inc. products listed on these pages is from the prescribing information in use as of July 31, 2014. For more information, please visit rxabbvie.com or call 1-800-633-9110.

Misuse Abuse and Diversion of Opioids

VICODIN ES contains hydrocodone an opioid agonist, and is a Schedule III controlled substance. Opioid agonists have the potential for being abused and are sought by abusers and people with addiction disorders, and are subject to diversion.

VICODIN ES can be abused in a manner similar to other opioid agonists, legal or illicit. This should be considered when prescribing or dispensing VICODIN ES in situations where the physician or pharmacist is concerned about an increased risk of misuse, abuse or diversion (see **DRUG ABUSE AND DEPENDENCE**).

PRECAUTIONS
General
Special Risk Patients
As with any narcotic analgesic agent, VICODIN ES Tablets should be used with caution in elderly or debilitated patients and those with severe impairment of hepatic or renal function, hypothyroidism, Addison's disease, prostatic hypertrophy or urethral stricture. The usual precautions should be observed and the possibility of respiratory depression should be kept in mind.

Cough Reflex
Hydrocodone suppresses the cough reflex; as with all narcotics, caution should be exercised when VICODIN ES Tablets are used postoperatively and in patients with pulmonary disease.

Information for Patients/Caregivers
• Do not take VICODIN ES Tablets if you are allergic to any of its ingredients.
• If you develop signs of allergy such as a rash or difficulty breathing stop taking VICODIN ES Tablets and contact your healthcare provider immediately.
• Do not take more than 4000 milligrams of acetaminophen per day. Call your doctor if you took more than the recommended dose.

Hydrocodone, like all narcotics, may impair the mental and/or physical abilities required for the performance of potentially hazardous tasks such as driving a car or operating machinery; patients should be cautioned accordingly.
Alcohol and other CNS depressants may produce an additive CNS depression, when taken with this combination product, and should be avoided.
Hydrocodone may be habit forming. Patients should take the drug only for as long as it is prescribed, in the amounts prescribed, and no more frequently than prescribed.

Laboratory Tests
In patients with severe hepatic or renal disease, effects of therapy should be monitored with serial liver and/or renal function tests.

Drug Interactions
Patients receiving other narcotic analgesics, antihistamines, antipsychotics, antianxiety agents, or other CNS depressants (including alcohol) concomitantly with VICODIN ES Tablets may exhibit an additive CNS depression. When combined therapy is contemplated, the dose of one or both agents should be reduced.
The use of MAO inhibitors or tricyclic antidepressants with hydrocodone preparations may increase the effect of either the antidepressant or hydrocodone.

Drug/Laboratory Test Interactions
Acetaminophen may produce false-positive test results for urinary 5-hydroxyindoleacetic acid.

Carcinogenesis, Mutagenesis, Impairment of Fertility
No adequate studies have been conducted in animals to determine whether hydrocodone or acetaminophen have a potential for carcinogenesis, mutagenesis, or impairment of fertility.

Pregnancy
Teratogenic Effects
Pregnancy Category C
There are no adequate and well-controlled studies in pregnant women. VICODIN ES Tablets should be used during pregnancy only if the potential benefit justifies the potential risk to the fetus.
Nonteratogenic Effects
Babies born to mothers who have been taking opioids regularly prior to delivery will be physically dependent. The withdrawal signs include irritability and excessive crying, tremors, hyperactive reflexes, increased respiratory rate, increased stools, sneezing, yawning, vomiting, and fever. The intensity of the syndrome does not always correlate with the duration of maternal opioid use or dose. There is no consensus on the best method of managing withdrawal.

Labor and Delivery
As with all narcotics, administration of VICODIN ES Tablets to the mother shortly before delivery may result in some degree of respiratory depression in the newborn, especially if higher doses are used.

Nursing Mothers
Acetaminophen is excreted in breast milk in small amounts, but the significance of its effects on nursing infants is not known. It is not known whether hydrocodone is excreted in

human milk. Because many drugs are excreted in human milk and because of the potential for serious adverse reactions in nursing infants from hydrocodone and acetaminophen, a decision should be made whether to discontinue nursing or to discontinue the drug, taking into account the importance of the drug to the mother.

Pediatric Use
Safety and effectiveness in the pediatric population have not been established.

Geriatric Use
Clinical studies of VICODIN ES (hydrocodone bitartrate 7.5 mg and acetaminophen 750 mg) did not include sufficient numbers of subjects aged 65 and over to determine whether they respond differently from younger subjects. Other reported clinical experience has not identified differences in responses between the elderly and younger patients. In general, dose selection for an elderly patient should be cautious, usually starting at the low end of the dosing range, reflecting the greater frequency of decreased hepatic, renal, or cardiac function, and of concomitant disease or other drug therapy.
Hydrocodone and the major metabolites of acetaminophen are known to be substantially excreted by the kidney. Thus the risk of toxic reactions may be greater in patients with impaired renal function due to accumulation of the parent compound and/or metabolites in the plasma. Because elderly patients are more likely to have decreased renal function, care should be taken in dose selection, and it may be useful to monitor renal function.
Hydrocodone may cause confusion and over-sedation in the elderly; elderly patients generally should be started on low doses of hydrocodone bitartrate and acetaminophen tablets and observed closely.

ADVERSE REACTIONS
The most frequently reported adverse reactions include: lightheadedness, dizziness, sedation, nausea and vomiting. These effects seem to be more prominent in ambulatory than in nonambulatory patients and some of these adverse reactions may be alleviated if the patient lies down.
Other adverse reactions include:
Central Nervous System
Drowsiness, mental clouding, lethargy, impairment of mental and physical performance, anxiety, fear, dysphoria, psychic dependence, mood changes.
Gastrointestinal System
Prolonged administration of VICODIN ES Tablets may produce constipation.
Genitourinary System
Ureteral spasm, spasm of vesical sphincters and urinary retention have been reported with opiates.
Respiratory Depression
Hydrocodone bitartrate may produce dose-related respiratory depression by acting directly on the brain stem respiratory center. (see **OVERDOSAGE**).
Special Senses
Cases of hearing impairment or permanent loss have been reported predominantly in patients with chronic overdose.
Dermatological
Skin rash, pruritus.
The following adverse drug events may be borne in mind as potential effects of acetaminophen: allergic reactions, rash, thrombocytopenia, agranulocytosis, Stevens-Johnson syndrome, toxic epidermal necrolysis.
Potential effects of high dosage are listed in the **OVERDOSAGE** section.

DRUG ABUSE AND DEPENDENCE
Misuse Abuse and Diversion of Opioids
VICODIN ES contains hydrocodone, an opioid agonist, and is a Schedule III controlled substance. VICODIN ES, and other opioids used in analgesia can be abused and are subject to criminal diversion.
Addiction is a primary, chronic, neurobiologic disease, with genetic, psychosocial, and environmental factors influencing its development and manifestations. It is characterized by behaviors that include one or more of the following: impaired control over drug use, compulsive use, continued use despite harm, and craving. Drug addiction is a treatable disease utilizing a multidisciplinary approach, but relapse is common.
"Drug seeking" behavior is very common in addicts and drug abusers. Drug-seeking tactics include emergency calls or visits near the end of office hours, refusal to undergo appropriate examination, testing or referral, repeated "loss" of prescriptions, tampering with prescriptions and reluctance to provide prior medical records or contact information for other treating physician(s). "Doctor shopping" to obtain additional prescriptions is common among drug abusers and people suffering from untreated addiction.
Abuse and addiction are separate and distinct from physical dependence and tolerance. Physical dependence usually assumes clinically significant dimensions only after several weeks of continued opioid use, although a mild degree of

physical dependence may develop after a few days of opioid therapy. Tolerance, in which increasingly large doses are required in order to produce the same degree of analgesia, is manifested initially by a shortened duration of analgesic effect, and subsequently by decreases in the intensity of analgesia. The rate of development of tolerance varies among patients. Physicians should be aware that abuse of opioids can occur in the absence of true addiction and is characterized by misuse for non-medical purposes, often in combination with other psychoactive substances. VICODIN ES, like other opioids, may be diverted for non-medical use. Record-keeping of prescribing information, including quantity, frequency, and renewal requests is strongly advised.
Proper assessment of the patient, proper prescribing practices, periodic re-evaluation of therapy, and proper dispensing and storage are appropriate measures that help to limit abuse of opioid drugs.

OVERDOSAGE
Following an acute overdosage, toxicity may result from hydrocodone or acetaminophen.
Signs and Symptoms
Hydrocodone: Serious overdose with hydrocodone is characterized by respiratory depression (a decrease in respiratory rate and/or tidal volume, Cheyne-Stokes respiration, cyanosis), extreme somnolence progressing to stupor or coma, skeletal muscle flaccidity, cold and clammy skin, and sometimes bradycardia and hypotension. In severe overdosage, apnea, circulatory collapse, cardiac arrest and death may occur.
Acetaminophen: In acetaminophen overdosage: dose-dependent, potentially fatal hepatic necrosis is the most serious adverse effect. Renal tubular necrosis, hypoglycemic coma, and coagulation defects may also occur.
Early symptoms following a potentially hepatotoxic overdose may include: nausea, vomiting, diaphoresis and general malaise. Clinical and laboratory evidence of hepatic toxicity may not be apparent until 48 to 72 hours post-ingestion.
Treatment
A single or multiple drug overdose with hydrocodone and acetaminophen is a potentially lethal polydrug overdose, and consultation with a regional poison control center is recommended.
Immediate treatment includes support of cardiorespiratory function and measures to reduce drug absorption.
Oxygen, intravenous fluids, vasopressors, and other supportive measures should be employed as indicated. Assisted or controlled ventilation should also be considered.
For hydrocodone overdose, primary attention should be given to the reestablishment of adequate respiratory exchange through provision of a patent airway and the institution of assisted or controlled ventilation. The narcotic antagonist naloxone hydrochloride is a specific antidote against respiratory depression which may result from overdose or unusual sensitivity to narcotics, including hydrocodone. Since the duration of action of hydrocodone may exceed that of the antagonist, the patient should be kept under continued surveillance, and repeated doses of the antagonist should be administered as needed to maintain adequate respiration. A narcotic antagonist should not be administered in the absence of clinically significant respiratory or cardiovascular depression.
Gastric decontamination with activated charcoal should be administered just prior to N-acetylcysteine (NAC) to decrease systemic absorption if acetaminophen ingestion is known or suspected to have occurred within a few hours of presentation. Serum acetaminophen levels should be obtained immediately if the patient presents 4 hours or more after ingestion to assess potential risk of hepatotoxicity; acetaminophen levels drawn less than 4 hours post-ingestion may be misleading. To obtain the best possible outcome, NAC should be administered as soon as possible where impending or evolving liver injury is suspected. Intravenous NAC may be administered when circumstances preclude oral administration.
Vigorous supportive therapy is required in severe intoxication. Procedures to limit the continuing absorption of the drug must be readily performed since the hepatic injury is dose dependent and occurs early in the course of intoxication.

DOSAGE AND ADMINISTRATION
Dosage should be adjusted according to the severity of the pain and the response of the patient. However, it should be kept in mind that tolerance to hydrocodone can develop with continued use and that the incidence of untoward effects is dose related. The usual adult dosage is one tablet every four to six hours as needed for pain. The total daily dosage should not exceed 5 tablets.

HOW SUPPLIED
White, oval-shaped, faceted edged tablet bisected on one side and imprinted with "VICODIN ES" on the other side.
Bottles of 100-NDC #0074-1973-14
Bottles of 500-NDC #0074-1973-54
Hospital Unit Dosage Package-100 tablets (4 × 25 tablets)-NDC #0074-1973-12.

Storage

Store at 25°C (77°F); excursions permitted to 15°-30°C (59°-86°F). [See USP Controlled Room Temperature].
Dispense in a tight, light-resistant container as defined in the USP.
A Schedule Ⅲ Controlled Drug Substance.
©AbbVie Inc. 2013
Manufactured for
AbbVie Inc.
North Chicago, IL 60064 U.S.A.
by Halo Pharmaceutical Inc.
Whippany, NJ 07981 U.S.A.
Ref. DN2844V2-Rev. October, 2013
Shown in Product Identification Guide, page 304

VICODIN HP®   Ⅲ ℞

[vĭkō-dĭn]
(hydrocodone bitartrate and acetaminophen tablets, USP)
10 mg/660 mg

BOXED WARNING

Hepatotoxicity

Acetaminophen has been associated with cases of acute liver failure, at times resulting in liver transplant and death. Most of the cases of liver injury are associated with the use of acetaminophen at doses that exceed 4000 milligrams per day, and often involve more than one acetaminophen-containing product.

DESCRIPTION

Hydrocodone bitartrate and acetaminophen is supplied in tablet form for oral administration.
Hydrocodone bitartrate is an opioid analgesic and antitussive and occurs as fine, white crystals or as a crystalline powder. It is affected by light. The chemical name is 4,5α-epoxy-3-methoxy-17-methylmorphinan-6-one tartrate (1:1) hydrate (2:5). It has the following structural formula:

$C_{18}H_{21}NO_3 \cdot C_4H_6O_6 \cdot 2\frac{1}{2}H_2O$ M.W. = 494.50

Acetaminophen, 4'-hydroxyacetanilide, a slightly bitter, white, odorless, crystalline powder, is a non-opiate, nonsalicylate analgesic and antipyretic. It has the following structural formula:

$C_8H_9NO_2$ M.W. = 151.17

Each VICODIN HP Tablet contains:
Hydrocodone Bitartrate 10 mg
Acetaminophen 660 mg
In addition each tablet contains the following inactive ingredients: colloidal silicon dioxide, croscarmellose sodium, magnesium stearate, microcrystalline cellulose, povidone, pregelatinized starch, and stearic acid.
Meets USP Dissolution Test 2.

CLINICAL PHARMACOLOGY

Hydrocodone is a semisynthetic narcotic analgesic and antitussive with multiple actions qualitatively similar to those of codeine. Most of these involve the central nervous system and smooth muscle. The precise mechanism of action of hydrocodone and other opiates is not known, although it is believed to relate to the existence of opiate receptors in the central nervous system. In addition to analgesia, narcotics may produce drowsiness, changes in mood and mental clouding.
The analgesic action of acetaminophen involves peripheral influences, but the specific mechanism is as yet undetermined. Antipyretic activity is mediated through hypothalamic heat regulating centers. Acetaminophen inhibits prostaglandin synthetase. Therapeutic doses of acetaminophen have negligible effects on the cardiovascular or respiratory systems; however, toxic doses may cause circulatory failure and rapid, shallow breathing.

Pharmacokinetics

The behavior of the individual components is described below.
Hydrocodone
Following a 10 mg oral dose of hydrocodone administered to five adult male subjects, the mean peak concentration was 23.6 ± 5.2 ng/mL. Maximum serum levels were achieved at 1.3 ± 0.3 hours and the half-life was determined to be 3.8 ± 0.3 hours. Hydrocodone exhibits a complex pattern of metabolism including O-demethylation, N-demethylation and 6-keto reduction to the corresponding 6-α- and 6-β-hydroxymetabolites. See **OVERDOSAGE** for toxicity information.
Acetaminophen
Acetaminophen is rapidly absorbed from the gastrointestinal tract and is distributed throughout most body tissues. The plasma half-life is 1.25 to 3 hours, but may be increased by liver damage and following overdosage. Elimination of acetaminophen is principally by liver metabolism (conjugation) and subsequent renal excretion of metabolites. Approximately 85% of an oral dose appears in the urine within 24 hours of administration, most as the glucuronide conjugate, with small amounts of other conjugates and unchanged drug. See **OVERDOSAGE** for toxicity information.

INDICATIONS AND USAGE

VICODIN HP Tablets are indicated for the relief of moderate to moderately severe pain.

CONTRAINDICATIONS

This product should not be administered to patients who have previously exhibited hypersensitivity to hydrocodone or acetaminophen.
Patients known to be hypersensitive to other opioids may exhibit cross-sensitivity to hydrocodone.

WARNINGS

Hepatotoxicity

Acetaminophen has been associated with cases of acute liver failure, at times resulting in liver transplant and death. Most of the cases of liver injury are associated with the use of acetaminophen at doses that exceed 4000 milligrams per day, and often involve more than one acetaminophen-containing product. The excessive intake of acetaminophen may be intentional to cause self-harm or unintentional as patients attempt to obtain more pain relief or unknowingly take other acetaminophen-containing products.
The risk of acute liver failure is higher in individuals with underlying liver disease and in individuals who ingest alcohol while taking acetaminophen.
Instruct patients to look for acetaminophen or APAP on package labels and not to use more than one product that contains acetaminophen. Instruct patients to seek medical attention immediately upon ingestion of more than 4000 milligrams of acetaminophen per day, even if they feel well.

Serious skin reactions

Rarely, acetaminophen may cause serious skin reactions such as acute generalized exanthematous pustulosis (AGEP), Stevens-Johnson Syndrome (SJS), and toxic epidermal necrolysis (TEN), which can be fatal. Patients should be informed about the signs of serious skin reactions, and use of the drug should be discontinued at the first appearance of skin rash or any other sign of hypersensitivity.

Hypersensitivity/anaphylaxis

There have been post-marketing reports of hypersensitivity and anaphylaxis associated with use of acetaminophen. Clinical signs included swelling of the face, mouth and throat, respiratory distress, urticaria, rash, pruritus, and vomiting. There were infrequent reports of life-threatening anaphylaxis requiring emergency medical attention. Instruct patients to discontinue VICODIN HP Tablets immediately and seek medical care if they experience these symptoms. Do not prescribe VICODIN HP Tablets for patients with acetaminophen allergy.

Respiratory Depression

At high doses or in sensitive patients, hydrocodone may produce dose-related respiratory depression by acting directly on the brain stem respiratory center. Hydrocodone also affects the center that controls respiratory rhythm, and may produce irregular and periodic breathing.

Head Injury and Increased Intracranial Pressure

The respiratory depressant effects of narcotics and their capacity to elevate cerebrospinal fluid pressure may be markedly exaggerated in the presence of head injury, other intracranial lesions or a preexisting increase in intracranial pressure. Furthermore, narcotics produce adverse reactions which may obscure the clinical course of patients with head injuries.

Acute Abdominal Conditions

The administration of narcotics may obscure the diagnosis or clinical course of patients with acute abdominal conditions.

Misuse Abuse and Diversion of Opioids

VICODIN HP contains hydrocodone an opioid agonist, and is a Schedule III controlled substance. Opioid agonists have the potential for being abused and are sought by abusers and people with addiction disorders, and are subject to diversion.
VICODIN HP can be abused in a manner similar to other opioid agonists, legal or illicit. This should be considered when prescribing or dispensing VICODIN HP in situations where the physician or pharmacist is concerned about an increased risk of misuse, abuse or diversion (see DRUG ABUSE AND DEPENDENCE).

PRECAUTIONS

General

Special Risk Patients

As with any narcotic analgesic agent, VICODIN HP Tablets should be used with caution in elderly or debilitated patients, and those with severe impairment of hepatic or renal function, hypothyroidism, Addison's disease, prostatic hypertrophy or urethral stricture. The usual precautions should be observed and the possibility of respiratory depression should be kept in mind.
Cough Reflex

Hydrocodone suppresses the cough reflex; as with all narcotics, caution should be exercised when VICODIN HP Tablets are used postoperatively and in patients with pulmonary disease.

Information for Patients/Caregivers

- Do not take VICODIN HP Tablets if you are allergic to any of its ingredients.
- If you develop signs of allergy such as a rash or difficulty breathing stop taking VICODIN HP Tablets and contact your healthcare provider immediately.
- Do not take more than 4000 milligrams of acetaminophen per day. Call your doctor if you took more than the recommended dose.

Hydrocodone, like all narcotics, may impair the mental and/or physical abilities required for the performance of potentially hazardous tasks such as driving a car or operating machinery; patients should be cautioned accordingly. Alcohol and other CNS depressants may produce an additive CNS depression, when taken with this combination product, and should be avoided.
Hydrocodone may be habit forming. Patients should take the drug only for as long as it is prescribed, in the amounts prescribed, and no more frequently than prescribed.

Laboratory Tests

In patients with severe hepatic or renal disease, effects of therapy should be monitored with serial liver and/or renal function tests.

Drug Interactions

Patients receiving narcotics, antihistamines, antipsychotics, antianxiety agents, or other CNS depressants (including alcohol) concomitantly with VICODIN HP Tablets may exhibit an additive CNS depression. When combined therapy is contemplated, the dose of one or both agents should be reduced.
The use of MAO inhibitors or tricyclic antidepressants with hydrocodone preparations may increase the effect of either the antidepressant or hydrocodone.

Drug/Laboratory Test Interactions

Acetaminophen may produce false-positive test results for urinary 5-hydroxyindoleacetic acid.

Carcinogenesis, Mutagenesis, Impairment of Fertility

No adequate studies have been conducted in animals to determine whether hydrocodone or acetaminophen have a potential for carcinogenesis, mutagenesis, or impairment of fertility.

Pregnancy

Teratogenic Effects

Pregnancy Category C

There are no adequate and well-controlled studies in pregnant women. VICODIN HP Tablets should be used during pregnancy only if the potential benefit justifies the potential risk to the fetus.

Nonteratogenic Effects

Babies born to mothers who have been taking opioids regularly prior to delivery will be physically dependent. The withdrawal signs include irritability and excessive crying, tremors, hyperactive reflexes, increased respiratory rate, increased stools, sneezing, yawning, vomiting, and fever. The intensity of the syndrome does not always correlate with the duration of maternal opioid use or dose. There is no consensus on the best method of managing withdrawal.

Labor and Delivery

As with all narcotics, administration of VICODIN HP Tablets to the mother shortly before delivery may result in some degree of respiratory depression in the newborn, especially if higher doses are used.

Information on the AbbVie, Inc. products listed on these pages is from the prescribing information in use as of July 31, 2014. For more information, please visit rxabbvie.com or call 1-800-633-9110.

Nursing Mothers
Acetaminophen is excreted in breast milk in small amounts, but the significance of its effects on nursing infants is not known. It is not known whether hydrocodone is excreted in human milk. Because many drugs are excreted in human milk and because of the potential for serious adverse reactions in nursing infants from hydrocodone and acetaminophen, a decision should be made whether to discontinue nursing or to discontinue the drug, taking into account the importance of the drug to the mother.

Pediatric Use
Safety and effectiveness in the pediatric population have not been established.

Geriatric Use
Clinical studies of VICODIN HP (hydrocodone bitartrate and acetaminophen 10 mg/660 mg) did not include sufficient numbers of subjects aged 65 and over to determine whether they respond differently from younger subjects. Other reported clinical experience has not identified differences in responses between the elderly and younger patients. In general, dose selection for an elderly patient should be cautious, usually starting at the low end of the dosing range, reflecting the greater frequency of decreased hepatic, renal, or cardiac function, and of concomitant disease or other drug therapy.

Hydrocodone and the major metabolites of acetaminophen are known to be substantially excreted by the kidney. Thus the risk of toxic reactions may be greater in patients with impaired renal function due to accumulation of the parent compound and/or metabolites in the plasma. Because elderly patients are more likely to have decreased renal function, care should be taken in dose selection, and it may be useful to monitor renal function.

Hydrocodone may cause confusion and over-sedation in the elderly; elderly patients generally should be started on low doses of hydrocodone bitartrate and acetaminophen tablets and observed closely.

ADVERSE REACTIONS
The most frequently reported adverse reactions are lightheadedness, dizziness, sedation, nausea and vomiting. These effects seem to be more prominent in ambulatory than in nonambulatory patients, and some of these adverse reactions may be alleviated if the patient lies down. Other adverse reactions include:

Central Nervous System
Drowsiness, mental clouding, lethargy, impairment of mental and physical performance, anxiety, fear, dysphoria, psychic dependence, mood changes.

Gastrointestinal System
Prolonged administration of VICODIN HP Tablets may produce constipation.

Genitourinary System
Ureteral spasm, spasm of vesical sphincters and urinary retention have been reported with opiates.

Respiratory Depression
Hydrocodone bitartrate may produce dose-related respiratory depression by acting directly on the brain stem respiratory centers (see OVERDOSAGE).

Special Senses
Cases of hearing impairment or permanent loss have been reported predominantly in patients with chronic overdose.

Dermatological
Skin rash, pruritus.

The following adverse drug events may be borne in mind as potential effects of acetaminophen: allergic reactions, rash, thrombocytopenia, agranulocytosis, Stevens-Johnson syndrome, toxic epidermal necrolysis.

Potential effects of high dosage are listed in the OVERDOSAGE section.

DRUG ABUSE AND DEPENDENCE
Misuse Abuse and Diversion of Opioids
VICODIN HP contains hydrocodone, an opioid agonist, and is a Schedule III controlled substance. VICODIN HP, and other opioids used in analgesia can be abused and are subject to criminal diversion.

Addiction is a primary, chronic, neurobiologic disease, with genetic, psychosocial, and environmental factors influencing its development and manifestations. It is characterized by behaviors that include one or more of the following: impaired control over drug use, compulsive use, continued use despite harm, and craving. Drug addiction is a treatable disease utilizing a multidisciplinary approach, but relapse is common.

"Drug seeking" behavior is very common in addicts and drug abusers. Drug-seeking tactics include emergency calls or visits near the end of office hours, refusal to undergo appropriate examination, testing or referral, repeated "loss" of prescriptions, tampering with prescriptions and reluctance to provide prior medical records or contact information for other treating physician(s). "Doctor shopping" to obtain additional prescriptions is common among drug abusers and people suffering from untreated addiction.

Abuse and addiction are separate and distinct from physical dependence and tolerance. Physical dependence usually assumes clinically significant dimensions only after several weeks of continued opioid use, although a mild degree of physical dependence may develop after a few days of opioid therapy. Tolerance, in which increasingly large doses are required in order to produce the same degree of analgesia, is manifested initially by a shortened duration of analgesic effect, and subsequently by decreases in the intensity of analgesia. The rate of development of tolerance varies among patients. Physicians should be aware that abuse of opioids can occur in the absence of true addiction and is characterized by misuse for non-medical purposes, often in combination with other psychoactive substances. VICODIN HP, like other opioids, may be diverted for non-medical use. Record-keeping of prescribing information, including quantity, frequency, and renewal requests is strongly advised.

Proper assessment of the patient, proper prescribing practices, periodic re-evaluation of therapy, and proper dispensing and storage are appropriate measures that help to limit abuse of opioid drugs.

OVERDOSAGE
Following an acute overdosage, toxicity may result from hydrocodone or acetaminophen.

Signs and Symptoms
Hydrocodone: Serious overdose with hydrocodone is characterized by respiratory depression (a decrease in respiratory rate and/or tidal volume, Cheyne-Stokes respiration, cyanosis), extreme somnolence progressing to stupor or coma, skeletal muscle flaccidity, cold and clammy skin, and sometimes bradycardia and hypotension. In severe overdosage, apnea, circulatory collapse, cardiac arrest and death may occur.

Acetaminophen: In acetaminophen overdosage: dose-dependent, potentially fatal hepatic necrosis is the most serious adverse effect. Renal tubular necrosis, hypoglycemic coma, and coagulation defects may also occur.

Early symptoms following a potentially hepatotoxic overdose may include: nausea, vomiting, diaphoresis and general malaise. Clinical and laboratory evidence of hepatic toxicity may not be apparent until 48 to 72 hours post-ingestion.

Treatment
A single or multiple drug overdose with hydrocodone and acetaminophen is a potentially lethal polydrug overdose, and consultation with a regional poison control center is recommended.

Immediate treatment includes support of cardiorespiratory function and measures to reduce drug absorption.

Oxygen, intravenous fluids, vasopressors, and other supportive measures should be employed as indicated. Assisted or controlled ventilation should also be considered.

For hydrocodone overdose, primary attention should be given to the reestablishment of adequate respiratory exchange through provision of a patent airway and the institution of assisted or controlled ventilation. The narcotic antagonist naloxone hydrochloride is a specific antidote against respiratory depression which may result from overdosage or unusual sensitivity to narcotics, including hydrocodone. Since the duration of action of hydrocodone may exceed that of the antagonist, the patient should be kept under continued surveillance, and repeated doses of the antagonist should be administered as needed to maintain adequate respiration. A narcotic antagonist should not be administered in the absence of clinically significant respiratory or cardiovascular depression.

Gastric decontamination with activated charcoal should be administered just prior to N-acetylcysteine (NAC) to decrease systemic absorption if acetaminophen ingestion is known or suspected to have occurred within a few hours of presentation. Serum acetaminophen levels should be obtained immediately if the patient presents 4 hours or more after ingestion to assess potential risk of hepatotoxicity; acetaminophen levels drawn less than 4 hours post-ingestion may be misleading. To obtain the best possible outcome, NAC should be administered as soon as possible where impending or evolving liver injury is suspected. Intravenous NAC may be administered when circumstances preclude oral administration.

Vigorous supportive therapy is required in severe intoxication. Procedures to limit the continuing absorption of the drug must be readily performed since the hepatic injury is dose dependent and occurs early in the course of intoxication.

DOSAGE AND ADMINISTRATION
Dosage should be adjusted according to severity of pain and the response of the patient. However, it should be kept in mind that tolerance to hydrocodone can develop with continued use and that the incidence of untoward effects is dose related.

The usual adult dosage is one tablet every four to six hours as needed for pain. The total daily dosage should not exceed 6 tablets.

HOW SUPPLIED
VICODIN HP (hydrocodone bitartrate and acetaminophen, 10 mg/660 mg) is supplied as a white, oval-shaped, tablet bisected on one side and debossed with "VICODIN HP" on the other side.
Bottles of 100-NDC #0074-2274-14
Bottles of 500-NDC #0074-2274-54

Storage
Store at 25°C (77°F); excursions permitted to 15°-30°C (59°-86°F). [see USP Controlled Room Temperature]. Dispense in a tight, light-resistant container as defined in the USP.
A Schedule Ⅲ Controlled Drug Substance.
©AbbVie Inc. 2013
Manufactured for
AbbVie Inc.
North Chicago, IL 60064 U.S.A.
by Halo Pharmaceutical Inc.
Whippany, NJ 07981 U.S.A.
Ref. DN2845V2 - Rev. October, 2013
Shown in Product Identification Guide, page 304

VICOPROFEN®   Ⅲ R
(hydrocodone bitartrate and ibuprofen tablets)
7.5 mg/200 mg

DESCRIPTION
Each VICOPROFEN tablet contains:
Hydrocodone Bitartrate, USP 7.5 mg
Ibuprofen, USP 200 mg
VICOPROFEN is supplied in a fixed combination tablet form for oral administration. VICOPROFEN combines the opioid analgesic agent, hydrocodone bitartrate, with the nonsteroidal anti-inflammatory (NSAID) agent, ibuprofen. Hydrocodone bitartrate is a semisynthetic and centrally acting opioid analgesic. Its chemical name is: 4,5 α-epoxy-3-methoxy-17-methylmorphinan-6-one tartrate (1:1) hydrate (2:5). Its chemical formula is: $C_{18}H_{21}NO_3 \cdot C_4H_6O_6 \cdot 2\frac{1}{2}H_2O$, and the molecular weight is 494.50. Its structural formula is:

Ibuprofen is a nonsteroidal anti-inflammatory agent [nonselective COX inhibitor] with analgesic and antipyretic properties. Its chemical name is: (±)-2-(p-isobutylphenyl) propionic acid. Its chemical formula is: $C_{13}H_{18}O_2$, and the molecular weight is: 206.29. Its structural formula is:

Inactive ingredients in VICOPROFEN tablets include: colloidal silicon dioxide, corn starch, croscarmellose sodium, hypromellose, magnesium stearate, microcrystalline cellulose, polyethylene glycol, polysorbate 80, propylene glycol and titanium dioxide.

CLINICAL PHARMACOLOGY
Hydrocodone Component
Hydrocodone is a semisynthetic opioid analgesic and antitussive with multiple actions qualitatively similar to those of codeine. Most of these involve the central nervous system and smooth muscle. The precise mechanism of action of hydrocodone and other opioids is not known, although it is believed to relate to the existence of opiate receptors in the central nervous system. In addition to analgesia, opioids may produce drowsiness, changes in mood, and mental clouding.

Ibuprofen Component
Ibuprofen is a non-steroidal anti-inflammatory agent that possesses analgesic and antipyretic activities. Its mode of action, like that of other NSAIDs, is not completely understood, but may be related to inhibition of cyclooxygenase activity and prostaglandin synthesis. Ibuprofen is a peripherally acting analgesic. Ibuprofen does not have any known effects on opiate receptors.

Pharmacokinetics
Absorption
After oral dosing with the VICOPROFEN tablet, a peak hydrocodone plasma level of 27 ng/mL is achieved at 1.7 hours, and a peak ibuprofen plasma level of 30 mcg/mL is achieved at 1.8 hours. The effect of food on the absorption of either component from the VICOPROFEN tablet has not been established.

Distribution

Ibuprofen is highly protein-bound (99%) like most other non-steroidal anti-inflammatory agents. Although the extent of protein binding of hydrocodone in human plasma has not been definitely determined, structural similarities to related opioid analgesics suggest that hydrocodone is not extensively protein bound. As most agents in the 5-ring morphinan group of semi-synthetic opioids bind plasma protein to a similar degree (range 19% [hydromorphone] to 45% [oxycodone]), hydrocodone is expected to fall within this range.

Metabolism

Hydrocodone exhibits a complex pattern of metabolism, including O-demethylation, N-demethylation, and 6-keto reduction to the corresponding 6-α-and 6-β-hydroxy metabolites. Hydromorphone, a potent opioid, is formed from the O-demethylation of hydrocodone and contributes to the total analgesic effect of hydrocodone. The O- and N- demethylation processes are mediated by separate P-450 isoenzymes: CYP2D6 and CYP3A4, respectively.

Ibuprofen is present in this product as a racemate, and following absorption it undergoes interconversion in the plasma from the R-isomer to the S-isomer. Both the R- and S- isomers are metabolized to two primary metabolites: (+)-2-4'-(2hydroxy-2-methyl-propyl) phenyl propionic acid and (+)-2-4'-(2carboxypropyl) phenyl propionic acid, both of which circulate in the plasma at low levels relative to the parent.

Elimination

Hydrocodone and its metabolites are eliminated primarily in the kidneys, with a mean plasma half-life of 4.5 hours. Ibuprofen is excreted in the urine, 50% to 60% as metabolites and approximately 15% as unchanged drug and conjugate. The plasma half-life is 2.2 hours.

Special Populations

No significant pharmacokinetic differences based on age or gender have been demonstrated. The pharmacokinetics of hydrocodone and ibuprofen from VICOPROFEN has not been evaluated in children.

Renal Impairment

The effect of renal insufficiency on the pharmacokinetics of the VICOPROFEN dosage form has not been determined.

CLINICAL STUDIES

In single-dose studies of post surgical pain (abdominal, gynecological, orthopedic), 940 patients were studied at doses of one or two tablets. VICOPROFEN produced greater efficacy than placebo and each of its individual components given at the same dose. No advantage was demonstrated for the two-tablet dose.

INDICATIONS AND USAGE

Carefully consider the potential benefits and risks of VICOPROFEN and other treatment options before deciding to use VICOPROFEN. Use the lowest effective dose for the shortest duration consistent with individual patient treatment goals (see **WARNINGS**).

VICOPROFEN tablets are indicated for the short-term (generally less than 10 days) management of acute pain. VICOPROFEN is not indicated for the treatment of such conditions as osteoarthritis or rheumatoid arthritis.

CONTRAINDICATIONS

VICOPROFEN is contraindicated in patients with known hypersensitivity to hydrocodone or ibuprofen. Patients known to be hypersensitive to other opioids may exhibit cross-sensitivity to hydrocodone.

VICOPROFEN should not be given to patients who have experienced asthma, urticaria, or allergic-type reactions after taking aspirin or other NSAIDs. Severe, rarely fatal, anaphylactic-like reactions to NSAIDs have been reported in such patients (see **WARNINGS – Anaphylactoid Reactions**, and **PRECAUTIONS - Preexisting Asthma**).

VICOPROFEN is contraindicated for the treatment of perioperative pain in the setting of coronary artery bypass graft (CABG) surgery (see **WARNINGS**).

WARNINGS
CARDIOVASCULAR EFFECTS
Cardiovascular Thrombotic Events

Clinical trials of several COX-2 selective and nonselective NSAIDs of up to three years duration have shown an increased risk of serious cardiovascular (CV) thrombotic events, myocardial infarction, and stroke, which can be fatal. All NSAIDs, both COX-2 selective and nonselective, may have a similar risk. Patients with known CV disease or risk factors for CV disease may be at greater risk. To minimize the potential risk for an adverse CV event in patients treated with an NSAID, the lowest effective dose should be used for the shortest duration possible. Physicians and patients should remain alert for the development of such events, even in the absence of previous CV symptoms. Patients should be informed about the signs and/or symptoms of serious CV events and the steps to take if they occur.

There is no consistent evidence that concurrent use of aspirin mitigates the increased risk of serious CV thrombotic events associated with NSAID use. The concurrent use of aspirin and an NSAID does increase the risk of serious GI events (see **GI WARNINGS**).

Two large, controlled, clinical trials of a COX-2 selective NSAID for the treatment of pain in the first 10-14 days following CABG surgery found an increased incidence of myocardial infarction and stroke (see **CONTRAINDICATIONS**).

Hypertension

NSAID-containing products, including VICOPROFEN, can lead to onset of new hypertension or worsening of preexisting hypertension, either of which may contribute to the increased incidence of CV events. Patients taking thiazides or loop diuretics may have impaired response to these therapies when taking NSAIDs. NSAID-containing products, including VICOPROFEN, should be used with caution in patients with hypertension. Blood pressure (BP) should be monitored closely during the initiation of NSAID treatment and throughout the course of therapy.

Congestive Heart Failure and Edema

Fluid retention and edema have been observed in some patients taking NSAIDs. VICOPROFEN should be used with caution in patients with fluid retention or heart failure.

Misuse Abuse and Diversion of Opioids

VICOPROFEN contains hydrocodone an opioid agonist, and is a Schedule III controlled substance. Opioid agonists have the potential for being abused and are sought by abusers and people with addiction disorders, and are subject to diversion.

VICOPROFEN can be abused in a manner similar to other opioid agonists, legal or illicit. This should be considered when prescribing or dispensing VICOPROFEN in situations where the physician or pharmacist is concerned about an increased risk of misuse, abuse or diversion (see **DRUG ABUSE AND DEPENDENCE**).

Respiratory Depression

At high doses or in opioid-sensitive patients, hydrocodone may produce dose-related respiratory depression by acting directly on the brain stem respiratory centers. Hydrocodone also affects the center that controls respiratory rhythm, and may produce irregular and periodic breathing.

Head Injury and Increased Intracranial Pressure

The respiratory depressant effects of opioids and their capacity to elevate cerebrospinal fluid pressure may be markedly exaggerated in the presence of head injury, intracranial lesions or a pre-existing increase in intracranial pressure. Furthermore, opioids produce adverse reactions, which may obscure the clinical course of patients with head injuries.

Acute Abdominal Conditions

The administration of opioids may obscure the diagnosis or clinical course of patients with acute abdominal conditions.

Gastrointestinal (GI) Effects - Risk of GI Ulceration, Bleeding and Perforation

NSAIDs, including VICOPROFEN, can cause serious gastrointestinal (GI) adverse events including inflammation, bleeding, ulceration, and perforation of the stomach, small intestine, or large intestine, which can be fatal. These serious adverse events can occur at any time, with or without warning symptoms, in patients treated with NSAIDs. Only one in five patients who develops a serious upper GI adverse event on NSAID therapy, is symptomatic. Upper GI ulcers, gross bleeding, or perforation caused by NSAIDs occur in approximately 1% of patients treated for 3-6 months, and in about 2-4% of patients treated for one year. These trends continue with longer duration of use, increasing the likelihood of developing a serious GI event at some time during the course of therapy. However, even short-term therapy is not without risk.

NSAIDs should be prescribed with extreme caution in those with a prior history of ulcer disease or gastrointestinal bleeding. Patients with a *prior history of peptic ulcer disease and/or gastrointestinal bleeding who* use NSAIDs have a greater than 10-fold increased risk for developing a GI bleed compared to patients with neither of these risk factors. Other factors that increase the risk for GI bleeding in patients treated with NSAIDs include concomitant use of oral corticosteroids or anticoagulants, longer duration of NSAID therapy, smoking, use of alcohol, older age, and poor general health status. Most spontaneous reports of fatal GI events are in elderly or debilitated patients and therefore, special care should be taken in treating this population.

To minimize the potential risk for an adverse GI event in patients treated with an NSAID, the lowest effective dose should be used for the shortest possible duration. Patients and physicians should remain alert for signs and symptoms of GI ulceration and bleeding during NSAID therapy and promptly initiate additional evaluation and treatment if a serious GI adverse event is suspected. This should include discontinuation of the NSAID until a serious GI adverse event is ruled out. For high-risk patients, alternate therapies that do not involve NSAIDs should be considered.

Renal Effects

Long-term administration of NSAIDs has resulted in renal papillary necrosis and other renal injury. Renal toxicity has also been seen in patients in whom renal prostaglandins have a compensatory role in the maintenance of renal perfusion. In these patients, administration of a nonsteroidal anti-inflammatory drug may cause a dose-dependent reduction in prostaglandin formation and, secondarily, in renal blood flow, which may precipitate overt renal decompensation. Patients at greatest risk of this reaction are those with impaired renal function, heart failure, liver dysfunction, those taking diuretics and ACE inhibitors, and the elderly. Discontinuation of NSAID therapy is usually followed by recovery to the pretreatment state.

Advanced Renal Disease

No information is available from controlled clinical studies regarding the use of VICOPROFEN in patients with advanced renal disease. Therefore, treatment with VICOPROFEN is not recommended in patients with advanced renal disease. If VICOPROFEN therapy must be initiated, close monitoring of the patient's renal function is advisable.

Anaphylactoid Reactions

As with other NSAID-containing products, anaphylactoid reactions may occur in patients without known prior exposure to VICOPROFEN. VICOPROFEN should not be given to patients with the aspirin triad. This symptom complex typically occurs in asthmatic patients who experience rhinitis with or without nasal polyps, or who exhibit severe, potentially fatal bronchospasm after taking aspirin or other NSAIDs. Fatal reactions to NSAIDs have been reported in such patients (see **CONTRAINDICATIONS** and **PRECAUTIONS** - Pre-existing Asthma). Emergency help should be sought in cases where an anaphylactoid reaction occurs.

Skin Reactions

Products containing NSAIDs, including VICOPROFEN, can cause serious skin adverse events such as exfoliative dermatitis, Stevens-Johnson Syndrome (SJS), and toxic epidermal necrolysis (TEN), which can be fatal. These serious events may occur without warning. Patients should be informed about the signs and symptoms of serious skin manifestations and use of the drug should be discontinued at the first appearance of skin rash or any other sign of hypersensitivity.

Pregnancy

As with other NSAID-containing products, VICOPROFEN should be avoided in late pregnancy because it may cause premature closure of the ductus arteriosus.

PRECAUTIONS
General

VICOPROFEN cannot be expected to substitute for corticosteroids or to treat corticosteroid insufficiency. Abrupt discontinuation of corticosteroids may lead to disease exacerbation. Patients on prolonged corticosteroid therapy should have their therapy tapered slowly if a decision is made to discontinue corticosteroids.

The pharmacological activity of VICOPROFEN in reducing fever and inflammation may diminish the utility of these diagnostic signs in detecting complications of presumed noninfectious, painful conditions.

Special Risk Patients

As with any opioid analgesic agent, VICOPROFEN tablets should be used with caution in elderly or debilitated patients, and those with severe impairment of hepatic or renal function, hypothyroidism, Addison's disease, prostatic hypertrophy or urethral stricture. The usual precautions should be observed and the possibility of respiratory depression should be kept in mind.

Cough Reflex

Hydrocodone suppresses the cough reflex; as with opioids, caution should be exercised when VICOPROFEN is used postoperatively and in patients with pulmonary disease.

Hepatic Effects

Borderline elevations of one or more liver enzymes may occur in up to 15% of patients taking NSAIDs including ibuprofen as found in VICOPROFEN. These laboratory abnormalities may progress, may remain essentially unchanged, or may be transient with continued therapy. Notable elevations of SGPT (ALT) or SGOT (AST) (approximately three or more times the upper limit of normal) have been reported in approximately 1% of patients in clinical trials with NSAIDS. In addition, rare cases of severe hepatic reactions, including jaundice and fatal fulminant hepatitis, liver necrosis and hepatic failure, some of them with fatal outcomes have been reported.

Information on the AbbVie, Inc. products listed on these pages is from the prescribing information in use as of July 31, 2014. For more information, please visit rxabbvie.com or call 1-800-633-9110.

A patient with symptoms and/or signs suggesting liver dysfunction, or in whom an abnormal liver test has occurred, should be evaluated for evidence of the development of more severe hepatic reactions while on VICOPROFEN therapy. If clinical signs and symptoms consistent with liver disease develop, or if systemic manifestations occur (e.g., eosinophilia, rash, etc.), VICOPROFEN should be discontinued.

Hematological Effects
Anemia is sometimes seen in patients receiving NSAIDs including ibuprofen as found in VICOPROFEN. This may be due to fluid retention, occult or gross GI blood loss, or an incompletely described effect upon erythropoiesis. Patients on long-term treatment with NSAIDs including ibuprofen, should have their hemoglobin or hematocrit checked if they exhibit any signs or symptoms of anemia.

NSAIDs inhibit platelet aggregation and have been shown to prolong bleeding time in some patients. Unlike aspirin, their effect on platelet function is quantitatively less, of shorter duration, and reversible. Patients receiving VICOPROFEN who may be adversely affected by alterations in platelet function, such as those with coagulation disorders or patients receiving anticoagulants, should be carefully monitored.

Pre-existing Asthma
Patients with asthma may have aspirin-sensitive asthma. The use of aspirin in patients with aspirin-sensitive asthma has been associated with severe bronchospasm, which may be fatal. Since cross-reactivity between aspirin and other NSAIDs has been reported in such aspirin-sensitive patients, VICOPROFEN should not be administered to patients with this form of aspirin sensitivity and should be used with caution in patients with pre-existing asthma.

Aseptic Meningitis
Aseptic meningitis with fever and coma has been observed on rare occasions in patients on ibuprofen therapy as found in VICOPROFEN. Although it is probably more likely to occur in patients with systemic lupus erythematosus and related connective tissue diseases, it has been reported in patients who do not have an underlying chronic disease. If signs or symptoms of meningitis develop in a patient on VICOPROFEN, the possibility of its being related to ibuprofen should be considered.

Information for Patients
Patients should be informed of the following information before initiating therapy with an NSAID and periodically during the course of ongoing therapy. Patients should also be encouraged to read the NSAID Medication Guide that accompanies each prescription dispensed.
1. VICOPROFEN® (hydrocodone bitartrate 7.5 mg and ibuprofen 200 mg), like other opioid-containing analgesics, may impair mental and/or physical abilities required for the performance of potentially hazardous tasks such as driving a car or operating machinery; patients should be cautioned accordingly.
2. Alcohol and other CNS depressants may produce an additive CNS depression, when taken with this combination product, and should be avoided.
3. VICOPROFEN can be abused in a manner similar to other opioid agonists, legal or illicit. VICOPROFEN may be habit-forming. Patients should take the drug only for as long as it is prescribed, in the amounts prescribed, and no more frequently than prescribed.
4. VICOPROFEN, like other NSAID-containing products, may cause serious CV side effects, such as MI or stroke, which may result in hospitalization and even death. Although serious CV events can occur without warning symptoms, patients should be alert for the signs and symptoms of chest pain, shortness of breath, weakness, slurring of speech, and should ask for medical advice when observing any indicative sign or symptoms. Patients should be apprised of the importance of this follow-up (see **WARNINGS, Cardiovascular Effects**).
5. VICOPROFEN, like other NSAID-containing products, can cause GI discomfort and serious GI side effects, such as ulcers and bleeding, which may result in hospitalization and even death. Although serious GI tract ulcerations and bleeding can occur without warning symptoms, patients should be alert for the signs and symptoms of ulcerations and bleeding, and should ask for medical advice when observing any indicative sign or symptoms including epigastric pain, dyspepsia, melena, and hematemesis. Patients should be apprised of the importance of this follow-up (see **WARNINGS, Gastrointestinal Effects: Risk of Ulceration, Bleeding, and Perforation**).
6. VICOPROFEN, like other NSAID-containing products, can cause serious skin side effects such as exfoliative dermatitis, SJS, and TEN, which may result in hospitalizations and even death. Although serious skin reactions may occur without warning, patients should be alert for the signs and symptoms of skin rash and blisters, fever, or other signs of hypersensitivity such as itching, and should ask for medical advice when observing any indicative signs or symptoms. Patients should

be advised to stop the drug immediately if they develop any type of rash and contact their physicians as soon as possible.
7. Patients should promptly report signs or symptoms of unexplained weight gain or edema to their physicians.
8. Patients should be informed of the warning signs and symptoms of hepatotoxicity (e.g., nausea, fatigue, lethargy, pruritus, jaundice, right upper quadrant tenderness, and "flu-like" symptoms). If these occur, patients should be instructed to stop therapy and seek immediate medical therapy.
9. Patients should be informed of the signs of an anaphylactoid reaction (e.g., difficulty breathing, swelling of the face or throat). If these occur, patients should be instructed to seek immediate emergency help (see **WARNINGS**).
10. In late pregnancy, as with other NSAIDs, VICOPROFEN should be avoided because it may cause premature closure of the ductus arteriosus.
11. Patients should be instructed to report any signs of blurred vision or other eye symptoms.

Laboratory Tests
Because serious GI tract ulcerations and bleeding can occur without warning symptoms, physicians should monitor for signs or symptoms of GI bleeding. Patients on long-term treatment with NSAIDs should have their CBC and a chemistry profile checked periodically. If clinical signs and symptoms consistent with liver or renal disease develop, systemic manifestations occur (e.g., eosinophilia, rash, etc.) or if abnormal liver tests persist or worsen, VICOPROFEN should be discontinued.

Drug Interactions
ACE-inhibitors
Reports suggest that NSAIDs may diminish the antihypertensive effect of ACE-inhibitors. This interaction should be given consideration in patients taking VICOPROFEN concomitantly with ACE-inhibitors.
Anticholinergics
The concurrent use of anticholinergics with hydrocodone preparations may produce paralytic ileus.
Antidepressants
The use of Monoamine Oxidase Inhibitors (MAOIs) or tricyclic antidepressants with VICOPROFEN may increase the effect of either the antidepressant or hydrocodone.
MAOIs have been reported to intensify the effects of at least one opioid drug causing anxiety, confusion and significant depression of respiration or coma. The use of hydrocodone is not recommended for patients taking MAOIs or within 14 days of stopping such treatment.
Aspirin
When VICOPROFEN is administered with aspirin, the protein binding of aspirin is reduced, although the clearance of free VICOPROFEN is not altered. The clinical significance of this interaction is not known; however, as with other NSAID-containing products, concomitant administration of VICOPROFEN and aspirin is not generally recommended because of the potential of increased adverse effects.
CNS Depressants
Patients receiving other opioids, antihistamines, antipsychotics, antianxiety agents, or other CNS depressants (including alcohol) concomitantly with VICOPROFEN may exhibit an additive CNS depression. When combined therapy is contemplated, the dose of one or both agents should be reduced.
Diuretics
Ibuprofen has been shown to reduce the natriuretic effect of furosemide and thiazides in some patients. This response has been attributed to inhibition of renal prostaglandin synthesis. During concomitant therapy with VICOPROFEN the patient should be observed closely for signs of renal failure (see **WARNINGS - Renal Effects**), as well as diuretic efficacy.
Lithium
Ibuprofen has been shown to elevate plasma lithium concentration and reduce renal lithium clearance. The mean minimum lithium concentration increased 15% and the renal clearance was decreased by approximately 20%. This effect has been attributed to inhibition of renal prostaglandin synthesis by ibuprofen. Thus, when VICOPROFEN and lithium are administered concurrently, patients should be observed for signs of lithium toxicity.
Methotrexate
Ibuprofen, as well as other NSAIDs, has been reported to competitively inhibit methotrexate accumulation in rabbit kidney slices. This may indicate that ibuprofen could enhance the toxicity of methotrexate. Caution should be used when VICOPROFEN is administered concomitantly with methotrexate.
Mixed Agonist/Antagonist Opioid Analgesics
Agonist/antagonist analgesics (i.e., pentazocine, nalbuphine, butorphanol and buprenorphine) should be administered with caution to patients who have received or are receiving a course of therapy with a pure opioid agonist analgesic such as hydrocodone. In this situation, mixed ag-

onist/antagonist analgesics may reduce the analgesic effect of hydrocodone and/or may precipitate withdrawal symptoms in these patients.
Neuromuscular Blocking Agents
Hydrocodone, as well as other opioid analgesics, may enhance the neuromuscular blocking action of skeletal muscle relaxants and produce an increased degree of respiratory depression.
Warfarin
The effects of warfarin and NSAIDs on GI bleeding are synergistic, such that users of both drugs together have a risk of serious GI bleeding higher than users of either drug alone.

Carcinogenicity, Mutagenicity, and Impairment of Fertility
The carcinogenic and mutagenic potential of VICOPROFEN has not been investigated. The ability of VICOPROFEN to impair fertility has not been assessed.

Pregnancy
Pregnancy Category C.
Teratogenic Effects
Reproductive studies conducted in rats and rabbits have not demonstrated evidence of developmental abnormalities. VICOPROFEN, administered to rabbits at 95 mg/kg (5.72 and 1.9 times the maximum clinical dose based on body weight and surface area, respectively), a maternally toxic dose, resulted in an increase in the percentage of litters and fetuses with any major abnormality and an increase in the number of litters and fetuses with one or more nonossified metacarpals (a minor abnormality). VICOPROFEN, administered to rats at 166 mg/kg (10.0 and 1.66 times the maximum clinical dose based on body weight and surface area, respectively), a maternally toxic dose, did not result in any reproductive toxicity. However, animal reproduction studies are not always predictive of human response. There are no adequate and well-controlled studies in pregnant women. VICOPROFEN should be used during pregnancy only if the potential benefit justifies the potential risk to the fetus.
Nonteratogenic Effects
Because of the known effects of nonsteroidal anti-inflammatory drugs on the fetal cardiovascular system (closure of the ductus arteriosus), use during pregnancy (particularly late pregnancy) should be avoided. Babies born to mothers who have been taking opioids regularly prior to delivery will be physically dependent. The withdrawal signs include irritability and excessive crying, tremors, hyperactive reflexes, increased respiratory rate, increased stools, sneezing, yawning, vomiting, and fever. The intensity of the syndrome does not always correlate with the duration of maternal opioid use or dose. There is no consensus on the best method of managing withdrawal.

Labor and Delivery
As with other drugs known to inhibit prostaglandin synthesis, an increased incidence of dystocia and delayed parturition occurred in rats. Administration of VICOPROFEN is not recommended during labor and delivery. The effects of VICOPROFEN on labor and delivery in pregnant women are unknown.

Nursing Mothers
It is not known whether hydrocodone is excreted in human milk. In limited studies, an assay capable of detecting 1 mcg/mL did not demonstrate ibuprofen in the milk of lactating mothers. However, because of the limited nature of the studies, and because of the potential for serious adverse reactions in nursing infants from VICOPROFEN, a decision should be made whether to discontinue nursing or to discontinue the drug, taking into account the importance of the drug to the mother.

Pediatric Use
The safety and effectiveness of VICOPROFEN in pediatric patients below the age of 16 have not been established.

Geriatric Use
In controlled clinical trials there was no difference in tolerability between patients < 65 years of age and those ≥ 65, apart from an increased tendency of the elderly to develop constipation. However, because the elderly may be more sensitive to the renal and gastrointestinal effects of nonsteroidal anti-inflammatory agents as well as possible increased risk of respiratory depression with opioids, extra caution and reduced dosages should be used when treating the elderly with VICOPROFEN.

ADVERSE REACTIONS
VICOPROFEN was administered to approximately 300 pain patients in a safety study that employed dosages and a duration of treatment sufficient to encompass the recommended usage (see **DOSAGE AND ADMINISTRATION**). Adverse event rates generally increased with increasing daily dose. The event rates reported below are from approximately 150 patients who were in a group that received one tablet of VICOPROFEN an average of three to four times daily. The overall incidence rates of adverse experiences in the trials were fairly similar for this patient group and those who received the comparison treatment, acetaminophen 600 mg with codeine 60 mg.

The following lists adverse events that occurred with an incidence of 1% or greater in clinical trials of VICOPROFEN, without regard to the causal relationship of the events to the drug. To distinguish different rates of occurrence in clinical studies, the adverse events are listed as follows:

name of adverse event = less than 3%
*adverse events marked with an asterisk * = 3% to 9%*
adverse event rates over 9% are in parentheses.

Body as a Whole
Abdominal pain*; Asthenia*; Fever; Flu syndrome; Headache (27%); Infection*; Pain.

Cardiovascular
Palpitations; Vasodilation.

Central Nervous System
Anxiety*; Confusion; Dizziness (14%); Hypertonia; Insomnia*; Nervousness*; Paresthesia; Somnolence (22%); Thinking abnormalities.

Digestive
Anorexia; Constipation (22%); Diarrhea*; Dry mouth*; Dyspepsia (12%); Flatulence*; Gastritis; Melena; Mouth ulcers; Nausea (21%); Thirst; Vomiting*.

Metabolic and Nutritional Disorders
Edema*.

Respiratory
Dyspnea; Hiccups; Pharyngitis; Rhinitis.

Skin and Appendages
Pruritus*; Sweating*.

Special Senses
Tinnitus.

Urogenital
Urinary frequency.

Incidence less than 1%
Body as a Whole
Allergic reaction.
Cardiovascular
Arrhythmia; Hypotension; Tachycardia.
Central Nervous System
Agitation; Abnormal dreams; Decreased libido; Depression; Euphoria; Mood changes; Neuralgia; Slurred speech; Tremor, Vertigo.
Digestive
Chalky stool; "Clenching teeth"; Dysphagia; Esophageal spasm; Esophagitis; Gastroenteritis; Glossitis; Liver enzyme elevation.
Metabolic and Nutritional
Weight decrease.
Musculoskeletal
Arthralgia; Myalgia.
Respiratory
Asthma; Bronchitis; Hoarseness; Increased cough; Pulmonary congestion; Pneumonia; Shallow breathing; Sinusitis.
Skin and Appendages
Rash; Urticaria.
Special Senses
Altered vision; Bad taste; Dry eyes.
Urogenital
Cystitis; Glycosuria; Impotence; Urinary incontinence; Urinary retention.

DRUG ABUSE AND DEPENDENCE
Misuse Abuse and Diversion of Opioids
VICOPROFEN contains hydrocodone, an opioid agonist, and is a Schedule III controlled substance. VICOPROFEN, and other opioids used in analgesia can be abused and are subject to criminal diversion.

Addiction is a primary, chronic, neurobiologic disease, with genetic, psychosocial, and environmental factors influencing its development and manifestations. It is characterized by behaviors that include one or more of the following: impaired control over drug use, compulsive use, continued use despite harm, and craving. Drug addiction is a treatable disease utilizing a multidisciplinary approach, but relapse is common.

"Drug seeking" behavior is very common in addicts and drug abusers. Drug-seeking tactics include emergency calls or visits near the end of office hours, refusal to undergo appropriate examination, testing or referral, repeated "loss" of prescriptions, tampering with prescriptions and reluctance to provide prior medical records or contact information for other treating physician(s). "Doctor shopping" to obtain additional prescriptions is common among drug abusers and people suffering from untreated addiction.

Abuse and addiction are separate and distinct from physical dependence and tolerance. Physical dependence usually assumes clinically significant dimensions only after several weeks of continued opioid use, although a mild degree of physical dependence may develop after a few days of opioid therapy. Tolerance, in which increasingly large doses are required in order to produce the same degree of analgesia, is manifested initially by a shortened duration of analgesic effect, and subsequently by decreases in the intensity of analgesia. The rate of development of tolerance varies among patients. Physicians should be aware that abuse of opioids can occur in the absence of true addiction and is character-

ized by misuse for non-medical purposes, often in combination with other psychoactive substances. VICOPROFEN, like other opioids, may be diverted for non-medical use. Record-keeping of prescribing information, including quantity, frequency, and renewal requests is strongly advised. Proper assessment of the patient, proper prescribing practices, periodic re-evaluation of therapy, and proper dispensing and storage are appropriate measures that help to limit abuse of opioid drugs.

OVERDOSAGE
Following an acute overdosage, toxicity may result from hydrocodone and/or ibuprofen.
Signs and Symptoms
Hydrocodone Component
Serious overdose with hydrocodone is characterized by respiratory depression (a decrease in respiratory rate and/or tidal volume, Cheyne-Stokes respiration, cyanosis) extreme somnolence progressing to stupor or coma, skeletal muscle flaccidity, cold and clammy skin, and sometimes bradycardia and hypotension. In severe overdosage, apnea, circulatory collapse, cardiac arrest and death may occur.
Ibuprofen Component
Symptoms include gastrointestinal irritation with erosion and hemorrhage or perforation, kidney damage, liver damage, heart damage, hemolytic anemia, agranulocytosis, thrombocytopenia, aplastic anemia, and meningitis. Other symptoms may include headache, dizziness, tinnitus, confusion, blurred vision, mental disturbances, skin rash, stomatitis, edema, reduced retinal sensitivity, corneal deposits, and hyperkalemia.
Treatment
Primary attention should be given to the re-establishment of adequate respiratory exchange through provision of a patent airway and the institution of assisted or controlled ventilation. Naloxone, a narcotic antagonist, can reverse respiratory depression and coma associated with opioid overdose or unusual sensitivity to opioids, including hydrocodone. Therefore, an appropriate dose of naloxone hydrochloride should be administered intravenously with simultaneous efforts at respiratory resuscitation. Since the duration of action of hydrocodone may exceed that of the naloxone, the patient should be kept under continuous surveillance and repeated doses of the antagonist should be administered as needed to maintain adequate respiration. Supportive measures should be employed as indicated. Gastric emptying may be useful in removing unabsorbed drug. In cases where consciousness is impaired it may be inadvisable to perform gastric lavage. If gastric lavage is performed, little drug will likely be recovered if more than an hour has elapsed since ingestion. Ibuprofen is acidic and is excreted in the urine; therefore, it may be beneficial to administer alkali and induce diuresis. In addition to supportive measures the use of oral activated charcoal may help to reduce the absorption and reabsorption of ibuprofen. Dialysis is not likely to be effective for removal of ibuprofen because it is very highly bound to plasma proteins.

DOSAGE AND ADMINISTRATION
Carefully consider the potential benefits and risks of VICOPROFEN and other treatment options before deciding to use VICOPROFEN. Use the lowest effective dose for the shortest duration consistent with individual patient treatment goals (see **WARNINGS**).
After observing the response to initial therapy with VICOPROFEN, the dose and frequency should be adjusted to suit an individual patient's needs.
For the short-term (generally less than 10 days) management of acute pain, the recommended dose of VICOPROFEN is one tablet every 4 to 6 hours, as necessary. Dosage should not exceed 5 tablets in a 24-hour period. It should be kept in mind that tolerance to hydrocodone can develop with continued use and that the incidence of untoward effects is dose related.
The lowest effective dose or the longest dosing interval should be sought for each patient (see **WARNINGS**), especially in the elderly. After observing the initial response to therapy with VICOPROFEN, the dose and frequency of dosing should be adjusted to suit the individual patient's need, without exceeding the total daily dose recommended.

HOW SUPPLIED
VICOPROFEN tablets are available as:
White film-coated round convex tablets, engraved with "VP" over "a" logo on one side and plain on the other side.
Bottles of 100-NDC 0074-2277-14
Bottles of 500-NDC 0074-2277-54
Hospital Unit Dosage Package-100 tablets
(4 × 25 tablets)-NDC 0074-2277-12
Storage
Store at 25°C (77°F); excursions permitted to 15°-30°C (59°-86°F). [See USP Controlled Room Temperature].
Dispense in a tight, light-resistant container.
A Schedule CS-III Controlled Substance.
© AbbVie Inc. 2013

Manufactured by Halo Pharmaceutical Inc.
Whippany, NJ 07981 U.S.A.
for AbbVie Inc.
North Chicago, IL 60064 U.S.A.
Ref. 03-A691-R5-Revised April, 2013

Medication Guide
for
Non-Steroidal Anti-Inflammatory Drugs (NSAIDs)
(See the end of this Medication Guide for a list of prescription NSAID medicines.)
What is the most important information I should know about medicines called Non-Steroidal Anti-Inflammatory Drugs (NSAIDs)?
NSAID medicines may increase the chance of a heart attack or stroke that can lead to death.
This chance increases:
• with longer use of NSAID medicines
• in people who have heart disease
NSAID medicines should never be used right before or after a heart surgery called a "coronary artery bypass graft (CABG)."
NSAID medicines can cause ulcers and bleeding in the stomach and intestines at any time during treatment. Ulcers and bleeding:
• can happen without warning symptoms
• may cause death
The chance of a person getting an ulcer or bleeding increases with:
• taking medicines called "corticosteroids" and "anticoagulants"
• longer use
• smoking
• drinking alcohol
• older age
• having poor health
NSAID medicines should only be used:
• exactly as prescribed
• at the lowest dose possible for your treatment
• for the shortest time needed
What are Non-Steroidal Anti-Inflammatory Drugs (NSAIDs)?
NSAID medicines are used to treat pain and redness, swelling, and heat (inflammation) from medical conditions such as:
• different types of arthritis
• menstrual cramps and other types of short-term pain
Who should not take a Non-Steroidal Anti-Inflammatory Drug (NSAID)?
Do not take an NSAID medicine:
• if you had an asthma attack, hives, or other allergic reaction with aspirin or any other NSAID medicine
• for pain right before or after heart bypass surgery
Tell your healthcare provider:
• about all your medical conditions.
• about all of the medicines you take. NSAIDs and some other medicines can interact with each other and cause serious side effects. **Keep a list of your medicines to show to your healthcare provider and pharmacist.**
• if you are pregnant. NSAID medicines should not be used by pregnant women late in their pregnancy.
• if you are breastfeeding. Talk to your doctor.
What are the possible side effects of Non-Steroidal Anti-Inflammatory Drugs (NSAIDs)?

Serious side effects include:	Other side effects include:
• heart attack	• stomach pain
• stroke	• constipation
• high blood pressure	• diarrhea
• heart failure from body swelling (fluid retention)	• gas
	• heartburn
• kidney problems including kidney failure	• nausea
	• vomiting
• bleeding and ulcers in the stomach and intestine	• dizziness
• low red blood cells (anemia)	
• life-threatening skin reactions	
• life-threatening allergic reactions	
• liver problems including liver failure	
• asthma attacks in people who have asthma	

Information on the AbbVie, Inc. products listed on these pages is from the prescribing information in use as of July 31, 2014. For more information, please visit rxabbvie.com or call 1-800-633-9110.

Get emergency help right away if you have any of the following symptoms:

- shortness of breath or trouble breathing
- chest pain
- weakness in one part or side of your body
- slurred speech
- swelling of the face or throat

Stop your NSAID medicine and call your healthcare provider right away if you have any of the following symptoms:

- nausea
- more tired or weaker than usual
- itching
- your skin or eyes look yellow
- stomach pain
- flu-like symptoms
- vomit blood
- there is blood in your bowel movement or it is black and sticky like tar
- unusual weight gain
- skin rash or blisters with fever
- swelling of the arms and legs, hands and feet

These are not all the side effects with NSAID medicines. Talk to your healthcare provider or pharmacist for more information about NSAID medicines. Call your doctor for medical advice about side effects. You may report side effects to FDA at 1–800–FDA–1088.

Other information about Non-Steroidal Anti-Inflammatory Drugs (NSAIDs)

- Aspirin is an NSAID medicine but it does not increase the chance of a heart attack. Aspirin can cause bleeding in the brain, stomach, and intestines. Aspirin can also cause ulcers in the stomach and intestines.
- Some of these NSAID medicines are sold in lower doses without a prescription (over the counter). Talk to your healthcare provider before using over the counter NSAIDs for more than 10 days.

NSAID medicines that need a prescription

Generic Name	Tradename
Celecoxib	Celebrex
Diclofenac	Cataflam, Voltaren, Arthrotec (combined with misoprostol)
Diflunisal	Dolobid
Etodolac	Lodine, Lodine XL
Fenoprofen	Nalfon, Nalfon 200
Flurbirofen	Ansaid
Ibuprofen	Motrin, Tab-Profen, Vicoprofen* (combined with hydrocodone), Combunox (combined with oxycodone)
Indomethacin	Indocin, Indocin SR, Indo-Lemmon, Indomethagan
Ketoprofen	Oruvail
Ketorolac	Toradol
Mefenamic Acid	Ponstel
Meloxicam	Mobic
Nabumetone	Relafen
Naproxen	Naprosyn, Anaprox, Anaprox DS, EC-Naproxyn, Naprelan, Naprapac (copackaged with lansoprazole)
Oxaprozin	Daypro
Piroxicam	Feldene
Sulindac	Clinoril
Tolmetin	Tolectin, Tolectin DS, Tolectin 600

* Vicoprofen contains the same dose of ibuprofen as over-the-counter (OTC) NSAIDs, and is usually used for less than 10 days to treat pain. The OTC NSAID label warns that long term continuous use may increase the risk of heart attack or stroke.

Manufactured by Halo Pharmaceutical Inc. Whippany, NJ 07981 U.S.A. for AbbVie Inc. North Chicago, IL 60064 U.S.A. Ref. 03-A691-R5-Revised April, 2013

This Medication Guide has been approved by the U.S. Food and Drug Administration.

- *Shown in Product Identification Guide, page 305*

ZEMPLAR®   ℞
[zĕm-plər]
(paricalcitol) capsules

HIGHLIGHTS OF PRESCRIBING INFORMATION
These highlights do not include all the information needed to use ZEMPLAR safely and effectively.
See full prescribing information for ZEMPLAR.
ZEMPLAR (paricalcitol) capsules
Initial U.S. Approval: 1998

———INDICATIONS AND USAGE———
Zemplar is a vitamin D analog indicated for the prevention and treatment of secondary hyperparathyroidism associated with
- Chronic kidney disease (CKD) Stages 3 and 4 (1.1).
- CKD Stage 5 in patients on hemodialysis (HD) or peritoneal dialysis (PD) (1.2).

———DOSAGE AND ADMINISTRATION———
- CKD Stages 3 and 4: Zemplar Capsules may be administered once daily or every other day, three times a week (2.1).
- CKD Stage 5: Zemplar Capsules are dosed every other day, three times a week (2.2). To minimize the risk of hypercalcemia patients should be treated only after their baseline serum calcium has been reduced to 9.5 mg/dL or lower.
[See first table at top of next page]
[See second table at top of next page]

———DOSAGE FORMS AND STRENGTHS———
Capsules: 1 mcg, 2 mcg, and 4 mcg (3).

———CONTRAINDICATIONS———
Evidence of hypercalcemia or vitamin D toxicity (4).

———WARNINGS AND PRECAUTIONS———
- Hypercalcemia: Excessive administration of Zemplar Capsules can cause over suppression of PTH, hypercalcemia, hypercalciuria, hyperphosphatemia, and adynamic bone disease. Prescription-based doses of vitamin D and its derivatives should be withheld during Zemplar treatment (5.1).
- Digitalis toxicity: Potentiated by hypercalcemia of any cause. Use caution when Zemplar Capsules are prescribed concomitantly with digitalis compounds (5.2).
- Laboratory tests: Monitor serum calcium, serum phosphorus, and serum or plasma iPTH during initial dosing or following any dose adjustment (5.3).
- Aluminum overload and toxicity: Avoid excessive use of aluminum containing compounds (5.4).

———ADVERSE REACTIONS———
The most common adverse reactions (> 5% and more frequent than placebo) include diarrhea, hypertension, dizziness and vomiting.
To report SUSPECTED ADVERSE REACTIONS, contact AbbVie Inc. at 1-800-633-9110 or FDA at 1-800-FDA-1088 or www.fda.gov/medwatch

———DRUG INTERACTIONS———
- Strong CYP3A inhibitors (e.g. ketoconazole) will increase the exposure of paricalcitol. Use with caution (7.1).
- Cholestyramine, Mineral Oil: Intestinal absorption of Zemplar may be reduced if administered simultaneously with mineral oil or cholestyramine (7.2,7.3).
See 17 for PATIENT COUNSELING INFORMATION
            Revised: 01/2013

FULL PRESCRIBING INFORMATION: CONTENTS*
* Sections or subsections omitted from the full prescribing information are not listed

---

FULL PRESCRIBING INFORMATION

1   INDICATIONS AND USAGE
1.1   Chronic Kidney Disease Stages 3 and 4
Zemplar Capsules are indicated for the prevention and treatment of secondary hyperparathyroidism associated with Chronic Kidney Disease (CKD) Stages 3 and 4.
1.2   Chronic Kidney Disease Stage 5
Zemplar Capsules are indicated for the prevention and treatment of secondary hyperparathyroidism associated with CKD Stage 5 in patients on hemodialysis (HD) or peritoneal dialysis (PD).

2   DOSAGE AND ADMINISTRATION
2.1   Chronic Kidney Disease Stages 3 and 4
Zemplar Capsules may be administered daily or three times a week. When dosing three times weekly, the dose should be administered not more frequently than every other day. The total weekly doses for both daily and three times a week dosage regimens are similar [*see Clinical Studies (14.1)*]. Zemplar Capsules may be taken without regard to food. No dosing adjustment is required in patients with mild and moderate hepatic impairment.
Initial Dose
The initial dose of Zemplar Capsules for CKD Stages 3 and 4 patients is based on baseline intact parathyroid hormone (iPTH) levels.

Baseline iPTH Level	Daily Dose	Three Times a Week Dose*
≤ 500 pg/mL	1 mcg	2 mcg
> 500 pg/mL	2 mcg	4 mcg

* To be administered not more often than every other day

Dose Titration
Dosing must be individualized and based on serum or plasma iPTH levels, with monitoring of serum calcium and serum phosphorus. The following is a suggested approach to dose titration.

	Dose Adjustment at 2 to 4 Week Intervals		
iPTH Level Relative to Baseline	Zemplar Capsule Dose	Daily Dosage	Three Times a Week Dosage*
The same, increased or decreased by < 30%	Increase dose by	1 mcg	2 mcg
Decreased by ≥ 30% and ≤ 60%	Maintain dose	-	-
Decreased by > 60% or iPTH < 60 pg/mL	Decrease dose by	1 mcg	2 mcg

* To be administered not more often than every other day

If a patient is taking the lowest dose, 1 mcg, on the daily regimen and a dose reduction is needed, the dose can be decreased to 1 mcg three times a week. If a further dose reduction is required, the drug should be withheld as needed and restarted at a lower dosing frequency. If a patient is on a calcium-based phosphate binder, the phosphate-binder dose may be decreased or withheld, or the patient may be switched to a non-calcium-based phosphate binder. If hypercalcemia or an elevated Ca × P is observed, the dose of Zemplar should be reduced or withheld until these parameters are normalized.

Serum calcium and phosphorus levels should be closely monitored after initiation of Zemplar Capsules, during dose titration periods and during co-administration with strong CYP3A inhibitors [see *Warnings and Precautions (5.3)*, *Drug Interactions (7)* and *Clinical Pharmacology (12.3)*].

2.2 Chronic Kidney Disease Stage 5

Zemplar Capsules are to be administered three times a week, not more frequently than every other day.

Zemplar Capsules may be taken without regard to food. No dosing adjustment is required in patients with mild and moderate hepatic impairment.

Initial Dose

The initial dose of Zemplar Capsules in micrograms is based on a baseline iPTH level (pg/mL)/80. To minimize the risk of hypercalcemia patients should be treated only after their baseline serum calcium has been adjusted to 9.5 mg/dL or lower [see *Clinical Pharmacology (12.2)* and *Clinical Studies (14.2)*].

Dose Titration

Subsequent dosing should be individualized and based on iPTH, serum calcium and phosphorus levels. A suggested dose titration of Zemplar Capsules is based on the following formula:

Titration dose (micrograms) = most recent iPTH level (pg/ml)/80

Serum calcium and phosphorus levels should be closely monitored after initiation, during dose titration periods, and with co-administration of strong P450 3A inhibitors. If an elevated serum calcium or elevated Ca × P is observed and the patient is on a calcium-based phosphate binder, the binder dose may be decreased or withheld, or the patient may be switched to a non-calcium-based phosphate binder. If serum calcium or Ca × P are elevated, the dose should be decreased by 2 to 4 micrograms lower than that calculated by the most recent iPTH/80. If further adjustment is required, the dose of paricalcitol capsules should be reduced or withheld until these parameters are normalized.

As iPTH approaches the target range, small, individualized dose adjustments may be necessary in order to achieve a stable iPTH. In situations where monitoring of iPTH, Ca or P occurs less frequently than once per week, a more modest initial and dose titration ratio (e.g., iPTH/100) may be warranted.

3 DOSAGE FORMS AND STRENGTHS

Zemplar Capsules are available as 1 mcg, 2 mcg, and 4 mcg soft gelatin capsules.

- 1 mcg: oval, gray capsule imprinted with the "a" logo and "ZA"
- 2 mcg: oval, orange-brown capsule imprinted with the "a" logo and "ZF"
- 4 mcg: oval, gold capsule imprinted with the "a" logo and "ZK"

4 CONTRAINDICATIONS

Zemplar Capsules should not be given to patients with evidence of
- hypercalcemia or
- vitamin D toxicity [see *Warnings and Precautions (5.1)*].

5 WARNINGS AND PRECAUTIONS

Excessive administration of vitamin D compounds, including Zemplar Capsules, can cause over suppression of PTH, hypercalcemia, hypercalciuria, hyperphosphatemia, and adynamic bone disease.

5.1 Hypercalcemia

Progressive hypercalcemia due to overdosage of vitamin D and its metabolites may be so severe as to require emergency attention [see *Overdosage (10)*]. Acute hypercalcemia may exacerbate tendencies for cardiac arrhythmias and seizures and may potentiate the action of digitalis. Chronic hypercalcemia can lead to generalized vascular calcification and other soft-tissue calcification. Concomitant administration of high doses of calcium-containing preparations or thiazide diueretics with Zemplar may increase the risk of hypercalcemia. High intake of calcium and phosphate concomitant with vitamin D compounds may lead to serum abnormalities requiring more frequent patient monitoring and individualized dose titration. Patients also should be informed about the symptoms of elevated calcium, which include feeling tired, difficulty thinking clearly, loss of appetite, nausea, vomiting, constipation, increased thirst, increased urination and weight loss.

Prescription-based doses of vitamin D and its derivatives should be withheld during Zemplar treatment to avoid hypercalcemia.

5.2 Digitalis Toxicity

Digitalis toxicity is potentiated by hypercalcemia of any cause. Use caution when Zemplar Capsules are prescribed concomitantly with digitalis compounds.

Initial Dosage

CKD Stages 3, 4		CKD Stage 5
Baseline intact parathyroid (iPTH) Level	Starting Dose	Dose in micrograms is based on baseline iPTH level (pg/mL)/80.
≤ 500 pg/mL	1 mcg daily or 2 mcg three times a week (e.g. every other day)	
> 500 pg/mL	2 mcg daily or 4 mcg three times a week (e.g. every other day)	Dose three times a week (e.g. every other day).

Dose Titration

CKD Stages 3, 4		CKD Stage 5
iPTH Level Relative to Baseline	Dosing Recommendation	
Decreased by < 30%	Increase dose by 1 mcg daily or 2 mcg three times a week (e.g. every other day)	Dose in micrograms is based on most recent iPTH level (pg/mL)/80 with adjustments based on serum calcium and phosphorous levels.
Decreased by ≥ 30% and ≤ 60%	Maintain dose	Dose three times a week (e.g. every other day).
Decreased by > 60% or iPTH < 60 pg/mL	Decrease dose by 1 mcg daily or 2 mcg three times a week (e.g. every other day)	

5.3 Laboratory Tests

During the initial dosing or following any dose adjustment of medication, serum calcium, serum phosphorus, and serum or plasma iPTH should be monitored at least every two weeks for 3 months, then monthly for 3 months, and every 3 months thereafter.

5.4 Aluminum Overload and Toxicity

Aluminum-containing preparations (e.g., antacids, phosphate binders) should not be administered chronically with Zemplar, as increased blood levels of aluminum and aluminum bone toxicity may occur.

6 ADVERSE REACTIONS

Because clinical studies are conducted under widely varying conditions, adverse reaction rates observed in the clinical studies of a drug cannot be directly compared to rates in the clinical studies of another drug and may not reflect the rates observed in practice.

6.1 Clinical Trials Experience

CKD Stages 3 and 4

The safety of Zemplar Capsules has been evaluated in three 24-week (approximately six-month), double-blind, placebo-controlled, multicenter clinical studies involving 220 CKD Stages 3 and 4 patients. Six percent (6%) of Zemplar Capsules treated patients and 4% of placebo treated patients discontinued from clinical studies due to an adverse event. Adverse events occurring in the Zemplar Capsules group at a frequency of 2% or greater and more frequently than in the placebo group are presented in Table 1:

Table 1. Treatment-Emergent Adverse Events by Body System Occurring in ≥ 2% of Subjects in the Zemplar-Treated Group of Three, Double-Blind, Placebo-Controlled, Phase 3, CKD Stages 3 and 4 Studies; All Treated Patients

Adverse Event[a]	Zemplar Capsules (n = 107)		Placebo (n = 113)	
Overall	88	(82%)	86	(76%)
Ear and Labyrinth Disorders				
Vertigo	5	(4.7%)	0	(0.0%)
Gastrointestinal Disorders				
Abdominal Discomfort	4	(3.7%)	1	(0.9%)
Constipation	4	(3.7%)	4	(3.5%)
Diarrhea	7	(6.5%)	5	(4.4%)
Nausea	6	(5.6%)	4	(3.5%)
Vomiting	5	(4.7%)	5	(4.4%)
General Disorders and Administration Site Conditions				
Chest Pain	3	(2.8%)	1	(0.9%)
Edema	6	(5.6%)	5	(4.4%)
Pain	4	(3.7%)	4	(3.5%)
Immune System Disorders				
Hypersensitivity	6	(5.6%)	2	(1.8%)
Infections and Infestations				
Fungal Infection	3	(2.8%)	0	(0.0%)
Gastroenteritis	3	(2.8%)	3	(2.7%)
Infection	3	(2.8%)	3	(2.7%)
Sinusitis	3	(2.8%)	1	(0.9%)
Urinary Tract Infection	3	(2.8%)	1	(0.9%)
Viral Infection	8	(7.5%)	8	(7.1%)
Metabolism and Nutrition Disorders				
Dehydration	3	(2.8%)	1	(0.9%)
Musculoskeletal and Connective Tissue Disorders				
Arthritis	5	(4.7%)	0	(0.0%)
Back Pain	3	(2.8%)	1	(0.9%)
Muscle Spasms	3	(2.8%)	0	(0.0%)
Nervous System Disorders				
Dizziness	5	(4.7%)	5	(4.4%)
Headache	5	(4.7%)	5	(4.4%)
Syncope	3	(2.8%)	1	(0.9%)

Information on the AbbVie, Inc. products listed on these pages is from the prescribing information in use as of July 31, 2014. For more information, please visit rxabbvie.com or call 1-800-633-9110.

Psychiatric Disorders

Depression	3	(2.8%)	0	(0.0%)

Respiratory, Thoracic and Mediastinal Disorders

Cough	3	(2.8%)	2	(1.8%)
Oropharyngeal Pain	4	(3.7%)	0	(0.0%)

Skin and Subcutaneous Tissue Disorders

Pruritus	3	(2.8%)	3	(2.7%)
Rash	4	(3.7%)	1	(0.9%)
Skin Ulcer	3	(2.8%)	0	(0.0%)

Vascular Disorders

Hypertension	7	(6.5%)	4	(3.5%)
Hypotension	5	(4.7%)	3	(2.7%)

a. Includes only events more common in the Zemplar treatment group.

The following adverse reactions, with a causal relationship to Zemplar, occurred in <2% of the Zemplar treated patients in the above double-blind, placebo-controlled clinical trial data set.

Gastrointestinal Disorders: Dry mouth
Investigations: Hepatic enzyme abnormal
Nervous System Disorders: Dysgeusia
Skin and Subcutaneous Tissue Disorders: Urticaria

CKD Stage 5

The safety of Zemplar Capsules has been evaluated in one 12-week, double-blind, placebo-controlled, multicenter clinical study involving 88 CKD Stage 5 patients. Sixty-one patients received Zemplar Capsules and 27 patients received placebo.

The proportion of patients who terminated prematurely from the study due to adverse events was 7% for Zemplar Capsules treated patients and 7% for placebo patients.

Adverse events occurring in the Zemplar Capsules group at a frequency of 2% or greater and more frequently than in the placebo group are as follows:

Table 2. Treatment-Emergent Adverse Events by Body System Occurring in ≥ 2% of Subjects in the Zemplar-Treated Group, Double-Blind, Placebo-Controlled, Phase 3, CKD Stage 5 Study; All Treated Patients

Adverse Events[a]	Number (%) of Subjects			
	Zemplar Capsules (n=61)		Placebo (n = 27)	
Overall	43	(70%)	19	(70%)
Gastrointestinal Disorders				
Constipation	3	(4.9%)	0	(0.0%)
Diarrhea	7	(11.5%)	3	(11.1%)
Vomiting	4	(6.6%)	0	(0.0%)
General Disorders and Administration Site Conditions				
Fatigue	2	(3.3%)	0	(0.0%)
Edema Peripheral	2	(3.3%)	0	(0.0%)
Infections and Infestations				
Nasopharyngitis	5	(8.2%)	2	(7.4%)
Peritonitis	3	(4.9%)	0	(0.0%)
Sinusitis	2	(3.3%)	0	(0.0%)
Urinary Tract Infection	2	(3.3%)	0	(0.0%)

Metabolism and Nutrition Disorders

Fluid Overload	3	(4.9%)	0	(0.0%)
Hypoglycemia	2	(3.3%)	0	(0.0%)

Nervous System Disorders

Dizziness	4	(6.6%)	0	(0.0%)
Headache	2	(3.3%)	0	(0.0%)

Psychiatric Disorders

Anxiety	2	(3.3%)	0	(0.0%)
Insomnia	3	(4.9%)	0	(0.0%)

Renal and Urinary Disorders

Renal Failure Chronic	2	(3.3%)	0	(0.0%)

a. Includes only events more common in the Zemplar treatment group.

The following adverse reactions, with a causal relationship to Zemplar, occurred in <2% of the Zemplar treated patients in the above double-blind, placebo-controlled clinical trial data set.
Gastrointestinal Disorders: Gastroesophageal reflux disease
Metabolism and Nutrition Disorders: Decreased appetite, hypercalcemia, hypocalcemia
Reproductive System and Breast Disorders: Breast tenderness
Skin and Subcutaneous Tissue Disorders: Acne

6.2   Postmarketing Experience
The following additional adverse reactions have been reported during post-approval use with the active ingredient in Zemplar capsules: angioedema (including laryngeal edema).

7   DRUG INTERACTIONS
7.1   CYP3A Inhibitors
Since paricalcitol is partially metabolized by CYP3A, exposure of paricalcitol will be increased while paricalcitol is co-administered with strong CYP3A inhibitors including the following drugs but not limited to: ketoconazole, atazanavir, clarithromycin, indinavir, itraconazole, nefazodone, nelfinavir, ritonavir, saquinavir, telithromycin or voriconazole. Dose adjustment of Zemplar Capsules may be required, and iPTH and serum calcium concentrations should be closely monitored if a patient initiates or discontinues therapy with a strong CYP3A4 inhibitor [see *Clinical Pharmacology (12.3)*].
7.2   Cholestyramine
Drugs that impair intestinal absorption of fat-soluble vitamins, such as cholestyramine, may interfere with the absorption of Zemplar Capsules.
7.3   Mineral Oil
The use of mineral oil or other substances that may affect absorption of fat may influence the absorption of Zemplar Capsules.

8   USE IN SPECIFIC POPULATIONS
8.1   Pregnancy
Pregnancy Category C.
Paricalcitol has been shown to cause minimal decreases in fetal viability (5%) when administered daily to rabbits at a dose 0.5 times a human dose of 14 mcg or 0.24 mcg/kg (based on body surface area, mcg/m^2), and when administered to rats at a dose two times the 0.24 mcg/kg human dose (based on body surface area, mcg/m^2). At the highest dose tested, 20 mcg/kg administered three times per week in rats (13 times the 14 mcg human dose based on surface area, mcg/m^2), there was a significant increase in the mortality of newborn rats at doses that were maternally toxic and are known to produce hypercalcemia in rats. No other effects on offspring development were observed.
Paricalcitol was not teratogenic at the doses tested.
Paricalcitol (20 mcg/kg) has been shown to cross the placental barrier in rats. There are no adequate and well-controlled clinical studies in pregnant women. Zemplar Capsules should be used during pregnancy only if the potential benefit to the mother justifies the potential risk to the fetus.
8.3   Nursing Mothers
Studies in rats have shown that paricalcitol is present in the milk. It is not known whether paricalcitol is excreted in human milk. In the nursing patient, a decision should be made whether to discontinue nursing or to discontinue the drug, taking into account the importance of the drug to the mother.
8.4   Pediatric Use
Safety and efficacy of Zemplar Capsules in pediatric patients have not been established.
8.5   Geriatric Use
Of the total number (n = 220) of CKD Stages 3 and 4 patients in clinical studies of Zemplar Capsules, 49% were age 65 and over, while 17% were age 75 and over. Of the total number (n = 88) of CKD Stage 5 patients in the pivotal study of Zemplar Capsules, 28% were age 65 and over, while 6% were age 75 and over. No overall differences in safety and effectiveness were observed between these patients and younger patients, and other reported clinical experience has not identified differences in responses between the elderly and younger patients, but greater sensitivity of some older individuals cannot be ruled out.

10   OVERDOSAGE
Excessive administration of Zemplar Capsules can cause hypercalcemia, hypercalciuria, and hyperphosphatemia, and over suppression of PTH [see *Warnings and Precautions (5.1)*].
Treatment of Overdosage
The treatment of acute overdosage of Zemplar Capsules should consist of general supportive measures. If drug ingestion is discovered within a relatively short time, induction of emesis or gastric lavage may be of benefit in preventing further absorption. If the drug has passed through the stomach, the administration of mineral oil may promote its fecal elimination. Serial serum electrolyte determinations (especially calcium), rate of urinary calcium excretion, and assessment of electrocardiographic abnormalities due to hypercalcemia should be obtained. Such monitoring is critical in patients receiving digitalis. Discontinuation of supplemental calcium and institution of a low-calcium diet are also indicated in accidental overdosage. Due to the relatively short duration of the pharmacological action of paricalcitol, further measures are probably unnecessary. If persistent and markedly elevated serum calcium levels occur, there are a variety of therapeutic alternatives that may be considered depending on the patient's underlying condition. These include the use of drugs such as phosphates and corticosteroids, as well as measures to induce an appropriate forced diuresis.
Zemplar is not significantly removed by dialysis.

11   DESCRIPTION
Paricalcitol, USP, the active ingredient in Zemplar Capsules, is a synthetically manufactured, metabolically active vitamin D analog of calcitriol with modifications to the side chain (D$_2$) and the A (19-nor) ring. Zemplar is indicated for the prevention and treatment of secondary hyperparathyroidism in chronic kidney disease. Zemplar is available as soft gelatin capsules for oral administration containing 1 microgram, 2 micrograms or 4 micrograms of paricalcitol. Each capsule also contains medium chain triglycerides, alcohol, and butylated hydroxytoluene. The medium chain triglycerides are fractionated from coconut oil or palm kernel oil. The capsule shell is composed of gelatin, glycerin, titanium dioxide, iron oxide red (2 microgram capsules only), iron oxide yellow (2 microgram and 4 microgram capsules), iron oxide black (1 microgram capsules only), and water.
Paricalcitol is a white, crystalline powder with the empirical formula of $C_{27}H_{44}O_3$, which corresponds to a molecular weight of 416.64. Paricalcitol is chemically designated as 19-nor-1α,3β,25-trihydroxy-9,10-secoergosta-5(Z),7(E), 22(E)-triene and has the following structural formula:

12   CLINICAL PHARMACOLOGY
Secondary hyperparathyroidism is characterized by an elevation in parathyroid hormone (PTH) associated with inadequate levels of active vitamin D hormone. The source of vitamin D in the body is from synthesis in the skin as vitamin D$_3$ and from dietary intake as either vitamin D$_2$ or D$_3$. Both vitamin D$_2$ and D$_3$ require two sequential hydroxylations in the liver and the kidney to bind to and activate the vitamin D receptor (VDR). The endogenous VDR activator, calcitriol [1,25(OH)$_2$D$_3$], is a hormone that binds to VDRs that are present in the parathyroid gland, intestine, kidney, and bone to maintain parathyroid function and calcium and phosphorus homeostasis, and to VDRs found in many other tissues, including prostate, endothelium and

immune cells. VDR activation is essential for the proper formation and maintenance of normal bone. In the diseased kidney, the activation of vitamin D is diminished, resulting in a rise of PTH, subsequently leading to secondary hyperparathyroidism and disturbances in the calcium and phosphorus homeostasis. Decreased levels of $1,25(OH)_2D_3$ have been observed in early stages of chronic kidney disease. The decreased levels of $1,25(OH)_2D_3$ and resultant elevated PTH levels, both of which often precede abnormalities in serum calcium and phosphorus, affect bone turnover rate and may result in renal osteodystrophy.

12.1 Mechanism of Action
Paricalcitol is a synthetic, biologically active vitamin D_2 analog of calcitriol. Preclinical and *in vitro* studies have demonstrated that paricalcitol's biological actions are mediated through binding of the VDR, which results in the selective activation of vitamin D responsive pathways. Vitamin D and paricalcitol have been shown to reduce parathyroid hormone levels by inhibiting PTH synthesis and secretion.

12.2 Pharmacodynamics
Paricalcitol decreases serum intact parathyroid hormone (iPTH) and increases serum calcium and serum phosphorous in both HD and PD patients. This observed relationship was quantified using a mathematical model for HD and PD patient populations separately. Computer-based simulations of 100 trials in HD or PD patients (N = 100) using these relationships predict slightly lower efficacy (at least two consecutive ≥ 30% reductions from baseline iPTH) with lower hypercalcemia rates (at least two consecutive serum calcium ≥ 10.5 mg/dL) for lower iPTH-based dosing regimens. Further lowering of hypercalcemia rates was predicted if the treatment with paricalcitol is initiated in patients with lower serum calcium levels at screening.

Based on these simulations, a dosing regimen of iPTH/80 with a screening serum calcium ≤ 9.5 mg/dL, approximately 76.5% (95% CI: 75.6% – 77.3%) of HD patients are predicted to achieve at least two consecutive weekly ≥ 30% reductions from baseline iPTH over a duration of 12 weeks. The predicted incidence of hypercalcemia is 0.8% (95% CI: 0.7% – 1.0%). In PD patients, with this dosing regimen, approximately 83.3% (95% CI: 82.6% – 84.0%) of patients are predicted to achieve at least two consecutive weekly ≥ 30% reductions from baseline iPTH. The predicted incidence of hypercalcemia is 12.4% (95% CI: 11.7% - 13.0%) [*see Clinical Studies (14.2) and Dosage and Administration (2.2)*].

12.3 Pharmacokinetics
Absorption
The mean absolute bioavailability of Zemplar Capsules under low-fat fed condition ranged from 72% to 86% in healthy subjects, CKD Stage 5 patients on HD, and CKD Stage 5 patients on PD. A food effect study in healthy subjects indicated that the C_{max} and $AUC_{0-\infty}$ were unchanged when paricalcitol was administered with a high fat meal compared to fasting. Food delayed T_{max} by about 2 hours. The $AUC_{0-\infty}$ of paricalcitol increased proportionally over the dose range of 0.06 to 0.48 mcg/kg in healthy subjects.

Distribution
Paricalcitol is extensively bound to plasma proteins (≥ 99.8%). The mean apparent volume of distribution following a 0.24 mcg/kg dose of paricalcitol in healthy subjects was 34 L. The mean apparent volume of distribution following a 4 mcg dose of paricalcitol in CKD Stage 3 and a 3 mcg dose in CKD Stage 4 patients is between 44 and 46 L.

Metabolism
After oral administration of a 0.48 mcg/kg dose of ^{3}H-paricalcitol, parent drug was extensively metabolized, with only about 2% of the dose eliminated unchanged in the feces, and no parent drug was found in the urine. Several metabolites were detected in both the urine and feces. Most of the systemic exposure was from the parent drug. Two minor metabolites, relative to paricalcitol, were detected in human plasma. One metabolite was identified as 24(R)-hydroxy paricalcitol, while the other metabolite was unidentified. The 24(R)-hydroxy paricalcitol is less active than paricalcitol in an *in vivo* rat model of PTH suppression.

In vitro data suggest that paricalcitol is metabolized by multiple hepatic and non-hepatic enzymes, including mitochondrial CYP24, as well as CYP3A4 and UGT1A4. The identified metabolites include the product of 24(R)-hydroxylation, 24,26- and 24,28-dihydroxylation and direct glucuronidation.

Elimination
Paricalcitol is eliminated primarily via hepatobiliary excretion; approximately 70% of the radiolabeled dose is recovered in the feces and 18% is recovered in the urine. While the mean elimination half-life of paricalcitol is 4 to 6 hours in healthy subjects, the mean elimination half-life of paricalcitol in CKD Stages 3, 4, and 5 (on HD and PD) patients ranged from 14 to 20 hours.
[See table 3 above]

Table 3. Paricalcitol Capsule Pharmacokinetic Characteristics in CKD Stages 3, 4, and 5 Patients

Pharmacokinetic Parameters	CKD Stage 3 n = 15*	CKD Stage 4 n = 14*	CKD Stage 5 HD** n = 14	CKD Stage 5 PD** n = 8
C_{max} (ng/mL)	0.11 ± 0.04	0.06 ± 0.01	0.575 ± 0.17	0.413 ± 0.06
$AUC_{0-\infty}$ (ng·h/mL)	2.42 ± 0.61	2.13 ± 0.73	11.67 ± 3.23	13.41 ± 5.48
CL/F (L/h)	1.77 ± 0.50	1.52 ± 0.36	1.82 ± 0.75	1.76 ± 0.77
V/F (L)	43.7 ± 14.4	46.4 ± 12.4	38 ± 16.4	48.7 ± 15.6
$t_{1/2}$	16.8 ± 2.65	19.7 ± 7.2	13.9 ± 5.1	17.7 ± 9.6

* Four mcg paricalcitol capsules were given to CKD Stage 3 patients; three mcg paricalcitol capsules were given to CKD Stage 4 patients.
** CKD Stage 5 HD and PD patients received a 0.24 mcg/kg dose of paricalcitol as capsules.

Specific Populations
Geriatric
The pharmacokinetics of paricalcitol has not been investigated in geriatric patients greater than 65 years [*see Use in Specific Populations (8.5)*].
Pediatric
The pharmacokinetics of paricalcitol has not been investigated in patients less than 18 years of age.
Gender
The pharmacokinetics of paricalcitol following single doses over the 0.06 to 0.48 mcg/kg dose range was gender independent.
Hepatic Impairment
The disposition of paricalcitol (0.24 mcg/kg) was compared in patients with mild (n = 5) and moderate (n = 5) hepatic impairment (as indicated by the Child-Pugh method) and subjects with normal hepatic function (n = 10). The pharmacokinetics of unbound paricalcitol was similar across the range of hepatic function evaluated in this study. No dose adjustment is required in patients with mild and moderate hepatic impairment. The influence of severe hepatic impairment on the pharmacokinetics of paricalcitol has not been evaluated.
Renal Impairment
Following administration of Zemplar Capsules, the pharmacokinetic profile of paricalcitol for CKD Stage 5 on HD or PD was comparable to that in CKD 3 or 4 patients. Therefore, no special dose adjustments are required other than those recommended in the Dosage and Administration section [*see Dosage and Administration (2)*].
Drug Interactions
An *in vitro* study indicates that paricalcitol is neither an inhibitor of CYP1A2, CYP2A6, CYP2B6, CYP2C8, CYP2C9, CYP2C19, CYP2D6, CYP2E1 or CYP3A nor an inducer of CYP2B6, CYP2C9 or CYP3A. Hence, paricalcitol is neither expected to inhibit nor induce the clearance of drugs metabolized by these enzymes.
Omeprazole
The effect of omeprazole (40 mg capsule), a strong inhibitor of CYP2C19, on paricalcitol (four 4 mcg capsules) pharmacokinetics was investigated in a single dose, crossover study in healthy subjects. The pharmacokinetics of paricalcitol was not affected when omeprazole was administered approximately 2 hours prior to the paricalcitol dose.
Ketoconazole
The effect of multiple doses of ketoconazole, a strong inhibitor of CYP3A, administered as 200 mg BID for 5 days on the pharmacokinetics of paricalcitol (4 mcg capsule) has been studied in healthy subjects. The C_{max} of paricalcitol was minimally affected, but $AUC_{0-\infty}$ approximately doubled in the presence of ketoconazole. The mean half-life of paricalcitol was 17.0 hours in the presence of ketoconazole as compared to 9.8 hours, when paricalcitol was administered alone [*see Drug Interactions (7)*].

13 NONCLINICAL TOXICOLOGY
13.1 Carcinogenesis, Mutagenesis and Impairment of Fertility
In a 104-week carcinogenicity study in CD-1 mice, an increased incidence of uterine leiomyoma and leiomyosarcoma was observed at subcutaneous doses of 1, 3, 10 mcg/kg given three times weekly (2 to 15 times the AUC at a human dose of 14 mcg, equivalent to 0.24 mcg/kg based on AUC). The incidence rate of uterine leiomyoma was significantly different than the control group at the highest dose of 10 mcg/kg. In a 104-week carcinogenicity study in rats, there was an increased incidence of benign adrenal pheochromocytoma at subcutaneous doses of 0.15, 0.5, 1.5 mcg/kg (< 1 to 7 times the exposure following a human dose of 14 mcg, equivalent to 0.24 mcg/kg based on AUC). The increased incidence of pheochromocytomas in rats may be related to the alteration of calcium homeostasis by paricalcitol. Paricalcitol did not exhibit genetic toxicity *in vitro* with or without metabolic activation in the microbial mutagenesis assay (Ames Assay), mouse lymphoma mutagenesis assay (L5178Y), or a human lymphocyte cell chromosomal aberration assay. There was also no evidence of genetic toxicity in an *in vivo* mouse micronucleus assay. Paricalcitol had no effect on fertility (male or female) in rats at intravenous doses up to 20 mcg/kg/dose (equivalent to 13 times a human dose of 14 mcg based on surface area, mcg/m^2).

14 CLINICAL STUDIES
14.1 Chronic Kidney Disease Stages 3 and 4
The safety and efficacy of Zemplar Capsules were evaluated in three, 24-week, double blind, placebo-controlled, randomized, multicenter, Phase 3 clinical studies in CKD Stages 3 and 4 patients. Two studies used an identical three times a week dosing design, and one study used a daily dosing design. A total of 107 patients received Zemplar Capsules and 113 patients received placebo. The mean age of the patients was 63 years, 68% were male, 71% were Caucasian, and 26% were African-American. The average baseline iPTH was 274 pg/mL (range: 145-856 pg/mL). The average duration of CKD prior to study entry was 5.7 years. At study entry 22% were receiving calcium based phosphate binders and/or calcium supplements. Baseline 25-hydroxyvitamin D levels were not measured.
The initial dose of Zemplar Capsules was based on baseline iPTH. If iPTH was ≤ 500 pg/mL, Zemplar Capsules were administered 1 mcg daily or 2 mcg three times a week, not more than every other day. If iPTH was > 500 pg/mL, Zemplar Capsules were administered 2 mcg daily or 4 mcg three times a week, not more than every other day. The dose was increased by 1 mcg daily or 2 mcg three times a week every 2 to 4 weeks until iPTH levels were reduced by at least 30% from baseline. The overall average weekly dose of Zemplar Capsules was 9.6 mcg/week in the daily regimen and 9.5 mcg/week in the three times a week regimen.
In the clinical studies, doses were titrated for any of the following reasons: if iPTH fell to < 60 pg/mL, or decreased > 60% from baseline, the dose was reduced or temporarily withheld; if iPTH decreased < 30% from baseline and serum calcium was ≤ 10.3 mg/dL and serum phosphorus was ≤ 5.5 mg/dL, the dose was increased; and if iPTH decreased between 30 to 60% from baseline and serum calcium and phosphorus were ≤ 10.3 mg/dL and ≤ 5.5 mg/dL, respectively, the dose was maintained. Additionally, if serum calcium was between 10.4 to 11.0 mg/dL, the dose was reduced irrespective of iPTH, and the dose was withheld if serum calcium was > 11.0 mg/dL. If serum phosphorus was > 5.5 mg/dL, dietary counseling was provided, and phosphate binders could have been initiated or increased. If the elevation persisted, the Zemplar Capsules dose was decreased. Seventy-seven percent (77%) of the Zemplar Capsules treated patients and 82% of the placebo treated patients completed the 24-week treatment. The primary efficacy endpoint of at least two consecutive ≥ 30% reductions from baseline iPTH was achieved by 91% of Zemplar Capsules treated patients and 13% of the placebo treated patients (p < 0.001). The proportion of Zemplar Capsules treated patients achieving two consecutive ≥ 30% reductions was similar between the daily and the three times a week regimens (daily: 30/33, 91%; three times a week: 62/68, 91%).
The incidence of hypercalcemia (defined as two consecutive serum calcium values > 10.5 mg/dL), hyperphosphatemia and elevated Ca × P product in Zemplar Capsules treated patients was similar to placebo. There were no treatment related adverse events associated with hypercalcemia or hyperphosphatemia in the Zemplar Capsules group. No increases in urinary calcium or phosphorous were detected in Zemplar Capsules treated patients compared to placebo.
The pattern of change in the mean values for serum iPTH during the studies is shown in Figure 1.

Information on the AbbVie, Inc. products listed on these pages is from the prescribing information in use as of July 31, 2014. For more information, please visit rxabbvie.com or call 1-800-633-9110.

Figure 1. Mean Values for Serum iPTH Over Time in the Three Double-Blind, Placebo-Controlled, Phase 3, CKD Stages 3 and 4 Studies Combined

The mean changes from baseline to final treatment visit in serum iPTH, calcium, phosphorus, calcium-phosphorus product (Ca × P), and bone-specific alkaline phosphatase are shown in Table 4.

Table 4. Mean Changes from Baseline to Final Treatment Visit in Serum iPTH, Bone Specific Alkaline Phosphatase, Calcium, Phosphorus, and Calcium × Phosphorus Product in Three Combined Double-Blind, Placebo-Controlled, Phase 3, CKD Stages 3 and 4 Studies

	Zemplar Capsules	Placebo
iPTH (pg/mL)	n = 104	n = 110
Mean Baseline Value	266	279
Mean Final Treatment Value	162	315
Mean Change from Baseline (SE)	-104 (9.2)	+35 (9.0)
Bone Specific Alkaline Phosphatase (mcg/L)	n = 101	n = 107
Mean Baseline	17.1	18.8
Mean Final Treatment Value	9.2	17.4
Mean Change from Baseline (SE)	-7.9 (0.76)	-1.4 (0.74)
Calcium (mg/dL)	n = 104	n = 110
Mean Baseline	9.3	9.4
Mean Final Treatment Value	9.5	9.3
Mean Change from Baseline (SE)	+0.2 (0.04)	-0.1 (0.04)
Phosphorus (mg/dL)	n = 104	n = 110
Mean Baseline	4.0	4.0
Mean Final Treatment Value	4.3	4.3
Mean Change from Baseline (SE)	+0.3 (0.08)	+0.3 (0.08)
Calcium × Phosphorus Product (mg²/dL²)	n = 104	n = 110
Mean Baseline	36.7	36.9
Mean Final Treatment Value	40.7	39.7
Mean Change from Baseline (SE)	+4.0 (0.74)	+2.9 (0.72)

14.2   Chronic Kidney Disease Stage 5

The safety and efficacy of Zemplar Capsules were evaluated in a Phase 3, 12-week, double blind, placebo-controlled, randomized, multicenter study in patients with CKD Stage 5 on HD or PD. The study used a three times a week dosing design. A total of 61 patients received Zemplar Capsules and 27 patients received placebo. The mean age of the patients was 57 years, 67% were male, 50% were Caucasian, 45% were African- American, and 53% were diabetic. The average baseline iPTH was 701 pg/mL (range: 216-1933 pg/mL). The average time since first dialysis across all subjects was 3.3 years.

The initial dose of Zemplar Capsules was based on baseline iPTH/60. Subsequent dose adjustments were based on iPTH/60 as well as primary chemistry results that were measured once a week. Starting at Treatment Week 2, study drug was maintained, increased or decreased weekly based on the results of the previous week's calculation of iPTH/60. Zemplar Capsules were administered three times a week, not more than every other day.

The proportion of patients achieving at least two consecutive weekly ≥ 30% reductions from baseline iPTH was 88% of Zemplar Capsules treated patients and 13% of the placebo treated patients. The proportion of patients achieving at least two consecutive weekly ≥ 30% reductions from baseline iPTH was similar for HD and PD patients.

The incidence of hypercalcemia (defined as two consecutive serum calcium values > 10.5 mg/dL) in patients treated with Zemplar Capsules was 6.6% as compared to 0% for patients given placebo. In PD patients the incidence of hypercalcemia in patients treated with Zemplar Capsules was 21% as compared to 0% for patients given placebo. The patterns of change in the mean values for serum iPTH are shown in Figure 2. The rate of hypercalcemia with Zemplar Capsules may be reduced with a lower dosing regimen based on the iPTH/80 formula as shown by computer simulations. The hypercalcemia rate can be further predicted to decrease, if the treatment is initiated in only those with baseline serum calcium ≤ 9.5 mg/dL [see *Clinical Pharmacology (12.2)* and *Dosage and Administration (2.2)*].

Figure 2. Mean Values for Serum iPTH Over Time in a Phase 3, Double-Blind, Placebo-Controlled CKD Stage 5 Study

16   HOW SUPPLIED/STORAGE AND HANDLING

Zemplar Capsules are available as 1 mcg, 2 mcg, and 4 mcg capsules.

The 1 mcg capsule is an oval, gray, soft gelatin capsule imprinted with the "a" logo and ZA, and is available in the following package size:
Bottles of 30 (NDC 0074-4317-30)
The 2 mcg capsule is an oval, orange-brown, soft gelatin capsule imprinted with the "a" logo and ZF, and is available in the following package size:
Bottles of 30 (NDC 0074-4314-30)
The 4 mcg capsule is an oval, gold soft gelatin capsule imprinted with the "a" logo and ZK, and is available in the following package size:
Bottles of 30 (NDC 0074-4315-30)

Storage

Store Zemplar Capsules at 25°C (77°F). Excursions permitted between 15°- 30°C (59°- 86°F). See USP Controlled Room Temperature.

17   PATIENT COUNSELING INFORMATION

Patients should be advised:
- of the most common adverse reactions with use of Zemplar Capsules, which include diarrhea, hypertension, dizziness and vomiting.
- to adhere to instructions regarding diet and phosphorus restriction.
- to contact a health care provider if you develop symptoms of elevated calcium, (e.g. feeling tired, difficulty thinking clearly, loss of appetite, nausea, vomiting, constipation, increased thirst, increased urination and weight loss).
- to return to the physician's office for routine monitoring. More frequent monitoring is necessary during the initiation of therapy, following dose changes or when potentially interacting medications are started or discontinued.
- to inform their physician of all medications, including prescription and nonprescription drugs, supplements, and herbal preparations they are taking and any change to their medical condition. Patients should also be advised to inform their physicians prescribing a new medication that they are taking Zemplar Capsules.

© AbbVie Inc.
Manufactured for
AbbVie Inc.
North Chicago, IL 60064, U.S.A.
03-A689-R8-Revised January, 2013
Shown in Product Identification Guide, page 305

ZEMPLAR®   ℞
[zĕm-plar]
(paricalcitol) Injection
Fliptop Vial

DESCRIPTION

Paricalcitol, USP, the active ingredient in Zemplar Injection, is a synthetically manufactured analog of calcitriol, the metabolically active form of vitamin D indicated for the prevention and treatment of secondary hyperparathyroidism associated with chronic kidney disease (CKD) Stage 5. Zemplar is available as a sterile, clear, colorless, aqueous solution for intravenous injection. Each mL contains paricalcitol, 2 mcg or 5 mcg and the following inactive ingredients: alcohol, 20% (v/v) and propylene glycol, 30% (v/v).

Paricalcitol is a white powder chemically designated as 19-nor-1α,3β,25-trihydroxy-9,10-secoergosta-5(Z),7(E),22(E)-triene and has the following structural formula:

Molecular formula is $C_{27}H_{44}O_3$.
Molecular weight is 416.64.

CLINICAL PHARMACOLOGY

Secondary hyperparathyroidism is characterized by an elevation in parathyroid hormone (PTH) associated with inadequate levels of active vitamin D hormone. The source of vitamin D in the body is from synthesis in the skin and from dietary intake. Vitamin D requires two sequential hydroxylations in the liver and the kidney to bind to and to activate the vitamin D receptor (VDR). The endogenous VDR activator, calcitriol $[1,25(OH)_2 D_3]$, is a hormone that binds to VDRs that are present in the parathyroid gland, intestine, kidney, and bone to maintain parathyroid function and calcium and phosphorus homeostasis, and to VDRs found in many other tissues, including prostate, endothelium and immune cells. VDR activation is essential for the proper formation and maintenance of normal bone. In the diseased kidney, the activation of vitamin D is diminished, resulting in a rise of PTH, subsequently leading to secondary hyperparathyroidism, and disturbances in the calcium and phosphorus homeostasis. The decreased levels of $1,25(OH)_2 D_3$ and resultant elevated PTH levels, both of which often precede abnormalities in serum calcium and phosphorus, affect bone turnover rate and may result in renal osteodystrophy.

Mechanism of Action

Paricalcitol is a synthetic, biologically active vitamin D analog of calcitriol with modifications to the side chain (D_2) and the A (19-nor) ring. Preclinical and *in vitro* studies have demonstrated that paricalcitol's biological actions are mediated through binding of the VDR, which results in the selective activation of vitamin D responsive pathways. Vitamin D and paricalcitol have been shown to reduce parathyroid hormone levels by inhibiting PTH synthesis and secretion.

Pharmacokinetics

Within two hours after administering Zemplar intravenous doses ranging from 0.04 to 0.24 mcg/kg, concentrations of paricalcitol decreased rapidly; thereafter, concentrations of paricalcitol declined log-linearly. No accumulation of paricalcitol was observed with three times a week dosing.

Distribution

Paricalcitol is extensively bound to plasma proteins (≥99.8%). In healthy subjects, the steady state volume of distribution is approximately 23.8 L. The mean volume of distribution following a 0.24 mcg/kg dose of paricalcitol in CKD Stage 5 subjects requiring hemodialysis (HD) and peritoneal dialysis (PD) is between 31 and 35 L.

Metabolism

After IV administration of a 0.48 mcg/kg dose of ³H-paricalcitol, parent drug was extensively metabolized, with only about 2% of the dose eliminated unchanged in the feces and no parent drug found in the urine. Several metabolites were detected in both the urine and feces. Most of the systemic exposure was from the parent drug. Two minor metabolites, relative to paricalcitol, were detected in human plasma. One metabolite was identified as 24(R)-hydroxy paricalcitol, while the other metabolite was unidentified. The 24(R)-hydroxy paricalcitol is less active than paricalcitol in an *in vivo* rat model of PTH suppression. *In vitro* data suggest that paricalcitol is metabolized by multiple hepatic and non-hepatic enzymes, including mitochondrial CYP24, as well as CYP3A4 and UGT1A4. The identified metabolites include the product of 24(R)-hydroxylation (present at low levels in plasma), as well as 24,26- and 24,28-dihydroxylation and direct glucuronidation.

Elimination
Paricalcitol is excreted primarily by hepatobiliary excretion. Approximately 63% of the radioactivity was eliminated in the feces and 19% was recovered in the urine in healthy subjects. In healthy subjects, the mean elimination half-life of paricalcitol is about five to seven hours over the studied dose range of 0.04 to 0.16 mcg/kg. The pharmacokinetics of paricalcitol has been studied in CKD Stage 5 subjects requiring hemodialysis (HD) and peritoneal dialysis (PD). The mean elimination half-life of paricalcitol after administration of 0.24 mcg/kg paricalcitol IV bolus dose in CKD Stage 5 HD and PD patients is 13.9 and 15.4 hours, respectively (Table 1).

Table 1 Mean ± SD Paricalcitol Pharmacokinetic Parameters in CKD Stage 5 Subjects Following Single 0.24 mcg/kg IV Bolus Dose

	CKD Stage 5-HD (n=14)	CKD Stage 5-PD (n=8)
C_{max} (ng/mL)	1.680 ± 0.511	1.832 ± 0.315
$AUC_{0-\infty}$ (ng•h/mL)	14.51 ± 4.12	16.01 ± 5.98
β (1/h)	0.050 ± 0.023	0.045 ± 0.026
$t_{1/2}$ (h)†	13.9 ± 7.3	15.4 ± 10.5
CL (L/h)	1.49 ± 0.60	1.54 ± 0.95
Vd_{β} (L)	30.8 ± 7.5	34.9 ± 9.5

† harmonic mean ± pseudo standard deviation, HD: hemodialysis, PD: peritoneal dialysis

No accumulation of paricalcitol was observed with three times a week dosing which is consistent with the observed half-life.

Special Populations
Geriatric
The pharmacokinetics of paricalcitol have not been investigated in geriatric patients greater than 65 years.
Pediatrics
The pharmacokinetics of paricalcitol have not been investigated in patients less than 18 years of age.
Gender
The pharmacokinetics of paricalcitol were gender independent.
Hepatic Impairment
The disposition of paricalcitol (0.24 mcg/kg) was compared in patients with mild (n=5) and moderate (n=5) hepatic impairment (as indicated by the Child-Pugh method) and subjects with normal hepatic function (n=10). The pharmacokinetics of unbound paricalcitol were similar across the range of hepatic function evaluated in this study. No dose adjustment is required in patients with mild and moderate hepatic impairment. The influence of severe hepatic impairment on the pharmacokinetics of paricalcitol has not been evaluated.
Renal Impairment
The pharmacokinetics of paricalcitol have been studied in CKD Stage 5 subjects requiring hemodialysis (HD) and peritoneal dialysis (PD). Hemodialysis procedure has essentially no effect on paricalcitol elimination. However, compared to healthy subjects, CKD Stage 5 subjects showed a decreased CL and increased half-life (see **Pharmacokinetics-Elimination**).

Drug Interactions
An *in vitro* study indicates that paricalcitol is not an inhibitor of CYP1A2, CYP2A6, CYP2B6, CYP2C8, CYP2C9, CYP2C19, CYP2D6, CYP2E1, or CYP3A at concentrations up to 50 nM (21 ng/mL) (approximately 20-fold greater than that obtained after highest tested dose). In fresh primary cultured hepatocytes, the induction observed at paricalcitol concentrations up to 50 nM was less than two-fold for CYP2B6, CYP2C9 or CYP3A, where the positive controls rendered a six- to nineteen-fold induction. Hence, paricalcitol is not expected to inhibit or induce the clearance of drugs metabolized by these enzymes.
Drug interactions with paricalcitol injection have not been studied.
Omeprazole
The pharmacokinetic interaction between paricalcitol capsule (16 mcg) and omeprazole (40 mg; oral), a strong inhibitor of CYP2C19, was investigated in a single dose, crossover study in healthy subjects. The pharmacokinetics of paricalcitol were unaffected when omeprazole was administrated approximately 2 hours prior to the paricalcitol dose.
Ketoconazole
Although no data are available for the drug interaction between paricalcitol injection and ketoconazole, a strong inhibitor of CYP3A, the effect of multiple doses of ketoconazole administered as 200 mg BID for 5 days on the

Group (No. of Pts.)		Baseline Mean (Range)	Mean (SE) Change From Baseline to Final Evaluation
PTH (pg/mL)	Zemplar (n = 40)	783 (291 – 2076)	-379 (43.7)
	placebo (n = 38)	745 (320 –1671)	-69.6 (44.8)
Alkaline Phosphatase (U/L)	Zemplar (n = 31)	150 (40 – 600)	-41.5 (10.6)
	placebo (n = 34)	169 (56 – 911)	+2.6 (10.1)
Calcium (mg/dL)	Zemplar (n = 40)	9.3 (7.2 – 10.4)	+0.47 (0.1)
	placebo (n = 38)	9.1 (7.8 – 10.7)	+0.02 (0.1)
Phosphorus (mg/dL)	Zemplar (n = 40)	5.8 (3.7 – 10.2)	+0.47 (0.3)
	placebo (n = 38)	6.0 (2.8 – 8.8)	-0.47 (0.3)
Calcium × Phosphorus Product	Zemplar (n = 40)	54 (32 – 106)	+7.9 (2.2)
	placebo (n = 38)	54 (26 – 77)	-3.9 (2.3)

pharmacokinetics of paricalcitol capsule has been studied in healthy subjects. The C_{max} of paricalcitol was minimally affected, but $AUC_{0-\infty}$ approximately doubled in the presence of ketoconazole. The mean half-life of paricalcitol was 17.0 hours in the presence of ketoconazole as compared to 9.8 hours, when paricalcitol was administered alone (See **PRECAUTIONS**).

CLINICAL STUDIES

In three 12-week, placebo-controlled, phase 3 studies in chronic kidney disease Stage 5 patients on dialysis, the dose of Zemplar was started at 0.04 mcg/kg 3 times per week. The dose was increased by 0.04 mcg/kg every 2 weeks until intact parathyroid hormone (iPTH) levels were decreased at least 30% from baseline or a fifth escalation brought the dose to 0.24 mcg/kg, or iPTH fell to less than 100 pg/mL, or the Ca × P product was greater than 75 within any 2 week period, or serum calcium became greater than 11.5 mg/dL at any time.
Patients treated with Zemplar achieved a mean iPTH reduction of 30% within 6 weeks. In these studies, there was no significant difference in the incidence of hypercalcemia or hyperphosphatemia between Zemplar and placebo-treated patients. The results from these studies are as follows:
[See table above]
A long-term, open-label safety study of 164 CKD Stage 5 patients (mean dose of 7.5 mcg three times per week), demonstrated that mean serum Ca, P, and Ca × P remained within clinically appropriate ranges with PTH reduction (mean decrease of 319 pg/mL at 13 months).

INDICATIONS AND USAGE

Zemplar is indicated for the prevention and treatment of secondary hyperparathyroidism associated with chronic kidney disease Stage 5.

CONTRAINDICATIONS

Zemplar should not be given to patients with evidence of vitamin D toxicity, hypercalcemia, or hypersensitivity to any ingredient in this product (see **WARNINGS**).

WARNINGS

Acute overdose of Zemplar may cause hypercalcemia, and require emergency attention (see **OVERDOSAGE**). During dose adjustment, serum calcium and phosphorus levels should be monitored closely (e.g., twice weekly). If clinically significant hypercalcemia develops, the dose should be reduced or interrupted. Chronic administration of Zemplar may place patients at risk of hypercalcemia, elevated Ca × P product, and metastatic calcification. Chronic hypercalcemia can lead to generalized vascular calcification and other soft-tissue calcification.
Concomitant administration of high doses of calcium-containing preparations or thiazide diuretics with Zemplar may increase the risk of hypercalcemia. High intake of calcium and phosphate concomitant with vitamin D compounds may lead to serum abnormalities requiring more frequent patient monitoring and individualized dose titration. Patients also should be informed about the symptoms of elevated calcium, which include feeling tired, difficulty

thinking clearly, loss of appetite, nausea, vomiting, constipation, increased thirst, increased urination and weight loss.
Prescription-based doses of vitamin D and its derivatives should be withheld during Zemplar treatment to avoid hypercalcemia.
Aluminum-containing preparations (e.g., antacids, phosphate binders) should not be administered chronically with Zemplar, as increased blood levels of aluminum and aluminum bone toxicity may occur.

PRECAUTIONS
General
Digitalis toxicity is potentiated by hypercalcemia of any cause, so caution should be applied when digitalis compounds are prescribed concomitantly with Zemplar. Adynamic bone lesions may develop if PTH levels are suppressed to abnormal levels.
Information for the Patient
The patient should be instructed that, to ensure effectiveness of Zemplar therapy, it is important to adhere to a dietary regimen of calcium supplementation and phosphorus restriction. Appropriate types of phosphate-binding compounds may be needed to control serum phosphorus levels in patients with chronic kidney disease (CKD) Stage 5, but excessive use of aluminum containing compounds should be avoided (see **WARNINGS**). Patients should also be carefully informed about the symptoms of elevated calcium (see **WARNINGS**).
Laboratory Tests
During the initial phase of medication, serum calcium and phosphorus should be determined frequently (e.g., twice weekly). Once dosage has been established, serum calcium and phosphorus should be measured at least monthly. Measurements of serum or plasma PTH are recommended every 3 months. During dose adjustment of Zemplar, laboratory tests may be required more frequently.
Drug Interactions
Specific interaction studies were not performed with Zemplar Injection. Paricalcitol is not expected to inhibit the clearance of drugs metabolized by cytochrome P450 enzymes CYP1A2, CYP2A6, CYP2B6, CYP2C8, CYP2C9, CYP2C19, CYP2D6, CYP2E1, or CYP3A nor induce the clearance of drug metabolized by CYP2B6, CYP2C9 or CYP3A.
A multiple dose drug-drug interaction study with ketoconazole and paricalcitol capsule demonstrated that ketoconazole approximately doubled paricalcitol $AUC_{0-\infty}$ (see **CLINICAL PHARMACOLOGY**). Since paricalcitol is partially metabolized by CYP3A and ketoconazole is known to be a strong inhibitor of cytochrome P450 3A enzyme, care should be taken while paricalcitol is co-administered with ketoconazole and other strong P450 3A inhibitors including the following drugs but not limited to: atazanavir, clarithromycin, indinavir, itraconazole, nefazodone, nelfinavir, ritonavir, saquinavir, telithromycin or voriconazole.
Digitalis toxicity is potentiated by hypercalcemia of any cause, so caution should be applied when digitalis compounds are prescribed concomitantly with Zemplar.
Carcinogenesis, Mutagenesis, Impairment of Fertility
In a 104-week carcinogenicity study in CD-1 mice, an increased incidence of uterine leiomyoma and leiomyosarcoma was observed at subcutaneous doses of 1, 3, 10 mcg/kg (2 to 15 times the AUC at a human dose of 14 mcg, equivalent to 0.24 mcg/kg based on AUC). The incidence rate of uterine leiomyoma was significantly different than the control group at the highest dose of 10 mcg/kg.
In a 104-week carcinogenicity study in rats, there was an increased incidence of benign adrenal pheochromocytoma at subcutaneous doses of 0.15, 0.5, 1.5 mcg/kg (< 1 to 7 times the exposure following a human dose of 14 mcg, equivalent to 0.24 mcg/kg based on AUC). The increased incidence of pheochromocytomas in rats may be related to the alteration of calcium homeostasis by paricalcitol.
Paricalcitol did not exhibit genetic toxicity *in vitro* with or without metabolic activation in the microbial mutagenesis

---

Information on the AbbVie, Inc. products listed on these pages is from the prescribing information in use as of July 31, 2014. For more information, please visit rxabbvie.com or call 1-800-633-9110.

List No.	Volume/Container	Concentration	Total Content	Vial Type
4637-01	1 mL/Fliptop Vial	2 mcg/mL	2 mcg	Single-dose
1658-01	1 mL/Fliptop Vial	5 mcg/mL	5 mcg	Single-dose
1658-05	2 mL/Fliptop Vial	5 mcg/mL	10 mcg	Multi-dose

assay (Ames Assay), mouse lymphoma mutagenesis assay (L5178Y), or a human lymphocyte cell chromosomal aberration assay. There was also no evidence of genetic toxicity in an *in vivo* mouse micronucleus assay. Zemplar had no effect on fertility (male or female) in rats at intravenous doses up to 20 mcg/kg/dose [equivalent to 13 times the highest recommended human dose (0.24 mcg/kg) based on surface area, mg/m^2].

Pregnancy
Pregnancy Category C
Paricalcitol has been shown to cause minimal decreases in fetal viability (5%) when administered daily to rabbits at a dose 0.5 times the 0.24 mcg/kg human dose (based on surface area, mg/m^2) and when administered to rats at a dose 2 times the 0.24 mcg/kg human dose (based on plasma levels of exposure). At the highest dose tested (20 mcg/kg 3 times per week in rats, 13 times the 0.24 mcg/kg human dose based on surface area), there was a significant increase of the mortality of newborn rats at doses that were maternally toxic (hypercalcemia). No other effects on offspring development were observed. Paricalcitol was not teratogenic at the doses tested.

There are no adequate and well-controlled studies in pregnant women. Zemplar should be used during pregnancy only if the potential benefit to the mother justifies the potential risk to the fetus.

Nursing Mothers
Studies in rats have shown that paricalcitol is present in the milk. It is not known whether paricalcitol is excreted in human milk. In the nursing patient, a decision should be made whether to discontinue nursing or to discontinue the drug, taking into account the importance of the drug to the mother.

Pediatric Use
The safety and effectiveness of Zemplar were examined in a 12-week randomized, double-blind, placebo-controlled study of 29 pediatric patients, aged 5-19 years, with end-stage renal disease on hemodialysis and nearly all had received some form of vitamin D prior to the study. Seventy-six percent of the patients were male, 52% were Caucasian and 45% were African-American. The initial dose of Zemplar was 0.04 mcg/kg 3 times per week based on baseline iPTH level of less than 500 pg/mL, or 0.08 mcg/kg 3 times a week, based on baseline iPTH level of ≥ 500 pg/mL, respectively. The dose of Zemplar was adjusted in 0.04 mcg/kg increments based on the levels of serum iPTH, calcium and Ca × P. The mean baseline levels of iPTH were 841 pg/mL for the 15 Zemplar-treated patients and 740 pg/mL for the 14 placebo-treated subjects. The mean dose of Zemplar administered was 4.6 mcg (range: 0.8 mcg – 9.6 mcg). Ten of the 15 (67%) Zemplar-treated patients and 2 of the 14 (14%) placebo-treated patients completed the trial. Ten of the placebo patients (71%) were discontinued due to excessive elevations in iPTH levels as defined by 2 consecutive iPTH levels > 700 pg/mL and greater than baseline after 4 weeks of treatment.

In the primary efficacy analysis, 9 of 15 (60%) subjects in the Zemplar group had 2 consecutive 30% decreases from baseline iPTH compared with 3 of 14 (21%) patients in the placebo group (95% CI for the difference between groups –1%, 63%). Twenty-three percent of Zemplar vs. 31% of placebo patients had at least one serum calcium level > 10.3 mg/dL, and 40% vs. 14% of Zemplar vs. placebo subjects had at least one Ca × P ion product > 72 (mg/dL)^2. The overall percentage of serum calcium measurements > 10.3 mg/dL was 7% in the Zemplar group and 7% in the placebo group; the overall percentage of patients with Ca × P product > 72 (mg/dL)^2 was 8% in the Zemplar group and 7% in the placebo group. No subjects in either the Zemplar group or placebo group developed hypercalcemia (defined as at least one calcium value > 11.2 mg/dL) during the study.

Geriatric Use
Of the 40 patients receiving Zemplar in the three phase 3 placebo-controlled CKD Stage 5 studies, 10 patients were 65 years or over. In these studies, no overall differences in efficacy or safety were observed between patients 65 years or older and younger patients.

ADVERSE REACTIONS
Zemplar has been evaluated for safety in clinical studies in 609 CKD Stage 5 patients. In four, placebo-controlled, double-blind, multicenter studies, discontinuation of therapy due to any adverse event occurred in 6.5% of 62 patients treated with Zemplar (dosage titrated as tolerated, see **CLINICAL PHARMACOLOGY - Clinical Studies**) and 2.0% of 51 patients treated with placebo for 1 to 3 months. Adverse events occurring in the Zemplar group at a fre-

quency of 2% or greater and with an incidence greater than that in the placebo group, regardless of causality, are presented in the following table:

Adverse Event Incidence Rates for All Treated Patients In All Placebo-Controlled Studies

Adverse Event	Zemplar (n = 62) %	Placebo (n = 51) %
Overall	71	78
Cardiac Disorders		
Palpitations	3.2	0.0
Gastrointestinal Disorders		
Dry Mouth	3.2	2.0
Gastrointestinal Hemorrhage	4.8	2.0
Nausea	12.9	7.8
Vomiting	8.1	5.9
General Disorders and Administration Site Conditions		
Chills	4.8	2.0
Edema	6.5	0.0
Malaise	3.2	0.0
Pyrexia	4.8	2.0
Infections and Infestations		
Influenza	4.8	3.9
Pneumonia	4.8	0.0
Sepsis	4.8	2.0
Musculoskeletal and Connective Tissue Disorders		
Arthralgia	4.8	3.9

A patient who reported the same medical term more than once was counted only once for that medical term.

Safety parameters (changes in mean Ca, P, Ca × P) in an open-label safety study up to 13 months in duration support the long-term safety of Zemplar in this patient population (see **CLINICAL STUDIES**).

Other Adverse Reactions Observed During Clinical Evaluation of Zemplar Injection
The following adverse reactions, with a causal relationship to Zemplar, occurred in <2% of the Zemplar treated patients in the above double-blind, placebo-controlled clinical trial data set. In addition, the following also includes adverse reactions reported in Zemplar-treated patients who participated in other studies (non placebo-controlled), including double-blind, active-controlled and open-label studies:
Blood and Lymphatic System Disorders:
Anemia, lymphadenopathy
Cardiac Disorders:
Arrhythmia, atrial flutter, cardiac arrest
Ear and Labyrinth Disorders:
Ear discomfort
Endocrine Disorders:
Hyperparathyroidism, hypoparathyroidism
Eye Disorders:
Conjunctivitis, glaucoma, ocular hyperemia
Gastrointestinal Disorders:
Abdominal discomfort, constipation, diarrhea, dysphagia, gastritis, intestinal ischemia, rectal hemorrhage
General Disorders and Administration Site Conditions:
Asthenia, chest discomfort, chest pain, condition aggravated, edema peripheral, fatigue, feeling abnormal, gait disturbance, injection site extravasation, injection site pain, pain, swelling, thirst
Infections and Infestations:
Nasopharyngitis, upper respiratory tract infection, vaginal infection
Investigations:
Aspartate aminotransferase increased, bleeding time prolonged, heart rate irregular, laboratory test abnormal, weight decreased
Metabolism and Nutrition Disorders:
Decreased appetite, hypercalcemia, hyperkalemia, hyperphosphatemia, hypocalcemia
Musculoskeletal and Connective Tissue Disorders:
Joint stiffness, muscle twitching, myalgia
Neoplasms Benign, Malignant and Unspecified:
Breast cancer
Nervous System Disorders:
Cerebrovascular accident, dizziness, dysgeusia, headache, hypoesthesia, myoclonus, paresthesia, syncope, unresponsive to stimuli
Psychiatric Disorders:
Agitation, confusional state, delirium, insomnia, nervousness, restlessness

Reproductive System and Breast Disorders:
Breast pain, erectile dysfunction
Respiratory, Thoracic and Mediastinal Disorders:
Cough, dyspnea, orthopnea, pulmonary edema, wheezing
Skin and Subcutaneous Tissue Disorders:
Alopecia, blister, hirsutism, night sweats, rash pruritic, pruritus, skin burning sensation
Vascular Disorders:
Hypertension, hypotension

Additional Adverse Events Reported During Postmarketing Experience
Allergic reactions, such as rash, urticaria, and angioedema (including laryngeal edema) have been reported.

OVERDOSAGE
Overdosage of Zemplar may lead to hypercalcemia, hypercalciuria, hyperphosphatemia, and over suppression of PTH. (see **WARNINGS**).

Treatment of Overdosage and Hypercalcemia
The treatment of acute overdosage should consist of general supportive measures. Serial serum electrolyte determinations (especially calcium), rate of urinary calcium excretion, and assessment of electrocardiographic abnormalities due to hypercalcemia should be obtained. Such monitoring is critical in patients receiving digitalis. Discontinuation of supplemental calcium and institution of a low calcium diet are also indicated in acute overdosage.

General treatment of hypercalcemia due to overdosage consists of immediate dose reduction or suspension of Zemplar therapy, institution of a low calcium diet, withdrawal of calcium supplements, patient mobilization, and attention to fluid and electrolyte imbalances. Serum calcium levels should be determined at least weekly until normocalcemia ensues. When serum calcium levels have returned to within normal limits, Zemplar may be reinitiated at a lower dose. If persistent and markedly elevated serum calcium levels occur, there are a variety of therapeutic alternatives that may be considered. These include the use of drugs such as phosphates and corticosteroids as well as measures to induce diuresis. Also, one may consider dialysis against a calcium-free dialysate.
Zemplar is not significantly removed by dialysis.

DOSAGE AND ADMINISTRATION
The currently accepted target range for iPTH levels in CKD Stage 5 patients is no more than 1.5 to 3 times the nonuremic upper limit of normal.
The recommended initial dose of Zemplar is 0.04 mcg/kg to 0.1 mcg/kg (2.8 – 7 mcg) administered as a bolus dose no more frequently than every other day at any time during dialysis.
If a satisfactory response is not observed, the dose may be increased by 2 to 4 mcg at 2- to 4-week intervals. During any dose adjustment period, serum calcium and phosphorus levels should be monitored more frequently, and if an elevated calcium level or a Ca × P product greater than 75 is noted, the drug dosage should be immediately reduced or interrupted until these parameters are normalized. Then, Zemplar should be reinitiated at a lower dose. If a patient is on a calcium-based phosphate binder, the dose may be decreased or withheld, or the patient may be switched to a non-calcium-based phosphate binder. Zemplar doses may need to be decreased as the PTH levels decrease in response to therapy. Thus, incremental dosing must be individualized.
The following table is a suggested approach in dose titration:

Suggested Dosing Guidelines

PTH Level	Zemplar Dose
the same or increasing	increase
decreasing by < 30%	increase
decreasing by > 30%, < 60%	maintain
decreasing by > 60%	decrease
one and one-half to three times upper limit of normal	maintain

The influence of mild to moderately impaired hepatic function on paricalcitol pharmacokinetics is sufficiently small that no dosing adjustment is required.
Parenteral drug products should be inspected visually for particulate matter and discoloration prior to administration whenever solution and container permit.
After initial vial use, the contents of the multi-dose vial remain stable up to seven days when stored at controlled room temperature (see **HOW SUPPLIED**). Discard unused portion of the single-dose vial.

HOW SUPPLIED
Zemplar Injection is available as 2 mcg/mL (**NDC** 0074-4637-01) and 5 mcg/mL (**NDC** 0074-1658-01 and **NDC** 0074-1658-05) in trays of 25 vials.
[See table above]

Store at 25°C (77°F). Excursions permitted between 15° - 30°C (59° - 86°F).
© AbbVie Inc.
Manufactured for
AbbVie Inc.
North Chicago, IL 60064, U.S.A.
Ref. EN-2945-Rev. January, 2013

Amgen
ONE AMGEN CENTER DRIVE
THOUSAND OAKS, CA 91320-1799

For Product Inquiries and Adverse Event Reporting Contact:
Amgen Medical Information
(800) 772-6436
FAX: (866) 292-6436
Sales and Ordering:
Amgen Trade Operations
(800) 282-6436
FAX: (866) 292-6436

PROLIA®
[PRÓ-lee-a]
(denosumab)
Injection, for subcutaneous use

℞

HIGHLIGHTS OF PRESCRIBING INFORMATION
These highlights do not include all the information needed to use PROLIA safely and effectively. See full prescribing information for PROLIA.
Prolia® (denosumab)
Injection, for subcutaneous use
Initial U.S. Approval: 2010

RECENT MAJOR CHANGES
- Contraindications (4.3)   07/2013
- Warnings and Precautions (5.2)   07/2013
- Warnings and Precautions (5.3)   06/2014
- Warnings and Precautions (5.8)   06/2014

INDICATIONS AND USAGE
Prolia is a RANK ligand (RANKL) inhibitor indicated for:
- Treatment of postmenopausal women with osteoporosis at high risk for fracture (1.1)
- Treatment to increase bone mass in men with osteoporosis at high risk for fracture (1.2)
- Treatment to increase bone mass in men at high risk for fracture receiving androgen deprivation therapy for non-metastatic prostate cancer (1.3)
- Treatment to increase bone mass in women at high risk for fracture receiving adjuvant aromatase inhibitor therapy for breast cancer (1.4)

DOSAGE AND ADMINISTRATION
- Prolia should be administered by a healthcare professional (2.1)
- Administer 60 mg every 6 months as a subcutaneous injection in the upper arm, upper thigh, or abdomen (2.1)
- Instruct patients to take calcium 1000 mg daily and at least 400 IU vitamin D daily (2.1)

DOSAGE FORMS AND STRENGTHS
- Single-use prefilled syringe containing 60 mg in a 1 mL solution (3)
- Single-use vial containing 60 mg in a 1 mL solution (3)

CONTRAINDICATIONS
- Hypocalcemia (4.1, 5.3)
- Pregnancy (4.2, 8.1)
- Known hypersensitivity to Prolia (4.3, 5.2)

WARNINGS AND PRECAUTIONS
- Same Active Ingredient: Patients receiving Prolia should not receive XGEVA® (5.1)
- Hypersensitivity including anaphylactic reactions may occur. Discontinue permanently if a clinically significant reaction occurs (5.2)
- Hypocalcemia: Must be corrected before initiating Prolia. May worsen, especially in patients with renal impairment. Adequately supplement patients with calcium and vitamin D (5.3)
- Osteonecrosis of the jaw: Has been reported with Prolia. Monitor for symptoms (5.4)
- Atypical femoral fractures: Have been reported. Evaluate patients with thigh or groin pain to rule out a femoral fracture (5.5)

- Serious infections including skin infections: May occur, including those leading to hospitalization. Advise patients to seek prompt medical attention if they develop signs or symptoms of infection, including cellulitis (5.6)
- Dermatologic reactions: Dermatitis, rashes, and eczema have been reported. Consider discontinuing Prolia if severe symptoms develop (5.7)
- Severe Bone, Joint, Muscle Pain may occur. Discontinue use if severe symptoms develop (5.8)
- Suppression of bone turnover: Significant suppression has been demonstrated. Monitor for consequences of bone oversuppression (5.9)

ADVERSE REACTIONS
- Postmenopausal osteoporosis: Most common adverse reactions (> 5% and more common than placebo) were: back pain, pain in extremity, hypercholesterolemia, musculoskeletal pain, and cystitis. Pancreatitis has been reported in clinical trials (6.1)
- Male Osteoporosis: Most common adverse reactions (> 5% and more common than placebo) were: back pain, arthralgia, and nasopharyngitis (6.1)
- Bone loss due to hormone ablation for cancer: Most common adverse reactions (≥ 10% and more common than placebo) were: arthralgia and back pain. Pain in extremity and musculoskeletal pain have also been reported in clinical trials (6.1)

To report SUSPECTED ADVERSE REACTIONS, contact Amgen Inc. at 1-800-77-AMGEN (1-800-772-6436) or FDA at 1-800-FDA-1088 or www.fda.gov/medwatch.

USE IN SPECIFIC POPULATIONS
- Nursing mothers: Discontinue drug or nursing taking into consideration importance of drug to mother (8.3)
- Pediatric patients: Safety and efficacy not established (8.4)
- Renal impairment: No dose adjustment is necessary in patients with renal impairment. Patients with creatinine clearance < 30 mL/min or receiving dialysis are at risk for hypocalcemia. Supplement with calcium and vitamin D, and consider monitoring serum calcium (8.6)

See 17 for PATIENT COUNSELING INFORMATION and Medication Guide

Revised: 06/2014

FULL PRESCRIBING INFORMATION: CONTENTS*

FULL PRESCRIBING INFORMATION

1   INDICATIONS AND USAGE
1.1   Treatment of Postmenopausal Women with Osteoporosis at High Risk for Fracture
Prolia is indicated for the treatment of postmenopausal women with osteoporosis at high risk for fracture, defined as a history of osteoporotic fracture, or multiple risk factors for fracture; or patients who have failed or are intolerant to other available osteoporosis therapy. In postmenopausal women with osteoporosis, Prolia reduces the incidence of vertebral, nonvertebral, and hip fractures *[see Clinical Studies (14.1)]*.

1.2   Treatment to Increase Bone Mass in Men with Osteoporosis
Prolia is indicated for treatment to increase bone mass in men with osteoporosis at high risk for fracture, defined as a history of osteoporotic fracture, or multiple risk factors for fracture; or patients who have failed or are intolerant to other available osteoporosis therapy *[see Clinical Studies (14.2)]*.

1.3   Treatment of Bone Loss in Men Receiving Androgen Deprivation Therapy for Prostate Cancer
Prolia is indicated as a treatment to increase bone mass in men at high risk for fracture receiving androgen deprivation therapy for nonmetastatic prostate cancer. In these patients Prolia also reduced the incidence of vertebral fractures *[see Clinical Studies (14.3)]*.

1.4   Treatment of Bone Loss in Women Receiving Adjuvant Aromatase Inhibitor Therapy for Breast Cancer
Prolia is indicated as a treatment to increase bone mass in women at high risk for fracture receiving adjuvant aromatase inhibitor therapy for breast cancer *[see Clinical Studies (14.4)]*.

2   DOSAGE AND ADMINISTRATION
2.1   Recommended Dosage
Prolia should be administered by a healthcare professional. The recommended dose of Prolia is 60 mg administered as a single subcutaneous injection once every 6 months. Administer Prolia via subcutaneous injection in the upper arm, the upper thigh, or the abdomen. All patients should receive calcium 1000 mg daily and at least 400 IU vitamin D daily *[see Warnings and Precautions (5.3)]*.
If a dose of Prolia is missed, administer the injection as soon as the patient is available. Thereafter, schedule injections every 6 months from the date of the last injection.

2.2   Preparation and Administration
Visually inspect Prolia for particulate matter and discoloration prior to administration whenever solution and container permit. Prolia is a clear, colorless to pale yellow solution that may contain trace amounts of translucent to white proteinaceous particles. Do not use if the solution is discolored or cloudy or if the solution contains many particles or foreign particulate matter.
Latex Allergy: People sensitive to latex should not handle the grey needle cap on the single-use prefilled syringe, which contains dry natural rubber (a derivative of latex).
Prior to administration, Prolia may be removed from the refrigerator and brought to room temperature (up to 25°C/77°F) by standing in the original container. This generally takes 15 to 30 minutes. Do not warm Prolia in any other way *[see How Supplied/Storage and Handling (16)]*.
Instructions for Prefilled Syringe with Needle Safety Guard
IMPORTANT: In order to minimize accidental needle-

sticks, the Prolia single-use prefilled syringe will have a green safety guard; manually activate the safety guard <u>after</u> the injection is given.

DO NOT slide the green safety guard forward over the needle before administering the injection; it will lock in place and prevent injection.

Activate the green safety guard (slide over the needle) <u>after</u> the injection.

The grey needle cap on the single-use prefilled syringe contains dry natural rubber (a derivative of latex); people sensitive to latex should not handle the cap.

Step 1: Remove Grey Needle Cap

Remove needle cap.

Step 2: Administer Subcutaneous Injection

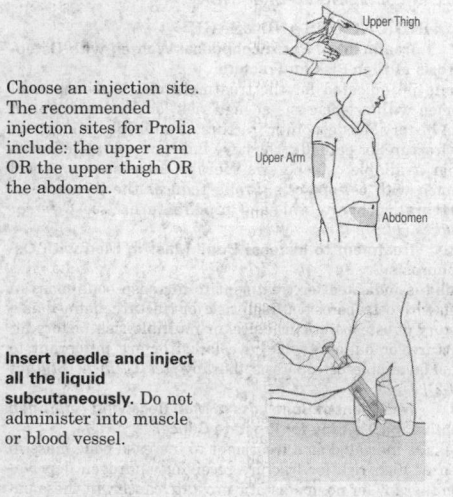

Choose an injection site. The recommended injection sites for Prolia include: the upper arm OR the upper thigh OR the abdomen.

Insert needle and inject **all the liquid subcutaneously.** Do not administer into muscle or blood vessel.

DO NOT put grey needle cap back on needle.

Step 3: Immediately Slide Green Safety Guard Over Needle
With the *needle pointing away from you...*
Hold the prefilled syringe by the clear plastic finger grip with one hand. Then, with the other hand, grasp the green safety guard by its base and gently slide it towards the needle until the green safety guard locks securely in place and/or you hear a "click." **DO NOT** grip the green safety guard too firmly – it will move easily if you hold and slide it gently.

Hold clear finger grip.

Gently slide green safety guard over needle and lock securely in place. Do not grip green safety guard too firmly when sliding over needle.

Immediately dispose of the syringe and needle cap in the nearest sharps container. **DO NOT** put the needle cap back on the used syringe.
Instructions for Single-use Vial
For administration of Prolia from the single-use vial, use a 27-gauge needle to withdraw and inject the 1 mL dose. Do not re-enter the vial. Discard vial and any liquid remaining in the vial.

3 DOSAGE FORMS AND STRENGTHS
• 1 mL of a 60 mg/mL solution in a single-use prefilled syringe
• 1 mL of a 60 mg/mL solution in a single-use vial

4 CONTRAINDICATIONS
4.1 Hypocalcemia
Pre-existing hypocalcemia must be corrected prior to initiating therapy with Prolia *[see Warnings and Precautions (5.3)].*
4.2 Pregnancy
Prolia may cause fetal harm when administered to a pregnant woman. In utero denosumab exposure in cynomolgus monkeys resulted in increased fetal loss, stillbirths, and postnatal mortality, along with evidence of absent lymph nodes, abnormal bone growth and decreased neonatal growth. Prolia is contraindicated in women who are pregnant. If this drug is used during pregnancy, or if the patient becomes pregnant while taking this drug, the patient should be apprised of the potential hazard to a fetus *[see Use in Specific Populations (8.1)].*
4.3 Hypersensitivity
Prolia is contraindicated in patients with a history of systemic hypersensitivity to any component of the product. Reactions have included anaphylaxis, facial swelling and urticaria *[see Warnings and Precautions (5.2), Adverse Reactions (6.2)].*

5 WARNINGS AND PRECAUTIONS
5.1 Drug Products with Same Active Ingredient
Prolia contains the same active ingredient (denosumab) found in Xgeva. Patients receiving Prolia should not receive Xgeva.
5.2 Hypersensitivity
Clinically significant hypersensitivity including anaphylaxis has been reported with Prolia. Symptoms have included hypotension, dyspnea, throat tightness, facial and upper airway edema, pruritus, and urticaria. If an anaphylactic or other clinically significant allergic reaction occurs, initiate appropriate therapy and discontinue further use of Prolia. *[see Contraindications (4.3), Adverse Reactions (6.2)].*
5.3 Hypocalcemia and Mineral Metabolism
Hypocalcemia may be exacerbated by the use of Prolia. Pre-existing hypocalcemia must be corrected prior to initiating therapy with Prolia. In patients predisposed to hypocalcemia and disturbances of mineral metabolism (e.g. history of hypoparathyroidism, thyroid surgery, parathyroid surgery, malabsorption syndromes, excision of small intestine, severe renal impairment [creatinine clearance <30 mL/min] or receiving dialysis), clinical monitoring of calcium and mineral levels (phosphorus and magnesium) is highly recommended.
Hypocalcemia following Prolia administration is a significant risk in patients with severe renal impairment [creatinine clearance <30 mL/min] or receiving dialysis. These patients may also develop marked elevations of serum parathyroid hormone (PTH). Instruct all patients with severe renal impairment, including those receiving dialysis, about the symptoms of hypocalcemia and the importance of maintaining calcium levels with adequate calcium and vitamin D supplementation.
Adequately supplement all patients with calcium and vitamin D *[see Dosage and Administration (2.1), Contraindications (4.1), Adverse Reactions (6.1), and Patient Counseling Information (17.3)].*
5.4 Osteonecrosis of the Jaw
Osteonecrosis of the jaw (ONJ), which can occur spontaneously, is generally associated with tooth extraction and/or local infection with delayed healing. ONJ has been reported in patients receiving denosumab *[see Adverse Reactions (6.1)].* A routine oral exam should be performed by the prescriber prior to initiation of Prolia treatment. A dental examination with appropriate preventive dentistry should be considered prior to treatment with Prolia in patients with risk factors for ONJ such as invasive dental procedures (e.g. tooth extraction, dental implants, oral surgery), diagnosis of cancer, concomitant therapies (e.g. chemotherapy, corticosteroids), poor oral hygiene, and co-morbid disorders (e.g. periodontal and/or other pre-existing dental disease, anemia, coagulopathy, infection, ill-fitting dentures). Good oral hygiene practices should be maintained during treatment with Prolia.
For patients requiring invasive dental procedures, clinical judgment of the treating physician and/or oral surgeon should guide the management plan of each patient based on individual benefit-risk assessment.
Patients who are suspected of having or who develop ONJ while on Prolia should receive care by a dentist or an oral surgeon. In these patients, extensive dental surgery to treat ONJ may exacerbate the condition. Discontinuation of Prolia therapy should be considered based on individual benefit-risk assessment.
5.5 Atypical Subtrochanteric and Diaphyseal Femoral Fractures
Atypical low-energy or low trauma fractures of the shaft have been reported in patients receiving Prolia *[see Adverse Reactions (6.1)].* These fractures can occur anywhere in the femoral shaft from just below the lesser trochanter to above the supracondylar flare and are transverse or short oblique in orientation without evidence of comminution. Causality has not been established as these fractures also occur in osteoporotic patients who have not been treated with antiresorptive agents.
Atypical femoral fractures most commonly occur with minimal or no trauma to the affected area. They may be bilateral and many patients report prodromal pain in the affected area, usually presenting as dull, aching thigh pain, weeks to months before a complete fracture occurs. A number of reports note that patients were also receiving treatment with glucocorticoids (e.g. prednisone) at the time of fracture.
During Prolia treatment, patients should be advised to report new or unusual thigh, hip, or groin pain. Any patient who presents with thigh or groin pain should be suspected of having an atypical fracture and should be evaluated to rule out an incomplete femur fracture. Patient presenting with an atypical femur fracture should also be assessed for symptoms and signs of fracture in the contralateral limb. Interruption of Prolia therapy should be considered, pending a risk/benefit assessment, on an individual basis.
5.6 Serious Infections
In a clinical trial of over 7800 women with postmenopausal osteoporosis, serious infections leading to hospitalization were reported more frequently in the Prolia group than in the placebo group *[see Adverse Reactions (6.1)].* Serious skin infections, as well as infections of the abdomen, urinary tract, and ear, were more frequent in patients treated with Prolia. Endocarditis was also reported more frequently in Prolia-treated patients. The incidence of opportunistic infections was similar between placebo and Prolia groups, and the overall incidence of infections was similar between the treatment groups. Advise patients to seek prompt medical attention if they develop signs or symptoms of severe infection, including cellulitis.
Patients on concomitant immunosuppressant agents or with impaired immune systems may be at increased risk for serious infections. Consider the benefit-risk profile in such patients before treating with Prolia. In patients who develop serious infections while on Prolia, prescribers should assess the need for continued Prolia therapy.
5.7 Dermatologic Adverse Reactions
In a large clinical trial of over 7800 women with postmenopausal osteoporosis, epidermal and dermal adverse events such as dermatitis, eczema, and rashes occurred at a significantly higher rate in the Prolia group compared to the placebo group. Most of these events were not specific to the injection site *[see Adverse Reactions (6.1)].* Consider discontinuing Prolia if severe symptoms develop.
5.8 Musculoskeletal Pain
In post-marketing experience, severe and occasionally incapacitating bone, joint, and/or muscle pain has been reported in patients taking Prolia *[see Adverse Reactions (6.2)].* The time to onset of symptoms varied from one day to several months after starting Prolia. Consider discontinuing use if severe symptoms develop *[see Patient Counseling Information (17.8)].*
5.9 Suppression of Bone Turnover
In clinical trials in women with postmenopausal osteoporosis, treatment with Prolia resulted in significant suppression of bone remodeling as evidenced by markers of bone turnover and bone histomorphometry *[see Clinical Pharmacology (12.2) and Clinical Studies (14.1)].* The significance of these findings and the effect of long-term treatment with Prolia are unknown. The long-term consequences of the degree of suppression of bone remodeling observed with Prolia may contribute to adverse outcomes such as osteonecrosis of the jaw, atypical fractures, and delayed fracture healing. Monitor patients for these consequences.

6 ADVERSE REACTIONS
The following serious adverse reactions are discussed below and also elsewhere in the labeling:
• Hypocalcemia *[see Warnings and Precautions (5.3)]*
• Serious Infections *[see Warnings and Precautions (5.6)]*
• Dermatologic Adverse Reactions *[see Warnings and Precautions (5.7)]*
• Osteonecrosis of the Jaw *[see Warnings and Precautions (5.4)]*
• Atypical Subtrochanteric and Diaphyseal Femoral Fractures *[see Warnings and Precautions (5.5)]*
The most common adverse reactions reported with Prolia in patients with postmenopausal osteoporosis are back pain, pain in extremity, musculoskeletal pain, hypercholesterolemia, and cystitis.
The most common adverse reactions reported with Prolia in men with osteoporosis are back pain, arthralgia, and nasopharyngitis.
The most common (per patient incidence ≥ 10%) adverse reactions reported with Prolia in patients with bone loss receiving androgen deprivation therapy for prostate cancer or

adjuvant aromatase inhibitor therapy for breast cancer are arthralgia and back pain. Pain in extremity and musculo-skeletal pain have also been reported in clinical trials.

The most common adverse reactions leading to discontinuation of Prolia in patients with postmenopausal osteoporosis are back pain and constipation.

The Prolia Postmarketing Active Safety Surveillance Program is available to collect information from prescribers on specific adverse events. Please see www.proliasafety.com or call 1-800-772-6436 for more information about this program.

6.1 Clinical Trials Experience

Because clinical studies are conducted under widely varying conditions, adverse reaction rates observed in the clinical studies of a drug cannot be directly compared to rates in the clinical studies of another drug and may not reflect the rates observed in clinical practice.

Treatment of Postmenopausal Women with Osteoporosis

The safety of Prolia in the treatment of postmenopausal osteoporosis was assessed in a 3-year, randomized, double-blind, placebo-controlled, multinational study of 7808 post-menopausal women aged 60 to 91 years. A total of 3876 women were exposed to placebo and 3886 women were exposed to Prolia administered subcutaneously once every 6 months as a single 60 mg dose. All women were instructed to take at least 1000 mg of calcium and 400 IU of vitamin D supplementation per day.

The incidence of all-cause mortality was 2.3% (n = 90) in the placebo group and 1.8% (n = 70) in the Prolia group. The incidence of nonfatal serious adverse events was 24.2% in the placebo group and 25.0% in the Prolia group. The percentage of patients who withdrew from the study due to adverse events was 2.1% and 2.4% for the placebo and Prolia groups, respectively.

Adverse reactions reported in ≥ 2% of postmenopausal women with osteoporosis and more frequently in the Prolia-treated women than in the placebo-treated women are shown in the table below.

Table 1. Adverse Reactions Occurring in ≥ 2% of Patients with Osteoporosis and More Frequently than in Placebo-treated Patients

SYSTEM ORGAN CLASS Preferred Term	Prolia (N = 3886) n (%)	Placebo (N = 3876) n (%)
BLOOD AND LYMPHATIC SYSTEM DISORDERS		
Anemia	129 (3.3)	107 (2.8)
CARDIAC DISORDERS		
Angina pectoris	101 (2.6)	87 (2.2)
Atrial fibrillation	79 (2.0)	77 (2.0)
EAR AND LABYRINTH DISORDERS		
Vertigo	195 (5.0)	187 (4.8)
GASTROINTESTINAL DISORDERS		
Abdominal pain upper	129 (3.3)	111 (2.9)
Flatulence	84 (2.2)	53 (1.4)
Gastroesophageal reflux disease	80 (2.1)	66 (1.7)
GENERAL DISORDERS AND ADMINISTRATION SITE CONDITIONS		
Edema peripheral	189 (4.9)	155 (4.0)
Asthenia	90 (2.3)	73 (1.9)
INFECTIONS AND INFESTATIONS		
Cystitis	228 (5.9)	225 (5.8)
Upper respiratory tract infection	190 (4.9)	167 (4.3)
Pneumonia	152 (3.9)	150 (3.9)
Pharyngitis	91 (2.3)	78 (2.0)
Herpes zoster	79 (2.0)	72 (1.9)
METABOLISM AND NUTRITION DISORDERS		
Hypercholesterolemia	280 (7.2)	236 (6.1)
MUSCULOSKELETAL AND CONNECTIVE TISSUE DISORDERS		
Back pain	1347 (34.7)	1340 (34.6)
Pain in extremity	453 (11.7)	430 (11.1)
Musculoskeletal pain	297 (7.6)	291 (7.5)
Bone pain	142 (3.7)	117 (3.0)
Myalgia	114 (2.9)	94 (2.4)
Spinal osteoarthritis	82 (2.1)	64 (1.7)
NERVOUS SYSTEM DISORDERS		
Sciatica	178 (4.6)	149 (3.8)
PSYCHIATRIC DISORDERS		
Insomnia	126 (3.2)	122 (3.1)
SKIN AND SUBCUTANEOUS TISSUE DISORDERS		
Rash	96 (2.5)	79 (2.0)
Pruritus	87 (2.2)	82 (2.1)

Hypocalcemia

Decreases in serum calcium levels to less than 8.5 mg/dL at any visit were reported in 0.4% women in the placebo group and 1.7% women in the Prolia group. The nadir in serum calcium level occurs at approximately day 10 after Prolia dosing in subjects with normal renal function.

In clinical studies, subjects with impaired renal function were more likely to have greater reductions in serum calcium levels compared to subjects with normal renal function. In a study of 55 subjects with varying degrees of renal function, serum calcium levels < 7.5 mg/dL or symptomatic hypocalcemia were observed in 5 subjects. These included no subjects in the normal renal function group, 10% of subjects in the creatinine clearance 50 to 80 mL/min group, 29% of subjects in the creatinine clearance < 30 mL/min group, and 29% of subjects in the hemodialysis group. These subjects did not receive calcium and vitamin D supplementation. In a study of 4550 postmenopausal women with osteoporosis, the mean change from baseline in serum calcium level 10 days after Prolia dosing was -5.5% in subjects with creatinine clearance < 30 mL/min vs. -3.1% in subjects with creatinine clearance ≥ 30 mL/min.

Serious Infections

Receptor activator of nuclear factor kappa-B ligand (RANKL) is expressed on activated T and B lymphocytes and in lymph nodes. Therefore, a RANKL inhibitor such as Prolia may increase the risk of infection.

In the clinical study of 7808 postmenopausal women with osteoporosis, the incidence of infections resulting in death was 0.2% in both placebo and Prolia treatment groups. However, the incidence of nonfatal serious infections was 3.3% in the placebo and 4.0% in the Prolia groups. Hospitalizations due to serious infections in the abdomen (0.7% placebo vs. 0.9% Prolia), urinary tract (0.5% placebo vs. 0.7% Prolia), and ear (0.0% placebo vs. 0.1% Prolia) were reported. Endocarditis was reported in no placebo patients and 3 patients receiving Prolia.

Skin infections, including erysipelas and cellulitis, leading to hospitalization were reported more frequently in patients treated with Prolia (< 0.1% placebo vs. 0.4% Prolia).

The incidence of opportunistic infections was similar to that reported with placebo.

Dermatologic Reactions

A significantly higher number of patients treated with Prolia developed epidermal and dermal adverse events (such as dermatitis, eczema, and rashes), with these events reported in 8.2% of the placebo and 10.8% of the Prolia groups (p < 0.0001). Most of these events were not specific to the injection site [see Warnings and Precautions (5.7)].

Osteonecrosis of the Jaw

ONJ has been reported in the osteoporosis clinical trial program in patients treated with Prolia [see Warnings and Precautions (5.4)].

Atypical Subtrochanteric and Diaphyseal Fractures

In the osteoporosis clinical trial program, atypical femoral fractures were reported in patients treated with Prolia. The duration of Prolia exposure to time of atypical femoral fracture diagnosis was as early as 2½ years [see Warnings and Precautions (5.5)].

Pancreatitis

Pancreatitis was reported in 4 patients (0.1%) in the placebo and 8 patients (0.2%) in the Prolia groups. Of these reports, 1 patient in the placebo group and all 8 patients in the Prolia group had serious events, including one death in the Prolia group. Several patients had a prior history of pancreatitis. The time from product administration to event occurrence was variable.

New Malignancies

The overall incidence of new malignancies was 4.3% in the placebo and 4.8% in the Prolia groups. New malignancies related to the breast (0.7% placebo vs. 0.9% Prolia), reproductive system (0.2% placebo vs. 0.5% Prolia), and gastrointestinal system (0.6% placebo vs. 0.9% Prolia) were reported. A causal relationship to drug exposure has not been established.

Treatment to Increase Bone Mass in Men with Osteoporosis

The safety of Prolia in the treatment of men with osteoporosis was assessed in a 1-year randomized, double-blind, placebo-controlled study. A total of 120 men were exposed to placebo and 120 men were exposed to Prolia administered subcutaneously once every 6 months as a single 60 mg dose. All men were instructed to take at least 1000 mg of calcium and 800 IU of vitamin D supplementation per day.

The incidence of all-cause mortality was 0.8% (n = 1) in the placebo group and 0.8% (n = 1) in the Prolia group. The incidence of nonfatal serious adverse events was 7.5% in the placebo group and 8.3% in the Prolia group. The percentage of patients who withdrew from the study due to adverse events was 0% and 2.5% for the placebo and Prolia groups, respectively.

Adverse reactions reported in ≥ 5% of men with osteoporosis and more frequently with Prolia than in the placebo-treated patients were: back pain (6.7% placebo vs. 8.3% Prolia), arthralgia (5.8% placebo vs. 6.7% Prolia), and nasopharyngitis (5.8% placebo vs. 6.7% Prolia).

Serious Infections

Serious infection was reported in 1 patient (0.8%) in the placebo group and no patients in the Prolia group.

Dermatologic Reactions

Epidermal and dermal adverse events (such as dermatitis, eczema, and rashes) were reported in 4 patients (3.3%) in the placebo group and 5 patients (4.2%) in the Prolia group.

Osteonecrosis of the Jaw

No cases of ONJ were reported.

Pancreatitis

Pancreatitis was reported in 1 patient (0.8%) in the placebo group and 1 patient (0.8%) in the Prolia group.

New Malignancies

New malignancies were reported in no patients in the placebo group and 4 (3.3%) patients (3 prostate cancers, 1 basal cell carcinoma) in the Prolia group.

Treatment of Bone Loss in Patients Receiving Androgen Deprivation Therapy for Prostate Cancer or Adjuvant Aromatase Inhibitor Therapy for Breast Cancer

The safety of Prolia in the treatment of bone loss in men with nonmetastatic prostate cancer receiving androgen deprivation therapy (ADT) was assessed in a 3-year, randomized, double-blind, placebo-controlled, multinational study of 1468 men aged 48 to 97 years. A total of 725 men were exposed to placebo and 731 men were exposed to Prolia administered once every 6 months as a single 60 mg subcutaneous dose. All men were instructed to take at least 1000 mg of calcium and 400 IU of vitamin D supplementation per day.

The incidence of serious adverse events was 30.6% in the placebo group and 34.6% in the Prolia group. The percentage of patients who withdrew from the study due to adverse events was 6.1% and 7.0% for the placebo and Prolia groups, respectively.

The safety of Prolia in the treatment of bone loss in women with nonmetastatic breast cancer receiving aromatase inhibitor (AI) therapy was assessed in a 2-year, randomized, double-blind, placebo-controlled, multinational study of 252 postmenopausal women aged 35 to 84 years. A total of 120 women were exposed to placebo and 129 women were exposed to Prolia administered once every 6 months as a single 60 mg subcutaneous dose. All women were instructed to take at least 1000 mg of calcium and 400 IU of vitamin D supplementation per day.

The incidence of serious adverse events was 9.2% in the placebo group and 14.7% in the Prolia group. The percentage of patients who withdrew from the study due to adverse events was 4.2% and 0.8% for the placebo and Prolia groups, respectively.

Adverse reactions reported in ≥ 10% of Prolia-treated patients receiving ADT for prostate cancer or adjuvant AI therapy for breast cancer, and more frequently than in the placebo-treated patients were: arthralgia (13.0% placebo vs. 14.3% Prolia) and back pain (10.5% placebo vs. 11.5% Prolia). Pain in extremity (7.7% placebo vs. 9.9% Prolia) and musculoskeletal pain (3.8% placebo vs. 6.0% Prolia) have also been reported in clinical trials. Additionally in Prolia-treated men with nonmetastatic prostate cancer receiving ADT, a greater incidence of cataracts was observed (1.2% placebo vs. 4.7% Prolia). Hypocalcemia (serum calcium < 8.4 mg/dL) was reported only in Prolia-treated patients (2.4% vs. 0%) at the month 1 visit.

6.2 Postmarketing Experience

Because postmarketing reactions are reported voluntarily from a population of uncertain size, it is not always possible to reliably estimate their frequency or establish a causal relationship to drug exposure.

The following adverse reactions have been identified during post approval use of Prolia:
- Drug-related hypersensitivity reactions: anaphylaxis, rash, urticaria, facial swelling, and erythema
- Hypocalcemia: severe symptomatic hypocalcemia
- Musculoskeletal pain, including severe cases
- Parathyroid Hormone (PTH): Marked elevation in serum PTH in patients with severe renal impairment (creatinine clearance < 30 mL/min) or receiving dialysis.

6.3 Immunogenicity

Denosumab is a human monoclonal antibody. As with all therapeutic proteins, there is potential for immunogenicity. Using an electrochemiluminescent bridging immunoassay, less than 1% (55 out of 8113) of patients treated with Prolia for up to 5 years tested positive for binding antibodies (including pre-existing, transient, and developing antibodies). None of the patients tested positive for neutralizing antibodies, as was assessed using a chemiluminescent cell-based in vitro biological assay. No evidence of altered pharmacokinetic profile, toxicity profile, or clinical response was associated with binding antibody development.

The incidence of antibody formation is highly dependent on the sensitivity and specificity of the assay. Additionally, the observed incidence of a positive antibody (including neutralizing antibody) test result may be influenced by several factors, including assay methodology, sample handling, timing of sample collection, concomitant medications, and underlying disease. For these reasons, comparison of antibodies to denosumab with the incidence of antibodies to other products may be misleading.

7 DRUG INTERACTIONS

In subjects with postmenopausal osteoporosis, Prolia (60 mg subcutaneous injection) did not affect the pharmacokinetics of midazolam, which was metabolized by cytochrome P450 3A4 (CYP3A4), indicating that it should not affect the pharmacokinetics of drugs metabolized by this enzyme in this population [see Clinical Pharmacology (12.3)].

8 USE IN SPECIFIC POPULATIONS

8.1 Pregnancy

Pregnancy Category X

Risk Summary

Prolia may cause fetal harm when administered to a pregnant woman based on findings in animals. In utero denosumab exposure in cynomolgus monkeys resulted in increased fetal loss, stillbirths, and postnatal mortality, along with evidence of absent lymph nodes, abnormal bone growth and decreased neonatal growth. Prolia is contraindicated in women who are pregnant. If this drug is used during pregnancy, or if the patient becomes pregnant while taking this drug, the patient should be apprised of the potential hazard to a fetus.

Women who become pregnant during Prolia treatment are encouraged to enroll in Amgen's Pregnancy Surveillance Program. Patients or their physicians should call 1-800-77-AMGEN (1-800-772-6436) to enroll.

Clinical Considerations

The effects of Prolia on the fetus are likely to be greater during the second and third trimesters of pregnancy. Monoclonal antibodies, such as denosumab, are transported across the placenta in a linear fashion as pregnancy progresses, with the largest amount transferred during the third trimester. If the patient becomes pregnant during Prolia therapy, treatment should be discontinued and the patient should consult their physician.

Animal Data

The effects of denosumab on prenatal development have been studied in both cynomolgus monkeys and genetically engineered mice in which RANK ligand (RANKL) expression was turned off by gene removal (a "knockout mouse"). In cynomolgus monkeys dosed subcutaneously with denosumab throughout pregnancy at a pharmacologically active dose, there was increased fetal loss during gestation, stillbirths, and postnatal mortality. Other findings in offspring included absence of axillary, inguinal, mandibular, and mesenteric lymph nodes; abnormal bone growth, reduced bone strength, reduced hematopoiesis, dental dysplasia and tooth malalignment; and decreased neonatal growth. At birth out to 1 month of age, infants had measurable blood levels of denosumab (22-621% of maternal levels).

Following a recovery period from birth out to 6 months of age, the effects on bone quality and strength returned to normal; there were no adverse effects on tooth eruption, though dental dysplasia was still apparent; axillary and inguinal lymph nodes remained absent, while mandibular and mesenteric lymph nodes were present, though small; and minimal to moderate mineralization in multiple tissues was seen in one recovery animal. There was no evidence of maternal harm prior to labor; adverse maternal effects occurred infrequently during labor. Maternal mammary gland development was normal. There was no fetal NOAEL (no observable adverse effect level) established for this study because only one dose of 50 mg/kg was evaluated.

In RANKL knockout mice, absence of RANKL (the target of denosumab) also caused fetal lymph node agenesis and led to postnatal impairment of dentition and bone growth. Pregnant RANKL knockout mice showed altered maturation of the maternal mammary gland, leading to impaired lactation [see Use in Specific Populations (8.3) and Nonclinical Toxicology (13.2)].

8.3 Nursing Mothers

It is not known whether Prolia is excreted into human milk. Measurable concentrations of denosumab were present in the maternal milk of cynomolgus monkeys up to 1 month after the last dose of denosumab (≤ 0.5% milk:serum ratio). Because many drugs are excreted in human milk and because of the potential for serious adverse reactions in nursing infants from Prolia, a decision should be made whether to discontinue nursing or discontinue the drug, taking into account the importance of the drug to the mother.

Maternal exposure to Prolia during pregnancy may impair mammary gland development and lactation based on animal studies in pregnant mice lacking the RANK/RANKL signaling pathway that have shown altered maturation of the maternal mammary gland, leading to impaired lactation postpartum. However in cynomolgus monkeys treated with denosumab throughout pregnancy, maternal mammary gland development was normal, with no impaired lactation. Mammary gland histopathology at 6 months of age was normal in female offspring exposed to denosumab in utero; however, development and lactation have not been fully evaluated [see Use in Specific Populations (8.1) and Nonclinical Toxicology (13.2)].

8.4 Pediatric Use

Prolia is not recommended in pediatric patients. The safety and effectiveness of Prolia in pediatric patients have not been established.

Treatment with Prolia may impair bone growth in children with open growth plates and may inhibit eruption of dentition. In neonatal rats, inhibition of RANKL (the target of Prolia therapy) with a construct of osteoprotegerin bound to Fc (OPG-Fc) at doses ≤ 10 mg/kg was associated with inhibition of bone growth and tooth eruption. Adolescent primates treated with denosumab at doses 10 and 50 times (10 and 50 mg/kg dose) higher than the recommended human dose of 60 mg administered every 6 months, based on body weight (mg/kg), had abnormal growth plates, considered to be consistent with the pharmacological activity of denosumab.

Cynomolgus monkeys exposed in utero to denosumab exhibited bone abnormalities, an absence of axillary, inguinal, mandibular, and mesenteric lymph nodes, reduced hematopoiesis, tooth malalignment, and decreased neonatal growth. Some bone abnormalities recovered once exposure was ceased following birth; however, axillary and inguinal lymph nodes remained absent 6 months post-birth [see Use in Specific Populations (8.1)].

8.5 Geriatric Use

Of the total number of patients in clinical studies of Prolia, 9943 patients (76%) were ≥ 65 years old, while 3576 (27%) were ≥ 75 years old. Of the patients in the osteoporosis study in men, 133 patients (55%) were ≥ 65 years old, while 39 patients (16%) were ≥ 75 years old. No overall differences in safety or efficacy were observed between these patients and younger patients and other reported clinical experience has not identified differences in responses between the elderly and younger patients, but greater sensitivity of some older individuals cannot be ruled out.

8.6 Renal Impairment

No dose adjustment is necessary in patients with renal impairment.

In clinical studies, patients with severe renal impairment (creatinine clearance < 30 mL/min) or receiving dialysis were at greater risk of developing hypocalcemia. Consider the benefit-risk profile when administering Prolia to patients with severe renal impairment or receiving dialysis. Clinical monitoring of calcium and mineral levels (phosphorus and magnesium) is highly recommended. Adequate intake of calcium and vitamin D is important in patients with severe renal impairment or receiving dialysis [see Warnings and Precautions (5.3), Adverse Reactions (6.1), and Clinical Pharmacology (12.3)].

8.7 Hepatic Impairment

No clinical studies have been conducted to evaluate the effect of hepatic impairment on the pharmacokinetics of Prolia.

8.8 Males

Prolia may cause fetal harm [see Use in Specific Populations (8.1)].

The extent to which denosumab is present in seminal fluid is unknown. There is a potential for fetal exposure to denosumab when a man treated with Prolia has unprotected sexual intercourse with a pregnant partner. The risk of fetal harm is likely to be low. Advise men being treated with Prolia who have a pregnant partner of this potential risk.

10 OVERDOSAGE

There is no experience with overdosage with Prolia.

11 DESCRIPTION

Prolia (denosumab) is a human IgG2 monoclonal antibody with affinity and specificity for human RANKL (receptor activator of nuclear factor kappa-B ligand). Denosumab has an approximate molecular weight of 147 kDa and is produced in genetically engineered mammalian (Chinese hamster ovary) cells.

Prolia is a sterile, preservative-free, clear, colorless to pale yellow solution.

Each 1 mL single-use prefilled syringe of Prolia contains 60 mg denosumab (60 mg/mL solution), 4.7% sorbitol, 17 mM acetate, 0.01% polysorbate 20, Water for Injection (USP), and sodium hydroxide to a pH of 5.2.

Each 1 mL single-use vial of Prolia contains 60 mg denosumab (60 mg/mL solution), 4.7% sorbitol, 17 mM acetate, Water for Injection (USP), and sodium hydroxide to a pH of 5.2.

12 CLINICAL PHARMACOLOGY

12.1 Mechanism of Action

Prolia binds to RANKL, a transmembrane or soluble protein essential for the formation, function, and survival of osteoclasts, the cells responsible for bone resorption. Prolia prevents RANKL from activating its receptor, RANK, on the surface of osteoclasts and their precursors. Prevention of the RANKL/RANK interaction inhibits osteoclast formation, function, and survival, thereby decreasing bone resorption and increasing bone mass and strength in both cortical and trabecular bone.

12.2 Pharmacodynamics

In clinical studies, treatment with 60 mg of Prolia resulted in reduction in the bone resorption marker serum type 1 C-telopeptide (CTX) by approximately 85% by 3 days, with maximal reductions occurring by 1 month. CTX levels were below the limit of assay quantitation (0.049 ng/mL) in 39% to 68% of patients 1 to 3 months after dosing of Prolia. At the end of each dosing interval, CTX reductions were partially attenuated from a maximal reduction of ≥ 87% to ≥ 45% (range: 45% to 80%), as serum denosumab levels diminished, reflecting the reversibility of the effects of Prolia on bone remodeling. These effects were sustained with continued treatment. Upon reinitiation, the degree of inhibition of CTX by Prolia was similar to that observed in patients initiating Prolia treatment.

Consistent with the physiological coupling of bone formation and resorption in skeletal remodeling, subsequent reductions in bone formation markers (i.e. osteocalcin and procollagen type 1 N-terminal peptide [P1NP]) were observed starting 1 month after the first dose of Prolia. After discontinuation of Prolia therapy, markers of bone resorption increased to levels 40% to 60% above pretreatment values but returned to baseline levels within 12 months.

12.3 Pharmacokinetics

In a study conducted in healthy male and female volunteers (n = 73, age range: 18 to 64 years) following a single subcutaneously administered Prolia dose of 60 mg after fasting (at least for 12 hours), the mean maximum denosumab concentration (C_{max}) was 6.75 mcg/mL (standard deviation [SD] = 1.89 mcg/mL). The median time to maximum denosumab concentration (T_{max}) was 10 days (range: 3 to 21 days). After C_{max}, serum denosumab concentrations declined over a period of 4 to 5 months with a mean half-life of 25.4 days (SD = 8.5 days; n = 46). The mean area-under-the-concentration-time curve up to 16 weeks ($AUC_{0-16\ weeks}$) of denosumab was 316 mcg×day/mL (SD = 101 mcg×day/mL). No accumulation or change in denosumab pharmacokinetics with time was observed upon multiple dosing of 60 mg subcutaneously administered once every 6 months.

Prolia pharmacokinetics were not affected by the formation of binding antibodies.

A population pharmacokinetic analysis was performed to evaluate the effects of demographic characteristics. This analysis showed no notable differences in pharmacokinetics with age (in postmenopausal women), race, or body weight (36 to 140 kg).

Drug Interactions

In a study of 17 postmenopausal women with osteoporosis, midazolam (2 mg oral) was administered two weeks after a single dose of denosumab (60 mg subcutaneous injection), which approximates the T_{max} of denosumab. Denosumab did not affect the pharmacokinetics of midazolam, which is metabolized by cytochrome P450 3A4 (CYP3A4). This indicates that denosumab should not alter the pharmacokinetics of drugs metabolized by CYP3A4 in postmenopausal women with osteoporosis.

Specific Populations

Gender: Mean serum denosumab concentration-time profiles observed in a study conducted in healthy men ≥ 50 years were similar to those observed in a study conducted in postmenopausal women using the same dose regimen.

Age: The pharmacokinetics of denosumab were not affected by age across all populations studied whose ages ranged from 28 to 87 years.

Race: The pharmacokinetics of denosumab were not affected by race.

Renal Impairment: In a study of 55 patients with varying degrees of renal function, including patients on dialysis, the degree of renal impairment had no effect on the pharmacokinetics of denosumab; thus, dose adjustment for renal impairment is not necessary.

Hepatic Impairment: No clinical studies have been conducted to evaluate the effect of hepatic impairment on the pharmacokinetics of denosumab.

13 NONCLINICAL TOXICOLOGY

13.1 Carcinogenesis, Mutagenesis, Impairment of Fertility

Carcinogenicity

The carcinogenic potential of denosumab has not been evaluated in long-term animal studies.

Mutagenicity

The genotoxic potential of denosumab has not been evaluated.

Impairment of Fertility

Denosumab had no effect on female fertility or male reproductive organs in monkeys at doses that were 13- to 50-fold higher than the recommended human dose of 60 mg subcutaneously administered once every 6 months, based on body weight (mg/kg).

13.2 Animal Toxicology and/or Pharmacology

Denosumab is an inhibitor of osteoclastic bone resorption via inhibition of RANKL.

In ovariectomized monkeys, once-monthly treatment with denosumab suppressed bone turnover and increased bone mineral density (BMD) and strength of cancellous and cortical bone at doses 50-fold higher than the recommended human dose of 60 mg administered once every 6 months, based on body weight (mg/kg). Bone tissue was normal with no evidence of mineralization defects, accumulation of osteoid, or woven bone.

Because the biological activity of denosumab in animals is specific to nonhuman primates, evaluation of genetically engineered ("knockout") mice or use of other biological inhibitors of the RANK/RANKL pathway, namely OPG-Fc, provided additional information on the pharmacodynamic properties of denosumab. RANK/RANKL knockout mice exhibited absence of lymph node formation, as well as an absence of lactation due to inhibition of mammary gland maturation (lobulo-alveolar gland development during pregnancy). Neonatal RANK/RANKL knockout mice exhibited reduced bone growth and lack of tooth eruption. A corroborative study in 2-week-old rats given the RANKL inhibitor OPG-Fc also showed reduced bone growth, altered growth plates, and impaired tooth eruption. These changes were partially reversible in this model when dosing with the RANKL inhibitors was discontinued.

14 CLINICAL STUDIES

14.1 Postmenopausal Women with Osteoporosis

The efficacy and safety of Prolia in the treatment of postmenopausal osteoporosis was demonstrated in a 3-year, randomized, double-blind, placebo-controlled trial. Enrolled women had a baseline BMD T–score between -2.5 and -4.0 at either the lumbar spine or total hip. Women with other diseases (such as rheumatoid arthritis, osteogenesis imperfecta, and Paget's disease) or on therapies that affect bone were excluded from this study. The 7808 enrolled women were aged 60 to 91 years with a mean age of 72 years. Overall, the mean baseline lumbar spine BMD T-score was -2.8, and 23% of women had a vertebral fracture at baseline. Women were randomized to receive subcutaneous injections of either placebo (N = 3906) or Prolia 60 mg (N = 3902) once every 6 months. All women received at least 1000 mg calcium and 400 IU vitamin D supplementation daily.

The primary efficacy variable was the incidence of new morphometric (radiologically-diagnosed) vertebral fractures at 3 years. Vertebral fractures were diagnosed based on lateral spine radiographs (T4-L4) using a semiquantitative scoring method. Secondary efficacy variables included the incidence of hip fracture and nonvertebral fracture, assessed at 3 years.

Effect on Vertebral Fractures

Prolia significantly reduced the incidence of new morphometric vertebral fractures at 1, 2, and 3 years (p < 0.0001), as shown in Table 2. The incidence of new vertebral fractures at year 3 was 7.2% in the placebo-treated women compared to 2.3% for the Prolia-treated women. The absolute risk reduction was 4.8% and relative risk reduction was 68% for new morphometric vertebral fractures at year 3. [See table 2 above]

Prolia was effective in reducing the risk for new morphometric vertebral fractures regardless of age, baseline rate of bone turnover, baseline BMD, baseline history of fracture, or prior use of a drug for osteoporosis.

Effect on Hip Fractures

The incidence of hip fracture was 1.2% for placebo-treated women compared to 0.7% for Prolia-treated women at year 3. The age-adjusted absolute risk reduction of hip fractures was 0.3% with a relative risk reduction of 40% at 3 years (p = 0.04) (Figure 1).

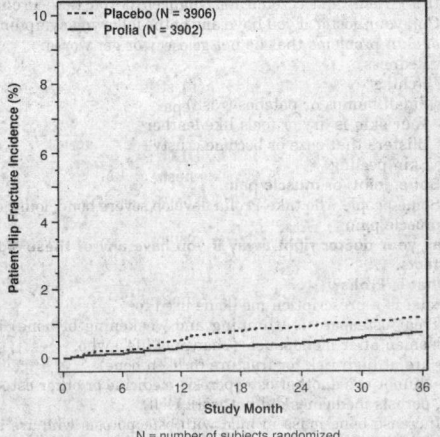

Figure 1. Cumulative Incidence of Hip Fractures Over 3 Years

Effect on Nonvertebral Fractures

Treatment with Prolia resulted in a significant reduction in the incidence of nonvertebral fractures (Table 3). [See table 3 above]

Effect on Bone Mineral Density (BMD)

Treatment with Prolia significantly increased BMD at all anatomic sites measured at 3 years. The treatment differences in BMD at 3 years were 8.8% at the lumbar spine,

Table 2. The Effect of Prolia on the Incidence of New Vertebral Fractures in Postmenopausal Women

	Proportion of Women With Fracture (%)*		Absolute Risk Reduction (%)[†] (95% CI)	Relative Risk Reduction (%)[†] (95% CI)
	Placebo N = 3691 (%)	Prolia N = 3702 (%)		
0-1 Year	2.2	0.9	1.4 (0.8, 1.9)	61 (42, 74)
0-2 Years	5.0	1.4	3.5 (2.7, 4.3)	71 (61, 79)
0-3 Years	7.2	2.3	4.8 (3.9, 5.8)	68 (59, 74)

* Event rates based on crude rates in each interval.
† Absolute risk reduction and relative risk reduction based on Mantel-Haenszel method adjusting for age group variable.

Table 3. The Effect of Prolia on the Incidence of Nonvertebral Fractures at Year 3

	Proportion of Women With Fracture (%)*		Absolute Risk Reduction (%) (95% CI)	Relative Risk Reduction (%) (95% CI)
	Placebo N = 3906 (%)	Prolia N = 3902 (%)		
Nonvertebral fracture[†]	8.0	6.5	1.5 (0.3, 2.7)	20 (5, 33)[‡]

* Event rates based on Kaplan-Meier estimates at 3 years.
† Excluding those of the vertebrae (cervical, thoracic, and lumbar), skull, facial, mandible, metacarpus, and finger and toe phalanges.
‡ p-value = 0.01.

6.4% at the total hip, and 5.2% at the femoral neck. Consistent effects on BMD were observed at the lumbar spine, regardless of baseline age, race, weight/body mass index (BMI), baseline BMD, and level of bone turnover.

After Prolia discontinuation, BMD returned to approximately baseline levels within 12 months.

Bone Histology and Histomorphometry

A total of 115 transiliac crest bone biopsy specimens were obtained from 92 postmenopausal women with osteoporosis at either month 24 and/or month 36 (53 specimens in Prolia group, 62 specimens in placebo group). Of the biopsies obtained, 115 (100%) were adequate for qualitative histology and 7 (6%) were adequate for full quantitative histomorphometry assessment.

Qualitative histology assessments showed normal architecture and quality with no evidence of mineralization defects, woven bone, or marrow fibrosis in patients treated with Prolia.

The presence of double tetracycline labeling in a biopsy specimen provides an indication of active bone remodeling, while the absence of tetracycline label suggests suppressed bone formation. In patients treated with Prolia, 35% had no tetracycline label present at the month 24 biopsy and 38% had no tetracycline label present at the month 36 biopsy, while 100% of placebo-treated patients had double label present at both time points. When compared to placebo, treatment with Prolia resulted in virtually absent activation frequency and markedly reduced bone formation rates. However, the long-term consequences of this degree of suppression of bone remodeling are unknown.

14.2 Treatment to Increase Bone Mass in Men with Osteoporosis

The efficacy and safety of Prolia in the treatment to increase bone mass in men with osteoporosis was demonstrated in a 1-year, randomized, double-blind, placebo-controlled trial. Enrolled men had a baseline BMD T-score between -2.0 and -3.5 at the lumbar spine or femoral neck. Men with a BMD T-score between -1.0 and -3.5 at the lumbar spine or femoral neck were also enrolled if there was a history of prior fragility fracture. Men with other diseases (such as rheumatoid arthritis, osteogenesis imperfecta, and Paget's disease) or on therapies that may affect bone were excluded from this study. The 242 men enrolled in the study ranged in age from 31 to 84 years with a mean age of 65 years. Men were randomized to receive SC injections of either placebo (n = 121) or Prolia 60 mg (n = 121) once every 6 months. All men received at least 1000 mg calcium and at least 800 IU vitamin D supplementation daily.

Effect on Bone Mineral Density (BMD)

The primary efficacy variable was percent change in lumbar spine BMD from baseline to 1 year. Secondary efficacy variables included percent change in total hip, and femoral neck BMD from baseline to 1 year.

Treatment with Prolia significantly increased BMD at 1 year. The treatment differences in BMD at 1 year were 4.8% (+0.9% placebo, +5.7% Prolia; (95% CI: 4.0, 5.6); p < 0.0001) at the lumbar spine, 2.0% (+0.3% placebo, +2.4% Prolia) at the total hip, and 2.2% (0.0% placebo, +2.1% Prolia) at femoral neck. Consistent effects on BMD were observed at the lumbar spine regardless of baseline age, race, BMD, testosterone concentrations and level of bone turnover.

Bone Histology and Histomorphometry

A total of 29 transiliac crest bone biopsy specimens were obtained from men with osteoporosis at 12 months (17 specimens in Prolia group, 12 specimens in placebo group). Of the biopsies obtained, 29 (100%) were adequate for qualitative histology and, in Prolia patients, 6 (35%) were adequate for full quantitative histomorphometry assessment. Qualitative histology assessments showed normal architecture and quality with no evidence of mineralization defects, woven bone, or marrow fibrosis in patients treated with Prolia. The presence of double tetracycline labeling in a biopsy specimen provides an indication of active bone remodeling, while the absence of tetracycline label suggests suppressed bone formation. In patients treated with Prolia, 6% had no tetracycline label present at the month 12 biopsy, while 100% of placebo-treated patients had double label present. When compared to placebo, treatment with Prolia resulted in markedly reduced bone formation rates. However, the long-term consequences of this degree of suppression of bone remodeling are unknown.

14.3 Treatment of Bone Loss in Men with Prostate Cancer

The efficacy and safety of Prolia in the treatment of bone loss in men with nonmetastatic prostate cancer receiving androgen deprivation therapy (ADT) were demonstrated in a 3–year, randomized (1:1), double-blind, placebo-controlled, multinational study. Men less than 70 years of age had either a BMD T–score at the lumbar spine, total hip, or femoral neck between –1.0 and -4.0, or a history of an osteoporotic fracture. The mean baseline lumbar spine BMD T-score was -0.4, and 22% of men had a vertebral fracture at baseline. The 1468 men enrolled ranged in age from 48 to 97 years (median 76 years). Men were randomized to receive subcutaneous injections of either placebo (n = 734) or Prolia 60 mg (n = 734) once every 6 months for a total of 6 doses. Randomization was stratified by age (< 70 years vs. ≥ 70 years) and duration of ADT at trial entry (≤ 6 months vs. > 6 months). Seventy-nine percent of patients received ADT for more than 6 months at study entry. All men received at least 1000 mg calcium and 400 IU vitamin D supplementation daily.

Effect on Bone Mineral Density (BMD)

The primary efficacy variable was percent change in lumbar spine BMD from baseline to month 24. An additional key secondary efficacy variable was the incidence of new vertebral fracture through month 36 diagnosed based on x-ray evaluation by two independent radiologists. Lumbar spine BMD was higher at 2 years in Prolia-treated patients as compared to placebo-treated patients [-1.0% placebo, +5.6% Prolia; treatment difference 6.7% (95% CI: 6.2, 7.1); p < 0.0001].

With approximately 62% of patients followed for 3 years, treatment differences in BMD at 3 years were 7.9% (-1.2% placebo, +6.8% Prolia) at the lumbar spine, 5.7% (-2.6% placebo, +3.2% Prolia) at the total hip, and 4.9% (-1.8% placebo, +3.0% Prolia) at the femoral neck. Consistent effects on BMD were observed at the lumbar spine in relevant subgroups defined by baseline age, BMD, and baseline history of vertebral fracture.

Effect on Vertebral Fractures

Prolia significantly reduced the incidence of new vertebral fractures at 3 years (p = 0.0125), as shown in Table 4.

Table 4. The Effect of Prolia on the Incidence of New Vertebral Fractures in Men with Nonmetastatic Prostate Cancer

	Proportion of Men With Fracture (%)*		Absolute Risk Reduction (%)[†] (95% CI)	Relative Risk Reduction (%)[†] (95% CI)
	Placebo N = 673 (%)	Prolia N = 679 (%)		
0-1 Year	1.9	0.3	1.6 (0.5, 2.8)	85 (33, 97)
0-2 Years	3.3	1.0	2.2 (0.7, 3.8)	69 (27, 86)
0-3 Years	3.9	1.5	2.4 (0.7, 4.1)	62 (22, 81)

* Event rates based on crude rates in each interval.
† Absolute risk reduction and relative risk reduction based on Mantel-Haenszel method adjusting for age group and ADT duration variables.

[See table 4 above]

14.4 Treatment of Bone Loss in Women with Breast Cancer

The efficacy and safety of Prolia in the treatment of bone loss in women receiving adjuvant aromatase inhibitor (AI) therapy for breast cancer was assessed in a 2–year, randomized (1:1), double-blind, placebo-controlled, multinational study. Women had baseline BMD T-scores between –1.0 to –2.5 at the lumbar spine, total hip, or femoral neck, and had not experienced fracture after age 25. The mean baseline lumbar spine BMD T-score was -1.1, and 2.0% of women had a vertebral fracture at baseline. The 252 women enrolled ranged in age from 35 to 84 years (median 59 years). Women were randomized to receive subcutaneous injections of either placebo (n = 125) or Prolia 60 mg (n = 127) once every 6 months for a total of 4 doses. Randomization was stratified by duration of adjuvant AI therapy at trial entry (≤ 6 months vs. > 6 months). Sixty-two percent of patients received adjuvant AI therapy for more than 6 months at study entry. All women received at least 1000 mg calcium and 400 IU vitamin D supplementation daily.

Effect on Bone Mineral Density (BMD)
The primary efficacy variable was percent change in lumbar spine BMD from baseline to month 12. Lumbar spine BMD was higher at 12 months in Prolia-treated patients as compared to placebo-treated patients [-0.7% placebo, +4.8% Prolia; treatment difference 5.5% (95% CI: 4.8, 6.3); p < 0.0001].

With approximately 81% of patients followed for 2 years, treatment differences in BMD at 2 years were 7.6% (-1.4% placebo, +6.2% Prolia) at the lumbar spine, 4.7 % (-1.0% placebo, +3.8% Prolia) at the total hip, and 3.6% (-0.8% placebo, +2.8% Prolia) at the femoral neck.

16 HOW SUPPLIED/STORAGE AND HANDLING

Prolia is supplied in a single-use prefilled syringe with a safety guard or in a single-use vial. The grey needle cap on the single-use prefilled syringe contains dry natural rubber (a derivative of latex).

60 mg/1 mL in a single-use prefilled syringe	1 per carton	NDC 55513-710-01
60 mg/1 mL in a single-use vial	1 per carton	NDC 55513-720-01

Store Prolia in a refrigerator at 2°C to 8°C (36°F to 46°F) in the original carton. Do not freeze. Prior to administration, Prolia may be allowed to reach room temperature (up to 25°C/77°F) in the original container. Once removed from the refrigerator, Prolia must not be exposed to temperatures above 25°C/77°F and must be used within 14 days. If not used within the 14 days, Prolia should be discarded. Do not use Prolia after the expiry date printed on the label.
Protect Prolia from direct light and heat.
Avoid vigorous shaking of Prolia.

17 PATIENT COUNSELING INFORMATION

See FDA-approved patient labeling (Medication Guide).

17.1 Drug Products with Same Active Ingredient
Advise patients that denosumab is also marketed as Xgeva, and if taking Prolia, they should not receive Xgeva [see Warnings and Precautions (5.1)].

17.2 Hypersensitivity
Advise patients to seek prompt medical attention if signs or symptoms of hypersensitivity reactions occur. Advise patients who have had signs or symptoms of systemic hypersensitivity reactions that they should not receive denosumab (Prolia or Xgeva) [see Warnings & Precautions (5.2), Contraindications (4.3)].

17.3 Hypocalcemia
Adequately supplement patients with calcium and vitamin D and instruct them on the importance of maintaining serum calcium levels while receiving Prolia [see Warnings

and Precautions (5.3) and Use in Specific Populations (8.6)]. Advise patients to seek prompt medical attention if they develop signs or symptoms of hypocalcemia.

17.4 Osteonecrosis of the Jaw
Advise patients to maintain good oral hygiene during treatment with Prolia and to inform their dentist prior to dental procedures that they are receiving Prolia. Patients should inform their physician or dentist if they experience persistent pain and/or slow healing of the mouth or jaw after dental surgery [see Warnings and Precautions (5.4)].

17.5 Atypical Subtrochanteric and Diaphyseal Femoral Fractures
Advise patients to report new or unusual thigh, hip, or groin pain [see Warnings and Precautions (5.5)].

17.6 Serious Infections
Advise patients to seek prompt medical attention if they develop signs or symptoms of infections, including cellulitis [see Warnings and Precautions (5.6)].

17.7 Dermatologic Reactions
Advise patients to seek prompt medical attention if they develop signs or symptoms of dermatological reactions (dermatitis, rashes, and eczema) [see Warnings and Precautions (5.7)].

17.8 Musculoskeletal Pain
Inform patients that severe bone, joint, and/or muscle pain have been reported in patients taking Prolia. Patients should report severe symptoms if they develop [see Warnings and Precautions (5.8)].

17.9 Embryo-Fetal Toxicity
Pregnancy
Advise patients that Prolia is contraindicated in women who are pregnant and may cause fetal harm [see Contraindications (4.2), Use in Specific Populations (8.1)].
Males
Advise patients of a potential for fetal exposure to denosumab when a man treated with Prolia has unprotected sexual intercourse with a pregnant partner [see Use in Specific Populations (8.8)]

17.10 Nursing Mothers
Advise patients that because many drugs are excreted in human milk and because of the potential for serious adverse reactions in nursing infants from Prolia, a decision should be made whether to discontinue nursing or discontinue the drug, taking into account the importance of the drug to the mother [see Use in Specific Populations (8.3)].

17.11 Schedule of Administration
If a dose of Prolia is missed, administer the injection as soon as convenient. Thereafter, schedule injections every 6 months from the date of the last injection.

[Amgen Logo]
Manufactured by:
Amgen Manufacturing Limited, a subsidiary of Amgen Inc.
One Amgen Center Drive
Thousand Oaks, California 91320-1799
Patent: http://pat.amgen.com/prolia/
© 2010-2014 Amgen Inc. All rights reserved.
1xxxxxx - v7

MEDICATION GUIDE
Prolia® (PRŌ-lee-a)
(denosumab)
Injection, for subcutaneous use

Read the Medication Guide that comes with Prolia before you start taking it and each time you get a refill. There may be new information. This Medication Guide does not take the place of talking with your doctor about your medical condition or treatment. Talk to your doctor if you have any questions about Prolia.

What is the most important information I should know about Prolia?
If you receive Prolia, you should not receive XGEVA®. Prolia contains the same medicine as Xgeva (denosumab).
Prolia can cause serious side effects including:
• **Serious allergic reactions.**
  Serious allergic reactions have happened in people who take Prolia. Call your doctor or go to your nearest emer-

gency room right away if you have any symptoms of a serious allergic reaction. Symptoms of a serious allergic reaction may include:
  ○ low blood pressure (hypotension)
  ○ trouble breathing
  ○ throat tightness
  ○ swelling of your face, lips, or tongue
  ○ rash
  ○ itching
  ○ hives
• **Low calcium levels in your blood (hypocalcemia).**
  Prolia may lower the calcium levels in your blood. If you have low blood calcium before you start receiving Prolia, it may get worse during treatment. Your low blood calcium must be treated before you receive Prolia. Most people with low blood calcium levels do not have symptoms, but some people may have symptoms. Call your doctor right away if you have symptoms of low blood calcium such as:
  ○ Spasms, twitches, or cramps in your muscles
  ○ Numbness or tingling in your fingers, toes, or around your mouth
  Your doctor may prescribe calcium and vitamin D to help prevent low calcium levels in your blood while you take Prolia.
  Take calcium and vitamin D as your doctor tells you to.
• **Severe jaw bone problems (osteonecrosis).**
  Severe jaw bone problems may happen when you take Prolia. Your doctor should examine your mouth before you start Prolia. Your doctor may tell you to see your dentist before you start Prolia. It is important for you to practice good mouth care during treatment with Prolia. Ask your doctor or dentist about good mouth care if you have any questions
• **Unusual thigh bone fractures.**
  Some people have developed unusual fractures in their thigh bone. Symptoms of a fracture include new or unusual pain in your hip, groin, or thigh.
• **Serious infections.**
  Serious infections in your skin, lower stomach area (abdomen), bladder, or ear may happen if you take Prolia. Inflammation of the inner lining of the heart (endocarditis) due to an infection also may happen more often in people who take Prolia. You may need to go to the hospital for treatment if you develop an infection.
  Prolia is a medicine that may affect the ability of your body to fight infections. People who have weakened immune system or take medicines that affect the immune system may have an increased risk for developing serious infections.
  Call your doctor right away if you have any of the following symptoms of infection:
  • Fever or chills
  • Skin that looks red or swollen and is hot or tender to touch
  • Fever, shortness of breath, cough that will not go away
  • Severe abdominal pain
  • Frequent or urgent need to urinate or burning feeling when you urinate
• **Skin problems.**
  Skin problems such as inflammation of your skin (dermatitis), rash, and eczema may happen if you take Prolia. Call your doctor if you have any of the following symptoms of skin problems that do not go away or get worse:
  ○ Redness
  ○ Itching
  ○ Small bumps or patches (rash)
  ○ Your skin is dry or feels like leather
  ○ Blisters that ooze or become crusty
  ○ Skin peeling
• **Bone, joint, or muscle pain.**
  Some people who take Prolia develop severe bone, joint, or muscle pain.
Call your doctor right away if you have any of these side effects.
What is Prolia?
Prolia is a prescription medicine used to:
• Treat osteoporosis (thinning and weakening of bone) in women after menopause ("change of life") who:
  ○ are at high risk for fracture (broken bone)
  ○ cannot use another osteoporosis medicine or other osteoporosis medicines did not work well
• Increase bone mass in men with osteoporosis who are at high risk for fracture
• Treat bone loss in men who are at high risk for fracture receiving certain treatments for prostate cancer that has not spread to other parts of the body
• Treat bone loss in women who are at high risk for fracture receiving certain treatments for breast cancer that has not spread to other parts of the body
It is not known if Prolia is safe and effective in children.
Who should not take Prolia?
Do not take Prolia if you:
• have been told by your doctor that your blood calcium level is too low.

- are pregnant or plan to become pregnant
- are allergic to denosumab or any of the ingredients in Prolia. See the end of this leaflet for a complete list of ingredients in Prolia.

What should I tell my doctor before taking Prolia?
Before taking Prolia, tell your doctor if you:
- Are taking a medicine called Xgeva (denosumab). Xgeva contains the same medicine as Prolia.
- Have low blood calcium
- Cannot take daily calcium and vitamin D
- Had parathyroid or thyroid surgery (glands located in your neck)
- Have been told you have trouble absorbing minerals in your stomach or intestines (malabsorption syndrome)
- Have kidney problems or are on kidney dialysis
- Plan to have dental surgery or teeth removed.
- Are pregnant or plan to become pregnant. Prolia may harm your unborn baby. Tell your doctor right away if you become pregnant while taking Prolia.
  ◦ Pregnancy Surveillance Program: Prolia is not intended for use in pregnant women. If you become pregnant while taking Prolia, talk to your doctor about enrolling in Amgen's Pregnancy Surveillance Program or call 1-800-772-6436 (1-800-77-AMGEN). The purpose of this program is to collect information about women who have become pregnant while taking Prolia.
  ◦ If you are a man and you receive Prolia: Small amounts of Prolia may be in semen. If your sexual partner is pregnant, some Prolia from your semen may reach the unborn baby. While the risk is likely to be low, it is important to talk to your doctor if your partner becomes pregnant while you are taking Prolia.
- Are breastfeeding or plan to breastfeed. It is not known if Prolia passes into your breast milk. You and your doctor should decide if you will take Prolia or breastfeed. You should not do both.

Tell your doctor about all the medicines you take, including prescription and nonprescription drugs, vitamins, and herbal supplements.
Know the medicines you take. Keep a list of medicines with you to show to your doctor or pharmacist when you get a new medicine.

How will I receive Prolia?
- Prolia is an injection that will be given to you by a healthcare professional. Prolia is injected under your skin (subcutaneous).
- You will receive Prolia 1 time every 6 months.
- You should take calcium and vitamin D as your doctor tells you to while you receive Prolia.
- If you miss a dose of Prolia, you should receive your injection as soon as you can.
- Take good care of your teeth and gums while you receive Prolia. Brush and floss your teeth regularly.
- Tell your dentist that you are receiving Prolia before you have dental work.

What are the possible side effects of Prolia?
Prolia may cause serious side effects.
- See "What is the most important information I should know about Prolia?"
- It is not known if the use of Prolia over a long period of time may cause slow healing of broken bones.
The most common side effects of Prolia in women who are being treated for osteoporosis after menopause are:
- back pain
- pain in your arms and legs
- high cholesterol
- muscle pain
- bladder infection
The most common side effects of Prolia in men with osteoporosis are:
- back pain
- joint pain
- common cold (runny nose or sore throat)
The most common side effects of Prolia in patients receiving certain treatments for prostate or breast cancer are:
- joint pain
- back pain
- pain in your arms and legs
- muscle pain
Tell your doctor if you have any side effect that bothers you or that does not go away.
These are not all the possible side effects of Prolia. For more information, ask your doctor or pharmacist.
Call your doctor for medical advice about side effects. You may report side effects to FDA at 1-800-FDA-1088.

How should I store Prolia if I need to pick it up from a pharmacy?
- Keep Prolia in a refrigerator at 36°F to 46°F (2°C to 8°C) in the original carton.
- Do not freeze Prolia.
- When you remove Prolia from the refrigerator, Prolia must be kept at room temperature [up to 77°F (25°C)] in the original carton and must be used within 14 days.

- Do not keep Prolia at temperatures above 77°F (25°C). Warm temperatures will affect how Prolia works.
- Do not shake Prolia.
- Keep Prolia in the original carton to protect from light.
Keep Prolia and all medicines out of reach of children.
General information about Prolia.
Do not give Prolia to other people even if they have the same symptoms that you have. It may harm them.
This Medication Guide summarizes the most important information about Prolia. If you would like more information, talk with your doctor. You can ask your doctor or pharmacist for information about Prolia that is written for health professionals.
For more information, go to www.Prolia.com or call Amgen at 1-800-772-6436.
What are the ingredients in Prolia?
Active ingredient: denosumab
Inactive ingredients: sorbitol, acetate, polysorbate 20 (prefilled syringe only), Water for Injection (USP), and sodium hydroxide
[Amgen Logo]
Amgen Manufacturing Limited, a subsidiary of Amgen Inc.
One Amgen Center Drive
Thousand Oaks, California 91320-1799
This Medication Guide has been approved by the U.S. Food and Drug Administration.
1xxxxxx - v7
Revised: 06/2014
Shown in Product Identification Guide, page 305

Bayer HealthCare LLC
100 Bayer Boulevard
Whippany, NJ 07981

Direct Inquiries to:
Phone: 1-888-84-BAYER
(1-888-842-2937)
http//www.bayerhealthcare.com

For Medical Information contact:
Vice President, Medical Communications
1-888-84-Bayer (1-888-842-2937)

NEXAVAR
(sorafenib)
tablets, oral   ℞

HIGHLIGHTS OF PRESCRIBING INFORMATION
These highlights do not include all the information needed to use NEXAVAR safely and effectively.
See full prescribing information for NEXAVAR.
NEXAVAR (sorafenib) tablets, oral
Initial U.S. Approval: 2005

——————RECENT MAJOR CHANGES——————
Indications and Usage
- Differentiated Thyroid Carcinoma (DTC) (1.3) 11/2013
Dosage and Administration
- Patients with DTC (2) 11/2013
Warnings and Precautions
- Impairment of Thyroid Stimulating Hormone (TSH) Suppression in DTC (5.12) 11/2013

——————INDICATIONS AND USAGE——————
NEXAVAR is a kinase inhibitor indicated for the treatment of
- Unresectable hepatocellular carcinoma (1.1)
- Advanced renal cell carcinoma (1.2)
- Locally recurrent or metastatic, progressive, differentiated thyroid carcinoma refractory to radioactive iodine treatment (1.3)

——————DOSAGE FORMS AND STRENGTHS——————
200 mg Tablets (3)

——————CONTRAINDICATIONS——————
- NEXAVAR is contraindicated in patients with known severe hypersensitivity to sorafenib or any other component of NEXAVAR. (4)
- NEXAVAR in combination with carboplatin and paclitaxel is contraindicated in patients with squamous cell lung cancer. (4)

——————WARNINGS AND PRECAUTIONS——————
- Cardiac Ischemia and/or Infarction: Consider temporary or permanent discontinuation of NEXAVAR. (5.1)
- Bleeding: Discontinue NEXAVAR if needed. (5.2)
- Hypertension: Monitor blood pressure weekly during the first 6 weeks and periodically thereafter. (5.3)

- Dermatologic Toxicities: Interrupt and/or decrease dose. Discontinue for severe or persistent reactions, or if Stevens-Johnson syndrome and toxic epidermal necrolysis is suspected. (5.4)
- Gastrointestinal Perforation: Discontinue NEXAVAR. (5.5)
- QT Prolongation: Monitor electrocardiograms and electrolytes in patients at increased risk for ventricular arrhythmias. (5.9, 12.2)
- Drug-Induced Hepatitis: Monitor liver function tests regularly; discontinue for unexplained transaminase elevations. (5.10)
- Embryofetal Toxicity: Advise women of potential risk to fetus and to avoid becoming pregnant. (5.11, 8.1)
- Impairment of TSH suppression in DTC: Monitor TSH monthly and adjust thyroid replacement therapy in patients with thyroid cancer. (5.12)

——————ADVERSE REACTIONS——————
The most common adverse reactions (≥20%) for NEXAVAR are diarrhea, fatigue, infection, alopecia, hand-foot skin reaction, rash, weight loss, decreased appetite, nausea, gastrointestinal and abdominal pains, hypertension, and hemorrhage. (6)
To report SUSPECTED ADVERSE REACTIONS, contact Bayer HealthCare Pharmaceuticals Inc. at 1-888-842-2937, or FDA at 1-800-FDA-1088 or www.fda.gov/medwatch

——————DRUG INTERACTIONS——————
- Avoid strong CYP3A4 inducers. (7.1)
See 17 for PATIENT COUNSELING INFORMATION and FDA-approved patient labeling
Revised: 11/2013

FULL PRESCRIBING INFORMATION: CONTENTS*
1   **INDICATIONS AND USAGE**
   1.1   Hepatocellular Carcinoma
   1.2   Renal Cell Carcinoma
   1.3   Differentiated Thyroid Carcinoma
2   **DOSAGE AND ADMINISTRATION**
   2.1   Recommended Dose for Hepatocellular Carcinoma, Renal Cell Carcinoma, and Differentiated Thyroid Carcinoma
   2.2   Dose Modifications for Suspected Adverse Drug Reactions
3   **DOSAGE FORMS AND STRENGTHS**
4   **CONTRAINDICATIONS**
5   **WARNINGS AND PRECAUTIONS**
   5.1   Risk of Cardiac Ischemia and/or Infarction
   5.2   Risk of Hemorrhage
   5.3   Risk of Hypertension
   5.4   Risk of Dermatologic Toxicities
   5.5   Risk of Gastrointestinal Perforation
   5.6   Warfarin
   5.7   Wound Healing Complications
   5.8   Increased Mortality Observed with NEXAVAR Administered in Combination with Carboplatin/Paclitaxel and Gemcitabine/Cisplatin in Squamous Cell Lung Cancer
   5.9   Risk of QT Interval Prolongation
   5.10   Drug-Induced Hepatitis
   5.11   Embryofetal Risk
   5.12   Impairment of Thyroid Stimulating Hormone Suppression in Differentiated Thyroid Carcinoma
6   **ADVERSE REACTIONS**
   6.1   Adverse Reactions in HCC Study
   6.2   Adverse Reactions in RCC Study 1
   6.3   Adverse Reactions in DTC Study
   6.4   Additional Data from Multiple Clinical Trials
   6.5   Postmarketing Experience
7   **DRUG INTERACTIONS**
   7.1   Effect of Strong CYP3A4 Inducers on Sorafenib
   7.2   Effect of Strong CYP3A4 Inhibitors on Sorafenib
   7.3   Effect of Sorafenib on Other Drugs
   7.4   Neomycin
   7.5   Drugs that Increase Gastric pH
8   **USE IN SPECIFIC POPULATIONS**
   8.1   Pregnancy
   8.3   Nursing Mothers
   8.4   Pediatric Use
   8.5   Geriatric Use
   8.6   Patients with Hepatic Impairment
   8.7   Patients with Renal Impairment
10   **OVERDOSAGE**
11   **DESCRIPTION**
12   **CLINICAL PHARMACOLOGY**
   12.1   Mechanism of Action
   12.2   Pharmacodynamics
   12.3   Pharmacokinetics
13   **NONCLINICAL TOXICOLOGY**
   13.1   Carcinogenesis, Mutagenesis, Impairment of Fertility

14   CLINICAL STUDIES
    14.1   Hepatocellular Carcinoma
    14.2   Renal Cell Carcinoma
    14.3   Differentiated Thyroid Carcinoma
16   HOW SUPPLIED/STORAGE AND HANDLING
17   PATIENT COUNSELING INFORMATION
Patient Information
* Sections or subsections omitted from the full prescribing information are not listed

FULL PRESCRIBING INFORMATION

1   INDICATIONS AND USAGE
1.1   Hepatocellular Carcinoma
NEXAVAR® is indicated for the treatment of patients with unresectable hepatocellular carcinoma (HCC).
1.2   Renal Cell Carcinoma
NEXAVAR is indicated for the treatment of patients with advanced renal cell carcinoma (RCC).
1.3   Differentiated Thyroid Carcinoma
NEXAVAR is indicated for the treatment of patients with locally recurrent or metastatic, progressive, differentiated thyroid carcinoma (DTC) that is refractory to radioactive iodine treatment.

2   DOSAGE AND ADMINISTRATION
2.1   Recommended Dose for Hepatocellular Carcinoma, Renal Cell Carcinoma, and Differentiated Thyroid Carcinoma
The recommended daily dose of NEXAVAR is 400 mg (2 × 200 mg tablets) taken twice daily without food (at least 1 hour before or 2 hours after a meal). Treatment should continue until the patient is no longer clinically benefiting from therapy or until unacceptable toxicity occurs.
2.2   Dose Modifications for Suspected Adverse Drug Reactions
Temporary interruption of NEXAVAR is recommended in patients undergoing major surgical procedures [see Warnings and Precautions (5.7)].
Temporary interruption or permanent discontinuation of NEXAVAR may be required for the following:
• Cardiac ischemia or infarction [see Warnings and Precautions (5.1)];
• Hemorrhage requiring medical intervention [see Warnings and Precautions (5.2)]
• Severe or persistent hypertension despite adequate antihypertensive therapy [see Warnings and Precautions (5.3)]
• Gastrointestinal perforation [see Warnings and Precautions (5.5)]
• QTc prolongation [see Warnings and Precautions (5.9)]
• Severe drug-induced liver injury [see Warnings and Precautions (5.10)]
Dose modifications for Hepatocellular Carcinoma and Renal Cell Carcinoma
When dose reduction is necessary, the NEXAVAR dose may be reduced to 400 mg once daily. If additional dose reduction is required, NEXAVAR may be reduced to a single 400 mg dose every other day [see Warnings and Precautions (5)].
Suggested dose modifications for dermatologic toxicities are outlined in Table 1.
[See table 1 above]
Dose modifications for Differentiated Thyroid Carcinoma

Table 2: Recommended Doses for Patients with Differentiated Thyroid Carcinoma Requiring Dose Reduction

Dose Reduction	NEXAVAR Dose	
First Dose Reduction	600 mg daily dose	400 mg and 200 mg 12 hours apart (2 tablets and 1 tablet 12 hours apart — either dose can come first)
Second Dose Reduction	400 mg daily dose	200 mg twice daily (1 tablet twice daily)
Third Dose Reduction	200 mg daily dose	200 mg once daily (1 tablet once daily)

When dose reduction is necessary for dermatologic toxicities, reduce the NEXAVAR dose as indicated in Table 3 below.
[See table 3 above]
Following improvement of Grade 2 or 3 dermatologic toxicity to Grade 0–1 after at least 28 days of treatment on a reduced dose of NEXAVAR, the dose of NEXAVAR may be increased one dose level from the reduced dose. Approximately 50% of patients requiring a dose reduction for dermatologic toxicity are expected to meet these criteria for resumption of the higher dose and roughly 50% of patients resuming the previous dose are expected to tolerate the higher dose (that is, maintain the higher dose level without recurrent Grade 2 or higher dermatologic toxicity)

Table 1: Suggested Dose Modifications for Dermatologic Toxicities in Patients with Hepatocellular or Renal Cell Carcinoma

Dermatologic Toxicity Grade	Occurrence	Suggested Dose Modification
Grade 1: Numbness, dysesthesia, paresthesia, tingling, painless swelling, erythema or discomfort of the hands or feet which does not disrupt the patient's normal activities	Any occurrence	Continue treatment with NEXAVAR and consider topical therapy for symptomatic relief
Grade 2: Painful erythema and swelling of the hands or feet and/or discomfort affecting the patient's normal activities	1st occurrence	Continue treatment with NEXAVAR and consider topical therapy for symptomatic relief. If no improvement within 7 days, see below
	No improvement within 7 days or 2nd or 3rd occurrence	Interrupt NEXAVAR treatment until toxicity resolves to Grade 0–1. When resuming treatment, decrease NEXAVAR dose by one dose level (400 mg daily or 400 mg every other day)
	4th occurrence	Discontinue NEXAVAR treatment
Grade 3: Moist desquamation, ulceration, blistering or severe pain of the hands or feet, or severe discomfort that causes the patient to be unable to work or perform activities of daily living	1st or 2nd occurrence	Interrupt NEXAVAR treatment until toxicity resolves to Grade 0–1. When resuming treatment, decrease NEXAVAR dose by one dose level (400 mg daily or 400 mg every other day)
	3rd occurrence	Discontinue NEXAVAR treatment

Table 3: Recommended Dose Modifications for Dermatologic Toxicities for Patients with Differentiated Thyroid Carcinoma

Dermatologic Toxicity Grade	Occurrence	NEXAVAR Dose Modification
Grade 1: Numbness, dysesthesia, paresthesia, tingling, painless swelling, erythema or discomfort of the hands or feet which does not disrupt the patient's normal activities	Any occurrence	Continue treatment with NEXAVAR
Grade 2: Painful erythema and swelling of the hands or feet and/or discomfort affecting the patient's normal activities	1st occurrence	Decrease NEXAVAR dose to 600 mg daily. If no improvement within 7 days, see below
	No improvement within 7 days at reduced dose or 2nd occurrence	Interrupt NEXAVAR until resolved or improved to grade 1. If NEXAVAR is resumed, decrease dose (see Table 2)
	3rd occurrence	Interrupt NEXAVAR until resolved or improved to grade 1. If NEXAVAR is resumed, decrease dose (see Table 2)
	4th occurrence	Discontinue NEXAVAR permanently
Grade 3: Moist desquamation, ulceration, blistering, or severe pain of the hands or feet, resulting in inability to work or perform activities of daily living	1st occurrence	Interrupt NEXAVAR until resolved or improved to grade 1. If NEXAVAR is resumed, decrease dose by one dose level (see Table 2)
	2nd occurrence	Interrupt NEXAVAR until resolved or improved to grade 1. When NEXAVAR is resumed, decrease dose by 2 dose levels (see Table 2)
	3rd occurrence	Discontinue NEXAVAR permanently

3   DOSAGE FORMS AND STRENGTHS
Tablets containing sorafenib tosylate (274 mg) equivalent to 200 mg of sorafenib.
NEXAVAR tablets are round, biconvex, red film-coated tablets, debossed with the "Bayer cross" on one side and "200" on the other side.

4   CONTRAINDICATIONS
NEXAVAR is contraindicated in patients with known severe hypersensitivity to sorafenib or any other component of NEXAVAR.
NEXAVAR in combination with carboplatin and paclitaxel is contraindicated in patients with squamous cell lung cancer [see Warnings and Precautions (5.8)].

5   WARNINGS AND PRECAUTIONS
5.1   Risk of Cardiac Ischemia and/or Infarction
In the HCC study, the incidence of cardiac ischemia/infarction was 2.7% in NEXAVAR-treated patients compared with 1.3% in the placebo-treated group, in RCC Study 1, the incidence of cardiac ischemia/infarction was higher in the NEXAVAR-treated group (2.9%) compared with the placebo-treated group (0.4%), and in the DTC study, the incidence of cardiac ischemia/infarction was 1.9% in the NEXAVAR-treated group compared with 0% in the placebo-treated group. Patients with unstable coronary artery disease or recent myocardial infarction were excluded from this study. Temporary or permanent discontinuation of NEXAVAR should be considered in patients who develop cardiac ischemia and/or infarction.
5.2   Risk of Hemorrhage
An increased risk of bleeding may occur following NEXAVAR administration. In the HCC study, an excess of bleeding regardless of causality was not apparent and the rate of bleeding from esophageal varices was 2.4% in NEXAVAR-treated patients and 4% in placebo-treated patients. Bleeding with a fatal outcome from any site was reported in 2.4% of NEXAVAR-treated patients and 4% in placebo-treated patients. In RCC Study 1, bleeding regardless of causality was reported in 15.3% of patients in the NEXAVAR-treated group and 8.2% of patients in the placebo-treated group. The incidence of CTCAE Grade 3 and 4 bleeding was 2% and 0%, respectively, in NEXAVAR-treated patients, and 1.3% and 0.2%, respectively, in

placebo-treated patients. There was one fatal hemorrhage in each treatment group in RCC Study 1. In the DTC study, bleeding was reported in 17.4% of NEXAVAR-treated patients and 9.6% of placebo-treated patients; however the incidence of CTCAE Grade 3 bleeding was 1% in NEXAVAR-treated patients and 1.4% in placebo-treated patients. There was no Grade 4 bleeding reported and there was one fatal hemorrhage in a placebo-treated patient. If any bleeding necessitates medical intervention, permanent discontinuation of NEXAVAR should be considered. Due to the potential risk of bleeding, tracheal, bronchial, and esophageal infiltration should be treated with local therapy prior to administering NEXAVAR in patients with DTC.

5.3 Risk of Hypertension

Monitor blood pressure weekly during the first 6 weeks of NEXAVAR. Thereafter, monitor blood pressure and treat hypertension, if required, in accordance with standard medical practice. In the HCC study, hypertension was reported in approximately 9.4% of NEXAVAR-treated patients and 4.3% of patients in the placebo-treated group. In RCC Study 1, hypertension was reported in approximately 16.9% of NEXAVAR-treated patients and 1.8% of patients in the placebo-treated group. In the DTC study, hypertension was reported in 40.6% of NEXAVAR-treated patients and 12.4% of placebo-treated patients. Hypertension was usually mild to moderate, occurred early in the course of treatment, and was managed with standard antihypertensive therapy. In cases of severe or persistent hypertension despite institution of antihypertensive therapy, consider temporary or permanent discontinuation of NEXAVAR. Permanent discontinuation due to hypertension occurred in 1 of 297 NEXAVAR-treated patients in the HCC study, 1 of 451 NEXAVAR-treated patients in RCC Study 1, and 1 of 207 NEXAVAR-treated patients in the DTC study.

5.4 Risk of Dermatologic Toxicities

Hand-foot skin reaction and rash represent the most common adverse reactions attributed to NEXAVAR. Rash and hand-foot skin reaction are usually CTCAE Grade 1 and 2 and generally appear during the first six weeks of treatment with NEXAVAR. Management of dermatologic toxicities may include topical therapies for symptomatic relief, temporary treatment interruption and/or dose modification of NEXAVAR, or in severe or persistent cases, permanent discontinuation of NEXAVAR [see Dosage and Administration (2.2)]. Permanent discontinuation of therapy due to hand-foot skin reaction occurred in 4 (1.3%) of 297 NEXAVAR-treated patients with HCC, 3 (0.7%) of 451 NEXAVAR-treated patients with RCC, and 11 (5.3%) of 207 NEXAVAR-treated patients with DTC.

There have been reports of severe dermatologic toxicities, including Stevens-Johnson syndrome (SJS) and toxic epidermal necrolysis (TEN). These cases may be life-threatening. Discontinue NEXAVAR if SJS or TEN are suspected.

5.5 Risk of Gastrointestinal Perforation

Gastrointestinal perforation is an uncommon adverse reaction and has been reported in less than 1% of patients taking NEXAVAR. In some cases this was not associated with apparent intra-abdominal tumor. In the event of a gastrointestinal perforation, discontinue NEXAVAR.

5.6 Warfarin

Infrequent bleeding or elevations in the International Normalized Ratio (INR) have been reported in some patients taking warfarin while on NEXAVAR. Monitor patients taking concomitant warfarin regularly for changes in prothrombin time (PT), INR or clinical bleeding episodes.

5.7 Wound Healing Complications

No formal studies of the effect of NEXAVAR on wound healing have been conducted. Temporary interruption of NEXAVAR is recommended in patients undergoing major surgical procedures. There is limited clinical experience regarding the timing of reinitiation of NEXAVAR following major surgical intervention. Therefore, the decision to resume NEXAVAR following a major surgical intervention should be based on clinical judgment of adequate wound healing.

5.8 Increased Mortality Observed with NEXAVAR Administered in Combination with Carboplatin/Paclitaxel and Gemcitabine/Cisplatin in Squamous Cell Lung Cancer

In a subset analysis of two randomized controlled trials in chemo-naive patients with Stage IIIB-IV non-small cell lung cancer, patients with squamous cell carcinoma experienced higher mortality with the addition of NEXAVAR compared to those treated with carboplatin/paclitaxel alone (HR 1.81, 95% CI 1.19–2.74) and gemcitabine/cisplatin alone (HR 1.22, 95% CI 0.82-1.80). The use of NEXAVAR in combination with carboplatin/paclitaxel is contraindicated in patients with squamous cell lung cancer. NEXAVAR in combination with gemcitabine/cisplatin is not recommended in patients with squamous cell lung cancer. The safety and effectiveness of NEXAVAR has not been established in patients with non-small cell lung cancer.

5.9 Risk of QT Interval Prolongation

NEXAVAR can prolong the QT/QTc interval. QT/QTc interval prolongation increases the risk for ventricular arrhythmias. Avoid NEXAVAR in patients with congenital long QT syndrome. Monitor electrolytes and electrocardiograms in patients with congestive heart failure, bradyarrhythmias, drugs known to prolong the QT interval, including Class Ia and III antiarrhythmics. Correct electrolyte abnormalities (magnesium, potassium, calcium). Interrupt NEXAVAR if QTc interval is greater than 500 milliseconds or for an increase from baseline of 60 milliseconds or greater [see Clinical Pharmacology (12.2)].

5.10 Drug-Induced Hepatitis

Sorafenib-induced hepatitis is characterized by a hepatocellular pattern of liver damage with significant increases of transaminases which may result in hepatic failure and death. Increases in bilirubin and INR may also occur. The incidence of severe drug-induced liver injury, defined as elevated transaminase levels above 20 times the upper limit of normal or transaminase elevations with significant clinical sequelae (for example, elevated INR, ascites, fatal, or transplantation), was two of 3,357 patients (0.06%) in a global monotherapy database. Monitor liver function tests regularly. In case of significantly increased transaminases without alternative explanation, such as viral hepatitis or progressing underlying malignancy, discontinue NEXAVAR.

5.11 Embryofetal Risk

Based on its mechanism of action and findings in animals, NEXAVAR may cause fetal harm when administered to a pregnant woman. Sorafenib caused embryo-fetal toxicities in animals at maternal exposures that were significantly lower than the human exposures at the recommended dose of 400 mg twice daily. Advise women of childbearing potential to avoid becoming pregnant while on NEXAVAR because of the potential hazard to the fetus [see Use in Specific Populations (8.1)].

5.12 Impairment of Thyroid Stimulating Hormone Suppression in Differentiated Thyroid Carcinoma

NEXAVAR impairs exogenous thyroid suppression. In the DTC study, 99% of patients had a baseline thyroid stimulating hormone (TSH) level less than 0.5 mU/L. Elevation of TSH level above 0.5 mU/L was observed in 41% of NEXAVAR-treated patients as compared with 16% of placebo-treated patients. For patients with impaired TSH suppression while receiving NEXAVAR, the median maximal TSH was 1.6 mU/L and 25% had TSH levels greater than 4.4 mU/L. Monitor TSH levels monthly and adjust thyroid replacement medication as needed in patients with DTC

6 ADVERSE REACTIONS

The following serious adverse reactions are discussed elsewhere in the labeling:

Cardiac ischemia, infarction [see Warnings and Precautions (5.1)]

Hemorrhage [see Warnings and Precautions (5.2)]

Hypertension [see Warnings and Precautions (5.3)]

Hand-foot skin reaction, rash, Stevens-Johnson syndrome, and toxic epidermal necrolysis [see Warnings and Precautions (5.4)]

Gastrointestinal perforation [see Warnings and Precautions (5.5)]

QT Interval Prolongation [see Warnings and Precautions (5.9) and Clinical Pharmacology (12.2)]

Drug-Induced Hepatitis [see Warnings and Precautions (5.10)]

Impairment of TSH suppression in DTC [see Warnings and Precautions (5.12)]

Because clinical trials are conducted under widely varying conditions, adverse reaction rates observed in the clinical trials of a drug cannot be directly compared to rates in the clinical trials of another drug and may not reflect the rates observed in practice.

The data described in sections 6.1, 6.2 and 6.3 reflect exposure to NEXAVAR in 955 patients who participated in placebo controlled studies in hepatocellular carcinoma (N=297), advanced renal cell carcinoma (N=451), or differentiated thyroid carcinoma (N = 207).

The most common adverse reactions (≥20%), which were considered to be related to NEXAVAR, in patients with HCC, RCC or DTC are diarrhea, fatigue, infection, alopecia, hand-foot skin reaction, rash, weight loss, decreased appetite, nausea, gastrointestinal and abdominal pains, hypertension, and hemorrhage.

6.1 Adverse Reactions in HCC Study

Table 4 shows the percentage of patients with HCC experiencing adverse reactions that were reported in at least 10% of patients and at a higher rate in the NEXAVAR arm than the placebo arm. CTCAE Grade 3 adverse reactions were reported in 39% of patients receiving NEXAVAR compared to 24% of patients receiving placebo. CTCAE Grade 4 ad-

Table 4: Adverse Reactions Reported in at Least 10% of Patients and at a Higher Rate in NEXAVAR Arm than the Placebo Arm – HCC Study

Adverse Reaction NCI- CTCAE v3 Category/Term	NEXAVAR N=297			Placebo N=302		
	All Grades %	Grade 3 %	Grade 4 %	All Grades %	Grade 3 %	Grade 4 %
Any Adverse Reaction	98	39	6	96	24	8
Constitutional symptoms						
Fatigue	46	9	1	45	12	2
Weight loss	30	2	0	10	1	0
Dermatology/skin						
Rash/desquamation	19	1	0	14	0	0
Pruritus	14	<1	0	11	<1	0
Hand-foot skin reaction	21	8	0	3	<1	0
Dry skin	10	0	0	6	0	0
Alopecia	14	0	0	2	0	0
Gastrointestinal						
Diarrhea	55	10	<1	25	2	0
Anorexia	29	3	0	18	3	<1
Nausea	24	1	0	20	3	0
Vomiting	15	2	0	11	2	0
Constipation	14	0	0	10	0	0
Hepatobiliary/pancreas						
Liver dysfunction	11	2	1	8	2	1
Pain						
Pain, abdomen	31	9	0	26	5	1

Table 5: Adverse Reactions Reported in at Least 10% of Patients and at a Higher Rate in NEXAVAR Arm than the Placebo Arm – RCC Study 1

Adverse Reactions NCI- CTCAE v3 Category/Term	NEXAVAR N=451			Placebo N=451		
	All Grades %	Grade 3 %	Grade 4 %	All Grades %	Grade 3 %	Grade 4 %
Any Adverse Reactions	95	31	7	86	22	6
Cardiovascular, General						
Hypertension	17	3	<1	2	<1	0
Constitutional symptoms						
Fatigue	37	5	<1	28	3	<1
Weight loss	10	<1	0	6	0	0
Dermatology/skin						
Rash/desquamation	40	<1	0	16	<1	0
Hand-foot skin reaction	30	6	0	7	0	0
Alopecia	27	<1	0	3	0	0
Pruritus	19	<1	0	6	0	0
Dry skin	11	0	0	4	0	0
Gastrointestinal symptoms						
Diarrhea	43	2	0	13	<1	0
Nausea	23	<1	0	19	<1	0
Anorexia	16	<1	0	13	1	0
Vomiting	16	<1	0	12	1	0
Constipation	15	<1	0	11	<1	0
Hemorrhage/bleeding						
Hemorrhage – all sites	15	2	0	8	1	<1
Neurology						
Neuropathy-sensory	13	<1	0	6	<1	0
Pain						
Pain, abdomen	11	2	0	9	2	0
Pain, joint	10	2	0	6	<1	0
Pain, headache	10	<1	0	6	0	0
Pulmonary						
Dyspnea	14	3	<1	12	2	<1

verse reactions were reported in 6% of patients receiving NEXAVAR compared to 8% of patients receiving placebo.
[See table 4 at top of previous page]
Hypertension was reported in 9% of patients treated with NEXAVAR and 4% of those treated with placebo. CTCAE Grade 3 hypertension was reported in 4% of NEXAVAR-treated patients and 1% of placebo-treated patients. No patients were reported with CTCAE Grade 4 reactions in either treatment group.
Hemorrhage/bleeding was reported in 18% of those receiving NEXAVAR and 20% of placebo-treated patients. The rates of CTCAE Grade 3 and 4 bleeding were also higher in the placebo-treated group (CTCAE Grade 3 – 3% NEXAVAR and 5% placebo and CTCAE Grade 4 – 2% NEXAVAR and 4% placebo). Bleeding from esophageal varices was reported in 2.4% in NEXAVAR-treated patients and 4% of placebo-treated patients.
Renal failure was reported in <1% of patients treated with NEXAVAR and 3% of placebo-treated patients.
The rate of adverse reactions (including those associated with progressive disease) resulting in permanent discontinuation was similar in both the NEXAVAR and placebo-treated groups (32% of NEXAVAR-treated patients and 35% of placebo-treated patients).
Laboratory Abnormalities
The following laboratory abnormalities were observed in patients with HCC:
Hypophosphatemia was a common laboratory finding, observed in 35% of NEXAVAR-treated patients compared to 11% of placebo-treated patients; CTCAE Grade 3 hypophosphatemia (1–2 mg/dL) occurred in 11% of NEXAVAR-treated patients and 2% of patients in the placebo-treated group; there was 1 case of CTCAE Grade 4 hypophosphatemia (<1 mg/dL) reported in the placebo-treated group. The etiology of hypophosphatemia associated with NEXAVAR is not known.
Elevated lipase was observed in 40% of patients treated with NEXAVAR compared to 37% of patients in the placebo-treated group. CTCAE Grade 3 or 4 lipase elevations occurred in 9% of patients in each group. Elevated amylase was observed in 34% of patients treated with NEXAVAR compared to 29% of patients in the placebo-treated group. CTCAE Grade 3 or 4 amylase elevations were reported in 2% of patients in each group. Many of the lipase and amylase elevations were transient, and in the majority of cases NEXAVAR treatment was not interrupted. Clinical pancreatitis was reported in 1 of 297 NEXAVAR-treated patients (CTCAE Grade 2).
Elevations in liver function tests were comparable between the 2 arms of the study. Hypoalbuminemia was observed in 59% of NEXAVAR-treated patients and 47% of placebo-treated patients; no CTCAE Grade 3 or 4 hypoalbuminemia was observed in either group.
INR elevations were observed in 42% of NEXAVAR-treated patients and 34% of placebo-treated patients; CTCAE Grade 3 INR elevations were reported in 4% of NEXAVAR-treated patients and 2% of placebo-treated patients; there was no CTCAE Grade 4 INR elevation in either group.

Lymphopenia was observed in 47% of NEXAVAR-treated patients and 42% of placebo-treated patients.
Thrombocytopenia was observed in 46% of NEXAVAR-treated patients and 41% of placebo-treated patients; CTCAE Grade 3 or 4 thrombocytopenia was reported in 4% of NEXAVAR-treated patients and less than 1% of placebo-treated patients.
Hypocalcemia was reported in 27% of NEXAVAR-treated patients and 15% of placebo-treated patients. CTCAE Grade 3 hypocalcemia (6–7 mg /dL) occurred in 2% of NEXAVAR-treated patients and 1% of placebo-treated patients. CTCAE Grade 4 hypocalcemia (<6 mg/dL) occurred in 0.4% of NEXAVAR-treated patients and in no placebo-treated patients.
Hypokalemia was reported in 9.5% of NEXAVAR- treated patients compared to 5.9% of placebo-treated patients. Most reports of hypokalemia were low grade (CTCAE Grade 1). CTCAE Grade 3 hypokalemia occurred in 0.4% of NEXAVAR-treated patients and 0.7% of placebo-treated patients. There were no reports of Grade 4 hypokalemia.

6.2   Adverse Reactions in RCC Study 1
Table 5 shows the percentage of patients with RCC experiencing adverse reactions that were reported in at least 10% of patients and at a higher rate in the NEXAVAR arm than the placebo arm. CTCAE Grade 3 adverse reactions were reported in 31% of patients receiving NEXAVAR compared to 22% of patients receiving placebo. CTCAE Grade 4 adverse reactions were reported in 7% of patients receiving NEXAVAR compared to 6% of patients receiving placebo.
[See table 5 above]
The rate of adverse reactions (including those associated with progressive disease) resulting in permanent discontinuation was similar in both the NEXAVAR and placebo-treated groups (10% of NEXAVAR-treated patients and 8% of placebo-treated patients).
Laboratory Abnormalities
The following laboratory abnormalities were observed in patients with RCC in Study 1:
Hypophosphatemia was a common laboratory finding, observed in 45% of NEXAVAR-treated patients compared to 11% of placebo-treated patients. CTCAE Grade 3 hypophosphatemia (1–2 mg/dL) occurred in 13% of NEXAVAR-treated patients and 3% of patients in the placebo-treated group. There were no cases of CTCAE Grade 4 hypophosphatemia (<1 mg/dL) reported in either NEXAVAR or placebo-treated patients. The etiology of hypophosphatemia associated with NEXAVAR is not known.
Elevated lipase was observed in 41% of patients treated with NEXAVAR compared to 30% of patients in the placebo-treated group. CTCAE Grade 3 or 4 lipase elevations occurred in 12% of patients in the NEXAVAR-treated group compared to 7% of patients in the placebo-treated group. Elevated amylase was observed in 30% of patients treated with NEXAVAR compared to 23% of patients in the placebo-treated group. CTCAE Grade 3 or 4 amylase elevations were reported in 1% of patients in the NEXAVAR-treated group compared to 3% of patients in the placebo-treated group. Many of the lipase and amylase elevations were transient, and in the majority of cases NEXAVAR treatment was not interrupted. Clinical pancreatitis was reported in 3 of 451 NEXAVAR-treated patients (one CTCAE Grade 2 and two Grade 4) and 1 of 451 patients (CTCAE Grade 2) in the placebo-treated group.
Lymphopenia was observed in 23% of NEXAVAR-treated patients and 13% of placebo-treated patients. CTCAE Grade 3 or 4 lymphopenia was reported in 13% of NEXAVAR-treated patients and 7% of placebo-treated patients. Neutropenia was observed in 18% of NEXAVAR-treated patients and 10% of placebo-treated patients. CTCAE Grade 3 or 4 neutropenia was reported in 5% of NEXAVAR-treated patients and 2% of placebo-treated patients.
Anemia was observed in 44% of NEXAVAR-treated patients and 49% of placebo-treated patients. CTCAE Grade 3 or 4 anemia was reported in 2% of NEXAVAR-treated patients and 4% of placebo-treated patients.
Thrombocytopenia was observed in 12% of NEXAVAR-treated patients and 5% of placebo-treated patients. CTCAE Grade 3 or 4 thrombocytopenia was reported in 1% of NEXAVAR-treated patients and in no placebo-treated patients.
Hypocalcemia was reported in 12% of NEXAVAR-treated patients and 8% of placebo-treated patients. CTCAE Grade 3 hypocalcemia (6–7 mg/dL) occurred in 1% of NEXAVAR-treated patients and 0.2% of placebo-treated patients, and CTCAE Grade 4 hypocalcemia (<6 mg/dL) occurred in 1% of NEXAVAR-treated patients and 0.5% of placebo-treated patients.
Hypokalemia was reported in 5.4% of NEXAVAR-treated patients compared to 0.7% of placebo-treated patients. Most reports of hypokalemia were low grade (CTCAE Grade 1). CTCAE Grade 3 hypokalemia occurred in 1.1% of NEXAVAR-treated patients and 0.2% of placebo-treated patients. There were no reports of Grade 4 hypokalemia.

6.3 Adverse Reactions in DTC Study

The safety of NEXAVAR was evaluated in 416 patients with locally recurrent or metastatic, progressive differentiated thyroid carcinoma (DTC) refractory to radioactive iodine (RAI) treatment randomized to receive 400 mg twice daily NEXAVAR (n=207) or matching placebo (n=209) until disease progression or intolerable toxicity in a double-blind trial [see Clinical Studies (14.3)]. The data described below reflect a median exposure to NEXAVAR for 46 weeks (range 0.3 to 135). The population exposed to NEXAVAR was 50% male, and had a median age of 63 years.

Dose interruptions for adverse reactions were required in 66% of patients receiving NEXAVAR and 64% of patients had their dose reduced. Drug-related adverse reactions that resulted in treatment discontinuation were reported in 14% of NEXAVAR-treated patients compared to 1.4% of placebo-treated patients.

Table 6 shows the percentage of DTC patients experiencing adverse reactions at a higher rate in NEXAVAR-treated patients than placebo-treated patients in the double-blind phase of the DTC study. CTCAE Grade 3 adverse reactions occurred in 53% of NEXAVAR-treated patients compared to 23% of placebo-treated patients. CTCAE Grade 4 adverse reactions occurred in 12% of NEXAVAR-treated patients compared to 7% of placebo-treated patients.
[See table 6 above]

Laboratory Abnormalities

Elevated TSH levels are discussed elsewhere in the labeling [see Warnings and Precautions (5.12)]. The relative increase for the following laboratory abnormalities observed in NEXAVAR-treated DTC patients as compared to placebo-treated patients is similar to that observed in the RCC and HCC studies: lipase, amylase, hypokalemia, hypophosphatemia, neutropenia, lymphopenia, anemia, and thrombocytopenia [see Adverse Reactions (6.1, 6.2)].

Serum ALT and AST elevations were observed in 59% and 54% of the NEXAVAR-treated patients as compared to 24% and 15% of placebo-treated patients, respectively. High grade (≥ 3) ALT and AST elevations were observed in 4% and 2%, respectively, in the NEXAVAR-treated patients as compared to none of the placebo-treated patients.

Hypocalcemia was more frequent and more severe in patients with DTC, especially those with a history of hypoparathyroidism, compared to patients with RCC or HCC. Hypocalcemia was observed in 36% of DTC patients receiving NEXAVAR (with 10% ≥ Grade 3) as compared with 11% of placebo-treated patients (3% ≥ Grade 3). In the DTC study, serum calcium levels were monitored monthly.

6.4 Additional Data from Multiple Clinical Trials

The following additional drug-related adverse reactions and laboratory abnormalities were reported from clinical trials of NEXAVAR (*very common* 10% or greater, *common* 1 to less than 10%, *uncommon* 0.1% to less than 1%, *rare* less than 0.1 %):

Cardiovascular: *Common:* congestive heart failure[1][2], myocardial ischemia and/or infarction *Uncommon:* hypertensive crisis[1] *Rare:* QT prolongation[1]

Dermatologic: *Very common:* erythema *Common:* exfoliative dermatitis, acne, flushing, folliculitis, hyperkeratosis *Uncommon:* eczema, erythema multiforme

Digestive: *Very common:* increased lipase, increased amylase *Common:* mucositis, stomatitis (including dry mouth and glossodynia), dyspepsia, dysphagia, gastrointestinal reflux *Uncommon:* pancreatitis, gastritis, gastrointestinal perforations[1], cholecystitis, cholangitis
Note that elevations in lipase are very common (41%, see below); a diagnosis of pancreatitis should not be made solely on the basis of abnormal laboratory values.

General Disorders: *Very common:* infection, hemorrhage (including gastrointestinal[1] and respiratory tract[1] and uncommon cases of cerebral hemorrhage[1]), asthenia, pain (including mouth, bone, and tumor pain), pyrexia, decreased appetite *Common:* influenza-like illness

Hematologic: *Very common:* leukopenia, lymphopenia *Common:* anemia, neutropenia, thrombocytopenia *Uncommon:* INR abnormal

Hepatobiliary disorders: *Rare:* drug-induced hepatitis (including hepatic failure and death)

Hypersensitivity: *Uncommon:* hypersensitivity reactions (including skin reactions and urticaria), anaphylactic reaction

Metabolic and Nutritional: *Very common:* hypophosphatemia *Common:* transient increases in transaminases, hypocalcemia, hypokalemia, hyponatremia, hypothyroidism *Uncommon:* dehydration, transient increases in alkaline phosphatase, increased bilirubin (including jaundice), hyperthyroidism

Musculoskeletal: *Very common:* arthralgia *Common:* myalgia, muscle spasms

Nervous System and Psychiatric: *Common:* depression, dysgeusia *Uncommon:* tinnitus, reversible posterior leukoencephalopathy[1]

Table 6: Per-Patient Incidence of Selected Adverse Reactions Occurring at a Higher Incidence in NEXAVAR-Treated Patients [Between Arm Difference of ≥ 5% (All Grades)1 or ≥ 2% (Grades 3 and 4)]

MedDRA Primary System Organ Class & Preferred Term	NEXAVAR N = 207		Placebo N = 209	
	All Grades (%)	Grades 3 and 4 (%)	All Grades (%)	Grades 3 and 4 (%)
Gastrointestinal disorders				
Diarrhea	68	6	15	1
Nausea	21	0	12	0
Abdominal pain[2]	20	1	7	1
Constipation	16	0	8	0.5
Stomatitis[3]	24	2	3	0
Vomiting	11	0.5	6	0
Oral pain[4]	14	0	3	0
General disorders and administration site conditions				
Fatigue	41	5	20	1
Asthenia	12	0	7	0
Pyrexia	11	1	5	0
Investigations				
Weight loss	49	6	14	1
Metabolism and nutrition disorders				
Decreased appetite	30	2	5	0
Musculoskeletal and connective tissue disorders				
Pain in extremity	15	1	7	0
Muscle spasms	10	0	3	0
Neoplasms benign, malignant and unspecified				
Squamous cell carcinoma of skin	3	3	0	0
Nervous system disorders				
Headache	17	0	6	0
Dysgeusia	6	0	0	0
Respiratory, thoracic and mediastinal disorders				
Dysphonia	13	0.5	3	0
Epistaxis	7	0	1	0
Skin and subcutaneous tissue disorders				
PPES[5]	69	19	8	0
Alopecia	67	0	8	0
Rash	35	5	7	0
Pruritus	20	0.5	11	0
Dry skin	13	0.5	5	0
Erythema	10	0	0.5	0
Hyperkeratosis	7	0	0	0
Vascular disorders				
Hypertension[6]	41	10	12	2

[1] National Cancer Institute Common Terminology Criteria for Adverse Events Version 3.0
[2] Includes the following terms: abdominal pain, abdominal discomfort, hepatic pain, esophageal pain, esophageal discomfort, abdominal pain lower, abdominal pain upper, abdominal tenderness, abdominal rigidity
[3] Includes the following terms: stomatitis, aphthous stomatitis, mouth ulceration, mucosal inflammation
[4] Includes the following terms: oral pain, oropharyngeal discomfort, glossitis, burning mouth syndrome, glossodynia
[5] Palmar-plantar erythrodysesthesia syndrome (Hand-foot skin reaction)
[6] Includes the following terms: hypertension, blood pressure increased, blood pressure systolic increased

Renal and Genitourinary: *Common:* renal failure, proteinuria *Rare:* nephrotic syndrome
Reproductive: *Common:* erectile dysfunction *Uncommon:* gynecomastia
Respiratory: *Common:* rhinorrhea *Uncommon:* interstitial lung disease-like events (includes reports of pneumonitis, radiation pneumonitis, acute respiratory distress, interstitial pneumonia, pulmonitis and lung inflammation)
In addition, the following medically significant adverse reactions were uncommon during clinical trials of NEXAVAR: transient ischemic attack, arrhythmia, and thromboembolism. For these adverse reactions, the causal relationship to NEXAVAR has not been established.

---

[1]adverse reactions may have a life-threatening or fatal outcome.
[2]reported in 1.9% of patients treated with NEXAVAR (N= 2276).

6.5   Postmarketing Experience
The following adverse drug reactions have been identified during post-approval use of NEXAVAR. Because these reactions are reported voluntarily from a population of uncertain size, it is not always possible to reliably estimate their frequency or establish a causal relationship to drug exposure.
Dermatologic: Stevens-Johnson syndrome and toxic epidermal necrolysis (TEN)
Hypersensitivity: Angioedema
Musculoskeletal: Rhabdomyolysis, osteonecrosis of the jaw
Respiratory: Interstitial lung disease-like events (which may have a life-threatening or fatal outcome)

7   DRUG INTERACTIONS
7.1   Effect of Strong CYP3A4 Inducers on Sorafenib
Rifampin, a strong CYP3A4 inducer, administered at a dose of 600 mg once daily for 5 days with a single oral dose of NEXAVAR 400 mg in healthy volunteers resulted in a 37% decrease in the mean AUC of sorafenib [see Clinical Pharmacology (12.3)]. Avoid concomitant use of strong CYP3A4 inducers (such as, carbamazepine, dexamethasone, phenobarbital, phenytoin, rifampin, rifabutin, St. John's wort), when possible, because these drugs can decrease the systemic exposure to sorafenib.
7.2   Effect of Strong CYP3A4 Inhibitors on Sorafenib
Ketoconazole, a strong inhibitor of CYP3A4 and P-glycoprotein, administered at a dose of 400 mg once daily for 7 days did not alter the mean AUC of a single oral dose of NEXAVAR 50 mg in healthy volunteers.
7.3   Effect of Sorafenib on Other Drugs
NEXAVAR 400 mg twice daily for 28 days did not increase the systemic exposure of concomitantly administered midazolam (CYP3A4 substrate), dextromethorphan (CYP2D6 substrate), and omeprazole (CYP2C19 substrate) [see Clinical Pharmacology (12.3)].
7.4   Neomycin
Neomycin administered as an oral dose of 1 g three times daily for 5 days decreased the mean AUC of sorafenib by 54% in healthy volunteers administered a single oral dose of NEXAVAR 400 mg. The effects of other antibiotics on the pharmacokinetics of sorafenib have not been studied [see Clinical Pharmacology (12.3)].
7.5   Drugs that Increase Gastric pH
The aqueous solubility of sorafenib is pH dependent, with higher pH resulting in lower solubility. However, omeprazole, a proton pump inhibitor, administered at a dose of 40 mg once daily for 5 days, did not result in a clinically meaningful change in sorafenib single dose exposure. No dose adjustment for NEXAVAR is necessary.

8   USE IN SPECIFIC POPULATIONS
8.1   Pregnancy
Pregnancy Category D [see Warnings and Precautions (5.11)].
Based on its mechanism of action and findings in animals, NEXAVAR may cause fetal harm when administered to a pregnant woman. Sorafenib caused embryo-fetal toxicities in animals at maternal exposures that were significantly lower than the human exposures at the recommended dose of 400 mg twice daily. There are no adequate and well-controlled studies in pregnant women using NEXAVAR. Inform patients of childbearing potential that NEXAVAR can cause birth defects or fetal loss. Instruct both men and women of childbearing potential to use effective birth control during treatment with NEXAVAR and for at least 2 weeks after stopping treatment. Counsel female patients to contact their healthcare provider if they become pregnant while taking NEXAVAR.
When administered to rats and rabbits during the period of organogenesis, sorafenib was teratogenic and induced embryo-fetal toxicity (including increased post-implantation loss, resorptions, skeletal retardations, and retarded fetal weight). The effects occurred at doses considerably below the recommended human dose of 400 mg twice daily (approximately 500 mg/m²/day on a body surface area basis).

Adverse intrauterine development effects were seen at doses ≥0.2 mg/kg/day (1.2 mg/m²/day) in rats and 0.3 mg/kg/day (3.6 mg/m²/day) in rabbits. These doses result in exposures (AUC) approximately 0.008 times the AUC seen in patients at the recommended human dose. A NOAEL (no observed adverse effect level) was not defined for either species, since lower doses were not tested.
8.3   Nursing Mothers
It is not known whether sorafenib is excreted in human milk. Because many drugs are excreted in human milk and because of the potential for serious adverse reactions in nursing infants from NEXAVAR, a decision should be made whether to discontinue nursing or to discontinue the drug, taking into account the importance of the drug to the mother.
Following administration of radiolabeled sorafenib to lactating Wistar rats, approximately 27% of the radioactivity was secreted into the milk. The milk to plasma AUC ratio was approximately 5:1.
8.4   Pediatric Use
The safety and effectiveness of NEXAVAR in pediatric patients have not been studied.
Repeat dosing of sorafenib to young and growing dogs resulted in irregular thickening of the femoral growth plate at daily sorafenib doses ≥ 600 mg/m² (approximately 0.3 times the AUC at the recommended human dose), hypocellularity of the bone marrow adjoining the growth plate at 200 mg/m²/day (approximately 0.1 times the AUC at the recommended human dose), and alterations of the dentin composition at 600 mg/m²/day. Similar effects were not observed in adult dogs when dosed for 4 weeks or less.
8.5   Geriatric Use
In total, 59% of HCC patients treated with NEXAVAR were age 65 years or older, and 19% were 75 and older. In total, 32% of RCC patients treated with NEXAVAR were age 65 years or older, and 4% were 75 and older. No differences in safety or efficacy were observed between older and younger patients, and other reported clinical experience has not identified differences in responses between the elderly and younger patients, but greater sensitivity of some older individuals cannot be ruled out.
8.6   Patients with Hepatic Impairment
In a trial of HCC patients with mild (Child-Pugh A) or moderate (Child-Pugh B) hepatic impairment, the systemic exposure (AUC) of sorafenib was within the range observed in patients without hepatic impairment. In another trial in subjects without HCC, the mean AUC was similar for subjects with mild (n=15) and moderate (n=14) hepatic impairment compared to subjects (n=15) with normal hepatic function. No dose adjustment is necessary for patients with mild or moderate hepatic impairment. The pharmacokinetics of sorafenib have not been studied in patients with severe (Child-Pugh C) hepatic impairment [see Clinical Pharmacology (12.3)].
8.7   Patients with Renal Impairment
No correlation between sorafenib exposure and renal function was observed following administration of a single oral dose of NEXAVAR 400 mg to subjects with normal renal function and subjects with mild (CLcr 50–80 mL/min), moderate (CLcr 30–<50 mL/min), or severe (CLcr <30 mL/min) renal impairment who are not on dialysis. No dose adjustment is necessary for patients with mild, moderate or severe renal impairment who are not on dialysis. The pharmacokinetics of sorafenib have not been studied in patients who are on dialysis [see Clinical Pharmacology (12.3)].

10   OVERDOSAGE
There is no specific treatment for NEXAVAR overdose. The highest dose of NEXAVAR studied clinically was 800 mg twice daily. The adverse reactions observed at this dose were primarily diarrhea and dermatologic. No information is available on symptoms of acute overdose in animals because of the saturation of absorption in oral acute toxicity studies conducted in animals.
In cases of suspected overdose, NEXAVAR should be withheld and supportive care instituted.

11   DESCRIPTION
NEXAVAR, a kinase inhibitor, is the tosylate salt of sorafenib.
Sorafenib tosylate has the chemical name 4-(4-{3-[4-Chloro-3-(trifluoromethyl)phenyl]ureido}phenoxy)N2-methylpyridine-2-carboxamide 4-methylbenzenesulfonate and its structural formula is:
[See chemical structure at top of next column]
Sorafenib tosylate is a white to yellowish or brownish solid with a molecular formula of $C_{21}H_{16}ClF_3N_4O_3 \times C_7H_8O_3S$ and a molecular weight of 637.0 g/mole. Sorafenib tosylate is practically insoluble in aqueous media, slightly soluble in ethanol and soluble in PEG 400.
Each red, round NEXAVAR film-coated tablet contains sorafenib tosylate (274 mg) equivalent to 200 mg of sorafenib and the following inactive ingredients: croscarmellose sodium, microcrystalline cellulose, hypromellose, sodium lauryl sulphate, magnesium stearate, polyethylene glycol, titanium dioxide and ferric oxide red.

12   CLINICAL PHARMACOLOGY
12.1   Mechanism of Action
Sorafenib is a kinase inhibitor that decreases tumor cell proliferation in vitro.
Sorafenib was shown to inhibit multiple intracellular (c-CRAF, BRAF and mutant BRAF) and cell surface kinases (KIT, FLT- 3, RET, RET/PTC, VEGFR-1, VEGFR- 2, VEGFR- 3, and PDGFR-ß). Several of these kinases are thought to be involved in tumor cell signaling, angiogenesis and apoptosis. Sorafenib inhibited tumor growth of HCC, RCC, and DTC human tumor xenografts in immunocompromised mice. Reductions in tumor angiogenesis were seen in models of HCC and RCC upon sorafenib treatment, and increases in tumor apoptosis were observed in models of HCC, RCC, and DTC.
12.2   Pharmacodynamics
Cardiac Electrophysiology
The effect of NEXAVAR 400 mg twice daily on the QTc interval was evaluated in a multi-center, open-label, non-randomized trial in 53 patients with advanced cancer. No large changes in the mean QTc intervals (that is, >20 ms) from baseline were detected in the trial. After one 28-day treatment cycle, the largest mean QTc interval change of 8.5 ms (upper bound of two-sided 90% confidence interval, 13.3 ms) was observed at 6 hours post-dose on day 1 of cycle 2 [see Warnings and Precautions (5.9)].
12.3   Pharmacokinetics
The mean elimination half-life of sorafenib was approximately 25 to 48 hours. Multiple doses of NEXAVAR for 7 days resulted in a 2.5- to 7-fold accumulation compared to a single dose. Steady-state plasma sorafenib concentrations were achieved within 7 days, with a peak-to-trough ratio of mean concentrations of less than 2.
The steady-state concentrations of sorafenib following administration of 400 mg NEXAVAR twice daily were evaluated in DTC, RCC and HCC patients. Patients with DTC have mean steady-state concentrations that are 1.8-fold higher than patients with HCC and 2.3-fold higher than those with RCC. The reason for increased sorafenib concentrations in DTC patients is unknown.
Absorption and Distribution: After administration of NEXAVAR tablets, the mean relative bioavailability was 38–49% when compared to an oral solution. Following oral administration, sorafenib reached peak plasma levels in approximately 3 hours. With a moderate-fat meal (30% fat; 700 calories), bioavailability was similar to that in the fasted state. With a high-fat meal (50% fat; 900 calories), bioavailability was reduced by 29% compared to that in the fasted state. It is recommended that NEXAVAR be administered without food [see Dosage and Administration (2.1)]. Mean C_{max} and AUC increased less than proportionally beyond oral doses of 400 mg administered twice daily. In vitro binding of sorafenib to human plasma proteins was 99.5%.
Metabolism and Elimination: Sorafenib undergoes oxidative metabolism by hepatic CYP3A4, as well as glucuronidation by UGT1A9. Inducers of CYP3A4 activity can decrease the systemic exposure of sorafenib [see Drug Interactions (7.1)].
Sorafenib accounted for approximately 70–85% of the circulating analytes in plasma at steady-state. Eight metabolites of sorafenib have been identified, of which 5 have been detected in plasma. The main circulating metabolite of sorafenib, the pyridine N-oxide that comprises approximately 9–16% of circulating analytes at steady-state, showed in vitro potency similar to that of sorafenib.
Following oral administration of a 100 mg dose of a solution formulation of sorafenib, 96% of the dose was recovered within 14 days, with 77% of the dose excreted in feces and 19% of the dose excreted in urine as glucuronidated metabolites. Unchanged sorafenib, accounting for 51% of the dose, was found in feces but not in urine.
Effects of Age, Gender and Race: A study of the pharmacokinetics of sorafenib indicated that the mean AUC of sorafenib in Asians (N=78) was 30% lower than in Caucasians (N=40). Gender and age do not have a clinically meaningful effect on the pharmacokinetics of sorafenib.
Renal Impairment: Mild (CLcr 50-80 mL/min), moderate (CLcr 30 - <50 mL/min), and severe (CLcr <30 mL/min) renal impairment do not affect the pharmacokinetics of sorafenib. No dose adjustment is necessary [see Use in Specific Populations (8.7)].

Hepatic Impairment: Mild (Child-Pugh A) and moderate (Child-Pugh B) hepatic impairment do not affect the pharmacokinetics of sorafenib. No dose adjustment is necessary *[see Use in Specific Populations (8.6)].*

Drug-Drug Interactions: Studies in human liver microsomes demonstrated that sorafenib competitively inhibited CYP2B6, CYP2C8, CYP2C9, CYP2C19, CYP2D6, and CYP3A4. However, NEXAVAR 400 mg twice daily for 28 days with substrates of CYP3A4, CYP2D6 and CYP2C19 did not increase the systemic exposure of these substrates *[see Drug Interactions (7.3)].*

Studies with cultured human hepatocytes demonstrated that sorafenib did not increase CYP1A2 and CYP3A4 activities, suggesting that sorafenib is unlikely to induce CYP1A2 or CYP3A4 in humans.

Sorafenib inhibits glucuronidation by UGT1A1 and UGT1A9 *in vitro.* NEXAVAR could increase the systemic exposure of concomitantly administered drugs that are UGT1A1 or UGT1A9 substrates.

Sorafenib inhibited P-glycoprotein *in vitro.* NEXAVAR could increase the concentrations of concomitantly administered drugs that are P-glycoprotein substrates.

13 NONCLINICAL TOXICOLOGY
13.1 Carcinogenesis, Mutagenesis, Impairment of Fertility

Carcinogenicity studies have not been performed with sorafenib.

Sorafenib was clastogenic when tested in an *in vitro* mammalian cell assay (Chinese hamster ovary) in the presence of metabolic activation. Sorafenib was not mutagenic in the *in vitro* Ames bacterial cell assay or clastogenic in an *in vivo* mouse micronucleus assay. One intermediate in the manufacturing process, which is also present in the final drug substance (<0.15%), was positive for mutagenesis in an *in vitro* bacterial cell assay (Ames test) when tested independently.

No specific studies with sorafenib have been conducted in animals to evaluate the effect on fertility. However, results from the repeat-dose toxicity studies suggest there is a potential for sorafenib to impair reproductive function and fertility. Multiple adverse effects were observed in male and female reproductive organs, with the rat being more susceptible than mice or dogs. Typical changes in rats consisted of testicular atrophy or degeneration, degeneration of epididymis, prostate, and seminal vesicles, central necrosis of the corpora lutea and arrested follicular development. Sorafenib-related effects on the reproductive organs of rats were manifested at daily oral doses ≥ 5 mg/kg (30 mg/m^2). This dose results in an exposure (AUC) that is approximately 0.5 times the AUC in patients at the recommended human dose. Dogs showed tubular degeneration in the testes at 30 mg/kg/day (600 mg/m^2/day). This dose results in an exposure that is approximately 0.3 times the AUC at the recommended human dose. Oligospermia was observed in dogs at 60 mg/kg/day (1200 mg/m^2/day) of sorafenib. Adequate contraception should be used during therapy and for at least 2 weeks after completing therapy.

14 CLINICAL STUDIES

The clinical safety and efficacy of NEXAVAR have been studied in patients with hepatocellular carcinoma (HCC), renal cell carcinoma (RCC), and differentiated thyroid carcinoma (DTC).

14.1 Hepatocellular Carcinoma

The **HCC Study** was a Phase 3, international, multicenter, randomized, double blind, placebo-controlled trial in patients with unresectable hepatocellular carcinoma. Overall survival was the primary endpoint. A total of 602 patients were randomized; 299 to NEXAVAR 400 mg twice daily and 303 to matching placebo.

Demographics and baseline disease characteristics were similar between the NEXAVAR and placebo-treated groups with regard to age, gender, race, performance status, etiology (including hepatitis B, hepatitis C and alcoholic liver disease), TNM stage (stage I: <1% vs. <1%; stage II: 10.4% vs. 8.3%; stage III: 37.8% vs. 43.6%; stage IV: 50.8% vs. 46.9%), absence of both macroscopic vascular invasion and extrahepatic tumor spread (30.1% vs. 30.0%), and Barcelona Clinic Liver Cancer stage (stage B: 18.1% vs. 16.8%; stage C: 81.6% vs. 83.2%; stage D: <1% vs. 0%). Liver impairment by Child-Pugh score was comparable between the NEXAVAR and placebo-treated groups (Class A: 95% vs. 98%; B: 5% vs. 2%). Only one patient with Child-Pugh class C was entered. Prior treatments included surgical resection procedures (19.1% vs. 20.5%), locoregional therapies (including radiofrequency ablation, percutaneous ethanol injection and transarterial chemoembolization; 38.8% vs. 40.6%), radiotherapy (4.3% vs. 5.0%) and systemic therapy (3.0% vs. 5.0%).

The trial was stopped for efficacy following a pre-specified second interim analysis for survival showing a statistically significant advantage for NEXAVAR over placebo for overall survival (HR: 0.69, p= 0.00058) (see Table 4 and Figure 1). This advantage was consistent across all subsets analyzed.

Table 7: Efficacy Results from HCC Study

Efficacy Parameter	NEXAVAR (N=299)	Placebo (N=303)	Hazard Ratio* (95% CI)	P-value (log-rank test)[†]
Overall Survival Median, months (95% CI) No. of events	10.7 (9.4, 13.3) 143	7.9 (6.8, 9.1) 178	0.69 (0.55, 0.87)	0.00058
Time to Progression[‡] Median, months (95% CI) No. of events	5.5 (4.1, 6.9) 107	2.8 (2.7, 3.9) 156	0.58 (0.45, 0.74)	0.000007

CI=Confidence interval

* Hazard ratio, sorafenib/placebo, stratified Cox model
† Stratified log rank (for the interim analysis of survival, the stopping boundary one-sided alpha = 0.0077)
‡ The time-to-progression (TTP) analysis, based on independent radiologic review, was based on data from an earlier time point than the survival analysis

Final analysis of time to tumor progression (TTP) based on data from an earlier time point (by independent radiologic review) also was significantly longer in the NEXAVAR arm (HR: 0.58, p=0.000007) (see Table 7).
[See table 7 above]

Figure 1: Kaplan-Meier Curve of Overall Survival in HCC Study (Intent-to-Treat Population)

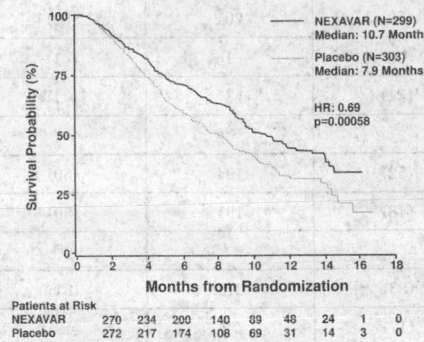

Patients at Risk										
NEXAVAR	270	234	200	140	89	48	24	1	0
Placebo	272	217	174	108	69	31	14	3	0

14.2 Renal Cell Carcinoma

The safety and efficacy of NEXAVAR in the treatment of advanced renal cell carcinoma (RCC) were studied in the following two randomized controlled clinical trials.

RCC Study 1 was a Phase 3, international, multicenter, randomized, double blind, placebo-controlled trial in patients with advanced renal cell carcinoma who had received one prior systemic therapy. Primary study endpoints included overall survival and progression-free survival (PFS). Tumor response rate was a secondary endpoint. The PFS analysis included 769 patients stratified by MSKCC (Memorial Sloan Kettering Cancer Center) prognostic risk category (low or intermediate) and country and randomized to NEXAVAR 400 mg twice daily (N=384) or to placebo (N=385).

Table 8 summarizes the demographic and disease characteristics of the study population analyzed. Baseline demographics and disease characteristics were well balanced for both treatment groups. The median time from initial diagnosis of RCC to randomization was 1.6 and 1.9 years for the NEXAVAR and placebo-treated groups, respectively.
[See table 8 at top of next page]

Progression-free survival, defined as the time from randomization to progression or death from any cause, whichever occurred earlier, was evaluated by blinded independent radiological review using RECIST criteria.

Figure 2 depicts Kaplan-Meier curves for PFS. The PFS analysis was based on a two-sided Log-Rank test stratified by MSKCC prognostic risk category and country.
[See figure 2 at top of next column]

NOTE: HR is from Cox regression model with the following covariates: MSKCC prognostic risk category and country. P-value is from two-sided Log-Rank test stratified by MSKCC prognostic risk category and country.

The median PFS for patients randomized to NEXAVAR was 167 days compared to 84 days for patients randomized to placebo. The estimated hazard ratio (risk of progression with NEXAVAR compared to placebo) was 0.44 (95% CI: 0.35, 0.55).

A series of patient subsets were examined in exploratory univariate analyses of PFS. The subsets included age above or below 65 years, ECOG PS 0 or 1, MSKCC prognostic risk category, whether the prior therapy was for progressive metastatic disease or for an earlier disease setting and time

Figure 2: Kaplan-Meier Curves for Progression-free Survival – RCC Study 1

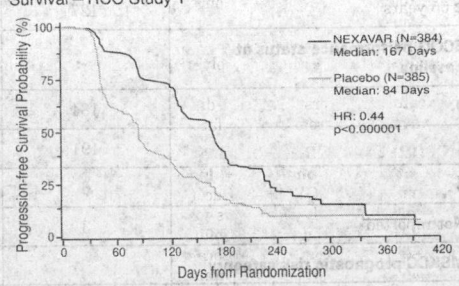

from diagnosis of less than or greater than 1.5 years. The effect of NEXAVAR on PFS was consistent across these subsets, including patients with no prior IL-2 or interferon therapy (N=137; 65 patients receiving NEXAVAR and 72 placebo), for whom the median PFS was 172 days on NEXAVAR compared to 85 days on placebo.

Tumor response was determined by independent radiologic review according to RECIST criteria. Overall, of 672 patients who were evaluable for response, 7 (2%) NEXAVAR-treated patients and 0 (0%) placebo-treated patients had a confirmed partial response. Thus the gain in PFS in NEXAVAR-treated patients primarily reflects the stable disease population.

At the time of a planned interim survival analysis, based on 220 deaths, overall survival was longer for NEXAVAR than placebo with a hazard ratio (NEXAVAR over placebo) of 0.72. This analysis did not meet the prespecified criteria for statistical significance. Additional analyses are planned as the survival data mature.

RCC Study 2 was a Phase 2 randomized discontinuation trial in patients with metastatic malignancies, including RCC. The primary endpoint was the percentage of randomized patients remaining progression-free at 24 weeks. All patients received NEXAVAR for the first 12 weeks. Radiologic assessment was repeated at week 12. Patients with <25% change in bi-dimensional tumor measurements from baseline were randomized to NEXAVAR or placebo for a further 12 weeks. Patients who were randomized to placebo were permitted to cross over to open-label NEXAVAR upon progression. Patients with tumor shrinkage ≥25% continued NEXAVAR, whereas patients with tumor growth ≥25% discontinued treatment.

A total of 202 patients with advanced RCC were enrolled into RCC Study 2, including patients who had received no prior therapy and patients with tumor histology other than clear cell carcinoma. After the initial 12 weeks of NEXAVAR, 79 patients with RCC continued on open-label NEXAVAR, and 65 patients were randomized to NEXAVAR or placebo. After an additional 12 weeks, at week 24, for the 65 randomized patients, the progression-free rate was significantly higher in patients randomized to NEXAVAR (16/32, 50%) than in patients randomized to placebo (6/33, 18%) (p=0.0077). Progression-free survival was significantly longer in the NEXAVAR-treated group (163 days) than in the placebo-treated group (41 days) (p=0.0001, HR=0.29).

14.3 Differentiated Thyroid Carcinoma

The safety and effectiveness of NEXAVAR was established in a multicenter, randomized (1:1), double-blind, placebo-controlled trial conducted in 417 patients with locally recurrent or metastatic, progressive differentiated thyroid carcinoma (DTC) refractory to radioactive iodine (RAI) treatment. Randomization was stratified by age (< 60 years versus ≥ 60 years) and geographical region (North America, Europe, and Asia).

Table 8: Demographic and Disease Characteristics – RCC Study 1

Characteristics	NEXAVAR N=384		Placebo N=385	
	N	(%)	N	(%)
Gender				
Male	267	(70)	287	(75)
Female	116	(30)	98	(25)
Race				
White	276	(72)	278	(73)
Black/Asian/ Hispanic/Other	11	(3)	10	(2)
Not reported *	97	(25)	97	(25)
Age group				
< 65 years	255	(67)	280	(73)
≥ 65 years	127	(33)	103	(27)
ECOG performance status at baseline				
0	184	(48)	180	(47)
1	191	(50)	201	(52)
2	6	(2)	1	(<1)
Not reported	3	(<1)	3	(<1)
MSKCC prognostic risk category				
Low	200	(52)	194	(50)
Intermediate	184	(48)	191	(50)
Prior IL-2 and/or interferon				
Yes	319	(83)	313	(81)
No	65	(17)	72	(19)

* Race was not collected from the 186 patients enrolled in France due to local regulations. In 8 other patients, race was not available at the time of analysis.

All patients were required to have actively progressing disease defined as progression within 14 months of enrollment. RAI-refractory disease was defined based on four criteria that were not mutually exclusive. All RAI treatments and diagnostic scans were to be performed under conditions of a low iodine diet and adequate TSH stimulation. Following are the RAI-refractory criteria and the proportion of patients in the study that met each one: a target lesion with no iodine uptake on RAI scan (68%); tumors with iodine uptake and progression after RAI treatment within 16 months of enrollment (12%); tumors with iodine uptake and multiple RAI treatments with the last treatment greater than 16 months prior to enrollment, and disease progression after each of two RAI treatments administered within 16 months of each other (7%); cumulative RAI dose ≥ 600 mCi administered (34%). The major efficacy outcome measure was progression-free survival (PFS) as determined by a blinded, independent radiological review using a modified Response Evaluation Criteria in Solid Tumors v. 1.0 (RECIST). RECIST was modified by inclusion of clinical progression of bone lesions based on the need for external beam radiation (4.4% of progression events). Additional efficacy outcomes measures included overall survival (OS), tumor response rate, and duration of response.

Patients were randomized to receive NEXAVAR 400 mg twice daily (n=207) or placebo (n=210). Of the 417 patients randomized, 48% were male, the median age was 63 years, 61% were 60 years or older, 60% were white, 62% had an ECOG performance status of 0, and 99% had undergone thyroidectomy. The histological diagnoses were papillary carcinoma in 57%, follicular carcinoma (including Hürthle cell) in 25%, and poorly differentiated carcinoma in 10%, and other in 8% of the study population. Metastases were present in 96% of the patients: lungs in 86%, lymph nodes in 51%, and bone in 27%. The median cumulative RAI activity administered prior to study entry was 400 mCi.

A statistically significant prolongation in PFS was demonstrated among NEXAVAR-treated patients compared to those receiving placebo. Following investigator-determined disease progression, 157 (75%) patients randomized to placebo crossed over to open-label NEXAVAR, and 61 (30%) patients randomized to NEXAVAR received open-label NEXAVAR. There was no statistically significant difference in overall survival between the two treatment arms (see Table 9 and Figure 3).

Table 9: Efficacy Results from Study in Differentiated Thyroid Carcinoma

	NEXAVAR N=207	Placebo N=210
Progression-free Survival[1]		
Number of Deaths or Progression	113 (55%)	136 (65%)
Median PFS in Months (95% CI)	10.8 (9.1, 12.9)	5.8 (5.3, 7.8)
Hazard Ratio (95% CI)	0.59 (0.46, 0.76)	
P-value [2]	<0.001	
Overall Survival[3]		
Number of Deaths	66 (32%)	72 (34%)
Median OS in Months (95% CI)	NR	36.5 (32.2, NR)
Hazard Ratio (95% CI)	0.88 (0.63, 1.24)	
P-value[2]	0.47	

Objective Response

Number of Objective Responders [4]	24 (12%)	1 (0.5%)
(95%CI)	(7.6%, 16.8%)	(0.01%, 2.7%)
Median Duration of Response in Months (95% CI)	10.2 (7.4, 16.6)	NE

[1] Independent radiological review
[2] Two-sided log-rank test stratified by age (< 60 years, ≥ 60 years) and geographic region (North America, Europe, Asia)
[3] Conducted 9 months after the data cut-off for the final PFS analysis
[4] All objective responses were partial responses
NR = Not Reached, CI = Confidence interval, NE = Not Estimable

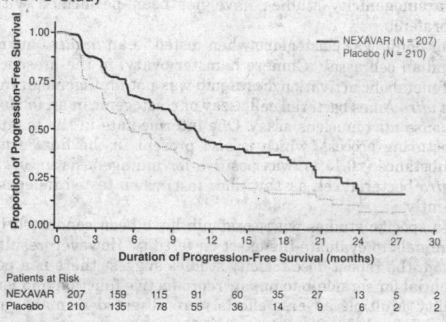

Figure 3: Kaplan-Meier Curve of Progression-Free Survival in DTC Study

16 HOW SUPPLIED/STORAGE AND HANDLING

NEXAVAR tablets are supplied as round, biconvex, red film-coated tablets, debossed with the "Bayer cross" on one side and "200" on the other side, each containing sorafenib tosylate equivalent to 200 mg of sorafenib.
Bottles of 120 tablets NDC 50419-488-58
Storage
Store at 25°C (77°F); excursions permitted to 15–30°C (59–86°F) (see USP controlled room temperature). Store in a dry place.

17 PATIENT COUNSELING INFORMATION

See FDA-approved Patient Labeling
Cardiac Ischemia; Infarction
Discuss with patients that cardiac ischemia and/or infarction has been reported during NEXAVAR treatment, and that they should immediately report any episodes of chest pain or other symptoms of cardiac ischemia *[see Warnings and Precautions (5.1)]*.
Bleeding
Inform patients that NEXAVAR can increase the risk of bleeding and that they should promptly report any episodes of bleeding *[see Warnings and Precautions (5.2)]*.
Inform patients that bleeding or elevations in the International Normalized Ratio (INR) have been reported in some patients taking warfarin while on NEXAVAR and that their INR should be monitored regularly *[see Warnings and Precautions (5.6)]*.
Hypertension
Inform patients that hypertension can develop during NEXAVAR treatment, especially during the first six weeks of therapy, and that blood pressure should be monitored regularly during treatment *[see Warnings and Precautions (5.3)]*.
Skin Reactions
Advise patients of the possible occurrence of hand-foot skin reaction and rash during NEXAVAR treatment and appropriate countermeasures *[see Warnings and Precautions (5.4)]*.
Gastrointestinal Perforation
Advise patients that cases of gastrointestinal perforation have been reported in patients taking NEXAVAR *[see Warnings and Precautions (5.5)]*.
Wound Healing Complications
Inform patients that temporary interruption of NEXAVAR is recommended in patients undergoing major surgical procedures *[see Warnings and Precautions (5.7)]*.
QT Interval Prolongation
Inform patients with a history of prolonged QT interval that NEXAVAR can worsen the condition *[see Warnings and Precautions (5.9) and Clinical Pharmacology (12.2)]*.

Drug-Induced Hepatitis
Inform patients that NEXAVAR can cause hepatitis which may result in hepatic failure and death. Advise patients that liver function tests should be monitored regularly during treatment and to report signs and symptoms of hepatitis *[see Warnings and Precautions (5.10)].*

Birth Defects and Fetal Loss
Inform patients that NEXAVAR can cause birth defects or fetal loss. Counsel both male and female patients to use effective birth control during treatment with NEXAVAR and for at least 2 weeks after stopping treatment. Inform female patients to contact their healthcare provider if they become pregnant while taking NEXAVAR *[see Warnings and Precautions (5.11), Use in Specific Populations (8.1)].*

Nursing Mothers
Advise mothers not to breast-feed while taking NEXAVAR *[see Use in Specific Populations (8.3)].*

Missed Doses
Instruct patients that if a dose of NEXAVAR is missed, the next dose should be taken at the regularly scheduled time, and not double the dose. Instruct patients to contact their healthcare provider immediately if they take too much NEXAVAR.

Patient Information

NEXAVAR® (NEX-A-VAR)
(sorafenib)
tablets, oral
Read this Patient Information before you start taking NEXAVAR and each time you get a refill. There may be new information. This information does not take the place of talking with your doctor about your medical condition or your treatment.

What is NEXAVAR?
NEXAVAR is an anticancer medicine used to treat a certain type of liver, kidney or thyroid cancer called:
• Hepatocellular carcinoma (HCC, a type of liver cancer), when it cannot be treated with surgery
• Renal cell carcinoma (RCC, a type of kidney cancer)
• Differentiated thyroid carcinoma (DTC, a type of thyroid cancer) that can no longer be treated with radioactive iodine and is progressing
NEXAVAR has not been studied in children.

Who should not take NEXAVAR?
Do not take NEXAVAR if you:
• are allergic to sorafenib or any of the other ingredients in NEXAVAR. See the end of this leaflet for a complete list of ingredients in NEXAVAR.
• have a specific type of lung cancer (squamous cell) and receive carboplatin and paclitaxel.

What should I tell my doctor before taking NEXAVAR?
Before you take NEXAVAR, tell your doctor if you:
• have any allergies
• have heart problems, including a problem called "congenital long QT syndrome"
• have chest pain
• have bleeding problems
• have high blood pressure
• plan to have any surgical procedures
• have lung cancer or are being treated for lung cancer
• have kidney problems in addition to kidney cancer
• have liver problems in addition to liver cancer
• are pregnant or plan to become pregnant. See **"What are the possible side effects of NEXAVAR?"**
• are breast-feeding or plan to breast-feed. It is not known if NEXAVAR passes into your breast milk. You and your doctor should decide if you will take NEXAVAR or breast-feed. You should not do both.
Tell your doctor about all the medicines you take, including prescription and over-the-counter medicines, vitamins, and herbal supplements.
NEXAVAR and certain other medicines can interact with each other and cause serious side effects.
Especially tell your doctor if you are taking the following medicines:
• warfarin (Coumadin, Jantoven®)
• neomycin
• St. Johns Wort
• dexamethasone
• phenytoin (Fosphenytoin sodium, Dilantin, Phenytek)
• carbamazepine (Carbatrol, Equetro, Tegretol, Teril, Epitol)
• rifampin (Rifater, Rifamate, Rifadin, Rimactane)
• rifabutin (Mycobutin)
• phenobarbital
Know the medicines you take. Keep a list of your medicines and show it to your doctor and pharmacist when you get a new medicine. Do not take other medicines with NEXAVAR until you have talked with your doctor.

How should I take NEXAVAR?
• Take NEXAVAR exactly as prescribed by your doctor.
• The usual dose of NEXAVAR is 2 tablets taken 2 times a day (for a total of 4 tablets each day). Your doctor may change your dose during treatment, stop treatment for some time or completely stop treatment with NEXAVAR if you have side effects.

• Take NEXAVAR without food (at least 1 hour before or 2 hours after a meal).
• If you miss a dose of NEXAVAR, skip the missed dose, and take your next dose at your regular time. Do not double your dose of NEXAVAR.
• If you take too much NEXAVAR call your doctor or go to the nearest hospital emergency room right away.

What are the possible side effects of NEXAVAR?
NEXAVAR may cause serious side effects, including:
• **decreased blood flow to the heart and heart attack.** Get emergency help right away and call your doctor if you get symptoms such as chest pain, shortness of breath, feel lightheaded or faint, nausea, vomiting, or sweat a lot.
• **bleeding problems. Bleeding is a common side effect of NEXAVAR** that can be serious and sometimes lead to death. Tell your doctor if you have any bleeding while taking NEXAVAR.
• **high blood pressure. High blood pressure is a common side effect of NEXAVAR and can be serious.** Your blood pressure should be checked every week during the first 6 weeks of starting NEXAVAR. Your blood pressure should be checked regularly and any high blood pressure should be treated while you are taking NEXAVAR.
• **a skin problem called hand-foot skin reaction.** This causes redness, pain, swelling, or blisters on the palms of your hands or soles of your feet. If you get this side effect, your doctor may change your dose or stop treatment for some time.
• **serious skin and mouth reactions.** NEXAVAR can cause serious skin reactions which can be life-threatening. Tell your doctor if you have any of the following symptoms:
• skin rash
• blistering and peeling of the skin
• blistering and peeling on the inside of your mouth
• **an opening in the wall of your stomach or intestines (perforation of the bowel).** Tell your doctor right away if you get high fever, nausea, vomiting or severe stomach (abdominal) pain.
• **possible wound healing problems.** If you need to have a surgical procedure, tell your doctor that you are taking NEXAVAR. NEXAVAR may need to be stopped until your wound heals after some types of surgery.
• **changes in the electrical activity of your heart called QT prolongation.** QT prolongation can cause irregular heartbeats that can be life-threatening. Your doctor may do tests during your treatment with NEXAVAR to check the levels of potassium, magnesium, and calcium in your blood, and check the electrical activity of your heart with an ECG. Tell your doctor right away if you feel faint, lightheaded, dizzy or feel your heart beating irregularly or fast while taking NEXAVAR.
• **inflammation of your liver (drug-induced hepatitis).** NEXAVAR may cause liver problems that may lead to liver failure and death. Your doctor may stop your treatment with NEXAVAR if you develop changes in certain liver function tests. Call your doctor right away if you develop any of the following symptoms:
• your skin or the white part of your eyes turns yellow (jaundice)
• dark "tea-colored" urine
• light-colored bowel movements (stools)
• worsening nausea
• worsening vomiting
• abdominal pain
• **birth defects or death of an unborn baby.** Women should not get pregnant during treatment with NEXAVAR and for at least 2 weeks after stopping treatment. Men and women should use effective birth control during treatment with NEXAVAR and for at least 2 weeks after stopping treatment. Talk with your doctor about effective birth control methods. Call your doctor right away if you become pregnant during treatment with NEXAVAR.
• **change in thyroid hormone levels.** If you have differentiated thyroid cancer, you can have changes in your thyroid hormone levels when taking NEXAVAR. Your doctor may need to increase your dose of thyroid medicine while you are taking NEXAVAR. Your doctor should check your thyroid hormone levels every month during treatment with NEXAVAR.

The most common side effects of NEXAVAR include:
• diarrhea (frequent or loose bowel movements)
• tiredness
• infection
• hair thinning or patchy hair loss
• rash
• weight loss
• loss of appetite
• nausea
• stomach (abdominal) pain
• low blood calcium levels in people with differentiated thyroid cancer
Tell your doctor if you have any side effect that bothers you or that does not go away. These are not all the possible side effects of NEXAVAR. Ask your doctor or pharmacist for more information.
Call your doctor for medical advice about side effects. You may report side effects to FDA at 1-800-FDA-1088.

How should I store NEXAVAR?
• Store NEXAVAR tablets at room temperature between 68° F to 77° F (20° C to 25° C).
• Store NEXAVAR tablets in a dry place.
Keep NEXAVAR and all medicines out of the reach of children.

General information about NEXAVAR
Medicines are sometimes prescribed for purposes other than those listed in a Patient Information leaflet. Do not use NEXAVAR for a condition for which it is not prescribed. Do not give NEXAVAR to other people even if they have the same symptoms you have. It may harm them.
This Patient Information leaflet summarizes the most important information about NEXAVAR. If you would like more information, talk with your doctor. You can ask your doctor or pharmacist for information about NEXAVAR that is written for health professionals.
For more information, go to www.NEXAVAR.com, or call 1-866-639-2827.

What are the ingredients in NEXAVAR?
Active Ingredient: sorafenib tosylate
Inactive Ingredients: croscarmellose sodium, microcrystalline cellulose, hypromellose, sodium lauryl sulphate, magnesium stearate, polyethylene glycol, titanium dioxide and ferric oxide red.
This Patient Information has been approved by the U.S. Food and Drug Administration.
Manufactured for:
Bayer HealthCare Pharmaceuticals Inc.,
Whippany, NJ 07981
Manufactured in Germany
Onyx Pharmaceuticals, Inc.,
249 East Grand Avenue, South San Francisco, CA 94080
Distributed and marketed by:
Bayer HealthCare Pharmaceuticals Inc.,
Whippany, NJ 07981
Marketed by:
Onyx Pharmaceuticals, Inc.
249 East Grand Avenue, South San Francisco, CA 94080
© 2013 Bayer HealthCare Pharmaceuticals Inc. Printed in U.S.A.
Revised 11/2013
Shown in Product Identification Guide, page 305

STIVARGA   ℞
(regorafenib)
tablets, for oral use

HIGHLIGHTS OF PRESCRIBING INFORMATION
These highlights do not include all the information needed to use STIVARGA safely and effectively. See full prescribing information for STIVARGA.
STIVARGA® (regorafenib) tablets, for oral use
Initial U.S. Approval: 2012

WARNING: HEPATOTOXICITY
See full prescribing information for complete boxed warning.
• **Severe and sometimes fatal hepatotoxicity has been observed in clinical trials. (5.1)**
• **Monitor hepatic function prior to and during treatment. (5.1)**
• **Interrupt and then reduce or discontinue Stivarga for hepatotoxicity as manifested by elevated liver function tests or hepatocellular necrosis, depending upon severity and persistence. (2.2)**

——————RECENT MAJOR CHANGES——————
Indications and Usage (1.2)   02/2013
Warnings and Precautions (5.1, 5.2, 5.3, 5.4, 5.5)   02/2013

——————INDICATIONS AND USAGE——————
Stivarga is a kinase inhibitor indicated for the treatment of patients with:
• Metastatic colorectal cancer (CRC) who have been previously treated with fluoropyrimidine-, oxaliplatin- and irinotecan-based chemotherapy, an anti-VEGF therapy, and, if KRAS wild type, an anti-EGFR therapy. (1.1)
• Locally advanced, unresectable or metastatic gastrointestinal stromal tumor (GIST) who have been previously treated with imatinib mesylate and sunitinib malate. (1.2)

——————DOSAGE AND ADMINISTRATION——————
• Recommended Dose: 160 mg orally, once daily for the first 21 days of each 28-day cycle. (2.1)
• Take Stivarga with food (a low-fat breakfast). (2.1, 12.3)

——————DOSAGE FORMS AND STRENGTHS——————
40 mg film-coated tablets (3)

——————CONTRAINDICATIONS——————
None. (4)

WARNINGS AND PRECAUTIONS

- Hemorrhage: Permanently discontinue Stivarga for severe or life-threatening hemorrhage. (5.2)
- Dermatological toxicity: Interrupt and then reduce or discontinue Stivarga depending on severity and persistence of dermatologic toxicity. (5.3)
- Hypertension: Temporarily or permanently discontinue Stivarga for severe or uncontrolled hypertension. (5.4)
- Cardiac ischemia and infarction: Withhold Stivarga for new or acute cardiac ischemia/infarction and resume only after resolution of acute ischemic events. (5.5)
- Reversible Posterior Leukoencephalopathy Syndrome (RPLS): Discontinue Stivarga. (5.6)
- Gastrointestinal perforation or fistulae: Discontinue Stivarga. (5.7)
- Wound healing complications: Stop Stivarga before surgery. Discontinue in patients with wound dehiscence. (5.8)
- Embryofetal toxicity: Can cause fetal harm. Advise women of potential risk to a fetus. (5.9, 8.1)

ADVERSE REACTIONS

The most common adverse reactions (≥20%) are asthenia/fatigue, HFSR, diarrhea, decreased appetite/food intake, hypertension, mucositis, dysphonia, and infection, pain (not otherwise specified), decreased weight, gastrointestinal and abdominal pain, rash, fever, and nausea. (6)

To report SUSPECTED ADVERSE REACTIONS, contact Bayer HealthCare Pharmaceuticals Inc. at 1-888-842-2937 or FDA at 1-800-FDA-1088 or www.fda.gov/medwatch.

DRUG INTERACTIONS

- Strong CYP3A4 inducers: Avoid strong CYP3A4 inducers. (7.1)
- Strong CYP3A4 inhibitors: Avoid strong CYP3A4 inhibitors. (7.2)

USE IN SPECIFIC POPULATIONS

Nursing Mothers: Discontinue drug or nursing, taking into consideration the importance of the drug to the mother. (8.3)

See 17 for PATIENT COUNSELING INFORMATION and FDA-approved patient labeling

Revised: 08/2013

FULL PRESCRIBING INFORMATION

> **WARNING: HEPATOTOXICITY**
> - Severe and sometimes fatal hepatotoxicity has been observed in clinical trials *[see Warnings and Precautions (5.1)]*.
> - Monitor hepatic function prior to and during treatment *[see Warnings and Precautions (5.1)]*.
> - Interrupt and then reduce or discontinue Stivarga for hepatotoxicity as manifested by elevated liver function tests or hepatocellular necrosis, depending upon severity and persistence *[see Dosage and Administration (2.2)]*.

1   INDICATIONS AND USAGE

1.1   Colorectal Cancer

Stivarga® is indicated for the treatment of patients with metastatic colorectal cancer (CRC) who have been previously treated with fluoropyrimidine-, oxaliplatin- and irinotecan-based chemotherapy, an anti-VEGF therapy, and, if KRAS wild type, an anti-EGFR therapy.

1.2   Gastrointestinal Stromal Tumors

Stivarga is indicated for the treatment of patients with locally advanced, unresectable or metastatic gastrointestinal stromal tumor (GIST) who have been previously treated with imatinib mesylate and sunitinib malate.

2   DOSAGE AND ADMINISTRATION

2.1   Recommended Dose

The recommended dose is 160 mg regorafenib (four 40 mg tablets) taken orally once daily for the first 21 days of each 28-day cycle. Continue treatment until disease progression or unacceptable toxicity.

Take Stivarga at the same time each day. Swallow tablet whole with a low-fat breakfast that contains less than 30% fat *[see Clinical Pharmacology (12.3)]*. Examples of a low-fat breakfast include 2 slices of white toast with 1 tablespoon of low-fat margarine and 1 tablespoon of jelly, and 8 ounces of skim milk (319 calories and 8.2 g fat); or 1 cup of cereal, 8 ounces of skim milk, 1 slice of toast with jam, apple juice, and 1 cup of coffee or tea (520 calories and 2 g fat). Do not take two doses of Stivarga on the same day to make up for a missed dose from the previous day.

2.2   Dose Modifications

Interrupt Stivarga for the following:
- NCI CTCAE Grade 2 hand-foot skin reaction (HFSR) [palmar-plantar erythrodysesthesia (PPE)] that is recurrent or does not improve within 7 days despite dose reduction; interrupt therapy for a minimum of 7 days for Grade 3 HFSR
- Symptomatic Grade 2 hypertension
- Any NCI CTCAE Grade 3 or 4 adverse reaction

Reduce the dose of Stivarga to 120 mg:
- For the first occurrence of Grade 2 HFSR of any duration
- After recovery of any Grade 3 or 4 adverse reaction
- For Grade 3 aspartate aminotransferase (AST)/alanine aminotransferase (ALT) elevation; only resume if the potential benefit outweighs the risk of hepatotoxicity

Reduce the dose of Stivarga to 80 mg:
- For re-occurrence of Grade 2 HFSR at the 120 mg dose
- After recovery of any Grade 3 or 4 adverse reaction at the 120 mg dose (except hepatotoxicity)

Discontinue Stivarga permanently for the following:
- Failure to tolerate 80 mg dose
- Any occurrence of AST or ALT more than 20 times the upper limit of normal (ULN)
- Any occurrence of AST or ALT more than 3 times ULN with concurrent bilirubin more than 2 times ULN
- Re-occurrence of AST or ALT more than 5 times ULN despite dose reduction to 120 mg
- For any Grade 4 adverse reaction; only resume if the potential benefit outweighs the risks

3   DOSAGE FORMS AND STRENGTHS

Stivarga is a 40 mg, light pink, oval shaped, film-coated tablet, debossed with 'BAYER' on one side and '40' on the other side.

4   CONTRAINDICATIONS

None

5   WARNINGS AND PRECAUTIONS

5.1   Hepatotoxicity

Severe drug induced liver injury with fatal outcome occurred in 0.3% of 1200 Stivarga-treated patients across all clinical trials. Liver biopsy results, when available, showed hepatocyte necrosis with lymphocyte infiltration. In Study 1, fatal hepatic failure occurred in 1.6% of patients in the regorafenib arm and in 0.4% of patients in the placebo arm; all the patients with hepatic failure had metastatic disease in the liver. In Study 2, fatal hepatic failure occurred in 0.8% of patients in the regorafenib arm *[see Adverse Reactions (6.1)]*.

Obtain liver function tests (ALT, AST and bilirubin) before initiation of Stivarga and monitor at least every two weeks during the first 2 months of treatment. Thereafter, monitor monthly or more frequently as clinically indicated. Monitor liver function tests weekly in patients experiencing elevated liver function tests until improvement to less than 3 times the ULN or baseline.

Temporarily hold and then reduce or permanently discontinue Stivarga depending on the severity and persistence of hepatotoxicity as manifested by elevated liver function tests or hepatocellular necrosis *[see Dosage and Administration (2.2)]*.

5.2   Hemorrhage

Stivarga caused an increased incidence of hemorrhage. The overall incidence (Grades 1-5) was 21% and 11% in Stivarga-treated patients compared to 8% and 3% in placebo-treated patients in Studies 1 and 2. Fatal hemorrhage occurred in 4 of 632 (0.6%) of Stivarga-treated patients in Studies 1 and 2 and involved the respiratory, gastrointestinal, or genitourinary tracts.

Permanently discontinue Stivarga in patients with severe or life-threatening hemorrhage. Monitor INR levels more frequently in patients receiving warfarin *[see Clinical Pharmacology (12.3)]*.

5.3   Dermatological Toxicity

Stivarga caused increased incidences of adverse reactions involving the skin and subcutaneous tissues (72% versus 24% in Study 1 and 78% versus 24% in Study 2), including hand-foot skin reaction (HFSR) also known as palmar-plantar erythrodysesthesia (PPE), and severe rash requiring dose modification.

The overall incidence of HFSR was higher in Stivarga-treated patients, (45% versus 7% in Study 1 and 67% versus 12% in Study 2), than in the placebo-treated patients. Most cases of HFSR in Stivarga-treated patients appeared during the first cycle of treatment (69% and 71% of patients who developed HFSR in Study 1 and Study 2, respectively). The incidence of Grade 3 HFSR (17% versus 0% in Study 1 and 22% versus 0% in Study 2), Grade 3 rash (6% versus <1% in Study 1 and 7% versus 0% in Study 2), serious adverse reactions of erythema multiforme (0.2% vs. 0% in Study 1) and Stevens Johnson Syndrome (0.2% vs. 0% in Study 1) was higher in Stivarga-treated patients *[see Adverse Reactions (6.1)]*.

Toxic epidermal necrolysis occurred in 0.17% of 1200 Stivarga-treated patients across all clinical trials.

Withhold Stivarga, reduce the dose, or permanently discontinue Stivarga depending on the severity and persistence of dermatologic toxicity *[see Dosage and Administration (2.2)]*. Institute supportive measures for symptomatic relief.

5.4   Hypertension

Stivarga caused an increased incidence of hypertension (30% versus 8% in Study 1 and 59% versus 27% in Study 2) *[see Adverse Reactions (6.1)]*. Hypertensive crisis occurred in 0.25% of 1200 Stivarga-treated patients across all clinical trials. The onset of hypertension occurred during the first cycle of treatment in most patients who developed hypertension (72% in Study 1 and Study 2).

Do not initiate Stivarga unless blood pressure is adequately controlled. Monitor blood pressure weekly for the first 6 weeks of treatment and then every cycle, or more frequently, as clinically indicated. Temporarily or permanently withhold Stivarga for severe or uncontrolled hypertension *[see Dosage and Administration (2.2)]*.

5.5   Cardiac Ischemia and Infarction

Stivarga increased the incidence of myocardial ischemia and infarction in Study 1 (1.2% versus 0.4 %) *[see Adverse Reactions (6.1)]*. Withhold Stivarga in patients who develop new or acute onset cardiac ischemia or infarction. Resume Stivarga only after resolution of acute cardiac ischemic events, if the potential benefits outweigh the risks of further cardiac ischemia.

5.6   Reversible Posterior Leukoencephalopathy Syndrome (RPLS)

Reversible Posterior Leukoencephalopathy Syndrome (RPLS), a syndrome of subcortical vasogenic edema diagnosed by characteristic finding on MRI, occurred in one of 1200 Stivarga-treated patients across all clinical trials. Perform an evaluation for RPLS in any patient presenting with seizures, headache, visual disturbances, confusion or altered mental function. Discontinue Stivarga in patients who develop RPLS.

5.7   Gastrointestinal Perforation or Fistula

Gastrointestinal perforation or fistula occurred in 0.6% of 1200 patients treated with Stivarga across all clinical trials; this included four fatal events. In Study 2, 2.1 % (4/188) of Stivarga-treated patients who were treated during the blinded or open-label portion of the study developed gastrointestinal fistula or perforation; of these, two cases of gastrointestinal perforation were fatal. Permanently discontinue Stivarga in patients who develop gastrointestinal perforation or fistula.

5.8 Wound Healing Complications

No formal studies of the effect of regorafenib on wound healing have been conducted. Since vascular endothelial growth factor receptor (VEGFR) inhibitors such as regorafenib can impair wound healing, treatment with regorafenib should be stopped at least 2 weeks prior to scheduled surgery. The decision to resume regorafenib after surgery should be based on clinical judgment of adequate wound healing. Regorafenib should be discontinued in patients with wound dehiscence.

5.9 Embryo-Fetal Toxicity

Stivarga can cause fetal harm when administered to a pregnant woman. Regorafenib was embryolethal and teratogenic in rats and rabbits at exposures lower than human exposures at the recommended dose, with increased incidences of cardiovascular, genitourinary, and skeletal malformations. If this drug is used during pregnancy, or if the patient becomes pregnant while taking this drug, the patient should be apprised of the potential *hazard to a fetus [see Use in Specific Populations (8.1)].*

6 ADVERSE REACTIONS

The following serious adverse reactions are discussed elsewhere in the labeling:

- Hepatotoxicity *[See Warnings and Precautions (5.1)]*
- Hemorrhage *[See Warnings and Precautions (5.2)]*
- Dermatological Toxicity *[See Warnings and Precautions (5.3)]*
- Hypertension *[See Warnings and Precautions (5.4)]*
- Cardiac Ischemia and Infarction *[See Warnings and Precautions (5.5)]*
- Reversible Posterior Leukoencephalopathy Syndrome (RPLS) *[See Warnings and Precautions (5.6)]*
- Gastrointestinal Perforation or Fistula *[See Warnings and Precautions (5.7)]*

Because clinical trials are conducted under widely varying conditions, adverse reaction rates observed in the clinical trials of a drug cannot be directly compared to rates in the clinical trials of another drug and may not reflect the rate observed in practice.

The most frequently observed adverse drug reactions (≥20%) in patients receiving Stivarga are asthenia/fatigue, HFSR, diarrhea, decreased appetite/food intake, hypertension, mucositis, dysphonia, infection, pain (not otherwise specified), decreased weight, gastrointestinal and abdominal pain, rash, fever, and nausea.

The most serious adverse drug reactions in patients receiving Stivarga are hepatotoxicity, hemorrhage, and gastrointestinal perforation.

6.1 Clinical Trials Experience

Colorectal Cancer

The safety data described below, except where noted, are derived from a randomized (2:1), double-blind, placebo-controlled trial (Study 1) in which 500 patients (median age 61 years; 61% men) with previously treated metastatic colorectal cancer received Stivarga as a single agent at the dose of 160 mg daily for the first 3 weeks of each 4 week treatment cycle and 253 patients (median age 61 years; 60% men) received placebo. The median duration of therapy was 7.3 (range 0.3, 47.0) weeks for patients receiving Stivarga. Due to adverse reactions, 61% of the patients receiving Stivarga required a dose interruption and 38% of the patients had their dose reduced. Drug-related adverse reactions that resulted in treatment discontinuation were reported in 8.2% of Stivarga-treated patients compared to 1.2% of patients who received placebo. Hand-foot skin reaction (HFSR) and rash were the most common reasons for permanent discontinuation of Stivarga.

Table 1 compares the incidence of adverse reactions (≥10%) in patients receiving Stivarga and reported more commonly than in patients receiving placebo (Study 1).

[See table 1 above]

Laboratory Abnormalities

Laboratory abnormalities observed in Study 1 are shown in Table 2.

[See table 2 above]

Gastrointestinal Stromal Tumors

The safety data described below are derived from a randomized (2:1), double-blind, placebo-controlled trial (Study 2) in which 132 patients (median age 60 years; 64% men) with previously treated GIST received Stivarga as a single agent at a dose of 160 mg daily for the first 3 weeks of each 4 week treatment cycle and 66 patients (median age 61 years; 64% men) received placebo. The median duration of therapy was 22.9 (range 0.1, 50.9) weeks for patients receiving Stivarga. Dose interruptions for adverse events were required in 58% of patients receiving Stivarga and 50% of patients had their dose reduced. Drug-related adverse reactions that resulted in treatment discontinuation were reported in 2.3% of Stivarga-treated patients compared to 1.5% of patients who received placebo.

Table 3 compares the incidence of adverse reactions (≥10%) in GIST patients receiving Stivarga and reported more commonly than in patients receiving placebo (Study 2).

[See table 3 at top of next page]

Laboratory abnormalities observed in Study 2 are shown in Table 4.

[See table 4 at top of next page]

Table 1 Adverse drug reactions (≥10%) reported in patients treated with Stivarga in Study 1 and reported more commonly than in patients receiving placebo

Adverse Reactions	Stivarga (N=500)		Placebo (N=253)	
	Grade		Grade	
	All %	≥ 3 %	All %	≥ 3 %
General disorders and administration site conditions				
Asthenia/fatigue	64	15	46	9
Pain	29	3	21	2
Fever	28	2	15	0
Metabolism and nutrition disorders				
Decreased appetite and food intake	47	5	28	4
Skin and subcutaneous tissue disorders				
HFSR/PPE	45	17	7	0
Rash *	26	6	4	<1
Gastrointestinal disorders				
Diarrhea	43	8	17	2
Mucositis	33	4	5	0
Investigations				
Weight loss	32	<1	10	0
Infections and infestations				
Infection	31	9	17	6
Vascular disorders				
Hypertension	30	8	8	<1
Hemorrhage †	21	2	8	<1
Respiratory, thoracic and mediastinal disorders				
Dysphonia	30	0	6	0
Nervous system disorders				
Headache	10	<1	7	0

* The term rash represents reports of events of drug eruption, rash, erythematous rash, generalized rash, macular rash, maculo-papular rash, papular rash, and pruritic rash.
† Fatal outcomes observed.

Table 2 Laboratory test abnormalities reported in Study 1

Laboratory Parameter	Stivarga (N=500 *)			Placebo (N=253 *)		
	Grade †			Grade †		
	All %	3 %	4 %	All %	3 %	4 %
Blood and lymphatic system disorders						
Anemia	79	5	1	66	3	0
Thrombocytopenia	41	2	<1	17	<1	0
Neutropenia	3	1	0	0	0	0
Lymphopenia	54	9	0	34	3	0
Metabolism and nutrition disorders						
Hypocalcemia	59	1	<1	18	1	0
Hypokalemia	26	4	0	8	<1	0
Hyponatremia	30	7	1	22	4	0
Hypophosphatemia	57	31	1	11	4	0
Hepatobiliary disorders						
Hyperbilirubinemia	45	10	3	17	5	3
Increased AST	65	5	1	46	4	1
Increased ALT	45	5	1	30	3	<1
Renal and urinary disorders						
Proteinuria	60	<1	0	34	<1	0
Investigations						
Increased INR ‡	24	4	N/A	17	2	N/A
Increased Lipase	46	9	2	19	3	2
Increased Amylase	26	2	<1	17	2	<1

* % based on number of patients with post-baseline samples which may be less than 500 (regorafenib) or 253 (placebo).
† Common Terminology Criteria for Adverse Events (CTCAE), v3.0.
‡ International normalized ratio: No Grade 4 denoted in CTCAE, v3.0.

7 DRUG INTERACTIONS

7.1 Effect of Strong CYP3A4 Inducers on Regorafenib

Co-administration of a strong CYP3A4 inducer (rifampin) with a single 160 mg dose of Stivarga decreased the mean exposure of regorafenib, increased the mean exposure of the active metabolite M-5, and resulted in no change in the mean exposure of the active metabolite M-2. Avoid concomitant use of Stivarga with strong CYP3A4 inducers (e.g. rifampin, phenytoin, carbamazepine, phenobarbital, and St. John's Wort) [see Clinical Pharmacology (12.3)].

7.2   Effect of Strong CYP3A4 Inhibitors on Regorafenib
Co-administration of a strong CYP3A4 inhibitor (ketoconazole) with a single 160 mg dose of Stivarga increased the mean exposure of regorafenib and decreased the mean exposure of the active metabolites M-2 and M-5. Avoid concomitant use of Stivarga with strong inhibitors of CYP3A4 activity (e.g. clarithromycin, grapefruit juice, itraconazole, ketoconazole, nefazadone, posaconazole, telithromycin, and voriconazole) [see Clinical Pharmacology (12.3)].

8   USE IN SPECIFIC POPULATIONS

8.1   Pregnancy
Pregnancy Category D [see Warnings and Precautions (5.9)]
Risk Summary
Based on its mechanism of action, Stivarga can cause fetal harm when administered to a pregnant woman. There are no adequate and well-controlled studies with Stivarga in pregnant women. Regorafenib was embryolethal and teratogenic in rats and rabbits at exposures lower than human exposures at the recommended dose, with increased incidences of cardiovascular, genitourinary, and skeletal malformations. If this drug is used during pregnancy or if the patient becomes pregnant while taking this drug, the patient should be apprised of the potential hazard to a fetus.
Animal Data
In embryo-fetal development studies, a total loss of pregnancy (100% resorption of litter) was observed in rats at doses as low as 1 mg/kg (approximately 6% of the recommended human dose, based on body surface area) and in rabbits at doses as low as 1.6 mg/kg (approximately 25% of the human exposure at the clinically recommended dose measured by AUC).
In a single dose distribution study in pregnant rats, there was increased penetration of regorafenib across the blood-brain barrier in fetuses compared to dams. In a repeat dose study with daily administration of regorafenib to pregnant rats during organogenesis, findings included delayed ossification in fetuses at doses ≥ 0.8 mg/kg (approximately 5% of the recommended human dose based on body surface area) with dose-dependent increases in skeletal malformations including cleft palate and enlarged fontanelle at doses ≥ 1 mg/kg (approximately 10% of the clinical exposure based on AUC). At doses ≥ 1.6 mg/kg (approximately 11% of the recommended human dose based on body surface area), there were dose-dependent increases in the incidence of cardiovascular malformations, external abnormalities, diaphragmatic hernia, and dilation of the renal pelvis.
In pregnant rabbits administered regorafenib daily during organogenesis, there were findings of ventricular septal defects evident at the lowest tested dose of 0.4 mg/kg (approximately 7% of the AUC in patients at the recommended dose). At doses of ≥ 0.8 mg/kg (approximately 15% of the human exposure at the recommended human dose based on AUC), administration of regorafenib resulted in dose-dependent increases in the incidence of additional cardiovascular malformations and skeletal anomalies as well as significant adverse effects on the urinary system including missing kidney/ureter; small, deformed and malpositioned kidney; and hydronephrosis. The proportion of viable fetuses that were male decreased with increasing dose in two rabbit embryo-fetal toxicity studies.

8.3   Nursing Mothers
It is unknown whether regorafenib or its metabolites are excreted in human milk. In rats, regorafenib and its metabolites are excreted in milk. Because many drugs are excreted in human milk and because of the potential for serious adverse reactions in nursing infants from Stivarga, a decision should be made whether to discontinue nursing or discontinue the drug, taking into account the importance of the drug to the mother.

8.4   Pediatric Use
The safety and efficacy of Stivarga in pediatric patients less than 18 years of age have not been established.
In 28-day repeat dose studies in rats there were dose-dependent findings of dentin alteration and angiectasis. These findings were observed at regorafenib doses as low as 4 mg/kg (approximately 25% of the AUC in humans at the recommended dose). In 13-week repeat dose studies in dogs there were similar findings of dentin alteration at doses as low as 20 mg/kg (approximately 43% of the AUC in humans at the recommended dose). Administration of regorafenib in these animals also led to persistent growth and thickening of the femoral epiphyseal growth plate.

8.5   Geriatric Use
Of the 632 Stivarga-treated patients enrolled in Studies 1 and 2, 37% were 65 years of age or older and over, while 8% were 75 and over. No overall differences in safety or efficacy were observed between these patients and younger patients.

8.6   Hepatic Impairment
No clinically important differences in the mean exposure of regorafenib or the active metabolites M-2 and M-5 were observed in patients with hepatocellular carcinoma and mild (Child-Pugh A) or moderate (Child-Pugh B) hepatic impairment compared to patients with normal hepatic function [see Clinical Pharmacology (12.3)]. No dose adjustment is

Table 3 Adverse reactions (≥10%) reported in patients treated with Stivarga in Study 2 and reported more commonly than in patients receiving placebo

Adverse Reactions	Stivarga (N=132)		Placebo (N=66)	
	Grade		Grade	
	All %	≥ 3 %	All %	≥ 3 %
Skin and subcutaneous tissue disorders				
HFSR/PPE	67	22	15	2
Rash *	30	7	3	0
Alopecia	24	2	2	0
General disorders and administration site conditions				
Asthenia/Fatigue	52	4	39	2
Fever	21	0	11	2
Vascular disorders				
Hypertension	59	28	27	5
Hemorrhage	11	4	3	0
Gastrointestinal disorders				
Diarrhea	47	8	9	0
Mucositis	40	2	8	2
Nausea	20	2	12	2
Vomiting	17	<1	8	0
Respiratory, thoracic and mediastinal disorders				
Dysphonia	39	0	9	0
Infections and infestations				
Infection	32	5	5	0
Metabolism and nutrition disorders				
Decreased appetite and food intake	31	<1	21	3
Hypothyroidism †	18	0	6	0
Nervous system disorders				
Headache	16	0	9	0
Investigations				
Weight loss	14	0	8	0
Musculoskeletal and connective tissue disorders				
Musculoskeletal stiffness	14	0	3	0

* The term rash represents reports of events of rash, erythematous rash, macular rash, maculo-papular rash, papular rash and pruritic rash.
† Hypothyroidism incidence based on subset of patients with normal TSH and no thyroid supplementation at baseline.

Table 4 Laboratory test abnormalities reported in Study 2

Laboratory Parameter	Stivarga (N=132*)			Placebo (N=66 *)		
	Grade †			Grade †		
	All %	3 %	4 %	All %	3 %	4 %
Blood and lymphatic system disorders						
Thrombocytopenia	13	1	0	2	0	2
Neutropenia	16	2	0	12	3	0
Lymphopenia	30	8	0	24	3	0
Metabolism and nutrition disorders						
Hypocalcemia	17	2	0	5	0	0
Hypokalemia	21	3	0	3	0	0
Hypophosphatemia	55	20	2	3	0	2
Hepatobiliary disorders						
Hyperbilirubinemia	33	3	1	12	2	0
Increased AST	58	3	1	47	3	0
Increased ALT	39	4	1	39	2	0
Renal and urinary disorders						
Proteinuria	33	3	- ‡	30	3	- ‡
Investigations						
Increased Lipase	14	0	1	5	0	0

* % based on number of patients with post-baseline samples which may be less than 132 (regorafenib) or 66 (placebo).
† CTCAE, v4.0.
‡ No Grade 4 denoted in CTCAE, v4.0.

recommended in patients with mild or moderate hepatic impairment. Closely monitor patients with hepatic impairment for adverse reactions *[see Warnings and Precautions (5.1)]*.

Stivarga is not recommended for use in patients with severe hepatic impairment (Child-Pugh Class C), as it has not been studied in this population.

8.7 Renal Impairment

No clinically relevant differences in the mean exposure of regorafenib and the active metabolites M-2 and M-5 were observed in patients with mild renal impairment (CLcr 60-89 mL/min) compared to patients with normal renal function following regorafenib 160 mg daily for 21 days *[see Clinical Pharmacology (12.3)]*. No dose adjustment is recommended for patients with mild renal impairment. Limited pharmacokinetic data are available from patients with moderate renal impairment (CLcr 30-59 mL/min). Stivarga has not been studied in patients with severe renal impairment or end-stage renal disease.

8.8 Females and Males of Reproductive Potential

Contraception

Use effective contraception during treatment and up to 2 months after completion of therapy.

Infertility

There are no data on the effect of Stivarga on human fertility. Results from animal studies indicate that regorafenib can impair male and female fertility *[see Nonclinical Toxicology (13.1)]*.

10 OVERDOSAGE

The highest dose of Stivarga studied clinically is 220 mg per day. In the event of suspected overdose, interrupt Stivarga, institute supportive care, and observe until clinical stabilization.

11 DESCRIPTION

Stivarga (regorafenib) has the chemical name 4-[4-({[4-chloro-3-(trifluoromethyl) phenyl] carbamoyl] amino)-3-fluorophenoxy]-N-methylpyridine-2-carboxamide monohydrate. Regorafenib has the following structural formula:

Regorafenib is a monohydrate and it has a molecular formula $C_{21}H_{15}ClF_4N_4O_3 \cdot H_2O$ and a molecular weight of 500.83. Regorafenib is practically insoluble in water, slightly soluble in acetonitrile, methanol, ethanol, and ethyl acetate and sparingly soluble in acetone.

Stivarga tablets for oral administration are formulated as light pink oval shaped tablets debossed with "BAYER" on one side and "40" on the other. Each tablet contains 40 mg of regorafenib in the anhydrous state, which corresponds to 41.49 mg of regorafenib monohydrate, and the following inactive ingredients: cellulose microcrystalline, croscarmellose sodium, magnesium stearate, povidone, and colloidal silicon dioxide. The film-coating contains the following inactive ingredients: ferric oxide red, ferric oxide yellow, lecithin (soy), polyethylene glycol 3350, polyvinyl alcohol, talc, and titanium dioxide.

12 CLINICAL PHARMACOLOGY

12.1 Mechanism of Action

Regorafenib is a small molecule inhibitor of multiple membrane-bound and intracellular kinases involved in normal cellular functions and in pathologic processes such as oncogenesis, tumor angiogenesis, and maintenance of the tumor microenvironment. In *in vitro* biochemical or cellular assays, regorafenib or its major human active metabolites M-2 and M-5 inhibited the activity of RET, VEGFR1, VEGFR2, VEGFR3, KIT, PDGFR-alpha, PDGFR-beta, FGFR1, FGFR2, TIE2, DDR2, TrkA, Eph2A, RAF-1, BRAF, BRAF^{V600E}, SAPK2, PTK5, and Abl at concentrations of regorafenib that have been achieved clinically. In *in vivo* models, regorafenib demonstrated anti-angiogenic activity in a rat tumor model, and inhibition of tumor growth as well as anti-metastatic activity in several mouse xenograft models including some for human colorectal carcinoma.

12.3 Pharmacokinetics

Absorption

Following a single 160 mg dose of Stivarga in patients with advanced solid tumors, regorafenib reaches a geometric mean peak plasma level (C_{max}) of 2.5 µg/mL at a median time of 4 hours and a geometric mean area under the plasma concentration vs. time curve (AUC) of 70.4 µg*h/mL. The AUC of regorafenib at steady-state increases less than dose proportionally at doses greater than 60 mg. At steady-state, regorafenib reaches a geometric mean C_{max} of 3.9 µg/mL and a geometric mean AUC of 58.3 µg*h/mL. The coefficient of variation of AUC and C_{max} is between 35% and 44%.

The mean relative bioavailability of tablets compared to an oral solution is 69% to 83%.

In a food-effect study, 24 healthy men received a single 160 mg dose of Stivarga on three separate occasions: under a fasted state, with a high-fat meal and with a low-fat meal. A high-fat meal (945 calories and 54.6 g fat) increased the mean AUC of regorafenib by 48% and decreased the mean AUC of the M-2 and M-5 metabolites by 20% and 51%, respectively, as compared to the fasted state. A low-fat meal (319 calories and 8.2 g fat) increased the mean AUC of regorafenib, M-2 and M-5 by 36%, 40% and 23%, respectively as compared to fasted conditions. Stivarga was administered with a low-fat meal in Studies 1 and 2 *[see Dosage and Administration (2.1), Clinical Studies (14)]*.

Distribution

Regorafenib undergoes enterohepatic circulation with multiple plasma concentration peaks observed across the 24-hour dosing interval. Regorafenib is highly bound (99.5%) to human plasma proteins.

Metabolism

Regorafenib is metabolized by CYP3A4 and UGT1A9. The main circulating metabolites of regorafenib measured at steady-state in human plasma are M-2 (N-oxide) and M-5 (N-oxide and N-desmethyl), both of them having similar *in vitro* pharmacological activity and steady-state concentrations as regorafenib. M-2 and M-5 are highly protein bound (99.8% and 99.95%, respectively).

Elimination

Following a single 160 mg oral dose of Stivarga, the geometric mean (range) elimination half-lives for regorafenib and the M-2 metabolite in plasma are 28 hours (14 to 58 hours) and 25 hours (14 to 32 hours), respectively. M-5 has a longer mean (range) elimination half-life of 51 hours (32 to 70 hours).

Approximately 71% of a radiolabeled dose was excreted in feces (47% as parent compound, 24% as metabolites) and 19% of the dose was excreted in urine (17% as glucuronides) within 12 days after administration of a radiolabeled oral solution at a dose of 120 mg.

Age, Gender, and Weight

Based on the population pharmacokinetic analysis, there is no clinically relevant effect of age, gender or weight on the pharmacokinetics of regorafenib.

Hepatic Impairment

The pharmacokinetics of regorafenib, M-2, and M-5 was evaluated in 14 patients with hepatocellular carcinoma (HCC) and mild hepatic impairment (Child-Pugh A); 4 patients with HCC and moderate hepatic impairment (Child-Pugh B); and 10 patients with solid tumors and normal hepatic function after the administration of a single 100 mg dose of Stivarga. No clinically important differences in the mean exposure of regorafenib, M-2, or M-5 were observed in patients with mild or moderate hepatic impairment compared to the patients with normal hepatic function. The pharmacokinetics of regorafenib has not been studied in patients with severe hepatic impairment (Child-Pugh C).

Renal Impairment

The pharmacokinetics of regorafenib, M-2, and M-5 was evaluated in 10 patients with mild renal impairment (CLcr 60-89 mL/min) and 18 patients with normal renal function following the administration of Stivarga at a dose of 160 mg daily for 21 days. No differences in the mean steady-state exposure of regorafenib, M-2, or M-5 were observed in patients with mild renal impairment compared to patients with normal renal function. Limited pharmacokinetic data are available from patients with moderate renal impairment (CLcr 30-59 mL/min). The pharmacokinetics of regorafenib has not been studied in patients with severe renal impairment or end-stage renal disease.

Drug-Drug Interactions

Effect of Regorafenib on Cytochrome P450 Substrates: In vitro studies suggested that regorafenib is an inhibitor of CYP2C8, CYP2C9, CYP2B6, CYP3A4 and CYP2C19; M-2 metabolite is an inhibitor of CYP2C9, CYP2C8, CYP3A4 and CYP2D6, and M-5 metabolite is an inhibitor of CYP2C8. In vitro studies suggested that regorafenib is not an inducer of CYP1A2, CYP2B6, CYP2C19, and CYP3A4 enzyme activity.

Patients with advanced solid tumors received single oral doses of CYP substrates, 2 mg of midazolam (CYP3A4), 40 mg of omeprazole (CYP2C19) and 10 mg of warfarin (CYP2C9) or 4 mg of rosiglitazone (CYP2C8) one week before and two weeks before and after Stivarga at a dose of 160 mg once daily. No clinically relevant change was observed in the mean AUC of rosiglitazone (N=12) or the mean omeprazole (N=11) plasma concentrations measured 6 hours after dosing or the mean AUC of midazolam (N=15). The mean AUC of warfarin (N=8) increased by 25% *[see Warnings and Precautions (5.2)]*.

Effect of CYP3A4 Strong Inducers on Regorafenib: Twenty-two healthy men received a single 160 mg dose of Stivarga alone and then 7 days after starting rifampin. Rifampin, a strong CYP3A4 inducer, was administered at a dose of 600 mg daily for 9 days. The mean AUC of regorafenib decreased by 50% and mean AUC of M-5 increased by 264%. No change in the mean AUC of M-2 was observed *[see Drug Interactions (7.1)]*.

Effect of CYP3A4 Strong Inhibitors on Regorafenib: Eighteen healthy men received a single 160 mg dose of Stivarga alone and then 5 days after starting ketoconazole. Ketoconazole, a strong CYP3A4 inhibitor, was administered at a dose of 400 mg daily for 18 days. The mean AUC of regorafenib increased by 33% and the mean AUC of M-2 and M-5 both decreased by 93% *[see Drug Interactions (7.2)]*.

Effect of Regorafenib on UGT1A1 Substrates: In vitro studies showed that regorafenib, M-2, and M-5 competitively inhibit UGT1A9 and UGT1A1 at therapeutically relevant concentrations. Eleven patients received irinotecan-containing combination chemotherapy with Stivarga at a dose of 160 mg. The mean AUC of irinotecan increased 28% and the mean AUC of SN-38 increased by 44% when irinotecan was administered 5 days after the last of 7 daily doses of Stivarga.

In vitro screening of transporters: In vitro data suggested that regorafenib is an inhibitor of ABCG2 (Breast Cancer Resistance Protein) and ABCB1 (P-glycoprotein).

12.6 Cardiac Electrophysiology

The effect of multiple doses of Stivarga (160 mg once daily for 21 days) on the QTc interval was evaluated in an open label, single arm study in 25 patients with advanced solid tumors. No large changes in the mean QTc interval (i.e., > 20 msec) were detected in the study.

13 NONCLINICAL TOXICOLOGY

13.1 Carcinogenesis, Mutagenesis, Impairment of Fertility

Studies examining the carcinogenic potential of regorafenib have not been conducted. Regorafenib itself did not demonstrate genotoxicity in *in vitro* or *in vivo* assays; however, a major human active metabolite of regorafenib, (M-2), was positive for clastogenicity, causing chromosome aberration in Chinese hamster V79 cells.

Dedicated studies to examine the effects of regorafenib on fertility have not been conducted; however, there were histological findings of tubular atrophy and degeneration in the testes, atrophy in the seminal vesicle, and cellular debris and oligospermia in the epididymides in male rats at doses similar to those in human at the clinical recommended dose based on AUC. In female rats, there were increased findings of necrotic corpora lutea in the ovaries at the same exposures. There were similar findings in dogs of both sexes in repeat dose studies at exposures approximately 83% of the human exposure at the recommended human dose based on AUC. These findings suggest that regorafenib may adversely affect fertility in humans.

13.2 Animal Toxicology and/or Pharmacology

In a chronic 26 week repeat dose study in rats there was a dose-dependent increase in the finding of thickening of the atrioventricular valve. At a dose that resulted in an exposure of approximately 12% of the human exposure at the recommended dose, this finding was present in half of the examined animals.

14 CLINICAL STUDIES

14.1 Colorectal Cancer

The clinical efficacy and safety of Stivarga were evaluated in an international, multi-center, randomized (2:1), double-blind, placebo-controlled trial (Study 1) in 760 patients with previously treated metastatic colorectal cancer. The major efficacy outcome measure was overall survival (OS); supportive efficacy outcome measures included progression-free survival (PFS) and objective tumor response rate.

Patients were randomized to receive 160 mg regorafenib orally once daily (N=505) plus Best Supportive Care (BSC) or placebo (N=255) plus BSC for the first 21 days of each 28-day cycle. Stivarga was administered with a low-fat breakfast that contains less than 30% fat *[see Dosage and Administration (2.1), Clinical Pharmacology (12.3)]*. Treatment continued until disease progression or unacceptable toxicity.

In the all-randomized population, median age was 61 years, 61% were men, 78% were White, and all patients had baseline ECOG performance status of 0 or 1. The primary site of disease was colon (65%), rectum (29%), or both (6%). History of KRAS evaluation was reported for 729 (96%) patients; 430 (59%) of these patients were reported to have KRAS mutation. The median number of prior lines of therapy for metastatic disease was 3. All patients received prior treatment with fluoropyrimidine-, oxaliplatin-, and irinotecan-based chemotherapy, and with bevacizumab. All but one patient with KRAS mutation-negative tumors received panitumumab or cetuximab.

The addition of Stivarga to BSC resulted in a statistically significant improvement in survival compared to placebo plus BSC (see Table 5 and Figure 1).

Table 5 Efficacy Results from Study 1

	Stivarga (N=505)	Placebo (N=255)
Overall Survival		
Number of deaths, N (%)	275 (55%)	157 (62%)
Median Overall Survival (months)	6.4	5.0
95% CI	(5.8, 7.3)	(4.4, 5.8)
HR (95% CI)	0.77 (0.64, 0.94)	
Stratified Log-Rank Test P-value*,†	0.0102	
Progression-free Survival		
Number of Death or Progression, N (%)	417 (83%)	231 (91%)
Median Progression-free Survival (months)	2.0	1.7
95% CI	(1.9, 2.3)	(1.7, 1.8)
HR (95% CI)	0.49 (0.42, 0.58)	
Stratified Log-Rank Test P-value*	<0.0001	
Overall Response Rate		
Overall response, N (%)	5 (1%)	1 (0.4%)
95% CI	0.3%, 2.3%	0%, 2.2%

* Stratified by geographic region and time from diagnosis of metastatic disease.
† Crossed the O'Brien-Fleming boundary (two-sided p-value < 0.018) at second interim analysis.

Figure 1 Kaplan-Meier Curves of Overall Survival

Patients at Risk						
Stivarga	452	352	187	93	33	7
Placebo	221	150	75	32	9	3

14.2 Gastrointestinal Stromal Tumors

The efficacy and safety of Stivarga were evaluated in an international, multi-center, randomized (2:1), double-blind, placebo-controlled trial (Study 2) in 199 patients with unresectable, locally advanced or metastatic gastrointestinal stromal tumor (GIST), who had been previously treated with imatinib mesylate and sunitinib malate. Randomization was stratified by line of therapy (third vs. four or more) and geographic region (Asia vs. rest of the world).

The major efficacy outcome measure of Study 2 was progression-free survival (PFS) based on disease assessment by independent radiological review using modified RECIST 1.1 criteria, in which lymph nodes and bone lesions were not target lesions and progressively growing new tumor nodule within a pre-existing tumor mass was progression. The key secondary outcome measure was overall survival.

Patients were randomized to receive 160 mg regorafenib orally once daily (N=133) plus best supportive care (BSC) or placebo (N=66) plus BSC for the first 21 days of each 28-day cycle. Treatment continued until disease progression or unacceptable toxicity. In Study 2, the median age of patients was 60 years, 64% were men, 68% were White, and all patients had baseline ECOG performance status of 0 (55%) or 1 (45%). At the time of disease progression as assessed by central review, the study blind was broken and all patients were offered the opportunity to take Stivarga at the investigator's discretion. Fifty-six (85%) patients randomized to placebo and 41 (31%) patients randomized to Stivarga received open-label Stivarga.

A statistically significant improvement in PFS was demonstrated among patients treated with Stivarga compared to placebo (see Table 6 and Figure 2). There was no statistically significant difference in overall survival at the time of the planned interim analysis based on 29% of the total events for the final analysis.

Table 6 Efficacy Results for Study 2

	Stivarga (N=133)	Placebo (N=66)
Progression-free Survival		
Number of Death or Progression, N (%)	82 (62%)	63 (96%)
Median Progression-free Survival (months)	4.8	0.9
95% CI	(3.9, 5.7)	(0.9, 1.1)
HR (95% CI)	0.27 (0.19, 0.39)	
Stratified Log-Rank Test P-value*	<0.0001	
Overall Survival		
Number of Deaths, N (%)	29 (22%)	17 (26%)
Median Overall Survival (months)	NR†	NR†
HR (95% CI)	0.77 (0.42, 1.41)	
Stratified Log-Rank Test P-value*,†	0.2	

* Stratified by line of treatment and geographical region
† NR: Not Reached.

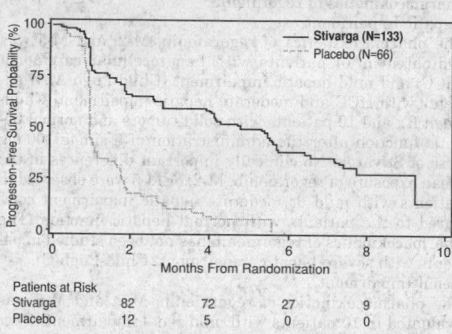

Figure 2 Kaplan-Meier Curves of Progression-free Survival for Study 2

Patients at Risk					
Stivarga	82	72	27	9	0
Placebo	12	5	0	0	0

16 HOW SUPPLIED/STORAGE AND HANDLING

16.1 How Supplied

Stivarga tablets are supplied in packages containing three bottles, with each bottle containing 28 tablets, for a total of 84 tablets per package (NDC 50419-171-03).

16.2 Storage and Handling

Store Stivarga at 25°C (77°F); excursions are permitted from 15 to 30°C (59 to 86°F) [See USP Controlled Room Temperature].

Store tablets in the original bottle and do not remove the desiccant. Keep the bottle tightly closed after first opening. Discard any unused tablets 28 days after opening the bottle. Dispose of unused tablets in accordance with local requirements.

17 PATIENT COUNSELING INFORMATION

See FDA-Approved Patient Labeling (Patient Information).
Inform your patients of the following:
- Stivarga may cause severe or life-threatening liver damage. Inform patients that they will need to undergo monitoring for liver damage and to immediately report any signs or symptoms of severe liver damage to their health care provider.
- Stivarga can cause severe bleeding. Advise patients to contact their health care provider for any episode of bleeding.
- Stivarga can cause hand-foot skin reactions or rash elsewhere. Advise patients to contact their health care provider if they experience skin changes associated with redness, pain, blisters, bleeding, or swelling.
- Stivarga can cause or exacerbate existing hypertension. Advise patients they will need to undergo blood pressure monitoring and to contact their health care provider if blood pressure is elevated or if symptoms from hypertension occur including severe headache, lightheadedness, or neurologic symptoms.
- Stivarga increased the risk for myocardial ischemia and infarction. Advise patients to seek immediate emergency help if they experience chest pain, shortness of breath, or feel dizzy or like passing out.
- Contact a healthcare provider immediately if they experience severe pains in their abdomen, persistent swelling of the abdomen, high fever, chills, nausea, vomiting, severe diarrhea (frequent or loose bowel movements), or dehydration.
- Stivarga may complicate wound healing. Advise patients to inform their health care provider if they plan to undergo a surgical procedure or had recent surgery.
- Inform patients that regorafenib can cause fetal harm. Advise women of reproductive potential and men of the need for effective contraception during Stivarga treatment and for up to 2 months after completion of treatment. Instruct women of reproductive potential to immediately contact her health care provider if pregnancy is suspected or confirmed during or within 2 months of completing treatment with Stivarga.
- Advise nursing mothers that it is not known whether regorafenib is present in breast milk and discuss whether to discontinue nursing or to discontinue regorafenib.
- Inform patients to take any missed dose on the same day, as soon as they remember, and that they must not take two doses on the same day to make up for a dose missed on the previous day.
- Inform patients to store medicine in the original container. Do not place medication in daily or weekly pill boxes . Any remaining tablets should be discarded 28 days after opening the bottle. Tightly close bottle after each opening and keep the desiccant in the bottle.

Patient Package Insert
Stivarga® (sti-VAR-gah)
(regorafenib)
tablets

Read this Patient Information before you start taking Stivarga and each time you get a refill. There may be new information. This information does not take the place of talking to your healthcare provider about your medical condition or treatment.

What is the most important information I should know about Stivarga?

Stivarga can cause serious side effects, including:

Liver problems. Stivarga can cause liver problems which can be serious and sometimes lead to death. Your healthcare provider will do blood tests to check your liver function before you start taking Stivarga and during your treatment with Stivarga to check for liver problems. Tell your healthcare provider right away if you get any of these symptoms of liver problems during treatment:
- yellowing of your skin or the white part of your eyes (jaundice)
- nausea or vomiting
- dark "tea-colored" urine
- change in sleep pattern

What is Stivarga?

Stivarga is a prescription medicine used to treat people with:

colon or rectal cancer that has spread to other parts of the body and for which they have received previous treatment with certain chemotherapy medicines

a rare stomach, bowel, or esophagus cancer called GIST (gastrointestinal stromal tumors) that cannot be treated with surgery or that has spread to other parts of the body and for which they have received previous treatment with certain medicines

Stivarga has not been used to treat children less than 18 years of age.

What should I tell my healthcare provider before taking Stivarga?

Before you take Stivarga, tell your healthcare provider if you:
- have liver problems
- have bleeding problems
- have high blood pressure
- have heart problems or chest pain
- plan to have any surgical procedures
- have any other medical conditions
- are pregnant or plan to become pregnant. Stivarga can harm your unborn baby. Females and males should use effective birth control during treatment with Stivarga and for 2 months after your last dose of Stivarga. Tell your healthcare provider right away if you or your partner becomes pregnant either while taking Stivarga or within 2 months after your last dose of Stivarga.
- are breastfeeding or plan to breastfeed. It is not known if Stivarga passes into your breast milk. You and your healthcare provider should decide if you will take Stivarga or breastfeed.

Tell your healthcare provider about all the medicines you take, including prescription and non-prescription medicines, vitamins and herbal supplements. Stivarga may affect the way other medicines work, and other medicines may affect how Stivarga works.

Know the medicines you take. Keep a list of your medicines and show it to your healthcare provider and pharmacist when you get a new medicine.

How should I take Stivarga?
• Take Stivarga exactly as your healthcare provider tells you.
• You will usually take Stivarga 1 time a day for 21 days (3 weeks) and then stop for 7 days (1 week). This is 1 cycle of treatment. Repeat this cycle for as long as your healthcare provider tells you to.
• Swallow Stivarga tablets whole.
• Take Stivarga at the same time each day with a low-fat breakfast.
Examples of a low-fat breakfast include:
• 2 slices of white toast with 1 tablespoon of low-fat margarine and 1 tablespoon of jelly, and 8 ounces of skim milk (319 calories and 8.2 grams fat), **or**
• 1 cup of cereal, 8 ounces of skim milk, 1 slice of toast with jelly, apple juice, and 1 cup of coffee or tea (520 calories and 2 grams fat).
• Your healthcare provider may stop your treatment or change the dose of your treatment if you get side effects.
• If you miss a dose, take it as soon as you remember on that day. Do not take two doses on the same day to make up for a missed dose.
• If you take too much Stivarga call your healthcare provider or go to the nearest emergency room right away.

What should I avoid while taking Stivarga?
• Avoid drinking grapefruit juice and taking St. John's Wort while taking Stivarga. These can affect the way Stivarga works.

What are the possible side effects of Stivarga?
Stivarga can cause serious side effects including:
• See "What is the most important information I should know about Stivarga?"
• **severe bleeding.** Stivarga can cause bleeding which can be serious and sometimes lead to death. Tell your healthcare provider if you have any signs of bleeding while taking Stivarga including:
 • vomiting blood or if your vomit looks like coffee-grounds
 • pink or brown urine
 • red or black (looks like tar) stools
 • coughing up blood or blood clots
 • menstrual bleeding that is heavier than normal
 • unusual vaginal bleeding
 • nose bleeds that happen often
• **a skin problem called hand-foot skin reaction and severe skin rash.** Hand-foot skin reactions can cause redness, pain, blisters, bleeding, or swelling on the palms of your hands or soles of your feet. If you get this side effect or a severe skin rash, your healthcare provider may stop your treatment for some time.
• **high blood pressure.** Your blood pressure should be checked every week for the first 6 weeks of starting Stivarga. Your blood pressure should be checked regularly and any high blood pressure should be treated while you are receiving Stivarga. Tell your healthcare provider if you have severe headaches, lightheadedness, or changes in your vision.
• **decreased blood flow to the heart and heart attack.** Get emergency help right away and call your healthcare provider if you get symptoms such as chest pain, shortness of breath, feel dizzy or feel like passing out.
• **a condition called Reversible Posterior Leukoencephalopathy Syndrome (RPLS).** Call your healthcare provider right away if you get: severe headaches, seizure, confusion, change in vision, or problems thinking.
• **a tear in your stomach or intestinal wall (bowel perforation).** Stivarga may cause a tear in your stomach or bowel perforation that can be serious and sometimes lead to death. Tell your healthcare provider right away if you get:
 • severe pain in your stomach-area (abdomen)
 • swelling of the abdomen
 • high fever
• **wound healing problems.** If you need to have a surgical procedure, tell your healthcare provider that you are taking Stivarga. You should stop taking Stivarga at least 2 weeks before any planned surgery.

The most common side effects of Stivarga include:
• tiredness, weakness, fatigue
• frequent or loose bowel movements (diarrhea)
• loss of appetite
• swelling, pain and redness of the lining in your mouth, throat, stomach and bowel (mucositis)
• voice changes or hoarseness
• infection
• pain in other parts of your body
• weight loss
• nausea
Tell your healthcare provider if you have any side effect that bothers you or that does not go away.

These are not all of the possible side effects of Stivarga. For more information, ask your healthcare provider or pharmacist.
Call your doctor for medical advice about side effects. You may report side effects to FDA at 1-800-FDA-1088.

How do I store Stivarga?
• Store Stivarga tablets at room temperature between 68° F to 77° F (20° C to 25° C).
• Keep Stivarga in the bottle that it comes in. Do not put Stivarga tablets in a daily or weekly pill box.
• The Stivarga bottle contains a desiccant to help keep your medicine dry. Keep the desiccant in the bottle.
• Keep the bottle of Stivarga tightly closed.
• Safely throw away (discard) any unused Stivarga tablets after 28 days of opening the bottle.
Keep Stivarga and all medicines out of the reach of children.

General information about Stivarga.
Medicines are sometimes prescribed for purposes other than those listed in a Patient Information leaflet. Do not use Stivarga for a condition for which it was not prescribed. Do not give Stivarga to other people even if they have the same symptoms you have. It may harm them.
This leaflet summarizes the most important information about Stivarga. If you would like more information, talk with your healthcare provider. You can ask your healthcare provider or pharmacist for information about Stivarga this is written for health professionals.
For more information, go to www.STIVARGA-US.com or call 1-888-842-2937.

What are the ingredients in Stivarga?
Active ingredient: regorafenib
Inactive ingredients: cellulose microcrystalline, croscarmellose sodium, magnesium stearate, povidone and colloidal silicon dioxide.
Film coat: ferric oxide red, ferric oxide yellow, lecithin (soy), polyethylene glycol 3350, polyvinyl alcohol, talc and titanium dioxide.
This Patient Information has been approved by the U.S. Food and Drug Administration.
Manufactured in Germany
Distributed and marketed by:
Bayer HealthCare Pharmaceuticals Inc.
Wayne, NJ 07470
© 2013 Bayer HealthCare Pharmaceuticals Inc.
Revised: 8/2013
Shown in Product Identification Guide, page 305

XOFIGO ℞
(radium Ra 223 dichloride)
Injection, for intravenous use

HIGHLIGHTS OF PRESCRIBING INFORMATION
These highlights do not include all the information needed to use XOFIGO safely and effectively. See full prescribing information for XOFIGO.
Xofigo (radium Ra 223 dichloride) Injection, for intravenous use
Initial U.S. Approval: 2013

————INDICATIONS AND USAGE————
Xofigo is an alpha particle-emitting radioactive therapeutic agent indicated for the treatment of patients with castration-resistant prostate cancer, symptomatic bone metastases and no known visceral metastatic disease. (1)

————DOSAGE AND ADMINISTRATION————
The dose regimen of Xofigo is 50 kBq (1.35 microcurie) per kg body weight, given at 4 week intervals for 6 injections. (2.1)

————DOSAGE FORMS AND STRENGTHS————
Single-use vial at a concentration of 1,000 kBq/mL (27 microcurie/mL) at the reference date with a total radioactivity of 6,000 kBq/vial (162 microcurie/vial) at the reference date (3)

————CONTRAINDICATIONS————
Pregnancy (4, 8.1)

————WARNINGS AND PRECAUTIONS————
Bone Marrow Suppression: Measure blood counts prior to treatment initiation and before every dose of Xofigo. Discontinue Xofigo if hematologic values do not recover within 6 to 8 weeks after treatment. Monitor patients with compromised bone marrow reserve closely. Discontinue Xofigo in patients who experience life-threatening complications despite supportive care measures. (5.1)

————ADVERSE REACTIONS————
The most common adverse drug reactions (≥ 10%) in patients receiving Xofigo were nausea, diarrhea, vomiting, and peripheral edema.

The most common hematologic laboratory abnormalities (≥ 10%) were anemia, lymphocytopenia, leukopenia, thrombocytopenia, and neutropenia (6.1).
To report SUSPECTED ADVERSE REACTIONS, contact Bayer HealthCare Pharmaceuticals Inc. at 1-888-842-2937 or FDA at 1-800-FDA-1088 or www.fda.gov/medwatch
See 17 for PATIENT COUNSELING INFORMATION
Revised: 05/2013

FULL PRESCRIBING INFORMATION

1 INDICATIONS AND USAGE
Xofigo is indicated for the treatment of patients with castration-resistant prostate cancer, symptomatic bone metastases and no known visceral metastatic disease.

2 DOSAGE AND ADMINISTRATION
2.1 Recommended Dosage
The dose regimen of Xofigo is 50 kBq (1.35 microcurie) per kg body weight, given at 4 week intervals for 6 injections. Safety and efficacy beyond 6 injections with Xofigo have not been studied.
The volume to be administered to a given patient should be calculated using:
• Patient's body weight (kg)
• Dosage level 50 kBq/kg body weight or 1.35 microcurie/kg body weight
• Radioactivity concentration of the product (1,000 kBq/mL; 27 microcurie/mL) at the reference date
• Decay correction factor to correct for physical decay of radium-223.
The total volume to be administered to a patient is calculated as follows:

$$\text{Volume to be administered (mL)} = \frac{\text{Body weight in kg} \times 50 \text{ kBq/kg body weight}}{\text{Decay factor} \times 1,000 \text{ kBq/mL}}$$

or

$$\text{Volume to be administered (mL)} = \frac{\text{Body weight in kg} \times 1.35 \text{ microcurie/kg body weight}}{\text{Decay factor} \times 27 \text{ microcurie/mL}}$$

Table 1: Decay Correction Factor Table

Days from Reference Date	Decay Factor	Days from Reference Date	Decay Factor
-14	2.296	0	0.982
-13	2.161	1	0.925

-12	2.034	2	0.870
-11	1.914	3	0.819
-10	1.802	4	0.771
-9	1.696	5	0.725
-8	1.596	6	0.683
-7	1.502	7	0.643
-6	1.414	8	0.605
-5	1.330	9	0.569
-4	1.252	10	0.536
-3	1.178	11	0.504
-2	1.109	12	0.475
-1	1.044	13	0.447
		14	0.420

The Decay Correction Factor Table is corrected to 12 noon Central Standard Time (CST). To determine the decay correction factor, count the number of days before or after the reference date. The Decay Correction Factor Table includes a correction to account for the 7 hour time difference between 12 noon Central European Time (CET) at the site of manufacture and 12 noon US CST, which is 7 hours earlier than CET.

Immediately before and after administration, the net patient dose of administered Xofigo should be determined by measurement in an appropriate radioisotope dose calibrator that has been calibrated with a National Institute of Standards and Technology (NIST) traceable radium-223 standard (available upon request from Bayer) and corrected for decay using the date and time of calibration. The dose calibrator must be calibrated with nationally recognized standards, carried out at the time of commissioning, after any maintenance procedure that could affect the dosimetry and at intervals not to exceed one year.

2.2   Administration
Administer Xofigo by slow intravenous injection over 1 minute.
Flush the intravenous access line or cannula with isotonic saline before and after injection of Xofigo.

2.3   Instructions for Use / Handling
General warning
Xofigo (an alpha particle-emitting pharmaceutical) should be received, used and administered only by authorized persons in designated clinical settings. The receipt, storage, use, transfer and disposal Xofigo are subject to the regulations and/or appropriate licenses of the competent official organization.
Xofigo should be handled by the user in a manner which satisfies both radiation safety and pharmaceutical quality requirements. Appropriate aseptic precautions should be taken.

Radiation protection
The administration of Xofigo is associated with potential risks to other persons (e.g., medical staff, caregivers and patient's household members) from radiation or contamination from spills of bodily fluids such as urine, feces, or vomit. Therefore, radiation protection precautions must be taken in accordance with national and local regulations.

For drug handling
Follow the normal working procedures for the handling of radiopharmaceuticals and use universal precautions for handling and administration such as gloves and barrier gowns when handling blood and bodily fluids to avoid contamination. In case of contact with skin or eyes, the affected area should be flushed immediately with water. In the event of spillage of Xofigo, the local radiation safety officer should be contacted immediately to initiate the necessary measurements and required procedures to decontaminate the area. A complexing agent such as 0.01 M ethylene-diamine-tetraacetic acid (EDTA) solution is recommended to remove contamination.

For patient care
Whenever possible, patients should use a toilet and the toilet should be flushed several times after each use. When handling bodily fluids, simply wearing gloves and hand washing will protect caregivers. Clothing soiled with Xofigo or patient fecal matter or urine should be washed promptly and separately from other clothing.
Radium-223 is primarily an alpha emitter, with a 95.3% fraction of energy emitted as alpha-particles. The fraction emitted as beta-particles is 3.6%, and the fraction emitted as gamma-radiation is 1.1%. The external radiation expo-

sure associated with handling of patient doses is expected to be low, because the typical treatment activity will be below 8,000 kBq (216 microcurie). In keeping with the **A**s **L**ow **A**s **R**easonably **A**chievable (ALARA) principle for minimization of radiation exposure, it is recommended to minimize the time spent in radiation areas, to maximize the distance to radiation sources, and to use adequate shielding. Any unused product or materials used in connection with the preparation or administration are to be treated as radioactive waste and should be disposed of in accordance with local regulations.
The gamma radiation associated with the decay of radium-223 and its daughters allows for the radioactivity measurement of Xofigo and the detection of contamination with standard instruments.

Instructions for preparation
Parenteral drug products should be inspected visually for particulate matter and discoloration prior to administration, whenever solution and container permit.
Xofigo is a ready-to-use solution and should not be diluted or mixed with any solutions. Each vial is for single use only.

Dosimetry
The absorbed radiation doses in major organs were calculated based on clinical biodistribution data in five patients with castration-resistant prostate cancer. Calculations of absorbed radiation doses were performed using OLINDA/EXM (**O**rgan **L**evel **IN**ternal **D**ose **A**ssessment/**EX**ponential **M**odeling), a software program based on the Medical Internal Radiation Dose (MIRD) algorithm, which is widely used for established beta and gamma emitting radionuclides. For radium-223, which is primarily an alpha particle-emitter, assumptions were made for intestine, red marrow and bone/osteogenic cells to provide the best possible absorbed radiation dose calculations for Xofigo, considering its observed biodistribution and specific characteristics.
The calculated absorbed radiation doses to different organs are listed in Table 2. The organs with highest absorbed radiation doses were bone (osteogenic cells), red marrow, upper large intestine wall, and lower large intestine wall. The calculated absorbed doses to other organs are lower.

Table 2: Calculated Absorbed Radiation Doses to Organs

Target Organ	Mean (Gy/MBq)	Mean (rad/mCi)	Coefficient of Variation (%)
Adrenals	0.00012	0.44	56
Brain	0.00010	0.37	80
Breasts	0.00005	0.18	120
Gallbladder wall	0.00023	0.85	14
LLI* wall	0.04645	171.88	83
Small intestine wall	0.00726	26.87	45
Stomach wall	0.00014	0.51	22
ULI† wall	0.03232	119.58	50
Heart wall	0.00173	6.40	42
Kidneys	0.00320	11.86	36
Liver	0.00298	11.01	36
Lungs	0.00007	0.27	90
Muscle	0.00012	0.44	41
Ovaries	0.00049	1.80	40
Pancreas	0.00011	0.41	43
Red marrow	0.13879	513.51	41
Osteogenic cells	1.15206	4262.60	41
Skin	0.00007	0.27	79
Spleen	0.00009	0.33	54
Testes	0.00008	0.31	59
Thymus	0.00006	0.21	109
Thyroid	0.00007	0.26	96
Urinary bladder wall	0.00403	14.90	63
Uterus	0.00026	0.94	28

Whole body	0.02311	85.50	16

* LLI: lower large intestine
† ULI: upper large intestine

3   DOSAGE FORMS AND STRENGTHS
Xofigo (radium Ra 223 dichloride injection) is available in single-use vials containing 6 mL of solution at a concentration of 1,000 kBq/mL (27 microcurie/mL) at the reference date with a total radioactivity of 6,000 kBq/vial (162 microcurie/vial) at the reference date.

4   CONTRAINDICATIONS
Xofigo is contraindicated in pregnancy.
Xofigo can cause fetal harm when administered to a pregnant woman based on its mechanism of action. Xofigo is not indicated for use in women. Xofigo is contraindicated in women who are or may become pregnant. If this drug is used during pregnancy, or if the patient becomes pregnant while taking this drug, apprise the patient of the potential hazard to the fetus [see Use in Specific Populations (8.1)].

5   WARNINGS AND PRECAUTIONS
5.1   Bone Marrow Suppression
In the randomized trial, 2% of patients on the Xofigo arm experienced bone marrow failure or ongoing pancytopenia compared to no patients treated with placebo. There were two deaths due to bone marrow failure and for 7 of 13 patients treated with Xofigo, bone marrow failure was ongoing at the time of death. Among the 13 patients who experienced bone marrow failure, 54% required blood transfusions. Four percent (4%) of patients on the Xofigo arm and 2% on the placebo arm permanently discontinued therapy due to bone marrow suppression.
In the randomized trial, deaths related to vascular hemorrhage in association with myelosuppression were observed in 1% of Xofigo-treated patients compared to 0.3% of patients treated with placebo. The incidence of infection-related deaths (2%), serious infections (10%), and febrile neutropenia (<1%) were similar for patients treated with Xofigo and placebo. Myelosuppression; notably thrombocytopenia, neutropenia, pancytopenia, and leukopenia; has been reported in patients treated with Xofigo. In the randomized trial, complete blood counts (CBCs) were obtained every 4 weeks prior to each dose and the nadir CBCs and times of recovery were not well characterized. In a separate single-dose phase 1 study of Xofigo, neutrophil and platelet count nadirs occurred 2 to 3 weeks after Xofigo administration at doses that were up to 1 to 5 times the recommended dose, and most patients recovered approximately 6 to 8 weeks after administration [see Adverse Reactions (6)].
Hematologic evaluation of patients must be performed at baseline and prior to every dose of Xofigo. Before the first administration of Xofigo, the absolute neutrophil count (ANC) should be ≥ 1.5 × 10⁹/L, the platelet count ≥ 100 × 10⁹/L and hemoglobin ≥ 10 g/dL. Before subsequent administrations of Xofigo, the ANC should be ≥ 1 × 10⁹/L and the platelet count ≥ 50 × 10⁹/L. If there is no recovery to these values within 6 to 8 weeks after the last administration of Xofigo, despite receiving supportive care, further treatment with Xofigo should be discontinued. Patients with evidence of compromised bone marrow reserve should be monitored closely and provided with supportive care measures when clinically indicated. Discontinue Xofigo in patients who experience life-threatening complications despite supportive care for bone marrow failure.
The safety and efficacy of concomitant chemotherapy with Xofigo have not been established. Outside of a clinical trial, concomitant use with chemotherapy is not recommended due to the potential for additive myelosuppression. If chemotherapy, other systemic radioisotopes or hemibody external radiotherapy are administered during the treatment period, Xofigo should be discontinued.

6   ADVERSE REACTIONS
The following serious adverse reactions are discussed in greater detail in another section of the label:
• Bone Marrow Suppression [see Warnings and Precautions (5.1)]

6.1   Clinical Trials Experience
Because clinical trials are conducted under widely varying conditions, adverse reaction rates observed in the clinical trials of a drug cannot be directly compared to rates in the clinical trials of another drug and may not reflect the rates observed in practice.
In the randomized clinical trial in patients with metastatic castration-resistant prostate cancer with bone metastases, 600 patients received intravenous injections of 50 kBq/kg (1.35 microcurie/kg) of Xofigo and best standard of care and 301 patients received placebo and best standard of care once every 4 weeks for up to 6 injections. Prior to randomization, 58% and 57% of patients had received docetaxel in the Xofigo and placebo arms, respectively. The median duration of treatment was 20 weeks (6 cycles) for Xofigo and 18 weeks (5 cycles) for placebo.

The most common adverse reactions (≥ 10%) in patients receiving Xofigo were nausea, diarrhea, vomiting, and peripheral edema (Table 3). Grade 3 and 4 adverse events were reported among 57% of Xofigo-treated patients and 63% of placebo-treated patients. The most common hematologic laboratory abnormalities in Xofigo-treated patients (≥ 10%) were anemia, lymphocytopenia, leukopenia, thrombocytopenia, and neutropenia (Table 4).

Treatment discontinuations due to adverse events occurred in 17% of patients who received Xofigo and 21% of patients who received placebo. The most common hematologic laboratory abnormalities leading to discontinuation for Xofigo were anemia (2%) and thrombocytopenia (2%).

Table 3 shows adverse reactions occurring in ≥ 2% of patients and for which the incidence for Xofigo exceeds the incidence for placebo.
[See table 3 above]

Laboratory Abnormalities
Table 4 shows hematologic laboratory abnormalities occurring in ≥ 10% of patients and for which the incidence for Xofigo exceeds the incidence for placebo.
[See table 4 above]

As an adverse reaction, grade 3-4 thrombocytopenia was reported in 6% of patients on Xofigo and in 2% of patients on placebo. Among patients who received Xofigo, the laboratory abnormality grade 3-4 thrombocytopenia occurred in 1% of docetaxel naïve patients and in 4% of patients who had received prior docetaxel. Grade 3-4 neutropenia occurred in 1% of docetaxel naïve patients and in 3% of patients who have received prior docetaxel.

Fluid Status
Dehydration occurred in 3% of patients on Xofigo and 1% of patients on placebo. Xofigo increases adverse reactions such as diarrhea, nausea, and vomiting which may result in dehydration. Monitor patients' oral intake and fluid status carefully and promptly treat patients who display signs or symptoms of dehydration or hypovolemia.

Injection Site Reactions
Erythema, pain, and edema at the injection site were reported in 1% of patients on Xofigo.

Secondary Malignant Neoplasms
Xofigo contributes to a patient's overall long-term cumulative radiation exposure. Long-term cumulative radiation exposure may be associated with an increased risk of cancer and hereditary defects. Due to its mechanism of action and neoplastic changes, including osteosarcomas, in rats following administration of radium-223 dichloride, Xofigo may increase the risk of osteosarcoma or other secondary malignant neoplasms *[see Nonclinical Toxicology (13.1)]*. However, the overall incidence of new malignancies in the randomized trial was lower on the Xofigo arm compared to placebo (<1% vs. 2%; respectively), but the expected latency period for the development of secondary malignancies exceeds the duration of follow up for patients on the trial.

Subsequent Treatment with Cytotoxic Chemotherapy
In the randomized clinical trial, 16% patients in the Xofigo group and 18% patients in the placebo group received cytotoxic chemotherapy after completion of study treatments. Adequate safety monitoring and laboratory testing was not performed to assess how patients treated with Xofigo will tolerate subsequent cytotoxic chemotherapy.

7 DRUG INTERACTIONS

No formal clinical drug interaction studies have been performed.

Subgroup analyses indicated that the concurrent use of bisphosphonates or calcium channel blockers did not affect the safety and efficacy of Xofigo in the randomized clinical trial.

8 USE IN SPECIFIC POPULATIONS

8.1 Pregnancy
Category X *[see Contraindications (4)]*
Xofigo can cause fetal harm when administered to a pregnant woman based on its mechanism of action. While there are no human or animal data on the use of Xofigo in pregnancy and Xofigo is not indicated for use in women, maternal use of a radioactive therapeutic agent could affect development of a fetus. Xofigo is contraindicated in women who are or may become pregnant while receiving the drug. If this drug is used during pregnancy, or if the patient becomes pregnant while taking this drug, apprise the patient of the potential hazard to the fetus and the potential risk for pregnancy loss. Advise females of reproductive potential to avoid becoming pregnant during treatment with Xofigo.

8.3 Nursing Mothers
Xofigo is not indicated for use in women. It is not known whether radium-223 dichloride is excreted in human milk. Because many drugs are excreted in human milk, and because of the potential for serious adverse reactions in nursing infants from Xofigo, a decision should be made whether to discontinue nursing, or discontinue the drug taking into account the importance of the drug to the mother.

Table 3: Adverse Reactions in the Randomized Trial

System/Organ Class Preferred Term	Xofigo (n=600)		Placebo (n=301)	
	Grades 1-4 %	Grades 3-4 %	Grades 1-4 %	Grades 3-4 %
Blood and lymphatic system disorders				
Pancytopenia	2	1	0	0
Gastrointestinal disorders				
Nausea	36	2	35	2
Diarrhea	25	2	15	2
Vomiting	19	2	14	2
General disorders and administration site conditions				
Peripheral edema	13	2	10	1
Renal and urinary disorders				
Renal failure and impairment	3	1	1	1

Table 4: Hematologic Laboratory Abnormalities

Hematologic Laboratory Abnormalities	Xofigo (n=600)		Placebo (n=301)	
	Grades 1-4 %	Grades 3-4 %	Grades 1-4 %	Grades 3-4 %
Anemia	93	6	88	6
Lymphocytopenia	72	20	53	7
Leukopenia	35	3	10	<1
Thrombocytopenia	31	3	22	<1
Neutropenia	18	2	5	<1

Laboratory values were obtained at baseline and prior to each 4-week cycle.

8.4 Pediatric Use
The safety and efficacy of Xofigo in pediatric patients have not been established.

In single- and repeat-dose toxicity studies in rats, findings in the bones (depletion of osteocytes, osteoblasts, osteoclasts, fibro-osseous lesions, disruption/disorganization of the physis/growth line) and teeth (missing, irregular growth, fibro-osseous lesions in bone socket) correlated with a reduction of osteogenesis that occurred at clinically relevant doses beginning in the range of 20 – 80 kBq (0.541 - 2.16 microcurie) per kg body weight.

8.5 Geriatric Use
Of the 600 patients treated with Xofigo in the randomized trial, 75% were 65 years of age and over and while 33% were 75 years of age and over. No dosage adjustment is considered necessary in elderly patients. No overall differences in safety or effectiveness were observed between these subjects and younger subjects, and other reported clinical experience has not identified differences in responses between the elderly and younger patients, but greater sensitivity of some older individuals cannot be ruled out.

8.6 Patients with Hepatic Impairment
No dedicated hepatic impairment trial for Xofigo has been conducted. Since radium-223 is neither metabolized by the liver nor eliminated via the bile, hepatic impairment is unlikely to affect the pharmacokinetics of radium-223 dichloride *[see Clinical Pharmacology (12.3)]*. Based on subgroup analyses in the randomized clinical trial, dose adjustment is not needed in patients with mild hepatic impairment. No dose adjustments can be recommended for patients with moderate or severe hepatic impairment due to lack of clinical data.

8.7 Patients with Renal Impairment
No dedicated renal impairment trial for Xofigo has been conducted. Based on subgroup analyses in the randomized clinical trial, dose adjustment is not needed in patients with existing mild (creatinine clearance [CrCl] 60 to 89 mL/min) or moderate (CrCl 30 to 59 mL/min) renal impairment. No dose adjustment can be recommended for patients with severe renal impairment (CrCl less than 30 mL/min) due to limited data available (n = 2) *[see Clinical Pharmacology (12.3)]*.

8.8 Males of Reproductive Potential
Contraception
Because of potential effects on spermatogenesis associated with radiation, advise men who are sexually active to use condoms and their female partners of reproductive potential to use a highly effective contraceptive method during and for 6 months after completing treatment with Xofigo.

Infertility
There are no data on the effects of Xofigo on human fertility. There is a potential risk that radiation by Xofigo could impair human fertility *[see Nonclinical Toxicology (13.1)]*.

10 OVERDOSAGE

There have been no reports of inadvertent overdosing of Xofigo during clinical studies.

There is no specific antidote. In the event of an inadvertent overdose of Xofigo, utilize general supportive measures, including monitoring for potential hematological and gastrointestinal toxicity, and consider using medical countermeasures such as aluminum hydroxide, barium sulfate, calcium carbonate, calcium gluconate, calcium phosphate, or sodium alginate.[1]

Single Xofigo doses up to 250 kBq (6.76 microcurie) per kg body weight were evaluated in a phase 1 clinical trial and no dose-limiting toxicities were observed.

11 DESCRIPTION

Radium Ra 223 dichloride, an alpha particle-emitting pharmaceutical, is a radiotherapeutic drug.

Xofigo is supplied as a clear, colorless, isotonic, and sterile solution to be administered intravenously with pH between 6 and 8.

Each milliliter of solution contains 1,000 kBq radium-223 dichloride (27 microcurie), corresponding to 0.53 ng radium-223, at the reference date. Radium is present in the solution as a free divalent cation.

Each vial contains 6 mL of solution (6,000 kBq (162 microcurie) radium-223 dichloride at the reference date). The inactive ingredients are 6.3 mg/mL sodium chloride USP (tonicity agent), 7.2 mg/mL sodium citrate USP (for pH adjustment), 0.2 mg/mL hydrochloric acid USP (for pH adjustment), and water for injection USP.

The molecular weight of radium-223 dichloride, $^{223}RaCl_2$, is 293.9 g/mol.

Radium-223 has a half-life of 11.4 days. The specific activity of radium-223 is 1.9 MBq (51.4 microcurie)/ng.

The six-stage-decay of radium-223 to stable lead-207 occurs via short-lived daughters, and is accompanied predominantly by alpha emissions. There are also beta and gamma emissions with different energies and emission probabilities. The fraction of energy emitted from radium-223 and its daughters as alpha-particles is 95.3% (energy range of 5 - 7.5 MeV). The fraction emitted as beta-particles is 3.6% (average energies are 0.445 MeV and 0.492 MeV), and the fraction emitted as gamma-radiation is 1.1% (energy range of 0.01 - 1.27 MeV).

12 CLINICAL PHARMACOLOGY
12.1 Mechanism of Action
The active moiety of Xofigo is the alpha particle-emitting isotope radium-223 (as radium Ra 223 dichloride), which mimics calcium and forms complexes with the bone mineral hydroxyapatite at areas of increased bone turnover, such as bone metastases (see Table 2). The high linear energy transfer of alpha emitters (80 keV/micrometer) leads to a high frequency of double-strand DNA breaks in adjacent cells, resulting in an anti-tumor effect on bone metastases. The alpha particle range from radium-223 dichloride is less than 100 micrometers (less than 10 cell diameters) which limits damage to the surrounding normal tissue.

12.2 Pharmacodynamics
Compared with placebo, there was a significant difference in favor of Xofigo for all five serum biomarkers for bone turnover studied in a phase 2 randomized study (bone formation markers: bone alkaline phosphatase [ALP], total ALP and procollagen I N propeptide [PINP], bone resorption markers: C-terminal crosslinking telopeptide of type I collagen [S-CTX-I] and type I collagen crosslinked C-telopeptide [ICTP]).

12.3 Pharmacokinetics
The pharmacokinetics of radium-223 dichloride in blood was linear in terms of dose proportionality and time independence in the dose range investigated (46 to 250 kBq [1.24 to 6.76 microcurie] per kg body weight).
Distribution
After intravenous injection, radium-223 is rapidly cleared from the blood and is distributed primarily into bone or is excreted into intestine. Fifteen minutes post-injection, about 20% of the injected radioactivity remained in blood. At 4 hours, about 4% of the injected radioactivity remained in blood, decreasing to less than 1% at 24 hours after the injection. At 10 minutes post-injection, radioactivity was observed in bone and in intestine. At 4 hours post-injection, the percentage of the radioactive dose present in bone and intestine was approximately 61% and 49%, respectively. No significant uptake was seen in other organs such as heart, liver, kidneys, urinary bladder, and spleen at 4 hours post-injection *[see Dosage and Administration (2.3)]*.
Metabolism
Radium-223 is an isotope that decays and is not metabolized.
Elimination
Special Populations
Pediatric patients
Safety and effectiveness of Xofigo have not been established in children and adolescents below 18 years of age.

Patients with hepatic impairment
No dedicated pharmacokinetic study in patients with hepatic impairment has been conducted. However, since radium-223 is not metabolized and there is no evidence of hepato-biliary excretion based on imaging data, hepatic impairment is not expected to affect the pharmacokinetics of radium-223 dichloride.

Patients with renal impairment
No dedicated pharmacokinetic study in patients with renal impairment has been conducted. However, since excretion in urine is minimal and the major route of elimination is via the feces, renal impairment is not expected to affect the pharmacokinetics of radium-223 dichloride.

12.6 Cardiac Electrophysiology
The effect of a single dose of 50 kBq/kg of radium-223 dichloride on the QTc interval was evaluated in a subgroup of 29 patients (21 received Xofigo and 8 received placebo) in the randomized clinical trial. No large changes in the mean QTc interval (i.e., greater than 20 ms) were detected up to 6 hours post-dose. The potential for delayed effects on the QT interval after 6 hours was not evaluated.

13 NONCLINICAL TOXICOLOGY
13.1 Carcinogenesis, Mutagenesis, Impairment of Fertility
Animal studies have not been conducted to evaluate the carcinogenic potential of radium-223 dichloride. However, in repeat-dose toxicity studies in rats, osteosarcomas, a known effect of bone-seeking radionuclides, were observed at clinically relevant doses 7 to 12 months after the start of treatment. The presence of other neoplastic changes, including

lymphoma and mammary gland carcinoma, was also reported in 12- to 15-month repeat-dose toxicity studies in rats.
Genetic toxicology studies have not been conducted with radium-223 dichloride. However, the mechanism of action of radium-223 dichloride involves induction of double-strand DNA breaks, which is a known effect of radiation.
Animal studies have not been conducted to evaluate the effects of radium-223 dichloride on male or female fertility or reproductive function. Xofigo may impair fertility and reproductive function in humans based on its mechanism of action.

14 CLINICAL STUDIES
The efficacy and safety of Xofigo were evaluated in a double-blind, randomized, placebo-controlled phase 3 clinical trial of patients with castration-resistant prostate cancer with symptomatic bone metastases. Patients with visceral metastases and malignant lymphadenopathy exceeding 3 cm were excluded. The primary efficacy endpoint was overall survival. A key secondary efficacy endpoint was time to first symptomatic skeletal event (SSE) defined as external beam radiation therapy (EBRT) to relieve skeletal symptoms, new symptomatic pathologic bone fracture, occurrence of spinal cord compression, or tumor-related orthopedic surgical intervention. There were no scheduled radiographic assessments performed on study. All patients were to continue androgen deprivation therapy. At the cut-off date of the pre-planned interim analysis, a total of 809 patients had been randomized 2:1 to receive Xofigo 50 kBq (1.35 microcurie)/kg intravenously every 4 weeks for 6 cycles (n = 541) plus best standard of care or matching placebo plus best standard of care (n = 268). Best standard of care included local EBRT, corticosteroids, antiandrogens, estrogens, estramustine or ketoconazole. Therapy was continued until unacceptable toxicity or initiation of cytotoxic chemotherapy, other systemic radioisotope, hemi-body EBRT or other investigational drug. Patients with Crohn's disease, ulcerative colitis, prior hemibody radiation or untreated imminent spinal cord compression were excluded from the study. In patients with bone fractures, orthopedic stabilization was performed before starting or resuming treatment with Xofigo.
The following patient demographics and baseline disease characteristics were balanced between the arms. The median age was 71 (range 44-94) with a racial distribution of 94% Caucasian, 4% Asian, 2% Black and <1% Other. Patients were enrolled predominantly from Europe (85%) with 4% of patients enrolled from North America. ECOG performance status was 0-1 in 86% of patients. Eighty-five percent of patients had 6 or more bone scan lesions and of those 40% had > 20 lesions or a superscan. Opiate pain medications were used for cancer-related pain in 54% of patients, non-opiate pain medications in 44% of patients and no pain medications in 2% of patients. Patients were stratified by baseline ALP, bisphosphonate use, and prior docetaxel exposure. Prior bisphosphonates were used by 41% of patients and 58% had received prior docetaxel. During the treatment period, 83% of Xofigo patients and 82% of placebo patients received gonadotropin-releasing hormone agonists and 21% of Xofigo patients and 34% of placebo patients received concomitant antiandrogens. Use of systemic steroids (41%) and bisphosphonates (40%) was balanced between the arms.
The pre-specified interim analysis of overall survival revealed a statistically significant improvement in patients receiving XOFIGO plus best standard of care compared with patients receiving placebo plus best standard of care.
An exploratory updated overall survival analysis performed before patient crossover with an additional 214 events resulted in findings consistent with the interim analysis (Table 5).

Table 5: Overall Survival Results from the Phase 3 Clinical Trial

	Xofigo	Placebo
Interim Analysis		
Subjects randomized	541	268
Number of deaths	191 (35.3%)	123 (45.9%)
Censored	350 (64.7%)	145 (54.1%)
Median survival (months)*	14.0	11.2
(95% CI)	(12.1, 15.8)	(9.0, 13.2)
p-value†	0.00185	
Hazard ratio (95% CI)‡	0.695 (0.552, 0.875)	
Updated Analysis		
Subjects randomized	614	307
Number of deaths	333 (54.2%)	195 (63.5%)
Censored	281 (45.8%)	112 (36.5%)
Median survival (months)*	14.9	11.3
(95% CI)	(13.9, 16.1)	(10.4, 12.8)
Hazard ratio (95% CI)‡	0.695 (0.581, 0.832)	

* Survival time is calculated as months from date of randomization to date of death from any cause. Subjects who are not deceased at time of analysis are censored on the last date subject was known to be alive or lost to follow-up.

† p-value is from a log-rank test stratified by total ALP, current use of bisphosphonates, and prior use of docetaxel.

‡ Hazard ratio is from a Cox proportional hazards model adjusted for total ALP, current use of bisphosphonates, and prior use of docetaxel. Hazard ratio < 1 favors radium-223 dichloride.

The Kaplan-Meier curves for overall survival based on the updated survival results are shown in Figure 1.

Figure 1: Kaplan-Meier Overall Survival Curves from the Phase 3 Clinical Trial

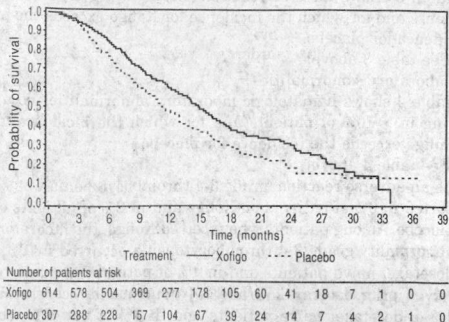

Number of patients at risk														
Xofigo	614	578	504	369	277	178	105	60	41	18	7	1	0	0
Placebo	307	288	228	157	104	67	39	24	14	7	4	2	1	0

The survival results were supported by a delay in the time to first SSE favoring the Xofigo arm. The majority of events consisted of external beam radiotherapy to bone metastases.

15 REFERENCES
1. 1. Radiation Emergency Medical Management. [REMM/ National Library of Medicine Website.] http://www.remm.nlm.gov/ int_contamination.htm#blockingagents

16 HOW SUPPLIED/STORAGE AND HANDLING
Xofigo (radium Ra 223 dichloride injection) is supplied in single-use vials containing 6 mL of solution at a concentration of 1,000 kBq/mL (27 microcurie/mL) with a total radioactivity of 6,000 kBq/vial (162 microcurie/vial) at the reference date (NDC 50419-208-01).
Store at room temperature, below 40° C (104° F). Store Xofigo in the original container or equivalent radiation shielding.
This preparation is approved for use by persons under license by the Nuclear Regulatory Commission or the relevant regulatory authority of an Agreement State.
Follow procedures for proper handling and disposal of radioactive pharmaceuticals *[see Dosage and Administration (2.3)]*.

17 PATIENT COUNSELING INFORMATION
Advise patients:
- To be compliant with blood cell count monitoring appointments while receiving Xofigo. Explain the importance of routine blood cell counts. Instruct patients to report signs of bleeding or infections.
- To stay well hydrated and to monitor oral intake, fluid status, and urine output while being treated with Xofigo. Instruct patients to report signs of dehydration, hypovolemia, urinary retention, or renal failure / insufficiency.
- There are no restrictions regarding contact with other people after receiving Xofigo. Follow good hygiene practices while receiving Xofigo and for at least 1 week after the last injection in order to minimize radiation exposure from bodily fluids to household members and caregivers. Whenever possible, patients should use a toilet and the toilet should be flushed several times after each use. Clothing soiled with patient fecal matter or urine should be washed promptly and separately from other clothing. Caregivers should use universal precautions for patient care such as gloves and barrier gowns when handling bodily fluids to avoid contamination. When handling bodily fluids, wearing gloves and hand washing will protect caregivers.
- Who are sexually active to use condoms and their female partners of reproductive potential to use a highly effective method of birth control during treatment and for 6 months following completion of Xofigo treatment.
Manufactured for:
Bayer HealthCare Pharmaceuticals Inc.
Wayne, NJ 07470
Manufactured in Norway
Xofigo is a trademark of Bayer Aktiengesellschaft.
© 2013, Bayer HealthCare Pharmaceuticals Inc.
All rights reserved.
Revised: 05/2013
Shown in Product Identification Guide, page 305

Bristol-Myers Squibb Company
P.O. BOX 4500
PRINCETON, NJ 08543-4500

For Medical Information Contact:
Generally:
Bristol-Myers Squibb Medical Information Department
P.O. Box 4500
Princeton, NJ 08543-4500
(800) 321-1335 between 8:00 AM-8:00 PM EST
To report SUSPECTED ADVERSE REACTIONS,
Contact Bristol-Myers Squibb Company at
(800) 721-5072 between 8:00 AM-8:00 PM EST
Sales and Ordering:
Orders may be placed by:
Calling your purchase orders in toll-free between
9:00 AM-5:00 PM EST:
(800) 631-5244
E-mailing your purchase orders to:
customerserviceoperations@BMS.com
Faxing your purchase orders in:
(800) 277-0988

ATRIPLA®   Rx
[uh TRIP luh]
(efavirenz/emtricitabine/tenofovir disoproxil fumarate)
tablets, for oral use

HIGHLIGHTS OF PRESCRIBING INFORMATION
These highlights do not include all the information needed
to use ATRIPLA safely and effectively. See full prescribing
information for ATRIPLA.
ATRIPLA® (efavirenz/emtricitabine/tenofovir disoproxil
fumarate) tablets, for oral use
Initial U.S. Approval: 2006

WARNING: LACTIC ACIDOSIS/SEVERE HEPATO-
MEGALY WITH STEATOSIS and POST TREATMENT
EXACERBATION OF HEPATITIS B
See full prescribing information for complete boxed
warning.
- **Lactic acidosis and severe hepatomegaly with stea-**
tosis, including fatal cases, have been reported with
the use of nucleoside analogs, including tenofovir
disoproxil fumarate, a component of ATRIPLA. (5.1)
- **ATRIPLA is not approved for the treatment of**
chronic hepatitis B virus (HBV) infection. Severe
acute exacerbations of hepatitis B have been re-
ported in patients coinfected with HBV and HIV-1
who have discontinued EMTRIVA or VIREAD, two of
the components of ATRIPLA. Hepatic function
should be monitored closely in these patients. If ap-
propriate, initiation of anti-hepatitis B therapy may
be warranted. (5.2)

RECENT MAJOR CHANGES
Warnings and Precautions
Coadministration with Related Products   04/2013
(5.4)
New Onset or Worsening Renal   10/2013
Impairment (5.7)
Rash (5.9)   04/2013
Bone Effects of Tenofovir DF (5.11)   10/2013

INDICATIONS AND USAGE
ATRIPLA, a combination of 2 nucleoside analog HIV-1 reverse transcriptase inhibitors and 1 non-nucleoside HIV-1
reverse transcriptase inhibitor, is indicated for use alone as
a complete regimen or in combination with other antiretroviral agents for the treatment of HIV-1 infection in adults
and pediatric patients 12 years of age and older. (1)

DOSAGE AND ADMINISTRATION
- Recommended dose in adults and pediatric patients (12
years of age and older and weighing at least 40 kg): One
tablet once daily taken orally on an empty stomach, preferably at bedtime. (2)
- Dose in renal impairment: Should not be administered
in patients with estimated creatinine clearance below
50 mL/min. (2)
- With rifampin coadministration, an additional 200 mg/day
of efavirenz is recommended for patients weighing 50 kg
or more. (2)

DOSAGE FORMS AND STRENGTHS
Tablet containing 600 mg of efavirenz, 200 mg of
emtricitabine and 300 mg of tenofovir disoproxil fumarate.
(3)

CONTRAINDICATIONS
- Previously demonstrated hypersensitivity (e.g., Stevens-
Johnson syndrome, erythema multiforme, or toxic skin
eruptions) to efavirenz, a component of ATRIPLA
(efavirenz/emtricitabine/tenofovir disoproxil fumarate).
(4.1)
- For some drugs, competition for CYP3A by efavirenz could
result in inhibition of their metabolism and create the potential for serious and/or life-threatening adverse reactions (e.g., cardiac arrhythmias, prolonged sedation, or
respiratory depression). (4.2)

WARNINGS AND PRECAUTIONS
- Serious psychiatric symptoms: Immediate medical evaluation is recommended. (5.5, 6.1)
- Nervous system symptoms (NSS): NSS are frequent,
usually begin 1–2 days after initiating therapy and resolve
in 2–4 weeks. Dosing at bedtime may improve tolerability.
NSS are not predictive of onset of psychiatric symptoms.
(2, 5.6)
- New onset or worsening renal impairment: Can include
acute renal failure and Fanconi syndrome. Assess estimated creatinine clearance before initiating treatment
with ATRIPLA. In patients at risk for renal dysfunction,
assess estimated creatinine clearance, serum phosphorus,
urine glucose and urine protein before initiating treatment with ATRIPLA and periodically during treatment.
Avoid administering ATRIPLA with concurrent or recent
use of nephrotoxic drugs. (5.7)
- Pregnancy: Fetal harm can occur when administered to
a pregnant woman during the first trimester. Women
should be apprised of the potential harm to the fetus. A
pregnancy registry is available. (5.8, 8.1)
- Rash: Discontinue if severe rash develops. (5.9, 6.1)
- Hepatotoxicity: Monitor liver function tests before and
during treatment in patients with underlying hepatic disease, including hepatitis B or C coinfection, marked transaminase elevations, or who are taking medications associated with liver toxicity. Among reported cases of hepatic
failure, a few occurred in patients with no pre-existing hepatic disease. (5.10, 6.3, 8.6)
- Decreases in bone mineral density (BMD): Consider assessment of BMD in patients with a history of pathological
fracture or other risk factors for osteoporosis or bone loss.
(5.11)
- Convulsions: Use caution in patients with a history of
seizures. (5.12)
- Immune reconstitution syndrome: May necessitate further evaluation and treatment. (5.13)
- Redistribution/accumulation of body fat: Observed in patients receiving antiretroviral therapy. (5.14)
- Coadministration with other products: Do not use with
drugs containing emtricitabine or tenofovir disoproxil
fumarate including COMPLERA, EMTRIVA, STRIBILD,
TRUVADA, or VIREAD; or with drugs containing lamivudine. SUSTIVA (efavirenz) should not be coadministered
with ATRIPLA unless required for dose-adjustment when
coadministered with rifampin. (5.4) Do not administer in
combination with HEPSERA. (5.2)

ADVERSE REACTIONS
Most common adverse reactions (incidence greater than or
equal to 10%) observed in an active-controlled clinical trial
of efavirenz, emtricitabine, and tenofovir DF are diarrhea,
nausea, fatigue, headache, dizziness, depression, insomnia,
abnormal dreams, and rash. (6)
To report SUSPECTED ADVERSE REACTIONS, contact
Gilead Sciences, Inc. at 1-800-GILEAD-5 or FDA at
1-800-FDA-1088 or www.fda.gov/medwatch

DRUG INTERACTIONS
- Efavirenz: Coadministration of efavirenz can alter the
concentrations of other drugs and other drugs may alter
the concentrations of efavirenz. The potential for drug-
drug interactions must be considered before and during
therapy. (4.2, 7.1, 12.3)
- Didanosine: Tenofovir disoproxil fumarate increases didanosine concentrations. Use with caution and monitor for
evidence of didanosine toxicity (e.g., pancreatitis, neuropathy) when coadministered. Consider dose reductions or
discontinuations of didanosine if warranted. (7.2)
- HIV-1 protease inhibitors: Coadministration of
ATRIPLA with either lopinavir/ritonavir or darunavir and
ritonavir increases tenofovir concentrations. Monitor for
evidence of tenofovir toxicity. Coadministration of
ATRIPLA with either atazanavir or atazanavir and ritonavir is not recommended. (7.3)

USE IN SPECIFIC POPULATIONS
- Pregnancy: Women should avoid pregnancy while receiving ATRIPLA and for 12 weeks after discontinuation.
(5.8)
- Nursing mothers: Women infected with HIV should be
instructed not to breastfeed. (8.3)
- Hepatic impairment: ATRIPLA is not recommended for
patients with moderate or severe hepatic impairment. Use
caution in patients with mild hepatic impairment. (5.10,
8.6)

- Pediatrics: The incidence of rash was higher than in
adults. (5.9, 6.1)
See 17 for PATIENT COUNSELING INFORMATION
and FDA-approved patient labeling

Revised: 10/2013

FULL PRESCRIBING INFORMATION

WARNING: LACTIC ACIDOSIS/SEVERE HEPATO-
MEGALY WITH STEATOSIS and POST-TREATMENT
EXACERBATION OF HEPATITIS B
Lactic acidosis and severe hepatomegaly with steato-
sis, including fatal cases, have been reported with the
use of nucleoside analogs, including tenofovir
disoproxil fumarate, a component of ATRIPLA
(efavirenz/emtricitabine/tenofovir   disoproxil
fumarate), in combination with other antiretrovirals
[See Warnings and Precautions (5.1)].
ATRIPLA is not approved for the treatment of chronic
hepatitis B virus (HBV) infection and the safety and
efficacy of ATRIPLA have not been established in pa-

Table 1: Drugs That Are Contraindicated or Not Recommended for Use With ATRIPLA

Drug Class: Drug Name	Clinical Comment
Antifungal: voriconazole	Efavirenz significantly decreases voriconazole plasma concentrations, and coadministration may decrease the therapeutic effectiveness of voriconazole. Also, voriconazole significantly increases efavirenz plasma concentrations, which may increase the risk of efavirenz-associated side effects. Because ATRIPLA is a fixed-dose combination product, the dose of efavirenz cannot be altered. [See Clinical Pharmacology (12.3) Tables 5 and 6]
Ergot derivatives (dihydroergotamine, ergonovine, ergotamine, methylergonovine)	Potential for serious and/or life-threatening reactions such as acute ergot toxicity characterized by peripheral vasospasm and ischemia of the extremities and other tissues.
Benzodiazepines: midazolam, triazolam	Potential for serious and/or life-threatening reactions such as prolonged or increased sedation or respiratory depression.
Calcium channel blocker: bepridil	Potential for serious and/or life-threatening reactions such as cardiac arrhythmias.
GI motility agent: cisapride	Potential for serious and/or life-threatening reactions such as cardiac arrhythmias.
Neuroleptic: pimozide	Potential for serious and/or life-threatening reactions such as cardiac arrhythmias.
St. John's wort (Hypericum perforatum)	May lead to loss of virologic response and possible resistance to efavirenz or to the class of non-nucleoside reverse transcriptase inhibitors (NNRTIs).

tients coinfected with HBV and HIV-1. Severe acute exacerbations of hepatitis B have been reported in patients who have discontinued EMTRIVA or VIREAD, which are components of ATRIPLA. Hepatic function should be monitored closely with both clinical and laboratory follow-up for at least several months in patients who are coinfected with HIV-1 and HBV and discontinue ATRIPLA. If appropriate, initiation of anti-hepatitis B therapy may be warranted [See Warnings and Precautions (5.2)].

1   INDICATIONS AND USAGE

ATRIPLA® (efavirenz/emtricitabine/tenofovir disoproxil fumarate) is indicated for use alone as a complete regimen or in combination with other antiretroviral agents for the treatment of HIV-1 infection in adults and pediatric patients 12 years of age and older.

2   DOSAGE AND ADMINISTRATION

Adults and pediatric patients 12 years of age and older with body weight at least 40 kg (at least 88 lbs): The dose of ATRIPLA is one tablet once daily taken orally on an empty stomach. Dosing at bedtime may improve the tolerability of nervous system symptoms.

Renal Impairment: Because ATRIPLA is a fixed-dose combination, it should not be prescribed for patients requiring dosage adjustment such as those with moderate or severe renal impairment (estimated creatinine clearance below 50 mL/min).

Rifampin Coadministration: When ATRIPLA is administered with rifampin to patients weighing 50 kg or more, an additional 200 mg/day of efavirenz is recommended [See Drug Interactions (7.3), Table 4, and Clinical Pharmacology (12.3), Table 5].

3   DOSAGE FORMS AND STRENGTHS

ATRIPLA is available as tablets. Each tablet contains 600 mg of efavirenz, 200 mg of emtricitabine and 300 mg of tenofovir disoproxil fumarate (tenofovir DF, which is equivalent to 245 mg of tenofovir disoproxil). The tablets are pink, capsule-shaped, film-coated, debossed with "123" on one side and plain-faced on the other side.

4   CONTRAINDICATIONS

4.1   Hypersensitivity

ATRIPLA is contraindicated in patients with previously demonstrated clinically significant hypersensitivity (e.g., Stevens-Johnson syndrome, erythema multiforme, or toxic skin eruptions) to efavirenz, a component of ATRIPLA.

4.2   Contraindicated Drugs

For some drugs, competition for CYP3A by efavirenz could result in inhibition of their metabolism and create the potential for serious and/or life-threatening adverse reactions (e.g., cardiac arrhythmias, prolonged sedation, or respiratory depression). Drugs that are contraindicated with ATRIPLA are listed in Table 1.

[See table 1 above]

5   WARNINGS AND PRECAUTIONS

5.1   Lactic Acidosis/Severe Hepatomegaly with Steatosis

Lactic acidosis and severe hepatomegaly with steatosis, including fatal cases, have been reported with the use of nucleoside analogs including tenofovir DF, a component of ATRIPLA, in combination with other antiretrovirals. A majority of these cases have been in women. Obesity and prolonged nucleoside exposure may be risk factors. Particular caution should be exercised when administering nucleoside analogs to any patient with known risk factors for liver disease; however, cases have also been reported in patients with no known risk factors. Treatment with ATRIPLA should be suspended in any patient who develops clinical or laboratory findings suggestive of lactic acidosis or pronounced hepatotoxicity (which may include hepatomegaly and steatosis even in the absence of marked transaminase elevations).

5.2   Patients Coinfected with HIV-1 and HBV

It is recommended that all patients with HIV-1 be tested for the presence of chronic HBV before initiating antiretroviral therapy. ATRIPLA is not approved for the treatment of chronic HBV infection, and the safety and efficacy of ATRIPLA have not been established in patients coinfected with HBV and HIV-1. Severe acute exacerbations of hepatitis B have been reported in patients who are coinfected with HBV and HIV-1 and have discontinued emtricitabine or tenofovir DF, two of the components of ATRIPLA. In some patients infected with HBV and treated with emtricitabine, the exacerbations of hepatitis B were associated with liver decompensation and liver failure. Patients who are coinfected with HIV-1 and HBV should be closely monitored with both clinical and laboratory follow-up for at least several months after stopping treatment with ATRIPLA. If appropriate, initiation of anti-hepatitis B therapy may be warranted.

ATRIPLA (efavirenz/emtricitabine/tenofovir disoproxil fumarate) should not be administered with HEPSERA® (adefovir dipivoxil) [See Drug Interactions (7.2)].

5.3   Drug Interactions

Efavirenz plasma concentrations may be altered by substrates, inhibitors, or inducers of CYP3A. Likewise, efavirenz may alter plasma concentrations of drugs metabolized by CYP3A or CYP2B6 [See Contraindications (4.2), Drug Interactions (7.1)].

5.4   Coadministration with Related Products

Related drugs not for coadministration with ATRIPLA include COMPLERA® (emtricitabine/rilpivirine/tenofovir DF), EMTRIVA® (emtricitabine), STRIBILD® (elvitegravir/cobicistat/emtricitabine/tenofovir DF), TRUVADA® (emtricitabine/tenofovir DF), and VIREAD® (tenofovir DF), which contain the same active components as ATRIPLA. SUSTIVA® (efavirenz) should not be coadministered with ATRIPLA unless needed for dose-adjustment (e.g., with rifampin) [See Dosage and Administration (2), Drug Interactions (7.1)]. Due to similarities between emtricitabine and lamivudine, ATRIPLA should not be coadministered with drugs containing lamivudine, including Combivir (lamivudine/zidovudine), Epivir, or Epivir-HBV (lamivudine), Epzicom (abacavir sulfate/lamivudine), or Trizivir (abacavir sulfate/lamivudine/zidovudine).

5.5   Psychiatric Symptoms

Serious psychiatric adverse experiences have been reported in patients treated with efavirenz. In controlled trials of 1008 subjects treated with regimens containing efavirenz for a mean of 2.1 years and 635 subjects treated with control regimens for a mean of 1.5 years, the frequency (regardless of causality) of specific serious psychiatric events among subjects who received efavirenz or control regimens, respectively, were: severe depression (2.4%, 0.9%), suicidal ideation (0.7%, 0.3%), nonfatal suicide attempts (0.5%, 0%), aggressive behavior (0.4%, 0.5%), paranoid reactions (0.4%, 0.3%), and manic reactions (0.2%, 0.3%). When psychiatric symptoms similar to those noted above were combined and evaluated as a group in a multifactorial analysis of data from Study AI266006 (006), treatment with efavirenz was associated with an increase in the occurrence of these selected psychiatric symptoms. Other factors associated with an increase in the occurrence of these psychiatric symptoms were history of injection drug use, psychiatric history, and receipt of psychiatric medication at trial entry; similar associations were observed in both the efavirenz and control treatment groups. In Study 006, onset of new serious psychiatric symptoms occurred throughout the trial for both efavirenz-treated and control-treated subjects. One percent of efavirenz-treated subjects discontinued or interrupted treatment because of one or more of these selected psychiatric symptoms. There have also been occasional post-marketing reports of death by suicide, delusions, and psychosis-like behavior, although a causal relationship to the use of efavirenz cannot be determined from these reports. Patients with serious psychiatric adverse experiences should seek immediate medical evaluation to assess the possibility that the symptoms may be related to the use of efavirenz, and if so, to determine whether the risks of continued therapy outweigh the benefits [See Adverse Reactions (6)].

5.6   Nervous System Symptoms

Fifty-three percent (531/1008) of subjects receiving efavirenz in controlled trials reported central nervous system symptoms (any grade, regardless of causality) compared to 25% (156/635) of subjects receiving control regimens. These symptoms included dizziness (28.1% of the 1008 subjects), insomnia (16.3%), impaired concentration (8.3%), somnolence (7.0%), abnormal dreams (6.2%), and hallucinations (1.2%). Other reported symptoms were euphoria, confusion, agitation, amnesia, stupor, abnormal thinking, and depersonalization. The majority of these symptoms were mild-to-moderate (50.7%); symptoms were severe in 2.0% of subjects. Overall, 2.1% of subjects discontinued therapy as a result. These symptoms usually begin during the first or second day of therapy and generally resolve after the first 2–4 weeks of therapy. After 4 weeks of therapy, the prevalence of nervous system symptoms of at least moderate severity ranged from 5% to 9% in subjects treated with regimens containing efavirenz and from 3% to 5% in subjects treated with a control regimen. Patients should be informed that these common symptoms were likely to improve with continued therapy and were not predictive of subsequent onset of the less frequent psychiatric symptoms [See Warnings and Precautions (5.5)]. Dosing at bedtime may improve the tolerability of these nervous system symptoms [See Dosage and Administration (2)].

Analysis of long-term data from Study 006 (median follow-up 180 weeks, 102 weeks, and 76 weeks for subjects treated with efavirenz + zidovudine + lamivudine, efavirenz + indinavir, and indinavir + zidovudine + lamivudine, respectively) showed that, beyond 24 weeks of therapy, the incidences of new-onset nervous system symptoms among efavirenz-treated subjects were generally similar to those in the indinavir-containing control arm.

Patients receiving ATRIPLA (efavirenz/emtricitabine/tenofovir disoproxil fumarate) should be alerted to the potential for additive central nervous system effects when ATRIPLA is used concomitantly with alcohol or psychoactive drugs.

Patients who experience central nervous system symptoms such as dizziness, impaired concentration, and/or drowsiness should avoid potentially hazardous tasks such as driving or operating machinery.

5.7   New Onset or Worsening Renal Impairment

Emtricitabine and tenofovir are principally eliminated by the kidney; however, efavirenz is not. Since ATRIPLA is a combination product and the dose of the individual components cannot be altered, patients with estimated creatinine clearance below 50 mL/min should not receive ATRIPLA.

Renal impairment, including cases of acute renal failure and Fanconi syndrome (renal tubular injury with severe hypophosphatemia), has been reported with the use of tenofovir DF [See Adverse Reactions (6.3)].

It is recommended that estimated creatinine clearance be assessed in all patients prior to initiating therapy and as clinically appropriate during therapy with ATRIPLA. In patients at risk of renal dysfunction, including patients who have previously experienced renal events while receiving HEPSERA, it is recommended that estimated creatinine clearance, serum phosphorus, urine glucose, and urine protein be assessed prior to initiation of ATRIPLA, and periodically during ATRIPLA therapy.

ATRIPLA should be avoided with concurrent or recent use of a nephrotoxic agent (e.g., high-dose or multiple nonsteroidal anti-inflammatory drugs (NSAIDs)) [See Drug Interactions (7.2)]. Cases of acute renal failure after initiation of high dose or multiple NSAIDs have been reported in HIV-infected patients with risk factors for renal dysfunction who appeared stable on tenofovir DF. Some patients required hospitalization and renal replacement therapy. Alternatives to NSAIDs should be considered, if needed, in patients at risk for renal dysfunction.

Persistent or worsening bone pain, pain in extremities, fractures and/or muscular pain or weakness may be manifestations of proximal renal tubulopathy and should prompt an evaluation of renal function in at-risk patients.

5.8 Reproductive Risk Potential

Pregnancy Category D: Efavirenz may cause fetal harm when administered during the first trimester to a pregnant woman. Pregnancy should be avoided in women receiving ATRIPLA (efavirenz/emtricitabine/tenofovir disoproxil fumarate). Barrier contraception must always be used in combination with other methods of contraception (e.g., oral or other hormonal contraceptives). Because of the long half-life of efavirenz, use of adequate contraceptive measures for 12 weeks after discontinuation of ATRIPLA is recommended. Women of childbearing potential should undergo pregnancy testing before initiation of ATRIPLA. If this drug is used during the first trimester of pregnancy, or if the patient becomes pregnant while taking this drug, the patient should be apprised of the potential harm to the fetus.

There are no adequate and well-controlled trials of ATRIPLA in pregnant women. ATRIPLA should be used during pregnancy only if the potential benefit justifies the potential risk to the fetus, such as in pregnant women without other therapeutic options [See Use in Specific Populations (8.1)].

5.9 Rash

In controlled clinical trials, 26% (266/1008) of subjects treated with 600 mg efavirenz experienced new-onset skin rash compared with 17% (111/635) of subjects treated in control groups. Rash associated with blistering, moist desquamation, or ulceration occurred in 0.9% (9/1008) of subjects treated with efavirenz. The incidence of Grade 4 rash (e.g., erythema multiforme, Stevens-Johnson syndrome) in subjects treated with efavirenz in all trials and expanded access was 0.1%. Rashes are usually mild-to-moderate maculopapular skin eruptions that occur within the first 2 weeks of initiating therapy with efavirenz (median time to onset of rash in adults was 11 days) and, in most subjects continuing therapy with efavirenz, rash resolves within 1 month (median duration, 16 days). The discontinuation rate for rash in clinical trials was 1.7% (17/1008). ATRIPLA can be reinitiated in patients interrupting therapy because of rash. ATRIPLA should be discontinued in patients developing severe rash associated with blistering, desquamation, mucosal involvement, or fever. Appropriate antihistamines and/or corticosteroids may improve the tolerability and hasten the resolution of rash. For patients who have had a life-threatening cutaneous reaction (e.g., Stevens-Johnson syndrome), alternative therapy should be considered [See also Contraindications (4.1)].

Experience with efavirenz in subjects who discontinued other antiretroviral agents of the NNRTI class is limited. Nineteen subjects who discontinued nevirapine because of rash have been treated with efavirenz. Nine of these subjects developed mild-to-moderate rash while receiving therapy with efavirenz, and two of these subjects discontinued because of rash.

Rash was reported in 26 of 57 pediatric subjects (46%) treated with efavirenz [See Adverse Reactions (6.1)]. One pediatric subject experienced Grade 3 rash (confluent rash with fever), and two subjects had Grade 4 rash (erythema multiforme). The median time to onset of rash in pediatric subjects was 8 days. Prophylaxis with appropriate antihistamines before initiating therapy with ATRIPLA in pediatric patients should be considered.

5.10 Hepatotoxicity

Monitoring of liver enzymes before and during treatment is recommended for patients with underlying hepatic disease, including hepatitis B or C infection; patients with marked transaminase elevations; and patients treated with other medications associated with liver toxicity [See also Warnings and Precautions (5.2)]. A few of the postmarketing reports of hepatic failure occurred in patients with no pre-existing hepatic disease or other identifiable risk factors [See Adverse Reactions (6.3)]. Liver enzyme monitoring should also be considered for patients without pre-existing hepatic dysfunction or other risk factors. In patients with persistent elevations of serum transaminases to greater than five times the upper limit of the normal range, the benefit of continued therapy with ATRIPLA needs to be weighed against the unknown risks of significant liver toxicity [See Adverse Reactions (6.2)].

5.11 Bone Effects of Tenofovir DF

Bone Mineral Density:
In clinical trials in HIV-1 infected adults, tenofovir DF was associated with slightly greater decreases in bone mineral density (BMD) and increases in biochemical markers of bone metabolism, suggesting increased bone turnover relative to comparators. Serum parathyroid hormone levels and 1,25 Vitamin D levels were also higher in subjects receiving tenofovir DF.

Clinical trials evaluating tenofovir DF in pediatric and adolescent subjects were conducted. Under normal circumstances, BMD increases rapidly in pediatric patients. In HIV-1 infected subjects aged 2 years to less than 18 years, bone effects were similar to those observed in adult subjects and suggest increased bone turnover. Total body BMD gain was less in the tenofovir DF treated HIV-1 infected pediatric subjects as compared to the control groups. Similar trends were observed in chronic hepatitis B infected adolescent subjects aged 12 years to less than 18 years. In all pediatric trials, skeletal growth (height) appeared to be unaffected. For more information, consult the VIREAD prescribing information.

The effects of tenofovir DF-associated changes in BMD and biochemical markers on long-term bone health and future fracture risk are unknown. Assessment of BMD should be considered for adult and pediatric patients who have a history of pathologic bone fracture or other risk factors for osteoporosis or bone loss. Although the effect of supplementation with calcium and vitamin D was not studied, such supplementation may be beneficial for all patients. If bone abnormalities are suspected then appropriate consultation should be obtained.

Mineralization Defects:
Cases of osteomalacia associated with proximal renal tubulopathy, manifested as bone pain or pain in extremities and which may contribute to fractures, have been reported in association with the use of tenofovir DF [See Adverse Reactions (6.3)]. Arthralgias and muscle pain or weakness have also been reported in cases of proximal renal tubulopathy. Hypophosphatemia and osteomalacia secondary to proximal renal tubulopathy should be considered in patients at risk of renal dysfunction who present with persistent or worsening bone or muscle symptoms while receiving products containing tenofovir DF [See Warnings and Precautions (5.7)].

5.12 Convulsions

Convulsions have been observed in patients receiving efavirenz, generally in the presence of known medical history of seizures. Caution must be taken in any patient with a history of seizures.

Patients who are receiving concomitant anticonvulsant medications primarily metabolized by the liver, such as phenytoin and phenobarbital, may require periodic monitoring of plasma levels [See Drug Interactions (7.3)].

5.13 Immune Reconstitution Syndrome

Immune reconstitution syndrome has been reported in patients treated with combination antiretroviral therapy, including the components of ATRIPLA (efavirenz/emtricitabine/tenofovir disoproxil fumarate). During the initial phase of combination antiretroviral treatment, patients whose immune system responds may develop an inflammatory response to indolent or residual opportunistic infections [such as *Mycobacterium avium* infection, cytomegalovirus, *Pneumocystis jirovecii* pneumonia (PCP), or tuberculosis], which may necessitate further evaluation and treatment.

Autoimmune disorders (such as Graves' disease, polymyositis, and Guillain-Barré syndrome) have also been reported to occur in the setting of immune reconstitution, however, the time to onset is more variable, and can occur many months after initiation of treatment.

5.14 Fat Redistribution

Redistribution/accumulation of body fat including central obesity, dorsocervical fat enlargement (buffalo hump), peripheral wasting, facial wasting, breast enlargement, and "cushingoid appearance" have been observed in patients receiving antiretroviral therapy. The mechanism and long-term consequences of these events are currently unknown. A causal relationship has not been established.

6 ADVERSE REACTIONS

Efavirenz, Emtricitabine and Tenofovir Disoproxil Fumarate: The following adverse reactions are discussed in other sections of the labeling:

- Lactic Acidosis/Severe Hepatomegaly with Steatosis [See Boxed Warning, Warnings and Precautions (5.1)].
- Severe Acute Exacerbations of Hepatitis B [See Boxed Warning, Warnings and Precautions (5.2)].
- Psychiatric Symptoms [See Warnings and Precautions (5.5)].
- Nervous System Symptoms [See Warnings and Precautions (5.6)].
- New Onset or Worsening Renal Impairment [See Warnings and Precautions (5.7)].
- Rash [See Warnings and Precautions (5.9)].
- Hepatotoxicity [See Warnings and Precautions (5.10)].
- Bone Effects of Tenofovir DF [See Warnings and Precautions (5.11)].
- Immune Reconstitution Syndrome [See Warnings and Precautions (5.13)].
- Drug Interactions [See Contraindications (4.2), Warnings and Precautions (5.3) and Drug Interactions (7)].

For additional safety information about SUSTIVA (efavirenz), EMTRIVA (emtricitabine), or VIREAD (tenofovir DF) in combination with other antiretroviral agents, consult the prescribing information for these products.

6.1 Adverse Reactions from Clinical Trials Experience

Because clinical trials are conducted under widely varying conditions, adverse reaction rates observed in the clinical trials of a drug cannot be directly compared to rates in the clinical trials of another drug and may not reflect the rates observed in practice.

Clinical Trials in Adult Subjects
Study 934
Study 934 was an open-label active-controlled trial in which 511 antiretroviral-naive subjects received either emtricitabine + tenofovir DF administered in combination with efavirenz (N=257) or zidovudine/lamivudine administered in combination with efavirenz (N=254).

The most common adverse reactions (incidence greater than or equal to 10%, any severity) occurring in Study 934 include diarrhea, nausea, fatigue, headache, dizziness, depression, insomnia, abnormal dreams, and rash. Adverse reactions observed in Study 934 were generally consistent with those seen in previous trials of the individual components (Table 2).

Table 2: Selected Treatment-Emergent Adverse Reactions* (Grades 2–4) Reported in ≥5% in Either Treatment Group in Study 934 (0–144 Weeks)

	FTC + TDF + EFV[†]	AZT/3TC + EFV
	N=257	N=254
Gastrointestinal Disorder		
Diarrhea	9%	5%
Nausea	9%	7%
Vomiting	2%	5%
General Disorders and Administration Site Condition		
Fatigue	9%	8%
Infections and Infestations		
Sinusitis	8%	4%
Upper respiratory tract infections	8%	5%
Nasopharyngitis	5%	3%
Nervous System Disorders		
Headache	6%	5%
Dizziness	8%	7%
Psychiatric Disorders		
Anxiety	5%	4%
Depression	9%	7%
Insomnia	5%	7%
Skin and Subcutaneous Tissue Disorders		
Rash Event[‡]	7%	9%

* Frequencies of adverse reactions are based on all treatment-emergent adverse events, regardless of relationship to study drug.

† From Weeks 96 to 144 of the trial, subjects received emtricitabine/tenofovir DF administered in combination with efavirenz in place of emtricitabine + tenofovir DF with efavirenz.

‡ Rash event includes rash, exfoliative rash, rash generalized, rash macular, rash maculopapular, rash pruritic, and rash vesicular.

Study 073
In Study 073, subjects with stable, virologic suppression on antiretroviral therapy and no history of virologic failure were randomized to receive ATRIPLA (efavirenz/emtricitabine/tenofovir disoproxil fumarate) or to stay on their baseline regimen. The adverse reactions observed in Study 073 were generally consistent with those seen in Study 934 and those seen with the individual components of ATRIPLA when each was administered in combination with other antiretroviral agents.

Efavirenz, Emtricitabine, or Tenofovir Disoproxil Fumarate
In addition to the adverse reactions in Study 934 and Study 073, the following adverse reactions were observed in clinical trials of efavirenz, emtricitabine, or tenofovir DF in combination with other antiretroviral agents.

Efavirenz: The most significant adverse reactions observed in subjects treated with efavirenz are nervous system symptoms [See Warnings and Precautions (5.6)], psychiatric symptoms [See Warnings and Precautions (5.5)], and rash [See Warnings and Precautions (5.9)].

Selected adverse reactions of moderate-to-severe intensity observed in greater than or equal to 2% of efavirenz-treated subjects in two controlled clinical trials included pain, impaired concentration, abnormal dreams, somnolence, anorexia, dyspepsia, abdominal pain, nervousness, and pruritus.

Pancreatitis has also been reported, although a causal relationship with efavirenz has not been established. Asymptomatic increases in serum amylase levels were observed in a significantly higher number of subjects treated with efavirenz 600 mg than in control subjects.

Emtricitabine and Tenofovir Disoproxil Fumarate: Adverse reactions that occurred in at least 5% of treatment-experienced or treatment-naive subjects receiving emtricitabine or tenofovir DF with other antiretroviral agents in clinical trials include arthralgia, increased cough, dyspepsia, fever, myalgia, pain, abdominal pain, back pain, paresthesia, peripheral neuropathy (including peripheral neuritis and neuropathy), pneumonia, rhinitis and rash event (including rash, pruritus, maculopapular rash, urticaria, vesiculobullous rash, pustular rash, and allergic reaction).

Skin discoloration has been reported with higher frequency among emtricitabine-treated subjects; it was manifested by hyperpigmentation on the palms and/or soles and was generally mild and asymptomatic. The mechanism and clinical significance are unknown.

Clinical Trials in Pediatric Subjects

Efavirenz: In a pediatric clinical trial in 57 NRTI-experienced subjects aged 3 to 16 years, the type and frequency of adverse experiences was generally similar to that of adult subjects with the exception of a higher incidence of rash, which was reported in 46% (26/57) of pediatric subjects compared to 26% of adults, and a higher frequency of Grade 3 or 4 rash reported in 5% (3/57) of pediatric subjects compared to 0.9% of adults [See Warnings and Precautions (5.9)]. For additional information, please consult the SUSTIVA prescribing information.

Emtricitabine: In addition to the adverse reactions reported in adults, anemia and hyperpigmentation were observed in 7% and 32%, respectively, of pediatric subjects (3 months to less than 18 years of age) who received treatment with emtricitabine in the larger of two open-label, uncontrolled pediatric trials (N=116). For additional information, please consult the EMTRIVA prescribing information.

Tenofovir Disoproxil Fumarate: In a pediatric clinical trial conducted in subjects 12 to less than 18 years of age, the adverse reactions observed in pediatric subjects who received treatment with tenofovir DF were consistent with those observed in clinical trials of tenofovir DF in adults [See Warnings and Precautions (5.11)].

6.2 Laboratory Abnormalities

Efavirenz, Emtricitabine and Tenofovir Disoproxil Fumarate: Laboratory abnormalities observed in Study 934 were generally consistent with those seen in previous trials (Table 3).

Table 3: Significant Laboratory Abnormalities Reported in ≥1% of Subjects in Either Treatment Group in Study 934 (0–144 Weeks)

	FTC + TDF + EFV*	AZT/3TC + EFV
	N=257	N=254
Any ≥ Grade 3 Laboratory Abnormality	30%	26%
Fasting Cholesterol (>240 mg/dL)	22%	24%
Creatine Kinase (M: >990 U/L) (F: >845 U/L)	9%	7%
Serum Amylase (>175 U/L)	8%	4%
Alkaline Phosphatase (>550 U/L)	1%	0%
AST (M: >180 U/L) (F: >170 U/L)	3%	3%
ALT (M: >215 U/L) (F: >170 U/L)	2%	3%
Hemoglobin (<8.0 mg/dL)	0%	4%
Hyperglycemia (>250 mg/dL)	2%	1%
Hematuria (>75 RBC/HPF)	3%	2%
Glycosuria (≥3+)	<1%	1%
Neutrophils (<750/mm³)	3%	5%
Fasting Triglycerides (>750 mg/dL)	4%	2%

* From Weeks 96 to 144 of the trial, subjects received emtricitabine/tenofovir DF administered in combination with efavirenz in place of emtricitabine + tenofovir DF with efavirenz.

Laboratory abnormalities observed in Study 073 were generally consistent with those in Study 934.

In addition to the laboratory abnormalities described for Study 934 (Table 3), Grade 3/4 laboratory abnormalities of increased bilirubin (greater than 2.5 × upper limit of normal (ULN)), increased pancreatic amylase (greater than 2.0 × ULN), increased or decreased serum glucose (less than 40 or greater than 250 mg/dL), and increased serum lipase (greater than 2.0 × ULN) occurred in up to 3% of subjects treated with emtricitabine or tenofovir DF with other antiretroviral agents in clinical trials.

Hepatic Events: In Study 934, 19 subjects treated with efavirenz, emtricitabine, and tenofovir DF and 20 subjects treated with efavirenz and fixed-dose zidovudine/lamivudine were hepatitis B surface antigen or hepatitis C antibody positive. Among these coinfected subjects, one subject (1/19) in the efavirenz, emtricitabine and tenofovir DF arm had elevations in transaminases to greater than five times ULN through 144 weeks. In the fixed-dose zidovudine/lamivudine arm, two subjects (2/20) had elevations in transaminases to greater than five times ULN through 144 weeks. No HBV and/or HCV coinfected subject discontinued from the trial due to hepatobiliary disorders [See Warnings and Precautions (5.10)].

6.3 Postmarketing Experience

The following adverse reactions have been identified during postapproval use of efavirenz, emtricitabine, or tenofovir DF. Because postmarketing reactions are reported voluntarily from a population of uncertain size, it is not always possible to reliably estimate their frequency or establish a causal relationship to drug exposure.

Efavirenz:

Cardiac Disorders
Palpitations
Ear and Labyrinth Disorders
Tinnitus, vertigo
Endocrine Disorders
Gynecomastia
Eye Disorders
Abnormal vision
Gastrointestinal Disorders
Constipation, malabsorption
General Disorders and Administration Site Conditions
Asthenia
Hepatobiliary Disorders
Hepatic enzyme increase, hepatic failure, hepatitis. A few of the postmarketing reports of hepatic failure, including cases in patients with no pre-existing hepatic disease or other identifiable risk factors, were characterized by a fulminant course, progressing in some cases to transplantation or death.
Immune System Disorders
Allergic reactions
Metabolism and Nutrition Disorders
Redistribution/accumulation of body fat [See Warnings and Precautions (5.14)], hypercholesterolemia, hypertriglyceridemia
Musculoskeletal and Connective Tissue Disorders
Arthralgia, myalgia, myopathy
Nervous System Disorders
Abnormal coordination, ataxia, cerebellar coordination and balance disturbances, convulsions, hypoesthesia, paresthesia, neuropathy, tremor
Psychiatric Disorders
Aggressive reactions, agitation, delusions, emotional lability, mania, neurosis, paranoia, psychosis, suicide
Respiratory, Thoracic and Mediastinal Disorders
Dyspnea
Skin and Subcutaneous Tissue Disorders
Flushing, erythema multiforme, photoallergic dermatitis, Stevens-Johnson syndrome
Emtricitabine: No postmarketing adverse reactions have been identified for inclusion in this section.
Tenofovir Disoproxil Fumarate:
Immune System Disorders
Allergic reaction, including angioedema
Metabolism and Nutrition Disorders
Lactic acidosis, hypokalemia, hypophosphatemia
Respiratory, Thoracic, and Mediastinal Disorders
Dyspnea
Gastrointestinal Disorders
Pancreatitis, increased amylase, abdominal pain

Hepatobiliary Disorders
Hepatic steatosis, hepatitis, increased liver enzymes (most commonly AST, ALT, gamma GT)
Skin and Subcutaneous Tissue Disorders
Rash
Musculoskeletal and Connective Tissue Disorders
Rhabdomyolysis, osteomalacia (manifested as bone pain and which may contribute to fractures), muscular weakness, myopathy
Renal and Urinary Disorders
Acute renal failure, renal failure, acute tubular necrosis, Fanconi syndrome, proximal renal tubulopathy, interstitial nephritis (including acute cases), nephrogenic diabetes insipidus, renal insufficiency, increased creatinine, proteinuria, polyuria
General Disorders and Administration Site Conditions
Asthenia
The following adverse reactions, listed under the body system headings above, may occur as a consequence of proximal renal tubulopathy: rhabdomyolysis, osteomalacia, hypokalemia, muscular weakness, myopathy, hypophosphatemia.

7 DRUG INTERACTIONS

This section describes clinically relevant drug interactions with ATRIPLA (efavirenz/emtricitabine/tenofovir disoproxil fumarate). Drug interaction trials are described elsewhere in the labeling [See Clinical Pharmacology (12.3)].

7.1 Efavirenz

Efavirenz has been shown *in vivo* to induce CYP3A and CYP2B6. Other compounds that are substrates of CYP3A or CYP2B6 may have decreased plasma concentrations when coadministered with efavirenz. *In vitro* studies have demonstrated that efavirenz inhibits CYP2C9, 2C19, and 3A4 isozymes in the range of observed efavirenz plasma concentrations. Coadministration of efavirenz with drugs primarily metabolized by these isozymes may result in altered plasma concentrations of the coadministered drug. Therefore, appropriate dose adjustments may be necessary for these drugs.

Drugs that induce CYP3A activity (e.g., phenobarbital, rifampin, rifabutin) would be expected to increase the clearance of efavirenz, resulting in lowered plasma concentrations [See Dosage and Administration (2)].

7.2 Emtricitabine and Tenofovir Disoproxil Fumarate

Since emtricitabine and tenofovir are primarily eliminated by the kidneys, coadministration of ATRIPLA with drugs that reduce renal function or compete for active tubular secretion may increase serum concentrations of emtricitabine, tenofovir, and/or other renally eliminated drugs. Some examples include, but are not limited to, acyclovir, adefovir dipivoxil, cidofovir, ganciclovir, valacyclovir, valganciclovir, aminoglycosides (e.g., gentamicin), and high-dose or multiple NSAIDs [See Warnings and Precautions (5.7)].

Coadministration of tenofovir DF and didanosine should be undertaken with caution and patients receiving this combination should be monitored closely for didanosine-associated adverse reactions. Didanosine should be discontinued in patients who develop didanosine-associated adverse reactions [for didanosine dosing adjustment recommendations, see Table 4]. Suppression of CD4+ cell counts has been observed in patients receiving tenofovir DF with didanosine 400 mg daily.

Darunavir with ritonavir and lopinavir/ritonavir have been shown to increase tenofovir concentrations. Tenofovir DF is a substrate of P-glycoprotein (Pgp) and breast cancer resistance protein (BCRP) transporters. When tenofovir DF is co-administered with an inhibitor of these transporters, an increase in absorption may be observed. Patients receiving darunavir with ritonavir and ATRIPLA, or lopinavir/ritonavir with ATRIPLA, should be monitored for tenofovir-associated adverse reactions. ATRIPLA should be discontinued in patients who develop tenofovir-associated adverse reactions [See Table 4].

Coadministration of atazanavir with ATRIPLA is not recommended since coadministration of atazanavir with either efavirenz or tenofovir DF has been shown to decrease plasma concentrations of atazanavir. Also, atazanavir has been shown to increase tenofovir concentrations. There are insufficient data to support dosing recommendations for atazanavir or atazanavir/ritonavir in combination with ATRIPLA [See Table 4].

7.3 Efavirenz, Emtricitabine and Tenofovir Disoproxil Fumarate

Other important drug interaction information for ATRIPLA is summarized in Table 1 and Table 4. The drug interactions described are based on trials conducted with efavirenz, emtricitabine or tenofovir DF as individual agents or are potential drug interactions; no drug interaction trials have been conducted using ATRIPLA [for pharmacokinetics data see Clinical Pharmacology (12.3), Tables 5–8]. The tables include potentially significant interactions, but are not all inclusive.

[See table 4 on pages 649 and 650]

Table 4: Established and Other Potentially Significant* Drug Interactions: Alteration in Dose or Regimen May Be Recommended Based on Drug Interaction Trials or Predicted Interaction

Concomitant Drug Class: Drug Name	Effect	Clinical Comment
HIV antiviral agents		
Protease inhibitor: atazanavir	↓atazanavir ↑ tenofovir	Coadministration of atazanavir with ATRIPLA is not recommended. Coadministration of atazanavir with either efavirenz or tenofovir DF decreases plasma concentrations of atazanavir. The combined effect of efavirenz plus tenofovir DF on atazanavir plasma concentrations is not known. Also, atazanavir has been shown to increase tenofovir concentrations. There are insufficient data to support dosing recommendations for atazanavir or atazanavir/ritonavir in combination with ATRIPLA.
Protease inhibitor: fosamprenavir calcium	↓ amprenavir	Fosamprenavir (unboosted): Appropriate doses of fosamprenavir and ATRIPLA with respect to safety and efficacy have not been established. Fosamprenavir/ritonavir: An additional 100 mg/day (300 mg total) of ritonavir is recommended when ATRIPLA is administered with fosamprenavir/ritonavir once daily. No change in the ritonavir dose is required when ATRIPLA is administered with fosamprenavir plus ritonavir twice daily.
Protease inhibitor: indinavir	↓ indinavir	The optimal dose of indinavir, when given in combination with efavirenz, is not known. Increasing the indinavir dose to 1000 mg every 8 hours does not compensate for the increased indinavir metabolism due to efavirenz.
Protease inhibitor: lopinavir/ritonavir	↓ lopinavir ↑ tenofovir	Do not use once daily administration of lopinavir/ritonavir. Dose adjustment of lopinavir/ritonavir is recommended when coadministered with efavirenz. Refer to the full prescribing information for lopinavir/ritonavir for guidance on coadministration with efavirenz- or tenofovir-containing regimens, such as ATRIPLA. **Patients should be monitored for tenofovir-associated adverse reactions.**
Protease inhibitor: ritonavir	↑ ritonavir ↑ efavirenz	When ritonavir 500 mg every 12 hours was coadministered with efavirenz 600 mg once daily, the combination was associated with a higher frequency of adverse clinical experiences (e.g., dizziness, nausea, paresthesia) and laboratory abnormalities (elevated liver enzymes). Monitoring of liver enzymes is recommended when ATRIPLA is used in combination with ritonavir.
Protease inhibitor: saquinavir	↓ saquinavir	Appropriate doses of the combination of efavirenz and saquinavir/ritonavir with respect to safety and efficacy have not been established.
CCR5 co-receptor antagonist: maraviroc	↓ maraviroc	Efavirenz decreases plasma concentrations of maraviroc. Refer to the full prescribing information for maraviroc for guidance on coadministration with ATRIPLA.
NRTI: didanosine	↑ didanosine	Coadministration of ATRIPLA and didanosine should be undertaken with caution and patients receiving this combination should be monitored closely for didanosine-associated adverse reactions including pancreatitis, lactic acidosis, and neuropathy. A dose reduction of didanosine is recommended when coadministered with tenofovir DF. For additional information on coadministration with tenofovir DF-containing products, please refer to the didanosine prescribing information.
NNRTI: Other NNRTIs	↑ or ↓ efavirenz and/or NNRTI	Combining two NNRTIs has not been shown to be beneficial. ATRIPLA contains efavirenz and should not be coadministered with other NNRTIs.
Integrase strand transfer inhibitor: raltegravir	↓ raltegravir	Efavirenz reduces plasma concentrations of raltegravir. The clinical significance of this interaction has not been directly assessed.
Hepatitis C antiviral agents		
Protease inhibitor: boceprevir	↓ boceprevir	Plasma trough concentrations of boceprevir were decreased when boceprevir was coadministered with efavirenz, which may result in loss of therapeutic effect. The combination should be avoided.
Protease inhibitor: telaprevir	↓ telaprevir ↓ efavirenz	Concomitant administration of telaprevir and efavirenz resulted in reduced steady-state exposures to telaprevir and efavirenz.
Other agents		
Anticoagulant: warfarin	↑ or ↓ warfarin	Plasma concentrations and effects potentially increased or decreased by efavirenz.

(Table continued on next page)

7.4 Efavirenz Assay Interference

Cannabinoid Test Interaction: Efavirenz does not bind to cannabinoid receptors. False-positive urine cannabinoid test results have been observed in non-HIV-infected volunteers receiving efavirenz when the Microgenics Cedia DAU Multi-Level THC assay was used for screening. Negative results were obtained when more specific confirmatory testing was performed with gas chromatography/mass spectrometry. For more information, please consult the SUSTIVA prescribing information.

8 USE IN SPECIFIC POPULATIONS

8.1 Pregnancy

Pregnancy Category D *[See Warnings and Precautions (5.8)].*

Antiretroviral Pregnancy Registry: To monitor fetal outcomes of pregnant women, an Antiretroviral Pregnancy Registry has been established. Physicians are encouraged to register patients who become pregnant by calling (800) 258-4263.

Efavirenz: As of July 2010, the Antiretroviral Pregnancy Registry has received prospective reports of 792 pregnancies exposed to efavirenz-containing regimens, nearly all of which were first-trimester exposures (718 pregnancies). Birth defects occurred in 17 of 604 live births (first-trimester exposure) and 2 of 69 live births (second/third-trimester exposure). One of these prospectively reported defects with first-trimester exposure was a neural tube defect. A single case of anophthalmia with first-trimester exposure to efavirenz has also been prospectively reported; however, this case included severe oblique facial clefts and amniotic banding, a known association with anophthalmia. There have been six retrospective reports of findings consistent with neural tube defects, including meningomyelocele. All mothers were exposed to efavirenz-containing regimens in the first trimester. Although a causal relationship of these events to the use of efavirenz has not been established, similar defects have been observed in preclinical studies of efavirenz.

Animal Data

Effects of efavirenz on embryo-fetal development have been studied in three nonclinical species (cynomolgus monkeys, rats, and rabbits). In monkeys, efavirenz 60 mg/kg/day was administered to pregnant females throughout pregnancy (gestation Days 20 through 150). The maternal systemic drug exposures (AUC) were 1.3 times the exposure in humans at the recommended clinical dose (600 mg/day), with fetal umbilical venous drug concentrations approximately 0.7 times the maternal values. Three fetuses of 20 fetuses/infants had one or more malformations; there were no malformed fetuses or infants from placebo-treated mothers. The malformations that occurred in these three monkey fetuses included anencephaly and unilateral anophthalmia in one fetus, microphthalmia in a second, and cleft palate in the third. There was no NOAEL (no observable adverse effect level) established for this study because only one dosage was evaluated. In rats, efavirenz was administered either during organogenesis (gestation Days 7 to 18) or from gestation Day 7 through lactation Day 21 at 50, 100, or 200 mg/kg/day. Administration of 200 mg/kg/day in rats was associated with an increase in the incidence of early resorptions, and doses 100 mg/kg/day and greater were associated with early neonatal mortality. The AUC at the NOAEL (50 mg/kg/day) in this rat study was 0.1 times that in humans at the recommended rat clinical dose. Drug concentrations in the milk on lactation Day 10 were approximately 8 times higher than those in maternal plasma. In pregnant rabbits, efavirenz was neither embryo lethal nor teratogenic when administered at doses of 25, 50, and 75 mg/kg/day over the period of organogenesis (gestation Days 6 through 18). The AUC at the NOAEL (75 mg/kg/day) in rabbits was 0.4 times that in humans at the recommended clinical dose.

8.3 Nursing Mothers

The Centers for Disease Control and Prevention recommend that HIV-1 infected mothers not breastfeed their infants to avoid risking postnatal transmission of HIV-1. Studies in rats have demonstrated that efavirenz is secreted in milk. Studies in humans have shown that both tenofovir and emtricitabine are excreted in human milk. Because the risks of low level exposure to emtricitabine and tenofovir to infants are unknown, and because of the potential for HIV-1 transmission, **mothers should be instructed not to breastfeed if they are receiving ATRIPLA (efavirenz/emtricitabine/ tenofovir disoproxil fumarate).**

Emtricitabine

Samples of breast milk obtained from five HIV-1 infected mothers show that emtricitabine is secreted in human milk. Breastfeeding infants whose mothers are being treated with emtricitabine may be at risk for developing viral resistance to emtricitabine. Other emtricitabine-associated risks in infants breastfed by mothers being treated with emtricitabine are unknown.

Tenofovir Disoproxil Fumarate

Samples of breast milk obtained from five HIV-1 infected mothers show that tenofovir is secreted in human milk. Tenofovir-associated risks, including the risk of viral resistance to tenofovir, in infants breastfed by mothers being treated with tenofovir disoproxil fumarate are unknown.

8.4 Pediatric Use

ATRIPLA should only be administered to pediatric patients 12 years of age and older with a body weight greater than or equal to 40 kg (greater than or equal to 88 lbs). Because

Table 4 *(cont.)*: Established and Other Potentially Significant* Drug Interactions: Alteration in Dose or Regimen May Be Recommended Based on Drug Interaction Trials or Predicted Interaction

Concomitant Drug Class: Drug Name	Effect	Clinical Comment
Other agents (cont.)		
Anticonvulsants: carbamazepine phenytoin phenobarbital	↓ carbamazepine ↓ efavirenz ↓ anticonvulsant ↓ efavirenz	There are insufficient data to make a dose recommendation for ATRIPLA. Alternative anticonvulsant treatment should be used. Potential for reduction in anticonvulsant and/or efavirenz plasma levels; periodic monitoring of anticonvulsant plasma levels should be conducted.
Antidepressants: bupropion	↓ buproprion	The effect of efavirenz on bupropion exposure is thought to be due to the induction of bupropion metabolism. Increases in bupropion dosage should be guided by clinical response, but the maximum recommended dose of bupropion should not be exceeded.
sertraline	↓ sertraline	Increases in sertraline dose should be guided by clinical response.
Antifungals: itraconazole ketoconazole posaconazole	↓ itraconazole ↓ hydroxy-itraconazole ↓ ketoconazole ↓ posaconazole	Since no dose recommendation for itraconazole can be made, alternative antifungal treatment should be considered. Drug interaction trials with ATRIPLA and ketoconazole have not been conducted. Efavirenz has the potential to decrease plasma concentrations of ketoconazole. Avoid concomitant use unless the benefit outweighs the risks.
Anti-infective: clarithromycin	↓ clarithromycin ↑ 14-OH metabolite	Clinical significance unknown. In uninfected volunteers, 46% developed rash while receiving efavirenz and clarithromycin. No dose adjustment of ATRIPLA is recommended when given with clarithromycin. Alternatives to clarithromycin, such as azithromycin, should be considered. Other macrolide antibiotics, such as erythromycin, have not been studied in combination with ATRIPLA.
Antimycobacterial: rifabutin	↓ rifabutin	Increase daily dose of rifabutin by 50%. Consider doubling the rifabutin dose in regimens where rifabutin is given 2 or 3 times a week.
rifampin	↓ efavirenz	If ATRIPLA is coadministered with rifampin to patients weighing 50 kg or more, an additional 200 mg/day of efavirenz is recommended.
Calcium channel blockers: diltiazem Others (e.g., felodipine, nicardipine, nifedipine, verapamil)	↓ diltiazem ↓ desacetyl diltiazem ↓ N-monodes-methyl diltiazem ↓ calcium channel blocker	Diltiazem dose adjustments should be guided by clinical response (refer to the full prescribing information for diltiazem). No dose adjustment of ATRIPLA is necessary when administered with diltiazem. No data are available on the potential interactions of efavirenz with other calcium channel blockers that are substrates of CYP3A. The potential exists for reduction in plasma concentrations of the calcium channel blocker. Dose adjustments should be guided by clinical response (refer to the full prescribing information for the calcium channel blocker).
HMG-CoA reductase inhibitors: atorvastatin pravastatin simvastatin	↓ atorvastatin ↓ pravastatin ↓ simvastatin	Plasma concentrations of atorvastatin, pravastatin, and simvastatin decreased with efavirenz. Consult the full prescribing information for the HMG-CoA reductase inhibitor for guidance on individualizing the dose.
Hormonal contraceptives: Oral: ethinyl estradiol/norgestimate	↓ active metabolites of norgestimate	A reliable method of barrier contraception must be used in addition to hormonal contraceptives. Efavirenz had no effect on ethinyl estradiol concentrations, but progestin levels (norelgestromin and levonorgestrel) were markedly decreased. No effect of ethinyl estradiol/norgestimate on efavirenz plasma concentrations was observed.
Implant: etonogestrel	↓ etonogestrel	A reliable method of barrier contraception must be used in addition to hormonal contraceptives. The interaction between etonogestrel and efavirenz has not been studied. Decreased exposure of etonogestrel may be expected. There have been postmarketing reports of contraceptive failure with etonogestrel in efavirenz-exposed patients.
Immunosuppressants: cyclosporine, tacrolimus, sirolimus, and others metabolized by CYP3A	↓ immuno-suppressant	Decreased exposure of the immunosuppressant may be expected due to CYP3A induction by efavirenz. These immunosuppressants are not anticipated to affect exposure of efavirenz. Dose adjustments of the immunosuppressant may be required. Close monitoring of immunosuppressant concentrations for at least 2 weeks (until stable concentrations are reached) is recommended when starting or stopping treatment with ATRIPLA.
Narcotic analgesic: methadone	↓ methadone	Coadministration of efavirenz in HIV-1 infected individuals with a history of injection drug use resulted in decreased plasma levels of methadone and signs of opiate withdrawal. Methadone dose was increased by a mean of 22% to alleviate withdrawal symptoms. Patients should be monitored for signs of withdrawal and their methadone dose increased as required to alleviate withdrawal symptoms.

* This table is not all inclusive.

ATRIPLA (efavirenz/emtricitabine/tenofovir disoproxil fumarate) is a fixed-dose combination tablet, the dose adjustments recommended for pediatric patients younger than 12 years of age for each individual component cannot be made with ATRIPLA *[See Warnings and Precautions (5.9, 5.11), Adverse Reactions (6.1) and Clinical Pharmacology (12.3)]*.

8.5   Geriatric Use

Clinical trials of efavirenz, emtricitabine, or tenofovir DF did not include sufficient numbers of subjects aged 65 and over to determine whether they respond differently from younger subjects. In general, dose selection for elderly patients should be cautious, keeping in mind the greater frequency of decreased hepatic, renal, or cardiac function, and of concomitant disease or other drug therapy.

8.6   Hepatic Impairment

ATRIPLA is not recommended for patients with moderate or severe hepatic impairment because there are insufficient data to determine an appropriate dose. Patients with mild hepatic impairment may be treated with ATRIPLA at the approved dose. Because of the extensive cytochrome P450-mediated metabolism of efavirenz and limited clinical experience in patients with hepatic impairment, caution should be exercised in administering ATRIPLA to these patients *[See Warnings and Precautions (5.10) and Clinical Pharmacology (12.3)]*.

8.7   Renal Impairment

Because ATRIPLA is a fixed-dose combination, it should not be prescribed for patients requiring dosage adjustment such as those with moderate or severe renal impairment (estimated creatinine clearance below 50 mL/min) *[See Warnings and Precautions (5.7)]*.

10   OVERDOSAGE

If overdose occurs, the patient should be monitored for evidence of toxicity, including monitoring of vital signs and observation of the patient's clinical status; standard supportive treatment should then be applied as necessary. Administration of activated charcoal may be used to aid removal of unabsorbed efavirenz. Hemodialysis can remove both emtricitabine and tenofovir DF (refer to detailed information below), but is unlikely to significantly remove efavirenz from the blood.

Efavirenz: Some patients accidentally taking 600 mg twice daily have reported increased nervous system symptoms. One patient experienced involuntary muscle contractions.

Emtricitabine: Limited clinical experience is available at doses higher than the therapeutic dose of emtricitabine. In one clinical pharmacology trial single doses of emtricitabine 1200 mg were administered to 11 subjects. No severe adverse reactions were reported.

Hemodialysis treatment removes approximately 30% of the emtricitabine dose over a 3-hour dialysis period starting within 1.5 hours of emtricitabine dosing (blood flow rate of 400 mL/min and a dialysate flow rate of 600 mL/min). It is not known whether emtricitabine can be removed by peritoneal dialysis.

Tenofovir Disoproxil Fumarate: Limited clinical experience at doses higher than the therapeutic dose of tenofovir DF 300 mg is available. In one trial, 600 mg tenofovir DF was administered to 8 subjects orally for 28 days, and no severe adverse reactions were reported. The effects of higher doses are not known.

Tenofovir is efficiently removed by hemodialysis with an extraction coefficient of approximately 54%. Following a single 300 mg dose of tenofovir DF, a 4-hour hemodialysis session removed approximately 10% of the administered tenofovir dose.

11   DESCRIPTION

ATRIPLA is a fixed-dose combination tablet containing efavirenz, emtricitabine, and tenofovir disoproxil fumarate (tenofovir DF). SUSTIVA is the brand name for efavirenz, a non-nucleoside reverse transcriptase inhibitor. EMTRIVA is the brand name for emtricitabine, a synthetic nucleoside analog of cytidine. VIREAD is the brand name for tenofovir DF, which is converted *in vivo* to tenofovir, an acyclic nucleoside phosphonate (nucleotide) analog of adenosine 5'-monophosphate. VIREAD and EMTRIVA are the components of TRUVADA.

ATRIPLA tablets are for oral administration. Each tablet contains 600 mg of efavirenz, 200 mg of emtricitabine, and 300 mg of tenofovir DF (which is equivalent to 245 mg of tenofovir disoproxil) as active ingredients. The tablets include the following inactive ingredients: croscarmellose sodium, hydroxypropyl cellulose, magnesium stearate, microcrystalline cellulose, and sodium lauryl sulfate. The tablets are film-coated with a coating material containing black iron oxide, polyethylene glycol, polyvinyl alcohol, red iron oxide, talc, and titanium dioxide.

Efavirenz: Efavirenz is chemically described as (S)-6-chloro-4-(cyclopropylethynyl)-1,4-dihydro-4-(trifluoromethyl)-2H-3,1-benzoxazin-2-one. Its molecular formula is $C_{14}H_9ClF_3NO_2$ and its structural formula is:

Efavirenz is a white to slightly pink crystalline powder with a molecular mass of 315.68. It is practically insoluble in water (less than 10 μg/mL).

Emtricitabine: The chemical name of emtricitabine is 5-fluoro-1-(2R,5S)-[2-(hydroxymethyl)-1,3-oxathiolan-5-yl]cytosine. Emtricitabine is the (-) enantiomer of a thio analog of cytidine, which differs from other cytidine analogs in that it has a fluorine in the 5-position.

It has a molecular formula of $C_8H_{10}FN_3O_3S$ and a molecular weight of 247.24. It has the following structural formula:

Emtricitabine is a white to off-white crystalline powder with a solubility of approximately 112 mg/mL in water at 25 °C.

Tenofovir Disoproxil Fumarate: Tenofovir DF is a fumaric acid salt of the *bis*-isopropoxycarbonyloxymethyl ester derivative of tenofovir. The chemical name of tenofovir disoproxil fumarate is 9-[(R)-2-[[bis[[(isopropoxycarbonyl)oxy]-methoxy]phosphinyl]methoxy]propyl]adenine fumarate (1:1). It has a molecular formula of $C_{19}H_{30}N_5O_{10}P \cdot C_4H_4O_4$ and a molecular weight of 635.52. It has the following structural formula:

Tenofovir DF is a white to off-white crystalline powder with a solubility of 13.4 mg/mL in water at 25 °C.

12   CLINICAL PHARMACOLOGY
For additional information on Mechanism of Action, Antiviral Activity, Resistance and Cross Resistance, please consult the SUSTIVA, EMTRIVA and VIREAD prescribing information.

12.1   Mechanism of Action
ATRIPLA (efavirenz/emtricitabine/tenofovir disoproxil fumarate) is a fixed-dose combination of antiviral drugs efavirenz, emtricitabine and tenofovir disoproxil fumarate *[See Clinical Pharmacology (12.4)].*

12.3   Pharmacokinetics
ATRIPLA: One ATRIPLA tablet is bioequivalent to one SUSTIVA tablet (600 mg) plus one EMTRIVA capsule (200 mg) plus one VIREAD tablet (300 mg) following single-dose administration to fasting healthy subjects (N=45).

Efavirenz: In HIV-1 infected subjects time-to-peak plasma concentrations were approximately 3–5 hours and steady-state plasma concentrations were reached in 6–10 days. In 35 HIV-1 infected subjects receiving efavirenz 600 mg once daily, steady-state C_{max} was 12.9 ± 3.7 μM (mean ± SD), C_{min} was 5.6 ± 3.2 μM, and AUC was 184 ± 73 μM•hr. Efavirenz is highly bound (approximately 99.5–99.75%) to human plasma proteins, predominantly albumin. Following administration of ^{14}C-labeled efavirenz, 14–34% of the dose was recovered in the urine (mostly as metabolites) and 16–61% was recovered in feces (mostly as parent drug). *In vitro* studies suggest CYP3A and CYP2B6 are the major isozymes responsible for efavirenz metabolism. Efavirenz has been shown to induce CYP enzymes, resulting in induction of its own metabolism. Efavirenz has a terminal half-life of 52–76 hours after single doses and 40–55 hours after multiple doses.

Emtricitabine: Following oral administration, emtricitabine is rapidly absorbed, with peak plasma concentrations occurring at 1–2 hours post-dose. Following multiple dose oral administration of emtricitabine to 20 HIV-1 infected subjects, the steady-state plasma emtricitabine C_{max} was 1.8 ± 0.7 μg/mL (mean ± SD) and the AUC over a 24-hour dosing interval was 10.0 ± 3.1 μg•hr/mL. The mean steady-state plasma trough concentration at 24 hours post-dose was 0.09 μg/mL. The mean absolute bioavailability of emtricitabine was 93%. Less than 4% of emtricitabine binds to human plasma proteins *in vitro* and the binding is independent of concentration over the range of 0.02–200 μg/mL. Following administration of radiolabelled emtricitabine, approximately 86% is recovered in the urine and 13% is recovered as metabolites. The metabolites of emtricitabine include 3'-sulfoxide diastereomers and their glucuronic acid conjugate. Emtricitabine is eliminated by a combination of glomerular filtration and active tubular secretion with a renal clearance in adults with normal renal function of 213 ± 89 mL/min (mean ± SD). Following a single oral dose, the plasma emtricitabine half-life is approximately 10 hours.

Tenofovir Disoproxil Fumarate: Following oral administration of a single 300 mg dose of tenofovir DF to HIV-1 infected subjects in the fasted state, maximum serum concentrations (C_{max}) were achieved in 1.0 ± 0.4 hrs (mean ± SD) and C_{max} and AUC values were 296 ± 90 ng/mL and 2287 ± 685 ng•hr/mL, respectively. The oral bioavailability of tenofovir from tenofovir DF in fasted subjects is approximately 25%. Less than 0.7% of tenofovir binds to human plasma proteins *in vitro* and the binding is independent of concentration over the range of 0.01–25 μg/mL. Approximately 70–80% of the intravenous dose of tenofovir is recovered as unchanged drug in the urine. Tenofovir is eliminated by a combination of glomerular filtration and active tubular secretion with a renal clearance in adults with normal renal function of 243 ± 33 mL/min (mean ± SD). Following a single oral dose, the terminal elimination half-life of tenofovir is approximately 17 hours.

Effects of Food on Oral Absorption
ATRIPLA (efavirenz/emtricitabine/tenofovir disoproxil fumarate) has not been evaluated in the presence of food. Administration of efavirenz tablets with a high fat meal increased the mean AUC and C_{max} of efavirenz by 28% and 79%, respectively, compared to administration in the fasted state. Compared to fasted administration, dosing of tenofovir DF and emtricitabine in combination with either a high fat meal or a light meal increased the mean AUC and C_{max} of tenofovir by 35% and 15%, respectively, without affecting emtricitabine exposures *[See Dosage and Administration (2) and Patient Counseling Information (17.7)].*

Special Populations
Race
Efavirenz: The pharmacokinetics of efavirenz in HIV-1 infected subjects appear to be similar among the racial groups studied.
Emtricitabine: No pharmacokinetic differences due to race have been identified following the administration of emtricitabine.
Tenofovir Disoproxil Fumarate: There were insufficient numbers from racial and ethnic groups other than Caucasian to adequately determine potential pharmacokinetic differences among these populations following the administration of tenofovir DF.

Gender
Efavirenz, Emtricitabine, and Tenofovir Disoproxil Fumarate: Efavirenz, emtricitabine, and tenofovir pharmacokinetics are similar in male and female subjects.

Pediatric Patients
ATRIPLA should only be administered to pediatric patients 12 years of age and weighing greater than or equal to 40 kg (greater than or equal to 88 lb).
Efavirenz: In an open-label trial in NRTI-experienced pediatric subjects (mean age 8 years, range 3–16), the pharmacokinetics of efavirenz in pediatric subjects were similar to the pharmacokinetics in adults who received a 600 mg daily dose of efavirenz. In 48 pediatric subjects, receiving the equivalent of a 600 mg dose of efavirenz, mean (± SD) steady-state C_{max} was 14.2 ± 5.8 μM, steady-state C_{min} was 5.6 ± 4.1 μM, and AUC was 218 ± 104 μM•hr.
Emtricitabine: The pharmacokinetics of emtricitabine at steady state were determined in 27 HIV-1-infected pediatric subjects 13 to 17 years of age receiving a daily dose of 6 mg/kg up to a maximum dose of 240 mg oral solution or a 200 mg capsule; 26 of 27 subjects in this age group received the 200 mg EMTRIVA capsule. Mean (± SD) C_{max} and AUC were 2.7 ± 0.9 μg/mL and 12.6 ± 5.4 μg•hr/mL, respectively. Exposures achieved in pediatric subjects 12 to less than 18 years of age were similar to those achieved in adults receiving a once daily dose of 200 mg.
Tenofovir Disoproxil Fumarate: Steady-state pharmacokinetics of tenofovir were evaluated in 8 HIV-1 infected pediatric subjects (12 to less than 18 years). Mean (± SD) C_{max} and AUC_{tau} are 0.38 ± 0.13 μg/mL and 3.39 ± 1.22 μg•hr/mL, respectively. Tenofovir exposure achieved in these pediatric subjects receiving oral daily doses of VIREAD 300 mg was similar to exposures achieved in adults receiving once-daily doses of VIREAD 300 mg.

Geriatric Patients
Pharmacokinetics of efavirenz, emtricitabine and tenofovir have not been fully evaluated in the elderly (65 years of age and older) *[See Use in Specific Populations (8.5)].*

Patients with Impaired Renal Function
Efavirenz: The pharmacokinetics of efavirenz have not been studied in subjects with renal insufficiency; however, less than 1% of efavirenz is excreted unchanged in the urine, so the impact of renal impairment on efavirenz elimination should be minimal.
Emtricitabine and Tenofovir Disoproxil Fumarate: The pharmacokinetics of emtricitabine and tenofovir DF are altered in subjects with renal impairment. In subjects with creatinine clearance below 50 mL/min, C_{max} and $AUC_{0-∞}$ of emtricitabine and tenofovir were increased *[See Warnings and Precautions (5.7)].*

Patients with Hepatic Impairment
Efavirenz: A multiple-dose trial showed no significant effect on efavirenz pharmacokinetics in subjects with mild hepatic impairment (Child-Pugh Class A) compared with controls. There were insufficient data to determine whether moderate or severe hepatic impairment (Child-Pugh Class B or C) affects efavirenz pharmacokinetics *[See Warnings and Precautions (5.10) and Use in Specific Populations (8.6)].*
Emtricitabine: The pharmacokinetics of emtricitabine have not been studied in subjects with hepatic impairment; however, emtricitabine is not significantly metabolized by liver enzymes, so the impact of liver impairment should be limited.
Tenofovir Disoproxil Fumarate: The pharmacokinetics of tenofovir following a 300 mg dose of tenofovir DF have been studied in non-HIV infected subjects with moderate to severe hepatic impairment. There were no substantial alterations in tenofovir pharmacokinetics in subjects with hepatic impairment compared with unimpaired subjects.

Assessment of Drug Interactions
The drug interaction trials described were conducted with efavirenz, emtricitabine, or tenofovir DF as individual agents; no drug interaction trials have been conducted using ATRIPLA (efavirenz/emtricitabine/tenofovir disoproxil fumarate).
Efavirenz: The steady-state pharmacokinetics of efavirenz and tenofovir were unaffected when efavirenz and tenofovir DF were administered together versus each agent dosed alone. Specific drug interaction trials have not been performed with efavirenz and NRTIs other than tenofovir, lamivudine, and zidovudine. Clinically significant interactions would not be expected based on NRTIs elimination pathways.
Efavirenz has been shown *in vivo* to cause hepatic enzyme induction, thus increasing the biotransformation of some drugs metabolized by CYP3A and CYP2B6. *In vitro* studies have shown that efavirenz inhibited CYP isozymes 2C9, 2C19, and 3A4 with K_i values (8.5–17 μM) in the range of observed efavirenz plasma concentrations. In *in vitro* studies, efavirenz did not inhibit CYP2E1 and inhibited CYP2D6 and CYP1A2 (K_i values 82–160 μM) only at concentrations well above those achieved clinically. Coadministration of efavirenz with drugs primarily metabolized by 2C9, 2C19, and 3A4 isozymes may result in altered plasma concentrations of the coadministered drug. Drugs which induce CYP3A activity would be expected to increase the clearance of efavirenz resulting in lowered plasma concentrations.
Drug interaction trials were performed with efavirenz and other drugs likely to be coadministered or drugs commonly used as probes for pharmacokinetic interaction. There was no clinically significant interaction observed between efavirenz and zidovudine, lamivudine, azithromycin, fluconazole, lorazepam, cetirizine, or paroxetine. Single doses of famotidine or an aluminum and magnesium antacid with simethicone had no effects on efavirenz exposures. The effects of coadministration of efavirenz on C_{max}, AUC, and C_{min} are summarized in Table 5 (effect of other drugs on efavirenz) and Table 6 (effect of efavirenz on other drugs). For information regarding clinical recommendations see *Drug Interactions (7).*

[See table 5 on pages 652 and 653]
[See table 6 on pages 654 through 656]

Emtricitabine and Tenofovir Disoproxil Fumarate: The steady-state pharmacokinetics of emtricitabine and tenofovir were unaffected when emtricitabine and tenofovir DF were administered together versus each agent dosed alone.
In vitro and clinical pharmacokinetic drug-drug interaction studies have shown that the potential for CYP mediated interactions involving emtricitabine and tenofovir with other medicinal products is low.
Emtricitabine and tenofovir are primarily excreted by the kidneys by a combination of glomerular filtration and active tubular secretion. No drug-drug interactions due to competition for renal excretion have been observed; however, coadministration of emtricitabine and tenofovir DF with drugs that are eliminated by active tubular secretion may increase concentrations of emtricitabine, tenofovir, and/or the coadministered drug.
Drugs that decrease renal function may increase concentrations of emtricitabine and/or tenofovir.
No clinically significant drug interactions have been observed between emtricitabine and famciclovir, indinavir, stavudine, tenofovir DF and zidovudine. Similarly, no clinically significant drug interactions have been observed between tenofovir DF and abacavir, efavirenz, emtricitabine, entecavir, indinavir, lamivudine, lopinavir/ritonavir, methadone, nelfinavir, oral contraceptives, ribavirin, saquinavir/ritonavir or tacrolimus in trials conducted in healthy volunteers.

Table 5: Drug Interactions: Changes in Pharmacokinetic Parameters for Efavirenz in the Presence of the Coadministered Drug

Coadministered Drug	Dose of Coadministered Drug (mg)	Efavirenz Dose (mg)	N	Mean % Change of Efavirenz Pharmacokinetic Parameters* (90% CI)		
				C_{max}	AUC	C_{min}
Indinavir	800 mg q8h × 14 days	200 mg qd × 14 days	11	↔	↔	↔
Lopinavir/ ritonavir	400/100 mg q12h × 9 days	600 mg qd × 9 days	11, 12†	↔	↓ 16 (↓ 38 to ↑ 15)	↓ 16 (↓ 42 to ↑ 20)
Nelfinavir	750 mg q8h × 7 days	600 mg qd × 7 days	10	↓ 12 (↓ 32 to ↑ 13)‡	↓ 12 (↓ 35 to ↑ 18)‡	↓ 21 (↓ 53 to ↑ 33)
Ritonavir	500 mg q12h × 8 days	600 mg qd × 10 days	9	↑ 14 (↑ 4 to ↑ 26)	↑ 21 (↑ 10 to ↑ 34)	↑ 25 (↑ 7 to ↑ 46)‡
Saquinavir SGC§	1200 mg q8h × 10 days	600 mg qd × 10 days	13	↓ 13 (↓ 5 to ↓ 20)	↓ 12 (↓ 4 to ↓ 19)	↓ 14 (↓ 2 to ↓ 24)‡
Boceprevir	800 mg tid × 6 days	600 mg qd × 16 days	NA	↑ 11 (↑ 2 to ↑ 20)	↑ 20 (↑ 15 to ↑ 26)	NA
Telaprevir	750 mg q8h × 10 days	600 mg qd × 20 days	21	↓ 16 (↓ 7 to ↓ 24)	↓ 7 (↓ 2 to ↓ 13)	↓ 2 (↓ 6 to ↑ 2)
Telaprevir, coadministered with tenofovir disoproxil fumarate (TDF)	1125 mg q8h × 7 days	600 mg efavirenz/ 300 mg TDF qd × 7 days	15	↓ 24 (↓ 15 to ↓ 32)	↓ 18 (↓ 10 to ↓ 26)	↓ 10 (↓ 19 to ↑ 1)
	1500 mg q12h × 7 days	600 mg efavirenz/ 300 mg TDF qd × 7 days	16	↓ 20 (↓ 14 to ↓ 26)	↓ 15 (↓ 9 to ↓ 21)	↓ 11 (↓ 4 to ↓ 18)
Clarithromycin	500 mg q12h × 7 days	400 mg qd × 7 days	12	↑ 11 (↑ 3 to ↑ 19)	↔	↔
Itraconazole	200 mg q12h × 14 days	600 mg qd × 28 days	16	↔	↔	↔
Rifabutin	300 mg qd × 14 days	600 mg qd × 14 days	11			↓ 12 (↓ 24 to ↑ 1)
Rifampin	600 mg × 7 days	600 mg qd × 7 days	12	↓ 20 (↓ 11 to ↓ 28)	↓ 26 (↓ 15 to ↓ 36)	↓ 32 (↓ 15 to ↓ 46)
Atorvastatin	10 mg qd × 4 days	600 mg qd × 15 days	14	↔	↔	↔
Pravastatin	40 mg qd × 4 days	600 mg qd × 15 days	11	↔	↔	↔
Simvastatin	40 mg qd × 4 days	600 mg qd × 15 days	14	↓ 12 (↓ 28 to ↑ 8)	↔	↓ 12 (↓ 25 to ↑ 3)
Carbamazepine	200 mg qd × 3 days, 200 mg bid × 3 days, then 400 mg qd × 15 days	600 mg qd × 35 days	14	↓ 21 (↓ 15 to ↓ 26)	↓ 36 (↓ 32 to ↓ 40)	↓ 47 (↓ 41 to ↓ 53)
Diltiazem	240 mg × 14 days	600 mg qd × 28 days	12	↑ 16 (↑ 6 to ↑ 26)	↑ 11 (↑ 5 to ↑ 18)	↑ 13 (↑ 1 to ↑ 26)

(Table continued on next page)

Following multiple dosing to HIV-negative subjects receiving either chronic methadone maintenance therapy, oral contraceptives, or single doses of ribavirin, steady-state tenofovir pharmacokinetics were similar to those observed in previous trials, indicating a lack of clinically significant drug interactions between these agents and tenofovir DF. The effects of coadministered drugs on the C_{max}, AUC, and C_{min} of tenofovir are shown in Table 7. The effects of coadministration of tenofovir DF on C_{max}, AUC, and C_{min} of coadministered drugs are shown in Table 8.

[See table 7 at top of page 656]
[See table 8 at top of page 657]
Coadministration of tenofovir DF with didanosine results in changes in the pharmacokinetics of didanosine that may be of clinical significance. Concomitant dosing of tenofovir DF with didanosine enteric-coated capsules significantly increases the C_{max} and AUC of didanosine. When didanosine 250 mg enteric-coated capsules were administered with tenofovir DF, systemic exposures of didanosine were similar to those seen with the 400 mg enteric-coated capsules alone

under fasted conditions. The mechanism of this interaction is unknown [for didanosine dosing adjustment recommendations see *Drug Interactions (7.3)*, Table 4].

12.4 Microbiology
Mechanism of Action
Efavirenz: Efavirenz is a non-nucleoside reverse transcriptase (RT) inhibitor of HIV-1. Efavirenz activity is mediated predominantly by noncompetitive inhibition of HIV-1 reverse transcriptase (RT). HIV-2 RT and human cellular DNA polymerases α, β, γ, and σ are not inhibited by efavirenz.

Emtricitabine: Emtricitabine, a synthetic nucleoside analog of cytidine, is phosphorylated by cellular enzymes to form emtricitabine 5′-triphosphate. Emtricitabine 5′-triphosphate inhibits the activity of the HIV-1 RT by competing with the natural substrate deoxycytidine 5′-triphosphate and by being incorporated into nascent viral DNA which results in chain termination. Emtricitabine 5′-triphosphate is a weak inhibitor of mammalian DNA polymerase α, β, ε, and mitochondrial DNA polymerase γ.

Tenofovir Disoproxil Fumarate: Tenofovir DF is an acyclic nucleoside phosphonate diester analog of adenosine monophosphate. Tenofovir DF requires initial diester hydrolysis for conversion to tenofovir and subsequent phosphorylations by cellular enzymes to form tenofovir diphosphate. Tenofovir diphosphate inhibits the activity of HIV-1 RT by competing with the natural substrate deoxyadenosine 5′-triphosphate and, after incorporation into DNA, by DNA chain termination. Tenofovir diphosphate is a weak inhibitor of mammalian DNA polymerases α, β, and mitochondrial DNA polymerase γ.

Antiviral Activity
Efavirenz, Emtricitabine, and Tenofovir Disoproxil Fumarate: In combination studies evaluating the antiviral activity in cell culture of emtricitabine and efavirenz together, efavirenz and tenofovir together, and emtricitabine and tenofovir together, additive to synergistic antiviral effects were observed.

Efavirenz: The concentration of efavirenz inhibiting replication of wild-type laboratory adapted strains and clinical isolates in cell culture by 90–95% (EC_{90-95}) ranged from 1.7–25 nM in lymphoblastoid cell lines, peripheral blood mononuclear cells, and macrophage/monocyte cultures. Efavirenz demonstrated additive antiviral activity against HIV-1 in cell culture when combined with non-nucleoside reverse transcriptase inhibitors (NNRTIs) (delavirdine and nevirapine), nucleoside reverse transcriptase inhibitors (NRTIs) (abacavir, didanosine, lamivudine, stavudine, zalcitabine, and zidovudine), protease inhibitors (PIs) (amprenavir, indinavir, lopinavir, nelfinavir, ritonavir, and saquinavir), and the fusion inhibitor enfuvirtide. Efavirenz demonstrated additive to antagonistic antiviral activity in cell culture with atazanavir. Efavirenz demonstrated antiviral activity against clade B and most non-clade B isolates (subtypes A, AE, AG, C, D, F, G, J, and N), but had reduced antiviral activity against group O viruses. Efavirenz is not active against HIV-2.

Emtricitabine: The antiviral activity in cell culture of emtricitabine against laboratory and clinical isolates of HIV-1 was assessed in lymphoblastoid cell lines, the MAGI-CCR5 cell line, and peripheral blood mononuclear cells. The 50% effective concentration (EC_{50}) values for emtricitabine were in the range of 0.0013–0.64 μM (0.0003–0.158 μg/mL). In drug combination studies of emtricitabine with NRTIs (abacavir, lamivudine, stavudine, zalcitabine, and zidovudine), NNRTIs (delavirdine, efavirenz, and nevirapine), and PIs (amprenavir, nelfinavir, ritonavir, and saquinavir), additive to synergistic effects were observed. Emtricitabine displayed antiviral activity in cell culture against HIV-1 clades A, B, C, D, E, F, and G (EC_{50} values ranged from 0.007–0.075 μM) and showed strain specific activity against HIV-2 (EC_{50} values ranged from 0.007–1.5 μM).

Tenofovir Disoproxil Fumarate: The antiviral activity in cell culture of tenofovir against laboratory and clinical isolates of HIV-1 was assessed in lymphoblastoid cell lines, primary monocyte/macrophage cells and peripheral blood lymphocytes. The EC_{50} values for tenofovir were in the range of 0.04–8.5 μM. In drug combination studies of tenofovir with NRTIs (abacavir, didanosine, lamivudine, stavudine, zalcitabine, and zidovudine), NNRTIs (delavirdine, efavirenz, and nevirapine), and PIs (amprenavir, indinavir, nelfinavir, ritonavir, and saquinavir), additive to synergistic effects were observed. Tenofovir displayed antiviral activity in cell culture against HIV-1 clades A, B, C, D, E, F, G and O (EC_{50} values ranged from 0.5–2.2 μM) and showed strain specific activity against HIV-2 (EC_{50} values ranged from 1.6 μM–5.5 μM).

Resistance
Efavirenz, Emtricitabine, and Tenofovir Disoproxil Fumarate: HIV-1 isolates with reduced susceptibility to the combination of emtricitabine and tenofovir have been selected in cell culture and in clinical trials. Genotypic analysis of these isolates identified the M184V/I and/or K65R amino acid substitutions in the viral RT.

In a clinical trial of treatment-naive subjects [*Study 934, see Clinical Studies (14)*] resistance analysis was performed on HIV-1 isolates from all confirmed virologic failure subjects with greater than 400 copies/mL of HIV-1 RNA at Week 144 or early discontinuations. Genotypic resistance to efavirenz, predominantly the K103N substitution, was the most common form of resistance that developed. Resistance to efavirenz occurred in 13/19 analyzed subjects in the emtricitabine + tenofovir DF group and in 21/29 analyzed subjects in the zidovudine/lamivudine fixed-dose combination group. The M184V amino acid substitution, associated with resistance to emtricitabine and lamivudine, was observed in 2/19 analyzed subject isolates in the emtricitabine + tenofovir DF group and in 10/29 analyzed subject isolates in the zidovudine/lamivudine group. Through 144 weeks of Study 934, no subjects developed a detectable K65R substitution in their HIV-1 as analyzed through standard genotypic analysis.

In a clinical trial of treatment-naive subjects, isolates from 8/47 (17%) analyzed subjects receiving tenofovir DF developed the K65R substitution through 144 weeks of therapy; 7 of these occurred in the first 48 weeks of treatment and one at Week 96. In treatment experienced subjects, 14/304 (5%) of tenofovir DF treated subjects with virologic failure through Week 96 showed greater than 1.4-fold (median 2.7) reduced susceptibility to tenofovir. Genotypic analysis of the resistant isolates showed a substitution in the HIV-1 RT gene resulting in the K65R amino acid substitution.

Efavirenz: Clinical isolates with reduced susceptibility in cell culture to efavirenz have been obtained. The most frequently observed amino acid substitution in clinical trials with efavirenz is K103N (54%). One or more RT substitutions at amino acid positions 98, 100, 101, 103, 106, 108, 188, 190, 225, 227, and 230 were observed in subjects failing treatment with efavirenz in combination with other antiretrovirals. Other resistance substitutions observed to emerge commonly included L100I (7%), K101E/Q/R (14%), V108I (11%), G190S/T/A (7%), P225H (18%), and M230L (11%). HIV-1 isolates with reduced susceptibility to efavirenz (greater than 380-fold increase in EC_{90} value) emerged rapidly under selection in cell culture. Genotypic characterization of these viruses identified substitutions resulting in single amino acid substitutions L100I or V179D, double substitutions L100I/V108I, and triple substitutions L100I/V179D/Y181C in RT.

Emtricitabine: Emtricitabine-resistant isolates of HIV-1 have been selected in cell culture and in clinical trials. Genotypic analysis of these isolates showed that the reduced susceptibility to emtricitabine was associated with a substitution in the HIV-1 RT gene at codon 184 which resulted in an amino acid substitution of methionine by valine or isoleucine (M184V/I).

Tenofovir Disoproxil Fumarate: HIV-1 isolates with reduced susceptibility to tenofovir have been selected in cell culture. These viruses expressed a K65R substitution in RT and showed a 2- to 4-fold reduction in susceptibility to tenofovir.

Cross Resistance

Efavirenz, Emtricitabine, and Tenofovir Disoproxil Fumarate: Cross-resistance has been recognized among NNRTIs. Cross resistance has also been recognized among certain NRTIs. The M184V/I and/or K65R substitutions selected in cell culture by the combination of emtricitabine and tenofovir are also observed in some HIV-1 isolates from subjects failing treatment with tenofovir in combination with either lamivudine or emtricitabine, and either abacavir or didanosine. Therefore, cross-resistance among these drugs may occur in patients whose virus harbors either or both of these amino acid substitutions.

Efavirenz: Clinical isolates previously characterized as efavirenz-resistant were also phenotypically resistant in cell culture to delavirdine and nevirapine compared to baseline. Delavirdine- and/or nevirapine-resistant clinical viral isolates with NNRTI resistance-associated substitutions (A98G, L100I, K101E/P, K103N/S, V106A, Y181X, Y188X, G190X, P225H, F227L, or M230L) showed reduced susceptibility to efavirenz in cell culture. Greater than 90% of NRTI-resistant isolates tested in cell culture retained susceptibility to efavirenz.

Emtricitabine: Emtricitabine-resistant isolates (M184V/I) were cross-resistant to lamivudine and zalcitabine but retained susceptibility in cell culture to didanosine, stavudine, tenofovir, zidovudine, and NNRTIs (delavirdine, efavirenz, and nevirapine). HIV-1 isolates containing the K65R substitution, selected *in vivo* by abacavir, didanosine, tenofovir, and zalcitabine, demonstrated reduced susceptibility to inhibition by emtricitabine. Viruses harboring substitutions conferring reduced susceptibility to stavudine and zidovudine (M41L, D67N, K70R, L210W, T215Y/F, and K219Q/E) or didanosine (L74V) remained sensitive to emtricitabine.

Tenofovir Disoproxil Fumarate: The K65R substitution selected by tenofovir is also selected in some HIV-1 infected patients treated with abacavir, didanosine, or zalcitabine. HIV-1 isolates with the K65R substitution also showed reduced susceptibility to emtricitabine and lamivudine.

Therefore, cross-resistance among these drugs may occur in patients whose virus harbors the K65R substitution. HIV-1 isolates from subjects (N=20) whose HIV-1 expressed a mean of 3 zidovudine-associated RT amino acid substitutions (M41L, D67N, K70R, L210W, T215Y/F, or K219Q/E/N) showed a 3.1-fold decrease in the susceptibility to tenofovir. Subjects whose virus expressed an L74V substitution without zidovudine resistance associated substitutions (N=8) had reduced response to VIREAD. Limited data are available for patients whose virus expressed a Y115F substitution (N=3), Q151M substitution (N=2), or T69 insertion (N=4), all of whom had a reduced response.

13 NONCLINICAL TOXICOLOGY

13.1 Carcinogenesis, Mutagenesis, Impairment of Fertility

Efavirenz: Long-term carcinogenicity studies in mice and rats were carried out with efavirenz. Mice were dosed with 0, 25, 75, 150, or 300 mg/kg/day for 2 years. Incidences of hepatocellular adenomas and carcinomas and pulmonary alveolar/bronchiolar adenomas were increased above background in females. No increases in tumor incidence above background were seen in males. In studies in which rats were administered efavirenz at doses of 0, 25, 50, or 100 mg/kg/day for 2 years, no increases in tumor incidence above background were observed. The systemic exposure (based on AUCs) in mice was approximately 1.7-fold that in humans receiving the 600-mg/day dose. The exposure in rats was lower than that in humans. The mechanism of the carcinogenic potential is unknown. However, in genetic toxicology assays, efavirenz showed no evidence of mutagenic or clastogenic activity in a battery of *in vitro* and *in vivo* studies. These included bacterial mutation assays in *S. typhimurium* and *E. coli*, mammalian mutation assays in Chinese hamster ovary cells, chromosome aberration assays in human peripheral blood lymphocytes or Chinese hamster ovary cells, and an *in vivo* mouse bone marrow micronucleus assay. Given the lack of genotoxic activity of efavirenz, the relevance to humans of neoplasms in efavirenz-treated mice is not known.

Efavirenz did not impair mating or fertility of male or female rats, and did not affect sperm of treated male rats. The reproductive performance of offspring born to female rats given efavirenz was not affected. As a result of the rapid clearance of efavirenz in rats, systemic drug exposures achieved in these studies were equivalent to or below those achieved in humans given therapeutic doses of efavirenz.

Emtricitabine: In long-term carcinogenicity studies of emtricitabine, no drug-related increases in tumor incidence were found in mice at doses up to 750 mg/kg/day (26 times the human systemic exposure at the therapeutic dose of 200 mg/day) or in rats at doses up to 600 mg/kg/day (31 times the human systemic exposure at the therapeutic dose). Emtricitabine was not genotoxic in the reverse mutation bacterial test (Ames test), mouse lymphoma or mouse micronucleus assays.

Emtricitabine did not affect fertility in male rats at approximately 140-fold or in male and female mice at approximately 60-fold higher exposures (AUC) than in humans given the recommended 200 mg daily dose. Fertility was normal in the offspring of mice exposed daily from before birth (*in utero*) through sexual maturity at daily exposures (AUC) of approximately 60-fold higher than human exposures at the recommended 200 mg daily dose.

Tenofovir Disoproxil Fumarate: Long-term oral carcinogenicity studies of tenofovir DF in mice and rats were carried out at exposures up to approximately 16 times (mice) and 5 times (rats) those observed in humans at the therapeutic dose for HIV-1 infection. At the high dose in female mice, liver adenomas were increased at exposures 16 times that in humans. In rats, the study was negative for carcinogenic findings at exposures up to 5 times that observed in humans at the therapeutic dose.

Tenofovir DF was mutagenic in the *in vitro* mouse lymphoma assay and negative in an *in vitro* bacterial mutagenicity test (Ames test). In an *in vivo* mouse micronucleus assay, tenofovir DF was negative when administered to male mice.

There were no effects on fertility, mating performance or early embryonic development when tenofovir DF was administered to male rats at a dose equivalent to 10 times the human dose based on body surface area comparisons for 28 days prior to mating and to female rats for 15 days prior to mating through Day seven of gestation. There was, however, an alteration of the estrous cycle in female rats.

13.2 Animal Toxicology and/or Pharmacology

Efavirenz: Nonsustained convulsions were observed in 6 of 20 monkeys receiving efavirenz at doses yielding plasma AUC values 4- to 13-fold greater than those in humans given the recommended dose.

Tenofovir Disoproxil Fumarate: Tenofovir and tenofovir DF administered in toxicology studies to rats, dogs and monkeys at exposures (based on AUCs) greater than or equal to 6-fold those observed in humans caused bone toxicity. In monkeys the bone toxicity was diagnosed as osteomalacia. Osteomalacia observed in monkeys appeared to be reversible upon dose reduction or discontinuation of tenofovir. In rats and dogs, the bone toxicity manifested as reduced bone mineral density. The mechanism(s) underlying bone toxicity is unknown.

Evidence of renal toxicity was noted in 4 animal species administered tenofovir and tenofovir DF. Increases in serum creatinine, BUN, glycosuria, proteinuria, phosphaturia and/or calciuria and decreases in serum phosphate were observed to varying degrees in these animals. These toxicities were noted at exposures (based on AUCs) 2- to 20-times higher than those observed in humans. The relationship of the renal abnormalities, particularly the phosphaturia, to the bone toxicity is not known.

14 CLINICAL STUDIES

Clinical Study 934 supports the use of ATRIPLA tablets in antiretroviral treatment-naive HIV-1 infected patients. Additional data in support of the use of ATRIPLA in treatment-naive patients can be found in the prescribing information for VIREAD.

Clinical Study 073 provides clinical experience in subjects with stable, virologic suppression and no history of virologic failure who switched from their current regimen to ATRIPLA (efavirenz/emtricitabine/tenofovir disoproxil fumarate).

Table 5 *(cont.)*: Drug Interactions: Changes in Pharmacokinetic Parameters for Efavirenz in the Presence of the Coadministered Drug

Coadministered Drug	Dose of Coadministered Drug (mg)	Efavirenz Dose (mg)	N	C_{max}	AUC	C_{min}
Sertraline	50 mg qd × 14 days	600 mg qd × 14 days	13	↑ 11 (↑ 6 to ↑ 16)	↔	↔
Voriconazole	400 mg po q12h × 1 day then 200 mg po q12h × 8 days	400 mg qd × 9 days	NA	↑ 38¶	↑ 44¶	NA
	300 mg po q12h days 2–7	300 mg qd × 7 days	NA	↓ 14# (↓ 7 to ↓ 21)	↔#	NA
	400 mg po q12h days 2–7	300 mg qd × 7 days	NA	↔#	↑ 17# (↑ 6 to ↑ 29)	NA

NA = not available
* Increase = ↑; Decrease = ↓; No Effect = ↔
† Parallel-group design; N for efavirenz + lopinavir/ritonavir, N for efavirenz alone.
‡ 95% CI
§ Soft Gelatin Capsule
¶ 90% CI not available
# Relative to steady-state administration of efavirenz (600 mg once daily for 9 days).

Table 6: Drug Interactions: Changes in Pharmacokinetic Parameters for Coadministered Drug in the Presence of Efavirenz

Coadministered Drug	Dose of Coadministered Drug (mg)	Efavirenz Dose (mg)	N	Mean % Change of Coadministered Drug Pharmacokinetic Parameters* (90% CI)		
				C_{max}	AUC	C_{min}
Atazanavir	400 mg qd with a light meal d 1–20	600 mg qd with a light meal d 7–20	27	↓59 (↓49 to ↓67)	↓74 (↓68 to ↓78)	↓93 (↓90 to ↓95)
	400 mg qd d 1–6, then 300 mg qd d 7–20 with ritonavir 100 mg qd and a light meal	600 mg qd 2 h after atazanavir and ritonavir d 7–20	13	↑14[†] (↓17 to ↓58)	↑39[†] (↑2 to ↑88)	↑48[†] (↑24 to ↑76)
	300 mg qd/ritonavir 100 mg qd d 1–10 (pm), then 400 mg qd/ritonavir 100 mg qd d 11–24 (pm) (simultaneous with efavirenz)	600 mg qd with a light snack d 11–24 (pm)	14	↑17 (↑8 to ↑27)	↔	↓42 (↓31 to ↓51)
Indinavir	1000 mg q8h × 10 days	600 mg qd × 10 days	20			
	After morning dose			↔[‡]	↓33[‡] (↓26 to ↓39)	↓39[‡] (↓24 to ↓51)
	After afternoon dose			↔[‡]	↓37[‡] (↓26 to ↓46)	↓52[‡] (↓47 to ↓57)
	After evening dose			↓29[‡] (↓11 to ↓43)	↓46[‡] (↓37 to ↓54)	↓57[‡] (↓50 to ↓63)
Lopinavir/ ritonavir	400/100 mg q12h × 9 days	600 mg qd × 9 days	11, 7[§]	↔[¶]	↓19[¶] (↓36 to ↑3)	↓39[¶] (↓3 to ↓62)
Nelfinavir	750 mg q8h × 7 days	600 mg qd × 7 days	10	↑21 (↑10 to ↑33)	↑20 (↑8 to ↑34)	↔
Metabolite AG-1402				↓40 (↓30 to ↓48)	↓37 (↓25 to ↓48)	↓43 (↓21 to ↓59)
Ritonavir	500 mg q12h × 8 days	600 mg qd × 10 days	11			
	After AM dose			↑24 (↑12 to ↑38)	↑18 (↑6 to ↑33)	↑42 (↑9 to ↑86)[#]
	After PM dose			↔	↔	↑24 (↑3 to ↑50)[#]
Saquinavir SGC[b]	1200 mg q8h × 10 days	600 mg qd × 10 days	12	↓50 (↓28 to ↓66)	↓62 (↓45 to ↓74)	↓56 (↓16 to ↓77)[#]
Maraviroc	100 mg bid	600 mg qd	12	↓51 (↓37 to ↓62)	↓45 (↓38 to ↓51)	↓45 (↓28 to ↓57)
Raltegravir	400 mg single dose	600 mg qd	9	↓36 (↓2 to ↓59)	↓36 (↓20 to ↓48)	↓21 (↓51 to ↑28)
Boceprevir	800 mg tid × 6 days	600 mg qd × 16 days	NA	↓8 (↓22 to ↑8)	↓19 (↓11 to ↓25)	↓44 (↓26 to ↓58)
Telaprevir	750 mg q8h × 10 days	600 mg qd × 20 days	21	↓9 (↓18 to ↑2)	↓26 (↓16 to ↓35)	↓47 (↓35 to ↓56)

(Table continued on next page)

In antiretroviral treatment-experienced patients, the use of ATRIPLA (efavirenz/emtricitabine/tenofovir disoproxil fumarate) tablets may be considered for patients with HIV-1 strains that are expected to be susceptible to the components of ATRIPLA as assessed by treatment history or by genotypic or phenotypic testing *[See Clinical Pharmacology (12.4)]*.

Study 934: Data through 144 weeks are reported for Study 934, a randomized, open-label, active-controlled multicenter trial comparing emtricitabine + tenofovir DF administered in combination with efavirenz versus zidovudine/lamivudine fixed-dose combination administered in combination with efavirenz in 511 antiretroviral-naive subjects. From Weeks 96 to 144 of the trial, subjects received emtricitabine/tenofovir DF fixed-dose combination with efavirenz in place of emtricitabine + tenofovir DF with efavirenz. Subjects had a mean age of 38 years (range 18–80), 86% were male, 59% were Caucasian and 23% were Black. The mean baseline CD4+ cell count was 245 cells/mm^3 (range 2–1191) and median baseline plasma HIV-1 RNA was 5.01 log$_{10}$ copies/mL (range 3.56–6.54). Subjects were stratified by baseline CD4+ cell count (< or ≥200 cells/mm^3) and 41% had CD4+ cell counts <200 cells/mm^3. Fifty-one percent (51%) of subjects had baseline viral loads >100,000 copies/mL. Treatment outcomes through 48 and 144 weeks for those subjects who did not have efavirenz resistance at baseline (N=487) are presented in Table 9.

[See table 9 at top of page 657]

Through Week 48, 84% and 73% of subjects in the emtricitabine + tenofovir DF group and the zidovudine/lamivudine group, respectively, achieved and maintained HIV-1 RNA <400 copies/mL (71% and 58% through Week 144). The difference in the proportion of subjects who achieved and maintained HIV-1 RNA <400 copies/mL through 48 weeks largely results from the higher number of discontinuations due to adverse events and other reasons in the zidovudine/lamivudine group in this open-label trial. In addition, 80% and 70% of subjects in the emtricitabine + tenofovir DF group and the zidovudine/lamivudine group, respectively, achieved and maintained HIV-1 RNA <50 copies/mL through Week 48 (64% and 56% through Week 144). The mean increase from baseline in CD4+ cell count was 190 cells/mm^3 in the emtricitabine + tenofovir DF group and 158 cells/mm^3 in the zidovudine/lamivudine group at Week 48 (312 and 271 cells/mm^3 at Week 144).

Through 48 weeks, 7 subjects in the emtricitabine + tenofovir DF group and 5 subjects in the zidovudine/lamivudine group experienced a new CDC Class C event (10 and 6 subjects through 144 weeks).

Study 073: Study 073 was a 48-week open-label, randomized clinical trial in subjects with stable virologic suppression on combination antiretroviral therapy consisting of at least two nucleoside reverse transcriptase inhibitors (NRTIs) administered in combination with a protease inhibitor (with or without ritonavir) or a non-nucleoside reverse transcriptase inhibitor (NNRTI).

To be enrolled, subjects were to have HIV-1 RNA <200 copies/mL for at least 12 weeks on their current regimen prior to trial entry with no known HIV-1 substitutions conferring resistance to the components of ATRIPLA (efavirenz/emtricitabine/tenofovir disoproxil fumarate) and no history of virologic failure.

The trial compared the efficacy of switching to ATRIPLA or staying on the baseline antiretroviral regimen (SBR). Subjects were randomized in a 2:1 ratio to switch to ATRIPLA (N=203) or stay on SBR (N=97). Subjects had a mean age of 43 years (range 22–73 years), 88% were male, 68% were white, 29% were Black or African-American, and 3% were of other races. At baseline, median CD4+ cell count was 516 cells/mm^3 and 96% had HIV-1 RNA <50 copies/mL. The median time since onset of antiretroviral therapy was 3 years and 88% of subjects were receiving their first antiretroviral regimen at trial enrollment.

At Week 48, 89% and 87% of subjects who switched to ATRIPLA maintained HIV RNA <200 copies/mL and <50 copies/mL, respectively, compared to 88% and 85% who remained on SBR; this difference was not statistically significant. No changes in CD4+ cell counts from baseline to Week 48 were observed in either treatment arm.

16 HOW SUPPLIED/STORAGE AND HANDLING

ATRIPLA tablets are pink, capsule-shaped, film-coated, debossed with "123" on one side and plain-faced on the other side. Each bottle contains 30 tablets (NDC 15584-0101-1) and silica gel desiccant, and is closed with a child-resistant closure.

Store at 25 °C (77 °F); excursions permitted to 15–30 °C (59–86 °F) *[See USP Controlled Room Temperature]*.
• Keep container tightly closed.
• Dispense only in original container.
• Do not use if seal over bottle opening is broken or missing.

17 PATIENT COUNSELING INFORMATION

See FDA-approved patient labeling (Patient Information)

17.1 Drug Interactions

A statement to patients and healthcare providers is included on the product's bottle labels: *ALERT: Find out about medicines that should NOT be taken with ATRIPLA.* ATRIPLA may interact with some drugs; therefore, patients should be advised to report to their doctor the use of any other prescription, nonprescription medication, or herbal products, particularly St. John's wort.

17.2 General Information for Patients

Patients should be advised that:
• ATRIPLA is not a cure for HIV-1 infection and patients may continue to experience illnesses associated with HIV-1 infection, including opportunistic infections. Patients should remain under the care of a physician when using ATRIPLA.
• Patients should avoid doing things that can spread HIV-1 to others.
• **Do not share needles or other injection equipment.**
• **Do not share personal items that can have blood or body fluids on them, like toothbrushes and razor blades.**

- **Do not have any kind of sex without protection.** Always practice safe sex by using a latex or polyurethane condom to lower the chance of sexual contact with semen, vaginal secretions, or blood.
- **Do not breastfeed.** Some of the medicines in ATRIPLA can be passed to your baby in your breast milk. We do not know whether it could harm your baby. Also, mothers with HIV-1 should not breastfeed because HIV-1 can be passed to the baby in the breast milk.
- The long-term effects of ATRIPLA (efavirenz/emtricitabine/tenofovir disoproxil fumarate) are unknown.
- Redistribution or accumulation of body fat may occur in patients receiving antiretroviral therapy and that the cause and long-term health effects of these conditions are not known.
- ATRIPLA should not be coadministered with COMPLERA, EMTRIVA, STRIBILD, TRUVADA, or VIREAD; or drugs containing lamivudine, including Combivir, Epivir, Epivir-HBV, Epzicom, or Trizivir. SUSTIVA should not be coadministered with ATRIPLA unless needed for dose adjustment *[See Warnings and Precautions (5.4)].*
- ATRIPLA should not be administered with HEPSERA *[See Warnings and Precautions (5.2)].*

17.3   Lactic Acidosis/Severe Hepatomegaly with Steatosis
Patients should be informed that lactic acidosis and severe hepatomegaly with steatosis, including fatal cases, have been reported. Treatment will be suspended in any patients who develop clinical symptoms suggestive of lactic acidosis or pronounced hepatotoxicity (including nausea, vomiting, unusual or unexpected stomach discomfort, and weakness) *[See Warnings and Precautions (5.1)].*

17.4   Patients Coinfected with HIV-1 and HBV
Patients with HIV-1 should be tested for hepatitis B virus (HBV) before initiating antiretroviral therapy.
Patients should be advised that severe acute exacerbations of hepatitis B have been reported in patients who are coinfected with HBV and HIV-1 and have discontinued EMTRIVA (emtricitabine) or VIREAD (tenofovir DF), which are components of ATRIPLA.

17.5   New Onset or Worsening Renal Impairment
Renal impairment, including cases of acute renal failure and Fanconi syndrome, has been reported. ATRIPLA should be avoided with concurrent or recent use of a nephrotoxic agent (e.g. high-dose or multiple NSAIDs) *[See Warnings and Precautions (5.7)].*

17.6   Decreases in Bone Mineral Density
Patients should be informed that decreases in bone mineral density have been observed with the use of tenofovir DF. Bone mineral density monitoring may be performed in patients who have a history of pathologic bone fracture or other risk factors for osteoporosis or bone loss *[See Warnings and Precautions (5.11)].*

17.7   Dosing Instructions
Patients should be advised to take ATRIPLA orally on an empty stomach and that it is important to take ATRIPLA on a regular dosing schedule to avoid missing doses.

17.8   Nervous System Symptoms
Patients should be informed that central nervous system symptoms (NSS) including dizziness, insomnia, impaired concentration, drowsiness, and abnormal dreams are commonly reported during the first weeks of therapy with efavirenz. Dosing at bedtime may improve the tolerability of these symptoms, which are likely to improve with continued therapy. Patients should be alerted to the potential for additive effects when ATRIPLA is used concomitantly with alcohol or psychoactive drugs. Patients should be instructed that if they experience NSS they should avoid potentially hazardous tasks such as driving or operating machinery *[See Warnings and Precautions (5.6) and Dosage and Administration (2)].*

17.9   Psychiatric Symptoms
Patients should be informed that serious psychiatric symptoms including severe depression, suicide attempts, aggressive behavior, delusions, paranoia, and psychosis-like symptoms have been reported in patients receiving efavirenz. If they experience severe psychiatric adverse experiences they should seek immediate medical evaluation. Patients should be advised to inform their physician of any history of mental illness or substance abuse *[See Warnings and Precautions (5.5)].*

17.10   Rash
Patients should be informed that a common side effect is rash. Rashes usually go away without any change in treatment. However, since rash may be serious, patients should be advised to contact their physician promptly if rash occurs.

17.11   Reproductive Risk Potential
Women receiving ATRIPLA should be instructed to avoid pregnancy *[See Warnings and Precautions (5.8)].* A reliable form of barrier contraception must always be used in combination with other methods of contraception, including oral or other hormonal contraception. Because of the long half-life of efavirenz, use of adequate contraceptive measures for 12 weeks after discontinuation of ATRIPLA (efavirenz/emtricitabine/tenofovir disoproxil fumarate) is recommended. Women should be advised to notify their physician if they become pregnant or plan to become pregnant while taking ATRIPLA (efavirenz/emtricitabine/tenofovir disoproxil fumarate). If this drug is used during the first trimester of pregnancy, or if the patient becomes pregnant while taking this drug, she should be apprised of the potential harm to the fetus.

Table 6 (cont.): Drug Interactions: Changes in Pharmacokinetic Parameters for Coadministered Drug in the Presence of Efavirenz

Coadministered Drug	Dose of Coadministered Drug (mg)	Efavirenz Dose (mg)	N	Mean % Change of Coadministered Drug Pharmacokinetic Parameters* (90% CI)		
				C_{max}	AUC	C_{min}
Clarithromycin	500 mg q12h × 7 days	400 mg qd × 7 days	11	↓ 26 (↓ 15 to ↓ 35)	↓ 39 (↓ 30 to ↓ 46)	↓ 53 (↓ 42 to ↓ 63)
14-OH metabolite				↑ 49 (↑ 32 to ↑ 69)	↑ 34 (↑ 18 to ↑ 53)	↑ 26 (↑ 9 to ↑ 45)
Itraconazole	200 mg q12h × 28 days	600 mg qd × 14 days	18	↓ 37 (↓ 20 to ↓ 51)	↓ 39 (↓ 21 to ↓ 53)	↓ 44 (↓ 27 to ↓ 58)
Hydroxy-itraconazole				↓ 35 (↓ 12 to ↓ 52)	↓ 37 (↓ 14 to ↓ 55)	↓ 43 (↓ 18 to ↓ 60)
Posaconazole	400 mg (oral suspension) bid × 10 and 20 days	400 mg qd × 10 and 20 days	11	↓ 45 (↓ 34 to ↓ 53)	↓ 50 (↓ 40 to ↓ 57)	NA
Rifabutin	300 mg qd × 14 days	600 mg qd × 14 days	9	↓ 32 (↓ 15 to ↓ 46)	↓ 38 (↓ 28 to ↓ 47)	↓ 45 (↓ 31 to ↓ 56)
Atorvastatin	10 mg qd × 4 days	600 mg qd × 15 days	14	↓ 14 (↓ 1 to ↓ 26)	↓ 43 (↓ 34 to ↓ 50)	↓ 69 (↓ 49 to ↓ 81)
Total active (including metabolites)				↓ 15 (↓ 2 to ↓ 26)	↓ 32 (↓ 21 to ↓ 41)	↓ 48 (↓ 23 to ↓ 64)
Pravastatin	40 mg qd × 4 days	600 mg qd × 15 days	13	↓ 32 (↓ 59 to ↑ 12)	↓ 44 (↓ 26 to ↓ 57)	↓ 19 (↓ 0 to ↓ 35)
Simvastatin	40 mg qd × 4 days	600 mg qd × 15 days	14	↓ 72 (↓ 63 to ↓ 79)	↓ 68 (↓ 62 to ↓ 73)	↓ 45 (↓ 20 to ↓ 62)
Total active (including metabolites)				↓ 68 (↓ 55 to ↓ 78)	↓ 60 (↓ 52 to ↓ 68)	NA[§]
Carbamazepine	200 mg qd × 3 days, 200 mg bid × 3 days, then 400 mg qd × 29 days	600 mg qd × 14 days	12	↓ 20 (↓ 15 to ↓ 24)	↓ 27 (↓ 20 to ↓ 33)	↓ 35 (↓ 24 to ↓ 44)
Epoxide metabolite				↔	↔	↓ 13 (↓ 30 to ↑ 7)
Diltiazem	240 mg × 21 days	600 mg qd × 14 days	13	↓ 60 (↓ 50 to ↓ 68)	↓ 69 (↓ 55 to ↓ 79)	↓ 63 (↓ 44 to ↓ 75)
Desacetyl diltiazem				↓ 64 (↓ 57 to ↓ 69)	↓ 75 (↓ 59 to ↓ 84)	↓ 62 (↓ 44 to ↓ 75)
N-monodesmethyl diltiazem				↓ 28 (↓ 7 to ↓ 44)	↓ 37 (↓ 17 to ↓ 52)	↓ 37 (↓ 17 to ↓ 52)
Ethinyl estradiol/ Norgestimate	0.035 mg/0.25 mg × 14 days	600 mg qd × 14 days				
Ethinyl estradiol			21	↔	↔	↔
Norelgestromin			21	↓ 46 (↓ 39 to ↓ 52)	↓ 64 (↓ 62 to ↓ 67)	↓ 82 (↓ 79 to ↓ 85)
Levonorgestrel			6	↓ 80 (↓ 77 to ↓ 83)	↓ 83 (↓ 79 to ↓ 87)	↓ 86 (↓ 80 to ↓ 90)
Methadone	Stable maintenance 35–100 mg daily	600 mg qd × 14–21 days	11	↓ 45 (↓ 25 to ↓ 59)	↓ 52 (↓ 33 to ↓ 66)	NA

(Table continued on next page)

Patient Information
ATRIPLA® (uh TRIP luh) Tablets
ALERT: Find out about medicines that should NOT be taken with ATRIPLA.
Please also read the section **"MEDICINES YOU SHOULD NOT TAKE WITH ATRIPLA."**
Generic name: efavirenz, emtricitabine and tenofovir disoproxil fumarate (eh FAH vih renz, em tri SIT uh bean and te NOE' fo veer dye soe PROX il FYOU mar ate)
Read the Patient Information that comes with ATRIPLA before you start taking it and each time you get a refill since there may be new information. This information does not take the place of talking to your healthcare provider about your medical condition or treatment. You should stay under a healthcare provider's care when taking ATRIPLA (efavirenz/emtricitabine/tenofovir disoproxil fumarate). **Do not change or stop your medicine without first talking with your healthcare provider.** Talk to your healthcare provider or pharmacist if you have any questions about ATRIPLA.

What is the most important information I should know about ATRIPLA?
- **Some people who have taken medicine like ATRIPLA (which contains nucleoside analogs) have developed a serious condition called lactic acidosis** (build up of an acid in the blood). Lactic acidosis can be a medical emergency and may need to be treated in the hospital. **Call your healthcare provider right away if you get the following signs or symptoms of lactic acidosis:**
  - You feel very weak or tired.
  - You have unusual (not normal) muscle pain.
  - You have trouble breathing.
  - You have stomach pain with nausea and vomiting.
  - You feel cold, especially in your arms and legs.
  - You feel dizzy or lightheaded.
  - You have a fast or irregular heartbeat.
- **Some people who have taken medicines like ATRIPLA have developed serious liver problems called hepatotoxicity,** with liver enlargement (hepatomegaly) and fat in the liver (steatosis). **Call your healthcare provider right away if you get the following signs or symptoms of liver problems:**
  - Your skin or the white part of your eyes turns yellow (jaundice).
  - Your urine turns dark.
  - Your bowel movements (stools) turn light in color.
  - You don't feel like eating food for several days or longer.
  - You feel sick to your stomach (nausea).
  - You have lower stomach area (abdominal) pain.
- **You may be more likely to get lactic acidosis or liver problems** if you are female, very overweight (obese), or have been taking nucleoside analog-containing medicines, like ATRIPLA, for a long time.
- **If you also have hepatitis B virus (HBV) infection and you stop taking ATRIPLA, you may get a "flare-up" of your hepatitis.** A "flare-up" is when the disease suddenly returns in a worse way than before. Patients with HBV who stop taking ATRIPLA need close medical follow-up for several months, including medical exams and blood tests to check for hepatitis that could be getting worse. ATRIPLA is not approved for the treatment of HBV, so you must discuss your HBV therapy with your healthcare provider.

What is ATRIPLA?
ATRIPLA contains 3 medicines, SUSTIVA® (efavirenz), EMTRIVA® (emtricitabine) and VIREAD® (tenofovir disoproxil fumarate also called tenofovir DF) combined in one pill. EMTRIVA and VIREAD are HIV-1 (human immunodeficiency virus) nucleoside analog reverse transcriptase inhibitors (NRTIs) and SUSTIVA is an HIV-1 non-nucleoside analog reverse transcriptase inhibitor (NNRTI). VIREAD and EMTRIVA are the components of TRUVADA®. ATRIPLA can be used alone as a complete regimen, or in combination with other anti-HIV-1 medicines to treat people with HIV-1 infection. ATRIPLA is for adults and children 12 years of age and older who weigh at least 40 kg (at least 88 lbs). ATRIPLA is not recommended for children younger than 12 years of age. ATRIPLA has not been studied in adults over 65 years of age.
HIV infection destroys CD4+ T cells, which are important to the immune system. The immune system helps fight infection. After a large number of T cells are destroyed, acquired immune deficiency syndrome (AIDS) develops.
ATRIPLA helps block HIV-1 reverse transcriptase, a viral chemical in your body (enzyme) that is needed for HIV-1 to multiply. ATRIPLA lowers the amount of HIV-1 in the blood (viral load). ATRIPLA may also help to increase the number of T cells (CD4+ cells), allowing your immune system to improve. Lowering the amount of HIV-1 in the blood lowers the chance of death or infections that happen when your immune system is weak (opportunistic infections).

Does ATRIPLA cure HIV-1 or AIDS?
ATRIPLA does not cure HIV-1 infection or AIDS and you may continue to experience illnesses associated with HIV-1 infection, including opportunistic infections. You should remain under the care of a doctor when using ATRIPLA.

Who should not take ATRIPLA?
Together with your healthcare provider, you need to decide whether ATRIPLA is right for you.
Do not take ATRIPLA if you are allergic to ATRIPLA or any of its ingredients. The active ingredients of ATRIPLA are

efavirenz, emtricitabine, and tenofovir DF. See the end of this leaflet for a complete list of ingredients.
What should I tell my healthcare provider before taking ATRIPLA?
Tell your healthcare provider if you:
- **Are pregnant or planning to become pregnant** (see "What should I avoid while taking ATRIPLA?").
- **Are breastfeeding** (see "What should I avoid while taking ATRIPLA?").

- **Have kidney problems or are undergoing kidney dialysis treatment.**
- **Have bone problems.**
- **Have liver problems, including hepatitis B virus infection.** Your healthcare provider may want to do tests to check your liver while you take ATRIPLA (efavirenz/emtricitabine/tenofovir disoproxil fumarate) or may switch you to another medicine.
- **Have ever had mental illness or are using drugs or alcohol.**

Table 6 (cont.): Drug Interactions: Changes in Pharmacokinetic Parameters for Coadministered Drug in the Presence of Efavirenz

Coadministered Drug	Dose of Coadministered Drug (mg)	Efavirenz Dose (mg)	N	Mean % Change of Coadministered Drug Pharmacokinetic Parameters* (90% CI)		
				C_{max}	AUC	C_{min}
Bupropion	150 mg single dose (sustained-release)	600 mg qd × 14 days	13	↓ 34 (↓21 to ↓47)	↓ 55 (↓48 to ↓62)	NA
Hydroxybupropion				↑ 50 (↑ 20 to ↑ 80)	↔	NA
Sertraline	50 mg qd × 14 days	600 mg qd × 14 days	13	↓ 29 (↓ 15 to ↓ 40)	↓ 39 (↓ 27 to ↓ 50)	↓ 46 (↓ 31 to ↓ 58)
Voriconazole	400 mg po q12h × 1 day then 200 mg po q12h × 8 days	400 mg qd × 9 days	NA	↓ 61[a]	↓ 77[a]	NA
	300 mg po q12h days 2–7	300 mg qd × 7 days	NA	↓ 36[è] (↓ 21 to ↓ 49)	↓ 55[è] (↓ 45 to ↓ 62)	NA
	400 mg po q12h days 2–7	300 mg qd × 7 days	NA	↑ 23[è] (↓ 1 to ↑ 53)	↓ 7[è] (↓ 23 to ↑ 13)	NA

NA = not available
* Increase = ↑; Decrease = ↓; No Effect = ↔
† Compared with atazanavir 400 mg qd alone.
‡ Comparator dose of indinavir was 800 mg q8h × 10 days.
§ Parallel-group design; N for efavirenz + lopinavir/ritonavir, N for lopinavir/ritonavir alone.
¶ Values are for lopinavir. The pharmacokinetics of ritonavir 100 mg q12h are unaffected by concurrent efavirenz.
# 95% CI
Þ Soft Gelatin Capsule
ß Not available because of insufficient data.
à 90% CI not available
è Relative to steady-state administration of voriconazole (400 mg for 1 day, then 200 mg po q12h for 2 days).

Table 7: Drug Interactions: Changes in Pharmacokinetic Parameters for Tenofovir in the Presence of the Coadministered Drug*,†

Coadministered Drug	Dose of Coadministered Drug (mg)	N	Mean % Change of Tenofovir Pharmacokinetic Parameters‡ (90% CI)		
			C_{max}	AUC	C_{min}
Atazanavir§	400 once daily × 14 days	33	↑ 14 (↑ 8 to ↑ 20)	↑ 24 (↑ 21 to ↑ 28)	↑ 22 (↑ 15 to ↑ 30)
Atazanavir/ ritonavir§	300/100 once daily	12	↑ 34 (↑ 20 to ↑ 51)	↑ 37 (↑ 30 to ↑ 45)	↑ 29 (↑ 21 to ↑ 36)
Darunavir/ ritonavir¶	300/100 twice daily	12	↑ 24 (↑ 8 to ↑ 42)	↑ 22 (↑ 10 to ↑ 35)	↑ 37 (↑ 19 to ↑ 57)
Didanosine#	250 or 400 once daily × 7 days	14	↔	↔	↔
Lopinavir/ ritonavir	400/100 twice daily × 14 days	24	↔	↑ 32 (↑ 25 to ↑ 38)	↑ 51 (↑ 37 to ↑ 66)
Tipranavir/ ritonavirÞ	500/100 twice daily	22	↓ 23 (↓ 32 to ↓ 13)	↓ 2 (↓ 9 to ↑ 5)	↑ 7 (↓ 2 to ↑ 17)
	750/200 twice daily (23 doses)	20	↓ 38 (↓ 46 to ↓ 29)	↑ 2 (↓ 6 to ↑ 10)	↑ 14 (↑ 1 to ↑ 27)

* All interaction trials conducted in healthy volunteers.
† Subjects received tenofovir DF 300 mg once daily.
‡ Increase = ↑; Decrease = ↓; No Effect = ↔
§ Reyataz Prescribing Information.
¶ Prezista Prescribing Information.
# Subjects received didanosine buffered tablets.
Þ Aptivus Prescribing Information.

- Have ever had seizures or are taking medicine for seizures.

What important information should I know about taking other medicines with ATRIPLA (efavirenz/emtricitabine/tenofovir disoproxil fumarate)?

ATRIPLA may change the effect of other medicines, including the ones for HIV-1, and may cause serious side effects. Your healthcare provider may change your other medicines or change their doses. Other medicines, including herbal products, may affect ATRIPLA. For this reason, **it is very important to** let all your healthcare providers and pharmacists know what medications, herbal supplements, or vitamins you are taking.

MEDICINES YOU SHOULD NOT TAKE WITH ATRIPLA

- The following medicines may cause serious and life-threatening side effects when taken with ATRIPLA. You should not take any of these medicines while taking ATRIPLA: Vascor (bepridil), Propulsid (cisapride), Versed (midazolam), Orap (pimozide), Halcion (triazolam), ergot medications (for example, Wigraine and Cafergot).
- ATRIPLA also should not be used with Combivir (lamivudine/zidovudine), COMPLERA®, EMTRIVA, Epivir, Epivir-HBV (lamivudine), Epzicom (abacavir sulfate/lamivudine), STRIBILD® Trizivir (abacavir sulfate/lamivudine/zidovudine), TRUVADA, or VIREAD. ATRIPLA also should not be used with SUSTIVA unless recommended by your healthcare provider.
- Vfend (voriconazole) should not be taken with ATRIPLA since it may lose its effect or may increase the chance of having side effects from ATRIPLA.
- **Do not take St. John's wort (***Hypericum perforatum***), or products containing St. John's wort with ATRIPLA.** St. John's wort is an herbal product sold as a dietary supplement. Talk with your healthcare provider if you are taking or are planning to take St. John's wort. Taking St. John's wort may decrease ATRIPLA levels and lead to increased viral load and possible resistance to ATRIPLA or cross-resistance to other anti-HIV-1 drugs.
- ATRIPLA should not be used with HEPSERA® (adefovir dipivoxil).

It is also important to tell your healthcare provider if you are taking any of the following:

- Fortovase, Invirase (saquinavir), Biaxin (clarithromycin), Noxafil (posaconazole), Sporanox (itraconazole), or Victrelis (boceprevir); **these medicines may need to be replaced with another medicine when taken with ATRIPLA.**
- Calcium channel blockers such as Cardizem or Tiazac (diltiazem), Covera HS or Isoptin (verapamil) and others; Crixivan (indinavir), Selzentry (maraviroc); the immunosuppressant medicines cyclosporine (Gengraf, Neoral, Sandimmune, and others), Prograf (tacrolimus), or Rapamune (sirolimus); Methadone; Mycobutin (rifabutin); Rifampin; cholesterol-lowering medicines such as Lipitor (atorvastatin), Pravachol (pravastatin sodium), and Zocor (simvastatin); or the anti-depressant medications bupropion (Wellbutrin, Wellbutrin SR, Wellbutrin XL, and Zyban) or Zoloft (sertraline); **dose changes may be needed when these drugs are taken with ATRIPLA.**
- Videx, Videx EC (didanosine); tenofovir DF (a component of ATRIPLA) may increase the amount of didanosine in your blood, which could result in more side effects. **You may need to be monitored more carefully** if you are taking ATRIPLA and didanosine together. Also, the dose of didanosine may need to be changed.
- Reyataz (atazanavir sulfate), Prezista (darunavir) with Norvir (ritonavir), or Kaletra (lopinavir/ritonavir); these medicines may increase the amount of tenofovir DF (a component of ATRIPLA) in your blood, which could result in more side effects. Reyataz is not recommended with ATRIPLA. **You may need to be monitored more carefully** if you are taking ATRIPLA, Prezista, and Norvir together, or if you are taking ATRIPLA and Kaletra together. Also, the dose of Kaletra may need to be changed.
- Medicine for seizures [for example, Dilantin (phenytoin), Tegretol (carbamazepine), or phenobarbital]; your healthcare provider may want to switch you to another medicine or check drug levels in your blood from time to time.

These are not all the medicines that may cause problems if you take ATRIPLA. Be sure to tell your healthcare provider about all medicines that you take.

Keep a complete list of all the prescription and nonprescription medicines as well as any herbal remedies that you are taking, how much you take, and how often you take them. Make a new list when medicines or herbal remedies are added or stopped, or if the dose changes. Give copies of this list to all of your healthcare providers and pharmacists **every** time you visit your healthcare provider or fill a prescription. This will give your healthcare provider a complete picture of the medicines you use. Then he or she can decide the best approach for your situation.

How should I take ATRIPLA?

- Take the exact amount of ATRIPLA your healthcare provider prescribes. Never change the dose on your own. Do not stop this medicine unless your healthcare provider tells you to stop.
- You should take ATRIPLA on an empty stomach.

Table 8: Drug Interactions: Changes in Pharmacokinetic Parameters for Coadministered Drug in the Presence of Tenofovir Disoproxil Fumarate[*,†]

Coadministered Drug	Dose of Coadministered Drug (mg)	N	Mean % Change of Coadministered Drug Pharmacokinetic Parameters[‡] (90% CI)		
			C_{max}	AUC	C_{min}
Atazanavir[§]	400 once daily × 14 days	34	↓ 21 (↓ 27 to ↓ 14)	↓ 25 (↓ 30 to ↓ 19)	↓ 40 (↓ 48 to ↓ 32)
	Atazanavir/ritonavir 300/100 once daily × 42 days	10	↓ 28 (↓ 50 to ↑ 5)	↓ 25[¶] (↓ 42 to ↓ 3)	↓ 23[¶] (↓ 46 to ↑ 10)
Darunavir[#]	Darunavir/ritonavir 300/100 mg once daily	12	↑ 16 (↓ 6 to ↑ 42)	↑ 21 (↓ 5 to ↑ 54)	↑ 24 (↓ 10 to ↑ 69)
Didanosine[Þ]	250 once, simultaneously with tenofovir DF and a light meal[ß]	33	↓ 20[à] (↓ 32 to ↓ 7)	↔[à]	NA
Lopinavir	Lopinavir/ritonavir 400/100 twice daily × 14 days	24	↔	↔	↔
Ritonavir	Lopinavir/ritonavir 400/100 twice daily × 14 days	24	↔	↔	↔
Tipranavir[è]	Tipranavir/ritonavir 500/100 twice daily	22	↓ 17 (↓ 26 to ↓ 6)	↓ 18 (↓ 25 to ↓ 9)	↓ 21 (↓ 30 to ↓ 10)
	Tipranavir/ritonavir 750/200 twice daily (23 doses)	20	↓ 11 (↓ 16 to ↓ 4)	↓ 9 (↓ 15 to ↓ 3)	↓ 12 (↓ 22 to 0)

* All interaction trials conducted in healthy volunteers.
† Subjects received tenofovir DF 300 mg once daily.
‡ Increase = ↑; Decrease = ↓; No Effect = ↔
§ Reyataz Prescribing Information.
¶ In HIV-infected patients, addition of tenofovir DF to atazanavir 300 mg plus ritonavir 100 mg, resulted in AUC and C_{min} values of atazanavir that were 2.3- and 4-fold higher than the respective values observed for atazanavir 400 mg when given alone.
# Prezista Prescribing Information.
Þ Videx EC Prescribing Information. Subjects received didanosine enteric-coated capsules.
ß 373 kcal, 8.2 g fat.
à Compared with didanosine (enteric-coated) 400 mg administered alone under fasting conditions.
è Aptivus Prescribing Information.

Table 9: Outcomes of Randomized Treatment at Weeks 48 and 144 (Study 934)

Outcomes	At Week 48		At Week 144	
	FTC + TDF + EFV (N=244)	AZT/3TC + EFV (N=243)	FTC + TDF + EFV (N=227)*	AZT/3TC + EFV (N=229)*
Responder[†]	84%	73%	71%	58%
Virologic failure[‡]	2%	4%	3%	6%
Rebound	1%	3%	2%	5%
Never suppressed	0%	0%	0%	0%
Change in antiretroviral regimen	1%	1%	1%	1%
Death	<1%	1%	1%	1%
Discontinued due to adverse event	4%	9%	5%	12%
Discontinued for other reasons[§]	10%	14%	20%	22%

* Subjects who were responders at Week 48 or Week 96 (HIV-1 RNA <400 copies/mL) but did not consent to continue trial after Week 48 or Week 96 were excluded from analysis.
† Subjects achieved and maintained confirmed HIV-1 RNA <400 copies/mL through Weeks 48 and 144.
‡ Includes confirmed viral rebound and failure to achieve confirmed HIV-1 RNA <400 copies/mL through Weeks 48 and 144.
§ Includes lost to follow-up, patient withdrawal, noncompliance, protocol violation and other reasons.

- Swallow ATRIPLA (efavirenz/emtricitabine/tenofovir disoproxil fumarate) with water.
- Taking ATRIPLA at bedtime may make some side effects less bothersome.
- Do not miss a dose of ATRIPLA. If you forget to take ATRIPLA, take the missed dose right away, unless it is almost time for your next dose. Do not double the next dose. Carry on with your regular dosing schedule. If you need help in planning the best times to take your medicine, ask your healthcare provider or pharmacist.

- If you believe you took more than the prescribed amount of ATRIPLA (efavirenz/emtricitabine/tenofovir disoproxil fumarate), contact your local poison control center or emergency room right away.
- Tell your healthcare provider if you start any new medicine or change how you take old ones. Your doses may need adjustment.
- When your ATRIPLA supply starts to run low, get more from your healthcare provider or pharmacy. This is very important because the amount of virus in your blood may

increase if the medicine is stopped for even a short time. The virus may develop resistance to ATRIPLA and become harder to treat.

- Your healthcare provider may want to do blood tests to check for certain side effects while you take ATRIPLA (efavirenz/emtricitabine/tenofovir disoproxil fumarate).

What should I avoid while taking ATRIPLA?

- **Women should not become pregnant while taking ATRIPLA and for 12 weeks after stopping it.** Serious birth defects have been seen in the babies of animals and women treated with efavirenz (a component of ATRIPLA) during pregnancy. It is not known whether efavirenz caused these defects. **Tell your healthcare provider right away if you are pregnant.** Also talk with your healthcare provider if you want to become pregnant.
- Women should not rely only on hormone-based birth control, such as pills, injections, or implants, because ATRIPLA may make these contraceptives ineffective. Women must use a reliable form of barrier contraception, such as a condom or diaphragm, even if they also use other methods of birth control. Efavirenz, a component of ATRIPLA, may remain in your blood for a time after therapy is stopped. Therefore, you should continue to use contraceptive measures for 12 weeks after you stop taking ATRIPLA.
- **Do not breastfeed if you are taking ATRIPLA.** Some of the medicines in ATRIPLA can be passed to your baby in your breast milk. We do not know whether it could harm your baby. Also, mothers with HIV-1 should not breastfeed because HIV-1 can be passed to the baby in the breast milk. Talk with your healthcare provider if you are breastfeeding. You should stop breastfeeding or may need to use a different medicine.
- Taking ATRIPLA with alcohol or other medicines causing similar side effects as ATRIPLA, such as drowsiness, may increase those side effects.
- Do not take any other medicines, including prescription and nonprescription medicines and herbal products, without checking with your healthcare provider.
- Avoid doing things that can spread HIV-1 to others.
  - **Do not share needles or other injection equipment.**
  - **Do not share personal items that can have blood or body fluids on them, like toothbrushes and razor blades.**
  - **Do not have any kind of sex without protection.** Always practice safe sex by using a latex or polyurethane condom to lower the chance of sexual contact with semen, vaginal secretions, or blood.

What are the possible side effects of ATRIPLA?
ATRIPLA may cause the following serious side effects:

- **Lactic acidosis** (buildup of an acid in the blood). Lactic acidosis can be a medical emergency and may need to be treated in the hospital. **Call your healthcare provider right away if you get signs of lactic acidosis.** (See "What is the most important information I should know about ATRIPLA?")
- **Serious liver problems (hepatotoxicity),** with liver enlargement (hepatomegaly) and fat in the liver (steatosis). Call your healthcare provider right away if you get any signs of liver problems. (See "What is the most important information I should know about ATRIPLA?")
- **"Flare-ups" of hepatitis B virus (HBV) infection,** in which the disease suddenly returns in a worse way than before, can occur if you have HBV and you stop taking ATRIPLA. Your healthcare provider will monitor your condition for several months after stopping ATRIPLA if you have both HIV-1 and HBV infection and may recommend treatment for your HBV. ATRIPLA is not approved for the treatment of hepatitis B virus infection. If you have advanced liver disease and stop treatment with ATRIPLA, the "flare-up" of hepatitis B may cause your liver function to decline.
- **Serious psychiatric problems.** A small number of patients may experience severe depression, strange thoughts, or angry behavior while taking ATRIPLA. Some patients have thoughts of suicide and a few have actually committed suicide. These problems may occur more often in patients who have had mental illness. Contact your healthcare provider right away if you think you are having these psychiatric symptoms, so your healthcare provider can decide if you should continue to take ATRIPLA.
- **Kidney problems** (including decline or failure of kidney function). If you have had kidney problems in the past or take other medicines that can cause kidney problems, your healthcare provider should do regular blood tests to check your kidneys. Symptoms that may be related to kidney problems include a high volume of urine, thirst, muscle pain, and muscle weakness.
- **Other serious liver problems.** Some patients have experienced serious liver problems including liver problems resulting in transplantation or death. Most of these serious side effects occurred in patients with a chronic liver disease such as hepatitis infection, but there have also been a few reports in patients without any existing liver disease.
- **Changes in bone mineral density (thinning bones).** Laboratory tests show changes in the bones of patients treated

with tenofovir DF, a component of ATRIPLA (efavirenz/emtricitabine/tenofovir disoproxil fumarate). Some HIV patients treated with tenofovir DF developed thinning of the bones (osteopenia) which could lead to fractures. If you have had bone problems in the past, your healthcare provider may need to do tests to check your bone mineral density or may prescribe medicines to help your bone mineral density. Additionally, bone pain and softening of the bone (which may contribute to fractures) may occur as a consequence of kidney problems.

Common side effects:
Patients may have dizziness, headache, trouble sleeping, drowsiness, trouble concentrating, and/or unusual dreams during treatment with ATRIPLA. These side effects may be reduced if you take ATRIPLA at bedtime on an empty stomach. They also tend to go away after you have taken the medicine for a few weeks. If you have these common side effects, such as dizziness, it does not mean that you will also have serious psychiatric problems, such as severe depression, strange thoughts, or angry behavior. Tell your healthcare provider right away if any of these side effects continue or if they bother you. It is possible that these symptoms may be more severe if ATRIPLA is used with alcohol or mood altering (street) drugs.
If you are dizzy, have trouble concentrating, or are drowsy, avoid activities that may be dangerous, such as driving or operating machinery.
Rash may be common. Rashes usually go away without any change in treatment. In a small number of patients, rash may be serious. If you develop a rash, call your healthcare provider right away. **Rash may be a serious problem in some children.** Tell your child's healthcare provider right away if you notice rash or any other side effects while your child is taking ATRIPLA.
Other common side effects include tiredness, upset stomach, vomiting, gas, and diarrhea.

Other possible side effects with ATRIPLA:

- Changes in body fat. Changes in body fat develop in some patients taking anti HIV-1 medicine. These changes may include an increased amount of fat in the upper back and neck ("buffalo hump"), in the breasts, and around the trunk. Loss of fat from the legs, arms, and face may also happen. The cause and long-term health effects of these fat changes are not known.
- Skin discoloration (small spots or freckles) may also happen with ATRIPLA.
- In some patients with advanced HIV infection (AIDS), signs and symptoms of inflammation from previous infections may occur soon after anti-HIV treatment is started. It is believed that these symptoms are due to an improvement in the body's immune response, enabling the body to fight infections that may have been present with no obvious symptoms. If you notice any symptoms of infection, please inform your doctor immediately.
- Additional side effects are inflammation of the pancreas, allergic reaction (including swelling of the face, lips, tongue, or throat), shortness of breath, pain, stomach pain, weakness and indigestion.

Tell your healthcare provider or pharmacist if you notice any side effects while taking ATRIPLA.
Contact your healthcare provider before stopping ATRIPLA because of side effects or for any other reason.
This is not a complete list of side effects possible with ATRIPLA. Ask your healthcare provider or pharmacist for a more complete list of side effects of ATRIPLA and all the medicines you will take.

How do I store ATRIPLA?

- **Keep ATRIPLA and all other medicines out of reach of children.**
- Store ATRIPLA at room temperature 77 °F (25 °C).
- Keep ATRIPLA in its original container and keep the container tightly closed.
- Do not keep medicine that is out of date or that you no longer need. If you throw any medicines away make sure that children will not find them.

General information about ATRIPLA:
Medicines are sometimes prescribed for conditions that are not mentioned in patient information leaflets. Do not use ATRIPLA for a condition for which it was not prescribed. Do not give ATRIPLA to other people, even if they have the same symptoms you have. It may harm them.
This leaflet summarizes the most important information about ATRIPLA. If you would like more information, talk with your healthcare provider. You can ask your healthcare provider or pharmacist for information about ATRIPLA that is written for health professionals.
Do not use ATRIPLA if the seal over bottle opening is broken or missing.

What are the ingredients of ATRIPLA?
Active Ingredients: efavirenz, emtricitabine, and tenofovir disoproxil fumarate
Inactive Ingredients: croscarmellose sodium, hydroxypropyl cellulose, microcrystalline cellulose, magnesium stea-

rate, sodium lauryl sulfate. The film coating contains black iron oxide, polyethylene glycol, polyvinyl alcohol, red iron oxide, talc, and titanium dioxide.
October 2013
ATRIPLA (efavirenz/emtricitabine/tenofovir disoproxil fumarate) is a trademark of Bristol-Myers Squibb & Gilead Sciences, LLC. COMPLERA, EMTRIVA, HEPSERA, STRIBILD, TRUVADA, and VIREAD are trademarks of Gilead Sciences, Inc., or its related companies. SUSTIVA is a trademark of Bristol-Myers Squibb Pharma Company. Reyataz and Videx are trademarks of Bristol-Myers Squibb Company. Pravachol is a trademark of ER Squibb & Sons, LLC. Other brands listed are the trademarks of their respective owners.
21-937-GS-013
Shown in Product Identification Guide, page 306

BARACLUDE®   ℞
[*BEAR ah klude*]
(entecavir)
tablets, for oral use
BARACLUDE®
(entecavir)
oral solution

HIGHLIGHTS OF PRESCRIBING INFORMATION
These highlights do not include all the information needed to use BARACLUDE safely and effectively. See full prescribing information for BARACLUDE.
BARACLUDE® (entecavir) tablets, for oral use
BARACLUDE® (entecavir) oral solution
Initial U.S. Approval: 2005

WARNING: SEVERE ACUTE EXACERBATIONS OF HEPATITIS B, PATIENTS CO-INFECTED WITH HIV AND HBV, and LACTIC ACIDOSIS AND HEPATOMEGALY
See full prescribing information for complete boxed warning.

- **Severe acute exacerbations of hepatitis B have been reported in patients who have discontinued anti-hepatitis B therapy, including entecavir. Hepatic function should be monitored closely for at least several months after discontinuation. Initiation of anti-hepatitis B therapy may be warranted. (5.1)**
- **BARACLUDE is not recommended for patients co-infected with human immunodeficiency virus (HIV) and hepatitis B virus (HBV) who are not also receiving highly active antiretroviral therapy (HAART), because of the potential for the development of resistance to HIV nucleoside reverse transcriptase inhibitors. (5.2)**
- **Lactic acidosis and severe hepatomegaly with steatosis, including fatal cases, have been reported with the use of nucleoside analogue inhibitors. (5.3)**

———RECENT MAJOR CHANGES———
Indications and Usage (1)   3/2014
Dosage and Administration
  Recommended Dosage in Pediatric Patients (2.3) 3/2014
  Renal Impairment (2.4)   3/2014

———INDICATIONS AND USAGE———
BARACLUDE is a hepatitis B virus nucleoside analogue reverse transcriptase inhibitor indicated for the treatment of chronic hepatitis B virus infection in adults and children at least 2 years of age with evidence of active viral replication and either evidence of persistent elevations in serum aminotransferases (ALT or AST) or histologically active disease. (1)

———DOSAGE AND ADMINISTRATION———

- Nucleoside-inhibitor-treatment-naïve with compensated liver disease (greater than or equal to 16 years old): 0.5 mg once daily. (2.2)
- Nucleoside-inhibitor-treatment-naïve and lamivudine-experienced pediatric patients at least 2 years of age and weighing at least 10 kg: dosing is based on weight. (2.3)
- Lamivudine-refractory or known lamivudine or telbivudine resistance substitutions (greater than or equal to 16 years old): 1 mg once daily. (2.2)
- Decompensated liver disease (adults): 1 mg once daily. (2.2)
- Renal impairment: Dosage adjustment is recommended if creatinine clearance is less than 50 mL/min. (2.4)
- BARACLUDE should be administered on an empty stomach. (2.1)

———DOSAGE FORMS AND STRENGTHS———

- Tablets: 0.5 mg and 1 mg (3, 16)
- Oral solution: 0.05 mg/mL (3, 16)

———CONTRAINDICATIONS———

- None. (4)

WARNINGS AND PRECAUTIONS

- Severe acute exacerbations of hepatitis B virus infection after discontinuation: Monitor hepatic function closely for at least several months. (5.1, 6.1)
- Co-infection with HIV: BARACLUDE (entecavir) is not recommended unless the patient is also receiving HAART. (5.2)
- Lactic acidosis and severe hepatomegaly with steatosis: If suspected, treatment should be suspended. (5.3)

ADVERSE REACTIONS

- Most common adverse reactions (≥3%, all severity grades) are headache, fatigue, dizziness, and nausea. (6.1)

To report SUSPECTED ADVERSE REACTIONS, contact Bristol-Myers Squibb at 1-800-721-5072 or FDA at 1-800-FDA-1088 or www.fda.gov/medwatch

USE IN SPECIFIC POPULATIONS

- Nursing mothers: Discontinue nursing or BARACLUDE taking into consideration the importance of BARACLUDE to the mother. (8.3)
- Liver transplant recipients: Limited data on safety and efficacy are available. (8.8)

See 17 for PATIENT COUNSELING INFORMATION and FDA-approved patient labeling

Revised: 05/2014

FULL PRESCRIBING INFORMATION: CONTENTS*

WARNING: SEVERE ACUTE EXACERBATIONS OF HEPATITIS B, PATIENTS CO-INFECTED WITH HIV AND HBV, and LACTIC ACIDOSIS AND HEPATO-MEGALY

FULL PRESCRIBING INFORMATION

WARNING: SEVERE ACUTE EXACERBATIONS OF HEPATITIS B, PATIENTS CO-INFECTED WITH HIV AND HBV, and LACTIC ACIDOSIS AND HEPATOMEGALY

Severe acute exacerbations of hepatitis B have been reported in patients who have discontinued anti-hepatitis B therapy, including entecavir. Hepatic function should be monitored closely with both clinical and laboratory follow-up for at least several months in patients who discontinue anti-hepatitis B therapy. If appropriate, initiation of anti-hepatitis B therapy may be warranted [see Warnings and Precautions (5.1)].

Limited clinical experience suggests there is a potential for the development of resistance to HIV (human immunodeficiency virus) nucleoside reverse transcriptase inhibitors if BARACLUDE is used to treat chronic hepatitis B virus (HBV) infection in patients with HIV infection that is not being treated. Therapy with BARACLUDE is not recommended for HIV/HBV co-infected patients who are not also receiving highly active antiretroviral therapy (HAART) [see Warnings and Precautions (5.2)].

Lactic acidosis and severe hepatomegaly with steatosis, including fatal cases, have been reported with the use of nucleoside analogue inhibitors alone or in combination with antiretrovirals [see Warnings and Precautions (5.3)].

1   INDICATIONS AND USAGE

BARACLUDE® (entecavir) is indicated for the treatment of chronic hepatitis B virus infection in adults and pediatric patients 2 years of age and older with evidence of active viral replication and either evidence of persistent elevations in serum aminotransferases (ALT or AST) or histologically active disease.

The following points should be considered when initiating therapy with BARACLUDE:
- In adult patients, this indication is based on clinical trial data in nucleoside-inhibitor-treatment-naïve and lamivudine-resistant subjects with HBeAg-positive and HBeAg-negative HBV infection and compensated liver disease and a more limited number of subjects with decompensated liver disease [see Clinical Studies (14.1)].
- In pediatric patients 2 years of age and older, this indication is based on clinical trial data in nucleoside-inhibitor-treatment-naïve and in a limited number of lamivudine-experienced subjects with HBeAg-positive chronic HBV infection and compensated liver disease [see Clinical Studies (14.2)].

2   DOSAGE AND ADMINISTRATION

2.1   Timing of Administration

BARACLUDE should be administered on an empty stomach (at least 2 hours after a meal and 2 hours before the next meal).

2.2   Recommended Dosage in Adults

Compensated Liver Disease

The recommended dose of BARACLUDE for chronic hepatitis B virus infection in nucleoside-inhibitor-treatment-naïve adults and adolescents 16 years of age and older is 0.5 mg once daily.

The recommended dose of BARACLUDE in adults and adolescents (at least 16 years of age) with a history of hepatitis B viremia while receiving lamivudine or known lamivudine or telbivudine resistance substitutions rtM204I/V with or without rtL180M, rtL80I/V, or rtV173L is 1 mg once daily.

Decompensated Liver Disease

The recommended dose of BARACLUDE for chronic hepatitis B virus infection in adults with decompensated liver disease is 1 mg once daily.

2.3   Recommended Dosage in Pediatric Patients

Table 1 describes the recommended dose of BARACLUDE for pediatric patients 2 years of age or older and weighing at least 10 kg. The oral solution should be used for patients with body weight up to 30 kg.

Table 1: Dosing Schedule for Pediatric Patients

| Body Weight (kg) | Recommended Once-Daily Dose of Oral Solution (mL) | |
	Treatment-Naïve Patients[a]	Lamivudine-Experienced Patients[b]
10 to 11	3	6
greater than 11 to 14	4	8
greater than 14 to 17	5	10
greater than 17 to 20	6	12
greater than 20 to 23	7	14
greater than 23 to 26	8	16
greater than 26 to 30	9	18
greater than 30	10	20

[a] Children with body weight greater than 30 kg should receive 10 mL (0.5 mg) of oral solution or one 0.5 mg tablet once daily.
[b] Children with body weight greater than 30 kg should receive 20 mL (1 mg) of oral solution or one 1 mg tablet once daily.

2.4   Renal Impairment

In adult subjects with renal impairment, the apparent oral clearance of entecavir decreased as creatinine clearance decreased [see Clinical Pharmacology (12.3)]. Dosage adjust-

ment is recommended for patients with creatinine clearance less than 50 mL/min, including patients on hemodialysis or continuous ambulatory peritoneal dialysis (CAPD), as shown in Table 2. The once-daily dosing regimens are preferred.

Table 2: Recommended Dosage of BARACLUDE in Adult Patients with Renal Impairment

Creatinine Clearance (mL/min)	Usual Dose (0.5 mg)	Lamivudine-Refractory or Decompensated Liver Disease (1 mg)
50 or greater	0.5 mg once daily	1 mg once daily
30 to less than 50	0.25 mg once daily[a] OR 0.5 mg every 48 hours	0.5 mg once daily OR 1 mg every 48 hours
10 to less than 30	0.15 mg once daily[a] OR 0.5 mg every 72 hours	0.3 mg once daily[a] OR 1 mg every 72 hours
Less than 10 Hemodialysis[b] or CAPD	0.05 mg once daily[a] OR 0.5 mg every 7 days	0.1 mg once daily[a] OR 1 mg every 7 days

[a] For doses less than 0.5 mg, BARACLUDE Oral Solution is recommended.
[b] If administered on a hemodialysis day, administer BARACLUDE after the hemodialysis session.

Although there are insufficient data to recommend a specific dose adjustment of BARACLUDE (entecavir) in pediatric patients with renal impairment, a reduction in the dose or an increase in the dosing interval similar to adjustments for adults should be considered.

2.5   Hepatic Impairment

No dosage adjustment is necessary for patients with hepatic impairment.

2.6   Duration of Therapy

The optimal duration of treatment with BARACLUDE for patients with chronic hepatitis B virus infection and the relationship between treatment and long-term outcomes such as cirrhosis and hepatocellular carcinoma are unknown.

3   DOSAGE FORMS AND STRENGTHS

- BARACLUDE 0.5 mg film-coated tablets are white to off-white, triangular-shaped, and debossed with "BMS" on one side and "1611" on the other side.
- BARACLUDE 1 mg film-coated tablets are pink, triangular-shaped, and debossed with "BMS" on one side and "1612" on the other side.
- BARACLUDE oral solution, 0.05 mg/mL, is a ready-to-use, orange-flavored, clear, colorless to pale yellow, aqueous solution. Ten milliliters of the oral solution provides a 0.5 mg dose and 20 mL provides a 1 mg dose of entecavir.

4   CONTRAINDICATIONS

None.

5   WARNINGS AND PRECAUTIONS

5.1   Severe Acute Exacerbations of Hepatitis B

Severe acute exacerbations of hepatitis B have been reported in patients who have discontinued anti-hepatitis B therapy, including entecavir [see Adverse Reactions (6.1)]. Hepatic function should be monitored closely with both clinical and laboratory follow-up for at least several months in patients who discontinue anti-hepatitis B therapy. If appropriate, initiation of anti-hepatitis B therapy may be warranted.

5.2   Patients Co-infected with HIV and HBV

BARACLUDE has not been evaluated in HIV/HBV co-infected patients who were not simultaneously receiving effective HIV treatment. Limited clinical experience suggests there is a potential for the development of resistance to HIV nucleoside reverse transcriptase inhibitors if BARACLUDE is used to treat chronic hepatitis B virus infection in patients with HIV infection that is not being treated [see Microbiology (12.4)]. Therefore, therapy with BARACLUDE is not recommended for HIV/HBV co-infected patients who are not also receiving HAART. Before initiating BARACLUDE therapy, HIV antibody testing should be offered to all patients. BARACLUDE has not been studied as a treatment for HIV infection and is not recommended for this use.

5.3   Lactic Acidosis and Severe Hepatomegaly with Steatosis

Lactic acidosis and severe hepatomegaly with steatosis, including fatal cases, have been reported with the use of nucleoside analogue inhibitors, alone or in combination with antiretrovirals. A majority of these cases have been in women. Obesity and prolonged nucleoside inhibitor exposure may be risk factors. Particular cau-

Table 3: Clinical Adverse Reactions[a] of Moderate-Severe Intensity (Grades 2–4) Reported in Four Entecavir Clinical Trials Through 2 Years

Body System/ Adverse Reaction	Nucleoside-Inhibitor-Naïve[b]		Lamivudine-Refractory[c]	
	BARACLUDE 0.5 mg n=679	Lamivudine 100 mg n=668	BARACLUDE 1 mg n=183	Lamivudine 100 mg n=190
Any Grade 2–4 adverse reaction[a]	15%	18%	22%	23%
Gastrointestinal				
Diarrhea	<1%	0	1%	0
Dyspepsia	<1%	<1%	1%	0
Nausea	<1%	<1%	<1%	2%
Vomiting	<1%	<1%	<1%	0
General				
Fatigue	1%	1%	3%	3%
Nervous System				
Headache	2%	2%	4%	1%
Dizziness	<1%	<1%	0	1%
Somnolence	<1%	<1%	0	0
Psychiatric				
Insomnia	<1%	<1%	0	<1%

[a] Includes events of possible, probable, certain, or unknown relationship to treatment regimen.
[b] Studies AI463022 and AI463027.
[c] Includes Study AI463014 and the BARACLUDE 1 mg and lamivudine treatment arms of Study AI463014, a Phase 2 multinational, randomized, double-blind study of three doses of BARACLUDE (0.1, 0.5, and 1 mg) once daily versus continued lamivudine 100 mg once daily for up to 52 weeks in subjects who experienced recurrent viremia on lamivudine therapy.

Table 4: Selected Treatment-Emergent[a] Laboratory Abnormalities Reported in Four Entecavir Clinical Trials Through 2 Years

Test	Nucleoside-Inhibitor-Naïve[b]		Lamivudine-Refractory[c]	
	BARACLUDE 0.5 mg n=679	Lamivudine 100 mg n=668	BARACLUDE 1 mg n=183	Lamivudine 100 mg n=190
Any Grade 3–4 laboratory abnormality[d]	35%	36%	37%	45%
ALT >10 × ULN and >2 × baseline	2%	4%	2%	11%
ALT >5 × ULN	11%	16%	12%	24%
Albumin <2.5 g/dL	<1%	<1%	0	2%
Total bilirubin >2.5 × ULN	2%	2%	3%	2%
Lipase ≥2.1 × ULN	7%	6%	7%	7%
Creatinine >3 × ULN	0	0	0	0
Confirmed creatinine increase ≥0.5 mg/dL	1%	1%	2%	1%
Hyperglycemia, fasting >250 mg/dL	2%	1%	3%	1%
Glycosuria[e]	4%	3%	4%	6%
Hematuria[f]	9%	10%	9%	6%
Platelets <50,000/mm³	<1%	<1%	<1%	<1%

[a] On-treatment value worsened from baseline to Grade 3 or Grade 4 for all parameters except albumin (any on-treatment value <2.5 g/dL), confirmed creatinine increase ≥0.5 mg/dL, and ALT >10 × ULN and >2 × baseline.
[b] Studies AI463022 and AI463027.
[c] Includes Study AI463026 and the BARACLUDE 1 mg and lamivudine treatment arms of Study AI463014, a Phase 2 multinational, randomized, double-blind study of three doses of BARACLUDE (0.1, 0.5, and 1 mg) once daily versus continued lamivudine 100 mg once daily for up to 52 weeks in subjects who experienced recurrent viremia on lamivudine therapy.
[d] Includes hematology, routine chemistries, renal and liver function tests, pancreatic enzymes, and urinalysis.
[e] Grade 3 = 3+, large, ≥500 mg/dL; Grade 4 = 4+, marked, severe.
[f] Grade 3 = 3+, large; Grade 4 = ≥4+, marked, severe, many.
ULN=upper limit of normal.

tion should be exercised when administering nucleoside analogue inhibitors to any patient with known risk factors for liver disease; however, cases have also been reported in patients with no known risk factors.

Lactic acidosis with BARACLUDE (entecavir) use has been reported, often in association with hepatic decompensation, other serious medical conditions, or drug exposures. Patients with decompensated liver disease may be at higher risk for lactic acidosis. Treatment with BARACLUDE should be suspended in any patient who develops clinical or laboratory findings suggestive of lactic acidosis or pronounced hepatotoxicity (which may include hepatomegaly and steatosis even in the absence of marked transaminase elevations).

6 ADVERSE REACTIONS

The following adverse reactions are discussed in other sections of the labeling:
• Exacerbations of hepatitis after discontinuation of treatment [see Boxed Warning, Warnings and Precautions (5.1)].
• Lactic acidosis and severe hepatomegaly with steatosis [see Boxed Warning, Warnings and Precautions (5.3)].

6.1 Clinical Trial Experience in Adults

Because clinical trials are conducted under widely varying conditions, adverse reaction rates observed in the clinical trials of a drug cannot be directly compared to rates in the clinical trials of another drug and may not reflect the rates observed in practice.

Compensated Liver Disease

Assessment of adverse reactions is based on four studies (AI463014, AI463022, AI463026, and AI463027) in which 1720 subjects with chronic hepatitis B virus infection and compensated liver disease received double-blind treatment with BARACLUDE 0.5 mg/day (n=679), BARACLUDE 1 mg/day (n=183), or lamivudine (n=858) for up to 2 years. Median duration of therapy was 69 weeks for BARACLUDE-treated subjects and 63 weeks for lamivudine-treated subjects in Studies AI463022 and AI463027 and 73 weeks for BARACLUDE-treated subjects and 51 weeks for lamivudine-treated subjects in Studies AI463026 and AI463014. The safety profiles of BARACLUDE (entecavir) and lamivudine were comparable in these studies.

The most common adverse reactions of any severity (≥3%) with at least a possible relation to study drug for BARACLUDE-treated subjects were headache, fatigue, dizziness, and nausea. The most common adverse reactions among lamivudine-treated subjects were headache, fatigue, and dizziness. One percent of BARACLUDE-treated sub-

jects in these four studies compared with 4% of lamivudine-treated subjects discontinued for adverse events or abnormal laboratory test results.

Clinical adverse reactions of moderate-severe intensity and considered at least possibly related to treatment occurring during therapy in four clinical studies in which BARACLUDE was compared with lamivudine are presented in Table 3.
[See table 3 above]

Laboratory Abnormalities

Frequencies of selected treatment-emergent laboratory abnormalities reported during therapy in four clinical trials of BARACLUDE (entecavir) compared with lamivudine are listed in Table 4.
[See table 4 above]

Among BARACLUDE-treated subjects in these studies, on-treatment ALT elevations greater than 10 times the upper limit of normal (ULN) and greater than 2 times baseline generally resolved with continued treatment. A majority of these exacerbations were associated with a ≥2 log₁₀/mL reduction in viral load that preceded or coincided with the ALT elevation. Periodic monitoring of hepatic function is recommended during treatment.

Exacerbations of Hepatitis after Discontinuation of Treatment

An exacerbation of hepatitis or ALT flare was defined as ALT greater than 10 times ULN and greater than 2 times the subject's reference level (minimum of the baseline or last measurement at end of dosing). For all subjects who discontinued treatment (regardless of reason), Table 5 presents the proportion of subjects in each study who experienced post-treatment ALT flares. In these studies, a subset of subjects was allowed to discontinue treatment at or after 52 weeks if they achieved a protocol-defined response to therapy. If BARACLUDE is discontinued without regard to treatment response, the rate of post-treatment flares could be higher. [See Warnings and Precautions (5.1).]

Table 5: Exacerbations of Hepatitis During Off-Treatment Follow-up, Subjects in Studies AI463022, AI463027, and AI463026

	Subjects with ALT Elevations >10 × ULN and >2 × Reference[a]	
	BARACLUDE	Lamivudine
Nucleoside-inhibitor-naïve		
HBeAg-positive	4/174 (2%)	13/147 (9%)
HBeAg-negative	24/302 (8%)	30/270 (11%)
Lamivudine-refractory	6/52 (12%)	0/16

[a] Reference is the minimum of the baseline or last measurement at end of dosing. Median time to off-treatment exacerbation was 23 weeks for BARACLUDE-treated subjects and 10 weeks for lamivudine-treated subjects.

Decompensated Liver Disease

Study AI463048 was a randomized, open-label study of BARACLUDE 1 mg once daily versus adefovir dipivoxil 10 mg once daily given for up to 48 weeks in adult subjects with chronic HBV infection and evidence of hepatic decompensation, defined as a Child-Turcotte-Pugh (CTP) score of 7 or higher [see Clinical Studies (14.1)]. Among the 102 subjects receiving BARACLUDE, the most common treatment-emergent adverse events of any severity, regardless of causality, occurring through Week 48 were peripheral edema (16%), ascites (15%), pyrexia (14%), hepatic encephalopathy (10%), and upper respiratory infection (10%). Clinical adverse reactions not listed in Table 3 that were observed through Week 48 include blood bicarbonate decreased (2%) and renal failure (<1%).

Eighteen of 102 (18%) subjects treated with BARACLUDE and 18/89 (20%) subjects treated with adefovir dipivoxil died during the first 48 weeks of therapy. The majority of deaths (11 in the BARACLUDE group and 16 in the adefovir dipivoxil group) were due to liver-related causes such as hepatic failure, hepatic encephalopathy, hepatorenal syndrome, and upper gastrointestinal hemorrhage. The rate of hepatocellular carcinoma (HCC) through Week 48 was 6% (6/102) for subjects treated with BARACLUDE and 8% (7/89) for subjects treated with adefovir dipivoxil. Five percent of subjects in either treatment arm discontinued therapy due to an adverse event through Week 48.

No subject in either treatment arm experienced an on-treatment hepatic flare (ALT >2 × baseline and >10 × ULN) through Week 48. Eleven of 102 (11%) subjects treated with BARACLUDE and 11/89 (13%) subjects treated with adefovir dipivoxil had a confirmed increase in serum creatinine of 0.5 mg/dL through Week 48.

HIV/HBV Co-infected

The safety profile of BARACLUDE 1 mg (n=51) in HIV/HBV co-infected subjects enrolled in Study AI463038 was similar to that of placebo (n=17) through 24 weeks of blinded treatment and similar to that seen in non-HIV infected subjects *[see Warnings and Precautions (5.2)]*.

Liver Transplant Recipients
Among 65 subjects receiving BARACLUDE (entecavir) in an open-label, post-liver transplant trial *[see Use in Specific Populations (8.8)]*, the frequency and nature of adverse events were consistent with those expected in patients who have received a liver transplant and the known safety profile of BARACLUDE (entecavir).

6.2 Clinical Trial Experience in Pediatric Subjects
Because clinical trials are conducted under widely varying conditions, adverse reaction rates observed in the clinical trials of a drug cannot be directly compared to rates in the clinical trials of another drug and may not reflect the rates observed in practice.

The safety of BARACLUDE in pediatric subjects 2 to less than 18 years of age is based on two ongoing clinical trials in subjects with chronic HBV infection (one Phase 2 pharmacokinetic trial [AI463028] and one Phase 3 trial [AI463189]). These trials provide experience in 168 HBeAg-positive subjects treated with BARACLUDE for a median duration of 72 weeks. The adverse reactions observed in pediatric subjects who received treatment with BARACLUDE were consistent with those observed in clinical trials of BARACLUDE in adults. Adverse drug reactions reported in greater than 1% of pediatric subjects included abdominal pain, rash events, poor palatability ("product taste abnormal"), nausea, diarrhea, and vomiting.

6.3 Postmarketing Experience
The following adverse reactions have been reported during postmarketing use of BARACLUDE. Because these reactions were reported voluntarily from a population of unknown size, it is not possible to reliably estimate their frequency or establish a causal relationship to BARACLUDE exposure.
Immune system disorders: Anaphylactoid reaction.
Metabolism and nutrition disorders: Lactic acidosis.
Hepatobiliary disorders: Increased transaminases.
Skin and subcutaneous tissue disorders: Alopecia, rash.

7 DRUG INTERACTIONS
Since entecavir is primarily eliminated by the kidneys *[see Clinical Pharmacology (12.3)]*, coadministration of BARACLUDE with drugs that reduce renal function or compete for active tubular secretion may increase serum concentrations of either entecavir or the coadministered drug. Coadministration of entecavir with lamivudine, adefovir dipivoxil, or tenofovir disoproxil fumarate did not result in significant drug interactions. The effects of coadministration of BARACLUDE with other drugs that are renally eliminated or are known to affect renal function have not been evaluated, and patients should be monitored closely for adverse events when BARACLUDE is coadministered with such drugs.

8 USE IN SPECIFIC POPULATIONS
8.1 Pregnancy
Pregnancy Category C
There are no adequate and well-controlled studies of BARACLUDE in pregnant women. Because animal reproduction studies are not always predictive of human response, BARACLUDE should be used during pregnancy only if the potential benefit justifies the potential risk to the fetus.

Antiretroviral Pregnancy Registry: To monitor fetal outcomes of pregnant women exposed to BARACLUDE, an **Antiretroviral Pregnancy Registry** has been established. Healthcare providers are encouraged to register patients by calling 1-800-258-4263.

Animal Data
Animal reproduction studies with entecavir in rats and rabbits revealed no evidence of teratogenicity. Developmental toxicity studies were performed in rats and rabbits. There were no signs of embryofetal or maternal toxicity when pregnant animals received oral entecavir at approximately 28 (rat) and 212 (rabbit) times the human exposure achieved at the highest recommended human dose of 1 mg/day. In rats, maternal toxicity, embryofetal toxicity (resorptions), lower fetal body weights, tail and vertebral malformations, reduced ossification (vertebrae, sternebrae, and phalanges), and extra lumbar vertebrae and ribs were observed at exposures 3100 times those in humans. In rabbits, embryofetal toxicity (resorptions), reduced ossification (hyoid), and an increased incidence of 13th rib were observed at exposures 883 times those in humans. In a peripostnatal study, no adverse effects on offspring occurred when rats received oral entecavir at exposures greater than 94 times those in humans.

8.2 Labor and Delivery
There are no studies in pregnant women and no data on the effect of BARACLUDE on transmission of HBV from mother to infant. Therefore, appropriate interventions should be used to prevent neonatal acquisition of HBV.

8.3 Nursing Mothers
It is not known whether BARACLUDE is excreted into human milk; however, entecavir is excreted into the milk of rats. Because many drugs are excreted into human milk and because of the potential for serious adverse reactions in nursing infants from BARACLUDE, a decision should be made to discontinue nursing or to discontinue BARACLUDE taking into consideration the importance of continued hepatitis B therapy to the mother and the known benefits of breastfeeding.

8.4 Pediatric Use
BARACLUDE (entecavir) was evaluated in two clinical trials of pediatric subjects 2 years of age and older with HBeAg-positive chronic HBV infection and compensated liver disease. The exposure of BARACLUDE in nucleoside-inhibitor-treatment-naive and lamivudine-experienced pediatric subjects 2 years of age and older with HBeAg-positive chronic HBV infection and compensated liver disease receiving 0.015 mg/kg (up to 0.5 mg once daily) or 0.03 mg/kg (up to 1 mg once daily), respectively, was evaluated in Study AI463028. Safety and efficacy of the selected dose in treatment-naive pediatric subjects were confirmed in Study AI463189, a randomized, placebo-controlled treatment trial *[see Indications and Usage (1), Dosage and Administration (2.3), Adverse Reactions (6.2), Clinical Pharmacology (12.3), and Clinical Studies (14.2)]*.

There are limited data available on the use of BARACLUDE in lamivudine-experienced pediatric patients; BARACLUDE should be used in these patients only if the potential benefit justifies the potential risk to the child. Since some pediatric patients may require long-term or even lifetime management of chronic active hepatitis B, consideration should be given to the impact of BARACLUDE on future treatment options *[see Microbiology (12.4)]*.

The efficacy and safety of BARACLUDE have not been established in patients less than 2 years of age. Use of BARACLUDE in this age group has not been evaluated because treatment of HBV in this age group is rarely required.

8.5 Geriatric Use
Clinical studies of BARACLUDE did not include sufficient numbers of subjects aged 65 years and over to determine whether they respond differently from younger subjects. Entecavir is substantially excreted by the kidney, and the risk of toxic reactions to this drug may be greater in patients with impaired renal function. Because elderly patients are more likely to have decreased renal function, care should be taken in dose selection, and it may be useful to monitor renal function *[see Dosage and Administration (2.4)]*.

8.6 Racial/Ethnic Groups
There are no significant racial differences in entecavir pharmacokinetics. The safety and efficacy of BARACLUDE 0.5 mg once daily were assessed in a single-arm, open-label trial of HBeAg-positive or -negative, nucleoside-inhibitor-naive, Black/African American (n=40) and Hispanic (n=6) subjects with chronic HBV infection. In this trial, 76% of subjects were male, the mean age was 42 years, 57% were HBeAg-positive, the mean baseline HBV DNA was 7.0 $\log_{10}$ IU/mL, and the mean baseline ALT was 162 U/L. At Week 48 of treatment, 32 of 46 (70%) subjects had HBV DNA <50 IU/mL (approximately 300 copies/mL), 31 of 46 (67%) subjects had ALT normalization ($\leq 1 \times$ ULN), and 12 of 26 (46%) HBeAg-positive subjects had HBe seroconversion. Safety data were similar to those observed in the larger controlled clinical trials.

Because of low enrollment, safety and efficacy have not been established in the US Hispanic population.

8.7 Renal Impairment
Dosage adjustment of BARACLUDE is recommended for patients with creatinine clearance less than 50 mL/min, including patients on hemodialysis or CAPD *[see Dosage and Administration (2.4) and Clinical Pharmacology (12.3)]*.

8.8 Liver Transplant Recipients
The safety and efficacy of BARACLUDE were assessed in a single-arm, open-label trial in 65 subjects who received a liver transplant for complications of chronic HBV infection. Eligible subjects who had HBV DNA less than 172 IU/mL (approximately 1000 copies/mL) at the time of transplant were treated with BARACLUDE 1 mg once daily in addition to usual post-transplantation management, including hepatitis B immune globulin. The trial population was 82% male, 39% Caucasian, and 37% Asian, with a mean age of 49 years; 89% of subjects had HBeAg-negative disease at the time of transplant.

Four of the 65 subjects received 4 weeks or less of BARACLUDE (2 deaths, 1 retransplantation, and 1 protocol violation) and were not considered evaluable. Of the 61 subjects who received more than 4 weeks of BARACLUDE, 60 received hepatitis B immune globulin post-transplant. Fifty-three subjects (82% of all 65 subjects treated) completed the trial and had HBV DNA measurements at or after 72 weeks treatment post-transplant. All 53 subjects had HBV DNA <50 IU/mL (approximately 300 copies/mL). Eight

evaluable subjects did not have HBV DNA data available at 72 weeks, including 3 subjects who died prior to study completion. No subjects had HBV DNA values ≥ 50 IU/mL while receiving BARACLUDE (plus hepatitis B immune globulin). All 61 evaluable subjects lost HBsAg post-transplant; 2 of these subjects experienced recurrence of measurable HBsAg without recurrence of HBV viremia. This trial was not designed to determine whether addition of BARACLUDE to hepatitis B immune globulin decreased the proportion of subjects with measurable HBV DNA post-transplant compared to hepatitis B immune globulin alone.

If BARACLUDE treatment is determined to be necessary for a liver transplant recipient who has received or is receiving an immunosuppressant that may affect renal function, such as cyclosporine or tacrolimus, renal function must be carefully monitored both before and during treatment with BARACLUDE *[see Dosage and Administration (2.4) and Clinical Pharmacology (12.3)]*.

10 OVERDOSAGE
There is limited experience of entecavir overdosage reported in patients. Healthy subjects who received single entecavir doses up to 40 mg or multiple doses up to 20 mg/day for up to 14 days had no increase in or unexpected adverse events. If overdose occurs, the patient must be monitored for evidence of toxicity, and standard supportive treatment applied as necessary.

Following a single 1 mg dose of entecavir, a 4-hour hemodialysis session removed approximately 13% of the entecavir dose.

11 DESCRIPTION
BARACLUDE® (entecavir) is the tradename for entecavir, a guanosine nucleoside analogue with selective activity against HBV. The chemical name for entecavir is 2-amino-1,9-dihydro-9-[(1S,3R,4S)-4-hydroxy-3-(hydroxymethyl)-2-methylenecyclopentyl]-6H-purin-6-one, monohydrate. Its molecular formula is $C_{12}H_{15}N_5O_3 \bullet H_2O$, which corresponds to a molecular weight of 295.3. Entecavir has the following structural formula:

Entecavir is a white to off-white powder. It is slightly soluble in water (2.4 mg/mL), and the pH of the saturated solution in water is 7.9 at 25° C ± 0.5° C.
BARACLUDE film-coated tablets are available for oral administration in strengths of 0.5 mg and 1 mg of entecavir. BARACLUDE 0.5 mg and 1 mg film-coated tablets contain the following inactive ingredients: lactose monohydrate, microcrystalline cellulose, crospovidone, povidone, and magnesium stearate. The tablet coating contains titanium dioxide, hypromellose, polyethylene glycol 400, polysorbate 80 (0.5 mg tablet only), and iron oxide red (1 mg tablet only). BARACLUDE Oral Solution is available for oral administration as a ready-to-use solution containing 0.05 mg of entecavir per milliliter. BARACLUDE Oral Solution contains the following inactive ingredients: maltitol, sodium citrate, citric acid, methylparaben, propylparaben, and orange flavor.

12 CLINICAL PHARMACOLOGY
12.1 Mechanism of Action
Entecavir is an antiviral drug *[see Microbiology (12.4)]*.
12.3 Pharmacokinetics
The single- and multiple-dose pharmacokinetics of entecavir were evaluated in healthy subjects and subjects with chronic hepatitis B virus infection.

Absorption
Following oral administration in healthy subjects, entecavir peak plasma concentrations occurred between 0.5 and 1.5 hours. Following multiple daily doses ranging from 0.1 to 1 mg, C_{max} and area under the concentration-time curve (AUC) at steady state increased in proportion to dose. Steady state was achieved after 6 to 10 days of once-daily administration with approximately 2-fold accumulation. For a 0.5 mg oral dose, C_{max} at steady state was 4.2 ng/mL and trough plasma concentration (C_{trough}) was 0.3 ng/mL. For a 1 mg oral dose, C_{max} was 8.2 ng/mL and C_{trough} was 0.5 ng/mL.
In healthy subjects, the bioavailability of the tablet was 100% relative to the oral solution. The oral solution and tablet may be used interchangeably.
Effects of food on oral absorption: Oral administration of 0.5 mg of entecavir with a standard high-fat meal (945 kcal, 54.6 g fat) or a light meal (379 kcal, 8.2 g fat) resulted in a

delay in absorption (1.0–1.5 hours fed vs. 0.75 hours fasted), a decrease in C_{max} of 44%–46%, and a decrease in AUC of 18%–20% [see Dosage and Administration (2)].

Distribution

Based on the pharmacokinetic profile of entecavir after oral dosing, the estimated apparent volume of distribution is in excess of total body water, suggesting that entecavir is extensively distributed into tissues.

Binding of entecavir to human serum proteins in vitro was approximately 13%.

Metabolism and Elimination

Following administration of ^{14}C-entecavir in humans and rats, no oxidative or acetylated metabolites were observed. Minor amounts of phase II metabolites (glucuronide and sulfate conjugates) were observed. Entecavir is not a substrate, inhibitor, or inducer of the cytochrome P450 (CYP450) enzyme system. See Drug Interactions, below.

After reaching peak concentration, entecavir plasma concentrations decreased in a bi-exponential manner with a terminal elimination half-life of approximately 128–149 hours. The observed drug accumulation index is approximately 2-fold with once-daily dosing, suggesting an effective accumulation half-life of approximately 24 hours.

Entecavir is predominantly eliminated by the kidney with urinary recovery of unchanged drug at steady state ranging from 62% to 73% of the administered dose. Renal clearance is independent of dose and ranges from 360 to 471 mL/min suggesting that entecavir undergoes both glomerular filtration and net tubular secretion [see Drug Interactions (7)].

Special Populations

Gender: There are no significant gender differences in entecavir pharmacokinetics.

Race: There are no significant racial differences in entecavir pharmacokinetics.

Elderly: The effect of age on the pharmacokinetics of entecavir was evaluated following administration of a single 1 mg oral dose in healthy young and elderly volunteers. Entecavir AUC was 29.3% greater in elderly subjects compared to young subjects. The disparity in exposure between elderly and young subjects was most likely attributable to differences in renal function. Dosage adjustment of BARACLUDE (entecavir) should be based on the renal function of the patient, rather than age [see Dosage and Administration (2.4)].

Pediatrics: The steady-state pharmacokinetics of entecavir was evaluated in nucleoside-inhibitor-naïve and lamivudine-experienced HBeAg-positive pediatric subjects 2 to less than 18 years of age with compensated liver disease. Results are shown in Table 6. Entecavir exposure among nucleoside-inhibitor-naïve subjects was similar to the exposure achieved in adults receiving once-daily doses of 0.5 mg. Entecavir exposure among lamivudine-experienced subjects was similar to the exposure achieved in adults receiving once-daily doses of 1 mg.

Table 6: Pharmacokinetic Parameters in Pediatric Subjects

	Nucleoside-Inhibitor-Naïve[a] n=24	Lamivudine-Experienced[b] n=19
C_{max} (ng/mL)	6.31	14.48
(CV%)	(30)	(31)
$AUC_{(0-24)}$ (ng•h/mL)	18.33	38.58
(CV%)	(27)	(26)
C_{min} (ng/mL)	0.28	0.47
(CV%)	(22)	(23)

[a] Subjects received once-daily doses of 0.015 mg/kg up to a maximum of 0.5 mg.
[b] Subjects received once-daily doses of 0.030 mg/kg up to a maximum of 1 mg.

Renal impairment: The pharmacokinetics of entecavir following a single 1 mg dose were studied in subjects (without chronic hepatitis B virus infection) with selected degrees of renal impairment, including subjects whose renal impairment was managed by hemodialysis or continuous ambulatory peritoneal dialysis (CAPD). Results are shown in Table 7 [see Dosage and Administration (2.4)].

[See table 7 above]

Following a single 1 mg dose of entecavir administered 2 hours before the hemodialysis session, hemodialysis removed approximately 13% of the entecavir dose over 4 hours. CAPD removed approximately 0.3% of the dose over 7 days [see Dosage and Administration (2.4)].

Hepatic impairment: The pharmacokinetics of entecavir following a single 1 mg dose were studied in adult subjects (without chronic hepatitis B virus infection) with moderate or severe hepatic impairment (Child-Turcotte-Pugh Class B or C). The pharmacokinetics of entecavir were similar between hepatically impaired and healthy control subjects; therefore, no dosage adjustment of BARACLUDE is recom-

Table 7: Pharmacokinetic Parameters in Subjects with Selected Degrees of Renal Function

	Renal Function Group					
	Baseline Creatinine Clearance (mL/min)					
	Unimpaired >80 n=6	Mild >50–≤80 n=6	Moderate 30–50 n=6	Severe <30 n=6	Severe Managed with Hemodialysis[a] n=6	Severe Managed with CAPD n=4
C_{max} (ng/mL)	8.1	10.4	10.5	15.3	15.4	16.6
(CV%)	(30.7)	(37.2)	(22.7)	(33.8)	(56.4)	(29.7)
$AUC_{(0-T)}$ (ng•h/mL)	27.9	51.5	69.5	145.7	233.9	221.8
(CV)	(25.6)	(22.8)	(22.7)	(31.5)	(28.4)	(11.6)
CLR (mL/min)	383.2	197.9	135.6	40.3	NA	NA
(SD)	(101.8)	(78.1)	(31.6)	(10.1)		
CLT/F (mL/min)	588.1	309.2	226.3	100.6	50.6	35.7
(SD)	(153.7)	(62.6)	(60.1)	(29.1)	(16.5)	(19.6)

[a] Dosed immediately following hemodialysis.
CLR = renal clearance; CLT/F = apparent oral clearance.

mended for patients with hepatic impairment. The pharmacokinetics of entecavir have not been studied in pediatric subjects with hepatic impairment.

Post-liver transplant: Limited data are available on the safety and efficacy of BARACLUDE (entecavir) in liver transplant recipients. In a small pilot study of entecavir use in HBV-infected liver transplant recipients on a stable dose of cyclosporine A (n=5) or tacrolimus (n=4), entecavir exposure was approximately 2-fold the exposure in healthy subjects with normal renal function. Altered renal function contributed to the increase in entecavir exposure in these subjects. The potential for pharmacokinetic interactions between entecavir and cyclosporine A or tacrolimus was not formally evaluated [see Use in Specific Populations (8.8)].

Drug Interactions

The metabolism of entecavir was evaluated in in vitro and in vivo studies. Entecavir is not a substrate, inhibitor, or inducer of the cytochrome P450 (CYP450) enzyme system. At concentrations up to approximately 10,000-fold higher than those obtained in humans, entecavir inhibited none of the major human CYP450 enzymes 1A2, 2C9, 2C19, 2D6, 3A4, 2B6, and 2E1. At concentrations up to approximately 340-fold higher than those observed in humans, entecavir did not induce the human CYP450 enzymes 1A2, 2C9, 2C19, 3A4, 3A5, and 2B6. The pharmacokinetics of entecavir are unlikely to be affected by coadministration with agents that are either metabolized by, inhibit, or induce the CYP450 system. Likewise, the pharmacokinetics of known CYP substrates are unlikely to be affected by coadministration of entecavir.

The steady-state pharmacokinetics of entecavir and coadministered drug were not altered in interaction studies of entecavir with lamivudine, adefovir dipivoxil, and tenofovir disoproxil fumarate [see Drug Interactions (7)].

12.4 Microbiology

Mechanism of Action

Entecavir, a guanosine nucleoside analogue with activity against HBV reverse transcriptase (rt), is efficiently phosphorylated to the active triphosphate form, which has an intracellular half-life of 15 hours. By competing with the natural substrate deoxyguanosine triphosphate, entecavir triphosphate functionally inhibits all three activities of the HBV reverse transcriptase: (1) base priming, (2) reverse transcription of the negative strand from the pregenomic messenger RNA, and (3) synthesis of the positive strand of HBV DNA. Entecavir triphosphate is a weak inhibitor of cellular DNA polymerases α, β, and δ and mitochondrial DNA polymerase γ with K_i values ranging from 18 to >160 μM.

Antiviral Activity

Entecavir inhibited HBV DNA synthesis (50% reduction, EC_{50}) at a concentration of 0.004 μM in human HepG2 cells transfected with wild-type HBV. The median EC_{50} value for entecavir against lamivudine-resistant (rtL180M, rtM204V) was 0.026 μM (range 0.010–0.059 μM).

The coadministration of HIV nucleoside/nucleotide reverse transcriptase inhibitors (NRTIs) with BARACLUDE is unlikely to reduce the antiviral efficacy of BARACLUDE against HBV or of any of these agents against HIV. In HBV combination assays in cell culture, abacavir, didanosine, lamivudine, stavudine, tenofovir, or zidovudine were not antagonistic to the anti-HBV activity of entecavir over a wide range of concentrations. In HIV antiviral assays, entecavir was not antagonistic to the cell culture anti-HIV activity of these six NRTIs or emtricitabine at concentrations greater than 100 times the C_{max} of entecavir using the 1 mg dose.

Antiviral Activity Against HIV

A comprehensive analysis of the inhibitory activity of entecavir against a panel of laboratory and clinical HIV type 1 (HIV-1) isolates using a variety of cells and assay con-

ditions yielded EC_{50} values ranging from 0.026 to >10 μM; the lower EC_{50} values were observed when decreased levels of virus were used in the assay. In cell culture, entecavir selected for an M184I substitution in HIV reverse transcriptase at micromolar concentrations, confirming inhibitory pressure at high entecavir concentrations. HIV variants containing the M184V substitution showed loss of susceptibility to entecavir.

Resistance

In Cell Culture

In cell-based assays, 8- to 30-fold reductions in entecavir phenotypic susceptibility were observed for lamivudine-resistant strains. Further reductions (>70-fold) in entecavir phenotypic susceptibility required the presence of amino acid substitutions rtM204I/V with or without rtL180M along with additional substitutions at residues rtT184, rtS202, or rtM250, or a combination of these substitutions with or without an rtI169 substitution in the HBV reverse transcriptase.

Clinical Studies

Nucleoside-inhibitor-naïve subjects: Genotypic evaluations were performed on evaluable samples (>300 copies/mL serum HBV DNA) from 562 subjects who were treated with BARACLUDE (entecavir) for up to 96 weeks in nucleoside-inhibitor-naïve studies (AI463022, AI463027, and rollover study AI463901). By Week 96, evidence of emerging amino acid substitution rtS202G with rtM204V and rtL180M substitutions was detected in the HBV of 2 subjects (2/562=<1%), and 1 of them experienced virologic rebound (≥1 log_{10} increase above nadir). In addition, emerging amino acid substitutions at rtM204I/V and rtL180M, rtL80I, or rtV173L, which conferred decreased phenotypic susceptibility to entecavir in the absence of rtT184, rtS202, or rtM250 changes, were detected in the HBV of 3 subjects (3/562=<1%) who experienced virologic rebound. For subjects who continued treatment beyond 48 weeks, 75% (202/269) had HBV DNA <300 copies/mL at end of dosing (up to 96 weeks).

HBeAg-positive (n=243) and -negative (n=39) treatment-naïve subjects who failed to achieve the study-defined complete response by 96 weeks were offered continued entecavir treatment in a rollover study. Complete response for HBeAg-positive was <0.7 MEq/mL (approximately 7×10^5 copies/mL) serum HBV DNA and HBeAg loss and, for HBeAg-negative was <0.7 MEq/mL HBV DNA and ALT normalization. Subjects received 1 mg entecavir once daily for up to an additional 144 weeks. Of these 282 subjects, 141 HBeAg-positive and 8 HBeAg-negative subjects entered the long-term follow-up rollover study and were evaluated for entecavir resistance. Of the 149 subjects entering the rollover study, 88% (131/149), 92% (137/149), and 92% (137/149) attained serum HBV DNA <300 copies/mL by Weeks 144, 192, and 240 (including end of dosing), respectively. No novel entecavir resistance-associated substitutions were identified in a comparison of the genotypes of evaluable isolates with their respective baseline isolates. The cumulative probability of developing rtT184, rtS202, or rtM250 entecavir resistance-associated substitutions (in the presence of rtM204V and rtL180M substitutions) at Weeks 48, 96, 144, 192, and 240 was 0.2%, 0.5%, 1.2%, 1.2%, and 1.2%, respectively.

Lamivudine-refractory subjects: Genotypic evaluations were performed on evaluable samples from 190 subjects treated with BARACLUDE for up to 96 weeks in studies of lamivudine-refractory HBV (AI463026, AI463014, AI463015, and rollover study AI463901). By Week 96, resistance-associated amino acid substitutions at rtS202, rtT184, or rtM250, with or without rtI169 changes, in the presence of amino acid substitutions rtM204I/V with or without rtL180M, rtL80V, or rtV173L/M emerged in the HBV from 22 subjects (22/190=12%), 16 of whom experienced virologic rebound (≥1 log$_{10}$ increase above nadir) and 4 of whom were never suppressed <300 copies/mL. The HBV from 4 of these subjects had entecavir resistance substitutions at baseline and acquired further changes on entecavir treatment. In addition to the 22 subjects, 3 subjects experienced virologic rebound with the emergence of rtM204I/V and rtL180M, rtL80V, or rtV173L/M. For isolates from subjects who experienced virologic rebound with the emergence of resistance substitutions (n=19), the median fold-change in entecavir EC$_{50}$ values from reference was 19-fold at baseline and 106-fold at the time of virologic rebound. For subjects who continued treatment beyond 48 weeks, 40% (31/77) had HBV DNA <300 copies/mL at end of dosing (up to 96 weeks).

Lamivudine-refractory subjects (n=157) who failed to achieve the study-defined complete response by Week 96 were offered continued entecavir treatment. Subjects received 1 mg entecavir once daily for up to an additional 144 weeks. Of these subjects, 80 subjects entered the long-term follow-up study and were evaluated for entecavir resistance. By Weeks 144, 192, and 240 (including end of dosing), 34% (27/80), 35% (28/80), and 36% (29/80), respectively, attained HBV DNA <300 copies/mL. The cumulative probability of developing rtT184, rtS202, or rtM250 entecavir resistance-associated substitutions (in the presence of rtM204I/V with or without rtL180M substitutions) at Weeks 48, 96, 144, 192, and 240 was 6.2%, 15%, 36.3%, 46.6%, and 51.5%, respectively. The HBV of 6 subjects developed rtA181C/G/S/T amino acid substitutions while receiving entecavir, and of these, 4 developed entecavir resistance-associated substitutions at rtT184, rtS202, or rtM250 and 1 had an rtT184S substitution at baseline. Of 7 subjects whose HBV had an rtA181 substitution at baseline, 2 also had substitutions at rtT184, rtS202, or rtM250 at baseline and another 2 developed them while on treatment with entecavir.

Cross-resistance

Cross-resistance has been observed among HBV nucleoside analogue inhibitors. In cell-based assays, entecavir had 8- to 30-fold less inhibition of HBV DNA synthesis for HBV containing lamivudine and telbivudine resistance substitutions rtM204I/V with or without rtL180M than for wild-type HBV. Substitutions rtM204I/V with or without rtL180M, rtL80I/V, or rtV173L, which are associated with lamivudine and telbivudine resistance, also confer decreased phenotypic susceptibility to entecavir. The efficacy of entecavir against HBV harboring adefovir resistance-associated substitutions has not been established in clinical trials. HBV isolates from lamivudine-refractory subjects failing entecavir therapy were susceptible in cell culture to adefovir but remained resistant to lamivudine. Recombinant HBV genomes encoding adefovir resistance-associated substitutions at either rtN236T or rtA181V had 0.3- and 1.1-fold shifts in susceptibility to entecavir in cell culture, respectively.

13 NONCLINICAL TOXICOLOGY

13.1 Carcinogenesis, Mutagenesis, Impairment of Fertility

Carcinogenesis

Long-term oral carcinogenicity studies of entecavir in mice and rats were carried out at exposures up to approximately 42 times (mice) and 35 times (rats) those observed in humans at the highest recommended dose of 1 mg/day. In mouse and rat studies, entecavir was positive for carcinogenic findings.

In mice, lung adenomas were increased in males and females at exposures 3 and 40 times those in humans. Lung carcinomas in both male and female mice were increased at exposures 40 times those in humans. Combined lung adenomas and carcinomas were increased in male mice at exposures 3 times and in female mice at exposures 40 times those in humans. Tumor development was preceded by pneumocyte proliferation in the lung, which was not observed in rats, dogs, or monkeys administered entecavir, supporting the conclusion that lung tumors in mice may be a species-specific event. Hepatocellular carcinomas were increased in males and combined liver adenomas and carcinomas were also increased at exposures 42 times those in humans. Vascular tumors in female mice (hemangiomas of ovaries and uterus and hemangiosarcomas of spleen) were increased at exposures 40 times those in humans. In rats, hepatocellular adenomas were increased in females at exposures 24 times those in humans; combined adenomas and carcinomas were also increased in females at exposures 24 times those in humans. Brain gliomas were induced in both males and females at exposures 35 and 24 times those in humans. Skin fibromas were induced in females at exposures 4 times those in humans.

It is not known how predictive the results of rodent carcinogenicity studies may be for humans.

Mutagenesis

Entecavir was clastogenic to human lymphocyte cultures. Entecavir was not mutagenic in the Ames bacterial reverse mutation assay using *S. typhimurium* and *E. coli* strains in the presence or absence of metabolic activation, a mammalian-cell gene mutation assay, and a transformation assay with Syrian hamster embryo cells. Entecavir was also negative in an oral micronucleus study and an oral DNA repair study in rats.

Impairment of Fertility

In reproductive toxicology studies, in which animals were administered entecavir at up to 30 mg/kg for up to 4 weeks, no evidence of impaired fertility was seen in male or female rats at systemic exposures greater than 90 times those achieved in humans at the highest recommended dose of 1 mg/day. In rodent and dog toxicology studies, seminiferous tubular degeneration was observed at exposures 35 times or greater than those achieved in humans. No testicular changes were evident in monkeys.

14 CLINICAL STUDIES

14.1 Outcomes in Adults

At 48 Weeks

The safety and efficacy of BARACLUDE (entecavir) in adults were evaluated in three Phase 3 active-controlled trials. These studies included 1633 subjects 16 years of age or older with chronic hepatitis B virus infection (serum HBsAg-positive for at least 6 months) accompanied by evidence of viral replication (detectable serum HBV DNA, as measured by the bDNA hybridization or PCR assay). Subjects had persistently elevated ALT levels at least 1.3 times ULN and chronic inflammation on liver biopsy compatible with a diagnosis of chronic viral hepatitis. The safety and efficacy of BARACLUDE were also evaluated in a study of 191 HBV-infected subjects with decompensated liver disease and in a study of 68 subjects co-infected with HBV and HIV.

Nucleoside-inhibitor-naïve Subjects with Compensated Liver Disease

HBeAg-positive: Study AI463022 was a multinational, randomized, double-blind study of BARACLUDE 0.5 mg once daily versus lamivudine 100 mg once daily for a minimum of 52 weeks in 709 (of 715 randomized) nucleoside-inhibitor-naïve subjects with chronic hepatitis B virus infection, compensated liver disease, and detectable HBeAg. The mean age of subjects was 35 years, 75% were male, 57% were Asian, 40% were Caucasian, and 13% had previously received interferon-α. At baseline, subjects had a mean Knodell Necroinflammatory Score of 7.8, mean serum HBV DNA as measured by Roche COBAS Amplicor® PCR assay

was 9.66 log$_{10}$ copies/mL, and mean serum ALT level was 143 U/L. Paired, adequate liver biopsy samples were available for 89% of subjects.

HBeAg-negative (anti-HBe-positive/HBV DNA-positive): Study AI463027 was a multinational, randomized, double-blind study of BARACLUDE (entecavir) 0.5 mg once daily versus lamivudine 100 mg once daily for a minimum of 52 weeks in 638 (of 648 randomized) nucleoside-inhibitor-naïve subjects with HBeAg-negative (HBeAb-positive) chronic hepatitis B virus infection and compensated liver disease. The mean age of subjects was 44 years, 76% were male, 39% were Asian, 58% were Caucasian, and 13% had previously received interferon-α. At baseline, subjects had a mean Knodell Necroinflammatory Score of 7.8, mean serum HBV DNA as measured by Roche COBAS Amplicor PCR assay was 7.58 log$_{10}$ copies/mL, and mean serum ALT level was 142 U/L. Paired, adequate liver biopsy samples were available for 88% of subjects.

In Studies AI463022 and AI463027, BARACLUDE was superior to lamivudine on the primary efficacy endpoint of Histologic Improvement, defined as a 2-point or greater reduction in Knodell Necroinflammatory Score with no worsening in Knodell Fibrosis Score at Week 48, and on the secondary efficacy measures of reduction in viral load and ALT normalization. Histologic Improvement and change in Ishak Fibrosis Score are shown in Table 8. Selected virologic, biochemical, and serologic outcome measures are shown in Table 9.

[See table 8 above]

[See table 9 above]

Histologic Improvement was independent of baseline levels of HBV DNA or ALT.

Lamivudine-refractory Subjects with Compensated Liver Disease

Study AI463026 was a multinational, randomized, double-blind study of BARACLUDE in 286 (of 293 randomized) subjects with lamivudine-refractory chronic hepatitis B virus infection and compensated liver disease. Subjects receiving lamivudine at study entry either switched to BARACLUDE 1 mg once daily (with neither a washout nor an overlap period) or continued on lamivudine 100 mg for a minimum of 52 weeks. The mean age of subjects was 39 years, 76% were male, 37% were Asian, 62% were Caucasian, and 52% had previously received interferon-α. The mean duration of prior lamivudine therapy was 2.7 years, and 85% had lamivudine resistance substitutions at baseline by an investigational line probe assay. At baseline, subjects had a mean Knodell Necroinflammatory Score of 6.5,

Table 8: Histologic Improvement and Change in Ishak Fibrosis Score at Week 48, Nucleoside-Inhibitor-Naïve Subjects in Studies AI463022 and AI463027

	Study AI463022 (HBeAg-Positive)		Study AI463027 (HBeAg-Negative)	
	BARACLUDE 0.5 mg n=314[a]	Lamivudine 100 mg n=314[a]	BARACLUDE 0.5 mg n=296[a]	Lamivudine 100 mg n=287[a]
Histologic Improvement (Knodell Scores)				
Improvement[b]	72%	62%	70%	61%
No improvement	21%	24%	19%	26%
Ishak Fibrosis Score				
Improvement[c]	39%	35%	36%	38%
No change[c]	46%	40%	41%	34%
Worsening[c]	8%	10%	12%	15%
Missing Week 48 biopsy	7%	14%	10%	13%

[a] Subjects with evaluable baseline histology (baseline Knodell Necroinflammatory Score ≥2).
[b] ≥2-point decrease in Knodell Necroinflammatory Score from baseline with no worsening of the Knodell Fibrosis Score.
[c] For Ishak Fibrosis Score, improvement = ≥1-point decrease from baseline and worsening = ≥1-point increase from baseline.

Table 9: Selected Virologic, Biochemical, and Serologic Endpoints at Week 48, Nucleoside-Inhibitor-Naïve Subjects in Studies AI463022 and AI463027

	Study AI463022 (HBeAg-Positive)		Study AI463027 (HBeAg-Negative)	
	BARACLUDE 0.5 mg n=354	Lamivudine 100 mg n=355	BARACLUDE 0.5 mg n=325	Lamivudine 100 mg n=313
HBV DNA[a]				
Proportion undetectable (<300 copies/mL)	67%	36%	90%	72%
Mean change from baseline (log$_{10}$ copies/mL)	−6.86	−5.39	−5.04	−4.53
ALT normalization (≤1 × ULN)	68%	60%	78%	71%
HBeAg seroconversion	21%	18%	NA	NA

[a] Roche COBAS Amplicor PCR assay [lower limit of quantification (LLOQ) = 300 copies/mL].

mean serum HBV DNA as measured by Roche COBAS Amplicor PCR assay was 9.36 log10 copies/mL, and mean serum ALT level was 128 U/L. Paired, adequate liver biopsy samples were available for 87% of subjects.

BARACLUDE (entecavir) was superior to lamivudine on a primary endpoint of Histologic Improvement (using the Knodell Score at Week 48). These results and change in Ishak Fibrosis Score are shown in Table 10. Table 11 shows selected virologic, biochemical, and serologic endpoints.

Table 10: Histologic Improvement and Change in Ishak Fibrosis Score at Week 48, Lamivudine-Refractory Subjects in Study AI463026

	BARACLUDE 1 mg n=124[a]	Lamivudine 100 mg n=116[a]
Histologic Improvement (Knodell Scores)		
Improvement[b]	55%	28%
No improvement	34%	57%
Ishak Fibrosis Score		
Improvement[c]	34%	16%
No change	44%	42%
Worsening[c]	11%	26%
Missing Week 48 biopsy	11%	16%

[a] Subjects with evaluable baseline histology (baseline Knodell Necroinflammatory Score ≥2).
[b] ≥2-point decrease in Knodell Necroinflammatory Score from baseline with no worsening of the Knodell Fibrosis Score.
[c] For Ishak Fibrosis Score, improvement = ≥1-point decrease from baseline and worsening = ≥1-point increase from baseline.

Table 11: Selected Virologic, Biochemical, and Serologic Endpoints at Week 48, Lamivudine-Refractory Subjects in Study AI463026

	BARACLUDE 1 mg n=141	Lamivudine 100 mg n=145
HBV DNA[a]		
Proportion undetectable (<300 copies/mL)	19%	1%
Mean change from baseline (log10 copies/mL)	−5.11	−0.48
ALT normalization (≤1 × ULN)	61%	15%
HBeAg seroconversion	8%	3%

[a] Roche COBAS Amplicor PCR assay (LLOQ = 300 copies/mL).

Histologic Improvement was independent of baseline levels of HBV DNA or ALT.

Subjects with Decompensated Liver Disease

Study AI463048 was a randomized, open-label study of BARACLUDE 1 mg once daily versus adefovir dipivoxil 10 mg once daily in 191 (of 195 randomized) adult subjects with HBeAg-positive or -negative chronic HBV infection and evidence of hepatic decompensation, defined as a Child-Turcotte-Pugh (CTP) score of 7 or higher. Subjects were either HBV-treatment-naïve or previously treated, predominantly with lamivudine or interferon-α.

In Study AI463048, 100 subjects were randomized to treatment with BARACLUDE and 91 subjects to treatment with adefovir dipivoxil. Two subjects randomized to treatment with adefovir dipivoxil actually received treatment with BARACLUDE for the duration of the study. The mean age of subjects was 52 years, 74% were male, 54% were Asian, 33% were Caucasian, and 5% were Black/African American. At baseline, subjects had a mean serum HBV DNA by PCR of 7.83 log10 copies/mL and mean ALT level of 100 U/L; 54% of subjects were HBeAg-positive; 35% had genotypic evidence of lamivudine resistance. The baseline mean CTP score was 8.6. Results for selected study endpoints at Week 48 are shown in Table 12.

Table 12: Selected Endpoints at Week 48, Subjects with Decompensated Liver Disease, Study AI463048

	BARACLUDE 1 mg n=100[a]	Adefovir Dipivoxil 10 mg n=91[a]
HBV DNA[b]		
Proportion undetectable (<300 copies/mL)	57%	20%

Stable or improved CTP score[c]	61%	67%
HBsAg loss	5%	0
Normalization of ALT (≤1 × ULN)[d]	49/78 (63%)	33/71 (46%)

[a] Endpoints were analyzed using intention-to-treat (ITT) method, treated subjects as randomized.
[b] Roche COBAS Amplicor PCR assay (LLOQ = 300 copies/mL).
[c] Defined as decrease or no change from baseline in CTP score.
[d] Denominator is subjects with abnormal values at baseline.
ULN=upper limit of normal.

Subjects Co-infected with HIV and HBV

Study AI463038 was a randomized, double-blind, placebo-controlled study of BARACLUDE (entecavir) versus placebo in 68 subjects co-infected with HIV and HBV who experienced recurrence of HBV viremia while receiving a lamivudine-containing highly active antiretroviral (HAART) regimen. Subjects continued their lamivudine-containing HAART regimen (lamivudine dose 300 mg/day) and were assigned to add either BARACLUDE 1 mg once daily (51 subjects) or placebo (17 subjects) for 24 weeks followed by an open-label phase for an additional 24 weeks where all subjects received BARACLUDE. At baseline, subjects had a mean serum HBV DNA level by PCR of 9.13 log10 copies/mL. Ninety-nine percent of subjects were HBeAg-positive at baseline, with a mean baseline ALT level of 71.5 U/L. Median HIV RNA level remained stable at approximately 2 log10 copies/mL through 24 weeks of blinded therapy. Virologic and biochemical endpoints at Week 24 are shown in Table 13. There are no data in patients with HIV/HBV co-infection who have not received prior lamivudine therapy. BARACLUDE has not been evaluated in HIV/HBV co-infected patients who were not simultaneously receiving effective HIV treatment [see Warnings and Precautions (5.2)].

Table 13: Virologic and Biochemical Endpoints at Week 24, Study AI463038

	BARACLUDE 1 mg[a] n=51	Placebo[a] n=17
HBV DNA[b]		
Proportion undetectable (<300 copies/mL)	6%	0
Mean change from baseline (log10 copies/mL)	−3.65	+0.11
ALT normalization (≤1 × ULN)	34%[c]	8%[c]

[a] All subjects also received a lamivudine-containing HAART regimen.
[b] Roche COBAS Amplicor PCR assay (LLOQ = 300 copies/mL).
[c] Percentage of subjects with abnormal ALT (>1 × ULN) at baseline who achieved ALT normalization (n=35 for BARACLUDE and n=12 for placebo).

For subjects originally assigned to BARACLUDE, at the end of the open-label phase (Week 48), 8% of subjects had HBV DNA <300 copies/mL by PCR, the mean change from baseline HBV DNA by PCR was −4.20 log10 copies/mL, and 37% of subjects with abnormal ALT at baseline had ALT normalization (≤1 × ULN).

Beyond 48 Weeks

The optimal duration of therapy with BARACLUDE is unknown. According to protocol-mandated criteria in the Phase 3 clinical trials, subjects discontinued BARACLUDE or lamivudine treatment after 52 weeks according to a definition of response based on HBV virologic suppression (<0.7 MEq/mL by bDNA assay) and loss of HBeAg (in HBeAg-positive subjects) or ALT <1.25 × ULN (in HBeAg-negative subjects) at Week 48. Subjects who achieved virologic suppression but did not have serologic response (HBeAg-positive) or did not achieve ALT <1.25 × ULN (HBeAg-negative) continued blinded dosing through 96 weeks or until the response criteria were met. These protocol-specified subject management guidelines are not intended as guidance for clinical practice.

Nucleoside-inhibitor-naïve Subjects

Among nucleoside-inhibitor-naïve, HBeAg-positive subjects (Study AI463022), 243 (69%) BARACLUDE-treated subjects and 164 (46%) lamivudine-treated subjects continued blinded treatment for up to 96 weeks. Of those continuing blinded treatment in Year 2, 180 (74%) BARACLUDE subjects and 60 (37%) lamivudine subjects achieved HBV DNA <300 copies/mL by PCR at the end of dosing (up to 96 weeks). 193 (79%) BARACLUDE subjects achieved ALT ≤1

× ULN compared to 112 (68%) lamivudine subjects, and HBeAg seroconversion occurred in 26 (11%) BARACLUDE (entecavir) subjects and 20 (12%) lamivudine subjects. Among nucleoside-inhibitor-naïve, HBeAg-positive subjects, 74 (21%) BARACLUDE subjects and 67 (19%) lamivudine subjects met the definition of response at Week 48, discontinued study drugs, and were followed off treatment for 24 weeks. Among BARACLUDE responders, 26 (35%) subjects had HBV DNA <300 copies/mL, 55 (74%) subjects had ALT ≤1 × ULN, and 56 (76%) subjects sustained HBeAg seroconversion at the end of follow-up. Among lamivudine responders, 20 (30%) subjects had HBV DNA <300 copies/mL, 41 (61%) had ALT ≤1 × ULN, and 47 (70%) subjects sustained HBeAg seroconversion at the end of follow-up.

Among nucleoside-inhibitor-naïve, HBeAg-negative subjects (Study AI463027), 26 (8%) BARACLUDE-treated subjects and 28 (9%) lamivudine-treated subjects continued blinded treatment for up to 96 weeks. In this small cohort continuing treatment in Year 2, 22 BARACLUDE and 16 lamivudine subjects had HBV DNA <300 copies/mL by PCR, and 7 and 6 subjects, respectively, had ALT ≤1 × ULN at end of dosing (up to 96 weeks).

Among nucleoside-inhibitor-naïve, HBeAg-negative subjects, 275 (85%) BARACLUDE subjects and 245 (78%) lamivudine subjects met the definition of response at Week 48, discontinued study drugs, and were followed off treatment for 24 weeks. In this cohort, very few subjects in each treatment arm had HBV DNA <300 copies/mL by PCR at the end of follow-up. At the end of follow-up, 126 (46%) BARACLUDE subjects and 84 (34%) lamivudine subjects had ALT ≤1 × ULN.

Lamivudine-refractory Subjects

Among lamivudine-refractory subjects (Study AI463026), 77 (55%) BARACLUDE-treated subjects and 3 (2%) lamivudine subjects continued blinded treatment for up to 96 weeks. In this cohort of BARACLUDE subjects, 31 (40%) subjects achieved HBV DNA <300 copies/mL, 62 (81%) subjects had ALT ≤1 × ULN, and 8 (10%) subjects demonstrated HBeAg seroconversion at the end of dosing.

14.2   Outcomes in Pediatric Subjects

The pharmacokinetics, safety and antiviral activity of BARACLUDE in pediatric subjects were initially assessed in Study AI463028. Twenty-four treatment-naïve and 19 lamivudine-experienced HBeAg-positive pediatric subjects 2 to less than 18 years of age with compensated CHB and elevated ALT were treated with BARACLUDE 0.015 mg/kg (up to 0.5 mg) or 0.03 mg/kg (up to 1 mg) once daily. Fifty-eight percent (14/24) of treatment-naïve subjects and 47% (9/19) of lamivudine-experienced subjects achieved HBV DNA <50 IU/mL at Week 48 and ALT normalized in 83% (20/24) of treatment-naïve and 95% (18/19) of lamivudine-experienced subjects.

Safety and antiviral efficacy were confirmed in Study AI463189, an ongoing study of BARACLUDE (entecavir) among 180 nucleoside-inhibitor-treatment-naïve pediatric subjects 2 to less than 18 years of age with HBeAg-positive chronic hepatitis B infection, compensated liver disease, and elevated ALT. Subjects were randomized 2:1 to receive blinded treatment with BARACLUDE 0.015 mg/kg up to 0.5 mg/day (N=120) or placebo (N=60). The randomization was stratified by age group (2 to 6 years; >6 to 12 years; and >12 to <18 years). Baseline demographics and HBV disease characteristics were comparable between the 2 treatment arms and across age cohorts. At study entry, the mean HBV DNA was 8.1 log10 IU/mL and mean ALT was 103 U/L. The primary efficacy endpoint was a composite of HBeAg seroconversion and serum HBV DNA <50 IU/mL at Week 48 assessed in the first 123 subjects reaching 48 weeks of blinded treatment. Twenty-four percent (20/82) of subjects in the BARACLUDE-treated group and 2% (1/41) of subjects in the placebo-treated group met the primary endpoint. Forty-six percent (38/82) of BARACLUDE-treated subjects and 2% (1/41) of placebo-treated subjects achieved HBV DNA <50 IU/mL at Week 48. ALT normalization occurred in 67% (55/82) of BARACLUDE-treated subjects and 22% (9/41) of placebo-treated subjects; 24% (20/82) of BARACLUDE-treated subjects and 12% (5/41) of placebo-treated subjects had HBeAg seroconversion.

16   HOW SUPPLIED/STORAGE AND HANDLING

BARACLUDE® Tablets and Oral Solution are available in the following strengths and configurations of plastic bottles with child-resistant closures:

[See table at top of next page]

BARACLUDE Oral Solution is a ready-to-use product; dilution or mixing with water or any other solvent or liquid product is not recommended. Each bottle of the oral solution is accompanied by a dosing spoon that is calibrated in 0.5 mL increments up to 10 mL.

Storage

BARACLUDE Tablets should be stored in a tightly closed container at 25°C (77°F); excursions permitted between 15°C and 30°C (59°F and 86°F) [see USP Controlled Room Temperature]. Store in the outer carton to protect from light.

BARACLUDE (entecavir) Oral Solution should be stored in the outer carton at 25°C (77°F); excursions permitted between 15°C and 30°C (59°F and 86°F) [see USP Controlled Room Temperature]. Protect from light. After opening, the oral solution can be used up to the expiration date on the bottle. The bottle and its contents should be discarded after the expiration date.

17 PATIENT COUNSELING INFORMATION

See FDA-approved patient labeling (Patient Information).

Information about Treatment

Physicians should inform their patients of the following important points when initiating BARACLUDE treatment:

• Patients should remain under the care of a physician while taking BARACLUDE. They should discuss any new symptoms or concurrent medications with their physician.

• Patients should be advised that treatment with BARACLUDE has not been shown to reduce the risk of transmission of HBV to others through sexual contact or blood contamination.

• Patients should be advised to take BARACLUDE on an empty stomach (at least 2 hours after a meal and 2 hours before the next meal).

• Patients using the oral solution should be instructed to hold the dosing spoon in a vertical position and fill it gradually to the mark corresponding to the prescribed dose. Rinsing of the dosing spoon with water is recommended after each daily dose. Some patients may find it difficult to accurately measure the prescribed dose using the provided dosing spoon; therefore, patients/caregivers should refer to the steps in the Patient Information section that demonstrate the correct technique of using the provided dosing spoon to measure the prescribed BARACLUDE dose.

• Patients should be advised to take a missed dose as soon as remembered unless it is almost time for the next dose. Patients should not take two doses at the same time.

• Patients should be advised that treatment with BARACLUDE will not cure HBV.

• Patients should be informed that BARACLUDE may lower the amount of HBV in the body, may lower the ability of HBV to multiply and infect new liver cells, and may improve the condition of the liver.

• Patients should be informed that it is not known whether BARACLUDE will reduce their chances of getting liver cancer or cirrhosis.

Post-treatment Exacerbation of Hepatitis

Patients should be informed that deterioration of liver disease may occur in some cases if treatment is discontinued, and that they should discuss any change in regimen with their physician.

HIV/HBV Co-infection

Patients should be offered HIV antibody testing before starting BARACLUDE therapy. They should be informed that if they have HIV infection and are not receiving effective HIV treatment, BARACLUDE may increase the chance of HIV resistance to HIV medication.

Patient Information

BARACLUDE® (BEAR ah klude)
(entecavir)
Tablets

BARACLUDE® (BEAR ah klude)
(entecavir)
Oral Solution

Read this Patient Information before you start taking BARACLUDE and each time you get a refill. There may be new information. This information does not take the place of talking with your healthcare provider about your medical condition or treatment.

What is the most important information I should know about BARACLUDE?

1. **Your hepatitis B virus (HBV) infection may get worse if you stop taking BARACLUDE.** This usually happens within 6 months after stopping BARACLUDE.

• Take BARACLUDE exactly as prescribed.
• Do not run out of BARACLUDE.
• Do not stop BARACLUDE without talking to your healthcare provider.
• Your healthcare provider should monitor your health and do regular blood tests to check your liver if you stop taking BARACLUDE.

2. **If you have or get HIV that is not being treated with medicines while taking BARACLUDE, the HIV virus may develop resistance to certain HIV medicines and become harder to treat.** You should get an HIV test before you start taking BARACLUDE and anytime after that when there is a chance you were exposed to HIV.

BARACLUDE can cause serious side effects including:

3. **Lactic acidosis (buildup of acid in the blood). Some people who have taken BARACLUDE or medicines like BARACLUDE (a nucleoside analogue) have developed a serious condition called lactic acidosis.** Lactic acidosis is a serious medical emergency that can cause death. Lactic acidosis must be treated in the hospital. Reports of lactic acidosis with BARACLUDE generally involved patients

Product Strength and Dosage Form	Description	Quantity	NDC Number
0.5 mg film-coated tablet	White to off-white, triangular-shaped tablet, debossed with "BMS" on one side and "1611" on the other side.	30 tablets 90 tablets	0003-1611-12 0003-1611-13
1 mg film-coated tablet	Pink, triangular-shaped tablet, debossed with "BMS" on one side and "1612" on the other side.	30 tablets	0003-1612-12
0.05 mg/mL oral solution	Ready-to-use, orange-flavored, clear, colorless to pale yellow, aqueous solution in a 260 mL bottle.	210 mL	0003-1614-12

• If you are taking BARACLUDE Oral Solution, or giving it to your child, carefully measure the dose with the dosing spoon provided, as follows:

• Hold the dosing spoon in an upright (vertical) position and slowly fill it to the measurement line on the dosing spoon that is the same as the prescribed dose. Bring the dosing spoon to eye level to be sure that the level of the BARACLUDE Oral Solution is at the correct measurement line (see Figure 1).

Hold spoon upright (as shown). Measure the medicine at eye level.

Figure 1

• With the dosing spoon at eye level, holding it with the measurement lines facing you, check that it has been filled to the correct measurement line. The top of the BARACLUDE Oral Solution in the dosing spoon will look curved, not flat. Measure the dose of BARACLUDE Oral Solution at the bottom of the curve. Your dose of BARACLUDE Oral Solution is measured correctly when the bottom of the curve is lined up with the measurement line of the prescribed dose. As an example, Figure 2 shows the right way to measure a 5 mL dose of BARACLUDE (see Figure 2).

Figure 2

who were seriously ill due to their liver disease or other medical condition.

Call your healthcare provider right away if you get any of the following signs or symptoms of lactic acidosis:

• You feel very weak or tired.
• You have unusual (not normal) muscle pain.
• You have trouble breathing.
• You have stomach pain with nausea and vomiting.
• You feel cold, especially in your arms and legs.
• You feel dizzy or light-headed.
• You have a fast or irregular heartbeat.

4. **Serious liver problems. Some people who have taken medicines like BARACLUDE have developed serious liver problems called hepatotoxicity, with liver enlargement (hepatomegaly) and fat in the liver (steatosis). Hepatomegaly with steatosis is a serious medical emergency that can cause death.**

Call your healthcare provider right away if you get any of the following signs or symptoms of liver problems:

• Your skin or the white part of your eyes turns yellow (jaundice).
• Your urine turns dark.
• Your bowel movements (stools) turn light in color.
• You don't feel like eating food for several days or longer.
• You feel sick to your stomach (nausea).
• You have lower stomach pain.

You may be more likely to get lactic acidosis or serious liver problems if you are female, very overweight, or have been taking nucleoside analogue medicines, like BARACLUDE, for a long time.

What is BARACLUDE?

BARACLUDE (entecavir) is a prescription medicine used to treat chronic hepatitis B virus (HBV) in adults and children 2 years of age and older who have active liver disease.

• BARACLUDE will not cure HBV.
• BARACLUDE may lower the amount of HBV in the body.
• BARACLUDE may lower the ability of HBV to multiply and infect new liver cells.
• BARACLUDE may improve the condition of your liver.
• It is not known whether BARACLUDE will reduce your chances of getting liver cancer or liver damage (cirrhosis), which may be caused by chronic HBV infection.

• It is not known if BARACLUDE is safe and effective for use in children less than 2 years of age.

What should I tell my healthcare provider before taking BARACLUDE?

Before you take BARACLUDE (entecavir), tell your healthcare provider if you:

• have kidney problems. Your BARACLUDE dose or schedule may need to be changed.

• have received medicine for HBV before. Some people, especially those who have already been treated with certain other medicines for HBV infection, may develop resistance to BARACLUDE. These people may have less benefit from treatment with BARACLUDE and may have worsening of hepatitis after resistant virus appears. Your healthcare provider will test the level of the hepatitis B virus in your blood regularly.

• have any other medical conditions.

• are pregnant or plan to become pregnant. It is not known if BARACLUDE will harm your unborn baby. Talk to your healthcare provider if you are pregnant or plan to become pregnant.

Antiretroviral Pregnancy Registry. If you take BARACLUDE while you are pregnant, talk to your healthcare provider about how you can take part in the BARACLUDE Antiretroviral Pregnancy Registry. The purpose of the pregnancy registry is to collect information about the health of you and your baby.

• are breastfeeding or plan to breastfeed. It is not known if BARACLUDE can pass into your breast milk. You and your healthcare provider should decide if you will take BARACLUDE or breastfeed.

Tell your healthcare provider about all the medicines you take, including prescription and over-the-counter medicines, vitamins, and herbal supplements. Especially tell your healthcare provider if you have taken a medicine to treat HBV in the past.

Know the medicines you take. Keep a list of your medicines with you to show your healthcare provider and pharmacist when you get a new medicine.

How should I take BARACLUDE?

• Take BARACLUDE exactly as your healthcare provider tells you to.

- Your healthcare provider will tell you how much BARACLUDE (entecavir) to take.
- Your healthcare provider will tell you when and how often to take BARACLUDE.
- **Take BARACLUDE on an empty stomach,** at least 2 hours after a meal and at least 2 hours before the next meal. [See table at top of previous page]
  - BARACLUDE Oral Solution should be swallowed directly from the dosing spoon.
  - BARACLUDE Oral Solution should not be mixed with water or any other liquid.
  - After each use, rinse the dosing spoon with water and allow it to air dry.
  - If you lose the dosing spoon, call your pharmacist or healthcare provider for instructions.
- **Do not change your dose or stop taking BARACLUDE without talking to your healthcare provider.**
- **If you miss a dose of BARACLUDE,** take it as soon as you remember and then take your next dose at its regular time. If it is almost time for your next dose, skip the missed dose. Do not take two doses at the same time. Call your healthcare provider or pharmacist if you are not sure what to do.
- When your supply of BARACLUDE starts to run low, call your healthcare provider or pharmacy for a refill. **Do not run out of BARACLUDE.**
- **If you take too much BARACLUDE,** call your healthcare provider or go to the nearest emergency room right away.

What are the possible side effects of BARACLUDE?
BARACLUDE may cause serious side effects. See "What is the most important information I should know about BARACLUDE?"
The most common side effects of BARACLUDE include:
- headache
- tiredness
- dizziness
- nausea

Tell your healthcare provider if you have any side effect that bothers you or that does not go away.
These are not all the possible side effects of BARACLUDE. For more information, ask your healthcare provider or pharmacist.
Call your doctor for medical advice about side effects. You may report side effects to the FDA at 1-800-FDA-1088.

How should I store BARACLUDE?
- Store BARACLUDE Tablets or Oral Solution at room temperature, between 68°F to 77°F (20°C to 25°C).
- Keep BARACLUDE Tablets in a tightly closed container.
- Store BARACLUDE Tablets or BARACLUDE Oral Solution in the original carton, and keep the carton out of the light.
- Safely throw away BARACLUDE that is out of date or no longer needed. Dispose of unused medicines through community take-back disposal programs when available or place BARACLUDE in an unrecognizable closed container in the household trash.

Keep BARACLUDE and all medicines out of the reach of children.

General information about the safe and effective use of BARACLUDE
BARACLUDE does not stop you from spreading the hepatitis B virus (HBV) to others by sex, sharing needles, or being exposed to your blood. Talk with your healthcare provider about safe sexual practices that protect your partner. Never share needles. Do not share personal items that can have blood or body fluids on them, like toothbrushes or razor blades. A shot (vaccine) is available to protect people at risk from becoming infected with HBV.
Medicines are sometimes prescribed for purposes other than those listed in a Patient Information leaflet. Do not use BARACLUDE for a condition for which it was not prescribed. Do not give BARACLUDE to other people, even if they have the same symptoms you have. It may harm them.
This Patient Information leaflet summarizes the most important information about BARACLUDE. If you would like more information, talk with your healthcare provider. You can ask your healthcare provider or pharmacist for information about BARACLUDE that is written for health professionals.
For more information, go to *www.Baraclude.com* or call 1-800-321-1335.

What are the ingredients in BARACLUDE?
Active ingredient: entecavir
Inactive ingredients in BARACLUDE Tablets: lactose monohydrate, microcrystalline cellulose, crospovidone, povidone, magnesium stearate.
Tablet film-coat: titanium dioxide, hypromellose, polyethylene glycol 400, polysorbate 80 (0.5 mg tablet only), and iron oxide red (1 mg tablet only).
Inactive ingredients in BARACLUDE Oral Solution: maltitol, sodium citrate, citric acid, methylparaben, propylparaben, and orange flavor.
Bristol-Myers Squibb Company
Princeton, NJ 08543 USA

Product of Ireland
1323583
Revised: May 2014
This Patient Information has been approved by the U.S. Food and Drug Administration.
Shown in Product Identification Guide, page 306

COUMADIN ℞
[*COU-ma-din*]
(warfarin sodium)
tablets, for oral use
COUMADIN
(warfarin sodium)
for injection, for intravenous use

HIGHLIGHTS OF PRESCRIBING INFORMATION
These highlights do not include all the information needed to use COUMADIN safely and effectively. See full prescribing information for COUMADIN.
COUMADIN (warfarin sodium) tablets, for oral use
COUMADIN (warfarin sodium) for injection, for intravenous use
Initial U.S. Approval: 1954

WARNING: BLEEDING RISK
See full prescribing information for complete boxed warning.
• **COUMADIN can cause major or fatal bleeding. (5.1)**
• **Perform regular monitoring of INR in all treated patients. (2.1)**
• **Drugs, dietary changes, and other factors affect INR levels achieved with COUMADIN therapy. (7)**
• **Instruct patients about prevention measures to minimize risk of bleeding and to report signs and symptoms of bleeding. (17)**

—————RECENT MAJOR CHANGES—————
Contraindications (4)   10/2011
Warnings and Precautions, Use in Pregnant
  Women with Mechanical Heart Valves (5.5)   10/2011

—————INDICATIONS AND USAGE—————
COUMADIN is a vitamin K antagonist indicated for:
- Prophylaxis and treatment of venous thrombosis and its extension, pulmonary embolism (1)
- Prophylaxis and treatment of thromboembolic complications associated with atrial fibrillation and/or cardiac valve replacement (1)
- Reduction in the risk of death, recurrent myocardial infarction, and thromboembolic events such as stroke or systemic embolization after myocardial infarction (1)

Limitation of Use
COUMADIN has no direct effect on an established thrombus, nor does it reverse ischemic tissue damage. (1)

—————DOSAGE AND ADMINISTRATION—————
- Individualize dosing regimen for each patient, and adjust based on INR response. (2.1, 2.2)
- Knowledge of genotype can inform initial dose selection. (2.3)
- Monitoring: Obtain daily INR determinations upon initiation until stable in the therapeutic range. Obtain subsequent INR determinations every 1 to 4 weeks. (2.4)
- Review conversion instructions from other anticoagulants. (2.8)

—————DOSAGE FORMS AND STRENGTHS—————
- Scored tablets: 1, 2, 2-1/2, 3, 4, 5, 6, 7-1/2, or 10 mg (3)
- For injection: Vial containing 5 mg lyophilized powder (3)

—————CONTRAINDICATIONS—————
- Pregnancy, except in women with mechanical heart valves (4)
- Hemorrhagic tendencies or blood dyscrasias (4)
- Recent or contemplated surgery of the central nervous system (CNS) or eye, or traumatic surgery resulting in large open surfaces (4, 5.7)
- Bleeding tendencies associated with certain conditions (4)
- Threatened abortion, eclampsia, and preeclampsia (4)
- Unsupervised patients with potential high levels of noncompliance (4)
- Spinal puncture and other diagnostic or therapeutic procedures with potential for uncontrollable bleeding (4)
- Hypersensitivity to warfarin or any component of the product (4)
- Major regional or lumbar block anesthesia (4)
- Malignant hypertension (4)

—————WARNINGS AND PRECAUTIONS—————
- Tissue necrosis: Necrosis or gangrene of skin or other tissues can occur, with severe cases requiring debridement or amputation. Discontinue COUMADIN and consider alternative anticoagulants if necessary. (5.2)
- Systemic atheroemboli and cholesterol microemboli: Some cases have progressed to necrosis or death. Discontinue COUMADIN if such emboli occur. (5.3)

- Heparin-induced thrombocytopenia (HIT): Initial therapy with COUMADIN in HIT has resulted in cases of amputation and death. COUMADIN (warfarin sodium) may be considered after platelet count has normalized. (5.4)
- Pregnant women with mechanical heart valves: COUMADIN may cause fetal harm; however, the benefits may outweigh the risks. (5.5)

—————ADVERSE REACTIONS—————
Most common adverse reactions to COUMADIN are fatal and nonfatal hemorrhage from any tissue or organ. (6)
To report SUSPECTED ADVERSE REACTIONS, contact Bristol-Myers Squibb at 1-800-721-5072 or FDA at 1-800-FDA-1088 or *www.fda.gov/medwatch*.

—————DRUG INTERACTIONS—————
- Consult labeling of all concurrently used drugs for complete information about interactions with COUMADIN or increased risks for bleeding. (7)
- Inhibitors and inducers of CYP2C9, 1A2, or 3A4: May alter warfarin exposure. Monitor INR closely when any such drug is used with COUMADIN. (7.1)
- Drugs that increase bleeding risk: Closely monitor patients receiving any such drug (e.g., other anticoagulants, antiplatelet agents, nonsteroidal anti-inflammatory drugs, serotonin reuptake inhibitors). (7.2)
- Antibiotics and antifungals: Closely monitor INR when initiating or stopping an antibiotic or antifungal course of therapy. (7.3)
- Botanical (herbal) products: Some may influence patient response to COUMADIN necessitating close INR monitoring. (7.4)

—————USE IN SPECIFIC POPULATIONS—————
- Nursing mothers: Use with caution in a nursing woman. Monitor breast-feeding infants for bruising or bleeding. (8.3)

See 17 for PATIENT COUNSELING INFORMATION and Medication Guide

Revised: 10/2011

15 REFERENCES
16 HOW SUPPLIED/STORAGE AND HANDLING
17 PATIENT COUNSELING INFORMATION
* Sections or subsections omitted from the full prescribing information are not listed

FULL PRESCRIBING INFORMATION

> **WARNING: BLEEDING RISK**
> * COUMADIN can cause major or fatal bleeding [see *Warnings and Precautions (5.1)*].
> * Perform regular monitoring of INR in all treated patients [see *Dosage and Administration (2.1)*].
> * Drugs, dietary changes, and other factors affect INR levels achieved with COUMADIN therapy [see *Drug Interactions (7)*].
> * Instruct patients about prevention measures to minimize risk of bleeding and to report signs and symptoms of bleeding [see *Patient Counseling Information (17)*].

1 INDICATIONS AND USAGE

COUMADIN® (warfarin sodium) is indicated for:
* Prophylaxis and treatment of venous thrombosis and its extension, pulmonary embolism (PE).
* Prophylaxis and treatment of thromboembolic complications associated with atrial fibrillation (AF) and/or cardiac valve replacement.
* Reduction in the risk of death, recurrent myocardial infarction (MI), and thromboembolic events such as stroke or systemic embolization after myocardial infarction.

Limitations of Use

COUMADIN has no direct effect on an established thrombus, nor does it reverse ischemic tissue damage. Once a thrombus has occurred, however, the goals of anticoagulant treatment are to prevent further extension of the formed clot and to prevent secondary thromboembolic complications that may result in serious and possibly fatal sequelae.

2 DOSAGE AND ADMINISTRATION
2.1 Individualized Dosing

The dosage and administration of COUMADIN must be individualized for each patient according to the patient's INR response to the drug. Adjust the dose based on the patient's INR and the condition being treated. Consult the latest evidence-based clinical practice guidelines from the American College of Chest Physicians (ACCP) to assist in the determination of the duration and intensity of anticoagulation with COUMADIN [see *References (15)*].

2.2 Recommended Target INR Ranges and Durations for Individual Indications

An INR of greater than 4.0 appears to provide no additional therapeutic benefit in most patients and is associated with a higher risk of bleeding.

Venous Thromboembolism (including deep venous thrombosis [DVT] and PE)

Adjust the warfarin dose to maintain a target INR of 2.5 (INR range, 2.0-3.0) for all treatment durations. The duration of treatment is based on the indication as follows:
* For patients with a DVT or PE secondary to a transient (reversible) risk factor, treatment with warfarin for 3 months is recommended.
* For patients with an unprovoked DVT or PE, treatment with warfarin is recommended for at least 3 months. After 3 months of therapy, evaluate the risk-benefit ratio of long-term treatment for the individual patient.
* For patients with two episodes of unprovoked DVT or PE, long-term treatment with warfarin is recommended. For a patient receiving long-term anticoagulant treatment, periodically reassess the risk-benefit ratio of continuing such treatment in the individual patient.

Atrial Fibrillation

In patients with non-valvular AF, anticoagulate with warfarin to target INR of 2.5 (range, 2.0-3.0).
* In patients with non-valvular AF that is persistent or paroxysmal and at high risk of stroke (i.e., having any of the following features: prior ischemic stroke, transient ischemic attack, or systemic embolism, or 2 of the following risk factors: age greater than 75 years, moderately or severely impaired left ventricular systolic function and/or heart failure, history of hypertension, or diabetes mellitus), long-term anticoagulation with warfarin is recommended.
* In patients with non-valvular AF that is persistent or paroxysmal and at an intermediate risk of ischemic stroke (i.e., having 1 of the following risk factors: age greater than 75 years, moderately or severely impaired left ventricular systolic function and/or heart failure, history of hypertension, or diabetes mellitus), long-term anticoagulation with warfarin is recommended.
* For patients with AF and mitral stenosis, long-term anticoagulation with warfarin is recommended.

* For patients with AF and prosthetic heart valves, long-term anticoagulation with warfarin is recommended; the target INR may be increased and aspirin added depending on valve type and position, and on patient factors.

Mechanical and Bioprosthetic Heart Valves
* For patients with a bileaflet mechanical valve or a Medtronic Hall (Minneapolis, MN) tilting disk valve in the aortic position who are in sinus rhythm and without left atrial enlargement, therapy with warfarin to a target INR of 2.5 (range, 2.0-3.0) is recommended.
* For patients with tilting disk valves and bileaflet mechanical valves in the mitral position, therapy with warfarin to a target INR of 3.0 (range, 2.5-3.5) is recommended.
* For patients with caged ball or caged disk valves, therapy with warfarin to a target INR of 3.0 (range, 2.5-3.5) is recommended.
* For patients with a bioprosthetic valve in the mitral position, therapy with warfarin to a target INR of 2.5 (range, 2.0-3.0) for the first 3 months after valve insertion is recommended. If additional risk factors for thromboembolism are present (AF, previous thromboembolism, left ventricular dysfunction), a target INR of 2.5 (range, 2.0-3.0) is recommended.

Post-Myocardial Infarction
* For high-risk patients with MI (e.g., those with a large anterior MI, those with significant heart failure, those with intracardiac thrombus visible on transthoracic echocardiography, those with AF, and those with a history of a thromboembolic event), therapy with combined moderate-intensity (INR, 2.0-3.0) warfarin plus low-dose aspirin (≤100 mg/day) for at least 3 months after the MI is recommended.

Recurrent Systemic Embolism and Other Indications

Oral anticoagulation therapy with warfarin has not been fully evaluated by clinical trials in patients with valvular disease associated with AF, patients with mitral stenosis, and patients with recurrent systemic embolism of unknown etiology. However, a moderate dose regimen (INR 2.0-3.0) may be used for these patients.

2.3 Initial and Maintenance Dosing

The appropriate initial dosing of COUMADIN (warfarin sodium) varies widely for different patients. Not all factors responsible for warfarin dose variability are known, and the initial dose is influenced by:
* Clinical factors including age, race, body weight, sex, concomitant medications, and comorbidities
* Genetic factors (CYP2C9 and VKORC1 genotypes) [see *Clinical Pharmacology (12.5)*]

Select the initial dose based on the expected maintenance dose, taking into account the above factors. Modify this dose based on consideration of patient-specific clinical factors. Consider lower initial and maintenance doses for elderly and/or debilitated patients and in Asian patients [see *Use in Specific Populations (8.5)* and *Clinical Pharmacology (12.3)*]. Routine use of loading doses is not recommended as this practice may increase hemorrhagic and other complications and does not offer more rapid protection against clot formation.

Individualize the duration of therapy for each patient. In general, anticoagulant therapy should be continued until the danger of thrombosis and embolism has passed [see *Dosage and Administration (2.2)*].

Dosing Recommendations without Consideration of Genotype

If the patient's CYP2C9 and VKORC1 genotypes are not known, the initial dose of COUMADIN is usually 2 to 5 mg once daily. Determine each patient's dosing needs by close monitoring of the INR response and consideration of the indication being treated. Typical maintenance doses are 2 to 10 mg once daily.

Dosing Recommendations with Consideration of Genotype

Table 1 displays three ranges of expected maintenance COUMADIN doses observed in subgroups of patients having different combinations of CYP2C9 and VKORC1 gene variants [see *Clinical Pharmacology (12.5)*]. If the patient's CYP2C9 and/or VKORC1 genotype are known, consider these ranges in choosing the initial dose. Patients with CYP2C9 *1/*3, *2/*2, *2/*3, and *3/*3 may require more

prolonged time (>2 to 4 weeks) to achieve maximum INR effect for a given dosage regimen than patients without these CYP variants.
[See table 1 above]

2.4 Monitoring to Achieve Optimal Anticoagulation

COUMADIN (warfarin sodium) is a narrow therapeutic range (index) drug, and its action may be affected by factors such as other drugs and dietary vitamin K. Therefore, anticoagulation must be carefully monitored during COUMADIN therapy. Determine the INR daily after the administration of the initial dose until INR results stabilize in the therapeutic range. After stabilization, maintain dosing within the therapeutic range by performing periodic INRs. The frequency of performing INR should be based on the clinical situation but generally acceptable intervals for INR determinations are 1 to 4 weeks. Perform additional INR tests when other warfarin products are interchanged with COUMADIN, as well as whenever other medications are initiated, discontinued, or taken irregularly. Heparin, a common concomitant drug, increases the INR [see *Dosage and Administration (2.8)* and *Drug Interactions (7)*]. Determinations of whole blood clotting and bleeding times are not effective measures for monitoring of COUMADIN (warfarin sodium) therapy.

2.5 Missed Dose

The anticoagulant effect of COUMADIN persists beyond 24 hours. If a patient misses a dose of COUMADIN at the intended time of day, the patient should take the dose as soon as possible on the same day. The patient should not double the dose the next day to make up for a missed dose.

2.6 Intravenous Route of Administration

The intravenous dose of COUMADIN is the same as the oral dose. After reconstitution, COUMADIN for injection should be administered as a slow bolus injection into a peripheral vein over 1 to 2 minutes. COUMADIN for injection is not recommended for intramuscular administration.
Reconstitute the vial with 2.7 mL of Sterile Water for Injection. The resulting yield is 2.5 mL of a 2 mg per mL solution (5 mg total). Parenteral drug products should be inspected visually for particulate matter and discoloration prior to administration. Do not use if particulate matter or discoloration is noted.
After reconstitution, COUMADIN for injection is stable for 4 hours at room temperature. It does not contain any antimicrobial preservative and, thus, care must be taken to assure the sterility of the prepared solution. The vial is for single use only, and any unused solution should be discarded.

2.7 Treatment During Dentistry and Surgery

Some dental or surgical procedures may necessitate the interruption or change in the dose of COUMADIN therapy. Consider the benefits and risks when discontinuing COUMADIN even for a short period of time. Determine the INR immediately prior to any dental or surgical procedure. In patients undergoing minimally invasive procedures who must be anticoagulated prior to, during, or immediately following these procedures, adjusting the dosage of COUMADIN to maintain the INR at the low end of the therapeutic range may safely allow for continued anticoagulation.

2.8 Conversion From Other Anticoagulants

Heparin

Since the full anticoagulant effect of COUMADIN is not achieved for several days, heparin is preferred for initial rapid anticoagulation. During initial therapy with COUMADIN, the interference with heparin anticoagulation is of minimal clinical significance. Conversion to COUMADIN may begin concomitantly with heparin therapy or may be delayed 3 to 6 days. To ensure therapeutic anticoagulation, continue full dose heparin therapy and overlap COUMADIN therapy with heparin for 4 to 5 days and until COUMADIN has produced the desired therapeutic response as determined by INR, at which point heparin may be discontinued.
As heparin may affect the INR, patients receiving both heparin and COUMADIN should have INR monitoring at least:

Table 1: Three Ranges of Expected Maintenance COUMADIN Daily Doses Based on CYP2C9 and VKORC1 Genotypes†

VKORC1	CYP2C9					
	*1/*1	*1/*2	*1/*3	*2/*2	*2/*3	*3/*3
GG	5-7 mg	5-7 mg	3-4 mg	3-4 mg	3-4 mg	0.5-2 mg
AG	5-7 mg	3-4 mg	3-4 mg	3-4 mg	0.5-2 mg	0.5-2 mg
AA	3-4 mg	3-4 mg	0.5-2 mg	0.5-2 mg	0.5-2 mg	0.5-2 mg

†Ranges are derived from multiple published clinical studies. VKORC1 –1639G>A (rs9923231) variant is used in this table. Other co-inherited VKORC1 variants may also be important determinants of warfarin dose.

- 5 hours after the last intravenous bolus dose of heparin, or
- 4 hours after cessation of a continuous intravenous infusion of heparin, or
- 24 hours after the last subcutaneous heparin injection.

COUMADIN (warfarin sodium) may increase the activated partial thromboplastin time (aPTT) test, even in the absence of heparin. A severe elevation (>50 seconds) in aPTT with an INR in the desired range has been identified as an indication of increased risk of postoperative hemorrhage.

Other Anticoagulants
Consult the labeling of other anticoagulants for instructions on conversion to COUMADIN.

3 DOSAGE FORMS AND STRENGTHS

COUMADIN tablets are single scored with one face imprinted numerically with 1, 2, 2-1/2, 3, 4, 5, 6, 7-1/2, or 10 superimposed and inscribed with "COUMADIN" and with the opposite face plain.
COUMADIN tablets are supplied in the following strengths:

COUMADIN Tablets

Strength	Color
1 mg	pink
2 mg	lavender
2-1/2 mg	green
3 mg	tan
4 mg	blue
5 mg	peach
6 mg	teal
7-1/2 mg	yellow
10 mg	white (dye-free)

COUMADIN for injection is available in a vial containing 5 mg of lyophilized powder.

4 CONTRAINDICATIONS

- Pregnancy

COUMADIN is contraindicated in women who are pregnant except in pregnant women with mechanical heart valves, who are at high risk of thromboembolism [see *Warnings and Precautions (5.5)* and *Use in Specific Populations (8.1)*]. COUMADIN can cause fetal harm when administered to a pregnant woman. COUMADIN exposure during pregnancy causes a recognized pattern of major congenital malformations (warfarin embryopathy and fetotoxicity), fatal fetal hemorrhage, and an increased risk of spontaneous abortion and fetal mortality. If COUMADIN is used during pregnancy or if the patient becomes pregnant while taking this drug, the patient should be apprised of the potential hazard to a fetus [see *Warnings and Precautions (5.6)* and *Use in Specific Populations (8.1)*].
- Hemorrhagic tendencies or blood dyscrasias
- Recent or contemplated surgery of the central nervous system or eye, or traumatic surgery resulting in large open surfaces [see *Warnings and Precautions (5.7)*]
- Bleeding tendencies associated with:
  – Active ulceration or overt bleeding of the gastrointestinal, genitourinary, or respiratory tract
  – Central nervous system hemorrhage
  – Cerebral aneurysms, dissecting aorta
  – Pericarditis and pericardial effusions
  – Bacterial endocarditis
- Threatened abortion, eclampsia, and preeclampsia
- Unsupervised patients with conditions associated with potential high level of non-compliance
- Spinal puncture and other diagnostic or therapeutic procedures with potential for uncontrollable bleeding
- Hypersensitivity to warfarin or to any other components of this product (e.g., anaphylaxis) [see *Adverse Reactions (6)*]
- Major regional or lumbar block anesthesia
- Malignant hypertension

5 WARNINGS AND PRECAUTIONS

5.1 Hemorrhage
COUMADIN can cause major or fatal bleeding. Bleeding is more likely to occur within the first month. Risk factors for bleeding include high intensity of anticoagulation (INR >4.0), age greater than or equal to 65, history of highly variable INRs, history of gastrointestinal bleeding, hypertension, cerebrovascular disease, anemia, malignancy, trauma, renal impairment, certain genetic factors [see *Clinical Pharmacology (12.5)*], certain concomitant drugs [see *Drug Interactions (7)*], and long duration of warfarin therapy.
Perform regular monitoring of INR in all treated patients. Those at high risk of bleeding may benefit from more frequent INR monitoring, careful dose adjustment to desired INR, and a shortest duration of therapy appropriate for the clinical condition. However, maintenance of INR in the therapeutic range does not eliminate the risk of bleeding.
Drugs, dietary changes, and other factors affect INR levels achieved with COUMADIN therapy. Perform more frequent INR monitoring when starting or stopping other drugs, including botanicals, or when changing dosages of other drugs [see *Drug Interactions (7)*].
Instruct patients about prevention measures to minimize risk of bleeding and to report signs and symptoms of bleeding [see *Patient Counseling Information (17)*].

5.2 Tissue Necrosis
Necrosis and/or gangrene of skin and other tissues is an uncommon but serious risk (<0.1%). Necrosis may be associated with local thrombosis and usually appears within a few days of the start of COUMADIN therapy. In severe cases of necrosis, treatment through debridement or amputation of the affected tissue, limb, breast, or penis has been reported. Careful clinical evaluation is required to determine whether necrosis is caused by an underlying disease. Although various treatments have been attempted, no treatment for necrosis has been considered uniformly effective. Discontinue COUMADIN therapy if necrosis occurs. Consider alternative drugs if continued anticoagulation therapy is necessary.

5.3 Systemic Atheroemboli and Cholesterol Microemboli
Anticoagulation therapy with COUMADIN (warfarin sodium) may enhance the release of atheromatous plaque emboli. Systemic atheroemboli and cholesterol microemboli can present with a variety of signs and symptoms depending on the site of embolization. The most commonly involved visceral organs are the kidneys followed by the pancreas, spleen, and liver. Some cases have progressed to necrosis or death. A distinct syndrome resulting from microemboli to the feet is known as "purple toes syndrome." Discontinue COUMADIN therapy if such phenomena are observed. Consider alternative drugs if continued anticoagulation therapy is necessary.

5.4 Heparin-Induced Thrombocytopenia
Do not use COUMADIN as initial therapy in patients with heparin-induced thrombocytopenia (HIT) and with heparin-induced thrombocytopenia with thrombosis syndrome (HITTS). Cases of limb ischemia, necrosis, and gangrene have occurred in patients with HIT and HITTS when heparin treatment was discontinued and warfarin therapy was started or continued. In some patients, sequelae have included amputation of the involved area and/or death. Treatment with COUMADIN may be considered after the platelet count has normalized.

5.5 Use in Pregnant Women with Mechanical Heart Valves
COUMADIN can cause fetal harm when administered to a pregnant woman. While COUMADIN is contraindicated during pregnancy, the potential benefits of using COUMADIN may outweigh the risks for pregnant women with mechanical heart valves at high risk of thromboembolism. In those individual situations, the decision to initiate or continue COUMADIN should be reviewed with the patient, taking into consideration the specific risks and benefits pertaining to the individual patient's medical situation, as well as the most current medical guidelines. COUMADIN exposure during pregnancy causes a recognized pattern of major congenital malformations (warfarin embryopathy and fetotoxicity), fatal fetal hemorrhage, and an increased risk of spontaneous abortion and fetal mortality. If this drug is used during pregnancy, or if the patient becomes pregnant while taking this drug, the patient should be apprised of the potential hazard to a fetus [see *Use in Specific Populations (8.1)*].

5.6 Females of Reproductive Potential
COUMADIN exposure during pregnancy can cause pregnancy loss, birth defects, or fetal death. Discuss pregnancy planning with females of reproductive potential who are on COUMADIN therapy [see *Contraindications (4)* and *Use in Specific Populations (8.8)*].

5.7 Other Clinical Settings with Increased Risks
In the following clinical settings, the risks of COUMADIN therapy may be increased:
- Moderate to severe hepatic impairment
- Infectious diseases or disturbances of intestinal flora (e.g., sprue, antibiotic therapy)
- Use of an indwelling catheter
- Severe to moderate hypertension
- Deficiency in protein C-mediated anticoagulant response: COUMADIN reduces the synthesis of the naturally occurring anticoagulants, protein C and protein S. Hereditary or acquired deficiencies of protein C or its cofactor, protein S, have been associated with tissue necrosis following warfarin administration. Concomitant anticoagulation therapy with heparin for 5 to 7 days during initiation of therapy with COUMADIN may minimize the incidence of tissue necrosis in these patients.
- Eye surgery: In cataract surgery, COUMADIN use was associated with a significant increase in minor complications of sharp needle and local anesthesia block but not associated with potentially sight-threatening operative hemorrhagic complications. As COUMADIN cessation or reduction may lead to serious thromboembolic complications, the decision to discontinue COUMADIN before a relatively less invasive and complex eye surgery, such as lens surgery, should be based upon the risks of anticoagulant therapy weighed against the benefits.
- Polycythemia vera
- Vasculitis
- Diabetes mellitus

5.8 Endogenous Factors Affecting INR
The following factors may be responsible for **increased** INR response: diarrhea, hepatic disorders, poor nutritional state, steatorrhea, or vitamin K deficiency.

The following factors may be responsible for **decreased** INR response: increased vitamin K intake or hereditary warfarin resistance.

6 ADVERSE REACTIONS

The following serious adverse reactions to COUMADIN are discussed in greater detail in other sections of the labeling:
- Hemorrhage [see *Boxed Warning*, *Warnings and Precautions (5.1)*, and *Overdosage (10)*]
- Necrosis of skin and other tissues [see *Warnings and Precautions (5.2)*]
- Systemic atheroemboli and cholesterol microemboli [see *Warnings and Precautions (5.3)*]
Other adverse reactions to COUMADIN include:
- Immune system disorders: hypersensitivity/allergic reactions (including urticaria and anaphylactic reactions)
- Vascular disorders: vasculitis
- Hepatobiliary disorders: hepatitis, elevated liver enzymes. Cholestatic hepatitis has been associated with concomitant administration of COUMADIN and ticlopidine.
- Gastrointestinal disorders: nausea, vomiting, diarrhea, taste perversion, abdominal pain, flatulence, bloating
- Skin disorders: rash, dermatitis (including bullous eruptions), pruritus, alopecia
- Respiratory disorders: tracheal or tracheobronchial calcification
- General disorders: chills

7 DRUG INTERACTIONS

Drugs may interact with COUMADIN (warfarin sodium) through pharmacodynamic or pharmacokinetic mechanisms. Pharmacodynamic mechanisms for drug interactions with COUMADIN are synergism (impaired hemostasis, reduced clotting factor synthesis), competitive antagonism (vitamin K), and alteration of the physiologic control loop for vitamin K metabolism (hereditary resistance). Pharmacokinetic mechanisms for drug interactions with COUMADIN are mainly enzyme induction, enzyme inhibition, and reduced plasma protein binding. It is important to note that some drugs may interact by more than one mechanism.
More frequent INR monitoring should be performed when starting or stopping other drugs, including botanicals, or when changing dosages of other drugs, including drugs intended for short-term use (e.g., antibiotics, antifungals, corticosteroids) [see *Boxed Warning*].
Consult the labeling of all concurrently used drugs to obtain further information about interactions with COUMADIN or adverse reactions pertaining to bleeding.

7.1 CYP450 Interactions
CYP450 isozymes involved in the metabolism of warfarin include CYP2C9, 2C19, 2C8, 2C18, 1A2, and 3A4. The more potent warfarin S-enantiomer is metabolized by CYP2C9 while the R-enantiomer is metabolized by CYP1A2 and 3A4.
- Inhibitors of CYP2C9, 1A2, and/or 3A4 have the potential to increase the effect (increase INR) of warfarin by increasing the exposure of warfarin.
- Inducers of CYP2C9, 1A2, and/or 3A4 have the potential to decrease the effect (decrease INR) of warfarin by decreasing the exposure of warfarin.

Examples of inhibitors and inducers of CYP2C9, 1A2, and 3A4 are below in Table 2; however, this list should not be considered all-inclusive. Consult the labeling of all concurrently used drugs to obtain further information about CYP450 interaction potential. The CYP450 inhibition and induction potential should be considered when starting, stopping, or changing dose of concomitant mediations. Closely monitor INR if a concomitant drug is a CYP2C9, 1A2, and/or 3A4 inhibitor or inducer.

Table 2: Examples of CYP450 Interactions with Warfarin

Enzyme	Inhibitors	Inducers
CYP2C9	amiodarone, capecitabine, cotrimoxazole, etravirine, fluconazole, fluvastatin, fluvoxamine, metronidazole, miconazole, oxandrolone, sulfinpyrazone, tigecycline, voriconazole, zafirlukast	aprepitant, bosentan, carbamazepine, phenobarbital, rifampin
CYP1A2	acyclovir, allopurinol, caffeine, cimetidine, ciprofloxacin, disulfiram, enoxacin, famotidine, fluvoxamine, methoxsalen, mexiletine, norfloxacin, oral contraceptives, phenylpropanolamine, propafenone, propranolol, terbinafine, thiabendazole, ticlopidine, verapamil, zileuton	montelukast, moricizine, omeprazole, phenobarbital, phenytoin, cigarette smoking

CYP3A4	alprazolam, amiodarone, amlodipine, amprenavir, aprepitant, atorvastatin, atazanavir, bicalutamide, cilostazol, cimetidine, ciprofloxacin, clarithromycin, conivaptan, cyclosporine, darunavir/ritonavir, diltiazem, erythromycin, fluconazole, fluoxetine, fluvoxamine, fosamprenavir, imatinib, indinavir, isoniazid, itraconazole, ketoconazole, lopinavir/ritonavir, nefazodone, nelfinavir, nilotinib, oral contraceptives, posaconazole, ranitidine, ranolazine, ritonavir, saquinavir, telithromycin, tipranavir, voriconazole, zileuton	armodafinil, amprenavir, aprepitant, bosentan, carbamazepine, efavirenz, etravirine, modafinil, nafcillin, phenytoin, pioglitazone, prednisone, rifampin, rufinamide

7.2 Drugs that Increase Bleeding Risk

Examples of drugs known to increase the risk of bleeding are presented in Table 3. Because bleeding risk is increased when these drugs are used concomitantly with warfarin, closely monitor patients receiving any such drug with warfarin.

Table 3: Drugs that Can Increase the Risk of Bleeding

Drug Class	Specific Drugs
Anticoagulants	argatroban, dabigatran, bivalirudin, desirudin, heparin, lepirudin
Antiplatelet Agents	aspirin, cilostazol, clopidogrel, dipyridamole, prasugrel, ticlopidine
Nonsteroidal Anti-Inflammatory Agents	celecoxib, diclofenac, diflunisal, fenoprofen, ibuprofen, indomethacin, ketoprofen, ketorolac, mefenamic acid, naproxen, oxaprozin, piroxicam, sulindac
Serotonin Reuptake Inhibitors	citalopram, desvenlafaxine, duloxetine, escitalopram, fluoxetine, fluvoxamine, milnacipran, paroxetine, sertraline, venlafaxine, vilazodone

7.3 Antibiotics and Antifungals

There have been reports of changes in INR in patients taking warfarin and antibiotics or antifungals, but clinical pharmacokinetic studies have not shown consistent effects of these agents on plasma concentrations of warfarin.

Closely monitor INR when starting or stopping any antibiotic or antifungal in patients taking warfarin.

7.4 Botanical (Herbal) Products and Foods

Exercise caution when botanical (herbal) products are taken concomitantly with COUMADIN (warfarin sodium). Few adequate, well-controlled studies evaluating the potential for metabolic and/or pharmacologic interactions between botanicals and COUMADIN exist. Due to a lack of manufacturing standardization with botanical medicinal preparations, the amount of active ingredients may vary. This could further confound the ability to assess potential interactions and effects on anticoagulation.

Some botanicals may cause bleeding events when taken alone (e.g., garlic and Ginkgo biloba) and may have anticoagulant, antiplatelet, and/or fibrinolytic properties. These effects would be expected to be additive to the anticoagulant effects of COUMADIN. Conversely, some botanicals may decrease the effects of COUMADIN (e.g., co-enzyme Q_{10}, St. John's wort, ginseng). Some botanicals and foods can interact with COUMADIN through CYP450 interactions (e.g., echinacea, grapefruit juice, ginkgo, goldenseal, St. John's wort).

Monitor the patient's response with additional INR determinations when initiating or discontinuing any botanicals.

8 USE IN SPECIFIC POPULATIONS

8.1 Pregnancy

Pregnancy Category D for women with mechanical heart valves [see *Warnings and Precautions (5.5)*] and **Pregnancy Category X** for other pregnant populations [see *Contraindications (4)*].

COUMADIN is contraindicated in women who are pregnant except in pregnant women with mechanical heart valves, who are at high risk of thromboembolism, and for whom the benefits of COUMADIN may outweigh the risks.

COUMADIN (warfarin sodium) can cause fetal harm when administered to a pregnant woman. COUMADIN exposure during pregnancy causes a recognized pattern of major congenital malformations (warfarin embryopathy), fetal hemorrhage, and an increased risk of spontaneous abortion and fetal mortality. The reproductive and developmental effects of COUMADIN have not been evaluated in animals. If this drug is used during pregnancy or if the patient becomes pregnant while taking this drug, the patient should be apprised of the potential hazard to the fetus.

In humans, warfarin crosses the placenta, and concentrations in fetal plasma approach the maternal values. Exposure to warfarin during the first trimester of pregnancy caused a pattern of congenital malformations in about 5% of exposed offspring. Warfarin embryopathy is characterized by nasal hypoplasia with or without stippled epiphyses (chondrodysplasia punctata) and growth retardation (including low birth weight). Central nervous system and eye abnormalities have also been reported, including dorsal midline dysplasia characterized by agenesis of the corpus callosum, Dandy-Walker malformation, midline cerebellar atrophy, and ventral midline dysplasia characterized by optic atrophy. Mental retardation, blindness, schizencephaly, microcephaly, hydrocephalus, and other adverse pregnancy outcomes have been reported following warfarin exposure during the second and third trimesters of pregnancy [see *Contraindications (4)* and *Warnings and Precautions (5.6)*].

8.3 Nursing Mothers

Based on published data in 15 nursing mothers, warfarin was not detected in human milk. Among the 15 full-term newborns, 6 nursing infants had documented prothrombin times within the expected range. Prothrombin times were not obtained for the other 9 nursing infants. Monitor breastfeeding infants for bruising or bleeding. Effects in premature infants have not been evaluated. Caution should be exercised when COUMADIN is administered to a nursing woman.

8.4 Pediatric Use

Adequate and well-controlled studies with COUMADIN have not been conducted in any pediatric population, and the optimum dosing, safety, and efficacy in pediatric patients is unknown. Pediatric use of COUMADIN is based on adult data and recommendations, and available limited pediatric data from observational studies and patient registries. Pediatric patients administered COUMADIN should avoid any activity or sport that may result in traumatic injury.

The developing hemostatic system in infants and children results in a changing physiology of thrombosis and response to anticoagulants. Dosing of warfarin in the pediatric population varies by patient age, with infants generally having the highest, and adolescents having the lowest milligram per kilogram dose requirements to maintain target INRs. Because of changing warfarin requirements due to age, concomitant medications, diet, and existing medical condition, target INR ranges may be difficult to achieve and maintain in pediatric patients, and more frequent INR determinations are recommended. Bleeding rates varied by patient population and clinical care center in pediatric observational studies and patient registries.

Infants and children receiving vitamin K-supplemented nutrition, including infant formulas, may be resistant to warfarin therapy, while human milk-fed infants may be sensitive to warfarin therapy.

8.5 Geriatric Use

Of the total number of patients receiving warfarin sodium in controlled clinical trials for which data were available for analysis, 1885 patients (24.4%) were 65 years and older, while 185 patients (2.4%) were 75 years and older. No overall differences in effectiveness or safety were observed between these patients and younger patients, but greater sensitivity of some older individuals cannot be ruled out.

Patients 60 years or older appear to exhibit greater than expected INR response to the anticoagulant effects of warfarin [see *Clinical Pharmacology (12.3)*]. COUMADIN is contraindicated in any unsupervised patient with senility. Observe caution with administration of COUMADIN to elderly patients in any situation or with any physical condition where added risk of hemorrhage is present. Consider lower initiation and maintenance doses of COUMADIN in elderly patients [see *Dosage and Administration (2.2, 2.3)*].

8.6 Renal Impairment

Renal clearance is considered to be a minor determinant of anticoagulant response to warfarin. No dosage adjustment is necessary for patients with renal impairment.

8.7 Hepatic Impairment

Hepatic impairment can potentiate the response to warfarin through impaired synthesis of clotting factors and decreased metabolism of warfarin. Use caution when using COUMADIN in these patients.

8.8 Females of Reproductive Potential

COUMADIN exposure during pregnancy can cause spontaneous abortion, birth defects, or fetal death. Females of reproductive potential who are candidates for COUMADIN therapy should be counseled regarding the benefits of therapy and potential reproductive risks. Discuss pregnancy planning with females of reproductive potential who are on COUMADIN (warfarin sodium) therapy. If the patient becomes pregnant while taking COUMADIN, she should be apprised of the potential risks to the fetus.

10 OVERDOSAGE

10.1 Signs and Symptoms

Bleeding (e.g., appearance of blood in stools or urine, hematuria, excessive menstrual bleeding, melena, petechiae, excessive bruising or persistent oozing from superficial injuries, unexplained fall in hemoglobin) is a manifestation of excessive anticoagulation.

10.2 Treatment

The treatment of excessive anticoagulation is based on the level of the INR, the presence or absence of bleeding, and clinical circumstances. Reversal of COUMADIN anticoagulation may be obtained by discontinuing COUMADIN therapy and, if necessary, by administration of oral or parenteral vitamin K_1.

The use of vitamin K_1 reduces response to subsequent COUMADIN therapy and patients may return to a pretreatment thrombotic status following the rapid reversal of a prolonged INR. Resumption of COUMADIN administration reverses the effect of vitamin K, and a therapeutic INR can again be obtained by careful dosage adjustment. If rapid re-anticoagulation is indicated, heparin may be preferable for initial therapy.

Prothrombin complex concentrate (PCC), fresh frozen plasma, or activated Factor VII treatment may be considered if the requirement to reverse the effects of COUMADIN is urgent. A risk of hepatitis and other viral diseases is associated with the use of blood products; PCC and activated Factor VII are also associated with an increased risk of thrombosis. Therefore, these preparations should be used only in exceptional or life-threatening bleeding episodes secondary to COUMADIN overdosage.

11 DESCRIPTION

COUMADIN (warfarin sodium) is an anticoagulant that acts by inhibiting vitamin K-dependent coagulation factors. Chemically, it is 3-(α-acetonylbenzyl)-4-hydroxycoumarin and is a racemic mixture of the *R*- and *S*-enantiomers. Crystalline warfarin sodium is an isopropanol clathrate. Its empirical formula is $C_{19}H_{15}NaO_4$, and its structural formula is represented by the following:

Crystalline warfarin sodium occurs as a white, odorless, crystalline powder that is discolored by light. It is very soluble in water, freely soluble in alcohol, and very slightly soluble in chloroform and ether.

COUMADIN tablets for oral use also contain:

All strengths:	Lactose, starch, and magnesium stearate
1 mg:	D&C Red No. 6 Barium Lake
2 mg:	FD&C Blue No. 2 Aluminum Lake and FD&C Red No. 40 Aluminum Lake
2-1/2 mg:	D&C Yellow No. 10 Aluminum Lake and FD&C Blue No. 1 Aluminum Lake
3 mg:	FD&C Yellow No. 6 Aluminum Lake, FD&C Blue No. 2 Aluminum Lake, and FD&C Red No. 40 Aluminum Lake
4 mg:	FD&C Blue No. 1 Aluminum Lake
5 mg:	FD&C Yellow No. 6 Aluminum Lake
6 mg:	FD&C Yellow No. 6 Aluminum Lake and FD&C Blue No. 1 Aluminum Lake
7-1/2 mg:	D&C Yellow No. 10 Aluminum Lake and FD&C Yellow No. 6 Aluminum Lake
10 mg:	Dye-free

COUMADIN for injection for intravenous use is supplied as a sterile, lyophilized powder, which, after reconstitution with 2.7 mL Sterile Water for Injection, contains:

Warfarin sodium	2 mg per mL
Sodium phosphate, dibasic, heptahydrate	4.98 mg per mL
Sodium phosphate, monobasic, monohydrate	0.194 mg per mL
Sodium chloride	0.1 mg per mL
Mannitol	38.0 mg per mL
Sodium hydroxide, as needed for pH adjustment to 8.1 to 8.3	

12 CLINICAL PHARMACOLOGY

12.1 Mechanism of Action

Warfarin acts by inhibiting the synthesis of vitamin K-dependent clotting factors, which include Factors II, VII, IX, and X, and the anticoagulant proteins C and S. Vitamin K is an essential cofactor for the post ribosomal synthesis of the vitamin K-dependent clotting factors. Vitamin K pro-

Table 4: Clinical Studies of Warfarin in Non-Rheumatic AF Patients*

	N				Thromboembolism			% Major Bleeding	
Study	Warfarin-Treated Patients	Control Patients	PT Ratio	INR	% Risk Reduction	p-value		Warfarin-Treated Patients	Control Patients
AFASAK	335	336	1.5-2.0	2.8-4.2	60	0.027		0.6	0.0
SPAF	210	211	1.3-1.8	2.0-4.5	67	0.01		1.9	1.9
BAATAF	212	208	1.2-1.5	1.5-2.7	86	<0.05		0.9	0.5
CAFA	187	191	1.3-1.6	2.0-3.0	45	0.25		2.7	0.5
SPINAF	260	265	1.2-1.5	1.4-2.8	79	0.001		2.3	1.5

*All study results of warfarin vs. control are based on intention-to-treat analysis and include ischemic stroke and systemic thromboembolism, excluding hemorrhagic stroke and transient ischemic attacks.

Table 5: Prospective, Randomized, Open-Label, Positive-Controlled Clinical Study of Warfarin in Patients with Mechanical Prosthetic Heart Valves

	Patients Treated With		
Event	Warfarin	Dipyridamole/Aspirin	Pentoxifylline/Aspirin
Thromboembolism	2.2/100 py	8.6/100 py	7.9/100 py
Major Bleeding	2.5/100 py	0.0/100 py	0.9/100 py

py=patient years

Table 6: Prospective, Open-Label Clinical Study of Warfarin in Patients with Mechanical Prosthetic Heart Valves

Event	Moderate Warfarin Therapy INR 2.65	High Intensity Warfarin Therapy INR 9.0
Thromboembolism	4.0/100 py	3.7/100 py
Major Bleeding	0.95/100 py	2.1/100 py

py=patient years

motes the biosynthesis of γ-carboxyglutamic acid residues in the proteins that are essential for biological activity. Warfarin is thought to interfere with clotting factor synthesis by inhibition of the C1 subunit of vitamin K epoxide reductase (VKORC1) enzyme complex, thereby reducing the regeneration of vitamin K_1 epoxide [see *Clinical Pharmacology (12.5)*].

12.2   Pharmacodynamics

An anticoagulation effect generally occurs within 24 hours after warfarin administration. However, peak anticoagulant effect may be delayed 72 to 96 hours. The duration of action of a single dose of racemic warfarin is 2 to 5 days. The effects of COUMADIN may become more pronounced as effects of daily maintenance doses overlap. This is consistent with the half-lives of the affected vitamin K-dependent clotting factors and anticoagulation proteins: Factor II - 60 hours, VII - 4 to 6 hours, IX - 24 hours, X - 48 to 72 hours, and proteins C and S are approximately 8 hours and 30 hours, respectively.

12.3   Pharmacokinetics

COUMADIN (warfarin sodium) is a racemic mixture of the *R*- and *S*-enantiomers of warfarin. The *S*-enantiomer exhibits 2 to 5 times more anticoagulant activity than the *R*-enantiomer in humans, but generally has a more rapid clearance.

Absorption

Warfarin is essentially completely absorbed after oral administration, with peak concentration generally attained within the first 4 hours.

Distribution

Warfarin distributes into a relatively small apparent volume of distribution of about 0.14 L/kg. A distribution phase lasting 6 to 12 hours is distinguishable after rapid intravenous or oral administration of an aqueous solution. Approximately 99% of the drug is bound to plasma proteins.

Metabolism

The elimination of warfarin is almost entirely by metabolism. Warfarin is stereoselectively metabolized by hepatic cytochrome P-450 (CYP450) microsomal enzymes to inactive hydroxylated metabolites (predominant route) and by reductases to reduced metabolites (warfarin alcohols) with minimal anticoagulant activity. Identified metabolites of warfarin include dehydrowarfarin, two diastereoisomer alcohols, and 4'-, 6-, 7-, 8-, and 10-hydroxywarfarin. The CYP450 isozymes involved in the metabolism of warfarin include CYP2C9, 2C19, 2C8, 2C18, 1A2, and 3A4. CYP2C9, a polymorphic enzyme, is likely to be the principal form of human liver CYP450 that modulates the *in vivo* anticoagulant activity of warfarin. Patients with one or more variant CYP2C9 alleles have decreased S-warfarin clearance [see *Clinical Pharmacology (12.5)*].

Excretion

The terminal half-life of warfarin after a single dose is approximately 1 week; however, the effective half-life ranges from 20 to 60 hours, with a mean of about 40 hours. The clearance of R-warfarin is generally half that of S-warfarin, thus as the volumes of distribution are similar, the half-life of R-warfarin is longer than that of S-warfarin. The half-life of R-warfarin ranges from 37 to 89 hours, while that of S-warfarin ranges from 21 to 43 hours. Studies with radiolabeled drug have demonstrated that up to 92% of the orally administered dose is recovered in urine. Very little warfarin is excreted unchanged in urine. Urinary excretion is in the form of metabolites.

Geriatric Patients

Patients 60 years or older appear to exhibit greater than expected INR response to the anticoagulant effects of warfarin. The cause of the increased sensitivity to the anticoagulant effects of warfarin in this age group is unknown but may be due to a combination of pharmacokinetic and pharmacodynamic factors. Limited information suggests there is no difference in the clearance of S-warfarin; however, there may be a slight decrease in the clearance of R-warfarin in the elderly as compared to the young. Therefore, as patient age increases, a lower dose of warfarin is usually required to produce a therapeutic level of anticoagulation [see *Dosage and Administration (2.3, 2.4)*].

Asian Patients

Asian patients may require lower initiation and maintenance doses of warfarin. A non-controlled study of 151 Chinese outpatients stabilized on warfarin for various indications reported a mean daily warfarin requirement of 3.3 ± 1.4 mg to achieve an INR of 2 to 2.5. Patient age was the most important determinant of warfarin requirement in these patients, with a progressively lower warfarin requirement with increasing age.

12.5   Pharmacogenomics

CYP2C9 and VKORC1 Polymorphisms

The *S*-enantiomer of warfarin is mainly metabolized to 7-hydroxywarfarin by CYP2C9, a polymorphic enzyme. The variant alleles, CYP2C9*2 and CYP2C9*3, result in decreased *in vitro* CYP2C9 enzymatic 7-hydroxylation of S-warfarin. The frequencies of these alleles in Caucasians are approximately 11% and 7% for CYP2C9*2 and CYP2C9*3, respectively.

Other CYP2C9 alleles associated with reduced enzymatic activity occur at lower frequencies, including *5, *6, and *11 alleles in populations of African ancestry and *5, *9, and *11 alleles in Caucasians.

Warfarin reduces the regeneration of vitamin K from vitamin K epoxide in the vitamin K cycle through inhibition of VKOR, a multiprotein enzyme complex. Certain single nucleotide polymorphisms in the VKORC1 gene (e.g., −1639G>A) have been associated with variable warfarin dose requirements. VKORC1 and CYP2C9 gene variants generally explain the largest proportion of known variability in warfarin dose requirements.

CYP2C9 and VKORC1 genotype information, when available, can assist in selection of the initial dose of warfarin [see *Dosage and Administration (2.3)*].

13   NONCLINICAL TOXICOLOGY

13.1   Carcinogenesis, Mutagenesis, Impairment of Fertility

Carcinogenicity, mutagenicity, or fertility studies have not been performed with warfarin.

14   CLINICAL STUDIES

14.1   Atrial Fibrillation

In five prospective, randomized, controlled clinical trials involving 3711 patients with non-rheumatic AF, warfarin significantly reduced the risk of systemic thromboembolism including stroke (see Table 4). The risk reduction ranged from 60% to 86% in all except one trial (CAFA: 45%), which was stopped early due to published positive results from two of these trials. The incidence of major bleeding in these trials ranged from 0.6% to 2.7% (see Table 4).

[See table 4 above]

Trials in patients with both AF and mitral stenosis suggest a benefit from anticoagulation with COUMADIN (warfarin sodium) [see *Dosage and Administration (2.2)*].

14.2   Mechanical and Bioprosthetic Heart Valves

In a prospective, randomized, open-label, positive-controlled study in 254 patients with mechanical prosthetic heart valves, the thromboembolic-free interval was found to be significantly greater in patients treated with warfarin alone compared with dipyridamole/aspirin-treated patients (p<0.005) and pentoxifylline/aspirin-treated patients (p<0.05). The results of this study are presented in Table 5.

[See table 5 above]

In a prospective, open-label, clinical study comparing moderate (INR 2.65) vs. high intensity (INR 9.0) warfarin therapies in 258 patients with mechanical prosthetic heart valves, thromboembolism occurred with similar frequency in the two groups (4.0 and 3.7 events per 100 patient years, respectively). Major bleeding was more common in the high intensity group. The results of this study are presented in Table 6.

[See table 6 above]

In a randomized trial in 210 patients comparing two intensities of warfarin therapy (INR 2.0-2.25 vs. INR 2.5-4.0) for a three-month period following tissue heart valve replacement, thromboembolism occurred with similar frequency in the two groups (major embolic events 2.0% vs. 1.9%, respectively, and minor embolic events 10.8% vs. 10.2%, respectively). Major hemorrhages occurred in 4.6% of patients in the higher intensity INR group compared to zero in the lower intensity INR group.

14.3   Myocardial Infarction

WARIS (The Warfarin Re-Infarction Study) was a double-blind, randomized study of 1214 patients 2 to 4 weeks postinfarction treated with warfarin to a target INR of 2.8 to 4.8. The primary endpoint was a composite of total mortality and recurrent infarction. A secondary endpoint of cerebrovascular events was assessed. Mean follow-up of the patients was 37 months. The results for each endpoint separately, including an analysis of vascular death, are provided in Table 7.

[See table 7 at top of next page]

WARIS II (The Warfarin, Aspirin, Re-Infarction Study) was an open-label, randomized study of 3630 patients hospitalized for acute myocardial infarction treated with warfarin to a target INR 2.8 to 4.2, aspirin 160 mg per day, or warfarin to a target INR 2.0 to 2.5 plus aspirin 75 mg per day prior to hospital discharge. The primary endpoint was a composite of death, nonfatal reinfarction, or thromboembolic stroke. The mean duration of observation was approximately 4 years. The results for WARIS II are provided in Table 8.

[See table 8 at top of next page]

There were approximately four times as many major bleeding episodes in the two groups receiving warfarin than in the group receiving aspirin alone. Major bleeding episodes were not more frequent among patients receiving aspirin plus warfarin than among those receiving warfarin alone, but the incidence of minor bleeding episodes was higher in the combined therapy group.

15   REFERENCES

• Ansell J, Hirsh J, Hylek E, Jacobson A, Crowther M, Palareti G. Pharmacology and management of the vitamin

K antagonists. American College of Chest Physicians Evidence-Based Clinical Practice Guidelines. 8th Ed. *Chest.* 2008;133:160S-198S.

- Kearon C, Kahn SR, Agnelli G, Goldhaber S, Raskob GE, Comerota AJ. Antithrombotic therapy for venous thrombo-embolic disease. American College of Chest Physicians Evidence-Based Clinical Practice Guidelines. 8th Ed. *Chest.* 2008;133:454S-545S.
- Singer DE, Albers GW, Dalen JE, et al. Antithrombotic therapy in atrial fibrillation. American College of Chest Physicians Evidence-Based Clinical Practice Guidelines. 8th Ed. *Chest.* 2008;133:546S-592S.
- Becker RC, Meade TW, Berger PB, et al. The primary and secondary prevention of coronary artery disease. American College of Chest Physicians Evidence-Based Clinical Practice Guidelines. 8th Ed. *Chest.* 2008;133:776S-814S.
- Salem DN, O'Gara PT, Madias C, Pauker SG. Valvular and structural heart disease. American College of Chest Physicians Evidence-Based Clinical Practice Guidelines. 8th Ed. *Chest.* 2008;133:593S-629S.
- Monagle P, Chalmers E, Chan A, et al. Antithrombotic therapy in neonates and children. American College of Chest Physicians Evidence-Based Clinical Practice Guidelines. 8th Ed. *Chest.* 2008;133:887S-968S.

16   HOW SUPPLIED/STORAGE AND HANDLING

Tablets

COUMADIN (warfarin sodium) tablets are single-scored, with one face imprinted numerically with 1, 2, 2-1/2, 3, 4, 5, 6, 7-1/2, or 10 superimposed and inscribed with "COUMADIN" and with the opposite face plain. COUMADIN is available in bottles and hospital unit-dose blister packages with potencies and colors as follows: [See third table above]

Protect from light and moisture. Store at controlled room temperature (59°-86°F, 15°-30°C). Dispense in a tight, light-resistant container as defined in the USP.

Store the hospital unit-dose blister packages in the carton until contents have been used.

Injection

COUMADIN for injection vials yield 5 mg of warfarin after reconstitution with 2.7 mL of Sterile Water for Injection (maximum yield is 2.5 mL of a 2 mg/mL solution). Net content of vial is 5.4 mg lyophilized powder.

5-mg vial (box of 6)   NDC 0590-0324-35

Protect from light. Keep vial in box until used. Store at controlled room temperature (59°-86°F, 15°-30°C).

After reconstitution, store at controlled room temperature (59°-86°F, 15°-30°C) and use within 4 hours. Do not refrigerate. Discard any unused solution.

17   PATIENT COUNSELING INFORMATION

See FDA-approved patient labeling (Medication Guide).

Advise patients to:

- Tell their physician if they fall often as this may increase their risk for complications.
- Strictly adhere to the prescribed dosage schedule. Do not take or discontinue any other drug, including salicylates (e.g., aspirin and topical analgesics), other over-the-counter drugs, and botanical (herbal) products except on advice of your physician.
- Notify their physician immediately if any unusual bleeding or symptoms occur. Signs and symptoms of bleeding include: pain, swelling or discomfort, prolonged bleeding from cuts, increased menstrual flow or vaginal bleeding, nosebleeds, bleeding of gums from brushing, unusual bleeding or bruising, red or dark brown urine, red or tar black stools, headache, dizziness, or weakness.
- Contact their doctor
  – immediately if they think they are pregnant
  – to discuss pregnancy planning
  – if they are considering breast-feeding
- Avoid any activity or sport that may result in traumatic injury.
- Obtain prothrombin time tests and make regular visits to their physician or clinic to monitor therapy.
- Carry identification stating that they are taking COUMADIN.
- If the prescribed dose of COUMADIN is missed, take the dose as soon as possible on the same day but do not take a double dose of COUMADIN the next day to make up for missed doses.
- Eat a normal, balanced diet to maintain a consistent intake of vitamin K. Avoid drastic changes in dietary habits, such as eating large amounts of leafy, green vegetables.
- Contact their physician to report any serious illness, such as severe diarrhea, infection, or fever.
- Be aware that if therapy with COUMADIN is discontinued, the anticoagulant effects of COUMADIN may persist for about 2 to 5 days.

Distributed by:
Bristol-Myers Squibb Company
Princeton, New Jersey 08543 USA

Table 7: WARIS – Endpoint Analysis of Separate Events

Event	Warfarin (N=607)	Placebo (N=607)	RR (95% CI)	% Risk Reduction (p-value)
Total Patient Years of Follow-up	2018	1944		
Total Mortality	94 (4.7/100 py)	123 (6.3/100 py)	0.76 (0.60, 0.97)	24 (p=0.030)
Vascular Death	82 (4.1/100 py)	105 (5.4/100 py)	0.78 (0.60, 1.02)	22 (p=0.068)
Recurrent MI	82 (4.1/100 py)	124 (6.4/100 py)	0.66 (0.51, 0.85)	34 (p=0.001)
Cerebrovascular Event	20 (1.0/100 py)	44 (2.3/100 py)	0.46 (0.28, 0.75)	54 (p=0.002)

RR=Relative risk; Risk reduction=(1 - RR); CI=Confidence interval; MI=Myocardial infarction; py=patient years

Table 8: WARIS II - Distribution of Events According to Treatment Group

Event	Aspirin (N=1206)	Warfarin (N=1216)	Aspirin plus Warfarin (N=1208)	Rate Ratio (95% CI)	p-value
	No. of Events				
Major Bleeding[a]	8	33	28	3.35[b] (ND)	ND
				4.00[c] (ND)	ND
Minor Bleeding[d]	39	103	133	3.21[b] (ND)	ND
				2.55[c] (ND)	ND
Composite Endpoints[e]	241	203	181	0.81 (0.69-0.95)[b]	0.03
				0.71 (0.60-0.83)[c]	0.001
Reinfarction	117	90	69	0.56 (0.41-0.78)[b]	<0.001
				0.74 (0.55-0.98)[c]	0.03
Thromboembolic Stroke	32	17	17	0.52 (0.28-0.98)[b]	0.03
				0.52 (0.28-0.97)[c]	0.03
Death	92	96	95		0.82

[a] Major bleeding episodes were defined as nonfatal cerebral hemorrhage or bleeding necessitating surgical intervention or blood transfusion.
[b] The rate ratio is for aspirin plus warfarin as compared with aspirin.
[c] The rate ratio is for warfarin as compared with aspirin.
[d] Minor bleeding episodes were defined as non-cerebral hemorrhage not necessitating surgical intervention or blood transfusion.
[e] Includes death, nonfatal reinfarction, and thromboembolic cerebral stroke.
CI=confidence interval
ND=not determined

	Bottles of 100	Bottles of 1000	Hospital Unit-Dose Blister Package of 100
1 mg pink	NDC 0056-0169-70	NDC 0056-0169-90	NDC 0056-0169-75
2 mg lavender	NDC 0056-0170-70	NDC 0056-0170-90	NDC 0056-0170-75
2-1/2 mg green	NDC 0056-0176-70	NDC 0056-0176-90	NDC 0056-0176-75
3 mg tan	NDC 0056-0188-70	NDC 0056-0188-90	NDC 0056-0188-75
4 mg blue	NDC 0056-0168-70	NDC 0056-0168-90	NDC 0056-0168-75
5 mg peach	NDC 0056-0172-70	NDC 0056-0172-90	NDC 0056-0172-75
6 mg teal	NDC 0056-0189-70	NDC 0056-0189-90	NDC 0056-0189-75
7-1/2 mg yellow	NDC 0056-0173-70		NDC 0056-0173-75
10 mg white (dye-free)	NDC 0056-0174-70		NDC 0056-0174-75

COUMADIN® is a trademark of Bristol-Myers Squibb Pharma Company.
Copyright © Bristol-Myers Squibb Company 2011
Printed in USA
1274054A0 / 1274029A0 / 1274055A0 / 1274053A0
Rev October 2011

MEDICATION GUIDE
COUMADIN® (COU-ma-din)
(warfarin sodium)

Read this Medication Guide before you start taking COUMADIN (warfarin sodium) and each time you get a refill. There may be new information. This Medication Guide does not take the place of talking to your healthcare provider about your medical condition or treatment. You and your healthcare provider should talk about COUMADIN when you start taking it and at regular checkups.

What is the most important information I should know about COUMADIN?

COUMADIN can cause bleeding which can be serious and sometimes lead to death. This is because COUMADIN is a blood thinner medicine that lowers the chance of blood clots forming in your body.

- You may have a higher risk of bleeding if you take COUMADIN:
- are 65 years of age or older
- have a history of stomach or intestinal bleeding
- have high blood pressure (hypertension)
- have a history of stroke, or "mini-stroke" (transient ischemic attack or TIA)
- have serious heart disease
- have a low blood count or cancer
- have had trauma, such as an accident or surgery
- have kidney problems
- take other medicines that increase your risk of bleeding, including:
  - a medicine that contains heparin
  - other medicines to prevent or treat blood clots
  - nonsteroidal anti-inflammatory drugs (NSAIDs)
- take warfarin sodium for a long time. Warfarin sodium is the active ingredient in COUMADIN (warfarin sodium).

Tell your healthcare provider if you take any of these medicines. Ask your healthcare provider if you are not sure if your medicine is listed above.

Many other medicines can interact with COUMADIN and affect the dose you need or increase COUMADIN side effects. Do not change or stop any of your medicines or start any new medicines before you talk to your healthcare provider.

Do not take other medicines that contain warfarin sodium while taking COUMADIN.

- **Get your regular blood test to check for your response to COUMADIN.** This blood test is called an INR test. The INR test checks to see how fast your blood clots. Your healthcare provider will decide what INR numbers are best for you. Your dose of COUMADIN will be adjusted to keep your INR in a target range for you.
- **Call your healthcare provider right away if you get any of the following signs or symptoms of bleeding problems:**
  - pain, swelling, or discomfort
  - headaches, dizziness, or weakness

- unusual bruising (bruises that develop without known cause or grow in size)
- nosebleeds
- bleeding gums
- bleeding from cuts takes a long time to stop
- menstrual bleeding or vaginal bleeding that is heavier than normal
- pink or brown urine
- red or black stools
- coughing up blood
- vomiting blood or material that looks like coffee grounds
- **Some foods and beverages can interact with COUMADIN and affect your treatment and dose.**
  - Eat a normal, balanced diet. Talk to your healthcare provider before you make any diet changes. Do not eat large amounts of leafy, green vegetables. Leafy, green vegetables contain vitamin K. Certain vegetable oils also contain large amounts of vitamin K. Too much vitamin K can lower the effect of COUMADIN (warfarin sodium).
- Always tell all of your healthcare providers that you take COUMADIN.
- Wear or carry information that you take COUMADIN.

See "What are the possible side effects of COUMADIN?" for more information about side effects.

What is COUMADIN?
COUMADIN is prescription medicine used to treat blood clots and to lower the chance of blood clots forming in your body. Blood clots can cause a stroke, heart attack, or other serious conditions if they form in the legs or lungs.
It is not known if COUMADIN is safe and effective in children.

Who should not take COUMADIN?
Do not take COUMADIN if:
- **your chance of having bleeding problems is higher than the possible benefit of treatment.** Your healthcare provider will decide if COUMADIN is right for you. Talk to your healthcare provider about all of your health conditions.
- **you are pregnant unless you have a mechanical heart valve.** COUMADIN may cause birth defects, miscarriage, or death of your unborn baby.
- **you are allergic to warfarin or any of the other ingredients in COUMADIN. See the end of this leaflet for a complete list of ingredients in COUMADIN.**

What should I tell my healthcare provider before taking COUMADIN?
Before you take COUMADIN, tell your healthcare provider if you:
- have bleeding problems
- fall often
- have liver or kidney problems
- have high blood pressure
- have a heart problem called congestive heart failure
- have diabetes
- plan to have any surgery or a dental procedure
- have any other medical conditions
- are pregnant or plan to become pregnant. See **"Who should not take COUMADIN?"**
- are breast-feeding. You and your healthcare provider should decide if you will take COUMADIN and breast-feed.

Tell all of your healthcare providers and dentists that you are taking COUMADIN. They should talk to the healthcare provider who prescribed COUMADIN for you before you have **any** surgery or dental procedure. Your COUMADIN may need to be stopped for a short time or you may need your dose adjusted.
Tell your healthcare provider about all the medicines you take, including prescription and non-prescription medicines, vitamins, and herbal supplements. Some of your other medicines may affect the way COUMADIN works. Certain medicines may increase your risk of bleeding. See **"What is the most important information I should know about COUMADIN?"**
Know the medicines you take. Keep a list of them to show your healthcare provider and pharmacist when you get a new medicine.

How should I take COUMADIN?
- **Take COUMADIN exactly as prescribed.** Your healthcare provider will adjust your dose from time to time depending on your response to COUMADIN.
- **You must have regular blood tests and visits with your healthcare provider to monitor your condition.**
- **If you miss a dose of COUMADIN, call your healthcare provider.** Take the dose as soon as possible on the same day. **Do not** take a double dose of COUMADIN the next day to make up for a missed dose.
- Call your healthcare provider right away if you:
  - take too much COUMADIN
  - are sick with diarrhea, an infection, or have a fever
  - fall or injure yourself, especially if you hit your head. Your healthcare provider may need to check you

What should I avoid while taking COUMADIN?
- Do not do any activity or sport that may cause a serious injury.

What are the possible side effects of COUMADIN?
COUMADIN may cause serious side effects including:
- See **"What is the most important information I should know about COUMADIN?"**
- **Death of skin tissue (skin necrosis or gangrene).** This can happen soon after starting COUMADIN. It happens because blood clots form and block blood flow to an area of your body. Call your healthcare provider right away if you have pain, color, or temperature change to any area of your body. You may need medical care right away to prevent death or loss (amputation) of your affected body part.
- **"Purple toes syndrome."** Call your healthcare provider right away if you have pain in your toes and they look purple in color or dark in color.

Tell your healthcare provider if you have any side effect that bothers you or does not go away.
These are not all of the side effects of COUMADIN (warfarin sodium). For more information, ask your healthcare provider or pharmacist.
Call your doctor for medical advice about side effects. You may report side effects to FDA at 1-800-FDA-1088.

How should I store COUMADIN?
- Store COUMADIN at 59°F to 86°F (15°C to 30°C).
- Keep COUMADIN in a tightly closed container, and keep COUMADIN out of the light.

Keep COUMADIN and all medicines out of the reach of children.

General Information about COUMADIN.
Medicines are sometimes prescribed for purposes other than those listed in a Medication Guide. Do not use COUMADIN for a condition for which it was not prescribed. Do not give COUMADIN to other people, even if they have the same symptoms that you have. It may harm them.
This Medication Guide summarizes the most important information about COUMADIN. If you would like more information, talk with your healthcare provider. You can ask your healthcare provider or pharmacist for information about COUMADIN that is written for healthcare professionals.
If you would like more information, go to www.coumadin.com or call 1-800-321-1335.

What are the ingredients in COUMADIN?
Active ingredient: Warfarin Sodium
Inactive ingredients: Lactose, starch, and magnesium stearate. The following tablets contain:

1 mg:	D&C Red No. 6 Barium Lake
2 mg:	FD&C Blue No. 2 Aluminum Lake and FD&C Red No. 40 Aluminum Lake
2-1/2 mg:	D&C Yellow No. 10 Aluminum Lake and FD&C Blue No. 1 Aluminum Lake
3 mg:	FD&C Yellow No. 6 Aluminum Lake, FD&C Blue No. 2 Aluminum Lake, and FD&C Red No. 40 Aluminum Lake
4 mg:	FD&C Blue No. 1 Aluminum Lake
5 mg:	FD&C Yellow No. 6 Aluminum Lake
6 mg:	FD&C Yellow No. 6 Aluminum Lake and FD&C Blue No. 1 Aluminum Lake
7-1/2 mg:	D&C Yellow No. 10 Aluminum Lake and FD&C Yellow No. 6 Aluminum Lake

This Medication Guide has been approved by the U.S. Food and Drug Administration.
COUMADIN is distributed by:
Bristol-Myers Squibb Company
Princeton, New Jersey 08543 USA
COUMADIN® is a registered trademark of Bristol-Myers Squibb Pharma Company.
**The brands listed (other than COUMADIN®) are registered trademarks of their respective owners and are not trademarks of Bristol-Myers Squibb Company.
1258498A3 / 1215385A4 / 1205734A4 / 1205736A4
Rev October 2011
Shown in Product Identification Guide, page 306

ELIQUIS®
[*ELL eh kwiss*]
(apixaban)
tablets for oral use

HIGHLIGHTS OF PRESCRIBING INFORMATION
These highlights do not include all the information needed to use ELIQUIS safely and effectively. See full prescribing information for ELIQUIS.
ELIQUIS® (apixaban) tablets for oral use
Initial U.S. Approval: 2012

WARNING: (A) PREMATURE DISCONTINUATION OF ELIQUIS INCREASES THE RISK OF THROMBOTIC EVENTS
(B) SPINAL/EPIDURAL HEMATOMA
See full prescribing information for complete boxed warning.

(A) PREMATURE DISCONTINUATION OF ELIQUIS INCREASES THE RISK OF THROMBOTIC EVENTS: Premature discontinuation of any oral anticoagulant, including ELIQUIS, increases the risk of thrombotic events. To reduce this risk, consider coverage with another anticoagulant if ELIQUIS is discontinued for a reason other than pathological bleeding or completion of a course of therapy. (2.5, 5.1, 14.1)
(B) SPINAL/EPIDURAL HEMATOMA: Epidural or spinal hematomas may occur in patients treated with ELIQUIS who are receiving neuraxial anesthesia or undergoing spinal puncture. These hematomas may result in long-term or permanent paralysis. Consider these risks when scheduling patients for spinal procedures. (5.3)

————RECENT MAJOR CHANGES————

Boxed Warning	8/2014
Indications and Usage (1.2)	3/2014
Indications and Usage (1.3, 1.4, 1.5)	8/2014
Dosage and Administration (2.1)	8/2014
Dosage and Administration (2.8)	3/2014
Warnings and Precautions (5.1)	8/2014
Warnings and Precautions (5.3)	3/2014
Warnings and Precautions (5.5)	8/2014

————INDICATIONS AND USAGE————
ELIQUIS (apixaban) is a factor Xa inhibitor anticoagulant indicated:
- to reduce the risk of stroke and systemic embolism in patients with nonvalvular atrial fibrillation. (1.1)
- for the prophylaxis of deep vein thrombosis (DVT), which may lead to pulmonary embolism (PE), in patients who have undergone hip or knee replacement surgery. (1.2)
- for the treatment of DVT and PE, and for the reduction in the risk of recurrent DVT and PE following initial therapy. (1.3, 1.4, 1.5)

————DOSAGE AND ADMINISTRATION————
- Reduction of risk of stroke and systemic embolism in nonvalvular atrial fibrillation:
  - The recommended dose is 5 mg orally twice daily. (2.1)
  - In patients with at least 2 of the following characteristics: age ≥80 years, body weight ≤60 kg, or serum creatinine ≥1.5 mg/dL, the recommended dose is 2.5 mg orally twice daily. (2.2)
- Prophylaxis of DVT following hip or knee replacement surgery:
  - The recommended dose is 2.5 mg orally twice daily. (2.1)
- Treatment of DVT and PE:
  - The recommended dose is 10 mg taken orally twice daily for 7 days, followed by 5 mg taken orally twice daily. (2.1)
- Reduction in the risk of recurrent DVT and PE following initial therapy:
  - The recommended dose is 2.5 mg taken orally twice daily. (2.1)

————DOSAGE FORMS AND STRENGTHS————
- Tablets: 2.5 mg and 5 mg (3)

————CONTRAINDICATIONS————
- Active pathological bleeding (4)
- Severe hypersensitivity to ELIQUIS (4)

————WARNINGS AND PRECAUTIONS————
- ELIQUIS can cause serious, potentially fatal bleeding. Promptly evaluate signs and symptoms of blood loss. (5.2)
- Prosthetic heart valves: ELIQUIS use not recommended. (5.4)

————ADVERSE REACTIONS————
Most common adverse reactions (>1%) are related to bleeding. (6.1)
To report SUSPECTED ADVERSE REACTIONS, contact Bristol-Myers Squibb at 1-800-721-5072 or FDA at 1-800-FDA-1088 or *www.fda.gov/medwatch*.

————DRUG INTERACTIONS————
- Strong dual inhibitors of CYP3A4 and P-gp increase blood levels of apixaban. Reduce dose or avoid coadministration. (2.2, 7.1, 12.3)
- Simultaneous use of strong dual inducers of CYP3A4 and P-gp reduces blood levels of apixaban: Avoid concomitant use. (2.2, 7.2, 12.3)

————USE IN SPECIFIC POPULATIONS————
- *Pregnancy:* Not recommended. (8.1)
- *Nursing Mothers:* Discontinue drug or discontinue nursing. (8.3)
- *Severe Hepatic Impairment:* Not recommended. (12.2)

See 17 for PATIENT COUNSELING INFORMATION and Medication Guide.

Revised: 8/2014

FULL PRESCRIBING INFORMATION: CONTENTS*
WARNING: (A) PREMATURE DISCONTINUATION OF ELIQUIS INCREASES THE RISK OF THROMBOTIC EVENTS (B) SPINAL/EPIDURAL HEMATOMA
1 INDICATIONS AND USAGE
  1.1 Reduction of Risk of Stroke and Systemic Embolism in Nonvalvular Atrial Fibrillation

℞

1.2 Prophylaxis of Deep Vein Thrombosis Following Hip or Knee Replacement Surgery
1.3 Treatment of Deep Vein Thrombosis
1.4 Treatment of Pulmonary Embolism
1.5 Reduction in the Risk of Recurrence of DVT and PE
2 DOSAGE AND ADMINISTRATION
2.1 Recommended Dose
2.2 Dosage Adjustments
2.3 Missed Dose
2.4 Temporary Interruption for Surgery and Other Interventions
2.5 Converting from or to ELIQUIS
2.6 Hepatic Impairment
2.7 Renal Impairment
2.8 Administration Options
3 DOSAGE FORMS AND STRENGTHS
4 CONTRAINDICATIONS
5 WARNINGS AND PRECAUTIONS
5.1 Increased Risk of Thrombotic Events after Premature Discontinuation
5.2 Bleeding
5.3 Spinal/Epidural Anesthesia or Puncture
5.4 Patients with Prosthetic Heart Valves
5.5 Acute PE in Hemodynamically Unstable Patients or Patients who Require Thrombolysis or Pulmonary Embolectomy
6 ADVERSE REACTIONS
6.1 Clinical Trials Experience
7 DRUG INTERACTIONS
7.1 Strong Dual Inhibitors of CYP3A4 and P-gp
7.2 Strong Dual Inducers of CYP3A4 and P-gp
7.3 Anticoagulants and Antiplatelet Agents
8 USE IN SPECIFIC POPULATIONS
8.1 Pregnancy
8.2 Labor and Delivery
8.3 Nursing Mothers
8.4 Pediatric Use
8.5 Geriatric Use
8.6 End-Stage Renal Disease Patients Maintained with Hemodialysis
10 OVERDOSAGE
11 DESCRIPTION
12 CLINICAL PHARMACOLOGY
12.1 Mechanism of Action
12.2 Pharmacodynamics
12.3 Pharmacokinetics
13 NONCLINICAL TOXICOLOGY
13.1 Carcinogenesis, Mutagenesis, Impairment of Fertility
14 CLINICAL STUDIES
14.1 Reduction of Risk of Stroke and Systemic Embolism in Nonvalvular Atrial Fibrillation
14.2 Prophylaxis of Deep Vein Thrombosis Following Hip or Knee Replacement Surgery
14.3 Treatment of DVT and PE and Reduction in the Risk of Recurrence of DVT and PE
16 HOW SUPPLIED/STORAGE AND HANDLING
17 PATIENT COUNSELING INFORMATION
* Sections or subsections omitted from the full prescribing information are not listed.

FULL PRESCRIBING INFORMATION

WARNING: (A) PREMATURE DISCONTINUATION OF ELIQUIS INCREASES THE RISK OF THROMBOTIC EVENTS (B) SPINAL/EPIDURAL HEMATOMA

(A) PREMATURE DISCONTINUATION OF ELIQUIS INCREASES THE RISK OF THROMBOTIC EVENTS
Premature discontinuation of any oral anticoagulant, including ELIQUIS (apixaban), increases the risk of thrombotic events. If anticoagulation with ELIQUIS is discontinued for a reason other than pathological bleeding or completion of a course of therapy, consider coverage with another anticoagulant [see Dosage and Administration (2.5), Warnings and Precautions (5.1), and Clinical Studies (14.1)].
(B) SPINAL/EPIDURAL HEMATOMA
Epidural or spinal hematomas may occur in patients treated with ELIQUIS who are receiving neuraxial anesthesia or undergoing spinal puncture. These hematomas may result in long-term or permanent paralysis. Consider these risks when scheduling patients for spinal procedures. Factors that can increase the risk of developing epidural or spinal hematomas in these patients include:
• use of indwelling epidural catheters
• concomitant use of other drugs that affect hemostasis, such as nonsteroidal antiinflammatory drugs (NSAIDs), platelet inhibitors, other anticoagulants
• a history of traumatic or repeated epidural or spinal punctures
• a history of spinal deformity or spinal surgery

• optimal timing between the administration of ELIQUIS and neuraxial procedures is not known [see Warnings and Precautions (5.3)]
Monitor patients frequently for signs and symptoms of neurological impairment. If neurological compromise is noted, urgent treatment is necessary [see Warnings and Precautions (5.3)].
Consider the benefits and risks before neuraxial intervention in patients anticoagulated or to be anticoagulated [see Warnings and Precautions (5.3)].

1 INDICATIONS AND USAGE
1.1 Reduction of Risk of Stroke and Systemic Embolism in Nonvalvular Atrial Fibrillation
ELIQUIS® (apixaban) is indicated to reduce the risk of stroke and systemic embolism in patients with nonvalvular atrial fibrillation.
1.2 Prophylaxis of Deep Vein Thrombosis Following Hip or Knee Replacement Surgery
ELIQUIS is indicated for the prophylaxis of deep vein thrombosis (DVT), which may lead to pulmonary embolism (PE), in patients who have undergone hip or knee replacement surgery.
1.3 Treatment of Deep Vein Thrombosis
ELIQUIS is indicated for the treatment of DVT.
1.4 Treatment of Pulmonary Embolism
ELIQUIS is indicated for the treatment of PE.
1.5 Reduction in the Risk of Recurrence of DVT and PE
ELIQUIS is indicated to reduce the risk of recurrent DVT and PE following initial therapy.
2 DOSAGE AND ADMINISTRATION
2.1 Recommended Dose
Reduction of Risk of Stroke and Systemic Embolism in Patients with Nonvalvular Atrial Fibrillation
The recommended dose of ELIQUIS for most patients is 5 mg taken orally twice daily.
Prophylaxis of Deep Vein Thrombosis Following Hip or Knee Replacement Surgery
The recommended dose of ELIQUIS is 2.5 mg taken orally twice daily. The initial dose should be taken 12 to 24 hours after surgery.
• In patients undergoing hip replacement surgery, the recommended duration of treatment is 35 days.
• In patients undergoing knee replacement surgery, the recommended duration of treatment is 12 days.
Treatment of DVT and PE
The recommended dose of ELIQUIS is 10 mg taken orally twice daily for 7 days, followed by 5 mg taken orally twice daily.
Reduction in the Risk of Recurrence of DVT and PE
The recommended dose of ELIQUIS is 2.5 mg taken orally twice daily after at least 6 months of treatment for DVT or PE [see Clinical Studies (14.3)].
2.2 Dosage Adjustments
In patients with nonvalvular atrial fibrillation: The recommended dose of ELIQUIS is 2.5 mg twice daily in patients with any 2 of the following characteristics:
• age ≥80 years
• body weight ≤60 kg
• serum creatinine ≥1.5 mg/dL
Coadministration with strong dual CYP3A4 and P-gp inhibitors: For patients receiving ELIQUIS doses greater than 2.5 mg twice daily, reduce the dose by 50% when ELIQUIS is coadministered with drugs that are strong dual inhibitors of cytochrome P450 3A4 (CYP3A4) and P-glycoprotein (P-gp) (e.g., ketoconazole, itraconazole, ritonavir, clarithromycin) [see Clinical Pharmacology (12.3)].
In patients already taking 2.5 mg twice daily, avoid coadministration of ELIQUIS with strong dual inhibitors of CYP3A4 and P-gp [see Drug Interactions (7.1)].
2.3 Missed Dose
If a dose of ELIQUIS is not taken at the scheduled time, the dose should be taken as soon as possible on the same day and twice-daily administration should be resumed. The dose should not be doubled to make up for a missed dose.
2.4 Temporary Interruption for Surgery and Other Interventions
ELIQUIS should be discontinued at least 48 hours prior to elective surgery or invasive procedures with a moderate or high risk of unacceptable or clinically significant bleeding. ELIQUIS should be discontinued at least 24 hours prior to elective surgery or invasive procedures with a low risk of bleeding or where the bleeding would be non-critical in location and easily controlled. Bridging anticoagulation during the 24 to 48 hours after stopping ELIQUIS and prior to the intervention is not generally required. ELIQUIS should be restarted after the surgical or other procedures as soon as adequate hemostasis has been established.
2.5 Converting from or to ELIQUIS
Switching from warfarin to ELIQUIS: Warfarin should be discontinued and ELIQUIS started when the international normalized ratio (INR) is below 2.0.

Switching from ELIQUIS to warfarin: ELIQUIS (apixaban) affects INR, so that initial INR measurements during the transition to warfarin may not be useful for determining the appropriate dose of warfarin. If continuous anticoagulation is necessary, discontinue ELIQUIS and begin both a parenteral anticoagulant and warfarin at the time the next dose of ELIQUIS would have been taken, discontinuing the parenteral anticoagulant when INR reaches an acceptable range.
Switching between ELIQUIS and anticoagulants other than warfarin: Discontinue one being taken and begin the other at the next scheduled dose.
2.6 Hepatic Impairment
No dose adjustment is required in patients with mild hepatic impairment.
Because patients with moderate hepatic impairment may have intrinsic coagulation abnormalities and there is limited clinical experience with ELIQUIS in these patients, dosing recommendations cannot be provided [see Clinical Pharmacology (12.2)].
ELIQUIS is not recommended in patients with severe hepatic impairment [see Clinical Pharmacology (12.3)].
2.7 Renal Impairment
The dosing adjustment for patients with moderate renal impairment and nonvalvular atrial fibrillation is described above [see Dosage and Administration (2.2)]. The recommended dose for nonvalvular atrial fibrillation patients with end-stage renal disease (ESRD) maintained on hemodialysis is 5 mg twice daily. Reduce dose to 2.5 mg twice daily if one of the following patient characteristics (age ≥80 years or body weight ≤60 kg) is present [see Use in Specific Populations (8.6) and Clinical Pharmacology (12.3)].
No dose adjustment is required for the following indications:
• for the prophylaxis of DVT, which may lead to PE, in patients who have undergone hip or knee replacement surgery.
• for the treatment of DVT and PE, and for the reduction in the risk of recurrent DVT and PE.
2.8 Administration Options
For patients who are unable to swallow whole tablets, 5 mg and 2.5 mg ELIQUIS tablets may be crushed and suspended in 60 mL D5W and immediately delivered through a nasogastric tube (NGT) [see Clinical Pharmacology (12.3)]. Information regarding the administration of crushed and suspended ELIQUIS tablets swallowed by mouth is not available.

3 DOSAGE FORMS AND STRENGTHS
• 2.5 mg, yellow, round, biconvex, film-coated tablets with "893" debossed on one side and "2½" on the other side.
• 5 mg, pink, oval-shaped, biconvex, film-coated tablets with "894" debossed on one side and "5" on the other side.

4 CONTRAINDICATIONS
ELIQUIS is contraindicated in patients with the following conditions:
• Active pathological bleeding [see Warnings and Precautions (5.2) and Adverse Reactions (6.1)]
• Severe hypersensitivity reaction to ELIQUIS (e.g., anaphylactic reactions) [see Adverse Reactions (6.1)]

5 WARNINGS AND PRECAUTIONS
5.1 Increased Risk of Thrombotic Events after Premature Discontinuation
Premature discontinuation of any oral anticoagulant, including ELIQUIS, in the absence of adequate alternative anticoagulation increases the risk of thrombotic events. An increased rate of stroke was observed during the transition from ELIQUIS to warfarin in clinical trials in atrial fibrillation patients. If ELIQUIS is discontinued for a reason other than pathological bleeding or completion of a course of therapy, consider coverage with another anticoagulant [see Dosage and Administration (2.5) and Clinical Studies (14.1)].
5.2 Bleeding
ELIQUIS increases the risk of bleeding and can cause serious, potentially fatal, bleeding [see Dosage and Administration (2.2) and Adverse Reactions (6.1)].
Concomitant use of drugs affecting hemostasis increases the risk of bleeding. These include aspirin and other antiplatelet agents, other anticoagulants, heparin, thrombolytic agents, selective serotonin reuptake inhibitors, serotonin norepinephrine reuptake inhibitors, and nonsteroidal antiinflammatory drugs (NSAIDs) [see Drug Interactions (7.3)]. Advise patients of signs and symptoms of blood loss and to report them immediately or go to an emergency room. Discontinue ELIQUIS in patients with active pathological hemorrhage.
There is no established way to reverse the anticoagulant effect of apixaban, which can be expected to persist for at

Table 1: Bleeding Events in Patients with Nonvalvular Atrial Fibrillation in ARISTOTLE

	ELIQUIS N=9088 n (%/year)	Warfarin N=9052 n (%/year)	Hazard Ratio (95% CI*)	P-value
Major[†]	327 (2.13)	462 (3.09)	0.69 (0.60, 0.80)	<0.0001
Gastrointestinal (GI)[‡]	128 (0.83)	141 (0.93)	0.89 (0.70, 1.14)	-
Intracranial	52 (0.33)	125 (0.82)	0.41 (0.30, 0.57)	-
Intraocular[§]	32 (0.21)	22 (0.14)	1.42 (0.83, 2.45)	-
Fatal[¶]	10 (0.06)	37 (0.24)	0.27 (0.13, 0.53)	-
CRNM**	318 (2.08)	444 (3.00)	0.70 (0.60, 0.80)	<0.0001

* Confidence interval.
[†] International Society on Thrombosis and Hemostasis (ISTH) major bleed assessed by sequential testing strategy for superiority designed to control the overall type I error in the trial.
[‡] GI bleed includes upper GI, lower GI, and rectal bleeding.
[§] Intraocular bleed is within the corpus of the eye (a conjunctival bleed is not an intraocular bleed).
[¶] Fatal bleed is an adjudicated death because of bleeding during the treatment period and includes both fatal extracranial bleeds and fatal hemorrhagic stroke.
** CRNM = clinically relevant nonmajor bleeding.
Events associated with each endpoint were counted once per subject, but subjects may have contributed events to multiple endpoints.

Figure 1: Major Bleeding Hazard Ratios by Baseline Characteristics – ARISTOTLE Study

Subgroup	No. of Patients	No. of Events (% per yr) Apixaban	No. of Events (% per yr) Warfarin	Hazard Ratio (95% CI)	P-value for Interaction
All Patients	18140	327 (2.13)	462 (3.09)		
Prior Warfarin/VKA Status					0.50
Experienced	10376	185 (2.1)	274 (3.2)		
Naïve	7764	142 (2.2)	188 (3.0)		
Age					0.64
<65 yrs old	5455	56 (1.2)	72 (1.5)		
≥65 to <75 yrs old	7030	120 (2.0)	166 (2.8)		
≥75 yrs old	5655	151 (3.3)	224 (5.2)		
Gender					0.08
Male	11747	225 (2.3)	294 (3.0)		
Female	6393	102 (1.9)	168 (3.3)		
Weight					0.22
≤60 kg	1978	36 (2.3)	62 (4.3)		
>60 kg	16102	290 (2.1)	398 (3.0)		
Type of Atrial Fibrillation					0.75
Permanent/Persistent	15361	283 (2.2)	402 (3.2)		
Paroxysmal	2776	44 (1.9)	60 (2.6)		
Prior Stroke or TIA					0.71
Yes	3422	77 (2.8)	106 (3.9)		
No	14718	250 (2.0)	356 (2.9)		
Diabetes Mellitus					0.003
Yes	4526	112 (3.0)	114 (3.1)		
No	13614	215 (1.9)	348 (3.1)		
Heart Failure					0.30
Yes	5527	87 (1.9)	137 (3.1)		
No	12613	240 (2.2)	325 (3.1)		
CHADS$_2$ Score					0.40
≤1	6169	76 (1.4)	126 (2.3)		
=2	6492	125 (2.3)	163 (3.0)		
≥3	5479	126 (2.9)	173 (4.2)		
Level of Renal Impairment					0.03
Severe or Moderate	3005	73 (3.2)	142 (6.4)		
Mild	7565	157 (2.5)	199 (3.2)		
Normal	7496	96 (1.5)	119 (1.8)		
Apixaban Dose					0.21
2.5 mg BID or placebo	826	20 (3.3)	37 (6.7)		
5 mg BID or placebo	17314	307 (2.1)	425 (3.0)		
Geographic Region					0.16
North America	4463	106 (2.8)	137 (3.6)		
Latin America	3460	60 (2.1)	94 (3.5)		
Europe	7313	110 (1.7)	135 (2.2)		
Asia/Pacific	2904	51 (2.1)	96 (4.1)		
Aspirin at Randomization					0.40
Yes	5608	129 (2.7)	164 (3.7)		
No	12532	198 (1.9)	298 (2.8)		

Hazard Ratio scale: 0.25 0.5 1 2
Apixaban Better — Warfarin Better

least 24 hours after the last dose, i.e., for about two drug half-lives. A specific antidote for ELIQUIS (apixaban) is not available. Hemodialysis does not appear to have a substantial impact on apixaban exposure *[see Clinical Pharmacology (12.3)]*. Protamine sulfate and vitamin K are not expected to affect the anticoagulant activity of apixaban. There is no experience with antifibrinolytic agents (tranexamic acid, aminocaproic acid) in individuals receiving apixaban. There is neither scientific rationale for reversal nor experience with systemic hemostatics (desmopressin and aprotinin) in individuals receiving apixaban. Use of procoagulant reversal agents such as prothrombin complex concentrate, activated prothrombin complex concentrate, or recombinant factor VIIa may be considered but has not been evaluated in clinical studies. Activated oral charcoal reduces absorption of apixaban, thereby lowering apixaban plasma concentration *[see Overdosage (10)]*.

5.3 Spinal/Epidural Anesthesia or Puncture
When neuraxial anesthesia (spinal/epidural anesthesia) or spinal/epidural puncture is employed, patients treated with antithrombotic agents for prevention of thromboembolic complications are at risk of developing an epidural or spinal hematoma which can result in long-term or permanent paralysis.

The risk of these events may be increased by the postoperative use of indwelling epidural catheters or the concomitant use of medicinal products affecting hemostasis. Indwelling epidural or intrathecal catheters should not be removed earlier than 24 hours after the last administration of ELIQUIS (apixaban). The next dose of ELIQUIS should not be administered earlier than 5 hours after the removal of the catheter. The risk may also be increased by traumatic or repeated epidural or spinal puncture. If traumatic puncture occurs, delay the administration of ELIQUIS for 48 hours.

Monitor patients frequently for signs and symptoms of neurological impairment (e.g., numbness or weakness of the legs, bowel, or bladder dysfunction). If neurological compromise is noted, urgent diagnosis and treatment is necessary. Prior to neuraxial intervention the physician should consider the potential benefit versus the risk in anticoagulated patients or in patients to be anticoagulated for thromboprophylaxis.

5.4 Patients with Prosthetic Heart Valves
The safety and efficacy of ELIQUIS have not been studied in patients with prosthetic heart valves. Therefore, use of ELIQUIS is not recommended in these patients.

5.5 Acute PE in Hemodynamically Unstable Patients or Patients who Require Thrombolysis or Pulmonary Embolectomy
Initiation of ELIQUIS is not recommended as an alternative to unfractionated heparin for the initial treatment of patients with PE who present with hemodynamic instability or who may receive thrombolysis or pulmonary embolectomy.

6 ADVERSE REACTIONS
The following serious adverse reactions are discussed in greater detail in other sections of the prescribing information.
- Increased risk of thrombotic events after premature discontinuation *[see Warnings and Precautions (5.1)]*
- Bleeding *[see Warnings and Precautions (5.2)]*
- Spinal/epidural anesthesia or puncture *[see Warnings and Precautions (5.3)]*

6.1 Clinical Trials Experience
Because clinical trials are conducted under widely varying conditions, adverse reaction rates observed in the clinical trials of a drug cannot be directly compared to rates in the clinical trials of another drug and may not reflect the rates observed in practice.

Reduction of Risk of Stroke and Systemic Embolism in Nonvalvular Atrial Fibrillation
The safety of ELIQUIS was evaluated in the ARISTOTLE and AVERROES studies *[see Clinical Studies (14)]*, including 11,284 patients exposed to ELIQUIS 5 mg twice daily and 602 patients exposed to ELIQUIS 2.5 mg twice daily. The duration of ELIQUIS exposure was ≥12 months for 9375 patients and ≥24 months for 3369 patients in the two studies. In ARISTOTLE, the mean duration of exposure was 89 weeks (>15,000 patient-years). In AVERROES, the mean duration of exposure was approximately 59 weeks (>3000 patient-years).

The most common reason for treatment discontinuation in both studies was for bleeding-related adverse reactions; in ARISTOTLE this occurred in 1.7% and 2.5% of patients treated with ELIQUIS and warfarin, respectively, and in AVERROES, in 1.5% and 1.3% on ELIQUIS and aspirin, respectively.

Bleeding in Patients with Nonvalvular Atrial Fibrillation in ARISTOTLE and AVERROES
Tables 1 and 2 show the number of patients experiencing major bleeding during the treatment period and the bleeding rate (percentage of subjects with at least one bleeding event per year) in ARISTOTLE and AVERROES.

Major bleeding was defined as clinically overt bleeding that was accompanied by one or more of the following: a decrease in hemoglobin of 2 g/dL or more; a transfusion of 2 or more units of packed red blood cells; bleeding that occurred in at least one of the following critical sites: intracranial, intraspinal, intraocular, pericardial, intra-articular, intramuscular with compartment syndrome, retroperitoneal; or bleeding that was fatal. Intracranial hemorrhage included intracerebral (hemorrhagic stroke), subarachnoid, and subdural bleeds.

[See table 1 above]
In ARISTOTLE, the results for major bleeding were generally consistent across most major subgroups including age, weight, CHADS$_2$ score (a scale from 0 to 6 used to estimate risk of stroke, with higher scores predicting greater risk), prior warfarin use, geographic region, ELIQUIS dose, type of atrial fibrillation (AF), and aspirin use at randomization (Figure 1). Subjects treated with apixaban with diabetes bled more (3.0% per year) than did subjects without diabetes (1.9% per year).
[See figure 1 above]

[See table 2 above]
Other Adverse Reactions
Hypersensitivity reactions (including drug hypersensitivity, such as skin rash, and anaphylactic reactions, such as allergic edema) and syncope were reported in <1% of patients receiving ELIQUIS (apixaban).
Prophylaxis of Deep Vein Thrombosis Following Hip or Knee Replacement Surgery
The safety of ELIQUIS has been evaluated in 1 Phase II and 3 Phase III studies including 5924 patients exposed to ELIQUIS 2.5 mg twice daily undergoing major orthopedic surgery of the lower limbs (elective hip replacement or elective knee replacement) treated for up to 38 days.
In total, 11% of the patients treated with ELIQUIS 2.5 mg twice daily experienced adverse reactions.
Bleeding results during the treatment period in the Phase III studies are shown in Table 3. Bleeding was assessed in each study beginning with the first dose of double-blind study drug.
[See table 3 above]
Adverse reactions occurring in ≥1% of patients undergoing hip or knee replacement surgery in the 1 Phase II study and the 3 Phase III studies are listed in Table 4.
[See table 4 above]
Less common adverse reactions in apixaban-treated patients undergoing hip or knee replacement surgery occurring at a frequency of ≥0.1% to <1%:
Blood and lymphatic system disorders: thrombocytopenia (including platelet count decreases)
Vascular disorders: hypotension (including procedural hypotension)
Respiratory, thoracic, and mediastinal disorders: epistaxis
Gastrointestinal disorders: gastrointestinal hemorrhage (including hematemesis and melena), hematochezia
Hepatobiliary disorders: liver function test abnormal, blood alkaline phosphatase increased, blood bilirubin increased
Renal and urinary disorders: hematuria (including respective laboratory parameters)
Injury, poisoning, and procedural complications: wound secretion, incision-site hemorrhage (including incision-site hematoma), operative hemorrhage
Less common adverse reactions in apixaban-treated patients undergoing hip or knee replacement surgery occurring at a frequency of <0.1%:
Gingival bleeding, hemoptysis, hypersensitivity, muscle hemorrhage, ocular hemorrhage (including conjunctival hemorrhage), rectal hemorrhage
Treatment of DVT and PE and Reduction in the Risk of Recurrence of DVT or PE
The safety of ELIQUIS has been evaluated in the AMPLIFY and AMPLIFY-EXT studies, including 2676 patients exposed to ELIQUIS 10 mg twice daily, 3359 patients exposed to ELIQUIS 5 mg twice daily, and 840 patients exposed to ELIQUIS 2.5 mg twice daily.
Common adverse reactions (≥1%) were gingival bleeding, epistaxis, contusion, hematuria, rectal hemorrhage, hematoma, menorrhagia, and hemoptysis.
AMPLIFY Study
The mean duration of exposure to ELIQUIS was 154 days and to enoxaparin/warfarin was 152 days in the AMPLIFY study. Adverse reactions related to bleeding occurred in 417 (15.6%) ELIQUIS-treated patients compared to 661 (24.6%) enoxaparin/warfarin-treated patients. The discontinuation rate due to bleeding events was 0.7% in the ELIQUIS-treated patients compared to 1.7% in enoxaparin/warfarin-treated patients in the AMPLIFY study.
In the AMPLIFY study, ELIQUIS was statistically superior to enoxaparin/warfarin in the primary safety endpoint of major bleeding (relative risk 0.31, 95% CI [0.17, 0.55], P-value <0.0001).
Bleeding results from the AMPLIFY study are summarized in Table 5.
[See table 5 at top of next page]
Adverse reactions occurring in ≥1% of patients in the AMPLIFY study are listed in Table 6.
[See table 6 at top of next page]
AMPLIFY-EXT Study
The mean duration of exposure to ELIQUIS was approximately 330 days and to placebo was 312 days in the AMPLIFY-EXT study. Adverse reactions related to bleeding occurred in 219 (13.3%) ELIQUIS-treated patients compared to 72 (8.7%) placebo-treated patients. The discontinuation rate due to bleeding events was approximately 1% in the ELIQUIS-treated patients compared to 0.4% in those patients in the placebo group in the AMPLIFY-EXT study.
Bleeding results from the AMPLIFY-EXT study are summarized in Table 7.
[See table 7 at top of next page]
Adverse reactions occurring in ≥1% of patients in the AMPLIFY-EXT study are listed in Table 8.
[See table 8 at top of next page]

Table 2: Bleeding Events in Patients with Nonvalvular Atrial Fibrillation in AVERROES

	ELIQUIS N=2798 n (%/year)	Aspirin N=2780 n (%/year)	Hazard Ratio (95% CI)	P-value
Major	45 (1.41)	29 (0.92)	1.54 (0.96, 2.45)	0.07
Fatal	5 (0.16)	5 (0.16)	0.99 (0.23, 4.29)	-
Intracranial	11 (0.34)	11 (0.35)	0.99 (0.39, 2.51)	-

Events associated with each endpoint were counted once per subject, but subjects may have contributed events to multiple endpoints.

Table 3: Bleeding During the Treatment Period in Patients Undergoing Elective Hip or Knee Replacement Surgery

Bleeding Endpoint*	ADVANCE-3 Hip Replacement Surgery		ADVANCE-2 Knee Replacement Surgery		ADVANCE-1 Knee Replacement Surgery	
	ELIQUIS 2.5 mg po bid 35±3 days	Enoxaparin 40 mg sc qd 35±3 days	ELIQUIS 2.5 mg po bid 12±2 days	Enoxaparin 40 mg sc qd 12±2 days	ELIQUIS 2.5 mg po bid 12±2 days	Enoxaparin 30 mg sc q12h 12±2 days
	First dose 12 to 24 hours post surgery	First dose 9 to 15 hours prior to surgery	First dose 12 to 24 hours post surgery	First dose 9 to 15 hours prior to surgery	First dose 12 to 24 hours post surgery	First dose 12 to 24 hours post surgery
All treated	N=2673	N=2659	N=1501	N=1508	N=1596	N=1588
Major (including surgical site)	22 (0.82%)†	18 (0.68%)	9 (0.60%)‡	14 (0.93%)	11 (0.69%)	22 (1.39%)
Fatal	0	0	0	0	0	1 (0.06%)
Hgb decrease ≥2 g/dL	13 (0.49%)	10 (0.38%)	8 (0.53%)	9 (0.60%)	10 (0.63%)	16 (1.01%)
Transfusion of ≥2 units RBC	16 (0.60%)	14 (0.53%)	5 (0.33%)	9 (0.60%)	9 (0.56%)	18 (1.13%)
Bleed at critical site§	1 (0.04%)	1 (0.04%)	1 (0.07%)	2 (0.13%)	1 (0.06%)	4 (0.25%)
Major + CRNM¶	129 (4.83%)	134 (5.04%)	53 (3.53%)	72 (4.77%)	46 (2.88%)	68 (4.28%)
All	313 (11.71%)	334 (12.56%)	104 (6.93%)	126 (8.36%)	85 (5.33%)	108 (6.80%)

* All bleeding criteria included surgical site bleeding.
† Includes 13 subjects with major bleeding events that occurred before the first dose of apixaban (administered 12 to 24 hours post surgery).
‡ Includes 5 subjects with major bleeding events that occurred before the first dose of apixaban (administered 12 to 24 hours post surgery).
§ Intracranial, intraspinal, intraocular, pericardial, an operated joint requiring re-operation or intervention, intramuscular with compartment syndrome, or retroperitoneal. Bleeding into an operated joint requiring re-operation or intervention was present in all patients with this category of bleeding. Events and event rates include one enoxaparin-treated patient in ADVANCE-1 who also had intracranial hemorrhage.
¶ CRNM = clinically relevant nonmajor.

Table 4: Adverse Reactions Occurring in ≥1% of Patients in Either Group Undergoing Hip or Knee Replacement Surgery

	ELIQUIS, n (%) 2.5 mg po bid N=5924	Enoxaparin, n (%) 40 mg sc qd or 30 mg sc q12h N=5904
Nausea	153 (2.6)	159 (2.7)
Anemia (including postoperative and hemorrhagic anemia, and respective laboratory parameters)	153 (2.6)	178 (3.0)
Contusion	83 (1.4)	115 (1.9)
Hemorrhage (including hematoma, and vaginal and urethral hemorrhage)	67 (1.1)	81 (1.4)
Postprocedural hemorrhage (including postprocedural hematoma, wound hemorrhage, vessel puncture site hematoma and catheter site hemorrhage)	54 (0.9)	60 (1.0)
Transaminases increased (including alanine aminotransferase increased and alanine aminotransferase abnormal)	50 (0.8)	71 (1.2)
Aspartate aminotransferase increased	47 (0.8)	69 (1.2)
Gamma-glutamyltransferase increased	38 (0.6)	65 (1.1)

Other Adverse Reactions
Less common adverse reactions in ELIQUIS (apixaban)-treated patients in the AMPLIFY or AMPLIFY-EXT studies occurring at a frequency of ≥0.1% to <1%:
Blood and lymphatic system disorders: hemorrhagic anemia
Gastrointestinal disorders: hematochezia, hemorrhoidal hemorrhage, gastrointestinal hemorrhage, hematemesis, melena, anal hemorrhage
Injury, poisoning, and procedural complications: wound hemorrhage, postprocedural hemorrhage, traumatic hematoma, periorbital hematoma

Table 5: Bleeding Results in the AMPLIFY Study

	ELIQUIS N=2676 n (%)	Enoxaparin/Warfarin N=2689 n (%)	Relative Risk (95% CI)
Major	15 (0.6)	49 (1.8)	0.31 (0.17, 0.55) p<0.0001
CRNM*	103 (3.9)	215 (8.0)	
Major + CRNM	115 (4.3)	261 (9.7)	
Minor	313 (11.7)	505 (18.8)	
All	402 (15.0)	676 (25.1)	

* CRNM = clinically relevant nonmajor bleeding.
Events associated with each endpoint were counted once per subject, but subjects may have contributed events to multiple endpoints.

Table 6: Adverse Reactions Occurring in ≥1% of Patients Treated for DVT and PE in the AMPLIFY Study

	ELIQUIS N=2676 n (%)	Enoxaparin/Warfarin N=2689 n (%)
Epistaxis	77 (2.9)	146 (5.4)
Contusion	49 (1.8)	97 (3.6)
Hematuria	46 (1.7)	102 (3.8)
Menorrhagia	38 (1.4)	30 (1.1)
Hematoma	35 (1.3)	76 (2.8)
Hemoptysis	32 (1.2)	31 (1.2)
Rectal hemorrhage	26 (1.0)	39 (1.5)
Gingival bleeding	26 (1.0)	50 (1.9)

Table 7: Bleeding Results in the AMPLIFY-EXT Study

	ELIQUIS 2.5 mg N=840 n (%)	ELIQUIS 5 mg N=811 n (%)	Placebo N=826 n (%)
Major	2 (0.2)	1 (0.1)	4 (0.5)
CRNM*	25 (3.0)	34 (4.2)	19 (2.3)
Major + CRNM	27 (3.2)	35 (4.3)	22 (2.7)
Minor	75 (8.9)	98 (12.1)	58 (7.0)
All	94 (11.2)	121 (14.9)	74 (9.0)

* CRNM = clinically relevant nonmajor bleeding.
Events associated with each endpoint were counted once per subject, but subjects may have contributed events to multiple endpoints.

Table 8: Adverse Reactions Occurring in ≥1% of Patients Undergoing Extended Treatment for DVT and PE in the AMPLIFY-EXT Study

	ELIQUIS 2.5 mg N=840 n (%)	ELIQUIS 5 mg N=811 n (%)	Placebo N=826 n (%)
Epistaxis	13 (1.5)	29 (3.6)	9 (1.1)
Hematuria	12 (1.4)	17 (2.1)	9 (1.1)
Hematoma	13 (1.5)	16 (2.0)	10 (1.2)
Contusion	18 (2.1)	18 (2.2)	18 (2.2)
Gingival bleeding	12 (1.4)	9 (1.1)	3 (0.4)

Musculoskeletal and connective tissue disorders: muscle hemorrhage
Reproductive system and breast disorders: vaginal hemorrhage, metrorrhagia, menometrorrhagia, genital hemorrhage
Vascular disorders: hemorrhage
Skin and subcutaneous tissue disorders: ecchymosis, skin hemorrhage, petechiae
Eye disorders: conjunctival hemorrhage, retinal hemorrhage, eye hemorrhage
Investigations: blood urine present, occult blood positive, occult blood, red blood cells urine positive
General disorders and administration-site conditions: injection-site hematoma, vessel puncture-site hematoma

7   DRUG INTERACTIONS

Apixaban is a substrate of both CYP3A4 and P-gp. Inhibitors of CYP3A4 and P-gp increase exposure to apixaban and increase the risk of bleeding. Inducers of CYP3A4 and P-gp decrease exposure to apixaban and increase the risk of stroke and other thromboembolic events.

7.1   Strong Dual Inhibitors of CYP3A4 and P-gp

For patients receiving ELIQUIS (apixaban) doses greater than 2.5 mg twice daily, the dose of ELIQUIS should be decreased by 50% when it is coadministered with drugs that are strong dual inhibitors of CYP3A4 and P-gp (e.g., ketoconazole, itraconazole, ritonavir, or clarithromycin) [see Dosage and Administration (2.2) and Clinical Pharmacology (12.3)].

For patients receiving ELIQUIS (apixaban) at a dose of 2.5 mg twice daily, avoid coadministration with strong dual inhibitors of CYP3A4 and P-gp [see Dosage and Administration (2.2) and Clinical Pharmacology (12.3)].

7.2   Strong Dual Inducers of CYP3A4 and P-gp

Avoid concomitant use of ELIQUIS with strong dual inducers of CYP3A4 and P-gp (e.g., rifampin, carbamazepine, phenytoin, St. John's wort) because such drugs will decrease exposure to apixaban [see Clinical Pharmacology (12.3)].

7.3   Anticoagulants and Antiplatelet Agents

Coadministration of antiplatelet agents, fibrinolytics, heparin, aspirin, and chronic NSAID use increases the risk of bleeding.
APPRAISE-2, a placebo-controlled clinical trial of apixaban in high-risk, post-acute coronary syndrome patients treated with aspirin or the combination of aspirin and clopidogrel, was terminated early due to a higher rate of bleeding with apixaban compared to placebo. The rate of ISTH major bleeding was 2.77% per year with apixaban versus 0.62% per year with placebo in patients receiving single antiplatelet therapy and was 5.91% per year with apixaban versus 2.50% per year with placebo in those receiving dual antiplatelet therapy.
In ARISTOTLE, concomitant use of aspirin increased the bleeding risk on ELIQUIS from 1.8% per year to 3.4% per year and the bleeding risk on warfarin from 2.7% per year to 4.6% per year. In this clinical trial, there was limited (2.3%) use of dual antiplatelet therapy with ELIQUIS.

8   USE IN SPECIFIC POPULATIONS

8.1   Pregnancy

Pregnancy Category B
There are no adequate and well-controlled studies of ELIQUIS (apixaban) in pregnant women. Treatment is likely to increase the risk of hemorrhage during pregnancy and delivery. ELIQUIS should be used during pregnancy only if the potential benefit outweighs the potential risk to the mother and fetus.
Treatment of pregnant rats, rabbits, and mice after implantation until the end of gestation resulted in fetal exposure to apixaban, but was not associated with increased risk for fetal malformations or toxicity. No maternal or fetal deaths were attributed to bleeding. Increased incidence of maternal bleeding was observed in mice, rats, and rabbits at maternal exposures that were 19, 4, and 1 times, respectively, the human exposure of unbound drug, based on area under plasma-concentration time curve (AUC) comparisons at the maximum recommended human dose (MRHD) of 10 mg (5 mg twice daily).

8.2   Labor and Delivery

Safety and effectiveness of ELIQUIS during labor and delivery have not been studied in clinical trials. Consider the risks of bleeding and of stroke in using ELIQUIS in this setting [see Warnings and Precautions (5.2)].
Treatment of pregnant rats from implantation (gestation Day 7) to weaning (lactation Day 21) with apixaban at a dose of 1000 mg/kg (about 5 times the human exposure based on unbound apixaban) did not result in death of offspring or death of mother rats during labor in association with uterine bleeding. However, increased incidence of maternal bleeding, primarily during gestation, occurred at apixaban doses of ≥25 mg/kg, a dose corresponding to ≥1.3 times the human exposure.

8.3   Nursing Mothers

It is unknown whether apixaban or its metabolites are excreted in human milk. Rats excrete apixaban in milk (12% of the maternal dose).
Women should be instructed either to discontinue breastfeeding or to discontinue ELIQUIS therapy, taking into account the importance of the drug to the mother.

8.4   Pediatric Use

Safety and effectiveness in pediatric patients have not been established.

8.5   Geriatric Use

Of the total subjects in the ARISTOTLE and AVERROES clinical studies, >69% were 65 and older, and >31% were 75 and older. In the ADVANCE-1, ADVANCE-2, and ADVANCE-3 clinical studies, 50% of subjects were 65 and older, while 16% were 75 and older. In the AMPLIFY and AMPLIFY-EXT clinical studies, >32% of subjects were 65 and older and >13% were 75 and older. No clinically significant differences in safety or effectiveness were observed when comparing subjects in different age groups.

8.6   End-Stage Renal Disease Patients Maintained with Hemodialysis

Patients with ESRD with or without hemodialysis were not studied in clinical efficacy and safety studies with ELIQUIS; therefore, the dosing recommendation for patients with nonvalvular atrial fibrillation is based on pharmacokinetic and pharmacodynamic (anti-Factor Xa activity) data in subjects with ESRD maintained on dialysis. The recommended dose for ESRD patients maintained with hemodialysis is 5 mg orally twice daily. For ESRD patients maintained with hemodialysis with one of the following patient characteristics, age ≥80 years or body weight ≤60 kg, reduce dose to 2.5 mg twice daily [see Dosage and Administration (2.7) and Clinical Pharmacology (12.2, 12.3)].

10   OVERDOSAGE

There is no antidote to ELIQUIS. Overdose of ELIQUIS increases the risk of bleeding [see Warnings and Precautions (5.2)].
In controlled clinical trials, orally administered apixaban in healthy subjects at doses up to 50 mg daily for 3 to 7 days (25 mg twice daily for 7 days or 50 mg once daily for 3 days) had no clinically relevant adverse effects.
In healthy subjects, administration of activated charcoal 2 and 6 hours after ingestion of a 20-mg dose of apixaban reduced mean apixaban AUC by 50% and 27%, respectively. Thus, administration of activated charcoal may be useful in the management of apixaban overdose or accidental ingestion.

11   DESCRIPTION

ELIQUIS (apixaban), a factor Xa (FXa) inhibitor, is chemically described as 1-(4-methoxyphenyl)-7-oxo-6-[4-(2-oxopiperidin-1-yl)phenyl]-4,5,6,7-tetrahydro-1*H*-pyrazolo-[3,4-*c*]pyridine-3-carboxamide. Its molecular formula is $C_{25}H_{25}N_5O_4$, which corresponds to a molecular weight of 459.5. Apixaban has the following structural formula:

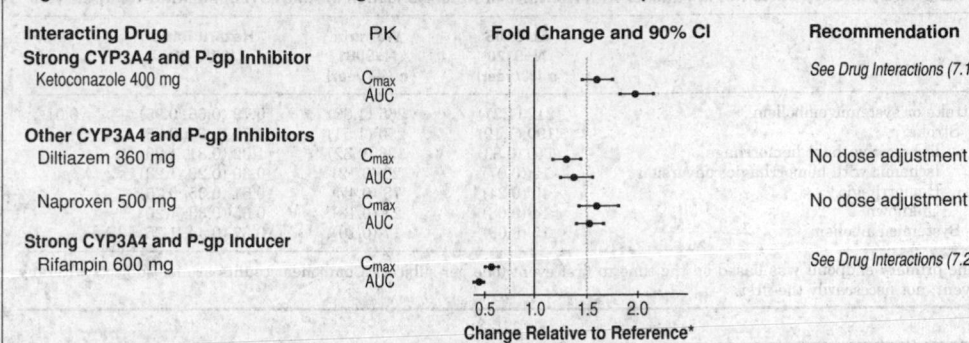

Apixaban is a white to pale-yellow powder. At physiological pH (1.2–6.8), apixaban does not ionize; its aqueous solubility across the physiological pH range is ~0.04 mg/mL. ELIQUIS (apixaban) tablets are available for oral administration in strengths of 2.5 mg and 5 mg of apixaban with the following inactive ingredients: anhydrous lactose, microcrystalline cellulose, croscarmellose sodium, sodium lauryl sulfate, and magnesium stearate. The film coating contains lactose monohydrate, hypromellose, titanium dioxide, triacetin, and yellow iron oxide (2.5 mg tablets) or red iron oxide (5 mg tablets).

12 CLINICAL PHARMACOLOGY

12.1 Mechanism of Action

Apixaban is a selective inhibitor of FXa. It does not require antithrombin III for antithrombotic activity. Apixaban inhibits free and clot-bound FXa, and prothrombinase activity. Apixaban has no direct effect on platelet aggregation, but indirectly inhibits platelet aggregation induced by thrombin. By inhibiting FXa, apixaban decreases thrombin generation and thrombus development.

12.2 Pharmacodynamics

As a result of FXa inhibition, apixaban prolongs clotting tests such as prothrombin time (PT), INR, and activated partial thromboplastin time (aPTT). Changes observed in these clotting tests at the expected therapeutic dose, however, are small, subject to a high degree of variability, and not useful in monitoring the anticoagulation effect of apixaban.

The Rotachrom® Heparin chromogenic assay was used to measure the effect of apixaban on FXa activity in humans during the apixaban development program. A concentration-dependent increase in anti-FXa activity was observed in the dose range tested and was similar in healthy subjects and patients with AF.

This test is not recommended for assessing the anticoagulant effect of apixaban.

Pharmacodynamic Drug Interaction Studies

Pharmacodynamic drug interaction studies with aspirin, clopidogrel, aspirin and clopidogrel, prasugrel, enoxaparin, and naproxen were conducted. No pharmacodynamic interactions were observed with aspirin, clopidogrel, or prasugrel *[see Warnings and Precautions (5.2)]*. A 50% to 60% increase in anti-FXa activity was observed when apixaban was coadministered with enoxaparin or naproxen.

Specific Populations

Renal impairment: Anti-FXa activity adjusted for exposure to apixaban was similar across renal function categories.

Hepatic impairment: Changes in anti-FXa activity were similar in patients with mild-to-moderate hepatic impairment and healthy subjects. However, in patients with moderate hepatic impairment, there is no clear understanding of the impact of this degree of hepatic function impairment on the coagulation cascade and its relationship to efficacy and bleeding. Patients with severe hepatic impairment were not studied.

Cardiac Electrophysiology

Apixaban has no effect on the QTc interval in humans at doses up to 50 mg.

12.3 Pharmacokinetics

Apixaban demonstrates linear pharmacokinetics with dose-proportional increases in exposure for oral doses up to 10 mg.

Absorption

The absolute bioavailability of apixaban is approximately 50% for doses up to 10 mg of ELIQUIS. Food does not affect the bioavailability of apixaban. Maximum concentrations (C_{max}) of apixaban appear 3 to 4 hours after oral administration of ELIQUIS. At doses ≥25 mg, apixaban displays dissolution-limited absorption with decreased bioavailability. Following administration of a crushed 5 mg ELIQUIS tablet that was suspended in 60 mL D5W and delivered through a nasogastric tube (NGT), exposure was similar to that seen in other clinical trials involving healthy volunteers receiving a single oral 5 mg tablet dose.

Distribution

Plasma protein binding in humans is approximately 87%. The volume of distribution (Vss) is approximately 21 liters.

Metabolism

Approximately 25% of an orally administered apixaban dose is recovered in urine and feces as metabolites. Apixaban is metabolized mainly via CYP3A4 with minor contributions from CYP1A2, 2C8, 2C9, 2C19, and 2J2. O-demethylation and hydroxylation at the 3-oxopiperidinyl moiety are the major sites of biotransformation.

Unchanged apixaban is the major drug-related component in human plasma; there are no active circulating metabolites.

Elimination

Apixaban is eliminated in both urine and feces. Renal excretion accounts for about 27% of total clearance. Biliary and direct intestinal excretion contributes to elimination of apixaban in the feces.

Apixaban has a total clearance of approximately 3.3 L/hour and an apparent half-life of approximately 12 hours following oral administration.

Apixaban is a substrate of transport proteins: P-gp and breast cancer resistance protein.

Drug Interaction Studies

In vitro apixaban studies at concentrations significantly greater than therapeutic exposures, no inhibitory effect on the activity of CYP1A2, CYP2A6, CYP2B6, CYP2C8, CYP2C9, CYP2D6, CYP3A4/5, or CYP2C19, nor induction effect on the activity of CYP1A2, CYP2B6, or CYP3A4/5 were observed. Therefore, apixaban is not expected to alter the metabolic clearance of coadministered drugs that are metabolized by these enzymes. Apixaban is not a significant inhibitor of P-gp.

The effects of coadministered drugs on the pharmacokinetics of apixaban and associated dose recommendations are summarized in Figure 2 *[see also Warnings and Precautions (5.2) and Drug Interactions (7)]*.

[See figure 2 above]

In dedicated studies conducted in healthy subjects, famotidine, atenolol, prasugrel, and enoxaparin did not meaningfully alter the pharmacokinetics of apixaban.

In studies conducted in healthy subjects, apixaban did not meaningfully alter the pharmacokinetics of digoxin, naproxen, atenolol, prasugrel, or acetylsalicylic acid.

Specific Populations

The effects of level of renal impairment, age, body weight, and level of hepatic impairment on the pharmacokinetics of apixaban are summarized in Figure 3.

[See figure 3 above]

A study in healthy subjects comparing the pharmacokinetics in males and females showed no meaningful difference. The results across pharmacokinetic studies in normal subjects showed no differences in apixaban pharmacokinetics among White/Caucasian, Asian, and Black/African American subjects. No dose adjustment is required based on race/ethnicity.

In subjects with ESRD, a 4-hour hemodialysis session with a dialysate flow rate of 500 mL/min and a blood flow rate in the range of 350 to 500 mL/min started 2 hours after administration of a single 5 mg dose of apixaban, the AUC of apixaban was 17% greater compared to those with normal renal function. The dialysis clearance of apixaban is approximately 18 mL/min resulting in a 14% decrease in exposure due to hemodialysis compared to off-dialysis period.

Protein binding was similar (92%-94%) between healthy controls and the on-dialysis and off-dialysis periods.

Figure 2: Effect of Coadministered Drugs on the Pharmacokinetics of Apixaban

Interacting Drug	PK	Fold Change and 90% CI	Recommendation
Strong CYP3A4 and P-gp Inhibitor			
Ketoconazole 400 mg	C_{max}		*See Drug Interactions (7.1)*
	AUC		
Other CYP3A4 and P-gp Inhibitors			
Diltiazem 360 mg	C_{max}		No dose adjustment
	AUC		
Naproxen 500 mg	C_{max}		No dose adjustment
	AUC		
Strong CYP3A4 and P-gp Inducer			
Rifampin 600 mg	C_{max}		*See Drug Interactions (7.2)*
	AUC		

Change Relative to Reference*

* Dashed vertical lines illustrate pharmacokinetic changes that were used to inform dosing recommendations. Dosing recommendations were also informed by clinical considerations *[see Warnings and Precautions (5.2) and Drug Interactions (7)]*.

Figure 3: Effect of Specific Populations on the Pharmacokinetics of Apixaban

Population Description	PK	Fold Change and 90% CI	Recommendation
End-Stage Renal Disease*/Normal	C_{max}		No dose adjustment
	AUC		
Renal Impairment: Severe†/Normal	C_{max}		No dose adjustment
	AUC		
Renal Impairment: Moderate/Normal	C_{max}		No dose adjustment
	AUC		
Renal Impairment: Mild/Normal	C_{max}		No dose adjustment
	AUC		
Age: ≥65 years/18-40 years	C_{max}		No dose adjustment
	AUC		
Body Weight: ≥120 kg/65-85 kg	C_{max}		No dose adjustment
	AUC		
Body Weight: ≤50 kg/65-85 kg	C_{max}		No dose adjustment
	AUC		
Hepatic Impairment: Moderate/Normal	C_{max}		Dosing recommendation cannot be provided
	AUC		
Hepatic Impairment: Mild/Normal	C_{max}		No dose adjustment
	AUC		

Change Relative to Reference‡

* ESRD subjects maintained with chronic and stable hemodialysis; reported PK findings are following single dose of apixaban post hemodialysis.
† Creatinine clearance 15 to 29 mL/min.
‡ Dashed vertical lines illustrate pharmacokinetic changes that were used to inform dosing recommendations.

Table 9: Key Efficacy Outcomes in Patients with Nonvalvular Atrial Fibrillation in ARISTOTLE (Intent-to-Treat Analysis)

	ELIQUIS N=9120 n (%/year)	Warfarin N=9081 n (%/year)	Hazard Ratio (95% CI)	P-value
Stroke or systemic embolism	212 (1.27)	265 (1.60)	0.79 (0.66, 0.95)	0.01
Stroke	199 (1.19)	250 (1.51)	0.79 (0.65, 0.95)	
Ischemic without hemorrhage	140 (0.83)	136 (0.82)	1.02 (0.81, 1.29)	
Ischemic with hemorrhagic conversion	12 (0.07)	20 (0.12)	0.60 (0.29, 1.23)	
Hemorrhagic	40 (0.24)	78 (0.47)	0.51 (0.35, 0.75)	
Unknown	14 (0.08)	21 (0.13)	0.65 (0.33, 1.29)	
Systemic embolism	15 (0.09)	17 (0.10)	0.87 (0.44, 1.75)	

The primary endpoint was based on the time to first event (one per subject). Component counts are for subjects with any event, not necessarily the first.

Figure 4: Kaplan-Meier Estimate of Time to First Stroke or Systemic Embolism in ARISTOTLE (Intent-to-Treat Population)

Number of Subjects at Risk

ELIQUIS	9120	8726	8440	6051	3464	1754	600
Warfarin	9081	8620	8301	5972	3405	1768	572

13 NONCLINICAL TOXICOLOGY

13.1 Carcinogenesis, Mutagenesis, Impairment of Fertility

Carcinogenesis: Apixaban was not carcinogenic when administered to mice and rats for up to 2 years. The systemic exposures (AUCs) of unbound apixaban in male and female mice at the highest doses tested (1500 and 3000 mg/kg/day) were 9 and 20 times, respectively, the human exposure of unbound drug at the MRHD of 10 mg/day. Systemic exposures of unbound apixaban in male and female rats at the highest dose tested (600 mg/kg/day) were 2 and 4 times, respectively, the human exposure.

Mutagenesis: Apixaban was neither mutagenic in the bacterial reverse mutation (Ames) assay, nor clastogenic in Chinese hamster ovary cells *in vitro*, in a 1-month *in vivo/in vitro* cytogenetics study in rat peripheral blood lymphocytes, or in a rat micronucleus study *in vivo*.

Impairment of Fertility: Apixaban had no effect on fertility in male or female rats when given at doses up to 600 mg/kg/day, a dose resulting in exposure levels that are 3 and 4 times, respectively, the human exposure.

Apixaban administered to female rats at doses up to 1000 mg/kg/day from implantation through the end of lactation produced no adverse findings in male offspring (F_1 generation) at doses up to 1000 mg/kg/day, a dose resulting in exposure that is 5 times the human exposure. Adverse effects in the F_1-generation female offspring were limited to decreased mating and fertility indices at 1000 mg/kg/day.

14 CLINICAL STUDIES

14.1 Reduction of Risk of Stroke and Systemic Embolism in Nonvalvular Atrial Fibrillation

ARISTOTLE

Evidence for the efficacy and safety of ELIQUIS (apixaban) was derived from ARISTOTLE, a multinational, double-blind study in patients with nonvalvular AF comparing the effects of ELIQUIS and warfarin on the risk of stroke and non-central nervous system (CNS) systemic embolism. In ARISTOTLE, patients were randomized to ELIQUIS 5 mg orally twice daily (or 2.5 mg twice daily in subjects with at least 2 of the following characteristics: age ≥80 years, body weight ≤60 kg, or serum creatinine ≥1.5 mg/dL) or to warfarin (targeted to an INR range of 2.0–3.0). Patients had to have one or more of the following additional risk factors for stroke:

- prior stroke or transient ischemic attack (TIA)
- prior systemic embolism
- age ≥75 years
- arterial hypertension requiring treatment
- diabetes mellitus
- heart failure ≥New York Heart Association Class 2
- left ventricular ejection fraction ≤40%

The primary objective of ARISTOTLE was to determine whether ELIQUIS (apixaban) 5 mg twice daily (or 2.5 mg twice daily) was effective (noninferior to warfarin) in reducing the risk of stroke (ischemic or hemorrhagic) and systemic embolism. Superiority of ELIQUIS to warfarin was also examined for the primary endpoint (rate of stroke and systemic embolism), major bleeding, and death from any cause.

A total of 18,201 patients were randomized and followed on study treatment for a median of 89 weeks. Forty-three percent of patients were vitamin K antagonist (VKA) "naive," defined as having received ≤30 consecutive days of treatment with warfarin or another VKA before entering the study. The mean age was 69 years and the mean CHADS₂ score (a scale from 0 to 6 used to estimate risk of stroke, with higher scores predicting greater risk) was 2.1. The population was 65% male, 83% Caucasian, 14% Asian, and 1% Black. There was a history of stroke, TIA, or non-CNS systemic embolism in 19% of patients. Concomitant diseases of patients in this study included hypertension 88%, diabetes 25%, congestive heart failure (or left ventricular ejection fraction ≤40%) 35%, and prior myocardial infarction 14%. Patients treated with warfarin in ARISTOTLE had a mean percentage of time in therapeutic range (INR 2.0–3.0) of 62%.

ELIQUIS was superior to warfarin for the primary endpoint of reducing the risk of stroke and systemic embolism (Table 9 and Figure 4). Superiority to warfarin was primarily attributable to a reduction in hemorrhagic stroke and ischemic strokes with hemorrhagic conversion compared to

warfarin. Purely ischemic strokes occurred with similar rates on both drugs.

ELIQUIS (apixaban) also showed significantly fewer major bleeds than warfarin *[see Adverse Reactions (6.1)]*.

[See table 9 above]

[See figure 4 above]

All-cause death was assessed using a sequential testing strategy that allowed testing for superiority if effects on earlier endpoints (stroke plus systemic embolus and major bleeding) were demonstrated. ELIQUIS treatment resulted in a significantly lower rate of all-cause death (p = 0.046) than did treatment with warfarin, primarily because of a reduction in cardiovascular death, particularly stroke deaths. Non-vascular death rates were similar in the treatment arms.

In ARISTOTLE, the results for the primary efficacy endpoint were generally consistent across most major subgroups including weight, CHADS₂ score (a scale from 0 to 6 used to predict risk of stroke in patients with AF, with higher scores predicting greater risk), prior warfarin use, level of renal impairment, geographic region, ELIQUIS dose, type of AF, and aspirin use at randomization (Figure 5).

[See figure 5 at top of next page]

At the end of the ARISTOTLE study, warfarin patients who completed the study were generally maintained on a VKA with no interruption of anticoagulation. ELIQUIS patients who completed the study were generally switched to a VKA with a 2-day period of coadministration of ELIQUIS and VKA, so that some patients may not have been adequately anticoagulated after stopping ELIQUIS until attaining a stable and therapeutic INR. During the 30 days following the end of the study, there were 21 stroke or systemic embolism events in the 6791 patients (0.3%) in the ELIQUIS arm compared to 5 in the 6569 patients (0.1%) in the warfarin arm *[see Dosage and Administration (2.5)]*.

AVERROES

In AVERROES, patients with nonvalvular atrial fibrillation thought not to be candidates for warfarin therapy were randomized to treatment with ELIQUIS 5 mg orally twice daily (or 2.5 mg twice daily in selected patients) or aspirin 81 to 324 mg once daily. The primary objective of the study was to determine if ELIQUIS was superior to aspirin for preventing the composite outcome of stroke or systemic embolism. AVERROES was stopped early on the basis of a prespecified interim analysis showing a significant reduction in stroke and systemic embolism for ELIQUIS compared to aspirin that was associated with a modest increase in major bleeding (Table 10) *[see Adverse Reactions (6.1)]*.

[See table 10 at top of next page]

14.2 Prophylaxis of Deep Vein Thrombosis Following Hip or Knee Replacement Surgery

The clinical evidence for the effectiveness of ELIQUIS is derived from the ADVANCE-1, ADVANCE-2, and ADVANCE-3 clinical trials in adult patients undergoing elective hip (ADVANCE-3) or knee (ADVANCE-2 and ADVANCE-1) replacement surgery. A total of 11,659 patients were randomized in 3 double-blind, multi-national studies. Included in this total were 1866 patients age 75 or older, 1161 patients with low body weight (≤60 kg), 2528 patients with Body Mass Index ≥33 kg/m², and 625 patients with severe or moderate renal impairment.

In the ADVANCE-3 study, 5407 patients undergoing elective hip replacement surgery were randomized to receive either ELIQUIS 2.5 mg orally twice daily or enoxaparin 40 mg subcutaneously once daily. The first dose of ELIQUIS was given 12 to 24 hours post surgery, whereas enoxaparin was started 9 to 15 hours prior to surgery. Treatment duration was 32 to 38 days.

In patients undergoing elective knee replacement surgery, ELIQUIS 2.5 mg orally twice daily was compared to enoxaparin 40 mg subcutaneously once daily (ADVANCE-2, N=3057) or enoxaparin 30 mg subcutaneously every 12 hours (ADVANCE-1, N=3195). In the ADVANCE-2 study, the first dose of ELIQUIS was given 12 to 24 hours post surgery, whereas enoxaparin was started 9 to 15 hours prior to surgery. In the ADVANCE-1 study, both ELIQUIS and enoxaparin were initiated 12 to 24 hours post surgery. Treatment duration in both ADVANCE-2 and ADVANCE-1 was 10 to 14 days.

In all 3 studies, the primary endpoint was a composite of adjudicated asymptomatic and symptomatic DVT, nonfatal PE, and all-cause death at the end of the double-blind intended treatment period. In ADVANCE-3 and ADVANCE-2, the primary endpoint was tested for noninferiority, then superiority, of ELIQUIS to enoxaparin. In ADVANCE-1, the primary endpoint was tested for noninferiority of ELIQUIS to enoxaparin.

The efficacy data are provided in Tables 11 and 12.

Table 11: Summary of Key Efficacy Analysis Results During the Intended Treatment Period for Patients Undergoing Elective Hip Replacement Surgery*

Events During 35-Day Treatment Period	ADVANCE-3		Relative Risk (95% CI) P-value
	ELIQUIS 2.5 mg po bid	Enoxaparin 40 mg sc qd	
Number of Patients	N=1949	N=1917	
Total VTE[†]/ All-cause death	27 (1.39%) (0.95, 2.02)	74 (3.86%) (3.08, 4.83)	0.36 (0.22, 0.54) p<0.0001
Number of Patients	N=2708	N=2699	
All-cause death	3 (0.11%) (0.02, 0.35)	1 (0.04%) (0.00, 0.24)	
PE	3 (0.11%) (0.02, 0.35)	5 (0.19%) (0.07, 0.45)	
Symptomatic DVT	1 (0.04%) (0.00, 0.24)	5 (0.19%) (0.07, 0.45)	
Number of Patients	N=2196	N=2190	
Proximal DVT[‡]	7 (0.32%) (0.14, 0.68)	20 (0.91%) (0.59, 1.42)	
Number of Patients	N=1951	N=1908	
Distal DVT[‡]	20 (1.03%) (0.66, 1.59)	57 (2.99%) (2.31, 3.86)	

* Events associated with each endpoint were counted once per subject but subjects may have contributed events to multiple endpoints.
† Total VTE includes symptomatic and asymptomatic DVT and PE.
‡ Includes symptomatic and asymptomatic DVT.

[See table 12 at top of next page]

The efficacy profile of ELIQUIS (apixaban) was generally consistent across subgroups of interest for this indication (e.g., age, gender, race, body weight, renal impairment).

14.3 Treatment of DVT and PE and Reduction in the Risk of Recurrence of DVT and PE

Efficacy and safety of ELIQUIS for the treatment of DVT and PE, and for the reduction in the risk of recurrent DVT and PE following 6 to 12 months of anticoagulant treatment was derived from the AMPLIFY and AMPLIFY-EXT studies. Both studies were randomized, parallel-group, double-blind trials in patients with symptomatic proximal DVT and/or symptomatic PE. All key safety and efficacy endpoints were adjudicated in a blinded manner by an independent committee.

AMPLIFY

The primary objective of AMPLIFY was to determine whether ELIQUIS was noninferior to enoxaparin/warfarin for the incidence of recurrent VTE (venous thromboembolism) or VTE-related death. Patients with an objectively confirmed symptomatic DVT and/or PE were randomized to treatment with ELIQUIS 10 mg twice daily orally for 7 days followed by ELIQUIS 5 mg twice daily orally for 6 months, or enoxaparin 1 mg/kg twice daily subcutaneously for at least 5 days (until INR ≥2) followed by warfarin (target INR range 2.0-3.0) orally for 6 months. Patients who required thrombectomy, insertion of a caval filter, or use of a fibrinolytic agent, and patients with creatinine clearance <25 mL/min, significant liver disease, an existing heart valve or atrial fibrillation, or active bleeding were excluded from the AMPLIFY study. Patients were allowed to enter the study with or without prior parenteral anticoagulation (up to 48 hours).

A total of 5244 patients were evaluable for efficacy and were followed for a mean of 154 days in the ELIQUIS group and 152 days in the enoxaparin/warfarin group. The mean age was 57 years. The AMPLIFY study population was 59% male, 83% Caucasian, 8% Asian, and 4% Black. For patients randomized to warfarin, the mean percentage of time in therapeutic range (INR 2.0-3.0) was 60.9%.

Approximately 90% of patients enrolled in AMPLIFY had an unprovoked DVT or PE at baseline. The remaining 10% of patients with a provoked DVT or PE were required to have an additional ongoing risk factor in order to be randomized, which included previous episode of DVT or PE, immobilization, history of cancer, active cancer, and known prothrombotic genotype.

Figure 5: Stroke and Systemic Embolism Hazard Ratios by Baseline Characteristics — ARISTOTLE Study

Subgroup	No. of Patients	No. of Events (% per yr) Apixaban	No. of Events (% per yr) Warfarin	Hazard Ratio (95% CI)	P-value for Interaction
All Patients	18201	212 (1.27)	265 (1.60)		
Prior Warfarin/VKA Status					0.39
Experienced	10401	102 (1.1)	138 (1.5)		
Naïve	7800	110 (1.5)	127 (1.8)		
Age					0.12
<65 yrs old	5471	51 (1.0)	44 (0.9)		
≥65 to <75 yrs old	7052	82 (1.3)	112 (1.7)		
≥75 yrs old	5678	79 (1.6)	109 (2.2)		
Gender					0.60
Male	11785	132 (1.2)	160 (1.5)		
Female	6416	80 (1.4)	105 (1.8)		
Weight					0.26
≤60 kg	1985	34 (2.0)	52 (3.2)		
>60 kg	16154	177 (1.2)	212 (1.4)		
Type of Atrial Fibrillation					0.70
Permanent/Persistent	15412	191 (1.4)	235 (1.7)		
Paroxysmal	2786	21 (0.8)	30 (1.1)		
Prior Stroke or TIA					0.71
Yes	3436	73 (2.5)	98 (3.2)		
No	14765	139 (1.0)	167 (1.2)		
Diabetes Mellitus					0.71
Yes	4547	57 (1.4)	75 (1.9)		
No	13654	155 (1.2)	190 (1.5)		
Heart Failure					0.50
Yes	5541	70 (1.4)	79 (1.6)		
No	12660	142 (1.2)	186 (1.6)		
CHADS₂ Score					0.45
≤1	6183	44 (0.7)	51 (0.9)		
=2	6516	74 (1.2)	82 (1.4)		
≥3	5502	94 (1.9)	132 (2.8)		
Level of Renal Impairment					0.72
Severe or Moderate	3017	54 (2.1)	69 (2.7)		
Mild	7587	87 (1.2)	116 (1.7)		
Normal	7518	70 (1.0)	79 (1.1)		
Apixaban Dose					0.22
2.5 mg BID or placebo	831	12 (1.7)	22 (3.3)		
5 mg BID or placebo	17370	200 (1.3)	243 (1.5)		
Geographic Region					0.44
North America	4474	42 (1.0)	56 (1.3)		
Latin America	3468	43 (1.4)	52 (1.8)		
Europe	7343	75 (1.1)	77 (1.1)		
Asia/Pacific	2916	52 (2.0)	80 (3.1)		
Aspirin at Randomization					0.44
Yes	5632	70 (1.3)	94 (1.9)		
No	12569	142 (1.2)	171 (1.5)		

0.25 0.5 1 2
← Apixaban Better   Warfarin Better →

ELIQUIS (apixaban) was shown to be noninferior to enoxaparin/warfarin in the AMPLIFY study for the primary endpoint of recurrent symptomatic VTE (nonfatal DVT or nonfatal PE) or VTE-related death over 6 months of therapy (Table 13).

[See table 13 at top of next page]

In the AMPLIFY study, patients were stratified according to their index event of PE (with or without DVT) or DVT (without PE). Efficacy in the initial treatment of VTE was consistent between the two subgroups.

AMPLIFY-EXT

Patients who had been treated for DVT and/or PE for 6 to 12 months with anticoagulant therapy without having a recurrent event were randomized to treatment with ELIQUIS 2.5 mg orally twice daily, ELIQUIS 5 mg orally twice daily, or placebo for 12 months. Approximately one-third of patients participated in the AMPLIFY study prior to enrollment in the AMPLIFY-EXT study.

A total of 2482 patients were randomized to study treatment and were followed for a mean of approximately 330 days in the ELIQUIS (apixaban) group and 312 days in the placebo group. The mean age in the AMPLIFY-EXT study was 57 years. The study population was 57% male, 85% Caucasian, 5% Asian, and 3% Black.

The AMPLIFY-EXT study enrolled patients with either an unprovoked DVT or PE at baseline (approximately 92%) or patients with a provoked baseline event and one additional risk factor for recurrence (approximately 8%). However, patients who had experienced multiple episodes of unprovoked DVT or PE were excluded from the AMPLIFY-EXT study. In the AMPLIFY-EXT study, both doses of ELIQUIS were superior to placebo in the primary endpoint of symptomatic, recurrent VTE (nonfatal DVT or nonfatal PE), or all-cause death (Table 14).

Table 10: Key Efficacy Outcomes in Patients with Nonvalvular Atrial Fibrillation in AVERROES

	ELIQUIS N=2807 n (%/year)	Aspirin N=2791 n (%/year)	Hazard Ratio (95% CI)	P-value
Stroke or systemic embolism	51 (1.62)	113 (3.63)	0.45 (0.32, 0.62)	<0.0001
Stroke				
Ischemic or undetermined	43 (1.37)	97 (3.11)	0.44 (0.31, 0.63)	-
Hemorrhagic	6 (0.19)	9 (0.28)	0.67 (0.24, 1.88)	-
Systemic embolism	2 (0.06)	13 (0.41)	0.15 (0.03, 0.68)	-
MI	24 (0.76)	28 (0.89)	0.86 (0.50, 1.48)	-
All-cause death	111 (3.51)	140 (4.42)	0.79 (0.62, 1.02)	0.068
Vascular death	84 (2.65)	96 (3.03)	0.87 (0.65, 1.17)	

Table 12: Summary of Key Efficacy Analysis Results During the Intended Treatment Period for Patients Undergoing Elective Knee Replacement Surgery*

Events during 12-day treatment period	ADVANCE-1			ADVANCE-2		
	ELIQUIS 2.5 mg po bid	Enoxaparin 30 mg sc q12h	Relative Risk (95% CI) P-value	ELIQUIS 2.5 mg po bid	Enoxaparin 40 mg sc qd	Relative Risk (95% CI) P-value
Number of Patients	N=1157	N=1130		N=976	N=997	
Total VTE[†]/ All-cause death	104 (8.99%) (7.47, 10.79)	100 (8.85%) (7.33, 10.66)	1.02 (0.78, 1.32) NS	147 (15.06%) (12.95, 17.46)	243 (24.37%) (21.81, 27.14)	0.62 (0.51, 0.74) p<0.0001
Number of Patients	N=1599	N=1596		N=1528	N=1529	
All-cause death	3 (0.19%) (0.04, 0.59)	3 (0.19%) (0.04, 0.59)		2 (0.13%) (0.01, 0.52)	0 (0%) (0.00, 0.31)	
PE	16 (1.0%) (0.61, 1.64)	7 (0.44%) (0.20, 0.93)		4 (0.26%) (0.08, 0.70)	0 (0%) (0.00, 0.31)	
Symptomatic DVT	3 (0.19%) (0.04, 0.59)	7 (0.44%) (0.20, 0.93)		3 (0.20%) (0.04, 0.61)	7 (0.46%) (0.20, 0.97)	
Number of Patients	N=1254	N=1207		N=1192	N=1199	
Proximal DVT[‡]	9 (0.72%) (0.36, 1.39)	11 (0.91%) (0.49, 1.65)		9 (0.76%) (0.38, 1.46)	26 (2.17%) (1.47, 3.18)	
Number of Patients	N=1146	N=1133		N=978	N=1000	
Distal DVT[‡]	83 (7.24%) (5.88, 8.91)	91 (8.03%) (6.58, 9.78)		142 (14.52%) (12.45, 16.88)	239 (23.9%) (21.36, 26.65)	

* Events associated with each endpoint were counted once per subject but subjects may have contributed events to multiple endpoints.
† Total VTE includes symptomatic and asymptomatic DVT and PE.
‡ Includes symptomatic and asymptomatic DVT.

Table 13: Efficacy Results in the AMPLIFY Study

	ELIQUIS N=2609 n	Enoxaparin/Warfarin N=2635 n	Relative Risk (95% CI)
VTE or VTE-related death*	59 (2.3%)	71 (2.7%)	0.84 (0.60, 1.18)
DVT†	22 (0.8%)	35 (1.3%)	
PE†	27 (1.0%)	25 (0.9%)	
VTE-related death†	12 (0.4%)	16 (0.6%)	
VTE or all-cause death	84 (3.2%)	104 (4.0%)	0.82 (0.61, 1.08)
VTE or CV-related death	61 (2.3%)	77 (2.9%)	0.80 (0.57, 1.11)

* Noninferior compared to enoxaparin/warfarin (P-value <0.0001).
† Events associated with each endpoint were counted once per subject, but subjects may have contributed events to multiple endpoints.

Table 14: Efficacy Results in the AMPLIFY-EXT Study

	ELIQUIS 2.5 mg N=840	ELIQUIS 5 mg N=813	Placebo N=829	Relative Risk (95% CI) ELIQUIS 2.5 mg vs Placebo	ELIQUIS 5 mg vs Placebo
	n (%)				
Recurrent VTE or all-cause death	32 (3.8)	34 (4.2)	96 (11.6)	0.33 (0.22, 0.48) p<0.0001	0.36 (0.25, 0.53) p<0.0001
DVT*	19 (2.3)	28 (3.4)	72 (8.7)		
PE*	23 (2.7)	25 (3.1)	37 (4.5)		
All-cause death	22 (2.6)	25 (3.1)	33 (4.0)		

* Patients with more than one event are counted in multiple rows.

[See table 14 above]

16 HOW SUPPLIED/STORAGE AND HANDLING

How Supplied
ELIQUIS (apixaban) tablets are available as listed in the table below.
[See table at top of next page]

Storage and Handling
Store at 20°C to 25°C (68°F-77°F); excursions permitted between 15°C and 30°C (59°F-86°F) [see USP Controlled Room Temperature].

17 PATIENT COUNSELING INFORMATION

See FDA-approved patient labeling (Medication Guide).
Advise patients of the following:
• They should not discontinue ELIQUIS (apixaban) without talking to their physician first.
• They should be informed that it might take longer than usual for bleeding to stop, and they may bruise or bleed more easily when treated with ELIQUIS. Advise patients about how to recognize bleeding or symptoms of hypovolemia and of the urgent need to report any unusual bleeding to their physician.

• They should tell their physicians and dentists they are taking ELIQUIS, and/or any other product known to affect bleeding (including nonprescription products, such as aspirin or NSAIDs), before any surgery or medical or dental procedure is scheduled and before any new drug is taken.
• If the patient is having neuraxial anesthesia or spinal puncture, inform the patient to watch for signs and symptoms of spinal or epidural hematomas, such as numbness or weakness of the legs, or bowel or bladder dysfunction [see Warnings and Precautions (5.3)]. If any of these symptoms occur, the patient should contact his or her physician immediately.
• They should tell their physicians if they are pregnant or plan to become pregnant or are breastfeeding or intend to breastfeed during treatment with ELIQUIS [see Use in Specific Populations (8.1, 8.3)].
• If a dose is missed, the dose should be taken as soon as possible on the same day and twice-daily administration should be resumed. The dose should not be doubled to make up for a missed dose.

Manufactured by:
Bristol-Myers Squibb Company
Princeton, New Jersey 08543 USA
Marketed by:
Bristol-Myers Squibb Company
Princeton, New Jersey 08543 USA
and
Pfizer Inc
New York, New York 10017 USA
Rotachrom® is a registered trademark of Diagnostica Stago.
1289808A1 / 1289807A1 / 1298500A1

MEDICATION GUIDE
ELIQUIS® (ELL eh kwiss)
(apixaban)
tablets
What is the most important information I should know about ELIQUIS?
• **For people taking ELIQUIS for atrial fibrillation:**
People with atrial fibrillation (a type of irregular heartbeat) are at an increased risk of forming a blood clot in the heart, which can travel to the brain, causing a stroke, or to other parts of the body. ELIQUIS lowers your chance of having a stroke by helping to prevent clots from forming. If you stop taking ELIQUIS, you may have increased risk of forming a clot in your blood.
Do not stop taking ELIQUIS without talking to the doctor who prescribes it for you. Stopping ELIQUIS increases your risk of having a stroke.
ELIQUIS may need to be stopped, if possible, prior to surgery or a medical or dental procedure. Ask the doctor who prescribed ELIQUIS for you when you should stop taking it. Your doctor will tell you when you may start taking ELIQUIS again after your surgery or procedure. If you have to stop taking ELIQUIS, your doctor may prescribe another medicine to help prevent a blood clot from forming.
• **ELIQUIS can cause bleeding** which can be serious and rarely may lead to death. This is because ELIQUIS is a blood thinner medicine that reduces blood clotting.
You may have a higher risk of bleeding if you take ELIQUIS and take other medicines that increase your risk of bleeding, including:
• aspirin or aspirin-containing products
• long-term (chronic) use of nonsteroidal anti-inflammatory drugs (NSAIDs)
• warfarin sodium (COUMADIN®, JANTOVEN®)
• any medicine that contains heparin
• selective serotonin reuptake inhibitors (SSRIs) or serotonin norepinephrine reuptake inhibitors (SNRIs)
• other medicines to help prevent or treat blood clots
Tell your doctor if you take any of these medicines. Ask your doctor or pharmacist if you are not sure if your medicine is one listed above.
While taking ELIQUIS:
• you may bruise more easily
• it may take longer than usual for any bleeding to stop
Call your doctor or get medical help right away if you have any of these signs or symptoms of bleeding when taking ELIQUIS:
• unexpected bleeding, or bleeding that lasts a long time, such as:
  • unusual bleeding from the gums
  • nosebleeds that happen often
  • menstrual bleeding or vaginal bleeding that is heavier than normal
• bleeding that is severe or you cannot control
• red, pink, or brown urine
• red or black stools (looks like tar)
• cough up blood or blood clots
• vomit blood or your vomit looks like coffee grounds
• unexpected pain, swelling, or joint pain
• headaches, feeling dizzy or weak
• **ELIQUIS is not for patients with artificial heart valves.**
• **Spinal or epidural blood clots (hematoma).** People who take a blood thinner medicine (anticoagulant) like ELIQUIS, and have medicine injected into their spinal

Tablet Strength	Tablet Color/Shape	Tablet Markings	Package Size	NDC Code
2.5 mg	Yellow, round, biconvex	Debossed with "893" on one side and "2½" on the other side	Bottles of 60	0003-0893-21
			Bottles of 180	0003-0893-41
			Hospital Unit-Dose Blister Package of 100	0003-0893-31
5 mg	Pink, oval, biconvex	Debossed with "894" on one side and "5" on the other side	Bottles of 60	0003-0894-21
			Bottles of 180	0003-0894-41
			Hospital Unit-Dose Blister Package of 100	0003-0894-31

and epidural area, or have a spinal puncture have a risk of forming a blood clot that can cause long-term or permanent loss of the ability to move (paralysis). Your risk of developing a spinal or epidural blood clot is higher if:
• a thin tube called an epidural catheter is placed in your back to give you certain medicine
• you take NSAIDs or a medicine to prevent blood from clotting
• you have a history of difficult or repeated epidural or spinal punctures
• you have a history of problems with your spine or have had surgery on your spine
If you take ELIQUIS and receive spinal anesthesia or have a spinal puncture, your doctor should watch you closely for symptoms of spinal or epidural blood clots or bleeding. Tell your doctor right away if you have tingling, numbness, or muscle weakness, especially in your legs and feet.

What is ELIQUIS?
ELIQUIS (apixaban) is a prescription medicine used to:
• reduce the risk of stroke and blood clots in people who have atrial fibrillation.
• reduce the risk of forming a blood clot in the legs and lungs of people who have just had hip or knee replacement surgery.
• treat blood clots in the veins of your legs (deep vein thrombosis) or lungs (pulmonary embolism), and reduce the risk of them occurring again.
It is not known if ELIQUIS is safe and effective in children.
Who should not take ELIQUIS?
Do not take ELIQUIS if you:
• currently have certain types of abnormal bleeding.
• have had a serious allergic reaction to ELIQUIS. Ask your doctor if you are not sure.
What should I tell my doctor before taking ELIQUIS?
Before you take ELIQUIS, tell your doctor if you:
• have kidney or liver problems
• have any other medical condition
• have ever had bleeding problems
• are pregnant or plan to become pregnant. It is not known if ELIQUIS will harm your unborn baby.
• are breastfeeding or plan to breastfeed. It is not known if ELIQUIS passes into your breast milk. You and your doctor should decide if you will take ELIQUIS or breastfeed. You should not do both.
Tell all of your doctors and dentists that you are taking ELIQUIS. They should talk to the doctor who prescribed ELIQUIS for you, before you have **any** surgery, medical or dental procedure.
Tell your doctor about all the medicines you take, including prescription and over-the-counter medicines, vitamins, and herbal supplements. Some of your other medicines may affect the way ELIQUIS works. Certain medicines may increase your risk of bleeding or stroke when taken with ELIQUIS. See "**What is the most important information I should know about ELIQUIS?**"
Know the medicines you take. Keep a list of them to show your doctor and pharmacist when you get a new medicine.
How should I take ELIQUIS?
• **Take ELIQUIS exactly as prescribed by your doctor.**
• Take ELIQUIS twice every day with or without food.
• Do not change your dose or stop taking ELIQUIS unless your doctor tells you to.
• If you miss a dose of ELIQUIS, take it as soon as you remember. Do not take more than one dose of ELIQUIS at the same time to make up for a missed dose.
• Your doctor will decide how long you should take ELIQUIS. **Do not stop taking it without first talking with your doctor. If you are taking ELIQUIS for atrial fibrillation, stopping ELIQUIS may increase your risk of having a stroke.**
• **Do not run out of ELIQUIS. Refill your prescription before you run out.** When leaving the hospital following hip or knee replacement, be sure that you will have ELIQUIS available to avoid missing any doses.
• If you take too much ELIQUIS, call your doctor or go to the nearest hospital emergency room right away.

• Call your doctor or healthcare provider right away if you fall or injure yourself, especially if you hit your head. Your doctor or healthcare provider may need to check you.
What are the possible side effects of ELIQUIS?
• See "**What is the most important information I should know about ELIQUIS?**"
• ELIQUIS (apixaban) can cause a skin rash or severe allergic reaction. Call your doctor or get medical help right away if you have any of the following symptoms:
 • chest pain or tightness
 • swelling of your face or tongue
 • trouble breathing or wheezing
 • feeling dizzy or faint
Tell your doctor if you have any side effect that bothers you or that does not go away.
These are not all of the possible side effects of ELIQUIS. For more information, ask your doctor or pharmacist.
Call your doctor for medical advice about side effects. You may report side effects to FDA at 1-800-FDA-1088.
How should I store ELIQUIS?
Store ELIQUIS at room temperature between 68°F to 77°F (20°C to 25°C).
Keep ELIQUIS and all medicines out of the reach of children.
General Information about ELIQUIS
Medicines are sometimes prescribed for purposes other than those listed in a Medication Guide. Do not use ELIQUIS for a condition for which it was not prescribed. Do not give ELIQUIS to other people, even if they have the same symptoms that you have. It may harm them.
If you would like more information, talk with your doctor. You can ask your pharmacist or doctor for information about ELIQUIS that is written for health professionals.
For more information, call 1-855-354-7847 (1-855-ELIQUIS) or go to www.ELIQUIS.com.
What are the ingredients in ELIQUIS?
Active ingredient: apixaban.
Inactive ingredients: anhydrous lactose, microcrystalline cellulose, croscarmellose sodium, sodium lauryl sulfate, and magnesium stearate. The film coating contains lactose monohydrate, hypromellose, titanium dioxide, triacetin, and yellow iron oxide (2.5 mg tablets) or red iron oxide (5 mg tablets).
This Medication Guide has been approved by the U.S. Food and Drug Administration.
Manufactured by:
Bristol-Myers Squibb Company
Princeton, New Jersey 08543 USA
Marketed by:
Bristol-Myers Squibb Company
Princeton, New Jersey 08543 USA
and
Pfizer Inc
New York, New York 10017 USA
COUMADIN® is a registered trademark of Bristol-Myers Squibb Pharma Company.
All other trademarks are property of their respective companies.
1289808A1 / 1289807A1 / 1298500A1
1295958A1
Revised August 2014
Shown in Product Identification Guide, page 306

ERBITUX®   ℞
[ER-be-tux]
(cetuximab)
injection, for intravenous infusion

HIGHLIGHTS OF PRESCRIBING INFORMATION
These highlights do not include all the information needed to use ERBITUX safely and effectively. See full prescribing information for ERBITUX.
ERBITUX® (cetuximab)
injection, for intravenous infusion
Initial U.S. Approval: 2004

> **WARNING: SERIOUS INFUSION REACTIONS and CARDIOPULMONARY ARREST**
> *See full prescribing information for complete boxed warning.*
> • **Serious infusion reactions, some fatal, occurred in approximately 3% of patients. (5.1)**
> • **Cardiopulmonary arrest and/or sudden death occurred in 2% of patients with squamous cell carcinoma of the head and neck treated with Erbitux and radiation therapy and in 3% of patients with squamous cell carcinoma of the head and neck treated with cetuximab in combination with platinum-based therapy with 5-fluorouracil (5-FU). Closely monitor serum electrolytes, including serum magnesium, potassium, and calcium, during and after Erbitux administration. (5.2, 5.6)**

———**RECENT MAJOR CHANGES**———
Warnings and Precautions
Use of Erbitux in Combination With
Radiation and Cisplatin (5.5)   03/2013

———**INDICATIONS AND USAGE**———
Erbitux® (cetuximab) is an epidermal growth factor receptor (EGFR) antagonist indicated for treatment of:
Head and Neck Cancer
• Locally or regionally advanced squamous cell carcinoma of the head and neck in combination with radiation therapy. (1.1, 14.1)
• Recurrent locoregional disease or metastatic squamous cell carcinoma of the head and neck in combination with platinum-based therapy with 5-FU. (1.1, 14.1)
• Recurrent or metastatic squamous cell carcinoma of the head and neck progressing after platinum-based therapy. (1.1, 14.1)
Colorectal Cancer
K-Ras mutation-negative (wild-type), EGFR-expressing, metastatic colorectal cancer as determined by FDA-approved tests
• in combination with FOLFIRI for first-line treatment,
• in combination with irinotecan in patients who are refractory to irinotecan-based chemotherapy,
• as a single agent in patients who have failed oxaliplatin- and irinotecan-based chemotherapy or who are intolerant to irinotecan. (1.2, 5.7, 12.1, 14.2)
Limitation of Use: Erbitux is not indicated for treatment of K-Ras mutation-positive colorectal cancer. (5.7, 14.2)

———**DOSAGE AND ADMINISTRATION**———
• Premedicate with an H_1 antagonist. (2.3)
• Administer 400 mg/m² initial dose as a 120-minute intravenous infusion followed by 250 mg/m² weekly infused over 60 minutes. (2.1, 2.2)
• Initiate Erbitux one week prior to initiation of radiation therapy. Complete Erbitux administration 1 hour prior to platinum-based therapy with 5-FU (2.1) and FOLFIRI (2.2).
• Reduce the infusion rate by 50% for NCI CTC Grade 1 or 2 infusion reactions and non-serious NCI CTC Grade 3 infusion reaction. (2.4)
• Permanently discontinue for serious infusion reactions. (2.4)
• Withhold infusion for severe, persistent acneiform rash. Reduce dose for recurrent, severe rash. (2.4)

———**DOSAGE FORMS AND STRENGTHS**———
• 100 mg/50 mL, single-use vial (3)
• 200 mg/100 mL, single-use vial (3)

———**CONTRAINDICATIONS**———
None. (4)

———**WARNINGS AND PRECAUTIONS**———
• **Infusion Reactions:** Immediately stop and permanently discontinue Erbitux for serious infusion reactions. Monitor patients following infusion. (5.1)
• **Cardiopulmonary Arrest:** Closely monitor serum electrolytes during and after Erbitux. (5.2, 5.6)
• **Pulmonary Toxicity:** Interrupt therapy for acute onset or worsening of pulmonary symptoms. (5.3)
• **Dermatologic Toxicity:** Limit sun exposure. Monitor for inflammatory or infectious sequelae. (2.4, 5.4)
• **Hypomagnesemia:** Periodically monitor during and for at least 8 weeks following the completion of Erbitux. Replete electrolytes as necessary. (5.6)

———**ADVERSE REACTIONS**———
The most common adverse reactions (incidence ≥25%) are: cutaneous adverse reactions (including rash, pruritus, and nail changes), headache, diarrhea, and infection. (6)
To report SUSPECTED ADVERSE REACTIONS, contact Bristol-Myers Squibb at 1-800-721-5072 or FDA at 1-800-FDA-1088 or www.fda.gov/medwatch.

Table 1: Erbitux Dose Modification Guidelines for Rash

Severe Acneiform Rash	Erbitux	Outcome	Erbitux Dose Modification
1st occurrence	Delay infusion 1 to 2 weeks	Improvement No Improvement	Continue at 250 mg/m^2 Discontinue Erbitux
2nd occurrence	Delay infusion 1 to 2 weeks	Improvement No Improvement	Reduce dose to 200 mg/m^2 Discontinue Erbitux
3rd occurrence	Delay infusion 1 to 2 weeks	Improvement No Improvement	Reduce dose to 150 mg/m^2 Discontinue Erbitux
4th occurrence	Discontinue Erbitux		

USE IN SPECIFIC POPULATIONS

- **Pregnancy:** Administer Erbitux to a pregnant woman only if the potential benefit justifies the potential risk to the fetus. (8.1)
- **Nursing Mothers:** Discontinue nursing during and for 60 days following treatment with Erbitux (cetuximab). (8.3)

See 17 for PATIENT COUNSELING INFORMATION
Revised: 08/2013

FULL PRESCRIBING INFORMATION: CONTENTS*
WARNING: SERIOUS INFUSION REACTIONS and CARDIOPULMONARY ARREST

FULL PRESCRIBING INFORMATION

WARNING: SERIOUS INFUSION REACTIONS and CARDIOPULMONARY ARREST

Infusion Reactions: Serious infusion reactions occurred with the administration of Erbitux in approximately 3% of patients in clinical trials, with fatal outcome reported in less than 1 in 1000. [See *Warn-*

---

ings and Precautions (5.1), Adverse Reactions (6).]
Immediately interrupt and permanently discontinue Erbitux infusion for serious infusion reactions. [See *Dosage and Administration (2.4), Warnings and Precautions (5.1).*]
Cardiopulmonary Arrest: Cardiopulmonary arrest and/or sudden death occurred in 2% of patients with squamous cell carcinoma of the head and neck treated with Erbitux and radiation therapy in Study 1 and in 3% of patients with squamous cell carcinoma of the head and neck treated with European Union (EU)-approved cetuximab in combination with platinum-based therapy with 5-fluorouracil (5-FU) in Study 2. Closely monitor serum electrolytes, including serum magnesium, potassium, and calcium, during and after Erbitux administration. [See *Warnings and Precautions (5.2, 5.6), Clinical Studies (14.1).*]

1 INDICATIONS AND USAGE

1.1 Squamous Cell Carcinoma of the Head and Neck (SCCHN)

Erbitux® (cetuximab) is indicated in combination with radiation therapy for the initial treatment of locally or regionally advanced squamous cell carcinoma of the head and neck. [See *Clinical Studies (14.1).*]

Erbitux is indicated in combination with platinum-based therapy with 5-FU for the first-line treatment of patients with recurrent locoregional disease or metastatic squamous cell carcinoma of the head and neck. [See *Clinical Studies (14.1).*]

Erbitux, as a single agent, is indicated for the treatment of patients with recurrent or metastatic squamous cell carcinoma of the head and neck for whom prior platinum-based therapy has failed. [See *Clinical Studies (14.1).*]

1.2 *K-Ras* Mutation-negative, EGFR-expressing Colorectal Cancer

Erbitux is indicated for the treatment of *K-Ras* mutation-negative (wild-type), epidermal growth factor receptor (EGFR)-expressing, metastatic colorectal cancer (mCRC) as determined by FDA-approved tests for this use [see *Dosage and Administration (2.2), Warnings and Precautions (5.7), Clinical Studies (14.2)*]

- in combination with FOLFIRI (irinotecan, 5-fluorouracil, leucovorin) for first-line treatment,
- in combination with irinotecan in patients who are refractory to irinotecan-based chemotherapy,
- as a single agent in patients who have failed oxaliplatin- and irinotecan-based chemotherapy or who are intolerant to irinotecan. [See *Warnings and Precautions (5.7), Clinical Pharmacology (12.1), Clinical Studies (14.2).*]

Limitation of Use: Erbitux is not indicated for treatment of *K-Ras* mutation-positive colorectal cancer [see *Warnings and Precautions (5.7), Clinical Studies (14.2).*]

2 DOSAGE AND ADMINISTRATION

2.1 Squamous Cell Carcinoma of the Head and Neck

Erbitux in combination with radiation therapy or in combination with platinum-based therapy with 5-FU:
- The recommended initial dose is 400 mg/m^2 administered one week prior to initiation of a course of radiation therapy or on the day of initiation of platinum-based therapy with 5-FU as a 120-minute intravenous infusion (maximum infusion rate 10 mg/min). Complete Erbitux administration 1 hour prior to platinum-based therapy with 5-FU.
- The recommended subsequent weekly dose (all other infusions) is 250 mg/m^2 infused over 60 minutes (maximum infusion rate 10 mg/min) for the duration of radiation therapy (6–7 weeks) or until disease progression or unacceptable toxicity when administered in combination with platinum-based therapy with 5-FU. Complete Erbitux administration 1 hour prior to radiation therapy or platinum-based therapy with 5-FU.

Erbitux monotherapy:
- The recommended initial dose is 400 mg/m^2 administered as a 120-minute intravenous infusion (maximum infusion rate 10 mg/min).

- The recommended subsequent weekly dose (all other infusions) is 250 mg/m^2 infused over 60 minutes (maximum infusion rate 10 mg/min) until disease progression or unacceptable toxicity.

2.2 Colorectal Cancer

- Determine *K-Ras* mutation and EGFR-expression status using FDA-approved tests prior to initiating treatment. Only patients whose tumors are *K-Ras* mutation-negative (wild-type) should receive Erbitux (cetuximab).
- The recommended initial dose, either as monotherapy or in combination with irinotecan or FOLFIRI (irinotecan, 5-fluorouracil, leucovorin), is 400 mg/m^2 administered as a 120-minute intravenous infusion (maximum infusion rate 10 mg/min). Complete Erbitux administration 1 hour prior to FOLFIRI.
- The recommended subsequent weekly dose, either as monotherapy or in combination with irinotecan or FOLFIRI, is 250 mg/m^2 infused over 60 minutes (maximum infusion rate 10 mg/min) until disease progression or unacceptable toxicity. Complete Erbitux administration 1 hour prior to FOLFIRI.

2.3 Recommended Premedication

Premedicate with an H$_1$ antagonist (eg, 50 mg of diphenhydramine) intravenously 30–60 minutes prior to the first dose; premedication should be administered for subsequent Erbitux doses based upon clinical judgment and presence/severity of prior infusion reactions.

2.4 Dose Modifications

Infusion Reactions
Reduce the infusion rate by 50% for NCI CTC Grade 1 or 2 and non-serious NCI CTC Grade 3 infusion reaction.
Immediately and permanently discontinue Erbitux for serious infusion reactions, requiring medical intervention and/or hospitalization. [See *Warnings and Precautions (5.1).*]

Dermatologic Toxicity
Recommended dose modifications for severe (NCI CTC Grade 3 or 4) acneiform rash are specified in Table 1. [See *Warnings and Precautions (5.4).*]
[See table 1 above]

2.5 Preparation for Administration

Do not administer Erbitux as an intravenous push or bolus. Administer via infusion pump or syringe pump. Do not exceed an infusion rate of 10 mg/min.

Administer through a low protein binding 0.22-micrometer in-line filter.

Parenteral drug products should be inspected visually for particulate matter and discoloration prior to administration, whenever solution and container permit.

The solution should be clear and colorless and may contain a small amount of easily visible, white, amorphous, cetuximab particulates. **Do not shake or dilute.**

3 DOSAGE FORMS AND STRENGTHS

100 mg/50 mL, single-use vial
200 mg/100 mL, single-use vial

4 CONTRAINDICATIONS

None.

5 WARNINGS AND PRECAUTIONS

5.1 Infusion Reactions

Serious infusion reactions, requiring medical intervention and immediate, permanent discontinuation of Erbitux included rapid onset of airway obstruction (bronchospasm, stridor, hoarseness), hypotension, shock, loss of consciousness, myocardial infarction, and/or cardiac arrest. Severe (NCI CTC Grades 3 and 4) infusion reactions occurred in 2–5% of 1373 patients in Studies 1, 3, 5, and 6 receiving Erbitux, with fatal outcome in 1 patient. [See *Clinical Studies (14.1, 14.2).*]

Approximately 90% of severe infusion reactions occurred with the first infusion despite premedication with antihistamines.

Monitor patients for 1 hour following Erbitux infusions in a setting with resuscitation equipment and other agents necessary to treat anaphylaxis (eg, epinephrine, corticosteroids, intravenous antihistamines, bronchodilators, and oxygen). Monitor longer to confirm resolution of the event in patients requiring treatment for infusion reactions.

Immediately and permanently discontinue Erbitux in patients with serious infusion reactions. [See *Boxed Warning, Dosage and Administration (2.4).*]

5.2 Cardiopulmonary Arrest

Cardiopulmonary arrest and/or sudden death occurred in 4 (2%) of 208 patients treated with radiation therapy and Erbitux as compared to none of 212 patients treated with radiation therapy alone in Study 1. Three patients with prior history of coronary artery disease died at home, with myocardial infarction as the presumed cause of death. One of these patients had arrhythmia and one had congestive heart failure. Death occurred 27, 32, and 43 days after the last dose of Erbitux. One patient with no prior history of coronary artery disease died one day after the last dose of Erbitux. In Study 2, fatal cardiac disorders and/or sudden death occurred in 7 (3%) of 219 patients treated with EU-approved cetuximab and platinum-based therapy with 5-FU as compared to 4 (2%) of 215 patients treated with chemotherapy alone. Five of these 7 patients in the chemotherapy plus cetuximab arm received concomitant cisplatin and 2 patients received concomitant carboplatin. All 4 patients in the chemotherapy-alone arm received cisplatin. Carefully consider use of Erbitux in combination with radiation therapy or platinum-based therapy with 5-FU in head and neck cancer patients with a history of coronary artery disease, congestive heart failure, or arrhythmias in light of these risks. Closely monitor serum electrolytes, including serum magnesium, potassium, and calcium, during and after Erbitux (cetuximab). [See *Boxed Warning, Warnings and Precautions (5.6)*.]

5.3 Pulmonary Toxicity
Interstitial lung disease (ILD), including 1 fatality, occurred in 4 of 1570 (<0.5%) patients receiving Erbitux in Studies 1, 3, and 6, as well as other studies, in colorectal cancer and head and neck cancer. Interrupt Erbitux for acute onset or worsening of pulmonary symptoms. Permanently discontinue Erbitux for confirmed ILD.

5.4 Dermatologic Toxicity
Dermatologic toxicities, including acneiform rash, skin drying and fissuring, paronychial inflammation, infectious sequelae (for example, *S. aureus* sepsis, abscess formation, cellulitis, blepharitis, conjunctivitis, keratitis/ulcerative keratitis with decreased visual acuity, cheilitis), and hypertrichosis occurred in patients receiving Erbitux therapy. Acneiform rash occurred in 76–88% of 1373 patients receiving Erbitux in Studies 1, 3, 5, and 6. Severe acneiform rash occurred in 1–17% of patients.

Acneiform rash usually developed within the first two weeks of therapy and resolved in a majority of the patients after cessation of treatment, although in nearly half, the event continued beyond 28 days. Monitor patients receiving Erbitux for dermatologic toxicities and infectious sequelae. Instruct patients to limit sun exposure during Erbitux therapy. [See *Dosage and Administration (2.4)*.]

5.5 Use of Erbitux in Combination With Radiation and Cisplatin
In a controlled study, 940 patients with locally advanced SCCHN were randomized 1:1 to receive either Erbitux in combination with radiation therapy and cisplatin or radiation therapy and cisplatin alone. The addition of Erbitux resulted in an increase in the incidence of Grade 3–4 mucositis, radiation recall syndrome, acneiform rash, cardiac events, and electrolyte disturbances compared to radiation and cisplatin alone. Adverse reactions with fatal outcome were reported in 20 patients (4.4%) in the Erbitux combination arm and 14 patients (3.0%) in the control arm. Nine patients in the Erbitux arm (2.0%) experienced myocardial ischemia compared to 4 patients (0.9%) in the control arm. The main efficacy outcome of the study was progression-free survival (PFS). The addition of Erbitux to radiation and cisplatin did not improve PFS.

5.6 Hypomagnesemia and Electrolyte Abnormalities
In patients evaluated during clinical trials, hypomagnesemia occurred in 55% of 365 patients receiving Erbitux in Study 5 and two other clinical trials in colorectal cancer and head and neck cancer, respectively, and was severe (NCI CTC Grades 3 and 4) in 6–17%.

In Study 2, where EU-approved cetuximab was administered in combination with platinum-based therapy, the addition of cetuximab to cisplatin and 5-FU resulted in an increased incidence of hypomagnesemia (14% vs. 6%) and of Grade 3–4 hypomagnesemia (7% vs. 2%) compared to cisplatin and 5-FU alone. In contrast, the incidences of hypomagnesemia were similar for those who received cetuximab, carboplatin, and 5-FU compared to carboplatin and 5-FU (4% vs. 4%). No patient experienced Grade 3–4 hypomagnesemia in either arm in the carboplatin subgroup.

The onset of hypomagnesemia and accompanying electrolyte abnormalities occurred days to months after initiation of Erbitux. Periodically monitor patients for hypomagnesemia, hypocalcemia, and hypokalemia, during and for at least 8 weeks following the completion of Erbitux. Replete electrolytes as necessary.

5.7 K-Ras Testing in Metastatic or Advanced Colorectal Cancer Patients
Determination of *K-Ras* mutational status in colorectal tumors using an FDA-approved test indicated for this use is necessary for selection of patients for treatment with Erbitux. Erbitux is indicated only for patients with EGFR-expressing *K-Ras* mutation-negative (wild-type) mCRC. Erbitux is not an effective treatment for patients with colorectal cancer that harbor somatic mutations in codons 12 and 13 (exon 2). Studies 4 and 5, conducted in patients with colorectal cancer, demonstrated a benefit with Erbitux treatment only in the subset of patients whose tumors were *K-Ras* mutation-negative (wild-type). Erbitux is not effective for the treatment of *K-Ras* mutation-positive colorectal cancer as determined by an FDA-approved test for this use. [See *Indications and Usage (1.2), Clinical Pharmacology (12.1), Clinical Studies (14.2)*.]

Perform the assessment for *K-Ras* mutation status in colorectal cancer in laboratories with demonstrated proficiency in the specific technology being utilized. Improper assay performance can lead to unreliable test results.

Refer to an FDA-approved test's package insert for instructions on the identification of patients eligible for the treatment of Erbitux (cetuximab).

5.8 Epidermal Growth Factor Receptor (EGFR) Expression and Response
Because expression of EGFR has been detected in nearly all SCCHN tumor specimens, patients enrolled in the head and neck cancer clinical studies were not required to have immunohistochemical evidence of EGFR tumor expression prior to study entry.

Patients enrolled in the colorectal cancer clinical studies were required to have immunohistochemical evidence of EGFR tumor expression. Primary tumor or tumor from a metastatic site was tested with the DakoCytomation EGFR pharmDx™ test kit. Specimens were scored based on the percentage of cells expressing EGFR and intensity (barely/faint, weak-to-moderate, and strong). Response rate did not correlate with either the percentage of positive cells or the intensity of EGFR expression.

6 ADVERSE REACTIONS
The following adverse reactions are discussed in greater detail in other sections of the label:
- Infusion reactions [See *Boxed Warning, Warnings and Precautions (5.1)*.]
- Cardiopulmonary arrest [See *Boxed Warning, Warnings and Precautions (5.2)*.]
- Pulmonary toxicity [See *Warnings and Precautions (5.3)*.]
- Dermatologic toxicity [See *Warnings and Precautions (5.4)*.]
- Hypomagnesemia and Electrolyte Abnormalities [See *Warnings and Precautions (5.6)*.]

The most common adverse reactions in Erbitux clinical trials (incidence ≥25%) include cutaneous adverse reactions (including rash, pruritus, and nail changes), headache, diarrhea, and infection.

The most serious adverse reactions with Erbitux are infusion reactions, cardiopulmonary arrest, dermatologic toxicity and radiation dermatitis, sepsis, renal failure, interstitial lung disease, and pulmonary embolus.

Across Studies 1, 3, 5, and 6, Erbitux was discontinued in 3–10% of patients because of adverse reactions.

6.1 Clinical Trials Experience
Because clinical trials are conducted under widely varying conditions, adverse reaction rates observed in the clinical

trials of a drug cannot be directly compared to rates in the clinical trials of another drug and may not reflect the rates observed in practice.

The data below reflect exposure to Erbitux (cetuximab) in 1373 patients with SCCHN or colorectal cancer in randomized Phase 3 (Studies 1 and 5) or Phase 2 (Studies 3 and 6) trials treated at the recommended dose and schedule for medians of 7 to 14 weeks. [See *Clinical Studies (14)*.]

Infusion reactions: Infusion reactions, which included pyrexia, chills, rigors, dyspnea, bronchospasm, angioedema, urticaria, hypertension, and hypotension occurred in 15–21% of patients across studies. Grades 3 and 4 infusion reactions occurred in 2–5% of patients; infusion reactions were fatal in 1 patient.

Infections: The incidence of infection was variable across studies, ranging from 13–35%. Sepsis occurred in 1–4% of patients.

Renal: Renal failure occurred in 1% of patients with colorectal cancer.

Squamous Cell Carcinoma of the Head and Neck
Erbitux in Combination with Radiation Therapy
Table 2 contains selected adverse reactions in 420 patients receiving radiation therapy either alone or with Erbitux for locally or regionally advanced SCCHN in Study 1. Erbitux was administered at the recommended dose and schedule (400 mg/m² initial dose, followed by 250 mg/m² weekly). Patients received a median of 8 infusions (range 1–11).

[See table 2 above]

The incidence and severity of mucositis, stomatitis, and xerostomia were similar in both arms of the study.

Late Radiation Toxicity
The overall incidence of late radiation toxicities (any grade) was higher in Erbitux in combination with radiation therapy compared with radiation therapy alone. The following sites were affected: salivary glands (65% versus 56%), larynx (52% versus 36%), subcutaneous tissue (49% versus 45%), mucous membrane (48% versus 39%), esophagus (44% versus 35%), skin (42% versus 33%). The incidence of Grade 3 or 4 late radiation toxicities was similar between the radiation therapy alone and the Erbitux plus radiation treatment groups.

Study 2: EU-Approved Cetuximab in Combination with Platinum-based Therapy with 5-Fluorouracil
Study 2 used EU-approved cetuximab. Since U.S.-licensed Erbitux provides approximately 22% higher exposure relative to the EU-approved cetuximab, the data provided below may underestimate the incidence and severity of adverse reactions anticipated with Erbitux for this indication. How-

Table 2: Incidence of Selected Adverse Reactions (≥10%) in Patients with Locoregionally Advanced SCCHN

Body System Preferred Term	Erbitux plus Radiation (n=208)		Radiation Therapy Alone (n=212)	
	Grades 1–4	Grades 3 and 4	Grades 1–4	Grades 3 and 4
	% of Patients			
Body as a Whole				
Asthenia	56	4	49	5
Fever[a]	29	1	13	1
Headache	19	<1	8	<1
Infusion Reaction[b]	15	3	2	0
Infection	13	1	9	1
Chills[a]	16	0	5	0
Digestive				
Nausea	49	2	37	2
Emesis	29	2	23	4
Diarrhea	19	2	13	1
Dyspepsia	14	0	9	1
Metabolic/Nutritional				
Weight Loss	84	11	72	7
Dehydration	25	6	19	8
Alanine Transaminase, high[c]	43	2	21	1
Aspartate Transaminase, high[c]	38	1	24	1
Alkaline Phosphatase, high[c]	33	<1	24	0
Respiratory				
Pharyngitis	26	3	19	4
Skin/Appendages				
Acneiform Rash[d]	87	17	10	1
Radiation Dermatitis	86	23	90	18
Application Site Reaction	18	0	12	1
Pruritus	16	0	4	0

[a] Includes cases also reported as infusion reaction.

[b] Infusion reaction is defined as any event described at any time during the clinical study as "allergic reaction" or "anaphylactoid reaction", or any event occurring on the first day of dosing described as "allergic reaction", "anaphylactoid reaction", "fever", "chills", "chills and fever", or "dyspnea".

[c] Based on laboratory measurements, not on reported adverse reactions, the number of subjects with tested samples varied from 205–206 for Erbitux plus Radiation arm; 209–210 for Radiation alone.

[d] Acneiform rash is defined as any event described as "acne", "rash", "maculopapular rash", "pustular rash", "dry skin", or "exfoliative dermatitis".

Table 3: Incidence of Selected Adverse Reactions (≥10%) in Patients with Recurrent Locoregional Disease or Metastatic SCCHN

System Organ Class Preferred Term	EU-Approved Cetuximab plus Platinum-based Therapy with 5-FU (n=219)		Platinum-based Therapy with 5-FU Alone (n=215)	
	Grades 1–4	Grades 3 and 4	Grades 1–4	Grades 3 and 4
	% of Patients			
Eye Disorders				
Conjunctivitis	10	0	0	0
Gastrointestinal Disorders				
Nausea	54	4	47	4
Diarrhea	26	5	16	1
General Disorders and Administration Site Conditions				
Pyrexia	22	0	13	1
Infusion Reaction[a]	10	2	<1	0
Infections and Infestations				
Infection[b]	44	11	27	8
Metabolism and Nutrition Disorders				
Anorexia	25	5	14	1
Hypocalcemia	12	4	5	1
Hypokalemia	12	7	7	5
Hypomagnesemia	11	5	5	1
Skin and Subcutaneous Tissue Disorders				
Acneiform Rash[c]	70	9	2	0
Rash	28	5	2	0
Acne	22	2	0	0
Dermatitis Acneiform	15	2	0	0
Dry Skin	14	0	<1	0
Alopecia	12	0	7	0

[a] Infusion reaction defined as any event of "anaphylactic reaction", "hypersensitivity", "fever and/or chills", "dyspnea", or "pyrexia" on the first day of dosing.
[b] Infection – this term excludes sepsis-related events which are presented separately.
[c] Acneiform rash defined as any event described as "acne", "dermatitis acneiform", "dry skin", "exfoliative rash", "rash", "rash erythematous", "rash macular", "rash papular", or "rash pustular".
Chemotherapy = cisplatin + 5-fluorouracil or carboplatin + 5-fluorouracil

ever, the tolerability of the recommended dose is supported by safety data from additional studies of Erbitux (cetuximab) [see *Clinical Pharmacology (12.3)*].

Table 3 contains selected adverse reactions in 434 patients with recurrent locoregional disease or metastatic SCCHN receiving EU-approved cetuximab in combination with platinum-based therapy with 5-FU or platinum-based therapy with 5-FU alone in Study 2. Cetuximab was administered at 400 mg/m² for the initial dose, followed by 250 mg/m² weekly. Patients received a median of 17 infusions (range 1–89).

[See table 3 above]

For cardiac disorders, approximately 9% of subjects in both the EU-approved cetuximab plus chemotherapy and chemotherapy-only treatment arms in Study 2 experienced a cardiac event. The majority of these events occurred in patients who received cisplatin/5-FU, with or without cetuximab as follows: 11% and 12% in patients who received cisplatin/5-FU with or without cetuximab, respectively, and 6% or 4% in patients who received carboplatin/5-FU with or without cetuximab, respectively. In both arms, the incidence of cardiovascular events was higher in the cisplatin with 5-FU containing subgroup. Death attributed to cardiovascular event or sudden death was reported in 3% of the patients in the cetuximab plus platinum-based therapy with 5-FU arm and 2% in the platinum-based chemotherapy with 5-FU alone arm.

Colorectal Cancer

Study 4: EU-Approved Cetuximab in Combination with FOLFIRI

Study 4 used EU-approved cetuximab. U.S.-licensed Erbitux provides approximately 22% higher exposure to cetuximab relative to the EU-approved cetuximab. The data provided below for Study 4 is consistent in incidence and severity of adverse reactions with those seen for Erbitux in this indication. The tolerability of the recommended dose is supported by safety data from additional studies of Erbitux [see *Clinical Pharmacology (12.3)*].

Table 4 contains selected adverse reactions in 667 patients with *K-Ras* mutation-negative (wild-type), EGFR-expressing, metastatic colorectal cancer receiving EU-approved cetuximab plus FOLFIRI or FOLFIRI alone in Study 4 [see *Warnings and Precautions (5.8)*]. Cetuximab was administered at the recommended dose and schedule (400 mg/m² initial dose, followed by 250 mg/m² weekly). Patients received a median of 26 infusions (range 1–224).

[See table 4 at top of next page]

Erbitux Monotherapy

Table 5 contains selected adverse reactions in 242 patients with *K-Ras* mutation-negative (wild-type), EGFR-expressing, metastatic colorectal cancer who received best supportive care (BSC) alone or with Erbitux in Study 5 [see *Warnings and Precautions (5.8)*]. Erbitux was administered at the recommended dose and schedule (400 mg/m² initial dose, followed by 250 mg/m² weekly). Patients received a median of 17 infusions (range 1–51).

[See table 5 at top of page 686]

Erbitux in Combination with Irinotecan

The most frequently reported adverse reactions in 354 patients treated with Erbitux (cetuximab) plus irinotecan in clinical trials were acneiform rash (88%), asthenia/malaise (73%), diarrhea (72%), and nausea (55%). The most common Grades 3–4 adverse reactions included diarrhea (22%), leukopenia (17%), asthenia/malaise (16%), and acneiform rash (14%).

6.2   Immunogenicity

As with all therapeutic proteins, there is potential for immunogenicity. Immunogenic responses to cetuximab were assessed using either a double antigen radiometric assay or an ELISA assay. Due to limitations in assay performance and sampling timing, the incidence of antibody development in patients receiving Erbitux has not been adequately determined. Non-neutralizing anti-cetuximab antibodies were detected in 5% (49 of 1001) of evaluable patients without apparent effect on the safety or antitumor activity of Erbitux.

The incidence of antibody formation is highly dependent on the sensitivity and specificity of the assay. Additionally, the observed incidence of antibody (including neutralizing antibody) positivity in an assay may be influenced by several factors including assay methodology, sample handling, timing of sample collection, concomitant medications, and underlying disease. For these reasons, comparison of the incidence of antibodies to Erbitux with the incidence of antibodies to other products may be misleading.

6.3   Postmarketing Experience

The following adverse reactions have been identified during post-approval use of Erbitux. Because these reactions are reported from a population of uncertain size, it is not always possible to reliably estimate their frequency or establish a causal relationship to drug exposure.

• Aseptic meningitis
• Mucosal inflammation

7   DRUG INTERACTIONS

A drug interaction study was performed in which Erbitux was administered in combination with irinotecan. There was no evidence of any pharmacokinetic interactions between Erbitux and irinotecan.

8   USE IN SPECIFIC POPULATIONS

8.1   Pregnancy

Pregnancy Category C

There are no adequate and well-controlled studies of Erbitux (cetuximab) in pregnant women. Based on animal models, EGFR has been implicated in the control of prenatal development and may be essential for normal organogenesis, proliferation, and differentiation in the developing embryo. Human IgG is known to cross the placental barrier; therefore, Erbitux may be transmitted from the mother to the developing fetus, and has the potential to cause fetal harm when administered to pregnant women. Erbitux should be used during pregnancy only if the potential benefit justifies the potential risk to the fetus.

Pregnant cynomolgus monkeys were treated weekly with 0.4 to 4 times the recommended human dose of cetuximab (based on body surface area) during the period of organogenesis (gestation day [GD] 20–48). Cetuximab was detected in the amniotic fluid and in the serum of embryos from treated dams at GD 49. No fetal malformations or other teratogenic effects occurred in offspring. However, significant increases in embryolethality and abortions occurred at doses of approximately 1.6 to 4 times the recommended human dose of cetuximab (based on total body surface area).

8.3   Nursing Mothers

It is not known whether Erbitux is secreted in human milk. IgG antibodies, such as Erbitux, can be excreted in human milk. Because many drugs are excreted in human milk and because of the potential for serious adverse reactions in nursing infants from Erbitux, a decision should be made whether to discontinue nursing or to discontinue the drug, taking into account the importance of the drug to the mother. If nursing is interrupted, based on the mean half-life of cetuximab [see *Clinical Pharmacology (12.3)*], nursing should not be resumed earlier than 60 days following the last dose of Erbitux.

8.4   Pediatric Use

The safety and effectiveness of Erbitux in pediatric patients have not been established. The pharmacokinetics of cetuximab, in combination with irinotecan, were evaluated in pediatric patients with refractory solid tumors in an open-label, single-arm, dose-finding study. Erbitux was administered once-weekly, at doses up to 250 mg/m², to 27 patients ranging from 1 to 12 years old; and in 19 patients ranging from 13 to 18 years old. No new safety signals were identified in pediatric patients. The pharmacokinetic profiles of cetuximab between the two age groups were similar at the 75 and 150 mg/m² single dose levels. The volume of the distribution appeared to be independent of dose and approximated the vascular space of 2–3 L/m². Following a single dose of 250 mg/m², the geometric mean $AUC_{0\text{-inf}}$ (CV%) value was 17.7 mg•h/mL (34%) in the younger age group (1–12 years, n=9) and 13.4 mg•h/mL (38%) in the adolescent group (13–18 years, n=6). The mean half-life of cetuximab was 110 hours (range 69 to 188 hours) for the younger age group, and 82 hours (range 55 to 117 hours) for the adolescent age group.

8.5   Geriatric Use

Of the 1662 patients who received Erbitux with irinotecan, FOLFIRI or Erbitux monotherapy in six studies of advanced colorectal cancer, 588 patients were 65 years of age or older. No overall differences in safety or efficacy were observed between these patients and younger patients.

Clinical studies of Erbitux conducted in patients with head and neck cancer did not include sufficient number of subjects aged 65 and over to determine whether they respond differently from younger subjects.

10   OVERDOSAGE

The maximum single dose of Erbitux administered is 1000 mg/m² in one patient. No adverse events were reported for this patient.

11   DESCRIPTION

Erbitux® (cetuximab) is a recombinant, human/mouse chimeric monoclonal antibody that binds specifically to the extracellular domain of the human epidermal growth factor receptor (EGFR). Cetuximab is composed of the Fv regions of a murine anti-EGFR antibody with human IgG1 heavy and kappa light chain constant regions and has an approximate molecular weight of 152 kDa. Cetuximab is produced in mammalian (murine myeloma) cell culture.

Erbitux is a sterile, clear, colorless liquid of pH 7.0 to 7.4, which may contain a small amount of easily visible, white, amorphous cetuximab particulates. Erbitux is supplied at a concentration of 2 mg/mL in either 100 mg (50 mL) or 200 mg (100 mL), single-use vials. Cetuximab is formulated in a solution with no preservatives, which contains 8.48 mg/mL sodium chloride, 1.88 mg/mL sodium phosphate dibasic heptahydrate, 0.41 mg/mL sodium phosphate monobasic monohydrate, and Water for Injection, USP.

12   CLINICAL PHARMACOLOGY

12.1   Mechanism of Action

The epidermal growth factor receptor (EGFR, HER1, c-ErbB-1) is a transmembrane glycoprotein that is a member of a subfamily of type I receptor tyrosine kinases including EGFR, HER2, HER3, and HER4. The EGFR is constitutively expressed in many normal epithelial tissues, including the skin and hair follicle. Expression of EGFR is also detected in many human cancers including those of the head and neck, colon, and rectum.

Cetuximab binds specifically to the EGFR on both normal and tumor cells, and competitively inhibits the binding of epidermal growth factor (EGF) and other ligands, such as transforming growth factor-alpha. *In vitro* assays and *in vivo* animal studies have shown that binding of cetuximab to the EGFR blocks phosphorylation and activation of receptor-associated kinases, resulting in inhibition of cell growth, induction of apoptosis, and decreased matrix metalloproteinase and vascular endothelial growth factor production. Signal transduction through the EGFR results in activation of wild-type *K-Ras* protein. However, in cells with activating *K-Ras* somatic mutations, the mutant *K-Ras* protein is continuously active and appears independent of EGFR regulation.

In vitro, cetuximab can mediate antibody-dependent cellular cytotoxicity (ADCC) against certain human tumor types. *In vitro* assays and *in vivo* animal studies have shown that cetuximab inhibits the growth and survival of tumor cells that express the EGFR. No anti-tumor effects of cetuximab were observed in human tumor xenografts lacking EGFR expression. The addition of cetuximab to radiation therapy or irinotecan in human tumor xenograft models in mice resulted in an increase in anti-tumor effects compared to radiation therapy or chemotherapy alone.

12.2 Pharmacodynamics

Effects on Electrocardiogram (ECG)

The effect of cetuximab on QT interval was evaluated in an open-label, single-arm, monotherapy trial in 37 subjects with advanced malignancies who received an initial dose of 400 mg/m^2, followed by weekly infusions of 250 mg/m^2 for a total of 5 weeks. No large changes in the mean QT interval of >20 ms from baseline were detected in the trial based on the Fridericia correction method. A small increase in the mean QTc interval of <10 ms cannot be excluded because of the limitations in the trial design.

12.3 Pharmacokinetics

Erbitux (cetuximab) administered as monotherapy or in combination with concomitant chemotherapy or radiation therapy exhibits nonlinear pharmacokinetics. The area under the concentration time curve (AUC) increased in a greater than dose proportional manner while clearance of cetuximab decreased from 0.08 to 0.02 L/h/m^2 as the dose increased from 20 to 200 mg/m^2, and at doses >200 mg/m^2, it appeared to plateau. The volume of the distribution for cetuximab appeared to be independent of dose and approximated the vascular space of 2–3 L/m^2.

Following the recommended dose regimen (400 mg/m^2 initial dose; 250 mg/m^2 weekly dose), concentrations of cetuximab reached steady-state levels by the third weekly infusion with mean peak and trough concentrations across studies ranging from 168 to 235 and 41 to 85 µg/mL, respectively. The mean half-life of cetuximab was approximately 112 hours (range 63–230 hours). The pharmacokinetics of cetuximab were similar in patients with SCCHN and those with colorectal cancer.

Erbitux had an approximately 22% (90% confidence interval; 6%, 38%) higher systemic exposure relative to the EU-approved cetuximab used in Studies 2 and 4 based on a population pharmacokinetic analysis. [See *Clinical Studies (14.1)*.]

13 NONCLINICAL TOXICOLOGY

13.1 Carcinogenesis, Mutagenesis, Impairment of Fertility

Long-term animal studies have not been performed to test cetuximab for carcinogenic potential, and no mutagenic or clastogenic potential of cetuximab was observed in the *Salmonella-Escherichia coli* (Ames) assay or in the *in vivo* rat micronucleus test. Menstrual cyclicity was impaired in female cynomolgus monkeys receiving weekly doses of 0.4 to 4 times the human dose of cetuximab (based on total body surface area). Cetuximab-treated animals exhibited increased incidences of irregular or absent cycles, as compared to control animals. These effects were initially noted beginning week 25 of cetuximab treatment and continued through the 6-week recovery period. In this same study, there were no effects of cetuximab treatment on measured male fertility parameters (ie, serum testosterone levels and analysis of sperm counts, viability, and motility) as compared to control male monkeys. It is not known if cetuximab can impair fertility in humans.

13.2 Animal Pharmacology and/or Toxicology

In cynomolgus monkeys, cetuximab, when administered at doses of approximately 0.4 to 4 times the weekly human exposure (based on total body surface area), resulted in dermatologic findings, including inflammation at the injection site and desquamation of the external integument. At the highest dose level, the epithelial mucosa of the nasal passage, esophagus, and tongue were similarly affected, and degenerative changes in the renal tubular epithelium occurred. Deaths due to sepsis were observed in 50% (5/10) of the animals at the highest dose level beginning after approximately 13 weeks of treatment.

14 CLINICAL STUDIES

Studies 2 and 4 were conducted outside the U.S. using an EU-approved cetuximab as the clinical trial material. Erbitux (cetuximab) provides approximately 22% higher exposure relative to the EU-approved cetuximab used in Studies 2 and 4; these pharmacokinetic data, together with the results of Studies 2, 4, and other clinical trial data establish the efficacy of Erbitux at the recommended dose in SCCHN and mCRC. [see *Clinical Pharmacology (12.3)*].

14.1 Squamous Cell Carcinoma of the Head and Neck (SCCHN)

Study 1 was a randomized, multicenter, controlled trial of 424 patients with locally or regionally advanced SCCHN. Patients with Stage III/IV SCCHN of the oropharynx, hypopharynx, or larynx with no prior therapy were randomized (1:1) to receive either Erbitux plus radiation therapy or radiation therapy alone. Stratification factors were Karnofsky performance status (60–80 versus 90–100), nodal stage (N0 versus N+), tumor stage (T1–3 versus T4 using American Joint Committee on Cancer 1998 staging criteria), and radiation therapy fractionation (concomitant boost versus once-daily versus twice-daily). Radiation therapy was administered for 6–7 weeks as once-daily, twice-daily, or concomitant boost. Erbitux was administered as a 400 mg/m^2 initial dose beginning one week prior to initiation of radiation therapy, followed by 250 mg/m^2 weekly administered 1 hour prior to radiation therapy for the duration of radiation therapy (6–7 weeks).

Of the 424 randomized patients, the median age was 57 years, 80% were male, 83% were Caucasian, and 90% had baseline Karnofsky performance status ≥80. There were 258 patients enrolled in U.S. sites (61%). Sixty percent of patients had oropharyngeal, and 15% laryngeal, and 15% hypopharyngeal primary tumors; 28% had AJCC T4 tumor stage. Fifty-six percent of the patients received radiation therapy with concomitant boost, 26% received once-daily regimen, and 18% twice-daily regimen.

The main outcome measure of this trial was duration of locoregional control. Overall survival was also assessed. Results are presented in Table 6.

[See table 6 at top of next page]

Study 2 was an open-label, randomized, multicenter, controlled trial of 442 patients with recurrent locoregional disease or metastatic SCCHN.

Patients with no prior therapy for recurrent locoregional disease or metastatic SCCHN were randomized (1:1) to receive EU-approved cetuximab plus cisplatin or carboplatin and 5-FU, or cisplatin or carboplatin and 5-FU alone. Choice of cisplatin or carboplatin was at the discretion of the treating physician. Stratification factors were Karnofsky performance status (<80 versus ≥80) and previous chemotherapy. Cisplatin (100 mg/m^2, Day 1) or carboplatin (AUC 5, Day 1) plus intravenous 5-FU (1000 mg/m^2/day, Days 1–4) were administered every 3 weeks (1 cycle) for a maximum of 6 cycles in the absence of disease progression or unacceptable toxicity. Cetuximab was administered at a 400 mg/m^2 initial dose, followed by a 250 mg/m^2 weekly dose in combination with chemotherapy. Patients demonstrating at least stable disease on cetuximab in combination with chemotherapy were to continue cetuximab monotherapy at 250 mg/m^2 weekly, in the absence of disease progression or unacceptable toxicity after completion of 6

Table 4: Incidence of Selected Adverse Reactions Occurring in ≥10% of Patients with *K-Ras* Mutation-negative (Wild-type) and EGFR-expressing, Metastatic Colorectal Cancer[a]

Body System Preferred Term	EU-Approved Cetuximab plus FOLFIRI (n=317)		FOLFIRI Alone (n=350)	
	Grades 1–4[b]	Grades 3 and 4	Grades 1–4	Grades 3 and 4
	% of Patients			
Blood and Lymphatic System Disorders				
Neutropenia	49	31	42	24
Eye Disorders				
Conjunctivitis	18	<1	3	0
Gastrointestinal Disorders				
Diarrhea	66	16	60	10
Stomatitis	31	3	19	1
Dyspepsia	16	0	9	0
General Disorders and Administration Site Conditions				
Infusion-related Reaction[c]	14	2	<1	0
Pyrexia	26	1	14	1
Infections and Infestations				
Paronychia	20	4	<1	0
Investigations				
Weight Decreased	15	1	9	1
Metabolism and Nutrition Disorders				
Anorexia	30	3	23	2
Skin and Subcutaneous Tissue Disorders				
Acne-like Rash[d]	86	18	13	<1
Rash	44	9	4	0
Dermatitis Acneiform	26	5	<1	0
Dry Skin	22	0	4	0
Acne	14	2	0	0
Pruritus	14	0	3	0
Palmar-plantar Erythrodysesthesia Syndrome	19	4	4	<1
Skin Fissures	19	2	1	0

[a] Adverse reactions occurring in at least 10% of Erbitux combination arm with a frequency at least 5% greater than that seen in the FOLFIRI arm.

[b] Adverse reactions were graded using the NCI CTC, V 2.0.

[c] Infusion related reaction is defined as any event meeting the medical concepts of allergy/anaphylaxis at any time during the clinical study or any event occurring on the first day of dosing and meeting the medical concepts of dyspnea and fever or by the following events using MedDRA preferred terms: "acute myocardial infarction", "angina pectoris", "angioedema", "autonomic seizure", "blood pressure abnormal", "blood pressure decreased", "blood pressure increased", "cardiac failure", "cardiopulmonary failure", "cardiovascular insufficiency", "clonus", "convulsion", "coronary no-reflow phenomenon", "epilepsy", "hypertension", "hypertensive crisis", "hypertensive emergency", "hypotension", "infusion related reaction", "loss of consciousness", "myocardial infarction", "myocardial ischaemia", "prinzmetal angina", "shock", "sudden death", "syncope", or "systolic hypertension".

[d] Acne-like rash is defined by the events using MedDRA preferred terms and included "acne", "acne pustular", "butterfly rash", "dermatitis acneiform", "drug rash with eosinophilia and systemic symptoms", "dry skin", "erythema", "exfoliative rash", "folliculitis", "genital rash", "mucocutaneous rash", "pruritus", "rash", "rash erythematous", "rash follicular", "rash generalized", "rash macular", "rash maculopapular", "rash maculovesicular", "rash morbilliform", "rash papular", "rash papulosquamous", "rash pruritic", "rash pustular", "rash rubelliform", "rash scarlatiniform", "rash vesicular", "skin exfoliation", "skin hyperpigmentation", "skin plaque", "telangiectasia", or "xerosis".

planned courses of platinum-based therapy. For patients where treatment was delayed because of the toxic effects of chemotherapy, weekly cetuximab was continued. If chemotherapy was discontinued for toxicity, cetuximab could be continued as monotherapy until disease progression or unacceptable toxicity.

Of the 442 randomized patients, the median age was 57 years, 90% were male, 98% were Caucasian, and 88% had baseline Karnofsky performance status ≥80. Thirty-four percent of patients had oropharyngeal, 25% laryngeal, 20% oral cavity, and 14% hypopharyngeal primary tumors. Fifty-three percent of patients had recurrent locoregional disease only and 47% had metastatic disease. Fifty-eight percent had AJCC Stage IV disease and 21% had Stage III disease. Sixty-four percent of patients received cisplatin therapy and 34% received carboplatin as initial therapy. Approximately fifteen percent of the patients in the cisplatin alone arm switched to carboplatin during the treatment period.

The main outcome measure of this trial was overall survival. Results are presented in Table 7 and Figure 1.

[See table 7 at top of next page]

Figure 1: Kaplan-Meier Curve for Overall Survival in Patients with Recurrent Locoregional Disease or Metastatic Squamous Cell Carcinoma of the Head and Neck

Patients at Risk

CET+CT	222	184	153	118	82	57	30	15	3	0
CT	220	173	127	83	65	47	19	8	1	0

CT = Platinum-based therapy with 5-FU
CET = EU-approved cetuximab

In exploratory subgroup analyses of Study 2 by initial platinum therapy (cisplatin or carboplatin), for patients (N=284) receiving cetuximab plus cisplatin with 5-FU compared to cisplatin with 5-FU alone, the difference in median overall survival was 3.3 months (10.6 versus 7.3 months, respectively; HR 0.71; 95% CI 0.54, 0.93). The difference in median progression-free survival was 2.1 months (5.6 versus 3.5 months, respectively; HR 0.55; 95% CI 0.41, 0.73). The objective response rate was 39% and 23%, respectively (OR 2.18; 95% CI 1.29, 3.69). For patients (N=149) receiving cetuximab plus carboplatin with 5-FU compared to carboplatin with 5-FU alone, the difference in median overall survival was 1.4 months (9.7 versus 8.3 months; HR 0.99; 95% CI 0.69, 1.43). The difference in median progression-free survival was 1.7 months (4.8 versus 3.1 months, respectively; HR 0.61; 95% CI 0.42, 0.89). The objective response rate was 30% and 15%, respectively (OR 2.45; 95% CI 1.10, 5.46).

Study 3 was a single-arm, multicenter clinical trial in 103 patients with recurrent or metastatic SCCHN. All patients had documented disease progression within 30 days of a platinum-based chemotherapy regimen. Patients received a 20-mg test dose of Erbitux (cetuximab) on Day 1, followed by a 400 mg/m^2 initial dose, and 250 mg/m^2 weekly until disease progression or unacceptable toxicity.

The median age was 57 years, 82% were male, 100% Caucasian, and 62% had a Karnofsky performance status of ≥80.

The objective response rate was 13% (95% confidence interval 7%–21%). Median duration of response was 5.8 months (range 1.2–5.8 months).

14.2 Colorectal Cancer

Erbitux Clinical Trials in K-Ras Mutation-negative (Wild-type), EGFR-expressing, Metastatic Colorectal Cancer

Study 4 was a randomized, open-label, multicenter, study of 1217 patients with EGFR-expressing, metastatic colorectal cancer. Patients were randomized (1:1) to receive either EU-approved cetuximab in combination with FOLFIRI or FOLFIRI alone as first-line treatment. Stratification factors were Eastern Cooperative Oncology Group (ECOG) performance status (0 and 1 versus 2) and region (sites in Western Europe versus Eastern Europe versus other).

FOLFIRI regimen included 14-day cycles of irinotecan (180 mg/m^2 administered intravenously on Day 1), folinic acid (400 mg/m^2 [racemic] or 200 mg/m^2 [L-form] administered intravenously on Day 1), and 5-FU (400 mg/m^2 bolus on Day 1 followed by 2400 mg/m^2 as a 46-hour continuous infusion). Cetuximab was administered as a 400 mg/m^2 initial dose on Day 1, Week 1, followed by 250 mg/m^2 weekly

administered 1 hour prior to chemotherapy. Study treatment continued until disease progression or unacceptable toxicity occurred.

Of the 1217 randomized patients, the median age was 61 years, 60% were male, 86% were Caucasian, and 96% had a baseline ECOG performance status 0–1, 60% had primary tumor localized in colon, 84% had 1–2 metastatic sites and 20% had received prior adjuvant and/or neoadjuvant chemotherapy. Demographics and baseline characteristics were similar between study arms.

K-Ras mutation status was available for 1079/1217 (89%) of the patients: 676 (63%) patients had K-Ras mutation-negative (wild-type) tumors and 403 (37%) patients had K-Ras mutation-positive tumors where testing assessed for the following somatic mutations in codons 12 and 13 (exon 2): G12A, G12D, G12R, G12C, G12S, G12V, G13D [see Warnings and Precautions (5.7)].

Baseline characteristics and demographics in the K-Ras mutation-negative (wild-type) subset were similar to that seen in the overall population [see Warnings and Precautions (5.7)].

The main outcome measure of this trial was progression-free survival assessed by an independent review committee (IRC). Overall survival and response rate were also assessed. A statistically significant improvement in PFS was observed for the cetuximab plus FOLFIRI arm compared with the FOLFIRI arm (median PFS 8.9 vs 8.1 months, HR 0.85 [95% CI 0.74, 0.99], p-value=0.036). Overall survival was not significantly different at the planned, final analysis based on 838 events [HR=0.93, 95% CI (0.8, 1.1), p-value 0.327].

Results of the planned PFS and ORR analysis in all randomized patients and post-hoc PFS and ORR analysis in subgroups of patients defined by K-Ras mutation status, and post-hoc analysis of updated OS based on additional follow-up (1000 events) in all randomized patients and in subgroups of patients defined by K-Ras mutation status are presented in Table 8 and Figure 2. The treatment effect in the all-randomized population for PFS was driven by treatment effects limited to patients who have K-Ras mutation-negative (wild-type) tumors. There is no evidence of effectiveness in the subgroup of patients with K-Ras mutation-positive tumors.

Table 5: Incidence of Selected Adverse Reactions Occurring in ≥10% of Patients with K-Ras Mutation-negative (Wild-type), EGFR-expressing, Metastatic Colorectal Cancer Treated with Erbitux Monotherapy[a]

Body System Preferred Term	Erbitux plus BSC (n=118)		BSC alone (n=124)	
	Grades 1–4[b]	Grades 3 and 4	Grades 1–4	Grades 3 and 4
	% of Patients			
Dermatology/Skin				
Rash/Desquamation	95	16	21	1
Dry Skin	57	0	15	0
Pruritus	47	2	11	0
Other-Dermatology	35	0	7	2
Nail Changes	31	0	4	0
Constitutional Symptoms				
Fatigue	91	31	79	29
Fever	25	3	16	0
Infusion Reactions[c]	18	3	0	0
Rigors, Chills	16	1	3	0
Pain				
Pain-Other	59	18	37	10
Headache	38	2	11	0
Bone Pain	15	4	8	2
Pulmonary				
Dyspnea	49	16	44	13
Cough	30	2	19	2
Gastrointestinal				
Nausea	64	6	50	6
Constipation	53	3	38	3
Diarrhea	42	2	23	2
Vomiting	40	5	26	5
Stomatitis	32	1	10	0
Other-Gastrointestinal	22	12	16	5
Dehydration	13	5	3	0
Mouth Dryness	12	0	6	0
Taste Disturbance	10	0	5	0
Infection				
Infection without neutropenia	38	11	19	5
Musculoskeletal				
Arthralgia	14	3	6	0
Neurology				
Neuropathy-sensory	45	1	38	2
Insomnia	27	0	13	0
Confusion	18	6	10	2
Anxiety	14	1	5	1
Depression	14	0	5	0

[a] Adverse reactions occurring in at least 10% of Erbitux plus BSC arm with a frequency at least 5% greater than that seen in the BSC alone arm.
[b] Adverse reactions were graded using the NCI CTC, V 2.0.
[c] Infusion reaction is defined as any event (chills, rigors, dyspnea, tachycardia, bronchospasm, chest tightness, swelling, urticaria, hypotension, flushing, rash, hypertension, nausea, angioedema, pain, sweating, tremors, shaking, drug fever, or other hypersensitivity reaction) recorded by the investigator as infusion-related.

Table 6: Study 1: Clinical Efficacy in Locoregionally Advanced SCCHN

	Erbitux + Radiation (n=211)	Radiation Alone (n=213)	Hazard Ratio (95% CI[a])	Stratified Log-rank p-value
Locoregional Control				
Median duration (months)	24.4	14.9	0.68 (0.52–0.89)	0.005
Overall Survival				
Median duration (months)	49.0	29.3	0.74 (0.57–0.97)	0.03

[a] CI = confidence interval

[See table 8 above]

Figure 2: Kaplan-Meier Curve for Overall Survival in the *K-Ras* Mutation-negative (Wild-type) Population in Study 4

Patients at Risk										
CET+CT	320	282	237	198	144	108	82	65	21	4
CT	356	313	247	179	132	92	64	48	18	2

Study 5 was a multicenter, open-label, randomized, clinical trial conducted in 572 patients with EGFR-expressing, previously treated, recurrent mCRC. Patients were randomized (1:1) to receive either Erbitux plus best supportive care (BSC) or BSC alone. Erbitux (cetuximab) was administered as a 400 mg/m^2 initial dose, followed by 250 mg/m^2 weekly until disease progression or unacceptable toxicity.

Of the 572 randomized patients, the median age was 63 years, 64% were male, 89% were Caucasian, and 77% had baseline ECOG performance status of 0–1. Demographics and baseline characteristics were similar between study arms. All patients were to have received and progressed on prior therapy including an irinotecan-containing regimen and an oxaliplatin-containing regimen.

K-Ras status was available for 453/572 (79%) of the patients: 245 (54%) patients had *K-Ras* mutation-negative (wild-type) tumors and 208 (46%) patients had *K-Ras* mutation-positive tumors where testing assessed for the following somatic mutations in codons 12 and 13 (exon 2): G12A, G12D, G12R, G12C, G12S, G12V, G13D [see *Warnings and Precautions (5.7)*].

The main outcome measure of the study was overall survival. Results are presented in Table 9 and Figure 3.
[See table 9 above]

Figure 3: Kaplan-Meier Curve for Overall Survival in Patients with *K-Ras* Mutation-negative (Wild-type) Metastatic Colorectal Cancer in Study 5

Patients at Risk								
ERB+BSC	117	100	76	44	20	7	2	0	0
BSC	128	89	45	24	15	7	5	1	0

Study 6 was a multicenter, clinical trial conducted in 329 patients with EGFR-expressing recurrent mCRC. Tumor specimens were not available for testing for *K-Ras* mutation status. Patients were randomized (2:1) to receive either Erbitux plus irinotecan (218 patients) or Erbitux monotherapy (111 patients). Erbitux was administered as a 400 mg/m^2 initial dose, followed by 250 mg/m^2 weekly until disease progression or unacceptable toxicity. In the Erbitux plus irinotecan arm, irinotecan was added to Erbitux using the same dose and schedule for irinotecan as the patient had previously failed. Acceptable irinotecan schedules were 350 mg/m^2 every 3 weeks, 180 mg/m^2 every 2 weeks, or 125 mg/m^2 weekly times four doses every 6 weeks. Of the 329 patients, the median age was 59 years, 63% were male, 98% were Caucasian, and 88% had baseline Karnofsky performance status ≥80. Approximately two-thirds had previously failed oxaliplatin treatment.

The efficacy of Erbitux plus irinotecan or Erbitux monotherapy, based on durable objective responses, was evaluated in all randomized patients and in two pre-specified subpopulations: irinotecan refractory patients, and irinotecan and oxaliplatin failures. In patients receiving Erbitux plus irinotecan, the objective response rate was 23% (95% confidence interval 18%–29%), median duration of response was 5.7 months, and median time to progression was 4.1 months. In patients receiving Erbitux monotherapy, the objective response rate was 11% (95% confidence interval 6%–18%), median duration of response was 4.2 months, and me-

dian time to progression was 1.5 months. Similar response rates were observed in the pre-defined subsets in both the combination arm and monotherapy arm of the study.

Table 7: Study 2: Clinical Efficacy in Recurrent Locoregional Disease or Metastatic SCCHN

	EU-Approved Cetuximab + Platinum-based Therapy + 5-FU (n=222)	Platinum-based Therapy + 5-FU (n=220)	Hazard Ratio (95% CI[a])	Stratified Log-rank p-value
Overall Survival				
Median duration (months)	10.1	7.4	0.80 (0.64, 0.98)	0.034
Progression-free Survival				
Median duration (months)	5.5	3.3	0.57 (0.46, 0.72)	<0.0001
	EU-Approved Cetuximab + Platinum-based Therapy + 5-FU (n=222)	Platinum-based Therapy + 5-FU (n=220)	Odds Ratio (95% CI[a])	CMH[b] test p-value
Objective Response Rate	35.6%	19.5%	2.33 (1.50, 3.60)	0.0001

[a] CI = confidence interval
[b] CMH = Cochran-Mantel-Haenszel

Table 8: Clinical Efficacy in First-line EGFR-expressing, Metastatic Colorectal Cancer (All Randomized and *K-Ras* Status)

	All Randomized		*K-Ras* Mutation-negative (Wild-type)		*K-Ras* Mutation-positive	
	EU-Approved Cetuximab plus FOLFIRI (n=608)	FOLFIRI (n=609)	EU-Approved Cetuximab plus FOLFIRI (n=320)	FOLFIRI (n=356)	EU-Approved Cetuximab plus FOLFIRI (n=216)	FOLFIRI (n=187)
Progression-Free Survival						
Number of Events (%)	343 (56)	371 (61)	165 (52)	214 (60)	138 (64)	112 (60)
Median (months)	8.9	8.1	9.5	8.1	7.5	8.2
(95% CI)	(8.0, 9.4)	(7.6, 8.8)	(8.9, 11.1)	(7.4, 9.2)	(6.7, 8.7)	(7.4, 9.2)
HR (95% CI)	0.85 (0.74, 0.99)		0.70 (0.57, 0.86)		1.13 (0.88, 1.46)	
p-value[a]	0.0358					
Overall Survival[b]						
Number of Events (%)	491 (81)	509 (84)	244 (76)	292 (82)	189 (88)	159 (85)
Median (months)	19.6	18.5	23.5	19.5	16.0	16.7
(95% CI)	(18, 21)	(17, 20)	(21, 26)	(17, 21)	(15, 18)	(15, 19)
HR (95% CI)	0.88 (0.78, 1.0)		0.80 (0.67, 0.94)		1.04 (0.84, 1.29)	
Objective Response Rate						
ORR (95% CI)	46% (42, 50)	38% (34, 42)	57% (51, 62)	39% (34, 44)	31% (25, 38)	35% (28, 43)

[a] Based on the Stratified Log-rank test.
[b] Post-hoc updated OS analysis, results based on an additional 162 events.

Table 9: Overall Survival in Previously Treated EGFR-expressing, Metastatic Colorectal Cancer (All Randomized and *K-Ras* Status)

	All Randomized		*K-Ras* Mutation-negative (Wild-type)		*K-Ras* Mutation-positive	
	Erbitux plus BSC (N=287)	BSC (N=285)	Erbitux plus BSC (N=117)	BSC (N=128)	Erbitux plus BSC (N=108)	BSC (N=100)
Median (months)	6.1	4.6	8.6	5.0	4.8	4.6
(95% CI)	(5.4, 6.7)	(4.2, 4.9)	(7.0, 10.3)	(4.3, 5.7)	(3.9, 5.6)	(3.6, 4.9)
HR	0.77		0.63		0.91	
(95% CI)	(0.64, 0.92)		(0.47, 0.84)		(0.67, 1.24)	
p-value[a]	0.0046					

[a] Based on the Stratified Log-rank test.

16 HOW SUPPLIED/STORAGE AND HANDLING

Erbitux® (cetuximab) is supplied at a concentration of 2 mg/mL as a 100 mg/50 mL, single-use vial or as a 200 mg/100 mL, single-use vial as a sterile, injectable liquid containing no preservatives.

NDC 66733-948-23   100 mg/50 mL, single-use vial, individually packaged in a carton
NDC 66733-958-23   200 mg/100 mL, single-use vial, individually packaged in a carton

Store vials under refrigeration at 2° C to 8° C (36° F to 46° F). **Do not freeze.** Increased particulate formation may occur at temperatures at or below 0° C. This product contains no preservatives. Preparations of Erbitux in infusion containers are chemically and physically stable for up to 12 hours at 2° C to 8° C (36° F to 46° F) and up to 8 hours at controlled room temperature (20° C to 25° C; 68° F to 77° F). Discard any remaining solution in the infusion container after 8 hours at controlled room temperature or after 12 hours at 2° C to 8° C. Discard any unused portion of the vial.

17 PATIENT COUNSELING INFORMATION

Advise patients:
- To report signs and symptoms of infusion reactions such as fever, chills, or breathing problems.
- Of the potential risks of using Erbitux during pregnancy or nursing and of the need to use adequate contraception in both males and females during and for 6 months following the last dose of Erbitux (cetuximab) therapy.
- That nursing is not recommended during, and for 2 months following the last dose of Erbitux therapy.
- To limit sun exposure (use sunscreen, wear hats) while receiving and for 2 months following the last dose of Erbitux.

Help Patients Save on Rx Drugs: PDR.net/PharmacyDiscountCard

Erbitux® (cetuximab) is a registered trademark of ImClone LLC a wholly-owned subsidiary of Eli Lilly and Company. Manufactured by ImClone LLC a wholly-owned subsidiary of Eli Lilly and Company, Branchburg, NJ 08876 USA Distributed and marketed by Bristol-Myers Squibb Company, Princeton, NJ 08543 USA Co-marketed by Eli Lilly and Company, Indianapolis, IN 46285 USA
Copyright © 2004–2013 ImClone LLC a wholly-owned subsidiary of Eli Lilly and Company, and Bristol-Myers Squibb Company. All rights reserved.
1236886B3
Rev August 2013
Shown in Product Identification Guide, page 306

IXEMPRA® Kit

[ĭk-sĕm-prä]
(ixabepilone)
for Injection, for intravenous infusion only

HIGHLIGHTS OF PRESCRIBING INFORMATION
These highlights do not include all the information needed to use IXEMPRA® safely and effectively. See full prescribing information for IXEMPRA®.

IXEMPRA® Kit (ixabepilone) for Injection, for intravenous infusion only
Initial U.S. Approval: 2007

WARNING: TOXICITY IN HEPATIC IMPAIRMENT
See full prescribing information for complete boxed warning.
IXEMPRA® in combination with capecitabine must not be given to patients with AST or ALT >2.5 × ULN or bilirubin >1 × ULN due to increased risk of toxicity and neutropenia-related death. (4, 5.3)

INDICATIONS AND USAGE

- IXEMPRA, a microtubule inhibitor, in combination with capecitabine is indicated for the treatment of metastatic or locally advanced breast cancer in patients after failure of an anthracycline and a taxane (1).
- IXEMPRA as monotherapy is indicated for the treatment of metastatic or locally advanced breast cancer in patients after failure of an anthracycline, a taxane, and capecitabine (1).

DOSAGE AND ADMINISTRATION

- The recommended dose of IXEMPRA is 40 mg/m² infused intravenously over 3 hours every 3 weeks (2.1).
- Dose reduction is required in certain patients with elevated AST, ALT, or bilirubin (2.2, 8.6).

IXEMPRA (ixabepilone) for injection must be constituted with supplied DILUENT. The ixabepilone concentration in constituted solution is 2 mg/mL.
Constituted solution must be diluted with one of the specified fluids, to a final ixabepilone concentration of 0.2 mg/mL to 0.6 mg/mL. The final solution must be used within 6 hours of preparation (2.4).

DOSAGE FORMS AND STRENGTHS

- IXEMPRA for injection, 15 mg supplied with DILUENT for IXEMPRA, 8 mL (3)
- IXEMPRA for injection, 45 mg supplied with DILUENT for IXEMPRA, 23.5 mL (3)

CONTRAINDICATIONS

- Hypersensitivity to drugs formulated with Cremophor® EL (4).
- Baseline neutrophil count <1500 cells/mm³ or a platelet count <100,000 cells/mm³ (4).
- Patients with AST or ALT >2.5 × ULN or bilirubin >1 × ULN must not be treated with IXEMPRA in combination with capecitabine (4).

WARNINGS AND PRECAUTIONS

- Peripheral Neuropathy: Monitor for symptoms of neuropathy, primarily sensory. Neuropathy is cumulative, generally reversible, and should be managed by dose adjustment and delays (2.2, 5.1).
- Myelosuppression: Primarily neutropenia. Monitor with peripheral blood cell counts and adjust dose as appropriate (2.2, 5.2).
- Hypersensitivity reaction: Must premedicate all patients with an H₁ antagonist and an H₂ antagonist before treatment (2.3, 5.4).
- Fetal harm can occur when administered to a pregnant woman. Women should be advised not to become pregnant when taking IXEMPRA (5.5, 8.1).

ADVERSE REACTIONS

- The most common adverse reactions (≥20%) are peripheral sensory neuropathy, fatigue/asthenia, myalgia/arthralgia, alopecia, nausea, vomiting, stomatitis/mucositis, diarrhea, and musculoskeletal pain. Additional reactions occurred in ≥20% in combination treatment: palmar-plantar erythrodysesthesia syndrome, anorexia, abdominal pain, nail disorder, and constipation (6).

- Drug-associated hematologic abnormalities (>40%) include neutropenia, leukopenia, anemia, and thrombocytopenia (6).

To report SUSPECTED ADVERSE REACTIONS, contact Bristol-Myers Squibb at 1-800-721-5072 or FDA at 1-800-FDA-1088 or www.fda.gov/medwatch

DRUG INTERACTIONS

- Inhibitors of CYP3A4 may increase plasma concentrations of ixabepilone; dose of IXEMPRA (ixabepilone) must be reduced with strong CYP3A4 inhibitors (7.1).
- Inducers of CYP3A4 may decrease plasma concentrations of ixabepilone; alternative therapeutic agents with low enzyme induction potential should be considered (7.1).

See 17 for PATIENT COUNSELING INFORMATION and FDA-Approved Patient Labeling

Revised: 10/2011

FULL PRESCRIBING INFORMATION: CONTENTS*
WARNING: TOXICITY IN HEPATIC IMPAIRMENT

* Sections or subsections omitted from the full prescribing information are not listed

---

FULL PRESCRIBING INFORMATION

WARNING: TOXICITY IN HEPATIC IMPAIRMENT

IXEMPRA in combination with capecitabine is contraindicated in patients with AST or ALT >2.5 × ULN or bilirubin >1 × ULN due to increased risk of toxicity and neutropenia-related death *[see Contraindications (4) and Warnings and Precautions (5.3)]*.

---

1 INDICATIONS AND USAGE

IXEMPRA (ixabepilone) is indicated in combination with capecitabine for the treatment of patients with metastatic or locally advanced breast cancer resistant to treatment with an anthracycline and a taxane, or whose cancer is taxane resistant and for whom further anthracycline therapy is contraindicated. Anthracycline resistance is defined as progression while on therapy or within 6 months in the adjuvant setting or 3 months in the metastatic setting. Taxane resistance is defined as progression while on therapy or within 12 months in the adjuvant setting or 4 months in the metastatic setting.
IXEMPRA (ixabepilone) is indicated as monotherapy for the treatment of metastatic or locally advanced breast cancer in patients whose tumors are resistant or refractory to anthracyclines, taxanes, and capecitabine.

2 DOSAGE AND ADMINISTRATION

2.1 General Dosing Information
The recommended dosage of IXEMPRA is 40 mg/m² administered intravenously over 3 hours every 3 weeks. Doses for patients with body surface area (BSA) greater than 2.2 m² should be calculated based on 2.2 m².

2.2 Dose Modification
Dose Adjustments During Treatment
Patients should be evaluated during treatment by periodic clinical observation and laboratory tests including complete blood cell counts. If toxicities are present, treatment should be delayed to allow recovery. Dosing adjustment guidelines for monotherapy and combination therapy are shown in Table 1. If toxicities recur, an additional 20% dose reduction should be made.
[See table 1 at top of next page]
Re-treatment Criteria: Dose adjustments at the start of a cycle should be based on nonhematologic toxicity or blood counts from the preceding cycle following the guidelines in Table 1. Patients should not begin a new cycle of treatment unless the neutrophil count is at least 1500 cells/mm³, the platelet count is at least 100,000 cells/mm³, and nonhematologic toxicities have improved to grade 1 (mild) or resolved.
Dose Adjustments in Special Populations - Hepatic Impairment
Combination Therapy:
IXEMPRA in combination with capecitabine is contraindicated in patients with AST or ALT >2.5 × ULN or bilirubin >1 × ULN. Patients receiving combination treatment who have AST and ALT ≤2.5 × ULN and bilirubin ≤1 × ULN may receive the standard dose of ixabepilone (40 mg/m²) *[see Boxed Warning, Contraindications (4), Warnings and Precautions (5.3), and Use in Specific Populations (8.6)]*.
Monotherapy:
Patients with hepatic impairment should be dosed with IXEMPRA based on the guidelines in Table 2. Patients with moderate hepatic impairment should be started at 20 mg/m², the dosage in subsequent cycles may be escalated up to, but not exceeding, 30 mg/m² if tolerated. Use in patients with AST or ALT >10 × ULN or bilirubin >3 × ULN is not recommended. Limited data are available for patients with baseline AST or ALT >5 × ULN. Caution should be used when treating these patients *[see Warnings and Precautions (5.3) and Use in Specific Populations (8.6)]*.
[See table 2 at top of next page]
Strong CYP3A4 Inhibitors
The use of concomitant strong CYP3A4 inhibitors should be avoided (eg, ketoconazole, itraconazole, clarithromycin, atazanavir, nefazodone, saquinavir, telithromycin, ritonavir, amprenavir, indinavir, nelfinavir, delavirdine, or voriconazole). Grapefruit juice may also increase plasma concentrations of IXEMPRA and should be avoided. Based on pharmacokinetic studies, if a strong CYP3A4 inhibitor must be coadministered, a dose reduction to 20 mg/m² is predicted to adjust the ixabepilone AUC to the range observed without inhibitors and should be considered. If the strong inhibitor is discontinued, a washout period of approximately 1 week should be allowed before the IXEMPRA dose is adjusted upward to the indicated dose *[see Drug Interactions (7.1)]*.
Strong CYP3A4 Inducers
The use of concomitant strong CYP3A4 inducers should be avoided (eg, phenytoin, carbamazepine, rifampin, rifabutin, dexamethasone, and phenobarbital). Selection of an alternative concomitant medication with no or minimal enzyme induction potential should be considered. Based on extrapolation from a drug interaction study with rifampin, the following guidance may be considered for dosing in patients requiring coadministration of a strong CYP3A4 inducer, if no alternatives are feasible. Once patients have been maintained on a strong CYP3A4 inducer, the dose of IXEMPRA may be gradually increased from 40 mg/m² to 60 mg/m² depending on tolerance. If the dose is increased, IXEMPRA should be given as a 4-hour intravenous infusion. This 60 mg/m² dose given intravenously over 4 hours is predicted to adjust the AUC to the range observed without inducers. However, there are no clinical data with this dose adjustment in patients receiving strong CYP3A4 inducers. Patients whose dose is increased above 40 mg/m² should be monitored carefully for toxicities associated with IXEMPRA. If the strong inducer is discontinued, the IXEMPRA dose should be returned to the dose used prior to initiation of the strong CYP3A4 inducer *[see Drug Interactions (7.1)]*.

2.3 Premedication

To minimize the chance of occurrence of a hypersensitivity reaction, all patients must be premedicated approximately 1 hour before the infusion of IXEMPRA (ixabepilone) with:

- An H₁ antagonist (eg, diphenhydramine 50 mg orally or equivalent) and
- An H₂ antagonist (eg, ranitidine 150 - 300 mg orally or equivalent).

Patients who experienced a hypersensitivity reaction to IXEMPRA require premedication with corticosteroids (eg, dexamethasone 20 mg intravenously, 30 minutes before infusion or orally, 60 minutes before infusion) in addition to pretreatment with H₁ and H₂ antagonists.

2.4 Instructions for Preparation and IV Administration

IXEMPRA *Kit* contains two vials, a vial labeled IXEMPRA (ixabepilone) for injection which contains ixabepilone powder and a vial containing DILUENT for IXEMPRA. Only supplied DILUENT must be used for constituting IXEMPRA (ixabepilone) for injection. IXEMPRA *Kit* must be stored in a refrigerator at 2° C - 8° C (36° F - 46° F) in the original package to protect from light. Prior to constituting IXEMPRA for injection, the *Kit* should be removed from the refrigerator and allowed to stand at room temperature for approximately 30 minutes. When the vials are first removed from the refrigerator, a white precipitate may be observed in the DILUENT vial. This precipitate will dissolve to form a clear solution once the DILUENT warms to room temperature. To allow for withdrawal losses, the vial labeled as 15 mg IXEMPRA for injection contains 16 mg of ixabepilone and the vial labeled as 45 mg IXEMPRA for injection contains 47 mg of ixabepilone. The 15-mg IXEMPRA *Kit* is supplied with a vial providing 8 mL of the DILUENT and the 45-mg IXEMPRA *Kit* is supplied with a vial providing 23.5 mL of the DILUENT. After constituting the DILUENT, the concentration of ixabepilone is 2 mg/mL.

Please refer to Preparation and Handling Precautions [see Dosage and Administration (2.5)] before preparation.

A. To constitute:

1. With a suitable syringe, aseptically withdraw the DILUENT and slowly inject it into the IXEMPRA for injection vial. The 15-mg IXEMPRA is constituted with 8 mL of DILUENT and the 45-mg IXEMPRA is constituted with 23.5 mL of DILUENT.
2. Gently swirl and invert the vial until the powder in IXEMPRA is completely dissolved.

B. To dilute:

Before administration, the constituted solution must be further diluted with one of the specified infusion fluids listed below. The IXEMPRA infusion must be prepared in a DEHP [di-(2-ethylhexyl) phthalate] free bag.

The following infusion fluids have been qualified for use in the dilution of IXEMPRA:

- Lactated Ringer's Injection, USP
- 0.9% Sodium Chloride Injection, USP (pH adjusted with Sodium Bicarbonate Injection, USP)
  - When using a 250 mL or a 500 mL bag of 0.9% Sodium Chloride Injection to prepare the infusion, the pH must be adjusted to a pH between 6.0 and 9.0 by adding 2 mEq (ie, 2 mL of an 8.4% w/v solution or 4 mL of a 4.2% w/v solution) of Sodium Bicarbonate Injection, prior to the addition of the constituted IXEMPRA solution.
- PLASMA-LYTE A Injection pH 7.4®

For most doses, a 250 mL bag of infusion fluid is sufficient. However, it is necessary to check the final IXEMPRA infusion concentration of each dose based on the volume of infusion fluid to be used.

The final concentration for infusion must be between 0.2 mg/mL and 0.6 mg/mL. To calculate the final infusion concentration, use the following formulas:

Total Infusion Volume = mL of Constituted Solution + mL of infusion fluid

Final Infusion Concentration = Dose of IXEMPRA (mg)/ Total Infusion Volume (mL)

1. Aseptically withdraw the appropriate volume of constituted solution containing 2 mg of ixabepilone per mL.
2. Aseptically transfer to an intravenous (IV) bag containing an appropriate volume of infusion fluid to achieve the final desired concentration of IXEMPRA.
3. Thoroughly mix the infusion bag by manual rotation.

The infusion solution must be administered through an appropriate in-line filter with a microporous membrane of 0.2 to 1.2 microns. DEHP-free infusion containers and administration sets must be used. Any remaining solution should be discarded according to institutional procedures for antineoplastics.

Stability

After constituting IXEMPRA, the constituted solution should be further diluted with infusion fluid as soon as possible, but may be stored in the vial (not the syringe) for a maximum of 1 hour at room temperature and room light. Once diluted with infusion fluid, the solution is stable at room temperature and room light for a maximum of 6 hours. Administration of diluted IXEMPRA must be completed within this 6-hour period. The infusion fluids previously mentioned are specified because their pH is in the range of 6.0 to 9.0, which is required to maintain IXEMPRA stability. Other infusion fluids should not be used with IXEMPRA (ixabepilone).

2.5 Preparation and Handling Precautions

Procedures for proper handling and disposal of antineoplastic drugs *[see References (15)]* should be followed. To minimize the risk of dermal exposure, impervious gloves should be worn when handling vials containing IXEMPRA, regardless of the setting, including unpacking and inspection, transport within a facility, and dose preparation and administration.

3 DOSAGE FORMS AND STRENGTHS

IXEMPRA for injection, 15 mg supplied with DILUENT for IXEMPRA, 8 mL.

IXEMPRA for injection, 45 mg supplied with DILUENT for IXEMPRA, 23.5 mL.

4 CONTRAINDICATIONS

IXEMPRA is contraindicated in patients with a history of a severe (CTC grade 3/4) hypersensitivity reaction to agents containing Cremophor® EL or its derivatives (eg, polyoxyethylated castor oil) *[see Warnings and Precautions (5.4)]*. IXEMPRA is contraindicated in patients who have a neutrophil count <1500 cells/mm³ or a platelet count <100,000 cells/mm³ *[see Warnings and Precautions (5.2)]*. IXEMPRA in combination with capecitabine is contraindicated in patients with AST or ALT >2.5 × ULN or bilirubin >1 × ULN *[see Boxed Warning and Warnings and Precautions (5.3)]*.

5 WARNINGS AND PRECAUTIONS

5.1 Peripheral Neuropathy

Peripheral neuropathy was common (see Table 3). Patients treated with IXEMPRA should be monitored for symptoms of neuropathy, such as burning sensation, hyperesthesia, hypoesthesia, paresthesia, discomfort, or neuropathic pain. Neuropathy occurred early during treatment; ~75% of new onset or worsening neuropathy occurred during the first 3 cycles. Patients experiencing new or worsening symptoms may require a reduction or delay in the dose of IXEMPRA *[see Dosage and Administration (2.2)]*. In clinical studies, peripheral neuropathy was managed through dose reductions, dose delays, and treatment discontinuation. Neuropathy was the most frequent cause of treatment discontinuation due to drug toxicity. In Studies 046 and 081, 80% and 87%, respectively, of patients with peripheral neuropathy

who received IXEMPRA (ixabepilone) had improvement or no worsening of their neuropathy following dose reduction. For patients with grade 3/4 neuropathy in Studies 046 and 081, 76% and 79%, respectively, had documented improvement to baseline or grade 1, twelve weeks after onset.

Table 1: Dose Adjustment Guidelines[a]

IXEMPRA (Monotherapy or Combination Therapy)	IXEMPRA Dose Modification
Nonhematologic:	
Grade 2 neuropathy (moderate) lasting ≥7 days	Decrease the dose by 20%
Grade 3 neuropathy (severe) lasting <7 days	Decrease the dose by 20%
Grade 3 neuropathy (severe) lasting ≥7 days or disabling neuropathy	Discontinue treatment
Any grade 3 toxicity (severe) other than neuropathy	Decrease the dose by 20%
Transient grade 3 arthralgia/myalgia or fatigue	No change in dose of IXEMPRA
Grade 3 hand-foot syndrome (palmar-plantar erythrodysesthesia)	
Any grade 4 toxicity (disabling)	Discontinue treatment
Hematologic:	
Neutrophil <500 cells/mm³ for ≥7 days	Decrease the dose by 20%
Febrile neutropenia	Decrease the dose by 20%
Platelets <25,000/mm³ or platelets <50,000/mm³ with bleeding	Decrease the dose by 20%

Capecitabine (when used in combination with IXEMPRA)	Capecitabine Dose Modification
Nonhematologic:	Follow Capecitabine Label
Hematologic:	
Platelets <25,000/mm³ or <50,000/mm³ with bleeding	Hold for concurrent diarrhea or stomatitis until platelet count >50,000/mm³, then continue at same dose.
Neutrophils <500 cells/mm³ for ≥7 days or febrile neutropenia	Hold for concurrent diarrhea or stomatitis until neutrophil count >1,000 cells/mm³, then continue at same dose.

[a] Toxicities graded in accordance with National Cancer Institute (NCI) Common Terminology Criteria for Adverse Events (CTCAE v3.0).

Table 2: Dose Adjustments for IXEMPRA as Monotherapy in Patients with Hepatic Impairment

	Transaminase Levels		Bilirubin Levels[a]	IXEMPRA[b] (mg/m²)
Mild	AST and ALT ≤2.5 × ULN	and	≤1 × ULN	40
	AST and ALT ≤10 × ULN	and	≤1.5 × ULN	32
Moderate	AST and ALT ≤10 × ULN	and	>1.5 × ULN - ≤3 × ULN	20 - 30

[a] Excluding patients whose total bilirubin is elevated due to Gilbert's disease.
[b] Dosage recommendations are for first course of therapy; further decreases in subsequent courses should be based on individual tolerance.

Table 3: Treatment-related Peripheral Neuropathy

	IXEMPRA with capecitabine Study 046	IXEMPRA as monotherapy Study 081
Peripheral neuropathy (all grades)[a,b]	67%	63%
Peripheral neuropathy (grade 3/4)[a,b]	23%	14%
Discontinuation due to neuropathy	21%	6%
Median number of cycles to onset of grade 3/4 neuropathy	4	4
Median time to improvement of grade 3/4 neuropathy to baseline or to grade 1	6.0 weeks	4.6 weeks

[a] Sensory and motor neuropathy combined.
[b] 24% and 27% of patients in 046 and 081, respectively, had preexisting neuropathy (grade 1).

A pooled analysis of 1540 cancer patients treated with IXEMPRA indicated that patients with diabetes mellitus or preexisting peripheral neuropathy may be at increased risk of severe neuropathy. Prior therapy with neurotoxic chemotherapy agents did not predict the development of neuropathy. Patients with moderate to severe neuropathy (grade 2 or greater) were excluded from studies with IXEMPRA. Caution should be used when treating patients with diabetes mellitus or preexisting peripheral neuropathy.

5.2 Myelosuppression

Myelosuppression is dose-dependent and primarily manifested as neutropenia. In clinical studies, grade 4 neutropenia (<500 cells/mm³) occurred in 36% of patients treated with IXEMPRA in combination with capecitabine and 23% of patients treated with IXEMPRA monotherapy. Febrile

Table 4: Nonhematologic Drug-related Adverse Reactions Occurring in at Least 5% of Patients with Metastatic or Locally Advanced Breast Cancer Treated with IXEMPRA

System Organ Class[a]/ Preferred Term	Study 046 IXEMPRA with capecitabine n=369 Total (%)	Grade 3/4 (%)	Capecitabine n=368 Total (%)	Grade 3/4 (%)	Study 081 IXEMPRA monotherapy n=126 Total (%)	Grade 3/4 (%)
Infections and Infestations						
Upper respiratory tract infection[b]	4	0	3	0	6	0
Blood and Lymphatic System Disorders						
Febrile neutropenia	5	4[c]	1	1[d]	3	3[d]
Immune System Disorders						
Hypersensitivity[b]	2	1[d]	0	0	5	1[d]
Metabolism and Nutrition Disorders						
Anorexia[b]	34	3[d]	15	1[d]	19	2[d]
Dehydration[b]	5	2	2	<1[d]	2	1[d]
Psychiatric Disorders						
Insomnia[b]	9	<1[d]	2	0	5	0
Nervous System Disorders						
Peripheral neuropathy						
Sensory neuropathy[b,e]	65	21	16	0	62	14
Motor neuropathy[b]	16	5[d]	<1	0	10	1[d]
Headache	8	<1[d]	3	0	11	0
Taste disorder[b]	12	0	4	0	6	0
Dizziness	8	0	5	1[d]	7	0
Eye Disorders						
Lacrimation increased	5	0	4	<1[d]	4	0
Vascular Disorders						
Hot flush[b]	5	0	2	0	6	0
Respiratory, Thoracic, and Mediastinal Disorders						
Dyspnea[b]	7	1	4	1	9	1[d]
Cough[b]	6	0	2	0	2	0
Gastrointestinal Disorders						
Nausea	53	3[d]	40	2[d]	42	2[d]
Vomiting[b]	39	4[d]	24	2	29	1[d]
Stomatitis/mucositis[b]	31	4	20	3[d]	29	6
Diarrhea[b]	44	6[d]	39	9	22	1[d]
Constipation	22	0	6	<1[d]	16	2[d]
Abdominal pain[b]	24	2[d]	14	1[d]	13	2[d]
Gastroesophageal reflux disease[b]	7	1[d]	8	0	6	0
Skin and Subcutaneous Tissue Disorders						
Alopecia[b]	31	0	3	0	48	0
Skin rash[b]	17	1[d]	7	0	9	2[d]
Nail disorder[b]	24	2[d]	10	<1[d]	9	0
Palmar-plantar erythrodysesthesia syndrome[b,f]	64	18[d]	63	17[d]	8	2[d]
Pruritus[b]	5	0	2	0	6	1[d]
Skin exfoliation[b]	5	<1[d]	3	0	2	0
Skin hyperpigmentation[b]	11	0	14	0	2	0
Musculoskeletal, Connective Tissue, and Bone Disorders						
Myalgia/arthralgia[b]	39	8[d]	5	<1[d]	49	8[d]
Musculoskeletal pain[b]	23	2[d]	5	0	20	3[d]
General Disorders and Administration Site Conditions						
Fatigue/asthenia[b]	60	16	29	4	56	13
Edema[b]	8	0	5	<1[d]	9	1[d]
Pyrexia	10	1[d]	4	0	8	1[d]
Pain[b]	9	1[d]	2	0	8	3[d]
Chest pain[b]	4	1[d]	<1	0	5	1[d]
Investigations						
Weight decreased	11	0	3	0	6	0

[a] System organ class presented as outlined in Guidelines for Preparing Core Clinical Safety Information on Drugs by the Council for International Organizations of Medical Sciences (CIOMS).

[b] A composite of multiple MedDRA Preferred Terms.

[c] NCI CTC grading for febrile neutropenia ranges from Grade 3 to 5. Three patients (1%) experienced Grade 5 (fatal) febrile neutropenia. Other neutropenia-related deaths (9) occurred in the absence of reported febrile neutropenia [see Warnings and Precautions (5.2)].

[d] No grade 4 reports.

[e] Peripheral sensory neuropathy (graded with the NCI CTC scale) was defined as the occurrence of any of the following: areflexia, burning sensation, dysesthesia, hyperesthesia, hypoesthesia, hyporeflexia, neuralgia, neuritis, neuropathy, neuropathy peripheral, neurotoxicity, painful response to normal stimuli, paresthesia, pallanesthesia, peripheral sensory neuropathy, polyneuropathy, polyneuropathy toxic and sensorimotor disorder. Peripheral motor neuropathy was defined as the occurrence of any of the following: multifocal motor neuropathy, neuromuscular toxicity, peripheral motor neuropathy, and peripheral sensorimotor neuropathy.

[f] Palmar-plantar erythrodysesthesia (hand-foot syndrome) was graded on a 1-3 severity scale in Study 046.

neutropenia and infection with neutropenia were reported in 5% and 6% of patients treated with IXEMPRA (ixabepilone) in combination with capecitabine, respectively, and 3% and 5% of patients treated with IXEMPRA as monotherapy, respectively. Neutropenia-related death occurred in 1.9% of 414 patients with normal hepatic function or mild hepatic impairment treated with IXEMPRA in combination with capecitabine. The rate of neutropenia-related deaths was higher (29%, 5 out of 17) in patients with AST or ALT >2.5 × ULN or bilirubin >1.5 × ULN [see Boxed Warning, Contraindications (4), and Warnings and Precautions (5.3)]. Neutropenia-related death occurred in 0.4% of 240 patients treated with IXEMPRA (ixabepilone) as monotherapy. No neutropenia-related deaths were reported in 24 patients with AST or ALT >2.5 × ULN or bilirubin >1.5 × ULN treated with IXEMPRA monotherapy. IXEMPRA must not be administered to patients with a neutrophil count <1500 cells/mm³. To monitor for myelosuppression, frequent peripheral blood cell counts are recommended for all patients receiving IXEMPRA (ixabepilone). Patients who experience severe neutropenia or thrombocytopenia should have their dose reduced [see Dosage and Administration (2.2)].

5.3 Hepatic Impairment

Patients with baseline AST or ALT >2.5 × ULN or bilirubin >1.5 × ULN experienced greater toxicity than patients with baseline AST or ALT ≤2.5 × ULN or bilirubin ≤1.5 × ULN when treated with IXEMPRA at 40 mg/m² in combination with capecitabine or as monotherapy in breast cancer studies. In combination with capecitabine, the overall frequency of grade 3/4 adverse reactions, febrile neutropenia, serious adverse reactions, and toxicity-related deaths was greater [see Warnings and Precautions (5.2)]. With monotherapy, grade 4 neutropenia, febrile neutropenia, and serious adverse reactions were more frequent. The safety and pharmacokinetics of IXEMPRA as monotherapy were evaluated in a dose escalation study in 56 patients with varying degrees of hepatic impairment. Exposure was increased in patients with elevated AST or bilirubin [see Use in Specific Populations (8.6)].

IXEMPRA in combination with capecitabine is contraindicated in patients with AST or ALT >2.5 × ULN or bilirubin >1 × ULN due to increased risk of toxicity- and neutropenia-related death [see Boxed Warning, Contraindications (4), and Warnings and Precautions (5.2)]. Patients who are treated with IXEMPRA as monotherapy should receive a reduced dose depending on the degree of hepatic impairment [see Dosage and Administration (2.2)]. Use in patients with AST or ALT >10 × ULN or bilirubin >3 × ULN is not recommended. Limited data are available for patients with AST or ALT >5 × ULN. Caution should be used when treating these patients [see Dosage and Administration (2.2)].

5.4 Hypersensitivity Reactions

Patients with a history of a severe hypersensitivity reaction to agents containing Cremophor® EL or its derivatives (eg, polyoxyethylated castor oil) should not be treated with IXEMPRA. All patients should be premedicated with an H₁ and an H₂ antagonist approximately 1 hour before IXEMPRA infusion and be observed for hypersensitivity reactions (eg, flushing, rash, dyspnea, and bronchospasm). In case of severe hypersensitivity reactions, infusion of IXEMPRA should be stopped and aggressive supportive treatment (eg, epinephrine, corticosteroids) started. Of the 1323 patients treated with IXEMPRA in clinical studies, 9 patients (1%) had experienced severe hypersensitivity reactions (including anaphylaxis). Three of the 9 patients were able to be retreated. Patients who experience a hypersensitivity reaction in one cycle of IXEMPRA must be premedicated in subsequent cycles with a corticosteroid in addition to the H₁ and H₂ antagonists, and extension of the infusion time should be considered [see Dosage and Administration (2.3) and Contraindications (4)].

5.5 Pregnancy

Pregnancy Category D.

IXEMPRA may cause fetal harm when administered to pregnant women. There are no adequate and well-controlled studies with IXEMPRA in pregnant women. Women should be advised not to become pregnant when taking IXEMPRA. If this drug is used during pregnancy, or if the patient becomes pregnant while taking this drug, the patient should be apprised of the potential hazard to the fetus.

Ixabepilone was studied for effects on embryo-fetal development in pregnant rats and rabbits given IV doses of 0.02, 0.08, and 0.3 mg/kg/day and 0.01, 0.03, 0.11, and 0.3 mg/kg/day, respectively. There were no teratogenic effects. In rats, an increase in resorptions and post-implantation loss and a decrease in the number of live fetuses and fetal weight was observed at the maternally toxic dose of 0.3 mg/kg/day (approximately one-tenth the human clinical exposure based on AUC). Abnormalities included a reduced ossification of caudal vertebrae, sternebrae, and metacarpals. In rabbits, ixabepilone caused maternal toxicity (death) and embryo-fetal toxicity (resorptions) at 0.3 mg/kg/day (approximately one-tenth the human clinical dose based on body surface area). No fetuses were available at this dose for evaluation.

5.6 Cardiac Adverse Reactions

The frequency of cardiac adverse reactions (myocardial ischemia and ventricular dysfunction) was higher in the IXEMPRA in combination with capecitabine (1.9%) than in the capecitabine alone (0.3%) treatment group. Supraventricular arrhythmias were observed in the combination arm (0.5%) and not in the capecitabine alone arm. Caution should be exercised in patients with a history of cardiac disease. Discontinuation of IXEMPRA should be considered in patients who develop cardiac ischemia or impaired cardiac function.

5.7 Potential for Cognitive Impairment from Excipients

Since IXEMPRA contains dehydrated alcohol USP, consideration should be given to the possibility of central nervous system and other effects of alcohol [see Description (11)].

6 ADVERSE REACTIONS

The following adverse reactions are discussed in greater detail in other sections.
- Peripheral neuropathy [see Warnings and Precautions (5.1)]
- Myelosuppression [see Warnings and Precautions (5.2)]
- Hypersensitivity reactions [see Warnings and Precautions (5.4)]

6.1 Clinical Trials Experience

Because clinical trials are conducted under widely varying conditions, the adverse reaction rates observed in the clinical trials of a drug cannot be directly compared to rates in other clinical trials and may not reflect the rates observed in clinical practice.

Unless otherwise specified, assessment of adverse reactions is based on one randomized study (Study 046) and one single-arm study (Study 081). In Study 046, 369 patients with metastatic breast cancer were treated with IXEMPRA (ixabepilone) 40 mg/m^2 administered intravenously over 3 hours every 21 days, combined with capecitabine 1000 mg/m^2 twice daily for 2 weeks followed by a 1-week rest period. Patients treated with capecitabine as monotherapy (n=368) in this study received 1250 mg/m^2 twice daily for 2 weeks every 21 days. In Study 081, 126 patients with metastatic or locally advanced breast cancer were treated with IXEMPRA 40 mg/m^2 administered intravenously over 3 hours every 3 weeks.

The most common adverse reactions (≥20%) reported by patients receiving IXEMPRA were peripheral sensory neuropathy, fatigue/asthenia, myalgia/arthralgia, alopecia, nausea, vomiting, stomatitis/mucositis, diarrhea, and musculoskeletal pain. The following additional reactions occurred in ≥20% in combination treatment: palmar-plantar erythrodysesthesia (hand-foot) syndrome, anorexia, abdominal pain, nail disorder, and constipation. The most common hematologic abnormalities (>40%) include neutropenia, leukopenia, anemia, and thrombocytopenia.

Table 4 presents nonhematologic adverse reactions reported in 5% or more of patients. Hematologic abnormalities are presented separately in Table 5.

[See table 4 at top of previous page]

[See table 5 above]

The following serious adverse reactions were also reported in 1323 patients treated with IXEMPRA as monotherapy or in combination with other therapies in Phase 2 and 3 studies.

Infections and Infestations: sepsis, pneumonia, infection, neutropenic infection, urinary tract infection, bacterial infection, enterocolitis, laryngitis, lower respiratory tract infection

Blood and Lymphatic System Disorders: coagulopathy, lymphopenia

Metabolism and Nutrition Disorders: hyponatremia, metabolic acidosis, hypokalemia, hypovolemia

Nervous System Disorders: cognitive disorder, syncope, cerebral hemorrhage, abnormal coordination, lethargy

Cardiac Disorders: myocardial infarction, supraventricular arrhythmia, left ventricular dysfunction, angina pectoris, atrial flutter, cardiomyopathy, myocardial ischemia

Vascular Disorders: hypotension, thrombosis, embolism, hemorrhage, hypovolemic shock, vasculitis

Respiratory, Thoracic, and Mediastinal Disorders: pneumonitis, hypoxia, respiratory failure, acute pulmonary edema, dysphonia, pharyngolaryngeal pain

Gastrointestinal Disorders: ileus, colitis, impaired gastric emptying, esophagitis, dysphagia, gastritis, gastrointestinal hemorrhage

Hepatobiliary Disorders: acute hepatic failure, jaundice

Skin and Subcutaneous Tissue Disorders: erythema multiforme

Musculoskeletal, Connective Tissue, and Bone Disorders: muscular weakness, muscle spasms, trismus

Renal and Urinary Disorders: nephrolithiasis, renal failure

General Disorders and Administration Site Conditions: chills

Investigations: increased transaminases, increased blood alkaline phosphatase, increased gamma-glutamyltransferase

6.2 Postmarketing Experience

Radiation recall has been reported during postmarketing use of IXEMPRA. Because this reaction was reported voluntarily from a population of uncertain size, it is not always possible to reliably estimate the frequency or establish a causal relationship to drug exposure.

7 DRUG INTERACTIONS

7.1 Effect of Other Drugs on Ixabepilone

Drugs That May Increase Ixabepilone Plasma Concentrations

CYP3A4 Inhibitors: Coadministration of ixabepilone with ketoconazole, a potent CYP3A4 inhibitor, increased ixabepilone AUC by 79% compared to ixabepilone treatment alone. If alternative treatment cannot be administered, a dose adjustment should be considered. The effect of mild or

Table 5: Hematologic Abnormalities in Patients with Metastatic or Locally Advanced Breast Cancer Treated with IXEMPRA

| Hematology Parameter | Study 046 | | | | Study 081 | |
| | IXEMPRA with capecitabine n=369 | | Capecitabine n=368 | | IXEMPRA monotherapy n=126 | |
	Grade 3 (%)	Grade 4 (%)	Grade 3 (%)	Grade 4 (%)	Grade 3 (%)	Grade 4 (%)
Neutropenia[a]	32	36	9	2	31	23
Leukopenia (WBC)	41	16	5	1	36	13
Anemia (Hgb)	8	2	4	1	6	2
Thrombocytopenia	5	3	2	2	5	2

[a] G-CSF (granulocyte colony stimulating factor) or GM-CSF (granulocyte macrophage colony stimulating factor) was used in 20% and 17% of patients who received IXEMPRA in Study 046 and Study 081, respectively.

moderate inhibitors (eg, erythromycin, fluconazole, or verapamil) on exposure to ixabepilone has not been studied. Therefore, caution should be used when administering mild or moderate CYP3A4 inhibitors during treatment with IXEMPRA (ixabepilone), and alternative therapeutic agents that do not inhibit CYP3A4 should be considered. Patients receiving CYP3A4 inhibitors during treatment with IXEMPRA should be monitored closely for acute toxicities (eg, frequent monitoring of peripheral blood counts between cycles of IXEMPRA) [see Dosage and Administration (2.2)].

Drugs That May Decrease Ixabepilone Plasma Concentrations

CYP3A4 Inducers: IXEMPRA is a CYP3A4 substrate. Coadministration of IXEMPRA with rifampin, a potent CYP3A4 inducer, decreased ixabepilone AUC by 43% compared to IXEMPRA treatment alone. Other strong CYP3A4 inducers (eg, dexamethasone, phenytoin, carbamazepine, rifabutin, and phenobarbital) may also decrease ixabepilone concentrations leading to subtherapeutic levels. Therefore, therapeutic agents with low enzyme induction potential should be considered for coadministration with IXEMPRA. St. John's Wort may decrease ixabepilone plasma concentrations unpredictably and should be avoided. If patients must be coadministered a strong CYP3A4 inducer, a gradual dose adjustment may be considered [see Dosage and Administration (2.2)].

7.2 Effect of Ixabepilone on Other Drugs

Ixabepilone does not inhibit CYP enzymes at relevant clinical concentrations and is not expected to alter the plasma concentrations of other drugs [see Clinical Pharmacology (12.3)].

7.3 Capecitabine

In patients with cancer who received ixabepilone (40 mg/m^2) in combination with capecitabine (1000 mg/m^2), ixabepilone C_{max} decreased by 19%, capecitabine C_{max} decreased by 27%, and 5-fluorouracil AUC increased by 14%, as compared to ixabepilone or capecitabine administered separately. The interaction is not clinically significant given that the combination treatment is supported by efficacy data.

8 USE IN SPECIFIC POPULATIONS

8.1 Pregnancy

Pregnancy Category D [see Warnings and Precautions (5.5)].

8.3 Nursing Mothers

It is not known whether ixabepilone is excreted into human milk. Following intravenous administration of radiolabeled ixabepilone to rats on days 7 to 9 postpartum, concentrations of radioactivity in milk were comparable with those in plasma and declined in parallel with the plasma concentrations. Because many drugs are excreted in human milk and because of the potential for serious adverse reactions in nursing infants from ixabepilone, a decision must be made whether to discontinue nursing or to discontinue IXEMPRA taking into account the importance of the drug to the mother.

8.4 Pediatric Use

The effectiveness of IXEMPRA in pediatric patients has not been established. IXEMPRA was evaluated in one Phase 1 and one Phase 2 trial. The pediatric patients had a safety profile consistent with that seen in adults, and no new safety signals were identified.

In the Phase 1 open-label, dose-finding trial, the safety of IXEMPRA was evaluated in 19 pediatric patients with advanced or refractory solid tumors and 2 with acute leukemias. IXEMPRA was administered as a one-hour IV infusion daily for the first five days of a 21-day cycle at one of 5 dose levels, ranging from 3 to 10 mg/m^2. Among the 21 patients, 12 ranged in age from 2 to 12 years and 9 ranged from 13 to 18 years. The maximum tolerated dose was 8 mg/m^2 IV daily for 5 days every 21 days. No significant activity was observed. The pharmacokinetics of ixabepilone were characterized by population pharmacokinetic analysis of data for 16 patients from this trial, who were aged 2 to 18

years (median 12 years). The pharmacokinetic parameters of ixabepilone in these pediatric patients were compared to the corresponding parameters of 130 adult patients enrolled in clinical trials using the same dosing schedule. The median BSA normalized clearance of ixabepilone in pediatric patients (17 $L/h/m^2$) was similar to that in adult patients (20 $L/h/m^2$).

In the Phase 2 trial of 59 patients with advanced or refractory solid tumors, 28 ranged in age from 3 to 12 years and 19 ranged in age from 13 to 18 years. Twelve additional patients over the age of 18 were treated in this trial. IXEMPRA (ixabepilone) was administered at a dose of 8 mg/m^2 IV for 5 days every 21 days. This trial was terminated early due to lack of efficacy.

8.5 Geriatric Use

Clinical studies of IXEMPRA did not include sufficient numbers of subjects aged sixty-five and over to determine whether they respond differently from younger subjects.

Forty-five of 431 patients treated with IXEMPRA in combination with capecitabine were ≥65 years of age and 3 patients were ≥75. Overall, the incidence of grade 3/4 adverse reactions was higher in patients ≥65 years of age versus those <65 years of age (82% versus 68%) including grade 3/4 stomatitis (9% versus 1%), diarrhea (9% versus 6%), palmar-plantar erythrodysesthesia syndrome (27% versus 20%), peripheral neuropathy (24% versus 22%), febrile neutropenia (9% versus 3%), fatigue (16% versus 12%), and asthenia (11% versus 6%). Toxicity-related deaths occurred in 2 (4.7%) of 43 patients ≥65 years with normal baseline hepatic function or mild impairment.

Thirty-two of 240 breast cancer patients treated with IXEMPRA as monotherapy were ≥65 years of age and 6 patients were ≥75. No overall differences in safety were observed in these patients compared to those <65 years of age.

8.6 Hepatic Impairment

IXEMPRA was evaluated in 56 patients with mild to severe hepatic impairment defined by bilirubin levels and AST levels. Compared to patients with normal hepatic function (n=17), the area under the curve ($AUC_{0-infinity}$) of ixabepilone increased by:
- 22% in patients with a) bilirubin >1 – 1.5 × ULN **or** b) AST >ULN but bilirubin <1.5 × ULN;
- 30% in patients with bilirubin >1.5 – 3 × ULN and any AST level; and
- 81% in patients with bilirubin >3 × ULN and any AST level.

Doses of 10 and 20 mg/m^2 as monotherapy were tolerated in 17 patients with severe hepatic impairment (bilirubin >3 × ULN).

IXEMPRA in combination with capecitabine must not be given to patients with AST or ALT >2.5 × ULN or bilirubin >1 × ULN [see Boxed Warning, Contraindications (4), and Warnings and Precautions (5.3)]. Dose reduction is recommended when administering IXEMPRA as monotherapy to patients with hepatic impairment [see Dosage and Administration (2.3)]. Because there is a need for dosage adjustment based upon hepatic function, assessment of hepatic function is recommended before initiation of IXEMPRA and periodically thereafter.

8.7 Renal Impairment

Ixabepilone is minimally excreted via the kidney. No controlled pharmacokinetic studies were conducted with IXEMPRA in patients with renal impairment. IXEMPRA in combination with capecitabine has not been evaluated in patients with calculated creatinine clearance of <50 mL/min. IXEMPRA as monotherapy has not been evaluated in patients with creatinine >1.5 times ULN. In a population pharmacokinetic analysis of IXEMPRA as monotherapy, there was no meaningful effect of mild and moderate renal insufficiency (CrCL >30 mL/min) on the pharmacokinetics of ixabepilone.

10 OVERDOSAGE

Experience with overdose of IXEMPRA is limited to isolated cases. The adverse reactions reported in these cases included peripheral neuropathy, fatigue, musculoskeletal pain/myalgia, and gastrointestinal symptoms (nausea, anorexia, diarrhea, abdominal pain, stomatitis). The highest dose mistakenly received was 100 mg/m^2 (total dose 185 mg).

There is no known antidote for overdosage of IXEMPRA (ixabepilone). In case of overdosage, the patient should be closely monitored and supportive treatment should be administered. Management of overdose should include supportive medical interventions to treat the presenting clinical manifestations.

11 DESCRIPTION

IXEMPRA (ixabepilone) is a microtubule inhibitor belonging to a class of antineoplastic agents, the epothilones and their analogs. The epothilones are isolated from the myxobacterium *Sorangium cellulosum*. Ixabepilone is a semisynthetic analog of epothilone B, a 16-membered polyketide macrolide, with a chemically modified lactam substitution for the naturally existing lactone.

The chemical name for ixabepilone is (1S,3S,7S,10R, 11S,12S,16R)-7,11-dihydroxy-8,8,10,12,16-pentamethyl-3-[(1E)-1-methyl-2-(2-methyl-4-thiazolyl)ethenyl]-17-oxa-4-azabicyclo[14.1.0] heptadecane-5,9-dione, and it has a molecular weight of 506.7. Ixabepilone has the following structural formula:

IXEMPRA (ixabepilone) for injection is intended for intravenous infusion only after constitution with the supplied DILUENT and after further dilution with a specified infusion fluid *[see Instructions for Preparation and IV Administration (2.4)]*. IXEMPRA (ixabepilone) for injection is supplied as a sterile, non-pyrogenic, single-use vial providing 15 mg or 45 mg ixabepilone as a lyophilized white powder. The DILUENT for IXEMPRA is a sterile, non-pyrogenic solution of 52.8% (w/v) purified polyoxyethylated castor oil and 39.8% (w/v) dehydrated alcohol, USP. The IXEMPRA (ixabepilone) for injection and the DILUENT for IXEMPRA are copackaged and supplied as IXEMPRA *Kit*.

12 CLINICAL PHARMACOLOGY

12.1 Mechanism of Action

Ixabepilone is a semi-synthetic analog of epothilone B. Ixabepilone binds directly to β-tubulin subunits on microtubules, leading to suppression of microtubule dynamics. Ixabepilone suppresses the dynamic instability of αβ–II and αβ–III microtubules. Ixabepilone possesses low *in vitro* susceptibility to multiple tumor resistance mechanisms including efflux transporters, such as MRP-1 and P-glycoprotein (P-gp). Ixabepilone blocks cells in the mitotic phase of the cell division cycle, leading to cell death.

12.2 Pharmacodynamics

In cancer patients, ixabepilone has a plasma concentration-dependent effect on tubulin dynamics in peripheral blood mononuclear cells that is observed as the formation of microtubule bundles. Ixabepilone has antitumor activity *in vivo* against multiple human tumor xenografts, including drug-resistant types that overexpress P-gp, MRP-1, and βIII tubulin isoforms, or harbor tubulin mutations. Ixabepilone is active in xenografts that are resistant to multiple agents including taxanes, anthracyclines, and vinca alkaloids. Ixabepilone demonstrated synergistic antitumor activity in combination with capecitabine *in vivo*. In addition to direct antitumor activity, ixabepilone has antiangiogenic activity.

12.3 Pharmacokinetics

Absorption

Following administration of a single 40 mg/m^2 dose of IXEMPRA in patients with cancer, the mean C_{max} was 252 ng/mL (coefficient of variation, CV 56%) and the mean AUC was 2143 ng•hr/mL (CV 48%). Typically C_{max} occurred at the end of the 3-hour infusion. In cancer patients, the pharmacokinetics of ixabepilone were linear at doses of 15 to 57 mg/m^2.

Distribution

The mean volume of distribution of 40 mg/m^2 ixabepilone at steady-state was in excess of 1000 L. *In vitro*, the binding of ixabepilone to human serum proteins ranged from 67 to 77%, and the blood-to-plasma concentration ratios in human blood ranged from 0.65 to 0.85 over a concentration range of 50 to 5000 ng/mL.

Metabolism

Ixabepilone is extensively metabolized in the liver. *In vitro* studies indicated that the main route of oxidative metabolism of ixabepilone is via CYP3A4. More than 30 metabolites of ixabepilone are excreted into human urine and feces. No single metabolite accounted for more than 6% of the administered dose. The biotransformation products generated

from ixabepilone by human liver microsomes were not active when tested for *in vitro* cytotoxicity against a human tumor cell line.

In vitro studies using human liver microsomes indicate that clinically relevant concentrations of ixabepilone do not inhibit CYP3A4, CYP1A2, CYP2A6, CYP2B6, CYP2C8, CYP2C9, CYP2C19, or CYP2D6. Ixabepilone does not induce the activity or the corresponding mRNA levels of CYP1A2, CYP2B6, CYP2C9, or CYP3A4 in cultured human hepatocytes at clinically relevant concentrations. Therefore, it is unlikely that ixabepilone will affect the plasma levels of drugs that are substrates of CYP enzymes.

Elimination

Ixabepilone is eliminated primarily as metabolized drug. After an intravenous ^{14}[C]-ixabepilone dose to patients, approximately 86% of the dose was eliminated within 7 days in feces (65% of the dose) and in urine (21% of the dose). Unchanged ixabepilone accounted for approximately 1.6% and 5.6% of the dose in feces and urine, respectively. Ixabepilone has a terminal elimination half-life of approximately 52 hours. No accumulation in plasma is expected for ixabepilone administered every 3 weeks.

Drug Transport Systems

Ixabepilone is a substrate and a weak inhibitor for the drug efflux transporter P-glycoprotein (P-gp) *in vitro*.

Ixabepilone is not a substrate for the breast cancer resistance protein (BCRP) *in vitro*.

Effects of Age, Gender, and Race

Based upon a population pharmacokinetic analysis in 676 cancer patients, gender, race, and age do not have meaningful effects on the pharmacokinetics of ixabepilone.

12.4 Effect of Ixabepilone on QT/QTc Interval

The QT prolongation potential of ixabepilone was assessed as part of an uncontrolled, open-label, single-dose study in advanced cancer patients. Fourteen patients received a single dose of IXEMPRA (ixabepilone) 40 mg/m^2 intravenously over 3 hours and serial ECGs were collected over 24 hours. The maximum mean ΔQTcF was observed 1 hour after the end of infusion and was 8 ms (upper 95% CI: 12 ms). No patients had a QTcF interval >450 ms or ΔQTcF >30 ms after IXEMPRA administration. However, small increases in QTc interval with the use of ixabepilone cannot be excluded due to study design limitations.

13 NONCLINICAL TOXICOLOGY

13.1 Carcinogenesis, Mutagenesis, Impairment of Fertility

Carcinogenicity studies with ixabepilone have not been conducted. Ixabepilone did not induce mutations in the microbial mutagenesis (Ames) assay and was not clastogenic in an *in vitro* cytogenetic assay using primary human lymphocytes. Ixabepilone was clastogenic (induction of micronuclei) in the *in vivo* rat micronucleus assay at doses ≥0.625 mg/kg/day.

There were no effects on male or female rat mating or fertility at doses up to 0.2 mg/kg/day in both males and females (approximately one-fifteenth the expected human clinical exposure based on AUC). The effect of ixabepilone on human fertility is unknown. However, when rats were given an IV infusion of ixabepilone during breeding and through the first 7 days of gestation, a significant increase in resorptions and pre- and post-implantation loss and a decrease in the number of corpora lutea was observed at 0.2 mg/kg/day. Testicular atrophy or degeneration was observed in 6-month rat and 9-month dog studies when ixabepilone was given every 21 days at intravenous doses of 6.7 mg/kg (40 mg/m^2) in rats (approximately 2.1 times the expected clinical exposure based on AUC) and 0.5 and 0.75 mg/kg (10 and 15 mg/m^2) in dogs (approximately 0.2 and 0.4 times the expected clinical exposure based on AUC).

13.2 Animal Toxicology

Overdose

In rats, single intravenous doses of ixabepilone from 60 to 180 mg/m^2 (mean AUC values ≥8156 ng·h/mL) were associated with mortality occurring between 5 and 14 days after dosing, and toxicity was principally manifested in the gastrointestinal, hematopoietic (bone-marrow), lymphatic, peripheral-nervous, and male-reproductive systems. In dogs, a single intravenous dose of 100 mg/m^2 (mean AUC value of 6925 ng·h/mL) was markedly toxic, inducing severe gastrointestinal toxicity and death 3 days after dosing.

14 CLINICAL STUDIES

Combination Therapy

In an open-label, multicenter, multinational, randomized trial of 752 patients with metastatic or locally advanced breast cancer, the efficacy and safety of IXEMPRA (40 mg/m^2 every 3 weeks) in combination with capecitabine (at 1000 mg/m^2 twice daily for 2 weeks followed by 1 week rest) were assessed in comparison with capecitabine as monotherapy (at 1250 mg/m^2 twice daily for 2 weeks followed by 1 week rest). Patients were previously treated with anthracyclines and taxanes. Patients were required to have demonstrated tumor progression or resistance to taxanes and anthracyclines as follows:

- tumor progression within 3 months of the last anthracycline dose in the metastatic setting or recurrence within 6 months in the adjuvant or neoadjuvant setting, and
- tumor progression within 4 months of the last taxane dose in the metastatic setting or recurrence within 12 months in the adjuvant or neoadjuvant setting.

For anthracyclines, patients who received a minimum cumulative dose of 240 mg/m^2 of doxorubicin or 360 mg/m^2 of epirubicin were also eligible.

Sixty-seven percent of patients were White, 23% were Asian, and 3% were Black. Both arms were evenly matched with regards to race, age (median 53 years), baseline performance status (Karnofsky 70-100%), and receipt of prior adjuvant or neo-adjuvant chemotherapy (75%). Tumors were ER-positive in 47% of patients, ER-negative in 43%, HER2-positive in 15%, HER2-negative in 61%, and ER-negative, PR-negative, HER2-negative in 25%. The baseline disease characteristics and previous therapies for all patients (n=752) are shown in Table 6.

Table 6: Baseline Disease Characteristics and Previous Therapies

	IXEMPRA with capecitabine n=375	Capecitabine n=377
Site of disease		
Visceral disease (liver or lung)	316 (84%)	315 (84%)
Liver	245 (65%)	228 (61%)
Lung	180 (48%)	174 (46%)
Lymph node	250 (67%)	249 (66%)
Bone	168 (45%)	162 (43%)
Skin/soft tissue	60 (16%)	62 (16%)
Number of prior chemotherapy regimens in metastatic setting[a]		
0	27 (7%)	33 (9%)
1	179 (48%)	184 (49%)
2	152 (41%)	138 (37%)
≥3	17 (5%)	22 (6%)
Anthracycline resistance[b]	164 (44%)	165 (44%)
Taxane Resistance[c]		
Neoadjuvant/adjuvant setting	40 (11%)	44 (12%)
Metastatic setting	327 (87%)	319 (85%)

[a] For IXEMPRA (ixabepilone) plus capecitabine versus capecitabine only, prior treatment in the metastatic setting included cyclophosphamide (25% vs. 23%), fluorouracil (22% vs. 16%), vinorelbine (11% vs. 12%), gemcitabine (9% each arm), carboplatin (9% vs. 7%), liposomal doxorubicin (3% each arm), and cisplatin (2% vs. 3%).
[b] Tumor progression within 3 months in the metastatic setting or recurrence within 6 months in the adjuvant or neoadjuvant setting.
[c] 24% and 21% of patients had received 2 or more taxane-containing regimens in the combination and single agent treatment groups, respectively.

The patients in the combination treatment group received a median of 5 cycles of treatment and patients in the capecitabine monotherapy treatment group received a median of 4 cycles of treatment.

The primary endpoint of the study was progression-free survival (PFS) defined as time from randomization to radiologic progression as determined by Independent Radiologic Review (IRR), clinical progression of measurable skin lesions or death from any cause. Other study endpoints included objective tumor response based on Response Evaluation Criteria in Solid Tumors (RECIST), time to response, response duration, and overall survival.

IXEMPRA in combination with capecitabine resulted in a statistically significant improvement in PFS compared to capecitabine. The results of the study are presented in Table 7 and Figure 1.

Table 7: Efficacy of IXEMPRA in Combination with Capecitabine vs Capecitabine Alone – Intent-to-Treat Analysis

Efficacy Parameter	IXEMPRA with capecitabine n=375	Capecitabine n=377
PFS		
Number of events[a]	242	256
Median	5.7 months	4.1 months
(95% CI)	(4.8 - 6.7)	(3.1 - 4.3)

Hazard Ratio[b] (95% CI)	0.69 (0.58 - 0.83)	
p-value[c] (Log rank)	<0.0001	
Objective Tumor Response Rate	34.7%	14.3%
(95% CI)	(29.9 - 39.7)	(10.9 - 18.3)
p-value[c] (CMH)[d]	<0.0001	
Duration of Response, Median	6.4 months	5.6 months
(95% CI)	(5.6 - 7.1)	(4.2 - 7.5)

[a] Patients were censored for PFS at the last date of tumor assessment prior to the start of subsequent therapy. In patients where independent review was not available PFS was censored at the randomization date.
[b] For the hazard ratio, a value less than 1.00 favors combination treatment.
[c] Stratified by visceral metastasis in liver/lung, prior chemotherapy in metastatic setting, and anthracycline resistance.
[d] Cochran-Mantel-Haenszel test

Figure 1: Progression-free Survival Kaplan Meier Curves

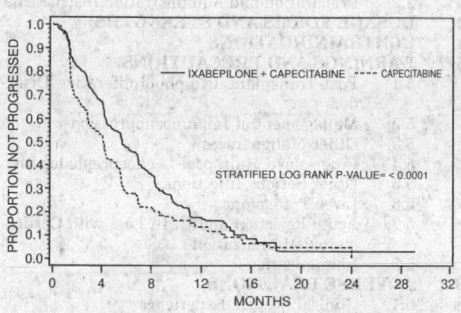

STRATIFIED LOG RANK P-VALUE= < 0.0001

There was no statistically significant difference in overall survival between treatment arms in this study, as well as in a second similar study. In the study described above, the median overall survivals were 12.9 months (95% CI: 11.5, 14.2) in the combination therapy arm and 11.1 months (95% CI: 10.0, 12.5) in the capecitabine alone arm [Hazard Ratio 0.90 (95% CI: 0.77, 1.05), p-value=0.19].

In the second trial, comparing IXEMPRA in combination with capecitabine versus capecitabine alone, conducted in 1221 patients pretreated with an anthracycline and a taxane, the median overall survivals were 16.4 months (95% CI: 15.0, 17.9) in the combination therapy arm and 15.6 months (95% CI: 13.9, 17.0), in the capecitabine alone arm [Hazard Ratio 0.90 (95% CI: 0.78, 1.03), p-value=0.12].

Monotherapy
IXEMPRA (ixabepilone) was evaluated as a single agent in a multicenter single-arm study in 126 women with metastatic or locally advanced breast cancer. The study enrolled patients whose tumors had recurred or had progressed following two or more chemotherapy regimens including an anthracycline, a taxane, and capecitabine. Patients who had received a minimum cumulative dose of 240 mg/m^2 of doxorubicin or 360 mg/m^2 of epirubicin were also eligible. Tumor progression or recurrence were prospectively defined as follows:
- Disease progression while on therapy in the metastatic setting (defined as progression while on treatment or within 8 weeks of last dose),
- Recurrence within 6 months of the last dose in the adjuvant or neoadjuvant setting (only for anthracycline and taxane),
- HER2-positive patients must also have progressed during or after discontinuation of trastuzumab.

In this study, the median age was 51 years (range, 30-78), and 79% were White, 5% Black, and 2% Asian, Karnofsky performance status was 70-100%, 88% had received two or more prior chemotherapy regimens for metastatic disease, and 86% had liver and/or lung metastases. Tumors were ER-positive in 48% of patients, ER-negative in 44%, HER2-positive in 7%, HER2-negative in 72%, and ER-negative, PR-negative, HER2-negative in 33%.

IXEMPRA was administered at a dose of 40 mg/m^2 intravenously over 3 hours every 3 weeks. Patients received a median of 4 cycles (range 1 to 18) of IXEMPRA therapy.

Objective tumor response was determined by independent radiologic and investigator review using RECIST. Efficacy results are presented in Table 8.

Table 8: Efficacy of IXEMPRA in Metastatic and Locally Advanced Breast Cancer

Endpoint	Result
Objective tumor response rate (95% CI)	
IRR Assessment[a] (n=113)	12.4% (6.9 - 19.9)
Investigator Assessment (n=126)	18.3% (11.9 - 26.1)
Time to response[b] (n=14)	
Median, weeks (min - max)	6.1 (5 - 54.4)
Duration of response[b] (n=14)	
Median, months (95% CI)	6.0 (5.0 - 7.6)

[a] All responses were partial.
[b] As assessed by IRR.

15 REFERENCES

1. Preventing Occupational Exposures to Antineoplastic and Other Hazardous Drugs in Health Care Settings. NIOSH Alert 2004-165.
2. OSHA Technical Manual, TED 1-0.15A, Section VI: Chapter 2. Controlling Occupational Exposure to Hazardous Drugs. OSHA, 1999. http://www.osha.gov/dts/osta/otm/otm_vi/otm_vi_2.html
3. American Society of Health-System Pharmacists. ASHP guidelines on handling hazardous drugs. *Am J Health-Syst Pharm.* 2006;63:1172-1193.
4. Polovich, M., White, J.M., & Kelleher, L.O. (eds.) 2005. Chemotherapy and biotherapy guidelines and recommendations for practice (2nd. ed.) Pittsburgh, PA: Oncology Nursing Society.

16 HOW SUPPLIED/STORAGE AND HANDLING

IXEMPRA is supplied as a *Kit* containing one vial of IXEMPRA® (ixabepilone) for injection and one vial of DILUENT for IXEMPRA.

| NDC 0015-1910-12 | IXEMPRA®*Kit* containing one vial of IXEMPRA® (ixabepilone) for injection, 15 mg and one vial of DILUENT for IXEMPRA, 8 mL |
| NDC 0015-1911-13 | IXEMPRA®*Kit* containing one vial of IXEMPRA® (ixabepilone) for injection, 45 mg and one vial of DILUENT for IXEMPRA, 23.5 mL |

IXEMPRA (ixabepilone) *Kit* must be stored in a refrigerator at 2° C to 8° C (36° F to 46° F). Retain in original package until time of use to protect from light.

Procedures for proper handling and disposal of antineoplastic drugs *[see References (15)]* should be followed. To minimize the risk of dermal exposure, impervious gloves should be worn when handling vials containing IXEMPRA, regardless of the setting, including unpacking and inspection, transport within a facility, and dose preparation and administration.

17 PATIENT COUNSELING INFORMATION

[see FDA-Approved Patient Labeling]

17.1 Peripheral Neuropathy
Patients should be advised to report to their physician any numbness and tingling of the hands or feet *[see Warnings and Precautions (5.1)]*.

17.2 Fever/Neutropenia
Patients should be instructed to call their physician if a fever of 100.5° F or greater or other evidence of potential infection such as chills, cough, or burning or pain on urination develops *[see Warnings and Precautions (5.2)]*.

17.3 Hypersensitivity Reactions
Patients should be advised to call their physician if they experience urticaria, pruritus, rash, flushing, swelling, dyspnea, chest tightness, or other hypersensitivity-related symptoms following an infusion of IXEMPRA *[see Warnings and Precautions (5.4)]*.

17.4 Pregnancy
Patients should be advised to use effective contraceptive measures to prevent pregnancy and to avoid nursing during treatment with IXEMPRA *[see Warnings and Precautions (5.5) and Use in Specific Populations (8.1, 8.3)]*.

17.5 Cardiac Adverse Reactions
Patients should be advised to report to their physician chest pain, difficulty breathing, palpitations, or unusual weight gain *[see Warnings and Precautions (5.6)]*.

FDA-Approved Patient Labeling
Patient Information
IXEMPRA®*Kit* (pronounced as ĭk-'sĕm-prä)
(ixabepilone)
for Injection, for intravenous infusion only

Read the Patient Information that comes with IXEMPRA before you start receiving it and before each injection. There

may be new information. This leaflet does not take the place of talking with your healthcare provider about your medical condition or your treatment.

What is the most important information I should know about IXEMPRA?
Your healthcare provider should do blood tests to check your liver function:
- before you begin receiving IXEMPRA (ixabepilone)
- as needed while you are receiving IXEMPRA

If blood tests show that you have liver problems, do not receive injections of IXEMPRA along with the medicine capecitabine. Taking these two medicines together if you have liver problems increases your chance of serious problems. These include: serious infection and death due to a very low white blood cell count (neutropenia).

What is IXEMPRA?
IXEMPRA is a cancer medicine. IXEMPRA is used alone or with another cancer medicine called capecitabine. IXEMPRA is used to treat breast cancer, when certain other medicines have not worked or no longer work.

Who should not receive IXEMPRA?
Do not receive injections of IXEMPRA if you:
- are allergic to a medicine, such as TAXOL®, that contains Cremophor® EL or polyoxyethylated castor oil.
- have low white blood cell or platelet counts. Your healthcare provider will check your blood counts.
- are also taking a cancer medicine called capecitabine and you have liver problems. **See "What is the most important information I should know about IXEMPRA?"**

What should I tell my healthcare provider before receiving IXEMPRA?
IXEMPRA may not be right for you. Before you receive IXEMPRA, tell your healthcare provider about all of your medical conditions, including if you:
- have liver problems
- have heart problems or a history of heart problems
- have had an allergic reaction to IXEMPRA. You will receive medicines before each injection of IXEMPRA to decrease the chance of an allergic reaction. **See "How will I receive IXEMPRA?"**
- are pregnant or plan to become pregnant. You should not receive IXEMPRA during pregnancy because it may harm your unborn baby. Talk with your healthcare provider about how to prevent pregnancy while receiving IXEMPRA. Tell your healthcare provider right away if you become pregnant or think you are pregnant while receiving IXEMPRA.
- are breast-feeding. It is not known if IXEMPRA passes into breast milk. You and your healthcare provider should decide if you will receive IXEMPRA or breast-feed. You should not do both.

Tell your healthcare provider about all the medicines you take, including prescription and non-prescription medicines, vitamins, and herbal supplements.

IXEMPRA and certain other medicines may affect each other causing side effects. IXEMPRA may affect the way other medicines work, and other medicines may affect how IXEMPRA works. Know the medicines you take. Keep a list of your medicines with you to show your healthcare provider.

How will I receive IXEMPRA?
IXEMPRA is given by an injection directly into your vein (intravenous infusion). IXEMPRA is usually given once every three weeks. Each treatment with IXEMPRA will take about 3 hours.

Your healthcare provider will decide how much IXEMPRA you will receive and how often you will receive it.

To lower the chance of allergic reaction, you will receive other medicines about 1 hour before each treatment with IXEMPRA. **See "What are the possible side effects of IXEMPRA?"**

If you have an allergic reaction to IXEMPRA, you will receive a steroid medicine before future doses of IXEMPRA. You may also need to receive your doses of IXEMPRA more slowly.

What should I avoid while receiving IXEMPRA?
IXEMPRA contains alcohol. If you are dizzy or drowsy, avoid activities that may be dangerous, such as driving or operating machinery.

Do not drink grapefruit juice while receiving IXEMPRA. Drinking grapefruit juice may cause you to have too much IXEMPRA in your blood and lead to side effects.

What are the possible side effects of IXEMPRA?
IXEMPRA may cause serious side effects including:
- **Numbness, tingling, or burning in the hands or feet can occur while receiving IXEMPRA (neuropathy).** These symptoms may be new or get worse while you are receiving IXEMPRA. These symptoms often occur early during treatment with IXEMPRA. Tell your healthcare provider if you have any of these symptoms. Your dose of IXEMPRA may need to be decreased, stopped until your symptoms get better, or totally stopped.
- **Low white blood cell count (neutropenia).** White blood cells help protect the body from infections caused by bacteria. If you get a fever or infection when your white blood cells are very low, you can become seriously ill and die. You may need treatment in the hospital with antibiotic medicines. Your healthcare provider will monitor your white blood cell count often with blood tests. Tell your healthcare

provider right away or go to the nearest hospital emergency room if you have a fever (temperature above 100.5° F) or other sign of infection, such as chills, cough, burning or pain when you urinate, any time between treatments with IXEMPRA (ixabepilone).

• **Allergic Reactions.** Severe allergic reactions can occur with IXEMPRA and may cause death in rare cases. Allergic reactions are most likely to occur while IXEMPRA is being injected into your vein. Tell your healthcare provider right away if you get any of the following signs and symptoms of an allergic reaction:
  • itching, hives (raised itchy welts), rash
  • flushed face
  • sudden swelling of face, throat or tongue
  • chest tightness, trouble breathing
  • feel dizzy or faint
  • feel your heart beating (palpitations)
  • **Harm to an unborn child. See "What should I tell my healthcare provider before receiving IXEMPRA?"**
  • **Heart problems.** IXEMPRA might cause decreased blood flow to the heart, problems with heart function, and abnormal heart beat. This is seen more often in patients who also take capecitabine. **Tell your healthcare provider right away if you have any of the following symptoms:**
  • chest pain,
  • difficulty breathing,
  • feel your heart beating (palpitations), or
  • unusual weight gain.

The most common side effects with IXEMPRA used alone or with capecitabine may include:
  • tiredness
  • loss of appetite
  • disorders of toenails and fingernails
  • hair loss
  • fever
  • decreased red blood cells (anemia)
  • joint and muscle pain
  • headache
  • decreased platelets (thrombocytopenia)
  • nausea, vomiting, diarrhea, constipation, and abdominal pain
  • sores on the lip, in the mouth and esophagus
  • tender, red palms and soles of feet (hand-foot syndrome) that looks like a sunburn; the skin may become dry and peel. There may also be numbness and tingling.

Tell your healthcare provider about any side effect that bothers you or that does not go away.

These are not all the side effects of IXEMPRA. Ask your healthcare provider or pharmacist for more information if you have questions or concerns.

General information about IXEMPRA

This patient information leaflet summarizes the most important information about IXEMPRA. Medicines are sometimes prescribed for purposes other than those listed in a Patient Information Leaflet. If you would like more information about IXEMPRA, talk with your healthcare provider. You can ask your healthcare provider or pharmacist for information about IXEMPRA that is written for health professionals. For more information about IXEMPRA, call 1–888–IXEMPRA.

IXEMPRA® (ixabepilone) for injection Manufactured by: Baxter Oncology GmbH, 33790 Halle/Westfalen, Germany DILUENT for IXEMPRA Manufactured by: Baxter Oncology GmbH, 33790 Halle/Westfalen, Germany Distributed by Bristol-Myers Squibb Company, Princeton, NJ 08543 USA

1236925A7
5645-0006
Rev October 2011

Shown in Product Identification Guide, page 306

NULOJIX   ℞
[noo-LOJ-jiks]
(belatacept)
For injection, for intravenous use

HIGHLIGHTS OF PRESCRIBING INFORMATION
These highlights do not include all the information needed to use NULOJIX safely and effectively. See full prescribing information for NULOJIX.
NULOJIX (belatacept)
For injection, for intravenous use
Initial U.S. Approval: 2011

WARNING: POST-TRANSPLANT LYMPHOPROLIFERATIVE DISORDER, OTHER MALIGNANCIES, AND SERIOUS INFECTIONS
See full prescribing information for complete boxed warning.
• **Increased risk for developing post-transplant lymphoproliferative disorder (PTLD), predominantly involving the central nervous system (CNS). Recipi-**

ents without immunity to Epstein-Barr virus (EBV) are at a particularly increased risk; therefore, use in EBV seropositive patients only. Do not use NULOJIX in transplant recipients who are EBV seronegative or with unknown serostatus. (4, 5.1)
• **Only physicians experienced in immunosuppressive therapy and management of kidney transplant patients should prescribe NULOJIX. (5.2)**
• **Increased susceptibility to infection and the possible development of malignancies may result from immunosuppression. (5.1, 5.3, 5.4, 5.5)**
• **Use in liver transplant patients is not recommended due to an increased risk of graft loss and death. (5.6)**

INDICATIONS AND USAGE
• NULOJIX (belatacept) is a selective T-cell costimulation blocker indicated for prophylaxis of organ rejection in adult patients receiving a kidney transplant. (1.1)
• Use in combination with basiliximab induction, mycophenolate mofetil, and corticosteroids. (1.1)
Limitations of Use:
• Use only in patients who are EBV seropositive. (1.2, 4, 5.1)
• Use has not been established for the prophylaxis of organ rejection in transplanted organs other than the kidney. (1.2, 5.6)

DOSAGE AND ADMINISTRATION
• Use of higher than recommended or more frequent dosing is not recommended due to increased risk of serious infections and malignancy. (5.1, 5.4, 6.1)
• For complete dosing instructions, see full prescribing information. (2.1)

Dosing of NULOJIX for Kidney Transplant Recipients (2.1)

Dosing for Initial Phase	Dose
Day 1 (day of transplantation, prior to implantation) and Day 5 (approximately 96 hours after Day 1 dose)	10 mg per kg
End of Week 2 and Week 4 after transplantation	10 mg per kg
End of Week 8 and Week 12 after transplantation	10 mg per kg

Dosing for Maintenance Phase	Dose
End of Week 16 after transplantation and every 4 weeks (plus or minus 3 days) thereafter	5 mg per kg

• For intravenous infusion only; administer over 30 minutes. (2.1, 2.2)
• Only use the enclosed *silicone-free disposable syringe* to prepare for administration. (2.2)

DOSAGE FORMS AND STRENGTHS
• Lyophilized powder for injection: 250 mg per vial (3)

CONTRAINDICATIONS
• Patients who are EBV seronegative or with unknown EBV serostatus. (4)

WARNINGS AND PRECAUTIONS
• Post-Transplant Lymphoproliferative Disorder (PTLD): increased risk, predominantly involving the CNS; monitor for new or worsening neurological, cognitive, or behavioral signs and symptoms. (Boxed Warning, 4, 5.1, 5.6)
• Other malignancies: increased risk with all immunosuppressants; appears related to intensity and duration of use. Avoid prolonged exposure to UV light and sunlight. (5.3)
• Progressive Multifocal Leukoencephalopathy (PML): increased risk; consider in the diagnosis of patients reporting new or worsening neurological, cognitive, or behavioral signs and symptoms. Recommended doses of immunosuppressants should not be exceeded. (5.4)
• Other serious infections: increased risk of bacterial, viral, fungal, and protozoal infections, including opportunistic infections and tuberculosis. Some infections were fatal. Polyoma virus-associated nephropathy can lead to kidney graft loss; consider reduction in immunosuppression. Evaluate for tuberculosis and initiate treatment for latent infection prior to NULOJIX use. Cytomegalovirus and pneumocystis prophylaxis are recommended after transplantation. (5.1, 5.4, 5.5)
• Liver transplant: use is not recommended. (5.6)
• Acute Rejection and Graft Loss with Corticosteroid Minimization: corticosteroid utilization should be consistent with the NULOJIX clinical trial experience. (2.1, 5.7, 14.1)
• Immunizations: avoid use of live vaccines during treatment. (5.8)

ADVERSE REACTIONS
Most common adverse reactions (≥20% on NULOJIX (belatacept) treatment) are anemia, diarrhea, urinary tract infection, peripheral edema, constipation, hypertension, pyrexia, graft dysfunction, cough, nausea, vomiting, headache, hypokalemia, hyperkalemia, and leukopenia. (6.1)
To report SUSPECTED ADVERSE REACTIONS, contact Bristol-Myers Squibb at 1-800-721-5072 or FDA at 1-800-FDA-1088 or *www.fda.gov/medwatch*

USE IN SPECIFIC POPULATIONS
• Pregnancy: Based on animal data, may cause fetal harm; pregnancy registry available. (8.1)
• Nursing Mothers: Discontinue drug or nursing, taking into consideration importance of drug to mother. (8.3)

See 17 for PATIENT COUNSELING INFORMATION and Medication Guide

Revised: 05/2014

FULL PRESCRIBING INFORMATION: CONTENTS*
WARNING: POST-TRANSPLANT LYMPHOPROLIFERATIVE DISORDER, OTHER MALIGNANCIES, AND SERIOUS INFECTIONS

FULL PRESCRIBING INFORMATION

WARNING: POST-TRANSPLANT LYMPHOPROLIFERATIVE DISORDER, OTHER MALIGNANCIES, AND SERIOUS INFECTIONS

Increased risk for developing post-transplant lymphoproliferative disorder (PTLD), predominantly involving the central nervous system (CNS). Recipients without immunity to Epstein-Barr virus (EBV) are at a particularly increased risk; therefore, use in EBV seropositive patients only. Do not use NULOJIX in transplant recipients who are EBV seronegative or with unknown EBV serostatus [see *Contraindications (4)* and *Warnings and Precautions (5.1)*].

Only physicians experienced in immunosuppressive therapy and management of kidney transplant patients should prescribe NULOJIX. Patients receiving the drug should be managed in facilities equipped and staffed with adequate laboratory and supportive medical resources. The physician responsible for maintenance therapy should have complete information requisite for the follow-up of the patient [see *Warnings and Precautions (5.2)*].

Increased susceptibility to infection and the possible development of malignancies may result from immunosuppression [see *Warnings and Precautions (5.1, 5.3, 5.4, 5.5)*].

Use in liver transplant patients is not recommended due to an increased risk of graft loss and death [see *Warnings and Precautions (5.6)*].

1 INDICATIONS AND USAGE

1.1 Adult Kidney Transplant Recipients
NULOJIX® (belatacept) is indicated for prophylaxis of organ rejection in adult patients receiving a kidney transplant. NULOJIX is to be used in combination with basiliximab induction, mycophenolate mofetil, and corticosteroids.

1.2 Limitations of Use
Use NULOJIX only in patients who are EBV seropositive [see *Contraindications (4)* and *Warnings and Precautions (5.1)*].

Use of NULOJIX for the prophylaxis of organ rejection in transplanted organs other than kidney has not been established [see *Warnings and Precautions (5.6)*].

2 DOSAGE AND ADMINISTRATION

2.1 Dosage in Adult Kidney Transplant Recipients
NULOJIX should be administered in combination with basiliximab induction, mycophenolate mofetil (MMF), and corticosteroids. In clinical trials the median (25th-75th percentile) corticosteroid doses were tapered to approximately 15 mg (10-20 mg) per day by the first 6 weeks and remained at approximately 10 mg (5-10 mg) per day for the first 6 months post-transplant. Corticosteroid utilization should be consistent with the NULOJIX clinical trial experience [see *Warnings and Precautions (5.7)* and *Clinical Studies (14.1)*]. Due to an increased risk of post-transplant lymphoproliferative disorder (PTLD) predominantly involving the central nervous system (CNS), progressive multifocal leukoencephalopathy (PML), and serious CNS infections, administration of higher than the recommended doses or more frequent dosing of NULOJIX is not recommended [see *Warnings and Precautions (5.1, 5.4, 5.5)* and *Adverse Reactions (6.1)*].

NULOJIX is for intravenous infusion only. Patients do not require premedication prior to administration of NULOJIX. Dosing instructions are provided in Table 1.

- The total infusion dose of NULOJIX should be based on the actual body weight of the patient at the time of transplantation, and should not be modified during the course of therapy, unless there is a change in body weight of greater than 10%.
- The prescribed dose of NULOJIX must be evenly divisible by 12.5 mg in order for the dose to be prepared accurately using the reconstituted solution and the *silicone-free disposable syringe* provided. Evenly divisible increments are 0, 12.5, 25, 37.5, 50, 62.5, 75, 87.5, and 100. For example:
  - *A patient weighs 64 kg. The dose is 10 mg per kg.*
  - *Calculated Dose: 64 kg × 10 mg per kg = 640 mg*
  - *The closest doses evenly divisible by 12.5 mg below and above 640 mg are 637.5 mg and 650 mg.*
  - *The nearest dose to 640 mg is 637.5 mg.*
  - *Therefore, the actual prescribed dose for the patient should be 637.5 mg.*

Table 1: Dosing*,† of NULOJIX for Kidney Transplant Recipients

Dosing for Initial Phase	Dose
Day 1 (day of transplantation, prior to implantation) and Day 5 (approximately 96 hours after Day 1 dose)	10 mg per kg
End of Week 2 and Week 4 after transplantation	10 mg per kg
End of Week 8 and Week 12 after transplantation	10 mg per kg

Dosing for Maintenance Phase	Dose
End of Week 16 after transplantation and every 4 weeks (plus or minus 3 days) thereafter	5 mg per kg

* [See *Clinical Studies (14.1)*.]
† The dose prescribed for the patient must be evenly divisible by 12.5 mg (see instructions above; e.g., evenly divisible increments are 0, 12.5, 25, 37.5, 50, 62.5, 75, 87.5, and 100).

2.2 Preparation and Administration Instructions
NULOJIX is for intravenous infusion only.

Caution: NULOJIX (belatacept) must be reconstituted/prepared using only the *silicone-free disposable syringe* provided with each vial.

If the *silicone-free disposable syringe* is dropped or becomes contaminated, use a new *silicone-free disposable syringe* from inventory. For information on obtaining additional *silicone-free disposable syringes*, contact Bristol-Myers Squibb at 1-888-NULOJIX.

Preparation for Administration
1. Calculate the number of NULOJIX vials required to provide the total infusion dose. Each vial contains 250 mg of belatacept lyophilized powder.
2. Reconstitute the contents of each vial of NULOJIX with 10.5 mL of a suitable diluent using the *silicone-free disposable syringe* provided with each vial and an 18- to 21-gauge needle. Suitable diluents include: sterile water for injection (SWFI), 0.9% sodium chloride (NS), or 5% dextrose in water (D5W).
   Note: If the NULOJIX powder is accidentally reconstituted using a different syringe than the one provided, the solution may develop a few translucent particles. Discard any solutions prepared using siliconized syringes.
3. To reconstitute the NULOJIX powder, remove the flip-top from the vial and wipe the top with an alcohol swab. Insert the syringe needle into the vial through the center of the rubber stopper and direct the stream of diluent (10.5 mL of SWFI, NS, or D5W) to the glass wall of the vial.
4. To minimize foam formation, rotate the vial and invert with gentle swirling until the contents are completely dissolved. Avoid prolonged or vigorous agitation. Do not shake.
5. The reconstituted solution contains a belatacept concentration of 25 mg/mL and should be clear to slightly opalescent and colorless to pale yellow. Do not use if opaque particles, discoloration, or other foreign particles are present.
6. Calculate the total volume of the reconstituted 25 mg/mL NULOJIX solution required to provide the total infusion dose.
   Volume of 25 mg/mL NULOJIX solution (in mL) = Prescribed Dose (in mg) ÷ 25 mg/mL
7. Prior to intravenous infusion, the required volume of the reconstituted NULOJIX solution must be further diluted with a suitable infusion fluid (NS or D5W). NULOJIX reconstituted with:
   - SWFI should be further diluted with either NS or D5W
   - NS should be further diluted with NS
   - D5W should be further diluted with D5W
8. From the appropriate size infusion bag or bottle, withdraw a volume of infusion fluid that is equal to the volume of the reconstituted NULOJIX solution required to provide the prescribed dose. With the same *silicone-free disposable syringe* used for reconstitution, withdraw the required amount of belatacept solution from the vial, inject it into the infusion bag or bottle, and gently rotate the infusion bag or bottle to ensure mixing.
   The final belatacept concentration in the infusion bag or bottle should range from 2 mg/mL to 10 mg/mL. Typically, an infusion volume of 100 mL will be appropriate for most patients and doses, but total infusion volumes ranging from 50 mL to 250 mL may be used. Any unused solution remaining in the vials must be discarded.
9. Prior to administration, the NULOJIX infusion should be inspected visually for particulate matter and discoloration. Discard the infusion if any particulate matter or discoloration is observed.
10. The entire NULOJIX infusion should be administered over a period of 30 minutes and must be administered with an infusion set and a sterile, non-pyrogenic, low-protein-binding filter (with a pore size of 0.2-1.2 µm).
    - The reconstituted solution should be transferred from the vial to the infusion bag or bottle immediately. The NULOJIX infusion must be completed within 24 hours of reconstitution of the NULOJIX lyophilized powder. If not used immediately, the infusion solution may be stored under refrigeration conditions: 2°-8°C (36°-46°F) and protected from light for up to 24 hours (a maximum of 4 hours of the total 24 hours can be at room temperature: 20°-25°C [68°-77°F] and room light).
    - Infuse NULOJIX in a separate line from other concomitantly infused agents. NULOJIX should not be infused concomitantly in the same intravenous line with other agents. No physical or biochemical compatibility studies have been conducted to evaluate the coadministration of NULOJIX with other agents.

3 DOSAGE FORMS AND STRENGTHS
Lyophilized powder for injection: 250 mg per vial.

4 CONTRAINDICATIONS
NULOJIX is contraindicated in transplant recipients who are Epstein-Barr virus (EBV) seronegative or with un-

known EBV serostatus due to the risk of post-transplant lymphoproliferative disorder (PTLD), predominantly involving the central nervous system (CNS) [see *Boxed Warning* and *Warnings and Precautions (5.1)*].

5 WARNINGS AND PRECAUTIONS

5.1 Post-Transplant Lymphoproliferative Disorder
NULOJIX (belatacept)-treated patients have an increased risk for developing post-transplant lymphoproliferative disorder (PTLD), predominantly involving the CNS, compared to patients on a cyclosporine-based regimen [see *Adverse Reactions (6.1)* and *Table 2*]. As the total burden of immunosuppression is a risk factor for PTLD, higher than the recommended doses or more frequent dosing of NULOJIX and higher than recommended doses of concomitant immunosuppressive agents are not recommended [see *Dosage and Administration (2.1)* and *Warnings and Precautions (5.6)*]. Physicians should consider PTLD in patients reporting new or worsening neurological, cognitive, or behavioral signs or symptoms.

EBV Serostatus
The risk of PTLD was higher in EBV seronegative patients compared to EBV seropositive patients. EBV seropositive patients are defined as having evidence of acquired immunity shown by the presence of IgG antibodies to viral capsid antigen (VCA) and EBV nuclear antigen (EBNA).

Epstein-Barr virus serology should be ascertained before starting administration of NULOJIX, and only patients who are EBV seropositive should receive NULOJIX. Transplant recipients who are EBV seronegative, or with unknown serostatus, should not receive NULOJIX [see *Boxed Warning* and *Contraindications (4)*].

Other Risk Factors
Other known risk factors for PTLD include cytomegalovirus (CMV) infection and T-cell-depleting therapy. T-cell-depleting therapies to treat acute rejection should be used cautiously. CMV prophylaxis is recommended for at least 3 months after transplantation [see *Warnings and Precautions (5.5)*].

Patients who are EBV seropositive and CMV seronegative may be at increased risk for PTLD compared to patients who are EBV seropositive and CMV seropositive [see *Adverse Reactions (6.1)*]. Since CMV seronegative patients are at increased risk for CMV disease (a known risk factor for PTLD), the clinical significance of CMV serology for PTLD remains to be determined; however, these findings should be considered when prescribing NULOJIX.

5.2 Management of Immunosuppression
Only physicians experienced in management of systemic immunosuppressant therapy in transplantation should prescribe NULOJIX. Patients receiving the drug should be managed in facilities equipped and staffed with adequate laboratory and supportive medical resources. The physician responsible for the maintenance therapy should have complete information requisite for the follow-up of the patient [see *Boxed Warning*].

5.3 Other Malignancies
Patients receiving immunosuppressants, including NULOJIX, are at increased risk of developing malignancies, in addition to PTLD, including the skin [see *Boxed Warning* and *Warnings and Precautions (5.1)*]. Exposure to sunlight and ultraviolet (UV) light should be limited by wearing protective clothing and using a sunscreen with a high protection factor.

5.4 Progressive Multifocal Leukoencephalopathy
Progressive multifocal leukoencephalopathy (PML) is an often rapidly progressive and fatal opportunistic infection of the CNS that is caused by the JC virus, a human polyoma virus. In clinical trials with NULOJIX, two cases of PML were reported in patients receiving NULOJIX at higher cumulative doses and more frequently than the recommended regimen, along with mycophenolate mofetil (MMF) and corticosteroids; one case occurred in a kidney transplant recipient and the second case occurred in a liver transplant recipient [see *Warnings and Precautions (5.6)*]. As PML has been associated with high levels of overall immunosuppression, the recommended doses and frequency of NULOJIX and concomitant immunosuppressives, including MMF, should not be exceeded.

Physicians should consider PML in the differential diagnosis in patients with new or worsening neurological, cognitive, or behavioral signs or symptoms. PML is usually diagnosed by brain imaging, cerebrospinal fluid (CSF) testing for JC viral DNA by polymerase chain reaction (PCR), and/or brain biopsy. Consultation with a specialist (e.g., neurologist and/or infectious disease) should be considered for any suspected or confirmed cases of PML.

If PML is diagnosed, consideration should be given to reduction or withdrawal of immunosuppression taking into account the risk to the allograft.

5.5 Other Serious Infections
Patients receiving immunosuppressants, including NULOJIX, are at increased risk of developing bacterial, viral (cytomegalovirus [CMV] and herpes), fungal, and proto-

Table 2: Summary of PTLD Reported in Studies 1, 2, and 3 Through Three Years of Treatment

Trial	NULOJIX Non-Recommended Regimen* (N=477)			NULOJIX Recommended Regimen† (N=472)			Cyclosporine (N=476)		
	EBV Positive (n=406)	EBV Negative (n=43)	EBV Unknown (n=28)	EBV Positive (n=404)	EBV Negative (n=48)	EBV Unknown (n=20)	EBV Positive (n=399)	EBV Negative (n=57)	EBV Unknown (n=20)
Study 1									
CNS PTLD	1	1							
Non-CNS PTLD		1		2				1	
Study 2									
CNS PTLD	1	1		1	1				
Non-CNS PTLD									
Study 3									
CNS PTLD		2							
Non-CNS PTLD			1						
Total (%)	2 (0.5)	5 (11.6)	1 (3.6)	3 (0.7)	2 (4.1)	0	0	1 (1.8)	0

* Regimen with higher cumulative dose and more frequent dosing than the recommended NULOJIX regimen.
† In Studies 1 and 2 the NULOJIX regimen is identical to the recommended regimen, but is slightly different in Study 3.

zoal infections, including opportunistic infections. These infections may lead to serious, including fatal, outcomes [see *Boxed Warning* and *Adverse Reactions (6.1)*].
Prophylaxis for cytomegalovirus is recommended for at least 3 months after transplantation. Prophylaxis for *Pneumocystis jiroveci* is recommended after transplantation.

Tuberculosis
Tuberculosis was more frequently observed in patients receiving NULOJIX (belatacept) than cyclosporine in clinical trials [see *Adverse Reactions (6.1)*]. Patients should be evaluated for tuberculosis and tested for latent infection prior to initiating NULOJIX. Treatment of latent tuberculosis infection should be initiated prior to NULOJIX use.

Polyoma Virus Nephropathy
In addition to cases of JC virus-associated PML [see *Warnings and Precautions (5.4)*], cases of polyoma virus-associated nephropathy (PVAN), mostly due to BK virus infection, have been reported. PVAN is associated with serious outcomes; including deteriorating renal function and kidney graft loss [see *Adverse Reactions (6.1)*]. Patient monitoring may help detect patients at risk for PVAN. Reductions in immunosuppression should be considered for patients who develop evidence of PVAN. Physicians should also consider the risk that reduced immunosuppression represents to the functioning allograft.

5.6   Liver Transplant
Use of NULOJIX in liver transplant patients is not recommended [see *Boxed Warning*]. In a clinical trial of liver transplant patients, use of NULOJIX regimens with more frequent administration of belatacept than any of those studied in kidney transplant, along with mycophenolate mofetil (MMF) and corticosteroids, was associated with a higher rate of graft loss and death compared to the tacrolimus control arms. In addition, two cases of PTLD involving the liver allograft (one fatal) and one fatal case of PML were observed among the 147 patients randomized to NULOJIX. The two cases of PTLD were reported among the 140 EBV seropositive patients (1.4%). The fatal case of PML was reported in a patient receiving higher than recommended doses of NULOJIX and MMF [see *Warnings and Precautions (5.4)*].

5.7   Acute Rejection and Graft Loss with Corticosteroid Minimization
In postmarketing experience, use of NULOJIX in conjunction with basiliximab induction, MMF, and corticosteroid minimization to 5 mg per day between Day 3 and Week 6 post-transplant was associated with an increased rate and grade of acute rejection, particularly Grade III rejection. These Grade III rejections occurred in patients with 4 to 6 HLA mismatches. Graft loss was a consequence of Grade III rejection in some patients.
Corticosteroid utilization should be consistent with the NULOJIX clinical trial experience [see *Dosage and Administration (2.1)* and *Clinical Studies (14.1)*].

5.8   Immunizations
The use of live vaccines should be avoided during treatment with NULOJIX, including but not limited to the following: intranasal influenza, measles, mumps, rubella, oral polio, BCG, yellow fever, varicella, and TY21a typhoid vaccines.

6   ADVERSE REACTIONS
The most serious adverse reactions reported with NULOJIX (belatacept) are:
• PTLD, predominantly CNS PTLD, and other malignancies [see *Boxed Warning* and *Warnings and Precautions (5.1, 5.3)*]
• Serious infections, including JC virus-associated PML and polyoma virus nephropathy [see *Warnings and Precautions (5.4, 5.5, 5.6)*]

6.1   Clinical Studies Experience
The data described below primarily derive from two randomized, active-controlled three-year trials of NULOJIX in *de novo* kidney transplant patients. In Study 1 and Study 2, NULOJIX was studied at the recommended dose and frequency [see *Dosage and Administration (2.1)*] in a total of 401 patients compared to a cyclosporine control regimen in a total of 405 patients. These two trials also included a total of 403 patients treated with a NULOJIX regimen of higher cumulative dose and more frequent dosing than recommended [see *Clinical Studies (14.1)*]. All patients also received basiliximab induction, mycophenolate mofetil, and corticosteroids. Patients were treated and followed for 3 years.
CNS PTLD, PML, and other CNS infections were more frequently observed in association with a NULOJIX regimen of higher cumulative dose and more frequent dosing compared to the recommended regimen; therefore, administration of higher than the recommended doses and/or more frequent dosing of NULOJIX is not recommended [see *Dosage and Administration (2.1)*].
The average age of patients in Studies 1 and 2 in the NULOJIX recommended dose and cyclosporine control regimens was 49 years, ranging from 18 to 79 years. Approximately 70% of patients were male; 67% were white, 11% were black, and 22% other races. About 25% of patients were from the United States and 75% from other countries. Because clinical trials are conducted under widely varying conditions, the adverse reaction rates observed cannot be directly compared to rates in other trials and may not reflect the rates observed in clinical practice.
The most commonly reported adverse reactions occurring in ≥20% of patients treated with the recommended dose and frequency of NULOJIX were anemia, diarrhea, urinary tract infection, peripheral edema, constipation, hypertension, pyrexia, graft dysfunction, cough, nausea, vomiting, headache, hypokalemia, hyperkalemia, and leukopenia.
The proportion of patients who discontinued treatment due to adverse reactions was 13% for the recommended NULOJIX regimen and 19% for the cyclosporine control arm through three years of treatment. The most common adverse reactions leading to discontinuation in NULOJIX-treated patients were cytomegalovirus infection (1.5%) and complications of transplanted kidney (1.5%).
Information on selected significant adverse reactions observed during clinical trials is summarized below.

Post-Transplant Lymphoproliferative Disorder
Reported cases of post-transplant lymphoproliferative disorder (PTLD) up to 36 months post transplant were obtained

for NULOJIX (belatacept) by pooling both dosage regimens of NULOJIX in Studies 1 and 2 (804 patients) with data from a third study in kidney transplantation (Study 3, 145 patients) which evaluated two NULOJIX dosage regimens similar, but slightly different, from those of Studies 1 and 2 (see Table 2). The total number of NULOJIX patients from these three studies (949) was compared to the pooled cyclosporine control groups from all three studies (476 patients). Among 401 patients in Studies 1 and 2 treated with the recommended regimen of NULOJIX and the 71 patients in Study 3 treated with a very similar (but non-identical) NULOJIX regimen, there were 5 cases of PTLD: 3 in EBV seropositive patients and 2 in EBV seronegative patients. Two of the 5 cases presented with CNS involvement.
Among the 477 patients in Studies 1, 2, and 3 treated with the NULOJIX regimen of higher cumulative dose and more frequent dosing than recommended, there were 8 cases of PTLD: 2 in EBV seropositive patients and 6 in EBV seronegative or serostatus unknown patients. Six of the 8 cases presented with CNS involvement. Therefore, administration of higher than the recommended doses or more frequent dosing of NULOJIX is not recommended. [See *Dosage and Administration (2.1)* and *Warnings and Precautions (5.1)*.]
One of the 476 patients treated with cyclosporine developed PTLD, without CNS involvement.
All cases of PTLD reported up to 36 months post transplant in NULOJIX- or cyclosporine-treated patients presented within 18 months of transplantation.
Overall, the rate of PTLD in 949 patients treated with any of the NULOJIX regimens was 9-fold higher in those who were EBV seronegative or EBV serostatus unknown (8/139) compared to those who were EBV seropositive (5/810 patients). Therefore NULOJIX is recommended for use only in patients who are EBV seropositive [see *Boxed Warning* and *Contraindications (4)*].

[See table 2 above]

EBV Seropositive Subpopulation
Among the 806 EBV seropositive patients with known CMV serostatus treated with either NULOJIX regimen in Studies 1, 2, and 3, two percent (2%; 4/210) of CMV seronegative patients developed PTLD compared to 0.2% (1/596) of CMV seropositive patients. Among the 404 EBV seropositive recipients treated with the recommended dosage regimen of NULOJIX, three PTLD cases were detected among 99 CMV seronegative patients (3%) and there was no case detected among 303 CMV seropositive patients. The clinical significance of CMV serology as a risk factor for PTLD remains to be determined; however, these findings should be considered when prescribing NULOJIX [see *Warnings and Precautions (5.1)*].

Other Malignancies
Malignancies, excluding non-melanoma skin cancer and PTLD, were reported in Study 1 and Study 2 in 3.5% (14/401) of patients treated with the recommended NULOJIX regimen and 3.7% (15/405) of patients treated with the cyclosporine control regimen. Non-melanoma skin cancer was reported in 1.5% (6/401) of patients treated with the recommended NULOJIX regimen and in 3.7% (15/405) of patients treated with cyclosporine [see *Warnings and Precautions (5.3)*].

Progressive Multifocal Leukoencephalopathy
Two fatal cases of progressive multifocal leukoencephalopathy (PML) have been reported among 1096 patients treated with a NULOJIX-containing regimen: one patient in clinical trials of kidney transplant (Studies 1, 2, and 3 described above) and one patient in a trial of liver transplant (trial of 250 patients). No cases of PML were reported in patients treated with the recommended NULOJIX regimen or the control regimen in these trials.
The kidney transplant recipient was treated with the NULOJIX regimen of higher cumulative dose and more frequent dosing than recommended, mycophenolate mofetil (MMF), and corticosteroids for 2 years. The liver transplant recipient was treated with 6 months of a NULOJIX dosage regimen that was more intensive than that studied in kidney transplant recipients, MMF at doses higher than the recommended dose, and corticosteroids [see *Warnings and Precautions (5.4)*].

Bacterial, Mycobacterial, Viral, and Fungal Infections
Adverse reactions of infectious etiology were reported based on clinical assessment by physicians. The causative organisms for these reactions are identified when provided by the physician. The overall number of infections, serious infections, and select infections with identified etiology reported in patients treated with the NULOJIX recommended regimen or the cyclosporine control in Studies 1 and 2 are shown in Table 3. Fungal infections were reported in 18% of patients receiving NULOJIX compared to 22% receiving cyclosporine, primarily due to skin and mucocutaneous fungal infections. Tuberculosis and herpes infections were reported more frequently in patients receiving NULOJIX than cyclosporine. Of the patients who developed tuberculosis through

3 years, all but one NULOJIX (belatacept) patient lived in countries with a high prevalence of tuberculosis [see *Warnings and Precautions (5.5)*].
[See table 3 above]

Infections Reported in the CNS

Following three years of treatment in Studies 1 and 2, cryptococcal meningitis was reported in one patient out of 401 patients treated with the NULOJIX recommended regimen (0.2%) and one patient out of the 405 treated with the cyclosporine control (0.2%).

Six patients out of the 403 who were treated with the NULOJIX regimen of higher cumulative dose and more frequent dosing than recommended in Studies 1 and 2 (1.5%) were reported to have developed CNS infections, including 2 cases of cryptococcal meningitis, one case of Chagas encephalitis with cryptococcal meningitis, one case of cerebral aspergillosis, one case of West Nile encephalitis, and one case of PML (discussed above).

Infusion Reactions

There were no reports of anaphylaxis or drug hypersensitivity in patients treated with NULOJIX in Studies 1 and 2 through three years.

Infusion-related reactions within one hour of infusion were reported in 5% of patients treated with the recommended dose of NULOJIX, similar to the placebo rate. No serious events were reported through Year 3. The most frequent reactions were hypotension and hypertension.

Proteinuria

At Month 1 after transplantation in Studies 1 and 2, the frequency of 2+ proteinuria on urine dipstick in patients treated with the NULOJIX recommended regimen was 33% (130/390) and 28% (107/384) in patients treated with the cyclosporine control regimen. The frequency of 2+ proteinuria was similar between the two treatment groups between one and three years after transplantation (<10% in both studies). There were no differences in the occurrence of 3+ proteinuria (<4% in both studies) at any time point, and no patients experienced 4+ proteinuria. The clinical significance of this increase in early proteinuria is unknown.

Immunogenicity

Antibodies directed against the belatacept molecule were assessed in 398 patients treated with the NULOJIX recommended regimen in Studies 1 and 2 (212 of these patients were treated for at least 2 years). Of the 372 patients with immunogenicity assessment at baseline (prior to receiving belatacept treatment), 29 patients tested positive for anti-belatacept antibodies; 13 of these patients had antibodies to the modified cytotoxic T-lymphocyte-associated antigen 4 (CTLA-4). Anti-belatacept antibody titers did not increase during treatment in these 29 patients.

Eight (2%) patients developed antibodies during treatment with the NULOJIX recommended regimen. In the patients who developed antibodies during treatment, the median titer (by dilution method) was 8, with a range of 5 to 80. Of 56 patients who tested negative for antibodies during treatment and reassessed approximately 7 half-lives after discontinuation of NULOJIX, 1 tested antibody positive. Anti-belatacept antibody development was not associated with altered clearance of belatacept.

Samples from 6 patients with confirmed binding activity to the modified cytotoxic T-lymphocyte-associated antigen 4 (CTLA-4) region of the belatacept molecule were assessed by an *in vitro* bioassay for the presence of neutralizing antibodies. Three of these 6 patients tested positive for neutralizing antibodies. However, the development of neutralizing antibodies may be underreported due to lack of assay sensitivity.

The clinical impact of anti-belatacept antibodies (including neutralizing anti-belatacept antibodies) could not be determined in the studies.

The data reflect the percentage of patients whose test results were positive for antibodies to belatacept in specific assays. The observed incidence of antibody (including neutralizing antibody) positivity in an assay may be influenced by several factors including assay sensitivity and specificity, assay methodology, sample handling, timing of sample collection, concomitant medications, and underlying disease. For these reasons, comparison of the incidence of antibodies to belatacept with the incidence of antibodies to other products may be misleading.

New-Onset Diabetes After Transplantation

The incidence of new-onset diabetes after transplantation (NODAT) was defined in Studies 1 and 2 as use of an anti-diabetic agent for ≥30 days or ≥2 fasting plasma glucose values ≥126 mg/dL (7.0 mmol/L) post-transplantation. Of the patients treated with the NULOJIX recommended regimen, 5% (14/304) developed NODAT by the end of one year compared to 10% (27/280) of patients on the cyclosporine control regimen. However, by the end of the third year, the cumulative incidence of NODAT was 8% (24/304) in patients treated with the NULOJIX recommended regimen and 10% (29/280) in patients treated with the cyclosporine regimen.

Table 3: Overall Infections and Select Infections with Identified Etiology by Treatment Group following One and Three Years of Treatment in Studies 1 and 2*

	Up to Year 1		Up to Year 3[†]	
	NULOJIX Recommended Regimen N=401 n (%)	Cyclosporine N=405 n (%)	NULOJIX Recommended Regimen N=401 n (%)	Cyclosporine N=405 n (%)
All infections[‡]	287 (72)	299 (74)	329 (82)	327 (81)
Serious infections[§]	98 (24)	113 (28)	144 (36)	157 (39)
CMV	44 (11)	52 (13)	53 (13)	56 (14)
Polyoma virus[¶]	10 (3)	23 (6)	17 (4)	27 (7)
Herpes[#]	27 (7)	26 (6)	55 (14)	46 (11)
Tuberculosis	2 (1)	1 (<1)	6 (2)	1 (<1)

* Studies 1 and 2 were not designed to support comparative claims for NULOJIX for the adverse reactions reported in this table.
[†] Median exposure in days for pooled studies: 1203 for NULOJIX recommended regimen and 1163 for cyclosporine in Studies 1 and 2.
[‡] All infections include bacterial, viral, fungal, and other organisms. For infectious adverse reactions, the causative organism is reported if specified by the physician in the clinical trials.
[§] A medically important event that may be life-threatening or result in death or hospitalization or prolongation of existing hospitalization. Infections not meeting these criteria are considered non-serious.
[¶] BK virus-associated nephropathy was reported in 6 NULOJIX patients (4 of which resulted in graft loss) and 6 cyclosporine patients (none of which resulted in graft loss) by Year 3.
[#] Most herpes infections were non-serious and 1 led to treatment discontinuation.

Hypertension

Blood pressure and use of antihypertensive medications were reported in Studies 1 and 2. By Year 3, one or more antihypertensive medications were used in 85% of NULOJIX-treated patients and 92% of cyclosporine-treated patients. At one year after transplantation, systolic blood pressures were 8 mmHg lower and diastolic blood pressures were 3 mmHg lower in patients treated with the NULOJIX (belatacept) recommended regimen compared to the cyclosporine control regimen. At three years after transplantation, systolic blood pressures were 6 mmHg lower and diastolic blood pressures were 3 mmHg lower in NULOJIX-treated patients compared to cyclosporine-treated patients. Hypertension was reported as an adverse reaction in 32% of NULOJIX-treated patients and 37% of cyclosporine-treated patients (see Table 4).

Dyslipidemia

Mean values of total cholesterol, HDL, LDL, and triglycerides were reported in Studies 1 and 2. At one year after transplantation these values were 183 mg/dL, 50 mg/dL, 102 mg/dL, and 151 mg/dL, respectively, in 401 patients treated with the NULOJIX recommended regimen and 196 mg/dL, 48 mg/dL, 108 mg/dL, and 195 mg/dL, respectively, in 405 patients treated with the cyclosporine control regimen. At three years after transplantation, the total cholesterol, HDL, LDL, and triglycerides were 176 mg/dL, 49 mg/dL, 100 mg/dL, and 141 mg/dL, respectively, in NULOJIX-treated patients compared to 193 mg/dL, 48 mg/dL, 106 mg/dL, and 180 mg/dL in cyclosporine-treated patients.

The clinical significance of the lower mean triglyceride values in NULOJIX-treated patients at one and three years is unknown.

Other Adverse Reactions

Adverse reactions that occurred at a frequency of ≥10% in patients treated with the NULOJIX recommended regimen or cyclosporine control regimen in Studies 1 and 2 through three years are summarized by preferred term in decreasing order of frequency within Table 4.

Table 4: Adverse Reactions Reported by ≥10% of Patients Treated with Either the NULOJIX Recommended Regimen or Control in Studies 1 and 2 Through Three Years*,[†]

Adverse Reaction	NULOJIX Recommended Regimen N=401 %	Cyclosporine N=405 %
Infections and Infestations		
Urinary tract infection	37	36
Upper respiratory infection	15	16
Nasopharyngitis	13	16
Cytomegalovirus infection	12	12
Influenza	11	8
Bronchitis	10	7
Gastrointestinal Disorders		
Diarrhea	39	36
Constipation	33	35
Nausea	24	27
Vomiting	22	20
Abdominal pain	19	16
Abdominal pain upper	9	10
Metabolism and Nutrition Disorders		
Hyperkalemia	20	20
Hypokalemia	21	14
Hypophosphatemia	19	13
Dyslipidemia	19	24
Hyperglycemia	16	17
Hypocalcemia	13	11
Hypercholesterolemia	11	11
Hypomagnesemia	7	10
Hyperuricemia	5	12
Procedural Complications		
Graft dysfunction	25	34
General Disorders		
Peripheral edema	34	42
Pyrexia	28	26
Blood and Lymphatic System Disorders		
Anemia	45	44

Leukopenia	20	23
Renal and Urinary Disorders		
Hematuria	16	18
Proteinuria	16	12
Dysuria	11	11
Renal tubular necrosis	9	13
Vascular Disorders		
Hypertension	32	37
Hypotension	18	12
Respiratory, Thoracic, and Mediastinal Disorders		
Cough	24	18
Dyspnea	12	15
Investigations		
Blood creatinine increased	15	20
Musculoskeletal and Connective Tissue Disorders		
Arthralgia	17	13
Back pain	13	13
Nervous System Disorders		
Headache	21	18
Dizziness	9	10
Tremor	8	17
Skin and Subcutaneous Tissue Disorders		
Acne	8	11
Psychiatric Disorders		
Insomnia	15	18
Anxiety	10	11

* All randomized and transplanted patients in Studies 1 and 2.

† Studies 1 and 2 were not designed to support comparative claims for NULOJIX for the adverse reactions reported in this table.

Selected adverse reactions occurring in <10% from NULOJIX (belatacept)-treated patients in either regimen through three years in Studies 1 and 2 are listed below:
Immune System Disorders: Guillain-Barré syndrome
Infections and Infestations: see Table 3
Gastrointestinal Disorders: stomatitis, including aphthous stomatitis
Injury, Poisoning, and Procedural Complications: chronic allograft nephropathy, complications of transplanted kidney, including wound dehiscence, arteriovenous fistula thrombosis
Blood and Lymphatic System Disorders: neutropenia
Renal and Urinary Disorders: renal impairment, including acute renal failure, renal artery stenosis, urinary incontinence, hydronephrosis
Vascular Disorders: hematoma, lymphocele
Musculoskeletal and Connective Tissue Disorders: musculoskeletal pain
Skin and Subcutaneous Tissue Disorders: alopecia, hyperhidrosis
Cardiac Disorders: atrial fibrillation

7   DRUG INTERACTIONS
7.1   Cytochrome P450 Substrates
No formal drug interaction studies have been conducted with NULOJIX. Other biologic therapies that are cytokines or cytokine modulators have been shown to affect the expression and/or functional activities of cytochrome P450 (CYP450) enzymes *in vitro* and/or *in vivo*. *In vitro* studies have shown that NULOJIX (belatacept) inhibits the production of certain cytokines during an alloimmune response. No studies in kidney transplant patients have been conducted to assess if NULOJIX inhibits cytokine production *in vivo*. The potential for NULOJIX to alter the systemic concentrations of drugs that are CYP450 substrates has not been studied; however, in the event that kidney transplant patients receiving NULOJIX exhibit signs and symptoms of altered efficacy or adverse events associated with coadministered drugs which are known to be metabolized by CYP450, the clinician should be aware of potentially altered CYP450 metabolism of these drugs.

7.2   Use with Mycophenolate Mofetil
In a pharmacokinetic substudy of Studies 1 and 2, the plasma concentrations of mycophenolic acid (MPA) were measured in 41 patients who received fixed mycophenolate mofetil (MMF) doses of 500 mg to 1500 mg twice daily with either 5 mg per kg of NULOJIX or cyclosporine. The mean dose-normalized MPA C_{max} and AUC_{0-12} were approximately 20% and 40% higher, respectively, with NULOJIX coadministration than with cyclosporine coadministration. Clinicians should be aware that there is also a potential change of MPA exposure after crossover from cyclosporine to NULOJIX or from NULOJIX to cyclosporine in patients concomitantly receiving MMF.

8   USE IN SPECIFIC POPULATIONS
8.1   Pregnancy
Pregnancy Category C
NULOJIX should not be used in pregnancy unless the potential benefit to the mother outweighs the potential risk to the fetus. There are no studies of NULOJIX treatment in pregnant women. Belatacept is known to cross the placenta of animals. Belatacept was not teratogenic in pregnant rats and rabbits at doses approximately 16 and 19 times greater than the exposure associated with the maximum recommended human dose (MRHD) of 10 mg per kg administered over the first month of treatment, based on area under the concentration-time curve (AUC).

Belatacept administered to female rats daily during gestation and throughout the lactation period was associated with maternal toxicity (infections) in a small percentage of dams at doses of ≥20 mg per kg (≥3 times the MRHD exposure based on AUC) resulting in increased pup mortality (up to 100% pup mortality in some dams). In pups that survived, there were no abnormalities or malformations at doses up to 200 mg per kg (19 times the MRHD exposure). *In vitro* data indicate that belatacept has lower binding affinity to CD80/CD86 and lower potency in rodents than in humans. Although the rat toxicity studies with belatacept were done at pharmacologically saturating doses, the *in vivo* difference in potency between rats and humans is unknown. Therefore, the relevance of the rat toxicities to humans and the significance of the magnitude of the relative exposures (rats: humans) are unknown.

Abatacept, a fusion protein that differs from belatacept by 2 amino acids, binds to the same ligands (CD80/CD86) and blocks T-cell costimulation like belatacept, but is more active than belatacept in rodents. Therefore, toxicities identified with abatacept in rodents, including infections and autoimmunity, may be predictive of adverse effects in humans treated with belatacept [see *Nonclinical Toxicology (13.2)*]. Autoimmunity was observed in one rat offspring exposed to abatacept *in utero* and/or during lactation and in juvenile rats after treatment with abatacept. However, the clinical relevance of autoimmunity in rats to patients or a fetus exposed *in utero* is unknown [see *Nonclinical Toxicology (13.2)*].

Pregnancy Registry: To monitor maternal-fetal outcomes of pregnant women who have received NULOJIX or whose partners have received NULOJIX, healthcare providers are strongly encouraged to register pregnant patients in the National Transplant Pregnancy Registry (NTPR) by calling 1-877-955-6877.

8.3   Nursing Mothers
It is not known whether belatacept is excreted in human milk or absorbed systemically after ingestion by a nursing infant. However, belatacept is excreted in rat milk. Because many drugs are excreted in human milk and because of the potential for serious adverse reactions from NULOJIX in nursing infants, a decision should be made whether to discontinue nursing or to discontinue the drug, taking into account the importance of the drug to the mother.

8.4   Pediatric Use
The safety and efficacy of NULOJIX in patients under 18 years of age have not been established. Because T cell development continues into the teenage years, the potential concern for autoimmunity in neonates applies to pediatric use as well [see *Use in Specific Populations (8.1)*].

8.5   Geriatric Use
Of 401 patients treated with the recommended dosage regimen of NULOJIX, 15% were 65 years of age and older, while 3% were 75 and older. No overall differences in safety or effectiveness were observed between these subjects and younger subjects, but greater sensitivity or less efficacy in older individuals cannot be ruled out.

10   OVERDOSAGE
Single doses up to 20 mg per kg of NULOJIX (belatacept) have been administered to healthy subjects without apparent toxic effect. The administration of NULOJIX of higher cumulative dose and more frequent dosing than recommended in kidney transplant patients resulted in a higher frequency of CNS-related adverse reactions [see *Adverse Reactions (6.1)*]. In case of overdosage, it is recommended that the patient be monitored for any signs or symptoms of adverse reactions and appropriate symptomatic treatment instituted.

11   DESCRIPTION
NULOJIX® (belatacept), a selective T-cell costimulation blocker, is a soluble fusion protein consisting of the modified extracellular domain of CTLA-4 fused to a portion (hinge-CH2-CH3 domains) of the Fc domain of a human immunoglobulin G1 antibody. Belatacept is produced by recombinant DNA technology in a mammalian cell expression system. Two amino acid substitutions (L104 to E; A29 to Y) were made in the ligand binding region of CTLA-4. As a result of these modifications, belatacept binds CD80 and CD86 more avidly than abatacept, the parent CTLA4-Immunoglobulin (CTLA4-Ig) molecule from which it is derived. The molecular weight of belatacept is approximately 90 kilodaltons.

NULOJIX is supplied as a sterile, white or off-white lyophilized powder for intravenous administration. Prior to use, the lyophile is reconstituted with a suitable fluid to obtain a clear to slightly opalescent, colorless to pale yellow solution, with a pH in the range of 7.2 to 7.8. Suitable fluids for constitution of the lyophile include SWFI, 0.9% NS, or D5W [see *Dosage and Administration (2.2)*]. Each 250 mg single-use vial of NULOJIX also contains: monobasic sodium phosphate (34.5 mg), sodium chloride (5.8 mg), and sucrose (500 mg).

12   CLINICAL PHARMACOLOGY
12.1   Mechanism of Action
Belatacept, a selective T-cell (lymphocyte) costimulation blocker, binds to CD80 and CD86 on antigen-presenting cells thereby blocking CD28 mediated costimulation of T lymphocytes. *In vitro*, belatacept inhibits T lymphocyte proliferation and the production of the cytokines interleukin-2, interferon-γ, interleukin-4, and TNF-α. Activated T lymphocytes are the predominant mediators of immunologic rejection.

In non-human primate models of renal transplantation, belatacept monotherapy prolonged graft survival and decreased the production of anti-donor antibodies, compared to vehicle.

12.2   Pharmacodynamics
Belatacept-mediated costimulation blockade results in the inhibition of cytokine production by T cells required for antigen-specific antibody production by B cells. In clinical trials, greater reductions in mean immunoglobulin (IgG, IgM, and IgA) concentrations were observed from baseline to Month 6 and Month 12 post-transplant in belatacept-treated patients compared to cyclosporine-treated patients. In an exploratory subset analysis, a trend of decreasing IgG concentrations with increasing belatacept trough concentrations was observed at Month 6. Also in this exploratory subset analysis, belatacept-treated patients with CNS PTLD, CNS infections including PML, other serious infections, and malignancies were observed to have a higher incidence of IgG concentrations below the lower limit of the normal range (<694 mg/dL) at Month 6 than those patients who did not experience these adverse events. This observation was more pronounced with the higher than recommended dose of belatacept. A similar trend was also observed for cyclosporine-treated patients with serious infections and malignancies.

However, it is unclear whether any causal relationship between an IgG concentration below the lower level of normal and these adverse events exists, as the analysis may have been confounded by other factors (e.g., age greater than 60 years, receipt of an extended criteria donor kidney, exposure to lymphocyte depleting agents) which were also associated with IgG below the lower level of normal at Month 6 in these trials.

12.3   Pharmacokinetics
Table 5 summarizes the pharmacokinetic parameters of belatacept in healthy adult subjects after a single 10 mg per kg intravenous infusion; and in kidney transplant patients after the 10 mg per kg intravenous infusion at Week 12, and after 5 mg per kg intravenous infusion every 4 weeks at Month 12 post-transplant or later.
[See table 5 at top of next page]
In healthy subjects, the pharmacokinetics of belatacept was linear and the exposure to belatacept increased proportionally after a single intravenous infusion dose of 1 to 20 mg per kg. The pharmacokinetics of belatacept in *de novo* kid-

Table 5: Pharmacokinetic Parameters (Mean±SD [Range]) of Belatacept in Healthy Subjects and Kidney Transplant Patients After 5 and 10 mg per kg Intravenous Infusions Administered Over 30 Minutes

Pharmacokinetic Parameter	Healthy Subjects (After 10 mg per kg Single Dose) N=15	Kidney Transplant Patients (After 10 mg per kg Multiple Doses) N=10	Kidney Transplant Patients (After 5 mg per kg Multiple Doses) N=14
Peak concentration (C_{max}) [µg/mL]	300±77 (190-492)	247±68 (161-340)	139±28 (80-176)
AUC* [µg•h/mL]	26398±5175 (18964-40684)	22252±7868 (13575-42144)	14090±3860 (7906-20510)
Terminal half-life ($t_{1/2}$) [days]	9.8±2.8 (6.4-15.6)	9.8±3.2 (6.1-15.1)	8.2±2.4 (3.1-11.9)
Systemic clearance (CL) [mL/h/kg]	0.39±0.07 (0.25-0.53)	0.49±0.13 (0.23-0.70)	0.51±0.14 (0.33-0.75)
Volume of distribution (Vss) [L/kg]	0.09±0.02 (0.07-0.15)	0.11±0.03 (0.067-0.17)	0.12±0.03 (0.09-0.17)

* AUC=AUC (INF) after single dose and AUC (TAU) after multiple dose, where TAU=4 weeks

Table 6: Actual Corticosteroid* Dosing in Studies 1 and 2

Day of Dosing	Median (Q1–Q3) Daily Dose[†,‡]	
	Study 1	Study 2
Week 1	31.7 mg (26.7-50 mg)	30 mg (26.7-50 mg)
Week 2	25 mg (20-30 mg)	25 mg (20-30 mg)
Week 4	20 mg (15-20 mg)	20 mg (15-22.5 mg)
Week 6	15 mg (10-20 mg)	16.7 mg (12.5-20 mg)
Month 6	10 mg (5-10 mg)	10 mg (5-12.5 mg)

* Corticosteroid = prednisone or prednisolone.
[†] The protocols allowed for flexibility in determining corticosteroid dose and rapidity of taper after Day 15. It is not possible to distinguish corticosteroid doses used to treat acute rejection versus doses used in a maintenance regimen.
[‡] Q1 and Q3 are the 25th and 75th percentiles of daily corticosteroid doses, respectively.

ney transplant patients and healthy subjects are comparable. Following the recommended regimen, the mean belatacept serum concentration reached steady-state by Week 8 in the initial phase following transplantation and by Month 6 during the maintenance phase. Following once monthly intravenous infusion of 10 mg per kg and 5 mg per kg, there was about 20% and 10% systemic accumulation of belatacept in kidney transplant patients, respectively.

Based on population pharmacokinetic analysis of 924 kidney transplant patients up to 1 year post-transplant, the pharmacokinetics of belatacept were similar at different time periods post-transplant. In clinical trials, trough concentrations of belatacept were consistently maintained from Month 6 up to 3 years post-transplant. Population pharmacokinetic analyses in kidney transplant patients revealed that there was a trend toward higher clearance of belatacept with increasing body weight. Age, gender, race, renal function (measured by calculated glomerular filtration rate [GFR]), hepatic function (measured by albumin), diabetes, and concomitant dialysis did not affect the clearance of belatacept.

13 NONCLINICAL TOXICOLOGY

13.1 Carcinogenesis, Mutagenesis, Impairment of Fertility

A carcinogenicity study was not conducted with belatacept. However, a murine carcinogenicity study was conducted with abatacept (a more active analog in rodents) to determine the carcinogenic potential of CD28 blockade. Weekly subcutaneous injections of 20, 65, or 200 mg per kg of abatacept were associated with increases in the incidence of malignant lymphomas (all doses) and mammary gland tumors (intermediate- and high-dose in females) at clinically relevant exposures. The mice in this study were infected with endogenous murine leukemia and mouse mammary tumor viruses which are associated with an increased incidence of lymphomas and mammary gland tumors, respectively, in immunosuppressed mice. Although the precise relevance of these findings to the clinical use of NULOJIX (belatacept) is unknown, cases of PTLD (a premalignant or malignant proliferation of B lymphocytes) were reported in clinical trials. Genotoxicity testing is not required for protein therapeutics; therefore, no genotoxicity studies were conducted with belatacept.

Belatacept had no adverse effects on male or female fertility in rats at doses up to 200 mg per kg daily (25 times the MRHD exposure).

13.2 Animal Toxicology and/or Pharmacology

Abatacept, a fusion protein that differs from belatacept by 2 amino acids, binds to the same ligands (CD80/CD86) and blocks T-cell costimulation like belatacept, but is more active than belatacept in rodents. Therefore, toxicities identified with abatacept in rodents may be predictive of adverse effects in humans treated with belatacept.

Studies in rats exposed to abatacept have shown immune system abnormalities including a low incidence of infections leading to death (observed in juvenile rats and pregnant rats) as well as autoimmunity of the thyroid and pancreas (observed in rats exposed in utero, as juveniles or as adults). Studies of abatacept in adult mice and monkeys, as well as belatacept in adult monkeys, have not demonstrated similar findings.

The increased susceptibility to opportunistic infections observed in juvenile rats is likely associated with the exposure to abatacept before the complete development of memory immune responses. In pregnant rats, the increased susceptibility to opportunistic infections may be due to the inherent lapses in immunity that occur in rats during late pregnancy/lactation. Infections related to NULOJIX (belatacept) have been observed in human clinical trials [see Warnings and Precautions (5.5)].

Administration of abatacept to rats was associated with a significant decrease in T-regulatory cells (up to 90%). Deficiency of T-regulatory cells in humans has been associated with autoimmunity. The occurrence of autoimmune events across the core clinical trials was infrequent. However, the possibility that patients administered NULOJIX could develop autoimmunity (or that fetuses exposed to NULOJIX in utero could develop autoimmunity) cannot be excluded.

In a 6-month toxicity study with belatacept in cynomolgus monkeys administered weekly doses up to 50 mg per kg (6 times the MRHD exposure) and in a 1-year toxicity study with abatacept in adult cynomolgus monkeys administered weekly doses up to 50 mg per kg, no significant drug-related toxicities were observed. Reversible pharmacological effects consisted of minimal transient decreases in serum IgG and minimal to severe lymphoid depletion of germinal centers in the spleen and/or lymph nodes.

Following 5 doses (10 mg per kg or 50 mg per kg, once a week for 5 weeks) of systemic administration, belatacept was not detected in brain tissue of normal healthy cynomolgus monkeys. The number of cells expressing major histocompatibility complex (MHC) class-II antigens (potential marker of immune cell activation) in the brain were increased in monkeys administered belatacept compared to vehicle control. However, distribution of some other cells expressing CD68, CD20, CD80, and CD86, typically expressed on MHC class II-positive cells, was not altered and there were no other histological changes in the brain. The clinical relevance of the findings is unknown.

14 CLINICAL STUDIES

14.1 Prevention of Organ Rejection in Kidney Transplant Recipients

The efficacy and safety of NULOJIX in de novo kidney transplantation were assessed in two open-label, randomized, multicenter, active-controlled trials (Study 1 and Study 2). These trials evaluated two dose regimens of NULOJIX, the recommended dosage regimen [see Dosage and Administration (2.1)] and a regimen with higher cumulative doses and more frequent dosing than the recommended dosage regimen, compared to a cyclosporine control regimen. All treatment groups also received basiliximab induction, mycophenolate mofetil (MMF), and corticosteroids.

Treatment Regimen

The NULOJIX recommended regimen consisted of a 10 mg per kg dose administered on Day 1 (the day of transplantation, prior to implantation), Day 5 (approximately 96 hours after the Day 1 dose), end of Weeks 2 and 4; then every 4 weeks through Week 12 after transplantation. Starting at Week 16 after transplantation, NULOJIX was administered at the maintenance dose of 5 mg per kg every 4 weeks (plus or minus 3 days). NULOJIX was administered as an intravenous infusion over 30 minutes [see Dosage and Administration (2.1)].

Basiliximab 20 mg was administered intravenously on the day of transplantation and 4 days later.

The initial dose of MMF was 1 gram twice daily and was adjusted, as needed based on clinical signs of adverse events or efficacy failure.

The protocol-specified dosing of corticosteroids in Studies 1 and 2 at Day 1 was methylprednisolone (as sodium succinate) 500 mg IV on arrival in the operating room, Day 2, methylprednisolone 250 mg IV, and Day 3, prednisone 100 mg orally. Actual median corticosteroid doses used with the NULOJIX recommended regimen from Week 1 through Month 6 are summarized in the table below (Table 6).

Study 1 enrolled recipients of living donor and standard criteria deceased donor organs and Study 2 enrolled recipients of extended criteria donor organs. Standard criteria donor organs were defined as organs from a deceased donor with anticipated cold ischemia time of <24 hours and not meeting the definition of extended criteria donor organs. Extended criteria donors were defined as deceased donors with at least one of the following: (1) donor age ≥60 years; (2) donor age ≥50 years and other donor comorbidities (≥2 of the following: stroke, hypertension, serum creatinine >1.5 mg/dL); (3) donation of organ after cardiac death; or (4) anticipated cold ischemia time of the organ of ≥24 hours. Study 1 excluded recipients undergoing a first transplant whose current Panel Reactive Antibodies (PRA) were ≥50% and recipients undergoing a retransplantation whose current PRA were ≥30%; Study 2 excluded recipients with a current PRA ≥30%. Both studies excluded recipients with HIV, hepatitis C, or evidence of current hepatitis B infection; recipients with active tuberculosis; and recipients in whom intravenous access was difficult to obtain.

Efficacy data are presented for the NULOJIX (belatacept) recommended regimen and cyclosporine regimen in Studies 1 and 2.

The NULOJIX regimen with higher cumulative doses and more frequent dosing of belatacept was associated with more efficacy failures. Higher doses and/or more frequent dosing of NULOJIX are not recommended [see Dosage and Administration (2.1), Warnings and Precautions (5.1), and Adverse Reactions (6.1)].

Study 1: Recipients of Living Donor and Standard Criteria Deceased Donor Kidneys

In Study 1, 666 patients were enrolled, randomized, and transplanted: 226 to the NULOJIX recommended regimen, 219 to the NULOJIX regimen with higher cumulative doses and more frequent dosing than recommended, and 221 to cyclosporine control regimen. The median age was 45 years; 58% of organs were from living donors; 3% were retransplanted; 69% of the study population was male; 61% of patients were white, 8% were black/African-American, 31% were categorized as of other races; 16% had PRA ≥10%; 41% had 4 to 6 HLA mismatches; and 27% had diabetes prior to transplant. The incidence of delayed graft function was similar in all treatment arms (14% to 18%).

Premature discontinuation from treatment at the end of the first year occurred in 19% of patients receiving the NULOJIX recommended regimen and 19% of patients on the cyclosporine regimen. Among the patients who received the NULOJIX recommended regimen, 10% discontinued due to lack of efficacy, 5% due to adverse events, and 4% for other reasons. Among the patients who received the cyclosporine regimen, 9% discontinued due to adverse events, 5% due to lack of efficacy, and 5% for other reasons.

At the end of three years, 25% of patients receiving the NULOJIX recommended regimen and 34% of patients receiving the cyclosporine regimen had discontinued from treatment. Among the patients who received the NULOJIX recommended regimen, 12% discontinued due to lack of efficacy, 7% due to adverse events, and 6% for other reasons. Among the patients who received the cyclosporine regimen, 15% discontinued due to adverse events, 8% due to lack of efficacy, and 11% for other reasons.

Assessment of Efficacy

Table 7 summarizes the results of Study 1 following one and three years of treatment with the NULOJIX recommended dosage regimen and the cyclosporine control regimen. Efficacy failure at one year was defined as the occurrence of biopsy proven acute rejection (BPAR), graft loss, death, or lost

Table 7: Efficacy Outcomes by Years 1 and 3 for Study 1: Recipients of Living and Standard Criteria Deceased Donor Kidneys

Parameter	NULOJIX Recommended Regimen N=226 n (%)	Cyclosporine CSA N=221 n (%)	NULOJIX-CSA (97.3% CI)
Efficacy Failure by Year 1	49 (21.7)	37 (16.7)	4.9 (−3.3, 13.2)
Components of Efficacy Failure*			
Biopsy Proven Acute Rejection	45 (19.9)	23 (10.4)	
Graft Loss	5 (2.2)	8 (3.6)	
Death	4 (1.8)	7 (3.2)	
Lost to follow-up	0	1 (0.5)	
Efficacy Failure by Year 3	58 (25.7)	57 (25.8)	−0.1 (−9.3, 9)
Components of Efficacy Failure*			
Biopsy Proven Acute Rejection	50 (22.1)	31 (14)	
Graft Loss	9 (4)	10 (4.5)	
Death	10 (4.4)	15 (6.8)	
Lost to follow-up	2 (0.9)	5 (2.3)	
Patient and graft survival[†]			
Year 1	218 (96.5)	206 (93.2)	3.2 (−1.5, 8.4)
Year 3	206 (91.2)	192 (86.9)	4.3 (−2.2, 10.8)

* Patients may have experienced more than one event.
[†] Patients known to be alive with a functioning graft.

Table 8: Measured and Calculated GFR for Study 1: Recipients of Living and Standard Criteria Deceased Donor Kidneys

Parameter	NULOJIX Recommended Regimen N=226	Cyclosporine (CSA) N=221	NULOJIX-CSA (97.3% CI)
Measured GFR* mL/min/1.73 m² mean (SD)			
Year 1	63.4 (27.7) (n=206)	50.4 (18.7) (n=199)	13.0 (7.3, 18.7)
Year 2[†]	67.9 (29.9) (n=199)	50.5 (20.5) (n=185)	17.4 (11.5, 23.4)
Calculated GFR[‡] mL/min/1.73 m² mean (SD)			
Year 1	65.4 (22.9) (n=200)	50.1 (21.1) (n=199)	15.3 (10.3, 20.3)
Year 2	65.4 (25.2) (n=201)	47.9 (23) (n=182)	17.5 (12, 23.1)
Year 3	65.8 (27) (n=190)	44.4 (23.6) (n=171)	21.4 (15.4, 27.4)

* GFR was measured using the cold-iothalamate method.
[†] Measured GFR was not assessed at Year 3.
[‡] GFR was calculated using the MDRD formula.

to follow-up. BPAR was defined as histologically confirmed acute rejection by a central pathologist on a biopsy done for any reason, whether or not accompanied by clinical signs of rejection. Patient and graft survival was also assessed separately.
[See table 7 above]
In Study 1, the rate of BPAR at one year and three years was higher in patients treated with the NULOJIX (belatacept) recommended regimen than the cyclosporine regimen. Of the patients who experienced BPAR with NULOJIX, 70% experienced BPAR by Month 3, and 84% experienced BPAR by Month 6. By three years, recurrent BPAR occurred with similar frequency across treatment groups (<3%). The component of BPAR determined by biopsy only (subclinical protocol-defined acute rejection) was 5% in both treatment groups.
Patients treated with the NULOJIX recommended regimen experienced episodes of BPAR classified as Banff grade IIb or higher (6% [14/226] at one year and 7% [15/226] at three years) more frequently compared to patients treated with the cyclosporine regimen (2% [4/221] at one year and 2% [5/221] at three years). Also, T-cell depleting therapy was used more frequently to treat episodes of BPAR in NULOJIX-treated patients (10%; 23/226) compared to cyclosporine-treated patients (2%; 5/221). At Month 12, the difference in mean calculated glomerular filtration rate (GFR) between patients with and without history of BPAR was 19 mL/min/1.73 m² among NULOJIX-treated patients compared to 7 mL/min/1.73 m² among cyclosporine-treated patients. By three years, 22% (11/50) of NULOJIX-treated patients with a history of BPAR experienced graft loss and/or death compared to 10% (3/31) of cyclosporine-treated patients with a history of BPAR; at that time point, 10% (5/50) of NULOJIX-treated patients experienced graft loss and 12% (6/50) of NULOJIX-treated patients had died following an episode of BPAR, whereas 7% (2/31) of cyclosporine-treated patients experienced graft loss and 7% (2/31) of cyclosporine-treated patients had died following an episode of BPAR. The overall prevalence of donor-specific

antibodies was 5% and 11% for the NULOJIX (belatacept) recommended regimen and cyclosporine, respectively, up to 36 months post-transplant.
While the difference in GFR in patients with BPAR versus those without BPAR was greater in patients treated with NULOJIX than cyclosporine, the mean GFR following BPAR was similar in NULOJIX (49 mL/min/1.73 m²) and cyclosporine treated patients (43 mL/min/1.73 m²) at one year. The relationship between BPAR, GFR, and patient and graft survival is unclear due to the limited number of patients who experienced BPAR, differences in renal hemodynamics (and, consequently, GFR) across maintenance immunosuppression regimens, and the high rate of switching treatment regimens after BPAR.

Assessment of Efficacy in the EBV Seropositive Subpopulation
NULOJIX is recommended for use only in EBV seropositive patients [see *Indications and Usage (1.2)*].
In Study 1, approximately 87% of patients were EBV seropositive prior to transplant. Efficacy results in the EBV seropositive subpopulation were consistent with those in the total population studied.
By one year, the efficacy failure rate in the EBV seropositive population was 21% (42/202) in patients treated with the NULOJIX recommended regimen and 17% (31/184) in patients treated with cyclosporine (difference=4%, 97.3% CI [−4.8, 12.8]). Patient and graft survival was 98% (198/202) in NULOJIX-treated patients and 92% (170/184) in cyclosporine-treated patients (difference=5.6%, 97.3% CI [0.8, 10.4]).
By three years, efficacy failure was 25% in both treatment groups and patient and graft survival was 94% (187/202) in NULOJIX-treated patients compared with 88% (162/184) in cyclosporine-treated patients (difference=4.6%, 97.3% CI [−2.1, 11.3]).

Assessment of Glomerular Filtration Rate (GFR)
Glomerular Filtration Rate (GFR) was measured at one and two years and was calculated using the Modification of Diet in Renal Disease (MDRD) formula at one, two, and three

years after transplantation. As shown in Table 8, both measured and calculated GFR was higher in patients treated with the NULOJIX (belatacept) recommended regimen compared to patients treated with the cyclosporine control regimen at all time points. As shown in Figure 1, the differences in GFR were apparent in the first month after transplant and were maintained up to three years (36 months). An analysis of change of calculated mean GFR between three and 36 months demonstrated an increase of 0.8 mL/min/year (95% CI [−0.2, 1.8]) for NULOJIX-treated patients and a decrease of 2.2 mL/min/year (95% CI [−3.2, −1.2]) for cyclosporine-treated patients.
[See table 8 above]

Figure 1: Calculated (MDRD) GFR through Month 36; Study 1: Recipients of Living and Standard Criteria Deceased Donor Kidneys

Assessment of Chronic Allograft Nephropathy (CAN)
The prevalence of chronic allograft nephropathy (CAN) at one year, as defined by the Banff '97 classification system, was 24% (54/226) in patients treated with the NULOJIX recommended regimen and in 32% (71/219) of patients treated with the cyclosporine control regimen. CAN was not evaluated after the first year following transplantation. The clinical significance of this finding is unknown.
Study 2: Recipients of Extended Criteria Donor Kidneys
In Study 2, 543 patients were enrolled, randomized, and transplanted: 175 to the NULOJIX recommended regimen, 184 to the NULOJIX regimen with higher cumulative doses and more frequent dosing than recommended, and 184 to the cyclosporine control regimen. The median age was 58 years; 67% of the study population was male; 75% of patients were white, 13% were black/African-American, 12% were categorized as of other races; 3% had PRA ≥10%; 53% had 4 to 6 HLA mismatches; and 29% had diabetes prior to transplantation. The incidence of delayed graft function was similar in all treatment arms (47% to 49%).
Premature discontinuation from treatment at the end of the first year occurred in 25% of patients receiving the NULOJIX recommended regimen and 30% of patients receiving the cyclosporine control regimen. Among the patients who received the NULOJIX recommended regimen, 14% discontinued due to adverse events, 9% due to lack of efficacy, and 2% for other reasons. Among the patients who received the cyclosporine regimen, 17% discontinued due to adverse events, 7% due to lack of efficacy, and 6% for other reasons.
At the end of three years, 35% of patients receiving the NULOJIX recommended regimen and 44% of patients receiving the cyclosporine regimen had discontinued from treatment. Among the patients who received the NULOJIX recommended regimen, 20% discontinued due to adverse events, 9% due to lack of efficacy, and 6% for other reasons. Among the patients who received the cyclosporine regimen, 25% discontinued due to adverse events, 10% due to lack of efficacy, and 10% for other reasons.
Assessment of Efficacy
Table 9 summarizes the results of Study 2 following one and three years of treatment with the NULOJIX recommended dosage regimen and the cyclosporine control regimen. Efficacy failure at one year was defined as the occurrence of biopsy proven acute rejection (BPAR), graft loss, death, or lost to follow-up. BPAR was defined as histologically confirmed acute rejection by a central pathologist on a biopsy done for any reason, whether or not accompanied by clinical signs of rejection. Patient and graft survival was also assessed.
[See table 9 at top of next page]
In Study 2, the rate of BPAR at one year and three years was similar in patients treated with NULOJIX and cyclosporine. Of the patients who experienced BPAR with NULOJIX, 62% experienced BPAR by Month 3, and 76% experienced BPAR by Month 6. By three years, recurrent BPAR occurred with similar frequency across treatment groups (<3%). The component of BPAR determined by biopsy only (subclinical protocol-defined acute rejection) was 5% in both treatment groups.

A similar proportion of patients in the NULOJIX (belatacept) recommended regimen group experienced BPAR classified as Banff grade IIb or higher (5% [9/175] at one year and 6% [10/175] at three years) compared to patients treated with the cyclosporine regimen (4% [7/184] at one year and 5% [9/184] at three years). Also, T-cell depleting therapy was used with similar frequency to treat any episode of BPAR in NULOJIX-treated patients (5% or 9/175) compared to cyclosporine-treated patients (4% or 7/184). At Month 12, the difference in mean calculated GFR between patients with and without a history of BPAR was 10 mL/min/1.73 m^2 among NULOJIX-treated patients compared to 14 mL/min/1.73 m^2 among cyclosporine-treated patients. By three years, 24% (10/42) of NULOJIX-treated patients with a history of BPAR experienced graft loss and/or death compared to 31% (13/42) of cyclosporine-treated patients with a history of BPAR; at that time point, 17% (7/42) of NULOJIX-treated patients experienced graft loss and 14% (6/42) of NULOJIX-treated patients had died following an episode of BPAR, whereas 19% (8/42) of cyclosporine-treated patients experienced graft loss and 19% (8/42) of cyclosporine-treated patients had died following an episode of BPAR. The overall prevalence of donor-specific antibodies was 6% and 15% for the NULOJIX recommended regimen and cyclosporine, respectively, up to 36 months post-transplant.

The mean GFR following BPAR was 36 mL/min/1.73 m^2 in NULOJIX patients and 24 mL/min/1.73 m^2 in cyclosporine-treated patients at one year. The relationship between BPAR, GFR, and patient and graft survival is unclear due to the limited number of patients who experienced BPAR, differences in renal hemodynamics (and, consequently, GFR) across maintenance immunosuppression regimens, and the high rate of switching treatment regimens after BPAR.

Assessment of Efficacy in the EBV Seropositive Subpopulation

NULOJIX is recommended for use only in EBV seropositive patients [see *Indications and Usage (1.2)*].

In Study 2, approximately 91% of the patients were EBV seropositive prior to transplant. Efficacy results in the EBV seropositive subpopulation were consistent with those in the total population studied.

By one year, the efficacy failure rate in the EBV seropositive population was 29% (45/156) in patients treated with the NULOJIX recommended regimen and 28% (47/168) in patients treated with cyclosporine (difference=0.8%, 97.3% CI [–10.3, 11.9]). Patient and graft survival rate in the EBV seropositive population was 89% (139/156) in the NULOJIX-treated patients and 86% (144/168) in cyclosporine-treated patients (difference=3.4%, 97.3% CI [–4.7, 11.5]).

By three years, efficacy failure was 35% (54/156) in NULOJIX-treated patients and 36% (61/168) in cyclosporine-treated patients. Patient and graft survival was 83% (130/156) in NULOJIX-treated patients compared with 77% (130/168) in cyclosporine-treated patients (difference=5.9%, 97.3% CI [–3.8, 15.6]).

Assessment of Glomerular Filtration Rate (GFR)

Glomerular Filtration Rate (GFR) was measured at one and two years and was calculated using the Modification of Diet in Renal Disease (MDRD) formula at one, two, and three years after transplantation. As shown in Table 10, both measured and calculated GFR was higher in patients treated with the NULOJIX recommended regimen compared to patients treated with the cyclosporine control regimen at all time points. As shown in Figure 2, the differences in GFR were apparent in the first month after transplant and were maintained up to three years (36 months). An analysis of change of calculated mean GFR between Month 3 and Month 36 demonstrated a decrease of 0.8 mL/min/year (95% CI [–1.9, 0.3]) for NULOJIX-treated patients and a decrease of 2.0 mL/min/year (95% CI [–3.1, –0.8]) for cyclosporine-treated patients.

[See table 10 above]

Figure 2: Calculated (MDRD) GFR through Month 36; Study 2: Recipients of Extended Criteria Donor Kidneys

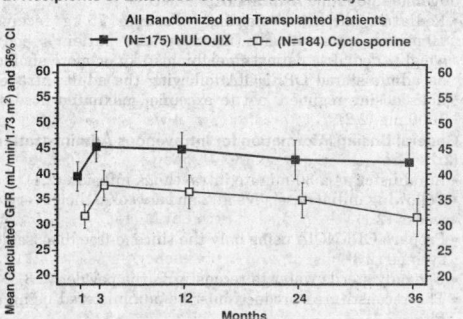

All Randomized and Transplanted Patients
■ (N=175) NULOJIX   □ (N=184) Cyclosporine

Table 9: Efficacy Outcomes by Years 1 and 3 for Study 2: Recipients of Extended Criteria Donor Kidneys

Parameter	NULOJIX Recommended Regimen N=175 n (%)	Cyclosporine (CSA) N=184 n (%)	NULOJIX-CSA (97.3% CI)
Efficacy Failure by Year 1	51 (29.1)	52 (28.3)	0.9 (–9.7, 11.5)
Components of Efficacy Failure*			
Biopsy Proven Acute Rejection	37 (21.1)	34 (18.5)	
Graft Loss	16 (9.1)	20 (10.9)	
Death	5 (2.9)	8 (4.3)	
Lost to follow-up	0	2 (1.1)	
Efficacy Failure by Year 3	63 (36)	68 (37)	–1.0 (–12.1, 10.3)
Components of Efficacy Failure*			
Biopsy Proven Acute Rejection	42 (24)	42 (22.8)	
Graft Loss	21 (12)	23 (12.5)	
Death	15 (8.6)	17 (9.2)	
Lost to follow-up	1 (0.6)	5 (2.7)	
Patient and graft survival†			
Year 1	155 (88.6)	157 (85.3)	3.2 (–4.8, 11.3)
Year 3	143 (81.7)	143 (77.7)	4.0 (–5.4, 13.4)

* Patients may have experienced more than one event.
† Patients known to be alive with a functioning graft.

Table 10: Measured and Calculated GFR for Study 2: Recipients of Extended Criteria Donor Kidneys

Parameter	NULOJIX Recommended Regimen N=175	Cyclosporine (CSA) N=184	NULOJIX-CSA (97.3% CI)
Measured GFR* mL/min/1.73 m^2 mean (SD)			
Year 1	49.6 (25.8) (n=151)	45.2 (21.1) (n=154)	4.3 (–1.5, 10.2)
Year 2†	49.7 (23.7) (n=139)	45.0 (27.2) (n=136)	4.7 (–1.8, 11.3)
Calculated GFR‡ mL/min/1.73 m^2 mean (SD)			
Year 1	44.5 (21.8) (n=158)	36.5 (21.1) (n=159)	8.0 (2.5, 13.4)
Year 2	42.8 (24.1) (n=158)	34.9 (21.6) (n=154)	8.0 (1.9, 14)
Year 3	42.2 (25.2) (n=154)	31.5 (22.1) (n=143)	10.7 (4.3, 17.2)

* GFR was measured using the cold-iothalamate method.
† Measured GFR was not assessed at Year 3.
‡ GFR was calculated using the MDRD formula.

Assessment of Chronic Allograft Nephropathy (CAN)

The prevalence of chronic allograft nephropathy (CAN) at one year, as defined by the Banff '97 classification system, was 46% (80/174) in patients treated with the NULOJIX recommended regimen and 52% (95/184) of patients treated with the cyclosporine control regimen. CAN was not evaluated after the first year following transplantation. The clinical significance of this finding is unknown.

16   HOW SUPPLIED/STORAGE AND HANDLING

NULOJIX® (belatacept) lyophilized powder for intravenous infusion is supplied as a single-use vial with a *silicone-free disposable syringe* in the following packaging configuration:

Description	NDC Number
One 250-mg vial One 12 mL Syringe	0003-0371-13

16.1   Storage

NULOJIX lyophilized powder is stored refrigerated at 2°-8°C (36°-46°F). Protect NULOJIX from light by storing in the original package until time of use.

The reconstituted solution should be transferred from the vial to the infusion bag or bottle immediately. The NULOJIX infusion must be completed within 24 hours of constitution of the NULOJIX lyophilized powder. If not used immediately, the infusion solution may be stored under refrigeration conditions: 2°-8°C (36°-46°F) and protected from light for up to 24 hours (a maximum of 4 hours of the total 24 hours can be at room temperature: 20°-25°C [68°-77°F] and room light) [see *Dosage and Administration (2.2)*].

17   PATIENT COUNSELING INFORMATION

See FDA-approved patient labeling (Medication Guide).

17.1   Post-Transplant Lymphoproliferative Disorder

The overall risk of PTLD, especially CNS PTLD, was elevated in NULOJIX-treated patients. Instruct patients to immediately report any of the following neurological, cognitive, or behavioral signs and symptoms during and after therapy with NULOJIX [see *Boxed Warning* and *Warnings and Precautions (5.1)*]:

- changes in mood or usual behavior
- confusion, problems thinking, loss of memory
- changes in walking or talking
- decreased strength or weakness on one side of the body
- changes in vision

17.2   Other Malignancies

Inform patients about the increased risk of malignancies, in addition to PTLD, while taking immunosuppressive therapy, especially skin cancer. Instruct patients to limit exposure to sunlight and UV light by wearing protective clothing and using a sunscreen with a high protection factor. Instruct patients to look for any signs and symptoms of skin cancer, such as suspicious moles or lesions [see *Warnings and Precautions (5.3)*].

17.3   Progressive Multifocal Leukoencephalopathy

Cases of PML have been reported in NULOJIX-treated patients. Instruct patients to immediately report any of the following neurological, cognitive, or behavioral signs and symptoms during and after therapy with NULOJIX (belatacept) [see *Warnings and Precautions (5.4)*]:

- changes in mood or usual behavior
- confusion, problems thinking, loss of memory
- changes in walking or talking
- decreased strength or weakness on one side of the body
- changes in vision

17.4   Other Serious Infections

Inform patients about the increased risk of infection while taking immunosuppressive therapy. Instruct patients to adhere to antimicrobial prophylaxis regimens as prescribed. Tell patients to immediately report any signs and symptoms of infection during therapy with NULOJIX [see *Warnings and Precautions (5.5)*].

17.5   Immunizations

Inform patients that vaccinations may be less effective while they are being treated with NULOJIX. Advise patients that live vaccines should be avoided [see *Warnings and Precautions (5.8)*].

17.6   Pregnant Women and Nursing Mothers

Inform patients that NULOJIX has not been studied in pregnant women or nursing mothers so the effects of NULOJIX on pregnant women or nursing infants are not known. Instruct patients to tell their healthcare provider if they are pregnant, become pregnant, or are thinking about becoming pregnant [see *Use in Specific Populations (8.1)*]. Instruct patients to tell their healthcare provider if they plan to breast-feed their infant [see *Use in Specific Populations (8.3)*].

Bristol-Myers Squibb Company
Princeton, New Jersey 08543
1274492A1
Rev May 2014

MEDICATION GUIDE
NULOJIX® (noo-LOJ-jiks)
(belatacept)
For Injection, For Intravenous Use

Read this Medication Guide before you start receiving NULOJIX and before each treatment. There may be new information. This Medication Guide does not take the place of talking with your doctor about your medical condition or your treatment.

What is the most important information I should know about NULOJIX?

NULOJIX increases your risk of serious side effects, including:

• **Post-transplant lymphoproliferative disorder (PTLD).** PTLD is a condition that can happen if certain white blood cells grow out of control after an organ transplant because your immune system is weak. PTLD can get worse and become a type of cancer. PTLD can lead to death.

People treated with NULOJIX have a higher risk of getting PTLD. If you get PTLD with NULOJIX you are at especially high risk of getting it in your brain. Your risk for PTLD is also higher if you:
  • have never been exposed to the Epstein-Barr virus (EBV). Your doctor should test you for EBV. Do not receive NULOJIX unless you are EBV positive (you have been exposed to EBV).
  • get an infection with a virus called cytomegalovirus (CMV).
  • receive treatment for transplant rejection that lowers certain white blood cells called T lymphocytes.

• **Increased risk of getting cancers other than PTLD.** People who take medicines that weaken the immune system, including NULOJIX, have a higher risk of getting other cancers, including skin cancer. Talk to your doctor about your risk for cancer. See "**What should I avoid while receiving NULOJIX?**"

• **Progressive multifocal leukoencephalopathy (PML).** PML is a rare, serious brain infection caused by JC virus. People with weakened immune systems are at risk for getting PML. PML can result in death or severe disability. There is no known prevention, treatment, or cure for PML.

• **Increased risk of getting other serious infections, including tuberculosis (TB) and other infections caused by bacteria, viruses, or fungi.** These serious infections may lead to death. Also, a virus called BK virus can affect how your kidney works and cause your transplanted kidney to fail.

Tell your doctor right away if you get any of the following symptoms during treatment with NULOJIX:
• change in mood or your usual behavior
• confusion or problems thinking or with memory
• change in the way you walk or talk
• decreased strength or weakness on one side of your body
• change in vision
• fever, night sweats, or tiredness that does not go away
• weight loss
• swollen glands
• flu, cold symptoms, or cough
• stomach-area pain
• vomiting or diarrhea
• tenderness over your transplanted kidney
• change in the amount of urine that you make, blood in your urine, pain or burning on urination
• a new skin lesion or bump, or change in size or color of a mole

See "**What are the possible side effects of NULOJIX?**" for more information about side effects.

Liver transplant patients should not receive NULOJIX because of an increased risk of losing the transplanted liver (graft loss) and death. Talk to your doctor if you would like more information about this risk.

What is NULOJIX?

NULOJIX is a prescription medicine used in adults to prevent transplant rejection in people who have received a kidney transplant. Transplant rejection happens when the body's immune system senses that the new transplanted kidney is different or foreign, and attacks it. NULOJIX is used with corticosteroids and certain other medicines to help prevent rejection of your new kidney.

It is not known if NULOJIX is safe and effective in children under 18 years of age.

NULOJIX is only used in people who have been exposed to the EBV virus.

It is not known if NULOJIX (belatacept) is safe and effective in people who receive an organ transplant other than a kidney transplant.

Who should not receive NULOJIX?

Do not receive treatment with NULOJIX if you are EBV negative. Your doctor will do a test to see if you were exposed to EBV in the past.

What should I tell my doctor before receiving NULOJIX?

Before receiving NULOJIX, tell your doctor if you:
• plan to receive any vaccines. Talk to your doctor about which vaccines are safe for you to receive during your treatment with NULOJIX. See "**What should I avoid while receiving NULOJIX?**"
• have any other medical conditions
• are pregnant or plan to become pregnant. It is not known if NULOJIX will harm your unborn baby. If you become pregnant while taking NULOJIX:
  • **Tell your doctor right away.** You and your doctor should decide if you will keep receiving NULOJIX while you are pregnant.
  • Talk with your doctor about enrolling in the National Transplant Pregnancy Registry (NTPR). This Registry collects information about pregnancies in women who have received NULOJIX or if their partner has received NULOJIX, and had a transplant. You can also enroll by calling 1-877-955-6877.
• are breast-feeding or plan to breast-feed. It is not known if NULOJIX passes into your breast milk. You and your doctor should decide if you will receive NULOJIX or breast-feed. You should not do both.

Tell your doctor about all of the medicines you take, including prescription and non-prescription medicines, vitamins, and herbal supplements.

Know the medicines you take. Keep a list of them to show your doctor and pharmacist when you get a new medicine. Do not take any new medicine without talking with your transplant doctor first.

How will I receive NULOJIX?
• To help prevent rejection of your new kidney, you will receive NULOJIX regularly as prescribed by your doctor. It is important for you to keep all your appointments for NULOJIX treatment and follow up.
• You will receive NULOJIX as an intravenous (IV) infusion in your arm. Each IV infusion takes about 30 minutes.
• During treatment with NULOJIX, your doctor will test your blood and urine to check how your kidney is working.
• Take all the medicines prescribed by your doctor to prevent infection or transplant rejection. Take them exactly as your doctor tells you. Talk to your doctor or pharmacist if you have any questions about how to take your medicines.

What should I avoid while receiving NULOJIX?
• Limit the amount of time you spend in sunlight. Avoid using tanning beds or sunlamps. People who take medicines that weaken the immune system, including NULOJIX, have a higher risk of getting cancer, including skin cancer. Wear protective clothing and use sunscreen with a high protection factor (SPF) when you have to be in the sun.
• **Avoid receiving live vaccines during treatment with NULOJIX.** Talk to your doctor to find out which vaccines are safe for you during this time. Some vaccines may not work as well while you are receiving NULOJIX. See "**What should I tell my doctor before receiving NULOJIX?**"

What are the possible side effects of NULOJIX?

NULOJIX increases your risk of serious side effects that can cause death. See "**What is the most important information I should know about NULOJIX?**"

Common side effects of NULOJIX include:
• low red blood count (anemia)
• diarrhea
• kidney or bladder infection
• swollen legs, feet, or ankles
• constipation
• high blood pressure
• fever
• new kidney not working well
• cough
• nausea or vomiting
• headache
• low potassium or high potassium in your blood
• low white blood cell count

Tell your doctor about any side effect that bothers you or that does not go away. These are not all the possible side effects of NULOJIX. For more information, ask your doctor or pharmacist.

Call your doctor for medical advice about side effects. You may report side effects to FDA at 1-800-FDA-1088.

You may also report side effects to BMS at 1-800-321-1335.

General information about NULOJIX

Medicines are sometimes prescribed for purposes other than those listed in a Medication Guide. This Medication Guide summarizes the most important information about NULOJIX. If you would like more information about

NULOJIX (belatacept), talk with your doctor. You can ask your pharmacist or doctor for information about NULOJIX that is written for healthcare professionals.

For more information, go to www.NULOJIX.com or call 1-800-321-1335.

What are the ingredients in NULOJIX?

Active ingredient: belatacept
Inactive ingredients: monobasic sodium phosphate, sodium chloride, and sucrose

This Medication Guide has been approved by the U.S. Food and Drug Administration.

Bristol-Myers Squibb Company
Princeton, New Jersey 08543
1274492A1
1275358A1
Rev May 2014

Shown in Product Identification Guide, page 306

ORENCIA
[oh-REN-see-ah]
(abatacept)
for injection for intravenous use
injection, for subcutaneous use

Ŗ

HIGHLIGHTS OF PRESCRIBING INFORMATION
These highlights do not include all the information needed to use ORENCIA safely and effectively. See full prescribing information for ORENCIA.
ORENCIA (abatacept)
for injection for intravenous use
injection, for subcutaneous use
Initial U.S. Approval: 2005

-------RECENT MAJOR CHANGES-------

Dosage and Administration, Adult Rheumatoid Arthritis (2.1)   12/2013

-------INDICATIONS AND USAGE-------

ORENCIA is a selective T cell costimulation modulator indicated for:

Adult Rheumatoid Arthritis (RA) (1.1)
• moderately to severely active RA in adults. ORENCIA may be used as monotherapy or concomitantly with DMARDs other than TNF antagonists (1.1).

Juvenile Idiopathic Arthritis (1.2)
• moderately to severely active polyarticular juvenile idiopathic arthritis in pediatric patients 6 years of age and older. ORENCIA may be used as monotherapy or concomitantly with methotrexate (1.2).

Important Limitations of Use (1.3)
• should not be given concomitantly with TNF antagonists (1.3, 5.1).

-------DOSAGE AND ADMINISTRATION-------

Intravenous Administration for Adult RA (2.1)

Body Weight of Patient	Dose	Number of Vials
Less than 60 kg	500 mg	2
60 to 100 kg	750 mg	3
More than 100 kg	1000 mg	4

Subcutaneous Administration for Adult RA (2.1)
• Administer by subcutaneous injection once weekly with or without an intravenous loading dose. For patients initiating therapy with an intravenous loading dose, administer a single intravenous infusion (as per body weight categories above), followed by the first 125 mg subcutaneous injection given within a day of the intravenous infusion.
• Patients transitioning from ORENCIA intravenous therapy to subcutaneous administration should administer the first subcutaneous dose instead of the next scheduled intravenous dose.

Juvenile Idiopathic Arthritis (2.2)
• Pediatric patients weighing less than 75 kg receive 10 mg/kg intravenously based on the patient's body weight. Pediatric patients weighing 75 kg or more should be administered ORENCIA following the adult intravenous dosing regimen, not to exceed a maximum dose of 1000 mg (2.2).

General Dosing Information for Intravenous Administration (2.1)
• Administer as a 30-minute intravenous infusion (2.1)
• Following initial dose, give at 2 and 4 weeks, then every 4 weeks (2.1)
• Prepare ORENCIA using only the silicone-free disposable syringe (2.3)
• Use only sterile water to reconstitute the powder (2.3)
• The reconstituted product must be administered using a filter (2.3)

DOSAGE FORMS AND STRENGTHS

- 250 mg lyophilized powder in a single-use vial for intravenous infusion (3)
- 125 mg/mL solution in a single-dose prefilled syringe (3)

CONTRAINDICATIONS

- None (4)

WARNINGS AND PRECAUTIONS

- Concomitant use with a TNF antagonist can increase the risk of infections and serious infections (5.1)
- Hypersensitivity, anaphylaxis, and anaphylactoid reactions (5.2)
- Patients with a history of recurrent infections or underlying conditions predisposing to infections may experience more infections (5.3, 8.5)
- Discontinue if a serious infection develops (5.3)
- Screen for latent TB infection prior to initiating therapy. Patients testing positive should be treated prior to initiating ORENCIA (abatacept) (5.3)
- Live vaccines should not be given concurrently or within 3 months of discontinuation (5.4)
- Patients with juvenile idiopathic arthritis should be brought up to date with all immunizations prior to ORENCIA therapy (5.4)
- Based on its mechanism of action, ORENCIA may blunt the effectiveness of some immunizations (5.4)
- COPD patients may develop more frequent respiratory adverse events (5.5)

ADVERSE REACTIONS

Most common adverse events (≥10%) are headache, upper respiratory tract infection, nasopharyngitis, and nausea (6.1).

To report SUSPECTED ADVERSE REACTIONS, contact Bristol-Myers Squibb at 1-800-721-5072 or FDA at 1-800-FDA-1088 or www.fda.gov/medwatch.

USE IN SPECIFIC POPULATIONS

- Pregnancy: Registry available. Based on animal data, may cause fetal harm (8.1).

See 17 for PATIENT COUNSELING INFORMATION and FDA-approved patient labeling

Revised: 12/2013

FULL PRESCRIBING INFORMATION: CONTENTS*

* Sections or subsections omitted from the full prescribing information are not listed

FULL PRESCRIBING INFORMATION

1 INDICATIONS AND USAGE

1.1 Adult Rheumatoid Arthritis (RA)

ORENCIA® (abatacept) is indicated for reducing signs and symptoms, inducing major clinical response, inhibiting the progression of structural damage, and improving physical function in adult patients with moderately to severely active rheumatoid arthritis. ORENCIA may be used as monotherapy or concomitantly with disease-modifying antirheumatic drugs (DMARDs) other than tumor necrosis factor (TNF) antagonists.

1.2 Juvenile Idiopathic Arthritis

ORENCIA is indicated for reducing signs and symptoms in pediatric patients 6 years of age and older with moderately to severely active polyarticular juvenile idiopathic arthritis. ORENCIA may be used as monotherapy or concomitantly with methotrexate (MTX).

1.3 Important Limitations of Use

ORENCIA should not be administered concomitantly with TNF antagonists. ORENCIA is not recommended for use concomitantly with other biologic rheumatoid arthritis (RA) therapy, such as anakinra.

2 DOSAGE AND ADMINISTRATION

2.1 Adult Rheumatoid Arthritis

For adult patients with RA, ORENCIA may be administered as an intravenous infusion or a subcutaneous injection.

ORENCIA may be used as monotherapy or concomitantly with DMARDs other than TNF antagonists.

For pediatric juvenile idiopathic arthritis, a dose calculated based on each patient's body weight is used [see Dosage and Administration (2.2)].

Intravenous Dosing Regimen

ORENCIA intravenous should be administered as a 30-minute intravenous infusion utilizing the weight range-based dosing specified in Table 1. Following the initial intravenous administration, an intravenous infusion should be given at 2 and 4 weeks after the first infusion and every 4 weeks thereafter.

Table 1: Dose of ORENCIA for Intravenous Infusion in Adult RA Patients

Body Weight of Patient	Dose	Number of Vials[a]
Less than 60 kg	500 mg	2
60 to 100 kg	750 mg	3
More than 100 kg	1000 mg	4

[a] Each vial provides 250 mg of abatacept for administration.

Subcutaneous Dosing Regimen

ORENCIA 125 mg should be administered by subcutaneous injection once weekly and may be initiated with or without an intravenous loading dose. For patients initiating therapy with an intravenous loading dose, ORENCIA should be initiated with a single intravenous infusion (as per body weight categories listed in Table 1), followed by the first 125 mg subcutaneous injection administered within a day of the intravenous infusion.

Patients transitioning from ORENCIA intravenous therapy to subcutaneous administration should administer the first subcutaneous dose instead of the next scheduled intravenous dose.

2.2 Juvenile Idiopathic Arthritis

The recommended dose of ORENCIA for patients 6 to 17 years of age with juvenile idiopathic arthritis who weigh less than 75 kg is 10 mg/kg intravenously calculated based on the patient's body weight at each administration. Pediatric patients weighing 75 kg or more should be administered ORENCIA following the adult intravenous dosing regimen, not to exceed a maximum dose of 1000 mg. ORENCIA should be administered as a 30-minute intravenous infusion. Following the initial administration, ORENCIA should be given at 2 and 4 weeks after the first infusion and every 4 weeks thereafter. Any unused portions in the vials must be immediately discarded.

The safety and efficacy of subcutaneous ORENCIA (abatacept) injection has not been studied in patients under 18 years of age.

2.3 Preparation and Administration Instructions for Intravenous Infusion

Use aseptic technique.

ORENCIA is provided as a lyophilized powder in preservative-free, single-use vials. Each ORENCIA vial provides 250 mg of abatacept for administration. The ORENCIA powder in each vial must be reconstituted with 10 mL of Sterile Water for Injection, USP, using *only the silicone-free disposable syringe provided with each vial* and an 18- to 21-gauge needle. After reconstitution, the concentration of abatacept in the vial will be 25 mg/mL. If the ORENCIA powder is accidentally reconstituted using a siliconized syringe, the solution may develop a few translucent particles. Discard any solutions prepared using siliconized syringes.

If the *silicone-free disposable syringe* is dropped or becomes contaminated, use a new *silicone-free disposable syringe* from inventory. For information on obtaining additional *silicone-free disposable syringes*, contact Bristol-Myers Squibb 1-800-ORENCIA.

1) Use 10 mL of Sterile Water for Injection, USP to reconstitute the ORENCIA powder. To reconstitute the ORENCIA powder, remove the flip-top from the vial and wipe the top with an alcohol swab. Insert the syringe needle into the vial through the center of the rubber stopper and direct the stream of Sterile Water for Injection, USP, to the glass wall of the vial. Do not use the vial if the vacuum is not present. Rotate the vial with gentle swirling to minimize foam formation, until the contents are completely dissolved. Do not shake. Avoid prolonged or vigorous agitation.

2) Upon complete dissolution of the lyophilized powder, the vial should be vented with a needle to dissipate any foam that may be present. After reconstitution, each milliliter will contain 25 mg (250 mg/10 mL). The solution should be clear and colorless to pale yellow. Do not use if opaque particles, discoloration, or other foreign particles are present.

3) The reconstituted ORENCIA solution must be further diluted to 100 mL as follows. From a 100 mL infusion bag or bottle, withdraw a volume of 0.9% Sodium Chloride Injection, USP, equal to the volume of the reconstituted ORENCIA solution required for the patient's dose. Slowly add the reconstituted ORENCIA solution into the infusion bag or bottle using the same *silicone-free disposable syringe provided with each vial*. Gently mix. *Do not shake the bag or bottle.* The final concentration of abatacept in the bag or bottle will depend upon the amount of drug added, but will be no more than 10 mg/mL. Any unused portions in the vials must be immediately discarded.

4) Prior to administration, the ORENCIA solution should be inspected visually for particulate matter and discoloration. Discard the solution if any particulate matter or discoloration is observed.

5) The entire, fully diluted ORENCIA solution should be administered over a period of 30 minutes and must be administered with an infusion set and a *sterile, non-pyrogenic, low-protein-binding filter* (pore size of 0.2 μm to 1.2 μm).

6) The infusion of the fully diluted ORENCIA solution must be completed within 24 hours of reconstitution of the ORENCIA vials. The fully diluted ORENCIA solution may be stored at room temperature or refrigerated at 2°C to 8°C (36°F to 46°F) before use. Discard the fully diluted solution if not administered within 24 hours.

7) ORENCIA should not be infused concomitantly in the same intravenous line with other agents. No physical or biochemical compatibility studies have been conducted to evaluate the coadministration of ORENCIA with other agents.

2.4 General Considerations for Subcutaneous Administration

ORENCIA Injection, 125 mg/syringe is not intended for intravenous infusion.

ORENCIA Injection is intended for use under the guidance of a physician or healthcare practitioner. After proper training in subcutaneous injection technique, a patient may self-inject with ORENCIA if a physician/healthcare practitioner determines that it is appropriate. Patients should be instructed to follow the directions provided in the Instructions for Use for additional details on medication administration. Parenteral drug products should be inspected visually for particulate matter and discoloration prior to administration, whenever solution and container permit. Do not use ORENCIA prefilled syringes exhibiting particulate matter or discoloration. ORENCIA should be clear and colorless to pale yellow.

Patients using ORENCIA for subcutaneous administration should be instructed to inject the full amount in the syringe (1 mL), which provides 125 mg of ORENCIA, according to the directions provided in the Instructions for Use.

Injection sites should be rotated and injections should never be given into areas where the skin is tender, bruised, red, or hard.

3 DOSAGE FORMS AND STRENGTHS

- Lyophilized Powder for Intravenous Infusion
  250 mg single-use vial
- Solution for Subcutaneous Injection
  125 mg/mL single-dose prefilled glass syringe

4 CONTRAINDICATIONS

None.

5 WARNINGS AND PRECAUTIONS

5.1 Concomitant Use with TNF Antagonists

In controlled clinical trials in patients with adult RA, patients receiving concomitant intravenous ORENCIA (abatacept) and TNF antagonist therapy experienced more infections (63%) and serious infections (4.4%) compared to patients treated with only TNF antagonists (43% and 0.8%, respectively) [see Adverse Reactions (6.1)]. These trials failed to demonstrate an important enhancement of efficacy with concomitant administration of ORENCIA with TNF antagonist; therefore, concurrent therapy with ORENCIA and a TNF antagonist is not recommended. While transitioning from TNF antagonist therapy to ORENCIA therapy, patients should be monitored for signs of infection.

5.2 Hypersensitivity

In controlled, double-blind and open-label clinical trials, the occurrence of anaphylaxis and anaphylactoid reactions was rare (<0.1%) and was only observed in patients dosed with intravenous ORENCIA. Other reactions potentially associated with drug hypersensitivity, such as hypotension, urticaria, and dyspnea that occurred within 24 hours of ORENCIA infusion, were uncommon (<1%). Of the 190 patients with juvenile idiopathic arthritis treated with ORENCIA in clinical trials, there was one case of a hypersensitivity reaction (0.5%). Appropriate medical support measures for the treatment of hypersensitivity reactions should be available for immediate use in the event of a reaction [see Adverse Reactions (6.1, 6.3)]. Anaphylaxis or anaphylactoid reactions can occur after the first infusion and can be life threatening. In postmarketing experience, a case of fatal anaphylaxis following the first infusion of ORENCIA has been reported. If an anaphylactic or other serious allergic reaction occurs, administration of ORENCIA should be stopped immediately with appropriate therapy instituted, and the use of ORENCIA should be permanently discontinued.

5.3 Infections

Serious infections, including sepsis and pneumonia, have been reported in patients receiving ORENCIA. Some of these infections have been fatal. Many of the serious infections have occurred in patients on concomitant immunosuppressive therapy which in addition to their underlying disease, could further predispose them to infection. Physicians should exercise caution when considering the use of ORENCIA in patients with a history of recurrent infections, underlying conditions which may predispose them to infections, or chronic, latent, or localized infections. Patients who develop a new infection while undergoing treatment with ORENCIA should be monitored closely. Administration of ORENCIA should be discontinued if a patient develops a serious infection [see Adverse Reactions (6.1)]. A higher rate of serious infections has been observed in adult RA patients treated with concurrent TNF antagonists and ORENCIA [see Warnings and Precautions (5.1)].

Prior to initiating immunomodulatory therapies, including ORENCIA, patients should be screened for latent tuberculosis infection with a tuberculin skin test. ORENCIA has not been studied in patients with a positive tuberculosis screen, and the safety of ORENCIA in individuals with latent tuberculosis infection is unknown. Patients testing positive in tuberculosis screening should be treated by standard medical practice prior to therapy with ORENCIA.

Antirheumatic therapies have been associated with hepatitis B reactivation. Therefore, screening for viral hepatitis should be performed in accordance with published guidelines before starting therapy with ORENCIA. In clinical studies with ORENCIA, patients who screened positive for hepatitis were excluded from study.

5.4 Immunizations

Live vaccines should not be given concurrently with ORENCIA or within 3 months of its discontinuation. No data are available on the secondary transmission of infection from persons receiving live vaccines to patients receiving ORENCIA. The efficacy of vaccination in patients receiving ORENCIA is not known. Based on its mechanism of action, ORENCIA may blunt the effectiveness of some immunizations.

It is recommended that patients with juvenile idiopathic arthritis be brought up to date with all immunizations in agreement with current immunization guidelines prior to initiating ORENCIA therapy.

5.5 Use in Patients with Chronic Obstructive Pulmonary Disease (COPD)

Adult COPD patients treated with ORENCIA developed adverse events more frequently than those treated with pla-

cebo, including COPD exacerbations, cough, rhonchi, and dyspnea. Use of ORENCIA in patients with RA and COPD should be undertaken with caution and such patients should be monitored for worsening of their respiratory status [see Adverse Reactions (6.1)].

5.6 Immunosuppression

The possibility exists for drugs inhibiting T cell activation, including ORENCIA (abatacept), to affect host defenses against infections and malignancies since T cells mediate cellular immune responses. The impact of treatment with ORENCIA on the development and course of malignancies is not fully understood [see Adverse Reactions (6.1)]. In clinical trials in patients with adult RA, a higher rate of infections was seen in ORENCIA-treated patients compared to placebo [see Adverse Reactions (6.1)].

6 ADVERSE REACTIONS

6.1 Clinical Studies Experience in Adult RA Patients Treated with Intravenous ORENCIA

Because clinical trials are conducted under widely varying and controlled conditions, adverse reaction rates observed in clinical trials of a drug cannot be directly compared to rates in the clinical trials of another drug and may not predict the rates observed in a broader patient population in clinical practice.

The data described herein reflect exposure to ORENCIA administered intravenously in patients with active RA in placebo-controlled studies (1955 patients with ORENCIA, 989 with placebo). The studies had either a double-blind, placebo-controlled period of 6 months (258 patients with ORENCIA, 133 with placebo) or 1 year (1697 patients with ORENCIA, 856 with placebo). A subset of these patients received concomitant biologic DMARD therapy, such as a TNF blocking agent (204 patients with ORENCIA, 134 with placebo).

The majority of patients in RA clinical studies received one or more of the following concomitant medications with ORENCIA: methotrexate, nonsteroidal anti-inflammatory drugs (NSAIDs), corticosteroids, TNF blocking agents, azathioprine, chloroquine, gold, hydroxychloroquine, leflunomide, sulfasalazine, and anakinra.

The most serious adverse reactions were serious infections and malignancies.

The most commonly reported adverse events (occurring in ≥10% of patients treated with ORENCIA) were headache, upper respiratory tract infection, nasopharyngitis, and nausea.

The adverse events most frequently resulting in clinical intervention (interruption or discontinuation of ORENCIA) were due to infection. The most frequently reported infections resulting in dose interruption were upper respiratory tract infection (1.0%), bronchitis (0.7%), and herpes zoster (0.7%). The most frequent infections resulting in discontinuation were pneumonia (0.2%), localized infection (0.2%), and bronchitis (0.1%).

Infections

In the placebo-controlled trials, infections were reported in 54% of ORENCIA-treated and 48% of placebo-treated patients. The most commonly reported infections (reported in 5%-13% of patients) were upper respiratory tract infection, nasopharyngitis, sinusitis, urinary tract infection, influenza, and bronchitis. Other infections reported in fewer than 5% of patients at a higher frequency (>0.5%) with ORENCIA compared to placebo, were rhinitis, herpes simplex, and pneumonia [see Warnings and Precautions (5.3)].

Serious infections were reported in 3.0% of patients treated with ORENCIA and 1.9% of patients treated with placebo. The most common (0.2%-0.5%) serious infections reported with ORENCIA were pneumonia, cellulitis, urinary tract infection, bronchitis, diverticulitis, and acute pyelonephritis [see Warnings and Precautions (5.3)].

Malignancies

In the placebo-controlled portions of the clinical trials (1955 patients treated with ORENCIA for a median of 12 months), the overall frequencies of malignancies were similar in the ORENCIA- and placebo-treated patients (1.3% and 1.1%, respectively). However, more cases of lung cancer were observed in ORENCIA-treated patients (4, 0.2%) than placebo-treated patients (0). In the cumulative ORENCIA clinical trials (placebo-controlled and uncontrolled, open-label) a total of 8 cases of lung cancer (0.21 cases per 100 patient-years) and 4 lymphomas (0.10 cases per 100 patient-years) were observed in 2688 patients (3827 patient-years). The rate observed for lymphoma is approximately 3.5-fold higher than expected in an age- and gender-matched general population based on the National Cancer Institute's Surveillance, Epidemiology, and End Results Database. Patients with RA, particularly those with highly active disease, are at a higher risk for the development of lymphoma. Other malignancies included skin, breast, bile duct, bladder, cervical, endometrial, lymphoma, melanoma, myelodysplastic syndrome, ovarian, prostate, renal, thyroid,

and uterine cancers [see Warnings and Precautions (5.6)]. The potential role of ORENCIA (abatacept) in the development of malignancies in humans is unknown.

Infusion-Related Reactions and Hypersensitivity Reactions

Acute infusion-related reactions (adverse reactions occurring within 1 hour of the start of the infusion) in Studies III, IV, and V [see Clinical Studies (14.1)] were more common in the ORENCIA-treated patients than the placebo patients (9% for ORENCIA, 6% for placebo). The most frequently reported events (1%-2%) were dizziness, headache, and hypertension.

Acute infusion-related events that were reported in >0.1% and ≤1% of patients treated with ORENCIA included cardiopulmonary symptoms, such as hypotension, increased blood pressure, and dyspnea; other symptoms included nausea, flushing, urticaria, cough, hypersensitivity, pruritus, rash, and wheezing. Most of these reactions were mild (68%) to moderate (28%). Fewer than 1% of ORENCIA-treated patients discontinued due to an acute infusion-related event. In controlled trials, 6 ORENCIA-treated patients compared to 2 placebo-treated patients discontinued study treatment due to acute infusion-related events.

Anaphylaxis was observed in patients dosed with ORENCIA administered intravenously in controlled and open-label clinical trials, and the occurrence was rare (<0.1%). Other reactions potentially associated with drug hypersensitivity, such as hypotension, urticaria, and dyspnea that occurred within 24 hours of ORENCIA infusion, were uncommon (<1%). Appropriate medical support measures for the treatment of hypersensitivity reactions should be available for immediate use in the event of a reaction [see Warnings and Precautions (5.2)].

Adverse Reactions in Patients with COPD

In Study V [see Clinical Studies (14.1)], there were 37 patients with chronic obstructive pulmonary disease (COPD) who were treated with ORENCIA and 17 COPD patients who were treated with placebo. The COPD patients treated with ORENCIA developed adverse events more frequently than those treated with placebo (97% vs 88%, respectively). Respiratory disorders occurred more frequently in ORENCIA-treated patients compared to placebo-treated patients (43% vs 24%, respectively) including COPD exacerbation, cough, rhonchi, and dyspnea. A greater percentage of ORENCIA-treated patients developed a serious adverse event compared to placebo-treated patients (27% vs 6%), including COPD exacerbation (3 of 37 patients [8%]) and pneumonia (1 of 37 patients [3%]) [see Warnings and Precautions (5.5)].

Other Adverse Reactions

Adverse events occurring in 3% or more of patients and at least 1% more frequently in ORENCIA-treated patients during placebo-controlled RA studies are summarized in Table 2.

Table 2: Adverse Events Occurring in 3% or More of Patients and at Least 1% More Frequently in ORENCIA-Treated Patients During Placebo-Controlled RA Studies

Adverse Event (Preferred Term)	ORENCIA (n=1955)[a] Percentage	Placebo (n=989)[b] Percentage
Headache	18	13
Nasopharyngitis	12	9
Dizziness	9	7
Cough	8	7
Back pain	7	6
Hypertension	7	4
Dyspepsia	6	4
Urinary tract infection	6	5
Rash	4	3
Pain in extremity	3	2

[a] Includes 204 patients on concomitant biologic DMARDs (adalimumab, anakinra, etanercept, or infliximab).

[b] Includes 134 patients on concomitant biologic DMARDs (adalimumab, anakinra, etanercept, or infliximab).

Immunogenicity

Antibodies directed against the entire abatacept molecule or to the CTLA-4 portion of abatacept were assessed by ELISA assays in RA patients for up to 2 years following repeated treatment with ORENCIA. Thirty-four of 1993 (1.7%) patients developed binding antibodies to the entire abatacept molecule or to the CTLA-4 portion of abatacept. Because trough levels of abatacept can interfere with assay results, a subset analysis was performed. In this analysis it was observed that 9 of 154 (5.8%) patients that had discontinued treatment with ORENCIA for over 56 days developed antibodies.

Samples with confirmed binding activity to CTLA-4 were assessed for the presence of neutralizing antibodies in a cell-based luciferase reporter assay. Six of 9 (67%) evaluable patients were shown to possess neutralizing antibodies. However, the development of neutralizing antibodies may be underreported due to lack of assay sensitivity.

No correlation of antibody development to clinical response or adverse events was observed.

The data reflect the percentage of patients whose test results were positive for antibodies to abatacept in specific assays. The observed incidence of antibody (including neutralizing antibody) positivity in an assay is highly dependent on several factors, including assay sensitivity and specificity, assay methodology, sample handling, timing of sample collection, concomitant medication, and underlying disease. For these reasons, comparison of the incidence of antibodies to abatacept with the incidence of antibodies to other products may be misleading.

Clinical Experience in Methotrexate-Naive Patients

Study VI was an active-controlled clinical trial in methotrexate-naive patients [see *Clinical Studies (14.1)*]. The safety experience in these patients was consistent with Studies I-V.

6.2 Clinical Experience in Adult RA Patients Treated with Subcutaneous ORENCIA (abatacept)

Because clinical trials are conducted under widely varying and controlled conditions, adverse reaction rates observed in clinical trials of a drug cannot be directly compared to rates in the clinical trials of another drug and may not predict the rates observed in a broader patient population in clinical practice.

Study SC-1 was a randomized, double-blind, double-dummy, non-inferiority study that compared the efficacy and safety of abatacept administered subcutaneously (SC) and intravenously (IV) in 1457 subjects with rheumatoid arthritis, receiving background methotrexate, and experiencing an inadequate response to methotrexate (MTX-IR) [see *Clinical Studies (14.1)*]. The safety experience and immunogenicity for ORENCIA administered subcutaneously was consistent with intravenous Studies I-VI. Due to the route of administration, injection site reactions and immunogenicity were evaluated in Study SC-1 and two other smaller studies discussed in the sections below.

Injection Site Reactions in Adult RA Patients Treated with Subcutaneous ORENCIA

Study SC-1 compared the safety of abatacept including injection site reactions following subcutaneous or intravenous administration. The overall frequency of injection site reactions was 2.6% (19/736) and 2.5% (18/721) for the subcutaneous abatacept group and the intravenous abatacept group (subcutaneous placebo), respectively. All these injection site reactions (including hematoma, pruritus, and erythema) were mild (83%) to moderate (17%) in severity, and none necessitated drug discontinuation.

Immunogenicity in Adult RA Patients Treated with Subcutaneous ORENCIA

Study SC-1 compared the immunogenicity to abatacept following subcutaneous or intravenous administration. The overall immunogenicity frequency to abatacept was 1.1% (8/725) and 2.3% (16/710) for the subcutaneous and intravenous groups, respectively. The rate is consistent with previous experience, and there was no correlation of immunogenicity with effects on pharmacokinetics, safety, or efficacy.

Immunogenicity and Safety of Subcutaneous ORENCIA administration as Monotherapy without an Intravenous Loading Dose

Study SC-2 was conducted to determine the effect of monotherapy use of ORENCIA on immunogenicity following subcutaneous administration without an intravenous load in 100 RA patients, who had not previously received abatacept or other CTLA4Ig, who received either subcutaneous ORENCIA plus methotrexate (n=51) or subcutaneous ORENCIA monotherapy (n=49). No patients in either group developed anti-product antibodies after 4 months of treatment. The safety observed in this study was consistent with that observed in the other subcutaneous studies.

Immunogenicity and Safety of Subcutaneous ORENCIA upon Withdrawal (Three Months) and Restart of Treatment

Study SC-3 in the subcutaneous program was conducted to investigate the effect of withdrawal (three months) and restart of ORENCIA subcutaneous treatment on immunogenicity in RA patients treated concomitantly with methotrexate. One hundred sixty-seven patients were enrolled in the first 3-month treatment period and responders (n=120) were randomized to either subcutaneous ORENCIA or placebo for the second 3-month period (withdrawal period). Patients from this period then received open-label ORENCIA treatment in the final 3-month period of the study (period 3). At the end of the withdrawal period, 0/38 patients who continued to receive subcutaneous ORENCIA developed anti-product antibodies compared to 7/73 (9.6%) of patients who had subcutaneous ORENCIA withdrawn during this period. Half of the patients receiving subcutaneous placebo during the withdrawal period received a single intravenous infusion of ORENCIA at the start of period 3 and half received intravenous placebo. At the end of period 3, when all patients again received subcutaneous ORENCIA, the im-

munogenicity rates were 1/38 (2.6%) in the group receiving subcutaneous ORENCIA (abatacept) throughout, and 2/73 (2.7%) in the group that had received placebo during the withdrawal period. Upon reinitiating therapy, there were no injection reactions and no differences in response to therapy in patients who were withdrawn from subcutaneous therapy for up to 3 months relative to those who remained on subcutaneous therapy, whether therapy was reintroduced with or without an intravenous loading dose. The safety observed in this study was consistent with that observed in the other studies.

6.3 Clinical Studies Experience in Juvenile Idiopathic Arthritis

Because clinical trials are conducted under widely varying conditions, adverse reaction rates observed in the clinical trials of a drug cannot be directly compared to rates in the clinical trials of another drug and may not reflect the rates observed in practice.

In general, the adverse events in pediatric patients were similar in frequency and type to those seen in adult patients [see *Warnings and Precautions (5)*, *Adverse Reactions (6)*]. ORENCIA has been studied in 190 pediatric patients, 6 to 17 years of age, with polyarticular juvenile idiopathic arthritis. Overall frequency of adverse events in the 4-month, lead-in, open-label period of the study was 70%; infections occurred at a frequency of 36% [see *Clinical Studies (14.2)*]. The most common infections were upper respiratory tract infection and nasopharyngitis. The infections resolved without sequelae, and the types of infections were consistent with those commonly seen in outpatient pediatric populations. Other events that occurred at a prevalence of at least 5% were headache, nausea, diarrhea, cough, pyrexia, and abdominal pain.

A total of 6 serious adverse events (acute lymphocytic leukemia, ovarian cyst, varicella infection, disease flare [2], and joint wear) were reported during the initial 4 months of treatment with ORENCIA.

Of the 190 patients with juvenile idiopathic arthritis treated with ORENCIA in clinical trials, there was one case of a hypersensitivity reaction (0.5%). During Periods A, B, and C, acute infusion-related reactions occurred at a frequency of 4%, 2%, and 3%, respectively, and were consistent with the types of events reported in adults.

Upon continued treatment in the open-label extension period, the types of adverse events were similar in frequency and type to those seen in adult patients, except for a single patient diagnosed with multiple sclerosis while on open-label treatment.

Immunogenicity

Antibodies directed against the entire abatacept molecule or to the CTLA-4 portion of abatacept were assessed by ELISA assays in patients with juvenile idiopathic arthritis following repeated treatment with ORENCIA throughout the open-label period. For patients who were withdrawn from therapy for up to 6 months during the double-blind period, the rate of antibody formation to the CTLA-4 portion of the molecule was 41% (22/54), while for those who remained on therapy the rate was 13% (7/54). Twenty of these patients had samples that could be tested for antibodies with neutralizing activity; of these, 8 (40%) patients were shown to possess neutralizing antibodies.

The presence of antibodies was generally transient and titers were low. The presence of antibodies was not associated with adverse events, changes in efficacy, or an effect on serum concentrations of abatacept. For patients who were withdrawn from ORENCIA during the double-blind period for up to 6 months, no serious acute infusion-related events were observed upon re-initiation of ORENCIA therapy.

6.4 Postmarketing Experience

Adverse reactions have been reported during the postapproval use of ORENCIA. Because these reactions are reported voluntarily from a population of uncertain size, it is not always possible to reliably estimate their frequency or establish a causal relationship to ORENCIA. Based on the postmarketing experience in adult RA patients, the following adverse reaction has been identified during postapproval use with ORENCIA.

• Vasculitis (including cutaneous vasculitis and leukocytoclastic vasculitis)

7 DRUG INTERACTIONS

7.1 TNF Antagonists

Concurrent administration of a TNF antagonist with ORENCIA has been associated with an increased risk of serious infections and no significant additional efficacy over use of the TNF antagonists alone. Concurrent therapy with ORENCIA and TNF antagonists is not recommended [see *Warnings and Precautions (5.1)*].

7.2 Other Biologic RA Therapy

There is insufficient experience to assess the safety and efficacy of ORENCIA administered concurrently with other biologic RA therapy, such as anakinra, and therefore such use is not recommended.

7.3 Blood Glucose Testing

Parenteral drug products containing maltose can interfere with the readings of blood glucose monitors that use test strips with glucose dehydrogenase pyrroloquinolinequinone (GDH-PQQ). The GDH-PQQ based glucose monitoring systems may react with the maltose present in ORENCIA (abatacept) for intravenous administration, resulting in falsely elevated blood glucose readings on the day of infusion. When receiving ORENCIA through intravenous administration, patients that require blood glucose monitoring should be advised to consider methods that do not react with maltose, such as those based on glucose dehydrogenase nicotine adenine dinucleotide (GDH-NAD), glucose oxidase, or glucose hexokinase test methods.

ORENCIA for subcutaneous administration does not contain maltose; therefore, patients do not need to alter their glucose monitoring.

8 USE IN SPECIFIC POPULATIONS

8.1 Pregnancy

Pregnancy Category C

There are no adequate and well-controlled studies of ORENCIA use in pregnant women. Abatacept has been shown to cross the placenta in animals, and in animal reproduction studies alterations in immune function occurred. ORENCIA should be used during pregnancy only if the potential benefit to the mother justifies the potential risk to the fetus.

Abatacept was not teratogenic when administered to pregnant mice at doses up to 300 mg/kg and in pregnant rats and rabbits at doses up to 200 mg/kg daily representing approximately 29 times the exposure associated with the maximum recommended human dose (MRHD) of 10 mg/kg based on AUC (area under the time-concentration curve). Abatacept administered to female rats every three days during early gestation and throughout the lactation period, produced no adverse effects in offspring at doses up to 45 mg/kg, representing 3 times the exposure associated with the MRHD of 10 mg/kg based on AUC. However, at 200 mg/kg, 11 times the MRHD exposure, alterations in immune function were observed consisting of a 9-fold increase in T-cell dependent antibody response in female pups and thyroid inflammation in one female pup. It is not known whether these findings indicate a risk for development of autoimmune diseases in humans exposed *in utero* to abatacept. However, exposure to abatacept in the juvenile rat, which may be more representative of the fetal immune system state in the human, resulted in immune system abnormalities including inflammation of the thyroid and pancreas [see *Nonclinical Toxicology (13.2)*].

Pregnancy Registry: To monitor maternal-fetal outcomes of pregnant women exposed to ORENCIA, a pregnancy registry has been established. Healthcare professionals are encouraged to register patients and pregnant women are encouraged to enroll themselves by calling 1-877-311-8972.

8.3 Nursing Mothers

It is not known whether ORENCIA is excreted into human milk or absorbed systemically after ingestion by a nursing infant. However, abatacept was excreted in rat milk. Because many drugs are excreted in human milk, and because of the potential for serious adverse reactions in nursing infants from ORENCIA, a decision should be made whether to discontinue nursing or to discontinue the drug, taking into account the importance of the drug to the mother.

8.4 Pediatric Use

Intravenous ORENCIA is indicated for reducing signs and symptoms in pediatric patients with moderately to severely active polyarticular juvenile idiopathic arthritis ages 6 years and older. ORENCIA may be used as monotherapy or concomitantly with methotrexate.

Studies in juvenile rats exposed to ORENCIA prior to immune system maturity have shown immune system abnormalities including an increase in the incidence of infections leading to death as well as inflammation of the thyroid and pancreas [see *Nonclinical Toxicology (13.2)*]. Studies in adult mice and monkeys have not demonstrated similar findings. As the immune system of the rat is undeveloped in the first few weeks after birth, the relevance of these results to humans greater than 6 years of age (where the immune system is largely developed) is unknown.

ORENCIA is not recommended for use in patients below the age of 6 years.

The safety and effectiveness of ORENCIA in pediatric patients below 6 years of age have not been established. The safety and efficacy of ORENCIA in pediatric patients for uses other than juvenile idiopathic arthritis have not been established.

The safety and efficacy of subcutaneous ORENCIA has not been studied in patients under 18 years of age.

8.5 Geriatric Use

A total of 323 patients 65 years of age and older, including 53 patients 75 years and older, received ORENCIA in clinical studies. No overall differences in safety or effectiveness were observed between these patients and younger patients, but these numbers are too low to rule out differences. The frequency of serious infection and malignancy among ORENCIA-treated patients over age 65 was higher than for those under age 65. Because there is a higher incidence of infections and malignancies in the elderly population in general, caution should be used when treating the elderly.

10   OVERDOSAGE

Doses up to 50 mg/kg have been administered intravenously without apparent toxic effect. In case of overdosage, it is recommended that the patient be monitored for any signs or symptoms of adverse reactions and appropriate symptomatic treatment instituted.

11   DESCRIPTION

ORENCIA® (abatacept) is a soluble fusion protein that consists of the extracellular domain of human cytotoxic T-lymphocyte-associated antigen 4 (CTLA-4) linked to the modified Fc (hinge, CH2, and CH3 domains) portion of human immunoglobulin G1 (IgG1). Abatacept is produced by recombinant DNA technology in a mammalian cell expression system. The apparent molecular weight of abatacept is 92 kilodaltons.

ORENCIA lyophilized powder for intravenous infusion is supplied as a sterile, white, preservative-free, lyophilized powder for intravenous administration. Following reconstitution of the lyophilized powder with 10 mL of Sterile Water for Injection, USP, the solution of ORENCIA is clear, colorless to pale yellow, with a pH range of 7.2 to 7.8. Each single-use vial of ORENCIA provides 250 mg abatacept, maltose (500 mg), monobasic sodium phosphate (17.2 mg), and sodium chloride (14.6 mg) for administration.

ORENCIA solution for subcutaneous administration is supplied as a sterile, preservative-free, clear, colorless to pale-yellow solution with a pH of 6.8 to 7.4. Each single dose of subcutaneous injection provides 125 mg abatacept, dibasic sodium phosphate anhydrous (0.838 mg), monobasic sodium phosphate monohydrate (0.286 mg), poloxamer 188 (8 mg), sucrose (170 mg), and quantity sufficient to 1 mL with water for injection. Unlike the intravenous formulation, ORENCIA solution for subcutaneous administration contains no maltose.

12   CLINICAL PHARMACOLOGY

12.1   Mechanism of Action

Abatacept, a selective costimulation modulator, inhibits T cell (T lymphocyte) activation by binding to CD80 and CD86, thereby blocking interaction with CD28. This interaction provides a costimulatory signal necessary for full activation of T lymphocytes. Activated T lymphocytes are implicated in the pathogenesis of RA and are found in the synovium of patients with RA.

In vitro, abatacept decreases T cell proliferation and inhibits the production of the cytokines TNF alpha (TNFα), interferon-γ, and interleukin-2. In a rat collagen-induced arthritis model, abatacept suppresses inflammation, decreases anti-collagen antibody production, and reduces antigen specific production of interferon-γ. The relationship of these biological response markers to the mechanisms by which ORENCIA exerts its effects in RA is unknown.

12.2   Pharmacodynamics

In clinical trials with ORENCIA at doses approximating 10 mg/kg, decreases were observed in serum levels of soluble interleukin-2 receptor (sIL-2R), interleukin-6 (IL-6), rheumatoid factor (RF), C-reactive protein (CRP), matrix metalloproteinase-3 (MMP3), and TNFα. The relationship of these biological response markers to the mechanisms by which ORENCIA exerts its effects in RA is unknown.

12.3   Pharmacokinetics

Healthy Adults and Adult RA - Intravenous Administration

The pharmacokinetics of abatacept were studied in healthy adult subjects after a single 10 mg/kg intravenous infusion and in RA patients after multiple 10 mg/kg intravenous infusions (see Table 3).

Table 3: Pharmacokinetic Parameters (Mean, Range) in Healthy Subjects and RA Patients After 10 mg/kg Intravenous Infusion(s)

PK Parameter	Healthy Subjects (After 10 mg/kg Single Dose) n=13	RA Patients (After 10 mg/kg Multiple Doses[a]) n=14
Peak Concentration (C_{max}) [mcg/mL]	292 (175-427)	295 (171-398)
Terminal half-life ($t_{1/2}$) [days]	16.7 (12-23)	13.1 (8-25)
Systemic clearance (CL) [mL/h/kg]	0.23 (0.16-0.30)	0.22 (0.13-0.47)
Volume of distribution (Vss) [L/kg]	0.09 (0.06-0.13)	0.07 (0.02-0.13)

[a] Multiple intravenous infusions were administered at days 1, 15, 30, and monthly thereafter.

The pharmacokinetics of abatacept in RA patients and healthy subjects appeared to be comparable. In RA patients, after multiple intravenous infusions, the pharmacokinetics of abatacept showed proportional increases of C_{max} and AUC over the dose range of 2 mg/kg to 10 mg/kg. At 10 mg/kg, serum concentration appeared to reach a steady-state by day 60 with a mean (range) trough concentration of 24 mcg/mL (1 to 66 mcg/mL). No systemic accumulation of abatacept occurred upon continued repeated treatment with 10 mg/kg at monthly intervals in RA patients.

Population pharmacokinetic analyses in RA patients revealed that there was a trend toward higher clearance of abatacept with increasing body weight. Age and gender (when corrected for body weight) did not affect clearance. Concomitant methotrexate, NSAIDs, corticosteroids, and TNF blocking agents did not influence abatacept clearance. No formal studies were conducted to examine the effects of either renal or hepatic impairment on the pharmacokinetics of abatacept.

Juvenile Idiopathic Arthritis

In patients 6 to 17 years of age, the mean (range) steady-state serum peak and trough concentrations of abatacept were 217 mcg/mL (57 to 700 mcg/mL) and 11.9 mcg/mL (0.15 to 44.6 mcg/mL). Population pharmacokinetic analyses of the serum concentration data showed that clearance of abatacept increased with baseline body weight. The estimated mean (range) clearance of abatacept in the juvenile idiopathic arthritis patients was 0.4 mL/h/kg (0.20 to 1.12 mL/h/kg). After accounting for the effect of body weight, the clearance of abatacept was not related to age and gender. Concomitant methotrexate, corticosteroids, and NSAIDs were also shown not to influence abatacept clearance.

Adult RA - Subcutaneous Administration

Abatacept exhibited linear pharmacokinetics following subcutaneous administration. The mean (range) for C_{min} and C_{max} at steady state observed after 85 days of treatment was 32.5 mcg/mL (6.6 to 113.8 mcg/mL) and 48.1 mcg/mL (9.8 to 132.4 mcg/mL), respectively. The bioavailability of abatacept following subcutaneous administration relative to intravenous administration is 78.6%. Mean estimates for systemic clearance (0.28 mL/h/kg), volume of distribution (0.11 L/kg), and terminal half-life (14.3 days) were comparable between subcutaneous and intravenous administration.

Study SC-2 was conducted to determine the effect of monotherapy use of ORENCIA (abatacept) on immunogenicity following subcutaneous administration without an intravenous load. When the intravenous loading dose was not administered, a mean trough concentration of 12.6 mcg/mL was achieved after 2 weeks of dosing.

Consistent with the intravenous data, population pharmacokinetic analyses for subcutaneous abatacept in RA patients revealed that there was a trend toward higher clearance of abatacept with increasing body weight. Age and gender (when corrected for body weight) did not affect apparent clearance. Concomitant medication, such as methotrexate, corticosteroids, and NSAIDs, did not influence abatacept apparent clearance.

13   NONCLINICAL TOXICOLOGY

13.1   Carcinogenesis, Mutagenesis, Impairment of Fertility

In a mouse carcinogenicity study, weekly subcutaneous injections of 20, 65, or 200 mg/kg of abatacept administered for up to 84 weeks in males and 88 weeks in females were associated with increases in the incidence of malignant lymphomas (all doses) and mammary gland tumors (intermediate- and high-dose in females). The mice from this study were infected with murine leukemia virus and mouse mammary tumor virus. These viruses are associated with an increased incidence of lymphomas and mammary gland tumors, respectively, in immunosuppressed mice. The doses used in these studies produced exposures 0.8, 2.0, and 3.0 times higher, respectively, than the exposure associated with the maximum recommended human dose (MRHD) of 10 mg/kg based on AUC (area under the time-concentration curve). The relevance of these findings to the clinical use of ORENCIA is unknown.

In a one-year toxicity study in cynomolgus monkeys, abatacept was administered intravenously once weekly at doses up to 50 mg/kg (producing 9 times the MRHD exposure based on AUC). Abatacept was not associated with any significant drug-related toxicity. Reversible pharmacological effects consisted of minimal transient decreases in serum IgG and minimal to severe lymphoid depletion of germinal centers in the spleen and/or lymph nodes. No evidence of lymphomas or preneoplastic morphologic changes was observed, despite the presence of a virus (lymphocryptovirus) known to cause these lesions in immunosuppressed monkeys within the time frame of this study. The relevance of these findings to the clinical use of ORENCIA (abatacept) is unknown.

No mutagenic potential of abatacept was observed in the *in vitro* bacterial reverse mutation (Ames) or Chinese hamster ovary/hypoxanthine guanine phosphoribosyltransferase (CHO/HGPRT) forward point mutation assays with or without metabolic activation, and no chromosomal aberrations were observed in human lymphocytes treated with abatacept with or without metabolic activation.

Abatacept had no adverse effects on male or female fertility in rats at doses up to 200 mg/kg every three days (11 times the MRHD exposure based on AUC).

13.2   Animal Toxicology and/or Pharmacology

A juvenile animal study was conducted in rats dosed with abatacept from 4 to 94 days of age in which an increase in the incidence of infections leading to death occurred at all doses compared with controls. Altered T-cell subsets including increased T-helper cells and reduced T-regulatory cells were observed. In addition, inhibition of T-cell-dependent antibody responses (TDAR) was observed. Upon following these animals into adulthood, lymphocytic inflammation of the thyroid and pancreatic islets was observed.

In studies of adult mice and monkeys, inhibition of TDAR was apparent. However, infection and mortality, altered T-helper cells, and inflammation of thyroid and pancreas were not observed.

14   CLINICAL STUDIES

14.1   Adult Rheumatoid Arthritis

The efficacy and safety of ORENCIA for intravenous administration were assessed in six randomized, double-blind, controlled studies (five placebo-controlled and one active-controlled) in patients ≥18 years of age with active RA diagnosed according to American College of Rheumatology (ACR) criteria. Studies I, II, III, IV, and VI required patients to have at least 12 tender and 10 swollen joints at randomization. Study V did not require any specific number of tender or swollen joints. ORENCIA or placebo treatment was given intravenously at weeks 0, 2, and then every 4 weeks thereafter in intravenous Studies I, II, III, IV, and VI. The safety and efficacy of ORENCIA for subcutaneous administration were assessed in Study SC-1, which was a randomized, double-blind, double-dummy, non-inferiority study that compared abatacept administered subcutaneously and intravenously in 1457 subjects with rheumatoid arthritis (RA), receiving background methotrexate (MTX), and experiencing an inadequate response to methotrexate (MTX-IR). Study I evaluated ORENCIA as monotherapy in 122 patients with active RA who had failed at least one non-biologic DMARD or etanercept. In Study II and Study III, the efficacy and safety of ORENCIA were assessed in patients with an inadequate response to methotrexate and who were continued on their stable dose of methotrexate. In Study IV, the efficacy and safety of ORENCIA were assessed in patients with an inadequate response to a TNF blocking agent, with the TNF blocking agent discontinued prior to randomization; other DMARDs were permitted. Study V primarily assessed safety in patients with active RA requiring additional intervention in spite of current therapy with DMARDs; all DMARDs used at enrollment were continued. Patients in Study V were not excluded for comorbid medical conditions. In Study VI, the efficacy and safety of ORENCIA were assessed in methotrexate-naive patients with RA of less than 2 years disease duration. In Study VI, patients previously naive to methotrexate were randomized to receive ORENCIA plus methotrexate or methotrexate plus placebo. In Study SC-1, the goal was to demonstrate the efficacy and safety of ORENCIA subcutaneous relative to ORENCIA intravenous administration in subjects with moderate to severely active RA and experiencing inadequate response to methotrexate, using a non-inferiority study design.

Study I patients were randomized to receive one of three doses of ORENCIA (0.5, 2, or 10 mg/kg) or placebo ending at week 8. Study II patients were randomized to receive ORENCIA 2 or 10 mg/kg or placebo for 12 months. Study III, IV, V, and VI patients were randomized to receive a dose of ORENCIA based on weight range or placebo for 12 months (Studies III, V, and VI) or 6 months (Study IV). The dose of ORENCIA was 500 mg for patients weighing less than 60 kg, 750 mg for patients weighing 60 to 100 kg, and 1000 mg for patients weighing greater than 100 kg. In Study SC-1, patients were randomized with stratification by body weight (<60 kg, 60 to 100 kg, >100 kg) to receive ORENCIA 125 mg subcutaneous injections weekly, after a single intravenous loading dose of ORENCIA based on body weight or ORENCIA intravenously on Days 1, 15, 29, and every four weeks thereafter. Subjects continued taking their current dose of methotrexate from the day of randomization.

Clinical Response

The percent of ORENCIA (abatacept)-treated patients achieving ACR 20, 50, and 70 responses and major clinical response in Studies I, III, IV, and VI are shown in Table 4. ORENCIA-treated patients had higher ACR 20, 50, and 70 response rates at 6 months compared to placebo-treated patients. Month 6 ACR response rates in Study II for the 10 mg/kg group were similar to the ORENCIA group in Study III.

In Studies III and IV, improvement in the ACR 20 response rate versus placebo was observed within 15 days in some patients and within 29 days versus methotrexate in Study VI. In Studies II, III, and VI, ACR response rates were maintained to 12 months in ORENCIA-treated patients. ACR responses were maintained up to three years in the open-label extension of Study II. In Study III, ORENCIA-treated patients experienced greater improvement than placebo-treated patients in morning stiffness.

In Study VI, a greater proportion of patients treated with ORENCIA plus methotrexate achieved a low level of disease activity as measured by a DAS28-CRP less than 2.6 at 12 months compared to those treated with methotrexate plus placebo (Table 4). Of patients treated with ORENCIA plus methotrexate who achieved DAS28-CRP less than 2.6, 54% had no active joints, 17% had one active joint, 7% had two active joints, and 22% had three or more active joints, where an active joint was a joint that was rated as tender or swollen or both.

In Study SC-1, the main outcome measure was ACR 20 at 6 months. The pre-specified non-inferiority margin was a treatment difference of −7.5%. As shown in Table 4, the study demonstrated non-inferiority of ORENCIA administered subcutaneously to intravenous infusions of ORENCIA with respect to ACR 20 responses up to 6 months of treatment. ACR 50 and 70 responses are also shown in Table 4. No major differences in ACR responses were observed between intravenous and subcutaneous treatment groups in subgroups based on weight categories (less than 60 kg, 60 to 100 kg, and more than 100 kg; data not shown).

[See table 4 above]

The results of the components of the ACR response criteria for Studies III, IV, and SC-1 are shown in Table 5 (results at Baseline [BL] and 6 months [6 M]). In ORENCIA-treated patients, greater improvement was seen in all ACR response criteria components through 6 and 12 months than in placebo-treated patients.

[See table 5 above]

The percent of patients achieving the ACR 50 response for Study III by visit is shown in Figure 1. The time course for the ORENCIA group in Study VI was similar to that in Study III.

Figure 1: Percent of Patients Achieving ACR 50 Response by Visit* (Study III)

Time Course of ACR 50 Response
Inadequate Response to MTX (Study III)

*The same patients may not have responded at each time point.

The percent of patients achieving the ACR 50 response for Study SC-1 in the ORENCIA subcutaneous (SC) and intravenous (IV) treatment arms at each treatment visit was as follows: Day 15—SC 3%, IV 5%; Day 29—SC 11%, IV 14%; Day 57—SC 24%, IV 30%; Day 85—SC 33%, IV 38%; Day 113—SC 39%, IV 41%; Day 141—SC 46%, IV 47%; Day 169—SC 51%, IV 50%.

Radiographic Response

In Study III and Study VI, structural joint damage was assessed radiographically and expressed as change from baseline in the Genant-modified Total Sharp Score (TSS) and its components, the Erosion Score (ES) and Joint Space Narrowing (JSN) score. ORENCIA/methotrexate slowed the progression of structural damage compared to placebo/methotrexate after 12 months of treatment as shown in Table 6.

[See table 6 at top of next page]

In the open-label extension of Study III, 75% of patients initially randomized to ORENCIA/methotrexate and 65% of patients initially randomized to placebo/methotrexate were evaluated radiographically at Year 2. As shown in Table 6, progression of structural damage in ORENCIA (abatacept)/methotrexate-treated patients was further reduced in the second year of treatment.

Following 2 years of treatment with ORENCIA/methotrexate, 51% of patients had no progression of structural damage as defined by a change in the TSS of zero or less compared with baseline. Fifty-six percent (56%) of ORENCIA/methotrexate-treated patients had no progression during the first year compared to 45% of placebo/methotrexate-treated patients. In their second year of treatment with ORENCIA/methotrexate, more patients had no progression than in the first year (65% vs 56%).

Physical Function Response and Health-Related Outcomes

Improvement in physical function was measured by the Health Assessment Questionnaire Disability Index (HAQ-DI). In the HAQ-DI, ORENCIA (abatacept) demonstrated greater improvement from baseline versus placebo in Studies II-V and versus methotrexate in Study VI. In Study

Table 4: Clinical Responses in Controlled Trials

	Percent of Patients									
	Intravenous Administration								Subcutaneous Administration	
	Inadequate Response to DMARDs		Inadequate Response to Methotrexate (MTX)		Inadequate Response to TNF Blocking Agent		MTX-Naive		Inadequate Response to MTX	
	Study I		Study III		Study IV		Study VI		Study SC-1	
Response Rate	ORN[a] n=32	PBO n=32	ORN[b] +MTX n=424	PBO +MTX n=214	ORN[b] + DMARDs n=256	PBO + DMARDs n=133	ORN[b] +MTX n=256	PBO +MTX n=253	ORN[e] SC +MTX n=693	ORN[e] IV +MTX n=678
ACR 20										
Month 3	53%	31%	62%‡	37%	46%‡	18%	64%*	53%	68%	69%
Month 6	NA	NA	68%‡	40%	50%‡	20%	75%‡	62%	76%§	76%
Month 12	NA	NA	73%‡	40%	NA	NA	76%‡	62%	NA	NA
ACR 50										
Month 3	16%	6%	32%‡	8%	18%†	6%	40%‡	23%	33%	39%
Month 6	NA	NA	40%‡	17%	20%‡	4%	53%‡	38%	52%	50%
Month 12	NA	NA	48%‡	18%	NA	NA	57%‡	42%	NA	NA
ACR 70										
Month 3	6%	0	13%‡	3%	6%*	1%	19%†	10%	13%	16%
Month 6	NA	NA	20%‡	7%	10%†	2%	32%†	20%	26%	25%
Month 12	NA	NA	29%‡	6%	NA	NA	43%‡	27%	NA	NA
Major Clinical Response[e]	NA	NA	14%‡	2%	NA	NA	27%‡	12%	NA	NA
DAS28-CRP <2.6[d]										
Month 12	NA	NA	NA	NA	NA	NA	41%‡	23%	NA	NA

* $p<0.05$, ORENCIA (ORN) vs placebo (PBO) or MTX.
† $p<0.01$, ORENCIA vs placebo or MTX.
‡ $p<0.001$, ORENCIA vs placebo or MTX.
§ 95% CI: −4.2, 4.8 (based on prespecified margin for non-inferiority of −7.5%).
[a] 10 mg/kg.
[b] Dosing based on weight range [see Dosage and Administration (2.1)].
[c] Major clinical response is defined as achieving an ACR 70 response for a continuous 6-month period.
[d] Refer to text for additional description of remaining joint activity.
[e] Per protocol data is presented in table. For ITT; n=736, 721 for SC and IV ORENCIA, respectively.

Table 5: Components of ACR Responses at 6 Months

	Intravenous Administration						Subcutaneous Administration			
	Inadequate Response to Methotrexate (MTX)				Inadequate Response to TNF Blocking Agent				Inadequate Response to MTX	
	Study III				Study IV				Study SC-1[c]			
	ORN +MTX n=424		PBO +MTX n=214		ORN +DMARDs n=256		PBO +DMARDs n=133		ORN SC +MTX n=693		ORN IV +MTX n=678	
Component (median)	BL	6 M	BL	6 M	BL	6 M	BL	6 M	BL	6 M	BL	6 M
Number of tender joints (0-68)	28	7‡	31	14	30	13‡	31	24	27	5	27	6
Number of swollen joints (0-66)	19	5‡	20	11	21	10‡	20	14	18	4	18	3
Pain[a]	67	27‡	70	50	73	43†	74	64	71	25	70	28
Patient global assessment[a]	66	29‡	64	48	71	44†	73	63	70	26	68	27
Disability index[b]	1.75	1.13‡	1.75	1.38	1.88	1.38‡	2.00	1.75	1.88	1.00	1.75	1.00
Physician global assessment[a]	69	21‡	68	40	71	32‡	69	54	65	16	65	15
CRP (mg/dL)	2.2	0.9‡	2.1	1.8	3.4	1.3‡	2.8	2.3	1.6	0.7	1.8	0.7

† $p<0.01$, ORENCIA (ORN) vs placebo (PBO), based on mean percent change from baseline.
‡ $p<0.001$, ORENCIA vs placebo, based on mean percent change from baseline.
[a] Visual analog scale: 0 = best, 100 = worst.
[b] Health Assessment Questionnaire: 0 = best, 3 = worst; 20 questions; 8 categories: dressing and grooming, arising, eating, walking, hygiene, reach, grip, and activities.
[c] SC-I is a non-inferiority study. Per protocol data is presented in table.

Table 6: Mean Radiographic Changes in Study III[a] and Study VI[b]

Parameter	ORENCIA/MTX	Placebo/MTX	Differences	P-value[d]
Study III				
First Year				
TSS	1.07	2.43	1.36	<0.01
ES	0.61	1.47	0.86	<0.01
JSN score	0.46	0.97	0.51	<0.01
Second Year				
TSS	0.48	0.74[c]	-	-
ES	0.23	0.22[c]	-	-
JSN score	0.25	0.51[c]	-	-
Study VI				
First Year				
TSS	0.6	1.1	0.5	0.04

[a] Patients with an inadequate response to MTX.
[b] MTX-naive patients.
[c] Patients received 1 year of placebo/MTX followed by 1 year of ORENCIA/MTX.
[d] Based on a nonparametric ANCOVA model.

Table 7: Mean Improvement from Baseline in Health Assessment Questionnaire Disability Index (HAQ-DI)

	Inadequate Response to Methotrexate			
	Study II		**Study III**	
HAQ Disability Index	ORENCIA[a] +MTX (n=115)	Placebo +MTX (n=119)	ORENCIA[b] +MTX (n=422)	Placebo +MTX (n=212)
Baseline (Mean)	0.98[c]	0.97[c]	1.69[d]	1.69[d]
Mean Improvement Year 1	0.40[c,***]	0.15[c]	0.66[d,***]	0.37[d]

*** $p<0.001$, ORENCIA vs placebo.
[a] 10 mg/kg.
[b] Dosing based on weight range [see Dosage and Administration (2.1)].
[c] Modified Health Assessment Questionnaire: 0 = best, 3 = worst; 8 questions; 8 categories: dressing and grooming, arising, eating, walking, hygiene, reach, grip, and activities.
[d] Health Assessment Questionnaire: 0 = best, 3 = worst; 20 questions; 8 categories: dressing and grooming, arising, eating, walking, hygiene, reach, grip, and activities.

SC-1, improvement from baseline as measured by HAQ-DI at 6 months and over time was similar between subcutaneous and intravenous administration. The results from Studies II and III are shown in Table 7. Similar results were observed in Study V compared to placebo and in Study VI compared to methotrexate. During the open-label period of Study II, the improvement in physical function has been maintained for up to 3 years.

[See table 7 above]

Health-related quality of life was assessed by the SF-36 questionnaire at 6 months in Studies II, III, and IV and at 12 months in Studies II and III. In these studies, improvement was observed in the ORENCIA (abatacept) group as compared with the placebo group in all 8 domains of the SF-36 as well as the Physical Component Summary (PCS) and the Mental Component Summary (MCS).

14.2   Juvenile Idiopathic Arthritis

The safety and efficacy of ORENCIA were assessed in a three-part study including an open-label extension in children with polyarticular juvenile idiopathic arthritis (JIA). Patients 6 to 17 years of age (n=190) with moderately to severely active polyarticular JIA who had an inadequate response to one or more DMARDs, such as methotrexate or TNF antagonists, were treated. Patients had a disease duration of approximately 4 years with moderately to severely active disease at study entry, as determined by baseline counts of active joints (mean, 16) and joints with loss of motion (mean, 16); patients had elevated C-reactive protein (CRP) levels (mean, 3.2 mg/dL) and ESR (mean, 32 mm/h). The patients enrolled had subtypes of JIA that at disease onset included Oligoarticular (16%), Polyarticular (64%; 20% were rheumatoid factor positive), and Systemic (20%). At study entry, 74% of patients were receiving methotrexate (mean dose, 13.2 mg/m² per week) and remained on a stable dose of methotrexate (those not receiving methotrexate did not initiate methotrexate treatment during the study).

In Period A (open-label, lead-in), patients received 10 mg/kg (maximum 1000 mg per dose) intravenously on days 1, 15, 29, and monthly thereafter. Response was assessed utilizing the ACR Pediatric 30 definition of improvement, defined as ≥30% improvement in at least 3 of the 6 JIA core set variables and ≥30% worsening in not more than 1 of the 6 JIA core set variables. Patients demonstrating an ACR Pedi 30 response at the end of Period A were randomized into the double-blind phase (Period B) and received either ORENCIA (abatacept) or placebo for 6 months or until disease flare. Disease flare was defined as a ≥30% worsening in at least 3 of the 6 JIA core set variables with ≥30% improvement in not more than 1 of the 6 JIA core set variables; ≥2 cm of worsening of the Physician or Parent Global Assessment was necessary if used as 1 of the 3 JIA core set variables used to define flare, and worsening in ≥2 joints was necessary if the number of active joints or joints with limitation of motion was used as 1 of the 3 JIA core set variables used to define flare.

At the conclusion of Period A, pediatric ACR 30/50/70 responses were 65%, 50%, and 28%, respectively. Pediatric ACR 30 responses were similar in all subtypes of JIA studied.

During the double-blind randomized withdrawal phase (Period B), ORENCIA-treated patients experienced significantly fewer disease flares compared to placebo-treated patients (20% vs 53%); 95% CI of the difference (15%, 52%). The risk of disease flare among patients continuing on ORENCIA was less than one-third than that for patients withdrawn from ORENCIA treatment (hazard ratio=0.31, 95% CI [0.16, 0.59]). Among patients who received ORENCIA throughout the study (Period A, Period B, and the open-label extension Period C), the proportion of pediatric ACR 30/50/70 responders has remained consistent for 1 year.

16   HOW SUPPLIED/STORAGE AND HANDLING

For Intravenous Infusion

ORENCIA® (abatacept) lyophilized powder for intravenous infusion is supplied as an individually packaged, single-use vial with a silicone-free disposable syringe, providing 250 mg of abatacept in a 15-mL vial: NDC 0003-2187-10

For Subcutaneous Injection

ORENCIA® (abatacept) injection solution for subcutaneous administration is supplied either as a single-dose disposable prefilled glass syringe with UltraSafe Passive® needle guard with flange extenders or as a single-dose disposable prefilled glass syringe with flange extender. The Type I glass syringe has a coated stopper and fixed stainless steel needle (5 bevel, 29-gauge thin wall, ½-inch needle) covered with a rigid needle shield. The prefilled syringe provides 125 mg of abatacept in 1 mL and is provided in the following packages:

NDC 0003-2188-11: pack of 4 syringes with a passive needle safety guard
NDC 0003-2188-31: pack of 4 syringes without a passive needle safety guard

Storage

ORENCIA (abatacept) lyophilized powder supplied in a vial should be refrigerated at 2°C to 8°C (36°F to 46°F). Do not use beyond the expiration date on the vial. Protect the vials from light by storing in the original package until time of use.

ORENCIA solution supplied in a prefilled syringe should be refrigerated at 2°C to 8°C (36°F to 46°F). Do not use beyond the expiration date on the prefilled syringe. Protect from light by storing in the original package until time of use. Do not allow the prefilled syringe to freeze.

17   PATIENT COUNSELING INFORMATION

See FDA-approved patient labeling (Patient Information and Instructions for Use)

17.1   Concomitant Use With Biologic Medications for RA

Patients should be informed that they should not receive ORENCIA treatment concomitantly with a TNF antagonist, such as adalimumab, etanercept, and infliximab because such combination therapy may increase their risk for infections [see Indications and Usage (1.3), Warnings and Precautions (5.1), and Drug Interactions (7.1)], and that they should not receive ORENCIA concomitantly with other biologic RA therapy, such as anakinra because there is not enough information to assess the safety and efficacy of such combination therapy [see Indications and Usage (1.3), Drug Interactions (7.2)].

17.2   Hypersensitivity

Patients should be instructed to immediately tell their healthcare professional if they experience symptoms of an allergic reaction during or for the first day after the administration of ORENCIA [see Warnings and Precautions (5.2)].

17.3   Infections

Patients should be asked if they have a history of recurrent infections, have underlying conditions which may predispose them to infections, or have chronic, latent, or localized infections. Patients should be asked if they have had tuberculosis (TB), a positive skin test for TB, or recently have been in close contact with someone who has had TB. Patients should be instructed that they may be tested for TB before they receive ORENCIA. Patients should be informed to tell their healthcare professional if they develop an infection during therapy with ORENCIA [see Warnings and Precautions (5.3)].

17.4   Immunizations

Patients should be informed that live vaccines should not be given concurrently with ORENCIA or within 3 months of its discontinuation. Caregivers of patients with juvenile idiopathic arthritis should be informed that the patient should be brought up to date with all immunizations in agreement with current immunization guidelines prior to initiating ORENCIA therapy and to discuss with their healthcare provider how best to handle future immunizations once ORENCIA therapy has been initiated [see Warnings and Precautions (5.4)].

17.5   Pregnancy and Nursing Mothers

Patients should be informed that ORENCIA has not been studied in pregnant women or nursing mothers so the effects of ORENCIA on pregnant women or nursing infants are not known. Patients should be instructed to tell their healthcare professional if they are pregnant, become pregnant, or are thinking about becoming pregnant [see Use in Specific Populations (8.1)]. Patients should be instructed to tell their healthcare professional if they plan to breastfeed their infant [see Use in Specific Populations (8.3)].

17.6   Blood Glucose Testing

Intravenous Administration

Patients should be asked if they have diabetes. Maltose is contained in ORENCIA for intravenous administration and can give falsely elevated blood glucose readings with certain blood glucose monitors on the day of ORENCIA infusion. If a patient is using such a monitor, the patient should be advised to discuss with their healthcare professional methods that do not react with maltose [see Drug Interactions (7.3)].

Subcutaneous Administration

ORENCIA for subcutaneous administration does not contain maltose; therefore, patients do not need to alter their glucose monitoring.

Bristol-Myers Squibb Company
Princeton, New Jersey 08543 USA
1292618A3 / 1294018A2
Rev December 2013

PATIENT INFORMATION

ORENCIA® (oh-REN-see-ah)

(abatacept)

Lyophilized Powder for Intravenous Infusion

ORENCIA® (oh-REN-see-ah)

(abatacept)

Injection, Solution for Subcutaneous Administration

Read this Patient Information before you start using ORENCIA and each time you get a refill. There may be new information. This information does not take the place of talking with your healthcare provider about your medical condition or your treatment.

What is ORENCIA?

ORENCIA (abatacept) is a prescription medicine that reduces signs and symptoms in:

• adults with moderate to severe rheumatoid arthritis (RA), including those who have not been helped enough by other medicines for RA. ORENCIA may prevent further damage to your bones and joints and may help your ability to perform daily activities. In adults, ORENCIA may be used alone or with other RA treatments other than tumor necrosis factor (TNF) antagonists.

• children and adolescents 6 years of age and older with moderate to severe polyarticular juvenile idiopathic arthritis (JIA). ORENCIA may be used alone or with methotrexate.

It is not known if ORENCIA is safe and effective in children under 6 years of age.

It is not known if ORENCIA is safe and effective in children for uses other than juvenile idiopathic arthritis.

ORENCIA for subcutaneous injection has not been studied in children under 18 years of age; therefore, it is not known if ORENCIA for subcutaneous injection is safe and effective in children under 18 years of age.

What should I tell my healthcare provider before using ORENCIA?

Before you use ORENCIA, tell your healthcare provider if you:

• have any kind of infection even if it is small (such as an open cut or sore), or an infection that is in your whole body (such as the flu). If you have an infection when taking ORENCIA, you may have a higher chance for getting serious side effects.

• have an infection that will not go away or an infection that keeps coming back.

• are allergic to abatacept or any of the ingredients in ORENCIA. See the end of this leaflet for a list of the ingredients in ORENCIA.

• have or have had inflammation of your liver due to an infection (viral hepatitis). Before you use ORENCIA, your healthcare provider may examine you for hepatitis.

• have had a lung infection called tuberculosis (TB), a positive skin test for TB, or you recently have been in close contact with someone who has had TB. Before you use ORENCIA, your healthcare provider may examine you for TB or perform a skin test. Symptoms of TB may include:
  • a cough that does not go away
  • weight loss
  • fever
  • night sweats

• are scheduled to have surgery.

• recently received a vaccination or are scheduled for a vaccination. If you are receiving ORENCIA, and for 3 months after you stop receiving ORENCIA, you should not receive live vaccines.

• have a history of a breathing problem called chronic obstructive pulmonary disease (COPD).

• have diabetes and use a blood glucose monitor to check your blood sugar (blood glucose) levels. ORENCIA for intravenous infusion (given through a needle placed in a vein) contains maltose, a type of sugar that can give false high blood sugar readings with certain types of blood glucose monitors, on the day of ORENCIA infusion. Your doctor may tell you to use a different way to monitor your blood sugar levels.

• ORENCIA for subcutaneous injection (injected under the skin) does not contain maltose. You do not need to change your blood sugar monitoring if you are taking ORENCIA subcutaneously.

• have any other medical conditions.

• are pregnant or planning to become pregnant. It is not known if ORENCIA can harm your unborn baby. Bristol-Myers Squibb Company has a registry for pregnant women exposed to ORENCIA. The purpose of this registry is to check the health of the pregnant mother and her child. Women are encouraged to call the registry themselves or ask their doctors to contact the registry for them by calling 1-877-311-8972.

• are breastfeeding or plan to breastfeed. It is not known if ORENCIA passes into your breast milk. You and your healthcare provider should decide if you will use ORENCIA or breastfeed. You should not do both.

Tell your healthcare provider about all the medicines you take, including prescription and non-prescription medicines, vitamins, and herbal supplements.

ORENCIA may affect the way other medicines work, and other medicines may affect the way ORENCIA works causing serious side effects.

Especially tell your healthcare provider if you take other biologic medicines to treat RA or JIA that may affect your immune system, such as:

• Enbrel® (etanercept)
• Humira® (adalimumab)
• Remicade® (infliximab)
• Kineret® (anakinra)
• Rituxan® (rituximab)
• Simponi® (golimumab)
• Cimzia® (certolizumab pegol)
• Actemra® (tocilizumab)

You may have a higher chance of getting a serious infection if you take ORENCIA (abatacept) with other biologic medicines for your RA or JIA.

Know the medicines you take. Keep a list of your medicines and show it to your healthcare provider and pharmacist when you get a new prescription.

How should I use ORENCIA?

• You may receive ORENCIA given by a healthcare provider through a vein in your arm (IV or intravenous infusion). It takes about 30 minutes to give you the full dose of medicine. You will then receive ORENCIA 2 weeks and 4 weeks after the first dose and then every 4 weeks.

• You may also receive ORENCIA as an injection under your skin (subcutaneous). If your healthcare provider decides that you or a caregiver can give your injections of ORENCIA at home, you or your caregiver should receive training on the right way to prepare and inject ORENCIA. Do not try to inject ORENCIA until you have been shown the right way to give the injections by your healthcare provider.

• Your healthcare provider will tell you how much ORENCIA to use and when to use it.

• **See the Instructions for Use at the end of this Patient Information leaflet for instructions about the right way to prepare and give your ORENCIA injections at home.**

What are the possible side effects of ORENCIA?

ORENCIA can cause serious side effects including:

• **infections.** ORENCIA can make you more likely to get infections or make the infection that you have get worse. Some patients have died from these infections. Call your healthcare provider right away if you have any symptoms of an infection. Symptoms of an infection may include:
  • fever
  • feel very tired
  • have a cough
  • have flu-like symptoms
  • warm, red, or painful skin

• **allergic reactions.** Allergic reactions can happen to people who use ORENCIA. Call your healthcare provider or go to the emergency room right away if you have any symptoms of an allergic reaction. Symptoms of an allergic reaction may include:
  • hives
  • swollen face, eyelids, lips, or tongue
  • trouble breathing

• **hepatitis B infection** in people who carry the virus in their blood. If you are a carrier of the hepatitis B virus (a virus that affects the liver), the virus can become active while you use ORENCIA. Your healthcare provider may do a blood test before you start treatment with ORENCIA while you use ORENCIA.

• **vaccinations.** You should not receive ORENCIA with certain types of vaccines (live vaccines). ORENCIA may also cause some vaccinations to be less effective. Talk with your healthcare provider about your vaccination plans.

• **breathing problems in patients with Chronic Obstructive Pulmonary Disease (COPD).** Some people may get certain respiratory problems more often if you receive ORENCIA and have COPD. Symptoms of respiratory problems include:
  • COPD that becomes worse
  • cough
  • trouble breathing

• **cancer (malignancies).** Certain kinds of cancer have been reported in people using ORENCIA. It is not known if ORENCIA increases your chance of getting certain kinds of cancer.

Common side effects of ORENCIA include:
• headache
• upper respiratory tract infection
• sore throat
• nausea

In children and adolescents, other side effects may include:
• diarrhea
• cough
• fever
• abdominal pain

Tell your healthcare provider if you have any side effect that bothers you or that does not go away.

These are not all the possible side effects of ORENCIA. For more information, ask your healthcare provider or pharmacist.

Call your doctor for medical advice about side effects. You may report side effects to FDA at 1-800-FDA-1088.

How should I store ORENCIA?

• Store ORENCIA (abatacept) in the refrigerator at 36°F to 46°F (2°C to 8°C).

• Keep ORENCIA in the original package and out of the light.

• Do not freeze ORENCIA.

• Safely throw away medicine that is out of date or no longer needed.

Keep ORENCIA and all medicines out of the reach of children.

General information about the safe and effective use of ORENCIA

Medicines are sometimes prescribed for purposes other than those listed in this Patient Information leaflet. Do not use ORENCIA for a condition for which it was not prescribed. Do not give ORENCIA to other people, even if they have the same symptoms that you have. It may harm them.

This Patient Information leaflet summarizes the most important information about ORENCIA. If you would like more information, talk to your healthcare provider.

You can ask your pharmacist or healthcare provider for information about ORENCIA that is written for health professionals.

For more information, go to www.ORENCIA.com or call 1-800-ORENCIA.

What are the ingredients in ORENCIA?

Active ingredient: abatacept

Intravenous inactive ingredients: maltose, monobasic sodium phosphate, sodium chloride for administration

Subcutaneous inactive ingredients: sucrose, poloxamer 188, monobasic sodium phosphate monohydrate, dibasic sodium phosphate anhydrous, water for injection

This Patient Information has been approved by the U.S. Food and Drug Administration.

Bristol-Myers Squibb Company
Princeton, NJ 08543 USA

All other trademarks are property of their respective companies.

1292618A3 / 1294018A2
Rev December 2013

INSTRUCTIONS FOR USE
ORENCIA® (oh-REN-see-ah)
(abatacept)
Prefilled Syringe

Read and follow these Instructions for Use that come with your ORENCIA prefilled syringe before you start using it and each time you get a refill. Before you use ORENCIA prefilled syringe for the first time, make sure your healthcare provider shows you the right way to use it.

Do not remove the needle cover (the cap) until you are ready to inject ORENCIA. Do not put the needle cover back on the needle once removed.

Figure A

• The ORENCIA prefilled syringe has a flange extender that makes it easier to hold the syringe and inject (**see Figure A**).

Supplies needed for your ORENCIA Prefilled Syringe Injection (see Figure B):
• a new ORENCIA prefilled syringe
• alcohol swab
• cotton ball or gauze
• adhesive bandage
• puncture resistant container (sharps container)

Figure B

STEP 1: Preparing for an ORENCIA Injection

Find a comfortable space with a clean, flat, working surface.

- Check the expiration date on the ORENCIA (abatacept) prefilled syringe (**see Figure A**). **Do not** use it if the expiration date has passed. Throw it away and get a new one.
- Remove 1 single-use ORENCIA prefilled syringe from the refrigerator and let it warm up for 30 to 60 minutes to allow it to reach room temperature.
  - **Do not** speed up the warming process in any way, such as using the microwave or placing the syringe in warm water.

Do not remove the needle cover while allowing ORENCIA prefilled syringe to reach room temperature.

- Keep your unused syringes in their original carton and keep in the refrigerator at 36°F to 46°F (2°C to 8°C). **Do not** freeze.
- Hold your ORENCIA prefilled syringe by the barrel with the covered needle pointing down (**see Figure C**).

Air Bubble
Fill Lines
Fluid Level
Fluid

Figure C

- Check the liquid in the ORENCIA prefilled syringe. It should be clear and colorless to pale yellow. **Do not** inject ORENCIA if the liquid is cloudy, discolored, or has lumps or particles in it. Throw the syringe away and get a new one.
- Check that the amount of liquid in your ORENCIA prefilled syringe is the correct amount. The liquid should be between the two lines on the syringe barrel (**see Figure C**).
- **Do not** inject ORENCIA if it does not have the correct amount of liquid. Throw the ORENCIA prefilled syringe away and get a new one. It is normal to see an air bubble. There is no reason to remove it.
- Wash your hands well with soap and water.

STEP 2: Choose and Prepare an Injection Site

Choose an Injection Site

- The front of your thigh is a recommended injection area. You may use your abdomen except for the 2-inch area around your navel (**see Figure D**).
- The outer area of the upper arms may also be used only if the injection is being given by a caregiver. Do not attempt to use the upper arm area by yourself (**see Figure E**).

Rotate Injection Site

- Choose a different injection site for each new injection. You may use the same thigh for weekly injections, as long as each injection is at least 1 inch away from the last area you injected.
- Do not inject into areas where your skin is tender, bruised, red, scaly, or hard. Avoid any areas with scars or stretch marks.

Areas for self-injection and caregiver injection	Additional injection area for caregivers only
Injection Area	Injection Area
Figure D	**Figure E**

Prepare the Injection Site

- Wipe the injection site with an alcohol swab in a circular motion and let it air dry. **Do not** touch the injection site again before giving the injection.
- **Do not** fan or blow on the clean area.

STEP 3: Inject ORENCIA

- Remove the needle cover only when you are ready to administer the injection. Hold the barrel of the ORENCIA (abatacept) prefilled syringe with one hand and pull the needle cover straight off with your other hand (**see Figure F**). **Do not** touch the plunger while you remove the needle cover.

Figure F

- **Do not** put the needle cover back on the needle once removed. Throw away the needle cover in your household trash.
- **Do not** use the syringe if there are visible signs of needle damage or bending.
- There may be a small air bubble in the ORENCIA prefilled syringe barrel. You do not need to remove it.
- You may notice a drop of fluid leaving the needle. This is normal and will not affect your dose.
- **Do not** touch the needle or let it touch any surfaces.
- **Do not** use the prefilled syringe if it is dropped without the needle cover in place.
- Hold the barrel of your ORENCIA prefilled syringe in one hand between the thumb and index finger (**see Figure G**).

Figure G

- **Do not** pull back on the plunger of the syringe.
- Use your other hand and gently pinch the area of skin you cleaned. Hold firmly.
- Insert the needle with a quick motion into the pinched skin at a 45° angle (**see Figure H**).

Figure H

- To inject all of the medicine, use your thumb to push down on the plunger head until the plunger head is pushed in as far as it will go (**see Figure I**).

Figure I

- Remove the needle from the skin and let go of the surrounding skin.

After the Injection

- There may be a little bleeding at the injection site. You can press a cotton ball or gauze over the injection site.
- **Do not** rub the injection site.
- If needed, you may cover the injection site with a small bandage.

STEP 4: Disposal and Recordkeeping

- The ORENCIA prefilled syringe should not be reused.
- Put the used syringe into your puncture resistant container (see **"How do I throw away used syringes?"**).
- **Do not** put the needle cover back on the needle.
- **If your injection is given by another person, this person must also be careful when removing the syringe and disposing of the syringe to prevent accidental needle stick injury and passing infection.**

How do I throw away used syringes?

Check with your healthcare provider or pharmacist for instructions about the right way to throw away used syringes. There may be special local or state laws about how to throw away used syringes.

- **Do not** throw away used syringes in the household trash and do not recycle them.
- Put used and empty ORENCIA prefilled syringes in a biohazard container made specifically for disposing of used syringes (called a "sharps" container) or in a hard plastic container with a screw-on cap (such as an empty detergent bottle) or in a metal container with a plastic lid (such as a coffee can). Sharps containers can be purchased at your local pharmacy or many retail outlets.
- When the container is full, tape around the cap or lid to make sure the cap or lid does not come off.
- **Keep ORENCIA (abatacept) prefilled syringes and the disposal container out of the reach of children.**

Record your Injection

- Write the date, time, and specific part of your body where you injected yourself. It may also be helpful to write any questions or concerns about the injection so you can ask your healthcare provider.

If you have questions or concerns about your ORENCIA prefilled syringe, please contact a healthcare provider familiar with ORENCIA or call our toll-free help line at 1-800-ORENCIA (1-800-673-6242).

Frequently Asked Questions

Injecting with the ORENCIA prefilled syringe

I feel a little bit of burning or pain during injection. Is this normal?

- When giving yourself an injection, you may feel a prick from the needle. Sometimes, the medicine can cause slight irritation near the injection site. This may happen and the discomfort should be mild to moderate. If you have any side effects, including pain, swelling, or discoloration near the injection site, contact your healthcare provider.

Traveling with ORENCIA prefilled syringes

How should I keep my prefilled syringes cool while traveling?

- If you need to take your prefilled syringes with you, store them in a cool carrier between 36°F to 46°F (2°C to 8°C) until you are ready to use.
- **Do not** freeze ORENCIA.
- Keep ORENCIA in the original carton and protected from light. Your healthcare provider may know about special carrying cases for injectable medicines.

Can I take my prefilled syringes on an airplane?

- Generally you are allowed to carry ORENCIA prefilled syringes with you on an airplane. **Be sure to carry the prefilled syringes with you on board the plane, and do not put them in your "checked" luggage.** You should carry ORENCIA prefilled syringes with you in your travel cooler at a temperature of 36°F to 46°F (2°C to 8°C) until you are ready to use.
- Keep ORENCIA in the original carton, with its original preprinted labels and protected from light.

What if my syringe does not stay cool for an extended period of time? Is it dangerous to use?

- Contact 1-800-ORENCIA (1-800-673-6242) for details.

If you have questions or concerns about your ORENCIA prefilled syringe, please contact a healthcare provider familiar with ORENCIA or call our toll-free help line at 1-800-ORENCIA (1-800-673-6242).

Bristol-Myers Squibb Company
Princeton, NJ 08543 USA

This Instructions for Use has been approved by the U.S. Food and Drug Administration.

All other trademarks are property of their respective companies.

Rev December 2013

INSTRUCTIONS FOR USE
ORENCIA® (oh-REN-see-ah)
(abatacept)
Prefilled Syringe with UltraSafe Passive® Needle Guard

Read and follow these Instructions for Use that come with your ORENCIA prefilled syringe before you start using it and each time you get a refill. Before you use ORENCIA prefilled syringe for the first time, make sure your healthcare provider shows you the right way to use it.

Do not remove the needle cover (the cap) until you are ready to inject ORENCIA. Do not put the needle cover back on the needle once removed.

Flange Extender
Air Bubble
Viewing Window
Needle
Plunger Head
Plunger
Drug Level
Needle Cover
EXP 12 2023
Label
Housing
Needle Guard Activation Clips
Fluid Level Indicator Line
Needle Guard Activation Spring
Needle Guard Activation Wings

Figure A

- The ORENCIA prefilled syringe has a flange extender that makes it easier to hold the syringe and inject, and a needle guard that automatically extends over the needle after the injection is complete (**see Figure A**).

Supplies needed for your ORENCIA Prefilled Syringe Injection (see Figure B):
- a new ORENCIA (abatacept) prefilled syringe
- alcohol swab
- cotton ball or gauze
- adhesive bandage
- puncture resistant container (sharps container)

Figure B

STEP 1: Preparing for an ORENCIA Injection
Find a comfortable space with a clean, flat, working surface.
- Check the expiration date on the ORENCIA prefilled syringe (**see Figure A**). **Do not** use it if the expiration date has passed. Throw it away and get a new one.
- Remove 1 single-use ORENCIA prefilled syringe from the refrigerator and let it warm up for 30 to 60 minutes to allow it to reach room temperature.
  - **Do not** speed up the warming process in any way, such as using the microwave or placing the syringe in warm water.

Do not remove the needle cover while allowing ORENCIA prefilled syringe to reach room temperature.
- Keep your unused syringes in their original carton and keep in the refrigerator at 36°F to 46°F (2°C to 8°C). **Do not** freeze.
- Hold your ORENCIA prefilled syringe by the housing with the covered needle pointing down (**see Figure C**).

Figure C

- Check the liquid in the ORENCIA prefilled syringe. It should be clear and colorless to pale yellow. **Do not** inject ORENCIA if the liquid is cloudy, discolored, or has lumps or particles in it. Throw the syringe away and get a new one.
- Check that the amount of liquid in your ORENCIA prefilled syringe is the correct amount. Confirm the drug level is above the fluid level indicator line (**see Figure C**).
- **Do not** inject ORENCIA if it does not have the correct amount of liquid. Throw the ORENCIA prefilled syringe away and get a new one. It is normal to see an air bubble. There is no reason to remove it.
- Wash your hands well with soap and water.

STEP 2: Choose and Prepare an Injection Site
Choose an Injection Site
- The front of your thigh is a recommended injection area. You may use your abdomen except for the 2-inch area around your navel (**see Figure D**).
- The outer area of the upper arms may also be used only if the injection is being given by a caregiver. Do not attempt to use the upper arm area by yourself (**see Figure E**).

Rotate Injection Site
- Choose a different injection site for each new injection. You may use the same thigh for weekly injections, as long as each injection is at least 1 inch away from the last area you injected.
- Do not inject into areas where your skin is tender, bruised, red, scaly, or hard. Avoid any areas with scars or stretch marks.

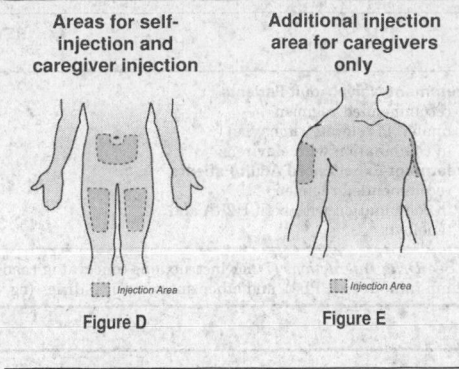

Areas for self-injection and caregiver injection

Additional injection area for caregivers only

▨ *Injection Area*   ▨ *Injection Area*

Figure D   **Figure E**

Prepare the Injection Site
- Wipe the injection site with an alcohol swab in a circular motion and let it air dry. **Do not** touch the injection site again before giving the injection.
- **Do not** fan or blow on the clean area.

STEP 3: Inject ORENCIA
- Remove the needle cover only when you are ready to administer the injection. Hold the housing of the ORENCIA (abatacept) prefilled syringe with one hand and pull the needle cover straight off with your other hand (**see Figure F**). **Do not** touch the plunger while you remove the needle cover.

Figure F

- **Do not** put the needle cover back on the needle once removed. Throw away the needle cover in your household trash.
- **Do not** use the syringe if there are visible signs of needle damage or bending.
- There may be a small air bubble in the ORENCIA prefilled syringe housing. You do not need to remove it.
- You may notice a drop of fluid leaving the needle. This is normal and will not affect your dose.
- **Do not** touch the needle or let it touch any surfaces.
- **Do not** use the prefilled syringe if it is dropped without the needle cover in place.
- Hold the housing of your ORENCIA prefilled syringe in one hand between the thumb and index finger (**see Figure G**).

Figure G

- **Do not** pull back on the plunger of the syringe.
- Use your other hand and gently pinch the area of skin you cleaned. Hold firmly.
- Insert the needle with a quick motion into the pinched skin at a 45° angle (**see Figure H**).

Figure H

- To inject all of the medicine, use your thumb to push the plunger until the plunger head is pushed in as far as it will go.
- Slowly lift your thumb from the plunger head. This allows the needle to be completely covered by the needle guard as it is removed from the skin (**see Figure I**).

Figure I

- Remove the prefilled syringe and let go of the surrounding skin (**see Figure J**).

Figure J

After the Injection
- There may be a little bleeding at the injection site. You can press a cotton ball or gauze over the injection site.
- **Do not** rub the injection site.
- If needed, you may cover the injection site with a small bandage.

STEP 4: Disposal and Recordkeeping
- The ORENCIA (abatacept) prefilled syringe should not be reused.
- Put the used syringe into your puncture resistant container (see "How do I throw away used syringes?").
- **Do not** put the needle cover back on the needle.
- **If your injection is given by another person, this person must also be careful when removing the syringe and disposing of the syringe to prevent accidental needle stick injury and passing infection.**

How do I throw away used syringes?
Check with your healthcare provider or pharmacist for instructions about the right way to throw away used syringes. There may be special local or state laws about how to throw away used syringes.
- **Do not** throw away used syringes in the household trash and do not recycle them.
- Put used and empty ORENCIA prefilled syringes in a biohazard container made specifically for disposing of used syringes (called a "sharps" container) or in a hard plastic container with a screw-on cap (such as an empty detergent bottle) or in a metal container with a plastic lid (such as a coffee can). Sharps containers can be purchased at your local pharmacy or many retail outlets.
- When the container is full, tape around the cap or lid to make sure the cap or lid does not come off.
- **Keep ORENCIA prefilled syringes and the disposal container out of the reach of children.**

Record your Injection
- Write the date, time, and specific part of your body where you injected yourself. It may also be helpful to write any questions or concerns about the injection so you can ask your healthcare provider.

If you have questions or concerns about your ORENCIA prefilled syringe, please contact a healthcare provider familiar with ORENCIA or call our toll-free help line at 1-800-ORENCIA (1-800-673-6242).

Frequently Asked Questions
Injecting with the ORENCIA prefilled syringe
I feel a little bit of burning or pain during injection. Is this normal?
- When giving yourself an injection, you may feel a prick from the needle. Sometimes, the medicine can cause slight irritation near the injection site. This may happen and the discomfort should be mild to moderate. If you have any side effects, including pain, swelling, or discoloration near the injection site, contact your healthcare provider.

Traveling with ORENCIA prefilled syringes
How should I keep my prefilled syringes cool while traveling?
- If you need to take your prefilled syringes with you, store them in a cool carrier between 36°F to 46°F (2°C to 8°C) until you are ready to use.
- **Do not** freeze ORENCIA.
- Keep ORENCIA in the original carton and protected from light. Your healthcare provider may know about special carrying cases for injectable medicines.

Can I take my prefilled syringes on an airplane?
- Generally you are allowed to carry ORENCIA prefilled syringes with you on an airplane. **Be sure to carry the prefilled syringes with you on board the plane, and do not put them in your "checked" luggage.** You should carry ORENCIA prefilled syringes with you in your travel cooler at a temperature of 36°F to 46°F (2°C to 8°C) until you are ready to use.
- Keep ORENCIA in the original carton, with its original preprinted labels and protected from light.

What if my syringe does not stay cool for an extended period of time? Is it dangerous to use?
- Contact 1-800-ORENCIA (1-800-673-6242) for details.

If you have questions or concerns about your ORENCIA prefilled syringe, please contact a healthcare provider familiar with ORENCIA or call our toll-free help line at 1-800-ORENCIA (1-800-673-6242).

Bristol-Myers Squibb Company
Princeton, NJ 08543 USA
This Instructions for Use has been approved by the U.S. Food and Drug Administration.

UltraSafe Passive® is a registered trademark of Safety Syringes, Inc.
All other trademarks are property of their respective companies.
1292618A3 / 1294018A2
Rev December 2013
Shown in Product Identification Guide, page 306

REYATAZ®
[RAY-ah-taz]
(atazanavir)
Capsules

REYATAZ®
(atazanavir)
Oral powder

R

HIGHLIGHTS OF PRESCRIBING INFORMATION
These highlights do not include all the information needed to use REYATAZ safely and effectively. See full prescribing information for REYATAZ.
REYATAZ® (atazanavir) capsules, for oral use
REYATAZ® (atazanavir) oral powder
Initial U.S. Approval: 2003

RECENT MAJOR CHANGES

Indications and Usage (1)	6/2014
Dosage and Administration, Overview (2.1)	6/2014
Dosage and Administration of REYATAZ Oral Powder in Pediatric Patients (2.4)	6/2014
Contraindications (4)	6/2014
Warnings and Precautions, Patients with Phenylketonuria (5.4)	6/2014

INDICATIONS AND USAGE
REYATAZ is a protease inhibitor indicated for use in combination with other antiretroviral agents for the treatment of HIV-1 infection for patients 3 months and older weighing at least 10 kg. (1)

DOSAGE AND ADMINISTRATION
• *Treatment-naive adults:* REYATAZ 300 mg with ritonavir 100 mg once daily with food or REYATAZ 400 mg once daily with food. (2.2)
• *Treatment-experienced adults:* REYATAZ 300 mg with ritonavir 100 mg once daily with food. (2.2)
• *Pediatric patients:* REYATAZ capsule dosage is based on body weight not to exceed the adult dose and must be taken with food. (2.3)
• *REYATAZ oral powder:* Must be taken with ritonavir and food and should not be used in children who weigh less than 10 kg or who weigh 25 kg or more. (2.4)
• *Pregnancy:* REYATAZ 300 mg with ritonavir 100 mg once daily with food, with dosing modifications for some concomitant medications. (2.5)
• *Concomitant therapy:* Dosing modifications may be required. (2.2, 2.3, 2.4, 2.4, 7)
• *Renal impairment:* Dosing modifications may be required. (2.6)
• *Hepatic impairment:* Dosing modifications may be required. (2.7)

DOSAGE FORMS AND STRENGTHS
• Capsules: 150 mg, 200 mg, 300 mg. (3, 16)
• Oral powder: 50 mg packet. (3, 16)

CONTRAINDICATIONS
• REYATAZ is contraindicated in patients with previously demonstrated hypersensitivity (eg, Stevens-Johnson syndrome, erythema multiforme, or toxic skin eruptions) to any of the components of this product. (4)
• Coadministration with alfuzosin, triazolam, orally administered midazolam, ergot derivatives, rifampin, irinotecan, lovastatin, simvastatin, indinavir, cisapride, pimozide, St. John's wort, nevirapine, and sildenafil when dosed as REVATIO®. (4)

WARNINGS AND PRECAUTIONS
• *Cardiac conduction abnormalities:* PR interval prolongation may occur in some patients. ECG monitoring should be considered in patients with preexisting conduction system disease or when administered with other drugs that may prolong the PR interval. (5.1, 7.3, 12.2, 17)
• *Rash:* Discontinue if severe rash develops. (5.2, 17)
• *Hyperbilirubinemia:* Most patients experience asymptomatic increases in indirect bilirubin, which is reversible upon discontinuation. Do not dose reduce. If a concomitant transaminase increase occurs, evaluate for alternative etiologies. (5.3)
• *Hepatotoxicity:* Patients with hepatitis B or C infection are at risk of increased transaminases or hepatic decompensation. Monitor hepatic laboratory tests prior to therapy and during treatment. (2.5, 5.5, 8.8)
• *Nephrolithiasis and cholelithiasis* have been reported. Consider temporary interruption or discontinuation. (5.6)
• Patients receiving REYATAZ (atazanavir) may develop new onset or exacerbations of diabetes mellitus/hyperglycemia (5.7), immune reconstitution syndrome (5.8), and redistribution/accumulation of body fat (5.9).
• *Hemophilia:* Spontaneous bleeding may occur and additional factor VIII may be required. (5.10)
• *Phenylketonuria:* REYATAZ oral powder contains phenylalanine which can be harmful to patients with phenylketonuria. (5.4)

ADVERSE REACTIONS
Most common adverse reactions (≥2%) are nausea, jaundice/scleral icterus, rash, headache, abdominal pain, vomiting, insomnia, peripheral neurologic symptoms, dizziness, myalgia, diarrhea, depression, and fever. (6.1, 6.2)
To report SUSPECTED ADVERSE REACTIONS, contact Bristol-Myers Squibb at 1-800-721-5072 or FDA at 1-800-FDA-1088 or www.fda.gov/medwatch.

DRUG INTERACTIONS
Coadministration of REYATAZ can alter the concentration of other drugs and other drugs may alter the concentration of atazanavir. The potential drug-drug interactions must be considered prior to and during therapy. (4, 7, 12.3)

USE IN SPECIFIC POPULATIONS
• *Pregnancy:* Use only if the potential benefit justifies the potential risk. (8.1)
• *Nursing mothers* should be instructed not to breastfeed due to the potential for postnatal HIV transmission. (8.3)
• *Hepatitis B or C co-infection:* Monitor liver enzymes. (5.5, 6.3)
• *Renal impairment:* REYATAZ is not recommended for use in treatment-experienced patients with end stage renal disease managed with hemodialysis. (2.6, 8.7)
• *Hepatic impairment:* REYATAZ is not recommended in patients with severe hepatic impairment. REYATAZ/ritonavir is not recommended in patients with any degree of hepatic impairment. (2.7, 8.8)

See 17 for PATIENT COUNSELING INFORMATION and FDA-approved patient labeling
Revised: 06/2014

Table 1: Recommended REYATAZ and Ritonavir Dosage in Adults[a]

	REYATAZ Once Daily Dosage	Ritonavir Once Daily Dosage
Treatment-Naive Adult Patients		
recommended regimen	300 mg	100 mg
unable to tolerate ritonavir	400 mg	N/A
in combination with efavirenz	400 mg	100 mg
Treatment-Experienced Adult Patients		
recommended regimen	300 mg	100 mg
in combination with both H2RA and tenofovir	400 mg	100 mg

[a] See *Drug Interactions* (7) for instructions concerning coadministration of acid reducing medications (eg, H2RA or proton pump inhibitors [PPIs]), and other antiretroviral drugs (eg, efavirenz, tenofovir, and didanosine).

Table 2: Recommended Dosage of REYATAZ Capsules and Ritonavir in Pediatric Patients (6 to less than 18 years of age)[a,b]

Body Weight	REYATAZ Daily Dosage	Ritonavir Daily Dosage
Treatment-Naive and Treatment-Experienced[c]		
Less than 15 kg	Capsules not recommended	N/A
15 kg to less than 20 kg	150 mg	100 mg
20 kg to less than 40 kg	200 mg	100 mg
At least 40 kg	300 mg	100 mg
Treatment-Naive, at least 13 years old and cannot tolerate ritonavir[c]		
At least 40 kg	400 mg	N/A

[a] Administer REYATAZ capsules and ritonavir simultaneously with food.
[b] The same recommendations regarding the timing and maximum doses of concomitant PPIs and H2RAs in adults also apply to pediatric patients. See *Drug Interactions* (7) for instructions concerning coadministration of acid reducing medications (eg, H2RA or PPIs), and other antiretroviral drugs (eg, efavirenz, tenofovir, and didanosine).
[c] In treatment-experienced patients, REYATAZ capsules must be administered with ritonavir.

FULL PRESCRIBING INFORMATION: CONTENTS*

14 CLINICAL STUDIES
14.1 Adult Patients without Prior Antiretroviral Therapy
14.2 Adult Patients with Prior Antiretroviral Therapy
14.3 Pediatric Patients
16 HOW SUPPLIED/STORAGE AND HANDLING
17 PATIENT COUNSELING INFORMATION
* Sections or subsections omitted from the full prescribing information are not listed.

FULL PRESCRIBING INFORMATION

1 INDICATIONS AND USAGE

REYATAZ® (atazanavir) is indicated in combination with other antiretroviral agents for the treatment of HIV-1 infection for patients 3 months and older weighing at least 10 kg. Limitations of Use:
• REYATAZ is not recommended for use in pediatric patients below the age of 3 months due to the risk of kernicterus.
• Use of REYATAZ/ritonavir in treatment-experienced patients should be guided by the number of baseline primary protease inhibitor resistance substitutions [see Microbiology (12.4)].

2 DOSAGE AND ADMINISTRATION

2.1 Overview
• REYATAZ capsules and oral powder must be taken with food.
• Do not open the capsules.
• The recommended oral dosage of REYATAZ depends on the treatment history of the patient and the use of other coadministered drugs. When coadministered with H_2-receptor antagonists or proton-pump inhibitors, dose separation may be required [see Dosage and Administration (2.2, 2.3, 2.4, 2.5) and Drug Interactions (7)].
• REYATAZ capsules without ritonavir are not recommended for treatment-experienced adult or pediatric patients with prior virologic failure [see Clinical Studies (14)].
• REYATAZ oral powder must be taken with ritonavir and is not recommended for use in children who weigh less than 10 kg or who weigh 25 kg or more. [See Dosage and Administration (2.4).]
• Efficacy and safety of REYATAZ with ritonavir when ritonavir is administered in doses greater than 100 mg once daily have not been established. The use of higher ritonavir doses may alter the safety profile of atazanavir (cardiac effects, hyperbilirubinemia) and, therefore, is not recommended. Prescribers should consult the complete prescribing information for ritonavir when using ritonavir.

2.2 Dosage in Adult Patients
Table 1 displays the recommended dosage of REYATAZ capsules in treatment-naive and treatment-experienced adults. Table 1 also displays recommended dosage of REYATAZ and ritonavir when given concomitantly with other antiretroviral drugs and H_2-receptor antagonists (H2RA). Ritonavir is required with several REYATAZ dosage regimens (see the ritonavir complete prescribing information about the safe and effective use of ritonavir). The use of REYATAZ in treatment-experienced adult patients without ritonavir is not recommended.
[See table 1 at top of previous page]

2.3 Dosage of REYATAZ Capsules in Pediatric Patients
The recommended daily dosage of REYATAZ capsules and ritonavir in pediatric patients (6 years of age to less than 18 years of age) is based on body weight (see Table 2).
[See table 2 at top of previous page]

2.4 Dosage and Administration of REYATAZ Oral Powder in Pediatric Patients
REYATAZ oral powder is for use in treatment-naive or treatment-experienced pediatric patients who are at least 3 months of age and weighing at least 10 kg and less than 25 kg. REYATAZ oral powder must be mixed with food or beverage for administration and ritonavir must be given immediately afterwards. Table 3 displays the recommended dosage of REYATAZ oral powder and ritonavir.

Table 3: Recommended Dosage of REYATAZ Oral Powder and Ritonavir in Pediatric Patients (at least 3 months of age and weighing at least 10 kg and less than 25 kg)[a]

Body Weight	Daily Dosage of REYATAZ Oral Powder	Daily Dosage of Ritonavir Oral Solution
10 kg to less than 15 kg	200 mg (4 packets)[b]	80 mg
15 kg to less than 25 kg	250 mg (5 packets)[b]	80 mg

[a] The same recommendations regarding the timing and maximum doses of concomitant PPIs and H2RAs in adults also apply to pediatric patients. See Drug Interactions (7) for instructions concerning coadministration of acid reducing medications (eg, H2RA or PPIs), and other antiretroviral drugs (eg, efavirenz, tenofovir, and didanosine).
[b] Each packet contains 50 mg of REYATAZ (atazanavir).

Instructions for Mixing REYATAZ Oral Powder [see FDA-approved Instructions for Use]
• It is preferable to mix REYATAZ oral powder with food such as applesauce or yogurt. Mixing REYATAZ oral powder with a beverage (milk, infant formula, or water) may be used for infants who can drink from a cup. For young infants (less than 6 months) who cannot eat solid food or drink from a cup, REYATAZ oral powder should be mixed with infant formula and given using an oral dosing syringe. Administration of REYATAZ and infant formula using an infant bottle is not recommended because full dose may not be delivered.
• Determine the number of packets (4 or 5 packets) that are needed.
• Prior to mixing, tap the packet to settle the powder. Use a clean pair of scissors to cut each packet along the dotted line.
• **Mixing with food:** Using a spoon, mix the recommended number of REYATAZ oral powder packets with a minimum of one tablespoon of food (such as applesauce or yogurt). Feed the mixture to the infant or young child. Add an additional one tablespoon of food to the small container, mix, and feed the child the residual mixture.
• **Mixing with a beverage such as milk or water in a small drinking cup:** Using a spoon, mix the recommended number of REYATAZ oral powder packets with a minimum of 30 mL of the beverage. Have the child drink the mixture. Add an additional 15 mL more of beverage to the drinking cup, mix, and have the child drink the residual mixture. If water is used, food should also be taken at the same time.
• **Mixing with liquid infant formula using an oral dosing syringe and a small medicine cup:** Using a spoon, mix the recommended number of REYATAZ oral powder packets with 10 mL of prepared liquid infant formula. Draw up the full amount of the mixture into an oral syringe and administer into either right or left inner cheek of infant. Pour another 10 mL of formula into the medicine cup to rinse off remaining REYATAZ oral powder in cup. Draw up residual mixture into the syringe and administer into either right or left inner cheek of infant.
• Administer ritonavir immediately following REYATAZ powder administration.
• Administer the entire dosage of REYATAZ oral powder (mixed in the food or beverage) within one hour of preparation (may leave the mixture at room temperature during this one hour period). Ensure that the patient eats or drinks all the food or beverage that contains the powder. Additional food may be given after consumption of the entire mixture.

2.5 Dosage Adjustments in Pregnant Patients
Table 4 includes the recommended dosage of REYATAZ capsules and ritonavir in treatment-naive and treatment-experienced pregnant patients. In these patients, REYATAZ must be administered with ritonavir. There are no dosage adjustments for postpartum patients (see Table 1 for the recommended REYATAZ dosage in adults). [See Use in Specific Populations (8.1).]

Table 4: Recommended Dosage of REYATAZ and Ritonavir in Pregnant Patients[a]

	REYATAZ Once Daily Dosage	Ritonavir Once Daily Dosage
Treatment-Naive and Treatment-Experienced		
Recommended Regimen	300 mg	100 mg
Treatment-Experienced During the Second or Third Trimester When Coadministered with either H2RA or Tenofovir[b]		
In combination with either H2RA or tenofovir	400 mg	100 mg

[a] See Drug Interactions (7) for instructions concerning coadministration of acid reducing medications (eg, H2RA or PPIs), and other antiretroviral drugs (eg, efavirenz, tenofovir, and didanosine).
[b] REYATAZ (atazanavir) is not recommended for treatment-experienced pregnant patients during the second and third trimester taking REYATAZ with both tenofovir and H2RA.

2.6 Renal Impairment
For patients with renal impairment, including those with severe renal impairment who are not managed with hemodialysis, no dose adjustment is required for REYATAZ. Treatment-naive patients with end stage renal disease managed with hemodialysis should receive REYATAZ 300 mg with ritonavir 100 mg. REYATAZ should not be administered to HIV-treatment-experienced patients with end stage renal disease managed with hemodialysis. [See Use in Specific Populations (8.7).]

2.7 Dosage Adjustments in Patients with Hepatic Impairment
Table 5 displays the recommended REYATAZ dosage in treatment-naive patients with hepatic impairment. The use of REYATAZ in patients with severe hepatic impairment (Child-Pugh Class C) is not recommended. The coadministration of REYATAZ with ritonavir in patients with any degree of hepatic impairment is not recommended.
[See table 5 above]

Table 5: Recommended Dosage of REYATAZ Capsules in Treatment-Naive Adults with Hepatic Impairment

	REYATAZ Once Daily Dosage
Mild hepatic impairment (Child-Pugh Class A)	400 mg
Moderate hepatic impairment (Child-Pugh Class B)	300 mg
Severe hepatic impairment (Child-Pugh Class C)	REYATAZ with or without ritonavir is not recommended

3 DOSAGE FORMS AND STRENGTHS

REYATAZ Capsules:
• 150 mg capsule with blue cap and powder blue body, printed with white ink "BMS 150 mg" on the cap and with blue ink "3624" on the body.
• 200 mg capsule with blue cap and blue body, printed with white ink "BMS 200 mg" on the cap and with white ink "3631" on the body.
• 300 mg capsule with red cap and blue body, printed with white ink "BMS 300 mg" on the cap and with white ink "3622" on the body.
REYATAZ Oral Powder:
• 50 mg of atazanavir as an oral powder in a packet.

4 CONTRAINDICATIONS

REYATAZ is contraindicated:
• in patients with previously demonstrated clinically significant hypersensitivity (eg, Stevens-Johnson syndrome, erythema multiforme, or toxic skin eruptions) to any of the components of REYATAZ capsules or REYATAZ oral powder [see Warnings and Precautions (5.2)].
• when coadministered with drugs that are highly dependent on CYP3A or UGT1A1 for clearance, and for which elevated plasma concentrations of the interacting drugs are associated with serious and/or life-threatening events (see Table 6).
• when coadministered with drugs that strongly induce CYP3A and may lead to lower exposure and loss of efficacy of REYATAZ (see Table 6).
Table 6 displays drugs that are contraindicated with REYATAZ.
[See table 6 at top of next page]

5 WARNINGS AND PRECAUTIONS
5.1 Cardiac Conduction Abnormalities
REYATAZ has been shown to prolong the PR interval of the electrocardiogram in some patients. In healthy volunteers and in patients, abnormalities in atrioventricular (AV) con-

Table 6: Drugs that are Contraindicated with REYATAZ (Information in the table applies to REYATAZ with or without ritonavir, unless otherwise indicated)

Drug Class	Drugs within class that are contraindicated with REYATAZ	Clinical Comment
Alpha 1-Adrenoreceptor Antagonist	Alfuzosin	Potential for increased alfuzosin concentrations, which can result in hypotension.
Antimycobacterials	Rifampin	Rifampin substantially decreases plasma concentrations of atazanavir, which may result in loss of therapeutic effect and development of resistance.
Antineoplastics	Irinotecan	Atazanavir inhibits UGT1A1 and may interfere with the metabolism of irinotecan, resulting in increased irinotecan toxicities.
Benzodiazepines	Triazolam, orally administered midazolam[a]	Triazolam and orally administered midazolam are extensively metabolized by CYP3A4. Coadministration of triazolam or orally administered midazolam with REYATAZ may cause large increases in the concentration of these benzodiazepines. Potential for serious and/or life-threatening events such as prolonged or increased sedation or respiratory depression.
Ergot Derivatives	Dihydroergotamine, ergotamine, ergonovine, methylergonovine	Potential for serious and/or life-threatening events such as acute ergot toxicity characterized by peripheral vasospasm and ischemia of the extremities and other tissues.
GI Motility Agent	Cisapride	Potential for serious and/or life-threatening reactions such as cardiac arrhythmias.
Herbal Products	St. John's wort (*Hypericum perforatum*)	Coadministration of St. John's wort and REYATAZ may result in loss of therapeutic effect and development of resistance.
HMG-CoA Reductase Inhibitors	Lovastatin, simvastatin	Potential for serious reactions such as myopathy, including rhabdomyolysis.
Neuroleptic	Pimozide	Potential for serious and/or life-threatening reactions such as cardiac arrhythmias.
PDE5 Inhibitor	Sildenafil[b] when dosed as REVATIO® for the treatment of pulmonary arterial hypertension	Potential for sildenafil-associated adverse events (which include visual disturbances, hypotension, priapism, and syncope).
Protease Inhibitors	Indinavir	Both REYATAZ and indinavir are associated with indirect (unconjugated) hyperbilirubinemia.
Non-nucleoside Reverse Transcriptase Inhibitors	Nevirapine	Nevirapine substantially decreases atazanavir exposure which may result in loss of therapeutic effect and development of resistance. Potential risk for nevirapine-associated adverse reactions due to increased nevirapine exposures.

[a] See *Drug Interactions, Table 16 (7)* for parenterally administered midazolam.
[b] See *Drug Interactions, Table 16 (7)* for sildenafil when dosed as VIAGRA® for erectile dysfunction.

duction were asymptomatic and generally limited to first-degree AV block. There have been reports of second-degree AV block and other conduction abnormalities *[see Adverse Reactions (6.4) and Overdosage (10)].* In clinical trials that included electrocardiograms, asymptomatic first-degree AV block was observed in 5.9% of atazanavir-treated patients (n=920), 5.2% of lopinavir/ritonavir-treated patients (n=252), 10.4% of nelfinavir-treated patients (n=48), and 3.0% of efavirenz-treated patients (n=329). In Study AI424-045, asymptomatic first-degree AV block was observed in 5% (6/118) of atazanavir/ritonavir-treated patients and 5% (6/116) of lopinavir/ritonavir-treated patients who had on-study electrocardiogram measurements. Because of limited clinical experience in patients with preexisting conduction system disease (eg, marked first-degree AV block or second- or third-degree AV block). ECG monitoring should be considered in these patients. *[See Clinical Pharmacology (12.2).]*

5.2   Rash
In controlled clinical trials, rash (all grades, regardless of causality) occurred in approximately 20% of patients treated with REYATAZ (atazanavir). The median time to onset of rash in clinical studies was 7.3 weeks and the median duration of rash was 1.4 weeks. Rashes were generally mild-to-moderate maculopapular skin eruptions. Treatment-emergent adverse reactions of moderate or severe rash (occurring at a rate of ≥2%) are presented for the individual clinical studies *[see Adverse Reactions (6.1)].* Dosing with REYATAZ was often continued without interruption in patients who developed rash. The discontinuation rate for rash in clinical trials was <1%. Cases of Stevens-Johnson syndrome, erythema multiforme, and toxic skin eruptions, including drug rash, eosinophilia, and systemic symptoms (DRESS) syndrome, have been reported in pa-

tients receiving REYATAZ. *[See Contraindications (4) and Adverse Reactions (6.1).]* REYATAZ should be discontinued if severe rash develops.

5.3   Hyperbilirubinemia
Most patients taking REYATAZ (atazanavir) experience asymptomatic elevations in indirect (unconjugated) bilirubin related to inhibition of UDP-glucuronosyl transferase (UGT). This hyperbilirubinemia is reversible upon discontinuation of REYATAZ. Hepatic transaminase elevations that occur with hyperbilirubinemia should be evaluated for alternative etiologies. No long-term safety data are available for patients experiencing persistent elevations in total bilirubin >5 times the upper limit of normal (ULN). Alternative antiretroviral therapy to REYATAZ may be considered if jaundice or scleral icterus associated with bilirubin elevations presents cosmetic concerns for patients. Dose reduction of atazanavir is not recommended since long-term efficacy of reduced doses has not been established. *[See Adverse Reactions (6.1, 6.2).]*

5.4   Patients with Phenylketonuria
Phenylalanine can be harmful to patients with phenylketonuria (PKU). REYATAZ oral powder contains phenylalanine (a component of aspartame). Each packet of REYATAZ oral powder contains 35 mg of phenylalanine. REYATAZ capsules do not contain phenylalanine.

5.5   Hepatotoxicity
Patients with underlying hepatitis B or C viral infections or marked elevations in transaminases before treatment may be at increased risk for developing further transaminase elevations or hepatic decompensation. In these patients, hepatic laboratory testing should be conducted prior to initiating therapy with REYATAZ and during treatment. *[See Adverse Reactions (6.3) and Use in Specific Populations (8.8).]*

5.6   Nephrolithiasis and Cholelithiasis
Cases of nephrolithiasis and/or cholelithiasis have been reported during postmarketing surveillance in HIV-infected patients receiving REYATAZ (atazanavir) therapy. Some patients required hospitalization for additional management and some had complications. Because these events were reported voluntarily during clinical practice, estimates of frequency cannot be made. If signs or symptoms of nephrolithiasis and/or cholelithiasis occur, temporary interruption or discontinuation of therapy may be considered. *[See Adverse Reactions (6.4).]*

5.7   Diabetes Mellitus/Hyperglycemia
New-onset diabetes mellitus, exacerbation of preexisting diabetes mellitus, and hyperglycemia have been reported during postmarketing surveillance in HIV-infected patients receiving protease inhibitor therapy. Some patients required either initiation or dose adjustments of insulin or oral hypoglycemic agents for treatment of these events. In some cases, diabetic ketoacidosis has occurred. In those patients who discontinued protease inhibitor therapy, hyperglycemia persisted in some cases. Because these events have been reported voluntarily during clinical practice, estimates of frequency cannot be made and a causal relationship between protease inhibitor therapy and these events has not been established. *[See Adverse Reactions (6.4).]*

5.8   Immune Reconstitution Syndrome
Immune reconstitution syndrome has been reported in patients treated with combination antiretroviral therapy, including REYATAZ. During the initial phase of combination antiretroviral treatment, patients whose immune system responds may develop an inflammatory response to indolent or residual opportunistic infections (such as *Mycobacterium avium* infection, cytomegalovirus, *Pneumocystis jiroveci* pneumonia, or tuberculosis), which may necessitate further evaluation and treatment.
Autoimmune disorders (such as Graves' disease, polymyositis, and Guillain-Barré syndrome) have also been reported to occur in the setting of immune reconstitution; however, the time to onset is more variable, and can occur many months after initiation of treatment.

5.9   Fat Redistribution
Redistribution/accumulation of body fat including central obesity, dorsocervical fat enlargement (buffalo hump), peripheral wasting, facial wasting, breast enlargement, and "cushingoid appearance" have been observed in patients receiving antiretroviral therapy. The mechanism and long-term consequences of these events are currently unknown. A causal relationship has not been established.

5.10   Hemophilia
There have been reports of increased bleeding, including spontaneous skin hematomas and hemarthrosis, in patients with hemophilia type A and B treated with protease inhibitors. In some patients additional factor VIII was given. In more than half of the reported cases, treatment with protease inhibitors was continued or reintroduced. A causal relationship between protease inhibitor therapy and these events has not been established.

5.11   Resistance/Cross-Resistance
Various degrees of cross-resistance among protease inhibitors have been observed. Resistance to atazanavir may not preclude the subsequent use of other protease inhibitors. *[See Microbiology (12.4).]*

6   ADVERSE REACTIONS
The following adverse reactions are discussed in greater detail in other sections of the labeling:
• cardiac conduction abnormalities *[see Warnings and Precautions (5.1)]*
• rash *[see Warnings and Precautions (5.2)]*
• hyperbilirubinemia *[see Warnings and Precautions (5.3)]*
• nephrolithiasis and cholelithiasis *[see Warnings and Precautions (5.6)]*
Because clinical trials are conducted under widely varying conditions, adverse reaction rates observed in the clinical trials of a drug cannot be directly compared to rates in the clinical trials of another drug and may not reflect the rates observed in practice.

6.1   Clinical Trial Experience in Adults
Treatment-Emergent Adverse Reactions in Treatment-Naive Patients
The safety profile of REYATAZ in treatment-naive adults is based on 1625 HIV-1 infected patients in clinical trials. 536 patients received REYATAZ 300 mg with ritonavir 100 mg and 1089 patients received REYATAZ 400 mg or higher (without ritonavir).
The most common adverse reactions were nausea, jaundice/scleral icterus, and rash.
Selected clinical adverse reactions of moderate or severe intensity reported in ≥2% of treatment-naive patients receiving combination therapy including REYATAZ 300 mg with ritonavir 100 mg and REYATAZ 400 mg (without ritonavir) are presented in Tables 7 and 8, respectively.
[See table 7 at top of next page]
[See table 8 at top of next page]

Treatment-Emergent Adverse Reactions in Treatment-Experienced Patients

The safety profile of REYATAZ (atazanavir) in treatment-experienced adults is based on 119 HIV-1 infected patients in clinical trials.

The most common adverse reactions are jaundice/scleral icterus and myalgia.

Selected clinical adverse reactions of moderate or severe intensity reported in ≥2% of treatment-experienced patients receiving REYATAZ/ritonavir are presented in Table 9.

Table 9: Selected Treatment-Emergent Adverse Reactions[a] of Moderate or Severe Intensity Reported in ≥2% of Adult Treatment-Experienced Patients,[b] Study AI424-045

	48 weeks[c] REYATAZ/ritonavir 300/100 mg once daily + tenofovir + NRTI (n=119)	48 weeks[c] lopinavir/ritonavir 400/100 mg twice daily[d] + tenofovir + NRTI (n=118)
Body as a Whole		
Fever	2%	*
Digestive System		
Jaundice/scleral icterus	9%	*
Diarrhea	3%	11%
Nausea	3%	2%
Nervous System		
Depression	2%	<1%
Musculoskeletal System		
Myalgia	4%	*

* None reported in this treatment arm.
[a] Includes events of possible, probable, certain, or unknown relationship to treatment regimen.
[b] Based on the regimen containing REYATAZ.
[c] Median time on therapy.
[d] As a fixed-dose combination.

Laboratory Abnormalities in Treatment-Naive Patients

The percentages of adult treatment-naive patients treated with combination therapy including REYATAZ 300 mg with ritonavir 100 mg and REYATAZ 400 mg (without ritonavir) with Grade 3–4 laboratory abnormalities are presented in Tables 10 and 11, respectively.

[See table 10 above]

[See table 11 at top of next page]

Laboratory Abnormalities in Treatment-Experienced Patients

The percentages of adult treatment-experienced patients treated with combination therapy including REYATAZ/ritonavir with Grade 3–4 laboratory abnormalities are presented in Table 12.

[See table 12 at top of next page]

Lipids, Change from Baseline in Treatment-Naive Patients

For Study AI424-138 and Study AI424-034, changes from baseline in LDL-cholesterol, HDL-cholesterol, total cholesterol, and triglycerides are shown in Tables 13 and 14, respectively.

[See table 13 at top of page 717]

[See table 14 on page 717]

Lipids, Change from Baseline in Treatment-Experienced Patients

For Study AI424-045, changes from baseline in LDL-cholesterol, HDL-cholesterol, total cholesterol, and triglycerides are shown in Table 15. The observed magnitude of dyslipidemia was less with REYATAZ/ritonavir than with lopinavir/ritonavir. However, the clinical impact of such findings has not been demonstrated.

[See table 15 at top of page 718]

6.2   Clinical Trial Experience in Pediatric Patients

Adverse Reactions in Pediatric Patients: REYATAZ Capsules

The safety and tolerability of REYATAZ Capsules with and without ritonavir have been established in pediatric patients at least 6 years of age from the open-label, multicenter clinical trial PACTG 1020A.

The safety profile of REYATAZ in pediatric patients (6 to less than 18 years of age) taking the capsule formulation was generally similar to that observed in clinical studies of REYATAZ in adults. The most common Grade 2–4 adverse events (≥5%, regardless of causality) reported in pediatric patients were cough (21%), fever (18%), jaundice/scleral icterus (15%), rash (14%), vomiting (12%), diarrhea (9%), headache (8%), peripheral edema (7%), extremity pain (6%), nasal congestion (6%), oropharyngeal pain (6%), wheezing (6%), and rhinorrhea (6%). Asymptomatic second-degree atrioventricular block was reported in <2% of patients. The most common Grade 3–4 laboratory abnormalities occurring in pediatric patients taking the capsule formulation were elevation of total bilirubin (≥3.2 mg/dL, 58%), neutropenia (9%), and hypoglycemia (4%). All other Grade 3–4 laboratory abnormalities occurred with a frequency of less than 3%.

Table 7: Selected Treatment-Emergent Adverse Reactions[a] of Moderate or Severe Intensity Reported in ≥2% of Adult Treatment-Naive Patients,[b] Study AI424-138

	96 weeks[c] REYATAZ 300 mg with ritonavir 100 mg (once daily) and tenofovir with emtricitabine[d] (n=441)	96 weeks[c] lopinavir 400 mg with ritonavir 100 mg (twice daily) and tenofovir with emtricitabine[d] (n=437)
Digestive System		
Nausea	4%	8%
Jaundice/scleral icterus	5%	*
Diarrhea	2%	12%
Skin and Appendages		
Rash	3%	2%

* None reported in this treatment arm.
[a] Includes events of possible, probable, certain, or unknown relationship to treatment regimen.
[b] Based on the regimen containing REYATAZ.
[c] Median time on therapy.
[d] As a fixed-dose combination: 300 mg tenofovir, 200 mg emtricitabine once daily.

Table 8: Selected Treatment-Emergent Adverse Reactions[a] of Moderate or Severe Intensity Reported in ≥2% of Adult Treatment-Naive Patients,[b] Studies AI424-034, AI424-007, and AI424-008

	Study AI424-034		Studies AI424-007, -008	
	64 weeks[c] REYATAZ 400 mg once daily + lamivudine + zidovudine[e] (n=404)	64 weeks[c] efavirenz 600 mg once daily + lamivudine + zidovudine[e] (n=401)	120 weeks[c,d] REYATAZ 400 mg once daily + stavudine + lamivudine or didanosine (n=279)	73 weeks[c,d] nelfinavir 750 mg TID or 1250 mg BID + stavudine + lamivudine or didanosine (n=191)
Body as a Whole				
Headache	6%	6%	1%	2%
Digestive System				
Nausea	14%	12%	6%	4%
Jaundice/scleral icterus	7%	*	7%	*
Vomiting	4%	7%	3%	3%
Abdominal pain	4%	4%	4%	2%
Diarrhea	1%	2%	3%	16%
Nervous System				
Insomnia	3%	3%	<1%	*
Dizziness	2%	7%	<1%	*
Peripheral neurologic symptoms	<1%	1%	4%	3%
Skin and Appendages				
Rash	7%	10%	5%	1%

* None reported in this treatment arm.
[a] Includes events of possible, probable, certain, or unknown relationship to treatment regimen.
[b] Based on regimens containing REYATAZ.
[c] Median time on therapy.
[d] Includes long-term follow-up.
[e] As a fixed-dose combination: 150 mg lamivudine, 300 mg zidovudine twice daily.

Table 10: Grade 3–4 Laboratory Abnormalities Reported in ≥2% of Adult Treatment-Naive Patients,[a] Study AI424-138

Variable	Limit[c]	96 weeks[b] REYATAZ 300 mg with ritonavir 100 mg (once daily) and tenofovir with emtricitabine[d] (n=441)	96 weeks[b] lopinavir 400 mg with ritonavir 100 mg (twice daily) and tenofovir with emtricitabine[d] (n=437)
Chemistry	High		
SGOT/AST	≥5.1 × ULN	3%	1%
SGPT/ALT	≥5.1 × ULN	3%	2%
Total Bilirubin	≥2.6 × ULN	44%	<1%
Lipase	≥2.1 × ULN	2%	2%
Creatine Kinase	≥5.1 × ULN	8%	7%
Total Cholesterol	≥240 mg/dL	11%	25%
Hematology	Low		
Neutrophils	<750 cells/mm³	5%	2%

[a] Based on the regimen containing REYATAZ.
[b] Median time on therapy.
[c] ULN = upper limit of normal.
[d] As a fixed-dose combination: 300 mg tenofovir, 200 mg emtricitabine once daily.

Table 11: Grade 3–4 Laboratory Abnormalities Reported in ≥2% of Adult Treatment-Naive Patients,[a] Studies AI424-034, AI424-007, and AI424-008

		Study AI424-034		Studies AI424-007, -008	
		64 weeks[b] REYATAZ 400 mg once daily + lamivudine + zidovudine[e]	64 weeks[b] efavirenz 600 mg once daily + lamivudine + zidovudine[e]	120 weeks[b,c] REYATAZ 400 mg once daily + stavudine + lamivudine or + stavudine + didanosine	73 weeks[b,c] nelfinavir 750 mg TID or 1250 mg BID + stavudine + lamivudine or + stavudine + didanosine
Variable	Limit[d]	(n=404)	(n=401)	(n=279)	(n=191)
Chemistry	High				
SGOT/AST	≥5.1 × ULN	2%	2%	7%	5%
SGPT/ALT	≥5.1 × ULN	4%	3%	9%	7%
Total Bilirubin	≥2.6 × ULN	35%	<1%	47%	3%
Amylase	≥2.1 × ULN	*	*	14%	10%
Lipase	≥2.1 × ULN	<1%	1%	4%	5%
Creatine Kinase	≥5.1 × ULN	6%	6%	11%	9%
Total Cholesterol	≥240 mg/dL	6%	24%	19%	48%
Triglycerides	≥751 mg/dL	<1%	3%	4%	2%
Hematology	Low				
Hemoglobin	<8.0 g/dL	5%	3%	<1%	4%
Neutrophils	<750 cells/mm³	7%	9%	3%	7%

* None reported in this treatment arm.
[a] Based on regimen(s) containing REYATAZ.
[b] Median time on therapy.
[c] Includes long-term follow-up.
[d] ULN = upper limit of normal.
[e] As a fixed-dose combination: 150 mg lamivudine, 300 mg zidovudine twice daily.

Table 12: Grade 3–4 Laboratory Abnormalities Reported in ≥2% of Adult Treatment-Experienced Patients, Study AI424-045[a]

		48 weeks[b] REYATAZ/ritonavir 300/100 mg once daily + tenofovir + NRTI (n=119)	48 weeks[b] lopinavir/ritonavir 400/100 mg twice daily[d] + tenofovir + NRTI (n=118)
Variable	Limit[c]		
Chemistry	High		
SGOT/AST	≥5.1 × ULN	3%	3%
SGPT/ALT	≥5.1 × ULN	4%	3%
Total Bilirubin	≥2.6 × ULN	49%	<1%
Lipase	≥2.1 × ULN	5%	6%
Creatine Kinase	≥5.1 × ULN	8%	8%
Total Cholesterol	≥240 mg/dL	25%	26%
Triglycerides	≥751 mg/dL	8%	12%
Glucose	≥251 mg/dL	5%	<1%
Hematology	Low		
Platelets	<50,000 cells/mm³	2%	3%
Neutrophils	<750 cells/mm³	7%	8%

[a] Based on regimen(s) containing REYATAZ.
[b] Median time on therapy.
[c] ULN = upper limit of normal.
[d] As a fixed-dose combination.

Adverse Reactions in Pediatric Patients: REYATAZ Oral Powder
The data described below reflect exposure to REYATAZ (atazanavir) oral powder in 89 subjects weighing from 10 kg to less than 25 kg, including 65 patients exposed for 48 weeks. These data are from two pooled open-label, multicenter clinical trials in treatment-naive and treatment-experienced pediatric patients (AI424-397 [PRINCE I] and AI424-451 [PRINCE II]). Age ranged from 15 months to less than 7.5 years of age. In these studies 53% were female and 47% were male. All patients received ritonavir and 2 nucleoside reverse transcriptase inhibitors (NRTIs).
The safety profile of REYATAZ in pediatric patients taking REYATAZ oral powder was generally similar to that observed in clinical studies of REYATAZ in pediatric patients taking REYATAZ capsules. The most common Grade 3–4 laboratory abnormalities occurring in pediatric patients weighing 10 kg to less than 25 kg taking REYATAZ oral powder were increased amylase (19%), neutropenia (12%), increased SGPT/ALT (5%), elevation of total bilirubin (≥2.6 times ULN, 12%), increased lipase (5%), and decreased hemoglobin (3%). All other Grade 3–4 laboratory abnormalities occurred with a frequency of less than 3%.

6.3 Patients Co-Infected with Hepatitis B and/or Hepatitis C Virus
In study AI424-138, 60 patients treated with REYATAZ (atazanavir)/ritonavir 300 mg/100 mg once daily, and 51 patients treated with lopinavir/ritonavir 400 mg/100 mg once daily, each with fixed dose tenofovir-emtricitabine, were seropositive for hepatitis B and/or C at study entry. ALT levels >5 times ULN developed in 10% (6/60) of the REYATAZ/ritonavir-treated patients and 8% (4/50) of the lopinavir/ritonavir-treated patients. AST levels >5 times ULN developed in 10% (6/60) of the REYATAZ/ritonavir-treated patients and none (0/50) of the lopinavir/ritonavir-treated patients.
In study AI424-045, 20 patients treated with REYATAZ/ritonavir 300 mg/100 mg once daily, and 18 patients treated with lopinavir/ritonavir 400 mg/100 mg twice daily, were seropositive for hepatitis B and/or C at study entry. ALT levels >5 times ULN developed in 25% (5/20) of the REYATAZ/

ritonavir-treated patients and 6% (1/18) of the lopinavir/ritonavir-treated patients. AST levels >5 times ULN developed in 10% (2/20) of the REYATAZ/ritonavir-treated patients and 6% (1/18) of the lopinavir/ritonavir-treated patients.
In studies AI424-008 and AI424-034, 74 patients treated with 400 mg of REYATAZ (atazanavir) once daily, 58 who received efavirenz, and 12 who received nelfinavir were seropositive for hepatitis B and/or C at study entry. ALT levels >5 times ULN developed in 15% of the REYATAZ-treated patients, 14% of the efavirenz-treated patients, and 17% of the nelfinavir-treated patients. AST levels >5 times ULN developed in 9% of the REYATAZ-treated patients, 5% of the efavirenz-treated patients, and 17% of the nelfinavir-treated patients. Within REYATAZ and control regimens, no difference in frequency of bilirubin elevations was noted between seropositive and seronegative patients. [See Warnings and Precautions (5.3).]

6.4 Postmarketing Experience
The following events have been identified during postmarketing use of REYATAZ. Because these reactions are reported voluntarily from a population of unknown size, it is not always possible to reliably estimate their frequency or establish a causal relationship to drug exposure.
Body as a Whole: edema
Cardiovascular System: second-degree AV block, third-degree AV block, left bundle branch block, QTc prolongation [see Warnings and Precautions (5.1)]
Gastrointestinal System: pancreatitis
Hepatic System: hepatic function abnormalities
Hepatobiliary Disorders: cholelithiasis [see Warnings and Precautions (5.5)], cholecystitis, cholestasis
Metabolic System and Nutrition Disorders: diabetes mellitus, hyperglycemia [see Warnings and Precautions (5.7)]
Musculoskeletal System: arthralgia
Renal System: nephrolithiasis [see Warnings and Precautions (5.6)], interstitial nephritis
Skin and Appendages: alopecia, maculopapular rash [see Contraindications (4) and Warnings and Precautions (5.2)], pruritus, angioedema

7 DRUG INTERACTIONS
See also *Contraindications (4)* and *Clinical Pharmacology (12.3)*.
7.1 Potential for REYATAZ to Affect Other Drugs
Atazanavir is an inhibitor of CYP3A and UGT1A1. Coadministration of REYATAZ and drugs primarily metabolized by CYP3A or UGT1A1 may result in increased plasma concentrations of the other drug that could increase or prolong its therapeutic and adverse effects.
Atazanavir is a weak inhibitor of CYP2C8. Use of REYATAZ without ritonavir is not recommended when coadministered with drugs highly dependent on CYP2C8 with narrow therapeutic indices (eg, paclitaxel, repaglinide). When REYATAZ with ritonavir is coadministered with substrates of CYP2C8, clinically significant interactions are not expected. [See Clinical Pharmacology, Table 22 (12.3).]
The magnitude of CYP3A-mediated drug interactions on coadministered drug may change when REYATAZ is coadministered with ritonavir. See the complete prescribing information for ritonavir for information on drug interactions with ritonavir.
7.2 Potential for Other Drugs to Affect REYATAZ
Atazanavir is a CYP3A4 substrate; therefore, drugs that induce CYP3A4 may decrease atazanavir plasma concentrations and reduce REYATAZ's therapeutic effect.
Atazanavir solubility decreases as pH increases. Reduced plasma concentrations of atazanavir are expected if proton-pump inhibitors, antacids, buffered medications, or H_2-receptor antagonists are administered with REYATAZ [see Dosage and Administration (2.2, 2.3, 2.4, and 2.5)].
7.3 Established and Other Potentially Significant Drug Interactions
Table 16 provides dosing recommendations as a result of drug interactions with REYATAZ. These recommendations are based on either drug interaction studies or predicted interactions due to the expected magnitude of interaction and potential for serious events or loss of efficacy.
[See table 16 on pages 719 through 724]
7.4 Drugs with No Observed or Predicted Interactions with REYATAZ
Clinically significant interactions are not expected between atazanavir and substrates of CYP2C19, CYP2C9, CYP2D6, CYP2B6, CYP2A6, CYP1A2, or CYP2E1. Clinically significant interactions are not expected between atazanavir when administered with ritonavir and substrates of CYP2C8. See the complete prescribing information for ritonavir for information on other potential drug interactions with ritonavir. Based on known metabolic profiles, clinically significant

drug interactions are not expected between REYATAZ (atazanavir) and dapsone, trimethoprim/sulfamethoxazole, azithromycin, or erythromycin. REYATAZ does not interact with substrates of CYP2D6 (eg, nortriptyline, desipramine, metoprolol). Additionally, no clinically significant drug interactions were observed when REYATAZ was coadministered with methadone, fluconazole, acetaminophen, or atenolol. [See Clinical Pharmacology, Tables 21 and 22 (12.3).]

8 USE IN SPECIFIC POPULATIONS

8.1 Pregnancy

Pregnancy Category B

Antiretroviral Pregnancy Registry: To monitor maternal-fetal outcomes of pregnant women exposed to REYATAZ, an Antiretroviral Pregnancy Registry has been established. Physicians are encouraged to register patients by calling 1-800-258-4263.

Risk Summary

Atazanavir has been evaluated in a limited number of women during pregnancy and postpartum. Available human and animal data suggest that atazanavir does not increase the risk of major birth defects overall compared to the background rate. However, because the studies in humans cannot rule out the possibility of harm, REYATAZ should be used during pregnancy only if clearly needed.

Cases of lactic acidosis syndrome, sometimes fatal, and symptomatic hyperlactatemia have occurred in pregnant women using REYATAZ in combination with nucleoside analogues. Nucleoside analogues are associated with an increased risk of lactic acidosis syndrome.

Hyperbilirubinemia occurs frequently in patients who take REYATAZ, including pregnant women. All infants, including neonates exposed to REYATAZ in utero, should be monitored for the development of severe hyperbilirubinemia during the first few days of life.

Clinical Considerations

Dosing During Pregnancy and the Postpartum Period:

• REYATAZ should not be administered without ritonavir.

• REYATAZ should only be administered to pregnant women with HIV-1 strains susceptible to atazanavir.

• For pregnant patients, no dose adjustment is required for REYATAZ with the following exceptions:

 • For treatment-experienced pregnant women during the second or third trimester, when REYATAZ is coadministered with either an H₂-receptor antagonist **or** tenofovir, REYATAZ 400 mg with ritonavir 100 mg once daily is recommended. There are insufficient data to recommend a REYATAZ dose for use with both an H₂-receptor antagonist *and* tenofovir in treatment-experienced pregnant women.

• No dose adjustment is required for postpartum patients. However, patients should be closely monitored for adverse events because atazanavir exposures could be higher during the first 2 months after delivery. [See Dosage and Administration (2.5) and Clinical Pharmacology (12.3).]

Human Data

Clinical Trials: In clinical trial AI424-182, REYATAZ/ritonavir (300/100 mg or 400/100 mg) in combination with zidovudine/lamivudine was administered to 41 HIV-infected pregnant women during the second or third trimester. Among the 39 women who completed the study, 38 women achieved an HIV RNA <50 copies/mL at time of delivery. Six of 20 (30%) women on REYATAZ/ritonavir 300/100 mg and 13 of 21 (62%) women on REYATAZ/ritonavir 400/100 mg experienced hyperbilirubinemia (total bilirubin greater than or equal to 2.6 times ULN). There were no cases of lactic acidosis observed in clinical trial AI424-182.

Atazanavir drug concentrations in fetal umbilical cord blood were approximately 12% to 19% of maternal concentrations. Among the 40 infants born to 40 HIV-infected pregnant women, all had test results that were negative for HIV-1 DNA at the time of delivery and/or during the first 6 months postpartum. All 40 infants received antiretroviral prophylactic treatment containing zidovudine. No evidence of severe hyperbilirubinemia (total bilirubin levels greater than 20 mg/dL) or acute or chronic bilirubin encephalopathy was observed among neonates in this study. However, 10/36 (28%) infants (6 greater than or equal to 38 weeks gestation and 4 less than 38 weeks gestation) had bilirubin levels of 4 mg/dL or greater within the first day of life.

Lack of ethnic diversity was a study limitation. In the study population, 33/40 (83%) infants were Black/African American, who have a lower incidence of neonatal hyperbilirubinemia than Caucasians and Asians. In addition, women with Rh incompatibility were excluded, as well as women who had a previous infant who developed hemolytic disease and/or had neonatal pathologic jaundice (requiring phototherapy).

Additionally, of the 38 infants who had glucose samples collected in the first day of life, 3 had adequately collected serum glucose samples with values of <40 mg/dL that could not be attributed to maternal glucose intolerance, difficult delivery, or sepsis.

Antiretroviral Pregnancy Registry Data: As of January 2010, the Antiretroviral Pregnancy Registry (APR) has received prospective reports of 635 exposures to atazanavir-containing regimens (425 exposed in the first trimester and 160 and 50 exposed in second and third trimester, respectively). Birth defects occurred in 9 of 393 (2.3%) live births (first trimester exposure) and 5 of 212 (2.4%) live births (second/third trimester exposure). Among pregnant women in the U.S. reference population, the background rate of birth defects is 2.7%. There was no association between atazanavir and overall birth defects observed in the APR.

Pharmacokinetics of Atazanavir in Pregnancy

[See Clinical Pharmacology (12.3).]

Animal Data

In animal reproduction studies, there was no evidence of teratogenicity in offspring born to animals at systemic drug exposure levels (AUC) 0.7 (in rabbits) to 1.2 (in rats) times those observed at the human clinical dose (300 mg/day atazanavir boosted with 100 mg/day ritonavir). In pre- and postnatal development studies in the rat, atazanavir caused body weight loss or weight gain suppression in the animal offspring with maternal drug exposure (AUC) 1.3 times the human exposure at this clinical dose. However, maternal toxicity also occurred at this exposure level.

8.3 Nursing Mothers

The Centers for Disease Control and Prevention recommend that HIV-infected mothers not breastfeed their infants to avoid risking postnatal transmission of HIV. It is not known whether atazanavir is present in human milk. Because of both the potential for HIV transmission and the potential for serious adverse reactions in nursing infants, **mothers should be instructed not to breastfeed if they are taking REYATAZ.**

8.4 Pediatric Use

REYATAZ (atazanavir) is indicated in combination with other antiretroviral agents for the treatment of HIV-1 infection in pediatric patients 3 months of age and older weighing at least 10 kg. REYATAZ is not recommended for use in pediatric patients below the age of 3 months due to the risk of kernicterus [see Indications and Usage (1)]. All REYATAZ contraindications, warnings, and precautions apply to pediatric patients [see Contraindications (4) and Warnings and Precautions (5)].

The safety, pharmacokinetic profile, and virologic response of REYATAZ in pediatric patients at least 3 months of age and older weighing at least 10 kg were established in three open-label, multicenter clinical trials: PACTG 1020A, AI424-451, and AI424-397 [see Clinical Pharmacology (12.3) and Clinical Studies (14.3)]. The safety profile in pediatric patients was generally similar to that observed in adults [see Adverse Reactions (6.2)]. See Dosage and Administration (2.3, 2.4) for dosing recommendations for the use of REYATAZ capsules and REYATAZ oral powder in pediatric patients.

8.5 Geriatric Use

Clinical studies of REYATAZ did not include sufficient numbers of patients aged 65 and over to determine whether they respond differently from younger patients. Based on a comparison of mean single-dose pharmacokinetic values for C_{max} and AUC, a dose adjustment based upon age is not recommended. In general, appropriate caution should be exercised in the administration and monitoring of REYATAZ in elderly patients reflecting the greater frequency of decreased hepatic, renal, or cardiac function, and of concomitant disease or other drug therapy.

Table 13: Lipid Values, Mean Change from Baseline, Study AI424-138

	REYATAZ/ritonavir[a,b]					lopinavir/ritonavir[b,c]				
	Baseline mg/dL (n=428[e])	Week 48 mg/dL (n=372[e])	Week 48 Change[d] (n=372[e])	Week 96 mg/dL (n=342[e])	Week 96 Change[d] (n=342[e])	Baseline mg/dL (n=424[e])	Week 48 mg/dL (n=335[e])	Week 48 Change[d] (n=335[e])	Week 96 mg/dL (n=291[e])	Week 96 Change[d] (n=291[e])
LDL-Cholesterol[f]	92	105	+14%	105	+14%	93	111	+19%	110	+17%
HDL-Cholesterol[f]	37	46	+29%	44	+21%	36	48	+37%	46	+29%
Total Cholesterol[f]	149	169	+13%	169	+13%	150	187	+25%	186	+25%
Triglycerides[f]	126	145	+15%	140	+13%	129	194	+52%	184	+50%

[a] REYATAZ 300 mg with ritonavir 100 mg once daily with the fixed-dose combination: 300 mg tenofovir, 200 mg emtricitabine once daily.

[b] Values obtained after initiation of serum lipid-reducing agents were not included in these analyses. At baseline, serum lipid-reducing agents were used in 1% in the lopinavir/ritonavir treatment arm and 1% in the REYATAZ/ritonavir arm. Through Week 48, serum lipid-reducing agents were used in 8% in the lopinavir/ritonavir treatment arm and 2% in the REYATAZ/ritonavir arm. Through Week 96, serum lipid-reducing agents were used in 10% in the lopinavir/ritonavir treatment arm and 3% in the REYATAZ/ritonavir arm.

[c] Lopinavir 400 mg with ritonavir 100 mg twice daily with the fixed-dose combination 300 mg tenofovir, 200 mg emtricitabine once daily.

[d] The change from baseline is the mean of within-patient changes from baseline for patients with both baseline and Week 48 or Week 96 values and is not a simple difference of the baseline and Week 48 or Week 96 mean values, respectively.

[e] Number of patients with LDL-cholesterol measured.

[f] Fasting.

Table 14: Lipid Values, Mean Change from Baseline, Study AI424-034

	REYATAZ[a,b]			efavirenz[b,c]		
	Baseline mg/dL (n=383[e])	Week 48 mg/dL (n=283[e])	Week 48 Change[d] (n=272[e])	Baseline mg/dL (n=378[e])	Week 48 mg/dL (n=264[e])	Week 48 Change[d] (n=253[e])
LDL-Cholesterol[f]	98	98	+1%	98	114	+18%
HDL-Cholesterol	39	43	+13%	38	46	+24%
Total Cholesterol	164	168	+2%	162	195	+21%
Triglycerides[f]	138	124	−9%	129	168	+23%

[a] REYATAZ 400 mg once daily with the fixed-dose combination: 150 mg lamivudine, 300 mg zidovudine twice daily.

[b] Values obtained after initiation of serum lipid-reducing agents were not included in these analyses. At baseline, serum lipid-reducing agents were used in 0% in the efavirenz treatment arm and <1% in the REYATAZ arm. Through Week 48, serum lipid-reducing agents were used in 3% in the efavirenz treatment arm and 1% in the REYATAZ arm.

[c] Efavirenz 600 mg once daily with the fixed-dose combination: 150 mg lamivudine, 300 mg zidovudine twice daily.

[d] The change from baseline is the mean of within-patient changes from baseline for patients with both baseline and Week 48 values and is not a simple difference of the baseline and Week 48 mean values.

[e] Number of patients with LDL-cholesterol measured.

[f] Fasting.

Help Patients Save on Rx Drugs: PDR.net/PharmacyDiscountCard

Table 15: Lipid Values, Mean Change from Baseline, Study AI424-045

	REYATAZ/ritonavir[a,b]			lopinavir/ritonavir[b,c]		
	Baseline mg/dL (n=111[e])	Week 48 mg/dL (n=75[e])	Week 48 Change[d] (n=74[e])	Baseline mg/dL (n=108[e])	Week 48 mg/dL (n=76[e])	Week 48 Change[d] (n=73[e])
LDL-Cholesterol[f]	108	98	−10%	104	103	+1%
HDL-Cholesterol	40	39	−7%	39	41	+2%
Total Cholesterol	188	170	−8%	181	187	+6%
Triglycerides[f]	215	161	−4%	196	224	+30%

[a] REYATAZ 300 mg once daily + ritonavir + tenofovir + 1 NRTI.
[b] Values obtained after initiation of serum lipid-reducing agents were not included in these analyses. At baseline, serum lipid-reducing agents were used in 4% in the lopinavir/ritonavir treatment arm and 4% in the REYATAZ/ritonavir arm. Through Week 48, serum lipid-reducing agents were used in 19% in the lopinavir/ritonavir treatment arm and 8% in the REYATAZ/ritonavir arm.
[c] Lopinavir/ritonavir (400/100 mg) BID + tenofovir + 1 NRTI.
[d] The change from baseline is the mean of within-patient changes from baseline for patients with both baseline and Week 48 values and is not a simple difference of the baseline and Week 48 mean values.
[e] Number of patients with LDL-cholesterol measured.
[f] Fasting.

8.6 Age/Gender
A study of the pharmacokinetics of atazanavir was performed in young (n=29; 18-40 years) and elderly (n=30; ≥65 years) healthy subjects. There were no clinically significant pharmacokinetic differences observed due to age or gender.

8.7 Impaired Renal Function
REYATAZ (atazanavir) is not recommended for use in HIV-treatment-experienced patients with end stage renal disease managed with hemodialysis. *[See Dosage and Administration (2.6) and Clinical Pharmacology (12.3).]*

8.8 Impaired Hepatic Function
REYATAZ is not recommended for use in patients with severe hepatic impairment. REYATAZ/ritonavir is not recommended in patients with any degree of hepatic impairment. *[See Dosage and Administration (2.7) and Clinical Pharmacology (12.3).]*

10 OVERDOSAGE
Human experience of acute overdose with REYATAZ is limited. Single doses up to 1200 mg (three times the 400 mg maximum recommended dose) have been taken by healthy volunteers without symptomatic untoward effects. A single self-administered overdose of 29.2 g of REYATAZ in an HIV-infected patient (73 times the 400-mg recommended dose) was associated with asymptomatic bifascicular block and PR interval prolongation. These events resolved spontaneously. At REYATAZ doses resulting in high atazanavir exposures, jaundice due to indirect (unconjugated) hyperbilirubinemia (without associated liver function test changes) or PR interval prolongation may be observed. *[See Warnings and Precautions (5.1, 5.3) and Clinical Pharmacology (12.2).]*
Treatment of overdosage with REYATAZ should consist of general supportive measures, including monitoring of vital signs and ECG, and observations of the patient's clinical status. If indicated, elimination of unabsorbed atazanavir should be achieved by emesis or gastric lavage. Administration of activated charcoal may also be used to aid removal of unabsorbed drug. There is no specific antidote for overdose with REYATAZ. Since atazanavir is extensively metabolized by the liver and is highly protein bound, dialysis is unlikely to be beneficial in significant removal of this medicine.

11 DESCRIPTION
The active ingredient in REYATAZ capsules and oral powder is atazanavir sulfate, which is an HIV-1 protease inhibitor.
The chemical name for atazanavir sulfate is (3S,8S,9S,12S)-3,12-Bis(1,1-dimethylethyl)-8-hydroxy-4,11-dioxo-9-(phenylmethyl)-6-[[4-(2-pyridinyl)phenyl]methyl]-2,5,6,10,13-pentaazatetradecanedioic acid dimethyl ester, sulfate (1:1). Its molecular formula is $C_{38}H_{52}N_6O_7 \cdot H_2SO_4$, which corresponds to a molecular weight of 802.9 (sulfuric acid salt). The free base molecular weight is 704.9. Atazanavir sulfate has the following structural formula:
[See chemical structure at top of next column]
Atazanavir sulfate is a white to pale-yellow crystalline powder. It is slightly soluble in water (4-5 mg/mL, free base equivalent) with the pH of a saturated solution in water being about 1.9 at 24 ± 3°C.

REYATAZ (atazanavir) Capsules are available for oral administration in strengths of 150 mg, 200 mg, or 300 mg of atazanavir, which are equivalent to 170.8 mg, 227.8 mg, or 341.69 mg of atazanavir sulfate, respectively. The capsules also contain the following inactive ingredients: crospovidone, lactose monohydrate, and magnesium stearate. The capsule shells contain the following inactive ingredients: gelatin, FD&C Blue No. 2, titanium dioxide, black iron oxide, red iron oxide, and yellow iron oxide. The capsules are printed with ink containing shellac, titanium dioxide, FD&C Blue No. 2, isopropyl alcohol, ammonium hydroxide, propylene glycol, n-butyl alcohol, simethicone, and dehydrated alcohol.
REYATAZ oral powder comes in a packet containing 50 mg of atazanavir equivalent to 56.9 mg of atazanavir sulfate in 1.5 g of powder. The powder is off-white to pale yellow and contains the following inactive ingredients: aspartame, sucrose, and orange-vanilla flavor.

12 CLINICAL PHARMACOLOGY
12.1 Mechanism of Action
Atazanavir is an HIV-1 antiviral drug *[see Microbiology (12.4)]*.

12.2 Pharmacodynamics
Effects on Electrocardiogram
Concentration- and dose-dependent prolongation of the PR interval in the electrocardiogram has been observed in healthy volunteers receiving atazanavir. In a placebo-controlled study (AI424-076), the mean (±SD) maximum change in PR interval from the predose value was 24 (±15) msec following oral dosing with 400 mg of atazanavir (n=65) compared to 13 (±11) msec following dosing with placebo (n=67). The PR interval prolongations in this study were asymptomatic. There is limited information on the potential for a pharmacodynamic interaction in humans between atazanavir and other drugs that prolong the PR interval of the electrocardiogram. *[See Warnings and Precautions (5.1).]*
Electrocardiographic effects of atazanavir were determined in a clinical pharmacology study of 72 healthy subjects. Oral doses of 400 mg (maximum recommended dosage) and 800 mg (twice the maximum recommended dosage) were compared with placebo; there was no concentration-dependent effect of atazanavir on the QTc interval (using Fridericia's correction). In 1793 HIV-infected patients receiving antiretroviral regimens, QTc prolongation was comparable in the atazanavir and comparator regimens. No

atazanavir-treated healthy subject or HIV-infected patient in clinical trials had a QTc interval >500 msec. *[See Warnings and Precautions (5.1).]*

12.3 Pharmacokinetics
The pharmacokinetics of atazanavir were evaluated in healthy adult volunteers and in HIV-infected patients after administration of REYATAZ (atazanavir) 400 mg once daily and after administration of REYATAZ 300 mg with ritonavir 100 mg once daily (see Table 17).
[See table 17 on page 724]
Figure 1 displays the mean plasma concentrations of atazanavir at steady state after REYATAZ 400 mg once daily (as two 200-mg capsules) with a light meal and after REYATAZ 300 mg (as two 150-mg capsules) with ritonavir 100 mg once daily with a light meal in HIV-infected adult patients.

Figure 1: Mean (SD) Steady-State Plasma Concentrations of Atazanavir 400 mg (n=13) and 300 mg with Ritonavir (n=10) for HIV-Infected Adult Patients

Absorption
Atazanavir is rapidly absorbed with a T_{max} of approximately 2.5 hours. Atazanavir demonstrates nonlinear pharmacokinetics with greater than dose-proportional increases in AUC and C_{max} values over the dose range of 200 to 800 mg once daily. Steady state is achieved between Days 4 and 8, with an accumulation of approximately 2.3 fold.

Food Effect
Administration of REYATAZ with food enhances bioavailability and reduces pharmacokinetic variability. Administration of a single 400-mg dose of REYATAZ with a light meal (357 kcal, 8.2 g fat, 10.6 g protein) resulted in a 70% increase in AUC and 57% increase in C_{max} relative to the fasting state. Administration of a single 400-mg dose of REYATAZ with a high-fat meal (721 kcal, 37.3 g fat, 29.4 g protein) resulted in a mean increase in AUC of 35% with no change in C_{max} relative to the fasting state. Administration of REYATAZ with either a light meal or high-fat meal decreased the coefficient of variation of AUC and C_{max} by approximately one-half compared to the fasting state.
Coadministration of a single 300-mg dose of REYATAZ and a 100-mg dose of ritonavir with a light meal (336 kcal, 5.1 g fat, 9.3 g protein) resulted in a 33% increase in the AUC and a 40% increase in both the C_{max} and the 24-hour concentration of atazanavir relative to the fasting state. Coadministration with a high-fat meal (951 kcal, 54.7 g fat, 35.9 g protein) did not affect the AUC of atazanavir relative to fasting conditions and the C_{max} was within 11% of fasting values. The 24-hour concentration following a high-fat meal was increased by approximately 33% due to delayed absorption; the median T_{max} increased from 2.0 to 5.0 hours. Coadministration of REYATAZ with ritonavir with either a light or a high-fat meal decreased the coefficient of variation of AUC and C_{max} by approximately 25% compared to the fasting state.

Distribution
Atazanavir is 86% bound to human serum proteins and protein binding is independent of concentration. Atazanavir binds to both alpha-1-acid glycoprotein (AAG) and albumin to a similar extent (89% and 86%, respectively). In a multiple-dose study in HIV-infected patients dosed with REYATAZ 400 mg once daily with a light meal for 12 weeks, atazanavir was detected in the cerebrospinal fluid and semen. The cerebrospinal fluid/plasma ratio for atazanavir (n=4) ranged between 0.0021 and 0.0226 and seminal fluid/plasma ratio (n=5) ranged between 0.11 and 4.42.

Metabolism
Atazanavir is extensively metabolized in humans. The major biotransformation pathways of atazanavir in humans consisted of monooxygenation and dioxygenation. Other minor biotransformation pathways for atazanavir or its metabolites consisted of glucuronidation, N-dealkylation, hy-

Table 16: Established and Other Potentially Significant Drug Interactions: Alteration in Dose or Regimen May Be Recommended Based on Drug Interaction Studies[a] or Predicted Interactions (Information in the table applies to REYATAZ with or without ritonavir, unless otherwise indicated)

Concomitant Drug Class: Specific Drugs	Effect on Concentration of Atazanavir or Concomitant Drug	Clinical Comment
HIV Antiviral Agents		
Nucleoside Reverse Transcriptase Inhibitors (NRTIs): didanosine buffered formulations enteric-coated (EC) capsules	↓ atazanavir ↓ didanosine	Coadministration of REYATAZ with didanosine buffered tablets resulted in a marked decrease in atazanavir exposure. It is recommended that REYATAZ be given (with food) 2 h before or 1 h after didanosine buffered formulations. Simultaneous administration of didanosine EC and REYATAZ with food results in a decrease in didanosine exposure. Thus, REYATAZ and didanosine EC should be administered at different times.
Nucleotide Reverse Transcriptase Inhibitors: tenofovir disoproxil fumarate	↓ atazanavir ↑ tenofovir	Tenofovir may decrease the AUC and C_{min} of atazanavir. When coadministered with tenofovir, it is recommended that REYATAZ 300 mg be given with ritonavir 100 mg and tenofovir 300 mg (all as a single daily dose with food). REYATAZ increases tenofovir concentrations. The mechanism of this interaction is unknown. Higher tenofovir concentrations could potentiate tenofovir-associated adverse reactions, including renal disorders. Patients receiving REYATAZ and tenofovir should be monitored for tenofovir-associated adverse reactions. For pregnant women taking REYATAZ with ritonavir *and* tenofovir, see *Dosage and Administration (2.5).*
Non-nucleoside Reverse Transcriptase Inhibitors (NNRTIs): efavirenz	↓ atazanavir	Efavirenz decreases atazanavir exposure. ***In treatment-naive patients:*** If REYATAZ is combined with efavirenz, REYATAZ 400 mg (two 200-mg capsules) should be administered with ritonavir 100 mg simultaneously once daily with food, and efavirenz 600 mg should be administered once daily on an empty stomach, preferably at bedtime. ***In treatment-experienced patients:*** Coadministration of REYATAZ with efavirenz in treatment-experienced patients is not recommended due to decreased atazanavir exposure.
Protease Inhibitors: saquinavir (soft gelatin capsules)	↑ saquinavir	Appropriate dosing recommendations for this combination, with or without ritonavir, with respect to efficacy and safety have not been established. In a clinical study, saquinavir 1200 mg coadministered with REYATAZ 400 mg and tenofovir 300 mg (all given once daily) plus nucleoside analogue reverse transcriptase inhibitors did not provide adequate efficacy *[see Clinical Studies (14.2)].*
ritonavir	↑ atazanavir	If REYATAZ is coadministered with ritonavir, it is recommended that REYATAZ 300 mg once daily be given with ritonavir 100 mg once daily with food. See the complete prescribing information for ritonavir for information on drug interactions with ritonavir.
others	↑ other protease inhibitor	Although not studied, the coadministration of REYATAZ/ritonavir and an additional protease inhibitor would be expected to increase exposure to the other protease inhibitor. Such coadministration is not recommended.
HCV Antiviral Agents		
Protease Inhibitors: boceprevir	↓ atazanavir ↓ ritonavir	Concomitant administration of boceprevir and atazanavir/ritonavir resulted in reduced steady-state exposures to atazanavir and ritonavir. Coadministration of REYATAZ/ritonavir and boceprevir is not recommended.
telaprevir	↓ telaprevir ↑ atazanavir	Concomitant administration of telaprevir and atazanavir/ritonavir resulted in reduced steady-state telaprevir exposure, while steady-state atazanavir exposure was increased.
Other Agents		
Antacids and buffered medications	↓ atazanavir	Reduced plasma concentrations of atazanavir are expected if antacids, including buffered medications, are administered with REYATAZ. REYATAZ should be administered 2 hours before or 1 hour after these medications.
Antiarrhythmics: amiodarone, bepridil, lidocaine (systemic), quinidine	↑ amiodarone, bepridil, lidocaine (systemic), quinidine	Coadministration with REYATAZ has the potential to produce serious and/or life-threatening adverse events and has not been studied. Caution is warranted and therapeutic concentration monitoring of these drugs is recommended if they are used concomitantly with REYATAZ.

(Table continued on next page)

drolysis, and oxygenation with dehydrogenation. Two minor metabolites of atazanavir in plasma have been characterized. Neither metabolite demonstrated *in vitro* antiviral activity. *In vitro* studies using human liver microsomes suggested that atazanavir is metabolized by CYP3A.

Elimination
Following a single 400-mg dose of ^{14}C-atazanavir, 79% and 13% of the total radioactivity was recovered in the feces and urine, respectively. Unchanged drug accounted for approximately 20% and 7% of the administered dose in the feces and urine, respectively. The mean elimination half-life of atazanavir in healthy volunteers (n=214) and HIV-infected adult patients (n=13) was approximately 7 hours at steady state following a dose of 400 mg daily with a light meal.

Specific Populations
Renal Impairment
In healthy subjects, the renal elimination of unchanged atazanavir was approximately 7% of the administered dose. REYATAZ (atazanavir) has been studied in adult subjects with severe renal impairment (n=20), including those on hemodialysis, at multiple doses of 400 mg once daily. The mean atazanavir C_{max} was 9% lower, AUC was 19% higher, and C_{min} was 96% higher in subjects with severe renal impairment not undergoing hemodialysis (n=10), than in age-, weight-, and gender-matched subjects with normal renal function. In a 4-hour dialysis session, 2.1% of the administered dose was removed. When atazanavir was administered either prior to, or following hemodialysis (n=10), the geometric means for C_{max}, AUC, and C_{min} were approximately 25% to 43% lower compared to subjects with normal renal function. The mechanism of this decrease is unknown. REYATAZ is not recommended for use in HIV-treatment-experienced patients with end stage renal disease managed with hemodialysis. *[See Dosage and Administration (2.6).]*

Hepatic Impairment
REYATAZ has been studied in adult subjects with moderate-to-severe hepatic impairment (14 Child-Pugh B and 2 Child-Pugh C subjects) after a single 400-mg dose. The mean AUC(0–∞) was 42% greater in subjects with impaired hepatic function than in healthy volunteers. The mean half-life of atazanavir in hepatically impaired subjects was 12.1 hours compared to 6.4 hours in healthy volunteers. A dose reduction to 300 mg is recommended for patients with moderate hepatic impairment (Child-Pugh Class B) who have not experienced prior virologic failure as increased concentrations of atazanavir are expected. REYATAZ is not recommended for use in patients with severe hepatic impairment. The pharmacokinetics of REYATAZ in combination with ritonavir has not been studied in subjects with hepatic impairment; thus, coadministration of REYATAZ with ritonavir is not recommended for use in patients with any degree of hepatic impairment. *[See Dosage and Administration (2.7).]*

Pediatrics
The pharmacokinetic parameters for atazanavir at steady state in pediatric patients taking the powder formulation are summarized in Table 18 by weight ranges that correspond to the recommended doses. *[See Dosage and Administration (2.4).]*
[See table 18 at bottom of page 724]
The pharmacokinetic parameters for atazanavir at steady state in pediatric patients taking the capsule formulation were predicted by a population pharmacokinetic model and are summarized in Table 19 by weight ranges that correspond to the recommended doses. *[See Dosage and Administration (2.4).]*
[See table 19 at bottom of page 724]

Pregnancy
The pharmacokinetic data from HIV-infected pregnant women receiving REYATAZ Capsules with ritonavir are presented in Table 20.

Table 20: Steady-State Pharmacokinetics of Atazanavir with Ritonavir in HIV-Infected Pregnant Women in the Fed State

Pharmacokinetic Parameter	Atazanavir 300 mg with ritonavir 100 mg		
	2nd Trimester (n=5[a])	3rd Trimester (n=20)	Postpartum[b] (n=34)
C_{max} ng/mL Geometric mean (CV%)	3078.85 (50)	3291.46 (48)	5721.21 (31)
AUC ng•h/mL Geometric mean (CV%)	27657.1 (43)	34251.5 (43)	61990.4 (32)

C_{min} ng/mL[c]	538.70	668.48	1462.59
Geometric mean	(46)	(50)	(45)
(CV%)			

[a] Available data during the 2nd trimester are limited.
[b] Atazanavir peak concentrations and AUCs were found to be approximately 28% to 43% higher during the postpartum period (4-12 weeks) than those observed historically in HIV-infected, non-pregnant patients. Atazanavir plasma trough concentrations were approximately 2.2-fold higher during the postpartum period when compared to those observed historically in HIV-infected, non-pregnant patients.
[c] C_{min} is concentration 24 hours post-dose.

Drug Interaction Data

Atazanavir is a metabolism-dependent CYP3A inhibitor, with a K_{inact} value of 0.05 to 0.06 min^{-1} and K_i value of 0.84 to 1.0 μM. Atazanavir is also a direct inhibitor for UGT1A1 (K_i=1.9 μM) and CYP2C8 (K_i=2.1 μM).

Atazanavir has been shown *in vivo* not to induce its own metabolism nor to increase the biotransformation of some drugs metabolized by CYP3A. In a multiple-dose study, REYATAZ (atazanavir) decreased the urinary ratio of endogenous 6β-OH cortisol to cortisol versus baseline, indicating that CYP3A production was not induced.

Drug interaction studies were performed with REYATAZ and other drugs likely to be coadministered and some drugs commonly used as probes for pharmacokinetic interactions. The effects of coadministration of REYATAZ on the AUC, C_{max}, and C_{min} are summarized in Tables 21 and 22. For information regarding clinical recommendations, see *Drug Interactions (7)*.

[See table 21 on pages 725 through 727]
[See table 22 on pages 728 and 729]

12.4   Microbiology

Mechanism of Action

Atazanavir (ATV) is an azapeptide HIV-1 protease inhibitor (PI). The compound selectively inhibits the virus-specific processing of viral Gag and Gag-Pol polyproteins in HIV-1 infected cells, thus preventing formation of mature virions.

Antiviral Activity in Cell Culture

Atazanavir exhibits anti-HIV-1 activity with a mean 50% effective concentration (EC_{50}) in the absence of human serum of 2 to 5 nM against a variety of laboratory and clinical HIV-1 isolates grown in peripheral blood mononuclear cells, macrophages, CEM-SS cells, and MT-2 cells. ATV has activity against HIV-1 Group M subtype viruses A, B, C, D, AE, AG, F, G, and J isolates in cell culture. ATV has variable activity against HIV-2 isolates (1.9-32 nM), with EC_{50} values above the EC_{50} values of failure isolates. Two-drug combination antiviral activity studies with ATV showed no antagonism in cell culture with NNRTIs (delavirdine, efavirenz, and nevirapine), PIs (amprenavir, indinavir, lopinavir, nelfinavir, ritonavir, and saquinavir), NRTIs (abacavir, didanosine, emtricitabine, lamivudine, stavudine, tenofovir, zalcitabine, and zidovudine), the HIV-1 fusion inhibitor enfuvirtide, and two compounds used in the treatment of viral hepatitis, adefovir and ribavirin, without enhanced cytotoxicity.

Resistance

In Cell Culture: HIV-1 isolates with a decreased susceptibility to ATV have been selected in cell culture and obtained from patients treated with ATV or atazanavir/ritonavir (ATV/RTV). HIV-1 isolates with 93- to 183-fold reduced susceptibility to ATV from three different viral strains were selected in cell culture by 5 months. The substitutions in these HIV-1 viruses that contributed to ATV resistance include I50L, N88S, I84V, A71V, and M46I. Changes were also observed at the protease cleavage sites following drug selection. Recombinant viruses containing the I50L substitution without other major PI substitutions were growth impaired and displayed increased susceptibility in cell culture to other PIs (amprenavir, indinavir, lopinavir, nelfinavir, ritonavir, and saquinavir). The I50L and I50V substitutions yielded selective resistance to ATV and amprenavir, respectively, and did not appear to be cross-resistant.

Clinical Studies of Treatment-Naive Patients: Comparison of Ritonavir-Boosted REYATAZ vs. Unboosted REYATAZ: Study AI424-089 compared REYATAZ 300 mg once daily with ritonavir 100 mg vs. REYATAZ 400 mg once daily when administered with lamivudine and extended-release stavudine in HIV-infected treatment-naive patients. A summary of the number of virologic failures and virologic failure isolates with ATV resistance in each arm is shown in Table 23.

[See 23 table at top of page 730]

Clinical Studies of Treatment-Naive Patients Receiving REYATAZ 300 mg with Ritonavir 100 mg: In Phase III study AI424-138, an as-treated genotypic and phenotypic analysis was conducted on samples from patients who experienced virologic failure (HIV-1 RNA ≥400 copies/mL) or discontinued before achieving suppression on ATV/RTV (n=39; 9%) and LPV/RTV (n=39; 9%) through 96 weeks of treatment. In the ATV/RTV arm, one of the virologic failure isolates had a 56-fold decrease in ATV susceptibility emerge on therapy with the development of PI resistance-associated substitutions L10F, V32I, K43T, M46I, A71I, G73S, I85I/V, and L90M. The NRTI resistance-associated substitution M184V also emerged on treatment in this isolate conferring

---

Table 16 *(cont.)*: Established and Other Potentially Significant Drug Interactions: Alteration in Dose or Regimen May Be Recommended Based on Drug Interaction Studies[a] or Predicted Interactions (Information in the table applies to REYATAZ with or without ritonavir, unless otherwise indicated)

Concomitant Drug Class: Specific Drugs	Effect on Concentration of Atazanavir or Concomitant Drug	Clinical Comment
Other Agents (cont.)		
Anticoagulants: warfarin	↑ warfarin	Coadministration with REYATAZ has the potential to produce serious and/or life-threatening bleeding and has not been studied. It is recommended that International Normalized Ratio (INR) be monitored.
Antidepressants: tricyclic antidepressants	↑ tricyclic antidepressants	Coadministration with REYATAZ has the potential to produce serious and/or life-threatening adverse events and has not been studied. Concentration monitoring of these drugs is recommended if they are used concomitantly with REYATAZ.
trazodone	↑ trazodone	Concomitant use of trazodone and REYATAZ with or without ritonavir may increase plasma concentrations of trazodone. Nausea, dizziness, hypotension, and syncope have been observed following coadministration of trazodone and ritonavir. If trazodone is used with a CYP3A4 inhibitor such as REYATAZ, the combination should be used with caution and a lower dose of trazodone should be considered.
Antiepileptics: carbamazepine	↓ atazanavir ↑ carbamazepine	Plasma concentrations of atazanavir may be decreased when carbamazepine is administered with REYATAZ without ritonavir. Coadministration of carbamazepine and REYATAZ without ritonavir is not recommended. Ritonavir may increase plasma levels of carbamazepine. If patients beginning treatment with REYATAZ/ritonavir have been titrated to a stable dose of carbamazepine, a dose reduction for carbamazepine may be necessary.
phenytoin, phenobarbital	↓ atazanavir ↓ phenytoin ↓ phenobarbital	Plasma concentrations of atazanavir may be decreased when phenytoin or phenobarbital is administered with REYATAZ without ritonavir. Coadministration of phenytoin or phenobarbital and REYATAZ without ritonavir is not recommended. Ritonavir may decrease plasma levels of phenytoin and phenobarbital. When REYATAZ with ritonavir is coadministered with either phenytoin or phenobarbital, a dose adjustment of phenytoin or phenobarbital may be required.
lamotrigine	↓ lamotrigine	Coadministration of lamotrigine and REYATAZ **with** ritonavir may decrease lamotrigine plasma concentrations. Dose adjustment of lamotrigine may be required when coadministered with REYATAZ and ritonavir. Coadministration of lamotrigine and REYATAZ **without** ritonavir is not expected to decrease lamotrigine plasma concentrations. No dose adjustment of lamotrigine is required when coadministered with REYATAZ without ritonavir.
Antifungals: ketoconazole, itraconazole	**REYATAZ/ritonavir:** ↑ ketoconazole ↑ itraconazole	Coadministration of ketoconazole has only been studied with REYATAZ without ritonavir (negligible increase in atazanavir AUC and C_{max}). Due to the effect of ritonavir on ketoconazole, high doses of ketoconazole and itraconazole (>200 mg/day) should be used cautiously with REYATAZ/ritonavir.
voriconazole	**REYATAZ/ritonavir in subjects with a functional CYP2C19 allele:** ↓ voriconazole ↓ atazanavir **REYATAZ/ritonavir in subjects without a functional CYP2C19 allele:** ↑ voriconazole ↓ atazanavir	The use of voriconazole in patients receiving REYATAZ/ritonavir is not recommended unless an assessment of the benefit/risk to the patient justifies the use of voriconazole. Patients should be carefully monitored for voriconazole-associated adverse reactions and loss of either voriconazole or atazanavir efficacy during the coadministration of voriconazole and REYATAZ/ritonavir. Coadministration of voriconazole with REYATAZ (without ritonavir) may affect atazanavir concentrations; however, no data are available.

(Table continued on next page)

emtricitabine resistance. Two ATV/RTV-virologic failure isolates had baseline phenotypic ATV resistance and IAS-defined major PI resistance-associated substitutions at baseline. The I50L substitution emerged on study in one of these failure isolates and was associated with a 17-fold decrease in ATV susceptibility from baseline and the other failure isolate with baseline ATV resistance and PI substitutions (M46M/I and I84I/V) had additional IAS-defined major PI substitutions (V32I, M46I, and I84V) emerge on ATV treatment associated with a 3-fold decrease in ATV susceptibility from baseline. Five of the treatment failure isolates in the ATV/RTV arm developed phenotypic emtricitabine resistance with the emergence of either the M184I (n=1) or the M184V (n=4) substitution on therapy and none developed phenotypic tenofovir disoproxil resistance. In the LPV/RTV arm, one of the virologic failure patient isolates had a 69-fold decrease in LPV susceptibility emerge on therapy with the development of PI substitutions L10V, V11I, I54V, G73S, and V82A in addition to baseline PI substitutions L10L/I, V32I, I54I/V, A71I, G73G/S, V82V/A, L89V, and L90M. Six LPV/RTV virologic failure isolates developed the M184V substitution and phenotypic emtricitabine resistance and two developed phenotypic tenofovir disoproxil resistance.

Clinical Studies of Treatment-Naive Patients Receiving REYATAZ (atazanavir) 400 mg without Ritonavir: ATV-resistant clinical isolates from treatment-naive patients who experienced virologic failure on REYATAZ 400 mg treatment without ritonavir often developed an I50L substitution (after an average of 50 weeks of ATV therapy), often in combination with an A71V substitution, but also developed one or more other PI substitutions (eg, V32I, L33F, G73S, V82A, I85V, or N88S) with or without the I50L substitution. In treatment-naive patients, viral isolates that developed the I50L substitution, without other major PI substitutions, showed phenotypic resistance to ATV but retained in cell culture susceptibility to other PIs (amprenavir, indinavir, lopinavir, nelfinavir, ritonavir, and saquinavir); however, there are no clinical data available to demonstrate the effect of the I50L substitution on the efficacy of subsequently administered PIs.

Clinical Studies of Treatment-Experienced Patients: In studies of treatment-experienced patients treated with ATV or ATV/RTV, most ATV-resistant isolates from patients who experienced virologic failure developed substitutions that were associated with resistance to multiple PIs and displayed decreased susceptibility to multiple PIs. The most common protease substitutions to develop in the viral isolates of patients who failed treatment with ATV 300 mg once daily and RTV 100 mg once daily (together with tenofovir and an NRTI) included V32I, L33F/V/I, E35D/G, M46I/L, I50L, F53L/V, I54V, A71V/T/I, G73S/T/C, V82A/T/L, I85V, and L89V/Q/M/T. Other substitutions that developed on ATV/RTV treatment including E34K/A/Q, G48V, I84V, N88S/D/T, and L90M occurred in less than 10% of patient isolates. Generally, if multiple PI resistance substitutions were present in the HIV-1 virus of the patient at baseline, ATV resistance developed through substitutions associated with resistance to other PIs and could include the development of the I50L substitution. The I50L substitution has been detected in treatment-experienced patients experiencing virologic failure after long-term treatment. Protease cleavage site changes also emerged on ATV treatment but their presence did not correlate with the level of ATV resistance.

Clinical Studies of Pediatric Subjects in AI424-397 (PRINCE I) and AI424-451(PRINCE II): No treatment-emergent ATV-associated substitutions were detected among treatment failures in AI424-397, and four known resistance-associated substitutions to other PIs arose in the viruses from one subject each (L19I/R, M36M/I, H69K/R, and I72I/V). None of these viruses acquired phenotypic resistance to ATV, ATV/RTV, or any NNRTI or NRTI. In AI424-451, ATV-associated resistance substitution (I84V) and other PI substitutions arose in the virus of one subject, including M46M/V, V82V/I, I84I/V, and L90L/M; however, these substitutions did not result in phenotypic resistance to ATV (ATV phenotypic fold change: 1.74, using a commercial investigational assay with an ATV cutoff of 2.2 fold change). Secondary PI substitutions also arose in the viruses of one subject each, including V11V/I, G16G/E, D30D/G, E35E/D, K45K/R, L63P/S, and I72I/T. Q61D and Q61E/G emerged in the viruses of two subjects who failed treatment with ATV/RTV. Viruses from three subjects developed M184V in the reverse transcriptase, and all three exhibited phenotypic resistance to emtricitabine and lamivudine.

Cross-Resistance
Cross-resistance among PIs has been observed. Baseline phenotypic and genotypic analyses of clinical isolates from ATV clinical trials of PI-experienced patients showed that

isolates cross-resistant to multiple PIs were cross-resistant to ATV. Greater than 90% of the isolates with substitutions that included I84V or G48V were resistant to ATV. Greater than 60% of isolates containing L90M, G73S/T/C, A71V/T, I54V, M46I/L, or a change at V82 were resistant to ATV, and 38% of isolates containing a D30N substitution in addition to other changes were resistant to ATV. Isolates resistant to ATV were also cross-resistant to other PIs with >90% of the isolates resistant to indinavir, lopinavir, nelfinavir, ritonavir, and saquinavir, and 80% resistant to amprenavir. In treatment-experienced patients, PI-resistant viral isolates

that developed the I50L substitution in addition to other PI resistance-associated substitution were also cross-resistant to other PIs.

Baseline Genotype/Phenotype and Virologic Outcome Analyses
Genotypic and/or phenotypic analysis of baseline virus may aid in determining ATV susceptibility before initiation of ATV/RTV therapy. An association between virologic response at 48 weeks and the number and type of primary PI resistance-associated substitutions detected in baseline HIV-1 isolates from antiretroviral-experienced patients re-

Table 16 *(cont.)*: Established and Other Potentially Significant Drug Interactions: Alteration in Dose or Regimen May Be Recommended Based on Drug Interaction Studies[a] or Predicted Interactions (Information in the table applies to REYATAZ with or without ritonavir, unless otherwise indicated)

Concomitant Drug Class: Specific Drugs	Effect on Concentration of Atazanavir or Concomitant Drug	Clinical Comment
Other Agents (cont.)		
Antigout: colchicine	↑ colchicine	The coadministration of REYATAZ with colchicine in patients with renal or hepatic impairment is not recommended. *Recommended dosage of colchicine when administered with REYATAZ:* *Treatment of gout flares:* 0.6 mg (1 tablet) for 1 dose, followed by 0.3 mg (half tablet) 1 hour later. Not to be repeated before 3 days. *Prophylaxis of gout flares:* If the original regimen was 0.6 mg *twice* a day, the regimen should be adjusted to 0.3 mg *once a day.* If the original regimen was 0.6 mg *once* a day, the regimen should be adjusted to 0.3 mg *once every other day.* *Treatment of familial Mediterranean fever (FMF):* Maximum daily dose of 0.6 mg (may be given as 0.3 mg twice a day).
Antimycobacterials: rifabutin	↑ rifabutin	A rifabutin dose reduction of up to 75% (eg, 150 mg every other day or 3 times per week) is recommended. Increased monitoring for rifabutin-associated adverse reactions including neutropenia is warranted.
Benzodiazepines: parenterally administered midazolam[b]	↑ midazolam	Concomitant use of parenteral midazolam with REYATAZ may increase plasma concentrations of midazolam. Coadministration should be done in a setting which ensures close clinical monitoring and appropriate medical management in case of respiratory depression and/or prolonged sedation. Dosage reduction for midazolam should be considered, especially if more than a single dose of midazolam is administered. Coadministration of oral midazolam with REYATAZ is CONTRAINDICATED.
Calcium channel blockers: diltiazem	↑ diltiazem and desacetyl-diltiazem	Caution is warranted. A dose reduction of diltiazem by 50% should be considered. ECG monitoring is recommended. Coadministration of REYATAZ/ritonavir with diltiazem has not been studied.
felodipine, nifedipine, nicardipine, and verapamil	↑ calcium channel blocker	Caution is warranted. Dose titration of the calcium channel blocker should be considered. ECG monitoring is recommended.
Endothelin receptor antagonists: bosentan	↓ atazanavir ↑ bosentan	Plasma concentrations of atazanavir may be decreased when bosentan is administered with REYATAZ without ritonavir. Coadministration of bosentan and REYATAZ without ritonavir is not recommended. *Coadministration of bosentan in patients on REYATAZ/ritonavir:* For patients who have been receiving REYATAZ/ritonavir for at least 10 days, start bosentan at 62.5 mg once daily or every other day based on individual tolerability. *Coadministration of REYATAZ/ritonavir in patients on bosentan:* Discontinue bosentan at least 36 hours before starting REYATAZ/ritonavir. At least 10 days after starting REYATAZ/ritonavir, resume bosentan at 62.5 mg once daily or every other day based on individual tolerability.
HMG-CoA reductase inhibitors: atorvastatin, rosuvastatin	↑ atorvastatin ↑ rosuvastatin	Titrate atorvastatin dose carefully and use the lowest necessary dose. Rosuvastatin dose should not exceed 10 mg/day. The risk of myopathy, including rhabdomyolysis, may be increased when HIV protease inhibitors, including REYATAZ, are used in combination with these drugs.

(Table continued on next page)

ceiving ATV/RTV once daily or lopinavir (LPV)/RTV twice daily in Study AI424-045 is shown in Table 24.

Overall, both the number and type of baseline PI substitutions affected response rates in treatment-experienced patients. In the ATV/RTV group, patients had lower response rates when 3 or more baseline PI substitutions, including a substitution at position 36, 71, 77, 82, or 90, were present compared to patients with 1–2 PI substitutions, including one of these substitutions.

[See table 24 at top of page 730]

The response rates of antiretroviral-experienced patients in Study AI424-045 were analyzed by baseline phenotype (shift in susceptibility in cell culture relative to reference, Table 25). The analyses are based on a select patient population with 62% of patients receiving an NNRTI-based regimen before study entry compared to 35% receiving a PI-based regimen. Additional data are needed to determine clinically relevant break points for REYATAZ (atazanavir).

Table 25: Baseline Phenotype by Outcome, Antiretroviral-Experienced Patients in Study AI424-045, As-Treated Analysis

Baseline Phenotype[a]	Virologic Response = HIV RNA <400 copies/mL[b]	
	ATV/RTV (n=111)	LPV/RTV (n=111)
0–2	71% (55/78)	70% (56/80)
>2–5	53% (8/15)	44% (4/9)
>5–10	13% (1/8)	33% (3/9)
>10	10% (1/10)	23% (3/13)

[a] Fold change susceptibility in cell culture relative to the wild-type reference.

[b] Results should be interpreted with caution because the subgroups were small.

13 NONCLINICAL TOXICOLOGY

13.1 Carcinogenesis, Mutagenesis, Impairment of Fertility

Carcinogenesis

Long-term carcinogenicity studies in mice and rats were carried out with atazanavir for two years. In the mouse study, drug-related increases in hepatocellular adenomas were found in females at 360 mg/kg/day. The systemic drug exposure (AUC) at the NOAEL (no observable adverse effect level) in females, (120 mg/kg/day) was 2.8 times and in males (80 mg/kg/day) was 2.9 times higher than those in humans at the clinical dose (300 mg/day atazanavir boosted with 100 mg/day ritonavir, non-pregnant patients). In the rat study, no drug-related increases in tumor incidence were observed at doses up to 1200 mg/kg/day, for which AUCs were 1.1 (males) or 3.9 (females) times those measured in humans at the clinical dose.

Mutagenesis

Atazanavir tested positive in an in vitro clastogenicity test using primary human lymphocytes, in the absence and presence of metabolic activation. Atazanavir tested negative in the in vitro Ames reverse-mutation assay, in vivo micronucleus and DNA repair tests in rats, and in vivo DNA damage test in rat duodenum (comet assay).

Impairment of Fertility

At the systemic drug exposure levels (AUC) 0.9 (in male rats) or 2.3 (in female rats) times that of the human clinical dose, (300 mg/day atazanavir boosted with 100 mg/day ritonavir) significant effects on mating, fertility, or early embryonic development were not observed.

14 CLINICAL STUDIES

14.1 Adult Patients without Prior Antiretroviral Therapy

Study AI424-138: a 96-week study comparing the antiviral efficacy and safety of REYATAZ/ritonavir with lopinavir/ritonavir, each in combination with fixed-dose tenofovir-emtricitabine in HIV-1 infected treatment-naive subjects. Study AI424-138 was a 96-week, open-label, randomized, multicenter study, comparing REYATAZ (300 mg once daily) with ritonavir (100 mg once daily) to lopinavir with ritonavir (400/100 mg twice daily), each in combination with fixed-dose tenofovir with emtricitabine (300/200 mg once daily), in 878 antiretroviral treatment-naive patients. Patients had a mean age of 36 years (range: 19-72), 49% were Caucasian, 18% Black, 9% Asian, 23% Hispanic/Mestizo/mixed race, and 68% were male. The median baseline plasma CD4+ cell count was 204 cells/mm³ (range: 2 to 810 cells/mm³) and the mean baseline plasma HIV-1 RNA level was 4.94 log₁₀ copies/mL (range: 2.60 to 5.88 log₁₀ cop-

ies/mL). Treatment response and outcomes through Week 96 are presented in Table 26.

[See table 26 at bottom of page 730]

Through 96 weeks of therapy, the proportion of responders among patients with high viral loads (ie, baseline HIV RNA ≥100,000 copies/mL) was comparable for the REYATAZ (atazanavir)/ritonavir (165 of 223 patients, 74%) and lopinavir/ritonavir (148 of 222 patients, 67%) arms. At 96 weeks, the median increase from baseline in CD4+ cell count was 261 cells/mm³ for the REYATAZ/ritonavir arm and 273 cells/mm³ for the lopinavir/ritonavir arm.

Table 16 (cont.): Established and Other Potentially Significant Drug Interactions: Alteration in Dose or Regimen May Be Recommended Based on Drug Interaction Studies[a] or Predicted Interactions (Information in the table applies to REYATAZ with or without ritonavir, unless otherwise indicated)

Concomitant Drug Class: Specific Drugs	Effect on Concentration of Atazanavir or Concomitant Drug	Clinical Comment
Other Agents (cont.)		
H₂-Receptor antagonists	↓ atazanavir	Plasma concentrations of atazanavir were substantially decreased when REYATAZ 400 mg once daily was administered simultaneously with famotidine 40 mg twice daily, which may result in loss of therapeutic effect and development of resistance. **In treatment-naive patients:** REYATAZ 300 mg with ritonavir 100 mg once daily with food should be administered simultaneously with, and/or at least 10 hours after, a dose of the H₂-receptor antagonist (H2RA). An H2RA dose comparable to famotidine 20 mg once daily up to a dose comparable to famotidine 40 mg twice daily can be used with REYATAZ 300 mg with ritonavir 100 mg in treatment-naive patients. OR For patients unable to tolerate ritonavir, REYATAZ 400 mg once daily with food should be administered at least 2 hours before and at least 10 hours after a dose of the H2RA. No single dose of the H2RA should exceed a dose comparable to famotidine 20 mg, and the total daily dose should not exceed a dose comparable to famotidine 40 mg. The use of REYATAZ without ritonavir in pregnant women is not recommended. **In treatment-experienced patients:** Whenever an H2RA is given to a patient receiving REYATAZ with ritonavir, the H2RA dose should not exceed a dose comparable to famotidine 20 mg twice daily, and the REYATAZ and ritonavir doses should be administered simultaneously with, and/or at least 10 hours after, the dose of the H2RA. • REYATAZ 300 mg with ritonavir 100 mg once daily (all as a single dose with food) if taken with an H2RA. • REYATAZ 400 mg with ritonavir 100 mg once daily (all as a single dose with food) if taken with both tenofovir and an H2RA. • REYATAZ 400 mg with ritonavir 100 mg once daily (all as a single dose with food) if taken with either tenofovir or an H2RA for pregnant women during the second and third trimester. REYATAZ is not recommended for pregnant women during the second and third trimester taking REYATAZ with both tenofovir and an H2RA.
Hormonal contraceptives: ethinyl estradiol and norgestimate or norethindrone	↓ ethinyl estradiol ↑ norgestimate[c] ↑ ethinyl estradiol ↑ norethindrone[d]	Use with caution if coadministration of REYATAZ or REYATAZ/ritonavir with oral contraceptives is considered. If an oral contraceptive is administered with REYATAZ plus ritonavir, it is recommended that the oral contraceptive contain at least 35 mcg of ethinyl estradiol. If REYATAZ is administered without ritonavir, the oral contraceptive should contain no more than 30 mcg of ethinyl estradiol. Potential safety risks include substantial increases in progesterone exposure. The long-term effects of increases in concentration of the progestational agent are unknown and could increase the risk of insulin resistance, dyslipidemia, and acne. Coadministration of REYATAZ or REYATAZ/ritonavir with other hormonal contraceptives (eg, contraceptive patch, contraceptive vaginal ring, or injectable contraceptives) or oral contraceptives containing progestogens other than norethindrone or norgestimate, or less than 25 mcg of ethinyl estradiol, has not been studied; therefore, alternative methods of contraception are recommended.
Immunosuppressants: cyclosporin, sirolimus, tacrolimus	↑ immunosuppressants	Therapeutic concentration monitoring is recommended for these immunosuppressants when coadministered with REYATAZ.

(Table continued on next page)

Study AI424-034: REYATAZ (atazanavir) once daily compared to efavirenz once daily, each in combination with fixed-dose lamivudine + zidovudine twice daily. Study AI424-034 was a randomized, double-blind, multicenter trial comparing REYATAZ (400 mg once daily) to efavirenz (600 mg once daily), each in combination with a fixed-dose combination of lamivudine (3TC) (150 mg) and zidovudine (ZDV) (300 mg) given twice daily, in 810 antiretroviral treatment-naive patients. Patients had a mean age of 34 years (range: 18 to 73), 36% were Hispanic, 33% were Caucasian, and 65% were

male. The mean baseline CD4+ cell count was 321 cells/mm³ (range: 64 to 1424 cells/mm³) and the mean baseline plasma HIV-1 RNA level was 4.8 $\log_{10}$ copies/mL (range: 2.2 to 5.9 $\log_{10}$ copies/mL). Treatment response and outcomes through Week 48 are presented in Table 27.
[See table 27 at top of page 731]

Through 48 weeks of therapy, the proportion of responders among patients with high viral loads (ie, baseline HIV RNA ≥100,000 copies/mL) was comparable for the REYATAZ (atazanavir) and efavirenz arms. The mean increase from baseline in CD4+ cell count was 176 cells/mm³ for the REYATAZ arm and 160 cells/mm³ for the efavirenz arm.

Study AI424-008: REYATAZ 400 mg once daily compared to REYATAZ 600 mg once daily, and compared to nelfinavir 1250 mg twice daily, each in combination with stavudine and lamivudine twice daily. Study AI424-008 was a 48-week, randomized, multicenter trial, blinded to dose of REYATAZ, comparing REYATAZ at two dose levels (400 mg and 600 mg once daily) to nelfinavir (1250 mg twice daily), each in combination with stavudine (40 mg) and lamivudine (150 mg) given twice daily, in 467 antiretroviral treatment-naive patients. Patients had a mean age of 35 years (range: 18 to 69), 55% were Caucasian, and 63% were male. The mean baseline CD4+ cell count was 295 cells/mm³ (range: 4 to 1003 cells/mm³) and the mean baseline plasma HIV-1 RNA level was 4.7 $\log_{10}$ copies/mL (range: 1.8 to 5.9 $\log_{10}$ copies/mL). Treatment response and outcomes through Week 48 are presented in Table 28.
[See table 28 on page 731]

Through 48 weeks of therapy, the mean increase from baseline in CD4+ cell count was 234 cells/mm³ for the REYATAZ 400-mg arm and 211 cells/mm³ for the nelfinavir arm.

14.2   Adult Patients with Prior Antiretroviral Therapy

Study AI424-045: REYATAZ once daily + ritonavir once daily compared to REYATAZ once daily + saquinavir (soft gelatin capsules) once daily, and compared to lopinavir + ritonavir twice daily, each in combination with tenofovir + one NRTI. Study AI424-045 was a randomized, multicenter trial comparing REYATAZ (300 mg once daily) with ritonavir (100 mg once daily) to REYATAZ (400 mg once daily) with saquinavir soft gelatin capsules (1200 mg once daily), and to lopinavir + ritonavir (400/100 mg twice daily), each in combination with tenofovir and one NRTI, in 347 (of 358 randomized) patients who experienced virologic failure on HAART regimens containing PIs, NNRTIs, and NRTIs. The mean time of prior exposure to antiretrovirals was 139 weeks for PIs, 85 weeks for NNRTIs, and 283 weeks for NRTIs. The mean age was 41 years (range: 24 to 74); 60% were Caucasian, and 78% were male. The mean baseline CD4+ cell count was 338 cells/mm³ (range: 14 to 1543 cells/mm³) and the mean baseline plasma HIV-1 RNA level was 4.4 $\log_{10}$ copies/mL (range: 2.6 to 5.88 $\log_{10}$ copies/mL).

Treatment outcomes through Week 48 for the REYATAZ/ritonavir and lopinavir/ritonavir treatment arms are presented in Table 29. REYATAZ/ritonavir and lopinavir/ritonavir were similar for the primary efficacy outcome measure of time-averaged difference in change from baseline in HIV RNA level. Study AI424-045 was not large enough to reach a definitive conclusion that REYATAZ/ritonavir and lopinavir/ritonavir are equivalent on the secondary efficacy outcome measure of proportions below the HIV RNA lower limit of quantification. *[See Microbiology, Tables 24 and 25 (12.4).]*
[See table 29 on page 731]

No patients in the REYATAZ/ritonavir treatment arm and three patients in the lopinavir/ritonavir treatment arm experienced a new-onset CDC Category C event during the study.

In Study AI424-045, the mean change from baseline in plasma HIV-1 RNA for REYATAZ 400 mg with saquinavir (n=115) was −1.55 $\log_{10}$ copies/mL, and the time-averaged difference in change in HIV-1 RNA levels versus lopinavir/ritonavir was 0.33. The corresponding mean increase in CD4+ cell count was 72 cells/mm³. Through 48 weeks of treatment, the proportion of patients in this treatment arm with plasma HIV-1 RNA <400 (<50) copies/mL was 38% (26%). In this study, coadministration of REYATAZ and saquinavir did not provide adequate efficacy *[see Drug Interactions (7)]*.

Study AI424-045 also compared changes from baseline in lipid values. *[See Adverse Reactions (6.1).]*

Study AI424-043: Study AI424-043 was a randomized, open-label, multicenter trial comparing REYATAZ (400 mg once daily) to lopinavir/ritonavir (400/100 mg twice daily), each in combination with two NRTIs, in 300 patients who expe-

Table 16 *(cont.)*: **Established and Other Potentially Significant Drug Interactions: Alteration in Dose or Regimen May Be Recommended Based on Drug Interaction Studies[a] or Predicted Interactions (Information in the table applies to REYATAZ with or without ritonavir, unless otherwise indicated)**

Concomitant Drug Class: Specific Drugs	Effect on Concentration of Atazanavir or Concomitant Drug	Clinical Comment
Other Agents *(cont.)*		
Inhaled beta agonist: salmeterol	↑ salmeterol	Coadministration of salmeterol with REYATAZ is not recommended. Concomitant use of salmeterol and REYATAZ may result in increased risk of cardiovascular adverse reactions associated with salmeterol, including QT prolongation, palpitations, and sinus tachycardia.
Inhaled/nasal steroid: fluticasone	***REYATAZ*** ↑ fluticasone	Concomitant use of fluticasone propionate and REYATAZ (without ritonavir) may increase plasma concentrations of fluticasone propionate. Use with caution. Consider alternatives to fluticasone propionate, particularly for long-term use.
	REYATAZ/ritonavir ↑ fluticasone	Concomitant use of fluticasone propionate and REYATAZ/ritonavir may increase plasma concentrations of fluticasone propionate, resulting in significantly reduced serum cortisol concentrations. Systemic corticosteroid effects, including Cushing's syndrome and adrenal suppression, have been reported during postmarketing use in patients receiving ritonavir and inhaled or intranasally administered fluticasone propionate. Coadministration of fluticasone propionate and REYATAZ/ritonavir is not recommended unless the potential benefit to the patient outweighs the risk of systemic corticosteroid side effects *[see Warnings and Precautions (5.1)]*.
Macrolide antibiotics: clarithromycin	↑ clarithromycin ↓ 14-OH clarithromycin ↑ atazanavir	Increased concentrations of clarithromycin may cause QTc prolongations; therefore, a dose reduction of clarithromycin by 50% should be considered when it is coadministered with REYATAZ. In addition, concentrations of the active metabolite 14-OH clarithromycin are significantly reduced; consider alternative therapy for indications other than infections due to *Mycobacterium avium* complex. Coadministration of REYATAZ/ritonavir with clarithromycin has not been studied.
Opioids: Buprenorphine	↑ buprenorphine ↑ norbuprenorphine	Coadministration of buprenorphine and REYATAZ with or without ritonavir increases the plasma concentration of buprenorphine and norbuprenorphine. Coadministration of REYATAZ plus ritonavir with buprenorphine warrants clinical monitoring for sedation and cognitive effects. A dose reduction of buprenorphine may be considered. Coadministration of buprenorphine and REYATAZ with ritonavir is not expected to decrease atazanavir plasma concentrations. Coadministration of buprenorphine and REYATAZ without ritonavir may decrease atazanavir plasma concentrations. The coadministration of REYATAZ and buprenorphine without ritonavir is not recommended.
PDE5 inhibitors: sildenafil, tadalafil, vardenafil	↑ sildenafil ↑ tadalafil ↑ vardenafil	Coadministration with REYATAZ has not been studied but may result in an increase in PDE5 inhibitor-associated adverse reactions, including hypotension, syncope, visual disturbances, and priapism. ***Use of PDE5 inhibitors for pulmonary arterial hypertension (PAH):*** Use of REVATIO® (sildenafil) for the treatment of pulmonary hypertension (PAH) is contraindicated with REYATAZ *[see Contraindications (4)]*. The following dose adjustments are recommended for the use of ADCIRCA® (tadalafil) with REYATAZ: Coadministration of ADCIRCA® in patients on REYATAZ (with or without ritonavir): • For patients receiving REYATAZ (with or without ritonavir) for at least one week, start ADCIRCA® at 20 mg once daily. Increase to 40 mg once daily based on individual tolerability. Coadministration of REYATAZ (with or without ritonavir) in patients on ADCIRCA®: • Avoid the use of ADCIRCA® when starting REYATAZ (with or without ritonavir). Stop ADCIRCA® at least 24 hours before starting REYATAZ (with or without ritonavir). At least one week after starting REYATAZ (with or without ritonavir), resume ADCIRCA® at 20 mg once daily. Increase to 40 mg once daily based on individual tolerability. ***Use of PDE5 inhibitors for erectile dysfunction:*** Use VIAGRA® (sildenafil) with caution at reduced doses of 25 mg every 48 hours with increased monitoring for adverse events. Use CIALIS® (tadalafil) with caution at reduced doses of 10 mg every 72 hours with increased monitoring for adverse events.

(Table continued on next page)

Table 16 (cont.): Established and Other Potentially Significant Drug Interactions: Alteration in Dose or Regimen May Be Recommended Based on Drug Interaction Studies[a] or Predicted Interactions (Information in the table applies to REYATAZ with or without ritonavir, unless otherwise indicated)

Concomitant Drug Class: Specific Drugs	Effect on Concentration of Atazanavir or Concomitant Drug	Clinical Comment
Other Agents (cont.)		
Proton-pump inhibitors: omeprazole	↓ atazanavir	**REYATAZ/ritonavir:** Use vardenafil with caution at reduced doses of no more than 2.5 mg every 72 hours with increased monitoring for adverse reactions. **REYATAZ:** Use vardenafil with caution at reduced doses of no more than 2.5 mg every 24 hours with increased monitoring for adverse reactions. Plasma concentrations of atazanavir were substantially decreased when REYATAZ 400 mg or REYATAZ 300 mg/ritonavir 100 mg once daily was administered with omeprazole 40 mg once daily, which may result in loss of therapeutic effect and development of resistance. *In treatment-naive patients:* The proton-pump inhibitor (PPI) dose should not exceed a dose comparable to omeprazole 20 mg and must be taken approximately 12 hours prior to the REYATAZ 300 mg with ritonavir 100 mg dose. *In treatment-experienced patients:* The use of PPIs in treatment-experienced patients receiving REYATAZ is not recommended.

[a] For magnitude of interactions see *Clinical Pharmacology*, Tables 21 and 22 (12.3).
[b] See *Contraindications (4)*, *Table 6* for orally administered midazolam.
[c] In combination with atazanavir 300 mg and ritonavir 100 mg once daily.
[d] In combination with atazanavir 400 mg once daily.

Table 17: Steady-State Pharmacokinetics of Atazanavir in Healthy Subjects or HIV-Infected Patients in the Fed State

Parameter	400 mg once daily		300 mg with ritonavir 100 mg once daily	
	Healthy Subjects (n=14)	HIV-Infected Patients (n=13)	Healthy Subjects (n=28)	HIV-Infected Patients (n=10)
C_{max} (ng/mL)				
Geometric mean (CV%)	5199 (26)	2298 (71)	6129 (31)	4422 (58)
Mean (SD)	5358 (1371)	3152 (2231)	6450 (2031)	5233 (3033)
T_{max} (h)				
Median	2.5	2.0	2.7	3.0
AUC (ng•h/mL)				
Geometric mean (CV%)	28132 (28)	14874 (91)	57039 (37)	46073 (66)
Mean (SD)	29303 (8263)	22262 (20159)	61435 (22911)	53761 (35294)
T-half (h)				
Mean (SD)	7.9 (2.9)	6.5 (2.6)	18.1 (6.2)[a]	8.6 (2.3)
C_{min} (ng/mL)				
Geometric mean (CV%)	159 (88)	120 (109)	1227 (53)	636 (97)
Mean (SD)	218 (191)	273 (298)[b]	1441 (757)	862 (838)

[a] n=26.
[b] n=12.

Table 18: Steady-State Pharmacokinetics of Atazanavir (powder formulation) with Ritonavir in HIV-Infected Pediatric Patients

Body Weight (range in kg) [n]	atazanavir/ritonavir Dose (mg)	Cmax ng/mL Geometric Mean (CV%)	AUC ng•h/mL Geometric Mean (CV%)	C_{min} ng/mL Geometric Mean (CV%)
10 to <15 [18]	200/80	5197 (53%)	50305 (67%)	572 (111%)
15 to <25 [31]	250/80	5386 (47%)	55525 (46%)	678 (69%)

Table 19: Predicted Steady-State Pharmacokinetics of Atazanavir (capsule formulation) with Ritonavir in HIV-Infected Pediatric Patients

Body Weight (range in kg)	atazanavir/ritonavir Dose (mg)	C_{max} ng/mL Geometric Mean (CV%)	AUC ng•h/mL Geometric Mean (CV%)	C_{min} ng/mL Geometric Mean (CV%)
15 to <20	150/100	5213 (78.7%)	42902 (77.0%)	504 (99.5%)
20 to <40	200/100	4954 (81.7%)	42999 (78.5%)	562 (98.9%)
≥40	300/100	5040 (84.6%)	46777 (80.6%)	691 (98.5%)

rienced virologic failure to only one prior PI-containing regimen. Through 48 weeks, the proportion of patients with plasma HIV-1 RNA <400 (<50) copies/mL was 49% (35%) for patients randomized to REYATAZ (atazanavir) (n=144) and 69% (53%) for patients randomized to lopinavir/ritonavir (n=146). The mean change from baseline was −1.59 $\log_{10}$ copies/mL in the REYATAZ without ritonavir was inferior to lopinavir/ritonavir in PI-experienced patients with prior virologic failure and is not recommended for such patients.

14.3 Pediatric Patients
Pediatric Trials with REYATAZ Capsules
Assessment of the pharmacokinetics, safety, tolerability, and virologic response of REYATAZ capsules was based on REYATAZ treatment arm and −2.02 $\log_{10}$ copies/mL in the lopinavir arm. Based on the results of this study, data from the open-label, multicenter clinical trial PACTG 1020A which included patients from 6 years to 21 years of age. In this study, 105 patients (43 antiretroviral-naive and 62 antiretroviral-experienced) received once daily REYATAZ capsule formulation, with or without ritonavir, in combination with two NRTIs.

One-hundred five (105) patients (6 to less than 18 years of age) treated with the REYATAZ capsule formulation, with or without ritonavir, were evaluated. Using an ITT analysis, the overall proportions of antiretroviral-naive and -experienced patients with HIV RNA <400 copies/mL at Week 96 were 51% (22/43) and 34% (21/62), respectively. The overall proportions of antiretroviral-naive and -experienced patients with HIV RNA <50 copies/mL at Week 96 were 47% (20/43) and 24% (15/62), respectively. The median increase from baseline in absolute CD4 count at 96 weeks of therapy was 335 cells/mm[3] in antiretroviral-naive patients and 220 cells/mm[3] in antiretroviral-experienced patients.

Pediatric Trials with REYATAZ Oral Powder
Assessment of the pharmacokinetics, safety, tolerability, and virologic response of REYATAZ oral powder was based on data from two open-label, multicenter clinical trials.
• AI424-397 (PRINCE I): In pediatric patients from 3 months to less than 6 years of age
• AI424-451 (PRINCE II): In pediatric patients from 3 months to less than 11 years of age
In these studies 134 patients (73 antiretroviral-naive and 61 antiretroviral-experienced) received once daily REYATAZ oral powder and ritonavir, in combination with two NRTIs.

For inclusion in both trials, treatment-naive patients had to have genotypic sensitivity to REYATAZ and two NRTIs, and treatment-experienced patients had to have documented genotypic and phenotypic sensitivity at screening to REYATAZ and at least 2 NRTIs. Patients exposed only to antiretrovirals *in utero* or intrapartum were considered treatment-naive. Patients who received REYATAZ or REYATAZ/ritonavir at any time prior to study enrollment or who had a history of treatment failure on two or more protease inhibitors were excluded from the trials.

Sixty-five (65) patients from both studies weighing 10 kg to less than 25 kg treated with REYATAZ oral powder with ritonavir were evaluated. Patients 10 kg to less than 15 kg received 200 mg REYATAZ and 80 mg ritonavir oral solution, and patients 15 kg to less than 25 kg received 250 mg REYATAZ and 80 mg ritonavir oral solution. Using a modified ITT analysis, the overall proportions of antiretroviral-naive and antiretroviral-experienced patients with HIV RNA <400 copies/mL at Week 48 were 78% (32/41) and 71% (17/24), respectively in patients who received REYATAZ oral powder with ritonavir. The overall proportions of antiretroviral-naive and antiretroviral-experienced patients with HIV RNA <50 copies/mL at Week 48 were 66% (27/41) and 58% (14/24), respectively in patients who received REYATAZ oral powder with ritonavir. The median increase from baseline in absolute CD4 count (percent) at 48 weeks of therapy was 412 cells/mm[3] (10.5%) in antiretroviral-naive patients and 228 cells/mm[3] (6%) in antiretroviral-experienced patients who received REYATAZ oral powder with ritonavir.

16 HOW SUPPLIED/STORAGE AND HANDLING
REYATAZ Capsules
REYATAZ® (atazanavir) capsules are available in the following strengths and configurations of plastic bottles with child-resistant closures.
[See fourth table on page 731]
Store REYATAZ capsules at 25°C (77°F); excursions permitted to 15°C-30°C (59°F-86°F) [see USP Controlled Room Temperature].

Table 21: Drug Interactions: Pharmacokinetic Parameters for Atazanavir in the Presence of Coadministered Drugs[a]

Coadministered Drug	Coadministered Drug Dose/Schedule	REYATAZ Dose/Schedule	Ratio (90% Confidence Interval) of Atazanavir Pharmacokinetic Parameters with/without Coadministered Drug; No Effect = 1.00		
			C_{max}	AUC	C_{min}
atenolol	50 mg QD, d 7-11 (n=19) and d 19-23	400 mg QD, d 1-11 (n=19)	1.00 (0.89, 1.12)	0.93 (0.85, 1.01)	0.74 (0.65, 0.86)
boceprevir	800 mg TID, d 1-6, 25-31	300 mg QD/ritonavir 100 mg QD, d 10-31	atazanavir: 0.75 (0.64-0.88) ritonavir: 0.73 (0.64-0.83)	atazanavir: 0.65 (0.55-0.78) ritonavir: 0.64 (0.58-0.72)	atazanavir: 0.51 (0.44-0.61) ritonavir: 0.55 (0.45-0.67)
clarithromycin	500 mg BID, d 7-10 (n=29) and d 18-21	400 mg QD, d 1-10 (n=29)	1.06 (0.93, 1.20)	1.28 (1.16, 1.43)	1.91 (1.66, 2.21)
didanosine (ddI) (buffered tablets) plus stavudine (d4T)[b]	ddI: 200 mg × 1 dose, d4T: 40 mg × 1 dose (n=31)	400 mg × 1 dose simultaneously with ddI and d4T (n=31)	0.11 (0.06, 0.18)	0.13 (0.08, 0.21)	0.16 (0.10, 0.27)
	ddI: 200 mg × 1 dose, d4T: 40 mg × 1 dose (n=32)	400 mg × 1 dose 1 h after ddI + d4T (n=32)	1.12 (0.67, 1.18)	1.03 (0.64, 1.67)	1.03 (0.61, 1.73)
ddI (enteric-coated [EC] capsules)[c]	400 mg d 8 (fed) (n=34) 400 mg d 19 (fed) (n=31)	400 mg QD, d 2-8 (n=34) 300 mg/ritonavir 100 mg QD, d 9-19 (n=31)	1.03 (0.93, 1.14) 1.04 (1.01, 1.07)	0.99 (0.91, 1.08) 1.00 (0.96, 1.03)	0.98 (0.89, 1.08) 0.87 (0.82, 0.92)
diltiazem	180 mg QD, d 7-11 (n=30) and d 19-23	400 mg QD, d 1-11 (n=30)	1.04 (0.96, 1.11)	1.00 (0.95, 1.05)	0.98 (0.90, 1.07)
efavirenz	600 mg QD, d 7-20 (n=27)	400 mg QD, d 1-20 (n=27)	0.41 (0.33, 0.51)	0.26 (0.22, 0.32)	0.07 (0.05, 0.10)
	600 mg QD, d 7-20 (n=13)	400 mg QD, d 1-6 (n=23) then 300 mg/ritonavir 100 mg QD, 2 h before efavirenz, d 7-20 (n=13)	1.14 (0.83, 1.58)	1.39 (1.02, 1.88)	1.48 (1.24, 1.76)
	600 mg QD, d 11-24 (pm) (n=14)	300 mg QD/ritonavir 100 mg QD, d 1-10 (pm) (n=22), then 400 mg QD/ritonavir 100 mg QD, d 11-24 (pm), (simultaneously with efavirenz) (n=14)	1.17 (1.08, 1.27)	1.00 (0.91, 1.10)	0.58 (0.49, 0.69)
famotidine	40 mg BID, d 7-12 (n=15)	400 mg QD, d 1-6 (n=45), d 7-12 (simultaneous administration) (n=15)	0.53 (0.34, 0.82)	0.59 (0.40, 0.87)	0.58 (0.37, 0.89)
	40 mg BID, d 7-12 (n=14)	400 mg QD (pm), d 1-6 (n=14), d 7-12 (10 h after, 2 h before famotidine) (n=14)	1.08 (0.82, 1.41)	0.95 (0.74, 1.21)	0.79 (0.60, 1.04)
	40 mg BID, d 11-20 (n=14)[d]	300 mg QD/ritonavir 100 mg QD, d 1-10 (n=46), d 11-20[d] (simultaneous administration) (n=14)	0.86 (0.79, 0.94)	0.82 (0.75, 0.89)	0.72 (0.64, 0.81)
	20 mg BID, d 11-17 (n=18)	300 mg QD/ritonavir 100 mg QD/tenofovir 300 mg QD, d 1-10 (am) (n=39), d 11-17 (am) (simultaneous administration with am famotidine) (n=18)[e,f]	0.91 (0.84, 0.99)	0.90 (0.82, 0.98)	0.81 (0.69, 0.94)
	40 mg QD (pm), d 18-24 (n=20)	300 mg QD/ritonavir 100 mg QD/tenofovir 300 mg QD, d 1-10 (am) (n=39), d 18-24 (am) (12 h after pm famotidine) (n=20)[f]	0.89 (0.81, 0.97)	0.88 (0.80, 0.96)	0.77 (0.63, 0.93)
	40 mg BID, d 18-24 (n=18)	300 mg QD/ritonavir 100 mg QD/tenofovir 300 mg QD, d 1-10 (am) (n=39), d 18-24 (am) (10 h after pm famotidine and 2 h before am famotidine) (n=18)[f]	0.74 (0.66, 0.84)	0.79 (0.70, 0.88)	0.72 (0.63, 0.83)
	40 mg BID, d 11-20 (n=15)	300 mg QD/ritonavir 100 mg QD, d 1-10 (am) (n=46), then 400 mg QD/ritonavir 100 mg QD, d 11-20 (am) (n=15)	1.02 (0.87, 1.18)	1.03 (0.86, 1.22)	0.86 (0.68, 1.08)

(Table continued on next page)

REYATAZ Oral Powder

REYATAZ (atazanavir) oral powder is an orange-vanilla flavored powder, packed in child-resistant packets. Each packet contains 50 mg of atazanavir equivalent to 56.9 mg of atazanavir sulfate in 1.5 g of powder. REYATAZ oral powder is supplied in cartons (NDC 0003-3638-10) of 30 packets each. *[See Dosage and Administration (2.4).]*

Store REYATAZ oral powder below 30°C (86°F). Once the REYATAZ oral powder is mixed with food or beverage, it may be kept at room temperature 20°C to 30°C (68°F-86°F) for up to 1 hour prior to administration. Store REYATAZ oral powder in the original packet and do not open until ready to use.

17 PATIENT COUNSELING INFORMATION

See FDA-approved patient labeling *(Patient Information and Instructions for Use)*.

A statement to patients and healthcare providers is included on the product's label: **ALERT: Find out about medicines that should NOT be taken with REYATAZ®.**

REYATAZ is not a cure for HIV infection and patients may continue to experience illnesses associated with HIV infection, including opportunistic infections. Patients should remain under the care of a healthcare provider when using REYATAZ.

Patients should be advised to avoid doing things that can spread HIV infection to others.

- **Do not share or reuse needles or other injection equipment.**
- **Do not share personal items that can have blood or body fluids on them, like toothbrushes and razor blades.**
- **Do not have any kind of sex without protection.** Always practice safer sex by using a latex or polyurethane condom to lower the chance of sexual contact with semen, vaginal secretions, or blood.
- **Do not breastfeed.** It is not known if REYATAZ can be passed to your baby in your breast milk and whether it could harm your baby. Also, mothers with HIV should not breastfeed because HIV can be passed to the baby in breast milk.

Dosing Instructions

Patients should be told that sustained decreases in plasma HIV RNA have been associated with a reduced risk of progression to AIDS and death. Patients should remain under the care of a healthcare provider while using REYATAZ. Patients should be advised to take REYATAZ with food every day and take other concomitant antiretroviral therapy as prescribed. REYATAZ must always be used in combination with other antiretroviral drugs. Patients should not alter the dose or discontinue therapy without consulting with their healthcare provider. If a dose of REYATAZ is missed, patients should take the dose as soon as possible and then return to their normal schedule. However, if a dose is skipped the patient should not double the next dose.

REYATAZ oral powder is available for pediatric patients who are 3 months and older weighing 10 kg to less than 25 kg. Caregivers should be advised on how to mix the REYATAZ oral powder with a food or beverage such as milk or water for infants and young children who can take solid foods or drink liquids from a cup. For infants who cannot take solid food or drink from a cup, the powder formulation mixed in liquid infant formula should be given with an oral dosing syringe. Caregivers should carefully follow the *Instructions for Use* and storage of the powder *[see Dosage and Administration (2.4) and FDA-approved patient labeling (Patient Information and Instructions for Use)]*.

Caregivers of patients with phenylketonuria should be advised that REYATAZ oral powder contains phenylalanine.

Patients or caregivers should call their healthcare provider or pharmacist if they have any questions.

Drug Interactions

REYATAZ may interact with some drugs; therefore, patients should be advised to report to their healthcare provider the use of any other prescription, nonprescription medication, or herbal products, particularly St. John's wort. Patients receiving a PDE5 inhibitor and atazanavir should be advised that they may be at an increased risk of PDE5 inhibitor-associated adverse events including hypotension, syncope, visual disturbances, and priapism, and should promptly report any symptoms to their doctor.

Patients should be informed that REVATIO® (used to treat pulmonary arterial hypertension) is contraindicated with REYATAZ and that dose adjustments are necessary when REYATAZ is used with CIALIS®, LEVITRA®, or VIAGRA® (used to treat erectile dysfunction), or ADCIRCA® (used to treat pulmonary arterial hypertension).

Table 21 (cont.): Drug Interactions: Pharmacokinetic Parameters for Atazanavir in the Presence of Coadministered Drugs[a]

Coadministered Drug	Coadministered Drug Dose/Schedule	REYATAZ Dose/Schedule	C_{max}	AUC	C_{min}
fluconazole	200 mg QD, d 11–20 (n=29)	300 mg QD/ritonavir 100 mg QD, d 1–10 (n=19), d 11–20 (n=29)	1.03 (0.95, 1.11)	1.04 (0.95, 1.13)	0.98 (0.85, 1.13)
ketoconazole	200 mg QD, d 7–13 (n=14)	400 mg QD, d 1–13 (n=14)	0.99 (0.77, 1.28)	1.10 (0.89, 1.37)	1.03 (0.53, 2.01)
nevirapine[g,h]	200 mg BID, d 1–23 (n=23)	300 mg QD/ritonavir 100 mg QD, d 4–13, then 400 mg QD/ritonavir 100 mg QD, d 14–23 (n=23)[i]	0.72 (0.60, 0.86) / 1.02 (0.85, 1.24)	0.58 (0.48, 0.71) / 0.81 (0.65, 1.02)	0.28 (0.20, 0.40) / 0.41 (0.27, 0.60)
omeprazole	40 mg QD, d 7–12 (n=16)[j]	400 mg QD, d 1–6 (n=48), d 7–12 (n=16)	0.04 (0.04, 0.05)	0.06 (0.05, 0.07)	0.05 (0.03, 0.07)
	40 mg QD, d 11–20 (n=15)[j]	300 mg QD/ritonavir 100 mg QD, d 1–20 (n=15)	0.28 (0.24, 0.32)	0.24 (0.21, 0.27)	0.22 (0.19, 0.26)
	20 mg QD, d 17–23 (am) (n=13)	300 mg QD/ritonavir 100 mg QD, d 7–16 (pm) (n=27), d 17–23 (pm) (n=13)[k,l]	0.61 (0.46, 0.81)	0.58 (0.44, 0.75)	0.54 (0.41, 0.71)
	20 mg QD, d 17–23 (am) (n=14)	300 mg QD/ritonavir 100 mg QD, d 7–16 (am) (n=27), then 400 mg QD/ritonavir 100 mg QD, d 17–23 (am) (n=14)[m,n]	0.69 (0.58, 0.83)	0.70 (0.57, 0.86)	0.69 (0.54, 0.88)
pitavastatin	4 mg QD for 5 days	300 mg QD for 5 days	1.13 (0.96, 1.32)	1.06 (0.90, 1.26)	NA
rifabutin	150 mg QD, d 15–28 (n=7)	400 mg QD, d 1–28 (n=7)	1.34 (1.14, 1.59)	1.15 (0.98, 1.34)	1.13 (0.68, 1.87)
rifampin	600 mg QD, d 17–26 (n=16)	300 mg QD/ritonavir 100 mg QD, d 7–16 (n=48), d 17–26 (n=16)	0.47 (0.41, 0.53)	0.28 (0.25, 0.32)	0.02 (0.02, 0.03)
ritonavir[o]	100 mg QD, d 11–20 (n=28)	300 mg QD, d 1–20 (n=28)	1.86 (1.69, 2.05)	3.38 (3.13, 3.63)	11.89 (10.23, 13.82)
telaprevir	750 mg q8h for 10 days	300 mg QD/ritonavir 100 mg QD for 20 days (n=7)	0.85 (0.73, 0.98)	1.17 (0.97, 1.43)	1.85 (1.40, 2.44)
tenofovir[p]	300 mg QD, d 9–16 (n=34)	400 mg QD, d 2–16 (n=34)	0.79 (0.73, 0.86)	0.75 (0.70, 0.81)	0.60 (0.52, 0.68)
	300 mg QD, d 15–42 (n=10)	300 mg/ritonavir 100 mg QD, d 1–42 (n=10)	0.72[q] (0.50, 1.05)	0.75[q] (0.58, 0.97)	0.77[q] (0.54, 1.10)

(Table continued on next page)

Cardiac Conduction Abnormalities
Patients should be informed that atazanavir may produce changes in the electrocardiogram (eg, PR prolongation). Patients should consult their healthcare provider if they are experiencing symptoms such as dizziness or lightheadedness.

Rash
Patients should be informed that mild rashes without other symptoms have been reported with REYATAZ (atazanavir) use. These rashes go away within two weeks with no change in treatment. However, there have been reports of severe skin reactions (eg, Stevens-Johnson syndrome, erythema multiforme, and toxic skin eruptions) with REYATAZ use. Patients developing signs or symptoms of severe skin reactions or hypersensitivity reactions (including, but not limited to, severe rash or rash accompanied by one or more of the following: fever, general malaise, muscle or joint aches, blisters, oral lesions, conjunctivitis, facial edema, hepatitis, eosinophilia, granulocytopenia, lymphadenopathy, and renal dysfunction) must discontinue REYATAZ and seek medical evaluation immediately.

Hyperbilirubinemia
Patients should be informed that asymptomatic elevations in indirect bilirubin have occurred in patients receiving REYATAZ. This may be accompanied by yellowing of the skin or whites of the eyes and alternative antiretroviral therapy may be considered if the patient has cosmetic concerns.

Nephrolithiasis and Cholelithiasis
Patients should be informed that kidney stones and/or gallstones have been reported with REYATAZ use. Some patients with kidney stones and/or gallstones required hospitalization for additional management and some had complications. Discontinuation of REYATAZ may be necessary as part of the medical management of these adverse events.

Fat Redistribution
Patients should be informed that redistribution or accumulation of body fat may occur in patients receiving antiretroviral therapy including protease inhibitors and that the cause and long-term health effects of these conditions are not known at this time.

PATIENT INFORMATION
REYATAZ® (RAY-ah-taz)
(atazanavir)
capsules
REYATAZ® (RAY-ah-taz)
(atazanavir)
oral powder
Important: Ask your healthcare provider or pharmacist about medicines that should not be taken with REYATAZ. For more information, see "Who should not take REYATAZ?" and "What should I tell my healthcare provider before taking REYATAZ?"
Read this Patient Information before you start taking REYATAZ and each time you get a refill. There may be new information. This information does not take the place of talking with your healthcare provider about your medical condition or treatment.

What is REYATAZ?
REYATAZ (atazanavir) is a prescription HIV-1 (Human Immunodeficiency Virus) medicine that is used with other antiretroviral medicines to treat HIV-1 infection in adults and children 3 months of age and older and who weigh at least 22 pounds (10 kg).
HIV is the virus that causes AIDS (Acquired Immunodeficiency Syndrome).
REYATAZ should not be used in children younger than 3 months of age.
When used with other antiretroviral medicines to treat HIV infection, REYATAZ may help:
• reduce the amount of HIV in your blood. This is called viral load.
• increase the number of CD4+ (T) cells in your blood that help fight off other infections.
Reducing the amount of HIV and increasing the CD4+ (T) cells in your blood may help improve your immune system. This may reduce your risk of death or getting infections that can happen when your immune system is weak (opportunistic infections).
REYATAZ does not cure HIV infection or AIDS. You must stay on continuous HIV therapy to control HIV infection and decrease HIV-related illnesses.
Avoid doing things that can spread HIV infection to others:
• Do not share or reuse needles or other injection equipment.
• Do not share personal items that can have blood or body fluids on them, like toothbrushes and razor blades.
• Do not have any kind of sex without protection. Always practice safer sex by using a latex or polyurethane condom to lower the chance of sexual contact with any body fluids such as semen, vaginal secretions, or blood.
Ask your healthcare provider if you have any questions about how to prevent passing HIV to other people.
Who should not take REYATAZ?
Do not take REYATAZ if you:
• are allergic to atazanavir or any of the ingredients in REYATAZ. See the end of this leaflet for a complete list of ingredients in REYATAZ.
• are taking any of the following medicines. Taking REYATAZ with these medicines may affect how REYATAZ works. REYATAZ may cause serious life-threatening side effects or death when used with these medicines:
• alfuzosin (UROXATRAL®)
• cisapride (PROPULSID®)
• ergot medicines including:
  • ergotamine tartrate (CAFERGOT®, MIGERGOT®, ERGOMAR®, ERGOSTAT®, MEDIHALER®, Ergotamine, WIGRAINE®, WIGRETTES®)
  • dihydroergotamine mesylate (D.H.E. 45®, MIGRANAL®)
  • methylergonovine (METHERGINE®)
• indinavir (CRIXIVAN®)
• irinotecan (CAMPTOSAR®)
• lovastatin (ADVICOR®, ALTOPREV®, MEVACOR®)
• midazolam (VERSED®), when taken by mouth for sedation
• nevirapine (VIRAMUNE®, VIRAMUNE XR®)
• pimozide (ORAP®)
• rifampin (RIMACTANE®, RIFADIN®, RIFATER®, RIFAMATE®)
• sildenafil (REVATIO®), when used for the treatment of pulmonary arterial hypertension
• simvastatin (ZOCOR®, VYTORIN, SIMCOR)
• St. John's wort (Hypericum perforatum)
• triazolam (HALCION®)
Serious problems can happen if you or your child take any of the medicines listed above with REYATAZ.
What should I tell my healthcare provider before taking REYATAZ?
Before taking REYATAZ, tell your healthcare provider if you:
• have heart problems
• have liver problems, including hepatitis B or C virus infection
• have phenylketonuria (PKU). REYATAZ oral powder contains phenylalanine as part of the artificial sweetener aspartame. The artificial sweetener can be harmful to people with PKU.
• are receiving dialysis treatment
• have diabetes
• have hemophilia
• have any other medical conditions
• are pregnant or plan to become pregnant. It is not known if REYATAZ will harm your unborn baby. Pregnant women have developed a serious condition called lactic acidosis (a build-up of lactic acid in the blood) when taking REYATAZ with other HIV medicines called nucleoside analogues.

- Hormonal forms of birth control, such as injections, vaginal rings or implants, contraceptive patch, and some birth control pills may not work during treatment with REYATAZ (atazanavir). Talk to your healthcare provider about forms of birth control that may be used during treatment with REYATAZ.
- **Pregnancy Registry.** There is a pregnancy registry for women who take antiviral medicines during pregnancy. The purpose of this registry is to collect information about the health of you and your baby. Talk to your healthcare provider about how you can take part in this registry.
- **After your baby is born,** tell your healthcare provider if your baby's skin or the white part of his/her eyes turns yellow.
- are breastfeeding or plan to breastfeed. Do not breastfeed if you are taking REYATAZ. You should not breastfeed if you have HIV because of the risk of passing HIV to your baby. It is not known if REYATAZ passes into your breast milk. Talk to your healthcare provider about the best way to feed your baby.

Tell your healthcare provider about all the medicines you take, including prescription and over-the-counter medicines, vitamins, and herbal supplements.

REYATAZ may affect the way other medicines work, and other medicines may affect how REYATAZ works and may cause serious side effects. If you take certain medicines with REYATAZ, the amount of REYATAZ in your body may be too low and it may not work to help control your HIV infection. The HIV virus in your body may become resistant to REYATAZ or other HIV medicines that are like it. Especially tell your healthcare provider if you take any of the medicines below:

The following medicines should not be taken during your treatment with REYATAZ:
- boceprevir (VICTRELIS®)
- salmeterol (SEREVENT DISKUS®) and salmeterol with fluticasone (ADVAIR DISKUS®, ADVAIR HFA®)
- voriconazole (VFEND®)

If you take any of the following medicines during treatment with REYATAZ, your healthcare provider may need to change the dose of the medicine or change the dose of REYATAZ, or your healthcare provider may need to monitor you more closely:
- medicines used to treat abnormal heart rhythm:
  - amiodarone (CORDARONE®, NEXTERONE®, PACERONE®)
  - lidocaine
  - quinidine
- allergy or asthma medicines (nasal spray or inhaled treatment):
  - fluticasone propionate (FLONASE®, FLOVENT DISKUS®, FLOVENT HFA®)
- an antibiotic used to treat tuberculosis (TB):
  - rifabutin (MYCOBUTIN®)
- the anticoagulant (blood thinner) medicine:
  - warfarin (COUMADIN®, JANTOVEN®)
- antidepressant medicines:
  - amitriptyline
  - desipramine (NORPRAMIN®)
  - doxepin (SILENOR®)
  - trazodone (OLEPTRO®)
  - trimipramine (SURMONTIL®)
  - imipramine (TOFRANIL®, TOFRANIL-PM®)
  - protriptyline (VIVACTIL®)
- the chest pain medicine:
  - bepridil (VASCOR®)
- cholesterol-lowering medicines:
  - atorvastatin (LIPITOR®)
  - rosuvastatin (CRESTOR®)
- erectile dysfunction medicines:
  - sildenafil (VIAGRA®)
  - tadalafil (CIALIS®)
  - vardenafil (LEVITRA®, STAXYN®)
- a medicine for gout or treatment of familial Mediterranean fever:
  - colchicine (COLCRYS®)
- organ transplant rejection medicines:
  - cyclosporine (SANDIMMUNE®, NEORAL®, GENGRAF®)
  - sirolimus (RAPAMUNE®)
  - tacrolimus (PROGRAF®, ASTAGRAF XL®)
- pain and addiction medicines:
  - buprenorphine or buprenorphine/naloxone (BUPRENEX®, BUTRANS®, ZUBSOLV®, SUBOXONE®)
- pulmonary arterial hypertension medicines:
  - bosentan (TRACLEER®)
  - tadalafil (ADCIRCA®)
- medicine to treat fungal infections
  - ketoconazole (NIZORAL®)
  - itraconazole (SPORANOX®, ONMEL®)

Table 21 (cont.): Drug Interactions: Pharmacokinetic Parameters for Atazanavir in the Presence of Coadministered Drugs[a]

Coadministered Drug	Coadministered Drug Dose/Schedule	REYATAZ Dose/Schedule	Ratio (90% Confidence Interval) of Atazanavir Pharmacokinetic Parameters with/without Coadministered Drug; No Effect = 1.00		
			C_{max}	AUC	C_{min}
voriconazole (Subjects with at least one functional CYP2C19 allele)	200 mg BID, d 2–3, 22–30; 400 mg BID, d 1, 21 (n=20)	300 mg/ritonavir 100 mg QD, d 11–30 (n=20)	0.87 (0.80, 0.96)	0.88 (0.82, 0.95)	0.80 (0.72, 0.90)
voriconazole (Subjects without a functional CYP2C19 allele)	50 mg BID, d 2–3, 22–30; 100 mg BID, d 1, 21 (n=8)	300 mg/ritonavir 100 mg QD, d 11–30 (n=8)	0.81 (0.66, 1.00)	0.80 (0.65, 0.97)	0.69 (0.54, 0.87)

[a] Data provided are under fed conditions unless otherwise noted.
[b] All drugs were given under fasted conditions.
[c] 400 mg ddI EC and REYATAZ were administered together with food on Days 8 and 19.
[d] REYATAZ 300 mg plus ritonavir 100 mg once daily coadministered with famotidine 40 mg twice daily resulted in atazanavir geometric mean C_{max} that was similar and AUC and C_{min} values that were 1.79- and 4.46-fold higher relative to REYATAZ 400 mg once daily alone.
[e] Similar results were noted when famotidine 20 mg BID was administered 2 hours after and 10 hours before atazanavir 300 mg and ritonavir 100 mg plus tenofovir 300 mg.
[f] Atazanavir/ritonavir/tenofovir was administered after a light meal.
[g] Study was conducted in HIV-infected individuals.
[h] Compared with atazanavir 400 mg historical data without nevirapine (n=13), the ratio of geometric means (90% confidence intervals) for C_{max}, AUC, and C_{min} were 1.42 (0.98, 2.05), 1.64 (1.11, 2.42), and 1.25 (0.66, 2.36), respectively, for atazanavir/ritonavir 300/100 mg; and 2.02 (1.42, 2.87), 2.28 (1.54, 3.38), and 1.80 (0.94, 3.45), respectively, for atazanavir/ritonavir 400/100 mg.
[i] Parallel group design; n=23 for atazanavir/ritonavir plus nevirapine, n=22 for atazanavir 300 mg/ritonavir 100 mg without nevirapine. Subjects were treated with nevirapine prior to study entry.
[j] Omeprazole 40 mg was administered on an empty stomach 2 hours before REYATAZ.
[k] Omeprazole 20 mg was administered 30 minutes prior to a light meal in the morning and REYATAZ 300 mg plus ritonavir 100 mg in the evening after a light meal, separated by 12 hours from omeprazole.
[l] REYATAZ 300 mg plus ritonavir 100 mg once daily separated by 12 hours from omeprazole 20 mg daily resulted in increases in atazanavir geometric mean AUC (10%) and C_{min} (2.4-fold), with a decrease in C_{max} (29%) relative to REYATAZ 400 mg once daily in the absence of omeprazole (study days 1–6).
[m] Omeprazole 20 mg was given 30 minutes prior to a light meal in the morning and REYATAZ 400 mg plus ritonavir 100 mg once daily after a light meal, 1 hour after omeprazole. Effects on atazanavir concentrations were similar when REYATAZ 400 mg plus ritonavir 100 mg was separated from omeprazole 20 mg by 12 hours.
[n] REYATAZ 400 mg plus ritonavir 100 mg once daily administered with omeprazole 20 mg once daily resulted in increases in atazanavir geometric mean AUC (32%) and C_{min} (3.3-fold), with a decrease in C_{max} (26%) relative to REYATAZ 400 mg once daily in the absence of omeprazole (study days 1–6).
[o] Compared with atazanavir 400 mg QD historical data, administration of atazanavir/ritonavir 300/100 mg QD increased the atazanavir geometric mean values of C_{max}, AUC, and C_{min} by 18%, 103%, and 671%, respectively.
[p] Note that similar results were observed in studies where administration of tenofovir and REYATAZ was separated by 12 hours.
[q] Ratio of atazanavir plus ritonavir plus tenofovir to atazanavir plus ritonavir. Atazanavir 300 mg plus ritonavir 100 mg results in higher atazanavir exposure than atazanavir 400 mg (see footnote o). The geometric mean values of atazanavir pharmacokinetic parameters when coadministered with ritonavir and tenofovir were: C_{max} = 3190 ng/mL, AUC = 34459 ng•h/mL, and C_{min} = 491 ng/mL. Study was conducted in HIV-infected individuals.
NA = not available.

People who take sildenafil (VIAGRA®), tadalafil (CIALIS®, ADCIRCA®) or vardenafil (LEVITRA®, STAXYN®) with REYATAZ (atazanavir) may have a higher risk of certain side effects. Tell your healthcare provider right away if you take any of these medicines and have any of the following side effects:
- lightheadedness, especially when standing
- fainting
- changes in your vision
- an erection that lasts more than 4 hours

If you take any of the following medicines, your healthcare provider may change the dose or the time you take REYATAZ or the other medicine:
- antiepileptic medicines:
  - carbamazepine (CARBATROL®, EPITOL®, TEGRETOL®, TEGRETOL-XR®, EQUETRO®, TERIL®)
  - phenytoin (DILANTIN®)
  - lamotrigine (LAMICTAL®, LAMICTAL CD®, LAMICTAL XR®, LAMICTAL ODT®)
- calcium channel blockers such as:
  - diltiazem (CARDIZEM®, CARDIZEM CD®, CARDIZEM LA®, TIAZAC®, CARTIA XT®, DILACOR XR®, DILT-CD®, DILTZAC®, TAZTIA XT®)
  - verapamil (COVERA-HS®, CALAN®, CALAN SR®, VERALAN®, VERELAN PM®)
  - felodipine (PLENDIL®)
  - nifedipine (ADALAT CC®, AFEDITAB CR®, PROCARDIA®, PROCARDIA XL®)
  - nicardipine (CARDENE®, CARDENE SR®)

- indigestion, heartburn, or ulcer medicines:
  - cimetidine (TAGAMET®)
  - esomeprazole (NEXIUM®)
  - famotidine (PEPCID®, PEPCID AC®)
  - rabeprazole (ACIPHEX®, ACIPHEX SPRINKLE™)
  - nizatidine (AXID®)
  - lansoprazole (PREVACID®)
  - omeprazole (PRILOSEC®)
  - pantoprazole (PROTONIX®)
  - ranitidine (ZANTAC®)
- antacids or buffered medicines
- antibiotics or antiviral medicines
  - clarithromycin (BIAXIN®, BIAXIN XL®)
  - didanosine (VIDEX®, VIDEX EC®)
  - efavirenz (SUSTIVA®)
  - rifabutin (MYCOBUTIN®)
  - ritonavir (NORVIR®)
  - saquinavir (INVIRASE®)
  - tenofovir disoproxil fumarate (VIREAD®)

Ask your healthcare provider or pharmacist if you are not sure if your medicine is one that is listed above.

Know the medicines you take. Keep a list of your medicines and show it to your healthcare provider and pharmacist when you get a new medicine.

Your healthcare provider and your pharmacist can tell you if you can take these medicines with REYATAZ (atazanavir). Do not start any new medicines while you are taking REYATAZ without first talking with your healthcare provider or pharmacist. You can ask your healthcare provider or pharmacist for a list of medicines that can interact with REYATAZ.

Table 22: Drug Interactions: Pharmacokinetic Parameters for Coadministered Drugs in the Presence of REYATAZ[a]

Coadministered Drug	Coadministered Drug Dose/Schedule	REYATAZ Dose/Schedule	Ratio (90% Confidence Interval) of Coadministered Drug Pharmacokinetic Parameters with/without REYATAZ; No Effect = 1.00		
			C_{max}	AUC	C_{min}
acetaminophen	1 gm BID, d 1–20 (n=10)	300 mg QD/ritonavir 100 mg QD, d 11–20 (n=10)	0.87 (0.77, 0.99)	0.97 (0.91, 1.03)	1.26 (1.08, 1.46)
atenolol	50 mg QD, d 7–11 and d 19–23 (n=19)	400 mg QD, d 1–11 (n=19)	1.34 (1.26, 1.42)	1.25 (1.16, 1.34)	1.02 (0.88, 1.19)
boceprevir	800 mg TID, d 1–6, 25–31	300 mg QD/ritonavir 100 mg QD, d 10–31	0.93 (0.80, 1.08)	0.95 (0.87, 1.05)	0.82 (0.68, 0.98)
clarithromycin	500 mg BID, d 7–10 (n=21) and d 18–21	400 mg QD, d 1–10 (n=21)	1.50 (1.32, 1.71) OH-clarithromycin: 0.28 (0.24, 0.33)	1.94 (1.75, 2.16) OH-clarithromycin: 0.30 (0.26, 0.34)	2.60 (2.35, 2.88) OH-clarithromycin: 0.38 (0.34, 0.42)
didanosine (ddI) (buffered tablets) plus stavudine (d4T)[b]	ddI: 200 mg × 1 dose, d4T: 40 mg × 1 dose (n=31)	400 mg × 1 dose simultaneous with ddI and d4T (n=31)	ddI: 0.92 (0.84, 1.02) d4T: 1.08 (0.96, 1.22)	ddI: 0.98 (0.92, 1.05) d4T: 1.00 (0.97, 1.03)	NA d4T: 1.04 (0.94, 1.16)
ddI (enteric-coated [EC] capsules)[c]	400 mg d 1 (fasted), d 8 (fed) (n=34)	400 mg QD, d 2–8 (n=34)	0.64 (0.55, 0.74)	0.66 (0.60, 0.74)	1.13 (0.91, 1.41)
	400 mg d 1 (fasted), d 19 (fed) (n=31)	300 mg QD/ritonavir 100 mg QD, d 9–19 (n=31)	0.62 (0.52, 0.74)	0.66 (0.59, 0.73)	1.25 (0.92, 1.69)
diltiazem	180 mg QD, d 7–11 (n=28) and d 19–23	400 mg QD, d 1–11 (n=28)	1.98 (1.78, 2.19) desacetyl-diltiazem: 2.72 (2.44, 3.03)	2.25 (2.09, 2.16) desacetyl-diltiazem: 2.65 (2.45, 2.87)	2.42 (2.14, 2.73) desacetyl-diltiazem: 2.21 (2.02, 2.42)
ethinyl estradiol & norethindrone[d]	Ortho-Novum® 7/7/7 QD, d 1–29 (n=19)	400 mg QD, d 16–29 (n=19)	ethinyl estradiol: 1.15 (0.99, 1.32) norethindrone: 1.67 (1.42, 1.96)	ethinyl estradiol: 1.48 (1.31, 1.68) norethindrone: 2.10 (1.68, 2.62)	ethinyl estradiol: 1.91 (1.57, 2.33) norethindrone: 3.62 (2.57, 5.09)
ethinyl estradiol & norgestimate[e]	Ortho Tri-Cyclen® QD, d 1–28 (n=18), then Ortho Tri-Cyclen® LO QD, d 29–42[f] (n=14)	300 mg QD/ritonavir 100 mg QD, d 29–42 (n=14)	ethinyl estradiol: 0.84 (0.74, 0.95) 17-deacetyl norgestimate:[g] 1.68 (1.51, 1.88)	ethinyl estradiol: 0.81 (0.75, 0.87) 17-deacetyl norgestimate:[g] 1.85 (1.67, 2.05)	ethinyl estradiol: 0.63 (0.55, 0.71) 17-deacetyl norgestimate:[g] 2.02 (1.77, 2.31)
fluconazole	200 mg QD, d 1–10 (n=11) and 200 mg QD, d 11–20 (n=29)	300 mg QD/ritonavir 100 mg QD, d 11–20 (n=29)	1.05 (0.99, 1.10)	1.08 (1.02, 1.15)	1.07 (1.00, 1.15)
methadone	Stable maintenance dose, d 1–15 (n=16)	400 mg QD, d 2–15 (n=16)	(R)-methadone[h] 0.91 (0.84, 1.0) total: 0.85 (0.78, 0.93)	(R)-methadone[h] 1.03 (0.95, 1.10) total: 0.94 (0.87, 1.02)	(R)-methadone[h] 1.11 (1.02, 1.20) total: 1.02 (0.93, 1.12)
nevirapine[i,j]	200 mg BID, d 1–23 (n=23)	300 mg QD/ritonavir 100 mg QD, d 4–13, then 400 mg QD/ritonavir 100 mg QD, d 14–23 (n=23)	1.17 (1.09, 1.25) 1.21 (1.11, 1.32)	1.25 (1.17, 1.34) 1.26 (1.17, 1.36)	1.32 (1.22, 1.43) 1.35 (1.25, 1.47)
omeprazole[k]	40 mg single dose, d 7 and d 20 (n=16)	400 mg QD, d 1–12 (n=16)	1.24 (1.04, 1.47)	1.45 (1.20, 1.76)	NA
rifabutin	300 mg QD, d 1–10 then 150 mg QD, d 11–20 (n=3)	600 mg QD,[l] d 11–20 (n=3)	1.18 (0.94, 1.48) 25-O-desacetyl-rifabutin: 8.20 (5.90, 11.40)	2.10 (1.57, 2.79) 25-O-desacetyl-rifabutin: 22.01 (15.97, 30.34)	3.43 (1.98, 5.96) 25-O-desacetyl-rifabutin: 75.6 (30.1, 190.0)
	150 mg twice weekly, d 1–15 (n=7)	300 mg QD/ritonavir 100 mg QD, d 1–17 (n=7)	2.49[m] (2.03, 3.06) 25-O-desacetyl-rifabutin: 7.77 (6.13, 9.83)	1.48[m] (1.19, 1.84) 25-O-desacetyl-rifabutin: 10.90 (8.14, 14.61)	1.40[m] (1.05, 1.87) 25-O-desacetyl-rifabutin: 11.45 (8.15, 16.10)

(Table continued on next page)

How should I take REYATAZ (atazanavir)?
- **Take REYATAZ exactly as your healthcare provider tells you to.**
- **Do not change your dose or stop taking REYATAZ unless your healthcare provider tells you to.**
- Stay under the care of your healthcare provider during treatment with REYATAZ.

- REYATAZ (atazanavir) must be used with other antiretroviral medicines.
- Take REYATAZ 1 time each day.
- REYATAZ comes as capsules and oral powder.
- **Take REYATAZ capsules and oral powder with food.**
- Swallow the capsules whole. **Do not open the capsules.**

- REYATAZ (atazanavir) oral powder must be mixed with food or liquid. Your child's healthcare provider will prescribe the right dose of REYATAZ based on your child's weight.
- REYATAZ oral powder must be taken with ritonavir.
- If you miss a dose of REYATAZ, take it as soon as you remember. Then take the next dose at your regular time. Do not take 2 doses at the same time.
- **If you take too much REYATAZ,** call your healthcare provider or go to the nearest hospital emergency room right away.

When your supply of REYATAZ starts to run low, get more from your healthcare provider or pharmacy. It is important not to run out of REYATAZ. The amount of HIV-1 in your blood may increase if the medicine is stopped for even a short time. The virus may become resistant to REYATAZ and harder to treat.

What are the possible side effects of REYATAZ?
REYATAZ can cause serious side effects, including:
- **A change in the way your heart beats (heart rhythm change).** Tell your healthcare provider right away if you get dizzy or lightheaded. These could be symptoms of a heart problem.
- **Skin rash.** Skin rash is common with REYATAZ but can sometimes be severe. Skin rash usually goes away within 2 weeks without any change in treatment. Severe rash may develop in association with other symptoms which could be serious. **If you develop a severe rash or a rash with any of the following symptoms, stop taking REYATAZ and call your healthcare provider right away:**
  - general feeling of discomfort or "flu-like" symptoms
  - fever
  - muscle or joint aches
  - red or inflamed eyes, like "pink eye" (conjunctivitis)
  - blisters
  - mouth sores
  - swelling of your face
  - painful, warm, or red lump under your skin
- **Yellowing of your skin or the white part of your eyes** is common with REYATAZ but may be a symptom of a serious problem. These effects may be due to increases in bilirubin levels in your blood (bilirubin is made by the liver). Although these effects may not be damaging to your liver, skin, or eyes, tell your healthcare provider right away if your skin or the white part of your eyes turns yellow.
- **Liver problems.** If you have liver problems, including hepatitis B or C infection, your liver problems may get worse when you take REYATAZ. Your healthcare provider will do blood tests to check your liver before you start REYATAZ and during treatment. Tell your healthcare provider right away if you get any of the following symptoms:
  - your skin or the white part of your eyes turns yellow
  - dark "tea-colored" urine
  - light colored stools
  - nausea
  - itching
  - stomach-area pain
- **Kidney stones** have happened in some people who take REYATAZ. Tell your healthcare provider right away if you get symptoms of kidney stones which may include, pain in your low back or low stomach-area, blood in your urine, or pain when you urinate.
- **Gallbladder problems** have happened in some people who take REYATAZ. Tell your healthcare provider right away if you get symptoms of gallbladder problems which may include:
  - pain in the right or middle upper stomach area
  - fever
  - nausea and vomiting
  - your skin or the white part of your eyes turns yellow
- **Diabetes and high blood sugar (hyperglycemia)** have happened or have worsened in some people who take protease inhibitor medicines like REYATAZ. Some people have had to start taking medicine to treat diabetes or have had to change their diabetes medicine.
- **Changes in your immune system (Immune Reconstitution Syndrome)** can happen when you start taking HIV medicines. Your immune system may get stronger and begin to fight infections that have been hidden in your body for a long time. Tell your healthcare provider if you start having new symptoms after starting your HIV medicine.
- **Changes in body fat** can happen in people taking HIV medicine. These changes may include increased amount of fat in the upper back and neck ("buffalo hump"), breast, and around the main part of your body (trunk). Loss of fat from the legs, arms, and face may also happen. The cause and long-term health effects of these conditions are not known.
- **Increased bleeding problems in people with hemophilia** have happened when taking protease inhibitors like REYATAZ.

The most common side effects of REYATAZ include:
- nausea
- headache
- stomach-area pain
- vomiting
- trouble sleeping
- numbness, tingling, or burning of hands or feet
- dizziness
- muscle pain
- diarrhea
- depression
- fever

Table 22 *(cont.)*: Drug Interactions: Pharmacokinetic Parameters for Coadministered Drugs in the Presence of REYATAZ[a]

Coadministered Drug	Coadministered Drug Dose/Schedule	REYATAZ Dose/Schedule	Ratio (90% Confidence Interval) of Coadministered Drug Pharmacokinetic Parameters with/without REYATAZ; No Effect = 1.00		
			C_{max}	AUC	C_{min}
pitavastatin	4 mg QD for 5 days	300 mg QD for 5 days	1.60 (1.39, 1.85)	1.31 (1.23, 1.39)	NA
rosiglitazone[n]	4 mg single dose, d 1, 7, 17 (n=14)	400 mg QD, d 2–7, then 300 mg QD/ ritonavir 100 mg QD, d 8–17 (n=14)	1.08 (1.03, 1.13) 0.97 (0.91, 1.04)	1.35 (1.26, 1.44) 0.83 (0.77, 0.89)	NA NA
rosuvastatin	10 mg single dose	300 mg QD/ ritonavir 100 mg QD for 7 days	↑ 7-fold[o]	↑ 3-fold[o]	NA
saquinavir[p] (soft gelatin capsules)	1200 mg QD, d 1–13 (n=7)	400 mg QD, d 7–13 (n=7)	4.39 (3.24, 5.95)	5.49 (4.04, 7.47)	6.86 (5.29, 8.91)
telaprevir	750 mg q8h for 10 days (n=14)	300 mg QD/ ritonavir 100 mg QD for 20 days (n=14)	0.79 (0.74, 0.84)	0.80 (0.76, 0.85)	0.85 (0.75, 0.98)
tenofovir[q]	300 mg QD, d 9–16 (n=33) and d 24–30 (n=33)	400 mg QD, d 2–16 (n=33)	1.14 (1.08, 1.20)	1.24 (1.21, 1.28)	1.22 (1.15, 1.30)
	300 mg QD, d 1–7 (pm) (n=14) d 25–34 (pm) (n=12)	300 mg QD/ritonavir 100 mg QD, d 25–34 (am) (n=12)[r]	1.34 (1.20, 1.51)	1.37 (1.30, 1.45)	1.29 (1.21, 1.36)
voriconazole (Subjects with at least one functional CYP2C19 allele)	200 mg BID, d 2–3, 22–30; 400 mg BID, d 1, 21 (n=20)	300 mg/ritonavir 100 mg QD, d 11–30 (n=20)	0.90 (0.78, 1.04)	0.67 (0.58, 0.78)	0.61 (0.51, 0.72)
voriconazole (Subjects without a functional CYP2C19 allele)	50 mg BID, d 2–3, 22–30; 100 mg BID, d 1, 21 (n=8)	300 mg/ritonavir 100 mg QD, d 11–30 (n=8)	4.38 (3.55, 5.39)	5.61 (4.51, 6.99)	7.65 (5.71, 10.2)
lamivudine + zidovudine	150 mg lamivudine + 300 mg zidovudine BID, d 1–12 (n=19)	400 mg QD, d 7–12 (n=19)	lamivudine: 1.04 (0.92, 1.16) zidovudine: 1.05 (0.88, 1.24) zidovudine glucuronide: 0.95 (0.88, 1.02)	lamivudine: 1.03 (0.98, 1.08) zidovudine: 1.05 (0.96, 1.14) zidovudine glucuronide: 1.00 (0.97, 1.03)	lamivudine: 1.12 (1.04, 1.21) zidovudine: 0.69 (0.57, 0.84) zidovudine glucuronide: 0.82 (0.62, 1.08)

[a] Data provided are under fed conditions unless otherwise noted.
[b] All drugs were given under fasted conditions.
[c] 400 mg ddI EC and REYATAZ were administered together with food on Days 8 and 19.
[d] Upon further dose normalization of ethinyl estradiol 25 mcg with atazanavir relative to ethinyl estradiol 35 mcg without atazanavir, the ratio of geometric means (90% confidence intervals) for C_{max}, AUC, and C_{min} were 0.82 (0.73, 0.92), 1.06 (0.95, 1.17), and 1.35 (1.11, 1.63), respectively.
[e] Upon further dose normalization of ethinyl estradiol 35 mcg with atazanavir/ritonavir relative to ethinyl estradiol 25 mcg without atazanavir/ritonavir, the ratio of geometric means (90% confidence intervals) for C_{max}, AUC, and C_{min} were 1.17 (1.03, 1.34), 1.13 (1.05, 1.22), and 0.88 (0.77, 1.00), respectively.
[f] All subjects were on a 28 day lead-in period; one full cycle of Ortho Tri-Cyclen®. Ortho Tri-Cyclen® contains 35 mcg of ethinyl estradiol. Ortho Tri-Cyclen® LO contains 25 mcg of ethinyl estradiol. Results were dose normalized to an ethinyl estradiol dose of 35 mcg.
[g] 17-deacetyl norgestimate is the active component of norgestimate.
[h] (R)-methadone is the active isomer of methadone.
[i] Study was conducted in HIV-infected individuals.
[j] Subjects were treated with nevirapine prior to study entry.
[k] Omeprazole was used as a metabolic probe for CYP2C19. Omeprazole was given 2 hours after REYATAZ on Day 7; and was given alone 2 hours after a light meal on Day 20.
[l] Not the recommended therapeutic dose of atazanavir.
[m] When compared to rifabutin 150 mg QD alone d1–10 (n=14). Total of Rifabutin + 25-O-desacetyl-rifabutin: AUC 2.19 (1.78, 2.69).
[n] Rosiglitazone used as a probe substrate for CYP2C8.
[o] Mean ratio (with/without coadministered drug). ↑ indicates an increase in rosuvastatin exposure.
[p] The combination of atazanavir and saquinavir 1200 mg QD produced daily saquinavir exposures similar to the values produced by the standard therapeutic dosing of saquinavir at 1200 mg TID. However, the C_{max} is about 79% higher than that for the standard dosing of saquinavir (soft gelatin capsules) alone at 1200 mg TID.
[q] Note that similar results were observed in a study where administration of tenofovir and REYATAZ was separated by 12 hours.
[r] Administration of tenofovir and REYATAZ was temporally separated by 12 hours.
NA = not available.

Tell your healthcare provider if you have any side effect that bothers you or that does not go away.
These are not all the possible side effects of REYATAZ (atazanavir). For more information, ask your healthcare provider or pharmacist.
Call your doctor for medical advice about side effects. You may report side effects to FDA at 1-800-FDA-1088.

How should I store REYATAZ (atazanavir)?
REYATAZ capsules:
• Store REYATAZ capsules at room temperature, between 68°F to 77°F (20°C to 25°C).
• Keep capsules in a tightly closed container.
REYATAZ oral powder:
• Store REYATAZ oral powder below 86°F (30°C).

• Store REYATAZ (atazanavir) oral powder in the original packet. Do not open until ready to use.
• After REYATAZ oral powder is mixed with food or liquid it may be kept at room temperature 68°F to 86°F (20°C to 30°C) for up to 1 hour. Take REYATAZ oral powder within 1 hour after mixing with food or liquid.

Keep REYATAZ and all medicines out of the reach of children.

General information about REYATAZ
Medicines are sometimes prescribed for purposes other than those listed in a Patient Information leaflet. Do not use REYATAZ for a condition for which it was not prescribed. Do not give REYATAZ to other people, even if they have the same symptoms that you have. It may harm them. If you would like more information, talk with your healthcare provider. You can ask your pharmacist or healthcare provider for information about REYATAZ that is written for health professionals.

For more information, go to www.reyataz.com or call 1-800-321-1335.

What are the ingredients in REYATAZ?
Active ingredient: atazanavir sulfate
Inactive ingredients:
REYATAZ capsules: crospovidone, lactose monohydrate, and magnesium stearate. The capsule shells contain gelatin, FD&C Blue No. 2, titanium dioxide, black iron oxide, red iron oxide, and yellow iron oxide. The capsules are printed with ink containing shellac, titanium dioxide, FD&C Blue No. 2, isopropyl alcohol, ammonium hydroxide, propylene glycol, n-butyl alcohol, simethicone, and dehydrated alcohol.
REYATAZ oral powder: aspartame, sucrose, and orange-vanilla flavor.

This Patient Information has been approved by the U.S. Food and Drug Administration.

Distributed by:
Bristol-Myers Squibb Company
Princeton, NJ 08543 USA
Product of Ireland
1341313
Revised: June 2014
VIDEX® and REYATAZ® are registered trademarks of Bristol-Myers Squibb Company. COUMADIN® and SUSTIVA® are registered trademarks of Bristol-Myers Squibb Pharma Company. Other brands listed are the trademarks of their respective owners and are not trademarks of Bristol-Myers Squibb Company.

Instructions for Use
REYATAZ® (RAY-ah-taz)
(atazanavir)
oral powder
Read this Instructions for Use before you prepare your child's first dose of REYATAZ oral powder, each time you get a refill, and as needed. There may be new information. This information does not take the place of talking to your child's healthcare provider about their medical condition or treatment. Ask your child's healthcare provider or pharmacist if you have questions about how to mix or give a dose of REYATAZ oral powder.

Important information:
• For more information about REYATAZ oral powder, see the Patient Information leaflet.
• REYATAZ oral powder must be mixed with food or liquid. If REYATAZ oral powder is mixed with water, the child must eat food right after taking REYATAZ oral powder.
• REYATAZ oral powder must be taken with ritonavir.
• Talk with your child's healthcare provider to help decide the best schedule for giving your child REYATAZ oral powder.

Instructions for mixing REYATAZ oral powder:
REYATAZ oral powder should be mixed with food such as applesauce or yogurt, instead of a liquid (milk, infant formula, or water) in young children and infants who can take food.
• Infants less than 6 months old and who cannot eat solid food or drink from a cup should be given REYATAZ oral powder mixed with infant formula using an oral dosing syringe.
• REYATAZ oral powder that is mixed in infant formula or liquid should not be given using a baby bottle.
When preparing REYATAZ oral powder with either food or liquid, choose a clean, flat work surface. Place a clean paper towel on the work surface. Place the supplies you will need on the paper towel.
Wash and dry your hands before and after preparing REYATAZ oral powder.

Preparing a dose of REYATAZ oral powder mixed with food:
Before you prepare a dose of REYATAZ oral powder mixed with food, gather the following supplies:
• paper towel
• tablespoon

- **small** clean container (such as a **small** cup or bowl)
- a food such as applesauce or yogurt
- the correct number of packets of REYATAZ (atazanavir) oral powder needed for the prescribed dose

Step 1. Place at least 1 tablespoon of a food such as applesauce or yogurt in the small container (see Figure A).

Figure A

Step 2. Tap the packet of REYATAZ oral powder to settle the contents to the bottom of the packet (see Figure B).

Figure B

Step 3. Using a clean pair of scissors, cut open the packet on the dotted line (see Figure C).

Figure C

Step 4. Empty the contents of the packet into the small container onto the food (see Figure D).

Figure D

Repeat Steps 2 through 4 for each packet of REYATAZ oral powder needed for the total prescribed dose.

Step 5. Use a tablespoon to gently mix the powder and the food together (see Figure E).

Figure E

Table 23: Summary of Virologic Failures[a] at Week 96 in Study AI424-089: Comparison of Ritonavir Boosted REYATAZ vs. Unboosted REYATAZ: Randomized Patients

	REYATAZ 300 mg + ritonavir 100 mg (n=95)	REYATAZ 400 mg (n=105)
Virologic Failure (≥50 copies/mL) at Week 96	15 (16%)	34 (32%)
Virologic Failure with Genotypes and Phenotypes Data	5	17
Virologic Failure Isolates with ATV-resistance at Week 96	0/5 (0%)[b]	4/17 (24%)[b]
Virologic Failure Isolates with I50L Emergence at Week 96[c]	0/5 (0%)[b]	2/17 (12%)[b]
Virologic Failure Isolates with Lamivudine Resistance at Week 96	2/5 (40%)[b]	11/17 (65%)[b]

[a] Virologic failure includes patients who were never suppressed through Week 96 and on study at Week 96, had virologic rebound or discontinued due to insufficient viral load response.
[b] Percentage of Virologic Failure Isolates with genotypic and phenotypic data.
[c] Mixture of I50I/L emerged in 2 other ATV 400 mg-treated patients. Neither isolate was phenotypically resistant to ATV.

Table 24: HIV RNA Response by Number and Type of Baseline PI Substitution, Antiretroviral-Experienced Patients in Study AI424-045, As-Treated Analysis

	Virologic Response = HIV RNA <400 copies/mL[b]	
Number and Type of Baseline PI Substitutions[a]	ATV/RTV (n=110)	LPV/RTV (n=113)
3 or more primary PI substitutions including[c]:		
D30N	75% (6/8)	50% (3/6)
M36I/V	19% (3/16)	33% (6/18)
M46I/L/T	24% (4/17)	23% (5/22)
I54V/L/T/M/A	31% (5/16)	31% (5/16)
A71V/T/I/G	34% (10/29)	39% (12/31)
G73S/A/C/T	14% (1/7)	38% (3/8)
V77I	47% (7/15)	44% (7/16)
V82A/F/T/S/I	29% (6/21)	27% (7/26)
I84V/A	11% (1/9)	33% (2/6)
N88D	63% (5/8)	67% (4/6)
L90M	10% (2/21)	44% (11/25)
Number of baseline primary PI substitutions[a]		
All patients, as-treated	58% (64/110)	59% (67/113)
0–2 PI substitutions	75% (50/67)	75% (50/67)
3–4 PI substitutions	41% (14/34)	43% (12/28)
5 or more PI substitutions	0% (0/9)	28% (5/18)

[a] Primary substitutions include any change at D30, V32, M36, M46, I47, G48, I50, I54, A71, G73, V77, V82, I84, N88, and L90.
[b] Results should be interpreted with caution because the subgroups were small.
[c] There were insufficient data (n<3) for PI substitutions V32I, I47V, G48V, I50V, and F53L.

Table 26: Outcomes of Treatment Through Week 96 in Treatment-Naive Adults (Study AI424-138)

Outcome	REYATAZ 300 mg + ritonavir 100 mg (once daily) with tenofovir/emtricitabine (once daily)[a] (n=441) 96 Weeks	lopinavir 400 mg + ritonavir 100 mg (twice daily) with tenofovir/emtricitabine (once daily)[a] (n=437) 96 Weeks
Responder[b,c,d]	75%	68%
Virologic failure[e]	17%	19%
Rebound	8%	10%
Never suppressed through Week 96	9%	9%
Death	1%	1%
Discontinued due to adverse event	3%	5%
Discontinued for other reasons[f]	4%	7%

[a] As a fixed-dose combination: 300 mg tenofovir, 200 mg emtricitabine once daily.
[b] Patients achieved HIV RNA <50 copies/mL at Week 96. Roche Amplicor®, v1.5 ultra-sensitive assay.
[c] Pre-specified ITT analysis at Week 48 using as-randomized cohort: ATV/RTV 78% and LPV/RTV 76% (difference estimate: 1.7% [95% confidence interval: –3.8%, 7.1%]).
[d] Pre-specified ITT analysis at Week 96 using as-randomized cohort: ATV/RTV 74% and LPV/RTV 68% (difference estimate: 6.1% [95% confidence interval: 0.3%, 12.0%]).
[e] Includes viral rebound and failure to achieve confirmed HIV RNA <50 copies/mL through Week 96.
[f] Includes lost to follow-up, patient's withdrawal, noncompliance, protocol violation, and other reasons.

Steps 6 through 8 must be completed **within 1 hour** of mixing the medicine.

Step 6. Use the tablespoon or a small spoon to feed the REYATAZ (atazanavir) oral powder and food mixture to your child. Look in your child's mouth to make sure that all of the mixture is swallowed.

Step 7. Add 1 tablespoon more of food to the empty container and gently stir to mix with any contents that may still be in the container.

Step 8. Use the tablespoon or a small spoon to feed your child the mixture, making sure your child has swallowed all of the mixture.

Table 27: Outcomes of Randomized Treatment Through Week 48 in Treatment-Naive Adults (Study AI424-034)

Outcome	REYATAZ 400 mg once daily + lamivudine + zidovudine[d] (n=405)	efavirenz 600 mg once daily + lamivudine + zidovudine[d] (n=405)
Responder[a]	67% (32%)	62% (37%)
Virologic failure[b]	20%	21%
Rebound	17%	16%
Never suppressed through Week 48	3%	5%
Death	–	<1%
Discontinued due to adverse event	5%	7%
Discontinued for other reasons[c]	8%	10%

[a] Patients achieved and maintained confirmed HIV RNA <400 copies/mL (<50 copies/mL) through Week 48. Roche Amplicor® HIV-1 Monitor™ Assay, test version 1.0 or 1.5 as geographically appropriate.
[b] Includes viral rebound and failure to achieve confirmed HIV RNA <400 copies/mL through Week 48.
[c] Includes lost to follow-up, patient's withdrawal, noncompliance, protocol violation, and other reasons.
[d] As a fixed-dose combination: 150 mg lamivudine, 300 mg zidovudine twice daily.

Table 28: Outcomes of Randomized Treatment Through Week 48 in Treatment-Naive Adults (Study AI424-008)

Outcome	REYATAZ 400 mg once daily + lamivudine + stavudine (n=181)	nelfinavir 1250 mg twice daily + lamivudine + stavudine (n=91)
Responder[a]	67% (33%)	59% (38%)
Virologic failure[b]	24%	27%
Rebound	14%	14%
Never suppressed through Week 48	10%	13%
Death	<1%	–
Discontinued due to adverse event	1%	3%
Discontinued for other reasons[c]	7%	10%

[a] Patients achieved and maintained confirmed HIV RNA <400 copies/mL (<50 copies/mL) through Week 48. Roche Amplicor® HIV-1 Monitor™ Assay, test version 1.0 or 1.5 as geographically appropriate.
[b] Includes viral rebound and failure to achieve confirmed HIV RNA <400 copies/mL through Week 48.
[c] Includes lost to follow-up, patient's withdrawal, noncompliance, protocol violation, and other reasons.

Table 29: Outcomes of Treatment Through Week 48 in Study AI424-045 (Patients with Prior Antiretroviral Experience)

Outcome	REYATAZ 300 mg + ritonavir 100 mg once daily + tenofovir + 1 NRTI (n=119)	lopinavir/ritonavir (400/100 mg) twice daily + tenofovir + 1 NRTI (n=118)	Difference[a] (REYATAZ-lopinavir/ ritonavir) (CI)
HIV RNA Change from Baseline ($\log_{10}$ copies/mL)[b]	−1.58	−1.70	+0.12[c] (−0.17, 0.41)
CD4+ Change from Baseline (cells/mm^3)[d]	116	123	−7 (−67, 52)
Percent of Patients Responding[e]			
HIV RNA <400 copies/mL[b]	55%	57%	−2.2% (−14.8%, 10.5%)
HIV RNA <50 copies/mL[b]	38%	45%	−7.1% (−19.6%, 5.4%)

[a] Time-averaged difference through Week 48 for HIV RNA; Week 48 difference in HIV RNA percentages and CD4+ mean changes, REYATAZ/ritonavir vs lopinavir/ritonavir; CI = 97.5% confidence interval for change in HIV RNA; 95% confidence interval otherwise.
[b] Roche Amplicor® HIV-1 Monitor™ Assay, test version 1.5.
[c] Protocol-defined primary efficacy outcome measure.
[d] Based on patients with baseline and Week 48 CD4+ cell count measurements (REYATAZ/ritonavir, n=85; lopinavir/ ritonavir, n=93).
[e] Patients achieved and maintained confirmed HIV-1 RNA <400 copies/mL (<50 copies/mL) through Week 48.

Product Strength*	Capsule Shell Color (cap/body)	Markings on Capsule (ink color)		Capsules per Bottle	NDC Number
		cap	body		
150 mg	blue/powder blue	BMS 150 mg (white)	3624 (blue)	60	0003-3624-12
200 mg	blue/blue	BMS 200 mg (white)	3631 (white)	60	0003-3631-12
300 mg	red/blue	BMS 300 mg (white)	3622 (white)	30	0003-3622-12

* 150 mg atazanavir equivalent to 170.8 mg atazanavir sulfate.
200 mg atazanavir equivalent to 227.8 mg atazanavir sulfate.
300 mg atazanavir equivalent to 341.69 mg atazanavir sulfate.

Step 9. Give your child ritonavir as prescribed right after taking REYATAZ (atazanavir) oral powder.

Step 10. Wash the container and tablespoon. Allow the container and spoon to dry. Throw away the paper towel and clean the work surface.

Preparing a dose of REYATAZ oral powder mixed with liquid in a small drinking cup:
Before you prepare a dose of REYATAZ oral powder mixed with liquid in a small drinking cup, gather the following supplies:

- paper towel
- spoon
- 30 milliliter (mL) medicine cup (ask your pharmacist for this). See Figure F.
- small drinking cup
- liquid such as milk or water
- the correct number of packets of REYATAZ oral powder needed for the prescribed dose

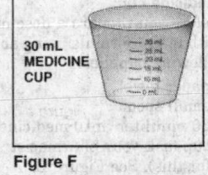

Figure F

Step 1. Using the 30 mL medicine cup, pour at least 30 mL of liquid into the small drinking cup (see Figure G).

Figure G

Step 2. Tap the packet of REYATAZ oral powder to settle the contents to the bottom of the packet (see Figure H).

Figure H

Step 3. Using a clean pair of scissors, cut open the packet on the dotted line (see Figure I).

Figure I

Step 4. Empty the contents of the packet into the small drinking cup (see Figure J).

Figure J

Repeat Steps 2 through 4 for each packet of REYATAZ oral powder needed for the total prescribed dose.

Step 5. Hold the small drinking cup with one hand. With your other hand, use the spoon to gently mix the powder and the liquid (see Figure K).

Figure K

Steps 6 and 7 must be completed **within 1 hour** of mixing the medicine.

Step 6. Have your child drink all of the mixture in the small drinking cup.

Step 7. To make sure there is no mixture left in the small drinking cup add 15 mL more liquid to the small drinking cup:

- Stir with the spoon.

• Repeat Step 6 above.

If REYATAZ (atazanavir) oral powder is mixed with water, your child must eat food right after taking REYATAZ oral powder.

Step 8. Give your child ritonavir as prescribed right after taking REYATAZ oral powder.

Step 9. Wash the small drinking cup, medicine cup, and spoon. Allow the small drinking cup, medicine cup, and spoon to dry. Throw away the paper towel and clean the work surface.

Preparing a dose of REYATAZ oral powder mixed with liquid infant formula using an oral dosing syringe and a small medicine cup:

Before you prepare a dose of REYATAZ oral powder mixed with infant formula using an oral dosing syringe, gather the following supplies:

• paper towel
• small spoon
• 30 milliliter (mL) medicine cup (ask your pharmacist for this). See Figure L.
• 10 mL oral dosing syringe (ask your pharmacist for this). See Figure L.
• infant formula
• the correct number of packets of REYATAZ oral powder needed for the prescribed dose

Figure L

Step 1. Prepare the infant formula according to the directions on the infant formula package.

Step 2. Pour 10 mL of infant formula into the medicine cup (see Figure M).

Figure M

Step 3. Tap the packet of REYATAZ oral powder to settle the contents to the bottom of the packet (see Figure N).

Figure N

Step 4. Using a clean pair of scissors, cut open the packet on the dotted line (see Figure O).

Figure O

Step 5. Empty the contents of the packet into the medicine cup (see Figure P).

Figure P

Repeat Steps 3 through 5 for each packet of REYATAZ oral powder needed for the total prescribed dose.

Step 6. Hold the medicine cup with one hand. With your other hand, use the small spoon to gently mix the powder and the infant formula (see Figure Q).

Figure Q

Steps 7 through 9 must be completed **within 1 hour** of mixing the medicine.

Step 7. Draw up the powder and infant formula mixture into the oral dosing syringe as follows:

• Check that the plunger is completely pushed into barrel of the syringe (see Figure R).

Figure R

• Place the tip of the syringe into the powder and infant formula mixture in the medicine cup (see Figure S).

Figure S

• Slowly pull back on the plunger and draw up 10 mL of the mixture (see Figure T).

Figure T

Step 8. Place the tip of the oral dosing syringe in your baby's mouth along the inner cheek on either the right or left side (see Figure U). Slowly push on the plunger to give your baby all of the REYATAZ oral powder and infant formula mixture.

• Draw up any remaining mixture with the oral dosing syringe and repeat until all of the mixture has been given to the baby.

Figure U

Step 9. To make sure there is no mixture left in the medicine cup or syringe:

• Repeat Step 1 above to add 10 mL more infant formula to the medicine cup
• Stir with a small spoon.
• **Then repeat Steps 7 through 8 above.**

To make sure that your baby gets all of the medicine, do not give REYATAZ oral powder in a baby bottle.

Step 10. Give your baby ritonavir as prescribed right after taking REYATAZ (atazanavir) oral powder.

Step 11. Remove the plunger from the oral dosing syringe. Wash the medicine cup, spoon, and oral dosing syringe. Allow the medicine cup, spoon, and oral dosing syringe to dry. Throw away the paper towel and clean the work surface.

How should I store REYATAZ oral powder?

• Store REYATAZ oral powder below 86°F (30°C).
• Store REYATAZ oral powder in the original packet. Do not open until ready to use.
• After REYATAZ oral powder is mixed with food or liquid, it may be kept at room temperature 68°F to 86°F (20°C to 30°C) for up to 1 hour. Take REYATAZ oral powder within 1 hour after mixing with food or liquid.

Keep REYATAZ (atazanavir) oral powder and all medicines out of the reach of children.

This Instructions for Use has been approved by the U.S. Food and Drug Administration.

Distributed by:
Bristol-Myers Squibb Company
Princeton, NJ 08543 USA
Product of Ireland
1341313
Issued: June 2014

Shown in Product Identification Guide, page 306

SPRYCEL®   ℞
[*Spry-sell*]
(dasatinib)
Tablet for Oral Use

HIGHLIGHTS OF PRESCRIBING INFORMATION

These highlights do not include all the information needed to use SPRYCEL safely and effectively. See full prescribing information for SPRYCEL.

SPRYCEL® (dasatinib) Tablet for Oral Use
Initial U.S. Approval: 2006

───────INDICATIONS AND USAGE───────

SPRYCEL is a kinase inhibitor indicated for the treatment of

• newly diagnosed adults with Philadelphia chromosome-positive (Ph+) chronic myeloid leukemia (CML) in chronic phase. The trial is ongoing and further data will be required to determine long-term outcome. (1, 14)
• adults with chronic, accelerated, or myeloid or lymphoid blast phase Ph+ CML with resistance or intolerance to prior therapy including imatinib. (1, 14)
• adults with Philadelphia chromosome-positive acute lymphoblastic leukemia (Ph+ ALL) with resistance or intolerance to prior therapy. (1, 14)

───────DOSAGE AND ADMINISTRATION───────

• Chronic phase CML: 100 mg once daily. (2)
• Accelerated phase CML, myeloid or lymphoid blast phase CML, or Ph+ ALL: 140 mg once daily. (2)
Administer orally, with or without a meal. Do not crush or cut. (2)

───────DOSAGE FORMS AND STRENGTHS───────

Tablets: 20 mg, 50 mg, 70 mg, 80 mg, 100 mg, and 140 mg. (3, 16)

───────CONTRAINDICATIONS───────

None. (4)

───────WARNINGS AND PRECAUTIONS───────

• *Myelosuppression and Bleeding Events:* Severe thrombocytopenia, neutropenia, and anemia may occur. Use caution if used concomitantly with medications that inhibit platelet function or anticoagulants. Monitor complete blood counts regularly. Transfuse and interrupt SPRYCEL when indicated. (2.3, 5.1, 5.2, 6.1)
• *Fluid Retention:* Fluid retention, sometimes severe, including ascites, edema, and pleural and pericardial effusions. Manage with appropriate supportive care measures. (5.3, 6.1)
• *QT Prolongation:* Use SPRYCEL with caution in patients who have or may develop prolongation of the QT interval. (5.4)
• *Cardiac Dysfunction:* Monitor patients for signs or symptoms and treat appropriately. (5.5, 6.1)
• *Pulmonary Arterial Hypertension (PAH):* SPRYCEL may increase the risk of developing PAH which may be reversible on discontinuation. Consider baseline risk and evaluate patients for signs and symptoms of PAH during treatment. Stop SPRYCEL if PAH is confirmed. (5.6)
• *Embryo-fetal Toxicity:* SPRYCEL can cause fetal harm. Advise females of the potential risk to the fetus. (5.7, 8.1, 8.8)

───────ADVERSE REACTIONS───────

Most common adverse reactions (≥15%) in patients with newly diagnosed chronic phase CML included myelosuppression, fluid retention, and diarrhea. Most common adverse reactions (≥20%) in patients with resistance or intolerance to prior imatinib therapy included myelosuppression, fluid retention events, diarrhea, headache, dyspnea, skin rash, fatigue, nausea, and hemorrhage. (6)

To report SUSPECTED ADVERSE REACTIONS, contact Bristol-Myers Squibb at 1-800-721-5072 or FDA at 1-800-FDA-1088 or www.fda.gov/medwatch.

───────DRUG INTERACTIONS───────

• *CYP3A4 Inhibitors:* May increase dasatinib drug levels and should be avoided. If coadministration cannot be avoided, monitor closely and consider reducing SPRYCEL dose. (2.1, 7.1)

- *CYP3A4 Inducers:* May decrease dasatinib drug levels. If coadministration cannot be avoided, consider increasing SPRYCEL (dasatinib) dose. (2.1, 7.2)
- *Antacids:* May decrease dasatinib drug levels. Avoid simultaneous administration. If needed, administer the antacid at least 2 hours prior to or 2 hours after the dose of SPRYCEL. (7.2)
- *H_2 Antagonists/Proton Pump Inhibitors:* May decrease dasatinib drug levels. Consider antacids in place of H_2 antagonists or proton pump inhibitors. (7.2)

---USE IN SPECIFIC POPULATIONS---

- *Nursing Mothers:* Discontinue drug or nursing taking into consideration the importance of the drug to the mother. (8.3)
- *Hepatic Impairment:* Use SPRYCEL with caution in patients with hepatic impairment. (8.6)

See 17 for PATIENT COUNSELING INFORMATION and FDA-approved patient labeling

Revised: 05/2014

FULL PRESCRIBING INFORMATION: CONTENTS*

FULL PRESCRIBING INFORMATION

1   INDICATIONS AND USAGE

SPRYCEL® (dasatinib) is indicated for the treatment of adults with

- newly diagnosed Philadelphia chromosome-positive (Ph+) chronic myeloid leukemia (CML) in chronic phase. The effectiveness of SPRYCEL (dasatinib) is based on cytogenetic response and major molecular response rates *[see Clinical Studies (14.1)].* The trial is ongoing and further data will be required to determine long-term outcome.
- chronic, accelerated, or myeloid or lymphoid blast phase Ph+ CML with resistance or intolerance to prior therapy including imatinib.
- Philadelphia chromosome-positive acute lymphoblastic leukemia (Ph+ ALL) with resistance or intolerance to prior therapy.

2   DOSAGE AND ADMINISTRATION

The recommended starting dosage of SPRYCEL for chronic phase CML is 100 mg administered orally once daily. The recommended starting dosage of SPRYCEL for accelerated phase CML, myeloid or lymphoid blast phase CML, or Ph+ ALL is 140 mg administered orally once daily. Tablets should not be crushed or cut; they should be swallowed whole. SPRYCEL can be taken with or without a meal, either in the morning or in the evening.

In clinical studies, treatment with SPRYCEL was continued until disease progression or until no longer tolerated by the patient. The effect of stopping treatment after the achievement of a complete cytogenetic response (CCyR) has not been investigated.

2.1   Dose Modification

Concomitant Strong CYP3A4 inducers: The use of concomitant strong CYP3A4 inducers may decrease dasatinib plasma concentrations and should be avoided (eg, dexamethasone, phenytoin, carbamazepine, rifampin, rifabutin, phenobarbital). St. John's Wort may decrease dasatinib plasma concentrations unpredictably and should be avoided. If patients must be coadministered a strong CYP3A4 inducer, based on pharmacokinetic studies, a SPRYCEL dose increase should be considered. If the dose of SPRYCEL is increased, the patient should be monitored carefully for toxicity *[see Drug Interactions (7.2)].*

Concomitant Strong CYP3A4 inhibitors: CYP3A4 inhibitors (eg, ketoconazole, itraconazole, clarithromycin, atazanavir, indinavir, nefazodone, nelfinavir, ritonavir, saquinavir, telithromycin, and voriconazole) may increase dasatinib plasma concentrations. Grapefruit juice may also increase plasma concentrations of dasatinib and should be avoided. Selection of an alternate concomitant medication with no or minimal enzyme inhibition potential, if possible, is recommended. If SPRYCEL must be administered with a strong CYP3A4 inhibitor, a dose decrease should be considered. Based on pharmacokinetic studies, a dose decrease to 20 mg daily should be considered for patients taking SPRYCEL 100 mg daily. For patients taking SPRYCEL 140 mg daily, a dose decrease to 40 mg daily should be considered. These reduced doses of SPRYCEL are predicted to adjust the area under the curve (AUC) to the range observed without CYP3A4 inhibitors. However, there are no clinical data with these dose adjustments in patients receiving strong CYP3A4 inhibitors. If SPRYCEL is not tolerated after dose reduction, either the strong CYP3A4 inhibitor must be discontinued, or SPRYCEL should be stopped until treatment with the inhibitor has ceased. When the strong inhibitor is discontinued, a washout period of approximately 1 week should be allowed before the SPRYCEL dose is increased. *[See Drug Interactions (7.1).]*

Table 1:   Dose Adjustments for Neutropenia and Thrombocytopenia

Chronic Phase CML (starting dose 100 mg once daily)	ANC* $<0.5 \times 10^9$/L or Platelets $<50 \times 10^9$/L	1. Stop SPRYCEL until ANC $\geq 1.0 \times 10^9$/L and platelets $\geq 50 \times 10^9$/L. 2. Resume treatment with SPRYCEL at the original starting dose if recovery occurs in ≤7 days. 3. If platelets $<25 \times 10^9$/L or recurrence of ANC $<0.5 \times 10^9$/L for >7 days, repeat Step 1 and resume SPRYCEL at a reduced dose of 80 mg once daily for second episode. For third episode, further reduce dose to 50 mg once daily (for newly diagnosed patients) or discontinue SPRYCEL (for patients resistant or intolerant to prior therapy including imatinib).
Accelerated Phase CML, Blast Phase CML and Ph+ ALL (starting dose 140 mg once daily)	ANC* $<0.5 \times 10^9$/L or Platelets $<10 \times 10^9$/L	1. Check if cytopenia is related to leukemia (marrow aspirate or biopsy). 2. If cytopenia is unrelated to leukemia, stop SPRYCEL until ANC $\geq 1.0 \times 10^9$/L and platelets $\geq 20 \times 10^9$/L and resume at the original starting dose. 3. If recurrence of cytopenia, repeat Step 1 and resume SPRYCEL at a reduced dose of 100 mg once daily (second episode) or 80 mg once daily (third episode). 4. If cytopenia is related to leukemia, consider dose escalation to 180 mg once daily.

* ANC: absolute neutrophil count

2.2   Dose Escalation

In clinical studies of adult CML and Ph+ ALL patients, dose escalation to 140 mg once daily (chronic phase CML) or 180 mg once daily (advanced phase CML and Ph+ ALL) was allowed in patients who did not achieve a hematologic or cytogenetic response at the recommended starting dosage.

2.3   Dose Adjustment for Adverse Reactions
Myelosuppression

In clinical studies, myelosuppression was managed by dose interruption, dose reduction, or discontinuation of study therapy. Hematopoietic growth factor has been used in patients with resistant myelosuppression. Guidelines for dose modifications are summarized in Table 1.

[See table 1 above]

Non-hematological adverse reactions

If a severe non-hematological adverse reaction develops with SPRYCEL use, treatment must be withheld until the event has resolved or improved. Thereafter, treatment can be resumed as appropriate at a reduced dose depending on the initial severity of the event.

3   DOSAGE FORMS AND STRENGTHS

SPRYCEL (dasatinib) Tablets are available as 20-mg, 50-mg, 70-mg, 80-mg, 100-mg, and 140-mg white to off-white, biconvex, film-coated tablets *[see How Supplied (16.1)].*

4   CONTRAINDICATIONS

None.

5   WARNINGS AND PRECAUTIONS

5.1   Myelosuppression

Treatment with SPRYCEL is associated with severe (NCI CTC Grade 3 or 4) thrombocytopenia, neutropenia, and anemia. Their occurrence is more frequent in patients with advanced phase CML or Ph+ ALL than in chronic phase CML. In a dose-optimization trial in patients with resistance or intolerance to prior imatinib therapy and chronic phase CML, Grade 3 or 4 myelosuppression was reported less frequently in patients treated with 100 mg once daily than in patients treated with other dosing regimens.

Perform complete blood counts weekly for the first 2 months and then monthly thereafter, or as clinically indicated. Myelosuppression was generally reversible and usually managed by withholding SPRYCEL temporarily or dose reduction *[see Dosage and Administration (2.3) and Adverse Reactions (6.1)].*

5.2   Bleeding Related Events

In addition to causing thrombocytopenia in human subjects, dasatinib caused platelet dysfunction *in vitro.* In all clinical studies, severe central nervous system (CNS) hemorrhages, including fatalities, occurred in 1% of patients receiving SPRYCEL. Severe gastrointestinal hemorrhage, including fatalities, occurred in 4% of patients and generally required treatment interruptions and transfusions. Other cases of severe hemorrhage occurred in 2% of patients. Most bleeding events were associated with severe thrombocytopenia.

Patients were excluded from participation in initial SPRYCEL clinical studies if they took medications that inhibit platelet function or anticoagulants. In subsequent trials, the use of anticoagulants, aspirin, and non-steroidal anti-inflammatory drugs (NSAIDs) was allowed concurrently with SPRYCEL if the platelet count was >50,000–75,000 per microliter. Exercise caution if patients are required to take medications that inhibit platelet function or anticoagulants.

Table 2: Adverse Reactions Reported in ≥10% of Patients with Newly Diagnosed Chronic Phase CML (minimum of 36 months follow up)

| | All Grades | | Grade 3/4 | |
| | SPRYCEL (n=258) | Imatinib (n=258) | SPRYCEL (n=258) | Imatinib (n=258) |
Preferred Term	Percent (%) of Patients			
Fluid retention	31	44	3	1
Pleural effusion	19	<1	2	0
Superficial localized edema	13	37	0	<1
Generalized edema	3	7	0	0
Congestive heart failure/cardiac dysfunction[a]	2	1	<1	<1
Pericardial effusion	3	1	1	0
Pulmonary hypertension	2	0	<1	0
Pulmonary edema	1	0	0	0
Diarrhea	21	22	1	1
Headache	13	11	0	0
Musculoskeletal pain	13	17	0	<1
Rash[b]	13	18	0	2
Nausea	10	24	0	0
Fatigue	9	11	<1	0
Myalgia	6	12	0	0
Hemorrhage[c]	7	7	1	1
Gastrointestinal bleeding	2	1	1	0
Other bleeding[d]	6	5	0	1
CNS bleeding	0	<1	0	<1
Vomiting	5	11	0	0
Muscle spasms	5	21	0	<1

[a] Includes cardiac failure acute, cardiac failure congestive, cardiomyopathy, diastolic dysfunction, ejection fraction decreased, and left ventricular dysfunction.
[b] Includes erythema, erythema multiforme, rash, rash generalized, rash macular, rash papular, rash pustular, skin exfoliation, and rash vesicular.
[c] Adverse reaction of special interest with <10% frequency.
[d] Includes conjunctival hemorrhage, ear hemorrhage, ecchymosis, epistaxis, eye hemorrhage, gingival bleeding, hematoma, hematuria, hemoptysis, intra-abdominal hematoma, petechiae, scleral hemorrhage, uterine hemorrhage, and vaginal hemorrhage.

5.3 Fluid Retention

SPRYCEL (dasatinib) is associated with fluid retention. In clinical trials, severe fluid retention was reported in up to 10% of patients. Severe ascites, pulmonary edema, and generalized edema were each reported in ≤1% of patients. Patients who develop symptoms suggestive of pleural effusion, such as dyspnea or dry cough, should be evaluated by chest x-ray. Severe pleural effusion may require thoracentesis and oxygen therapy. Fluid retention events were typically managed by supportive care measures that include diuretics or short courses of steroids. In dose-optimization studies, fluid retention events were reported less frequently with once daily dosing than with other dosing regimens.

5.4 QT Prolongation

In vitro data suggest that dasatinib has the potential to prolong cardiac ventricular repolarization (QT interval). Of the 2440 patients treated with SPRYCEL in clinical studies, 16 patients (1%) had QTc prolongation reported as an adverse reaction. Twenty-two patients (1%) experienced a QTcF >500 ms. In 865 patients with leukemia treated with SPRYCEL in five Phase 2 single-arm studies, the maximum mean changes in QTcF (90% upper bound CI) from baseline ranged from 7.0 ms to 13.4 ms.

Administer SPRYCEL with caution to patients who have or may develop prolongation of QTc. These include patients with hypokalemia or hypomagnesemia, patients with congenital long QT syndrome, patients taking anti-arrhythmic medicines or other medicinal products that lead to QT prolongation, and cumulative high-dose anthracycline therapy. Correct hypokalemia or hypomagnesemia prior to SPRYCEL administration.

5.5 Congestive Heart Failure, Left Ventricular Dysfunction, and Myocardial Infarction

Cardiac adverse reactions were reported in 7% of 258 patients taking SPRYCEL, including, 1.6% of patients with cardiomyopathy, heart failure congestive, diastolic dysfunction, fatal myocardial infarction, and left ventricular dysfunction. Monitor patients for signs or symptoms consistent with cardiac dysfunction and treat appropriately.

5.6 Pulmonary Arterial Hypertension

SPRYCEL may increase the risk of developing pulmonary arterial hypertension (PAH) which may occur any time after initiation, including after more than one year of treatment. Manifestations include dyspnea, fatigue, hypoxia, and fluid retention. PAH may be reversible on discontinuation of SPRYCEL. Evaluate patients for signs and symptoms of underlying cardiopulmonary disease prior to initiating SPRYCEL and during treatment. If PAH is confirmed, SPRYCEL should be permanently discontinued.

5.7 Embryo-fetal Toxicity

SPRYCEL (dasatinib) can cause fetal harm when administered to a pregnant woman. Adverse fetal and infant outcomes have been reported from women who have taken SPRYCEL during pregnancy. In animal reproduction studies, embryo-fetal toxicities, including skeletal malformations, were observed in rats and rabbits at plasma concentrations below those in humans receiving therapeutic doses of dasatinib. If SPRYCEL is used during pregnancy, or if the patient becomes pregnant while taking SPRYCEL, the patient should be apprised of the potential hazard to the fetus *[see Use in Specific Populations (8.1)]*.

Advise females of reproductive potential to avoid pregnancy, which may include the use of contraception, during treatment with SPRYCEL *[see Use in Specific Populations (8.8)]*.

6 ADVERSE REACTIONS

The following adverse reactions are discussed in greater detail in other sections of the labeling:
- Myelosuppression *[see Dosage and Administration (2.3) and Warnings and Precautions (5.1)]*.
- Bleeding related events *[see Warnings and Precautions (5.2)]*.
- Fluid retention *[see Warnings and Precautions (5.3)]*.
- QT prolongation *[see Warnings and Precautions (5.4)]*.
- Congestive heart failure, left ventricular dysfunction, and myocardial infarction *[see Warnings and Precautions (5.5)]*.
- Pulmonary Arterial Hypertension *[see Warnings and Precautions (5.6)]*.

Because clinical trials are conducted under widely varying conditions, adverse reaction rates observed in the clinical trials of a drug cannot be directly compared to rates in the clinical trials of another drug and may not reflect the rates observed in practice.

The data described below reflect exposure to SPRYCEL in clinical studies including 258 patients with newly diagnosed chronic phase CML and in 2182 patients with imatinib resistant or intolerant CML or Ph+ ALL.

In the newly diagnosed chronic phase CML trial with a minimum of 36 months follow up and median duration of therapy of 37 months, the median average daily dose was 99 mg.

In the imatinib resistant or intolerant CML or Ph+ ALL clinical trials, 1520 patients had a minimum of 2 years follow up and 662 patients with chronic phase CML had a minimum of 60 months follow up (starting dosage 100 mg once daily, 140 mg once daily, 50 mg twice daily, or 70 mg twice daily). Among patients with chronic phase CML and resistance or intolerance to prior imatinib therapy, the median

duration of treatment with SPRYCEL (dasatinib) 100 mg once daily was 37 months (range 1–65 months). The median duration of treatment with SPRYCEL 140 mg once daily was 15 months (range 0.03–36 months) for accelerated phase CML, 3 months (range 0.03–29 months) for myeloid blast phase CML, and 3 months (range 0.1–10 months) for lymphoid blast CML.

The majority of SPRYCEL-treated patients experienced adverse reactions at some time. In the newly diagnosed chronic phase CML trial, drug was discontinued for adverse reactions in 6% of SPRYCEL-treated patients with a minimum of 12 months follow up. After a minimum of 36 months follow up, the cumulative discontinuation rate was 9%. Among patients with resistance or intolerance to prior imatinib therapy, the rates of discontinuation for adverse reactions at 2 years were 15% in chronic phase CML for all dosages, 16% in accelerated phase CML, 15% in myeloid blast phase CML, 8% in lymphoid blast phase CML, and 8% in Ph+ ALL. In a dose-optimization trial in patients with resistance or intolerance to prior imatinib therapy and chronic phase CML with a minimum of 60 months follow up, the rate of discontinuation for adverse reactions was 18% in patients treated with 100 mg once daily.

The most frequently reported adverse reactions reported in ≥10% of patients in newly diagnosed chronic phase CML included myelosuppression, fluid retention events (pleural effusion, superficial localized edema, generalized edema), diarrhea, headache, musculoskeletal pain, rash, and nausea. Pleural effusions were reported in 50 patients (see Table 2). The most frequently reported adverse reactions reported in ≥20% of patients with resistance or intolerance to prior imatinib therapy included myelosuppression, fluid retention events, diarrhea, headache, dyspnea, skin rash, fatigue, nausea, and hemorrhage.

The most frequently reported serious adverse reactions in patients with newly diagnosed chronic phase CML included pleural effusion (4%), hemorrhage (2%), congestive heart failure (1%), pulmonary hypertension (1%), and pyrexia (1%). The most frequently reported serious adverse reactions in patients with resistance or intolerance to prior imatinib therapy included pleural effusion (11%), gastrointestinal bleeding (4%), febrile neutropenia (4%), dyspnea (3%), pneumonia (3%), pyrexia (3%), diarrhea (3%), infection (2%), congestive heart failure/cardiac dysfunction (2%), pericardial effusion (1%), and CNS hemorrhage (1%).

6.1 Chronic Myeloid Leukemia (CML)

Adverse reactions (excluding laboratory abnormalities) that were reported in at least 10% of patients are shown in Table 2 for newly diagnosed patients with chronic phase CML and Tables 3 and 4 for CML patients with resistance or intolerance to prior imatinib therapy.

[See table 2 above]

The cumulative rates of the majority of adverse reactions (all grades) in newly diagnosed patients with chronic phase CML were similar after 12 and 36 months minimum follow up including congestive heart failure/cardiac dysfunction (2% vs 2%), pericardial effusion (2% vs 3%), pulmonary edema (<1% vs 1%), gastrointestinal bleeding (2% vs 2%), diarrhea (18% vs 21%), and generalized edema (3% vs 3%). Cumulative adverse reaction rates (all grades) that increased between 12 months and 36 months minimum follow up included overall fluid retention (23% vs 31%), pleural effusion (12% vs 19%), and superficial edema (10% vs 13%). A total of 9 patients (3.5%) discontinued due to pleural effusion in the trial.

At 36 months, there were 17 deaths in the dasatinib-treated patients (6.6%) and 20 deaths in the imatinib-treated patients (7.7%); 1 in each group was judged by the investigator as related to study therapy.

Table 3: Adverse Reactions Reported in ≥10% of Patients with Chronic Phase CML Resistant or Intolerant to Prior Imatinib Therapy (minimum of 36 months follow up)

	100 mg Once Daily	
	Chronic (n=165)	
	All Grades	Grade 3/4
Preferred Term	Percent (%) of Patients	
Fluid retention	42	5
Superficial localized edema	21	0
Pleural effusion	24	4
Generalized edema	4	0
Pericardial effusion	2	1
Congestive heart failure/ cardiac dysfunction[a]	0	0
Pulmonary edema	0	0
Headache	33	1
Diarrhea	28	2
Fatigue	26	4

Dyspnea	24	2
Musculoskeletal pain	22	2
Nausea	18	1
Skin rash[b]	18	2
Myalgia	13	0
Arthralgia	12	1
Infection (including bacterial, viral, fungal, and non-specified)	13	1
Abdominal pain	12	1
Hemorrhage	11	1
Gastrointestinal bleeding	2	1
CNS bleeding	0	0
Pruritus	10	1
Pain	10	1

[a] Includes ventricular dysfunction, cardiac failure, cardiac failure congestive, cardiomyopathy, congestive cardiomyopathy, diastolic dysfunction, ejection fraction decreased, and ventricular failure.

[b] Includes drug eruption, erythema, erythema multiforme, erythrosis, exfoliative rash, generalized erythema, genital rash, heat rash, milia, rash, rash erythematous, rash follicular, rash generalized, rash macular, rash maculopapular, rash papular, rash pruritic, rash pustular, skin exfoliation, skin irritation, urticaria vesiculosa, and rash vesicular.

With a minimum follow up of 60 months (see Table 3), the cumulative rates of the majority of adverse reactions (all grades) in patients with chronic phase CML treated with a starting dose of 100 mg once daily were identical with a minimum follow up of 24 and 60 months including congestive heart failure/cardiac dysfunction, pericardial effusion, pulmonary edema, and gastrointestinal bleeding or similar for diarrhea (27% vs 28%), and generalized edema (3% vs 4%). Cumulative adverse reaction rates (all grades) that increased between 24 months and 60 months minimum follow up included: overall fluid retention (34% vs 42%), pleural effusion (18% vs 24%), and superficial edema (18% vs 21%). The cumulative rate of Grade 3 or 4 pleural effusion was 2% versus 4%, respectively.

[See table 4 above]

Laboratory Abnormalities

Myelosuppression was commonly reported in all patient populations. The frequency of Grade 3 or 4 neutropenia, thrombocytopenia, and anemia was higher in patients with advanced phase CML than in chronic phase CML (Tables 5 and 6). Myelosuppression was reported in patients with normal baseline laboratory values as well as in patients with pre-existing laboratory abnormalities.

In patients who experienced severe myelosuppression, recovery generally occurred following dose interruption or reduction; permanent discontinuation of treatment occurred in 2% of patients with newly diagnosed chronic phase CML and 5% of patients with resistance or intolerance to prior imatinib therapy [see Warnings and Precautions (5.1)].

Grade 3 or 4 elevations of transaminase or bilirubin and Grade 3 or 4 hypocalcemia, hypokalemia, and hypophosphatemia were reported in patients with all phases of CML but were reported with an increased frequency in patients with myeloid or lymphoid blast phase CML. Elevations in transaminase or bilirubin were usually managed with dose reduction or interruption. Patients developing Grade 3 or 4 hypocalcemia during the course of SPRYCEL (dasatinib) therapy often had recovery with oral calcium supplementation.

Laboratory abnormalities reported in patients with newly diagnosed chronic phase CML are shown in Table 5. There were no discontinuations of SPRYCEL therapy in this patient population due to biochemical laboratory parameters.

Table 5: CTC Grade 3/4 Laboratory Abnormalities in Patients with Newly Diagnosed Chronic Phase CML (minimum of 36 months follow up)

	SPRYCEL (n=258)	Imatinib (n=258)
	Percent (%) of Patients	
Hematology Parameters		
Neutropenia	24	21
Thrombocytopenia	19	11
Anemia	12	9
Biochemistry Parameters		
Hypophosphatemia	7	28
Hypokalemia	0	2
Hypocalcemia	3	2
Elevated SGPT (ALT)	<1	2
Elevated SGOT (AST)	<1	1
Elevated Bilirubin	1	0
Elevated Creatinine	1	1

CTC grades: neutropenia (Grade 3 ≥0.5–<1.0 × 10^9/L, Grade 4 <0.5 × 10^9/L); thrombocytopenia (Grade 3 ≥25–<50 × 10^9/L, Grade 4 <25 × 10^9/L); anemia (hemoglobin Grade 3 ≥65–<80 g/L, Grade 4 <65 g/L); elevated creatinine (Grade 3 >3–6 × upper limit of normal range (ULN), Grade 4 >6 × ULN); elevated bilirubin (Grade 3 >3–10 × ULN, Grade 4 >10 × ULN); elevated SGOT or SGPT (Grade 3 >5–20 × ULN, Grade 4 >20 × ULN); hypocalcemia (Grade 3 <7.0–6.0 mg/dL, Grade 4 <6.0 mg/dL); hypophosphatemia (Grade 3 <2.0–1.0 mg/dL, Grade 4 <1.0 mg/dL); hypokalemia (Grade 3 <3.0–2.5 mmol/L, Grade 4 <2.5 mmol/L).

Table 4: Adverse Reactions Reported in ≥10% of Patients with Advanced Phase CML Resistant or Intolerant to Prior Imatinib Therapy

	140 mg Once Daily					
	Accelerated (n=157)		Myeloid Blast (n=74)		Lymphoid Blast (n=33)	
	All Grades	Grade 3/4	All Grades	Grade 3/4	All Grades	Grade 3/4
Preferred Term	Percent (%) of Patients					
Fluid retention	35	8	34	7	21	6
Superficial localized edema	18	1	14	0	3	0
Pleural effusion	21	7	20	7	21	6
Generalized edema	1	0	3	0	0	0
Pericardial effusion	3	1	0	0	0	0
Congestive heart failure/cardiac dysfunction[a]	0	0	4	0	0	0
Pulmonary edema	1	0	4	3	0	0
Headache	27	1	18	1	15	3
Diarrhea	31	3	20	5	18	0
Fatigue	19	2	20	1	9	3
Dyspnea	20	3	15	3	3	3
Musculoskeletal pain	11	0	8	1	0	0
Nausea	19	1	23	4	21	3
Skin rash[b]	15	0	16	1	21	0
Arthralgia	10	0	5	1	0	0
Infection (including bacterial, viral, fungal, and non-specified)	10	6	14	7	9	0
Hemorrhage	26	8	19	9	24	9
Gastrointestinal bleeding	8	6	9	7	9	3
CNS bleeding	1	1	0	0	3	3
Vomiting	11	1	12	0	15	0
Pyrexia	11	2	18	3	6	0
Febrile neutropenia	4	4	12	12	12	12

[a] Includes ventricular dysfunction, cardiac failure, cardiac failure congestive, cardiomyopathy, congestive cardiomyopathy, diastolic dysfunction, ejection fraction decreased, and ventricular failure.

[b] Includes drug eruption, erythema, erythema multiforme, erythrosis, exfoliative rash, generalized erythema, genital rash, heat rash, milia, rash, rash erythematous, rash follicular, rash generalized, rash macular, rash maculopapular, rash papular, rash pruritic, rash pustular, skin exfoliation, skin irritation, urticaria vesiculosa, and rash vesicular.

Table 6: CTC Grade 3/4 Laboratory Abnormalities in Clinical Studies of CML: Resistance or Intolerance to Prior Imatinib Therapy

	Chronic Phase CML 100 mg Once Daily	Advanced Phase CML 140 mg Once Daily		
		Accelerated Phase (n=157)	Myeloid Blast Phase (n=74)	Lymphoid Blast Phase (n=33)
	(n=165)	Percent (%) of Patients		
Hematology Parameters*				
Neutropenia	36	58	77	79
Thrombocytopenia	24	63	78	85
Anemia	13	47	74	52
Biochemistry Parameters				
Hypophosphatemia	10	13	12	18
Hypokalemia	2	7	11	15
Hypocalcemia	<1	4	9	12
Elevated SGPT (ALT)	0	2	5	3
Elevated SGOT (AST)	<1	0	4	3
Elevated Bilirubin	<1	1	3	6
Elevated Creatinine	0	2	8	0

CTC grades: neutropenia (Grade 3 ≥0.5–<1.0 × 10^9/L, Grade 4 <0.5 × 10^9/L); thrombocytopenia (Grade 3 ≥25–<50 × 10^9/L, Grade 4 <25 × 10^9/L); anemia (hemoglobin Grade 3 ≥65–<80 g/L, Grade 4 <65 g/L); elevated creatinine (Grade 3 >3–6 × upper limit of normal range (ULN), Grade 4 >6 × ULN); elevated bilirubin (Grade 3 >3–10 × ULN, Grade 4 >10 × ULN); elevated SGOT or SGPT (Grade 3 >5–20 × ULN, Grade 4 >20 × ULN); hypocalcemia (Grade 3 <7.0–6.0 mg/dL, Grade 4 <6.0 mg/dL); hypophosphatemia (Grade 3 <2.0–1.0 mg/dL, Grade 4 <1.0 mg/dL); hypokalemia (Grade 3 <3.0–2.5 mmol/L, Grade 4 <2.5 mmol/L).

* Hematology parameters for 100 mg once-daily dosing in chronic phase CML reflects 60 month minimum follow up.

Laboratory abnormalities reported in patients with CML resistant or intolerant to imatinib who received the recommended starting doses of SPRYCEL (dasatinib) are shown by disease phase in Table 6.

[See table 6 above]

Among chronic phase CML patients with resistance or intolerance to prior imatinib therapy, cumulative Grade 3 or 4 cytopenias were similar at 2 and 5 years including: neutropenia (36% vs 36%), thrombocytopenia (23% vs 24%), and anemia (13% vs 13%).

6.2 Philadelphia Chromosome-Positive Acute Lymphoblastic Leukemia (Ph+ ALL)

A total of 135 patients with Ph+ ALL were treated with SPRYCEL in clinical studies. The median duration of treatment was 3 months (range 0.03–31 months). The safety profile of patients with Ph+ ALL was similar to those with lymphoid blast phase CML. The most frequently reported adverse reactions included fluid retention events, such as pleural effusion (24%) and superficial edema (19%), and gastrointestinal disorders, such as diarrhea (31%), nausea (24%), and vomiting (16%). Hemorrhage (19%), pyrexia (17%), rash (16%), and dyspnea (16%) were also frequently reported. The most frequently reported serious adverse reactions included pleural effusion (11%), gastrointestinal bleeding (7%), febrile neutropenia (6%), infection (5%), pyrexia (4%), pneumonia (3%), diarrhea (3%), nausea (2%), vomiting (2%), and colitis (2%).

6.3 Additional Data From Clinical Trials
The following adverse reactions were reported in patients in the SPRYCEL (dasatinib) clinical studies at a frequency of ≥10%, 1%–<10%, 0.1%–<1%, or <0.1%. These events are included on the basis of clinical relevance.

Gastrointestinal Disorders: 1%–<10% – mucosal inflammation (including mucositis/stomatitis), dyspepsia, abdominal distension, constipation, gastritis, colitis (including neutropenic colitis), oral soft tissue disorder; 0.1%–<1% – ascites, dysphagia, anal fissure, upper gastrointestinal ulcer, esophagitis, pancreatitis; <0.1% – protein losing gastroenteropathy, ileus.

General Disorders and Administration Site Conditions: 1%–<10% – asthenia, pain, chest pain, chills; 0.1%–<1% – malaise, temperature intolerance.

Skin and Subcutaneous Tissue Disorders: 1%–<10% – pruritus, alopecia, acne, dry skin, hyperhidrosis, urticaria, dermatitis (including eczema); 0.1%–<1% – pigmentation disorder, skin ulcer, bullous conditions, photosensitivity, nail disorder, acute febrile neutrophilic dermatosis, panniculitis, palmar-plantar erythrodysesthesia syndrome.

Respiratory, Thoracic, and Mediastinal Disorders: ≥10% – cough; 1%–<10% – lung infiltration, pneumonitis, pulmonary hypertension; 0.1%–<1% – asthma, bronchospasm; <0.1% – acute respiratory distress syndrome.

Nervous System Disorders: 1%–<10% – neuropathy (including peripheral neuropathy), dizziness, dysgeusia, somnolence; 0.1%–<1% – amnesia, tremor, syncope; <0.1% – convulsion, cerebrovascular accident, transient ischemic attack, optic neuritis, VIIth nerve paralysis.

Blood and Lymphatic System Disorders: 1%–<10% – pancytopenia; <0.1% – aplasia pure red cell.

Musculoskeletal and Connective Tissue Disorders: 1%–<10% – muscular weakness, musculoskeletal stiffness, muscle spasm; 0.1%–<1% – rhabdomyolysis, tendonitis, muscle inflammation.

Investigations: 1%–<10% – weight increased, weight decreased; 0.1%–<1% – blood creatine phosphokinase increased.

Infections and Infestations: 1%–<10% – pneumonia (including bacterial, viral, and fungal), upper respiratory tract infection/inflammation, herpes virus infection, enterocolitis infection, sepsis (including fatal outcomes [0.2%]).

Metabolism and Nutrition Disorders: 1%–<10% – anorexia, appetite disturbances, hyperuricemia; 0.1%–<1% – hypoalbuminemia.

Cardiac Disorders: 1%–<10% – arrhythmia (including tachycardia), palpitations; 0.1%–<1% – angina pectoris, cardiomegaly, pericarditis, ventricular arrhythmia (including ventricular tachycardia); <0.1% – cor pulmonale, myocarditis, acute coronary syndrome.

Eye Disorders: 1%–<10% – visual disorder (including visual disturbance, vision blurred, and visual acuity reduced), dry eye; 0.1%–<1% – conjunctivitis; <0.1% – visual impairment.

Vascular Disorders: 1%–<10% – flushing, hypertension; 0.1%–<1% – hypotension, thrombophlebitis; <0.1% – livedo reticularis.

Psychiatric Disorders: 1%–<10% – insomnia, depression; 0.1%–<1% – anxiety, affect lability, confusional state, libido decreased.

Reproductive System and Breast Disorders: 0.1%–<1% – gynecomastia, menstruation irregular.

Injury, Poisoning, and Procedural Complications: 1%–<10% – contusion.

Ear and Labyrinth Disorders: 1%–<10% – tinnitus; 0.1%–<1% – vertigo.

Hepatobiliary Disorders: 0.1%–<1% – cholestasis, cholecystitis, hepatitis.

Renal and Urinary Disorders: 0.1%–<1% – urinary frequency, renal failure, proteinuria.

Neoplasms Benign, Malignant, and Unspecified: 0.1%–<1% – tumor lysis syndrome.

Immune System Disorders: 0.1%–<1% – hypersensitivity (including erythema nodosum).

6.4 Postmarketing Experience
The following additional adverse reactions have been identified during post approval use of SPRYCEL. Because these reactions are reported voluntarily from a population of uncertain size, it is not always possible to reliably estimate their frequency or establish a causal relationship to drug exposure.

Cardiac disorders: atrial fibrillation/atrial flutter
Vascular disorders: thrombosis/embolism (including pulmonary embolism, deep vein thrombosis)
Respiratory, thoracic, and mediastinal disorders: interstitial lung disease, pulmonary arterial hypertension

7 DRUG INTERACTIONS
7.1 Drugs That May Increase Dasatinib Plasma Concentrations
CYP3A4 Inhibitors: Dasatinib is a CYP3A4 substrate. In a trial of 18 patients with solid tumors, 20-mg SPRYCEL (dasatinib) once daily coadministered with 200 mg of ketoconazole twice daily increased the dasatinib C_{max} and AUC by four- and five-fold, respectively. Concomitant use of SPRYCEL and drugs that inhibit CYP3A4 may increase exposure to dasatinib and should be avoided. In patients receiving treatment with SPRYCEL, close monitoring for toxicity and a SPRYCEL dose reduction should be considered if systemic administration of a potent CYP3A4 inhibitor cannot be avoided [see Dosage and Administration (2.1)].

7.2 Drugs That May Decrease Dasatinib Plasma Concentrations
CYP3A4 Inducers: When a single morning dose of SPRYCEL was administered following 8 days of continuous evening administration of 600 mg of rifampin, a potent CYP3A4 inducer, the mean C_{max} and AUC of dasatinib were decreased by 81% and 82%, respectively. Alternative agents with less enzyme induction potential should be considered. If SPRYCEL must be administered with a CYP3A4 inducer, a dose increase in SPRYCEL should be considered [see Dosage and Administration (2.1)].

Antacids: Nonclinical data demonstrate that the solubility of dasatinib is pH dependent. In a trial of 24 healthy subjects, administration of 30 mL of aluminum hydroxide/magnesium hydroxide 2 hours prior to a single 50-mg dose of SPRYCEL was associated with no relevant change in dasatinib AUC; however, the dasatinib C_{max} increased 26%. When 30 mL of aluminum hydroxide/magnesium hydroxide was administered to the same subjects concomitantly with a 50-mg dose of SPRYCEL, a 55% reduction in dasatinib AUC and a 58% reduction in C_{max} were observed. Simultaneous administration of SPRYCEL with antacids should be avoided. If antacid therapy is needed, the antacid dose should be administered at least 2 hours prior to or 2 hours after the dose of SPRYCEL.

H₂ Antagonists/Proton Pump Inhibitors: Long-term suppression of gastric acid secretion by H_2 antagonists or proton pump inhibitors (eg, famotidine and omeprazole) is likely to reduce dasatinib exposure. In a trial of 24 healthy subjects, administration of a single 50-mg dose of SPRYCEL 10 hours following famotidine reduced the AUC and C_{max} of dasatinib by 61% and 63%, respectively. In a trial of 14 healthy subjects, administration of a single 100-mg dose of SPRYCEL 22 hours following a 40-mg omeprazole dose at steady state reduced the AUC and C_{max} of dasatinib by 43% and 42%, respectively. The concomitant use of H_2 antagonists or proton pump inhibitors with SPRYCEL is not recommended. The use of antacids (at least 2 hours prior to or 2 hours after the dose of SPRYCEL) should be considered in place of H_2 antagonists or proton pump inhibitors in patients receiving SPRYCEL therapy.

7.3 Drugs That May Have Their Plasma Concentration Altered By Dasatinib
CYP3A4 Substrates: Single-dose data from a trial of 54 healthy subjects indicate that the mean C_{max} and AUC of simvastatin, a CYP3A4 substrate, were increased by 37% and 20%, respectively, when simvastatin was administered in combination with a single 100-mg dose of SPRYCEL. Therefore, CYP3A4 substrates known to have a narrow therapeutic index such as alfentanil, astemizole, terfenadine, cisapride, cyclosporine, fentanyl, pimozide, quinidine, sirolimus, tacrolimus, or ergot alkaloids (ergotamine, dihydroergotamine) should be administered with caution in patients receiving SPRYCEL.

8 USE IN SPECIFIC POPULATIONS
8.1 Pregnancy
Pregnancy Category D
Risk Summary
SPRYCEL can cause fetal harm when administered to a pregnant woman. There are no studies with SPRYCEL in pregnant women. However, in animal reproduction studies, embryo-fetal toxicities, including skeletal malformations, were observed at dasatinib doses producing plasma concentrations below those in humans receiving therapeutic doses of dasatinib. If SPRYCEL is used during pregnancy, or if the patient becomes pregnant while taking SPRYCEL, the patient should be apprised of the potential risk to the fetus. [See Warnings and Precautions (5.7).]
Data
Based on human experience, dasatinib is suspected to cause congenital malformations, including neural tube defects, and harmful pharmacological effects on the fetus when administered during pregnancy.

Clinical Considerations
Fetal / Neonatal Adverse Reactions
Transplacental transfer of dasatinib has been reported. Dasatinib has been measured in fetal plasma and amniotic fluid and concentrations were found to be comparable to those in maternal plasma. Hydrops fetalis and fetal bicytopenia have been reported with maternal exposure to dasatinib. There have been other reports of maternal dasatinib exposure with no adverse fetal outcomes noted.
Animal Data
In nonclinical studies, at plasma concentrations below those observed in humans receiving therapeutic doses of dasatinib, embryo-fetal toxicities were observed in rats and rabbits. Fetal death was observed in rats. In both rats and rabbits, the lowest doses of dasatinib tested (rat: 2.5 mg/kg/day [15 mg/m²/day] and rabbit: 0.5 mg/kg/day [6 mg/m²/day]) resulted in embryo-fetal toxicities. These doses produced maternal AUCs of 105 ng•hr/mL and 44 ng•hr/mL (0.1-fold the human AUC) in rats and rabbits, respectively. Embryo-fetal toxicities included skeletal malformations at multiple sites (scapula, humerus, femur, radius, ribs, and clavicle), reduced ossification (sternum; thoracic, lumbar, and sacral vertebrae; forepaw phalanges; pelvis; and hyoid body), edema, and microhepatia. In a pre- and postnatal development study in rats, administration of dasatinib from gestation day (GD) 16 through lactation day (LD) 20, GD 21 through LD 20, or LD 4 through LD 20 resulted in extensive pup mortality at maternal exposures that were below the exposures in patients treated with dasatinib at the recommended labeling dose.

8.3 Nursing Mothers
It is unknown whether SPRYCEL (dasatinib) is present in human milk. However, dasatinib was present in the milk of lactating rats. Because many drugs are excreted in human milk and because of the potential for serious adverse reactions in nursing infants from SPRYCEL, a decision should be made whether to discontinue nursing or to discontinue the drug, taking into account the importance of the drug to the mother.

8.4 Pediatric Use
The safety and efficacy of SPRYCEL in patients less than 18 years of age have not been established.

8.5 Geriatric Use
In the newly diagnosed chronic phase CML trial, 25 patients (10%) were 65 years of age and over and 7 patients (3%) were 75 years of age and over. Of the 2182 patients in clinical studies of SPRYCEL with resistance or intolerance to imatinib therapy, 547 (25%) were 65 years of age and over and 105 (5%) were 75 years of age and over. No differences in efficacy were observed between older and younger patients. Compared to patients under age 65 years, patients aged 65 years and older are more likely to experience toxicity.

8.6 Hepatic Impairment
The effect of hepatic impairment on the pharmacokinetics of dasatinib was evaluated in healthy volunteers with normal liver function and patients with moderate (Child-Pugh class B) and severe (Child-Pugh class C) hepatic impairment. Compared to the healthy volunteers with normal hepatic function, the dose-normalized pharmacokinetic parameters were decreased in the patients with hepatic impairment. No dosage adjustment is necessary in patients with hepatic impairment [see Clinical Pharmacology (12.3)]. Caution is recommended when administering SPRYCEL to patients with hepatic impairment.

8.7 Renal Impairment
There are currently no clinical studies with SPRYCEL in patients with impaired renal function. Less than 4% of dasatinib and its metabolites are excreted via the kidney.

8.8 Females of Reproductive Potential
SPRYCEL can cause fetal harm when administered during pregnancy. Advise female patients of reproductive potential to avoid pregnancy, which may include the use of contraception, during treatment. Advise patients to contact their healthcare provider if they become pregnant, or if pregnancy is suspected, while taking SPRYCEL [see Use in Specific Populations (8.1)].

10 OVERDOSAGE
Experience with overdose of SPRYCEL in clinical studies is limited to isolated cases. The highest overdosage of 280 mg per day for 1 week was reported in two patients and both developed severe myelosuppression and bleeding. Since SPRYCEL is associated with severe myelosuppression [see Warnings and Precautions (5.1) and Adverse Reactions (6.1)], patients who ingested more than the recommended dosage should be closely monitored for myelosuppression and given appropriate supportive treatment.
Acute overdose in animals was associated with cardiotoxicity. Evidence of cardiotoxicity included ventricular necrosis and valvular/ventricular/atrial hemorrhage at single doses ≥100 mg/kg (600 mg/m²) in rodents. There was a tendency for increased systolic and diastolic blood pressure in monkeys at single doses ≥10 mg/kg (120 mg/m²).

11 DESCRIPTION
SPRYCEL (dasatinib) is a kinase inhibitor. The chemical name for dasatinib is N-(2-chloro-6-methylphenyl)-

2-[[6-[4-(2-hydroxyethyl)-1-piperazinyl]-2-methyl-4-pyrimidinyl]amino]-5-thiazolecarboxamide, monohydrate. The molecular formula is $C_{22}H_{26}ClN_7O_2S \cdot H_2O$, which corresponds to a formula weight of 506.02 (monohydrate). The anhydrous free base has a molecular weight of 488.01. Dasatinib has the following chemical structure:

Dasatinib is a white to off-white powder. The drug substance is insoluble in water and slightly soluble in ethanol and methanol. SPRYCEL (dasatinib) tablets are white to off-white, biconvex, film-coated tablets containing dasatinib, with the following inactive ingredients: lactose monohydrate, microcrystalline cellulose, croscarmellose sodium, hydroxypropyl cellulose, and magnesium stearate. The tablet coating consists of hypromellose, titanium dioxide, and polyethylene glycol.

12 CLINICAL PHARMACOLOGY

12.1 Mechanism of Action

Dasatinib, at nanomolar concentrations, inhibits the following kinases: BCR-ABL, SRC family (SRC, LCK, YES, FYN), c-KIT, EPHA2, and PDGFRβ. Based on modeling studies, dasatinib is predicted to bind to multiple conformations of the ABL kinase.

In vitro, dasatinib was active in leukemic cell lines representing variants of imatinib mesylate sensitive and resistant disease. Dasatinib inhibited the growth of chronic myeloid leukemia (CML) and acute lymphoblastic leukemia (ALL) cell lines overexpressing BCR-ABL. Under the conditions of the assays, dasatinib was able to overcome imatinib resistance resulting from BCR-ABL kinase domain mutations, activation of alternate signaling pathways involving the SRC family kinases (LYN, HCK), and multi-drug resistance gene overexpression.

12.3 Pharmacokinetics

Absorption

Maximum plasma concentrations (C_{max}) of dasatinib are observed between 0.5 and 6 hours (T_{max}) following oral administration. Dasatinib exhibits dose proportional increases in AUC and linear elimination characteristics over the dose range of 15 mg to 240 mg/day. The overall mean terminal half-life of dasatinib is 3 to 5 hours.

Data from a trial of 54 healthy subjects administered a single, 100-mg dose of dasatinib 30 minutes following consumption of a high-fat meal resulted in a 14% increase in the mean AUC of dasatinib. The observed food effects were not clinically relevant.

Distribution

In patients, dasatinib has an apparent volume of distribution of 2505 L, suggesting that the drug is extensively distributed in the extravascular space. Binding of dasatinib and its active metabolite to human plasma proteins *in vitro* was approximately 96% and 93%, respectively, with no concentration dependence over the range of 100 to 500 ng/mL.

Metabolism

Dasatinib is extensively metabolized in humans, primarily by the cytochrome P450 enzyme 3A4. CYP3A4 was the primary enzyme responsible for the formation of the active metabolite. Flavin-containing monooxygenase 3 (FMO-3) and uridine diphosphate-glucuronosyltransferase (UGT) enzymes are also involved in the formation of dasatinib metabolites.

The exposure of the active metabolite, which is equipotent to dasatinib, represents approximately 5% of the dasatinib AUC. This indicates that the active metabolite is unlikely to play a major role in the observed pharmacology of the drug. Dasatinib also had several other inactive oxidative metabolites.

Dasatinib is a weak time-dependent inhibitor of CYP3A4. At clinically relevant concentrations, dasatinib does not inhibit CYP1A2, 2A6, 2B6, 2C8, 2C9, 2C19, 2D6, or 2E1. Dasatinib is not an inducer of human CYP enzymes.

Elimination

Elimination is primarily via the feces. Following a single oral dose of [^{14}C]-labeled dasatinib, approximately 4% and 85% of the administered radioactivity was recovered in the urine and feces, respectively, within 10 days. Unchanged dasatinib accounted for 0.1% and 19% of the administered dose in urine and feces, respectively, with the remainder of the dose being metabolites.

Effects of Age and Gender

Pharmacokinetic analyses of demographic data indicate that there are no clinically relevant effects of age and gender on the pharmacokinetics of dasatinib.

Hepatic Impairment

Dasatinib doses of 50 mg and 20 mg were evaluated in eight patients with moderate (Child-Pugh class B) and seven patients with severe (Child-Pugh class C) hepatic impairment, respectively. Matched controls with normal hepatic function (n=15) were also evaluated and received a dasatinib dose of 70 mg. Compared to subjects with normal liver function, patients with moderate hepatic impairment had decreases in dose-normalized C_{max} and AUC by 47% and 8%, respectively. Patients with severe hepatic impairment had dose-normalized C_{max} decreased by 43% and AUC decreased by 28% compared to the normal controls.

These differences in C_{max} and AUC are not clinically relevant. Dose adjustment is not necessary in patients with hepatic impairment.

13 NONCLINICAL TOXICOLOGY

13.1 Carcinogenesis, Mutagenesis, Impairment of Fertility

In a two-year carcinogenicity study, rats were administered oral doses of dasatinib at 0.3, 1, and 3 mg/kg/day. The highest dose resulted in a plasma drug exposure (AUC) level approximately 60% of the human exposure at 100 mg once daily. Dasatinib induced a statistically significant increase in the combined incidence of squamous cell carcinomas and papillomas in the uterus and cervix of high-dose females and prostate adenoma in low-dose males.

Dasatinib was clastogenic when tested *in vitro* in Chinese hamster ovary cells, with and without metabolic activation. Dasatinib was not mutagenic when tested in an *in vitro* bacterial cell assay (Ames test) and was not genotoxic in an *in vivo* rat micronucleus study.

Dasatinib did not affect mating or fertility in male and female rats at plasma drug exposure (AUC) similar to the human exposure at 100 mg daily; however, dasatinib induced embryo lethality. In repeat dose studies, administration of dasatinib resulted in reduced size and secretion of seminal vesicles, and immature prostate, seminal vesicle, and testis. The administration of dasatinib resulted in uterine inflammation and mineralization in monkeys, and cystic ovaries and ovarian hypertrophy in rodents.

14 CLINICAL STUDIES

14.1 Newly Diagnosed Chronic Phase CML

An open-label, multicenter, international, randomized trial was conducted in adult patients with newly diagnosed chronic phase CML. A total of 519 patients were randomized to receive either SPRYCEL (dasatinib) 100 mg once daily or imatinib 400 mg once daily. Patients with a history of cardiac disease were included in this trial except those which had a myocardial infarction within 6 months, congestive heart failure within 3 months, significant arrhythmias, or QTc prolongation. The primary endpoint was the rate of confirmed complete cytogenetic response (CCyR) within 12 months. Confirmed CCyR was defined as a CCyR noted on two consecutive occasions (at least 28 days apart).

Median age was 46 years in the SPRYCEL group and 49 years in the imatinib groups, with 10% and 11% of patients ≥65 years of age. There were slightly more male than female patients in both groups (59% vs 41%). Fifty-three percent of all patients were Caucasian and 39% were Asian. At baseline, the distribution of Hasford Scores was similar in the SPRYCEL and imatinib treatment groups (low risk: 33% and 34%; intermediate risk: 48% and 47%; high risk: 19% and 19%, respectively). With a minimum of 12 months follow-up, 85% of patients randomized to SPRYCEL and 81% of patients randomized to imatinib were still on study. With a minimum of 24 months follow up, 77% of patients randomized to SPRYCEL and 75% of patients randomized to imatinib were still on study and with a minimum of 36 months follow up, 71% and 69% of patients, respectively, were still on study.

Efficacy results are summarized in Table 7.

[See table 7 above]

After 36 months follow up, median time to confirmed CCyR was 3.1 months in 214 SPRYCEL (dasatinib) responders and 5.8 months in 201 imatinib responders. Median time to MMR after 36 months follow up was 8.9 months in 179 SPRYCEL responders and 13.4 months in 146 imatinib responders.

At 36 months, 8 patients (3%) on the dasatinib arm progressed to either accelerated phase or blast crisis while 13 patients (5%) on the imatinib arm progressed to either accelerated phase or blast crisis.

The rate of MMR at any time in each risk group determined by Hasford score was higher in the SPRYCEL group compared with the imatinib group (low risk: 81% and 64%; intermediate risk: 64% and 56%; high risk: 61% and 42%, respectively).

BCR-ABL sequencing was performed on blood samples from patients in the newly diagnosed trial who discontinued dasatinib or imatinib therapy. Among dasatinib-treated patients the mutations detected were T315I, F317I/L, and V299L.

Dasatinib does not appear to be active against the T315I mutation, based on *in vitro* data.

14.2 Imatinib-resistant or Intolerant CML or Ph+ ALL

The efficacy and safety of SPRYCEL were investigated in adult patients with CML or Ph+ ALL whose disease was resistant to or who were intolerant to imatinib: 1158 patients had chronic phase CML, 858 patients had accelerated phase, myeloid blast phase, or lymphoid blast phase CML, and 130 patients had Ph+ ALL. In a clinical trial in chronic phase CML, resistance to imatinib was defined as failure to achieve a complete hematologic response (CHR; after 3 months), major cytogenetic response (MCyR; after 6 months), or complete cytogenetic response (CCyR; after 12 months); or loss of a previous molecular response (with concurrent ≥10% increase in Ph+ metaphases), cytogenetic response, or hematologic response. Imatinib intolerance was defined as inability to tolerate 400 mg or more of imatinib per day or discontinuation of imatinib because of toxicity.

Results described below are based on a minimum of 2 years follow up after the start of SPRYCEL therapy in patients with a median time from initial diagnosis of approximately 5 years. Across all studies, 48% of patients were women, 81% were white, 15% were black or Asian, 25% were 65 years of age or older, and 5% were 75 years of age or older. Most patients had long disease histories with extensive prior treatment, including imatinib, cytotoxic chemotherapy, interferon, and stem cell transplant. Overall, 80% of patients had imatinib-resistant disease and 20% of patients were intolerant to imatinib. The maximum imatinib dose had been 400–600 mg/day in about 60% of the patients and >600 mg/day in 40% of the patients.

The primary efficacy endpoint in chronic phase CML was MCyR, defined as elimination (CCyR) or substantial diminution (by at least 65%, partial cytogenetic response) of Ph+ hematopoietic cells. The primary efficacy endpoint in accelerated phase, myeloid blast phase, lymphoid blast phase CML, and Ph+ ALL was major hematologic response (MaHR), defined as either a CHR or no evidence of leukemia (NEL).

Table 7: Efficacy Results in Newly Diagnosed Patients with Chronic Phase CML

	SPRYCEL (n=259)	Imatinib (n=260)	p-value
	Response Rate (95% CI)		
Confirmed CCyR[a]			
within 12 months	76.8% (71.2–81.8)	66.2% (60.1–71.9)	p=0.007*
within 24 months	80.3%	74.2%	_**
within 36 months	82.6%	77.3%	_**
Major Molecular Response[b]			
12 months	52.1% (45.9–58.3)	33.8% (28.1–39.9)	p<0.0001*
24 months	64.5% (58.3–70.3)	50% (43.8–56.2)	_**
36 months	69.1% (63.1–74.7)	56.2% (49.9–62.3)	_**

[a] Confirmed CCyR is defined as a CCyR noted on two consecutive occasions at least 28 days apart.
[b] Major molecular response (at any time) was defined as BCR-ABL ratios ≤0.1% by RQ-PCR in peripheral blood samples standardized on the International scale. These are cumulative rates representing minimum follow up for the time frame specified.
* Adjusted for Hasford Score and indicated statistical significance at a pre-defined nominal level of significance.
** Formal statistical comparison of cCCyR and MMR rates was only performed at the time of the primary endpoint (cCCyR within 12 months).
CI = confidence interval.

Chronic Phase CML

Dose-Optimization Trial: A randomized, open-label trial was conducted in patients with chronic phase CML to evaluate the efficacy and safety of SPRYCEL (dasatinib) administered once daily compared with SPRYCEL administered twice daily. Patients with significant cardiac diseases, including myocardial infarction within 6 months, congestive heart failure within 3 months, significant arrhythmias, or QTc prolongation were excluded from the trial. The primary efficacy endpoint was MCyR in patients with imatinib-resistant CML. A total of 670 patients, of whom 497 had imatinib-resistant disease, were randomized to the SPRYCEL 100 mg once daily, 140 mg once daily, 50 mg twice daily, or 70 mg twice daily group. Median duration of treatment was 22 months.

Efficacy was achieved across all SPRYCEL treatment groups with the once daily schedule demonstrating comparable efficacy (non-inferiority) to the twice daily schedule on the primary efficacy endpoint (difference in MCyR 1.9%; 95% CI [−6.8%–10.6%]).

Efficacy results are presented in Table 8 for patients with chronic phase CML who received the recommended starting dose of 100 mg once daily. Additional efficacy results in this patient population are described after the table. Results for all patients with chronic phase CML, regardless of dosage (a starting dosage of 100 mg once daily, 140 mg once daily, 50 mg twice daily, or 70 mg twice daily), were consistent with those for patients treated with 100 mg once daily.

Table 8: Efficacy of SPRYCEL in Imatinib Resistant or Intolerant Chronic Phase CML (minimum of 24 months follow up)

	100 mg Once Daily (n=167)
CHR[a]% (95% CI)	92% (86–95)
MCyR[b]% (95% CI)	63% (56–71)
CCyR% (95% CI)	50% (42–58)

[a] CHR (response confirmed after 4 weeks): WBC ≤ institutional ULN, platelets <450,000/mm^3, no blasts or promyelocytes in peripheral blood, <5% myelocytes plus metamyelocytes in peripheral blood, basophils in peripheral blood <20%, and no extramedullary involvement.
[b] MCyR combines both complete (0% Ph+ metaphases) and partial (>0%–35%) responses.

In the SPRYCEL 100 mg once daily group, median time to MCyR was 2.9 months (95% CI: [2.8%–3.0%]) with a minimum of 24 months follow up. Based on the Kaplan-Meier estimates, 93% (95% CI: [88%–98%]) of patients who had achieved an MCyR maintained that response for 18 months. In the 100 mg once daily group, MMR was achieved in 43% of all randomized patients within 5 years. The estimated rate of progression-free survival and overall survival at 2 years in all patients treated with 100 mg once daily was 80% (95% CI: [73%–87%]) and 91% (95% CI: [86%–96%]), respectively. Based on data six years after the last patient was enrolled in the trial, 64% were known to be alive at 5 years, 22% were known to have died prior to 5 years and 14% had an unknown 5-year survival status.

By 5 years, transformation to either accelerated or blast phase occurred in eight patients on treatment.

Advanced Phase CML and Ph+ ALL

Dose-Optimization Trial: One randomized open-label trial was conducted in patients with advanced phase CML (accelerated phase CML, myeloid blast phase CML, or lymphoid blast phase CML) to evaluate the efficacy and safety of SPRYCEL administered once daily compared with SPRYCEL administered twice daily. The primary efficacy endpoint was MaHR. A total of 611 patients were randomized to either the SPRYCEL 140 mg once daily or 70 mg twice daily group. Median duration of treatment was approximately 6 months for both treatment groups. The once daily schedule demonstrated comparable efficacy (non-inferiority) to the twice daily schedule on the primary efficacy endpoint.

The efficacy and safety of SPRYCEL were also investigated in patients with Ph+ ALL in one randomized trial (starting dosage 140 mg once daily or 70 mg twice daily) and one single-arm trial (starting dosage 70 mg twice daily). The primary efficacy endpoint was MaHR. A total of 130 patients were enrolled in these studies. The median duration of therapy was 3 months.

Response rates are presented in Table 9.

[See table 9 above]

In the SPRYCEL 140 mg once daily group, the median time to MaHR was 1.9 months for patients with accelerated phase CML, 1.9 months for patients with myeloid blast phase CML, and 1.8 months for patients with lymphoid blast phase CML.

In patients with myeloid blast phase CML, the median duration of MaHR was 8 months and 9 months for the 140 mg

Table 9: Efficacy of SPRYCEL in Imatinib Resistant or Intolerant Advanced Phase CML and Ph+ ALL

	140 mg Once Daily			
	Accelerated (n=158)	Myeloid Blast (n=75)	Lymphoid Blast (n=33)	Ph+ALL (n=40)
MaHR[a]	66%	28%	42%	38%
(95% CI)	(59–74)	(18–40)	(26–61)	(23–54)
CHR[a]	47%	17%	21%	33%
(95% CI)	(40–56)	(10–28)	(9–39)	(19–49)
NEL[a]	19%	11%	21%	5%
(95% CI)	(13–26)	(5–20)	(9–39)	(1–17)
MCyR[b]	39%	28%	52%	70%
(95% CI)	(31–47)	(18–40)	(34–69)	(54–83)
CCyR	32%	17%	39%	50%
(95% CI)	(25–40)	(10–28)	(23–58)	(34–66)

[a] Hematologic response criteria (all responses confirmed after 4 weeks): Major hematologic response: (MaHR) = complete hematologic response (CHR) + no evidence of leukemia (NEL).
CHR: WBC ≤ institutional ULN, ANC ≥1000/mm^3, platelets ≥100,000/mm^3, no blasts or promyelocytes in peripheral blood, bone marrow blasts ≤5%, <5% myelocytes plus metamyelocytes in peripheral blood, basophils in peripheral blood <20%, and no extramedullary involvement.
NEL: same criteria as for CHR but ANC ≥500/mm^3 and <1000/mm^3, or platelets ≥20,000/mm^3 and ≤100,000/mm^3.
[b] MCyR combines both complete (0% Ph+ metaphases) and partial (>0%–35%) responses.
CI = confidence interval ULN = upper limit of normal range.

Table 10: SPRYCEL Trade Presentations

NDC Number	Strength	Description	Tablets per Bottle
0003-0527-11	20 mg	white to off-white, biconvex, round, film-coated tablet with "BMS" debossed on one side and "527" on the other side	60
0003-0528-11	50 mg	white to off-white, biconvex, oval, film-coated tablet with "BMS" debossed on one side and "528" on the other side	60
0003-0524-11	70 mg	white to off-white, biconvex, round, film-coated tablet with "BMS" debossed on one side and "524" on the other side	60
0003-0855-22	80 mg	white to off-white, biconvex, triangle, film-coated tablet with "BMS" and "80" (BMS over 80) debossed on one side and "855" on the other side	30
0003-0852-22	100 mg	white to off-white, biconvex, oval, film-coated tablet with "BMS 100" debossed on one side and "852" on the other side	30
0003-0857-22	140 mg	white to off-white, biconvex, round, film-coated tablet with "BMS" and "140" (BMS over 140) debossed on one side and "857" on the other side	30

once daily group and the 70 mg twice daily group, respectively. In patients with lymphoid blast phase CML, the median duration of MaHR was 5 months and 8 months for the 140 mg once daily group and the 70 mg twice daily group, respectively. In patients with Ph+ ALL who were treated with SPRYCEL 140 mg once daily, the median duration of MaHR was 4.6 months. The medians of progression-free survival for patients with Ph+ ALL treated with SPRYCEL 140 mg once daily and 70 mg twice daily were 4.0 months and 3.5 months, respectively.

16 HOW SUPPLIED/STORAGE AND HANDLING

16.1 How Supplied

SPRYCEL® (dasatinib) tablets are available as described in Table 10.

[See table 10 above]

16.2 Storage

SPRYCEL® tablets should be stored at 20°C to 25°C (68°F to 77°F); excursions permitted between 15°C and 30°C (59°F and 86°F) [see USP Controlled Room Temperature].

16.3 Handling and Disposal

SPRYCEL is an antineoplastic product. Follow special handling and disposal procedures.

SPRYCEL (dasatinib) tablets consist of a core tablet (containing the active drug substance), surrounded by a film coating to prevent exposure of pharmacy and clinical personnel to the active drug substance. However, if tablets are inadvertently crushed or broken, pharmacy and clinical personnel should wear disposable chemotherapy gloves. Personnel who are pregnant should avoid exposure to crushed or broken tablets.

17 PATIENT COUNSELING INFORMATION

See FDA-Approved Patient Labeling.

17.1 Bleeding

Patients should be informed of the possibility of serious bleeding and to report immediately any signs or symptoms suggestive of hemorrhage (unusual bleeding or easy bruising).

17.2 Myelosuppression

Patients should be informed of the possibility of developing low blood cell counts; they should be instructed to report immediately should fever develop, particularly in association with any suggestion of infection.

17.3 Fluid Retention

Patients should be informed of the possibility of developing fluid retention (swelling, weight gain, or shortness of breath) and to seek medical attention if those symptoms arise.

17.4 Embryo-fetal Toxicity

Patients should be informed that SPRYCEL (dasatinib) can cause fetal harm when administered to a pregnant woman. Women should be advised of the potential hazard to the fetus and to avoid becoming pregnant. If SPRYCEL is used during pregnancy, or if the patient becomes pregnant while taking SPRYCEL, the patient should be apprised of the potential hazard to the fetus [*see Warnings and Precautions (5.7)* and *Use in Specific Populations (8.1, 8.8)*].

17.5 Gastrointestinal Complaints

Patients should be informed that they may experience nausea, vomiting, or diarrhea with SPRYCEL. If these symptoms are significant, they should seek medical attention.

17.6 Pain

Patients should be informed that they may experience headache or musculoskeletal pain with SPRYCEL (dasatinib). If these symptoms are significant, they should seek medical attention.

17.7 Fatigue

Patients should be informed that they may experience fatigue with SPRYCEL. If this symptom is significant, they should seek medical attention.

17.8 Rash

Patients should be informed that they may experience skin rash with SPRYCEL. If this symptom is significant, they should seek medical attention.

17.9 Lactose

Patients should be informed that SPRYCEL contains 135 mg of lactose monohydrate in a 100-mg daily dose and 189 mg of lactose monohydrate in a 140-mg daily dose.

17.10 Missed Dose

If the patient misses a dose of SPRYCEL, the patient should take the next scheduled dose at its regular time. The patient should not take two doses at the same time.

PATIENT INFORMATION

SPRYCEL® (Spry-sell)
(dasatinib)
Tablets

Read the Patient Information that comes with SPRYCEL before you start taking it and each time you get a refill. There may be new information. This leaflet does not take the place of talking with your healthcare provider about your medical condition or treatment.

What is SPRYCEL?

SPRYCEL® is a prescription medicine used to treat adults who have:

- newly diagnosed Philadelphia chromosome-positive (Ph+) chronic myeloid leukemia (CML) in chronic phase.
- Ph+ CML who no longer benefit from, or did not tolerate, other treatment, including Gleevec® (imatinib mesylate).
- Philadelphia chromosome-positive acute lymphoblastic leukemia (Ph+ ALL) who no longer benefit from, or did not tolerate, other treatment.

It is not known if SPRYCEL is safe and effective in children younger than 18 years old.

What should I tell my healthcare provider before taking SPRYCEL?

Before you take SPRYCEL, tell your healthcare provider if you:

- have problems with your immune system
- have liver problems
- have heart problems
- are lactose intolerant
- have any other medical conditions
- are pregnant or planning to become pregnant. SPRYCEL can harm your unborn baby. Sexually active female patients of childbearing potential taking SPRYCEL should avoid pregnancy. Talk to your healthcare provider right away if you are pregnant or plan to become pregnant.
- are breastfeeding or plan to breastfeed. It is not known if SPRYCEL passes into your breast milk or if it can harm your baby. You and your healthcare provider should decide if you will take SPRYCEL or breastfeed. You should not do both.

Tell your healthcare provider about all the medicines you take, including prescription and non-prescription medicines, vitamins, antacids, and herbal supplements.

Especially tell your healthcare provider if you take:

- **medicines that increase the amount of SPRYCEL in your bloodstream, such as:**

Nizoral® (ketoconazole),	Nefazodone (serzone,
Sporanox® (itraconazole),	nefadar),
Norvir® (ritonavir),	Invirase® (saquinavir),
Reyataz® (atazanavir	Ketek® (telithromycin),
sulfate),	E-mycin® (erythromycin),
Crixivan® (indinavir),	Biaxin® (clarithromycin).
Viracept® (nelfinavir),	

- **medicines that decrease the amount of SPRYCEL in your bloodstream, such as:**

Decadron®	Rimactane® (rifampin),
(dexamethasone),	Luminal® (phenobarbital).
Dilantin® (phenytoin),	
Tegretol®	
(carbamazepine),	

- **medicines whose blood levels might change by taking SPRYCEL, such as:**

Sandimmune®	Rapamune® (sirolimus),
(cyclosporine),	Prograf® (tacrolimus),
Alfenta® (alfentanil),	Ergomar® (ergotamine).
Fentanyl® (fentanyl),	
Orap® (pimozide),	

SPRYCEL is best absorbed from your stomach into your bloodstream in the presence of stomach acid. You should avoid taking medicines that reduce stomach acid, such as:

Tagamet® (cimetidine),	Protonix® (pantoprazole
Pepcid® (famotidine),	sodium),
Zantac® (ranitidine),	Nexium® (esomeprazole),
Prilosec® (omeprazole),	AcipHex® (rabeprazole),
	Prevacid® (lansoprazole).

Medicines that neutralize stomach acid, such as Maalox® (aluminum hydroxide/magnesium hydroxide), Tums® (calcium carbonate), or Rolaids® (calcium carbonate and magnesia), may be taken up to 2 hours before or 2 hours after SPRYCEL (dasatinib).

Since SPRYCEL therapy may cause bleeding, tell your healthcare provider if you are using blood thinner medicine, such as Coumadin® (warfarin sodium) or aspirin.

Know the medicines you take. Keep a list of your medicines and show it to your healthcare provider and pharmacist when you get a new medicine.

How should I take SPRYCEL?

Take SPRYCEL exactly as prescribed by your healthcare provider.

- Take SPRYCEL with or without food. Try to take SPRYCEL at the same time each day.
- Swallow SPRYCEL tablets whole. Do not break, cut, or crush the tablets.
- You should not drink grapefruit juice while taking SPRYCEL.
- **Your healthcare provider may:**
  - **change your dose of SPRYCEL or**
  - **tell you to temporarily stop taking SPRYCEL.**
- **Do not change your dose or stop taking SPRYCEL without first talking with your healthcare provider.**
- **If you miss a dose of SPRYCEL,** take your next scheduled dose at its regular time. Do not take two doses at the same time. Call your healthcare provider or pharmacist if you are not sure what to do.
- **If you take too much SPRYCEL,** call your healthcare provider or go to the nearest hospital emergency room right away.

What are the possible side effects of SPRYCEL?

SPRYCEL may cause serious side effects, including:

- **Low Blood Cell Counts:** SPRYCEL may cause low red blood cell counts (anemia), low white blood cell counts (neutropenia), and low platelet counts (thrombocytopenia). Your healthcare provider will do blood tests to check your blood cell counts regularly during your treatment with SPRYCEL. Call your healthcare provider right away if you have a fever or any signs of an infection while taking SPRYCEL.
- **Bleeding:** SPRYCEL may cause severe bleeding that can lead to death. Call your healthcare provider right away if you have:
  - unusual bleeding or bruising of your skin
  - bright red or dark tar-like stools
  - a decrease in your level of consciousness, headache, or change in speech.
- **Your body may hold too much fluid (fluid retention):** In severe cases, fluid may build up in the lining of your lungs, the sac around your heart, or your stomach cavity. Call your healthcare provider right away if you get any of these symptoms during treatment with SPRYCEL:
  - swelling all over your body
  - weight gain
  - shortness of breath and cough.
- **Heart problems.** SPRYCEL may cause an abnormal heart rate, heart problems or a heart attack. Your healthcare provider will monitor the potassium and magnesium levels in your blood, and your heart function.
- **Pulmonary Arterial Hypertension (PAH).** SPRYCEL may cause high blood pressure in the vessels of your lungs. PAH may happen at any time during your treatment with SPRYCEL. Your healthcare provider should check your heart and lungs before and during your treatment with SPRYCEL. Call your healthcare provider right away if you have shortness of breath, tiredness, or swelling all over your body (fluid retention).

Other common side effects of SPRYCEL therapy include:

• diarrhea	• tiredness
• headache	• vomiting
• cough	• muscle pain
• skin rash	• weakness
• fever	• infections
• nausea	

Tell your healthcare provider if you have any side effect that bothers you or that does not go away.

These are not all of the possible side effects of SPRYCEL. For more information, ask your healthcare provider or pharmacist.

Call your doctor for medical advice about side effects. You may report side effects to FDA at 1-800-FDA-1088.

How should I store SPRYCEL?

- Store SPRYCEL at room temperature, between 68°F to 77°F (20°C to 25°C).

- Ask your healthcare provider or pharmacist about the right way to throw away outdated or unused SPRYCEL (dasatinib).
- Women who are pregnant should not handle crushed or broken SPRYCEL tablets.
- **Keep SPRYCEL and all medicines out of the reach of children and pets.**

General information about SPRYCEL

Medicines are sometimes prescribed for purposes other than those listed in the Patient Information leaflet. Do not use SPRYCEL for a condition for which it is not prescribed. Do not give SPRYCEL to other people even if they have the same symptoms you have. It may harm them.

This Patient Information leaflet summarizes the most important information about SPRYCEL. If you would like more information, talk with your healthcare provider. You can ask your healthcare provider or pharmacist for information about SPRYCEL that is written for healthcare professionals.

For more information, go to www.sprycel.com or call 1-800-332-2056.

What are the ingredients in SPRYCEL?

Active ingredient: dasatinib

Inactive ingredients: lactose monohydrate, microcrystalline cellulose, croscarmellose sodium, hydroxypropyl cellulose, and magnesium stearate. The tablet coating consists of hypromellose, titanium dioxide, and polyethylene glycol.

This Patient Package Insert has been approved by the U.S. Food and Drug Administration.

Manufactured by:
Bristol-Myers Squibb Company
Princeton, NJ 08543 USA
Bristol-Myers Squibb Company
Princeton, NJ 08543 USA
Product of Ireland
Rev May 2014
1284903A3

Shown in Product Identification Guide, page 306

SUSTIVA® ℞

[sus-TEE-vah]
(efavirenz)
capsules for oral use
SUSTIVA®
(efavirenz)
tablets for oral use

HIGHLIGHTS OF PRESCRIBING INFORMATION
These highlights do not include all the information needed to use SUSTIVA safely and effectively. See full prescribing information for SUSTIVA.
SUSTIVA® (efavirenz) capsules for oral use
SUSTIVA® (efavirenz) tablets for oral use
Initial U.S. Approval: 1998

────── **RECENT MAJOR CHANGES** ──────

Contraindications,	
Contraindicated Drugs (4.2)	Removed 5/2014
Warnings and Precautions,	
Drug Interactions (5.1)	5/2014

────── **INDICATIONS AND USAGE** ──────

SUSTIVA is a non-nucleoside reverse transcriptase inhibitor indicated in combination with other antiretroviral agents for the treatment of human immunodeficiency virus type 1 infection in adults and in pediatric patients at least 3 months old and weighing at least 3.5 kg. (1)

────── **DOSAGE AND ADMINISTRATION** ──────

- SUSTIVA should be taken orally once daily on an empty stomach, preferably at bedtime. (2)
- Recommended adult dose: 600 mg. (2.1)
- With voriconazole, increase voriconazole maintenance dose to 400 mg every 12 hours and decrease SUSTIVA dose to 300 mg once daily using the capsule formulation. (2.1)
- With rifampin, increase SUSTIVA dose to 800 mg once daily for patients weighing 50 kg or more. (2.1)
- Pediatric dosing is based on weight. (2.2)

────── **DOSAGE FORMS AND STRENGTHS** ──────

- Capsules: 200 mg and 50 mg (3)
- Tablets: 600 mg (3)

────── **CONTRAINDICATIONS** ──────

SUSTIVA is contraindicated in patients with previously demonstrated hypersensitivity (eg, Stevens-Johnson syndrome, erythema multiforme, or toxic skin eruptions) to any of the components of this product. (4.1)

────── **WARNINGS AND PRECAUTIONS** ──────

- *Do not use as a single agent* or add on as a sole agent to a failing regimen. Consider potential for cross-resistance when choosing other agents. (5.2)

- Not recommended with ATRIPLA, which contains efavirenz, emtricitabine, and tenofovir disoproxil fumarate, unless needed for dose adjustment when coadministered with rifampin. (5.3)
- *Serious psychiatric symptoms:* Immediate medical evaluation is recommended for serious psychiatric symptoms such as severe depression or suicidal ideation. (5.4, 17)
- *Nervous system symptoms (NSS):* NSS are frequent, usually begin 1-2 days after initiating therapy and resolve in 2-4 weeks. Dosing at bedtime may improve tolerability. NSS are not predictive of onset of psychiatric symptoms. (5.5, 5.6.1, 17)
- *Pregnancy:* Fetal harm may occur when administered to a pregnant woman during the first trimester. Women should be apprised of the potential harm to the fetus. (5.6, 17) Pregnancy registry is available. (8.1)
- *Hepatotoxicity:* Monitor liver function tests before and during treatment in patients with underlying hepatic disease, including hepatitis B or C coinfection, marked transaminase elevations, or who are taking medications associated with liver toxicity. Among reported cases of hepatic failure, a few occurred in patients with no pre-existing hepatic disease. (5.8, 6.1, 8.6)
- *Rash:* Rash usually begins within 1-2 weeks after initiating therapy and resolves within 4 weeks. Discontinue if severe rash develops. (5.7, 6.1, 17)
- *Convulsions:* Use caution in patients with a history of seizures. (5.9)
- *Lipids:* Total cholesterol and triglyceride elevations. Monitor before therapy and periodically thereafter. (5.10)
- *Immune reconstitution syndrome:* May necessitate further evaluation and treatment. (5.11)
- *Redistribution/accumulation of body fat:* Observed in patients receiving antiretroviral therapy. (5.12, 17)

————ADVERSE REACTIONS————

Most common adverse reactions (>5%, moderate-severe) are impaired concentration, abnormal dreams, rash, dizziness, nausea, headache, fatigue, insomnia, and vomiting. (5.5, 6)
To report SUSPECTED ADVERSE REACTIONS, contact Bristol-Myers Squibb at 1-800-721-5072 or FDA at 1-800-FDA-1088 or www.fda.gov/medwatch.

————DRUG INTERACTIONS————

Coadministration of efavirenz can alter the concentrations of other drugs and other drugs may alter the concentrations of efavirenz. The potential for drug-drug interactions must be considered before and during therapy. (7.1, 12.3)

————USE IN SPECIFIC POPULATIONS————

- *Pregnancy:* Women should avoid pregnancy during SUSTIVA (efavirenz) therapy and for 12 weeks after discontinuation. (5.6)
- *Nursing mothers:* Women infected with HIV should be instructed not to breastfeed. (8.3)
- *Hepatic impairment:* SUSTIVA is not recommended for patients with moderate or severe hepatic impairment. Use caution in patients with mild hepatic impairment. (8.6)
- *Pediatric patients:* The incidence of rash was higher than in adults. (5.7, 6.2, 8.4)

See 17 for PATIENT COUNSELING INFORMATION and FDA-approved patient labeling

Revised: 05/2014

FULL PRESCRIBING INFORMATION

1   INDICATIONS AND USAGE

SUSTIVA® (efavirenz) in combination with other antiretroviral agents is indicated for the treatment of human immunodeficiency virus type 1 (HIV-1) infection in adults and in pediatric patients at least 3 months old and weighing at least 3.5 kg.

2   DOSAGE AND ADMINISTRATION
2.1   Adults
The recommended dosage of SUSTIVA (efavirenz) is 600 mg orally, once daily, in combination with a protease inhibitor and/or nucleoside analogue reverse transcriptase inhibitors (NRTIs). It is recommended that SUSTIVA be taken on an empty stomach, preferably at bedtime. The increased efavirenz concentrations observed following administration of SUSTIVA with food may lead to an increase in frequency of adverse reactions [*see Clinical Pharmacology (12.3)*]. Dosing at bedtime may improve the tolerability of nervous system symptoms [*see Warnings and Precautions (5.5), Adverse Reactions (6.1), and Patient Counseling Information (17)*]. SUSTIVA capsules or tablets should be swallowed intact with liquid. For patients who cannot swallow capsules or tablets, the capsule sprinkle method of administration is recommended [*see Dosage and Administration (2.3)*].
Concomitant Antiretroviral Therapy
SUSTIVA must be given in combination with other antiretroviral medications [*see Indications and Usage (1), Warnings and Precautions (5.2), Drug Interactions (7.1), and Clinical Pharmacology (12.3)*].

Dosage Adjustment
If SUSTIVA (efavirenz) is coadministered with voriconazole, the voriconazole maintenance dose should be increased to 400 mg every 12 hours and the SUSTIVA dose should be decreased to 300 mg once daily using the capsule formulation (one 200 mg and two 50 mg capsules or six 50 mg capsules). SUSTIVA tablets should not be broken. [*See Drug Interactions (7.1, Table 5) and Clinical Pharmacology (12.3, Tables 7 and 8).*]
If SUSTIVA is coadministered with rifampin to patients weighing 50 kg or more, an increase in the dose of SUSTIVA to 800 mg once daily is recommended [*see Drug Interactions (7.1, Table 5) and Clinical Pharmacology (12.3, Table 8)*].

2.2   Pediatric Patients
It is recommended that SUSTIVA be taken on an empty stomach, preferably at bedtime. Table 1 describes the recommended dose of SUSTIVA for pediatric patients 3 months of age or older and weighing between 3.5 kg and 40 kg [*see Clinical Pharmacology (12.3)*]. The recommended dosage of SUSTIVA for pediatric patients weighing 40 kg or greater is 600 mg once daily. For pediatric patients who cannot swallow capsules, the capsule contents can be administered with a small amount of food or infant formula using the capsule sprinkle method of administration [*see Dosage and Administration (2.3)*].
[See table 1 below]

2.3   Capsule Sprinkle Method of Administration
For pediatric patients at least 3 months old and weighing at least 3.5 kg and adults who cannot swallow capsules or tablets, the capsule contents may be administered with a small amount (1 to 2 teaspoons) of food. Use of infant formula for mixing should only be considered for those young infants who cannot reliably consume solid foods. Patients and caregivers must be instructed to open the capsule carefully to avoid spillage or dispersion of the capsule contents into the air. The capsule should be held horizontally over a small container and carefully twisted to open. For patients able to tolerate solid foods, the entire capsule contents should be gently mixed with an age-appropriate soft food, such as applesauce, grape jelly, or yogurt, in the small container. For young infants receiving the capsule sprinkle-infant formula mixture, the entire capsule contents should be gently mixed into 2 teaspoons (10 mL) of reconstituted room temperature infant formula in a medicine cup by carefully stirring with a small spoon, and then drawing up the mixture into a 10 mL oral dosing syringe for administration. After administration of the SUSTIVA-food or -formula mixture, an additional small amount (approximately 2 teaspoons) of food or formula must be added to the empty mixing container, stirred to disperse any remaining SUSTIVA residue, and administered to the patient. The SUSTIVA-food or -formula mixture should be administered within 30 minutes of mixing. No additional food should be consumed for 2 hours after administration of SUSTIVA.
Further patient instructions on the capsule sprinkle method of administration are provided in the FDA-approved patient labeling (see Patient Information and Instructions for Use).

3   DOSAGE FORMS AND STRENGTHS
- *Capsules*
  200 mg capsules are gold color, reverse printed with "SUSTIVA" on the body and imprinted "200 mg" on the cap.
  50 mg capsules are gold color and white, printed with "SUSTIVA" on the gold color cap and reverse printed "50 mg" on the white body.
- *Tablets*
  600 mg tablets are yellow, capsular-shaped, film-coated tablets, with "SUSTIVA" printed on both sides.

4   CONTRAINDICATIONS
4.1   Hypersensitivity
SUSTIVA is contraindicated in patients with previously demonstrated clinically significant hypersensitivity (eg, Stevens-Johnson syndrome, erythema multiforme, or toxic skin eruptions) to any of the components of this product.

5   WARNINGS AND PRECAUTIONS
5.1   Drug Interactions
Efavirenz plasma concentrations may be altered by substrates, inhibitors, or inducers of CYP3A. Likewise, efavirenz may alter plasma concentrations of drugs metabolized by CYP3A or CYP2B6. The most prominent effect of efavirenz at steady-state is induction of CYP3A and CYP2B6. [*See Dosage and Administration (2.1) and Drug Interactions (7.1).*]
5.2   Resistance
SUSTIVA must not be used as a single agent to treat HIV-1 infection or added on as a sole agent to a failing regimen. Resistant virus emerges rapidly when efavirenz is administered as monotherapy. The choice of new antiretroviral agents to be used in combination with efavirenz should take into consideration the potential for viral cross-resistance.
5.3   Coadministration with Related Products
Coadministration of SUSTIVA with ATRIPLA (efavirenz 600 mg/emtricitabine 200 mg/tenofovir disoproxil fumarate

Table 1: SUSTIVA Dosing in Pediatric Patients

Patient Body Weight	SUSTIVA Daily Dose	Number of Capsules[a] or Tablets[b] and Strength to Administer
3.5 kg to less than 5 kg	100 mg	two 50 mg capsules
5 kg to less than 7.5 kg	150 mg	three 50 mg capsules
7.5 kg to less than 15 kg	200 mg	one 200 mg capsule
15 kg to less than 20 kg	250 mg	one 200 mg + one 50 mg capsule
20 kg to less than 25 kg	300 mg	one 200 mg + two 50 mg capsules
25 kg to less than 32.5 kg	350 mg	one 200 mg + three 50 mg capsules
32.5 kg to less than 40 kg	400 mg	two 200 mg capsules
at least 40 kg	600 mg	one 600 mg tablet OR three 200 mg capsules

[a] Capsules can be administered intact or as sprinkles [*see Dosage and Administration (2.3)*].
[b] Tablets must not be crushed.

300 mg) is not recommended unless needed for dose adjustment (eg, with rifampin), since efavirenz is one of its active ingredients.

5.4 Psychiatric Symptoms

Serious psychiatric adverse experiences have been reported in patients treated with SUSTIVA (efavirenz). In controlled trials of 1008 patients treated with regimens containing SUSTIVA for a mean of 2.1 years and 635 patients treated with control regimens for a mean of 1.5 years, the frequency (regardless of causality) of specific serious psychiatric events among patients who received SUSTIVA or control regimens, respectively, were severe depression (2.4%, 0.9%), suicidal ideation (0.7%, 0.3%), nonfatal suicide attempts (0.5%, 0), aggressive behavior (0.4%, 0.5%), paranoid reactions (0.4%, 0.3%), and manic reactions (0.2%, 0.3%). When psychiatric symptoms similar to those noted above were combined and evaluated as a group in a multifactorial analysis of data from Study 006, treatment with efavirenz was associated with an increase in the occurrence of these selected psychiatric symptoms. Other factors associated with an increase in the occurrence of these psychiatric symptoms were history of injection drug use, psychiatric history, and receipt of psychiatric medication at study entry; similar associations were observed in both the SUSTIVA and control treatment groups. In Study 006, onset of new serious psychiatric symptoms occurred throughout the study for both SUSTIVA-treated and control-treated patients. One percent of SUSTIVA-treated patients discontinued or interrupted treatment because of one or more of these selected psychiatric symptoms. There have also been occasional postmarketing reports of death by suicide, delusions, and psychosis-like behavior, although a causal relationship to the use of SUSTIVA cannot be determined from these reports. Patients with serious psychiatric adverse experiences should seek immediate medical evaluation to assess the possibility that the symptoms may be related to the use of SUSTIVA, and if so, to determine whether the risks of continued therapy outweigh the benefits. [See Adverse Reactions (6.1).]

5.5 Nervous System Symptoms

Fifty-three percent (531/1008) of patients receiving SUSTIVA in controlled trials reported central nervous system symptoms (any grade, regardless of causality) compared to 25% (156/635) of patients receiving control regimens [see Adverse Reactions (6.1, Table 3)]. These symptoms included, but were not limited to, dizziness (28.1% of the 1008 patients), insomnia (16.3%), impaired concentration (8.3%), somnolence (7.0%), abnormal dreams (6.2%), and hallucinations (1.2%). These symptoms were severe in 2.0% of patients, and 2.1% of patients discontinued therapy as a result. These symptoms usually begin during the first or second day of therapy and generally resolve after the first 2-4 weeks of therapy. After 4 weeks of therapy, the prevalence of nervous system symptoms of at least moderate severity ranged from 5% to 9% in patients treated with regimens containing SUSTIVA and from 3% to 5% in patients treated with a control regimen. Patients should be informed that these common symptoms were likely to improve with continued therapy and were not predictive of subsequent onset of the less frequent psychiatric symptoms [see Warnings and Precautions (5.4)]. Dosing at bedtime may improve the tolerability of these nervous system symptoms [see Dosage and Administration (2)].

Analysis of long-term data from Study 006 (median follow-up 180 weeks, 102 weeks, and 76 weeks for patients treated with SUSTIVA + zidovudine + lamivudine, SUSTIVA + indinavir, and indinavir + zidovudine + lamivudine, respectively) showed that, beyond 24 weeks of therapy, the incidences of new-onset nervous system symptoms among SUSTIVA-treated patients were generally similar to those in the indinavir-containing control arm.

Patients receiving SUSTIVA should be alerted to the potential for additive central nervous system effects when SUSTIVA is used concomitantly with alcohol or psychoactive drugs.

Patients who experience central nervous system symptoms such as dizziness, impaired concentration, and/or drowsiness should avoid potentially hazardous tasks such as driving or operating machinery.

5.6 Reproductive Risk Potential

Pregnancy Category D. Efavirenz may cause fetal harm when administered during the first trimester to a pregnant woman. Pregnancy should be avoided in women receiving SUSTIVA. Barrier contraception must always be used in combination with other methods of contraception (eg, oral or other hormonal contraceptives). Because of the long half-life of efavirenz, use of adequate contraceptive measures for 12 weeks after discontinuation of SUSTIVA is recommended. Women of childbearing potential should undergo pregnancy testing before initiation of SUSTIVA. If this drug is used during the first trimester of pregnancy, or if the patient becomes pregnant while taking this drug, the patient should be apprised of the potential harm to the fetus.

There are no adequate and well-controlled studies in pregnant women. SUSTIVA should be used during pregnancy only if the potential benefit justifies the potential risk to the fetus, such as in pregnant women without other therapeutic options. [See Use in Specific Populations (8.1).]

5.7 Rash

In controlled clinical trials, 26% (266/1008) of adult patients treated with 600 mg SUSTIVA (efavirenz) experienced new-onset skin rash compared with 17% (111/635) of those treated in control groups [see Adverse Reactions (6.1)]. Rash associated with blistering, moist desquamation, or ulceration occurred in 0.9% (9/1008) of patients treated with SUSTIVA. The incidence of Grade 4 rash (eg, erythema multiforme, Stevens-Johnson syndrome) in adult patients treated with SUSTIVA in all studies and expanded access was 0.1%. Rashes are usually mild-to-moderate maculopapular skin eruptions that occur within the first 2 weeks of initiating therapy with efavirenz (median time to onset of rash in adults was 11 days) and, in most patients continuing therapy with efavirenz, rash resolves within 1 month (median duration, 16 days). The discontinuation rate for rash in adult clinical trials was 1.7% (17/1008).

Rash was reported in 59 of 182 pediatric patients (32%) treated with SUSTIVA [see Adverse Reactions (6.2)]. Two pediatric patients experienced Grade 3 rash (confluent rash with fever, generalized rash), and four patients had Grade 4 rash (erythema multiforme). The median time to onset of rash in pediatric patients was 28 days (range 3-1642 days). Prophylaxis with appropriate antihistamines before initiating therapy with SUSTIVA in pediatric patients should be considered.

SUSTIVA can be reinitiated in patients interrupting therapy because of rash. SUSTIVA should be discontinued in patients developing severe rash associated with blistering, desquamation, mucosal involvement, or fever. Appropriate antihistamines and/or corticosteroids may improve the tolerability and hasten the resolution of rash. For patients who have had a life-threatening cutaneous reaction (eg, Stevens-Johnson syndrome), alternative therapy should be considered [see also Contraindications (4.1)].

5.8 Hepatotoxicity

Monitoring of liver enzymes before and during treatment is recommended for patients with underlying hepatic disease, including hepatitis B or C infection; patients with marked transaminase elevations; and patients treated with other medications associated with liver toxicity [see Adverse Reactions (6.1) and Use in Specific Populations (8.6)]. A few of the postmarketing reports of hepatic failure occurred in patients with no pre-existing hepatic disease or other identifiable risk factors [see Adverse Reactions (6.3)]. Liver enzyme monitoring should also be considered for patients without pre-existing hepatic dysfunction or other risk factors. In patients with persistent elevations of serum transaminases to greater than five times the upper limit of the normal range, the benefit of continued therapy with SUSTIVA (efavirenz) needs to be weighed against the unknown risks of significant liver toxicity.

5.9 Convulsions

Convulsions have been observed in adult and pediatric patients receiving efavirenz, generally in the presence of known medical history of seizures [see Nonclinical Toxicology (13.2)]. Caution must be taken in any patient with a history of seizures. Patients who are receiving concomitant anticonvulsant medications primarily metabolized by the liver, such as phenytoin and phenobarbital, may require periodic monitoring of plasma levels [see Drug Interactions (7.1)].

5.10 Lipid Elevations

Treatment with SUSTIVA has resulted in increases in the concentration of total cholesterol and triglycerides [see Adverse Reactions (6.1)]. Cholesterol and triglyceride testing should be performed before initiating SUSTIVA therapy and at periodic intervals during therapy.

5.11 Immune Reconstitution Syndrome

Immune reconstitution syndrome has been reported in patients treated with combination antiretroviral therapy, including SUSTIVA. During the initial phase of combination antiretroviral treatment, patients whose immune system responds may develop an inflammatory response to indolent or residual opportunistic infections [such as Mycobacterium avium infection, cytomegalovirus, Pneumocystis jiroveci pneumonia (PCP), or tuberculosis], which may necessitate further evaluation and treatment.

Autoimmune disorders (such as Graves' disease, polymyositis, and Guillain-Barré syndrome) have also been reported to occur in the setting of immune reconstitution; however, the time to onset is more variable, and can occur many months after initiation of treatment.

5.12 Fat Redistribution

Redistribution/accumulation of body fat including central obesity, dorsocervical fat enlargement (buffalo hump), peripheral wasting, facial wasting, breast enlargement, and

---

Table 2: Selected Treatment-Emergent[a] Adverse Reactions of Moderate or Severe Intensity Reported in ≥2% of SUSTIVA-Treated Patients in Studies 006 and ACTG 364

Adverse Reactions	Study 006 LAM-, NNRTI-, and Protease Inhibitor-Naive Patients			Study ACTG 364 NRTI-experienced, NNRTI-, and Protease Inhibitor-Naive Patients		
	SUSTIVA[b] + ZDV/LAM (n=412) 180 weeks[c]	SUSTIVA[b] + Indinavir (n=415) 102 weeks[c]	Indinavir + ZDV/LAM (n=401) 76 weeks[c]	SUSTIVA[b] + Nelfinavir + NRTIs (n=64) 71.1 weeks[c]	SUSTIVA[b] + NRTIs (n=65) 70.9 weeks[c]	Nelfinavir + NRTIs (n=66) 62.7 weeks[c]
Body as a Whole						
Fatigue	8%	5%	9%	0	2%	3%
Pain	1%	2%	8%	13%	6%	17%
Central and Peripheral Nervous System						
Dizziness	9%	9%	2%	2%	6%	6%
Headache	8%	5%	3%	5%	2%	3%
Insomnia	7%	7%	2%	0	0	2%
Concentration impaired	5%	3%	<1%	0	0	0
Abnormal dreams	3%	1%	0	—	—	—
Somnolence	2%	2%	<1%	0	0	0
Anorexia	1%	<1%	<1%	0	2%	2%
Gastrointestinal						
Nausea	10%	6%	24%	3%	2%	2%
Vomiting	6%	3%	14%	0	0	—
Diarrhea	3%	5%	6%	14%	3%	9%
Dyspepsia	4%	4%	6%	0	0	2%
Abdominal pain	2%	2%	5%	3%	3%	3%
Psychiatric						
Anxiety	2%	4%	<1%	—	—	—
Depression	5%	4%	<1%	3%	0	5%
Nervousness	2%	2%	0	2%	0	2%
Skin & Appendages						
Rash[d]	11%	16%	5%	9%	5%	9%
Pruritus	<1%	1%	1%	9%	5%	9%

[a] Includes adverse events at least possibly related to study drug or of unknown relationship for Study 006. Includes all adverse events regardless of relationship to study drug for Study ACTG 364.
[b] SUSTIVA provided as 600 mg once daily.
[c] Median duration of treatment.
[d] Includes erythema multiforme, rash, rash erythematous, rash follicular, rash maculopapular, rash petechial, rash pustular, and urticaria for Study 006 and macules, papules, rash, erythema, redness, inflammation, allergic rash, urticaria, welts, hives, itchy, and pruritus for ACTG 364.
— = Not Specified.
ZDV = zidovudine, LAM = lamivudine.

Table 4: Selected Grade 3-4 Laboratory Abnormalities Reported in ≥2% of SUSTIVA-Treated Patients in Studies 006 and ACTG 364

		Study 006 LAM-, NNRTI-, and Protease Inhibitor-Naive Patients			Study ACTG 364 NRTI-experienced, NNRTI-, and Protease Inhibitor-Naive Patients		
Variable	Limit	SUSTIVA[a] + ZDV/LAM (n=412) 180 weeks[b]	SUSTIVA[a] + Indinavir (n=415) 102 weeks[b]	Indinavir + ZDV/LAM (n=401) 76 weeks[b]	SUSTIVA[a] + Nelfinavir + NRTIs (n=64) 71.1 weeks[b]	SUSTIVA[a] + NRTIs (n=65) 70.9 weeks[b]	Nelfinavir + NRTIs (n=66) 62.7 weeks[b]
Chemistry							
ALT	>5 × ULN	5%	8%	5%	2%	6%	3%
AST	>5 × ULN	5%	6%	5%	6%	8%	8%
GGT[c]	>5 × ULN	8%	7%	3%	5%	0	5%
Amylase	>2 × ULN	4%	4%	1%	0	6%	2%
Glucose	>250 mg/dL	3%	3%	3%	5%	3%	3%
Triglycerides[d]	≥751 mg/dL	9%	6%	6%	11%	8%	17%
Hematology							
Neutrophils	<750/mm³	10%	3%	5%	2%	3%	2%

[a] SUSTIVA provided as 600 mg once daily.
[b] Median duration of treatment.
[c] Isolated elevations of GGT in patients receiving SUSTIVA may reflect enzyme induction not associated with liver toxicity.
[d] Nonfasting.
ZDV = zidovudine, LAM = lamivudine, ULN = Upper limit of normal, ALT = alanine aminotransferase, AST = aspartate aminotransferase, GGT = gamma-glutamyltransferase.

"cushingoid appearance" have been observed in patients receiving antiretroviral therapy. The mechanism and long-term consequences of these events are currently unknown. A causal relationship has not been established.

6 ADVERSE REACTIONS

6.1 Clinical Trials Experience in Adults

Because clinical studies are conducted under widely varying conditions, the adverse reaction rates reported cannot be directly compared to rates in other clinical studies and may not reflect the rates observed in clinical practice.

The most significant adverse reactions observed in patients treated with SUSTIVA (efavirenz) are:
- psychiatric symptoms [see *Warnings and Precautions (5.4)*],
- nervous system symptoms [see *Warnings and Precautions (5.5)*],
- rash [see *Warnings and Precautions (5.7)*].

The most common (>5% in either efavirenz treatment group) adverse reactions of at least moderate severity among patients in Study 006 treated with SUSTIVA in combination with zidovudine/lamivudine or indinavir were rash, dizziness, nausea, headache, fatigue, insomnia, and vomiting.

Selected clinical adverse reactions of moderate or severe intensity observed in ≥2% of SUSTIVA-treated patients in two controlled clinical trials are presented in Table 2.
[See table 2 at top of previous page]

Pancreatitis has been reported, although a causal relationship with efavirenz has not been established. Asymptomatic increases in serum amylase levels were observed in a significantly higher number of patients treated with efavirenz 600 mg than in control patients (see *Laboratory Abnormalities*).

Nervous System Symptoms

For 1008 patients treated with regimens containing SUSTIVA and 635 patients treated with a control regimen in controlled trials, Table 3 lists the frequency of symptoms of different degrees of severity and gives the discontinuation rates for one or more of the following nervous system symptoms: dizziness, insomnia, impaired concentration, somnolence, abnormal dreaming, euphoria, confusion, agitation, amnesia, hallucinations, stupor, abnormal thinking, and depersonalization [see *Warnings and Precautions (5.5)*]. The frequencies of specific central and peripheral nervous system symptoms are provided in Table 2.

Table 3: Percent of Patients with One or More Selected Nervous System Symptoms[a,b]

Percent of Patients with:	SUSTIVA 600 mg Once Daily (n=1008) %	Control Groups (n=635) %
Symptoms of any severity	52.7	24.6
Mild symptoms[c]	33.3	15.6
Moderate symptoms[d]	17.4	7.7
Severe symptoms[e]	2.0	1.3

Treatment discontinuation as a result of symptoms	2.1	1.1

[a] Includes events reported regardless of causality.
[b] Data from Study 006 and three Phase 2/3 studies.
[c] "Mild" = Symptoms which do not interfere with patient's daily activities.
[d] "Moderate" = Symptoms which may interfere with daily activities.
[e] "Severe" = Events which interrupt patient's usual daily activities.

Psychiatric Symptoms

Serious psychiatric adverse experiences have been reported in patients treated with SUSTIVA (efavirenz). In controlled trials, psychiatric symptoms observed at a frequency greater than 2% among patients treated with SUSTIVA or control regimens, respectively, were depression (19%, 16%), anxiety (13%, 9%), and nervousness (7%, 2%).

Rash

In controlled clinical trials, the frequency of rash (all grades, regardless of causality) was 26% for 1008 adults treated with regimens containing SUSTIVA and 17% for 635 adults treated with a control regimen. Most reports of rash were mild or moderate in severity. The frequency of Grade 3 rash was 0.8% for SUSTIVA-treated patients and 0.3% for control groups, and the frequency of Grade 4 rash was 0.1% for SUSTIVA and 0 for control groups. The discontinuation rates as a result of rash were 1.7% for SUSTIVA-treated patients and 0.3% for control groups [see *Warnings and Precautions (5.7)*].

Experience with SUSTIVA in patients who discontinued other antiretroviral agents of the NNRTI class is limited. Nineteen patients who discontinued nevirapine because of rash have been treated with SUSTIVA. Nine of these patients developed mild-to-moderate rash while receiving therapy with SUSTIVA, and two of these patients discontinued because of rash.

Laboratory Abnormalities

Selected Grade 3-4 laboratory abnormalities reported in ≥2% of SUSTIVA-treated patients in two clinical trials are presented in Table 4.
[See table 4 above]

Patients Coinfected with Hepatitis B or C

Liver function tests should be monitored in patients with a history of hepatitis B and/or C. In the long-term data set from Study 006, 137 patients treated with SUSTIVA-containing regimens (median duration of therapy, 68 weeks) and 84 treated with a control regimen (median duration, 56 weeks) were seropositive at screening for hepatitis B (surface antigen positive) and/or C (hepatitis C antibody positive). Among these coinfected patients, elevations in AST to greater than five times ULN developed in 13% of patients in the SUSTIVA arms and 7% of those in the control arm, and elevations in ALT to greater than five times ULN developed in 20% of patients in the SUSTIVA arms and 7% of patients in the control arm. Among coinfected patients, 3% of those treated with SUSTIVA-containing regimens and 2% in the

control arm discontinued from the study because of liver or biliary system disorders [see *Warnings and Precautions (5.8)*].

Lipids

Increases from baseline in total cholesterol of 10-20% have been observed in some uninfected volunteers receiving SUSTIVA (efavirenz). In patients treated with SUSTIVA + zidovudine + lamivudine, increases from baseline in non-fasting total cholesterol and HDL of approximately 20% and 25%, respectively, were observed. In patients treated with SUSTIVA + indinavir, increases from baseline in nonfasting cholesterol and HDL of approximately 40% and 35%, respectively, were observed. Nonfasting total cholesterol levels ≥240 mg/dL and ≥300 mg/dL were reported in 34% and 9%, respectively, of patients treated with SUSTIVA + zidovudine + lamivudine; 54% and 20%, respectively, of patients treated with SUSTIVA + indinavir; and 28% and 4%, respectively, of patients treated with indinavir + zidovudine + lamivudine. The effects of SUSTIVA on triglycerides and LDL in this study were not well characterized since samples were taken from nonfasting patients. The clinical significance of these findings is unknown [see *Warnings and Precautions (5.10)*].

6.2 Clinical Trial Experience in Pediatric Patients

Because clinical studies are conducted under widely varying conditions, the adverse reaction rates reported cannot be directly compared to rates in other clinical studies and may not reflect the rates observed in clinical practice.

Assessment of adverse reactions is based on three clinical trials in 182 HIV-1 infected pediatric patients (3 months to 21 years of age) who received SUSTIVA in combination with other antiretroviral agents for a median of 123 weeks. The adverse reactions observed in the three trials were similar to those observed in clinical trials in adults except that rash was more common in pediatric patients (32% for all grades regardless of causality) and more often of higher grade (ie, more severe). Two (1.1%) pediatric patients experienced Grade 3 rash (confluent rash with fever, generalized rash), and four (2.2%) pediatric patients had Grade 4 rash (all erythema multiforme). Five pediatric patients (2.7%) discontinued from the study because of rash [see *Warnings and Precautions (5.7)*].

6.3 Postmarketing Experience

The following adverse reactions have been identified during postapproval use of SUSTIVA. Because these reactions are reported voluntarily from a population of unknown size, it is not always possible to reliably estimate their frequency or establish a causal relationship to drug exposure.

Body as a Whole: allergic reactions, asthenia, redistribution/accumulation of body fat [see *Warnings and Precautions (5.12)*]

Central and Peripheral Nervous System: abnormal coordination, ataxia, cerebellar coordination and balance disturbances, convulsions, hypoesthesia, paresthesia, neuropathy, tremor, vertigo

Endocrine: gynecomastia

Gastrointestinal: constipation, malabsorption

Cardiovascular: flushing, palpitations

Liver and Biliary System: hepatic enzyme increase, hepatic failure, hepatitis. A few of the postmarketing reports of hepatic failure, including cases in patients with no pre-existing hepatic disease or other identifiable risk factors, were characterized by a fulminant course, progressing in some cases to transplantation or death.

Metabolic and Nutritional: hypercholesterolemia, hypertriglyceridemia

Musculoskeletal: arthralgia, myalgia, myopathy

Psychiatric: aggressive reactions, agitation, delusions, emotional lability, mania, neurosis, paranoia, psychosis, suicide

Respiratory: dyspnea

Skin and Appendages: erythema multiforme, photoallergic dermatitis, Stevens-Johnson syndrome

Special Senses: abnormal vision, tinnitus

7 DRUG INTERACTIONS

7.1 Drug-Drug Interactions

Efavirenz has been shown *in vivo* to induce CYP3A and CYP2B6. Other compounds that are substrates of CYP3A or CYP2B6 may have decreased plasma concentrations when coadministered with SUSTIVA. Drugs that induce CYP3A activity (eg, phenobarbital, rifampin, rifabutin) would be expected to increase the clearance of efavirenz resulting in lowered plasma concentrations [see *Dosage and Administration (2.1)*]. Drug interactions with SUSTIVA are summarized in Table 5 [for pharmacokinetics data see *Clinical Pharmacology (12.3, Tables 7 and 8)*]. This table includes potentially significant interactions, but is not all inclusive.
[See table 5 on pages 743 through 745]

Other Drugs

Based on the results of drug interaction studies [see *Clinical Pharmacology (12.3, Tables 7 and 8)*], no dosage adjustment is recommended when SUSTIVA is given with the following: aluminum/magnesium hydroxide antacids, azithromycin,

Table 5: Established and Other Potentially Significant Drug Interactions: Alteration in Dose or Regimen May Be Recommended Based on Drug Interaction Studies or Predicted Interaction

Concomitant Drug Class: Drug Name	Effect	Clinical Comment
HIV antiviral agents		
Protease inhibitor: Fosamprenavir calcium	↓ amprenavir	Fosamprenavir (unboosted): Appropriate doses of the combinations with respect to safety and efficacy have not been established. Fosamprenavir/ritonavir: An additional 100 mg/day (300 mg total) of ritonavir is recommended when SUSTIVA is administered with fosamprenavir/ritonavir once daily. No change in the ritonavir dose is required when SUSTIVA is administered with fosamprenavir plus ritonavir twice daily.
Protease inhibitor: Atazanavir sulfate	↓ atazanavir*	*Treatment-naive patients:* When coadministered with SUSTIVA, the recommended dose of atazanavir is 400 mg with ritonavir 100 mg (together once daily with food) and SUSTIVA 600 mg (once daily on an empty stomach, preferably at bedtime). *Treatment-experienced patients:* Coadministration of SUSTIVA and atazanavir is not recommended.
Protease inhibitor: Indinavir	↓ indinavir*	The optimal dose of indinavir, when given in combination with SUSTIVA, is not known. Increasing the indinavir dose to 1000 mg every 8 hours does not compensate for the increased indinavir metabolism due to SUSTIVA. When indinavir at an increased dose (1000 mg every 8 hours) was given with SUSTIVA (600 mg once daily), the indinavir AUC and C_{min} were decreased on average by 33-46% and 39-57%, respectively, compared to when indinavir (800 mg every 8 hours) was given alone.
Protease inhibitor: Lopinavir/ritonavir	↓ lopinavir*	Dose increase of lopinavir/ritonavir is recommended for all patients. Lopinavir/ritonavir tablets should not be administered once daily in combination with SUSTIVA. See the lopinavir/ritonavir prescribing information for dose adjustments of lopinavir/ritonavir when coadministered with efavirenz in adult and pediatric patients.
Protease inhibitor: Ritonavir	↑ ritonavir* ↑ efavirenz*	When ritonavir 500 mg q12h was coadministered with SUSTIVA 600 mg once daily, the combination was associated with a higher frequency of adverse clinical experiences (eg, dizziness, nausea, paresthesia) and laboratory abnormalities (elevated liver enzymes). Monitoring of liver enzymes is recommended when SUSTIVA is used in combination with ritonavir.
Protease inhibitor: Saquinavir	↓ saquinavir*	Appropriate doses of the combination of SUSTIVA and saquinavir/ritonavir with respect to safety and efficacy have not been established.
NNRTI: Other NNRTIs	↑ or ↓ efavirenz and/or NNRTI	Combining two NNRTIs has not been shown to be beneficial. SUSTIVA should not be coadministered with other NNRTIs.
CCR5 co-receptor antagonist: Maraviroc	↓ maraviroc*	Refer to the full prescribing information for maraviroc for guidance on coadministration with efavirenz.
Integrase strand transfer inhibitor: Raltegravir	↓ raltegravir*	SUSTIVA reduces plasma concentrations of raltegravir. The clinical significance of this interaction has not been directly assessed.
Hepatitis C antiviral agents		
Protease inhibitor: Boceprevir	↓ boceprevir*	Plasma trough concentrations of boceprevir were decreased when boceprevir was coadministered with SUSTIVA, which may result in loss of therapeutic effect. The combination should be avoided.
Protease inhibitor: Telaprevir	↓ telaprevir* ↓ efavirenz*	Concomitant administration of telaprevir and SUSTIVA resulted in reduced steady-state exposures to telaprevir and efavirenz.
Other agents		
Anticoagulant: Warfarin	↑ or ↓ warfarin	Plasma concentrations and effects potentially increased or decreased by SUSTIVA.
Anticonvulsants: Carbamazepine	↓ carbamazepine* ↓ efavirenz*	There are insufficient data to make a dose recommendation for efavirenz. Alternative anticonvulsant treatment should be used. Potential for reduction in anticonvulsant and/or efavirenz plasma levels; periodic monitoring of anticonvulsant plasma levels should be conducted.
Phenytoin Phenobarbital	↓ anticonvulsant ↓ efavirenz	
Antidepressants: Bupropion	↓ bupropion*	The effect of efavirenz on bupropion exposure is thought to be due to the induction of bupropion metabolism. Increases in bupropion dosage should be guided by clinical response, but the maximum recommended dose of bupropion should not be exceeded.
Sertraline	↓ sertraline*	Increases in sertraline dosage should be guided by clinical response.

(Table continued on next page)

cetirizine, famotidine, fluconazole, lamivudine, lorazepam, nelfinavir, paroxetine, tenofovir disoproxil fumarate, and zidovudine.

Specific drug interaction studies have not been performed with SUSTIVA (efavirenz) and NRTIs other than lamivudine and zidovudine. Clinically significant interactions would not be expected since the NRTIs are metabolized via a different route than efavirenz and would be unlikely to compete for the same metabolic enzymes and elimination pathways.

7.2 Cannabinoid Test Interaction

Efavirenz does not bind to cannabinoid receptors. False-positive urine cannabinoid test results have been reported with some screening assays in uninfected and HIV-infected subjects receiving efavirenz. Confirmation of positive screening tests for cannabinoids by a more specific method is recommended.

8 USE IN SPECIFIC POPULATIONS

8.1 Pregnancy

Pregnancy Category D: See *Warnings and Precautions (5.6)*.

Antiretroviral Pregnancy Registry: To monitor fetal outcomes of pregnant women exposed to SUSTIVA, an Antiretroviral Pregnancy Registry has been established. Physicians are encouraged to register patients by calling 1-800-258-4263.

As of July 2010, the Antiretroviral Pregnancy Registry has received prospective reports of 792 pregnancies exposed to efavirenz-containing regimens, nearly all of which were first-trimester exposures (718 pregnancies). Birth defects occurred in 17 of 604 live births (first-trimester exposure) and 2 of 69 live births (second/third-trimester exposure). One of these prospectively reported defects with first-trimester exposure was a neural tube defect. A single case of anophthalmia with first-trimester exposure to efavirenz has also been prospectively reported; however, this case included severe oblique facial clefts and amniotic banding, a known association with anophthalmia. There have been six retrospective reports of findings consistent with neural tube defects, including meningomyelocele. All mothers were exposed to efavirenz-containing regimens in the first trimester. Although a causal relationship of these events to the use of SUSTIVA has not been established, similar defects have been observed in preclinical studies of efavirenz.

Animal Data

Effects of efavirenz on embryo-fetal development have been studied in three nonclinical species (cynomolgus monkeys, rats, and rabbits). In monkeys, efavirenz 60 mg/kg/day was administered to pregnant females throughout pregnancy (gestation days 20 through 150). The maternal systemic drug exposures (AUC) were 1.3 times the exposure in humans at the recommended clinical dose (600 mg/day), with fetal umbilical venous drug concentrations approximately 0.7 times the maternal values. Three fetuses of 20 fetuses/infants had one or more malformations; there were no malformed fetuses or infants from placebo-treated mothers. The malformations that occurred in these three monkey fetuses included anencephaly and unilateral anophthalmia in one fetus, microphthalmia in a second, and cleft palate in the third. There was no NOAEL (no observable adverse effect level) established for this study because only one dosage was evaluated. In rats, efavirenz was administered either during organogenesis (gestation days 7 to 18) or from gestation day 7 through lactation day 21 at 50, 100, or 200 mg/kg/day. Administration of 200 mg/kg/day in rats was associated with increase in the incidence of early resorptions; and doses 100 mg/kg/day and greater were associated with early neonatal mortality. The AUC at the NOAEL (50 mg/kg/day) in this rat study was 0.1 times that in humans at the recommended clinical dose. Drug concentrations in the milk on lactation day 10 were approximately 8 times higher than those in maternal plasma. In pregnant rabbits, efavirenz was neither embryo lethal nor teratogenic when administered at doses of 25, 50, and 75 mg/kg/day over the period of organogenesis (gestation days 6 through 18). The AUC at the NOAEL (75 mg/kg/day) in rabbits was 0.4 times that in humans at the recommended clinical dose.

8.3 Nursing Mothers

The Centers for Disease Control and Prevention recommend that HIV-infected mothers not breastfeed their infants to avoid risking postnatal transmission of HIV. Efavirenz has been shown to pass into human breast milk. Because of the potential for HIV transmission and the potential for serious adverse effects in nursing infants, mothers should be instructed not to breastfeed if they are receiving SUSTIVA.

8.4 Pediatric Use

The safety, pharmacokinetic profile, and virologic and immunologic responses of SUSTIVA were evaluated in antiretroviral-naive and -experienced HIV-1 infected pediatric patients 3 months to 21 years of age in three open-label clinical trials [see *Adverse Reactions (6.2)*, *Clinical Pharmacology (12.3)*, and *Clinical Studies (14.2)*]. The type and frequency of adverse reactions in these trials were generally similar to those of adult patients with the exception of a higher frequency of rash, including a higher frequency of Grade 3 or 4 rash, in pediatric patients compared to adults [see *Warnings and Precautions (5.7)* and *Adverse Reactions (6.2)*].

Use of SUSTIVA (efavirenz) in patients younger than 3 months of age OR less than 3.5 kg body weight is not recommended because the safety, pharmacokinetics, and antiviral activity of SUSTIVA have not been evaluated in this age group and there is a risk of developing HIV resistance if SUSTIVA is underdosed. See *Dosage and Administration (2.2)* for dosing recommendations for pediatric patients.

8.5 Geriatric Use

Clinical studies of SUSTIVA did not include sufficient numbers of subjects aged 65 years and over to determine whether they respond differently from younger subjects. In general, dose selection for an elderly patient should be cautious, reflecting the greater frequency of decreased hepatic, renal, or cardiac function and of concomitant disease or other therapy.

8.6 Hepatic Impairment

SUSTIVA is not recommended for patients with moderate or severe hepatic impairment because there are insufficient data to determine whether dose adjustment is necessary. Patients with mild hepatic impairment may be treated with efavirenz without any adjustment in dose. Because of the extensive cytochrome P450-mediated metabolism of efavirenz and limited clinical experience in patients with hepatic impairment, caution should be exercised in administering SUSTIVA to these patients [see *Warnings and Precautions (5.8)* and *Clinical Pharmacology (12.3)*].

10 OVERDOSAGE

Some patients accidentally taking 600 mg twice daily have reported increased nervous system symptoms. One patient experienced involuntary muscle contractions.

Treatment of overdose with SUSTIVA should consist of general supportive measures, including monitoring of vital signs and observation of the patient's clinical status. Administration of activated charcoal may be used to aid removal of unabsorbed drug. There is no specific antidote for overdose with SUSTIVA. Since efavirenz is highly protein bound, dialysis is unlikely to significantly remove the drug from blood.

11 DESCRIPTION

SUSTIVA® (efavirenz) is an HIV-1 specific, non-nucleoside, reverse transcriptase inhibitor (NNRTI). Efavirenz is chemically described as (S)-6-chloro-4-(cyclopropylethynyl)-1,4-dihydro-4-(trifluoromethyl)-2H-3,1-benzoxazin-2-one. Its empirical formula is $C_{14}H_9ClF_3NO_2$ and its structural formula is:

Efavirenz is a white to slightly pink crystalline powder with a molecular mass of 315.68. It is practically insoluble in water (<10 microgram/mL).

Capsules: SUSTIVA is available as capsules for oral administration containing either 50 mg or 200 mg of efavirenz and the following inactive ingredients: lactose monohydrate, magnesium stearate, sodium lauryl sulfate, and sodium starch glycolate. The capsule shell contains the following inactive ingredients and dyes: gelatin, sodium lauryl sulfate, titanium dioxide, and/or yellow iron oxide. The capsule shells may also contain silicon dioxide. The capsules are printed with ink containing carmine 40 blue, FD&C Blue No. 2, and titanium dioxide.

Tablets: SUSTIVA is available as film-coated tablets for oral administration containing 600 mg of efavirenz and the following inactive ingredients: croscarmellose sodium, hydroxypropyl cellulose, lactose monohydrate, magnesium stearate, microcrystalline cellulose, and sodium lauryl sulfate. The film coating contains Opadry Yellow and Opadry Clear. The tablets are polished with carnauba wax and printed with purple ink, Opacode WB.

12 CLINICAL PHARMACOLOGY

12.1 Mechanism of Action

Efavirenz is an antiviral drug [see *Microbiology (12.4)*].

12.3 Pharmacokinetics

Absorption

Peak efavirenz plasma concentrations of 1.6-9.1 µM were attained by 5 hours following single oral doses of 100 mg to 1600 mg administered to uninfected volunteers. Dose-related increases in C_{max} and AUC were seen for doses up to 1600 mg; the increases were less than proportional suggesting diminished absorption at higher doses.

Table 5 *(cont.)*: Established and Other Potentially Significant Drug Interactions: Alteration in Dose or Regimen May Be Recommended Based on Drug Interaction Studies or Predicted Interaction

Concomitant Drug Class: Drug Name	Effect	Clinical Comment
Other agents (cont.)		
Antifungals: Voriconazole	↓ voriconazole* ↑ efavirenz*	SUSTIVA and voriconazole must not be coadministered at standard doses. Efavirenz significantly decreases voriconazole plasma concentrations, and coadministration may decrease the therapeutic effectiveness of voriconazole. Also, voriconazole significantly increases efavirenz plasma concentrations, which may increase the risk of SUSTIVA-associated side effects. When voriconazole is coadministered with SUSTIVA, voriconazole maintenance dose should be increased to 400 mg every 12 hours and SUSTIVA dose should be decreased to 300 mg once daily using the capsule formulation. SUSTIVA tablets should not be broken. [*See Dosage and Administration (2.1)* and *Clinical Pharmacology (12.3, Tables 7 and 8).*]
Itraconazole	↓ itraconazole* ↓ hydroxyitraconazole*	Since no dose recommendation for itraconazole can be made, alternative antifungal treatment should be considered.
Ketoconazole	↓ ketoconazole	Drug interaction studies with SUSTIVA and ketoconazole have not been conducted. SUSTIVA has the potential to decrease plasma concentrations of ketoconazole.
Posaconazole	↓ posaconazole*	Avoid concomitant use unless the benefit outweighs the risks.
Anti-infective: Clarithromycin	↓ clarithromycin* ↑ 14-OH metabolite*	Plasma concentrations decreased by SUSTIVA; clinical significance unknown. In uninfected volunteers, 46% developed rash while receiving SUSTIVA and clarithromycin. No dose adjustment of SUSTIVA is recommended when given with clarithromycin. Alternatives to clarithromycin, such as azithromycin, should be considered (see *Other Drugs*, following table). Other macrolide antibiotics, such as erythromycin, have not been studied in combination with SUSTIVA.
Antimycobacterials: Rifabutin	↓ rifabutin*	Increase daily dose of rifabutin by 50%. Consider doubling the rifabutin dose in regimens where rifabutin is given 2 or 3 times a week.
Rifampin	↓ efavirenz*	If SUSTIVA is coadministered with rifampin to patients weighing 50 kg or more, an increase in the dose of SUSTIVA to 800 mg once daily is recommended.
Antimalarials: Artemether/lumefantrine	↓ artemether* ↓ dihydroartemisinin* ↓ lumefantrine*	Artemether/lumefantrine should be used cautiously with efavirenz because decreased artemether, dihydroartemisinin (active metabolite of artemether), and/or lumefantrine concentrations may result in a decrease of antimalarial efficacy of artemether/lumefantrine.
Calcium channel blockers: Diltiazem	↓ diltiazem* ↓ desacetyl diltiazem* ↓ N-monodesmethyl diltiazem*	Diltiazem dose adjustments should be guided by clinical response (refer to the full prescribing information for diltiazem). No dose adjustment of efavirenz is necessary when administered with diltiazem.
Others (eg, felodipine, nicardipine, nifedipine, verapamil)	↓ calcium channel blocker	No data are available on the potential interactions of efavirenz with other calcium channel blockers that are substrates of CYP3A. The potential exists for reduction in plasma concentrations of the calcium channel blocker. Dose adjustments should be guided by clinical response (refer to the full prescribing information for the calcium channel blocker).
HMG-CoA reductase inhibitors: Atorvastatin Pravastatin Simvastatin	↓ atorvastatin* ↓ pravastatin* ↓ simvastatin*	Plasma concentrations of atorvastatin, pravastatin, and simvastatin decreased. Consult the full prescribing information for the HMG-CoA reductase inhibitor for guidance on individualizing the dose.
Hormonal contraceptives: Oral Ethinyl estradiol/ Norgestimate	↓ active metabolites of norgestimate*	A reliable method of barrier contraception must be used in addition to hormonal contraceptives. Efavirenz had no effect on ethinyl estradiol concentrations, but progestin levels (norelgestromin and levonorgestrel) were markedly decreased. No effect of ethinyl estradiol/norgestimate on efavirenz plasma concentrations was observed.
Implant Etonogestrel	↓ etonogestrel	A reliable method of barrier contraception must be used in addition to hormonal contraceptives. The interaction between etonogestrel and efavirenz has not been studied. Decreased exposure of etonogestrel may be expected. There have been postmarketing reports of contraceptive failure with etonogestrel in efavirenz-exposed patients.

(Table continued on next page)

In HIV-1-infected patients at steady state, mean C_{max}, mean C_{min}, and mean AUC were dose proportional following 200 mg, 400 mg, and 600 mg daily doses. Time-to-peak plasma concentrations were approximately 3-5 hours and steady-state plasma concentrations were reached in 6-10 days. In 35 patients receiving SUSTIVA 600 mg once daily, steady-state C_{max} was 12.9 ± 3.7 µM (mean ± SD), steady-state C_{min} was 5.6 ± 3.2 µM, and AUC was 184 ± 73 µM•h.

Effect of Food on Oral Absorption:
Capsules: Administration of a single 600 mg dose of efavirenz capsules with a high-fat/high-caloric meal (894 kcal, 54 g fat, 54% calories from fat) or a reduced-fat/normal-caloric meal (440 kcal, 2 g fat, 4% calories from fat) was associated with a mean increase of 22% and 17% in efavirenz AUC_∞ and a mean increase of 39% and 51% in efavirenz C_{max}, respectively, relative to the exposures

achieved when given under fasted conditions. [*See Dosage and Administration (2)* and *Patient Counseling Information (17).*]

Tablets: Administration of a single 600 mg efavirenz tablet with a high-fat/high-caloric meal (approximately 1000 kcal, 500-600 kcal from fat) was associated with a 28% increase in mean $AUC_∞$ of efavirenz and a 79% increase in mean C_{max} of efavirenz relative to the exposures achieved under fasted conditions. [*See Dosage and Administration (2)* and *Patient Counseling Information (17).*]

Bioavailability of capsule contents mixed with food vehicles: In healthy adult subjects, the efavirenz AUC when administered as the contents of three 200 mg capsules mixed with 2 teaspoons of certain food vehicles (applesauce, grape jelly or yogurt, or infant formula) met bioequivalence criteria for the AUC of the intact capsule formulation administered under fasted conditions.

Distribution
Efavirenz is highly bound (approximately 99.5-99.75%) to human plasma proteins, predominantly albumin. In HIV-1 infected patients (n=9) who received SUSTIVA (efavirenz) 200 to 600 mg once daily for at least one month, cerebrospinal fluid concentrations ranged from 0.26 to 1.19% (mean 0.69%) of the corresponding plasma concentration. This proportion is approximately 3-fold higher than the non-protein-bound (free) fraction of efavirenz in plasma.

Metabolism
Studies in humans and *in vitro* studies using human liver microsomes have demonstrated that efavirenz is principally metabolized by the cytochrome P450 system to hydroxylated metabolites with subsequent glucuronidation of these hydroxylated metabolites. These metabolites are essentially inactive against HIV-1. The *in vitro* studies suggest that CYP3A and CYP2B6 are the major isozymes responsible for efavirenz metabolism.

Efavirenz has been shown to induce CYP enzymes, resulting in the induction of its own metabolism. Multiple doses of 200-400 mg per day for 10 days resulted in a lower than predicted extent of accumulation (22-42% lower) and a shorter terminal half-life of 40-55 hours (single dose half-life 52-76 hours).

Elimination
Efavirenz has a terminal half-life of 52-76 hours after single doses and 40-55 hours after multiple doses. A one-month mass balance/excretion study was conducted using 400 mg per day with a ^{14}C-labeled dose administered on Day 8. Approximately 14-34% of the radiolabel was recovered in the urine and 16-61% was recovered in the feces. Nearly all of the urinary excretion of the radiolabeled drug was in the form of metabolites. Efavirenz accounted for the majority of the total radioactivity measured in feces.

Special Populations
Pediatric: The pharmacokinetic parameters for efavirenz at steady state in pediatric patients were predicted by a population pharmacokinetic model and are summarized in Table 6 by weight ranges that correspond to the recommended doses.

[See table 6 above]

Gender and race: The pharmacokinetics of efavirenz in patients appear to be similar between men and women and among the racial groups studied.

Renal impairment: The pharmacokinetics of efavirenz have not been studied in patients with renal insufficiency; however, less than 1% of efavirenz is excreted unchanged in the urine, so the impact of renal impairment on efavirenz elimination should be minimal.

Hepatic impairment: A multiple-dose study showed no significant effect on efavirenz pharmacokinetics in patients with mild hepatic impairment (Child-Pugh Class A) compared with controls. There were insufficient data to determine whether moderate or severe hepatic impairment (Child-Pugh Class B or C) affects efavirenz pharmacokinetics.

Drug Interaction Studies
Efavirenz has been shown *in vivo* to cause hepatic enzyme induction, thus increasing the biotransformation of some drugs metabolized by CYP3A and CYP2B6. *In vitro* studies have shown that efavirenz inhibited CYP isozymes 2C9 and 2C19 with K_i values (8.5-17 µM) in the range of observed efavirenz plasma concentrations. *In vitro* studies, efavirenz did not inhibit CYP2E1 and inhibited CYP2D6 and CYP1A2 (K_i values 82-160 µM) only at concentrations well above those achieved clinically. Coadministration of efavirenz with drugs primarily metabolized by CYP2C9, CYP2C19, CYP3A, or CYP2B6 isozymes may result in altered plasma concentrations of the coadministered drug. Drugs which induce CYP3A and CYP2B6 activity would be expected to increase the clearance of efavirenz resulting in lowered plasma concentrations.

Drug interaction studies were performed with efavirenz and other drugs likely to be coadministered or drugs commonly used as probes for pharmacokinetic interaction. The effects of coadministration of efavirenz on the C_{max}, AUC, and C_{min} are summarized in Table 7 (effect of efavirenz on other drugs) and Table 8 (effect of other drugs on efavirenz). For information regarding clinical recommendations see *Drug Interactions (7.1).*

Table 5 *(cont.)*: Established and Other Potentially Significant Drug Interactions: Alteration in Dose or Regimen May Be Recommended Based on Drug Interaction Studies or Predicted Interaction

Concomitant Drug Class: Drug Name	Effect	Clinical Comment
Other agents (cont.)		
Immunosuppressants: Cyclosporine, tacrolimus, sirolimus, and others metabolized by CYP3A	↓ immunosuppressant	Decreased exposure of the immunosuppressant may be expected due to CYP3A induction. These immunosuppressants are not anticipated to affect exposure of efavirenz. Dose adjustments of the immunosuppressant may be required. Close monitoring of immunosuppressant concentrations for at least 2 weeks (until stable concentrations are reached) is recommended when starting or stopping treatment with efavirenz.
Narcotic analgesic: Methadone	↓ methadone*	Coadministration in HIV-infected individuals with a history of injection drug use resulted in decreased plasma levels of methadone and signs of opiate withdrawal. Methadone dose was increased by a mean of 22% to alleviate withdrawal symptoms. Patients should be monitored for signs of withdrawal and their methadone dose increased as required to alleviate withdrawal symptoms.

* The interaction between SUSTIVA and the drug was evaluated in a clinical study. All other drug interactions shown are predicted.
This table is not all-inclusive.

Table 6: Predicted Steady-State Pharmacokinetics of Recommended Doses of Efavirenz (Capsules/Capsule Sprinkles) in HIV-Infected Pediatric Patients

Body Weight	Dose	Mean $AUC_{(0-24)}$ µM·h	Mean C_{max} µg/mL	Mean C_{min} µg/mL
3.5-5 kg	100 mg	220.52	5.81	2.43
5-7.5 kg	150 mg	262.62	7.07	2.71
7.5-10 kg	200 mg	284.28	7.75	2.87
10-15 kg	200 mg	238.14	6.54	2.32
15-20 kg	250 mg	233.98	6.47	2.3
20-25 kg	300 mg	257.56	7.04	2.55
25-32.5 kg	350 mg	262.37	7.12	2.68
32.5-40 kg	400 mg	259.79	6.96	2.69
>40 kg	600 mg	254.78	6.57	2.82

[See table 7 on pages 746 through 748]
[See table 8 on pages 749 and 750]

12.4   Microbiology
Mechanism of Action
Efavirenz is an NNRTI of HIV-1. Efavirenz activity is mediated predominantly by noncompetitive inhibition of HIV-1 reverse transcriptase. HIV-2 reverse transcriptase and human cellular DNA polymerases α, β, γ, and δ are not inhibited by efavirenz.

Antiviral Activity in Cell Culture
The concentration of efavirenz inhibiting replication of wild-type laboratory adapted strains and clinical isolates in cell culture by 90-95% (EC_{90-95}) ranged from 1.7 to 25 nM in lymphoblastoid cell lines, peripheral blood mononuclear cells (PBMCs), and macrophage/monocyte cultures. Efavirenz demonstrated antiviral activity against clade B and most non-clade B isolates (subtypes A, AE, AG, C, D, F, G, J, N), but had reduced antiviral activity against group O viruses. Efavirenz demonstrated additive antiviral activity without cytotoxicity against HIV-1 in cell culture when combined with the NNRTIs delavirdine and nevirapine, NRTIs (abacavir, didanosine, emtricitabine, lamivudine, stavudine, tenofovir, zalcitabine, zidovudine), PIs (amprenavir, indinavir, lopinavir, nelfinavir, ritonavir, saquinavir), and the fusion inhibitor enfuvirtide. Efavirenz demonstrated additive to antagonistic antiviral activity in cell culture with atazanavir. Efavirenz was not antagonistic with adefovir, used for the treatment of hepatitis B virus infection, or ribavirin, used in combination with interferon for the treatment of hepatitis C virus infection.

Resistance
In cell culture
In cell culture, HIV-1 isolates with reduced susceptibility to efavirenz (>380-fold increase in EC_{90} value) emerged rapidly in the presence of drug. Genotypic characterization of these viruses identified single amino acid substitutions L100I or V179D, double substitutions L100I/V108I, and triple substitutions L100I/V179D/Y181C in reverse transcriptase.

Clinical studies
Clinical isolates with reduced susceptibility in cell culture to efavirenz have been obtained. One or more substitutions at amino acid positions 98, 100, 101, 103, 106, 108, 188, 190, 225, and 227 in reverse transcriptase were observed in patients failing treatment with efavirenz in combination with indinavir, or with zidovudine plus lamivudine. The K103N substitution was the most frequently observed. Long-term resistance surveillance (average 52 weeks, range 4-106 weeks) analyzed 28 matching baseline and virologic failure isolates. Sixty-one percent (17/28) of these failure isolates had decreased efavirenz susceptibility in cell culture with a median 88-fold change in efavirenz susceptibility (EC_{50} value) from reference. The most frequent NNRTI substitution to develop in these patient isolates was K103N (54%). Other NNRTI substitutions that developed included L100I (7%), K101E/Q/R (14%), V108I (11%), G190S/T/A (7%), P225H (18%), and M230I/L (11%).

Cross-Resistance
Cross-resistance among NNRTIs has been observed. Clinical isolates previously characterized as efavirenz-resistant were also phenotypically resistant in cell culture to delavirdine and nevirapine compared to baseline. Delavirdine-and/or nevirapine-resistant clinical viral isolates with NNRTI resistance-associated substitutions (A98G, L100I, K101E/P, K103N/S, V106A, Y181X, Y188X, G190X, P225H, F227L, or M230L) showed reduced susceptibility to efavirenz in cell culture. Greater than 90% of NRTI-resistant clinical isolates tested in cell culture retained susceptibility to efavirenz.

13   NONCLINICAL TOXICOLOGY
13.1   Carcinogenesis, Mutagenesis, Impairment of Fertility
Carcinogenesis
Long-term carcinogenicity studies in mice and rats were carried out with efavirenz. Mice were dosed with 0, 25, 75, 150, or 300 mg/kg/day for 2 years. Incidences of hepatocellular adenomas and carcinomas and pulmonary alveolar/bronchiolar adenomas were increased above background in females. No increases in tumor incidence above background were seen in males. There was no NOAEL in females established for this study because tumor findings occurred at all doses. AUC at the NOAEL (150 mg/kg) in the males was approximately 0.9 times that in humans at the recommended clinical dose. In the rat study, no increases in tumor incidence were observed at doses up to 100 mg/kg/day, for which AUCs were 0.1 (males) or 0.2 (females) times those in humans at the recommended clinical dose.

Mutagenesis
Efavirenz tested negative in a battery of *in vitro* and *in vivo* genotoxicity assays. These included bacterial mutation assays in *S. typhimurium* and *E. coli*, mammalian mutation assays in Chinese hamster ovary cells, chromosome aberration assays in human peripheral blood lymphocytes or Chinese hamster ovary cells, and an *in vivo* mouse bone marrow micronucleus assay.

Table 7: Effect of Efavirenz on Coadministered Drug Plasma C_{max}, AUC, and C_{min}

Coadministered Drug	Dose	Efavirenz Dose	Number of Subjects	Coadministered Drug (mean % change)		
				C_{max} (90% CI)	AUC (90% CI)	C_{min} (90% CI)
Atazanavir	400 mg qd with a light meal d 1-20	600 mg qd with a light meal d 7-20	27	↓ 59% (49-67%)	↓ 74% (68-78%)	↓ 93% (90-95%)
	400 mg qd d 1-6, then 300 mg qd d 7-20 with ritonavir 100 mg qd and a light meal	600 mg qd 2 h after atazanavir and ritonavir d 7-20	13	↑ 14%[a] (↓ 17-↑ 58%)	↑ 39%[a] (2-88%)	↑ 48%[a] (24-76%)
	300 mg qd/ritonavir 100 mg qd d 1-10 (pm), then 400 mg qd/ritonavir 100 mg qd d 11-24 (pm) (simultaneous with efavirenz)	600 mg qd with a light snack d 11-24 (pm)	14	↑ 17% (8-27%)	↔	↓ 42% (31-51%)
Indinavir	1000 mg q8h × 10 days	600 mg qd × 10 days	20			
	After morning dose			↔[b]	↓ 33%[b] (26-39%)	↓ 39%[b] (24-51%)
	After afternoon dose			↔[b]	↓ 37%[b] (26-46%)	↓ 52%[b] (47-57%)
	After evening dose			↓ 29%[b] (11-43%)	↓ 46%[b] (37-54%)	↓ 57%[b] (50-63%)
Lopinavir/ ritonavir	400/100 mg capsule q12h × 9 days	600 mg qd × 9 days	11,7[c]	↔[d]	↓ 19%[d] (↓ 36-↑ 3%)	↓ 39%[d] (3-62%)
	500/125 mg tablet q12h × 10 days with efavirenz compared to 400/100 mg q12h alone	600 mg qd × 9 days	19	↑ 12%[d] (2-23%)	↔[d]	↓ 10%[d] (↓ 22-↑ 4%)
	600/150 mg tablet q12h × 10 days with efavirenz compared to 400/100 mg q12h alone	600 mg qd × 9 days	23	↑ 36%[d] (28-44%)	↑ 36%[d] (28-44%)	↑ 32%[d] (21-44%)
Nelfinavir	750 mg q8h × 7 days	600 mg qd × 7 days	10	↑ 21% (10-33%)	↑ 20% (8-34%)	↔
Metabolite AG-1402				↓ 40% (30-48%)	↓ 37% (25-48%)	↓ 43% (21-59%)
Ritonavir	500 mg q12h × 8 days	600 mg qd × 10 days	11			
	After AM dose			↑ 24% (12-38%)	↑ 18% (6-33%)	↑ 42% (9-86%)[e]
	After PM dose			↔	↔	↑ 24% (3-50%)[e]
Saquinavir SGC[f]	1200 mg q8h × 10 days	600 mg qd × 10 days	12	↓ 50% (28-66%)	↓ 62% (45-74%)	↓ 56% (16-77%)[e]
Lamivudine	150 mg q12h × 14 days	600 mg qd × 14 days	9	↔	↔	↑ 265% (37-873%)
Tenofovir[g]	300 mg qd	600 mg qd × 14 days	29	↔	↔	↔
Zidovudine	300 mg q12h × 14 days	600 mg qd × 14 days	9	↔	↔	↑ 225% (43-640%)
Maraviroc	100 mg bid	600 mg qd	12	↓ 51% (37-62%)	↓ 45% (38-51%)	↓ 45% (28-57%)
Raltegravir	400 mg single dose	600 mg qd	9	↓ 36% (2-59%)	↓ 36% (20-48%)	↓ 21% (↓ 51-↑ 28%)
Boceprevir	800 mg tid × 6 days	600 mg qd × 16 days	NA	↓ 8% (↓ 22-↑ 8%)	↓ 19% (11-25%)	↓ 44% (26-58%)
Telaprevir	750 mg q8h × 10 days	600 mg qd × 20 days	21	↓ 9% (↓ 18-↑ 2%)	↓ 26% (16-35%)	↓ 47% (35-56%)
Azithromycin	600 mg single dose	400 mg qd × 7 days	14	↑ 22% (4-42%)	↔	NA
Clarithromycin	500 mg q12h × 7 days	400 mg qd × 7 days	11	↓ 26% (15-35%)	↓ 39% (30-46%)	↓ 53% (42-63%)
14-OH metabolite				↑ 49% (32-69%)	↑ 34% (18-53%)	↑ 26% (9-45%)

(Table continued on next page)

13.2 Animal Toxicology

Nonsustained convulsions were observed in 6 of 20 monkeys receiving efavirenz at doses yielding plasma AUC values 4- to 13-fold greater than those in humans given the recommended dose [see *Warnings and Precautions (5.9)*].

14 CLINICAL STUDIES

14.1 Adults

Study 006, a randomized, open-label trial, compared SUSTIVA (efavirenz) (600 mg once daily) + zidovudine (ZDV, 300 mg q12h) + lamivudine (LAM, 150 mg q12h) or SUSTIVA (600 mg once daily) + indinavir (IDV, 1000 mg q8h) with indinavir (800 mg q8h) + zidovudine (300 mg q12h) + lamivudine (150 mg q12h). Twelve hundred sixty-six patients (mean age 36.5 years [range 18-81], 60% Caucasian, 83% male) were enrolled. All patients were efavirenz-, lamivudine-, NNRTI-, and PI-naive at study entry. The median baseline CD4+ cell count was 320 cells/mm³ and the median baseline HIV-1 RNA level was 4.8 log₁₀ copies/mL. Treatment outcomes with standard assay (assay limit

400 copies/mL) through 48 and 168 weeks are shown in Table 9. Plasma HIV RNA levels were quantified with standard (assay limit 400 copies/mL) and ultrasensitive (assay limit 50 copies/mL) versions of the AMPLICOR HIV-1 MONITOR assay. During the study, version 1.5 of the assay was introduced in Europe to enhance detection of non-clade B virus.

[See table 9 at top of page 750]

For patients treated with SUSTIVA + zidovudine + lamivudine, SUSTIVA + indinavir, or indinavir + zidovudine + lamivudine, the percentage of responders with HIV-1 RNA <50 copies/mL was 65%, 50%, and 45%, respectively, through 48 weeks, and 43%, 31%, and 23%, respectively, through 168 weeks. A Kaplan-Meier analysis of time to loss of virologic response (HIV RNA <400 copies/mL) suggests that both the trends of virologic response and differences in response continue through 4 years.

ACTG 364 is a randomized, double-blind, placebo-controlled, 48-week study in NRTI-experienced patients who had completed two prior ACTG studies. One-hundred ninety-six patients (mean age 41 years [range 18-76], 74% Caucasian, 88% male) received NRTIs in combination with SUSTIVA (600 mg once daily), or nelfinavir (NFV, 750 mg three times daily), or SUSTIVA (600 mg once daily) + nelfinavir in a randomized, double-blinded manner. The mean baseline CD4+ cell count was 389 cells/mm³ and mean baseline HIV-1 RNA level was 8130 copies/mL. Upon entry into the study, all patients were assigned a new open-label NRTI regimen, which was dependent on their previous NRTI treatment experience. There was no significant difference in the mean CD4+ cell count among treatment groups; the overall mean increase was approximately 100 cells at 48 weeks among patients who continued on study regimens. Treatment outcomes are shown in Table 10. Plasma HIV RNA levels were quantified with the AMPLICOR HIV-1 MONITOR assay using a lower limit of quantification of 500 copies/mL.

[See table 10 on page 750]

A Kaplan-Meier analysis of time to treatment failure through 72 weeks demonstrates a longer duration of virologic suppression (HIV RNA <500 copies/mL) in the SUSTIVA-containing treatment arms.

14.2 Pediatric Patients

Study AI266922 is an open-label study to evaluate the pharmacokinetics, safety, tolerability, and antiviral activity of SUSTIVA in combination with didanosine and emtricitabine in antiretroviral-naive and -experienced pediatric patients. Thirty-seven patients 3 months to 6 years of age (median 0.7 years) were treated with SUSTIVA. At baseline, median plasma HIV-1 RNA was 5.88 log₁₀ copies/mL, median CD4+ cell count was 1144 cells/mm³, and median CD4+ percentage was 25%. The median time on study therapy was 60 weeks; 27% of patients discontinued before Week 48. Using an ITT analysis, the overall proportions of patients with HIV RNA <400 copies/mL and <50 copies/mL at Week 48 were 57% (21/37) and 46% (17/37), respectively. The median increase from baseline in CD4+ count at 48 weeks was 196 cells/mm³ and the median increase in CD4+ percentage was 6%.

Study PACTG 1021 was an open-label study to evaluate the pharmacokinetics, safety, tolerability, and antiviral activity of SUSTIVA in combination with didanosine and emtricitabine in pediatric patients who were antiretroviral therapy naive. Forty-three patients 3 months to 21 years of age (median 9.6 years) were dosed with SUSTIVA. At baseline, median plasma HIV-1 RNA was 4.8 log₁₀ copies/mL, median CD4+ cell count was 367 cells/mm³, and median CD4+ percentage was 18%. The median time on study therapy was 181 weeks; 16% of patients discontinued before Week 48. Using an ITT analysis, the overall proportions of patients with HIV RNA <400 copies/mL and <50 copies/mL at Week 48 were 77% (33/43) and 70% (30/43), respectively. The median increase from baseline in CD4+ count at 48 weeks of therapy was 238 cells/mm³ and the median increase in CD4+ percentage was 13%.

Study PACTG 382 was an open-label study to evaluate the pharmacokinetics, safety, tolerability, and antiviral activity of SUSTIVA in combination with nelfinavir and an NRTI in

Impairment of Fertility

Efavirenz did not impair mating or fertility of male or female rats, and did not affect sperm of treated male rats. The reproductive performance of offspring born to female rats given efavirenz was not affected. The AUCs at the NOAEL values in male (200 mg/kg) and female (100 mg/kg) rats were approximately ≤0.15 times that in humans at the recommended clinical dose.

antiretroviral-naive and NRTI-experienced pediatric patients. One hundred two patients 3 months to 16 years of age (median 5.7 years) were treated with SUSTIVA. Eighty-seven percent of patients had received prior antiretroviral therapy. At baseline, median plasma HIV-1 RNA was 4.57 $\log_{10}$ copies/mL, median CD4+ cell count was 755 cells/mm³, and median CD4+ percentage was 30%. The median time on study therapy was 118 weeks; 25% of patients discontinued before Week 48. Using an ITT analysis, the overall proportion of patients with HIV RNA <400 copies/mL and <50 copies/mL at Week 48 were 57% (58/102) and 43% (44/102), respectively. The median increase from baseline in CD4+ count at 48 weeks of therapy was 128 cells/mm³ and the median increase in CD4+ percentage was 5%.

16 HOW SUPPLIED/STORAGE AND HANDLING

16.1 Capsules
SUSTIVA® (efavirenz) capsules are available as follows:
Capsules 200 mg are gold color, reverse printed with "SUSTIVA" on the body and imprinted "200 mg" on the cap.
  Bottles of 90   NDC 0056-0474-92
Capsules 50 mg are gold color and white, printed with "SUSTIVA" on the gold color cap and reverse printed "50 mg" on the white body.
  Bottles of 30   NDC 0056-0470-30

16.2 Tablets
SUSTIVA® (efavirenz) tablets are available as follows:
Tablets 600 mg are yellow, capsular-shaped, film-coated tablets, with "SUSTIVA" printed on both sides.
  Bottles of 30   NDC 0056-0510-30

16.3 Storage
SUSTIVA capsules and SUSTIVA tablets should be stored at 25°C (77°F); excursions permitted to 15°C–30°C (59°F–86°F) [see USP Controlled Room Temperature].

17 PATIENT COUNSELING INFORMATION
Advise the patient to read the FDA-approved patient labeling (Patient Information and Instructions for Use).
Drug Interactions
A statement to patients and healthcare providers is included on the product's bottle labels:
ALERT: Find out about medicines that should NOT be taken with SUSTIVA.
SUSTIVA may interact with some drugs; therefore, patients should be advised to report to their doctor the use of any other prescription, or nonprescription medication
General Information for Patients
Patients should be informed that SUSTIVA is not a cure for HIV-1 infection and patients may continue to experience illnesses associated with HIV-1 infection, including opportunistic infections. Patients should remain under the care of a physician while taking SUSTIVA.
Patients should be advised to avoid doing things that can spread HIV-1 infection to others.
• **Do not share or reuse needles or other injection equipment.**
• **Do not share personal items that can have blood or body fluids on them, like toothbrushes and razor blades.**
• **Do not have any kind of sex without protection.** Always practice safer sex by using a latex or polyurethane condom to lower the chance of sexual contact with semen, vaginal secretions, or blood.
• **Do not breastfeed.** It is not known if SUSTIVA can be passed to your baby in your breast milk and whether it could harm your baby. Also, mothers with HIV-1 should not breastfeed because HIV-1 can be passed to the baby in breast milk.
Dosing Instructions
Patients should be advised to take SUSTIVA every day as prescribed. If a patient forgets to take SUSTIVA, tell the patient to take the missed dose right away, unless it is almost time for the next dose. Advise the patient not to take 2 doses at one time and to take the next dose at the regularly scheduled time. Advise the patient to ask a healthcare provider if he/she needs help in planning the best times to take his/her medicine.
SUSTIVA must always be used in combination with other antiretroviral drugs. Patients should be advised to take SUSTIVA on an empty stomach, preferably at bedtime. Taking SUSTIVA with food increases efavirenz concentrations and may increase the frequency of adverse reactions. Dosing at bedtime may improve the tolerability of nervous system symptoms [see Dosage and Administration (2) and Adverse Reactions (6.1)]. Healthcare providers should assist parents or caregivers in determining the best SUSTIVA dosing schedule for infants and young children.
For adult and pediatric patients who cannot swallow capsules or tablets, patients or their caregivers should be advised to read and carefully follow the instructions for administering the capsule contents in a small amount of food or infant formula [see Dosage and Administration (2.3) and FDA-approved patient labeling (Patient Information and Instructions for Use)]. Patients should call their healthcare provider or pharmacist if they have any questions.

Nervous System Symptoms
Patients should be informed that central nervous system symptoms (NSS) including dizziness, insomnia, impaired concentration, drowsiness, and abnormal dreams are commonly reported during the first weeks of therapy with SUSTIVA (efavirenz) [see Warnings and Precautions (5.5)]. Dosing at bedtime may improve the tolerability of these symptoms, which are likely to improve with continued therapy. Patients should be alerted to the potential for additive effects when SUSTIVA is used concomitantly with alcohol or psychoactive drugs. Patients should be instructed that if they experience NSS they should avoid potentially hazardous tasks such as driving or operating machinery.
Psychiatric Symptoms
Patients should be informed that serious psychiatric symptoms including severe depression, suicide attempts, aggressive behavior, delusions, paranoia, and psychosis-like symptoms have been reported in patients receiving SUSTIVA (efavirenz) [see Warnings and Precautions (5.4)]. If they experience severe psychiatric adverse experiences they should

Table 7 (cont.): Effect of Efavirenz on Coadministered Drug Plasma C_{max}, AUC, and C_{min}

Coadministered Drug	Dose	Efavirenz Dose	Number of Subjects	Coadministered Drug (mean % change)		
				C_{max} (90% CI)	AUC (90% CI)	C_{min} (90% CI)
Fluconazole	200 mg × 7 days	400 mg qd × 7 days	10	↔	↔	↔
Itraconazole	200 mg q12h × 28 days	600 mg qd × 14 days	18	↓ 37% (20-51%)	↓ 39% (21-53%)	↓ 44% (27-58%)
Hydroxy-itraconazole				↓ 35% (12-52%)	↓ 37% (14-55%)	↓ 43% (18-60%)
Posaconazole	400 mg (oral suspension) bid × 10 and 20 days	400 mg qd × 10 and 20 days	11	↓ 45% (34-53%)	↓ 50% (40-57%)	NA
Rifabutin	300 mg qd × 14 days	600 mg qd × 14 days	9	↓ 32% (15-46%)	↓ 38% (28-47%)	↓ 45% (31-56%)
Voriconazole	400 mg po q12h × 1 day, then 200 mg po q12h × 8 days	400 mg qd × 9 days	NA	↓ 61%[h]	↓ 77%[h]	NA
	300 mg po q12h days 2-7	300 mg qd × 7 days	NA	↓ 36%[i] (21-49%)	↓ 55%[i] (45-62%)	NA
	400 mg po q12h days 2-7	300 mg qd × 7 days	NA	↑ 23%[i] (↓ 1-↑ 53%)	↓ 7%[i] (↓ 23-↑ 13%)	NA
Artemether/lumefantrine	Artemether 20 mg/lumefantrine 120 mg tablets (6 4-tablet doses over 3 days)	600 mg qd × 26 days	12			
Artemether				↓ 21%	↓ 51%	NA
dihydroartemisinin				↓ 38%	↓ 46%	NA
lumefantrine				↔	↓ 21%	NA
Atorvastatin	10 mg qd × 4 days	600 mg qd × 15 days	14	↓ 14% (1-26%)	↓ 43% (34-50%)	↓ 69% (49-81%)
Total active (including metabolites)				↓ 15% (2-26%)	↓ 32% (21-41%)	↓ 48% (23-64%)
Pravastatin	40 mg qd × 4 days	600 mg qd × 15 days	13	↓ 32% (↓ 59-↑ 12%)	↓ 44% (26-57%)	↓ 19% (0-35%)
Simvastatin	40 mg qd × 4 days	600 mg qd × 15 days	14	↓ 72% (63-79%)	↓ 68% (62-73%)	↓ 45% (20-62%)
Total active (including metabolites)				↓ 68% (55-78%)	↓ 60% (52-68%)	NA[j]
Carbamazepine	200 mg qd × 3 days, 200 mg bid × 3 days, then 400 mg qd × 29 days	600 mg qd × 14 days	12	↓ 20% (15-24%)	↓ 27% (20-33%)	↓ 35% (24-44%)
Epoxide metabolite				↔	↔	↓ 13% (↓ 30-↑ 7%)
Cetirizine	10 mg single dose	600 mg qd × 10 days	11	↓ 24% (18-30%)	↔	NA
Diltiazem	240 mg × 21 days	600 mg qd × 14 days	13	↓ 60% (50-68%)	↓ 69% (55-79%)	↓ 63% (44-75%)
Desacetyl diltiazem				↓ 64% (57-69%)	↓ 75% (59-84%)	↓ 62% (44-75%)
N-monodesmethyl diltiazem				↓ 28% (7-44%)	↓ 37% (17-52%)	↓ 37% (17-52%)
Ethinyl estradiol/Norgestimate	0.035 mg/0.25 mg × 14 days	600 mg qd × 14 days				
Ethinyl estradiol			21	↔	↔	↔
Norelgestromin			21	↓ 46% (39-52%)	↓ 64% (62-67%)	↓ 82% (79-85%)
Levonorgestrel			6	↓ 80% (77-83%)	↓ 83% (79-87%)	↓ 86% (80-90%)

(Table continued on next page)

Table 7 *(cont.)*: Effect of Efavirenz on Coadministered Drug Plasma C_{max}, AUC, and C_{min}

Coadministered Drug	Dose	Efavirenz Dose	Number of Subjects	Coadministered Drug (mean % change)		
				C_{max} (90% CI)	AUC (90% CI)	C_{min} (90% CI)
Lorazepam	2 mg single dose	600 mg qd × 10 days	12	↑ 16% (2-32%)	↔	NA
Methadone	Stable maintenance 35-100 mg daily	600 mg qd × 14-21 days	11	↓ 45% (25-59%)	↓ 52% (33-66%)	NA
Bupropion	150 mg single dose (sustained-release)	600 mg qd × 14 days	13	↓ 34% (21-47%)	↓ 55% (48-62%)	NA
Hydroxy-bupropion				↑ 50% (20-80%)	↔	NA
Paroxetine	20 mg qd × 14 days	600 mg qd × 14 days	16	↔	↔	↔
Sertraline	50 mg qd × 14 days	600 mg qd × 14 days	13	↓ 29% (15-40%)	↓ 39% (27-50%)	↓ 46% (31-58%)

↑ Indicates increase   ↓ Indicates decrease   ↔ Indicates no change or a mean increase or decrease of <10%.
[a] Compared with atazanavir 400 mg qd alone.
[b] Comparator dose of indinavir was 800 mg q8h × 10 days.
[c] Parallel-group design; n for efavirenz + lopinavir/ritonavir, n for lopinavir/ritonavir alone.
[d] Values are for lopinavir, the pharmacokinetics of ritonavir in this study were unaffected by concurrent efavirenz.
[e] 95% CI.
[f] Soft Gelatin Capsule.
[g] Tenofovir disoproxil fumarate.
[h] 90% CI not available.
[i] Relative to steady-state administration of voriconazole (400 mg for 1 day, then 200 mg po q12h for 2 days).
[j] Not available because of insufficient data.
NA = not available.

seek immediate medical evaluation. Patients should be advised to inform their physician of any history of mental illness or substance abuse.

Rash
Patients should be informed that a common side effect is rash [see *Warnings and Precautions (5.7)*]. Rashes usually go away without any change in treatment. However, since rash may be serious, patients should be advised to contact their physician promptly if rash occurs.

Reproductive Risk Potential
Women receiving SUSTIVA (efavirenz) should be instructed to avoid pregnancy [see *Warnings and Precautions (5.6)*]. A reliable form of barrier contraception must always be used in combination with other methods of contraception, including oral or other hormonal contraception. Because of the long half-life of efavirenz, use of adequate contraceptive measures for 12 weeks after discontinuation of SUSTIVA is recommended. Women should be advised to notify their physician if they become pregnant or plan to become pregnant while taking SUSTIVA. If this drug is used during the first trimester of pregnancy, or if the patient becomes pregnant while taking this drug, she should be apprised of the potential harm to the fetus.

Fat Redistribution
Patients should be informed that redistribution or accumulation of body fat may occur in patients receiving antiretroviral therapy and that the cause and long-term health effects of these conditions are not known [see *Warnings and Precautions (5.12)*].

SUSTIVA is a registered trademark of Bristol-Myers Squibb Pharma Company, ATRIPLA is a trademark of Bristol-Myers Squibb & Gilead Sciences, LLC, PRAVACHOL is a registered trademark of ER Squibb & Sons, LLC, and REYATAZ is a registered trademark of Bristol-Myers Squibb Company. Other brands listed are the trademarks of their respective owners.
Distributed by:
Bristol-Myers Squibb Company
Princeton, NJ 08543 USA
SUSTIVA® (efavirenz) capsules made in India.
© Bristol-Myers Squibb Company 2014
Patient Information
SUSTIVA® (sus-TEE-vah)
(efavirenz)
capsules
SUSTIVA® (sus-TEE-vah)
(efavirenz)
tablets
Important: Ask your doctor or pharmacist about medicines that should not be taken with SUSTIVA. For more information, see the section "What should I tell my doctor before taking SUSTIVA?"
Read this Patient Information before you start taking SUSTIVA and each time you get a refill. There may be new

information. This information does not take the place of talking with your doctor about your medical condition or treatment.

What is SUSTIVA?
SUSTIVA (efavirenz) is a prescription HIV-1 (Human Immunodeficiency Virus type 1) medicine used with other antiretroviral medicines to treat HIV-1 infection in adults and in children who are at least 3 months old and who weigh at least 7 pounds 12 ounces (3.5 kg). HIV is the virus that causes AIDS (Acquired Immune Deficiency Syndrome).
It is not known if SUSTIVA is safe and effective in children younger than 3 months of age or who weigh less than 7 pounds 12 ounces (3.5 kg).
When used with other antiretroviral medicines to treat HIV-1 infection, SUSTIVA may help:
• reduce the amount of HIV-1 in your blood. This is called viral load.
• increase the number of CD4+ (T) cells in your blood that help fight off other infections.
Reducing the amount of HIV-1 and increasing the CD4+ (T) cells in your blood may help improve your immune system. This may reduce your risk of death or getting infections that can happen when your immune system is weak (opportunistic infections).
SUSTIVA does not cure HIV-1 infection or AIDS. You must keep taking HIV-1 medicines to control HIV-1 infection and decrease HIV-related illnesses.
Avoid doing things that can spread HIV-1 infection to others:
• Do not share or reuse needles or other injection equipment.
• Do not share personal items that can have blood or body fluids on them, like toothbrushes and razor blades.
• Do not have any kind of sex without protection. Always practice safer sex by using a latex or polyurethane condom to lower the chance of sexual contact with any body fluids such as semen, vaginal secretions, or blood.
Ask your doctor if you have any questions about how to prevent passing HIV to other people.
Who should not take SUSTIVA?
Do not take SUSTIVA if you are allergic to efavirenz or any of the ingredients in SUSTIVA. See the end of this leaflet for a complete list of ingredients in SUSTIVA.
What should I tell my doctor before taking SUSTIVA?
Before taking SUSTIVA, tell your doctor if you have any medical conditions and in particular, if you:
• have ever had a mental health problem
• have ever used street drugs or large amounts of alcohol
• have liver problems, including hepatitis B or C virus infection
• have a history of seizures
• are pregnant or plan to become pregnant. SUSTIVA may harm your unborn baby. You should not become pregnant

while taking SUSTIVA (efavirenz) and for 12 weeks after stopping treatment with SUSTIVA.
Females who are able to become pregnant must use 2 effective forms of birth control during treatment and for 12 weeks after stopping treatment with SUSTIVA. A barrier form of birth control must be used along with another type of birth control.
• Barrier forms of birth control may include latex or polyurethane condom, contraceptive sponge, diaphragm with spermicide, and cervical cap.
• Hormonal forms of birth control, such as birth control pills, injections, vaginal rings, or implants may not work during treatment with SUSTIVA.
• Talk to your doctor about forms of birth control that may be used during treatment with SUSTIVA.
Pregnancy Registry. There is a pregnancy registry for women who take antiretroviral medicines during pregnancy. The purpose of this registry is to collect information about the health of you and your baby. Talk to your doctor about how you can take part in this registry.
• are breastfeeding or plan to breastfeed. You should not breastfeed if you have HIV because of the risk of passing HIV to your baby. Do not breastfeed if you take SUSTIVA. SUSTIVA can pass into your breast milk. It is not known if this could harm your baby. Talk with your doctor about the best way to feed your baby.
Tell your doctor about all the medicines you take, including prescription and over-the-counter medicines, vitamins, and herbal supplements.
SUSTIVA may affect the way other medicines work, and other medicines may affect how SUSTIVA works, and may cause serious side effects. If you take certain medicines with SUSTIVA, the amount of SUSTIVA in your body may be too low and it may not work to help control your HIV infection. The HIV virus in your body may become resistant to SUSTIVA or other HIV medicines that are like it.
You should not take SUSTIVA if you take ATRIPLA (efavirenz, emtricitabine, tenofovir-disoproxil fumarate) unless your doctor tells you to.
Especially tell your doctor if you take any of the medicines below:
The following medicines may need to be replaced with another medicine during your treatment with SUSTIVA:
• boceprevir (Victrelis)
• carbamazepine (Carbatrol, Tegretol, Tegretol-XR, Equetro, Teril, Epitol)
• clarithromycin (Biaxin, Biaxin XL)
• itraconazole (Sporanox, Onmel)
• posaconazole (Noxafil)
• saquinavir mesylate (Invirase)
• atazanavir sulfate (REYATAZ)
If you take any of the following medicines during treatment with SUSTIVA, your doctor may need to change the dose of the medicine or change the dose of SUSTIVA, or your doctor may need to monitor you more closely:
• calcium channel blockers such as diltiazem (Cardizem, Cardizem CD, Cardizem LA, Tiazac, Cartia XT, Dilacor XR, Dilt-CD, Diltzac, Taztia XT), verapamil (Covera-HS, Calan, Calan SR, Verelan, Verelan PM), felodipine (Plendil), nicardipine (Cardene, Cardene SR), or nifedipine (Adalat CC, Afeditab CR, Procardia, Procardia XL)
• the cholesterol-lowering medicines atorvastatin (Lipitor), pravastatin sodium (PRAVACHOL), or simvastatin (Zocor)
• immunosuppressant medicines such as cyclosporine (Gengraf, Neoral, Sandimmune), tacrolimus (Prograf, Astagraf XL), or sirolimus (Rapamune)
• artemether/lumefantrine (Coartem)
• atazanavir sulfate (REYATAZ)
• bupropion (Wellbutrin, Wellbutrin SR, Wellbutrin XL, Forfivo XL, Zyban)
• indinavir (Crixivan)
• lopinavir/ritonavir (Kaletra)
• ritonavir (Norvir)
• maraviroc (Selzentry)
• methadone (Dolophine, Methadose)
• rifabutin (Mycobutin)
• rifampin (Rifadin, Rimactane, Rifamate, Rifater)
• sertraline (Zoloft)
• voriconazole (Vfend). Your doses of both Vfend and SUSTIVA may need to be changed.
• raltegravir (Isentress)
• telaprevir (Incivek)
• warfarin (Coumadin, Jantoven)
• phenytoin (Dilantin)
• ketoconazole (Nizoral)
Ask your doctor or pharmacist if you are not sure if your medicine is one that is listed above.
Know the medicines you take. Keep a list of your medicines and show it to your doctor and pharmacist when you get a new medicine.
Your doctor and your pharmacist can tell you if you can take these medicines with SUSTIVA. Do not start any new medicines while you are taking SUSTIVA without first talking with your doctor or pharmacist. You can ask your doctor or pharmacist for a list of medicines that can interact with SUSTIVA.

How should I take SUSTIVA?

- Take SUSTIVA (efavirenz) exactly as your doctor tells you to.
- Do not change your dose or stop taking SUSTIVA unless your doctor tells you to.
- Stay under the care of your doctor during treatment with SUSTIVA.
- SUSTIVA must be used with other antiretroviral medicines.
- Take SUSTIVA 1 time each day.
- SUSTIVA comes as tablets or capsules.
- SUSTIVA tablets should not be broken.
- Swallow SUSTIVA tablets or capsules whole with liquid.

How and when to take SUSTIVA

- You should take SUSTIVA on an empty stomach at bedtime. Taking SUSTIVA with food increases the amount of medicine in your body. Some side effects may bother you less if you take SUSTIVA on an empty stomach and at bedtime.
- Your child's doctor will prescribe the right dose of SUSTIVA based on your child's weight.
- If you have difficulty swallowing tablets or capsules, tell your doctor. Your doctor may recommend opening the SUSTIVA capsule and mixing the contents with food or infant formula. **See the detailed "Instructions for Use" at the end of this Patient Information to learn the right way to take SUSTIVA using the capsule sprinkle method.**
- Adults and children who take SUSTIVA using the capsule sprinkle method should not eat for 2 hours after taking a dose of SUSTIVA.
- Babies should not be given infant formula for 2 hours after taking a dose of SUSTIVA using the capsule sprinkle method.
- Do not miss a dose of SUSTIVA. If you forget to take SUSTIVA, take the missed dose right away, unless it is almost time for your next dose. Do not take 2 doses at one time. Just take your next dose at your regularly scheduled time. If you need help in planning the best times to take your medicine, ask your doctor or pharmacist.
- If you take too much SUSTIVA, call your doctor or go to the nearest hospital emergency room right away.
- When your SUSTIVA supply starts to run low, get more from your doctor or pharmacy. It is important not to run out of SUSTIVA. The amount of HIV in your blood may increase if the medicine is stopped for even a short time. The virus may become resistant to SUSTIVA and harder to treat.

What are the possible side effects of SUSTIVA?

SUSTIVA may cause serious side effects, including:

- **Serious mental health problems** can happen in people who take SUSTIVA. Tell your doctor right away if you have any of the following symptoms:
  - feel sad or hopeless
  - feel anxious or restless
  - have thoughts of hurting yourself (suicide) or have tried to hurt yourself or others
  - are not able to tell the difference between what is true or real and what is false or unreal
  - do not trust other people
  - hear or see things that are not real
- **Nervous system symptoms** are common in people who take SUSTIVA and can be severe. These symptoms usually begin during the first or second day of treatment with SUSTIVA and usually go away after 2 to 4 weeks of treatment. These symptoms may become worse if you drink alcohol, take a medicine for mental health problems, or use certain street drugs during treatment with SUSTIVA. Symptoms may include:
  - dizziness
  - trouble sleeping
  - trouble concentrating
  - drowsiness
  - unusual dreams

  If you have dizziness, trouble concentrating or drowsiness, do not drive a car, use machinery, or do anything that needs you to be alert.
- **Skin rash** is common with SUSTIVA but can sometimes be severe. Skin rash usually goes away without any change in treatment. If you develop a rash with any of the following symptoms, tell your doctor right away:
  - skin rash, with or without itching
  - fever
  - swelling of your face
  - blisters or skin lesions
  - peeling skin
  - mouth sores
  - red or inflamed eyes, like "pink eye" (conjunctivitis)
- **Liver problems, including liver failure and death.** If you have liver problems, including hepatitis B or C infection or take another medicine that can cause liver problems, your doctor may do blood tests to check your liver before you start SUSTIVA and during treatment. Liver problems can also happen in people without a history of liver problems. Tell your doctor right away if you get any of the following symptoms:

- your skin or the white part of your eyes turns yellow (jaundice)
- your urine turns dark
- your bowel movements (stools) turn light in color
- you don't feel like eating food for several days or longer
- you feel sick to your stomach (nausea)
- you have lower stomach area (abdominal) pain

- **Seizures** can happen in people who take SUSTIVA (efavirenz). Seizures are more likely to happen if you have had seizures in the past. Tell your doctor if you have had a seizure or if you take a medicine to help prevent seizures.
- **Changes in your immune system (Immune Reconstitution Syndrome)** can happen when you start taking HIV-1 medicines. Your immune system may get stronger and be-

Table 8: Effect of Coadministered Drug on Efavirenz Plasma C$_{max}$, AUC, and C$_{min}$

Coadministered Drug	Dose	Efavirenz Dose	Number of Subjects	Efavirenz (mean % change)		
				C$_{max}$ (90% CI)	AUC (90% CI)	C$_{min}$ (90% CI)
Indinavir	800 mg q8h × 14 days	200 mg qd × 14 days	11	↔	↔	↔
Lopinavir/ ritonavir	400/100 mg q12h × 9 days	600 mg qd × 9 days	11,12[a]	↔	↓ 16% (↓ 38-↑ 15%)	↓ 16% (↓ 42-↑ 20%)
Nelfinavir	750 mg q8h × 7 days	600 mg qd × 7 days	10	↓ 12% (↓ 32-↑ 13%)[b]	↓ 12% (↓ 35-↑ 18%)[b]	↓ 21% (↓ 53-↑ 33%)
Ritonavir	500 mg q12h × 8 days	600 mg qd × 10 days	9	↑ 14% (4-26%)	↑ 21% (10-34%)	↑ 25% (7-46%)[b]
Saquinavir SGC[c]	1200 mg q8h × 10 days	600 mg qd × 10 days	13	↓ 13% (5-20%)	↓ 12% (4-19%)	↓ 14% (2-24%)[b]
Tenofovir[d]	300 mg qd	600 mg qd × 14 days	30	↔	↔	↔
Boceprevir	800 mg tid × 6 days	600 mg qd × 16 days	NA	↑ 11% (2-20%)	↑ 20% (15-26%)	NA
Telaprevir	750 mg q8h × 10 days	600 mg qd × 20 days	21	↓ 16% (7-24%)	↓ 7% (2-13%)	↓ 2% (↓ 6-↑ 2%)
Telaprevir, coadministered with tenofovir disoproxil fumarate (TDF)	1125 mg q8h × 7 days	600 mg efavirenz/300 mg TDF qd × 7 days	15	↓ 24% (15-32%)	↓ 18% (10-26%)	↓ 10% (↓ 19-↑ 1%)
	1500 mg q12h × 7 days	600 mg efavirenz/300 mg TDF qd × 7 days	16	↓ 20% (14-26%)	↓ 15% (9-21%)	↓ 11% (4-18%)
Azithromycin	600 mg single dose	400 mg qd × 7 days	14	↔	↔	↔
Clarithromycin	500 mg q12h × 7 days	400 mg qd × 7 days	12	↑ 11% (3-19%)	↔	↔
Fluconazole	200 mg × 7 days	400 mg qd × 7 days	10	↔	↑ 16% (6-26%)	↑ 22% (5-41%)
Itraconazole	200 mg q12h × 14 days	600 mg qd × 28 days	16	↔	↔	↔
Rifabutin	300 mg qd × 14 days	600 mg qd × 14 days	11	↔	↔	↓ 12% (↓ 24-↑ 1%)
Rifampin	600 mg × 7 days	600 mg qd × 7 days	12	↓ 20% (11-28%)	↓ 26% (15-36%)	↓ 32% (15-46%)
Voriconazole	400 mg po q12h × 1 day, then 200 mg po q12h × 8 days	400 mg qd × 9 days	NA	↑ 38%[e]	↑ 44%[e]	NA
	300 mg po q12h days 2-7	300 mg qd × 7 days	NA	↓ 14%[f] (7-21%)	↔[f]	NA
	400 mg po q12h days 2-7	300 mg qd × 7 days	NA	↔[f]	↑ 17%[f] (6-29%)	NA
Artemether/ Lumefantrine	Artemether 20 mg/ lumefantrine 120 mg tablets (6 4-tablet doses over 3 days)	600 mg qd × 26 days	12	↔	↓ 17%	NA
Atorvastatin	10 mg qd × 4 days	600 mg qd × 15 days	14	↔	↔	↔
Pravastatin	40 mg qd × 4 days	600 mg qd × 15 days	11	↔	↔	↔
Simvastatin	40 mg qd × 4 days	600 mg qd × 15 days	14	↓ 12% (↓ 28-↑ 8%)	↔	↓ 12% (↓ 25-↑ 3%)

(Table continued on next page)

gin to fight infections that have been hidden in your body for a long time. Tell your doctor if you start having new symptoms after starting your HIV-1 medicine.

- **Changes in body fat** can happen in people who take HIV-1 medicine. These changes may include increased amount of fat in the upper back and neck ("buffalo hump"), breast, and around the main part of your body (trunk). Loss of fat from the legs, arms, and face may also happen. The cause and long-term health effects of these conditions are not known.

The most common side effects of SUSTIVA (efavirenz) include:

- rash
- dizziness
- nausea
- headache
- difficulty concentrating
- abnormal dreams
- tiredness
- trouble sleeping
- vomiting

Some patients taking SUSTIVA have experienced increased levels of lipids (cholesterol and triglycerides) in the blood. Tell your doctor if you have any side effect that bothers you or that does not go away.

These are not all the possible side effects of SUSTIVA. For more information, ask your doctor or pharmacist.

Call your doctor for medical advice about side effects. You may report side effects to FDA at 1-800-FDA-1088.

How should I store SUSTIVA?

- Store SUSTIVA capsules and tablets at room temperature between 68°F to 77°F (20°C to 25°C).

Keep SUSTIVA and all medicines out of the reach of children.

General information about SUSTIVA

Medicines are sometimes prescribed for purposes other than those listed in a Patient Information leaflet. Do not use SUSTIVA for a condition for which it was not prescribed. Do not give SUSTIVA to other people, even if they have the same symptoms that you have. It may harm them.

If you would like more information, talk with your doctor. You can ask your pharmacist or doctor for information about SUSTIVA that is written for health professionals. For more information, go to www.sustiva.com or call 1–800–321–1335.

What are the ingredients in SUSTIVA?

Active ingredient: efavirenz

Inactive ingredients:

SUSTIVA capsules: lactose monohydrate, magnesium stearate, sodium lauryl sulfate, and sodium starch glycolate. The capsule shell contains gelatin, sodium lauryl sulfate, titanium dioxide, and/or yellow iron oxide. The capsule shell may also contain silicon dioxide. The capsules are printed with ink containing carmine 40 blue, FD&C Blue No. 2, and titanium dioxide.

SUSTIVA tablets: croscarmellose sodium, hydroxypropyl cellulose, lactose monohydrate, magnesium stearate, microcrystalline cellulose, and sodium lauryl sulfate. The tablet film coating contains Opadry Yellow and Opadry Clear. The tablets are polished with carnauba wax and printed with purple ink, Opacode WB.

This Patient Information has been approved by the U.S. Food and Drug Administration.

Distributed by:
Bristol-Myers Squibb Company
Princeton, NJ 08543 USA
SUSTIVA® (efavirenz) capsules made in India.
© Bristol-Myers Squibb Company 2014
Revised: May 2014
1320416A0
510230013IN12

SUSTIVA is a registered trademark of Bristol-Myers Squibb Pharma Company, ATRIPLA is a registered trademark of Bristol-Myers Squibb & Gilead Sciences, LLC, PRAVACHOL is a registered trademark of ER Squibb & Sons, LLC, and REYATAZ is a registered trademark of Bristol-Myers Squibb Company. Other brands listed are the trademarks of their respective owners.

Instructions for Use

SUSTIVA (sus-TEE-vah)

efavirenz

capsules

Preparing a dose of SUSTIVA using the capsule sprinkle method

Read this Instructions for Use before you prepare your first dose of SUSTIVA mixed with food or infant formula using the capsule sprinkle method, each time you get a refill, and as needed. There may be new information. This information does not take the place of talking to your doctor about your medical condition or treatment. Ask your doctor or pharmacist if you have any questions about how to mix or give a dose of SUSTIVA using the capsule sprinkle method.

Important Information:

- For more information about SUSTIVA capsules, see the Patient Information leaflet.

Table 8 (cont.): Effect of Coadministered Drug on Efavirenz Plasma C_{max}, AUC, and C_{min}

Coadministered Drug	Dose	Efavirenz Dose	Number of Subjects	Efavirenz (mean % change)		
				C_{max} (90% CI)	AUC (90% CI)	C_{min} (90% CI)
Aluminum hydroxide 400 mg, magnesium hydroxide 400 mg, plus simethicone 40 mg	30 mL single dose	400 mg single dose	17	↔	↔	NA
Carbamazepine	200 mg qd × 3 days, 200 mg bid × 3 days, then 400 mg qd × 15 days	600 mg qd × 35 days	14	↓ 21% (15-26%)	↓ 36% (32-40%)	↓ 47% (41-53%)
Cetirizine	10 mg single dose	600 mg qd × 10 days	11	↔	↔	↔
Diltiazem	240 mg × 14 days	600 mg qd × 28 days	12	↑ 16% (6-26%)	↑ 11% (5-18%)	↑ 13% (1-26%)
Famotidine	40 mg single dose	400 mg single dose	17	↔	↔	NA
Paroxetine	20 mg qd × 14 days	600 mg qd × 14 days	12	↔	↔	↔
Sertraline	50 mg qd × 14 days	600 mg qd × 14 days	13	↑ 11% (6-16%)	↔	↔

↑ Indicates increase   ↓ Indicates decrease   ↔ Indicates no change or a mean increase or decrease of <10%.

[a] Parallel-group design; n for efavirenz + lopinavir/ritonavir, n for efavirenz alone.
[b] 95% CI.
[c] Soft Gelatin Capsule.
[d] Tenofovir disoproxil fumarate.
[e] 90% CI not available.
[f] Relative to steady-state administration of efavirenz (600 mg once daily for 9 days).
NA = not available.

Table 9: Outcomes of Randomized Treatment Through 48 and 168 Weeks, Study 006

Outcome	SUSTIVA + ZDV + LAM (n=422)		SUSTIVA + IDV (n=429)		IDV + ZDV + LAM (n=415)	
	Week 48	Week 168	Week 48	Week 168	Week 48	Week 168
Responder[a]	69%	48%	57%	40%	50%	29%
Virologic failure[b]	6%	12%	15%	20%	13%	19%
Discontinued for adverse events	7%	8%	6%	8%	16%	20%
Discontinued for other reasons[c]	17%	31%	22%	32%	21%	32%
CD4+ cell count (cells/mm³)						
Observed subjects (n)	(279)	(205)	(256)	(158)	(228)	(129)
Mean change from baseline	190	329	191	319	180	329

[a] Patients achieved and maintained confirmed HIV-1 RNA <400 copies/mL through Week 48 or Week 168.
[b] Includes patients who rebounded, patients who were on study at Week 48 and failed to achieve confirmed HIV-1 RNA <400 copies/mL at time of discontinuation, and patients who discontinued due to lack of efficacy.
[c] Includes consent withdrawn, lost to follow-up, noncompliance, never treated, missing data, protocol violation, death, and other reasons. Patients with HIV-1 RNA levels <400 copies/mL who chose not to continue in the voluntary extension phases of the study were censored at date of last dose of study medication.

Table 10: Outcomes of Randomized Treatment Through 48 Weeks, Study ACTG 364*

Outcome	SUSTIVA + NFV + NRTIs (n=65)	SUSTIVA + NRTIs (n=65)	NFV + NRTIs (n=66)
HIV-1 RNA <500 copies/mL[a]	71%	63%	41%
HIV-1 RNA ≥500 copies/mL[b]	17%	34%	54%
CDC Category C Event	2%	0%	0%
Discontinuations for adverse events[c]	3%	3%	5%
Discontinuations for other reasons[d]	8%	0%	0%

* For some patients, Week 56 data were used to confirm the status at Week 48.
[a] Subjects achieved virologic response (two consecutive viral loads <500 copies/mL) and maintained it through Week 48.
[b] Includes viral rebound and failure to achieve confirmed <500 copies/mL by Week 48.
[c] See Adverse Reactions (6.1) for a safety profile of these regimens.
[d] Includes loss to follow-up, consent withdrawn, noncompliance.

- The capsule sprinkle method for mixing the contents of SUSTIVA (efavirenz) capsules with soft food or infant formula may be used for adults or children who cannot swallow capsules or tablets.
- You should take SUSTIVA on an empty stomach at bedtime.
- You should not eat for 2 hours after taking SUSTIVA mixed with food.
- Babies who are old enough to swallow food should be given SUSTIVA using the capsule sprinkle method mixed with food instead of with infant formula.
- Talk with your doctor to help decide the best schedule for giving your baby SUSTIVA mixed with infant formula using the capsule sprinkle method.

Preparing a dose of SUSTIVA mixed with food using the capsule sprinkle method.

Before you prepare a dose of SUSTIVA mixed with food using the capsule sprinkle method, gather the following supplies:
- paper towels
- small spoon
- **small** clean container (such as a **small** cup or bowl)
- soft food such as applesauce, grape jelly, or yogurt

Step 1. Choose a clean, flat work surface. Place a clean paper towel on the work surface. Then place the other supplies on the paper towel.

Step 2. Wash and dry your hands well.

Step 3. Place 1 to 2 teaspoons of soft food such as applesauce, grape jelly, or yogurt in the small container (see Figure A). The color and thickness of the food may change when mixed with the medicine.

Figure A

Step 4. There are 2 parts of the SUSTIVA capsule. Look at the SUSTIVA capsule to see which part of the capsule overlaps the other part (see Figure B).

Figure B

Step 5. Turn the SUSTIVA capsule so that you are holding it in a sideways (horizontal) position directly over the container of food. Hold each end of the SUSTIVA capsule between your thumbs and index (pointer) fingers (see Figure C).

Figure C

Step 6. Use your thumb and index finger to pinch near the end of the overlapping part of the SUSTIVA capsule (see Figure D).

Figure D

Then, carefully twist both ends of the SUSTIVA capsule in opposite directions to open it (see Figure E). Be careful not to spill the capsule contents or spread it in the air.

Figure E

Step 7. Sprinkle the contents of the SUSTIVA capsule onto the food (see Figure F). Throw away the empty capsule shells.

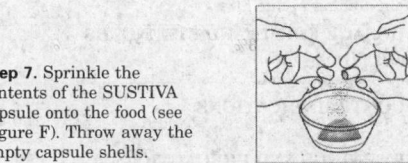

Figure F

If the total prescribed dose is more than 1 capsule, follow Steps 4 through 7 for each capsule. Do not add more food.

Steps 8 through 11 must be completed **within 30 minutes** of mixing the medicine.

Step 8. Use a spoon to gently mix the capsule contents and food together (see Figure G).

Figure G

Step 9. Use the spoon to take the food and capsule contents mixture or feed it to your child. Swallow all of the mixture. If you are giving the mixture to your child, look in your child's mouth to make sure that all of the mixture is swallowed.

Step 10. Add about 2 teaspoons more of the food to the empty container and gently stir to mix with any capsule contents that may still be in the container.

Step 11. Use the spoon to take the mixture or feed it to your child. Swallow all of the mixture. If you are giving the mixture to your child, look in your child's mouth to make sure that all of the mixture is swallowed.

Step 12. Wash the container and spoon. Throw away the paper towel and clean the work surface.

Step 13. Wash your hands.

Preparing a dose of SUSTIVA (efavirenz) mixed with infant formula using the capsule sprinkle method

Before you prepare a dose of SUSTIVA mixed with infant formula using the capsule sprinkle method, gather the following supplies:
- paper towels
- small spoon
- 30 milliliter (mL) medicine cup (ask your pharmacist for this). See Figure H.
- 10 mL oral dosing syringe (ask your pharmacist for this). See Figure H.
- infant formula at room temperature. If you are using powdered formula, you should prepare the formula according to the formula directions before mixing with SUSTIVA capsule contents.

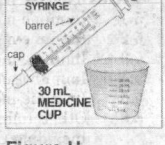

Figure H

Step 1. Choose a clean, flat work surface. Place a clean paper towel on the work surface. Place the supplies you will need on the paper towel.

Step 2. Wash and dry your hands well.

Step 3. Pour 10 mL of room temperature infant formula into the 30 mL medicine cup (see Figure I).

Figure I

Step 4. There are 2 parts of the SUSTIVA capsule. Look at the SUSTIVA capsule to see which part of the capsule overlaps the other part (see Figure J).

Figure J

Step 5. Turn the SUSTIVA capsule so that you are holding it in a sideways (horizontal) position directly over the medicine cup that contains the infant formula. Hold each end of the SUSTIVA capsule between your thumbs and index (pointer) fingers (see Figure K).

Figure K

Step 6. Use your thumb and index finger to pinch near the end of the overlapping part of the SUSTIVA (efavirenz) capsule (see Figure L).

Figure L

Then, carefully twist both ends of the SUSTIVA capsule in opposite directions to open it (see Figure M). Be careful not to spill the capsule contents or spread it in the air.

Figure M

Step 7. Sprinkle the contents of the SUSTIVA capsule onto the infant formula (see Figure N). Throw away the empty capsule shells.

Figure N

If the total prescribed dose is more than 1 capsule, follow Steps 4 through 7 for each capsule. Do not add more infant formula.

Steps 8 through 11 must be completed **within 30 minutes** of mixing the medicine.

Step 8. Hold the medicine cup with one hand. With your other hand, use the small spoon to gently mix the capsule contents and the infant formula (see Figure O).

Figure O

Step 9. Draw up the capsule contents and infant formula mixture into the 10 mL oral dosing syringe as follows:
- Check that the plunger is completely pushed into barrel of the syringe (see Figure P).

Figure P

- Place the tip of the syringe into the capsule contents and infant formula mixture in the medicine cup (see Figure Q).

Figure Q

- Slowly pull back on the plunger and draw up all of the mixture (see Figure R).

Figure R

Step 10. Place the tip of the oral dosing syringe in your baby's mouth along the inner cheek on either the right or left side (see Figure S). Slowly push on the plunger to give your baby all of the SUSTIVA capsule contents and infant formula mixture.

Figure S

To make sure that your baby gets all of the medicine, do not give SUSTIVA (efavirenz) capsule contents to your baby in a bottle.

Step 11. To make sure there is no capsule contents and formula mixture left in the medicine cup or syringe:

• **Repeat Step 3 above** to add 10 mL more infant formula into the medicine cup.
• Stir with a small spoon.
• Then, repeat **Steps 9 and 10 above.**

Step 12. Remove the plunger from the oral dosing syringe. Wash the medicine cup, spoon, and oral dosing syringe. Allow the medicine cup, spoon, and oral dosing syringe to dry. Throw away the paper towel and clean the work surface.

Step 13. Wash your hands.

How should I store SUSTIVA capsules?

• Store SUSTIVA capsules at room temperature between 68°F to 77°F (20°C to 25°C).

Keep SUSTIVA capsules and all medicines out of the reach of children.

This Instructions for Use has been approved by the U.S. Food and Drug Administration.

Distributed by:
Bristol-Myers Squibb Company
Princeton, NJ 08543 USA
SUSTIVA® (efavirenz) capsules made in India.
Issued: May 2013
1320416A0
510230013IN12

Shown in Product Identification Guide, page 306

YERVOY®   ℞

[yur-voi]
(ipilimumab)
Injection, for intravenous infusion

HIGHLIGHTS OF PRESCRIBING INFORMATION
These highlights do not include all the information needed to use YERVOY safely and effectively. See full prescribing information for YERVOY.
YERVOY ® (ipilimumab)
Injection, for intravenous infusion
Initial U.S. Approval: 2011

WARNING: IMMUNE-MEDIATED ADVERSE REACTIONS

See full prescribing information for complete boxed warning.

YERVOY can result in severe and fatal immune-mediated adverse reactions due to T-cell activation and proliferation. These immune-mediated reactions may involve any organ system; however, the most common severe immune-mediated adverse reactions are enterocolitis, hepatitis, dermatitis (including toxic epidermal necrolysis), neuropathy, and endocrinopathy. The majority of these immune-mediated reactions initially manifested during treatment; however, a minority occurred weeks to months after discontinuation of YERVOY.

Permanently discontinue YERVOY and initiate systemic high-dose corticosteroid therapy for severe immune-mediated reactions. (2.2)

Assess patients for signs and symptoms of enterocolitis, dermatitis, neuropathy, and endocrinopathy and evaluate clinical chemistries including liver function tests and thyroid function tests at baseline and before each dose. (5.1, 5.2, 5.3, 5.4, 5.5)

———RECENT MAJOR CHANGES———
Warnings and Precautions (5.2) 12/2013

———INDICATIONS AND USAGE———
YERVOY is a human cytotoxic T-lymphocyte antigen 4 (CTLA-4)-blocking antibody indicated for the treatment of unresectable or metastatic melanoma. (1)

———DOSAGE AND ADMINISTRATION———
• YERVOY 3 mg/kg administered intravenously over 90 minutes every 3 weeks for a total of four doses. (2.1)
• Permanently discontinue for severe adverse reactions. (2.2)

———DOSAGE FORMS AND STRENGTHS———
• 50 mg/10 mL (5 mg/mL) (3)
• 200 mg/40 mL (5 mg/mL) (3)

———CONTRAINDICATIONS———
None. (4)

———WARNINGS AND PRECAUTIONS———
Immune-mediated adverse reactions: Permanently discontinue for severe reactions. Withhold dose for moderate immune-mediated adverse reactions until return to baseline, improvement to mild severity, or complete resolution, and patient is receiving less than 7.5 mg prednisone or equivalent per day. Administer systemic high-dose corticosteroids for severe, persistent, or recurring immune-mediated reactions. (5.1, 5.2, 5.3, 5.4, 5.5)
• Immune-mediated hepatitis: Evaluate liver function tests before each dose of YERVOY (ipilimumab). (5.2)
• Immune-mediated endocrinopathies: Monitor thyroid function tests and clinical chemistries prior to each dose. Evaluate at each visit for signs and symptoms of endocrinopathy. Institute hormone replacement therapy as needed. (5.5)

———ADVERSE REACTIONS———
Most common adverse reactions (≥5%) are fatigue, diarrhea, pruritus, rash, and colitis. (6.1)
To report SUSPECTED ADVERSE REACTIONS, contact Bristol-Myers Squibb at 1-800-721-5072 or FDA at 1-800-FDA-1088 or www.fda.gov/medwatch.

———USE IN SPECIFIC POPULATIONS———
• Pregnancy: Based on animal data, YERVOY may cause fetal harm. (8.1)
• Nursing mothers: Discontinue nursing or discontinue YERVOY. (8.3)

See 17 for PATIENT COUNSELING INFORMATION and Medication Guide

Revised: 12/2013

FULL PRESCRIBING INFORMATION: CONTENTS*
WARNING: IMMUNE-MEDIATED ADVERSE REACTIONS

FULL PRESCRIBING INFORMATION

WARNING: IMMUNE-MEDIATED ADVERSE REACTIONS

YERVOY can result in severe and fatal immune-mediated adverse reactions due to T-cell activation and proliferation. These immune-mediated reactions may involve any organ system; however, the most common severe immune-mediated adverse reactions are enterocolitis, hepatitis, dermatitis (including toxic epidermal necrolysis), neuropathy, and endocrinopathy. The majority of these immune-mediated reactions initially manifested during treatment; however, a minority occurred weeks to months after discontinuation of YERVOY.

Permanently discontinue YERVOY and initiate systemic high-dose corticosteroid therapy for severe immune-mediated reactions. [See Dosage and Administration (2.2).]

Assess patients for signs and symptoms of enterocolitis, dermatitis, neuropathy, and endocrinopathy and evaluate clinical chemistries including liver function tests and thyroid function tests at baseline and before each dose. [See Warnings and Precautions (5.1, 5.2, 5.3, 5.4, 5.5).]

1   INDICATIONS AND USAGE
YERVOY (ipilimumab) is indicated for the treatment of unresectable or metastatic melanoma.

2   DOSAGE AND ADMINISTRATION
2.1   Recommended Dosing
The recommended dose of YERVOY is 3 mg/kg administered intravenously over 90 minutes every 3 weeks for a total of 4 doses.

2.2   Recommended Dose Modifications
• Withhold scheduled dose of YERVOY for any moderate immune-mediated adverse reactions or for symptomatic endocrinopathy. For patients with complete or partial resolution of adverse reactions (Grade 0-1), and who are receiving less than 7.5 mg prednisone or equivalent per day, resume YERVOY at a dose of 3 mg/kg every 3 weeks until administration of all 4 planned doses or 16 weeks from first dose, whichever occurs earlier.
• Permanently discontinue YERVOY for any of the following:
  ◦ Persistent moderate adverse reactions or inability to reduce corticosteroid dose to 7.5 mg prednisone or equivalent per day.
  ◦ Failure to complete full treatment course within 16 weeks from administration of first dose.
  ◦ Severe or life-threatening adverse reactions, including any of the following:
    ■ Colitis with abdominal pain, fever, ileus, or peritoneal signs; increase in stool frequency (7 or more over baseline), stool incontinence, need for intravenous hydration for more than 24 hours, gastrointestinal hemorrhage, and gastrointestinal perforation
    ■ Aspartate aminotransferase (AST) or alanine aminotransferase (ALT) >5 times the upper limit of normal or total bilirubin >3 times the upper limit of normal
    ■ Stevens-Johnson syndrome, toxic epidermal necrolysis, or rash complicated by full thickness dermal ulceration, or necrotic, bullous, or hemorrhagic manifestations
    ■ Severe motor or sensory neuropathy, Guillain-Barré syndrome, or myasthenia gravis
    ■ Severe immune-mediated reactions involving any organ system (eg, nephritis, pneumonitis, pancreatitis, non-infectious myocarditis)
    ■ Immune-mediated ocular disease that is unresponsive to topical immunosuppressive therapy

2.3   Preparation and Administration
• Do not shake product.
• Inspect parenteral drug products visually for particulate matter and discoloration prior to administration. Discard vial if solution is cloudy, there is pronounced discoloration (solution may have pale-yellow color), or there is foreign particulate matter other than translucent-to-white, amorphous particles.

Preparation of Solution
• Allow the vials to stand at room temperature for approximately 5 minutes prior to preparation of infusion.
• Withdraw the required volume of YERVOY and transfer into an intravenous bag.
• Dilute with 0.9% Sodium Chloride Injection, USP or 5% Dextrose Injection, USP to prepare a diluted solution with a final concentration ranging from 1 mg/mL to 2 mg/mL. Mix diluted solution by gentle inversion.
• Store the diluted solution for no more than 24 hours under refrigeration (2°C to 8°C, 36°F to 46°F) or at room temperature (20°C to 25°C, 68°F to 77°F).
• Discard partially used vials or empty vials of YERVOY.

Administration Instructions
• Do not mix YERVOY with, or administer as an infusion with, other medicinal products.
• Flush the intravenous line with 0.9% Sodium Chloride Injection, USP or 5% Dextrose Injection, USP after each dose.
• Administer diluted solution over 90 minutes through an intravenous line containing a sterile, non-pyrogenic, low-protein-binding in-line filter.

3   DOSAGE FORMS AND STRENGTHS
50 mg/10 mL (5 mg/mL)
200 mg/40 mL (5 mg/mL)

4   CONTRAINDICATIONS
None.

5   WARNINGS AND PRECAUTIONS
YERVOY can result in severe and fatal immune-mediated reactions due to T-cell activation and proliferation. [See Boxed Warning.]

5.1 Immune-mediated Enterocolitis

In Study 1, severe, life-threatening, or fatal (diarrhea of 7 or more stools above baseline, fever, ileus, peritoneal signs; Grade 3-5) immune-mediated enterocolitis occurred in 34 (7%) YERVOY (ipilimumab)-treated patients, and moderate (diarrhea with up to 6 stools above baseline, abdominal pain, mucus or blood in stool; Grade 2) enterocolitis occurred in 28 (5%) YERVOY-treated patients. Across all YERVOY-treated patients (n=511), 5 (1%) patients developed intestinal perforation, 4 (0.8%) patients died as a result of complications, and 26 (5%) patients were hospitalized for severe enterocolitis.

The median time to onset was 7.4 weeks (range: 1.6-13.4) and 6.3 weeks (range: 0.3-18.9) after the initiation of YERVOY for patients with Grade 3-5 enterocolitis and with Grade 2 enterocolitis, respectively.

Twenty-nine patients (85%) with Grade 3-5 enterocolitis were treated with high-dose (≥40 mg prednisone equivalent per day) corticosteroids, with a median dose of 80 mg/day of prednisone or equivalent; the median duration of treatment was 2.3 weeks (ranging up to 13.9 weeks) followed by corticosteroid taper. Of the 28 patients with moderate enterocolitis, 46% were not treated with systemic corticosteroids, 29% were treated with <40 mg prednisone or equivalent per day for a median duration of 5.1 weeks, and 25% were treated with high-dose corticosteroids for a median duration of 10 days prior to corticosteroid taper. Infliximab was administered to 5 of the 62 patients (8%) with moderate, severe, or life-threatening immune-mediated enterocolitis following inadequate response to corticosteroids.

Of the 34 patients with Grade 3-5 enterocolitis, 74% experienced complete resolution, 3% experienced improvement to Grade 2 severity, and 24% did not improve. Among the 28 patients with Grade 2 enterocolitis, 79% experienced complete resolution, 11% improved, and 11% did not improve.

Monitor patients for signs and symptoms of enterocolitis (such as diarrhea, abdominal pain, mucus or blood in stool, with or without fever) and of bowel perforation (such as peritoneal signs and ileus). In symptomatic patients, rule out infectious etiologies and consider endoscopic evaluation for persistent or severe symptoms.

Permanently discontinue YERVOY in patients with severe enterocolitis and initiate systemic corticosteroids at a dose of 1 to 2 mg/kg/day of prednisone or equivalent. Upon improvement to Grade 1 or less, initiate corticosteroid taper and continue to taper over at least 1 month. In clinical trials, rapid corticosteroid tapering resulted in recurrence or worsening symptoms of enterocolitis in some patients.

Withhold YERVOY dosing for moderate enterocolitis; administer anti-diarrheal treatment and, if persistent for more than 1 week, initiate systemic corticosteroids at a dose of 0.5 mg/kg/day prednisone or equivalent. [See Dosage and Administration (2.2).]

5.2 Immune-mediated Hepatitis

In Study 1, severe, life-threatening, or fatal hepatotoxicity (AST or ALT elevations of more than 5 times the upper limit of normal or total bilirubin elevations more than 3 times the upper limit of normal; Grade 3-5) occurred in 8 (2%) YERVOY-treated patients, with fatal hepatic failure in 0.2% and hospitalization in 0.4% of YERVOY-treated patients. An additional 13 (2.5%) patients experienced moderate hepatotoxicity manifested by liver function test abnormalities (AST or ALT elevations of more than 2.5 times but not more than 5 times the upper limit of normal or total bilirubin elevation of more than 1.5 times but not more than 3 times the upper limit of normal; Grade 2). The underlying pathology was not ascertained in all patients but in some instances included immune-mediated hepatitis. There were insufficient numbers of patients with biopsy-proven hepatitis to characterize the clinical course of this event.

Monitor liver function tests (hepatic transaminase and bilirubin levels) and assess patients for signs and symptoms of hepatotoxicity before each dose of YERVOY. In patients with hepatotoxicity, rule out infectious or malignant causes and increase frequency of liver function test monitoring until resolution.

Permanently discontinue YERVOY in patients with Grade 3-5 hepatotoxicity and administer systemic corticosteroids at a dose of 1 to 2 mg/kg/day of prednisone or equivalent. When liver function tests show sustained improvement or return to baseline, initiate corticosteroid tapering and continue to taper over 1 month. Across the clinical development program for YERVOY, mycophenolate treatment has been administered in patients who have persistent severe hepatitis despite high-dose corticosteroids. Withhold YERVOY in patients with Grade 2 hepatotoxicity. [See Dosage and Administration (2.2).]

Concurrent Administration with Vemurafenib

In a dose-finding trial, Grade 3 increases in transaminases with or without concomitant increases in total bilirubin occurred in 6 of 10 patients who received concurrent YERVOY (3 mg/kg) and vemurafenib (960 mg BID or 720 mg BID).

5.3 Immune-mediated Dermatitis

In Study 1, severe, life-threatening, or fatal immune-mediated dermatitis (eg, Stevens-Johnson syndrome, toxic epidermal necrolysis, or rash complicated by full thickness dermal ulceration, or necrotic, bullous, or hemorrhagic manifestations; Grade 3-5) occurred in 13 (2.5%) YERVOY-treated patients. One (0.2%) patient died as a result of toxic epidermal necrolysis and one additional patient required hospitalization for severe dermatitis. There were 63 (12%) patients with moderate (Grade 2) dermatitis.

The median time to onset of moderate, severe, or life-threatening immune-mediated dermatitis was 3.1 weeks and ranged up to 17.3 weeks from the initiation of YERVOY (ipilimumab).

Seven (54%) YERVOY-treated patients with severe dermatitis received high-dose corticosteroids (median dose 60 mg prednisone/day or equivalent) for up to 14.9 weeks followed by corticosteroid taper. Of these 7 patients, 6 had complete resolution; time to resolution ranged up to 15.6 weeks.

Of the 63 patients with moderate dermatitis, 25 (40%) were treated with systemic corticosteroids (median of 60 mg/day of prednisone or equivalent) for a median of 2.1 weeks, 7 (11%) were treated with only topical corticosteroids, and 31 (49%) did not receive systemic or topical corticosteroids. Forty-four (70%) patients with moderate dermatitis were reported to have complete resolution, 7 (11%) improved to mild (Grade 1) severity, and 12 (19%) had no reported improvement.

Monitor patients for signs and symptoms of dermatitis such as rash and pruritus. Unless an alternate etiology has been identified, signs or symptoms of dermatitis should be considered immune-mediated.

Permanently discontinue YERVOY in patients with Stevens-Johnson syndrome, toxic epidermal necrolysis, or rash complicated by full thickness dermal ulceration, or necrotic, bullous, or hemorrhagic manifestations. Administer systemic corticosteroids at a dose of 1 to 2 mg/kg/day of prednisone or equivalent. When dermatitis is controlled, corticosteroid tapering should occur over a period of at least 1 month. Withhold YERVOY dosing in patients with moderate to severe signs and symptoms. [See Dosage and Administration (2.2).]

For mild to moderate dermatitis, such as localized rash and pruritus, treat symptomatically. Administer topical or systemic corticosteroids if there is no improvement of symptoms within 1 week.

5.4 Immune-mediated Neuropathies

In Study 1, 1 case of fatal Guillain-Barré syndrome and 1 case of severe (Grade 3) peripheral motor neuropathy were reported. Across the clinical development program of YERVOY, myasthenia gravis and additional cases of Guillain-Barré syndrome have been reported.

Monitor for symptoms of motor or sensory neuropathy such as unilateral or bilateral weakness, sensory alterations, or paresthesia. Permanently discontinue YERVOY in patients with severe neuropathy (interfering with daily activities) such as Guillain-Barré-like syndromes. Institute medical intervention as appropriate for management of severe neuropathy. Consider initiation of systemic corticosteroids at a dose of 1 to 2 mg/kg/day prednisone or equivalent for severe neuropathies. Withhold YERVOY dosing in patients with moderate neuropathy (not interfering with daily activities). [See Dosage and Administration (2.2).]

5.5 Immune-mediated Endocrinopathies

In Study 1, severe to life-threatening immune-mediated endocrinopathies (requiring hospitalization, urgent medical intervention, or interfering with activities of daily living; Grade 3-4) occurred in 9 (1.8%) YERVOY-treated patients. All 9 patients had hypopituitarism and some had additional concomitant endocrinopathies such as adrenal insufficiency, hypogonadism, and hypothyroidism. Six of the 9 patients were hospitalized for severe endocrinopathies. Moderate endocrinopathy (requiring hormone replacement or medical intervention; Grade 2) occurred in 12 (2.3%) patients and consisted of hypothyroidism, adrenal insufficiency, hypopituitarism, and 1 case each of hyperthyroidism and Cushing's syndrome. The median time to onset of moderate to severe immune-mediated endocrinopathy was 11 weeks and ranged up to 19.3 weeks after the initiation of YERVOY (ipilimumab).

Of the 21 patients with moderate to life-threatening endocrinopathy, 17 patients required long-term hormone replacement therapy including, most commonly, adrenal hormones (n=10) and thyroid hormones (n=13).

Monitor patients for clinical signs and symptoms of hypophysitis, adrenal insufficiency (including adrenal crisis), and hyper- or hypothyroidism. Patients may present with fatigue, headache, mental status changes, abdominal pain, unusual bowel habits, and hypotension, or nonspecific symptoms which may resemble other causes such as brain metastasis or underlying disease. Unless an alternate etiology has been identified, signs or symptoms of endocrinopathies should be considered immune-mediated.

Monitor thyroid function tests and clinical chemistries at the start of treatment, before each dose, and as clinically indicated based on symptoms. In a limited number of patients, hypophysitis was diagnosed by imaging studies through enlargement of the pituitary gland.

Withhold YERVOY dosing in symptomatic patients. Initiate systemic corticosteroids at a dose of 1 to 2 mg/kg/day of prednisone or equivalent, and initiate appropriate hormone replacement therapy. [See Dosage and Administration (2.2).]

5.6 Other Immune-mediated Adverse Reactions, Including Ocular Manifestations

The following clinically significant immune-mediated adverse reactions were seen in less than 1% of YERVOY-treated patients in Study 1: nephritis, pneumonitis, meningitis, pericarditis, uveitis, iritis, and hemolytic anemia.

Across the clinical development program for YERVOY, the following likely immune-mediated adverse reactions were also reported with less than 1% incidence: myocarditis, angiopathy, temporal arteritis, vasculitis, polymyalgia rheumatica, conjunctivitis, blepharitis, episcleritis, scleritis, leukocytoclastic vasculitis, erythema multiforme, psoriasis, pancreatitis, arthritis, autoimmune thyroiditis, sarcoidosis, neurosensory hypoacusis, autoimmune central neuropathy (encephalitis), myositis, polymyositis, and ocular myositis.

Permanently discontinue YERVOY for clinically significant or severe immune-mediated adverse reactions. Initiate systemic corticosteroids at a dose of 1 to 2 mg/kg/day prednisone or equivalent for severe immune-mediated adverse reactions.

Administer corticosteroid eye drops to patients who develop uveitis, iritis, or episcleritis. Permanently discontinue YERVOY for immune-mediated ocular disease that is unresponsive to local immunosuppressive therapy. [See Dosage and Administration (2.2).]

6 ADVERSE REACTIONS

The following adverse reactions are discussed in greater detail in other sections of the labeling.

- Immune-mediated enterocolitis [see Warnings and Precautions (5.1)].
- Immune-mediated hepatitis [see Warnings and Precautions (5.2)].
- Immune-mediated dermatitis [see Warnings and Precautions (5.3)].
- Immune-mediated neuropathies [see Warnings and Precautions (5.4)].
- Immune-mediated endocrinopathies [see Warnings and Precautions (5.5)].
- Other immune-mediated adverse reactions, including ocular manifestations [see Warnings and Precautions (5.6)].

Table 1: Selected Adverse Reactions in Study 1

System Organ Class/ Preferred Term	YERVOY 3 mg/kg n=131		YERVOY 3 mg/kg+gp100 n=380		gp100 n=132	
	Any Grade	Grade 3-5	Any Grade	Grade 3-5	Any Grade	Grade 3-5
Gastrointestinal Disorders						
Diarrhea	32	5	37	4	20	1
Colitis	8	5	5	3	2	0
Skin and Subcutaneous Tissue Disorders						
Pruritus	31	0	21	<1	11	0
Rash	29	2	25	2	8	0
General Disorders and Administration Site Conditions						
Fatigue	41	7	34	5	31	3

[a] Incidences presented in this table are based on reports of adverse events regardless of causality.

6.1 Clinical Trials Experience

Because clinical trials are conducted under widely varying conditions, the adverse reaction rates observed cannot be directly compared with rates in other clinical trials or experience with therapeutics in the same class and may not reflect the rates observed in clinical practice.

The clinical development program excluded patients with active autoimmune disease or those receiving systemic immunosuppression for organ transplantation. Exposure to YERVOY (ipilimumab) 3 mg/kg for 4 doses given by intravenous infusion in previously treated patients with unresectable or metastatic melanoma was assessed in a randomized, double-blind clinical study (Study 1). [See Clinical Studies (14).] One hundred thirty-one patients (median age 57 years, 60% male) received YERVOY as a single agent, 380 patients (median age 56 years, 61% male) received YERVOY with an investigational gp100 peptide vaccine (gp100), and 132 patients (median age 57 years, 54% male) received gp100 peptide vaccine alone. Patients in the study received a median of 4 doses (range: 1-4 doses). YERVOY was discontinued for adverse reactions in 10% of patients. The most common adverse reactions (≥5%) in patients who received YERVOY at 3 mg/kg were fatigue, diarrhea, pruritus, rash, and colitis.

Table 1 presents selected adverse reactions from Study 1, which occurred in at least 5% of patients in the YERVOY-containing arms and with at least 5% increased incidence over the control gp100 arm for all-grade events and at least 1% incidence over the control group for Grade 3-5 events.

[See table 1 at top of previous page]

Table 2 presents the per-patient incidence of severe, life-threatening, or fatal immune-mediated adverse reactions from Study 1.

Table 2: Severe to Fatal Immune-mediated Adverse Reactions in Study 1

	Percentage (%) of Patients	
	YERVOY 3 mg/kg n=131	YERVOY 3 mg/kg+gp100 n=380
Any Immune-mediated Adverse Reaction	15	12
Enterocolitis[a,b]	7	7
Hepatotoxicity[a]	1	2
Dermatitis[a]	2	3
Neuropathy[a]	1	<1
Endocrinopathy	4	1
Hypopituitarism	4	1
Adrenal insufficiency	0	1
Other		
Pneumonitis	0	<1
Meningitis	0	<1
Nephritis	1	0
Eosinophilia[c]	1	0
Pericarditis[a,c]	0	<1

[a] Including fatal outcome.
[b] Including intestinal perforation.
[c] Underlying etiology not established.

Across clinical studies that utilized YERVOY doses ranging from 0.3 to 10 mg/kg, the following adverse reactions were also reported (incidence less than 1% unless otherwise noted): urticaria (2%), large intestinal ulcer, esophagitis, acute respiratory distress syndrome, renal failure, and infusion reaction.

Based on the experience in the entire clinical program for melanoma, the incidence and severity of enterocolitis and hepatitis appear to be dose dependent.

6.2 Immunogenicity

In clinical studies, 1.1% of 1024 evaluable patients tested positive for binding antibodies against ipilimumab in an electrochemiluminescent (ECL) based assay. This assay has substantial limitations in detecting anti-ipilimumab antibodies in the presence of ipilimumab. Infusion-related or peri-infusional reactions consistent with hypersensitivity or anaphylaxis were not reported in these 11 patients nor were neutralizing antibodies against ipilimumab detected.

Because trough levels of ipilimumab interfere with the ECL assay results, a subset analysis was performed in the dose cohort with the lowest trough levels. In this analysis, 6.9% of 58 evaluable patients, who were treated with 0.3 mg/kg dose, tested positive for binding antibodies against ipilimumab.

Immunogenicity assay results are highly dependent on several factors including assay sensitivity and specificity, assay methodology, sample handling, timing of sample collection, concomitant medications, and underlying disease. For these reasons, comparison of incidence of antibodies to YERVOY with the incidences of antibodies to other products may be misleading.

7 DRUG INTERACTIONS

No formal pharmacokinetic drug interaction studies have been conducted with YERVOY (ipilimumab).

8 USE IN SPECIFIC POPULATIONS

8.1 Pregnancy

Pregnancy Category C

There are no adequate and well-controlled studies of YERVOY in pregnant women. Use YERVOY during pregnancy only if the potential benefit justifies the potential risk to the fetus.

In a combined study of embryo-fetal and peri-postnatal development, pregnant cynomolgus monkeys received ipilimumab every 3 weeks from the onset of organogenesis in the first trimester through parturition, at exposure levels either 2.6 or 7.2 times higher by AUC than the exposures at the clinical dose of 3 mg/kg of ipilimumab. No treatment-related adverse effects on reproduction were detected during the first two trimesters of pregnancy. Beginning in the third trimester, the ipilimumab treated groups experienced higher incidences of severe toxicities including abortion, stillbirth, premature delivery (with corresponding lower birth weight), and higher incidences of infant mortality in a dose-related manner compared to controls. [See Nonclinical Toxicology (13.2).]

Human IgG1 is known to cross the placental barrier and ipilimumab is an IgG1; therefore, ipilimumab has the potential to be transmitted from the mother to the developing fetus.

8.3 Nursing Mothers

It is not known whether ipilimumab is secreted in human milk. In monkeys treated at dose levels resulting in exposures 2.6 and 7.2 times higher than those in humans at the recommended dose, ipilimumab was present in milk at concentrations of 0.1 and 0.4 mcg/mL, representing a ratio of up to 0.3% of the serum concentration of the drug. Because many drugs are secreted in human milk and because of the potential for serious adverse reactions in nursing infants from YERVOY, a decision should be made whether to discontinue nursing or to discontinue YERVOY, taking into account the importance of YERVOY to the mother.

8.4 Pediatric Use

Safety and effectiveness of YERVOY have not been established in pediatric patients.

8.5 Geriatric Use

Of the 511 patients treated with YERVOY at 3 mg/kg, 28% were 65 years and over. No overall differences in safety or efficacy were reported between the elderly patients (65 years and over) and younger patients (less than 65 years).

8.6 Renal Impairment

No dose adjustment is needed for patients with renal impairment. [See Clinical Pharmacology (12.3).]

8.7 Hepatic Impairment

No dose adjustment is needed for patients with mild hepatic impairment (total bilirubin [TB] >1.0 × to 1.5 × the upper limit of normal [ULN] or AST >ULN). YERVOY has not been studied in patients with moderate (TB >1.5 × to 3.0 × ULN and any AST) or severe (TB >3 × ULN and any AST) hepatic impairment. [See Clinical Pharmacology (12.3).]

10 OVERDOSAGE

There is no information on overdosage with YERVOY.

11 DESCRIPTION

YERVOY (ipilimumab) is a recombinant, human monoclonal antibody that binds to the cytotoxic T-lymphocyte-associated antigen 4 (CTLA-4). Ipilimumab is an IgG1 kappa immunoglobulin with an approximate molecular weight of 148 kDa. Ipilimumab is produced in mammalian (Chinese hamster ovary) cell culture.

YERVOY is a sterile, preservative-free, clear to slightly opalescent, colorless to pale-yellow solution for intravenous infusion, which may contain a small amount of visible translucent-to-white, amorphous ipilimumab particulates. It is supplied in single-use vials of 50 mg/10 mL and 200 mg/40 mL. Each milliliter contains 5 mg of ipilimumab and the following inactive ingredients: diethylene triamine pentaacetic acid (DTPA) (0.04 mg), mannitol (10 mg), polysorbate 80 (vegetable origin) (0.1 mg), sodium chloride (5.85 mg), tris hydrochloride (3.15 mg), and Water for Injection, USP at a pH of 7.

12 CLINICAL PHARMACOLOGY

12.1 Mechanism of Action

CTLA-4 is a negative regulator of T-cell activation. Ipilimumab binds to CTLA-4 and blocks the interaction of CTLA-4 with its ligands, CD80/CD86. Blockade of CTLA-4 has been shown to augment T-cell activation and proliferation. The mechanism of action of ipilimumab's effect in patients with melanoma is indirect, possibly through T-cell mediated anti-tumor immune responses.

12.3 Pharmacokinetics

The pharmacokinetics of ipilimumab were studied in 785 patients with unresectable or metastatic melanoma who received doses of 0.3, 3, or 10 mg/kg once every 3 weeks for 4

doses. Peak concentration (C_{max}), trough concentration (C_{min}), and area under the plasma concentration versus time curve (AUC) of ipilimumab increased dose proportionally within the dose range examined. Upon repeated dosing every 3 weeks, the clearance (CL) of ipilimumab was found to be time-invariant, and systemic accumulation was 1.5-fold or less. Steady-state concentrations of ipilimumab were reached by the third dose; the mean C_{min} at steady-state was 19.4 mcg/mL following repeated doses of 3 mg/kg. The mean value (% coefficient of variation) generated through population pharmacokinetic analysis for the terminal half-life ($t_{1/2}$) was 15.4 days (34%) and for CL was 16.8 mL/h (38%).

Specific Populations: The effects of various covariates on the pharmacokinetics of ipilimumab were assessed in population pharmacokinetic analyses. The CL of ipilimumab increased with increasing body weight; however, no dose adjustment is recommended for body weight after administration on a mg/kg basis. The following factors had no clinically important effect on the CL of ipilimumab: age (range: 23-88 years), gender, performance status, renal impairment, mild hepatic impairment, previous cancer therapy, and baseline lactate dehydrogenase (LDH) levels. The effect of race was not examined due to limited data available in non-Caucasian ethnic groups.

Renal Impairment: The effect of renal impairment on the CL of ipilimumab was evaluated in patients with mild (GFR <90 and ≥60 mL/min/1.73 m²; n=349), moderate (GFR <60 and ≥30 mL/min/1.73 m²; n=82), or severe (GFR <30 and ≥15 mL/min/1.73 m²; n=4) renal impairment compared to patients with normal renal function (GFR ≥90 mL/min/1.73 m²; n=350) in population pharmacokinetic analyses. No clinically important differences in the CL of ipilimumab were found between patients with renal impairment and patients with normal renal function. [See Use in Specific Populations (8.6).]

Hepatic Impairment: The effect of hepatic impairment on the CL of ipilimumab was evaluated in patients with mild hepatic impairment (TB 1.0 × to 1.5 × ULN or AST >ULN as defined using the National Cancer Institute criteria of hepatic dysfunction; n=76) compared to patients with normal hepatic function (TB and AST ≤ULN; n=708) in the population pharmacokinetic analyses. No clinically important differences in the CL of ipilimumab were found between patients with mild hepatic impairment and normal hepatic function. YERVOY (ipilimumab) has not been studied in patients with moderate (TB >1.5 × to 3 × ULN and any AST) or severe hepatic impairment (TB >3 × ULN and any AST). [See Use in Specific Populations (8.7).]

13 NONCLINICAL TOXICOLOGY

13.1 Carcinogenesis, Mutagenesis, Impairment of Fertility

Carcinogenesis

The carcinogenic potential of ipilimumab has not been evaluated in long-term animal studies.

Mutagenesis

The genotoxic potential of ipilimumab has not been evaluated.

Impairment of Fertility

Fertility studies have not been performed with ipilimumab.

13.2 Animal Toxicology and/or Pharmacology

In addition to the severe findings of abortion, stillbirths, and postnatal deaths observed in pregnant cynomolgus monkeys that received ipilimumab every 3 weeks from the onset of organogenesis in the first trimester through parturition [see Use in Specific Populations (8.1)], developmental abnormalities were identified in the urogenital system of 2 infant monkeys exposed in utero to 30 mg/kg of ipilimumab (7.2 times the AUC in humans at the clinically recommended dose). One female infant monkey had unilateral renal agenesis of the left kidney and ureter, and 1 male infant monkey had an imperforate urethra with associated urinary obstruction and subcutaneous scrotal edema.

Genetically engineered mice heterozygous for CTLA-4 (CTLA-4+/−), the target for ipilimumab, appeared healthy and gave birth to healthy CTLA-4+/− heterozygous offspring. Mated CTLA-4+/− heterozygous mice also produced offspring deficient in CTLA-4 (homozygous negative, CTLA-4−/−). The CTLA-4−/− homozygous negative offspring appeared healthy at birth, exhibited signs of multiorgan lymphoproliferative disease by 2 weeks of age, and all died by 3-4 weeks of age with massive lymphoproliferation and multiorgan tissue destruction.

14 CLINICAL STUDIES

The safety and efficacy of YERVOY were investigated in a randomized (3:1:1), double-blind, double-dummy study (Study 1) that included 676 randomized patients with unresectable or metastatic melanoma previously treated with one or more of the following: aldesleukin, dacarbazine, temozolomide, fotemustine, or carboplatin. Of these 676 patients, 403 were randomized to receive YERVOY at 3 mg/kg in combination with an investigational peptide vaccine with incomplete Freund's adjuvant (gp100), 137 were randomized to receive YERVOY (ipilimumab) at 3 mg/kg, and 136 were randomized to receive gp100 alone. The study enrolled only patients with HLA-A2*0201 genotype; this HLA genotype facilitates the immune presentation of the investigational peptide vaccine. The study excluded patients with active autoimmune disease or those receiving systemic immunosuppression for organ transplantation. YERVOY/placebo was administered at 3 mg/kg as an intravenous infusion every 3 weeks for 4 doses. Gp100/placebo was administered at a dose of 2 mg peptide by deep subcutaneous injection every 3 weeks for 4 doses. Assessment of tumor response was conducted at weeks 12 and 24, and every 3 months thereafter. Patients with evidence of objective tumor response at 12 or 24 weeks had assessment for confirmation of durability of response at 16 or 28 weeks, respectively.

The major efficacy outcome measure was overall survival (OS) in the YERVOY+gp100 arm compared to that in the gp100 arm. Secondary efficacy outcome measures were OS in the YERVOY+gp100 arm compared to the YERVOY arm, OS in the YERVOY arm compared to the gp100 arm, best overall response rate (BORR) at week 24 between each of the study arms, and duration of response.

Of the randomized patients, 61%, 59%, and 54% in the YERVOY+gp100, YERVOY, and gp100 arms, respectively, were men. Twenty-nine percent were ≥65 years of age, the median age was 57 years, 71% had M1c stage, 12% had a history of previously treated brain metastasis, 98% had ECOG performance status of 0 and 1, 23% had received aldesleukin, and 38% had elevated LDH level. Sixty-one percent of patients randomized to either YERVOY-containing arm received all 4 planned doses. The median duration of follow-up was 8.9 months.

The OS results are shown in Table 3 and Figure 1.
[See table 3 above]
[See figure 1 above]
The best overall response rate (BORR) as assessed by the investigator was 5.7% (95% CI: 3.7%, 8.4%) in the YERVOY+gp100 arm, 10.9% (95% CI: 6.3%, 17.4%) in the YERVOY arm, and 1.5% (95% CI: 0.2%, 5.2%) in the gp100 arm. The median duration of response was 11.5 months in the YERVOY+gp100 arm and has not been reached in the YERVOY or gp100 arm.

16   HOW SUPPLIED/STORAGE AND HANDLING

YERVOY is available as follows:

Carton Contents	NDC
One 50 mg vial (5 mg/mL), single-use vial	NDC 0003-2327-11
One 200 mg vial (5 mg/mL), single-use vial	NDC 0003-2328-22

Store YERVOY under refrigeration at 2°C to 8°C (36°F to 46°F). Do not freeze. Protect vials from light.

17   PATIENT COUNSELING INFORMATION

See MEDICATION GUIDE.
• Inform patients of the potential risk of immune-mediated adverse reactions.
• Advise patients to read the YERVOY Medication Guide before each YERVOY infusion.
• Advise women that YERVOY may cause fetal harm.
• Advise nursing mothers not to breastfeed while taking YERVOY.

Manufactured by:
Bristol-Myers Squibb Company
Princeton, NJ 08543 USA
U.S. License No. 1713
1321675A0
Rev December 2013

MEDICATION GUIDE
YERVOY®(yur-voi)
(ipilimumab)
Read this Medication Guide before you start receiving YERVOY and before each infusion. There may be new information. This Medication Guide does not take the place of talking with your healthcare provider about your medical condition or your treatment.

What is the most important information I should know about YERVOY?
YERVOY can cause serious side effects in many parts of your body which can lead to death. These side effects are most likely to begin during treatment; however, side effects can show up months after your last infusion.
These side effects may include:
1. **Inflammation of the intestines (colitis) that can cause tears or holes (perforation) in the intestines.** Signs and symptoms of colitis may include:
   • diarrhea (loose stools) or more bowel movements than usual

---

• blood in your stools or dark, tarry, sticky stools
• stomach pain (abdominal pain) or tenderness
2. **Inflammation of the liver (hepatitis) that can lead to liver failure.** Signs and symptoms of hepatitis may include:
   • yellowing of your skin or the whites of your eyes
   • dark urine (tea colored)
   • nausea or vomiting
   • pain on the right side of your stomach
   • bleeding or bruise more easily than normal
3. **Inflammation of the skin that can lead to severe skin reaction (toxic epidermal necrolysis).** Signs and symptoms of severe skin reactions may include:
   • skin rash with or without itching
   • sores in your mouth
   • your skin blisters and/or peels
4. **Inflammation of the nerves that can lead to paralysis.** Symptoms of nerve problems may include:
   • unusual weakness of legs, arms, or face
   • numbness or tingling in hands or feet
5. **Inflammation of hormone glands (especially the pituitary, adrenal, and thyroid glands) that may affect how these glands work.** Signs and symptoms that your glands are not working properly may include:
   • persistent or unusual headaches
   • unusual sluggishness, feeling cold all the time, or weight gain
   • changes in mood or behavior such as decreased sex drive, irritability, or forgetfulness
   • dizziness or fainting
6. **Inflammation of the eyes.** Symptoms may include:
   • blurry vision, double vision, or other vision problems
   • eye pain or redness

Call your healthcare provider if you have any of these signs or symptoms or they get worse. Do not try to treat symptoms yourself.
Getting medical treatment right away may keep the problem from becoming more serious. Your oncologist may decide to delay or stop YERVOY (ipilimumab).

What is YERVOY?
YERVOY is a prescription medicine used in adults to treat melanoma (a kind of skin cancer) that has spread or cannot be removed by surgery.
It is not known if YERVOY is safe and effective in children less than 18 years of age.

What should I tell my healthcare provider before getting YERVOY?
Before you are given YERVOY, tell your healthcare provider about all your health problems if you:

• have an active condition where your immune system attacks your body (autoimmune disease), such as ulcerative colitis, Crohn's disease, lupus, or sarcoidosis
• had an organ transplant, such as a kidney transplant
• have liver damage from diseases or drugs
• have any other medical conditions
• are pregnant or plan to become pregnant. YERVOY (ipilimumab) may cause stillbirth, premature delivery, and/or death of your unborn baby
• are breastfeeding

Tell your healthcare provider about all the medicines you take, including all prescription and non-prescription medicines, steroids or other medicines that lower your immune response, vitamins, and herbal supplements.
Know the medicines you take. Keep a list to show your doctors and pharmacists each time you get a new medicine.
You should not start a new medicine before you talk with the healthcare provider who prescribes you YERVOY.

How will I receive YERVOY?
You will get YERVOY through an intravenous line in your vein (infusion). It takes about 90 minutes to get a full dose.
• YERVOY is usually given every 3 weeks for up to 4 doses. Your healthcare provider may change how often you receive YERVOY or how long the infusion may take.
• Your healthcare provider should perform blood tests before starting and during treatment with YERVOY.
It is important for you to keep all appointments with your healthcare provider. Call your healthcare provider if you miss an appointment. There may be special instructions for you.

What are the possible side effects of YERVOY?
YERVOY can cause serious side effects. See "What is the most important information I should know about YERVOY?"

The most common side effects of YERVOY include:
• tiredness
• diarrhea
• itching
• rash
These are not all of the possible side effects of YERVOY. For more information, ask your healthcare provider.
Call your healthcare provider for medical advice about side effects. You may report side effects to FDA at 1-800-FDA-1088.
You may also report side effects to Bristol-Myers Squibb at 1-800-721-5072.

Table 3:   Overall Survival Results

	YERVOY n=137	YERVOY+gp100 n=403	gp100 n=136
Hazard Ratio (vs. gp100)	0.66	0.68	
(95% CI)	(0.51, 0.87)	(0.55, 0.85)	
p-value	p=0.0026[a]	p=0.0004	
Hazard Ratio (vs. YERVOY)		1.04	
(95% CI)		(0.83, 1.30)	
Median (months)	10	10	6
(95% CI)	(8.0, 13.8)	(8.5, 11.5)	(5.5, 8.7)

[a] Not adjusted for multiple comparisons.

Figure 1:   Overall Survival

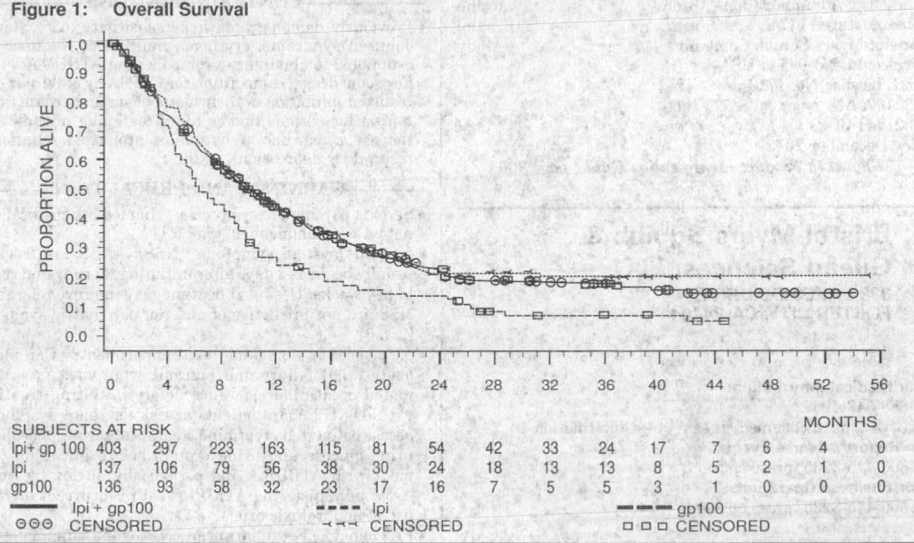

SUBJECTS AT RISK													MONTHS
Ipi+ gp 100	403	297	223	163	115	81	54	42	33	24	17	7	6	4	0
Ipi	137	106	79	56	38	30	24	18	13	13	8	5	2	1	0
gp100	136	93	58	32	23	17	16	7	5	3	1	0	0	0	0

Ipi + gp100   - - - - Ipi   □ □ □ gp100
⊙⊙⊙ CENSORED   ⊰⊣⊢⊣ CENSORED   □ □ □ CENSORED

General information about the safe and effective use of YERVOY (ipilimumab).

Medicines are sometimes prescribed for purposes other than those listed in a Medication Guide.

This Medication Guide summarizes the most important information about YERVOY. If you would like more information, talk with your healthcare provider. You can ask your healthcare provider for information about YERVOY that is written for healthcare professionals.

For more information, call 1-800-321-1335.

What are the ingredients of YERVOY?
Active ingredient: ipilimumab
Inactive ingredients: diethylene triamine pentaacetic acid (DTPA), mannitol, polysorbate 80, sodium chloride, tris hydrochloride, and Water for Injection, USP

This Medication Guide has been approved by the U.S. Food and Drug Administration.

Manufactured by:
Bristol-Myers Squibb Company
Princeton, NJ 08543 USA
U.S. License No. 1713
1321675A0
1321744A0
Rev December 2013
Shown in Product Identification Guide, page 306

Bristol-Myers Squibb & Gilead Sciences, LLC

333 LAKESIDE DRIVE
FOSTER CITY, CA 94404

For Medical Information:
1-888-547-4267
or www.gilead.com/medicines/request-information
To Report Adverse Events:
1-800-445-3235, press option 3
For Business Operations:
1-800-445-3235, press option 8

ATRIPLA® ℞
[uh TRIP luh]
(efavirenz/emtricitabine/tenofovir disoproxil fumarate) tablets, for oral use

HIGHLIGHTS OF PRESCRIBING INFORMATION
These highlights do not include all the information needed to use ATRIPLA safely and effectively. See full prescribing information for ATRIPLA.
ATRIPLA® (efavirenz/emtricitabine/tenofovir disoproxil fumarate) tablets, for oral use
Initial U.S. Approval: 2006

WARNING: LACTIC ACIDOSIS/SEVERE HEPATO-MEGALY WITH STEATOSIS and POST TREATMENT EXACERBATION OF HEPATITIS B
See full prescribing information for complete boxed warning.
- **Lactic acidosis and severe hepatomegaly with steatosis, including fatal cases, have been reported with the use of nucleoside analogs, including tenofovir disoproxil fumarate, a component of ATRIPLA. (5.1)**
- **ATRIPLA is not approved for the treatment of chronic hepatitis B virus (HBV) infection. Severe acute exacerbations of hepatitis B have been reported in patients coinfected with HBV and HIV-1 who have discontinued EMTRIVA or VIREAD, two of the components of ATRIPLA. Hepatic function should be monitored closely in these patients. If appropriate, initiation of anti-hepatitis B therapy may be warranted. (5.2)**

RECENT MAJOR CHANGES

INDICATIONS AND USAGE
ATRIPLA, a combination of 2 nucleoside analog HIV-1 reverse transcriptase inhibitors and 1 non-nucleoside HIV-1 reverse transcriptase inhibitor, is indicated for use alone as a complete regimen or in combination with other antiretroviral agents for the treatment of HIV-1 infection in adults and pediatric patients 12 years of age and older. (1)

DOSAGE AND ADMINISTRATION
- Recommended dose in adults and pediatric patients (12 years of age and older and weighing at least 40 kg): One tablet once daily taken orally on an empty stomach, preferably at bedtime. (2)
- Dose in renal impairment: Should not be administered in patients with estimated creatinine clearance below 50 mL/min. (2)
- With rifampin coadministration, an additional 200 mg/day of efavirenz is recommended for patients weighing 50 kg or more. (2)

DOSAGE FORMS AND STRENGTHS
Tablet containing 600 mg of efavirenz, 200 mg of emtricitabine and 300 mg of tenofovir disoproxil fumarate. (3)

CONTRAINDICATIONS
- Previously demonstrated hypersensitivity (e.g., Stevens-Johnson syndrome, erythema multiforme, or toxic skin eruptions) to efavirenz, a component of ATRIPLA. (4.1)
- For some drugs, competition for CYP3A by efavirenz could result in inhibition of their metabolism and create the potential for serious and/or life-threatening adverse reactions (e.g., cardiac arrhythmias, prolonged sedation, or respiratory depression). (4.2)

WARNINGS AND PRECAUTIONS
- Serious psychiatric symptoms: Immediate medical evaluation is recommended. (5.5, 6.1)
- Nervous system symptoms (NSS): NSS are frequent, usually begin 1–2 days after initiating therapy and resolve in 2–4 weeks. Dosing at bedtime may improve tolerability. NSS are not predictive of onset of psychiatric symptoms. (2, 5.6)
- New onset or worsening renal impairment: Can include acute renal failure and Fanconi syndrome. Assess estimated creatinine clearance before initiating treatment with ATRIPLA. In patients at risk for renal dysfunction, assess estimated creatinine clearance, serum phosphorus, urine glucose and urine protein before initiating treatment with ATRIPLA and periodically during treatment. Avoid administering ATRIPLA with concurrent or recent use of nephrotoxic drugs. (5.7)
- Pregnancy: Fetal harm can occur when administered to a pregnant woman during the first trimester. Women should be apprised of the potential harm to the fetus. A pregnancy registry is available. (5.8, 8.1)
- Rash: Discontinue if severe rash develops. (5.9, 6.1)
- Hepatotoxicity: Monitor liver function tests before and during treatment in patients with underlying hepatic disease, including hepatitis B or C coinfection, marked transaminase elevations, or who are taking medications associated with liver toxicity. Among reported cases of hepatic failure, a few occurred in patients with no pre-existing hepatic disease. (5.10, 6.3, 8.6)
- Decreases in bone mineral density (BMD): Consider assessment of BMD in patients with a history of pathological fracture or other risk factors for osteoporosis or bone loss. (5.11)
- Convulsions: Use caution in patients with a history of seizures. (5.12)
- Immune reconstitution syndrome: May necessitate further evaluation and treatment. (5.13)
- Redistribution/accumulation of body fat: Observed in patients receiving antiretroviral therapy. (5.14)
- Coadministration with other products: Do not use with drugs containing emtricitabine or tenofovir disoproxil fumarate including COMPLERA, EMTRIVA, STRIBILD, TRUVADA, or VIREAD; or with drugs containing lamivudine. SUSTIVA (efavirenz) should not be coadministered with ATRIPLA unless required for dose-adjustment when coadministered with rifampin. (5.4) Do not administer in combination with HEPSERA. (5.2)

ADVERSE REACTIONS
Most common adverse reactions (incidence greater than or equal to 10%) observed in an active-controlled clinical trial of efavirenz, emtricitabine, and tenofovir DF are diarrhea, nausea, fatigue, headache, dizziness, depression, insomnia, abnormal dreams, and rash. (6)
To report SUSPECTED ADVERSE REACTIONS, contact Gilead Sciences, Inc. at 1-800-GILEAD-5 or FDA at 1-800-FDA-1088 or www.fda.gov/medwatch

DRUG INTERACTIONS
- Efavirenz: Coadministration of efavirenz can alter the concentrations of other drugs and other drugs may alter the concentrations of efavirenz. The potential for drug-drug interactions must be considered before and during therapy. (4.2, 7.1, 12.3)
- Didanosine: Tenofovir disoproxil fumarate increases didanosine concentrations. Use with caution and monitor for evidence of didanosine toxicity (e.g., pancreatitis, neuropathy) when coadministered. Consider dose reductions or discontinuations of didanosine if warranted. (7.2)

- HIV-1 protease inhibitors: Coadministration of ATRIPLA with either lopinavir/ritonavir or darunavir and ritonavir increases tenofovir concentrations. Monitor for evidence of tenofovir toxicity. Coadministration of ATRIPLA with either atazanavir or atazanavir and ritonavir is not recommended. (7.3)

USE IN SPECIFIC POPULATIONS
- Pregnancy: Women should avoid pregnancy while receiving ATRIPLA and for 12 weeks after discontinuation. (5.8)
- Nursing mothers: Women infected with HIV should be instructed not to breastfeed. (8.3)
- Hepatic impairment: ATRIPLA is not recommended for patients with moderate or severe hepatic impairment. Use caution in patients with mild hepatic impairment. (5.10, 8.6)
- Pediatrics: The incidence of rash was higher than in adults. (5.9, 6.1)

See 17 for PATIENT COUNSELING INFORMATION and FDA-approved patient labeling

Revised: 10/2013

FULL PRESCRIBING INFORMATION: CONTENTS*
* Sections or subsections omitted from the full prescribing information are not listed

FULL PRESCRIBING INFORMATION

> **WARNING: LACTIC ACIDOSIS/SEVERE HEPATOMEGALY WITH STEATOSIS and POST TREATMENT EXACERBATION OF HEPATITIS B**
>
> Lactic acidosis and severe hepatomegaly with steatosis, including fatal cases, have been reported with the use of nucleoside analogs, including tenofovir disoproxil fumarate, a component of ATRIPLA, in combination with other antiretrovirals [See Warnings and Precautions (5.1)].
>
> ATRIPLA is not approved for the treatment of chronic hepatitis B virus (HBV) infection and the safety and efficacy of ATRIPLA have not been established in patients coinfected with HBV and HIV-1. Severe acute exacerbations of hepatitis B have been reported in patients who have discontinued EMTRIVA or VIREAD, which are components of ATRIPLA. Hepatic function should be monitored closely with both clinical and laboratory follow-up for at least several months in patients who are coinfected with HIV-1 and HBV and discontinue ATRIPLA. If appropriate, initiation of anti-hepatitis B therapy may be warranted [See Warnings and Precautions (5.2)].

1 INDICATIONS AND USAGE

ATRIPLA® is indicated for use alone as a complete regimen or in combination with other antiretroviral agents for the treatment of HIV-1 infection in adults and pediatric patients 12 years of age and older.

2 DOSAGE AND ADMINISTRATION

Adults and pediatric patients 12 years of age and older with body weight at least 40 kg (at least 88 lbs): The dose of ATRIPLA is one tablet once daily taken orally on an empty stomach. Dosing at bedtime may improve the tolerability of nervous system symptoms.

Renal Impairment: Because ATRIPLA is a fixed-dose combination, it should not be prescribed for patients requiring dosage adjustment such as those with moderate or severe renal impairment (estimated creatinine clearance below 50 mL/min).

Rifampin Coadministration: When ATRIPLA is administered with rifampin to patients weighing 50 kg or more, an additional 200 mg/day of efavirenz is recommended [See Drug Interactions (7.3), Table 4, and Clinical Pharmacology (12.3), Table 5].

3 DOSAGE FORMS AND STRENGTHS

ATRIPLA is available as tablets. Each tablet contains 600 mg of efavirenz, 200 mg of emtricitabine and 300 mg of tenofovir disoproxil fumarate (tenofovir DF, which is equivalent to 245 mg of tenofovir disoproxil). The tablets are pink, capsule-shaped, film-coated, debossed with "123" on one side and plain-faced on the other side.

4 CONTRAINDICATIONS

4.1 Hypersensitivity

ATRIPLA is contraindicated in patients with previously demonstrated clinically significant hypersensitivity (e.g., Stevens-Johnson syndrome, erythema multiforme, or toxic skin eruptions) to efavirenz, a component of ATRIPLA.

4.2 Contraindicated Drugs

For some drugs, competition for CYP3A by efavirenz could result in inhibition of their metabolism and create the potential for serious and/or life-threatening adverse reactions (e.g., cardiac arrhythmias, prolonged sedation, or respiratory depression). Drugs that are contraindicated with ATRIPLA are listed in Table 1.

[See table 1 above]

5 WARNINGS AND PRECAUTIONS

5.1 Lactic Acidosis/Severe Hepatomegaly with Steatosis

Lactic acidosis and severe hepatomegaly with steatosis, including fatal cases, have been reported with the use of nucleoside analogs including tenofovir DF, a component of ATRIPLA, in combination with other antiretrovirals. A majority of these cases have been in women. Obesity and prolonged nucleoside exposure may be risk factors. Particular caution should be exercised when administering nucleoside analogs to any patient with known risk factors for liver disease; however, cases have also been reported in patients with no known risk factors. Treatment with ATRIPLA should be suspended in any patient who develops clinical or laboratory findings suggestive of lactic acidosis or pronounced hepatotoxicity (which may include hepatomegaly and steatosis even in the absence of marked transaminase elevations).

5.2 Patients Coinfected with HIV-1 and HBV

It is recommended that all patients with HIV-1 be tested for the presence of chronic HBV before initiating antiretroviral therapy. ATRIPLA is not approved for the treatment of chronic HBV infection, and the safety and efficacy of ATRIPLA have not been established in patients coinfected with HBV and HIV-1. Severe acute exacerbations of hepatitis B have been reported in patients who are coinfected with HBV and HIV-1 and have discontinued emtricitabine or tenofovir DF, two of the components of ATRIPLA. In some patients infected with HBV and treated with emtricitabine, the exacerbations of hepatitis B were associated with liver decompensation and liver failure. Patients who are coinfected with HIV-1 and HBV should be closely monitored with both clinical and laboratory follow-up for at least several months after stopping treatment with ATRIPLA. If appropriate, initiation of anti-hepatitis B therapy may be warranted.

ATRIPLA should not be administered with HEPSERA® (adefovir dipivoxil) [See Drug Interactions (7.2)].

5.3 Drug Interactions

Efavirenz plasma concentrations may be altered by substrates, inhibitors, or inducers of CYP3A. Likewise, efavirenz may alter plasma concentrations of drugs metabolized by CYP3A or CYP2B6 [See Contraindications (4.2), Drug Interactions (7.1)].

5.4 Coadministration with Related Products

Related drugs not for coadministration with ATRIPLA include COMPLERA® (emtricitabine/rilpivirine/tenofovir DF), EMTRIVA® (emtricitabine), STRIBILD® (elvitegravir/cobicistat/emtricitabine/tenofovir DF), TRUVADA® (emtricitabine/tenofovir DF), and VIREAD® (tenofovir DF), which contain the same active components as ATRIPLA. SUSTIVA® (efavirenz) should not be coadministered with ATRIPLA unless needed for dose-adjustment (e.g., with rifampin) [See Dosage and Administration (2), Drug Interactions (7.1)]. Due to similarities between emtricitabine and lamivudine, ATRIPLA should not be coadministered with drugs containing lamivudine, including Combivir (lamivudine/zidovudine), Epivir, or Epivir-HBV (lamivudine), Epzicom (abacavir sulfate/lamivudine), or Trizivir (abacavir sulfate/lamivudine/zidovudine).

5.5 Psychiatric Symptoms

Serious psychiatric adverse experiences have been reported in patients treated with efavirenz. In controlled trials of 1008 subjects treated with regimens containing efavirenz for a mean of 2.1 years and 635 subjects treated with control regimens for a mean of 1.5 years, the frequency (regardless of causality) of specific serious psychiatric events among subjects who received efavirenz or control regimens, respectively, were: severe depression (2.4%, 0.9%), suicidal ideation (0.7%, 0.3%), nonfatal suicide attempts (0.5%, 0%), aggressive behavior (0.4%, 0.5%), paranoid reactions (0.4%, 0.3%), and manic reactions (0.2%, 0.3%). When psychiatric symptoms similar to those noted above were combined and evaluated as a group in a multifactorial analysis of data from Study AI266006 (006), treatment with efavirenz was associated with an increase in the occurrence of these selected psychiatric symptoms. Other factors associated with an increase in the occurrence of these psychiatric symptoms were history of injection drug use, psychiatric history, and receipt of psychiatric medication at trial entry; similar associations were observed in both the efavirenz and control treatment groups. In Study 006, onset of new serious psychiatric symptoms occurred throughout the trial for both efavirenz-treated and control-treated subjects. One percent of efavirenz-treated subjects discontinued or interrupted treatment because of one or more of these selected psychiatric symptoms. There have also been occasional post-marketing reports of death by suicide, delusions, and psychosis-like behavior, although a causal relationship to the use of efavirenz cannot be determined from these reports. Patients with serious psychiatric adverse experiences should seek immediate medical evaluation to assess the possibility that the symptoms may be related to the use of efavirenz, and if so, to determine whether the risks of continued therapy outweigh the benefits [See Adverse Reactions (6)].

5.6 Nervous System Symptoms

Fifty-three percent (531/1008) of subjects receiving efavirenz in controlled trials reported central nervous system symptoms (any grade, regardless of causality) compared to 25% (156/635) of subjects receiving control regimens. These symptoms included dizziness (28.1% of the 1008 subjects), insomnia (16.3%), impaired concentration (8.3%), somnolence (7.0%), abnormal dreams (6.2%), and hallucinations (1.2%). Other reported symptoms were euphoria, confusion, agitation, amnesia, stupor, abnormal thinking, and depersonalization. The majority of these symptoms were mild-to-moderate (50.7%); symptoms were severe in 2.0% of subjects. Overall, 2.1% of subjects discontinued therapy as a result. These symptoms usually begin during the first or second day of therapy and generally resolve after the first 2–4 weeks of therapy. After 4 weeks of therapy, the prevalence of nervous system symptoms of at least moderate severity ranged from 5% to 9% in subjects treated with regimens containing efavirenz and from 3% to 5% in subjects treated with a control regimen. Patients should be informed that these common symptoms were likely to improve with continued therapy and were not predictive of subsequent onset of the less frequent psychiatric symptoms [See Warnings and Precautions (5.5)]. Dosing at bedtime may improve the tolerability of these nervous system symptoms [See Dosage and Administration (2)].

Analysis of long-term data from Study 006 (median follow-up 180 weeks, 102 weeks, and 76 weeks for subjects treated with efavirenz + zidovudine + lamivudine, efavirenz + indinavir, and indinavir + zidovudine + lamivudine, respectively) showed that, beyond 24 weeks of therapy, the incidences of new-onset nervous system symptoms among efavirenz-treated subjects were generally similar to those in the indinavir-containing control arm.

Patients receiving ATRIPLA should be alerted to the potential for additive central nervous system effects when ATRIPLA is used concomitantly with alcohol or psychoactive drugs.

Patients who experience central nervous system symptoms such as dizziness, impaired concentration, and/or drowsiness should avoid potentially hazardous tasks such as driving or operating machinery.

5.7 New Onset or Worsening Renal Impairment

Emtricitabine and tenofovir are principally eliminated by the kidney; however, efavirenz is not. Since ATRIPLA is a

Table 1 Drugs That Are Contraindicated or Not Recommended for Use With ATRIPLA

Drug Class: Drug Name	Clinical Comment
Antifungal: voriconazole	Efavirenz significantly decreases voriconazole plasma concentrations, and coadministration may decrease the therapeutic effectiveness of voriconazole. Also, voriconazole significantly increases efavirenz plasma concentrations, which may increase the risk of efavirenz-associated side effects. Because ATRIPLA is a fixed-dose combination product, the dose of efavirenz cannot be altered. [See Clinical Pharmacology (12.3) Tables 5 and 6]
Ergot derivatives (dihydroergotamine, ergonovine, ergotamine, methylergonovine)	Potential for serious and/or life-threatening reactions such as acute ergot toxicity characterized by peripheral vasospasm and ischemia of the extremities and other tissues.
Benzodiazepines: midazolam, triazolam	Potential for serious and/or life-threatening reactions such as prolonged or increased sedation or respiratory depression.
Calcium channel blocker: bepridil	Potential for serious and/or life-threatening reactions such as cardiac arrhythmias.
GI motility agent: cisapride	Potential for serious and/or life-threatening reactions such as cardiac arrhythmias.
Neuroleptic: pimozide	Potential for serious and/or life-threatening reactions such as cardiac arrhythmias.
St. John's wort (*Hypericum perforatum*)	May lead to loss of virologic response and possible resistance to efavirenz or to the class of non-nucleoside reverse transcriptase inhibitors (NNRTIs).

combination product and the dose of the individual components cannot be altered, patients with estimated creatinine clearance below 50 mL/min should not receive ATRIPLA. Renal impairment, including cases of acute renal failure and Fanconi syndrome (renal tubular injury with severe hypophosphatemia), has been reported with the use of tenofovir DF [See Adverse Reactions (6.3)].

It is recommended that estimated creatinine clearance be assessed in all patients prior to initiating therapy and as clinically appropriate during therapy with ATRIPLA. In patients at risk of renal dysfunction, including patients who have previously experienced renal events while receiving HEPSERA, it is recommended that estimated creatinine clearance, serum phosphorus, urine glucose, and urine protein be assessed prior to initiation of ATRIPLA, and periodically during ATRIPLA therapy.

ATRIPLA should be avoided with concurrent or recent use of a nephrotoxic agent (e.g., high-dose or multiple nonsteroidal anti-inflammatory drugs (NSAIDs)) [See Drug Interactions (7.2)]. Cases of acute renal failure after initiation of high dose or multiple NSAIDs have been reported in HIV-infected patients with risk factors for renal dysfunction who appeared stable on tenofovir DF. Some patients required hospitalization and renal replacement therapy. Alternatives to NSAIDs should be considered, if needed, in patients at risk for renal dysfunction.

Persistent or worsening bone pain, pain in extremities, fractures and/or muscular pain or weakness may be manifestations of proximal renal tubulopathy and should prompt an evaluation of renal function in at-risk patients.

5.8 Reproductive Risk Potential

Pregnancy Category D: Efavirenz may cause fetal harm when administered during the first trimester to a pregnant woman. Pregnancy should be avoided in women receiving ATRIPLA. Barrier contraception must always be used in combination with other methods of contraception (e.g., oral or other hormonal contraceptives). Because of the long half-life of efavirenz, use of adequate contraceptive measures for 12 weeks after discontinuation of ATRIPLA is recommended. Women of childbearing potential should undergo pregnancy testing before initiation of ATRIPLA. If this drug is used during the first trimester of pregnancy, or if the patient becomes pregnant while taking this drug, the patient should be apprised of the potential harm to the fetus.

There are no adequate and well-controlled trials of ATRIPLA in pregnant women. ATRIPLA should be used during pregnancy only if the potential benefit justifies the potential risk to the fetus, such as in pregnant women without other therapeutic options [See Use in Specific Populations (8.1)].

5.9 Rash

In controlled clinical trials, 26% (266/1008) of subjects treated with 600 mg efavirenz experienced new-onset skin rash compared with 17% (111/635) of subjects treated in control groups. Rash associated with blistering, moist desquamation, or ulceration occurred in 0.9% (9/1008) of subjects treated with efavirenz. The incidence of Grade 4 rash (e.g., erythema multiforme, Stevens-Johnson syndrome) in subjects treated with efavirenz in all trials and expanded access was 0.1%. Rashes are usually mild-to-moderate maculopapular skin eruptions that occur within the first 2 weeks of initiating therapy with efavirenz (median time to onset of rash in adults was 11 days) and, in most subjects continuing therapy with efavirenz, rash resolves within 1 month (median duration, 16 days). The discontinuation rate for rash in clinical trials was 1.7% (17/1008). ATRIPLA can be reinitiated in patients interrupting therapy because of rash. ATRIPLA should be discontinued in patients developing severe rash associated with blistering, desquamation, mucosal involvement, or fever. Appropriate antihistamines and/or corticosteroids may improve the tolerability and hasten the resolution of rash. For patients who have had a life-threatening cutaneous reaction (e.g., Stevens-Johnson syndrome), alternative therapy should be considered [See also Contraindications (4.1)].

Experience with efavirenz in subjects who discontinued other antiretroviral agents of the NNRTI class is limited. Nineteen subjects who discontinued nevirapine because of rash have been treated with efavirenz. Nine of these subjects developed mild-to-moderate rash while receiving therapy with efavirenz, and two of these subjects discontinued because of rash.

Rash was reported in 26 of 57 pediatric subjects (46%) treated with efavirenz [See Adverse Reactions (6.1)]. One pediatric subject experienced Grade 3 rash (confluent rash with fever), and two subjects had Grade 4 rash (erythema multiforme). The median time to onset of rash in pediatric subjects was 8 days. Prophylaxis with appropriate antihistamines before initiating therapy with ATRIPLA in pediatric patients should be considered.

5.10 Hepatotoxicity

Monitoring of liver enzymes before and during treatment is recommended for patients with underlying hepatic disease, including hepatitis B or C infection; patients with marked transaminase elevations; and patients treated with other medications associated with liver toxicity [See also Warnings and Precautions (5.2)]. A few of the postmarketing reports of hepatic failure occurred in patients with no pre-existing hepatic disease or other identifiable risk factors [See Adverse Reactions (6.3)]. Liver enzyme monitoring should also be considered for patients without pre-existing hepatic dysfunction or other risk factors. In patients with persistent elevations of serum transaminases to greater than five times the upper limit of the normal range, the benefit of continued therapy with ATRIPLA needs to be weighed against the unknown risks of significant liver toxicity [See Adverse Reactions (6.2)].

5.11 Bone Effects of Tenofovir DF

Bone Mineral Density:
In clinical trials in HIV-1 infected adults, tenofovir DF was associated with slightly greater decreases in bone mineral density (BMD) and increases in biochemical markers of bone metabolism, suggesting increased bone turnover relative to comparators. Serum parathyroid hormone levels and 1,25 Vitamin D levels were also higher in subjects receiving tenofovir DF.

Clinical trials evaluating tenofovir DF in pediatric and adolescent subjects were conducted. Under normal circumstances, BMD increases rapidly in pediatric subjects. In HIV-1 infected subjects aged 2 years to less than 18 years, bone effects were similar to those observed in adult subjects and suggest increased bone turnover. Total body BMD gain was less in the tenofovir DF treated HIV-1 infected pediatric subjects as compared to the control groups. Similar trends were observed in chronic hepatitis B infected adolescent subjects aged 12 years to less than 18 years. In all pediatric trials, skeletal growth (height) appeared to be unaffected. For more information, consult the VIREAD prescribing information.

The effects of tenofovir DF-associated changes in BMD and biochemical markers on long-term bone health and future fracture risk are unknown. Assessment of BMD should be considered for adult and pediatric patients who have a history of pathologic bone fracture or other risk factors for osteoporosis or bone loss. Although the effect of supplementation with calcium and vitamin D was not studied, such supplementation may be beneficial for all patients. If bone abnormalities are suspected then appropriate consultation should be obtained.

Mineralization Defects:
Cases of osteomalacia associated with proximal renal tubulopathy, manifested as bone pain or pain in extremities and which may contribute to fractures, have been reported in association with the use of tenofovir DF [See Adverse Reactions (6.3)]. Arthralgias and muscle pain or weakness have also been reported in cases of proximal renal tubulopathy. Hypophosphatemia and osteomalacia secondary to proximal renal tubulopathy should be considered in patients at risk of renal dysfunction who present with persistent or worsening bone or muscle symptoms while receiving products containing tenofovir DF [See Warnings and Precautions (5.7)].

5.12 Convulsions

Convulsions have been observed in patients receiving efavirenz, generally in the presence of known medical history of seizures. Caution must be taken in any patient with a history of seizures.

Patients who are receiving concomitant anticonvulsant medications primarily metabolized by the liver, such as phenytoin and phenobarbital, may require periodic monitoring of plasma levels [See Drug Interactions (7.3)].

5.13 Immune Reconstitution Syndrome

Immune reconstitution syndrome has been reported in patients treated with combination antiretroviral therapy, including the components of ATRIPLA. During the initial phase of combination antiretroviral treatment, patients whose immune system responds may develop an inflammatory response to indolent or residual opportunistic infections [such as *Mycobacterium avium* infection, cytomegalovirus, *Pneumocystis jirovecii* pneumonia (PCP) or tuberculosis], which may necessitate further evaluation and treatment.

Autoimmune disorders (such as Graves' disease, polymyositis, and Guillain-Barré syndrome) have also been reported to occur in the setting of immune reconstitution, however, the time to onset is more variable, and can occur many months after initiation of treatment.

5.14 Fat Redistribution

Redistribution/accumulation of body fat including central obesity, dorsocervical fat enlargement (buffalo hump), peripheral wasting, facial wasting, breast enlargement, and "cushingoid appearance" have been observed in patients receiving antiretroviral therapy. The mechanism and long-term consequences of these events are currently unknown. A causal relationship has not been established.

6 ADVERSE REACTIONS

Efavirenz, Emtricitabine and Tenofovir Disoproxil Fumarate: The following adverse reactions are discussed in other sections of the labeling:

- Lactic Acidosis/Severe Hepatomegaly with Steatosis [See Boxed Warning, Warnings and Precautions (5.1)].
- Severe Acute Exacerbations of Hepatitis B [See Boxed Warning, Warnings and Precautions (5.2)].
- Psychiatric Symptoms [See Warnings and Precautions (5.5)].
- Nervous System Symptoms [See Warnings and Precautions (5.6)].
- New Onset or Worsening Renal Impairment [See Warnings and Precautions (5.7)].
- Rash [See Warnings and Precautions (5.9)].
- Hepatotoxicity [See Warnings and Precautions (5.10)].
- Bone Effects of Tenofovir DF [See Warnings and Precautions (5.11)].
- Immune Reconstitution Syndrome [See Warnings and Precautions (5.13)].
- Drug Interactions [See Contraindications (4.2), Warnings and Precautions (5.3) and Drug Interactions (7)].

For additional safety information about SUSTIVA (efavirenz), EMTRIVA (emtricitabine), or VIREAD (tenofovir DF) in combination with other antiretroviral agents, consult the prescribing information for these products.

6.1 Adverse Reactions from Clinical Trials Experience

Because clinical trials are conducted under widely varying conditions, adverse reaction rates observed in the clinical trials of a drug cannot be directly compared to rates in the clinical trials of another drug and may not reflect the rates observed in practice.

Clinical Trials in Adult Subjects
Study 934
Study 934 was an open-label active-controlled trial in which 511 antiretroviral-naive subjects received either emtricitabine + tenofovir DF administered in combination with efavirenz (N=257) or zidovudine/lamivudine administered in combination with efavirenz (N=254).

The most common adverse reactions (incidence greater than or equal to 10%, any severity) occurring in Study 934 include diarrhea, nausea, fatigue, headache, dizziness, depression, insomnia, abnormal dreams, and rash. Adverse reactions observed in Study 934 were generally consistent with those seen in previous trials of the individual components (Table 2).

Table 2 Selected Treatment-Emergent Adverse Reactions* (Grades 2–4) Reported in ≥5% in Either Treatment Group in Study 934 (0–144 Weeks)

	FTC + TDF + EFV[†]	AZT/3TC + EFV
	N=257	N=254
Gastrointestinal Disorder		
Diarrhea	9%	5%
Nausea	9%	7%
Vomiting	2%	5%
General Disorders and Administration Site Condition		
Fatigue	9%	8%
Infections and Infestations		
Sinusitis	8%	4%
Upper respiratory tract infections	8%	5%
Nasopharyngitis	5%	3%
Nervous System Disorders		
Headache	6%	5%
Dizziness	8%	7%
Psychiatric Disorders		
Anxiety	5%	4%
Depression	9%	7%
Insomnia	5%	7%
Skin and Subcutaneous Tissue Disorders		
Rash Event[‡]	7%	9%

* Frequencies of adverse reactions are based on all treatment-emergent adverse events, regardless of relationship to study drug.

† From Weeks 96 to 144 of the trial, subjects received emtricitabine/tenofovir DF administered in combination with efavirenz in place of emtricitabine + tenofovir DF with efavirenz.

‡ Rash event includes rash, exfoliative rash, rash generalized, rash macular, rash maculopapular, rash pruritic, and rash vesicular.

Study 073
In Study 073, subjects with stable, virologic suppression on antiretroviral therapy and no history of virologic failure were randomized to receive ATRIPLA or to stay on their

baseline regimen. The adverse reactions observed in Study 073 were generally consistent with those seen in Study 934 and those seen with the individual components of ATRIPLA when each was administered in combination with other antiretroviral agents.

Efavirenz, Emtricitabine, or Tenofovir Disoproxil Fumarate In addition to the adverse reactions in Study 934 and Study 073, the following adverse reactions were observed in clinical trials of efavirenz, emtricitabine, or tenofovir DF in combination with other antiretroviral agents.

Efavirenz: The most significant adverse reactions observed in subjects treated with efavirenz are nervous system symptoms [See Warnings and Precautions (5.6)], psychiatric symptoms [See Warnings and Precautions (5.5)], and rash [See Warnings and Precautions (5.9)].

Selected adverse reactions of moderate-to-severe intensity observed in greater than or equal to 2% of efavirenz-treated subjects in two controlled clinical trials included pain, impaired concentration, abnormal dreams, somnolence, anorexia, dyspepsia, abdominal pain, nervousness, and pruritus.

Pancreatitis has also been reported, although a causal relationship with efavirenz has not been established. Asymptomatic increases in serum amylase levels were observed in a significantly higher number of subjects treated with efavirenz 600 mg than in control subjects.

Emtricitabine and Tenofovir Disoproxil Fumarate: Adverse reactions that occurred in at least 5% of treatment-experienced or treatment-naive subjects receiving emtricitabine or tenofovir DF with other antiretroviral agents in clinical trials include arthralgia, increased cough, dyspepsia, fever, myalgia, pain, abdominal pain, back pain, paresthesia, peripheral neuropathy (including peripheral neuritis and neuropathy), pneumonia, rhinitis and rash event (including rash, pruritus, maculopapular rash, urticaria, vesiculobullous rash, pustular rash, and allergic reaction).

Skin discoloration has been reported with higher frequency among emtricitabine-treated subjects; it was manifested by hyperpigmentation on the palms and/or soles and was generally mild and asymptomatic. The mechanism and clinical significance are unknown.

Clinical Trials in Pediatric Subjects

Efavirenz: In a pediatric clinical trial in 57 NRTI-experienced subjects aged 3 to 16 years, the type and frequency of adverse experiences was generally similar to that of adult subjects with the exception of a higher incidence of rash, which was reported in 46% (26/57) of pediatric subjects compared to 26% of adults, and a higher frequency of Grade 3 or 4 rash reported in 5% (3/57) of pediatric subjects compared to 0.9% of adults [See Warnings and Precautions (5.9)]. For additional information, please consult the SUSTIVA prescribing information.

Emtricitabine: In addition to the adverse reactions reported in adults, anemia and hyperpigmentation were observed in 7% and 32%, respectively, of pediatric subjects (3 months to less than 18 years of age) who received treatment with emtricitabine in the larger of two open-label, uncontrolled pediatric trials (N=116). For additional information, please consult the EMTRIVA prescribing information.

Tenofovir Disoproxil Fumarate: In a pediatric clinical trial conducted in subjects 12 to less than 18 years of age, the adverse reactions observed in pediatric subjects who received treatment with tenofovir DF were consistent with those observed in clinical trials of tenofovir DF in adults [See Warnings and Precautions (5.11)].

6.2 Laboratory Abnormalities

Efavirenz, Emtricitabine and Tenofovir Disoproxil Fumarate: Laboratory abnormalities observed in Study 934 were generally consistent with those seen in previous trials (Table 3).

Table 3 Significant Laboratory Abnormalities Reported in ≥1% of Subjects in Either Treatment Group in Study 934 (0–144 Weeks)

	FTC + TDF + EFV*	AZT/3TC + EFV
	N=257	N=254
Any ≥ Grade 3 Laboratory Abnormality	30%	26%
Fasting Cholesterol (>240 mg/dL)	22%	24%
Creatine Kinase (M: >990 U/L) (F: >845 U/L)	9%	7%
Serum Amylase (>175 U/L)	8%	4%
Alkaline Phosphatase (>550 U/L)	1%	0%
AST (M: >180 U/L) (F: >170 U/L)	3%	3%
ALT (M: >215 U/L) (F: >170 U/L)	2%	3%
Hemoglobin (<8.0 mg/dL)	0%	4%
Hyperglycemia (>250 mg/dL)	2%	1%
Hematuria (>75 RBC/HPF)	3%	2%
Glycosuria (≥3+)	<1%	1%
Neutrophils (<750/mm^3)	3%	5%
Fasting Triglycerides (>750 mg/dL)	4%	2%

* From Weeks 96 to 144 of the trial, subjects received emtricitabine/tenofovir DF administered in combination with efavirenz in place of emtricitabine + tenofovir DF with efavirenz.

Laboratory abnormalities observed in Study 073 were generally consistent with those in Study 934.

In addition to the laboratory abnormalities described for Study 934 (Table 3), Grade 3/4 laboratory abnormalities of increased bilirubin (greater than 2.5 × upper limit of normal (ULN)), increased pancreatic amylase (greater than 2.0 × ULN), increased or decreased serum glucose (less than 40 or greater than 250 mg/dL), and increased serum lipase (greater than 2.0 × ULN) occurred in up to 3% of subjects treated with emtricitabine or tenofovir DF with other antiretroviral agents in clinical trials.

Hepatic Events: In Study 934, 19 subjects treated with efavirenz, emtricitabine, and tenofovir DF and 20 subjects treated with efavirenz and fixed-dose zidovudine/lamivudine were hepatitis B surface antigen or hepatitis C antibody positive. Among these coinfected subjects, one subject (1/19) in the efavirenz, emtricitabine and tenofovir DF arm had elevations in transaminases to greater than five times ULN through 144 weeks. In the fixed-dose zidovudine/lamivudine arm, two subjects (2/20) had elevations in transaminases to greater than five times ULN through 144 weeks. No HBV and/or HCV coinfected subject discontinued from the trial due to hepatobiliary disorders [See Warnings and Precautions (5.10)].

6.3 Postmarketing Experience

The following adverse reactions have been identified during postapproval use of efavirenz, emtricitabine, or tenofovir DF. Because postmarketing reactions are reported voluntarily from a population of uncertain size, it is not always possible to reliably estimate their frequency or establish a causal relationship to drug exposure.

Efavirenz:

Cardiac Disorders
Palpitations

Ear and Labyrinth Disorders
Tinnitus, vertigo

Endocrine Disorders
Gynecomastia

Eye Disorders
Abnormal vision

Gastrointestinal Disorders
Constipation, malabsorption

General Disorders and Administration Site Conditions
Asthenia

Hepatobiliary Disorders
Hepatic enzyme increase, hepatic failure, hepatitis. A few of the postmarketing reports of hepatic failure, including cases in patients with no pre-existing hepatic disease or other identifiable risk factors, were characterized by a fulminant course, progressing in some cases to transplantation or death.

Immune System Disorders
Allergic reactions

Metabolism and Nutrition Disorders
Redistribution/accumulation of body fat [See Warnings and Precautions (5.14)], hypercholesterolemia, hypertriglyceridemia

Musculoskeletal and Connective Tissue Disorders
Arthralgia, myalgia, myopathy

Nervous System Disorders
Abnormal coordination, ataxia, cerebellar coordination and balance disturbances, convulsions, hypoesthesia, paresthesia, neuropathy, tremor

Psychiatric Disorders
Aggressive reactions, agitation, delusions, emotional lability, mania, neurosis, paranoia, psychosis, suicide

Respiratory, Thoracic and Mediastinal Disorders
Dyspnea

Skin and Subcutaneous Tissue Disorders
Flushing, erythema multiforme, photoallergic dermatitis, Stevens-Johnson syndrome

Emtricitabine: No postmarketing adverse reactions have been identified for inclusion in this section.

Tenofovir Disoproxil Fumarate:

Immune System Disorders
Allergic reaction, including angioedema

Metabolism and Nutrition Disorders
Lactic acidosis, hypokalemia, hypophosphatemia

Respiratory, Thoracic, and Mediastinal Disorders
Dyspnea

Gastrointestinal Disorders
Pancreatitis, increased amylase, abdominal pain

Hepatobiliary Disorders
Hepatic steatosis, hepatitis, increased liver enzymes (most commonly AST, ALT, gamma GT)

Skin and Subcutaneous Tissue Disorders
Rash

Musculoskeletal and Connective Tissue Disorders
Rhabdomyolysis, osteomalacia (manifested as bone pain and which may contribute to fractures), muscular weakness, myopathy

Renal and Urinary Disorders
Acute renal failure, renal failure, acute tubular necrosis, Fanconi syndrome, proximal renal tubulopathy, interstitial nephritis (including acute cases), nephrogenic diabetes insipidus, renal insufficiency, increased creatinine, proteinuria, polyuria

General Disorders and Administration Site Conditions
Asthenia

The following adverse reactions, listed under the body system headings above, may occur as a consequence of proximal renal tubulopathy: rhabdomyolysis, osteomalacia, hypokalemia, muscular weakness, myopathy, hypophosphatemia.

7 DRUG INTERACTIONS

This section describes clinically relevant drug interactions with ATRIPLA. Drug interaction trials are described elsewhere in the labeling [See Clinical Pharmacology (12.3)].

7.1 Efavirenz

Efavirenz has been shown *in vivo* to induce CYP3A and CYP2B6. Other compounds that are substrates of CYP3A or CYP2B6 may have decreased plasma concentrations when coadministered with efavirenz. *In vitro* studies have demonstrated that efavirenz inhibits CYP2C9, 2C19, and 3A4 isozymes in the range of observed efavirenz plasma concentrations. Coadministration of efavirenz with drugs primarily metabolized by these isozymes may result in altered plasma concentrations of the coadministered drug. Therefore, appropriate dose adjustments may be necessary for these drugs.

Drugs that induce CYP3A activity (e.g., phenobarbital, rifampin, rifabutin) would be expected to increase the clearance of efavirenz, resulting in lowered plasma concentrations [See Dosage and Administration (2)].

7.2 Emtricitabine and Tenofovir Disoproxil Fumarate

Since emtricitabine and tenofovir are primarily eliminated by the kidneys, coadministration of ATRIPLA with drugs that reduce renal function or compete for active tubular secretion may increase serum concentrations of emtricitabine, tenofovir, and/or other renally eliminated drugs. Some examples include, but are not limited to, acyclovir, adefovir dipivoxil, cidofovir, ganciclovir, valacyclovir, valganciclovir, aminoglycosides (e.g., gentamicin), and high-dose or multiple NSAIDs [See Warnings and Precautions (5.7)].

Coadministration of tenofovir DF and didanosine should be undertaken with caution and patients receiving this combination should be monitored closely for didanosine-associated adverse reactions. Didanosine should be discontinued in patients who develop didanosine-associated adverse reactions [for didanosine dosing adjustment recommendations, see *Table 4*]. Suppression of CD4$^+$ cell counts has been observed in patients receiving tenofovir DF with didanosine 400 mg daily.

Darunavir with ritonavir and lopinavir/ritonavir have been shown to increase tenofovir concentrations. Tenofovir DF is a substrate of P-glycoprotein (Pgp) and breast cancer resistance protein (BCRP) transporters. When tenofovir DF is co-administered with an inhibitor of these transporters, an increase in absorption may be observed. Patients receiving darunavir with ritonavir and ATRIPLA, or lopinavir/ritonavir with ATRIPLA, should be monitored for tenofovir-associated adverse reactions. ATRIPLA should be discontinued in patients who develop tenofovir-associated adverse reactions [See Table 4].

Coadministration of atazanavir with ATRIPLA is not recommended since coadministration of atazanavir with either

Table 4 Established and Other Potentially Significant* Drug Interactions: Alteration in Dose or Regimen May Be Recommended Based on Drug Interaction Trials or Predicted Interaction

Concomitant Drug Class: Drug Name	Effect	Clinical Comment
HIV antiviral agents		
Protease inhibitor: atazanavir	↓atazanavir ↑ tenofovir	Coadministration of atazanavir with ATRIPLA is not recommended. Coadministration of atazanavir with either efavirenz or tenofovir DF decreases plasma concentrations of atazanavir. The combined effect of efavirenz plus tenofovir DF on atazanavir plasma concentrations is not known. Also, atazanavir has been shown to increase tenofovir concentrations. There are insufficient data to support dosing recommendations for atazanavir or atazanavir/ritonavir in combination with ATRIPLA.
Protease inhibitor: fosamprenavir calcium	↓ amprenavir	Fosamprenavir (unboosted): Appropriate doses of fosamprenavir and ATRIPLA with respect to safety and efficacy have not been established. Fosamprenavir/ritonavir: An additional 100 mg/day (300 mg total) of ritonavir is recommended when ATRIPLA is administered with fosamprenavir/ritonavir once daily. No change in the ritonavir dose is required when ATRIPLA is administered with fosamprenavir plus ritonavir twice daily.
Protease inhibitor: indinavir	↓ indinavir	The optimal dose of indinavir, when given in combination with efavirenz, is not known. Increasing the indinavir dose to 1000 mg every 8 hours does not compensate for the increased indinavir metabolism due to efavirenz.
Protease inhibitor: lopinavir/ritonavir	↓ lopinavir ↑ tenofovir	Do not use once daily administration of lopinavir/ritonavir. Dose adjustment of lopinavir/ritonavir is recommended when coadministered with efavirenz. Refer to the full prescribing information for lopinavir/ritonavir for guidance on coadministration with efavirenz- or tenofovir-containing regimens, such as ATRIPLA. **Patients should be monitored for tenofovir-associated adverse reactions.**
Protease inhibitor: ritonavir	↑ ritonavir ↑ efavirenz	When ritonavir 500 mg every 12 hours was coadministered with efavirenz 600 mg once daily, the combination was associated with a higher frequency of adverse clinical experiences (e.g., dizziness, nausea, paresthesia) and laboratory abnormalities (elevated liver enzymes). Monitoring of liver enzymes is recommended when ATRIPLA is used in combination with ritonavir.
Protease inhibitor: saquinavir	↓ saquinavir	Appropriate doses of the combination of efavirenz and saquinavir/ritonavir with respect to safety and efficacy have not been established.
CCR5 co-receptor antagonist: maraviroc	↓ maraviroc	Efavirenz decreases plasma concentrations of maraviroc. Refer to the full prescribing information for maraviroc for guidance on coadministration with ATRIPLA.
NRTI: didanosine	↑ didanosine	Coadministration of ATRIPLA and didanosine should be undertaken with caution and patients receiving this combination should be monitored closely for didanosine-associated adverse reactions including pancreatitis, lactic acidosis, and neuropathy. A dose reduction of didanosine is recommended when coadministered with tenofovir DF. For additional information on coadministration with tenofovir DF-containing products, please refer to the didanosine prescribing information.
NNRTI: Other NNRTIs	↑ or ↓ efavirenz and/or NNRTI	Combining two NNRTIs has not been shown to be beneficial. ATRIPLA contains efavirenz and should not be coadministered with other NNRTIs.
Integrase strand transfer inhibitor: raltegravir	↓ raltegravir	Efavirenz reduces plasma concentrations of raltegravir. The clinical significance of this interaction has not been directly assessed.
Hepatitis C antiviral agents		
Protease inhibitor: boceprevir	↓ boceprevir	Plasma trough concentrations of boceprevir were decreased when boceprevir was coadministered with efavirenz, which may result in loss of therapeutic effect. The combination should be avoided.
Protease inhibitor: telaprevir	↓ telaprevir ↓ efavirenz	Concomitant administration of telaprevir and efavirenz resulted in reduced steady-state exposures to telaprevir and efavirenz.
Other agents		
Anticoagulant: warfarin	↑ or ↓ warfarin	Plasma concentrations and effects potentially increased or decreased by efavirenz.

(Table continued on next page)

efavirenz or tenofovir DF has been shown to decrease plasma concentrations of atazanavir. Also, atazanavir has been shown to increase tenofovir concentrations. There are insufficient data to support dosing recommendations for atazanavir/ritonavir in combination with ATRIPLA [See Table 4].

7.3 Efavirenz, Emtricitabine and Tenofovir Disoproxil Fumarate

Other important drug interaction information for ATRIPLA is summarized in Table 1 and Table 4. The drug interactions described are based on trials conducted with efavirenz, emtricitabine or tenofovir DF as individual agents or are potential drug interactions; no drug interaction trials have been conducted using ATRIPLA [for pharmacokinetics data see *Clinical Pharmacology (12.3)*, Tables 5–8]. The tables include potentially significant interactions, but are not all inclusive.

[See table 4 above and on next page]

7.4 Efavirenz Assay Interference

Cannabinoid Test Interaction: Efavirenz does not bind to cannabinoid receptors. False-positive urine cannabinoid test results have been observed in non-HIV-infected volunteers receiving efavirenz when the Microgenics Cedia DAU Multi-Level THC assay was used for screening. Negative results were obtained when more specific confirmatory testing was performed with gas chromatography/mass spectrometry. For more information, please consult the SUSTIVA prescribing information.

8 USE IN SPECIFIC POPULATIONS

8.1 Pregnancy

Pregnancy Category D *[See Warnings and Precautions (5.8)]*

Antiretroviral Pregnancy Registry: To monitor fetal outcomes of pregnant women, an Antiretroviral Pregnancy Registry has been established. Physicians are encouraged to register patients who become pregnant by calling (800) 258-4263.

Efavirenz: As of July 2010, the Antiretroviral Pregnancy Registry has received prospective reports of 792 pregnancies exposed to efavirenz-containing regimens, nearly all of which were first-trimester exposures (718 pregnancies). Birth defects occurred in 17 of 604 live births (first-trimester exposure) and 2 of 69 live births (second/third-trimester exposure). One of these prospectively reported defects with first-trimester exposure was a neural tube defect. A single case of anophthalmia with first-trimester exposure to efavirenz has also been prospectively reported; however, this case included severe oblique facial clefts and amniotic banding, a known association with anophthalmia. There have been six retrospective reports of findings consistent with neural tube defects, including meningomyelocele. All mothers were exposed to efavirenz-containing regimens in the first trimester. Although a causal relationship of these events to the use of efavirenz has not been established, similar defects have been observed in preclinical studies of efavirenz.

Animal Data

Effects of efavirenz on embryo-fetal development have been studied in three nonclinical species (cynomolgus monkeys, rats, and rabbits). In monkeys, efavirenz 60 mg/kg/day was administered to pregnant females throughout pregnancy (gestation Days 20 through 150). The maternal systemic drug exposures (AUC) were 1.3 times the exposure in humans at the recommended clinical dose (600 mg/day), with fetal umbilical venous drug concentrations approximately 0.7 times the maternal values. Three fetuses of 20 fetuses/infants had one or more malformations; there were no malformed fetuses or infants from placebo-treated mothers. The malformations that occurred in these three monkey fetuses included anencephaly and unilateral anophthalmia in one fetus, microophthalmia in a second, and cleft palate in the third. There was no NOAEL (no observable adverse effect level) established for this study because only one dosage was evaluated. In rats, efavirenz was administered either during organogenesis (gestation Days 7 to 18) or from gestation Day 7 through lactation Day 21 at 50, 100, or 200 mg/kg/day. Administration of 200 mg/kg/day in rats was associated with an increase in the incidence of early resorptions, and doses 100 mg/kg/day and greater were associated with early neonatal mortality. The AUC at the NOAEL (50 mg/kg/day) in this rat study was 0.1 times that in humans at the recommended clinical dose. Drug concentrations in the milk on lactation Day 10 were approximately 8 times higher than those in maternal plasma. In pregnant rabbits, efavirenz was neither embryo lethal nor teratogenic when administered at doses of 25, 50, and 75 mg/kg/day over the period of organogenesis (gestation Days 6 through 18). The AUC at the NOAEL (75 mg/kg/day) in rabbits was 0.4 times that in humans at the recommended clinical dose.

8.3 Nursing Mothers

The Centers for Disease Control and Prevention recommend that HIV-1 infected mothers not breastfeed their infants to avoid risking postnatal transmission of HIV-1. Studies in rats have demonstrated that efavirenz is secreted in milk. Studies in humans have shown that both tenofovir and emtricitabine are excreted in human milk. Because the risks of low level exposure to emtricitabine and tenofovir to infants are unknown, and because of the potential for HIV-1 transmission, **mothers should be instructed not to breastfeed if they are receiving ATRIPLA.**

Table 4 *(cont.)* Established and Other Potentially Significant* Drug Interactions: Alteration in Dose or Regimen May Be Recommended Based on Drug Interaction Trials or Predicted Interaction

Concomitant Drug Class: Drug Name	Effect	Clinical Comment
Other agents (cont.)		
Anticonvulsants: carbamazepine phenytoin phenobarbital	↓ carbamazepine ↓ efavirenz ↓ anticonvulsant ↓ efavirenz	There are insufficient data to make a dose recommendation for ATRIPLA. Alternative anticonvulsant treatment should be used. Potential for reduction in anticonvulsant and/or efavirenz plasma levels; periodic monitoring of anticonvulsant plasma levels should be conducted.
Antidepressants: buproprion	↓ buproprion	The effect of efavirenz on bupropion exposure is thought to be due to the induction of bupropion metabolism. Increases in bupropion dosage should be guided by clinical response, but the maximum recommended dose of bupropion should not be exceeded.
sertraline	↓ sertraline	Increases in sertraline dose should be guided by clinical response.
Antifungals: itraconazole ketoconazole posaconazole	↓ itraconazole ↓ hydroxy-itraconazole ↓ ketoconazole ↓ posaconazole	Since no dose recommendation for itraconazole can be made, alternative antifungal treatment should be considered. Drug interaction trials with ATRIPLA and ketoconazole have not been conducted. Efavirenz has the potential to decrease plasma concentrations of ketoconazole. Avoid concomitant use unless the benefit outweighs the risks.
Anti-infective: clarithromycin	↓ clarithromycin ↑ 14-OH metabolite	Clinical significance unknown. In uninfected volunteers, 46% developed rash while receiving efavirenz and clarithromycin. No dose adjustment of ATRIPLA is recommended when given with clarithromycin. Alternatives to clarithromycin, such as azithromycin, should be considered. Other macrolide antibiotics, such as erythromycin, have not been studied in combination with ATRIPLA.
Antimycobacterial: rifabutin	↓ rifabutin	Increase daily dose of rifabutin by 50%. Consider doubling the rifabutin dose in regimens where rifabutin is given 2 or 3 times a week.
rifampin	↓ efavirenz	If ATRIPLA is coadministered with rifampin to patients weighing 50 kg or more, an additional 200 mg/day of efavirenz is recommended.
Calcium channel blockers: diltiazem	↓ diltiazem ↓ desacetyl diltiazem ↓ N-monodes-methyl diltiazem	Diltiazem dose adjustments should be guided by clinical response (refer to the full prescribing information for diltiazem). No dose adjustment of ATRIPLA is necessary when administered with diltiazem.
Others (e.g., felodipine, nicardipine, nifedipine, verapamil)	↓ calcium channel blocker	No data are available on the potential interactions of efavirenz with other calcium channel blockers that are substrates of CYP3A. The potential exists for reduction in plasma concentrations of the calcium channel blocker. Dose adjustments should be guided by clinical response (refer to the full prescribing information for the calcium channel blocker).
HMG-CoA reductase inhibitors: atorvastatin pravastatin simvastatin	↓ atorvastatin ↓ pravastatin ↓ simvastatin	Plasma concentrations of atorvastatin, pravastatin, and simvastatin decreased with efavirenz. Consult the full prescribing information for the HMG-CoA reductase inhibitor for guidance on individualizing the dose.
Hormonal contraceptives: Oral: ethinyl estradiol/norgestimate	↓ active metabolites of norgestimate	A reliable method of barrier contraception must be used in addition to hormonal contraceptives. Efavirenz had no effect on ethinyl estradiol concentrations, but progestin levels (norelgestromin and levonorgestrel) were markedly decreased. No effect of ethinyl estradiol/norgestimate on efavirenz plasma concentrations was observed.
Implant: etonogestrel	↓ etonogestrel	A reliable method of barrier contraception must be used in addition to hormonal contraceptives. The interaction between etonogestrel and efavirenz has not been studied. Decreased exposure of etonogestrel may be expected. There have been postmarketing reports of contraceptive failure with etonogestrel in efavirenz-exposed patients.
Immunosuppressants: cyclosporine, tacrolimus, sirolimus, and others metabolized by CYP3A	↓ immuno-suppressant	Decreased exposure of the immunosuppressant may be expected due to CYP3A induction by efavirenz. These immunosuppressants are not anticipated to affect exposure of efavirenz. Dose adjustments of the immunosuppressant may be required. Close monitoring of immunosuppressant concentrations for at least 2 weeks (until stable concentrations are reached) is recommended when starting or stopping treatment with ATRIPLA.
Narcotic analgesic: methadone	↓ methadone	Coadministration of efavirenz in HIV-1 infected individuals with a history of injection drug use resulted in decreased plasma levels of methadone and signs of opiate withdrawal. Methadone dose was increased by a mean of 22% to alleviate withdrawal symptoms. Patients should be monitored for signs of withdrawal and their methadone dose increased as required to alleviate withdrawal symptoms.

* This table is not all inclusive.

Emtricitabine
Samples of breast milk obtained from five HIV-1 infected mothers show that emtricitabine is secreted in human milk. Breastfeeding infants whose mothers are being treated with emtricitabine may be at risk for developing viral resistance to emtricitabine. Other emtricitabine-associated risks in infants breastfed by mothers being treated with emtricitabine are unknown.

Tenofovir Disoproxil Fumarate
Samples of breast milk obtained from five HIV-1 infected mothers show that tenofovir is secreted in human milk. Tenofovir-associated risks, including the risk of viral resistance to tenofovir, in infants breastfed by mothers being treated with tenofovir disoproxil fumarate are unknown.

8.4 Pediatric Use
ATRIPLA should only be administered to pediatric patients 12 years of age and older with a body weight greater than or equal to 40 kg (greater than or equal to 88 lbs). Because ATRIPLA is a fixed-dose combination tablet, the dose adjustments recommended for pediatric patients younger than 12 years of age for each individual component cannot be made with ATRIPLA [*See Warnings and Precautions (5.9, 5.11), Adverse Reactions (6.1) and Clinical Pharmacology (12.3)*].

8.5 Geriatric Use
Clinical trials of efavirenz, emtricitabine, or tenofovir DF did not include sufficient numbers of subjects aged 65 and over to determine whether they respond differently from younger subjects. In general, dose selection for elderly patients should be cautious, keeping in mind the greater frequency of decreased hepatic, renal, or cardiac function, and of concomitant disease or other drug therapy.

8.6 Hepatic Impairment
ATRIPLA is not recommended for patients with moderate or severe hepatic impairment because there are insufficient data to determine an appropriate dose. Patients with mild hepatic impairment may be treated with ATRIPLA at the approved dose. Because of the extensive cytochrome P450-mediated metabolism of efavirenz and limited clinical experience in patients with hepatic impairment, caution should be exercised in administering ATRIPLA to these patients [*See Warnings and Precautions (5.10) and Clinical Pharmacology (12.3)*].

8.7 Renal Impairment
Because ATRIPLA is a fixed-dose combination, it should not be prescribed for patients requiring dosage adjustment such as those with moderate or severe renal impairment (estimated creatinine clearance below 50 mL/min) [*See Warnings and Precautions (5.7)*].

10 OVERDOSAGE
If overdose occurs, the patient should be monitored for evidence of toxicity, including monitoring of vital signs and observation of the patient's clinical status; standard supportive treatment should then be applied as necessary. Administration of activated charcoal may be used to aid removal of unabsorbed efavirenz. Hemodialysis can remove both emtricitabine and tenofovir DF (refer to detailed information below), but is unlikely to significantly remove efavirenz from the blood.
Efavirenz: Some patients accidentally taking 600 mg twice daily have reported increased nervous system symptoms. One patient experienced involuntary muscle contractions.
Emtricitabine: Limited clinical experience is available at doses higher than the therapeutic dose of emtricitabine. In one clinical pharmacology trial single doses of emtricitabine 1200 mg were administered to 11 subjects. No severe adverse reactions were reported.
Hemodialysis treatment removes approximately 30% of the emtricitabine dose over a 3-hour dialysis period starting within 1.5 hours of emtricitabine dosing (blood flow rate of 400 mL/min and a dialysate flow rate of 600 mL/min). It is not known whether emtricitabine can be removed by peritoneal dialysis.
Tenofovir Disoproxil Fumarate: Limited clinical experience at doses higher than the therapeutic dose of tenofovir DF 300 mg is available. In one trial, 600 mg tenofovir DF was administered to 8 subjects orally for 28 days, and no severe adverse reactions were reported. The effects of higher doses are not known.
Tenofovir is efficiently removed by hemodialysis with an extraction coefficient of approximately 54%. Following a single 300 mg dose of tenofovir DF, a 4-hour hemodialysis session removed approximately 10% of the administered tenofovir dose.

11 DESCRIPTION
ATRIPLA is a fixed-dose combination tablet containing efavirenz, emtricitabine, and tenofovir disoproxil fumarate (tenofovir DF). SUSTIVA is the brand name for efavirenz, a non-nucleoside reverse transcriptase inhibitor. EMTRIVA is the brand name for emtricitabine, a synthetic nucleoside analog of cytidine. VIREAD is the brand name for tenofovir DF, which is converted *in vivo* to tenofovir, an acyclic nucle-

oside phosphonate (nucleotide) analog of adenosine 5'-monophosphate. VIREAD and EMTRIVA are the components of TRUVADA.

ATRIPLA tablets are for oral administration. Each tablet contains 600 mg of efavirenz, 200 mg of emtricitabine, and 300 mg of tenofovir DF (which is equivalent to 245 mg of tenofovir disoproxil) as active ingredients. The tablets include the following inactive ingredients: croscarmellose sodium, hydroxypropyl cellulose, magnesium stearate, microcrystalline cellulose, and sodium lauryl sulfate. The tablets are film-coated with a coating material containing black iron oxide, polyethylene glycol, polyvinyl alcohol, red iron oxide, talc, and titanium dioxide.

Efavirenz: Efavirenz is chemically described as (S)-6-chloro-4-(cyclopropylethynyl)-1,4-dihydro-4-(trifluoromethyl)-2H-3,1-benzoxazin-2-one. Its molecular formula is $C_{14}H_9ClF_3NO_2$ and its structural formula is:

Efavirenz is a white to slightly pink crystalline powder with a molecular mass of 315.68. It is practically insoluble in water (less than 10 µg/mL).

Emtricitabine: The chemical name of emtricitabine is 5-fluoro-1-(2R,5S)-[2-(hydroxymethyl)-1,3-oxathiolan-5-yl]cytosine. Emtricitabine is the (-) enantiomer of a thio analog of cytidine, which differs from other cytidine analogs in that it has a fluorine in the 5-position.

It has a molecular formula of $C_8H_{10}FN_3O_3S$ and a molecular weight of 247.24. It has the following structural formula:

Emtricitabine is a white to off-white crystalline powder with a solubility of approximately 112 mg/mL in water at 25 °C.

Tenofovir Disoproxil Fumarate: Tenofovir DF is a fumaric acid salt of the *bis*-isopropoxycarbonyloxymethyl ester derivative of tenofovir. The chemical name of tenofovir disoproxil fumarate is 9-[(R)-2[[bis[[(isopropoxycarbonyl)oxy]- methoxy]phosphinyl]methoxy]propyl]adenine fumarate (1:1). It has a molecular formula of $C_{19}H_{30}N_5O_{10}P$ • $C_4H_4O_4$ and a molecular weight of 635.52. It has the following structural formula:

Tenofovir DF is a white to off-white crystalline powder with a solubility of 13.4 mg/mL in water at 25 °C.

12   CLINICAL PHARMACOLOGY

For additional information on Mechanism of Action, Antiviral Activity, Resistance and Cross Resistance, please consult the SUSTIVA, EMTRIVA and VIREAD prescribing information.

12.1   Mechanism of Action

ATRIPLA is a fixed-dose combination of antiviral drugs efavirenz, emtricitabine and tenofovir disoproxil fumarate *[See Clinical Pharmacology (12.4)]*.

12.3   Pharmacokinetics

ATRIPLA: One ATRIPLA tablet is bioequivalent to one SUSTIVA tablet (600 mg) plus one EMTRIVA capsule (200 mg) plus one VIREAD tablet (300 mg) following single-dose administration to fasting healthy subjects (N=45).

Efavirenz: In HIV-1 infected subjects time-to-peak plasma concentrations were approximately 3–5 hours and steady-state plasma concentrations were reached in 6–10 days. In 35 HIV-1 infected subjects receiving efavirenz 600 mg once daily, steady-state C_{max} was 12.9 ± 3.7 µM (mean ± SD), C_{min} was 5.6 ± 3.2 µM, and AUC was 184 ± 73 µM•hr. Efavirenz is highly bound (approximately 99.5–99.75%) to human plasma proteins, predominantly albumin. Following administration of ^{14}C-labeled efavirenz, 14–34% of the dose was recovered in the urine (mostly as metabolites) and 16–61% was recovered in feces (mostly as parent drug). *In vitro* studies suggest CYP3A and CYP2B6 are the major isozymes responsible for efavirenz metabolism. Efavirenz has been shown to induce CYP enzymes, resulting in induc-

tion of its own metabolism. Efavirenz has a terminal half-life of 52–76 hours after single doses and 40–55 hours after multiple doses.

Emtricitabine: Following oral administration, emtricitabine is rapidly absorbed, with peak plasma concentrations occurring at 1–2 hours post-dose. Following multiple dose oral administration of emtricitabine to 20 HIV-1 infected subjects, the steady-state plasma emtricitabine C_{max} was 1.8 ± 0.7 µg/mL (mean ± SD) and the AUC over a 24-hour dosing interval was 10.0 ± 3.1 µg•hr/mL. The mean steady-state plasma trough concentration at 24 hours post-dose was 0.09 µg/mL. The mean absolute bioavailability of emtricitabine was 93%. Less than 4% of emtricitabine binds

to human plasma proteins *in vitro* and the binding is independent of concentration over the range of 0.02–200 µg/mL. Following administration of radiolabelled emtricitabine, approximately 86% is recovered in the urine and 13% is recovered as metabolites. The metabolites of emtricitabine include 3'-sulfoxide diastereomers and their glucuronic acid conjugate. Emtricitabine is eliminated by a combination of glomerular filtration and active tubular secretion with a renal clearance in adults with normal renal function of 213 ± 89 mL/min (mean ± SD). Following a single oral dose, the plasma emtricitabine half-life is approximately 10 hours.

Tenofovir Disoproxil Fumarate: Following oral administration of a single 300 mg dose of tenofovir DF to HIV-1 in-

Table 5 Drug Interactions: Changes in Pharmacokinetic Parameters for Efavirenz in the Presence of the Coadministered Drug

Coadministered Drug	Dose of Coadministered Drug (mg)	Efavirenz Dose (mg)	N	Mean % Change of Efavirenz Pharmacokinetic Parameters* (90% CI)		
				C_{max}	AUC	C_{min}
Indinavir	800 mg q8h × 14 days	200 mg qd × 14 days	11	↔	↔	↔
Lopinavir/ ritonavir	400/100 mg q12h × 9 days	600 mg qd × 9 days	11, 12†	↔	↓ 16 (↓ 38 to ↑ 15)	↓ 16 (↓ 42 to ↑ 20)
Nelfinavir	750 mg q8h × 7 days	600 mg qd × 7 days	10	↓ 12 (↓ 32 to ↑ 13)‡	↓ 12 (↓ 35 to ↑ 18)‡	↓ 21 (↓ 53 to ↓ 33)
Ritonavir	500 mg q12h × 8 days	600 mg qd × 10 days	9	↑ 14 (↑ 4 to ↑ 26)	↑ 21 (↑ 10 to ↑ 34)	↑ 25 (↑ 7 to ↑ 46)‡
Saquinavir SGC§	1200 mg q8h × 10 days	600 mg qd × 10 days	13	↓ 13 (↓ 5 to ↓ 20)	↓ 12 (↓ 4 to ↓ 19)	↓ 14 (↓ 2 to ↓ 24)‡
Boceprevir	800 mg tid × 6 days	600 mg qd × 16 days	NA	↑ 11 (↑ 2 to ↑ 20)	↑ 20 (↑ 15 to ↑ 26)	NA
Telaprevir	750 mg q8h × 10 days	600 mg qd × 20 days	21	↓ 16 (↓ 7 to ↓ 24)	↓ 7 (↓ 2 to ↓ 13)	↓ 2 (↓ 6 to ↑ 2)
Telaprevir, coadministered with tenofovir disoproxil fumarate (TDF)	1125 mg q8h × 7 days	600 mg efavirenz/ 300 mg TDF qd × 7 days	15	↓ 24 (↓ 15 to ↓ 32)	↓ 18 (↓ 10 to ↓ 26)	↓ 10 (↓ 19 to ↑ 1)
	1500 mg q12h × 7 days	600 mg efavirenz/ 300 mg TDF qd × 7 days	16	↓ 20 (↓ 14 to ↓ 26)	↓ 15 (↓ 9 to ↓ 21)	↓ 11 (↓ 4 to ↓ 18)
Clarithromycin	500 mg q12h × 7 days	400 mg qd × 7 days	12	↑ 11 (↑ 3 to ↑ 19)	↔	↔
Itraconazole	200 mg q12h × 14 days	600 mg qd × 28 days	16	↔	↔	↔
Rifabutin	300 mg qd × 14 days	600 mg qd × 14 days	11	↔	↔	↓ 12 (↓ 24 to ↑ 1)
Rifampin	600 mg × 7 days	600 mg qd × 7 days	12	↓ 20 (↓ 11 to ↓ 28)	↓ 26 (↓ 15 to ↓ 36)	↓ 32 (↓ 15 to ↓ 46)
Atorvastatin	10 mg qd × 4 days	600 mg qd × 15 days	14	↔	↔	↔
Pravastatin	40 mg qd × 4 days	600 mg qd × 15 days	11	↔	↔	↔
Simvastatin	40 mg qd × 4 days	600 mg qd × 15 days	14	↓ 12 (↓ 28 to ↑ 8)	↔	↓ 12 (↓ 25 to ↑ 3)
Carbamazepine	200 mg qd × 3 days, 200 mg bid × 3 days, then 400 mg qd × 15 days	600 mg qd × 35 days	14	↓ 21 (↓ 15 to ↓ 26)	↓ 36 (↓ 32 to ↓ 40)	↓ 47 (↓ 41 to ↓ 53)
Diltiazem	240 mg × 14 days	600 mg qd × 28 days	12	↑ 16 (↑ 6 to ↑ 26)	↑ 11 (↑ 5 to ↑ 18)	↑ 13 (↑ 1 to ↑ 26)

(Table continued on next page)

fected subjects in the fasted state, maximum serum concentrations (C_{max}) were achieved in 1.0 ± 0.4 hrs (mean $\pm$ SD) and C_{max} and AUC values were 296 ± 90 ng/mL and 2287 ± 685 ng•hr/mL, respectively. The oral bioavailability of tenofovir from tenofovir DF in fasted subjects is approximately 25%. Less than 0.7% of tenofovir binds to human plasma proteins *in vitro* and the binding is independent of concentration over the range of 0.01–25 μg/mL. Approximately 70–80% of the intravenous dose of tenofovir is recovered as unchanged drug in the urine. Tenofovir is eliminated by a combination of glomerular filtration and active tubular secretion with a renal clearance in adults with normal renal function of 243 ± 33 mL/min (mean $\pm$ SD). Following a single oral dose, the terminal elimination half-life of tenofovir is approximately 17 hours.

Effects of Food on Oral Absorption
ATRIPLA has not been evaluated in the presence of food. Administration of efavirenz tablets with a high fat meal increased the mean AUC and C_{max} of efavirenz by 28% and 79%, respectively, compared to administration in the fasted state. Compared to fasted administration, dosing of tenofovir DF and emtricitabine in combination with either a high fat meal or a light meal increased the mean AUC and C_{max} of tenofovir by 35% and 15%, respectively, without affecting emtricitabine exposures *[See Dosage and Administration (2) and Patient Counseling Information (17.7)]*.

Special Populations
Race
Efavirenz: The pharmacokinetics of efavirenz in HIV-1 infected subjects appear to be similar among the racial groups studied.
Emtricitabine: No pharmacokinetic differences due to race have been identified following the administration of emtricitabine.
Tenofovir Disoproxil Fumarate: There were insufficient numbers from racial and ethnic groups other than Caucasian to adequately determine potential pharmacokinetic differences among these populations following the administration of tenofovir DF.
Gender
Efavirenz, Emtricitabine, and Tenofovir Disoproxil Fumarate: Efavirenz, emtricitabine, and tenofovir pharmacokinetics are similar in male and female subjects.
Pediatric Patients
ATRIPLA should only be administered to pediatric patients 12 years of age and weighing greater than or equal to 40 kg (greater than or equal to 88 lb).
Efavirenz: In an open-label trial in NRTI-experienced pediatric subjects (mean age 8 years, range 3–16), the pharmacokinetics of efavirenz in pediatric subjects were similar to the pharmacokinetics in adults who received a 600 mg daily dose of efavirenz. In 48 pediatric subjects, receiving the equivalent of a 600 mg dose of efavirenz, mean ($\pm$ SD) steady-state C_{max} was 14.2 ± 5.8 μM, steady-state C_{min} was 5.6 ± 4.1 μM, and AUC was 218 ± 104 μM•hr.
Emtricitabine: The pharmacokinetics of emtricitabine at steady state were determined in 27 HIV-1-infected pediatric subjects 13 to 17 years of age receiving a daily dose of 6 mg/kg up to a maximum of 240 mg oral solution or a 200 mg capsule; 26 of 27 subjects in this age group received the 200 mg EMTRIVA capsule. Mean ($\pm$ SD) C_{max} and AUC were 2.7 ± 0.9 μg/mL and 12.6 ± 5.4 μg•hr/mL, respectively. Exposures achieved in pediatric subjects 12 to less than 18 years of age were similar to those achieved in adults receiving a once daily dose of 200 mg.
Tenofovir Disoproxil Fumarate: Steady-state pharmacokinetics of tenofovir were evaluated in 8 HIV-1 infected pediatric subjects (12 to less than 18 years). Mean ($\pm$ SD) C_{max} and AUC_{tau} were 0.38 ± 0.13 μg/mL and 3.39 ± 1.22 μg•hr/mL, respectively. Tenofovir exposure achieved in these pediatric subjects receiving oral daily doses of VIREAD 300 mg was similar to exposures achieved in adults receiving once-daily doses of VIREAD 300 mg.
Geriatric Patients
Pharmacokinetics of efavirenz, emtricitabine and tenofovir have not been fully evaluated in the elderly (65 years of age and older) *[See Use in Specific Populations (8.5)]*.
Patients with Impaired Renal Function
Efavirenz: The pharmacokinetics of efavirenz have not been studied in subjects with renal insufficiency; however, less than 1% of efavirenz is excreted unchanged in the urine, so the impact of renal impairment on efavirenz elimination should be minimal.
Emtricitabine and Tenofovir Disoproxil Fumarate: The pharmacokinetics of emtricitabine and tenofovir DF are altered in subjects with renal impairment. In subjects with creatinine clearance below 50 mL/min, C_{max} and $AUC_{0-\infty}$ of emtricitabine and tenofovir were increased *[See Warnings and Precautions (5.7)]*.
Patients with Hepatic Impairment
Efavirenz: A multiple-dose trial showed no significant effect on efavirenz pharmacokinetics in subjects with mild hepatic impairment (Child-Pugh Class A) compared with controls. There were insufficient data to determine whether

Table 5 (cont.) Drug Interactions: Changes in Pharmacokinetic Parameters for Efavirenz in the Presence of the Coadministered Drug

Coadministered Drug	Dose of Coadministered Drug (mg)	Efavirenz Dose (mg)	N	Mean % Change of Efavirenz Pharmacokinetic Parameters* (90% CI)		
				C_{max}	AUC	C_{min}
Sertraline	50 mg qd × 14 days	600 mg qd × 14 days	13	↑ 11 (↑ 6 to ↑ 16)	↔	↔
Voriconazole	400 mg po q12h × 1 day then 200 mg po q12h × 8 days	400 mg qd × 9 days	NA	↑ 38¶	↑ 44¶	NA
	300 mg po q12h days 2–7	300 mg qd × 7 days	NA	↓ 14# (↓ 7 to ↓ 21)	↔#	NA
	400 mg po q12h days 2–7	300 mg qd × 7 days	NA	↔#	↑ 17# (↑ 6 to ↑ 29)	NA

NA = not available
* Increase = ↑; Decrease = ↓; No Effect = ↔
† Parallel-group design; N for efavirenz + lopinavir/ritonavir, N for efavirenz alone.
‡ 95% CI
§ Soft Gelatin Capsule
¶ 90% CI not available
# Relative to steady-state administration of efavirenz (600 mg once daily for 9 days).

moderate or severe hepatic impairment (Child-Pugh Class B or C) affects efavirenz pharmacokinetics *[See Warnings and Precautions (5.10) and Use in Specific Populations (8.6)]*.
Emtricitabine: The pharmacokinetics of emtricitabine have not been studied in subjects with hepatic impairment; however, emtricitabine is not significantly metabolized by liver enzymes, so the impact of liver impairment should be limited.
Tenofovir Disoproxil Fumarate: The pharmacokinetics of tenofovir following a 300 mg dose of tenofovir DF have been studied in non-HIV infected subjects with moderate to severe hepatic impairment. There were no substantial alterations in tenofovir pharmacokinetics in subjects with hepatic impairment compared with unimpaired subjects.
Assessment of Drug Interactions
The drug interaction trials described were conducted with efavirenz, emtricitabine, or tenofovir DF as individual agents; no drug interaction trials have been conducted using ATRIPLA.
Efavirenz: The steady-state pharmacokinetics of efavirenz and tenofovir were unaffected when efavirenz and tenofovir DF were administered together versus each agent dosed alone. Specific drug interaction trials have not been performed with efavirenz and NRTIs other than tenofovir, lamivudine, and zidovudine. Clinically significant interactions would not be expected based on NRTIs elimination pathways.
Efavirenz has been shown *in vivo* to cause hepatic enzyme induction, thus increasing the biotransformation of some drugs metabolized by CYP3A and CYP2B6. *In vitro* studies have shown that efavirenz inhibited CYP isozymes 2C9, 2C19, and 3A4 with K_i values (8.5–17 μM) in the range of observed efavirenz plasma concentrations. In *in vitro* studies, efavirenz did not inhibit CYP2E1 and inhibited CYP2D6 and CYP1A2 (K_i values 82–160 μM) only at concentrations well above those achieved clinically. Coadministration of efavirenz with drugs primarily metabolized by 2C9, 2C19, and 3A4 isozymes may result in altered plasma concentrations of the coadministered drug. Drugs which induce CYP3A activity would be expected to increase the clearance of efavirenz resulting in lowered plasma concentrations.
Drug interaction trials were performed with efavirenz and other drugs likely to be coadministered or drugs commonly used as probes for pharmacokinetic interaction. There was no clinically significant interaction observed between efavirenz and zidovudine, lamivudine, azithromycin, fluconazole, lorazepam, cetirizine, or paroxetine. Single doses of famotidine or an aluminum and magnesium antacid with simethicone had no effects on efavirenz exposures. The effects of coadministration of efavirenz on C_{max}, AUC, and C_{min} are summarized in Table 5 (effect of other drugs on efavirenz) and Table 6 (effect of efavirenz on other drugs). For information regarding clinical recommendations see *Drug Interactions (7)*.
[See table 5 on previous page and above]
[See table 6 on pages 764 through 766]

Emtricitabine and Tenofovir Disoproxil Fumarate: The steady-state pharmacokinetics of emtricitabine and tenofovir were unaffected when emtricitabine and tenofovir DF were administered together versus each agent dosed alone.
In vitro and clinical pharmacologic drug-drug interaction studies have shown that the potential for CYP mediated interactions involving emtricitabine and tenofovir with other medicinal products is low.
Emtricitabine and tenofovir are primarily excreted by the kidneys by a combination of glomerular filtration and active tubular secretion. No drug-drug interactions due to competition for renal excretion have been observed; however, coadministration of emtricitabine and tenofovir DF with drugs that are eliminated by active tubular secretion may increase concentrations of emtricitabine, tenofovir, and/or the coadministered drug.
Drugs that decrease renal function may increase concentrations of emtricitabine and/or tenofovir.
No clinically significant drug interactions have been observed between emtricitabine and famciclovir, indinavir, stavudine, tenofovir DF and zidovudine. Similarly, no clinically significant drug interactions have been observed between tenofovir DF and abacavir, efavirenz, emtricitabine, entecavir, indinavir, lamivudine, lopinavir/ritonavir, methadone, nelfinavir, oral contraceptives, ribavirin, saquinavir/ritonavir or tacrolimus in trials conducted in healthy volunteers.
Following multiple dosing to HIV-negative subjects receiving either chronic methadone maintenance therapy, oral contraceptives, or single doses of ribavirin, steady-state tenofovir pharmacokinetics were similar to those observed in previous trials, indicating a lack of clinically significant drug interactions between these agents and tenofovir DF. The effects of coadministered drugs on the C_{max}, AUC, and C_{min} of tenofovir are shown in Table 7. The effects of coadministration of tenofovir DF on C_{max}, AUC, and C_{min} of coadministered drugs are shown in Table 8.
[See table 7 at top of page 766]
[See table 8 at top of page 767]
Coadministration of tenofovir DF with didanosine results in changes in the pharmacokinetics of didanosine that may be of clinical significance. Concomitant dosing of tenofovir DF with didanosine enteric-coated capsules significantly increases the C_{max} and AUC of didanosine. When didanosine 250 mg enteric-coated capsules were administered with tenofovir DF, systemic exposures of didanosine were similar to those seen with the 400 mg enteric-coated capsules alone under fasted conditions. The mechanism of this interaction is unknown [for didanosine dosing adjustment recommendations see *Drug Interactions (7.3)*; Table 4].

12.4   Microbiology
Mechanism of Action
Efavirenz: Efavirenz is a non-nucleoside reverse transcriptase (RT) inhibitor of HIV-1. Efavirenz activity is mediated predominantly by noncompetitive inhibition of HIV-1 reverse transcriptase (RT). HIV-2 RT and human cellular DNA polymerases α, β, γ, and σ are not inhibited by efavirenz.

Emtricitabine: Emtricitabine, a synthetic nucleoside analog of cytidine, is phosphorylated by cellular enzymes to form emtricitabine 5'-triphosphate. Emtricitabine 5'-triphosphate inhibits the activity of the HIV-1 RT by competing with the natural substrate deoxycytidine 5'-triphosphate and by being incorporated into nascent viral DNA which results in chain termination. Emtricitabine 5'-triphosphate is a weak inhibitor of mammalian DNA polymerase α, β, ϵ, and mitochondrial DNA polymerase γ.

Tenofovir Disoproxil Fumarate: Tenofovir DF is an acyclic nucleoside phosphonate diester analog of adenosine monophosphate. Tenofovir DF requires initial diester hydrolysis for conversion to tenofovir and subsequent phosphorylations by cellular enzymes to form tenofovir diphosphate. Tenofovir diphosphate inhibits the activity of HIV-1 RT by competing with the natural substrate deoxyadenosine 5'-triphosphate and, after incorporation into DNA, by DNA chain termination. Tenofovir diphosphate is a weak inhibitor of mammalian DNA polymerases α, β, and mitochondrial DNA polymerase γ.

Antiviral Activity

Efavirenz, Emtricitabine, and Tenofovir Disoproxil Fumarate: In combination studies evaluating the antiviral activity in cell culture of emtricitabine and efavirenz together, efavirenz and tenofovir together, and emtricitabine and tenofovir together, additive to synergistic antiviral effects were observed.

Efavirenz: The concentration of efavirenz inhibiting replication of wild-type laboratory adapted strains and clinical isolates in cell culture by 90–95% (EC_{90-95}) ranged from 1.7–25 nM in lymphoblastoid cell lines, peripheral blood mononuclear cells, and macrophage/monocyte cultures. Efavirenz demonstrated additive antiviral activity against HIV-1 in cell culture when combined with non-nucleoside reverse transcriptase inhibitors (NNRTIs) (delavirdine and nevirapine), nucleoside reverse transcriptase inhibitors (NRTIs) (abacavir, didanosine, lamivudine, stavudine, zalcitabine, and zidovudine), protease inhibitors (PIs) (amprenavir, indinavir, lopinavir, nelfinavir, ritonavir, and saquinavir), and the fusion inhibitor enfuvirtide. Efavirenz demonstrated additive to antagonistic antiviral activity in cell culture with atazanavir. Efavirenz demonstrated antiviral activity against clade B and most non-clade B isolates (subtypes A, AE, AG, C, D, F, G, J, and N), but had reduced antiviral activity against group O viruses. Efavirenz is not active against HIV-2.

Emtricitabine: The antiviral activity in cell culture of emtricitabine against laboratory and clinical isolates of HIV-1 was assessed in lymphoblastoid cell lines, the MAGI-CCR5 cell line, and peripheral blood mononuclear cells. The 50% effective concentration (EC_{50}) values for emtricitabine were in the range of 0.0013–0.64 μM (0.0003–0.158 μg/mL). In drug combination studies of emtricitabine with NRTIs (abacavir, lamivudine, stavudine, zalcitabine, and zidovudine), NNRTIs (delavirdine, efavirenz, and nevirapine), and PIs (amprenavir, nelfinavir, ritonavir, and saquinavir), additive to synergistic effects were observed. Emtricitabine displayed antiviral activity in cell culture against HIV-1 clades A, B, C, D, E, F, and G (EC_{50} values ranged from 0.007–0.075 μM) and showed strain specific activity against HIV-2 (EC_{50} values ranged from 0.007–1.5 μM).

Tenofovir Disoproxil Fumarate: The antiviral activity in cell culture of tenofovir against laboratory and clinical isolates of HIV-1 was assessed in lymphoblastoid cell lines, primary monocyte/macrophage cells and peripheral blood lymphocytes. The EC_{50} values for tenofovir were in the range of 0.04–8.5 μM. In drug combination studies of tenofovir with NRTIs (abacavir, didanosine, lamivudine, stavudine, zalcitabine, and zidovudine), NNRTIs (delavirdine, efavirenz, and nevirapine), and PIs (amprenavir, indinavir, nelfinavir, ritonavir, and saquinavir), additive to synergistic effects were observed. Tenofovir displayed antiviral activity in cell culture against HIV-1 clades A, B, C, D, E, F, G and O (EC_{50} values ranged from 0.5–2.2 μM) and showed strain specific activity against HIV-2 (EC_{50} values ranged from 1.6 μM–5.5 μM).

Resistance

Efavirenz, Emtricitabine, and Tenofovir Disoproxil Fumarate: HIV-1 isolates with reduced susceptibility to the combination of emtricitabine and tenofovir have been selected in cell culture and in clinical trials. Genotypic analysis of these isolates identified the M184V/I and/or K65R amino acid substitutions in the viral RT.

In a clinical trial of treatment-naive subjects *[Study 934, see Clinical Studies (14)]* resistance analysis was performed on HIV-1 isolates from all confirmed virologic failure subjects with greater than 400 copies/mL of HIV-1 RNA at Week 144 or early discontinuations. Genotypic resistance to efavirenz, predominantly the K103N substitution, was the most common form of resistance that developed. Resistance to efavirenz occurred in 13/19 analyzed subjects in the emtricitabine + tenofovir DF group and in 21/29 analyzed subjects in the zidovudine/lamivudine fixed-dose combina-

tion group. The M184V amino acid substitution, associated with resistance to emtricitabine and lamivudine, was observed in 2/19 analyzed subject isolates in the emtricitabine + tenofovir DF group and in 10/29 analyzed subject isolates

Table 6 Drug Interactions: Changes in Pharmacokinetic Parameters for Coadministered Drug in the Presence of Efavirenz

Coadministered Drug	Dose of Coadministered Drug (mg)	Efavirenz Dose (mg)	N	Mean % Change of Coadministered Drug Pharmacokinetic Parameters* (90% CI)		
				C_{max}	AUC	C_{min}
Atazanavir	400 mg qd with a light meal d 1–20	600 mg qd with a light meal d 7–20	27	↓ 59 (↓ 49 to ↓ 67)	↓ 74 (↓ 68 to ↓ 78)	↓ 93 (↓ 90 to ↓ 95)
	400 mg qd d 1–6, then 300 mg qd d 7–20 with ritonavir 100 mg qd and a light meal	600 mg qd 2 h after atazanavir and ritonavir d 7–20	13	↑ 14[†] (↓ 17 to ↑ 58)	↑ 39[†] (↑ 2 to ↑ 88)	↑ 48[†] (↑ 24 to ↑ 76)
	300 mg qd/ritonavir 100 mg qd d 1–10 (pm), then 400 mg qd/ritonavir 100 mg qd d 11–24 (pm) (simultaneous with efavirenz)	600 mg qd with a light snack d 11–24 (pm)	14	↑ 17 (↑ 8 to ↑ 27)	↔	↓ 42 (↓ 31 to ↓ 51)
Indinavir	1000 mg q8h × 10 days	600 mg qd × 10 days	20			
	After morning dose			↔[‡]	↓ 33[‡] (↓ 26 to ↓ 39)	↓ 39[‡] (↓ 24 to ↓ 51)
	After afternoon dose			↔[‡]	↓ 37[‡] (↓ 26 to ↓ 46)	↓ 52[‡] (↓ 47 to ↓ 57)
	After evening dose			↓ 29[‡] (↓ 11 to ↓ 43)	↓ 46[‡] (↓ 37 to ↓ 54)	↓ 57[‡] (↓ 50 to ↓ 63)
Lopinavir/ritonavir	400/100 mg q12h × 9 days	600 mg qd × 9 days	11, 7[§]	↔[¶]	↓ 19[¶] (↓ 36 to ↑ 3)	↓ 39[¶] (↓ 3 to ↓ 62)
Nelfinavir	750 mg q8h × 7 days	600 mg qd × 7 days	10	↑ 21 (↑ 10 to ↑ 33)	↑ 20 (↑ 8 to ↑ 34)	↔
Metabolite AG-1402				↓ 40 (↓ 30 to ↓ 48)	↓ 37 (↓ 25 to ↓ 48)	↓ 43 (↓ 21 to ↓ 59)
Ritonavir	500 mg q12h × 8 days	600 mg qd × 10 days	11			
	After AM dose			↑ 24 (↑ 12 to ↑ 38)	↑ 18 (↑ 6 to ↑ 33)	↑ 42 (↑ 9 to ↑ 86)[#]
	After PM dose			↔	↔	↑ 24 (↑ 3 to ↑ 50)[#]
Saquinavir SGC[b]	1200 mg q8h × 10 days	600 mg qd × 10 days	12	↓ 50 (↓ 28 to ↓ 66)	↓ 62 (↓ 45 to ↓ 74)	↓ 56 (↓ 16 to ↓ 77)[#]
Maraviroc	100 mg bid	600 mg qd	12	↓ 51 (↓ 37 to ↓ 62)	↓ 45 (↓ 38 to ↓ 51)	↓ 45 (↓ 28 to ↓ 57)
Raltegravir	400 mg single dose	600 mg qd	9	↓ 36 (↓ 2 to ↓ 59)	↓ 36 (↓ 20 to ↓ 48)	↓ 21 (↓ 51 to ↑ 28)
Boceprevir	800 mg tid × 6 days	600 mg qd × 16 days	NA	↓ 8 (↓ 22 to ↑ 8)	↓ 19 (↓ 11 to ↓ 25)	↓ 44 (↓ 26 to ↓ 58)
Telaprevir	750 mg q8h × 10 days	600 mg qd × 20 days	21	↓ 9 (↓18 to ↑ 2)	↓ 26 (↓16 to ↓ 35)	↓ 47 (↓ 35 to ↓ 56)
Clarithromycin	500 mg q12h × 7 days	400 mg qd × 7 days	11	↓ 26 (↓ 15 to ↓ 35)	↓ 39 (↓ 30 to ↓ 46)	↓ 53 (↓ 42 to ↓ 63)
14-OH metabolite				↑ 49 (↑ 32 to ↑ 69)	↑ 34 (↑ 18 to ↑ 53)	↑ 26 (↑ 9 to ↑ 45)

(Table continued on next page)

in the zidovudine/lamivudine group. Through 144 weeks of Study 934, no subjects developed a detectable K65R substitution in their HIV-1 as analyzed through standard genotypic analysis.

In a clinical trial of treatment-naive subjects, isolates from 8/47 (17%) analyzed subjects receiving tenofovir DF developed the K65R substitution through 144 weeks of therapy; 7 of these occurred in the first 48 weeks of treatment and one at Week 96. In treatment experienced subjects, 14/304 (5%) of tenofovir DF treated subjects with virologic failure through Week 96 showed greater than 1.4-fold (median 2.7) reduced susceptibility to tenofovir. Genotypic analysis of the resistant isolates showed a substitution in the HIV-1 RT gene resulting in the K65R amino acid substitution.

Efavirenz: Clinical isolates with reduced susceptibility in cell culture to efavirenz have been obtained. The most frequently observed amino acid substitution in clinical trials with efavirenz is K103N (54%). One or more RT substitutions at amino acid positions 98, 100, 101, 103, 106, 108, 188, 190, 225, 227, and 230 were observed in subjects failing treatment with efavirenz in combination with other antiretrovirals. Other resistance substitutions observed to emerge commonly included L100I (7%), K101E/Q/R (14%), V108I (11%), G190S/T/A (7%), P225H (18%), and M230I/L (11%). HIV-1 isolates with reduced susceptibility to efavirenz (greater than 380-fold increase in EC_{90} value) emerged rapidly under selection in cell culture. Genotypic characterization of these viruses identified substitutions resulting in single amino acid substitutions L100I or V179D, double substitutions L100I/V108I, and triple substitutions L100I/V179D/Y181C in RT.

Emtricitabine: Emtricitabine-resistant isolates of HIV-1 have been selected in cell culture and in clinical trials. Genotypic analysis of these isolates showed that the reduced susceptibility to emtricitabine was associated with a substitution in the HIV-1 RT gene at codon 184 which resulted in an amino acid substitution of methionine by valine or isoleucine (M184V/I).

Tenofovir Disoproxil Fumarate: HIV-1 isolates with reduced susceptibility to tenofovir have been selected in cell culture. These viruses expressed a K65R substitution in RT and showed a 2- to 4-fold reduction in susceptibility to tenofovir.

Cross Resistance

Efavirenz, Emtricitabine, and Tenofovir Disoproxil Fumarate: Cross-resistance has been recognized among NNRTIs. Cross resistance has also been recognized among certain NRTIs. The M184V/I and/or K65R substitutions selected in cell culture by the combination of emtricitabine and tenofovir are also observed in some HIV-1 isolates from subjects failing treatment with tenofovir in combination with either lamivudine or emtricitabine, and either abacavir or didanosine. Therefore, cross-resistance among these drugs may occur in patients whose virus harbors either or both of these amino acid substitutions.

Efavirenz: Clinical isolates previously characterized as efavirenz-resistant were also phenotypically resistant in cell culture to delavirdine and nevirapine compared to baseline. Delavirdine- and/or nevirapine-resistant clinical viral isolates with NNRTI resistance-associated substitutions (A98G, L100I, K101E/P, K103N/S, V106A, Y181X, Y188X, G190X, P225H, F227L, or M230L) showed reduced susceptibility to efavirenz in cell culture. Greater than 90% of NRTI-resistant isolates tested in cell culture retained susceptibility to efavirenz.

Emtricitabine: Emtricitabine-resistant isolates (M184V/I) were cross-resistant to lamivudine and zalcitabine but retained susceptibility in cell culture to didanosine, stavudine, tenofovir, zidovudine, and NNRTIs (delavirdine, efavirenz, and nevirapine). HIV-1 isolates containing the K65R substitution, selected *in vivo* by abacavir, didanosine, tenofovir, and zalcitabine, demonstrated reduced susceptibility to inhibition by emtricitabine. Viruses harboring substitutions conferring reduced susceptibility to stavudine and zidovudine (M41L, D67N, K70R, L210W, T215Y/F, and K219Q/E) or didanosine (L74V) remained sensitive to emtricitabine.

Tenofovir Disoproxil Fumarate: The K65R substitution selected by tenofovir is also selected in some HIV-1 infected patients treated with abacavir, didanosine, or zalcitabine. HIV-1 isolates with the K65R substitution also showed reduced susceptibility to emtricitabine and lamivudine. Therefore, cross-resistance among these drugs may occur in patients whose virus harbors the K65R substitution. HIV-1 isolates from subjects (N=20) whose HIV-1 expressed a mean of 3 zidovudine-associated RT amino acid substitutions (M41L, D67N, K70R, L210W, T215Y/F, or K219Q/E/N) showed a 3.1-fold decrease in the susceptibility to tenofovir. Subjects whose virus expressed an L74V substitution without zidovudine resistance associated substitutions (N=8) had reduced response to VIREAD. Limited data are available for patients whose virus expressed a Y115F substitution (N=3), Q151M substitution (N=2), or T69 insertion (N=4), all of whom had a reduced response.

Table 6 *(cont.)* Drug Interactions: Changes in Pharmacokinetic Parameters for Coadministered Drug in the Presence of Efavirenz

Coadministered Drug	Dose of Coadministered Drug (mg)	Efavirenz Dose (mg)	N	C_{max}	AUC	C_{min}
				Mean % Change of Coadministered Drug Pharmacokinetic Parameters* (90% CI)		
Itraconazole	200 mg q12h × 28 days	600 mg qd × 14 days	18	↓ 37 (↓ 20 to ↓ 51)	↓ 39 (↓ 21 to ↓ 53)	↓ 44 (↓ 27 to ↓ 58)
Hydroxy-itraconazole				↓ 35 (↓ 12 to ↓ 52)	↓ 37 (↓ 14 to ↓ 55)	↓ 43 (↓ 18 to ↓ 60)
Posaconazole	400 mg (oral suspension) bid × 10 and 20 days	400 mg qd × 10 and 20 days	11	↓ 45 (↓ 34 to ↓ 53)	↓ 50 (↓ 40 to ↓ 57)	NA
Rifabutin	300 mg qd × 14 days	600 mg qd × 14 days	9	↓ 32 (↓ 15 to ↓ 46)	↓ 38 (↓ 28 to ↓ 47)	↓ 45 (↓ 31 to ↓ 56)
Atorvastatin	10 mg qd × 4 days	600 mg qd × 15 days	14	↓ 14 (↓ 1 to ↓ 26)	↓ 43 (↓ 34 to ↓ 50)	↓ 69 (↓ 49 to ↓ 81)
Total active (including metabolites)				↓ 15 (↓ 2 to ↓ 26)	↓ 32 (↓ 21 to ↓ 41)	↓ 48 (↓ 23 to ↓ 64)
Pravastatin	40 mg qd × 4 days	600 mg qd × 15 days	13	↓ 32 (↓ 59 to ↑ 12)	↓ 44 (↓ 26 to ↓ 57)	↓ 19 (↓ 0 to ↓ 35)
Simvastatin	40 mg qd × 4 days	600 mg qd × 15 days	14	↓ 72 (↓ 63 to ↓ 79)	↓ 68 (↓ 62 to ↓ 73)	↓ 45 (↓ 20 to ↓ 62)
Total active (including metabolites)				↓ 68 (↓ 55 to ↓ 78)	↓ 60 (↓ 52 to ↓ 68)	NAᵝ
Carbamazepine	200 mg qd × 3 days, 200 mg bid × 3 days, then 400 mg qd × 29 days	600 mg qd × 14 days	12	↓ 20 (↓ 15 to ↓ 24)	↓ 27 (↓ 20 to ↓ 33)	↓ 35 (↓ 24 to ↓ 44)
Epoxide metabolite				↔	↔	↓ 13 (↓ 30 to ↑ 7)
Diltiazem	240 mg × 21 days	600 mg qd × 14 days	13	↓ 60 (↓ 50 to ↓ 68)	↓ 69 (↓ 55 to ↓ 79)	↓ 63 (↓ 44 to ↓ 75)
Desacetyl diltiazem				↓ 64 (↓ 57 to ↓ 69)	↓ 75 (↓ 59 to ↓ 84)	↓ 62 (↓ 44 to ↓ 75)
N-monodesmethyl diltiazem				↓ 28 (↓ 7 to ↓ 44)	↓ 37 (↓ 17 to ↓ 52)	↓ 37 (↓ 17 to ↓ 52)
Ethinyl estradiol/ Norgestimate	0.035 mg/0.25 mg × 14 days	600 mg qd × 14 days				
Ethinyl estradiol			21	↔	↔	↔
Norelgestromin			21	↓ 46 (↓39 to ↓ 52)	↓ 64 (↓ 62 to ↓ 67)	↓ 82 (↓ 79 to ↓ 85)
Levonorgestrel			6	↓ 80 (↓77 to ↓ 83)	↓ 83 (↓79 to ↓ 87)	↓ 86 (↓80 to ↓ 90)
Methadone	Stable maintenance 35–100 mg daily	600 mg qd × 14–21 days	11	↓ 45 (↓ 25 to ↓ 59)	↓ 52 (↓ 33 to ↓ 66)	NA

(Table continued on next page)

13 NONCLINICAL TOXICOLOGY

13.1 Carcinogenesis, Mutagenesis, Impairment of Fertility

Efavirenz: Long-term carcinogenicity studies in mice and rats were carried out with efavirenz. Mice were dosed with 0, 25, 75, 150, or 300 mg/kg/day for 2 years. Incidences of hepatocellular adenomas and carcinomas and pulmonary alveolar/bronchiolar adenomas were increased above background in females. No increases in tumor incidence above background were seen in males. In studies in which rats were administered efavirenz at doses of 0, 25, 50, or 100 mg/kg/day for 2 years, no increases in tumor incidence above background were observed. The systemic exposure (based on AUCs) in mice was approximately 1.7-fold that in humans receiving the 600-mg/day dose. The exposure in rats was lower than that in humans. The mechanism of the carcinogenic potential is unknown. However, in genetic toxicology assays, efavirenz showed no evidence of mutagenic or clastogenic activity in a battery of *in vitro* and *in vivo* studies. These included bacterial mutation assays in *S. typhimurium* and *E. coli*, mammalian mutation assays in Chinese hamster ovary cells, chromosome aberration assays in human peripheral blood lymphocytes or Chinese hamster ovary cells, and an *in vivo* mouse bone marrow micronu-

Table 6 (cont.) Drug Interactions: Changes in Pharmacokinetic Parameters for Coadministered Drug in the Presence of Efavirenz

Coadministered Drug	Dose of Coadministered Drug (mg)	Efavirenz Dose (mg)	N	C_max	AUC	C_min
Bupropion	150 mg single dose (sustained-release)	600 mg qd × 14 days	13	↓ 34 (↓21 to ↓47)	↓ 55 (↓48 to ↓62)	NA
Hydroxybupropion				↑ 50 (↑ 20 to ↑ 80)	↔	NA
Sertraline	50 mg qd × 14 days	600 mg qd × 14 days	13	↓ 29 (↓ 15 to ↓ 40)	↓ 39 (↓ 27 to ↓ 50)	↓ 46 (↓ 31 to ↓ 58)
Voriconazole	400 mg po q12h × 1 day then 200 mg po q12h × 8 days	400 mg qd × 9 days	NA	↓ 61[a]	↓ 77[a]	NA
	300 mg po q12h days 2–7	300 mg qd × 7 days	NA	↓ 36[e] (↓ 21 to ↓ 49)	↓ 55[e] (↓ 45 to ↓ 62)	NA
	400 mg po q12h days 2–7	300 mg qd × 7 days	NA	↑ 23[e] (↓ 1 to ↑ 53)	↓ 7[e] (↓ 23 to ↑ 13)	NA

NA = not available
* Increase = ↑; Decrease = ↓; No Effect = ↔
† Compared with atazanavir 400 mg qd alone.
‡ Comparator dose of indinavir was 800 mg q8h × 10 days.
§ Parallel-group design; N for efavirenz + lopinavir/ritonavir, N for lopinavir/ritonavir alone.
¶ Values are for lopinavir. The pharmacokinetics of ritonavir 100 mg q12h are unaffected by concurrent efavirenz.
# 95% CI
Þ Soft Gelatin Capsule
ß Not available because of insufficient data.
à 90% CI not available
è Relative to steady-state administration of voriconazole (400 mg for 1 day, then 200 mg po q12h for 2 days).

Table 7 Drug Interactions: Changes in Pharmacokinetic Parameters for Tenofovir in the Presence of the Coadministered Drug*,†

Coadministered Drug	Dose of Coadministered Drug (mg)	N	C_max	AUC	C_min
Atazanavir[§]	400 once daily × 14 days	33	↑ 14 (↑ 8 to ↑ 20)	↑ 24 (↑ 21 to ↑ 28)	↑ 22 (↑ 15 to ↑ 30)
Atazanavir/ ritonavir[§]	300/100 once daily	12	↑ 34 (↑ 20 to ↑ 51)	↑ 37 (↑ 30 to ↑ 45)	↑ 29 (↑ 21 to ↑ 36)
Darunavir/ ritonavir[¶]	300/100 twice daily	12	↑ 24 (↑ 8 to ↑ 42)	↑ 22 (↑ 10 to ↑ 35)	↑ 37 (↑ 19 to ↑ 57)
Didanosine[#]	250 or 400 once daily × 7 days	14	↔	↔	↔
Lopinavir/ ritonavir	400/100 twice daily × 14 days	24	↔	↑ 32 (↑ 25 to ↑ 38)	↑ 51 (↑ 37 to ↑ 66)
Tipranavir/ ritonavir[Þ]	500/100 twice daily	22	↓ 23 (↓ 32 to ↓ 13)	↓ 2 (↓ 9 to ↑ 5)	↑ 7 (↓ 2 to ↑ 17)
	750/200 twice daily (23 doses)	20	↓ 38 (↓ 46 to ↓ 29)	↑ 2 (↓ 6 to ↑ 10)	↑ 14 (↑ 1 to ↑ 27)

* All interaction trials conducted in healthy volunteers.
† Subjects received tenofovir DF 300 mg once daily.
‡ Increase = ↑; Decrease = ↓; No Effect = ↔
§ Reyataz Prescribing Information.
¶ Prezista Prescribing Information.
# Subjects received didanosine buffered tablets.
Þ Aptivus Prescribing Information.

cleus assay. Given the lack of genotoxic activity of efavirenz, the relevance to humans of neoplasms in efavirenz-treated mice is not known. Efavirenz did not impair mating or fertility of male or female rats, and did not affect sperm of treated male rats. The reproductive performance of offspring born to female rats given efavirenz was not affected. As a result of the rapid clearance of efavirenz in rats, systemic drug exposures

achieved in these studies were equivalent to or below those achieved in humans given therapeutic doses of efavirenz.
Emtricitabine: In long-term carcinogenicity studies of emtricitabine, no drug-related increases in tumor incidence were found in mice at doses up to 750 mg/kg/day (26 times the human systemic exposure at the therapeutic dose of 200 mg/day) or in rats at doses up to 600 mg/day (31 times the human systemic exposure at the therapeutic dose).

Emtricitabine was not genotoxic in the reverse mutation bacterial test (Ames test), mouse lymphoma or mouse micronucleus assays.

Emtricitabine did not affect fertility in male rats at approximately 140-fold or in male and female mice at approximately 60-fold higher exposures (AUC) than in humans given the recommended 200 mg daily dose. Fertility was normal in the offspring of mice exposed daily from before birth *(in utero)* through sexual maturity at daily exposures (AUC) of approximately 60-fold higher than human exposures at the recommended 200 mg daily dose.

Tenofovir Disoproxil Fumarate: Long-term oral carcinogenicity studies of tenofovir DF in mice and rats were carried out at exposures up to approximately 16 times (mice) and 5 times (rats) those observed in humans at the therapeutic dose for HIV-1 infection. At the high dose in female mice, liver adenomas were increased at exposures 16 times that in humans. In rats, the study was negative for carcinogenic findings at exposures up to 5 times that observed in humans at the therapeutic dose.

Tenofovir DF was mutagenic in the *in vitro* mouse lymphoma assay and negative in an in vitro bacterial mutagenicity test (Ames test). In an *in vivo* mouse micronucleus assay, tenofovir DF was negative when administered to male mice.

There were no effects on fertility, mating performance or early embryonic development when tenofovir DF was administered to male rats at a dose equivalent to 10 times the human dose based on body surface area comparisons for 28 days prior to mating and to female rats for 15 days prior to mating through Day seven of gestation. There was, however, an alteration of the estrous cycle in female rats.

13.2 Animal Toxicology and/or Pharmacology

Efavirenz: Nonsustained convulsions were observed in 6 of 20 monkeys receiving efavirenz at doses yielding plasma AUC values 4- to 13-fold greater than those in humans given the recommended dose.

Tenofovir Disoproxil Fumarate: Tenofovir and tenofovir DF administered in toxicology studies to rats, dogs and monkeys at exposures (based on AUCs) greater than or equal to 6-fold those observed in humans caused bone toxicity. In monkeys the bone toxicity was diagnosed as osteomalacia. Osteomalacia observed in monkeys appeared to be reversible upon dose reduction or discontinuation of tenofovir. In rats and dogs, the bone toxicity manifested as reduced bone mineral density. The mechanism(s) underlying bone toxicity is unknown.

Evidence of renal toxicity was noted in 4 animal species administered tenofovir and tenofovir DF. Increases in serum creatinine, BUN, glycosuria, proteinuria, phosphaturia and/or calciuria and decreases in serum phosphate were observed to varying degrees in these animals. These toxicities were noted at exposures (based on AUCs) 2- to 20-times higher than those observed in humans. The relationship of the renal abnormalities, particularly the phosphaturia, to the bone toxicity is not known.

14 CLINICAL STUDIES

Clinical Study 934 supports the use of ATRIPLA tablets in antiretroviral treatment-naive HIV-1 infected patients. Additional data in support of the use of ATRIPLA in treatment- naive patients can be found in the prescribing information for VIREAD.

Clinical Study 073 provides clinical experience in subjects with stable, virologic suppression and no history of virologic failure who switched from their current regimen to ATRIPLA.

In antiretroviral treatment-experienced patients, the use of ATRIPLA tablets may be considered for patients with HIV-1 strains that are expected to be susceptible to the components of ATRIPLA as assessed by treatment history or by genotypic or phenotypic testing *[See Clinical Pharmacology (12.4)]*.

Study 934: Data through 144 weeks are reported for Study 934, a randomized, open-label, active-controlled multicenter trial comparing emtricitabine + tenofovir DF administered in combination with efavirenz versus zidovudine/lamivudine fixed-dose combination administered in combination with efavirenz in 511 antiretroviral-naive subjects. From Weeks 96 to 144 of the trial, subjects received emtricitabine/tenofovir DF fixed-dose combination with efavirenz in place of emtricitabine + tenofovir DF with efavirenz. Subjects had a mean age of 38 years (range 18–80), 86% were male, 59% were Caucasian and 23% were Black. The mean baseline CD4+ cell count was 245 cells/mm³ (range 2–1191) and median baseline plasma HIV-1 RNA was 5.01 log₁₀ copies/mL (range 3.56–6.54). Subjects were stratified by baseline CD4+ cell count (< or ≥200 cells/mm³) and 41% had CD4+ cell counts <200 cells/mm³. Fifty-one percent (51%) of subjects had baseline viral loads >100,000 copies/mL. Treatment outcomes through 48 and 144 weeks for those subjects who did not have efavirenz resistance at baseline (N=487) are presented in Table 9.

[See table 9 at top of next page]

Through Week 48, 84% and 73% of subjects in the emtricitabine + tenofovir DF group and the zidovudine/lamivudine group, respectively, achieved and maintained HIV-1 RNA <400 copies/mL (71% and 58% through Week 144). The difference in the proportion of subjects who achieved and maintained HIV-1 RNA <400 copies/mL through 48 weeks largely results from the higher number of discontinuations due to adverse events and other reasons in the zidovudine/lamivudine group in this open-label trial. In addition, 80% and 70% of subjects in the emtricitabine + tenofovir DF group and the zidovudine/lamivudine group, respectively, achieved and maintained HIV-1 RNA <50 copies/mL through Week 48 (64% and 56% through Week 144). The mean increase from baseline in $CD4^+$ cell count was 190 cells/mm^3 in the emtricitabine + tenofovir DF group and 158 cells/mm^3 in the zidovudine/lamivudine group at Week 48 (312 and 271 cells/mm^3 at Week 144).

Through 48 weeks, 7 subjects in the emtricitabine + tenofovir DF group and 5 subjects in the zidovudine/lamivudine group experienced a new CDC Class C event (10 and 6 subjects through 144 weeks).

Study 073: Study 073 was a 48-week open-label, randomized clinical trial in subjects with stable virologic suppression on combination antiretroviral therapy consisting of at least two nucleoside reverse transcriptase inhibitors (NRTIs) administered in combination with a protease inhibitor (with or without ritonavir) or a non-nucleoside reverse transcriptase inhibitor (NNRTI).

To be enrolled, subjects were to have HIV-1 RNA <200 copies/mL for at least 12 weeks on their current regimen prior to trial entry with no known HIV-1 substitutions conferring resistance to the components of ATRIPLA and no history of virologic failure.

The trial compared the efficacy of switching to ATRIPLA or staying on the baseline antiretroviral regimen (SBR). Subjects were randomized in a 2:1 ratio to switch to ATRIPLA (N=203) or stay on SBR (N=97). Subjects had a mean age of 43 years (range 22–73 years), 88% were male, 68% were white, 29% were Black or African-American, and 3% were of other races. At baseline, median $CD4^+$ cell count was 516 cells/mm^3 and 96% had HIV-1 RNA <50 copies/mL. The median time since onset of antiretroviral therapy was 3 years and 88% of subjects were receiving their first antiretroviral regimen at trial enrollment.

At Week 48, 89% and 87% of subjects who switched to ATRIPLA maintained HIV RNA <200 copies/mL and <50 copies/mL, respectively, compared to 88% and 85% who remained on SBR; this difference was not statistically significant. No changes in $CD4^+$ cell counts from baseline to Week 48 were observed in either treatment arm.

16 HOW SUPPLIED/STORAGE AND HANDLING

ATRIPLA tablets are pink, capsule-shaped, film-coated, debossed with "123" on one side and plain-faced on the other side. Each bottle contains 30 tablets (NDC 15584-0101-1) and silica gel desiccant, and is closed with a child-resistant closure.

Store at 25 °C (77 °F); excursions permitted to 15–30 °C (59–86 °F) *[See USP Controlled Room Temperature]*.

• Keep container tightly closed.
• Dispense only in original container.
• Do not use if seal over bottle opening is broken or missing.

17 PATIENT COUNSELING INFORMATION

See FDA-approved patient labeling (Patient Information)

17.1 Drug Interactions

A statement to patients and healthcare providers is included on the product's bottle labels: *ALERT: Find out about medicines that should NOT be taken with ATRIPLA.* ATRIPLA may interact with some drugs; therefore, patients should be advised to report to their doctor the use of any other prescription, nonprescription medication, or herbal products, particularly St. John's wort.

17.2 General Information for Patients

Patients should be advised that:

• ATRIPLA is not a cure for HIV-1 infection and patients may continue to experience illnesses associated with HIV-1 infection, including opportunistic infections. Patients should remain under the care of a physician when using ATRIPLA.
• Patients should avoid doing things that can spread HIV-1 to others.
  • **Do not share needles or other injection equipment.**
  • **Do not share personal items that can have blood or body fluids on them, like toothbrushes and razor blades.**
  • **Do not have any kind of sex without protection.** Always practice safe sex by using a latex or polyurethane condom to lower the chance of sexual contact with semen, vaginal secretions, or blood.
  • **Do not breastfeed.** Some of the medicines in ATRIPLA can be passed to your baby in your breast milk. We do not know whether it could harm your baby. Also, mothers with HIV-1 should not breastfeed because HIV-1 can be passed to the baby in the breast milk.

Table 8 Drug Interactions: Changes in Pharmacokinetic Parameters for Coadministered Drug in the Presence of Tenofovir Disoproxil Fumarate*,†

Coadministered Drug	Dose of Coadministered Drug (mg)	N	Mean % Change of Coadministered Drug Pharmacokinetic Parameters‡ (90% CI)		
			C_{max}	AUC	C_{min}
Atazanavir§	400 once daily × 14 days	34	↓ 21 (↓ 27 to ↓ 14)	↓ 25 (↓ 30 to ↓ 19)	↓ 40 (↓ 48 to ↓ 32)
	Atazanavir/ritonavir 300/100 once daily × 42 days	10	↓ 28 (↓ 50 to ↑ 5)	↓ 25¶ (↓ 42 to ↓ 3)	↓ 23¶ (↓ 46 to ↑ 10)
Darunavir#	Darunavir/ritonavir 300/100 mg once daily	12	↑ 16 (↓ 6 to ↑ 42)	↑ 21 (↓ 5 to ↑ 54)	↑ 24 (↓ 10 to ↑ 69)
Didanosine Þ	250 once, simultaneously with tenofovir DF and a light meal ß	33	↓ 20ª (↓ 32 to ↓ 7)	↔ª	NA
Lopinavir	Lopinavir/ritonavir 400/100 twice daily × 14 days	24	↔	↔	↔
Ritonavir	Lopinavir/ritonavir 400/100 twice daily × 14 days	24	↔	↔	↔
Tipranavir è	Tipranavir/ritonavir 500/100 twice daily	22	↓ 17 (↓ 26 to ↓ 6)	↓ 18 (↓ 25 to ↓ 9)	↓ 21 (↓ 30 to ↓ 10)
	Tipranavir/ritonavir 750/200 twice daily (23 doses)	20	↓ 11 (↓ 16 to ↓ 4)	↓ 9 (↓ 15 to ↓ 3)	↓ 12 (↓ 22 to 0)

* All interaction trials conducted in healthy volunteers.
† Subjects received tenofovir DF 300 mg once daily.
‡ Increase = ↑; Decrease = ↓; No Effect = ↔
§ Reyataz Prescribing Information.
¶ In HIV-infected patients, addition of tenofovir DF to atazanavir 300 mg plus ritonavir 100 mg, resulted in AUC and C_{min} values of atazanavir that were 2.3- and 4-fold higher than the respective values observed for atazanavir 400 mg when given alone.
# Prezista Prescribing Information.
Þ Videx EC Prescribing Information. Subjects received didanosine enteric-coated capsules.
ß 373 kcal, 8.2 g fat.
à Compared with didanosine (enteric-coated) 400 mg administered alone under fasting conditions.
è Aptivus Prescribing Information.

Table 9 Outcomes of Randomized Treatment at Weeks 48 and 144 (Study 934)

Outcomes	At Week 48		At Week 144	
	FTC + TDF + EFV (N=244)	AZT/3TC + EFV (N=243)	FTC + TDF + EFV (N=227)*	AZT/3TC + EFV (N=229)*
Responder†	84%	73%	71%	58%
Virologic failure‡	2%	4%	3%	6%
Rebound	1%	3%	2%	5%
Never suppressed	0%	0%	0%	0%
Change in antiretroviral regimen	1%	1%	1%	1%
Death	<1%	1%	1%	1%
Discontinued due to adverse event	4%	9%	5%	12%
Discontinued for other reasons§	10%	14%	20%	22%

* Subjects who were responders at Week 48 or Week 96 (HIV-1 RNA <400 copies/mL) but did not consent to continue trial after Week 48 or Week 96 were excluded from analysis.
† Subjects achieved and maintained confirmed HIV-1 RNA <400 copies/mL through Weeks 48 and 144.
‡ Includes confirmed viral rebound and failure to achieve confirmed HIV-1 RNA <400 copies/mL through Weeks 48 and 144.
§ Includes lost to follow-up, patient withdrawal, noncompliance, protocol violation and other reasons.

• The long-term effects of ATRIPLA are unknown.
• Redistribution or accumulation of body fat may occur in patients receiving antiretroviral therapy and that the cause and long-term health effects of these conditions are not known.
• ATRIPLA should not be coadministered with COMPLERA, EMTRIVA, STRIBILD, TRUVADA, or VIREAD; or drugs containing lamivudine, including Combivir, Epivir, Epivir-HBV, Epzicom, or Trizivir.

SUSTIVA should not be coadministered with ATRIPLA unless needed for dose adjustment *[See Warnings and Precautions (5.4)]*.
• ATRIPLA should not be administered with HEPSERA *[See Warnings and Precautions (5.2)]*.

17.3 Lactic Acidosis/Severe Hepatomegaly with Steatosis

Patients should be informed that lactic acidosis and severe hepatomegaly with steatosis, including fatal cases, have been reported. Treatment will be suspended in any patients who develop clinical symptoms suggestive of lactic acidosis or pronounced hepatotoxicity (including nausea, vomiting, unusual or unexpected stomach discomfort, and weakness) *[See Warnings and Precautions (5.1)].*

17.4   Patients Coinfected with HIV-1 and HBV

Patients with HIV-1 should be tested for hepatitis B virus (HBV) before initiating antiretroviral therapy.

Patients should be advised that severe acute exacerbations of hepatitis B have been reported in patients who are coinfected with HBV and HIV-1 and have discontinued EMTRIVA (emtricitabine) or VIREAD (tenofovir DF), which are components of ATRIPLA.

17.5   New Onset or Worsening Renal Impairment

Renal impairment, including cases of acute renal failure and Fanconi syndrome, has been reported. ATRIPLA should be avoided with concurrent or recent use of a nephrotoxic agent (e.g. high-dose or multiple NSAIDs) *[See Warnings and Precautions (5.7)].*

17.6   Decreases in Bone Mineral Density

Patients should be informed that decreases in bone mineral density have been observed with the use of tenofovir DF. Bone mineral density monitoring may be performed in patients who have a history of pathologic bone fracture or other risk factors for osteoporosis or bone loss *[See Warnings and Precautions (5.11)].*

17.7   Dosing Instructions

Patients should be advised to take ATRIPLA orally on an empty stomach and that it is important to take ATRIPLA on a regular dosing schedule to avoid missing doses.

17.8   Nervous System Symptoms

Patients should be informed that central nervous system symptoms (NSS) including dizziness, insomnia, impaired concentration, drowsiness, and abnormal dreams are commonly reported during the first weeks of therapy with efavirenz. Dosing at bedtime may improve the tolerability of these symptoms, which are likely to improve with continued therapy. Patients should be alerted to the potential for additive effects when ATRIPLA is used concomitantly with alcohol or psychoactive drugs. Patients should be instructed that if they experience NSS they should avoid potentially hazardous tasks such as driving or operating machinery *[See Warnings and Precautions (5.6) and Dosage and Administration (2)].*

17.9   Psychiatric Symptoms

Patients should be informed that serious psychiatric symptoms including severe depression, suicide attempts, aggressive behavior, delusions, paranoia, and psychosis-like symptoms have been reported in patients receiving efavirenz. If they experience severe psychiatric adverse experiences they should seek immediate medical evaluation. Patients should be advised to inform their physician of any history of mental illness or substance abuse *[See Warnings and Precautions (5.5)].*

17.10   Rash

Patients should be informed that a common side effect is rash. Rashes usually go away without any change in treatment. However, since rash may be serious, patients should be advised to contact their physician promptly if rash occurs.

17.11   Reproductive Risk Potential

Women receiving ATRIPLA should be instructed to avoid pregnancy *[See Warnings and Precautions (5.8)].* A reliable form of barrier contraception must always be used in combination with other methods of contraception, including oral or other hormonal contraception. Because of the long half-life of efavirenz, use of adequate contraceptive measures for 12 weeks after discontinuation of ATRIPLA is recommended. Women should be advised to notify their physician if they become pregnant or plan to become pregnant while taking ATRIPLA. If this drug is used during the first trimester of pregnancy, or if the patient becomes pregnant while taking this drug, she should be apprised of the potential harm to the fetus.

Patient Information

ATRIPLA® (uh TRIP luh) Tablets

ALERT: Find out about medicines that should NOT be taken with ATRIPLA.

Please also read the section **"MEDICINES YOU SHOULD NOT TAKE WITH ATRIPLA."**

Generic name: efavirenz, emtricitabine and tenofovir disoproxil fumarate (eh FAH vih renz, em tri SIT uh bean and te NOE' fo veer dye soe PROX il FYOU mar ate)

Read the Patient Information that comes with ATRIPLA before you start taking it and each time you get a refill since there may be new information. This information does not take the place of talking to your healthcare provider about your medical condition or treatment. You should stay under a healthcare provider's care when taking ATRIPLA. **Do not change or stop your medicine without first talking with your healthcare provider.** Talk to your healthcare provider or pharmacist if you have any questions about ATRIPLA.

What is the most important information I should know about ATRIPLA?
- **Some people who have taken medicine like ATRIPLA (which contains nucleoside analogs) have developed a serious condition called lactic acidosis** (build up of an acid in the blood). Lactic acidosis can be a medical emergency and may need to be treated in the hospital. **Call your healthcare provider right away if you get the following signs or symptoms of lactic acidosis:**
  - You feel very weak or tired.
  - You have unusual (not normal) muscle pain.
  - You have trouble breathing.
  - You have stomach pain with nausea and vomiting.
  - You feel cold, especially in your arms and legs.
  - You feel dizzy or lightheaded.
  - You have a fast or irregular heartbeat.
- **Some people who have taken medicines like ATRIPLA have developed serious liver problems called hepatotoxicity,** with liver enlargement (hepatomegaly) and fat in the liver (steatosis). **Call your healthcare provider right away if you get the following signs or symptoms of liver problems:**
  - Your skin or the white part of your eyes turns yellow (jaundice).
  - Your urine turns dark.
  - Your bowel movements (stools) turn light in color.
  - You don't feel like eating food for several days or longer.
  - You feel sick to your stomach (nausea).
  - You have lower stomach area (abdominal) pain.
- **You may be more likely to get lactic acidosis or liver problems** if you are female, very overweight (obese), or have been taking nucleoside analog-containing medicines, like ATRIPLA, for a long time.
- **If you also have hepatitis B virus (HBV) infection and you stop taking ATRIPLA, you may get a "flare-up" of your hepatitis. A "flare-up" is when the disease suddenly returns in a worse way than before.** Patients with HBV who stop taking ATRIPLA need close medical follow-up for several months, including medical exams and blood tests to check for hepatitis that could be getting worse. ATRIPLA is not approved for the treatment of HBV, so you must discuss your HBV therapy with your healthcare provider.

What is ATRIPLA?
ATRIPLA contains 3 medicines, SUSTIVA® (efavirenz), EMTRIVA® (emtricitabine) and VIREAD® (tenofovir disoproxil fumarate also called tenofovir DF) combined in one pill. EMTRIVA and VIREAD are HIV-1 (human immunodeficiency virus) nucleoside analog reverse transcriptase inhibitors (NRTIs) and SUSTIVA is an HIV-1 non-nucleoside analog reverse transcriptase inhibitor (NNRTI). VIREAD and EMTRIVA are the components of TRUVADA®. ATRIPLA can be used alone as a complete regimen, or in combination with other anti-HIV-1 medicines to treat people with HIV-1 infection. ATRIPLA is for adults and children 12 years of age and older who weigh at least 40 kg (at least 88 lbs). ATRIPLA is not recommended for children younger than 12 years of age. ATRIPLA has not been studied in adults over 65 years of age.

HIV infection destroys CD4+ T cells, which are important to the immune system. The immune system helps fight infection. After a large number of T cells are destroyed, acquired immune deficiency syndrome (AIDS) develops.
ATRIPLA helps block HIV-1 reverse transcriptase, a viral chemical in your body (enzyme) that is needed for HIV-1 to multiply. ATRIPLA lowers the amount of HIV-1 in the blood (viral load). ATRIPLA may also help to increase the number of T cells (CD4+ cells), allowing your immune system to improve. Lowering the amount of HIV-1 in the blood lowers the chance of death or infections that happen when your immune system is weak (opportunistic infections).

Does ATRIPLA cure HIV-1 or AIDS?
ATRIPLA does not cure HIV-1 infection or AIDS and you may continue to experience illnesses associated with HIV-1 infection, including opportunistic infections. You should remain under the care of a doctor when using ATRIPLA.

Who should not take ATRIPLA?
Together with your healthcare provider, you need to decide whether ATRIPLA is right for you.
Do not take ATRIPLA if you are allergic to ATRIPLA or any of its ingredients. The active ingredients of ATRIPLA are efavirenz, emtricitabine, and tenofovir DF. See the end of this leaflet for a complete list of ingredients.

What should I tell my healthcare provider before taking ATRIPLA?
Tell your healthcare provider if you:
- **Are pregnant or planning to become pregnant** (see "What should I avoid while taking ATRIPLA?").
- **Are breastfeeding** (see "What should I avoid while taking ATRIPLA?").
- **Have kidney problems or are undergoing kidney dialysis treatment.**
- **Have bone problems.**
- **Have liver problems, including hepatitis B virus infection.** Your healthcare provider may want to do tests to check your liver while you take ATRIPLA or may switch you to another medicine.

- **Have ever had mental illness or are using drugs or alcohol.**
- **Have ever had seizures or are taking medicine for seizures.**

What important information should I know about taking other medicines with ATRIPLA?
ATRIPLA may change the effect of other medicines, including the ones for HIV-1, and may cause serious side effects. Your healthcare provider may change your other medicines or change their doses. Other medicines, including herbal products, may affect ATRIPLA. For this reason, **it is very important** to let all your healthcare providers and pharmacists know what medications, herbal supplements, or vitamins you are taking.

MEDICINES YOU SHOULD NOT TAKE WITH ATRIPLA
- The following medicines may cause serious and life-threatening side effects when taken with ATRIPLA. You should not take any of these medicines while taking ATRIPLA: Vascor (bepridil), Propulsid (cisapride), Versed (midazolam), Orap (pimozide), Halcion (triazolam), ergot medications (for example, Wigraine and Cafergot).
- ATRIPLA also should not be used with Combivir (lamivudine/zidovudine), COMPLERA®, EMTRIVA, Epivir, Epivir-HBV (lamivudine), Epzicom (abacavir sulfate/lamivudine), STRIBILD®, Trizivir (abacavir sulfate/lamivudine/zidovudine), TRUVADA, or VIREAD. ATRIPLA also should not be used with SUSTIVA unless recommended by your healthcare provider.
- Vfend (voriconazole) should not be taken with ATRIPLA since it may lose its effect or may increase the chance of having side effects from ATRIPLA.
- **Do not take St. John's wort (*Hypericum perforatum*), or products containing St. John's wort with ATRIPLA.** St. John's wort is an herbal product sold as a dietary supplement. Talk with your healthcare provider if you are taking or are planning to take St. John's wort. Taking St. John's wort may decrease ATRIPLA levels and lead to increased viral load and possible resistance to ATRIPLA or cross-resistance to other anti-HIV-1 drugs.
- ATRIPLA should not be used with HEPSERA® (adefovir dipivoxil).

It is also important to tell your healthcare provider if you are taking any of the following medicines:
- Fortovase, Invirase (saquinavir), Biaxin (clarithromycin), Noxafil (posaconazole), Sporanox (itraconazole), or Victrelis (boceprevir); **these medicines may need to be replaced with another medicine when taken with ATRIPLA.**
- Calcium channel blockers such as Cardizem or Tiazac (diltiazem), Covera HS or Isoptin (verapamil) and others; Crixivan (indinavir), Selzentry (maraviroc); the immunosuppressant medicines cyclosporine (Gengraf, Neoral, Sandimmune, and others), Prograf (tacrolimus), or Rapamune (sirolimus); Methadone; Mycobutin (rifabutin); Rifampin; cholesterol-lowering medicines such as Lipitor (atorvastatin), Pravachol (pravastatin sodium), and Zocor (simvastatin); or the anti-depressant medications bupropion (Wellbutrin, Wellbutrin SR, Wellbutrin XL, and Zyban) or Zoloft (sertraline); **dose changes may be needed when these drugs are taken with ATRIPLA.**
- Videx, Videx EC (didanosine); tenofovir DF (a component of ATRIPLA) may increase the amount of didanosine in your blood, which could result in more side effects. **You may need to be monitored more carefully** if you are taking ATRIPLA and didanosine together. Also, the dose of didanosine may need to be changed.
- Reyataz (atazanavir sulfate), Prezista (darunavir) with Norvir (ritonavir), or Kaletra (lopinavir/ritonavir); these medicines may increase the amount of tenofovir DF (a component of ATRIPLA) in your blood, which could result in more side effects. Reyataz is not recommended with ATRIPLA. **You may need to be monitored more carefully** if you are taking ATRIPLA, Prezista, and Norvir together, or if you are taking ATRIPLA and Kaletra together. Also, the dose of Kaletra may need to be changed.
- Medicine for seizures [for example, Dilantin (phenytoin), Tegretol (carbamazepine), or phenobarbital]; your healthcare provider may want to switch you to another medicine or check drug levels in your blood from time to time.

These are not all the medicines that may cause problems if you take ATRIPLA. Be sure to tell your healthcare provider about all medicines that you take.
Keep a complete list of all the prescription and nonprescription medicines as well as any herbal remedies that you are taking, how much you take, and how often you take them. Make a new list when medicines or herbal remedies are added or stopped, or if the dose changes. Give copies of this list to all of your healthcare providers and pharmacists **every time you visit your healthcare provider or fill a prescription. This will give your healthcare provider a complete picture of the medicines you use. Then he or she can decide the best approach for your situation.

How should I take ATRIPLA?
- Take the exact amount of ATRIPLA your healthcare provider prescribes. Never change the dose on your own. Do not stop this medicine unless your healthcare provider tells you to stop.

- You should take ATRIPLA on an empty stomach.
- Swallow ATRIPLA with water.
- Taking ATRIPLA at bedtime may make some side effects less bothersome.
- Do not miss a dose of ATRIPLA. If you forget to take ATRIPLA, take the missed dose right away, unless it is almost time for your next dose. Do not double the next dose. Carry on with your regular dosing schedule. If you need help in planning the best times to take your medicine, ask your healthcare provider or pharmacist.
- If you believe you took more than the prescribed amount of ATRIPLA, contact your local poison control center or emergency room right away.
- Tell your healthcare provider if you start any new medicine or change how you take old ones. Your doses may need adjustment.
- When your ATRIPLA supply starts to run low, get more from your healthcare provider or pharmacy. This is very important because the amount of virus in your blood may increase if the medicine is stopped for even a short time. The virus may develop resistance to ATRIPLA and become harder to treat.
- Your healthcare provider may want to do blood tests to check for certain side effects while you take ATRIPLA.

What should I avoid while taking ATRIPLA?
- **Women should not become pregnant while taking ATRIPLA and for 12 weeks after stopping it.** Serious birth defects have been seen in the babies of animals and women treated with efavirenz (a component of ATRIPLA) during pregnancy. It is not known whether efavirenz caused these defects. **Tell your healthcare provider right away if you are pregnant.** Also talk with your healthcare provider if you want to become pregnant.
- Women should not rely only on hormone-based birth control, such as pills, injections, or implants, because ATRIPLA may make these contraceptives ineffective. Women must use a reliable form of barrier contraception, such as a condom or diaphragm, even if they also use other methods of birth control. Efavirenz, a component of ATRIPLA, may remain in your blood for a time after therapy is stopped. Therefore, you should continue to use contraceptive measures for 12 weeks after you stop taking ATRIPLA.
- **Do not breastfeed if you are taking ATRIPLA.** Some of the medicines in ATRIPLA can be passed to your baby in your breast milk. We do not know whether it could harm your baby. Also, mothers with HIV-1 should not breastfeed because HIV-1 can be passed to the baby in the breast milk. Talk with your healthcare provider if you are breastfeeding. You should stop breastfeeding or may need to use a different medicine.
- Taking ATRIPLA with alcohol or other medicines causing similar side effects as ATRIPLA, such as drowsiness, may increase those side effects.
- Do not take any other medicines, including prescription and nonprescription medicines and herbal products, without checking with your healthcare provider.
- Avoid doing things that can spread HIV-1 to others.
  - **Do not share needles or other injection equipment.**
  - **Do not share personal items that can have blood or body fluids on them, like toothbrushes and razor blades.**
  - **Do not have any kind of sex without protection.** Always practice safe sex by using a latex or polyurethane condom to lower the chance of sexual contact with semen, vaginal secretions, or blood.

What are the possible side effects of ATRIPLA?
ATRIPLA may cause the following serious side effects:
- **Lactic acidosis** (buildup of an acid in the blood). Lactic acidosis can be a medical emergency and may need to be treated in the hospital. **Call your healthcare provider right away if you get signs of lactic acidosis.** (See "What is the most important information I should know about ATRIPLA?")
- **Serious liver problems (hepatotoxicity)**, with liver enlargement (hepatomegaly) and fat in the liver (steatosis). Call your healthcare provider right away if you get any signs of liver problems. (See "What is the most important information I should know about ATRIPLA?")
- **"Flare-ups" of hepatitis B virus (HBV) infection**, in which the disease suddenly returns in a worse way than before, can occur if you have HBV and you stop taking ATRIPLA. Your healthcare provider will monitor your condition for several months after stopping ATRIPLA if you have both HIV-1 and HBV infection and may recommend treatment for your HBV. ATRIPLA is not approved for the treatment of hepatitis B virus infection. If you have advanced liver disease and stop treatment with ATRIPLA, the "flare-up" of hepatitis B may cause your liver function to decline.
- **Serious psychiatric problems.** A small number of patients may experience severe depression, strange thoughts, or angry behavior while taking ATRIPLA. Some patients have thoughts of suicide and a few have actually committed suicide. These problems may occur more often in pa-

tients who have had mental illness. Contact your healthcare provider right away if you think you are having these psychiatric symptoms, so your healthcare provider can decide if you should continue to take ATRIPLA.
- **Kidney problems** (including decline or failure of kidney function). If you have had kidney problems in the past or take other medicines that can cause kidney problems, your healthcare provider should do regular blood tests to check your kidneys. Symptoms that may be related to kidney problems include a high volume of urine, thirst, muscle pain, and muscle weakness.
- **Other serious liver problems.** Some patients have experienced serious liver problems including liver failure resulting in transplantation or death. Most of these serious side effects occurred in patients with a chronic liver disease such as hepatitis infection, but there have also been a few reports in patients without any existing liver disease.
- **Changes in bone mineral density (thinning bones).** Laboratory tests show changes in the bones of patients treated with tenofovir DF, a component of ATRIPLA. Some HIV patients treated with tenofovir DF developed thinning of the bones (osteopenia) which could lead to fractures. If you have had bone problems in the past, your healthcare provider may need to do tests to check your bone mineral density or may prescribe medicines to help your bone mineral density. Additionally, bone pain and softening of the bone (which may contribute to fractures) may occur as a consequence of kidney problems.

Common side effects:
Patients may have dizziness, headache, trouble sleeping, drowsiness, trouble concentrating, and/or unusual dreams during treatment with ATRIPLA. These side effects may be reduced if you take ATRIPLA at bedtime on an empty stomach. They also tend to go away after you have taken the medicine for a few weeks. If you have these common side effects, such as dizziness, it does not mean that you will also have serious psychiatric problems, such as severe depression, strange thoughts, or angry behavior. Tell your healthcare provider right away if any of these side effects continue or if they bother you. It is possible that these symptoms may be more severe if ATRIPLA is used with alcohol or mood altering (street) drugs.

If you are dizzy, have trouble concentrating, or are drowsy, avoid activities that may be dangerous, such as driving or operating machinery.

Rash may be common. Rashes usually go away without any change in treatment. In a small number of patients, rash may be serious. If you develop a rash, call your healthcare provider right away. **Rash may be a serious problem in some children.** Tell your child's healthcare provider right away if you notice rash or any other side effects while your child is taking ATRIPLA.

Other common side effects include tiredness, upset stomach, vomiting, gas, and diarrhea.

Other possible side effects with ATRIPLA:
- Changes in body fat. Changes in body fat develop in some patients taking anti HIV-1 medicine. These changes may include an increased amount of fat in the upper back and neck ("buffalo hump"), in the breasts, and around the trunk. Loss of fat from the legs, arms, and face may also happen. The cause and long-term health effects of these fat changes are not known.
- Skin discoloration (small spots or freckles) may also happen with ATRIPLA.
- In some patients with advanced HIV infection (AIDS), signs and symptoms of inflammation from previous infections may occur soon after anti-HIV treatment is started. It is believed that these symptoms are due to an improvement in the body's immune response, enabling the body to fight infections that may have been present with no obvious symptoms. If you notice any symptoms of infection, please inform your doctor immediately.
- Additional side effects are inflammation of the pancreas, allergic reaction (including swelling of the face, lips, tongue, or throat), shortness of breath, pain, stomach pain, weakness and indigestion.

Tell your healthcare provider or pharmacist if you notice any side effects while taking ATRIPLA.

Contact your healthcare provider before stopping ATRIPLA because of side effects or for any other reason.

This is not a complete list of side effects possible with ATRIPLA. Ask your healthcare provider or pharmacist for a more complete list of side effects of ATRIPLA and all the medicines you will take.

How do I store ATRIPLA?
- **Keep ATRIPLA and all other medicines out of reach of children.**
- Store ATRIPLA at room temperature 77 °F (25 °C).
- Keep ATRIPLA in its original container and keep the container tightly closed.
- Do not keep medicine that is out of date or that you no longer need. If you throw any medicines away make sure that children will not find them.

General information about ATRIPLA:
Medicines are sometimes prescribed for conditions that are not mentioned in patient information leaflets. Do not use ATRIPLA for a condition for which it was not prescribed. Do not give ATRIPLA to other people, even if they have the same symptoms you have. It may harm them.

This leaflet summarizes the most important information about ATRIPLA. If you would like more information, talk with your healthcare provider. You can ask your healthcare provider or pharmacist for information about ATRIPLA that is written for health professionals.

Do not use ATRIPLA if the seal over bottle opening is broken or missing.

What are the ingredients of ATRIPLA?
Active Ingredients: efavirenz, emtricitabine, and tenofovir disoproxil fumarate
Inactive Ingredients: croscarmellose sodium, hydroxypropyl cellulose, microcrystalline cellulose, magnesium stearate, sodium lauryl sulfate. The film coating contains black iron oxide, polyethylene glycol, polyvinyl alcohol, red iron oxide, talc, and titanium dioxide.
October 2013
ATRIPLA is a trademark of Bristol-Myers Squibb & Gilead Sciences, LLC. COMPLERA, EMTRIVA, HEPSERA, STRIBILD, TRUVADA, and VIREAD are trademarks of Gilead Sciences, Inc., or its related companies. SUSTIVA is a trademark of Bristol-Myers Squibb Pharma Company. Reyataz and Videx are trademarks of Bristol-Myers Squibb Company. Pravachol is a trademark of ER Squibb & Sons, LLC. Other brands listed are the trademarks of their respective owners.
21-937-GS-013

Fleet Laboratories
Division of C. B. Fleet Company, Incorporated
LYNCHBURG, VA 24502

Direct Inquiries to:
Sherrie McNamara, RN, MSN, MBA
Director, Global Medical Affairs and Pharmacovigilance
1-888-999-9711
www.fleetlabs.com

BOUDREAUX'S BUTT PASTE®   OTC
ORIGINAL FORMULA OINTMENT
ALL NATURAL FORMULA OINTMENT
MAXIMUM STRENGTH FORMULA OINTMENT
DIAPER RASH SKIN PROTECTANT

COMPOSITION
Original: 16% Zinc Oxide
All-Natural: 16% Zinc Oxide
Maximum Strength: 40% Zinc Oxide

ACTIONS AND USES
Zinc oxide is a skin protectant used to help treat and prevent diaper rash. It protects chafed skin due to diaper rash and helps seal out wetness. Zinc oxide is effective as a skin protectant due to its absorbent and lubricant properties. It has a low range of sensitization, and has cooling, slightly astringent, antiseptic, antibacterial and protective actions.

GENERAL SKIN PROTECTANT WARNINGS
For external use only. When using this product avoid contact with the eyes. Stop use and ask a doctor if condition worsens or does not improve after seven (7) days.
Keep this and all drugs out of the reach of children to prevent accidental ingestion. In case of accidental ingestion, get medical help or contact a Poison Control Center right away.

DIRECTIONS FOR USE
Change wet and soiled diaper immediately. Cleanse the diaper area and allow to dry. Remove foil seal from the jar or the tube's tip. Apply ointment liberally and as often as necessary, with each diaper change and especially when exposed to wet diapers for a prolonged period of time, such as bedtime.

INACTIVE INGREDIENTS
Original formula: castor oil, mineral oil, paraffin, Peruvian balsam, white petrolatum.
All Natural formula: Aloe Vera, beeswax, carnauba wax, castor oil, citric acid, hydrogenated castor oil, Peruvian balsam oil.
Maximum Strength formula: castor oil, mineral oil, paraffin, Peruvian balsam, white petrolatum.

HOW SUPPLIED

Original formula is available in 2 oz (NDC 0132033322), 4 oz (NDC 0132033344) and 16 oz (NDC 0132033316) containers. **All Natural formula** is available in 2 oz (NDC 0132033422) and 4 oz (NDC 0132033444) containers. **Maximum Strength formula** is available in 2 oz (NDC 0132032322) and 4 oz (NDC 0132032344) containers.
IS THIS PRODUCT OTC?
Yes.
QUESTIONS? Call 1-855-785-2888 or visit www.buttpaste.com

FLEET® GLYCERIN LAXATIVES: OTC
FLEET® GLYCERIN SUPPOSITORIES,
FLEET® PEDIA-LAX® GLYCERIN SUPPOSITORIES,
FLEET® BABYLAX® AND
FLEET® PEDIA-LAX® LIQUID GLYCERIN SUPPOSITORIES AND
FLEET® LIQUID GLYCERIN SUPPOSITORIES
A HYPEROSMOTIC LAXATIVE

COMPOSITION

FLEET® Pedia-Lax® and Babylax® Liquid Glycerin Suppositories for Children 2 to under 6 years—Each 4 mL rectal applicator delivers on average 2.7 mL of an 80% solution (about 2.8 g glycerin).
FLEET® Liquid Glycerin Suppositories for Adults and Children 6 years of age and over—Each 7.5 mL rectal applicator delivers on average 5.4 mL of an 80% solution (about 5.4 g glycerin).
FLEET® Pedia-Lax® Glycerin Suppositories for Children 2 to under 6 years—Each suppository contains 1 g of glycerin.
FLEET® Glycerin Suppositories for Adults—Each suppository contains 2 g of glycerin.

ACTIONS AND USES

Glycerin is a hyperosmotic laxative, given rectally, which usually produces a bowel movement within 15 minutes to 1 hour. Hyperosmotic laxatives encourage bowel movements by drawing water into the bowel from surrounding tissues. This produces a softer stool mass and increased bowel action. These products are used for fast, predictable relief of occasional constipation. However, rectal irritation may occur with its use.

INFORMATION FOR PATIENT

WARNINGS

This product may cause rectal discomfort or a burning sensation.

GENERAL LAXATIVE WARNINGS

Ask a doctor before using any laxative if you have (or your child has):
• abdominal pain, nausea or vomiting
• a sudden change in bowel habits lasting more than 2 weeks
• already used a laxative for more than 1 week
Stop using this product and consult a doctor if you have (or your child has):
• rectal bleeding
• no bowel movement within 1 hour of using this product
• if constipation continues after one week of use
These symptoms may be signs of a serious condition.
Keep this and all drugs out of the reach of children to prevent accidental ingestion. In case of accidental overdose or ingestion, seek professional assistance or contact a Poison Control Center right away.

DOSAGE AND ADMINISTRATION

FLEET® Pedia-Lax® and Babylax® Liquid Glycerin Suppositories—Children 2 to under 6 years: only 1 suppository per 24 hours or as directed by a physician. Children under 2 years: Consult a physician.
Professional Labeling: Dosage and Administration for children less than 2 years of age: 2 to 5 mL glycerin (as an 80% solution) in a single daily dose (per 24 hours).
Positions for using the liquid suppository:
• **Left-side position:** Place child on left side with knees bent, and arms resting comfortably.
• **Knee-chest position:** Have child kneel, then lower head and chest forward until left side of face is resting on surface with left arm folded comfortably.
REMOVE ORANGE PROTECTIVE SHIELD FROM TIP BEFORE INSERTING. Hold the unit upright, grasping the bulb with fingers. Grasp the orange protective shield with the other hand; pull gently to remove.
• With steady pressure, gently insert tip into rectum with a slight side-to-side movement, with tip pointing toward navel. Insertion may be easier if child receiving the liquid suppository bears down, as if having a bowel movement. This helps relax the muscles around the anus.

• **DISCONTINUE USE IF RESISTANCE IS ENCOUNTERED. FORCING THE TIP INTO RECTUM CAN CAUSE INJURY.**
• Squeeze bulb until nearly all liquid is gone. It is not necessary to empty the bulb completely, as it contains more liquid than needed. A small amount of liquid will remain in the bulb after squeezing.
• Remove tip from rectum and discard the bulb. The liquid suppository will usually cause a bowel movement after 15 minutes but may take up to 1 hour. Do not allow child to retain liquid suppository for more than 1 hour.
• Stop using this product and consult a doctor if your child doesn't have a bowel movement within 1 hour of using this product.
FLEET® Liquid Glycerin Suppositories for Adults and Children 6 years of age and older: only 1 suppository per 24 hours or as directed by a physician. Children 2 to under 6 years use Fleet® Pedia-Lax® or Fleet® Babylax® Liquid Glycerin Suppositories. Children under 2 years, consult a physician.
Positions for using the liquid suppository:
• **Left-side position:** Lie on left side with knee bent, and arms resting comfortably.
• **Knee-chest position:** Kneel, then lower head and chest forward until left side of face is resting on surface with left arm folded comfortably.
REMOVE ORANGE PROTECTIVE SHIELD FROM TIP BEFORE INSERTING. Hold the unit upright, grasping the bulb with fingers. Grasp the orange protective shield with the other hand; pull gently to remove.
• With steady pressure, gently insert tip into rectum with a slight side-to-side movement, with tip pointing toward navel. Insertion may be easier if person receiving the liquid suppository bears down, as if having a bowel movement. This helps relax the muscles around the anus.
• **DISCONTINUE USE IF RESISTANCE IS ENCOUNTERED. FORCING THE TIP INTO RECTUM CAN CAUSE INJURY.**
• Squeeze bulb until nearly all liquid is gone. It is not necessary to empty the bulb completely, as it contains more liquid than needed. A small amount of liquid will remain in the bulb after squeezing.
• Remove tip from rectum and discard the bulb. The liquid suppository will usually cause a bowel movement after 15 minutes but may take up to 1 hour. Do not retain liquid suppository for more than 1 hour.
• Stop using this product and consult a doctor if you don't have a bowel movement within 1 hour of using this product.
Professional Labeling and Dosage Limit: Single Daily Dosage (per 24 hours)

Adults and children 6 years of age and older	5-15 mL
Children 2 to under 6 years of age	2-5 mL
Children less than 2 years of age	2-5 mL

FLEET® Pedia-Lax® Glycerin Suppositories—Children 2 to under 6 years: only 1 suppository per 24 hours or as directed by a physician.
Children under 2 years: Consult a physician.
Professional Labeling: Dosage and Administration for children less than 2 years of age: 1.0 to 1.7 grams glycerin in a single daily dose (per 24 hours).
Positions for using the suppository:
• **Left-side position:** Place child on left side with knees bent, and arms resting comfortably.
• **Knee-chest position:** Have child kneel, then lower head and chest forward until left side of face is resting on surface with left arm folded comfortably.
• Insert one suppository fully into the rectum. The suppository need not melt completely to produce laxative action. The suppository is designed to partially dissolve which may or may not be noticeable.
• The suppository will usually cause a bowel movement after 15 minutes but may take up to 1 hour. Do not allow child to retain suppository for more than 1 hour.
• Stop using this product and consult a doctor if your child doesn't have a bowel movement within 1 hour of using this product.
Store the container tightly closed and keep away from excessive heat.
FLEET® Glycerin Suppositories—Adults and Children 6 years of age and older: only 1 suppository per 24 hours or as directed by a physician.
Positions for using the suppository:
• **Left-side position:** Lie on left side with knee bent, and arms resting comfortably.
• **Knee-chest position:** Kneel, then lower head and chest forward until left side of face is resting on surface with left arm folded comfortably.

• Insert one suppository fully into the rectum. The suppository need not melt completely to produce laxative action. The suppository is designed to partially dissolve which may or may not be noticeable.
• The suppository will usually cause a bowel movement after 15 minutes but may take up to 1 hour.
• Do not retain suppository for more than 1 hour.
• Stop using this product and consult a doctor if you don't have a bowel movement within 1 hour of using this product.
Store the container tightly closed and keep away from excessive heat.
Professional Labeling and Dosage Limit: Single Daily Dosage (per 24 hours)

Adults and children 6 years of age and older	2-3 gm
Children 2 to under 6 years of age	1.0-1.7 gm
Children less than 2 years of age	1.0-1.7 gm

HOW SUPPLIED

FLEET® Pedia-Lax® and Babylax® Liquid Glycerin Suppositories for children 2 to under 6 years—Each box contains 6 child rectal applicators (4 mL each). NDC code: 0132019012 or 0132019024 (8×3 bundle)
FLEET® Liquid Glycerin Suppositories for Adults and Children 6 years of age and over—Each box contains 4 adult rectal applicators (7.5 mL each). NDC code: 0132018582
FLEET® Pedia-Lax® Glycerin Suppositories—Available in jars of 12. NDC code: 0132008112.
FLEET® Glycerin Suppositories—Available in jars of 12, 24, 50 and 100 adult suppositories. NDC code: 0132007912 (12 count); NDC code: 0132007924 (24 count); NDC code: 0132007950 (50 count) or 0132007953 (2×6 bundle); NDC code: 0132007900 (100 count)
IS THIS PRODUCT OTC? Yes.
QUESTIONS? Call 1-866-255-6960 or visit www.fleetlabs.com or www.pedia-lax.com.

FLEET® BISACODYL LAXATIVES: OTC
ENEMA AND TABLETS
A STIMULANT LAXATIVE

COMPOSITION

FLEET® Bisacodyl Enema - 10 mg bisacodyl enema solution in a 37-mL ready-to-use squeeze bottle which is **not made with natural rubber latex**, with a 2-inch, pre-lubricated Comfortip®. It is disposable after a single use.
FLEET® Stimulant Laxative Tablets - Enteric-coated 5 mg bisacodyl each tablet.

ACTION AND USES

Bisacodyl is a stimulant laxative given either orally or rectally, acting directly on the colonic mucosa where it stimulates sensory nerve endings to produce parasympathetic reflexes resulting in increased peristaltic contractions of the colon. The contact action of the drug is restricted to the colon, and motility in the small intestine is not appreciably influenced. FLEET® Stimulant Laxative Tablets usually work within 6-12 hours, and the FLEET® Bisacodyl Enema produces a bowel movement within 5–20 minutes. Bisacodyl is useful as a laxative for relief of occasional constipation and in bowel cleansing in preparation for x-ray or endoscopic examination. Bisacodyl may be used as a laxative in postoperative, antepartum, or postpartum care or in preparation for delivery under guidance of a healthcare professional.
Store at controlled room temperature 68-77°F (20-25°C).
WARNINGS: Do not administer Fleet® Bisacodyl Enema to children under 12 years of age.

GENERAL LAXATIVE WARNINGS
INFORMATION FOR PATIENT
Ask a doctor before using any laxative if you have
• abdominal pain, nausea or vomiting
• a sudden change in bowel habits lasting more than 2 weeks
• already used a laxative for more than 1 week
Stop using this product and consult a doctor if you have
• rectal bleeding
• no bowel movement within 20 minutes of using the rectal product
• if constipation continues after one week of use
These symtoms may be signs of a serious condition.
All bisacodyl products may cause
• abdominal discomfort
• faintness
• mild cramps

Rectal products may also cause rectal burning.

As with any drug, if you are pregnant or nursing a baby, seek the advice of a healthcare professional before using this product.

Keep this and all drugs out of the reach of children to prevent accidental ingestion. In case of accidental overdose or ingestion, seek professional assistance or contact a Poison Control Center right away.

DOSAGE AND ADMINISTRATION
Enema
SHAKE BEFORE USING.

Dosage:

Adults and children 12 years of age and over: Use one 1.25 fl. oz. bottle (30-mL delivered dose) as a single daily dose (per 24 hours).

Children under 12 years of age: DO NOT USE.

Positions for using this enema:

• **Left-side position:** Lie on left side with knee bent, and arms resting comfortably.

• **Knee-chest position:** Kneel, then lower head and chest forward until left side of face is resting on surface with left arm folded comfortably.

Fleet® Bisacodyl Enema should be used at room temperature.

How to use this enema:

• Shake bottle well before removing protective shield.

• REMOVE ORANGE PROTECTIVE SHIELD FROM ENEMA COMFORTIP® BEFORE INSERTING.

• With steady pressure, gently insert enema tip into rectum with a slight side-to-side movement, with tip pointing toward navel. Insertion may be easier if person receiving enema bears down, as if having a bowel movement. This helps relax the muscles around the anus.

• DO NOT FORCE THE ENEMA TIP INTO RECTUM AS THIS CAN CAUSE INJURY.

• Squeeze bottle until nearly all liquid is gone. It is not necessary to empty the bottle completely, as it contains more liquid than needed. A small amount of liquid will remain in the bottle after squeezing.

• Remove Comfortip® from rectum and discard bottle.

• Maintain position until urge to evacuate is strong (usually 5 to 20 minutes). Do not retain enema solution for more than 20 minutes.

• Stop using this product and consult a doctor if you don't have a bowel movement within 20 minutes of using this product.

The diaphragm at the base of the nozzle prevents reflux and assures controlled flow of the enema solution.

IMPORTANT: FLEET® Bisacodyl Enema IS NOT INTENDED FOR ORAL CONSUMPTION in any dosage size.

PROFESSIONAL ADMINISTRATION

FLEET® Bisacodyl Enema should not be used in children under 12 years of age. Careful consideration of the use of enemas in children in general is recommended. Proper and safe use of FLEET® enemas also requires that the products be administered according to the directions. Healthcare professionals should remember when administering the product to gently insert the enema into the rectum with the tip pointing toward the navel. Insertion may be made easier by having the patient bear down as if having a bowel movement. Care during insertion is necessary due to lack of sensory innervation of the rectum and due to the possibility of bowel perforation. Once inserted, squeeze the bottle until nearly all the liquid is expelled. If resistance is encountered on insertion of the nozzle or in administering the solution, the procedure should be discontinued. **Forcing the enema can result in perforation and/or abrasion of the rectum.**

Tablets

Adults and children 12 years of age and over: Take 1 to 3 tablets (usually 2) in a single dose once daily (per 24 hours).

Children 6 to under 12 years of age: Take 1 tablet once daily (per 24 hours).

Children under 6 years of age: Consult a physician.

Expect results in 6–12 hours if taken at bedtime or within 6 hours if taken before breakfast. Swallow tablets whole. Do not chew or crush tablets. Do not administer tablets within 1 hour after taking an antacid, milk, or milk products.

HOW SUPPLIED
Enema
FLEET® Bisacodyl Enema is supplied in a 1.25 fl. oz. (37-mL) ready-to-use squeeze bottle.

NDC code: 0132070336.

Tablets
FLEET® Stimulant Laxative Tablets are supplied in cartons of 25 tablets (5 mg bisacodyl in each tablet) wrapped in a foil seal.

NDC code: 0132070402

IS THIS PRODUCT OTC? Yes.

QUESTIONS? Call 1-866-255-6960 or visit www.fleetlabs.com

FLEET® ENEMA, A SALINE LAXATIVE   OTC
FLEET® ENEMA EXTRA®, A SALINE LAXATIVE
FLEET® PEDIA-LAX® ENEMA, A SALINE LAXATIVE, FLEET® ENEMA FOR CHILDREN, A SALINE LAXATIVE

FLEET® enemas are designed for quick, convenient administration by nurse, patient or caregiver according to instructions. Each is disposable after a single use.

COMPOSITION
FLEET® ENEMA: Each FLEET® Enema unit, with a 2-inch, pre-lubricated Comfortip®, contains 4.5 fl. oz. (133 mL) of enema solution in a ready-to-use squeeze bottle which is **not made with natural rubber latex.** Each enema unit delivers a dose of 118 mL, which contains 19 g monobasic sodium phosphate monohydrate and 7 g dibasic sodium phosphate heptahydrate. Each Fleet® Enema 118 mL delivered dose contains 4.4 grams sodium.

FLEET® ENEMA EXTRA®: Each FLEET® Enema EXTRA® unit, with a 2-inch, pre-lubricated Comfortip®, contains 7.8 fl. oz. (230 mL) of enema solution in a ready-to-use squeeze bottle which is **not made with natural rubber latex.** Each enema unit delivers a dose of 197 mL, which contains 19 g monobasic sodium phosphate monohydrate and 7 g dibasic sodium phosphate heptahydrate. Each Fleet® Enema EXTRA® 197 mL delivered dose contains 4.4 grams sodium.

FLEET® PEDIA-LAX® ENEMA and FLEET® ENEMA FOR CHILDREN: Each Fleet® Pedia-Lax® Enema and FLEET® Enema for Children unit, with a 2-inch, pre-lubricated Comfortip®, contains 2.25 fl. oz. (66 mL) of enema solution in a ready-to-use squeeze bottle which is **not made with natural rubber latex.** Each enema unit delivers a dose of 59 mL, which contains 9.5 g monobasic sodium phosphate monohydrate and 3.5 g dibasic sodium phosphate heptahydrate. Each Fleet® Enema for Children and Fleet® Pedia-Lax® Enema 59 mL delivered dose contains 2.2 grams sodium.

ELEMENTAL AND ELECTROLYTIC CONTENT (Fleet® Enema, Fleet® Pedia-Lax® Enema and Fleet® Enema for Children)

mEq Phosphate (PO_4) per mL	4.15
mEq Sodium (Na) per mL	1.61
mg Sodium (Na) per mL	37
mmole Phosphorus (P) per mL	1.38

ELEMENTAL AND ELECTROLYTIC CONTENT (Fleet® Enema EXTRA®)

mEq Phosphate (PO_4) per mL	2.484
mEq Sodium (Na) per mL	0.961
mg Sodium (Na) per mL	22.1
mmole Phosphorus (P) per mL	0.828

ACTION AND USES

FLEET® Enema, FLEET® Enema EXTRA®, Fleet® Pedia-Lax® Enema and FLEET® Enema for Children are useful as laxatives in the relief of occasional constipation and as part of a bowel cleansing regimen in preparing the colon for surgery, x-ray or endoscopic examination.

When used as directed, FLEET® Enema, FLEET® Enema EXTRA®, Fleet® Pedia-Lax® Enema and FLEET® Enema for Children provide thorough yet safe cleansing action and induce complete emptying of the left colon, usually within 1 to 5 minutes, without pain or spasm.

INFORMATION FOR PATIENT
WARNINGS
Using more than one enema in 24 hours can be harmful.

AFTER THE ENEMA SOLUTION IS ADMINISTERED, THE RETENTION TIME SHOULD NOT EXCEED 10 MINUTES. IF THE RETENTION TIME EXCEEDS 10 MINUTES OR THERE IS NO RETURN OF ENEMA SOLUTION, CONTACT A PHYSICIAN IMMEDIATELY, AS ELECTROLYTE DISTURBANCES AND CONSEQUENT SERIOUS SIDE EFFECTS COULD OCCUR.

DO NOT USE ANY FLEET® ENEMA IN CHILDREN UNDER 2 YEARS OF AGE.

DO NOT ADMINISTER THE 4.5 FL. OZ. (133 mL) ADULT SIZE OR THE 7.8 FL.OZ. (230 mL) EXTRA® SIZE TO CHILDREN UNDER 12 YEARS OF AGE.

DO NOT ADMINISTER A FULL 2.25 FL. OZ. (66 mL) CHILDREN'S SIZE TO CHILDREN UNDER 5 YEARS OF AGE.

FOR CHILDREN 2 TO UNDER 5 YEARS, USE ONE-HALF BOTTLE OF 2.25 FL. OZ. (66 mL) CHILDREN'S SIZE. (SEE **DOSAGE AND ADMINISTRATION**).

IMPORTANT: FLEET® Enema (Adult size), FLEET® Enema EXTRA®, Fleet® Pedia-Lax® Enema and Fleet® Enema for Children ARE NOT INTENDED FOR ORAL CONSUMPTION in any dosage size.

When using any of these Fleet® enemas, patient may experience anal discomfort.

GENERAL LAXATIVE WARNINGS

Ask a doctor before using any laxative if you have (or your child has)

• abdominal pain, nausea or vomiting

• a sudden change in bowel habits lasting more than 2 weeks

• already used a laxative for more than 1 week

Stop using this product and consult a doctor if you have (or your child has)

• rectal bleeding

• no bowel movement within 30 minutes of using this product

• if constipation continues after one week of use

• symptoms that your body (or your child's body) is losing more fluids than you (or your child) are drinking. This is called dehydration. Early symptoms of dehydration include feeling thirsty, dizziness, urinating less often than normal and vomiting.

These symptoms may be signs of a serious condition.

Fleet enemas should be administered according to the instructions for use and handling. Stop use if resistance is encountered as forced administration of the enema may cause injury.

As with any drug, if you are pregnant or nursing a baby, seek the advice of a healthcare professional before using this product. As sodium phosphate may pass into the breast milk, it is advised that breast milk is expressed and discarded for at least 24 hours after receiving the Fleet® enema.

Keep this and all drugs out of the reach of children to prevent accidental ingestion. In case of accidental overdose or ingestion, seek professional assistance or contact a Poison Control Center right away.

PROFESSIONAL USE INFORMATION
CONTRAINDICATIONS
Do not use in patients with

• Congestive heart failure

• Clinically significant impairment of renal function

• Known or suspected gastrointestinal obstruction

• Megacolon (congenital or acquired)

• Paralytic ileus

• Perforation

• Active inflammatory bowel disease

• Imperforate anus

• Dehydration

• Generally in all cases where absorption capacity is increased or elimination capacity is decreased

• Children under 2 years of age

• Hypersensitivity to active ingredients or to any of the excipients of the product

PRECAUTIONS
Use with caution in patients

• With impaired renal function

• Taking medications known to affect renal perfusion or function, or hydration status

• With pre-existing electrolyte disturbances or who are taking diuretics or other medications which may affect electrolyte levels

• Who are taking medications known to prolong the QT interval

• Ascites

• With a colostomy

• In children 2-11 years of age

• 65 or older and under a doctor's care for any medical condition

• Who are pregnant or nursing a baby

Patients with conditions that may predispose to dehydration or those taking medications which may decrease glomerular filtration rate, such as diuretics, angiotensin converting enzyme inhibitors (ACE-Is), angiotensin receptor blockers (ARBs), or non-steroidal anti-inflammatory drugs (NSAIDs), should be assessed for hydration status prior to use and managed appropriately.

Fleet® Pedia-Lax® Enema and Fleet® Enema for Children should be used with caution in children of any age. Careful consideration of the use of enemas in children in general is recommended.

Careful consideration of the use of sodium phosphates enemas in the elderly with co-morbidities is also recommended. See PROFESSIONAL USE WARNINGS. In those cases where complications have been reported, elderly patients with co-morbidities are often involved.

Since FLEET® enemas contain sodium phosphates, in all patients there is a risk of elevated serum levels of sodium and phosphate and decreased levels of calcium and potassium, and consequently hypernatremia, hyperphosphatemia, hypocalcemia and hypokalemia may occur which could result in metabolic acidosis, tetany, renal failure, QT prolongation and/or, in more severe cases, multi-organ failure, cardiac arrhythmia/arrest and death. This is of particular concern in children with megacolon or any other condition where there is retention of enema solution, and in patients with co-morbidities, particularly gastrointestinal, renal and neurological disorders. If any patient develops vomiting and/or signs of dehydration, measure post-administration labs (phosphate, calcium, potassium, sodium, creatinine, GFR and BUN).

SINCE FLEET® BRAND ENEMAS ARE AVAILABLE IN ADULT, ADULT EXTRA, AND CHILDREN'S SIZES, PRESCRIBE CAREFULLY.

DRUG INTERACTIONS

NO OTHER SODIUM PHOSPHATES PREPARATIONS INCLUDING SODIUM PHOSPHATES ORAL SOLUTION OR TABLETS SHOULD BE GIVEN CONCOMITANTLY. Electrolyte disturbances and hypovolemia from purgation may be exacerbated by inadequate oral fluid intake, nausea, vomiting, loss of appetite, or use of diuretics, angiotensin converting enzyme inhibitors (ACE-Is), angiotensin receptor blockers (ARBs), non-steroidal anti-inflammatory drugs (NSAIDs), and lithium or other medications that may affect electrolyte levels, and may result in metabolic acidosis, tetany, renal failure, QT prolongation and, in more severe cases, multi-organ failure, cardiac arrhythmia/arrest and death.

As hypernatremia is associated with lower lithium levels, concomitant use of Fleet® enemas and lithium therapy could lead to a fall in serum lithium levels with a lessening of effectiveness.

POSSIBLE SIDE EFFECTS

Hypersensitivity
Pruritis
Dehydration
Hyperphosphatemia
Hypocalcemia
Hypokalemia
Hypernatremia
Metabolic Acidosis
Nausea
Vomiting
Abdominal Pain
Abdominal Distension
Diarrhea
Gastrointestinal Pain
Chills
Blistering
Stinging
Anal Discomfort
Proctalgia

HYDRATION

Additional liquids by mouth are recommended.
Encourage patients to drink large amounts of clear liquids to prevent dehydration. Inadequate fluid intake when using any effective purgative may lead to excessive fluid loss, possibly producing dehydration and hypovolemia.

OVERDOSAGE OR RETENTION

Overdosage (more than one enema in a 24-hour period), no return of enema solution, retention time greater than 10 minutes or failure to have a bowel movement within 30 minutes of enema use may lead to severe electrolyte disturbances, including hypernatremia, hyperphosphatemia, hypocalcemia, and hypokalemia, as well as dehydration and hypovolemia, with attendant signs and symptoms of these disturbances (such as metabolic acidosis, renal failure, and tetany), QT prolongation and/or, in more severe cases, multi-organ failure, cardiac arrhythmia/arrest and death. The patient who has taken an overdose or who has retained the product for more than 10 minutes should be monitored carefully. If any patient develops vomiting and/or signs of dehydration, measure post-procedure labs (phosphate, calcium, potassium, sodium, creatinine, GFR and BUN). **Treatment of electrolyte imbalance may require immediate medical intervention with appropriate electrolyte and fluid replacement therapy.**

DOSAGE AND ADMINISTRATION

Dosage: FLEET® Enema (Adult size) and FLEET® Enema EXTRA®:
Use only 1 enema per 24 hours.
Do not use more unless directed by a doctor. See Warnings. Do not use if taking another sodium phosphates product.

Age	Daily Dose (per 24 hours)
adults and children 12 years and older	one bottle
children 2 to 11 years	use Fleet® Pedia-Lax® Enema or FLEET® Enema for Children (See below)
children under 2 years	DO NOT USE

How to use this enema:
- **REMOVE ORANGE PROTECTIVE SHIELD FROM ENEMA COMFORTIP® BEFORE INSERTING.**
- With steady pressure, gently insert enema tip into rectum with a slight side-to-side movement, with tip pointing toward navel. Insertion may be easier if person receiving enema bears down, as if having a bowel movement. This helps relax the muscles around the anus.
- **DO NOT FORCE THE ENEMA TIP INTO RECTUM AS THIS CAN CAUSE INJURY.**
- Squeeze bottle until nearly all liquid is gone. It is not necessary to empty the bottle completely, as it contains more liquid than needed.
- Remove Comfortip® from rectum and maintain position until urge to evacuate is strong (usually 1 to 5 minutes). Do not retain enema solution for more than 10 minutes. Contact a doctor if there is no bowel movement within 30 minutes of enema use.

Positions for using this enema:
- **Left-side position:** Lie on left side with knee bent, and arms resting comfortably.
- **Knee-chest position:** Kneel, then lower head and chest forward until left side of face is resting on surface with left arm folded comfortably.

The diaphragm at base of nozzle prevents reflux and assures controlled flow of the enema solution. Fleet® Enema should be used at room temperature.

Dosage: Fleet® Pedia-Lax® Enema and FLEET® Enema for Children:
Use only 1 enema per 24 hours.
Do not use more unless directed by a doctor. See Warnings. **Do not use if child is taking another sodium phosphates product.**

Age	Daily Dose (per 24 hours)
children 5 to 11 years	one bottle or as directed by a doctor
children 2 to under 5 years	one-half bottle (see below) or as directed by a doctor
children under 2 years	DO NOT USE

One-half bottle preparation: Unscrew cap and remove 2 Tablespoons of liquid with a measuring spoon. Replace cap and follow DIRECTIONS on back of carton.
How to use this enema:
- **REMOVE ORANGE PROTECTIVE SHIELD FROM ENEMA COMFORTIP® BEFORE INSERTING.**
- With steady pressure, gently insert enema tip into rectum with a slight side-to-side movement, with tip pointing toward navel. Insertion may be easier if child receiving enema bears down, as if having a bowel movement. This helps relax the muscles around the anus.
- **DO NOT FORCE THE ENEMA TIP INTO RECTUM AS THIS CAN CAUSE INJURY.**
- Squeeze bottle until nearly all liquid is gone. It is not necessary to empty the bottle completely, as it contains more liquid than needed.
- Remove Comfortip® from rectum and keep child in position until urge to evacuate is strong (usually 1 to 5 minutes). Do not allow child to retain enema solution for more than 10 minutes. Contact a doctor if the child doesn't have a bowel movement within 30 minutes of enema use.

Positions for using this enema:
- **Left-side position:** Place child on left side with knees bent, and arms resting comfortably.
- **Knee-chest position:** Have child kneel, then lower head and chest forward until left side of face is resting on surface with left arm folded comfortably.

The diaphragm at base of nozzle prevents reflux and assures controlled flow of the enema solution. Fleet® Pedia-Lax® Enema and FLEET® Enema for Children should be used at room temperature.

PROFESSIONAL DOSAGE AND ADMINISTRATION

Administration of more than one enema in 24 hours can be harmful. In those cases where complications have been reported, overdoses are often involved.
NO OTHER SODIUM PHOSPHATES PREPARATIONS INCLUDING SODIUM PHOSPHATES ORAL SOLUTION OR TABLETS SHOULD BE GIVEN CONCOMITANTLY. FLEET® Enema (Adult size) and FLEET® Enema EXTRA® should not be used in children under 12 years of age. In those cases where complications have been reported, infants and young children are often involved. Fleet® Pedia-Lax® Enema and FLEET® Enema for Children should be used with caution in children of any age. Careful consideration of the use of enemas in children in general is recommended.
Careful consideration of the use of sodium phosphates enemas in the elderly with co-morbidities is also recommended. See PROFESSIONAL USE WARNINGS. In those cases where complications have been reported, elderly patients with co-morbidities are often involved.
See **DOSAGE AND ADMINISTRATION** for dosing detail.

Proper and safe use of FLEET® Enemas also requires that the products be administered according to the Directions. Healthcare professionals should remember when administering the product to gently insert the enema into the rectum with the tip pointing toward the navel. Insertion may be made easier by having the patient bear down as if having a bowel movement. Care during insertion is necessary due to lack of sensory innervation of the rectum and due to possibility of bowel perforation. Once inserted, squeeze the bottle until nearly all the liquid is expelled. If resistance is encountered on insertion of the nozzle or in administering the solution, the procedure should be discontinued. **Forcing the enema can result in perforation and/or abrasion of the rectum.**

If an enema containing phosphate or sodium is not advised, consider using FLEET® Bisacodyl Enema.

HOW SUPPLIED

FLEET® Enema is supplied in a 4.5 fl. oz. (133-mL) ready-to-use squeeze bottle. NDC code: 0132020140 (single), 0132020142 (twin), 0132020145 (4-pack), 0132011946 (6-pack), Fleet® Enema EXTRA® is supplied in a 7.8 fl. oz. (230-mL) ready-to-use squeeze bottle. NDC code: 0132020110 Fleet® Pedia-Lax® Enema and Fleet® Enema for Children are supplied in a 2.25 fl. oz. (66 mL) ready-to-use squeeze bottle. NDC code: 0132020220
IS THIS PRODUCT OTC? Yes.
QUESTIONS? Call 1-866-255-6960 or visit www.fleetlabs.com

FLEET® MINERAL OIL ENEMA   OTC
A LUBRICANT LAXATIVE

COMPOSITION

FLEET® Mineral Oil Enema unit, with a 2-inch, pre-lubricated Comfortip®, delivers 118 mL of mineral oil, 100%, in a ready-to-use squeeze bottle **not made with natural rubber latex.** FLEET® Mineral Oil Enema is sodium-free. The unit is disposable after a single use.

ACTION AND USES

FLEET® Mineral Oil Enema serves to soften and lubricate hard stools, easing their passage without irritating the mucosa. Results approximate a normal bowel movement in that only the rectum, sigmoid, and part or all of the descending colon are evacuated. FLEET® Mineral Oil Enema is indicated for relief of fecal impaction; is valuable in relief of occasional constipation when straining must be avoided (in hypertension, coronary occlusion, proctologic procedures, or postoperative care); is indicated for removal of barium sulfate residues from the colon after barium administration and is indicated for obtaining the laxative benefits of mineral oil while avoiding possible untoward effects of oral administration such as (1) interference with intestinal absorption of fat-soluble vitamins A, D, E and K and other nutrients, (2) danger of systemic absorption, or (3) possible risk of lipid pneumonia due to aspiration. It is generally effective in 2 to 15 minutes.

WARNINGS

DO NOT ADMINISTER TO CHILDREN UNDER 2 YEARS OF AGE.

GENERAL LAXATIVE WARNINGS
INFORMATION FOR PATIENT
Ask a doctor before using any laxative if you have
- abdominal pain, nausea or vomiting
- a sudden change in bowel habits lasting more than 2 weeks
- already used a laxative for more than 1 week
Stop using this product and consult a doctor if you have
- rectal bleeding
- no bowel movement within 15 minutes of using this product
- if constipation continues after one week of use
These symptoms may be signs of a serious condition.
As with any drug, if you are pregnant or nursing a baby, seek the advice of a healthcare professional before using this product.
Keep this and all drugs out of the reach of children to prevent accidental ingestion. In case of accidental overdose or ingestion, seek professional assistance or contact a Poison Control Center right away.

DOSAGE AND ADMINISTRATION

Use only 1 enema per 24 hours.

Adults & children 12 years of age and over	1 bottle
Children 2 to 11 years of age	One-half bottle
Children under 2 years of age	DO NOT USE

One-half bottle preparation: Unscrew cap and remove 4 Tablespoons of liquid with a measuring spoon. Replace cap and follow DIRECTIONS on back of carton.

Positions for using this enema:
- **Left-side position:** Lie on left side with knee bent, and arms resting comfortably.
- **Knee-chest position:** Kneel, then lower head and chest forward until left side of face is resting on surface with left arm folded comfortably.

REMOVE ORANGE PROTECTIVE SHIELD FROM ENEMA COMFORTIP® BEFORE INSERTING.
- With steady pressure, gently insert enema tip into rectum with a slight side-to-side movement, with tip pointing toward navel. Insertion may be easier if person receiving enema bears down, as if having a bowel movement. This helps relax the muscles around the anus.
- **DISCONTINUE USE IF RESISTANCE IS ENCOUNTERED. FORCING THE TIP INTO RECTUM CAN CAUSE INJURY**
- Squeeze bottle until nearly all liquid is gone. It is not necessary to empty the bottle completely, as it contains more liquid than needed. A small amount of liquid will remain in the bottle after squeezing.
- Remove tip from rectum and discard bottle. The enema will usually cause a bowel movement within 2 to 15 minutes. Do not retain liquid for more than 15 minutes.
- Stop using this product and consult a doctor if you don't have a bowel movement within 15 minutes of using this product.

The diaphragm at base of nozzle prevents reflux and assures controlled flow of the enema solution. The enema should be used at room temperature.

PROFESSIONAL DOSAGE AND ADMINISTRATION

FLEET® Mineral Oil Enema should not be used in children under 2 years of age and should be used with caution in children of any age. In general, careful consideration of the use of enemas in children is recommended.

Proper and safe use of FLEET® Mineral Oil Enema also requires that the product be administered according to the Directions. Healthcare professionals should remember when administering the product to gently insert the enema into the rectum with the tip pointing toward the navel. Insertion may be made easier by having the patient bear down as if having a bowel movement. Care during insertion is necessary due to lack of sensory innervation of the rectum and due to the possibility of bowel perforation. Once inserted, squeeze the bottle until nearly all the liquid is expelled. If resistance is encountered on insertion of the nozzle or in administering the solution, the procedure should be discontinued. **Forcing the enema can result in perforation and/or abrasion of the rectum.**

HOW SUPPLIED

FLEET® Mineral Oil Enema is supplied in 4.5 fl. oz. (133-mL) ready-to-use squeeze bottle.
NDC code: 0132030140.
IS THIS PRODUCT OTC? Yes.
QUESTIONS? Call 1-866-255-6960 or visit www.fleetlabs.com

FLEET® PEDIA-LAX® DOCUSATE SODIUM LIQUID STOOL SOFTENER   OTC
Stool softener laxative

COMPOSITION

Active ingredient (in each tablespoon – 15 mL)	Purpose
Docusate sodium 50 mg	Stool softener

Each tablespoon (15 mL) contains 13 mg sodium.

USES
- to help prevent dry, hard stools
- to relieve occasional constipation

DESCRIPTION

Docusate sodium is a stool softener laxative, given orally, which usually produces a bowel movement within 12 to 72 hours. Stool softener laxatives penetrate and soften the stool, thereby promoting bowel movement.

INFORMATION FOR PATIENT

DRUG INTERACTION PRECAUTION: Do not give this product to child if child is presently taking mineral oil, unless directed by a doctor.

WARNINGS

Ask a doctor before using any laxative if your child has
- abdominal pain, nausea or vomiting
- a sudden change in bowel habits lasting more than 2 weeks
- already used a laxative for more than 1 week

Stop using this product and consult a doctor if your child has
- rectal bleeding

- no bowel movement within 72 hours of using this product
- if constipation continues after one week of use, contact your child's doctor.

These symptoms may be signs of a serious condition.

Keep this and all drugs out of the reach of children to prevent accidental ingestion. In case of overdose, get medical help or contact a Poison Control Center right away.

DIRECTIONS

Doses may be taken as a single daily dose or in divided doses in a 24-hour period.

Doses can be given in a glass of juice to prevent throat irritation and to help mask the naturally tart flavor of the active ingredient.

Dosing Chart

Age	Starting Dose	Maximum Dose per Day (24 hours)
Children 2 to 11 years	1–3 tablespoons	3 tablespoons
Children under 2	Ask a doctor	Ask a doctor

Professional Labeling: Dosage and Administration for children less than 2 years of age: 20 to 50 mg in a single daily dose or in divided doses (per 24 hours).

Inactive ingredients: citric acid, edetate disodium, FD&C Red #3, flavor, methylparaben, polyethylene glycol, povidone, propylene glycol, propylparaben, sodium citrate, sorbitol, sucralose, water, xanthan gum, xylitol.

HOW SUPPLIED

4 fl.oz. (118 mL) bottles with child-resistant cap, and sealed for your protection. Fruit punch flavor.
NDC code: 0132010624
IS THIS PRODUCT OTC? Yes.
QUESTIONS? Call 1-866-255-6960 or visit www.Pedia-Lax.com

FLEET® PEDIA-LAX® MAGNESIUM HYDROXIDE CHEWABLE TABLETS   OTC
Saline laxative

COMPOSITION

Active ingredient (in each tablet):	Purpose
Magnesium hydroxide 400 mg	Saline laxative

Each tablet contains 170 mg magnesium.

USE
- to relieve occasional constipation

DESCRIPTION

Magnesium hydroxide is a saline laxative, given orally, which usually produces a bowel movement within 30 minutes to 6 hours. Saline laxatives increase water in the intestine thereby promoting bowel movement.

INFORMATION FOR PATIENT
WARNINGS

Ask a physician before using this product if child has a magnesium-restricted diet or kidney disease.

Ask a doctor before using any laxative if your child has
- abdominal pain, nausea or vomiting
- a sudden change in bowel habits lasting more than 2 weeks
- already used a laxative for more than 1 week

Stop using this product and consult a doctor if your child has
- rectal bleeding
- no bowel movement within 6 hours of taking this product
- if constipation continues after one week of use, contact your child's doctor.

These symptoms may be signs of a serious condition.

Keep this and all drugs out of the reach of children to prevent accidental ingestion. In case of overdose, get medical help or contact a Poison Control Center right away.

DIRECTIONS

Doses may be taken as a single daily dose or in divided doses in a 24-hour period. **Have child drink a full glass (8 fluid ounces) of liquid with each dose.**

Dosing Chart

Age	Starting Dose	Maximum Dose per Day (24 hours)
Children 6 to 11 years	3–6 tablets	6 tablets
Children 2 to 5 years	1–3 tablets	3 tablets
Children under 2	Ask a doctor	Ask a doctor

Inactive ingredients: colloidal silicon dioxide, FD&C Red #40 aluminum lake, flavor, magnesium stearate, maltodextrin, mannitol, sorbitol, stearic acid, sucralose

HOW SUPPLIED

30 Pedia-Lax Chewable Tablets per bottle with child-resistant cap, sealed for your protection. Watermelon flavor.
NDC code: 0132065501
IS THIS PRODUCT OTC? Yes
QUESTIONS?
Call 1-866-255-6960 or visit www.Pedia-Lax.com

PHAZYME® ANTIGAS   OTC
SIMETHICONE SOFTGEL

COMPOSITION

Each Phazyme® Maximum Strength softgel contains 250 mg of Simethicone

Each Phazyme® Ultra Strength softgel contains 180 mg of Simethicone

ACTIONS AND USES

Simethicone is used to relieve bloating, pressure or fullness commonly referred to as gas. Simethicone reduces the surface tension of gas bubbles in the stomach, allowing them to break up or create a larger gas mass which is more easily expelled from the gastrointestinal tract.

INFORMATION FOR PATIENT
GENERAL WARNINGS
Stop use and ask a doctor if condition persists.
Keep out of the reach of children.

Due to the low potential for acute toxicity resulting from accidental ingestion, the labeling for antiflatulent drug products containing simethicone is exempt from the requirement that the labeling bear the general warning statement "In case of accidental overdose, seek professional assistance or contact a poison control center immediately."

DOSAGE AND ADMINISTRATION

The maximum daily dose for Simethicone is 500 mg. Swallow one or two softgels as symptoms occur. Do not exceed two softgels per day except under the advice and supervision of a physician.

PROFESSIONAL DOSAGE AND ADMINISTRATION

There is no dosage limitation at this time for professional labeling.

Maximum Strength Phazyme® 250 mg and **Ultra Strength Phazyme® 180 mg** may be used to relieve postoperative gas pain or for use in endoscopic examination.

INACTIVE INGREDIENTS

Phazyme® 250 mg
DC red no. 33, FD&C blue no. 1, gelatin, glycerin, purified water, white edible ink.
Phazyme® 180 mg
FD&C yellow no. 6, gelatin, glycerin, purified water, white edible ink.

HOW SUPPLIED

Maximum Strength Phazyme® 250 mg is available in 12 (NDC 0132021112), 24 (NDC 0132021424) and 36 (NDC 0132021537) count blister packs.
Ultra Strength Phazyme® 180 mg is available in 12 (NDC 0132020812) count blister packs, 48 (NDC 0132020848) count blister packs and 60 (NDC 0132020860) count bottles.
IS THIS PRODUCT OTC?
Yes.

QUESTIONS?

Call 1-855-727-4277 or visit www.phazyme.com

Help your patients save on prescription drugs with the PDR® Pharmacy Discount Card.
For more, visit PDR.net/PharmacyDiscountCard.

Help Patients Save on Rx Drugs: PDR.net/PharmacyDiscountCard

Gilead Sciences, Inc.

333 LAKESIDE DRIVE
FOSTER CITY, CA 94404
www.gilead.com

For Medical Information:
1-800-445-3235, press option 2
or www.gilead.com/medicines/request-information
To Report Adverse Events:
1-800-445-3235, press option 3
For Business Operations:
1-800-445-3235, press option 8

ATRIPLA®

ATRIPLA® is co-marketed by Bristol-Myers Squibb and Gilead Sciences. Please see Bristol-Myers Squibb & Gilead Sciences, LLC for full prescribing information.
Shown in Product Identification Guide, page 306

CAYSTON®   ℞

[*kay-stun*]
(aztreonam for inhalation solution)

HIGHLIGHTS OF PRESCRIBING INFORMATION
These highlights do not include all the information needed to use CAYSTON safely and effectively. See full prescribing information for CAYSTON.

CAYSTON® (aztreonam for inhalation solution)
Initial U.S. Approval: 1986

To reduce the development of drug-resistant bacteria and maintain the effectiveness of CAYSTON and other antibacterial drugs, CAYSTON should be used only to treat patients with cystic fibrosis (CF) known to have *Pseudomonas aeruginosa* in the lungs.

——————INDICATIONS AND USAGE——————
CAYSTON is a monobactam antibacterial indicated to improve respiratory symptoms in cystic fibrosis (CF) patients with *Pseudomonas aeruginosa*. Safety and effectiveness have not been established in pediatric patients below the age of 7 years, patients with FEV_1 <25% or >75% predicted, or patients colonized with *Burkholderia cepacia*. (1)

——————DOSAGE AND ADMINISTRATION——————
• Administer one dose (one single use vial and one ampule of diluent) 3 times a day for 28 days. (2.1)
• Use dose immediately after reconstitution. (2.2)
• Administer only with the Altera® Nebulizer System. Do not administer with any other type of nebulizer. (2.3)

——————DOSAGE FORMS AND STRENGTHS——————
• Lyophilized aztreonam (75 mg/vial) (3)
• Diluent (0.17% sodium chloride): 1 mL/ampule (3)

——————CONTRAINDICATIONS——————
• Do not administer to patients with a known allergy to aztreonam. (4)

——————WARNINGS AND PRECAUTIONS——————
• Allergic reaction to CAYSTON was seen in clinical trials. Stop treatment if an allergic reaction occurs. Use caution when CAYSTON is administered to patients with a known allergic reaction to beta-lactams. (5.1)
• Bronchospasm has been reported with CAYSTON. Stop treatment if chest tightness develops during nebulizer use. (5.2)

——————ADVERSE REACTIONS——————
• Common adverse reactions (more than 5%) occurring more frequently in CAYSTON patients are cough, nasal congestion, wheezing, pharyngolaryngeal pain, pyrexia, chest discomfort, abdominal pain and vomiting. (6.1)

To report SUSPECTED ADVERSE REACTIONS, contact Gilead Sciences, Inc. at 1-800-GILEAD5, option 3 or FDA at 1-800-FDA-1088 or www.fda.gov/medwatch.
See 17 for PATIENT COUNSELING INFORMATION and FDA-approved patient labeling
Revised: 05/2014

FULL PRESCRIBING INFORMATION: CONTENTS*

FULL PRESCRIBING INFORMATION

1   INDICATIONS AND USAGE

CAYSTON® is indicated to improve respiratory symptoms in cystic fibrosis (CF) patients with *Pseudomonas aeruginosa*. Safety and effectiveness have not been established in pediatric patients below the age of 7 years, patients with FEV_1 <25% or >75% predicted, or patients colonized with *Burkholderia cepacia [see Clinical Studies (14)]*.
To reduce the development of drug-resistant bacteria and maintain the effectiveness of CAYSTON and other antibacterial drugs, CAYSTON should be used only to treat patients with CF known to have *Pseudomonas aeruginosa* in the lungs.

2   DOSAGE AND ADMINISTRATION
2.1   Dosing Information
The recommended dose of CAYSTON for both adults and pediatric patients 7 years of age and older is one single-use vial (75 mg of aztreonam) reconstituted with 1 mL of sterile diluent administered 3 times a day for a 28-day course (followed by 28 days off CAYSTON therapy). Dosage is not based on weight or adjusted for age. Doses should be taken at least 4 hours apart.
CAYSTON is administered by inhalation using an Altera® Nebulizer System. Patients should use a bronchodilator before administration of CAYSTON.

2.2   Instructions for CAYSTON Reconstitution
CAYSTON should be administered immediately after reconstitution. Do not reconstitute CAYSTON until ready to administer a dose.
Take one amber glass vial containing CAYSTON and one diluent ampule from the carton. To open the glass vial, carefully remove the metal ring by lifting or pulling the tab and remove the gray rubber stopper. Twist the tip off the diluent ampule and squeeze the liquid into the glass vial. Replace the rubber stopper, then gently swirl the vial until contents have completely dissolved.
The empty vial, stopper, and diluent ampule should be disposed of properly upon completion of dosing.

2.3   Instructions for CAYSTON Administration
CAYSTON is administered by inhalation using an Altera Nebulizer System. CAYSTON should not be administered with any other nebulizer. CAYSTON should not be mixed with any other drugs in the Altera Nebulizer Handset.
CAYSTON is not for intravenous or intramuscular administration.
Patients should use a bronchodilator before administration of CAYSTON. Short-acting bronchodilators can be taken between 15 minutes and 4 hours prior to each dose of CAYSTON. Alternatively, long-acting bronchodilators can be taken between 30 minutes and 12 hours prior to administration of CAYSTON. For patients taking multiple inhaled therapies, the recommended order of administration is as follows: bronchodilator, mucolytics, and lastly, CAYSTON.
To administer CAYSTON, pour the reconstituted solution into the handset of the nebulizer system. Turn the unit on. Place the mouthpiece of the handset in your mouth and breathe normally only through your mouth. Administration typically takes between 2 and 3 minutes. Further patient

instructions on how to administer CAYSTON are provided in the FDA-approved patient labeling. Instructions on testing nebulizer functionality and cleaning the handset are provided in the Instructions for Use included with the nebulizer system.

3   DOSAGE FORMS AND STRENGTHS
A dose of CAYSTON consists of a single-use vial of sterile, lyophilized aztreonam (75 mg) reconstituted with a 1 mL ampule of sterile diluent (0.17% sodium chloride). Reconstituted CAYSTON is administered by inhalation.

4   CONTRAINDICATIONS
CAYSTON is contraindicated in patients with a known allergy to aztreonam.

5   WARNINGS AND PRECAUTIONS
5.1   Allergic Reactions
Severe allergic reactions have been reported following administration of aztreonam for injection to patients with no known history of exposure to aztreonam. In addition, allergic reaction with facial rash, facial swelling, and throat tightness was reported with CAYSTON in clinical trials. If an allergic reaction to CAYSTON occurs, stop administration of CAYSTON and initiate treatment as appropriate. Caution is advised when administering CAYSTON to patients if they have a history of beta-lactam allergy, although patients with a known beta-lactam allergy have received CAYSTON in clinical trials and no severe allergic reactions were reported. A history of allergy to beta-lactam antibiotics, such as penicillins, cephalosporins, and/or carbapenems, may be a risk factor, since cross-reactivity may occur.

5.2   Bronchospasm
Bronchospasm is a complication associated with nebulized therapies, including CAYSTON. Reduction of 15% or more in forced expiratory volume in 1 second (FEV_1) immediately following administration of study medication after pretreatment with a bronchodilator was observed in 3% of patients treated with CAYSTON.

5.3   Decreases in FEV_1 After 28-Day Treatment Cycle
In clinical trials, patients with increases in FEV_1 during a 28-day course of CAYSTON were sometimes treated for pulmonary exacerbations when FEV_1 declined after the treatment period. Healthcare providers should consider a patient's baseline FEV_1 measured prior to CAYSTON therapy and the presence of other symptoms when evaluating whether post-treatment changes in FEV_1 are caused by a pulmonary exacerbation.

5.4   Development of Drug-Resistant Bacteria
Prescribing CAYSTON in the absence of known *Pseudomonas aeruginosa* infection in patients with CF is unlikely to provide benefit and increases the risk of development of drug-resistant bacteria.

6   ADVERSE REACTIONS
6.1   Clinical Trials Experience
Because clinical trials are conducted under widely varying conditions, adverse reaction rates observed in the clinical trials of drugs cannot be directly compared to rates in the clinical trials of another drug and may not reflect the rates observed in practice.
The safety of CAYSTON was evaluated in 344 patients from two placebo-controlled trials and one open-label follow-on trial. In controlled trials, 146 patients with CF received 75 mg CAYSTON 3 times a day for 28 days.
Table 1 displays adverse reactions reported in more than 5% of patients treated with CAYSTON 3 times a day in placebo-controlled trials. The listed adverse reactions occurred more frequently in CAYSTON-treated patients than in placebo-treated patients.

Table 1 Adverse Reactions Reported in more than 5% of Patients Treated with CAYSTON in the Placebo-Controlled Trials

Event (Preferred Term)	Placebo (N=160) n (%)	CAYSTON 75 mg 3 times a day (N=146) n (%)
Cough	82 (51%)	79 (54%)
Nasal congestion	19 (12%)	23 (16%)
Wheezing	16 (10%)	23 (16%)
Pharyngolaryngeal pain	17 (11%)	18 (12%)
Pyrexia	9 (6%)	19 (13%)
Chest discomfort	10 (6%)	11 (8%)
Abdominal Pain	8 (5%)	10 (7%)
Vomiting	7 (4%)	9 (6%)

Adverse reactions that occurred in less than 5% of patients treated with CAYSTON were bronchospasm (3%) [see *Warnings and Precautions (5.2)*] and rash (2%).

6.2 Postmarketing Experience

In addition to adverse reactions reported from clinical trials, the following possible adverse reactions have been identified during post-approval use of CAYSTON. Because these events have been reported voluntarily from a population of unknown size, estimates of frequency cannot be made.
MUSCULOSKELETAL AND CONNECTIVE TISSUE DISORDERS
Arthralgia, joint swelling

7 DRUG INTERACTIONS

No formal clinical studies of drug interactions with CAYSTON have been conducted.

8 USE IN SPECIFIC POPULATIONS

8.1 Pregnancy

Pregnancy Category B
No reproductive toxicology studies have been conducted with CAYSTON. However, studies were conducted with aztreonam for injection. Aztreonam has been shown to cross the placenta and enter fetal circulation. No evidence of embryo or fetotoxicity or teratogenicity has been shown in studies with pregnant rats and rabbits. In rats receiving aztreonam for injection during late gestation and lactation, no drug induced changes in maternal, fetal or neonatal parameters were observed. These animal reproduction and developmental toxicity studies used parenteral routes of administration that would provide systemic exposures far in excess of the average peak plasma levels measured in humans following CAYSTON therapy.

No adequate and well-controlled studies of aztreonam for injection or CAYSTON in pregnant women have been conducted. Because animal reproduction studies are not always predictive of human response, CAYSTON should be used during pregnancy only if clearly needed.

8.3 Nursing Mothers

Following administration of aztreonam for injection, aztreonam is excreted in human milk at concentrations that are less than one percent of those determined in simultaneously obtained maternal serum. Peak plasma concentrations of aztreonam following administration of CAYSTON (75 mg) are approximately 1% of peak concentrations observed following IV aztreonam (500 mg). Therefore, use of CAYSTON during breastfeeding is unlikely to pose a risk to infants.

8.4 Pediatric Use

Patients 7 years and older were included in clinical trials with CAYSTON. Fifty-five patients under 18 years of age received CAYSTON in placebo-controlled trials. No dose adjustments were made for pediatric patients. Pyrexia was more commonly reported in pediatric patients than in adult patients. Safety and effectiveness in pediatric patients below the age of 7 years have not been established.

8.5 Geriatric Use

Clinical trials of CAYSTON did not include CAYSTON-treated patients aged 65 years of age and older to determine whether they respond differently from younger patients.

8.6 Use in Patients with Renal Impairment

Aztreonam is known to be excreted by the kidney. Placebo-controlled clinical trials with CAYSTON excluded patients with abnormal baseline renal function (defined as serum creatinine greater than 2 times the upper limit of normal range). Given the low systemic exposure of aztreonam following administration of CAYSTON, clinically relevant accumulation of aztreonam is unlikely to occur in patients with renal impairment. Therefore, CAYSTON may be administered to patients with mild, moderate and severe renal impairment with no dosage adjustment.

10 OVERDOSAGE

No overdoses have been reported with CAYSTON in clinical trials to date. In clinical trials, 225 mg doses of CAYSTON via inhalation were associated with higher rates of drug-related respiratory adverse reactions, particularly cough. Since the peak plasma concentration of aztreonam following administration of CAYSTON (75 mg) is approximately 0.6 mcg/mL, compared to a serum concentration of 54 mcg/mL following administration of aztreonam for injection (500 mg), no systemic safety issues associated with CAYSTON overdose are anticipated.

11 DESCRIPTION

A dose of CAYSTON consists of a 2 mL amber glass vial containing lyophilized aztreonam (75 mg) and lysine (46.7 mg), and a low-density polyethylene ampule containing 1 mL sterile diluent (0.17% sodium chloride). The reconstituted solution is for inhalation. The formulation contains no preservatives or arginine.

The active ingredient in CAYSTON is aztreonam, a monobactam antibacterial. The monobactams are structurally different from beta-lactam antibiotics (e.g., penicillins, cephalosporins, carbapenems) due to a monocyclic nucleus. This nucleus contains several side chains; sulfonic acid in the 1-position activates the nucleus, an aminothiazolyl oxime side chain in the 3-position confers specificity for aerobic Gram-negative bacteria including *Pseudomonas spp.*, and a methyl group in the 4-position enhances beta-lactamase stability.

Aztreonam is designated chemically as (Z)-2-[[[(2-amino-4-thiazolyl)][(2S,3S)-2-methyl-4-oxo-1-sulfo-3-azetidinyl]carbamoyl]methylene]amino]oxy]-2-methylpropionic acid. The structural formula is presented below:

CAYSTON is a white to off-white powder. CAYSTON is sterile, hygroscopic, and light sensitive. Once reconstituted with the supplied diluent, the pH range is 4.5 to 6.0.

12 CLINICAL PHARMACOLOGY

12.1 Mechanism of Action

Aztreonam is an antibacterial drug [*see Clinical Pharmacology (12.4)*].

12.3 Pharmacokinetics

Sputum Concentrations
Sputum aztreonam concentrations exhibited considerable variability between patients receiving CAYSTON (75 mg) in clinical trials. The mean sputum concentration 10 minutes following the first dose of CAYSTON (n = 195 patients with CF) was 726 mcg/g. Mean sputum concentrations of aztreonam in patients receiving CAYSTON 3 times a day for 28 days were 984 mcg/g, 793 mcg/g, and 715 mcg/g 10 minutes after dose administration on Days 0, 14, and 28, respectively, indicating no accumulation of aztreonam in sputum.

Plasma Concentrations
Plasma aztreonam concentrations exhibited considerable variability between patients receiving CAYSTON (75 mg) in the clinical trials. The mean plasma concentration one hour following the first dose of CAYSTON (at approximately the peak plasma concentration) was 0.59 mcg/mL. Mean peak plasma concentrations in patients receiving CAYSTON 3 times a day for 28 days were 0.55 mcg/mL, 0.67 mcg/mL, and 0.65 mcg/mL on Days 0, 14, and 28, respectively, indicating no systemic accumulation of aztreonam. In contrast, the serum concentration of aztreonam following administration of aztreonam for injection (500 mg) is approximately 54 mcg/mL.

Absorption
Evaluation of plasma and urine aztreonam concentrations following administration of CAYSTON indicates low systemic absorption of aztreonam. Approximately 10% of the total CAYSTON dose is excreted in the urine as unchanged drug, as compared to 60–65% following intravenous administration of aztreonam for injection.

Distribution
The protein binding of aztreonam in serum is approximately 56% and is independent of dose.

Metabolism
Following intramuscular administration of aztreonam for injection 500 mg every 8 hours for 7 days, approximately 6% of the dose was excreted as a microbiologically inactive open β-lactam ring hydrolysis product in an 8-hour urine collection on the last day of multiple dosing.

Excretion
The elimination half-life of aztreonam from plasma is approximately 2.1 hours following administration of CAYSTON to adult patients with CF, similar to what has been reported for aztreonam for injection. Approximately 10% of the total CAYSTON dose is excreted in the urine as unchanged drug. Systemically absorbed aztreonam is eliminated about equally by active tubular secretion and glomerular filtration. Following administration of a single intravenous dose of radiolabeled aztreonam for injection, about 12% of the dose was recovered in the feces.

12.4 Microbiology

Mechanism of Action
Aztreonam exhibits activity *in vitro* against Gram-negative aerobic pathogens including *P. aeruginosa*. Aztreonam binds to penicillin-binding proteins of susceptible bacteria, which leads to inhibition of bacterial cell wall synthesis and death of the cell. Aztreonam activity is not decreased in the presence of CF lung secretions.

Susceptibility Testing
A single sputum sample from a patient with CF may contain multiple morphotypes of *P. aeruginosa* and each morphotype may have a different level of *in vitro* susceptibility to aztreonam. There are no *in vitro* susceptibility test interpretive criteria for isolates of *P. aeruginosa* obtained from the sputum of CF patients.[1]

Development of Resistance
No changes in the susceptibility of *P. aeruginosa* to aztreonam were observed following a 28-day course of CAYSTON in the placebo-controlled trials.

Cross-Resistance
No cross-resistance to other classes of antibiotics, including aminoglycosides, quinolones, and beta-lactams, was observed following a 28-day course of CAYSTON in the Phase 3 placebo-controlled trials or in an open-label follow-on trial of up to nine 28-day courses of 75 mg CAYSTON 3 times a day.

Other
No trends in the treatment-emergent isolation of other bacterial respiratory pathogens (*Burkholderia cepacia*, *Stenotrophomonas maltophilia*, *Achromobacter xylosoxidans*, and *Staphylococcus aureus*) were observed in clinical trials. There was a slight increase in the isolation of *Candida spp.* following up to nine 28-day courses of CAYSTON therapy.

13 NONCLINICAL TOXICOLOGY

13.1 Carcinogenesis, Mutagenesis, Impairment of Fertility

A 104-week rat inhalation toxicology study to assess the carcinogenic potential of aztreonam demonstrated no drug-related increase in the incidence of tumors. Rats were exposed to aztreonam for up to 4 hours per day. Peak plasma levels of aztreonam averaging approximately 6.8 mcg/mL were measured in rats at the highest dose level. This is approximately 12-fold higher than the average peak plasma level measured in humans following CAYSTON therapy.

Genetic toxicology studies performed *in vitro* demonstrated that aztreonam did not induce structural chromosome aberrations in CHO cells and did not induce mutations at the TK locus in mouse lymphoma L5178Y TK$^{+/-}$ cells. Likewise, genetic toxicology studies performed *in vivo* did not reveal evidence of mutagenic potential.

Aztreonam did not impair the fertility of rats when administered at doses that would provide systemic exposures far in excess of peak plasma levels measured in humans following CAYSTON therapy.

14 CLINICAL STUDIES

CAYSTON was evaluated over a period of 28 days of treatment in a randomized, double-blind, placebo-controlled, multicenter trial that enrolled patients with CF and *P. aeruginosa*. This trial was designed to evaluate improvement in respiratory symptoms. Patients 7 years of age and older and with FEV_1 of 25% to 75% predicted were enrolled. All patients received CAYSTON or placebo on an outpatient basis administered with the Altera Nebulizer System. All patients were required to take a dose of an inhaled bronchodilator (beta-agonist) prior to taking a dose of CAYSTON or placebo. Patients were receiving standard care for CF, including drugs for obstructive airway diseases.

The trial enrolled 164 patients with CF and *P. aeruginosa*. The mean age was 30 years, and the mean baseline FEV_1 % predicted was 55%; 43% were females and 96% were Caucasian. These patients were randomized in a 1:1 ratio to receive either CAYSTON (75 mg) or volume-matched placebo administered by inhalation 3 times a day for 28 days. Patients were required to have been off antibiotics for at least 28 days before treatment with study drug. The primary efficacy endpoint was improvement in respiratory symptoms on the last day of treatment with CAYSTON or placebo. Respiratory symptoms were also assessed two weeks after the completion of treatment with CAYSTON or placebo. Changes in respiratory symptoms were assessed using a questionnaire that asks patients to report on symptoms like cough, wheezing, and sputum production.

Improvement in respiratory symptoms was noted for CAYSTON-treated patients relative to placebo-treated patients on the last day of drug treatment. Statistically significant improvements were seen in both adult and pediatric patients, but were substantially smaller in adult patients. Two weeks after completion of treatment, a difference in respiratory symptoms between treatment groups was still present, though the difference was smaller.

Pulmonary function, as measured by FEV_1 (L), increased from baseline in patients treated with CAYSTON (see Figure 1). The treatment difference at Day 28 between CAYSTON-treated and placebo-treated patients for percent change in FEV_1 (L) was statistically significant at 10% (95% CI: 6%, 14%). Improvements in FEV_1 were comparable between adult and pediatric patients. Two weeks after completion of drug treatment, the difference in FEV_1 between CAYSTON and placebo groups had decreased to 6% (95% CI: 2%, 9%).

Figure 1 Adjusted Mean Percent Change in FEV₁ from Baseline to Study End (Days 0–42)

15   REFERENCES

1. Clinical and Laboratory Standards Institute (CLSI). Methods for Dilution Antimicrobial Susceptibility Tests for Bacteria that Grow Aerobically—Eighth Edition; Approved Standard. CLSI Document M7-A8. CLSI, Wayne, PA 19087. January, 2009.

16   HOW SUPPLIED/STORAGE AND HANDLING

Each kit for a 28-day course of CAYSTON contains 84 sterile vials of CAYSTON and 88 ampules of sterile diluent packed in 2 cartons, each carton containing a 14-day supply. The four additional diluent ampules are provided in case of spillage.

Package Configuration	Dosage Strength	NDC
28-Day Kit	75 mg	61958-0901-1

CAYSTON vials and diluent ampules should be stored in the refrigerator at 2 °C to 8 °C (36 °F to 46 °F) until needed. Once removed from the refrigerator, CAYSTON and diluent may be stored at room temperature (up to 25 °C / 77 °F) for up to 28 days. Do not separate the CAYSTON vials from the diluent ampules. CAYSTON should be protected from light. Do not use CAYSTON if it has been stored at room temperature for more than 28 days. Do not use CAYSTON beyond the expiration date stamped on the vial. Do not use diluent beyond the expiration date embossed on the ampule. CAYSTON should be used immediately upon reconstitution. Do not reconstitute more than one dose at a time.
Do not use diluent or reconstituted CAYSTON if it is cloudy or if there are particles in the solution.

17   PATIENT COUNSELING INFORMATION

See FDA-Approved Patient Labeling
Patients should be advised that CAYSTON is for inhalation use only and that CAYSTON should only be administered using the Altera Nebulizer System. Patients should be instructed only to reconstitute CAYSTON with the provided diluent and not mix other drugs with CAYSTON in the Altera Nebulizer System.
Patients should be advised to complete the full 28-day course of CAYSTON even if they are feeling better. Inform the patient that if they miss a dose, they should take all 3 daily doses as long as the doses are at least 4 hours apart. Patients should be advised to use a bronchodilator prior to administration of CAYSTON. Patients taking several inhaled medications should be advised to use the medications in the following order of administration: bronchodilator, mucolytics, and lastly, CAYSTON.
Patients should be advised to tell their doctor if they have new or worsening symptoms. Patients who believe they are experiencing an allergic reaction to CAYSTON should be advised to contact their doctor immediately.
Patients should be counseled that antibacterial drugs including CAYSTON should only be used to treat bacterial infections. They do not treat viral infection (e.g., the common cold). When CAYSTON is prescribed to treat a bacterial infection, patients should be told that although it is common to feel better early in the course of therapy, the medication should be taken as directed. Skipping doses or not completing the full course of therapy may (1) decrease the effectiveness of the immediate treatment and (2) increase the likelihood that bacteria will develop resistance and will not be treatable by CAYSTON or other antibacterial drugs in the future.
Manufactured by: Gilead Sciences, Inc., Foster City, CA 94404
CAYSTON is a trademark of Gilead Sciences, Inc. All other trademarks referenced herein are the property of their respective owners.

© 2014 Gilead Sciences, Inc. All rights reserved.
50-814-GS-002
FDA-Approved Patient Labeling
PATIENT INFORMATION
CAYSTON® (kay-stun)
(aztreonam for inhalation solution)
Read this Patient Information before you start taking CAYSTON and each time you get a refill. This information does not take the place of talking with your doctor about your medical condition or your treatment.
What is CAYSTON?
CAYSTON is a prescription inhaled antibiotic. CAYSTON is used to improve breathing symptoms in people with cystic fibrosis (CF) who have *Pseudomonas aeruginosa (P. aeruginosa)* in their lungs.
CAYSTON is only for infections caused by bacteria. It is not for infections caused by viruses, such as the common cold. CAYSTON is used only with the Altera® Nebulizer System. It is not known if CAYSTON is safe and effective in children under the age of 7.
Who should not take CAYSTON?
Do not take CAYSTON if you are allergic to aztreonam (AZACTAM®).
What should I tell my doctor before taking CAYSTON?
Before taking CAYSTON, tell your doctor if you:
• are allergic to any antibiotics.
• are pregnant or plan to become pregnant.
• are breast-feeding or plan to breast feed. Talk to your doctor about the best way to breast feed your baby if you take CAYSTON.
Tell your doctor about all the medicine you take, including prescription and non-prescription medicines, vitamins and herbal supplements.
Know the medicines you take. Keep a list of them to show your doctor and pharmacist when you get a new medicine.
How should I take CAYSTON?
• Take CAYSTON exactly as prescribed by your doctor.
• The dose of CAYSTON for both adults and children 7 years of age and older is one vial of CAYSTON, mixed with one ampule of saline (diluent) 3 times a day.
• Doses of CAYSTON should be taken at least 4 hours apart (for example: morning, after school, and before bed).
• CAYSTON should be taken for 28 days.
• CAYSTON is taken as a breathing treatment (inhalation) with the Altera Nebulizer System. Do not use any other nebulizer for your CAYSTON treatment.
• You should use an inhaled bronchodilator (a type of medicine used to relax and open your airways) before taking a dose of CAYSTON. If you do not have an inhaled bronchodilator, ask your doctor to prescribe one for you.
• If you are taking several medicines or treatments to treat your cystic fibrosis, you should take your medicines or other treatments in this order:
  1) bronchodilator
  2) mucolytics (medicines to help clear mucus from your lungs)
  3) CAYSTON
• You should take CAYSTON as prescribed, in courses of 28 days on CAYSTON, followed by at least 28 days off CAYSTON, as directed by your doctor.
• Do not mix CAYSTON with any other medicines in your Altera Nebulizer System.
• Do not mix CAYSTON with the saline until right before you are ready to use it. Do not mix more than one dose of CAYSTON at a time.
• Each treatment should take about 2 to 3 minutes.
• If you miss a dose of CAYSTON, you can still take all 3 daily doses as long as they are at least 4 hours apart.
• It is important for you to finish taking the full 28-day course of CAYSTON even if you are feeling better. If you skip doses or do not finish the full 28-day course of CAYSTON, your infection may not be fully treated and CAYSTON may not work as well as a treatment for infections in the future.
• See the end of this Patient Information leaflet for the Patient Instructions for Use on how to take CAYSTON the right way.
What are the possible side effects of CAYSTON?
CAYSTON can cause serious side effects, including:
• **Severe allergic reactions. Stop your treatment with CAYSTON and call your doctor right away if you have any symptoms of an allergic reaction, including:**
  ◦ Rash or swelling of your face
  ◦ Throat tightness
• **Trouble breathing right after treatment with CAYSTON (bronchospasm).** To decrease the chance of this happening, be sure to use your inhaled bronchodilator medicine before each treatment with CAYSTON. See "How should I take CAYSTON?"
Common side effects of CAYSTON include:
• Cough
• Nasal congestion
• Wheezing
• Sore throat

• Fever. Fever may be more common in children than in adults.
• Chest discomfort
• Stomach area (abdominal) pain
• Vomiting
Other possible side effects of CAYSTON include:
• Swelling or pain of joints
Tell your doctor if you have any new or worsening symptoms while taking CAYSTON. Tell your doctor about any side effect that bothers you or that does not go away.
These are not all the possible side effects of CAYSTON. For more information, ask your doctor or pharmacist.
Call your doctor for medical advice about side effects. You may report side effects to FDA at 1-800-FDA-1088.
How should I store CAYSTON?
• Each CAYSTON kit contains enough vials of CAYSTON and ampules of saline for 28 days of treatment. There are 4 extra saline ampules in case some saline spills.
• Always keep your CAYSTON and saline together.
• Store CAYSTON and saline in the refrigerator at 36 °F to 46°F (2 °C to 8 °C) until needed.
• When you remove CAYSTON and saline from the refrigerator, they may be stored at room temperature (less than 77 °F) for up to 28 days. Do not use any CAYSTON that has been stored at room temperature for more than 28 days.
• Keep CAYSTON away from light.
• Do not use CAYSTON after the expiration date on the vial. Do not use the saline after the expiration date on the ampule.
Keep CAYSTON and all medicines out of the reach of children.
General information about CAYSTON
Medicines are sometimes prescribed for purposes other than those listed in a Patient Information leaflet. Do not use CAYSTON for a condition for which it was not prescribed. Do not give CAYSTON to other people, even if they have the same symptoms that you have. It may harm them.
This Patient Information leaflet summarizes the most important information about CAYSTON. If you would like more information, talk with your doctor. You can ask your pharmacist or doctor for information about CAYSTON that is written for health professionals.
For more information, call 1-877-7CAYSTON (1-877-722-9786).
What are the ingredients in CAYSTON?
Active ingredient: aztreonam
Inactive ingredient: lysine, sodium chloride (diluent)

PATIENT INSTRUCTIONS FOR USE
CAYSTON®
(aztreonam for inhalation solution)
Be sure that you read, understand and follow the Patient Instructions for Use below for the right way to take CAYSTON. If you have any questions, ask your doctor or pharmacist.
You will need the following supplies (Figure 1):
• 1 amber colored CAYSTON vial covered by a metal seal with a blue cap or a metal seal only
• 1 ampule of saline (diluent)
• Altera Nebulizer System

Figure 1

Check to make sure that your Altera Nebulizer System works properly before starting your treatment with CAYSTON. See the manufacturer's instructions for use that comes with your Altera Nebulizer System. This should have complete information about how to put together (assemble), prepare, use, and care for your Altera Nebulizer System.
Step 1 Preparing your CAYSTON for inhalation
1. Mix (reconstitute) CAYSTON with the saline only when ready to take a dose. Take one amber vial of CAYSTON and one ampule of saline from the carton. Separate the saline ampules by gently pulling apart.

2. Look at the ampule of saline. If it looks cloudy do not use it. Throw away this ampule and get another ampule of saline.
3. Gently tap the vial so that the powder settles to the bottom of the vial. This helps you get the proper dose of medicine. Open the amber drug vial by lifting up the metal flap or blue cap on the top (Figure 2) and pulling down (Figure 3) to carefully remove the entire metal ring from the vial (Figure 4). Safely dispose of the ring in household garbage. Carefully remove the rubber stopper (Figure 5).

METAL FLAP   BLUE CAP   METAL FLAP   BLUE CAP

Figure 2   *Figure 3*

METAL RING   METAL RING   RUBBER STOPPER

Figure 4   *Figure 5*

4. Open the ampule of saline by twisting off the tip. Squeeze out the contents completely into the vial (Figure 6). Next, close the vial with the rubber stopper and gently swirl the vial until the powder has completely dissolved and the liquid is clear.

SALINE AMPULE

Figure 6

5. After mixing CAYSTON with the saline, check to make sure the diluted medicine is clear. If it is cloudy or has particles in it, do not use this medicine. Throw away this dose of medicine and start over again with a new vial of CAYSTON and a new ampule of saline.
6. Use CAYSTON right away after you mix with the saline.

Step 2 Taking your CAYSTON treatment
See the manufacturer's instructions for use that comes with your Altera Nebulizer System for complete instructions on taking a treatment, and how to clean and disinfect your Altera Nebulizer Handset.

7. Make sure the handset is on a flat, stable surface.
8. Remove the rubber stopper from the vial, then pour all of the mixed CAYSTON and saline into the Medication Reservoir of the handset (Figure 7). Be sure to completely empty the vial, gently tapping the vial against the side of the Medication Reservoir if necessary. Close the Medication Reservoir (Figure 8).

MEDICATION RESERVOIR

MOUTHPIECE   TAB

TAB SLOT

Figure 7   *Figure 8*

9. Begin your treatment by sitting in a relaxed, upright position. Hold the handset level, and place the Mouthpiece in your mouth. Close your lips around the Mouthpiece (Figure 9).

Figure 9

10. Breathe in and out normally (inhale and exhale) through the Mouthpiece. **Avoid breathing through your nose.** Continue to inhale and exhale comfortably until the treatment is finished.
11. The empty vial, stopper and saline ampule should be disposed of in household garbage upon completion of dosing.

Manufactured by: Gilead Sciences, Inc., Foster City, CA 94404
CAYSTON is a trademark of Gilead Sciences, Inc. All other trademarks referenced herein are the property of their respective owners.
© 2014 Gilead Sciences, Inc. All rights reserved.
50-814-GS-002

Shown in Product Identification Guide, page 306

COMPLERA®

[kom-PLEH-rah]
(emtricitabine, rilpivirine, tenofovir disoproxil fumarate) tablets, for oral use

℞

HIGHLIGHTS OF PRESCRIBING INFORMATION
These highlights do not include all the information needed to use COMPLERA safely and effectively. See full prescribing information for COMPLERA.
COMPLERA®(emtricitabine, rilpivirine, tenofovir disoproxil fumarate) tablets, for oral use
Initial U.S. Approval: 2011

WARNING: LACTIC ACIDOSIS/SEVERE HEPATO-MEGALY WITH STEATOSIS and POST TREATMENT ACUTE EXACERBATION OF HEPATITIS B
See full prescribing information for complete boxed warning.
- **Lactic acidosis and severe hepatomegaly with steatosis, including fatal cases, have been reported with the use of nucleoside analogs, including tenofovir disoproxil fumarate, a component of COMPLERA. (5.1)**
- **COMPLERA is not approved for the treatment of chronic hepatitis B virus (HBV) infection. Severe acute exacerbations of hepatitis B have been reported in patients coinfected with HIV-1 and HBV who have discontinued EMTRIVA or VIREAD, two of the components of COMPLERA. Hepatic function should be monitored closely in these patients. If appropriate, initiation of anti-hepatitis B therapy may be warranted. (5.2)**

RECENT MAJOR CHANGES

Indications and Usage (1)	12/2013
Dosage and Administration (2)	06/2014
Contraindications (4)	06/2014
Warnings and Precautions (5.3, 5.7)	10/2013
Warnings and Precautions (5.8)	06/2014

INDICATIONS AND USAGE

COMPLERA, a combination of two nucleoside analog HIV-1 reverse transcriptase inhibitors (emtricitabine and tenofovir disoproxil fumarate) and one non-nucleoside reverse transcriptase inhibitor (rilpivirine), is indicated for use as a complete regimen for the treatment of HIV-1 infection in (1) adult patients with no antiretroviral treatment history and with HIV-1 RNA less than or equal to 100,000 copies/mL at the start of therapy, and (2) in certain virologically-suppressed (HIV-1 RNA <50 copies/mL) adult patients on a stable antiretroviral regimen at start of therapy in order to replace their current antiretroviral treatment regimen (see below). (1, 14)

The following points should be considered when initiating therapy with COMPLERA in adult patients with no antiretroviral treatment history (1, 12.4, 14).
- More rilpivirine-treated subjects with HIV-1 RNA greater than 100,000 copies/mL at the start of therapy experienced virologic failure (HIV-1 RNA ≥50 copies/mL) compared to rilpivirine-treated subjects with HIV-1 RNA less than or equal to 100,000 copies/mL.
- Regardless of HIV-1 RNA level at the start of therapy, more rilpivirine-treated subjects with CD4+ cell count less than 200 cells/mm³ at the start of therapy experienced virologic failure compared to subjects with CD4+ cell count greater than or equal to 200 cells/mm³.
- The observed virologic failure rate in rilpivirine-treated subjects conferred a higher rate of overall treatment resistance and cross-resistance to the NNRTI class compared to efavirenz.
- More subjects treated with rilpivirine developed tenofovir and lamivudine/emtricitabine associated resistance compared to efavirenz.

The efficacy of COMPLERA was established in patients who were virologically-suppressed (HIV-1 RNA <50 copies/mL) on stable ritonavir-boosted protease inhibitor-containing regimen. The following points should be met when considering replacing the current regimen with COMPLERA in virologically-suppressed (HIV-1 RNA <50 copies/mL) adults (1,14):
- Patients should have no history of virologic failure.
- Patients should have been suppressed (HIV-1 RNA <50 copies/mL) for at least 6 months prior to switching therapy.
- Patients should currently be on their first or second antiretroviral regimen prior to switching therapy.
- Patients should have no current or past history of resistance to any of the three components of COMPLERA.

Additional monitoring of HIV-1 RNA and regimen tolerability is recommended after replacing therapy to assess for potential virologic failure or rebound. (1)

COMPLERA is not recommended for patients less than 18 years of age. (1, 8.4)

DOSAGE AND ADMINISTRATION
- Recommended dose: One tablet (containing 200 mg of emtricitabine, 25 mg of rilpivirine, and 300 mg of tenofovir disoproxil fumarate) taken once daily with food. (2)
- Dose in renal impairment: Should not be administered in patients with estimated creatinine clearance below 50 mL per minute. (2)
- With rifabutin coadministration, an additional 25 mg tablet of rilpivirine (Edurant) once per day is recommended to be taken concomitantly with COMPLERA and with a meal for the duration of the rifabutin coadministration. (2,7.5,12.3)

DOSAGE FORMS AND STRENGTHS
Tablets: 200 mg of emtricitabine, 25 mg of rilpivirine, and 300 mg of tenofovir disoproxil fumarate. (3)

CONTRAINDICATIONS
Coadministration of COMPLERA is contraindicated with drugs where significant decreases in rilpivirine plasma concentrations may occur, which may result in loss of virologic response and possible resistance and cross-resistance. (4)

WARNINGS AND PRECAUTIONS
- New onset or worsening renal impairment: Can include acute renal failure and Fanconi syndrome. Assess estimated creatinine clearance before initiating treatment with COMPLERA. In patients at risk for renal dysfunction, assess estimated creatinine clearance, serum phosphorus, urine glucose and urine protein before initiating treatment with COMPLERA and periodically during treatment. Avoid administering COMPLERA with concurrent or recent use of nephrotoxic drugs. (5.3)
- Caution should be given to prescribing COMPLERA with drugs that may reduce the exposure of rilpivirine. (5.4)
- Caution should be given to prescribing COMPLERA with drugs with a known risk of Torsade de Pointes. (5.4)
- Depressive disorders: Severe depressive disorders have been reported. Immediate medical evaluation is recommended for severe depressive disorders. (5.5)
- Hepatotoxicity: Hepatic adverse events have been reported in patients receiving a rilpivirine-containing regimen. Monitor liver-associated tests before and during treatment with COMPLERA in patients with underlying hepatic disease or marked elevations in liver-associated tests. Also consider monitoring liver-associated tests in patients without risk factors. (5.6)
- Decreases in bone mineral density (BMD): Consider monitoring BMD in patients with a history of pathologic fracture or other risk factors of osteoporosis or bone loss. (5.7)

• Coadministration with other products: Do not use with drugs containing emtricitabine, rilpivirine or tenofovir disoproxil fumarate including ATRIPLA, EMTRIVA, STRIBILD, TRUVADA, VIREAD, or with drugs containing lamivudine. Do not administer in combination with HEPSERA. Do not coadminister in combination with rilpivirine (Edurant) unless required for dose adjustment when coadministered with rifabutin. (5.8)
• Redistribution/accumulation of body fat: Observed in patients receiving antiretroviral therapy. (5.9)
• Immune reconstitution syndrome: May necessitate further evaluation and treatment. (5.10)

————————ADVERSE REACTIONS————————

Most common adverse drug reactions to rilpivirine (incidence greater than or equal to 2%, Grades 2–4) are depressive disorders, insomnia, and headache. (6.1)
Most common adverse drug reactions to emtricitabine and tenofovir disoproxil fumarate (incidence ≥10%) are diarrhea, nausea, fatigue, headache, dizziness, depression, insomnia, abnormal dreams, and rash. (6.1)
To report SUSPECTED ADVERSE REACTIONS, contact Gilead Sciences, Inc. at 1-800-GILEAD-5 or FDA at 1-800-FDA-1088 or www.fda.gov/medwatch

————————DRUG INTERACTIONS————————

• COMPLERA is a complete regimen for the treatment of HIV-1 infection; therefore, COMPLERA should not be administered with other antiretroviral medications for treatment of HIV-1 infection.
• CYP3A4 inducers or inhibitors: Drugs that induce or inhibit CYP3A4 may affect the plasma concentrations of rilpivirine. (7.1)
• Drugs that increase gastric pH: Drugs that increase gastric pH may decrease plasma concentrations of rilpivirine. (7.2)

————————USE IN SPECIFIC POPULATIONS————————

• Pregnancy: Use during pregnancy only if the potential benefit justifies the potential risk. (8.1)
• Nursing mothers: Women infected with HIV should be instructed not to breastfeed due to the potential for HIV transmission. (8.3)
• Pediatrics: Not recommended for patients less than 18 years of age. (8.4)

See 17 for PATIENT COUNSELING INFORMATION and FDA-approved patient labeling

Revised: 06/2014

FULL PRESCRIBING INFORMATION: CONTENTS*
WARNING: LACTIC ACIDOSIS/SEVERE HEPATOMEGALY WITH STEATOSIS and POST TREATMENT ACUTE EXACERBATION OF HEPATITIS B

FULL PRESCRIBING INFORMATION

> **WARNING: LACTIC ACIDOSIS/SEVERE HEPATOMEGALY WITH STEATOSIS and POST TREATMENT ACUTE EXACERBATION OF HEPATITIS B**
>
> Lactic acidosis and severe hepatomegaly with steatosis, including fatal cases, have been reported with the use of nucleoside analogs, including tenofovir disoproxil fumarate, a component of COMPLERA, in combination with other antiretrovirals [See Warnings and Precautions (5.1)].
>
> COMPLERA is not approved for the treatment of chronic hepatitis B virus (HBV) infection and the safety and efficacy of COMPLERA have not been established in patients coinfected with HBV and HIV-1. Severe acute exacerbations of hepatitis B have been reported in patients who are coinfected with HBV and HIV-1 and have discontinued EMTRIVA or VIREAD, which are components of COMPLERA. Hepatic function should be monitored closely with both clinical and laboratory follow-up for at least several months in patients who are coinfected with HIV-1 and HBV and discontinue COMPLERA. If appropriate, initiation of anti-hepatitis B therapy may be warranted [See Warnings and Precautions (5.2)].

1   INDICATIONS AND USAGE

COMPLERA, a combination of two nucleoside analog HIV 1 reverse transcriptase inhibitors (emtricitabine and tenofovir disoproxil fumarate) and one non-nucleoside reverse transcriptase inhibitor (rilpivirine), is indicated for use as a complete regimen for the treatment of HIV-1 infection in adult patients with no antiretroviral treatment history and with HIV-1 RNA less than or equal to 100,000 copies/mL at the start of therapy, and in certain virologically-suppressed (HIV-1 RNA <50 copies/mL) adult patients on a stable antiretroviral regimen at start of therapy in order to replace their current antiretroviral treatment regimen (see below).

• The following points should be considered when initiating therapy with COMPLERA in adult patients with no antiretroviral treatment history:
   • More rilpivirine-treated subjects with HIV-1 RNA greater than 100,000 copies/mL at the start of therapy experienced virologic failure (HIV-1 RNA ≥50 copies/mL) compared to rilpivirine-treated subjects with HIV-1 RNA less than or equal to 100,000 copies/mL [See Clinical Studies (14)].
   • Regardless of HIV-1 RNA level at the start of therapy, more rilpivirine-treated subjects with CD4+ cell count less than 200 cells/mm³ experienced virologic failure compared to rilpivirine-treated subjects with CD4+ cell count greater than or equal to 200 cells/mm³ [See Clinical Studies (14)].
   • The observed virologic failure rate in rilpivirine-treated subjects conferred a higher rate of overall treatment resistance and cross-resistance to the NNRTI class compared to efavirenz [See Microbiology (12.4)].
   • More subjects treated with rilpivirine developed tenofovir and lamivudine/emtricitabine associated resistance compared to efavirenz [See Microbiology (12.4)].
• The efficacy of COMPLERA was established in patients who were virologically-suppressed (HIV-1 RNA <50 copies/mL) on stable ritonavir-boosted protease inhibitor-containing regimen. The following points should be met when considering replacing the current regimen with COMPLERA in virologically-suppressed adults [See Clinical Studies (14)]:
   • Patients should have no history of virologic failure.
   • Patients should have been stably suppressed (HIV-1 RNA <50 copies/mL) for at least 6 months prior to switching therapy.
   • Patients should currently be on their first or second antiretroviral regimen prior to switching therapy.
   • Patients should have no current or past history of resistance to any of the three components of COMPLERA.
Additional monitoring of HIV-1 RNA and regimen tolerability is recommended after replacing therapy to assess for potential virologic failure or rebound.

COMPLERA is not recommended for patients less than 18 years of age [See Use in Specific Populations (8.4)].

2   DOSAGE AND ADMINISTRATION

Adults: The recommended dose of COMPLERA is one tablet taken orally once daily with food [See Clinical Pharmacology (12.3)].
Renal Impairment: Because COMPLERA is a fixed-dose combination, it should not be prescribed for patients requiring dose reduction such as those with moderate or severe renal impairment (estimated creatinine clearance below 50 mL per minute).
Rifabutin Coadministration: If COMPLERA is coadministered with rifabutin, an additional 25 mg tablet of rilpivirine (Edurant®) once per day is recommended to be taken concomitantly with COMPLERA and with a meal for the duration of the rifabutin coadministration [See Drug Interactions (7.5) and Clinical Pharmacology (12.3)].

3   DOSAGE FORMS AND STRENGTHS

COMPLERA is available as tablets. Each tablet contains 200 mg of emtricitabine (FTC), 27.5 mg of rilpivirine hydrochloride (equivalent to 25 mg of rilpivirine) and 300 mg of tenofovir disoproxil fumarate (tenofovir DF or TDF, equivalent to 245 mg of tenofovir disoproxil).
The tablets are purplish-pink, capsule-shaped, film-coated, debossed with "GSI" on one side and plain-faced on the other side.

4   CONTRAINDICATIONS

COMPLERA should not be coadministered with the following drugs, as significant decreases in rilpivirine plasma concentrations may occur due to CYP3A enzyme induction or gastric pH increase, which may result in loss of virologic response and possible resistance to COMPLERA or to the class of NNRTIs [See Drug Interactions (7) and Clinical Pharmacology (12.3)]:
• the anticonvulsants carbamazepine, oxcarbazepine, phenobarbital, phenytoin
• the antimycobacterials rifampin, rifapentine
• proton pump inhibitors, such as dexlansoprazole, esomeprazole, lansoprazole, omeprazole, pantoprazole, rabeprazole
• the glucocorticoid systemic dexamethasone (more than a single dose)
• St. John's wort (*Hypericum perforatum*)

5   WARNINGS AND PRECAUTIONS

5.1   Lactic Acidosis/Severe Hepatomegaly with Steatosis

Lactic acidosis and severe hepatomegaly with steatosis, including fatal cases, have been reported with the use of nucleoside analogs, including tenofovir DF, a component of COMPLERA, in combination with other antiretrovirals. A majority of these cases have been in women. Obesity and prolonged nucleoside exposure may be risk factors. Particular caution should be exercised when administering nucleoside analogs to any patient with known risk factors for liver disease; however, cases have also been reported in patients with no known risk factors. Treatment with COMPLERA should be suspended in any patient who develops clinical or laboratory findings suggestive of lactic acidosis or pronounced hepatotoxicity (which may include hepatomegaly and steatosis even in the absence of marked transaminase elevations).

5.2   Patients Coinfected with HIV-1 and HBV

It is recommended that all patients with HIV-1 be tested for the presence of chronic hepatitis B virus before initiating antiretroviral therapy. COMPLERA is not approved for the treatment of chronic HBV infection and the safety and efficacy of COMPLERA have not been established in patients coinfected with HBV and HIV-1. Severe acute exacerbations of hepatitis B have been reported in patients who are coinfected with HBV and HIV-1 and have discontinued emtricitabine or tenofovir DF, two of the components of COMPLERA. In some patients infected with HBV and treated with EMTRIVA®, the exacerbations of hepatitis B were associated with liver decompensation and liver failure. Patients who are coinfected with HIV-1 and HPV should be closely monitored with both clinical and laboratory follow-up for at least several months after stopping treatment with COMPLERA. If appropriate, initiation of anti-hepatitis B therapy may be warranted.

5.3   New Onset or Worsening Renal Impairment

Renal impairment, including cases of acute renal failure and Fanconi syndrome (renal tubular injury with severe hypophosphatemia), has been reported with the use of tenofovir DF [See Adverse Reactions (6.2)].
It is recommended that estimated creatinine clearance be assessed in all patients prior to initiating therapy and as clinically appropriate during therapy with COMPLERA. In patients at risk of renal dysfunction, including patients who have previously experienced renal events while receiving HEPSERA®, it is recommended that estimated creatinine clearance, serum phosphorus, urine glucose, and urine protein be assessed prior to initiation of COMPLERA, and periodically during COMPLERA therapy.

COMPLERA should be avoided with concurrent or recent use of a nephrotoxic agent (e.g., high-dose or multiple non-steroidal anti-inflammatory drugs (NSAIDs)) *[See Drug Interactions (7.3)]*. Cases of acute renal failure after initiation of high dose or multiple NSAIDs have been reported in HIV-infected patients with risk factors for renal dysfunction who appeared stable on tenofovir DF. Some patients required hospitalization and renal replacement therapy. Alternatives to NSAIDs should be considered, if needed, in patients at risk for renal dysfunction.

Persistent or worsening bone pain, pain in extremities, fractures and/or muscular pain or weakness may be manifestations of proximal renal tubulopathy and should prompt an evaluation of renal function in at-risk patients.

Emtricitabine and tenofovir are principally eliminated by the kidney; however, rilpivirine is not. Since COMPLERA is a combination product and the dose of the individual components cannot be altered, patients with estimated creatinine clearance below 50 mL per minute should not receive COMPLERA.

5.4 Drug Interactions

Caution should be given to prescribing COMPLERA with drugs that may reduce the exposure of rilpivirine *[See Contraindications (4), Drug Interactions (7), and Clinical Pharmacology (12.3)]*.

In healthy subjects, supratherapeutic doses of rilpivirine (75 mg once daily and 300 mg once daily) have been shown to prolong the QTc interval of the electrocardiogram *[See Drug Interactions (7) and Clinical Pharmacology (12.2)]*. COMPLERA should be used with caution when coadministered with a drug with a known risk of Torsade de Pointes.

5.5 Depressive Disorders

The adverse reaction depressive disorders (depressed mood, depression, dysphoria, major depression, mood altered, negative thoughts, suicide attempt, suicidal ideation) has been reported with rilpivirine. During the Phase 3 trials (N=1368) through 96 weeks, the incidence of depressive disorders (regardless of causality, severity) reported among rilpivirine (N=686) or efavirenz (N=682) was 9% and 8%, respectively. Most events were mild or moderate in severity. The incidence of Grades 3 and 4 depressive disorders (regardless of causality) was 1% for both rilpivirine and efavirenz. The incidence of discontinuation due to depressive disorders among rilpivirine or efavirenz was 1% in each arm. Suicidal ideation was reported in 4 subjects in each arm while suicide attempt was reported in 2 subjects in the rilpivirine arm. Patients with severe depressive symptoms should seek immediate medical evaluation to assess the possibility that the symptoms are related to COMPLERA, and if so, to determine whether the risks of continued therapy outweigh the benefits.

5.6 Hepatotoxicity

Hepatic adverse events have been reported in patients receiving a rilpivirine containing regimen. Patients with underlying hepatitis B or C, or marked elevations in liver-associated tests prior to treatment may be at increased risk for worsening or development of liver-associated test elevations with use of COMPLERA. A few cases of hepatic toxicity have been reported in patients receiving a rilpivirine containing regimen who had no pre-existing hepatic disease or other identifiable risk factors. Appropriate laboratory testing prior to initiating therapy and monitoring for hepatotoxicity during therapy with COMPLERA is recommended in patients with underlying hepatic disease such as hepatitis B or C, or in patients with marked elevations in liver-associated tests prior to treatment initiation. Liver-associated test monitoring should also be considered for patients without pre-existing hepatic dysfunction or other risk factors.

5.7 Bone Effects of Tenofovir DF

Bone Mineral Density:

In clinical trials in HIV-1-infected adults, tenofovir DF was associated with slightly greater decreases in bone mineral density (BMD) and increases in biochemical markers of bone metabolism, suggesting increased bone turnover relative to comparators. Serum parathyroid hormone levels and 1,25 Vitamin D levels were also higher in subjects receiving tenofovir DF. For more information, please consult the VIREAD prescribing information.

The effects of tenofovir DF-associated changes in BMD and biochemical markers on long-term bone health and future fracture risk are unknown. Assessment of BMD should be considered for patients who have a history of pathologic bone fracture or other risk factors for osteoporosis or bone loss. Although the effect of supplementation with calcium and Vitamin D was not studied, such supplementation may be beneficial for all patients. If bone abnormalities are suspected then appropriate consultation should be obtained.

Mineralization Defects:

Cases of osteomalacia associated with proximal renal tubulopathy, manifested as bone pain or pain in extremities and which may contribute to fractures, have been reported in association with the use of tenofovir DF *[See Adverse Reactions (6.2)]*. Arthralgias and muscle pain or weakness have

also been reported in cases of proximal renal tubulopathy. Hypophosphatemia and osteomalacia secondary to proximal renal tubulopathy should be considered in patients at risk of renal dysfunction who present with persistent or worsening bone or muscle symptoms while receiving products containing tenofovir DF *[See Warnings and Precautions (5.3)]*.

5.8 Coadministration with Other Products

COMPLERA should not be administered concurrently with other medicinal products containing the active components emtricitabine or tenofovir DF (ATRIPLA®, EMTRIVA, STRIBILD®, TRUVADA®, VIREAD), with medicinal products containing lamivudine (Epivir®, Epivir-HBV®, Epzicom®, Combivir®, Trizivir®), or with adefovir dipivoxil (HEPSERA). COMPLERA should not be administered with rilpivirine (Edurant) unless needed for dose adjustment (e.g., with rifabutin) *[See Dosage and Administration (2) and Drug Interactions (7.5)]*.

5.9 Fat Redistribution

Redistribution/accumulation of body fat including central obesity, dorsocervical fat enlargement (buffalo hump), peripheral wasting, facial wasting, breast enlargement, and "cushingoid appearance" have been observed in patients receiving antiretroviral therapy. The mechanism and long-term consequences of these events are unknown. A causal relationship has not been established.

5.10 Immune Reconstitution Syndrome

Immune reconstitution syndrome has been reported in patients treated with combination antiretroviral therapy, including the components of COMPLERA. During the initial phase of combination antiretroviral treatment, patients whose immune system responds may develop an inflammatory response to indolent or residual opportunistic infections [such as *Mycobacterium avium* infection, cytomegalovirus, *Pneumocystis jirovecii* pneumonia (PCP), or tuberculosis], which may necessitate further evaluation and treatment.

Autoimmune disorders (such as Graves' disease, polymyositis, and Guillain-Barré syndrome) have also been reported to occur in the setting of immune reconstitution, however, the time to onset is more variable, and can occur many months after initiation of treatment.

6   ADVERSE REACTIONS

The following adverse drug reactions are discussed in other sections of the labeling:

- Lactic Acidosis/Severe Hepatomegaly with Steatosis *[See Boxed Warning, Warnings and Precautions (5.1)]*.
- Severe Acute Exacerbations of Hepatitis B *[See Boxed Warning, Warnings and Precautions (5.2)]*.
- New Onset or Worsening Renal Impairment *[See Warnings and Precautions (5.3)]*.
- Depressive Disorders *[See Warnings and Precautions (5.5)]*.
- Hepatotoxicity *[See Warnings and Precautions (5.6)]*.
- Bone Effects of Tenofovir DF *[See Warnings and Precautions (5.7)]*.
- Immune Reconstitution Syndrome *[See Warnings and Precautions (5.10)]*.

6.1   Adverse Reactions from Clinical Trials Experience

Because clinical trials are conducted under widely varying conditions, adverse reaction rates observed in the clinical trials of a drug cannot be directly compared to rates in the clinical trials of another drug and may not reflect the rates observed in practice.

In HIV-1-Infected Subjects With No Antiretroviral Treatment History

Studies C209 and C215 – Treatment-Emergent Adverse Drug Reactions: The safety assessment of rilpivirine, used in combination with other antiretroviral drugs, is based on the Week 96 pooled data from 1368 subjects in the Phase 3 trials TMC278-C209 (ECHO) and TMC278-C215 (THRIVE) in antiretroviral treatment-naive HIV-1-infected adult subjects. A total of 686 subjects received rilpivirine in combination with other antiretroviral drugs as background regimen; most (N=550) received emtricitabine/tenofovir DF as background regimen. The number of subjects randomized to the control arm efavirenz was 682, of which 546 received emtricitabine/tenofovir DF as background regimen *[See Clinical Studies (14)]*. The median duration of exposure for subjects in either treatment arm was 104 weeks.

Adverse drug reactions (ADR) observed at Week 96 in subjects who received rilpivirine or efavirenz plus emtricitabine/tenofovir DF as background regimen are shown in Table 1. No new types of adverse reactions were identified between Week 48 and Week 96. The adverse drug reactions observed in this subset of subjects were generally consistent with those seen for the overall patient population participating in these studies (refer to the prescribing information for Edurant).

The proportion of subjects who discontinued treatment with rilpivirine or efavirenz + emtricitabine/tenofovir DF due to ADR, regardless of severity, was 2% and 5%, respectively. The most common ADRs leading to discontinuation were psychiatric disorders: 9 (1.6%) subjects in the rilpivirine +

emtricitabine/tenofovir DF arm and 12 (2.2%) subjects in the efavirenz + emtricitabine/tenofovir DF arm. Rash led to discontinuation in 1 (0.2%) subject in the rilpivirine + emtricitabine/tenofovir DF arm and 10 (1.8%) subjects in the efavirenz + emtricitabine/tenofovir DF arm.

Common Adverse Drug Reactions

Clinical ADRs to rilpivirine or efavirenz of at least moderate intensity (≥ Grade 2) reported in at least 2% of adult subjects are shown in Table 1.

Table 1 Selected Treatment-Emergent Adverse Drug Reactions* (Grades 2–4) Reported in ≥2% of Subjects Receiving Rilpivirine or Efavirenz in Combination with Emtricitabine/Tenofovir DF in Studies C209 and C215 (Week 96 analysis)

	Rilpivirine + FTC/TDF	Efavirenz + FTC/TDF
	N=550	N=546
Gastrointestinal Disorder		
Nausea	1%	2%
Nervous System Disorders		
Headache	2%	2%
Dizziness	1%	7%
Psychiatric Disorders		
Depressive disorders[†]	2%	2%
Insomnia	2%	2%
Abnormal dreams	1%	3%
Skin and Subcutaneous Tissue Disorders		
Rash	1%	5%

*   Frequencies of adverse reactions are based on all Grades 2–4 treatment-emergent adverse events assessed to be related to study drug.

†   Includes adverse drug reactions reported as depressed mood, depression, dysphoria, major depression, mood altered, negative thoughts, suicide attempt, suicide ideation.

Rilpivirine: Treatment-emergent adverse drug reactions of at least moderate intensity (≥ Grade 2) that occurred in less than 2% of subjects treated with rilpivirine plus any of the allowed background regimens (N=686) in clinical studies C209 and C215 include (grouped by Body System): vomiting, diarrhea, abdominal discomfort, abdominal pain, fatigue, cholecystitis, cholelithiasis, decreased appetite, somnolence, sleep disorders, anxiety, glomerulonephritis membranous, glomerulonephritis mesangioproliferative, and nephrolithiasis.

In Virologically-Suppressed HIV-1-Infected Subjects

No new adverse reactions to COMPLERA were identified in stable, virologically-suppressed subjects switching to COMPLERA from a regimen containing a ritonavir-boosted protease inhibitor; however the frequency of adverse reactions increased by 20% (Study 106) after switching to COMPLERA.

Emtricitabine and Tenofovir Disoproxil Fumarate: The following adverse reactions were observed in clinical trials of emtricitabine or tenofovir DF in combination with other antiretroviral agents:

The most common adverse drug reactions occurring in at least 10% of HIV-1-infected treatment-naive adult subjects in a Phase 3 clinical trial of emtricitabine and tenofovir DF in combination with another antiretroviral agent are diarrhea, nausea, fatigue, headache, dizziness, depression, insomnia, abnormal dreams, and rash. In addition, adverse drug reactions that occurred in at least 5% of treatment-experienced or treatment-naive subjects receiving emtricitabine or tenofovir DF with other antiretroviral agents in clinical trials include abdominal pain, dyspepsia, vomiting, fever, pain, nasopharyngitis, pneumonia, sinusitis, upper respiratory tract infection, arthralgia, back pain, myalgia, paresthesia, peripheral neuropathy (including peripheral neuritis and neuropathy), anxiety, increased cough, and rhinitis.

Skin discoloration has been reported with higher frequency among emtricitabine-treated subjects; it was manifested by hyperpigmentation on the palms and/or soles and was generally mild and asymptomatic. The mechanism and clinical significance are unknown.

Laboratory Abnormalities: The percentage of subjects treated with rilpivirine + emtricitabine/tenofovir DF or efavirenz + emtricitabine/tenofovir DF in studies C209 and C215 with selected treatment-emergent laboratory abnormalities (Grades 1 to 4), representing worst grade toxicity, are presented in Table 2.

Table 2 Selected Laboratory Abnormalities (Grades 1–4) Reported in Subjects Who Received Rilpivirine or Efavirenz in Combination with Emtricitabine/Tenofovir DF in Studies C209 and C215 (Week 96 Analysis)

Laboratory Parameter Abnormality, (%)	DAIDS Toxicity Range	Rilpivirine + FTC/TDF N=550	Efavirenz + FTC/TDF N=546
BIOCHEMISTRY			
Increased Creatinine			
Grade 1	1.1–1.3 × ULN*	6%	1%
Grade 2	>1.3–1.8 × ULN	1%	1%
Grade 3	>1.8–3.4 × ULN	<1%	0
Grade 4	>3.4 × ULN	0	<1%
Increased AST			
Grade 1	1.25–2.5 × ULN	16%	19%
Grade 2	>2.5–5.0 × ULN	4%	7%
Grade 3	>5.0–10.0 × ULN	2%	3%
Grade 4	>10.0 × ULN	1%	1%
Increased ALT			
Grade 1	1.25–2.5 × ULN	19%	22%
Grade 2	>2.5–5.0 × ULN	5%	7%
Grade 3	>5.0–10.0 × ULN	1%	2%
Grade 4	>10.0 × ULN	1%	1%
Increased Total Bilirubin			
Grade 1	1.1–1.5 × ULN	6%	<1%
Grade 2	>1.5–2.5 × ULN	3%	1%
Grade 3	>2.5–5.0 × ULN	1%	<1%
Increased Total Cholesterol (fasted)			
Grade 1	200–239 mg/dL	14%	31%
Grade 2	240–300 mg/dL	6%	18%
Grade 3	>300 mg/dL	<1%	2%
Increased LDL Cholesterol (fasted)			
Grade 1	130–159 mg/dL	13%	28%
Grade 2	160–190 mg/dL	5%	13%
Grade 3	>190 mg/dL	1%	4%
Increased Triglycerides (fasted)			
Grade 2	500–750 mg/dL	1%	2%
Grade 3	751–1,200 mg/dL	1%	2%
Grade 4	>1,200 mg/dL	0	1%

N = number of subjects per treatment group
Note: Percentages were calculated versus the number of subjects in ITT population with emtricitabine + tenofovir DF as background regimen.
* ULN = Upper limit of normal value.

Emtricitabine or Tenofovir Disoproxil Fumarate: The following laboratory abnormalities have been previously reported in subjects treated with emtricitabine or tenofovir DF with other antiretroviral agents in other clinical trials: Grade 3 or 4 laboratory abnormalities of increased pancreatic amylase (>2.0 × ULN), increased serum amylase (>175 U/L), increased lipase (>3.0 × ULN), increased alkaline phosphatase (>550 U/L), increased or decreased serum glucose (<40 or >250 mg/dL), increased glycosuria (≥3+), in-

creased creatine kinase (M: >990 U/L; F: >845 U/L), decreased neutrophils (<750/mm³) and increased hematuria (>75 RBC/HPF) occurred.
Adrenal Function
In the pooled Phase 3 trials of C209 and C215, in subjects treated with rilpivirine plus any of the allowed background regimen (N=686), at Week 96, there was an overall mean change from baseline in basal cortisol of -19.1 (95% CI: -30.9; -7.4) nmol/L in the rilpivirine group, and of -0.6 (95% CI: -13.3; 12.2) nmol/L in the efavirenz group. At Week 96, the mean change from baseline in ACTH-stimulated cortisol levels was lower in the rilpivirine group (+18.4 ± 8.36 nmol/L) than in the efavirenz group (+54.1 ± 7.24 nmol/L). Mean values for both basal and ACTH-stimulated cortisol values at Week 96 were within the normal range. Overall, there were no serious adverse events, deaths, or treatment discontinuations that could clearly be attributed to adrenal insufficiency. Effects on adrenal function were comparable by background N(t)RTIs.
Serum Creatinine
In the pooled Phase 3 trials of C209 and C215 trials in subjects treated with rilpivirine plus any of the allowed background regimen (N=686), there was a small increase in serum creatinine over 96 weeks of treatment with rilpivirine. Most of this increase occurred within the first four weeks of treatment with a mean change of 0.1 mg/dL (range: -0.3 mg/dL to 0.6 mg/dL) observed through Week 96. In subjects who entered the trial with mild or moderate renal impairment, the serum creatinine increase observed was similar to that seen in subjects with normal renal function. These changes are not considered to be clinically relevant and no subject discontinued treatment due to increases in serum creatinine. Creatinine increases were comparable by background N(t)RTIs.
Serum Lipids
Changes from baseline in total cholesterol, LDL-cholesterol and triglycerides are presented in Table 3.
[See table 3 below]
Subjects Coinfected with Hepatitis B and/or Hepatitis C Virus
In patients coinfected with hepatitis B or C virus receiving rilpivirine in studies C209 and C215, the incidence of hepatic enzyme elevation was higher than in subjects receiving rilpivirine who were not coinfected. The same increase was also observed in the efavirenz arm. The pharmacokinetic exposure of rilpivirine in coinfected subjects was comparable to that in subjects without coinfection.
6.2   Postmarketing Experience
The following adverse reactions have been identified during postapproval use of rilpivirine- or tenofovir DF-containing regimens . Because postmarketing reactions are reported voluntarily from a population of uncertain size, it is not always possible to reliably estimate their frequency or establish a causal relationship to drug exposure.
Rilpivirine:
Renal and Urinary Disorders
nephrotic syndrome
Emtricitabine:
No postmarketing adverse reactions have been identified for inclusion in this section.
Tenofovir Disoproxil Fumarate:
Immune System Disorders
allergic reaction, including angioedema
Metabolism and Nutrition Disorders
lactic acidosis, hypokalemia, hypophosphatemia
Respiratory, Thoracic, and Mediastinal Disorders
dyspnea
Gastrointestinal Disorders
pancreatitis, increased amylase, abdominal pain
Hepatobiliary Disorders
hepatic steatosis, hepatitis, increased liver enzymes (most commonly AST, ALT gamma GT)
Skin and Subcutaneous Tissue Disorders
rash
Musculoskeletal and Connective Tissue Disorders
rhabdomyolysis, osteomalacia (manifested as bone pain and which may contribute to fractures), muscular weakness, myopathy
Renal and Urinary Disorders
acute renal failure, renal failure, acute tubular necrosis, Fanconi syndrome, proximal renal tubulopathy, interstitial nephritis (including acute cases), nephrogenic diabetes insipidus, renal insufficiency, increased creatinine, proteinuria, polyuria
General Disorders and Administration Site Conditions
asthenia
The following adverse reactions, listed under the body system headings above, may occur as a consequence of proximal renal tubulopathy: rhabdomyolysis, osteomalacia, hypokalemia, muscular weakness, myopathy, hypophosphatemia.

Table 3 Lipid Values Reported in Subjects Receiving Rilpivirine or Efavirenz in Combination with Emtricitabine/Tenofovir DF in Studies C209 and C215*

	Pooled Data from the Week 96 Analysis of C209 and C215 Trials							
	Rilpivirine + FTC/TDF N=550				Efavirenz + FTC/TDF N=546			
Mean	N	Baseline Mean (mg/dL)	Week 96 Mean (mg/dL)	Mean Change† (mg/dL)	N	Baseline Mean (mg/dL)	Week 96 Mean (mg/dL)	Mean Change† (mg/dL)
Total Cholesterol (fasted)	430	162	164	2	401	160	186	26
HDL-cholesterol (fasted)	429	42	45	4	399	40	50	11
LDL-cholesterol (fasted)	427	97	97	-1	397	96	110	14
Triglycerides (fasted)	430	123	109	-14	401	127	133	6

N = number of subjects per treatment group
*   Excludes subjects who received lipid lowering agents during the treatment period.
†   The change from baseline is the mean of within-patient changes from baseline for patients with both baseline and Week 96 values.

7 DRUG INTERACTIONS

COMPLERA is a complete regimen for the treatment of HIV-1 infection; therefore, COMPLERA should not be administered with other antiretroviral medications. Information regarding potential drug-drug interactions with other antiretroviral medications is not provided. Please refer to the Edurant, VIREAD and EMTRIVA prescribing information as needed.

There were no drug-drug interaction trials conducted with the fixed-dose combination tablet. Drug interaction studies were conducted with emtricitabine, rilpivirine, or tenofovir DF, the components of COMPLERA. This section describes clinically relevant drug interactions with COMPLERA *[See Dosage and Administration (2), Contraindications (4), and Clinical Pharmacology (12.3)]*.

7.1 Drugs Inducing or Inhibiting CYP3A Enzymes

Rilpivirine is primarily metabolized by cytochrome P450 (CYP) 3A, and drugs that induce or inhibit CYP3A may thus affect the clearance of rilpivirine *[See Clinical Pharmacology (12.3), Contraindications (4)]*. Coadministration of rilpivirine and drugs that induce CYP3A may result in decreased plasma concentrations of rilpivirine and loss of virologic response and possible resistance to rilpivirine or to the class of NNRTIs. Coadministration of rilpivirine and drugs that inhibit CYP3A may result in increased plasma concentrations of rilpivirine.

Rilpivirine at a dose of 25 mg once daily is not likely to have a clinically relevant effect on the exposure of drugs metabolized by CYP enzymes.

7.2 Drugs Increasing Gastric pH

Coadministration of rilpivirine with drugs that increase gastric pH may decrease plasma concentrations of rilpivirine and loss of virologic response and possible resistance to rilpivirine or to the class of NNRTIs *[See Table 4]*.

7.3 Drugs Affecting Renal Function

Because emtricitabine and tenofovir are primarily eliminated by the kidneys through a combination of glomerular filtration and active tubular secretion, coadministration of COMPLERA with drugs that reduce renal function or compete for active tubular secretion may increase serum concentrations of emtricitabine, tenofovir, and/or other renally eliminated drugs. Some examples of drugs that are eliminated by active tubular secretion include, but are not limited to, acyclovir, adefovir dipivoxil, cidofovir, ganciclovir, valacyclovir, valganciclovir, aminoglycosides (e.g., gentamicin), and high-dose or multiple NSAIDs *[See Warnings and Precautions (5.3)]*.

7.4 QT Prolonging Drugs

There is limited information available on the potential for a pharmacodynamic interaction between rilpivirine and drugs that prolong the QTc interval of the electrocardiogram. In a study of healthy subjects, supratherapeutic doses of rilpivirine (75 mg once daily and 300 mg once daily) have been shown to prolong the QTc interval of the electrocardiogram *[See Clinical Pharmacology (12.2)]*. COMPLERA should be used with caution when coadministered with a drug with a known risk of Torsade de Pointes.

7.5 Established and Other Potentially Significant Drug Interactions

Important drug interaction information for COMPLERA is summarized in Table 4. The drug interactions described are based on studies conducted with emtricitabine, rilpivirine, or tenofovir DF as individual medications that may occur with COMPLERA or are potential drug interactions; no drug interaction studies have been conducted using COMPLERA [for pharmacokinetic data see *Clinical Pharmacology (12.3)*, Tables 6–7]. The tables include potentially significant interactions, but are not all inclusive.

[See table 4 above]

7.6 Drugs with No Observed or Predicted Interactions with COMPLERA

No clinically significant drug interactions have been observed between emtricitabine and the following medications: famciclovir or tenofovir DF. Similarly, no clinically significant drug interactions have been observed between tenofovir DF and the following medications: entecavir, methadone, oral contraceptives, ribavirin, or tacrolimus in studies conducted in healthy subjects.

No clinically significant drug interactions have been observed between rilpivirine and the following medications: acetaminophen, atorvastatin, chlorzoxazone, ethinyl estradiol, norethindrone, sildenafil, telaprevir, or tenofovir DF. Rilpivirine did not have a clinically significant effect on the pharmacokinetics of digoxin or metformin. No clinically relevant drug-drug interaction is expected when rilpivirine is coadministered with ribavirin.

8 USE IN SPECIFIC POPULATIONS

8.1 Pregnancy

Pregnancy Category B

Emtricitabine: The incidence of fetal variations and malformations was not increased in embryofetal toxicity studies performed with emtricitabine in mice at exposures (AUC)

approximately 60 times higher and in rabbits at approximately 120 times higher than human exposures at the recommended daily dose.

Rilpivirine: Studies in animals have shown no evidence of embryonic or fetal toxicity or an effect on reproductive function. In offspring from rat and rabbit dams treated with rilpivirine during pregnancy and lactation, there were no toxicologically significant effects on developmental endpoints. The exposures at the embryo-fetal No Observed Adverse Effects Levels in rats and rabbits were respectively 15 and 70 times higher than the exposure in humans at the recommended dose of 25 mg once daily.

Tenofovir Disoproxil Fumarate: Reproduction studies have been performed in rats and rabbits at doses up to 14 and 19 times the human dose based on body surface area comparisons and revealed no evidence of impaired fertility or harm to the fetus due to tenofovir.

There are, however, no adequate and well-controlled studies in pregnant women. Because animal reproduction studies are not always predictive of human response, COMPLERA should be used during pregnancy only if the potential benefit justifies the potential risk to the fetus.

Antiretroviral Pregnancy Registry: To monitor fetal outcomes of pregnant women exposed to COMPLERA, an Antiretroviral Pregnancy Registry has been established. Healthcare providers are encouraged to register patients by calling 1-800-258-4263.

8.3 Nursing Mothers

The Centers for Disease Control and Prevention recommend that HIV infected mothers not breastfeed their infants to avoid risking postnatal transmission of HIV.

Emtricitabine: Samples of breast milk obtained from five HIV-1-infected mothers show that emtricitabine is secreted in human milk. Breastfeeding infants whose mothers are being treated with emtricitabine may be at risk for developing viral resistance to emtricitabine. Other emtricitabine-associated risks in infants breastfed by mothers being treated with emtricitabine are unknown.

Rilpivirine: Studies in lactating rats and their offspring indicate that rilpivirine was present in rat milk. It is not known whether rilpivirine is secreted in human milk.

Tenofovir Disoproxil Fumarate: Samples of breast milk obtained from five HIV-1-infected mothers in the first postpartum week show that tenofovir is excreted in human milk. The impact of this exposure in breastfed infants is unknown.

Because of both the potential for HIV transmission and the potential for serious adverse reactions in nursing infants, **mothers should be instructed not to breastfeed if they are receiving COMPLERA.**

8.4 Pediatric Use

COMPLERA is not recommended for patients less than 18 years of age because not all the individual components of COMPLERA have safety, efficacy and dosing recommendations available for all pediatric age groups *[See Clinical Pharmacology (12.3)]*.

8.5 Geriatric Use

Clinical studies of emtricitabine, rilpivirine, or tenofovir DF did not include sufficient numbers of subjects aged 65 and over to determine whether they respond differently from younger subjects. In general, dose selection for the elderly patients should be cautious, keeping in mind the greater frequency of decreased hepatic, renal, or cardiac function, and of concomitant disease or other drug therapy *[See Clinical Pharmacology (12.3)]*.

8.6 Renal Impairment

Because COMPLERA is a fixed-dose combination, it should not be prescribed for patients requiring dosage adjustment such as those with moderate, severe or end stage renal impairment (estimated creatinine clearance below 50 mL per minute) or that require dialysis *[See Warnings and Precautions (5.3), Clinical Pharmacology (12.3)]*.

Table 4 Established and Other Potentially Significant* Drug Interactions: Alteration in Dose or Regimen May Be Recommended Based on Drug Interaction Studies or Predicted Interaction

Concomitant Drug Class: Drug Name	Effect on Concentration[†]	Clinical Comment
Antacids: antacids (e.g., aluminium, magnesium hydroxide, or calcium carbonate)	↔ rilpivirine (antacids taken at least 2 hours before or at least 4 hours after rilpivirine) ↓ rilpivirine (concomitant intake)	The combination of COMPLERA and antacids should be used with caution as coadministration may cause significant decreases in rilpivirine plasma concentrations (increase in gastric pH). Antacids should only be administered either at least 2 hours before or at least 4 hours after COMPLERA.
Antimycobacterials: rifabutin	↓ rilpivirine[‡]	Concomitant use of COMPLERA with rifabutin may cause significant decreases in rilpivirine plasma concentrations (induction of CYP3A enzymes). If COMPLERA is coadministered with rifabutin, an additional 25 mg tablet of rilpivirine (Edurant) once per day is recommended to be taken concomitantly with COMPLERA and with a meal for the duration of rifabutin coadministration.
Azole Antifungal Agents: fluconazole itraconazole ketoconazole posaconazole voriconazole	↑ rilpivirine[‡,§] ↓ ketoconazole[‡,§]	Concomitant use of COMPLERA with azole antifungal agents may cause an increase in the plasma concentrations of rilpivirine (inhibition of CYP3A enzymes). No dose adjustment is required when COMPLERA is coadministered with azole antifungal agents. Clinically monitor for breakthrough fungal infections when azole antifungals are coadministered with COMPLERA.
H₂-Receptor Antagonists: cimetidine famotidine nizatidine ranitidine	↔ rilpivirine[‡,§] (famotidine taken 12 hours before rilpivirine or 4 hours after rilpivirine) ↓ rilpivirine[‡] (famotidine taken 2 hours before rilpivirine)	The combination of COMPLERA and H₂-receptor antagonists should be used with caution as coadministration may cause significant decreases in rilpivirine plasma concentrations (increase in gastric pH). H₂-receptor antagonists should only be administered at least 12 hours before or at least 4 hours after COMPLERA.
Macrolide or Ketolide Antibiotics: clarithromycin erythromycin telithromycin	↑ rilpivirine ↔ clarithromycin ↔ erythromycin ↔ telithromycin	Concomitant use of COMPLERA with clarithromycin, erythromycin or telithromycin may cause an increase in the plasma concentrations of rilpivirine (inhibition of CYP3A enzymes). Where possible, alternatives such as azithromycin should be considered.
Narcotic Analgesics: methadone	↓ R(−) methadone[‡] ↓ S(+) methadone[‡] ↔ rilpivirine[‡] ↔ methadone[‡] (when used with tenofovir)	No dose adjustments are required when initiating coadministration of methadone with COMPLERA. However, clinical monitoring is recommended as methadone maintenance therapy may need to be adjusted in some patients.

* This table is not all inclusive.
† Increase = ↑; Decrease = ↓; No Effect = ↔
‡ The interaction was evaluated in a clinical study. All other drug-drug interactions shown are predicted.
§ This interaction study has been performed with a dose higher than the recommended dose for rilpivirine. The dosing recommendation is applicable to the recommended dose of rilpivirine 25 mg once daily.

8.7 Hepatic Impairment

No dose adjustment of COMPLERA is required in patients with mild (Child-Pugh Class A) or moderate (Child-Pugh Class B) hepatic impairment. COMPLERA has not been studied in patients with severe hepatic impairment (Child-Pugh Class C) [See Clinical Pharmacology (12.3)].

10 OVERDOSAGE

If overdose occurs the patient must be monitored for evidence of toxicity. Treatment of overdose with COMPLERA consists of general supportive measures including monitoring of vital signs and ECG (QT interval) as well as observation of the clinical status of the patient.

Emtricitabine: Limited clinical experience is available at doses higher than the therapeutic dose of EMTRIVA. In one clinical pharmacology study, single doses of emtricitabine 1200 mg were administered to 11 subjects. No severe adverse reactions were reported. The effects of higher doses are not known.

Hemodialysis treatment removes approximately 30% of the emtricitabine dose over a 3-hour dialysis period starting within 1.5 hours of emtricitabine dosing (blood flow rate of 400 mL per minute and a dialysate flow rate of 600 mL per minute). It is not known whether emtricitabine can be removed by peritoneal dialysis.

Rilpivirine: There is no specific antidote for overdose with rilpivirine. Human experience of overdose with rilpivirine is limited. Since rilpivirine is highly bound to plasma protein, dialysis is unlikely to result in significant removal of rilpivirine.

Administration of activated charcoal may be used to aid in removal of unabsorbed active substance.

Tenofovir Disoproxil Fumarate: Limited clinical experience at doses higher than the therapeutic dose of VIREAD 300 mg is available. In one study, 600 mg tenofovir DF was administered to 8 subjects orally for 28 days, and no severe adverse reactions were reported. The effects of higher doses are not known.

Tenofovir is efficiently removed by hemodialysis with an extraction coefficient of approximately 54%. Following a single 300 mg dose of VIREAD, a four-hour hemodialysis session removed approximately 10% of the administered tenofovir dose.

11 DESCRIPTION

COMPLERA is a fixed-dose combination tablet containing emtricitabine, rilpivirine hydrochloride, and tenofovir DF. EMTRIVA is the brand name for emtricitabine, a synthetic nucleoside analog of cytidine. Edurant is the brand name for rilpivirine, a non-nucleoside reverse transcriptase inhibitor. VIREAD is the brand name for tenofovir DF, which is converted *in vivo* to tenofovir, an acyclic nucleoside phosphonate (nucleotide) analog of adenosine 5'-monophosphate. VIREAD and EMTRIVA are the components of TRUVADA.

COMPLERA tablets are for oral administration. Each tablet contains 200 mg of emtricitabine, 27.5 mg of rilpivirine hydrochloride (equivalent to 25 mg of rilpivirine), and 300 mg of tenofovir DF (equivalent to 245 mg of tenofovir disoproxil) as active ingredients. The tablets include the following inactive ingredients: pregelatinized starch, lactose monohydrate, microcrystalline cellulose, croscarmellose sodium, magnesium stearate, povidone, polysorbate 20. The tablets are film-coated with a coating material containing polyethylene glycol, hypromellose, lactose monohydrate, triacetin, titanium dioxide, iron oxide red, FD&C Blue #2 aluminum lake, FD&C Yellow #6 aluminum lake.

Emtricitabine: The chemical name of emtricitabine is 5-fluoro-1-[(2R,5S)-2-(hydroxymethyl)-1,3-oxathiolan-5-yl]cytosine. Emtricitabine is the (–) enantiomer of a thio analog of cytidine, which differs from other cytidine analogs in that it has a fluorine in the 5-position.

It has a molecular formula of $C_8H_{10}FN_3O_3S$ and a molecular weight of 247.24. It has the following structural formula:

Emtricitabine is a white to off-white crystalline powder with a solubility of approximately 112 mg per mL in water at 25 °C.

Rilpivirine: Rilpivirine is available as the hydrochloride salt. The chemical name for rilpivirine hydrochloride is 4-[[4-[[4-[(E)-2-cyanoethenyl]-2,6-dimethylphenyl]amino]-2-pyrimidinyl]amino]benzonitrile monohydrochloride. Its molecular formula is $C_{22}H_{18}N_6$ • HCl and its molecular weight is 402.88. Rilpivirine hydrochloride has the following structural formula:

[See chemical structure at top of next column]

Rilpivirine hydrochloride is a white to almost white powder. Rilpivirine hydrochloride is practically insoluble in water over a wide pH range.

Tenofovir Disoproxil Fumarate: Tenofovir DF is a fumaric acid salt of the bis-isopropoxycarbonyloxymethyl ester de-

rivative of tenofovir. The chemical name of tenofovir DF is 9-[(R)-2 [[bis[[(isopropoxycarbonyl)oxy]-methoxy] phosphinyl]methoxy]propyl]adenine fumarate (1:1). It has a molecular formula of $C_{19}H_{30}N_5O_{10}P$ • $C_4H_4O_4$, and a molecular weight of 635.52. It has the following structural formula:

Tenofovir DF is a white to off-white crystalline powder with a solubility of 13.4 mg per mL in water at 25 °C. All dosages are expressed in terms of tenofovir DF except where otherwise noted.

12 CLINICAL PHARMACOLOGY

12.1 Mechanism of Action

COMPLERA is a fixed-dose combination of the antiretroviral drugs emtricitabine, rilpivirine and tenofovir disoproxil fumarate [See Microbiology (12.4)].

12.2 Pharmacodynamics

Effects on Electrocardiogram

The effect of rilpivirine at the recommended dose of 25 mg once daily on the QTcF interval was evaluated in a randomized, placebo and active (moxifloxacin 400 mg once daily) controlled crossover study in 60 healthy adults, with 13 measurements over 24 hours at steady state. The maximum mean time-matched (95% upper confidence bound) differences in QTcF interval from placebo after baseline-correction was 2.0 (5.0) milliseconds (i.e., below the threshold of clinical concern).

When supratherapeutic doses of 75 mg once daily and 300 mg once daily of rilpivirine were studied in healthy adults, the maximum mean time-matched (95% upper confidence bound) differences in QTcF interval from placebo after baseline-correction were 10.7 (15.3) and 23.3 (28.4) milliseconds, respectively. Steady-state administration of rilpivirine 75 mg once daily and 300 mg once daily resulted in a mean steady-state C_{max} approximately 2.6-fold and 6.7-fold, respectively, higher than the mean C_{max} observed with the recommended 25 mg once daily dose of rilpivirine [See Warnings and Precautions (5.4)].

12.3 Pharmacokinetics

COMPLERA: Under fed conditions (total calorie content of the meal was approximately 400 kcal with approximately 13 grams of fat), rilpivirine, emtricitabine and tenofovir exposures were bioequivalent when comparing COMPLERA to EMTRIVA capsules (200 mg) plus Edurant tablets (25 mg) plus VIREAD tablets (300 mg) following single-dose administration to healthy subjects (N=34).

Single-dose administration of COMPLERA tablet to healthy subjects under fasted conditions provided approximately 25% higher exposure of rilpivirine compared to administration of EMTRIVA capsules (200 mg) plus Edurant tablets (25 mg) plus VIREAD tablets (300 mg), while exposures of emtricitabine and tenofovir were comparable (N=15).

Emtricitabine: Following oral administration, emtricitabine is absorbed with peak plasma concentrations occurring at 1–2 hours post-dose. Following multiple dose oral administration of EMTRIVA to 20 HIV-1-infected subjects, the mean steady-state plasma emtricitabine C_{max} was 1.8 ± 0.7 µg per mL and the AUC over a 24-hour dosing interval was 10.0 ± 3.1 µg·hr per mL. The mean steady state plasma trough concentration at 24 hours post-dose was 0.09 µg per mL. The mean absolute bioavailability of EMTRIVA capsules was 93%. Less than 4% of emtricitabine binds to human plasma proteins *in vitro* over the range of 0.02 to 200 µg per mL. Following administration of radiolabelled emtricitabine, approximately 86% is recovered in the urine, approximately 14% in the feces and 13% is recovered as metabolites in the urine. The metabolites of emtricitabine include 3'-sulfoxide diastereomers (approximately 9% of the dose) and the glucuronic acid conjugate (approximately 4% of the dose). Emtricitabine is eliminated by a combination of glomerular filtration and active tubular secretion with a renal clearance in adults with creatinine clearance >80 mL per minute of 213 ± 89 mL per minute (mean ± SD). The plasma emtricitabine half-life is approximately 10 hours.

Rilpivirine: The pharmacokinetic properties of rilpivirine have been evaluated in adult healthy subjects and in adult antiretroviral treatment-naive HIV-1-infected subjects. Exposure to rilpivirine was generally lower in HIV-1-infected

subjects than in healthy subjects. After oral administration, the C_{max} of rilpivirine is achieved within 4–5 hours. The absolute bioavailability of rilpivirine is unknown.

Table 5 Population Pharmacokinetic Estimates of Rilpivirine 25 mg Once Daily in Antiretroviral Treatment-Naive HIV-1-infected Subjects (Pooled Data from Phase 3 Trials through Week 96)

Parameter	Rilpivirine 25 mg once daily N=679
AUC_{24h} (ng·h/mL)	
Mean ± Standard Deviation	2235 ± 851
Median (Range)	2096 (198 – 7307)
C_{0h} (ng/mL)	
Mean ± Standard Deviation	79 ± 35
Median (Range)	73 (2 – 288)

Rilpivirine is approximately 99.7% bound to plasma proteins *in vitro*, primarily to albumin. *In vitro* experiments indicate that rilpivirine primarily undergoes oxidative metabolism by the cytochrome CYP3A system. The terminal elimination half-life of rilpivirine is approximately 50 hours. After single dose oral administration of ^{14}C-rilpivirine, on average 85% and 6.1% of the radioactivity could be retrieved in feces and urine, respectively. In feces, unchanged rilpivirine accounted for on average 25% of the administered dose. Only trace amounts of unchanged rilpivirine (less than 1% of dose) were detected in urine.

Tenofovir Disoproxil Fumarate: Following oral administration of a single 300 mg dose of VIREAD to HIV-1-infected subjects in the fasted state, C_{max} was achieved in one hour. C_{max} and AUC values were 0.30 ± 0.09 µg per mL and 2.29 ± 0.69 µg·hr per mL, respectively. The oral bioavailability of tenofovir from VIREAD in fasted subjects is approximately 25%. Less than 0.7% of tenofovir binds to human plasma proteins *in vitro* over the range of 0.01 to 25 µg per mL. Approximately 70–80% of the intravenous dose of tenofovir is recovered as unchanged drug in the urine within 72 hours of dosing. Tenofovir is eliminated by a combination of glomerular filtration and active tubular secretion with a renal clearance in adults with creatinine clearance >80 mL per minute of 243.5 ± 33.3 mL per minute (mean ± SD). Following a single oral dose, the terminal elimination half-life of tenofovir is approximately 17 hours.

Effects of Food on Oral Absorption

The food effect trial for COMPLERA evaluated two types of meals. The trial defined a meal with 390 kcal containing 12 g fat as a light meal, and a meal with 540 kcal containing 21 g fat as a standard meal. Relative to fasting conditions, the administration of COMPLERA to healthy adult subjects with both types of meals resulted in increased exposures of rilpivirine and tenofovir. The C_{max} and AUC of rilpivirine increased 34% and 9% with a light meal, while increasing 26% and 16% with a standard meal, respectively. The C_{max} and AUC of tenofovir increased 12% and 28% with a light meal, while increasing 32% and 38% with a standard meal, respectively. Emtricitabine exposures were not affected by food.

The effects on rilpivirine, emtricitabine and tenofovir exposure when COMPLERA is administered with a high fat meal were not evaluated.

COMPLERA should be taken with food.

Special Populations

Race

Emtricitabine: No pharmacokinetic differences due to race have been identified following the administration of EMTRIVA.

Rilpivirine: Population pharmacokinetic analysis of rilpivirine in HIV-1-infected subjects indicated that race had no clinically relevant effect on the exposure to rilpivirine.

Tenofovir Disoproxil Fumarate: There were insufficient numbers from racial and ethnic groups other than Caucasian to adequately determine potential pharmacokinetic differences among these populations following the administration of VIREAD.

Gender

No clinically relevant pharmacokinetic differences have been observed between men and women for emtricitabine, rilpivirine, and tenofovir DF.

Pediatric Patients

Emtricitabine has been studied in pediatric subjects from 3 months to 17 years of age. Tenofovir DF has been studied in adolescent subjects (12 to less than 18 years of age). The pharmacokinetics of rilpivirine in pediatric subjects have not been established.

Geriatric Patients
Pharmacokinetics of emtricitabine, rilpivirine and tenofovir have not been fully evaluated in the elderly (65 years of age and older) [See Use in Specific Populations (8.5)].

Patients with Renal Impairment
Emtricitabine and Tenofovir Disoproxil Fumarate: The pharmacokinetics of emtricitabine and tenofovir DF are altered in subjects with renal impairment. In subjects with creatinine clearance below 50 mL per minute or with end stage renal disease requiring dialysis, C_{max}, and AUC of emtricitabine and tenofovir were increased [See Warnings and Precautions (5.3) and Use in Specific Populations (8.6)].

Rilpivirine: Population pharmacokinetic analysis indicated that rilpivirine exposure was similar in HIV-1-infected subjects with mild renal impairment relative to HIV-1-infected subjects with normal renal function. There is limited or no information regarding the pharmacokinetics of rilpivirine in patients with moderate or severe renal impairment or in patients with end-stage renal disease, and rilpivirine concentrations may be increased due to alteration of drug absorption, distribution, and metabolism secondary to renal dysfunction [See Use in Specific Populations (8.6)].

Patients with Hepatic Impairment
Emtricitabine: The pharmacokinetics of emtricitabine have not been studied in subjects with hepatic impairment; however, emtricitabine is not significantly metabolized by liver enzymes, so the impact of liver impairment should be limited.

Rilpivirine: Rilpivirine is primarily metabolized and eliminated by the liver. In a study comparing 8 subjects with mild hepatic impairment (Child-Pugh score A) to 8 matched controls and 8 subjects with moderate hepatic impairment (Child-Pugh score B) to 8 matched controls, the multiple dose exposure of rilpivirine was 47% higher in subjects with mild hepatic impairment and 5% higher in subjects with moderate hepatic impairment [See Use in Specific Populations (8.7)].

Tenofovir Disoproxil Fumarate: The pharmacokinetics of tenofovir following a 300 mg dose of VIREAD have been studied in non-HIV-infected subjects with moderate to severe hepatic impairment. There were no substantial alterations in tenofovir pharmacokinetics in subjects with hepatic impairment compared with unimpaired subjects.

Hepatitis B and/or Hepatitis C Virus Coinfection
Pharmacokinetics of emtricitabine and tenofovir DF have not been fully evaluated in hepatitis B and/or C virus-coinfected patients. Population pharmacokinetic analysis indicated that hepatitis B and/or C virus coinfection had no clinically relevant effect on the exposure to rilpivirine.

Assessment of Drug Interactions
COMPLERA is a complete regimen for the treatment of HIV-1 infection; therefore, COMPLERA should not be administered with other HIV antiretroviral medications. Information regarding potential drug-drug interactions with other antiretroviral medications is not provided. Please refer to the Edurant, VIREAD and EMTRIVA prescribing information as needed.

The drug interaction studies described were conducted with emtricitabine, rilpivirine, or tenofovir DF as individual agents; no drug interaction studies have been conducted using COMPLERA.

Emtricitabine and Tenofovir Disoproxil Fumarate: In vitro and clinical pharmacokinetic drug-drug interaction studies have shown that the potential for CYP mediated interactions involving emtricitabine and tenofovir with other medicinal products is low.

Emtricitabine and tenofovir are primarily excreted by the kidneys by a combination of glomerular filtration and active tubular secretion. No drug-drug interactions due to competition for renal excretion have been observed; however, coadministration of emtricitabine and tenofovir DF with drugs that are eliminated by active tubular secretion may increase concentrations of emtricitabine, tenofovir, and/or the coadministered drug [See Drug Interactions (7.6)].

Drugs that decrease renal function may increase concentrations of emtricitabine and/or tenofovir.

Drug interaction studies were performed for emtricitabine and the following medications: tenofovir DF and famciclovir. Tenofovir increased the C_{min} of emtricitabine by 20% (90% confidence interval [CI]: [↑12 to ↑29]) and had no effect on emtricitabine C_{max} and AUC. Emtricitabine had no effect on the C_{max}, AUC and C_{min} of tenofovir. Coadministration of emtricitabine and famciclovir had no effect on the C_{max} or AUC of either medication.

Drug interaction studies were performed for tenofovir DF and the following medications: entecavir, methadone, oral contraceptives (ethinyl estradiol/norgestimate), ribavirin, and tacrolimus. Tacrolimus increased the C_{max} of tenofovir by 13% (90% CI: [↑1 to ↑27]) and had no effect on the tenofovir AUC and C_{min}. Tenofovir had no effect on the C_{max}, AUC and C_{min} of tacrolimus.

The C_{max}, AUC and C_{min} of tenofovir were not affected in the presence of entecavir. Tenofovir increased the AUC of entecavir by 13% (90% CI: [↑11 to ↑15]) and had no effect on the entecavir C_{max} and C_{min}.
Tenofovir had no effect on the C_{max}, AUC and C_{min} of methadone or ethinyl estradiol/norgestimate or the C_{max} and AUC of ribavirin.

Rilpivirine: Rilpivirine is primarily metabolized by cytochrome CYP3A, and drugs that induce or inhibit CYP3A may thus affect the clearance of rilpivirine. Coadministration of COMPLERA and drugs that induce CYP3A may result in decreased plasma concentrations of rilpivirine and loss of virologic response and possible resistance. Coadministration of COMPLERA and drugs that inhibit CYP3A may result in increased plasma concentrations of rilpivirine. Coadministration of COMPLERA with drugs that increase gastric pH may result in decreased plasma concentrations of rilpivirine and loss of virologic response and possible resistance to rilpivirine and to the class of NNRTIs.

Rilpivirine at a dose of 25 mg once daily is not likely to have a clinically relevant effect on the exposure of medicinal products metabolized by CYP enzymes.
The effects of coadministration of other drugs on the AUC, C_{max} and C_{min} values of rilpivirine are summarized in Table 6. The effect of coadministration of rilpivirine on the AUC, C_{max} and C_{min} values of other drugs are summarized in Table 7. For information regarding clinical recommendations, see *Drug Interactions (7)*.
[See table 6 above]
[See table 7 at top of next page]

12.4   Microbiology
Mechanism of Action
Emtricitabine: Emtricitabine, a synthetic nucleoside analog of cytidine, is phosphorylated by cellular enzymes to form emtricitabine 5'-triphosphate. Emtricitabine 5'-triphosphate inhibits the activity of the HIV-1 RT by competing with the natural substrate deoxycytidine 5'-triphosphate and by being incorporated into nascent viral DNA which results in chain termination. Emtricitabine 5'-triphosphate is a weak inhibitor of mammalian DNA polymerase α, β, ϵ, and mitochondrial DNA polymerase γ.
Rilpivirine: Rilpivirine is a diarylpyrimidine non-nucleoside reverse transcriptase inhibitor of HIV-1 and inhibits HIV-1 replication by non-competitive inhibition of HIV-1 RT. Rilpivirine does not inhibit the human cellular DNA polymerases α, β, and mitochondrial DNA polymerase γ.
Tenofovir Disoproxil Fumarate: Tenofovir DF is an acyclic nucleoside phosphonate diester analog of adenosine mono-

Table 6 Drug Interactions: Changes in Pharmacokinetic Parameters for Rilpivirine in the Presence of the Coadministered Drugs

Coadministered Drug	Dose of Coadministered Drug (mg)	Dose of Rilpivirine	N*	Mean % Change of Rilpivirine Pharmacokinetic Parameters† (90% CI)		
				C_{max}	AUC	C_{min}
Acetaminophen	500 mg single dose	150 mg once daily‡	16	↑9 (↑1 to ↑18)	↑16 (↑10 to ↑22)	↑26 (↑16 to ↑38)
Atorvastatin	40 mg once daily	150 mg once daily‡	16	↓9 (↓21 to ↑6)	↓10 (↓19 to ↓1)	↓10 (↓16 to ↓4)
Chlorzoxazone	500 mg single dose taken 2 hours after rilpivirine	150 mg once daily‡	16	↑17 (↑8 to ↑27)	↑25 (↑16 to ↑35)	↑18 (↑9 to ↑28)
Ethinyl estradiol/ Norethindrone	0.035 mg once daily/1 mg once daily	25 mg once daily	16	↔§	↔§	↔§
Famotidine	40 mg single dose taken 12 hours before rilpivirine	150 mg single dose‡	24	↓1 (↓16 to ↑16)	↓9 (↓22 to ↑7)	NA
Famotidine	40 mg single dose taken 2 hours before rilpivirine	150 mg single dose‡	23	↓85 (↓88 to ↓81)	↓76 (↓80 to ↓72)	NA
Famotidine	40 mg single dose taken 4 hours after rilpivirine	150 mg single dose‡	24	↑21 (↑6 to ↑39)	↑13 (↑1 to ↑27)	NA
Ketoconazole	400 mg once daily	150 mg once daily‡	15	↑30 (↑13 to ↑48)	↑49 (↑31 to ↑70)	↑76 (↑57 to ↑97)
Methadone	60–100 mg once daily individualized dose	25 mg once daily	12	↔§	↔§	↔§
Omeprazole	20 mg once daily	150 mg once daily‡	16	↓40 (↓52 to ↓27)	↓40 (↓49 to ↓29)	↓33 (↓42 to ↓22)
Rifabutin	300 mg once daily	25 mg once daily	18	↓31 (↓38 to ↓24)	↓42 (↓48 to ↓35)	↓48 (↓54 to ↓41)
Rifabutin	300 mg once daily	50 mg once daily	18	↑43 (↑30 to ↑56)¶	↑16 (↑6 to ↑26)¶	↓7 (↓15 to ↑1)¶
Rifampin	600 mg once daily	150 mg once daily‡	16	↓69 (↓73 to ↓64)	↓80 (↓82 to ↓77)	↓89 (↓90 to ↓87)
Sildenafil	50 mg single dose	75 mg once daily	16	↓8 (↓15 to ↓1)	↓2 (↓8 to ↑5)	↑4 (↓2 to ↑9)
Telaprevir	750 mg every 8 hours	25 mg once daily	16	↑49 (↑20 to ↑84)	↑78 (↑44 to ↑120)	↑93 (↑55 to ↑141)
Tenofovir Disoproxil Fumarate	300 mg once daily	150 mg once daily‡	16	↓4 (↓19 to ↑13)	↑1 (↓13 to ↑18)	↓1 (↓17 to ↑16)

NA = not available
*   N=maximum number of subjects for C_{max}, AUC, or C_{min}
†   Increase = ↑; Decrease = ↓; No Effect = ↔
‡   The Interaction study has been performed with a dose higher than the recommended dose for rilpivirine (25 mg once daily) assessing the maximal effect on the coadministered drug.
§   Comparison based on historic controls.
¶   Reference arm for comparison was 25 mg q.d. rilpivirine administered alone.

Table 7 Drug Interactions: Changes in Pharmacokinetic Parameters for Coadministered Drugs in the Presence of Rilpivirine

Coadministered Drug	Dose of Coadministered Drug (mg)	Dose of Rilpivirine	N*	Mean % Change of Coadministered Drug Pharmacokinetic Parameters[†] (90% CI)		
				C_{max}	AUC	C_{min}
Acetaminophen	500 mg single dose	150 mg once daily[‡]	16	↓ 3 (↓ 14 to ↑ 10)	↓ 9 (↓ 14 to ↓ 3)	NA
Atorvastatin	40 mg once daily		16	↑ 35 (↑ 8 to ↑ 68)	↑ 4 (↓ 3 to ↑ 12)	↓ 15 (↓ 31 to ↑ 3)
2-hydroxy-atorvastatin		150 mg once daily[‡]	16	↑ 58 (↑ 33 to ↑ 87)	↑ 39 (↑ 29 to ↑ 50)	↑ 32 (↑ 10 to ↑ 58)
4-hydroxy-atorvastatin			16	↑ 28 (↑ 15 to ↑ 43)	↑ 23 (↑ 13 to ↑ 33)	NA
Chlorzoxazone	500 mg single dose taken 2 hours after rilpivirine	150 mg once daily[‡]	16	↓ 2 (↓ 15 to ↑ 13)	↓ 3 (↓ 5 to ↑ 13)	NA
Digoxin	0.5 mg single dose	25 mg once daily	22	↑ 6 (↓ 3 to ↑ 17)	↓ 2 (↓ 7 to ↑ 4)[§]	NA
Ethinyl estradiol	0.035 mg once daily		17	↑ 17 (↑ 6 to ↑ 30)	↑ 14 (↑ 10 to ↑ 19)	↑ 9 (↑ 3 to ↑ 16)
Norethindrone	1 mg once daily	25 mg once daily	17	↓ 6 (↓ 17 to ↑ 6)	↓ 11 (↓ 16 to ↑ 6)	↓ 1 (↓ 10 to ↑ 8)
Ketoconazole	400 mg once daily	150 mg once daily[‡]	14	↓ 15 (↓ 20 to ↓ 10)	↓ 24 (↓ 30 to ↓ 18)	↓ 66 (↓ 75 to ↓ 54)
R(−) methadone	60–100 mg once daily individualized dose	25 mg once daily	13	↓ 14 (↓ 22 to ↓ 5)	↓ 16 (↓ 26 to ↓ 5)	↓ 22 (↓ 33 to ↓ 9)
S(+) methadone			13	↓ 13 (↓ 22 to ↓ 3)	↓ 16 (↓ 26 to ↓ 4)	↓ 21 (↓ 33 to ↓ 8)
Metformin	850 mg single dose	25 mg once daily	20	↑ 2 (↓ 5 to ↑ 10)	↓ 3 (↓ 10 to ↑ 6)[¶]	NA
Omeprazole	20 mg once daily	150 mg once daily[‡]	15	↓ 14 (↓ 32 to ↑ 9)	↓ 14 (↓ 24 to ↓ 3)	NA
Rifampin	600 mg once daily	150 mg once daily[‡]	16	↑ 2 (↓ 7 to ↑ 12)	↓ 1 (↓ 8 to ↑ 7)	NA
25-desacetylrifampin			16	↔ (↓ 13 to ↑ 15)	↓ 9 (↓ 23 to ↑ 7)	NA
Sildenafil	50 mg single dose	75 mg once daily[‡]	16	↓ 7 (↓ 20 to ↑ 8)	↓ 3 (↓ 13 to ↑ 8)	NA
N-desmethyl-sildenafil			16	↓ 10 (↓ 20 to ↑ 2)	↓ 8 (↓ 15 to ↑ 1)[§]	NA
Telaprevir	750 mg every 8 hours	25 mg once daily	13	↓ 3 (↓ 21 to ↑ 21)	↓ 5 (↓ 24 to ↑ 18)	↓ 11 (↓ 33 to ↑ 18)
Tenofovir Disoproxil Fumarate	300 mg once daily	150 mg once daily[‡]	16	↑19 (↑6 to ↑34)	↑23 (↑16 to ↑31)	↑24 (↑10 to ↑38)

NA = not available
* N=maximum number of subjects for C_{max}, AUC, or C_{min}
† Increase = ↑; Decrease = ↓; No Effect = ↔
‡ The Interaction study has been performed with a dose higher than the recommended dose for rilpivirine (25 mg once daily).
§ $AUC_{(0-last)}$
¶ N (maximum number of subjects with data) for $AUC_{(0-∞)}$=15

phosphate. Tenofovir DF requires initial diester hydrolysis for conversion to tenofovir and subsequent phosphorylations by cellular enzymes to form tenofovir diphosphate. Tenofovir diphosphate inhibits the activity of HIV-1 RT by competing with the natural substrate deoxyadenosine 5′-triphosphate and, after incorporation into DNA, by DNA chain termination. Tenofovir diphosphate is a weak inhibitor of mammalian DNA polymerases α, β, and mitochondrial DNA polymerase γ.

Antiviral Activity

Emtricitabine, Rilpivirine, and Tenofovir Disoproxil Fumarate: The triple combination of emtricitabine, rilpivirine, and tenofovir was not antagonistic in cell culture.

Emtricitabine: The antiviral activity of emtricitabine against laboratory and clinical isolates of HIV-1 was assessed in lymphoblastoid cell lines, the MAGI-CCR5 cell line, and peripheral blood mononuclear cells. The 50% effective concentration (EC_{50}) values for emtricitabine were in the range of 0.0013–0.64 μM. Emtricitabine displayed antiviral activity in cell culture against HIV-1 clades A, B, C, D, E, F, and G (EC_{50} values ranged from 0.007–0.075 μM) and showed strain specific activity against HIV-2 (EC_{50} values ranged from 0.007–1.5 μM). In drug combination studies of emtricitabine with nucleoside reverse transcriptase inhibitors (abacavir, lamivudine, stavudine, tenofovir, zidovudine), non-nucleoside reverse transcriptase inhibitors (delavirdine, efavirenz, nevirapine, and rilpivirine), and protease inhibitors (amprenavir, nelfinavir, ritonavir, saquinavir), no antagonistic effects were observed.

Rilpivirine: Rilpivirine exhibited activity against laboratory strains of wild-type HIV-1 in an acutely infected T-cell line with a median EC_{50} value for HIV-1IIIB of 0.73 nM. Rilpivirine demonstrated limited activity in cell culture against HIV-2 with a median EC_{50} value of 5220 nM (range 2510 to 10830 nM). Rilpivirine demonstrated antiviral activity against a broad panel of HIV-1 group M (subtype A, B, C, D, F, G, H) primary isolates with EC_{50} values ranging from 0.07 to 1.01 nM and was less active against group O primary isolates with EC_{50} values ranging from 2.88 to 8.45 nM. The antiviral activity of rilpivirine was not antagonistic when combined with the NNRTIs efavirenz, etravirine or nevirapine; N(t)RTIs abacavir, didanosine, emtricitabine, lamivudine, stavudine, tenofovir or zidovudine; the PIs amprenavir, atazanavir, darunavir, indinavir, lopinavir, nelfinavir, ritonavir, saquinavir or tipranavir; the fusion inhibitor enfuvirtide; the CCR5 co-receptor antagonist maraviroc or the integrase strand transfer inhibitor raltegravir.

Tenofovir Disoproxil Fumarate: The antiviral activity of tenofovir against laboratory and clinical isolates of HIV-1 was assessed in lymphoblastoid cell lines, primary monocyte/macrophage cells and peripheral blood lymphocytes. The EC_{50} values for tenofovir were in the range of 0.04–8.5 μM. Tenofovir displayed antiviral activity in cell culture against HIV-1 clades A, B, C, D, E, F, G, and O (EC_{50} values ranged from 0.5–2.2 μM) and showed strain specific activity against HIV-2 (EC_{50} values ranged from 1.6 μM–5.5 μM). In drug combination studies of tenofovir with NRTIs (abacavir, didanosine, emtricitabine, lamivudine, stavudine, and zidovudine), NNRTIs (delavirdine, efavirenz, nevirapine, and rilpivirine), and PIs (amprenavir, indinavir, nelfinavir, ritonavir, saquinavir), no antagonistic effects were observed.

Resistance

In Cell Culture

Emtricitabine and Tenofovir Disoproxil Fumarate: HIV-1 isolates with reduced susceptibility to emtricitabine or tenofovir have been selected in cell culture. Reduced susceptibility to emtricitabine was associated with M184V/I substitutions in HIV-1 RT. HIV-1 isolates selected by tenofovir expressed a K65R substitution in HIV-1 RT and showed a 2–4 fold reduction in susceptibility to tenofovir.

Rilpivirine: Rilpivirine-resistant strains were selected in cell culture starting from wild-type HIV-1 of different origins and subtypes as well as NNRTI resistant HIV-1. The frequently observed amino acid substitutions that emerged and conferred decreased phenotypic susceptibility to rilpivirine included: L100I, K101E, V106I and A, V108I, E138K and G, Q, R, V179F and I, Y181C and I, V189I, G190E, H221Y, F227C and M230I and L.

In HIV-1-Infected Subjects With No Antiretroviral Treatment History

In the Week 96 pooled resistance analysis for subjects receiving rilpivirine or efavirenz in combination with emtricitabine/tenofovir DF in the Phase 3 clinical trials C209 and C215, the emergence of resistance was greater among subjects' viruses in the rilpivirine plus emtricitabine/tenofovir DF arm compared to the efavirenz plus emtricitabine/tenofovir DF arm and was dependent on baseline viral load. In the pooled resistance analysis, 61% (47/77) of the subjects who qualified for resistance analysis (resistance analysis subjects) in the rilpivirine plus emtricitabine/tenofovir DF arm had virus with genotypic and/or phenotypic resistance to rilpivirine compared to 42% (18/43) of the resistance analysis subjects in the efavirenz plus emtricitabine/tenofovir DF arm who had genotypic and/or phenotypic resistance to efavirenz. Moreover, genotypic and/or phenotypic resistance to emtricitabine or tenofovir emerged in viruses from 57% (44/77) of the resistance analysis subjects in the rilpivirine arm compared to 26% (11/43) in the efavirenz arm.

Emerging NNRTI substitutions in the rilpivirine resistance analysis of subjects' viruses included V90I, K101E/P/T, E138K/A/Q/G, V179I/L, Y181C/I, V189I, H221Y, F227C/L and M230L, which were associated with a rilpivirine phenotypic fold change range of 2.6–621. The E138K substitution emerged most frequently during rilpivirine treatment commonly in combination with the M184I substitution. The emtricitabine and lamivudine resistance-associated substitutions M184I or V and NRTI resistance-associated substitutions (K65R/N, A62V, D67N/G, K70E, Y115F, K219E/R) emerged more frequently in the rilpivirine resistance analysis subjects than in efavirenz resistance analysis subjects (See Table 8).

NNRTI- and NRTI-resistance substitutions emerged less frequently in the resistance analysis of viruses from subjects with baseline viral loads of ≤100,000 copies/mL compared to viruses from subjects with baseline viral loads of >100,000 copies/mL: 23% (10/44) compared to 77% (34/44) of NNRTI-resistance substitutions and 20% (9/44) compared to 80% (35/44) of NRTI-resistance substitutions. This difference was also observed for the individual emtricitabine/lamivudine and tenofovir resistance substitutions: 22% (9/41) compared to 78% (32/41) for M184I/V and 0% (0/8) compared to 100% (8/8) for K65R/N. Additionally, NNRTI and/or NRTI-resistance substitutions emerged less frequently in the resistance analysis of the viruses from subjects with baseline CD4+ cell counts ≥200 cells/mm³ compared to the viruses from subjects with baseline CD4+ cell counts <200 cells/mm^3: 32% (14/44) compared to 68% (30/44) of NNRTI-resistance substitutions and 27% (12/44) compared to 73% (32/44) of NRTI-resistance substitutions.

Table 8 Proportion of Frequently Emerging Reverse Transcriptase Substitutions in the HIV-1 Virus of Resistance Analysis Subjects* Who Received Rilpivirine or Efavirenz in Combination with Emtricitabine/Tenofovir DF from Pooled Phase 3 TMC278-C209 and TMC278-C215 Trials in the Week 96 Analysis

	C209 and C215 N=1096	
	Rilpivirine + FTC/TDF	Efavirenz + FTC/TDF
	N=550	N=546
Subjects who Qualified for Resistance Analysis	14% (77/550)	8% (43/546)
Subjects with Evaluable Post-Baseline Resistance Data	70	31
Emergent NNRTI Substitutions†		
Any	63% (44/70)	55% (17/31)
V90I	14% (10/70)	0
K101E/P/T/Q	19% (13/70)	10% (3/31)
K103N	1% (1/70)	39% (12/31)
E138K/A/Q/G	40% (28/70)	0
E138K+M184I‡	30% (21/70)	0
V179I/D	6% (4/70)	10% (3/31)
Y181C/I/S	13% (9/70)	3% (1/31)
V189I	9% (6/70)	0
H221Y	10% (7/70)	0
Emergent NRTI Substitutions§		
Any	63% (44/70)	32% (10/31)
M184I/V	59% (41/70)	26% (8/31)
K65R/N	11% (8/70)	6% (2/31)
A62V, D67N/G, K70E, Y115F, or K219E/R¶	20% (14/70)	3% (1/31)

* Subjects who qualified for resistance analysis
† V90, L100, K101, K103, V106, V108, E138, V179, Y181, Y188, V189, G190, H221, P225, F227, and M230
‡ This combination of NRTI and NNRTI substitutions is a subset of those with the E138K.
§ A62V, K65R/N, D67N/G, K70E, L74I, Y115F, M184V/I, L210F, K219E/R
¶ These substitutions emerged in addition to the primary substitutions M184V/I or K65R; A62V (n=2), D67N/G (n=3), K70E (n=4), Y115F (n=2), K219E/R (n=8) in rilpivirine resistance analysis subjects.

In Virologically-Suppressed HIV-1-Infected Subjects
Study 106: Through Week 48, four subjects who switched to COMPLERA (4 of 469 subjects, 0.9%) and one subject who maintained their ritonavir-boosted protease inhibitor-based regimen (1 of 159 subjects, 0.6%) developed genotypic and/or phenotypic resistance to a study drug. All four of the subjects who had resistance emergence on COMPLERA had evidence of emtricitabine resistance and three of the subjects had evidence of rilpivirine resistance.
Cross Resistance
Rilpivirine, Emtricitabine, and Tenofovir Disoproxil Fumarate:
In Cell Culture
No significant cross-resistance has been demonstrated between rilpivirine-resistant HIV-1 variants and emtricitabine or tenofovir, or between emtricitabine- or tenofovir-resistant variants and rilpivirine.
Rilpivirine:
Site-Directed NNRTI Mutant Virus
Cross-resistance has been observed among NNRTIs. The single NNRTI substitutions K101P, Y181I and Y181V con-

ferred 52-fold, 15-fold and 12-fold decreased susceptibility to rilpivirine, respectively. The combination of E138K and M184I showed 6.7-fold reduced susceptibility to rilpivirine compared to 2.8-fold for E138K alone. The K103N substitution did not show reduced susceptibility to rilpivirine by itself. However, the combination of K103N and L100I resulted in a 7-fold reduced susceptibility to rilpivirine. In another study, the Y188L substitution resulted in a reduced susceptibility to rilpivirine of 9-fold for clinical isolates and 6-fold for site-directed mutants. Combinations of 2 or 3 NNRTI resistance-associated substitutions gave decreased susceptibility to rilpivirine (fold change range of 3.7–554) in 38% and 66% of mutants, respectively.
In HIV-1-Infected Subjects With No Antiretroviral Treatment History
Considering all of the available cell culture and clinical data, any of the following amino acid substitutions, when present at baseline, are likely to decrease the antiviral activity of rilpivirine: K101E, K101P, E138A, E138G, E138K, E138R, E138Q, V179L, Y181C, Y181I, Y181V, Y188L, H221Y, F227C, M230I or M230L.
Cross-resistance to efavirenz, etravirine and/or nevirapine is likely after virologic failure and development of rilpivirine resistance. In a pooled 96-Week analysis for subjects receiving rilpivirine in combination with emtricitabine/tenofovir DF in the Phase 3 clinical trials TMC278-C209 and TMC278-C215, 43 of the 70 (61%) rilpivirine resistance analysis subjects with post-baseline resistance data had virus with decreased susceptibility to rilpivirine (≥2.5-fold). Of these, 84% (n=36/43) were resistant to efavirenz (≥3.3 fold change), 88% (n=38/43) were resistant to etravirine (≥3.2 fold change) and 60% (n=26/43) were resistant to nevirapine (≥6 fold change). In the efavirenz arm, 3 of the 15 (20%) efavirenz resistance analysis subjects had viruses with resistance to etravirine and rilpivirine, and 93% (14/15) had resistance to nevirapine. Virus from subjects experiencing virologic failure on rilpivirine in combination with emtricitabine/tenofovir DF developed more NNRTI resistance-associated substitutions conferring more cross-resistance to the NNRTI class and had a higher likelihood of cross-resistance to all NNRTIs in the class than subjects who failed on efavirenz.
Emtricitabine: Emtricitabine-resistant isolates (M184V/I) were cross-resistant to lamivudine but retained susceptibility in cell culture to didanosine, stavudine, tenofovir, zidovudine, and NNRTIs (delavirdine, efavirenz, nevirapine, and rilpivirine). HIV-1 isolates containing the K65R substitution, selected *in vivo* by abacavir, didanosine, and tenofovir, demonstrated reduced susceptibility to inhibition by emtricitabine. Viruses harboring substitutions conferring reduced susceptibility to stavudine and zidovudine (M41L, D67N, K70R, L210W, T215Y/F, K219Q/E), or didanosine (L74V) remained sensitive to emtricitabine. HIV-1 containing the substitutions associated with NNRTI resistance K103N or rilpivirine-associated substitutions were susceptible to emtricitabine.
Tenofovir Disoproxil Fumarate: The K65R substitution selected by tenofovir is also selected in some HIV-1-infected patients treated with abacavir or didanosine. HIV-1 isolates with the K65R substitution also showed reduced susceptibility to emtricitabine and lamivudine. Therefore, cross-resistance among these NRTIs may occur in patients whose virus harbors the K65R substitution. HIV-1 isolates from patients (N=20) whose HIV-1 expressed a mean of 3 zidovudine-associated RT amino acid substitutions (M41L, D67N, K70R, L210W, T215Y/F, or K219Q/E/N) showed a 3.1-fold decrease in the susceptibility to tenofovir.
Subjects whose virus expressed an L74V substitution without zidovudine resistance associated substitutions (N=8) had reduced response to VIREAD. Limited data are available for patients whose virus expressed a Y115F substitution (N=3), Q151M substitution (N=2), or T69 insertion (N=4), all of whom had a reduced response.
HIV-1 containing the substitutions associated with NNRTI resistance K103N and Y181C, or rilpivirine-associated substitutions were susceptible to tenofovir.

13 NONCLINICAL TOXICOLOGY
13.1 Carcinogenesis, Mutagenesis, Impairment of Fertility
Emtricitabine: In long-term carcinogenicity studies of emtricitabine, no drug-related increases in tumor incidence were found in mice at doses up to 750 mg per kg per day (26 times the human systemic exposure at the therapeutic dose of 200 mg per day) or in rats at doses up to 600 mg per kg per day (31 times the human systemic exposure at the therapeutic dose).
Emtricitabine was not genotoxic in the reverse mutation bacterial test (Ames test), mouse lymphoma or mouse micronucleus assays.
Emtricitabine did not affect fertility in male rats at approximately 140-fold or in male and female mice at approximately 60-fold higher exposures (AUC) than in humans given the recommended 200 mg daily dose. Fertility was

normal in the offspring of mice exposed daily from before birth (in utero) through sexual maturity at daily exposures (AUC) of approximately 60-fold higher than human exposures at the recommended 200 mg daily dose.
Rilpivirine: Rilpivirine was evaluated for carcinogenic potential by oral gavage administration to mice and rats up to 104 weeks. Daily doses of 20, 60 and 160 mg per kg per day were administered to mice and doses of 40, 200, 500 and 1500 mg per kg per day were administered to rats. In rats, there were no drug related neoplasms. In mice, rilpivirine was positive for hepatocellular neoplasms in both males and females. The observed hepatocellular findings in mice may be rodent-specific. At the lowest tested doses in the carcinogenicity studies, the systemic exposures (based on AUC) to rilpivirine were 21 fold (mice) and 3 fold (rats), relative to those observed in humans at the recommended dose (25 mg once daily).
Rilpivirine has tested negative in the absence and presence of a metabolic activation system, in the *in vitro* Ames reverse mutation assay and *in vitro* clastogenicity mouse lymphoma assay. Rilpivirine did not induce chromosomal damage in the *in vivo* micronucleus test in mice.
In a study conducted in rats, there were no effects on mating or fertility with rilpivirine up to 400 mg per kg per day, a dose of rilpivirine that showed maternal toxicity. This dose is associated with an exposure that is approximately 40 times higher than the exposure in humans at the recommended dose of 25 mg once daily.
Tenofovir Disoproxil Fumarate: Long-term oral carcinogenicity studies of tenofovir DF in mice and rats were carried out at exposures up to approximately 16 times (mice) and 5 times (rats) those observed in humans at the therapeutic dose for HIV-1 infection. At the high dose in female mice, liver adenomas were increased at exposures 16 times that in humans. In rats, the study was negative for carcinogenic findings at exposures up to 5 times that observed in humans at the therapeutic dose.
Tenofovir DF was mutagenic in the *in vitro* mouse lymphoma assay and negative in an *in vitro* bacterial mutagenicity test (Ames test). In an *in vivo* mouse micronucleus assay, tenofovir DF was negative when administered to male mice.
There were no effects on fertility, mating performance or early embryonic development when tenofovir DF was administered to male rats at a dose equivalent to 10 times the human dose based on body surface area comparisons for 28 days prior to mating and to female rats for 15 days prior to mating through day seven of gestation. There was, however, an alteration of the estrous cycle in female rats.
13.2 Animal Toxicology and/or Pharmacology
Tenofovir Disoproxil Fumarate: Tenofovir and tenofovir DF administered in toxicology studies to rats, dogs and monkeys at exposures (based on AUCs) greater than or equal to 6-fold those observed in humans caused bone toxicity. In monkeys the bone toxicity was diagnosed as osteomalacia. Osteomalacia observed in monkeys appeared to be reversible upon dose reduction or discontinuation of tenofovir. In rats and dogs, the bone toxicity manifested as reduced bone mineral density. The mechanism(s) underlying bone toxicity is unknown.
Evidence of renal toxicity was noted in 4 animal species. Increases in serum creatinine, BUN, glycosuria, proteinuria, phosphaturia, and/or calciuria and decreases in serum phosphate were observed to varying degrees in these animals. These toxicities were noted at exposures (based on AUCs) 2–20 times higher than those observed in humans. The relationship of the renal abnormalities, particularly the phosphaturia, to the bone toxicity is not known.

14 CLINICAL STUDIES
In HIV-1-Infected Subjects With No Antiretroviral Treatment History
The efficacy of COMPLERA is based on the analyses of 48- and 96-week data from two randomized, double-blind, controlled studies C209 (ECHO) and C215 (THRIVE) in treatment-naive, HIV-1-infected subjects (N=1368). The studies are identical in design with the exception of the background regimen (BR). Subjects were randomized in a 1:1 ratio to receive either rilpivirine 25 mg (N=686) once daily or efavirenz 600 mg (N=682) once daily in addition to a BR. In Study C209 (N=690), the BR was emtricitabine/tenofovir DF. In Study C215 (N=678), the BR consisted of 2 NRTIs: emtricitabine/tenofovir DF (60%, N=406) or lamivudine/zidovudine (30%, N=204) or abacavir plus lamivudine (10%, N=68).
For subjects who received emtricitabine/tenofovir DF (N=1096) in C209 and C215, the mean age was 37 years (range 18–78), 78% were male, 62% were White, 24% were Black, and 11% were Asian. The mean baseline CD4+ cell count was 265 cells/mm^3 (range 1–888) and 31% had CD4+ cell counts <200 cells/mm^3. The median baseline plasma HIV-1 RNA was 5 log$_{10}$ copies/mL (range 2–7). Subjects were stratified by baseline HIV-1 RNA. Fifty percent of subjects had baseline viral loads ≤100,000 copies/mL, 39% of

subjects had baseline viral load between 100,000 copies/mL to 500,000 copies/mL and 11% of subjects had baseline viral load >500,000 copies/mL.

Treatment outcomes through 96 weeks for the subset of subjects receiving emtricitabine/tenofovir DF in studies C209 and C215 (Table 9) are generally consistent with treatment outcomes for all participating subjects (presented in the prescribing information for Edurant). The incidence of virologic failure was higher in the rilpivirine arm than the efavirenz arm at Week 96. Virologic failures and discontinuations due to adverse events mostly occurred in the first 48 weeks of treatment.

Table 9 Virologic Outcome of Randomized Treatment of Studies C209 and C215 (Pooled Data for Subjects Receiving Rilpivirine or Efavirenz in Combination with Emtricitabine/Tenofovir DF) at Week 96*

	Rilpivirine + FTC/TDF N=550	Efavirenz + FTC/TDF N=546
HIV-1 RNA <50 copies/mL[†]	77%	77%
HIV-1 RNA ≥50 copies/mL[‡]	14%	8%
No virologic data at Week 96 window Reasons		
Discontinued study due to adverse event or death[§]	4%	9%
Discontinued study for other reasons[¶] and the last available HIV-1 RNA <50 copies/mL (or missing)	4%	6%
Missing data during window but on study	<1%	<1%
HIV-1 RNA <50 copies/mL by Baseline HIV-1 RNA (copies/mL)		
≤100,000	83%	80%
>100,000	71%	74%
HIV-1 RNA ≥50 copies/mL[‡] **by Baseline HIV-1 RNA (copies/mL)**		
≤100,000	7%	5%
>100,000	22%	12%
HIV-1 RNA <50 copies/mL by Baseline CD4+ Cell Count (cells/mm³)		
<200	68%	72%
≥200	82%	79%
HIV-1 RNA ≥50 copies/mL[‡] **by Baseline CD4+ Cell Count (cells/mm³)**		
<200	27%	12%
≥200	8%	7%

* Analyses were based on the last observed viral load data within the Week 96 window (Week 90–103).
† Predicted difference (95% CI) of response rate is 0.5% (-4.5% to 5.5%) at Week 96.
‡ Includes subjects who had ≥50 copies/mL in the Week 96 window, subjects who discontinued early due to lack or loss of efficacy, subjects who discontinued for reasons other than an adverse event, death or lack or loss of efficacy and at the time of discontinuation had a viral load value of ≥50 copies/mL, and subjects who had a switch in background regimen that was not permitted by the protocol.
§ Includes subjects who discontinued due to an adverse event or death if this resulted in no on-treatment virologic data in the Week 96 window.
¶ Includes subjects who discontinued for reasons other than an adverse event, death or lack or loss of efficacy, e.g., withdrew consent, loss to follow-up, etc.

Based on the pooled data from studies C209 and C215, the mean CD4+ cell count increase from baseline at Week 96 was 226 cells/mm³ for rilpivirine plus emtricitabine/

tenofovir DF-treated subjects and 223 cells/mm³ for efavirenz plus emtricitabine/tenofovir DF-treated subjects.

In Virologically-Suppressed HIV-1-Infected subjects

The efficacy and safety of switching from a ritonavir-boosted protease inhibitor in combination with two NRTIs to COMPLERA was evaluated in Study 106, a randomized, open-label study in virologically-suppressed HIV-1-infected adults. Subjects had to be on either their first or second antiretroviral regimen with no history of virologic failure, have no current or past history of resistance to any of the three components of COMPLERA, and must have been suppressed (HIV-1 RNA <50 copies/mL) for at least 6 months prior to screening. Subjects were randomized in a 2:1 ratio to either switch to COMPLERA at baseline (COMPLERA arm, N = 317), or stay on their baseline antiretroviral regimen for 24 weeks (SBR arm, N = 159) and then switch to COMPLERA for an additional 24 weeks (N = 152). Subjects had a mean age of 42 years (range 19–73), 88% were male, 77% were White, 17% were Black, and 17% were Hispanic/Latino. The mean baseline CD4+ cell count was 584 cells/mm³ (range 42–1484). Randomization was stratified by use of tenofovir DF and/or lopinavir/ritonavir in the baseline regimen.

Treatment outcomes are presented in Table 10.

Table 10 Virologic Outcomes of Randomized Treatment in Study GS-US-264-0106

	COMPLERA Week 48* N = 317	Stayed on Baseline Regimen (SBR) Week 24[†] N = 159
HIV-1 RNA <50 copies/mL[‡]	89% (283/317)	90% (143/159)
HIV-1 RNA ≥50 copies/mL[§]	3% (8/317)	5% (8/159)
No Virologic Data at Week 24 Window		
Discontinued Study Drug Due to AE or Death[¶]	2% (7/317)	0%
Discontinued Study Drug Due to Other Reasons and Last Available HIV-1 RNA <50 copies/mL[#]	5% (16/317)	3% (5/159)
Missing Data During Window but on Study Drug	1% (3/317)	2% (3/159)

* Week 48 window is between Day 295 and 378 (inclusive).
† For subjects in the SBR arm who maintained their baseline regimen for 24 weeks and then switched to COMPLERA, the Week 24 window is between Day 127 and first dose day on COMPLERA.
‡ Predicted difference (95% CI) of response rate for switching to COMPLERA at Week 48 compared to staying on baseline regimen at Week 24 (in absence of Week 48 results from the SBR group by study design) is -0.7% (-6.4% to 5.1%).
§ Includes subjects who had HIV-1 RNA ≥50 copies/mL in the time window, subjects who discontinued early due to lack or loss of efficacy, and subjects who discontinued for reasons other than an adverse event or death and at the time of discontinuation had a viral load value of ≥50 copies/mL.
¶ Includes subjects who discontinued due to adverse event or death at any time point from Day 1 through the time window if this resulted in no virologic data on treatment during the specified window.
# Includes subjects who discontinued for reasons other than an adverse event, death or lack or loss of efficacy, e.g., withdrew consent, loss to follow-up, etc.

16 HOW SUPPLIED/STORAGE AND HANDLING

COMPLERA tablets are purplish-pink, capsule-shaped, film-coated, debossed with "GSI" on one side and plain-faced on the other side. Each bottle contains 30 tablets (NDC 61958-1101-1), a silica gel desiccant, polyester fiber coil, and is closed with a child-resistant closure.

Store at 25 °C (77 °F), excursions permitted to 15 °C–30 °C (59 °F–86 °F) (see USP Controlled Room Temperature).

- Keep container tightly closed
- Dispense only in original container
- Do not use if seal over bottle opening is broken or missing.

17 PATIENT COUNSELING INFORMATION

Advise the patient to read the FDA-approved patient labeling (Patient Information).

A statement to patients and healthcare providers is included on the product's bottle label: **ALERT: Find out about medicines that should NOT be taken with COMPLERA.** A Patient Package Insert for COMPLERA is available for patient information.

Information for Patients

Patients should be advised that:
- Patients should remain under the care of a healthcare provider when using COMPLERA.
- Patients should be informed that COMPLERA is not a cure for HIV infection. Patients should stay on continuous HIV therapy to control HIV infection and decrease HIV-related illnesses. Patients should be told that sustained decreases in plasma HIV RNA have been associated with a reduced risk of progression to AIDS and death.
- Patients should be advised to continue to practice safer sex and to use latex or polyurethane condoms to lower the chance of sexual contact with any body fluids such as semen, vaginal secretions or blood. Patients should be advised never to re-use or share needles.
- Patients should be advised not to breastfeed because at least two of the drugs contained in COMPLERA can be passed to the baby in breast milk. It is not known whether this could harm the baby. Also, mothers with HIV-1 should not breastfeed because HIV-1 can be passed to the baby in breast milk.
- It is important to take COMPLERA on a regular dosing schedule with food and to avoid missing doses. A protein drink is not a substitute for food. If the healthcare provider decides to stop COMPLERA and the patient is switched to new medicines to treat HIV that includes rilpivirine tablets, the rilpivirine tablets should be taken only with a meal.
- If the patient misses a dose of COMPLERA within 12 hours of the time it is usually taken, the patient should take COMPLERA with food as soon as possible and then take the next dose of COMPLERA at the regularly scheduled time. If a patient misses a dose of COMPLERA by more than 12 hours, the patient should not take the missed dose, but resume the usual dosing schedule. Inform the patient that he or she should not take more or less than the prescribed dose of COMPLERA at any one time.
- Lactic acidosis and severe hepatomegaly with steatosis, including fatal cases, have been reported. Treatment with COMPLERA should be suspended in any patients who develop clinical symptoms suggestive of lactic acidosis or pronounced hepatotoxicity (including nausea, vomiting, unusual or unexpected stomach discomfort, and weakness) *[See Warnings and Precautions (5.1)].*
- Patients with HIV-1 should be tested for hepatitis B virus (HBV) before initiating antiretroviral therapy. Severe acute exacerbations of hepatitis B have been reported in patients who are coinfected with HBV and HIV-1 and have discontinued EMTRIVA or VIREAD *[See Warnings and Precautions (5.2)].* COMPLERA should not be discontinued without first informing their healthcare provider.
- Renal impairment, including cases of acute renal failure and Fanconi syndrome, has been reported in association with the use of VIREAD. COMPLERA should be avoided with concurrent or recent use of a nephrotoxic agent (e.g., high-dose or multiple NSAIDs) *[See Warnings and Precautions (5.3)].*
- COMPLERA may interact with many drugs; therefore, patients should be advised to report to their healthcare provider the use of any other prescription or nonprescription medication or herbal products, including St. John's wort *[See Warnings and Precautions (5.4)].*
- COMPLERA should not be coadministered with the following drugs, as significant decreases in rilpivirine plasma concentrations may occur due to CYP3A enzyme induction or gastric pH increase, which may result in loss of virologic response and possible resistance to COMPLERA or to the class of NNRTIs: the anticonvulsants carbamazepine, oxcarbazepine, phenobarbital, phenytoin; the antimycobacterials rifampin, rifapentine; proton pump inhibitors, such as esomeprazole, lansoprazole, omeprazole, pantoprazole, rabeprazole; the glucocorticoid systemic dexamethasone (more than a single dose); or St. John's wort (*Hypericum perforatum*) *[See Contraindications (4)].*
- For patients receiving rifabutin, an additional 25 mg tablet of rilpivirine (Edurant) once per day is recommended to be taken concomitantly with COMPLERA and with a meal for the duration of rifabutin coadministration.
- Patients should be informed that depressive disorders (depressed mood, depression, dysphoria, major depression,

mood altered, negative thoughts, suicide attempt, suicidal ideation) have been reported with COMPLERA. If they experience depressive symptoms, they should seek immediate medical evaluation [See Warnings and Precautions (5.5)].

• Patients should be informed that hepatotoxicity has been reported with COMPLERA [See Warnings and Precautions (5.6)].

• Decreases in bone mineral density have been observed with the use of VIREAD. Bone mineral density (BMD) monitoring should be considered in patients who have a history of pathologic bone fracture or other risk factors for osteoporosis or bone loss [See Warnings and Precautions (5.7)].

• COMPLERA should not be coadministered with ATRIPLA, EMTRIVA, STRIBILD, TRUVADA, or VIREAD; or with drugs containing lamivudine, including Combivir, Epivir or Epivir-HBV, Epzicom, or Trizivir; or with HEPSERA. COMPLERA should not be coadministered with rilpivirine (Edurant) unless needed for dose adjustment (e.g., with rifabutin) [See Warnings and Precautions (5.8)].

• Redistribution or accumulation of body fat may occur in patients receiving antiretroviral therapy and that the cause and long-term health effects of these conditions are not known [See Warnings and Precautions (5.9)].

• In some patients with advanced HIV infection (AIDS), signs and symptoms of inflammation from previous infections may occur soon after anti-HIV treatment is started. It is believed that these symptoms are due to an improvement in the body's immune response, enabling the body to fight infections that may have been present with no obvious symptoms. Patients should be advised to inform their healthcare provider immediately of any symptoms of infection [See Warnings and Precautions (5.10)].

Manufactured and distributed by:
Gilead Sciences, Inc.
Foster City, CA 94404

Patient Information
COMPLERA® (kom-PLEH-rah)
(emtricitabine, rilpivirine, tenofovir disoproxil fumarate)
Tablets
Important: Ask your healthcare provider or pharmacist about medicines that should not be taken with COMPLERA. For more information, see the section "What should I tell my healthcare provider before taking COMPLERA?"

Read this Patient Information before you start taking COMPLERA and each time you get a refill. There may be new information. This information does not take the place of talking to your healthcare provider about your medical condition or treatment.
What is the most important information I should know about COMPLERA?
COMPLERA can cause serious side effects, including:
1. Build-up of an acid in your blood (lactic acidosis). Lactic acidosis can happen in some people who take COMPLERA or similar (nucleoside analogs) medicines. **Lactic acidosis is a serious medical emergency that can lead to death.**

Lactic acidosis can be hard to identify early, because the symptoms could seem like symptoms of other health problems. **Call your healthcare provider right away if you get any of the following symptoms which could be signs of lactic acidosis:**
• feeling very weak or tired
• have unusual (not normal) muscle pain
• have trouble breathing
• have stomach pain with
  • nausea (feel sick to your stomach)
  • vomiting
• feel cold, especially in your arms and legs
• feel dizzy or lightheaded
• have a fast or irregular heartbeat

2. Severe liver problems. Severe liver problems can happen in people who take COMPLERA or similar medicines. In some cases these liver problems can lead to death. Your liver may become large (hepatomegaly) and you may develop fat in your liver (steatosis) when you take COMPLERA.

Call your healthcare provider right away if you have any of the following symptoms of liver problems:
• your skin or the white part of your eyes turns yellow (jaundice)
• dark "tea-colored" urine
• light-colored bowel movements (stools)
• loss of appetite for several days or longer
• nausea
• stomach pain

You may be more likely to get lactic acidosis or severe liver problems if you are female, very overweight (obese), or have been taking COMPLERA or a similar medicine containing nucleoside analogs for a long time.

3. Worsening of Hepatitis B infection. If you also have hepatitis B virus (HBV) infection and you stop taking COMPLERA, your HBV infection may become worse (flare-up). A "flare-up" is when your HBV infection suddenly returns in a worse way than before. COMPLERA is not approved for the treatment of HBV, so you must discuss your HBV therapy with your healthcare provider.
• Do not let your COMPLERA run out. Refill your prescription or talk to your healthcare provider before your COMPLERA is all gone.
• Do not stop taking COMPLERA without first talking to your healthcare provider.
• If you stop taking COMPLERA, your healthcare provider will need to check your health often and do blood tests regularly to check your HBV infection. Tell your healthcare provider about any new or unusual symptoms you may have after you stop taking COMPLERA.

What is COMPLERA?
COMPLERA is a prescription HIV (Human Immunodeficiency Virus) medicine. HIV is the virus that causes AIDS (Acquired Immunodeficiency Syndrome).
COMPLERA is used to treat HIV-1 infection in:
• adults who have **never** taken HIV medicines before, **and** who have an amount of HIV in their blood (this is called 'viral load') that is no more than 100,000 copies/mL before they start taking COMPLERA,
  and
• certain adults who have a viral load that is less than 50 copies/mL when they start taking COMPLERA, to replace their current HIV medicines.
Your healthcare provider will measure your viral load.
COMPLERA contains 3 medicines, (rilpivirine, emtricitabine, tenofovir disoproxil fumarate) combined in one tablet. Emtricitabine (EMTRIVA®) and tenofovir disoproxil fumarate (VIREAD®) are HIV-1 (human immunodeficiency virus) nucleoside analog reverse transcriptase inhibitors (NRTIs). Rilpivirine (Edurant®) is an HIV-1 non-nucleoside analog reverse transcriptase inhibitor (NNRTI). It is not known if COMPLERA is safe and effective in children under the age of 18 years.
COMPLERA may help:
• Reduce the amount of HIV in your blood.
• Increase the number of white blood cells called CD4+ (T) cells in your blood that help fight off other infections.
Reducing the amount of HIV and increasing the CD4+ (T) cells in your blood may help improve your immune system. This may reduce your risk of death or getting infections that can happen when your immune system is weak (opportunistic infections).
COMPLERA does not cure HIV infections or AIDS.
You must stay on continuous HIV therapy to control HIV infection and decrease HIV-related illnesses.
Avoid doing things that can spread HIV-1 infection to others.
• Do not share or re-use needles or other injection equipment.
• Do not share personal items that can have blood or body fluids on them, like toothbrushes and razor blades.
• Do not have any kind of sex without protection. Always practice safer sex by using a latex or polyurethane condom to lower the chance of sexual contact with any body fluids such as semen, vaginal secretions, or blood.
Ask your healthcare provider if you have any questions about how to prevent passing HIV to other people.
Who should not take COMPLERA?
Do not take COMPLERA if:
• you are taking any of the following medicines:
  • anti-seizure medicines:
    • carbamazepine (Carbatrol®, Equetro®, Tegretol®, Tegretol-XR®, Teril®, Epitol®)
    • oxcarbazepine (Trileptal®)
    • phenobarbital (Luminal®)
    • phenytoin (Dilantin®, Dilantin-125®, Phenytek®)
  • anti-tuberculosis (anti-TB) medicines:
    • rifampin (Rifater®, Rifamate®, Rimactane®, Rifadin®)
    • rifapentine (Priftin®)
  • proton pump inhibitor (PPI) medicine for certain stomach or intestinal problems:
    • dexlansoprazole (Dexilant®)
    • esomeprazole (Nexium®, Vimovo®)
    • lansoprazole (Prevacid®)
    • omeprazole (Prilosec®, Zegerid®)
    • pantoprazole sodium (Protonix®)
    • rabeprazole (Aciphex®)
  • more than 1 dose of the steroid medicine dexamethasone or dexamethasone sodium phosphate
  • St. John's wort (Hypericum perforatum)
What should I tell my healthcare provider before taking COMPLERA?
Before you take COMPLERA, tell your healthcare provider if you:
• have liver problems, including hepatitis B or C virus infection
• have kidney problems
• have ever had a mental health problem
• have bone problems

• are pregnant or plan to become pregnant. It is not known if COMPLERA can harm your unborn child.
Pregnancy Registry. There is a pregnancy registry for women who take antiretroviral medicines during pregnancy. The purpose of this registry is to collect information about the health of you and your baby. Talk to your healthcare provider about how you can take part in this registry.
• are breast-feeding or plan to breast-feed. You should not breastfeed if you have HIV because of the risk of passing HIV to your baby. Do not breastfeed if you are taking COMPLERA. At least two of the medicines contained in COMPLERA can be passed to your baby in your breast milk. We do not know whether this could harm your baby. Talk to your healthcare provider about the best way to feed your baby.
Tell your healthcare provider about all the medicines you take, including prescription and nonprescription medicines, vitamins, and herbal supplements.
COMPLERA may affect the way other medicines work, and other medicines may affect how COMPLERA works, and may cause serious side effects. If you take certain medicines with COMPLERA, the amount of COMPLERA in your body may be too low and it may not work to help control your HIV infection. The HIV virus in your body may become resistant to COMPLERA or other HIV medicines that are like it.
COMPLERA provides a complete treatment for HIV infection. Do not take other HIV medicines with COMPLERA.
If you take COMPLERA, you should not take:
• other medicines that contain tenofovir (VIREAD, TRUVADA®, STRIBILD®, ATRIPLA®)
• other medicines that contain emtricitabine or lamivudine (EMTRIVA, Combivir®, Epivir® or Epivir-HBV®, Epzicom®, Trizivir®, ATRIPLA, TRUVADA, STRIBILD)
• rilpivirine (Edurant), unless recommended by your healthcare provider and you are taking rifabutin (Mycobutin®)
• adefovir (HEPSERA®)
Especially tell your healthcare provider if you take:
• rifabutin (Mycobutin), a medicine to treat some bacterial infections. Talk to your doctor or pharmacist about the right amount of rilpivirine you should take.
• an antacid medicine that contains aluminum, magnesium hydroxide, or calcium carbonate. If you take an antacid during treatment with COMPLERA, take the antacid **at least 2 hours before or at least 4 hours after** you take COMPLERA.
• a medicine to block the acid in your stomach, including cimetidine (Tagamet®), famotidine (Pepcid®), nizatidine (Axid®), or ranitidine hydrochloride (Zantac®). If you take one of these medicines during treatment with COMPLERA, take the acid blocker **at least 12 hours before or at least 4 hours after** you take COMPLERA.
• any of these medicines (if taken by mouth or injection):
  • clarithromycin (Biaxin®)
  • erythromycin (E-Mycin®, Eryc®, Ery-Tab®, PCE®, Pediazole®, Ilosone®)
  • fluconazole (Diflucan®)
  • itraconazole (Sporanox®)
  • ketoconazole (Nizoral®)
  • methadone (Dolophine®)
  • posaconazole (Noxafil®)
  • telithromycin (Ketek®)
  • voriconazole (Vfend®)
• certain medicines that can affect how your kidneys work, including acyclovir (Zovirax®), cidofovir (VISTIDE®), ganciclovir (Cytovene IV®, Vitrasert®), valacyclovir (Valtrex®), and valganciclovir (Valcyte®)
Ask your healthcare provider or pharmacist if you are not sure if your medicine is one that is listed above.
Know the medicines you take. Keep a list of your medicines and show it to your healthcare provider and pharmacist when you get a new medicine. Your healthcare provider and your pharmacist can tell you if you can take these medicines with COMPLERA. Do not start any new medicines while you are taking COMPLERA without first talking with your healthcare provider or pharmacist. You can ask your healthcare provider or pharmacist for a list of medicines that can interact with COMPLERA.
How should I take COMPLERA?
• **Stay under the care of your healthcare provider during treatment with COMPLERA.**
• **Take COMPLERA exactly as your healthcare provider tells you to take it.**
• **Always take COMPLERA with food.** Taking COMPLERA with food is important to help get the right amount of medicine in your body. A protein drink does not replace food. If your healthcare provider decides to stop COMPLERA and you are switched to new medicines to treat HIV that includes rilpivirine tablets, the rilpivirine tablets should be taken only with a meal.
• Do not change your dose or stop taking COMPLERA without first talking with your healthcare provider. See your healthcare provider regularly while taking COMPLERA.

- If you miss a dose of COMPLERA within 12 hours of the time you usually take it, take your dose of COMPLERA **with food** as soon as possible. Then, take your next dose of COMPLERA at the regularly scheduled time. If you miss a dose of COMPLERA by more than 12 hours of the time you usually take it, wait and then take the next dose of COMPLERA at the regularly scheduled time.
- Do not take more than your prescribed dose to make up for a missed dose.
- When your COMPLERA supply starts to run low, get more from your healthcare provider or pharmacy. It is very important not to run out of COMPLERA. The amount of virus in your blood may increase if the medicine is stopped for even a short time.
- If you take too much COMPLERA, contact your local poison control center or go to the nearest hospital emergency room right away.

What are the possible side effects of COMPLERA?
COMPLERA can cause serious side effects, including:
- **See "What is the most important information I should know about COMPLERA?"**
- **New or worse kidney problems, including kidney failure,** can happen in some people who take COMPLERA. Your healthcare provider should do blood tests to check your kidneys before starting treatment with COMPLERA. If you have had kidney problems in the past or need to take another medicine that can cause kidney problems, your healthcare provider may need to do blood tests to check your kidneys during your treatment with COMPLERA.
- **Depression or mood changes. Tell your healthcare provider right away if you have any of the following symptoms:**
  - feeling sad or hopeless
  - feeling anxious or restless
  - have thoughts of hurting yourself (suicide) or have tried to hurt yourself
- **Change in liver enzymes.** People with a history of hepatitis B or C virus infection or who have certain liver enzyme changes may have an increased risk of developing new or worsening liver problems during treatment with COMPLERA. Liver problems can also happen during treatment with COMPLERA in people without a history of liver disease. Your healthcare provider may need to do tests to check your liver enzymes before and during treatment with COMPLERA.
- **Bone problems** can happen in some people who take COMPLERA. Bone problems include bone pain, softening or thinning (which may lead to fractures). Your healthcare provider may need to do additional tests to check your bones.
- **Changes in body fat** can happen in people taking HIV medicine. These changes may include increased amount of fat in the upper back and neck ("buffalo hump"), breast, and around the main part of your body (trunk). Loss of fat from the legs, arms and face may also happen. The cause and long term health effect of these conditions are not known.
- **Changes in your immune system (Immune Reconstitution Syndrome)** can happen when you start taking HIV medicines. Your immune system may get stronger and begin to fight infections that have been hidden in your body for a long time. Tell your healthcare provider if you start having new symptoms after starting your HIV medicine.

The most common side effects of COMPLERA include:
- trouble sleeping (insomnia)
- abnormal dreams
- headache
- dizziness
- diarrhea
- nausea
- rash
- tiredness
- depression

Additional common side effects include:
- vomiting
- stomach pain or discomfort
- skin discoloration (small spots or freckles)
- pain

Tell your healthcare provider if you have any side effect that bothers you or that does not go away.

These are not all the possible side effects of COMPLERA. For more information, ask your healthcare provider or pharmacist.

Call your doctor for medical advice about side effects. You may report side effects to FDA at 1-800-FDA-1088.

How do I store COMPLERA?
- Store COMPLERA at room temperature between 68 °F to 77 °F (20 °C to 25 °C).
- Keep COMPLERA in its original container and keep the container tightly closed.
- Do not use COMPLERA if the seal over the bottle opening is broken or missing.

Keep COMPLERA and all other medicines out of reach of children.

General information about COMPLERA:
Medicines are sometimes prescribed for purposes other than those listed in a Patient Information leaflet. Do not use COMPLERA for a condition for which it was not prescribed. Do not give COMPLERA to other people, even if they have the same symptoms you have. It may harm them.

This leaflet summarizes the most important information about COMPLERA. If you would like more information, talk with your healthcare provider. You can ask your healthcare provider or pharmacist for information about COMPLERA that is written for health professionals. For more information, call 1-800-445-3235 or go to www.COMPLERA.com.

What are the ingredients of COMPLERA?
Active ingredients: emtricitabine, rilpivirine hydrochloride, and tenofovir disoproxil fumarate.
Inactive ingredients: pregelatinized starch, lactose monohydrate, microcrystalline cellulose, croscarmellose sodium, magnesium stearate, povidone, polysorbate 20. The tablet film coating contains polyethylene glycol, hypromellose, lactose monohydrate, triacetin, titanium dioxide, iron oxide red, FD&C Blue #2 aluminum lake, FD&C Yellow #6 aluminum lake.

This Patient Information has been approved by the U.S. Food and Drug Administration

Manufactured and distributed by:
Gilead Sciences, Inc.
Foster City, CA 94404
Revised: June 2014
COMPLERA, EMTRIVA, HEPSERA, STRIBILD, TRUVADA, VIREAD, and VISTIDE are trademarks of Gilead Sciences, Inc., or its related companies. Edurant is a trademark of Janssen Pharmaceuticals, Inc. ATRIPLA is a trademark of Bristol-Myers Squibb & Gilead Sciences, LLC. All other trademarks referenced herein are the property of their respective owners.
202123-GS-006
Shown in Product Identification Guide, page 306

LETAIRIS®
[le-TAIR-is]
(ambrisentan)
tablets, for oral use

℞

HIGHLIGHTS OF PRESCRIBING INFORMATION
These highlights do not include all the information needed to use LETAIRIS® safely and effectively. See full prescribing information for LETAIRIS.
Letairis (ambrisentan) tablets, for oral use
Initial U.S. Approval: 2007

> **WARNING: EMBRYO-FETAL TOXICITY**
> *See full prescribing information for complete boxed warning.*
> - Do not administer Letairis to a pregnant female because it may cause fetal harm (4.1, 5.1, 8.1).
> - Females of reproductive potential: Exclude pregnancy before the start of treatment, monthly during treatment, and 1 month after stopping treatment. Prevent pregnancy during treatment and for one month after stopping treatment by using acceptable methods of contraception (2.2, 8.6).
> - For all female patients, Letairis is available only through a restricted program called the Letairis Risk Evaluation and Mitigation Strategy (REMS). (5.2)

RECENT MAJOR CHANGES
• Boxed Warning	08/2013
• Dosage and Administration (2.2)	08/2013
• Warnings and Precautions, Embryo-fetal Toxicity (5.1)	08/2013
• Warnings and Precautions, Letairis REMS Program (5.2)	08/2013

INDICATIONS AND USAGE
Letairis is an endothelin receptor antagonist indicated for the treatment of pulmonary arterial hypertension (PAH) (WHO Group 1) to improve exercise ability and delay clinical worsening. Studies establishing effectiveness included predominantly patients with WHO Functional Class II–III symptoms and etiologies of idiopathic or heritable PAH (64%) or PAH associated with connective tissue diseases (32%) (1).

DOSAGE AND ADMINISTRATION
- Initiate treatment at 5 mg once daily with or without food, and consider increasing the dose to 10 mg once daily if 5 mg is tolerated (2.1).
- Tablets should not be split, crushed, or chewed (2.1).

DOSAGE FORMS AND STRENGTHS
Tablet: 5 mg and 10 mg (3)

CONTRAINDICATIONS
- Pregnancy (4.1)
- Idiopathic Pulmonary Fibrosis (4.2)

WARNINGS AND PRECAUTIONS
- Fluid retention may require intervention (5.3).
- If patients develop acute pulmonary edema during initiation of therapy with Letairis, consider underlying pulmonary veno-occlusive disease and discontinue treatment if necessary (5.4).
- Decreases in sperm count have been observed in patients taking endothelin receptor antagonists (5.5).
- Decreases in hemoglobin have been observed within the first few weeks; measure hemoglobin at initiation, at 1 month, and periodically thereafter (5.6).

ADVERSE REACTIONS
Most common adverse reactions (>3% compared to placebo) are peripheral edema, nasal congestion, sinusitis, and flushing (6.1).
To report SUSPECTED ADVERSE REACTIONS, contact Gilead Sciences, Inc. at (1-800-445-3235, Option 3) or FDA at 1-800-FDA-1088 or www.fda.gov/medwatch.

DRUG INTERACTIONS
Multiple dose coadministration of ambrisentan and cyclosporine resulted in an about 2-fold increase in ambrisentan exposure in healthy volunteers. When coadministered with cyclosporine, limit the dose to 5 mg once daily (7).

USE IN SPECIFIC POPULATIONS
- Breastfeeding: Choose Letairis or breastfeeding (8.3).
- Not recommended in patients with moderate or severe hepatic impairment (8.8).

See 17 for PATIENT COUNSELING INFORMATION and Medication Guide

Revised: 05/2014

FULL PRESCRIBING INFORMATION

> **WARNING: EMBRYO-FETAL TOXICITY**
>
> **Do not administer Letairis to a pregnant female because it may cause fetal harm. Letairis is very likely to produce serious birth defects if used by pregnant females, as this effect has been seen consistently when it is administered to animals** *[see Contraindications (4.1), Warnings and Precautions (5.1), and Use in Specific Populations (8.1)].*
>
> **Exclude pregnancy before the initiation of treatment with Letairis. Females of reproductive potential must use acceptable methods of contraception during treatment with Letairis and for one month after treatment. Obtain monthly pregnancy tests during treatment and 1 month after discontinuation of treatment** *[see Dosage and Administration (2.2) and Use in Specific Populations (8.6)].*
>
> **Because of the risk of embryo-fetal toxicity, females can only receive Letairis through a restricted program called the Letairis REMS program** *[see Warnings and Precautions (5.2)].*

1 INDICATIONS AND USAGE

Letairis is indicated for the treatment of pulmonary arterial hypertension (PAH) (WHO Group 1) to improve exercise ability and delay clinical worsening. Studies establishing effectiveness included predominantly patients with WHO Functional Class II–III symptoms and etiologies of idiopathic or heritable PAH (64%) or PAH associated with connective tissue diseases (32%).

2 DOSAGE AND ADMINISTRATION

2.1 Adult Dosage

Initiate treatment at 5 mg once daily, and consider increasing the dose to 10 mg once daily if 5 mg is tolerated.

Tablets may be administered with or without food. Tablets should not be split, crushed, or chewed. Doses higher than 10 mg once daily have not been studied in patients with pulmonary arterial hypertension (PAH).

2.2 Pregnancy Testing in Females of Reproductive Potential

Initiate treatment with Letairis in females of reproductive potential only after a negative pregnancy test. Obtain monthly pregnancy tests during treatment *[see Use in Specific Populations (8.6)].*

3 DOSAGE FORMS AND STRENGTHS

5 mg and 10 mg film-coated tablets for oral administration
- Each 5 mg tablet is square convex, pale pink, with "5" on one side and "GSI" on the other side.
- Each 10 mg tablet is oval convex, deep pink, with "10" on one side and "GSI" on the other side.

4 CONTRAINDICATIONS

4.1 Pregnancy

Letairis may cause fetal harm when administered to a pregnant female. Letairis is contraindicated in females who are pregnant. Letairis was consistently shown to have teratogenic effects when administered to animals. If this drug is used during pregnancy, or if the patient becomes pregnant while taking this drug, the patient should be apprised of the potential hazard to a fetus *[see Warnings and Precautions (5.1, 5.2) and Use in Specific Populations (8.1)].*

4.2 Idiopathic Pulmonary Fibrosis

Letairis is contraindicated in patients with Idiopathic Pulmonary Fibrosis (IPF), including IPF patients with pulmonary hypertension (WHO Group 3) *[see Clinical Studies (14.3)].*

5 WARNINGS AND PRECAUTIONS

5.1 Embryo-fetal Toxicity

Letairis may cause fetal harm when administered during pregnancy and is contraindicated for use in females who are pregnant. In females of reproductive potential, exclude pregnancy prior to initiation of therapy, ensure use of acceptable contraceptive methods, and obtain monthly pregnancy tests *[see Dosage and Administration (2.2), and Use in Specific Populations (8.1, 8.6)].*

Letairis is only available for females through a restricted program under a REMS *[see Warnings and Precautions (5.2)].*

5.2 Letairis REMS Program

For all females, Letairis is available only through a restricted program called the Letairis REMS, because of the risk of embryo-fetal toxicity *[see Contraindications (4.1), Warnings and Precautions (5.1), and Use in Specific Populations (8.1, 8.6)].*

Notable requirements of the Letairis REMS program include the following:
- Prescribers must be certified with the program by enrolling and completing training.

- All females, regardless of reproductive potential, must enroll in the Letairis REMS program prior to initiating Letairis. Male patients are not enrolled in the REMS.
  - Females of reproductive potential must comply with the pregnancy testing and contraception requirements *[see Use in Specific Populations (8.6)].*
- Pharmacies that dispense Letairis must be certified with the program and must dispense to female patients who are authorized to receive Letairis.

Further information is available at www.letairisrems.com or 1-866-664-5327.

5.3 Fluid Retention

Peripheral edema is a known class effect of endothelin receptor antagonists, and is also a clinical consequence of PAH and worsening PAH. In the placebo-controlled studies, there was an increased incidence of peripheral edema in patients treated with doses of 5 or 10 mg Letairis compared to placebo *[see Adverse Reactions (6.1)].* Most edema was mild to moderate in severity, and it occurred with greater frequency and severity in elderly patients.

In addition, there have been postmarketing reports of fluid retention in patients with pulmonary hypertension, occurring within weeks after starting Letairis. Patients required intervention with a diuretic, fluid management, or, in some cases, hospitalization for decompensating heart failure.

If clinically significant fluid retention develops, with or without associated weight gain, further evaluation should be undertaken to determine the cause, such as Letairis or underlying heart failure, and the possible need for specific treatment or discontinuation of Letairis therapy.

5.4 Pulmonary Edema with Pulmonary Veno-occlusive Disease (PVOD)

If patients develop acute pulmonary edema during initiation of therapy with vasodilating agents such as Letairis, the possibility of PVOD should be considered, and if confirmed Letairis should be discontinued.

5.5 Decreased Sperm Counts

Decreased sperm counts have been observed in human and animal studies with another endothelin receptor antagonist and in animal fertility studies with ambrisentan. Letairis may have an adverse effect on spermatogenesis. Counsel patients about potential effects on fertility *[see Use in Specific Populations (8.6) and Nonclinical Toxicology (13.1)].*

5.6 Hematological Changes

Decreases in hemoglobin concentration and hematocrit have followed administration of other endothelin receptor antagonists and were observed in clinical studies with Letairis. These decreases were observed within the first few weeks of treatment with Letairis, and stabilized thereafter. The mean decrease in hemoglobin from baseline to end of treatment for those patients receiving Letairis in the 12-week placebo-controlled studies was 0.8 g/dL.

Marked decreases in hemoglobin (>15% decrease from baseline resulting in a value below the lower limit of normal) were observed in 7% of all patients receiving Letairis (and 10% of patients receiving 10 mg) compared to 4% of patients receiving placebo. The cause of the decrease in hemoglobin is unknown, but it does not appear to result from hemorrhage or hemolysis.

In the long-term open-label extension of the two pivotal clinical studies, mean decreases from baseline (ranging from 0.9 to 1.2 g/dL) in hemoglobin concentrations persisted for up to 4 years of treatment.

There have been postmarketing reports of decreases in hemoglobin concentration and hematocrit that have resulted in anemia requiring transfusion.

Measure hemoglobin prior to initiation of Letairis, at one month, and periodically thereafter. Initiation of Letairis therapy is not recommended for patients with clinically significant anemia. If a clinically significant decrease in hemoglobin is observed and other causes have been excluded, consider discontinuing Letairis.

6 ADVERSE REACTIONS

Clinically significant adverse reactions that appear in other sections of the labeling include:
- Embryo-fetal Toxicity *[see Warnings and Precautions (5.1), Use in Specific Populations (8.1)]*
- Fluid Retention *[see Warnings and Precautions (5.3)]*
- Pulmonary Edema with PVOD *[see Warnings and Precautions (5.4)]*
- Decreased Sperm Count *[see Warnings and Precautions (5.5)]*
- Hematologic Changes *[see Warnings and Precautions (5.6)]*

6.1 Clinical Trials Experience

Because clinical trials are conducted under widely varying conditions, adverse reaction rates observed in the clinical trials of a drug cannot be directly compared to rates in the clinical trials of another drug and may not reflect the rates observed in practice.

Safety data for Letairis were obtained from two 12-week, placebo-controlled studies in patients with pulmonary arterial hypertension (PAH) (ARIES-1 and ARIES-2) and four

nonplacebo-controlled studies in 483 patients with PAH who were treated with doses of 1, 2.5, 5, or 10 mg once daily. The exposure to Letairis in these studies ranged from 1 day to 4 years (N = 418 for at least 6 months and N = 343 for at least 1 year).

In ARIES-1 and ARIES-2, a total of 261 patients received Letairis at doses of 2.5, 5, or 10 mg once daily and 132 patients received placebo. The adverse reactions that occurred in >3% more patients receiving Letairis than receiving placebo are shown in Table 1.

Table 1 Adverse Reactions with Placebo-Adjusted Rates >3%

Adverse Reaction	Placebo (N = 132) n (%)	Letairis (N = 261) n (%)	Letairis (N = 261) Placebo-adjusted (%)
Peripheral edema	14 (11)	45 (17)	6
Nasal congestion	2 (2)	15 (6)	4
Sinusitis	0 (0)	8 (3)	3
Flushing	1 (1)	10 (4)	3

Most adverse drug reactions were mild to moderate and only nasal congestion was dose-dependent.

Few notable differences in the incidence of adverse reactions were observed for patients by age or sex. Peripheral edema was similar in younger patients (<65 years) receiving Letairis (14%; 29/205) or placebo (13%; 13/104), and was greater in elderly patients (≥65 years) receiving Letairis (29%; 16/56) compared to placebo (4%; 1/28). The results of such subgroup analyses must be interpreted cautiously.

The incidence of treatment discontinuations due to adverse events other than those related to PAH during the clinical trials in patients with PAH was similar for Letairis (2%; 5/261 patients) and placebo (2%; 3/132 patients). The incidence of patients with serious adverse events other than those related to PAH during the clinical trials in patients with PAH was similar for placebo (7%; 9/132 patients) and for Letairis (5%; 13/261 patients).

During 12-week controlled clinical trials, the incidence of aminotransferase elevations >3 × upper limit of normal (ULN) were 0% on Letairis and 2.3% on placebo. In practice, cases of hepatic injury should be carefully evaluated for cause.

Use in Patients with Prior Endothelin Receptor Antagonist (ERA) Related Serum Liver Enzyme Abnormalities

In an uncontrolled, open-label study, 36 patients who had previously discontinued endothelin receptor antagonists (ERAs: bosentan, an investigational drug, or both) due to aminotransferase elevations >3 × ULN were treated with Letairis. Prior elevations were predominantly moderate, with 64% of the ALT elevations <5 × ULN, but 9 patients had elevations >8 × ULN. Eight patients had been rechallenged with bosentan and/or the investigational ERA and all eight had a recurrence of aminotransferase abnormalities that required discontinuation of ERA therapy. All patients had to have normal aminotransferase levels on entry to this study. Twenty-five of the 36 patients were also receiving prostanoid and/or phosphodiesterase type 5 (PDE5) inhibitor therapy. Two patients discontinued early (including one of the patients with a prior 8 × ULN elevation). Of the remaining 34 patients, one patient experienced a mild aminotransferase elevation at 12 weeks on Letairis 5 mg that resolved with decreasing the dosage to 2.5 mg, and that did not recur with later escalations to 10 mg. With a median follow-up of 13 months and with 50% of patients increasing the dose of Letairis to 10 mg, no patients were discontinued for aminotransferase elevations. While the uncontrolled study design does not provide information about what would have occurred with re-administration of previously used ERAs or show that Letairis led to fewer aminotransferase elevations than would have been seen with those drugs, the study indicates that Letairis may be tried in patients who have experienced asymptomatic aminotransferase elevations on other ERAs after aminotransferase levels have returned to normal.

6.2 Postmarketing Experience

The following adverse reactions were identified during postapproval use of Letairis. Because these reactions are reported voluntarily from a population of uncertain size, it is not possible to estimate reliably the frequency or to establish a causal relationship to drug exposure: anemia *[see Warnings and Precautions (5.6)],* asthenia, dizziness, fatigue, fluid retention *[see Warnings and Precautions (5.3)],* heart failure (associated with fluid retention), hypersensitivity (eg, angioedema, rash), nausea, and vomiting.

Elevations of liver aminotransferases (ALT, AST) have been reported with Letairis use; in most cases alternative causes

Help Patients Save on Rx Drugs: PDR.net/PharmacyDiscountCard

of the liver injury could be identified (heart failure, hepatic congestion, hepatitis, alcohol use, hepatotoxic medications). Other endothelin receptor antagonists have been associated with elevations of aminotransferases, hepatotoxicity, and cases of liver failure [see Adverse Reactions (6.1)].

7   DRUG INTERACTIONS
Multiple dose coadministration of ambrisentan and cyclosporine resulted in an approximately 2-fold increase in ambrisentan exposure in healthy volunteers; therefore, limit the dose of ambrisentan to 5 mg once daily when coadministered with cyclosporine [see Clinical Pharmacology (12.3)].

8   USE IN SPECIFIC POPULATIONS
8.1   Pregnancy
Pregnancy Category X
Risk Summary
Letairis may cause fetal harm when administered to a pregnant woman and is contraindicated during pregnancy. Letairis was teratogenic in rats and rabbits at doses which resulted in exposures of 3.5 and 1.7 times, respectively, the human dose of 10 mg per day. If this drug is used during pregnancy, or if the patient becomes pregnant while taking this drug, advise the patient of the potential hazard to a fetus [see Contraindications (4.1), Warnings and Precautions (5.1)].
Animal Data
Letairis was teratogenic at oral doses of $\geq$ 15 mg/kg/day (AUC 51.7 h•µg/mL) in rats and $\geq$ 7 mg/kg/day (24.7 h•µg/mL) in rabbits; it was not studied at lower doses. These doses are of 3.5 and 1.7 times, respectively, the human dose of 10 mg per day (14.8 h•µg/mL) based on AUC. In both species, there were abnormalities of the lower jaw and hard and soft palate, malformation of the heart and great vessels, and failure of formation of the thymus and thyroid.
A preclinical study in rats has shown decreased survival of newborn pups (mid and high doses) and effects on testicle size and fertility of pups (high dose) following maternal treatment with ambrisentan from late gestation through weaning. Doses tested were 17 ×, 51 ×, and 170 × (on a mg/kg:mg/m² basis) the maximum oral human dose of 10 mg and an average adult body weight of 70 kg.
8.3   Nursing Mothers
It is not known whether ambrisentan is present in human milk. Because many drugs are present in human milk and because of the potential for serious adverse reactions in nursing infants from Letairis, a decision should be made whether to discontinue nursing or discontinue Letairis, taking into account the importance of the drug to the mother.
8.4   Pediatric Use
Safety and effectiveness of Letairis in pediatric patients have not been established.
8.5   Geriatric Use
In one placebo-controlled clinical studies of Letairis, 21% of patients were ≥65 years old and 5% were ≥75 years old. The elderly (age ≥65 years) showed less improvement in walk distances with Letairis than younger patients did, but the results of such subgroup analyses must be interpreted cautiously. Peripheral edema was more common in the elderly than in younger patients.
8.6   Females and Males of Reproductive Potential
Pregnancy Testing
Female patients of reproductive potential must have a negative pregnancy test prior to initiation of treatment, monthly pregnancy test during treatment, and 1 month after stopping treatment with Letairis. Advise patients to contact their healthcare provider if they become pregnant or suspect they may be pregnant. Perform a pregnancy test if pregnancy is suspected for any reason. For positive pregnancy tests, counsel patient on the potential risk to the fetus and patient options [see Boxed Warning and Dosage and Administration (2.2)].
Contraception
Female patients of reproductive potential must use acceptable methods of contraception during treatment with Letairis and for 1 month after stopping treatment with Letairis. Patients may choose one highly effective form of contraception (intrauterine device (IUD), contraceptive implant, or tubal sterilization) or a combination of methods (hormone method with a barrier method or two barrier methods). If a partner's vasectomy is the chosen method of contraception, a hormone or barrier method must be used along with this method. Counsel patients on pregnancy planning and prevention, including emergency contraception, or designate counseling by another healthcare provider trained in contraceptive counseling [see Boxed Warning].
Infertility
Males
In a 6-month study of another endothelin receptor antagonist, bosentan, 25 male patients with WHO functional class III and IV PAH and normal baseline sperm count were evaluated for effects on testicular function. There was a decline in sperm count of at least 50% in 25% of the patients after 3

or 6 months of treatment with bosentan. One patient developed marked oligospermia at 3 months, and the sperm count remained low with 2 follow-up measurements over the subsequent 6 weeks. Bosentan was discontinued and after 2 months the sperm count had returned to baseline levels. In 22 patients who completed 6 months of treatment, sperm count remained within the normal range and no changes in sperm morphology, sperm motility, or hormone levels were observed. Based on these findings and preclinical data [see Nonclinical Toxicology (13.1)] from endothelin receptor antagonists, it cannot be excluded that endothelin receptor antagonists such as Letairis have an adverse effect on spermatogenesis. Counsel patients about the potential effects on fertility [see Warnings and Precautions (5.5)].
8.7   Renal Impairment
The impact of renal impairment on the pharmacokinetics of ambrisentan has been examined using a population pharmacokinetic approach in PAH patients with creatinine clearances ranging between 20 and 150 mL/min. There was no significant impact of mild or moderate renal impairment on exposure to ambrisentan [see Clinical Pharmacology (12.3)]. Dose adjustment of Letairis in patients with mild or moderate renal impairment is therefore not required. There is no information on the exposure to ambrisentan in patients with severe renal impairment.
The impact of hemodialysis on the disposition of ambrisentan has not been investigated.
8.8   Hepatic Impairment
Pre-existing Hepatic Impairment
The influence of pre-existing hepatic impairment on the pharmacokinetics of ambrisentan has not been evaluated. Because there is in vitro and in vivo evidence of significant metabolic and biliary contribution to the elimination of ambrisentan, hepatic impairment might be expected to have significant effects on the pharmacokinetics of ambrisentan [see Clinical Pharmacology (12.3)]. Letairis is not recommended in patients with moderate or severe hepatic impairment. There is no information on the use of Letairis in patients with mild pre-existing impaired liver function; however, exposure to ambrisentan may be increased in these patients.
Elevation of Liver Transaminases
Other endothelin receptor antagonists (ERAs) have been associated with aminotransferase (AST, ALT) elevations, hepatotoxicity, and cases of liver failure [see Adverse Reactions (6.1, 6.2)]. In patients who develop hepatic impairment after Letairis initiation, the cause of liver injury should be fully investigated. Discontinue Letairis if elevations of liver aminotransferases are >5 × ULN or if elevations are accompanied by bilirubin >2 × ULN, or by signs or symptoms of liver dysfunction and other causes are excluded.

10   OVERDOSAGE
There is no experience with overdosage of Letairis. The highest single dose of Letairis administered to healthy volunteers was 100 mg, and the highest daily dose administered to patients with PAH was 10 mg once daily. In healthy volunteers, single doses of 50 mg and 100 mg (5 to 10 times the maximum recommended dose) were associated with headache, flushing, dizziness, nausea, and nasal congestion. Massive overdosage could potentially result in hypotension that may require intervention.

11   DESCRIPTION
Letairis is the brand name for ambrisentan, an endothelin receptor antagonist that is selective for the endothelin type-A (ETA) receptor. The chemical name of ambrisentan is (+)-(2S)-2-[(4,6-dimethylpyrimidin-2-yl)oxy]-3-methoxy-3,3-diphenylpropanoic acid. It has a molecular formula of $C_{22}H_{22}N_2O_4$ and a molecular weight of 378.42. It contains a single chiral center determined to be the (S) configuration and has the following structural formula:

Figure 1 Ambrisentan Structural Formula

Ambrisentan is a white to off-white, crystalline solid. It is a carboxylic acid with a pKa of 4.0. Ambrisentan is practically insoluble in water and in aqueous solutions at low pH. Solubility increases in aqueous solutions at higher pH. In the solid state ambrisentan is very stable, is not hygroscopic, and is not light sensitive.
Letairis is available as 5 mg and 10 mg film-coated tablets for once daily oral administration. The tablets include the following inactive ingredients: croscarmellose sodium, lactose monohydrate, magnesium stearate and microcrystalline cellulose. The tablets are film-coated with a coating material containing FD&C Red #40 aluminum lake, lecithin,

polyethylene glycol, polyvinyl alcohol, talc, and titanium dioxide. Each square, pale pink Letairis tablet contains 5 mg of ambrisentan. Each oval, deep pink Letairis tablet contains 10 mg of ambrisentan. Letairis tablets are unscored.

12   CLINICAL PHARMACOLOGY
12.1   Mechanism of Action
Endothelin-1 (ET-1) is a potent autocrine and paracrine peptide. Two receptor subtypes, ETA and ETB, mediate the effects of ET-1 in the vascular smooth muscle and endothelium. The primary actions of ETA are vasoconstriction and cell proliferation, while the predominant actions of ETB are vasodilation, antiproliferation, and ET-1 clearance.
In patients with PAH, plasma ET-1 concentrations are increased as much as 10-fold and correlate with increased mean right atrial pressure and disease severity. ET-1 and ET-1 mRNA concentrations are increased as much as 9-fold in the lung tissue of patients with PAH, primarily in the endothelium of pulmonary arteries. These findings suggest that ET-1 may play a critical role in the pathogenesis and progression of PAH.
Ambrisentan is a high-affinity (K_i=0.011 nM) ETA receptor antagonist with a high selectivity for the ETA versus ETB receptor (>4000-fold). The clinical impact of high selectivity for ETA is not known.
12.2   Pharmacodynamics
Cardiac Electrophysiology
In a randomized, positive- and placebo-controlled, parallel-group study, healthy subjects received either Letairis 10 mg daily followed by a single dose of 40 mg, placebo followed by a single dose of moxifloxacin 400 mg, or placebo alone. Letairis 10 mg daily had no significant effect on the QTc interval. The 40 mg dose of Letairis increased mean QTc at t_{max} by 5 ms with an upper 95% confidence limit of 9 ms. For patients receiving Letairis 5–10 mg daily and not taking metabolic inhibitors, no significant QT prolongation is expected.
12.3   Pharmacokinetics
The pharmacokinetics of ambrisentan (S-ambrisentan) in healthy subjects is dose proportional. The absolute bioavailability of ambrisentan is not known. Ambrisentan is absorbed with peak concentrations occurring approximately 2 hours after oral administration in healthy subjects and PAH patients. Food does not affect its bioavailability. In vitro studies indicate that ambrisentan is a substrate of P-gp. Ambrisentan is highly bound to plasma proteins (99%). The elimination of ambrisentan is predominantly by non-renal pathways, but the relative contributions of metabolism and biliary elimination have not been well characterized. In plasma, the AUC of 4-hydroxymethyl ambrisentan accounts for approximately 4% relative to parent ambrisentan AUC. The in vivo inversion of S-ambrisentan to R-ambrisentan is negligible. The mean oral clearance of ambrisentan is 38 mL/min and 19 mL/min in healthy subjects and in PAH patients, respectively. Although ambrisentan has a 15-hour terminal half-life, the mean trough concentration of ambrisentan at steady-state is about 15% of the mean peak concentration and the accumulation factor is about 1.2 after long-term daily dosing, indicating that the effective half-life of ambrisentan is about 9 hours.
Drug Interactions
In Vitro Studies
Studies with human liver tissue indicate that ambrisentan is metabolized by CYP3A, CYP2C19, and uridine 5'-diphosphate glucuronosyltransferases (UGTs) 1A9S, 2B7S, and 1A3S. In vitro studies suggest that ambrisentan is a substrate of the Organic Anion Transporting Polypeptides OATP1B1 and OATP1B3, and P-glycoprotein (P-gp). Drug interactions might be expected because of these factors; however, a clinically relevant interaction has been demonstrated only with cyclosporine [see Drug Interactions (7)]. In vitro studies found ambrisentan to have little to no inhibition of human hepatic transporters. Ambrisentan demonstrated weak dose-dependent inhibition of OATP1B1, OATP1B3, and NTCP (IC_{50} of 47 µM, 45 µM, and approximately 100 µM, respectively) and no transporter-specific inhibition of BSEP, BRCP, P-gp, or MRP2. Ambrisentan does not inhibit or induce drug metabolizing enzymes at clinically relevant concentrations.
In Vivo Studies
The effects of other drugs on ambrisentan pharmacokinetics and the effects of ambrisentan on the exposure to other drugs are shown in Figure 2 and Figure 3, respectively.
[See figure 2 at top of next column]
[See figure 3 at top of next column]

13   NONCLINICAL TOXICOLOGY
13.1   Carcinogenesis, Mutagenesis, Impairment of Fertility
Oral carcinogenicity studies of up to two years duration were conducted at starting doses of 10, 30, and 60 mg/kg/day in rats (8 to 48 times the maximum recommended human dose [MRHD] on a mg/m² basis) and at 50, 150, and 250 mg/kg/day in mice (28 to 140 times the MRHD). In the rat study, the high- and mid-dose male and female groups had their doses lowered to 40 and 20 mg/kg/day, respectively, in week 51 because of effects on survival. The high-

Figure 2 Effects of Other Drugs on Ambrisentan Pharmacokinetics

Interacting Drug	PK	Fold Change and 90% CI	Recommendation
Cyclosporine	Cmax AUC		Limit ambrisentan to 5 mg once daily
Mycophenolate Mofetil	Cmax AUC		No dose adjustment
Ketoconazole	Cmax AUC		No dose adjustment
Omeprazole*	Cmax AUC		No dose adjustment
Rifampin**	Cmax AUC		No dose adjustment
Ritonavir	Cmax AUC		No dose adjustment
Sildenafil	Cmax AUC		No dose adjustment
Tacrolimus	Cmax AUC		No dose adjustment
Tadalafil	Cmax AUC		No dose adjustment
Warfarin	Cmax AUC		No dose adjustment

0.0 0.5 1.0 1.5 2.0 2.5 3.0
Change relative to ambrisentan alone

* Omeprazole: based on population pharmacokinetic analysis in PAH patients

** Rifampin: AUC and C_{max} were measured at steady-state. On Day 3 of coadministration a transient 2-fold increase in AUC was noted that was no longer evident by Day 7. Day 7 results are presented.

Figure 3 Effects of Ambrisentan on Other Drugs

Interacting Drug	PK	Fold Change and 90% CI	Recommendation
Cyclosporine	Cmax AUC		No dose adjustment
Digoxin	Cmax AUC		No dose adjustment
Ethinylestradiol	Cmax AUC		No dose adjustment
Norethindrone	Cmax AUC		No dose adjustment
Mycophenolic acid*	Cmax AUC		No dose adjustment
Ritonavir	Cmax AUC		No dose adjustment
Sildenafil	Cmax AUC		No dose adjustment
- Desmethylsildenafil	Cmax AUC		
Tadalafil	Cmax AUC		No dose adjustment
Warfarin	Emax** AUEC**		No dose adjustment
- S-Warfarin	Cmax AUC		
- R-Warfarin	Cmax AUC		

0.0 0.5 1.0 1.5 2.0 2.5 3.0
Change relative to interacting drug alone

* Active metabolite of mycophenolate mofetil

** GMR (95% CI) for INR

dose males and females were taken off drug completely in weeks 69 and 93, respectively. The only evidence of ambrisentan-related carcinogenicity was a positive trend in male rats, for the combined incidence of benign basal cell tumor and basal cell carcinoma of skin/subcutis in the mid-dose group (high-dose group excluded from analysis), and the occurrence of mammary fibroadenomas in males in the high-dose group. In the mouse study, high-dose male and female groups had their doses lowered to 150 mg/kg/day in week 39 and were taken off drug completely in week 96 (males) or week 76 (females). In mice, ambrisentan was not associated with excess tumors in any dosed group.

Positive findings of clastogenicity were detected, at drug concentrations producing moderate to high toxicity, in the chromosome aberration assay in cultured human lymphocytes. There was no evidence for genetic toxicity of ambrisentan when tested in vitro in bacteria (Ames test) or in vivo in rats (micronucleus assay, unscheduled DNA synthesis assay).

Table 2 Changes from Baseline in 6-Minute Walk Distance (meters)

	ARIES-1			ARIES-2		
	Placebo (N = 67)	5 mg (N = 67)	10 mg (N = 67)	Placebo (N = 65)	2.5 mg (N = 64)	5 mg (N = 63)
Baseline	342 ± 73	340 ± 77	342 ± 78	343 ± 86	347 ± 84	355 ± 84
Mean change from baseline	-8 ± 79	23 ± 83	44 ± 63	-10 ± 94	22 ± 83	49 ± 75
Placebo-adjusted mean change from baseline	–	31	51	–	32	59
Placebo-adjusted median change from baseline	–	27	39	–	30	45
p-value*	–	0.008	<0.001	–	0.022	<0.001

Mean ± standard deviation

* p-values are Wilcoxon rank sum test comparisons of Letairis to placebo at Week 12 stratified by idiopathic or heritable PAH and non-idiopathic, non-heritable PAH patients

The development of testicular tubular atrophy and impaired fertility has been linked to the chronic administration of endothelin receptor antagonists in rodents. Testicular tubular degeneration was observed in rats treated with ambrisentan for two years at doses ≥10 mg/kg/day (8-fold MRHD). Increased incidences of testicular findings were also observed in mice treated for two years at doses ≥50 mg/kg/day (28-fold MRHD). Effects on sperm count, sperm morphology, mating performance, and fertility were observed in fertility studies in which male rats were treated with ambrisentan at oral doses of 300 mg/kg/day (236-fold MRHD). At doses of ≥10 mg/kg/day, observations of testicular histopathology in the absence of fertility and sperm effects were also present.

14 CLINICAL STUDIES

14.1 Pulmonary Arterial Hypertension (PAH)

Two 12-week, randomized, double-blind, placebo-controlled, multicenter studies were conducted in 393 patients with PAH (WHO Group 1). The two studies were identical in design except for the doses of Letairis and the geographic region of the investigational sites. ARIES-1 compared once-daily doses of 5 mg and 10 mg Letairis to placebo, while ARIES-2 compared once-daily doses of 2.5 mg and 5 mg Letairis to placebo. In both studies, Letairis or placebo was added to current therapy, which could have included a combination of anticoagulants, diuretics, calcium channel blockers, or digoxin, but not epoprostenol, treprostinil, iloprost, bosentan, or sildenafil. The primary study endpoint was 6-minute walk distance. In addition, clinical worsening, WHO functional class, dyspnea, and SF-36® Health Survey were assessed.

Patients had idiopathic or heritable PAH (64%) or PAH associated with connective tissue diseases (32%), HIV infection (3%), or anorexigen use (1%). There were no patients with PAH associated with congenital heart disease.

Patients had WHO functional class I (2%), II (38%), III (55%), or IV (5%) symptoms at baseline. The mean age of patients was 50 years, 79% of patients were female, and 77% were Caucasian.

Submaximal Exercise Ability

Results of the 6-minute walk distance at 12 weeks for the ARIES-1 and ARIES-2 studies are shown in Table 2 and Figure 4.

[See table 2 above]

[See figure 4 at top of next column]

In both studies, treatment with Letairis resulted in a significant improvement in 6-minute walk distance for each dose of Letairis and the improvements increased with dose. An increase in 6-minute walk distance was observed after 4 weeks of treatment with Letairis, with a dose-response observed after 12 weeks of treatment. Improvements in walk distance with Letairis were smaller for elderly patients (age ≥65) than younger patients and for patients with secondary PAH than for patients with idiopathic or heritable PAH. The results of such subgroup analyses must be interpreted cautiously.

The effects of Letairis on walk distances at trough drug levels are not known. Because only once-daily dosing was studied in the clinical trials, the efficacy and safety of more frequent dosing regimens for Letairis are not known. If exercise ability is not sustained throughout the day in a patient, consider other PAH treatments that have been studied with more-frequent dosing regimens.

Clinical Worsening

Time to clinical worsening of PAH was defined as the first occurrence of death, lung transplantation, hospitalization for PAH, atrial septostomy, study withdrawal due to the addition of other PAH therapeutic agents, or study withdrawal

Figure 4 Mean Change in 6-Minute Walk Distance

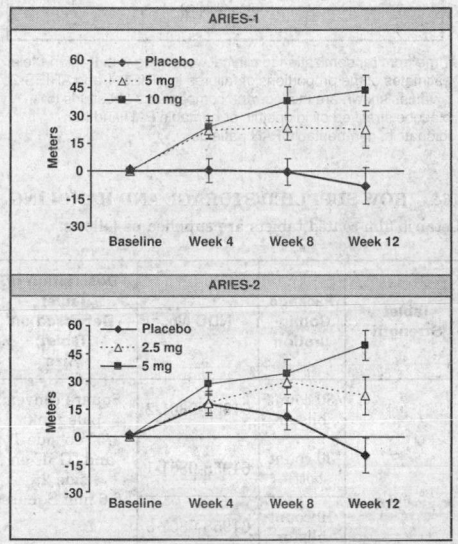

Mean change from baseline in 6-minute walk distance in the placebo and Letairis groups

Values are expressed as mean ± standard error of the mean.

due to early escape. Early escape was defined as meeting two or more of the following criteria: a 20% decrease in the 6-minute walk distance; an increase in WHO functional class; worsening right ventricular failure; rapidly progressing cardiogenic, hepatic, or renal failure; or refractory systolic hypotension. The clinical worsening events during the 12-week treatment period of the Letairis clinical trials are shown in Table 3 and Figure 5.

[See table 3 at top of next page]

There was a significant delay in the time to clinical worsening for patients receiving Letairis compared to placebo. Results in subgroups such as the elderly were also favorable.

[See figure 5 at top of next column]

14.2 Long-term Treatment of PAH

In long-term follow-up of patients who were treated with Letairis (2.5 mg, 5 mg, or 10 mg once daily) in the two pivotal studies and their open-label extension (N = 383), Kaplan-Meier estimates of survival at 1, 2, and 3 years were 93%, 85%, and 79%, respectively. Of the patients who remained on Letairis for up to 3 years, the majority received no other treatment for PAH. These uncontrolled observations do not allow comparison with a group not given Letairis and cannot be used to determine the long-term effect of Letairis on mortality.

14.3 Adverse Effects in Idiopathic Pulmonary Fibrosis (IPF)

A randomized controlled study in patients with IPF, with or without pulmonary hypertension (WHO Group 3), compared Letairis (N = 329) to placebo (N = 163). The study was terminated after 34 weeks for lack of efficacy, and was found to demonstrate a greater risk of disease progression or death on Letairis. More patients taking Letairis died (8% vs. 4%), had a respiratory hospitalization (13% vs. 6%), and had a decrease in FVC/DLCO (17% vs. 12%) [see Contraindications (4.2)].

Figure 5 Time to Clinical Worsening

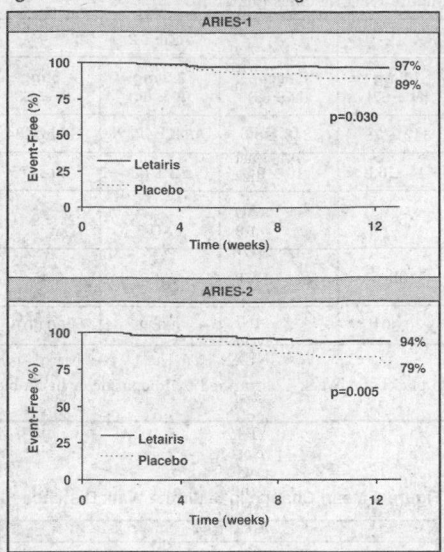

Time from randomization to clinical worsening with Kaplan-Meier estimates of the proportions of failures in ARIES-1 and ARIES-2. p-values shown are the log-rank comparisons of Letairis to placebo stratified by idiopathic or heritable PAH and non-idiopathic, non-heritable PAH patients

Table 3 Time to Clinical Worsening

	ARIES-1		ARIES-2	
	Placebo (N = 67)	Letairis (N = 134)	Placebo (N = 65)	Letairis (N = 127)
Clinical worsening, no. (%)	7 (10%)	4 (3%)	13 (22%)	8 (6%)
Hazard ratio	–	0.28	–	0.30
p-value, Fisher exact test	–	0.044	–	0.006
p-value, Log-rank test	–	0.030	–	0.005

Intention-to-treat population
Note: Patients may have had more than one reason for clinical worsening.
Nominal p-values

Acceptable Birth Control Options

Option 1
One method from this list:
- Standard intrauterine device (Copper T 380A IUD)
- Intrauterine system (LNg 20 IUS – progesterone IUD)
- Tubal sterilization
- Progesterone implant

OR

Option 2
One method from this list:
- Estrogen and progesterone oral contraceptives ("the pill")
- Estrogen and progesterone transdermal patch
- Vaginal ring
- Progesterone injection

PLUS
One method from this list:
- Male condom
- Diaphragm with spermicide
- Cervical cap with spermicide

OR

Option 3
One method from this list:
- Diaphragm with spermicide
- Cervical cap with spermicide

PLUS
One method from this list:
- Male condom

OR

Option 4
One method from this list:
- Partner's vasectomy

PLUS
One method from this list:
- Male condom
- Diaphragm with spermicide
- Cervical cap with spermicide
- Estrogen and progesterone oral contraceptive ("the pill")
- Estrogen and progesterone transdermal patch
- Vaginal ring
- Progesterone injection

16   HOW SUPPLIED/STORAGE AND HANDLING

Letairis film-coated tablets are supplied as follows:

Tablet Strength	Package Configuration	NDC No.	Description of Tablet; Debossed on Tablet; Size
5 mg	30 count blister	61958-0801-2	Square convex; pale pink; "5" on side 1 and "GSI" on side 2; 6.6 mm Square
	30 count bottle	61958-0801-1	
	10 count blister	61958-0801-3	
	10 count bottle	61958-0801-5	
10 mg	30 count blister	61958-0802-2	Oval convex; deep pink; "10" on side 1 and "GSI" on side 2; 9.8 mm × 4.9 mm Oval
	30 count bottle	61958-0802-1	
	10 count blister	61958-0802-3	
	10 count bottle	61958-0802-5	

Store at 25° C (77° F); excursions permitted to 15–30° C (59–86° F) [see USP controlled room temperature]. Store Letairis in its original packaging.

17   PATIENT COUNSELING INFORMATION

See FDA-approved patient labeling (Medication Guide).

17.1   Embryo-fetal Toxicity

Instruct patients on the risk of fetal harm when Letairis is used in pregnancy [see Warnings and Precautions (5.1) and Use in Specific Populations (8)]. Female patients must enroll in the Letairis REMS program. Instruct females of reproductive potential to immediately contact their physician if they suspect they may be pregnant.

17.2   Letairis REMS Program

For female patients, Letairis is only available through a restricted program called the Letairis REMS [see Contraindications (4.1), Warnings and Precautions (5.2)]. Male patients are not enrolled in the Letairis REMS.
Inform female patients (and their guardians, if applicable) of the following notable requirements:
- All female patients must sign an enrollment form.
- Advise female patients of reproductive potential that they must comply with the pregnancy testing and contraception requirements [see Use in Specific Populations (8.6)].

- Educate and counsel females of reproductive potential on the use of emergency contraception in the event of unprotected sex or known or suspected contraceptive failure.
- Advise pre-pubertal females to report any changes in their reproductive status immediately to their prescriber.

Review the Letairis Medication Guide and REMS educational material with female patients.
A limited number of pharmacies are certified to dispense Letairis. Therefore, provide patients with the telephone number and website for information on how to obtain the product.

17.3   Hepatic Effects

Some members of this pharmacological class are hepatotoxic. Patients should be educated on the symptoms of potential liver injury (such as anorexia, nausea, vomiting, fever, malaise, fatigue, right upper quadrant abdominal discomfort, jaundice, dark urine, or itching) and instructed to report any of these symptoms to their physician.

17.4   Hematological Change

Patients should be advised of the importance of hemoglobin testing.

17.5   Other Risks Associated with Letairis

Instruct patients that the risks associated with Letairis also include the following:
- Decreases in hemoglobin and hematocrit
- Decreases in sperm count
- Fluid overload

17.6   Administration

Patients should be advised not to split, crush, or chew tablets.

Gilead Sciences, Inc., Foster City, CA 94404
Letairis is a registered trademark of Gilead Sciences, Inc. Gilead and the Gilead logo are trademarks of Gilead Sciences, Inc. Other brands noted herein are the property of their respective owners.
© 2014 Gilead Sciences, Inc.
GS22-081-014-PI

Medication Guide

Letairis® (le-TAIR-is)
(ambrisentan)
Tablets

Read this Medication Guide before you start taking Letairis and each time you get a refill. There may be new information. This Medication Guide does not take the place of talking with your doctor about your medical condition or your treatment.

What is the most important information I should know about Letairis?
- **Serious birth defects.**
Letairis can cause serious birth defects if taken during pregnancy.
  ■ **Females must not be pregnant when they start taking Letairis or become pregnant during treatment with Letairis.**
  ■ Females who are able to get pregnant must have a negative pregnancy test before beginning treatment with Letairis, each month during treatment with Letairis, and one month after stopping Letairis. Talk to your doctor about your menstrual cycle. Your doctor will decide when to do the tests, and order the tests for you depending on your menstrual cycle.
    ○ Females who are able to get pregnant are females who:
      ■ Have entered puberty, even if they have not started their period, **and**
      ■ Have a uterus, **and**
      ■ Have not gone through menopause (have not had a period for at least 12 months for natural reasons, or who have had their ovaries removed)
    ○ Females who are not able to get pregnant are females who:
      ■ Have not yet entered puberty, **or**
      ■ Do not have a uterus, **or**
      ■ Have gone through menopause (have not had a period for at least 12 months for natural reasons, or who have had their ovaries removed)

Females who are able to get pregnant must use two acceptable forms of birth control, during treatment with Letairis, and for one month after stopping Letairis because the medicine may still be in the body.
  ■ If you have had a tubal sterilization or have an IUD (intrauterine device) or progesterone implant, these methods can be used alone and no other form of birth control is needed.
  ■ Talk with your doctor or gynecologist (a doctor who specializes in female reproduction) to find out about options for acceptable forms of birth control that you may use to prevent pregnancy during treatment with Letairis.
  ■ If you decide that you want to change the form of birth control that you use, talk with your doctor or gynecologist to be sure that you choose another acceptable form of birth control.

See the chart below for Acceptable Birth Control Options during treatment with Letairis.
[See figure above]
  ■ **Do not have unprotected sex. Talk to your doctor or pharmacist right away if you have unprotected sex or if you think your birth control has failed. Your doctor may tell you to use emergency birth control.**

- Tell your doctor right away if you miss a menstrual period or think you may be pregnant for any reason.

If you are the parent or caregiver of a female child who started taking Letairis before reaching puberty, you should check your child regularly to see if she is developing signs of puberty. Tell your doctor right away if you notice that she is developing breast buds or any pubic hair. Your doctor should decide if your child has reached puberty. Your child may reach puberty before having her first menstrual period.

Females can only receive Letairis through a restricted program called the Letairis Risk Evaluation and Mitigation Strategy (REMS) program. If you are a female who can get pregnant, you must talk to your doctor, understand the benefits and risks of Letairis, and agree to all of the instructions in the Letairis REMS program.

Males can receive Letairis without taking part in the Letairis REMS program.

What is Letairis?
- Letairis is a prescription medicine to treat pulmonary arterial hypertension (PAH), which is high blood pressure in the arteries of your lungs.
- Letairis can improve your ability to exercise and it can help slow down the worsening of your physical condition and symptoms.
- It is not known if Letairis is safe and effective in children.

Who should not take Letairis?
Do not take Letairis if:
- **you are pregnant, plan to become pregnant, or become pregnant during treatment with Letairis.** Letairis can cause serious birth defects. (See the Medication Guide section above called "What is the most important information I should know about Letairis?") Serious birth defects from Letairis happen early in pregnancy.
- you have a condition called Idiopathic Pulmonary Fibrosis (IPF).

Tell your doctor about all your medical conditions and all the medicines you take including prescription and nonprescription medicines. Letairis and other medicines may affect each other causing side effects. Do not start any new medicines until you check with your doctor.

Especially tell your doctor if you take the medicine cyclosporine (Gengraf, Neoral, Sandimmune). Your doctor may need to change your dose of Letairis. You should not take more than 5 mg of Letairis each day if you also take cyclosporine.

How should I take Letairis?
Letairis will be mailed to you by a certified pharmacy. Your doctor will give you complete details.
- Take Letairis exactly as your doctor tells you. Do not stop taking Letairis unless your doctor tells you.
- You can take Letairis with or without food.
- Do not split, crush or chew Letairis tablets.
- It will be easier to remember to take Letairis if you take it at the same time each day.
- If you take more than your regular dose of Letairis, call your doctor right away.
- If you miss a dose, take it as soon as you remember that day. Take your next dose at the regular time. Do not take two doses at the same time to make up for a missed dose.

What should I avoid while taking Letairis?
- **Do not get pregnant** while taking Letairis. (See the serious birth defects section of the Medication Guide above called "What is the most important information I should know about Letairis?") If you miss a menstrual period, or think you might be pregnant, call your doctor right away.

It is not known if Letairis passes into your breast milk. You should not breastfeed if you are taking Letairis. Talk to your doctor about the best way to feed your baby if you take Letairis.

What are the possible side effects of Letairis?
Letairis can cause serious side effects including:
- **Serious birth defects.** (See "What is the most important information I should know about Letairis?")
- **Swelling all over the body** (fluid retention) can happen within weeks after starting Letairis. Tell your doctor right away if you have any unusual weight gain, tiredness, or trouble breathing while taking Letairis. These may be symptoms of a serious health problem. You may need to be treated with medicine or need to go to the hospital.
- **Sperm count reduction.** Reduced sperm counts have been observed in some men taking a drug similar to Letairis, an effect which might impair their ability to father a child. Tell your doctor if remaining fertile is important to you.
- **Low red blood cell levels** (anemia) can happen during the first weeks after starting Letairis. If this happens, you may need a blood transfusion. Your doctor will do blood tests to check your red blood cells before starting Letairis. Your doctor may also do these tests during treatment with Letairis.

The most common side effects of Letairis are:
- Swelling of hands, legs, ankles and feet (peripheral edema)
- Stuffy nose (nasal congestion)

- Inflamed nasal passages (sinusitis)
- Hot flashes or getting red in the face (flushing)

Some medicines that are like Letairis can cause liver problems. Tell your doctor if you get any of these symptoms of a liver problem while taking Letairis:

- loss of appetite
- nausea or vomiting
- fever
- achiness
- generally do not feel well
- pain in the upper right stomach (abdominal) area
- yellowing of your skin or the whites of your eyes
- dark urine
- itching

Tell your doctor if you have any side effect that bothers you or that does not go away. These are not all of the possible side effects of Letairis. For more information, ask your doctor or pharmacist.

Call your doctor for medical advice about side effects. You may report side effects to FDA at 1-800-FDA-1088.

How should I store Letairis?
Store Letairis at room temperature between 68 °F to 77 °F (20 °C to 25 °C), in the package it comes in.

Keep Letairis and all medicines out of the reach of children.
General information about Letairis
Medicines are sometimes prescribed for purposes other than those listed in a Medication Guide. Do not use Letairis for a condition for which it was not prescribed. Do not give Letairis to other people, even if they have the same symptoms that you have. It may harm them.

This Medication Guide summarizes the most important information about Letairis. If you would like more information, ask your doctor. You can ask your doctor or pharmacist for information about Letairis that is written for health professionals.

For more information, call 1-866-664-5327 or visit www.letairis.com or www.gilead.com.

What are the ingredients in Letairis?
Active ingredient : ambrisentan.
Inactive Ingredients: croscarmellose sodium, lactose monohydrate, magnesium stearate and microcrystalline cellulose. The tablets are film-coated with a coating material containing FD&C Red #40 aluminum lake, lecithin, polyethylene glycol, polyvinyl alcohol, talc, and titanium dioxide.

This Medication Guide has been approved by the U.S. Food and Drug Administration.
Gilead Sciences, Inc., Foster City, CA 94404
Revised January 2014
Letairis is a registered trademark of Gilead Sciences, Inc. Gilead and the Gilead logo are trademarks of Gilead Sciences, Inc. Other brands noted herein are the property of their respective owners.
© 2014 Gilead Sciences, Inc.
GS22-081-013-MG
Shown in Product Identification Guide, page 307

RANEXA® ℞
[rAn-ex-a]
(ranolazine)
extended-release tablets

HIGHLIGHTS OF PRESCRIBING INFORMATION
These highlights do not include all the information needed to use RANEXA safely and effectively. See full prescribing information for RANEXA.

RANEXA® (ranolazine) extended-release tablets
Initial U.S. Approval: 2006

------RECENT MAJOR CHANGES------
- Warnings and Precautions
  Renal Failure (5.2)   12/2013

------INDICATIONS AND USAGE------
RANEXA is indicated for the treatment of chronic angina. (1)

------DOSAGE AND ADMINISTRATION------
- 500 mg twice daily and increase to 1000 mg twice daily, based on clinical symptoms (2.1)

------DOSAGE FORMS AND STRENGTHS------
Extended-release tablets: 500 mg, 1000 mg (3)

------CONTRAINDICATIONS------
- Strong CYP3A inhibitors (e.g., ketoconazole, clarithromycin, nelfinavir) (4, 7.1)
- CYP3A inducers (e.g., rifampin, phenobarbital, St. John's wort) (4, 7.1)
- Liver cirrhosis (4, 8.6)

------WARNINGS AND PRECAUTIONS------
- QT interval prolongation: Can occur with ranolazine. Little data available on high doses, long exposure, use with QT interval-prolonging drugs, potassium channel variants causing prolonged QT interval, in patients with a family history of (or congenital) long QT syndrome, or in patients with known acquired QT interval prolongation. (5.1)
- Renal failure: Monitor renal function after initiation and periodically in patients with moderate to severe renal impairment (CrCL < 60 mL/min). If acute renal failure develops, discontinue RANEXA. (5.2)

------ADVERSE REACTIONS------
Most common adverse reactions (> 4% and more common than with placebo) are dizziness, headache, constipation, nausea. (6.1)
To report SUSPECTED ADVERSE REACTIONS, contact Gilead Sciences, Inc., at 1-800-GILEAD-5 or FDA at 1-800-FDA-1088 or www.fda.gov/medwatch.

------DRUG INTERACTIONS------
- Moderate CYP3A inhibitors (e.g., diltiazem, verapamil, erythromycin): Limit RANEXA to 500 mg twice daily. (7.1)
- P-gp inhibitors (e.g., cyclosporine): Ranolazine exposure increased. Titrate RANEXA based on clinical response. (7.1)
- CYP3A substrates: Limit simvastatin to 20 mg when used with RANEXA. Doses of other sensitive CYP3A substrates (e.g., lovastatin) and CYP3A substrates with narrow therapeutic range (e.g., cyclosporine, tacrolimus, sirolimus) may need to be reduced with RANEXA. (7.2)
- OCT2 substrates: Limit the dose of metformin to 1700 mg daily when used with RANEXA 1000 mg twice daily. Doses of other OCT2 substrates may require adjusted doses. (7.2)
- Drugs transported by P-gp (e.g., digoxin), or drugs metabolized by CYP2D6 (e.g., tricyclic antidepressants) may need reduced doses when used with RANEXA. (7.2)
See 17 for PATIENT COUNSELING INFORMATION and FDA-approved patient labeling

Revised: 12/2013

FULL PRESCRIBING INFORMATION: CONTENTS*
* Sections or subsections omitted from the full prescribing information are not listed

FULL PRESCRIBING INFORMATION

1   INDICATIONS AND USAGE
RANEXA® is indicated for the treatment of chronic angina. RANEXA may be used with beta-blockers, nitrates, calcium channel blockers, anti-platelet therapy, lipid-lowering therapy, ACE inhibitors, and angiotensin receptor blockers.

2   DOSAGE AND ADMINISTRATION
2.1   Dosing Information
Initiate RANEXA dosing at 500 mg twice daily and increase to 1000 mg twice daily, as needed, based on clinical symptoms. Take RANEXA with or without meals. Swallow RANEXA tablets whole; do not crush, break, or chew.

The maximum recommended daily dose of RANEXA is 1000 mg twice daily.

If a dose of RANEXA is missed, take the prescribed dose at the next scheduled time; do not double the next dose.

2.2 Dose Modification

Dose adjustments may be needed when RANEXA is taken in combination with certain other drugs [see Drug Interactions (7.1)]. Limit the maximum dose of RANEXA to 500 mg twice daily in patients on moderate CYP3A inhibitors such as diltiazem, verapamil, and erythromycin. Use of RANEXA with strong CYP3A inhibitors is contraindicated [see Contraindications (4), Drug Interactions (7.1)].

Use of P-gp inhibitors, such as cyclosporine, may increase exposure to RANEXA. Titrate RANEXA based on clinical response [see Drug Interactions (7.1)].

3 DOSAGE FORMS AND STRENGTHS

RANEXA is supplied as film-coated, oblong-shaped, extended-release tablets in the following strengths:
• 500 mg tablets are light orange, with GSI500 on one side
• 1000 mg tablets are pale yellow, with GSI1000 on one side

4 CONTRAINDICATIONS

RANEXA is contraindicated in patients:
• Taking strong inhibitors of CYP3A [see Drug Interactions (7.1)]
• Taking inducers of CYP3A [see Drug Interactions (7.1)]
• With liver cirrhosis [see Use in Specific Populations (8.6)]

5 WARNINGS AND PRECAUTIONS

5.1 QT Interval Prolongation

Ranolazine blocks I_{Kr} and prolongs the QTc interval in a dose-related manner.

Clinical experience in an acute coronary syndrome population did not show an increased risk of proarrhythmia or sudden death [see Clinical Studies (14.2)]. However, there is little experience with high doses (> 1000 mg twice daily) or exposure, other QT-prolonging drugs, potassium channel variants resulting in a long QT interval, in patients with a family history of (or congenital) long QT syndrome, or in patients with known acquired QT interval prolongation.

5.2 Renal Failure

Acute renal failure has been observed in some patients with severe renal impairment (creatinine clearance [CrCL] < 30 mL/min) while taking RANEXA. If acute renal failure develops (e.g., marked increase in serum creatinine associated with an increase in blood urea nitrogen [BUN]), discontinue RANEXA and treat appropriately [see Use in Specific Populations (8.7)].

Monitor renal function after initiation and periodically in patients with moderate to severe renal impairment (CrCL < 60 mL/min) for increases in serum creatinine accompanied by an increase in BUN.

6 ADVERSE REACTIONS

6.1 Clinical Trial Experience

Because clinical trials are conducted under widely varying conditions, adverse reaction rates observed in the clinical trials of a drug cannot be directly compared to rates in the clinical trials of another drug and may not reflect the rates observed in practice.

A total of 2,018 patients with chronic angina were treated with ranolazine in controlled clinical trials. Of the patients treated with RANEXA, 1,026 were enrolled in three double-blind, placebo-controlled, randomized studies (CARISA, ERICA, MARISA) of up to 12 weeks' duration. In addition, upon study completion, 1,251 patients received treatment with RANEXA in open-label, long-term studies; 1,227 patients were exposed to RANEXA for more than 1 year, 613 patients for more than 2 years, 531 patients for more than 3 years, and 326 patients for more than 4 years.

At recommended doses, about 6% of patients discontinued treatment with RANEXA because of an adverse event in controlled studies in angina patients compared to about 3% on placebo. The most common adverse events that led to discontinuation more frequently on RANEXA than placebo were dizziness (1.3% versus 0.1%), nausea (1% versus 0%), asthenia, constipation, and headache (each about 0.5% versus 0%). Doses above 1000 mg twice daily are poorly tolerated.

In controlled clinical trials of angina patients, the most frequently reported treatment-emergent adverse reactions (> 4% and more common on RANEXA than on placebo) were dizziness (6.2%), headache (5.5%), constipation (4.5%), and nausea (4.4%). Dizziness may be dose-related. In open-label, long-term treatment studies, a similar adverse reaction profile was observed.

The following additional adverse reactions occurred at an incidence of 0.5 to 4.0% in patients treated with RANEXA and were more frequent than the incidence observed in placebo-treated patients:

Cardiac Disorders – bradycardia, palpitations
Ear and Labyrinth Disorders – tinnitus, vertigo
Eye Disorders – blurred vision

Gastrointestinal Disorders – abdominal pain, dry mouth, vomiting, dyspepsia
General Disorders and Administrative Site Adverse Events – asthenia, peripheral edema
Metabolism and Nutrition Disorders – anorexia
Nervous System Disorders – syncope (vasovagal)
Psychiatric Disorders – confusional state
Renal and Urinary Disorders – hematuria
Respiratory, Thoracic, and Mediastinal Disorders – dyspnea
Skin and Subcutaneous Tissue Disorders – hyperhidrosis
Vascular Disorders – hypotension, orthostatic hypotension
Other (< 0.5%) but potentially medically important adverse reactions observed more frequently with RANEXA than placebo treatment in all controlled studies included: angioedema, renal failure, eosinophilia, chromaturia, blood urea increased, hypoesthesia, paresthesia, tremor, pulmonary fibrosis, thrombocytopenia, leukopenia, and pancytopenia.

A large clinical trial in acute coronary syndrome patients was unsuccessful in demonstrating a benefit for RANEXA, but there was no apparent proarrhythmic effect in these high-risk patients [see Clinical Studies (14.2)].

Laboratory Abnormalities

RANEXA produces small reductions in hemoglobin A1c. RANEXA is not a treatment for diabetes.

RANEXA produces elevations of serum creatinine by 0.1 mg/dL, regardless of previous renal function, likely because of inhibition of creatinine's tubular secretion. In general, the elevation has a rapid onset, shows no signs of progression during long-term therapy, is reversible after discontinuation of RANEXA, and is not accompanied by changes in BUN. In healthy volunteers, RANEXA 1000 mg twice daily had no effect upon the glomerular filtration rate. More marked and progressive increases in serum creatinine, associated with increases in BUN or potassium, indicating acute renal failure, have been reported after initiation of RANEXA in patients with severe renal impairment [see Warnings and Precautions (5.2), Use in Specific Populations (8.7)].

6.2 Postmarketing Experience

The following adverse reactions have been identified during postapproval use of RANEXA. Because these reactions are reported voluntarily from a population of uncertain size, it is not always possible to reliably estimate their frequency or establish a causal relationship to drug exposure:

Nervous System Disorders

Tremor, paresthesia, abnormal coordination, and other serious neurologic adverse events have been reported to occur, sometimes concurrently, in patients taking ranolazine. The onset of events was often associated with an increase in ranolazine dose or exposure. Many patients reported symptom resolution following drug discontinuation or dose decrease.

Psychiatric Disorders – hallucination

Renal and Urinary Disorders – dysuria, urinary retention
Skin and Subcutaneous Tissue Disorders – angioedema, pruritus, rash

7 DRUG INTERACTIONS

7.1 Effects of Other Drugs on Ranolazine

Strong CYP3A Inhibitors

Do not use RANEXA with strong CYP3A inhibitors, including ketoconazole, itraconazole, clarithromycin, nefazodone, nelfinavir, ritonavir, indinavir, and saquinavir [see Contraindications (4), Clinical Pharmacology (12.3)].

Moderate CYP3A Inhibitors

Limit the dose of RANEXA to 500 mg twice daily in patients on moderate CYP3A inhibitors, including diltiazem, verapamil, erythromycin, fluconazole, and grapefruit juice or grapefruit-containing products [see Dosage and Administration (2.2), Clinical Pharmacology (12.3)].

P-gp Inhibitors

Concomitant use of RANEXA and P-gp inhibitors, such as cyclosporine, may result in increases in ranolazine concentrations. Titrate RANEXA based on clinical response in patients concomitantly treated with predominant P-gp inhibitors such as cyclosporine [see Dosage and Administration (2.2)].

CYP3A Inducers

Do not use RANEXA with CYP3A inducers such as rifampin, rifabutin, rifapentine, phenobarbital, phenytoin, carbamazepine, and St. John's wort [see Contraindications (4), Clinical Pharmacology (12.3)].

7.2 Effects of Ranolazine on Other Drugs

Drugs Metabolized by CYP3A

Limit the dose of simvastatin in patients on any dose of RANEXA to 20 mg once daily, when ranolazine is co-administered. Dose adjustment of other sensitive CYP3A substrates (e.g., lovastatin) and CYP3A substrates with a narrow therapeutic range (e.g., cyclosporine, tacrolimus, sirolimus) may be required as RANEXA may increase plasma concentrations of these drugs [see Clinical Pharmacology (12.3)].

Drugs Transported by P-gp

Concomitant use of ranolazine and digoxin results in increased exposure to digoxin. The dose of digoxin may have to be adjusted [see Clinical Pharmacology (12.3)].

Drugs Metabolized by CYP2D6

The exposure to CYP2D6 substrates, such as tricyclic antidepressants and antipsychotics, may be increased during co-administration with RANEXA, and lower doses of these drugs may be required.

Drugs Transported by OCT2

In subjects with type 2 diabetes mellitus, concomitant use of RANEXA 1000 mg twice daily and metformin results in increased plasma levels of metformin. When RANEXA 1000 mg twice daily is co-administered with metformin, metformin dose should not exceed 1700 mg/day. Monitor blood glucose levels and risks associated with high exposures of metformin. Metformin exposure was not significantly increased when given with RANEXA 500 mg twice daily [see Clinical Pharmacology (12.3)].

8 USE IN SPECIFIC POPULATIONS

8.1 Pregnancy

Pregnancy Category C

In animal studies, ranolazine at exposures 1.5 (rabbit) to 2 (rat) times the usual human exposure caused maternal toxicity and misshapen sternebrae and reduced ossification in offspring. These doses in rats and rabbits were associated with an increased maternal mortality rate [see Nonclinical Toxicology (13.3)]. There are no adequate well-controlled studies in pregnant women. RANEXA should be used during pregnancy only when the potential benefit to the patient justifies the potential risk to the fetus.

8.3 Nursing Mothers

It is not known whether ranolazine is excreted in human milk. Because many drugs are excreted in human milk and because of the potential for serious adverse reactions from ranolazine in nursing infants, decide whether to discontinue nursing or to discontinue RANEXA, taking into account the importance of the drug to the mother.

8.4 Pediatric Use

Safety and effectiveness have not been established in pediatric patients.

8.5 Geriatric Use

Of the chronic angina patients treated with RANEXA in controlled studies, 496 (48%) were ≥ 65 years of age, and 114 (11%) were ≥ 75 years of age. No overall differences in efficacy were observed between older and younger patients. There were no differences in safety for patients ≥ 65 years compared to younger patients, but patients ≥ 75 years of age on RANEXA, compared to placebo, had a higher incidence of adverse events, serious adverse events, and drug discontinuations due to adverse events. In general, dose selection for an elderly patient should usually start at the low end of the dosing range, reflecting the greater frequency of decreased hepatic, renal, or cardiac function, and of concomitant disease, or other drug therapy.

8.6 Use in Patients with Hepatic Impairment

RANEXA is contraindicated in patients with liver cirrhosis. In a study of cirrhotic patients, the C_{max} of ranolazine was increased 30% in cirrhotic patients with mild (Child-Pugh Class A) hepatic impairment, but increased 80% in cirrhotic patients with moderate (Child-Pugh Class B) hepatic impairment compared to patients without hepatic impairment. This increase was not enough to account for the 3-fold increase in QT prolongation seen in cirrhotic patients with mild to moderate hepatic impairment [see Clinical Pharmacology (12.2)].

8.7 Use in Patients with Renal Impairment

A pharmacokinetic study of RANEXA in subjects with severe renal impairment (CrCL < 30 mL/min) was stopped when 2 of 4 subjects developed acute renal failure after receiving RANEXA 500 mg twice daily for 5 days (lead-in phase) followed by 1000 mg twice a day (1 dose in one subject and 11 doses in the other). Increases in creatinine, BUN, and potassium were observed in 3 subjects during the 500 mg lead-in phase. One subject required hemodialysis, while the other 2 subjects improved upon drug discontinuation [see Warnings and Precautions (5.2)]. Monitor renal function periodically in patients with moderate to severe renal impairment. Discontinue RANEXA if acute renal failure develops.

In a separate study, C_{max} was increased between 40% and 50% in patients with mild, moderate or severe renal impairment compared to patients with no renal impairment, suggesting a similar increase in exposure in patients with renal failure independent of the degree of impairment. The pharmacokinetics of ranolazine has not been assessed in patients on dialysis.

8.8 Use in Patients with Heart Failure

Heart failure (NYHA Class I to IV) had no significant effect on ranolazine pharmacokinetics. RANEXA had minimal effects on heart rate and blood pressure in patients with angina and heart failure NYHA Class I to IV. No dose adjustment of RANEXA is required in patients with heart failure.

8.9   Use in Patients with Diabetes Mellitus

A population pharmacokinetic evaluation of data from angina patients and healthy subjects showed no effect of diabetes on ranolazine pharmacokinetics. No dose adjustment is required in patients with diabetes.

RANEXA produces small reductions in HbA1c in patients with diabetes, the clinical significance of which is unknown. RANEXA should not be considered a treatment for diabetes.

10   OVERDOSAGE

High oral doses of ranolazine produce dose-related increases in dizziness, nausea, and vomiting. High intravenous exposure also produces diplopia, paresthesia, confusion, and syncope. In addition to general supportive measures, continuous ECG monitoring may be warranted in the event of overdose. Severe tremor, unsteady gait/incoordination, dysphasia, and hallucinations have been reported in cases of overdose with RANEXA.

Since ranolazine is about 62% bound to plasma proteins, hemodialysis is unlikely to be effective in clearing ranolazine.

11   DESCRIPTION

RANEXA (ranolazine) is available as a film-coated, non-scored, extended-release tablet for oral administration. Ranolazine is a racemic mixture, chemically described as 1-piperazineacetamide, N-(2,6-dimethylphenyl)-4-[2-hydroxy-3-(2-methoxyphenoxy)propyl]-, (±)-. It has an empirical formula of $C_{24}H_{33}N_3O_4$, a molecular weight of 427.54 g/mole, and the following structural formula:

Ranolazine is a white to off-white solid. Ranolazine is soluble in dichloromethane and methanol; sparingly soluble in tetrahydrofuran, ethanol, acetonitrile, and acetone; slightly soluble in ethyl acetate, isopropanol, toluene, and ethyl ether; and very slightly soluble in water.

RANEXA tablets contain 500 mg or 1000 mg of ranolazine and the following inactive ingredients: carnauba wax, hypromellose, magnesium stearate, methacrylic acid copolymer (Type C), microcrystalline cellulose, polyethylene glycol, sodium hydroxide, and titanium dioxide. Additional inactive ingredients for the 500 mg tablet include polyvinyl alcohol, talc, Iron Oxide Yellow, and Iron Oxide Red; additional inactive ingredients for the 1000 mg tablet include lactose monohydrate, triacetin, and Iron Oxide Yellow.

12   CLINICAL PHARMACOLOGY

12.1   Mechanism of Action

The mechanism of action of ranolazine's antianginal effects has not been determined. Ranolazine has anti-ischemic and antianginal effects that do not depend upon reductions in heart rate or blood pressure. It does not affect the rate-pressure product, a measure of myocardial work, at maximal exercise. Ranolazine at therapeutic levels can inhibit the cardiac late sodium current (I_{Na}). However, the relationship of this inhibition to angina symptoms is uncertain.

The QT prolongation effect of ranolazine on the surface electrocardiogram is the result of inhibition of I_{Kr}, which prolongs the ventricular action potential.

12.2   Pharmacodynamics

Hemodynamic Effects

Patients with chronic angina treated with RANEXA in controlled clinical studies had minimal changes in mean heart rate (< 2 bpm) and systolic blood pressure (< 3 mm Hg). Similar results were observed in subgroups of patients with CHF NYHA Class I or II, diabetes, or reactive airway disease, and in elderly patients.

Electrocardiographic Effects

Dose and plasma concentration-related increases in the QTc interval [see Warnings and Precautions (5.1)], reductions in T wave amplitude, and, in some cases, notched T waves, have been observed in patients treated with RANEXA. These effects are believed to be caused by ranolazine and not by its metabolites. The relationship between the change in QTc and ranolazine plasma concentrations is linear, with a slope of about 2.6 msec/1000 ng/mL, through exposures corresponding to doses several-fold higher than the maximum recommended dose of 1000 mg twice daily. The variable blood levels attained after a given dose of ranolazine give a wide range of effects on QTc. At T_{max} following repeat dosing at 1000 mg twice daily, the mean change in QTc is about 6 msec, but in the 5% of the population with the highest plasma concentrations, the prolongation of QTc is at least 15 msec. In cirrhotic subjects with mild or moderate hepatic impairment, the relationship between plasma level of ranolazine and QTc is much steeper [see Contraindications (4)].

Age, weight, gender, race, heart rate, congestive heart failure, diabetes, and renal impairment did not alter the slope of the QTc-concentration relationship of ranolazine.

No proarrhythmic effects were observed on 7-day Holter recordings in 3,162 acute coronary syndrome patients treated with RANEXA. There was a significantly lower incidence of arrhythmias (ventricular tachycardia, bradycardia, supraventricular tachycardia, and new atrial fibrillation) in patients treated with RANEXA (80%) versus placebo (87%), including ventricular tachycardia ≥ 3 beats (52% versus 61%). However, this difference in arrhythmias did not lead to a reduction in mortality, a reduction in arrhythmia hospitalization, or a reduction in arrhythmia symptoms.

12.3   Pharmacokinetics

Ranolazine is extensively metabolized in the gut and liver and its absorption is highly variable. For example, at a dose of 1000 mg twice daily, the mean steady-state C_{max} was 2600 ng/mL with 95% confidence limits of 400 and 6100 ng/mL. The pharmacokinetics of the (+) R- and (-) S-enantiomers of ranolazine are similar in healthy volunteers. The apparent terminal half-life of ranolazine is 7 hours. Steady state is generally achieved within 3 days of twice-daily dosing with RANEXA. At steady state over the dose range of 500 to 1000 mg twice daily, C_{max} and $AUC_{0-\tau}$ increase slightly more than proportionally to dose, 2.2- and 2.4-fold, respectively. With twice-daily dosing, the trough:peak ratio of the ranolazine plasma concentration is 0.3 to 0.6. The pharmacokinetics of ranolazine is unaffected by age, gender, or food.

Absorption and Distribution

After oral administration of RANEXA, peak plasma concentrations of ranolazine are reached between 2 and 5 hours. After oral administration of ^{14}C-ranolazine as a solution, 73% of the dose is systemically available as ranolazine or metabolites. The bioavailability of ranolazine from RANEXA tablets relative to that from a solution of ranolazine is 76%. Because ranolazine is a substrate of P-gp, inhibitors of P-gp may increase the absorption of ranolazine.

Food (high-fat breakfast) has no important effect on the C_{max} and AUC of ranolazine. Therefore, RANEXA may be taken without regard to meals. Over the concentration range of 0.25 to 10 μg/mL, ranolazine is approximately 62% bound to human plasma proteins.

Metabolism and Excretion

Ranolazine is metabolized mainly by CYP3A and, to a lesser extent, by CYP2D6. Following a single oral dose of ranolazine solution, approximately 75% of the dose is excreted in urine and 25% in feces. Ranolazine is metabolized rapidly and extensively in the liver and intestine; less than 5% is excreted unchanged in urine and feces. The pharmacologic activity of the metabolites has not been well characterized. After dosing to steady state with 500 mg to 1500 mg twice daily, the four most abundant metabolites in plasma have AUC values ranging from about 5 to 33% that of ranolazine, and display apparent half-lives ranging from 6 to 22 hours.

Drug Interactions

Effect of other drugs on ranolazine

In vitro data indicate that ranolazine is a substrate of CYP3A and, to a lesser degree, of CYP2D6. Ranolazine is also a substrate of P-glycoprotein.

Strong CYP3A Inhibitors

Plasma levels of ranolazine with RANEXA 1000 mg twice daily are increased by 220% when coadministered with ketoconazole 200 mg twice daily [see Contraindications (4)].

Moderate CYP3A Inhibitors

Plasma levels of ranolazine with RANEXA 1000 mg twice daily are increased by 50 to 130% by diltiazem 180 to 360 mg, respectively. Plasma levels of ranolazine with RANEXA 750 mg twice daily are increased by 100% by verapamil 120 mg three times daily [see Drug Interactions (7.1)].

Weak CYP3A Inhibitors

The weak CYP3A inhibitors simvastatin (20 mg once daily) and cimetidine (400 mg three times daily) do not increase the exposure to ranolazine in healthy volunteers.

CYP3A Inducers

Rifampin 600 mg once daily decreases the plasma concentrations of ranolazine (1000 mg twice daily) by approximately 95% [see Contraindications (4)].

CYP2D6 Inhibitors

Paroxetine 20 mg once daily increased ranolazine concentrations by 20% in healthy volunteers receiving RANEXA 1000 mg twice daily. No dose adjustment of RANEXA is required in patients treated with CYP2D6 inhibitors.

Digoxin

Plasma concentrations of ranolazine are not significantly altered by concomitant digoxin at 0.125 mg once daily.

Effect of ranolazine on other drugs

In vitro ranolazine and its O-demethylated metabolite are weak inhibitors of CYP3A and moderate inhibitors of CYP2D6 and P-gp. In vitro ranolazine is an inhibitor of OCT2.

CYP3A Substrates

The plasma levels of simvastatin, a CYP3A substrate, and its active metabolite are increased by 100% in healthy vol-

unteers receiving 80 mg once daily and RANEXA 1000 mg twice daily [see Drug Interactions (7.2)]. Mean exposure to atorvastatin (80 mg daily) is increased by 40% following co-administration with RANEXA (1000 mg twice daily) in healthy volunteers. However, in one subject the exposure to atorvastatin and metabolites was increased by ~400% in the presence of RANEXA.

Diltiazem

The pharmacokinetics of diltiazem is not affected by ranolazine in healthy volunteers receiving diltiazem 60 mg three times daily and RANEXA 1000 mg twice daily.

P-gp Substrates

Ranolazine increases digoxin concentrations by 50% in healthy volunteers receiving RANEXA 1000 mg twice daily and digoxin 0.125 mg once daily [see Drug Interactions (7.2)].

CYP2D6 Substrates

RANEXA 750 mg twice daily increases the plasma concentrations of a single dose of immediate release metoprolol (100 mg), a CYP2D6 substrate, by 80% in extensive CYP2D6 metabolizers with no need for dose adjustment of metoprolol. In extensive metabolizers of dextromethorphan, a substrate of CYP2D6, ranolazine inhibits partially the formation of the main metabolite dextrorphan.

OCT2 Substrates

In subjects with type 2 diabetes mellitus, the exposure to metformin is increased by 40% and 80% following administration of ranolazine 500 mg twice daily and 1000 mg twice daily, respectively. If co-administered with RANEXA 1000 mg twice daily, do not exceed metformin doses of 1700 mg/day [see Drug Interactions (7.2)].

13   NONCLINICAL TOXICOLOGY

13.1   Carcinogenesis, Mutagenesis, Impairment of Fertility

Ranolazine tested negative for genotoxic potential in the following assays: Ames bacterial mutation assay, Saccharomyces assay for mitotic gene conversion, chromosomal aberrations assay in Chinese hamster ovary (CHO) cells, mammalian CHO/HGPRT gene mutation assay, and mouse and rat bone marrow micronucleus assays.

There was no evidence of carcinogenic potential in mice or rats. The highest oral doses used in the carcinogenicity studies were 150 mg/kg/day for 21 months in rats (900 mg/m²/day) and 50 mg/kg/day for 24 months in mice (150 mg/m²/day). These maximally tolerated doses are 0.8 and 0.1 times, respectively, the maximum recommended human dose (MRHD) of 2 grams on a surface area basis. A published study reported that ranolazine promoted tumor formation and progression to malignancy when given to transgenic APC (min/+) mice at a dose of 30 mg/kg twice daily [see References (15)]. The clinical significance of this finding is unclear.

13.3   Reproductive Toxicology Studies

Animal reproduction studies with ranolazine were conducted in rats and rabbits.

There was an increased incidence of misshapen sternebrae and reduced ossification of pelvic and cranial bones in fetuses of pregnant rats dosed at 400 mg/kg/day (2 times the MRHD on a surface area basis). Reduced ossification of sternebrae was observed in fetuses of pregnant rabbits dosed at 150 mg/kg/day (1.5 times the MRHD on a surface area basis). These doses in rats and rabbits were associated with an increased maternal mortality rate.

14   CLINICAL STUDIES

14.1   Chronic Stable Angina

CARISA (Combination Assessment of Ranolazine In Stable Angina) was a study in 823 chronic angina patients randomized to receive 12 weeks of treatment with twice-daily RANEXA 750 mg, 1000 mg, or placebo, who also continued on daily doses of atenolol 50 mg, amlodipine 5 mg, or diltiazem CD 180 mg. Sublingual nitrates were used in this study as needed.

In this trial, statistically significant (p < 0.05) increases in modified Bruce treadmill exercise duration and time to angina were observed for each RANEXA dose versus placebo, at both trough (12 hours after dosing) and peak (4 hours after dosing) plasma levels, with minimal effects on blood pressure and heart rate. The changes versus placebo in exercise parameters are presented in Table 1. Exercise treadmill results showed no increase in effect on exercise at the 1000 mg dose compared to the 750 mg dose.

Table 1 Exercise Treadmill Results (CARISA)

Study	Mean Difference from Placebo (sec)	
	CARISA (N = 791)	
RANEXA Twice-daily Dose	**750 mg**	**1000 mg**
Exercise Duration Trough	24*	24*

Peak	34[†]	26*
Time to Angina		
Trough	30*	26*
Peak	38[†]	38[†]
Time to 1 mm ST-Segment Depression		
Trough	20	21
Peak	41[†]	35[†]

* p-value ≤ 0.05
[†] p-value ≤ 0.005

The effects of RANEXA on angina frequency and nitroglycerin use are shown in Table 2.
[See table 2 below]
Tolerance to RANEXA did not develop after 12 weeks of therapy. Rebound increases in angina, as measured by exercise duration, have not been observed following abrupt discontinuation of RANEXA.

RANEXA has been evaluated in patients with chronic angina who remained symptomatic despite treatment with the maximum dose of an antianginal agent. In the ERICA (Efficacy of Ranolazine In Chronic Angina) trial, 565 patients were randomized to receive an initial dose of RANEXA 500 mg twice daily or placebo for 1 week, followed by 6 weeks of treatment with RANEXA 1000 mg twice daily or placebo, in addition to concomitant treatment with amlodipine 10 mg once daily. In addition, 45% of the study population also received long-acting nitrates. Sublingual nitrates were used as needed to treat angina episodes. Results are shown in Table 3. Statistically significant decreases in angina attack frequency (p = 0.028) and nitroglycerin use (p = 0.014) were observed with RANEXA compared to placebo. These treatment effects appeared consistent across age and use of long-acting nitrates.

Table 3 Angina Frequency and Nitroglycerin Use (ERICA)

		Placebo	RANEXA*
Angina Frequency (attacks/week)	N	281	277
	Mean	4.3	3.3
	Median	2.4	2.2
Nitroglycerin Use (doses/week)	N	281	277
	Mean	3.6	2.7
	Median	1.7	1.3

* 1000 mg twice daily

Gender
Effects on angina frequency and exercise tolerance were considerably smaller in women than in men. In CARISA, the improvement in Exercise Tolerance Test (ETT) in females was about 33% of that in males at the 1000 mg twice-daily dose level. In ERICA, where the primary endpoint was angina attack frequency, the mean reduction in weekly angina attacks was 0.3 for females and 1.3 for males.

Race
There were insufficient numbers of non-Caucasian patients to allow for analyses of efficacy or safety by racial subgroup.

14.2 Lack of Benefit in Acute Coronary Syndrome
In a large (n = 6,560) placebo-controlled trial (MERLIN-TIMI 36) in patients with acute coronary syndrome, there was no benefit shown on outcome measures. However, the study is somewhat reassuring regarding proarrhythmic risks, as ventricular arrhythmias were less common on ranolazine [see Clinical Pharmacology (12.2)], and there

was no difference between RANEXA and placebo in the risk of all-cause mortality (relative risk ranolazine:placebo 0.99 with an upper 95% confidence limit of 1.22).

15 REFERENCES
M.A. Suckow et al. The anti-ischemia agent ranolazine promotes the development of intestinal tumors in APC (min/+) mice. Cancer Letters 209(2004):165–9.

16 HOW SUPPLIED/STORAGE AND HANDLING
RANEXA is supplied as film-coated, oblong-shaped, extended-release tablets in the following strengths:
• 500 mg tablets are light orange, with GSI500 on one side
• 1000 mg tablets are pale yellow, with GSI1000 on one side
RANEXA (ranolazine) extended-release tablets are available in:

	Strength	NDC
Unit-of-Use Bottle (60 Tablets)	500 mg	61958-1003-1
Unit-of-Use Bottle (60 Tablets)	1000 mg	61958-1004-1

Store RANEXA tablets at 25°C (77°F) with excursions permitted to 15° to 30°C (59° to 86°F).

17 PATIENT COUNSELING INFORMATION
See FDA-Approved Patient Labeling (Patient Information)
To ensure safe and effective use of RANEXA, the following information and instructions should be communicated to the patient when appropriate.
Patients should be advised:
• that RANEXA will not abate an acute angina episode
• to inform their physician of any other medications when taken concurrently with RANEXA, including over-the-counter medications
• that RANEXA may produce changes in the electrocardiogram (QTc interval prolongation)
• to inform their physician of any personal or family history of QTc prolongation, congenital long QT syndrome, or if they are receiving drugs that prolong the QTc interval such as Class Ia (e.g., quinidine) or Class III (e.g., dofetilide, sotalol, amiodarone) antiarrhythmic agents, erythromycin, and certain antipsychotics (e.g., thioridazine, ziprasidone)
• to inform their physician if they have impaired renal function before or while taking RANEXA
• that patients with severe renal impairment may be at risk of renal failure while on RANEXA
• that RANEXA should not be used in patients who are receiving drugs that are strong CYP3A inhibitors (e.g., ketoconazole, clarithromycin, nefazodone, ritonavir)
• that initiation of treatment with RANEXA should be avoided during administration of inducers of CYP3A (e.g., rifampin, rifabutin, rifapentine, barbiturates, carbamazepine, phenytoin, St. John's wort)
• to inform their physician if they are receiving drugs that are moderate CYP3A inhibitors (e.g., diltiazem, verapamil, erythromycin)
• to inform their physician if they are receiving P-gp inhibitors (e.g., cyclosporine)
• that grapefruit juice or grapefruit products should be limited when taking RANEXA
• that RANEXA should not be used in patients with liver cirrhosis
• that doses of RANEXA higher than 1000 mg twice daily should not be used
• that if a dose is missed, the usual dose should be taken at the next scheduled time. The next dose should not be doubled
• that RANEXA may be taken with or without meals
• that RANEXA tablets should be swallowed whole and not crushed, broken, or chewed

• to contact their physician if they experience fainting spells while taking RANEXA
• that RANEXA may cause dizziness and lightheadedness; therefore, patients should know how they react to this drug before they operate an automobile, or machinery, or engage in activities requiring mental alertness or coordination
Manufactured for:
Gilead Sciences, Inc.
Foster City, CA 94404
RANEXA is a registered trademark of Gilead Sciences, Inc.
© 2013 Gilead Sciences, Inc.
21-526-GS-013
PATIENT INFORMATION
RANEXA® (rah NEX ah)
(ranolazine)
extended-release tablets
Dosing Strengths:
500 mg tablets
1000 mg tablets
Read this Patient Information before you start taking RANEXA and each time you get a refill. There may be new information. This information does not take the place of talking with your doctor about your medical condition or treatment.
What is RANEXA?
RANEXA is a prescription medicine used to treat angina that keeps coming back (chronic angina).
RANEXA may be used with other medicines that are used for heart problems and blood pressure control.
It is not known if RANEXA is safe and effective in children.
Who should not take RANEXA?
Do not take RANEXA if:
• you take any of the following medicines:
 • for fungus infection: ketoconazole (Nizoral®), itraconazole (Sporanox®, Onmel™)
 • for infection: clarithromycin (Biaxin®)
 • for depression: nefazodone
 • for HIV: nelfinavir (Viracept®), ritonavir (Norvir®), lopinavir and ritonavir (Kaletra®), indinavir (Crixivan®), saquinavir (Invirase®)
 • for tuberculosis (TB): rifampin (Rifadin®), rifabutin (Mycobutin®), rifapentine (Priftin®)
 • for seizures: phenobarbital, phenytoin (Phenytek®, Dilantin®, Dilantin-125®), carbamazepine (Tegretol®)
 • St. John's wort (Hypericum perforatum)
• you have scarring (cirrhosis) of your liver
What should I tell my doctor before taking RANEXA?
Before you take RANEXA, tell your doctor if you:
• have or have a family history of a heart problem, called 'QT prolongation' or 'long QT syndrome'.
• have liver problems.
• have kidney problems.
• are pregnant or plan to become pregnant. It is not known if RANEXA will harm your unborn baby.
• are breast-feeding or plan to breast-feed. It is not known if RANEXA passes into your breast milk. You and your doctor should decide if you will take RANEXA or breast-feed. You should not do both.
Tell your doctor about all the medicines you take, including all prescription and non-prescription medicines, vitamins and herbal supplements. RANEXA may affect the way other medicines work and other medicines may affect how RANEXA works.
Tell your doctor if you take medicines:
• for your heart
• for cholesterol
• for diabetes
• for infection
• for fungus
• for transplant
• for nausea and vomiting because of cancer treatments
• for mental problems
Know the medicines you take. Keep a list of them to show your doctor or pharmacist when you get a new medicine.
How should I take RANEXA?
• Take RANEXA exactly as your doctor tells you.
• Your doctor will tell you how much RANEXA to take and when to take it.
• Do not change your dose unless your doctor tells you to.
• Tell your doctor if you still have symptoms of angina after starting RANEXA.
• Take RANEXA by mouth, with or without food.
• Swallow the RANEXA tablets whole. Do not crush, break, or chew RANEXA tablets before swallowing.
• If you miss a dose of RANEXA, wait to take the next dose of RANEXA at your regular time. Do not make up for the missed dose. Do not take more than 1 dose at a time.
• If you take too much RANEXA, call your doctor, or go to the nearest emergency room right away.

Table 2 Angina Frequency and Nitroglycerin Use (CARISA)

		Placebo	RANEXA 750 mg*	RANEXA 1000 mg*
Angina Frequency (attacks/week)	N	258	272	261
	Mean	3.3	2.5	2.1
	p-value vs placebo	—	0.006	< 0.001
Nitroglycerin Use (doses/week)	N	252	262	244
	Mean	3.1	2.1	1.8
	p-value vs placebo	—	0.016	< 0.001

* Twice daily

What should I avoid while taking RANEXA?

- Grapefruit and grapefruit juice. Limit products that have grapefruit in them. They can cause your blood levels of RANEXA to increase.
- RANEXA can cause dizziness, lightheadedness, or fainting. If you have these symptoms, do not drive a car, use machinery, or do anything that needs you to be alert.

What are the possible side effects of RANEXA?

RANEXA may cause serious side effects, including:

- changes in the electrical activity of your heart called QT prolongation. Your doctor may check the electrical activity of your heart with an ECG. Tell your doctor right away if you feel faint, lightheaded, or feel your heart beating irregularly or fast while taking RANEXA. These may be symptoms related to QT prolongation.
- kidney failure in people who already have severe kidney problems. Your doctor may need to do tests to check how your kidneys are working.

The most common side effects of RANEXA include:

- dizziness
- headache
- constipation
- nausea

Tell your doctor if you have any side effect that bothers you or does not go away.

These are not all the possible side effects of RANEXA. For more information, ask your doctor or pharmacist.

Call your doctor for medical advice about side effects. You may report side effects to FDA at 1-800-FDA-1088.

How should I store RANEXA?

Store RANEXA tablets at room temperature between 59° to 86°F (15° to 30°C).

Keep RANEXA and all medicines out of the reach of children.

General information about RANEXA

Medicines are sometimes prescribed for purposes other than those listed in the Patient Information. Do not use RANEXA for a condition for which it was not prescribed. Do not give RANEXA to other people, even if they have the same condition you have. It may harm them.

The Patient Information summarizes the most important information about RANEXA. If you would like more information, talk with your doctor. You can ask your pharmacist or doctor for information about RANEXA that is written for health professionals.

For more information, go to www.ranexa.com or call Gilead Sciences, Inc. at 1-800-445-3235.

What is chronic angina?

Chronic angina means pain or discomfort in the chest, jaw, shoulder, back, or arm that keeps coming back. There are other possible signs and symptoms of angina including shortness of breath. Angina usually comes on when you are active or under stress. Chronic angina is a symptom of a heart problem called coronary heart disease (CHD), also known as coronary artery disease (CAD). When you have CHD, the blood vessels in your heart become stiff and narrow. Oxygen-rich blood cannot reach your heart muscle easily. Angina comes on when too little oxygen reaches your heart muscle.

What are the ingredients in RANEXA?

Active ingredient: ranolazine

Inactive ingredients:

500 mg tablet: carnauba wax, hypromellose, magnesium stearate, methacrylic acid copolymer (Type C), microcrystalline cellulose, polyethylene glycol, sodium hydroxide, titanium dioxide, polyvinyl alcohol, talc, Iron Oxide Yellow, and Iron Oxide Red.

1000 mg tablet: carnauba wax, hypromellose, magnesium stearate, methacrylic acid copolymer (Type C), microcrystalline cellulose, polyethylene glycol, sodium hydroxide, titanium dioxide, lactose monohydrate, triacetin, and Iron Oxide Yellow.

This Patient Information has been approved by the U.S. Food and Drug Administration.

Manufactured for:
Gilead Sciences, Inc.
Foster City, CA 94404
Issued December 2013
RANEXA is a registered trademark of Gilead Sciences, Inc.
© 2013 Gilead Sciences, Inc.
All other trademarks are the property of their respective owners.
21-526-GS-013

Shown in Product Identification Guide, page 307

SOVALDI®
(sofosbuvir)
tablets, for oral use   ℞

HIGHLIGHTS OF PRESCRIBING INFORMATION

These highlights do not include all the information needed to use SOVALDI safely and effectively. See full prescribing information for SOVALDI.

SOVALDI® (sofosbuvir) tablets, for oral use

Initial U.S. Approval: 2013

——INDICATIONS AND USAGE——

SOVALDI is a hepatitis C virus (HCV) nucleotide analog NS5B polymerase inhibitor indicated for the treatment of chronic hepatitis C (CHC) infection as a component of a combination antiviral treatment regimen. (1)

- SOVALDI efficacy has been established in subjects with HCV genotype 1, 2, 3 or 4 infection, including those with hepatocellular carcinoma meeting Milan criteria (awaiting liver transplantation) and those with HCV/HIV-1 co-infection. (1)

——DOSAGE AND ADMINISTRATION——

- One 400 mg tablet taken once daily with or without food. (2.1)
- Should be used in combination with ribavirin or in combination with pegylated interferon and ribavirin for the treatment of CHC. Recommended combination therapy: (2.1)

HCV Mono-infected and HCV/HIV-1 Co-infected	Treatment	Duration
Genotype 1 or 4	SOVALDI + peg-interferon alfa + ribavirin	12 weeks
Genotype 2	SOVALDI + ribavirin	12 weeks
Genotype 3	SOVALDI + ribavirin	24 weeks

- SOVALDI in combination with ribavirin for 24 weeks can be considered for CHC patients with genotype 1 infection who are interferon ineligible. (2.1)
- Should be used in combination with ribavirin for treatment of CHC in patients with hepatocellular carcinoma awaiting liver transplantation for up to 48 weeks or until liver transplantation, whichever occurs first. (2.1)
- A dose recommendation cannot be made for patients with severe renal impairment or end stage renal disease. (2.4, 8.6)

——DOSAGE FORMS AND STRENGTHS——

Tablets: 400 mg. (3)

——CONTRAINDICATIONS——

- When used in combination with peginterferon alfa/ribavirin or ribavirin alone, all contraindications to peginterferon alfa and/or ribavirin also apply to SOVALDI combination therapy. (4)
- Because ribavirin may cause birth defects and fetal death, SOVALDI in combination with peginterferon alfa/ribavirin or ribavirin is contraindicated in pregnant women and in men whose female partners are pregnant. (4)

——WARNINGS AND PRECAUTIONS——

- Pregnancy: Ribavirin may cause birth defects and fetal death and animal studies have shown interferons have abortifacient effects; avoid pregnancy in female patients and female partners of male patients. Patients must have a negative pregnancy test prior to initiating therapy, use at least 2 effective non-hormonal methods of contraception and have monthly pregnancy tests. (5.1)

——ADVERSE REACTIONS——

The most common adverse events (incidence greater than or equal to 20%, all grades) observed with SOVALDI in combination with ribavirin were fatigue and headache. The most common adverse events observed with SOVALDI in combination with peginterferon alfa and ribavirin were fatigue, headache, nausea, insomnia and anemia. (6.1)

To report SUSPECTED ADVERSE REACTIONS, contact Gilead Sciences, Inc. at 1-800-GILEAD-5 or FDA at 1-800-FDA-1088 or www.fda.gov/medwatch.

——DRUG INTERACTIONS——

Drugs that are potent intestinal P-gp inducers (e.g., rifampin, St. John's wort) may alter the concentrations of sofosbuvir. Consult the full prescribing information prior to use for potential drug-drug interactions. (5.2, 7, 12.3)

——USE IN SPECIFIC POPULATIONS——

- Patients with HCV/HIV-1 co-infection: Safety and efficacy have been studied. (8.8, 14.4)
- Patients with hepatocellular carcinoma awaiting liver transplantation: Safety and efficacy have been studied. (8.9)

See 17 for PATIENT COUNSELING INFORMATION and FDA-approved patient labeling

Revised: 12/2013

FULL PRESCRIBING INFORMATION

1   INDICATIONS AND USAGE

SOVALDI is a hepatitis C virus (HCV) nucleotide analog NS5B polymerase inhibitor indicated for the treatment of chronic hepatitis C (CHC) infection as a component of a combination antiviral treatment regimen.

- SOVALDI efficacy has been established in subjects with HCV genotype 1, 2, 3 or 4 infection, including those with hepatocellular carcinoma meeting Milan criteria (awaiting liver transplantation) and those with HCV/HIV-1 co-infection *[See Dosage and Administration (2), Use in Specific Populations (8) and Clinical Studies (14)].*

The following points should be considered when initiating treatment with SOVALDI:

- Monotherapy of SOVALDI is not recommended for treatment of CHC.
- Treatment regimen and duration are dependent on both viral genotype and patient population *[See Dosage and Administration (2)].*
- Treatment response varies based on baseline host and viral factors *[See Use in Specific Populations (8) and Clinical Studies (14)].*

2   DOSAGE AND ADMINISTRATION

2.1   Recommended Dose in Adults

The recommended dose of SOVALDI is one 400 mg tablet, taken orally, once daily with or without food *[See Clinical Pharmacology (12.3)].*

SOVALDI should be used in combination with ribavirin or in combination with pegylated interferon and ribavirin for the treatment of CHC in adults. The recommended regimen and treatment duration for SOVALDI combination therapy is provided in Table 1.

Table 1 Recommended Regimens and Treatment Duration for SOVALDI Combination Therapy in HCV Mono-infected and HCV/HIV-1 Co-infected Patients

	Treatment	Duration
Patients with genotype 1 or 4 CHC	SOVALDI + peginterferon alfa* + ribavirin	12 weeks
Patients with genotype 2 CHC	SOVALDI + ribavirin†	12 weeks
Patients with genotype 3 CHC	SOVALDI + ribavirin†	24 weeks

*See peginterferon alfa prescribing information for dosing recommendation for patients with genotype 1 or 4 CHC.
†Dose of ribavirin is weight-based (<75 kg = 1000 mg and ≥75 kg = 1200 mg). The daily dose of ribavirin is administered orally.in two divided doses with food. Patients with renal impairment (CrCl ≤ 50 mL/min) require ribavirin dose reduction; refer to ribavirin prescribing information.

SOVALDI in combination with ribavirin for 24 weeks can be considered as a therapeutic option for CHC patients with genotype 1 infection who are ineligible to receive an interferon-based regimen [See Use in Specific Populations (8.8) and Clinical Studies (14.4)]. Treatment decision should be guided by an assessment of the potential benefits and risks for the individual patient.
Patients with Hepatocellular Carcinoma Awaiting Liver Transplantation
SOVALDI in combination with ribavirin is recommended for up to 48 weeks or until the time of liver transplantation, whichever occurs first, to prevent post-transplant HCV re-infection [See Use in Specific Populations (8.9)].

2.2   Dose Modification
Dose reduction of SOVALDI is not recommended.
Genotype 1 and 4:
If a patient has a serious adverse reaction potentially related to peginterferon alfa and/or ribavirin, the peginterferon alfa and/or ribavirin dose should be reduced or discontinued. Refer to the peginterferon alfa and ribavirin prescribing information for additional information about how to reduce and/or discontinue the peginterferon alfa and/or ribavirin dose.
Genotype 2 and 3:
If a patient has a serious adverse reaction potentially related to ribavirin, the ribavirin dose should be modified or discontinued, if appropriate, until the adverse reaction abates or decreases in severity. Table 2 provides guidelines for dose modifications and discontinuation based on the patient's hemoglobin concentration and cardiac status.

Table 2 Ribavirin Dose Modification Guideline for Coadministration with SOVALDI

Laboratory Values	Reduce Ribavirin Dose to 600 mg/ day* If:	Discontinue Ribavirin If:†
Hemoglobin in patients with no cardiac disease	<10 g/dL	<8.5 g/dL
Hemoglobin in patients with history of stable cardiac disease	≥2 g/dL decrease in hemoglobin during any 4 week treatment period	<12 g/dL despite 4 weeks at reduced dose

*The daily dose of ribavirin is administered orally in two divided doses with food.
†Once ribavirin has been withheld due to either a laboratory abnormality or clinical manifestation, an attempt may be made to restart ribavirin at 600 mg daily and further increase the dose to 800 mg daily. However, it is not recommended that ribavirin be increased to the original assigned dose (1000 mg to 1200 mg daily).

2.3   Discontinuation of Dosing
If the other agents used in combination with SOVALDI are permanently discontinued, SOVALDI should also be discontinued.
2.4   Severe Renal Impairment and End Stage Renal Disease
No dose recommendation can be given for patients with severe renal impairment (estimated Glomerular Filtration Rate (eGFR) <30 mL/min/1.73m²) or with end stage renal disease (ESRD) due to higher exposures (up to 20-fold) of the predominant sofosbuvir metabolite [See Use in Specific Populations (8.6) and Clinical Pharmacology (12.3)].

Table 3 Treatment-Emergent Adverse Events (All Grades) Reported in ≥ 15% of Subjects in Any Treatment Arm

	Interferon-free Regimens			Interferon-containing Regimens	
	PBO 12 weeks	SOVALDI + RBV* 12 weeks	SOVALDI + RBV* 24 weeks	Peg-IFN alfa + RBV† 24 weeks	SOVALDI + Peg-IFN alfa + RBV* 12 weeks
	N=71	N=650	N=250	N=243	N=327
Fatigue	24%	38%	30%	55%	59%
Headache	20%	24%	30%	44%	36%
Nausea	18%	22%	13%	29%	34%
Insomnia	4%	15%	16%	29%	25%
Pruritus	8%	11%	27%	17%	17%
Anemia	0%	10%	6%	12%	21%
Asthenia	3%	6%	21%	3%	5%
Rash	8%	8%	9%	18%	18%
Decreased Appetite	10%	6%	6%	18%	18%
Chills	1%	2%	2%	18%	17%
Influenza Like Illness	3%	3%	6%	18%	16%
Pyrexia	0%	4%	4%	14%	18%
Diarrhea	6%	9%	12%	17%	12%
Neutropenia	0%	<1%	<1%	12%	17%
Myalgia	0%	6%	9%	16%	14%
Irritability	1%	10%	10%	16%	13%

*Subjects received weight-based ribavirin (1000 mg per day if weighing < 75 kg or 1200 mg per day if weighing ≥ 75 kg).
†Subjects received 800 mg ribavirin per day regardless of weight.

3   DOSAGE FORMS AND STRENGTHS
SOVALDI is available as a yellow colored, capsule-shaped, film-coated tablet debossed with "GSI" on one side and "7977" on the other side. Each tablet contains 400 mg sofosbuvir.
4   CONTRAINDICATIONS
When SOVALDI is used in combination with ribavirin or peginterferon alfa/ribavirin, the contraindications applicable to those agents are applicable to combination therapies. Refer to the prescribing information of peginterferon alfa and ribavirin for a list of their contraindications.
SOVALDI combination treatment with ribavirin or peginterferon alfa/ribavirin is contraindicated in women who are pregnant or may become pregnant and men whose female partners are pregnant because of the risks for birth defects and fetal death associated with ribavirin [See Warnings and Precautions (5.1) and Use in Specific Populations (8.1)].
5   WARNINGS AND PRECAUTIONS
5.1   Pregnancy: Use with Ribavirin or Peginterferon Alfa/Ribavirin
Ribavirin may cause birth defects and/or death of the exposed fetus and animal studies have shown that interferons have abortifacient effects [See Contraindications (4)]. Extreme care must be taken to avoid pregnancy in female patients and in female partners of male patients. Ribavirin therapy should not be started unless a report of a negative pregnancy test has been obtained immediately prior to initiation of therapy.
When SOVALDI is used in combination with ribavirin or peginterferon alfa/ribavirin, women of childbearing potential and their male partners must use two forms of effective contraception during treatment and for at least 6 months after treatment has concluded. Routine monthly pregnancy tests must be performed during this time. There are no data on the effectiveness of systemic hormonal contraceptives in women taking SOVALDI, therefore, two non-hormonal methods of contraception should be used during treatment with SOVALDI and concomitant ribavirin [See Contraindications (4) and Use in Specific Populations (8.1)]. Refer also to the prescribing information for ribavirin.
5.2   Use with Potent P-gp Inducers
Drugs that are potent P-gp inducers in the intestine (e.g., rifampin, St. John's wort) may significantly decrease sofosbuvir plasma concentrations and may lead to a reduced therapeutic effect of SOVALDI. Rifampin and St. John's wort should not be used with SOVALDI [See Drug Interactions (7.2)].
6   ADVERSE REACTIONS
6.1   Adverse Reactions from Clinical Trials Experience
SOVALDI should be administered with ribavirin or peginterferon alfa/ribavirin. Refer to the prescribing information of peginterferon alfa and ribavirin for a description of adverse reactions associated with their use.
Because clinical trials are conducted under widely varying conditions, adverse reaction rates observed in the clinical trials of a drug cannot be directly compared to rates in the clinical trials of another drug and may not reflect the rates observed in practice.
The safety assessment of SOVALDI is based on pooled Phase 3 clinical trial data (both controlled and uncontrolled) including 650 subjects who received SOVALDI + ribavirin (RBV) combination therapy for 12 weeks, 98 subjects who received SOVALDI + ribavirin combination therapy for 16 weeks, 250 subjects who received SOVALDI + ribavirin combination therapy for 24 weeks, 327 subjects who received SOVALDI + peginterferon (Peg-IFN) alfa + ribavirin combination therapy for 12 weeks, 243 subjects who received peginterferon alfa + ribavirin for 24 weeks and 71 subjects who received placebo (PBO) for 12 weeks.
The proportion of subjects who permanently discontinued treatment due to adverse events was 4% for subjects receiving placebo, 1% for subjects receiving SOVALDI + ribavirin for 12 weeks, <1% for subjects receiving SOVALDI + ribavirin for 24 weeks, 11% for subjects receiving peginterferon alfa + ribavirin for 24 weeks and 2% for subjects receiving SOVALDI + peginterferon alfa + ribavirin for 12 weeks.
Treatment-emergent adverse events observed in ≥15% of subjects in clinical trials are provided in Table 3. A side-by-side tabulation is to simplify presentation; direct comparison across trials should not be made due to differing trial designs.
The most common adverse events (≥ 20%) for SOVALDI + ribavirin combination therapy were fatigue and headache.
The most common adverse events (≥ 20%) for SOVALDI + peginterferon alfa + ribavirin combination therapy were fatigue, headache, nausea, insomnia and anemia.
[See table 3 above]

With the exception of anemia and neutropenia, the majority of events presented in Table 3 occurred at severity of grade 1 in SOVALDI-containing regimens.

Less Common Adverse Reactions Reported in Clinical Trials (<1%): The following ADRs occurred in <1% of subjects receiving SOVALDI in a combination regimen in any one trial. These events have been included because of their seriousness or assessment of potential causal relationship.

Hematologic Effects: pancytopenia (particularly in subjects receiving concomitant pegylated interferon).

Psychiatric Disorders: severe depression (particularly in subjects with pre-existing history of psychiatric illness), including suicidal ideation and suicide.

Laboratory Abnormalities:

Changes in selected hematological parameters are described in Table 4. A side-by-side tabulation is to simplify presentation; direct comparison across trials should not be made due to differing trial designs.

[See table 4 above]

Bilirubin Elevations

Total bilirubin elevation of more than 2.5×ULN was observed in none of the subjects in the SOVALDI + peginterferon alfa + ribavirin 12 weeks group and in 1%, 3% and 3% of subjects in the peginterferon alfa + ribavirin 24 weeks, SOVALDI + ribavirin 12 weeks and SOVALDI + ribavirin 24 weeks groups, respectively. Bilirubin levels peaked during the first 1 to 2 weeks of treatment and subsequently decreased and returned to baseline levels by post-treatment Week 4. These bilirubin elevations were not associated with transaminase elevations.

Creatine Kinase Elevations

Creatine kinase was assessed in the FISSION and NEUTRINO trials. Isolated, asymptomatic creatine kinase elevation of greater than or equal to 10×ULN was observed in <1%, 1% and 2% of subjects in the peginterferon alfa + ribavirin 24 weeks, SOVALDI + peginterferon alfa + ribavirin 12 weeks and SOVALDI + ribavirin 12 weeks groups, respectively.

Lipase Elevations

Isolated, asymptomatic lipase elevation of greater than 3×ULN was observed in <1%, 2%, 2%, and 2% of subjects in the SOVALDI + peginterferon alfa + ribavirin 12 weeks, SOVALDI + ribavirin 12 weeks, SOVALDI + ribavirin 24 weeks and peginterferon alfa + ribavirin 24 weeks groups, respectively.

7   DRUG INTERACTIONS
7.1   Potential for Drug Interactions
After oral administration of SOVALDI, sofosbuvir is rapidly converted to the predominant circulating metabolite GS-331007 that accounts for greater than 90% of drug related material systemic exposure, while the parent sofosbuvir accounts for approximately 4% of drug related material *[See Clinical Pharmacology (12.3)].* In clinical pharmacology studies, both sofosbuvir and GS-331007 were monitored for purposes of pharmacokinetic analyses.

Sofosbuvir is a substrate of drug transporter P-gp and breast cancer resistance protein (BCRP) while GS-331007 is not. Drugs that are potent P-gp inducers in the intestine (e.g., rifampin or St. John's wort) may decrease sofosbuvir plasma concentration leading to reduced therapeutic effect of SOVALDI and thus should not be used with SOVALDI *[See Warnings and Precautions (5.2)].* Coadministration of SOVALDI with drugs that inhibit P-gp and/or BCRP may increase sofosbuvir plasma concentration without increasing GS-331007 plasma concentration; accordingly, SOVALDI may be coadministered with P-gp and/or BCRP inhibitors. Sofosbuvir and GS-331007 are not inhibitors of P-gp and BCRP and thus are not expected to increase exposures of drugs that are substrates of these transporters.

The intracellular metabolic activation pathway of sofosbuvir is mediated by generally low affinity and high capacity hydrolase and nucleotide phosphorylation pathways that are unlikely to be affected by concomitant drugs *[See Clinical Pharmacology 12.3].*

7.2   Potentially Significant Drug Interactions
Drug interaction information for SOVALDI with potential concomitant drugs is summarized in Table 5. The drug interactions described are based on potential drug interactions that may occur with SOVALDI. The table is not all-inclusive *[See Warnings and Precautions (5.2) and Clinical Pharmacology (12.3)].*

[See table 5 above]

7.3   Drugs without Clinically Significant Interactions with SOVALDI
In addition to the drugs included in Table 5, the interaction between SOVALDI and the following drugs was evaluated in clinical trials and no dose adjustment is needed for either drug *[See Clinical Pharmacology (12.3)]:* cyclosporine, darunavir/ritonavir, efavirenz, emtricitabine, methadone, raltegravir, rilpivirine, tacrolimus, or tenofovir disoproxil fumarate.

Table 4 Percentage of Subjects Reporting Selected Hematological Parameters

Hematological Parameters	Interferon-free Regimens			Interferon-containing Regimens	
	PBO 12 weeks	SOVALDI + RBV* 12 weeks	SOVALDI+ RBV* 24 weeks	Peg-IFN + RBV† 24 weeks	SOVALDI + Peg-IFN + RBV* 12 weeks
	N=71	N=647	N=250	N=242	N=327
Hemoglobin (g/dL)					
< 10	0	8%	6%	14%	23%
< 8.5	0	1%	<1%	2%	2%
Neutrophils (×10⁹/L)					
≥0.5 – < 0.75	1%	<1%	0	12%	15%
< 0.5	0	<1%	0	2%	5%
Platelets (×10⁹/L)					
≥25 – < 50	3%	<1%	1%	7%	<1%
< 25	0	0	0	0	0

*Subjects received weight-based ribavirin (1000 mg per day if weighing < 75 kg or 1200 mg per day if weighing ≥ 75 kg).
†Subjects received 800 mg ribavirin per day regardless of weight.

Table 5 Potentially Significant Drug Interactions: Alteration in Dose or Regimen May Be Recommended Based on Drug Interaction Studies or Predicted Interaction*

Concomitant Drug Class: Drug Name	Effect on Concentration†	Clinical Comment
Anticonvulsants: carbamazepine phenytoin phenobarbital oxcarbazepine	↓ sofosbuvir ↓ GS-331007	Coadministration of SOVALDI with carbamazepine, phenytoin, phenobarbital or oxcarbazepine is expected to decrease the concentration of sofosbuvir, leading to reduced therapeutic effect of SOVALDI. Coadministration is not recommended.
Antimycobacterials: rifabutin rifampin rifapentine	↓ sofosbuvir ↓ GS-331007	Coadministration of SOVALDI with rifabutin or rifapentine is expected to decrease the concentration of sofosbuvir, leading to reduced therapeutic effect of SOVALDI. Coadministration is not recommended. SOVALDI should not be used with rifampin, a potent intestinal P-gp inducer *[See Warnings and Precautions (5.2)].*
Herbal Supplements: St. John's wort (*Hypericum perforatum*)	↓ sofosbuvir ↓ GS-331007	SOVALDI should not be used with St. John's wort, a potent intestinal P-gp inducer *[See Warnings and Precautions (5.2)].*
HIV Protease Inhibitors: tipranavir/ritonavir	↓ sofosbuvir ↓ GS-331007	Coadministration of SOVALDI with tipranavir/ritonavir is expected to decrease the concentration of sofosbuvir, leading to reduced therapeutic effect of SOVALDI. Coadministration is not recommended.

*This table is not all inclusive.
†↓ = decrease.

8   USE IN SPECIFIC POPULATIONS
8.1   Pregnancy
Pregnancy Category X: Use with Ribavirin or Peginterferon Alfa/Ribavirin

Extreme caution must be taken to avoid pregnancy in female patients and female partners of male patients while taking this combination. Women of childbearing potential and their male partners should not receive ribavirin unless they are using two forms of effective contraception during treatment with ribavirin and for 6 months after treatment has concluded. There are no data on the effectiveness of systemic hormonal contraceptives in women taking SOVALDI. Therefore, two effective non-hormonal methods of contraception should be used during treatment with SOVALDI and concomitant ribavirin *[See Warnings and Precautions (5.1)].*

In case of exposure during pregnancy, a Ribavirin Pregnancy Registry has been established to monitor maternal-fetal outcomes of pregnancies in female patients and female partners of male patients exposed to ribavirin during treatment and for 6 months following cessation of treatment. Healthcare providers and patients are encouraged to report such cases by calling Ribavirin Pregnancy Registry at 1-800-593-2214. For patients who are HCV/HIV-1 co-infected and taking concomitant antiretrovirals, an Antiretroviral Pregnancy Registry is also available at 1-800-258-4263.

Animal Data

Significant teratogenic and/or embryocidal effects have been demonstrated in all animal species exposed to ribavirin; and therefore ribavirin is contraindicated in women who are pregnant and in the male partners of women who are pregnant *[See Contraindications (4), Warnings and Precautions (5.1) and ribavirin Package Insert].* Interferons have abortifacient effects in animals and should be assumed to have abortifacient potential in humans *[See peginterferon alfa Package Insert].*

Pregnancy Category B: SOVALDI

There are no adequate and well-controlled studies with SOVALDI in pregnant women.

Animal Data

No effects on fetal development have been observed in rats and rabbits at the highest doses tested. In the rat and rabbit, AUC exposure to the predominant circulating metabolite GS-331007 increased over the course of gestation from approximately 5- to 10-fold and 12- to 28-fold the exposure in humans at the recommended clinical dose, respectively.

8.3   Nursing Mothers
It is not known whether SOVALDI and its metabolites are present in human breast milk. The predominant circulating metabolite GS-331007 was the primary component observed in the milk of lactating rats, without effect on nursing pups. Because of the potential for adverse reactions from the drug in nursing infants, a decision must be made whether to discontinue nursing or discontinue treatment with ribavirin-containing regimens, taking into account the importance of the therapy to the mother. See also the prescribing information for ribavirin.

8.4   Pediatric Use
Safety and effectiveness of SOVALDI in children less than 18 years of age have not been established.

8.5 Geriatric Use

SOVALDI was administered to 90 subjects aged 65 and over. The response rates observed for subjects over 65 years of age were similar to that of younger subjects across treatment groups. No dose adjustment of SOVALDI is warranted in geriatric patients [See Clinical Pharmacology (12.3)].

8.6 Renal Impairment

No dose adjustment of SOVALDI is required for patients with mild or moderate renal impairment. The safety and efficacy of SOVALDI have not been established in patients with severe renal impairment (eGFR <30 mL/min/1.73m^2) or end stage renal disease (ESRD) requiring hemodialysis. No dose recommendation can be given for patients with severe renal impairment or ESRD [See Dosage and Administration (2.4) and Clinical Pharmacology (12.3)]. Refer also to ribavirin and peginterferon alfa prescribing information for patients with CrCl <50 mL/min.

8.7 Hepatic Impairment

No dose adjustment of SOVALDI is required for patients with mild, moderate or severe hepatic impairment (Child-Pugh Class A, B or C). Safety and efficacy of SOVALDI have not been established in patients with decompensated cirrhosis [See Clinical Pharmacology (12.3)]. See peginterferon alfa prescribing information for contraindication in hepatic decompensation.

8.8 Patients with HCV/HIV-1 Co-infection

The safety and efficacy of SOVALDI was assessed in 223 HCV/HIV-1 co-infected subjects [See Clinical Studies (14.4)]. See Dosage and Administration (2.1) for dosing recommendations in HCV/HIV-1 co-infected patients. The safety profile in HCV/HIV-1 co-infected subjects was similar to that observed in HCV mono-infected subjects. Elevated total bilirubin (grade 3 or 4) was observed in 30/32 (94%) subjects receiving atazanavir as part of the antiretroviral regimen. None of the subjects had concomitant transaminase increases. Among subjects not taking atazanavir, grade 3 or 4 elevated total bilirubin was observed in 2 (1.5%) subjects, similar to the rate observed with HCV mono-infected subjects receiving SOVALDI + ribavirin in Phase 3 trials [See Adverse Reactions (6.1)].

8.9 Patients with Hepatocellular Carcinoma Awaiting Liver Transplantation

SOVALDI was studied in HCV-infected subjects with hepatocellular carcinoma prior to undergoing liver transplantation in an open-label clinical trial evaluating the safety and efficacy of SOVALDI and ribavirin administered pretransplant to prevent post-transplant HCV reinfection. The primary endpoint of the trial was post-transplant virologic response (pTVR) as HCV RNA < lower limit of quantification (LLOQ) at 12 weeks post-transplant. HCV-infected subjects, regardless of genotype, with hepatocellular carcinoma (HCC) meeting the MILAN criteria (defined as the presence of a tumor 5 cm or less in diameter in patients with single hepatocellular carcinomas and no more than three tumor nodules, each 3 cm or less in diameter in patients with multiple tumors and no extrahepatic manifestations of the cancer or evidence of vascular invasion of tumor) received 400 mg SOVALDI and weight-based 1000–1200 mg ribavirin daily for 24–48 weeks or until the time of liver transplantation, whichever occurred first. An interim analysis was conducted on 61 subjects who received SOVALDI and ribavirin; 45 subjects had HCV genotype 1; 44 subjects had a baseline CPT score less than 7 and all subjects had a baseline unadjusted MELD score ≤14. Of these 61 subjects, 41 subjects underwent liver transplantation following up to 48 weeks of treatment with SOVALDI and ribavirin; 37 had HCV RNA < LLOQ at the time of transplantation. Of the 37 subjects, the post-transplant virologic response (pTVR) rate is 64% (23/36) in the 36 evaluable subjects who have reached the 12 week post-transplant time point. The safety profile of SOVALDI and ribavirin in HCV-infected subjects prior to liver transplantation was comparable to that observed in subjects treated with SOVALDI and ribavirin in Phase 3 clinical trials.

8.10 Post-Liver Transplant Patients

The safety and efficacy of SOVALDI have not been established in post-liver transplant patients.

8.11 CHC Patients with Genotype 5 or 6 HCV Infection

Available data on subjects with genotype 5 or 6 HCV infection are insufficient for dosing recommendations.

10 OVERDOSAGE

The highest documented dose of sofosbuvir was a single supratherapeutic dose of sofosbuvir 1200 mg administered to 59 healthy subjects. In that trial, there were no untoward effects observed at this dose level, and adverse events were similar in frequency and severity to those reported in the placebo and sofosbuvir 400 mg treatment groups. The effects of higher doses are not known.

No specific antidote is available for overdose with SOVALDI. If overdose occurs the patient must be monitored for evidence of toxicity. Treatment of overdose with SOVALDI consists of general supportive measures including monitoring of vital signs as well as observation of the clinical status of the patient. A 4-hour hemodialysis session removed 18% of the administered dose.

11 DESCRIPTION

SOVALDI is the brand name for sofosbuvir, a nucleotide analog inhibitor of HCV NS5B polymerase.

The IUPAC name for sofosbuvir is (S)-Isopropyl 2-((S)-(((2R,3R,4R,5R)-5-(2,4-dioxo-3,4-dihydropyrimidin-1(2H)-yl)-4-fluoro-3-hydroxy-4-methyltetrahydrofuran-2-yl)methoxy)-(phenoxy)phosphorylamino)propanoate. It has a molecular formula of $C_{22}H_{29}FN_3O_9P$ and a molecular weight of 529.45. It has the following structural formula:

Sofosbuvir is a white to off-white crystalline solid with a solubility of ≥ 2 mg/mL across the pH range of 2–7.7 at 37 °C and is slightly soluble in water.

SOVALDI tablets are for oral administration. Each tablet contains 400 mg of sofosbuvir. The tablets include the following inactive ingredients: colloidal silicon dioxide, croscarmellose sodium, magnesium stearate, mannitol, and microcrystalline cellulose. The tablets are film-coated with a coating material containing the following inactive ingredients: polyethylene glycol, polyvinyl alcohol, talc, titanium dioxide, and yellow iron oxide.

12 CLINICAL PHARMACOLOGY

12.1 Mechanism of Action

Sofosbuvir is a direct-acting antiviral agent against the hepatitis C virus [See Microbiology (12.4)].

12.2 Pharmacodynamics

Effect on Electrocardiogram

The effect of sofosbuvir 400 and 1200 mg on QTc interval was evaluated in a randomized, single-dose, placebo-, and active-controlled (moxifloxacin 400 mg) four period crossover thorough QT trial in 59 healthy subjects. At a dose three times the maximum recommended dose, SOVALDI does not prolong QTc to any clinically relevant extent.

12.3 Pharmacokinetics

Absorption

The pharmacokinetic properties of sofosbuvir and the predominant circulating metabolite GS-331007 have been evaluated in healthy adult subjects and in subjects with chronic hepatitis C. Following oral administration of SOVALDI, sofosbuvir was absorbed with a peak plasma concentration observed at ~0.5–2 hour post-dose, regardless of dose level. Peak plasma concentration of GS-331007 was observed between 2 to 4 hours post-dose. Based on population pharmacokinetic analysis in subjects with genotype 1 to 6 HCV infection who were coadministered ribavirin (with or without pegylated interferon), geometric mean steady state sofosbuvir (N=838) and GS-331007 (N=1695) AUC_{0-24} were 828 ng·hr/mL and 6790 ng·hr/mL, respectively. Relative to healthy subjects administered sofosbuvir alone (N = 272), the sofosbuvir AUC_{0-24} was 39% higher and GS-331007 AUC_{0-24} was 39% lower, respectively, in HCV-infected subjects. Sofosbuvir and GS-331007 AUCs are near dose proportional over the dose range of 200 mg to 1200 mg.

Effect of Food

Relative to fasting conditions, the administration of a single dose of SOVALDI with a standardized high fat meal did not substantially affect the sofosbuvir C_{max} or AUC_{0-inf}. The exposure of GS-331007 was not altered in the presence of a high-fat meal. Therefore, SOVALDI can be administered without regard to food.

Distribution

Sofosbuvir is approximately 61–65% bound to human plasma proteins and the binding is independent of drug concentration over the range of 1 µg/mL to 20 µg/mL. Protein binding of GS-331007 was minimal in human plasma. After a single 400 mg dose of [^{14}C]-sofosbuvir in healthy subjects, the blood to plasma ratio of ^{14}C-radioactivity was approximately 0.7.

Metabolism

Sofosbuvir is extensively metabolized in the liver to form the pharmacologically active nucleoside analog triphosphate GS-461203. The metabolic activation pathway involves sequential hydrolysis of the carboxyl ester moiety catalyzed by human cathepsin A (CatA) or carboxylesterase 1 (CES1) and phosphoramidate cleavage by histidine triad nucleotide-binding protein 1 (HINT1) followed by phosphorylation by the pyrimidine nucleotide biosynthesis pathway. Dephosphorylation results in the formation of nucleoside metabolite GS-331007 that cannot be efficiently rephosphorylated and lacks anti-HCV activity in vitro.

After a single 400 mg oral dose of [^{14}C]-sofosbuvir, sofosbuvir and GS-331007 accounted for approximately 4% and >90% of drug related material (sum of molecular weight-adjusted AUC of sofosbuvir and its metabolites) systemic exposure, respectively.

Elimination

Following a single 400 mg oral dose of [^{14}C]-sofosbuvir, mean total recovery of the dose was greater than 92%, consisting of approximately 80%, 14%, and 2.5% recovered in urine, feces, and expired air, respectively. The majority of the sofosbuvir dose recovered in urine was GS-331007 (78%) while 3.5% was recovered as sofosbuvir. These data indicate that renal clearance is the major elimination pathway for GS-331007. The median terminal half-lives of sofosbuvir and GS-331007 were 0.4 and 27 hours, respectively.

Specific Populations

Race

Population pharmacokinetics analysis in HCV-infected subjects indicated that race had no clinically relevant effect on the exposure of sofosbuvir and GS-331007.

Gender

No clinically relevant pharmacokinetic differences have been observed between men and women for sofosbuvir and GS-331007.

Pediatric Patients

The pharmacokinetics of sofosbuvir in pediatric patients have not been established [See Use in Specific Populations (8.4)].

Geriatric Patients

Population pharmacokinetic analysis in HCV-infected subjects showed that within the age range (19 to 75 years) analyzed, age did not have a clinically relevant effect on the exposure to sofosbuvir and GS-331007 [See Use in Specific Populations (8.5)].

Patients with Renal Impairment

The pharmacokinetics of sofosbuvir were studied in HCV negative subjects with mild (eGFR ≥ 50 and < 80 mL/min/1.73m^2), moderate (eGFR ≥30 and <50 mL/min/1.73m^2), severe renal impairment (eGFR <30 mL/min/1.73m^2) and subjects with end stage renal disease (ESRD) requiring hemodialysis following a single 400 mg dose of sofosbuvir. Relative to subjects with normal renal function (eGFR >80 mL/min/1.73m^2), the sofosbuvir AUC_{0-inf} was 61%, 107% and 171% higher in mild, moderate and severe renal impairment, while the GS-331007 AUC_{0-inf} was 55%, 88% and 451% higher, respectively. In subjects with ESRD, relative to subjects with normal renal function, sofosbuvir and GS-331007 AUC_{0-inf} was 28% and 1280% higher when sofosbuvir was dosed 1 hour before hemodialysis compared with 60% and 2070% higher when sofosbuvir was dosed 1 hour after hemodialysis, respectively. A 4 hour hemodialysis session removed approximately 18% of administered dose. No dose adjustment is required for patients with mild or moderate renal impairment. The safety and efficacy of SOVALDI have not been established in patients with severe renal impairment or ESRD. No dose recommendation can be given for patients with severe renal impairment or ESRD [See Dosage and Administration (2.4) and Use in Specific Populations (8.6)].

Patients with Hepatic Impairment

The pharmacokinetics of sofosbuvir were studied following 7-day dosing of 400 mg sofosbuvir in HCV-infected subjects with moderate and severe hepatic impairment (Child-Pugh Class B and C). Relative to subjects with normal hepatic function, the sofosbuvir AUC_{0-24} were 126% and 143% higher in moderate and severe hepatic impairment, while the GS-331007 AUC_{0-24} were 18% and 9% higher, respectively. Population pharmacokinetics analysis in HCV-infected subjects indicated that cirrhosis had no clinically relevant effect on the exposure of sofosbuvir and GS-331007. No dose adjustment of SOVALDI is recommended for patients with mild, moderate and severe hepatic impairment [See Use in Specific Populations (8.7)].

Assessment of Drug Interactions

The effects of coadministered drugs on the exposure of sofosbuvir and GS-331007 are shown in Table 6. The effects of sofosbuvir on the exposure of coadministered drugs are shown in Table 7 [See Drug Interactions (7.3)].

[See table 6 at top of next page]

No effect on the pharmacokinetic parameters of sofosbuvir and GS-331007 was observed with raltegravir.

[See table 7 on next page]

No effect on the pharmacokinetic parameters of the following coadministered drugs was observed with sofosbuvir: cyclosporine, darunavir/ritonavir, efavirenz, emtricitabine, methadone or rilpivirine.

12.4 Microbiology

Mechanism of Action

Sofosbuvir is an inhibitor of the HCV NS5B RNA-dependent RNA polymerase, which is essential for viral replication. Sofosbuvir is a nucleotide prodrug that undergoes intracellular metabolism to form the pharmacologically active uridine analog triphosphate (GS-461203), which can be incorporated into HCV RNA by the NS5B polymerase and acts as a chain terminator. In a biochemical assay, GS-461203 inhibited the polymerase activity of the recombinant NS5B from HCV genotype 1b, 2a, 3a and 4a with IC$_{50}$ values ranging from 0.7 to 2.6 μM. GS-461203 is not an inhibitor of human DNA and RNA polymerases nor an inhibitor of mitochondrial RNA polymerase.

Antiviral Activity
In HCV replicon assays, the EC_{50} values of sofosbuvir against full-length replicons from genotype 1a, 1b, 2a, 3a and 4a, and chimeric 1b replicons encoding NS5B from genotype 2b, 5a or 6a ranged from 0.014 to 0.11 μM. The median EC_{50} value of sofosbuvir against chimeric replicons encoding NS5B sequences from clinical isolates was 0.062 μM for genotype 1a (range 0.029–0.128 μM; N=67), 0.102 μM for genotype 1b (range 0.045–0.170 μM; N=29), 0.029 μM for genotype 2 (range 0.014–0.081 μM; N=15) and 0.081 μM for genotype 3a (range 0.024–0.181 μM; N=106). In infectious virus assays, the EC_{50} values of sofosbuvir against genotype 1a and 2a were 0.03 and 0.02 μM, respectively. The presence of 40% human serum had no effect on the anti-HCV activity of sofosbuvir. Evaluation of sofosbuvir in combination with interferon alpha or ribavirin showed no antagonistic effect in reducing HCV RNA levels in replicon cells.

Resistance
In Cell Culture
HCV replicons with reduced susceptibility to sofosbuvir have been selected in cell culture for multiple genotypes including 1b, 2a, 2b, 3a, 4a, 5a and 6a. Reduced susceptibility to sofosbuvir was associated with the primary NS5B substitution S282T in all replicon genotypes examined. An M289L substitution developed along with the S282T substitution in genotype 2a, 5 and 6 replicons. Site-directed mutagenesis of the S282T substitution in replicons of 8 genotypes conferred 2- to 18-fold reduced susceptibility to sofosbuvir and reduced the replication viral capacity by 89% to 99% compared to the corresponding wild-type. In biochemical assays, recombinant NS5B polymerase from genotypes 1b, 2a, 3a and 4a expressing the S282T substitution showed reduced susceptibility to GS-461203 compared to respective wild-types.

In Clinical Trials
In a pooled analysis of 982 subjects who received SOVALDI in Phase 3 trials, 224 subjects had post-baseline NS5B genotypic data from next generation nucleotide sequencing (assay cutoff of 1%).
Treatment-emergent substitutions L159F (n= 6) and V321A (n= 5) were detected in post-baseline samples from GT3a-infected subjects across the Phase 3 trials. No detectable shift in the phenotypic susceptibility to sofosbuvir of subject isolates with L159F or V321A substitutions was seen. The sofosbuvir-associated resistance substitution S282T was not detected at baseline or in the failure isolates from Phase 3 trials. However, an S282T substitution was detected in one genotype 2b subject who relapsed at Week 4 post-treatment after 12 weeks of sofosbuvir monotherapy in the Phase 2 trial P7977-0523 [ELECTRON]. The isolate from this subject displayed a mean 13.5-fold reduced susceptibility to sofosbuvir. For this subject, the S282T substitution was no longer detectable at Week 12 post-treatment by next generation sequencing with an assay cut off of 1%.
In the trial done in subjects with hepatocellular carcinoma awaiting liver transplantation where subjects received up to 48 weeks of sofosbuvir and ribavirin, the L159F substitution emerged in multiple subjects with GT1a or GT2b HCV who experienced virologic failure (breakthrough and relapse). Furthermore, the presence of substitutions L159F and/or C316N at baseline was associated with sofosbuvir breakthrough and relapse post-transplant in multiple subjects infected with GT1b HCV. In addition, S282R and L320F substitutions were detected on-treatment by next generation sequencing in a subject infected with GT1a HCV with a partial treatment response.
The clinical significance of these substitutions is not known.

Cross Resistance
HCV replicons expressing the sofosbuvir-associated resistance substitution S282T were susceptible to NS5A inhibitors and ribavirin. HCV replicons expressing the ribavirin-associated substitutions T390I and F415Y were susceptible to sofosbuvir. Sofosbuvir was active against HCV replicons with NS3/4A protease inhibitor, NS5B non-nucleoside inhibitor and NS5A inhibitor resistant variants.

13 NONCLINICAL TOXICOLOGY
13.1 Carcinogenesis, Mutagenesis, Impairment of Fertility
Carcinogenesis and Mutagenesis
Use with Ribavirin and/or Peginterferon alfa: Ribavirin was shown to be genotoxic in several *in vitro* and *in vivo* assays. Ribavirin was not oncogenic in a 6-month p53+/- transgenic mouse study or a 2-year carcinogenicity study in rats. See the prescribing information for ribavirin.
Carcinogenicity studies of sofosbuvir in mice and rats are ongoing.
Sofosbuvir was not genotoxic in a battery of *in vitro* or *in vivo* assays, including bacterial mutagenicity, chromosome aberration using human peripheral blood lymphocytes and *in vivo* mouse micronucleus assays.

Table 6 Drug Interactions: Changes in Pharmacokinetic Parameters for Sofosbuvir and the Predominant Circulating Metabolite GS-331007 in the Presence of the Coadministered Drug*

Co-administered Drug	Dose of Coadministered Drug (mg)	Sofosbuvir Dose (mg)	N		Mean Ratio (90% CI) of Sofosbuvir and GS-331007 PK With/Without Coadministered Drug No Effect=1.00	
					C_{max}	AUC	C_{min}
Cyclosporine	600 single dose	400 single dose	19	sofosbuvir	2.54 (1.87, 3.45)	4.53 (3.26, 6.30)	NA
				GS-331007	0.60 (0.53, 0.69)	1.04 (0.90, 1.20)	NA
Darunavir (boosted with ritonavir)	800/100 once daily	400 single dose	18	sofosbuvir	1.45 (1.10, 1.92)	1.34 (1.12, 1.59)	NA
				GS-331007	0.97 (0.90, 1.05)	1.24 (1.18, 1.30)	NA
Efavirenz[†]	600 once daily	400 single dose	16	sofosbuvir	0.81 (0.60, 1.10)	0.94 (0.76, 1.16)	NA
Emtricitabine[†]	200 once daily						
Tenofovir disoproxil fumarate[†]	300 once daily			GS-331007	0.77 (0.70, 0.84)	0.84 (0.76, 0.92)	NA
Methadone	30 to 130 once daily	400 once daily	14	sofosbuvir	0.95[‡] (0.68, 1.33)	1.30[‡] (1.00, 1.69)	NA
				GS-331007	0.73[‡] (0.65, 0.83)	1.04[‡] (0.89, 1.22)	NA
Rilpivirine	25 once daily	400 single dose	17	sofosbuvir	1.21 (0.90, 1.62)	1.09 (0.94, 1.27)	NA
				GS-331007	1.06 (0.99, 1.14)	1.01 (0.97, 1.04)	NA
Tacrolimus	5 single dose	400 single dose	16	sofosbuvir	0.97 (0.65, 1.43)	1.13 (0.81, 1.57)	NA
				GS-331007	0.97 (0.83, 1.14)	1.00 (0.87, 1.13)	NA

NA = not available/not applicable
*All interaction studies conducted in healthy volunteers
†Administered as ATRIPLA
‡Comparison based on historic control

Table 7 Drug Interactions: Changes in Pharmacokinetic Parameters for Coadministered Drug in the Presence of Sofosbuvir*

Coadministered Drug	Dose of Coadministered Drug (mg)	Sofosbuvir Dose (mg)	N	Mean Ratio (90% CI) of Coadministered drug PK With/Without Coadministered Drug No Effect=1.00		
				C_{max}	AUC	C_{min}
Tenofovir disoproxil fumarate[†]	300 once daily	400 single dose	16	1.25 (1.08, 1.45)	0.98 (0.91, 1.05)	0.99 (0.91, 1.07)
Raltegravir	400 once daily	400 single dose	19	0.57 (0.44, 0.75)	0.73 (0.59, 0.91)	0.95 (0.81, 1.12)
Tacrolimus	5 single dose	400 single dose	16	0.73 (0.59, 0.90)	1.09 (0.84, 1.40)	NA

NA = not available/not applicable
*All interaction studies conducted in healthy volunteers
†Administered as ATRIPLA

Impairment of Fertility
Use with Ribavirin and/or Peginterferon alfa: In fertility studies in male animals, ribavirin induced reversible testicular toxicity, while peginterferon alfa may impair fertility in females. Refer to prescribing information for ribavirin and peginterferon alfa for additional information.
Sofosbuvir had no effects on embryo-fetal viability or on fertility when evaluated in rats. At the highest dose tested, AUC exposure to the predominant circulating metabolite GS-331007 was approximately 8-fold the exposure in humans at the recommended clinical dose.

13.2 Animal Toxicology and/or Pharmacology
Heart degeneration and inflammation were observed in rats following GS-9851 (a stereoisomeric mixture containing approximately 50% sofosbuvir) doses of 2000 mg/kg/day for up to 5 days. At this dose, AUC exposure to the predominant metabolite GS-331007 is approximately 29-fold higher than human exposure at the recommended clinical dose. No heart degeneration or inflammation was observed in rats

following sofosbuvir doses of up to 500 mg/kg/day for 6 months at a GS-331007 AUC exposure approximately 9-fold higher than human exposure at the recommended clinical dose. In dogs and mice, heart degeneration and inflammation were not observed following sofosbuvir doses of up to 500 and 1000 mg/kg/day for 9 and 3 months, respectively, the highest doses tested. At these doses, GS-331007 AUC exposures are approximately 27- and 41-fold higher, respectively, than human exposure at the recommended clinical dose.

14 CLINICAL STUDIES
14.1 Description of Clinical Trials
The safety and efficacy of SOVALDI was evaluated in five Phase 3 trials in a total of 1724 HCV mono-infected subjects with genotypes 1 to 6 chronic hepatitis C (CHC) and one Phase 3 trial in 223 HCV/HIV-1 co-infected subjects with genotype 1, 2 or 3 CHC. Among the five trials in HCV mono-infected subjects, one was conducted in treatment-naïve subjects with genotype 1, 4, 5 or 6 CHC in combination with

Table 11 SVR Rates by Cirrhosis and Genotype in Study FISSION

	Genotype 2		Genotype 3	
	SOVALDI + RBV 12 weeks	Peg-IFN alfa + RBV 24 weeks	SOVALDI + RBV 12 weeks	Peg-IFN alfa + RBV 24 weeks
	N=73	N=67	N=183	N=176
Cirrhosis				
No	97% (59/61)	81% (44/54)	61% (89/145)	71% (99/139)
Yes	83% (10/12)	62% (8/13)	34% (13/38)	30% (11/37)

peginterferon alfa 2a and ribavirin and the other four were conducted in subjects with genotype 2 or 3 CHC in combination with ribavirin, including one in treatment-naïve subjects, one in interferon intolerant, ineligible or unwilling subjects, one in subjects previously treated with an interferon-based regimen, and one in all subjects irrespective of prior treatment history or ability to take interferon. The trial in HCV/HIV-1 co-infected subjects was conducted in combination with ribavirin in treatment-naïve subjects with genotype 1 CHC and all subjects with genotype 2 or 3 CHC irrespective of prior treatment history or ability to take interferon. Subjects in these trials had compensated liver disease including cirrhosis. SOVALDI was administered at a dose of 400 mg once daily. The ribavirin (RBV) dose was weight-based at 1000–1200 mg daily administered in two divided doses when used in combination with SOVALDI, and the peginterferon alfa 2a dose, where applicable, was 180 micrograms per week. Treatment duration was fixed in each trial and was not guided by subjects' HCV RNA levels (no response guided algorithm). Plasma HCV RNA values were measured during the clinical trials using the COBAS TaqMan HCV test (version 2.0), for use with the High Pure System. The assay had a lower limit of quantification (LLOQ) of 25 IU per mL. Sustained virologic response (SVR) was the primary endpoint which was defined as HCV RNA less than LLOQ at 12 weeks after the end of treatment.

14.2 Clinical Trials in Subjects with Genotype 1 or 4 CHC

Treatment-Naïve Adults — NEUTRINO (Study 110)
NEUTRINO was an open-label, single-arm trial that evaluated 12 weeks of treatment with SOVALDI in combination with peginterferon alfa 2a and ribavirin in treatment-naïve subjects with genotype 1, 4, 5 or 6 HCV infection compared to pre-specified historical control.
Treated subjects (N=327) had a median age of 54 years (range: 19 to 70); 64% of the subjects were male; 79% were White, 17% were Black; 14% were Hispanic or Latino; mean body mass index was 29 kg/m^2 (range: 18 to 56 kg/m^2); 78% had baseline HCV RNA greater than 6 log$_{10}$ IU per mL; 17% had cirrhosis; 89% had HCV genotype 1; 9% had HCV genotype 4 and 2% had HCV genotype 5 or 6. Table 8 presents the response rates for the treatment group of SOVALDI + peginterferon alfa + ribavirin.

Table 8 Response Rates in Study NEUTRINO

	SOVALDI + Peg-IFN alfa + RBV 12 weeks
	N=327*
Overall SVR	90% (295/327)
Genotype 1†	89% (261/292)
Genotype 1a	92% (206/225)
Genotype 1b	82% (54/66)
Genotype 4	96% (27/28)
Outcome for subjects without SVR	
On-treatment virologic failure	0/327
Relapse‡	9% (28/326)
Other§	1% (4/327)

*Including seven subjects with genotype 5 or 6 infection.
†One subject had genotype 1a/1b mixed infection.
‡The denominator for relapse is the number of subjects with HCV RNA <LLOQ at their last on-treatment assessment.
§Other includes subjects who did not achieve SVR and did not meet virologic failure criteria (e.g., lost to follow-up).

Response rates for selected subgroups are presented in Table 9.

Table 9 SVR Rates for Selected Subgroups in NEUTRINO

	SOVALDI + Peg-IFN alfa + RBV 12 weeks
Cirrhosis	
No	92% (252/273)
Yes	80% (43/54)
Race	
Black	87% (47/54)
Non-black	91% (248/273)
Multiple Baseline Factors	
Genotype 1, Metavir F3/F4 fibrosis, IL28B non-C/C, HCV RNA >800,000 IU/mL	71% (37/52)

SVR rates were 98% (93/95) in subjects with baseline IL28B C/C allele and 87% (202/232) in subjects with baseline IL28B non-C/C alleles.
It is estimated that the response rate in patients who previously failed pegylated interferon and ribavirin therapy will approximate the observed response rate in NEUTRINO subjects with multiple baseline factors traditionally associated with a lower response to interferon-based treatment (Table 9). The SVR rate in the NEUTRINO trial in genotype 1 subjects with IL28B non-C/C alleles, HCV RNA >800,000 IU/mL and Metavir F3/F4 fibrosis was 71% (37/52).

14.3 Clinical Trials in Subjects with Genotype 2 or 3 CHC

Treatment-Naïve Adults — FISSION (Study 1231)
FISSION was a randomized, open-label, active-controlled trial that evaluated 12 weeks of treatment with SOVALDI and ribavirin compared to 24 weeks of treatment with peginterferon alfa 2a and ribavirin in treatment-naïve subjects with genotype 2 and 3 HCV. The ribavirin doses used in the SOVALDI + ribavirin and peginterferon alfa 2a + ribavirin arms were weight-based 1000–1200 mg per day and 800 mg per day regardless of weight, respectively. Subjects were randomized in a 1:1 ratio and stratified by cirrhosis (presence vs. absence), HCV genotype (2 vs. 3) and baseline HCV RNA level (<6 log$_{10}$IU/mL vs. ≥6 log$_{10}$IU/mL). Subjects with genotype 2 or 3 HCV were enrolled in an approximately 1:3 ratio.
Treated subjects (N=499) had a median age of 50 years (range: 19 to 77); 66% of the subjects were male; 87% were White, 3% were Black; 14% were Hispanic or Latino; mean body mass index was 28 kg/m^2 (range: 17 to 52 kg/m^2); 57% had baseline HCV RNA levels greater than 6 log$_{10}$ IU per mL; 20% had cirrhosis; 72% had HCV genotype 3. Table 10 presents the response rates for the treatment groups of SOVALDI + ribavirin and peginterferon alfa + ribavirin.

Table 10 Response Rates in Study FISSION

	SOVALDI + RBV 12 weeks	Peg-IFN alfa + RBV 24 weeks
	N=256*	N=243*
Overall SVR	67% (171/256)	67% (162/243)
Treatment difference†	0.3% (95% CI: -7.5% to 8.0%)	
Genotype 2	95% (69/73)	78% (52/67)
Genotype 3	56% (102/183)	63% (110/176)

Outcome for subjects without SVR		
On-treatment virologic failure	<1% (1/256)	7% (18/243)
Relapse‡	30% (76/252)	21% (46/217)
Genotype 2	5% (4/73)	15% (9/62)
Genotype 3	40% (72/179)	24% (37/155)
Other§	3% (8/256)	7% (17/243)

*Including three subjects with recombinant genotype 2/1 HCV infection.
†Adjusted for pre-specified stratification factors.
‡The denominator for relapse is the number of subjects with HCV RNA <LLOQ at their last on-treatment assessment.
§Other includes subjects who did not achieve SVR and did not meet virologic failure criteria (e.g., lost to follow-up).

Response rates for subjects with cirrhosis at baseline are presented in Table 11 by genotype.
[See table 11 above]
Interferon Intolerant, Ineligible or Unwilling Adults — POSITRON (Study 107)
POSITRON was a randomized, double-blinded, placebo-controlled trial that evaluated 12 weeks of treatment with SOVALDI and ribavirin (N=207) compared to placebo (N=71) in subjects who are interferon intolerant, ineligible or unwilling. Subjects were randomized in 3:1 ratio and stratified by cirrhosis (presence vs. absence).
Treated subjects (N=278) had a median age of 54 years (range: 21 to 75); 54% of the subjects were male; 91% were White, 5% were Black; 11% were Hispanic or Latino; mean body mass index was 28 kg/m^2 (range: 18 to 53 kg/m^2); 70% had baseline HCV RNA levels greater than 6 log$_{10}$ IU per mL; 16% had cirrhosis; 49% had HCV genotype 3. The proportions of subjects who were interferon intolerant, ineligible, or unwilling were 9%, 44%, and 47%, respectively. Most subjects had no prior HCV treatment (81%). Table 12 presents the response rates for the treatment groups of SOVALDI + ribavirin and placebo.

Table 12 Response Rates in Study POSITRON

	SOVALDI + RBV 12 weeks	Placebo 12 weeks
	N=207	N=71
Overall SVR	78% (161/207)	0/71
Genotype 2	93% (101/109)	0/34
Genotype 3	61% (60/98)	0/37
Outcome for subjects without SVR		
On-treatment virologic failure	0/207	97% (69/71)
Relapse*	20% (42/205)	0/0
Genotype 2	5% (5/107)	0/0
Genotype 3	38% (37/98)	0/0
Other†	2% (4/207)	3% (2/71)

*The denominator for relapse is the number of subjects with HCV RNA <LLOQ at their last on-treatment assessment.
†Other includes subjects who did not achieve SVR and did not meet virologic failure criteria (e.g., lost to follow-up).

Table 13 presents the subgroup analysis by genotype for cirrhosis and interferon classification.

Table 13 SVR Rates for Selected Subgroups by Genotype in POSITRON

	SOVALDI + RBV 12 weeks	
	Genotype 2	Genotype 3
	N=109	N=98
Cirrhosis		
No	92% (85/92)	68% (57/84)
Yes	94% (16/17)	21% (3/14)

Interferon Classification

Ineligible	88% (36/41)	70% (33/47)
Intolerant	100% (9/9)	50% (4/8)
Unwilling	95% (56/59)	53% (23/43)

Previously Treated Adults — FUSION (Study 108)
FUSION was a randomized, double-blinded trial that evaluated 12 or 16 weeks of treatment with SOVALDI and ribavirin in subjects who did not achieve SVR with prior interferon-based treatment (relapsers and nonresponders). Subjects were randomized in a 1:1 ratio and stratified by cirrhosis (presence vs. absence) and HCV genotype (2 vs. 3). Treated subjects (N=201) had a median age of 56 years (range: 24 to 70); 70% of the subjects were male; 87% were White; 3% were Black; 9% were Hispanic or Latino; mean body mass index was 29 kg/m^2 (range: 19 to 44 kg/m^2); 73% had baseline HCV RNA levels greater than 6log$_{10}$ IU per mL; 34% had cirrhosis; 63% had HCV genotype 3; 75% were prior relapsers. Table 14 presents the response rates for the treatment groups of SOVALDI + ribavirin for 12 weeks and 16 weeks.

Table 14 Response Rates in Study FUSION

	SOVALDI + RBV 12 weeks	SOVALDI + RBV 16 weeks
	N= 103*	N=98*
Overall SVR	50% (51/103)	71% (70/98)
Genotype 2	82% (32/39)	89% (31/35)
Genotype 3	30% (19/64)	62% (39/63)
Outcome for subjects without SVR		
On-treatment virologic failure	0/103	0/98
Relapse†	48% (49/103)	29% (28/98)
Genotype 2	18% (7/39)	11% (4/35)
Genotype 3	66% (42/64)	38% (24/63)
Other‡	3% (3/103)	0/98

*Including six subjects with recombinant genotype 2/1 HCV infection.
†The denominator for relapse is the number of subjects with HCV RNA <LLOQ at their last on-treatment assessment.
‡Other includes subjects who did not achieve SVR and did not meet virologic failure criteria (e.g., lost to follow-up).

Table 15 presents the subgroup analysis by genotype for cirrhosis and response to prior HCV treatment.
[See table 15 above]

Treatment-Naïve and Previously Treated Adults — VALENCE (Study 133)
The VALENCE trial evaluated SOVALDI in combination with weight-based ribavirin for the treatment of genotype 2 or 3 HCV infection in treatment-naïve subjects or subjects who did not achieve SVR with prior interferon-based treatment, including subjects with compensated cirrhosis. The original trial design was a 4 to 1 randomization to SOVALDI + ribavirin for 12 weeks or placebo. Based on emerging data, this trial was unblinded and all genotype 2 HCV-infected subjects continued the original planned treatment and received SOVALDI + ribavirin for 12 weeks, and duration of treatment with SOVALDI + ribavirin in genotype 3 HCV-infected subjects was extended to 24 weeks. Eleven genotype 3 subjects had already completed SOVALDI + ribavirin for 12 weeks at the time of the amendment.
Treated subjects (N=419) had a median age of 51 years (range: 19 to 74); 60% of the subjects were male; mean body mass index was 26 kg/m^2 (range: 17 to 44 kg/m^2); the mean baseline HCV RNA level was 6.4 log$_{10}$ IU per mL; 78% had HCV genotype 3; 58% of the subjects were treatment-experienced and 65% of those subjects experienced relapse/breakthrough to prior HCV treatment.
Table 16 presents the response rates for the treatment groups of SOVALDI + ribavirin for 12 weeks and 24 weeks.

Table 15 SVR Rates for Selected Subgroups by Genotype in Study FUSION

	Genotype 2		Genotype 3	
	SOVALDI + RBV 12 weeks	SOVALDI + RBV 16 weeks	SOVALDI + RBV 12 weeks	SOVALDI + RBV 16 weeks
	N=39	N=35	N=64	N=63
Cirrhosis				
No	90% (26/29)	92% (24/26)	37% (14/38)	63% (25/40)
Yes	60% (6/10)	78% (7/9)	19% (5/26)	61% (14/23)
Response to prior HCV treatment				
Relapser/ breakthrough	86% (25/29)	89% (24/27)	31% (15/49)	65% (30/46)
Nonresponder	70% (7/10)	88% (7/8)	27% (4/15)	53% (9/17)

Table 16 Response Rates in Study VALENCE*

	Genotype 2 SOVALDI + RBV 12 weeks	Genotype 3 SOVALDI + RBV 24 weeks
	N=73	N=250
Overall SVR	93% (68/73)	84% (210/250)
Outcome for subjects without SVR		
On-treatment virologic failure	0% (0/73)	<1% (1/250)
Relapse†	7% (5/73)	14% (34/249)
Treatment-naïve	3% (1/32)	5% (5/105)
Treatment-experienced	10% (4/41)	20% (29/144)
Other‡	0% (0/73)	2% (5/250)

*Placebo subjects (N=85) were not included as none achieved SVR12. Eleven genotype 3 subjects who received SOVALDI + ribavirin for 12 weeks were not included.
†The denominator for relapse is the number of subjects with HCV RNA <LLOQ at their last on treatment assessment.
‡Other includes subjects who did not achieve SVR12 and did not meet virologic failure criteria (e.g., lost to follow up).

Table 17 presents the subgroup analysis by genotype for cirrhosis and prior HCV treatment experience.

Table 17 SVR Rates for Selected Subgroup by Genotype in Study VALENCE

	Genotype 2 SOVALDI + RBV 12 weeks	Genotype 3 SOVALDI + RBV 24 weeks
	N=73	N=250
Treatment-naïve	97% (31/32)	93% (98/105)
Non-cirrhotic	97% (29/30)	93% (86/92)
Cirrhotic	100% (2/2)	92% (12/13)
Treatment-experienced	90% (37/41)	77% (112/145)
Non-cirrhotic	91% (30/33)	85% (85/100)
Cirrhotic	88% (7/8)	60% (27/45)

14.4   Clinical Trials in Subjects Co-infected with HCV and HIV-1
SOVALDI was studied in an open-label clinical trial (Study PHOTON-1) evaluating the safety and efficacy of 12 or 24 weeks of treatment with SOVALDI and ribavirin in subjects with genotype 1, 2 or 3 chronic hepatitis C co-infected with HIV-1. Genotype 2 and 3 subjects were either HCV treatment-naïve or experienced, whereas genotype 1 subjects were all treatment-naïve. Subjects received 400 mg SOVALDI and weight-based ribavirin (1000 mg for subjects weighing <75 kg or 1200 mg for subjects weighing ≥75kg) daily for 12 or 24 weeks based on genotype and prior treatment history. Subjects were either not on antiretroviral therapy with a CD4+ cell count >500 cells/mm^3 or had virologically suppressed HIV-1 with a CD4+ cell count >200 cells/mm^3. Efficacy data 12 weeks post treatment are available for 210 subjects (see Table 18).

Table 18 Response Rates in Study PHOTON-1*

	HCV genotype 1	HCV genotype 2	HCV genotype 3
	SOVALDI + RBV 24 weeks TN (N=114)	SOVALDI + RBV 12 weeks TN (N=26)	SOVALDI + RBV 24 weeks TE (N=13)
Overall	76% (87/114)	88% (23/26)	92% (12/13)
Outcome for subjects without SVR12			
On-treatment virologic failure	1% (1/114)	4% (1/26)	0/13
Relapse†	22% (25/113)	0/25	8% (1/13)
Other‡	1% (1/114)	8% (2/26)	0/13

TN = Treatment-naïve; TE = Treatment-experienced
*Subjects with genotype 2 CHC treated with SOVALDI + RBV for 24 weeks (N=15) and subjects with genotype 3 CHC treated with SOVALDI + RBV for 12 weeks (N=42) are not included in the table.
†The denominator for relapse is the number of subjects with HCV RNA <LLOQ at their last on treatment assessment.
‡Other includes subjects who did not achieve SVR12 and did not meet virologic failure criteria (e.g., lost to follow up).

In subjects with HCV genotype 1 infection, the SVR rate was 82% (74/90) in subjects with genotype 1a infection and 54% (13/24) in subjects with genotype 1b infection, with relapse accounting for the majority of treatment failures. SVR rates in subjects with HCV genotype 1 infection were 80% (24/30) in subjects with baseline IL28B C/C allele and 75% (62/83) in subjects with baseline IL28B non-C/C alleles.
In the 223 CHC subjects with HIV-1 co-infection, the percentage of CD4+ cells did not change during treatment. Median CD4+ cell count decreases of 85 cells/mm^3 and 84 cells/mm^3 were observed at the end of treatment with SOVALDI + ribavirin for 12 or 24 weeks, respectively. HIV-1 rebound during SOVALDI + ribavirin treatment occurred in 2 subjects (0.9%) on antiretroviral therapy.

16   HOW SUPPLIED/STORAGE AND HANDLING
SOVALDI tablets are yellow, capsule-shaped, film-coated tablets containing 400 mg sofosbuvir debossed with "GSI" on one side and "7977" on the other side. Each bottle contains 28 tablets (NDC 61958-1501-1), a silica gel desiccant, polyester coil and is closed with a child-resistant closure. Store at room temperature below 30 °C (86 °F).
• Dispense only in original container
• Do not use if seal over bottle opening is broken or missing

17   PATIENT COUNSELING INFORMATION
Advise the patient to read the FDA-approved patient labeling (Patient Information).

Pregnancy

Ribavirin must not be used by women who are pregnant or by men whose female partners are pregnant. Ribavirin therapy should not be initiated until a report of a negative pregnancy test has been obtained immediately before starting therapy. When SOVALDI is used in combination with peginterferon/ribavirin or ribavirin, patients must be advised of the teratogenic/embryocidal risks of ribavirin and should be advised that extreme care must be taken to avoid pregnancy in female patients and in female partners of male patients both during treatment and for 6 months after the completion of treatment [See Contraindications (4) and Warnings and Precautions (5.1)].

Women of childbearing potential and their male partners must use at least two forms of effective contraception during treatment and for 6 months after the treatment has been stopped; routine monthly pregnancy tests must be performed during this time. There is no data on the effectiveness of systemic hormonal contraceptives in women taking SOVALDI; therefore, two alternative non-hormonal methods of contraception should be used.

Patients should be advised to notify their health care provider immediately in the event of a pregnancy. There is a Ribavirin Pregnancy Registry established to monitor maternal and fetal outcomes of pregnant women exposed to ribavirin. Patients should be encouraged to register by calling 1-800-593-2214. For patients who are HCV/HIV-1 coinfected and taking concomitant antiretrovirals, an Antiretroviral Pregnancy Registry is also available at 1-800-258-4263.

Hepatitis C Virus Transmission

Patients should be informed that the effect of treatment of hepatitis C infection on transmission is not known, and that appropriate precautions to prevent transmission of the hepatitis C virus during treatment or in the event of treatment failure should be taken.

Administration

Patients should be advised that the recommended regimen for patients with genotype 1 or 4 HCV infection is SOVALDI administered in combination with peginterferon alfa and ribavirin and the recommended regimen for patients with genotype 2 or 3 HCV infection is SOVALDI administered in combination with ribavirin. If peginterferon and/or ribavirin are permanently discontinued, SOVALDI should also be discontinued.

Patients should be advised that the dose of SOVALDI must not be reduced and it should be taken on a regular dosing schedule with or without food. If a patient did not take the SOVALDI at the regular time, it could be taken later in the day. However, no more than 400 mg of SOVALDI should be taken on any calendar day. The patient should resume the regular dosing schedule on the next day.

Manufactured and distributed by:
Gilead Sciences, Inc.
Foster City, CA 94404
SOVALDI is a trademark of Gilead Sciences, Inc., or its related companies. ATRIPLA is a trademark of Bristol-Myers Squibb & Gilead Sciences, LLC. All other trademarks referenced herein are the property of their respective owners.
©2013 Gilead Sciences, Inc. All rights reserved.
204671-GS-000

Patient Information
SOVALDI™ (soh-VAHL-dee)
(sofosbuvir)
tablets

Read this Patient Information before you start taking SOVALDI and each time you get a refill. There may be new information. This information does not take the place of talking with your healthcare provider about your medical condition or your treatment.

SOVALDI is used in combination with other antiviral medicines. When taking SOVALDI with ribavirin or in combination with peginterferon alfa and ribavirin you should also read those Medication Guides.

The information in this Patient Information Leaflet talks about SOVALDI when it is used with ribavirin and in combination with peginterferon alfa and ribavirin.

What is the most important information I should know about SOVALDI?

SOVALDI, in combination with ribavirin or peginterferon alfa and ribavirin, may cause birth defects or death of your unborn baby. If you are pregnant or your sexual partner is pregnant or plans to become pregnant, do not take these medicines. You or your sexual partner should not become pregnant while taking SOVALDI with ribavirin or in combination with peginterferon alfa and ribavirin, and for 6 months after treatment is over.

• **Females and males must use 2 effective forms of birth control during treatment and for the 6 months after treatment with SOVALDI and ribavirin or in combination with peginterferon alfa and ribavirin.** Talk to your healthcare provider about forms of birth control that may be used during this time.

• Females must have a negative pregnancy test before starting treatment with SOVALDI and ribavirin or in combination with peginterferon alfa and ribavirin, every month while being treated, and for 6 months after your treatment ends.

• If you or your female sexual partner becomes pregnant while taking or within 6 months after you stop taking SOVALDI and ribavirin, or SOVALDI in combination with peginterferon alfa and ribavirin, tell your healthcare provider right away. You or your healthcare provider should contact the Ribavirin Pregnancy Registry by calling 1-800-593-2214. The Ribavirin Pregnancy Registry collects information about what happens to mothers and their babies if the mother takes ribavirin while she is pregnant. If you are also infected with HIV and taking medicines to treat your HIV infection, an Antiretroviral Pregnancy Registry is also available at 1-800-258-4263.

You should not take SOVALDI alone. SOVALDI should be used together with ribavirin or in combination with peginterferon alfa and ribavirin to treat chronic hepatitis C infection.

What is SOVALDI?

• SOVALDI is a prescription medicine used with other antiviral medicines to treat chronic (lasting a long time) hepatitis C infection in adults.

• SOVALDI should not be taken alone.

It is not known if SOVALDI is safe and effective in children under 18 years of age.

Who should not take SOVALDI?

See "What is the most important information I should know about SOVALDI?"

What should I tell my healthcare provider before taking SOVALDI?

Before taking SOVALDI, tell your healthcare provider if you:

• have liver problems other than hepatitis C infection

• have had a liver transplant

• have severe kidney problems or you are on dialysis

• have HIV

• have any other medical condition

• are breastfeeding or plan to breastfeed. It is not known if SOVALDI passes into your breast milk. You and your healthcare provider should decide if you will take SOVALDI or breastfeed. You should not do both.

Tell your healthcare provider about all the medicines you take, including prescription and over-the-counter medicines, vitamins, and herbal supplements. Other medicines may affect how SOVALDI works.

Especially tell your healthcare provider if you take any of the following medicines:

• carbamazepine (Carbatrol®, Epitol®, Equetro®, Tegretol®)
• oxcarbazepine (Trileptal®, Oxtellar XR™)
• phenytoin (Dilantin®, Phenytek®)
• phenobarbital (Luminal®)
• rifabutin (Mycobutin®)
• rifampin (Rifadin®, Rifamate®, Rifater®, Rimactane®)
• rifapentine (Priftin®)
• St. John's wort (Hypericum perforatum) or a product that contains St. John's wort
• tipranavir (Aptivus®)

Know the medicines you take. Keep a list of your medicines and show it to your healthcare provider and pharmacist when you get a new medicine.

How should I take SOVALDI?

• Take SOVALDI exactly as your healthcare provider tells you to take it. Do not change your dose unless your healthcare provider tells you to.

• Do not stop taking SOVALDI without first talking with your healthcare provider. If you think there is a reason to stop taking SOVALDI, talk to your healthcare provider before doing so.

• Take SOVALDI 1 time each day with or without food.

• If you miss a dose of SOVALDI, take the missed dose as soon as you remember the same day. Do not take more than 1 tablet (400 mg) of SOVALDI in a day. Take your next dose of SOVALDI at your regular time the next day.

• If you take too much SOVALDI, call your healthcare provider or go to the nearest hospital emergency room right away.

What are the possible side effects of SOVALDI?

See "What is the most important information I should know about SOVALDI?"

The most common side effects of SOVALDI when used in combination with ribavirin include:

• tiredness
• headache

The most common side effects of SOVALDI when used in combination with peginterferon alfa and ribavirin include:

• tiredness
• headache
• nausea
• difficulty sleeping
• low red blood cell count

Tell your healthcare provider if you have any side effect that bothers you or that does not go away.

These are not all the possible side effects of SOVALDI. For more information, ask your healthcare provider or pharmacist.

Call your doctor for medical advice about side effects. You may report side effects to FDA at 1-800-FDA-1088.

How should I store SOVALDI?

• Store SOVALDI at room temperature below 86°F (30°C).

• Keep SOVALDI in its original container.

• Do not use SOVALDI if the seal over the bottle opening is broken or missing.

Keep SOVALDI and all medicines out of the reach of children.

General information about the safe and effective use of SOVALDI

It is not known if treatment with SOVALDI will prevent you from infecting another person with the hepatitis C virus during treatment. Talk with your healthcare provider about ways to prevent spreading the hepatitis C virus.

Medicines are sometimes prescribed for purposes other than those listed in a Patient Information leaflet. Do not use SOVALDI for a condition for which it was not prescribed. Do not give SOVALDI to other people, even if they have the same symptoms you have. It may harm them.

If you would like more information about SOVALDI, talk with your healthcare provider. You can ask your healthcare provider or pharmacist for information about SOVALDI that is written for health professionals.

For more information, call 1-800-445-3235 or go to www.SOVALDI.com.

What are the ingredients in SOVALDI?

Active ingredient: sofosbuvir

Inactive ingredients: colloidal silicon dioxide, croscarmellose sodium, magnesium stearate, mannitol, and microcrystalline cellulose.

The tablet film-coat contains: polyethylene glycol, polyvinyl alcohol, talc, titanium dioxide, and yellow iron oxide.

This Patient Information has been approved by the U.S. Food and Drug Administration.

Manufactured and distributed by:
Gilead Sciences, Inc.
Foster City, CA 94404
Issued: December 2013
SOVALDI is a trademark of Gilead Sciences, Inc., or its related companies. All other trademarks referenced herein are the property of their respective owners.
©2013 Gilead Sciences, Inc. All rights reserved.
204671-GS-000

Shown in Product Identification Guide, page 307

STRIBILD®   ℞
(elvitegravir, cobicistat, emtricitabine, tenofovir disoproxil fumarate)
Tablets, for oral use

HIGHLIGHTS OF PRESCRIBING INFORMATION

These highlights do not include all the information needed to use STRIBILD safely and effectively. See full prescribing information for STRIBILD.
STRIBILD® (elvitegravir, cobicistat, emtricitabine, tenofovir disoproxil fumarate) tablets, for oral use
Initial U.S. Approval: 2012

> **WARNING: LACTIC ACIDOSIS/SEVERE HEPATO-MEGALY WITH STEATOSIS and POST TREATMENT ACUTE EXACERBATION OF HEPATITIS B**
> *See full prescribing information for complete boxed warning.*
> • **Lactic acidosis and severe hepatomegaly with steatosis, including fatal cases, have been reported with the use of nucleoside analogs, including tenofovir disoproxil fumarate (DF), a component of STRIBILD. (5.1)**
> • **STRIBILD is not approved for the treatment of chronic hepatitis B virus (HBV) infection. Severe acute exacerbations of hepatitis B have been reported in patients coinfected with HIV-1 and HBV who have discontinued EMTRIVA or VIREAD, two of the components of STRIBILD. Hepatic function should be monitored closely in these patients. If appropriate, initiation of anti-hepatitis B therapy may be warranted. (5.2)**

---RECENT MAJOR CHANGES---

Dosage and Administration (2.1, 2.2, 2.3, 2.4)	10/2013
Warnings and Precautions	
New Onset or Worsening Renal Impairment (5.3)	10/2013
Bone Effects of Tenofovir DF (5.5)	10/2013

---INDICATIONS AND USAGE---

STRIBILD is a four-drug combination of elvitegravir, an HIV integrase strand transfer inhibitor (HIV-1 INSTI), cobicistat, a CYP3A inhibitor, and emtricitabine and tenofovir DF, both HIV nucleoside analog reverse transcriptase inhibitors (HIV NRTI) and is indicated as a complete regimen for the treatment of HIV-1 infection in adults who are antiretroviral treatment-naïve. (1)

DOSAGE AND ADMINISTRATION

- Recommended dosage: One tablet taken once daily with food. (2.1)
- Dosage in renal impairment: Initiation of STRIBILD in patients with estimated creatinine clearance below 70 mL per minute is not recommended. Discontinue in patients with estimated creatinine clearance below 50 mL per minute. (2.2)

DOSAGE FORMS AND STRENGTHS

Tablets: 150 mg of elvitegravir, 150 mg of cobicistat, 200 mg of emtricitabine, and 300 mg of tenofovir disoproxil fumarate. (3)

CONTRAINDICATIONS

Coadministration of STRIBILD is contraindicated with drugs that:
- Are highly dependent on CYP3A for clearance and for which elevated plasma concentrations are associated with serious adverse events. (4)
- Strongly induce CYP3A which may lead to lower exposure of one or more components and loss of efficacy of STRIBILD and possible resistance. (4)

WARNINGS AND PRECAUTIONS

- New onset or worsening renal impairment: Can include acute renal failure and Fanconi syndrome. Assess creatinine clearance (CLcr), urine glucose and urine protein before initiating treatment with STRIBILD. Monitor CLcr, urine glucose, and urine protein in all patients. Monitor serum phosphorus in patients at risk for renal impairment. Avoid administering STRIBILD with concurrent or recent use of nephrotoxic drugs. (5.3)
- Avoid coadministration with other anti-retroviral products: Do not use with drugs containing emtricitabine or tenofovir disoproxil fumarate including ATRIPLA, COMPLERA, EMTRIVA, TRUVADA, or VIREAD; with drugs containing lamivudine; or with drugs or regimens containing ritonavir. Do not administer in combination with HEPSERA. (5.4)
- Decreases in bone mineral density (BMD): Consider monitoring BMD in patients with a history of pathologic fracture or other risk factors of osteoporosis or bone loss. (5.5)
- Redistribution/accumulation of body fat: Observed in patients receiving antiretroviral therapy. (5.6)
- Immune reconstitution syndrome: May necessitate further evaluation and treatment. (5.7)

ADVERSE REACTIONS

Most common adverse drug reactions to STRIBILD (incidence greater than or equal to 10%, all grades) are nausea and diarrhea. (6.1)

To report SUSPECTED ADVERSE REACTIONS, contact Gilead Sciences, Inc. at 1-800-GILEAD-5 or FDA at 1-800-FDA-1088 or www.fda.gov/medwatch.

DRUG INTERACTIONS

- STRIBILD is a complete regimen for the treatment of HIV-1 infection; therefore, STRIBILD should not be administered with other antiretroviral medications for treatment of HIV-1 infection. (5.4, 7.1)
- STRIBILD can alter the concentration of drugs metabolized by CYP3A or CYP2D6. Drugs that induce CYP3A can alter the concentrations of one or more components of STRIBILD. Consult the full prescribing information prior to and during treatment for potential drug-drug interactions. (4, 7.2, 7.3, 12.3)

USE IN SPECIFIC POPULATIONS

- Pregnancy: Use during pregnancy only if the potential benefit justifies the potential risk. (8.1)
- Nursing mothers: Women infected with HIV should be instructed not to breastfeed due to the potential for HIV transmission. (8.3)

See 17 for PATIENT COUNSELING INFORMATION and FDA-approved patient labeling

Revised: 10/2013

FULL PRESCRIBING INFORMATION

WARNING: LACTIC ACIDOSIS/SEVERE HEPATOMEGALY WITH STEATOSIS and POST TREATMENT ACUTE EXACERBATION OF HEPATITIS B

Lactic acidosis and severe hepatomegaly with steatosis, including fatal cases, have been reported with the use of nucleoside analogs, including tenofovir disoproxil fumarate, a component of STRIBILD, in combination with other antiretrovirals *[see Warnings and Precautions (5.1)]*.
STRIBILD is not approved for the treatment of chronic hepatitis B virus (HBV) infection and the safety and efficacy of STRIBILD have not been established in patients coinfected with HBV and HIV-1. Severe acute exacerbations of hepatitis B have been reported in patients who are coinfected with HBV and human immunodeficiency virus-1 (HIV-1) and have discontinued EMTRIVA or VIREAD, which are components of STRIBILD. Hepatic function should be monitored closely with both clinical and laboratory follow-up for at least several months in patients who are coinfected with HIV-1 and HBV and discontinue STRIBILD. If appropriate, initiation of anti-hepatitis B therapy may be warranted *[see Warnings and Precautions (5.2)]*.

1   INDICATIONS AND USAGE

STRIBILD® is indicated as a complete regimen for the treatment of HIV-1 infection in adults who are antiretroviral treatment-naïve.

2   DOSAGE AND ADMINISTRATION

2.1   Dosage Information

The recommended dosage of STRIBILD is one tablet taken orally once daily with food *[see Clinical Pharmacology (12.3)]*.

2.2   Dosage Adjustment in Patients with Renal Impairment

Initiation of STRIBILD in patients with estimated creatinine clearance below 70 mL per minute is not recommended. Because STRIBILD is a fixed-dose combination tablet, STRIBILD should be discontinued if estimated creatinine clearance declines below 50 mL per min during treatment with STRIBILD as dose interval adjustment required for emtricitabine and tenofovir disoproxil fumarate (DF) cannot be achieved *[see Warnings and Precautions (5.3), Adverse Reactions (6.1), Use in Specific Populations (8.6), Clinical Pharmacology (12.3), and Clinical Studies (14)]*.

2.3   Dosage in Patients with Hepatic Impairment

No dosage adjustment of STRIBILD is required in patients with mild (Child-Pugh Class A) or moderate (Child-Pugh Class B) hepatic impairment. No pharmacokinetic or safety data are available regarding the use of STRIBILD in patients with severe hepatic impairment (Child-Pugh Class C). Therefore, STRIBILD is not recommended for use in patients with severe hepatic impairment *[see Use in Specific Populations (8.7) and Clinical Pharmacology (12.3)]*.

2.4   Testing Prior to Initiation of STRIBILD

Prior to initiation of STRIBILD, patients should be tested for hepatitis B infection *[see Warnings and Precautions (5.2)]* and estimated creatinine clearance, urine glucose and urine protein should be documented in all patients *[see Warnings and Precautions (5.3)]*.

3   DOSAGE FORMS AND STRENGTHS

Each STRIBILD tablet contains 150 mg of elvitegravir, 150 mg of cobicistat, 200 mg of emtricitabine, and 300 mg of tenofovir disoproxil fumarate (tenofovir DF, equivalent to 245 mg of tenofovir disoproxil).
The tablets are green, capsule-shaped, film-coated, debossed with "GSI" on one side and the number "1" surrounded by a square box (1) on the other side of the tablet.

4   CONTRAINDICATIONS

Coadministration of STRIBILD is contraindicated with drugs that are highly dependent on CYP3A for clearance and for which elevated plasma concentrations are associated with serious and/or life-threatening events. These drugs and other contraindicated drugs (which may lead to reduced efficacy of STRIBILD and possible resistance) are listed in Table 1 *[see Drug Interactions (7.5), Clinical Pharmacology (12.3)]*.
[See table 1 at top of next page]

5   WARNINGS AND PRECAUTIONS

5.1   Lactic Acidosis/Severe Hepatomegaly with Steatosis

Lactic acidosis and severe hepatomegaly with steatosis, including fatal cases, have been reported with the use of nucleoside analogs, including tenofovir DF, a component of STRIBILD, in combination with other antiretrovirals. A majority of these cases have been in women. Obesity and prolonged nucleoside exposure may be risk factors. Particular caution should be exercised when administering nucleoside analogs to any patient with known risk factors for liver disease; however, cases have also been reported in patients with no known risk factors. Treatment with STRIBILD should be suspended in any patient who develops clinical or laboratory findings suggestive of lactic acidosis or pronounced hepatotoxicity (which may include hepatomegaly and steatosis even in the absence of marked transaminase elevations).

5.2   Patients Coinfected with HIV-1 and HBV

It is recommended that all patients with HIV-1 be tested for the presence of chronic hepatitis B virus (HBV) before initiating antiretroviral therapy. STRIBILD is not approved for the treatment of chronic HBV infection and the safety and efficacy of STRIBILD have not been established in patients coinfected with HBV and HIV-1. Severe acute exacerbations of hepatitis B have been reported in patients who are coinfected with HBV and HIV-1 and have discontinued emtricitabine or tenofovir DF, two of the components of STRIBILD. In some patients infected with HBV and treated with EMTRIVA, the exacerbations of hepatitis B were associated with liver decompensation and liver failure. Patients who are coinfected with HIV-1 and HBV should be closely monitored with both clinical and laboratory follow-up for at least several months after stopping treatment with STRIBILD. If appropriate, initiation of anti-hepatitis B therapy may be warranted.

5.3   New Onset or Worsening Renal Impairment

Renal impairment, including cases of acute renal failure and Fanconi syndrome (renal tubular injury with severe hypophosphatemia), has been reported with the use of tenofovir DF, a component of STRIBILD, and with the use of STRIBILD *[see Adverse Reactions (6.2)]*.

Table 1 Drugs that are Contraindicated with STRIBILD

Drug Class	Drugs within class that are contraindicated with STRIBILD	Clinical Comment
Alpha 1-Adrenoreceptor Antagonist	Alfuzosin	Potential for increased alfuzosin concentrations, which can result in hypotension.
Antimycobacterial	Rifampin	Rifampin is a potent inducer of CYP450 metabolism and may cause significant decrease in the plasma concentration of elvitegravir and cobicistat. This may result in loss of therapeutic effect to STRIBILD.
Ergot Derivatives	Dihydroergotamine Ergotamine Methylergonovine	Potential for serious and/or life-threatening events such as acute ergot toxicity characterized by peripheral vasospasm and ischemia of the extremities and other tissues.
GI Motility Agent	Cisapride	Potential for serious and/or life-threatening events such as cardiac arrhythmias.
Herbal Products	St. John's wort (*Hypericum perforatum*)	Coadministration of products containing St. John's wort and STRIBILD may result in reduced plasma concentrations of elvitegravir and cobicistat. This may result in loss of therapeutic effect and development of resistance.
HMG-CoA Reductase Inhibitors	Lovastatin Simvastatin	Potential for serious reactions such as myopathy, including rhabdomyolysis.
Neuroleptic	Pimozide	Potential for serious and/or life-threatening events such as cardiac arrhythmias.
Phosphodiesterase-5 (PDE5) Inhibitor	Sildenafil* when dosed as REVATIO for the treatment of pulmonary arterial hypertension	There is increased potential for sildenafil-associated adverse events (which include visual disturbances, hypotension, priapism, and syncope).
Sedative/hypnotics	Triazolam Orally administered midazolam†	Triazolam and orally administered midazolam are extensively metabolized by CYP3A4. Coadministration of triazolam or orally administered midazolam with STRIBILD may cause large increases in the concentration of these benzodiazepines. The potential exists for serious and/or life threatening events such as prolonged or increased sedation or respiratory depression.

* See Drug Interactions (7), Table 6 for sildenafil when dosed as VIAGRA for erectile dysfunction.
† See Drug Interactions (7), Table 6 for parenterally administered midazolam.

In the clinical trials of STRIBILD over 96 weeks, 10 (1.4%) subjects in the STRIBILD group (N=701) and 2 (0.3%) subjects in the combined comparator groups (N = 707) discontinued study drug due to a renal adverse reaction. Of these discontinuations, 8 in the STRIBILD group and 1 in the combined comparator groups occurred during the first 48 week. Four (0.6%) of the subjects who received STRIBILD developed laboratory findings consistent with proximal renal tubular dysfunction leading to discontinuation of STRIBILD compared to none in the comparator groups. Two of these four subjects had renal impairment (i.e. estimated creatinine clearance less than 70 mL per minute) at baseline. The laboratory findings in these 4 subjects with evidence of proximal tubulopathy improved but did not completely resolve in all subjects upon discontinuation of STRIBILD. Renal replacement therapy was not required for these subjects.

Estimated creatinine clearance, urine glucose and urine protein should be documented in all patients prior to initiating therapy. Initiation of STRIBILD in patients with estimated creatinine clearance below 70 mL per minute is not recommended.

STRIBILD should be avoided with concurrent or recent use of a nephrotoxic agent (e.g., high-dose or multiple non-steroidal anti-inflammatory drugs (NSAIDs)) *[see Drug Interactions (7.4)].* Cases of acute renal failure after initiation of high dose or multiple NSAIDs have been reported in HIV-infected patients with risk factors for renal dysfunction who appeared stable on tenofovir DF. Some patients required hospitalization and renal replacement therapy. Alternatives to NSAIDs should be considered, if needed, in patients at risk for renal dysfunction.

Persistent or worsening bone pain, pain in extremities, fractures and/or muscular pain or weakness may be manifestations of proximal renal tubulopathy and should prompt an evaluation of renal function in at-risk patients.

Routine monitoring of estimated creatinine clearance, urine glucose, and urine protein should be performed during STRIBILD therapy in all patients. Additionally, serum phosphorus should be measured in patients at risk for renal impairment. Although cobicistat (a component of STRIBILD) may cause modest increases in serum creatinine and modest declines in estimated creatinine clearance without affecting renal glomerular function *[see Adverse Re-*

actions (6.1)], patients who experience a confirmed increase in serum creatinine of greater than 0.4 mg per dL from baseline should be closely monitored for renal safety.

The emtricitabine and tenofovir DF components of STRIBILD are primarily excreted by the kidney. STRIBILD should be discontinued if estimated creatinine clearance declines below 50 mL per minute as dose interval adjustment required for emtricitabine and tenofovir DF cannot be achieved with the fixed-dose combination tablet.

5.4 Avoid Use with Other Antiretroviral Products
STRIBILD is indicated for use as a complete regimen for the treatment of HIV-1 infection and coadministration with other antiretroviral products is not recommended.

STRIBILD is not recommended for coadministration with the following:

- emtricitabine or tenofovir DF (ATRIPLA, COMPLERA, EMTRIVA, TRUVADA, VIREAD);
- products containing lamivudine (COMBIVIR, EPIVIR, EPIVIR-HBV, EPZICOM, TRIZIVIR) or adefovir dipivoxil (HEPSERA);
- ritonavir (NORVIR, KALETRA).

5.5 Bone Effects of Tenofovir DF
Bone Mineral Density:
In clinical trials in HIV-1 infected adults, tenofovir DF (a component of STRIBILD) was associated with slightly greater decreases in bone mineral density (BMD) and increases in biochemical markers of bone metabolism, suggesting increased bone turnover relative to comparators. Serum parathyroid hormone levels and 1.25 Vitamin D levels were also higher in subjects receiving tenofovir DF. For additional information, see Adverse Reactions (6.1) and consult the VIREAD prescribing information.

The effects of tenofovir DF-associated changes in BMD and biochemical markers on long-term bone health and future fracture risk are unknown. Assessment of BMD should be considered for HIV-1 infected patients who have a history of pathologic bone fracture or other risk factors for osteoporosis or bone loss. Although the effect of supplementation with calcium and vitamin D was not studied, such supplementation may be beneficial in all patients. If bone abnormalities are suspected, then appropriate consultation should be obtained.

Mineralization Defects:
Cases of osteomalacia associated with proximal renal tubulopathy, manifested as bone pain or pain in extremities and

which may contribute to fractures, have been reported in association with the use of tenofovir DF *[see Adverse Reactions (6.2)].* Arthralgias and muscle pain or weakness have also been reported in cases of proximal renal tubulopathy. Hypophosphatemia and osteomalacia secondary to proximal renal tubulopathy should be considered in patients at risk of renal dysfunction who present with persistent or worsening bone or muscle symptoms while receiving products containing tenofovir DF *[see Warnings and Precautions (5.3)].*

5.6 Fat Redistribution
Redistribution/accumulation of body fat including central obesity, dorsocervical fat enlargement (buffalo hump), peripheral wasting, facial wasting, breast enlargement, and "cushingoid appearance" have been observed in patients receiving antiretroviral therapy. The mechanism and long-term consequences of these events are currently unknown. A causal relationship has not been established.

5.7 Immune Reconstitution Syndrome
Immune reconstitution syndrome has been reported in patients treated with combination antiretroviral therapy, including STRIBILD. During the initial phase of combination antiretroviral treatment, patients whose immune system responds may develop an inflammatory response to indolent or residual opportunistic infections [such as *Mycobacterium avium* infection, cytomegalovirus, *Pneumocystis jirovecii* pneumonia (PCP), or tuberculosis], which may necessitate further evaluation and treatment.

Autoimmune disorders (such as Graves' disease, polymyositis, and Guillain-Barré syndrome) have also been reported to occur in the setting of immune reconstitution, however, the time to onset is more variable, and can occur many months after initiation of treatment.

6 ADVERSE REACTIONS
The following adverse drug reactions are discussed in other sections of the labeling:

- Lactic Acidosis/Severe Hepatomegaly with Steatosis *[see Boxed Warning, Warnings and Precautions (5.1)].*
- Severe Acute Exacerbations of Hepatitis B *[see Boxed Warning, Warnings and Precautions (5.2)].*
- New Onset or Worsening Renal Impairment *[see Warnings and Precautions (5.3)].*
- Bone Effects of Tenofovir DF *[see Warnings and Precautions (5.5)].*
- Immune Reconstitution Syndrome *[see Warnings and Precautions (5.7)].*

6.1 Adverse Reactions from Clinical Trials Experience
Because clinical trials are conducted under widely varying conditions, adverse reaction rates observed in the clinical trials of a drug cannot be directly compared to rates in the clinical trials of another drug and may not reflect the rates observed in practice.

The safety assessment of STRIBILD is based on the Week 96 pooled data from 1408 subjects in two randomized, double-blind, active-controlled clinical trials, Study 102 and Study 103, in antiretroviral treatment-naïve HIV-1 infected adult subjects *[see Clinical Studies (14)].* A total of 701 subjects received STRIBILD once daily for at least 96 weeks.

The proportion of subjects who discontinued treatment with STRIBILD (elvitegravir 150 mg/cobicistat 150 mg/emtricitabine 200 mg/tenofovir DF 300 mg); ATRIPLA (efavirenz 600 mg/emtricitabine 200 mg/tenofovir DF 300 mg); or atazanavir (ATV) + ritonavir (RTV) + TRUVADA (emtricitabine 200 mg/tenofovir DF 300 mg) due to adverse events, regardless of severity, was 4.6%, 6.8% and 5.9%, respectively. Table 2 displays the frequency of adverse drug reactions greater than or equal to 5% of subjects in any treatment arm.

[See table 2 at top of next page]

See *Warnings and Precautions (5.3),* for a discussion of renal adverse reactions from clinical trials experience with STRIBILD.

Adverse Reactions from Clinical Trials of the Components of STRIBILD
Emtricitabine and Tenofovir Disoproxil Fumarate: In addition to the adverse reactions observed with STRIBILD, the following adverse reactions occurred in at least 5% of treatment-experienced or treatment-naïve subjects receiving emtricitabine or tenofovir DF with other antiretroviral agents in other clinical trials: depression, abdominal pain, dyspepsia, vomiting, fever, pain, nasopharyngitis, pneumonia, sinusitis, upper respiratory tract infection, arthralgia, back pain, myalgia, paresthesia, peripheral neuropathy (including peripheral neuritis and neuropathy), anxiety, increased cough, and rhinitis.

Skin discoloration has been reported with higher frequency among emtricitabine-treated subjects; it was manifested by hyperpigmentation on the palms and/or soles and was generally mild and asymptomatic. The mechanism and clinical significance are unknown.

Laboratory Abnormalities
The frequency of laboratory abnormalities (Grades 3–4) occurring in at least 2% of subjects receiving STRIBILD in Studies 102 and 103 are presented in Table 3.

Table 3 Laboratory Abnormalities (Grades 3–4) Reported in ≥ 2% of Subjects Receiving STRIBILD in Studies 102 and 103 (Week 96 analysis)

	STRIBILD	ATRIPLA	ATV + RTV + TRUVADA
Laboratory Parameter Abnormality*,†	N=701	N=352	N=355
AST (>5.0 × ULN)	2%	6%	6%
Amylase* (>2.0 × ULN)	3%	2%	4%
Creatine Kinase (≥ 10.0 × ULN)	7%	14%	10%
Urine RBC (Hematuria) (> 75 RBC/HPF)	3%	2%	4%

* Frequencies are based on treatment-emergent laboratory abnormalities.

† For subjects with serum amylase > 1.5 × upper limit of normal, lipase test was also performed. The frequency of increased lipase (Grades 3–4) occurring in STRIBILD (N=61), ATRIPLA (N=36), and ATV +RTV + TRUVADA (N=36) was 15%, 17%, and 25%, respectively.

In Study 103, BMD was assessed by DEXA in a non-random subset of 120 subjects. Mean percentage decreases in BMD from baseline to Week 96 in the STRIBILD group (N = 47) were comparable to the ATV + RTV + TRUVADA group (N = 53) at the lumbar spine (-2.0% versus -3.5%, respectively) and at the hip (-3.2% versus -4.2%, respectively). In Studies 102 and 103, bone fractures occurred in 14 subjects (2.0%) in the STRIBILD group, 8 subjects (2.3%) in the ATRIPLA group, and 14 subjects (3.9%) in the ATV + RTV + TRU-VADA group. These findings were consistent with data from an earlier 144-week trial of treatment-naïve subjects receiving tenofovir DF + lamivudine + efavirenz.

Proteinuria (all grades) occurred in 46% of subjects receiving STRIBILD, 38% of subjects receiving ATRIPLA, and 37% of subjects receiving ATV + RTV + TRUVADA.

The cobicistat component of STRIBILD has been shown to increase serum creatinine and decrease estimated creatinine clearance due to inhibition of tubular secretion of creatinine without affecting renal glomerular function. In Studies 102 and 103, increases in serum creatinine and decreases in estimated creatinine clearance occurred early in treatment with STRIBILD, after which they stabilized. Table 4 displays the mean changes in serum creatinine and eGFR levels at Week 96 and the percentage of subjects with elevations in serum creatinine (All Grades).

Table 4 Change from Baseline in Serum Creatinine and eGFR and Incidence of Elevated Serum Creatinine (All Grades) at Week 96

	STRIBILD (N=701)	ATRIPLA (N=352)	ATV + RTV + TRUVADA (N=355)
Serum Creatinine (mg/dL)*	0.13 (±0.13)	0.01 (±0.13)	0.08 (±0.14)
eGFR by Cockcroft-Gault (mL/min)*	-13.2 (±15.7)	-0.9 (±16.1)	-8.6 (±17.8)
Subjects with Elevations in Serum Creatinine (All Grades)(%)	10	1	5

* Mean change ±SD

Emtricitabine or Tenofovir DF: In addition to the laboratory abnormalities observed with STRIBILD, the following laboratory abnormalities have been previously reported in subjects treated with emtricitabine or tenofovir DF with other antiretroviral agents in other clinical trials: Grade 3 or 4 laboratory abnormalities of ALT (M: greater than 215 U per L; F: greater than 170 U per L), alkaline phosphatase (greater than 550 U per L), bilirubin (greater than 2.5 × ULN), serum glucose (less than 40 or greater than 250 mg per dL), glycosuria (greater than or equal to 3+), neutrophils (less than 750 per mm³), fasting cholesterol (greater than 240 mg per dL), and fasting triglycerides (greater than 750 mg per dL).

Serum Lipids: In the clinical trials of STRIBILD, a similar percentage of subjects receiving STRIBILD, ATRIPLA, and

Table 2 Adverse Drug Reactions* (all grades) Reported in ≥ 5% of Subjects in Any Treatment Arm in Studies 102 and 103 (Week 96 analysis).

	STRIBILD N=701	ATRIPLA N=352	ATV + RTV + TRUVADA N=355
EYE DISORDERS			
Ocular icterus	<1%	0%	13%
GASTROINTESTINAL DISORDERS			
Diarrhea	12%	11%	17%
Flatulence	2%	<1%	8%
Nausea	16%	9%	14%
GENERAL DISORDERS AND ADMINISTRATION SITE CONDITIONS			
Fatigue	4%	8%	6%
HEPATOBILIARY DISORDERS			
Jaundice	0%	<1%	9%
NERVOUS SYSTEM DISORDERS			
Somnolence	1%	7%	1%
Headache	7%	4%	6%
Dizziness	3%	21%	4%
PSYCHIATRIC DISORDERS			
Insomnia	3%	8%	1%
Abnormal dreams	9%	26%	4%
SKIN AND SUBCUTANEOUS TISSUE DISORDERS			
Rash†	3%	15%	6%

* Frequencies of adverse reactions are based on all treatment-emergent adverse events, attributed to study drugs.

† Rash event includes dermatitis, drug eruption, eczema, pruritus, pruritus generalized, rash, rash erythematous, rash generalized, rash macular, rash maculo-papular, rash morbilliform, rash papular, rash pruritic, and urticaria.

Table 5 Lipid Values, Mean Change from Baseline, Reported in Subjects Receiving STRIBILD or Comparator in Studies 102 and 103

	STRIBILD N=701		ATRIPLA N=352		ATV + RTV + TRUVADA N=355	
	Baseline	Week 96	Baseline	Week 96	Baseline	Week 96
	mg/dL	Change*	mg/dL	Change*	mg/dL	Change*
Total Cholesterol (fasted)	166 [N=675]	+12 [N=571]	161 [N=343]	+20 [N=288]	168 [N=337]	+11 [N=279]
HDL-cholesterol (fasted)	43 [N=675]	+7 [N=571]	43 [N=343]	+9 [N=288]	42 [N=335]	+6 [N=278]
LDL-cholesterol (fasted)	100 [N=675]	+12 [N=572]	97 [N=343]	+17 [N=287]	101 [N=337]	+13 [N=280]
Triglycerides (fasted)	122 [N=675]	+8 [N=571]	121 [N=343]	+17 [N=288]	132 [N=337]	+25 [N=279]

* The change from baseline is the mean of within-patient changes from baseline for patients with both baseline and Week 96 values.

ATV + RTV + TRUVADA were on lipid lowering agents at baseline (11%, 11%, and 12%, respectively). While receiving study drug through Week 96, an additional 8% of STRIBILD subjects were started on lipid lowering agents, compared to 9% of ATRIPLA and 8% of ATV + RTV + TRU-VADA subjects.

Changes from baseline in total cholesterol, HDL-cholesterol, LDL-cholesterol, and triglycerides are presented in Table 5.

[See table 5 above]

6.2   Postmarketing Experience

Because postmarketing reactions are reported voluntarily from a population of uncertain size, it is not always possible to reliably estimate their frequency or establish a causal relationship to drug exposure. The following adverse reactions have been identified during post approval use of tenofovir DF. No additional postmarketing adverse reactions specific for emtricitabine have been identified.

Immune System Disorders
allergic reaction, including angioedema
Metabolism and Nutrition Disorders
lactic acidosis, hypokalemia, hypophosphatemia
Respiratory, Thoracic, and Mediastinal Disorders
dyspnea
Gastrointestinal Disorders
pancreatitis, increased amylase, abdominal pain
Hepatobiliary Disorders
hepatic steatosis, hepatitis, increased liver enzymes (most commonly AST, ALT gamma GT)

Skin and Subcutaneous Tissue Disorders
rash
Musculoskeletal and Connective Tissue Disorders
rhabdomyolysis, osteomalacia (manifested as bone pain and which may contribute to fractures), muscular weakness, myopathy
Renal and Urinary Disorders
acute renal failure, renal failure, acute tubular necrosis, Fanconi syndrome, proximal renal tubulopathy, interstitial nephritis (including acute cases), nephrogenic diabetes insipidus, renal insufficiency, increased creatinine, proteinuria, polyuria
General Disorders and Administration Site Conditions
asthenia
The following adverse reactions, listed under the body system headings above, may occur as a consequence of proximal renal tubulopathy: rhabdomyolysis, osteomalacia, hypokalemia, muscular weakness, myopathy, hypophosphatemia.

7   DRUG INTERACTIONS

See also *Contraindications (4)* and *Clinical Pharmacology (12.3)*.

7.1   Other Antiretroviral Medications

STRIBILD is a complete regimen for the treatment of HIV-1 infection; therefore, STRIBILD should not be administered with other antiretroviral medications for treatment of HIV-1 infection. Complete information regarding potential drug-drug interactions with other antiretroviral medications is not provided.

Table 6 Established and Other Potentially Significant* Drug Interactions: Alteration in Dose or Regimen May Be Recommended Based on Drug Interaction Studies or Predicted Interaction

Concomitant Drug Class: Drug Name	Effect on Concentration†	Clinical Comment
Acid Reducing Agents: Antacids‡ (for example aluminum and magnesium hydroxide)	↓ elvitegravir	Elvitegravir plasma concentrations are lower when STRIBILD is administered simultaneously with antacids. It is recommended to separate STRIBILD and antacid administration by at least 2 hours.
Antiarrhythmics: e.g. amiodarone bepridil digoxin‡ disopyramide flecainide systemic lidocaine mexiletine propafenone quinidine	↑ antiarrhythmics ↑ digoxin	Concentrations of these antiarrhythmic drugs may be increased when coadministered with STRIBILD. Caution is warranted and therapeutic concentration monitoring, if available, is recommended for antiarrhythmics when coadministered with STRIBILD.
Antibacterials: clarithromycin telithromycin	↑ clarithromycin ↑ telithromycin ↑ cobicistat	Concentrations of clarithromycin and/or cobicistat may be altered when clarithromycin is coadministered with STRIBILD. Patients with CLcr greater than or equal to 60 mL/min: No dose adjustment of clarithromycin is required. Patients with CLcr between 50 mL/min and 60 mL/min: The dose of clarithromycin should be reduced by 50%. Concentrations of telithromycin and/or cobicistat may be increased when telithromycin is coadministered with STRIBILD.
Anticoagulants: warfarin	Effect on warfarin unknown	Concentrations of warfarin may be affected upon coadministration with STRIBILD. It is recommended that the international normalized ratio (INR) be monitored upon coadministration with STRIBILD.
Anticonvulsants: carbamazepine oxcarbazepine phenobarbital phenytoin clonazepam ethosuximide	↑ carbamazepine ↓ elvitegravir ↓ cobicistat ↑ clonazepam ↑ ethosuximide	Coadministration of carbamazepine, oxcarbazepine, phenobarbital, or phenytoin with STRIBILD may significantly decrease cobicistat and elvitegravir plasma concentrations, which may result in loss of therapeutic effect and development of resistance. Alternative anticonvulsants should be considered. Concentrations of clonazepam and ethosuximide may be increased when coadministered with STRIBILD. Clinical monitoring is recommended upon coadministration with STRIBILD.
Antidepressants: Selective Serotonin Reuptake Inhibitors (SSRIs) e.g. paroxetine Tricyclic Antidepressants (TCAs) e.g. amitriptyline desipramine imipramine nortriptyline buproprion trazodone	↑ SSRIs ↑ TCAs ↑ trazodone	Concentrations of these antidepressant agents may be increased when coadministered with STRIBILD. Careful dose titration of the antidepressant and monitoring for antidepressant response are recommended.
Antifungals: itraconazole ketoconazole‡ voriconazole	↑ elvitegravir ↑ cobicistat ↑ itraconazole ↑ ketoconazole ↑voriconazole	Concentrations of ketoconazole, itraconazole and voriconazole may increase upon coadministration with STRIBILD. When administering with STRIBILD, the maximum daily dose of ketoconazole or itraconazole should not exceed 200 mg per day. An assessment of benefit/risk ratio is recommended to justify use of voriconazole with STRIBILD.
Anti-gout: colchicine	↑ colchicine	STRIBILD is not recommended to be coadministered with colchicine to patients with renal or hepatic impairment. Treatment of gout-flares – coadministration of colchicine in patients receiving STRIBILD: 0.6 mg (1 tablet) × 1 dose, followed by 0.3 mg (half tablet) 1 hour later. Treatment course to be repeated no earlier than 3 days. Prophylaxis of gout-flares – coadministration of colchicine in patients receiving STRIBILD: If the original regimen was 0.6 mg twice a day, the regimen should be adjusted to 0.3 mg once a day. If the original regimen was 0.6 mg once a day, the regimen should be adjusted to 0.3 mg once every other day. Treatment of familial Mediterranean fever – coadministration of colchicine in patients receiving STRIBILD: Maximum daily dose of 0.6 mg (may be given as 0.3 mg twice a day).

(Table continued on next page)

7.2 Potential for STRIBILD to Affect Other Drugs
Cobicistat, a component of STRIBILD, is an inhibitor of CYP3A and CYP2D6 and an inhibitor of the following transporters: p-glycoprotein (P-gp), BCRP, OATP1B1 and OATP1B3. Thus, coadministration of STRIBILD with drugs that are primarily metabolized by CYP3A or CYP2D6, or are substrates of P-gp, BCRP, OATP1B1 or OATP1B3 may result in increased plasma concentrations of such drugs. Elvitegravir is a modest inducer of CYP2C9 and may decrease the plasma concentrations of CYP2C9 substrates.

7.3 Potential for Other Drugs to Affect One or More Components of STRIBILD
Elvitegravir and cobicistat, components of STRIBILD, are metabolized by CYP3A. Cobicistat is also metabolized, to a minor extent, by CYP2D6.

Drugs that induce CYP3A activity are expected to increase the clearance of elvitegravir and cobicistat, resulting in decreased plasma concentration of cobicistat and elvitegravir, which may lead to loss of therapeutic effect of STRIBILD and development of resistance (see Table 6).

Coadministration of STRIBILD with other drugs that inhibit CYP3A may decrease the clearance and increase the plasma concentration of cobicistat (see Table 6).

7.4 Drugs Affecting Renal Function
Because emtricitabine and tenofovir, components of STRIBILD are primarily excreted by the kidneys by a combination of glomerular filtration and active tubular secretion, coadministration of STRIBILD with drugs that reduce renal function or compete for active tubular secretion may increase concentrations of emtricitabine, tenofovir, and other renally eliminated drugs and this may increase the risk of adverse reactions. Some examples of drugs that are eliminated by active tubular secretion include, but are not limited to acyclovir, cidofovir, ganciclovir, valacyclovir, valganciclovir, aminoglycosides (e.g. gentamicin), and high-dose or multiple NSAIDs *[see Warnings and Precautions (5.3)]*.

7.5 Established and Other Potentially Significant Interactions
Table 6 provides a listing of established or potentially clinically significant drug interactions. The drug interactions described are based on studies conducted with either STRIBILD, the components of STRIBILD, (elvitegravir, cobicistat, emtricitabine, and tenofovir DF) as individual agents and/or in combination, or are predicted drug interactions that may occur with STRIBILD *[for magnitude of interaction, see Clinical Pharmacology (12.3)]*. The table includes potentially significant interactions but is not all inclusive.
[See table 6 above and on pages 809 and 810]

7.6 Drugs without Clinically Significant Interactions with STRIBILD
Based on drug interaction studies conducted with the components of STRIBILD, no clinically significant drug interactions have been either observed or are expected when STRIBILD is combined with the following drugs: entecavir, famciclovir, H₂ receptor antagonists, methadone, proton pump inhibitors and ribavirin.

8 USE IN SPECIFIC POPULATIONS
8.1 Pregnancy
Pregnancy Category B
There are no adequate and well-controlled studies in pregnant women. Because animal reproduction studies are not always predictive of human response, STRIBILD should be used during pregnancy only if the potential benefit justifies the potential risk to the fetus.

Antiretroviral Pregnancy Registry: To monitor fetal outcomes of pregnant women exposed to STRIBILD, an Antiretroviral Pregnancy Registry has been established. Healthcare providers are encouraged to register patients by calling 1-800-258-4263.

Animal Data
Elvitegravir: Studies in animals have shown no evidence of teratogenicity or an effect on reproductive function. In offspring from rat and rabbit dams treated with elvitegravir during pregnancy, there were no toxicologically significant effects on developmental endpoints. The exposures (AUC) at the embryo-fetal No Observed Adverse Effects Levels (NOAELs) in rats and rabbits were respectively 23 and 0.2 times higher than the exposure in humans at the recommended daily dose of 150 mg.

Cobicistat: Studies in animals have shown no evidence of teratogenicity or an effect on reproductive function. In offspring from rat and rabbit dams treated with cobicistat during pregnancy, there were no toxicologically significant effects on developmental endpoints. The exposures (AUC) at the embryo-fetal NOAELs in rats and rabbits were respectively 1.8 and 4.3 times higher than the exposure in humans at the recommended daily dose of 150 mg.

Emtricitabine: The incidence of fetal variations and malformations was not increased in embryo-fetal toxicity studies performed with emtricitabine in mice at exposures

(AUC) approximately 60 times higher and in rabbits at approximately 120 times higher than human exposures at the recommended daily dose.

Tenofovir DF: Reproduction studies have been performed in rats and rabbits at doses up to 14 and 19 times the human dose based on body surface area comparisons and revealed no evidence of impaired fertility or harm to the fetus due to tenofovir.

8.3 Nursing Mothers

The Centers for Disease Control and Prevention recommend that HIV-infected mothers not breastfeed their infants to avoid risking postnatal transmission of HIV. Studies in rats have demonstrated that elvitegravir, cobicistat, and tenofovir are secreted in milk. It is not known whether elvitegravir or cobicistat is excreted in human milk.

In humans, samples of breast milk obtained from five HIV-1 infected mothers show that emtricitabine is secreted in human milk. Breastfeeding infants whose mothers are being treated with emtricitabine may be at risk for developing viral resistance to emtricitabine. Other emtricitabine-associated risks in infants breastfed by mothers being treated with emtricitabine are unknown.

Samples of breast milk obtained from five HIV-1 infected mothers show that tenofovir is secreted in human milk. Tenofovir-associated risks, including the risk of viral resistance to tenofovir, in infants breastfed by mothers being treated with tenofovir disoproxil fumarate are unknown.

Because of both the potential for HIV transmission and the potential for serious adverse reactions in nursing infants, **mothers should be instructed not to breastfeed if they are receiving STRIBILD.**

8.4 Pediatric Use

Safety and effectiveness of STRIBILD in pediatric patients less than 18 years of age have not been established *[see Clinical Pharmacology (12.3)]*.

8.5 Geriatric Use

Clinical studies of STRIBILD did not include sufficient numbers of subjects aged 65 and over to determine whether they respond differently from younger subjects. In general, caution should be exercised in the administration of STRIBILD in elderly patients, keeping in mind the greater frequency of decreased hepatic, renal, or cardiac function, and of concomitant disease or other drug therapy *[see Clinical Pharmacology (12.3)]*.

8.6 Renal Impairment

Initiation of STRIBILD in patients with estimated creatinine clearance below 70 mL per min is not recommended. Because STRIBILD is a fixed-dose combination tablet, STRIBILD should be discontinued if estimated creatinine clearance declines below 50 mL per min during treatment with STRIBILD as dose interval adjustment required for emtricitabine and tenofovir DF cannot be achieved *[see Warnings and Precautions (5.3), Adverse Reactions (6.1), Clinical Pharmacology (12.3), and Clinical Studies (14)]*.

8.7 Hepatic Impairment

No dose adjustment of STRIBILD is required in patients with mild (Child-Pugh Class A) or moderate (Child-Pugh Class B) hepatic impairment. No pharmacokinetic or safety data are available regarding the use of STRIBILD in patients with severe hepatic impairment (Child-Pugh Class C). Therefore, STRIBILD is not recommended for use in patients with severe hepatic impairment *[see Dosage and Administration (2) and Clinical Pharmacology (12.3)]*.

10 OVERDOSAGE

No data are available on overdose of STRIBILD in patients. If overdose occurs the patient must be monitored for evidence of toxicity. Treatment of overdose with STRIBILD consists of general supportive measures including monitoring of vital signs as well as observation of the clinical status of the patient.

Elvitegravir: Limited clinical experience is available at doses higher than the therapeutic dose of elvitegravir. In one study, boosted elvitegravir equivalent to 2 times the therapeutic dose of 150 mg once daily for 10 days was administered to 42 healthy subjects. No severe adverse reactions were reported. The effects of higher doses are not known. As elvitegravir is highly bound to plasma proteins, it is unlikely that it will be significantly removed by hemodialysis or peritoneal dialysis.

Cobicistat: Limited clinical experience is available at doses higher than the therapeutic dose of cobicistat. In two studies, a single dose of cobicistat 400 mg (2.7 times the dose in STRIBILD) was administered to a total of 60 healthy subjects. No severe adverse reactions were reported. The effects of higher doses are not known. As cobicistat is highly bound to plasma proteins, it is unlikely that it will be significantly removed by hemodialysis or peritoneal dialysis.

Emtricitabine: Limited clinical experience is available at doses higher than the therapeutic dose of EMTRIVA. In one clinical pharmacology study, single doses of emtricitabine 1200 mg (6 times the dose in STRIBILD) were administered to 11 subjects. No severe adverse reactions were reported. The effects of higher doses are not known.

Table 6 *(cont.)* Established and Other Potentially Significant* Drug Interactions: Alteration in Dose or Regimen May Be Recommended Based on Drug Interaction Studies or Predicted Interaction

Concomitant Drug Class: Drug Name	Effect on Concentration†	Clinical Comment
Antimycobacterial: rifabutin‡ rifapentine	↓ elvitegravir ↓ cobicistat	Coadministration of rifabutin and rifapentine with STRIBILD may significantly decrease elvitegravir and cobicistat plasma concentrations, which may result in loss of therapeutic effect and development of resistance. Coadministration of STRIBILD with rifabutin or rifapentine is not recommended.
Beta-Blockers: e.g. metoprolol timolol	↑ beta-blockers	Concentrations of beta-blockers may be increased when coadministered with STRIBILD. Clinical monitoring is recommended and a dose decrease of the beta blocker may be necessary when these agents are coadministered with STRIBILD.
Calcium Channel Blockers: e.g. amlodipine diltiazem felodipine nicardipine nifedipine verapamil	↑ calcium channel blockers	Concentrations of calcium channel blockers may be increased when coadministered with STRIBILD. Caution is warranted and clinical monitoring is recommended upon coadministration with STRIBILD.
Corticosteroid: Systemic: dexamethasone	↓ elvitegravir ↓ cobicistat	Systemic dexamethasone, a CYP3A inducer, may significantly decrease elvitegravir and cobicistat plasma concentrations, which may result in loss of therapeutic effect and development of resistance.
Corticosteroid: Inhaled/Nasal: fluticasone	↑ fluticasone	Concomitant use of inhaled or nasal fluticasone and STRIBILD may increase plasma concentrations of fluticasone, resulting in reduced serum cortisol concentrations. Alternative corticosteroids should be considered, particularly for long term use.
Endothelin Receptor Antagonists: bosentan	↑ bosentan	Coadministration of bosentan in patients on STRIBILD: In patients who have been receiving STRIBILD for at least 10 days, start bosentan at 62.5 mg once daily or every other day based upon individual tolerability. Coadministration of STRIBILD in patients on bosentan: Discontinue use of bosentan at least 36 hours prior to initiation of STRIBILD. After at least 10 days following the initiation of STRIBILD, resume bosentan at 62.5 mg once daily or every other day based upon individual tolerability.
HMG-CoA Reductase Inhibitors: atorvastatin	↑ atorvastatin	Initiate with the lowest starting dose of atorvastatin and titrate carefully while monitoring for safety.
Hormonal Contraceptives: norgestimate/ethinyl estradiol‡	↑ norgestimate ↓ ethinyl estradiol	The effects of increases in the concentration of the progestational component norgestimate are not fully known and can include increased risk of insulin resistance, dyslipidemia, acne, and venous thrombosis. The potential risks and benefits associated with coadministration of norgestimate/ethinyl estradiol with STRIBILD should be considered, particularly in women who have risk factors for these events. Coadministration of STRIBILD with other hormonal contraceptives (e.g., contraceptive patch, contraceptive vaginal ring, or injectable contraceptives) or oral contraceptives containing progestogens other than norgestimate has not been studied; therefore, alternative (non-hormonal) methods of contraception can be considered.
Immuno-suppressants: e.g. cyclosporine sirolimus tacrolimus	↑ immuno-suppressants	Concentrations of these immunosuppressant agents may be increased when coadministered with STRIBILD. Therapeutic monitoring of the immunosuppressive agents is recommended upon coadministration with STRIBILD.
Narcotic Analgesics: buprenorphine/ naloxone‡	↑ buprenorphine ↑ norbuprenorphine ↓ naloxone	Concentrations of buprenorphine and norbuprenorphine are increased when coadministered with STRIBILD. No dose adjustment of buprenorphine/naloxone is required upon coadministration with STRIBILD. Patients should be closely monitored for sedation and cognitive effects.
Inhaled Beta Agonist: salmeterol	↑ salmeterol	Coadministration of salmeterol and STRIBILD is not recommended. Coadministration of salmeterol with STRIBILD may result in increased risk of cardiovascular adverse events associated with salmeterol, including QT prolongation, palpitations, and sinus tachycardia.

(Table continued on next page)

Hemodialysis treatment removes approximately 30% of the emtricitabine dose over a 3 hour dialysis period starting within 1.5 hours of emtricitabine dosing (blood flow rate of 400 mL per minute and a dialysate flow rate of 600 mL per minute). It is not known whether emtricitabine can be removed by peritoneal dialysis.

Tenofovir DF: Limited clinical experience at doses higher than the therapeutic dose of VIREAD 300 mg is available. In one study, 600 mg tenofovir DF (2 times the dosage in STRIBILD) was administered to 8 subjects orally for 28 days, and no severe adverse reactions were reported. The effects of higher doses are not known. Tenofovir is efficiently removed by hemodialysis with an extraction coefficient of approximately 54%. Following a single 300 mg dose of VIREAD, a 4-hour hemodialysis session removed approximately 10% of the administered tenofovir dose.

11 DESCRIPTION

STRIBILD is a fixed-dose combination tablet containing elvitegravir, cobicistat, emtricitabine, and tenofovir DF for oral administration.
- Elvitegravir is an HIV-1 integrase strand transfer inhibitor.
- Cobicistat is a mechanism-based inhibitor of cytochrome P450 (CYP) enzymes of the CYP3A family.
- Emtricitabine is a synthetic nucleoside analog of cytidine. EMTRIVA is the brand name for emtricitabine.
- Tenofovir DF is converted *in vivo* to tenofovir, an acyclic nucleoside phosphonate (nucleotide) analog of adenosine 5'-monophosphate. VIREAD is the brand name for tenofovir DF.

Each tablet contains 150 mg of elvitegravir, 150 mg of cobicistat, 200 mg of emtricitabine, and 300 mg of tenofovir DF (equivalent to 245 mg of tenofovir disoproxil). The tablets include the following inactive ingredients: lactose monohydrate, microcrystalline cellulose, silicon dioxide, croscarmellose sodium, hydroxypropyl cellulose, sodium lauryl sulfate, and magnesium stearate. The tablets are film-coated with a coating material containing indigo carmine (FD&C Blue #2) aluminum lake, polyethylene glycol, polyvinyl alcohol, talc, titanium dioxide, and yellow iron oxide.

Elvitegravir: The chemical name of elvitegravir is 6-(3-Chloro-2-fluorobenzyl)-1-[(2S)-1-hydroxy-3-methylbutan-2-yl]-7-methoxy-4-oxo-1,4-dihydroquinoline-3-carboxylic acid. It has a molecular formula of $C_{23}H_{23}ClFNO_5$ and a molecular weight of 447.9. It has the following structural formula:

Elvitegravir is a white to pale yellow powder with a solubility of less than 0.3 micrograms per mL in water at 20 °C.

Cobicistat: The chemical name for cobicistat is 1,3-thiazol-5-ylmethyl [(2R,5R)-5-[[(2S)-2-[(methyl[[2-(propan-2-yl)-1,3-thiazol-4-yl]methyl]carbamoyl)amino]-4-(morpholin-4-yl)butanoyl]amino]-1,6-diphenylhexan-2-yl]carbamate.
It has a molecular formula of $C_{40}H_{53}N_7O_5S_2$ and a molecular weight of 776.0. It has the following structural formula:

Cobicistat is adsorbed onto silicon dioxide. Cobicistat on silicon dioxide is a white to pale yellow solid with a solubility of 0.1 mg per mL in water at 20 °C.

Emtricitabine: The chemical name of emtricitabine is 5-fluoro-1-[(2R,5S)-2-(hydroxymethyl)-1,3-oxathiolan-5-yl]-cytosine. Emtricitabine is the (-)enantiomer of a thio analog of cytidine, which differs from other cytidine analogs in that it has a fluorine in the 5-position.
It has a molecular formula of $C_8H_{10}FN_3O_3S$ and a molecular weight of 247.25. It has the following structural formula:

Emtricitabine is a white to off-white crystalline powder with a solubility of approximately 112 mg per mL in water at 25 °C.

Tenofovir Disoproxil Fumarate: Tenofovir DF is a fumaric acid salt of the bis-isopropoxycarbonyloxymethyl ester derivative of tenofovir. The chemical name of tenofovir DF is 9-[(R)-2-[[bis[[(isopropoxycarbonyl)oxy]-methoxy]phosphinyl]methoxy]propyl]adenine fumarate (1:1). It has a molecular formula of $C_{19}H_{30}N_5O_{10}P \cdot C_4H_4O_4$ and a molecular weight of 635.51. It has the following structural formula:

Tenofovir DF is a white to off-white crystalline powder with a solubility of 13.4 mg per mL in water at 25 °C. All dosages are expressed in terms of tenofovir DF except where otherwise noted.

12 CLINICAL PHARMACOLOGY

12.1 Mechanism of Action

STRIBILD is a fixed-dose combination of antiviral drugs elvitegravir (boosted by the CYP3A inhibitor cobicistat), emtricitabine, and tenofovir DF *[see Microbiology (12.4)]*.

12.2 Pharmacodynamics

Effects on Electrocardiogram

Thorough QT studies have been conducted for elvitegravir and cobicistat. The effect of the other two components, tenofovir and emtricitabine, or the combination regimen STRIBILD on the QT interval is not known.

The effect of multiple doses of elvitegravir 125 and 250 mg (0.83 and 1.67 times the dose in STRIBILD) (coadministered with 100 mg RTV to boost the blood levels of elvitegravir) on QTc interval was evaluated in a randomized, placebo- and active-controlled (moxifloxacin 400 mg) parallel group thorough QT study in 126 healthy subjects. In a study with demonstrated ability to detect small effects, the upper bound of the one-sided 95% confidence interval for the largest placebo adjusted, baseline-corrected QTc based on Fridericia's correction method (QTcF) was below 10 msec. In this study, there was no clinically relevant prolongation of the QTc interval.

The effect of a single dose of cobicistat 250 mg and 400 mg (1.67 and 2.67 times the dose in STRIBILD) on QTc interval was evaluated in a randomized, placebo- and active-controlled (moxifloxacin 400 mg) four-period crossover thorough QT study in 48 healthy subjects. In a study with demonstrated ability to detect small effects, the upper bound of the one-sided 95% confidence interval for the largest placebo adjusted, baseline-corrected QTc based on individual correction method (QTc) was below 10 msec, the threshold for regulatory concern. Prolongation of the PR interval was noted in subjects receiving cobicistat in the same study. The maximum mean (95% upper confidence bound) difference in PR from placebo after baseline-correction was 9.5 (12.1) msec for 250 mg dose and 20.2 (22.8) for 400 mg dose cobicistat. Because the 150 mg cobicistat dose used in the STRIBILD fixed-dose combination tablet is lower than the lowest dose studied in the thorough QT study, it is unlikely that treatment with STRIBILD will result in clinically relevant PR prolongation.

12.3 Pharmacokinetics

Absorption and Bioavailability

STRIBILD: Following oral administration of STRIBILD with food in HIV-1 infected subjects, peak plasma concentrations were observed 4 hours post-dose for elvitegravir, 3 hours post-dose for cobicistat, 3 hours post-dose for

Table 6 (cont.) Established and Other Potentially Significant* Drug Interactions: Alteration in Dose or Regimen May Be Recommended Based on Drug Interaction Studies or Predicted Interaction

Concomitant Drug Class: Drug Name	Effect on Concentration[†]	Clinical Comment
Neuroleptics: e.g. perphenazine risperidone thioridazine	↑ neuroleptics	A decrease in dose of the neuroleptic may be needed when coadministered with STRIBILD.
Phosphodiesterase-5 (PDE5) Inhibitors: sildenafil tadalafil vardenafil	↑ PDE5 inhibitors	Coadministration with STRIBILD may result in an increase in PDE-5 inhibitor associated adverse reactions, including hypotension, syncope, visual disturbances, and priapism. Use of PDE-5 inhibitors for pulmonary arterial hypertension (PAH): • Use of sildenafil is contraindicated when used for the treatment of pulmonary arterial hypertension (PAH). • The following dose adjustments are recommended for the use of tadalafil with STRIBILD: *Coadministration of tadalafil in patients on STRIBILD:* In patients receiving STRIBILD for at least 1 week, start tadalafil at 20 mg once daily. Increase tadalafil dose to 40 mg once daily based upon individual tolerability. *Coadministration of STRIBILD in patients on tadalafil:* Avoid use of tadalafil during the initiation of STRIBILD. Stop tadalafil at least 24 hours prior to starting STRIBILD. After at least one week following initiation of STRIBILD, resume tadalafil at 20 mg once daily. Increase tadalafil dose to 40 mg once daily based upon individual tolerability. Use of PDE-5 inhibitors for erectile dysfunction: Sildenafil at a single dose not exceeding 25 mg in 48 hours, vardenafil at a single dose not exceeding 2.5 mg in 72 hours, or tadalafil at a single dose not exceeding 10 mg in 72 hours can be used with increased monitoring for PDE-5 inhibitor associated with adverse events.
Sedative/hypnotics: Benzodiazepines: e.g. Parenterally administered midazolam clorazepate diazepam estazolam flurazepam buspirone zolpidem	↑ sedatives/hypnotics	Concomitant use of parenteral midazolam with STRIBILD may increase plasma concentrations of midazolam. Coadministration should be done in a setting that ensures close clinical monitoring and appropriate medical management in case of respiratory depression and/or prolonged sedation. Dosage reduction for midazolam should be considered, especially if more than a single dose of midazolam is administered. Coadministration of oral midazolam with STRIBILD is contraindicated. With other sedative/hypnotics, dose reduction may be necessary and clinical monitoring is recommended.

* This table is not all inclusive.
† ↑ = Increase, ↓ = Decrease, ⇔ = No Effect
‡ Indicates that a drug-drug interaction trial was conducted.

emtricitabine, and 2 hours for tenofovir following the conversion of tenofovir DF (see Table 7 for additional pharmacokinetic parameters).

[See table 7 above]

Effect of Food on Oral Absorption

Relative to fasting conditions, the administration of single dose STRIBILD with a light meal (~373 kcal, 20% fat) increased the mean systemic exposure of elvitegravir and tenofovir by 34% and 24%, respectively. The alterations in mean systemic exposures of cobicistat and emtricitabine were not clinically significant.

Relative to fasting conditions, the administration of single dose STRIBILD with a high fat meal (~ 800 kcal, 50% fat) increased the mean systemic exposure of elvitegravir and tenofovir by 87% and 23%, respectively. The alterations in mean systemic exposures of cobicistat and emtricitabine were not clinically significant.

STRIBILD should be taken with food.

Distribution

Elvitegravir: Elvitegravir is 98–99% bound to human plasma proteins and binding is independent of drug concentration over the range of 1 ng per mL to 1.6 micrograms per mL. The mean blood-to-plasma ratio was 0.73.

Cobicistat: Cobicistat is 97–98% bound to human plasma proteins and the mean blood-to-plasma ratio was approximately 0.5.

Emtricitabine: In vitro binding of emtricitabine to human plasma proteins is less than 4% and is independent of drug concentration over the range of 0.02–200 micrograms per mL.

Tenofovir Disoproxil Fumarate: In vitro binding of tenofovir to human plasma proteins is less than 0.7% and is independent of concentration over the range of 0.01–25 micrograms per mL.

Metabolism

Elvitegravir: The majority of elvitegravir metabolism is mediated by CYP3A enzymes. Elvitegravir also undergoes glucuronidation via UGT1A1/3 enzymes.

Cobicistat: Cobicistat is metabolized by CYP3A and to a minor extent by CYP2D6 enzymes and does not undergo glucuronidation.

Emtricitabine and tenofovir are not significantly metabolized.

Elimination

Elvitegravir: The median terminal plasma half-life of elvitegravir following administration of STRIBILD is approximately 12.9 hours. After single dose administration of [^{14}C] elvitegravir (coadministered with 100 mg RTV), 94.8% and 6.7% of the administered dose was excreted in feces and urine, respectively.

Cobicistat: The median terminal plasma half-life of cobicistat following administration of STRIBILD is approximately 3.5 hours. With single dose administration of [^{14}C] cobicistat after multiple dosing of cobicistat for six days, 86.2% and 8.2% of the administered dose was excreted in feces and urine, respectively.

Emtricitabine and tenofovir are primarily excreted in the urine by a combination of glomerular filtration and active tubular secretion.

Special Populations

Patients with Renal Impairment

Elvitegravir and cobicistat: A study of the pharmacokinetics of cobicistat-boosted elvitegravir was performed in healthy subjects and subjects with severe renal impairment (estimated creatinine clearance less than 30 mL per min). No clinically relevant differences in elvitegravir or cobicistat pharmacokinetics were observed between healthy subjects and subjects with severe renal impairment.

Emtricitabine and Tenofovir Disoproxil Fumarate: The pharmacokinetics of emtricitabine and tenofovir are altered in subjects with estimated creatinine clearance below 50 mL per min or with end stage renal disease requiring dialysis *[see Warnings and Precautions (5.3) and Use in Specific Populations (8.6)]*.

Patients with Hepatic Impairment

Elvitegravir and cobicistat: A study of the pharmacokinetics of cobicistat-boosted elvitegravir was performed in healthy subjects and subjects with moderate hepatic impairment. No clinically relevant differences in elvitegravir or cobicistat pharmacokinetics were observed between subjects with moderate hepatic impairment (Child-Pugh Class B) and healthy subjects. No dosage adjustment of elvitegravir or cobicistat is necessary for patients with mild to moderate hepatic impairment. The effect of severe hepatic impairment (Child-Pugh Class C) on the pharmacokinetics of elvitegravir or cobicistat has not been studied *[see Use in Specific Populations (8.7)]*.

Emtricitabine: The pharmacokinetics of emtricitabine has not been studied in subjects with hepatic impairment; however, emtricitabine is not significantly metabolized by liver enzymes, so the impact of liver impairment should be limited.

Tenofovir Disoproxil Fumarate: The pharmacokinetics of tenofovir following a 300 mg dose of VIREAD has been studied in healthy subjects with moderate to severe hepatic impairment. No clinically relevant differences in tenofovir pharmacokinetics were observed between subjects with hepatic impairment and healthy subjects.

Hepatitis B and/or Hepatitis C Virus Co-infection

Elvitegravir: Limited data from population pharmacokinetic analysis (N=24) indicated that hepatitis B and/or C virus infection had no clinically relevant effect on the exposure of cobicistat-boosted elvitegravir.

Cobicistat: There were insufficient pharmacokinetic data in the clinical trials to determine the effect of hepatitis B and/or C virus infection on the pharmacokinetics of cobicistat.

Emtricitabine and Tenofovir: Pharmacokinetics of emtricitabine and tenofovir DF have not been fully evaluated in subjects coinfected with hepatitis B and/or C virus.

Race

Elvitegravir: Population pharmacokinetic analysis of elvitegravir in HIV-1 infected subjects indicated that race had no clinically relevant effect on the exposure of cobicistat-boosted elvitegravir.

Cobicistat: Population pharmacokinetics analysis of cobicistat in HIV-1 infected subjects indicated that race had no clinically relevant effect on the exposure of COBI.

Emtricitabine: No pharmacokinetic differences due to race have been identified following the administration of EMTRIVA.

Tenofovir Disoproxil Fumarate: There were insufficient numbers from racial and ethnic groups other than Caucasian to adequately determine potential pharmacokinetic differences among these populations following the administration of VIREAD.

Gender

No clinically relevant pharmacokinetic differences have been observed between men and women for cobicistat-boosted elvitegravir, emtricitabine and tenofovir DF.

Pediatric Patients

Emtricitabine has been studied in pediatric subjects from 3 months to 17 years of age. Tenofovir DF has been studied in pediatric subjects from 2 years to less than 18 years of age. The pharmacokinetics of elvitegravir or cobicistat in pediatric subjects have not been established *[see Use in Specific Populations (8.4)]*.

Geriatric Patients

Pharmacokinetics of elvitegravir, cobicistat, emtricitabine and tenofovir have not been fully evaluated in elderly (65 years of age and older) patients *[see Use in Specific Populations (8.5)]*.

Assessment of Drug Interactions

[see also Contraindications (4) and Drug Interactions (7)]

The drug-drug interaction studies described in Tables 8 and 9 were conducted with STRIBILD, elvitegravir (coadministered with cobicistat or RTV), or cobicistat administered alone.

As STRIBILD is indicated for use as a complete regimen for the treatment of HIV-1 infection and should not be administered with other antiretroviral medications, information regarding drug-drug interactions with other antiretrovirals agents is not provided *[see Warnings and Precautions (5.4)]*. The effects of coadministered drugs on the exposure of elvitegravir are shown in Table 8. The effects of elvitegravir or cobicistat on the exposure of coadministered drugs are shown in Table 9. For information regarding clinical recommendations, see *Drug Interactions (7)*.

[See table 8 at top of next page]

[See table 9 at top of page 813]

12.4   Microbiology

Mechanism of Action

Elvitegravir: Elvitegravir inhibits the strand transfer activity of HIV-1 integrase (integrase strand transfer inhibitor; INSTI), an HIV-1 encoded enzyme that is required for viral replication. Inhibition of integrase prevents the integration of HIV-1 DNA into host genomic DNA, blocking the formation of the HIV-1 provirus and propagation of the viral infection. Elvitegravir does not inhibit human topoisomerases I or II.

Cobicistat: Cobicistat is a selective, mechanism-based inhibitor of cytochromes P450 of the CYP3A subfamily. Inhibition of CYP3A-mediated metabolism by cobicistat enhances the systemic exposure of CYP3A substrates, such as elvitegravir, where bioavailability is limited and half-life is shortened by CYP3A-dependent metabolism.

Emtricitabine: Emtricitabine, a synthetic nucleoside analog of cytidine, is phosphorylated by cellular enzymes to form emtricitabine 5'-triphosphate. Emtricitabine 5'-triphosphate inhibits the activity of the HIV-1 RT by competing with the natural substrate deoxycytidine 5'-triphosphate and by being incorporated into nascent viral DNA which results in chain termination. Emtricitabine 5'-triphosphate is a weak inhibitor of mammalian DNA polymerases α, β, ε, and mitochondrial DNA polymerase γ.

Tenofovir DF: Tenofovir DF is an acyclic nucleoside phosphonate diester analog of adenosine monophosphate. Tenofovir DF requires initial diester hydrolysis for conversion to tenofovir and subsequent phosphorylations by cellular enzymes to form tenofovir diphosphate. Tenofovir diphosphate inhibits the activity of HIV-1 RT by competing with the natural substrate deoxyadenosine 5'-triphosphate and, after incorporation into DNA, by DNA chain termination. Tenofovir diphosphate is a weak inhibitor of mammalian DNA polymerases α, β, and mitochondrial DNA polymerase γ.

Antiviral Activity in Cell Culture

Elvitegravir, Cobicistat, Emtricitabine, and Tenofovir DF: The triple combination of elvitegravir, emtricitabine, and tenofovir was not antagonistic in cell culture combination antiviral activity assays and was not affected by the addition of cobicistat.

Elvitegravir: The antiviral activity of elvitegravir against laboratory and clinical isolates of HIV-1 was assessed in T lymphoblastoid cell lines, monocyte/macrophage cells, and primary peripheral blood lymphocytes. The 50% effective concentrations (EC_{50}) ranged from 0.02 to 1.7 nM. Elvitegravir displayed antiviral activity in cell culture against HIV-1 clades A, B, C, D, E, F, G, and O (EC_{50} values ranged from 0.1 to 1.3 nM) and activity against HIV-2 (EC_{50} value of 0.53 nM). Elvitegravir did not show inhibition of replication of HBV or HCV in cell culture.

Cobicistat: Cobicistat has no detectable antiviral activity in cell culture against HIV-1, HBV, or HCV and does not antagonize the antiviral activity of elvitegravir, emtricitabine, or tenofovir.

Emtricitabine: The antiviral activity of emtricitabine against laboratory and clinical isolates of HIV-1 was assessed in T lymphoblastoid cell lines, the MAGI-CCR5 cell line, and primary peripheral blood mononuclear cells. The EC_{50} values for emtricitabine were in the range of 0.0013–0.64 micromolar. Emtricitabine displayed antiviral activity in cell culture against HIV-1 clades A, B, C, D, E, F, and G (EC_{50} values ranged from 0.007–0.075 micromolar) and showed strain specific activity against HIV-2 (EC_{50} values ranged from 0.007–1.5 micromolar).

Tenofovir DF: The antiviral activity of tenofovir against laboratory and clinical isolates of HIV-1 was assessed in T lymphoblastoid cell lines, primary monocyte/macrophage cells and peripheral blood lymphocytes. The EC_{50} values for tenofovir were in the range of 0.04–8.5 micromolar. Tenofovir displayed antiviral activity in cell culture against HIV-1 clades A, B, C, D, E, F, G, and O (EC_{50} val-

Table 7 Pharmacokinetic Parameters of Elvitegravir, Cobicistat, Emtricitabine, and Tenofovir Exposure Following Oral Administration of STRIBILD in HIV-Infected Subjects

Parameter Mean ± SD [range: min:max]	Elvitegravir*	Cobicistat†	Emtricitabine†	Tenofovir†
C_{max} (microgram per mL)	1.7 ± 0.4 [0.4:3.7]	1.1 ± 0.4 [0.1:2.1]	1.9 ± 0.5 [0.6:3.6]	0.45 ± 0.2 [0.2:1.2]
AUC_{tau} (microgram·hour per mL)	23.0 ± 7.5 [4.4:69.8]	8.3 ± 3.8 [0.5:18.3]	12.7 ± 4.5 [5.2:34.1]	4.4 ± 2.2 [2.1:18.2]
C_{trough} (microgram per mL)	0.45 ± 0.26 [0.05:2.34]	0.05 ± 0.13 [0.01:0.92]	0.14 ± 0.25 [0.04:1.94]	0.10 ± 0.08 [0.04:0.58]

SD = Standard Deviation
* From Population Pharmacokinetic analysis, N=419.
† From Intensive Pharmacokinetic analysis, N=61–62, except cobicistat C_{trough} N=53.

Help Patients Save on Rx Drugs: PDR.net/PharmacyDiscountCard

Table 8 Drug Interactions: Changes in Pharmacokinetic Parameters for Elvitegravir in the Presence of the Coadministered Drug*

Coadministered Drug	Dose of Coadministered Drug (mg)	Elvitegravir Dose (mg)	Cobicistat or RTV Booster Dose (mg)	N	Mean Ratio of Elvitegravir Pharmacokinetic Parameters (90% CI); No effect = 1.00		
					C_{max}	AUC	C_{min}
Antacids	20 mL single dose given 4 hours before elvitegravir	50 single dose	RTV 100 single dose	8	0.95 (0.84,1.07)	0.96 (0.88,1.04)	1.04 (0.93,1.17)
	20 mL single dose given 4 hours after elvitegravir			10	0.98 (0.88,1.10)	0.98 (0.91,1.06)	1.00 (0.90,1.11)
	20 mL single dose given 2 hours before elvitegravir			11	0.82 (0.74,0.91)	0.85 (0.79,0.91)	0.90 (0.82,0.99)
	20 mL single dose given 2 hours after elvitegravir			10	0.79 (0.71,0.88)	0.80 (0.75,0.86)	0.80 (0.73,0.89)
Famotidine	40 once daily given 12 hours after elvitegravir	150 once daily	Cobicistat 150 once daily	10	1.02 (0.89,1.17)	1.03 (0.95,1.13)	1.18 (1.05,1.32)
	40 once daily given simultaneously with elvitegravir			16	1.00 (0.92,1.10)	1.03 (0.98,1.08)	1.07 (0.98,1.17)
Ketoconazole	200 twice daily	150 once daily	RTV 100 once daily	18	1.17 (1.04,1.33)	1.48 (1.36,1.62)	1.67 (1.48,1.88)
Omeprazole	40 once daily given 2 hours before elvitegravir	50 once daily	RTV 100 once daily	9	0.93 (0.83,1.04)	0.99 (0.91,1.07)	0.94 (0.85,1.04)
	20 once daily given 2 hours before elvitegravir	150 once daily	Cobicistat 150 once daily	11	1.16 (1.04,1.30)	1.10 (1.02,1.19)	1.13 (0.96,1.34)
	20 once daily given 12 hours after elvitegravir			11	1.03 (0.92,1.15)	1.05 (0.93,1.18)	1.10 (0.92,1.32)
Rifabutin	150 once every other day	150 once daily	Cobicistat 150 once daily	12	0.91 (0.84,0.99)	0.79 (0.74,0.85)	0.33 (0.27,0.40)
Rosuvastatin	10 single dose	150 once daily	Cobicistat 150 once daily	10	0.94 (0.83,1.07)	1.02 (0.91,1.14)	0.98 (0.83,1.16)

* All interaction studies conducted in healthy volunteers.

ues ranged from 0.5–2.2 micromolar) and showed strain specific activity against HIV-2 (EC_{50} values ranged from 1.6–5.5 micromolar).

Resistance

In Cell Culture:

Elvitegravir: HIV-1 isolates with reduced susceptibility to elvitegravir have been selected in cell culture. Reduced susceptibility to elvitegravir was associated with the primary integrase substitutions T66A/I, E92G/Q, S147G, and Q148R. Additional integrase substitutions observed in cell culture selection included D10E, S17N, H51Y, F121Y, S153F/Y, E157Q, D232N, R263K, and V281M.

Emtricitabine and Tenofovir DF: HIV-1 isolates with reduced susceptibility to emtricitabine or tenofovir have been selected in cell culture. Reduced susceptibility to emtricitabine was associated with M184V/I substitutions in HIV-1 RT. HIV-1 isolates selected by tenofovir expressed a K65R substitution in HIV-1 RT and showed a 2–4 fold reduction in susceptibility to tenofovir.

In Clinical Studies:

In Treatment-Naïve HIV-1-Infected Adult Subjects: In Studies 102 and 103 *[see Clinical Studies (14)]*, the development of one or more primary substitutions associated with resistance to elvitegravir (T66A/I/K, E92G/Q, T97A, S147G, Q148H/K/R, and N155H), emtricitabine, and/or tenofovir was observed in 53% (16/30) of the STRIBILD-treatment failure subjects with evaluable genotypic resistance data who received at least 8 weeks of STRIBILD

and had HIV-1 RNA greater than 400 copies per mL at Week 96 or at the time of early study drug discontinuation. The most common substitutions that emerged were M184V/I (N=15) in HIV-1 RT and the primary elvitegravir resistance-associated substitutions, E92Q (N=9), N155H (N=5), Q148R (N=3), and T66I (N=2) in integrase; K65R in RT was also detected (N=5). In virus isolates harboring the observed primary elvitegravir resistance substitutions, additional substitutions in integrase were detected including H51Y, L68I/V, G70R, I73V, G140C, S153A and E157Q. All subjects with evaluable data for RT and IN and who developed integrase substitutions associated with elvitegravir resistance (N=13) also developed the M184I/V RT substitutions, conferring reduced susceptibility to both elvitegravir and emtricitabine. In phenotypic analyses, HIV-1 isolates expressing M184V/I RT substitutions showed reduced susceptibility to emtricitabine (42- to greater than 152-fold); those expressing the primary elvitegravir resistance-associated integrase substitutions showed reduced susceptibility to elvitegravir (6- to greater than 198-fold); and those expressing the K65R RT substitution showed reduced susceptibility to tenofovir (0.8- to 1.6-fold), compared to wild-type reference HIV-1.

Cross Resistance

STRIBILD-treatment failure subject isolates exhibited varying degrees of cross resistance within the INSTI and NRTI drug classes depending on the specific substitutions observed. These isolates remained susceptible to all NNRTIs and protease inhibitors.

Elvitegravir: Cross-resistance has been observed among INSTIs. Elvitegravir-resistant viruses showed varying degrees of cross-resistance in cell culture to raltegravir depending on the type and number of substitutions in HIV-1 integrase. Of the primary elvitegravir resistance-associated substitutions tested (T66A/I/K, E92G/Q, T97A, S147G, Q148H/K/R, and N155H), all but three (T66I, E92G, and S147G) conferred greater than 1.5-fold reduced susceptibility to raltegravir (above the biological cutoff for raltegravir) when introduced individually into a wild-type virus by site-directed mutagenesis. Of the primary raltegravir resistance-associated substitutions (Y143C/H/R, Q148H/K/R, and N155H), all but Y143C/H conferred greater than 2.5-fold reductions in susceptibility to elvitegravir (above the biological cutoff for elvitegravir).

Emtricitabine: Cross-resistance has been observed among NRTIs. Emtricitabine-resistant isolates harboring an M184V/I substitution in HIV-1 RT were cross-resistant to lamivudine. HIV-1 isolates containing the K65R RT substitution, selected *in vivo* by abacavir, didanosine, and tenofovir, demonstrated reduced susceptibility to inhibition by emtricitabine.

Tenofovir DF: Cross-resistance has been observed among NRTIs. The K65R substitution in HIV-1 RT selected by tenofovir is also selected in some HIV-1-infected patients treated with abacavir or didanosine. HIV-1 isolates with the K65R substitution also showed reduced susceptibility to emtricitabine and lamivudine. Therefore, cross-resistance among these NRTIs may occur in patients whose virus harbors the K65R substitution. HIV-1 isolates from patients (N=20) whose HIV-1 expressed a mean of 3 zidovudine-associated RT amino acid substitutions (M41L, D67N, K70R, L210W, T215Y/F, or K219Q/E/N) showed a 3.1-fold decrease in the susceptibility to tenofovir. Subjects whose virus expressed an L74V RT substitution without zidovudine resistance-associated substitutions (N=8) had reduced response to VIREAD. Limited data are available for patients whose virus expressed a Y115F substitution (N=3), Q151M substitution (N=2), or T69 insertion (N=4) in HIV-1 RT, all of whom had a reduced response in clinical trials.

13 NONCLINICAL TOXICOLOGY

13.1 Carcinogenesis, Mutagenesis, Impairment of Fertility

Elvitegravir: Long-term carcinogenicity studies of elvitegravir were carried out in mice (104 weeks) and in rats for up to 88 weeks (males) and 90 weeks (females). No drug-related increases in tumor incidence were found in mice at doses up to 2000 mg per kg per day alone or in combination with 25 mg per kg per day RTV at exposures 3- and 14-fold, respectively, the human systemic exposure at the recommended daily dose of 150 mg. No drug-related increases in tumor incidence were found in rats at doses up to 2000 mg per kg per day at exposures 12- to 27-fold, respectively in male and female, the human systemic exposure.

Elvitegravir was not genotoxic in the reverse mutation bacterial test (Ames test) and the rat micronucleus assay. In an *in vitro* chromosomal aberration test, elvitegravir was negative with metabolic activation; however, an equivocal response was observed without activation.

Elvitegravir did not affect fertility in male and female rats at approximately 16- and 30-fold higher exposures (AUC), respectively, than in humans at the therapeutic 150 mg daily dose.

Fertility was normal in the offspring of rats exposed daily from before birth (*in utero*) through sexual maturity at daily exposures (AUC) of approximately 18-fold higher than human exposures at the recommended 150 mg daily dose.

Cobicistat: In a long-term carcinogenicity study in mice, no drug-related increases in tumor incidence were observed at doses up to 50 and 100 mg/kg/day (males and females, respectively). Cobicistat exposures at these doses were approximately 7 (male) and 16 (females) times, respectively, the human systemic exposure at the therapeutic daily dose. In a long-term carcinogenicity study of cobicistat in rats, an increased incidence of follicular cell adenomas and/or carcinomas in the thyroid gland was observed at doses of 25 and 50 mg/kg/day in males, and at 30 mg/kg/day in females. The follicular cell findings are considered to be rat-specific, secondary to hepatic microsomal enzyme induction and thyroid hormone imbalance, and are not relevant for humans. At the highest doses tested in the rat carcinogenicity study, systemic exposures were approximately 2 times the human systemic exposure at the therapeutic daily dose.

Cobicistat was not genotoxic in the reverse mutation bacterial test (Ames test), mouse lymphoma or rat micronucleus assays.

Cobicistat did not affect fertility in male or female rats at daily exposures (AUC) approximately 4-fold higher than human exposures at the recommended 150 mg daily dose.

Fertility was normal in the offspring of rats exposed daily from before birth (*in utero*) through sexual maturity at daily exposures (AUC) of approximately 1.2-fold higher than human exposures at the recommended 150 mg daily dose.

Emtricitabine: In long-term carcinogenicity studies of emtricitabine, no drug-related increases in tumor incidence were found in mice at doses up to 750 mg per kg per day (23 times the human systemic exposure at the therapeutic dose of 200 mg per day) or in rats at doses up to 600 mg per kg per day (28 times the human systemic exposure at the therapeutic dose).

Emtricitabine was not genotoxic in the reverse mutation bacterial test (Ames test), mouse lymphoma or mouse micronucleus assays.

Emtricitabine did not affect fertility in male rats at approximately 140-fold or in male and female mice at approximately 60-fold higher exposures (AUC) than in humans given the recommended 200 mg daily dose. Fertility was normal in the offspring of mice exposed daily from before birth (*in utero*) through sexual maturity at daily exposures (AUC) of approximately 60-fold higher than human exposures at the recommended 200 mg daily dose.

Tenofovir Disoproxil Fumarate: Long-term oral carcinogenicity studies of tenofovir DF in mice and rats were carried out at exposures up to approximately 10 times (mice) and 4 times (rats) those observed in humans at the therapeutic dose for HIV-1 infection. At the high dose in female mice, liver adenomas were increased at exposures 10 times of that in humans. In rats, the study was negative for carcinogenic findings at exposures up to 4 times that observed in humans at the therapeutic dose.

Tenofovir DF was mutagenic in the *in vitro* mouse lymphoma assay and negative in an *in vitro* bacterial mutagenicity test (Ames test). In an *in vivo* mouse micronucleus assay, tenofovir DF was negative when administered to male mice.

There were no effects on fertility, mating performance or early embryonic development when tenofovir DF was administered to male rats at a dose equivalent to 10 times the human dose based on body surface area comparisons for 28 days prior to mating and to female rats for 15 days prior to mating through day seven of gestation. There was, however, an alteration of the estrous cycle in female rats.

14   CLINICAL STUDIES

The efficacy of STRIBILD is based on the analyses of 96-week data from two randomized, double-blind, active-controlled trials, Study 102 and Study 103, in treatment-naïve, HIV-1 infected subjects (N=1408, randomized and dosed) with baseline estimated creatinine clearance above 70 mL per min.

In Study 102, subjects were randomized in a 1:1 ratio to receive either STRIBILD (N=348) once daily or ATRIPLA (efavirenz 600 mg/emtricitabine 200 mg/tenofovir DF 300 mg; N=352) once daily. The mean age was 38 years (range 18–67), 89% were male, 63% were White, 28% were Black, and 2% were Asian. Twenty-four percent of subjects identified as Hispanic/Latino. The mean baseline plasma HIV-1 RNA was 4.8 $\log_{10}$ copies per mL (range 2.6–6.5). The mean baseline CD4+ cell count was 386 cells per mm^3 (range 3–1348) and 13% had CD4+ cell counts less than 200 cells per mm^3. Thirty-three percent of subjects had baseline viral loads greater than 100,000 copies per mL.

In Study 103, subjects were randomized in a 1:1 ratio to receive either STRIBILD (N=353) once daily or ATV 300 mg + RTV 100 mg + TRUVADA (emtricitabine 200 mg/tenofovir DF 300 mg) (N=355) once daily. The mean age was 38 years (range 19–72), 90% were male, 74% were White, 17% were Black, and 5% were Asian. Sixteen percent of subjects identified as Hispanic/Latino. The mean baseline plasma HIV-1 RNA was 4.8 $\log_{10}$ copies per mL (range 1.7–6.6). The mean baseline CD4+ cell count was 370 cells per mm^3 (range 5–1132) and 13% had CD4+ cell count less than 200 cells per mm^3. Forty-one percent of subjects had baseline viral loads greater than 100,000 copies per mL.

In both studies, subjects were stratified by baseline HIV-1 RNA (less than or equal to 100,000 copies per mL or greater than 100,000 copies per mL).

Treatment outcomes of Study 102 and Study 103 through 96 weeks are presented in Table 10.

[See table 10 above]

In Study 102, the mean increase from baseline in CD4+ cell count at Week 96 was 278 cells per mm^3 in the STRIBILD-treated subjects and 247 cells per mm^3 in the ATRIPLA-treated subjects. In Study 103, the mean increase from baseline in CD4+ cell count at Week 96 was 242 cells per mm^3 in the STRIBILD-treated subjects and 240 cells per mm^3 in the ATV + RTV + TRUVADA-treated subjects.

16   HOW SUPPLIED/STORAGE AND HANDLING

STRIBILD tablets are green, capsule-shaped, film-coated, debossed with "GSI" on one side and the number "1" sur-

Table 9 Drug Interactions: Changes in Pharmacokinetic Parameters for Coadministered Drug in the Presence of Elvitegravir plus Cobicistat, Cobicistat, or STRIBILD*

Coadministered Drug	Dose of Coadministered Drug (mg)	Elvitegravir Dose[†] (mg)	Cobicistat Booster Dose (mg)	N	Mean Ratio of Coadministered Drug Pharmacokinetic Parameters[‡] (90% CI); No effect = 1.00		
					C_{max}	AUC	C_{min}
Buprenorphine	16 – 24 once daily	150 once daily	150 once daily	17	1.12 (0.98 to 1.27)	1.35 (1.18 to 1.55)	1.66 (1.43 to 1.93)
Norbuprenorphine					1.24 (1.03 to 1.49)	1.42 (1.22 to 1.67)	1.57 (1.31 to 1.88)
Desipramine	50 single dose	N/A	150 once daily	8	1.24 (1.08,1.44)	1.65 (1.36,2.02)	NC
Digoxin	0.5 single dose	N/A	150 once daily	22	1.41 (1.29,1.55)	1.08 (1.00,1.17)	NC
Naloxone	4 – 6 once daily	150 once daily	150 once daily	17	0.72 (0.61, 0.85)	0.72 (0.59, 0.87)	N/A
Norgestimate/ ethinyl estradiol	0.180/0.215/ 0.250 norgestimate once daily	150 once daily[§]	150 once daily[§]	13	2.08 (2.00,2.17)	2.26 (2.15,2.37)	2.67 (2.43,2.92)
	0.025 ethinyl estradiol once daily				0.94 (0.86,1.04)	0.75 (0.69,0.81)	0.56 (0.52,0.61)
R-Methadone	80–120 daily	150 once daily	150 once daily	11	1.01 (0.91, 1.13)	1.07 (0.96, 1.19)	1.10 (0.95, 1.28)
S-Methadone					0.96 (0.87, 1.06)	1.00 (0.89, 1.12)	1.02 (0.89, 1.17)
Rifabutin	150 once every other day	150 once daily	150 once daily	12	1.09 (0.98,1.20)[¶]	0.92 (0.83,1.03)[¶]	0.94 (0.85,1.04)[¶]
25-O-desacetyl-rifabutin				12	4.84 (4.09,5.74)[¶]	6.25 (5.08,7.69)[¶]	4.94 (4.04,6.04)[¶]
Rosuvastatin	10 single dose	150 single dose	150 single dose	10	1.89 (1.48,2.42)	1.38 (1.14,1.67)	NC

* All interaction studies conducted in healthy volunteers.
† N/A = Not Applicable
‡ NC = Not Calculated
§ Study conducted with STRIBILD.
¶ Comparison based on rifabutin 300 mg once daily.

Table 10 Virologic Outcome of Randomized Treatment of Study 102 and Study 103 at Week 96*

	Study 102		Study 103	
	STRIBILD (N=348)	ATRIPLA (N=352)	STRIBILD (N=353)	ATV + RTV + TRUVADA (N=355)
Virologic Success HIV-1 RNA < 50 copies/mL	84%	82%	83%	82%
Treatment Difference	2.7% (95% CI = -2.9%, 8.3%)		1.1% (95% CI = -4.5%, 6.7%)	
Virologic Failure[†]	6%	8%	7%	7%
No Virologic Data at Week 96 Window				
Discontinued Study Drug Due to AE or Death[‡]	5%	6%	4%	6%
Discontinued Study Drug Due to Other Reasons and Last Available HIV-1 RNA < 50 copies/mL[§]	5%	4%	5%	5%
Missing Data During Window but on Study Drug	0%	1%	1%	0 %

* Week 96 window is between Day 631 and 714 (inclusive).
† Includes subjects who had ≥50 copies/mL in the Week 96 window, subjects who discontinued early due to lack or loss of efficacy, subjects who discontinued for reasons other than an adverse event, death or lack or loss of efficacy and at the time of discontinuation had a viral value of ≥50 copies/mL.
‡ Includes patients who discontinued due to adverse event or death at any time point from Day 1 through the time window if this resulted in no virologic data on treatment during the specified window.
§ Includes subjects who discontinued for reasons other than an adverse event, death or lack or loss of efficacy, e.g., withdrew consent, loss to follow-up, etc.

rounded by a square box (1) on the other side. Each bottle contains 30 tablets (NDC 61958-1201-1), a silica gel desiccant and closed with a child-resistant closure.

Store at 25 °C (77 °F), excursions permitted to 15–30 °C (59–86 °F) (see USP Controlled Room Temperature).
• Keep container tightly closed.

- Dispense only in original container.
- Do not use if seal over bottle opening is broken or missing.

17 PATIENT COUNSELING INFORMATION

See FDA-Approved Patient Labeling (Patient Information) A statement to patients and healthcare providers is included on the product's bottle label: ALERT: Find out about medicines that should NOT be taken with STRIBILD. Patients should be advised that:

- STRIBILD may interact with many drugs; therefore, patients should be advised to report to their healthcare provider the use of any other prescription or non-prescription medication or herbal products including St. John's wort.
- Patients should remain under the care of a healthcare provider when using STRIBILD.
- Patients should be informed that STRIBILD is not a cure for HIV-1 infection. Patients should stay on continuous HIV therapy to control HIV-1 infection and decrease HIV-related illnesses. Patients should be told that sustained decreases in plasma HIV RNA have been associated with a reduced risk of progression to AIDS and death.
- Patients should avoid doing things that can spread HIV-1 infection to others.
  - Do not share needles or other injection equipment.
  - Do not share personal items that can have blood or body fluids on them, like toothbrushes and razor blades.
  - Do not have any kind of sex without protection. Always practice safer sex by using a latex or polyurethane condom to lower the chance of sexual contact with semen, vaginal secretions, or blood.
  - Do not breastfeed. At least two of the drugs contained in STRIBILD can be passed to the baby in breast milk. It is not known whether this could harm the baby. Also, mothers with HIV-1 should not breastfeed because HIV-1 can be passed to the baby in breast milk.
- It is important to take STRIBILD on a regular dosing schedule with food and to avoid missing doses.
- Do not miss a dose of STRIBILD. If a patient misses a dose of STRIBILD, the patient should take the missed dose as soon as they remember. If it is almost time for the next dose of STRIBILD, the patient should not take the missed dose, but resume the usual dosing schedule. Inform the patient that he or she should not take more or less than the prescribed dose of STRIBILD at any one time.
- Lactic acidosis and severe hepatomegaly with steatosis, including fatal cases, have been reported. Advise patients that treatment with STRIBILD should be suspended if they develop clinical symptoms suggestive of lactic acidosis or pronounced hepatotoxicity (including nausea, vomiting, unusual or unexpected stomach discomfort, and weakness) [see Warnings and Precautions (5.1)].
- Instruct the patient that hepatitis B testing is recommended prior to initiating antiretroviral therapy. Severe acute exacerbations of hepatitis B have been reported in patients who are coinfected with HBV and HIV-1 and have discontinued EMTRIVA or VIREAD [see Warnings and Precautions (5.2)]. STRIBILD should not be discontinued without first informing their healthcare provider.
- Renal impairment, including cases of acute renal failure and Fanconi syndrome, has been reported in association with the use of STRIBILD. STRIBILD should be avoided with concurrent or recent use of a nephrotoxic agent (e.g., high dose or multiple NSAIDs) [see Warnings and Precautions (5.3)].
- STRIBILD should not be coadministered with other antiretroviral products because it provides a complete treatment regimen and because of potential drug interactions [see Warnings and Precautions (5.4) and Drug Interactions (7)].
- STRIBILD should not be administered in combination with ATRIPLA, COMPLERA, EMTRIVA, TRUVADA, or VIREAD; with drugs containing lamivudine, including COMBIVIR, EPIVIR or EPIVIR-HBV, EPZICOM, or TRIZIVIR; with drugs containing RTV or regimens containing RTV; or with HEPSERA [see Warnings and Precautions (5.4)].
- Decreases in bone mineral density have been observed with the use of STRIBILD. Assessment of bone mineral density (BMD) should be considered in patients who have a history of pathologic bone fracture or other risk factors for osteoporosis or bone loss [see Warnings and Precautions (5.5)].
- Redistribution or accumulation of body fat may occur in patients receiving antiretroviral therapy and that the cause and long-term health effects of these conditions are not known [see Warnings and Precautions (5.6)].
- In some patients with advanced HIV infection (AIDS), signs and symptoms of inflammation from previous infections may occur soon after anti-HIV treatment is started. It is believed that these symptoms are due to an improvement in the body's immune response, enabling the body to fight infections that may have been present with no obvi-

ous symptoms. Patients should be advised to inform their healthcare provider immediately of any symptoms of infection [see Warnings and Precautions (5.7)].

Patient Information
STRIBILD® (STRY-bild)
(elvitegravir, cobicistat, emtricitabine, and tenofovir disoproxil fumarate)
Tablets
Important: Ask your healthcare provider or pharmacist about medicines that should not be taken with STRIBILD. For more information, see the section "What should I tell my healthcare provider before taking STRIBILD?"
Read this Patient Information before you start taking STRIBILD and each time you get a refill. There may be new information. This information does not take the place of talking with your healthcare provider about your medical condition or treatment.
What is the most important information I should know about STRIBILD?
STRIBILD can cause serious side effects, including:
1. **Build-up of lactic acid in your blood (lactic acidosis).** Lactic acidosis can happen in some people who take STRIBILD or similar (nucleoside analogs) medicines. Lactic acidosis is a serious medical emergency that can lead to death.
Lactic acidosis can be hard to identify early, because the symptoms could seem like symptoms of other health problems. **Call your healthcare provider right away if you get any of the following symptoms which could be signs of lactic acidosis:**
   - feel very weak or tired
   - have unusual (not normal) muscle pain
   - have trouble breathing
   - have stomach pain with
     - nausea
     - vomiting
   - feel cold, especially in your arms and legs
   - feel dizzy or lightheaded
   - have a fast or irregular heartbeat
2. **Severe liver problems.** Severe liver problems can happen in people who take STRIBILD. In some cases, these liver problems can lead to death. Your liver may become large (hepatomegaly) and you may develop fat in your liver (steatosis).
   Call your healthcare provider right away if you get any of the following symptoms of liver problems:
   - your skin or the white part of your eyes turns yellow (jaundice)
   - dark "tea-colored" urine
   - light-colored bowel movements (stools)
   - loss of appetite for several days or longer
   - nausea
   - stomach pain**You may be more likely to get lactic acidosis or severe liver problems if you are female, very overweight (obese), or have been taking STRIBILD for a long time.**
3. **Worsening of Hepatitis B infection. If you have hepatitis B virus (HBV) infection and take STRIBILD, your HBV may get worse (flare-up) if you stop taking STRIBILD. A "flare-up" is when your HBV infection suddenly returns in a worse way than before.**
   - Do not run out of STRIBILD. Refill your prescription or talk to your healthcare provider before your STRIBILD is all gone.
   - Do not stop taking STRIBILD without first talking to your healthcare provider.
   - If you stop taking STRIBILD, your healthcare provider will need to check your health often and do blood tests regularly for several months to check your HBV infection. Tell your healthcare provider about any new or unusual symptoms you may have after you stop taking STRIBILD.
For more information about side effects, see the section "What are the possible side effects of STRIBILD?"
What is STRIBILD?
STRIBILD is a prescription medicine that is used without other antiretroviral medicines to treat Human Immunodeficiency Virus-1 (HIV-1) in adults who have never taken HIV-1 medicines before. HIV-1 is the virus that causes AIDS (Acquired Immune Deficiency Syndrome).
STRIBILD contains the prescription medicines elvitegravir, cobicistat, emtricitabine (EMTRIVA®) and tenofovir disoproxil fumarate (VIREAD®).
It is not known if STRIBILD is safe and effective in children under 18 years of age.
When used to treat HIV-1 infection, STRIBILD may:
- Reduce the amount of HIV-1 in your blood. This is called "viral load".
- Increase the number of CD4+ (T) cells in your blood that help fight off other infections.
- Reduce the amount of HIV-1 and increasing the CD4+ (T) cells in your blood may help improve your immune system. This may reduce your risk of death or getting infections that can happen when your immune system is weak (opportunistic infections).

STRIBILD does not cure HIV-1 infections or AIDS. You must stay on continuous HIV-1 therapy to control HIV-1 infection and decrease HIV-related illnesses.
Avoid doing things that can spread HIV-1 infection to others.
- Do not share or re-use needles or other injection equipment.
- Do not share personal items that can have blood or body fluids on them, like toothbrushes and razor blades.
- Do not have any kind of sex without protection. Always practice safer sex by using a latex or polyurethane condom to lower the chance of sexual contact with semen, vaginal secretions, or blood.
Ask your healthcare provider if you have any questions about how to prevent passing HIV-1 to other people.
Who should not take STRIBILD?
Do not take STRIBILD if you also take a medicine that contains:
- alfuzosin hydrochloride (UROXATRAL®)
- cisapride (PROPULSID®, PROPULSID QUICKSOLV®)
- ergot-containing medicines, including:
  - dihydroergotamine mesylate (D.H.E. 45®, MIGRANAL®)
  - ergotamine tartrate (CAFERGOT®, MIGERGOT®, ERGOSTAT®, MEDIHALER ERGOTAMINE®, WIGRAINE®, WIGRETTES®)
  - methylergonovine maleate (ERGOTRATE®, METHERGINE®)
- lovastatin (ADVICOR®, ALTOPREV®, MEVACOR®)
- oral midazolam
- pimozide (ORAP®)
- rifampin (RIFADIN®, RIFAMATE®, RIFATER®, RIMACTANE®)
- sildenafil (REVATIO®), when used for treating the lung problem, pulmonary arterial hypertension (PAH)
- simvastatin (SIMCOR®, VYTORIN®, ZOCOR®)
- triazolam (HALCION®)
- St. John's wort (Hypericum perforatum) or a product that contains St. John's wort

What should I tell my healthcare provider before taking STRIBILD?
Before taking STRIBILD, tell your healthcare provider if you:
- have liver problems including hepatitis B infection
- have kidney problems
- have bone problems
- have any other medical conditions
- are pregnant or plan to become pregnant. It is not known if STRIBILD can harm your unborn baby. Tell your healthcare provider if you become pregnant while taking STRIBILD.
  Pregnancy Registry. There is a pregnancy registry for women who take antiviral medicines during pregnancy. The purpose of this registry is to collect information about the health of you and your baby. Talk with your healthcare provider about how you can take part in this registry.
- are breastfeeding or plan to breastfeed. Do not breastfeed if you take STRIBILD.
  - You should not breastfeed if you have HIV-1 because of the risk of passing HIV-1 to your baby.
  - At least two of the medicines in STRIBILD can pass to your baby in your breast milk. It is not known if the other medicines in STRIBILD can pass into your breast milk.
Talk with your healthcare provider about the best way to feed your baby.

Tell your healthcare provider about all the medicines you take, including prescription and nonprescription medicines, vitamins, and herbal supplements. STRIBILD may affect the way other medicines work, and other medicines may affect how STRIBILD works.
You should not take STRIBILD if you also take:
- any other medicines to treat HIV-1 infection
- other medicines that contain tenofovir (ATRIPLA®, COMPLERA®, VIREAD®, TRUVADA®)
- other medicines that contain emtricitabine or lamivudine (ATRIPLA®, COMPLERA®, TRUVADA®, COMBIVIR®, EMTRIVA®, EPIVIR® or EPIVIR-HBV®, EPZICOM®, TRIZIVIR®)
- adefovir (HEPSERA®)
- ritonavir (NORVIR®, KALETRA®)
Especially tell your healthcare provider if you take:
- hormone-based contraceptives (birth control pills and patches)
- an antacid medicine that contains aluminum, magnesium hydroxide, or calcium carbonate. Take antacids at least 2 hours before or after you take STRIBILD.
- medicines to treat depression
- medicines to prevent organ transplant rejection
- medicines to treat high blood pressure
- any of the following medicines:
  - amiodarone (CORDARONE®, PACERONE®)
  - atorvastatin (LIPITOR®, CADUET®)
  - bepridil hydrochloride (VASCOR®, BEPADIN®)
  - bosentan (TRACLEER®)

- buspirone
- carbamazepine (CARBATROL®, EPITOL®, EQUETRO®, TEGRETOL®)
- clarithromycin (BIAXIN®, PREVPAC®)
- clonazepam (KLONOPIN®)
- clorazepate (GEN-XENE®, TRANXENE®)
- colchicine (COLCRYS®)
- medicines that contain dexamethasone
- diazepam (VALIUM®)
- digoxin (LANOXIN®)
- disopyramide (NORPACE®)
- estazolam
- ethosuximide (ZARONTIN®)
- flecainide (TAMBOCOR®)
- flurazepam
- fluticasone (FLOVENT®, FLONASE®, FLOVENT® DISKUS®, FLOVENT® HFA, VERAMYST®)
- itraconazole (SPORANOX®)
- ketoconazole (NIZORAL®)
- lidocaine (XYLOCAINE®)
- mexiletine
- oxcarbazepine (TRILEPTAL®)
- perphenazine
- phenobarbital (LUMINAL®)
- phenytoin (DILANTIN®, PHENYTEK®)
- propafenone (RYTHMOL®)
- quinidine (NEUDEXTA®)
- rifabutin (MYCOBUTIN®)
- rifapentine (PRIFTIN®)
- risperidone (RISPERDAL®, RISPERDAL CONSTA®)
- salmeterol (SEREVENT®) or salmeterol when taken in combination with fluticasone (ADVAIR DISKUS®, ADVAIR HFA®)
- sildenafil (VIAGRA®), tadalafil (CIALIS®) or vardenafil (LEVITRA®, STAXYN®), for the treatment of erectile dysfunction (ED). If you get dizzy or faint (low blood pressure), have vision changes or have an erection that last longer than 4 hours, call your healthcare provider or get medical help right away.
- tadalafil (ADCIRCA®), for the treatment of pulmonary arterial hypertension
- telithromycin (KETEK®)
- thioridazine
- voriconazole (VFEND®)
- warfarin (COUMADIN®, JANTOVEN®)
- zolpidem (AMBIEN®, EDLULAR®, INTERMEZZO®, ZOLPIMIST®)

Ask your healthcare provider or pharmacist if you are not sure if your medicine is one that is listed above. Do not start any new medicines while you are taking STRIBILD without first talking with your healthcare provider or pharmacist. Know the medicines you take. Keep a list of your medicines and show it to your healthcare provider and pharmacist when you get a new medicine.

How should I take STRIBILD?
- Take STRIBILD exactly as your healthcare provider tells you to take it. **STRIBILD is taken by itself (not with other antiretroviral medicines) to treat HIV-1 infection.**
- STRIBILD is usually taken 1 time each day.
- Take STRIBILD with food.
- Do not change your dose or stop taking STRIBILD without first talking with your healthcare provider. Stay under a healthcare provider's care when taking STRIBILD.
- Do not miss a dose of STRIBILD. If you miss a dose of STRIBILD, take the missed dose as soon as you remember. If it is almost time for your next dose of STRIBILD, do not take the missed dose. Take the next dose of STRIBILD at your regular time. Do not take 2 doses at the same time to make up for a missed dose.
- If you take too much STRIBILD, call your healthcare provider or go to the nearest hospital emergency room right away.
- When your STRIBILD supply starts to run low, get more from your healthcare provider or pharmacy. This is very important because the amount of virus in your blood may increase if the medicine is stopped for even a short time. The virus may develop resistance to STRIBILD and become harder to treat.

What are the possible side effects of STRIBILD?
STRIBILD may cause the following serious side effects, including:
- **See "What is the most important information I should know about STRIBILD?"**
- **New or worse kidney problems, including kidney failure.** Your healthcare provider should do blood and urine tests to check your kidneys before you start and while you are taking STRIBILD. Your healthcare provider may tell you to stop taking STRIBILD if you develop new or worse kidney problems.
- **Bone problems** can happen in some people who take STRIBILD. Bone problems include bone pain, softening or thinning (which may lead to fractures). Your healthcare provider may need to do tests to check your bones.
- **Changes in body fat** can happen in people who take HIV-1 medicine. These changes may include increased amount of

fat in the upper back and neck ("buffalo hump"), breast, and around the middle of your body (trunk). Loss of fat from the legs, arms and face may also happen. The exact cause and long-term health effects of these conditions are not known.
- **Changes in your immune system (Immune Reconstitution Syndrome)** can happen when you start taking HIV-1 medicines. Your immune system may get stronger and begin to fight infections that have been hidden in your body for a long time. Tell your healthcare provider right away if you start having any new symptoms after starting your HIV-1 medicine.

The most common side effects of STRIBILD include:
- nausea
- diarrhea

Tell your healthcare provider if you have any side effect that bothers you or that does not go away.

These are not all the possible side effects of STRIBILD. For more information, ask your healthcare provider or pharmacist.

Call your healthcare provider for medical advice about side effects. You may report side effects to FDA at 1-800-FDA-1088.

How should I store STRIBILD?
- Store STRIBILD at room temperature between 68 °F to 77 °F (20 °C to 25 °C).
- Keep STRIBILD in its original container.
- Keep the container tightly closed.
- Do not use STRIBILD if the seal over the bottle opening is broken or missing.

Keep STRIBILD and all medicines out of reach of children.
General information about STRIBILD.
Medicines are sometimes prescribed for purposes other than those listed in a Patient Information leaflet. Do not use STRIBILD for a condition for which it was not prescribed. Do not give STRIBILD to other people, even if they have the same symptoms you have. It may harm them.
This leaflet summarizes the most important information about STRIBILD. If you would like more information, talk with your healthcare provider. You can ask your healthcare provider or pharmacist for information about STRIBILD that is written for health professionals.
For more information, call 1-800-445-3235 or go to www.STRIBILD.com.

What are the ingredients in STRIBILD?
Active ingredients: elvitegravir, cobicistat, emtricitabine, and tenofovir disoproxil fumarate
Inactive ingredients: lactose monohydrate, microcrystalline cellulose, silicon dioxide, croscarmellose sodium, hydroxypropyl cellulose, sodium lauryl sulfate, and magnesium stearate. The tablets are film-coated with a coating material containing indigo carmine (FD&C blue #2) aluminum lake, polyethylene glycol, polyvinyl alcohol, talc, titanium dioxide, and yellow iron oxide.
This Patient Information has been approved by the U.S. Food and Drug Administration.
Manufactured and distributed by:
Gilead Sciences, Inc.
Foster City, CA 94404
Issued: October 2013
COMPLERA, EMTRIVA, HEPSERA, STRIBILD, TRUVADA, and VIREAD are trademarks of Gilead Sciences, Inc., or its related companies. ATRIPLA is a trademark of Bristol-Myers Squibb & Gilead Sciences, LLC. All other trademarks referenced herein are the property of their respective owners.
203100-GS-002
Shown in Product Identification Guide, page 307

TRUVADA®   Rx
[tru-VAH-dah]
(emtricitabine/tenofovir disoproxil fumarate)
tablets, for oral use

HIGHLIGHTS OF PRESCRIBING INFORMATION
These highlights do not include all the information needed to use TRUVADA safely and effectively. See full prescribing information for TRUVADA.
TRUVADA® (emtricitabine/tenofovir disoproxil fumarate)
tablets, for oral use
Initial U.S. Approval: 2004

WARNING: LACTIC ACIDOSIS/SEVERE HEPATOMEGALY WITH STEATOSIS, POST-TREATMENT ACUTE EXACERBATION OF HEPATITIS B, and RISK OF DRUG RESISTANCE WITH USE OF TRUVADA FOR PrEP IN UNDIAGNOSED HIV-1 INFECTION
See full prescribing information for complete boxed warning.
- **Lactic acidosis and severe hepatomegaly with steatosis, including fatal cases, have been reported with the use of nucleoside analogs, including VIREAD, a component of TRUVADA. (5.1)**

- **TRUVADA is not approved for the treatment of chronic hepatitis B virus (HBV) infection. Severe acute exacerbations of hepatitis B have been reported in patients coinfected with HIV-1 and HBV who have discontinued TRUVADA. Therefore, hepatic function should be monitored closely in HBV-infected patients who discontinue TRUVADA. If appropriate, initiation of anti-hepatitis B therapy may be warranted. (5.2)**
- **TRUVADA used for a PrEP indication must only be prescribed to individuals confirmed to be HIV-negative immediately prior to initial use and periodically during use. Drug-resistant HIV-1 variants have been identified with the use of TRUVADA for a PrEP indication following undetected acute HIV-1 infection. Do not initiate TRUVADA for a PrEP indication if signs or symptoms of acute HIV infection are present unless negative infection status is confirmed. (5.9)**

RECENT MAJOR CHANGES

Indications and Usage
Treatment of HIV-1 infection (1.1)   06/2013
Dosage and Administration (2.3)   10/2013
Warnings and Precautions
New Onset or Worsening Renal Impairment
(5.3)   10/2013
Coadministration with Other Products (5.4)   06/2013
Bone Effects of Tenofovir DF (5.5)   10/2013

INDICATIONS AND USAGE

TRUVADA is a combination of EMTRIVA and VIREAD, both nucleoside analog HIV-1 reverse transcriptase inhibitors.
TRUVADA is indicated in combination with other antiretroviral agents for the treatment of HIV-1 infection in adults and pediatric patients 12 years of age and older. (1)
TRUVADA is indicated in combination with safer sex practices for pre-exposure prophylaxis (PrEP) to reduce the risk of sexually acquired HIV-1 in adults at high risk. (1)

DOSAGE AND ADMINISTRATION

Treatment of HIV-1 Infection (2.1)
- Recommended dose in adults and pediatric patients (12 years of age and older and weighing greater than or equal to 35 kg): One tablet once daily taken orally with or without food. (2.1)
- Recommended dose in renally impaired HIV-1 infected adult patients: Creatinine clearance 30–49 mL/min: 1 tablet every 48 hours. (2.3) CrCl below 30 mL/min or hemodialysis: Do not use TRUVADA. (2.3)
Pre-exposure Prophylaxis (2.2)
- Recommended dose in HIV-1 uninfected adults: One tablet once daily taken orally with or without food. (2.2)
- Recommended dose in renally impaired HIV-uninfected individuals: Do not use TRUVADA in HIV-uninfected individuals if CrCl is below 60 mL/min. If a decrease in CrCl is observed in uninfected individuals while using TRUVADA for PrEP, evaluate potential causes and reassess potential risks and benefits of continued use. (2.3)

DOSAGE FORMS AND STRENGTHS

Tablets: 200 mg of emtricitabine and 300 mg of tenofovir disoproxil fumarate. (3)

CONTRAINDICATIONS

Do not use TRUVADA for pre-exposure prophylaxis in individuals with unknown or positive HIV-1 status. TRUVADA should be used in HIV-infected patients only in combination with other antiretroviral agents. (4)

WARNINGS AND PRECAUTIONS

- New onset or worsening renal impairment: Can include acute renal failure and Fanconi syndrome. Assess estimated creatinine clearance before initiating treatment with TRUVADA. In patients at risk for renal dysfunction, assess estimated creatinine clearance, serum phosphorus, urine glucose and urine protein before initiating treatment with TRUVADA and periodically during treatment. Avoid administering Truvada with concurrent or recent use of nephrotoxic drugs. (5.3)
- Coadministration with Other Products: Do not use with drugs containing emtricitabine or tenofovir disoproxil fumarate including ATRIPLA, COMPLERA, EMTRIVA, STRIBILD, VIREAD; or with drugs containing lamivudine. Do not administer in combination with HEPSERA. (5.4)
- Decreases in bone mineral density (BMD): Consider assessment of BMD in patients with a history of pathologic fracture or other risk factors for osteoporosis or bone loss. (5.5)
- Redistribution/accumulation of body fat: Observed in patients receiving antiretroviral therapy. (5.6)

- Immune reconstitution syndrome: May necessitate further evaluation and treatment. (5.7)
- Triple nucleoside-only regimens: Early virologic failure has been reported in HIV-infected patients. Monitor carefully and consider treatment modification. (5.8)
- Comprehensive management to reduce the risk of acquiring HIV-1: Use as part of a comprehensive prevention strategy including other prevention measures; strictly adhere to dosing schedule. (5.9)
- Management to reduce the risk of acquiring HIV-1 drug resistance:

  Prior to initiating TRUVADA for PrEP - if clinical symptoms consistent with acute viral infection are present and recent (<1 month) exposures are suspected, delay starting PrEP for at least one month and reconfirm negative HIV-1 status or use a test approved by the FDA as an aid in the diagnosis of HIV-1 infection, including acute or primary HIV-1 infection.

  While using TRUVADA for PrEP - HIV-1 screening tests should be repeated at least every 3 months. (5.9)

―――――――ADVERSE REACTIONS―――――――

In HIV1 infected patients, the most common adverse reactions (incidence greater than or equal to 10%) are diarrhea, nausea, fatigue, headache, dizziness, depression, insomnia, abnormal dreams, and rash. (6.1)
In HIV-1 uninfected individuals in PrEP trials, adverse reactions that were reported by more than 2% of TRUVADA subjects and more frequently than by placebo subjects were headache, abdominal pain and weight decreased. (6.2)

To report SUSPECTED ADVERSE REACTIONS, contact Gilead Sciences, Inc. at 1-800-445-3235 or FDA at 1-800-FDA-1088 or www.fda.gov/medwatch

―――――――DRUG INTERACTIONS―――――――

- Didanosine: Tenofovir disoproxil fumarate increases didanosine concentrations. Use with caution and monitor for evidence of didanosine toxicity (e.g., pancreatitis, neuropathy) when coadministered. Consider dose reductions or discontinuations of didanosine if warranted. (7.1)
- HIV-1 protease inhibitors: Coadministration decreases atazanavir concentrations and increases tenofovir concentrations. When coadministered with TRUVADA, use atazanavir given with ritonavir. Coadministration of TRUVADA with atazanavir and ritonavir, darunavir and ritonavir, or lopinavir/ritonavir increases tenofovir concentrations. Monitor for evidence of tenofovir toxicity. (7.2)

―――――――USE IN SPECIFIC POPULATIONS―――――――

- Nursing mothers: Women infected with HIV-1 should be instructed not to breast feed. (8.3)

See 17 for PATIENT COUNSELING INFORMATION and Medication Guide

Revised: 12/2013

FULL PRESCRIBING INFORMATION: CONTENTS*
WARNING: LACTIC ACIDOSIS/SEVERE HEPATO-MEGALY WITH STEATOSIS, POST TREATMENT ACUTE EXACERBATION OF HEPATITIS B, and RISK OF DRUG RESISTANCE WITH USE OF TRUVADA FOR PRE-EXPOSURE PROPHYLAXIS (PrEP) IN UNDIAGNOSED EARLY HIV-1 INFECTION

FULL PRESCRIBING INFORMATION

> **WARNING: LACTIC ACIDOSIS/SEVERE HEPA-TOMEGALY WITH STEATOSIS, POST TREAT-MENT ACUTE EXACERBATION OF HEPATITIS B, and RISK OF DRUG RESISTANCE WITH USE OF TRUVADA FOR PRE-EXPOSURE PROPHY-LAXIS (PrEP) IN UNDIAGNOSED EARLY HIV-1 INFECTION**
>
> **Lactic acidosis and severe hepatomegaly with steatosis, including fatal cases, have been reported with the use of nucleoside analogs, including VIREAD, a component of TRUVADA, in combination with other antiretrovirals [See Warnings and Precautions (5.1)].**
>
> **TRUVADA is not approved for the treatment of chronic hepatitis B virus (HBV) infection and the safety and efficacy of TRUVADA have not been established in patients coinfected with HBV and HIV-1. Severe acute exacerbations of hepatitis B have been reported in patients who are coinfected with HBV and HIV-1 and have discontinued TRUVADA. Therefore, hepatic function should be monitored closely with both clinical and laboratory follow-up for at least several months in patients who are infected with HBV and discontinue TRUVADA. If appropriate, initiation of anti-hepatitis B therapy may be warranted [See Warnings and Precautions (5.2)].**
>
> **TRUVADA used for a PrEP indication must only be prescribed to individuals confirmed to be HIV-negative immediately prior to initiating and periodically (at least every 3 months) during use. Drug-resistant HIV-1 variants have been identified with use of TRUVADA for a PrEP indication following undetected acute HIV-1 infection. Do not initiate TRUVADA for a PrEP indication if signs or symptoms of acute HIV-1 infection are present unless negative infection status is confirmed [See Warnings and Precautions (5.9)].**

1   INDICATIONS AND USAGE
1.1   Treatment of HIV-1 Infection
TRUVADA®, a combination of EMTRIVA® and VIREAD®, is indicated in combination with other antiretroviral agents (such as non-nucleoside reverse transcriptase inhibitors or protease inhibitors) for the treatment of HIV-1 infection in adults and pediatric patients 12 years of age and older.
The following points should be considered when initiating therapy with TRUVADA for the treatment of HIV-1 infection:

- It is not recommended that TRUVADA be used as a component of a triple nucleoside regimen.
- TRUVADA should not be coadministered with ATRIPLA®, COMPLERA®, EMTRIVA, STRIBILD®, VIREAD or lamivudine-containing products [See Warnings and Precautions (5.4)].
- In treatment experienced patients, the use of TRUVADA should be guided by laboratory testing and treatment history [See Clinical Pharmacology (12.4)].

1.2   Pre-Exposure Prophylaxis
TRUVADA is indicated in combination with safer sex practices for pre-exposure prophylaxis (PrEP) to reduce the risk of sexually acquired HIV-1 in adults at high risk. This indi-

cation is based on clinical trials in men who have sex with men (MSM) at high risk for HIV-1 infection and in heterosexual serodiscordant couples [See Clinical Studies (14.2, 14.3)].
When considering TRUVADA for pre-exposure prophylaxis the following factors may help to identify individuals at high risk:

- has partner(s) known to be HIV-1 infected, or
- engages in sexual activity within a high prevalence area or social network and one or more of the following:
  - inconsistent or no condom use
  - diagnosis of sexually transmitted infections
  - exchange of sex for commodities (such as money, food, shelter, or drugs)
  - use of illicit drugs or alcohol dependence
  - incarceration
  - partner(s) of unknown HIV-1 status with any of the factors listed above

When prescribing TRUVADA for pre-exposure prophylaxis, healthcare providers must:

- prescribe TRUVADA as part of a comprehensive prevention strategy because TRUVADA is not always effective in preventing the acquisition of HIV-1 infection [See Warnings and Precautions (5.9)];
- counsel all uninfected individuals to strictly adhere to the recommended TRUVADA dosing schedule because the effectiveness of TRUVADA in reducing the risk of acquiring HIV-1 was strongly correlated with adherence as demonstrated by measurable drug levels in clinical trials [See Warnings and Precautions (5.9)];
- confirm a negative HIV-1 test immediately prior to initiating TRUVADA for a PrEP indication. If clinical symptoms consistent with acute viral infection are present and recent (<1 month) exposures are suspected, delay starting PrEP for at least one month and reconfirm negative HIV-1 status or use a test approved by the FDA as an aid in the diagnosis of HIV-1 infection, including acute or primary HIV-1 infection. [See Warnings and Precautions (5.9)]; and
- screen for HIV-1 infection at least once every 3 months while taking TRUVADA for PrEP.

2   DOSAGE AND ADMINISTRATION
2.1   Recommended Dose for Treatment of HIV-1 Infection
The recommended dose of TRUVADA in adults and in pediatric patients 12 years of age and older with body weight greater than or equal to 35 kg (greater than or equal to 77 lb) is one tablet (containing 200 mg of emtricitabine and 300 mg of tenofovir disoproxil fumarate) once daily taken orally with or without food.
2.2   Recommended Dose for Pre-exposure Prophylaxis
The dose of TRUVADA in HIV-1 uninfected adults is one tablet (containing 200 mg of emtricitabine and 300 mg of tenofovir disoproxil fumarate) once daily taken orally with or without food.
2.3   Dose Adjustment for Renal Impairment
Treatment of HIV-1 Infection
Significantly increased drug exposures occurred when EMTRIVA or VIREAD were administered to subjects with moderate to severe renal impairment [See EMTRIVA or VIREAD Package Insert]. Therefore, adjust the dosing interval of TRUVADA in HIV-1 infected adult patients with baseline creatinine clearance 30–49 mL/min using the recommendations in Table 1. These dosing interval recommendations are based on modeling of single-dose pharmacokinetic data in non-HIV infected subjects. The safety and effectiveness of these dosing interval adjustment recommendations have not been clinically evaluated in patients with moderate renal impairment, therefore clinical response to treatment and renal function should be closely monitored in these patients [See Warnings and Precautions (5.3)].
No dose adjustment is necessary for HIV-1 infected patients with mild renal impairment (creatinine clearance 50–80 mL/min). No data are available to make dose recommendations in pediatric patients with renal impairment.

Table 1 Dosage Adjustment for HIV-1 Infected Adult Patients with Altered Creatinine Clearance

	Creatinine Clearance (mL/min)*		
	≥50	30–49	<30 (Including Patients Requiring Hemodialysis)
Recommended Dosing Interval	Every 24 hours	Every 48 hours	TRUVADA should not be administered.

* Calculated using ideal (lean) body weight

Routine monitoring of estimated creatinine clearance, serum phosphorus, urine glucose, and urine protein should be performed in all individuals with mild renal impairment [See Warnings and Precautions (5.3)].

Pre-exposure Prophylaxis
Do not use TRUVADA for a PrEP indication in HIV-1 uninfected individuals with estimated creatinine clearance below 60 mL/min [See Warnings and Precautions (5.3)]. Routine monitoring of estimated creatinine clearance, serum phosphorus, urine glucose, and urine protein should be performed in all individuals with mild renal impairment. If a decrease in estimated creatinine clearance is observed in uninfected individuals while using TRUVADA for PrEP, evaluate potential causes and re-assess potential risks and benefits of continued use [See Warnings and Precautions (5.3)].

3 DOSAGE FORMS AND STRENGTHS

TRUVADA is available as tablets. Each tablet contains 200 mg of emtricitabine and 300 mg of tenofovir disoproxil fumarate (which is equivalent to 245 mg of tenofovir disoproxil). The tablets are blue, capsule-shaped, film-coated, debossed with "GILEAD" on one side and with "701" on the other side.

4 CONTRAINDICATIONS

Do not use TRUVADA for pre-exposure prophylaxis in individuals with unknown or positive HIV-1 status. TRUVADA should be used in HIV-infected patients only in combination with other antiretroviral agents.

5 WARNINGS AND PRECAUTIONS

5.1 Lactic Acidosis/Severe Hepatomegaly with Steatosis
Lactic acidosis and severe hepatomegaly with steatosis, including fatal cases, have been reported with the use of nucleoside analogs, including VIREAD, a component of TRUVADA, in combination with other antiretrovirals. A majority of these cases have been in women. Obesity and prolonged nucleoside exposure may be risk factors. Particular caution should be exercised when administering nucleoside analogs to any patient or uninfected individual with known risk factors for liver disease; however, cases have also been reported in HIV-1 infected patients with no known risk factors. Treatment with TRUVADA should be suspended in any patient or uninfected individual who develops clinical or laboratory findings suggestive of lactic acidosis or pronounced hepatotoxicity (which may include hepatomegaly and steatosis even in the absence of marked transaminase elevations).

5.2 HBV Infection
It is recommended that all individuals be tested for the presence of chronic hepatitis B virus (HBV) before initiating TRUVADA. TRUVADA is not approved for the treatment of chronic HBV infection and the safety and efficacy of TRUVADA have not been established in patients infected with HBV. Severe acute exacerbations of hepatitis B have been reported in patients who are coinfected with HBV and HIV-1 and have discontinued TRUVADA. In some patients infected with HBV and treated with EMTRIVA, the exacerbations of hepatitis B were associated with liver decompensation and liver failure. Patients who are infected with HBV should be closely monitored with both clinical and laboratory follow-up for at least several months after stopping treatment with TRUVADA. If appropriate, initiation of anti-hepatitis B therapy may be warranted. HBV -uninfected individuals should be offered vaccination.

5.3 New Onset or Worsening Renal Impairment
Emtricitabine and tenofovir are principally eliminated by the kidney. Renal impairment, including cases of acute renal failure and Fanconi syndrome (renal tubular injury with severe hypophosphatemia), has been reported with the use of VIREAD [See Adverse Reactions (6.3)].

It is recommended that estimated creatinine clearance be assessed in all individuals prior to initiating therapy and as clinically appropriate during therapy with TRUVADA. In patients at risk of renal dysfunction, including patients who have previously experienced renal events while receiving HEPSERA®, it is recommended that estimated creatinine clearance, serum phosphorus, urine glucose, and urine protein be assessed prior to initiation of TRUVADA, and periodically during TRUVADA therapy.
TRUVADA should be avoided with concurrent or recent use of a nephrotoxic agent (e.g., high-dose or multiple non-steroidal anti-inflammatory drugs (NSAIDs)) [See Drug Interactions (7.3)]. Cases of acute renal failure after initiation of high dose or multiple NSAIDs have been reported in HIV-infected patients with risk factors for renal dysfunction who appeared stable on tenofovir DF. Some patients required hospitalization and renal replacement therapy. Alternatives to NSAIDs should be considered, if needed, in patients at risk for renal dysfunction.
Persistent or worsening bone pain, pain in extremities, fractures and/or muscular pain or weakness may be manifestations of proximal renal tubulopathy and should prompt an evaluation of renal function in at-risk patients.
Treatment of HIV-1 Infection
Dosing interval adjustment of TRUVADA and close monitoring of renal function are recommended in all patients with estimated creatinine clearance 30–49 mL/min, [See Dosage and Administration (2.3)]. No safety or efficacy data are available in patients with renal impairment who received TRUVADA using these dosing guidelines, so the potential benefit of TRUVADA therapy should be assessed against the potential risk of renal toxicity. TRUVADA should not be administered to patients with estimated creatinine clearance below 30 mL/min or patients requiring hemodialysis.
Pre-exposure Prophylaxis
TRUVADA for a PrEP indication should not be used if estimated creatinine clearance is less than 60 mL/min. If a decrease in estimated creatinine clearance is observed in uninfected individuals while using TRUVADA for PrEP, evaluate potential causes and re-assess potential risks and benefits of continued use [See Dosage and Administration (2.3)].

5.4 Coadministration with Other Products
TRUVADA is a fixed-dose combination of emtricitabine and tenofovir disoproxil fumarate. Do not coadminister TRUVADA with ATRIPLA, COMPLERA, EMTRIVA, STRIBILD, or VIREAD. Due to similarities between emtricitabine and lamivudine, do not coadminister TRUVADA with other drugs containing lamivudine, including Combivir (lamivudine/zidovudine), Epivir or Epivir-HBV (lamivudine), Epzicom (abacavir sulfate/lamivudine), or Trizivir (abacavir sulfate/lamivudine/zidovudine).
Do not coadminister TRUVADA with HEPSERA (adefovir dipivoxil).

5.5 Bone Effects of Tenofovir DF
Bone Mineral Density:
In clinical trials in HIV-1 infected adults and in a clinical trial of HIV-1 uninfected individuals, tenofovir DF was associated with slightly greater decreases in bone mineral density (BMD) and increases in biochemical markers of bone metabolism, suggesting increased bone turnover relative to comparators [See Adverse Reactions (6.2) and VIREAD prescribing information]. Serum parathyroid hormone levels and 1,25 Vitamin D levels were also higher in subjects receiving tenofovir DF.
Clinical trials evaluating tenofovir DF in pediatric and adolescent subjects were conducted. Under normal circumstances, BMD increases rapidly in pediatric patients. In HIV-1 infected subjects aged 2 years to less than 18 years, bone effects were similar to those observed in adult subjects and suggest increased bone turnover. Total body BMD gain was less in the tenofovir DF treated HIV-1 infected pediatric subjects as compared to the control groups. Similar trends were observed in chronic hepatitis B infected adolescent subjects aged 12 years to less than 18 years. In all pediatric trials, skeletal growth (height) appeared to be unaffected. For more information, please consult the VIREAD prescribing information.
The effects of tenofovir DF-associated changes in BMD and biochemical markers on long-term bone health and future fracture risk are unknown. Assessment of BMD should be considered for adult and pediatric patients who have a history of pathologic bone fracture or other risk factors for osteoporosis or bone loss. Although the effect of supplementation with calcium and vitamin D was not studied, such supplementation may be beneficial. If bone abnormalities are suspected then appropriate consultation should be obtained.
Mineralization Defects:
Cases of osteomalacia associated with proximal renal tubulopathy, manifested as bone pain or pain in extremities and which may contribute to fractures, have been reported in association with the use of tenofovir DF [See Adverse Reactions (6.3)]. Arthralgias and muscle pain or weakness have also been reported in cases of proximal renal tubulopathy. Hypophosphatemia and osteomalacia secondary to proximal renal tubulopathy should be considered in patients at risk of renal dysfunction who present with persistent or worsening bone or muscle symptoms while receiving products containing tenofovir DF [See Warnings and Precautions (5.3)].

5.6 Fat Redistribution
Redistribution/accumulation of body fat including central obesity, dorsocervical fat enlargement (buffalo hump), peripheral wasting, facial wasting, breast enlargement, and "cushingoid appearance" have been observed in HIV-1 infected patients receiving antiretroviral therapy. The mechanism and long-term consequences of these events are currently unknown. A causal relationship has not been established.

5.7 Immune Reconstitution Syndrome
Immune reconstitution syndrome has been reported in HIV-1 infected patients treated with combination antiretroviral therapy, including TRUVADA. During the initial phase of combination antiretroviral treatment, HIV-1 infected patients whose immune system responds may develop an inflammatory response to indolent or residual opportunistic infections [such as *Mycobacterium avium* infection, cytomegalovirus, *Pneumocystis jirovecii* pneumonia (PCP), or tuberculosis], which may necessitate further evaluation and treatment.

Autoimmune disorders (such as Graves' disease, polymyositis, and Guillain-Barré syndrome) have also been reported to occur in the setting of immune reconstitution, however, the time to onset is more variable, and can occur many months after initiation of treatment.

5.8 Early Virologic Failure
Clinical trials in HIV-1 infected subjects have demonstrated that certain regimens that only contain three nucleoside reverse transcriptase inhibitors (NRTI) are generally less effective than triple drug regimens containing two NRTIs in combination with either a non-nucleoside reverse transcriptase inhibitor or a HIV-1 protease inhibitor. In particular, early virological failure and high rates of resistance substitutions have been reported. Triple nucleoside regimens should therefore be used with caution. Patients on a therapy utilizing a triple nucleoside-only regimen should be carefully monitored and considered for treatment modification.

5.9 Comprehensive Management to Reduce the Risk of Acquiring HIV-1
Use TRUVADA for pre-exposure prophylaxis only as part of a comprehensive prevention strategy that includes other prevention measures, such as safer sex practices, because TRUVADA is not always effective in preventing the acquisition of HIV-1 [See Clinical Studies (14.2 and 14.3)].

■ Counsel uninfected individuals about safer sex practices that include consistent and correct use of condoms, knowledge of their HIV-1 status and that of their partner(s), and regular testing for other sexually transmitted infections that can facilitate HIV-1 transmission (such as syphilis and gonorrhea).
■ Inform uninfected individuals about and support their efforts in reducing sexual risk behavior.

Use TRUVADA to reduce the risk of acquiring HIV-1 only in individuals confirmed to be HIV-negative. HIV-1 resistance substitutions may emerge in individuals with undetected HIV-1 infection who are taking only TRUVADA, because TRUVADA alone does not constitute a complete treatment regimen for HIV-1 treatment [See Microbiology: Resistance (12.4)]; therefore, care should be taken to minimize drug exposure in HIV-infected individuals.

■ Many HIV-1 tests, such as rapid tests, detect anti-HIV antibodies and may not identify HIV-1 during the acute stage of infection. Prior to initiating TRUVADA for a PrEP indication, evaluate seronegative individuals for current or recent signs or symptoms consistent with acute viral infections (e.g., fever, fatigue, myalgia, skin rash, etc.) and ask about potential exposure events (e.g., unprotected, or condom broke during sex with an HIV-1 infected partner) that may have occurred within the last month.
• If clinical symptoms consistent with acute viral infection are present and recent (<1 month) exposures are suspected, delay starting PrEP for at least one month and reconfirm HIV-1 status or use a test approved by the FDA as an aid in the diagnosis of HIV-1 infection, including acute or primary HIV-1 infection.
■ While using TRUVADA for a PrEP indication, HIV-1 screening tests should be repeated at least every 3 months. If symptoms consistent with acute HIV-1 infection develop following a potential exposure event, PrEP should be discontinued until negative infection status is confirmed using a test approved by the FDA as an aid in the diagnosis of HIV-1, including acute or primary HIV-1 infection.

Counsel uninfected individuals to strictly adhere to the recommended TRUVADA dosing schedule. The effectiveness of TRUVADA in reducing the risk of acquiring HIV-1 is strongly correlated with adherence as demonstrated by measurable drug levels in clinical trials [See Clinical Studies (14.2 and 14.3)].

6 ADVERSE REACTIONS

The following adverse reactions are discussed in other sections of the labeling:
• Lactic Acidosis/Severe Hepatomegaly with Steatosis [See Boxed Warning, Warnings and Precautions (5.1)].
• Severe Acute Exacerbations of hepatitis B [See Boxed Warning, Warnings and Precautions (5.2)].
• New Onset or Worsening Renal Impairment [See Warnings and Precautions (5.3)].
• Bone Effects of Tenofovir DF [See Warnings and Precautions (5.5)].
• Immune Reconstitution Syndrome [See Warnings and Precautions (5.7)].

6.1 Adverse Reactions from Clinical Trials Experience in HIV-1 Infected Subjects
Because clinical trials are conducted under widely varying conditions, adverse reaction rates observed in the clinical trials of a drug cannot be directly compared to rates in the clinical trials of another drug and may not reflect the rates observed in practice.
Clinical Trials in Adult Subjects
The most common adverse reactions (incidence greater than or equal to 10%, any severity) occurring in Study 934, an

active-controlled clinical trial of efavirenz, emtricitabine, and tenofovir disoproxil fumarate, include diarrhea, nausea, fatigue, headache, dizziness, depression, insomnia, abnormal dreams, and rash. See also Table 2 for the frequency of treatment-emergent adverse reactions (Grades 2–4) occurring in greater than or equal to 5% of subjects treated in any treatment group in this trial.

Skin discoloration, manifested by hyperpigmentation on the palms and/or soles, was generally mild and asymptomatic. The mechanism and clinical significance are unknown.

Study 934 - Treatment Emergent Adverse Reactions: In Study 934, 511 antiretroviral-naive subjects received either VIREAD + EMTRIVA administered in combination with efavirenz (N=257) or zidovudine/lamivudine administered in combination with efavirenz (N=254) for 144 weeks. Subjects had a mean age of 40 years (range 20 to 73 years) and were predominantly male (88%). Overall, 65% were White, 17% were Black, and 13% were Hispanic. Adverse reactions observed in this trial were generally consistent with those seen in other trials in treatment-experienced or treatment-naive subjects receiving VIREAD and/or EMTRIVA (Table 2).

Table 2 Selected Treatment-Emergent Adverse Reactions* (Grades 2–4) Reported in ≥5% in Any Treatment Group in Study 934 (0–144 Weeks)

	FTC + TDF + EFV[†]	AZT/3TC + EFV
	N=257	N=254
Gastrointestinal Disorder		
Diarrhea	9%	5%
Nausea	9%	7%
Vomiting	2%	5%
General Disorders and Administration Site Condition		
Fatigue	9%	8%
Infections and Infestations		
Sinusitis	8%	4%
Upper respiratory tract infections	8%	5%
Nasopharyngitis	5%	3%
Nervous System Disorders		
Headache	6%	5%
Dizziness	8%	7%
Psychiatric Disorders		
Depression	9%	7%

Insomnia	5%	7%
Skin and Subcutaneous Tissue Disorders		
Rash event[‡]	7%	9%

* Frequencies of adverse reactions are based on all treatment-emergent adverse events, regardless of relationship to study drug.

† From Weeks 96 to 144 of the trial, subjects received TRUVADA with efavirenz in place of VIREAD + EMTRIVA with efavirenz.

‡ Rash event includes rash, exfoliative rash, rash generalized, rash macular, rash maculo-papular, rash pruritic, and rash vesicular.

Laboratory Abnormalities: Laboratory abnormalities observed in this trial were generally consistent with those seen in other trials of VIREAD and/or EMTRIVA (Table 3).

Table 3 Significant Laboratory Abnormalities Reported in ≥1% of Subjects in Any Treatment Group in Study 934 (0–144 Weeks)

	FTC + TDF + EFV*	AZT/3TC + EFV
	N=257	N=254
Any ≥ Grade 3 Laboratory Abnormality	30%	26%
Fasting Cholesterol (>240 mg/dL)	22%	24%
Creatine Kinase (M: >990 U/L) (F: >845 U/L)	9%	7%
Serum Amylase (>175 U/L)	8%	4%
Alkaline Phosphatase (>550 U/L)	1%	0%
AST (M: >180 U/L) (F: >170 U/L)	3%	3%
ALT (M: >215 U/L) (F: >170 U/L)	2%	3%

Hemoglobin (<8.0 mg/dL)	0%	4%
Hyperglycemia (>250 mg/dL)	2%	1%
Hematuria (>75 RBC/HPF)	3%	2%
Glycosuria (≥3+)	<1%	1%
Neutrophils (<750/mm³)	3%	5%
Fasting Triglycerides (>750 mg/dL)	4%	2%

* From Weeks 96 to 144 of the trial, subjects received TRUVADA with efavirenz in place of VIREAD + EMTRIVA with efavirenz.

In addition to the events described above for Study 934, other adverse reactions that occurred in at least 5% of subjects receiving EMTRIVA or VIREAD with other antiretroviral agents in clinical trials include anxiety, arthralgia, increased cough, dyspepsia, fever, myalgia, pain, abdominal pain, back pain, paresthesia, peripheral neuropathy (including peripheral neuritis and neuropathy), pneumonia, and rhinitis.

In addition to the laboratory abnormalities described above for Study 934, Grades 3–4 laboratory abnormalities of increased bilirubin (>2.5 × ULN), increased pancreatic amylase (>2.0 × ULN), increased or decreased serum glucose (<40 or >250 mg/dL), and increased serum lipase (>2.0 × ULN) occurred in up to 3% of subjects treated with EMTRIVA or VIREAD with other antiretroviral agents in clinical trials.

Clinical Trials in Pediatric Subjects 12 Years of Age and Older

Emtricitabine: In addition to the adverse reactions reported in adults, anemia and hyperpigmentation were observed in 7% and 32%, respectively, of pediatric subjects (3 months to less than 18 years of age) who received treatment with EMTRIVA in the larger of two open-label, uncontrolled pediatric trials (N=116). For additional information, please consult the EMTRIVA prescribing information.

Tenofovir Disoproxil Fumarate: In a pediatric clinical trial conducted in subjects 12 to less than 18 years of age, the adverse reactions observed in pediatric subjects who received treatment with VIREAD were consistent with those observed in clinical trials of VIREAD in adults [*See Warnings and Precautions (5.5)*].

6.2   Adverse Reactions from Clinical Trial Experience in HIV-1 Uninfected Adult Subjects

No new adverse reactions to TRUVADA were identified from two randomized placebo-controlled clinical trials (iPrEx, Partners PrEP) in which 2830 HIV-1 uninfected adults received TRUVADA once daily for pre-exposure prophylaxis. Subjects were followed for a median of 71 weeks and 87 weeks, respectively. These trials enrolled HIV-negative individuals ranging in age from 18 to 67 years. The iPrEx trial enrolled only males or transgender females of Hispanic/Latino (72%), White (18%), Black (9%) and Asian (5%) race. The Partners PrEP trial enrolled both males (61–64% across treatment groups) and females in Kenya and Uganda. Table 4 provides a list of all adverse events that occurred ≥2% of subjects in any treatment group in the iPrEx and Partners PrEP trials.

Laboratory Abnormalities: Table 5 provides a list of laboratory abnormalities observed in both trials. Six subjects in the TDF-containing arms of the Partners PrEP trial discontinued participation in the study due to an increase in blood creatinine compared with no discontinuations in the placebo group. One subject in the TRUVADA arm of the iPrEx trial discontinued from the study due to an increase in blood creatinine and another due to low phosphorous.

In addition to the laboratory abnormalities described above, Grade 1 proteinuria (1+) occurred in 6% of subjects receiving TRUVADA in the iPrEx trial. Grades 2–3 proteinuria (2–4+) and glycosuria (3+) occurred in less than 1% of subjects treated with TRUVADA in the iPrEx trial and Partners PrEP trial.

[See table 4 below]

[See table 5 at top of next page]

Changes in Bone Mineral Density:

In clinical trials of HIV-1 uninfected individuals, decreases in BMD were observed. In the iPrEx trial, a substudy of 503 subjects found mean changes from baseline in BMD ranging from -0.4% to -1.0% across total hip, spine, femoral neck, and trochanter in the TRUVADA group compared with the placebo group, which returned toward baseline after discontinuation of treatment. Thirteen percent of subjects receiving TRUVADA vs. 6% of subjects receiving placebo lost at least 5% of BMD at the spine during treatment. Bone fractures were reported in 1.7% of the TRUVADA group compared with 1.4% in the placebo group. No correlation between BMD and fractures was noted [*See Clinical Studies*

Table 4 Selected Adverse Events (All Grades) Reported in ≥2% in Any Treatment Group in the iPrEx Trial and Partners PrEP Trial

	iPrEx Trial		Partners PrEP Trial	
	FTC/TDF (N=1251)	Placebo (N=1248)	FTC/TDF (N=1579)	Placebo (N= 1584)
Gastrointestinal Disorders				
Diarrhea	7%	8%	2%	3%
Abdominal pain	4%	2%	-*	-
Infections and Infestations				
Pharyngitis	13%	16%	-	-
Urethritis	5%	7%	-	-
Urinary tract infection	2%	2%	5%	7%
Syphilis	6%	5%	-	-
Secondary syphilis	6%	4%	-	-
Anogenital warts	2%	3%	-	-
Musculoskeletal and Connective Tissue Disorders				
Back pain	5%	5%	-	-
Nervous System Disorders				
Headache	7%	6%	-	-
Psychiatric Disorders				
Depression	6%	7%	-	-
Anxiety	3%	3%	-	-
Reproductive System and Breast Disorders				
Genital ulceration	2%	2%	2%	2%
Investigations				
Weight decreased	3%	2%	-	-

* Not reported or reported below 2%.

(14.2)]. The Partners PrEP trial found similar fracture rates between treatment and placebo groups (0.8% and 0.6%, respectively). No BMD evaluations were conducted during this trial *[See Clinical Studies (14.3)].*

6.3 Postmarketing Experience

The following adverse reactions have been identified during postapproval use of VIREAD. No additional adverse reactions have been identified during postapproval use of EMTRIVA. Because postmarketing reactions are reported voluntarily from a population of uncertain size, it is not always possible to reliably estimate their frequency or establish a causal relationship to drug exposure.

Immune System Disorders
allergic reaction, including angioedema
Metabolism and Nutrition Disorders
lactic acidosis, hypokalemia, hypophosphatemia
Respiratory, Thoracic, and Mediastinal Disorders
dyspnea
Gastrointestinal Disorders
pancreatitis, increased amylase, abdominal pain
Hepatobiliary Disorders
hepatic steatosis, hepatitis, increased liver enzymes (most commonly AST, ALT gamma GT)
Skin and Subcutaneous Tissue Disorders
rash
Musculoskeletal and Connective Tissue Disorders
rhabdomyolysis, osteomalacia (manifested as bone pain and which may contribute to fractures), muscular weakness, myopathy
Renal and Urinary Disorders
acute renal failure, renal failure, acute tubular necrosis, Fanconi syndrome, proximal renal tubulopathy, interstitial nephritis (including acute cases), nephrogenic diabetes insipidus, renal insufficiency, increased creatinine, proteinuria, polyuria
General Disorders and Administration Site Conditions
asthenia

The following adverse reactions, listed under the body system headings above, may occur as a consequence of proximal renal tubulopathy: rhabdomyolysis, osteomalacia, hypokalemia, muscular weakness, myopathy, hypophosphatemia.

7 DRUG INTERACTIONS

No drug interaction trials have been conducted using TRUVADA tablets. Drug interaction trials have been conducted with emtricitabine and tenofovir disoproxil fumarate, the components of TRUVADA. This section describes clinically relevant drug interactions observed with emtricitabine and tenofovir disoproxil fumarate *[See Clinical Pharmacology (12.3)].*

7.1 Didanosine

Coadministration of TRUVADA and didanosine should be undertaken with caution and patients receiving this combination should be monitored closely for didanosine-associated adverse reactions. Didanosine should be discontinued in patients who develop didanosine-associated adverse reactions.

When tenofovir disoproxil fumarate was administered with didanosine the C_{max} and AUC of didanosine increased significantly *[See Clinical Pharmacology (12.3)].* The mechanism of this interaction is unknown. Higher didanosine concentrations could potentiate didanosine-associated adverse reactions, including pancreatitis, and neuropathy. Suppression of CD4+ cell counts has been observed in patients receiving tenofovir DF with didanosine 400 mg daily.

In patients weighing greater than 60 kg, the didanosine dose should be reduced to 250 mg when it is coadministered with TRUVADA. Data are not available to recommend a dose adjustment of didanosine for adult or pediatric patients weighing less than 60 kg. When coadministered, TRUVADA and Videx EC may be taken under fasted conditions or with a light meal (less than 400 kcal, 20% fat).

7.2 HIV-1 Protease Inhibitors

Tenofovir decreases the AUC and C_{min} of atazanavir *[See Clinical Pharmacology (12.3)].* When coadministered with TRUVADA, it is recommended that atazanavir 300 mg is given with ritonavir 100 mg. TRUVADA should not be coadministered with atazanavir without ritonavir.

Lopinavir/ritonavir, atazanavir coadministered with ritonavir, and darunavir coadministered with ritonavir have been shown to increase tenofovir concentrations *[See Clinical Pharmacology (12.3)].* Tenofovir disoproxil fumarate is a substrate of P-glycoprotein (Pgp) and breast cancer resistance protein (BCRP) transporters. When tenofovir disoproxil fumarate is co-administered with an inhibitor of these transporters, an increase in absorption may be observed. Patients receiving TRUVADA concomitantly with lopinavir/ritonavir, ritonavir-boosted atazanavir, or ritonavir-boosted darunavir should be monitored for tenofovir-associated adverse reactions. TRUVADA should be discontinued in patients who develop tenofovir-associated adverse reactions.

Table 5 Laboratory Abnormalities (Highest Toxicity Grade) Reported for Each Subject in the iPrEx Trial and Partners PrEP Trial

	Grade*		iPrEx Trial FTC/TDF N= 1251	iPrEx Trial Placebo N= 1248	Partners PrEP Trial FTC/TDF N=1579	Partners PrEP Trial Placebo N=1584
Creatinine	1	(1.1–1.3 × ULN)	27 (2%)	21 (2%)	18 (1%)	12 (<1%)
	2–4	(> 1.4 × ULN)	5 (<1%)	3 (<1%)	2 (<1%)	1 (<1%)
Phosphorus	1	(2.5 – <LLN mg/dL)	81 (7%)	110 (9%)	NR †	NR †
	2–4	(<2.0 mg/dL)	123 (10%)	101 (8%)	140 (9%)	136 (9%)
AST	1	(1.25–<2.5 × ULN)	175 (14%)	175 (14%)	20 (1%)	25 (2%)
	2–4	(> 2.6 × ULN)	57 (5%)	61 (5%)	10 (<1%)	4 (<1%)
ALT	1	(1.25–<2.5 × ULN)	178 (14%)	194 (16%)	21 (1%)	13 (<1%)
	2–4	(> 2.6 × ULN)	84 (7%)	82 (7%)	4 (<1%)	6 (<1%)
Hemoglobin	1	(8.5 – 10 mg/dL)	49 (4%)	62 (5%)	56 (4%)	39 (2%)
	2–4	(<9.4 mg/dL)	13 (1%)	19 (2%)	28 (2%)	39 (2%)
Neutrophils	1	(1000–1300/mm³)	23 (2%)	25 (2%)	208 (13%)	163 (10%)
	2–4	(<750/mm³)	7 (<1%)	7 (<1%)	73 (5%)	56 (3%)

* Grading is per DAIDS criteria.
† Grade 1 phosphorus was not reported for the Partners PrEP trial.

7.3 Drugs Affecting Renal Function

Emtricitabine and tenofovir are primarily excreted by the kidneys by a combination of glomerular filtration and active tubular secretion *[See Clinical Pharmacology (12.3)].* No drug-drug interactions due to competition for renal excretion have been observed; however, coadministration of TRUVADA with drugs that are eliminated by active tubular secretion may increase concentrations of emtricitabine, tenofovir, and/or the coadministered drug. Some examples include, but are not limited to acyclovir, adefovir dipivoxil, cidofovir, ganciclovir, valacyclovir, valganciclovir, aminoglycosides (e.g., gentamicin), and high-dose or multiple NSAIDs *[See Warnings and Precautions (5.3)].* Drugs that decrease renal function may increase concentrations of emtricitabine and/or tenofovir.

8 USE IN SPECIFIC POPULATIONS

8.1 Pregnancy

Pregnancy Category B
Antiretroviral Pregnancy Registry: To monitor fetal outcomes of pregnant women exposed to TRUVADA, an Antiretroviral Pregnancy Registry (APR) has been established. Healthcare providers are encouraged to register patients by calling 1-800-258-4263.

Risk Summary
TRUVADA has been evaluated in a limited number of women during pregnancy and postpartum. Available human and animal data suggest that TRUVADA does not increase the risk of major birth defects overall compared to the background rate. There are, however, no adequate and well-controlled trials in pregnant women. Because the studies in humans cannot rule out the possibility of harm, TRUVADA should be used during pregnancy only if clearly needed. If an uninfected individual becomes pregnant while taking TRUVADA for a PrEP indication, careful consideration should be given to whether use of TRUVADA should be continued, taking into account the potential increased risk of HIV-1 infection during pregnancy.

Clinical Considerations
As of July 2011, the APR has received prospective reports of 764 and 1219 exposures to emtricitabine- and tenofovir-containing regimens, respectively in the first trimester, 321 and 455 exposures, respectively, in second trimester, and 140 and 257 exposures, respectively, in the third trimester. Birth defects occurred in 18 of 764 (2.4%) live births for emtricitabine-containing regimens and 27 of 1219 (2.2%) live births for tenofovir-containing regimens (first trimester exposure) and 10 of 461 (2.2%) live births for emtricitabine-containing regimens and 15 of 714 (2.1%) live births for tenofovir-containing regimens (second/third trimester exposure). Among pregnant women in the U.S. reference population, the background rate of birth defects is 2.7%. There was no association between emtricitabine or tenofovir and overall birth defects observed in the APR.

Animal Data
Emtricitabine:
The incidence of fetal variations and malformations was not increased in embryofetal toxicity studies performed with emtricitabine in mice at exposures (AUC) approximately 60-fold higher and in rabbits at approximately 120-fold higher than human exposures at the recommended daily dose.

Tenofovir Disoproxil Fumarate:
Reproduction studies have been performed in rats and rabbits at doses up to 14 and 19 times the human dose based on body surface area comparisons and revealed no evidence of impaired fertility or harm to the fetus due to tenofovir.

8.3 Nursing Mothers

Nursing Mothers: The Centers for Disease Control and Prevention recommend that HIV-1 infected mothers not breast-feed their infants to avoid risking postnatal transmission of HIV-1.

Studies in humans have shown that both tenofovir and emtricitabine are excreted in human milk. Because the risks of low level exposure to emtricitabine and tenofovir to infants are unknown, **mothers should be instructed not to breast-feed if they are receiving TRUVADA**, whether they are taking TRUVADA for treatment or to reduce the risk of acquiring HIV-1.

Emtricitabine
Samples of breast milk obtained from five HIV-1 infected mothers show that emtricitabine is secreted in human milk. Breastfeeding infants whose mothers are being treated with emtricitabine may be at risk for developing viral resistance to emtricitabine. Other emtricitabine-associated risks in infants breastfed by mothers being treated with emtricitabine are unknown.

Tenofovir Disoproxil Fumarate
Samples of breast milk obtained from five HIV-1 infected mothers show that tenofovir is secreted in human milk. Tenofovir-associated risks, including the risk of viral resistance to tenofovir, in infants breastfed by mothers being treated with tenofovir disoproxil fumarate are unknown.

8.4 Pediatric Use

TRUVADA should only be administered to HIV-1 infected pediatric patients 12 years of age and older with body weight greater than or equal to 35 kg. Because it is a fixed-dose combination tablet, TRUVADA cannot be adjusted for patients of lower age and weight. Safety and efficacy have not been established in pediatric patients less than 12 years of age or weighing less than 35 kg *[See Warnings and Precautions (5.5), Adverse Reactions (6.1) and Clinical Pharmacology (12.3)].*

8.5 Geriatric Use

Clinical trials of EMTRIVA or VIREAD did not include sufficient numbers of subjects aged 65 and over to determine whether they respond differently from younger subjects. In general, dose selection for the elderly patients should be cautious, keeping in mind the greater frequency of decreased hepatic, renal, or cardiac function, and of concomitant disease or other drug therapy.

8.6 Patients with Impaired Renal Function

Treatment of HIV-1 Infection
The dosing interval for TRUVADA should be modified in HIV-infected adult patients with estimated creatinine clearance of 30–49 mL/min. TRUVADA should not be used in patients with estimated creatinine clearance below 30 mL/min

and in patients with end-stage renal disease requiring dialysis. *[See Dosage and Administration (2.3)].*

Pre-exposure Prophylaxis
TRUVADA for a PrEP indication should not be used in HIV-1 uninfected individuals with estimated creatinine clearance below 60 mL/min. If a decrease in estimated creatinine clearance is observed in uninfected individuals while using TRUVADA for PrEP, evaluate potential causes and re-assess potential risks and benefits of continued use *[See Dosage and Administration (2.3)].*

10 OVERDOSAGE

If overdose occurs, the patient must be monitored for evidence of toxicity, and standard supportive treatment applied as necessary.

Emtricitabine: Limited clinical experience is available at doses higher than the therapeutic dose of EMTRIVA. In one clinical pharmacology trial, single doses of emtricitabine 1200 mg were administered to 11 subjects. No severe adverse reactions were reported.

Hemodialysis treatment removes approximately 30% of the emtricitabine dose over a 3-hour dialysis period starting within 1.5 hours of emtricitabine dosing (blood flow rate of 400 mL/min and a dialysate flow rate of 600 mL/min). It is not known whether emtricitabine can be removed by peritoneal dialysis.

Tenofovir Disoproxil Fumarate: Limited clinical experience at doses higher than the therapeutic dose of VIREAD 300 mg is available. In one trial, 600 mg tenofovir disoproxil fumarate was administered to 8 subjects orally for 28 days, and no severe adverse reactions were reported. The effects of higher doses are not known.

Tenofovir is efficiently removed by hemodialysis with an extraction coefficient of approximately 54%. Following a single 300 mg dose of VIREAD, a four-hour hemodialysis session removed approximately 10% of the administered tenofovir dose.

11 DESCRIPTION

TRUVADA tablets are fixed dose combination tablets containing emtricitabine and tenofovir disoproxil fumarate. EMTRIVA is the brand name for emtricitabine, a synthetic nucleoside analog of cytidine. Tenofovir disoproxil fumarate (tenofovir DF) is converted in vivo to tenofovir, an acyclic nucleoside phosphonate (nucleotide) analog of adenosine 5'-monophosphate. Both emtricitabine and tenofovir exhibit inhibitory activity against HIV-1 reverse transcriptase.

Emtricitabine: The chemical name of emtricitabine is 5-fluoro-1-(2R,5S)-[2-(hydroxymethyl)-1,3-oxathiolan-5-yl]cytosine. Emtricitabine is the (-) enantiomer of a thio analog of cytidine, which differs from other cytidine analogs in that it has a fluorine in the 5-position.

It has a molecular formula of $C_8H_{10}FN_3O_3S$ and a molecular weight of 247.24. It has the following structural formula:

Emtricitabine is a white to off-white crystalline powder with a solubility of approximately 112 mg/mL in water at 25 °C. The partition coefficient (log p) for emtricitabine is -0.43 and the pKa is 2.65.

Tenofovir Disoproxil Fumarate: Tenofovir disoproxil fumarate is a fumaric acid salt of the bis-isopropoxycarbonyloxymethyl ester derivative of tenofovir. The chemical name of tenofovir disoproxil fumarate is 9-[(R)-2[[bis[[(isopropoxycarbonyl)oxy]- methoxy]phosphinyl]methoxy]propyl]adenine fumarate (1:1). It has a molecular formula of $C_{19}H_{30}N_5O_{10}P • C_4H_4O_4$ and a molecular weight of 635.52. It has the following structural formula:

Tenofovir disoproxil fumarate is a white to off-white crystalline powder with a solubility of 13.4 mg/mL in water at 25 °C. The partition coefficient (log p) for tenofovir disoproxil is 1.25 and the pKa is 3.75. All dosages are expressed in terms of tenofovir disoproxil fumarate except where otherwise noted.

TRUVADA tablets are for oral administration. Each film-coated tablet contains 200 mg of emtricitabine and 300 mg of tenofovir disoproxil fumarate, (which is equivalent to 245 mg of tenofovir disoproxil), as active ingredients. The tablets also include the following inactive ingredients: cros-

carmellose sodium, lactose monohydrate, magnesium stearate, microcrystalline cellulose, and pregelatinized starch (gluten free). The tablets are coated with Opadry II Blue Y-30-10701, which contains FD&C Blue #2 aluminum lake, hydroxypropyl methylcellulose 2910, lactose monohydrate, titanium dioxide, and triacetin.

12 CLINICAL PHARMACOLOGY

For additional information on Mechanism of Action, Antiviral Activity, Resistance and Cross Resistance, please consult the EMTRIVA and VIREAD prescribing information.

12.1 Mechanism of Action
TRUVADA is a fixed-dose combination of antiviral drugs emtricitabine and tenofovir disoproxil fumarate *[See Clinical Pharmacology (12.4)].*

12.3 Pharmacokinetics
TRUVADA: One TRUVADA tablet was bioequivalent to one EMTRIVA capsule (200 mg) plus one VIREAD tablet (300 mg) following single-dose administration to fasting healthy subjects (N=39).

Emtricitabine: The pharmacokinetic properties of emtricitabine are summarized in Table 6. Following oral administration of EMTRIVA, emtricitabine is rapidly absorbed with peak plasma concentrations occurring at 1–2 hours post-dose. Less than 4% of emtricitabine binds to human plasma proteins in vitro and the binding is independent of concentration over the range of 0.02–200 μg/mL. Following administration of radiolabelled emtricitabine, approximately 86% is recovered in the urine and 13% is recovered as metabolites. The metabolites of emtricitabine include 3'-sulfoxide diastereomers and their glucuronic acid conjugate. Emtricitabine is eliminated by a combination of glomerular filtration and active tubular secretion. Following a single oral dose of EMTRIVA, the plasma emtricitabine half-life is approximately 10 hours.

Tenofovir Disoproxil Fumarate: The pharmacokinetic properties of tenofovir disoproxil fumarate are summarized in Table 6. Following oral administration of VIREAD, maximum tenofovir serum concentrations are achieved in 1.0 ± 0.4 hour. Less than 0.7% of tenofovir binds to human plasma proteins in vitro and the binding is independent of concentration over the range of 0.01–25 μg/mL. Approximately 70–80% of the intravenous dose of tenofovir is recovered as unchanged drug in the urine. Tenofovir is eliminated by a combination of glomerular filtration and active tubular secretion. Following a single oral dose of VIREAD, the terminal elimination half-life of tenofovir is approximately 17 hours.

Table 6 Single Dose Pharmacokinetic Parameters for Emtricitabine and Tenofovir in Adults*

	Emtricitabine	Tenofovir
Fasted Oral Bioavailability† (%)	92 (83.1–106.4)	25 (NC–45.0)
Plasma Terminal Elimination Half-Life† (hr)	10 (7.4–18.0)	17 (12.0–25.7)
C_{max}‡ (μg/mL)	1.8 ± 0.72§	0.30 ± 0.09
AUC‡ (μg·hr/mL)	10.0 ± 3.12§	2.29 ± 0.69
CL/F‡ (mL/min)	302 ± 94	1043 ± 115
CL_{renal}‡ (mL/min)	213 ± 89	243 ± 33

* NC = Not calculated
† Median (range)
‡ Mean (± SD)
§ Data presented as steady state values

Effects of Food on Oral Absorption
TRUVADA may be administered with or without food. Administration of TRUVADA following a high fat meal (784 kcal; 49 grams of fat) or a light meal (373 kcal; 8 grams of fat) delayed the time of tenofovir C_{max} by approximately 0.75 hour. The mean increases in tenofovir AUC and C_{max} were approximately 35% and 15%, respectively, when administered with a high fat or light meal, compared to administration in the fasted state. In previous safety and efficacy trials, VIREAD (tenofovir) was taken under fed conditions. Emtricitabine systemic exposures (AUC and C_{max}) were unaffected when TRUVADA was administered with either a high fat or a light meal.

Special Populations
Race
Emtricitabine: No pharmacokinetic differences due to race have been identified following the administration of EMTRIVA.

Tenofovir Disoproxil Fumarate: There were insufficient numbers from racial and ethnic groups other than Caucasian to adequately determine potential pharmacokinetic differences among these populations following the administration of VIREAD.

Gender
Emtricitabine and Tenofovir Disoproxil Fumarate: Emtricitabine and tenofovir pharmacokinetics are similar in male and female subjects.

Pediatric Patients
TRUVADA should not be administered to HIV-1 infected pediatric patients less than 12 years of age or weighing less than 35 kg (less than 77 lb).

Emtricitabine: The pharmacokinetics of emtricitabine at steady state were determined in 27 HIV-1-infected pediatric subjects 13 to 17 years of age receiving a daily dose of 6 mg/kg up to a maximum dose of 240 mg oral solution or a 200 mg capsule; 26 of 27 subjects in this age group received the 200 mg EMTRIVA capsule. Mean (± SD) C_{max} and AUC were 2.7 ± 0.9 μg/mL and 12.6 ± 5.4 μg•hr/mL, respectively. Exposures achieved in pediatric subjects 12 to less than 18 years of age were similar to those achieved in adults receiving a once daily dose of 200 mg.

Tenofovir Disoproxil Fumarate: Steady-state pharmacokinetics of tenofovir were evaluated in 8 HIV-1 infected pediatric subjects (12 to less than 18 years). Mean (± SD) C_{max} and AUC_{tau} are 0.38 ± 0.13 μg/mL and 3.39 ± 1.22 μg•hr/mL, respectively. Tenofovir exposure achieved in these pediatric subjects receiving oral daily doses of VIREAD 300 mg was similar to exposures achieved in adults receiving once-daily doses of VIREAD 300 mg.

Geriatric Patients
Pharmacokinetics of emtricitabine and tenofovir have not been fully evaluated in the elderly (65 years of age and older).

Patients with Impaired Renal Function
The pharmacokinetics of emtricitabine and tenofovir are altered in subjects with renal impairment *[See Warnings and Precautions (5.3)].* In adult subjects with creatinine clearance below 50 mL/min, C_{max} and $AUC_{0-∞}$ of emtricitabine and tenofovir were increased. It is recommended that the dosing interval for TRUVADA be modified in HIV-infected adult patients with estimated creatinine clearance 30–49 mL/min. No data are available to make dose recommendations in pediatric patients with renal impairment. TRUVADA should not be used in patients with estimated creatinine clearance below 30 mL/min and in patients with end-stage renal disease requiring dialysis *[See Dosage and Administration (2.3)].*

TRUVADA for a PrEP indication should not be used in HIV-1 uninfected individuals with estimated creatinine clearance below 60 mL/min. If a decrease in estimated creatinine clearance is observed in uninfected individuals while using TRUVADA for PrEP, evaluate potential causes and re-assess potential risks and benefits of continued use *[See Dosage and Administration (2.3)].*

Patients with Hepatic Impairment
The pharmacokinetics of tenofovir following a 300 mg dose of VIREAD have been studied in non-HIV infected subjects with moderate to severe hepatic impairment. There were no substantial alterations in tenofovir pharmacokinetics in subjects with hepatic impairment compared with unimpaired subjects. The pharmacokinetics of TRUVADA or emtricitabine have not been studied in subjects with hepatic impairment; however, emtricitabine is not significantly metabolized by liver enzymes, so the impact of liver impairment should be limited.

Assessment of Drug Interactions
The steady state pharmacokinetics of emtricitabine and tenofovir were unaffected when emtricitabine and tenofovir disoproxil fumarate were administered together versus each agent dosed alone.

In vitro studies and clinical pharmacokinetic drug-drug interaction trials have shown that the potential for CYP mediated interactions involving emtricitabine and tenofovir with other medicinal products is low.

No clinically significant drug interactions have been observed between emtricitabine and famciclovir, indinavir, stavudine, tenofovir disoproxil fumarate, and zidovudine (see Tables 7 and 8). Similarly, no clinically significant drug interactions have been observed between tenofovir disoproxil fumarate and efavirenz, methadone, nelfinavir, oral contraceptives, or ribavirin in trials conducted in healthy volunteers (see Tables 9 and 10).

[See table 7 at top of next page]
[See table 8 at top of next page]
[See table 9 at top of page 822]
[See table 10 at top of page 823]

Coadministration of tenofovir disoproxil fumarate with didanosine results in changes in the pharmacokinetics of didanosine that may be of clinical significance. Concomitant dosing of tenofovir disoproxil fumarate and didanosine enteric-coated capsules significantly increases the C_{max} and AUC of didanosine. When didanosine 250 mg enteric-coated capsules were administered with tenofovir disoproxil fumarate, systemic exposures of didanosine were similar to those seen with the 400 mg enteric-coated capsules alone under fasted conditions. The mechanism of this interaction is unknown. See *Drug Interactions (7.1)* regarding use of didanosine with VIREAD.

12.4 Microbiology

Mechanism of Action

Emtricitabine: Emtricitabine, a synthetic nucleoside analog of cytidine, is phosphorylated by cellular enzymes to form emtricitabine 5'-triphosphate. Emtricitabine 5'-triphosphate inhibits the activity of the HIV-1 reverse transcriptase (RT) by competing with the natural substrate deoxycytidine 5'-triphosphate and by being incorporated into nascent viral DNA which results in chain termination. Emtricitabine 5'-triphosphate is a weak inhibitor of mammalian DNA polymerase α, β, ϵ and mitochondrial DNA polymerase γ.

Tenofovir Disoproxil Fumarate: Tenofovir disoproxil fumarate is an acyclic nucleoside phosphonate diester analog of adenosine monophosphate. Tenofovir disoproxil fumarate requires initial diester hydrolysis for conversion to tenofovir and subsequent phosphorylations by cellular enzymes to form tenofovir diphosphate. Tenofovir diphosphate inhibits the activity of HIV-1 RT by competing with the natural substrate deoxyadenosine 5'-triphosphate and, after incorporation into DNA, by DNA chain termination. Tenofovir diphosphate is a weak inhibitor of mammalian DNA polymerases α, β, and mitochondrial DNA polymerase γ.

Antiviral Activity

Emtricitabine and Tenofovir Disoproxil Fumarate: In combination studies evaluating the cell culture antiviral activity of emtricitabine and tenofovir together, synergistic antiviral effects were observed.

Emtricitabine: The antiviral activity of emtricitabine against laboratory and clinical isolates of HIV-1 was assessed in lymphoblastoid cell lines, the MAGI-CCR5 cell line, and peripheral blood mononuclear cells. The 50% effective concentration (EC_{50}) values for emtricitabine were in the range of 0.0013–0.64 μM (0.0003–0.158 μg/mL). In drug combination studies of emtricitabine with nucleoside reverse transcriptase inhibitors (abacavir, lamivudine, stavudine, zalcitabine, zidovudine), non-nucleoside reverse transcriptase inhibitors (delavirdine, efavirenz, nevirapine), and protease inhibitors (amprenavir, nelfinavir, ritonavir, saquinavir), additive to synergistic effects were observed. Emtricitabine displayed antiviral activity in cell culture against HIV-1 clades A, B, C, D, E, F, and G (EC_{50} values ranged from 0.007–0.075 μM) and showed strain specific activity against HIV-2 (EC_{50} values ranged from 0.007–1.5 μM).

Tenofovir Disoproxil Fumarate: The antiviral activity of tenofovir against laboratory and clinical isolates of HIV-1 was assessed in lymphoblastoid cell lines, primary monocyte/macrophage cells and peripheral blood lymphocytes. The EC_{50} values for tenofovir were in the range of 0.04–8.5 μM. In drug combination studies of tenofovir with nucleoside reverse transcriptase inhibitors (abacavir, didanosine, lamivudine, stavudine, zalcitabine, zidovudine), nonnucleoside reverse transcriptase inhibitors (delavirdine, efavirenz, nevirapine), and protease inhibitors (amprenavir, indinavir, nelfinavir, ritonavir, saquinavir), additive to synergistic effects were observed. Tenofovir displayed antiviral activity in cell culture against HIV-1 clades A, B, C, D, E, F, G and O (EC_{50} values ranged from 0.5–2.2 μM) and showed strain specific activity against HIV-2 (EC_{50} values ranged from 1.6 μM to 5.5 μM).

Prophylactic Activity in a Nonhuman Primate Model of HIV Transmission

Emtricitabine and Tenofovir Disoproxil Fumarate: The prophylactic activity of the combination of daily oral emtricitabine (FTC) and tenofovir disoproxil fumarate (TDF) was evaluated in a controlled study of macaques inoculated once weekly for 14 weeks with SIV/HIV-1 chimeric virus (SHIV) applied to the rectal surface. Of the 18 control animals, 17 became infected after a median of 2 weeks. In contrast, 4 of the 6 animals treated daily with oral FTC and TDF remained uninfected and the two infections that did occur were significantly delayed until 9 and 12 weeks and exhibited reduced viremia. An M184I-expressing FTC-resistant variant emerged in 1 of the 2 macaques after 3 weeks of continued drug exposure.

Resistance

Emtricitabine and Tenofovir Disoproxil Fumarate: HIV-1 isolates with reduced susceptibility to the combination of emtricitabine and tenofovir have been selected in cell culture. Genotypic analysis of these isolates identified the M184V/I and/or K65R amino acid substitutions in the viral RT.

In a clinical trial of treatment-naive subjects [*Study 934, see Clinical Studies (14.1)*], resistance analysis was performed on HIV-1 isolates from all confirmed virologic failure subjects with greater than 400 copies/mL of HIV-1 RNA at Week 144 or early discontinuation. Development of efavirenz resistance-associated substitutions occurred most frequently and was similar between the treatment arms.

Table 7 Drug Interactions: Changes in Pharmacokinetic Parameters for Emtricitabine in the Presence of the Coadministered Drug*

Coadministered Drug	Dose of Coadministered Drug (mg)	Emtricitabine Dose (mg)	N	% Change of Emtricitabine Pharmacokinetic Parameters[†] (90% CI)		
				C_{max}	AUC	C_{min}
Tenofovir DF	300 once daily × 7 days	200 once daily × 7 days	17	⇔	⇔	↑ 20 (↑ 12 to ↑ 29)
Zidovudine	300 twice daily × 7 days	200 once daily × 7 days	27	⇔	⇔	⇔
Indinavir	800 × 1	200 × 1	12	⇔	⇔	NA
Famciclovir	500 × 1	200 × 1	12	⇔	⇔	NA
Stavudine	40 × 1	200 × 1	6	⇔	⇔	NA

* All interaction trials conducted in healthy volunteers
† ↑ = Increase; ↓ = Decrease; ⇔ = No Effect; NA = Not Applicable

---

Table 8 Drug Interactions: Changes in Pharmacokinetic Parameters for Coadministered Drug in the Presence of Emtricitabine*

Coadministered Drug	Dose of Coadministered Drug (mg)	Emtricitabine Dose (mg)	N	% Change of Coadministered Drug Pharmacokinetic Parameters[†] (90% CI)		
				C_{max}	AUC	C_{min}
Tenofovir DF	300 once daily × 7 days	200 once daily × 7 days	17	⇔	⇔	⇔
Zidovudine	300 twice daily × 7 days	200 once daily × 7 days	27	↑ 17 (↑ 0 to ↑ 38)	↑ 13 (↑ 5 to ↑ 20)	⇔
Indinavir	800 × 1	200 × 1	12	⇔	⇔	NA
Famciclovir	500 × 1	200 × 1	12	⇔	⇔	NA
Stavudine	40 × 1	200 × 1	6	⇔	⇔	NA

* All interaction trials conducted in healthy volunteers
† ↑ = Increase; ↓ = Decrease; ⇔ = No Effect; NA = Not Applicable

---

The M184V amino acid substitution, associated with resistance to EMTRIVA and lamivudine, was observed in 2/19 analyzed subject isolates in the EMTRIVA + VIREAD group and in 10/29 analyzed subject isolates in the zidovudine/lamivudine group. Through 144 weeks of Study 934, no subjects have developed a detectable K65R substitution in their HIV-1 as analyzed through standard genotypic analysis.

Emtricitabine: Emtricitabine-resistant isolates of HIV-1 have been selected in cell culture and in vivo. Genotypic analysis of these isolates showed that the reduced susceptibility to emtricitabine was associated with a substitution in the HIV-1 RT gene at codon 184 which resulted in an amino acid substitution of methionine by valine or isoleucine (M184V/I).

Tenofovir Disoproxil Fumarate: HIV-1 isolates with reduced susceptibility to tenofovir have been selected in cell culture. These viruses expressed a K65R substitution in RT and showed a 2–4 fold reduction in susceptibility to tenofovir.

In treatment-naive subjects, isolates from 8/47 (17%) analyzed subjects developed the K65R substitution in the VIREAD arm through 144 weeks; 7 occurred in the first 48 weeks of treatment and 1 at Week 96. In treatment-experienced subjects, 14/304 (5%) isolates from subjects failing VIREAD through Week 96 showed greater than 1.4 fold (median 2.7) reduced susceptibility to tenofovir. Genotypic analysis of the resistant isolates showed a substitution in the HIV-1 RT gene resulting in the K65R amino acid substitution.

iPrEx Trial: In a clinical study of HIV-1 seronegative subjects [*iPrEx Trial, see Clinical Studies (14.2)*], no amino acid substitutions associated with resistance to emtricitabine or tenofovir were detected at the time of seroconversion among 48 subjects in the TRUVADA group and 83 subjects in the placebo group who became infected with HIV-1 during the trial. Ten subjects were observed to be HIV-1 infected at time of enrollment. The M184V/I substitutions associated with resistance to emtricitabine were observed in 3 of the 10 subjects (2 of 2 in the TRUVADA group and 1 of 8 in the placebo group). One of the two subjects in the TRUVADA group harbored wild type virus at enrollment and developed the M184V substitution 4 weeks after enrollment. The other subject had indeterminate resistance at enrollment but was found to have the M184I substitution 4 weeks after enrollment.

Partners PrEP Trial: In a clinical study of HIV-1 seronegative subjects [*Partners PrEP Trial, see Clinical Studies (14.3)*], no variants expressing amino acid substitutions associated with resistance to emtricitabine or tenofovir were detected at the time of seroconversion among 12 subjects in the TRUVADA group, 15 subjects in the VIREAD group, and 51 subjects in the placebo group. Fourteen subjects were observed to be HIV-1 infected at the time of enrollment (3 in the TRUVADA group, 5 in the VIREAD group, and 6 in the placebo group). One of the three subjects in the TRUVADA group who was infected with wild type virus at enrollment selected an M184V expressing virus by week 12. Two of the five subjects in the VIREAD group had tenofovir-resistant viruses at the time of seroconversion; one subject infected with wild type virus at enrollment developed a K65R substitution by week 16, while the second subject had virus expressing the combination of D67N and K70R substitutions upon seroconversion at week 60, although baseline virus was not genotyped and it is unclear if the resistance emerged or was transmitted. Following enrollment, 4 subjects (2 in the VIREAD group, 1 in the TRUVADA group, and 1 in the placebo group) had virus expressing K103N or V106A substitutions, which confer high-level resistance to NNRTIs but have not been associated with tenofovir or emtricitabine and may have been present in the infecting virus.

Cross Resistance

Emtricitabine and Tenofovir Disoproxil Fumarate: Cross-resistance among certain nucleoside reverse transcriptase inhibitors (NRTIs) has been recognized. The M184V/I and/or K65R substitutions selected in cell culture by the combination of emtricitabine and tenofovir are also observed in some HIV-1 isolates from subjects failing treatment with tenofovir in combination with either lamivudine or emtricitabine, and either abacavir or didanosine. Therefore, cross-resistance among these drugs may occur in patients whose virus harbors either or both of these amino acid substitutions.

Emtricitabine: Emtricitabine-resistant isolates (M184V/I) were cross-resistant to lamivudine and zalcitabine but retained susceptibility in cell culture to didanosine, stavudine, tenofovir, zidovudine, and NNRTIs (delavirdine, efavirenz, and nevirapine). HIV-1 isolates containing the K65R substitution, selected in vivo by abacavir, didanosine, tenofovir, and zalcitabine, demonstrated reduced susceptibility to inhibition by emtricitabine. Viruses harboring substitutions conferring reduced susceptibility to stavudine

Table 9 Drug Interactions: Changes in Pharmacokinetic Parameters for Tenofovir* in the Presence of the Coadministered Drug

Coadministered Drug	Dose of Coadministered Drug (mg)	N	% Change of Tenofovir Pharmacokinetic Parameters[†] (90% CI)		
			C_{max}	AUC	C_{min}
Abacavir	300 once	8	⇔	⇔	NC
Atazanavir[‡]	400 once daily × 14 days	33	↑ 14 (↑ 8 to ↑ 20)	↑ 24 (↑ 21 to ↑ 28)	↑ 22 (↑ 15 to ↑ 30)
Atazanavir/ Ritonavir[‡]	300/100 once daily	12	↑ 34 (↑ 20 to ↑ 51)	↑ 37 (↑ 30 to ↑ 45)	↑ 29 (↑ 21 to ↑ 36)
Darunavir/ Ritonavir[§]	300/100 twice daily	12	↑ 24 (↑ 8 to ↑ 42)	↑ 22 (↑ 10 to ↑ 35)	↑ 37 (↑ 19 to ↑ 57)
Didanosine[¶]	250 or 400 once daily × 7 days	14	⇔	⇔	⇔
Emtricitabine	200 once daily × 7 days	17	⇔	⇔	⇔
Entecavir	1 mg once daily × 10 days	28	⇔	⇔	⇔
Indinavir	800 three times daily × 7 days	13	↑ 14 (↓ 3 to ↑ 33)	⇔	⇔
Lamivudine	150 twice daily × 7 days	15	⇔	⇔	⇔
Lopinavir/ Ritonavir	400/100 twice daily × 14 days	24	⇔	↑ 32 (↑ 25 to ↑ 38)	↑ 51 (↑ 37 to ↑ 66)
Saquinavir/ Ritonavir	1000/100 twice daily × 14 days	35	⇔	⇔	↑ 23 (↑ 16 to ↑ 30)
Tacrolimus	0.05 mg/kg twice daily × 7 days	21	↑ 13 (↑ 1 to ↑ 27)	⇔	⇔
Tipranavir/ Ritonavir[#]	500/100 twice daily	22	↓ 23 (↓ 32 to ↓ 13)	↓ 2 (↓ 9 to ↑ 5)	↑ 7 (↓ 2 to ↑ 17)
	750/200 twice daily (23 doses)	20	↓ 38 (↓ 46 to ↓ 29)	↑ 2 (↓ 6 to ↑ 10)	↑ 14 (↑ 1 to ↑ 27)

* Subjects received VIREAD 300 mg once daily
† Increase = ↑; Decrease = ↓; No Effect = ⇔; NC = Not Calculated
‡ Reyataz Prescribing Information
§ Prezista Prescribing Information
¶ Subjects received didanosine buffered tablets.
# Aptivus Prescribing Information

and zidovudine (M41L, D67N, K70R, L210W, T215Y/F, K219Q/E), or didanosine (L74V) remained sensitive to emtricitabine. HIV-1 containing the K103N substitution associated with resistance to NNRTIs was susceptible to emtricitabine.
Tenofovir Disoproxil Fumarate: HIV-1 isolates from subjects (N=20) whose HIV-1 expressed a mean of 3 zidovudine-associated RT amino acid substitutions (M41L, D67N, K70R, L210W, T215Y/F, or K219Q/E/N) showed a 3.1-fold decrease in the susceptibility to tenofovir. Subjects whose virus expressed an L74V substitution without zidovudine resistance associated substitutions (N=8) had reduced response to VIREAD. Limited data are available for patients whose virus expressed a Y115F substitution (N=3), Q151M substitution (N=2), or T69 insertion (N=4), all of whom had a reduced response.

13 NONCLINICAL TOXICOLOGY
13.1 Carcinogenesis, Mutagenesis, Impairment of Fertility
Emtricitabine: In long-term oral carcinogenicity studies of emtricitabine, no drug-related increases in tumor incidence were found in mice at doses up to 750 mg/kg/day (26 times the human systemic exposure at the therapeutic dose of 200 mg/day) or in rats at doses up to 600 mg/kg/day (31 times the human systemic exposure at the therapeutic dose).
Emtricitabine was not genotoxic in the reverse mutation bacterial test (Ames test), mouse lymphoma or mouse micronucleus assays.
Emtricitabine did not affect fertility in male rats at approximately 140-fold or in male and female mice at approximately 60-fold higher exposures (AUC) than in humans given the recommended 200 mg daily dose. Fertility was normal in the offspring of mice exposed daily from before birth (in utero) through sexual maturity at daily exposures (AUC) of approximately 60-fold higher than human exposures at the recommended 200 mg daily dose.

Tenofovir Disoproxil Fumarate: Long-term oral carcinogenicity studies of tenofovir disoproxil fumarate in mice and rats were carried out at exposures up to approximately 16 times (mice) and 5 times (rats) those observed in humans at the therapeutic dose for HIV-1 infection. At the high dose in female mice, liver adenomas were increased at exposures 16 times that in humans. In rats, the study was negative for carcinogenic findings at exposures up to 5 times that observed in humans at the therapeutic dose.
Tenofovir disoproxil fumarate was mutagenic in the in vitro mouse lymphoma assay and negative in an in vitro bacterial mutagenicity test (Ames test). In an in vivo mouse micronucleus assay, tenofovir disoproxil fumarate was negative when administered to male mice.
There were no effects on fertility, mating performance or early embryonic development when tenofovir disoproxil fumarate was administered to male rats at a dose equivalent to 10 times the human dose based on body surface area comparisons for 28 days prior to mating and to female rats for 15 days prior to mating through day seven of gestation. There was, however, an alteration of the estrous cycle in female rats.
13.2 Animal Toxicology and/or Pharmacology
Tenofovir and tenofovir disoproxil fumarate administered in toxicology studies to rats, dogs and monkeys at exposures (based on AUCs) greater than or equal to 6-fold those observed in humans caused bone toxicity. In monkeys the bone toxicity was diagnosed as osteomalacia. Osteomalacia observed in monkeys appeared to be reversible upon dose reduction or discontinuation of tenofovir. In rats and dogs, the bone toxicity manifested as reduced bone mineral density. The mechanism(s) underlying bone toxicity is unknown.
Evidence of renal toxicity was noted in 4 animal species. Increases in serum creatinine, BUN, glycosuria, proteinuria, phosphaturia, and/or calciuria and decreases in serum phosphate were observed to varying degrees in these animals. These toxicities were noted at exposures (based on

AUCs) 2–20 times higher than those observed in humans. The relationship of the renal abnormalities, particularly the phosphaturia, to the bone toxicity is not known.

14 CLINICAL STUDIES
Clinical Study 934 supports the use of TRUVADA tablets for the treatment of HIV-1 infection. Additional data in support of the use of TRUVADA are derived from clinical Study 903, in which lamivudine and tenofovir disoproxil fumarate (tenofovir DF) were used in combination in treatment-naive adults, and clinical Study 303 in which emtricitabine and lamivudine demonstrated comparable efficacy, safety and resistance patterns as part of multidrug regimens. For additional information about these trials, please consult the prescribing information for tenofovir DF and emtricitabine. The iPrEx study and Partners PrEP study support the use of TRUVADA to help reduce the risk of acquiring HIV-1.
14.1 Study 934
Data through 144 weeks are reported for Study 934, a randomized, open-label, active-controlled multicenter trial comparing emtricitabine + tenofovir DF administered in combination with efavirenz versus zidovudine/lamivudine fixed-dose combination administered in combination with efavirenz in 511 antiretroviral-naive subjects. From Weeks 96 to 144 of the trial, subjects received TRUVADA with efavirenz in place of emtricitabine + tenofovir DF with efavirenz. Subjects had a mean age of 38 years (range 18–80), 86% were male, 59% were Caucasian and 23% were Black. The mean baseline CD4+ cell count was 245 cells/mm[3] (range 2–1191) and median baseline plasma HIV-1 RNA was 5.01 $\log_{10}$ copies/mL (range 3.56–6.54). Subjects were stratified by baseline CD4+ cell count (< or ≥200 cells/mm[3]); 41% had CD4+ cell counts <200 cells/mm[3] and 51% of subjects had baseline viral loads >100,000 copies/mL. Treatment outcomes through 48 and 144 weeks for those subjects who did not have efavirenz resistance at baseline are presented in Table 11.
[See table 11 at top of page 824]
Through Week 48, 84% and 73% of subjects in the emtricitabine + tenofovir DF group and the zidovudine/lamivudine group, respectively, achieved and maintained HIV-1 RNA <400 copies/mL (71% and 58% through Week 144). The difference in the proportion of subjects who achieved and maintained HIV-1 RNA <400 copies/mL through 48 weeks largely results from the higher number of discontinuations due to adverse events and other reasons in the zidovudine/lamivudine group in this open-label trial. In addition, 80% and 70% of subjects in the emtricitabine + tenofovir DF group and the zidovudine/lamivudine group, respectively, achieved and maintained HIV-1 RNA <50 copies/mL through Week 48 (64% and 56% through Week 144). The mean increase from baseline in CD4+ cell count was 190 cells/mm[3] in the emtricitabine + tenofovir DF group and 158 cells/mm[3] in the zidovudine/lamivudine group at Week 48 (312 and 271 cells/mm[3] at Week 144).
Through 48 weeks, 7 subjects in the emtricitabine + tenofovir DF group and 5 subjects in the zidovudine/lamivudine group experienced a new CDC Class C event (10 and 6 subjects through 144 weeks).
14.2 iPrEx Trial
The iPrEx trial was a randomized double-blind placebo-controlled multinational study evaluating TRUVADA in 2499 HIV-seronegative men or transgender women who have sex with men and with evidence of high risk behavior for HIV-1 infection. Evidence of high risk behavior included any one of the following reported to have occurred up to six months prior to study screening: no condom use during anal intercourse with an HIV-1 positive partner or a partner of unknown HIV status; anal intercourse with more than 3 sex partners; exchange of money, gifts, shelter or drugs for anal sex; sex with male partner and diagnosis of sexually transmitted infection; no consistent use of condoms with sex partner known to be HIV-1 positive.
All subjects received monthly HIV-1 testing, risk-reduction counseling, condoms and management of sexually transmitted infections. Of the 2499 enrolled, 1251 received TRUVADA and 1248 received placebo. The mean age of subjects was 27 years, 5% were Asian, 9% Black, 18% White, and 72% Hispanic/Latino.
Subjects were followed for 4237 person-years. The primary outcome measure for the study was the incidence of documented HIV seroconversion. At the end of treatment, emergent HIV-1 seroconversion was observed in 131 subjects, of which 48 occurred in the TRUVADA group and 83 occurred in the placebo group, indicating a 42% (95% CI: 18% to 60%) reduction in risk. Risk reduction was found to be higher (53%; 95% CI: 34% to 72%) among subjects who reported previous unprotected anal intercourse (URAI) at screening (732 and 753 subjects reported URAI within the last 12 weeks at screening in the TRUVADA and placebo groups, respectively). In a post-hoc case control study of plasma and intracellular drug levels in about 10% of study subjects, risk reduction appeared to be the greatest in subjects with detectable intracellular tenofovir. Efficacy was therefore strongly correlated with adherence.
14.3 Partners PrEP Trial
The Partners PrEP trial was a randomized, double-blind, placebo-controlled 3 arm trial conducted in 4758 serodiscor-

dant heterosexual couples in Kenya and Uganda to evaluate the efficacy and safety of TDF (N=1589) and FTC/TDF (N=1583) versus (parallel comparison) placebo (N=1586), in preventing HIV-1 acquisition by the uninfected partner. All subjects received monthly HIV-1 testing, evaluation of adherence, assessment of sexual behavior, and safety evaluations. Women were also tested monthly for pregnancy. Women who became pregnant during the trial had study drug interrupted for the duration of the pregnancy and while breastfeeding. The uninfected partner subjects were predominantly male (61–64% across study drug groups), and had a mean age of 33–34 years.

Following 7827 person-years of follow up, 82 emergent HIV-1 seroconversions were reported, with an overall observed seroincidence rate of 1.05 per 100 person-years. Of the 82 seroconversions, 13 and 52 occurred in partner subjects randomized to TRUVADA and placebo, respectively. Two of the 13 seroconversions in the TRUVADA arm and 3 of the 52 seroconversions in the placebo arm occurred in women during treatment interruptions for pregnancy. The risk reduction for TRUVADA relative to placebo was 75% (95% CI: 55% to 87%). In a post-hoc case control study of plasma drug levels in about 10% of study subjects, risk reduction appeared to be the greatest in subjects with detectable plasma tenofovir. Efficacy was therefore strongly correlated with adherence.

16 HOW SUPPLIED/STORAGE AND HANDLING

The blue, capsule-shaped, film-coated, tablets contain 200 mg of emtricitabine and 300 mg of tenofovir disoproxil fumarate (which is equivalent to 245 mg of tenofovir disoproxil), are debossed with "GILEAD" on one side and with "701" on the other side, and are available in unit of use bottles [containing a dessicant (silica gel canister or sachet) and closed with a child-resistant closure] of:
• 30 tablets (NDC 61958-0701-1)
Store at 25 °C (77 °F), excursions permitted to 15 °C –30 °C (59 °F –86 °F) (see USP Controlled Room Temperature).
• Keep container tightly closed
• Dispense only in original container
• Do not use if seal over bottle opening is broken or missing

17 PATIENT COUNSELING INFORMATION

As a part of patient counseling, healthcare providers must review the TRUVADA Medication Guide with every uninfected individual taking TRUVADA to reduce the risk of acquiring HIV.

See FDA-approved patient labeling (Medication Guide)

17.1 Important Information for All Patients and Uninfected Individuals

Advise patients and uninfected individuals that:
• The long term effects of TRUVADA are unknown.
• TRUVADA tablets are for oral ingestion only.
• Patients and uninfected individuals should not discontinue TRUVADA without first informing their physicians.
• Patients and uninfected individuals should remain under the care of a physician when using TRUVADA.
• It is important to take TRUVADA on a regular dosing schedule to avoid missing doses.
• Lactic acidosis and severe hepatomegaly with steatosis, including fatal cases, have been reported. Treatment with TRUVADA should be suspended in patients or uninfected individuals who develop clinical symptoms suggestive of lactic acidosis or pronounced hepatotoxicity (including nausea, vomiting, unusual or unexpected stomach discomfort, and weakness) [See Warnings and Precautions (5.1)].
• Severe acute exacerbations of hepatitis B have been reported in patients who are coinfected with hepatitis B virus (HBV) and HIV-1 and have discontinued TRUVADA. Before initiating TRUVADA, test all patients and uninfected individuals for HBV. All patients who are infected with HBV need close medical follow-up for several months after stopping TRUVADA to monitor for exacerbations of hepatitis [See Warnings and Precautions (5.2)].
• Renal impairment, including cases of acute renal failure and Fanconi syndrome, has been reported in association with the use of VIREAD. TRUVADA should be avoided with concurrent or recent use of a nephrotoxic agent (e.g., high-dose or multiple NSAIDs) [See Warnings and Precautions (5.3)]. Dosing interval of TRUVADA may need adjustment in HIV-1 infected patients with renal impairment. TRUVADA for a PrEP indication should not be used in HIV-1 uninfected individuals if estimated creatinine clearance is less than 60 mL/min. If a decrease in estimated creatinine clearance is observed in uninfected individuals while using TRUVADA for PrEP, evaluate potential causes and re-assess potential risks and benefits of continued use [See Dosage and Administration (2.3)].
• Do not administer TRUVADA with ATRIPLA, COMPLERA, EMTRIVA, STRIBILD, or VIREAD; or with drugs containing lamivudine, including Combivir (lamivudine/zidovudine), Epivir or Epivir-HBV (lamivudine), Epzicom (abacavir sulfate/lamivudine), or Trizivir (abacavir sulfate/lamivudine/zidovudine) [See Warnings and Precautions (5.4)].

• Do not administer TRUVADA with HEPSERA [See Warnings and Precautions (5.4)].
• Decreases in bone mineral density have been observed with the use of VIREAD or TRUVADA. Consider bone monitoring in patients and uninfected individuals who have a history of pathologic bone fracture or at risk for osteopenia [See Warnings and Precautions (5.5)].
• Patients and uninfected individuals should avoid doing things that can spread HIV-1 or HBV infection.
• Do not share needles or other injection equipment.
• Do not share personal items that can have blood or body fluids on them, like toothbrushes and razor blades.
• Do not have any kind of sex without protection. Always practice safer sex by using a latex or polyurethane condom to lower the chance of sexual contact with semen, vaginal secretions, or blood.
• Patients and uninfected individuals should not breastfeed because the drugs in TRUVADA can be passed to the baby in breast milk, and it is not known whether they can harm the baby. HIV-positive women should also not breastfeed because of the risk of passing the HIV-1 virus to the baby.

17.2 Treatment of HIV-1 Infection

When TRUVADA is used in the treatment of HIV-infection, advise patients that:
• TRUVADA is not a cure for HIV-1 infection and patients may continue to experience illnesses associated with HIV-1 infection, including opportunistic infections.
• It is important to take TRUVADA in a regular dosing schedule with combination therapy to avoid missing doses.
• All patients with HIV-1 should be tested for hepatitis B virus (HBV) before initiating and monitored after discontinuing taking TRUVADA.

17.3 Pre-Exposure Prophylaxis

When TRUVADA is used to reduce the risk of acquiring HIV-1, advise uninfected individuals about the importance of the following:
• Confirming that they are HIV-negative before starting to take TRUVADA to reduce the risk of acquiring HIV-1.
• TRUVADA should only be used as part of a complete prevention strategy including other prevention measures. In clinical trials, TRUVADA only protected some subjects from acquiring HIV-1.

Table 10 Drug Interactions: Changes in Pharmacokinetic Parameters for Coadministered Drug in the Presence of Tenofovir

Coadministered Drug	Dose of Coadministered Drug (mg)	N	% Change of Coadministered Drug Pharmacokinetic Parameters* (90% CI)		
			C_{max}	AUC	C_{min}
Abacavir	300 once	8	↑ 12 (↓ 1 to ↑ 26)	⇔	NA
Atazanavir[†]	400 once daily × 14 days	34	↓ 21 (↓ 27 to ↓ 14)	↓ 25 (↓ 30 to ↓ 19)	↓ 40 (↓ 48 to ↓ 32)
Atazanavir[†]	Atazanavir/Ritonavir 300/100 once daily × 42 days	10	↓ 28 (↓ 50 to ↑ 5)	↓ 25[‡] (↓ 42 to ↓ 3)	↓ 23[‡] (↓ 46 to ↑ 10)
Darunavir[§]	Darunavir/Ritonavir 300/100 mg once daily	12	↑ 16 (↓ 6 to ↑ 42)	↑ 21 (↓ 5 to ↑ 54)	↑ 24 (↓ 10 to ↑ 69)
Didanosine[¶]	250 once, simultaneously with tenofovir DF and a light meal[#]	33	↓ 20[P] (↓ 32 to ↓ 7)	⇔[P]	NA
Emtricitabine	200 once daily × 7 days	17	⇔		↑ 20 (↑ 12 to ↑ 29)
Indinavir	800 three times daily × 7 days	12	↓ 11 (↓ 30 to ↑ 12)	⇔	⇔
Entecavir	1 mg once daily × 10 days	28	⇔	↑ 13 (↑ 11 to ↑ 15)	
Lamivudine	150 twice daily × 7 days	15	↓ 24 (↓ 34 to ↓ 12)	⇔	
Lopinavir Ritonavir	Lopinavir/Ritonavir 400/100 twice daily × 14 days	24	⇔	⇔	⇔
Saquinavir	Saquinavir/Ritonavir 1000/100 twice daily × 14 days	32	↑ 22 (↑ 6 to ↑41)	↑ 29[ß] (↑ 12 to ↑ 48)	↑ 47[ß] (↑ 23 to ↑ 76)
Ritonavir			⇔	⇔	↑ 23 (↑ 3 to ↑ 46)
Tacrolimus	0.05 mg/kg twice daily × 7 days	21	⇔	⇔	⇔
Tipranavir[à]	Tipranavir/Ritonavir 500/100 twice daily	22	↓ 17 (↓ 26 to ↓ 6)	↓ 18 (↓ 25 to ↓ 9)	↓ 21 (↓ 30 to ↓ 10)
	Tipranavir/Ritonavir 750/200 twice daily (23 doses)	20	↓ 11 (↓ 16 to ↓ 4)	↓ 9 (↓ 15 to ↓ 3)	↓ 12 (↓ 22 to 0)

* Increase = ↑; Decrease = ↓; No Effect = ⇔; NA = Not Applicable
† Reyataz Prescribing Information
‡ In HIV-infected subjects, addition of tenofovir DF to atazanavir 300 mg plus ritonavir 100 mg, resulted in AUC and C_{min} values of atazanavir that were 2.3 and 4-fold higher than the respective values observed for atazanavir 400 mg when given alone.
§ Prezista Prescribing Information.
¶ Videx EC Prescribing Information. Subjects received didanosine enteric-coated capsules.
# 373 kcal, 8.2 g fat
P Compared with didanosine (enteric-coated) 400 mg administered alone under fasting conditions.
ß Increases in AUC and C_{min} are not expected to be clinically relevant; hence no dose adjustments are required when tenofovir DF and ritonavir-boosted saquinavir are coadministered.
à Aptivus Prescribing Information.

Help Patients Save on Rx Drugs: PDR.net/PharmacyDiscountCard

Table 11 Outcomes of Randomized Treatment at Week 48 and 144 (Study 934)

Outcomes	At Week 48		At Week 144	
	FTC + TDF + EFV (N=244)	AZT/3TC + EFV (N=243)	FTC + TDF + EFV (N=227)*	AZT/3TC + EFV (N=229)*
Responder[†]	84%	73%	71%	58%
Virologic failure[‡]	2%	4%	3%	6%
Rebound	1%	3%	2%	5%
Never suppressed	0%	0%	0%	0%
Change in antiretroviral regimen	1%	1%	1%	1%
Death	<1%	1%	1%	1%
Discontinued due to adverse event	4%	9%	5%	12%
Discontinued for other reasons[§]	10%	14%	20%	22%

* Subjects who were responders at Week 48 or Week 96 (HIV-1 RNA <400 copies/mL) but did not consent to continue trial after Week 48 or Week 96 were excluded from analysis.
† Subjects achieved and maintained confirmed HIV-1 RNA <400 copies/mL through Weeks 48 and 144.
‡ Includes confirmed viral rebound and failure to achieve confirmed <400 copies/mL through Weeks 48 and 144.
§ Includes lost to follow-up, subject withdrawal, noncompliance, protocol violation and other reasons.

- Using condoms consistently and correctly to lower the chance of sexual contact with any body fluids such as semen, vaginal secretions, or blood.
- Knowing their HIV status and the status of their partner(s).
- Getting tested regularly (at least every 3 months) for HIV-1 and ask their partner(s) to get tested as well.
- HIV-1 resistance substitutions may emerge in individuals with undetected HIV-1 infection who are taking TRUVADA, because TRUVADA alone does not constitute a complete regimen for HIV-1 treatment *[See Warnings and Precautions (5.9)]*
- Reporting any symptoms of acute HIV-1 infection (flu-like symptoms) to their healthcare provider immediately.
  - Signs and symptoms of acute infection include: fever, headache, fatigue, arthralgia, vomiting, myalgia, diarrhea, pharyngitis, rash, night sweats, and adenopathy (cervical and inguinal).
- Getting tested for other sexually transmitted infections such as syphilis and gonorrhea that may facilitate HIV-1 transmission.
- Learning about sexual risk behavior and getting support to help reduce sexual risk behavior.
- Taking TRUVADA on a regular dosing schedule and strictly adhere to the recommended dosing schedule to reduce the risk of acquiring HIV-1. Uninfected individuals who miss doses are at greater risk of acquiring HIV-1 than those who do not miss doses. *[See Warnings and Precautions (5.9)].*
- Women who are pregnant should learn about the risks and benefits of TRUVADA to reduce the risk of acquiring HIV-1 during their pregnancy.
- Encourage use of the Agreement Form for Initiating TRUVADA for PrEP of Sexually Acquired HIV-1 Infection.

COMPLERA, EMTRIVA, HEPSERA, STRIBILD, TRUVADA, and VIREAD are trademarks of Gilead Sciences, Inc., or its related companies. ATRIPLA is a trademark of Bristol-Myers Squibb & Gilead Sciences, LLC. All other trademarks referenced herein are the property of their respective owners.

Manufactured for and distributed by:
Gilead Sciences, Inc.
Foster City, CA 94404
21-752-GS-027

Medication Guide
TRUVADA® (tru-VAH-dah)
(emtricitabine and tenofovir disoproxil fumarate)
tablets

Read this Medication Guide before you start taking TRUVADA and each time you get a refill. There may be new information. This information does not take the place of talking to your healthcare provider about your medical condition or your treatment.

This Medication Guide provides information about two different ways that TRUVADA may be used (See the Medication Guide section **"What is TRUVADA?"** for important information about how TRUVADA may be used):

- **to treat Human Immunodeficiency Virus-1 (HIV-1) infection, and**
- **to reduce the risk of getting HIV-1 infection in adults who are HIV-negative**

HIV is the virus that causes AIDS (Acquired Immune Deficiency Syndrome).

What is the most important information I should know about TRUVADA?
TRUVADA can cause serious side effects, including:
1. Too much lactic acid in your blood (lactic acidosis). Your body normally makes lactic acid, but too much lactic acid is a serious medical emergency. It can be treated, but it can also lead to death.
Call your healthcare provider right away if you get these symptoms:
- weakness or being more tired than usual
- unusual muscle pain
- being short of breath or fast breathing
- nausea, vomiting, and stomach-area pain
- cold or blue hands and feet
- feel dizzy or lightheaded
- fast or abnormal heartbeats

2. Severe liver problems. Severe liver problems can happen in people who take TRUVADA. In some cases these liver problems can lead to death. Your liver may become large and tender. You may develop fat in your liver when you take TRUVADA.
Call your healthcare provider right away if you get the following symptoms:
- your skin or the white part of your eyes turns yellow
- dark "tea-colored" urine
- light-colored stools
- loss of appetite for several days or longer
- nausea
- stomach-area pain

You may be more likely to get lactic acidosis or severe liver problems if you are female, if you are very overweight (obese), or if you have been taking TRUVADA for a long time.

3. If you also have hepatitis B virus (HBV) infection and take TRUVADA, your hepatitis B may become worse if you stop taking TRUVADA.
- Do not stop taking TRUVADA without first talking to your healthcare provider.
- Do not run out of TRUVADA. Refill your prescription or talk to your healthcare provider before your TRUVADA is all gone.
- If your healthcare provider stops TRUVADA, your healthcare provider will need to watch you closely for several months to check your hepatitis B infection, or give you a medication to treat hepatitis B.

Tell your healthcare provider about any new or unusual symptoms you may have after you stop taking TRUVADA.

For more information about side effects, see the section **"What are the possible side effects of TRUVADA?"** in this Medication Guide.

Other important information for people who take TRUVADA to help reduce their risk of getting HIV-1 infection:

Before taking TRUVADA to reduce your risk of getting HIV-1 infection:
- **You must be HIV-negative to start TRUVADA. You must get tested to make sure that you do not already have HIV-1 infection.**
- **Do not take TRUVADA to reduce the risk of getting HIV-1 unless you are confirmed to be HIV-negative.**
- Many HIV-1 tests can miss HIV-1 infection in a person who has recently become infected. If you have flu-like symptoms, you could have recently become infected with

HIV-1. Tell your healthcare provider if you had a flu-like illness within the last month before starting TRUVADA or at any time while taking TRUVADA. Symptoms of new HIV-1 infection include:
- tiredness
- vomiting or diarrhea
- fever
- rash
- joint or muscle aches
- night sweats
- headache
- enlarged lymph nodes in the neck or groin
- sore throat

While you are taking TRUVADA to reduce your risk of getting HIV-1:
- **Just taking TRUVADA may not keep you from getting HIV-1.**
- **You must continue using safer sex practices** while you are taking TRUVADA to reduce your risk of getting HIV-1.
- **You must stay HIV-negative to keep taking TRUVADA to reduce your risk of infection.**
  - Know your HIV-1 status and the HIV-1 status of your partners.
  - Get tested for HIV-1 at least every 3 months or when your healthcare provider tells you.
  - Get tested for other sexually transmitted infections such as syphilis and gonorrhea. These infections make it easier for HIV-1 to infect you.
  - If you think you were exposed to HIV-1, tell your healthcare provider right away. They may want to do more tests to be sure you are still HIV-negative.
  - Get information and support to help reduce risky sexual behavior.
  - Have fewer sex partners.
  - Do not miss any doses of TRUVADA. Missing doses may increase your risk of getting HIV-1 infection.
- If you become HIV-positive, you need more medicine than TRUVADA alone to treat HIV-1. TRUVADA by itself is not a complete treatment for HIV-1.
- If you have HIV-1 and take only TRUVADA, over time your HIV-1 may become harder to treat.

See the section **"What should I avoid while taking TRUVADA?"** and talk to your healthcare provider for more information about how to prevent HIV-1 infection.

What is TRUVADA?
TRUVADA contains the prescription medicines emtricitabine (EMTRIVA®) and tenofovir disoproxil fumarate (VIREAD®). TRUVADA is used:
- **to treat HIV-1 infection** when used with other HIV-1 medicines in adults and children age 12 years and older
- **to reduce the risk of getting HIV-1 infection** when used with safer sex practices in:
  - HIV-negative men who have sex with men, who are at high risk of getting infected with HIV-1 through sex.
  - Male-female sex partners when one partner has HIV-1 infection and the other does not.

Use of TRUVADA to treat HIV-1 infection:
- **When used with other HIV-1 medicines to treat HIV-1 infection, TRUVADA may help:**
  - Reduce the amount of HIV-1 in your blood. This is called "viral load".
  - Increase the number of CD4+ (T) cells in your blood that help fight off other infections. Reducing the amount of HIV-1 and increasing the CD4+ (T) cells in your blood may help improve your immune system. This may reduce your risk of death or infections that can happen when your immune system is weak.
- **TRUVADA does not cure HIV-1 or AIDS.** If you have HIV-1 infection, you must keep taking HIV-1 medicines to control HIV-1 infection and decrease HIV-related illnesses.

It is not known if TRUVADA is safe and effective in children with HIV-1 infection who are under 12 years of age or who weigh less than 77 pounds.

Use of TRUVADA to reduce the risk of HIV-1 infection:
- **When used with safer sex practices, TRUVADA may help** to reduce the risk of getting HIV-1 infection.
- TRUVADA works better to reduce the risk of getting HIV-1 when the medicines are in your bloodstream **before** you are exposed to HIV-1.

Who should not take TRUVADA?
For people using TRUVADA to reduce the risk of getting HIV-1 infection:
TRUVADA can only help reduce your risk of getting HIV-1 **before** you are infected. **Do not take TRUVADA to help reduce your risk of getting HIV-1 if:**
- **you already have HIV-1 infection.** If you are HIV-positive, you need to take other medicines with TRUVADA to treat HIV-1. TRUVADA by itself is not a complete treatment for HIV-1.
- **you do not know your HIV-1 infection status.** You may already be HIV-positive. You need to take other HIV-1 medicines with TRUVADA to treat HIV-1.

What should I tell my healthcare provider before taking TRUVADA?
Tell your healthcare provider if you:
- have liver problems including hepatitis B virus infection
- have kidney problems or receive kidney dialysis treatment
- have bone problems

- have any other medical conditions
- are pregnant or plan to become pregnant. It is not known if TRUVADA can harm your unborn baby.

If you are a female who is taking TRUVADA to reduce the risk of getting HIV-1 infection and you become pregnant while taking TRUVADA, talk to your healthcare provider to decide if you should keep taking TRUVADA.

Pregnancy Registry: A pregnancy registry collects information about your health and the health of your baby. There is a pregnancy registry for women who take medicines to treat or prevent HIV-1 during pregnancy. For more information about the registry and how it works, talk to your healthcare provider.

- are breastfeeding or plan to breastfeed.
  - You should not breastfeed if you have HIV-1. There is a risk you will pass HIV-1 to your baby.
  - Do not breastfeed if you take TRUVADA. TRUVADA can pass to your baby in your breast milk.
  - Talk to your healthcare provider about the best way to feed your baby.

Tell your healthcare provider about all the medicines you take, including prescription and over-the-counter medicines, vitamins, and herbal supplements.

Do not take TRUVADA if you also take any of the medicines listed below:

- tenofovir or emtricitabine (ATRIPLA®, COMPLERA®, EMTRIVA, STRIBILD®, or VIREAD). These medicines contain the same active ingredient as TRUVADA.
- medicines which contain lamivudine (Combivir, Epivir, Epivir-HBV, Epzicom, or Trizivir)
- adefovir (HEPSERA®)

TRUVADA may interact with other medicines. Especially tell your healthcare provider if you take:

- didanosine (Videx EC)
- darunavir (Prezista)
- atazanavir (Reyataz)
- lopinavir with ritonavir (Kaletra)

Your doctor may need to check you more often or change your dose if you take any of these medicines and TRUVADA. Know the medicines you take. Keep a list of them to show your healthcare provider or pharmacist when you get a new medicine.

How should I take TRUVADA?

- Take TRUVADA exactly as prescribed.
- Take TRUVADA by mouth, with or without food.
- TRUVADA is usually taken 1 time each day. Take TRUVADA at the same time each day to keep TRUVADA blood levels constant.
  - If you have kidney problems, your healthcare provider may tell you to take TRUVADA less often.
- Do not miss any doses of TRUVADA. Missing a dose lowers the amount of medicine in your blood.
- If you miss a dose of TRUVADA, take it as soon as you remember that day. Do not take more than 1 dose of TRUVADA in a day. Do not take 2 doses at the same time to make up for a missed dose. Call your healthcare provider or pharmacist if you are not sure what to do.
- Do not change your dose or stop taking TRUVADA without first talking with your healthcare provider. Stay under a healthcare provider's care when taking TRUVADA.
- Refill your TRUVADA prescription before you run out of medicine.
- If you take too much TRUVADA, call your healthcare provider or go to the nearest hospital emergency room right away.
- If you take TRUVADA to treat HIV-1 infection, you need to take other HIV-1 medicines. Your healthcare provider will tell you what medicines to take and how to take them.
- If you take TRUVADA to reduce your risk of getting HIV-1:
  - you must also use other methods to reduce your risk of getting HIV-1. See the section **"What should I avoid while taking TRUVADA?"** in this Medication Guide.
  - **Take TRUVADA every day,** not just when you think you have been exposed to HIV-1.

What should I avoid while taking TRUVADA?

While taking TRUVADA, avoid doing things that increase your risk of getting HIV-1 or spreading HIV-1 to other people.

- See the section **"What is the most important information I should know about TRUVADA?"** at the beginning of this Medication Guide.
- Do not have any kind of sex without protection. Always practice safer sex. Use latex or non-latex condoms, except lambskin, to reduce contact with semen, vaginal fluids, or blood.
- Do not share personal items that can have blood or body fluids on them, such as toothbrushes and razor blades.
- Do not share or re-use needles or other injection equipment.

Ask your healthcare provider if you have any questions about how to prevent getting HIV-1 or spreading HIV-1 to other people.

What are the possible side effects of TRUVADA?
TRUVADA may cause serious side effects, including:

- See **"What is the most important information I should know about TRUVADA?"**.
- **New or worse kidney problems,** including kidney failure. If you had kidney problems in the past or take another medicine that can cause kidney problems, your healthcare provider may do blood tests to check your kidneys before you start and while you are taking TRUVADA. Your healthcare provider may tell you to take TRUVADA less often, or to stop taking TRUVADA if you have kidney problems.
- **Bone problems** can happen in some people who take TRUVADA. Bone problems include bone pain, or softening or thinning of bones, which may lead to fractures. Your healthcare provider may need to do tests to check your bones.
- **Changes in body fat** can happen in people who take HIV-1 medicines. The exact cause and long-term health effects of these problems are not known. The changes may include:
  - increased amount of fat in the upper back and neck ("buffalo hump"), breast, and around the middle of your body (trunk)
  - loss of fat from the legs, arms, and face
- **Changes in your immune system (Immune Reconstitution Syndrome)** can happen when an HIV-1-infected person starts taking HIV-1 medicines. Your immune system may get stronger, and can then cause you to develop inflammation in areas of your body where infections may have been hiding for a long time. This inflammation may cause you to have minor symptoms, such as fever, but inflammation can also lead to serious problems. Tell your healthcare provider right away if you start having any new symptoms after starting TRUVADA for treatment of HIV-1 infection.

The most common side effects of TRUVADA in people taking TRUVADA to treat HIV-1 infection include:

- diarrhea
- nausea
- tiredness
- headache
- dizziness
- depression
- problems sleeping
- abnormal dreams
- rash

Common side effects in people who take TRUVADA to reduce the risk of getting HIV-1 infection include:

- stomach-area (abdomen) pain
- headache
- decreased weight

Tell your healthcare provider if you have any side effect that bothers you or that does not go away.

These are not all the possible side effects of TRUVADA. For more information, ask your healthcare provider or pharmacist.

Call your doctor for medical advice about side effects. You may report side effects to FDA at 1-800-FDA-1088.

How should I store TRUVADA?

- Store TRUVADA at room temperature between 68°F to 77°F (20°C to 25°C).
- Keep TRUVADA in its original container and keep the container tightly closed.
- Do not use TRUVADA if seal over bottle opening is broken or missing.

Keep TRUVADA and all other medicines out of reach of children.

General information about TRUVADA.

Medicines are sometimes prescribed for purposes other than those listed in a Medication Guide. Do not use TRUVADA for a condition for which it was not prescribed. Do not give TRUVADA to other people, even if they have the same symptoms you have. It may harm them.

This Medication Guide summarizes the most important information about TRUVADA. If you would like more information, talk with your healthcare provider. You can ask your healthcare provider or pharmacist for information about TRUVADA that is written for health professionals. For more information, call 1-800-445-3235 or go to www.TRUVADA.com.

What are the ingredients in TRUVADA?

Active ingredients: emtricitabine and tenofovir disoproxil fumarate.

Inactive ingredients: Croscarmellose sodium, lactose monohydrate, magnesium stearate, microcrystalline cellulose, and pregelatinized starch (gluten free). The tablets are coated with Opadry II Blue Y-30-10701 which contains FD&C Blue #2 aluminum lake, hydroxypropyl methylcellulose 2910, lactose monohydrate, titanium dioxide, and triacetin.

This Medication Guide has been approved by the U.S. Food and Drug Administration.

Manufactured for and distributed by:
Gilead Sciences, Inc.
Foster City, CA 94404
Revised December 2013
21-752-GS-028

Shown in Product Identification Guide, page 307

VIREAD®
[VEER-ee-ad]
(tenofovir disoproxil fumarate)
tablets, for oral use

VIREAD®
(tenofovir disoproxil fumarate)
powder, for oral use

HIGHLIGHTS OF PRESCRIBING INFORMATION
These highlights do not include all the information needed to use VIREAD safely and effectively. See full prescribing information for VIREAD.

VIREAD® (tenofovir disoproxil fumarate) tablets, for oral use
VIREAD® (tenofovir disoproxil fumarate) powder, for oral use

Initial U.S. Approval: 2001

WARNING: LACTIC ACIDOSIS/SEVERE HEPATOMEGALY WITH STEATOSIS and POST TREATMENT EXACERBATION OF HEPATITIS
See full prescribing information for complete boxed warning.

- Lactic acidosis and severe hepatomegaly with steatosis, including fatal cases, have been reported with the use of nucleoside analogs, including VIREAD. (5.1)
- Severe acute exacerbations of hepatitis have been reported in HBV-infected patients who have discontinued anti-hepatitis B therapy, including VIREAD. Hepatic function should be monitored closely in these patients. If appropriate, resumption of anti-hepatitis B therapy may be warranted. (5.2)

———————RECENT MAJOR CHANGES———————

Indications and Usage (1.1)	11/2012
Indications and Usage (1.2)	07/2013
Dosage and Administration (2.3)	10/2013
Warnings and Precautions	
New Onset or Worsening Renal Impairment (5.3)	10/2013
Coadministration with Other Products (5.4)	11/2012
Bone Effects (5.6)	10/2013

———————INDICATIONS AND USAGE———————

VIREAD is a nucleotide analog HIV-1 reverse transcriptase inhibitor and an HBV reverse transcriptase inhibitor.
VIREAD is indicated in combination with other antiretroviral agents for the treatment of HIV-1 infection in adults and pediatric patients 2 years of age and older. (1)
VIREAD is indicated for the treatment of chronic hepatitis B in adults and pediatric patients 12 years of age and older. (1)

———————DOSAGE AND ADMINISTRATION———————

- Recommended dose for the treatment of HIV-1 or chronic hepatitis B in adults and pediatric patients 12 years of age and older (35 kg or more): 300 mg once daily taken orally without regard to food. (2.1)
- Recommended dose for the treatment of HIV-1 in pediatric patients (2 to less than 12 years of age):
  Tablets: for pediatric patients weighing greater than or equal to 17 kg who can swallow an intact tablet, one VIREAD tablet (150, 200, 250 or 300 mg based on body weight) once daily taken orally without regard to food. (2.2)
  Oral powder: 8 mg/kg VIREAD oral powder (up to a maximum of 300 mg) once daily with food. (2.2)
- Dose recommended in renal impairment in adults:
  Creatinine clearance 30–49 mL/min: 300 mg every 48 hours. (2.3)
  Creatinine clearance 10–29 mL/min: 300 mg every 72 to 96 hours. (2.3)
  Hemodialysis: 300 mg every 7 days or after approximately 12 hours of dialysis. (2.3)

———————DOSAGE FORMS AND STRENGTHS———————

Tablets: 150, 200, 250 and 300 mg (3)
Oral Powder: 40 mg per 1 g of oral powder (3)

———————CONTRAINDICATIONS———————

None. (4)

———————WARNINGS AND PRECAUTIONS———————

- New onset or worsening renal impairment: Can include acute renal failure and Fanconi syndrome. Assess estimated creatinine clearance before initiating treatment with VIREAD. In patients at risk for renal dysfunction, assess estimated creatinine clearance, serum phosphorus, urine glucose and urine protein before initiating treat-

container and spoon to dry. Throw away the paper towel and clean the work surface.
ment with VIREAD and periodically during treatment. Avoid administering VIREAD with concurrent or recent use of nephrotoxic drugs. (5.3)

• Coadministration with Other Products: Do not use with other tenofovir-containing products (e.g., ATRIPLA, COMPLERA, STRIBILD and TRUVADA). Do not administer in combination with HEPSERA. (5.4)

• HIV testing: HIV antibody testing should be offered to all HBV-infected patients before initiating therapy with VIREAD. VIREAD should be used as part of an appropriate antiretroviral combination regimen in HIV-infected patients with or without HBV coinfection. (5.5)

• Decreases in bone mineral density (BMD): Consider assessment of BMD in patients with a history of pathologic fracture or other risk factors for osteoporosis or bone loss. (5.6)

• Redistribution/accumulation of body fat: Observed in HIV-infected patients receiving antiretroviral combination therapy. (5.7)

• Immune reconstitution syndrome: Observed in HIV-infected patients. May necessitate further evaluation and treatment. (5.8)

• Triple nucleoside-only regimens: Early virologic failure has been reported in HIV-infected patients. Monitor carefully and consider treatment modification. (5.9)

----ADVERSE REACTIONS----

In HIV-infected adult subjects: Most common adverse reactions (incidence greater than or equal to 10%, Grades 2–4) are rash, diarrhea, headache, pain, depression, asthenia, and nausea. (6.1)

In HBV-infected subjects with compensated liver disease: most common adverse reaction (all grades) was nausea (9%). (6.1)

In pediatric subjects: Adverse reactions in pediatric subjects were consistent with those observed in adults. (6.1)

In HBV-infected subjects with decompensated liver disease: most common adverse reactions (incidence greater than or equal to 10%, all grades) were abdominal pain, nausea, insomnia, pruritus, vomiting, dizziness, and pyrexia. (6.1)

To report SUSPECTED ADVERSE REACTIONS, contact Gilead Sciences, Inc. at 1-800-GILEAD-5 or FDA at 1-800-FDA-1088 or www.fda.gov/medwatch

----DRUG INTERACTIONS----

• Didanosine: Coadministration increases didanosine concentrations. Use with caution and monitor for evidence of didanosine toxicity (e.g., pancreatitis, neuropathy). Consider dose reductions or discontinuations of didanosine if warranted. (7.1)

• HIV-1 protease inhibitors: Coadministration decreases atazanavir concentrations and increases tenofovir concentrations. When coadministered with VIREAD, use atazanavir given with ritonavir. Coadministration of VIREAD with atazanavir and ritonavir, darunavir and ritonavir, or lopinavir/ritonavir increases tenofovir concentrations. Monitor for evidence of tenofovir toxicity. (7.2)

----USE IN SPECIFIC POPULATIONS----

• Nursing mothers: Women infected with HIV should be instructed not to breast feed. (8.3)

See 17 for PATIENT COUNSELING INFORMATION and FDA-approved patient labeling

Revised: 10/2013

FULL PRESCRIBING INFORMATION

> **WARNING: LACTIC ACIDOSIS/SEVERE HEPATOMEGALY WITH STEATOSIS and POST TREATMENT EXACERBATION OF HEPATITIS**
>
> **Lactic acidosis and severe hepatomegaly with steatosis, including fatal cases, have been reported with the use of nucleoside analogs, including VIREAD, in combination with other antiretrovirals [See Warnings and Precautions (5.1)].**
>
> **Severe acute exacerbations of hepatitis have been reported in HBV-infected patients who have discontinued anti-hepatitis B therapy, including VIREAD. Hepatic function should be monitored closely with both clinical and laboratory follow-up for at least several months in patients who discontinue anti-hepatitis B therapy, including VIREAD. If appropriate, resumption of anti-hepatitis B therapy may be warranted [See Warnings and Precautions (5.2)].**

1   INDICATIONS AND USAGE
1.1   HIV-1 Infection
VIREAD is indicated in combination with other antiretroviral agents for the treatment of HIV-1 infection in adults and pediatric patients 2 years of age and older.
The following points should be considered when initiating therapy with VIREAD for the treatment of HIV-1 infection:
• VIREAD should not be used in combination with ATRIPLA®, COMPLERA®, STRIBILD®, or TRUVADA® [See Warnings and Precautions (5.4)].

1.2   Chronic Hepatitis B
VIREAD is indicated for the treatment of chronic hepatitis B in adults and pediatric patients 12 years of age and older.
The following points should be considered when initiating therapy with VIREAD for the treatment of HBV infection:
• The indication in adults is based on safety and efficacy data from treatment of subjects who were nucleoside-treatment-naïve and subjects who were treatment-experienced with documented resistance to lamivudine. Subjects were adults with HBeAg-positive and HBeAg-negative chronic hepatitis B with compensated liver disease [See Clinical Studies (14.2)].
• VIREAD was evaluated in a limited number of subjects with chronic hepatitis B and decompensated liver disease [See Adverse Reactions (6.1), Clinical Studies (14.2)].
• The numbers of subjects in clinical trials who had adefovir resistance-associated substitutions at baseline were too small to reach conclusions of efficacy [See Microbiology (12.4), Clinical Studies (14.2)].

2   DOSAGE AND ADMINISTRATION
2.1   Recommended Dose in Adults and Pediatric Patients 12 Years of Age and Older (35 kg or more)
For the treatment of HIV-1 or chronic hepatitis B: The dose is one 300 mg VIREAD tablet once daily taken orally, without regard to food.
For patients unable to swallow VIREAD tablets, the oral powder formulation (7.5 scoops) may be used.

In the treatment of chronic hepatitis B, the optimal duration of treatment is unknown. Safety and efficacy in pediatric patients with chronic hepatitis B weighing less than 35 kg have not been established.

2.2   Recommended Dose in Pediatric Patients 2 Years to Less Than 12 Years of Age
HIV-1 Infection
For the treatment of HIV-1 in pediatric patients 2 years of age and older, the recommended oral dose of VIREAD is 8 mg of tenofovir disoproxil fumarate per kilogram of body weight (up to a maximum of 300 mg) once daily administered as oral powder or tablets.
VIREAD oral powder should be measured only with the supplied dosing scoop. One level scoop delivers 1 g of powder which contains 40 mg of tenofovir disoproxil fumarate. VIREAD oral powder should be mixed in a container with 2 to 4 ounces of soft food not requiring chewing (e.g., applesauce, baby food, yogurt). The entire mixture should be ingested immediately to avoid a bitter taste. Do not administer VIREAD oral powder in a liquid as the powder may float on top of the liquid even after stirring. Further patient instructions on how to administer VIREAD oral powder with the supplied dosing scoop are provided in the FDA-approved patient labeling (Patient Information).
VIREAD is also available as tablets in 150, 200, 250 and 300 mg strengths for pediatric patients who weigh greater than or equal to 17 kg and who are able to reliably swallow intact tablets. The dose is one tablet once daily taken orally, without regard to food.
Tables 1 and 2 contain dosing recommendations for VIREAD oral powder and tablets based on body weight. Weight should be monitored periodically and the VIREAD dose adjusted accordingly.

Table 1 Dosing Recommendations for Pediatric Patients ≥2 Years of Age Using VIREAD Oral Powder

Body Weight Kilogram (kg)	Oral Powder Once Daily Scoops of Powder
10 to <12	2
12 to <14	2.5
14 to <17	3
17 to <19	3.5
19 to <22	4
22 to <24	4.5
24 to <27	5
27 to <29	5.5
29 to <32	6
32 to <34	6.5
34 to <35	7
≥35	7.5

Table 2 Dosing Recommendations for Pediatric Patients ≥2 Years of Age and Weighing ≥17 kg Using VIREAD Tablets

Body Weight Kilogram (kg)	Tablets Once Daily
17 to <22	150 mg
22 to <28	200 mg
28 to <35	250 mg
≥35	300 mg

Chronic Hepatitis B
Safety and efficacy of VIREAD in patients younger than 12 years of age have not been established.

2.3   Dose Adjustment for Renal Impairment in Adults
Significantly increased drug exposures occurred when VIREAD was administered to subjects with moderate to severe renal impairment [See Clinical Pharmacology (12.3)]. Therefore, the dosing interval of VIREAD tablets 300 mg should be adjusted in patients with baseline creatinine clearance below 50 mL/min using the recommendations in Table 3. These dosing interval recommendations are based on modeling of single-dose pharmacokinetic data in non-HIV and non-HBV infected subjects with varying degrees of renal impairment, including end-stage renal disease requiring hemodialysis. The safety and effectiveness of these dos-

ing interval adjustment recommendations have not been clinically evaluated in patients with moderate or severe renal impairment, therefore clinical response to treatment and renal function should be closely monitored in these patients [See Warnings and Precautions (5.3)]. There are no data to recommend use of VIREAD tablets 150, 200 or 250 mg or VIREAD oral powder in patients with renal impairment.

No dose adjustment of VIREAD tablets 300 mg is necessary for patients with mild renal impairment (creatinine clearance 50–80 mL/min). Routine monitoring of estimated creatinine clearance, serum phosphorus, urine glucose, and urine protein should be performed in patients with mild renal impairment [See Warnings and Precautions (5.3)]. [See table 3 above]

The pharmacokinetics of tenofovir have not been evaluated in non-hemodialysis patients with creatinine clearance below 10 mL/min; therefore, no dosing recommendation is available for these patients.

No data are available to make dose recommendations in pediatric patients with renal impairment.

3 DOSAGE FORMS AND STRENGTHS

VIREAD is available as tablets or as an oral powder.
VIREAD tablets 150 mg contain 150 mg of tenofovir disoproxil fumarate, which is equivalent to 123 mg of tenofovir disoproxil. The tablets are triangle-shaped, white, film-coated, and debossed with "GSI" on one side and "150" on the other side.
VIREAD tablets 200 mg contain 200 mg of tenofovir disoproxil fumarate, which is equivalent to 163 mg of tenofovir disoproxil. The tablets are round-shaped, white, film-coated, and debossed with "GSI" on one side and "200" on the other side.
VIREAD tablets 250 mg contain 250 mg of tenofovir disoproxil fumarate, which is equivalent to 204 mg of tenofovir disoproxil. The tablets are capsule-shaped, white, film-coated, and debossed with "GSI" on one side and "250" on the other side.
VIREAD tablets 300 mg contain 300 mg of tenofovir disoproxil fumarate, which is equivalent to 245 mg of tenofovir disoproxil. The tablets are almond-shaped, light blue, film-coated, and debossed with "GILEAD" and "4331" on one side and with "300" on the other side.
The oral powder consists of white, taste-masked, coated granules containing 40 mg of tenofovir disoproxil fumarate, which is equivalent to 33 mg of tenofovir disoproxil, per level scoop. Each level scoop contains 1 gram of oral powder.

4 CONTRAINDICATIONS

None.

5 WARNINGS AND PRECAUTIONS

5.1 Lactic Acidosis/Severe Hepatomegaly with Steatosis

Lactic acidosis and severe hepatomegaly with steatosis, including fatal cases, have been reported with the use of nucleoside analogs, including VIREAD, in combination with other antiretrovirals. A majority of these cases have been in women. Obesity and prolonged nucleoside exposure may be risk factors. Particular caution should be exercised when administering nucleoside analogs to any patient with known risk factors for liver disease; however, cases have also been reported in patients with no known risk factors. Treatment with VIREAD should be suspended in any patient who develops clinical or laboratory findings suggestive of lactic acidosis or pronounced hepatotoxicity (which may include hepatomegaly and steatosis even in the absence of marked transaminase elevations).

5.2 Exacerbation of Hepatitis after Discontinuation of Treatment

Discontinuation of anti-HBV therapy, including VIREAD, may be associated with severe acute exacerbations of hepatitis. Patients infected with HBV who discontinue VIREAD should be closely monitored with both clinical and laboratory follow-up for at least several months after stopping treatment. If appropriate, resumption of anti-hepatitis B therapy may be warranted.

5.3 New Onset or Worsening Renal Impairment

Tenofovir is principally eliminated by the kidney. Renal impairment, including cases of acute renal failure and Fanconi syndrome (renal tubular injury with severe hypophosphatemia), has been reported with the use of VIREAD [See Adverse Reactions (6.2)].

It is recommended that estimated creatinine clearance be assessed in all patients prior to initiating therapy and as clinically appropriate during therapy with VIREAD. In patients at risk of renal dysfunction, including patients who have previously experienced renal events while receiving HEPSERA®, it is recommended that estimated creatinine clearance, serum phosphorus, urine glucose, and urine protein be assessed prior to initiation of VIREAD, and periodically during VIREAD therapy.

Dosing interval adjustment of VIREAD and close monitoring of renal function are recommended in all patients with

creatinine clearance below 50 mL/min [See Dosage and Administration (2.3)]. No safety or efficacy data are available in patients with renal impairment who received VIREAD using these dosing guidelines, so the potential benefit of VIREAD therapy should be assessed against the potential risk of renal toxicity.

VIREAD should be avoided with concurrent or recent use of a nephrotoxic agent (e.g., high-dose or multiple non-steroidal anti-inflammatory drugs (NSAIDs)) [See Drug Interactions (7.3)]. Cases of acute renal failure after initiation of high dose or multiple NSAIDs have been reported in HIV-infected patients with risk factors for renal dysfunction who appeared stable on tenofovir DF. Some patients required hospitalization and renal replacement therapy. Alternatives to NSAIDs should be considered, if needed, in patients at risk for renal dysfunction.

Persistent or worsening bone pain, pain in extremities, fractures and/or muscular pain or weakness may be manifestations of proximal renal tubulopathy and should prompt an evaluation of renal function in at-risk patients.

5.4 Coadministration with Other Products

VIREAD should not be used in combination with the fixed-dose combination products ATRIPLA, COMPLERA, STRIBILD, or TRUVADA since tenofovir disoproxil fumarate is a component of these products.

VIREAD should not be administered in combination with HEPSERA (adefovir dipivoxil) [See Drug Interactions (7.3)].

5.5 Patients Coinfected with HIV-1 and HBV

Due to the risk of development of HIV-1 resistance, VIREAD should only be used in HIV-1 and HBV coinfected patients as part of an appropriate antiretroviral combination regimen.

HIV-1 antibody testing should be offered to all HBV-infected patients before initiating therapy with VIREAD. It is also recommended that all patients with HIV-1 be tested for the presence of chronic hepatitis B before initiating treatment with VIREAD.

5.6 Bone Effects

Bone Mineral Density:
In clinical trials in HIV-1 infected adults, VIREAD was associated with slightly greater decreases in bone mineral density (BMD) and increases in biochemical markers of bone metabolism, suggesting increased bone turnover relative to comparators. Serum parathyroid hormone levels and 1,25 Vitamin D levels were also higher in subjects receiving VIREAD [See Adverse Reactions (6.1)].

Clinical trials evaluating VIREAD in pediatric and adolescent subjects were conducted. Under normal circumstances, BMD increases rapidly in pediatric patients. In HIV-1 infected subjects aged 2 years to less than 18 years, bone effects were similar to those observed in adult subjects and suggest increased bone turnover. Total body BMD gain was less in the VIREAD-treated HIV-1 infected pediatric subjects as compared to the control groups. Similar trends were observed in chronic hepatitis B infected adolescent subjects aged 12 years to less than 18 years. In all pediatric trials, skeletal growth (height) appeared to be unaffected. [See Adverse Reactions (6.1)].

The effects of VIREAD-associated changes in BMD and biochemical markers on long-term bone health and future fracture risk are unknown. Assessment of BMD should be considered for adults and pediatric patients who have a history of pathologic bone fracture or other risk factors for osteoporosis or bone loss. Although the effect of supplementation with calcium and vitamin D was not studied, such supplementation may be beneficial for all patients. If bone abnormalities are suspected then appropriate consultation should be obtained.

Mineralization Defects:
Cases of osteomalacia associated with proximal renal tubulopathy, manifested as bone pain or pain in extremities and which may contribute to fractures, have been reported in association with the use of VIREAD [See Adverse Reactions (6.2)]. Arthralgias and muscle pain or weakness have also been reported in cases of proximal renal tubulopathy. Hypophosphatemia and osteomalacia secondary to proximal renal tubulopathy should be considered in patients at risk of

renal dysfunction who present with persistent or worsening bone or muscle symptoms while receiving products containing tenofovir DF [See Warnings and Precautions (5.3)].

5.7 Fat Redistribution

In HIV-infected patients redistribution/accumulation of body fat including central obesity, dorsocervical fat enlargement (buffalo hump), peripheral wasting, facial wasting, breast enlargement, and "cushingoid appearance" have been observed in patients receiving combination antiretroviral therapy. The mechanism and long-term consequences of these events are currently unknown. A causal relationship has not been established.

5.8 Immune Reconstitution Syndrome

Immune reconstitution syndrome has been reported in HIV-infected patients treated with combination antiretroviral therapy, including VIREAD. During the initial phase of combination antiretroviral treatment, patients whose immune system responds may develop an inflammatory response to indolent or residual opportunistic infections [such as *Mycobacterium avium* infection, cytomegalovirus, *Pneumocystis jirovecii* pneumonia (PCP), or tuberculosis], which may necessitate further evaluation and treatment.

Autoimmune disorders (such as Graves' disease, polymyositis, and Guillain-Barré syndrome) have also been reported to occur in the setting of immune reconstitution, however, the time to onset is more variable, and can occur many months after initiation of treatment.

5.9 Early Virologic Failure

Clinical trials in HIV-infected subjects have demonstrated that certain regimens that only contain three nucleoside reverse transcriptase inhibitors (NRTI) are generally less effective than triple drug regimens containing two NRTIs in combination with either a non-nucleoside reverse transcriptase inhibitor or a HIV-1 protease inhibitor. In particular, early virological failure and high rates of resistance substitutions have been reported. Triple nucleoside regimens should therefore be used with caution. Patients on a therapy utilizing a triple nucleoside-only regimen should be carefully monitored and considered for treatment modification.

6 ADVERSE REACTIONS

The following adverse reactions are discussed in other sections of the labeling:
• Lactic Acidosis/Severe Hepatomegaly with Steatosis [See Boxed Warning, Warnings and Precautions (5.1)].
• Severe Acute Exacerbation of Hepatitis [See Boxed Warning, Warnings and Precautions (5.2)].
• New Onset or Worsening Renal Impairment [See Warnings and Precautions (5.3)].
• Bone Effects [See Warnings and Precautions (5.6)].
• Immune Reconstitution Syndrome [See Warnings and Precautions (5.8)].

6.1 Adverse Reactions from Clinical Trials Experience

Because clinical trials are conducted under widely varying conditions, adverse reaction rates observed in the clinical trials of a drug cannot be directly compared to rates in the clinical trials of another drug and may not reflect the rates observed in practice.

Clinical Trials in Adult Patients with HIV-1 Infection
More than 12,000 subjects have been treated with VIREAD alone or in combination with other antiretroviral medicinal products for periods of 28 days to 215 weeks in clinical trials and expanded access programs. A total of 1,544 subjects have received VIREAD 300 mg once daily in clinical trials; over 11,000 subjects have received VIREAD in expanded access programs.

The most common adverse reactions (incidence greater than or equal to 10%, Grades 2–4) identified from any of the 3 large controlled clinical trials include rash, diarrhea, headache, pain, depression, asthenia, and nausea.

Treatment-Naïve Patients
Study 903 - Treatment-Emergent Adverse Reactions: The most common adverse reactions seen in a double-blind comparative controlled trial in which 600 treatment-naïve subjects received VIREAD (N=299) or stavudine (N=301) in

Table 3 Dosage Adjustment for Patients with Altered Creatinine Clearance

	Creatinine Clearance (mL/min)*			
	≥50	30–49	10–29	Hemodialysis Patients
Recommended 300 mg Dosing Interval	Every 24 hours	Every 48 hours	Every 72 to 96 hours	Every 7 days or after a total of approximately 12 hours of dialysis†

* Calculated using ideal (lean) body weight.
† Generally once weekly assuming three hemodialysis sessions a week of approximately 4 hours duration. VIREAD should be administered following completion of dialysis.

combination with lamivudine and efavirenz for 144 weeks (Study 903) were mild to moderate gastrointestinal events and dizziness.

Mild adverse reactions (Grade 1) were common with a similar incidence in both arms, and included dizziness, diarrhea, and nausea. Selected treatment-emergent moderate to severe adverse reactions are summarized in Table 4.

Table 4 Selected Treatment-Emergent Adverse Reactions* (Grades 2–4) Reported in ≥5% in Any Treatment Group in Study 903 (0–144 Weeks)

	VIREAD + 3TC + EFV	d4T + 3TC + EFV
	N=299	N=301
Body as a Whole		
Headache	14%	17%
Pain	13%	12%
Fever	8%	7%
Abdominal pain	7%	12%
Back pain	9%	8%
Asthenia	6%	7%
Digestive System		
Diarrhea	11%	13%
Nausea	8%	9%
Dyspepsia	4%	5%
Vomiting	5%	9%
Metabolic Disorders		
Lipodystrophy†	1%	8%
Musculoskeletal		
Arthralgia	5%	7%
Myalgia	3%	5%
Nervous System		
Depression	11%	10%
Insomnia	5%	8%
Dizziness	3%	6%
Peripheral neuropathy‡	1%	5%
Anxiety	6%	6%
Respiratory		
Pneumonia	5%	5%
Skin and Appendages		
Rash event§	18%	12%

* Frequencies of adverse reactions are based on all treatment-emergent adverse events, regardless of relationship to study drug.
† Lipodystrophy represents a variety of investigator-described adverse events not a protocol-defined syndrome.
‡ Peripheral neuropathy includes peripheral neuritis and neuropathy.
§ Rash event includes rash, pruritus, maculopapular rash, urticaria, vesiculobullous rash, and pustular rash.

Laboratory Abnormalities: With the exception of fasting cholesterol and fasting triglyceride elevations that were more common in the stavudine group (40% and 9%) compared with VIREAD (19% and 1%) respectively, laboratory abnormalities observed in this trial occurred with similar frequency in the VIREAD and stavudine treatment arms. A summary of Grades 3–4 laboratory abnormalities is provided in Table 5.

Table 5 Grades 3–4 Laboratory Abnormalities Reported in ≥1% of VIREAD-Treated Subjects in Study 903 (0–144 Weeks)

	VIREAD + 3TC + EFV	d4T + 3TC + EFV
	N=299	N=301
Any ≥ Grade 3 Laboratory Abnormality	36%	42%
Fasting Cholesterol (>240 mg/dL)	19%	40%
Creatine Kinase (M: >990 U/L; F: >845 U/L)	12%	12%
Serum Amylase (>175 U/L)	9%	8%
AST (M: >180 U/L; F: >170 U/L)	5%	7%
ALT (M: >215 U/L; F: >170 U/L)	4%	5%

Hematuria (>100 RBC/HPF)	7%	7%
Neutrophils (<750/mm³)	3%	1%
Fasting Triglycerides (>750 mg/dL)	1%	9%

Study 934 - Treatment Emergent Adverse Reactions: In Study 934, 511 antiretroviral-naïve subjects received either VIREAD + EMTRIVA® administered in combination with efavirenz (N=257) or zidovudine/lamivudine administered in combination with efavirenz (N=254). Adverse reactions observed in this trial were generally consistent with those seen in previous studies in treatment-experienced or treatment-naïve subjects (Table 6).

Changes in Bone Mineral Density:
In HIV-1 infected adult subjects in Study 903, there was a significantly greater mean percentage decrease from baseline in BMD at the lumbar spine in subjects receiving VIREAD + lamivudine + efavirenz (-2.2% ± 3.9) compared with subjects receiving stavudine + lamivudine + efavirenz (-1.0% ± 4.6) through 144 weeks. Changes in BMD at the hip were similar between the two treatment groups (-2.8% ± 3.5 in the VIREAD group vs. -2.4% ± 4.5 in the stavudine group). In both groups, the majority of the reduction in BMD occurred in the first 24-48 weeks of the trial and this reduction was sustained through Week 144. Twenty-eight percent of VIREAD-treated subjects vs. 21% of the stavudine-treated subjects lost at least 5% of BMD at the spine or 7% of BMD at the hip. Clinically relevant fractures (excluding fingers and toes) were reported in 4 subjects in the VIREAD group and 6 subjects in the stavudine group. In addition, there were significant increases in biochemical markers of bone metabolism (serum bone-specific alkaline phosphatase, serum osteocalcin, serum C telopeptide, and urinary N telopeptide) and higher serum parathyroid hormone levels and 1,25 Vitamin D levels in the VIREAD group relative to the stavudine group; however, except for bone-specific alkaline phosphatase, these changes resulted in values that remained within the normal range *[See Warnings and Precautions (5.6)]*.

Table 6 Selected Treatment-Emergent Adverse Reactions* (Grades 2–4) Reported in ≥5% in Any Treatment Group in Study 934 (0–144 Weeks)

	VIREAD† + FTC + EFV	AZT/3TC + EFV
	N=257	N=254
Gastrointestinal Disorder		
Diarrhea	9%	5%
Nausea	9%	7%
Vomiting	2%	5%
General Disorders and Administration Site Condition		
Fatigue	9%	8%
Infections and Infestations		
Sinusitis	8%	4%
Upper respiratory tract infections	8%	5%
Nasopharyngitis	5%	3%
Nervous System Disorders		
Headache	6%	5%
Dizziness	8%	7%
Psychiatric Disorders		
Depression	9%	7%
Insomnia	5%	7%
Skin and Subcutaneous Tissue Disorders		
Rash event‡	7%	9%

* Frequencies of adverse reactions are based on all treatment-emergent adverse events, regardless of relationship to study drug.
† From Weeks 96 to 144 of the trial, subjects received TRUVADA with efavirenz in place of VIREAD + EMTRIVA with efavirenz.
‡ Rash event includes rash, exfoliative rash, rash generalized, rash macular, rash maculopapular, rash pruritic, and rash vesicular.

Laboratory Abnormalities: Laboratory abnormalities observed in this trial were generally consistent with those seen in previous trials (Table 7).

Table 7 Significant Laboratory Abnormalities Reported in ≥1% of Subjects in Any Treatment Group in Study 934 (0–144 Weeks)

	VIREAD* + FTC + EFV	AZT/3TC + EFV
	N=257	N=254
Any ≥ Grade 3 Laboratory Abnormality	30%	26%
Fasting Cholesterol (>240 mg/dL)	22%	24%
Creatine Kinase (M: >990 U/L; F: >845 U/L)	9%	7%
Serum Amylase (>175 U/L)	8%	4%
Alkaline Phosphatase (>550 U/L)	1%	0%
AST (M: >180 U/L; F: >170 U/L)	3%	3%
ALT (M: >215 U/L; F: >170 U/L)	2%	3%
Hemoglobin (<8.0 mg/dL)	0%	4%
Hyperglycemia (>250 mg/dL)	2%	1%
Hematuria (>75 RBC/HPF)	3%	2%
Glycosuria (≥3+)	<1%	1%
Neutrophils (<750/mm³)	3%	5%
Fasting Triglycerides (>750 mg/dL)	4%	2%

* From Weeks 96 to 144 of the trial, subjects received TRUVADA with efavirenz in place of VIREAD + EMTRIVA with efavirenz.

Treatment-Experienced Patients
Treatment-Emergent Adverse Reactions: The adverse reactions seen in treatment experienced subjects were generally consistent with those seen in treatment naïve subjects including mild to moderate gastrointestinal events, such as nausea, diarrhea, vomiting, and flatulence. Less than 1% of subjects discontinued participation in the clinical trials due to gastrointestinal adverse reactions (Study 907).
A summary of moderate to severe, treatment-emergent adverse reactions that occurred during the first 48 weeks of Study 907 is provided in Table 8.
[See table 8 at top of next page]
Laboratory Abnormalities: Laboratory abnormalities observed in this trial occurred with similar frequency in the VIREAD and placebo-treated groups. A summary of Grades 3–4 laboratory abnormalities is provided in Table 9.
[See table 9 on next page]
Clinical Trials in Pediatric Subjects 2 Years of Age and Older with HIV-1 Infection
Assessment of adverse reactions is based on two randomized trials (Studies 352 and 321) in 184 HIV-1 infected pediatric subjects (2 to less than 18 years of age) who received treatment with VIREAD (N=93) or placebo/active comparator (N=91) in combination with other antiretroviral agents for 48 weeks. The adverse reactions observed in subjects who received treatment with VIREAD were consistent with those observed in clinical trials in adults.
Eighty-nine pediatric subjects (2 to less than 12 years of age) received VIREAD in Study 352 for a median exposure of 104 weeks. Of these, 4 subjects discontinued from the trial due to adverse reactions consistent with proximal renal tubulopathy. Three of these 4 subjects presented with hypophosphatemia and also had decreases in total body or spine BMD Z score *[See Warnings and Precautions (5.6)]*.
Changes in Bone Mineral Density:
Clinical trials in HIV-1 infected children and adolescents evaluated BMD changes. In Study 321 (12 to less than 18 years), the mean rate of BMD gain at Week 48 was less in the VIREAD compared to the placebo treatment group. Six VIREAD treated subjects and one placebo treated subject had significant (greater than 4%) lumbar spine BMD loss at Week 48. Changes from baseline BMD Z-scores were −0.341 for lumbar spine and −0.458 for total body in the 28 subjects who were treated with VIREAD for 96 weeks. In Study 352 (2 to less than 12 years), the mean rate of BMD gain in lumbar spine at Week 48 was similar between the VIREAD and the d4T or AZT treatment groups. Total body BMD gain was less in the VIREAD compared to the d4T or AZT treatment groups. One VIREAD-treated subject and none of the d4T or AZT-treated subjects experienced significant (greater than

4%) lumbar spine BMD loss at Week 48. Changes from baseline in BMD Z scores were –0.012 for lumbar spine and –0.338 for total body in the 64 subjects who were treated with VIREAD for 96 weeks. In both trials, skeletal growth (height) appeared to be unaffected [See Warnings and Precautions (5.6)].

Clinical Trials in Adult Subjects with Chronic Hepatitis B and Compensated Liver Disease

Treatment-Emergent Adverse Reactions: In controlled clinical trials in 641 subjects with chronic hepatitis B (0102 and 0103), more subjects treated with VIREAD during the 48-week double-blind period experienced nausea: 9% with VIREAD versus 2% with HEPSERA. Other treatment-emergent adverse reactions reported in more than 5% of subjects treated with VIREAD included: abdominal pain, diarrhea, headache, dizziness, fatigue, nasopharyngitis, back pain and skin rash.

During the open-label phase of treatment with VIREAD (weeks 48–240) in Studies 0102 and 0103, less than 1% of subjects (5/585) experienced a confirmed increase in serum creatinine of 0.5 mg/dL from baseline. No significant change in the tolerability profile was observed with continued treatment for up to 240 weeks.

Laboratory Abnormalities: A summary of Grades 3–4 laboratory abnormalities through Week 48 is provided in Table 10. Grades 3–4 laboratory abnormalities were similar in subjects continuing VIREAD treatment for up to 240 weeks in these trials.

Table 10 Grades 3–4 Laboratory Abnormalities Reported in ≥1% of VIREAD-Treated Subjects in Studies 0102 and 0103 (0–48 Weeks)

	VIREAD (N=426)	HEPSERA (N=215)
Any ≥ Grade 3 Laboratory Abnormality	19%	13%
Creatine Kinase (M: >990 U/L; F: >845 U/L)	2%	3%
Serum Amylase (>175 U/L)	4%	1%
Glycosuria (≥3+)	3%	<1%
AST (M: >180 U/L; F: >170 U/L)	4%	4%
ALT (M: >215 U/L; F: >170 U/L)	10%	6%

The overall incidence of on-treatment ALT flares (defined as serum ALT greater than 2 × baseline and greater than 10 × ULN, with or without associated symptoms) was similar between VIREAD (2.6%) and HEPSERA (2%). ALT flares generally occurred within the first 4–8 weeks of treatment and were accompanied by decreases in HBV DNA levels. No subject had evidence of decompensation. ALT flares typically resolved within 4 to 8 weeks without changes in study medication.

The adverse reactions observed in subjects with chronic hepatitis B and lamivudine resistance who received treatment with VIREAD were consistent with those observed in other hepatitis B clinical trials in adults.

Clinical Trials in Adult Subjects with Chronic Hepatitis B and Decompensated Liver Disease

In a small randomized, double-blind, active-controlled trial (0108), subjects with CHB and decompensated liver disease received treatment with VIREAD or other antiviral drugs for up to 48 weeks [See Clinical Studies (14.2)]. Among the 45 subjects receiving VIREAD, the most frequently reported treatment-emergent adverse reactions of any severity were abdominal pain (22%), nausea (20%), insomnia (18%), pruritus (16%), vomiting (13%), dizziness (13%), and pyrexia (11%). Two of 45 (4%) subjects died through Week 48 of the trial due to progression of liver disease. Three of 45 (7%) subjects discontinued treatment due to an adverse event. Four of 45 (9%) subjects experienced a confirmed increase in serum creatinine of 0.5 mg/dL (1 subject also had a confirmed serum phosphorus less than 2 mg/dL through Week 48). Three of these subjects (each of whom had a Child-Pugh score greater than or equal to 10 and MELD score greater than or equal to 14 at entry) developed renal failure. Because both VIREAD and decompensated liver disease may have an impact on renal function, the contribution of VIREAD to renal impairment in this population is difficult to ascertain.

One of 45 subjects experienced an on-treatment hepatic flare during the 48 Week trial.

Clinical Trials in Pediatric Subjects 12 Years of Age and Older with Chronic Hepatitis B

Assessment of adverse reactions is based on one randomized study (Study GS-US-174-0115) in 106 pediatric subjects (12 to less than 18 years of age) infected with chronic hepatitis B receiving treatment with VIREAD (N = 52) or placebo (N = 54) for 72 weeks. The adverse reactions observed in pediatric subjects who received treatment with VIREAD were consistent with those observed in clinical trials of VIREAD in adults.

In this study, both the VIREAD and placebo treatment arms experienced an overall increase in mean lumbar spine BMD over 72 weeks, as expected for an adolescent population. The BMD gains from baseline to Week 72 in lumbar spine and total body BMD in VIREAD-treated subjects (+5% and +3%, respectively) were less than the BMD gains observed in placebo-treated subjects (+8% and +5%, respectively). Three subjects in the VIREAD group and two subjects in the placebo group had significant (greater than 4%) lumbar spine BMD loss at Week 72. At baseline, mean BMD Z-scores in subjects randomized to VIREAD were –0.43 for lumbar spine and –0.20 for total body, and mean BMD Z-scores in subjects randomized to placebo were –0.28 for lumbar spine and –0.26 for total body. In subjects receiving VIREAD for 72 weeks, the mean change in BMD Z-score was –0.05 for lumbar spine and –0.15 for total body compared to +0.07 and +0.06, respectively, in subjects receiving placebo. As observed in pediatric studies of HIV-infected patients, skeletal growth (height) appeared to be unaffected [See Warnings and Precautions (5.6)].

6.2 Postmarketing Experience

The following adverse reactions have been identified during postapproval use of VIREAD. Because postmarketing reactions are reported voluntarily from a population of uncertain size, it is not always possible to reliably estimate their frequency or establish a causal relationship to drug exposure.

Immune System Disorders
allergic reaction, including angioedema
Metabolism and Nutrition Disorders
lactic acidosis, hypokalemia, hypophosphatemia
Respiratory, Thoracic, and Mediastinal Disorders
dyspnea

Table 8 Selected Treatment-Emergent Adverse Reactions* (Grades 2–4) Reported in ≥3% in Any Treatment Group in Study 907 (0–48 Weeks)

	VIREAD (N=368) (Week 0–24)	Placebo (N=182) (Week 0–24)	VIREAD (N=368) (Week 0–48)	Placebo Crossover to VIREAD (N=170) (Week 24–48)
Body as a Whole				
Asthenia	7%	6%	11%	1%
Pain	7%	7%	12%	4%
Headache	5%	5%	8%	2%
Abdominal pain	4%	3%	7%	6%
Back pain	3%	3%	4%	2%
Chest pain	3%	1%	3%	2%
Fever	2%	2%	4%	2%
Digestive System				
Diarrhea	11%	10%	16%	11%
Nausea	8%	5%	11%	7%
Vomiting	4%	1%	7%	5%
Anorexia	3%	2%	4%	1%
Dyspepsia	3%	2%	4%	2%
Flatulence	3%	1%	4%	1%
Respiratory				
Pneumonia	2%	0%	3%	2%
Nervous System				
Depression	4%	3%	8%	4%
Insomnia	3%	2%	4%	4%
Peripheral neuropathy[†]	3%	3%	5%	2%
Dizziness	1%	3%	3%	1%
Skin and Appendage				
Rash event[‡]	5%	4%	7%	1%
Sweating	3%	2%	3%	1%
Musculoskeletal				
Myalgia	3%	3%	4%	1%
Metabolic				
Weight loss	2%	1%	4%	2%

* Frequencies of adverse reactions are based on all treatment-emergent adverse events, regardless of relationship to study drug.
† Peripheral neuropathy includes peripheral neuritis and neuropathy.
‡ Rash event includes rash, pruritus, maculopapular rash, urticaria, vesiculobullous rash, and pustular rash.

Table 9 Grades 3–4 Laboratory Abnormalities Reported in ≥1% of VIREAD-Treated Subjects in Study 907 (0–48 Weeks)

	VIREAD (N=368) (Week 0–24)	Placebo (N=182) (Week 0–24)	VIREAD (N=368) (Week 0–48)	Placebo Crossover to VIREAD (N=170) (Week 24–48)
Any ≥ Grade 3 Laboratory Abnormality	25%	38%	35%	34%
Triglycerides (>750 mg/dL)	8%	13%	11%	9%
Creatine Kinase (M: >990 U/L; F: >845 U/L)	7%	14%	12%	12%
Serum Amylase (>175 U/L)	6%	7%	7%	6%
Glycosuria (≥3+)	3%	3%	3%	2%
AST (M: >180 U/L; F: >170 U/L)	3%	3%	4%	5%
ALT (M: >215 U/L; F: >170 U/L)	2%	2%	4%	5%
Serum Glucose (>250 U/L)	2%	4%	3%	3%
Neutrophils (<750/mm^3)	1%	1%	2%	1%

Gastrointestinal Disorders
pancreatitis, increased amylase, abdominal pain
Hepatobiliary Disorders
hepatic steatosis, hepatitis, increased liver enzymes (most commonly AST, ALT gamma GT)
Skin and Subcutaneous Tissue Disorders
rash
Musculoskeletal and Connective Tissue Disorders
rhabdomyolysis, osteomalacia (manifested as bone pain and which may contribute to fractures), muscular weakness, myopathy
Renal and Urinary Disorders
acute renal failure, renal failure, acute tubular necrosis, Fanconi syndrome, proximal renal tubulopathy, interstitial nephritis (including acute cases), nephrogenic diabetes insipidus, renal insufficiency, increased creatinine, proteinuria, polyuria
General Disorders and Administration Site Conditions
asthenia

The following adverse reactions, listed under the body system headings above, may occur as a consequence of proximal renal tubulopathy: rhabdomyolysis, osteomalacia, hypokalemia, muscular weakness, myopathy, hypophosphatemia.

7   DRUG INTERACTIONS

This section describes clinically relevant drug interactions with VIREAD. Drug interactions trials are described elsewhere in the labeling *[See Clinical Pharmacology (12.3)]*.

7.1   Didanosine

Coadministration of VIREAD and didanosine should be undertaken with caution and patients receiving this combination should be monitored closely for didanosine-associated adverse reactions. Didanosine should be discontinued in patients who develop didanosine-associated adverse reactions. When administered with VIREAD, C_{max} and AUC of didanosine increased significantly *[See Clinical Pharmacology (12.3)]*. The mechanism of this interaction is unknown. Higher didanosine concentrations could potentiate didanosine-associated adverse reactions, including pancreatitis and neuropathy. Suppression of $CD4^+$ cell counts has been observed in patients receiving VIREAD with didanosine 400 mg daily.

In patients weighing greater than 60 kg, the didanosine dose should be reduced to 250 mg once daily when it is co-administered with VIREAD. In patients weighing less than 60 kg, the didanosine dose should be reduced to 200 mg once daily when it is coadministered with VIREAD. When coadministered, VIREAD and didanosine EC may be taken under fasted conditions or with a light meal (less than 400 kcal, 20% fat). For additional information on coadministration of VIREAD and didanosine, please refer to the full prescribing information for didanosine.

7.2   HIV-1 Protease Inhibitors

VIREAD decreases the AUC and C_{min} of atazanavir *[See Clinical Pharmacology (12.3)]*. When coadministered with VIREAD, it is recommended that atazanavir 300 mg is given with ritonavir 100 mg. VIREAD should not be coadministered with atazanavir without ritonavir.

Lopinavir/ritonavir, atazanavir coadministered with ritonavir, and darunavir coadministered with ritonavir have been shown to increase tenofovir concentrations *[See Clinical Pharmacology (12.3)]*. Tenofovir disoproxil fumarate is a substrate of P-glycoprotein (Pgp) and breast cancer resistance protein (BCRP) transporters. When tenofovir disoproxil fumarate is co-administered with an inhibitor of these transporters, an increase in absorption may be observed. Patients receiving VIREAD concomitantly with lopinavir/ritonavir, ritonavir-boosted atazanavir, or ritonavir-boosted darunavir should be monitored for VIREAD-associated adverse reactions. VIREAD should be discontinued in patients who develop VIREAD-associated adverse reactions.

7.3   Drugs Affecting Renal Function

Since tenofovir is primarily eliminated by the kidneys *[See Clinical Pharmacology (12.3)]*, coadministration of VIREAD with drugs that reduce renal function or compete for active tubular secretion may increase serum concentrations of tenofovir and/or increase the concentrations of other renally eliminated drugs. Some examples include, but are not limited to cidofovir, acyclovir, valacyclovir, ganciclovir, valganciclovir, aminoglycosides (e.g., gentamicin), and high-dose or multiple NSAIDs *[See Warnings and Precautions (5.3)]*.

In the treatment of chronic hepatitis B, VIREAD should not be administered in combination with HEPSERA (adefovir dipivoxil).

8   USE IN SPECIFIC POPULATIONS

8.1   Pregnancy

Pregnancy Category B

There are no adequate and well-controlled studies in pregnant women. Because animal reproduction studies are not always predictive of human response, VIREAD should be used during pregnancy only if clearly needed.

Antiretroviral Pregnancy Registry: To monitor fetal outcomes of pregnant women exposed to VIREAD, an Antiretroviral Pregnancy Registry has been established. Healthcare providers are encouraged to register patients by calling 1-800-258-4263.

Animal Data

Reproduction studies have been performed in rats and rabbits at doses up to 14 and 19 times the human dose based on body surface area comparisons and revealed no evidence of impaired fertility or harm to the fetus due to tenofovir.

8.3   Nursing Mothers

Nursing Mothers: The Centers for Disease Control and Prevention recommend that HIV-1-infected mothers not breast-feed their infants to avoid risking postnatal transmission of HIV-1. Samples of breast milk obtained from five HIV-1 infected mothers in the first post-partum week show that tenofovir is secreted in human milk. The impact of this exposure in breastfed infants is unknown. Because of both the potential for HIV-1 transmission and the potential for serious adverse reactions in nursing infants, **mothers should be instructed not to breast-feed if they are receiving VIREAD.**

8.4   Pediatric Use

Pediatric Patients 2 Years of Age and Older with HIV-1 infection

The safety of VIREAD in pediatric patients aged 2 to less than 18 years is supported by data from two randomized trials in which VIREAD was administered to HIV-1 infected treatment-experienced subjects. In addition, the pharmacokinetic profile of tenofovir in patients 2 to less than 18 years of age at the recommended doses was similar to that found to be safe and effective in adult clinical trials *[See Clinical Pharmacology (12.3)]*.

In Study 352, 92 treatment-experienced subjects 2 to less than 12 years of age with stable, virologic suppression on stavudine- or zidovudine-containing regimen were randomized to either replace stavudine or zidovudine with VIREAD (N = 44) or continue their original regimen (N = 48) for 48 weeks. Five additional subjects over the age of 12 were enrolled and randomized (VIREAD N=4, original regimen N=1) but are not included in the efficacy analysis. After 48 weeks, all eligible subjects were allowed to continue in the study receiving open-label VIREAD. At Week 48, 89% of subjects in the VIREAD treatment group and 90% of subjects in the stavudine or zidovudine treatment group had HIV-1 RNA concentrations less than 400 copies/mL. During the 48 week randomized phase of the study, 1 subject in the VIREAD group discontinued the study prematurely because of virologic failure/lack of efficacy and 3 subjects (2 subjects in the VIREAD group and 1 subject in the stavudine or zidovudine group) discontinued for other reasons.

In Study 321, 87 treatment-experienced subjects 12 to less than 18 years of age were treated with VIREAD (N=45) or placebo (N=42) in combination with an optimized background regimen (OBR) for 48 weeks. The mean baseline CD4 cell count was 374 cells/mm³ and the mean baseline plasma HIV-1 RNA was 4.6 $\log_{10}$ copies/mL. At baseline, 90% of subjects harbored NRTI resistance-associated substitutions in their HIV-1 isolates. Overall, the trial failed to show a difference in virologic response between the VIREAD and placebo treatment groups. Subgroup analyses suggest the lack of difference in virologic response may be attributable to imbalances between treatment arms in baseline viral susceptibility to VIREAD and OBR.

Although changes in HIV-1 RNA in these highly treatment-experienced subjects were less than anticipated, the comparability of the pharmacokinetic and safety data to that observed in adults supports the use of VIREAD in pediatric patients 12 years of age and older who weigh greater than or equal to 35 kg whose HIV-1 isolate is expected to be sensitive to VIREAD. *[See Warnings and Precautions (5.6), Adverse Reactions (6.1), and Clinical Pharmacology (12.3)]*.

Safety and effectiveness of VIREAD in pediatric patients younger than 2 years of age with HIV-1 infection have not been established.

Pediatric Patients 12 Years of Age and Older with Chronic Hepatitis B

In Study 115, 106 HBeAg negative (9%) and positive (91%) subjects aged 12 to less than 18 years with chronic HBV infection were randomized to receive blinded treatment with VIREAD 300 mg (N = 52) or placebo (N = 54) for 72 weeks. At study entry, the mean HBV DNA was 8.1 $\log_{10}$ copies/mL and mean ALT was 101 U/L. Of 52 subjects treated with VIREAD, 20 subjects were nucleos(t)ide-naïve and 32 subjects were nucleos(t)ide-experienced. Thirty-one of the 32 nucleos(t)ide-experienced subjects had prior lamivudine experience. At Week 72, 88% (46/52) of subjects in the VIREAD group and 0% (0/54) of subjects in the placebo group had HBV DNA <400 copies/mL. Among subjects with abnormal ALT at baseline, 74% (26/35) of subjects receiving VIREAD had normalized ALT at Week 72 compared to 31% (13/42) in the placebo group. One VIREAD-treated subject experienced sustained HBsAg-loss and seroconversion to anti-HBs during the first 72 weeks of study participation.

Safety and effectiveness of VIREAD in pediatric patients younger than 12 years of age or less than 35 kg with chronic hepatitis B have not been established.

8.5   Geriatric Use

Clinical trials of VIREAD did not include sufficient numbers of subjects aged 65 and over to determine whether they respond differently from younger subjects. In general, dose selection for the elderly patient should be cautious, keeping in mind the greater frequency of decreased hepatic, renal, or cardiac function, and of concomitant disease or other drug therapy.

8.6   Patients with Impaired Renal Function

It is recommended that the dosing interval for VIREAD be modified in patients with estimated creatinine clearance below 50 mL/min or in patients with ESRD who require dialysis *[See Dosage and Administration (2.3), Clinical Pharmacology (12.3)]*.

10   OVERDOSAGE

Limited clinical experience at doses higher than the therapeutic dose of VIREAD 300 mg is available. In Study 901, 600 mg tenofovir disoproxil fumarate was administered to 8 subjects orally for 28 days. No severe adverse reactions were reported. The effects of higher doses are not known. If overdose occurs the patient must be monitored for evidence of toxicity, and standard supportive treatment applied as necessary.

Tenofovir is efficiently removed by hemodialysis with an extraction coefficient of approximately 54%. Following a single 300 mg dose of VIREAD, a four-hour hemodialysis session removed approximately 10% of the administered tenofovir dose.

11   DESCRIPTION

VIREAD is the brand name for tenofovir disoproxil fumarate (a prodrug of tenofovir) which is a fumaric acid salt of bis-isopropoxycarbonyloxymethyl ester derivative of tenofovir. *In vivo* tenofovir disoproxil fumarate is converted to tenofovir, an acyclic nucleoside phosphonate (nucleotide) analog of adenosine 5'-monophosphate. Tenofovir exhibits activity against HIV-1 reverse transcriptase.

The chemical name of tenofovir disoproxil fumarate is 9-[(R)-2-[[bis[[(isopropoxycarbonyl)oxy]methoxy]phosphinyl]methoxy]propyl]adenine fumarate (1:1). It has a molecular formula of $C_{19}H_{30}N_5O_{10}P \cdot C_4H_4O_4$ and a molecular weight of 635.52. It has the following structural formula:

Tenofovir disoproxil fumarate is a white to off-white crystalline powder with a solubility of 13.4 mg/mL in distilled water at 25 °C. It has an octanol/phosphate buffer (pH 6.5) partition coefficient (log p) of 1.25 at 25 °C.

VIREAD is available as tablets or as an oral powder.

VIREAD tablets are for oral administration in strengths of 150, 200, 250, and 300 mg of tenofovir disoproxil fumarate, which are equivalent to 123, 163, 204 and 245 mg of tenofovir disoproxil, respectively. Each tablet contains the following inactive ingredients: croscarmellose sodium, lactose monohydrate, magnesium stearate, microcrystalline cellulose, and pregelatinized starch. The 300 mg tablets are coated with Opadry II Y–30–10671–A, which contains FD&C blue #2 aluminum lake, hypromellose 2910, lactose monohydrate, titanium dioxide, and triacetin. The 150, 200, and 250 mg tablets are coated with Opadry II 32K-18425, which contains hypromellose 2910, lactose monohydrate, titanium dioxide, and triacetin.

VIREAD oral powder is available for oral administration as white, taste-masked, coated granules containing 40 mg of tenofovir disoproxil fumarate per gram of oral powder, which is equivalent to 33 mg of tenofovir disoproxil. The oral powder contains the following inactive ingredients: mannitol, hydroxypropyl cellulose, ethylcellulose, and silicon dioxide.

In this insert, all dosages are expressed in terms of tenofovir disoproxil fumarate except where otherwise noted.

12   CLINICAL PHARMACOLOGY

12.1   Mechanism of Action

Tenofovir disoproxil fumarate is an antiviral drug *[See Microbiology (12.4)]*.

12.3   Pharmacokinetics

The pharmacokinetics of tenofovir disoproxil fumarate have been evaluated in healthy volunteers and HIV-1 infected individuals. Tenofovir pharmacokinetics are similar between these populations.

Absorption

VIREAD is a water soluble diester prodrug of the active ingredient tenofovir. The oral bioavailability of tenofovir from VIREAD in fasted subjects is approximately 25%. Following oral administration of a single dose of VIREAD 300 mg to HIV-1 infected subjects in the fasted state, maximum serum concentrations (C_{max}) are achieved in 1.0 ± 0.4 hrs. C_{max} and AUC values are 0.30 ± 0.09 µg/mL and 2.29 ± 0.69 µg•hr/mL, respectively.

The pharmacokinetics of tenofovir are dose proportional over a VIREAD dose range of 75 to 600 mg and are not affected by repeated dosing.

In a single-dose bioequivalence study conducted under non-fasted conditions (dose administered with 4 oz. applesauce) in healthy adult volunteers, the mean C_{max} of tenofovir was 26% lower for the oral powder relative to the tablet formulation. Mean AUC of tenofovir was similar between the oral powder and tablet formulations.

Distribution

In vitro binding of tenofovir to human plasma or serum proteins is less than 0.7 or 7.2%, respectively, over the tenofovir concentration range 0.01 to 25 µg/mL. The volume of distribution at steady-state is 1.3 ± 0.6 L/kg and 1.2 ± 0.4 L/kg, following intravenous administration of tenofovir 1.0 mg/kg and 3.0 mg/kg.

Metabolism and Elimination

In vitro studies indicate that neither tenofovir disoproxil nor tenofovir are substrates of CYP enzymes.

Following IV administration of tenofovir, approximately 70–80% of the dose is recovered in the urine as unchanged tenofovir within 72 hours of dosing. Following single dose, oral administration of VIREAD, the terminal elimination half-life of tenofovir is approximately 17 hours. After multiple oral doses of VIREAD 300 mg once daily (under fed conditions), 32 ± 10% of the administered dose is recovered in urine over 24 hours.

Tenofovir is eliminated by a combination of glomerular filtration and active tubular secretion. There may be competition for elimination with other compounds that are also renally eliminated.

Effects of Food on Oral Absorption

Administration of VIREAD 300 mg tablets following a high-fat meal (~700 to 1000 kcal containing 40 to 50% fat) increases the oral bioavailability, with an increase in tenofovir $AUC_{0-\infty}$ of approximately 40% and an increase in C_{max} of approximately 14%. However, administration of VIREAD with a light meal did not have a significant effect on the pharmacokinetics of tenofovir when compared to fasted administration of the drug. Food delays the time to tenofovir C_{max} by approximately 1 hour. C_{max} and AUC of tenofovir are 0.33 ± 0.12 µg/mL and 3.32 ± 1.37 µg•hr/mL following multiple doses of VIREAD 300 mg once daily in the fed state, when meal content was not controlled.

Special Populations

Race: There were insufficient numbers from racial and ethnic groups other than Caucasian to adequately determine potential pharmacokinetic differences among these populations.

Gender: Tenofovir pharmacokinetics are similar in male and female subjects.

Pediatric Patients 2 Years of Age and Older: Steady-state pharmacokinetics of tenofovir were evaluated in 31 HIV-1 infected pediatric subjects 2 to less than 18 years (Table 11). Tenofovir exposure achieved in these pediatric subjects receiving oral once daily doses of VIREAD 300 mg (tablet) or 8 mg/kg of body weight (powder) up to a maximum dose of 300 mg was similar to exposures achieved in adults receiving once-daily doses of VIREAD 300 mg.

Table 11 Mean (± SD) Tenofovir Pharmacokinetic Parameters by Age Groups for HIV–1–infected Pediatric Patients

Dose and Formulation	300 mg Tablet	8 mg/kg Oral Powder
	12 to <18 Year (N=8)	2 to <12 Years (N=23)
C_{max} (µg/mL)	0.38 ± 0.13	0.24 ± 0.13
AUC_{tau} (µg•hr/mL)	3.39 ± 1.22	2.59 ± 1.06

Tenofovir exposures in 52 HBV-infected pediatric subjects (12 to less than 18 years of age) receiving oral once-daily doses of VIREAD 300 mg tablet were comparable to exposures achieved in HIV-1-infected adults and adolescents receiving once-daily doses of 300 mg.

Geriatric Patients: Pharmacokinetic trials have not been performed in the elderly (65 years and older).

Patients with Impaired Renal Function: The pharmacokinetics of tenofovir are altered in subjects with renal impairment [See Warnings and Precautions (5.3)]. In subjects with

Table 12 Pharmacokinetic Parameters (Mean ± SD) of Tenofovir* in Subjects with Varying Degrees of Renal Function

Baseline Creatinine Clearance (mL/min)	>80 (N=3)	50–80 (N=10)	30–49 (N=8)	12–29 (N=11)
C_{max} (µg/mL)	0.34 ± 0.03	0.33 ± 0.06	0.37 ± 0.16	0.60 ± 0.19
$AUC_{0-\infty}$ (µg•hr/mL)	2.18 ± 0.26	3.06 ± 0.93	6.01 ± 2.50	15.98 ± 7.22
CL/F (mL/min)	1043.7 ± 115.4	807.7 ± 279.2	444.4 ± 209.8	177.0 ± 97.1
CL_{renal} (mL/min)	243.5 ± 33.3	168.6 ± 27.5	100.6 ± 27.5	43.0 ± 31.2

* 300 mg, single dose of VIREAD

Table 13 Drug Interactions: Changes in Pharmacokinetic Parameters for Tenofovir* in the Presence of the Coadministered Drug

Coadministered Drug	Dose of Coadministered Drug (mg)	N	% Change of Tenofovir Pharmacokinetic Parameters[†] (90% CI)		
			C_{max}	AUC	C_{min}
Abacavir	300 once	8	⇔	⇔	NC
Atazanavir[‡]	400 once daily × 14 days	33	↑ 14 (↑ 8 to ↑ 20)	↑ 24 (↑ 21 to ↑ 28)	↑ 22 (↑ 15 to ↑ 30)
Atazanavir/ Ritonavir[‡]	300/100 once daily	12	↑ 34 (↑ 20 to ↑ 51)	↑ 37 (↑ 30 to ↑ 45)	↑ 29 (↑ 21 to ↑ 36)
Darunavir/ Ritonavir[§]	300/100 twice daily	12	↑ 24 (↑ 8 to ↑ 42)	↑ 22 (↑ 10 to ↑ 35)	↑ 37 (↑ 19 to ↑ 57)
Didanosine[¶]	250 or 400 once daily × 7 days	14	⇔	⇔	⇔
Emtricitabine	200 once daily × 7 days	17	⇔	⇔	⇔
Entecavir	1 mg once daily × 10 days	28	⇔	⇔	⇔
Indinavir	800 three times daily × 7 days	13	↑ 14 (↓ 3 to ↑ 33)	⇔	⇔
Lamivudine	150 twice daily × 7 days	15	⇔	⇔	⇔
Lopinavir/Ritonavir	400/100 twice daily × 14 days	24	⇔	↑ 32 (↑ 25 to ↑ 38)	↑ 51 (↑ 37 to ↑ 66)
Saquinavir/Ritonavir	1000/100 twice daily × 14 days	35	⇔	⇔	↑ 23 (↑ 16 to ↑ 30)
Tacrolimus	0.05 mg/kg twice daily × 7 days	21	↑ 13 (↑ 1 to ↑ 27)	⇔	⇔
Tipranavir/ Ritonavir[#]	500/100 twice daily	22	↓ 23 (↓ 32 to ↓ 13)	↓ 2 (↓ 9 to ↑ 5)	↑ 7 (↓ 2 to ↑ 17)
	750/200 twice daily (23 doses)	20	↓ 38 (↓ 46 to ↓ 29)	↑ 2 (↓ 6 to ↑ 10)	↑ 14 (↑ 1 to ↑ 27)

* Subjects received VIREAD 300 mg once daily.
[†] Increase = ↑; Decrease = ↓; No Effect = ⇔; NC = Not Calculated
[‡] Reyataz Prescribing Information
[§] Prezista Prescribing Information
[¶] Subjects received didanosine buffered tablets.
[#] Aptivus Prescribing Information

creatinine clearance below 50 mL/min or with end-stage renal disease (ESRD) requiring dialysis, C_{max}, and $AUC_{0-\infty}$ of tenofovir were increased (Table 12). It is recommended that the dosing interval for VIREAD be modified in patients with estimated creatinine clearance below 50 mL/min or in patients with ESRD who require dialysis [See Dosage and Administration (2.3)].

[See table 12 above]

Tenofovir is efficiently removed by hemodialysis with an extraction coefficient of approximately 54%. Following a single 300 mg dose of VIREAD, a four-hour hemodialysis session removed approximately 10% of the administered tenofovir dose.

Patients with Hepatic Impairment: The pharmacokinetics of tenofovir following a 300 mg single dose of VIREAD have been studied in non-HIV infected subjects with moderate to severe hepatic impairment. There were no substantial alterations in tenofovir pharmacokinetics in subjects with hepatic impairment compared with unimpaired subjects. No change in VIREAD dosing is required in patients with hepatic impairment.

Assessment of Drug Interactions

At concentrations substantially higher (~300-fold) than those observed in vivo, tenofovir did not inhibit in vitro drug metabolism mediated by any of the following human CYP isoforms: CYP3A4, CYP2D6, CYP2C9, or CYP2E1. However, a small (6%) but statistically significant reduction in metabolism of CYP1A substrate was observed. Based on the results of in vitro experiments and the known elimination pathway of tenofovir, the potential for CYP mediated interactions involving tenofovir with other medicinal products is low.

VIREAD has been evaluated in healthy volunteers in combination with other antiretroviral and potential concomitant drugs. Tables 13 and 14 summarize pharmacokinetic effects of coadministered drug on tenofovir pharmacokinetics and effects of VIREAD on the pharmacokinetics of coadministered drug. Coadministration of VIREAD with didanosine results in changes in the pharmacokinetics of didanosine that may be of clinical significance. Concomitant dosing of VIREAD with didanosine significantly increases the Cmax and AUC of didanosine. When didanosine 250 mg

Table 14 Drug Interactions: Changes in Pharmacokinetic Parameters for Coadministered Drug in the Presence of VIREAD

Coadministered Drug	Dose of Coadministered Drug (mg)	N	% Change of Coadministered Drug Pharmacokinetic Parameters* (90% CI)		
			C_{max}	AUC	C_{min}
Abacavir	300 once	8	↑ 12 (↓ 1 to ↑ 26)	⇔	NA
Atazanavir[†]	400 once daily × 14 days	34	↓ 21 (↓ 27 to ↓ 14)	↓ 25 (↓ 30 to ↓ 19)	↓ 40 (↓ 48 to ↓ 32)
Atazanavir[†]	Atazanavir/ Ritonavir 300/100 once daily × 42 days	10	↓ 28 (↓ 50 to ↑ 5)	↓ 25[‡] (↓ 42 to ↓ 3)	↓ 23[‡] (↓ 46 to ↑ 10)
Darunavir[§]	Darunavir/Ritonavir 300/100 mg once daily	12	↑ 16 (↓ 6 to ↑ 42)	↑ 21 (↓ 5 to ↑ 54)	↑ 24 (↓ 10 to ↑ 69)
Didanosine[¶]	250 once, simultaneously with VIREAD and a light meal[#]	33	↓ 20[Þ] (↓ 32 to ↓ 7)	⇔[Þ]	NA
Emtricitabine	200 once daily × 7 days	17	⇔	⇔	↑ 20 (↑ 12 to ↑ 29)
Entecavir	1 mg once daily × 10 days	28	⇔	↑ 13 (↑ 11 to ↑ 15)	⇔
Indinavir	800 three times daily × 7 days	12	↓ 11 (↓ 30 to ↑ 12)	⇔	⇔
Lamivudine	150 twice daily × 7 days	15	↓ 24 (↓ 34 to ↓ 12)	⇔	⇔
Lopinavir Ritonavir	Lopinavir/Ritonavir 400/100 twice daily × 14 days	24	⇔ ⇔	⇔ ⇔	⇔ ⇔
Saquinavir Ritonavir	Saquinavir/Ritonavir 1000/100 twice daily × 14 days	32	↑ 22 (↑ 6 to ↑ 41)	↑ 29[ß] (↑ 12 to ↑ 48) ⇔	↑ 47[ß] (↑ 23 to ↑ 76) ↑ 23 (↑ 3 to ↑ 46)
Tacrolimus	0.05 mg/kg twice daily × 7 days	21	⇔	⇔	⇔
Tipranavir[à]	Tipranavir/Ritonavir 500/100 twice daily	22	↓ 17 (↓ 26 to ↓ 6)	↓ 18 (↓ 25 to ↓ 9)	↓ 21 (↓ 30 to ↓ 10)
	Tipranavir/Ritonavir 750/200 twice daily (23 doses)	20	↓ 11 (↓ 16 to ↓ 4)	↓ 9 (↓ 15 to ↓ 3)	↓ 12 (↓ 22 to 0)

* Increase = ↑; Decrease = ↓; No Effect = ⇔; NA = Not Applicable
† Reyataz Prescribing Information
‡ In HIV-infected subjects, addition of tenofovir DF to atazanavir 300 mg plus ritonavir 100 mg, resulted in AUC and C_{min} values of atazanavir that were 2.3- and 4-fold higher than the respective values observed for atazanavir 400 mg when given alone.
§ Prezista Prescribing Information
¶ Videx EC Prescribing Information. Subjects received didanosine enteric-coated capsules.
# 373 kcal, 8.2 g fat
Þ Compared with didanosine (enteric-coated) 400 mg administered alone under fasting conditions.
ß Increases in AUC and C_{min} are not expected to be clinically relevant; hence no dose adjustments are required when tenofovir DF and ritonavir-boosted saquinavir are coadministered.
à Aptivus Prescribing Information

enteric-coated capsules were administered with VIREAD, systemic exposures of didanosine were similar to those seen with the 400 mg enteric-coated capsules alone under fasted conditions (Table 14). The mechanism of this interaction is unknown.
No clinically significant drug interactions have been observed between VIREAD and efavirenz, methadone, nelfinavir, oral contraceptives, or ribavirin.
[See table 13 at top of previous page]
[See table 14 above]

12.4 Microbiology
Mechanism of Action
Tenofovir disoproxil fumarate is an acyclic nucleoside phosphonate diester analog of adenosine monophosphate. Tenofovir disoproxil fumarate requires initial diester hydrolysis for conversion to tenofovir and subsequent phosphorylations by cellular enzymes to form tenofovir diphosphate, an obligate chain terminator. Tenofovir diphosphate inhibits the activity of HIV-1 reverse transcriptase and HBV reverse transcriptase by competing with the natural substrate deoxyadenosine 5'-triphosphate and, after incor-

poration into DNA, by DNA chain termination. Tenofovir diphosphate is a weak inhibitor of mammalian DNA polymerases α, β, and mitochondrial DNA polymerase γ.
Activity against HIV
Antiviral Activity
The antiviral activity of tenofovir against laboratory and clinical isolates of HIV-1 was assessed in lymphoblastoid cell lines, primary monocyte/macrophage cells and peripheral blood lymphocytes. The EC_{50} (50% effective concentration) values for tenofovir were in the range of 0.04 µM to 8.5 µM. In drug combination studies, tenofovir was not antagonistic with nucleoside reverse transcriptase inhibitors (abacavir, didanosine, lamivudine, stavudine, zalcitabine, zidovudine), non-nucleoside reverse transcriptase inhibitors (delavirdine, efavirenz, nevirapine), and protease inhibitors (amprenavir, indinavir, nelfinavir, ritonavir, saquinavir). Tenofovir displayed antiviral activity in cell culture against HIV-1 clades A, B, C, D, E, F, G, and O (EC_{50} values ranged from 0.5 µM to 2.2 µM) and strain specific activity against HIV-2 (EC_{50} values ranged from 1.6 µM to 5.5 µM).

Resistance
HIV-1 isolates with reduced susceptibility to tenofovir have been selected in cell culture. These viruses expressed a K65R substitution in reverse transcriptase and showed a 2–4 fold reduction in susceptibility to tenofovir.
In Study 903 of treatment-naïve subjects (VIREAD + lamivudine + efavirenz versus stavudine + lamivudine + efavirenz) [See Clinical Studies (14.1)], genotypic analyses of isolates from subjects with virologic failure through Week 144 showed development of efavirenz and lamivudine resistance-associated substitutions to occur most frequently and with no difference between the treatment arms. The K65R substitution occurred in 8/47 (17%) analyzed patient isolates on the VIREAD arm and in 2/49 (4%) analyzed patient isolates on the stavudine arm. Of the 8 subjects whose virus developed K65R in the VIREAD arm through 144 weeks, 7 of these occurred in the first 48 weeks of treatment and one at Week 96. Other substitutions resulting in resistance to VIREAD were not identified in this trial.
In Study 934 of treatment-naïve subjects (VIREAD + EMTRIVA + efavirenz versus zidovudine (AZT)/lamivudine (3TC) + efavirenz) [See Clinical Studies (14.1)], genotypic analysis performed on HIV-1 isolates from all confirmed virologic failure subjects with greater than 400 copies/mL of HIV-1 RNA at Week 144 or early discontinuation showed development of efavirenz resistance-associated substitutions occurred most frequently and was similar between the two treatment arms. The M184V substitution, associated with resistance to EMTRIVA and lamivudine, was observed in 2/19 analyzed subject isolates in the VIREAD + EMTRIVA group and in 10/29 analyzed subject isolates in the zidovudine/lamivudine group. Through 144 weeks of Study 934, no subjects have developed a detectable K65R substitution in their HIV-1 as analyzed through standard genotypic analysis.
Cross-Resistance
Cross-resistance among certain reverse transcriptase inhibitors has been recognized. The K65R substitution selected by tenofovir is also selected in some HIV-1 infected subjects treated with abacavir, didanosine, or zalcitabine. HIV-1 isolates with this substitution also show reduced susceptibility to emtricitabine and lamivudine. Therefore, cross-resistance among these drugs may occur in patients whose virus harbors the K65R substitution. HIV-1 isolates from subjects (N=20) whose HIV-1 expressed a mean of 3 zidovudine-associated reverse transcriptase substitutions (M41L, D67N, K70R, L210W, T215Y/F, or K219Q/E/N), showed a 3.1-fold decrease in the susceptibility to tenofovir. In Studies 902 and 907 conducted in treatment-experienced subjects (VIREAD + Standard Background Therapy (SBT) compared to Placebo + SBT) [See Clinical Studies (14.1)], 14/304 (5%) of the VIREAD-treated subjects with virologic failure through Week 96 had greater than 1.4-fold (median 2.7-fold) reduced susceptibility to tenofovir. Genotypic analysis of the baseline and failure isolates showed the development of the K65R substitution in the HIV-1 reverse transcriptase gene.
The virologic response to VIREAD therapy has been evaluated with respect to baseline viral genotype (N=222) in treatment-experienced subjects participating in Studies 902 and 907. In these clinical trials, 94% of the participants evaluated had baseline HIV-1 isolates expressing at least one NRTI substitution. Virologic responses for subjects in the genotype substudy were similar to the overall trial results.
Several exploratory analyses were conducted to evaluate the effect of specific substitutions and substitutional patterns on virologic outcome. Because of the large number of potential comparisons, statistical testing was not conducted. Varying degrees of cross-resistance of VIREAD to pre-existing zidovudine resistance-associated substitutions (M41L, D67N, K70R, L210W, T215Y/F, or K219Q/E/N) were observed and appeared to depend on the type and number of specific substitutions. VIREAD-treated subjects whose HIV-1 expressed 3 or more zidovudine resistance-associated substitutions that included either the M41L or L210W reverse transcriptase substitution showed reduced responses to VIREAD therapy; however, these responses were still improved compared with placebo. The presence of the D67N, K70R, T215Y/F, or K219Q/E/N substitution did not appear to affect responses to VIREAD therapy. Subjects whose virus expressed an L74V substitution without zidovudine resistance associated substitutions (N=8) had reduced response to VIREAD. Limited data are available for subjects whose virus expressed a Y115F substitution (N=3), Q151M substitution (N=2), or T69 insertion (N=4), all of whom had a reduced response.
In the protocol defined analyses, virologic response to VIREAD was not reduced in subjects with HIV-1 that expressed the abacavir/emtricitabine/lamivudine resistance-associated M184V substitution. HIV-1 RNA responses among these subjects were durable through Week 48.

Studies 902 and 907 Phenotypic Analyses

Phenotypic analysis of baseline HIV-1 from treatment-experienced subjects (N=100) demonstrated a correlation between baseline susceptibility to VIREAD and response to VIREAD therapy. Table 15 summarizes the HIV-1 RNA response by baseline VIREAD susceptibility.

Table 15 HIV-1 RNA Response at Week 24 by Baseline VIREAD Susceptibility (Intent-To-Treat)*

Baseline VIREAD Susceptibility[†]	Change in HIV-1 RNA[‡] (N)
<1	-0.74 (35)
>1 and ≤3	-0.56 (49)
>3 and ≤4	-0.3 (7)
>4	-0.12 (9)

* Tenofovir susceptibility was determined by recombinant phenotypic Antivirogram assay (Virco).
† Fold change in susceptibility from wild-type.
‡ Average HIV-1 RNA change from baseline through Week 24 (DAVG$_{24}$) in log$_{10}$ copies/mL.

Activity against HBV

Antiviral Activity

The antiviral activity of tenofovir against HBV was assessed in the HepG2 2.2.15 cell line. The EC$_{50}$ values for tenofovir ranged from 0.14 to 1.5 µM, with CC$_{50}$ (50% cytotoxicity concentration) values greater than 100 µM. In cell culture combination antiviral activity studies of tenofovir with the nucleoside HBV reverse transcriptase inhibitors entecavir, lamivudine, and telbivudine, and with the nucleoside HIV-1 reverse transcriptase inhibitor emtricitabine, no antagonistic activity was observed.

Resistance

Cumulative VIREAD genotypic resistance has been evaluated annually for up to 240 weeks in Studies 0102, 0103, 0106, 0108, and 0121 with the paired HBV reverse transcriptase amino acid sequences of the pre-treatment and on-treatment isolates from subjects who received at least 24 weeks of VIREAD monotherapy and remained viremic with HBV DNA greater than or equal to 400 copies/mL at the end of each study year (or at discontinuation of VIREAD monotherapy) using an as-treated analysis. In the nucleotide-naïve population from Studies 0102 and 0103, HBeAg-positive subjects had a higher baseline viral load than HBeAg-negative subjects and a significantly higher proportion of the subjects remained viremic at their last time point on VIREAD monotherapy (15% versus 4%, respectively).

HBV isolates from these subjects who remained viremic showed treatment-emergent substitutions (Table 16); however, no specific substitutions occurred at a sufficient frequency to be associated with resistance to VIREAD (genotypic and phenotypic analyses).

[See table 16 above]

Cross-Resistance

Cross-resistance has been observed between HBV nucleoside/nucleotide analogue reverse transcriptase inhibitors. In cell based assays, HBV strains expressing the rtV173L, rtL180M, and rtM204I/V substitutions associated with resistance to lamivudine and telbivudine showed a susceptibility to tenofovir ranging from 0.7- to 3.4-fold that of wild type virus. The rtL180M and rtM204I/V double substitutions conferred 3.4-fold reduced susceptibility to tenofovir. HBV strains expressing the rtL180M, rtT184G, rtS202G/I, rtM204V, and rtM250V substitutions associated with resistance to entecavir showed a susceptibility to tenofovir ranging from 0.6- to 6.9-fold that of wild type virus. HBV strains expressing the adefovir resistance-associated substitutions rtA181V and/or rtN236T showed reductions in susceptibility to tenofovir ranging from 2.9- to 10-fold that of wild type virus. Strains containing the rtA181T substitution showed changes in susceptibility to tenofovir ranging from 0.9- to 1.5-fold that of wild type virus.

One hundred fifty-two subjects initiating VIREAD therapy in Studies 0102, 0103, 0106, 0108, and 0121 harbored HBV with known resistance substitutions to HBV nucleos(t)ide analogue reverse transcriptase inhibitors: 14 with adefovir resistance-associated substitutions (rtA181S/T/V and/or rtN236T), 135 with lamivudine resistance-associated substitutions (rtM204I/V), and 3 with both adefovir and lamivudine resistance-associated substitutions. Following up to 240 weeks of VIREAD treatment, 11 of the 14 subjects with adefovir-resistant HBV, 124 of the 135 subjects with lamivudine-resistant HBV, and 2 of the 3 subjects with both adefovir- and lamivudine-resistant HBV achieved and maintained virologic suppression (HBV DNA less than 400 copies/mL). Three of the 5 subjects whose virus harbored both the rtA181T/V and rtN236T substitutions remained viremic.

Table 16 Amino Acid Substitutions in Viremic Subjects Across HBV Trials of VIREAD

	Compensated Liver Disease			Decompensated Liver Disease (N=39)*
	Nucleotide-Naïve (N=417)[†]	HEPSERA-Experienced (N=247)[‡]	Lamivudine-Resistant (N=136)[§]	
Viremic at Last Time Point on VIREAD	35/417 (8%)	34/247 (14%)	9/136 (7%)	7/39 (18%)
Treatment-Emergent Amino Acid Substitutions[¶]	19[#]/33 (58%)	10[Þ]/27 (37%)	6[ß]/8 (75%)	3/5 (60%)

* Subjects with decompensated liver disease from Study 0108 (N=39) receiving up to 48 weeks of treatment with VIREAD.
† Nucleotide-naïve subjects from Studies 0102 (N=246) and 0103 (N=171) receiving up to 240 weeks of treatment with VIREAD.
‡ HEPSERA-experienced subjects from Studies 0102/0103 (N=195) and 0106 (N=52) receiving up to 192 weeks of treatment with VIREAD after switching to VIREAD from HEPSERA. Study 0106, a randomized, double-blind, 168-week Phase 2 trial, has been completed.
§ Lamivudine-resistant subjects from Study 0121 (N=136) receiving up to 96 weeks of treatment with VIREAD after switching to VIREAD from lamivudine.
¶ Denominator includes those subjects who were viremic at last time point on VIREAD monotherapy and had evaluable paired genotypic data.
# Of the 19 subjects with treatment-emergent amino acid substitutions during Studies 0102 and 0103, 5 subjects had substitutions at conserved sites and 14 subjects had substitutions only at polymorphic sites, and 8 subjects had only transient substitutions that were not detected at the last time point on VIREAD.
Þ Of the 10 HEPSERA-experienced subjects with treatment-emergent amino acid substitutions, 2 subjects had substitutions at conserved sites and 8 had substitutions only at polymorphic sites.
ß Of the 6 lamivudine-resistant subjects with treatment-emergent substitutions during Study 0121, 3 subjects had substitutions at conserved sites and 3 had substitutions only at polymorphic sites.

Table 17 Outcomes of Randomized Treatment at Week 48 and 144 (Study 903)

	At Week 48		At Week 144	
Outcomes	VIREAD+3TC +EFV (N=299)	d4T+3TC +EFV (N=301)	VIREAD+3TC +EFV (N=299)	d4T+3TC +EFV (N=301)
Responder*	79%	82%	68%	62%
Virologic failure[†]	6%	4%	10%	8%
Rebound	5%	3%	8%	7%
Never suppressed	0%	1%	0%	0%
Added an antiretroviral agent	1%	1%	2%	1%
Death	<1%	1%	<1%	2%
Discontinued due to adverse event	6%	6%	8%	13%
Discontinued for other reasons[‡]	8%	7%	14%	15%

* Subjects achieved and maintained confirmed HIV-1 RNA <400 copies/mL through Week 48 and 144.
† Includes confirmed viral rebound and failure to achieve confirmed <400 copies/mL through Week 48 and 144.
‡ Includes lost to follow-up, subject's withdrawal, noncompliance, protocol violation and other reasons.

13 NONCLINICAL TOXICOLOGY

13.1 Carcinogenesis, Mutagenesis, Impairment of Fertility

Carcinogenesis

Long-term oral carcinogenicity studies of tenofovir disoproxil fumarate in mice and rats were carried out at exposures up to approximately 16 times (mice) and 5 times (rats) those observed in humans at the therapeutic dose for HIV-1 infection. At the high dose in female mice, liver adenomas were increased at exposures 16 times that in humans. In rats, the study was negative for carcinogenic findings at exposures up to 5 times that observed in humans at the therapeutic dose.

Mutagenesis

Tenofovir disoproxil fumarate was mutagenic in the *in vitro* mouse lymphoma assay and negative in an *in vitro* bacterial mutagenicity test (Ames test). In an *in vivo* mouse micronucleus assay, tenofovir disoproxil fumarate was negative when administered to male mice.

Impairment of Fertility

There were no effects on fertility, mating performance or early embryonic development when tenofovir disoproxil fumarate was administered to male rats at a dose equivalent to 10 times the human dose based on body surface area comparisons for 28 days prior to mating and to female rats for 15 days prior to mating through day seven of gestation. There was, however, an alteration of the estrous cycle in female rats.

13.2 Animal Toxicology and/or Pharmacology

Tenofovir and tenofovir disoproxil fumarate administered in toxicology studies to rats, dogs, and monkeys at exposures (based on AUCs) greater than or equal to 6 fold those observed in humans caused bone toxicity. In monkeys the bone toxicity was diagnosed as osteomalacia. Osteomalacia observed in monkeys appeared to be reversible upon dose reduction or discontinuation of tenofovir. In rats and dogs, the bone toxicity manifested as reduced bone mineral density. The mechanism(s) underlying bone toxicity is unknown.

Evidence of renal toxicity was noted in 4 animal species. Increases in serum creatinine, BUN, glycosuria, proteinuria, phosphaturia, and/or calciuria and decreases in serum phosphate were observed to varying degrees in these animals. These toxicities were noted at exposures (based on AUCs) 2–20 times higher than those observed in humans. The relationship of the renal abnormalities, particularly the phosphaturia, to the bone toxicity is not known.

14 CLINICAL STUDIES

14.1 Clinical Efficacy in Adults with HIV-1 Infection

Treatment-Naïve Adult Patients

Study 903

Data through 144 weeks are reported for Study 903, a double-blind, active-controlled multicenter trial comparing VIREAD (300 mg once daily) administered in combination with lamivudine and efavirenz versus stavudine (d4T), lamivudine, and efavirenz in 600 antiretroviral-naïve subjects. Subjects had a mean age of 36 years (range 18–64), 74% were male, 64% were Caucasian and 20% were Black. The mean baseline CD4$^+$ cell count was 279 cells/mm^3 (range 3–956) and median baseline plasma HIV-1 RNA was 77,600 copies/mL (range 417–5,130,000). Subjects were stratified by baseline HIV-1 RNA and CD4$^+$ cell count.

Table 18 Outcomes of Randomized Treatment at Week 48 and 144 (Study 934)

Outcomes	At Week 48		At Week 144	
	FTC +VIREAD +EFV (N=244)	AZT/3TC +EFV (N=243)	FTC +VIREAD +EFV (N=227)*	AZT/3TC +EFV (N=229)*
Responder[†]	84%	73%	71%	58%
Virologic failure[‡]	2%	4%	3%	6%
Rebound	1%	3%	2%	5%
Never suppressed	0%	0%	0%	0%
Change in antiretroviral regimen	1%	1%	1%	1%
Death	<1%	1%	1%	1%
Discontinued due to adverse event	4%	9%	5%	12%
Discontinued for other reasons[§]	10%	14%	20%	22%

* Subjects who were responders at Week 48 or Week 96 (HIV-1 RNA <400 copies/mL) but did not consent to continue the trial after Week 48 or Week 96 were excluded from analysis.
† Subjects achieved and maintained confirmed HIV-1 RNA <400 copies/mL through Weeks 48 and 144.
‡ Includes confirmed viral rebound and failure to achieve confirmed <400 copies/mL through Weeks 48 and 144.
§ Includes lost to follow-up, subject withdrawal, noncompliance, protocol violation and other reasons.

Table 19 Outcomes of Randomized Treatment (Study 907)

Outcomes	0–24 weeks		0–48 weeks	24–48 weeks
	VIREAD (N=368)	Placebo (N=182)	VIREAD (N=368)	Placebo Crossover to VIREAD (N=170)
HIV-1 RNA <400 copies/mL*	40%	11%	28%	30%
Virologic failure[†]	53%	84%	61%	64%
Discontinued due to adverse event	3%	3%	5%	5%
Discontinued for other reasons[‡]	3%	3%	5%	1%

* Subjects with HIV-1 RNA <400 copies/mL and no prior study drug discontinuation at Week 24 and 48 respectively.
† Subjects with HIV-1 RNA ≥400 copies/mL efficacy failure or missing HIV-1 RNA at Week 24 and 48 respectively.
‡ Includes lost to follow-up, subject withdrawal, noncompliance, protocol violation and other reasons.

Forty-three percent of subjects had baseline viral loads >100,000 copies/mL and 39% had CD4+ cell counts <200 cells/mm³. Treatment outcomes through 48 and 144 weeks are presented in Table 17.
[See table 17 on previous page]
Achievement of plasma HIV-1 RNA concentrations of less than 400 copies/mL at Week 144 was similar between the two treatment groups for the population stratified at baseline on the basis of HIV-1 RNA concentration (> or ≤100,000 copies/mL) and CD4+ cell count (< or ≥200 cells/mm³). Through 144 weeks of therapy, 62% and 58% of subjects in the VIREAD and stavudine arms, respectively, achieved and maintained confirmed HIV-1 RNA <50 copies/mL. The mean increase from baseline in CD4+ cell count was 263 cells/mm³ for the VIREAD arm and 283 cells/mm³ for the stavudine arm.
Through 144 weeks, 11 subjects in the VIREAD group and 9 subjects in the stavudine group experienced a new CDC Class C event.
Study 934
Data through 144 weeks are reported for Study 934, a randomized, open-label, active-controlled multicenter trial comparing emtricitabine + VIREAD administered in combination with efavirenz versus zidovudine/lamivudine fixed-dose combination administered in combination with efavirenz in 511 antiretroviral-naïve subjects. From Weeks 96 to 144 of the trial, subjects received a fixed-dose combination of emtricitabine and tenofovir DF with efavirenz in place of emtricitabine + VIREAD with efavirenz. Subjects had a mean age of 38 years (range 18–80), 86% were male, 59% were Caucasian and 23% were Black. The mean baseline CD4+ cell count was 245 cells/mm³ (range 2–1191) and median baseline plasma HIV-1 RNA was 5.01 log10 copies/mL (range 3.56–6.54). Subjects were stratified by baseline CD4+ cell count (< or ≥200 cells/mm³); 41% had CD4+ cell counts <200 cells/mm³ and 51% of subjects had baseline viral loads >100,000 copies/mL. Treatment outcomes through 48 and

144 weeks for those subjects who did not have efavirenz resistance at baseline are presented in Table 18.
[See table 18 above]
Through Week 48, 84% and 73% of subjects in the emtricitabine + VIREAD group and the zidovudine/lamivudine group, respectively, achieved and maintained HIV-1 RNA <400 copies/mL (71% and 58% through Week 144). The difference in the proportion of subjects who achieved and maintained HIV-1 RNA <400 copies/mL through 48 weeks largely results from the higher number of discontinuations due to adverse events and other reasons in the zidovudine/lamivudine group in this open-label trial. In addition, 80% and 70% of subjects in the emtricitabine + VIREAD group and the zidovudine/lamivudine group, respectively, achieved and maintained HIV-1 RNA <50 copies/mL through Week 48 (64% and 56% through Week 144). The mean increase from baseline in CD4+ cell count was 190 cells/mm³ in the EMTRIVA + VIREAD group and 158 cells/mm³ in the zidovudine/lamivudine group at Week 48 (312 and 271 cells/mm³ at Week 144).
Through 48 weeks, 7 subjects in the emtricitabine + VIREAD group and 5 subjects in the zidovudine/lamivudine group experienced a new CDC Class C event (10 and 6 subjects through 144 weeks).
Treatment-Experienced Adult Patients
Study 907
Study 907 was a 24-week, double-blind placebo-controlled multicenter trial of VIREAD added to a stable background regimen of antiretroviral agents in 550 treatment-experienced subjects. After 24 weeks of blinded trial treatment, all subjects continuing on trial were offered open-label VIREAD for an additional 24 weeks. Subjects had a mean baseline CD4+ cell count of 427 cells/mm³ (range 23–1385), median baseline plasma HIV-1 RNA of 2340 (range 50–75,000) copies/mL, and mean duration of prior HIV-1 treatment was 5.4 years. Mean age of the subjects was 42 years, 85% were male and 69% were Caucasian, 17% Black and 12% Hispanic.
The percent of subjects with HIV-1 RNA <400 copies/mL and outcomes of subjects through 48 weeks are summarized in Table 19.

[See table 19 above]
At 24 weeks of therapy, there was a higher proportion of subjects in the VIREAD arm compared to the placebo arm with HIV-1 RNA <50 copies/mL (19% and 1%, respectively). Mean change in absolute CD4+ cell counts by Week 24 was +11 cells/mm³ for the VIREAD group and -5 cells/mm³ for the placebo group. Mean change in absolute CD4+ cell counts by Week 48 was +4 cells/mm³ for the VIREAD group. Through Week 24, one subject in the VIREAD group and no subjects in the placebo arm experienced a new CDC Class C event.

14.2 Clinical Efficacy in Adults with Chronic Hepatitis B
HBeAg-Negative Chronic Hepatitis B
Study 0102 was a Phase 3, randomized, double-blind, active-controlled trial of VIREAD 300 mg compared to HEPSERA 10 mg in 375 HBeAg- (anti-HBe+) subjects with compensated liver function, the majority of whom were nucleoside-naïve. The mean age of subjects was 44 years, 77% were male, 25% were Asian, 65% were Caucasian, 17% had previously received alpha-interferon therapy and 18% were nucleoside-experienced (16% had prior lamivudine experience). At baseline, subjects had a mean Knodell necroinflammatory score of 7.8; mean plasma HBV DNA was 6.9 log10 copies/mL; and mean serum ALT was 140 U/L.
HBeAg-Positive Chronic Hepatitis B
Study 0103 was a Phase 3, randomized, double-blind, active-controlled trial of VIREAD 300 mg compared to HEPSERA 10 mg in 266 HBeAg+ nucleoside-naïve subjects with compensated liver function. The mean age of subjects was 34 years, 69% were male, 36% were Asian, 52% were Caucasian, 16% had previously received alpha-interferon therapy, and <5% were nucleoside experienced. At baseline, subjects had a mean Knodell necroinflammatory score of 8.4; mean plasma HBV DNA was 8.7 log10 copies /mL; and mean serum ALT was 147 U/L.
The primary data analysis was conducted after all subjects reached 48 weeks of treatment and results are summarized below.
The primary efficacy endpoint in both trials was complete response to treatment defined as HBV DNA <400 copies/mL and Knodell necroinflammatory score improvement of at least 2 points, without worsening in Knodell fibrosis at Week 48 (Table 20).
[See table 20 at top of next page]
Treatment Beyond 48 Weeks
In Studies 0102 (HBeAg-negative) and 0103 (HBeAg-positive), subjects who completed double-blind treatment (389 and 196 subjects who were originally randomized to VIREAD and HEPSERA, respectively) were eligible to roll over to open-label VIREAD with no interruption in treatment.
In Study 0102, 304 of 375 subjects (81%) continued in the study through Week 240. Among subjects randomized to VIREAD followed by open-label treatment with VIREAD, 82% had HBV DNA < 400 copies/mL, and 69% had ALT normalization at Week 240. Among subjects randomized to HEPSERA followed by open-label treatment with VIREAD, 88% had HBV DNA < 400 copies/mL and 76% had ALT normalization through Week 240. No subject in either treatment group experienced HBsAg loss/seroconversion through Week 240.
In Study 0103, 185 of 266 subjects (69%) continued in the study through Week 240. Among subjects randomized to VIREAD, 63% had HBV DNA < 400 copies/mL, 44% had ALT normalization, and 34% had HBeAg loss (26% seroconversion to anti-HBe antibody) through Week 240. Among subjects randomized to HEPSERA followed by up to 192 weeks of open-label treatment with VIREAD, 64% had HBV DNA < 400 copies/mL, 54% had ALT normalization, and 34% had HBeAg loss (29% seroconversion to anti-HBe antibody) through Week 240. At Week 240, HBsAg loss was 9% in both treatment groups, and seroconversion to anti-HBs was 7% for the subjects initially randomized to VIREAD and 9% for subjects initially randomized to HEPSERA.
Of the originally randomized and treated 641 subjects in the two studies, liver biopsy data from 328 subjects who received continuing open-label treatment with VIREAD monotherapy were available for analysis at baseline, Week 48 and Week 240. There were no apparent differences between the subset of subjects who had liver biopsy data at Week 240 and those subjects remaining on open-label VIREAD without biopsy data that would be expected to affect histological outcomes at Week 240. Among the 328 subjects evaluated, the observed histological response rates were 80% and 88% at Week 48 and Week 240, respectively. In the subjects without cirrhosis at baseline (Ishak fibrosis score 0-4), 92% (216/235) and 95% (223/235) had either improvement or no change in Ishak fibrosis score at Week 48 and Week 240, respectively. In subjects with cirrhosis at baseline (Ishak fibrosis score 5-6), 97% (90/93) and 99% (92/93) had either improvement or no change in Ishak fibrosis

score at Week 48 and Week 240, respectively. Twenty-nine percent (27/93) and 72% (67/93) of subjects with cirrhosis at baseline experienced regression of cirrhosis by Week 48 and Week 240, respectively, with a reduction in Ishak fibrosis score of at least 2 points. No definitive conclusions can be established about the remaining study population who were not part of this subset analysis.

Patients with Lamivudine-Resistant Chronic Hepatitis B
Study 121 was a randomized, double-blind, active-controlled trial evaluating the safety and efficacy of VIREAD compared to an unapproved antiviral regimen in subjects with chronic hepatitis B, persistent viremia (HBV DNA ≥ 1,000 IU/mL), and genotypic evidence of lamivudine resistance (rtM204I/V +/- rtL180M). One hundred forty-one adult subjects were randomized to the VIREAD treatment arm. The mean age of subjects randomized to VIREAD was 47 years (range 18–73), 74% were male, 59% were Caucasian, and 37% were Asian. At baseline, 54% of subjects were HBeAg-negative, 46% were HBeAg-positive, and 56% had abnormal ALT. Subjects had a mean HBV DNA of 6.4 $\log_{10}$ copies/mL and mean serum ALT of 71 U/L at baseline.

After 96 weeks of treatment, 126 of 141 subjects (89%) randomized to VIREAD had HBV DNA < 400 copies/mL, and 49 of 79 subjects (62%) with abnormal ALT at baseline had ALT normalization. Among the HBeAg-positive subjects randomized to VIREAD, 10 of 65 subjects (15%) experienced HBeAg loss, and 7 of 65 subjects (11%) experienced anti-HBe seroconversion through Week 96. The proportion of subjects with HBV DNA concentrations below 400 copies/mL at Week 96 was similar between the VIREAD monotherapy and the comparator arms.

Across the combined chronic hepatitis B treatment trials, the number of subjects with adefovir-resistance associated substitutions at baseline was too small to establish efficacy in this subgroup.

Patients with Chronic Hepatitis B and Decompensated Liver Disease
VIREAD was studied in a small randomized, double-blind, active-controlled trial evaluating the safety of VIREAD compared to other antiviral drugs in subjects with chronic hepatitis B and decompensated liver disease through 48 weeks (Study 0108).

Forty-five adult subjects (37 males and 8 females) were randomized to the VIREAD treatment arm. At baseline, 69% subjects were HBeAg-negative, and 31% were HBeAg-positive. Subjects had a mean Child-Pugh score of 7, a mean MELD score of 12, mean HBV DNA of 5.8 $\log_{10}$ copies/mL and mean serum ALT of 61 U/L at baseline. Trial endpoints were discontinuation due to an adverse event and confirmed increase in serum creatinine ≥ 0.5 mg/dL or confirmed serum phosphorus of < 2 mg/dL *[See Adverse Reactions (6.1)]*.

At 48 weeks, 31/44 (70%) and 12/26 (46%) Viread-treated subjects achieved an HBV DNA < 400 copies/mL, and normalized ALT, respectively. The trial was not designed to evaluate treatment impact on clinical endpoints such as progression of liver disease, need for liver transplantation, or death.

16   HOW SUPPLIED/STORAGE AND HANDLING
Tablets
VIREAD tablets, 150 mg, are triangle-shaped, white, film-coated tablets containing 150 mg of tenofovir disoproxil fumarate, which is equivalent to 123 mg of tenofovir disoproxil, are debossed with "GSI" on one side and with "150" on the other side. Each bottle contains 30 tablets, a desiccant (silica gel canister or sachet), and closed with a child-resistant closure. (NDC 61958-0404-1)
VIREAD tablets, 200 mg, are round-shaped, white, film-coated tablets containing 200 mg of tenofovir disoproxil fumarate, which is equivalent to 163 mg of tenofovir disoproxil, are debossed with "GSI" on one side and with "200" on the other side. Each bottle contains 30 tablets, a desiccant (silica gel canister or sachet), and closed with a child-resistant closure. (NDC 61958-0405-1)
VIREAD tablets, 250 mg, are capsule-shaped, white, film-coated tablets containing 250 mg of tenofovir disoproxil fumarate, which is equivalent to 204 mg of tenofovir disoproxil, are debossed with "GSI" on one side and with "250" on the other side. Each bottle contains 30 tablets, a desiccant (silica gel canister or sachet), and closed with a child-resistant closure. (NDC 61958-0406-1)
VIREAD tablets, 300 mg, are almond-shaped, light blue, film-coated tablets containing 300 mg of tenofovir disoproxil fumarate, which is equivalent to 245 mg of tenofovir disoproxil, are debossed with "GILEAD" and "4331" on one side and with "300" on the other side. Each bottle contains 30 tablets, a desiccant (silica gel canister or sachet), and closed with a child-resistant closure. (NDC 61958-0401-1)

Table 20 Histological, Virological, Biochemical, and Serological Response at Week 48

	0102 (HBeAg-)		0103 (HBeAg+)	
	VIREAD (N=250)	HEPSERA (N=125)	VIREAD (N=176)	HEPSERA (N=90)
Complete Response	71%	49%	67%	12%
Histology Histological Response*	72%	69%	74%	68%
HBV DNA <400 copies/mL (<69 IU/mL)	93%	63%	76%	13%
ALT Normalized ALT†	76%	77%	68%	54%
Serology HBeAg Loss/Seroconversion	NA‡	NA‡	20%/19%	16%/16%
HBsAg Loss/Seroconversion	0/0	0/0	3%/1%	0/0

* Knodell necroinflammatory score improvement of at least 2 points without worsening in Knodell fibrosis.
† The population used for analysis of ALT normalization included only subjects with ALT above ULN at baseline.
‡ NA = Not Applicable

Oral Powder
VIREAD oral powder consists of white, coated granules containing 40 mg of tenofovir disoproxil fumarate, which is equivalent to 33 mg of tenofovir disoproxil, per gram of powder and is available in multi-use bottles containing 60 grams of oral powder, closed with a child-resistant closure, and co-packaged with a dosing scoop. (NDC 61958-0403-1)
Store VIREAD tablets and oral powder at 25 °C (77 °F), excursions permitted to 15–30 °C (59–86 °F) (see USP Controlled Room Temperature).
Keep the bottle tightly closed. Dispense only in original container. Do not use if seal over bottle opening is broken or missing.

17   PATIENT COUNSELING INFORMATION
See FDA-approved patient labeling (Patient Information and Instructions for Use).
Information for Patients
Patients should be advised that:
• VIREAD is not a cure for HIV-1 infection and patients may continue to experience illnesses associated with HIV-1 infection, including opportunistic infections. Patients should remain under the care of a physician when using VIREAD.
• Patients should avoid doing things that can spread HIV or HBV to others.
  • **Do not share needles or other injection equipment.**
  • **Do not share personal items that can have blood or body fluids on them, like toothbrushes and razor blades.**
  • **Do not have any kind of sex without protection.** Always practice safer sex by using a latex or polyurethane condom to lower the chance of sexual contact with semen, vaginal secretions, or blood.
  • **Do not breastfeed.** Tenofovir is excreted in breast milk and it is not known whether it can harm the baby. Mothers with HIV-1 should not breastfeed because HIV-1 can be passed to the baby in the breast milk.
• The long term effects of VIREAD are unknown.
• VIREAD tablets and oral powder are for oral ingestion only.
• VIREAD should not be discontinued without first informing their physician.
• If you have HIV-1 infection, with or without HBV coinfection, it is important to take VIREAD with combination therapy.
• It is important to take VIREAD on a regular dosing schedule and to avoid missing doses.
• Lactic acidosis and severe hepatomegaly with steatosis, including fatal cases, have been reported. Treatment with VIREAD should be suspended in any patient who develops clinical symptoms suggestive of lactic acidosis or pronounced hepatotoxicity (including nausea, vomiting, unusual or unexpected stomach discomfort, and weakness) *[See Warnings and Precautions (5.1)]*.
• Severe acute exacerbations of hepatitis have been reported in patients who are infected with HBV or coinfected with HBV and HIV-1 and have discontinued VIREAD *[See Warnings and Precautions (5.2)]*.
• Renal impairment, including cases of acute renal failure and Fanconi syndrome, has been reported. VIREAD should be avoided with concurrent or recent use of a nephrotoxic agent (e.g., high-dose or multiple NSAIDs) *[See Warnings and Precautions (5.3)]*. Dosing interval of VIREAD may need adjustment in patients with renal impairment *[See Dosage and Administration (2.3)]*.
• VIREAD should not be coadministered with the fixed-dose combination products ATRIPLA, COMPLERA, STRIBILD, and TRUVADA since it is a component of these products *[See Warnings and Precautions (5.4)]*.
• VIREAD should not be administered in combination with HEPSERA *[See Warnings and Precautions (5.4)]*.
• Patients with HIV-1 should be tested for Hepatitis B virus (HBV) before initiating antiretroviral therapy *[See Warnings and Precautions (5.5)]*.
• In patients with chronic hepatitis B, it is important to obtain HIV antibody testing prior to initiating VIREAD *[See Warnings and Precautions (5.5)]*.
• Decreases in bone mineral density have been observed with the use of VIREAD. Bone mineral density monitoring should be considered in patients who have a history of pathologic bone fracture or at risk for osteopenia *[See Warnings and Precautions (5.6)]*.
• In the treatment of chronic hepatitis B, the optimal duration of treatment is unknown. The relationship between response and long-term prevention of outcomes such as hepatocellular carcinoma is not known.

PATIENT INFORMATION
VIREAD® (VEER-ee-ad)
(tenofovir disoproxil fumarate)
tablets and oral powder
Read this Patient Information before you start taking VIREAD and each time you get a refill. There may be new information. This information does not take the place of talking with your healthcare provider about your medical condition or your treatment.
What is the most important information I should know about VIREAD?
VIREAD can cause serious side effects, including:
1. **Build-up of an acid in your blood (lactic acidosis).** Lactic acidosis can happen in some people who take VIREAD. **Lactic acidosis** is a serious medical emergency that can lead to death.
   Lactic acidosis can be hard to identify early, because the symptoms could seem like symptoms of other health problems. **Call your healthcare provider right away if you get the following symptoms which could be signs of lactic acidosis:**
   • feeling very weak or tired
   • have unusual (not normal) muscle pain
   • have trouble breathing
   • have stomach pain with
     • nausea (feel sick to your stomach)
     • vomiting
   • feel cold, especially in your arms and legs
   • feel dizzy or lightheaded
   • have a fast or irregular heartbeat
2. **Severe liver problems.** Severe liver problems can happen in people who take VIREAD or similar medicines. In some cases these liver problems can lead to death. Your liver may become large (hepatomegaly) and you may develop fat in your liver (steatosis) when you take VIREAD.

Call your healthcare provider right away if you have any of the following symptoms of liver problems:

- Your skin or the white part of your eyes turns yellow (jaundice).
- dark "tea-colored" urine
- light-colored bowel movements (stools)
- loss of appetite for several days or longer
- nausea
- stomach pain

You may be more likely to get lactic acidosis or severe liver problems if you are female, very overweight (obese), or have been taking VIREAD for a long time.

3. **Worsening of your Hepatitis B infection.** Your hepatitis B Virus (HBV) infection may become worse (flare-up) if you take VIREAD and then stop it. A "flare-up" is when your HBV infection suddenly returns in a worse way than before.

- Do not let your VIREAD run out. Refill your prescription or talk to your healthcare provider before your VIREAD is all gone.
- Do not stop taking VIREAD without first talking to your healthcare provider.
- If you stop taking VIREAD, your healthcare provider will need to check your health often and do blood tests regularly to check your HBV infection. Tell your healthcare provider about any new or unusual symptoms you may have after you stop taking VIREAD.

4. **Talk to your doctor about taking an HIV test before starting treatment with VIREAD for chronic hepatitis B. You should also get a test for HBV if you are taking VIREAD for treatment of HIV.**

What is VIREAD?

VIREAD is a prescription medicine used:

1. with other antiviral medicines to treat Human Immunodeficiency Virus-1 (HIV-1) in people 2 years of age and older. HIV is the virus that causes AIDS (Acquired Immune Deficiency Syndrome).

- When used with other HIV medicines, VIREAD may reduce the amount of HIV in your blood (called "viral load"). VIREAD may also help to increase the number of CD4 (T) cells in your blood which help fight off other infections. Reducing the amount of HIV and increasing the CD4 (T) cell count may improve your immune system. This may reduce your risk of death or infections that can happen when your immune system is weak (opportunistic infections).
- **VIREAD does not cure HIV infection or AIDS.** People taking VIREAD may still develop infections or other conditions associated with HIV infection.
- You must stay on continuous HIV therapy to control infection and decrease HIV-related illnesses.
- It is very important that you stay under the care of your healthcare provider.
- It is not known if VIREAD is safe and effective for the treatment of HIV-1 infection in children under the age of 2 years.

2. to treat chronic (long-lasting) hepatitis B virus (HBV) in people 12 years of age and older.

- VIREAD will not cure HBV.
- VIREAD may lower the amount of HBV in your body.
- VIREAD may improve the condition of your liver.
- The long-term effects of taking VIREAD for treatment of chronic hepatitis B infection are not known.
- It is not known if VIREAD is safe and effective for treatment of chronic hepatitis B in children under the age of 12 years.

What should I tell my healthcare provider before taking VIREAD?

Before you take VIREAD, tell your healthcare provider if you:

- have liver problems, including hepatitis B (HBV) infection.
- have kidney problems.
- have bone problems.
- have any other medical conditions, including HIV infection.
- are pregnant or plan to become pregnant. It is not known if VIREAD will harm your unborn baby.

  Pregnancy Registry. There is a pregnancy registry for women who take antiviral medicines during pregnancy. Its purpose is to collect information about the health of you and your baby. Talk to your healthcare provider about how you can take part in this registry.

- are breastfeeding or plan to breastfeed. **Do not breastfeed if you are taking VIREAD.** Tenofovir passes into your breast milk. You should not breastfeed because of the risk of passing HIV to your baby. Talk to your healthcare provider about the best way to feed your baby.

Tell your healthcare provider about all the medicines you take, including prescription and non-prescription medicines, vitamins and herbal supplements.

VIREAD may affect the way other medicines work, and other medicines may affect how VIREAD works.

Do not take VIREAD if you also take:

- other medicines that contain tenofovir (ATRIPLA®, COMPLERA®, STRIBILD®, TRUVADA®)
- adefovir (HEPSERA®)

Especially tell your healthcare provider if you take the following medications.

- didanosine (Videx, Videx EC)
- atazanavir (Reyataz)
- darunavir (Prezista)
- lopinavir with ritonavir (Kaletra)

Know the medicines you take. Keep a list of them to show your healthcare provider or pharmacist when you get a new medicine.

How should I take VIREAD?

- See "What is the most important information I should know about VIREAD?"
- Take VIREAD exactly as your healthcare provider tells you to take it.
- Take VIREAD at the same time every day.
- For adults and children 12 years of age and older, the usual dose of VIREAD is one 300 mg tablet each day.
- If you are an adult with kidney problems, your healthcare provider may tell you to take VIREAD less often.
- Adults and children 12 years of age and older who are unable to swallow VIREAD tablets whole may take 7½ scoops of VIREAD oral powder.
- For children 2 to 12 years of age, your healthcare provider will prescribe the right dose of VIREAD oral powder or tablets based on your child's body weight.
- Tell your healthcare provider if your child has problems with swallowing tablets.
- See the "Instructions for Use" section at the end of this Patient Information leaflet for information about the right way to measure and take VIREAD oral powder.
- Take VIREAD tablets by mouth, with or without food.
- Do not miss a dose of VIREAD. If you miss a dose of VIREAD, take the missed dose as soon as you remember. If it is almost time for your next dose, do not take the missed dose. Take the next dose of VIREAD at your regular time.
- If you take too much VIREAD, call your local poison control center or go right away to the nearest hospital emergency room.

What are the possible side effects of VIREAD?

VIREAD may cause serious side effects, including:

- See "What is the most important information I should know about VIREAD?"
- **New or worse kidney problems, including kidney failure,** can happen in some people who take VIREAD. Your healthcare provider should do blood tests to check your kidneys before you start treatment with VIREAD. If you have had kidney problems in the past or need to take another medicine that can cause kidney problems, your healthcare provider may need to do blood tests to check your kidneys during your treatment with VIREAD.
- **Bone problems** can happen in some people who take VIREAD. Bone problems include bone pain, softening or thinning (which may lead to fractures). Your healthcare provider may need to do additional tests to check your bones.
- **Changes in body fat** can happen in some people who take antiviral medicines. These changes may include increased amount of fat in the upper back and neck ("buffalo hump"), breast, and around the main part of your body (trunk). Loss of fat from the legs, arms, and face may also happen. The cause and long-term health effects of these conditions are not known.
- **Changes in your immune system (Immune Reconstitution Syndrome)** can happen when you start taking HIV medicines. Your immune system may get stronger and begin to fight infections that have been hidden in your body for a long time. Tell your healthcare provider if you start having new symptoms after starting your HIV medicine.

The most common side effects in all people who take VIREAD are:

- nausea
- rash
- diarrhea
- headache

- pain
- depression
- weakness

In some people with advanced HBV-infection, other common side effects may include:

- sleeping problems
- itching
- vomiting
- dizziness
- fever

Tell your healthcare provider if you have any side effect that bothers you or that does not go away.

These are not all the possible side effects of VIREAD. For more information, ask your healthcare provider or pharmacist.

Call your doctor for medical advice about side effects. You may report side effects to FDA at 1-800-FDA-1088.

How should I store VIREAD?

- Store VIREAD tablets or oral powder at room temperature between 68 °F to 77 °F (20 °C to 25 °C).
- Keep VIREAD in the original container.
- Do not use VIREAD if the seal over the bottle opening is broken or missing.
- Keep the bottle tightly closed.

Keep VIREAD and all medicines out of the reach of children.

General information about VIREAD:

Medicines are sometimes prescribed for purposes other than those listed in a Patient Information leaflet. Do not use VIREAD for a condition for which it was not prescribed. Do not give VIREAD to other people, even if they have the same condition you have. It may harm them.

Avoid doing things that can spread HIV-1 or HBV infection to others.

- **Do not share or re-use needles or other injection equipment.**
- **Do not share personal items that can have blood or body fluids on them, like toothbrushes and razor blades.**
- **Do not have any kind of sex without protection.** Always practice safe sex by using a latex or polyurethane condom to lower the chance of sexual contact with semen, vaginal secretions, or blood.

A vaccine is available to protect people at risk for becoming infected with HBV. You can ask your healthcare provider for information about this vaccine.

This leaflet summarizes the most important information about VIREAD. If you would like more information, talk with your healthcare provider. You can ask your pharmacist or healthcare provider for information about VIREAD that is written for health professionals.

For more information, go to www.viread.com or call Gilead Sciences, Inc. at 1-800-GILEAD-5 (1-800-445-3235).

What are the ingredients in VIREAD?

Active Ingredient: tenofovir disoproxil fumarate

Inactive Ingredients:

VIREAD tablets: croscarmellose sodium, lactose monohydrate, magnesium stearate, microcrystalline cellulose, and pregelatinized starch.

VIREAD Oral Powder: mannitol, hydroxypropyl cellulose, ethylcellulose, and silicon dioxide.

Tablet Coating:

VIREAD tablets 300 mg: Opadry II Y–30–10671–A, which contains FD&C blue #2 aluminum lake, hypromellose 2910, lactose monohydrate, titanium dioxide, and triacetin.

VIREAD tablets 150, 200 and 250 mg: Opadry II 32K-18425, which contains hypromellose 2910, lactose monohydrate, titanium dioxide, and triacetin.

Instructions for Use of VIREAD oral powder

Read the Instructions for Use below before you give VIREAD oral powder. Be sure you can understand and follow them. If you have any questions, ask your healthcare provider or pharmacist.

Important information

- VIREAD oral powder comes in a box that has a bottle of VIREAD and a dosing scoop (see Figure A).

Figure A

- **Only use the dosing scoop to measure VIREAD oral powder.**
- **Only mix VIREAD oral powder with soft foods** that can be swallowed without chewing. Examples of soft foods you can use are: applesauce, baby food, or yogurt.
- **Do not mix VIREAD oral powder with liquid.** The powder may float to the top even after stirring.
- **Give the entire dose right away after mixing** to avoid a bad taste.

How do I prepare and give VIREAD oral powder?

1. Wash and dry your hands.
2. Measure ¼ to ½ cup of soft food into a cup or bowl.
3. To open a new bottle of powder, press down on the bottle lid and turn to remove (see picture on the top of the bottle cap). Peel off the foil.
4. Measure the number of scoops prescribed by your healthcare provider.
   - For each full scoop prescribed:
     - Fill the dosing scoop to the top.
     - Use the flat edge of clean knife to make the powder even with the top of the scoop (see Figure B).

Figure B

- For ½ scoop:
  - Fill the dosing scoop up to the "½ line" on the side (see Figure C).

½ line ⟶ [½]   Figure C

5. Sprinkle the VIREAD oral powder on the soft food. Stir with a spoon until well mixed. **Give the entire dose right away after mixing** to avoid a bad taste.
6. Close the bottle of VIREAD tightly.
7. Wash and dry the dosing scoop. Do not store the dosing scoop in the bottle.

See the section "How should I store VIREAD?" for information about how to store VIREAD oral powder.

This Patient Information has been approved by the U.S. Food and Drug Administration.

Manufactured for and distributed by:
Gilead Sciences, Inc.
Foster City, CA 94404
Revised October 2013

COMPLERA, EMTRIVA, GSI, HEPSERA, STRIBILD, TRUVADA, and VIREAD are trademarks or registered trademarks of Gilead Sciences, Inc., or its related companies. ATRIPLA is a registered trademark of Bristol-Myers Squibb & Gilead Sciences, LLC. All other trademarks herein are the property of their respective owners.

21-356-GS-035

Shown in Product Identification Guide, page 307

ZYDELIG®   ℞
(idelalisib)
tablets, for oral use

HIGHLIGHTS OF PRESCRIBING INFORMATION
These highlights do not include all the information needed to use ZYDELIG safely and effectively. See full prescribing information for ZYDELIG.
ZYDELIG® (idelalisib) tablets, for oral use
Initial U.S. Approval: 2014

> **WARNING: FATAL AND SERIOUS TOXICITIES: HEPATIC, SEVERE DIARRHEA, COLITIS, PNEUMONITIS, and INTESTINAL PERFORATION**
> *See full prescribing information for complete boxed warning.*
> - Fatal and/or serious hepatotoxicity occurred in 14% of Zydelig-treated patients. Monitor hepatic function prior to and during treatment. Interrupt and then reduce or discontinue Zydelig. (5.1)
> - Fatal and/or serious and severe diarrhea or colitis occurred in 14% of Zydelig-treated patients. Monitor for the development of severe diarrhea or colitis. Interrupt and then reduce or discontinue Zydelig. (5.2)
> - Fatal and serious pneumonitis can occur in Zydelig-treated patients. Monitor for pulmonary symptoms and bilateral interstitial infiltrates. Interrupt or discontinue Zydelig. (5.3)
> - Fatal and serious intestinal perforation can occur in Zydelig-treated patients across clinical trials. Discontinue Zydelig if intestinal perforation is suspected. (5.4)

INDICATIONS AND USAGE
Zydelig is a kinase inhibitor indicated for the treatment of patients with:
- Relapsed chronic lymphocytic leukemia (CLL), in combination with rituximab, in patients for whom rituximab alone would be considered appropriate therapy due to other co-morbidities. (1.1)
- Relapsed follicular B-cell non-Hodgkin lymphoma (FL) in patients who have received at least two prior systemic therapies. (1.2)
- Relapsed small lymphocytic lymphoma (SLL) in patients who have received at least two prior systemic therapies. (1.3)

Accelerated approval was granted for FL and SLL based on overall response rate. Improvement in patient survival or disease related symptoms has not been established. Continued approval for these indications may be contingent upon verification of clinical benefit in confirmatory trials.

DOSAGE AND ADMINISTRATION
Recommended starting dose: 150 mg orally, twice daily. (2.1)

DOSAGE FORMS AND STRENGTHS
Tablets: 150 mg, 100 mg. (3)

CONTRAINDICATIONS
History of serious allergic reactions including anaphylaxis and toxic epidermal necrolysis. (4)

WARNINGS AND PRECAUTIONS
- Severe cutaneous reactions: Monitor patients for the development of severe cutaneous reactions and discontinue Zydelig. (5.5)
- Anaphylaxis: Monitor patients for anaphylaxis and discontinue Zydelig. (5.6)
- Neutropenia: monitor blood counts. (5.7)
- Embryo-fetal toxicity: may cause fetal harm. Advise women of potential risk to a fetus and to avoid pregnancy while taking Zydelig. (5.8)

ADVERSE REACTIONS
The most common adverse reactions (incidence ≥20%) are diarrhea, pyrexia, fatigue, nausea, cough, pneumonia, abdominal pain, chills, and rash (6.1).
The most common laboratory abnormalities (incidence ≥30%) are neutropenia, hypertriglyceridemia, hyperglycemia, ALT elevations, and AST elevations (6.1).
To report SUSPECTED ADVERSE REACTIONS, contact Gilead Sciences, Inc. at 1-800-GILEAD-5 or FDA at 1-800-FDA-1088 or www.fda.gov/medwatch

DRUG INTERACTIONS
- CYP3A inducers: Avoid coadministration of strong CYP3A inducers with Zydelig. (7.1)
- CYP3A substrates: Avoid coadministration of CYP3A substrates with Zydelig. (7.2)

USE IN SPECIFIC POPULATIONS
Nursing mothers: Discontinue drug or nursing. (8.3)
See 17 for PATIENT COUNSELING INFORMATION and Medication Guide

Revised: 07/2014

Table 1 Dose Modifications for Toxicities Due to Zydelig

Pneumonitis	Any symptomatic pneumonitis		
	Discontinue Zydelig in patients with any severity of symptomatic pneumonitis		
ALT/AST	**>3-5 × ULN**	**>5-20 × ULN**	**>20 × ULN**
	Maintain Zydelig dose. Monitor at least weekly until <1 × ULN.	Withhold Zydelig. Monitor at least weekly until ALT/AST are <1 × ULN, then may resume Zydelig at 100 mg BID.	Discontinue Zydelig permanently.
Bilirubin	**>1.5-3 × ULN**	**>3-10 × ULN**	**>10 × ULN**
	Maintain Zydelig dose. Monitor at least weekly until <1 × ULN.	Withhold Zydelig. Monitor at least weekly until bilirubin is <1 × ULN, then may resume Zydelig at 100 mg BID.	Discontinue Zydelig permanently.
Diarrhea*	**Moderate diarrhea**	**Severe diarrhea or hospitalization**	**Life-threatening diarrhea**
	Maintain Zydelig dose. Monitor at least weekly until resolved.	Withhold Zydelig. Monitor at least weekly until resolved, then may resume Zydelig at 100 mg BID.	Discontinue Zydelig permanently.
Neutropenia	**ANC 1.0 to <1.5 Gi/L**	**ANC 0.5 to <1.0 Gi/L**	**ANC <0.5 Gi/L**
	Maintain Zydelig dose.	Maintain Zydelig dose. Monitor ANC at least weekly.	Interrupt Zydelig. Monitor ANC at least weekly until ANC ≥0.5 Gi/L, then may resume Zydelig at 100 mg BID.
Thrombocytopenia	**Platelets 50 to <75 Gi/L**	**Platelets 25 to <50 Gi/L**	**Platelets <25 Gi/L**
	Maintain Zydelig dose.	Maintain Zydelig dose. Monitor platelet counts at least weekly.	Interrupt Zydelig. Monitor platelet count at least weekly. May resume Zydelig at 100 mg BID when platelets ≥25 Gi/L.

Abbreviations: ALT, alanine aminotransferase; AST, aspartate aminotransferase; BID, twice daily; ULN, upper limit of normal

*Moderate diarrhea: increase of 4–6 stools per day over baseline; severe diarrhea: increase of ≥7 stools per day over baseline.

FULL PRESCRIBING INFORMATION: CONTENTS*
WARNING: FATAL AND SERIOUS TOXICITIES: HEPATIC, SEVERE DIARRHEA, COLITIS, PNEUMONITIS, and INTESTINAL PERFORATION

13   NONCLINICAL TOXICOLOGY
13.1   Carcinogenesis, Mutagenesis, Impairment of Fertility
13.2   Animal Pharmacology and/or Toxicology
14   CLINICAL STUDIES
14.1   Relapsed Chronic Lymphocytic Leukemia
14.2   Relapsed Follicular B-cell non-Hodgkin Lymphoma
14.3   Relapsed Small Lymphocytic Lymphoma
16   HOW SUPPLIED/STORAGE AND HANDLING
17   PATIENT COUNSELING INFORMATION
* Sections or subsections omitted from the full prescribing information are not listed

FULL PRESCRIBING INFORMATION

> **WARNING: FATAL AND SERIOUS TOXICITIES: HEPATIC, SEVERE DIARRHEA, COLITIS, PNEUMONITIS, and INTESTINAL PERFORATION**
> • Fatal and/or serious hepatotoxicity occurred in 14% of Zydelig-treated patients. Monitor hepatic function prior to and during treatment. Interrupt and then reduce or discontinue Zydelig as recommended *[see Dosage and Administration (2.2), Warnings and Precautions (5.1)].*
> • Fatal and/or serious and severe diarrhea or colitis occurred in 14% of Zydelig-treated patients. Monitor for the development of severe diarrhea or colitis. Interrupt and then reduce or discontinue Zydelig as recommended *[see Dosage and Administration (2.2), Warnings and Precautions (5.2)].*
> • Fatal and serious pneumonitis can occur in Zydelig-treated patients. Monitor for pulmonary symptoms and bilateral interstitial infiltrates. Interrupt or discontinue Zydelig as recommended *[see Dosage and Administration (2.2), Warnings and Precautions (5.3)].*
> • Fatal and serious intestinal perforation can occur in Zydelig-treated patients across clinical trials. Discontinue Zydelig for intestinal perforation *[see Warnings and Precautions (5.4)].*

1   INDICATIONS AND USAGE
1.1   Relapsed Chronic Lymphocytic Leukemia
Zydelig is indicated, in combination with rituximab, for the treatment of patients with relapsed chronic lymphocytic leukemia (CLL) for whom rituximab alone would be considered appropriate therapy due to other co-morbidities.
1.2   Relapsed Follicular B-cell non-Hodgkin Lymphoma
Zydelig is indicated for the treatment of patients with relapsed follicular B-cell non-Hodgkin lymphoma (FL) who have received at least two prior systemic therapies.
Accelerated approval was granted for this indication based on Overall Response Rate *[see Clinical Studies (14.2)].* An improvement in patient survival or disease related symptoms has not been established. Continued approval for this indication may be contingent upon verification of clinical benefit in confirmatory trials.
1.3   Relapsed Small Lymphocytic Lymphoma
Zydelig is indicated for the treatment of patients with relapsed small lymphocytic lymphoma (SLL) who have received at least two prior systemic therapies.
Accelerated approval was granted for this indication based on Overall Response Rate *[see Clinical Studies (14.3)].* An improvement in patient survival or disease related symptoms has not been established. Continued approval for this indication may be contingent upon verification of clinical benefit in confirmatory trials.

2   DOSAGE AND ADMINISTRATION
2.1   Recommended Dose
The recommended maximum starting dose of Zydelig is 150 mg administered orally twice daily.
Zydelig can be taken with or without food. Tablets should be swallowed whole.
Continue treatment until disease progression or unacceptable toxicity. The optimal and safe dosing regimen for patients who receive treatment longer than several months is unknown.
2.2   Dose Modification
See the table below for dose modification instructions for specific toxicities related to Zydelig. For other severe or life-threatening toxicities related to Zydelig, withhold drug until toxicity is resolved. If resuming Zydelig after interruption for other severe or life-threatening toxicities, reduce the dose to 100 mg twice daily. Recurrence of other severe or life-threatening Zydelig-related toxicity upon rechallenge should result in permanent discontinuation of Zydelig.
[See table 1 at top of previous page]

3   DOSAGE FORMS AND STRENGTHS
150 mg tablets: pink, oval-shaped, film-coated tablet debossed with "GSI" on one side and "150" on the other side.

100 mg tablets: orange, oval-shaped, film-coated tablet debossed with "GSI" on one side and "100" on the other side.

4   CONTRAINDICATIONS
History of serious allergic reactions including anaphylaxis and toxic epidermal necrolysis.

5   WARNINGS AND PRECAUTIONS
5.1   Hepatotoxicity
Fatal and/or serious hepatotoxicity occurred in 14% of patients treated with Zydelig. Elevations in ALT or AST greater than 5 times the upper limit of normal have occurred *[see Adverse Reactions (6.1)].* These findings were generally observed within the first 12 weeks of treatment and were reversible with dose interruption. After resumption of treatment at a lower dose, 26% of patients had recurrence of ALT and AST elevations. Discontinue Zydelig for recurrent hepatotoxicity.
Avoid concurrent use of Zydelig with other drugs that may cause liver toxicity.
Monitor ALT and AST in all patients every 2 weeks for the first 3 months of treatment, every 4 weeks for the next 3 months, then every 1 to 3 months thereafter. Monitor weekly for liver toxicity if the ALT or AST rises above 3 times the upper limit of normal until resolved. Withhold Zydelig if the ALT or AST is greater than 5 times the upper limit of normal, and continue to monitor AST, ALT and total bilirubin weekly until the abnormality is resolved *[see Dosage and Administration (2.2)].*

5.2   Severe Diarrhea or Colitis
Severe diarrhea or colitis (Grade 3 or higher) occurred in 14% of Zydelig-treated patients across clinical trials *[see Adverse Reactions (6.1)].* Diarrhea can occur at any time. Avoid concurrent use of Zydelig and other drugs that cause diarrhea. Diarrhea due to Zydelig responds poorly to antimotility agents. Median time to resolution ranged between 1 week and 1 month across trials, following interruption of Zydelig therapy and in some instances, use of corticosteroids *[see Dosage and Administration (2.2)].*
5.3   Pneumonitis
Fatal and serious pneumonitis occurred in patients treated with Zydelig. Patients taking Zydelig who present with pulmonary symptoms such as cough, dyspnea, hypoxia, interstitial infiltrates on a radiologic exam, or a decline by more than 5% in oxygen saturation should be evaluated for pneumonitis. If pneumonitis is suspected, interrupt Zydelig until the etiology of the pulmonary symptoms has been determined. Patients with pneumonitis thought to be caused by Zydelig have been treated with discontinuation of Zydelig and administration of corticosteroids.
5.4   Intestinal Perforation
Fatal and serious intestinal perforation occurred in Zydelig-treated patients. At the time of perforation, some patients had moderate to severe diarrhea. Advise patients to promptly report any new or worsening abdominal pain, chills, fever, nausea, or vomiting. Discontinue Zydelig permanently in patients who experience intestinal perforation.

Table 2 Adverse Reactions Reported in ≥5% of CLL Patients and Occurred at ≥2% Higher Incidence in Subjects Receiving Zydelig

Adverse Reaction	Zydelig + R N=110 (%)		Placebo + R N=108 (%)	
	Any Grade	Grade ≥3	Any Grade	Grade ≥3
Gastrointestinal disorders				
nausea	28 (25)	0	23 (21)	0
vomiting	14 (13)	0	9 (8)	0
diarrhea [(a)]	23 (21)	6 (5)	17 (16)	0
gastroesophageal reflux disease	7 (6)	0	1 (1)	0
stomatitis	7 (6)	2 (2)	2 (2)	0
Nervous system disorders				
headache	11 (10)	1 (1)	5 (5)	0
General disorders and administration site conditions				
pyrexia	38 (35)	3 (3)	18 (17)	1 (1)
chills	23 (21)	2 (2)	17 (16)	0
pain	8 (7)	0	2 (2)	0
Skin and subcutaneous tissue disorders				
rash [(b)]	20 (18)	4 (4)	7 (6)	1 (1)
Respiratory, thoracic, and mediastinal disorders				
pneumonia [(c)]	25 (23)	18 (16)	19 (18)	14 (13)
nasal congestion	6 (5)	0	2 (2)	0
Infections and infestations				
sepsis [(d)]	9 (8)	8 (7)	4 (4)	4 (4)
bronchitis	7 (6)	1 (1)	3 (3)	1 (1)
sinusitis	9 (8)	0	4 (4)	0
urinary tract infection	6 (5)	0	3 (3)	2 (2)
Musculoskeletal and connective tissue disorders				
arthralgia	8 (7)	1 (1)	4 (4)	1 (1)

(a) Diarrhea includes the following preferred terms: diarrhea, colitis.
(b) Rash includes the following preferred terms: dermatitis exfoliative, rash, rash macular, rash maculo-papular, rash papular, rash pruritic, and skin disorder.
(c) Pneumonia includes the terms: pneumonia, pneumonitis, lung infection, lung infiltration, pneumocystis jiroveci pneumonia, pneumonia legionella, lung infection pseudomonal, pneumonia fungal, respiratory tract infection, lower respiratory tract infection, and lower respiratory tract infection bacterial.
(d) Sepsis includes the terms: sepsis, septic shock, neutropenic sepsis, and sepsis syndrome.
R: rituximab

Table 3 Treatment-emergent Laboratory Abnormalities Reported in ≥10% of CLL Patients Occurring at a ≥5% Higher Incidence in Subjects Receiving Zydelig

Laboratory Parameter	Zydelig + R N=110 (%)		Placebo + R N=108 (%)	
	Any Grade	Grade 3–4	Any Grade	Grade 3–4
Hematology abnormalities				
neutrophil count decreased	66 (60)	41 (37)	55 (51)	29 (27)
lymphocyte count decreased	22 (20)	10 (9)	13 (12)	4 (4)
lymphocyte count increased	27 (25)	20 (18)	10 (9)	5 (5)
Serum chemistry abnormalities				
ALT increased	38 (35)	9 (8)	11 (10)	1 (1)
AST increased	27 (25)	6 (5)	15 (14)	0
GGT increased	29 (26)	2 (2)	15 (14)	3 (3)
triglycerides (hypertriglyceridemia)	62 (56)	3 (3)	37 (34)	0
hyperglycemia	59 (54)	8 (7)	50 (46)	2 (2)
hypoglycemia	12 (11)	0	5 (5)	0
hyponatremia	22 (20)	2 (2)	16 (15)	7 (6)

Grades were obtained per CTCAE version 4.03.
R: rituximab

5.5 Severe Cutaneous Reactions

One case of toxic epidermal necrolysis (TEN) occurred in a study of Zydelig in combination with rituximab and bendamustine. Other severe or life-threatening (Grade ≥3) cutaneous reactions, including dermatitis exfoliative, rash, rash erythematous, rash generalized, rash macular, rash maculopapular, rash papular, rash pruritic, exfoliative rash, and skin disorder, have been reported in Zydelig-treated patients. Monitor patients for the development of severe cutaneous reactions and discontinue Zydelig.

5.6 Anaphylaxis

Serious allergic reactions, including anaphylaxis, have been reported in patients on Zydelig. In patients who develop serious allergic reactions, discontinue Zydelig permanently and institute appropriate supportive measures.

5.7 Neutropenia

Treatment-emergent Grade 3 or 4 neutropenia occurred in 31% of Zydelig-treated patients across clinical trials *[see Adverse Reactions (6.1)]*. Monitor blood counts at least every two weeks for the first 3 months of therapy, and at least weekly in patients while neutrophil counts are less than 1.0 Gi/L *[see Dosage and Administration (2.2)]*.

5.8 Embryo-fetal Toxicity

Based on findings in animals, Zydelig may cause fetal harm when administered to a pregnant woman. Idelalisib is teratogenic in rats, at systemic exposures 12 times those reported in patients at the recommended dose of 150 mg twice daily. If this drug is used during pregnancy, or if the patient becomes pregnant while taking this drug, the patient should be apprised of the potential hazard to a fetus *[see Use in Specific Populations (8.1)]*.

Advise females of reproductive potential to avoid becoming pregnant while taking Zydelig. If contraceptive methods are being considered, use effective contraception during treatment, and for at least 1 month after the last dose of Zydelig *[see Use in Specific Populations (8.6)]*.

6 ADVERSE REACTIONS

The following serious adverse reactions have been associated with Zydelig in clinical trials and are discussed in greater detail in other sections of the prescribing information.

- Hepatotoxicity *[see Warnings and Precautions (5.1)]*
- Severe Diarrhea or Colitis *[see Warnings and Precautions (5.2)]*
- Pneumonitis *[see Warnings and Precautions (5.3)]*
- Intestinal Perforation *[see Warnings and Precautions (5.4)]*
- Severe Cutaneous Reactions *[see Warnings and Precautions (5.5)]*
- Anaphylaxis *[see Warnings and Precautions (5.6)]*
- Neutropenia *[see Warnings and Precautions (5.7)]*

6.1 Clinical Trial Experience

Because clinical trials are conducted under widely varying conditions, adverse reaction rates observed in the clinical trials of a drug cannot be directly compared to rates in the clinical trials of another drug and may not reflect the rates observed in practice.

Summary of Clinical Trials in Chronic Lymphocytic Leukemia

The safety data reflect subject exposure to Zydelig from Study 1, in which 218 subjects with relapsed CLL received up to 8 doses of rituximab with or without Zydelig 150 mg twice daily. The median duration of exposure to Zydelig was 5 months.

Serious adverse reactions were reported in 54 (49%) subjects treated with Zydelig + rituximab. The most frequent (≥2%) serious adverse reactions reported for subjects treated with Zydelig were pneumonia (17%), pyrexia (9%), sepsis (8%), febrile neutropenia (5%) and diarrhea (5%). Adverse reactions that led to discontinuation of Zydelig occurred in 11 (10%) subjects. The most common adverse reactions that led to treatment discontinuations were hepatotoxicity and diarrhea/colitis.

Thirty-nine subjects (35%) had dose interruptions and sixteen subjects (15%) had dose reductions due to adverse reactions or laboratory abnormalities. The most common reasons for dose reductions were elevated transaminases, diarrhea or colitis, and rash.

Table 2 and Table 3 summarize common adverse reactions and laboratory abnormalities reported for Zydelig + rituximab and placebo + rituximab arms.

[See table 2 at top of previous page]
[See table 3 above]

Summary of Clinical Trials in Indolent Non-Hodgkin Lymphoma

The safety data reflect exposure to Zydelig in 146 adults with indolent non-Hodgkin lymphoma treated with Zydelig 150 mg twice daily in clinical trials. The median duration of exposure was 6.1 months (range 0.3 to 26.4 months).

Serious adverse reactions were reported in 73 (50%) subjects. The most frequent serious adverse reactions that occurred were pneumonia (15%), diarrhea (11%), and pyrexia (9%).

Adverse reactions resulted in interruption or discontinuation for 78 (53%) subjects. The most common reasons for interruption or discontinuations were diarrhea (11%), pneumonia (11%), and elevated transaminases (10%).

Table 4 provides the adverse reactions occurring in at least 10% of subjects receiving Zydelig monotherapy, and Table 5 provides the treatment-emergent laboratory abnormalities.

Table 4 Adverse Reactions (≥ 10% of Subjects) in Patients with Indolent non-Hodgkin Lymphoma Treated with Zydelig 150 mg BID

Adverse Reaction	Zydelig Monotherapy N=146 (%)	
	Any Grade	Grade ≥3
Gastrointestinal disorders		
diarrhea [a]	68 (47)	20 (14)
nausea	42 (29)	2 (1)
abdominal pain [b]	38 (26)	3 (2)
vomiting	22 (15)	2 (1)
General disorders and administration site conditions		
fatigue	44 (30)	2 (1)
pyrexia	41 (28)	3 (2)
asthenia	17 (12)	3 (2)
peripheral edema	15 (10)	3 (2)
Infections and infestations		
upper respiratory tract infection	18 (12)	0
Respiratory, thoracic, and mediastinal disorders		
pneumonia [c]	37 (25)	23 (16)
cough	42 (29)	1 (1)
dyspnea	25 (17)	6 (4)
Skin and subcutaneous disorders		
rash [d]	31 (21)	4 (3)
night sweats	18 (12)	0
Nervous system disorders		
headache	16 (11)	1 (1)
Metabolism and nutrition disorders		
decreased appetite	24 (16)	1 (1)
Psychiatric disorders		
insomnia	17 (12)	0

(a) Diarrhea includes the following preferred terms: diarrhea, colitis, enterocolitis, and gastrointestinal inflammation.

(b) Abdominal pain includes the following preferred terms: abdominal pain, abdominal pain upper, abdominal pain lower, and abdominal discomfort.

(c) Pneumonia includes the terms: pneumonia, pneumonitis, interstitial lung disease, lung infiltration, pneumonia aspiration, respiratory tract infection, atypical pneumonia, lung infection, pneumocystis jiroveci pneumonia, bronchopneumonia, pneumonia necrotizing, lower respiratory tract infection, pneumonia pneumococcal, pneumonia staphylococcal, pneumonia streptococcal, pneumonia cytomegaloviral, and respiratory syncytial virus infection.

(d) Rash includes the following preferred terms: dermatitis exfoliative, rash, rash erythematous, rash macular, rash maculo-papular, rash pruritic, and exfoliative rash.

Table 5 Treatment-emergent Laboratory Abnormalities in Patients with Indolent non-Hodgkin Lymphoma Treated with Zydelig 150 mg BID

Laboratory Abnormality	Zydelig Monotherapy N=146 (%)		
	Any Grade	Grade 3	Grade 4
Serum chemistry abnormalities			
ALT increased	73 (50)	20 (14)	7 (5)
AST increased	60 (41)	12 (8)	6 (4)
Hematology abnormalities			
neutrophils decreased	78 (53)	20 (14)	16 (11)
hemoglobin decreased	41 (28)	3 (2)	0

platelets decreased	38 (26)	4 (3)	5 (3)

Grades were obtained per CTCAE version 4.03.

7 DRUG INTERACTIONS

7.1 Effects of Other Drugs on Zydelig

CYP3A Inducers

The AUC of idelalisib was reduced by 75% when Zydelig was coadministered with a strong CYP3A inducer. Avoid coadministration of Zydelig with strong CYP3A inducers, such as rifampin, phenytoin, St. John's wort, or carbamazepine *[see Clinical Pharmacology (12.3)]*.

CYP3A Inhibitors

The AUC of idelalisib was increased 1.8-fold when Zydelig was coadministered with a strong CYP3A inhibitor *[see Clinical Pharmacology (12.3)]*. If patients are taking concomitant strong CYP3A inhibitors, monitor for signs of Zydelig toxicity *[see Warnings and Precautions (5)]*. Follow dose modifications for adverse reactions *[see Dosage and Administration (2.2)]*.

7.2 Effects of Zydelig on Other Drugs

CYP3A Substrates

Zydelig is a strong CYP3A inhibitor. The AUC of a sensitive CYP3A substrate was increased 5.4-fold when Zydelig was coadministered with a sensitive CYP3A substrate. Avoid coadministration of Zydelig with CYP3A substrates *[see Clinical Pharmacology (12.3)]*.

8 USE IN SPECIFIC POPULATIONS

8.1 Pregnancy

Pregnancy Category D *[see Warnings and Precautions (5.8)]*
Risk Summary
Based on findings in animals, Zydelig may cause fetal harm when administered to a pregnant woman. Idelalisib was teratogenic in animals. If this drug is used during pregnancy, or if the patient becomes pregnant while taking this drug, the patient should be apprised of the potential hazard to a fetus.
Animal Data
In an embryo-fetal development study, pregnant rats were administered oral doses of idelalisib during the period of organogenesis at 25, 75, and 150 mg/kg/day. Embryo-fetal toxicities were observed at the mid- and high-doses that also resulted in maternal toxicity, based on reductions in maternal body weight gain. Adverse findings at idelalisib doses ≥ 75 mg/kg/day included decreased fetal weights, external malformations (short tail), and skeletal variations (delayed ossification and/or unossification of the skull, vertebrae, and sternebrae). Additional findings were observed at 150 mg/kg/day dose of idelalisib and included urogenital blood loss, complete resorption, increased post-implantation loss, and malformations (vertebral agenesis with anury, hydrocephaly, and microphthalmia/anophthalmia). The dose of 75 and 150 mg/kg/day of idelalisib in rats resulted in exposures (AUC) of approximately 12 and 30 times, respectively, the human exposure at the recommended dose of 150 mg twice daily.

8.3 Nursing Mothers

It is not known whether idelalisib is excreted in human milk. Because many drugs are excreted in human milk and because of the potential for serious adverse reactions in nursing infants from Zydelig, a decision should be made whether to discontinue nursing or to discontinue the drug, taking into account the importance of the drug to the mother.

8.4 Pediatric Use

Safety and effectiveness of Zydelig in children less than 18 years of age have not been established.

8.5 Geriatric Use

In clinical trials of Zydelig in patients with FL, SLL, and CLL, 131/208 (63%) patients were age 65 and older. No major differences in effectiveness were observed. In patients 65 years of age or older with indolent non-Hodgkin lymphoma in comparison to younger patients, older patients had a higher incidence of discontinuation due to an adverse reaction (28% vs 20%), higher incidence of serious adverse reactions (64% vs 37%), and higher incidence of death (11% vs 5%). In patients 65 years of age or older with CLL in comparison to younger patients, older patients had a higher incidence of discontinuation due to an adverse reaction (11% vs 5%), higher incidence of serious adverse reactions (51% vs 43%), and higher incidence of death (3% vs 0%).

8.6 Females of Reproductive Potential

Contraception
Zydelig may cause fetal harm when administered during pregnancy. Advise females of reproductive potential to avoid becoming pregnant while taking Zydelig. If contraceptive methods are being considered, use effective contraception while taking Zydelig and for at least one month after taking the last dose of Zydelig. Advise patients to contact their healthcare provider if they become pregnant, or if pregnancy is suspected, while taking Zydelig *[see Use in Specific Populations (8.1)]*.

8.7 Renal Impairment

No dose adjustment of Zydelig is necessary for patients with creatinine clearance (CLcr) ≥ 15 mL/min *[see Clinical Pharmacology (12.3)]*.

8.8 Hepatic Impairment

The AUC of idelalisib increased up to 1.7-fold in subjects with ALT or AST or bilirubin greater than the upper limit of normal (ULN) compared to healthy subjects with normal ALT or AST or bilirubin values *[see Clinical Pharmacology (12.3)]*. Safety and efficacy data are not available in patients with baseline ALT or AST values greater than 2.5 × ULN or bilirubin values greater than 1.5 × ULN, as these patients were excluded from Studies 1 and 2. Patients with baseline hepatic impairment should be monitored for signs of Zydelig toxicity *[see Warnings and Precautions (5)]*. Follow dose modifications for adverse reactions *[see Dosage and Administration (2.2)]*.

11 DESCRIPTION

Idelalisib is an inhibitor of phosphatidylinositol 3-kinase, PI3Kδ.

The chemical name for idelalisib is 5-fluoro-3-phenyl-2-[(1S)-1-(9H-purin-6-ylamino)propyl]quinazolin-4(3H)-one. It has a molecular formula of $C_{22}H_{18}FN_7O$ and a molecular weight of 415.42 g/mol. Idelalisib has the following structural formula:

Idelalisib is a white to off-white solid with a pH-dependent aqueous solubility ranging from <0.1 mg/mL at pH 5-7 to over 1 mg/mL at pH 2 under ambient conditions.
Zydelig (idelalisib) tablets are for oral administration. Each tablet contains either 100 mg or 150 mg of idelalisib with the following inactive ingredients: microcrystalline cellulose, hydroxypropyl cellulose, croscarmellose sodium, sodium starch glycolate, magnesium stearate and a tablet coating. The tablet coating consists of polyethylene glycol, talc, polyvinyl alcohol, and titanium dioxide and of FD&C Yellow #6/Sunset Yellow FCF Aluminum Lake (for the 100 mg tablet) and red iron oxide (for the 150 mg tablet).

12 CLINICAL PHARMACOLOGY

12.1 Mechanism of Action

Idelalisib is an inhibitor of PI3Kδ kinase, which is expressed in normal and malignant B-cells. Idelalisib induced apoptosis and inhibited proliferation in cell lines derived from malignant B-cells and in primary tumor cells. Idelalisib inhibits several cell signaling pathways, including B-cell receptor (BCR) signaling and the CXCR4 and CXCR5 signaling, which are involved in trafficking and homing of B-cells to the lymph nodes and bone marrow. Treatment of lymphoma cells with idelalisib resulted in inhibition of chemotaxis and adhesion, and reduced cell viability.

12.2 Pharmacodynamics

Electrocardiographic Effects
The effect of Zydelig (150 mg and 400 mg) on the QT/QTc interval was evaluated in a placebo- and positive-controlled (moxifloxacin 400 mg) crossover study in 46 healthy subjects. At a dose 2.7 times the maximum recommended dose, Zydelig did not prolong the QT/QTc interval (i.e., not greater than or equal to 10 ms).

12.3 Pharmacokinetics

Absorption
Following oral administration of a single dose of Zydelig in the fasted state, the median T_{max} was observed at 1.5 hours. Idelalisib exposure increased in a less than dose-proportional manner over a dose range of 50 mg to 350 mg twice daily in the fasted state.
Relative to fasting conditions, the administration of a single dose of Zydelig with a high-fat meal increased idelalisib AUC 1.4-fold. Zydelig can be administered without regard to food.

Distribution
Idelalisib is greater than 84% bound to human plasma proteins with no concentration dependence. The mean blood-to-plasma ratio was 0.7. The population apparent central volume of distribution at steady state is 23 L.
Metabolism and Elimination
Idelalisib is metabolized to its major metabolite GS-563117 via aldehyde oxidase and CYP3A. GS-563117 is inactive against PI3Kδ in vitro. Idelalisib undergoes minor metabolism by UGT1A4.
The population apparent systemic clearance at steady-state is 14.9 L/hr. The population terminal elimination half-life of idelalisib is 8.2 hours. Following a single dose of 150 mg of [^{14}C] idelalisib, 78% and 14% of the radioactivity was excreted in feces and urine, respectively. GS-563117 accounted for 49% of the radioactivity in the urine and 44% in the feces.
Specific Populations
Age, Gender, Race, and Weight
Population pharmacokinetic analyses indicated that age, gender, race, and weight had no effect on idelalisib exposure.
Pediatric Patients
The pharmacokinetics of idelalisib has not been studied in pediatric patients.
Patients with Renal Impairment
A pharmacokinetic study following a single dose of 150 mg of Zydelig was performed in healthy subjects and subjects with severe renal impairment (CLcr 15 to 29 mL/min). Creatinine clearance had no effect on idelalisib exposure. No dose adjustment is needed for patients with CLcr ≥15 mL/min.
Patients with Hepatic Impairment
A pharmacokinetic study of Zydelig was performed in healthy subjects and subjects with hepatic impairment. The geometric mean AUC increased up to 1.7-fold in subjects with ALT or AST or bilirubin values greater than the upper limit of normal (ULN) compared to subjects with normal AST or ALT or bilirubin values. Limited safety and efficacy data are available for patients with baseline AST or ALT greater than 2.5 × ULN or bilirubin greater than 1.5 × ULN, as these patients were excluded from Studies 1 and 2. Patients with baseline hepatic impairment should be monitored for signs of Zydelig toxicity *[see Boxed Warning and Warnings and Precautions (5.1)]*. Follow dose modifications for adverse reactions *[see Dosage and Administration (2.2)]*.
Drug Interactions
In Vitro Studies
Idelalisib is a substrate for aldehyde oxidase, CYP3A, and UGT1A4 in vitro.
Idelalisib inhibits CYP2C8, CYP2C19, CYP3A, and UGT1A1 and GS-563117 inhibits CYP2C8, CYP2C9, CYP2C19, CYP3A and UGT1A1 in vitro. Idelalisib and GS-563117 are not likely to inhibit CYP1A, CYP2B6, and CYP2D6.
Idelalisib induces CYP2B6 and CYP3A4, but does not induce CYP1A2 in vitro. GS-563117 does not induce these enzymes.
Idelalisib and GS-563117 are substrates of P-glycoprotein (P-gp) and BCRP in vitro. Idelalisib is not a substrate of OATP1B1, OATP1B3, OAT1, OAT3, or OCT2. GS-563117 is not a substrate of OATP1B1 or OATP1B3.
Idelalisib inhibits P-gp, OATP1B1, and OATP1B3, and GS-563117 inhibits OATP1B1, OATP1B3 in vitro. Idelalisib is not likely to inhibit BCRP, OCT2, OAT1, or OAT3, and GS-563117 is not likely to inhibit P-gp, BCRP, OCT2, OAT1, or OAT3.
Effect of Other Drugs on Idelalisib
A single dose of 150 mg of Zydelig was administered alone and after rifampin (a strong CYP3A and P-gp inducer) 600 mg once daily for 8 days in healthy subjects. Rifampin decreased the geometric mean idelalisib AUC by 75% and the geometric mean C_{max} by 58%. Avoid coadministration of Zydelig with strong CYP3A and P-gp inducers.
A single dose of 400 mg of Zydelig was administered alone and after ketoconazole (a strong CYP3A and P-gp inhibitor) 400 mg daily for 4 days in healthy subjects. Ketoconazole increased the geometric mean idelalisib AUC by 1.8-fold. No changes in the geometric mean C_{max} were observed. Patients taking concomitant CYP3A inhibitors should be monitored for signs of Zydelig toxicity *[see Warnings and Precautions (5)]*. Follow dose modifications for adverse reactions *[see Dosage and Administration (2.2)]*.
Effect of Idelalisib on Other Drugs
A single oral dose of midazolam 5 mg was administered alone and after Zydelig 150 mg for 15 doses in healthy subjects. The geometric mean midazolam Cmax increased by 2.4-fold and the geometric mean midazolam AUC increased by 5.4-fold. Avoid coadministration of Zydelig with CYP3A substrates, as Zydelig is a strong CYP3A inhibitor.
A single dose of 10 mg of rosuvastatin (OATP1B1 and OATP1B3 substrate) was administered alone and after Zydelig 150 mg for 12 doses in healthy subjects. No changes in exposure to rosuvastatin were observed.

Figure 1 Kaplan-Meier Plot of Study 1 IRC-Assessed PFS

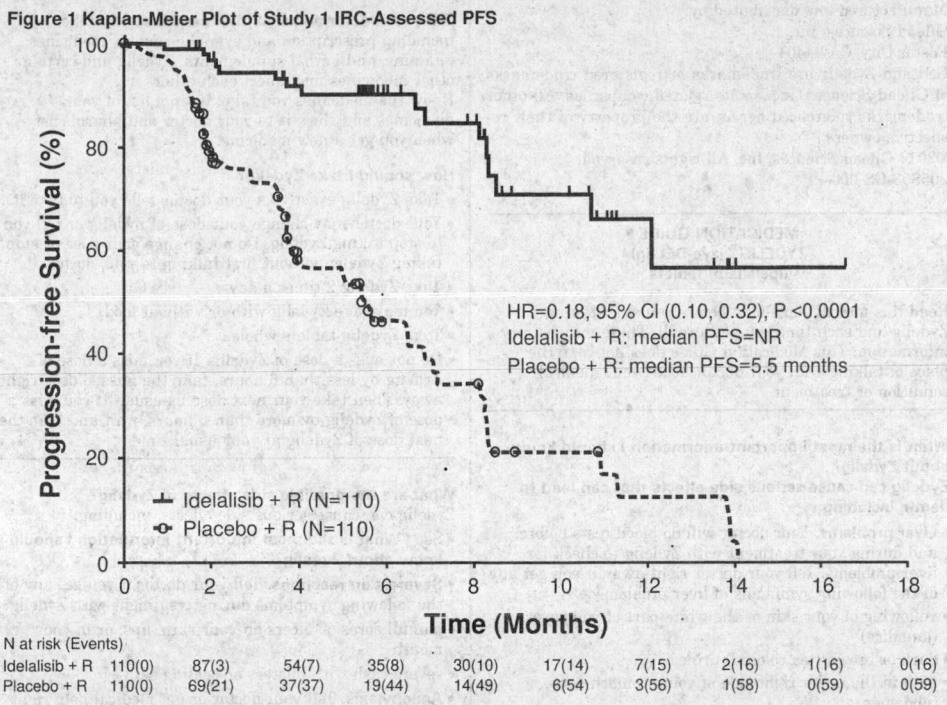

HR=0.18, 95% CI (0.10, 0.32), P <0.0001
Idelalisib + R: median PFS=NR
Placebo + R: median PFS=5.5 months

— Idelalisib + R (N=110)
-○- Placebo + R (N=110)

N at risk (Events)

Idelalisib + R	110(0)	87(3)	54(7)	35(8)	30(10)	17(14)	7(15)	2(16)	1(16)	0(16)
Placebo + R	110(0)	69(21)	37(37)	19(44)	14(49)	6(54)	3(56)	1(58)	0(59)	0(59)

Tablet Strength	Package Configuration	NDC No.	Description of Tablet; Debossed on Tablet
150 mg	High density polyethylene (HDPE) bottle with a polyester fiber coil, capped with a child-resistant closure. Each bottle contains 60 film-coated tablets.	61958-1702-1	Oval shaped; pink; "150" on one side and "GSI" on the other side
100 mg		61958-1701-1	Oval-shaped; orange; "100" on one side and "GSI" on the other side

A single dose of 0.5 mg of digoxin (P-gp substrate) was administered alone and after Zydelig 150 mg for 19 doses in healthy subjects. No changes in exposure to digoxin were observed.

13 NONCLINICAL TOXICOLOGY
13.1 Carcinogenesis, Mutagenesis, Impairment of Fertility
Carcinogenicity studies with idelalisib have not been conducted.

Idelalisib did not induce mutations in the bacterial mutagenesis (Ames) assay and was not clastogenic in the in vitro chromosome aberration assay using human peripheral blood lymphocytes. Idelalisib was genotoxic in males in the in vivo rat micronucleus study at a high dose of 2000 mg/kg. Idelalisib may impair fertility in humans. In a fertility study, treated male rats (25, 50, or 100 mg/kg/day of idelalisib) were mated with untreated females. Decreased epididymidal and testicular weights were observed at all dose levels and reduced sperm concentration at the mid- and high doses; however, there were no adverse effects on fertility parameters. The low dose in males resulted in an exposure (AUC) that is approximately 50% of the exposure in patients at the recommended dose of 150 mg twice daily. In a separate fertility study, treated female rats (25, 50, or 100 mg/kg/day of idelalisib) were mated with untreated males. There were no adverse effects on fertility parameters; however, there was a decrease in the number of live embryos at the high dose. The high dose in females resulted in an exposure (AUC) that is approximately 17-fold the exposure in patients at the recommended dose of 150 mg twice daily.

13.2 Animal Pharmacology and/or Toxicology
Toxicities observed in animals and not reported in patients include cardiac toxicity (cardiomyopathy, inflammation, and increased heart weight) and pancreatic findings (inflammation, hemorrhage, and low-incidence acinar degeneration and hyperplasia). These findings were observed in Sprague-Dawley rats in toxicology studies at exposures (AUCs) higher than those reported in patients at the recommended dose of 150 mg twice daily. Cardiac inflammation was mainly seen in a 28-day study in rats, the other findings were observed in the 13-week and/or 6-month studies.

14 CLINICAL STUDIES
14.1 Relapsed Chronic Lymphocytic Leukemia
Zydelig was evaluated in a randomized, double-blind, placebo-controlled study (Study 1) in 220 subjects with relapsed CLL who required treatment and were unable to tolerate standard chemoimmunotherapy due to coexisting medical conditions, reduced renal function as measured by creatinine clearance <60 mL/min, or NCI CTCAE Grade ≥3 neutropenia or Grade ≥3 thrombocytopenia resulting from myelotoxic effects of prior therapy with cytotoxic agents. Subjects were randomized 1:1 to receive 8 doses of rituximab (first dose at 375 mg/m², subsequent doses at 500 mg/m² every 2 weeks for 4 infusions and every 4 weeks for an additional 4 infusions) in combination with either an oral placebo twice daily or with Zydelig 150 mg taken twice daily until disease progression or unacceptable toxicity.
In Study 1, the median age was 71 (range 47, 92) with 78% over 65, 66% were male, and 90% were Caucasian. The median time since diagnosis was 8.5 years. The median number of prior therapies was 3. Nearly all (96%) subjects had received prior anti-CD20 monoclonal antibodies. The most common (>15%) prior regimens were: bendamustine + rituximab (98 subjects, 45%), fludarabine + cyclophosphamide + rituximab (75 subjects, 34%), single-agent rituximab (67 subjects, 31%), fludarabine + rituximab (37 subjects, 17%), and chlorambucil (36 subjects, 16%).
The primary endpoint was progression free survival (PFS), as assessed by an independent review committee (IRC). The trial was stopped for efficacy following the first pre-specified interim analysis. Results of a second interim analysis continued to show a statistically significant improvement for Zydelig + rituximab over placebo + rituximab for the primary endpoint of PFS (HR: 0.18, 95% CI [0.10, 0.32], p < 0.0001). The efficacy results are shown in Table 6 and the Kaplan-Meier curve for PFS is shown in Figure 1.

Table 6 Efficacy Results from Study 1

		Zydelig + R n=110	Placebo + R n=110
PFS	Median (months) (95% CI)	NR (10.7, NR)	5.5 (3.8, 7.1)

Hazard ratio (95% CI)	0.18 (0.10, 0.32)
P-value	< 0.0001 [†]

R: rituximab; PFS: progression-free survival; NR: not reached

[†] The p value for PFS was based on stratified log-rank test.

[See figure 1 above]

14.2 Relapsed Follicular B-cell non-Hodgkin Lymphoma
The safety and efficacy of Zydelig in patients with FL was evaluated in a single-arm, multicenter clinical trial which included 72 patients with follicular B-cell non-Hodgkin lymphoma who had relapsed within 6 months following rituximab and an alkylating agent and had received at least 2 prior treatments. The median age was 62 years (range 33 to 84), 54% were male, and 90% were Caucasian. At enrollment, 92% of patients had a baseline ECOG performance status of 0 or 1. The median time since diagnosis was 4.7 years and the median number of prior treatments was 4 (range 2 to 12). The most common prior combination regimens were R-CHOP (49%), BR (50%), and R-CVP (28%). At baseline, 33% of patients had extranodal involvement and 26% had bone marrow involvement.
Patients received 150 mg of Zydelig orally twice daily until evidence of disease progression or unacceptable toxicity. Tumor response was assessed according to the revised International Working Group response criteria for malignant lymphoma. The primary endpoint was Independent Review Committee-assessed overall response rate (ORR). Efficacy results are summarized in Table 7.

Table 7 Overall Response Rate (ORR) and Duration of Response (DOR) in Patients with Relapsed Follicular Lymphoma

	N=72
ORR	39 (54%)
95% CI	(42, 66%)
CR	6 (8%)
PR	33 (46%)
Median* DOR, months (range)	median not evaluable (0.0+, 14.8+)

CI = confidence interval; CR = complete response; PR = partial response

* Kaplan-Meier estimate

The median time to response was 1.9 months (range 1.6–8.3).

14.3 Relapsed Small Lymphocytic Lymphoma
The safety and efficacy of Zydelig in patients with SLL was evaluated in a single-arm, multicenter clinical trial which included 26 patients with small lymphocytic lymphoma who had relapsed within 6 months following rituximab and an alkylating agent and had received at least 2 prior treatments. The median age was 65 years (range 50 to 87), 73% were male, and 81% were Caucasian. At enrollment, 96% of patients had a baseline ECOG performance status of 0 or 1. The median time since diagnosis was 6.7 years and the median number of prior treatments was 4 (range 2 to 9). The most common prior combination regimens were BR (81%), FCR (62%) and R-CHOP (35%). At baseline, 27% of patients had extranodal involvement.
Subjects received 150 mg of Zydelig orally twice daily until evidence of disease progression or unacceptable toxicity. Tumor response was assessed according to the revised International Working Group response criteria for malignant lymphoma. The primary endpoint was Independent Review Committee-assessed overall response rate (ORR). Efficacy results are summarized in Table 8.

Table 8 Overall Response Rate (ORR) and Duration of Response (DOR) in Patients with Relapsed Small Lymphocytic Lymphoma

	N=26
ORR	15 (58%)
95% CI	(37, 77%)

Help Patients Save on Rx Drugs: PDR.net/PharmacyDiscountCard

CR	0
PR	15 (58%)
Median* DOR, months (range)	11.9 (0.0+, 14.7+)

CI = confidence interval; CR = complete response; PR = partial response
* Kaplan-Meier estimate

The median time to response was 1.9 months (range 1.6–8.3).

16 HOW SUPPLIED/STORAGE AND HANDLING

Zydelig tablets supplied as follows:
[See table at top of previous page]
Store between 20–30 °C (68–86 °F) with excursions permitted 15–30 °C (59–86 °F).
• Dispense only in original container.
• Do not use if seal over bottle opening is broken or missing.

17 PATIENT COUNSELING INFORMATION

Advise the patient to read the FDA-approved patient labeling (Medication Guide).
Physicians and health care professionals are advised to discuss the following with patients prior to treatment with Zydelig:

• Hepatotoxicity
Advise patients that Zydelig can cause significant elevations in liver enzymes, and that serial testing of serum liver tests (ALT, AST, and bilirubin) are recommended while taking Zydelig [see Warnings and Precautions (5.1)]. Advise patients to report symptoms of liver dysfunction including jaundice, bruising, abdominal pain, or bleeding.

• Severe Diarrhea or Colitis
Advise patients that Zydelig may cause severe diarrhea or colitis and to notify their healthcare provider immediately if the number of bowel movements in a day increases by six or more [see Warnings and Precautions (5.2)].

• Pneumonitis
Advise patients of the possibility of pneumonitis, and to report any new or worsening respiratory symptoms including cough or dyspnea [see Warnings and Precautions (5.3)].

• Intestinal Perforation
Advise patients of the possibility for intestinal perforation and to notify their healthcare provider immediately if they experience severe abdominal pain [see Warnings and Precautions (5.4)].

• Severe Cutaneous Reactions
Advise patients that Zydelig may cause severe cutaneous reactions and to notify their healthcare provider immediately if they develop a severe skin reaction [see Warnings and Precautions (5.5)].

• Anaphylaxis
Advise patients that anaphylaxis can occur during treatment with Zydelig and to notify their healthcare provider immediately if they experience symptoms of anaphylaxis [see Warnings and Precautions (5.6)].

• Neutropenia
Advise patients of the need for periodic monitoring of blood counts. Advise patients to notify their healthcare provider immediately if they develop a fever or any signs of infection [see Warnings and Precautions (5.7)].

• Pregnancy and Nursing
Advise women of the potential hazard to the fetus and to avoid pregnancy during treatment with Zydelig. If contraceptive methods are being considered, advise to use adequate contraception during therapy and for at least one month after completing therapy. Also advise patients not to breastfeed while taking Zydelig [see Warnings and Precautions (5.8) and Use in Specific Populations (8.1, 8.3, and 8.6)].

• Instructions for Taking Zydelig
Advise patients to take Zydelig exactly as prescribed and not to change their dose or to stop taking Zydelig unless they are told to do so by their healthcare provider. Zydelig may be taken with or without food. Zydelig tablets should be swallowed whole. Advise patients that if a dose of Zydelig is missed by less than 6 hours, to take the missed dose right away and take the next dose as usual. If a dose of Zydelig is missed by more than 6 hours, advise patients to wait and take the next dose at the usual time.

Manufactured and distributed by:
Gilead Sciences, Inc.
Foster City, CA 94404
GSI and Zydelig are trademarks or registered trademarks of Gilead Sciences, Inc., or its related companies. All other trademarks referenced herein are the property of their respective owners.
©2014 Gilead Sciences, Inc. All rights reserved.
205858-GS-000-PI

MEDICATION GUIDE
ZYDELIG® (zye-DEL-ig)
(idelalisib) tablets

Read this Medication Guide before you start taking Zydelig and each time you get a refill. There may be new information. This Medication Guide does not take the place of talking with your doctor about your medical condition or treatment.

What is the most important information I should know about Zydelig?
Zydelig can cause serious side effects that can lead to death, including:
• **Liver problems.** Your doctor will do blood tests before and during your treatment with Zydelig to check for liver problems. Tell your doctor right away if you get any of the following symptoms of liver problems:
• yellowing of your skin or the white part of your eyes (jaundice)
• dark or brown (tea colored) urine
• pain in the upper right side of your stomach area (abdomen)
• bleeding or bruising more easily than normal
• **Severe diarrhea.** Diarrhea is common with Zydelig and can sometimes be severe. Tell your doctor right away if the number of bowel movements you have in a day increases by six or more. Ask your doctor about medicines you can take to treat your diarrhea.
• **Lung or breathing problems.** Your doctor may do tests to check your lungs if you have breathing problems during treatment with Zydelig. Tell your doctor right away if you get new or worsening cough, shortness of breath, difficulty breathing, or wheezing.
• **Tear in intestinal wall (perforation).** Tell your doctor or get medical help right away if you get new or worsening stomach area (abdomen) pain, chills, fever, nausea, or vomiting.
If you have any of the above serious side effects during treatment with Zydelig, your doctor may completely stop your treatment, stop your treatment for a period of time, or change your dose of Zydelig.
See "What are the possible side effects of Zydelig?" for more information about side effects.

What is Zydelig?
Zydelig is a prescription medicine used to treat people with:
• **Chronic Lymphocytic Lymphoma (CLL)** in combination with rituximab when CLL comes back after prior cancer treatment when rituximab treatment alone may be used due to other health problems.
• **Follicular B-cell non-Hodgkin Lymphoma (FL)** when the disease has come back after treatment with at least two prior medicines.
• **Small Lymphocytic Lymphoma (SLL)** when the disease comes back after treatment with at least two prior medicines.
It is not known if Zydelig is safe and effective in children less than 18 years of age.

What should I tell my doctor before taking Zydelig?
Before taking Zydelig, tell your doctor about all of your medical conditions, including if you:
• have liver problems
• have lung or breathing problems
• are pregnant or plan to become pregnant. Zydelig may harm your unborn baby. Females who are able to become pregnant should use effective birth control (contraception) during treatment with Zydelig and for 1 month after stopping treatment. Talk to your doctor about birth control methods that may be right for you. Tell your doctor right away if you become pregnant during treatment with Zydelig.
• are breastfeeding or plan to breastfeed. It is not known if Zydelig passes into your breast milk. You and your doctor should decide if you will take Zydelig or breastfeed. You should not do both.

Tell your doctor about all the medicines you take, including prescription and over-the-counter medicines, vitamins, and herbal supplements. Zydelig and certain other medicines may affect each other.
Know the medicines you take. Keep a list of your medicines and show it to your doctor and pharmacist when you get a new medicine.

How should I take Zydelig?
• Take Zydelig exactly as your doctor tells you to take it.
• Your doctor may change your dose of Zydelig or tell you to stop taking Zydelig. Do not change your dose or stop taking Zydelig without first talking to your doctor.
• Take Zydelig 2 times a day.
• You may take Zydelig with or without food.
• Take Zydelig tablets whole.
• Do not miss a dose of Zydelig. If you miss a dose of Zydelig by less than 6 hours, take the missed dose right away. Then take your next dose as usual. If you miss a dose of Zydelig by more than 6 hours, wait and take the next dose of Zydelig at your usual time.

What are the possible side effects of Zydelig?
Zydelig can cause serious side effects, including:
• See "What is the most important information I should know about Zydelig?"
• **Severe skin reactions.** Tell your doctor if you get any of the following symptoms during treatment with Zydelig:
• painful sores or ulcers on your skin, lips, or in your mouth
• severe rash with blisters or peeling skin
• **Anaphylaxis.** Tell your doctor or get medical help right away if you have a serious allergic reaction while taking Zydelig.
• **Low white blood cell count (neutropenia).** Your doctor will check your blood counts regularly during treatment with Zydelig. Tell your doctor right away if you have a fever or any signs of an infection while taking Zydelig.

The most common side effects of Zydelig include fever, feeling tired, nausea, cough, stomach area (abdomen) pain, and chills.
Tell your doctor if you have any side effect that bothers you or that does not go away. These are not all the possible side effects of Zydelig. Call your doctor for medical advice about side effects. You may report side effects to FDA at 1-800-FDA-1088.

How should I store Zydelig?
• Store Zydelig between 68°F to 86°F (20°C to 30°C).
• Keep Zydelig in its original container.
• Do not use Zydelig if the seal over the bottle opening is broken or missing.

Keep Zydelig and all medicines out of reach of children.

General information about Zydelig
Medicines are sometimes prescribed for purposes other than those listed in a Medication Guide. Do not use Zydelig for a condition for which it was not prescribed. Do not give Zydelig to other people, even if they have the same symptoms you have. It may harm them. You can ask your doctor or pharmacist for information about Zydelig that is written for health professionals.

What are the ingredients in Zydelig?
Active ingredient: idelalisib
Inactive ingredients: microcrystalline cellulose, hydroxypropyl cellulose, croscarmellose sodium, sodium starch glycolate, and magnesium stearate.

The tablet coating contains polyethylene glycol, talc, polyvinyl alcohol, titanium dioxide and FD&C Yellow #6/Sunset Yellow (for the 100 mg tablet) and red iron oxide (for the 150 mg tablet).

Manufactured and distributed by: Gilead Sciences, Inc. Foster City, CA 94404
©2014 Gilead Sciences, Inc. All rights reserved
For more information, call 1-800-445-3235 or go to www.Zydelig.com.
205858-GS-000-MG

This Medication Guide has been approved by the U.S. Food and Drug Administration.

Issued: July 2014
Shown in Product Identification Guide, page 307

GlaxoSmithKline
FIVE MOORE DRIVE
RESEARCH TRIANGLE PARK, NC 27709

For all inquiries, including adverse event and quality assurance reporting, contact the GSK Response Center at 1-888-825-5249.

For updates to the product information listed below, also consult www.gsk.com.

ADVAIR DISKUS 100/50   ℞
[ad' vair disk' us]
(fluticasone propionate 100 mcg and salmeterol 50 mcg inhalation powder)
ADVAIR DISKUS 250/50
(fluticasone propionate 250 mcg and salmeterol 50 mcg inhalation powder)
ADVAIR DISKUS 500/50
(fluticasone propionate 500 mcg and salmeterol 50 mcg inhalation powder)
FOR ORAL INHALATION USE

HIGHLIGHTS OF PRESCRIBING INFORMATION
These highlights do not include all the information needed to use ADVAIR DISKUS safely and effectively. See full prescribing information for ADVAIR DISKUS.
ADVAIR DISKUS 100/50
(fluticasone propionate 100 mcg and salmeterol 50 mcg inhalation powder)
ADVAIR DISKUS 250/50
(fluticasone propionate 250 mcg and salmeterol 50 mcg inhalation powder)
ADVAIR DISKUS 500/50
(fluticasone propionate 500 mcg and salmeterol 50 mcg inhalation powder)
FOR ORAL INHALATION USE
Initial U.S. Approval: 2000

WARNING: ASTHMA-RELATED DEATH
See full prescribing information for complete boxed warning
- Long-acting beta$_2$-adrenergic agonists (LABA), such as salmeterol, one of the active ingredients in ADVAIR DISKUS, increase the risk of asthma-related death. A US trial showed an increase in asthma-related deaths in subjects receiving salmeterol (13 deaths out of 13,176 subjects treated for 28 weeks on salmeterol versus 3 out of 13,179 subjects on placebo). Currently available data are inadequate to determine whether concurrent use of inhaled corticosteroids or other long-term asthma control drugs mitigates the increased risk of asthma-related death from LABA. Available data from controlled clinical trials suggest that LABA increase the risk of asthma-related hospitalization in pediatric and adolescent patients. (5.1)
- When treating patients with asthma, only prescribe ADVAIR DISKUS for patients not adequately controlled on a long-term asthma control medication, such as an inhaled corticosteroid, or whose disease severity clearly warrants initiation of treatment with both an inhaled corticosteroid and a LABA. Once asthma control is achieved and maintained, assess the patient at regular intervals and step down therapy (e.g., discontinue ADVAIR DISKUS) if possible without loss of asthma control and maintain the patient on a long-term asthma control medication, such as an inhaled corticosteroid. Do not use ADVAIR DISKUS for patients whose asthma is adequately controlled on low- or medium-dose inhaled corticosteroids. (1.1, 5.1)

INDICATIONS AND USAGE
ADVAIR DISKUS is a combination product containing a corticosteroid and a LABA indicated for:
- Treatment of asthma in patients aged 4 years and older. (1.1)
- Maintenance treatment of airflow obstruction and reducing exacerbations in patients with chronic obstructive pulmonary disease (COPD). (1.2)
Important limitation:
- Not indicated for the relief of acute bronchospasm. (1.1, 1.2)

DOSAGE AND ADMINISTRATION
For oral inhalation only.
- Treatment of asthma in patients aged 12 years and older: 1 inhalation of ADVAIR DISKUS 100/50, ADVAIR DISKUS 250/50, or ADVAIR DISKUS 500/50 twice daily. Starting dosage is based on asthma severity. (2.1)
- Treatment of asthma in patients aged 4 to 11 years: 1 inhalation of ADVAIR DISKUS 100/50 twice daily. (2.1)
- Maintenance treatment of COPD: 1 inhalation of ADVAIR DISKUS 250/50 twice daily. (2.2)

DOSAGE FORMS AND STRENGTHS
Inhalation Powder. Inhaler containing a combination of fluticasone propionate (100, 250, or 500 mcg) and salmeterol (50 mcg) as a powder formulation for oral inhalation. (3)

CONTRAINDICATIONS
- Primary treatment of status asthmaticus or acute episodes of asthma or COPD requiring intensive measures. (4)
- Severe hypersensitivity to milk proteins. (4)

WARNINGS AND PRECAUTIONS
- LABA increase the risk of asthma-related death and asthma-related hospitalizations. Prescribe only for recommended patient populations. (5.1)
- Do not initiate in acutely deteriorating asthma or COPD. Do not use to treat acute symptoms. (5.2)
- Do not use in combination with an additional medicine containing LABA because of risk of overdose. (5.3)
- *Candida albicans* infection of the mouth and pharynx may occur. Monitor patients periodically. Advise the patient to rinse his/her mouth with water without swallowing after inhalation to help reduce the risk. (5.4)
- Increased risk of pneumonia in patients with COPD. Monitor patients for signs and symptoms of pneumonia. (5.5)
- Potential worsening of infections (e.g., existing tuberculosis; fungal, bacterial, viral, or parasitic infection; ocular herpes simplex). Use with caution in patients with these infections. More serious or even fatal course of chickenpox or measles can occur in susceptible patients. (5.6)
- Risk of impaired adrenal function when transferring from systemic corticosteroids. Taper patients slowly from systemic corticosteroids if transferring to ADVAIR DISKUS. (5.7)
- Hypercorticism and adrenal suppression may occur with very high dosages or at the regular dosage in susceptible individuals. If such changes occur, discontinue ADVAIR DISKUS slowly. (5.8)
- If paradoxical bronchospasm occurs, discontinue ADVAIR DISKUS and institute alternative therapy. (5.10)
- Use with caution in patients with cardiovascular or central nervous system disorders because of beta-adrenergic stimulation. (5.12)
- Assess for decrease in bone mineral density initially and periodically thereafter. (5.13)
- Monitor growth of pediatric patients. (5.14)
- Close monitoring for glaucoma and cataracts is warranted. (5.15)
- Be alert to eosinophilic conditions, hypokalemia, and hyperglycemia. (5.16, 5.18)
- Use with caution in patients with convulsive disorders, thyrotoxicosis, diabetes mellitus, and ketoacidosis. (5.17)

ADVERSE REACTIONS
Most common adverse reactions (incidence ≥3%) include:
- Asthma: Upper respiratory tract infection or inflammation, pharyngitis, dysphonia, oral candidiasis, bronchitis, cough, headaches, nausea and vomiting. (6.1)
- COPD: Pneumonia, oral candidiasis, throat irritation, dysphonia, viral respiratory infections, headaches, musculoskeletal pain. (6.2)

To report SUSPECTED ADVERSE REACTIONS, contact GlaxoSmithKline at 1-888-825-5249 or FDA at 1-800-FDA-1088 or www.fda.gov/medwatch.

DRUG INTERACTIONS
- Strong cytochrome P450 3A4 inhibitors (e.g., ritonavir, ketoconazole): Use not recommended. May increase risk of systemic corticosteroid and cardiovascular effects. (7.1)
- Monoamine oxidase inhibitors and tricyclic antidepressants: Use with extreme caution. May potentiate effect of salmeterol on vascular system. (7.2)
- Beta-blockers: Use with caution. May block bronchodilatory effects of beta-agonists and produce severe bronchospasm. (7.3)
- Diuretics: Use with caution. Electrocardiographic changes and/or hypokalemia associated with non-potassium-sparing diuretics may worsen with concomitant beta-agonists. (7.4)

USE IN SPECIFIC POPULATIONS
Hepatic impairment: Monitor patients for signs of increased drug exposure. (8.6)
See 17 for PATIENT COUNSELING INFORMATION and Medication Guide

Revised: 07/2014

FULL PRESCRIBING INFORMATION: CONTENTS*
WARNING: ASTHMA-RELATED DEATH

* Sections or subsections omitted from the full prescribing information are not listed

---

FULL PRESCRIBING INFORMATION

WARNING: ASTHMA-RELATED DEATH
Long-acting beta$_2$-adrenergic agonists (LABA), such as salmeterol, one of the active ingredients in ADVAIR DISKUS®, increase the risk of asthma-related death. Data from a large placebo-controlled US trial that compared the safety of salmeterol with placebo added to usual asthma therapy showed an increase in asthma-related deaths in subjects receiving salmeterol (13 deaths out of 13,176 subjects treated for 28 weeks on salmeterol versus 3 deaths out of 13,179 subjects on placebo). Currently available data are inadequate to determine whether concurrent use of inhaled corticosteroids or other long-term asthma control drugs mitigates the increased risk of asthma-related death from LABA. Available data from controlled clinical trials suggest that LABA increase the risk of asthma-related hospitalization in pediatric and adolescent patients.

Table 1. Asthma-Related Deaths in the 28-Week Salmeterol Multi-center Asthma Research Trial (SMART)

	Salmeterol n (%[a])	Placebo n (%[a])	Relative Risk[b] (95% Confidence Interval)	Excess Deaths Expressed per 10,000 Subjects[c] (95% Confidence Interval)
Total Population[d] Salmeterol: n = 13,176 Placebo: n = 13,179	13 (0.10%)	3 (0.02%)	4.37 (1.25, 15.34)	8 (3, 13)
Caucasian Salmeterol: n = 9,281 Placebo: n = 9,361	6 (0.07%)	1 (0.01%)	5.82 (0.70, 48.37)	6 (1, 10)
African American Salmeterol: n = 2,366 Placebo: n = 2,319	7 (0.31%)	1 (0.04%)	7.26 (0.89, 58.94)	27 (8, 46)

[a]Life-table 28-week estimate, adjusted according to the subjects' actual lengths of exposure to trial treatment to account for early withdrawal of subjects from the trial.
[b]Relative risk is the ratio of the rate of asthma-related death in the salmeterol group and the rate in the placebo group. The relative risk indicates how many more times likely an asthma-related death occurred in the salmeterol group than in the placebo group in a 28-week treatment period.
[c]Estimate of the number of additional asthma-related deaths in subjects treated with salmeterol in SMART, assuming 10,000 subjects received salmeterol for a 28-week treatment period. Estimate calculated as the difference between the salmeterol and placebo groups in the rates of asthma-related death multiplied by 10,000.
[d]The Total Population includes the following ethnic origins listed on the case report form: Caucasian, African American, Hispanic, Asian, and "Other." In addition, the Total Population includes those subjects whose ethnic origin was not reported. The results for Caucasian and African American subpopulations are shown above. No asthma-related deaths occurred in the Hispanic (salmeterol n = 996, placebo n = 999), Asian (salmeterol n = 173, placebo n = 149), or "Other" (salmeterol n = 230, placebo n = 224) subpopulations. One asthma-related death occurred in the placebo group in the subpopulation whose ethnic origin was not reported (salmeterol n = 130, placebo n = 127).

Therefore, when treating patients with asthma, physicians should only prescribe ADVAIR DISKUS for patients not adequately controlled on a long-term asthma control medication, such as an inhaled corticosteroid, or whose disease severity clearly warrants initiation of treatment with both an inhaled corticosteroid and a LABA. Once asthma control is achieved and maintained, assess the patient at regular intervals and step down therapy (e.g., discontinue ADVAIR DISKUS) if possible without loss of asthma control and maintain the patient on a long-term asthma control medication, such as an inhaled corticosteroid. Do not use ADVAIR DISKUS for patients whose asthma is adequately controlled on low- or medium-dose inhaled corticosteroids [see Warnings and Precautions (5.1)].

1 INDICATIONS AND USAGE
1.1 Treatment of Asthma
ADVAIR DISKUS is indicated for the treatment of asthma in patients aged 4 years and older.

LABA, such as salmeterol, one of the active ingredients in ADVAIR DISKUS, increase the risk of asthma-related death. Available data from controlled clinical trials suggest that LABA increase the risk of asthma-related hospitalization in pediatric and adolescent patients [see Warnings and Precautions (5.1)]. Therefore, when treating patients with asthma, physicians should only prescribe ADVAIR DISKUS for patients not adequately controlled on a long-term asthma control medication, such as an inhaled corticosteroid, or whose disease severity clearly warrants initiation of treatment with both an inhaled corticosteroid and a LABA. Once asthma control is achieved and maintained, assess the patient at regular intervals and step down therapy (e.g., discontinue ADVAIR DISKUS) if possible without loss of asthma control and maintain the patient on a long-term asthma control medication, such as an inhaled corticosteroid. Do not use ADVAIR DISKUS for patients whose asthma is adequately controlled on low- or medium-dose inhaled corticosteroids.

Important Limitation of Use: ADVAIR DISKUS is NOT indicated for the relief of acute bronchospasm.

1.2 Maintenance Treatment of Chronic Obstructive Pulmonary Disease
ADVAIR DISKUS 250/50 is indicated for the twice-daily maintenance treatment of airflow obstruction in patients with chronic obstructive pulmonary disease (COPD), including chronic bronchitis and/or emphysema. ADVAIR DISKUS 250/50 is also indicated to reduce exacerbations of COPD in patients with a history of exacerbations. ADVAIR DISKUS 250/50 twice daily is the only approved dosage for the treatment of COPD because an efficacy advantage of the higher strength ADVAIR DISKUS 500/50 over ADVAIR DISKUS 250/50 has not been demonstrated.

Important Limitation of Use: ADVAIR DISKUS is NOT indicated for the relief of acute bronchospasm.

2 DOSAGE AND ADMINISTRATION
ADVAIR DISKUS should be administered as 1 inhalation twice daily by the orally inhaled route only. After inhalation, the patient should rinse his/her mouth with water without swallowing to help reduce the risk of oropharyngeal candidiasis.

More frequent administration or a greater number of inhalations (more than 1 inhalation twice daily) of the prescribed strength of ADVAIR DISKUS is not recommended as some patients are more likely to experience adverse effects with higher doses of salmeterol. Patients using ADVAIR DISKUS should not use additional LABA for any reason. [See Warnings and Precautions (5.3, 5.12).]

2.1 Asthma
If asthma symptoms arise in the period between doses, an inhaled, short-acting beta2-agonist should be taken for immediate relief.

Adult and Adolescent Patients Aged 12 Years and Older: For patients aged 12 years and older, the dosage is 1 inhalation twice daily, approximately 12 hours apart.

The recommended starting dosages for ADVAIR DISKUS for patients aged 12 years and older are based upon patients' asthma severity.

The maximum recommended dosage is ADVAIR DISKUS 500/50 twice daily.

Improvement in asthma control following inhaled administration of ADVAIR DISKUS can occur within 30 minutes of beginning treatment, although maximum benefit may not be achieved for 1 week or longer after starting treatment. Individual patients will experience a variable time to onset and degree of symptom relief.

For patients who do not respond adequately to the starting dosage after 2 weeks of therapy, replacing the current strength of ADVAIR DISKUS with a higher strength may provide additional improvement in asthma control.

If a previously effective dosage regimen fails to provide adequate improvement in asthma control, the therapeutic regimen should be reevaluated and additional therapeutic options (e.g., replacing the current strength of ADVAIR DISKUS with a higher strength, adding additional inhaled corticosteroid, initiating oral corticosteroids) should be considered.

Pediatric Patients Aged 4 to 11 Years: For patients with asthma aged 4 to 11 years who are not controlled on an inhaled corticosteroid, the dosage is 1 inhalation of ADVAIR DISKUS 100/50 twice daily, approximately 12 hours apart.

2.2 Chronic Obstructive Pulmonary Disease
The recommended dosage for patients with COPD is 1 inhalation of ADVAIR DISKUS 250/50 twice daily, approximately 12 hours apart.

If shortness of breath occurs in the period between doses, an inhaled, short-acting beta2-agonist should be taken for immediate relief.

3 DOSAGE FORMS AND STRENGTHS
Inhalation Powder. Inhaler containing a foil blister strip of powder formulation for oral inhalation. The strip contains a combination of fluticasone propionate 100, 250, or 500 mcg and salmeterol 50 mcg per blister.

4 CONTRAINDICATIONS
The use of ADVAIR DISKUS is contraindicated in the following conditions:
- Primary treatment of status asthmaticus or other acute episodes of asthma or COPD where intensive measures are required [see Warnings and Precautions (5.2)]
- Severe hypersensitivity to milk proteins [see Warnings and Precautions (5.11), Adverse Reactions (6.3), Description (11)]

5 WARNINGS AND PRECAUTIONS
5.1 Asthma-Related Death
LABA, such as salmeterol, one of the active ingredients in ADVAIR DISKUS, increase the risk of asthma-related death. Currently available data are inadequate to determine whether concurrent use of inhaled corticosteroids or other long-term asthma control drugs mitigates the increased risk of asthma-related death from LABA. Available data from controlled clinical trials suggest that LABA increase the risk of asthma-related hospitalization in pediatric and adolescent patients. Therefore, when treating patients with asthma, physicians should only prescribe ADVAIR DISKUS for patients not adequately controlled on a long-term asthma control medication, such as an inhaled corticosteroid, or whose disease severity clearly warrants initiation of treatment with both an inhaled corticosteroid and a LABA. Once asthma control is achieved and maintained, assess the patient at regular intervals and step down therapy (e.g., discontinue ADVAIR DISKUS) if possible without loss of asthma control and maintain the patient on a long-term asthma control medication, such as an inhaled corticosteroid. Do not use ADVAIR DISKUS for patients whose asthma is adequately controlled on low- or medium-dose inhaled corticosteroids.

A large placebo-controlled US trial that compared the safety of salmeterol with placebo, each added to usual asthma therapy, showed an increase in asthma-related deaths in subjects receiving salmeterol. The Salmeterol Multi-center Asthma Research Trial (SMART) was a randomized double-blind trial that enrolled LABA-naive subjects with asthma to assess the safety of salmeterol 42 mcg twice daily over 28 weeks compared with placebo when added to usual asthma therapy. A planned interim analysis was conducted when approximately half of the intended number of subjects had been enrolled (N = 26,355), which led to premature termination of the trial. The results of the interim analysis showed that subjects receiving salmeterol were at increased risk for fatal asthma events (see Table 1 and Figure 1). In the total population, a higher rate of asthma-related death occurred in subjects treated with salmeterol than those treated with placebo (0.10% versus 0.02%; relative risk: 4.37 [95% CI: 1.25, 15.34]).

Post-hoc subpopulation analyses were performed. In Caucasians, asthma-related death occurred at a higher rate in subjects treated with salmeterol than in subjects treated with placebo (0.07% versus 0.01%; relative risk: 5.82 [95% CI: 0.70, 48.37]). In African Americans also, asthma-related death occurred at a higher rate in subjects treated with salmeterol than those treated with placebo (0.31% versus 0.04%; relative risk: 7.26 [95% CI: 0.89, 58.94]). Although the relative risks of asthma-related death were similar in Caucasians and African Americans, the estimate of excess deaths in subjects treated with salmeterol was greater in African Americans because there was a higher overall rate of asthma-related death in African American subjects (see Table 1). Given the similar basic mechanisms of action of beta2-agonists, the findings seen in the SMART trial are considered a class effect.

Post-hoc analyses in pediatric subjects aged 12 to 18 years were also performed. Pediatric subjects accounted for approximately 12% of subjects in each treatment arm. Respiratory-related death or life-threatening experience occurred at a similar rate in the salmeterol group (0.12% [2/1,653]) and the placebo group (0.12% [2/1,622]; relative risk: 1.0 [95% CI: 0.1, 7.2]). All-cause hospitalization, however, was increased in the salmeterol group (2% [35/1,653]) versus the placebo group (<1% [16/1,622]; relative risk: 2.1 [95% CI: 1.1, 3.7]).

The data from the SMART trial are not adequate to determine whether concurrent use of inhaled corticosteroids, such as fluticasone propionate, the other active ingredient in ADVAIR DISKUS, or other long-term asthma control therapy mitigates the risk of asthma-related death.

[See table 1 above]

[See figure 1 at top of next column]

A 16-week clinical trial performed in the United Kingdom, the Salmeterol Nationwide Surveillance (SNS) trial, showed results similar to the SMART trial. In the SNS trial, the rate of asthma-related death was numerically, though not statistically significantly, greater in subjects with asthma treated with salmeterol (42 mcg twice daily) than those treated with albuterol (180 mcg 4 times daily) added to usual asthma therapy.

The SNS and SMART trials enrolled subjects with asthma. No trials have been conducted that were primarily designed to determine whether the rate of death in patients with COPD is increased by LABA.

Figure 1. Cumulative Incidence of Asthma-Related Deaths in the 28-Week Salmeterol Multi-center Asthma Research Trial (SMART), by Duration of Treatment

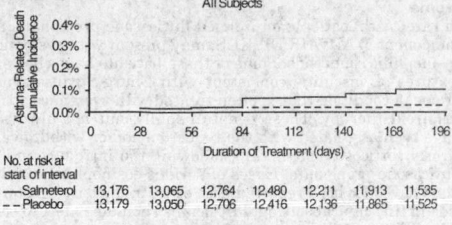

All Subjects

No. at risk at start of treatment							
Salmeterol	13,176	13,065	12,764	12,480	12,211	11,913	11,535
Placebo	13,179	13,050	12,706	12,416	12,136	11,865	11,525

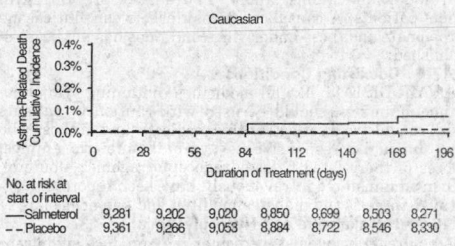

Caucasian

No. at risk at start of interval							
Salmeterol	9,281	9,202	9,020	8,850	8,699	8,503	8,271
Placebo	9,361	9,266	9,053	8,884	8,722	8,546	8,330

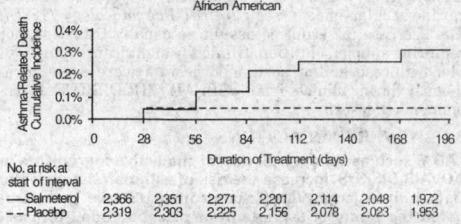

African American

No. at risk at start of interval							
Salmeterol	2,366	2,351	2,271	2,201	2,114	2,048	1,972
Placebo	2,319	2,303	2,225	2,156	2,078	2,023	1,953

5.2 Deterioration of Disease and Acute Episodes

ADVAIR DISKUS should not be initiated in patients during rapidly deteriorating or potentially life-threatening episodes of asthma or COPD. ADVAIR DISKUS has not been studied in subjects with acutely deteriorating asthma or COPD. The initiation of ADVAIR DISKUS in this setting is not appropriate.

Serious acute respiratory events, including fatalities, have been reported when salmeterol, a component of ADVAIR DISKUS, has been initiated in patients with significantly worsening or acutely deteriorating asthma. In most cases, these have occurred in patients with severe asthma (e.g., patients with a history of corticosteroid dependence, low pulmonary function, intubation, mechanical ventilation, frequent hospitalizations, previous life-threatening acute asthma exacerbations) and in some patients with acutely deteriorating asthma (e.g., patients with significantly increasing symptoms; increasing need for inhaled, short-acting beta₂-agonists; decreasing response to usual medications; increasing need for systemic corticosteroids; recent emergency room visits; deteriorating lung function). However, these events have occurred in a few patients with less severe asthma as well. It was not possible from these reports to determine whether salmeterol contributed to these events.

Increasing use of inhaled, short-acting beta₂-agonists is a marker of deteriorating asthma. In this situation, the patient requires immediate reevaluation with reassessment of the treatment regimen, giving special consideration to the possible need for replacing the current strength of ADVAIR DISKUS with a higher strength, adding additional inhaled corticosteroid, or initiating systemic corticosteroids. Patients should not use more than 1 inhalation twice daily of ADVAIR DISKUS.

ADVAIR DISKUS should not be used for the relief of acute symptoms, i.e., as rescue therapy for the treatment of acute episodes of bronchospasm. An inhaled, short-acting beta₂-agonist, not ADVAIR DISKUS, should be used to relieve acute symptoms such as shortness of breath. When prescribing ADVAIR DISKUS, the healthcare provider should also prescribe an inhaled, short-acting beta₂-agonist (e.g., albuterol) for treatment of acute symptoms, despite regular twice-daily use of ADVAIR DISKUS.

When beginning treatment with ADVAIR DISKUS, patients who have been taking oral or inhaled, short-acting beta₂-agonists on a regular basis (e.g., 4 times a day) should be instructed to discontinue the regular use of these drugs.

5.3 Excessive Use of ADVAIR DISKUS and Use With Other Long-Acting Beta₂-Agonists

ADVAIR DISKUS should not be used more often than recommended, at higher doses than recommended, or in conjunction with other medicines containing LABA, as an overdose may result. Clinically significant cardiovascular effects and fatalities have been reported in association with excessive use of inhaled sympathomimetic drugs. Patients using ADVAIR DISKUS should not use another medicine containing a LABA (e.g., salmeterol, formoterol fumarate, arformoterol tartrate, indacaterol) for any reason.

5.4 Local Effects of Inhaled Corticosteroids

In clinical trials, the development of localized infections of the mouth and pharynx with *Candida albicans* has occurred in subjects treated with ADVAIR DISKUS. When such an infection develops, it should be treated with appropriate local or systemic (i.e., oral) antifungal therapy while treatment with ADVAIR DISKUS continues, but at times therapy with ADVAIR DISKUS may need to be interrupted. Advise the patient to rinse his/her mouth with water without swallowing following inhalation to help reduce the risk of oropharyngeal candidiasis.

5.5 Pneumonia

Physicians should remain vigilant for the possible development of pneumonia in patients with COPD as the clinical features of pneumonia and exacerbations frequently overlap.

Lower respiratory tract infections, including pneumonia, have been reported in patients with COPD following the inhaled administration of corticosteroids, including fluticasone propionate and ADVAIR DISKUS. In 2 replicate 1-year trials in 1,579 subjects with COPD, there was a higher incidence of pneumonia reported in subjects receiving ADVAIR DISKUS 250/50 (7%) than in those receiving salmeterol 50 mcg (3%). The incidence of pneumonia in the subjects treated with ADVAIR DISKUS was higher in subjects older than 65 years (9%) compared with the incidence in subjects younger than 65 years (4%). [See Adverse Reactions (6.2), Use in Specific Populations (8.5).]

In a 3-year trial in 6,184 subjects with COPD, there was a higher incidence of pneumonia reported in subjects receiving ADVAIR DISKUS 500/50 compared with placebo (16% with ADVAIR DISKUS 500/50, 14% with fluticasone propionate 500 mcg, 11% with salmeterol 50 mcg, and 9% with placebo). Similar to what was seen in the 1-year trials with ADVAIR DISKUS 250/50, the incidence of pneumonia was higher in subjects older than 65 years (18% with ADVAIR DISKUS 500/50 versus 10% with placebo) compared with subjects younger than 65 years (14% with ADVAIR DISKUS 500/50 versus 8% with placebo). [See Adverse Reactions (6.2), Use in Specific Populations (8.5).]

5.6 Immunosuppression

Persons who are using drugs that suppress the immune system are more susceptible to infections than healthy individuals. Chickenpox and measles, for example, can have a more serious or even fatal course in susceptible children or adults using corticosteroids. In such children or adults who have not had these diseases or been properly immunized, particular care should be taken to avoid exposure. How the dose, route, and duration of corticosteroid administration affect the risk of developing a disseminated infection is not known. The contribution of the underlying disease and/or prior corticosteroid treatment to the risk is also not known. If a patient is exposed to chickenpox, prophylaxis with varicella zoster immune globulin (VZIG) may be indicated. If a patient is exposed to measles, prophylaxis with pooled intramuscular immunoglobulin (IG) may be indicated. (See the respective package inserts for complete VZIG and IG prescribing information.) If chickenpox develops, treatment with antiviral agents may be considered.

Inhaled corticosteroids should be used with caution, if at all, in patients with active or quiescent tuberculosis infections of the respiratory tract; systemic fungal, bacterial, viral, or parasitic infections; or ocular herpes simplex.

5.7 Transferring Patients From Systemic Corticosteroid Therapy

Particular care is needed for patients who have been transferred from systemically active corticosteroids to inhaled corticosteroids because deaths due to adrenal insufficiency have occurred in patients with asthma during and after transfer from systemic corticosteroids to less systemically available inhaled corticosteroids. After withdrawal from systemic corticosteroids, a number of months are required for recovery of hypothalamic-pituitary-adrenal (HPA) function.

Patients who have been previously maintained on 20 mg or more of prednisone (or its equivalent) may be most susceptible, particularly when their systemic corticosteroids have been almost completely withdrawn. During this period of HPA suppression, patients may exhibit signs and symptoms of adrenal insufficiency when exposed to trauma, surgery, or infection (particularly gastroenteritis) or other conditions associated with severe electrolyte loss. Although ADVAIR DISKUS may control asthma symptoms during these episodes, in recommended doses it supplies less than normal physiological amounts of glucocorticoid systemically and does NOT provide the mineralocorticoid activity that is necessary for coping with these emergencies.

During periods of stress or a severe asthma attack, patients who have been withdrawn from systemic corticosteroids should be instructed to resume oral corticosteroids (in large doses) immediately and to contact their physicians for further instruction. These patients should also be instructed to carry a warning card indicating that they may need supplementary systemic corticosteroids during periods of stress or a severe asthma attack.

Patients requiring oral corticosteroids should be weaned slowly from systemic corticosteroid use after transferring to ADVAIR DISKUS. Prednisone reduction can be accomplished by reducing the daily prednisone dose by 2.5 mg on a weekly basis during therapy with ADVAIR Diskus. Lung function (mean forced expiratory volume in 1 second [FEV₁] or morning peak expiratory flow [AM PEF]), beta-agonist use, and asthma symptoms should be carefully monitored during withdrawal of oral corticosteroids. In addition, patients should be observed for signs and symptoms of adrenal insufficiency, such as fatigue, lassitude, weakness, nausea and vomiting, and hypotension.

Transfer of patients from systemic corticosteroid therapy to ADVAIR DISKUS may unmask allergic conditions previously suppressed by the systemic corticosteroid therapy (e.g., rhinitis, conjunctivitis, eczema, arthritis, eosinophilic conditions).

During withdrawal from oral corticosteroids, some patients may experience symptoms of systemically active corticosteroid withdrawal (e.g., joint and/or muscular pain, lassitude, depression) despite maintenance or even improvement of respiratory function.

5.8 Hypercorticism and Adrenal Suppression

Fluticasone propionate, a component of ADVAIR DISKUS, will often help control asthma symptoms with less suppression of HPA function than therapeutically equivalent oral doses of prednisone. Since fluticasone propionate is absorbed into the circulation and can be systemically active at higher doses, the beneficial effects of ADVAIR DISKUS in minimizing HPA dysfunction may be expected only when recommended dosages are not exceeded and individual patients are titrated to the lowest effective dose. A relationship between plasma levels of fluticasone propionate and inhibitory effects on stimulated cortisol production has been shown after 4 weeks of treatment with fluticasone propionate inhalation aerosol. Since individual sensitivity to effects on cortisol production exists, physicians should consider this information when prescribing ADVAIR DISKUS.

Because of the possibility of significant systemic absorption of inhaled corticosteroids in sensitive patients, patients treated with ADVAIR DISKUS should be observed carefully for any evidence of systemic corticosteroid effects. Particular care should be taken in observing patients postoperatively or during periods of stress for evidence of inadequate adrenal response.

It is possible that systemic corticosteroid effects such as hypercorticism and adrenal suppression (including adrenal crisis) may appear in a small number of patients who are sensitive to these effects. If such effects occur, ADVAIR DISKUS should be reduced slowly, consistent with accepted procedures for reducing systemic corticosteroids, and other treatments for management of asthma symptoms should be considered.

5.9 Drug Interactions With Strong Cytochrome P450 3A4 Inhibitors

The use of strong cytochrome P450 3A4 (CYP3A4) inhibitors (e.g., ritonavir, atazanavir, clarithromycin, indinavir, itraconazole, nefazodone, nelfinavir, saquinavir, ketoconazole, telithromycin) with ADVAIR DISKUS is not recommended because increased systemic corticosteroid and increased cardiovascular adverse effects may occur [see Drug Interactions (7.1), Clinical Pharmacology (12.3)].

5.10 Paradoxical Bronchospasm and Upper Airway Symptoms

As with other inhaled medicines, ADVAIR DISKUS can produce paradoxical bronchospasm, which may be life threatening. If paradoxical bronchospasm occurs following dosing with ADVAIR DISKUS, it should be treated immediately with an inhaled, short-acting bronchodilator; ADVAIR DISKUS should be discontinued immediately; and alternative therapy should be instituted. Upper airway symptoms of laryngeal spasm, irritation, or swelling, such as stridor and choking, have been reported in patients receiving ADVAIR DISKUS.

5.11 Immediate Hypersensitivity Reactions

Immediate hypersensitivity reactions (e.g., urticaria, angioedema, rash, bronchospasm, hypotension), including anaphylaxis, may occur after administration of ADVAIR DISKUS. There have been reports of anaphylactic reactions in patients with severe milk protein allergy after inhalation of powder products containing lactose; therefore, patients with severe milk protein allergy should not use ADVAIR DISKUS [see Contraindications (4)].

5.12 Cardiovascular and Central Nervous System Effects

Excessive beta-adrenergic stimulation has been associated with seizures, angina, hypertension or hypotension, tachy-

Table 2. Adverse Reactions With ADVAIR DISKUS With ≥3% Incidence and More Common Than Placebo in Adult and Adolescent Subjects With Asthma

Adverse Event	ADVAIR DISKUS 100/50 (n = 92) %	ADVAIR DISKUS 250/50 (n = 84) %	Fluticasone Propionate 100 mcg (n = 90) %	Fluticasone Propionate 250 mcg (n = 84) %	Salmeterol 50 mcg (n = 180) %	Placebo (n = 175) %
Ear, nose, and throat						
Upper respiratory tract infection	27	21	29	25	19	14
Pharyngitis	13	10	7	12	8	6
Upper respiratory inflammation	7	6	7	8	8	5
Sinusitis	4	5	6	1	3	4
Hoarseness/dysphonia	5	2	2	4	<1	<1
Oral candidiasis	1	4	2	2	0	0
Lower respiratory						
Viral respiratory infections	4	4	4	10	6	3
Bronchitis	2	8	1	2	2	2
Cough	3	6	0	0	3	2
Neurology						
Headaches	12	13	14	8	10	7
Gastrointestinal						
Nausea and vomiting	4	6	3	4	1	1
Gastrointestinal discomfort and pain	4	1	0	2	1	1
Diarrhea	4	2	2	2	1	1
Viral gastrointestinal infections	3	0	3	1	2	2
Non-site specific						
Candidiasis unspecified site	3	0	1	4	0	1
Musculoskeletal						
Musculoskeletal pain	4	2	1	5	3	3

cardia with rates up to 200 beats/min, arrhythmias, nervousness, headache, tremor, palpitation, nausea, dizziness, fatigue, malaise, and insomnia *[see Overdosage (10)]*. Therefore, ADVAIR DISKUS, like all products containing sympathomimetic amines, should be used with caution in patients with cardiovascular disorders, especially coronary insufficiency, cardiac arrhythmias, and hypertension.
Salmeterol, a component of ADVAIR DISKUS, can produce a clinically significant cardiovascular effect in some patients as measured by pulse rate, blood pressure, and/or symptoms. Although such effects are uncommon after administration of salmeterol at recommended doses, if they occur, the drug may need to be discontinued. In addition, beta-agonists have been reported to produce electrocardiogram (ECG) changes, such as flattening of the T wave, prolongation of the QTc interval, and ST segment depression. The clinical significance of these findings is unknown. Large doses of inhaled or oral salmeterol (12 to 20 times the recommended dose) have been associated with clinically significant prolongation of the QTc interval, which has the potential for producing ventricular arrhythmias. Fatalities have been reported in association with excessive use of inhaled sympathomimetic drugs.

5.13   Reduction in Bone Mineral Density
Decreases in bone mineral density (BMD) have been observed with long-term administration of products containing inhaled corticosteroids. The clinical significance of small changes in BMD with regard to long-term consequences such as fracture is unknown. Patients with major risk factors for decreased bone mineral content, such as prolonged immobilization, family history of osteoporosis, postmenopausal status, tobacco use, advanced age, poor nutrition, or chronic use of drugs that can reduce bone mass (e.g., anticonvulsants, oral corticosteroids) should be monitored and treated with established standards of care. Since patients with COPD often have multiple risk factors for reduced BMD, assessment of BMD is recommended prior to initiating ADVAIR DISKUS and periodically thereafter. If significant reductions in BMD are seen and ADVAIR DISKUS is still considered medically important for that patient's COPD therapy, use of medicine to treat or prevent osteoporosis should be strongly considered.
2-Year Fluticasone Propionate Trial: A 2-year trial in 160 subjects (females aged 18 to 40 years, males 18 to 50) with asthma receiving CFC-propelled fluticasone propionate inhalation aerosol 88 or 440 mcg twice daily demonstrated no statistically significant changes in BMD at any time point (24, 52, 76, and 104 weeks of double-blind treatment) as assessed by dual-energy x-ray absorptiometry at lumbar regions L1 through L4.
3-Year Bone Mineral Density Trial: Effects of treatment with ADVAIR DISKUS 250/50 or salmeterol 50 mcg on BMD at the L_1-L_4 lumbar spine and total hip were evaluated in 186 subjects with COPD (aged 43 to 87 years) in a 3-year double-blind trial. Of those enrolled, 108 subjects (72

males and 36 females) were followed for the entire 3 years. BMD evaluations were conducted at baseline and at 6-month intervals. Conclusions cannot be drawn from this trial regarding BMD decline in subjects treated with ADVAIR DISKUS versus salmeterol due to the inconsistency of treatment differences across gender and between lumbar spine and total hip.
In this trial there were 7 non-traumatic fractures reported in 5 subjects treated with ADVAIR DISKUS and 1 non-traumatic fracture in 1 subject treated with salmeterol. None of the non-traumatic fractures occurred in the vertebrae, hip, or long bones.
3-Year Survival Trial: Effects of treatment with ADVAIR DISKUS 500/50, fluticasone propionate 500 mcg, salmeterol 50 mcg, or placebo on BMD was evaluated in a subset of 658 subjects (females and males aged 40 to 80 years) with COPD in the 3-year survival trial. BMD evaluations were conducted at baseline and at 48, 108, and 158 weeks. Conclusions cannot be drawn from this trial because of the large number of dropouts (>50%) before the end of the follow-up and the maldistribution of covariates among the treatment groups that can affect BMD.
Fracture risk was estimated for the entire population of subjects with COPD in the survival trial (N = 6,184). The probability of a fracture over 3 years was 6.3% for ADVAIR DISKUS, 5.4% for fluticasone propionate, 5.1% for salmeterol, and 5.1% for placebo.

5.14   Effect on Growth
Orally inhaled corticosteroids may cause a reduction in growth velocity when administered to pediatric patients. Monitor the growth of pediatric patients receiving ADVAIR DISKUS routinely (e.g., via stadiometry). To minimize the systemic effects of orally inhaled corticosteroids, including ADVAIR DISKUS, titrate each patient's dosage to the lowest dosage that effectively controls his/her symptoms *[see Dosage and Administration (2.1), Use in Specific Populations (8.4)]*.

5.15   Glaucoma and Cataracts
Glaucoma, increased intraocular pressure, and cataracts have been reported in patients with asthma and COPD following the long-term administration of inhaled corticosteroids, including fluticasone propionate, a component of ADVAIR DISKUS. Therefore, close monitoring is warranted in patients with a change in vision or with a history of increased intraocular pressure, glaucoma, and/or cataracts.
Effects of treatment with ADVAIR DISKUS 500/50, fluticasone propionate 500 mcg, salmeterol 50 mcg, or placebo on development of cataracts or glaucoma was evaluated in a subset of 658 subjects with COPD in the 3-year survival trial. Ophthalmic examinations were conducted at baseline and at 48, 108, and 158 weeks. Conclusions about cataracts cannot be drawn from this trial because the high incidence of cataracts at baseline (61% to 71%) resulted in an inadequate number of subjects treated with ADVAIR DISKUS 500/50 who were eligible and available for evalua-

tion of cataracts at the end of the trial (n = 53). The incidence of newly diagnosed glaucoma was 2% with ADVAIR DISKUS 500/50, 5% with fluticasone propionate, 0% with salmeterol, and 2% with placebo.
5.16   Eosinophilic Conditions and Churg-Strauss Syndrome
In rare cases, patients on inhaled fluticasone propionate, a component of ADVAIR DISKUS, may present with systemic eosinophilic conditions. Some of these patients have clinical features of vasculitis consistent with Churg-Strauss syndrome, a condition that is often treated with systemic corticosteroid therapy. These events usually, but not always, have been associated with the reduction and/or withdrawal of oral corticosteroid therapy following the introduction of fluticasone propionate. Cases of serious eosinophilic conditions have also been reported with other inhaled corticosteroids in this clinical setting. Physicians should be alert to eosinophilia, vasculitic rash, worsening pulmonary symptoms, cardiac complications, and/or neuropathy presenting in their patients. A causal relationship between fluticasone propionate and these underlying conditions has not been established.

5.17   Coexisting Conditions
ADVAIR DISKUS, like all medicines containing sympathomimetic amines, should be used with caution in patients with convulsive disorders or thyrotoxicosis and in those who are unusually responsive to sympathomimetic amines. Doses of the related beta$_2$-adrenoceptor agonist albuterol, when administered intravenously, have been reported to aggravate preexisting diabetes mellitus and ketoacidosis.
5.18   Hypokalemia and Hyperglycemia
Beta-adrenergic agonist medicines may produce significant hypokalemia in some patients, possibly through intracellular shunting, which has the potential to produce adverse cardiovascular effects *[see Clinical Pharmacology (12.2)]*. The decrease in serum potassium is usually transient, not requiring supplementation. Clinically significant changes in blood glucose and/or serum potassium were seen infrequently during clinical trials with ADVAIR DISKUS at recommended doses.

6   ADVERSE REACTIONS
LABA, such as salmeterol, one of the active ingredients in ADVAIR DISKUS, increase the risk of asthma-related death. Data from a large placebo-controlled US trial that compared the safety of salmeterol or placebo added to usual asthma therapy showed an increase in asthma-related deaths in subjects receiving salmeterol *[see Warnings and Precautions (5.1)]*. Currently available data are inadequate to determine whether concurrent use of inhaled corticosteroids or other long-term asthma control drugs mitigates the increased risk of asthma-related death from LABA. Available data from controlled clinical trials suggest that LABA increase the risk of asthma-related hospitalization in pediatric and adolescent patients *[see Warnings and Precautions (5.1)]*.
Systemic and local corticosteroid use may result in the following:
- *Candida albicans* infection *[see Warnings and Precautions (5.4)]*
- Pneumonia in patients with COPD *[see Warnings and Precautions (5.5)]*
- Immunosuppression *[see Warnings and Precautions (5.6)]*
- Hypercorticism and adrenal suppression *[see Warnings and Precautions (5.8)]*
- Reduction in bone mineral density *[see Warnings and Precautions (5.13)]*
- Growth effects *[see Warnings and Precautions (5.14)]*
- Glaucoma and cataracts *[see Warnings and Precautions (5.15)]*

Because clinical trials are conducted under widely varying conditions, adverse reaction rates observed in the clinical trials of a drug cannot be directly compared with rates in the clinical trials of another drug and may not reflect the rates observed in practice.

6.1   Clinical Trials Experience in Asthma
Adult and Adolescent Subjects Aged 12 Years and Older: The incidence of adverse reactions associated with ADVAIR DISKUS in Table 2 is based upon two 12-week, placebo-controlled, US clinical trials (Trials 1 and 2). A total of 705 adult and adolescent subjects (349 females and 356 males) previously treated with salmeterol or inhaled corticosteroids were treated twice daily with ADVAIR DISKUS (100/50- or 250/50-mcg doses), fluticasone propionate inhalation powder (100- or 250-mcg doses), salmeterol inhalation powder 50 mcg, or placebo. The average duration of exposure was 60 to 79 days in the active treatment groups compared with 42 days in the placebo group.
[See table 2 above]
The types of adverse reactions and events reported in Trial 3, a 28-week non-US clinical trial in 503 subjects previously treated with inhaled corticosteroids who were treated twice daily with ADVAIR DISKUS 500/50, fluticasone propionate inhalation powder 500 mcg and salmeterol inhalation powder 50 mcg used concurrently, or fluticasone propionate inhalation powder 500 mcg, were similar to those reported in Table 2.
Additional Adverse Reactions: Other adverse reactions not previously listed, whether considered drug-related or

not by the investigators, that were reported more frequently by subjects with asthma treated with ADVAIR DISKUS compared with subjects treated with placebo include the following: lymphatic signs and symptoms; muscle injuries; fractures; wounds and lacerations; contusions and hematomas; ear signs and symptoms; nasal signs and symptoms; nasal sinus disorders; keratitis and conjunctivitis; dental discomfort and pain; gastrointestinal signs and symptoms; oral ulcerations; oral discomfort and pain; lower respiratory signs and symptoms; pneumonia; muscle stiffness, tightness, and rigidity; bone and cartilage disorders; sleep disorders; compressed nerve syndromes; viral infections; pain; chest symptoms; fluid retention; bacterial infections; unusual taste; viral skin infections; skin flakiness and acquired ichthyosis; disorders of sweat and sebum.

Pediatric Subjects Aged 4 to 11 Years: The safety data for pediatric subjects aged 4 to 11 years is based upon 1 US trial of 12 weeks' treatment duration. A total of 203 subjects (74 females and 129 males) who were receiving inhaled corticosteroids at trial entry were randomized to either ADVAIR DISKUS 100/50 or fluticasone propionate inhalation powder 100 mcg twice daily. Common adverse reactions (≥3% and greater than placebo) seen in the pediatric subjects but not reported in the adult and adolescent clinical trials include: throat irritation and ear, nose, and throat infections.

Laboratory Test Abnormalities: Elevation of hepatic enzymes was reported in ≥1% of subjects in clinical trials. The elevations were transient and did not lead to discontinuation from the trials. In addition, there were no clinically relevant changes noted in glucose or potassium.

6.2 Clinical Trials Experience in Chronic Obstructive Pulmonary Disease

Short-Term (6 Months to 1 Year) Trials: The short-term safety data are based on exposure to ADVAIR DISKUS 250/50 twice daily in one 6-month and two 1-year clinical trials. In the 6-month trial, a total of 723 adult subjects (266 females and 457 males) were treated twice daily with ADVAIR DISKUS 250/50, fluticasone propionate inhalation powder 250 mcg, salmeterol inhalation powder, or placebo. The mean age of the subjects was 64, and the majority (93%) was Caucasian. In this trial, 70% of the subjects treated with ADVAIR DISKUS reported an adverse reaction compared with 64% on placebo. The average duration of exposure to Advair Diskus 250/50 was 141.3 days compared with 131.6 days for placebo. The incidence of adverse reactions in the 6-month trial is shown in Table 3.

[See table 3 above]

In the two 1-year trials, ADVAIR DISKUS 250/50 was compared with salmeterol in 1,579 subjects (863 males and 716 females). The mean age of the subjects was 65 years, and the majority (94%) was Caucasian. To be enrolled, all of the subjects had to have had a COPD exacerbation in the previous 12 months. In this trial, 88% of the subjects treated with ADVAIR DISKUS and 86% of the subjects treated with salmeterol reported an adverse event. The most common events that occurred with a frequency of >5% and more frequently in the subjects treated with ADVAIR DISKUS were nasopharyngitis, upper respiratory tract infection, nasal congestion, back pain, sinusitis, dizziness, nausea, pneumonia, candidiasis, and dysphonia. Overall, 55 (7%) of the subjects treated with ADVAIR DISKUS and 25 (3%) of the subjects treated with salmeterol developed pneumonia.

The incidence of pneumonia was higher in subjects older than 65 years, 9% in the subjects treated with ADVAIR DISKUS compared with 4% in the subjects treated with ADVAIR DISKUS younger than 65 years. In the subjects treated with salmeterol, the incidence of pneumonia was the same (3%) in both age-groups. [See Warnings and Precautions (5.5), Use in Specific Populations (8.5).]

Long-Term (3 Years) Trial: The safety of ADVAIR DISKUS 500/50 was evaluated in a randomized, double-blind, placebo-controlled, multicenter, international, 3-year trial in 6,184 adult subjects with COPD (4,684 males and 1,500 females). The mean age of the subjects was 65 years, and the majority (82%) was Caucasian. The distribution of adverse events was similar to that seen in the 1-year trials with ADVAIR DISKUS 250/50. In addition, pneumonia was reported in a significantly increased number of subjects treated with ADVAIR DISKUS 500/50 and fluticasone propionate 500 mcg (16% and 14%, respectively) compared with subjects treated with salmeterol 50 mcg or placebo (11% and 9%, respectively). When adjusted for time on treatment, the rates of pneumonia were 84 and 88 events per 1,000 treatment-years in the groups treated with fluticasone propionate 500 mcg and with ADVAIR DISKUS 500/50, respectively, compared with 52 events per 1,000 treatment-years in the salmeterol and placebo groups. Similar to what was seen in the 1-year trials with ADVAIR DISKUS 250/50, the incidence of pneumonia was higher in subjects older than 65 years (18% with ADVAIR DISKUS 500/50 versus 10% with placebo) compared with subjects younger than 65 years (14% with ADVAIR DISKUS 500/50 versus 8% with placebo). [See Warnings and Precautions (5.5), Use in Specific Populations (8.5).]

Table 3. Overall Adverse Reactions With ADVAIR DISKUS 250/50 With ≥3% Incidence in Subjects With Chronic Obstructive Pulmonary Disease Associated With Chronic Bronchitis

Adverse Event	ADVAIR DISKUS 250/50 (n = 178) %	Fluticasone Propionate 250 mcg (n = 183) %	Salmeterol 50 mcg (n = 177) %	Placebo (n = 185) %
Ear, nose, and throat				
Candidiasis mouth/throat	10	6	3	1
Throat irritation	8	5	4	7
Hoarseness/dysphonia	5	3	<1	0
Sinusitis	3	8	5	3
Lower respiratory				
Viral respiratory infections	6	4	3	3
Neurology				
Headaches	16	11	10	12
Dizziness	4	<1	3	2
Non-site specific				
Fever	4	3	0	3
Malaise and fatigue	3	2	2	3
Musculoskeletal				
Musculoskeletal pain	9	8	12	9
Muscle cramps and spasms	3	2	1	1

Additional Adverse Reactions: Other adverse reactions not previously listed, whether considered drug-related or not by the investigators, that were reported more frequently by subjects with COPD treated with ADVAIR DISKUS compared with subjects treated with placebo include the following: syncope; ear, nose, and throat infections; ear signs and symptoms; laryngitis; nasal congestion/blockage; nasal sinus disorders; pharyngitis/throat infection; hypothyroidism; dry eyes; eye infections; gastrointestinal signs and symptoms; oral lesions; abnormal liver function tests; bacterial infections; edema and swelling; viral infections.

Laboratory Abnormalities: There were no clinically relevant changes in these trials. Specifically, no increased reporting of neutrophilia or changes in glucose or potassium was noted.

6.3 Postmarketing Experience

In addition to adverse reactions reported from clinical trials, the following adverse reactions have been identified during postapproval use of any formulation of ADVAIR, fluticasone propionate, and/or salmeterol regardless of indication. Because these reactions are reported voluntarily from a population of uncertain size, it is not always possible to reliably estimate their frequency or establish a causal relationship to drug exposure. These events have been chosen for inclusion due to either their seriousness, frequency of reporting, or causal connection to ADVAIR DISKUS, fluticasone propionate, and/or salmeterol or a combination of these factors.

Cardiac Disorders: Arrhythmias (including atrial fibrillation, extrasystoles, supraventricular tachycardia), ventricular tachycardia.

Endocrine Disorders: Cushing's syndrome, Cushingoid features, growth velocity reduction in children/adolescents, hypercorticism.

Eye Disorders: Glaucoma.

Gastrointestinal Disorders: Abdominal pain, dyspepsia, xerostomia.

Immune System Disorders: Immediate and delayed hypersensitivity reaction (including very rare anaphylactic reaction). Very rare anaphylactic reaction in patients with severe milk protein allergy.

Infections and Infestations: Esophageal candidiasis.

Metabolic and Nutrition Disorders: Hyperglycemia, weight gain.

Musculoskeletal, Connective Tissue, and Bone Disorders: Arthralgia, cramps, myositis, osteoporosis.

Nervous System Disorders: Paresthesia, restlessness.

Psychiatric Disorders: Agitation, aggression, depression. Behavioral changes, including hyperactivity and irritability, have been reported very rarely and primarily in children.

Reproductive System and Breast Disorders: Dysmenorrhea.

Respiratory, Thoracic, and Mediastinal Disorders: Chest congestion; chest tightness; dyspnea; facial and oropharyngeal edema; immediate bronchospasm; paradoxical bronchospasm; tracheitis; wheezing; reports of upper respiratory symptoms of laryngeal spasm, irritation, or swelling such as stridor or choking.

Skin and Subcutaneous Tissue Disorders: Ecchymoses, photodermatitis.

Vascular Disorders: Pallor.

7   DRUG INTERACTIONS

ADVAIR DISKUS has been used concomitantly with other drugs, including short-acting beta₂-agonists, methylxan- thines, and intranasal corticosteroids, commonly used in patients with asthma or COPD without adverse drug reactions [see Clinical Pharmacology (12.2)]. No formal drug interaction trials have been performed with ADVAIR DISKUS.

7.1   Inhibitors of Cytochrome P450 3A4

Fluticasone propionate and salmeterol, the individual components of ADVAIR DISKUS, are substrates of CYP3A4. The use of strong CYP3A4 inhibitors (e.g., ritonavir, atazanavir, clarithromycin, indinavir, itraconazole, nefazodone, nelfinavir, saquinavir, ketoconazole, telithromycin) with ADVAIR DISKUS is not recommended because increased systemic corticosteroid and increased cardiovascular adverse effects may occur.

Ritonavir: Fluticasone Propionate: A drug interaction trial with fluticasone propionate aqueous nasal spray in healthy subjects has shown that ritonavir (a strong CYP3A4 inhibitor) can significantly increase plasma fluticasone propionate exposure, resulting in significantly reduced serum cortisol concentrations [see Clinical Pharmacology (12.3)]. During postmarketing use, there have been reports of clinically significant drug interactions in patients receiving fluticasone propionate and ritonavir, resulting in systemic corticosteroid effects including Cushing's syndrome and adrenal suppression.

Ketoconazole: Fluticasone Propionate: Coadministration of orally inhaled fluticasone propionate (1,000 mcg) and ketoconazole (200 mg once daily) resulted in a 1.9-fold increase in plasma fluticasone propionate exposure and a 45% decrease in plasma cortisol area under the curve (AUC), but had no effect on urinary excretion of cortisol.

Salmeterol: In a drug interaction trial in 20 healthy subjects, coadministration of inhaled salmeterol (50 mcg twice daily) and oral ketoconazole (400 mg once daily) for 7 days resulted in greater systemic exposure to salmeterol (AUC increased 16-fold and C_{max} increased 1.4-fold). Three (3) subjects were withdrawn due to beta₂-agonist side effects (2 with prolonged QTc and 1 with palpitations and sinus tachycardia). Although there was no statistical effect on the mean QTc, coadministration of salmeterol and ketoconazole was associated with more frequent increases in QTc duration compared with salmeterol and placebo administration.

7.2   Monoamine Oxidase Inhibitors and Tricyclic Antidepressants

ADVAIR DISKUS should be administered with extreme caution to patients being treated with monoamine oxidase inhibitors or tricyclic antidepressants, or within 2 weeks of discontinuation of such agents, because the action of salmeterol, a component of ADVAIR DISKUS, on the vascular system may be potentiated by these agents.

7.3   Beta-Adrenergic Receptor Blocking Agents

Beta-blockers not only block the pulmonary effect of beta-agonists, such as salmeterol, a component of ADVAIR DISKUS, but may also produce severe bronchospasm in patients with asthma or COPD. Therefore, patients with asthma or COPD should not normally be treated with beta-blockers. However, under certain circumstances, there may be no acceptable alternatives to the use of beta-adrenergic blocking agents for these patients; cardioselective beta-blockers could be considered, although they should be administered with caution.

7.4   Non-Potassium-Sparing Diuretics

The ECG changes and/or hypokalemia that may result from the administration of non–potassium-sparing diuretics (such as loop or thiazide diuretics) can be acutely worsened by beta-agonists, such as salmeterol, a component of ADVAIR DISKUS, especially when the recommended dose of the beta-agonist is exceeded. Although the clinical significance of these effects is not known, caution is advised in the coadministration of ADVAIR DISKUS with non–potassium–sparing diuretics.

8   USE IN SPECIFIC POPULATIONS

8.1   Pregnancy
Teratogenic Effects: Pregnancy Category C. There are no adequate and well-controlled trials with ADVAIR DISKUS in pregnant women. Corticosteroids and beta$_2$-agonists have been shown to be teratogenic in laboratory animals when administered systemically at relatively low dosage levels. Because animal reproduction studies are not always predictive of human response, ADVAIR DISKUS should be used during pregnancy only if the potential benefit justifies the potential risk to the fetus. Women should be advised to contact their physicians if they become pregnant while taking ADVAIR DISKUS.

Fluticasone Propionate and Salmeterol: In the mouse reproduction assay, fluticasone propionate by the subcutaneous route at a dose approximately 3/5 the maximum recommended human daily inhalation dose (MRHDID) (on a mg/m^2 basis at a maternal subcutaneous dose of 150 mcg/kg/day) combined with oral salmeterol at a dose approximately 410 times the MRHDID (on a mg/m^2 basis at a maternal oral dose of 10 mg/kg/day) produced cleft palate, fetal death, increased implantation loss, and delayed ossification. These observations are characteristic of glucocorticoids. No developmental toxicity was observed at combination doses of fluticasone propionate subcutaneously up to approximately 1/6 the MRHDID (on a mg/m^2 basis at a maternal subcutaneous dose of 40 mcg/kg/day) and doses of salmeterol up to approximately 55 times the MRHDID (on a mg/m^2 basis at a maternal oral dose of 1.4 mcg/kg/day). In rats, combining fluticasone propionate subcutaneously at a dose equivalent to the MRHDID (on a mg/m^2 basis at a maternal subcutaneous dose of 100 mcg/kg/day) and a dose of salmeterol at approximately 810 times the MRHDID (on a mg/m^2 basis at a maternal oral dose of 10 mg/kg/day) produced decreased fetal weight, umbilical hernia, delayed ossification, and changes in the occipital bone. No such effects were seen when combining fluticasone propionate subcutaneously at a dose less than the MRHDID (on a mg/m^2 basis at a maternal subcutaneous dose of 30 mcg/kg/day) and an oral dose of salmeterol at approximately 80 times the MRHDID (on a mg/m^2 basis at a maternal oral dose of 1 mg/kg/day).

Fluticasone Propionate: Mice and rats at fluticasone propionate doses less than or equivalent to the MRHDID (on a mg/m^2 basis at a maternal subcutaneous dose of 45 and 100 mcg/kg/day, respectively) showed fetal toxicity characteristic of potent corticosteroid compounds, including embryonic growth retardation, omphalocele, cleft palate, and retarded cranial ossification. No teratogenicity was seen in rats at doses approximately equivalent to the MRHDID (on a mg/m^2 basis at maternal inhaled doses up to 68.7 mg/kg/day).

In rabbits, fetal weight reduction and cleft palate were observed at a fluticasone propionate dose less than the MRHDID (on a mg/m^2 basis at a maternal subcutaneous dose of 4 mcg/kg/day). However, no teratogenic effects were reported at fluticasone propionate doses up to approximately 5 times the MRHDID (on a mg/m^2 basis at a maternal oral dose up to 300 mcg/kg/day). No fluticasone propionate was detected in the plasma in this study, consistent with the established low bioavailability following oral administration *[see Clinical Pharmacology (12.3)]*.

Fluticasone propionate crossed the placenta following subcutaneous administration to mice and rats and oral administration to rabbits.

Experience with oral corticosteroids since their introduction in pharmacologic, as opposed to physiologic, doses suggests that rodents are more prone to teratogenic effects from corticosteroids than humans. In addition, because there is a natural increase in corticosteroid production during pregnancy, most women will require a lower exogenous corticosteroid dose and many will not need corticosteroid treatment during pregnancy.

Salmeterol: No teratogenic effects occurred in rats at salmeterol doses approximately 160 times the MRHDID (on a mg/m^2 basis at maternal oral doses up to 2 mg/kg/day). In pregnant Dutch rabbits administered salmeterol doses approximately 50 times the MRHDID (on an AUC basis at maternal oral doses of 1 mg/kg/day and higher), fetal toxic effects were observed characteristically resulting from beta-adrenoceptor stimulation. These included precocious eyelid openings, cleft palate, sternebral fusion, limb and paw flexures, and delayed ossification of the frontal cranial bones. No such effects occurred at a salmeterol dose approximately 20 times the MRHDID (on an AUC basis at a maternal oral dose of 0.6 mg/kg/day).

New Zealand White rabbits were less sensitive since only delayed ossification of the frontal cranial bones was seen at

a salmeterol dose approximately 1,600 times the MRHDID on a mg/m^2 basis at a maternal oral dose of 10 mg/kg/day. Salmeterol xinafoate crossed the placenta following oral administration to mice and rats.

Nonteratogenic Effects: Hypoadrenalism may occur in infants born of mothers receiving corticosteroids during pregnancy. Such infants should be carefully monitored.

8.2   Labor and Delivery
There are no well-controlled human trials that have investigated effects of ADVAIR DISKUS on preterm labor or labor at term. Because of the potential for beta-agonist interference with uterine contractility, use of ADVAIR DISKUS during labor should be restricted to those patients in whom the benefits clearly outweigh the risks.

8.3   Nursing Mothers
Plasma levels of salmeterol, a component of ADVAIR DISKUS, after inhaled therapeutic doses are very low. In rats, salmeterol xinafoate is excreted in the milk. There are no data from controlled trials on the use of salmeterol by nursing mothers. It is not known whether fluticasone propionate, a component of ADVAIR DISKUS, is excreted in human breast milk. However, other corticosteroids have been detected in human milk. Subcutaneous administration to lactating rats of tritiated fluticasone propionate resulted in measurable radioactivity in milk.

Since there are no data from controlled trials on the use of ADVAIR DISKUS by nursing mothers, caution should be exercised when ADVAIR DISKUS is administered to a nursing woman.

8.4   Pediatric Use
Use of ADVAIR DISKUS 100/50 in patients aged 4 to 11 years is supported by extrapolation of efficacy data from older subjects and by safety and efficacy data from a trial of ADVAIR DISKUS 100/50 in children with asthma aged 4 to 11 years *[see Adverse Reactions (6.1), Clinical Pharmacology (12.3), Clinical Studies (14.1)]*. The safety and effectiveness of ADVAIR DISKUS in children with asthma younger than 4 years have not been established.

Inhaled corticosteroids, including fluticasone propionate, a component of ADVAIR DISKUS, may cause a reduction in growth velocity in children and adolescents *[see Warnings and Precautions (5.14)]*. The growth of pediatric patients receiving orally inhaled corticosteroids, including ADVAIR DISKUS, should be monitored.

A 52-week placebo-controlled trial to assess the potential growth effects of fluticasone propionate inhalation powder (FLOVENT® ROTADISK®) at 50 and 100 mcg twice daily was conducted in the US in 325 prepubescent children (244 males and 81 females) aged 4 to 11 years. The mean growth velocities at 52 weeks observed in the intent-to-treat population were 6.32 cm/year in the placebo group (n = 76), 6.07 cm/year in the 50-mcg group (n = 98), and 5.66 cm/year in the 100–mcg group (n = 89). An imbalance in the proportion of children entering puberty between groups and a higher dropout rate in the placebo group due to poorly controlled asthma may be confounding factors in interpreting these data. A separate subset analysis of children who remained prepubertal during the trial revealed growth rates at 52 weeks of 6.10 cm/year in the placebo group (n = 57), 5.91 cm/year in the 50–mcg group (n = 74), and 5.67 cm/year in the 100–mcg group (n = 79). In children aged 8.5 years, the mean age of children in this trial, the range for expected growth velocity is: boys – 3rd percentile = 3.8 cm/year, 50th percentile = 5.4 cm/year, and 97th percentile = 7.0 cm/year; girls – 3rd percentile = 4.2 cm/year, 50th percentile = 5.7 cm/year, and 97th percentile = 7.3 cm/year. The clinical relevance of these growth data is not certain.

If a child or adolescent on any corticosteroid appears to have growth suppression, the possibility that he/she is particularly sensitive to this effect of corticosteroids should be considered. The potential growth effects of prolonged treatment should be weighed against the clinical benefits obtained. To minimize the systemic effects of orally inhaled corticosteroids, including ADVAIR DISKUS, each patient should be titrated to the lowest strength that effectively controls his/her asthma *[see Dosage and Administration (2.1)]*.

8.5   Geriatric Use
Clinical trials of ADVAIR DISKUS for asthma did not include sufficient numbers of subjects aged 65 years and older to determine whether older subjects with asthma respond differently than younger subjects.

Of the total number of subjects in clinical trials receiving ADVAIR DISKUS for COPD, 1,621 were aged 65 years and older and 379 were aged 75 years and older. Subjects with COPD aged 65 years and older had a higher incidence of serious adverse events compared with subjects younger than 65 years. Although the distribution of adverse events was similar in the 2 age-groups, subjects older than 65 years experienced more severe events. In two 1-year trials, the excess risk of pneumonia that was seen in subjects treated with ADVAIR DISKUS compared with those treated with salmeterol was greater in subjects older than 65 years than in subjects younger than 65 years *[see Adverse Reactions (6.2)]*. As with other products containing beta$_2$-

agonists, special caution should be observed when using ADVAIR DISKUS in geriatric patients who have concomitant cardiovascular disease that could be adversely affected by beta$_2$-agonists. Based on available data for ADVAIR DISKUS or its active components, no adjustment of dosage of ADVAIR DISKUS in geriatric patients is warranted.

No relationship between fluticasone propionate systemic exposure and age was observed in 57 subjects with COPD (aged 40 to 82 years) given 250 or 500 mcg twice daily.

8.6   Hepatic Impairment
Formal pharmacokinetic studies using ADVAIR DISKUS have not been conducted in patients with hepatic impairment. However, since both fluticasone propionate and salmeterol are predominantly cleared by hepatic metabolism, impairment of liver function may lead to accumulation of fluticasone propionate and salmeterol in plasma. Therefore, patients with hepatic disease should be closely monitored.

8.7   Renal Impairment
Formal pharmacokinetic studies using ADVAIR DISKUS have not been conducted in patients with renal impairment.

10   OVERDOSAGE
No human overdosage data has been reported for ADVAIR DISKUS.

ADVAIR DISKUS contains both fluticasone propionate and salmeterol; therefore, the risks associated with overdosage for the individual components described below apply to ADVAIR DISKUS. Treatment of overdosage consists of discontinuation of ADVAIR DISKUS together with institution of appropriate symptomatic and/or supportive therapy. The judicious use of a cardioselective beta-receptor blocker may be considered, bearing in mind that such medication can produce bronchospasm. Cardiac monitoring is recommended in cases of overdosage.

10.1   Fluticasone Propionate
Chronic overdosage of fluticasone propionate may result in signs/symptoms of hypercorticism *[see Warnings and Precautions (5.7)]*. Inhalation by healthy volunteers of a single dose of 4,000 mcg of fluticasone propionate inhalation powder or single doses of 1,760 or 3,520 mcg of fluticasone propionate CFC inhalation aerosol was well tolerated. Fluticasone propionate given by inhalation aerosol at dosages of 1,320 mcg twice daily for 7 to 15 days to healthy human volunteers was also well tolerated. Repeat oral doses up to 80 mg daily for 10 days in healthy volunteers and repeat oral doses up to 20 mg daily for 42 days in subjects were well tolerated. Adverse reactions were of mild or moderate severity, and incidences were similar in active and placebo treatment groups.

10.2   Salmeterol
The expected signs and symptoms with overdosage of salmeterol are those of excessive beta–adrenergic stimulation and/or occurrence or exaggeration of any of the signs and symptoms of beta-adrenergic stimulation (e.g., seizures, angina, hypertension or hypotension, tachycardia with rates up to 200 beats/min, arrhythmias, nervousness, headache, tremor, muscle cramps, dry mouth, palpitation, nausea, dizziness, fatigue, malaise, insomnia, hyperglycemia, hypokalemia, metabolic acidosis). Overdosage with salmeterol can lead to clinically significant prolongation of the QTc interval, which can produce ventricular arrhythmias.

As with all inhaled sympathomimetic medicines, cardiac arrest and even death may be associated with an overdose of salmeterol.

11   DESCRIPTION
ADVAIR DISKUS 100/50, ADVAIR DISKUS 250/50, and ADVAIR DISKUS 500/50 are combinations of fluticasone propionate and salmeterol xinafoate.

One active component of ADVAIR DISKUS is fluticasone propionate, a corticosteroid having the chemical name *S*-(fluoromethyl) 6α,9-difluoro-11β,17-dihydroxy-16α-methyl-3-oxoandrosta-1,4-diene-17β-carbothioate, 17-propionate and the following chemical structure:

Fluticasone propionate is a white powder with a molecular weight of 500.6, and the empirical formula is $C_{25}H_{31}F_3O_5S$. It is practically insoluble in water, freely soluble in dimethyl sulfoxide and dimethylformamide, and slightly soluble in methanol and 95% ethanol.

The other active component of ADVAIR DISKUS is salmeterol xinafoate, a beta$_2$-adrenergic bronchodilator.

Salmeterol xinafoate is the racemic form of the 1-hydroxy-2-naphthoic acid salt of salmeterol. It has the chemical name 4-hydroxy-α^1-[[[6-(4-phenylbutoxy)hexyl]amino]methyl]-1,3-benzenedimethanol, 1-hydroxy-2-naphthalenecarboxylate and the following chemical structure:

Salmeterol xinafoate is a white powder with a molecular weight of 603.8, and the empirical formula is $C_{25}H_{37}NO_4 \bullet C_{11}H_8O_3$. It is freely soluble in methanol; slightly soluble in ethanol, chloroform, and isopropanol; and sparingly soluble in water.

ADVAIR DISKUS is a purple plastic inhaler containing a foil blister strip. Each blister on the strip contains a white powder mix of micronized fluticasone propionate (100, 250, or 500 mcg) and micronized salmeterol xinafoate (72.5 mcg, equivalent to 50 mcg of salmeterol base) in 12.5 mg of formulation containing lactose monohydrate (which contains milk proteins). After the inhaler is activated, the powder is dispersed into the airstream created by the patient inhaling through the mouthpiece.

Under standardized in vitro test conditions, ADVAIR DISKUS delivers 93, 233, and 465 mcg of fluticasone propionate and 45 mcg of salmeterol base per blister from ADVAIR DISKUS 100/50, ADVAIR DISKUS 250/50, and ADVAIR DISKUS 500/50, respectively, when tested at a flow rate of 60 L/min for 2 seconds.

In adult subjects with obstructive lung disease and severely compromised lung function (mean FEV_1 20% to 30% of predicted), mean peak inspiratory flow (PIF) through the DISKUS® inhaler was 82.4 L/min (range: 46.1 to 115.3 L/min).

Inhalation profiles for adolescent (N = 13, aged 12 to 17 years) and adult (N = 17, aged 18 to 50 years) subjects with asthma inhaling maximally through the DISKUS inhaler show mean PIF of 122.2 L/min (range: 81.6 to 152.1 L/min). Inhalation profiles for pediatric subjects with asthma inhaling maximally through the DISKUS inhaler show a mean PIF of 75.5 L/min (range: 49.0 to 104.8 L/min) for the 4–year–old subject set (N = 20) and 107.3 L/min (range: 82.8 to 125.6 L/min) for the 8–year–old subject set (N = 20). The actual amount of drug delivered to the lung will depend on patient factors, such as inspiratory flow profile.

12 CLINICAL PHARMACOLOGY

12.1 Mechanism of Action

ADVAIR DISKUS: ADVAIR DISKUS contains both fluticasone propionate and salmeterol. The mechanisms of action described below for the individual components apply to ADVAIR DISKUS. These drugs represent 2 different classes of medications (a synthetic corticosteroid and a LABA) that have different effects on clinical, physiologic, and inflammatory indices.

Fluticasone Propionate: Fluticasone propionate is a synthetic trifluorinated corticosteroid with anti–inflammatory activity. Fluticasone propionate has been shown in vitro to exhibit a binding affinity for the human glucocorticoid receptor that is 18 times that of dexamethasone, almost twice that of beclomethasone-17-monopropionate (BMP), the active metabolite of beclomethasone dipropionate, and over 3 times that of budesonide. Data from the McKenzie vasoconstrictor assay in man are consistent with these results. The clinical significance of these findings is unknown.

Inflammation is an important component in the pathogenesis of asthma. Corticosteroids have been shown to have a wide range of actions on multiple cell types (e.g., mast cells, eosinophils, neutrophils, macrophages, lymphocytes) and mediators (e.g., histamine, eicosanoids, leukotrienes, cytokines) involved in inflammation. These anti–inflammatory actions of corticosteroids contribute to their efficacy in asthma.

Inflammation is also a component in the pathogenesis of COPD. In contrast to asthma, however, the predominant inflammatory cells in COPD include neutrophils, CD8+ T-lymphocytes, and macrophages. The effects of corticosteroids in the treatment of COPD are not well defined and inhaled corticosteroids and fluticasone propionate when used apart from ADVAIR DISKUS are not indicated for the treatment of COPD.

Salmeterol Xinafoate: Salmeterol is a selective LABA. In vitro studies show salmeterol to be at least 50 times more selective for beta$_2$-adrenoceptors than albuterol. Although beta$_2$-adrenoceptors are the predominant adrenergic receptors in bronchial smooth muscle and beta$_1$-adrenoceptors are the predominant receptors in the heart, there are also beta$_2$-adrenoceptors in the human heart comprising 10% to 50% of the total beta-adrenoceptors. The precise function of these receptors has not been established, but their presence raises the possibility that even selective beta$_2$-agonists may have cardiac effects.

The pharmacologic effects of beta$_2$-adrenoceptor agonist drugs, including salmeterol, are at least in part attributable to stimulation of intracellular adenyl cyclase, the enzyme that catalyzes the conversion of adenosine triphosphate (ATP) to cyclic-3',5'-adenosine monophosphate (cyclic AMP). Increased cyclic AMP levels cause relaxation of bronchial smooth muscle and inhibition of release of mediators of immediate hypersensitivity from cells, especially from mast cells.

In vitro tests show that salmeterol is a potent and long-lasting inhibitor of the release of mast cell mediators, such as histamine, leukotrienes, and prostaglandin D$_2$, from human lung. Salmeterol inhibits histamine-induced plasma protein extravasation and inhibits platelet-activating factor-induced eosinophil accumulation in the lungs of guinea pigs when administered by the inhaled route. In humans, single doses of salmeterol administered via inhalation aerosol attenuate allergen-induced bronchial hyper-responsiveness.

12.2 Pharmacodynamics

ADVAIR DISKUS: *Healthy Subjects: Cardiovascular Effects:* Since systemic pharmacodynamic effects of salmeterol are not normally seen at the therapeutic dose, higher doses were used to produce measurable effects. Four (4) trials were conducted with healthy adult subjects: (1) a single–dose crossover trial using 2 inhalations of ADVAIR DISKUS 500/50, fluticasone propionate powder 500 mcg and salmeterol powder 50 mcg given concurrently, or fluticasone propionate powder 500 mcg given alone, (2) a cumulative dose trial using 50 to 400 mcg of salmeterol powder given alone or as ADVAIR DISKUS 500/50, (3) a repeat-dose trial for 11 days using 2 inhalations twice daily of ADVAIR DISKUS 250/50, fluticasone propionate powder 250 mcg, or salmeterol powder 50 mcg, and (4) a single-dose trial using 5 inhalations of ADVAIR DISKUS 100/50, fluticasone propionate powder 100 mcg alone, or placebo. In these trials no significant differences were observed in the pharmacodynamic effects of salmeterol (pulse rate, blood pressure, QTc interval, potassium, and glucose) whether the salmeterol was given as ADVAIR DISKUS, concurrently with fluticasone propionate from separate inhalers, or as salmeterol alone. The systemic pharmacodynamic effects of salmeterol were not altered by the presence of fluticasone propionate in ADVAIR DISKUS. The potential effect of salmeterol on the effects of fluticasone propionate on the HPA axis was also evaluated in these trials.

Hypothalamic-Pituitary-Adrenal Axis Effects: No significant differences across treatments were observed in 24–hour urinary cortisol excretion and, where measured, 24–hour plasma cortisol AUC. The systemic pharmacodynamic effects of fluticasone propionate were not altered by the presence of salmeterol in ADVAIR DISKUS in healthy subjects.

Subjects With Asthma: Adult and Adolescent Subjects: Cardiovascular Effects: In clinical trials with ADVAIR DISKUS in adult and adolescent subjects aged 12 years and older with asthma, no significant differences were observed in the systemic pharmacodynamic effects of salmeterol (pulse rate, blood pressure, QTc interval, potassium, and glucose) whether the salmeterol was given alone or as ADVAIR DISKUS. In 72 adult and adolescent subjects with asthma given either ADVAIR DISKUS 100/50 or ADVAIR DISKUS 250/50, continuous 24–hour electrocardiographic monitoring was performed after the first dose and after 12 weeks of therapy, and no clinically significant dysrhythmias were noted.

Hypothalamic-Pituitary-Adrenal Axis Effects: In a 28–week trial in adult and adolescent subjects with asthma, ADVAIR DISKUS 500/50 twice daily was compared with the concurrent use of salmeterol powder 50 mcg plus fluticasone propionate powder 500 mcg from separate inhalers or fluticasone propionate powder 500 mcg alone. No significant differences across treatments were observed in serum cortisol AUC after 12 weeks of dosing or in 24-hour urinary cortisol excretion after 12 and 28 weeks.

In a 12-week trial in adult and adolescent subjects with asthma, ADVAIR DISKUS 250/50 twice daily was compared with fluticasone propionate powder 250 mcg alone, salmeterol powder 50 mcg alone, and placebo. For most subjects, the ability to increase cortisol production in response to stress, as assessed by 30–minute cosyntropin stimulation, remained intact with ADVAIR DISKUS. One subject (3%) who received ADVAIR DISKUS 250/50 had an abnormal response (peak serum cortisol <18 mcg/dL) after dosing, compared with 2 subjects (6%) who received placebo, 2 subjects (6%) who received fluticasone propionate 250 mcg, and no subjects who received salmeterol.

In a repeat–dose, 3–way crossover trial, 1 inhalation twice daily of ADVAIR DISKUS 100/50, FLOVENT® DISKUS

100 mcg (fluticasone propionate inhalation powder, 100 mcg), or placebo was administered to 20 adult and adolescent subjects with asthma. After 28 days of treatment, geometric mean serum cortisol AUC over 12 hours showed no significant difference between ADVAIR DISKUS and FLOVENT DISKUS or between either active treatment and placebo.

Pediatric Subjects: Hypothalamic-Pituitary-Adrenal Axis Effects: In a 12–week trial in subjects with asthma aged 4 to 11 years who were receiving inhaled corticosteroids at trial entry, ADVAIR DISKUS 100/50 twice daily was compared with fluticasone propionate inhalation powder 100 mcg administered twice daily via the DISKUS. The values for 24-hour urinary cortisol excretion at trial entry and after 12 weeks of treatment were similar within each treatment group. After 12 weeks, 24–hour urinary cortisol excretion was also similar between the 2 groups.

Subjects With Chronic Obstructive Pulmonary Disease: Cardiovascular Effects: In clinical trials with ADVAIR DISKUS in subjects with COPD, no significant differences were seen in pulse rate, blood pressure, potassium, and glucose between ADVAIR DISKUS, the individual components of ADVAIR DISKUS, and placebo. In a trial of ADVAIR DISKUS 250/50, 8 subjects (2 [1.1%] in the group given ADVAIR DISKUS 250/50, 1 [0.5%] in the fluticasone propionate 250-mcg group, 3 [1.7%] in the salmeterol group, and 2 [1.1%] in the placebo group) had QTc intervals >470 msec at least 1 time during the treatment period. Five (5) of these 8 subjects had a prolonged QTc interval at baseline.

In a 24–week trial, 130 subjects with COPD received continuous 24–hour electrocardiographic monitoring prior to the first dose and after 4 weeks of twice–daily treatment with either ADVAIR DISKUS 500/50, fluticasone propionate powder 500 mcg, salmeterol powder 50 mcg, or placebo. No significant differences in ventricular or supraventricular arrhythmias and heart rate were observed among the groups treated with ADVAIR DISKUS 500/50, the individual components, or placebo. One (1) subject in the fluticasone propionate group experienced atrial flutter/atrial fibrillation, and 1 subject in the group given ADVAIR DISKUS 500/50 experienced heart block. There were 3 cases of nonsustained ventricular tachycardia (1 each in the placebo, salmeterol, and fluticasone propionate 500-mcg treatment groups).

In 24-week clinical trials in subjects with COPD, the incidence of clinically significant ECG abnormalities (myocardial ischemia, ventricular hypertrophy, clinically significant conduction abnormalities, clinically significant arrhythmias) was lower for subjects who received salmeterol (1%, 9 of 688 subjects who received either salmeterol 50 mcg or ADVAIR DISKUS) compared with placebo (3%, 10 of 370 subjects).

No significant differences with salmeterol 50 mcg alone or in combination with fluticasone propionate as ADVAIR DISKUS 500/50 were observed on pulse rate and systolic and diastolic blood pressure in a subset of subjects with COPD who underwent 12–hour serial vital sign measurements after the first dose (n = 183) and after 12 weeks of therapy (n = 149). Median changes from baseline in pulse rate and systolic and diastolic blood pressure were similar to those seen with placebo.

Hypothalamic-Pituitary-Adrenal Axis Effects: Short-cosyntropin stimulation testing was performed both at Day 1 and Endpoint in 101 subjects with COPD receiving twice-daily ADVAIR DISKUS 250/50, fluticasone propionate powder 250 mcg, salmeterol powder 50 mcg, or placebo. For most subjects, the ability to increase cortisol production in response to stress, as assessed by short cosyntropin stimulation, remained intact with ADVAIR DISKUS 250/50. One (1) subject (3%) who received ADVAIR DISKUS 250/50 had an abnormal stimulated cortisol response (peak cortisol <14.5 mcg/dL assessed by high–performance liquid chromatography) after dosing, compared with 2 subjects (9%) who received fluticasone propionate 250 mcg, 2 subjects (7%) who received salmeterol 50 mcg, and 1 subject (4%) who received placebo following 24 weeks of treatment or early discontinuation from trial.

After 36 weeks of dosing, serum cortisol concentrations in a subset of subjects with COPD (n = 83) were 22% lower in subjects receiving ADVAIR DISKUS 500/50 and 21% lower in subjects receiving fluticasone propionate 500 mcg than in subjects receiving placebo.

Other Fluticasone Propionate Products: Subjects With Asthma: Hypothalamic-Pituitary-Adrenal Axis Effects: In clinical trials with fluticasone propionate inhalation powder using dosages up to and including 250 mcg twice daily, occasional abnormal short cosyntropin tests (peak serum cortisol <18 mcg/dL assessed by radioimmunoassay) were noted both in subjects receiving fluticasone propionate and in subjects receiving placebo. The incidence of abnormal tests at 500 mcg twice daily was greater than placebo. In a 2–year trial carried out with the DISKHALER® inhalation device in 64 subjects with mild, persistent asthma (mean

FEV_1 91% of predicted) randomized to fluticasone propionate 500 mcg twice daily or placebo, no subject receiving fluticasone propionate had an abnormal response to 6-hour cosyntropin infusion (peak serum cortisol <18 mcg/dL). With a peak cortisol threshold of <35 mcg/dL, 1 subject receiving fluticasone propionate (4%) had an abnormal response at 1 year; repeat testing at 18 months and 2 years was normal. Another subject receiving fluticasone propionate (5%) had an abnormal response at 2 years. No subject on placebo had an abnormal response at 1 or 2 years.

Subjects With Chronic Obstructive Pulmonary Disease: Hypothalamic-Pituitary-Adrenal Axis Effects: After 4 weeks of dosing, the steady-state fluticasone propionate pharmacokinetics and serum cortisol levels were described in a subset of subjects with COPD (n = 86) randomized to twice-daily fluticasone propionate inhalation powder via the DISKUS 500 mcg, fluticasone propionate inhalation powder 250 mcg, or placebo. Serial serum cortisol concentrations were measured across a 12-hour dosing interval. Serum cortisol concentrations following 250- and 500-mcg twice-daily dosing were 10% and 21% lower than placebo, respectively, indicating a dose–dependent increase in systemic exposure to fluticasone propionate.

Other Salmeterol Xinafoate Products: *Subjects With Asthma: Cardiovascular Effects:* Inhaled salmeterol, like other beta-adrenergic agonist drugs, can produce dose-related cardiovascular effects and effects on blood glucose and/or serum potassium *[see Warnings and Precautions (5.12, 5.18)].* The cardiovascular effects (heart rate, blood pressure) associated with salmeterol inhalation occur with similar frequency, and are of similar type and severity, as those noted following albuterol administration.

The effects of rising inhaled doses of salmeterol and standard inhaled doses of albuterol were studied in volunteers and in subjects with asthma. Salmeterol doses up to 84 mcg administered as inhalation aerosol resulted in heart rate increases of 3 to 16 beats/min, about the same as albuterol dosed at 180 mcg by inhalation aerosol (4 to 10 beats/min). Adult and adolescent subjects receiving 50-mcg doses of salmeterol inhalation powder (N = 60) underwent continuous electrocardiographic monitoring during two 12-hour periods after the first dose and after 1 month of therapy, and no clinically significant dysrhythmias were noted.

Concomitant Use of ADVAIR DISKUS With Other Respiratory Medications: *Short-Acting Beta₂-Agonists:* In clinical trials in subjects with asthma, the mean daily need for albuterol by 166 adult and adolescent subjects aged 12 years and older using ADVAIR DISKUS was approximately 1.3 inhalations/day and ranged from 0 to 9 inhalations/day. Five percent (5%) of subjects using ADVAIR DISKUS in these trials averaged 6 or more inhalations per day over the course of the 12-week trials. No increase in frequency of cardiovascular adverse events was observed among subjects who averaged 6 or more inhalations per day.

In a clinical trial in subjects with COPD, the mean daily need for albuterol for subjects using ADVAIR DISKUS 250/50 was 4.1 inhalations/day. Twenty-six percent (26%) of subjects using ADVAIR DISKUS 250/50 averaged 6 or more inhalations of albuterol per day over the course of the 24-week trial. No increase in frequency of cardiovascular adverse reactions was observed among subjects who averaged 6 or more inhalations per day.

Methylxanthines: The concurrent use of intravenously or orally administered methylxanthines (e.g., aminophylline, theophylline) by adult and adolescent subjects aged 12 years and older receiving ADVAIR DISKUS has not been completely evaluated. In clinical trials in subjects with asthma, 39 subjects receiving ADVAIR DISKUS 100/50, ADVAIR DISKUS 250/50, or ADVAIR DISKUS 500/50 twice daily concurrently with a theophylline product had adverse event rates similar to those in 304 subjects receiving ADVAIR DISKUS without theophylline. Similar results were observed in subjects receiving salmeterol 50 mcg plus fluticasone propionate 500 mcg twice daily concurrently with a theophylline product (n = 39) or without theophylline (n = 132).

In a clinical trial in subjects with COPD, 17 subjects receiving ADVAIR DISKUS 250/50 twice daily concurrently with a theophylline product had adverse event rates similar to those in 161 subjects receiving ADVAIR DISKUS without theophylline. Based on the available data, the concomitant administration of methylxanthines with ADVAIR DISKUS did not alter the observed adverse event profile.

Fluticasone Propionate Nasal Spray: In adult and adolescent subjects aged 12 years and older taking ADVAIR DISKUS in clinical trials, no difference in the profile of adverse events or HPA axis effects was noted between subjects who were taking FLONASE® (fluticasone propionate) Nasal Spray, 50 mcg concurrently (n = 46) and those who were not (n = 130).

12.3 Pharmacokinetics

Absorption: *Fluticasone Propionate: Healthy Subjects:* Fluticasone propionate acts locally in the lung; therefore,

plasma levels do not predict therapeutic effect. Trials using oral dosing of labeled and unlabeled drug have demonstrated that the oral systemic bioavailability of fluticasone propionate is negligible (<1%), primarily due to incomplete absorption and presystemic metabolism in the gut and liver. In contrast, the majority of the fluticasone propionate delivered to the lung is systemically absorbed.

Following administration of ADVAIR DISKUS to healthy adult subjects, peak plasma concentrations of fluticasone propionate were achieved in 1 to 2 hours. In a single-dose crossover trial, a higher-than-recommended dose of ADVAIR DISKUS was administered to 14 healthy adult subjects. Two (2) inhalations of the following treatments were administered: ADVAIR DISKUS 500/50, fluticasone propionate powder 500 mcg and salmeterol powder 50 mcg given concurrently, and fluticasone propionate powder 500 mcg alone. Mean peak plasma concentrations of fluticasone propionate averaged 107, 94, and 120 pg/mL, respectively, indicating no significant changes in systemic exposures of fluticasone propionate.

In 15 healthy subjects, systemic exposure to fluticasone propionate from 4 inhalations of ADVAIR® HFA 230/21 (fluticasone propionate 230 mcg and salmeterol 21 mcg) Inhalation Aerosol (920/84 mcg) and 2 inhalations of ADVAIR DISKUS 500/50 (1,000/100 mcg) were similar between the 2 inhalers (i.e., 799 versus 832 pg•h/mL, respectively), but approximately half the systemic exposure from 4 inhalations of fluticasone propionate CFC inhalation aerosol 220 mcg (880 mcg, AUC = 1,543 pg•h/mL). Similar results were observed for peak fluticasone propionate plasma concentrations (186 and 182 pg/mL from ADVAIR HFA and ADVAIR DISKUS, respectively, and 307 pg/mL from the fluticasone propionate CFC inhalation aerosol). Absolute bioavailability of fluticasone propionate was 5.3% and 5.5% following administration of ADVAIR HFA and ADVAIR DISKUS, respectively.

Subjects With Asthma and COPD: Peak steady-state fluticasone propionate plasma concentrations in adult subjects with asthma (N = 11) ranged from undetectable to 266 pg/mL after a 500-mcg twice-daily dose of fluticasone propionate inhalation powder using the DISKUS inhaler. The mean fluticasone propionate plasma concentration was 110 pg/mL.

Full pharmacokinetic profiles were obtained from 9 female and 16 male subjects with asthma given fluticasone propionate inhalation powder 500 mcg twice daily using the DISKUS inhaler and from 14 female and 43 male subjects with COPD given 250 or 500 mcg twice daily. No overall differences in fluticasone propionate pharmacokinetics were observed.

Peak steady-state fluticasone propionate plasma concentrations in subjects with COPD averaged 53 pg/mL (range: 19.3 to 159.3 pg/mL) after treatment with 250 mcg twice daily (n = 30) and 84 pg/mL (range: 24.3 to 197.1 pg/mL) after treatment with 500 mcg twice daily (n = 27) via the fluticasone propionate DISKUS inhaler. In another trial in subjects with COPD, peak steady-state fluticasone propionate plasma concentrations averaged 115 pg/mL (range: 52.6 to 366.0 pg/mL) after treatment with 500 mcg twice daily via the fluticasone propionate DISKUS inhaler (n = 15) and 105 pg/mL (range: 22.5 to 299.0 pg/mL) via ADVAIR DISKUS (n = 24).

Salmeterol Xinafoate: Healthy Subjects: Salmeterol xinafoate, an ionic salt, dissociates in solution so that the salmeterol and 1-hydroxy-2-naphthoic acid (xinafoate) moieties are absorbed, distributed, metabolized, and eliminated independently. Salmeterol acts locally in the lung; therefore, plasma levels do not predict therapeutic effect.

Following administration of ADVAIR DISKUS to healthy adult subjects, peak plasma concentrations of salmeterol were achieved in about 5 minutes.

In 15 healthy subjects receiving ADVAIR HFA 230/21 Inhalation Aerosol (920/84 mcg) and ADVAIR DISKUS 500/50 (1,000/100 mcg), systemic exposure to salmeterol was higher (317 versus 169 pg•h/mL) and peak salmeterol concentrations were lower (196 versus 223 pg/mL) following ADVAIR HFA compared with ADVAIR DISKUS, although pharmacodynamic results were comparable.

Subjects With Asthma: Because of the small therapeutic dose, systemic levels of salmeterol are low or undetectable after inhalation of recommended doses (50 mcg of salmeterol inhalation powder twice daily). Following chronic administration of an inhaled dose of 50 mcg of salmeterol inhalation powder twice daily, salmeterol was detected in plasma within 5 to 45 minutes in 7 subjects with asthma; plasma concentrations were very low, with mean peak concentrations of 167 pg/mL at 20 minutes and no accumulation with repeated doses.

Distribution: *Fluticasone Propionate:* Following intravenous administration, the initial disposition phase for fluticasone propionate was rapid and consistent with its high lipid solubility and tissue binding. The volume of distribution averaged 4.2 L/kg.

The percentage of fluticasone propionate bound to human plasma proteins averages 99%. Fluticasone propionate is weakly and reversibly bound to erythrocytes and is not significantly bound to human transcortin.

Salmeterol: The percentage of salmeterol bound to human plasma proteins averages 96% in vitro over the concentration range of 8 to 7,722 ng of salmeterol base per milliliter, much higher concentrations than those achieved following therapeutic doses of salmeterol.

Metabolism: *Fluticasone Propionate:* The total clearance of fluticasone propionate is high (average, 1,093 mL/min), with renal clearance accounting for less than 0.02% of the total. The only circulating metabolite detected in man is the 17β-carboxylic acid derivative of fluticasone propionate, which is formed through the CYP3A4 pathway. This metabolite had less affinity (approximately 1/2,000) than the parent drug for the glucocorticoid receptor of human lung cytosol in vitro and negligible pharmacological activity in animal studies. Other metabolites detected in vitro using cultured human hepatoma cells have not been detected in man.

Salmeterol: Salmeterol base is extensively metabolized by hydroxylation, with subsequent elimination predominantly in the feces. No significant amount of unchanged salmeterol base was detected in either urine or feces.

An in vitro study using human liver microsomes showed that salmeterol is extensively metabolized to α-hydroxysalmeterol (aliphatic oxidation) by CYP3A4. Ketoconazole, a strong inhibitor of CYP3A4, essentially completely inhibited the formation of α-hydroxysalmeterol in vitro.

Elimination: *Fluticasone Propionate:* Following intravenous dosing, fluticasone propionate showed polyexponential kinetics and had a terminal elimination half-life of approximately 7.8 hours. Less than 5% of a radiolabeled oral dose was excreted in the urine as metabolites, with the remainder excreted in the feces as parent drug and metabolites. Terminal half-life estimates of fluticasone propionate for ADVAIR HFA, ADVAIR DISKUS, and fluticasone propionate CFC inhalation aerosol were similar and averaged 5.6 hours.

Salmeterol: In 2 healthy adult subjects who received 1 mg of radiolabeled salmeterol (as salmeterol xinafoate) orally, approximately 25% and 60% of the radiolabeled salmeterol was eliminated in urine and feces, respectively, over a period of 7 days. The terminal elimination half-life was about 5.5 hours (1 volunteer only).

The xinafoate moiety has no apparent pharmacologic activity. The xinafoate moiety is highly protein bound (greater than 99%) and has a long elimination half-life of 11 days. No terminal half-life estimates were calculated for salmeterol following administration of ADVAIR DISKUS.

Special Populations: A population pharmacokinetic analysis was performed for fluticasone propionate and salmeterol utilizing data from 9 controlled clinical trials that included 350 subjects with asthma aged 4 to 77 years who received treatment with ADVAIR DISKUS, the combination of HFA-propelled fluticasone propionate and salmeterol inhalation aerosol (ADVAIR HFA), fluticasone propionate inhalation powder (FLOVENT DISKUS), HFA-propelled fluticasone propionate inhalation aerosol (FLOVENT® HFA), or CFC-propelled fluticasone propionate inhalation aerosol. The population pharmacokinetic analyses for fluticasone propionate and salmeterol showed no clinically relevant effects of age, gender, race, body weight, body mass index, or percent of predicted FEV_1 on apparent clearance and apparent volume of distribution.

Age: When the population pharmacokinetic analysis for fluticasone propionate was divided into subgroups based on fluticasone propionate strength, formulation, and age (adolescents/adults and children), there were some differences in fluticasone propionate exposure. Higher fluticasone propionate exposure from ADVAIR DISKUS 100/50 compared with FLOVENT DISKUS 100 mcg was observed in adolescents and adults (ratio 1.52 [90% CI: 1.08, 2.13]). However, in clinical trials of up to 12 weeks' duration comparing ADVAIR DISKUS 100/50 and FLOVENT DISKUS 100 mcg in adolescents and adults, no differences in systemic effects of corticosteroid treatment (e.g., HPA axis effects) were observed. Similar fluticasone propionate exposure was observed from ADVAIR DISKUS 500/50 and FLOVENT DISKUS 500 mcg (ratio 0.83 [90% CI: 0.65, 1.07]) in adolescents and adults.

Steady-state systemic exposure to salmeterol when delivered as ADVAIR DISKUS 100/50, ADVAIR DISKUS 250/50, or ADVAIR HFA 115/21 (fluticasone propionate 115 mcg and salmeterol 21 mcg) Inhalation Aerosol was evaluated in 127 subjects aged 4 to 57 years. The geometric mean AUC was 325 pg•h/mL (90% CI: 309, 341) in adolescents and adults. The population pharmacokinetic analysis included 160 subjects with asthma aged 4 to 11 years who received ADVAIR DISKUS 100/50 or FLOVENT DISKUS 100 mcg. Higher fluticasone propionate exposure (AUC) was observed in children from ADVAIR DISKUS 100/50 compared with

FLOVENT DISKUS 100 mcg (ratio 1.20 [90% CI: 1.06, 1.37]). Higher fluticasone propionate exposure (AUC) from ADVAIR DISKUS 100/50 was observed in children compared with adolescents and adults (ratio 1.63 [90% CI: 1.35, 1.96]). However, in clinical trials of up to 12 weeks' duration comparing ADVAIR DISKUS 100/50 and FLOVENT DISKUS 100 mcg in both adolescents and adults and in children, no differences in systemic effects of corticosteroid treatment (e.g., HPA axis effects) were observed.

Exposure to salmeterol was higher in children compared with adolescents and adults who received ADVAIR DISKUS 100/50 (ratio 1.23 [90% CI: 1.10, 1.38]). However, in clinical trials of up to 12 weeks' duration with ADVAIR DISKUS 100/50 in both adolescents and adults and in children, no differences in systemic effects of beta$_2$-agonist treatment (e.g., cardiovascular effects, tremor) were observed.

Gender: The population pharmacokinetic analysis involved 202 males and 148 females with asthma who received fluticasone propionate alone or in combination with salmeterol and showed no gender differences for fluticasone propionate pharmacokinetics.

The population pharmacokinetic analysis involved 76 males and 51 females with asthma who received salmeterol in combination with fluticasone propionate and showed no gender differences for salmeterol pharmacokinetics.

Hepatic and Renal Impairment: Formal pharmacokinetic studies using ADVAIR DISKUS have not been conducted in patients with hepatic or renal impairment. However, since both fluticasone propionate and salmeterol are predominantly cleared by hepatic metabolism, impairment of liver function may lead to accumulation of fluticasone propionate and salmeterol in plasma. Therefore, patients with hepatic disease should be closely monitored.

Drug Interactions: In the repeat- and single–dose trials, there was no evidence of significant drug interaction in systemic exposure between fluticasone propionate and salmeterol when given alone or in combination via the DISKUS. The population pharmacokinetic analysis from 9 controlled clinical trials in 350 subjects with asthma showed no significant effects on fluticasone propionate or salmeterol pharmacokinetics following co–administration with beta$_2$-agonists, corticosteroids, antihistamines, or theophyllines.

Inhibitors of Cytochrome P450 3A4: Ritonavir: Fluticasone Propionate: Fluticasone propionate is a substrate of CYP3A4. Coadministration of fluticasone propionate and the strong CYP3A4 inhibitor ritonavir is not recommended based upon a multiple-dose, crossover drug interaction trial in 18 healthy subjects. Fluticasone propionate aqueous nasal spray (200 mcg once daily) was coadministered for 7 days with ritonavir (100 mg twice daily). Plasma fluticasone propionate concentrations following fluticasone propionate aqueous nasal spray alone were undetectable (<10 pg/mL) in most subjects, and when concentrations were detectable peak levels (C_{max}) averaged 11.9 pg/mL (range: 10.8 to 14.1 pg/mL) and $AUC_{(0-\tau)}$ averaged 8.43 pg•h/mL (range: 4.2 to 18.8 pg•h/mL). Fluticasone propionate C_{max} and $AUC_{(0-\tau)}$ increased to 318 pg/mL (range: 110 to 648 pg/mL) and 3,102.6 pg•h/mL (range: 1,207.1 to 5,662.0 pg•h/mL), respectively, after coadministration of ritonavir with fluticasone propionate aqueous nasal spray. This significant increase in plasma fluticasone propionate exposure resulted in a significant decrease (86%) in serum cortisol AUC.

Ketoconazole: Fluticasone Propionate: In a placebo-controlled, crossover trial in 8 healthy adult volunteers, coadministration of a single dose of orally inhaled fluticasone propionate (1,000 mcg) with multiple doses of ketoconazole (200 mg) to steady state resulted in increased plasma fluticasone propionate exposure, a reduction in plasma cortisol AUC, and no effect on urinary excretion of cortisol.

Salmeterol: In a placebo-controlled, crossover drug interaction trial in 20 healthy male and female subjects, coadministration of salmeterol (50 mcg twice daily) and the strong CYP3A4 inhibitor ketoconazole (400 mg once daily) for 7 days resulted in a significant increase in plasma salmeterol exposure as determined by a 16-fold increase in AUC (ratio with and without ketoconazole 15.76 [90% CI: 10.66, 23.31]) mainly due to increased bioavailability of the swallowed portion of the dose. Peak plasma salmeterol concentrations were increased by 1.4-fold (90% CI: 1.23, 1.68). Three (3) out of 20 subjects (15%) were withdrawn from salmeterol and ketoconazole coadministration due to beta-agonist–mediated systemic effects (2 with QTc prolongation and 1 with palpitations and sinus tachycardia). Coadministration of salmeterol and ketoconazole did not result in a clinically significant effect on mean heart rate, mean blood potassium, or mean blood glucose. Although there was no statistical effect on the mean QTc, coadministration of salmeterol and ketoconazole was associated with more frequent increases in QTc duration compared with salmeterol and placebo administration.

Erythromycin: Fluticasone Propionate: In a multiple-dose drug interaction trial, coadministration of orally inhaled fluticasone propionate (500 mcg twice daily) and erythromycin (333 mg 3 times daily) did not affect fluticasone propionate pharmacokinetics.

Salmeterol: In a repeat-dose trial in 13 healthy subjects, concomitant administration of erythromycin (a moderate CYP3A4 inhibitor) and salmeterol inhalation aerosol resulted in a 40% increase in salmeterol C_{max} at steady state (ratio with and without erythromycin 1.4 [90% CI: 0.96, 2.03], $P = 0.12$), a 3.6-beat/min increase in heart rate ([95% CI: 0.19, 7.03], $P<0.04$), a 5.8-msec increase in QTc interval ([95% CI: -6.14, 17.77], $P = 0.34$), and no change in plasma potassium.

13 NONCLINICAL TOXICOLOGY

13.1 Carcinogenesis, Mutagenesis, Impairment of Fertility

Fluticasone Propionate: Fluticasone propionate demonstrated no tumorigenic potential in mice at oral doses up to 1,000 mcg/kg (approximately 4 and 10 times the MRHDID for adults and children, respectively, on a mg/m² basis) for 78 weeks or in rats at inhalation doses up to 57 mcg/kg (less than and approximately equivalent to the MRHDID for adults and children, respectively, on a mg/m² basis) for 104 weeks.

Fluticasone propionate did not induce gene mutation in prokaryotic or eukaryotic cells in vitro. No significant clastogenic effect was seen in cultured human peripheral lymphocytes in vitro or in the in vivo mouse micronucleus test.

No evidence of impairment of fertility was observed in rats at subcutaneous doses up to 50 mcg/kg (less than the MRHDID on a mg/m² basis). Prostate weight was significantly reduced.

Salmeterol: In an 18-month carcinogenicity study in CD-mice, salmeterol at oral doses of 1.4 mg/kg and above (approximately 20 times the MRHDID for adults and children based on comparison of the plasma AUCs) caused a dose-related increase in the incidence of smooth muscle hyperplasia, cystic glandular hyperplasia, leiomyomas of the uterus, and ovarian cysts. No tumors were seen at 0.2 mg/kg (approximately 3 times the MRHDID for adults and children based on comparison of the AUCs).

In a 24–month oral and inhalation carcinogenicity study in Sprague Dawley rats, salmeterol caused a dose–related increase in the incidence of mesovarian leiomyomas and ovarian cysts at doses of 0.68 mg/kg and above (approximately 55 and 25 times the MRHDID for adults and children, respectively, on a mg/m² basis). No tumors were seen at 0.21 mg/kg (approximately 15 and 8 times the MRHDID for adults and children, respectively, on a mg/m² basis). These findings in rodents are similar to those reported previously for other beta–adrenergic agonist drugs. The relevance of these findings to human use is unknown.

Salmeterol produced no detectable or reproducible increases in microbial and mammalian gene mutation in vitro. No clastogenic activity occurred in vitro in human lymphocytes or in vivo in a rat micronucleus test. No effects on fertility were identified in rats treated with salmeterol at oral doses up to 2 mg/kg (approximately 160 times the MRHDID for adults on a mg/m² basis).

13.2 Animal Toxicology and/or Pharmacology

Preclinical: Studies in laboratory animals (minipigs, rodents, and dogs) have demonstrated the occurrence of cardiac arrhythmias and sudden death (with histologic evidence of myocardial necrosis) when beta-agonists and methylxanthines are administered concurrently. The clinical relevance of these findings is unknown.

14 CLINICAL STUDIES

14.1 Asthma

Adult and Adolescent Subjects Aged 12 Years and Older: In clinical trials comparing ADVAIR DISKUS with its individual components, improvements in most efficacy endpoints were greater with ADVAIR DISKUS than with the use of either fluticasone propionate or salmeterol alone. In addition, clinical trials showed similar results between ADVAIR DISKUS and the concurrent use of fluticasone propionate plus salmeterol at corresponding doses from separate inhalers.

Trials Comparing ADVAIR DISKUS With Fluticasone Propionate Alone or Salmeterol Alone: Three (3) double-blind, parallel–group clinical trials were conducted with ADVAIR DISKUS in 1,208 adult and adolescent subjects (aged 12 years and older) with asthma that was not optimally controlled on their current therapy. All treatments were inhalation powders given as 1 inhalation from the DISKUS inhaler twice daily, and other maintenance therapies were discontinued.

Trial 1: Clinical Trial With ADVAIR DISKUS 100/50: This placebo–controlled, 12–week, US trial compared ADVAIR DISKUS 100/50 with its individual components, fluticasone propionate 100 mcg and salmeterol 50 mcg. The trial was stratified according to baseline asthma maintenance therapy; subjects were using either inhaled corticosteroids (n = 250) (daily doses of beclomethasone

dipropionate 252 to 420 mcg; flunisolide 1,000 mcg; fluticasone propionate inhalation aerosol 176 mcg; or triamcinolone acetonide 600 to 1,000 mcg) or salmeterol (n = 106). Baseline FEV_1 measurements were similar across treatments: ADVAIR DISKUS 100/50, 2.17 L; fluticasone propionate 100 mcg, 2.11 L; salmeterol, 2.13 L; and placebo, 2.15 L.

Predefined withdrawal criteria for lack of efficacy, an indicator of worsening asthma, were utilized for this placebo-controlled trial. Worsening asthma was defined as a clinically important decrease in FEV_1 or PEF, increase in use of VENTOLIN® (albuterol, USP) Inhalation Aerosol, increase in night awakenings due to asthma, emergency intervention or hospitalization due to asthma, or requirement for asthma medication not allowed by the protocol. As shown in Table 4, statistically significantly fewer subjects receiving ADVAIR DISKUS 100/50 were withdrawn due to worsening asthma compared with fluticasone propionate, salmeterol, and placebo.

Table 4. Percent of Subjects Withdrawn Due to Worsening Asthma in Subjects Previously Treated With Either Inhaled Corticosteroids or Salmeterol (Trial 1)

ADVAIR DISKUS 100/50 (n = 87)	Fluticasone Propionate 100 mcg (n = 85)	Salmeterol 50 mcg (n = 86)	Placebo (n = 77)
3%	11%	35%	49%

The FEV_1 results are displayed in Figure 2. Because this trial used predetermined criteria for worsening asthma, which caused more subjects in the placebo group to be withdrawn, FEV_1 results at Endpoint (last available FEV_1 result) are also provided. Subjects receiving ADVAIR DISKUS 100/50 had significantly greater improvements in FEV_1 (0.51 L, 25%) compared with fluticasone propionate 100 mcg (0.28 L, 15%), salmeterol (0.11 L, 5%), and placebo (0.01 L, 1%). These improvements in FEV_1 with ADVAIR DISKUS were achieved regardless of baseline asthma maintenance therapy (inhaled corticosteroids or salmeterol).

Figure 2. Mean Percent Change From Baseline in FEV_1 in Subjects With Asthma Previously Treated With Either Inhaled Corticosteroids or Salmeterol (Trial 1)

Week	0	1	2	3	4	5	6	7	8	9	10	11	12	Endpoint
ADVAIR DISKUS 100/50	87					79							73	86
Fluticasone propionate 100 mcg	85					71							65	85
Salmeterol 50 mcg	86					59							51	86
Placebo	77					34							27	74

The effect of ADVAIR DISKUS 100/50 on morning and evening PEF endpoints is shown in Table 5.
[See table 5 at top of next page]

The subjective impact of asthma on subjects' perception of health was evaluated through use of an instrument called the Asthma Quality of Life Questionnaire (AQLQ) (based on a 7-point scale where 1 = maximum impairment and 7 = none). Subjects receiving ADVAIR DISKUS 100/50 had clinically meaningful improvements in overall asthma-specific quality of life as defined by a difference between groups of ≥0.5 points in change from baseline AQLQ scores (difference in AQLQ score of 1.25 compared with placebo).

Trial 2: Clinical Trial With ADVAIR DISKUS 250/50: This placebo-controlled, 12-week, US trial compared ADVAIR DISKUS 250/50 with its individual components, fluticasone propionate 250 mcg and salmeterol 50 mcg, in 349 subjects with asthma using inhaled corticosteroids (daily doses of beclomethasone dipropionate 462 to 672 mcg; flunisolide 1,250 to 2,000 mcg; fluticasone propionate inhalation aerosol 440 mcg; or triamcinolone acetonide 1,100 to 1,600 mcg). Baseline FEV_1 measurements were similar across treatments: ADVAIR DISKUS 250/50, 2.23 L; fluticasone propionate 250 mcg, 2.12 L; salmeterol, 2.20 L; and placebo, 2.19 L.

Efficacy results in this trial were similar to those observed in Trial 1. Subjects receiving ADVAIR DISKUS 250/50 had significantly greater improvements in FEV_1 (0.48 L, 23%) compared with fluticasone propionate 250 mcg (0.25 L,

13%), salmeterol (0.05 L, 4%), and placebo (decrease of 0.11 L, decrease of 5%). Statistically significantly fewer subjects receiving ADVAIR DISKUS 250/50 were withdrawn from this trial for worsening asthma (4%) compared with fluticasone propionate (22%), salmeterol (38%), and placebo (62%). In addition, ADVAIR DISKUS 250/50 was superior to fluticasone propionate, salmeterol, and placebo for improvements in morning and evening PEF. Subjects receiving ADVAIR DISKUS 250/50 also had clinically meaningful improvements in overall asthma–specific quality of life as described in Trial 1 (difference in AQLQ score of 1.29 compared with placebo).

Trial 3: Clinical Trial With ADVAIR DISKUS 500/50: This 28-week, non–US trial compared ADVAIR DISKUS 500/50 with fluticasone propionate 500 mcg alone and concurrent therapy (salmeterol 50 mcg plus fluticasone propionate 500 mcg administered from separate inhalers) twice daily in 503 subjects with asthma using inhaled corticosteroids (daily doses of beclomethasone dipropionate 1,260 to 1,680 mcg; budesonide 1,500 to 2,000 mcg; flunisolide 1,500 to 2,000 mcg; or fluticasone propionate inhalation aerosol 660 to 880 mcg [750 to 1,000 mcg inhalation powder]). The primary efficacy parameter, morning PEF, was collected daily for the first 12 weeks of the trial. The primary purpose of weeks 13 to 28 was to collect safety data. Baseline PEF measurements were similar across treatments: ADVAIR DISKUS 500/50, 359 L/min; fluticasone propionate 500 mcg, 351 L/min; and concurrent therapy, 345 L/min. Morning PEF improved significantly with ADVAIR DISKUS 500/50 compared with fluticasone propionate 500 mcg over the 12–week treatment period. Improvements in morning PEF observed with ADVAIR DISKUS 500/50 were similar to improvements observed with concurrent therapy.

Onset of Action and Progression of Improvement in Asthma Control: The onset of action and progression of improvement in asthma control were evaluated in the 2 placebo–controlled US trials. Following the first dose, the median time to onset of clinically significant bronchodilatation ($\geq$15% improvement in FEV_1) in most subjects was seen within 30 to 60 minutes. Maximum improvement in FEV_1 generally occurred within 3 hours, and clinically significant improvement was maintained for 12 hours (see Figure 3). Following the initial dose, predose FEV_1 relative to Day 1 baseline improved markedly over the first week of treatment and continued to improve over the 12 weeks of treatment in both trials. No diminution in the 12–hour bronchodilator effect was observed with either ADVAIR DISKUS 100/50 (Figures 3 and 4) or ADVAIR DISKUS 250/50 as assessed by FEV_1 following 12 weeks of therapy.

Figure 3. Percent Change in Serial 12-hour FEV_1 in Subjects With Asthma Previously Using Either Inhaled Corticosteroids or Salmeterol (Trial 1)

First Treatment Day

[See figure 4 at top of next column]

Reduction in asthma symptoms and use of rescue VENTOLIN Inhalation Aerosol and improvement in morning and evening PEF also occurred within the first day of treatment with ADVAIR DISKUS, and continued to improve over the 12 weeks of therapy in both trials.

Pediatric Subjects: In a 12-week US trial, ADVAIR DISKUS 100/50 twice daily was compared with fluticasone propionate inhalation powder 100 mcg twice daily in 203 children with asthma aged 4 to 11 years. At trial entry, the

Table 5. Peak Expiratory Flow Results for Subjects With Asthma Previously Treated With Either Inhaled Corticosteroids or Salmeterol (Trial 1)

Efficacy Variable[a]	ADVAIR DISKUS 100/50 (n = 87)	Fluticasone Propionate 100 mcg (n = 85)	Salmeterol 50 mcg (n = 86)	Placebo (n = 77)
AM PEF (L/min)				
Baseline	393	374	369	382
Change from baseline	53	17	-2	-24
PM PEF (L/min)				
Baseline	418	390	396	398
Change from baseline	35	18	-7	-13

[a]Change from baseline = change from baseline at Endpoint (last available data).

Figure 4. Percent Change in Serial 12-hour FEV_1 in Subjects With Asthma Previously Using Either Inhaled Corticosteroids or Salmeterol (Trial 1)

Last Treatment Day (Week 12)

children were symptomatic on low doses of inhaled corticosteroids (beclomethasone dipropionate 252 to 336 mcg/day; budesonide 200 to 400 mcg/day; flunisolide 1,000 mcg/day; triamcinolone acetonide 600 to 1,000 mcg/day; or fluticasone propionate 88 to 250 mcg/day). The primary objective of this trial was to determine the safety of ADVAIR DISKUS 100/50 compared with fluticasone propionate inhalation powder 100 mcg in this age-group; however, the trial also included secondary efficacy measures of pulmonary function. Morning predose FEV_1 was obtained at baseline and Endpoint (last available FEV_1 result) in children aged 6 to 11 years. In subjects receiving ADVAIR DISKUS 100/50, FEV_1 increased from 1.70 L at baseline (n = 79) to 1.88 L at Endpoint (n = 69) compared with an increase from 1.65 L at baseline (n = 83) to 1.77 L at Endpoint (n = 75) in subjects receiving fluticasone propionate 100 mcg.

The findings of this trial, along with extrapolation of efficacy data from subjects aged 12 years and older, support the overall conclusion that ADVAIR DISKUS 100/50 is efficacious in the treatment of asthma in subjects aged 4 to 11 years.

14.2   Chronic Obstructive Pulmonary Disease

The efficacy of ADVAIR DISKUS 250/50 and ADVAIR DISKUS 500/50 in the treatment of subjects with COPD was evaluated in 6 randomized, double-blind, parallel–group clinical trials in adult subjects aged 40 years and older. These trials were primarily designed to evaluate the efficacy of ADVAIR DISKUS on lung function (3 trials), exacerbations (2 trials), and survival (1 trial).

Lung Function: Two of the 3 clinical trials primarily designed to evaluate the efficacy of ADVAIR DISKUS on lung function were conducted in 1,414 subjects with COPD associated with chronic bronchitis. In these 2 trials, all the subjects had a history of cough productive of sputum that was not attributable to another disease process on most days for at least 3 months of the year for at least 2 years. The trials were randomized, double-blind, parallel-group, 24-week treatment duration. One trial evaluated the efficacy of ADVAIR DISKUS 250/50 compared with its components fluticasone propionate 250 mcg and salmeterol 50 mcg and with placebo, and the other trial evaluated the efficacy of ADVAIR DISKUS 500/50 compared with its components fluticasone propionate 500 mcg and salmeterol 50 mcg and with placebo. Trial treatments were inhalation powders

given as 1 inhalation from the DISKUS inhaler twice daily. Maintenance COPD therapies were discontinued, with the exception of theophylline. The subjects had a mean prebronchodilator FEV_1 of 41% and 20% reversibility at trial entry. Percent reversibility was calculated as 100 times (FEV_1 post-albuterol minus FEV_1 pre-albuterol)/FEV_1 pre-albuterol.

Improvements in lung function (as defined by predose and postdose FEV_1) were significantly greater with ADVAIR DISKUS than with fluticasone propionate, salmeterol, or placebo. The improvement in lung function with ADVAIR DISKUS 500/50 was similar to the improvement seen with ADVAIR DISKUS 250/50.

Figures 5 and 6 display predose and 2-hour postdose, respectively, FEV_1 results for the trial with ADVAIR DISKUS 250/50. To account for subject withdrawals during the trial, FEV_1 at Endpoint (last evaluable FEV_1) was evaluated. Subjects receiving ADVAIR DISKUS 250/50 had significantly greater improvements in predose FEV_1 at Endpoint (165 mL, 17%) compared with salmeterol 50 mcg (91 mL, 9%) and placebo (1 mL, 1%), demonstrating the contribution of fluticasone propionate to the improvement in lung function with ADVAIR DISKUS (Figure 5). Subjects receiving ADVAIR DISKUS 250/50 had significantly greater improvements in postdose FEV_1 at Endpoint (281 mL, 27% compared with fluticasone propionate 250 mcg (147 mL, 14%) and placebo (58 mL, 6%), demonstrating the contribution of salmeterol to the improvement in lung function with ADVAIR DISKUS (Figure 6).

Figure 5. Predose FEV_1: Mean Percent Change From Baseline in Subjects With Chronic Obstructive Pulmonary Disease

Figure 6. Two-Hour Postdose FEV_1: Mean Percent Changes From Baseline Over Time in Subjects With Chronic Obstructive Pulmonary Disease

The third trial was a 1-year trial that evaluated ADVAIR DISKUS 500/50, fluticasone propionate 500 mcg, salmeterol 50 mcg, and placebo in 1,465 subjects. The subjects had an established history of COPD and exacerbations, a pre-bronchodilator FEV_1 <70% of predicted at trial entry, and 8.3% reversibility. The primary endpoint was the comparison of pre-bronchodilator FEV_1 in the groups receiving ADVAIR DISKUS 500/50 or placebo. Subjects treated with ADVAIR DISKUS 500/50 had greater improvements in FEV_1 (113 mL, 10%) compared with fluticasone propionate 500 mcg (7 mL, 2%), salmeterol (15 mL, 2%), and placebo (-60 mL, -3%).

Exacerbations: Two trials were primarily designed to evaluate the effect of ADVAIR DISKUS 250/50 on exacerbations. In these 2 trials, exacerbations were defined as worsening of 2 or more major symptoms (dyspnea, sputum volume, and sputum purulence) or worsening of any 1 major symptom together with any 1 of the following minor symptoms: sore throat, colds (nasal discharge and/or nasal congestion), fever without other cause, and increased cough or wheeze for at least 2 consecutive days. COPD exacerbations were considered of moderate severity if treatment with systemic corticosteroids and/or antibiotics was required and were considered severe if hospitalization was required.

Exacerbations were also evaluated as a secondary outcome in the 1- and 3-year trials with ADVAIR DISKUS 500/50. There was not a symptomatic definition of exacerbation in these 2 trials. Exacerbations were defined in terms of severity requiring treatment with antibiotics and/or systemic corticosteroids (moderately severe) or requiring hospitalization (severe).

The 2 exacerbation trials with ADVAIR DISKUS 250/50 were identical trials designed to evaluate the effect of ADVAIR DISKUS 250/50 and salmeterol 50 mcg, each given twice daily, on exacerbations of COPD over a 12-month period. A total of 1,579 subjects had an established history of COPD (but no other significant respiratory disorders). Subjects had a pre-bronchodilator FEV_1 of 33% of predicted, a mean reversibility of 23% at baseline, and a history of ≥1 COPD exacerbation in the previous year that was moderate or severe. All subjects were treated with ADVAIR DISKUS 250/50 twice daily during a 4-week run-in period prior to being assigned trial treatment with twice-daily ADVAIR DISKUS 250/50 or salmeterol 50 mcg. In both trials, treatment with ADVAIR DISKUS 250/50 resulted in a significantly lower annual rate of moderate/severe COPD exacerbations compared with salmeterol (30.5% reduction [95% CI: 17.0, 41.8], P<0.001) in the first trial and (30.4% reduction [95% CI: 16.9, 41.7], P<0.001) in the second trial. Subjects treated with ADVAIR DISKUS 250/50 also had a significantly lower annual rate of exacerbations requiring treatment with oral corticosteroids compared with subjects treated with salmeterol (39.7% reduction [95% CI: 22.8, 52.9], P<0.001) in the first trial and (34.3% reduction [95% CI: 18.6, 47.0], P<0.001) in the second trial. Secondary endpoints including pulmonary function and symptom scores improved more in subjects treated with ADVAIR DISKUS 250/50 than with salmeterol 50 mcg in both trials.

Exacerbations were evaluated in the 1- and 3-year trials with ADVAIR DISKUS 500/50 as 1 of the secondary efficacy endpoints. In the 1-year trial, the group receiving ADVAIR DISKUS 500/50 had a significantly lower rate of moderate and severe exacerbations compared with placebo (25.4% reduction compared with placebo [95% CI: 13.5, 35.7]) but not when compared with its components (7.5% reduction compared with fluticasone propionate [95% CI: -7.3, 20.3] and 7% reduction compared with salmeterol [95% CI: -8.0, 19.9]). In the 3-year trial, the group receiving ADVAIR DISKUS 500/50 had a significantly lower rate of moderate and severe exacerbations compared with each of the other treatment groups (25.1% reduction compared with placebo [95% CI: 18.6, 31.1], 9.0% reduction compared with fluticasone propionate [95% CI: 1.2, 16.2], and 12.2% reduction compared with salmeterol [95% CI: 4.6, 19.2]).

There were no trials conducted to directly compare the efficacy of ADVAIR DISKUS 250/50 with ADVAIR DISKUS 500/50 on exacerbations. Across trials, the reduction in exacerbations seen with ADVAIR DISKUS 500/50 was not greater than the reduction in exacerbations seen with ADVAIR DISKUS 250/50.

Survival: A 3-year multicenter, international trial evaluated the efficacy of ADVAIR DISKUS 500/50 compared with fluticasone propionate 500 mcg, salmeterol 50 mcg, and placebo on survival in 6,112 subjects with COPD. During the trial subjects were permitted usual COPD therapy with the exception of other inhaled corticosteroids and long–acting bronchodilators. The subjects were aged 40 to 80 years with an established history of COPD, a pre-bronchodilator FEV_1 <60% of predicted at trial entry, and <10% of predicted reversibility. Each subject who withdrew from double–blind treatment for any reason was followed for the full 3-year trial period to determine survival status. The primary efficacy endpoint was all-cause mortality. Survival with ADVAIR DISKUS 500/50 was not significantly improved compared with placebo or the individual components (all-cause mortality rate 12.6% ADVAIR DISKUS versus 15.2% placebo). The rates for all-cause mortality were 13.5% and 16.0% in the groups treated with salmeterol

50 mcg and fluticasone propionate 500 mcg, respectively. Secondary outcomes, including pulmonary function (post-bronchodilator FEV_1), improved with ADVAIR DISKUS 500/50, salmeterol 50 mcg, and fluticasone propionate 500 mcg compared with placebo.

16   HOW SUPPLIED/STORAGE AND HANDLING

ADVAIR DISKUS 100/50 is supplied as a disposable purple plastic inhaler containing a foil blister strip with 60 blisters. The inhaler is packaged in a plastic-coated, moisture-protective foil pouch (NDC 0173-0695-00). ADVAIR DISKUS 100/50 is also supplied in an institutional pack containing 14 blisters (NDC 0173-0695-04).

ADVAIR DISKUS 250/50 is supplied as a disposable purple plastic inhaler containing a foil blister strip with 60 blisters. The inhaler is packaged in a plastic-coated, moisture-protective foil pouch (NDC 0173-0696-00). ADVAIR DISKUS 250/50 is also supplied in an institutional pack containing 14 blisters (NDC 0173-0696-04).

ADVAIR DISKUS 500/50 is supplied as a disposable purple plastic inhaler containing a foil blister strip with 60 blisters. The inhaler is packaged in a plastic-coated, moisture-protective foil pouch (NDC 0173-0697-00). ADVAIR DISKUS 500/50 is also supplied in an institutional pack containing 14 blisters (NDC 0173-0697-04).

Store at room temperature between 68°F and 77°F (20°C and 25°C); excursions permitted from 59°F to 86°F (15°C to 30°C) [See USP Controlled Room Temperature]. Store in a dry place away from direct heat or sunlight. Keep out of reach of children.

ADVAIR DISKUS should be stored inside the unopened moisture-protective foil pouch and only removed from the pouch immediately before initial use. Discard ADVAIR DISKUS 1 month after opening the foil pouch or when the counter reads "0" (after all blisters have been used), whichever comes first. The inhaler is not reusable. Do not attempt to take the inhaler apart.

17   PATIENT COUNSELING INFORMATION

Advise the patient to read the FDA-approved patient labeling (Medication Guide and Instructions for Use).

Asthma-Related Death: **Inform patients with asthma that salmeterol, one of the active ingredients in ADVAIR DISKUS, increases the risk of asthma-related death and may increase the risk of asthma-related hospitalization in pediatric and adolescent patients.Also inform them that currently available data are inadequate to determine whether concurrent use of inhaled corticosteroids or other long-term asthma control drugs mitigates the increased risk of asthma-related death from LABA.**

Not for Acute Symptoms: Inform patients that ADVAIR DISKUS is not meant to relieve acute asthma symptoms or exacerbations of COPD and extra doses should not be used for that purpose. Advise patients to treat acute symptoms with an inhaled, short-acting beta$_2$-agonist such as albuterol. Provide patients with such medication and instruct them in how it should be used.

Instruct patients to seek medical attention immediately if they experience any of the following:

- Decreasing effectiveness of inhaled, short-acting beta$_2$-agonists
- Need for more inhalations than usual of inhaled, short-acting beta$_2$-agonists
- Significant decrease in lung function as outlined by the physician

Tell patients they should not stop therapy with ADVAIR DISKUS without physician/provider guidance since symptoms may recur after discontinuation.

Do Not Use Additional Long-Acting Beta$_2$-Agonists: Instruct patients not to use other LABA for asthma and COPD.

Local Effects: Inform patients that localized infections with *Candida albicans* occurred in the mouth and pharynx in some patients. If oropharyngeal candidiasis develops, treat it with appropriate local or systemic (i.e., oral) antifungal therapy while still continuing therapy with ADVAIR DISKUS, but at times therapy with ADVAIR DISKUS may need to be temporarily interrupted under close medical supervision. Rinsing the mouth with water without swallowing after inhalation is advised to help reduce the risk of thrush.

Pneumonia: Patients with COPD have a higher risk of pneumonia; instruct them to contact their healthcare provider if they develop symptoms of pneumonia.

Immunosuppression: Warn patients who are on immunosuppressant doses of corticosteroids to avoid exposure to chickenpox or measles and, if exposed, to consult their physicians without delay. Inform patients of potential worsening of existing tuberculosis; fungal, bacterial, viral, or parasitic infections; or ocular herpes simplex.

Hypercorticism and Adrenal Suppression: Advise patients that ADVAIR DISKUS may cause systemic corticosteroid effects of hypercorticism and adrenal suppression. Additionally, inform patients that deaths due to adrenal insuffi-

ciency have occurred during and after transfer from systemic corticosteroids. Patients should taper slowly from systemic corticosteroids if transferring to ADVAIR DISKUS.

Immediate Hypersensitivity Reactions: Advise patients that immediate hypersensitivity reactions (e.g., urticaria, angioedema, rash, bronchospasm, hypotension), including anaphylaxis, may occur after administration of ADVAIR DISKUS. Patients should discontinue ADVAIR DISKUS if such reactions occur. There have been reports of anaphylactic reactions in patients with severe milk protein allergy after inhalation of powder products containing lactose; therefore, patients with severe milk protein allergy should not take ADVAIR DISKUS.

Reduction in Bone Mineral Density: Advise patients who are at an increased risk for decreased BMD that the use of corticosteroids may pose an additional risk.

Reduced Growth Velocity: Inform patients that orally inhaled corticosteroids, including fluticasone propionate, may cause a reduction in growth velocity when administered to pediatric patients. Physicians should closely follow the growth of children and adolescents taking corticosteroids by any route.

Ocular Effects: Long-term use of inhaled corticosteroids may increase the risk of some eye problems (cataracts or glaucoma); consider regular eye examinations.

Risks Associated With Beta-Agonist Therapy: Inform patients of adverse effects associated with beta$_2$–agonists, such as palpitations, chest pain, rapid heart rate, tremor, or nervousness.

ADVAIR, ADVAIR DISKUS, DISKHALER, DISKUS, FLONASE, FLOVENT, ROTADISK, and VENTOLIN are registered trademarks of the GSK group of companies.

GlaxoSmithKline

Research Triangle Park, NC 27709

©2014, the GSK group of companies. All rights reserved.

ADD:12PI

MEDICATION GUIDE

ADVAIR DISKUS® [*ad' vair disk' us*] **100/50**

(fluticasone propionate 100 mcg and salmeterol 50 mcg inhalation powder)

ADVAIR DISKUS® 250/50

(fluticasone propionate 250 mcg and salmeterol 50 mcg inhalation powder)

ADVAIR DISKUS® 500/50

(fluticasone propionate 500 mcg and salmeterol 50 mcg inhalation powder)

Read the Medication Guide that comes with ADVAIR DISKUS before you start using it and each time you get a refill. There may be new information. This Medication Guide does not take the place of talking to your healthcare provider about your medical condition or treatment.

What is the most important information I should know about ADVAIR DISKUS?

ADVAIR DISKUS can cause serious side effects, including:

- **People with asthma who take long-acting beta$_2$-adrenergic agonist (LABA) medicines, such as salmeterol (one of the medicines in ADVAIR DISKUS), have an increased risk of death from asthma problems.** It is not known whether fluticasone propionate, the other medicine in ADVAIR DISKUS, reduces the risk of death from asthma problems seen with LABA medicines.
- **It is not known if LABA medicines such as salmeterol increase the risk of death in people with COPD.**
- **Call your healthcare provider if breathing problems worsen over time while using ADVAIR DISKUS.** You may need different treatment.
- **Get emergency medical care if:**
  ○ your breathing problems worsen quickly.
  ○ you use your rescue inhaler, but it does not relieve your breathing problems.
- ADVAIR DISKUS should be used only if your healthcare provider decides that your asthma is not well controlled with a long-term asthma control medicine, such as an inhaled corticosteroid. When your asthma is well controlled, your healthcare provider may tell you to stop taking ADVAIR DISKUS. Your healthcare provider will decide if you can stop ADVAIR DISKUS without loss of asthma control. Your healthcare provider may prescribe a different asthma control medicine for you, such as an inhaled corticosteroid.
- Children and adolescents who take LABA medicines may have an increased risk of being hospitalized for asthma problems.

What is ADVAIR DISKUS?

- ADVAIR DISKUS combines the inhaled corticosteroid (ICS) medicine fluticasone propionate and the LABA medicine salmeterol.
- ICS medicines such as fluticasone propionate help to decrease inflammation in the lungs. Inflammation in the lungs can lead to breathing problems.
- LABA medicines such as salmeterol help the muscles around the airways in your lungs stay relaxed to prevent symptoms, such as wheezing, cough, chest tightness, and

shortness of breath. These symptoms can happen when the muscles around the airways tighten. This makes it hard to breathe.
- ADVAIR DISKUS is not used to relieve sudden breathing problems.
- It is not known if ADVAIR DISKUS is safe and effective in children younger than 4 years.
- ADVAIR DISKUS is used for asthma and COPD as follows:

Asthma:
ADVAIR DISKUS is a prescription medicine used to control symptoms of asthma and to prevent symptoms such as wheezing in adults and children aged 4 years and older. ADVAIR DISKUS contains salmeterol [the same medicine found in SEREVENT® DISKUS® (salmeterol xinafoate inhalation powder)]. LABA medicines such as salmeterol increase the risk of death from asthma problems.
ADVAIR DISKUS is not for adults and children with asthma who are well controlled with an asthma control medicine, such as a low to medium dose of an inhaled corticosteroid medicine.

COPD:
ADVAIR DISKUS 250/50 is a prescription medicine used to treat COPD. COPD is a chronic lung disease that includes chronic bronchitis, emphysema, or both. ADVAIR DISKUS 250/50 is used long term as 1 inhalation 2 times each day to improve symptoms of COPD for better breathing and to reduce the number of flare-ups (the worsening of your COPD symptoms for several days).

Who should not use ADVAIR DISKUS?
Do not use ADVAIR DISKUS if you:
- have a severe allergy to milk proteins. Ask your healthcare provider if you are not sure.
- are allergic to fluticasone propionate, salmeterol, or any of the ingredients in ADVAIR DISKUS. See "What are the ingredients in ADVAIR DISKUS?" below for a complete list of ingredients.

What should I tell my healthcare provider before using ADVAIR DISKUS?
Tell your healthcare provider about all of your health conditions, including if you:
- have heart problems.
- have high blood pressure.
- have seizures.
- have thyroid problems.
- have diabetes.
- have liver problems.
- have weak bones (osteoporosis).
- have an immune system problem.
- have eye problems such as glaucoma or cataracts.
- are allergic to any of the ingredients in ADVAIR DISKUS, any other medicines, or food products. See "What are the ingredients in ADVAIR DISKUS?" below for a complete list of ingredients.
- have any type of viral, bacterial, or fungal infection.
- are exposed to chickenpox or measles.
- have any other medical conditions.
- are pregnant or planning to become pregnant. It is not known if ADVAIR DISKUS may harm your unborn baby.
- are breastfeeding. It is not known if the medicines in ADVAIR DISKUS pass into your milk and if they can harm your baby.

Tell your healthcare provider about all the medicines you take, including prescription and over-the-counter medicines, vitamins, and herbal supplements. ADVAIR DISKUS and certain other medicines may interact with each other. This may cause serious side effects. Especially, tell your healthcare provider if you take antifungal or anti-HIV medicines.
Know the medicines you take. Keep a list of them to show your healthcare provider and pharmacist when you get a new medicine.

How should I use ADVAIR DISKUS?
Read the step-by-step instructions for using ADVAIR DISKUS at the end of this Medication Guide.
- **Do not** use ADVAIR DISKUS unless your healthcare provider has taught you how to use the inhaler and you understand how to use it correctly.
- Children should use ADVAIR DISKUS with an adult's help, as instructed by the child's healthcare provider.
- ADVAIR DISKUS comes in 3 different strengths. Your healthcare provider prescribed the strength that is best for you.
- Use ADVAIR DISKUS exactly as your healthcare provider tells you to use it. **Do not** use ADVAIR DISKUS more often than prescribed.
- Use 1 inhalation of ADVAIR DISKUS 2 times each day. Use ADVAIR DISKUS at the same time each day, about 12 hours apart.
- If you miss a dose of ADVAIR DISKUS, just skip that dose. Take your next dose at your usual time. Do not take 2 doses at 1 time.
- If you take too much ADVAIR DISKUS, call your healthcare provider or go to the nearest hospital emergency room

right away if you have any unusual symptoms, such as worsening shortness of breath, chest pain, increased heart rate, or shakiness.
- **Do not use other medicines that contain a LABA for any reason.** Ask your healthcare provider or pharmacist if any of your other medicines are LABA medicines.
- Do not stop using ADVAIR DISKUS unless told to do so by your healthcare provider because your symptoms might get worse. Your healthcare provider will change your medicines as needed.
- **ADVAIR DISKUS does not relieve sudden symptoms.** Always have a rescue inhaler with you to treat sudden symptoms. If you do not have a rescue inhaler, call your healthcare provider to have one prescribed for you.
- Call your healthcare provider or get medical care right away if:
  ○ your breathing problems get worse.
  ○ you need to use your rescue inhaler more often than usual.
  ○ your rescue inhaler does not work as well to relieve your symptoms.
  ○ you need to use 4 or more inhalations of your rescue inhaler in 24 hours for 2 or more days in a row.
  ○ you use 1 whole canister of your rescue inhaler in 8 weeks.
  ○ your peak flow meter results decrease. Your healthcare provider will tell you the numbers that are right for you.
  ○ you have asthma and your symptoms do not improve after using ADVAIR DISKUS regularly for 1 week.

What are the possible side effects with ADVAIR DISKUS?
ADVAIR DISKUS can cause serious side effects, including:
- **See "What is the most important information I should know about ADVAIR DISKUS?"**
- **fungal infection in your mouth or throat (thrush).** Rinse your mouth with water without swallowing after using ADVAIR DISKUS to help reduce your chance of getting thrush.
  ○ **pneumonia.** People with COPD have a higher chance of getting pneumonia. ADVAIR DISKUS may increase the chance of getting pneumonia. Call your healthcare provider if you notice any of the following symptoms:
    ○ increase in mucus (sputum) production
    ○ change in mucus color
    ○ fever
    ○ chills
    ○ increased cough
    ○ increased breathing problems
- **weakened immune system and increased chance of getting infections (immunosuppression)**
- **reduced adrenal function (adrenal insufficiency).** Adrenal insufficiency is a condition where the adrenal glands do not make enough steroid hormones. This can happen when you stop taking oral corticosteroid medicines (such as prednisone) and start taking a medicine containing an inhaled steroid (such as ADVAIR DISKUS). When your body is under stress such as from fever, trauma (such as a car accident), infection, surgery, or worse COPD symptoms, adrenal insufficiency can get worse and may cause death.
Symptoms of adrenal insufficiency include:
  ○ feeling tired
  ○ lack of energy
  ○ weakness
  ○ nausea and vomiting
  ○ low blood pressure
- **sudden breathing problems immediately after inhaling your medicine**
- **serious allergic reactions.** Call your healthcare provider or get emergency medical care if you get any of the following symptoms of a serious allergic reaction:
  ○ rash
  ○ hives
  ○ swelling of your face, mouth, and tongue
  ○ breathing problems
- **effects on heart**
  ○ increased blood pressure
  ○ a fast or irregular heartbeat
  ○ chest pain
- **effects on nervous system**
  ○ tremor
  ○ nervousness
- **bone thinning or weakness (osteoporosis)**
- **slowed growth in children.** A child's growth should be checked often.
- **eye problems including glaucoma and cataracts.** You should have regular eye exams while using ADVAIR DISKUS.
- **changes in laboratory blood values (sugar, potassium, certain types of white blood cells)**
Common side effects of ADVAIR DISKUS include:
Asthma:
- upper respiratory tract infection
- throat irritation
- hoarseness and voice changes

- thrush in your mouth or throat. Rinse your mouth with water without swallowing after use to help prevent this.
- bronchitis
- cough
- headache
- nausea and vomiting
In children with asthma, infections in the ear, nose, and throat are common.
COPD:
- thrush in your mouth or throat. Rinse your mouth with water without swallowing after use to help prevent this.
- throat irritation
- hoarseness and voice changes
- viral respiratory infections
- headache
- muscle and bone pain
Tell your healthcare provider about any side effect that bothers you or that does not go away.
These are not all the side effects with ADVAIR DISKUS. Ask your healthcare provider or pharmacist for more information.
Call your doctor for medical advice about side effects. You may report side effects to FDA at 1-800-FDA-1088.

How should I store ADVAIR DISKUS?
- Store ADVAIR DISKUS at room temperature between 68°F and 77°F (20°C and 25°C). Keep in a dry place away from heat and sunlight.
- Store ADVAIR DISKUS in the unopened foil pouch and only open when ready for use.
- Safely throw away ADVAIR DISKUS in the trash 1 month after you open the foil pouch or when the counter reads **0**, whichever comes first.
- **Keep ADVAIR DISKUS and all medicines out of the reach of children.**

General information about ADVAIR DISKUS
Medicines are sometimes prescribed for purposes not mentioned in a Medication Guide. Do not use ADVAIR DISKUS for a condition for which it was not prescribed. Do not give your ADVAIR DISKUS to other people, even if they have the same condition that you have. It may harm them.
This Medication Guide summarizes the most important information about ADVAIR DISKUS. If you would like more information, talk with your healthcare provider or pharmacist. You can ask your healthcare provider or pharmacist for information about ADVAIR DISKUS that was written for healthcare professionals.
For more information about ADVAIR DISKUS, call 1-888-825-5249 or visit our website at www.advair.com.

What are the ingredients in ADVAIR DISKUS?
Active ingredients: fluticasone propionate, salmeterol xinafoate
Inactive ingredient: lactose monohydrate (contains milk proteins)

Instructions for Use
For Oral Inhalation Only
Your ADVAIR Diskus inhaler

Figure A

Read this information before you start using your ADVAIR DISKUS inhaler:
- Take ADVAIR DISKUS out of the foil pouch just before you use it for the first time. Safely throw away the pouch. The DISKUS will be in the closed position.
- Write the date you opened the foil pouch in the first blank line on the label. **See Figure A.**
- Write the "use by" date in the second blank line on the label. **See Figure A.** That date is 1 month after the date you wrote in the first line.
- The counter should read **60**. If you have a sample (with "Sample" on the back label) or institutional (with "INSTITUTIONAL PACK" on the foil pouch) pack, the counter should read **14**.

How to use your ADVAIR Diskus inhaler
Follow these steps every time you use ADVAIR Diskus.
Step 1. Open your ADVAIR DISKUS.
- Hold the DISKUS in your left hand and place the thumb of your right hand in the thumb grip. Push the thumb grip away from you as far as it will go until the mouthpiece shows and snaps into place. **See Figure B.**
[See figure B at top of next page]

Figure B

Step 2. Slide the lever until you hear it click.
• **Hold the DISKUS in a level, flat position** with the mouthpiece towards you. Slide the lever away from the mouthpiece as far as it will go until it **clicks. See Figure C.**

Figure C

• The number on the counter will count down by 1. The DISKUS is now ready to use.
Follow the instructions below so you will not accidentally waste a dose:
• **Do not** close the DISKUS.
• **Do not** tilt the DISKUS.
• **Do not** move the lever on the DISKUS.
Step 3. Inhale your medicine.
• Before you breathe in your dose from the DISKUS, breathe out (exhale) as long as you can while you hold the DISKUS level and away from your mouth. **See Figure D.** Do not breathe into the mouthpiece.

Figure D

• Put the mouthpiece to your lips. **See Figure E.** Breathe in quickly and deeply through the DISKUS. Do not breathe in through your nose.

Figure E

• Remove the DISKUS from your mouth **and hold your breath for about 10 seconds,** or for as long as is comfortable for you.
• **Breathe out slowly as long as you can. See Figure D.**
• The DISKUS delivers your dose of medicine as a very fine powder that you may or may not taste or feel. **Do not** take an extra dose from the DISKUS even if you do not taste or feel the medicine.
Step 4. Close the DISKUS.
• Place your thumb in the thumb grip and slide it back towards you as far as it will go. **See Figure F.** Make sure the DISKUS clicks shut and you cannot see the mouthpiece.

Figure F

• The DISKUS is now ready for you to take your next scheduled dose in about 12 hours. **When you are ready to take your next dose, repeat Steps 1 through 4.**
Step 5. Rinse your mouth.
• **Rinse your mouth with water after breathing in the medicine.** Spit out the water. Do not swallow it. **See Figure G.**

Figure G

When should you get a refill?
The counter on top of the DISKUS shows you how many doses are left. After you have taken 55 doses (9 doses from the sample or institutional pack), the numbers 5 to 0 will show in red. **See Figure H.** These numbers warn you there are only a few doses left and are a reminder to get a refill.

Figure H

For correct use of the DISKUS, remember:
• Always use the DISKUS in a level, flat position.
• Make sure the lever firmly clicks into place.
• Hold your breath for about 10 seconds after inhaling. Then breathe out fully.
• After each dose, rinse your mouth with water and spit it out. Do not swallow the water.
• **Do not** take an extra dose, even if you did not taste or feel the powder.
• **Do not** take the DISKUS apart.
• **Do not** wash the DISKUS.
• Always keep the DISKUS in a dry place.
• **Do not** use the DISKUS with a spacer device.
If you have questions about ADVAIR DISKUS or how to use your inhaler, call GlaxoSmithKline (GSK) at 1-888-825-5249 or visit www.advair.com.
This Medication Guide and Instructions for Use have been approved by the U.S. Food and Drug Administration.
ADVAIR DISKUS, DISKUS, and SEREVENT are registered trademarks of the GSK group of companies.
GlaxoSmithKline
Research Triangle Park, NC 27709
©2014, the GSK group of companies. All rights reserved.
April 2014
ADD:8MG

ADVAIR HFA 45/21   ℞
[ad' vair]
(fluticasone propionate 45 mcg and salmeterol 21 mcg)
Inhalation Aerosol
ADVAIR HFA 115/21
(fluticasone propionate 115 mcg and salmeterol 21 mcg)
Inhalation Aerosol
ADVAIR HFA 230/21
(fluticasone propionate 230 mcg and salmeterol 21 mcg)
Inhalation Aerosol
FOR ORAL INHALATION

HIGHLIGHTS OF PRESCRIBING INFORMATION
These highlights do not include all the information needed to use ADVAIR HFA safely and effectively. See full prescribing information for ADVAIR HFA.
ADVAIR HFA 45/21
(fluticasone propionate 45 mcg and salmeterol 21 mcg)
Inhalation Aerosol
ADVAIR HFA 115/21
(fluticasone propionate 115 mcg and salmeterol 21 mcg)
Inhalation Aerosol
ADVAIR HFA 230/21
(fluticasone propionate 230 mcg and salmeterol 21 mcg)
Inhalation Aerosol
FOR ORAL INHALATION
Initial U.S. Approval: 2000

WARNING: ASTHMA-RELATED DEATH
See full prescribing information for complete boxed warning
• **Long-acting beta$_2$-adrenergic agonists (LABAs), such as salmeterol, one of the active ingredients in ADVAIR HFA, increase the risk of asthma-related death. A US study showed an increase in asthma-related deaths in patients receiving salmeterol (13 deaths out of 13,176 patients treated for 28 weeks on salmeterol versus 3 out of 13,179 patients on placebo). Currently available data are inadequate to determine whether concurrent use of inhaled corticosteroids or other long-term asthma control drugs mitigates the increased risk of asthma-related death from LABAs. Available data from controlled clinical trials suggest that LABAs increase the risk of asthma-related hospitalization in pediatric and adolescent patients. (5.1)**

• When treating patients with asthma, only prescribe ADVAIR HFA for patients not adequately controlled on a long-term asthma control medication, such as an inhaled corticosteroid, or whose disease severity clearly warrants initiation of treatment with both an inhaled corticosteroid and a LABA. Once asthma control is achieved and maintained, assess the patient at regular intervals and step down therapy (e.g., discontinue ADVAIR HFA) if possible without loss of asthma control and maintain the patient on a long-term asthma control medication, such as an inhaled corticosteroid. Do not use ADVAIR HFA for patients whose asthma is adequately controlled on low- or medium-dose inhaled corticosteroids. (1, 5.1)

---INDICATIONS AND USAGE---

ADVAIR HFA is a combination product containing a corticosteroid and a LABA indicated for treatment of asthma in patients aged 12 years and older.
Important limitation:
• Not indicated for the relief of acute bronchospasm. (1)

---DOSAGE AND ADMINISTRATION---

For oral inhalation only.
Treatment of asthma in patients ≥12 years: 2 inhalations of ADVAIR HFA 45/21, 115/21, or 230/21 twice daily. Starting dosage is based on asthma severity. (2)

---DOSAGE FORMS AND STRENGTHS---

Inhalation aerosol: delivers a combination of fluticasone propionate (45, 115, or 230 mcg) and salmeterol (21 mcg) from mouthpiece per actuation. (3)

---CONTRAINDICATIONS---

• Primary treatment of status asthmaticus or acute episodes of asthma requiring intensive measures. (4)
• Hypersensitivity to any ingredient. (4)

---WARNINGS AND PRECAUTIONS---

• Asthma-related death: LABAs increase the risk. Prescribe only for recommended patient populations. (5.1)
• Deterioration of disease and acute episodes: Do not initiate in acutely deteriorating asthma or to treat acute symptoms. (5.2)
• Use with additional LABA: Do not use in combination because of risk of overdose. (5.3)
• Localized infections: Candida albicans infection of the mouth and throat may occur. Monitor patients periodically for signs of adverse effects on the oral cavity. Advise patients to rinse the mouth following inhalation. (5.4)
• Pneumonia: Increased risk in patients with COPD. Monitor patients for signs and symptoms of pneumonia. (5.5)
• Immunosuppression: Potential worsening of infections (e.g., existing tuberculosis, fungal, bacterial, viral, or parasitic infection; ocular herpes simplex). Use with caution in patients with these infections. More serious or even fatal course of chickenpox or measles can occur in susceptible patients. (5.6)
• Transferring patients from systemic corticosteroids: Risk of impaired adrenal function when transferring from oral steroids. Taper patients slowly from systemic corticosteroids if transferring to ADVAIR HFA. (5.7)
• Hypercorticism and adrenal suppression: May occur with very high dosages or at the regular dosage in susceptible individuals. If such changes occur, discontinue ADVAIR HFA slowly. (5.8)
• Strong cytochrome P450 3A4 inhibitors (e.g., ritonavir): Risk of increased systemic corticosteroid and cardiovascular effects. Use not recommended with ADVAIR HFA. (5.9)
• Paradoxical bronchospasm: Discontinue ADVAIR HFA and institute alternative therapy if paradoxical bronchospasm occurs. (5.10)
• Patients with cardiovascular or central nervous system disorders: Use with caution because of beta-adrenergic stimulation. (5.12)
• Decreases in bone mineral density: Assess bone mineral density initially and periodically thereafter. (5.13)
• Effects on growth: Monitor growth of pediatric patients. (5.14)
• Glaucoma and cataracts: Close monitoring is warranted. (5.15)
• Metabolic effects: Be alert to eosinophilic conditions, hypokalemia, and hyperglycemia. (5.16, 5.18)
• Coexisting conditions: Use with caution in patients with convulsive disorders, thyrotoxicosis, diabetes mellitus, and ketoacidosis. (5.17)

---ADVERSE REACTIONS---

Most common adverse reactions (incidence ≥3%) are: upper respiratory tract infection or inflammation, throat irritation, dysphonia, headache, dizziness, nausea and vomiting. (6.1)

To report SUSPECTED ADVERSE REACTIONS, contact GlaxoSmithKline at 1-888-825-5249 or FDA at 1-800-FDA-1088 or www.fda.gov/medwatch.

---DRUG INTERACTIONS---

• Strong cytochrome P450 3A4 inhibitors (e.g., ritonavir): Use not recommended. May cause systemic corticosteroid and cardiovascular effects. (7.1)
• Monoamine oxidase inhibitors and tricyclic antidepressants: Use with extreme caution. May potentiate effect of salmeterol on vascular system. (7.2)
• Beta-blockers: Use with caution. May block bronchodilatory effects of beta-agonists and produce severe bronchospasm. (7.3)
• Diuretics: Use with caution. Electrocardiographic changes and/or hypokalemia associated with nonpotassium-sparing diuretics may worsen with concomitant beta-agonists. (7.4)

---USE IN SPECIFIC POPULATIONS---

Hepatic impairment: Monitor patients for signs of increased drug exposure. (8.6)
See 17 for PATIENT COUNSELING INFORMATION and Medication Guide

Revised: 05/2014

FULL PRESCRIBING INFORMATION: CONTENTS*
WARNING: ASTHMA-RELATED DEATH
* Sections or subsections omitted from the full prescribing information are not listed

FULL PRESCRIBING INFORMATION

WARNING: ASTHMA-RELATED DEATH

Long-acting beta₂-adrenergic agonists (LABAs), such as salmeterol, one of the active ingredients in ADVAIR® HFA, increase the risk of asthma-related death. Data from a large placebo-controlled US study that compared the safety of salmeterol (SEREVENT® Inhalation Aerosol) or placebo added to usual asthma therapy showed an increase in asthma-related deaths in patients receiving salmeterol (13 deaths out of 13,176 patients treated for 28 weeks on salmeterol versus 3 deaths out of 13,179 patients on placebo). Currently available data are inadequate to determine whether concurrent use of inhaled corticosteroids or other long-term asthma control drugs mitigates the increased risk of asthma-related death from LABAs. Available data from controlled clinical trials suggest that LABAs increase the risk of asthma-related hospitalization in pediatric and adolescent patients.
Therefore, when treating patients with asthma, physicians should only prescribe ADVAIR HFA for patients not adequately controlled on a long-term asthma control medication, such as an inhaled corticosteroid, or whose disease severity clearly warrants initiation of treatment with both an inhaled corticosteroid and a LABA. Once asthma control is achieved and maintained, assess the patient at regular intervals and step down therapy (e.g., discontinue ADVAIR HFA) if possible without loss of asthma control and maintain the patient on a long-term asthma control medication, such as an inhaled corticosteroid. Do not use ADVAIR HFA for patients whose asthma is adequately controlled on low- or medium-dose inhaled corticosteroids [see Warnings and Precautions (5.1)].

1   INDICATIONS AND USAGE

ADVAIR HFA is indicated for the treatment of asthma in patients aged 12 years and older.
Long-acting beta₂-adrenergic agonists (LABAs), such as salmeterol, one of the active ingredients in ADVAIR HFA, increase the risk of asthma-related death. Available data from controlled clinical trials suggest that LABAs increase the risk of asthma-related hospitalization in pediatric and adolescent patients [see Warnings and Precautions (5.1)]. Therefore, when treating patients with asthma, physicians should only prescribe ADVAIR HFA for patients not adequately controlled on a long-term asthma control medication, such as an inhaled corticosteroid, or whose disease severity clearly warrants initiation of treatment with both an inhaled corticosteroid and a LABA. Once asthma control is achieved and maintained, assess the patient at regular intervals and step down therapy (e.g., discontinue ADVAIR HFA) if possible without loss of asthma control and maintain the patient on a long-term asthma control medication, such as an inhaled corticosteroid. Do not use ADVAIR HFA for patients whose asthma is adequately controlled on low- or medium-dose inhaled corticosteroids.
Important Limitation of Use: ADVAIR HFA is NOT indicated for the relief of acute bronchospasm.

2   DOSAGE AND ADMINISTRATION

ADVAIR HFA should be administered twice daily every day by the orally inhaled route only. After inhalation, the patient should rinse the mouth with water without swallowing [see Patient Counseling Information (17.4)].
More frequent administration or a higher number of inhalations (more than 2 inhalations twice daily) of the prescribed strength of ADVAIR HFA is not recommended as some patients are more likely to experience adverse effects with higher doses of salmeterol. Patients using ADVAIR HFA should not use additional LABAs for any reason. [See Warnings and Precautions (5.3, 5.12).]
If asthma symptoms arise in the period between doses, an inhaled, short-acting beta₂-agonist should be taken for immediate relief.
For patients aged 12 years and older, the dosage is 2 inhalations twice daily (morning and evening, approximately 12 hours apart).
The recommended starting dosages for ADVAIR HFA for patients aged 12 years and older are based upon patients' asthma severity.

The maximum recommended dosage is 2 inhalations of ADVAIR HFA 230/21 twice daily.

Improvement in asthma control following inhaled administration of ADVAIR HFA can occur within 30 minutes of beginning treatment, although maximum benefit may not be achieved for 1 week or longer after starting treatment. Individual patients will experience a variable time to onset and degree of symptom relief.

For patients who do not respond adequately to the starting dosage after 2 weeks of therapy, replacing the current strength of ADVAIR HFA with a higher strength may provide additional improvement in asthma control.

If a previously effective dosage regimen of ADVAIR HFA fails to provide adequate improvement in asthma control, the therapeutic regimen should be reevaluated and additional therapeutic options (e.g., replacing the current strength of ADVAIR HFA with a higher strength, adding additional inhaled corticosteroid, initiating oral corticosteroids) should be considered.

ADVAIR HFA should be primed before using for the first time by releasing 4 test sprays into the air away from the face, shaking well for 5 seconds before each spray. In cases where the inhaler has not been used for more than 4 weeks or when it has been dropped, prime the inhaler again by releasing 2 test sprays into the air away from the face, shaking well for 5 seconds before each spray.

3   DOSAGE FORMS AND STRENGTHS

ADVAIR HFA is an inhalation aerosol. Each actuation delivers a combination of fluticasone propionate (45, 115, or 230 mcg) and salmeterol (21 mcg) from the actuator. ADVAIR HFA is supplied in 8- and 12-g pressurized aluminum canisters containing 60 and 120 metered inhalations, respectively. Each canister is fitted with a counter and a purple actuator with a light purple strapcap.

4   CONTRAINDICATIONS

The use of ADVAIR HFA is contraindicated in the following conditions:

• Primary treatment of status asthmaticus or other acute episodes of asthma where intensive measures are required.

• Hypersensitivity to any of the ingredients of these preparations contraindicates their use [see Description (11)].

5   WARNINGS AND PRECAUTIONS

5.1   Asthma-Related Death

LABAs, such as salmeterol, one of the active ingredients in ADVAIR HFA, increase the risk of asthma-related death. Currently available data are inadequate to determine whether concurrent use of inhaled corticosteroids or other long-term asthma control drugs mitigates the increased risk of asthma-related death from LABAs. Available data from controlled clinical trials suggest that LABAs increase the risk of asthma-related hospitalization in pediatric and adolescent patients. Therefore, when treating patients with asthma, physicians should only prescribe ADVAIR HFA for patients not adequately controlled on a long-term asthma control medication such as an inhaled corticosteroid, or whose disease severity clearly warrants initiation of treatment with both an inhaled corticosteroid and a LABA. Once asthma control is achieved and maintained, assess the patient at regular intervals and step down therapy (e.g., discontinue ADVAIR HFA) if possible without loss of asthma control and maintain the patient on a long-term asthma control medication, such as an inhaled corticosteroid. Do not use ADVAIR HFA for patients whose asthma is adequately controlled on low- or medium-dose inhaled corticosteroids.

A large placebo-controlled US study that compared the safety of salmeterol with placebo, each added to usual asthma therapy, showed an increase in asthma-related deaths in patients receiving salmeterol. The Salmeterol Multi-center Asthma Research Trial (SMART) was a randomized double-blind study that enrolled LABA-naive patients with asthma to assess the safety of salmeterol (SEREVENT Inhalation Aerosol) 42 mcg twice daily over 28 weeks compared with placebo when added to usual asthma therapy. A planned interim analysis was conducted when approximately half of the intended number of patients had been enrolled (N = 26,355), which led to premature termination of the study. The results of the interim analysis showed that patients receiving salmeterol were at increased risk for fatal asthma events (see Table 3 and Figure 5). In the total population, a higher rate of asthma-related death occurred in patients treated with salmeterol than those treated with placebo (0.10% versus 0.02%; relative risk: 4.37 [95% CI: 1.25, 15.34]).

Post-hoc subpopulation analyses were performed. In Caucasians, asthma-related death occurred at a higher rate in patients treated with salmeterol than in patients treated with placebo (0.07% versus 0.01%; relative risk: 5.82 [95% CI: 0.70, 48.37]). In African Americans also, asthma-related death occurred at a higher rate in patients treated with salmeterol than those treated with placebo (0.31% versus

Table 1. Asthma-Related Deaths in the 28-Week Salmeterol Multi-center Asthma Research Trial (SMART)

	Salmeterol n (%[a])	Placebo n (%[a])	Relative Risk[b] (95% Confidence Interval)	Excess Deaths Expressed per 10,000 Patients[c] (95% Confidence Interval)
Total Population[d]				
Salmeterol: n = 13,176	13 (0.10%)		4.37 (1.25, 15.34)	8 (3, 13)
Placebo: n = 13,179		3 (0.02%)		
Caucasian				
Salmeterol: n = 9,281	6 (0.07%)		5.82 (0.70, 48.37)	6 (1, 10)
Placebo: n = 9,361		1 (0.01%)		
African American				
Salmeterol: n = 2,366	7 (0.31%)		7.26 (0.89, 58.94)	27 (8, 46)
Placebo: n = 2,319		1 (0.04%)		

[a]Life-table 28-week estimate, adjusted according to the patients' actual lengths of exposure to study treatment to account for early withdrawal of patients from the study.

[b]Relative risk is the ratio of the rate of asthma-related death in the salmeterol group and the rate in the placebo group. The relative risk indicates how many more times likely an asthma-related death occurred in the salmeterol group than in the placebo group in a 28-week treatment period.

[c]Estimate of the number of additional asthma-related deaths in patients treated with salmeterol in SMART, assuming 10,000 patients received salmeterol for a 28-week treatment period. Estimate calculated as the difference between the salmeterol and placebo groups in the rates of asthma-related death multiplied by 10,000.

[d]The Total Population includes the following ethnic origins listed on the case report form: Caucasian, African American, Hispanic, Asian, and "Other." In addition, the Total Population includes those patients whose ethnic origin was not reported. The results for Caucasian and African American subpopulations are shown above. No asthma-related deaths occurred in the Hispanic (salmeterol n = 996, placebo n = 999), Asian (salmeterol n = 173, placebo n = 149), or "Other" (salmeterol n = 230, placebo n = 224) subpopulations. One asthma-related death occurred in the placebo group in the subpopulation whose ethnic origin was not reported (salmeterol n = 130, placebo n = 127).

0.04%; relative risk: 7.26 [95% CI: 0.89, 58.94]). Although the relative risks of asthma-related death were similar in Caucasians and African Americans, the estimate of excess deaths in patients treated with salmeterol was greater in African Americans because there was a higher overall rate of asthma-related death in African American patients (see Table 3). Given the similar basic mechanisms of action of beta$_2$-agonists, the findings seen in the SMART study are considered a class effect.

Post-hoc analyses in pediatric patients aged 12 to 18 years were also performed. Pediatric patients accounted for approximately 12% of patients in each treatment arm. Respiratory-related death or life-threatening experience occurred at a similar rate in the salmeterol group (0.12% [2/1,653]) and the placebo group (0.12% [2/1,622]; relative risk: 1.0 [95% CI: 0.1, 7.2]). All-cause hospitalization, however, was increased in the salmeterol group (2% [35/1,653]) versus the placebo group (<1% [16/1,622]; relative risk: 2.1 [95% CI: 1.1, 3.7]).

The data from the SMART study are not adequate to determine whether concurrent use of inhaled corticosteroids, such as fluticasone propionate, the other active ingredient in ADVAIR HFA, or other long-term asthma control therapy mitigates the risk of asthma-related death.

[See table 1 above]

[See figure 1 at top of next column]

A 16-week clinical study performed in the United Kingdom, the Salmeterol Nationwide Surveillance (SNS) study, showed results similar to the SMART study. In the SNS study, the rate of asthma-related death was numerically, though not statistically significantly, greater in patients with asthma treated with salmeterol (42 mcg twice daily) than those treated with albuterol (180 mcg 4 times daily) added to usual asthma therapy.

5.2   Deterioration of Disease and Acute Episodes

ADVAIR HFA should not be initiated in patients during rapidly deteriorating or potentially life-threatening episodes of asthma. ADVAIR HFA has not been studied in patients with acutely deteriorating asthma. The initiation of ADVAIR HFA in this setting is not appropriate.

Serious acute respiratory events, including fatalities, have been reported when salmeterol, a component of ADVAIR HFA, has been initiated in patients with significantly worsening or acutely deteriorating asthma. In most cases, these have occurred in patients with severe asthma (e.g., patients with a history of corticosteroid dependence, low pulmonary function, intubation, mechanical ventilation, frequent hospitalizations, previous life-threatening acute asthma exacerbations) and in some patients with acutely deteriorating asthma (e.g., patients with significantly increasing symptoms; increasing need for inhaled, short-acting beta$_2$-agonists; decreasing response to usual medications; increasing need for systemic corticosteroids; recent emergency room visits; deteriorating lung function). However, these events have occurred in a few patients with less severe asthma as well. It was not possible from these reports to determine whether salmeterol contributed to these events. Increasing use of inhaled, short-acting beta$_2$-agonists is a marker of deteriorating asthma. In this situation, the pa-

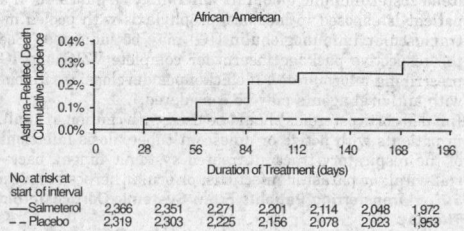

Figure 1. Cumulative Incidence of Asthma-Related Deaths in the 28-Week Salmeterol Multi-center Asthma Research Trial (SMART), by Duration of Treatment

tient requires immediate reevaluation with reassessment of the treatment regimen, giving special consideration to the possible need for replacing the current strength of ADVAIR HFA with a higher strength, adding additional inhaled corticosteroid, or initiating systemic corticosteroids. Patients should not use more than 2 inhalations twice daily (morning and evening) of ADVAIR HFA.

ADVAIR HFA should not be used for the relief of acute symptoms, i.e., as rescue therapy for the treatment of acute episodes of bronchospasm. An inhaled, short-acting beta$_2$-agonist, not ADVAIR HFA, should be used to relieve acute symptoms such as shortness of breath. When prescribing

ADVAIR HFA, the physician must also provide the patient with an inhaled, short-acting beta$_2$-agonist (e.g., albuterol) for treatment of acute symptoms, despite regular twice-daily (morning and evening) use of ADVAIR HFA.

When beginning treatment with ADVAIR HFA, patients who have been taking oral or inhaled, short-acting beta$_2$-agonists on a regular basis (e.g., 4 times a day) should be instructed to discontinue the regular use of these drugs.

5.3 Excessive Use of ADVAIR HFA and Use With Other Long-Acting Beta$_2$-Agonists

As with other inhaled drugs containing beta$_2$-adrenergic agents, ADVAIR HFA should not be used more often than recommended, at higher doses than recommended, or in conjunction with other medications containing LABAs, as an overdose may result. Clinically significant cardiovascular effects and fatalities have been reported in association with excessive use of inhaled sympathomimetic drugs. Patients using ADVAIR HFA should not use an additional LABA (e.g., salmeterol, formoterol fumarate, arformoterol tartrate) for any reason, including prevention of exercise-induced bronchospasm (EIB) or the treatment of asthma.

5.4 Local Effects

In clinical studies, the development of localized infections of the mouth and pharynx with *Candida albicans* has occurred in patients treated with ADVAIR HFA. When such an infection develops, it should be treated with appropriate local or systemic (i.e., oral antifungal) therapy while treatment with ADVAIR HFA continues, but at times therapy with ADVAIR HFA may need to be interrupted. Patients should rinse the mouth after inhalation of ADVAIR HFA.

5.5 Pneumonia

Lower respiratory tract infections, including pneumonia, have been reported in patients with chronic obstructive pulmonary disease (COPD) following the inhaled administration of corticosteroids, including fluticasone propionate and ADVAIR DISKUS® (fluticasone propionate and salmeterol inhalation powder). In 2 replicate 1-year studies of 1,579 patients with COPD, there was a higher incidence of pneumonia reported in patients receiving ADVAIR DISKUS 250/50 (7%) than in those receiving salmeterol 50 mcg (3%). The incidence of pneumonia in the patients treated with ADVAIR DISKUS was higher in patients over 65 years of age (9%) compared with the incidence in patients less than 65 years of age (4%).

In a 3-year study of 6,184 patients with COPD, there was a higher incidence of pneumonia reported in patients receiving ADVAIR DISKUS 500/50 compared with placebo (16% with ADVAIR DISKUS 500/50, 14% with fluticasone propionate 500 mcg, 11% with salmeterol 50 mcg, and 9% with placebo). Similar to what was seen in the 1-year studies with ADVAIR DISKUS 250/50, the incidence of pneumonia was higher in patients over 65 years of age (18% with ADVAIR DISKUS 500/50 versus 10% with placebo) compared with patients less than 65 years of age (14% with ADVAIR DISKUS 500/50 versus 8% with placebo).

5.6 Immunosuppression

Persons who are using drugs that suppress the immune system are more susceptible to infections than healthy individuals. Chickenpox and measles, for example, can have a more serious or even fatal course in susceptible children or adults using corticosteroids. In such children or adults who have not had these diseases or been properly immunized, particular care should be taken to avoid exposure. How the dose, route, and duration of corticosteroid administration affect the risk of developing a disseminated infection is not known. The contribution of the underlying disease and/or prior corticosteroid treatment to the risk is also not known. If a patient is exposed to chickenpox, prophylaxis with varicella zoster immune globulin (VZIG) may be indicated. If a patient is exposed to measles, prophylaxis with pooled intramuscular immunoglobulin (IG) may be indicated. (See the respective package inserts for complete VZIG and IG prescribing information.) If chickenpox develops, treatment with antiviral agents may be considered.

Inhaled corticosteroids should be used with caution, if at all, in patients with active or quiescent tuberculosis infections of the respiratory tract; untreated systemic fungal, bacterial, viral, or parasitic infections; or ocular herpes simplex.

5.7 Transferring Patients From Systemic Corticosteroid Therapy

Particular care is needed for patients who have been transferred from systemically active corticosteroids to inhaled corticosteroids because deaths due to adrenal insufficiency have occurred in patients with asthma during and after transfer from systemic corticosteroids to less systemically available inhaled corticosteroids. After withdrawal from systemic corticosteroids, a number of months are required for recovery of hypothalamic-pituitary-adrenal (HPA) function.

Patients who have been previously maintained on 20 mg or more per day of prednisone (or its equivalent) may be most susceptible, particularly when their systemic corticosteroids have been almost completely withdrawn. During this period of HPA suppression, patients may exhibit signs and symp-

toms of adrenal insufficiency when exposed to trauma, surgery, or infection (particularly gastroenteritis) or other conditions associated with severe electrolyte loss. Although ADVAIR HFA may provide control of asthma symptoms during these episodes, in recommended doses it supplies less than normal physiologic amounts of glucocorticoid systemically and does NOT provide the mineralocorticoid activity that is necessary for coping with these emergencies.

During periods of stress or a severe asthma attack, patients who have been withdrawn from systemic corticosteroids should be instructed to resume oral corticosteroids (in large doses) immediately and to contact their physicians for further instruction. These patients should also be instructed to carry a warning card indicating that they may need supplementary systemic corticosteroids during periods of stress or a severe asthma attack.

Patients requiring oral corticosteroids should be weaned slowly from systemic corticosteroid use after transferring to ADVAIR HFA. Prednisone reduction can be accomplished by reducing the daily prednisone dose by 2.5 mg on a weekly basis during therapy with ADVAIR HFA. Lung function (mean forced expiratory volume in 1 second [FEV$_1$] or morning peak expiratory flow [PEF]), beta-agonist use, and asthma symptoms should be carefully monitored during withdrawal of oral corticosteroids. In addition to monitoring asthma signs and symptoms, patients should be observed for signs and symptoms of adrenal insufficiency, such as fatigue, lassitude, weakness, nausea and vomiting, and hypotension.

Transfer of patients from systemic corticosteroid therapy to inhaled corticosteroids or ADVAIR HFA may unmask conditions previously suppressed by the systemic corticosteroid therapy (e.g., rhinitis, conjunctivitis, eczema, arthritis, eosinophilic conditions). Some patients may experience symptoms of systemically active corticosteroid withdrawal (e.g., joint and/or muscular pain, lassitude, depression) despite maintenance or even improvement of respiratory function.

5.8 Hypercorticism and Adrenal Suppression

Fluticasone propionate, a component of ADVAIR HFA, will often help control asthma symptoms with less suppression of HPA function than therapeutically equivalent oral doses of prednisone. Since fluticasone propionate is absorbed into the circulation and can be systemically active at higher doses, the beneficial effects of ADVAIR HFA in minimizing HPA dysfunction may be expected only when recommended dosages are not exceeded and individual patients are titrated to the lowest effective dose. A relationship between plasma levels of fluticasone propionate and inhibitory effects on stimulated cortisol production has been shown after 4 weeks of treatment with fluticasone propionate inhalation aerosol. Since individual sensitivity to effects on cortisol production exists, physicians should consider this information when prescribing ADVAIR HFA.

Because of the possibility of systemic absorption of inhaled corticosteroids, patients treated with ADVAIR HFA should be observed carefully for any evidence of systemic corticosteroid effects. Particular care should be taken in observing patients postoperatively or during periods of stress for evidence of inadequate adrenal response.

It is possible that systemic corticosteroid effects such as hypercorticism and adrenal suppression (including adrenal crisis) may appear in a small number of patients, particularly when fluticasone propionate is administered at higher than recommended doses over prolonged periods of time. If such effects occur, the dosage of ADVAIR HFA should be reduced slowly, consistent with accepted procedures for reducing systemic corticosteroids and for management of asthma symptoms.

5.9 Drug Interactions With Strong Cytochrome P450 3A4 Inhibitors

The use of strong cytochrome P450 3A4 (CYP3A4) inhibitors (e.g., ritonavir, atazanavir, clarithromycin, indinavir, itraconazole, nefazodone, nelfinavir, saquinavir, ketoconazole, telithromycin) with ADVAIR HFA is not recommended because increased systemic corticosteroid and increased cardiovascular adverse effects may occur [see Drug Interactions (7.1), Clinical Pharmacology (12.3)].

5.10 Paradoxical Bronchospasm and Upper Airway Symptoms

As with other inhaled medications, ADVAIR HFA can produce paradoxical bronchospasm, which may be life threatening. If paradoxical bronchospasm occurs following dosing with ADVAIR HFA, it should be treated immediately with an inhaled, short-acting bronchodilator; ADVAIR HFA should be discontinued immediately; and alternative therapy should be instituted. Upper airway symptoms of laryngeal spasm, irritation, or swelling, such as stridor and choking, have been reported in patients receiving fluticasone propionate and salmeterol.

5.11 Immediate Hypersensitivity Reactions

Immediate hypersensitivity reactions may occur after administration of ADVAIR HFA, as demonstrated by cases of urticaria, angioedema, rash, and bronchospasm [see Adverse Reactions (6.2)].

5.12 Cardiovascular and Central Nervous System Effects

Excessive beta-adrenergic stimulation has been associated with seizures, angina, hypertension or hypotension, tachycardia with rates up to 200 beats/min, arrhythmias, nervousness, headache, tremor, palpitation, nausea, dizziness, fatigue, malaise, and insomnia [see Overdosage (10)]. Therefore, ADVAIR HFA, like all products containing sympathomimetic amines, should be used with caution in patients with cardiovascular disorders, especially coronary insufficiency, cardiac arrhythmias, and hypertension.

Salmeterol, a component of ADVAIR HFA, can produce a clinically significant cardiovascular effect in some patients as measured by pulse rate, blood pressure, and/or symptoms. Although such effects are uncommon after administration of salmeterol at recommended doses, if they occur, the drug may need to be discontinued. In addition, beta-agonists have been reported to produce electrocardiogram (ECG) changes, such as flattening of the T wave, prolongation of the QTc interval, and ST segment depression. The clinical significance of these findings is unknown. Large doses of inhaled or oral salmeterol (12 to 20 times the recommended dose) have been associated with clinically significant prolongation of the QTc interval, which has the potential for producing ventricular arrhythmias. Fatalities have been reported in association with excessive use of inhaled sympathomimetic drugs.

5.13 Reduction in Bone Mineral Density

Decreases in bone mineral density (BMD) have been observed with long-term administration of products containing inhaled corticosteroids. The clinical significance of small changes in BMD with regard to long-term consequences such as fracture is unknown. Patients with major risk factors for decreased bone mineral content, such as prolonged immobilization, family history of osteoporosis, postmenopausal status, tobacco use, advanced age, poor nutrition, or chronic use of drugs that can reduce bone mass (e.g., anticonvulsants, oral corticosteroids) should be monitored and treated with established standards of care.

2-Year Fluticasone Propionate Study: A 2-year study of 160 patients (females aged 18 to 40 years, males 18 to 50) with asthma receiving CFC-propelled fluticasone propionate inhalation aerosol 88 or 440 mcg twice daily demonstrated no statistically significant changes in BMD at any time point (24, 52, 76, and 104 weeks of double-blind treatment) as assessed by dual-energy x-ray absorptiometry at lumbar regions L1 through L4.

5.14 Effect on Growth

Orally inhaled corticosteroids may cause a reduction in growth velocity when administered to pediatric patients. Monitor the growth of pediatric patients receiving ADVAIR HFA routinely (e.g., via stadiometry). To minimize the systemic effects of orally inhaled corticosteroids, including ADVAIR HFA, titrate each patient's dose to the lowest dosage that effectively controls his/her symptoms [see Use in Specific Populations (8.4)].

5.15 Glaucoma and Cataracts

Glaucoma, increased intraocular pressure, and cataracts have been reported in patients with asthma following the long-term administration of inhaled corticosteroids, including fluticasone propionate, a component of ADVAIR HFA. Therefore, close monitoring is warranted in patients with a change in vision or with a history of increased intraocular pressure, glaucoma, and/or cataracts.

5.16 Eosinophilic Conditions and Churg-Strauss Syndrome

In rare cases, patients on inhaled fluticasone propionate, a component of ADVAIR HFA, may present with systemic eosinophilic conditions. Some of these patients have clinical features of vasculitis consistent with Churg-Strauss syndrome, a condition that is often treated with systemic corticosteroid therapy. These events usually, but not always, have been associated with the reduction and/or withdrawal of oral corticosteroid therapy following the introduction of fluticasone propionate. Cases of serious eosinophilic conditions have also been reported with other inhaled corticosteroids in this clinical setting. Physicians should be alert to eosinophilia, vasculitic rash, worsening pulmonary symptoms, cardiac complications, and/or neuropathy presenting in their patients. A causal relationship between fluticasone propionate and these underlying conditions has not been established.

5.17 Coexisting Conditions

ADVAIR HFA, like all medications containing sympathomimetic amines, should be used with caution in patients with convulsive disorders or thyrotoxicosis and in those who are unusually responsive to sympathomimetic amines. Doses of the related beta$_2$-adrenoceptor agonist albuterol, when administered intravenously, have been reported to aggravate preexisting diabetes mellitus and ketoacidosis.

5.18 Hypokalemia and Hyperglycemia

Beta-adrenergic agonist medications may produce significant hypokalemia in some patients, possibly through intracellular shunting, which has the potential to produce adverse cardiovascular effects [see Clinical Pharmacology (12.2)]. The decrease in serum potassium is usually transient, not requiring supplementation. Clinically significant changes in blood glucose and/or serum potassium were seen infrequently during clinical studies with ADVAIR HFA at recommended doses.

6 ADVERSE REACTIONS

LABAs, such as salmeterol, one of the active ingredients in ADVAIR HFA, increase the risk of asthma-related death. Data from a large placebo-controlled US study that compared the safety of salmeterol (SEREVENT Inhalation Aerosol) or placebo added to usual asthma therapy showed an increase in asthma-related deaths in patients receiving salmeterol [see Warnings and Precautions (5.1)]. Currently available data are inadequate to determine whether concurrent use of inhaled corticosteroids or other long-term asthma control drugs mitigates the increased risk of asthma-related death from LABAs. Available data from controlled clinical trials suggest that LABAs increase the risk of asthma-related hospitalization in pediatric and adolescent patients.

Systemic and local corticosteroid use may result in the following:

- *Candida albicans* infection [see Warnings and Precautions (5.4)]
- Pneumonia in patients with COPD [see Warnings and Precautions (5.5)]
- Immunosuppression [see Warnings and Precautions (5.6)]
- Hypercorticism and adrenal suppression [see Warnings and Precautions (5.8)]
- Growth effects [see Warnings and Precautions (5.14)]
- Glaucoma and cataracts [see Warnings and Precautions (5.15)]

6.1 Clinical Trials Experience

Because clinical trials are conducted under widely varying conditions, adverse reaction rates observed in the clinical trials of a drug cannot be directly compared with rates in the clinical trials of another drug and may not reflect the rates observed in practice.

Adult and Adolescent Patients Aged 12 Years and Older: The incidence of adverse reactions associated with ADVAIR HFA in Table 2 is based upon 2 placebo-controlled 12-week US clinical studies (Studies 1 and 3) and 1 active-controlled 12-week US clinical study (Study 2). A total of 1,008 adult and adolescent patients with asthma (556 females and 452 males) previously treated with albuterol alone, salmeterol, or inhaled corticosteroids were treated twice daily with 2 inhalations of ADVAIR HFA 45/21 or ADVAIR HFA 115/21, fluticasone propionate chlorofluorocarbon (CFC) inhalation aerosol (44- or 110-mcg doses), salmeterol CFC inhalation aerosol 21 mcg, or placebo HFA inhalation aerosol. The average duration of exposure was 71 to 81 days in the active treatment groups compared with 51 days in the placebo group.

[See table 2 above]

The incidence of common adverse reactions reported in Study 4, a 12-week non-US clinical study of 509 patients previously treated with inhaled corticosteroids who were treated twice daily with 2 inhalations of ADVAIR HFA 230/21, fluticasone propionate CFC inhalation aerosol 220 mcg, or 1 inhalation of ADVAIR DISKUS 500/50 was similar to the incidences reported in Table 2.

Additional Adverse Reactions: Other adverse reactions not previously listed, whether considered drug-related or not by the investigators, that occurred in the groups receiving ADVAIR HFA with an incidence of 1% to 3% and that occurred at a greater incidence than with placebo include the following: tachycardia, arrhythmias, myocardial infarction, postoperative complications, wounds and lacerations, soft tissue injuries, ear signs and symptoms, rhinorrhea/postnasal drip, epistaxis, nasal congestion/blockage, laryngitis, unspecified oropharyngeal plaques, dryness of nose, weight gain, allergic eye disorders, eye edema and swelling, gastrointestinal discomfort and pain, dental discomfort and pain, candidiasis mouth/throat, hyposalivation, gastrointestinal infections, disorders of hard tissue of teeth, abdominal discomfort and pain, oral abnormalities, arthralgia and articular rheumatism, muscle cramps and spasms, musculoskeletal inflammation, bone and skeletal pain, muscle injuries, sleep disorders, migraines, allergies and allergic reactions, viral infections, bacterial infections, candidiasis unspecified site, congestion, inflammation, bacterial reproductive infections, lower respiratory signs and symptoms, lower respiratory infections, lower respiratory hemorrhage, eczema, dermatitis and dermatosis, urinary infections.

Laboratory Test Abnormalities: In Study 3, there were more reports of hyperglycemia among adults and adolescents receiving ADVAIR HFA, but this was not seen in Studies 1 and 2.

6.2 Postmarketing Experience

In addition to adverse reactions reported from clinical trials, the following adverse reactions have been identified during postmarketing use of any formulation of ADVAIR, fluticasone propionate, and/or salmeterol regardless of indication. Because these reactions are reported voluntarily from a population of uncertain size, it is not always possible to reliably estimate their frequency or establish a causal relationship to drug exposure. These events have been chosen for inclusion due to either their seriousness, frequency of reporting, or causal connection to ADVAIR, fluticasone propionate, and/or salmeterol or a combination of these factors.

Cardiovascular: Arrhythmias (including atrial fibrillation, extrasystoles, supraventricular tachycardia), hypertension, ventricular tachycardia.

Ear, Nose, and Throat: Aphonia, earache, facial and oropharyngeal edema, paranasal sinus pain, rhinitis, throat soreness, tonsillitis.

Endocrine and Metabolic: Cushing's syndrome, Cushingoid features, growth velocity reduction in children/adolescents, hypercorticism, osteoporosis.

Eye: Cataracts, glaucoma.

Gastrointestinal: Dyspepsia, xerostomia.

Hepatobiliary Tract and Pancreas: Abnormal liver function tests.

Immune System: Immediate and delayed hypersensitivity reactions, including rash and rare events of angioedema, bronchospasm, and anaphylaxis.

Infections and Infestations: Esophageal candidiasis.

Musculoskeletal: Back pain, myositis.

Neurology: Paresthesia, restlessness.

Non-Site Specific: Fever, pallor.

Psychiatry: Agitation, aggression, anxiety, depression. Behavioral changes, including hyperactivity and irritability, have been reported very rarely and primarily in children.

Respiratory: Asthma; asthma exacerbation; chest congestion; chest tightness; cough; dyspnea; immediate bronchospasm; influenza; paradoxical bronchospasm; tracheitis; wheezing; pneumonia; reports of upper respiratory symptoms of laryngeal spasm, irritation, or swelling such as stridor or choking.

Skin: Contact dermatitis, contusions, ecchymoses, photodermatitis, pruritus.

Urogenital: Dysmenorrhea, irregular menstrual cycle, pelvic inflammatory disease, vaginal candidiasis, vaginitis, vulvovaginitis.

7 DRUG INTERACTIONS

ADVAIR HFA has been used concomitantly with other drugs, including short-acting beta₂-agonists, methylxanthines, and intranasal corticosteroids, commonly used in patients with asthma, without adverse drug reactions [see Clinical Pharmacology (12.2)]. No formal drug interaction studies have been performed with ADVAIR HFA.

7.1 Inhibitors of Cytochrome P450 3A4

Fluticasone propionate and salmeterol, the individual components of ADVAIR HFA, are substrates of CYP3A4. The use of strong CYP3A4 inhibitors (e.g., ritonavir, atazanavir, clarithromycin, indinavir, itraconazole, nefazodone, nelfinavir, saquinavir, ketoconazole, telithromycin) with ADVAIR HFA is not recommended because increased systemic corticosteroid and increased cardiovascular adverse effects may occur.

Ritonavir: *Fluticasone Propionate:* A drug interaction study with fluticasone propionate aqueous nasal spray in healthy subjects has shown that ritonavir (a strong CYP3A4 inhibitor) can significantly increase plasma fluticasone propionate exposure, resulting in significantly reduced serum cortisol concentrations [see Clinical Pharmacology (12.3)]. During postmarketing use, there have been reports of clinically significant drug interactions in patients receiving fluticasone propionate and ritonavir, resulting in systemic corticosteroid effects including Cushing's syndrome and adrenal suppression.

Ketoconazole: *Fluticasone Propionate:* Coadministration of orally inhaled fluticasone propionate (1,000 mcg) and ketoconazole (200 mg once daily) resulted in increased plasma fluticasone propionate exposure and reduced plasma cortisol area under the curve (AUC), but had no effect on urinary excretion of cortisol.

Salmeterol: In a drug interaction study in 20 healthy subjects, coadministration of inhaled salmeterol (50 mcg twice daily) and oral ketoconazole (400 mg once daily) for 7 days resulted in greater systemic exposure to salmeterol (AUC increased 16-fold and C_{max} increased 1.4-fold). Three (3) subjects were withdrawn due to beta₂-agonist side effects (2 with prolonged QTc and 1 with palpitations and sinus tachycardia). Although there was no statistical effect on the mean QTc, coadministration of salmeterol and ketoconazole was associated with more frequent increases in QTc duration compared with salmeterol and placebo administration.

7.2 Monoamine Oxidase Inhibitors and Tricyclic Antidepressants

ADVAIR HFA should be administered with extreme caution to patients being treated with monoamine oxidase inhibitors or tricyclic antidepressants, or within 2 weeks of discontinuation of such agents, because the action of salmeterol, a component of ADVAIR HFA, on the vascular system may be potentiated by these agents.

7.3 Beta-Adrenergic Receptor Blocking Agents

Beta-blockers not only block the pulmonary effect of beta-agonists, such as salmeterol, a component of ADVAIR HFA, but may produce severe bronchospasm in patients with reversible obstructive airways disease. Therefore, patients with asthma should not normally be treated with beta-blockers. However, under certain circumstances, there may be no acceptable alternatives to the use of beta-adrenergic blocking agents for these patients; cardioselective beta-blockers could be considered, although they should be administered with caution.

7.4 Diuretics

The ECG changes and/or hypokalemia that may result from the administration of nonpotassium-sparing diuretics (such as loop or thiazide diuretics) can be acutely worsened by beta-agonists such as salmeterol, a component of ADVAIR HFA, especially when the recommended dose of the beta-agonist is exceeded. Although the clinical relevance of these effects is not known, caution is advised in the coadministration of ADVAIR HFA with nonpotassium-sparing diuretics.

8 USE IN SPECIFIC POPULATIONS

8.1 Pregnancy

Teratogenic Effects: Pregnancy Category C. There are no adequate and well-controlled studies with ADVAIR HFA in

Table 2. Adverse Reactions With ≥3% Incidence With ADVAIR HFA Inhalation Aerosol in Adult and Adolescent Patients With Asthma

Adverse Event	ADVAIR HFA Inhalation Aerosol		Fluticasone Propionate CFC Inhalation Aerosol		Salmeterol CFC Inhalation Aerosol	Placebo HFA Inhalation Aerosol
	45/21 (n = 187) %	115/21 (n = 94) %	44 mcg (n = 186) %	110 mcg (n = 91) %	21 mcg (n = 274) %	(n = 176) %
Ear, nose, and throat						
Upper respiratory tract infection	16	24	13	15	17	13
Throat irritation	9	7	12	13	9	7
Upper respiratory inflammation	4	4	3	7	5	3
Hoarseness/dysphonia	3	1	2	0	1	0
Lower respiratory						
Viral respiratory infection	3	5	4	5	3	4
Neurology						
Headache	21	15	24	16	20	11
Dizziness	4	1	4	1	<1	0
Gastrointestinal						
Nausea and vomiting	5	3	4	2	2	3
Viral gastrointestinal infection	4	2	2	0	1	2
Gastrointestinal signs and symptoms	3	2	2	1	1	1
Musculoskeletal						
Musculoskeletal pain	5	7	8	2	4	4
Muscle pain	4	1	1	1	3	<1

pregnant women. The combination of fluticasone propionate and salmeterol was teratogenic in mice and rats. Fluticasone propionate alone was teratogenic in mice, rats, and rabbits, and salmeterol alone was teratogenic in rabbits and not in rats. From the reproduction toxicity studies in mice and rats, no evidence of enhanced toxicity was seen using combinations of fluticasone propionate and salmeterol when compared with toxicity data from the components administered separately.

ADVAIR HFA should be used during pregnancy only if the potential benefit justifies the potential risk to the fetus.
Combination of Fluticasone Propionate and Salmeterol: In the mouse reproduction assay, fluticasone propionate by the subcutaneous route at a dose approximately equivalent to the maximum recommended human daily inhalation dose (MRHD) (on a mcg/m^2 basis at a maternal dose of 150 mcg/kg) combined with oral salmeterol at a dose approximately 580 times the MRHD (on a mg/m^2 basis at a maternal dose of 10 mg/kg) produced cleft palate, fetal death, increased implantation loss, and delayed ossification. These observations are characteristic of glucocorticoids. No developmental toxicity was observed at combination doses of fluticasone propionate subcutaneously up to approximately 1/5 the MRHD (on a mcg/m^2 basis at a maternal dose of 40 mcg/kg) and oral doses of salmeterol up to approximately 80 times the MRHD (on a mg/m^2 basis at a maternal dose of 1.4 mg/kg). In rats, combining fluticasone propionate subcutaneously at a dose equivalent to the MRHD (on a mcg/m^2 basis at a maternal dose of 100 mcg/kg) and an oral dose of salmeterol at approximately 1,200 times the MRHD (on a mg/m^2 basis at a maternal dose of 10 mg/kg) produced decreased fetal weight, umbilical hernia, delayed ossification, and changes in the occipital bone. No such effects were seen when combining fluticasone propionate subcutaneously at a dose less than the MRHD (on a mcg/m^2 basis at a maternal dose of 30 mcg/kg) and an oral dose of salmeterol at approximately 120 times the MRHD (on a mg/m^2 basis at a maternal dose of 1 mg/kg).
Fluticasone Propionate: Subcutaneous studies in mice at a dose less than the MRHD (on a mcg/m^2 basis at a maternal dose of 45 mcg/kg) and in rats at a dose equivalent to the MRHD (on a mcg/m^2 basis at a maternal dose of 100 mcg/kg) revealed fetal toxicity characteristic of potent corticosteroid compounds, including embryonic growth retardation, omphalocele, cleft palate, and retarded cranial ossification. No teratogenicity was seen in rats at inhalation doses approximately equivalent to the MRHD (on a mcg/m^2 basis at maternal doses up to 68.7 mg/kg).

In rabbits, fetal weight reduction and cleft palate were observed at a subcutaneous dose less than the MRHD (on a mcg/m^2 basis at a maternal dose of 4 mcg/kg). However, no teratogenic effects were reported at oral doses up to approximately 6 times the MRHD (on a mcg/m^2 basis at maternal doses up to 300 mcg/kg). No fluticasone propionate was detected in the plasma in this study, consistent with the established low bioavailability following oral administration *[see Clinical Pharmacology (12.3)]*.

Fluticasone propionate crossed the placenta following subcutaneous administration to mice and rats and oral administration to rabbits.

Experience with oral corticosteroids since their introduction in pharmacologic, as opposed to physiologic, doses suggests that rodents are more prone to teratogenic effects from corticosteroids than humans. In addition, because there is a natural increase in corticosteroid production during pregnancy, most women will require a lower exogenous corticosteroid dose and many will not need corticosteroid treatment during pregnancy.

Salmeterol: No teratogenic effects occurred in rats at oral doses approximately 230 times the MRHD (on a mg/m^2 basis at maternal doses up to 2 mg/kg). In Dutch rabbits administered oral doses approximately 25 times the MRHD (on an AUC basis at maternal doses of 1 mg/kg and higher), salmeterol exhibited fetal toxic effects characteristically resulting from beta-adrenoceptor stimulation. These included precocious eyelid openings, cleft palate, sternebral fusion, limb and paw flexures, and delayed ossification of the frontal cranial bones. No such effects occurred at an oral dose approximately 10 times the MRHD (on an AUC basis at a maternal dose of 0.6 mg/kg).

New Zealand White rabbits were less sensitive since only delayed ossification of the frontal cranial bones was seen at an oral dose approximately 2,300 times the MRHD (on a mg/m^2 basis at a maternal dose of 10 mg/kg). Extensive use of other beta-agonists has provided no evidence that these class effects in animals are relevant to their use in humans. Salmeterol xinafoate crossed the placenta following oral administration to mice and rats.

8.2 Labor and Delivery
There are no well-controlled human studies that have investigated effects of ADVAIR HFA on preterm labor or labor at term. Because of the potential for beta-agonist interference with uterine contractility, use of ADVAIR HFA during labor should be restricted to those patients in whom the benefits clearly outweigh the risks.

8.3 Nursing Mothers
Plasma levels of salmeterol, a component of ADVAIR HFA, after inhaled therapeutic doses are very low. In rats, salmeterol xinafoate is excreted in the milk. There are no data from controlled trials on the use of salmeterol by nursing mothers. It is not known whether fluticasone propionate is excreted in human breast milk. However, other corticosteroids have been detected in human milk. Subcutaneous administration to lactating rats of tritiated fluticasone propionate resulted in measurable radioactivity in milk.

Since there are no data from controlled trials on the use of ADVAIR HFA by nursing mothers, caution should be exercised when ADVAIR HFA is administered to a nursing woman.

8.4 Pediatric Use
Thirty-eight (38) patients aged 12 to 17 years were treated with ADVAIR HFA in US pivotal clinical trials. Patients in this age-group demonstrated efficacy results similar to those observed in patients aged 18 years and older. There were no obvious differences in the type or frequency of adverse events reported in this age-group compared with patients aged 18 years and older.

In a 12-week study, the safety of ADVAIR HFA 45/21 given as 2 inhalations twice daily was compared with that of fluticasone propionate 44 mcg HFA (FLOVENT® HFA) 2 inhalations twice daily in 350 subjects aged 4 to 11 years with persistent asthma currently being treated with inhaled corticosteroids. No new safety concerns were observed in children aged 4 to 11 years treated for 12 weeks with ADVAIR HFA 45/21 compared with adults and adolescents aged 12 years and older. Common adverse reactions (≥3%) seen in children aged 4 to 11 years treated with ADVAIR HFA 45/21 but not reported in the adult and adolescent clinical trials of ADVAIR HFA include: pyrexia, cough, pharyngolaryngeal pain, rhinitis, and sinusitis *[see Adverse Reactions (6.1)]*. This study was not designed to assess the effect of salmeterol, a component of ADVAIR HFA, on asthma hospitalizations and death in patients aged 4 to 11 years.

The pharmacokinetics and pharmacodynamic effect on serum cortisol of 21 days of treatment with ADVAIR HFA 45/21 (2 inhalations twice daily with or without a spacer) or ADVAIR DISKUS 100/50 (1 inhalation twice daily) was evaluated in a study of 31 children aged 4 to 11 years with mild asthma. Systemic exposure to salmeterol xinafoate was similar for ADVAIR HFA, ADVAIR HFA delivered with a spacer, and ADVAIR DISKUS while the systemic exposure to fluticasone propionate was lower with ADVAIR HFA compared with that of ADVAIR HFA delivered with a spacer or ADVAIR DISKUS. There were reductions in serum cortisol from baseline in all treatment groups (14%, 22%, and 13% for ADVAIR HFA, ADVAIR HFA delivered with a spacer, and ADVAIR DISKUS, respectively) *[see Clinical Pharmacology (12.2, 12.3)]*.

The safety and effectiveness of ADVAIR HFA in children less than 12 years have not been established.

Effects on Growth: Inhaled corticosteroids, including fluticasone propionate, a component of ADVAIR HFA, may cause a reduction in growth velocity in children and adolescents *[see Warnings and Precautions (5.14)]*. The growth of pediatric patients receiving orally inhaled corticosteroids, including ADVAIR HFA, should be monitored.

A 52-week placebo-controlled study to assess the potential growth effects of fluticasone propionate inhalation powder (FLOVENT® ROTADISK®) at 50 and 100 mcg twice daily was conducted in the US in 325 prepubescent children (244 males and 81 females) aged 4 to 11 years. The mean growth velocities at 52 weeks observed in the intent-to-treat population were 6.32 cm/year in the placebo group (n = 76), 6.07 cm/year in the 50-mcg group (n = 98), and 5.66 cm/year in the 100-mcg group (n = 89). An imbalance in the proportion of children entering puberty between groups and a higher dropout rate in the placebo group due to poorly controlled asthma may be confounding factors in interpreting these data. A separate subset analysis of children who remained prepubertal during the study revealed growth rates at 52 weeks of 6.10 cm/year in the placebo group (n = 57), 5.91 cm/year in the 50-mcg group (n = 74), and 5.67 cm/year in the 100-mcg group (n = 79). In children aged 8.5 years, the mean age of children in this study, the range for expected growth velocity is: boys – 3rd percentile = 3.8 cm/year, 50th percentile = 5.4 cm/year, and 97th percentile = 7.0 cm/year; girls – 3rd percentile = 4.2 cm/year, 50th percentile = 5.7 cm/year, and 97th percentile = 7.3 cm/year. The clinical relevance of these growth data is not certain.

If a child or adolescent on any corticosteroid appears to have growth suppression, the possibility that he/she is particularly sensitive to this effect of corticosteroids should be considered. The potential growth effects of prolonged treatment should be weighed against the clinical benefits obtained. To minimize the systemic effects of orally inhaled corticosteroids, including ADVAIR HFA, each patient should be titrated to the lowest strength that effectively controls his/her asthma.

8.5 Geriatric Use
Clinical studies of ADVAIR HFA did not include sufficient numbers of patients aged 65 years and older to determine whether older patients respond differently than younger patients. In general, dose selection for an elderly patient should be cautious, usually starting at the low end of the dosing range, reflecting the greater frequency of decreased hepatic, renal, or cardiac function, and of concomitant disease or other drug therapy. In addition, as with other products containing beta$_2$-agonists, special caution should be observed when using ADVAIR HFA in geriatric patients who have concomitant cardiovascular disease that could be adversely affected by beta$_2$-agonists.

8.6 Hepatic Impairment
Formal pharmacokinetic studies using ADVAIR HFA have not been conducted in patients with hepatic impairment. However, since both fluticasone propionate and salmeterol are predominantly cleared by hepatic metabolism, impairment of liver function may lead to accumulation of fluticasone propionate and salmeterol in plasma. Therefore, patients with hepatic disease should be closely monitored.

8.7 Renal Impairment
Formal pharmacokinetic studies using ADVAIR HFA have not been conducted in patients with renal impairment.

10 OVERDOSAGE
Fluticasone Propionate: Chronic overdosage with fluticasone propionate may result in signs/symptoms of hypercorticism *[see Warnings and Precautions (5.7)]*. Inhalation by healthy volunteers of a single dose of 4,000 mcg of fluticasone propionate inhalation powder or single doses of 1,760 or 3,520 mcg of fluticasone propionate CFC inhalation aerosol was well tolerated. Fluticasone propionate given by inhalation aerosol at dosages of 1,320 mcg twice daily for 7 to 15 days to healthy human volunteers was also well tolerated. Repeat oral doses up to 80 mg daily for 10 days in healthy volunteers and repeat oral doses up to 20 mg daily for 42 days in patients were well tolerated. Adverse reactions were of mild or moderate severity, and incidences were similar in active and placebo treatment groups.
Salmeterol: The expected signs and symptoms with overdosage of salmeterol are those of excessive beta-adrenergic stimulation and/or occurrence or exaggeration of any of the following: seizures, angina, hypertension or hypotension, tachycardia with rates up to 200 beats/min, arrhythmias, nervousness, headache, tremor, muscle cramps, dry mouth, palpitation, nausea, dizziness, fatigue, malaise, and insomnia. Overdosage with salmeterol can lead to clinically significant prolongation of the QTc interval, which can produce ventricular arrhythmias. Other signs of overdosage may include hypokalemia and hyperglycemia.

As with all sympathomimetic medications, cardiac arrest and even death may be associated with abuse of salmeterol. Treatment consists of discontinuation of salmeterol together with appropriate symptomatic therapy. The judicious use of a cardioselective beta-receptor blocker may be considered, bearing in mind that such medication can produce bronchospasm. There is insufficient evidence to determine if dialysis is beneficial for overdosage of salmeterol. Cardiac monitoring is recommended in cases of overdosage.

11 DESCRIPTION
ADVAIR HFA 45/21 Inhalation Aerosol, ADVAIR HFA 115/21 Inhalation Aerosol, and ADVAIR HFA 230/21 Inhalation Aerosol are combinations of fluticasone propionate and salmeterol xinafoate.

One active component of ADVAIR HFA is fluticasone propionate, a corticosteroid having the chemical name S-(fluoromethyl) 6α,9-difluoro-11β,17-dihydroxy-16α-methyl-3-oxoandrosta-1,4-diene-17β-carbothioate, 17-propionate and the following chemical structure:

Fluticasone propionate is a white powder with a molecular weight of 500.6, and the empirical formula is $C_{25}H_{31}F_3O_5S$. It is practically insoluble in water, freely soluble in dimethyl sulfoxide and dimethylformamide, and slightly soluble in methanol and 95% ethanol.

The other active component of ADVAIR HFA is salmeterol xinafoate, a beta$_2$-adrenergic bronchodilator. Salmeterol xinafoate is the racemic form of the 1-hydroxy-2-naphthoic acid salt of salmeterol. The chemical name of salmeterol xinafoate is 4-hydroxy-α^1-[[[6-(4-phenylbutoxy)hexyl] amino]methyl]-1,3-benzenedimethanol, 1-hydroxy-2-naphthalenecarboxylate, and it has the following chemical structure:

Salmeterol xinafoate is a white powder with a molecular weight of 603.8, and the empirical formula is $C_{25}H_{37}NO_4 \cdot C_{11}H_8O_3$. It is freely soluble in methanol; slightly soluble in ethanol, chloroform, and isopropanol; and sparingly soluble in water.

ADVAIR HFA 45/21 Inhalation Aerosol, ADVAIR HFA 115/21 Inhalation Aerosol, and ADVAIR HFA 230/21 Inhalation Aerosol are pressurized metered-dose aerosol units fitted with a counter. ADVAIR HFA is intended for oral inhalation only. Each unit contains a microcrystalline suspension of fluticasone propionate (micronized) and salmeterol xinafoate (micronized) in propellant HFA-134a (1,1,1,2-tetrafluoroethane). It contains no other excipients.

After priming, each actuation of the inhaler delivers 50, 125, or 250 mcg of fluticasone propionate and 25 mcg of salmeterol in 75 mg of suspension from the valve. Each actuation delivers 45, 115, or 230 mcg of fluticasone propionate and 21 mcg of salmeterol from the actuator. Twenty-one micrograms (21 mcg) of salmeterol base is equivalent to 30.45 mcg of salmeterol xinafoate. The actual amount of drug delivered to the lung may depend on patient factors, such as the coordination between the actuation of the device and inspiration through the delivery system.

Each 8-g canister contains 60 inhalations. Each 12-g canister provides 120 inhalations.

ADVAIR HFA should be primed before using for the first time by releasing 4 test sprays into the air away from the face, shaking well for 5 seconds before each spray. In cases where the inhaler has not been used for more than 4 weeks or when it has been dropped, prime the inhaler again by releasing 2 test sprays into the air away from the face, shaking well for 5 seconds before each spray.

12 CLINICAL PHARMACOLOGY

12.1 Mechanism of Action

ADVAIR HFA: Since ADVAIR HFA contains both fluticasone propionate and salmeterol, the mechanisms of action described below for the individual components apply to ADVAIR HFA. These drugs represent 2 classes of medications (a synthetic corticosteroid and a selective LABA) that have different effects on clinical, physiologic, and inflammatory indices of asthma.

Fluticasone Propionate: Fluticasone propionate is a synthetic trifluorinated corticosteroid with potent anti-inflammatory activity. In vitro assays using human lung cytosol preparations have established fluticasone propionate as a human glucocorticoid receptor agonist with an affinity 18 times greater than dexamethasone, almost twice that of beclomethasone-17-monopropionate (BMP), the active metabolite of beclomethasone dipropionate, and over 3 times that of budesonide. Data from the McKenzie vasoconstrictor assay in man are consistent with these results.

Inflammation is an important component in the pathogenesis of asthma. Corticosteroids have been shown to inhibit multiple cell types (e.g., mast cells, eosinophils, basophils, lymphocytes, macrophages, neutrophils) and mediator production or secretion (e.g., histamine, eicosanoids, leukotrienes, cytokines) involved in the asthmatic response. These anti-inflammatory actions of corticosteroids contribute to their efficacy in asthma.

Salmeterol Xinafoate: Salmeterol is a selective LABA. In vitro studies show salmeterol to be at least 50 times more selective for beta$_2$-adrenoceptors than albuterol. Although beta$_2$-adrenoceptors are the predominant adrenergic receptors in bronchial smooth muscle and beta$_1$-adrenoceptors are the predominant receptors in the heart, there are also beta$_2$-adrenoceptors in the human heart comprising 10% to 50% of the total beta-adrenoceptors. The precise function of these receptors has not been established, but their presence raises the possibility that even selective beta$_2$-agonists may have cardiac effects.

The pharmacologic effects of beta$_2$-adrenoceptor agonist drugs, including salmeterol, are at least in part attributable to stimulation of intracellular adenyl cyclase, the enzyme that catalyzes the conversion of adenosine triphosphate (ATP) to cyclic-3',5'-adenosine monophosphate (cyclic AMP). Increased cyclic AMP levels cause relaxation of bronchial smooth muscle and inhibition of release of mediators of immediate hypersensitivity from cells, especially from mast cells.

In vitro tests show that salmeterol is a potent and long-lasting inhibitor of the release of mast cell mediators, such as histamine, leukotrienes, and prostaglandin D$_2$, from human lung. Salmeterol inhibits histamine-induced plasma protein extravasation and inhibits platelet-activating factor-induced eosinophil accumulation in the lungs of guinea pigs when administered by the inhaled route. In humans, single doses of salmeterol administered via inhalation aerosol attenuate allergen-induced bronchial hyper-responsiveness.

12.2 Pharmacodynamics

ADVAIR HFA: Healthy Subjects: Cardiovascular Effects: Since systemic pharmacodynamic effects of salmeterol are not normally seen at the therapeutic dose, higher doses were used to produce measurable effects. Four (4) placebo-controlled crossover studies were conducted in healthy subjects: (1) a cumulative-dose study using 42 to 336 mcg of salmeterol CFC inhalation aerosol given alone or as ADVAIR HFA 115/21, (2) a single-dose study using 4 inhalations of ADVAIR HFA 230/21, salmeterol CFC inhalation aerosol 21 mcg, or fluticasone propionate CFC inhalation aerosol 220 mcg, (3) a single-dose study using 8 inhalations of ADVAIR HFA 45/21, ADVAIR HFA 115/21, or ADVAIR HFA 230/21, and (4) a single-dose study using 4 inhalations of ADVAIR HFA 230/21; 2 inhalations of ADVAIR DISKUS 500/50; 4 inhalations of fluticasone propionate CFC inhalation aerosol 220 mcg; or 1,010 mcg of fluticasone propionate given intravenously. In these studies pulse rate, blood pressure, QTc interval, glucose, and/or potassium were measured. Comparable or lower effects were observed for ADVAIR HFA compared with ADVAIR DISKUS or salmeterol alone. The effect of salmeterol on pulse rate and potassium was not altered by the presence of different amounts of fluticasone propionate in ADVAIR HFA.

Hypothalamic-Pituitary-Adrenal Axis Effects: The potential effect of salmeterol on the effects of fluticasone propionate on the HPA axis was also evaluated in 3 of these studies. Compared with fluticasone propionate CFC inhalation aerosol, ADVAIR HFA had less effect on 24-hour urinary cortisol excretion and less or comparable effect on 24-hour serum cortisol. In these crossover studies in healthy subjects, ADVAIR HFA and ADVAIR DISKUS had similar effects on urinary and serum cortisol.

Patients With Asthma: Cardiovascular Effects: In clinical studies with ADVAIR HFA in adult and adolescent patients aged 12 years and older with asthma, systemic pharmacodynamic effects of salmeterol (pulse rate, blood pressure, QTc interval, potassium, and glucose) were similar to or slightly lower in patients treated with ADVAIR HFA compared with patients treated with salmeterol CFC inhalation aerosol 21 mcg. In 61 adult and adolescent patients with asthma given ADVAIR HFA (45/21 or 115/21 mcg), continuous 24-hour electrocardiographic monitoring was performed after the first dose and after 12 weeks of twice-daily therapy, and no clinically significant dysrhythmias were noted. The effect of 21 days of treatment with ADVAIR HFA 45/21 (2 inhalations twice daily with or without a spacer) or ADVAIR DISKUS 100/50 (1 inhalation twice daily) was evaluated in 31 children aged 4 to 11 years with mild asthma. There were no notable changes from baseline for QTc, heart rate, or systolic and diastolic blood pressure.

Hypothalamic-Pituitary-Adrenal Axis Effects: A 4-way crossover study in 13 patients with asthma compared pharmacodynamics at steady state following 4 weeks of twice-daily treatment with 2 inhalations of ADVAIR HFA 115/21, 1 inhalation of ADVAIR DISKUS 250/50 mcg, 2 inhalations of fluticasone propionate HFA inhalation aerosol 110 mcg, and placebo. No significant differences in serum cortisol AUC were observed between active treatments and placebo. Mean 12-hour serum cortisol AUC ratios comparing active treatment with placebo ranged from 0.9 to 1.2. No statistically or clinically significant increases in heart rate or QTc interval were observed for any active treatment compared with placebo.

In a 12-week study in adult and adolescent patients with asthma, ADVAIR HFA 115/21 was compared with the individual components, fluticasone propionate CFC inhalation aerosol 110 mcg and salmeterol CFC inhalation aerosol 21 mcg, and placebo [see Clinical Studies (14.1)]. All treatments were administered as 2 inhalations twice daily. After 12 weeks of treatment with these therapeutic doses, the geometric mean ratio of urinary cortisol excretion compared with baseline was 0.9 for ADVAIR HFA and fluticasone propionate and 1.0 for placebo and salmeterol. In addition, the ability to increase cortisol production in response to stress, as assessed by 30-minute cosyntropin stimulation in 23 to 32 patients per treatment group, remained intact for the majority of patients and was similar across treatments. Three patients who received ADVAIR HFA 115/21 had an abnormal response (peak serum cortisol <18 mcg/dL) after dosing, compared with 1 patient who received placebo, 2 patients who received fluticasone propionate 110 mcg, and 1 patient who received salmeterol.

In another 12-week study in adult and adolescent patients with asthma, ADVAIR HFA 230/21 (2 inhalations twice daily) was compared with ADVAIR DISKUS 500/50 (1 inhalation twice daily) and fluticasone propionate CFC inhalation aerosol 220 mcg (2 inhalations twice daily) [see Clinical Studies (14.1)]. The geometric mean ratio of 24-hour urinary cortisol excretion at week 12 compared with baseline was 0.9 for all 3 treatment groups.

The effect of 21 days of treatment with ADVAIR HFA 45/21 (2 inhalations twice daily with or without a spacer) or ADVAIR DISKUS 100/50 (1 inhalation twice daily) on serum cortisol was evaluated in 31 children aged 4 to 11 years with mild asthma. There were reductions in serum cortisol from baseline in all treatment groups (14%, 22%, and 13% for ADVAIR HFA, ADVAIR HFA with spacer, and ADVAIR DISKUS, respectively).

Other Fluticasone Propionate Products: Patients With Asthma: Hypothalamic-Pituitary-Adrenal Axis Effects: In clinical trials with fluticasone propionate inhalation powder using dosages up to and including 250 mcg twice daily, occasional abnormal short cosyntropin tests (peak serum cortisol <18 mcg/dL assessed by radioimmunoassay) were noted both in patients receiving fluticasone propionate and in patients receiving placebo. The incidence of abnormal tests at 500 mcg twice daily was greater than placebo. In a 2-year study carried out with the DISKHALER® inhalation device in 64 patients with mild, persistent asthma (mean FEV$_1$ 91% of predicted) randomized to fluticasone propionate 500 mcg twice daily or placebo, no patient receiving fluticasone propionate had an abnormal response to 6-hour cosyntropin infusion (peak serum cortisol <18 mcg/dL). With a peak cortisol threshold of <35 mcg/dL, 1 patient receiving fluticasone propionate (4%) had an abnormal response at 1 year; repeat testing at 18 months and 2 years was normal. Another patient receiving fluticasone propionate (5%) had an abnormal response at 2 years. No patient on placebo had an abnormal response at 1 or 2 years.

Other Salmeterol Xinafoate Products: Patients With Asthma: Cardiovascular Effects: Inhaled salmeterol, like other beta-adrenergic agonist drugs, can produce dose-related cardiovascular effects and effects on blood glucose and/or serum potassium [see Warnings and Precautions (5.12, 5.18)]. The cardiovascular effects (heart rate, blood pressure) associated with salmeterol occur with similar frequency, and are of similar type and severity, as those noted following albuterol administration.

The effects of rising inhaled doses of salmeterol and standard inhaled doses of albuterol were studied in volunteers and in patients with asthma. Salmeterol doses up to 84 mcg administered as inhalation aerosol resulted in heart rate increases of 3 to 16 beats/min, about the same as albuterol dosed at 180 mcg by inhalation aerosol (4 to 10 beats/min). In 2 double-blind asthma studies, patients receiving either 42 mcg of salmeterol inhalation aerosol twice daily (n = 81) or 180 mcg of albuterol inhalation aerosol 4 times daily (n = 80) underwent continuous electrocardiographic monitoring during four 24-hour periods; no clinically significant dysrhythmias were noted.

Concomitant Use of ADVAIR HFA With Other Respiratory Medications: Short-Acting Beta$_2$-Agonists: In three 12-week US clinical trials, the mean daily need for additional beta$_2$-agonist use in 277 patients receiving ADVAIR HFA was approximately 1.2 inhalations/day and ranged from 0 to 9 inhalations/day. Two percent (2%) of patients receiving ADVAIR HFA in these trials averaged 6 or more inhalations per day over the course of the 12-week trials. No increase in frequency of cardiovascular adverse reactions was observed among patients who averaged 6 or more inhalations per day.

Methylxanthines: The concurrent use of intravenously or orally administered methylxanthines (e.g., aminophylline, theophylline) by patients receiving ADVAIR HFA has not been completely evaluated. In five 12-week clinical trials (3 US and 2 non-US), 45 patients receiving ADVAIR HFA 45/21, 115/21, or 230/21 twice daily concurrently with a theophylline product had adverse event rates similar to those in 577 patients receiving ADVAIR HFA without theophylline.

Fluticasone Propionate Nasal Spray: In patients receiving ADVAIR HFA in three 12-week US clinical trials, no difference in the profile of adverse events or HPA axis effects was noted between patients receiving FLONASE® (fluticasone propionate) Nasal Spray, 50 mcg concurrently (n = 89) and those who were not (n = 192).

12.3 Pharmacokinetics

Absorption: Fluticasone Propionate: Healthy Subjects: Fluticasone propionate acts locally in the lung; therefore, plasma levels do not predict therapeutic effect. Studies using oral dosing of labeled and unlabeled drug have demonstrated that the oral systemic bioavailability of fluticasone propionate is negligible (<1%), primarily due to incomplete absorption and presystemic metabolism in the gut and liver. In contrast, the majority of the fluticasone propionate delivered to the lung is systemically absorbed.

Three single-dose placebo-controlled crossover studies were conducted in healthy subjects: (1) a study using 4 inhalations of ADVAIR HFA 230/21, salmeterol CFC inhalation aerosol 21 mcg, or fluticasone propionate CFC inhalation aerosol 220 mcg, (2) a study using 8 inhalations of ADVAIR HFA 45/21, ADVAIR HFA 115/21, or ADVAIR HFA 230/21, and (3) a study using 4 inhalations of ADVAIR HFA 230/21; 2 inhalations of ADVAIR DISKUS 500/50; 4 inhalations of fluticasone propionate CFC inhalation aerosol 220 mcg; or 1,010 mcg of fluticasone propionate given intravenously. Peak plasma concentrations of fluticasone propionate were achieved in 0.33 to 1.5 hours and those of salmeterol were achieved in 5 to 10 minutes.

Peak plasma concentrations of fluticasone propionate (N = 20 subjects) following 8 inhalations of ADVAIR HFA 45/21, ADVAIR HFA 115/21, and ADVAIR HFA 230/21 averaged 41, 108, and 173 pg/mL, respectively.

Systemic exposure (N = 20 subjects) from 4 inhalations of ADVAIR HFA 230/21 was 53% of the value from the individual inhaler for fluticasone propionate CFC inhalation aerosol and 42% of the value from the individual inhaler for salmeterol CFC inhalation aerosol. Peak plasma concentrations from ADVAIR HFA for fluticasone propionate (86 versus 120 pg/mL) and salmeterol (170 versus 510 pg/mL) were significantly lower compared with individual inhalers.

In 15 healthy subjects, systemic exposure (AUC) to fluticasone propionate from 4 inhalations of ADVAIR HFA 230/21 (920/84 mcg) and 2 inhalations of ADVAIR DISKUS 500/50 (1,000/100 mcg) were similar between the 2 inhalers (i.e., 799 versus 832 pg•h/mL, respectively) but approximately half the systemic exposure from 4 inhalations of fluticasone propionate CFC inhalation aerosol 220 mcg (880 mcg, AUC = 1,543 pg•h/mL). Similar results were observed for peak fluticasone propionate plasma concentrations (186 and 182 pg/mL from ADVAIR HFA and ADVAIR DISKUS, respectively, and 307 pg/mL from the fluticasone propionate CFC inhalation aerosol). Absolute bioavailability of fluticasone propionate was 5.3% and 5.5% following administration of ADVAIR HFA and ADVAIR DISKUS, respectively.

Patients With Asthma: A double-blind crossover study was conducted in 13 adult patients with asthma to evaluate the steady-state pharmacokinetics of fluticasone propionate and salmeterol following administration of 2 inhalations of ADVAIR HFA 115/21 twice daily or 1 inhalation of ADVAIR DISKUS 250/50 twice daily for 4 weeks. Systemic exposure (AUC) to fluticasone propionate was similar for ADVAIR HFA (274 pg•h/mL [95% CI: 150, 502]) and ADVAIR DISKUS (338 pg•h/mL [95% CI: 197, 581]).

The effect of 21 days of treatment with ADVAIR HFA 45/21 (2 inhalations twice daily with or without a spacer) or ADVAIR DISKUS 100/50 (1 inhalation twice daily) was evaluated in a study of 31 children aged 4 to 11 years with mild asthma. Systemic exposure to fluticasone propionate was similar with ADVAIR DISKUS and ADVAIR HFA with a spacer (138 pg•h/mL [95% CI: 69, 273] and 107 pg•h/mL [95% CI: 46, 252], respectively) and lower with ADVAIR HFA without a spacer (24 pg•h/mL [95% CI: 10, 60]).

Salmeterol: Healthy Subjects: Salmeterol xinafoate, an ionic salt, dissociates in solution so that the salmeterol and 1-hydroxy-2-naphthoic acid (xinafoate) moieties are absorbed, distributed, metabolized, and eliminated independently. Salmeterol acts locally in the lung; therefore, plasma levels do not predict therapeutic effect.

Peak plasma concentrations of salmeterol (N = 20 subjects) following 8 inhalations of ADVAIR HFA 45/21, ADVAIR HFA 115/21, and ADVAIR HFA 230/21 ranged from 220 to 470 pg/mL.

In 15 healthy subjects receiving ADVAIR HFA 230/21 (920/84 mcg) and ADVAIR DISKUS 500/50 (1,000/100 mcg), systemic exposure to salmeterol was higher (317 versus 169 pg•h/mL) and peak salmeterol concentrations were lower (196 versus 223 pg/mL) following ADVAIR HFA compared with ADVAIR DISKUS, although pharmacodynamic results were comparable.

Patients With Asthma: Because of the small therapeutic dose, systemic levels of salmeterol are low or undetectable after inhalation of recommended dosages (42 mcg of salmeterol inhalation aerosol twice daily). Following chronic administration of an inhaled dosage of 42 mcg of salmeterol inhalation aerosol twice daily, salmeterol was detected in plasma within 5 to 10 minutes in 6 patients with asthma; plasma concentrations were very low, with mean peak concentrations of 150 pg/mL at 20 minutes and no accumulation with repeated doses.

A double-blind crossover study was conducted in 13 adult patients with asthma to evaluate the steady-state pharmacokinetics of fluticasone propionate and salmeterol following administration of 2 inhalations of ADVAIR HFA 115/21 twice daily or 1 inhalation of ADVAIR DISKUS 250/50 twice daily for 4 weeks. Systemic exposure to salmeterol was similar for ADVAIR HFA (53 pg•h/mL [95% CI: 17, 164]) and ADVAIR DISKUS (70 pg•h/mL [95% CI: 19, 254]).

The effect of 21 days of treatment with ADVAIR HFA 45/21 (2 inhalations twice daily with or without a spacer) or

ADVAIR DISKUS 100/50 (1 inhalation twice daily) was evaluated in 31 children aged 4 to 11 years with mild asthma. Systemic exposure to salmeterol was similar for ADVAIR HFA, ADVAIR HFA with spacer, and ADVAIR DISKUS (126 pg•h/mL [95% CI: 70, 225], 103 pg•h/mL [95% CI: 54, 200], and 110 pg•h/mL [95% CI: 55, 219], respectively).

Distribution: *Fluticasone Propionate:* Following intravenous administration, the initial disposition phase for fluticasone propionate was rapid and consistent with its high lipid solubility and tissue binding. The volume of distribution averaged 4.2 L/kg.

The percentage of fluticasone propionate bound to human plasma proteins averages 99%. Fluticasone propionate is weakly and reversibly bound to erythrocytes and is not significantly bound to human transcortin.

Salmeterol: The percentage of salmeterol bound to human plasma proteins averages 96% in vitro over the concentration range of 8 to 7,722 ng of salmeterol base per milliliter, much higher concentrations than those achieved following therapeutic doses of salmeterol.

Metabolism: *Fluticasone Propionate:* The total clearance of fluticasone propionate is high (average, 1,093 mL/min), with renal clearance accounting for less than 0.02% of the total. The only circulating metabolite detected in man is the 17β-carboxylic acid derivative of fluticasone propionate, which is formed through the CYP3A4 pathway. This metabolite had less affinity (approximately 1/2,000) than the parent drug for the glucocorticoid receptor of human lung cytosol in vitro and negligible pharmacological activity in animal studies. Other metabolites detected in vitro using cultured human hepatoma cells have not been detected in man.

Salmeterol: Salmeterol base is extensively metabolized by hydroxylation, with subsequent elimination predominantly in the feces. No significant amount of unchanged salmeterol base was detected in either urine or feces.

An in vitro study using human liver microsomes showed that salmeterol is extensively metabolized to α-hydroxysalmeterol (aliphatic oxidation) by CYP3A4. Ketoconazole, a strong inhibitor of CYP3A4, essentially completely inhibited the formation of α-hydroxysalmeterol in vitro.

Elimination: *Fluticasone Propionate:* Following intravenous dosing, fluticasone propionate showed polyexponential kinetics and had a terminal elimination half-life of approximately 7.8 hours. Less than 5% of a radiolabeled oral dose was excreted in the urine as metabolites, with the remainder excreted in the feces as parent drug and metabolites. Terminal half-life estimates of fluticasone propionate for ADVAIR HFA, ADVAIR DISKUS, and fluticasone propionate CFC inhalation aerosol were similar and averaged 5.6 hours.

Salmeterol: In 2 healthy adult subjects who received 1 mg of radiolabeled salmeterol (as salmeterol xinafoate) orally, approximately 25% and 60% of the radiolabeled salmeterol was eliminated in urine and feces, respectively, over a period of 7 days. The terminal elimination half-life was about 5.5 hours (1 volunteer only).

The xinafoate moiety has no apparent pharmacologic activity. The xinafoate moiety is highly protein bound (>99%) and has a long elimination half-life of 11 days. No terminal half-life estimates were calculated for salmeterol following administration of ADVAIR HFA.

Special Populations: A population pharmacokinetic analysis was performed for fluticasone propionate and salmeterol utilizing data from 9 controlled clinical trials that included 350 patients with asthma aged 4 to 77 years who received treatment with ADVAIR DISKUS, ADVAIR HFA, fluticasone propionate inhalation powder (FLOVENT® DISKUS®), HFA-propelled fluticasone propionate inhalation aerosol (FLOVENT HFA), or CFC-propelled fluticasone propionate inhalation aerosol. The population pharmacokinetic analyses for fluticasone propionate and salmeterol showed no clinically relevant effects of age, gender, race, body weight, body mass index, or percent of predicted FEV_1 on apparent clearance and apparent volume of distribution.

Hepatic and Renal Impairment: Formal pharmacokinetic studies using ADVAIR HFA have not been conducted in patients with hepatic or renal impairment. However, since both fluticasone propionate and salmeterol are predominantly cleared by hepatic metabolism, impairment of liver function may lead to accumulation of fluticasone propionate and salmeterol in plasma. Therefore, patients with hepatic disease should be closely monitored.

Drug Interactions: In the repeat- and single-dose studies, there was no evidence of significant drug interaction in systemic exposure between fluticasone propionate and salmeterol when given alone or in combination via the DISKUS. Similar definitive studies have not been performed with ADVAIR HFA. The population pharmacokinetic analysis from 9 controlled clinical trials in 350 patients with asthma showed no significant effects on

fluticasone propionate or salmeterol pharmacokinetics following co-administration with beta₂-agonists, corticosteroids, antihistamines, or theophyllines.

Inhibitors of Cytochrome P450 3A4: Ritonavir: Fluticasone Propionate: Fluticasone propionate is a substrate of CYP3A4. Coadministration of fluticasone propionate and the strong CYP3A4 inhibitor ritonavir is not recommended based upon a multiple-dose crossover drug interaction study in 18 healthy subjects. Fluticasone propionate aqueous nasal spray (200 mcg once daily) was coadministered for 7 days with ritonavir (100 mg twice daily). Plasma fluticasone propionate concentrations following fluticasone propionate aqueous nasal spray alone were undetectable (<10 pg/mL) in most subjects, and when concentrations were detectable peak levels (C_{max}) averaged 11.9 pg/mL (range: 10.8 to 14.1 pg/mL) and $AUC_{(0-\tau)}$ averaged 8.43 pg•h/mL (range: 4.2 to 18.8 pg•h/mL). Fluticasone propionate C_{max} and $AUC_{(0-\tau)}$ increased to 318 pg/mL (range: 110 to 648 pg/mL) and 3,102.6 pg•h/mL (range: 1,207.1 to 5,662.0 pg•h/mL), respectively, after coadministration of ritonavir with fluticasone propionate aqueous nasal spray. This significant increase in plasma fluticasone propionate exposure resulted in a significant decrease (86%) in serum cortisol AUC.

Ketoconazole: Fluticasone Propionate: In a placebo-controlled, crossover study in 8 healthy adult volunteers, coadministration of a single dose of orally inhaled fluticasone propionate (1,000 mcg) with multiple doses of ketoconazole (200 mg) to steady state resulted in increased plasma fluticasone propionate exposure, a reduction in plasma cortisol AUC, and no effect on urinary excretion of cortisol.

Salmeterol: In a placebo-controlled, crossover drug interaction study in 20 healthy male and female subjects, coadministration of salmeterol (50 mcg twice daily) and the strong CYP3A4 inhibitor ketoconazole (400 mcg once daily) for 7 days resulted in a significant increase in plasma salmeterol exposure as determined by a 16-fold increase in AUC (ratio with and without ketoconazole 15.76 [90% CI: 10.66, 23.31]) mainly due to increased bioavailability of the swallowed portion of the dose. Peak plasma salmeterol concentrations were increased by 1.4-fold (90% CI: 1.23, 1.68). Three (3) out of 20 subjects (15%) were withdrawn from salmeterol and ketoconazole coadministration due to beta-agonist–mediated systemic effects (2 with QTc prolongation and 1 with palpitations and sinus tachycardia). Coadministration of salmeterol and ketoconazole did not result in a clinically significant effect on mean heart rate, mean blood potassium, or mean blood glucose. Although there was no statistical effect on the mean QTc, coadministration of salmeterol and ketoconazole was associated with more frequent increases in QTc duration compared with salmeterol and placebo administration.

Erythromycin: Fluticasone Propionate: In a multiple-dose drug interaction study, coadministration of orally inhaled fluticasone propionate (500 mcg twice daily) and erythromycin (333 mg 3 times daily) did not affect fluticasone propionate pharmacokinetics.

Salmeterol: In a repeat-dose study in 13 healthy subjects, concomitant administration of erythromycin (a moderate CYP3A4 inhibitor) and salmeterol inhalation aerosol resulted in a 40% increase in salmeterol C_{max} at steady state (ratio with and without erythromycin 1.4 [90% CI: 0.96, 2.03], P = 0.12), a 3.6-beat/min increase in heart rate ([95% CI: 0.19, 7.03], P <0.04), a 5.8-msec increase in QTc interval ([95% CI: -6.14, 17.77], P = 0.34), and no change in plasma potassium.

13 NONCLINICAL TOXICOLOGY

13.1 Carcinogenesis, Mutagenesis, Impairment of Fertility

Fluticasone Propionate: Fluticasone propionate demonstrated no tumorigenic potential in mice at oral doses up to 1,000 mcg/kg (approximately 5 times the MRHD on a mcg/m² basis) for 78 weeks or in rats at inhalation doses up to 57 mcg/kg (less than the MRHD on a mcg/m² basis) for 104 weeks.

Fluticasone propionate did not induce gene mutation in prokaryotic or eukaryotic cells in vitro. No significant clastogenic effect was seen in cultured human peripheral lymphocytes in vitro or in the in vivo mouse micronucleus test.

No evidence of impairment of fertility was observed in reproductive studies conducted in rats at subcutaneous doses up to 50 mcg/kg (less than the MRHD on a mcg/m² basis). Prostate weight was significantly reduced.

Salmeterol: In an 18-month carcinogenicity study in CD-mice, salmeterol at oral doses of 1.4 mg/kg and above (approximately 10 times the MRHD based on comparison of the plasma AUCs) caused a dose-related increase in the incidence of smooth muscle hyperplasia, cystic glandular hyperplasia, leiomyomas of the uterus, and ovarian cysts. No tumors were seen at 0.2 mg/kg (approximately 2 times the MRHD for adults based on comparison of the AUCs).

In a 24-month oral and inhalation carcinogenicity study in Sprague Dawley rats, salmeterol caused a dose-related increase in the incidence of mesovarian leiomyomas and ovarian cysts at doses of 0.68 mg/kg and above (approximately 80 times the MRHD on a mg/m^2 basis). No tumors were seen at 0.21 mg/kg (approximately 25 times the MRHD on a mg/m^2 basis). These findings in rodents are similar to those reported previously for other beta-adrenergic agonist drugs. The relevance of these findings to human use is unknown. Salmeterol produced no detectable or reproducible increases in microbial and mammalian gene mutation in vitro. No clastogenic activity occurred in vitro in human lymphocytes or in vivo in a rat micronucleus test. No effects on fertility were identified in rats treated with salmeterol at oral doses up to 2 mg/kg (approximately 230 times the MRHD on a mg/m^2 basis).

13.2 Animal Toxicology and/or Pharmacology

Preclinical: Studies in laboratory animals (minipigs, rodents, and dogs) have demonstrated the occurrence of cardiac arrhythmias and sudden death (with histologic evidence of myocardial necrosis) when beta-agonists and methylxanthines are administered concurrently. The clinical relevance of these findings is unknown.

Propellant HFA-134a: In animals and humans, propellant HFA-134a was found to be rapidly absorbed and rapidly eliminated, with an elimination half-life of 3 to 27 minutes in animals and 5 to 7 minutes in humans. Time to maximum plasma concentration (T_{max}) and mean residence time are both extremely short, leading to a transient appearance of HFA-134a in the blood with no evidence of accumulation. Propellant HFA-134a is devoid of pharmacological activity except at very high doses in animals (i.e., 380 to 1,300 times the maximum human exposure based on comparisons of area under the plasma concentration versus time curve [AUC] values), primarily producing ataxia, tremors, dyspnea, or salivation. These events are similar to effects produced by the structurally related CFCs, which have been used extensively in metered-dose inhalers. In drug interaction studies in male and female dogs, there was a slight increase in the salmeterol-related effect on heart rate (a known effect of beta$_2$-agonists) when given in combination with high doses of fluticasone propionate. This effect was not observed in clinical studies.

14 CLINICAL STUDIES

ADVAIR HFA has been studied in patients with asthma aged 12 years and older. ADVAIR HFA has not been studied in patients less than 12 years of age or in patients with COPD. In clinical trials comparing ADVAIR HFA Inhalation Aerosol with its individual components, improvements in most efficacy endpoints were greater with ADVAIR HFA than with the use of either fluticasone propionate or salmeterol alone. In addition, clinical trials showed comparable results between Advair HFA and Advair Diskus.

14.1 Studies Comparing ADVAIR HFA With Fluticasone Propionate Alone or Salmeterol Alone

Four (4) double-blind parallel-group clinical trials were conducted with ADVAIR HFA in 1,517 adult and adolescent patients (≥12 years, mean baseline FEV$_1$ 65% to 75% of predicted normal) with asthma that was not optimally controlled on their current therapy. All metered-dose inhaler treatments were inhalation aerosols given as 2 inhalations twice daily, and other maintenance therapies were discontinued.

Study 1: Clinical Trial With ADVAIR HFA 45/21 Inhalation Aerosol: This placebo-controlled 12-week US study compared ADVAIR HFA 45/21 with fluticasone propionate CFC inhalation aerosol 44 mcg or salmeterol CFC inhalation aerosol 21 mcg, each given as 2 inhalations twice daily. The primary efficacy endpoints were predose FEV$_1$ and withdrawals due to worsening asthma. This study was stratified according to baseline asthma therapy: patients using beta-agonists (albuterol alone [n = 142], salmeterol [n = 84], or inhaled corticosteroids [n = 134] [daily doses of beclomethasone dipropionate 252 to 336 mcg; budesonide 400 to 600 mcg; flunisolide 1,000 mcg; fluticasone propionate inhalation aerosol 176 mcg; fluticasone propionate inhalation powder 200 mcg; or triamcinolone acetonide 600 to 800 mcg]). Baseline FEV$_1$ measurements were similar across treatments: ADVAIR HFA 45/21, 2.29 L; fluticasone propionate 44 mcg, 2.20 L; salmeterol, 2.33 L; and placebo, 2.27 L.

Predefined withdrawal criteria for lack of efficacy, an indicator of worsening asthma, were utilized for this placebo-controlled study. Worsening asthma was defined as a clinically important decrease in FEV$_1$ or PEF, increase in use of VENTOLIN® (albuterol, USP) Inhalation Aerosol, increase in night awakenings due to asthma, emergency intervention or hospitalization due to asthma, or requirement for asthma medication not allowed by the protocol. As shown in Table 3, statistically significantly fewer patients receiving ADVAIR HFA 45/21 were withdrawn due to worsening asthma compared with salmeterol and placebo. Fewer patients receiving ADVAIR HFA 45/21 were withdrawn due to worsening asthma compared with fluticasone propionate 44 mcg; however, the difference was not statistically significant.

Table 4. Secondary Efficacy Variable Results for Patients Previously Treated With Beta$_2$-Agonists (Albuterol or Salmeterol) or Inhaled Corticosteroids (Study 1)

Efficacy Variable[a]	ADVAIR HFA 45/21 Inhalation Aerosol (n = 92)	Fluticasone Propionate CFC Inhalation Aerosol 44 mcg (n = 89)	Salmeterol CFC Inhalation Aerosol 21 mcg (n = 92)	Placebo HFA Inhalation Aerosol (n = 87)
AM PEF (L/min)				
Baseline	377	369	381	382
Change from baseline	58	27	25	1
PM PEF (L/min)				
Baseline	397	387	402	407
Change from baseline	48	20	16	3
Use of VENTOLIN Inhalation Aerosol (inhalations/day)				
Baseline	3.1	2.4	2.7	2.7
Change from baseline	-2.1	-0.4	-0.8	0.2
Asthma symptom score/day				
Baseline	1.8	1.6	1.7	1.7
Change from baseline	-1.0	-0.3	-0.4	0.2

[a] Change from baseline = change from baseline at Endpoint (last available data).

Table 3. Percent of Patients Withdrawn Due to Worsening Asthma in Patients Previously Treated With Beta$_2$-Agonists (Albuterol or Salmeterol) or Inhaled Corticosteroids (Study 1)

ADVAIR HFA 45/21 Inhalation Aerosol (n = 92)	Fluticasone Propionate CFC Inhalation Aerosol 44 mcg (n = 89)	Salmeterol CFC Inhalation Aerosol 21 mcg (n = 92)	Placebo HFA Inhalation Aerosol (n = 87)
2%	8%	25%	28%

The FEV$_1$ results are displayed in Figure 2. Because this trial used predetermined criteria for worsening asthma, which caused more patients in the placebo group to be withdrawn, FEV$_1$ results at Endpoint (last available FEV$_1$ result) are also provided. Patients receiving ADVAIR HFA 45/21 had significantly greater improvements in FEV$_1$ (0.58 L, 27%) compared with fluticasone propionate 44 mcg (0.36 L, 18%), salmeterol (0.25 L, 12%), and placebo (0.14 L, 5%). These improvements in FEV$_1$ with ADVAIR HFA 45/21 were achieved regardless of baseline asthma therapy (albuterol alone, salmeterol, or inhaled corticosteroids).

Figure 2. Mean Percent Change From Baseline in FEV$_1$ in Patients Previously Treated With Either Beta$_2$-Agonists (Albuterol or Salmeterol) or Inhaled Corticosteroids (Study 1)

The effect of ADVAIR HFA 45/21 on the secondary efficacy parameters, including morning and evening PEF, usage of VENTOLIN Inhalation Aerosol, and asthma symptoms over 24 hours on a scale of 0 to 5 is shown in Table 4.
[See table 4 above]

The subjective impact of asthma on patients' perceptions of health was evaluated through use of an instrument called the Asthma Quality of Life Questionnaire (AQLQ) (based on a 7- point scale where 1 = maximum impairment and 7 = none). Patients receiving ADVAIR HFA 45/21 had clinically meaningful improvements in overall asthma-specific quality of life as defined by a difference between groups of ≥0.5 points in change from baseline AQLQ scores (difference in AQLQ score of 1.14 [95% CI: 0.85, 1.44] compared with placebo).

Study 2: Clinical Trial With ADVAIR HFA 45/21 Inhalation Aerosol: This active-controlled 12-week US study compared ADVAIR HFA 45/21 with fluticasone propionate CFC inhalation aerosol 44 mcg and salmeterol CFC inhalation aerosol 21 mcg, each given as 2 inhalations twice daily, in 283 patients using as-needed albuterol alone. The primary efficacy endpoint was predose FEV$_1$. Baseline FEV$_1$ measurements were similar across treatments: ADVAIR HFA 45/21, 2.37 L; fluticasone propionate 44 mcg, 2.31 L; and salmeterol, 2.34 L.

Efficacy results in this study were similar to those observed in Study 1. Patients receiving ADVAIR HFA 45/21 had significantly greater improvements in FEV$_1$ (0.69 L, 33%) compared with fluticasone propionate 44 mcg (0.51 L, 25%) and salmeterol (0.47 L, 22%).

Study 3: Clinical Trial With ADVAIR HFA 115/21 Inhalation Aerosol: This placebo-controlled 12-week US study compared ADVAIR HFA 115/21 with fluticasone propionate CFC inhalation aerosol 110 mcg or salmeterol CFC inhalation aerosol 21 mcg, each given as 2 inhalations twice daily, in 365 patients using inhaled corticosteroids (daily doses of beclomethasone dipropionate 378 to 840 mcg; budesonide 800 to 1,200 mcg; flunisolide 1,250 to 2,000 mcg; fluticasone propionate inhalation aerosol 440 to 660 mcg; fluticasone propionate inhalation powder 400 to 600 mcg; or triamcinolone acetonide 900 to 1,600 mcg). The primary efficacy endpoints were predose FEV$_1$ and withdrawals due to worsening asthma. Baseline FEV$_1$ measurements were similar across treatments: ADVAIR HFA 115/21, 2.23 L; fluticasone propionate 110 mcg, 2.18 L; salmeterol, 2.22 L; and placebo, 2.17 L.

Efficacy results in this study were similar to those observed in Studies 1 and 2. Patients receiving ADVAIR HFA 115/21 had significantly greater improvements in FEV$_1$ (0.41 L, 20%) compared with fluticasone propionate 110 mcg (0.19 L, 9%), salmeterol (0.15 L, 8%), and placebo (-0.12 L, -6%). Significantly fewer patients receiving ADVAIR HFA 115/21 were withdrawn from this study for worsening asthma (7%) compared with salmeterol (24%) and placebo (54%). Fewer patients receiving ADVAIR HFA 115/21 were withdrawn due to worsening asthma (7%) compared with fluticasone propionate 110 mcg (11%); however, the difference was not statistically significant.

Study 4: Clinical Trial With ADVAIR HFA 230/21 Inhalation Aerosol: This active-controlled 12-week non-US study compared ADVAIR HFA 230/21 with fluticasone propionate CFC inhalation aerosol 220 mcg, each given as 2 inhalations twice daily, and with ADVAIR DISKUS 500/50 given as 1 inhalation twice daily in 509 patients using inhaled corticosteroids (daily doses of beclomethasone dipropionate CFC inhalation aerosol 1,500 to 2,000 mcg; budesonide 1,500 to 2,000 mcg; flunisolide 1,500 to 2,000 mcg; fluticasone propionate inhalation aerosol 660 to 880 mcg; or fluticasone propionate inhalation powder 750 to 1,000 mcg). The primary efficacy endpoint was morning PEF.

Baseline morning PEF measurements were similar across treatments: ADVAIR HFA 230/21, 327 L/min; ADVAIR DISKUS 500/50, 341 L/min; and fluticasone propionate 220 mcg, 345 L/min. As shown in Figure 3, morning PEF improved significantly with ADVAIR HFA 230/21 compared with fluticasone propionate 220 mcg over the 12-week treatment period. Improvements in morning PEF observed with ADVAIR HFA 230/21 were similar to improvements observed with ADVAIR DISKUS 500/50.

Figure 3. Mean Percent Change From Baseline in Morning Peak Expiratory Flow in Patients Previously Treated With Inhaled Corticosteroids (Study 4)

	Week 0	N	N	N
ADVAIR HFA 230/21	176	159	130	
ADVAIR DISKUS 500/50	161	147	119	
Fluticasone propionate inhalation aerosol 220 mcg	172	155	133	

14.2 One-Year Safety Study

Clinical Trial With ADVAIR HFA 45/21, 115/21, and 230/21 Inhalation Aerosol: This 1-year open-label non-US study evaluated the safety of ADVAIR HFA 45/21, 115/21, and 230/21 given as 2 inhalations twice daily in 325 patients. This study was stratified into 3 groups according to baseline asthma therapy: patients using short-acting beta$_2$-agonists alone (n = 42), salmeterol (n = 91), or inhaled corticosteroids (n = 277). Patients treated with short-acting beta$_2$-agonists alone, salmeterol, or low doses of inhaled corticosteroids with or without concurrent salmeterol received ADVAIR HFA 45/21. Patients treated with moderate doses of inhaled corticosteroids with or without concurrent salmeterol received ADVAIR HFA 115/21. Patients treated with high doses of inhaled corticosteroids with or without concurrent salmeterol received ADVAIR HFA 230/21. Baseline FEV$_1$ measurements ranged from 2.3 to 2.6 L.

Improvements in FEV$_1$ (0.17 to 0.35 L at 4 weeks) were seen across all 3 treatments and were sustained throughout the 52-week treatment period. Few patients (3%) were withdrawn due to worsening asthma over 1 year.

14.3 Onset of Action and Progression of Improvement in Control

The onset of action and progression of improvement in asthma control were evaluated in 2 placebo-controlled US trials and 1 active-controlled US trial. Following the first dose, the median time to onset of clinically significant bronchodilatation (≥15% improvement in FEV$_1$) in most patients was seen within 30 to 60 minutes. Maximum improvement in FEV$_1$ occurred within 4 hours, and clinically significant improvement was maintained for 12 hours (see Figure 4). Following the initial dose, predose FEV$_1$ relative to Day 1 baseline improved markedly over the first week of treatment and continued to improve over the 12 weeks of treatment in all 3 studies.

No diminution in the 12-hour bronchodilator effect was observed with either ADVAIR HFA 45/21 (Figures 4 and 5) or ADVAIR HFA 230/21 as assessed by FEV$_1$ following 12 weeks of therapy.

[See figure 4 at top of next column]
[See figure 5 at top of next column]

Reduction in asthma symptoms and use of rescue VENTOLIN Inhalation Aerosol and improvement in morning and evening PEF also occurred within the first day of treatment with ADVAIR HFA, and continued to improve over the 12 weeks of therapy in all 3 studies.

16 HOW SUPPLIED/STORAGE AND HANDLING

ADVAIR HFA 45/21 Inhalation Aerosol is supplied in 12-g pressurized aluminum canisters containing 120 metered actuations in boxes of 1 (NDC 0173-0715-20) and 8-g pressurized aluminum canisters containing 60 metered actuations in institutional pack boxes of 1 (NDC 0173-0715-22).

ADVAIR HFA 115/21 Inhalation Aerosol is supplied in 12-g pressurized aluminum canisters containing 120 metered actuations in boxes of 1 (NDC 0173-0716-20) and 8-g pressurized aluminum canisters containing 60 metered actuations in institutional pack boxes of 1 (NDC 0173-0716-22).

ADVAIR HFA 230/21 Inhalation Aerosol is supplied in 12-g pressurized aluminum canisters containing 120 metered actuations in boxes of 1 (NDC 0173-0717-20) and 8-g pressurized aluminum canisters containing 60 metered actuations in institutional pack boxes of 1 (NDC 0173-0717-22).

Each canister is fitted with a counter, supplied with a purple actuator with a light purple strapcap, and sealed in a plastic-coated, moisture-protective foil pouch with a desiccant that should be discarded when the pouch is opened. Each canister is packaged with a Medication Guide leaflet.

Figure 4. Percent Change in Serial 12-Hour FEV$_1$ in Patients Previously Using Either Beta$_2$-Agonists (Albuterol or Salmeterol) or Inhaled Corticosteroids (Study 1)

First Treatment Day

Figure 5. Percent Change in Serial 12-Hour FEV$_1$ in Patients Previously Using Either Beta$_2$-Agonists (Albuterol or Salmeterol) or Inhaled Corticosteroids (Study 1)

Last Treatment Day (Week 12)

The purple actuator supplied with ADVAIR HFA Inhalation Aerosol should not be used with any other product canisters, and actuators from other products should not be used with an ADVAIR HFA Inhalation Aerosol canister.

The correct amount of medication in each actuation cannot be assured after the counter reads 000, even though the canister is not completely empty and will continue to operate. The inhaler should be discarded when the counter reads 000.

Keep out of reach of children. Avoid spraying in eyes. Contents Under Pressure: Do not puncture. Do not use or store near heat or open flame. Exposure to temperatures above 120°F may cause bursting. Never throw container into fire or incinerator.

Store at 25°C (77°F); excursions permitted to 15°-30°C (59°-86°F). Store the inhaler with the mouthpiece down. For best results, the inhaler should be at room temperature before use. SHAKE WELL FOR 5 SECONDS BEFORE USING.

17 PATIENT COUNSELING INFORMATION

See FDA-approved patient labeling (Medication Guide).

17.1 Asthma-Related Death

Patients should be informed that salmeterol, one of the active ingredients in ADVAIR HFA, increases the risk of asthma-related death and may increase the risk of asthma-related hospitalization in pediatric and adolescent patients. They should also be informed that currently available data are inadequate to determine whether concurrent use of in-haled corticosteroids or other long-term asthma control drugs mitigates the increased risk of asthma-related death from LABAs.

17.2 Not for Acute Symptoms

ADVAIR HFA is not meant to relieve acute asthma symptoms, and extra doses should not be used for that purpose. Acute symptoms should be treated with an inhaled, short-acting beta$_2$-agonist such as albuterol. The healthcare provider should provide the patient with such medication and instruct the patient in how it should be used.

Patients should be instructed to seek medical attention immediately if they experience any of the following:

- Decreasing effectiveness of inhaled, short-acting beta$_2$-agonists
- Need for more inhalations than usual of inhaled, short-acting beta$_2$-agonists
- Significant decrease in lung function as outlined by the physician

Patients should not stop therapy with ADVAIR HFA without physician/provider guidance since symptoms may recur after discontinuation.

17.3 Do Not Use Additional Long-Acting Beta$_2$-Agonists

When patients are prescribed ADVAIR HFA, other LABAs for asthma should not be used.

17.4 Risks Associated With Corticosteroid Therapy

Local Effects: Patients should be advised that localized infections with *Candida albicans* occurred in the mouth and pharynx in some patients. If oropharyngeal candidiasis develops, it should be treated with appropriate local or systemic (i.e., oral) antifungal therapy while still continuing therapy with ADVAIR HFA, but at times therapy with ADVAIR HFA may need to be temporarily interrupted under close medical supervision. Rinsing the mouth after inhalation is advised.

Pneumonia: Patients with COPD have a higher risk of pneumonia and should be instructed to contact their healthcare provider if they develop symptoms of pneumonia.

Immunosuppression: Patients who are on immunosuppressant doses of corticosteroids should be warned to avoid exposure to chickenpox or measles and if they are exposed to consult their physicians without delay. Patients should be informed of potential worsening of existing tuberculosis; fungal, bacterial, viral, or parasitic infections; or ocular herpes simplex.

Hypercorticism and Adrenal Suppression: Patients should be advised that ADVAIR HFA may cause systemic corticosteroid effects of hypercorticism and adrenal suppression. Additionally, patients should be instructed that deaths due to adrenal insufficiency have occurred during and after transfer from systemic corticosteroids. Patients should taper slowly from systemic corticosteroids if transferring to ADVAIR HFA.

Reduction in Bone Mineral Density: Patients who are at an increased risk for decreased BMD should be advised that the use of corticosteroids may pose an additional risk.

Reduced Growth Velocity: Patients should be informed that orally inhaled corticosteroids, including fluticasone propionate, may cause a reduction in growth velocity when administered to pediatric patients. Physicians should closely follow the growth of children and adolescents taking corticosteroids by any route.

Ocular Effects: Long-term use of inhaled corticosteroids may increase the risk of some eye problems (cataracts or glaucoma); regular eye examinations should be considered.

17.5 Risks Associated With Beta-Agonist Therapy

Patients should be informed of adverse effects associated with beta$_2$-agonists, such as palpitations, chest pain, rapid heart rate, tremor, or nervousness.

ADVAIR, ADVAIR DISKUS, DISKUS, FLONASE, FLOVENT, ROTADISK, SEREVENT, and VENTOLIN are registered trademarks of the GSK group of companies. The other brands listed are trademarks of their respective owners and are not trademarks of the GSK group of companies. The makers of these brands are not affiliated with and do not endorse GlaxoSmithKline or its products.

GlaxoSmithKline
Research Triangle Park, NC 27709
©2014, the GSK group of companies. All rights reserved.
ADH:9PI

PHARMACIST—DETACH HERE AND GIVE MEDICATION GUIDE TO PATIENT

MEDICATION GUIDE
ADVAIR® HFA [ad' vair] 45/21 Inhalation Aerosol (fluticasone propionate 45 mcg and salmeterol 21 mcg)
ADVAIR® HFA 115/21 Inhalation Aerosol (fluticasone propionate 115 mcg and salmeterol 21 mcg)
ADVAIR® HFA 230/21 Inhalation Aerosol (fluticasone propionate 230 mcg and salmeterol 21 mcg)
Read the Medication Guide that comes with ADVAIR HFA Inhalation Aerosol before you start using it and each time you get a refill. There may be new information. This Medication Guide does not take the place of talking to your healthcare provider about your medical condition or treatment.

What is the most important information I should know about ADVAIR HFA?

ADVAIR HFA can cause serious side effects, including:

1. **People with asthma who take long-acting beta$_2$-adrenergic agonist (LABA) medicines, such as salmeterol (one of the medicines in ADVAIR HFA), have an increased risk of death from asthma problems.** It is not known whether fluticasone propionate, the other medicine in ADVAIR HFA, reduces the risk of death from asthma problems seen with salmeterol.

• **Call your healthcare provider if breathing problems worsen over time while using ADVAIR HFA.** You may need different treatment.

• **Get emergency medical care if:**
   • breathing problems worsen quickly and
   • you use your rescue inhaler medicine, but it does not relieve your breathing problems.

2. ADVAIR HFA should be used only if your healthcare provider decides that your asthma is not well controlled with a long-term asthma control medicine, such as inhaled corticosteroids.

3. When your asthma is well controlled, your healthcare provider may tell you to stop taking ADVAIR HFA. Your healthcare provider will decide if you can stop ADVAIR HFA without loss of asthma control. Your healthcare provider may prescribe a different long-term asthma control medicine for you, such as an inhaled corticosteroid.

4. Children and adolescents who take LABA medicines may have an increased risk of being hospitalized for asthma problems.

What is ADVAIR HFA?

• ADVAIR HFA combines an inhaled corticosteroid medicine, fluticasone propionate (the same medicine found in FLOVENT®), and a LABA medicine, salmeterol (the same medicine found in SEREVENT®).
   • Inhaled corticosteroids help to decrease inflammation in the lungs. Inflammation in the lungs can lead to asthma symptoms.
   • LABA medicines are used in people with asthma and chronic obstructive pulmonary disease (COPD). LABA medicines help the muscles around the airways in your lungs stay relaxed to prevent symptoms, such as wheezing and shortness of breath. These symptoms can happen when the muscles around the airways tighten. This makes it hard to breathe. In severe cases, wheezing can stop your breathing and cause death if not treated right away.
• ADVAIR HFA is used to control symptoms of asthma and to prevent symptoms such as wheezing in adults and adolescents aged 12 years and older
• ADVAIR HFA should not be used as a rescue inhaler.
• ADVAIR HFA contains salmeterol (the same medicine found in SEREVENT). LABA medicines, such as salmeterol, increase the risk of death from asthma problems.

ADVAIR HFA is not for adults and adolescents with asthma who are well controlled with an asthma control medicine, such as a low to medium dose of an inhaled corticosteroid medicine.

Who should not use ADVAIR HFA?

Do not use ADVAIR HFA:

• to treat sudden, severe symptoms of asthma and
• if you are allergic to any of the ingredients in ADVAIR HFA. See the end of this Medication Guide for a list of ingredients in ADVAIR HFA.

What should I tell my healthcare provider before using ADVAIR HFA?

Tell your healthcare provider about all of your health conditions, including if you:
• **have heart problems**
• **have high blood pressure**
• **have seizures**
• **have thyroid problems**
• **have diabetes**
• **have liver problems**
• **have osteoporosis**
• **have an immune system problem**
• **have eye problems such as increased pressure in the eye (glaucoma) or cataracts**
• **are pregnant or planning to become pregnant.** It is not known if ADVAIR HFA may harm your unborn baby.
• **are breastfeeding.** It is not known if ADVAIR HFA passes into your milk and if it can harm your baby.
• **are allergic to ADVAIR HFA or any other medicines**
• **are exposed to chickenpox or measles**

Tell your healthcare provider about all the medicines you take including prescription and non-prescription medicines, vitamins, and herbal supplements. ADVAIR HFA and certain other medicines may interact with each other. This may cause serious side effects. Especially, tell your healthcare provider if you take ritonavir. The anti-HIV medicines NORVIR® (ritonavir capsules) Soft Gelatin, NORVIR (ritonavir oral solution), and KALETRA® (lopinavir/ritonavir) Tablets contain ritonavir.

Know the medicines you take. Keep a list and show it to your healthcare provider and pharmacist each time you get a new medicine.

How do I use ADVAIR HFA?

See the step-by-step instructions for using ADVAIR HFA at the end of this Medication Guide. Do not use ADVAIR HFA unless your healthcare provider has taught you and you understand everything. Ask your healthcare provider or pharmacist if you have any questions.

• Use ADVAIR HFA exactly as prescribed. **Do not use ADVAIR HFA more often than prescribed.** ADVAIR HFA comes in 3 strengths. Your healthcare provider has prescribed the one that is best for your condition.
• The usual dosage of ADVAIR HFA is 2 inhalations 2 times each day (morning and evening). The 2 doses should be about 12 hours apart. Rinse your mouth with water after using ADVAIR HFA.
• If you take more ADVAIR HFA than your doctor has prescribed, get medical help right away if you have any unusual symptom, such as worsening shortness of breath, chest pain, increased heart rate, or shakiness.
• If you miss a dose of ADVAIR HFA, just skip that dose. Take your next dose at your usual time. Do not take 2 doses at one time.
• **While you are using ADVAIR HFA 2 times each day, do not use other medicines that contain a LABA for any reason.** Ask your healthcare provider or pharmacist if any of your other medicines are LABA medicines.
• Do not stop using ADVAIR HFA or other asthma medicines unless told to do so by your healthcare provider because your symptoms might get worse. Your healthcare provider will change your medicines as needed.
• ADVAIR HFA does not relieve sudden symptoms. Always have a rescue inhaler medicine with you to treat sudden symptoms. If you do not have a short-acting bronchodilator rescue inhaler, call your healthcare provider to have one prescribed for you.
• Call your healthcare provider or get medical care right away if:
   • your breathing problems worsen with ADVAIR HFA
   • you need to use your rescue inhaler medicine more often than usual
   • your rescue inhaler medicine does not work as well for you at relieving symptoms
   • you need to use 4 or more inhalations of your rescue inhaler medicine for 2 or more days in a row
   • you use 1 whole canister of your rescue inhaler medicine in 8 weeks' time
   • your peak flow meter results decrease. Your healthcare provider will tell you the numbers that are right for you.
   • your asthma symptoms do not improve after using ADVAIR HFA regularly for 1 week

What are the possible side effects with ADVAIR HFA?

ADVAIR HFA can cause serious side effects, including:
• See "What is the most important information I should know about ADVAIR HFA?"
• **serious allergic reactions.** Call your healthcare provider or get emergency medical care if you get any of the following symptoms of a serious allergic reaction:
   • rash
   • hives
   • swelling of the face, mouth, and tongue
   • breathing problems
• **sudden breathing problems immediately after inhaling your medicine**
• **effects on heart**
   • increased blood pressure
   • a fast and irregular heartbeat
   • chest pain
• **effects on nervous system**
   • tremor
   • nervousness
• **reduced adrenal function (may result in loss of energy)**
• **changes in blood (sugar, potassium, certain types of white blood cells)**
• **weakened immune system and a higher chance of infections**
• **lower bone mineral density.** This may be a problem for people who already have a higher chance of low bone density (osteoporosis).
• **eye problems including glaucoma and cataracts.** You should have regular eye exams while using ADVAIR HFA.
• **slowed growth in children.** A child's growth should be checked often.
• **throat tightness**
• **pneumonia.** ADVAIR HFA contains the same medicine found in ADVAIR DISKUS®. ADVAIR DISKUS is used to treat people with asthma and people with chronic obstructive pulmonary disease (COPD). People with COPD have a higher chance of getting pneumonia. ADVAIR DISKUS may increase the chance of getting pneumonia. ADVAIR HFA has not been studied in people with COPD. Call your healthcare provider if you notice any of the following symptoms:

• increase in mucus (sputum) production
• change in mucus color
• fever
• chills
• increased cough
• increased breathing problems

Common side effects of ADVAIR HFA include:
• upper respiratory tract infection
• throat irritation
• hoarseness and voice changes
• headache
• dizziness
• nausea and vomiting

Tell your healthcare provider about any side effect that bothers you or that does not go away.

These are not all the side effects with ADVAIR HFA. Ask your healthcare provider or pharmacist for more information.

Call your doctor for medical advice about side effects. You may report side effects to FDA at 1-800-FDA-1088.

How do I store ADVAIR HFA?

• Store ADVAIR HFA at room temperature between 59°F to 86°F (15°C to 30°C), with the mouthpiece down.
• **Contents Under Pressure:** Do not puncture. Do not use or store near heat or open flame. Exposure to temperatures above 120°F may cause bursting.
• Do not throw into fire or an incinerator.
• Keep ADVAIR HFA and all medicines out of the reach of children.

General Information about ADVAIR HFA

Medicines are sometimes prescribed for purposes not mentioned in a Medication Guide. Do not use ADVAIR HFA for a condition for which it was not prescribed. Do not give your ADVAIR HFA to other people, even if they have the same condition that you have. It may harm them.

This Medication Guide summarizes the most important information about ADVAIR HFA. If you would like more information, talk with your healthcare provider or pharmacist. You can ask your healthcare provider or pharmacist for information about ADVAIR HFA that was written for healthcare professionals. You can also contact the company that makes ADVAIR HFA (toll free) at 1-888-825-5249 or at www.advair.com.

What are the ingredients in ADVAIR HFA?

Active ingredients: fluticasone propionate, salmeterol xinafoate

Inactive ingredient: propellant HFA-134a

Instructions for using your ADVAIR HFA

The parts of your ADVAIR HFA

There are 2 main parts to your ADVAIR HFA inhaler—the metal canister that holds the medicine and the purple plastic actuator that sprays the medicine from the canister (see Figure 1).

Figure 1

The canister has a counter to show how many sprays of medicine you have left. The number shows through a window in the back of the actuator. The counter starts at 124, or at 064 if you have a sample or institutional canister. The number will count down by 1 each time you spray the inhaler. The counter will stop counting at 000.

Never try to change the numbers or take the counter off the metal canister. The counter cannot be reset, and it is permanently attached to the canister.

The mouthpiece of the actuator is covered by a cap. The strap on the cap keeps it attached to the actuator.

Do not use the actuator with a canister of medicine from any other inhaler. Do not use an ADVAIR HFA canister with an actuator from any other inhaler.

Using your ADVAIR HFA

• The inhaler should be at room temperature before you use it.
• Take your ADVAIR HFA inhaler out of the moisture-protective pouch just before you use it for the first time. Safely throw away the foil pouch and the drying packet that comes inside the pouch.

Priming your ADVAIR HFA

Before you use ADVAIR HFA for the first time, you must prime the inhaler so that you will get the right amount of medicine when you use it. To prime the inhaler, take the cap off the mouthpiece and shake the inhaler well for 5 seconds. Then spray the inhaler 1 time into the air away from your face. **Avoid spraying in eyes.** Shake and spray the inhaler like this 3 more times to finish priming it. The counter should now read 120, or 060 if you have a sample or institutional canister.

You must prime your inhaler again if you have not used it in more than 4 weeks or if you drop it. Take the cap off the mouthpiece, shake the inhaler well for 5 seconds. Then spray it into the air away from your face. Shake and spray the inhaler like this 1 more time to finish priming it.

Read the following 7 steps before using ADVAIR HFA and follow them at each use. If you have any questions, ask your doctor or pharmacist.

1. **Take the cap off the mouthpiece of the actuator** (see Figure 2).

Look inside the mouthpiece for foreign objects, and take out any you see.

Make sure the canister fits firmly in the actuator.

Shake the inhaler well for 5 seconds.

Figure 2

2. Hold the inhaler with the mouthpiece down (see Figure 2).

Breathe out through your mouth and push as much air from your lungs as you can. Put the mouthpiece in your mouth and close your lips around it.

3. **Push the top of the canister all the way down while you breathe in deeply and slowly through your mouth** (see Figure 3).

Right after the spray comes out, take your finger off the canister. After you have breathed in all the way, take the inhaler out of your mouth and close your mouth.

Figure 3

4. **Hold your breath as long as you can** , up to 10 seconds, then breathe normally.

5. **Wait about 30 seconds and shake the inhaler** well for 5 seconds. Repeat steps 2 through 4.

6. After you finish taking this medicine, rinse your mouth with water. Spit out the water. Do not swallow it.

7. Put the cap back on the mouthpiece after every time you use the inhaler. Make sure it snaps firmly into place.

Cleaning your ADVAIR HFA

Clean your inhaler at least 1 time each week after your evening dose. It is important to keep the canister and plastic actuator clean so the medicine will not build-up and block the spray.

1. Take the cap off the mouthpiece. The strap on the cap will stay attached to the actuator. Do not take the canister out of the plastic actuator.

2. Use a dry cotton swab to clean the small circular opening where the medicine sprays out of the canister. Carefully twist the swab in a circular motion to take off any medicine (see Figure 4).

Figure 4

3. Wipe the inside of the mouthpiece with a clean tissue dampened with water. Let the actuator air-dry overnight.

4. Put the cap back on the mouthpiece after the actuator has dried.

Replacing your ADVAIR HFA

• **When the counter reads 020**, you should refill your prescription or ask your doctor if you need another prescription for ADVAIR HFA.

• **When the counter reads 000, throw the inhaler away.** You should not keep using the inhaler when the counter reads 000 because you will not receive the right amount of medicine.

• **Do not use the inhaler** after the expiration date, which is on the packaging it comes in.

This Medication Guide has been approved by the U.S. Food and Drug Administration.

ADVAIR, ADVAIR DISKUS, FLOVENT, and SEREVENT are registered trademarks of the GSK group of companies. The other brands listed are trademarks of their respective owners and are not trademarks of the GSK group of companies. The makers of these brands are not affiliated with and do not endorse GlaxoSmithKline or its products.

GlaxoSmithKline
Research Triangle Park, NC 27709
©2014, the GSK group of companies. All rights reserved.
May 2014
ADH:9MG

AMERGE ℞

[ə-merj']

(naratriptan hydrochloride)
Tablets, for oral use

HIGHLIGHTS OF PRESCRIBING INFORMATION

These highlights do not include all the information needed to use AMERGE safely and effectively. See full prescribing information for AMERGE.

AMERGE (naratriptan hydrochloride) Tablets, for oral use
Initial U.S. Approval: 1998

——INDICATIONS AND USAGE——

AMERGE is a serotonin (5-HT$_{1B/1D}$) receptor agonist (triptan) indicated for the acute treatment of migraine with or without aura in adults. (1)

Limitations of Use:

• Use only if a clear diagnosis of migraine has been established. (1)

• Not indicated for the prophylactic therapy of migraine attacks. (1)

• Not indicated for the treatment of cluster headache. (1)

——DOSAGE AND ADMINISTRATION——

• Recommended dose: 1 mg or 2.5 mg. (2.1)

• May repeat dose after 4 hours if needed; not to exceed 5 mg in any 24-hour period. (2.1)

• Mild or moderate renal or hepatic impairment: recommended starting dose is 1 mg not to exceed 2.5 mg in any 24-hour period. (2.2, 2.3)

——DOSAGE FORMS AND STRENGTHS——

Tablets: 1 mg and 2.5 mg. (3, 16)

——CONTRAINDICATIONS——

• History of coronary artery disease or coronary artery vasospasm (4)

• Wolff-Parkinson-White syndrome or other cardiac accessory conduction pathway disorders (4)

• History of stroke, transient ischemic attack, or hemiplegic or basilar migraine (4)

• Peripheral vascular disease (4)

• Ischemic bowel disease (4)

• Uncontrolled hypertension (4)

• Recent (within 24 hours) use of another 5-HT$_1$ agonist (e.g., another triptan) or an ergotamine-containing medication (4)

• Hypersensitivity to AMERGE (angioedema and anaphylaxis seen) (4)

• Severe renal or hepatic impairment (4)

——WARNINGS AND PRECAUTIONS——

• Myocardial ischemia/infarction and Prinzmetal's angina: Perform cardiac evaluation in patients with multiple cardiovascular risk factors. (5.1)

• Arrhythmias: Discontinue AMERGE if occurs. (5.2)

• Chest/throat/neck/jaw pain, tightness, pressure, or heaviness: Generally not associated with myocardial ischemia; evaluate for CAD in patients at high risk. (5.3)

• Cerebral hemorrhage, subarachnoid hemorrhage, and stroke: Discontinue AMERGE if occurs. (5.4)

• Gastrointestinal ischemic reactions and peripheral vasospastic reactions: Discontinue AMERGE if occurs. (5.5)

• Medication overuse headache: Detoxification may be necessary. (5.6)

• Serotonin syndrome: Discontinue AMERGE if occurs. (5.7)

——ADVERSE REACTIONS——

Most common adverse reactions (≥2 % and > placebo) were paresthesias, nausea, dizziness, drowsiness, malaise/fatigue, and throat/neck symptoms. (6.1)

To report SUSPECTED ADVERSE REACTIONS, contact GlaxoSmithKline at 1-888-825-5249 or FDA at 1-800-FDA-1088 or www.fda.gov/medwatch

——USE IN SPECIFIC POPULATIONS——

• Pregnancy: Based on animal data, may cause fetal harm (8.1)

See 17 for PATIENT COUNSELING INFORMATION and FDA-approved patient labeling

Revised: 10/2013

FULL PRESCRIBING INFORMATION

1   INDICATIONS AND USAGE

AMERGE® is indicated for the acute treatment of migraine with or without aura in adults.

Limitations of Use:

• Use only if a clear diagnosis of migraine has been established. If a patient has no response to the first migraine attack treated with AMERGE, reconsider the diagnosis of migraine before AMERGE is administered to treat any subsequent attacks.

• AMERGE is not indicated for the prevention of migraine attacks.

• Safety and effectiveness of AMERGE have not been established for cluster headache.

2   DOSAGE AND ADMINISTRATION

2.1   Dosing Information

The recommended dose of AMERGE is 1 mg or 2.5 mg. If the migraine returns or if the patient has only partial response, the dose may be repeated once after 4 hours, for a maximum dose of 5 mg in a 24-hour period.

The safety of treating an average of more than 4 migraine attacks in a 30-day period has not been established.

2.2   Dosage Adjustment in Patients With Renal Impairment

AMERGE is contraindicated in patients with severe renal impairment (creatinine clearance: <15 mL/min) because of decreased clearance of the drug [see Contraindications (4), Use in Specific Populations (8.6), Clinical Pharmacology (12.3)].

In patients with mild to moderate renal impairment, the maximum daily dose should not exceed 2.5 mg over a 24-hour period and a 1-mg starting dose is recommended [see Use in Specific Populations (8.6), Clinical Pharmacology (12.3)].

2.3 Dosage Adjustment in Patients With Hepatic Impairment

AMERGE is contraindicated in patients with severe hepatic impairment (Child-Pugh grade C) because of decreased clearance [see Contraindications (4), Use in Specific Populations (8.7), Clinical Pharmacology (12.3)].

In patients with mild or moderate hepatic impairment (Child-Pugh grade A or B), the maximum daily dose should not exceed 2.5 mg over a 24-hour period and a 1-mg starting dose is recommended [see Use in Specific Populations (8.7), Clinical Pharmacology (12.3)].

3 DOSAGE FORMS AND STRENGTHS

1-mg white tablets, D-shaped, film-coated, and debossed with "GX CE3".

2.5-mg green tablets, D-shaped, film-coated, and debossed with "GX CE5".

4 CONTRAINDICATIONS

AMERGE is contraindicated in patients with:
- Ischemic coronary artery disease (CAD) (angina pectoris, history of myocardial infarction, or documented silent ischemia) or coronary artery vasospasm, including Prinzmetal's angina [see Warnings and Precautions (5.1)]
- Wolff-Parkinson-White syndrome or arrhythmias associated with other cardiac accessory conduction pathway disorders [see Warnings and Precautions (5.2)]
- History of stroke or transient ischemic attack (TIA) or history of hemiplegic or basilar migraine because such patients are at a higher risk of stroke [see Warnings and Precautions (5.4)]
- Peripheral vascular disease [see Warnings and Precautions (5.5)]
- Ischemic bowel disease [see Warnings and Precautions (5.5)]
- Uncontrolled hypertension [see Warnings and Precautions (5.8)]
- Recent use (i.e., within 24 hours) of another 5-HT$_1$ agonist, ergotamine-containing medication, ergot-type medication (such as dihydroergotamine or methysergide) [see Drug Interactions (7.1, 7.2)]
- Hypersensitivity to AMERGE (angioedema and anaphylaxis seen) [see Warnings and Precautions (5.9)]
- Severe renal or hepatic impairment [see Use in Specific Populations (8.6, 8.7), Clinical Pharmacology (12.3)]

5 WARNINGS AND PRECAUTIONS

5.1 Myocardial Ischemia, Myocardial Infarction, and Prinzmetal's Angina

AMERGE is contraindicated in patients with ischemic or vasospastic CAD. There have been rare reports of serious cardiac adverse reactions, including acute myocardial infarction, occurring within a few hours following administration of AMERGE. Some of these reactions occurred in patients without known CAD. AMERGE may cause coronary artery vasospasm (Prinzmetal's angina), even in patients without a history of CAD.

Perform a cardiovascular evaluation in triptan-naive patients who have multiple cardiovascular risk factors (e.g., increased age, diabetes, hypertension, smoking, obesity, strong family history of CAD) prior to receiving AMERGE. If there is evidence of CAD or coronary artery vasospasm, AMERGE is contraindicated. For patients with multiple cardiovascular risk factors who have a negative cardiovascular evaluation, consider administering the first dose of AMERGE in a medically supervised setting and performing an electrocardiogram (ECG) immediately following administration of AMERGE. For such patients, consider periodic cardiovascular evaluation in intermittent long-term users of AMERGE.

5.2 Arrhythmias

Life-threatening disturbances of cardiac rhythm, including ventricular tachycardia and ventricular fibrillation leading to death, have been reported within a few hours following the administration of 5-HT$_1$ agonists. Discontinue AMERGE if these disturbances occur. AMERGE is contraindicated in patients with Wolff-Parkinson-White syndrome or arrhythmias associated with other cardiac accessory conduction pathway disorders.

5.3 Chest, Throat, Neck, and/or Jaw Pain/Tightness/Pressure

Sensations of tightness, pain, and pressure in the chest, throat, neck, and jaw commonly occur after treatment with AMERGE and are usually non-cardiac in origin. However, perform a cardiac evaluation if these patients are at high cardiac risk. 5-HT$_1$ agonists, including AMERGE, are contraindicated in patients with CAD and those with Prinzmetal's variant angina.

5.4 Cerebrovascular Events

Cerebral hemorrhage, subarachnoid hemorrhage, and stroke have occurred in patients treated with 5-HT$_1$ agonists, and some have resulted in fatalities. In a number of cases, it appears possible that the cerebrovascular events were primary, the 5-HT$_1$ agonist having been administered in the incorrect belief that the symptoms experienced were a consequence of migraine when they were not. Also, patients with migraine may be at increased risk of certain cerebrovascular events (e.g., stroke, hemorrhage, TIA). Discontinue AMERGE if a cerebrovascular event occurs.

Before treating headaches in patients not previously diagnosed as migraineurs, and in migraineurs who present with symptoms atypical for migraine, exclude other potentially serious neurological conditions. AMERGE is contraindicated in patients with a history of stroke or TIA.

5.5 Other Vasospasm Reactions

AMERGE may cause non-coronary vasospastic reactions, such as peripheral vascular ischemia, gastrointestinal vascular ischemia and infarction (presenting with abdominal pain and bloody diarrhea), splenic infarction, and Raynaud's syndrome. In patients who experience symptoms or signs suggestive of non-coronary vasospasm reaction following the use of any 5-HT$_1$ agonist, rule out a vasospastic reaction before receiving additional doses of AMERGE.

Reports of transient and permanent blindness and significant partial vision loss have been reported with the use of 5-HT$_1$ agonists. Since visual disorders may be part of a migraine attack, a causal relationship between these events and the use of 5-HT$_1$ agonists have not been clearly established.

5.6 Medication Overuse Headache

Overuse of acute migraine drugs (e.g., ergotamine, triptans, opioids, or combination of these drugs for 10 or more days per month) may lead to exacerbation of headache (medication overuse headache). Medication overuse headache may present as migraine-like daily headaches or as a marked increase in frequency of migraine attacks. Detoxification of patients, including withdrawal of the overused drugs, and treatment of withdrawal symptoms (which often includes a transient worsening of headache) may be necessary.

5.7 Serotonin Syndrome

Serotonin syndrome may occur with AMERGE, particularly during co-administration with selective serotonin reuptake inhibitors (SSRIs), serotonin norepinephrine reuptake inhibitors (SNRIs), tricyclic antidepressants (TCAs), and monoamine oxidase (MAO) inhibitors [see Drug Interactions (7.3)]. Serotonin syndrome symptoms may include mental status changes (e.g., agitation, hallucinations, coma), autonomic instability (e.g., tachycardia, labile blood pressure, hyperthermia), neuromuscular aberrations (e.g., hyperreflexia, incoordination), and/or gastrointestinal symptoms (e.g., nausea, vomiting, diarrhea). The onset of symptoms usually occurs within minutes to hours of receiving a new or a greater dose of a serotonergic medication. Discontinue AMERGE if serotonin syndrome is suspected.

5.8 Increase in Blood Pressure

Significant elevation in blood pressure, including hypertensive crisis with acute impairment of organ systems, has been reported on rare occasions in patients treated with 5-HT$_1$ agonists, including patients without a history of hypertension. Monitor blood pressure in patients treated with AMERGE. AMERGE is contraindicated in patients with uncontrolled hypertension.

5.9 Anaphylactic/Anaphylactoid Reactions

There have been reports of anaphylaxis and anaphylactoid and hypersensitivity reactions, including angioedema, in patients receiving AMERGE. Such reactions can be life threatening or fatal. In general, anaphylactic reactions to drugs are more likely to occur in individuals with a history of sensitivity to multiple allergens. AMERGE is contraindicated in patients with a history of hypersensitivity reaction to AMERGE.

6 ADVERSE REACTIONS

The following adverse reactions are discussed in more detail in other sections of the prescribing information:
- Myocardial ischemia, myocardial infarction, and Prinzmetal's angina [see Warnings and Precautions (5.1)]
- Arrhythmias [see Warnings and Precautions (5.2)]
- Chest, throat, neck, and/or jaw pain/tightness/pressure [see Warnings and Precautions (5.3)]
- Cerebrovascular events [see Warnings and Precautions (5.4)]
- Other vasospasm reactions [see Warnings and Precautions (5.5)]
- Medication overuse headache [see Warnings and Precautions (5.6)]
- Serotonin syndrome [see Warnings and Precautions (5.7)]
- Increase in blood pressure [see Warnings and Precautions (5.8)]
- Hypersensitivity reactions [see Contraindications (4), Warnings and Precautions (5.9)]

6.1 Clinical Trials Experience

Because clinical trials are conducted under widely varying conditions, adverse reaction rates observed in the clinical trials of a drug cannot be directly compared to rates in the clinical trials of another drug and may not reflect the rates observed in practice.

In a long-term open-label trial where patients were allowed to treat multiple migraine attacks for up to 1 year, 15 patients (3.6%) discontinued treatment due to adverse reactions.

In controlled clinical trials, the most common adverse reactions were paresthesias, dizziness, drowsiness, malaise/fatigue, and throat/neck symptoms, which occurred at a rate of 2% and at least 2 times placebo rate.

Table 1 lists the adverse reactions that occurred in 5 placebo-controlled clinical trials of approximately 1,752 exposures to placebo and AMERGE in adult patients with migraine. Only reactions that occurred at a frequency of 2% or more in groups treated with AMERGE 2.5 mg and that occurred at a frequency greater than the placebo group in the 5 pooled trials are included in Table 1.

Table 1. Adverse Reactions Reported by at Least 2% of Patients Treated With AMERGE and at a Frequency Greater Than Placebo

Adverse Reaction	Percent of Patients Reporting		
	AMERGE 1 mg (n = 627)	AMERGE 2.5 mg (n = 627)	Placebo (n = 498)
Atypical sensation	2	4	1
Paresthesias (all types)	1	2	<1
Gastrointestinal	6	7	5
Nausea	4	5	4
Neurological	4	7	3
Dizziness	1	2	1
Drowsiness	1	2	<1
Malaise/fatigue	2	2	1
Pain and pressure sensation	2	4	2
Throat/neck symptoms	1	2	1

The incidence of adverse reactions in controlled clinical trials was not affected by age or weight of the patients, duration of headache prior to treatment, presence of aura, use of prophylactic medications, or tobacco use. There were insufficient data to assess the impact of race on the incidence of adverse reactions.

7 DRUG INTERACTIONS

7.1 Ergot-Containing Drugs

Ergot-containing drugs have been reported to cause prolonged vasospastic reactions. Because these effects may be additive, use of ergotamine-containing or ergot-type medications (like dihydroergotamine or methysergide) and AMERGE within 24 hours of each other is contraindicated.

7.2 Other 5-HT$_1$ Agonists

Concomitant use of other 5-HT$_{1B/1D}$ agonists (including triptans) within 24 hours of treatment with AMERGE is contraindicated because the risk of vasospastic reactions may be additive.

7.3 Selective Serotonin Reuptake Inhibitors/Serotonin Norepinephrine Reuptake Inhibitors and Serotonin Syndrome

Cases of serotonin syndrome have been reported during co-administration of triptans and SSRIs, SNRIs, TCAs, and MAO inhibitors [see Warnings and Precautions (5.7)].

8 USE IN SPECIFIC POPULATIONS

8.1 Pregnancy

Pregnancy Category C: There are no adequate and well-controlled trials in pregnant women. AMERGE should be used during pregnancy only if the potential benefit justifies the potential risk to the fetus.

In reproductive toxicity studies in rats and rabbits, oral administration of naratriptan was associated with developmental toxicity (embryolethality, fetal abnormalities, pup mortality, offspring growth retardation) at doses producing maternal plasma drug exposures as low as 11 and 2.5 times, respectively, the exposure in humans receiving the maximum recommended daily dose (MRDD) of 5 mg.

When naratriptan was administered to pregnant rats during the period of organogenesis at doses of 10, 60, or 340 mg/kg/day, there was a dose-related increase in embryonic death; incidences of fetal structural variations (incomplete/irregular ossification of skull bones, sternebrae, ribs) were increased at all doses. The maternal plasma exposures (AUC) at these doses were approximately 11, 70, and 470 times the exposure in humans at the MRDD. The high dose was maternally toxic, as evidenced by decreased maternal body weight gain during gestation. A no-effect dose for developmental toxicity in rats exposed during organogenesis was not established.

When naratriptan was administered orally (1, 5, or 30 mg/kg/day) to pregnant Dutch rabbits throughout organogenesis, the incidence of a specific fetal skeletal malformation (fused sternebrae) was increased at the high dose, and increased incidences of embryonic death and fetal variations (major blood vessel variations, supernumerary ribs, incomplete skeletal ossification) were observed at all doses (4, 20, and 120 times, respectively, the MRDD on a body surface area basis). Maternal toxicity (decreased body weight gain) was evident at the high dose in this study. In a similar study in New Zealand White rabbits (1, 5, or 30 mg/kg/day throughout organogenesis), decreased fetal weights and increased incidences of fetal skeletal variations were observed at all doses (maternal exposures equivalent to 2.5, 19, and 140 times exposure in humans receiving the MRDD), while maternal body weight gain was reduced at 5 mg/kg or greater. A no-effect dose for developmental toxicity in rabbits exposed during organogenesis was not established.

When female rats were treated orally with naratriptan (10, 60, or 340 mg/kg/day) during late gestation and lactation, offspring behavioral impairment (tremors) and decreased offspring viability and growth were observed at doses of 60 mg/kg or greater, while maternal toxicity occurred only at the highest dose. Maternal exposures at the no-effect dose for developmental effects in this study were approximately 11 times the exposure in humans receiving the MRDD.

8.3 Nursing Mothers

Naratriptan is excreted in rat milk. It is not known whether naratriptan is excreted in human milk. Because many drugs are excreted in human milk, and because of the potential for serious adverse reactions in nursing infants from AMERGE, a decision should be made whether to discontinue nursing or to discontinue the drug, taking into account the importance of the drug to the mother.

8.4 Pediatric Use

Safety and effectiveness in pediatric patients have not been established. Therefore, AMERGE is not recommended for use in patients younger than 18 years of age.

One controlled clinical trial evaluated AMERGE (0.25 to 2.5 mg) in 300 adolescent migraineurs aged 12 to 17 years who received at least 1 dose of AMERGE for an acute migraine. In this study, 54% of the patients were female and 89% were Caucasian. There were no statistically significant differences between any of the treatment groups. The headache response rates at 4 hours (n) were 65% (n = 74), 67% (n = 78), and 64% (n = 70) for placebo, 1-mg, and 2.5-mg groups, respectively. This trial did not establish the efficacy of AMERGE compared with placebo in the treatment of migraine in adolescents. Adverse reactions observed in this clinical trial were similar in nature to those reported in clinical trials in adults.

8.5 Geriatric Use

Clinical trials of AMERGE did not include sufficient numbers of patients aged 65 and older to determine whether they respond differently from younger patients. Other reported clinical experience has not identified differences in responses between the elderly and younger patients. In general, dose selection for an elderly patient should be cautious, usually starting at the low end of the dosing range, reflecting the greater frequency of decreased hepatic, renal, or cardiac function and of concomitant disease or other drug therapy.

Naratriptan is known to be substantially excreted by the kidney, and the risk of adverse reactions to this drug may be greater in elderly patients who have reduced renal function. In addition, elderly patients are more likely to have decreased hepatic function, they are at higher risk for CAD, and blood pressure increases may be more pronounced in the elderly.

A cardiovascular evaluation is recommended for geriatric patients who have other cardiovascular risk factors (e.g., diabetes, hypertension, smoking, obesity, strong family history of CAD) prior to receiving AMERGE [see Warnings and Precautions (5.1)].

8.6 Renal Impairment

The use of AMERGE is contraindicated in patients with severe renal impairment (creatinine clearance: <15 mL/min) because of decreased clearance of the drug. In patients with mild to moderate renal impairment, the recommended starting dose is 1 mg, and the maximum daily dose should not exceed 2.5 mg over a 24-hour period [see Dosage and Administration (2.2), Clinical Pharmacology (12.3)].

8.7 Hepatic Impairment

The use of AMERGE is contraindicated in patients with severe hepatic impairment (Child-Pugh grade C) because of decreased clearance. In patients with mild or moderate hepatic impairment (Child-Pugh grade A or B), the recommendedstarting dose is 1 mg, and the maximum daily dose should not exceed 2.5 mg over a 24-hour period [see Dosage and Administration (2.3), Clinical Pharmacology (12.3)].

10 OVERDOSAGE

Adverse reactions observed after overdoses of up to 25 mg included increases in blood pressure resulting in lightheadedness, neck tension, tiredness, and loss of coordination. Also, ischemic ECG changes likely due to coronary artery vasospasm have been reported.

The elimination half-life of naratriptan is about 6 hours [see Clinical Pharmacology (12.3)], and therefore monitoring of patients after overdose with AMERGE should continue for at least 24 hours or while symptoms or signs persist. There is no specific antidote to naratriptan. It is unknown what effect hemodialysis or peritoneal dialysis has on the serum concentrations of naratriptan.

11 DESCRIPTION

AMERGE contains naratriptan hydrochloride, a selective $5\text{-HT}_{1B/1D}$ receptor agonist. Naratriptan hydrochloride is chemically designated as N-methyl-3-(1-methyl-4-piperidinyl)-1H-indole-5-ethanesulfonamide monohydrochloride, and it has the following structure:

The empirical formula is $C_{17}H_{25}N_3O_2S \bullet HCl$, representing a molecular weight of 371.93. Naratriptan hydrochloride is a white to pale yellow powder that is readily soluble in water. Each AMERGE tablet for oral administration contains 1.11 or 2.78 mg of naratriptan hydrochloride, equivalent to 1 or 2.5 mg of naratriptan, respectively. Each tablet also contains the inactive ingredients croscarmellose sodium; hypromellose; lactose; magnesium stearate; microcrystalline cellulose; triacetin; and titanium dioxide, iron oxide yellow (2.5-mg tablet only), and indigo carmine aluminum lake (FD&C Blue No. 2) (2.5-mg tablet only) for coloring.

12 CLINICAL PHARMACOLOGY

12.1 Mechanism of Action

Naratriptan binds with high affinity to human cloned $5\text{-HT}_{1B/1D}$ receptors. Migraines are likely due to local cranial vasodilatation and/or to the release of sensory neuropeptides (including substance P and calcitonin gene-related peptide) through nerve endings in the trigeminal system. The therapeutic activity of AMERGE for the treatment of migraine headache is thought to be due to the agonist effects at the $5\text{-HT}_{1B/1D}$ receptors on intracranial blood vessels (including the arterio-venous anastomoses) and sensory nerves of the trigeminal system, which result in cranial vessel constriction and inhibition of pro-inflammatory neuropeptide release.

12.2 Pharmacodynamics

In the anesthetized dog, naratriptan has been shown to reduce the carotid arterial blood flow with little or no effect on arterial blood pressure or total peripheral resistance. While the effect on blood flow was selective for the carotid arterial bed, increases in vascular resistance of up to 30% were seen in the coronary arterial bed. Naratriptan has also been shown to inhibit trigeminal nerve activity in rat and cat.

In 10 subjects with suspected CAD undergoing coronary artery catheterization, there was a 1% to 10% reduction in coronary artery diameter following subcutaneous injection of 1.5 mg of naratriptan [see Contraindications (4)].

12.3 Pharmacokinetics

Absorption: Naratriptan is well absorbed, with about 70% oral bioavailability. Following administration of a 2.5-mg tablet, the peak concentrations are obtained in 2 to 3 hours. After administration of 1- or 2.5-mg tablets, the C_{max} is somewhat (about 50%) higher in women (not corrected for milligram-per-kilogram dose) than in men. During a migraine attack, absorption is slower, with a T_{max} of 3 to 4 hours. Food does not affect the pharmacokinetics of naratriptan. Naratriptan displays linear kinetics over the therapeutic dose range.

Distribution: The steady-state volume of distribution of naratriptan is 170 L. Plasma protein binding is 28% to 31% over the concentration range of 50 to 1,000 ng/mL.

Metabolism: In vitro, naratriptan is metabolized by a wide range of cytochrome P450 isoenzymes into a number of inactive metabolites.

Elimination: Naratriptan is predominantly eliminated in urine, with 50% of the dose recovered unchanged and 30% as metabolites in urine. The mean elimination half-life of naratriptan is 6 hours. The systemic clearance of naratriptan is 6.6 mL/min/kg. The renal clearance of naratriptan (220 mL/min) exceeds glomerular filtration rate, indicating active tubular secretion. Repeat administration of naratriptan tablets does not result in drug accumulation.

Special Populations: Age: A small decrease in clearance (approximately 26%) was observed in healthy elderly subjects (65 to 77 years) compared with younger subjects, resulting in slightly higher exposure [see Use in Specific Populations (8.5)].

Race: The effect of race on the pharmacokinetics of naratriptan has not been examined.

Renal Impairment: Clearance of naratriptan was reduced by 50% in subjects with moderate renal impairment (creat-

inine clearance: 18 to 39 mL/min) compared with the normal group. Decrease in clearances resulted in an increase of mean half-life from 6 hours (healthy) to 11 hours (range: 7 to 20 hours). The mean C_{max} increased by approximately 40%. The effects of severe renal impairment (creatinine clearance:≤15 mL/min) on the pharmacokinetics of naratriptan have not been assessed [see Contraindications (4)].

Hepatic Impairment: Clearance of naratriptan was decreased by 30% in subjects with moderate hepatic impairment (Child-Pugh grade A or B). This resulted in an approximately 40% increase in the half-life (range: 8 to 16 hours). The effects of severe hepatic impairment (Child-Pugh grade C) on the pharmacokinetics of naratriptan have not been assessed [see Contraindications (4)].

Drug Interaction Studies: From population pharmacokinetic analyses, co-administration of naratriptan and fluoxetine, beta-blockers, or tricyclic antidepressants did not affect the clearance of naratriptan.

Oral Contraceptives: Oral contraceptives reduced clearance by 32% and volume of distribution by 22%, resulting in slightly higher concentrations of naratriptan. Hormone replacement therapy had no effect on pharmacokinetics in older female patients.

Monoamine Oxidase and P450 Inhibitors: Naratriptan does not inhibit monoamine oxidase (MAO) enzymes and is a poor inhibitor of P450; metabolic interactions between naratriptan and drugs metabolized by P450 or MAO are therefore unlikely.

Smoking: Smoking increased the clearance of naratriptan by 30%.

Alcohol: In normal volunteers, co-administration of single doses of naratriptan tablets and alcohol did not result in substantial modification of naratriptan pharmacokinetic parameters.

13 NONCLINICAL TOXICOLOGY

13.1 Carcinogenesis, Mutagenesis, Impairment of Fertility

Carcinogenesis: In carcinogenicity studies, mice and rats were given naratriptan by oral gavage for 104 weeks. There was no evidence of an increase in tumors related to naratriptan administration in mice receiving up to 200 mg/kg/day. That dose was associated with a plasma (AUC) exposure that was 110 times the exposure in humans receiving the maximum recommended daily dose (MRDD) of 5 mg. Two rat studies were conducted, one using a standard diet and the other a nitrite-supplemented diet (naratriptan can be nitrosated in vitro to form a mutagenic product that has been detected in the stomachs of rats fed a high-nitrite diet). Doses of 5, 20, and 90 mg/kg were associated with AUC exposures that in the standard-diet study were 7, 40, and 236 times, respectively, and in the nitrite-supplemented diet study were 7, 29, and 180 times, respectively, the exposure in humans at the MRDD. In both studies, there was an increase in the incidence of thyroid follicular hyperplasia in high-dose males and females and in thyroid follicular adenomas in high-dose males. In the standard-diet study only, there was also an increase in the incidence of benign c-cell adenomas in the thyroid of high-dose males and females. The exposures achieved at the no-effect dose for thyroid tumors were 40 (standard diet) and 29 (nitrite-supplemented diet) times the exposure achieved in humans at the MRDD. In the nitrite-supplemented diet study only, the incidence of benign lymphocytic thymoma was increased in all treated groups of females. It was not determined if the nitrosated product is systemically absorbed. However, no changes were seen in the stomachs of rats in that study.

Mutagenesis: Naratriptan was not mutagenic when tested in in vitro gene mutation (Ames and mouse lymphoma tk) assays. Naratriptan was also negative in the in vitro human lymphocyte assay and the in vivo mouse micronucleus assay. Naratriptan can be nitrosated in vitro to form a mutagenic product (WHO nitrosation assay) that has been detected in the stomachs of rats fed a nitrite-supplemented diet.

Impairment of Fertility: In a reproductive toxicity study in which male and female rats were administered naratriptan orally prior to and throughout the mating period (10, 60, 170, or 340 mg/kg/day; plasma exposures [AUC] approximately 11, 70, 230, and 470 times, respectively, the human exposure at the MRDD), there was a treatment-related decrease in the number of females exhibiting normal estrous cycles at doses of 170 mg/kg/day or greater and an increase in preimplantation loss at 60 mg/kg/day or greater. In high-dose males, testicular/epididymal atrophy accompanied by spermatozoa depletion reduced mating success and may have contributed to the observed preimplantation loss. The exposures achieved at the no-effect doses for preimplantation loss, anestrus, and testicular effects were approximately 11, 70, and 230 times, respectively, the exposures in humans at the MRDD.

In a study in which rats were dosed orally with naratriptan (10, 60, or 340 mg/kg/day) for 6 months, changes in the female reproductive tract including atrophic or cystic ovaries and anestrus were seen at the high dose. The exposure at the no-effect dose of 60 mg/kg was approximately 85 times that in humans at the MRDD.

14 CLINICAL STUDIES

The efficacy of AMERGE in the acute treatment of migraine headaches was evaluated in 3 randomized, double-blind, placebo-controlled trials in adult patients (Trials 1, 2, 3). These trials enrolled adult patients who were predominantly female (86%) and Caucasian (96%) with a mean age of 41 years (range: 18 to 65 years). In all studies, patients were instructed to treat at least 1 moderate to severe headache. Headache response, defined as a reduction in headache severity from moderate or severe pain to mild or no pain, was assessed up to 4 hours after dosing. Associated symptoms such as nausea, vomiting, photophobia, and phonophobia were also assessed. Maintenance of response was assessed for up to 24 hours postdose. A second dose of AMERGE or other rescue medication to treat migraines was allowed 4 to 24 hours after the initial treatment for recurrent headache.

In all 3 trials, the percentage of patients achieving headache response 4 hours after treatment, the primary outcome measure, was significantly greater among patients receiving AMERGE compared with those who received placebo. In all trials, response to 2.5 mg was numerically greater than response to 1 mg and in the largest of the 3 trials, there was a statistically significant greater percentage of patients with headache response at 4 hours in the 2.5-mg group compared with the 1-mg group. The results are summarized in Table 2.

Table 2. Percentage of Adult Patients With Headache Response (Mild or No Headache) 4 Hours Following Treatment

	AMERGE 1 mg (n = 491)	AMERGE 2.5 mg (n = 493)	Placebo (n = 395)
Trial 1	50%[a]	60%[a]	34%
Trial 2	52%[a]	66%[a,b]	27%
Trial 3	54%[a]	65%[a]	32%

[a]P<0.05 compared with placebo.
[b]P<0.05 compared with 1 mg.

The estimated probability of achieving an initial headache response in adults over the 4 hours following treatment in pooled Trials 1, 2, and 3 is depicted in Figure 1.

Figure 1. Estimated Probability of Achieving Initial Headache Response Within 4 Hoursin Pooled Trials 1, 2, and 3[a]

[a] The figure shows the probability over time of obtaining headache response (reduction in headache severity from moderate or severe pain to no or mild pain) following treatment with AMERGE. In this Kaplan-Meier plot, patients not achieving response within 240 minutes were censored at 240 minutes.

For patients with migraine-associated nausea, photophobia, and phonophobia at baseline, there was a lower incidence of these symptoms 4 hours following administration of 1-mg and 2.5-mg AMERGE compared with placebo.

Four to 24 hours following the initial dose of study treatment, patients were allowed to use additional treatment for pain relief in the form of a second dose of study treatment or other rescue medication. The estimated probability of patients taking a second dose or other rescue medication to treat migraine over the 24 hours following the initial dose of study treatment is summarized in Figure 2.

[See figure 2 at top of next column]

There is no evidence that doses of 5 mg provided a greater effect than 2.5 mg. There was no evidence to suggest that treatment with AMERGE was associated with an increase in the severity or frequency of migraine attacks. The efficacy of AMERGE was unaffected by presence of aura; gender, age, or weight of the subject; oral contraceptive use; or concomitant use of common migraine prophylactic drugs (e.g., beta-blockers, calcium channel blockers, tricyclic antidepressants). There was insufficient data to assess the impact of race on efficacy.

Figure 2. Estimated Probability of Patients Taking a Second Dose of AMERGE Tablets or Other Medication to Treat Migraine Over the 24 Hours Following the Initial Dose of Study Treatment in Pooled Trials 1, 2, and 3[a]

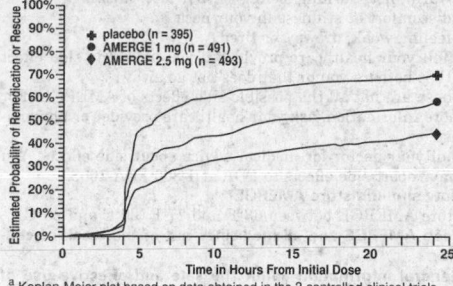

[a] Kaplan-Meier plot based on data obtained in the 3 controlled clinical trials (Trials 1, 2, and 3) providing evidence of efficacy with patients not using additional treatments censored at 24 hours. The plot also includes patients who had no response to the initial dose. Remediation is discouraged prior to 4 hours postdose.

16 HOW SUPPLIED/STORAGE AND HANDLING

AMERGE Tablets containing 1 mg and 2.5 mg of naratriptan (base) as the hydrochloride salt.
AMERGE Tablets, 1 mg, are white, D-shaped, film-coated tablets debossed with "GX CE3" on one side in blister packs of 9 tablets (NDC 0173-0561-00).
AMERGE Tablets, 2.5 mg, are green, D-shaped, film-coated tablets debossed with "GX CE5" on one side in blister packs of 9 tablets (NDC 0173-0562-00).
Store at controlled room temperature, 20° to 25°C (68° to 77°F) [see USP].

17 PATIENT COUNSELING INFORMATION

Advise the patient to read the FDA-approved patient labeling (Patient Information).
Risk of Myocardial Ischemia and/or Infarction, Prinzmetal's Angina, Other Vasospasm-Related Events, Arrhythmias, and Cerebrovascular Events: Inform patients that AMERGE may cause serious cardiovascular side effects such as myocardial infarction or stroke. Although serious cardiovascular events can occur without warning symptoms, patients should be alert for the signs and symptoms of chest pain, shortness of breath, irregular heartbeat, significant rise in blood pressure, weakness, and slurring of speech and should ask for medical advice if any indicative sign or symptoms are observed. Apprise patients of the importance of this follow-up [see Warnings and Precautions (5.1, 5.2, 5.4, 5.5, 5.8)].
Anaphylactic/Anaphylactoid Reactions: Inform patients that anaphylactic/anaphylactoid reactions have occurred in patients receiving AMERGE. Such reactions can be life threatening or fatal. In general, anaphylactic reactions to drugs are more likely to occur in individuals with a history of sensitivity to multiple allergens [see Contraindications (4), Warnings and Precautions (5.9)].
Concomitant Use With Other Triptans or Ergot Medications: Inform patients that use of AMERGE within 24 hours of another triptan or an ergot-type medication (including dihydroergotamine or methysergide) is contraindicated [see Contraindications (4), Drug Interactions (7.1, 7.2)].
Serotonin Syndrome: Caution patients about the risk of serotonin syndrome with the use of AMERGE or other triptans, particularly during combined use with SSRIs, SNRIs, TCAs, and MAO inhibitors [see Warnings and Precautions (5.7), Drug Interactions (7.3)].
Medication Overuse Headache: Inform patients that use of acute migraine drugs for 10 or more days per month may lead to an exacerbation of headache and encourage patients to record headache frequency and drug use (e.g., by keeping a headache diary) [see Warnings and Precautions (5.6)].
Pregnancy: Inform patients that AMERGE should not be used during pregnancy unless the potential benefit justifies the potential risk to the fetus [see Use in Specific Populations (8.1)].
Nursing Mothers: Advise patients to notify their healthcare provider if they are breastfeeding or plan to breastfeed [see Use in Specific Populations (8.3)].
Ability to Perform Complex Tasks: Treatment with AMERGE may cause somnolence and dizziness; instruct patients to evaluate their ability to perform complex tasks after administration of AMERGE.

AMERGE is a registered trademark of the GlaxoSmithKline group of companies.
GlaxoSmithKline
Research Triangle Park, NC 27709
©2013, GlaxoSmithKline group of companies. All rights reserved.
AMG:4PI

Patient Information
AMERGE® (a-MERJ)
(naratriptan hydrochloride)
Tablets

Read this Patient Information before you start taking AMERGE and each time you get a refill. There may be new information. This information does not take the place of talking with your healthcare provider about your medical condition or treatment.

What is the most important information I should know about AMERGE?
AMERGE can cause serious side effects, including:
Heart attack and other heart problems. Heart problems may lead to death.
Stop taking AMERGE and get emergency medical help right away if you have any of the following symptoms of a heart attack:
- discomfort in the center of your chest that lasts for more than a few minutes, or that goes away and comes back
- severe tightness, pain, pressure, or heaviness in your chest, throat, neck, or jaw
- pain or discomfort in your arms, back, neck, jaw, or stomach
- shortness of breath with or without chest discomfort
- breaking out in a cold sweat
- nausea or vomiting
- feeling lightheaded

AMERGE is not for people with risk factors for heart disease unless a heart exam is done and shows no problem. You have a higher risk for heart disease if you:
- have high blood pressure
- have high cholesterol levels
- smoke
- are overweight
- have diabetes
- have a family history of heart disease

What is AMERGE?
AMERGE is a prescription medicine used to treat acute migraine headaches with or without aura in adults who have been diagnosed with migraine headaches.
AMERGE is not used to prevent or decrease the number of migraine headaches you have.
AMERGE is not used to treat other types of headaches such as hemiplegic migraines (that make you unable to move on one side of your body) or basilar migraines (rare form of migraine with aura).
It is not known if AMERGE is safe and effective to treat cluster headaches.
It is not known if AMERGE is safe and effective in children under 18 years of age.

Who should not take AMERGE?
Do not take AMERGE if you have:
- heart problems or a history of heart problems
- narrowing of blood vessels to your legs, arms, stomach, or kidney (peripheral vascular disease)
- uncontrolled high blood pressure
- severe kidney problems
- severe liver problems
- hemiplegic migraines or basilar migraines. If you are not sure if you have these types of migraines, ask your healthcare provider
- had a stroke, transient ischemic attacks (TIAs), or problems with your blood circulation
- taken any of the following medicines in the last 24 hours:
- almotriptan (AXERT®)
- eletriptan (RELPAX®)
- frovatriptan (FROVA®)
- rizatriptan (MAXALT®, MAXALT-MLT®)
- sumatriptan (IMITREX®, SUMAVEL® DosePro®, ALSUMA®)
- sumatriptan and naproxen (TREXIMET®)
- ergotamines (CAFERGOT®, ERGOMAR®, MIGERGOT®)
- dihydroergotamine (D.H.E. 45®, MIGRANAL®)
Ask your healthcare provider if you are not sure if your medicine is listed above.
- an allergy to naratriptan or any of the ingredients in AMERGE. See the end of this leaflet for a complete list of ingredients in AMERGE.

What should I tell my healthcare provider before taking AMERGE?
Before you take AMERGE, tell your healthcare provider about all of your medical conditions, including if you:
- have high blood pressure
- have high cholesterol
- have diabetes
- smoke
- are overweight
- have heart problems or family history of heart problems or stroke
- have kidney problems
- have liver problems
- are not using effective birth control
- become pregnant while taking AMERGE

• are breastfeeding or plan to breastfeed. It is not known if AMERGE passes into your breast milk. Talk with your healthcare provider about the best way to feed your baby if you take AMERGE.

Tell your healthcare provider about all the medicines you take, including prescription and nonprescription medicines, vitamins, and herbal supplements.

Using AMERGE with certain other medicines can affect each other, causing serious side effects.

Especially tell your healthcare provider if you take antidepressant medicines called:

• selective serotonin reuptake inhibitors (SSRIs)
• serotonin norepinephrine reuptake inhibitors (SNRIs)
• tricyclic antidepressants (TCAs)
• monoamine oxidase inhibitors (MAOIs)

Ask your healthcare provider or pharmacist for a list of these medicines if you are not sure.

Know the medicines you take. Keep a list of them to show your healthcare provider or pharmacist when you get a new medicine.

How should I take AMERGE?

• Certain people should take their first dose of AMERGE in their healthcare provider's office or in another medical setting. Ask your healthcare provider if you should take your first dose in a medical setting.
• Take AMERGE exactly as your healthcare provider tells you to take it.
• Your healthcare provider may change your dose. Do not change your dose without first talking with your healthcare provider.
• Take AMERGE with water or other liquids.
• If you do not get any relief after your first AMERGE tablet, do not take a second tablet without first talking with your healthcare provider.
• If your headache comes back or you only get some relief from your headache, you can take a second tablet 4 hours after the first tablet.
• Do not take more than a total of 5 mg of AMERGE in a 24-hour period.
• Some people who take too many AMERGE tablets may have worse headaches (medication overuse headache). If your headaches get worse, your healthcare provider may decide to stop your treatment with AMERGE.
• If you take too much AMERGE, call your healthcare provider or go to the nearest hospital emergency room right away.
• You should write down when you have headaches and when you take AMERGE so you can talk with your healthcare provider about how AMERGE is working for you.

What should I avoid while taking AMERGE?

AMERGE can cause dizziness, weakness, or drowsiness. If you have these symptoms, do not drive a car, use machinery, or do anything where you need to be alert.

What are the possible side effects of AMERGE?

AMERGE may cause serious side effects. See "What is the most important information I should know about AMERGE?"

These serious side effects include:

• changes in color or sensation in your fingers and toes (Raynaud's syndrome)
• stomach and intestinal problems (gastrointestinal and colonic ischemic events). Symptoms of gastrointestinal and colonic ischemic events include:
  • sudden or severe stomach pain
  • stomach pain after meals
  • weight loss
  • nausea or vomiting
  • constipation or diarrhea
  • bloody diarrhea
  • fever
• problems with blood circulation to your legs and feet (peripheral vascular ischemia). Symptoms of peripheral vascular ischemia include:
  • cramping and pain in your legs or hips
  • feeling of heaviness or tightness in your leg muscles
  • burning or aching pain in your feet or toes while resting
  • numbness, tingling, or weakness in your legs
  • cold feeling or color changes in 1 or both legs or feet
• medication overuse headaches. Some people who use too many AMERGE Tablets may have worse headaches (medication overuse headache). If your headaches get worse, your healthcare provider may decide to stop your treatment with AMERGE.
• serotonin syndrome. Serotonin syndrome is a rare but serious problem that can happen in people using AMERGE, especially if AMERGE is used with anti-depressant medicines called SSRIs, SNRIs, TCAs, or MAOIs. Call your healthcare provider right away if you have any of the following symptoms of serotonin syndrome:
  • mental changes such as seeing things that are not there (hallucinations), agitation, or coma
  • fast heartbeat
  • changes in blood pressure
  • high body temperature

• tight muscles
• trouble walking

The most common side effects of AMERGE include:

• tingling or numbness in your fingers or toes
• dizziness
• warm, hot, burning feeling to your face (flushing)
• discomfort or stiffness in your neck
• feeling weak, drowsy, or tired
  Tell your healthcare provider if you have any side effect that bothers you or that does not go away.

These are not all the possible side effects of AMERGE. For more information, ask your healthcare provider or pharmacist.

Call your doctor for medical advice about side effects. You may report side effects to FDA at 1-800-FDA-1088.

How should I store AMERGE?

Store AMERGE between 68°F and 77°F (20°C and 25°C).

Keep AMERGE and all medicines out of the reach of children.

General information about the safe and effective use of AMERGE.

Medicines are sometimes prescribed for purposes other than those listed in Patient Information leaflets. Do not use AMERGE for a condition for which it was not prescribed. Do not give AMERGE to other people, even if they have the same symptoms you have. It may harm them.

This Patient Information leaflet summarizes the most important information about AMERGE. If you would like more information, talk with your healthcare provider. You can ask your healthcare provider or pharmacist for information about AMERGE that is written for healthcare professionals. For more information, go to www.gsk.com or call 1-888-825-5249.

What are the ingredients in AMERGE?

Active ingredient: naratriptan hydrochloride

Inactive ingredients: croscarmellose sodium, hypromellose, lactose, magnesium stearate, microcrystalline cellulose, triacetin, titanium dioxide

2.5-mg tablets also contain iron oxide yellow and indigo carmine aluminum lake (FD&C Blue No. 2) for coloring.

This Patient Information has been approved by the U.S. Food and Drug Administration.

AMERGE, IMITREX, and TREXIMET are registered trademarks of the GlaxoSmithKline group of companies. The other brands listed are trademarks of their respective owners and are not trademarks of the GlaxoSmithKline group of companies. The makers of these brands are not affiliated with and do not endorse GlaxoSmithKline or its products.

GlaxoSmithKline
Research Triangle Park, NC 27709
©2013, GlaxoSmithKline group of companies. All rights reserved.
October 2013
AMG:4PIL

ANORO ELLIPTA
(umeclidinium and vilanterol inhalation powder)
FOR ORAL INHALATION USE   ℞

HIGHLIGHTS OF PRESCRIBING INFORMATION
These highlights do not include all the information needed to use the ANORO ELLIPTA inhaler safely and effectively. See full prescribing information for ANORO ELLIPTA.
ANORO ELLIPTA (umeclidinium and vilanterol inhalation powder)
FOR ORAL INHALATION USE
Initial U.S. Approval: 2013

> **WARNING: ASTHMA-RELATED DEATH**
> *See full prescribing information for complete boxed warning.*
> • Long-acting beta₂-adrenergic agonists (LABA), such as vilanterol, one of the active ingredients in ANORO ELLIPTA, increase the risk of asthma-related death. A placebo-controlled trial with another LABA (salmeterol) showed an increase in asthma-related deaths in subjects receiving salmeterol. This finding with salmeterol is considered a class effect of all LABA, including vilanterol. (5.1)
> • The safety and efficacy of ANORO ELLIPTA in patients with asthma have not been established. ANORO ELLIPTA is not indicated for the treatment of asthma. (5.1)

—————INDICATIONS AND USAGE—————

ANORO ELLIPTA is a combination of umeclidinium, an anticholinergic, and vilanterol, a long-acting beta₂-adrenergic agonist (LABA), indicated for the long-term, once-daily, maintenance treatment of airflow obstruction in patients with chronic obstructive pulmonary disease (COPD). (1)

Important limitations: Not indicated for the relief of acute bronchospasm or for the treatment of asthma. (1, 5.2)

—————DOSAGE AND ADMINISTRATION—————

• For oral inhalation only. (2)
• Maintenance treatment of COPD: 1 inhalation of ANORO ELLIPTA once daily. (2)

—————DOSAGE FORMS AND STRENGTHS—————

Inhalation Powder. Inhaler containing 2 double-foil blister strips of powder formulation for oral inhalation. One strip contains umeclidinium 62.5 mcg per blister and the other contains vilanterol 25 mcg per blister. (3)

—————CONTRAINDICATIONS—————

• Severe hypersensitivity to milk proteins or any ingredients. (4)

—————WARNINGS AND PRECAUTIONS—————

• LABA increase the risk of asthma-related death. (5.1)
• Do not initiate in acutely deteriorating COPD or to treat acute symptoms. (5.2)
• Do not use in combination with an additional medicine containing LABA because of risk of overdose. (5.3)
• If paradoxical bronchospasm occurs, discontinue ANORO ELLIPTA and institute alternative therapy. (5.5)
• Use with caution in patients with cardiovascular disorders (5.7)
• Use with caution in patients with convulsive disorders, thyrotoxicosis, diabetes mellitus, and ketoacidosis. (5.8)
• Worsening of narrow-angle glaucoma may occur. Use with caution in patients with narrow-angle glaucoma and instruct patients to contact a physician immediately if symptoms occur. (5.9)
• Worsening of urinary retention may occur. Use with caution in patients with prostatic hyperplasia or bladder-neck obstruction and instruct patients to contact a physician immediately if symptoms occur. (5.10)
• Be alert to hypokalemia and hyperglycemia. (5.11)

—————ADVERSE REACTIONS—————

Most common adverse reactions (incidence ≥1% and more common than placebo) include pharyngitis, sinusitis, lower respiratory tract infection, constipation, diarrhea, pain in extremity, muscle spasms, neck pain, and chest pain. (6.1)
To report SUSPECTED ADVERSE REACTIONS, contact GlaxoSmithKline at 1-888-825-5249 or FDA at 1-800-FDA-1088 or www.fda.gov/medwatch.

—————DRUG INTERACTIONS—————

• Strong cytochrome P450 3A4 inhibitors (e.g., ketoconazole): Use with caution. May cause cardiovascular effects. (7.1)
• Monoamine oxidase inhibitors and tricyclic antidepressants: Use with extreme caution. May potentiate effect of vilanterol on cardiovascular system. (7.2)
• Beta-blockers: Use with caution. May block bronchodilatory effects of beta-agonists and produce severe bronchospasm. (7.3)
• Diuretics: Use with caution. Electrocardiographic changes and/or hypokalemia associated with non–potassium-sparing diuretics may worsen with concomitant beta-agonists. (7.4)
• Anticholinergics: May interact additively with concomitantly used anticholinergic medications. Avoid administration of ANORO ELLIPTA with other anticholinergic-containing drugs. (7.5)

See 17 for PATIENT COUNSELING INFORMATION and Medication Guide

Revised: 05/2014

FULL PRESCRIBING INFORMATION: CONTENTS*
WARNING: ASTHMA-RELATED DEATH

FULL PRESCRIBING INFORMATION

> **WARNING: ASTHMA-RELATED DEATH**
>
> Long-acting beta$_2$-adrenergic agonists (LABA) increase the risk of asthma-related death. Data from a large placebo-controlled US trial that compared the safety of another LABA (salmeterol) with placebo added to usual asthma therapy showed an increase in asthma-related deaths in subjects receiving salmeterol. This finding with salmeterol is considered a class effect of all LABA, including vilanterol, one of the active ingredients in ANORO™ ELLIPTA® *[see Warnings and Precautions (5.1)]*.
>
> The safety and efficacy of ANORO ELLIPTA in patients with asthma have not been established. ANORO ELLIPTA is not indicated for the treatment of asthma.

1 INDICATIONS AND USAGE

ANORO ELLIPTA is a combination anticholinergic/long-acting beta$_2$-adrenergic agonist (anticholinergic/LABA) indicated for the long-term, once-daily, maintenance treatment of airflow obstruction in patients with chronic obstructive pulmonary disease (COPD), including chronic bronchitis and/or emphysema.

Important Limitations of Use: ANORO ELLIPTA is NOT indicated for the relief of acute bronchospasm or for the treatment of asthma.

2 DOSAGE AND ADMINISTRATION

ANORO ELLIPTA (umeclidinium/vilanterol 62.5 mcg/25 mcg) should be administered as 1 inhalation once daily by the orally inhaled route only.

ANORO ELLIPTA should be taken at the same time every day. Do not use ANORO ELLIPTA more than 1 time every 24 hours.

No dosage adjustment is required for geriatric patients, patients with renal impairment, or patients with moderate hepatic impairment *[see Clinical Pharmacology (12.3)]*.

3 DOSAGE FORMS AND STRENGTHS

Inhalation Powder. Disposable light grey and red plastic inhaler containing 2 double-foil blister strips, each with 30 blisters containing powder intended for oral inhalation only. One strip contains umeclidinium (62.5 mcg per blister), and the other strip contains vilanterol (25 mcg per blister). An institutional pack containing 7 blisters per strip is also available.

4 CONTRAINDICATIONS

The use of ANORO ELLIPTA is contraindicated in patients with severe hypersensitivity to milk proteins or who have demonstrated hypersensitivity to umeclidinium, vilanterol, or any of the excipients *[see Warnings and Precautions (5.6), Description (11)]*.

5 WARNINGS AND PRECAUTIONS

5.1 Asthma-Related Death

• Data from a large placebo-controlled trial in subjects with asthma showed that LABA may increase the risk of asthma-related death. Data are not available to determine whether the rate of death in patients with COPD is increased by LABA.

• A 28-week, placebo-controlled, US trial comparing the safety of another LABA (salmeterol) with placebo, each added to usual asthma therapy, showed an increase in asthma-related deaths in subjects receiving salmeterol (13/13,176 in subjects treated with salmeterol vs. 3/13,179 in subjects treated with placebo; relative risk: 4.37 [95% CI: 1.25, 15.34]). The increased risk of asthma-related death is considered a class effect of LABA, including vilanterol, one of the active ingredients in ANORO ELLIPTA.

• No trial adequate to determine whether the rate of asthma-related death is increased in subjects treated with ANORO ELLIPTA has been conducted. The safety and efficacy of ANORO ELLIPTA in patients with asthma have not been established. ANORO ELLIPTA is not indicated for the treatment of asthma.

5.2 Deterioration of Disease and Acute Episodes

ANORO ELLIPTA should not be initiated in patients during rapidly deteriorating or potentially life-threatening episodes of COPD. ANORO ELLIPTA has not been studied in subjects with acutely deteriorating COPD. The initiation of ANORO ELLIPTA in this setting is not appropriate.

ANORO ELLIPTA should not be used for the relief of acute symptoms, i.e., as rescue therapy for the treatment of acute episodes of bronchospasm. ANORO ELLIPTA has not been studied in the relief of acute symptoms and extra doses should not be used for that purpose. Acute symptoms should be treated with an inhaled, short-acting beta$_2$-agonist.

When beginning treatment with ANORO ELLIPTA, patients who have been taking oral or inhaled, short-acting beta$_2$-agonists on a regular basis (e.g., 4 times a day) should be instructed to discontinue the regular use of these drugs and to use them only for symptomatic relief of acute respiratory symptoms. When prescribing ANORO ELLIPTA, the healthcare provider should also prescribe an inhaled, short-acting beta$_2$-agonist and instruct the patient on how it should be used. Increasing inhaled, short-acting beta$_2$-agonist use is a signal of deteriorating disease for which prompt medical attention is indicated.

COPD may deteriorate acutely over a period of hours or chronically over several days or longer. If ANORO ELLIPTA no longer controls symptoms of bronchoconstriction; the patient's inhaled, short-acting beta$_2$-agonist becomes less effective; or the patient needs more short-acting beta$_2$-agonist than usual, these may be markers of deterioration of disease. In this setting a re-evaluation of the patient and the COPD treatment regimen should be undertaken at once. Increasing the daily dose of ANORO ELLIPTA beyond the recommended dose is not appropriate in this situation.

5.3 Excessive Use of ANORO ELLIPTA and Use With Other Long-Acting Beta$_2$-Agonists

ANORO ELLIPTA should not be used more often than recommended, at higher doses than recommended, or in conjunction with other medicines containing LABA, as an overdose may result. Clinically significant cardiovascular effects and fatalities have been reported in association with excessive use of inhaled sympathomimetic drugs. Patients using ANORO ELLIPTA should not use another medicine containing a LABA (e.g., salmeterol, formoterol fumarate, arformoterol tartrate, indacaterol) for any reason.

5.4 Drug Interactions With Strong Cytochrome P450 3A4 Inhibitors

Caution should be exercised when considering the coadministration of ANORO ELLIPTA with long-term ketoconazole and other known strong cytochrome P450 3A4 (CYP3A4) inhibitors (e.g., ritonavir, clarithromycin, conivaptan, indinavir, itraconazole, lopinavir, nefazodone, nelfinavir, saquinavir, telithromycin, troleandomycin, voriconazole) because increased cardiovascular adverse effects may occur *[see Drug Interactions (7.1), Clinical Pharmacology (12.3)]*.

5.5 Paradoxical Bronchospasm

As with other inhaled medicines, ANORO ELLIPTA can produce paradoxical bronchospasm, which may be life threatening. If paradoxical bronchospasm occurs following dosing with ANORO ELLIPTA, it should be treated immediately with an inhaled, short-acting bronchodilator; ANORO ELLIPTA should be discontinued immediately; and alternative therapy should be instituted.

5.6 Hypersensitivity Reactions

Hypersensitivity reactions may occur after administration of ANORO ELLIPTA. There have been reports of anaphylactic reactions in patients with severe milk protein allergy after inhalation of other powder products containing lactose; therefore, patients with severe milk protein allergy should not use ANORO ELLIPTA *[see Contraindications (4)]*.

5.7 Cardiovascular Effects

Vilanterol, like other beta$_2$-agonists, can produce a clinically significant cardiovascular effect in some patients as measured by increases in pulse rate, systolic or diastolic blood pressure, or symptoms *[see Clinical Pharmacology (12.2)]*. If such effects occur, ANORO ELLIPTA may need to be discontinued. In addition, beta-agonists have been reported to produce electrocardiographic changes, such as flattening of the T wave, prolongation of the QTc interval, and ST segment depression, although the clinical significance of these findings is unknown.

Therefore, ANORO ELLIPTA should be used with caution in patients with cardiovascular disorders, especially coronary insufficiency, cardiac arrhythmias, and hypertension.

5.8 Coexisting Conditions

ANORO ELLIPTA, like all medicines containing sympathomimetic amines, should be used with caution in patients with convulsive disorders or thyrotoxicosis and in those who are unusually responsive to sympathomimetic amines. Doses of the related beta$_2$-adrenoceptor agonist albuterol, when administered intravenously, have been reported to aggravate preexisting diabetes mellitus and ketoacidosis.

5.9 Worsening of Narrow-Angle Glaucoma

ANORO ELLIPTA should be used with caution in patients with narrow-angle glaucoma. Prescribers and patients should be alert for signs and symptoms of acute narrow-angle glaucoma (e.g., eye pain or discomfort, blurred vision, visual halos or colored images in association with red eyes from conjunctival congestion and corneal edema). Instruct patients to consult a physician immediately if any of these signs or symptoms develops.

5.10 Worsening of Urinary Retention

ANORO ELLIPTA should be used with caution in patients with urinary retention. Prescribers and patients should be alert for signs and symptoms of urinary retention (e.g., difficulty passing urine, painful urination), especially in patients with prostatic hyperplasia or bladder-neck obstruction. Instruct patients to consult a physician immediately if any of these signs or symptoms develops.

5.11 Hypokalemia and Hyperglycemia

Beta-adrenergic agonist medicines may produce significant hypokalemia in some patients, possibly through intracellular shunting, which has the potential to produce adverse cardiovascular effects. The decrease in serum potassium is usually transient, not requiring supplementation. Beta-agonist medicines may produce transient hyperglycemia in some patients. In 4 clinical trials of 6-month duration evaluating ANORO ELLIPTA in subjects with COPD, there was no evidence of a treatment effect on serum glucose or potassium.

6 ADVERSE REACTIONS

LABA, such as vilanterol, one of the active ingredients in ANORO ELLIPTA, increase the risk of asthma-related death. ANORO ELLIPTA is not indicated for the treatment of asthma. *[See Boxed Warning and Warnings and Precautions (5.1).]*

The following adverse reactions are described in greater detail in other sections:

• Paradoxical bronchospasm *[see Warnings and Precautions (5.5)]*
• Cardiovascular effects *[see Warnings and Precautions (5.7)]*
• Worsening of narrow-angle glaucoma *[see Warnings and Precautions (5.9)]*
• Worsening of urinary retention *[see Warnings and Precautions (5.10)]*

6.1 Clinical Trials Experience

Because clinical trials are conducted under widely varying conditions, adverse reaction rates observed in the clinical trials of a drug cannot be directly compared with rates in the clinical trials of another drug and may not reflect the rates observed in practice.

The clinical program for ANORO ELLIPTA included 8,138 subjects with COPD in four 6-month lung function trials, one 12-month long-term safety study, and 9 other trials of shorter duration. A total of 1,124 subjects have received at least 1 dose of ANORO ELLIPTA (umeclidinium/vilanterol 62.5 mcg/25 mcg), and 1,330 subjects have received a higher dose of umeclidinium/vilanterol (125 mcg/25 mcg). The safety data described below are based on the four 6-month and the one 12-month trials. Adverse reactions observed in the other trials were similar to those observed in the confirmatory trials.

6-Month Trials: The incidence of adverse reactions associated with ANORO ELLIPTA in Table 1 is based on four 6-month trials: 2 placebo-controlled trials (Trials 1 and 2; n = 1,532 and n = 1,489, respectively) and 2 active-controlled trials (Trials 3 and 4; n = 843 and n = 869, respectively). Of the 4,733 subjects, 68% were male and 84% were Caucasian. They had a mean age of 63 years and an average smoking history of 45 pack-years, with 50% identified as current smokers. At screening, the mean post-bronchodilator percent predicted forced expiratory volume in 1 second (FEV$_1$) was 48% (range: 13% to 76%), the mean post-bronchodilator FEV$_1$/forced vital capacity (FVC) ratio was 0.47 (range: 0.13 to 0.78), and the mean percent reversibility was 14% (range: -45% to 109%).

Subjects received 1 dose once daily of the following: ANORO ELLIPTA, umeclidinium/vilanterol 125 mcg/25 mcg, umeclidinium 62.5 mcg, umeclidinium 125 mcg, vilanterol 25 mcg, active control, or placebo.

Table 1. Adverse Reactions With ANORO ELLIPTA With ≥1% Incidence and More Common Than With Placebo in Subjects With Chronic Obstructive Pulmonary Disease

Adverse Reaction	Placebo (n = 555) %	ANORO ELLIPTA (n = 842) %	Umeclidinium 62.5 mcg (n = 418) %	Vilanterol 25 mcg (n = 1,034) %
Infections and infestations				
Pharyngitis	<1	2	1	2
Sinusitis	<1	1	<1	1
Lower respiratory tract infection	<1	1	<1	<1
Gastrointestinal disorders				
Constipation	<1	1	<1	<1
Diarrhea	1	2	<1	2
Musculoskeletal and connective tissue disorders				
Pain in extremity	1	2	<1	2
Muscle spasms	<1	1	<1	<1
Neck pain	<1	1	<1	<1
General disorders and administration site conditions				
Chest pain	<1	1	<1	<1

[See table 1 above]
Other adverse reactions with ANORO ELLIPTA observed with an incidence less than 1% but more common than with placebo included the following: productive cough, dry mouth, dyspepsia, abdominal pain, gastroesophageal reflux disease, vomiting, musculoskeletal chest pain, chest discomfort, asthenia, atrial fibrillation, ventricular extrasystoles, supraventricular extrasystoles, myocardial infarction, pruritus, rash, and conjunctivitis.

12-Month Trial: In a long-term safety trial, 335 subjects were treated for up to 12 months with umeclidinium/vilanterol 125 mcg/25 mcg or placebo. The demographic and baseline characteristics of the long-term safety trial were similar to those of the placebo-controlled efficacy trials described above. Adverse reactions that occurred with a frequency of greater than or equal to 1% in the group receiving umeclidinium/vilanterol 125 mcg/25 mcg that exceeded that in placebo in this trial were: headache, back pain, sinusitis, cough, urinary tract infection, arthralgia, nausea, vertigo, abdominal pain, pleuritic pain, viral respiratory tract infection, toothache, and diabetes mellitus.

7 DRUG INTERACTIONS

7.1 Inhibitors of Cytochrome P450 3A4
Vilanterol, a component of ANORO ELLIPTA, is a substrate of CYP3A4. Concomitant administration of the strong CYP3A4 inhibitor ketoconazole increases the systemic exposure to vilanterol. Caution should be exercised when considering the coadministration of ANORO ELLIPTA with ketoconazole and other known strong CYP3A4 inhibitors (e.g., ritonavir, clarithromycin, conivaptan, indinavir, itraconazole, lopinavir, nefazodone, nelfinavir, saquinavir, telithromycin, troleandomycin, voriconazole) *[see Warnings and Precautions (5.4), Clinical Pharmacology (12.3)]*.

7.2 Monoamine Oxidase Inhibitors and Tricyclic Antidepressants
Vilanterol, like other beta₂-agonists, should be administered with extreme caution to patients being treated with monoamine oxidase inhibitors, tricyclic antidepressants, or drugs known to prolong the QTc interval or within 2 weeks of discontinuation of such agents, because the effect of adrenergic agonists on the cardiovascular system may be potentiated by these agents. Drugs that are known to prolong the QTc interval have an increased risk of ventricular arrhythmias.

7.3 Beta-Adrenergic Receptor Blocking Agents
Beta-blockers not only block the pulmonary effect of beta-agonists, such as vilanterol, a component of ANORO ELLIPTA, but may produce severe bronchospasm in patients with COPD. Therefore, patients with COPD should not normally be treated with beta-blockers. However, under certain circumstances, there may be no acceptable alternatives to the use of beta-adrenergic blocking agents for these patients; cardioselective beta-blockers could be considered, although they should be administered with caution.

7.4 Non–Potassium-Sparing Diuretics
The electrocardiographic changes and/or hypokalemia that may result from the administration of non–potassium-sparing diuretics (such as loop or thiazide diuretics) can be acutely worsened by beta-agonists, such as vilanterol, a component of ANORO ELLIPTA, especially when the recommended dose of the beta-agonist is exceeded. Although the clinical significance of these effects is not known, caution is advised in the coadministration of ANORO ELLIPTA with non–potassium-sparing diuretics.

7.5 Anticholinergics
There is potential for an additive interaction with concomitantly used anticholinergic medicines. Therefore, avoid coadministration of ANORO ELLIPTA with other anticholinergic-containing drugs as this may lead to an increase in anticholinergic adverse effects *[see Warnings and Precautions (5.9, 5.10), Adverse Reactions (6)]*.

8 USE IN SPECIFIC POPULATIONS

8.1 Pregnancy
Teratogenic Effects: Pregnancy Category C. There are no adequate and well-controlled trials of ANORO ELLIPTA or its individual components, umeclidinium and vilanterol, in pregnant women. Because animal reproduction studies are not always predictive of human response, ANORO ELLIPTA should be used during pregnancy only if the potential benefit justifies the potential risk to the fetus. Women should be advised to contact their physicians if they become pregnant while taking ANORO ELLIPTA.
Umeclidinium: There was no evidence of teratogenic effects in rats and rabbits at approximately 50 and 200 times, respectively, the MRHDID (maximum recommended human daily inhaled dose) in adults (on an AUC basis at maternal inhaled doses up to 278 mcg/kg/day in rats and at maternal subcutaneous doses up to 180 mcg/kg/day in rabbits).
Vilanterol: There were no teratogenic effects in rats and rabbits at approximately 13,000 and 70 times, respectively, the MRHDID in adults (on a mcg/m² basis at maternal inhaled doses up to 33,700 mcg/kg/day in rats and on an AUC basis at maternal inhaled doses up to 591 mcg/kg/day in rabbits). However, fetal skeletal variations were observed in rabbits at approximately 450 times the MRHDID in adults (on an AUC basis at maternal inhaled or subcutaneous doses of 5,740 or 300 mcg/kg/day, respectively). The skeletal variations included decreased or absent ossification in cervical vertebral centrum and metacarpals.
Nonteratogenic Effects: *Umeclidinium:* There were no effects on perinatal and postnatal developments in rats at approximately 80 times the MRHDID in adults (on an AUC basis at maternal subcutaneous doses up to 180 mcg/kg/day).
Vilanterol: There were no effects on perinatal and postnatal developments in rats at approximately 3,900 times the MRHDID in adults (on a mcg/m² basis at maternal oral doses up to 10,000 mcg/kg/day).

8.2 Labor and Delivery
There are no adequate and well-controlled human trials that have investigated the effects of ANORO ELLIPTA during labor and delivery.
Because beta-agonists may potentially interfere with uterine contractility, ANORO ELLIPTA should be used during labor only if the potential benefit justifies the potential risk.

8.3 Nursing Mothers
ANORO ELLIPTA: It is not known whether ANORO ELLIPTA is excreted in human breast milk. Because many drugs are excreted in human milk, caution should be exercised when ANORO ELLIPTA is administered to a nursing woman. Since there are no data from well-controlled human studies on the use of ANORO ELLIPTA by nursing mothers, based on the data for the individual components, a decision should be made whether to discontinue nursing or to discontinue ANORO ELLIPTA, taking into account the importance of ANORO ELLIPTA to the mother.
Umeclidinium: It is not known whether umeclidinium is excreted in human breast milk. However, administration to lactating rats at approximately 25 times the MRHDID in adults resulted in a quantifiable level of umeclidinium in 2 pups, which may indicate transfer of umeclidinium in milk. Vilanterol: It is not known whether vilanterol is excreted in human breast milk. However, other beta₂-agonists have been detected in human milk.

8.4 Pediatric Use
ANORO ELLIPTA is not indicated for use in children. The safety and efficacy in pediatric patients have not been established.

8.5 Geriatric Use
Based on available data, no adjustment of the dosage of ANORO ELLIPTA in geriatric patients is necessary, but greater sensitivity in some older individuals cannot be ruled out.
Clinical trials of ANORO ELLIPTA for COPD included 2,143 subjects aged 65 and older and, of those, 478 subjects were aged 75 and older. No overall differences in safety or effectiveness were observed between these subjects and younger subjects, and other reported clinical experience has not identified differences in responses between the elderly and younger subjects.

8.6 Hepatic Impairment
Patients with moderate hepatic impairment (Child-Pugh score of 7-9) showed no relevant increases in C_{max} or AUC, nor did protein binding differ between subjects with moderate hepatic impairment and their healthy controls. Studies in subjects with severe hepatic impairment have not been performed *[see Clinical Pharmacology (12.3)]*.

8.7 Renal Impairment
There were no significant increases in either umeclidinium or vilanterol exposure in subjects with severe renal impairment (CrCl<30 mL/min) compared with healthy subjects. No dosage adjustment is required in patients with renal impairment *[see Clinical Pharmacology (12.3)]*.

10 OVERDOSAGE
No case of overdose has been reported with ANORO ELLIPTA.
ANORO ELLIPTA contains both umeclidinium and vilanterol; therefore, the risks associated with overdosage for the individual components described below apply to ANORO ELLIPTA. Treatment of overdosage consists of discontinuation of ANORO ELLIPTA together with institution of appropriate symptomatic and/or supportive therapy. The judicious use of a cardioselective beta-receptor blocker may be considered, bearing in mind that such medicine can produce bronchospasm. Cardiac monitoring is recommended in cases of overdosage.

10.1 Umeclidinium
High doses of umeclidinium may lead to anticholinergic signs and symptoms. However, there were no systemic anticholinergic adverse effects following a once-daily inhaled dose of up to 1,000 mcg umeclidinium (16 times the maximum recommended daily dose) for 14 days in subjects with COPD.

10.2 Vilanterol
The expected signs and symptoms with overdosage of vilanterol are those of excessive beta-adrenergic stimulation and/or occurrence or exaggeration of any of the signs and symptoms of beta-adrenergic stimulation (e.g., angina, hypertension or hypotension, tachycardia with rates up to 200 beats/min, arrhythmias, nervousness, headache, tremor, seizures, muscle cramps, dry mouth, palpitation, nausea, dizziness, fatigue, malaise, insomnia, hyperglycemia, hypokalemia, metabolic acidosis). As with all inhaled sympathomimetic medicines, cardiac arrest and even death may be associated with an overdose of vilanterol.

11 DESCRIPTION
ANORO ELLIPTA is an inhalation powder drug product for delivery of a combination of umeclidinium (an anticholinergic) and vilanterol (a LABA) to patients by oral inhalation.
Umeclidinium bromide has the chemical name 1-[2-(benzyloxy)ethyl]-4-(hydroxydiphenylmethyl)-1-azoniabicyclo[2.2.2]octane bromide and the following chemical structure:

Umeclidinium bromide is a white powder with a molecular weight of 508.5, and the empirical formula is $C_{29}H_{34}NO_2 \cdot Br$ (as a quaternary ammonium bromide compound). It is slightly soluble in water.
Vilanterol trifenatate has the chemical name triphenylacetic acid-4-[(1R)-2-[(6-[2-[(2,6-dicholorobenzyl)oxy]ethoxy]hexyl)amino]-1-hydroxyethyl]-2-(hydroxymethyl)phenol (1:1) and the following chemical structure:

Vilanterol trifenatate is a white powder with a molecular weight of 774.8, and the empirical formula is $C_{24}H_{33}Cl_2NO_5 \cdot C_{20}H_{16}O_2$. It is practically insoluble in water.

ANORO ELLIPTA is a light grey and red plastic inhaler containing 2 double-foil blister strips. Each blister on one strip contains a white powder mix of micronized umeclidinium bromide (74.2 mcg equivalent to 62.5 mcg of umeclidinium), magnesium stearate (75 mcg), and lactose monohydrate (to 12.5 mg), and each blister on the other strip contains a white powder mix of micronized vilanterol trifenatate (40 mcg equivalent to 25 mcg of vilanterol), magnesium stearate (125 mcg), and lactose monohydrate (to 12.5 mg). The lactose monohydrate contains milk proteins. After the inhaler is activated, the powder within both blisters is exposed and ready for dispersion into the airstream created by the patient inhaling through the mouthpiece.

Under standardized *in vitro* test conditions, ANORO ELLIPTA delivers 55 mcg of umeclidinium and 22 mcg of vilanterol per dose when tested at a flow rate of 60 L/min for 4 seconds.

In adult subjects with obstructive lung disease and severely compromised lung function (COPD with FEV_1/FVC less than 70% and FEV_1 less than 30% predicted or FEV_1 less than 50% predicted plus chronic respiratory failure), mean peak inspiratory flow through the ELLIPTA inhaler was 66.5 L/min (range: 43.5 to 81.0 L/min).

The actual amount of drug delivered to the lung will depend on patient factors, such as inspiratory flow profile.

12   CLINICAL PHARMACOLOGY
12.1   Mechanism of Action
ANORO ELLIPTA: ANORO ELLIPTA contains both umeclidinium and vilanterol. The mechanisms of action described below for the individual components apply to ANORO ELLIPTA. These drugs represent 2 different classes of medications (an anticholinergic and a LABA) that have different effects on clinical and physiological indices.

Umeclidinium: Umeclidinium is a long-acting antimuscarinic agent, which is often referred to as an anticholinergic. It has similar affinity to the subtypes of muscarinic receptors M1 to M5. In the airways, it exhibits pharmacological effects through inhibition of M3 receptor at the smooth muscle leading to bronchodilation. The competitive and reversible nature of antagonism was shown with human and animal origin receptors and isolated organ preparations. In preclinical *in vitro* as well as *in vivo* studies, prevention of methacholine and acetylcholine-induced bronchoconstrictive effects was dose-dependent and lasted longer than 24 hours. The clinical relevance of these findings is unknown. The bronchodilation following inhalation of umeclidinium is predominantly a site-specific effect.

Vilanterol: Vilanterol is a LABA. *In vitro* tests have shown the functional selectivity of vilanterol was similar to salmeterol. The clinical relevance of this *in vitro* finding is unknown.

Although beta$_2$-receptors are the predominant adrenergic receptors in bronchial smooth muscle and beta$_1$-receptors are the predominant receptors in the heart, there are also beta$_2$-receptors in the human heart comprising 10% to 50% of the total beta-adrenergic receptors. The precise function of these receptors has not been established, but they raise the possibility that even highly selective beta$_2$-agonists may have cardiac effects.

The pharmacologic effects of beta$_2$-adrenergic agonist drugs, including vilanterol, are at least in part attributable to stimulation of intracellular adenyl cyclase, the enzyme that catalyzes the conversion of adenosine triphosphate (ATP) to cyclic-3',5'-adenosine monophosphate (cyclic AMP). Increased cyclic AMP levels cause relaxation of bronchial smooth muscle and inhibition of release of mediators of immediate hypersensitivity from cells, especially from mast cells.

12.2   Pharmacodynamics
Cardiovascular Effects: *Healthy Subjects:* QTc interval prolongation was studied in a double-blind, multiple dose, placebo- and positive-controlled crossover trial in 86 healthy subjects. The maximum mean (95% upper confidence bound) difference in QTcF from placebo after baseline correction was 4.6 (7.1) ms and 8.2 (10.7) ms for umeclidinium/vilanterol 125 mcg/25 mcg and umeclidinium/vilanterol 500 mcg/100 mcg (8/4 times the recommended dosage), respectively.

A dose-dependent increase in heart rate was also observed. The maximum mean (95% upper confidence bound) difference in heart rate from placebo after baseline correction was 8.8 (10.5) beats/min and 20.5 (22.3) beats/min seen 10 minutes after dosing for umeclidinium/vilanterol 125 mcg/25 mcg and umeclidinium/vilanterol 500 mcg/100 mcg, respectively.

Chronic Obstructive Pulmonary Disease: The effect of ANORO ELLIPTA on cardiac rhythm in subjects diagnosed with COPD was assessed using 24-hour Holter monitoring in 6- and 12-month trials: 53 subjects received ANORO ELLIPTA, 281 subjects received umeclidinium/vilanterol 125 mcg/25 mcg, and 182 subjects received placebo. No clinically meaningful effects on cardiac rhythm were observed.

12.3   Pharmacokinetics
Linear pharmacokinetics was observed for umeclidinium (62.5 to 500 mcg) and vilanterol (25 to 100 mcg).

Figure 1. Impact of Intrinsic Factors on the Pharmacokinetics (PK) of Umeclidinium and Vilanterol

[See figure 1 above]

Absorption: *Umeclidinium:* Umeclidinium plasma levels may not predict therapeutic effect. Following inhaled administration of umeclidinium in healthy subjects, C_{max} occurred at 5 to 15 minutes. Umeclidinium is mostly absorbed from the lung after inhaled doses with minimum contribution from oral absorption. Following repeat dosing of inhaled ANORO ELLIPTA, steady state was achieved within 14 days with up to 1.8-fold accumulation.

Vilanterol: Vilanterol plasma levels may not predict therapeutic effect. Following inhaled administration of vilanterol in healthy subjects, C_{max} occurred at 5 to 15 minutes. Vilanterol is mostly absorbed from the lung after inhaled doses with negligible contribution from oral absorption. Following repeat dosing of inhaled ANORO ELLIPTA, steady state was achieved within 14 days with up to 1.7-fold accumulation.

Distribution: *Umeclidinium:* Following intravenous administration to healthy subjects, the mean volume of distribution was 86 L. *In vitro* plasma protein binding in human plasma was on average 89%.

Vilanterol: Following intravenous administration to healthy subjects, the mean volume of distribution at steady state was 165 L. *In vitro* plasma protein binding in human plasma was on average 94%.

Metabolism: *Umeclidinium:* *In vitro* data showed that umeclidinium is primarily metabolized by the enzyme cytochrome P450 2D6 (CYP2D6) and is a substrate for the P-glycoprotein (P-gp) transporter. The primary metabolic routes for umeclidinium are oxidative (hydroxylation, O-dealkylation) followed by conjugation (e.g., glucuronidation), resulting in a range of metabolites with either reduced pharmacological activity or for which the pharmacological activity has not been established. Systemic exposure to the metabolites is low.

Vilanterol: *In vitro* data showed that vilanterol is metabolized principally by CYP3A4 and is a substrate for the P-gp transporter. Vilanterol is metabolized to a range of metabolites with significantly reduced β$_1$- and β$_2$-agonist activity.

Elimination: *Umeclidinium:* Following intravenous dosing with radio-labeled umeclidinium, mass balance showed 58% of the radio-label in the feces and 22% in the urine. The excretion of the drug-related material in the feces following intravenous dosing indicated elimination in the bile. Following oral dosing to healthy male subjects, radio-label recovered in feces was 92% of the total dose and that in urine was less than 1% of the total dose, suggesting negligible oral absorption. The effective half-life after once daily dosing is 11 hours.

Vilanterol: Following oral administration of radio-labeled vilanterol, mass balance showed 70% of the radio-label in the urine and 30% in the feces. The effective half-life for vilanterol, as determined from inhalation administration of multiple doses, is 11 hours.

Special Populations: The effects of renal and hepatic impairment and other intrinsic factors on the pharmacokinetics of umeclidinium and vilanterol are shown in Figure 1. Population pharmacokinetic analysis showed no evidence of a clinically significant effect of age (40 to 93 years) (see Figure 1), gender (69% male) (see Figure 1), inhaled corticosteroid use (48%), or weight (34 to 161 kg) on systemic exposure of either umeclidinium or vilanterol. In addition, there was no evidence of a clinically significant effect of race.

[See figure 1 above]

Hepatic Impairment: The impact of hepatic impairment on the pharmacokinetics of ANORO ELLIPTA has been evaluated in subjects with moderate hepatic impairment (Child-Pugh score of 7-9). There was no evidence of an increase in systemic exposure to either umeclidinium or vilanterol (C_{max} and AUC) (see Figure 1). There was no evidence of altered protein binding in subjects with moderate hepatic impairment compared with healthy subjects. ANORO ELLIPTA has not been evaluated in subjects with severe hepatic impairment.

Renal Impairment: The pharmacokinetics of ANORO ELLIPTA has been evaluated in subjects with severe renal impairment (creatinine clearance <30 mL/min). Umeclidinium systemic exposure was not increased and vilanterol systemic exposure ($AUC_{(0-24)}$) was 56% higher in subjects with severe renal impairment compared with healthy subjects (see Figure 1). There was no evidence of altered protein binding in subjects with severe renal impairment compared with healthy subjects.

Drug Interactions: When umeclidinium and vilanterol were administered in combination by the inhaled route, the pharmacokinetic parameters for each component were similar to those observed when each active substance was administered separately.

Inhibitors of Cytochrome P450 3A4: Vilanterol is a substrate of CYP3A4. A double-blind, repeat-dose, 2-way crossover drug interaction trial was conducted in healthy subjects to investigate the pharmacokinetic and pharmacodynamic effects of vilanterol 25 mcg as an inhalation powder with ketoconazole 400 mg. The plasma concentrations of vilanterol were higher after single and repeated doses when coadministered with ketoconazole than with placebo (see Figure 2). The increase in vilanterol exposure was not associated with an increase in beta-agonist–related systemic effects on heart rate or blood potassium.

Inhibitors of P-glycoprotein Transporter: Umeclidinium and vilanterol are both substrates of P-gp. The effect of the moderate P-gp transporter inhibitor verapamil (240 mg once daily) on the steady-state pharmacokinetics of umeclidinium and vilanterol was assessed in healthy subjects. No effect on umeclidinium or vilanterol C_{max} was observed; however, an approximately 1.4-fold increase in umeclidinium AUC was observed with no effect on vilanterol AUC (see Figure 2).

Inhibitors of Cytochrome P450 2D6: *In vitro* metabolism of umeclidinium is mediated primarily by CYP2D6. However, no clinically meaningful difference in systemic exposure to umeclidinium (500 mcg) (8 times the approved dose) was observed following repeat daily inhaled dosing in CYP2D6 normal (ultrarapid, extensive, and intermediate metabolizers) and poor metabolizer subjects (see Figure 1).

[See figure 2 at top of next page]

13   NONCLINICAL TOXICOLOGY
13.1   Carcinogenesis, Mutagenesis, Impairment of Fertility
ANORO ELLIPTA: No studies of carcinogenicity, mutagenicity, or impairment of fertility were conducted with ANORO ELLIPTA; however, studies are available for individual components, umeclidinium and vilanterol, as described below.

Umeclidinium: Umeclidinium produced no treatment-related increases in the incidence of tumors in 2-year

Figure 2. Impact of Extrinsic Factors on the Pharmacokinetics (PK) of Umeclidinium and Vilanterol

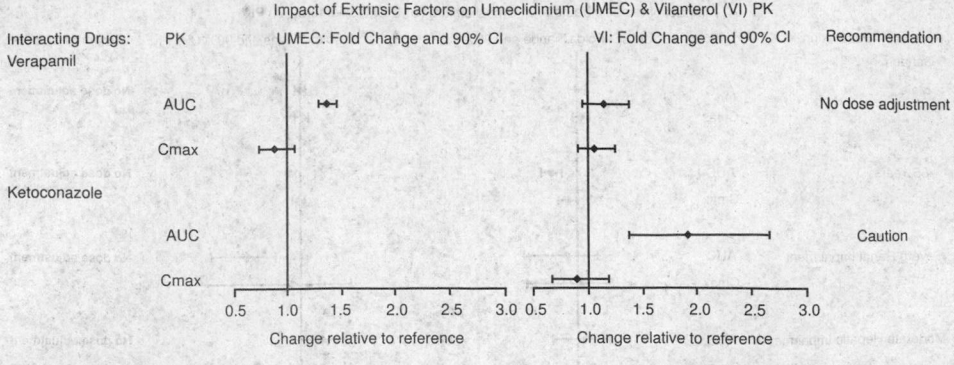

Impact of Extrinsic Factors on Umeclidinium (UMEC) & Vilanterol (VI) PK

Figure 4. Adjusted Mean Change From Baseline in Post-Dose Serial FEV₁ (0-24 hr, mL) on Days 1 and 28

inhalation studies in rats and mice at inhaled doses up to 137 mcg/kg/day and 295/200 mcg/kg/day (male/female), respectively (approximately 20 and 25/20 times the MRHDID in adults on an AUC basis, respectively).
Umeclidinium tested negative in the following genotoxicity assays: the *in vitro* Ames assay, *in vitro* mouse lymphoma assay, and *in vivo* rat bone marrow micronucleus assay.
No evidence of impairment of fertility was observed in male and female rats at subcutaneous doses up to 180 mcg/kg/day and inhaled doses up to 294 mcg/kg/day, respectively (approximately 100 and 50 times, respectively, the MRHDID in adults on an AUC basis).
Vilanterol: In a 2-year carcinogenicity study in mice, vilanterol caused a statistically significant increase in ovarian tubulostromal adenomas in females at an inhalation dose of 29,500 mcg/kg/day (approximately 7,800 times the MRHDID in adults on an AUC basis). No increase in tumors was seen at an inhalation dose of 615 mcg/kg/day (approximately 210 times the MRHDID in adults on an AUC basis).
In a 2-year carcinogenicity study in rats, vilanterol caused statistically significant increases in mesovarian leiomyomas in females and shortening of the latency of pituitary tumors at inhalation doses greater than or equal to 84.4 mcg/kg/day (greater than or equal to approximately 20 times the MRHDID in adults on an AUC basis). No tumors were seen at an inhalation dose of 10.5 mcg/kg/day (approximately 1 time the MRHDID in adults on an AUC basis).
These tumor findings in rodents are similar to those reported previously for other beta-adrenergic agonist drugs. The relevance of these findings to human use is unknown.
Vilanterol tested negative in the following genotoxicity assays: the *in vitro* Ames assay, *in vivo* rat bone marrow micronucleus assay, *in vivo* rat unscheduled DNA synthesis (UDS) assay, and *in vitro* Syrian hamster embryo (SHE) cell assay. Vilanterol tested equivocal in the *in vitro* mouse lymphoma assay.
No evidence of impairment of fertility was observed in reproductive studies conducted in male and female rats at inhaled vilanterol doses up to 31,500 and 37,100 mcg/kg/day, respectively (approximately 12,000 and 14,500 times, respectively, the MRHDID in adults on a mcg/m² basis).

14 CLINICAL STUDIES
The safety and efficacy of ANORO ELLIPTA were evaluated in a clinical development program that included 6 dose-ranging trials, 4 lung function trials of 6 months' duration (2 placebo-controlled and 2 active-controlled), two 12-week crossover trials, and a 12-month long-term safety trial. The efficacy of ANORO ELLIPTA is based primarily on the dose-ranging trials in 1,908 subjects with COPD or asthma and the 2 placebo-controlled confirmatory trials with additional support from the 2 active-controlled and 2 crossover trials in 5,388 subjects with COPD.

14.1 Dose-Ranging Trials
Dose selection for ANORO ELLIPTA for COPD was based on dose-ranging trials for the individual components, vilanterol and umeclidinium. Based on the findings from these studies, once-daily doses of umeclidinium/vilanterol 62.5 mcg/25 mcg and umeclidinium/vilanterol 125 mcg/25 mcg were evaluated in the confirmatory COPD trials.
ANORO ELLIPTA is not indicated for asthma.
Umeclidinium: Dose selection for umeclidinium in COPD was supported by a 7-day, randomized, double-blind, placebo-controlled, crossover trial evaluating 4 doses of umeclidinium (15.6 to 125 mcg) or placebo dosed once daily in the morning in 163 subjects with COPD. A dose ordering was observed, with the 62.5- and 125-mcg doses demonstrating larger improvements in FEV₁ over 24 hours compared with the lower doses of 15.6 and 31.25 mcg (Figure 3). The differences in trough FEV₁ from baseline after 7 days for placebo and the 15.6-, 31.25-, 62.5-, and 125-mcg doses were -74 mL (95% CI: -118, -31), 38 mL (95% CI: -6, 83), 27 mL (95% CI: -18, 72), 49 mL (95% CI: 6, 93), and 109 mL

(95% CI: 65, 152), respectively. Two additional dose-ranging trials in subjects with COPD demonstrated minimal additional benefit at doses above 125 mcg. The dose-ranging results supported the evaluation of 2 doses of umeclidinium, 62.5 and 125 mcg, in the confirmatory COPD trials to further assess dose response.
Evaluations of dosing interval by comparing once- and twice-daily dosing supported selection of a once-daily dosing interval for further evaluation in the confirmatory COPD trials.

Figure 3. Adjusted Mean Change From Baseline in Post-Dose Serial FEV₁ (mL) on Days 1 and 7

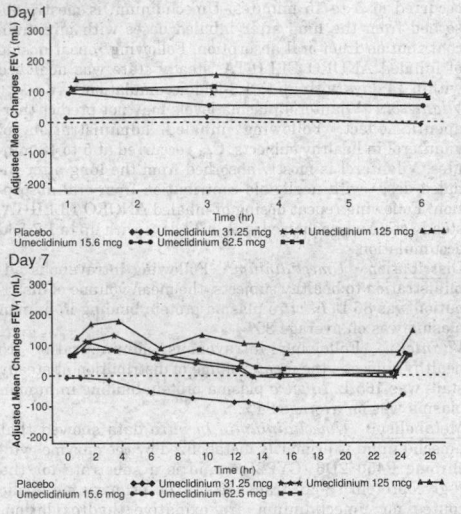

Vilanterol: Dose selection for vilanterol in COPD was supported by a 28-day, randomized, double-blind, placebo-controlled, parallel-group trial evaluating 5 doses of vilanterol (3 to 50 mcg) or placebo dosed in the morning in 602 subjects with COPD. Results demonstrated dose-related increases in FEV₁ compared with placebo at Day 1 and Day 28 (Figure 4).
[See figure 4 at top of next column]
The differences in trough FEV₁ after Day 28 from baseline for placebo and the 3-, 6.25-, 12.5-, 25-, and 50-mcg doses were 29 mL (95% CI: -8, 66), 120 mL (95% CI: 83, 158), 127 mL (95% CI: 90, 164), 138 mL (95% CI: 101, 176), 166 mL (95% CI: 129, 203), and 194 mL (95% CI: 156, 231), respectively. These results supported the evaluation of vilanterol 25 mcg in the confirmatory COPD trials.
Dose-ranging trials in subjects with asthma evaluated doses from 3 to 50 mcg and 12.5 mcg once-daily versus 6.25 mcg twice-daily dosing frequency. The results supported the selection of the vilanterol 25 mcg once-daily dose for further evaluation in the confirmatory COPD trials.

14.2 Confirmatory Trials
The clinical development program for ANORO ELLIPTA included two 6-month, randomized, double-blind, placebo-controlled, parallel-group trials; two 6-month active-controlled trials; and two 12-week crossover trials in subjects with COPD designed to evaluate the efficacy of ANORO ELLIPTA on lung function. The 6-month trials treated 4,733 subjects that had a clinical diagnosis of COPD, were 40 years of age or older, had a history of smoking greater than or equal to 10 pack-years, had a post-albuterol FEV₁ less than or equal to 70% of predicted normal values, had a ratio of FEV₁/FVC of less than 0.7, and had a Modified Medical Research Council (mMRC) score greater than or equal to 2. Of the 4,713 subjects included in

the efficacy analysis, 68% were male and 84% were Caucasian. They had a mean age of 63 years and an average smoking history of 45 pack-years, with 50% identified as current smokers. At screening, the mean post-bronchodilator percent predicted FEV₁ was 48% (range: 13% to 76%), the mean post-bronchodilator FEV₁/FVC ratio was 0.47 (range: 0.13 to 0.78), and the mean percent reversibility was 14% (range: -36% to 109%).
Trial 1 evaluated ANORO ELLIPTA (umeclidinium/vilanterol 62.5 mcg/25 mcg), umeclidinium 62.5 mcg, vilanterol 25 mcg, and placebo. The primary endpoint was change from baseline in trough (predose) FEV₁ at Day 169 (defined as the mean of the FEV₁ values obtained at 23 and 24 hours after the previous dose on Day 168) compared with placebo, umeclidinium 62.5 mcg, and vilanterol 25 mcg. The comparison of ANORO ELLIPTA with umeclidinium 62.5 mcg and vilanterol 25 mcg was assessed to evaluate the contribution of the individual comparators to ANORO ELLIPTA. ANORO ELLIPTA demonstrated a larger increase in mean change from baseline in trough (predose) FEV₁ relative to placebo, umeclidinium 62.5 mcg, and vilanterol 25 mcg (Table 2).

Table 2. Least Squares (LS) Mean Change From Baseline in Trough FEV₁ (mL) at Day 169 in the Intent-to-Treat Population (Trial 1)

Treatment	n	Trough FEV₁ (mL) at Day 169		
		Difference From		
		Placebo (95% CI) n = 280	Umeclidinium 62.5 mcg[a] (95% CI) n = 418	Vilanterol 25 mcg[a] (95% CI) n = 421
ANORO ELLIPTA	413	167 (128, 207)	52 (17, 87)	95 (60, 130)

n = Number in intent-to-treat population.
[a] The umeclidinium and vilanterol comparators used the same inhaler and excipients as ANORO ELLIPTA.

Trial 2 had a similar study design as Trial 1 but evaluated umeclidinium/vilanterol 125 mcg/25 mcg, umeclidinium 125 mcg, vilanterol 25 mcg, and placebo. Results for umeclidinium/vilanterol 125 mcg/25 mcg in Trial 2 were similar to those observed for ANORO ELLIPTA in Trial 1.
Results from the two active-controlled trials and the two 12-week trials provided additional support for the efficacy of ANORO ELLIPTA in terms of change from baseline in trough FEV₁ compared with the single-ingredient comparators and placebo.
Serial spirometric evaluations throughout the 24-hour dosing interval were performed in a subset of subjects (n = 197) at Days 1, 84, and 168 in Trial 1. Results from Trial 1 at Day 1 and Day 168 are shown in Figure 5.
[See figure 5 at top of next column]
The peak FEV₁ was defined as the maximum FEV₁ recorded within 6 hours after the dose of trial medicine on Days 1, 28, 84, and 168 (measurements recorded at 15 and 30 minutes and 1, 3, and 6 hours). The mean peak FEV₁ improvement from baseline for ANORO ELLIPTA compared with placebo at Day 1 and at Day 168 was 167 and 224 mL, respectively. The median time to onset on Day 1, defined as a 100-mL increase from baseline in FEV₁, was 27 minutes in subjects receiving ANORO ELLIPTA.

Figure 5. Least Squares (LS) Mean Change From Baseline in FEV$_1$ (mL) Over Time (0-24 h) on Days 1 and 168 (Trial 1 Subset Population)
Day 1

Day 168

16 HOW SUPPLIED/STORAGE AND HANDLING

ANORO ELLIPTA is supplied as a disposable light grey and red plastic inhaler containing 2 double-foil blister strips with 30 blisters each. The inhaler is packaged in a moisture-protective foil tray with a desiccant and a peelable lid (NDC 0173-0869-10).

ANORO ELLIPTA is also supplied in an institutional pack of a disposable light grey and red plastic inhaler containing 2 double-foil blister strips with 7 blisters each. The inhaler is packaged in a moisture protective foil tray with a desiccant and a peelable lid (NDC 0173-0869-06).

Store at room temperature between 68°F and 77°F (20°C and 25°C); excursions permitted from 59°F to 86°F (15°C to 30°C) [See USP Controlled Room Temperature]. Store in a dry place away from direct heat or sunlight. Keep out of reach of children.

ANORO ELLIPTA should be stored inside the unopened moisture-protective foil tray and only removed from the tray immediately before initial use. Discard ANORO ELLIPTA 6 weeks after opening the foil tray or when the counter reads "0" (after all blisters have been used), whichever comes first. The inhaler is not reusable. Do not attempt to take the inhaler apart.

17 PATIENT COUNSELING INFORMATION

Advise the patient to read the FDA-approved patient labeling (Medication Guide and Instructions for Use).

Asthma-Related Death: Inform patients that LABA, such as vilanterol, one of the active ingredients in ANORO ELLIPTA, increase the risk of asthma-related death. ANORO ELLIPTA is not indicated for the treatment of asthma.

Not for Acute Symptoms: Inform patients that ANORO ELLIPTA is not meant to relieve acute symptoms of COPD and extra doses should not be used for that purpose. Advise them to treat acute symptoms with a rescue inhaler such as albuterol. Provide patients with such medicine and instruct them in how it should be used.

Instruct patients to seek medical attention immediately if they experience any of the following:
• Symptoms get worse
• Need for more inhalations than usual of their rescue inhaler

Patients should not stop therapy with ANORO ELLIPTA without physician/provider guidance since symptoms may recur after discontinuation.

Do Not Use Additional Long-Acting Beta$_2$-Agonists: Instruct patients to not use other medicines containing a LABA. Patients should not use more than the recommended once-daily dose of ANORO ELLIPTA.

Instruct patients who have been taking inhaled, short-acting beta$_2$-agonists on a regular basis to discontinue the regular use of these products and use them only for the symptomatic relief of acute symptoms.

Paradoxical Bronchospasm: As with other inhaled medicines, ANORO ELLIPTA can cause paradoxical bronchospasm. If paradoxical bronchospasm occurs, instruct patients to discontinue ANORO ELLIPTA.

Risks Associated With Beta-Agonist Therapy: Inform patients of adverse effects associated with beta$_2$-agonists, such as palpitations, chest pain, rapid heart rate, tremor, or nervousness. Instruct patients to consult a physician immediately should any of these signs or symptoms develop.

Worsening of Narrow-Angle Glaucoma: Instruct patients to be alert for signs and symptoms of acute narrow-angle glaucoma (e.g., eye pain or discomfort, blurred vision, visual

halos or colored images in association with red eyes from conjunctival congestion and corneal edema). Instruct patients to consult a physician immediately if any of these signs or symptoms develops.

Worsening of Urinary Retention: Instruct patients to be alert for signs and symptoms of urinary retention (e.g., difficulty passing urine, painful urination). Instruct patients to consult a physician immediately if any of these signs or symptoms develops.

ANORO is a trademark and ELLIPTA is a registered trademark of the GSK group of companies.

ANORO ELLIPTA was developed in collaboration with Theravance.

GlaxoSmithKline
Research Triangle Park, NC 27709
©2014, the GSK group of companies. All rights reserved.
ANR:2PI

MEDICATION GUIDE
ANORO™ [a-nor′ oh] ELLIPTA®
(umeclidinium and vilanterol inhalation powder)

Read the Medication Guide that comes with ANORO ELLIPTA before you start using it and each time you get a refill. There may be new information. This Medication Guide does not take the place of talking to your healthcare provider about your medical condition or treatment.

What is the most important information I should know about ANORO ELLIPTA?

ANORO ELLIPTA is only approved for use in chronic obstructive pulmonary disease (COPD). ANORO ELLIPTA is NOT approved for use in asthma.

ANORO ELLIPTA can cause serious side effects, including:
• **People with asthma who take long-acting beta$_2$-adrenergic agonist (LABA) medicines, such as vilanterol (one of the medicines in ANORO ELLIPTA), have an increased risk of death from asthma problems.**
• **It is not known if LABA medicines, such as vilanterol (one of the medicines in ANORO ELLIPTA), increase the risk of death in people with COPD.**
• **Call your healthcare provider if breathing problems worsen over time while using ANORO ELLIPTA. You may need different treatment.**
• **Get emergency medical care if:**
  ○ your breathing problems worsen quickly
  ○ you use your rescue inhaler, but it does not relieve your breathing problems.

What is ANORO ELLIPTA?

ANORO ELLIPTA combines an anticholinergic, umeclidinium, and a LABA medicine, vilanterol.

Anticholinergic and LABA medicines help the muscles around the airways in your lungs stay relaxed to prevent symptoms such as wheezing, cough, chest tightness, and shortness of breath. These symptoms can happen when the muscles around the airways tighten. This makes it hard to breathe.

ANORO ELLIPTA is a prescription medicine used to treat COPD. COPD is a chronic lung disease that includes chronic bronchitis, emphysema, or both. ANORO ELLIPTA is used long term as 1 inhalation, 1 time each day, to improve symptoms of COPD for better breathing.

• **ANORO ELLIPTA is not for use to treat sudden symptoms of COPD.** Always have a rescue inhaler (an inhaled, short-acting bronchodilator) with you to treat sudden symptoms. If you do not have a rescue inhaler, contact your healthcare provider to have one prescribed for you.
• **ANORO ELLIPTA is not for the treatment of asthma.** It is not known if ANORO ELLIPTA is safe and effective in people with asthma.
• ANORO ELLIPTA should not be used in children. It is not known if ANORO ELLIPTA is safe and effective in children.

Who should not use ANORO ELLIPTA?

Do not use ANORO ELLIPTA if you:
• have a severe allergy to milk proteins. Ask your healthcare provider if you are not sure.
• are allergic to umeclidinium, vilanterol, or any of the ingredients in ANORO ELLIPTA. See "What are the ingredients in ANORO ELLIPTA?" below for a complete list of ingredients.

What should I tell my healthcare provider before using ANORO ELLIPTA?

Tell your healthcare provider about all of your health conditions, including if you:
• have heart problems
• have high blood pressure
• have seizures
• have thyroid problems
• have diabetes
• have liver problems
• have eye problems such as glaucoma. ANORO ELLIPTA may make your glaucoma worse.
• have prostate or bladder problems, or problems passing urine. ANORO ELLIPTA may make these problems worse.

• are allergic to any of the ingredients in ANORO ELLIPTA, any other medicines, or food products. See "What are the ingredients in ANORO ELLIPTA?" below for a complete list of ingredients.
• have any other medical conditions
• are pregnant or planning to become pregnant. It is not known if ANORO ELLIPTA may harm your unborn baby.
• are breastfeeding. It is not known if the medicines in ANORO ELLIPTA pass into your milk and if they can harm your baby.

Tell your healthcare provider about all the medicines you take, including prescription and over-the-counter medicines, vitamins, and herbal supplements. ANORO ELLIPTA and certain other medicines may interact with each other. This may cause serious side effects.

Especially tell your healthcare provider if you take:
• anticholinergics (including tiotropium, ipratropium, aclidinium)
• atropine

Know the medicines you take. Keep a list of them to show your healthcare provider and pharmacist when you get a new medicine.

How should I use ANORO ELLIPTA?

Read the step-by-step instructions for using ANORO ELLIPTA at the end of this Medication Guide.

• **Do not** use ANORO ELLIPTA unless your healthcare provider has taught you how to use the inhaler and you understand how to use it correctly.
• Use ANORO ELLIPTA exactly as your healthcare provider tells you to use it. **Do not** use ANORO ELLIPTA more often than prescribed.
• Use 1 inhalation of ANORO ELLIPTA 1 time each day. Use ANORO ELLIPTA at the same time each day.
• If you miss a dose of ANORO ELLIPTA, take it as soon as you remember. Do not take more than 1 inhalation each day. Take your next dose at your usual time. Do not take 2 doses at one time.
• If you take too much ANORO ELLIPTA, call your healthcare provider or go to the nearest hospital emergency room right away if you have any unusual symptoms, such as worsening shortness of breath, chest pain, increased heart rate, or shakiness.
• **Do not use other medicines that contain a LABA or an anticholinergic for any reason.** Ask your healthcare provider or pharmacist if any of your other medicines are LABA or anticholinergic medicines.
• Do not stop using ANORO ELLIPTA unless told to do so by your healthcare provider because your symptoms might get worse. Your healthcare provider will change your medicines as needed.
• **ANORO ELLIPTA does not relieve sudden symptoms.** Always have a rescue inhaler with you to treat sudden symptoms. If you do not have a rescue inhaler, call your healthcare provider to have one prescribed for you.
• Call your healthcare provider or get medical care right away if:
  ○ your breathing problems get worse
  ○ you need to use your rescue inhaler more often than usual
  ○ your rescue inhaler does not work as well to relieve your symptoms

What are the possible side effects with ANORO ELLIPTA?

ANORO ELLIPTA can cause serious side effects, including:
• See "What is the most important information I should know about ANORO ELLIPTA?"
• sudden breathing problems immediately after inhaling your medicine
• serious allergic reactions. Call your healthcare provider or get emergency medical care if you get any of the following symptoms of a serious allergic reaction:
  ○ rash
  ○ hives
  ○ swelling of the face, mouth, and tongue
  ○ breathing problems
• effects on your heart
  ○ increased blood pressure
  ○ a fast and/or irregular heartbeat
  ○ chest pain
• effects on your nervous system
  ○ tremor
  ○ nervousness
• new or worsened eye problems including acute narrow-angle glaucoma. Acute narrow-angle glaucoma can cause permanent loss of vision if not treated. Symptoms of acute narrow-angle glaucoma may include:
  ○ eye pain or discomfort
  ○ nausea or vomiting
  ○ blurred vision
  ○ seeing halos or bright colors around lights
  ○ red eyes
  If you have these symptoms, call your doctor right away before taking another dose.
• urinary retention. People who take ANORO ELLIPTA may develop new or worse urinary retention. Symptoms of urinary retention may include:

○ difficulty urinating
○ painful urination
○ urinating frequently
○ urination in a weak stream or drips
   If you have these symptoms of urinary retention, stop taking ANORO ELLIPTA and call your doctor right away before taking another dose.
● **changes in laboratory blood levels**, including high levels of blood sugar (hyperglycemia) and low levels of potassium (hypokalemia)

Common side effects of ANORO ELLIPTA include:
● sore throat
● sinus infection
● lower respiratory infection
● common cold symptoms
● constipation
● diarrhea
● pain in your arms or legs
● muscle spasms
● neck pain
● chest pain

Tell your healthcare provider about any side effect that bothers you or that does not go away.
These are not all the side effects with ANORO ELLIPTA. Ask your healthcare provider or pharmacist for more information.
Call your doctor for medical advice about side effects. You may report side effects to FDA at 1-800-FDA-1088.

How do I store ANORO ELLIPTA?
● Store ANORO ELLIPTA at room temperature between 68°F and 77°F (20°C and 25°C). Keep in a dry place away from heat and sunlight.
● Store ANORO ELLIPTA in the unopened foil tray and only open when ready for use.
● Safely throw away ANORO ELLIPTA in the trash 6 weeks after you open the foil tray or when the counter reads "0", whichever comes first. Write the date you open the tray on the label on the inhaler.
● **Keep ANORO ELLIPTA and all medicines out of the reach of children.**

General information about ANORO ELLIPTA
Medicines are sometimes prescribed for purposes not mentioned in a Medication Guide. Do not use ANORO ELLIPTA for a condition for which it was not prescribed. Do not give your ANORO ELLIPTA to other people, even if they have the same condition that you have. It may harm them.
This Medication Guide summarizes the most important information about ANORO ELLIPTA. If you would like more information, talk with your healthcare provider or pharmacist. You can ask your healthcare provider or pharmacist for information about ANORO ELLIPTA that was written for healthcare professionals.
For more information about ANORO ELLIPTA, call 1-888-825-5249 or visit our website at www.myANORO.com.

What are the ingredients in ANORO ELLIPTA?
Active ingredients: umeclidinium, vilanterol
Inactive ingredients: lactose monohydrate (contains milk proteins), magnesium stearate
Instructions for Use
For Oral Inhalation Only.
Read this before you start:
● **If you open and close the cover without inhaling the medicine, you will lose the dose.**
● **The lost dose will be securely held inside the inhaler, but it will no longer be available to be inhaled.**
● **It is not possible to accidentally take a double dose or an extra dose in one inhalation.**
Your ANORO ELLIPTA inhaler

How to use your inhaler
● ANORO ELLIPTA comes in a foil tray.
● Peel back the lid to open the tray. See Figure A.
● The tray contains a desiccant to reduce moisture. Do not eat or inhale. Throw it away in the household trash out of reach of children and pets. See Figure B.

Figure A

Figure B

Important Notes:
● Your inhaler contains 30 doses (7 doses if you have a sample or institutional pack).
● Each time you open the cover of the inhaler fully (you will hear a clicking sound), a dose is ready to be inhaled. This is shown by a decrease in the number on the counter.
● If you open and close the cover without inhaling the medicine, you will lose the dose. The lost dose will be held in the inhaler, but it will no longer be available to be inhaled. It is not possible to accidentally take a double dose or an extra dose in one inhalation.
● **Do not** open the cover of the inhaler until you are ready to use it. To avoid wasting doses after the inhaler is ready, **do not** close the cover until after you have inhaled the medicine.
● Write the "Tray opened" and "Discard" dates on the inhaler label. The "Discard" date is 6 weeks from the date you open the tray.
Check the counter. See Figure C.

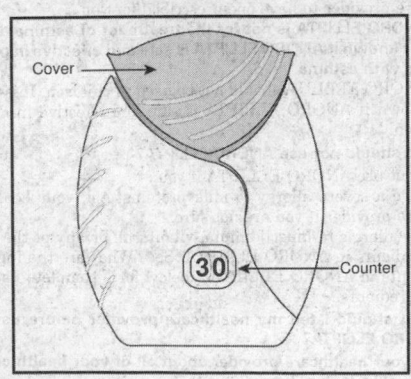

Figure C

● Before the inhaler is used for the first time, the counter should show the number 30 (7 if you have a sample or institutional pack). This is the number of doses in the inhaler.
● Each time you open the cover, you prepare 1 dose of medicine.
● The counter counts down by 1 each time you open the cover.

Prepare your dose:
Wait to open the cover until you are ready to take your dose.

Figure D

Step 1. Open the cover of the inhaler. See Figure D.
● Slide the cover down to expose the mouthpiece. You should hear a "click." The counter will count down by 1 number. You do not need to shake this kind of inhaler. **Your inhaler is now ready to use.**
● If the counter does not count down as you hear the click, the inhaler will not deliver the medicine. Call your healthcare provider or pharmacist if this happens.

Figure E

Step 2. Breathe out. See Figure E.
● While holding the inhaler away from your mouth, breathe out (exhale) fully. Do not breathe out into the mouthpiece.

Figure F

Step 3. Inhale your medicine. See Figure F.
● Put the mouthpiece between your lips, and close your lips firmly around it. Your lips should fit over the curved shape of the mouthpiece.
● Take one long, steady, deep breath in through your mouth. **Do not** breathe in through your nose.
[See figure G at top of next column]
● Do not block the air vent with your fingers. **See Figure G.**
[See figure G at top of next column]
● **Remove the inhaler from your mouth and hold your breath for about 3 to 4 seconds** (or as long as comfortable for you). **See Figure H.**
[See figure H at top of next column]

Do not block the air vent with your fingers.

Figure G

3-4 seconds

Figure H

Figure I

Step 4. Breathe out slowly and gently. See Figure I.
• You may not taste or feel the medicine, even when you are using the inhaler correctly.
• **Do not** take another dose from the inhaler even if you do not feel or taste the medicine.

Figure J

Step 5. Close the inhaler. See Figure J.
• You can clean the mouthpiece if needed, using a dry tissue, before you close the cover. Routine cleaning is not required.

• Slide the cover up and over the mouthpiece as far as it will go.
Important Note: When should you get a refill?

Red   **9**

Figure K

• **When you have less than 10 doses remaining** in your inhaler, the left half of the counter shows red as a reminder to get a refill. **See Figure K.**
• After you have inhaled the last dose, the counter will show "0" and will be empty.
• Throw the empty inhaler away in your household trash out of reach of children and pets.
If you have questions about ANORO ELLIPTA or how to use your inhaler, call GlaxoSmithKline (GSK) at 1-888-825-5249 or visit www.myANORO.com.
This Medication Guide and Instructions for Use have been approved by the U.S. Food and Drug Administration.
ANORO is a trademark and ELLIPTA is a registered trademark of the GSK group of companies.
ANORO ELLIPTA was developed in collaboration with Theravance.
GlaxoSmithKline
Research Triangle Park, NC 27709
©2014, the GSK group of companies. All rights reserved.
May 2014
ANR:2MG

ARGATROBAN INJECTION ℞
[är-ga' trō-ban]
for intravenous infusion only

HIGHLIGHTS OF PRESCRIBING INFORMATION
These highlights do not include all the information needed to use ARGATROBAN INJECTION safely and effectively. See full prescribing information for ARGATROBAN INJECTION.
ARGATROBAN INJECTION, for intravenous infusion only
Initial U.S. Approval: 2000

————INDICATIONS AND USAGE————
Argatroban is a direct thrombin inhibitor indicated:
• For prophylaxis or treatment of thrombosis in adult patients with heparin-induced thrombocytopenia (HIT) (1.1)
• As an anticoagulant in adults patients with or at risk for HIT undergoing percutaneous coronary intervention (PCI) (1.2)

————DOSAGE AND ADMINISTRATION————
Argatroban Injection must be diluted 100-fold by mixing with 0.9% Sodium Chloride Injection, 5% Dextrose Injection or Lactated Ringer's Injection to a final concentration of 1 mg/mL. (2.1). Argatroban dosage may be adjusted for Pediatric use (8.4)
Heparin-Induced Thrombocytopenia (2.1)
The dose for heparin-induced thrombocytopenia without hepatic impairment is 2 mcg/kg/min administered as a continuous infusion (2.1)
Percutaneous Coronary Intervention (2.2)
The dose for patients with or at risk for heparin-induced thrombocytopenia undergoing percutaneous coronary intervention is started at 25 mcg/kg/min and a bolus of 350 mcg/kg administered via a large bore intravenous line over 3 to 5 minutes (2.2)

————DOSAGE FORMS AND STRENGTHS————
250 mg/2.5 mL single use vial (3)

————CONTRAINDICATIONS————
• Major bleeding (4)
• History of hypersensitivity to this product (4)

————WARNINGS AND PRECAUTIONS————
• Hemorrhage can occur. Unexplained fall in hematocrit or blood pressure may indicate hemorrhage. (5.1)
• Hepatic impairment: Adjust starting dose and titrate carefully in patients with HIT who have moderate or severe hepatic impairment. Avoid use in PCI in patients with clinically significant hepatic impairment. (5.2)

————ADVERSE REACTIONS————
• HIT patients: The most common (> 5%) adverse reactions were dyspnea, hypotension, fever, diarrhea, sepsis, and cardiac arrest (6.1)
• PCI patients: The most common (> 5%) adverse reactions were chest pain, hypotension, back pain, nausea, vomiting and headache (6.2)
To report SUSPECTED ADVERSE REACTIONS, contact Pfizer, Inc at 1-800-438-1985 or FDA at 1-800-FDA-1088 or www.fda.gov/medwatch.

————DRUG INTERACTIONS————
• Heparin: Allow sufficient time for heparin's effect on aPTT to decrease before initiating Argatroban Injection therapy (7.1)
• Warfarin: Concomitant use results in increased prolongation of PT and INR (7.2)
• Thrombolytic agents or glycoprotein IIb/IIIa antagonists: Safety and effectiveness of concomitant use with argatroban have not been established (7.4, 7.5)

————USE IN SPECIFIC POPULATIONS————
• Nursing Mothers: Discontinue nursing or drug, taking into account the importance of the drug to the mother (8.3)
• Pediatric use: Safety and effectiveness have not been established; if used initial infusion doses are lower than in adult patients (2.4, 8.4, 12.3)
See 17 for PATIENT COUNSELING INFORMATION
Revised: 03/2014

FULL PRESCRIBING INFORMATION

1 INDICATIONS AND USAGE

1.1 Heparin-Induced Thrombocytopenia

Argatroban Injection is indicated for prophylaxis or treatment of thrombosis in adult patients with heparin- induced thrombocytopenia (HIT).

1.2 Percutaneous Coronary Intervention

Argatroban Injection is indicated as an anticoagulant in adult patients with or at risk for HIT undergoing percutaneous coronary intervention (PCI).

2 DOSAGE AND ADMINISTRATION

Argatroban Injection must be diluted 100-fold prior to infusion. Argatroban Injection should not be mixed with other drugs prior to dilution.

2.1 Preparation for Intravenous Administration

Argatroban Injection should be diluted in 0.9% Sodium Chloride Injection, 5% Dextrose Injection, or Lactated Ringer's Injection to a final concentration of 1 mg/mL. The contents of each 2.5-mL vial should be diluted 100-fold by mixing with 250 mL of diluent. Use 250 mg (2.5 mL) per 250 mL of diluent or 500 mg (5 mL) per 500 mL of diluent. The constituted solution must be mixed by repeated inversion of the diluent bag for 1 minute. Upon preparation, the solution may show slight but brief haziness due to the formation of microprecipitates that rapidly dissolve upon mixing. Use of diluent at room temperature is recommended. The final solution must be clear before use. The pH of the intravenous solution prepared as recommended is 3.2 to 7.5. Solutions prepared as recommended are stable at controlled room temperature, 20° to 25°C (68° to 77°F) (see USP) in ambient indoor light for 24 hours; therefore, light-resistant measures such as foil protection for intravenous lines are unnecessary. Solutions are physically and chemically stable for up to 96 hours when protected from light and stored at controlled room temperature, 20° to 25°C (68° to 77°F) (see USP), or at refrigerated conditions, 5° ± 3°C (41°± 5°F). Prepared solutions should not be exposed to direct sunlight. No significant potency losses have been noted following simulated delivery of the solution through intravenous tubing. Parenteral drug products should be inspected visually for particulate matter and discoloration prior to administration whenever solution and container permit.

2.2 Dosing in Patients with Heparin-Induced Thrombocytopenia

Initial Dosage:

Before administering argatroban, discontinue heparin therapy and obtain a baseline aPTT. The recommended initial dose of argatroban for adult patients without hepatic impairment is 2 mcg/kg/min, administered as a continuous infusion (see Table 1).

Table 1 Recommended Doses and Infusion Rates for 2 mcg/kg/min Dose of Argatroban for Patients With HIT* and Without Hepatic Impairment (1 mg/mL Final Concentration)

Body Weight (kg)	Dose (mcg/min)	Infusion Rate (mL/hr)
50	100	6
60	120	7
70	140	8
80	160	10
90	180	11
100	200	12
110	220	13
120	240	14
130	260	16
140	280	17

* with or without thrombosis

Monitoring Therapy:

For use in HIT, therapy with Argatroban Injection is monitored using the aPTT with a target range of 1.5 to 3 times the initial baseline value (not to exceed 100 seconds). Tests of anticoagulant effects (including the aPTT) typically attain steady-state levels within 1 to 3 hours following initiation of Argatroban Injection. Check the aPTT 2 hours after initiation of therapy and after any dose change to confirm that the patient has attained the desired therapeutic range.

Dosage Adjustment:

After the initiation of Argatroban Injection, adjust the dose (not to exceed 10 mcg/kg/min) as necessary to obtain a steady-state aPTT in the target range [*see Clinical Studies (14.1)*].

Table 2 Recommended Starting and Maintenance Doses (Within the Target ACT Range) of Argatroban Injection in Patients Undergoing PCI Without Hepatic Impairment (1 mg/mL Final Concentration)

Body Weight (kg)	Starting Bolus Dose (350 mcg/kg)		Starting and Maintenance Continuous Infusion Dosing For ACT 300–450 seconds 25 mcg/kg/min	
	Bolus Dose (mcg)	Bolus Volume (mL)	Continuous Infusion Dose (mg/min)	Continuous Infusion Rate (mL/hr)
50	17500	18	1250	75
60	21000	21	1500	90
70	24500	25	1750	105
80	28000	28	2000	120
90	31500	32	2250	135
100	35000	35	2500	150
110	38500	39	2750	165
120	42000	42	3000	180
130	45500	46	3250	195
140	49000	49	3500	210

NOTE: 1 mg = 1000 mcg; 1 kg = 2.2 lbs

Table 3 Recommended Dose Adjustments of Argatroban Injection for Patients Outside of ACT Target Range Undergoing PCI Without Hepatic Impairment (1 mg/mL Final Concentration)

Body Weight (kg)	If ACT Less than 300 seconds Dosage Adjustment* 30 mcg/kg/min				If ACT Greater than 450 seconds Dosage Adjustment† 15 mcg/kg/min	
	Additional Bolus Dose (mcg)	Bolus Volume (mL)	Continuous Infusion Dose (mcg/min)	Continuous Infusion Rate (mL/hr)	Continuous Infusion Dose (mcg/min)	Continuous Infusion Rate (mL/hr)
50	7500	8	1500	90	750	45
60	9000	9	1800	108	900	54
70	10500	11	2100	126	1050	63
80	12000	12	2400	144	1200	72
90	13500	14	2700	162	1350	81
100	15000	15	3000	180	1500	90
110	16500	17	3300	198	1650	99
120	18000	18	3600	216	1800	108
130	19500	20	3900	234	1950	117
140	21000	21	4200	252	2100	126

NOTE: 1 mg = 1000 mcg; 1 kg = 2.2 lbs

* Additional intravenous bolus dose of 150 mcg/kg should be administered if ACT less than 300 seconds.
† No bolus dose is given if ACT greater than 450 seconds

2.3 Dosing in Patients Undergoing Percutaneous Coronary Intervention

Initial Dosage:

Initiate an infusion of Argatroban Injection at 25 mcg/kg/min and administer a bolus of 350 mcg/kg via a large bore intravenous line over 3 to 5 minutes (see Table 2). Check an activated clotting time (ACT) 5 to 10 minutes after the bolus dose is completed. The PCI procedure may proceed if the ACT is greater than 300 seconds.

Dosage Adjustment:

If the ACT is less than 300 seconds, an additional intravenous bolus dose of 150 mcg/kg should be administered, the infusion dose increased to 30 mcg/kg/min, and the ACT checked 5 to 10 minutes later (see Table 2).

If the ACT is greater than 450 seconds, decrease the infusion rate to 15 mcg/kg/min, and check the ACT 5 to 10 minutes later (Table 3).

Continue titrating the dose until a therapeutic ACT (between 300 and 450 seconds) has been achieved; continue the same infusion rate for the duration of the PCI procedure.

In case of dissection, impending abrupt closure, thrombus formation during the procedure, or inability to achieve or maintain an ACT over 300 seconds, additional bolus doses of 150 mcg/kg may be administered and the infusion dose increased to 40 mcg/kg/min. Check the ACT after each additional bolus or change in the rate of infusion.

[See table 2 above]
[See table 3 above]

Monitoring Therapy:

For use in PCI, therapy with Argatroban Injection is monitored using ACT. Obtain ACTs before dosing, 5 to 10 minutes after bolus dosing, following adjustments in the infusion rate, and at the end of the PCI procedure.

Obtain additional ACTs every 20 to 30 minutes during a prolonged procedure.

Continued Anticoagulation after PCI:

If a patient requires anticoagulation after the procedure, Argatroban Injection may be continued, but at a rate of 2 mcg/kg/min and adjusted as needed to maintain the aPTT in the desired range [*see Dosage and Administration (2.1)*].

2.4 Dosing in Patients With Hepatic Impairment

Initial Dosage:

For adult patients with HIT and moderate or severe hepatic impairment (based on Child-Pugh classification), an initial dose of 0.5 mcg/kg/min is recommended, based on the approximately 4-fold decrease in argatroban clearance relative to those with normal hepatic function. Monitor the aPTT closely, and adjust the dosage as clinically indicated.

Monitoring Therapy:

Achievement of steady state aPTT levels may take longer and require more dose adjustments in patients with hepatic impairment compared to patients with normal hepatic function.

For patients with hepatic impairment undergoing PCI and who have HIT or are at risk for HIT, carefully titrate argatroban until the desired level of anticoagulation is achieved. Use of argatroban in PCI patients with clinically significant hepatic disease or AST/ALT levels ≥3 times the upper limit of normal should be avoided [see Warnings and Precautions (5.2)].

2.5 Dosing in Pediatric Patients With Heparin-Induced Thrombocytopenia/ Heparin-Induced Thrombocytopenia and Thrombosis Syndrome

Initial Dosage:
Initial argatroban infusion doses are lower for seriously ill pediatric patients compared to adults with normal hepatic function [see Use in Specific Populations (8.4)].

Monitoring Therapy:
In general, therapy with argatroban is monitored using the aPTT. Tests of anticoagulant effects (including the aPTT) typically attain steady-state levels within one to three hours following initiation of argatroban in patients without hepatic impairment [see Warnings and Precautions (5.2)]. Dose adjustment may be required to attain the target aPTT. Check the aPTT two hours after initiation of therapy and after any dose change to confirm that the patient has attained the desired therapeutic range.

Dosage Adjustment: [see Use in Specific Populations (8.4)].

2.6 Conversion to Oral Anticoagulant Therapy

Initiating Oral Anticoagulant Therapy:
When converting patients from argatroban to oral anticoagulant therapy, consider the potential for combined effects on INR with co-administration of argatroban and warfarin. A loading dose of warfarin should not be used. Initiate therapy using the expected daily dose of warfarin. To avoid prothrombotic effects and to ensure continuous anticoagulation when initiating warfarin, it is suggested that argatroban and warfarin therapy be overlapped. There are insufficient data available to recommend the duration of the overlap.

Co-Administration of Warfarin and Argatroban Injection at Doses up to 2 mcg/kg/min:
Measure INR daily while Argatroban Injection and warfarin are co-administered. In general, with doses of Argatroban Injection up to 2 mcg/kg/min, Argatroban Injection can be discontinued when the INR is >4 on combined therapy. After Argatroban Injection is discontinued, repeat the INR measurement in 4 to 6 hours. If the repeat INR is below the desired therapeutic range, resume the infusion of Argatroban Injection and repeat the procedure daily until the desired therapeutic range on warfarin alone is reached.

Co-Administration of Warfarin and Argatroban Injection at Doses Greater than 2 mcg/kg/min:
For doses of argatroban greater than 2 mcg/kg/min, the relationship of INR between warfarin alone to the INR on warfarin plus argatroban is less predictable. In this case, in order to predict the INR on warfarin alone, temporarily reduce the dose of Argatroban Injection to a dose of 2 mcg/kg/min. Repeat the INR on Argatroban Injection and warfarin 4 to 6 hours after reduction of the Argatroban Injection dose and follow the process outlined above for administering Argatroban Injection at doses up to 2 mcg/kg/min.

3 DOSAGE FORMS AND STRENGTHS

250 mg of argatroban in 2.5 ml of sterile solution for injection in a single use vial.

4 CONTRAINDICATIONS

Argatroban is contraindicated in
- Patients with major bleeding [see Warnings and Precautions (5.1)].
- Patients with history of hypersensitivity to argatroban. Airway, skin, and generalized hypersensitivity reactions have been reported [see Adverse Reactions (6.4)].

5 WARNINGS AND PRECAUTIONS

5.1 Risk of Hemorrhage

Hemorrhage can occur at any site in the body in patients receiving argatroban. Unexplained fall in hematocrit or blood pressure may indicate hemorrhage. Intracranial and retroperitoneal hemorrhage [see Adverse Reactions (6.2 and 6.3)] has been reported. The risk of hemorrhage with argatroban may be increased in severe hypertension, immediately following lumbar puncture, spinal anesthesia, major surgery (especially involving the brain, spinal cord, or eye), hematologic conditions associated with increased bleeding tendencies such as congenital or acquired bleeding disorders, and gastrointestinal lesions such as ulcerations.

Concomitant use of argatroban with antiplatelet agents, thrombolytics, and other anticoagulants may increase the risk of bleeding.

5.2 Use in Hepatic Impairment

When administering argatroban to patients with hepatic impairment, start with a lower dose and carefully titrate until the desired level of anticoagulation is achieved. Achievement of steady state aPTT levels may take longer and require more argatroban dose adjustments in patients with hepatic impairment compared to patients with normal hepatic function [see Use in Specific Populations (8.6)]. Also, upon cessation of argatroban infusion in the hepatically impaired patient, full reversal of anticoagulant effects may require longer than 4 hours due to decreased clearance and increased elimination half-life of argatroban [see Dosage and Administration (2.3) and Clinical Pharmacology (12.3)]. Avoid the use of high doses of argatroban in patients undergoing PCI who have clinically significant hepatic disease or AST/ALT levels ≥3 times the upper limit of normal.

5.3 Laboratory Tests

Anticoagulation effects associated with argatroban infusion at doses up to 40 mcg/kg/min correlate with increases of the activated partial thromboplastin time (aPTT). Although other global clot-based tests including prothrombin time (PT), the International Normalized Ratio (INR), and thrombin time (TT) are affected by argatroban, the therapeutic ranges for these tests have not been identified for argatroban therapy. In clinical trials in PCI, the activated clotting time (ACT) was used for monitoring argatroban anticoagulant activity during the procedure. The concomitant use of argatroban and warfarin results in prolongation of the PT and INR beyond that produced by warfarin alone [see Dosage and Administration (2.5) and Clinical Pharmacology (12.2)].

6 ADVERSE REACTIONS

Because clinical trials are conducted under widely varying conditions, adverse event rates observed in the clinical trials of a drug cannot be directly compared to rates in the clinical trials of another drug and may not reflect the rates observed in practice.

The following adverse reaction is also discussed in other sections of the labeling: Risk of Hemorrhage [see Warnings and Precautions (5.1)].

6.1 Adverse Events in Patients with HIT (With or Without Thrombosis)

The following safety information is based on all 568 patients treated with argatroban in Study 1 and Study 2. The safety profile of the patients from these studies is compared with that of 193 historical controls in which the adverse events were collected retrospectively. Adverse events are separated into hemorrhagic and non-hemorrhagic events.

Major bleeding was defined as bleeding that was overt and associated with a hemoglobin decrease ≥2 g/dL, that led to a transfusion of ≥2 units, or that was intracranial, retroperitoneal, or into a major prosthetic joint. Minor bleeding was overt bleeding that did not meet the criteria for major bleeding.

Table 4 gives an overview of the most frequently observed hemorrhagic events, presented separately by major and minor bleeding, sorted by decreasing occurrence among argatroban-treated patients with HIT(with or without thrombosis).

Table 4 Major and Minor Hemorrhagic Adverse Events in Patients With HIT*

Major Hemorrhagic Events[†]

	Argatroban-Treated Patients (Study 1 and Study 2) (n = 568) %	Historical Control[‡] (n = 193) %
Overall bleeding	5.3	6.7
Gastrointestinal	2.3	1.6
Genitourinary and hematuria	0.9	0.5
Decrease in hemoglobin and hematocrit	0.7	0
Multisystem hemorrhage and DIC	0.5	1
Limb and BKA stump	0.5	0
Intracranial hemorrhage	0[§]	0.5

Minor Hemorrhagic Events[†]

	Argatroban-Treated Patients (Study 1 and Study 2) (n = 568) %	Historical Control[‡] (n = 193) %
Gastrointestinal	14.4	18.1
Genitourinary and hematuria	11.6	0.8
Decrease in hemoglobin and hematocrit	10.4	0
Groin	5.4	3.1
Hemoptysis	2.9	0.8
Brachial	2.4	0.8

DIC = disseminated intravascular coagulation.
BKA = below-the-knee amputation.

* with or without thrombosis
† Patients may have experienced more than 1 adverse event.
‡ The historical control group consisted of patients with a clinical diagnosis of HIT (with or without thrombosis) that were considered eligible by an independent medical panel.
§ One patient experienced intracranial hemorrhage 4 days after discontinuation of argatroban and following therapy with urokinase and oral anticoagulation.

Table 5 gives an overview of the most frequently observed non-hemorrhagic events sorted by decreasing frequency of occurrence (≥2%) among argatroban-treated HIT/HITTS patients.

Table 5 Non-hemorrhagic Adverse Events in Patients* With HIT[†]

	Argatroban-Treated Patients (Study 1 and Study 2) (n = 568) %	Historical Control[‡] (n = 193) %
Dyspnea	8.1	8.8
Hypotension	7.2	2.6
Fever	6.9	2.1
Diarrhea	6.2	1.6
Sepsis	6.0	12.4
Cardiac arrest	5.8	3.1
Nausea	4.8	0.5
Ventricular tachycardia	4.8	3.1
Pain	4.6	3.1
Urinary tract infection	4.6	5.2
Vomiting	4.2	0
Infection	3.7	3.6
Pneumonia	3.3	9.3
Atrial fibrillation	3.0	11.4
Coughing	2.8	1.6
Abnormal renal function	2.8	4.7
Abdominal pain	2.6	1.6
Cerebrovascular disorder	2.3	4.1

* Patients may have experienced more than 1 adverse event.
† with or without thrombosis
‡ The historical control group consisted of patients with a clinical diagnosis of HIT (with or without thrombosis) that were considered eligible by an independent medical panel.

6.2 Adverse Events in Patients with or at Risk for HIT Patients Undergoing PCI

The following safety information is based on 91 patients initially treated with argatroban and 21 patients subsequently re-exposed to argatroban for a total of 112 PCIs with argatroban anticoagulation. Adverse events are separated into hemorrhagic (Table 6) and non-hemorrhagic (Table 7) events.

Major bleeding was defined as bleeding that was overt and associated with a hemoglobin decrease ≥5 g/dL, that led to a transfusion of ≥2 units, or that was intracranial, retroperitoneal, or into a major prosthetic joint.

The rate of major bleeding events in patients treated with argatroban in the PCI trials was 1.8%.

Table 6 Major and Minor Hemorrhagic Adverse Events in Patients With HIT Undergoing PCI

Major Hemorrhagic Events*	
	Argatroban-Treated Patients (n = 12)† %
Retroperitoneal	.0.9
Gastrointestinal	0.9
Intracranial	0

Minor Hemorrhagic Events*	
	Argatroban-Treated Patients (n = 12)† %
Groin (bleeding or hematoma)	3.6
Gastrointestinal (includes hematemesis)	2.6
Genitourinary (includes hematuria)	1.8
Decrease in hemoglobin and/or hematocrit	1.8
CABG (coronary arteries)	1.8
Access site	0.9
Hemoptysis	0.9
Other	0.9

CABG = coronary artery bypass graft.

* Patients may have experienced more than 1 adverse event.
† 91 patients who underwent 112 interventions.

Table 7 gives an overview of the most frequently observed non-hemorrhagic events (>2%), sorted by decreasing frequency of occurrence among argatroban-treated PCI patients.

Table 7 Non-hemorrhagic Adverse Events* in Patients With HIT Undergoing PCI

	Argatroban Procedures* (n = 112)† %
Chest pain	15.2
Hypotension	10.7
Back pain	8.0
Nausea	7.1
Vomiting	6.3
Headache	5.4
Bradycardia	4.5
Abdominal pain	3.6
Fever	3.6
Myocardial infarction	3.6

* Patients may have experienced more than 1 adverse event.
† 91 patients who underwent 112 interventions.

There were 22 serious adverse events in 17 PCI patients (19.6% in 112 interventions). Table 8 lists the serious adverse events occurring in argatroban-treated patients with or at risk for HIT undergoing PCI.

Table 8 Serious Adverse Events in Patients With HIT Undergoing PCI*

Coded Term	Argatroban Procedures† (n = 112)
Myocardial infarction	4 (3.5%)
Angina pectoris	2 (1.8%)
Coronary thrombosis	2 (1.8%)
Myocardial ischemia	2 (1.8%)
Occlusion coronary	2 (1.8%)
Chest pain	1 (0.9%)
Fever	1 (0.9%)
Retroperitoneal hemorrhage	1 (0.9%)
Aortic stenosis	1 (0.9%)
Arterial thrombosis	1 (0.9%)
Gastrointestinal hemorrhage	1 (0.9%)
Gastrointestinal disorder (GERD)	1 (0.9%)
Cerebrovascular disorder	1 (0.9%)
Lung edema	1 (0.9%)
Vascular disorder	1 (0.9%)

* Individual events may also have been reported elsewhere (see Table 6 and 7).
† 91 patients underwent 112 procedures. Some patients may have experienced more than 1 event.

6.3 Intracranial Bleeding in Other Populations

Increased risks for intracranial bleeding have been observed in investigational studies of argatroban for other uses. In a study of patients with acute myocardial infarction receiving both argatroban and thrombolytic therapy (streptokinase or tissue plasminogen activator), the overall frequency of intracranial bleeding was 1% (8 out of 810 patients). Intracranial bleeding was not observed in 317 subjects or patients who did not receive concomitant thrombolysis [see Drug Interactions (7.4)].

The safety and effectiveness of argatroban for cardiac indications other than PCI in patients with HIT have not been established. Intracranial bleeding was also observed in a prospective, placebo-controlled study of argatroban in patients who had onset of acute stroke within 12 hours of study entry. Symptomatic intracranial hemorrhage was reported in 5 of 117 patients (4.3%) who received argatroban at 1 to 3 mcg/kg/min and in none of the 54 patients who received placebo. Asymptomatic intracranial hemorrhage occurred in 5 (4.3%) and 2 (3.7%) of the patients, respectively.

6.4 Allergic Reactions

One hundred fifty-six allergic reactions or suspected allergic reactions were observed in 1,127 individuals who were treated with argatroban in clinical pharmacology studies or for various clinical indications. About 95% (148/156) of these reactions occurred in patients who concomitantly received thrombolytic therapy (e.g., streptokinase) or contrast media.

Allergic reactions or suspected allergic reactions in populations other than patients with HIT (with or without thrombosis) include (in descending order of frequency):
• Airway reactions (coughing, dyspnea): 10% or more
• Skin reactions (rash, bullous eruption): 1 to <10%
• General reactions (vasodilation): 1 to 10%
Limited data are available on the potential formation of drug-related antibodies. Plasma from 12 healthy volunteers treated with argatroban over 6 days showed no evidence of neutralizing antibodies. No loss of anticoagulant activity was noted with repeated administration of argatroban to more than 40 patients.

7 DRUG INTERACTIONS

7.1 Heparin

If argatroban is to be initiated after cessation of heparin therapy, allow sufficient time for heparin's effect on the aPTT to decrease prior to initiation of argatroban therapy.

7.2 Oral Anticoagulant Agents

Pharmacokinetic drug-drug interactions between argatroban and warfarin (7.5 mg single oral dose) have not been demonstrated. However, the concomitant use of argatroban and warfarin (5 to 7.5 mg initial oral dose, fol-

lowed by 2.5 to 6 mg/day orally for 6 to 10 days) results in prolongation of the prothrombin time (PT) and International Normalized Ratio (INR) [see Dosage and Administration (2.5) and Clinical Pharmacology (12.2)].

7.3 Aspirin/Acetaminophen

No drug-drug interactions have been demonstrated between argatroban and concomitantly administered aspirin or acetaminophen [see Clinical Pharmacology (12.3)].

7.4 Thrombolytic Agents

The safety and effectiveness of argatroban with thrombolytic agents have not been established [see Adverse Reactions (6.3)].

7.5 Glycoprotein IIb/IIIa Antagonists

The safety and effectiveness of argatroban with glycoprotein IIb/IIIa antagonists have not been established.

8 USE IN SPECIFIC POPULATIONS

8.1 Pregnancy

Pregnancy Category B
There are no adequate and well-controlled studies of argatroban use in pregnant women. Developmental studies performed in rats with argatroban at intravenous doses up to 27 mg/kg/day (0.3 times the maximum recommended human dose, based on body surface area) and in rabbits at intravenous doses up to 10.8 mg/kg/day (0.2 times the maximum recommended human dose, based on body surface area) have revealed no evidence of impaired fertility or harm to the fetus. Because animal reproductive studies are not always predictive of human response, this drug should be used during pregnancy only if clearly needed.

8.3 Nursing Mothers

It is not known whether argatroban is excreted in human milk. Argatroban is detected in rat milk. Because many drugs are excreted in human milk and because of the potential for serious adverse reactions in nursing infants from argatroban, a decision should be made whether to discontinue nursing or to discontinue the drug, taking into account the importance of the drug to the mother.

8.4 Pediatric Use

The safety and effectiveness of argatroban, including the appropriate anticoagulation goals and duration of therapy, have not been established among pediatric patients. Argatroban was studied among 18 seriously ill pediatric patients who required an alternative to heparin anticoagulation. Most patients were diagnosed with HIT or suspected HIT. Age ranges of patients were <6 months, n = 8; six months to <8 years, n = 6; 8 to 16 years, n = 4. All patients had serious underlying conditions and were receiving multiple concomitant medications. Thirteen patients received argatroban solely as a continuous infusion (no bolus dose). Dosing was initiated in the majority of these 13 patients at 1 mcg/kg/min. Dosing was titrated as needed to achieve and maintain an aPTT of 1.5 to 3 times the baseline value. Most patients required multiple dose adjustments to maintain anticoagulation parameters within the desired range. During the 30-day study period, thrombotic events occurred during argatroban administration to two patients and following argatroban discontinuation in three other patients. Major bleeding occurred among two patients; one patient experienced an intracranial hemorrhage after 4 days of argatroban therapy in the setting of sepsis and thrombocytopenia. Another patient completed 14 days of argatroban treatment in the study, but experienced an intracranial hemorrhage while receiving argatroban following completion of the study treatment period.

When argatroban is used among seriously ill pediatric patients with HIT/HITTS who require an alternative to heparin and who have normal hepatic function, initiate a continuous infusion of argatroban at a dose of 0.75 mcg/kg/min. Initiate the infusion at a dose of 0.2 mcg/kg/min among seriously ill pediatric patients with impaired hepatic function [see Clinical Pharmacology (12.3)]. Check the aPTT two hours after the initiation of the argatroban infusion and adjust the dose to achieve the target aPTT. Increments of 0.1 to 0.25 mcg/kg/min for pediatric patients with normal hepatic function and increments of 0.05 mcg/kg/min or lower for pediatric patients with impaired hepatic function may be considered but dose selection must take into account multiple factors including the current argatroban dose, the current aPTT, target aPTT, and the clinical status of the patient. These dose recommendations are based upon a goal of aPTT prolongation of 1.5 to 3 times the baseline value and avoidance of an aPTT >100 seconds.

8.5 Geriatric Use

Of the total number of subjects (1340) in clinical studies of argatroban, 35% were 65 and over. In the clinical studies of adult patients with HIT (with or without thrombosis), the effectiveness of argatroban was not affected by age. No trends were observed across age groups for both aPTT and the ACT. The safety analysis did suggest that older patients had increased underlying conditions, which may predispose them to events. The studies were not sized appropriately to detect differences in safety between age groups.

8.6 Hepatic Impairment

Dose reduction and careful titration are required when administering argatroban to patients with hepatic impairment. Reversal of anticoagulation effect may be prolonged in this population [see Dosage and Administration (2.3), Warning and Precautions (5.2), Clinical Pharmacology (12.3)].

10 OVERDOSAGE

Excessive anticoagulation, with or without bleeding, may be controlled by discontinuing argatroban or by decreasing the argatroban dose. In clinical studies, anticoagulation parameters generally returned from therapeutic levels to baseline within 2 to 4 hours after discontinuation of the drug. Reversal of anticoagulant effect may take longer in patients with hepatic impairment.

No specific antidote to argatroban is available; if life-threatening bleeding occurs and excessive plasma levels of argatroban are suspected, discontinue argatroban immediately and measure aPTT and other coagulation parameters. When argatroban was administered as a continuous infusion (2 mcg/kg/min) prior to and during a 4-hour hemodialysis session, approximately 20% of argatroban was cleared through dialysis.

Single intravenous doses of argatroban at 200, 124, 150, and 200 mg/kg were lethal to mice, rats, rabbits, and dogs, respectively. The symptoms of acute toxicity were loss of righting reflex, tremors, clonic convulsions, paralysis of hind limbs, and coma.

11 DESCRIPTION

Argatroban is a synthetic direct thrombin inhibitor and the chemical name is 1-[5-[(aminoiminomethyl)amino]- 1-oxo-2-[[(1,2,3,4-tetrahydro-3-methyl-8-quinolinyl)sulfonyl]amino]pentyl]-4-methyl-2-piperidinecarboxylic acid, monohydrate. Argatroban has 4 asymmetric carbons. One of the asymmetric carbons has an R configuration (stereoisomer Type I) and an S configuration (stereoisomer Type II). Argatroban consists of a mixture of R and S stereoisomers at a ratio of approximately 65:35.

The molecular formula of argatroban is $C_{23}H_{36}N_6O_5S \cdot H_2O$. Its molecular weight is 526.66 g/mol. The structural formula is:

Argatroban is a white, odorless crystalline powder that is freely soluble in glacial acetic acid, slightly soluble in ethanol, and insoluble in acetone, ethyl acetate, and ether.

Argatroban Injection is a sterile clear, colorless to pale yellow, slightly viscous solution in a single-use amber vial containing 250 mg/2.5 mL of argatroban. Each mL of sterile, nonpyrogenic solution contains 100 mg argatroban, 300 mg D-sorbitol, and 400 mg dehydrated alcohol in water for injection.

12 CLINICAL PHARMACOLOGY

12.1 Mechanism of Action

Argatroban is a direct thrombin inhibitor that reversibly binds to the thrombin active site. Argatroban does not require the co-factor antithrombin III for antithrombotic activity. Argatroban exerts its anticoagulant effects by inhibiting thrombin-catalyzed or -induced reactions, including fibrin formation; activation of coagulation factors V, VIII, and XIII; activation of protein C; and platelet aggregation. Argatroban inhibits thrombin with an inhibition constant (Ki) of 0.04 μM. At therapeutic concentrations, argatroban has little or no effect on related serine proteases (trypsin, factor Xa, plasmin, and kallikrein).

Argatroban is capable of inhibiting the action of both free and clot-associated thrombin.

12.2 Pharmacodynamics

When argatroban is administered by continuous infusion, anticoagulant effects and plasma concentrations of argatroban follow similar, predictable temporal response profiles, with low intersubject variability. Immediately upon initiation of argatroban infusion, anticoagulant effects are produced as plasma argatroban concentrations begin to rise. Steady-state levels of both drug and anticoagulant effect are typically attained within 1 to 3 hours and are maintained until the infusion is discontinued or the dosage adjusted. Steady-state plasma argatroban concentrations increase proportionally with dose (for infusion doses up to 40 mcg/kg/min in healthy subjects) and are well correlated with steady-state anticoagulant effects. For infusion doses up to 40 mcg/kg/min, argatroban increases in a dose-dependent fashion, the activated partial thromboplastin time (aPTT), the activated clotting time (ACT), the prothrombin time (PT), the International Normalized Ratio (INR), and the thrombin time (TT) in healthy volunteers

and cardiac patients. Representative steady-state plasma argatroban concentrations and anticoagulant effects are shown below for argatroban infusion doses up to 10 mcg/kg/min (see Figure 1).

Figure 1. Relationship at Steady State Between Argatroban Dose, Plasma Argatroban Concentration and Anticoagulant Effect

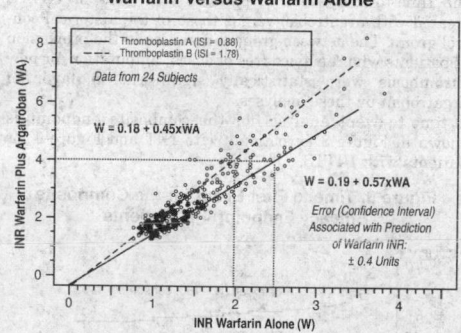

Effect on International Normalized Ratio (INR): Because argatroban is a direct thrombin inhibitor, co[82][c7e6] administration of argatroban and warfarin produces a combined effect on the laboratory measurement of the INR. However, concurrent therapy, compared to warfarin monotherapy, exerts no additional effect on vitamin K–dependent factor Xa activity.

The relationship between INR on co-therapy and warfarin alone is dependent on both the dose of argatroban and the thromboplastin reagent used. This relationship is influenced by the International Sensitivity Index (ISI) of the thromboplastin. Data for 2 commonly utilized thromboplastins with ISI values of 0.88 (Innovin, Dade) and 1.78 (Thromboplastin C Plus, Dade) are presented in Figure 2 for an argatroban dose of 2 mcg/kg/min. Thromboplastins with higher ISI values than shown result in higher INRs on combined therapy of warfarin and argatroban. These data are based on results obtained in normal individuals [see Drug Interactions (7.2), Dosage and Administration (2.5)].

Figure 2. INR Relationship of Argatroban Plus Warfarin Versus Warfarin Alone

Figure 2 demonstrates the relationship between INR for warfarin alone and INR for warfarin co-administered with argatroban at a dose of 2 mcg/kg/min. To calculate INR for warfarin alone (INR_W), based on INR for co[82][c7e6] therapy of warfarin and argatroban (INR_{WA}), when the argatroban dose is 2 mcg/kg/min, use the equation next to the appropriate curve. Example: At a dose of 2 mcg/kg/min and an INR performed with Thromboplastin A, the equation 0.19 + 0.57 (INR_{WA}) = INR_W would allow a prediction of the INR on warfarin alone (INR_W). Thus, using an INR_{WA} value of 4.0 obtained on combined therapy: INR_W = 0.19 + 0.57 (4) = 2.47 as the value for INR on warfarin alone. The error (confidence interval) associated with a prediction is ± 0.4 units. Similar linear relationships and prediction errors exist for argatroban at a dose of 1 mcg/kg/min. Thus, for argatroban doses of 1 or 2 mcg/kg/min, INR_W can be predicted from INR_{WA}. For argatroban doses greater than 2 mcg/kg/min, the error associated with predicting INR_W from INR_{WA} is ± 1. Thus, INR_W cannot be reliably predicted from INR_{WA} at doses greater than 2 mcg/kg/min.

12.3 Pharmacokinetics

Distribution:

Argatroban distributes mainly in the extra cellular fluid as evidenced by an apparent steady-state volume of distribution of 174 mL/kg (12.18 L in a 70 kg adult). Argatroban is 54% bound to human serum proteins, with binding to albumin and α_1-acid glycoprotein being 20% and 34%, respectively.

Metabolism:

The main route of argatroban metabolism is hydroxylation and aromatization of the 3-methyltetrahydroquinoline ring in the liver. The formation of each of the 4 known metabolites is catalyzed in vitro by the human liver microsomal cytochrome P450 enzymes CYP3A4/5. The primary metabolite (M1) exerts 3- to 5-fold weaker anticoagulant effects than argatroban. Unchanged argatroban is the major component

in plasma. The plasma concentrations of M1 range between 0% and 20% of that of the parent drug. The other metabolites (M2 to M4) are found only in very low quantities in the urine and have not been detected in plasma or feces. These data, together with the lack of effect of erythromycin (a potent CYP3A4/5 inhibitor) on argatroban pharmacokinetics, suggest that CYP3A4/5-mediated metabolism is not an important elimination pathway in vivo.

Total body clearance is approximately 5.1 mL/kg/min (0.31 L/kg/hr) for infusion doses up to 40 mcg/kg/min. The terminal elimination half-life of argatroban ranges between 39 and 51 minutes.

There is no interconversion of the 21–(R):21–(S) diastereoisomers. The plasma ratio of these diastereoisomers is unchanged by metabolism or hepatic impairment, remaining constant at 65:35 (± 2%).

Excretion:

Argatroban is excreted primarily in the feces, presumably through biliary secretion. In a study in which ^{14}C[82][c7e6] argatroban (5 mcg/kg/min) was infused for 4 hours into healthy subjects, approximately 65% of the radioactivity was recovered in the feces within 6 days of the start of infusion with little or no radioactivity subsequently detected. Approximately 22% of the radioactivity appeared in the urine within 12 hours of the start of infusion. Little or no additional urinary radioactivity was subsequently detected. Average percent recovery of unchanged drug, relative to total dose, was 16% in urine and at least 14% in feces.

Special Populations:

Hepatic Impairment: The dosage of argatroban should be decreased in patients with hepatic impairment [see Dosage and Administration (2.3) and Warnings and Precautions (5.2)]. Patients with hepatic impairment were not studied in percutaneous coronary intervention (PCI) trials. At a dose of 2.5 mcg/kg/min, hepatic impairment is associated with decreased clearance and increased elimination half-life of argatroban (to 1.9 mL/kg/min and 181 minutes, respectively, for patients with a Child-Pugh score >6).

Renal Impairment: No dosage adjustment is necessary in patients with renal dysfunction. The effect of renal disease on the pharmacokinetics of argatroban was studied in 6 subjects with normal renal function (mean Clcr = 95 ± 16 mL/min) and in 18 subjects with mild (mean Clcr = 64±10 mL/min), moderate (mean Clcr = 41 ± 5.8 mL/min), and severe (mean Clcr = 5 ± 7 mL/min) renal impairment. The pharmacokinetics and pharmacodynamics of argatroban at dosages up to 5 mcg/kg/min were not significantly affected by renal dysfunction.

Use of argatroban was evaluated in a study of 12 patients with stable end-stage renal disease undergoing chronic intermittent hemodialysis. Argatroban was administered at a rate of 2 to 3 mcg/kg/min (begun at least 4 hours prior to dialysis) or as a bolus dose of 250 mcg/kg at the start of dialysis followed by a continuous infusion of 2 mcg/kg/min. Although these regimens did not achieve the goal of maintaining ACT values at 1.8 times the baseline value throughout most of the hemodialysis period, the hemodialysis sessions were successfully completed with both of these regimens. The mean ACTs produced in this study ranged from 1.39 to 1.82 times baseline, and the mean aPTTs ranged from 1.96 to 3.4 times baseline. When argatroban was administered as a continuous infusion of 2 mcg/kg/min prior to and during a 4-hour hemodialysis session, approximately 20% was cleared through dialysis.

Age, Gender: There are no clinically significant effects of age or gender on the pharmacokinetics or pharmacodynamics (e.g., aPTT) of argatroban in adults.

Pediatric: Argatroban clearance is decreased in seriously ill pediatric patients. Pharmacokinetic parameters of argatroban were characterized in a population pharmacokinetic/pharmacodynamic analysis with sparse data from 15 seriously ill pediatric patients. Clearance in pediatric patients (0.16 L/hr/kg) was 50% lower compared to healthy adults (0.31 L/hr/kg). Four pediatric patients with elevated bilirubin (secondary to cardiac complications or hepatic impairment) had, on average, 80% lower clearance (0.03 L/hr/kg) when compared to pediatric patients with normal bilirubin levels. [see Use in Specific Populations (8.4)].

Drug-Drug Interactions:

Digoxin: In 12 healthy volunteers, intravenous infusion of argatroban (2 mcg/kg/min) over 5 days (study days 11 to 15) did not affect the steady-state pharmacokinetics of oral digoxin (0.375 mg daily for 15 days).

Erythromycin: In 10 healthy subjects, orally administered erythromycin (a potent inhibitor of CYP3A4/5) at 500 mg four times daily for 7 days had no effect on the pharmacokinetics of argatroban at a dose of 1 mcg/kg/min for 5 hours. These data suggest oxidative metabolism by CYP3A4/5 is not an important elimination pathway in vivo for argatroban.

Aspirin and Acetaminophen: Drug-drug interactions have not been demonstrated between argatroban and concomitantly administered aspirin (162.5 mg orally given 26 and 2

Table 9 Efficacy Results of Study 1: Composite Endpoint* and Individual Components, Ranked by Severity[†]

Parameter, N (%)	HIT		HITTS		HIT/HITTS	
	Control n = 147	Argatroban n = 160	Control n = 46	Argatroban n = 144	Control n = 193	Argatroban n = 304
Composite Endpoint	57 (38.8)	41 (25.6)	26 (56.5)	63 (43.8)	83 (43.0)	104 (34.2)
Individual Components[†]:						
Death	32 (21.8)	27 (16.9)	13 (28.3)	26 (18.1)	45 (23.3)	53 (17.4)
Amputation	3 (2.0)	3 (1.9)	4 (8.7)	16 (11.1)	7 (3.6)	19 (6.2)
New Thrombosis	22 (15.0)	11 (6.9)	9 (19.6)	21 (14.6)	31 (16.1)	32 (10.5)

* Death (all cause), amputation (all cause), or new thrombosis within 37-day study period
† Reported as the most severe outcome among the components of composite endpoint (severity ranking: death > amputation > new thrombosis); patients may have had multiple outcomes.

hours prior to initiation of argatroban 1 mcg/kg/min over 4 hours) or acetaminophen (1,000 mg orally given 12, 6, and 0 hours prior to, and 6 and 12 hours subsequent to, initiation of argatroban 1.5 mcg/kg/min over 18 hours).

13 NONCLINICAL TOXICOLOGY
13.1 Carcinogenesis, Mutagenesis, Impairment of Fertility
Carcinogenicity studies with argatroban have not been performed.
Argatroban was not genotoxic in the Ames test, the Chinese hamster ovary cell (CHO/HGPRT) forward mutation test, the Chinese hamster lung fibroblast chromosome aberration test, the rat hepatocyte, and WI-38 human fetal lung cell unscheduled DNA synthesis (UDS) tests, or the mouse micronucleus test.
Argatroban at intravenous doses up to 27 mg/kg/day (0.3 times the recommended maximum human dose based on body surface area) had no effect on fertility and reproductive function of male and female rats.

14 CLINICAL STUDIES
14.1 Heparin-Induced Thrombocytopenia
The safety and efficacy of argatroban were evaluated in a historically controlled efficacy and safety study (Study 1) and a follow-on efficacy and safety study (Study 2). These studies were comparable with regard to study design, study objectives, dosing regimens as well as study outline, conduct, and monitoring.
In these studies, 568 adult patients were treated with argatroban and 193 adult patients made up the historical control group. Patients had a clinical diagnosis of heparin-induced thrombocytopenia, either without thrombosis (HIT) or with thrombosis (HITTS [heparin-induced thrombocytopenia and thrombosis syndrome]) and were males or non-pregnant females between the age of 18 and 80 years old. HIT/HITTS was defined by a fall in platelet count to less than 100,000/μL or a 50% decrease in platelets after the initiation of heparin therapy with no apparent explanation other than HIT. Patients with HITTS also had an arterial or venous thrombosis documented by appropriate imaging techniques or supported by clinical evidence such as acute myocardial infarction, stroke, pulmonary embolism, or other clinical indications of vascular occlusion. Patients who had documented histories of positive heparin-dependent antibody tests without current thrombocytopenia or heparin challenge (e.g., patients with latent disease) were also included if they required anticoagulation.
These studies did not include patients with documented unexplained aPTT >200% of control at baseline, documented coagulation disorder or bleeding diathesis unrelated to HIT, a lumbar puncture within the past 7 days or a history of previous aneurysm, hemorrhagic stroke, or a thrombotic stroke within the past 6 months unrelated to HIT.
The initial dose of argatroban was 2 mcg/kg/min. Two hours after the start of the argatroban infusion, an aPTT level was obtained and dose adjustments were made (up to a maximum of 10 mcg/kg/min) to achieve a steady- state aPTT value that was 1.5 to 3.0 times the baseline value, not to exceed 100 seconds. Overall the mean aPTT level for HIT and HITTS patients during the argatroban infusion increased from baseline values of 34 and 38 seconds, respectively, to 62.5 and 64.5 seconds, respectively.
The primary efficacy analysis was based on a comparison of event rates for a composite endpoint that included death (all causes), amputation (all causes) or new thrombosis during the treatment and follow-up period (study days 0 to 37). Secondary analyses included evaluation of the event rates for the components of the composite endpoint as well as time-to-event analyses.
In Study 1, a total of 304 patients were enrolled as follows: active HIT (n=129), active HITTS (n=144), or latent disease (n=31). Among the 193 historical controls, 139 (72%) had ac-

tive HIT, 46 (24%) had active HITTS, and 8 (4%) had latent disease. Within each group, those with active HIT and those with latent disease were analyzed together. Positive laboratory confirmation of HIT/HITTS by the heparin-induced platelet aggregation test or serotonin release assay was demonstrated in 174 of 304 (57%) argatroban-treated patients (i.e., in 80 with HIT or latent disease and 94 with HITTS) and in 149 of 193 (77%) historical controls (i.e., in 119 with HIT or latent disease and 30 with HITTS). The test results for the remainder of the patients and controls were either negative or not determined.
There was a significant improvement in the composite outcome in patients with HIT and HITTS treated with argatroban versus those in the historical control group (see Table 9). The components of the composite endpoint are shown in Table 9.
[See table 9 above]
Time-to-event analyses showed significant improvements in the time-to-first event in patients with HIT or HITTS treated with argatroban versus those in the historical control group. The between-group differences in the proportion of patients who remained free of death, amputation, or new thrombosis were statistically significant in favor of argatroban by these analyses.
A time-to-event analysis for the composite endpoint is shown in Figure 3 for patients with HIT and Figure 4 for patients with HITTS.

Figure 3. Time to First Event for the Composite Efficacy Endpoint: HIT Patients

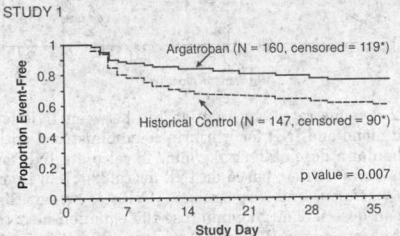

*Censored indicates no clinical endpoint (defined as death, amputation, or new thrombosis) was observed during the follow-up period (maximum period of follow-up was 37 days).

Figure 4. Time to First Event for the Composite Efficacy Endpoint: HITTS Patients

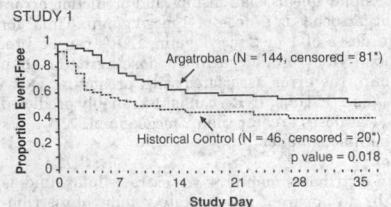

*Censored indicates no clinical endpoint (defined as death, amputation, or new thrombosis) was observed during the follow-up period (maximum period of follow-up was 37 days).

In Study 2, a total of 264 patients were enrolled as follows: HIT (n=125) or HITTS (n=139). There was a significant improvement in the composite efficacy outcome for argatroban-treated patients, versus the same historical control group from Study 1, among patients having HIT (25.6% vs. 38.8%), patients having HITTS (41.0% vs. 56.5%), and patients having either HIT or HITTS (33.7% vs. 43.0%). Time-to-event analyses showed significant improvements in the

time-to-first event in patients with HIT or HITTS treated with argatroban versus those in the historical control group. The between-group differences in the proportion of patients who remained free of death, amputation, or new thrombosis were statistically significant in favor of argatroban.
Anticoagulant Effect:
In Study 1, the mean (± SE) dose of argatroban administered was 2.0 ± 0.1 mcg/kg/min in the HIT arm and 1.9 ± 0.1 mcg/kg/min in the HITTS arm. Seventy-six percent of patients with HIT and 81% of patients with HITTS achieved a target aPTT at least 1.5-fold greater than the baseline aPTT at the first assessment occurring on average at 4.6 hours (HIT) and 3.9 hours (HITTS) following initiation of argatroban therapy.
No enhancement of aPTT response was observed in subjects receiving repeated administration of argatroban.
Platelet Count Recovery:
In Study 1, 53% of patients with HIT and 58% of patients with HITTS, had a recovery of platelet count by Day 3. Platelet Count Recovery was defined as an increase in platelet count to >100,000/μL or to at least 1.5-fold greater than the baseline count (platelet count at study initiation) by Day 3 of the study.

14.2 Percutaneous Coronary Intervention (PCI) Patients with or at Risk for HIT
In 3 similarly designed trials, argatroban was administered to 91 patients with current or previous clinical diagnosis of HIT or heparin-dependent antibodies, who underwent a total of 112 percutaneous coronary interventions (PCIs) including percutaneous transluminal coronary angioplasty (PTCA), coronary stent placement, or atherectomy. Among the 91 patients undergoing their first PCI with argatroban, notable ongoing or recent medical history included myocardial infarction (n = 35), unstable angina (n = 23), and chronic angina (n = 34). There were 33 females and 58 males. The average age was 67.6 years (median 70.7, range 44 to 86), and the average weight was 82.5 kg (median 81.0 kg, range 49 to 141).
Twenty-one of the 91 patients had a repeat PCI using argatroban an average of 150 days after their initial PCI. Seven of 91 patients received glycoprotein IIb/IIIa inhibitors. Safety and efficacy were assessed against historical control populations who had been anticoagulated with heparin.
All patients received oral aspirin (325 mg) 2 to 24 hours prior to the interventional procedure. After venous or arterial sheaths were in place, anticoagulation was initiated with a bolus of argatroban of 350 mcg/kg via a large-bore intravenous line or through the venous sheath over 3 to 5 minutes. Simultaneously, a maintenance infusion of 25 mcg/kg/min was initiated to achieve a therapeutic activated clotting time (ACT) of 300 to 450 seconds. If necessary to achieve this therapeutic range, the maintenance infusion dose was titrated (15 to 40 mcg/kg/min) and/or an additional bolus dose of 150 mcg/kg could be given. Each patient's ACT was checked 5 to 10 minutes following the bolus dose. The ACT was checked as clinically indicated. Arterial and venous sheaths were removed no sooner than 2 hours after discontinuation of argatroban and when the ACT was less than 160 seconds.
If a patient required anticoagulation after the procedure, argatroban could be continued, but at a lower infusion dose between 2.5 and 5 mcg/kg/min. An aPTT was drawn 2 hours after this dose reduction and the dose of argatroban then was adjusted as clinically indicated (not to exceed 10 mcg/kg/min), to reach an aPTT between 1.5 and 3 times baseline value (not to exceed 100 seconds).
In 92 of the 112 interventions (82%), the patient received the initial bolus of 350 mcg/kg and an initial infusion dose of 25 mcg/kg/min. The majority of patients did not require additional bolus dosing during the PCI procedure. The mean value for the initial ACT measurement after the start of dosing for all interventions was 379 sec (median 338 sec; 5th percentile-95th percentile 238 to 675 sec). The mean ACT value per intervention over all measurements taken during the procedure was 416 sec (median 390 sec; 5th percentile-95th percentile 261 to 698 sec). About 65% of patients had ACTs within the recommended range of 300 to 450 seconds throughout the procedure. The investigators did not achieve anticoagulation within the recommended range in about 23% of patients. However, in this small sample, patients with ACTs below 300 seconds did not have more coronary thrombotic events, and patients with ACTs over 450 seconds did not have higher bleeding rates.
Acute procedural success was defined as lack of death, emergent coronary artery bypass graft (CABG), or Q- wave myocardial infarction. Acute procedural success was reported in 98.2% of patients who underwent PCIs with argatroban anticoagulation compared with 94.3% of historical control patients anticoagulated with heparin (p = NS). Among the 112 interventions, 2 patients had emergency CABGs, 3 had repeat PTCAs, 4 had non-Q[82][c7e6] wave myocardial infarctions, 3 had myocardial ischemia, 1 had an abrupt closure, and 1 had an impending closure (some patients may have experienced more than 1 event). No patients died.

16 HOW SUPPLIED/STORAGE AND HANDLING

Argatroban Injection is supplied in 2.5 mL solution in single-use vials at the concentration of 100 mg/mL. Each vial contains 250 mg of argatroban.

NDC 0007-4407-01 (Package of 1)

Storage

Store the vials in original cartons at room temperature [25° C (77°F), with excursions permitted to 15°–30° C (59°–86°F)]. Do not freeze. Retain in the original carton to protect from light. If the solution is cloudy, or if an insoluble precipitate is noted, the vial should be discarded.

17 PATIENT COUNSELING INFORMATION

Inform patients of the risks associated with Argatroban Injection as well as the plan for regular monitoring during administration of the drug. Specifically, inform patients to report:

- the use of any other products known to affect bleeding.
- any medical history that may increase the risk for bleeding, including a history of severe hypertension; recent lumbar puncture or spinal anesthesia; major surgery, especially involving the brain, spinal cord, or eye; hematologic conditions associated with increased bleeding tendencies such as congenital or acquired bleeding disorders and gastrointestinal lesions such as ulcerations.
- any bleeding signs or symptoms.
- the occurrence of any signs or symptoms of allergic reactions (e.g., airway reactions, skin reactions and vasodilation reactions).

Manufactured, Distributed, and Marketed by **GlaxoSmithKline**
Research Triangle Park, NC 27709.
ARG:13PI

ARNUITY ELLIPTA   ℞
[ar-NEW-i-tee ee-LIP-ta]
(fluticasone furoate inhalation powder) 100 mcg

ARNUITY ELLIPTA
(fluticasone furoate inhalation powder) 200 mcg
FOR ORAL INHALATION

HIGHLIGHTS OF PRESCRIBING INFORMATION

These highlights do not include all the information needed to use ARNUITY ELLIPTA safely and effectively. See full prescribing information for ARNUITY ELLIPTA.

ARNUITY ELLIPTA (fluticasone furoate inhalation powder) 100 mcg
ARNUITY ELLIPTA (fluticasone furoate inhalation powder) 200 mcg
FOR ORAL INHALATION
Initial U.S. Approval: 2014

————INDICATIONS AND USAGE————

ARNUITY ELLIPTA is a corticosteroid indicated for:
- once-daily maintenance treatment of asthma as prophylactic therapy in patients aged 12 years and older. (1.1)
Important limitation:
- Not indicated for relief of acute bronchospasm. (1.1, 5.2)

————DOSAGE AND ADMINISTRATION————

For oral inhalation only. (2.1)
- Starting dosage is based on prior asthma therapy and disease severity. (2.2)
- Treatment of asthma in patients aged 12 years and older: 1 inhalation of ARNUITY ELLIPTA 100 mcg or ARNUITY ELLIPTA 200 mcg once daily. (2.2)

————DOSAGE FORMS AND STRENGTHS————

Inhalation powder containing 100 or 200 mcg of fluticasone furoate per actuation. (3)

————CONTRAINDICATIONS————

- Primary treatment of status asthmaticus or acute episodes of asthma requiring intensive measures. (4.1)
- Severe hypersensitivity to milk proteins or any ingredients of ARNUITY ELLIPTA. (4.2)

————WARNINGS AND PRECAUTIONS————

- Localized infections: *Candida albicans* infection of the mouth and throat may occur. Monitor patients periodically. Advise the patient to rinse his/her mouth with water without swallowing after inhalation. (5.1)
- Deterioration of asthma and acute episodes: Do not use for relief of acute symptoms. Patients require immediate re-evaluation during rapidly deteriorating asthma. (5.2)
- Immunosuppression: Potential worsening of existing tuberculosis, fungal, bacterial, viral, parasitic infections or ocular herpes simplex. Use with caution in patients with these infections. More serious or even fatal course of chickenpox or measles can occur in susceptible patients. (5.3)
- Transferring patients from systemic corticosteroids: Risk of impaired adrenal function when transfer-

ring from systemic corticosteroids. Wean patients slowly from systemic corticosteroids if transferring to ARNUITY ELLIPTA. (5.4)
- Hypercorticism and adrenal suppression: May occur with very high dosages or at the regular dosage in susceptible individuals. If such changes occur, discontinue ARNUITY ELLIPTA slowly. (5.5)
- Paradoxical bronchospasm: Discontinue ARNUITY ELLIPTA and institute alternative therapy if paradoxical bronchospasm occurs. (5.7)
- Decreases in bone mineral density: Monitor patients with major risk factors for decreased bone mineral content. (5.9)
- Monitor growth of adolescent patients. (5.10)
- Close monitoring for glaucoma and cataracts is warranted. (5.11)

————ADVERSE REACTIONS————

Most common adverse reactions (reported in greater than or equal to 5% of subjects) are:
- upper respiratory tract infection, nasopharyngitis, headache, and bronchitis. (6.1)

To report SUSPECTED ADVERSE REACTIONS, contact GlaxoSmithKline at 1-888-825-5249 or FDA at 1-800-FDA-1088 or www.fda.gov/medwatch.

————DRUG INTERACTIONS————

Strong cytochrome P450 3A4 inhibitors (e.g., ketoconazole): Use with caution. May cause systemic corticosteroid effects. (7.1)

————USE IN SPECIFIC POPULATIONS————

Hepatic impairment: Fluticasone furoate exposure may increase in patients with moderate or severe impairment. Monitor for systemic corticosteroid effects. (8.6, 12.3)

See 17 for PATIENT COUNSELING INFORMATION and FDA-approved patient labeling

Revised: 08/2014

FULL PRESCRIBING INFORMATION: CONTENTS*

FULL PRESCRIBING INFORMATION

1 INDICATIONS AND USAGE
1.1 Treatment of Asthma

ARNUITY™ ELLIPTA® is indicated for the once-daily maintenance treatment of asthma as prophylactic therapy in patients aged 12 years and older.

Important Limitation of Use: ARNUITY ELLIPTA is NOT indicated for the relief of acute bronchospasm.

2 DOSAGE AND ADMINISTRATION
2.1 General

ARNUITY ELLIPTA should be administered only by the orally inhaled route [see Instructions for Use in the Patient Information leaflet]. Advise the patient to rinse his/her mouth with water without swallowing after each dose.

2.2 Dosing

ARNUITY ELLIPTA should be administered as 1 inhalation once daily by the orally inhaled route. ARNUITY ELLIPTA should be used at the same time every day. Do not use ARNUITY ELLIPTA more than 1 time every 24 hours.

The starting dosage for ARNUITY ELLIPTA is based upon patients' asthma severity. The usual recommended starting dose for patients not on an inhaled corticosteroid is 100 mcg. For other patients, the starting dose should be based on previous asthma drug therapy and disease severity. For patients who do not respond to ARNUITY ELLIPTA 100 mcg after 2 weeks of therapy, replacement with ARNUITY ELLIPTA 200 mcg may provide additional asthma control.

If a dosage regimen of ARNUITY ELLIPTA fails to provide adequate control of asthma, the therapeutic regimen should be re-evaluated and additional therapeutic options, e.g., replacing the current strength of ARNUITY ELLIPTA with a higher strength, initiating an inhaled corticosteroid and long-acting beta$_2$-agonist (LABA) combination product, or initiating oral corticosteroids, should be considered.

The highest recommended daily dose is 200 mcg. If symptoms arise between doses, an inhaled short-acting beta$_2$-agonist should be used for immediate relief.

The maximum benefit may not be achieved for up to 2 weeks or longer after starting treatment. Individual patients may experience a variable time to onset and degree of symptom relief.

After asthma stability has been achieved, it is desirable to titrate to the lowest effective dosage to help reduce the possibility of side effects.

3 DOSAGE FORMS AND STRENGTHS

Inhalation Powder. Disposable light grey and orange plastic inhaler containing a foil blister strip of powder intended for oral inhalation only. Each blister contains fluticasone furoate 100 or 200 mcg.

4 CONTRAINDICATIONS
4.1 Status Asthmaticus

ARNUITY ELLIPTA is contraindicated in the primary treatment of status asthmaticus or other acute episodes of asthma where intensive measures are required [see Warnings and Precautions (5.2)].

4.2 Hypersensitivity

ARNUITY ELLIPTA is contraindicated in patients with known severe hypersensitivity to milk proteins or who have demonstrated hypersensitivity to fluticasone furoate or any of the excipients [see Warnings and Precautions (5.8), Description (11)].

5 WARNINGS AND PRECAUTIONS
5.1 Local Effects of Inhaled Corticosteroids

In clinical trials, the development of localized infections of the mouth and pharynx with *Candida albicans* has occurred in subjects treated with ARNUITY ELLIPTA. When such an infection develops, it should be treated with appropriate local or systemic (i.e., oral) antifungal therapy while treatment with ARNUITY ELLIPTA continues, but at times therapy with ARNUITY ELLIPTA may need to be interrupted. Advise the patient to rinse his/her mouth with water without swallowing following inhalation to help reduce the risk of oropharyngeal candidiasis.

5.2 Acute Asthma Episodes

ARNUITY ELLIPTA is not indicated for the relief of acute symptoms, i.e., as rescue therapy for treatment of acute episodes of bronchospasm. An inhaled, short-acting beta$_2$-agonist, not ARNUITY ELLIPTA, should be used to relieve acute symptoms such as shortness of breath. When prescribing ARNUITY ELLIPTA, the physician must provide the patient with an inhaled, short-acting beta$_2$-agonist (e.g., albuterol) for treatment of acute symptoms, despite regular once-daily use of ARNUITY ELLIPTA. Instruct patients to contact their physicians immediately if episodes of asthma not responsive to bronchodilators occur during the course of treatment with ARNUITY ELLIPTA. During such episodes, patients may require therapy with oral corticosteroids.

5.3 Immunosuppression

Persons using drugs that suppress the immune system are more susceptible to infections than healthy individuals.

Chickenpox and measles, for example, can have a more serious or even fatal course in susceptible children or adults using corticosteroids. In such patients who have not had these diseases or who have not been properly immunized, particular care should be taken to avoid exposure. How the dose, route, and duration of corticosteroid administration affect the risk of developing a disseminated infection is not known. The contribution of the underlying disease and/or prior corticosteroid treatment to the risk is also not known. If a patient is exposed to chickenpox, prophylaxis with varicella zoster immune globulin (VZIG) or pooled intravenous immunoglobulin (IVIG) may be indicated. If a patient is exposed to measles, prophylaxis with pooled intramuscular immunoglobulin (IG) may be indicated. (See the respective package inserts for complete VZIG and IG prescribing information.) If chickenpox develops, treatment with antiviral agents may be considered.

Inhaled corticosteroids should be used with caution, if at all, in patients with active or quiescent tuberculosis infections of the respiratory tract; untreated systemic fungal, bacterial, viral, or parasitic infections; or ocular herpes simplex.

5.4 Transferring Patients from Systemic Corticosteroid Therapy

Particular care is needed for patients who are transferred from systemically active corticosteroids to inhaled corticosteroids because deaths due to adrenal insufficiency have occurred in patients with asthma during and after transfer from systemic corticosteroids to less systemically available inhaled corticosteroids. After withdrawal from systemic corticosteroids, a number of months are required for recovery of hypothalamic–pituitary–adrenal (HPA) function.

Patients who have been previously maintained on 20 mg or more of prednisone (or its equivalent) may be most susceptible, particularly when their systemic corticosteroids have been almost completely withdrawn. During this period of HPA suppression, patients may exhibit signs and symptoms of adrenal insufficiency when exposed to trauma, surgery, or infection (particularly gastroenteritis) or other conditions associated with severe electrolyte loss. Although ARNUITY ELLIPTA may improve control of asthma symptoms during these episodes, in recommended doses it supplies less than normal physiological amounts of corticosteroid systemically and does NOT provide the mineralocorticoid activity that is necessary for coping with these emergencies.

During periods of stress or a severe asthma attack, patients who have been withdrawn from systemic corticosteroids should be instructed to resume oral corticosteroids (in large doses) immediately and to contact their physicians for further instruction. These patients should also be instructed to carry a medical identification warning card indicating that they may need supplementary systemic corticosteroids during periods of stress or a severe asthma attack.

Patients requiring systemic corticosteroids should be weaned slowly from systemic corticosteroid use after transferring to ARNUITY ELLIPTA. Lung function (forced expiratory volume in 1 second [FEV₁] or morning peak expiratory flow [AM PEF]), beta-agonist use, and asthma symptoms should be carefully monitored during withdrawal of systemic corticosteroids. In addition to monitoring asthma signs and symptoms, patients should be observed for signs and symptoms of adrenal insufficiency, such as fatigue, lassitude, weakness, nausea and vomiting, and hypotension.

Transfer of patients from systemic corticosteroid therapy to ARNUITY ELLIPTA may unmask allergic conditions previously suppressed by the systemic corticosteroid therapy (e.g., rhinitis, conjunctivitis, eczema, arthritis, eosinophilic conditions).

During withdrawal from oral corticosteroids, some patients may experience symptoms of systemically active corticosteroid withdrawal (e.g., joint and/or muscular pain, lassitude, depression), despite maintenance or even improvement of respiratory function.

5.5 Hypercorticism and Adrenal Suppression

ARNUITY ELLIPTA will often help control asthma symptoms with less suppression of HPA function than therapeutically equivalent oral doses of prednisone. Since ARNUITY ELLIPTA is absorbed into the circulation and can be systemically active at higher doses, the beneficial effects of ARNUITY ELLIPTA in minimizing HPA dysfunction may be expected only when recommended dosages are not exceeded and individual patients are titrated to the lowest effective dose.

Because of the possibility of significant systemic absorption of inhaled corticosteroids, patients treated with ARNUITY ELLIPTA should be observed carefully for any evidence of systemic corticosteroid effects. Particular care should be taken in observing patients postoperatively or during periods of stress for evidence of inadequate adrenal response.

It is possible that systemic corticosteroid effects such as hypercorticism and adrenal suppression (including adrenal crisis) may appear in a small number of patients, particularly when fluticasone furoate is administered at higher than recommended doses over prolonged periods of time. If

such effects occur, the dosage of ARNUITY ELLIPTA should be reduced slowly, consistent with accepted procedures for reducing systemic corticosteroids and for management of asthma symptoms.

5.6 Drug Interactions with Strong Cytochrome P450 3A4 Inhibitors

Caution should be exercised when considering the coadministration of ARNUITY ELLIPTA with long-term ketoconazole and other known strong CYP3A4 inhibitors (e.g., ritonavir, clarithromycin, conivaptan, indinavir, itraconazole, lopinavir, nefazodone, nelfinavir, saquinavir, telithromycin, troleandomycin, voriconazole) because increased systemic corticosteroid adverse effects may occur [see Drug Interactions (7.1), Clinical Pharmacology (12.3)].

5.7 Paradoxical Bronchospasm and Upper Airway Symptoms

As with other inhaled medicines, bronchospasm may occur with an immediate increase in wheezing after dosing. If bronchospasm occurs following dosing with ARNUITY ELLIPTA, it should be treated immediately with an inhaled, short-acting bronchodilator; ARNUITY ELLIPTA should be discontinued immediately; and alternative therapy should be instituted.

5.8 Hypersensitivity Reactions, Including Anaphylaxis

Hypersensitivity reactions such as urticaria, flushing, allergic dermatitis, and bronchospasm may occur after administration of ARNUITY ELLIPTA. Discontinue ARNUITY ELLIPTA if such reactions occur. There have been reports of anaphylactic reactions in patients with severe milk protein allergy after inhalation of other powder products containing lactose; therefore, patients with severe milk protein allergy should not use ARNUITY ELLIPTA [see Contraindications (4.2)].

5.9 Reduction in Bone Mineral Density

Decreases in bone mineral density (BMD) have been observed with long-term administration of products containing inhaled corticosteroids. The clinical significance of small changes in BMD with regard to long-term outcomes, such as fracture, is unknown. Patients with major risk factors for decreased bone mineral content, such as prolonged immobilization, family history of osteoporosis, or chronic use of drugs that can reduce bone mass (e.g., anticonvulsants, oral corticosteroids), should be monitored and treated with established standards of care.

5.10 Effect on Growth

Orally inhaled corticosteroids, including ARNUITY ELLIPTA, may cause a reduction in growth velocity when administered to children and adolescents.Monitor the growth of children and adolescents receiving ARNUITY ELLIPTA routinely (e.g., via stadiometry). To minimize the systemic effects of orally inhaled corticosteroids, including ARNUITY ELLIPTA, titrate each patient's dose to the lowest dosage that effectively controls his/her symptoms [see Use in Specific Populations (8.4)].

5.11 Glaucoma and Cataracts

Glaucoma, increased intraocular pressure, and cataracts have been reported in patients following the long–term administration of inhaled corticosteroids. Therefore, close monitoring is warranted in patients with a change in vision or with a history of increased intraocular pressure, glaucoma, and/or cataracts.

6 ADVERSE REACTIONS

Systemic and local corticosteroid use may result in the following:

- Candida albicans infection [see Warnings and Precautions (5.1)]
- Immunosuppression [see Warnings and Precautions (5.3)]
- Hypercorticism and adrenal suppression [see Warnings and Precautions (5.5)]
- Reduction in BMD [see Warnings and Precautions (5.9)]
- Growth effects in pediatrics [see Warnings and Precautions (5.10)]
- Glaucoma and cataracts [see Warnings and Precautions (5.11)]

6.1 Clinical Trials Experience

Because clinical trials are conducted under widely varying conditions, adverse reaction rates observed in the clinical trials of a drug cannot be directly compared with rates in the clinical trials of another drug and may not reflect the rates observed in practice.

The safety of ARNUITY ELLIPTA was evaluated in 10 double-blind, parallel-group, controlled trials (7 with placebo) of 8 to 76 weeks' duration, which enrolled 6,219 subjects with asthma. Doses of fluticasone furoate studied ranged from 25 to 800 mcg.

ARNUITY ELLIPTA 100 mcg was studied in 1,663 subjects, and ARNUITY ELLIPTA 200 mcg was studied in 608 subjects. Subject ages ranged from 12 to 84 years, 65% were female, and 75% were Caucasian.

In these trials, the proportion of subjects who discontinued study treatment early due to adverse reactions was 2% for subjects treated with both ARNUITY ELLIPTA 100 mcg and ARNUITY ELLIPTA 200 mcg and less than or equal to

1% for placebo-treated subjects. Serious adverse events, whether considered drug-related or not by the investigators, that occurred in more than 1 subject and in a greater percentage of subjects treated with ARNUITY ELLIPTA than placebo included hypertension, abscess, breast cancer, traumatic limb amputation, subarachnoid hemorrhage, and intervertebral disc protrusion; all events occurred at rates less than or equal to 1%.

The incidence of adverse reactions associated with ARNUITY ELLIPTA 100 mcg is shown in Table 1 and is based on one 24–week trial (Trial 1) in adolescent and adult subjects with asthma.

Table 1. Adverse Reactions with ARNUITY ELLIPTA 100 mcg with Greater than or Equal to 3% Incidence and More Common than Placebo (Trial 1, Intent-to-Treat Population)

Adverse Reaction	ARNUITY ELLIPTA 100 mcg n = 114 %	Placebo n = 115 %
Nasopharyngitis	8	5
Bronchitis	7	6
Upper respiratory tract infection	6	5
Headache	6	4
Pharyngitis	4	3
Sinusitis	4	<1
Toothache	3	<1
Gastroenteritis viral	3	0
Oral candidiasis	3	0
Oropharyngeal candidiasis	3	0
Oropharyngeal pain	3	0

The incidence of adverse reactions associated with ARNUITY ELLIPTA 200 mcg is shown in Table 2 and is based on one 24–week trial (Trial 3) in adolescent and adult subjects with asthma. This trial did not have a placebo arm.

Table 2. Adverse Reactions with ARNUITY ELLIPTA 200 mcg with Greater than or Equal to 3% Incidence (Trial 3, Safety Population)

Adverse Reaction	ARNUITY ELLIPTA 200 mcg n = 119 %	ARNUITY ELLIPTA 100 mcg n = 119 %
Nasopharyngitis	13	12
Headache	13	10
Bronchitis	7	12
Influenza	7	4
Upper respiratory tract infection	6	2
Sinusitis	4	7
Oropharyngeal pain	4	3
Pharyngitis	3	6
Back pain	3	3
Dysphonia	3	2
Oral candidiasis	3	<1
Procedural pain	3	<1
Rhinitis	3	<1
Throat irritation	3	<1
Abdominal pain	3	0
Cough	3	0

Adverse reactions observed in the other trials were consistent with those described in Tables 1 and 2.

Long-Term Safety: Long-term safety data are based on 2 trials in adolescent and adult subjects with asthma. In one 52-week trial, subjects received fluticasone furoate 100 mcg (n = 201) or fluticasone furoate 200 mcg (n = 202) in combination with a LABA. Subjects had a mean age of 39 years (adolescents made up 16% of the population), 63% were female, and 67% were Caucasian. In addition to the events shown in Table 1 and Table 2, adverse events occurring in greater than or equal to 3% of the subjects treated with fluticasone furoate 100 mcg or fluticasone furoate 200 mcg, in combination with a LABA, included pyrexia, extrasystoles, upper abdominal pain, respiratory tract infection, diarrhea, and allergic rhinitis.

In a second 24- to 76-week trial, subjects received fluticasone furoate 100 mcg (n = 1,010). Subjects participating in this trial had a history of one or more asthma exacerbations that required treatment with oral/systemic corticosteroids or emergency department visit or in-patient hospitalization for the treatment of asthma within the previous 12 months. Subjects had a mean age of 42 years (adolescents made up 14% of the population), 67% were female, and 73% were Caucasian. In addition to the events shown in Table 1 and Table 2, adverse events occurring in greater than or equal to 3% of subjects treated with fluticasone furoate 100 mcg for up to 76 weeks included allergic rhinitis, nasal congestion, and arthralgia.

7 DRUG INTERACTIONS

7.1 Inhibitors of Cytochrome P450 3A4

Fluticasone furoate is a substrate of CYP3A4. Concomitant administration of the strong CYP3A4 inhibitor ketoconazole increases the systemic exposure to fluticasone furoate. Caution should be exercised when considering the coadministration of ARNUITY ELLIPTA with long-term ketoconazole and other known strong CYP3A4 inhibitors (e.g., ritonavir, clarithromycin, conivaptan, indinavir, itraconazole, lopinavir, nefazodone, nelfinavir, saquinavir, telithromycin, troleandomycin, voriconazole) [see Warnings and Precautions (5.6), Clinical Pharmacology (12.3)].

8 USE IN SPECIFIC POPULATIONS

8.1 Pregnancy

Teratogenic Effects: Pregnancy Category C. There are no adequate and well-controlled trials with ARNUITY ELLIPTA in pregnant women. Corticosteroids have been shown to be teratogenic in laboratory animals when administered systemically at relatively low dosage levels. Because animal reproduction studies are not always predictive of human response, ARNUITY ELLIPTA should be used during pregnancy only if the potential benefit justifies the potential risk to the fetus. Women should be advised to contact their physicians if they become pregnant while taking ARNUITY ELLIPTA.

There were no teratogenic effects in rats and rabbits at approximately 4 times and equal to, respectively, the maximum recommended human daily inhalation dose (MRHDID) in adults (on a mcg/m^2 basis at maternal inhaled doses up to 91 and 8 mcg/kg/day in rats and rabbits, respectively). There were no effects on perinatal and postnatal development in rats at approximately equal to the MRHDID in adults (on a mcg/m^2 basis at maternal doses up to 27 mcg/kg/day).

Nonteratogenic Effects: Hypoadrenalism may occur in infants born of mothers receiving corticosteroids during pregnancy. Such infants should be carefully monitored.

8.2 Labor and Delivery

There are no adequate and well-controlled human trials that have investigated the effects of ARNUITY ELLIPTA during labor and delivery.

8.3 Nursing Mothers

It is not known whether fluticasone furoate is excreted in human breast milk. However, other corticosteroids have been detected in human milk. Since there are no data from controlled trials on the use of ARNUITY ELLIPTA by nursing mothers, caution should be exercised when it is administered to a nursing woman.

8.4 Pediatric Use

The safety and efficacy in pediatric patients younger than 12 years have not been established.

Effects on Growth: Orally inhaled corticosteroids may cause a reduction in growth velocity when administered to children and adolescents. A reduction of growth velocity in children and adolescents may occur as a result of poorly controlled asthma or from use of corticosteroids, including inhaled corticosteroids. The effects of long-term treatment of children and adolescents with inhaled corticosteroids, including fluticasone furoate, on final adult height are not known.

Controlled clinical trials have shown that inhaled corticosteroids may cause a reduction in growth in children. In these trials, the mean reduction in growth velocity was approximately 1 cm/year (range: 0.3 to 1.8 cm/year) and appears to be related to dose and duration of exposure. This effect has been observed in the absence of laboratory evidence of HPA axis suppression, suggesting that growth velocity is a more sensitive indicator of systemic corticosteroid exposure in children than some commonly used tests of HPA axis function. The long-term effects of this reduction in growth velocity associated with orally inhaled corticosteroids, including the impact on final adult height, are unknown. The potential for "catch-up" growth following discontinuation of treatment with orally inhaled corticosteroids has not been adequately studied. The growth of children and adolescents receiving orally inhaled corticosteroids, including ARNUITY ELLIPTA, should be monitored routinely (e.g., via stadiometry). The potential growth effects of prolonged treatment should be weighed against the clinical benefits obtained and the risks associated with alternative therapies. To minimize the systemic effects of orally inhaled corticosteroids, including ARNUITY ELLIPTA, each patient should be titrated to the lowest dose that effectively controls his/her symptoms.

A randomized, double-blind, parallel-group, multicenter, 1-year, placebo-controlled trial evaluated the effect of once-daily treatment with 110 mcg of fluticasone furoate in the nasal spray formulation on growth velocity assessed by stadiometry. The systemic exposure of fluticasone furoate in this trial is lower than that of ARNUITY ELLIPTA. The subjects were 474 prepubescent children (girls aged 5 to 7.5 years and boys aged 5 to 8.5 years). Mean growth velocity over the 52-week treatment period was lower in the subjects receiving fluticasone furoate nasal spray (5.19 cm/year) compared with placebo (5.46 cm/year). The mean reduction in growth velocity was 0.27 cm/year (95% CI: 0.06, 0.48) [see Warnings and Precautions (5.10)].

8.5 Geriatric Use

For the 4 confirmatory trials, 71 subjects were aged 65 and older (56 of which were treated with ARNUITY ELLIPTA) and 5 were aged 75 and older (1 of which was treated with ARNUITY ELLIPTA) [see Clinical Studies (14.2)]. Based on available data, no adjustment of the dosage of ARNUITY ELLIPTA in geriatric patients is necessary, but greater sensitivity in some older individuals cannot be ruled out. Clinical trials of ARNUITY ELLIPTA did not include sufficient numbers of subjects aged 65 and older to determine whether they respond differently from younger subjects. Other reported clinical experience has not identified differences in responses between the elderly and younger patients. In general, dose selection for an elderly patient should be cautious, usually starting at the low end of the dosing range, reflecting the greater frequency of decreased hepatic, renal, or cardiac function, and of concomitant disease or other drug therapy.

8.6 Hepatic Impairment

Fluticasone furoate systemic exposure increased by up to 3-fold in subjects with hepatic impairment compared with healthy subjects. Use ARNUITY ELLIPTA with caution in patients with moderate or severe hepatic impairment. Monitor patients for corticosteroid-related side effects [see Clinical Pharmacology (12.3)].

8.7 Renal Impairment

There were no significant increases in fluticasone furoate exposure in subjects with severe renal impairment (CrCl less than 30 mL/min) compared with healthy subjects. No dosage adjustment is required in patients with renal impairment [see Clinical Pharmacology (12.3)].

10 OVERDOSAGE

No human overdosage data have been reported for ARNUITY ELLIPTA. The potential for acute toxic corticosteroid effects following overdosage with ARNUITY ELLIPTA is low. Because of low systemic bioavailability (13.9%) and an absence of acute drug-related systemic findings in clinical trials, overdosage of fluticasone furoate is unlikely to require any treatment other than observation. If used at excessive doses for prolonged periods, systemic effects such as hypercorticism may occur [see Warnings and Precautions (5.5)].

Single- and repeat-dose trials of fluticasone furoate at doses of 50 to 4,000 mcg have been studied in human subjects. Decreases in mean serum cortisol were observed at dosages of 500 mcg or higher given once daily for 14 days.

11 DESCRIPTION

The active component of ARNUITY ELLIPTA is fluticasone furoate, a synthetic trifluorinated corticosteroid having the chemical name (6α,11β,16α,17α)-6,9-difluoro-17-{[(fluoro-methyl)thio]carbonyl}-11-hydroxy-16-methyl-3-oxoandrosta-1,4-dien-17-yl 2-furancarboxylate and the following chemical structure:

Fluticasone furoate is a white powder with a molecular weight of 538.6, and the empirical formula is $C_{27}H_{29}F_3O_6S$. It is practically insoluble in water.

ARNUITY ELLIPTA is a light grey and orange plastic inhaler containing a foil blister strip. Each blister on the strip contains a white powder mix of micronized fluticasone furoate (100 or 200 mcg) and lactose monohydrate (12.4 or 12.3 mg) for a total powder mix of 12.5 mg per blister. The lactose monohydrate contains milk proteins. After the inhaler is activated, the powder within the blister is exposed and ready for dispersion into the airstream created by the patient inhaling through the mouthpiece.

Under standardized in vitro test conditions, ARNUITY ELLIPTA 100 mcg and ARNUITY ELLIPTA 200 mcg deliver 90 and 182 mcg, respectively, of fluticasone furoate per blister when tested at a flow rate of 60 L/min for 4 seconds. In adult subjects with asthma and a mean FEV$_1$ of 2.55 L/sec (range: 1.63 to 3.97 L/sec), mean peak inspiratory flow through the ELLIPTA inhaler was 103.2 L/min (range: 71.2 to 133.1 L/min).

The actual amount of drug delivered to the lung will depend on patient factors, such as inspiratory flow profile.

12 CLINICAL PHARMACOLOGY

12.1 Mechanism of Action

Fluticasone furoate is a synthetic trifluorinated corticosteroid with anti-inflammatory activity. Fluticasone furoate has been shown in vitro to exhibit a binding affinity for the human glucocorticoid receptor that is approximately 29.9 times that of dexamethasone and 1.7 times that of fluticasone propionate. The clinical relevance of these findings is unknown.

The precise mechanism of corticosteroid action on asthma is not known. Inflammation is an important component in the pathogenesis of asthma. Corticosteroids have been shown to have a wide range of actions on multiple cell types (e.g., mast cells, eosinophils, neutrophils, macrophages, lymphocytes) and mediators (e.g., histamine, eicosanoids, leukotrienes, cytokines) involved in inflammation. These anti-inflammatory actions of corticosteroids contribute to their efficacy in asthma.

Though effective for the treatment of asthma, corticosteroids may not affect symptoms immediately. Individual patients will experience a variable time to onset and degree of symptom relief. Maximum benefit may not be achieved for 1 to 2 weeks or longer after starting treatment. When corticosteroids are discontinued, asthma stability may persist for several days or longer.

Trials in subjects with asthma have shown a favorable ratio between topical anti-inflammatory activity and systemic corticosteroid effects with recommended doses of orally inhaled fluticasone furoate. This is explained by a combination of a relatively high local anti-inflammatory effect, negligible oral systemic bioavailability (approximately 1.3%), and the minimal pharmacological activity of the metabolites detected in man.

12.2 Pharmacodynamics

The pharmacodynamics of fluticasone furoate were characterized in trials of fluticasone furoate given as a single component and also in trials of fluticasone furoate given in combination with vilanterol.

HPA Axis Effects: Healthy Subjects: Inhaled fluticasone furoate at repeat doses up to 400 mcg was not associated with statistically significant decreases in serum or urinary cortisol in healthy subjects. Decreases in serum and urine cortisol levels were observed at fluticasone furoate exposures several-fold higher than exposures observed at the therapeutic dose.

Subjects with Asthma: A randomized, double-blind, parallel-group trial in 185 subjects with asthma showed no difference between once-daily treatment with fluticasone furoate/vilanterol 100 mcg/25 mcg or fluticasone furoate/vilanterol 200 mcg/25 mcg compared with placebo on serum cortisol weighted mean (0 to 24 hours), serum cortisol AUC$_{(0-24)}$, and 24-hour urinary cortisol after 6 weeks of treatment, whereas prednisolone 10 mg given once daily for 7 days resulted in significant cortisol suppression.

Cardiac Effects: A QT/QTc trial did not demonstrate an effect of fluticasone furoate administration on the QTc interval. The effect of a single dose of 4,000 mcg of orally inhaled fluticasone furoate on the QTc interval was evaluated over 24 hours in 40 healthy male and female subjects in a placebo- and positive-controlled (a single dose of 400 mg oral moxifloxacin) cross-over trial. The QTcF maximal mean change from baseline following fluticasone furoate was similar to that observed with placebo with a treatment difference of 0.788 msec (90% CI: -1.802, 3.378). In contrast, moxifloxacin given as a 400-mg tablet resulted in prolongation of the QTcF maximal mean change from baseline compared with placebo with a treatment difference of 9.929 msec (90% CI: 7.339, 12.520).

12.3 Pharmacokinetics

The pharmacokinetics of fluticasone furoate were characterized in trials of fluticasone furoate given as a single component and also in trials of fluticasone furoate given in combination with vilanterol. Linear pharmacokinetics were observed for fluticasone furoate (200 to 800 mcg). On repeated once-daily inhalation administration, steady state of fluticasone furoate plasma concentration was achieved after 6 days, and the accumulation was up to 2.6-fold as compared with single dose.

Absorption: Fluticasone furoate plasma levels may not predict therapeutic effect. Peak plasma concentrations are reached within 0.5 to 1 hour. Absolute bioavailability of fluticasone furoate when administrated by inhalation was 13.9%, primarily due to absorption of the inhaled portion of the dose delivered to the lung. Oral bioavailability from the swallowed portion of the dose is low (approximately 1.3%) due to extensive first-pass metabolism. Systemic exposure (AUC) in subjects with asthma was 26% lower than observed in healthy subjects.

Distribution: Following intravenous administration to healthy subjects, the mean volume of distribution at steady state was 661 L. Binding of fluticasone furoate to human plasma proteins was high (99.6%).

Table 3. Change from Baseline in Trough FEV$_1$ (mL) at Week 24 – Trial 1

Trough FEV$_1$ (Week 24)	Placebo (n = 113)	ARNUITY ELLIPTA 100 mcg (n = 111)	Fluticasone Propionate 250 mcg Twice Daily (n = 107)
Least squares mean	2,372	2,519	2,517
Least squares mean change (SE)	15 (39.4)	161 (39.8)	159 (40.6)
Column vs. Placebo			
Difference	---	146	145
95% CI	---	36, 257	33, 257
P value	---	0.009	0.011

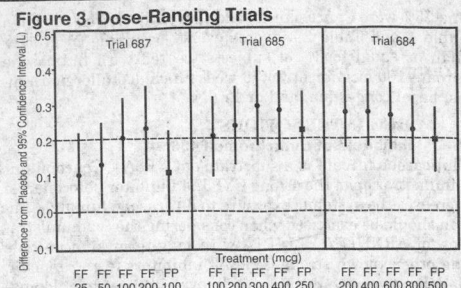

Figure 3. Dose-Ranging Trials

FF = Fluticasone furoate.
FP = Fluticasone propionate.
OD = Once daily.
BD = Twice daily.

Metabolism: Fluticasone furoate is cleared from systemic circulation principally by hepatic metabolism via CYP3A4 to metabolites with significantly reduced corticosteroid activity. There was no in vivo evidence for cleavage of the furoate moiety resulting in the formation of fluticasone.

Elimination: Fluticasone furoate and its metabolites are eliminated primarily in the feces, accounting for approximately 101% and 90% of the orally and intravenously administered doses, respectively. Urinary excretion accounted for approximately 1% and 2% of the orally and intravenously administered doses, respectively. Following repeat-dose inhaled administration, the plasma elimination phase half-life averaged 24 hours.

Special Populations: The effect of renal and hepatic impairment and other intrinsic factors on the pharmacokinetics of fluticasone furoate is shown in Figure 1.

Figure 1. Impact of Intrinsic Factors on the Pharmacokinetics (PK) of Fluticasone Furoate (FF)

[a] Age, gender, and ethnicity comparison for ARNUITY ELLIPTA in subjects with asthma.
[b] Renal groups (fluticasone furoate/vilanterol 200 mcg/25 mcg) and hepatic groups (fluticasone furoate/vilanterol 200 mcg/25 mcg or fluticasone furoate/vilanterol 100 mcg/12.5 mcg) compared with healthy control group.

Race: Systemic exposure (AUC$_{(0-24)}$) to inhaled fluticasone furoate 200 mcg was 27% to 49% higher in healthy subjects of Japanese, Korean, and Chinese heritage compared with Caucasian subjects. Similar differences were observed for subjects with asthma (Figure 1). There is no evidence that this higher exposure to fluticasone furoate results in clinically relevant effects on urinary cortisol excretion or on efficacy in these racial groups.

Hepatic Impairment: Following repeat dosing of fluticasone furoate/vilanterol 200 mcg/25 mcg (100 mcg/12.5 mcg in the severe impairment group) for 7 days, fluticasone furoate systemic exposure (AUC) increased 34%, 83%, and 75% in subjects with mild, moderate, and severe hepatic impairment, respectively, compared with healthy subjects (see Figure 1).

In subjects with moderate hepatic impairment receiving fluticasone furoate/vilanterol 200 mcg/25 mcg, mean serum cortisol (0 to 24 hours) was reduced by 34% (90% CI: 11%, 51%) compared with healthy subjects. In subjects with severe hepatic impairment receiving fluticasone furoate/vilanterol 100 mcg/12.5 mcg, mean serum cortisol (0 to 24 hours) was increased by 14% (90% CI: -16%, 55%) compared with healthy subjects. Patients with moderate to severe hepatic disease should be closely monitored.

Renal Impairment: Fluticasone furoate systemic exposure was not increased in subjects with severe renal impairment compared with healthy subjects (see Figure 1). There was no evidence of greater corticosteroid class-related systemic effects (assessed by serum cortisol) in subjects with severe renal impairment compared with healthy subjects.

Drug Interactions: The potential for fluticasone furoate to inhibit or induce metabolic enzymes and transporter systems is negligible at low inhalation doses.

Inhibitors of Cytochrome P450 3A4: The exposure (AUC) of fluticasone furoate was 36% higher after single and repeated doses when coadministered with ketoconazole 400 mg compared with placebo (see Figure 2). The increase in fluticasone furoate exposure was associated with a 27% reduction in weighted mean serum cortisol (0 to 24 hours).

Figure 2. Impact of Coadministered Ketoconazole[a] on the Pharmacokinetics (PK) of Fluticasone Furoate

[a] Compared with placebo group

13 NONCLINICAL TOXICOLOGY

13.1 Carcinogenesis, Mutagenesis, Impairment of Fertility

Fluticasone furoate produced no treatment-related increases in the incidence of tumors in 2-year inhalation studies in rats and mice at inhaled doses up to 9 and 19 mcg/kg/day, respectively (less than the MRHDID in adults on a mcg/m² basis).

Fluticasone furoate did not induce gene mutation in bacteria or chromosomal damage in a mammalian cell mutation test in mouse lymphoma L5178Y cells in vitro. There was also no evidence of genotoxicity in the in vivo micronucleus test in rats.

No evidence of impairment of fertility was observed in male and female rats at inhaled fluticasone furoate doses up to 29 and 91 mcg/kg/day, respectively (approximately equal to and 4 times, respectively, the MRHDID in adults on a mcg/m² basis).

14 CLINICAL STUDIES

The safety and efficacy of ARNUITY ELLIPTA were evaluated in 3,611 subjects with asthma. The development program included 4 confirmatory trials of 3 and 6 months' duration and 3 dose-ranging trials of 8 weeks' duration. The efficacy of ARNUITY ELLIPTA is based primarily on the dose-ranging trials and the confirmatory trials described below.

14.1 Dose-Ranging Trials

Eight doses of fluticasone furoate ranging from 25 to 800 mcg once daily were evaluated in 3 randomized, double-blind, placebo-controlled, 8-week trials in subjects with asthma. Across the 3 trials, subjects were uncontrolled at baseline on treatments of short-acting beta$_2$-agonist and/or non-inhaled corticosteroid controller medications (Trial 687), low-dose inhaled corticosteroid (Trial 685), or medium doses of inhaled corticosteroid (Trial 684). The trials in Figure 3 were dose-ranging trials of ARNUITY ELLIPTA not designed to provide comparative effectiveness data and should not be interpreted as evidence of superiority/inferiority to fluticasone propionate. A dose-related increase in trough FEV$_1$ at Week 8 was seen for doses from 25 to 200 mcg with no consistent additional benefit for doses above 200 mcg as seen in Figure 3. To evaluate dosing frequency, a separate trial compared fluticasone furoate 200 mcg once daily, fluticasone furoate 100 mcg twice daily, fluticasone propionate 100 mcg twice daily, and fluticasone propionate 200 mcg once daily. The results supported the selection of the once-daily dosing frequency.

[See figure 3 at top of next column]

14.2 Confirmatory Trials

The clinical development program for ARNUITY ELLIPTA included 4 confirmatory trials in adolescent and adult subjects aged 12 years and older with asthma. The trials were designed to evaluate the safety and efficacy of ARNUITY ELLIPTA given once daily in the evening on lung function in subjects who were not controlled on their current treatments of inhaled corticosteroids, or combination therapy consisting of an inhaled corticosteroid plus a LABA. Study treatments were delivered as inhalation powders. The primary endpoint in all trials was change from baseline in evening trough FEV$_1$ measured approximately 24 hours after the final dose of study medication. Trough FEV$_1$ (assessed at approximately 24 hours after the previous dose) was also

assessed at clinic visits throughout the trials. Trials 2 and 4 had a co-primary endpoint of change from baseline in weighted mean serial FEV$_1$ measured after the final dose of study medication at 5, 15, and 30 minutes and 1, 2, 3, 4, 5, 12, 16, 20, 23, and 24 hours post-dose.

Clinical Trials with ARNUITY ELLIPTA 100 mcg: Trial 1 was a 24-week trial that evaluated the efficacy of ARNUITY ELLIPTA 100 mcg compared with placebo on lung function in subjects with asthma. Inhaled fluticasone propionate 250 mcg twice daily was included as an active control. Of the 343 subjects, 59% were female and 79% were Caucasian. The mean age was 41 years. The trial included a 4-week run-in period during which the subjects were symptomatic while taking their usual low- to mid-dose inhaled corticosteroid therapy (i.e., fluticasone propionate 100 to 500 mcg daily or equivalent). Mean baseline percent predicted FEV$_1$ was approximately 73% overall and was similar across the 3 treatment groups. Thirty-five percent of subjects on placebo and 19% of subjects on ARNUITY ELLIPTA 100 mcg failed to complete the 24-week trial.

The change in trough FEV$_1$ from baseline to Week 24, or the last available on-treatment visit prior to Week 24, was assessed to evaluate the efficacy of ARNUITY ELLIPTA 100 mcg. The mean change from baseline in trough FEV$_1$ was greater among subjects receiving ARNUITY ELLIPTA 100 mcg than among those receiving placebo (mean treatment difference from placebo 146 mL; 95% CI: 36, 257) as shown in Table 3.

[See table 3 above]

Trial 2 was a 12-week trial that evaluated the efficacy of ARNUITY ELLIPTA 100 mcg on lung function in subjects with asthma compared with placebo. The combination of fluticasone furoate 100 mcg and vilanterol 25 mcg was also included as a treatment arm. Of the 609 subjects, 58% were female and 84% were Caucasian. The mean age was 40 years. The trial included a 4-week run-in period during which the subjects were symptomatic while taking their usual low- to mid-dose inhaled corticosteroid (fluticasone propionate 200 to 500 mcg/day or equivalent). If LABA were used prior to screening, their use was discontinued during the run-in. Mean baseline percent predicted FEV$_1$ was approximately 70% in both treatment groups. Twenty-six percent of subjects on placebo and 10% of subjects on ARNUITY ELLIPTA 100 mcg failed to complete the 12-week trial.

The co-primary efficacy endpoints in Trial 2 were change from baseline in trough FEV$_1$ at Week 12 and weighted mean FEV$_1$ (0-24 hours) at the end of the 12-week treatment period. Trough FEV$_1$ was assessed at clinic visits throughout the trial. Weighted mean FEV$_1$ (0-24 hours) was recorded at baseline and after the final study dose with serial measurements taken at frequent intervals (at 5, 15, and 30 minutes and 1, 2, 3, 4, 5, 12, 16, 20, 23, and 24 hours post-dose) in a subset of subjects (n = 201).

ARNUITY ELLIPTA 100 mcg once daily had greater mean changes from baseline in trough FEV$_1$ than placebo throughout the trial. At Week 12 or the last available on-treatment visit prior to Week 12, the mean change from baseline in trough FEV$_1$ was greater among subjects receiving ARNUITY ELLIPTA 100 mcg once daily than among those receiving placebo (mean treatment difference 136 mL; 95% CI: 51, 222).

Lung function improvements were sustained over the 24-hour period following the final dose of ARNUITY ELLIPTA 100 mcg (see Figure 4). Compared with placebo, at Week 12 the change from baseline in weighted mean FEV$_1$ was significantly greater for ARNUITY ELLIPTA 100 mcg (mean treatment difference 186 mL; 95% CI: 62, 310).

Figure 4. Mean Change from Baseline in Individual Serial FEV₁ (mL) Assessments after 12 Weeks of Treatment — Trial 2

Subjects in both Trials 1 and 2 receiving ARNUITY ELLIPTA 100 mcg once daily had a greater improvement from baseline in percentage of 24-hour periods without need of beta₂-agonist rescue medication use than subjects receiving placebo.

Clinical Trial with ARNUITY ELLIPTA 200 mcg: Trial 3 was a 24-week trial that evaluated the relative efficacy of ARNUITY ELLIPTA 100 mcg and ARNUITY ELLIPTA 200 mcg on lung function in subjects with asthma. Of the 219 subjects, 68% were female and 87% were Caucasian. The mean age was 46 years. The trial included a 4-week run-in period during which the subjects were symptomatic while taking their usual mid- to high-dose inhaled corticosteroid therapy (i.e., fluticasone propionate greater than 250 to 1,000 mcg/day or equivalent). If LABA were used prior to screening, their use was discontinued during the run-in. Mean baseline percent predicted FEV₁ was approximately 68% overall and similar in the 2 treatment groups. Sixteen percent of subjects on ARNUITY ELLIPTA 100 mcg and 13% of subjects on ARNUITY ELLIPTA 200 mcg failed to complete the 24-week trial.

The primary efficacy endpoint was mean change from baseline in trough FEV₁ at Week 24. There were trends toward greater mean changes from baseline in the group receiving ARNUITY ELLIPTA 200 mcg than the group receiving ARNUITY ELLIPTA 100 mcg throughout the trial (see Figure 5). At Week 24 or the last available on-treatment visit prior to Week 24, the mean change from baseline in trough FEV₁ was 208 mL for ARNUITY ELLIPTA 100 mcg, as compared to 284 mL for ARNUITY ELLIPTA 200 mcg (difference of 77 mL; 95% CI: -39, 192) as seen in Figure 5.

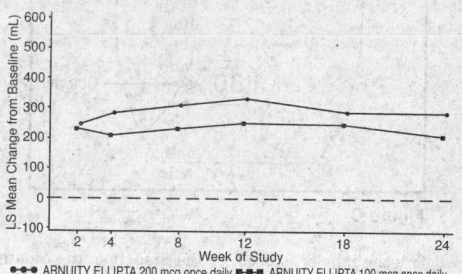

Figure 5. Mean Change from Baseline in Trough FEV₁ (mL) over Time — Trial 3

Trial 4 was a 24-week trial that evaluated the efficacy of ARNUITY ELLIPTA 200 mcg once daily and fluticasone propionate 500 mcg twice daily on lung function in subjects with asthma. The combination of fluticasone furoate 200 mcg and vilanterol 25 mcg was also included as a treatment arm (data not shown). Of the 586 subjects, 59% were female and 84% were Caucasian. The mean age was 46 years. The trial included a 4-week run-in period during which the subjects were symptomatic while taking their usual mid- to high-dose inhaled corticosteroid (fluticasone propionate 500 to 1,000 mcg/day or equivalent). If LABA were used prior to screening, their use was discontinued during the run-in. Mean baseline percent predicted FEV₁ was approximately 67% in both treatment groups.

Both ARNUITY ELLIPTA 200 mcg once daily and fluticasone propionate 500 mcg twice daily produced improvement from baseline in lung function. At Week 24 the mean change from baseline in trough FEV₁ was 201 mL for ARNUITY ELLIPTA 200 mcg once daily and 183 mL for fluticasone propionate 500 mcg twice daily (treatment difference of 18 mL, 95% CI: -66, 102).

Lung function improvements were sustained over the 24-hour period following the final dose of ARNUITY ELLIPTA 200 mcg (see Figure 6). At Week 24, the change from baseline in weighted mean FEV₁ was 328 mL for ARNUITY ELLIPTA 200 mcg once daily and 258 mL for fluticasone propionate 500 twice daily (difference of 70 mL; 95% CI: -67, 208).

Figure 6. Mean Change from Baseline in Individual Serial FEV₁ (mL) Assessments after 24 Weeks of Treatment — Trial 4

16 HOW SUPPLIED/STORAGE AND HANDLING

ARNUITY ELLIPTA 100 mcg is supplied as a disposable light grey and orange plastic inhaler containing a foil strip with 30 blisters (NDC 0173-0874-10) or 14 blisters (institutional pack) (NDC 0173-0874-14).

ARNUITY ELLIPTA 200 mcg is supplied as a disposable light grey and orange plastic inhaler containing a foil strip with 30 blisters (NDC 0173-0876-10) or 14 blisters (institutional pack) (NDC 0173-0876-14).

The inhaler is packaged in a moisture-protective foil tray with a desiccant and a peelable lid.

Store at room temperature between 68°F and 77°F (20°C and 25°C); excursions permitted from 59°F to 86°F (15°C to 30°C) [See USP Controlled Room Temperature]. Store in a dry place away from direct heat or sunlight. Keep out of reach of children.

ARNUITY ELLIPTA should be stored inside the unopened moisture-protective foil tray and only removed from the tray immediately before initial use. Discard ARNUITY ELLIPTA 6 weeks after opening the foil tray or when the counter reads "0" (after all blisters have been used), whichever comes first. The inhaler is not reusable. Do not attempt to take the inhaler apart.

17 PATIENT COUNSELING INFORMATION

Advise the patient to read the FDA-approved patient labeling (Patient Information and Instructions for Use).

Not for Acute Symptoms: Inform patients that ARNUITY ELLIPTA is not meant to relieve acute asthma symptoms and extra doses should not be used for that purpose. ARNUITY ELLIPTA is not a bronchodilator and should not be used to treat status asthmaticus or to relieve acute asthma symptoms. Advise patients to treat acute symptoms with an inhaled, short-acting beta₂-agonist such as albuterol. Provide patients with such medication and instruct them in how it should be used.

Instruct patients to seek medical attention immediately if they experience any of the following:
• Symptoms get worse
• Significant decrease in lung function as outlined by the physician
• Need for more inhalations than usual of inhaled, short-acting beta₂-agonists

Advise patients not to increase the dose or frequency of ARNUITY ELLIPTA. The daily dosage of ARNUITY ELLIPTA should not exceed 1 inhalation. If they miss a dose, instruct patients to take their next dose at the same time they normally do.

Tell patients they should not stop or reduce therapy with ARNUITY ELLIPTA without physician/provider guidance since symptoms may recur after discontinuation.

Local Effects: Inform patients that localized infections with Candida albicans occurred in the mouth and pharynx in some patients. If oropharyngeal candidiasis develops, treat it with appropriate local or systemic (i.e., oral) antifungal therapy while still continuing therapy with ARNUITY ELLIPTA therapy, but at times therapy with ARNUITY ELLIPTA may need to be temporarily interrupted under close medical supervision. Advise patients to rinse the mouth with water without swallowing after inhalation to help reduce the risk of thrush.

Immunosuppression: Warn patients who are on immunosuppressant doses of corticosteroids to avoid exposure to chickenpox or measles and, if exposed, to consult their physicians without delay. Inform patients of potential worsening of existing tuberculosis, fungal, bacterial, viral, or parasitic infections or ocular herpes simplex.

Hypercorticism and Adrenal Suppression: Advise patients that ARNUITY ELLIPTA may cause systemic corticosteroid effects of hypercorticism and adrenal suppression. Additionally, instruct that deaths due to adrenal insufficiency have occurred during and after transfer from systemic corticosteroids. Patients should taper slowly from systemic corticosteroids if transferring to ARNUITY ELLIPTA.

Reduction in Bone Mineral Density: Advise patients who are at an increased risk for decreased BMD that the use of corticosteroids may pose an additional risk.

Reduced Growth Velocity: Inform patients that orally inhaled corticosteroids, including ARNUITY ELLIPTA, may cause a reduction in growth velocity when administered to pediatric patients. Physicians should closely follow the growth of children and adolescents taking corticosteroids by any route.

Ocular Effects: Advise patients that long-term use of inhaled corticosteroids may increase the risk of some eye problems (cataracts or glaucoma); consider regular eye examinations.

Hypersensitivity Reactions Including Anaphylaxis: Advise patients that hypersensitivity reactions (e.g., urticaria, flushing, allergic dermatitis, bronchospasm), including anaphylaxis, may occur after administration of ARNUITY ELLIPTA. Instruct patients to discontinue ARNUITY ELLIPTA if such reactions occur. There have been reports of anaphylactic reactions in patients with severe milk protein allergy after inhalation of other powder medications containing lactose; therefore, patients with severe milk protein allergy should not use ARNUITY ELLIPTA.

Use Daily for Best Effect: Advise patients to use ARNUITY ELLIPTA at regular intervals, since its effectiveness depends on regular use. Maximum benefit may not be achieved for 1 week or longer after starting treatment. If symptoms do not improve after 2 weeks of therapy or if the condition worsens, instruct patients to contact their physicians.

ARNUITY is a trademark and ELLIPTA is a registered trademark of the GSK group of companies.

GlaxoSmithKline
Research Triangle Park, NC 27709
©2014, the GSK group of companies. All rights reserved.
ARN:2PI

Patient Information
ARNUITY™ ELLIPTA® *[ar-NEW-i-tee ee-LIP-ta]*
(fluticasone furoate inhalation powder) 100 mcg
ARNUITY™ ELLIPTA®
(fluticasone furoate inhalation powder) 200 mcg

Read the Patient Information that comes with ARNUITY ELLIPTA before you start using it and each time you get a refill. There may be new information. This Patient Information does not take the place of talking to your healthcare provider about your medical condition or treatment.

What is ARNUITY ELLIPTA?
ARNUITY ELLIPTA is an inhaled corticosteroid (ICS) medicine used for the control and prevention of asthma in adults and children aged 12 years and older.
• ARNUITY ELLIPTA helps to prevent and control symptoms of asthma.
• **ARNUITY ELLIPTA is not for use to treat sudden symptoms of an asthma attack, wheezing, cough, shortness of breath, and chest pain or tightness.** Always have a rescue inhaler (an inhaled, short-acting bronchodilator) with you to treat sudden symptoms. If you do not have a rescue inhaler, contact your healthcare provider to have one prescribed for you.
• It is not known if ARNUITY ELLIPTA is safe and effective in children younger than 12 years.

Who should not use ARNUITY ELLIPTA?
Do not use ARNUITY ELLIPTA:
• to treat sudden symptoms of asthma. **ARNUITY ELLIPTA is not a rescue inhaler and should not be used to give you fast relief from your asthma attack.** Always use a rescue inhaler, such as albuterol, during a sudden asthma attack.
• if you have a severe allergy to milk proteins. Ask your healthcare provider if you are not sure.
• are allergic to fluticasone furoate or any of the ingredients in ARNUITY ELLIPTA. See "What are the ingredients in ARNUITY ELLIPTA?" below for a complete list of ingredients.

What should I tell my healthcare provider before using ARNUITY ELLIPTA?
Tell your healthcare provider about all of your health conditions, including if you:
• have liver problems.
• have weak bones (osteoporosis).
• have an immune system problem.
• have eye problems such as glaucoma or cataracts.
• are allergic to any of the ingredients in ARNUITY ELLIPTA, any other medicines, or food products. See "What are the ingredients in ARNUITY ELLIPTA?" below for a complete list of ingredients.
• have any type of viral, bacterial, or fungal infection.
• are exposed to chickenpox or measles.
• have any other medical conditions.
• are pregnant or planning to become pregnant. It is not known if ARNUITY ELLIPTA may harm your unborn baby.
• are breastfeeding. It is not known if the medicine in ARNUITY ELLIPTA passes into your milk and if it can harm your baby.

Tell your healthcare provider about all the medicines you take, including prescription and over-the-counter medicines, vitamins, and herbal supplements. ARNUITY

ELLIPTA and certain other medicines may interact with each other. This may cause serious side effects. Especially, tell your healthcare provider if you take antifungal, anti-HIV, or any other corticosteroid medicines. Know the medicines you take. Keep a list of them to show your healthcare provider and pharmacist when you get a new medicine.

How should I use ARNUITY ELLIPTA?
Read the step-by-step instructions for using ARNUITY ELLIPTA at the end of this Patient Information.

- **Do not** use ARNUITY ELLIPTA unless your healthcare provider has taught you how to use the inhaler and you understand how to use it correctly.
- ARNUITY ELLIPTA comes in 2 different strengths. Your healthcare provider prescribed the strength that is best for you.
- Use ARNUITY ELLIPTA exactly as your healthcare provider tells you to use it. **Do not** use ARNUITY ELLIPTA more often than prescribed.
- Adolescents may need help to use ARNUITY ELLIPTA.
- Use 1 inhalation of ARNUITY ELLIPTA 1 time each day. Use ARNUITY ELLIPTA at the same time each day.
- If you miss a dose of ARNUITY ELLIPTA, take it as soon as you remember. Do not take more than 1 inhalation each day. Take your next dose at your usual time. Do not take 2 doses at one time.
- Do not stop using ARNUITY ELLIPTA unless told to do so by your healthcare provider because your symptoms might get worse. Your healthcare provider will change your medicines as needed.
- **ARNUITY ELLIPTA does not relieve sudden symptoms.** Always have a rescue inhaler with you to treat sudden symptoms. If you do not have a rescue inhaler, call your healthcare provider to have one prescribed for you.
- Call your healthcare provider or get medical care right away if:
  - your breathing problems get worse
  - you need to use your rescue inhaler more often than usual
  - your rescue inhaler does not work as well to relieve your symptoms
  - you need to use 4 or more inhalations of your rescue inhaler in 24 hours for 2 or more days in a row
  - you use 1 whole canister of your rescue inhaler in 8 weeks
  - your peak flow meter results decrease. Your healthcare provider will tell you the numbers that are right for you.

What are the possible side effects with ARNUITY ELLIPTA?
ARNUITY ELLIPTA can cause serious side effects, including:
- **fungal infection in your mouth or throat (thrush)**. Rinse your mouth with water without swallowing after using ARNUITY ELLIPTA to help reduce your chance of getting thrush.
- **weakened immune system and increased chance of getting infections (immunosuppression)**
- **reduced adrenal function (adrenal insufficiency)**. Adrenal insufficiency is a condition where the adrenal glands do not make enough steroid hormones. This can happen when you stop taking oral corticosteroid medicines (such as prednisone) and start taking a medicine containing an inhaled corticosteroid (such as ARNUITY ELLIPTA). When your body is under stress from fever, trauma (such as a car accident), infection, surgery, or worse asthma symptoms, adrenal insufficiency can get worse and may cause death.
  Symptoms of adrenal insufficiency include:
  - feeling tired
  - lack of energy
  - weakness
  - nausea and vomiting
  - low blood pressure
- **sudden breathing problems immediately after inhaling your medicine**
- **serious allergic reactions.** Call your healthcare provider or get emergency medical care if you get any of the following symptoms of a serious allergic reaction:
  - rash
  - hives
  - swelling of your face, mouth, and tongue
  - breathing problems
- **bone thinning or weakness (osteoporosis)**
- **slow growth in adolescents.** An adolescent's growth should be checked often.
- **eye problems including glaucoma and cataracts.** You should have regular eye exams while using ARNUITY ELLIPTA.

Common side effects of ARNUITY ELLIPTA include:
- runny nose and sore throat
- headache
- breathing problems (bronchitis)
- flu

Tell your healthcare provider about any side effect that bothers you or that does not go away.
These are not all the side effects with ARNUITY ELLIPTA. Ask your healthcare provider or pharmacist for more information.

Call your doctor for medical advice about side effects. You may report side effects to FDA at 1-800-FDA-1088.

How do I store ARNUITY ELLIPTA?
- Store ARNUITY ELLIPTA at room temperature between 68°F and 77°F (20°C and 25°C). Keep in a dry place away from heat and sunlight.
- Store ARNUITY ELLIPTA in the unopened foil tray and only open when ready for use.
- Safely throw away ARNUITY ELLIPTA in the trash 6 weeks after you open the foil tray or when the counter reads "0", whichever comes first. Write the date you open the tray on the label on the inhaler.
- **Keep ARNUITY ELLIPTA and all medicines out of the reach of children.**

General information about ARNUITY ELLIPTA
Medicines are sometimes prescribed for purposes not mentioned in a Patient Information leaflet. Do not use ARNUITY ELLIPTA for a condition for which it was not prescribed. Do not give your ARNUITY ELLIPTA to other people, even if they have the same condition that you have. It may harm them.
This Patient Information leaflet summarizes the most important information about ARNUITY ELLIPTA. If you would like more information, talk with your healthcare provider or pharmacist. You can ask your healthcare provider or pharmacist for information about ARNUITY ELLIPTA that was written for healthcare professionals.
For more information about ARNUITY ELLIPTA, call 1-888-825-5249 or visit our website at www.ARNUITY.com.

What are the ingredients in ARNUITY ELLIPTA?
Active ingredients: fluticasone furoate
Inactive ingredients: lactose monohydrate (contains milk proteins)

Instructions for Use
For Oral Inhalation Only.
Read this before you start:
- **If you open and close the cover without inhaling the medicine, you will lose the dose.**
- **The lost dose will be securely held inside the inhaler, but it will no longer be available to be inhaled.**
- **It is not possible to accidentally take a double dose or an extra dose in 1 inhalation.**
Your ARNUITY ELLIPTA inhaler

How to use your inhaler
- ARNUITY ELLIPTA comes in a foil tray.
- Peel back the lid to open the tray. See Figure A.
- The tray contains a desiccant to reduce moisture. Do not eat or inhale. Throw it away in the household trash out of reach of children and pets. See Figure B.

Figure A

Figure B

Important Notes:
- Your inhaler contains 30 doses (14 doses if you have a sample or institutional pack).
- Each time you fully open the cover of the inhaler (you will hear a clicking sound), a dose is ready to be inhaled. This is shown by a decrease in the number on the counter.
- If you open and close the cover without inhaling the medicine, you will lose the dose. The lost dose will be held in the inhaler, but it will no longer be available to be inhaled. It is not possible to accidentally take a double dose or an extra dose in 1 inhalation.
- **Do not** open the cover of the inhaler until you are ready to use it. To avoid wasting doses after the inhaler is ready, **do not** close the cover until after you have inhaled the medicine.
- Write the "Tray opened" and "Discard" dates on the inhaler label. The "Discard" date is 6 weeks from the date you open the tray.
Check the counter. See Figure C.

Figure C

- Before the inhaler is used for the first time, the counter should show the number 30 (14 if you have a sample or institutional pack). This is the number of doses in the inhaler.
- Each time you open the cover, you prepare 1 dose of medicine.
- The counter counts down by 1 each time you open the cover.
Prepare your dose:
Wait to open the cover until you are ready to take your dose.
Step 1. Open the cover of the inhaler. See Figure D.

Figure D

- Slide the cover down to expose the mouthpiece. You should hear a "click." The counter will count down by 1 number. You do not need to shake this kind of inhaler. **Your inhaler is now ready to use.**
- If the counter does not count down as you hear the click, the inhaler will not deliver the medicine. Call your healthcare provider or pharmacist if this happens.
Step 2. Breathe out. See Figure E.

Figure E

- While holding the inhaler away from your mouth, breathe out (exhale) fully. Do not breathe out into the mouthpiece.
Step 3. Inhale your medicine. See Figure F.

Figure F

- Put the mouthpiece between your lips, and close your lips firmly around it. Your lips should fit over the curved shape of the mouthpiece.
- Take 1 long, steady, deep breath in through your mouth. **Do not** breathe in through your nose.
- Do not block the air vent with your fingers. **See Figure G.**

Do not block the air vent with your fingers.

Figure G

- **Remove the inhaler from your mouth and hold your breath for about 3 to 4 seconds** (or as long as comfortable for you). **See Figure H.**
[See figure H at top of next column]
Figure H
Step 4. Breathe out slowly and gently. See Figures I.
[See figure I at top of next column]
- You may not taste or feel the medicine, even when you are using the inhaler correctly.

3-4 seconds

Figure H

Figure I

- **Do not** take another dose from the inhaler even if you do not feel or taste the medicine.
Step 5. Close the inhaler. See Figure J.

Figure J

- You can clean the mouthpiece if needed, using a dry tissue, before you close the cover. Routine cleaning is not required.
- Slide the cover up and over the mouthpiece as far as it will go.
Step 6. Rinse your mouth. See Figure K.

Figure K

- Rinse your mouth with water after you have used the inhaler and spit the water out. **Do not** swallow the water.
Important Note: When should you get a refill?
- **When you have less than 10 doses remaining** in your inhaler, the left half of the counter shows red as a reminder to get a refill. **See Figure L.**

Red

Figure L

- After you have inhaled the last dose, the counter will show "0" and will be empty.
- Throw the empty inhaler away in your household trash out of reach of children and pets.

If you have questions about ARNUITY ELLIPTA or how to use your inhaler, call GlaxoSmithKline (GSK) at 1-888-825-5249 or visit www.ARNUITY.com.

This Patient Information and Instructions for Use have been approved by the U.S. Food and Drug Administration. ARNUITY is a trademark and ELLIPTA is a registered trademark of the GSK group of companies.
GlaxoSmithKline
Research Triangle Park, NC 27709
©2014, the GSK group of companies. All rights reserved.
August 2014
ARN:1PIL

ARRANON   ℞
[air'ə-non]
(nelarabine)
injection

HIGHLIGHTS OF PRESCRIBING INFORMATION
These highlights do not include all the information needed to use ARRANON safely and effectively. See full prescribing information for ARRANON.
ARRANON (nelarabine) Injection
Initial U.S. Approval: 2005

WARNING: NEUROLOGIC ADVERSE REACTIONS
See full prescribing information for complete boxed warning.

Severe neurologic adverse reactions have been reported with the use of ARRANON. These adverse reactions have included altered mental states including severe somnolence, central nervous system effects including convulsions, and peripheral neuropathy ranging from numbness and paresthesias to motor weakness and paralysis. There have also been reports of adverse reactions associated with demyelination, and ascending peripheral neuropathies similar in appearance to Guillain-Barré syndrome. (5.1)

Full recovery from these adverse reactions has not always occurred with cessation of therapy with ARRANON. Close monitoring for neurologic adverse reactions is strongly recommended, and ARRANON should be discontinued for neurologic adverse reactions of NCI Common Toxicity Criteria grade 2 or greater. (5.1)

————INDICATIONS AND USAGE————
ARRANON is a nucleoside metabolic inhibitor indicated for the treatment of patients with T-cell acute lymphoblastic leukemia and T-cell lymphoblastic lymphoma whose disease has not responded to or has relapsed following treatment with at least two chemotherapy regimens. This use is based on the induction of complete responses. Randomized trials demonstrating increased survival or other clinical benefit have not been conducted. (1)

———DOSAGE AND ADMINISTRATION———

- Adult dose: 1,500 mg/m^2 administered intravenously over 2 hours on days 1, 3, and 5 repeated every 21 days. (2.1)
- Pediatric dose: 650 mg/m^2 administered intravenously over 1 hour daily for 5 consecutive days repeated every 21 days. (2.1)
- Discontinue treatment for ≥grade 2 neurologic reactions. (2.2)
- Dosage may be delayed for hematologic reactions (2.2)
- Take measures to prevent hyperuricemia. (2.4)

———DOSAGE FORMS AND STRENGTHS———

250 mg/50 mL (5 mg/mL) vial (3)

———CONTRAINDICATIONS———

None.

———WARNINGS AND PRECAUTIONS———

- Severe neurologic reactions have been reported. Monitor for signs and symptoms of neurologic toxicity. (5.1)
- Hematologic Reactions: Complete blood counts including platelets should be monitored regularly. (5.2)
- Fetal harm can occur if administered to a pregnant woman. Women should be advised not to become pregnant when taking ARRANON. (5.3)

———ADVERSE REACTIONS———

The most common (≥ 20%) adverse reactions were:
- Adult: anemia, thrombocytopenia, neutropenia, nausea, diarrhea, vomiting, constipation, fatigue, pyrexia, cough, and dyspnea (6.1)
- Pediatric: anemia, neutropenia, thrombocytopenia, and leukopenia (6.1)

The most common (>10%) neurological adverse reactions were:
- Adult: somnolence, dizziness, peripheral neurologic disorders, hypoesthesia, headache, and paresthesia (6.1)
- Pediatric: headache and peripheral neurologic disorders (6.1)

To report SUSPECTED ADVERSE REACTIONS, contact GlaxoSmithKline at 1-888-825-5249 or FDA at 1-800-FDA-1088 or www.fda.gov/medwatch.

———DRUG INTERACTIONS———

Administration in combination with adenosine deaminase inhibitors, such as pentostatin, is not recommended. (7, 12.3)

———USE IN SPECIFIC POPULATIONS———

- Renal Impairment: Closely monitor patients with moderate or severe renal impairment for toxicities. (8.6)
- Hepatic Impairment: Closely monitor patients with severe hepatic impairment for toxicities. (8.7)

See 17 for PATIENT COUNSELING INFORMATION and FDA-approved patient labeling

Revised: 12/2011

FULL PRESCRIBING INFORMATION

WARNING: NEUROLOGIC ADVERSE REACTIONS

Severe neurologic adverse reactions have been reported with the use of ARRANON. These adverse reactions have included altered mental states including severe somnolence, central nervous system effects including convulsions, and peripheral neuropathy ranging from numbness and paresthesias to motor weakness and paralysis. There have also been reports of adverse reactions associated with demyelination, and ascending peripheral neuropathies similar in appearance to Guillain-Barré syndrome [see Warnings and Precautions (5.1)].

Full recovery from these adverse reactions has not always occurred with cessation of therapy with ARRANON. Close monitoring for neurologic adverse reactions is strongly recommended, and ARRANON should be discontinued for neurologic adverse reactions of NCI Common Toxicity Criteria grade 2 or greater [see Warnings and Precautions (5.1)].

1   INDICATIONS AND USAGE

ARRANON® is indicated for the treatment of patients with T-cell acute lymphoblastic leukemia and T-cell lymphoblastic lymphoma whose disease has not responded to or has relapsed following treatment with at least two chemotherapy regimens. This use is based on the induction of complete responses. Randomized trials demonstrating increased survival or other clinical benefit have not been conducted.

2   DOSAGE AND ADMINISTRATION

2.1   Recommended Dosage

This product is for intravenous use only.

The recommended duration of treatment for adult and pediatric patients has not been clearly established. In clinical trials, treatment was generally continued until there was evidence of disease progression, the patient experienced unacceptable toxicity, the patient became a candidate for bone marrow transplant, or the patient no longer continued to benefit from treatment.

Adult Dosage: The recommended adult dose of ARRANON is 1,500 mg/m^2 administered intravenously over 2 hours on days 1, 3, and 5 repeated every 21 days. ARRANON is administered undiluted.

Pediatric Dosage: The recommended pediatric dose of ARRANON is 650 mg/m^2 administered intravenously over 1 hour daily for 5 consecutive days repeated every 21 days. ARRANON is administered undiluted.

2.2   Dosage Modification

ARRANON administration should be discontinued for neurologic adverse reactions of NCI Common Toxicity Criteria grade 2 or greater. Dosage may be delayed for other toxicity including hematologic toxicity. [See Boxed Warning and Warnings and Precautions (5.1, 5.2).]

2.3   Adjustment of Dose in Special Populations

ARRANON has not been studied in patients with renal or hepatic dysfunction [see Use in Specific Populations (8.6, 8.7)]. No dose adjustment is recommended for patients with a creatinine clearance (CL$_{cr}$) ≥50 mL/min [see Clinical Pharmacology (12.3)]. There are insufficient data to support a dose recommendation for patients with a CL$_{cr}$ <50 mL/min.

2.4   Prevention of Hyperuricemia

Appropriate measures (e.g., hydration, urine alkalinization, and prophylaxis with allopurinol) must be taken to prevent hyperuricemia [see Warnings and Precautions (5.4)].

2.5   Instructions for Handling, Preparation, and Administration

Handling: ARRANON is a cytotoxic agent. Caution should be used during handling and preparation. Use of gloves and other protective clothing to prevent skin contact is recom-

mended. Proper aseptic technique should be used. Guidelines for proper handling and disposal of anticancer drugs have been published.[1-4]

Preparation and Administration: Do not dilute ARRANON prior to administration. The appropriate dose of ARRANON is transferred into polyvinylchloride (PVC) infusion bags or glass containers and administered as a two-hour infusion in adult patients and as a one-hour infusion in pediatric patients.

Prior to administration, inspect the drug product visually for particulate matter and discoloration.

Stability: ARRANON Injection is stable in polyvinylchloride (PVC) infusion bags and glass containers for up to 8 hours at up to 30° C.

3   DOSAGE FORMS AND STRENGTHS

250 mg/50 mL (5 mg/mL) vial

4   CONTRAINDICATIONS

None.

5   WARNINGS AND PRECAUTIONS

5.1   Neurologic Adverse Reactions

Neurotoxicity is the dose-limiting toxicity of nelarabine. Patients undergoing therapy with ARRANON should be closely observed for signs and symptoms of neurologic toxicity [see Boxed Warning and Dosage and Administration (2.2)]. Common signs and symptoms of nelarabine-related neurotoxicity include somnolence, confusion, convulsions, ataxia, paresthesias, and hypoesthesia. Severe neurologic toxicity can manifest as coma, status epilepticus, craniospinal demyelination, or ascending neuropathy similar in presentation to Guillain-Barré syndrome.

Patients treated previously or concurrently with intrathecal chemotherapy or previously with craniospinal irradiation may be at increased risk for neurologic adverse events.

5.2   Hematologic Adverse Reactions

Leukopenia, thrombocytopenia, anemia, and neutropenia, including febrile neutropenia have been associated with nelarabine therapy. Complete blood counts including platelets should be monitored regularly [see Dosage and Administration (2.2) and Adverse Reactions (6.1)].

5.3   Pregnancy

Pregnancy Category D

ARRANON can cause fetal harm when administered to a pregnant woman.

Nelarabine administered during the period of organogenesis caused increased incidences of fetal malformations, anomalies, and variations in rabbits (see Use in Specific Populations (8.1)].

There are no adequate and well-controlled studies of ARRANON in pregnant women. If this drug is used during pregnancy, or if the patient becomes pregnant while taking this drug, the patient should be apprised of the potential hazard to the fetus. Women of child-bearing potential should be advised to avoid becoming pregnant while receiving treatment with ARRANON.

5.4   Hyperuricemia

Patients receiving ARRANON should receive intravenous hydration according to standard medical practice for the management of hyperuricemia in patients at risk for tumor lysis syndrome. Consideration should be given to the use of allopurinol in patients at risk of hyperuricemia [see Dosage and Administration (2.4)].

5.5   Vaccinations

Administration of live vaccines to immunocompromised patients should be avoided.

6   ADVERSE REACTIONS

The following serious adverse reactions are discussed in greater detail in other sections of the label:
- Neurologic [see Boxed Warning and Warnings and Precautions (5.1)]
- Hematologic [see Warnings and Precautions (5.2)]
- Hyperuricemia [see Warnings and Precautions (5.4)]

6.1   Clinical Trials Experience

Because clinical trials are conducted under widely varying conditions, adverse reaction rates observed in the clinical trials of a drug cannot be directly compared to rates in the clinical trials of another drug and may not reflect the rates observed in practice.

ARRANON was studied in 459 patients in Phase I and Phase II clinical trials.

Adults: The safety profile of ARRANON is based on data from 103 adult patients treated with the recommended dose and schedule in 2 studies: an adult T-cell acute lymphoblastic leukemia (T-ALL)/T-cell lymphoblastic lymphoma (T-LBL) study and an adult chronic lymphocytic leukemia study.

The most common adverse reactions in adults, regardless of causality, were fatigue; gastrointestinal (GI) disorders (nausea, diarrhea, vomiting, and constipation); hematologic disorders (anemia, neutropenia, and thrombocytopenia); respiratory disorders (cough and dyspnea); nervous system disorders (somnolence and dizziness); and pyrexia.

The most common adverse reactions in adults, by System Organ Class, regardless of causality, including severe or life threatening adverse reactions (NCI Common Toxicity Criteria grade 3 or grade 4) and fatal adverse reactions (grade 5) are shown in Table 1.

Table 1. Most Commonly Reported (≥5% Overall) Adverse Reactions Regardless of Causality in Adult Patients Treated with 1,500 mg/m^2 of ARRANON Administered Intravenously Over 2 Hours on Days 1, 3, and 5 Repeated Every 21 Days

| System Organ Class Preferred Term | Percentage of Patients (N = 103) | | |
| | Toxicity Grade | | |
	Grade 3 %	Grade 4 and 5^a %	All Grades %
Blood and Lymphatic System Disorders			
Anemia	20	14	99
Thrombocytopenia	37	22	86
Neutropenia	14	49	81
Febrile neutropenia	9	1	12
Cardiac Disorders			
Sinus tachycardia	1	0	8
Gastrointestinal Disorders			
Nausea	0	0	41
Diarrhea	1	0	22
Vomiting	1	0	22
Constipation	1	0	21
Abdominal pain	1	0	9
Stomatitis	1	0	8
Abdominal distension	0	0	6
General Disorders and Administration Site Conditions			
Fatigue	10	2	50
Pyrexia	5	0	23
Asthenia	0	1	17
Edema, peripheral	0	0	15
Edema	0	0	11
Pain	3	0	11
Rigors	0	0	8
Gait, abnormal	0	0	6
Chest pain	0	0	5
Non-cardiac chest pain	0	1	5
Infections			
Infection	2	1	9
Pneumonia	4	1	8
Sinusitis	1	0	7
Hepatobiliary Disorders			
AST increased	1	1	6
Metabolism and Nutrition Disorders			
Anorexia	0	0	9
Dehydration	3	1	7
Hyperglycemia	1	0	6
Musculoskeletal and Connective Tissue Disorders			
Myalgia	1	0	13
Arthralgia	1	0	9
Back pain	0	0	8
Muscular weakness	5	0	8
Pain in extremity	1	0	7
Nervous System Disorders (see Table 2)			
Psychiatric Disorders			
Confusional state	2	0	8
Insomnia	0	0	7
Depression	1	0	6
Respiratory, Thoracic, and Mediastinal Disorders			
Cough	0	0	25
Dyspnea	4	2	20
Pleural effusion	5	1	10
Epistaxis	0	0	8
Dyspnea, exertional	0	0	7
Wheezing	0	0	5
Vascular Disorders			
Petechiae	2	0	12
Hypotension	1	1	8

^{a} Five patients had a fatal adverse reaction. Fatal adverse reactions included hypotension (n = 1), respiratory arrest (n = 1), pleural effusion/pneumothorax (n = 1), pneumonia (n = 1), and cerebral hemorrhage/coma/leukoencephalopathy (n = 1).

Table 2. Neurologic Adverse Reactions (≥2%) Regardless of Causality in Adult Patients Treated with 1,500 mg/m^2 of ARRANON Administered Intravenously Over 2 Hours on Days 1, 3, and 5 Repeated Every 21 Days

| Nervous System Disorders Preferred Term | Percentage of Patients (N =103) | | | | |
	Grade 1 %	Grade 2 %	Grade 3 %	Grade 4 %	All Grades %
Somnolence	20	3	0	0	23
Dizziness	14	8	0	0	21
Peripheral neurologic disorders, any adverse reaction	8	12	2	0	21
Neuropathy	0	4	0	0	4
Peripheral neuropathy	2	2	1	0	5
Peripheral motor neuropathy	3	3	1	0	7
Peripheral sensory neuropathy	7	6	0	0	13
Hypoesthesia	5	10	2	0	17
Headache	11	3	1	0	15
Paresthesia	11	4	0	0	15
Ataxia	1	6	2	0	9
Depressed level of consciousness	4	1	0	1	6
Tremor	2	3	0	0	5
Amnesia	2	1	0	0	3
Dysgeusia	2	1	0	0	3
Balance disorder	1	1	0	0	2
Sensory loss	0	2	0	0	2

Other Adverse Events: Blurred vision was also reported in 4% of adult patients.

There was a single report of biopsy confirmed progressive multifocal leukoencephalopathy in the adult patient population.

Neurologic Adverse Reactions: Nervous system adverse reactions, regardless of drug relationship, were reported for 76% of adult patients across the Phase I and Phase II studies. The most common neurologic adverse reactions (≥2%) in adult patients, regardless of causality, including all grades (NCI Common Toxicity Criteria) are shown in Table 2. [See table 2 above]

One patient had a fatal neurologic adverse reaction, cerebral hemorrhage/coma/leukoencephalopathy.

Most nervous system adverse reactions in the adult patients were evaluated as grade 1 or 2. The additional grade 3 adverse reactions in adult patients, regardless of causality, were aphasia, convulsion, hemiparesis, and loss of consciousness, each reported in 1 patient (1%). The additional grade 4 adverse reactions, regardless of causality, were cerebral hemorrhage, coma, intracranial hemorrhage, leukoencephalopathy, and metabolic encephalopathy, each reported in one patient (1%).

The other neurologic adverse reactions, regardless of causality, reported as grade 1, 2, or unknown in adult patients were abnormal coordination, burning sensation, disturbance in attention, dysarthria, hyporeflexia, neuropathic pain, nystagmus, peroneal nerve palsy, sciatica, sensory disturbance, sinus headache, and speech disorder, each reported in one patient (1%).

Pediatrics: The safety profile for children is based on data from 84 pediatric patients treated with the recommended dose and schedule in a T-cell acute lymphoblastic leukemia (T-ALL)/T-cell lymphoblastic lymphoma (T-LBL) treatment study.

The most common adverse reactions in pediatric patients, regardless of causality, were hematologic disorders (anemia, leukopenia, neutropenia, and thrombocytopenia). Of the non-hematologic adverse reactions in pediatric patients, the most frequent adverse reactions reported were headache, increased transaminase levels, decreased blood potassium, decreased blood albumin, increased blood bilirubin, and vomiting.

The most common adverse reactions in pediatric patients, by System Organ Class, regardless of causality, including severe or life threatening adverse reactions (NCI Common Toxicity Criteria grade 3 or grade 4) and fatal adverse reactions (grade 5) are shown in Table 3.

Table 3. Most Commonly Reported (≥5% Overall) Adverse Reactions Regardless of Causality in Pediatric Patients Treated with 650 mg/m² of ARRANON Administered Intravenously Over 1 Hour Daily for 5 Consecutive Days Repeated Every 21 Days

System Organ Class Preferred Term	Percentage of Patients (N = 84)		
	Toxicity Grade		
	Grade 3 %	Grade 4 and 5ᵃ %	All Grades %
Blood and Lymphatic System Disorders			
Anemia	45	10	95
Neutropenia	17	62	94
Thrombocytopenia	27	32	88
Leukopenia	14	7	38
Hepatobiliary Disorders			
Transaminases increased	4	0	12
Blood albumin decreased	5	1	10
Blood bilirubin increased	7	2	10
Metabolic/Laboratory			
Blood potassium decreased	4	2	11
Blood calcium decreased	1	1	8
Blood creatinine increased	0	0	6
Blood glucose decreased	4	0	6
Blood magnesium decreased	2	0	6
Nervous System Disorders (see Table 4)			
Gastrointestinal Disorders			
Vomiting	0	0	10
General Disorders & Administration Site Conditions			
Asthenia	1	0	6
Infections & Infestations			
Infection	2	1	5

ᵃ Three patients had a fatal adverse reaction. Fatal adverse reactions included neutropenia and pyrexia (n = 1), status epilepticus/seizure (n = 1), and fungal pneumonia (n = 1).

Neurologic Adverse Reactions: Nervous system adverse reactions, regardless of drug relationship, were reported for 42% of pediatric patients across the Phase I and Phase II studies. The most common neurologic adverse reactions (≥2%) in pediatric patients, regardless of causality, including all grades (NCI Common Toxicity Criteria) are shown in Table 4.

[See table 4 above]

The other grade 3 neurologic adverse reaction in pediatric patients, regardless of causality, was hypertonia reported in 1 patient (1%). The additional grade 4 neurologic adverse reactions, regardless of causality, were 3rd nerve paralysis, and 6th nerve paralysis, each reported in 1 patient (1%).

The other neurologic adverse reactions, regardless of causality, reported as grade 1, 2, or unknown in pediatric patients were dysarthria, encephalopathy, hydrocephalus, hyporeflexia, lethargy, mental impairment, paralysis, and sensory loss, each reported in 1 patient (1%).

6.2 Postmarketing Experience

The following adverse reactions have been identified during post-approval use of ARRANON. Because these reactions are reported voluntarily from a population of uncertain size, it is not always possible to reliably estimate their frequency or establish a causal relationship to drug exposure.

Infections and Infestations: Fatal opportunistic infections.

Metabolism and Nutrition Disorders: Tumor lysis syndrome.

Nervous System Disorders: Demyelination and ascending peripheral neuropathies similar in appearance to Guillain-Barré syndrome.

Table 4. Neurologic Adverse Reactions (≥2%) Regardless of Causality in Pediatric Patients Treated with 650 mg/m² of ARRANON Administered Intravenously Over 1 Hour Daily for 5 Consecutive Days Repeated Every 21 Days

Nervous System Disorders Preferred Term	Percentage of Patients (N = 84)				
	Grade 1 %	Grade 2 %	Grade 3 %	Grade 4 and 5ᵃ %	All Grades %
Headache	8	2	4	2	17
Peripheral neurologic disorders, any adverse reaction	1	4	7	0	12
Peripheral neuropathy	0	4	2	0	6
Peripheral motor neuropathy	1	0	2	0	4
Peripheral sensory neuropathy	0	0	6	0	6
Somnolence	1	4	1	1	7
Hypoesthesia	1	1	4	0	6
Seizures	0	0	0	6	6
Convulsions	0	0	0	3	4
Grand mal convulsions	0	0	0	1	1
Status epilepticus	0	0	0	1	1
Motor dysfunction	1	1	1	0	4
Nervous system disorder	1	2	0	0	4
Paresthesia	0	2	1	0	4
Tremor	1	2	0	0	4
Ataxia	1	0	1	0	2

ᵃ One (1) patient had a fatal neurologic adverse reaction, status epilepticus.

Musculoskeletal and Connective Disorders: Rhabdomyolysis, blood creatine phosphokinase increased.

7 DRUG INTERACTIONS

Administration of nelarabine in combination with adenosine deaminase inhibitors, such as pentostatin, is not recommended *[see Clinical Pharmacology (12.3)]*.

8 USE IN SPECIFIC POPULATIONS

8.1 Pregnancy

Pregnancy Category D *[see Warnings and Precautions (5.3)]* ARRANON can cause fetal harm when administered to a pregnant woman. Nelarabine administered to rabbits during the period of organogenesis caused increased incidences of fetal malformations, anomalies, and variations at doses ≥360 mg/m²/day (8-hour IV infusion; approximately ¼ the adult dose compared on a mg/m² basis), which was the lowest dose tested. Cleft palate was seen in rabbits given 3,600 mg/m²/day (approximately 2-fold the adult dose), absent pollices (digits) in rabbits given ≥1,200 mg/m²/day (approximately ¾ the adult dose), while absent gall bladder, absent accessory lung lobes, fused or extra sternebrae and delayed ossification was seen at all doses. Maternal body weight gain and fetal body weights were reduced in rabbits given 3,600 mg/m²/day (approximately 2-fold the adult dose), but could not account for the increased incidence of malformations seen at this or lower administered doses.

There are no adequate and well-controlled studies of ARRANON in pregnant women. If this drug is used during pregnancy, or if the patient becomes pregnant while taking this drug, the patient should be apprised of the potential hazard to the fetus. Women of child-bearing potential should be advised to avoid becoming pregnant while receiving treatment with ARRANON.

8.3 Nursing Mothers

It is not known whether nelarabine or ara-G are excreted in human milk. Because many drugs are excreted in human milk and because of the potential for serious adverse reactions in nursing infants from ARRANON, a decision should be made whether to discontinue nursing or to discontinue the drug, taking into account the importance of the drug to the mother.

8.4 Pediatric Use

The safety and effectiveness of ARRANON has been established in pediatric patients *[see Dosage and Administration (2.1) and Clinical Studies (14.2)]*.

8.5 Geriatric Use

Clinical studies of ARRANON did not include sufficient numbers of patients aged 65 and over to determine whether they respond differently from younger patients. In an exploratory analysis, increasing age, especially age 65 years and older, appeared to be associated with increased rates of neurologic adverse reactions. Because elderly patients are more likely to have decreased renal function, care should be taken in dose selection, and it may be useful to monitor renal function.

8.6 Renal Impairment

Ara-G clearance decreased as renal function decreased *[see Clinical Pharmacology (12.3)]*. Because the risk of adverse reactions to this drug may be greater in patients with moderate (CL_{cr} 30 to 50 mL/min) or severe (CL_{cr} <30 mL/min) renal impairment, these patients should be closely monitored for toxicities when treated with ARRANON *[see Dosage and Administration (2.3)]*.

8.7 Hepatic Impairment

The influence of hepatic impairment on the pharmacokinetics of nelarabine has not been evaluated. Because the risk of adverse reactions to this drug may be greater in patients with severe hepatic impairment (total bilirubin >3 times upper limit of normal), these patients should be closely monitored for toxicities when treated with ARRANON.

10 OVERDOSAGE

There is no known antidote for overdoses of ARRANON. It is anticipated that overdosage would result in severe neurotoxicity (possibly including paralysis, coma), myelosuppression, and potentially death. In the event of overdose, supportive care consistent with good clinical practice should be provided.

Nelarabine has been administered in clinical trials up to a dose of 2,900 mg/m² on days 1, 3, and 5 to 2 adult patients. At a dose of 2,200 mg/m² given on days 1, 3, and 5 every 21 days, 2 patients developed a significant grade 3 ascending sensory neuropathy. MRI evaluations of the 2 patients demonstrated findings consistent with a demyelinating process in the cervical spine.

11 DESCRIPTION

ARRANON (nelarabine) is a pro-drug of the cytotoxic deoxyguanosine analogue, 9-β-D-arabinofuranosylguanine (ara-G).

The chemical name for nelarabine is 2-amino-9-β-D-arabinofuranosyl-6-methoxy-9H-purine. It has the molecular formula $C_{11}H_{15}N_5O_5$ and a molecular weight of 297.27. Nelarabine has the following structural formula:

Nelarabine is slightly soluble to soluble in water and melts with decomposition between 209° and 217° C.

ARRANON Injection is supplied as a clear, colorless, sterile solution in glass vials. Each vial contains 250 mg of nelarabine (5 mg nelarabine per mL) and the inactive ingredient sodium chloride (4.5 mg per mL) in 50 mL Water for Injection, USP. ARRANON is intended for intravenous infusion.

Hydrochloric acid and sodium hydroxide may have been used to adjust the pH. The solution pH ranges from 5.0 to 7.0.

12   CLINICAL PHARMACOLOGY

12.1   Mechanism of Action

Nelarabine is a pro-drug of the deoxyguanosine analogue 9-β-D-arabinofuranosylguanine (ara-G), a nucleoside metabolic inhibitor. Nelarabine is demethylated by adenosine deaminase (ADA) to ara-G, mono-phosphorylated by deoxyguanosine kinase and deoxycytidine kinase, and subsequently converted to the active 5'-triphosphate, ara-GTP. Accumulation of ara-GTP in leukemic blasts allows for incorporation into deoxyribonucleic acid (DNA), leading to inhibition of DNA synthesis and cell death. Other mechanisms may contribute to the cytotoxic and systemic toxicity of nelarabine.

12.3   Pharmacokinetics

Absorption: Following intravenous administration of nelarabine to adult patients with refractory leukemia or lymphoma, plasma ara-G C_{max} values generally occurred at the end of the nelarabine infusion and were generally higher than nelarabine C_{max} values, suggesting rapid and extensive conversion of nelarabine to ara-G. Mean plasma nelarabine and ara-G C_{max} values were 5.0 ± 3.0 µg/mL and 31.4 ± 5.6 µg/mL, respectively, after a 1,500 mg/m^2 nelarabine dose infused over 2 hours in adult patients. The area under the concentration-time curve (AUC) of ara-G is 37 times higher than that for nelarabine on Day 1 after nelarabine IV infusion of 1,500 mg/m^2 dose (162 ± 49 µg.h/mL versus 4.4 ± 2.2 µg.h/mL, respectively). Comparable C_{max} and AUC values were obtained for nelarabine between Days 1 and 5 at the nelarabine adult dosage of 1,500 mg/m^2, indicating that nelarabine does not accumulate after multiple-dosing. There are not enough ara-G data to make a comparison between Day 1 and Day 5. After a nelarabine adult dose of 1,500 mg/m^2, intracellular C_{max} for ara-GTP appeared within 3 to 25 hours on Day 1. Exposure (AUC) to intracellular ara-GTP was 532 times higher than that for nelarabine and 14 times higher than that for ara-G (2,339 ± 2,628 µg.h/mL versus 4.4 ± 2.2 µg.h/mL and 162 ± 49 µg.h/mL, respectively). Because the intracellular levels of ara-GTP were so prolonged, its elimination half-life could not be accurately estimated.

Distribution: Nelarabine and ara-G are extensively distributed throughout the body. For nelarabine, V_{SS} values were 197 ± 216 L/m^2 in adult patients. For ara-G, V_{SS}/F values were 50 ± 24 L/m^2 in adult patients.

Nelarabine and ara-G are not substantially bound to human plasma proteins (<25%) in vitro, and binding is independent of nelarabine or ara-G concentrations up to 600 µM.

Metabolism: The principal route of metabolism for nelarabine is O-demethylation by adenosine deaminase to form ara-G, which undergoes hydrolysis to form guanine. In addition, some nelarabine is hydrolyzed to form methylguanine, which is O-demethylated to form guanine. Guanine is N-deaminated to form xanthine, which is further oxidized to yield uric acid.

Excretion: Nelarabine and ara-G are partially eliminated by the kidneys. Mean urinary excretion of nelarabine and ara-G was 6.6 ± 4.7% and 27 ± 15% of the administered dose, respectively, in 28 adult patients over the 24 hours after nelarabine infusion on Day 1. Renal clearance averaged 24 ± 23 L/h for nelarabine and 6.2 ± 5.0 L/h for ara-G in 21 adult patients. Combined Phase 1 pharmacokinetic data at nelarabine doses of 199 to 2,900 mg/m^2 (n = 66 adult patients) indicate that the mean clearance (CL) of nelarabine is 197 ± 189 L/h/m^2 on Day 1. The apparent clearance of ara-G (CL/F) is 10.5 ± 4.5 L/h/m^2 on Day 1. Nelarabine and ara-G are rapidly eliminated from plasma with a mean half-life of 18 minutes and 3.2 hours, respectively, in adult patients.

Pediatrics: No pharmacokinetic data are available in pediatric patients at the once daily 650 mg/m^2 nelarabine dosage. Combined Phase 1 pharmacokinetic data at nelarabine doses of 104 to 2,900 mg/m^2 indicate that the mean clearance (CL) of nelarabine is about 30% higher in pediatric patients than in adult patients (259 ± 409 L/h/m^2 versus 197 ± 189 L/h/m^2, respectively; n = 66 adults, n = 22 pediatric patients) on Day 1. The apparent clearance of ara-G (CL/F) is comparable between the two groups (10.5 ± 4.5 L/h/m^2 in adult patients and 11.3 ± 4.2 L/h/m^2 in pediatric patients) on Day 1. Nelarabine and ara-G are extensively distributed

throughout the body. For nelarabine, V_{SS} values were 213 ± 358 L/m^2 in pediatric patients. For ara-G, V_{SS}/F values were 33 ± 9.3 L/m^2 in pediatric patients. Nelarabine and ara-G are rapidly eliminated from plasma in pediatric patients, with a half-life of 13 minutes and 2 hours, respectively.

Effect of Age: Age has no effect on the pharmacokinetics of nelarabine or ara-G in adults. Decreased renal function, which is more common in the elderly, may reduce ara-G clearance [see Use in Specific Populations (8.5)].

Effect of Gender: Gender has no effect on nelarabine or ara-G pharmacokinetics.

Effect of Race: In general, nelarabine mean clearance and volume of distribution values tend to be higher in Whites (n = 63) than in Blacks (by about 10%) (n = 15). The opposite is true for ara-G; mean apparent clearance and volume of distribution values tend to be lower in Whites than in Blacks (by about 15-20%). No differences in safety or effectiveness were observed between these groups.

Effect of Renal Impairment: The pharmacokinetics of nelarabine and ara-G have not been specifically studied in renally impaired or hemodialyzed patients. Nelarabine is excreted by the kidney to a small extent (5 to 10% of the administered dose). Ara-G is excreted by the kidney to a greater extent (20 to 30% of the administered nelarabine dose). In the combined Phase 1 studies, patients were categorized into 3 groups: normal with CL_{cr} >80 mL/min (n = 67), mild with CL_{cr} = 50-80 mL/min (n = 15), and moderate with CL_{cr} <50 mL/min (n = 3). The mean apparent clearance (CL/F) of ara-G was about 15% and 40% lower in patients with mild and moderate renal impairment, respectively, than in patients with normal renal function [see Use in Specific Populations (8.6) and Dosage and Administration (2.3)]. No differences in safety or effectiveness were observed.

Effect of Hepatic Impairment: The influence of hepatic impairment on the pharmacokinetics of nelarabine has not been evaluated [see Use in Specific Populations (8.7)].

Drug Interactions: Cytochrome P450: Nelarabine and ara-G did not significantly inhibit the activities of the human hepatic cytochrome P450 isoenzymes 1A2, 2A6, 2B6, 2C8, 2C9, 2C19, 2D6, or 3A4 in vitro at concentrations of nelarabine and ara-G up to 100 µM.

Fludarabine: Administration of fludarabine 30 mg/m^2 as a 30-minute infusion 4 hours before a 1,200 mg/m^2 infusion of nelarabine did not affect the pharmacokinetics of nelarabine, ara-G, or ara-GTP in 12 patients with refractory leukemia.

Pentostatin: There is in vitro evidence that pentostatin is a strong inhibitor of adenosine deaminase. Inhibition of adenosine deaminase may result in a reduction in the conversion of the pro-drug nelarabine to its active moiety and consequently in a reduction in efficacy of nelarabine and/or change in adverse reaction profile of either drug [see Drug Interactions (7)].

13   NONCLINICAL TOXICOLOGY

13.1   Carcinogenesis, Mutagenesis, Impairment of Fertility

Carcinogenicity testing of nelarabine has not been done. However, nelarabine was mutagenic when tested in vitro in L5178Y/TK mouse lymphoma cells with and without metabolic activation. No studies have been conducted in animals to assess genotoxic potential or effects on fertility. The effect on human fertility is unknown.

14   CLINICAL STUDIES

The safety and efficacy of ARRANON were evaluated in two open-label, single-arm, multicenter studies.

14.1   Adult Clinical Study

The safety and efficacy of ARRANON in adult patients were studied in a clinical trial which included 39 treated patients, 28 who had T-cell acute lymphoblastic leukemia (T-ALL) or T-cell lymphoblastic lymphoma (T-LBL) that had relapsed following or was refractory to at least two prior induction regimens. A 1,500 mg/m^2 dose of ARRANON was administered intravenously over 2 hours on days 1, 3, and 5 repeated every 21 days. Patients who experienced signs or symptoms of grade 2 or greater neurologic toxicity on therapy were to be discontinued from further therapy with ARRANON. Seventeen patients had a diagnosis of T-ALL and 11 had a diagnosis of T-LBL. For patients with ≥2 prior inductions, the age range was 16-65 years (mean 34 years) and most patients were male (82%) and Caucasian (61%). Patients with central nervous system (CNS) disease were not eligible.

Complete response (CR) in this study was defined as bone marrow blast counts ≤5%, no other evidence of disease, and full recovery of peripheral blood counts. Complete response without complete hematologic recovery (CR*) was also assessed. The results of the study for patients who had received ≥2 prior inductions are shown in Table 5.

Table 5. Efficacy Results in Adult Patients With ≥2 Prior Inductions Treated with 1,500 mg/m^2 of ARRANON Administered Intravenously Over 2 Hours on Days 1, 3, and 5 Repeated Every 21 Days

	N = 28
CR plus CR* % (n) [95% CI]	21% (6) [8%, 41%]
CR % (n) [95% CI]	18% (5) [6%, 37%]
CR* % (n) [95% CI]	4% (1) [0%, 18%]
Duration of CR plus CR* (range in weeks)[a]	4 to 195+
Median overall survival (weeks) [95% CI]	20.6 weeks [10.4, 36.4]

CR = Complete response
CR* = Complete response without hematologic recovery
[a] Does not include 1 patient who was transplanted (duration of response was 156+ weeks).

The mean number of days on therapy was 56 days (range of 10 to 136 days). Time to CR plus CR* ranged from 2.9 to 11.7 weeks.

14.2   Pediatric Clinical Study

The safety and efficacy of ARRANON in pediatric patients were studied in a clinical trial which included patients 21 years of age and younger, who had relapsed or refractory T-cell acute lymphoblastic leukemia (T-ALL) or T-cell lymphoblastic lymphoma (T-LBL). Eighty-four (84) patients, 39 of whom had received two or more prior induction regimens, were treated with 650 mg/m^2/day of ARRANON administered intravenously over 1 hour daily for 5 consecutive days repeated every 21 days (see Table 6). Patients who experienced signs or symptoms of grade 2 or greater neurologic toxicity on therapy were to be discontinued from further therapy with ARRANON.

Table 6. Pediatric Clinical Study - Patient Allocation

Patient Population	N
Patients treated at 650 mg/m^2/day × 5 days every 21 days.	84
Patients with T-ALL or T-LBL with two or more prior induction treated at 650 mg/m^2/day × 5 days every 21 days.	39
Patients with T-ALL or T-LBL with one prior induction treated at 650 mg/m^2/day × 5 days every 21 days.	31

The 84 patients ranged in age from 2.5-21.7 years (overall mean, 11.9 years), 52% were 3 to 12 years of age and most were male (74%) and Caucasian (62%). The majority (77%) of patients had a diagnosis of T-ALL.

Complete response (CR) in this study was defined as bone marrow blast counts ≤5%, no other evidence of disease, and full recovery of peripheral blood counts. Complete response without full hematologic recovery (CR*) was also assessed as a meaningful outcome in this heavily pretreated population. Duration of response is reported from date of response to date of relapse, and may include subsequent stem cell transplant. Efficacy results are presented in Table 7.

Table 7. Efficacy Results in Patients 21 Years of Age and Younger at Diagnosis With ≥2 Prior Inductions Treated with 650 mg/m^2 of ARRANON Administered Intravenously Over 1 Hour Daily for 5 Consecutive Days Repeated Every 21 Days

	N = 39
CR plus CR* % (n) [95% CI]	23% (9) [11%, 39%]
CR % (n) [95% CI]	13% (5) [4%, 27%]
CR* % (n) [95% CI]	10% (4) [3%, 24%]
Duration of CR plus CR* (range in weeks)[a]	3.3 to 9.3
Median overall survival (weeks) [95% CI]	13.1 [8.7, 17.4]

CR = Complete response
CR* = Complete response without hematologic recovery
[a] Does not include 5 patients who were transplanted or had subsequent systemic chemotherapy (duration of response in these 5 patients was 4.7 to 42.1 weeks).

The mean number of days on therapy was 46 days (range of 7 to 129 days). Median time to CR plus CR* was 3.4 weeks (95% CI: 3.0, 3.7).

15 REFERENCES

1. Preventing Occupational Exposures to Antineoplastic and Other Hazardous Drugs in Health Care Settings. NIOSH Alert 2004-165.
2. OSHA Technical Manual, TED 1-0.15A, Section VI: Chapter 2. Controlling Occupational Exposure to Hazardous Drugs. OSHA, 1999. http://www.osha.gov/dts/osta/otm/otm_vi/otm_vi_2.html
3. American Society of Health-System Pharmacists. ASHP Guidelines on Handling Hazardous Drugs. *Am J Health-Syst Pharm.* 2006;63:1172-1193.
4. Polovich M, White JM, Kelleher LO (eds.) 2005. Chemotherapy and Biotherapy Guidelines and Recommendations for Practice. (2nd ed) Pittsburgh, PA: Oncology Nursing Society.

16 HOW SUPPLIED/STORAGE AND HANDLING

ARRANON Injection is supplied as a clear, colorless, sterile solution in Type I, clear glass vials with a gray butyl rubber (latex-free) stopper and a red snap-off aluminum seal. Each vial contains 250 mg of nelarabine (5 mg nelarabine per mL) and the inactive ingredient sodium chloride (4.5 mg per mL) in 50 mL Water for Injection, USP. Vials are available in the following carton size:

NDC 0007-4401-06 (package of 6)

Store at 25° C (77° F); excursions permitted to 15° to 30° C (59° to 86° F) [see USP Controlled Room Temperature].

17 PATIENT COUNSELING INFORMATION

Patient labeling is provided as a tear-off leaflet at the end of this full prescribing information. However, inform the patients of the following:

- Since patients receiving nelarabine therapy may experience somnolence, they should be cautioned about operating hazardous machinery, including automobiles.
- Patients should be instructed to contact their physician if they experience new or worsening symptoms of peripheral neuropathy *(see Boxed Warning, Warnings and Precautions (5.1), and Dosage and Administration (2.3)].* These signs and symptoms include: tingling or numbness in fingers, hands, toes, or feet; difficulty with the fine motor coordination tasks such as buttoning clothing; unsteadiness while walking; weakness arising from a low chair; weakness in climbing stairs; increased tripping while walking over uneven surfaces.
- Patients should be instructed that seizures have been known to occur in patients who receive nelarabine. If a seizure occurs, the physician administering ARRANON should be promptly informed.
- Patients who develop fever or signs of infection while on therapy should notify their physician promptly.
- Patients should be advised to use effective contraceptive measures to prevent pregnancy and to avoid breast-feeding during treatment with ARRANON.

ARRANON is a registered trademark of GlaxoSmithKline.
GlaxoSmithKline
Research Triangle Park, NC 27709
©2011, GlaxoSmithKline. All rights reserved.
December 2011
ARR:2PI
PHARMACIST-DETACH HERE AND GIVE INSTRUCTIONS TO PATIENT

PATIENT INFORMATION LEAFLET
ARRANON® (AIR-ra-non)
Nelarabine Injection

Read the Patient Information that comes with ARRANON before you or your child start treatment with ARRANON. Read the information you get each time before each treatment with ARRANON. There may be new information. This information does not take the place of talking with the doctor about your or your child's medical condition or treatment. Talk to your or your child's doctor, if you have any questions.

What is the most important information I should know about ARRANON?

ARRANON may cause serious nervous system problems including:
- extreme sleepiness
- seizures
- coma
- numbness and tingling in the hands, fingers, feet, or toes (peripheral neuropathy)
- weakness and paralysis

Call the doctor right away if you or your child has the following symptoms:
- seizures
- numbness and tingling in the hands, fingers, feet, or toes
- problems with fine motor skills such as buttoning clothes
- unsteadiness while walking
- increased tripping while walking

- weakness when getting out of a chair or walking up stairs

These symptoms may not go away even when treatment with ARRANON is stopped.

What is ARRANON?

ARRANON is an anti-cancer medicine used to treat adults and children who have:
- T-cell acute lymphoblastic leukemia
- T-cell lymphoblastic lymphoma

What should you tell the doctor before you or your child starts ARRANON?

Tell the doctor about all health conditions you or your child have, including if you or your child:
- have any nervous system problems.
- have kidney problems.
- are breast-feeding or plan to breast-feed. It is not known whether ARRANON passes through breast milk. You should not breast-feed during treatment with ARRANON.
- are pregnant or plan to become pregnant. ARRANON may harm an unborn baby. You should use effective birth control to avoid getting pregnant. Talk with your doctor about your choices.

Tell the doctor about all the medicines you or your child take, including prescription and nonprescription medicines, vitamins, and herbal supplements.

How is ARRANON given?

ARRANON is an intravenous medicine. This means it is given through a tube in your vein.

What should you or your child avoid during treatment with ARRANON?

- You or your child should not drive or operate dangerous machines. ARRANON may cause sleepiness.
- You or your child should not receive vaccines made with live germs during treatment with ARRANON.

What are the possible side effects of ARRANON?

ARRANON may cause serious nervous system problems. See "What is the most important information I should know about ARRANON?"

ARRANON may also cause:
- decreased blood counts such as low red blood cells, low white blood cells, and low platelets. Blood tests should be done regularly to check blood counts. Call the doctor right away if you or your child:
  ○ is more tired than usual, pale, or has trouble breathing
  ○ has a fever or other signs of an infection
  ○ bruises easy or has any unusual bleeding
- stomach area problems such as nausea, vomiting, diarrhea, and constipation
- headache
- sleepiness
- blurry eyesight

Call your doctor right away if you experience unexplained muscle pain, tenderness, or weakness while taking ARRANON. This is because on rare occasions, muscle problems can be serious.

These are not all the side effects associated with ARRANON. Ask your doctor or pharmacist for more information.

General Advice about ARRANON

This leaflet summarizes important information about ARRANON. If you have questions or problems, talk with your or your child's doctor. You can ask your doctor or pharmacist for information about ARRANON that is written for healthcare providers or it is available at www.GSK.com.

ARRANON is a registered trademark of GlaxoSmithKline.
GlaxoSmithKline
Research Triangle Park, NC 27709
©2011, GlaxoSmithKline. All rights reserved.
December 2011
ARR:2PIL

ARZERRA®　　　　　　　　　　　　　　Ŗ
[ar-zer-ra]
(ofatumumab)
Injection, for intravenous infusion

HIGHLIGHTS OF PRESCRIBING INFORMATION

These highlights do not include all the information needed to use ARZERRA safely and effectively. See full prescribing information for ARZERRA.
ARZERRA (ofatumumab)
Injection, for intravenous infusion
Initial U.S. Approval: 2009

WARNING: HEPATITIS B VIRUS REACTIVATION AND PROGRESSIVE MULTIFOCAL LEUKOENCEPHALOPATHY

See full prescribing information for complete boxed warning.

- **Hepatitis B Virus (HBV) reactivation, in some cases resulting in fulminant hepatitis, hepatic failure, and death. (5.2)**

- **Progressive Multifocal Leukoencephalopathy(PML) resulting in death. (5.4)**

---RECENT MAJOR CHANGES---

Boxed Warning	09/2013
Indications and Usage (1)	04/2014
Dosage and Administration (2)	04/2014
Warnings and Precautions (5)	04/2014

---INDICATIONS AND USAGE---

ARZERRA (ofatumumab) is a CD20-directed cytolytic monoclonal antibody indicated:
- in combination with chlorambucil, for the treatment of previously untreated patients with chronic lymphocytic leukemia (CLL) for whom fludarabine-based therapy is considered inappropriate. (1.1)
- for the treatment of patients with CLL refractory to fludarabine and alemtuzumab. (1.2)

---DOSAGE AND ADMINISTRATION---

- Dilute and administer as an intravenous infusion. Do not administer subcutaneously or as an intravenous push or bolus. (2.1)
- Previously untreated CLL recommended dosage and schedule is:
  ○ 300 mg on Day 1 followed by 1,000 mg on Day 8 (Cycle 1)
  ○ 1,000 mg on Day 1 of subsequent 28-day cycles for a minimum of 3 cycles until best response or a maximum of 12 cycles. (2.1)
- Refractory CLL recommended dosage and schedule is:
  ○ 300 mg initial dose, followed 1 week later by
  ○ 2,000 mg weekly for 7 doses, followed 4 weeks later by
  ○ 2,000 mg every 4 weeks for 4 doses. (2.1)
- Administer where facilities to adequately monitor and treat infusion reactions are available. (2.2)
- Premedicate with acetaminophen, antihistamine, and corticosteroid. (2.4)

---DOSAGE FORMS AND STRENGTHS---

- 100 mg/5 mL single-use vial for intravenous infusion. (3)
- 1,000 mg/50 mL single-use vial for intravenous infusion. (3)

---CONTRAINDICATIONS---

None. (4)

---WARNINGS AND PRECAUTIONS---

- Infusion Reactions: Premedicate with corticosteroid, acetaminophen, and an antihistamine. Monitor patients during infusions. Interrupt infusion if infusion reactions occur. (2.3, 2.4, 5.1)
- Tumor Lysis Syndrome: Anticipate TLS in high-risk patients; premedicate with anti-hyperuricemics and hydration. (5.5)
- Cytopenias: Neutropenia, anemia, and thrombocytopenia occur. Late-onset and prolonged neutropenia can also occur. Monitor complete blood counts at regular intervals. (5.6)

---ADVERSE REACTIONS---

- Previously Untreated CLL: Common adverse reactions (≥10%) were infusion reactions and neutropenia. (6)
- Refractory CLL: Common adverse reactions (≥10%) were neutropenia, pneumonia, pyrexia, cough, diarrhea, anemia, fatigue, dyspnea, rash, nausea, bronchitis, and upper respiratory tract infections. (6)

To report SUSPECTED ADVERSE REACTIONS, contact GlaxoSmithKline at 1-888-825-5249 or FDA at 1-800-FDA-1088 or www.fda.gov/medwatch

---USE IN SPECIFIC POPULATIONS---

- Pregnancy: Based on animal data, may cause fetal harm. (8.1)
- Nursing Mothers: Published data suggest that consumption of breast milk does not result in substantial absorption of maternal antibodies into circulation. (8.3)

See 17 for PATIENT COUNSELING INFORMATION
Revised: 04/2014

FULL PRESCRIBING INFORMATION: CONTENTS*
WARNING: HEPATITIS B VIRUS (HBV) REACTIVATION AND PROGRESSIVE MULTIFOCAL LEUKOENCEPHALOPATHY

FULL PRESCRIBING INFORMATION

**WARNING: HEPATITIS B VIRUS (HBV) REAC-
TIVATION AND PROGRESSIVE MULTIFOCAL
LEUKOENCEPHALOPATHY**
- **Hepatitis B Virus Reactivation can occur in patients
  receiving CD20-directed cytolytic antibodies, includ-
  ing ARZERRA®, in some cases resulting in fulminant
  hepatitis, hepatic failure, and death** *[see Warnings
  and Precautions (5.2)]*.
- **Progressive Multifocal Leukoencephalopathy (PML)
  resulting in death can occur in patients receiving
  CD20-directed cytolytic antibodies, including
  ARZERRA** *[see Warnings and Precautions (5.4)]*.

---

1   INDICATIONS AND USAGE
**1.1   Previously Untreated Chronic Lymphocytic Leuke-
mia**
ARZERRA (ofatumumab) is indicated, in combination with
chlorambucil, for the treatment of previously untreated patients with chronic lymphocytic leukemia (CLL) for whom
fludarabine-based therapy is considered inappropriate *[see
Clinical Studies (14.1)]*.
1.2   Refractory CLL
ARZERRA is indicated for the treatment of patients with
CLL refractory to fludarabine and alemtuzumab *[see Clinical Studies (14.2)]*.

2   DOSAGE AND ADMINISTRATION
2.1   Recommended Dosage Regimen
- Dilute and administer as an intravenous infusion according to the following schedules.
- Do not administer as an intravenous push or bolus or as a
  subcutaneous injection.
- Premedicate before each infusion *[see Dosage and Administration (2.4)]*.
Previously Untreated CLL: The recommended dosage and
schedule is:
- 300 mg on Day 1 followed 1 week later by 1,000 mg on Day
  8 (Cycle 1) followed by
- 1,000 mg on Day 1 of subsequent 28-day cycles for a minimum of 3 cycles until best response or a maximum of 12
  cycles.
Refractory CLL: The recommended dosage and schedule
is 12 doses administered as follows:
- 300 mg initial dose (Dose 1), followed 1 week later by
- 2,000 mg weekly for 7 doses (Doses 2 through 8), followed
  4 weeks later by
- 2,000 mg every 4 weeks for 4 doses (Doses 9 through 12).
2.2   Administration
Administer ARZERRA in an environment where facilities to
adequately monitor and treat infusion reactions are available *[see Warnings and Precautions (5.1)]*.

Prepare all doses in 1,000 mL of 0.9% Sodium Chloride Injection, USP *[see Dosage and Administration (2.5)]*.
Previously Untreated CLL:
- Cycle 1, Day 1 (300-mg dose):   Initiate infusion at a rate
  of 3.6 mg/hour (12 mL/hour).
- Cycle 1, Day 8 and Cycles 2 through 12 (1,000-mg
  doses):   Initiate infusion at a rate of 25 mg/hour (25 mL/
  hour). Initiate infusion at a rate of 12 mg/hour if a Grade 3
  or greater infusion-related adverse event was experienced
  during the previous infusion.
In the absence of an infusion-related adverse event, the rate
of infusion may be increased every 30 minutes (Table 1). Do
not exceed the infusion rates in Table 1.

**Table 1. Infusion Rates for ARZERRA in Previously
Untreated CLL**

Interval After Start of Infusion (min)	Cycle 1, Day 1[a] (mL/hour)	Cycle 1, Day 8[b] and Cycles 2–12[c] (mL/hour)
0-30	12	25
31-60	25	50
61-90	50	100
91-120	100	200
121-150	200	400
151-180	300	400
>180	400	400

[a] Cycle 1, Day 1 = 300 mg; median duration of infusion =
5.2 hours.
[b] Cycle 1, Day 8 = 1,000 mg; median duration of infusion
= 4.4 hours.
[c] Cycles 2 through 12 = 1,000 mg; median durations of
infusion = 4.2 to 4.4 hours.

Refractory CLL:
- Dose 1 (300-mg dose):   Initiate infusion at a rate of
  3.6 mg/hour (12 mL/hour).
- Dose 2 (2,000-mg dose):   Initiate infusion at a rate of
  24 mg/hour (12 mL/hour).
- Doses 3 through 12 (2,000-mg doses):   Initiate infusion at
  a rate of 50 mg/hour (25 mL/hour).
In the absence of an infusion-related adverse event, the rate
of infusion may be increased every 30 minutes (Table 2). Do
not exceed the infusion rates in Table 2.

Table 2. Infusion Rates for ARZERRA in Refractory CLL

Interval After Start of Infusion (min)	Dose 1[a] (mL/hour)	Dose 2[b] (mL/hour)	Doses 3-12[b] (mL/hour)
0-30	12	12	25
31-60	25	25	50
61-90	50	50	100
91-120	100	100	200
>120	200	200	400

[a] Dose 1 = 300 mg; median duration of infusion = 6.8
hours.
[b] Doses 2 and 3 through 12 = 2,000 mg; median duration
of infusion for Dose 2 = 6.8 hours; median durations of
infusion for Doses 3 through 12 = 4.2 to 4.4 hours.

**2.3   Infusion Rate Dose Modification for Infusion Reac-
tions**
- Interrupt infusion for infusion reactions of any severity
  [see Warnings and Precautions (5.1)]. Treatment can be resumed at the discretion of the treating physician. The following infusion rate modifications can be used as a guide.
- If the infusion reaction resolves or remains less than or
  equal to Grade 2, resume infusion with the following modifications according to the initial Grade of the infusion reaction.
  ◦ Grade 1 or 2:   Infuse at one–half of the previous infu-
    sion rate.
  ◦ Grade 3 or 4:   Infuse at a rate of 12 mL/hour.
- After resuming the infusion, the infusion rate may be increased according to Tables 1 and 2 above, based on patient tolerance.
- Consider permanent discontinuation of ARZERRA if the
  severity of the infusion reaction does not resolve to less
  than or equal to Grade 2 despite adequate clinical intervention.

- Permanently discontinue therapy for patients who develop
  an anaphylactic reaction to ARZERRA.
2.4   Premedication
Patients should receive the following premedication 30 minutes to 2 hours prior to each infusion of ARZERRA:
Previously Untreated CLL:
- Oral acetaminophen 1,000 mg (or equivalent) plus
- Oral or intravenous antihistamine (diphenhydramine
  50 mg or cetirizine 10 mg or equivalent) plus
- Intravenous corticosteroid (prednisolone 50 mg or equiva-
  lent).
If the patient did not experience a Grade 3 or greater
infusion-related adverse event during the first 2 infusions of
ARZERRA, the dose of corticosteroid may be reduced or
omitted for subsequent infusions.
Refractory CLL:
- Oral acetaminophen 1,000 mg (or equivalent) plus
- Oral or intravenous antihistamine (diphenhydramine
  50 mg or cetirizine 10 mg or equivalent) plus
- Intravenous corticosteroid (prednisolone 100 mg or equivalent).
Do not reduce corticosteroid dose for Doses 1, 2, and 9. Corticosteroid dose may be reduced as follows:
- Doses 3 through 8:   Corticosteroid may be reduced or
  omitted with subsequent infusions if a Grade 3 or greater
  infusion reaction did not occur with the preceding dose.
- Doses 10 through 12:   Administer prednisolone 50 mg to
  100 mg or equivalent if a Grade 3 or greater infusion reaction did not occur with Dose 9.
2.5   Preparation and Administration
- Do not shake product.
- Inspect parenteral drug products visually for particulate
  matter and discoloration prior to administration.
  ARZERRA should be a clear to opalescent, colorless solution. The solution should not be used if discolored or
  cloudy, or if foreign particulate matter is present.
Preparation of Solution:
- 300-mg dose: Withdraw and discard 15 mL from a
  1,000-mL bag of 0.9% Sodium Chloride Injection, USP.
  Withdraw 5 mL from each of 3 single-use 100-mg vials of
  ARZERRA and add to the bag. Mix diluted solution by
  gentle inversion.
- 1,000-mg dose: Withdraw and discard 50 mL from a
  1,000-mL bag of 0.9% Sodium Chloride Injection, USP.
  Withdraw 50 mL from 1 single-use 1,000-mg vial of
  ARZERRA and add to the bag. Mix diluted solution by
  gentle inversion.
- 2,000-mg dose: Withdraw and discard 100 mL from a
  1,000-mL bag of 0.9% Sodium Chloride Injection, USP.
  Withdraw 50 mL from each of 2 single-use 1,000-mg vials
  of ARZERRA and add to the bag. Mix diluted solution by
  gentle inversion.
- Store diluted solution between 2° to 8°C (36° to 46°F).
- No incompatibilities between ARZERRA and polyvinyl-
  chloride or polyolefin bags and administration sets have
  been observed.
Administration Instructions:
- Do not mix ARZERRA with, or administer as an infusion
  with, other medicinal products.
- Administer using an infusion pump and an administration
  set.
- Flush the intravenous line with 0.9% Sodium Chloride In-
  jection, USP before and after each dose.
- Start infusion within 12 hours of preparation.
- Discard prepared solution after 24 hours.

3   DOSAGE FORMS AND STRENGTHS
- 100 mg/5 mL single–use vial for intravenous infusion.
- 1,000 mg/50 mL single–use vial for intravenous infusion.

4   CONTRAINDICATIONS
None.

5   WARNINGS AND PRECAUTIONS
5.1   Infusion Reactions
ARZERRA can cause serious, including fatal, infusion reactions manifesting as bronchospasm, dyspnea, laryngeal
edema, pulmonary edema, flushing, hypertension, hypotension, syncope, cardiac events (e.g., myocardial ischemia/
infarction, acute coronary syndrome, arrhythmia, bradycardia), back pain, abdominal pain, pyrexia, rash, urticaria,
angioedema, cytokine release syndrome, and anaphylactoid/
anaphylactic reactions. Infusion reactions occur more frequently with the first 2 infusions. These reactions may result in temporary interruption or withdrawal of treatment
[see Adverse Reactions (6.1)].
Premedicate with acetaminophen, an antihistamine, and a
corticosteroid *[see Dosage and Administration (2.1, 2.4)]*. Infusion reactions may occur despite premedication. Interrupt
infusion with ARZERRA for infusion reactions of any severity. Institute medical management for severe infusion reactions including angina or other signs and symptoms of myocardial ischemia *[see Dosage and Administration (2.3)]*. If
an anaphylactic reaction occurs, immediately and permanently discontinue ARZERRA and initiate appropriate medical treatment.

Table 3. Adverse Reactions With ≥5% Incidence in Patients Receiving ARZERRA Plus Chlorambucil and Also ≥2% More Than Patients Receiving Chlorambucil

Adverse Reactions	ARZERRA Plus Chlorambucil (N = 217)		Chlorambucil (N = 227)	
	All Grades %	Grade ≥3 %	All Grades %	Grade ≥3 %
Infusion reactions[a]	67	10	0	0
Neutropenia	27	26	18	14
Asthenia	8	<1	5	0
Headache	7	<1	3	0
Leukopenia	6	3	2	<1
Herpes simplex[b]	6	0	4	<1
Lower respiratory tract infection	5	1	3	<1
Arthralgia	5	<1	3	0
Upper abdominal pain	5	0	3	0

[a]Includes events which occurred on the day of an infusion or within 24 hours of the end of an infusion and resulted in an interruption or discontinuation of treatment. Infusion reactions may include, but are not limited to, chills, dyspnea, flushing, hypotension, nausea, pain, pruritus, pyrexia, rash, and urticaria.
[b] Includes oral herpes, herpes, herpes virus infection, genital herpes, and herpes simplex.

Table 4. Post-baseline Hematologic Laboratory Abnormalities Occurring With ≥5% Incidence in Patients Receiving ARZERRA Plus Chlorambucil and Also ≥2% More Than Patients Receiving Chlorambucil

	ARZERRA Plus Chlorambucil (N = 217)		Chlorambucil (N = 227)	
	All Grades %	Grade ≥3 %	All Grades %	Grade ≥3 %
Leukopenia	67	23	28	4
Neutropenia	66	29	56	24
Lymphopenia	52	29	20	7

5.2 Hepatitis B Virus Reactivation

Hepatitis B virus (HBV) reactivation, in some cases resulting in fulminant hepatitis, hepatic failure, and death, has occurred in patients treated with ARZERRA. Cases have been reported in patients who are hepatitis B surface antigen (HBsAg) positive and also in patients who are HBsAg negative but are hepatitis B core antibody (anti-HBc) positive. Reactivation also has occurred in patients who appear to have resolved hepatitis B infection (i.e., HBsAg negative, anti-HBc positive, and hepatitis B surface antibody [anti-HBs] positive).

HBV reactivation is defined as an abrupt increase in HBV replication manifesting as a rapid increase in serum HBV DNA level or detection of HBsAg in a person who was previously HBsAg negative and anti-HBc positive. Reactivation of HBV replication is often followed by hepatitis, i.e., increase in transaminase levels and, in severe cases, increase in bilirubin levels, liver failure, and death.

Screen all patients for HBV infection by measuring HBsAg and anti-HBc before initiating treatment with ARZERRA. For patients who show evidence of hepatitis B infection (HBsAg positive [regardless of antibody status] or HBsAg negative but anti-HBc positive), consult physicians with expertise in managing hepatitis B regarding monitoring and consideration for HBV antiviral therapy.

Monitor patients with evidence of current or prior HBV infection for clinical and laboratory signs of hepatitis or HBV reactivation during and for several months following treatment with ARZERRA. HBV reactivation has been reported for at least 12 months following completion of therapy.

In patients who develop reactivation of HBV while receiving ARZERRA, immediately discontinue ARZERRA and any concomitant chemotherapy, and institute appropriate treatment. Resumption of ARZERRA in patients whose HBV reactivation resolves should be discussed with physicians with expertise in managing hepatitis B. Insufficient data exist regarding the safety of resuming ARZERRA in patients who develop HBV reactivation.

5.3 Hepatitis B Virus Infection

Fatal infection due to hepatitis B in patients who have not been previously infected has been observed with ARZERRA. Monitor patients for clinical and laboratory signs of hepatitis.

5.4 Progressive Multifocal Leukoencephalopathy

Progressive multifocal leukoencephalopathy (PML) resulting in death has occurred with ARZERRA. Consider PML in any patient with new onset of or changes in pre-existing neurological signs or symptoms. If PML is suspected, discontinue ARZERRA and initiate evaluation for PML including neurology consultation.

5.5 Tumor Lysis Syndrome

Tumor lysis syndrome (TLS), including the need for hospitalization, has occurred in patients treated with ARZERRA. Patients with high tumor burden and/or high circulating lymphocyte counts (>25 × 10⁹/L) are at greater risk for developing TLS. Consider tumor lysis prophylaxis with antihyperuricemics and hydration beginning 12 to 24 hours prior to infusion of ARZERRA. For treatment of TLS, administer aggressive intravenous hydration and antihyperuricemic agents, correct electrolyte abnormalities, and monitor renal function.

5.6 Cytopenias

Severe cytopenias, including neutropenia, thrombocytopenia, and anemia, can occur with ARZERRA. Pancytopenia, agranulocytosis, and fatal neutropenic sepsis have occurred in patients who received ARZERRA in combination with chlorambucil. Grade 3 or 4 late-onset neutropenia (onset at least 42 days after last treatment dose) and/or prolonged neutropenia (not resolved between 24 and 42 days after last treatment dose) were reported in patients who received ARZERRA [see Adverse Reactions (6.1)]. Monitor complete blood counts at regular intervals during and after conclusion of therapy, and increase the frequency of monitoring in patients who develop Grade 3 or 4 cytopenias.

5.7 Immunizations

The safety of immunization with live viral vaccines during or following administration of ARZERRA has not been studied. Do not administer live viral vaccines to patients who have recently received ARZERRA. The ability to generate an immune response to any vaccine following administration of ARZERRA has not been studied.

6 ADVERSE REACTIONS

The following serious adverse reactions are discussed in greater detail in other sections of the labeling:
• Infusion Reactions [see Warnings and Precautions (5.1)]

• Hepatitis B Virus Reactivation [see Warnings and Precautions (5.2)]
• Hepatitis B Virus Infection [see Warnings and Precautions (5.3)]
• Progressive Multifocal Leukoencephalopathy [see Warnings and Precautions (5.4)]
• Tumor Lysis Syndrome [see Warnings and Precautions (5.5)]
• Cytopenias [see Warnings and Precautions (5.6)]

Previously Untreated CLL: The most common adverse reactions (≥10%) were infusion reactions and neutropenia (Table 3).

Refractory CLL: The most common adverse reactions (≥10%) were neutropenia, pneumonia, pyrexia, cough, diarrhea, anemia, fatigue, dyspnea, rash, nausea, bronchitis, and upper respiratory tract infections (Table 5). The most common serious adverse reactions were infections (including pneumonia and sepsis), neutropenia, and pyrexia. Infections were the most common adverse reactions leading to drug discontinuation.

6.1 Clinical Trials Experience

Because clinical trials are conducted under widely varying conditions, adverse reaction rates observed in the clinical trials of a drug cannot be directly compared with rates in the clinical trials of another drug and may not reflect the rates observed in practice.

Previously Untreated CLL: The safety of ARZERRA was evaluated in an open-label, parallel-arm, randomized trial (Study 1) in 444 patients with previously untreated CLL. Patients were randomized to receive either ARZERRA as an intravenous infusion every 28 days in combination with chlorambucil (n = 217) or chlorambucil as a single agent (n = 227). In both arms, patients received chlorambucil 10 mg/m2 orally on Days 1 to 7 every 28 days. The infusion schedule for ARZERRA was 300 mg administered on Cycle 1 Day 1, 1,000 mg administered on Cycle 1 Day 8, and 1,000 mg administered on Day 1 of subsequent 28-day cycles. The median number of cycles of ARZERRA completed was 6.

The data described in Table 3 include relevant adverse reactions occurring up to 60 days after the last dose of study medication; Table 4 includes relevant hematologic laboratory abnormalities.
[See table 3 above]
[See table 4 above]

Infusion Reactions: Overall, 67% of patients who received ARZERRA in combination with chlorambucil experienced one or more symptoms of infusion reactions (10% were Grade 3 or greater; none were fatal). Infusion reactions that were either Grade 3 or greater, serious, or led to treatment interruption or discontinuation occurred most frequently during Cycle 1 (56% on Day 1 [6% were Grade 3 or greater] and 23% on Day 8 [3% were Grade 3 or greater]) and decreased with subsequent infusions. Infusion reactions led to discontinuation of treatment in 3% of patients. Serious adverse events of infusion reactions occurred in 2% of patients.

Neutropenia: Overall, 3% of patients had neutropenia as a serious adverse event, reported up to 60 days after the last dose. One patient died with neutropenic sepsis and agranulocytosis. Prolonged neutropenia occurred in 6% of patients receiving ARZERRA in combination with chlorambucil compared with 4% of patients receiving chlorambucil. Late-onset neutropenia occurred in 6% of patients receiving ARZERRA in combination with chlorambucil compared with 1% of patients receiving chlorambucil alone.

Refractory CLL: The safety of monotherapy with ARZERRA was evaluated in 181 patients with relapsed or refractory CLL in 2 open–label, non–randomized, single–arm studies. In these studies, ARZERRA was administered at 2,000 mg beginning with the second dose for 11 doses (Study 2 [n = 154]) or 3 doses (Study 3 [n = 27]).

The data described in Table 5 and other sections below are derived from 154 patients in Study 2. All patients received 2,000 mg weekly from the second dose onward. Ninety percent of patients received at least 8 infusions of ARZERRA and 55% received all 12 infusions. The median age was 63 years (range: 41 to 86 years), 72% were male, and 97% were white.
[See table 5 at top of next page]

Infusion Reactions: Infusion reactions occurred in 44% of patients on the day of the first infusion (300 mg), 29% on the day of the second infusion (2,000 mg), and less frequently during subsequent infusions.

Infections: A total of 108 patients (70%) experienced bacterial, viral, or fungal infections. A total of 45 patients (29%) experienced Grade 3 or greater infections, of which 19 (12%) were fatal. The proportion of fatal infections in the fludarabine– and alemtuzumab–refractory group was 17%.

Neutropenia: Of 108 patients with normal neutrophil counts at baseline, 45 (42%) developed Grade 3 or greater neutropenia. Nineteen (18%) developed Grade 4 neutropenia. Some patients experienced new onset Grade 4 neutropenia >2 weeks in duration.

6.2 Immunogenicity

There is a potential for immunogenicity with therapeutic proteins such as ofatumumab. Serum samples from more than 300 patients with CLL were tested during and after treatment for antibodies to ARZERRA. There was no formation of anti–ofatumumab antibodies in patients with CLL after treatment with ofatumumab.

Immunogenicity assay results are highly dependent on several factors including assay sensitivity and specificity, assay methodology, sample handling, timing of sample collection, concomitant medications, and underlying disease. For these reasons, comparison of incidence of antibodies to ARZERRA with the incidence of antibodies to other products may be misleading.

6.3 Postmarketing Experience

The following adverse reactions have been identified during post-approval use of ARZERRA. Because these reactions are reported voluntarily from a population of uncertain size, it is not always possible to reliably estimate their frequency or establish a causal relationship to drug exposure.

Infusion-related Cardiac Events: Cardiac arrest.

Mucocutaneous Reactions: Stevens-Johnson syndrome, porphyria cutanea tarda.

7 DRUG INTERACTIONS

Coadministration of ARZERRA with chlorambucil did not result in clinically relevant effects on the pharmacokinetics of chlorambucil or its active metabolite, phenylacetic acid mustard.

8 USE IN SPECIFIC POPULATIONS

8.1 Pregnancy

Pregnancy Category C: There are no adequate or well–controlled studies of ofatumumab in pregnant women. A reproductive study in pregnant cynomolgus monkeys that received ofatumumab at doses up to 3.5 times the maximum recommended human dose (2,000 mg) of ofatumumab did not demonstrate maternal toxicity or teratogenicity. Ofatumumab crossed the placental barrier, and fetuses exhibited depletion of peripheral B cells and decreased spleen and placental weights. ARZERRA should be used during pregnancy only if the potential benefit to the mother justifies the potential risk to the fetus.

There are no human or animal data on the potential short- and long-term effects of perinatal B-cell depletion in offspring following in utero exposure to ofatumumab. Ofatumumab does not bind normal human tissues other than B lymphocytes. It is not known if binding occurs to unique embryonic or fetal tissue targets. In addition, the kinetics of B-lymphocyte recovery are unknown in offspring with B-cell depletion [see Nonclinical Toxicology (13.3)].

8.3 Nursing Mothers

It is not known whether ofatumumab is secreted in human milk; however, human IgG is secreted in human milk. Published data suggest that neonatal and infant consumption of breast milk does not result in substantial absorption of these maternal antibodies into circulation. Because the effects of local gastrointestinal and limited systemic exposure to ofatumumab are unknown, caution should be exercised when ARZERRA is administered to a nursing woman.

8.4 Pediatric Use

Safety and effectiveness of ARZERRA have not been established in children.

8.5 Geriatric Use

In Study 1, 68% of patients (148/217) receiving ARZERRA plus chlorambucil were 65 years and older. Patients age 65 years and older experienced a higher incidence of the following Grade 3 or greater adverse reactions compared with patients younger than 65 years of age: neutropenia (30% versus 17%) and pneumonia (5% versus 1%) [see Adverse Reactions (6.1)]. In patients 65 years and older, 29% experienced serious adverse events compared with 13% of patients younger than 65 years. No clinically meaningful differences in the effectiveness of ARZERRA plus chlorambucil were observed between older and younger patients [see Clinical Studies (14.1)].

In refractory CLL, clinical studies of ARZERRA did not include sufficient numbers of subjects aged 65 years and older to determine whether they respond differently from younger subjects [see Clinical Pharmacology (12.3)].

8.6 Renal Impairment

No formal studies of ARZERRA in patients with renal impairment have been conducted [see Clinical Pharmacology (12.3)].

8.7 Hepatic Impairment

No formal studies of ARZERRA in patients with hepatic impairment have been conducted.

10 OVERDOSAGE

No data are available regarding overdosage with ARZERRA.

11 DESCRIPTION

ARZERRA (ofatumumab) is an IgG1κ human monoclonal antibody with a molecular weight of approximately 149 kDa. The antibody was generated via transgenic mouse and hybridoma technology and is produced in a recombinant murine cell line (NS0) using standard mammalian cell cultivation and purification technologies.

Table 5. Incidence of All Adverse Reactions Occurring in ≥5% of Patients and in the Fludarabine– and Alemtuzumab–refractory Subset

Adverse Reaction	Total Population (N = 154)		Fludarabine– and Alemtuzumab–refractory (N = 59)	
	All Grades %	Grade ≥3 %	All Grades %	Grade ≥3 %
Pneumonia[a]	23	14	25	15
Pyrexia	20	3	25	5
Cough	19	0	19	0
Diarrhea	18	0	19	0
Anemia	16	5	17	8
Fatigue	15	0	15	0
Dyspnea	14	2	19	5
Rash[b]	14	<1	17	2
Bronchitis	11	<1	19	2
Nausea	11	0	12	0
Upper respiratory tract infection	11	0	3	0
Edema peripheral	9	<1	8	2
Back pain	8	1	12	2
Chills	8	0	10	0
Nasopharyngitis	8	0	8	0
Sepsis[c]	8	8	10	10
Urticaria	8	0	5	0
Insomnia	7	0	10	0
Headache	6	0	7	0
Herpes zoster	6	1	7	2
Hyperhidrosis	5	0	5	0
Hypertension	5	0	8	0
Hypotension	5	0	3	0
Muscle spasms	5	0	3	0
Sinusitis	5	2	3	2
Tachycardia	5	<1	7	2

[a] Includes pneumonia, lung infection, lobar pneumonia, and bronchopneumonia.
[b] Includes rash, rash macular, and rash vesicular.
[c] Includes sepsis, neutropenic sepsis, bacteremia, and septic shock.

ARZERRA is a sterile, clear to opalescent, colorless, preservative-free liquid concentrate for intravenous administration. ARZERRA is supplied at a concentration of 20 mg/mL in single-use vials. Each single-use vial contains either 100 mg ofatumumab in 5 mL of solution or 1,000 mg ofatumumab in 50 mL of solution.

Inactive ingredients include: 10 mg/mL arginine, diluted hydrochloric acid, 0.019 mg/mL edetate disodium, 0.2 mg/mL polysorbate 80, 6.8 mg/mL sodium acetate, 2.98 mg/mL sodium chloride, and Water for Injection, USP. The pH is 5.5.

12 CLINICAL PHARMACOLOGY

12.1 Mechanism of Action

Ofatumumab binds specifically to both the small and large extracellular loops of the CD20 molecule. The CD20 molecule is expressed on normal B lymphocytes (pre–B- to mature B-lymphocyte) and on B-cell CLL. The CD20 molecule is not shed from the cell surface and is not internalized following antibody binding.

The Fab domain of ofatumumab binds to the CD20 molecule and the Fc domain mediates immune effector functions to result in B-cell lysis in vitro. Data suggest that possible mechanisms of cell lysis include complement-dependent cytotoxicity and antibody-dependent, cell-mediated cytotoxicity.

12.2 Pharmacodynamics

B-Cell Depletion: In patients with previously untreated CLL, at 6 months after the last dose, the median reductions in CD19–positive B cells were >99% (n = 155) for ARZERRA in combination with chlorambucil and 94% (n = 121) for chlorambucil alone.

In patients with CLL refractory to fludarabine and alemtuzumab, the median decrease in circulating CD19–positive B cells was 91% (n = 50) with the 8th infusion and 85% (n = 32) with the 12th infusion. The time to recovery of lymphocytes, including CD19–positive B cells, to normal levels has not been determined.

Although the depletion of B-cells in the peripheral blood is a measurable pharmacodynamic effect, it is not directly correlated with the depletion of B cells in solid organs or in malignant deposits. B-cell depletion has not been shown to be directly correlated to clinical response.

Cardiac Electrophysiology: The effect of multiple doses of ARZERRA on the QTc interval was evaluated in a pooled analysis of 3 open-label studies in patients with CLL (N = 85). Patients received ARZERRA 300 mg on Day 1 followed by either 1,000 mg or 2,000 mg for subsequent doses. No large changes in the mean QTc interval (i.e., >20 milliseconds) were detected in the pooled analysis.

12.3 Pharmacokinetics

Ofatumumab is eliminated through both a target–independent route and a B cell–mediated route. Ofatumumab exhibited dose–dependent clearance in the dose range of 100 to 2,000 mg. Due to the depletion of B cells, the clearance of ofatumumab decreased substantially after subsequent infusions compared with the first infusion.

Pharmacokinetic data were obtained after repeated administration (4, 5, 8, or 12 infusions) of 1,000 mg or 2,000 mg

Table 6. IRC-assessed Efficacy Results in Previously Untreated CLL (ITT Population[a])

Primary and Key Secondary Endpoints	ARZERRA Plus Chlorambucil (N = 221)	Chlorambucil (N = 226)
Progression-free survival (PFS) Median, months (95% CI)	22.4 (19.0, 25.2)	13.1 (10.6, 13.8)
Hazard ratio[b] (95% CI) Stratified log rank P value	0.57 (0.45, 0.72) P <0.001	
Overall response, % (95% CI)	82.4 (76.7, 87.1)	68.6 (62.1, 74.6)
P value	P = 0.001	
Complete response, %	12	1
Duration of response Median, months (95% CI)	22.1 (19.1, 24.6)	13.2 (10.8, 16.4)

IRC = Independent Review Committee; ITT = intention to treat; CI = confidence interval.
[a] Intention-to-treat population includes all 447 randomized patients.
[b] Pike Estimator.

Figure 1. Kaplan-Meier Estimates of IRC-assessed Progression-free Survival

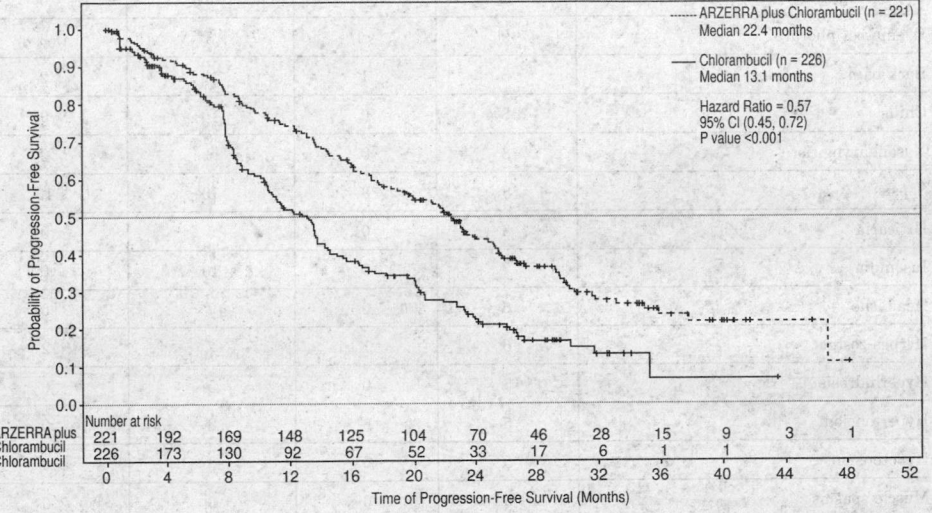

age was 69 years (range: 35 to 92 years) and 69% of patients in both arms were at least 65 years of age. In the overall trial population, 72% of patients had 2 or more co-morbidities, and 48% of patients had a creatinine clearance of less than 70 mL/min. Sixty-three percent of patients were male and 89% were white. Elevated beta-2 microglobulin (β2m) >3,500 mcg/L was present in 72% of patients at base-line.

The primary endpoint was progression-free-survival (PFS) as assessed by a blinded Independent Review Committee (IRC) using the International Workshop for Chronic Lymphocytic Leukemia (IWCLL) updated National Cancer Institute-sponsored Working Group (NCI-WG) guidelines (2008). ARZERRA plus chlorambucil resulted in statistically significant improvement in IRC-assessed median PFS compared with chlorambucil alone (22.4 months versus 13.1 months; hazard ratio: 0.57 [0.45, 0.72]) (Table 6; Figure 1). Secondary efficacy endpoints, including overall response (OR), complete response (CR), and duration of response, were also assessed by the IRC using the 2008 IWCLL Guidelines (Table 6).
[See table 6 above]
[See figure 1 above]

14.2 Refractory CLL
Study 2 was a single–arm, multicenter study in 154 patients with relapsed or refractory CLL. ARZERRA was administered by intravenous infusion according to the following schedule: 300 mg (Week 0), 2,000 mg weekly for 7 infusions (Weeks 1 through 7), and 2,000 mg every 4 weeks for 4 infusions (Weeks 12 through 24). Patients with CLL refractory to fludarabine and alemtuzumab (n = 59) comprised the efficacy population. Drug refractoriness was defined as failure to achieve at least a partial response to, or disease progression within 6 months of, the last dose of fludarabine or alemtuzumab. The main efficacy outcome was durable objective tumor response rate. Objective tumor responses were determined using the 1996 NCI-WG Guidelines for CLL.
In patients with CLL refractory to fludarabine and alemtuzumab, the median age was 64 years (range: 41 to 86 years), 75% were male, and 95% were white. The median number of prior therapies was 5; 93% received prior alkylating agents, 59% received prior rituximab, and all received prior fludarabine and alemtuzumab. Eighty-eight percent of patients received at least 8 infusions of ARZERRA and 54% received 12 infusions.
The investigator–determined overall response rate in patients with CLL refractory to fludarabine and alemtuzumab was 42% (99% CI: 26, 60) with a median duration of response of 6.5 months (95% CI: 5.8, 8.3). There were no complete responses. Anti–tumor activity was also observed in additional patients in Study 2 and in a multicenter, open–label, dose-escalation study (Study 3) conducted in patients with relapsed or refractory CLL.

16 HOW SUPPLIED/STORAGE AND HANDLING
ARZERRA (ofatumumab) is a sterile, clear to opalescent, colorless, preservative-free liquid concentrate (20 mg/mL) for dilution and intravenous administration provided in single-use glass vials with a rubber stopper (not made with natural rubber latex) and an aluminum overseal. Each vial contains either 100 mg ofatumumab in 5 mL of solution or 1,000 mg ofatumumab in 50 mL of solution.
ARZERRA is available as follows:

Carton Contents	NDC
3 single-use 100 mg/5 mL vials	Vial: NDC 0173-0821-02 Carton of 3 vials: NDC 0173-0821-33
1 single-use 1,000 mg/50 mL vial	Vial and Carton: NDC 0173-0821-01

Store ARZERRA refrigerated between 2° to 8°C (36° to 46°F). Do not freeze. Vials should be protected from light.

17 PATIENT COUNSELING INFORMATION
Advise patients to contact a healthcare professional for any of the following:
• Signs and symptoms of infusion reactions including fever, chills, rash, or breathing problems within 24 hours of infusion [see Warnings and Precautions (5.1), Adverse Reactions (6.1)]
• Symptoms of hepatitis including worsening fatigue or yellow discoloration of skin or eyes [see Warnings and Precautions (5.2, 5.3)]
• New neurological symptoms such as confusion, dizziness or loss of balance, difficulty talking or walking, or vision problems [see Warnings and Precautions (5.4)]
• Bleeding, easy bruising, petechiae, pallor, worsening weakness, or fatigue [see Warnings and Precautions (5.6)]
• Signs of infections including fever and cough [see Warnings and Precautions (5.6), Adverse Reactions (6.1)]

doses in 381 patients with CLL (Studies 1, 2, and 3). The geometric mean (%CV) values for clearance, volume of distribution at steady state (Vss), and half-life for ofatumumab in these patients were 12.9 mL/hour (76%), 5.7 L (65%), and 15.6 days (90%). The pharmacokinetic profile was similar across doses in patients with CLL.
Specific Populations: *Effects of Body Size, Gender, Age, and Renal Impairment:* Based on population pharmacokinetic analyses, body size, gender, age, and renal impairment (evaluated in patients with a calculated creatinine clearance ≥30 mL/min) do not have a clinically meaningful effect on the pharmacokinetics of ofatumumab.

13 NONCLINICAL TOXICOLOGY
13.1 Carcinogenesis, Mutagenesis, Impairment of Fertility
No carcinogenicity or mutagenicity studies of ofatumumab have been conducted. In a repeat–dose toxicity study, no tumorigenic or unexpected mitogenic responses were noted in cynomolgus monkeys treated for 7 months with up to 3.5 times the maximum human dose (2,000 mg) of ofatumumab. Effects on male and female fertility have not been evaluated in animal studies.
13.3 Reproductive and Developmental Toxicology
Pregnant cynomolgus monkeys dosed with 0.7 or 3.5 times the maximum human dose (2,000 mg) of ofatumumab weekly during the period of organogenesis (gestation days 20 to 50) had no maternal toxicity or teratogenicity. Both dose levels of ofatumumab depleted circulating B cells in the dams, with signs of initial B cell recovery 50 days after the final dose. Following Caesarean section at gestational day 100, fetuses from ofatumumab–treated dams exhibited decreases in mean peripheral B–cell counts (decreased to approximately 10% of control values), splenic B–cell counts (decreased to approximately 15% to 20% of control values), and spleen weights (decreased by 15% for the low–dose and by 30% for the high–dose group, compared with control val-

ues). Fetuses from treated dams exhibiting anti-ofatumumab antibody responses had higher B cell counts and higher spleen weights compared with the fetuses from other treated dams, indicating partial recovery in those animals developing anti–ofatumumab antibodies. When compared with control animals, fetuses from treated dams in both dose groups had a 10% decrease in mean placental weights. A 15% decrease in mean thymus weight compared with the controls was also observed in fetuses from dams treated with 3.5 times the human dose of ofatumumab. The biological significance of decreased placental and thymic weights is unknown.
The kinetics of B–lymphocyte recovery and the potential long-term effects of perinatal B–cell depletion in offspring from ofatumumab–treated dams have not been studied in animals.

14 CLINICAL STUDIES
14.1 Previously Untreated CLL
The efficacy of ARZERRA was evaluated in a randomized, open-label, parallel-arm study; 447 patients previously untreated for CLL were randomized to receive either ARZERRA as monthly intravenous infusions (Cycle 1: 300 mg on Day 1 and 1,000 mg on Day 8; subsequent cycles: 1,000 mg on Day 1 every 28 days) in combination with chlorambucil (10 mg/m2 orally on Days 1 to 7 every 28 days) or chlorambucil alone (10 mg/m2 orally on Days 1 to 7 every 28 days). Patients received treatment for a minimum of 3 cycles. Treatment was continued for 3 cycles beyond maximal response (2 consecutive response assessments of stable disease, partial response, or complete response) for up to 12 cycles. Approximately 60% of patients received 3 to 6 cycles of ARZERRA and 30% received 7 to 12 cycles.
This trial enrolled patients for whom fludarabine-based therapy was considered to be inappropriate by the investigator for reasons that included advanced age or presence of co-morbidities. In the overall trial population, the median

- Pregnancy or nursing *[see Use in Specific Populations (8.1, 8.3)]*

Advise patients of the need for:

- Monitoring and possible need for treatment if they have a history of hepatitis B infection (based on the blood test) *[see Warnings and Precautions (5.2)]*.
- Periodic monitoring for blood counts *[see Warnings and Precautions (5.6)]*
- Avoiding vaccination with live viral vaccines *[see Warnings and Precautions (5.7)]*

ARZERRA is a registered trademark of the GSK group of companies.
Manufactured by:
GLAXO GROUP LIMITED
Brentford, Middlesex, TW8 9GS, United Kingdom
U.S. License 1809
Distributed by:
GlaxoSmithKline
Research Triangle Park, NC 27709
©2014, the GSK group of companies. All rights reserved.
ARZ:8PI

AVANDAMET   Rx

[ə-van' də-met]

(rosiglitazone maleate and metformin hydrochloride) Tablets

HIGHLIGHTS OF PRESCRIBING INFORMATION
These highlights do not include all the information needed to use AVANDAMET safely and effectively. See full prescribing information for AVANDAMET.
AVANDAMET (rosiglitazone maleate and metformin hydrochloride) tablets
Initial U.S. Approval: 2002

RECENT MAJOR CHANGES

Boxed Warning, AVANDIA-Rosiglitazone Medicines Access Program removal	05/2014
Indications and Usage, patient population restrictions removal (1)	05/2014
Dosage and Administration (2.1)	05/2014
Contraindications (4)	05/2014
Warnings and Precautions, Cardiac Failure (5.2)	05/2014
Warnings and Precautions, Major Adverse Cardiovascular Events (5.3)	05/2014
Warnings and Precautions, Rosiglitazone REMS (Risk Evaluation and Mitigation Strategy) Program removal (formerly 5.4)	05/2014
Warnings and Precautions, Weight Gain (5.5)	05/2014

WARNINGS
See full prescribing information for complete boxed warning.
Rosiglitazone maleate: CONGESTIVE HEART FAILURE

- **Thiazolidinediones, including rosiglitazone, cause or exacerbate heart failure in some patients (5.2). After initiation of AVANDAMET, and after dose increases, observe patients carefully for signs and symptoms of heart failure (including excessive, rapid weight gain, dyspnea, and/or edema). If these signs and symptoms develop, the heart failure should be managed according to current standards of care. Furthermore, discontinuation or dose reduction must be considered. (5.2)**
- **AVANDAMET is not recommended in patients with symptomatic heart failure. Initiation of AVANDAMET in patients with established NYHA Class III or IV heart failure is contraindicated. (4, 5.2)**

Metformin hydrochloride: LACTIC ACIDOSIS

- **Lactic acidosis can occur due to metformin accumulation. The risk increases with conditions such as sepsis, dehydration, excess alcohol intake, hepatic insufficiency, renal impairment, and acute congestive heart failure. (5.1)**
- **Symptoms include malaise, myalgias, respiratory distress, increasing somnolence, and nonspecific abdominal distress. Laboratory abnormalities include low pH, increased anion gap and elevated blood lactate. (5.1)**
- **If acidosis is suspected, discontinue AVANDAMET and hospitalize the patient immediately. (5.1)**

INDICATIONS AND USAGE

AVANDAMET is a combination antidiabetic product containing a thiazolidinedione and a biguanide indicated as an adjunct to diet and exercise to improve glycemic control in adults with type 2 diabetes mellitus. (1)

Important Limitations of Use:

- Should not be used in patients with type 1 diabetes or for the treatment of diabetic ketoacidosis. (1)
- Coadministration with insulin is not recommended. (1, 5.2, 5.3)

DOSAGE AND ADMINISTRATION

- Individualize the starting dose based on the patient's current regimen. (2.1)
- Dose increases should be accompanied by careful monitoring for adverse events related to fluid retention. (2.1)
- Give in divided doses with meals and gradual dose escalation to reduce the gastrointestinal side effects. (2.2)
- Do not exceed the maximum recommended daily dose of 8 mg rosiglitazone and 2,000 mg metformin. (2.3)
- Do not initiate if the patient exhibits clinical evidence of active liver disease or increased serum transaminase levels. (2.4)

DOSAGE FORMS AND STRENGTHS

Oval, film-coated tablets containing rosiglitazone/metformin hydrochloride: 2 mg/500 mg, 4 mg/500 mg, 2 mg/1,000 mg, and 4 mg/1,000 mg (3)

CONTRAINDICATIONS

- Initiation in patients with established NYHA Class III or IV heart failure. (4)
- Use in significant renal disease or renal dysfunction. (4)
- Use in acute or chronic metabolic acidosis. (4)
- Use in patients undergoing radiologic studies involving intravascular administration of iodinated contrast materials. (4, 5.1)
- Hypersensitivity to rosiglitazone or any of the product's ingredients. (4)

WARNINGS AND PRECAUTIONS

- Fluid retention, which may exacerbate or lead to heart failure, may occur. Combination use with insulin and use in congestive heart failure NYHA Class I and II may increase risk of other cardiovascular effects. (5.2)
- Meta-analysis of 52 mostly short-term trials suggested a potential risk of ischemic cardiovascular (CV) events relative to placebo, not confirmed in a long-term CV outcome trial versus metformin or sulfonylurea. (5.3)
- Assess renal function before starting therapy and at least annually. (5.1)
- Avoid use in patients with evidence of hepatic disease. (2.4, 5.1)
- Warn patients against excessive alcohol intake. (5.1)
- Promptly evaluate patients who develop laboratory abnormalities or clinical illness for evidence of ketoacidosis or lactic acidosis. (5.1)
- Dose-related edema (5.4), weight gain (5.5), and anemia (5.9) may occur.
- Macular edema has been reported. (5.7)
- Increased incidence of bone fracture. (5.8)
- Measure hematologic parameters annually. (5.9)

ADVERSE REACTIONS

The most common adverse reactions (≥10%) include nausea/vomiting, diarrhea, headache, and dyspepsia. (6.1)
To report SUSPECTED ADVERSE REACTIONS, contact GlaxoSmithKline at 1-888-825-5249 or FDA at 1-800-FDA-1088 or www.fda.gov/medwatch.

DRUG INTERACTIONS

- Inhibitors of CYP2C8 (e.g., gemfibrozil) may increase rosiglitazone levels. (7.1)
- Inducers of CYP2C8 (e.g., rifampin) may decrease rosiglitazone levels. (7.1)
- Cationic drugs eliminated by renal tubular secretion; use with caution. (7.2)

USE IN SPECIFIC POPULATIONS

- Pregnancy: No adequate and well-controlled studies in pregnant women. Use during pregnancy only if the potential benefit justifies the potential risk to the fetus. (8.1)
- Nursing Mothers: Discontinue drug or nursing. (8.3)
- Safety and effectiveness in children younger than 18 years have not been established. (8.4)
- Because reduced renal function is associated with increasing age, use with caution in elderly patients. (8.5)

See 17 for PATIENT COUNSELING INFORMATION and Medication Guide

Revised: 05/2014

FULL PRESCRIBING INFORMATION

WARNINGS

Rosiglitazone maleate: CONGESTIVE HEART FAILURE

- Thiazolidinediones, including rosiglitazone, cause or exacerbate congestive heart failure in some patients *[see Warnings and Precautions (5.2)]*. After initiation of AVANDAMET®, and after dose increases, observe patients carefully for signs and symptoms of heart failure (including excessive, rapid weight gain, dyspnea, and/or edema). If these signs and symptoms develop, the heart failure should be managed according to current standards of care. Furthermore, discontinuation or dose reduction of AVANDAMET must be considered.
- AVANDAMET is not recommended in patients with symptomatic heart failure. Initiation of AVANDAMET in patients with established NYHA Class III or IV heart failure is contraindicated. *[See Contraindications (4), Warnings and Precautions (5.2).]*

Metformin hydrochloride: LACTIC ACIDOSIS

- Lactic acidosis is a rare, but serious complication that can occur due to metformin accumulation. The risk increases with conditions such as sepsis, dehydration, excess alcohol intake, hepatic insufficiency, renal impairment, and acute congestive heart failure. *[See Warnings and Precautions (5.1).]*
- Symptoms include malaise, myalgias, respiratory distress, increasing somnolence, and nonspecific abdominal distress. Laboratory abnormalities include low pH, increased anion gap and elevated blood lactate. *[See Warnings and Precautions (5.1).]*
- If acidosis is suspected, discontinue AVANDAMET and hospitalize the patient immediately *[see Warnings and Precautions (5.1)]*.

1 INDICATIONS AND USAGE

AVANDAMET is indicated as an adjunct to diet and exercise to improve glycemic control in adults with type 2 diabetes mellitus.

Important Limitations of Use:

- Due to its mechanism of action, rosiglitazone is active only in the presence of endogenous insulin. Therefore, AVANDAMET should not be used in patients with type 1 diabetes.

• Coadministration of AVANDAMET with insulin is not recommended [see Warnings and Precautions (5.2, 5.3)].

2 DOSAGE AND ADMINISTRATION

The dosage of antidiabetic therapy with AVANDAMET should be individualized on the basis of effectiveness and tolerability. The risk-benefit of initiating monotherapy versus dual therapy with AVANDAMET should be considered.

2.1 Starting Dose

AVANDAMET is generally given in divided doses with meals.

All patients should start the rosiglitazone component of AVANDAMET at the lowest recommended dose. Further increases in the dose of rosiglitazone should be accompanied by careful monitoring for adverse events related to fluid retention [see Boxed Warning, Warnings and Precautions (5.2)].

Patients Inadequately Controlled on Diet and Exercise: If therapy with a combination tablet containing rosiglitazone and metformin is considered appropriate for a patient with type 2 diabetes mellitus inadequately controlled on diet and exercise alone, the recommended starting dose of AVANDAMET is 2 mg/500 mg administered once or twice daily. For patients with HbA1c >11% or fasting plasma glucose (FPG) >270 mg/dL, a starting dose of 2 mg/500 mg twice daily may be considered. The dose of AVANDAMET may be increased in increments of 2 mg/500 mg per day given in divided doses if patients are not adequately controlled after 4 weeks. The maximum dose of AVANDAMET is 8 mg/2,000 mg per day.

Patients Inadequately Controlled on Rosiglitazone or Metformin Monotherapy: If therapy with a combination tablet containing rosiglitazone and metformin is considered appropriate for a patient with type 2 diabetes mellitus inadequately controlled on rosiglitazone or metformin monotherapy, then the selection of the dose of AVANDAMET should be based on the patient's current doses of rosiglitazone and/or metformin.

To switch to AVANDAMET for patients currently treated with metformin, the usual starting dose of AVANDAMET is 4 mg rosiglitazone (total daily dose) plus the dose of metformin already being taken (see Table 1).

To switch to AVANDAMET for patients currently treated with rosiglitazone, the usual starting dose of AVANDAMET is 1,000 mg metformin (total daily dose) plus the dose of rosiglitazone already being taken (see Table 1).

When switching from combination therapy of rosiglitazone plus metformin as separate tablets, the usual starting dose of AVANDAMET is the dose of rosiglitazone and metformin already being taken.

Table 1. AVANDAMET Starting Dose for Patients Treated With Metformin and/or Rosiglitazone

PRIOR THERAPY	Usual AVANDAMET Starting Dose	
Total Daily Dose	Tablet Strength	Number of Tablets
Metformin[a]		
1,000 mg/day	2 mg/500 mg	1 tablet twice a day
2,000 mg/day	2 mg/1,000 mg	1 tablet twice a day
Rosiglitazone		
4 mg/day	2 mg/500 mg	1 tablet twice a day
8 mg/day	4 mg/500 mg	1 tablet twice a day

[a] For patients on doses of metformin between 1,000 and 2,000 mg/day, initiation of AVANDAMET requires individualization of therapy.

2.2 Dose Titration

AVANDAMET is generally given in divided doses with meals, with gradual dose escalation. This reduces gastrointestinal side effects (largely due to metformin) and permits determination of the minimum effective dose for the individual patient.

Sufficient time should be given to assess adequacy of therapeutic response. FPG should be used initially to determine the therapeutic response to AVANDAMET. If additional glycemic control is needed, the daily dose of AVANDAMET may be increased by increments of 4 mg rosiglitazone and/or 500 mg metformin.

After an increase in metformin dosage, dose titration is recommended if patients are not adequately controlled after 1 to 2 weeks. After an increase in rosiglitazone dosage, dose titration is recommended if patients are not adequately controlled after 8 to 12 weeks.

2.3 Maximum Dose

The maximum recommended total daily dose of AVANDAMET is 8 mg rosiglitazone (taken as 4 mg twice daily) and 2,000 mg metformin (taken as 1,000 mg twice daily).

2.4 Specific Patient Populations

Renal Impairment: Any dosage adjustment should be based on a careful assessment of renal function. Generally, elderly, debilitated, and malnourished patients should not be titrated to the maximum dose of AVANDAMET. Monitoring of renal function is necessary to aid in prevention of metformin-associated lactic acidosis, particularly in the elderly [see Warnings and Precautions (5.1)].

Hepatic Impairment: Liver enzymes should be measured prior to initiating treatment with AVANDAMET. Therapy with AVANDAMET should not be initiated if the patient exhibits clinical evidence of active liver disease or increased serum transaminase levels (ALT >2.5× upper limit of normal at start of therapy). After initiation of AVANDAMET, liver enzymes should be monitored periodically per the clinical judgment of the healthcare professional [see Warnings and Precautions (5.6), Clinical Pharmacology (12.3)].

Geriatric: The initial and maintenance dosing of AVANDAMET should be conservative in patients with advanced age, due to the potential for decreased renal function in this population.

Pediatric: Safety and effectiveness of AVANDAMET in pediatric patients have not been established. AVANDAMET and rosiglitazone are not recommended for use in pediatric patients.

Pregnancy: AVANDAMET is not recommended for use in pregnancy.

3 DOSAGE FORMS AND STRENGTHS

Each film-coated oval tablet contains rosiglitazone as the maleate and metformin hydrochloride as follows:

• 2 mg/500 mg – pale pink, debossed with gsk on one side and 2/500 on the other
• 4 mg/500 mg – orange, debossed with gsk on one side and 4/500 on the other
• 2 mg/1,000 mg – yellow, debossed with gsk on one side and 2/1000 on the other
• 4 mg/1,000 mg – pink, debossed with gsk on one side and 4/1000 on the other

4 CONTRAINDICATIONS

• Initiation in patients with established New York Heart Association (NYHA) Class III or IV heart failure [see Boxed Warning].
• Use in patients with renal disease or renal dysfunction [e.g., as suggested by serum creatinine levels ≥1.5 mg/dL (males), ≥1.4 mg/dL (females), or abnormal creatinine clearance], which may also result from conditions such as cardiovascular collapse (shock), acute myocardial infarction, and septicemia [see Warnings and Precautions (5.1)].
• Use in patients with acute or chronic metabolic acidosis, including diabetic ketoacidosis, with or without coma.
• Use in patients undergoing radiologic studies involving intravascular administration of iodinated contrast materials, because use of such products may result in acute alteration of renal function. AVANDAMET should be temporarily discontinued in these patients. [See Warnings and Precautions (5.1).]
• Use in patients with a history of a hypersensitivity reaction to rosiglitazone or any of the product's ingredients.

5 WARNINGS AND PRECAUTIONS

5.1 Lactic Acidosis

Incidence and Management: Lactic acidosis is a rare, but serious, metabolic complication that can occur due to metformin accumulation during treatment with AVANDAMET; when it occurs, it is fatal in approximately 50% of cases. Lactic acidosis may also occur in association with a number of pathophysiologic conditions, including diabetes mellitus, and whenever there is significant tissue hypoperfusion and hypoxemia. Lactic acidosis is characterized by elevated blood lactate levels (>5 mmol/L), decreased blood pH, electrolyte disturbances with an increased anion gap, and an increased lactate/pyruvate ratio. When metformin is implicated as the cause of lactic acidosis, metformin plasma levels >5 mcg/mL are generally found.

The reported incidence of lactic acidosis in patients receiving metformin is very low (approximately 0.03 cases/1,000 patient-years of exposure, with approximately 0.015 fatal cases/1,000 patient-years of exposure). Reported cases have occurred primarily in diabetic patients with significant renal insufficiency, including both intrinsic renal disease and renal hypoperfusion, often in the setting of multiple concomitant medical/surgical problems and multiple concomitant medications. Patients with congestive heart failure requiring pharmacologic management, in particular those with unstable or acute congestive heart failure who are at risk of hypoperfusion and hypoxemia, are at increased risk of lactic acidosis. The risk of lactic acidosis increases with the degree of renal dysfunction and the patient's age. The

risk of lactic acidosis may, therefore, be significantly decreased by regular monitoring of renal function in patients taking AVANDAMET and by use of the minimum effective dose of AVANDAMET. In particular, treatment of the elderly should be accompanied by careful monitoring of renal function. Treatment with AVANDAMET should not be initiated in patients ≥80 years of age unless measurement of creatinine clearance demonstrates that renal function is not reduced, as these patients are more susceptible to developing lactic acidosis. In addition, AVANDAMET should be promptly withheld in the presence of any condition associated with hypoxemia, dehydration, or sepsis. Because impaired hepatic function may significantly limit the ability to clear lactate, AVANDAMET should generally be avoided in patients with clinical or laboratory evidence of hepatic disease. Patients should be cautioned against excessive alcohol intake, either acute or chronic, when taking AVANDAMET, since alcohol potentiates the effects of metformin on lactate metabolism. In addition, AVANDAMET should be temporarily discontinued prior to any intravascular radiocontrast study and for any surgical procedure.

The onset of lactic acidosis often is subtle, and accompanied only by nonspecific symptoms such as malaise, myalgias, respiratory distress, increasing somnolence, and nonspecific abdominal distress. There may be associated hypothermia, hypotension, and resistant bradyarrhythmias with more marked acidosis. The patient and the patient's physician must be aware of the possible importance of such symptoms and the patient should be instructed to notify the physician immediately if they occur. AVANDAMET should be withdrawn until the situation is clarified. Serum electrolytes, ketones, blood glucose, and, if indicated, blood pH, lactate levels, and even blood metformin levels may be useful. Once a patient is stabilized on any dose level of AVANDAMET, gastrointestinal symptoms, which are common during initiation of therapy, are unlikely to be drug related. Later occurrence of gastrointestinal symptoms could be due to lactic acidosis or other serious disease.

Levels of fasting venous plasma lactate above the upper limit of normal but less than 5 mmol/L in patients taking AVANDAMET do not necessarily indicate impending lactic acidosis and may be explainable by other mechanisms, such as poorly controlled diabetes or obesity, vigorous physical activity, or technical problems in sample handling.

Lactic acidosis should be suspected in any diabetic patient with metabolic acidosis lacking evidence of ketoacidosis (ketonuria and ketonemia).

Lactic acidosis is a medical emergency that must be treated in a hospital setting. In a patient with lactic acidosis who is taking AVANDAMET, the drug should be discontinued immediately and general supportive measures promptly instituted. Because metformin is dialyzable (with a clearance of up to 170 mL/min under good hemodynamic conditions), prompt hemodialysis is recommended to correct the acidosis and remove the accumulated metformin. Such management often results in prompt reversal of symptoms and recovery [see Contraindications (4)].

Factors That May Predispose Patients to Lactic Acidosis: Assessment of Renal Function: Metformin is known to be substantially excreted by the kidney, and the risk of metformin accumulation and lactic acidosis increases with the degree of impairment of renal function. Thus, patients with serum creatinine levels above the upper limit of normal for their age should not receive AVANDAMET. In patients with advanced age, AVANDAMET should be carefully titrated to establish the minimum dose for adequate glycemic effect, because aging is associated with reduced renal function. [See Dosage and Administration (2.4), Use in Specific Populations (8.5).]

Before initiation of therapy with AVANDAMET and at least annually thereafter, renal function should be assessed and verified as normal. In patients in whom development of renal dysfunction is anticipated, renal function should be assessed more frequently and AVANDAMET discontinued if evidence of renal impairment is present.

Medications That Affect Renal Function: Concomitant medication(s) that may affect renal function or result in significant hemodynamic change or may interfere with the disposition of metformin, such as cationic drugs that are eliminated by renal tubular secretion [see Drug Interactions (7.2), Clinical Pharmacology (12.4)], should be used with caution.

Hypoxic States: Cardiovascular collapse (shock) from whatever cause, acute congestive heart failure, acute myocardial infarction, and other conditions characterized by hypoxemia have been associated with lactic acidosis and may also cause prerenal azotemia. When such events occur in patients receiving AVANDAMET, the drug should be promptly discontinued.

Radiologic Studies With Intravascular Iodinated Contrast Materials: Intravascular contrast studies with iodinated materials can lead to acute alteration of renal function and have been associated with lactic acidosis in patients receiving metformin [see Contraindications (4)]. Therefore, in patients in whom any such study is planned, AVANDAMET should be temporarily discontinued at the time of or prior to the procedure, and withheld for 48 hours subsequent to the procedure and reinstituted only after renal function has been re-evaluated and found to be normal.

Surgical Procedures: Use of AVANDAMET should be temporarily suspended for any surgical procedure (except minor procedures not associated with restricted intake of food and fluids) and should not be restarted until the patient's oral intake has resumed and renal function has been evaluated as normal.

Alcohol Intake: Alcohol potentiates the effect of metformin on lactate metabolism. Patients, therefore, should be warned against excessive alcohol intake, acute or chronic, while receiving AVANDAMET.

Change in Clinical Status of Patients With Previously Controlled Diabetes: A patient with type 2 diabetes previously well-controlled on AVANDAMET who develops laboratory abnormalities or clinical illness (especially vague and poorly defined illness) should be evaluated promptly for evidence of ketoacidosis or lactic acidosis. Evaluation should include serum electrolytes and ketones, blood glucose, and, if indicated, blood pH, lactate, pyruvate, and metformin levels. If acidosis of either form occurs, AVANDAMET must be stopped immediately and other appropriate corrective measures initiated.

[See also Warnings and Precautions (5.6).]

5.2 Cardiac Failure

Rosiglitazone, like other thiazolidinediones, alone or in combination with other antidiabetic agents, can cause fluid retention, which may exacerbate or lead to heart failure. Patients should be observed for signs and symptoms of heart failure. If these signs and symptoms develop, the heart failure should be managed according to current standards of care. Furthermore, discontinuation or dose reduction of rosiglitazone must be considered *[see Boxed Warning].*

Patients with congestive heart failure (CHF) NYHA Class I and II treated with rosiglitazone have an increased risk of cardiovascular events. A 52-week, double-blind, placebo-controlled, echocardiographic trial was conducted in 224 patients with type 2 diabetes mellitus and NYHA Class I or II CHF (ejection fraction ≤45%) on background antidiabetic and CHF therapy. An independent committee conducted a blinded evaluation of fluid-related events (including congestive heart failure) and cardiovascular hospitalizations according to predefined criteria (adjudication). Separate from the adjudication, other cardiovascular adverse events were reported by investigators. Although no treatment difference in change from baseline of ejection fractions was observed, more cardiovascular adverse events were observed with rosiglitazone treatment compared with placebo during the 52-week trial. (See Table 2.)

Table 2. Emergent Cardiovascular Adverse Events in Patients With Congestive Heart Failure (NYHA Class I and II) Treated With Rosiglitazone or Placebo (in Addition to Background Antidiabetic and CHF Therapy)

Events	Rosiglitazone	Placebo
	N = 110 n (%)	N = 114 n (%)
Adjudicated		
Cardiovascular deaths	5 (5%)	4 (4%)
CHF worsening	7 (6%)	4 (4%)
– with overnight hospitalization	5 (5%)	4 (4%)
– without overnight hospitalization	2 (2%)	0 (0%)
New or worsening edema	28 (25%)	10 (9%)
New or worsening dyspnea	29 (26%)	19 (17%)
Increases in CHF medication	36 (33%)	20 (18%)
Cardiovascular hospitalization[a]	21 (19%)	15 (13%)
Investigator-reported, non-adjudicated		
Ischemic adverse events	10 (9%)	5 (4%)
– Myocardial infarction	5 (5%)	2 (2%)
– Angina	6 (5%)	3 (3%)

[a] Includes hospitalization for any cardiovascular reason.

In a long-term, cardiovascular outcome trial (RECORD) in patients with type 2 diabetes *[see Adverse Reactions (6.1)]*,

Figure 1. Hazard Ratios for the Risk of MACE, Myocardial Infarction, and Total Mortality With Rosiglitazone Compared With a Control Group in Long-term Trials

RSG = rosiglitazone; SU = sulfonylurea; MET = metformin; RAM = ramipril
* Myocardial infarction includes fatal and non-fatal MI plus sudden death

the incidence of heart failure was higher in patients treated with rosiglitazone [2.7% (61/2,220) compared with active control 1.3% (29/2,227), HR 2.10 (95% CI: 1.35, 3.27)].

Initiation of AVANDAMET in patients with established NYHA Class III or IV heart failure is contraindicated. AVANDAMET is not recommended in patients with symptomatic heart failure. *[see Boxed Warning.]*

Patients experiencing acute coronary syndromes have not been studied in controlled clinical trials. In view of the potential for development of heart failure in patients having an acute coronary event, initiation of AVANDAMET is not recommended for patients experiencing an acute coronary event, and discontinuation of AVANDAMET during this acute phase should be considered.

Patients with NYHA Class III and IV cardiac status (with or without CHF) have not been studied in controlled clinical trials. AVANDAMET is not recommended in patients with NYHA Class III and IV cardiac status.

Congestive Heart Failure During Coadministration of Rosiglitazone With Insulin: In trials in which rosiglitazone was added to insulin, rosiglitazone increased the risk of congestive heart failure. Coadministration of rosiglitazone and insulin is not recommended. *[See Indications and Usage (1), Warnings and Precautions (5.3).]*

In 7 controlled, randomized, double-blind trials which had durations from 16 to 26 weeks and which were included in a meta-analysis *[see Warnings and Precautions (5.3)]*, patients with type 2 diabetes mellitus were randomized to coadministration of rosiglitazone and insulin (N = 1,018) or insulin (N = 815). In these 7 trials, rosiglitazone was added to insulin. These trials included patients with long-standing diabetes (median duration of 12 years) and a high prevalence of pre-existing medical conditions, including peripheral neuropathy, retinopathy, ischemic heart disease, vascular disease, and congestive heart failure. The total number of patients with emergent congestive heart failure was 23 (2.3%) and 8 (1.0%) in the rosiglitazone plus insulin and insulin groups, respectively.

Heart Failure in Observational Studies of Elderly Diabetic Patients Comparing Rosiglitazone to Pioglitazone: Three observational studies in elderly diabetic patients (age 65 years and older) found that rosiglitazone statistically significantly increased the risk of hospitalized heart failure compared to use of pioglitazone. One other observational study in patients with a mean age of 54 years, which also included an analysis in a subpopulation of patients >65 years of age, found no statistically significant increase in emergency department visits or hospitalization for heart failure in patients treated with rosiglitazone compared to pioglitazone in the older subgroup.

5.3 Major Adverse Cardiovascular Events

Data from long-term, prospective, randomized, controlled clinical trials of rosiglitazone versus metformin or sulfonylureas, particularly a cardiovascular outcome trial (RECORD), observed no difference in overall mortality or in major adverse cardiovascular events (MACE) and its

components. A meta-analysis of mostly short-term trials suggested an increased risk for myocardial infarction with rosiglitazone compared with placebo.

Cardiovascular Events in Large, Long-term, Prospective, Randomized, Controlled Trials of Rosiglitazone: RECORD, a prospectively designed cardiovascular outcome trial (mean follow-up 5.5 years; 4,447 patients), compared the addition of rosiglitazone to metformin or a sulfonylurea (N = 2,220) with a control group of metformin plus sulfonylurea (N = 2,227) in patients with type 2 diabetes *[see Adverse Reactions (6.1)]*. Non-inferiority was demonstrated for the primary endpoint, cardiovascular hospitalization or cardiovascular death, for rosiglitazone compared with control [HR 0.99 (95% CI: 0.85, 1.16)] demonstrating no overall increased risk in cardiovascular morbidity or mortality. The hazard ratios for total mortality and MACE were consistent with the primary endpoint and the 95% CI similarly excluded a 20% increase in risk for rosiglitazone. The hazard ratios for the components of MACE were 0.72 (95% CI: 0.49, 1.06) for stroke, 1.14 (95% CI: 0.80, 1.63) for myocardial infarction, and 0.84 (95% CI: 0.59, 1.18) for cardiovascular death.

The results of RECORD are consistent with the findings of 2 earlier long-term, prospective, randomized, controlled clinical trials (each trial >3 years' duration; total of 9,620 patients) (see Figure 1). In patients with impaired glucose tolerance (DREAM trial), although the incidence of cardiovascular events was higher among subjects who were randomized to rosiglitazone in combination with ramipril than among subjects randomized to ramipril alone, no statistically significant differences were observed for MACE and its components between rosiglitazone and placebo. In type 2 diabetes patients who were initiating oral agent monotherapy (ADOPT trial), no statistically significant differences were observed for MACE and its components between rosiglitazone and metformin or a sulfonylurea.

[See figure 1 above]

Cardiovascular Events in a Group of 52 Clinical Trials: In a meta-analysis of 52 double-blind, randomized, controlled clinical trials designed to assess glucose-lowering efficacy in type 2 diabetes (mean duration 6 months), a statistically significant increased risk of myocardial infarction with rosiglitazone versus pooled comparators was observed [0.4% versus 0.3%; OR 1.8, (95% CI: 1.03, 3.25)]. A statistically non-significant increased risk of MACE was observed with rosiglitazone versus pooled comparators (OR 1.44, 95% CI: 0.95, 2.20). In the placebo-controlled trials, a statistically significant increased risk of myocardial infarction [0.4% versus 0.2%, OR 2.23 (95% CI: 1.14, 4.64)] and statistically non-significant increased risk of MACE [0.7% versus 0.5%, OR 1.53 (95% CI: 0.94, 2.54)] with rosiglitazone were observed. In the active-controlled trials, there was no increased risk of myocardial infarction or MACE.

Mortality in Observational Studies of Rosiglitazone Compared to Pioglitazone: Three observational studies in elderly diabetic patients (age 65 years and older) found that

Table 3. Weight Changes (kg) From Baseline at Endpoint During Clinical Trials [Median (25th, 75th Percentiles)]

	Monotherapy		
Duration	Control Group	Rosiglitazone 4 mg	Rosiglitazone 8 mg
26 weeks	Placebo	-0.9 (-2.8, 0.9) N = 210	1.0 (0.9, 3.6) N = 436	3.1 (1.1, 5.8) N = 439
52 weeks	Sulfonylurea	2.0 (0, 4.0) N = 173	2.0 (-0.6, 4.0) N = 150	2.6 (0, 5.3) N = 157

	Combination Therapy		
	Control Group	Rosiglitazone + Control Therapy	
Duration		Rosiglitazone 4 mg	Rosiglitazone 8 mg
24-26 weeks	Sulfonylurea	0 (-1.0, 1.3) N = 1,155	2.2 (0.5, 4.0) N = 613	3.5 (1.4, 5.9) N = 841
26 weeks	Metformin	-1.4 (-3.2, 0.2) N = 175	0.8 (-1.0, 2.6) N = 100	2.1 (0, 4.3) N = 184
26 weeks	Insulin	0.9 (-0.5, 2.7) N = 162	4.1 (1.4, 6.3) N = 164	5.4 (3.4, 7.3) N = 150

	AVANDAMET in Patients With Inadequate Control on Diet and Exercise	
Duration	Control Group	AVANDAMET
32 weeks	Metformin -2.2 (-5.5, -0.5) N = 123	0.05 kg (-3.45, 3.0) N = 136
	Rosiglitazone 1.7 (-1.2, 4.5) N = 136	

	AVANDAMET + Insulin	
Duration	Control Group	AVANDAMET + Insulin
24 weeks	Insulin 2.6 kg (0.3, 4.8) N = 145	3.3 kg (1.5, 6.0) N = 147

rosiglitazone statistically significantly increased the risk of all-cause mortality compared to use of pioglitazone. One observational study in patients with a mean age of 54 years found no difference in all-cause mortality between patients treated with rosiglitazone compared to pioglitazone and reported similar results in the subpopulation of patients >65 years of age. One additional small, prospective, observational study found no statistically significant differences for CV mortality and all-cause mortality in patients treated with rosiglitazone compared to pioglitazone.

5.4   Edema
AVANDAMET should be used with caution in patients with edema. In a clinical trial in healthy volunteers who received rosiglitazone 8 mg once daily for 8 weeks, there was a statistically significant increase in median plasma volume compared with placebo. Since thiazolidinediones, including rosiglitazone, can cause fluid retention, which can exacerbate or lead to congestive heart failure, AVANDAMET should be used with caution in patients at risk for heart failure. Patients should be monitored for signs and symptoms of heart failure [see Boxed Warning, Warnings and Precautions (5.2), Patient Counseling Information (17.1)].
In controlled clinical trials of patients with type 2 diabetes, mild to moderate edema was reported in patients treated with rosiglitazone, and may be dose-related. Patients with ongoing edema were more likely to have adverse events associated with edema if started on combination therapy with insulin and rosiglitazone [see Adverse Reactions (6.1)]. The use of AVANDAMET in combination with insulin is not recommended. [See Warnings and Precautions (5.2, 5.3).]

5.5   Weight Gain
Dose-related weight gain was seen with rosiglitazone alone and rosiglitazone together with other hypoglycemic agents (see Table 3). No overall change in median weight was observed with AVANDAMET in drug-naïve patients. The mechanism of weight gain with rosiglitazone is unclear but probably involves a combination of fluid retention and fat accumulation.
[See table 3 above]
In a 4- to 6-year, monotherapy, comparative trial (ADOPT) in patients recently diagnosed with type 2 diabetes not previously treated with antidiabetic medication, the median weight change (25th, 75th percentiles) from baseline at 4 years was 3.5 kg (0.0, 8.1) for rosiglitazone, 2.0 kg (-1.0, 4.8) for glyburide, and -2.4 kg (-5.4, 0.5) for metformin.
In postmarketing experience with rosiglitazone alone or in combination with other hypoglycemic agents, there have been rare reports of unusually rapid increases in weight and increases in excess of that generally observed in clinical trials. Patients who experience such increases should be as-

sessed for fluid accumulation and volume-related events such as excessive edema and congestive heart failure [see Boxed Warning].

5.6   Hepatic Effects
Metformin: Since impaired hepatic function has been associated with some cases of lactic acidosis, AVANDAMET should generally be avoided in patients with clinical or laboratory evidence of hepatic disease.
Rosiglitazone: Liver enzymes should be measured prior to the initiation of therapy with AVANDAMET in all patients and periodically thereafter per the clinical judgment of the healthcare professional. Therapy with AVANDAMET should not be initiated in patients with increased baseline liver enzyme levels (ALT >2.5× upper limit of normal). Patients with mildly elevated liver enzymes (ALT levels ≤2.5× upper limit of normal) at baseline or during therapy with AVANDAMET should be evaluated to determine the cause of the liver enzyme elevation. Initiation of, or continuation of, therapy with AVANDAMET in patients with mild liver enzyme elevations should proceed with caution and include close clinical follow-up, including more frequent liver enzyme monitoring, to determine if the liver enzyme elevations resolve or worsen. If at any time ALT levels increase to >3× the upper limit of normal in patients on therapy with AVANDAMET, liver enzyme levels should be rechecked as soon as possible. If ALT levels remain >3× the upper limit of normal, therapy with AVANDAMET should be discontinued.
If any patient develops symptoms suggesting hepatic dysfunction, which may include unexplained nausea, vomiting, abdominal pain, fatigue, anorexia, and/or dark urine, liver enzymes should be checked. The decision whether to continue the patient on therapy with AVANDAMET should be guided by clinical judgment pending laboratory evaluations. If jaundice is observed, drug therapy should be discontinued.
In addition, if the presence of hepatic disease or hepatic dysfunction of sufficient magnitude to predispose to lactic acidosis is confirmed, therapy with AVANDAMET should be discontinued.

5.7   Macular Edema
Macular edema has been reported in postmarketing experience in some diabetic patients who were taking rosiglitazone or another thiazolidinedione. Some patients presented with blurred vision or decreased visual acuity, but some patients appear to have been diagnosed on routine ophthalmologic examination. Most patients had peripheral edema at the time macular edema was diagnosed. Some patients had improvement in their macular edema after discontinuation of their thiazolidinedione. Patients with diabe-

tes should have regular eye exams by an ophthalmologist, per the Standards of Care of the American Diabetes Association. Additionally, any diabetic who reports any kind of visual symptom should be promptly referred to an ophthalmologist, regardless of the patient's underlying medications or other physical findings. [See Adverse Reactions (6.3).]

5.8   Fractures
Long-term trials (ADOPT and RECORD) show an increased incidence of bone fracture in patients, particularly female patients, taking rosiglitazone [see Adverse Reactions (6.1)]. This increased incidence was noted after the first year of treatment and persisted during the course of the trial. The majority of the fractures in the women who received rosiglitazone occurred in the upper arm, hand, and foot. These sites of fracture are different from those usually associated with postmenopausal osteoporosis (e.g., hip or spine). Other trials suggest that this risk may also apply to men, although the risk of fracture among women appears higher than that among men. The risk of fracture should be considered in the care of patients treated with rosiglitazone, and attention given to assessing and maintaining bone health according to current standards of care.

5.9   Hematologic Effects
Decreases in mean hemoglobin and hematocrit occurred in a dose-related fashion in adult patients treated with rosiglitazone [see Adverse Reactions (6.2)]. The observed changes may be related to the increased plasma volume observed with treatment with rosiglitazone and may be dose-related. The decrease in hemoglobin was seen more frequently in combination rosiglitazone and metformin therapy than in rosiglitazone therapy alone. Vitamin B_{12} deficiency may contribute to the observed reductions in hemoglobin [see Warnings and Precautions (5.10)]. Initial and periodic monitoring of hematologic parameters (e.g., hemoglobin/hematocrit and red blood cell indices) should be performed, at least on an annual basis.

5.10   Vitamin B_{12} Levels
In controlled clinical trials of metformin of 29 weeks' duration, a decrease to subnormal levels of previously normal serum vitamin B_{12} levels, without clinical manifestations, was observed in approximately 7% of patients. Such decrease, possibly due to interference with B_{12} absorption from the B_{12}-intrinsic factor complex, is, however, very rarely associated with anemia and appears to be rapidly reversible with discontinuation of metformin or vitamin B_{12} supplementation. Certain individuals (those with inadequate vitamin B_{12} or calcium intake or absorption) appear to be predisposed to developing subnormal vitamin B_{12} levels. In these patients, routine serum vitamin B_{12} measurements at 2- to 3-year intervals may be useful. Vitamin B_{12} deficiency should be excluded if megaloblastic anemia is suspected. [See Warnings and Precautions (5.9).]

5.11   Diabetes and Blood Glucose Control
Periodic fasting blood glucose and HbA1c measurements should be performed to monitor therapeutic response.
When a patient stabilized on any diabetic regimen is exposed to stress such as fever, trauma, infection, or surgery, a temporary loss of glycemic control may occur. At such times, it may be necessary to withhold AVANDAMET and temporarily administer insulin. AVANDAMET may be reinstituted after the acute episode is resolved.
Hypoglycemia does not occur in patients receiving metformin alone under usual circumstances of use but could occur when caloric intake is deficient, when strenuous exercise is not compensated by caloric supplementation, or during concomitant use with hypoglycemic agents (such as sulfonylureas or insulin) or ethanol. Elderly, debilitated or malnourished patients, and those with adrenal or pituitary insufficiency or alcohol intoxication are particularly susceptible to hypoglycemic effects. Hypoglycemia may be difficult to recognize in the elderly and in people who are taking β-adrenergic blocking drugs.
Patients receiving rosiglitazone in combination with other hypoglycemic agents may be at risk for hypoglycemia, and a reduction in the dose of the concomitant agent may be necessary.

5.12   Ovulation
Therapy with rosiglitazone, like other thiazolidinediones, may result in ovulation in some premenopausal anovulatory women. As a result, these patients may be at an increased risk for pregnancy while taking AVANDAMET [see Use in Specific Populations (8.1)]. Thus, adequate contraception in premenopausal women should be recommended. This possible effect has not been specifically investigated in clinical trials; therefore, the frequency of this occurrence is not known.
Although hormonal imbalance has been seen in preclinical studies [see Nonclinical Toxicology (13.1)], the clinical significance of this finding is not known. If unexpected menstrual dysfunction occurs, the benefits of continued therapy with AVANDAMET should be reviewed.

6   ADVERSE REACTIONS
The following adverse reactions are discussed in more detail elsewhere in the labeling:

- Lactic Acidosis *[see Warnings and Precautions (5.1)]*
- Cardiac Failure *[see Warnings and Precautions (5.2)]*
- Major Adverse Cardiovascular Events *[see Warnings and Precautions (5.3)]*
- Edema *[see Warnings and Precautions (5.4)]*
- Weight Gain *[see Warnings and Precautions (5.4)]*
- Hepatic Effects *[see Warnings and Precautions (5.6)]*
- Macular Edema *[see Warnings and Precautions (5.7)]*
- Fractures *[see Warnings and Precautions (5.8)]*
- Hematologic Effects *[see Warnings and Precautions (5.9)]*
- Vitamin B_{12} Levels *[see Warnings and Precautions (5.10)]*
- Ovulation *[see Warnings and Precautions (5.12)]*

6.1 Clinical Trial Experience

Because clinical trials are conducted under widely varying conditions, adverse reaction rates observed in the clinical trials of a drug cannot be directly compared with rates in the clinical trials of another drug and may not reflect the rates observed in practice.

Patients With Inadequate Glycemic Control on Diet and Exercise: Table 4 summarizes the incidence and types of adverse reactions without regard to causality reported in a controlled, 32-week, double-blind clinical trial of AVANDAMET in patients with inadequate glycemic control on diet and exercise (N = 468).

[See table 4 above]

Mild (no intervention required) to moderate (minor intervention required) symptomatic hypoglycemia was reported by 12% (18/155) of patients treated with AVANDAMET, 14/154 (9%) with metformin, and 8% (13/159) with rosiglitazone. Approximately half of these episodes were accompanied by a simultaneous capillary glucose measurement, and the rate of confirmed hypoglycemia (blood glucose ≤50 mg/dL) was low in this clinical trial: 0.6% (1/155) for AVANDAMET, 1.3% (2/154) for metformin, and 0% with rosiglitazone. No hypoglycemic episode led to withdrawal in patients treated with AVANDAMET, and no patients required medical intervention due to hypoglycemia.

The incidence of edema was 6% on AVANDAMET compared with 7% on rosiglitazone and 3% on metformin.

The incidence of anemia was 4% in patients treated with AVANDAMET compared with either rosiglitazone (2%) or metformin (0%).

Patients Inadequately Controlled on Rosiglitazone Monotherapy: The incidence and types of adverse events reported in controlled, 26-week clinical trials of rosiglitazone administered in combination with metformin 2,500 mg/day in comparison with adverse reactions reported in association with rosiglitazone and metformin monotherapies are shown in Table 5. Overall, the types of adverse reactions without regard to causality reported when rosiglitazone was used in combination with metformin were similar to those reported during monotherapy with rosiglitazone.

[See table 5 above]

Reports of hypoglycemia in patients treated with rosiglitazone added to maximum metformin therapy in double-blind trials were more frequent (3.0%) than in patients treated with rosiglitazone (0.6%) or metformin monotherapies (1.3%) or placebo (0.2%). Overall, anemia and edema were generally mild to moderate in severity and usually did not require discontinuation of treatment with rosiglitazone.

Edema was reported in 4.8% of patients receiving rosiglitazone compared with 1.3% on placebo, and 2.2% on metformin monotherapy and 4.4% on rosiglitazone in combination with maximum doses of metformin.

Reports of anemia (7.1%) were greater in patients treated with rosiglitazone added to metformin compared with monotherapy with rosiglitazone. Lower pre-treatment hemoglobin/hematocrit levels in patients enrolled in the metformin and rosiglitazone combination therapy clinical trials may have contributed to the higher reporting rate of anemia in these trials *[see Adverse Reactions (6.2)]*.

Combination With Insulin: The incidence of hypoglycemia (confirmed by fingerstick blood glucose concentration ≤50 mg/dL) was 14% for patients on AVANDAMET plus insulin compared to 10% for patients on insulin monotherapy. The incidence of edema was 7% when insulin was added to AVANDAMET compared with 3% with insulin monotherapy. This trial excluded patients with pre-existing heart failure or new or worsening edema on AVANDAMET. However, in 26-week, double-blind, fixed-dose trials of rosiglitazone added to insulin, edema was reported with higher frequency (rosiglitazone in combination with insulin, 14.7%; insulin, 5.4%) *[see Warnings and Precautions (5.2)]*.

In trials in which rosiglitazone was added to insulin, rosiglitazone increased the risk of congestive heart failure *[see Warnings and Precautions (5.2)]*.

In a trial in which insulin was added to AVANDAMET, no myocardial ischemia was observed in the insulin group (N = 158), and no congestive heart failure was reported in either group. There was one myocardial ischemic event and one sudden death in the group receiving AVANDAMET plus insulin (N = 161). *[See Warnings and Precautions (5.2).]*

Table 4. Adverse Events (≥5% for AVANDAMET) Reported by Patients With Inadequate Glycemic Control on Diet and Exercise in a 32-Week, Double-blind Clinical Trial of AVANDAMET

Preferred Term	AVANDAMET N = 155 %	Metformin N = 154 %	Rosiglitazone N = 159 %
Nausea/vomiting	16	13	8
Diarrhea	14	21	7
Headache	11	12	10
Dyspepsia	10	8	9
Upper respiratory tract infection	9	7	8
Dizziness	8	3	5
Edema	6	3	7
Nasopharyngitis	6	5	4
Abdominal pain	5	6	7
Arthralgia	5	3	7
Loose stools	5	6	1
Constipation	5	4	6

Table 5. Adverse Events (≥5% for Rosiglitazone Plus Metformin) Reported by Patients in 26-Week, Double-blind Clinical Trials of Rosiglitazone Added to Metformin Therapy

Preferred Term	Rosiglitazone + Metformin N = 338 %	Rosiglitazone N = 2,526 %	Placebo N = 601 %	Metformin N = 225 %
Upper respiratory tract infection	16.0	9.9	8.7	8.9
Diarrhea	12.7	2.3	3.3	15.6
Injury	8.0	7.6	4.3	7.6
Anemia	7.1	1.9	0.7	2.2
Headache	6.5	5.9	5.0	8.9
Sinusitis	6.2	3.2	4.5	5.3
Fatigue	5.9	3.6	5.0	4.0
Back pain	5.0	4.0	3.8	4.0
Viral infection	5.0	3.2	4.0	3.6
Arthralgia	5.0	3.0	4.0	2.2

The incidence of anemia was 2% for AVANDAMET in combination with insulin compared with 1% for insulin monotherapy.

Long-term Trial of Rosiglitazone as Monotherapy: A long-term, 4- to 6-year trial (ADOPT) compared the use of rosiglitazone (n = 1,456), glyburide (n = 1,441), and metformin (n = 1,454) as monotherapy in patients recently diagnosed with type 2 diabetes who were not previously treated with antidiabetic medication. Table 6 presents adverse reactions without regard to causality; rates are expressed per 100 patient-years (PY) exposure to account for the differences in exposure to trial medication across the 3 treatment groups.

In ADOPT, fractures were reported in a greater number of women treated with rosiglitazone (9.3%, 2.7/100 patient-years) compared with glyburide (3.5%, 1.3/100 patient-years) or metformin (5.1%, 1.5/100 patient-years). The majority of the fractures in the women who received rosiglitazone were reported in the upper arm, hand, and foot. *[See Warnings and Precautions (5.8).]* The observed incidence of fractures for male patients was similar among the 3 treatment groups.

[See table 6 at top of next page]

Long-term Trial of Rosiglitazone as Combination Therapy (RECORD): RECORD (Rosiglitazone Evaluated for Cardiac Outcomes and Regulation of Glycemia in Diabetes) was a multicenter, randomized, open-label, non-inferiority trial in subjects with type 2 diabetes inadequately controlled on maximum doses of metformin or sulfonylurea (glyburide, gliclazide, or glimepiride) to compare the time to reach the combined cardiovascular endpoint of cardiovascular death or cardiovascular hospitalization between patients randomized to the addition of rosiglitazone versus metformin or sulfonylurea. The trial included patients who have failed metformin or sulfonylurea monotherapy; those who failed metformin (n = 2,222) were randomized to receive either add-on rosiglitazone (n = 1,117) or add-on sulfonylurea (n = 1,105), and those who failed sulfonylurea (n = 2,225) were randomized to receive either add-on rosiglitazone (n = 1,103) or add-on metformin (n = 1,122). Patients were treated to target HbA1c ≤7% throughout the trial.

The mean age of patients in this trial was 58 years, 52% were male, and the mean duration of follow-up was 5.5 years. Rosiglitazone demonstrated non-inferiority to active control for the primary endpoint of cardiovascular hospitalization or cardiovascular death (HR 0.99, 95% CI: 0.85-1.16). There were no significant differences between groups for secondary endpoints with the exception of congestive heart failure (see Table 7). The incidence of congestive heart failure was significantly greater among patients randomized to rosiglitazone.

[See table 7 at top of next page]

There was an increased incidence of bone fracture for subjects randomized to rosiglitazone in addition to metformin or sulfonylurea compared with those randomized to metformin plus sulfonylurea (8.3% versus 5.3%) *[see Warnings and Precautions (5.8)]*. The majority of fractures were reported in the upper limbs and distal lower limbs. The risk of fracture appeared to be higher in females relative to control (11.5% versus 6.3%), than in males relative to control (5.3% versus 4.3%). Additional data are necessary to determine whether there is an increased risk of fracture in males after a longer period of follow-up.

6.2 Laboratory Abnormalities

Hematologic: Decreases in mean hemoglobin and hematocrit occurred in a dose-related fashion in adult patients treated with rosiglitazone (mean decreases in individual trials as much as 1.0 gram/dL hemoglobin and as much as 3.3% hematocrit). The changes occurred primarily during the first 3 months following initiation of rosiglitazone ther-

Help Patients Save on Rx Drugs: PDR.net/PharmacyDiscountCard

Table 6. On-therapy Adverse Events [≥5 Events/100 Patient-years (PY)] in any Treatment Group Reported in a 4- to 6-Year Clinical Trial of Rosiglitazone as Monotherapy (ADOPT)

Preferred Term	Rosiglitazone N = 1,456 PY = 4,954	Glyburide N = 1,441 PY = 4,244	Metformin N = 1,454 PY = 4,906
Nasopharyngitis	6.3	6.9	6.6
Back pain	5.1	4.9	5.3
Arthralgia	5.0	4.8	4.2
Hypertension	4.4	6.0	6.1
Upper respiratory tract infection	4.3	5.0	4.7
Hypoglycemia	2.9	13.0	3.4
Diarrhea	2.5	3.2	6.8

Table 7. Cardiovascular (CV) Outcomes for the RECORD Trial

Primary Endpoint	Rosiglitazone N = 2,220	Active Control N = 2,227	Hazard Ratio	95% CI
CV death or CV hospitalization	321	323	0.99	0.85-1.16
Secondary Endpoint				
All-cause death	136	157	0.86	0.68-1.08
CV death	60	71	0.84	0.59-1.18
Myocardial infarction	64	56	1.14	0.80-1.63
Stroke	46	63	0.72	0.49-1.06
CV death, myocardial infarction, or stroke	154	165	0.93	0.74-1.15
Heart failure	61	29	2.10	1.35-3.27

apy or following an increase in rosiglitazone dose. The time course and magnitude of decreases were similar in patients treated with a combination of rosiglitazone and other hypoglycemic agents or monotherapy with rosiglitazone. Pretreatment levels of hemoglobin and hematocrit were lower in patients in metformin combination trials and may have contributed to the higher reporting rate of anemia. In a single trial in pediatric patients, decreases in hemoglobin and hematocrit (mean decreases of 0.29 g/dL and 0.95%, respectively) were reported with rosiglitazone. White blood cell counts also decreased slightly in adult patients treated with rosiglitazone. Decreases in hematologic parameters may be related to increased plasma volume observed with rosiglitazone treatment.

In controlled clinical trials of metformin of 29 weeks' duration, a decrease to subnormal levels of previously normal serum vitamin B_{12} levels, without clinical manifestations, was observed in approximately 7% of patients. Such a decrease, possibly due to interference with B_{12} absorption from the B_{12}-intrinsic factor complex, is, however, very rarely associated with anemia and appears to be rapidly reversible with discontinuation of metformin or vitamin B_{12} supplementation.

Lipids: Changes in serum lipids have been observed following treatment with rosiglitazone in adults *[see Clinical Pharmacology (12.2)]*.

Serum Transaminase Levels: In pre-approval clinical trials in 4,598 patients treated with rosiglitazone encompassing approximately 3,600 patient-years of exposure, and in a long-term 4- to 6-year trial in 1,456 patients treated with rosiglitazone (4,954 patient-years exposure), there was no evidence of drug-induced hepatotoxicity.

In pre-approval controlled trials, 0.2% of patients treated with rosiglitazone had reversible elevations in ALT >3× the upper limit of normal compared with 0.2% on placebo and 0.5% on active comparators. The ALT elevations in patients treated with rosiglitazone were reversible. Hyperbilirubinemia was found in 0.3% of patients treated with rosiglitazone compared with 0.9% treated with placebo and 1% in patients treated with active comparators. In pre-approval clinical trials, there were no cases of idiosyncratic drug reactions leading to hepatic failure. *[See Warnings and Precautions (5.6).]*

In the 4- to 6-year ADOPT trial, patients treated with rosiglitazone (4,954 patient-years exposure), glyburide (4,244 patient-years exposure), or metformin (4,906 patient-years exposure) as monotherapy, had the same rate of ALT increase to >3× upper limit of normal (0.3 per 100 patient-years exposure).

In the RECORD trial, patients randomized to rosiglitazone in addition metformin or sulfonylurea and to metformin plus sulfonylurea (10,209 patient-years exposure) had a rate of ALT to ≥3× upper limit of normal of approximately 0.2 and 0.3 per 100 patient-years exposure, respectively.

6.3 Postmarketing Experience

In addition to adverse reactions reported from clinical trials, the events described below have been identified during post-approval use of AVANDAMET or its individual components. Because these events are reported voluntarily from a population of unknown size, it is not possible to reliably estimate their frequency or to always establish a causal relationship to drug exposure.

In patients receiving thiazolidinedione therapy, serious adverse events with or without a fatal outcome, potentially related to volume expansion (e.g., congestive heart failure, pulmonary edema, and pleural effusions) have been reported *[see Boxed Warning, Warnings and Precautions (5.2)]*.

There are postmarketing reports with rosiglitazone of hepatitis, hepatic enzyme elevations to 3 or more times the upper limit of normal, and hepatic failure with and without fatal outcome, although causality has not been established. There are postmarketing reports with rosiglitazone of rash, pruritus, urticaria, angioedema, anaphylactic reaction, Stevens-Johnson syndrome *[see Contraindications (4)]*, and new onset or worsening diabetic macular edema with decreased visual acuity *[see Warnings and Precautions (5.7)]*. (See also GLUCOPHAGE® prescribing information.)

7 DRUG INTERACTIONS

7.1 Drugs Metabolized by Cytochrome P450

An inhibitor of CYP2C8 (e.g., gemfibrozil) may increase the AUC of rosiglitazone and an inducer of CYP2C8 (e.g., rifampin) may decrease the AUC of rosiglitazone. Therefore, if an inhibitor or an inducer of CYP2C8 is started or stopped during treatment with rosiglitazone, changes in diabetes treatment may be needed based upon clinical response. *[See Clinical Pharmacology (12.4).]*

7.2 Cationic Drugs

Although drug interactions for metformin with cationic drugs (e.g., amiloride, digoxin, morphine, procainamide, quinidine, quinine, ranitidine, triamterene, trimethoprim, and vancomycin) remain theoretical (except for cimetidine), careful patient monitoring and dose adjustment of AVANDAMET and/or the interfering drug is recommended in patients who are taking cationic medications that are excreted via the proximal renal tubular secretory system. *[See Warnings and Precautions (5.1), Clinical Pharmacology (12.4).]*

7.3 Drugs That Produce Hyperglycemia

When drugs that produce hyperglycemia, which may lead to loss of glycemic control, are administered to a patient receiving AVANDAMET, the patient should be closely observed to maintain adequate glycemic control. *[See Clinical Pharmacology (12.4).]*

8 USE IN SPECIFIC POPULATIONS

8.1 Pregnancy

Pregnancy Category C.

All pregnancies have a background risk of birth defects, loss, or other adverse outcome regardless of drug exposure. This background risk is increased in pregnancies complicated by hyperglycemia and may be decreased with good metabolic control. It is essential for patients with diabetes or history of gestational diabetes to maintain good metabolic control before conception and throughout pregnancy. Careful monitoring of glucose control is essential in such patients. Most experts recommend that insulin monotherapy be used during pregnancy to maintain blood glucose levels as close to normal as possible. AVANDAMET should be used during pregnancy only if the potential benefit justifies the potential *risk to the fetus.*

Human Data: There are no adequate and well-controlled trials with AVANDAMET or its individual components in pregnant women. Rosiglitazone has been reported to cross the human placenta and be detectable in fetal tissue. The clinical significance of these findings is unknown.

Animal Studies: No animal studies have been conducted with AVANDAMET. The following data are based on findings in studies performed with rosiglitazone or metformin individually.

Rosiglitazone: There was no effect on implantation or the embryo with rosiglitazone treatment during early pregnancy in rats, but treatment during mid-late gestation was associated with fetal death and growth retardation in both rats and rabbits. Teratogenicity was not observed at doses up to 3 mg/kg in rats and 100 mg/kg in rabbits (approximately 20 and 75 times human AUC at the maximum recommended human daily dose of the rosiglitazone component of AVANDAMET, respectively). Rosiglitazone caused placental pathology in rats (3 mg/kg/day). Treatment of rats during gestation through lactation reduced litter size, neonatal viability, and postnatal growth, with growth retardation reversible after puberty. For effects on the placenta, embryo/fetus, and offspring, the no-effect dose was 0.2 mg/kg/day in rats and 15 mg/kg/day in rabbits. These no-effect levels are approximately 4 times human AUC at the maximum recommended human daily dose of the rosiglitazone component of AVANDAMET. Rosiglitazone reduced the number of uterine implantations and live offspring when juvenile female rats were treated at 40 mg/kg/day from 27 days of age through to sexual maturity (approximately 68 times human AUC at the maximum recommended daily dose). The no-effect level was 2 mg/kg/day (approximately 4 times human AUC at the maximum recommended daily dose). There was no effect on pre- or postnatal survival or growth.

Metformin: Metformin was not teratogenic in rats and rabbits at doses up to 600 mg/kg/day. This represents an exposure of about 2 and 6 times the maximum recommended human daily dose of 2,000 mg based on body surface area comparisons for rats and rabbits, respectively. Determination of fetal concentrations demonstrated a partial placental barrier to metformin.

8.2 Labor and Delivery

The effect of AVANDAMET or its components on labor and delivery in humans is unknown.

8.3 Nursing Mothers

No studies have been conducted with AVANDAMET. In studies performed with the individual components, both rosiglitazone-related material and metformin were detectable in milk from lactating rats. It is not known whether rosiglitazone or metformin is excreted in human milk. Because many drugs are excreted in human milk, a decision should be made whether to discontinue nursing or to discontinue AVANDAMET, taking into account the importance of the drug to the mother.

8.4 Pediatric Use

Safety and effectiveness of AVANDAMET in pediatric patients have not been established. AVANDAMET and rosiglitazone are not indicated for use in pediatric patients.

8.5 Geriatric Use

Metformin is known to be substantially excreted by the kidney and because the risk of serious adverse reactions to the drug is greater in patients with impaired renal function, AVANDAMET should only be used in patients with normal renal function *[see Contraindications (4), Warnings and Precautions (5.1), Clinical Pharmacology (12.3)]*. Because reduced renal function is associated with increasing age, AVANDAMET should be used with caution in elderly patients. Care should be taken in dose selection and should be based on careful and regular monitoring of renal function. Generally, elderly patients should not be titrated to the maximum dose of AVANDAMET *[see Dosage and Administration (2.4), Warnings and Precautions (5.1)]*.

Register at PDR.net to Receive Email Drug Alerts

10 OVERDOSAGE

Rosiglitazone: Limited data are available with regard to overdosage in humans. In clinical trials in volunteers, rosiglitazone has been administered at single oral doses of up to 20 mg and was well tolerated. In the event of an overdose, appropriate supportive treatment should be initiated as dictated by the patient's clinical status.

Metformin: Hypoglycemia has not been seen with ingestion of up to 85 grams of metformin, although lactic acidosis has occurred in such circumstances *[see Warnings and Precautions (5.1)]*. Metformin is dialyzable with a clearance of up to 170 mL/min under good hemodynamic conditions. Therefore, hemodialysis may be useful for removal of accumulated metformin from patients in whom metformin overdosage is suspected.

11 DESCRIPTION

AVANDAMET contains 2 oral antidiabetic drugs: rosiglitazone maleate and metformin hydrochloride. Rosiglitazone maleate is an oral antidiabetic agent, which acts primarily by increasing insulin sensitivity. Rosiglitazone improves glycemic control while reducing circulating insulin levels. Rosiglitazone maleate is not chemically or functionally related to the sulfonylureas, the biguanides, or the alpha-glucosidase inhibitors. Chemically, rosiglitazone maleate is (±)-5-[[4-[2-(methyl-2-pyridinyl-amino)ethoxy]phenyl]methyl]-2,4-thiazolidinedione, (Z)-2-butenedioate (1:1) with a molecular weight of 473.52 (357.44 free base). The molecule has a single chiral center and is present as a racemate. Due to rapid interconversion, the enantiomers are functionally indistinguishable. The molecular formula is $C_{18}H_{19}N_3O_3S \bullet C_4H_4O_4$. Rosiglitazone maleate is a white to off-white solid with a melting point range of 122° to 123°C. The pK_a values of rosiglitazone maleate are 6.8 and 6.1. It is readily soluble in ethanol and a buffered aqueous solution with pH of 2.3; solubility decreases with increasing pH in the physiological range. The structural formula of rosiglitazone maleate is:

Metformin hydrochloride (N,N-dimethylimidodi-carbonimidic diamide hydrochloride) is not chemically or pharmacologically related to any other classes of oral antidiabetic agents. Metformin hydrochloride is a white to off-white crystalline compound with a molecular formula of $C_4H_{11}N_5 \bullet HCl$ and a molecular weight of 165.63. Metformin hydrochloride is freely soluble in water and is practically insoluble in acetone, ether, and chloroform. The pK_a of metformin is 12.4. The pH of a 1% aqueous solution of metformin hydrochloride is 6.68. The structural formula of metformin hydrochloride is:

AVANDAMET is available for oral administration as film-coated tablets containing rosiglitazone maleate and metformin hydrochloride equivalent to: 2 mg rosiglitazone with 500 mg metformin hydrochloride (2 mg/500 mg), 4 mg rosiglitazone with 500 mg metformin hydrochloride (4 mg/500 mg), 2 mg rosiglitazone with 1,000 mg metformin hydrochloride (2 mg/1,000 mg), and 4 mg rosiglitazone with 1,000 mg metformin hydrochloride (4 mg/1,000 mg). Inactive ingredients are: hypromellose 2910, lactose monohydrate, magnesium stearate, microcrystalline cellulose, polyethylene glycol 400, povidone 29-32, sodium starch glycolate, titanium dioxide, and 1 or more of the following: red and yellow iron oxides.

12 CLINICAL PHARMACOLOGY

12.1 Mechanism of Action

AVANDAMET: AVANDAMET combines 2 antidiabetic agents with different mechanisms of action to improve glycemic control in patients with type 2 diabetes: Rosiglitazone, a member of the thiazolidinedione class, and metformin, a member of the biguanide class. Thiazolidinediones are insulin sensitizing agents that act primarily by enhancing peripheral glucose utilization, whereas biguanides act primarily by decreasing endogenous hepatic glucose production.

Rosiglitazone: Rosiglitazone improves glycemic control by improving insulin sensitivity. Rosiglitazone is a highly selective and potent agonist for the peroxisome proliferator-activated receptor-gamma (PPARγ). In humans, PPAR receptors are found in key target tissues for insulin action such as adipose tissue, skeletal muscle, and liver. Activation of PPARγ nuclear receptors regulates the transcription of insulin-responsive genes involved in the control of glucose production, transport, and utilization. In addition, PPARγ-responsive genes also participate in the regulation of fatty acid metabolism.

Insulin resistance is a common feature characterizing the pathogenesis of type 2 diabetes. The antidiabetic activity of rosiglitazone has been demonstrated in animal models of type 2 diabetes in which hyperglycemia and/or impaired glucose tolerance is a consequence of insulin resistance in target tissues. Rosiglitazone reduces blood glucose concentrations and reduces hyperinsulinemia in the ob/ob obese mouse, db/db diabetic mouse, and fa/fa fatty Zucker rat.

In animal models, the antidiabetic activity of rosiglitazone was shown to be mediated by increased sensitivity to insulin's action in the liver, muscle, and adipose tissue. Pharmacologic studies in animal models indicate that rosiglitazone improves sensitivity to insulin in muscle and adipose tissue and inhibits hepatic gluconeogenesis. The expression of the insulin-regulated glucose transporter GLUT-4 was increased in adipose tissue. Rosiglitazone did not induce hypoglycemia in animal models of type 2 diabetes and/or impaired glucose tolerance.

Metformin: Metformin is an antidiabetic agent, which improves glucose tolerance in patients with type 2 diabetes, lowering both basal and postprandial plasma glucose. Its pharmacologic mechanisms of action are different from other classes of oral antidiabetic agents. Metformin decreases hepatic glucose production, decreases intestinal absorption of glucose, and increases peripheral glucose uptake and utilization. Unlike sulfonylureas, metformin does not produce hypoglycemia in either patients with type 2 diabetes or normal subjects except in special circumstances *[see Warnings and Precautions (5.11)]* and does not cause hyperinsulinemia. With metformin therapy, insulin secretion remains unchanged while fasting insulin levels and day-long plasma insulin response may actually decrease.

12.2 Pharmacodynamics

In all 26-week controlled trials, across the recommended dose range, rosiglitazone as monotherapy was associated with increases in total cholesterol, LDL-cholesterol and HDL-cholesterol and decreases in free fatty acids.

The lipid profiles of AVANDAMET as well as rosiglitazone and metformin monotherapies in patients who have inadequate glycemic control on diet and exercise are shown in Table 8.

[See table 8 above]

The pattern of LDL, HDL, and total cholesterol changes following therapy with rosiglitazone added to metformin was generally similar to those seen with rosiglitazone monotherapy, and a small decrease in mean triglycerides was observed with the combination therapy.

12.3 Pharmacokinetics

Absorption: *AVANDAMET* In a bioequivalence and dose-proportionality trial of AVANDAMET 4 mg/500 mg, both the

Table 8. Summary of Mean[a] Lipid Changes in a 32-Week Trial of AVANDAMET in Patients With Type 2 Diabetes Mellitus who Have Inadequate Glycemic Control on Diet and Exercise

Parameter	AVANDAMET N[b] = 132	Rosiglitazone N[b] = 128	Metformin N[b] = 117
Total Cholesterol (mg/dL)			
Baseline (mean)	200.4	198.4	201.6
% Change from baseline (mean)	-2.2%	5.3%	-9.0%
LDL (mg/dL)			
Baseline (mean)	113.8	114.6	116.0
% Change from baseline (mean)	-0.2%	4.5%	-10.7%
HDL (mg/dL)			
Baseline (mean)	42.6	42.8	42.9
% Change from baseline (mean)	5.8%	3.1%	0.0%
Triglycerides (mg/dL)			
Baseline (mean)	180.3	166.6	175.7
% Change from baseline (mean)	-18.7%	-4.8%	-15.4%

[a] Data presented as geometric means throughout table.
[b] N = number of subjects with a baseline and end of treatment value.

Table 9. Mean (SD) Pharmacokinetic Parameters for Rosiglitazone and Metformin

Regimen	N	Pharmacokinetic Parameter			
		AUC_{0-inf} (ng.h/mL)	C_{max} (ng/mL)	T_{max}[a] (h)	$T_{½}$ (h)
Rosiglitazone					
A	25	1,442 (324)	242 (70)	0.95 (0.48-2.47)	4.26 (1.18)
B	25	1,398 (340)	254 (69)	0.57 (0.43-2.58)	3.95 (0.81)
C	24	349 (91)	63.0 (15.0)	0.57 (0.47-1.45)	3.87 (0.88)
Metformin					
A	25	7,116 (2,096)	1,106 (329)	2.97 (1.02-4.02)	3.46 (0.96)
B	25	7,413 (1,838)	1,135 (253)	2.50 (1.03-3.98)	3.36 (0.54)
C	24	6,945 (2,045)	1,080 (327)	2.97 (1.00-5.98)	3.35 (0.59)

[a] Median and range presented for T_{max}.
AUC = area under the curve; C_{max} = maximum concentration; $T_{½}$ = terminal half-life.
Regimen A = 4 mg/500 mg AVANDAMET; Regimen B = 4-mg rosiglitazone tablet + 500-mg metformin tablet; Regimen C = 1 mg/500 mg AVANDAMET.

rosiglitazone component and the metformin component were bioequivalent to coadministered 4-mg rosiglitazone tablet and 500-mg metformin tablet under fasted conditions (see Table 9). In this trial, dose proportionality of rosiglitazone in the combination formulations of 1 mg/500 mg and 4 mg/500 mg was demonstrated.

[See table 9 at top of previous page]

Administration of AVANDAMET 4 mg/500 mg with food resulted in no change in overall exposure (AUC) for either rosiglitazone or metformin. However, there were decreases in C_{max} of both components (22% for rosiglitazone and 15% for metformin, respectively) and a delay in T_{max} of both components (1.5 hours for rosiglitazone and 0.5 hours for metformin, respectively). These changes are not likely to be clinically significant. The pharmacokinetics of both the rosiglitazone component and the metformin component of AVANDAMET when taken with food were similar to the pharmacokinetics of rosiglitazone and metformin when administered concomitantly as separate tablets with food.

Absorption: _Rosiglitazone:_ The absolute bioavailability of rosiglitazone is 99%. Peak plasma concentrations are observed about 1 hour after dosing. Maximum plasma concentration (C_{max}) and the area under the curve (AUC) of rosiglitazone increase in a dose-proportional manner over the therapeutic dose range.

Absorption: _Metformin:_ The absolute bioavailability of a 500-mg metformin tablet given under fasting conditions is approximately 50% to 60%. Trials using single oral doses of metformin tablets of 500 mg to 1,500 mg, and 850 mg to 2,550 mg, indicate that there is a lack of dose proportionality with increasing doses, which is due to decreased absorption rather than an alteration in elimination.

Distribution: _Rosiglitazone:_ The mean (CV%) oral volume of distribution (V_{ss}/F) of rosiglitazone is approximately 17.6 (30%) liters, based on a population pharmacokinetic analysis. Rosiglitazone is approximately 99.8% bound to plasma proteins, primarily albumin.

Distribution: _Metformin:_ The apparent volume of distribution (V/F) of metformin following single oral doses of 850 mg metformin averaged 654 ± 358 L. Metformin is negligibly bound to plasma proteins. Metformin partitions into erythrocytes, most likely as a function of time. At usual clinical doses and dosing schedules of metformin, steady-state plasma concentrations of metformin are reached within 24 to 48 hours and are generally <1 mcg/mL. During controlled clinical trials, maximum metformin plasma levels did not exceed 5 mcg/mL, even at maximum doses.

Metabolism and Excretion: _Rosiglitazone:_ is extensively metabolized with no unchanged drug excreted in the urine. The major routes of metabolism were N-demethylation and hydroxylation, followed by conjugation with sulfate and glucuronic acid. All the circulating metabolites are considerably less potent than parent and, therefore, are not expected to contribute to the insulin-sensitizing activity of rosiglitazone. In vitro data demonstrate that rosiglitazone is predominantly metabolized by Cytochrome P450 (CYP) isoenzyme 2C8, with CYP2C9 contributing as a minor pathway. Following oral or intravenous administration of [^{14}C]rosiglitazone maleate, approximately 64% and 23% of the dose was eliminated in the urine and in the feces, respectively. The plasma half-life of [^{14}C]related material ranged from 103 to 158 hours. The elimination half-life is 3 to 4 hours and is independent of dose.

Metabolism and Excretion: _Metformin:_ Intravenous single-dose trials in normal subjects demonstrate that metformin is excreted unchanged in the urine and does not undergo hepatic metabolism (no metabolites have been identified in humans) nor biliary excretion. Renal clearance is approximately 3.5 times greater than creatinine clearance which indicates that tubular secretion is the major route of metformin elimination. Following oral administration, approximately 90% of the absorbed drug is eliminated via the renal route within the first 24 hours, with a plasma elimination half-life of approximately 6.2 hours. In blood, the elimination half-life is approximately 17.6 hours, suggesting that the erythrocyte mass may be a compartment of distribution.

Special Populations: _Renal Impairment:_ In subjects with decreased renal function (based on measured creatinine clearance), the plasma and blood half-life of metformin is prolonged and the renal clearance is decreased in proportion to the decrease in creatinine clearance [see Warnings and Precautions (5.1), GLUCOPHAGE prescribing information]. Since metformin is contraindicated in patients with renal impairment, administration of AVANDAMET is contraindicated in these patients.

Hepatic Impairment: Unbound oral clearance of rosiglitazone was significantly lower in patients with moderate or severe liver disease (Child-Pugh Class B/C) compared with healthy subjects. As a result, unbound C_{max} and AUC_{0-inf} were increased 2- and 3-fold, respectively. Elimination half-life for rosiglitazone was about 2 hours longer in patients with liver disease, compared with healthy subjects.

Therapy with AVANDAMET should not be initiated if the patient exhibits clinical evidence of active liver disease or increased serum transaminase levels (ALT >2.5× upper limit of normal) at baseline [see Warnings and Precautions (5.6)].

No pharmacokinetic trials of metformin have been conducted in subjects with hepatic insufficiency.

Geriatric: Results of the population pharmacokinetics analysis (N = 716 <65 years; N = 331 ≥65 years) showed that age does not significantly affect the pharmacokinetics of rosiglitazone. However, limited data from controlled pharmacokinetic trials of metformin in healthy elderly subjects suggest that total plasma clearance of metformin is decreased, the half-life is prolonged, and C_{max} is increased, compared with healthy young subjects. From these data, it appears that the change in metformin pharmacokinetics with aging is primarily accounted for by a change in renal function [see Use in Specific Populations (8.5), GLUCOPHAGE prescribing information]. Metformin treatment and therefore treatment with AVANDAMET should not be initiated in patients ≥80 years of age unless measurement of creatinine clearance demonstrates that renal function is not reduced [see Dosage and Administration (2), Warnings and Precautions (5.1)].

Gender: Results of the population pharmacokinetics analysis showed that the mean oral clearance of rosiglitazone in female patients (N = 405) was approximately 6% lower compared with male patients of the same body weight (N = 642). In rosiglitazone and metformin combination trials, efficacy was demonstrated with no gender differences in glycemic response.

Metformin pharmacokinetic parameters did not differ significantly between normal subjects and patients with type 2 diabetes when analyzed according to gender (males = 19, females = 16). Similarly, in controlled clinical trials in patients with type 2 diabetes, the antihyperglycemic effect of metformin tablets was comparable in males and females.

Race: Results of a population pharmacokinetic analysis including subjects of white, black, and other ethnic origins indicate that race has no influence on the pharmacokinetics of rosiglitazone.

No trials of metformin pharmacokinetic parameters according to race have been performed. In controlled clinical trials of metformin in patients with type 2 diabetes, the antihyperglycemic effect was comparable in whites (N = 249), blacks (N = 51), and Hispanics (N = 24).

Pediatric: No pharmacokinetic data from trials in pediatric subjects are available for AVANDAMET.

12.4   Drug-drug Interactions

Rosiglitazone: _Drugs That Inhibit, Induce, or are Metabolized by Cytochrome P450:_ In vitro drug metabolism studies suggest that rosiglitazone does not inhibit any of the major P450 enzymes at clinically relevant concentrations. In vitro data demonstrate that rosiglitazone is predominantly metabolized by CYP2C8, and to a lesser extent, 2C9. [See Drug Interactions (7.1).]

Rosiglitazone (4 mg twice daily) was shown to have no clinically relevant effect on the pharmacokinetics of nifedipine and oral contraceptives (ethinyl estradiol and norethindrone), which are predominantly metabolized by CYP3A4.

Gemfibrozil: Concomitant administration of gemfibrozil (600 mg twice daily), an inhibitor of CYP2C8, and rosiglitazone (4 mg once daily) for 7 days increased rosiglitazone AUC by 127%, compared with the administration of rosiglitazone (4 mg once daily) alone. Given the potential for dose-related adverse events with rosiglitazone, a decrease in the dose of rosiglitazone may be needed when gemfibrozil is introduced. [See Drug Interactions (7.1).]

Rifampin: Rifampin administration (600 mg once a day), an inducer of CYP2C8, for 6 days is reported to decrease rosiglitazone AUC by 66%, compared with the administration of rosiglitazone (8 mg) alone.[1] [See Drug Interactions (7.1).]

Metformin: _Cationic Drugs:_ Cationic drugs (e.g., amiloride, digoxin, morphine, procainamide, quinidine, quinine, ranitidine, triamterene, trimethoprim, and vancomycin) that are eliminated by renal tubular secretion theoretically have the potential for interaction with metformin by competing for common renal tubular transport systems. Such interaction between metformin and oral cimetidine has been observed in normal healthy volunteers in both single- and multiple-dose, metformin-cimetidine drug interaction trials, with a 60% increase in peak metformin plasma and whole blood concentrations and a 40% increase in plasma and whole blood metformin AUC. There was no change in elimination half-life in the single-dose trial. Metformin had no effect on cimetidine pharmacokinetics. [See Warnings and Precautions (5.1), Drug Interactions (7.2).]

Furosemide: A single-dose, metformin-furosemide drug interaction trial in healthy subjects demonstrated that pharmacokinetic parameters of both compounds were affected by coadministration. Furosemide increased the metformin plasma and blood C_{max} by 22% and blood AUC by 15%, with-

out any significant change in metformin renal clearance. When administered with metformin, the C_{max} and AUC of furosemide were 31% and 12% smaller, respectively, than when administered alone, and the terminal half-life was decreased by 32%, without any significant change in furosemide renal clearance. No information is available about the interaction of metformin and furosemide when coadministered chronically.

Nifedipine: A single-dose, metformin-nifedipine drug interaction trial in normal healthy volunteers demonstrated that coadministration of nifedipine increased plasma metformin C_{max} and AUC by 20% and 9%, respectively, and increased the amount excreted in the urine. T_{max} and half-life were unaffected. Nifedipine appears to enhance the absorption of metformin. Metformin had minimal effects on nifedipine.

Other: Certain drugs tend to produce hyperglycemia and may lead to loss of glycemic control. These drugs include thiazides and other diuretics, corticosteroids, phenothiazines, thyroid products, estrogens, oral contraceptives, phenytoin, nicotinic acid, sympathomimetics, calcium channel blocking drugs, and isoniazid.

In healthy volunteers, the pharmacokinetics of metformin and propranolol and metformin and ibuprofen were not affected when coadministered in single-dose interaction trials.

Metformin is negligibly bound to plasma proteins and is therefore, less likely to interact with highly protein-bound drugs such as salicylates, sulfonamides, chloramphenicol, and probenecid.

13   NONCLINICAL TOXICOLOGY

13.1   Carcinogenesis, Mutagenesis, Impairment of Fertility

No animal studies have been conducted with AVANDAMET. The following data are based on findings in studies performed with rosiglitazone or metformin individually.

Rosiglitazone: A 2-year carcinogenicity study was conducted in Charles River CD-1 mice at doses of 0.4, 1.5, and 6 mg/kg/day in the diet (highest dose equivalent to approximately 12 times human AUC at the maximum recommended human daily dose of the rosiglitazone component of AVANDAMET). Sprague-Dawley rats were dosed for 2 years by oral gavage at doses of 0.05, 0.3, and 2 mg/kg/day (highest dose equivalent to approximately 10 and 20 times human AUC at the maximum recommended human daily dose of the rosiglitazone component of AVANDAMET for male and female rats, respectively).

Rosiglitazone was not carcinogenic in the mouse. There was an increase in incidence of adipose hyperplasia in the mouse at doses ≥1.5 mg/kg/day (approximately 2 times human AUC at the maximum recommended human daily dose of the rosiglitazone component of AVANDAMET). In rats, there was a significant increase in the incidence of benign adipose tissue tumors (lipomas) at doses ≥0.3 mg/kg/day (approximately 2 times human AUC at the maximum recommended human daily dose of the rosiglitazone component of AVANDAMET). These proliferative changes in both species are considered due to the persistent pharmacological overstimulation of adipose tissue.

Rosiglitazone was not mutagenic or clastogenic in the in vitro bacterial assays for gene mutation, the in vitro chromosome aberration test in human lymphocytes, the in vivo mouse micronucleus test, and the in vivo/in vitro rat UDS assay. There was a small (about 2-fold) increase in mutation in the in vitro mouse lymphoma assay in the presence of metabolic activation.

Rosiglitazone had no effects on mating or fertility of male rats given up to 40 mg/kg/day (approximately 116 times human AUC at the maximum recommended human daily dose of the rosiglitazone component of AVANDAMET). Rosiglitazone altered estrous cyclicity (2 mg/kg/day) and reduced fertility (40 mg/kg/day) of female rats in association with lower plasma levels of progesterone and estradiol (approximately 20 and 200 times human AUC at the maximum recommended human daily dose of the rosiglitazone component of AVANDAMET, respectively). No such effects were noted at 0.2 mg/kg/day (approximately 3 times human AUC at the maximum recommended human daily dose of the rosiglitazone component of AVANDAMET). In juvenile rats dosed from 27 days of age through to sexual maturity (at up to 40 mg/kg/day), there was no effect on male reproductive performance, or on estrous cyclicity, mating performance or pregnancy incidence in females (approximately 68 times human AUC at the maximum recommended daily dose of rosiglitazone). In monkeys, rosiglitazone (0.6 and 4.6 mg/kg/day; approximately 3 and 15 times human AUC at the maximum recommended human daily dose of the rosiglitazone component of AVANDAMET, respectively) diminished the follicular phase rise in serum estradiol with consequential reduction in the luteinizing hormone surge, lower luteal phase progesterone levels, and amenorrhea. The mechanism for these effects appears to be direct inhibition of ovarian steroidogenesis.

Metformin: Long-term carcinogenicity studies have been performed in rats (dosing duration of 104 weeks) and mice (dosing duration of 91 weeks) at doses up to and including 900 mg/kg/day and 1,500 mg/kg/day, respectively. These doses are both approximately 4 times the maximum recommended human daily dose of 2,000 mg of the metformin component of AVANDAMET based on body surface area comparisons. No evidence of carcinogenicity with metformin was found in either male or female mice. Similarly, there was no tumorigenic potential observed with metformin in male rats. There was, however, an increased incidence of benign stromal uterine polyps in female rats treated with 900 mg/kg/day.

There was no evidence of mutagenic potential of metformin in the following in vitro tests: Ames test (*S. typhimurium*), gene mutation test (mouse lymphoma cells), or chromosomal aberrations test (human lymphocytes). Results in the in vivo mouse micronucleus test were also negative.

Fertility of male or female rats was unaffected by metformin when administered at doses as high as 600 mg/kg/day, which is approximately 3 times the maximum recommended human daily dose of the metformin component of AVANDAMET based on body surface area comparisons.

13.2 Animal Toxicology

Heart weights were increased in mice (3 mg/kg/day), rats (5 mg/kg/day), and dogs (2 mg/kg/day) with rosiglitazone treatments (approximately 5, 22, and 2 times human AUC at the maximum recommended human daily dose of the rosiglitazone component of AVANDAMET, respectively). Effects in juvenile rats were consistent with those seen in adults. Morphometric measurement indicated that there was hypertrophy in cardiac ventricular tissues, which may be due to increased heart work as a result of plasma volume expansion.

14 CLINICAL STUDIES

14.1 Patients who Have Inadequate Glycemic Control on Diet and Exercise

In a 32-week, randomized, double-blind clinical trial, 468 patients with type 2 diabetes mellitus inadequately controlled on diet and exercise alone (mean baseline FPG 198 mg/dL and mean baseline HbA1c 8.8%) were randomized to AVANDAMET 2 mg/500 mg, rosiglitazone 4 mg, or metformin 500 mg. Doses were increased at 4-week intervals up to a maximum of 8 mg/2,000 mg for AVANDAMET, 8 mg for rosiglitazone, and 2,000 mg for metformin to reach a target mean daily glucose of ≤110 mg/dL. Following the initial dosage level, AVANDAMET, rosiglitazone, and metformin were all administered as twice-daily regimens. Statistically significant improvements in FPG and HbA1c were observed in patients treated with AVANDAMET compared with either rosiglitazone or metformin alone (see Table 10). However, when considering the choice of therapy for drug-naïve patients, the risk-benefit of initiating monotherapy or dual therapy should be considered.

[See table 10 above]

Patients screened in the double-blind clinical trial described above with HbA1c >11% or FPG >270 mg/dL were not eligible for blinded treatment but were treated with open-label AVANDAMET (4 mg/1,000 mg up to a maximum dose of 8 mg/2,000 mg). Treatment with AVANDAMET reduced mean HbA1c from a baseline of 11.8% to 7.8% and mean FPG from a baseline of 305 mg/dL to 166 mg/dL. Given the lack of direct comparators in this evaluation, determination of the exact contribution of rosiglitazone and metformin as well as diet and exercise, to the observed improvement in glycemic control is not possible.

14.2 Patients Previously Treated With Metformin

AVANDAMET was not studied in patients previously treated with metformin monotherapy; however, the combination of rosiglitazone and metformin was compared with rosiglitazone and metformin monotherapies in clinical trials. Bioequivalence between AVANDAMET and coadministered rosiglitazone tablets and metformin tablets has been demonstrated [see Clinical Pharmacology (12.3)].

A total of 670 patients with type 2 diabetes participated in two 26-week, randomized, double-blind, placebo/active-controlled trials designed to assess the efficacy of rosiglitazone in combination with metformin. Rosiglitazone, administered in either once-daily or twice-daily dosing regimens, was added to the therapy of patients who were inadequately controlled on 2.5 grams/day of metformin.

In one trial, patients inadequately controlled on 2.5 grams/day of metformin (mean baseline FPG 216 mg/dL and mean baseline HbA1c 8.8%) were randomized to receive rosiglitazone 4 mg once daily, rosiglitazone 8 mg once daily, or placebo in addition to metformin. A statistically significant improvement in FPG and HbA1c was observed in patients treated with the combinations of metformin and rosiglitazone 4 mg once daily and rosiglitazone 8 mg once daily, versus patients continued on metformin alone (see Table 11).

[See table 11 above]

In a second 26-week trial, patients with type 2 diabetes inadequately controlled on 2.5 grams/day of metformin who were randomized to receive the combination of rosiglitazone 4 mg twice daily and metformin (N = 105) showed a statistically significant improvement in glycemic control with a mean treatment effect for FPG of -56 mg/dL and a mean treatment effect for HbA1c of -0.8% over metformin alone. The combination of metformin and rosiglitazone resulted in lower levels of FPG and HbA1c than either agent alone.

15 REFERENCES

1. Park JY, Kim KA, Kang MH, et al. Effect of rifampin on the pharmacokinetics of rosiglitazone in healthy subjects. *Clin Pharmacol Ther* 2004;75:157-162.

16 HOW SUPPLIED/STORAGE AND HANDLING

Each film-coated oval tablet contains rosiglitazone as the maleate and metformin hydrochloride as follows:
2 mg/500 mg – pale pink, tablet, debossed with gsk on one side and 2/500 on the other.
4 mg/500 mg – orange, tablet, debossed with gsk on one side and 4/500 on the other.
2 mg/1,000 mg – yellow, tablet, debossed with gsk on one side and 2/1000 on the other.
4 mg/1,000 mg – pink, tablet, debossed with gsk on one side and 4/1000 on the other.
2 mg/500 mg bottles of 60:   NDC 0173-0837-18
4 mg/500 mg bottles of 60:   NDC 0173-0839-18
2 mg/1,000 mg bottles of 60:   NDC 0173-0838-18
4 mg/1,000 mg bottles of 60:   NDC 0173-0840-18
Store at 25°C (77°F); excursions permitted to 15° to 30°C (59° to 86°F). Dispense in a tight, light-resistant container.

17 PATIENT COUNSELING INFORMATION

Advise the patient to read the FDA-approved patient labeling (Medication Guide).

There are multiple medications available to treat type 2 diabetes. The benefits and risks of each available diabetes medication should be taken into account when choosing a particular diabetes medication for a given patient.

Patients should be informed of the following:
- The risks of lactic acidosis, its symptoms, and conditions that predispose to its development, as noted in the WARNINGS and PRECAUTIONS sections, should be explained to patients. Patients should be advised to discontinue AVANDAMET immediately and to promptly notify their health practitioner if unexplained hyperventilation, myalgia, malaise, unusual somnolence, or other nonspecific symptoms occur. Once a patient is stabilized on any dose level of AVANDAMET, gastrointestinal symptoms, which are common during initiation of metformin therapy, are unlikely to be drug related. Later occurrence of gastrointestinal symptoms could be due to lactic acidosis or other serious disease.
- Avoid excessive alcohol intake, either acute or chronic, while receiving AVANDAMET.
- AVANDAMET is not recommended for patients with symptomatic heart failure.
- A meta-analysis of mostly short-term trials suggested an increased risk for myocardial infarction with rosiglitazone compared with placebo. Data from long-term clinical trials of rosiglitazone versus other antidiabetes agents (metformin or sulfonylureas), including a cardiovascular outcome trial (RECORD), observed no difference in overall mortality or in major adverse cardiovascular events (MACE) and its components.
- AVANDAMET is not recommended for patients who are taking insulin.
- Management of type 2 diabetes should include diet control. Caloric restriction, weight loss, and exercise are essential for the proper treatment of the diabetic patient because they help improve insulin sensitivity. This is important not only in the primary treatment of type 2 diabetes but also in maintaining the efficacy of drug therapy.
- It is important to adhere to dietary instructions and to regularly have blood glucose, glycosylated hemoglobin (HbA1c), renal function, and hematologic parameters tested. It can take 2 weeks to see a reduction in blood glucose and 2 to 3 months to see the full effect of AVANDAMET.
- Blood will be drawn to check their liver function prior to the start of therapy and periodically thereafter per the clinical judgment of the healthcare professional. Patients with unexplained symptoms of nausea, vomiting, abdominal pain, fatigue, anorexia, or dark urine should immediately report these symptoms to their physician.

Table 10. Glycemic Parameters in a 32-Week Trial of AVANDAMET in Patients With Type 2 Diabetes Mellitus Inadequately Controlled on Diet and Exercise

Parameter	AVANDAMET	Rosiglitazone	Metformin
Mean Final Dose	7.2 mg/1,799 mg	7.7 mg	1,847 mg
N	152	155	150
FPG (mg/dL)			
Baseline (mean)	201	194	199
Change from baseline (mean)	-74	-47	-51
Difference between AVANDAMET and monotherapy (adjusted mean)		-22[a]	-22[a]
% of patients with ≥30 mg/dL decrease from baseline	86%	68%	64%
HbA1c (%)			
Baseline (mean)	8.9%	8.8%	8.8%
Change from baseline (mean)	-2.3%	-1.6%	-1.8%
Difference between AVANDAMET and monotherapy (adjusted mean)		-0.6[a]	-0.4[a]
% of patients with HbA1c ≥0.7% decrease from baseline	92%	79%	84%
% of Patients with HbA1c <7.0%	77%	58%	57%

[a] <0.001 AVANDAMET compared with rosiglitazone or metformin.

Table 11. Glycemic Parameters in a 26-Week Trial of Rosiglitazone Added to Metformin Therapy

Parameter	Metformin	Rosiglitazone 4 mg Once Daily + Metformin	Rosiglitazone 8 mg Once Daily + Metformin
N	113	116	110
FPG (mg/dL)			
Baseline (mean)	214	215	220
Change from baseline (mean)	6	-33	-48
Difference from metformin alone (adjusted mean)		-40[a]	-53[a]
% of patients with ≥30 mg/dL decrease from baseline	20%	45%	61%
HbA1c (%)			
Baseline (mean)	8.6	8.9	8.9
Change from baseline (mean)	0.5	-0.6	-0.8
Difference from metformin alone (adjusted mean)		-1.0[a]	-1.2[a]
% of patients with HbA1c ≥0.7% decrease from baseline	11%	45%	52%

[a]P <0.0001 compared with metformin.

Help Patients Save on Rx Drugs: PDR.net/PharmacyDiscountCard

- Patients who experience an unusually rapid increase in weight or edema or who develop shortness of breath or other symptoms of heart failure while on AVANDAMET should immediately report these symptoms to their physician.
- Therapy with AVANDAMET, like other thiazolidinediones, may result in ovulation in some premenopausal anovulatory women. As a result, these patients may be at an increased risk for pregnancy while taking AVANDAMET. Thus, adequate contraception in premenopausal women should be recommended. This possible effect has not been specifically investigated in clinical trials so the frequency of this occurrence is not known.

AVANDAMET is a registered trademark of the GSK group of companies.
GLUCOPHAGE is a registered trademark of Merck Santé S.A.S. (an associate of Merck KGaA of Darmstadt, Germany; licensed to Bristol-Myers Squibb Company).
GlaxoSmithKline
Research Triangle Park, NC 27709
©2014, the GSK group of companies. All rights reserved.
AVM:22PI

MEDICATION GUIDE
AVANDAMET® (ah-VAN-duh-met)
(rosiglitazone maleate and metformin hydrochloride) tablets

Read this Medication Guide carefully before you start taking AVANDAMET and each time you get a refill. There may be new information. This information does not take the place of talking with your doctor about your medical condition or your treatment. If you have any questions about AVANDAMET, ask your doctor or pharmacist.

What is the most important information I should know about AVANDAMET?
AVANDAMET may cause serious side effects, including:
New or worse heart failure
- The risk of heart failure may be higher in people who take AVANDAMET with insulin. Most people who take insulin should not also take AVANDAMET.
- Rosiglitazone, one of the medicines in AVANDAMET, can cause your body to keep extra fluid (fluid retention), which leads to swelling (edema) and weight gain. Extra body fluid can make some heart problems worse or lead to heart failure. Heart failure means your heart does not pump blood well enough.
- If you have severe heart failure, you cannot start AVANDAMET.
- If you have heart failure with symptoms (such as shortness of breath or swelling), even if these symptoms are not severe, AVANDAMET may not be right for you.

Call your doctor right away if you have any of the following:
- swelling or fluid retention, especially in the ankles or legs
- shortness of breath or trouble breathing, especially when you lie down
- an unusually fast increase in weight
- unusual tiredness

Lactic acidosis
Metformin, one of the medicines in AVANDAMET, can cause a rare but serious condition called lactic acidosis (a build-up of an acid in the blood) that can cause death. Lactic acidosis is a medical emergency and must be treated in the hospital.
Most people who have had lactic acidosis with metformin have other things that, combined with the metformin, led to the lactic acidosis. Tell your doctor if you have any of the following, because you have a higher chance for getting lactic acidosis with AVANDAMET if you:
- have kidney problems or your kidneys are affected by certain X-ray tests that use injectable dye. People with kidney problems should not take AVANDAMET.
- have liver problems
- drink alcohol very often, or drink a lot of alcohol in short-term "binge" drinking
- get dehydrated (lose a large amount of body fluids). This can happen if you are sick with a fever, vomiting or diarrhea. Dehydration can also happen when you sweat a lot with activity or exercise and do not drink enough fluids.
- have surgery
- have a heart attack, severe infection, or stroke
- are 80 years of age or older, and your kidneys are not working properly

The best way to keep from having a problem with lactic acidosis from metformin is to tell your doctor if you have any of the problems in the list above. Your doctor may decide to stop your AVANDAMET for a while if you have any of these things.
Lactic acidosis can be hard to diagnose early, because the early symptoms could seem like the symptoms of many other health problems besides lactic acidosis. You should call your doctor right away if you get the following symptoms, which could be signs of lactic acidosis:
- you feel very weak or tired
- you have unusual (not normal) muscle pain
- you have stomach pains

- you have trouble breathing
- you feel dizzy or lightheaded
- you have a slow or irregular heartbeat

AVANDAMET can have other serious side effects. Be sure to read the section below "What are possible side effects of AVANDAMET?"

What is AVANDAMET?
AVANDAMET contains two prescription medicines for treating diabetes, rosiglitazone maleate (AVANDIA®) and metformin hydrochloride. AVANDAMET is used, with diet and exercise, to treat adults with type 2 ("adult-onset" or "non-insulin dependent") diabetes ("high blood sugar").
Metformin works mainly by decreasing the production of sugar by your liver. Rosiglitazone helps your body respond better to its natural insulin and does not cause your body to make more insulin. These medicines work together to help control your blood sugar. AVANDAMET may be used alone or with other diabetes medicines.
AVANDAMET is not for people with type 1 diabetes mellitus or to treat a condition called diabetic ketoacidosis.
It is not known if AVANDAMET is safe and effective in children younger than 18 years old.

Who should not take AVANDAMET?
Do not take AVANDAMET if you:
- have kidney problems. Before you take AVANDAMET and while you take it, your doctor should test your blood to check for signs of kidney problems.
- have a condition known as metabolic acidosis, including diabetic ketoacidosis.
- are going to have an X-ray procedure with an injection of dyes (contrast agents) in your vein with a needle. Talk to your doctor about when to stop AVANDAMET and when to start it again.

Many people with heart failure should not start taking AVANDAMET. See "What should I tell my doctor before taking AVANDAMET?"
Do not take AVANDAMET if you are allergic to rosiglitazone or any of the inactive ingredients in AVANDAMET. See the end of this leaflet for a complete list of ingredients in AVANDAMET.
Symptoms of a severe allergic reaction with AVANDAMET may include:
- swelling of your face, lips, tongue, or throat
- problems with breathing or swallowing
- skin rash or itching
- raised red areas on your skin (hives)
- blisters on your skin or in your mouth, nose, or eyes
- peeling of your skin
- fainting or feeling dizzy
- very rapid heartbeat

What should I tell my doctor before taking AVANDAMET?
Before starting AVANDAMET, ask your doctor about what the choices are for diabetes medicines, and what the expected benefits and possible risks are for you in particular.
Before taking AVANDAMET, tell your doctor about all of your medical conditions, including if you:
- **have heart problems or heart failure.**
- **have kidney problems.**
- **have type 1 ("juvenile") diabetes or had diabetic ketoacidosis.** These conditions should be treated with insulin.
- **are going to have dye injected into a vein for an X-ray, CAT scan, heart study, or other type of scanning.**
- **drink a lot of alcohol** (all the time or short binge drinking).
- **develop a serious condition such as a heart attack, severe infection, or a stroke.**
- **are 80 years old or older.** People who are older than 80 years should not take AVANDAMET unless their kidney function is checked and it is normal.
- **have a type of diabetic eye disease called macular edema** (swelling of the back of the eye).
- **have liver problems.** Your doctor should do blood tests to check your liver before you start taking AVANDAMET and during treatment as needed.
- **had liver problems while taking REZULIN™** (troglitazone), another medicine for diabetes.
- **are pregnant or plan to become pregnant.** It is not known if AVANDAMET can harm your unborn baby. You and your doctor should talk about the best way to control your diabetes during pregnancy. If you are a premenopausal woman (before the "change of life") who does not have regular monthly periods, AVANDAMET may increase your chances of becoming pregnant. Talk to your doctor about birth control choices while taking AVANDAMET. Tell your doctor right away if you become pregnant while taking AVANDAMET.
- **are breastfeeding or planning to breastfeed.** It is not known if AVANDAMET passes into breast milk. You and your doctor should decide if you will take AVANDAMET or breastfeed. You should not do both.

Tell your doctor about all of the medicines you take including prescription and non-prescription medicines, vitamins or herbal supplements. AVANDAMET and certain other medicines can affect each other and may lead to serious side effects including high or low blood sugar, or heart problems.

Your doctor may need to change your dose of AVANDAMET or your other medicines. Especially tell your doctor if you take:
- **insulin.**
- **any medicines for high blood pressure, high cholesterol or heart failure, or for prevention of heart disease or stroke.**

Know the medicines you take. Keep a list of all your medicines and show it to your doctor and pharmacist before you start a new medicine. They will tell you if it is alright to take AVANDAMET with other medicines.

How should I take AVANDAMET?
- Take AVANDAMET exactly as prescribed. Your doctor may need to change your dose until your blood sugar is better controlled.
- AVANDAMET should be taken by mouth and with meals.
- AVANDAMET may be prescribed alone or with other diabetes medicines. This will depend on how well your blood sugar is controlled.
- It can take 2 weeks for AVANDAMET to start lowering your blood sugar. It may take 2 to 3 months to see the full effect on your blood sugar level.
- If you miss a dose of AVANDAMET, take it as soon as you remember, unless it is time to take your next dose. Take your next dose at the usual time. Do not take double doses to make up for a missed dose.
- If you take too much AVANDAMET, call your doctor or poison control center right away.
- Test your blood sugar regularly as your doctor tells you.
- Diet and exercise can help your body use its blood sugar better. It is important to stay on your recommended diet, lose extra weight, and get regular exercise while taking AVANDAMET.
- Your doctor should do blood tests to check your liver and kidneys before you start AVANDAMET and during treatment as needed. Your doctor should also do regular blood sugar tests (for example, "A1C") to monitor your response to AVANDAMET.

There may be times when you will need to stop taking AVANDAMET for a short time. Tell your doctor if you:
- are sick with severe vomiting, diarrhea or fever, or if you drink a much lower amount of liquid than normal.
- are going to have dye injected into a vein for an X-ray, CAT scan, heart study or other type of scanning.
- plan to have surgery.

What should I avoid while taking AVANDAMET?
Do not drink a lot of alcohol while taking AVANDAMET. This means you should not "binge drink", and you should not drink a lot of alcohol on a regular basis. Drinking a lot of alcohol can increase the chance of getting lactic acidosis.

What are possible side effects of AVANDAMET?
AVANDAMET may cause serious side effects, including:
- **New or worse heart failure.** See "What is the most important information I should know about AVANDAMET?"
- **Heart attack.** AVANDAMET may increase the risk of a heart attack. Talk to your doctor about what this means to you.
  Symptoms of a heart attack can include the following:
  ○ chest discomfort in the center of your chest that lasts for more than a few minutes, or that goes away or comes back
  ○ chest discomfort that feels like uncomfortable pressure, squeezing, fullness, or pain
  ○ pain or discomfort in your arms, back, neck, jaw, or stomach
  ○ shortness of breath with or without chest discomfort
  ○ breaking out in a cold sweat
  ○ nausea or vomiting
  ○ feeling lightheaded
  Call your doctor or go to the nearest hospital emergency room right away if you think you are having a heart attack.
- **Swelling (edema).** AVANDAMET can cause swelling due to fluid retention. See "What is the most important information I should know about AVANDAMET?"
- **Weight gain.** Rosiglitazone, one of the medicines in AVANDAMET, can cause weight gain that may be due to fluid retention or extra body fat. Metformin, the other medicine in AVANDAMET, can cause weight loss. There is little change in weight with AVANDAMET. Weight gain can be a serious problem for people with certain conditions including heart problems. See "What is the most important information I should know about AVANDAMET?"
- **Liver problems.** It is important for your liver to be working normally when you take AVANDAMET. Your doctor should do blood tests to check your liver before you start taking AVANDAMET and during treatment as needed. Call your doctor right away if you have unexplained symptoms such as:
  ○ nausea or vomiting
  ○ stomach pain
  ○ unusual or unexplained tiredness
  ○ loss of appetite
  ○ dark urine
  ○ yellowing of your skin or the whites of your eyes.

- **Macular edema** (a diabetic eye disease with swelling in the back of the eye). Tell your doctor right away if you have any changes in your vision. Your doctor should check your eyes regularly. Very rarely, some people have had vision changes due to swelling in the back of the eye while taking rosiglitazone, one of the medicines in AVANDAMET.
- **Fractures (broken bones)**, usually in the hand, upper arm, or foot. Talk to your doctor for advice on how to keep your bones healthy.
- **Low red blood cell count (anemia)**.
- **Low blood sugar (hypoglycemia)**. Lightheadedness, dizziness, shakiness, or hunger may mean that your blood sugar is too low. This can happen if you skip meals, if you use another medicine that lowers blood sugar, or if you have certain medical problems. Call your doctor if low blood sugar levels are a problem for you.
- **Ovulation** (release of egg from an ovary in a woman) leading to pregnancy. Ovulation may happen in premenopausal women who do not have regular monthly periods. This can increase the chance of pregnancy. See "What should I tell my doctor before taking AVANDAMET?"

Common side effects of AVANDAMET include:
- **Diarrhea, nausea, and upset stomach.** These side effects usually happen during the first few weeks of treatment. Taking AVANDAMET with food can help lessen these side effects. If you have unusual or unexpected stomach problems, talk with your doctor. Stomach problems that start up later during treatment with AVANDAMET may be a sign of something more serious and should be discussed with your doctor.
- **Cold-like symptoms**
- **Headache**
- **Joint aches**
- **Dizziness**

Call your doctor for medical advice about side effects. You may report side effects to FDA at 1-800-FDA-1088.

How should I store AVANDAMET?
- Store AVANDAMET at room temperature, 59°F to 86°F (15°C to 30°C).
- Keep AVANDAMET in the container it comes in. Keep the container closed tightly.
- Safely, throw away AVANDAMET that is out of date or no longer needed.

Keep AVANDAMET and all medicines out of the reach of children.

General information about AVANDAMET
Medicines are sometimes prescribed for purposes other than those listed in a Medication Guide. Do not use AVANDAMET for a condition for which it was not prescribed. Do not give AVANDAMET to other people, even if they have the same symptoms you have. It may harm them. This Medication Guide summarizes important information about AVANDAMET. If you would like more information, talk with your doctor. You can ask your doctor or pharmacist for information about AVANDAMET that is written for healthcare professionals. You can also find out more about AVANDAMET by calling 1-888-825-5249.

What are the ingredients in AVANDAMET?
Active Ingredients: rosiglitazone maleate and metformin hydrochloride
Inactive Ingredients: hypromellose 2910, lactose monohydrate, magnesium stearate, microcrystalline cellulose, polyethylene glycol 400, povidone 29-32, sodium starch glycolate, titanium dioxide, and 1 or more of the following: red and yellow iron oxides.
Always check to make sure that the medicine you are taking is the correct one. AVANDAMET tablets are oval and look like this:
- 2 mg/500 mg – pale pink, with "gsk" on one side and "2/500" on the other.
- 4 mg/500 mg – orange, with "gsk" on one side and "4/500" on the other
- 2 mg/1,000 mg – yellow, with "gsk" on one side and "2/1000" on the other
- 4 mg/1,000 mg – pink, with "gsk" on one side and "4/1000" on the other

AVANDAMET and AVANDIA are registered trademarks of the GSK group of companies.
REZULIN is a trademark of its respective owner and is not a trademark of the GSK group of companies. The maker of this brand is not affiliated with and does not endorse the GSK group of companies or its products.

This Medication Guide has been approved by the U.S. Food and Drug Administration.
GlaxoSmithKline
Research Triangle Park, NC 27709
©2014, the GSK group of companies. All rights reserved.
May 2014
AVM:5MG

AVANDARYL®
[ə-van' də-ril]
(rosiglitazone maleate and glimepiride)
Tablets

℞

HIGHLIGHTS OF PRESCRIBING INFORMATION
These highlights do not include all the information needed to use AVANDARYL safely and effectively. See full prescribing information for AVANDARYL.
AVANDARYL (rosiglitazone maleate and glimepiride) tablets
Initial U.S. Approval: 2005

——————RECENT MAJOR CHANGES——————

Boxed Warning, AVANDIA-Rosiglitazone Medicines Access Program removal	05/2014
Indications and Usage, patient population restrictions removal (1)	05/2014
Dosage and Administration (2)	05/2014
Contraindications (4)	05/2014
Warnings and Precautions, Cardiac Failure (5.2)	05/2014
Warnings and Precautions, Major Adverse Cardiovascular Events (5.3)	05/2014
Warnings and Precautions, Rosiglitazone REMS (Risk Evaluation and Mitigation Strategy) Program removal (formerly 5.4)	05/2014
Warnings and Precautions, Weight Gain (5.6)	05/2014

WARNING: CONGESTIVE HEART FAILURE
See full prescribing information for complete boxed warning.
- Thiazolidinediones, including rosiglitazone, cause or exacerbate congestive heart failure in some patients (5.2). After initiation of AVANDARYL, and after dose increases, observe patients carefully for signs and symptoms of heart failure (including excessive, rapid weight gain, dyspnea, and/or edema). If these signs and symptoms develop, the heart failure should be managed according to current standards of care. Furthermore, discontinuation or dose reduction of AVANDARYL must be considered.
- AVANDARYL is not recommended in patients with symptomatic heart failure. Initiation of AVANDARYL in patients with established NYHA Class III or IV heart failure is contraindicated. (4, 5.2)

——————INDICATIONS AND USAGE——————
AVANDARYL is a combination antidiabetic product containing a thiazolidinedione and a sulfonylurea indicated as an adjunct to diet and exercise to improve glycemic control in adults with type 2 diabetes. (1)
Important Limitations of Use:
- Should not be used in patients with type 1 diabetes or for the treatment of diabetic ketoacidosis. (1, 4)
- Coadministration with insulin is not recommended. (1, 5.2, 5.3)

——————DOSAGE AND ADMINISTRATION——————
- Individualize the starting dose based on the patient's current regimen. (2.1)
- Dose increases should be accompanied by careful monitoring for adverse events related to fluid retention. (2.2)
- Do not exceed the maximum recommended daily dose of 8 mg rosiglitazone and 4 mg glimepiride. (2.3)
- Do not initiate if the patient exhibits clinical evidence of active liver disease or increased serum transaminase levels. (2.4)

——————DOSAGE FORMS AND STRENGTHS——————
Rounded triangular tablets containing rosiglitazone/glimepiride: 4 mg/1 mg, 4 mg/2 mg, 4 mg/4 mg, 8 mg/2 mg, and 8 mg/4 mg (3)

——————CONTRAINDICATIONS——————
- Initiation in patients with established NYHA Class III or IV heart failure. (4)
- Hypersensitivity to rosiglitazone or any of the product's ingredients. (4)

——————WARNINGS AND PRECAUTIONS——————
- One sulfonylurea has been shown to increase cardiovascular mortality; consider this risk when prescribing any sulfonylurea. (5.1)
- Fluid retention, which may exacerbate or lead to heart failure, may occur. Combination use with insulin and use in congestive heart failure NYHA Class I and II may increase risk of other cardiovascular effects. (5.2)

- Meta-analysis of 52 mostly short-term trials suggested a potential risk of ischemic cardiovascular (CV) events relative to placebo, not confirmed in a long-term CV outcome trial versus metformin or sulfonylurea. (5.3)
- Severe hypoglycemia may occur. Use particular care in elderly or debilitated patients and those with adrenal, pituitary, renal, or hepatic insufficiency. (5.4)
- Dose-related edema (5.5), weight gain (5.6), and anemia (5.10) may occur.
- Macular edema has been reported. (5.8)
- Increased incidence of bone fracture. (5.9)
- The glimepiride component may cause hemolytic anemia in patients with glucose 6-phosphate dehydrogenase (G6PD) deficiency. Consider a non-sulfonylurea alternative in these patients. (5.11)

——————ADVERSE REACTIONS——————
Common adverse reactions (≥5%) reported in clinical trials for AVANDARYL without regard to causality were headache, hypoglycemia, and nasopharyngitis. (6.1)
To report SUSPECTED ADVERSE REACTIONS, contact GlaxoSmithKline at 1-888-825-5249 or FDA at 1-800-FDA-1088 or www.fda.gov/medwatch.

——————DRUG INTERACTIONS——————
- Inhibitors of CYP2C8 (e.g., gemfibrozil) may increase rosiglitazone levels. (7.1)
- Inducers of CYP2C8 (e.g., rifampin) may decrease rosiglitazone levels. (7.1)
- Monitor patients for loss of control with drugs that cause hyperglycemia. (7.2)

——————USE IN SPECIFIC POPULATIONS——————
- Pregnancy: No adequate and well-controlled studies in pregnant women. Use during pregnancy only if the potential benefit justifies the potential risk to the fetus. (8.1)
- Nursing Mothers: Discontinue drug or nursing. (8.3)
- Safety and effectiveness in children younger than 18 years have not been established. (8.4)
- Elderly patients may be particularly susceptible to hypoglycemic effects. (8.5)

See 17 for PATIENT COUNSELING INFORMATION and Medication Guide

Revised: 05/2014

FULL PRESCRIBING INFORMATION: CONTENTS*
WARNING: CONGESTIVE HEART FAILURE

14   CLINICAL STUDIES
    14.1   Patients Inadequately Controlled on Diet and Exercise
    14.2   Patients Previously Treated With Sulfonylureas
15   REFERENCES
16   HOW SUPPLIED/STORAGE AND HANDLING
17   PATIENT COUNSELING INFORMATION
* Sections or subsections omitted from the full prescribing information are not listed

---

FULL PRESCRIBING INFORMATION

WARNING: CONGESTIVE HEART FAILURE
- Thiazolidinediones, including rosiglitazone, cause or exacerbate congestive heart failure in some patients *[see Warnings and Precautions (5.2)]*. After initiation of AVANDARYL®, and after dose increases, observe patients carefully for signs and symptoms of heart failure (including excessive, rapid weight gain, dyspnea, and/or edema). If these signs and symptoms develop, the heart failure should be managed according to current standards of care. Furthermore, discontinuation or dose reduction of AVANDARYL must be considered.
- AVANDARYL is not recommended in patients with symptomatic heart failure. Initiation of AVANDARYL in patients with established NYHA Class III or IV heart failure is contraindicated. *[See Contraindications (4), Warnings and Precautions (5.2).]*

---

1   INDICATIONS AND USAGE
AVANDARYL is indicated as an adjunct to diet and exercise to improve glycemic control in adults with type 2 diabetes mellitus.
Important Limitations of Use:
- Due to its mechanism of action, rosiglitazone is active only in the presence of endogenous insulin. Therefore, AVANDARYL should not be used in patients with type 1 diabetes or for the treatment of diabetic ketoacidosis.
- Coadministration of AVANDARYL with insulin is not recommended *[see Warnings and Precautions (5.2, 5.3)]*.

2   DOSAGE AND ADMINISTRATION
Therapy with AVANDARYL should be individualized for each patient. The risk-benefit of initiating monotherapy versus dual therapy with AVANDARYL should be considered. No studies have been performed specifically examining the safety and efficacy of AVANDARYL in patients previously treated with other oral hypoglycemic agents and switched to AVANDARYL. Any change in therapy of type 2 diabetes should be undertaken with care and appropriate monitoring as changes in glycemic control can occur. *[See Indications and Usage (1).]*
2.1   Starting Dose
The recommended starting dose is 4 mg/1 mg administered once daily with the first meal of the day. For adults already treated with a sulfonylurea or rosiglitazone, a starting dose of 4 mg/2 mg may be considered.
All patients should start the rosiglitazone component of AVANDARYL at the lowest recommended dose. Further increases in the dose of rosiglitazone should be accompanied by careful monitoring for adverse events related to fluid retention *[see Boxed Warning, Warnings and Precautions (5.2)]*.
When switching from combination therapy of rosiglitazone plus glimepiride as separate tablets, the usual starting dose of AVANDARYL is the dose of rosiglitazone and glimepiride already being taken.
2.2   Dose Titration
Dose increases should be individualized according to the glycemic response of the patient. Patients who may be more sensitive to glimepiride *[see Warnings and Precautions (5.4)]*, including the elderly, debilitated, or malnourished, and those with renal, hepatic, or adrenal insufficiency, should be carefully titrated to avoid hypoglycemia. If hypoglycemia occurs during up-titration of the dose or while maintained on therapy, a dosage reduction of the glimepiride component of AVANDARYL may be considered. Increases in the dose of rosiglitazone should be accompanied by careful monitoring for adverse events related to fluid retention *[see Boxed Warning, Warnings and Precautions (5.2)]*.
To switch to AVANDARYL for adults currently treated with rosiglitazone, dose titration of the glimepiride component of AVANDARYL is recommended if patients are not adequately controlled after 1 to 2 weeks. The glimepiride component may be increased in no more than 2 mg increments. After an increase in the dosage of the glimepiride component, dose titration of AVANDARYL is recommended if patients are not adequately controlled after 1 to 2 weeks.
To switch to AVANDARYL for adults currently treated with sulfonylurea, it may take 2 weeks to see a reduction in blood glucose and 2 to 3 months to see the full effect of the rosiglitazone component. Therefore, dose titration of the rosiglitazone component of AVANDARYL is recommended if patients are not adequately controlled after 8 to 12 weeks. Patients should be observed carefully (1 to 2 weeks) for hypoglycemia when being transferred from longer half-life sulfonylureas (e.g., chlorpropamide) to AVANDARYL due to potential overlapping of drug effect. After an increase in the dosage of the rosiglitazone component, dose titration of AVANDARYL is recommended if patients are not adequately controlled after 2 to 3 months.
2.3   Maximum Dose
The maximum recommended daily dose is 8 mg rosiglitazone and 4 mg glimepiride.
2.4   Specific Patient Populations
Elderly and Malnourished Patients and Those With Renal, Hepatic, or Adrenal Insufficiency: In elderly, debilitated, or malnourished patients, or in patients with renal, hepatic, or adrenal insufficiency, the starting dose, dose increments, and maintenance dosage of AVANDARYL should be conservative to avoid hypoglycemic reactions. *[See Warnings and Precautions (5.4), Clinical Pharmacology (12.3).]*
Hepatic Impairment: Liver enzymes should be measured prior to initiating treatment with AVANDARYL. Therapy with AVANDARYL should not be initiated if the patient exhibits clinical evidence of active liver disease or increased serum transaminase levels (ALT >2.5X upper limit of normal at start of therapy). After initiation of AVANDARYL, liver enzymes should be monitored periodically per the clinical judgment of the healthcare professional. *[See Warnings and Precautions (5.7), Clinical Pharmacology (12.3).]*
Pregnancy and Lactation: AVANDARYL should not be used during pregnancy or in nursing mothers.
Pediatric Use: Safety and effectiveness of AVANDARYL in pediatric patients have not been established. AVANDARYL and its components, rosiglitazone and glimepiride, are not recommended for use in pediatric patients.

3   DOSAGE FORMS AND STRENGTHS
Each rounded triangular tablet contains rosiglitazone maleate and glimepiride as follows:
- 4 mg/1 mg – yellow, gsk debossed on one side and 4/1 on the other.
- 4 mg/2 mg – orange, gsk debossed on one side and 4/2 on the other.
- 4 mg/4 mg – pink, gsk debossed on one side and 4/4 on the other.
- 8 mg/2 mg – pale pink, gsk debossed on one side and 8/2 on the other.
- 8 mg/4 mg – red, gsk debossed on one side and 8/4 on the other.

4   CONTRAINDICATIONS
Initiation of AVANDARYL in patients with established New York Heart Association (NYHA) Class III or IV heart failure is contraindicated *[see Boxed Warning]*.
AVANDARYL is contraindicated in patients with a history of a hypersensitivity reaction to rosiglitazone or any of the product's ingredients.

5   WARNINGS AND PRECAUTIONS
5.1   Increased Risk of Cardiovascular Mortality for Sulfonylurea Drugs
The administration of oral hypoglycemic drugs has been reported to be associated with increased cardiovascular mortality as compared with treatment with diet alone or diet plus insulin. This warning is based on the trial conducted by the University Group Diabetes Program (UGDP), a long-term, prospective clinical trial designed to evaluate the effectiveness of glucose-lowering drugs in preventing or delaying vascular complications in patients with non–insulin-dependent diabetes. The trial involved 823 patients who were randomly assigned to one of four treatment groups (*Diabetes* 1970;19[Suppl. 2]:747-830). UGDP reported that patients treated for 5 to 8 years with diet plus a fixed dose of tolbutamide (1.5 grams per day) had a rate of cardiovascular mortality approximately 2½ times that of patients treated with diet alone. A significant increase in total mortality was not observed, but the use of tolbutamide was discontinued based on the increase in cardiovascular mortality, thus limiting the opportunity for the trial to show an increase in overall mortality. Despite controversy regarding the interpretation of these results, the findings of the UGDP trial provide an adequate basis for this warning. The patient should be informed of the potential risks and advantages of glimepiride-containing tablets and of alternative modes of therapy.
Although only one drug in the sulfonylurea class (tolbutamide) was included in this trial, it is prudent from a safety standpoint to consider that this warning may also apply to other oral hypoglycemic drugs in this class, in view of their close similarities in mode of action and chemical structure.
5.2   Cardiac Failure With Rosiglitazone
Rosiglitazone, like other thiazolidinediones, alone or in combination with other antidiabetic agents, can cause fluid retention, which may exacerbate or lead to heart failure. Patients should be observed for signs and symptoms of heart failure. If these signs and symptoms develop, the heart failure should be managed according to current standards of care. Furthermore, discontinuation or dose reduction of AVANDARYL must be considered.
Patients with congestive heart failure (CHF) NYHA Class I and II treated with rosiglitazone have an increased risk of cardiovascular events. A 52-week, double-blind, placebo-controlled, echocardiographic trial was conducted in 224 patients with type 2 diabetes mellitus and NYHA Class I or II CHF (ejection fraction ≤45%) on background antidiabetic and CHF therapy. An independent committee conducted a blinded evaluation of fluid-related events (including congestive heart failure) and cardiovascular hospitalizations according to predefined criteria (adjudication). Separate from the adjudication, other cardiovascular adverse events were reported by investigators. Although no treatment difference in change from baseline of ejection fractions was observed, more cardiovascular adverse events were observed with rosiglitazone treatment compared with placebo during the 52-week trial. (See Table 1.)

Table 1. Emergent Cardiovascular Adverse Events in Patients With Congestive Heart Failure (NYHA Class I and II) Treated With Rosiglitazone or Placebo (in Addition to Background Antidiabetic and CHF Therapy)

Events	Rosiglitazone N = 110 n (%)	Placebo N = 114 n (%)
Adjudicated		
Cardiovascular deaths	5 (5%)	4 (4%)
CHF worsening	7 (6%)	4 (4%)
– with overnight hospitalization	5 (5%)	4 (4%)
– without overnight hospitalization	2 (2%)	0 (0%)
New or worsening edema	28 (25%)	10 (9%)
New or worsening dyspnea	29 (26%)	19 (17%)
Increases in CHF medication	36 (33%)	20 (18%)
Cardiovascular hospitalization[a]	21 (19%)	15 (13%)
Investigator-reported, non-adjudicated		
Ischemic adverse events	10 (9%)	5 (4%)
– Myocardial infarction	5 (5%)	2 (2%)
– Angina	6 (5%)	3 (3%)

[a] Includes hospitalization for any cardiovascular reason. In a long-term, cardiovascular outcome trial (RECORD) in patients with type 2 diabetes *[see Adverse Reactions (6.1)]*, the incidence of heart failure was higher in patients treated with rosiglitazone [2.7% (61/2,220) compared with active control 1.3% (29/2,227), HR 2.10 (95% CI: 1.35, 3.27)].
Initiation of AVANDARYL in patients with established NYHA Class III or IV heart failure is contraindicated. AVANDARYL is not recommended in patients with symptomatic heart failure. *[See Boxed Warning.]*
Patients experiencing acute coronary syndromes have not been studied in controlled clinical trials. In view of the potential for development of heart failure in patients having an acute coronary event, initiation of AVANDARYL is not recommended for patients experiencing an acute coronary event, and discontinuation of AVANDARYL during this acute phase should be considered.
Patients with NYHA Class III and IV cardiac status (with or without CHF) have not been studied in controlled clinical trials. AVANDARYL is not recommended in patients with NYHA Class III and IV cardiac status.
Congestive Heart Failure During Coadministration of Rosiglitazone With Insulin: In trials in which rosiglitazone was added to insulin, rosiglitazone increased the risk of congestive heart failure. Coadministration of rosiglitazone and insulin is not recommended. *[See Indications and Usage (1), Warnings and Precautions (5.3).]*
In 7 controlled, randomized, double-blind trials which had durations from 16 to 26 weeks and which were included in a meta-analysis *[see Warnings and Precautions (5.3)]*, pa-

tients with type 2 diabetes mellitus were randomized to co-administration of rosiglitazone and insulin (N = 1,018) or insulin (N = 815). In these 7 trials, rosiglitazone was added to insulin. These trials included patients with long-standing diabetes (median duration of 12 years) and a high prevalence of pre-existing medical conditions, including peripheral neuropathy, retinopathy, ischemic heart disease, vascular disease, and congestive heart failure. The total number of patients with emergent congestive heart failure was 23 (2.3%) and 8 (1.0%) in the rosiglitazone plus insulin and insulin groups, respectively.

Heart Failure in Observational Studies of Elderly Diabetic Patients Comparing Rosiglitazone to Pioglitazone: Three observational studies in elderly diabetic patients (age 65 years and older) found that rosiglitazone statistically significantly increased the risk of hospitalized heart failure compared to use of pioglitazone. One other observational study in patients with a mean age of 54 years, which also included an analysis in a subpopulation of patients >65 years of age, found no statistically significant increase in emergency department visits or hospitalization for heart failure in patients treated with rosiglitazone compared to pioglitazone in the older subgroup.

5.3 Major Adverse Cardiovascular Events

Data from long-term, prospective, randomized, controlled clinical trials of rosiglitazone versus metformin or sulfonylureas, particularly a cardiovascular outcome trial (RECORD), observed no difference in overall mortality or in major adverse cardiovascular events (MACE) and its components. A meta-analysis of mostly short-term trials suggested an increased risk for myocardial infarction with rosiglitazone compared with placebo.

Cardiovascular Events in Large, Long-term, Prospective, Randomized, Controlled Trials of Rosiglitazone: RECORD, a prospectively designed cardiovascular outcome trial (mean follow-up 5.5 years; 4,447 patients), compared the addition of rosiglitazone to metformin or a sulfonylurea (N = 2,220) with a control group of metformin plus sulfonylurea (N = 2,227) in patients with type 2 diabetes [see Adverse Reactions (6.1)]. Non-inferiority was demonstrated for the primary endpoint, cardiovascular hospitalization or cardiovascular death, for rosiglitazone compared with control [HR 0.99 (95% CI: 0.85, 1.16)] demonstrating no overall increased risk in cardiovascular morbidity or mortality. The hazard ratios for total mortality and MACE were consistent with the primary endpoint and the 95% CI similarly excluded a 20% increase in risk for rosiglitazone. The hazard ratios for the components of MACE were 0.72 (95% CI: 0.49, 1.06) for stroke, 1.14 (95% CI: 0.80, 1.63) for myocardial infarction, and 0.84 (95% CI: 0.59, 1.18) for cardiovascular death.

The results of RECORD are consistent with the findings of 2 earlier long-term, prospective, randomized, controlled clinical trials (each trial >3 years' duration; total of 9,620 patients) (see Figure 1). In patients with impaired glucose tolerance (DREAM trial), although the incidence of cardiovascular events was higher among subjects who were randomized to rosiglitazone in combination with ramipril than among subjects randomized to ramipril alone, no statistically significant differences were observed for MACE and its components between rosiglitazone and placebo. In type 2 diabetes patients who were initiating oral agent monotherapy (ADOPT trial), no statistically significant differences were observed for MACE and its components between rosiglitazone and metformin or a sulfonylurea.

[See figure 1 above]

Cardiovascular Events in a Group of 52 Clinical Trials: In a meta-analysis of 52 double-blind, controlled clinical trials designed to assess glucose-lowering efficacy in type 2 diabetes (mean duration 6 months), a statistically significant increased risk of myocardial infarction with rosiglitazone versus pooled comparators was observed [0.4% versus 0.3%; OR 1.8, (95% CI: 1.03, 3.25)]. A statistically non-significant increased risk of MACE was observed with rosiglitazone versus pooled comparators (OR 1.44, 95% CI: 0.95, 2.20). In the placebo-controlled trials, a statistically significant increased risk of myocardial infarction [0.4% versus 0.2%, OR 2.23 (95% CI: 1.14, 4.64)] and statistically non-significant increased risk of MACE [0.7% versus 0.5%, OR 1.53 (95% CI: 0.94, 2.54)] with rosiglitazone were observed. In the active-controlled trials, there was no increased risk of myocardial infarction or MACE.

Mortality in Observational Studies of Rosiglitazone Compared to Pioglitazone: Three observational studies in elderly diabetic patients (age 65 years and older) found that rosiglitazone statistically significantly increased the risk of all-cause mortality compared to use of pioglitazone. One observational study in patients with a mean age of 54 years found no difference in all-cause mortality between patients treated with rosiglitazone compared to pioglitazone and reported similar results in the subpopulation of patients >65 years of age. One additional small, prospective, observational study found no statistically significant differences for CV mortality and all-cause mortality in patients treated with rosiglitazone compared to pioglitazone.

Figure 1. Hazard Ratios for the Risk of MACE, Myocardial Infarction, and Total Mortality With Rosiglitazone Compared With a Control Group in Long-term Trials

Study	N	MACE n (%)	Myocardial Infarction * n (%)	Total Mortality n (%)
RECORD				
RSG+SU or MET	2220	154 (6.9%)	72 (3.2%)	136 (6.1%)
vs SU+MET	2227	165 (7.4%)	68 (3.1%)	157 (7.0%)
ADOPT				
RSG	1456	35 (2.4%)	20 (1.4%)	12 (0.8%)
vs. SU	1441	28 (1.9%)	15 (1.0%)	21 (1.5%)
vs. MET	1454	36 (2.5%)	17 (1.2%)	15 (1.0%)
DREAM				
RSG	1325	15 (1.1%)	5 (0.4%)	15 (1.1%)
vs. Placebo	1321	14 (1.1%)	7 (0.5%)	17 (1.3%)
RSG+RAM	1310	18 (1.4%)	12 (0.9%)	15 (1.1%)
vs. RAM	1313	9 (0.7%)	5 (0.4%)	16 (1.2%)
OVERALL				
RSG	6311	222 (3.5%)	109 (1.7%)	178 (2.8%)
vs control	7756	252 (3.3%)	112 (1.4%)	226 (2.9%)

Favors RSG Favors controls   Favors RSG Favors controls   Favors RSG Favors controls

RSG = rosiglitazone; SU = sulfonylurea; MET = metformin; RAM = ramipril
* Myocardial infarction includes fatal and non-fatal MI plus sudden death

---

Table 2. Weight Changes (kg) From Baseline at Endpoint During Clinical Trials [Median (25th, 75th Percentiles)]

Monotherapy

Duration	Control Group		Rosiglitazone 4 mg	Rosiglitazone 8 mg
• 26 weeks	Placebo	-0.9 (-2.8, 0.9) N = 210	1.0 (-0.9, 3.6) N = 436	3.1 (1.1, 5.8) N = 439
• 52 weeks	Sulfonylurea	2.0 (0, 4.0) N = 173	2.0 (-0.6, 4.0) N = 150	2.6 (0, 5.3) N = 157

Combination Therapy

Duration	Control Group		Rosiglitazone + Control Therapy	
			Rosiglitazone 4 mg	Rosiglitazone 8 mg
• 24-26 weeks	Sulfonylurea	0 (-1.0, 1.3) N = 1,155	2.2 (0.5, 4.0) N = 613	3.5 (1.4, 5.9) N = 841
• 26 weeks	Metformin	-1.4 (-3.2, 0.2) N = 175	0.8 (-1.0, 2.6) N = 100	2.1 (0, 4.3) N = 184
• 26 weeks	Insulin	0.9 (-0.5, 2.7) N = 162	4.1 (1.4, 6.3) N = 164	5.4 (3.4, 7.3) N = 150

AVANDARYL in Patients With Inadequate Control on Diet and Exercise

Duration	Control Group		AVANDARYL 4 mg/4 mg	AVANDARYL 8 mg/4 mg
• 28 weeks	Glimepiride	1.1 (-1.1, 3.2) N = 222	2.2 (0, 4.5) N = 221	2.9 (0, 5.8) N = 217
	Rosiglitazone	0.9 (-1.4, 3.2) N = 228		

5.4 Hypoglycemia

AVANDARYL is a combination tablet containing rosiglitazone and glimepiride, a sulfonylurea. All sulfonylurea drugs are capable of producing severe hypoglycemia. Proper patient selection, dosage, and instructions are important to avoid hypoglycemic episodes. Elderly patients are particularly susceptible to hypoglycemic action of glucose-lowering drugs. Debilitated or malnourished patients, and those with adrenal, pituitary, renal, or hepatic insufficiency are particularly susceptible to the hypoglycemic action of glucose-lowering drugs. A starting dose of 1 mg glimepiride, as contained in AVANDARYL 4 mg/1 mg, followed by appropriate dose titration is recommended in these patients. [See Clinical Pharmacology (12.3).] Hypoglycemia may be difficult to recognize in the elderly and in people who are taking beta-adrenergic blocking drugs or other sympatholytic agents. Hypoglycemia is more likely to occur when caloric intake is deficient, after severe or prolonged exercise, when alcohol is ingested, or when more than one glucose-lowering drug is used.

Patients receiving rosiglitazone in combination with a sulfonylurea may be at risk for hypoglycemia, and a reduction in the dose of the sulfonylurea may be necessary [see Dosage and Administration (2.2)].

5.5 Edema

AVANDARYL should be used with caution in patients with edema. In a clinical trial in healthy volunteers who received 8 mg of rosiglitazone once daily for 8 weeks, there was a statistically significant increase in median plasma volume compared with placebo.

Since thiazolidinediones, including rosiglitazone, can cause fluid retention, which can exacerbate or lead to congestive heart failure, AVANDARYL should be used with caution in patients at risk for heart failure. Patients should be moni-

Table 3. Adverse Events (≥5% in any Treatment Group) Reported by Patients With Inadequate Glycemic Control on Diet and Exercise in a 28-Week, Double-blind Clinical Trial of AVANDARYL

Preferred Term	Glimepiride Monotherapy N = 222 %	Rosiglitazone Monotherapy N = 230 %	AVANDARYL 4 mg/4 mg N = 224 %	AVANDARYL 8 mg/4 mg N = 218 %
Headache	2.3	6.1	3.1	6.0
Nasopharyngitis	3.6	5.2	4.0	4.6
Hypertension	3.6	5.2	3.1	2.3
Hypoglycemia[a]	4.1	0.4	3.6	5.5

tored for signs and symptoms of heart failure [see Boxed Warning, Warnings and Precautions (5.2), Patient Counseling Information (17.1)].

In controlled clinical trials of patients with type 2 diabetes, mild to moderate edema was reported in patients treated with rosiglitazone, and may be dose-related. Patients with ongoing edema were more likely to have adverse events associated with edema if started on combination therapy with insulin and rosiglitazone [see Adverse Reactions (6.1)]. The use of AVANDARYL in combination with insulin is not recommended [see Warnings and Precautions (5.2, 5.3)].

5.6   Weight Gain
Dose-related weight gain was seen with AVANDARYL, rosiglitazone alone, and rosiglitazone together with other hypoglycemic agents (see Table 2). The mechanism of weight gain is unclear but probably involves a combination of fluid retention and fat accumulation.
[See table 2 at top of previous page]
In a 4- to 6-year, monotherapy, comparative trial (ADOPT) in patients recently diagnosed with type 2 diabetes not previously treated with antidiabetic medication, the mean weight change (25th, 75th percentiles) from baseline at 4 years was 3.5 kg (0.0, 8.1) for rosiglitazone, 2.0 kg (-1.0, 4.8) for glyburide, and -2.4 kg (-5.4, 0.5) for metformin.
In postmarketing experience with rosiglitazone alone or in combination with other hypoglycemic agents, there have been rare reports of unusually rapid increases in weight and increases in excess of that generally observed in clinical trials. Patients who experience such increases should be assessed for fluid accumulation and volume-related events such as excessive edema and congestive heart failure [see Boxed Warning].

5.7   Hepatic Effects
With sulfonylureas, including glimepiride, there may be an elevation of liver enzyme levels in rare cases. In isolated instances, impairment of liver function (e.g., with cholestasis and jaundice), as well as hepatitis (which may also lead to liver failure) have been reported.
Liver enzymes should be measured prior to the initiation of therapy with AVANDARYL in all patients and periodically thereafter per the clinical judgment of the healthcare professional. Therapy with AVANDARYL should not be initiated in patients with increased baseline liver enzyme levels (ALT >2.5X upper limit of normal). Patients with mildly elevated liver enzymes (ALT levels ≤2.5X upper limit of normal) at baseline or during therapy with AVANDARYL should be evaluated to determine the cause of the liver enzyme elevation. Initiation of, or continuation of, therapy with AVANDARYL in patients with mild liver enzyme elevations should proceed with caution and include close clinical follow-up, including more frequent liver enzyme monitoring, to determine if the liver enzyme elevations resolve or worsen. If at any time ALT levels increase to >3X the upper limit of normal in patients on therapy with AVANDARYL, liver enzyme levels should be rechecked as soon as possible. If ALT levels remain >3X the upper limit of normal, therapy with AVANDARYL should be discontinued.
If any patient develops symptoms suggesting hepatic dysfunction, which may include unexplained nausea, vomiting, abdominal pain, fatigue, anorexia, and/or dark urine, liver enzymes should be checked. The decision whether to continue the patient on therapy with AVANDARYL should be guided by clinical judgment pending laboratory evaluations. If jaundice is observed, drug therapy should be discontinued.

5.8   Macular Edema
Macular edema has been reported in postmarketing experience in some diabetic patients who were taking rosiglitazone or another thiazolidinedione. Some patients presented with blurred vision or decreased visual acuity, but some patients appear to have been diagnosed on routine ophthalmologic examination. Most patients had peripheral edema at the time macular edema was diagnosed. Some patients had improvement in their macular edema after discontinuation of their thiazolidinedione. Patients with diabetes should have regular eye exams by an ophthalmologist,

per the Standards of Care of the American Diabetes Association. Additionally, any diabetic who reports any kind of visual symptom should be promptly referred to an ophthalmologist, regardless of the patient's underlying medications or other physical findings. [See Adverse Reactions (6.3).]

5.9   Fractures
Long-term trials (ADOPT and RECORD) show an increased incidence of bone fracture in patients, particularly female patients, taking rosiglitazone [see Adverse Reactions (6.1)]. This increased incidence was noted after the first year of treatment and persisted during the course of the trial. The majority of the fractures in the women who received rosiglitazone occurred in the upper arm, hand, and foot. These sites of fracture are different from those usually associated with postmenopausal osteoporosis (e.g., hip or spine). Other trials suggest that this risk may also apply to men, although the risk of fracture among women appears higher than that among men. The risk of fracture should be considered in the care of patients treated with rosiglitazone, and attention given to assessing and maintaining bone health according to current standards of care.

5.10   Hematologic Effects
Decreases in hemoglobin and hematocrit occurred in a dose-related fashion in adult patients treated with rosiglitazone [see Adverse Reactions (6.2)]. The observed changes may be related to the increased plasma volume observed with treatment with rosiglitazone.

5.11   Hemolytic Anemia
Treatment of patients with glucose 6-phosphate dehydrogenase (G6PD) deficiency with sulfonylurea agents can lead to hemolytic anemia. Because glimepiride, a component of AVANDARYL, belongs to the class of sulfonylurea agents, caution should be used in patients with G6PD deficiency and a non-sulfonylurea alternative should be considered. In postmarketing experience, hemolytic anemia has also been reported in patients receiving sulfonylureas who did not have known G6PD deficiency [see Adverse Reactions (6.1)].

5.12   Diabetes and Blood Glucose Control
When a patient stabilized on any antidiabetic regimen is exposed to stress such as fever, trauma, infection, or surgery, a temporary loss of glycemic control may occur. At such times, it may be necessary to withhold AVANDARYL and temporarily administer insulin. AVANDARYL may be reinstituted after the acute episode is resolved.
Periodic fasting glucose and HbA1c measurements should be performed to monitor therapeutic response.

5.13   Ovulation
Therapy with rosiglitazone, like other thiazolidinediones, may result in ovulation in some premenopausal anovulatory women. As a result, these patients may be at an increased risk for pregnancy while taking rosiglitazone [see Use in Specific Populations (8.1)]. Thus, adequate contraception in premenopausal women should be recommended. This possible effect has not been specifically investigated in clinical trials; therefore the frequency of this occurrence is not known.
Although hormonal imbalance has been seen in preclinical studies [see Nonclinical Toxicology (13.1)], the clinical significance of this finding is not known. If unexpected menstrual dysfunction occurs, the benefits of continued therapy with AVANDARYL should be reviewed.

6   ADVERSE REACTIONS
The following adverse reactions are discussed in more detail elsewhere in the labeling:
• Increased Risk of Cardiovascular Mortality for Sulfonylurea Drugs [see Warnings and Precautions (5.13)]
• Cardiac Failure With Rosiglitazone [see Warnings and Precautions (5.1)]
• Major Adverse Cardiovascular Events [see Warnings and Precautions (5.2)]
• Hypoglycemia [see Warnings and Precautions (5.4)]
• Edema [see Warnings and Precautions (5.5)]
• Weight Gain [see Warnings and Precautions (5.6)]
• Hepatic Effects [see Warnings and Precautions (5.7)]
• Macular Edema [see Warnings and Precautions (5.8)]

• Fractures [see Warnings and Precautions (5.9)]
• Hematologic Effects [see Warnings and Precautions (5.10)]
• Hemolytic Anemia [see Warnings and Precautions (5.11)]
• Ovulation [see Warnings and Precautions (5.13)]
6.1   Clinical Trial Experience
Because clinical trials are conducted under widely varying conditions, adverse reaction rates observed in the clinical trials of a drug cannot be directly compared with rates in the clinical trials of another drug and may not reflect the rates observed in practice.
Patients With Inadequate Glycemic Control on Diet and Exercise: Table 3 summarizes adverse events occurring at a frequency of ≥5% in any treatment group in the 28-week, double-blind trial of AVANDARYL in patients with type 2 diabetes mellitus inadequately controlled on diet and exercise. Patients in this trial were started on AVANDARYL 4 mg/1 mg, rosiglitazone 4 mg, or glimepiride 1 mg. Doses could be increased at 4-week intervals to reach a maximum total daily dose of either 4 mg/4 mg or 8 mg/4 mg for AVANDARYL, 8 mg for rosiglitazone monotherapy, or 4 mg for glimepiride monotherapy.
[See table 3 above]
[a]As documented by symptoms and a fingerstick blood glucose measurement of <50 mg/dL.
Hypoglycemia was reported to be generally mild to moderate in intensity and none of the reported events of hypoglycemia resulted in withdrawal from the trial. Hypoglycemia requiring parenteral treatment (i.e., intravenous glucose or glucagon injection) was observed in 3 (0.7%) patients treated with AVANDARYL. Edema was reported by 3.2% of patients on AVANDARYL, 3.0% on rosiglitazone alone, and 2.3% on glimepiride alone. Congestive heart failure was observed in 1 (0.2%) patient treated with AVANDARYL and in 1 (0.4%) patient treated with rosiglitazone monotherapy.
Patients Treated With Rosiglitazone Added to Sulfonylurea Monotherapy and Other Experience With Rosiglitazone or Glimepiride: Trials utilizing rosiglitazone in combination with a sulfonylurea provide support for the use of AVANDARYL. Adverse event data from these trials, in addition to adverse events reported with the use of rosiglitazone and glimepiride therapy, are presented below.
Rosiglitazone: The most common adverse experiences with rosiglitazone monotherapy (≥5%) were upper respiratory tract infection, injury, and headache. Overall, the types of adverse experiences reported when rosiglitazone was added to a sulfonylurea were similar to those during monotherapy with rosiglitazone. In controlled combination therapy trials with sulfonylureas, mild to moderate hypoglycemic symptoms, which appear to be dose-related, were reported. Few patients were withdrawn for hypoglycemia (<1%) and few episodes of hypoglycemia were considered to be severe (<1%).
Events of anemia and edema tended to be reported more frequently at higher doses, and were generally mild to moderate in severity and usually did not require discontinuation of treatment with rosiglitazone.
Edema was reported by 4.8% of patients receiving rosiglitazone compared with 1.3% on placebo, and 1.0% on sulfonylurea monotherapy. The reporting rate of edema was higher for rosiglitazone 8 mg added to a sulfonylurea (12.4%) compared with other combinations, with the exception of insulin. Anemia was reported by 1.9% of patients receiving rosiglitazone compared with 0.7% on placebo, 0.6% on sulfonylurea monotherapy, and 2.3% on rosiglitazone in combination with a sulfonylurea. Overall, the types of adverse experiences reported when rosiglitazone was added to a sulfonylurea were similar to those during monotherapy with rosiglitazone.
In 26-week double-blind, fixed-dose trials, edema was reported with higher frequency in the rosiglitazone plus insulin combination trials (insulin, 5.4%; and rosiglitazone in combination with insulin, 14.7%). Reports of new onset or exacerbation of congestive heart failure occurred at rates of 1% for insulin alone, and 2% (4 mg) and 3% (8 mg) for insulin in combination with rosiglitazone [see Boxed Warning, Warnings and Precautions (5.2)].
Glimepiride: Hypoglycemia: The incidence of hypoglycemia with glimepiride, as documented by blood glucose values <60 mg/dL, ranged from 0.9% to 1.7% in 2 large, well-controlled, 1-year trials. In patients treated with glimepiride in US placebo-controlled trials (N = 746), adverse events, other than hypoglycemia, considered to be possibly or probably related to trial drug that occurred in more than 1% of patients included dizziness (1.7%), asthenia (1.6%), headache (1.5%), and nausea (1.1%).
• Gastrointestinal Reactions: Vomiting, gastrointestinal pain, and diarrhea have been reported, but the incidence in placebo-controlled trials was less than 1%. In rare cases, there may be an elevation of liver enzyme levels. In isolated instances, impairment of liver function (e.g., with cholestasis and jaundice), as well as hepatitis, which may also lead to liver failure have been reported with sulfonylureas, including glimepiride.
• Dermatologic Reactions: Allergic skin reactions, e.g., pruritus, erythema, urticaria, and morbilliform or macu-

lopapular eruptions, occur in less than 1% of treated patients. These may be transient and may disappear despite continued use of glimepiride. If those hypersensitivity reactions persist or worsen, the drug should be discontinued. Porphyria cutanea tarda, photosensitivity reactions, and allergic vasculitis have been reported with sulfonylureas, including glimepiride.

- *Hematologic Reactions:* Leukopenia, agranulocytosis, thrombocytopenia, hemolytic anemia *[see Warnings and Precautions (5.11)]*, aplastic anemia, and pancytopenia have been reported with sulfonylureas, including glimepiride.
- *Metabolic Reactions:* Hepatic porphyria reactions and disulfiram-like reactions have been reported with sulfonylureas, including glimepiride. Cases of hyponatremia have been reported with glimepiride and all other sulfonylureas, most often in patients who are on other medications or have medical conditions known to cause hyponatremia or increase release of antidiuretic hormone. The syndrome of inappropriate antidiuretic hormone (SIADH) secretion has been reported with certain other sulfonylureas, including glimepiride, and it has been suggested that certain sulfonylureas may augment the peripheral (antidiuretic) action of ADH and/or increase release of ADH.
- *Other Reactions:* Changes in accommodation and/or blurred vision may occur with the use of glimepiride. This is thought to be due to changes in blood glucose, and may be more pronounced when treatment is initiated. This condition is also seen in untreated diabetic patients, and may actually be reduced by treatment. In placebo-controlled trials of glimepiride, the incidence of blurred vision was placebo, 0.7%, and glimepiride, 0.4%.
- *Human Ophthalmology Data:* Ophthalmic examinations were carried out in more than 500 subjects during long-term trials of glimepiride using the methodology of Taylor and West and Laties et al. No significant differences were seen between glimepiride and glyburide in the number of subjects with clinically important changes in visual acuity, intraocular tension, or in any of the 5 lens-related variables examined. Ophthalmic examinations were carried out during long-term trials using the method of Chylack et al. No significant or clinically meaningful differences were seen between glimepiride and glipizide with respect to cataract progression by subjective LOCS II grading and objective image analysis systems, visual acuity, intraocular pressure, and general ophthalmic examination *[see Nonclinical Toxicology (13.2)]*.

Long-term Trial of Rosiglitazone as Monotherapy: A 4- to 6-year trial (ADOPT) compared the use of rosiglitazone (n = 1,456), glyburide (n = 1,441), and metformin (n = 1,454) as monotherapy in patients recently diagnosed with type 2 diabetes who were not previously treated with antidiabetic medication. Table 4 presents adverse reactions without regard to causality; rates are expressed per 100 patient-years (PY) exposure to account for the differences in exposure to trial medication across the 3 treatment groups.

In ADOPT, fractures were reported in a greater number of women treated with rosiglitazone (9.3%, 2.7/100 patient-years) compared with glyburide (3.5%, 1.3/100 patient-years) or metformin (5.1%, 1.5/100 patient-years). The majority of the fractures in the women who received rosiglitazone were reported in the upper arm, hand, and foot. *[See Warnings and Precautions (5.9).]* The observed incidence of fractures for male patients was similar among the 3 treatment groups.

Table 4. On-therapy Adverse Events [≥5 Events/100 Patient-Years (PY)] in any Treatment Group Reported in a 4- to 6-Year Clinical Trial of Rosiglitazone as Monotherapy (ADOPT)

Preferred Term	Rosiglitazone N = 1,456 PY = 4,954	Glyburide N = 1,441 PY = 4,244	Metformin N = 1,454 PY = 4,906
Nasopharyngitis	6.3	6.9	6.6
Back pain	5.1	4.9	5.3
Arthralgia	5.0	4.8	4.2
Hypertension	4.4	6.0	6.1
Upper respiratory tract infection	4.3	5.0	4.7
Hypoglycemia	2.9	13.0	3.4
Diarrhea	2.5	3.2	6.8

Long-term Trial of Rosiglitazone as Combination Therapy (RECORD): RECORD (Rosiglitazone Evaluated for Cardiac Outcomes and Regulation of Glycemia in Diabetes) was

Table 5. Cardiovascular (CV) Outcomes for the RECORD Trial

Primary Endpoint	Rosiglitazone N = 2,220	Active Control N = 2,227	Hazard Ratio	95% CI
CV death or CV hospitalization	321	323	0.99	0.85-1.16
Secondary Endpoint				
All-cause death	136	157	0.86	0.68-1.08
CV death	60	71	0.84	0.59-1.18
Myocardial infarction	64	56	1.14	0.80-1.63
Stroke	46	63	0.72	0.49-1.06
CV death, myocardial infarction, or stroke	154	165	0.93	0.74-1.15
Heart failure	61	29	2.10	1.35-3.27

a multicenter, randomized, open-label, non-inferiority trial in subjects with type 2 diabetes inadequately controlled on maximum doses of metformin or sulfonylurea (glyburide, gliclazide, or glimepiride) to compare the time to reach the combined cardiovascular endpoint of cardiovascular death or cardiovascular hospitalization between patients randomized to the addition of rosiglitazone versus metformin or sulfonylurea. The trial included patients who have failed metformin or sulfonylurea monotherapy; those who failed metformin (n = 2,222) were randomized to receive either add-on rosiglitazone (n = 1,117) or add-on sulfonylurea (n = 1,105), and those who failed sulfonylurea (n = 2,225) were randomized to receive either add-on rosiglitazone (n = 1,103) or add-on metformin (n = 1,122). Patients were treated to target HbA1c ≤7% throughout the trial.

The mean age of patients in this trial was 58 years, 52% were male, and the mean duration of follow-up was 5.5 years. Rosiglitazone demonstrated non-inferiority to active control for the primary endpoint of cardiovascular hospitalization or cardiovascular death (HR 0.99, 95% CI: 0.85-1.16). There were no significant differences between groups for secondary endpoints with the exception of congestive heart failure (see Table 5). The incidence of congestive heart failure was significantly greater among patients randomized to rosiglitazone.

[See table 5 above]

There was an increased incidence of bone fracture for subjects randomized to rosiglitazone in addition to metformin or sulfonylurea compared with those randomized to metformin plus sulfonylurea (8.3% versus 5.3%) *[see Warnings and Precautions (5.9)]*. The majority of fractures were reported in the upper limbs and distal lower limbs. The risk of fracture appeared to be higher in females relative to control (11.5% versus 6.3%), than in males relative to control (5.3% versus 4.3%). Additional data are necessary to determine whether there is an increased risk of fracture in males after a longer period of follow-up.

6.2 Laboratory Abnormalities

Rosiglitazone: *Hematologic:* Decreases in mean hemoglobin and hematocrit occurred in a dose-related fashion in adult patients treated with rosiglitazone (mean decreases in individual trials as much as 1.0 g/dL hemoglobin and as much as 3.3% hematocrit). The changes occurred primarily during the first 3 months following initiation of therapy with rosiglitazone or following a dose increase in rosiglitazone. The time course and magnitude of decreases were similar in patients treated with a combination of rosiglitazone and other hypoglycemic agents or monotherapy with rosiglitazone. White blood cell counts also decreased slightly in adult patients treated with rosiglitazone. Decreases in hematologic parameters may be related to increased plasma volume observed with treatment with rosiglitazone.

Lipids: Changes in serum lipids have been observed following treatment with rosiglitazone in adults *[see Clinical Pharmacology (12.2)]*.

Serum Transaminase Levels: In pre-approval clinical trials in 4,598 patients treated with rosiglitazone encompassing approximately 3,600 patient-years of exposure, there was no evidence of drug-induced hepatotoxicity.

In pre-approval controlled trials, 0.2% of patients treated with rosiglitazone had reversible elevations in ALT >3X the upper limit of normal compared with 0.2% on placebo and 0.5% on active comparators. The ALT elevations in patients treated with rosiglitazone were reversible. Hyperbilirubinemia was found in 0.3% of patients treated with rosiglitazone compared with 0.9% treated with placebo and 1% in patients treated with active comparators. In preapproval clinical trials, there were no cases of idiosyncratic drug reactions leading to hepatic failure. *[See Warnings and Precautions (5.7).]*

In the 4- to 6-year ADOPT trial, patients treated with rosiglitazone (4,954 patient-years exposure), glyburide (4,244 patient-years exposure), or metformin (4,906 patient-years exposure) as monotherapy had the same rate of ALT increase to >3X upper limit of normal (0.3 per 100 patient-years exposure).

In the RECORD trial, patients randomized to rosiglitazone in addition to metformin or sulfonylurea (10,849 patient-years exposure) and to metformin plus sulfonylurea (10,209 patient-years exposure) had a rate of ALT increase to ≥3X upper limit of normal of approximately 0.2 and 0.3 per 100 patient-years exposure, respectively.

6.3 Postmarketing Experience

In addition to adverse reactions reported from clinical trials, the events described below have been identified during post-approval use of AVANDARYL or its individual components. Because these events are reported voluntarily from a population of unknown size, it is not possible to reliably estimate their frequency or to always establish a causal relationship to drug exposure.

In patients receiving thiazolidinedione therapy, serious adverse events with or without a fatal outcome, potentially related to volume expansion (e.g., congestive heart failure, pulmonary edema, and pleural effusions) have been reported *[see Boxed Warning, Warnings and Precautions (5.2)]*.

There are postmarketing reports with rosiglitazone of hepatitis, hepatic enzyme elevations to 3 or more times the upper limit of normal, and hepatic failure with and without fatal outcome, although causality has not been established. There are postmarketing reports with rosiglitazone of rash, pruritus, urticaria, angioedema, anaphylactic reaction, Stevens-Johnson syndrome *[see Contraindications (4)]*, and new onset or worsening diabetic macular edema with decreased visual acuity *[see Warnings and Precautions (5.8)]*.

7 DRUG INTERACTIONS

7.1 Drugs Metabolized by Cytochrome P450

An inhibitor of CYP2C8 (e.g., gemfibrozil) may increase the AUC of rosiglitazone and an inducer of CYP2C8 (e.g., rifampin) may decrease the AUC of rosiglitazone. Therefore, if an inhibitor or an inducer of CYP2C8 is started or stopped during treatment with rosiglitazone, changes in diabetes treatment may be needed based upon clinical response. *[See Clinical Pharmacology (12.4).]*

A potential interaction between oral miconazole and oral hypoglycemic agents leading to severe hypoglycemia has been reported. Whether this interaction also occurs with the IV, topical, or vaginal preparations of miconazole is not known. Potential interactions of glimepiride with other drugs metabolized by cytochrome P450 2C9 also include phenytoin, diclofenac, ibuprofen, naproxen, and mefenamic acid. *[See Clinical Pharmacology (12.4).]*

7.2 Drugs That Produce Hyperglycemia

Certain drugs tend to produce hyperglycemia and may lead to loss of control. These drugs include the thiazides and other diuretics, corticosteroids, phenothiazines, thyroid products, estrogens, oral contraceptives, phenytoin, nicotinic acid, sympathomimetics, and isoniazid. When these drugs are administered to a patient receiving glimepiride, the patient should be closely observed for loss of control. When these drugs are withdrawn from a patient receiving glimepiride, the patient should be observed closely for hypoglycemia.

8 USE IN SPECIFIC POPULATIONS

8.1 Pregnancy

Pregnancy Category C.

All pregnancies have a background risk of birth defects, loss, or other adverse outcome regardless of drug exposure. This background risk is increased in pregnancies complicated by hyperglycemia and may be decreased with good metabolic control. It is essential for patients with diabetes or history of gestational diabetes to maintain good metabolic control before conception and throughout pregnancy. Careful monitoring of glucose control is essential in such patients. Most experts recommend that insulin monotherapy be used during pregnancy to maintain blood glucose levels as close to normal as possible. AVANDARYL should be used during pregnancy only if the potential benefit justifies the potentialrisk to the fetus.

Human Data: There are no adequate and well-controlled trials with AVANDARYL or its individual components in pregnant women. Rosiglitazone has been reported to cross the human placenta and be detectable in fetal tissue. The clinical significance of these findings is unknown.

Animal Studies: No animal studies have been conducted with AVANDARYL. The following data are based on findings in studies performed with rosiglitazone or glimepiride individually.

Rosiglitazone: There was no effect on implantation or the embryo with rosiglitazone treatment during early pregnancy in rats, but treatment during mid-late gestation was associated with fetal death and growth retardation in both rats and rabbits. Teratogenicity was not observed at doses up to 3 mg/kg in rats and 100 mg/kg in rabbits (approximately 20 and 75 times human AUC at the maximum recommended human daily dose, respectively). Rosiglitazone caused placental pathology in rats (3 mg/kg/day). Treatment of rats during gestation through lactation reduced litter size, neonatal viability, and postnatal growth, with growth retardation reversible after puberty. For effects on the placenta, embryo/fetus, and offspring, the no-effect dose was 0.2 mg/kg/day in rats and 15 mg/kg/day in rabbits. These no-effect levels are approximately 4 times human AUC at the maximum recommended human daily dose. Rosiglitazone reduced the number of uterine implantations and live offspring when juvenile female rats were treated at 40 mg/kg/day from 27 days of age through to sexual maturity (approximately 68 times human AUC at the maximum recommended daily dose). The no-effect level was 2 mg/kg/day (approximately 4 times human AUC at the maximum recommended daily dose). There was no effect on pre- or post-natal survival or growth.

Glimepiride: Glimepiride did not produce teratogenic effects in rats exposed orally up to 4,000 mg/kg body weight (approximately 4,000 times the maximum recommended human dose based on surface area) or in rabbits exposed up to 32 mg/kg body weight (approximately 60 times the maximum recommended human dose based on surface area). Glimepiride has been shown to be associated with intrauterine fetal death in rats when given in doses as low as 50 times the human dose based on surface area and in rabbits when given in doses as low as 0.1 times the human dose based on surface area. This fetotoxicity, observed only at doses inducing maternal hypoglycemia, has been similarly noted with other sulfonylureas, and is believed to be directly related to the pharmacologic (hypoglycemic) action of glimepiride.

In some studies in rats, offspring of dams exposed to high levels of glimepiride during pregnancy and lactation developed skeletal deformities consisting of shortening, thickening, and bending of the humerus during the postnatal period. Significant concentrations of glimepiride were observed in the serum and breast milk of the dams as well as in the serum of the pups. These skeletal deformations were determined to be the result of nursing from mothers exposed to glimepiride. Prolonged severe hypoglycemia (4 to 10 days) has been reported in neonates born to mothers who were receiving a sulfonylurea drug at the time of delivery. This has been reported more frequently with the use of agents with prolonged half-lives.

8.2 Labor and Delivery
The effect of AVANDARYL or its components on labor and delivery in humans is unknown.

8.3 Nursing Mothers
No trials have been conducted with AVANDARYL. It is not known whether rosiglitazone or glimepiride is excreted in human milk. Because many drugs are excreted in human milk, a decision should be made whether to discontinue nursing or to discontinue AVANDARYL, taking into account the importance of the drug to the mother.

Rosiglitazone: Drug-related material was detected in milk from lactating rats.

Glimepiride: In rat reproduction studies, significant concentrations of glimepiride were observed in the serum and breast milk of the dams, as well as in the serum of the pups. Although it is not known whether glimepiride is excreted in human milk, other sulfonylureas are excreted in human milk.

8.4 Pediatric Use
Safety and effectiveness of AVANDARYL in pediatric patients have not been established. AVANDARYL and its components, rosiglitazone and glimepiride, are not indicated for use in pediatric patients.

8.5 Geriatric Use
Rosiglitazone: Results of the population pharmacokinetic analysis showed that age does not significantly affect the pharmacokinetics of rosiglitazone [see Clinical Pharmacology (12.3)]. Therefore, no dosage adjustments are required for the elderly. In controlled clinical trials, no overall differences in safety and effectiveness between older (≥65 years) and younger (<65 years) patients were observed.

Glimepiride: In US clinical trials of glimepiride, 608 of 1,986 patients were 65 and older. No overall differences in safety or effectiveness were observed between these subjects and younger subjects, but greater sensitivity of some older individuals cannot be ruled out.

Comparison of glimepiride pharmacokinetics in type 2 diabetes patients ≤65 years (N = 49) and those >65 years (N = 42) was performed in a trial using a dosing regimen of 6 mg daily. There were no significant differences in glimepiride pharmacokinetics between the 2 age groups [see Clinical Pharmacology (12.3)].

The drug is known to be substantially excreted by the kidney, and the risk of toxic reactions to this drug may be greater in patients with impaired renal function. Because elderly patients are more likely to have decreased renal function, care should be taken in dose selection, and it may be useful to monitor renal function.

Elderly patients are particularly susceptible to hypoglycemic action of glucose-lowering drugs. In elderly, debilitated, or malnourished patients, or in patients with renal, hepatic or adrenal insufficiency, the starting dose, dose increments, and maintenance dosage should be conservative based upon blood glucose levels prior to and after initiation of treatment to avoid hypoglycemic reactions. Hypoglycemia may be difficult to recognize in the elderly and in people who are taking beta-adrenergic blocking drugs or other sympatholytic agents [see Dosage and Administration (2.4), Warnings and Precautions (5.4), Clinical Pharmacology (12.3)].

10 OVERDOSAGE
Rosiglitazone: Limited data are available with regard to overdosage in humans. In clinical trials in volunteers, rosiglitazone has been administered at single oral doses of up to 20 mg and was well tolerated. In the event of an overdose, appropriate supportive treatment should be initiated as dictated by the patient's clinical status.

Glimepiride: Overdosage of sulfonylureas, including glimepiride, can produce hypoglycemia. Mild hypoglycemic symptoms without loss of consciousness or neurologic findings should be treated aggressively with oral glucose and adjustments in drug dosage and/or meal patterns. Close monitoring should continue until the physician is assured that the patient is out of danger. Severe hypoglycemic reactions with coma, seizure, or other neurological impairment occur infrequently, but constitute medical emergencies requiring immediate hospitalization. If hypoglycemic coma is diagnosed or suspected, the patient should be given a rapid IV injection of concentrated (50%) glucose solution. This should be followed by a continuous infusion of a more dilute (10%) glucose solution at a rate that will maintain the blood glucose level above 100 mg/dL. Patients should be closely monitored for a minimum of 24 to 48 hours, because hypoglycemia may recur after apparent clinical recovery.

11 DESCRIPTION
AVANDARYL contains 2 oral antidiabetic drugs used in the management of type 2 diabetes: rosiglitazone maleate and glimepiride.

Rosiglitazone maleate is an oral antidiabetic agent which acts primarily by increasing insulin sensitivity. Rosiglitazone maleate is not chemically or functionally related to the sulfonylureas, the biguanides, or the alpha-glucosidase inhibitors. Chemically, rosiglitazone maleate is (±)-5-[[4-[2-(methyl-2-pyridinylamino)ethoxy]phenyl]methyl]-2,4-thiazolidinedione, (Z)-2-butenedioate (1:1) with a molecular weight of 473.52 (357.44 free base). The molecule has a single chiral center and is present as a racemate. Due to rapid interconversion, the enantiomers are functionally indistinguishable. The molecular formula is $C_{18}H_{19}N_3O_3S\cdot C_4H_4O_4$. Rosiglitazone maleate is a white to off-white solid with a melting point range of 122° to 123°C. The pK_a values of rosiglitazone maleate are 6.8 and 6.1. It is readily soluble in ethanol and a buffered aqueous solution with pH of 2.3; solubility decreases with increasing pH in the physiological range. The structural formula of rosiglitazone maleate is:

Glimepiride is an oral antidiabetic drug of the sulfonylurea class. Glimepiride is a white to yellowish-white, crystalline, odorless to practically odorless powder. Chemically,

glimepiride is 1-[[p-[2-(3-ethyl-4-methyl-2-oxo-3-pyrroline-1-carboxamido)ethyl]phenyl]sulfonyl]-3-(trans-4-methylcyclohexyl)urea with a molecular weight of 490.62. The molecular formula for glimepiride is $C_{24}H_{34}N_4O_5S$. Glimepiride is practically insoluble in water. The structural formula of glimepiride is:

AVANDARYL is available for oral administration as tablets containing rosiglitazone maleate and glimepiride, respectively, in the following strengths (expressed as rosiglitazone maleate/glimepiride): 4 mg/1 mg, 4 mg/2 mg, 4 mg/4 mg, 8 mg/2 mg, and 8 mg/4 mg. Each tablet contains the following inactive ingredients: hypromellose 2910, lactose monohydrate, macrogol (polyethylene glycol), magnesium stearate, microcrystalline cellulose, sodium starch glycolate, titanium dioxide, and 1 or more of the following: yellow, red, or black iron oxides.

12 CLINICAL PHARMACOLOGY
12.1 Mechanism of Action
AVANDARYL combines 2 antidiabetic agents with different mechanisms of action to improve glycemic control in patients with type 2 diabetes: Rosiglitazone maleate, a member of the thiazolidinedione class, and glimepiride, a member of the sulfonylurea class. Thiazolidinediones are insulin-sensitizing agents that act primarily by enhancing peripheral glucose utilization, whereas sulfonylureas act primarily by stimulating release of insulin from functioning pancreatic beta cells.

Rosiglitazone: Rosiglitazone improves glycemic control by improving insulin sensitivity. Rosiglitazone is a highly selective and potent agonist for the peroxisome proliferator-activated receptor-gamma (PPARγ). In humans, PPAR receptors are found in key target tissues for insulin action such as adipose tissue, skeletal muscle, and liver. Activation of PPARγ nuclear receptors regulates the transcription of insulin-responsive genes involved in the control of glucose production, transport, and utilization. In addition, PPARγ-responsive genes also participate in the regulation of fatty acid metabolism.

Insulin resistance is a common feature characterizing the pathogenesis of type 2 diabetes. The antidiabetic activity of rosiglitazone has been demonstrated in animal models of type 2 diabetes in which hyperglycemia and/or impaired glucose tolerance is a consequence of insulin resistance in target tissues. Rosiglitazone reduces blood glucose concentrations and reduces hyperinsulinemia in the ob/ob obese mouse, db/db diabetic mouse, and fa/fa fatty Zucker rat.

In animal models, the antidiabetic activity of rosiglitazone was shown to be mediated by increased sensitivity to insulin's action in the liver, muscle, and adipose tissues. Pharmacologic studies in animal models indicate that rosiglitazone improves sensitivity to insulin in muscle and adipose tissue and inhibits hepatic gluconeogenesis. The expression of the insulin-regulated glucose transporter GLUT-4 was increased in adipose tissue. Rosiglitazone did not induce hypoglycemia in animal models of type 2 diabetes and/or impaired glucose tolerance.

Glimepiride: The primary mechanism of action of glimepiride in lowering blood glucose appears to be dependent on stimulating the release of insulin from functioning pancreatic beta cells. In addition, extrapancreatic effects may also play a role in the activity of sulfonylureas such as glimepiride. This is supported by both preclinical and clinical trials demonstrating that glimepiride administration can lead to increased sensitivity of peripheral tissues to insulin. These findings are consistent with the results of a long-term, randomized, placebo-controlled trial in which glimepiride therapy improved postprandial insulin/C-peptide responses and overall glycemic control without producing clinically meaningful increases in fasting insulin/C-peptide levels. However, as with other sulfonylureas, the mechanism by which glimepiride lowers blood glucose during long-term administration has not been clearly established.

12.2 Pharmacodynamics
The lipid profiles of rosiglitazone and glimepiride in a clinical trial of patients with inadequate glycemic control on diet and exercise were consistent with the known profile of each monotherapy. AVANDARYL was associated with increases in HDL and LDL (3% to 4% for each) and decreases in triglycerides (-4%), that were not considered to be clinically meaningful.

The pattern of LDL and HDL changes following therapy with rosiglitazone in patients previously treated with a sulfonylurea was generally similar to those seen with rosiglitazone in monotherapy. Rosiglitazone as monotherapy was associated with increases in total cholesterol, LDL, and HDL and decreases in free fatty acids. The changes in triglycerides during therapy with rosiglitazone were variable and were generally not statistically different from placebo or glyburide controls.

12.3 Pharmacokinetics

In a bioequivalence trial of AVANDARYL 4 mg/4 mg, the area under the curve (AUC) and maximum concentration (C_{max}) of rosiglitazone following a single dose of the combination tablet were bioequivalent to rosiglitazone 4 mg concomitantly administered with glimepiride 4 mg under fasted conditions. The AUC of glimepiride following a single fasted 4 mg/4 mg dose was equivalent to glimepiride concomitantly administered with rosiglitazone, while the C_{max} was 13% lower when administered as the combination tablet (see Table 6).

[See table 6 above]

AUC = area under the curve; C_{max} = maximum concentration; $T_{1/2}$ = terminal half-life; T_{max} = time of maximum concentration.

Regimen A = AVANDARYL 4 mg/4 mg tablet; Regimen B = Concomitant dosing of a rosiglitazone 4-mg tablet AND a glimepiride 4-mg tablet.

Data presented as geometric mean (range), except $T_{1/2}$ which is presented as arithmetic mean (range) and T_{max}, which is presented as median (range).

The rate and extent of absorption of both the rosiglitazone component and glimepiride component of AVANDARYL when taken with food were equivalent to the rate and extent of absorption of rosiglitazone and glimepiride when administered concomitantly as separate tablets with food.

Absorption: The AUC and C_{max} of glimepiride increased in a dose-proportional manner following administration of AVANDARYL 4 mg/1 mg, 4 mg/2 mg, and 4 mg/4 mg. Administration of AVANDARYL in the fed state resulted in no change in the overall exposure of rosiglitazone; however, the C_{max} of rosiglitazone decreased by 32% compared with the fasted state. There was an increase in both AUC (19%) and C_{max} (55%) of glimepiride in the fed state compared the fasted state.

Rosiglitazone: The absolute bioavailability of rosiglitazone is 99%. Peak plasma concentrations are observed about 1 hour after dosing. The C_{max} and AUC of rosiglitazone increase in a dose-proportional manner over the therapeutic dose range.

Glimepiride: After oral administration, glimepiride is completely (100%) absorbed from the gastrointestinal tract. Trials with single oral doses in normal subjects and with multiple oral doses in patients with type 2 diabetes have shown significant absorption of glimepiride within 1 hour after administration and C_{max} at 2 to 3 hours.

Distribution: Rosiglitazone: The mean (CV%) oral volume of distribution (V_{ss}/F) of rosiglitazone is approximately 17.6 (30%) liters, based on a population pharmacokinetic analysis. Rosiglitazone is approximately 99.8% bound to plasma proteins, primarily albumin.

Glimepiride: After intravenous (IV) dosing in normal subjects, the volume of distribution (Vd) was 8.8 L (113 mL/kg), and the total body clearance (CL) was 47.8 mL/min. Protein binding was greater than 99.5%.

Metabolism and Excretion: Rosiglitazone: Rosiglitazone is extensively metabolized with no unchanged drug excreted in the urine. The major routes of metabolism were N-demethylation and hydroxylation, followed by conjugation with sulfate and glucuronic acid. All the circulating metabolites are considerably less potent than parent and, therefore, are not expected to contribute to the insulin-sensitizing activity of rosiglitazone. In vitro data demonstrate that rosiglitazone is predominantly metabolized by cytochrome P450 (CYP) isoenzyme 2C8, with CYP2C9 contributing as a minor pathway. Following oral or IV administration of [14C]rosiglitazone maleate, approximately 64% and 23% of the dose was eliminated in the urine and in the feces, respectively. The plasma half-life of [14C]related material ranged from 103 to 158 hours. The elimination half-life is 3 to 4 hours and is independent of dose.

Glimepiride: Glimepiride is completely metabolized by oxidative biotransformation after either an IV or oral dose. The major metabolites are the cyclohexyl hydroxy methyl derivative (M1) and the carboxyl derivative (M2). Cytochrome P450 2C9 has been shown to be involved in the biotransformation of glimepiride to M1. M1 is further metabolized to M2 by one or several cytosolic enzymes. M1, but not M2, possesses about 1/3 of the pharmacological activity as compared with its parent in an animal model; however, whether the glucose-lowering effect of M1 is clinically meaningful is not clear.

When [14C]glimepiride was given orally, approximately 60% of the total radioactivity was recovered in the urine in 7 days and M1 (predominant) and M2 accounted for 80% to 90% of that recovered in the urine. Approximately 40% of the total radioactivity was recovered in feces and M1 and M2 (predominant) accounted for about 70% of that recovered in feces. No parent drug was recovered from urine or feces. After IV dosing in patients, no significant biliary excretion of glimepiride or its M1 metabolite has been observed.

Table 6. Pharmacokinetic Parameters for Rosiglitazone and Glimepiride (N = 28)

Parameter (Units)	Rosiglitazone		Glimepiride	
	Regimen A	Regimen B	Regimen A	Regimen B
AUC_{0-inf} • (ng.h/mL)	1,259 (833-2,060)	1,253 (756-2,758)	1,052 (643-2,117)	1,101 (648-2,555)
AUC_{0-t} • (ng.h/mL)	1,231 (810-2,019)	1,224 (744-2,654)	944 (511-1,898)	1,038 (606-2,337)
C_{max} • (ng/mL)	257 (157-352)	251 (77.3-434)	151 (63.2-345)	173 (70.5-329)
$T_{1/2}$ • (h)	3.53 (2.60-4.57)	3.54 (2.10-5.03)	7.63 (4.42-12.4)	5.08 (1.80-11.31)
T_{max} • (h)	1.00 (0.48-3.02)	0.98 (0.48-5.97)	3.02 (1.50-8.00)	2.53 (1.00-8.03)

Special Populations: No pharmacokinetic data are available for AVANDARYL in the following special populations. Information is provided for the individual components of AVANDARYL.

Gender: Rosiglitazone: Results of the population pharmacokinetics analysis showed that the mean oral clearance of rosiglitazone in female patients (N = 405) was approximately 6% lower compared with male patients of the same body weight (N = 642). Combination therapy with rosiglitazone and sulfonylureas improved glycemic control in both males and females with a greater therapeutic response observed in females. For a given body mass index (BMI), females tend to have a greater fat mass than males. Since the molecular target of rosiglitazone, PPARγ, is expressed in adipose tissues, this differentiating characteristic may account, at least in part, for the greater response to rosiglitazone in combination with sulfonylureas in females. Since therapy should be individualized, no dose adjustments are necessary based on gender alone.

• Glimepiride: There were no differences between males and females in the pharmacokinetics of glimepiride when adjustment was made for differences in body weight.

Geriatric: Rosiglitazone: Results of the population pharmacokinetics analysis (N = 716 <65 years; N = 331 ≥65 years) showed that age does not significantly affect the pharmacokinetics of rosiglitazone.

• Glimepiride: Comparison of glimepiride pharmacokinetics in type 2 diabetes patients 65 years and younger with those older than 65 years was performed in a trial using a dosing regimen of 6 mg daily. There were no significant differences in glimepiride pharmacokinetics between the 2 age groups. The mean AUC at steady state for the older patients was about 13% lower than that for the younger patients; the mean weight-adjusted clearance for the older patients was about 11% higher than that for the younger patients. [See Use in Specific Populations (8.5).]

Hepatic Impairment: Therapy with AVANDARYL should not be initiated if the patient exhibits clinical evidence of active liver disease or increased serum transaminase levels (ALT >2.5X upper limit of normal) at baseline [see Warnings and Precautions (5.7)].

• Rosiglitazone: Unbound oral clearance of rosiglitazone was significantly lower in patients with moderate to severe liver disease (Child-Pugh Class B/C) compared with healthy subjects. As a result, unbound C_{max} and AUC_{0-inf} were increased 2- and 3-fold, respectively. Elimination half-life for rosiglitazone was about 2 hours longer in patients with liver disease, compared with healthy subjects.

• Glimepiride: No trials of glimepiride have been conducted in patients with hepatic insufficiency.

Race: Rosiglitazone: Results of a population pharmacokinetic analysis including subjects of white, black, and other ethnic origins indicate that race has no influence on the pharmacokinetics of rosiglitazone.

• Glimepiride: No pharmacokinetic trials to assess the effects of race have been performed, but in placebo-controlled trials of glimepiride in patients with type 2 diabetes, the antihyperglycemic effect was comparable in whites (N = 536), blacks (N = 63), and Hispanics (N = 63).

Renal Impairment: Rosiglitazone: There are no clinically relevant differences in the pharmacokinetics of rosiglitazone in patients with mild to severe renal impairment or in hemodialysis-dependent patients compared with subjects with normal renal function.

• Glimepiride: A single-dose glimepiride, open-label trial was conducted in 15 patients with renal impairment. Glimepiride (3 mg) was administered to 3 groups of patients with different levels of mean creatinine clearance (CL_{cr}); (Group I, CL_{cr} = 77.7 mL/min, N = 5), (Group II, CL_{cr} = 27.7 mL/min, N = 3), and (Group III, CL_{cr} = 9.4 mL/min, N = 7). Glimepiride was found to be well tolerated in all 3 groups. The results showed that glimepiride serum levels decreased as renal function decreased. However, M1 and M2 serum levels (mean AUC values) increased 2.3 and 8.6 times from Group I to Group III. The apparent terminal half-life ($t_{1/2}$) for glimepiride did not change, while the half-lives for M1 and M2 increased as renal function decreased. Mean urinary excretion of M1 plus M2 as percent of dose, however, decreased (44.4%, 21.9%, and 9.3% for Groups I to III). A multiple-dose titration trial was also conducted in 16 type 2 diabetes patients with renal impairment using doses ranging from 1 to 8 mg daily for 3 months. The results were consistent with those observed after single doses. All patients with a CL_{cr} less than 22 mL/min had adequate control of their glucose levels with a dosage regimen of only 1 mg daily. The results from this trial suggest that a starting dose of 1 mg glimepiride, as contained in AVANDARYL 4 mg/1 mg, may be given to type 2 diabetes patients with kidney disease, and the dose may be titrated based on fasting glucose levels.

Pediatric: No pharmacokinetic data from trials in pediatric subjects are available for AVANDARYL.

• Rosiglitazone: Pharmacokinetic parameters of rosiglitazone in pediatric patients were established using a population pharmacokinetic analysis with sparse data from 96 pediatric patients in a single pediatric clinical trial including 33 males and 63 females with ages ranging from 10 to 17 years (weights ranging from 35 to 178.3 kg). Population mean CL/F and V/F of rosiglitazone were 3.15 L/h and 13.5 L, respectively. These estimates of CL/F and V/F were consistent with the typical parameter estimates from a prior adult population analysis.

• Glimepiride: The pharmacokinetics of glimepiride (1 mg) were evaluated in a single-dose trial conducted in 30 type 2 diabetic patients (male = 7; female = 23) between ages 10 and 17 years. The mean AUC_{0-last} (338.8 ± 203.1 ng.h/mL), C_{max} (102.4 ± 47.7 ng/mL), and $t_{1/2}$ (3.1 ± 1.7 hours) were comparable to those previously reported in adults (AUC_{0-last} 315.2 ± 95.9 ng.h/mL, C_{max} 103.2 ± 34.3 ng/mL, and $t_{1/2}$ 5.3 ± 4.1 hours).

12.4 Drug-drug Interactions

Single oral doses of glimepiride in 14 healthy adult subjects had no clinically significant effect on the steady-state pharmacokinetics of rosiglitazone. No clinically significant reductions in glimepiride AUC and C_{max} were observed after repeat doses of rosiglitazone (8 mg once daily) for 8 days in healthy adult subjects.

Rosiglitazone: Drugs That Inhibit, Induce, or are Metabolized by Cytochrome P450: In vitro drug metabolism studies suggest that rosiglitazone does not inhibit any of the major P450 enzymes at clinically relevant concentrations. In vitro data demonstrate that rosiglitazone is predominantly metabolized by CYP2C8, and to a lesser extent, 2C9. [See Drug Interactions (7.1).]

Rosiglitazone (4 mg twice daily) was shown to have no clinically relevant effect on the pharmacokinetics of nifedipine and oral contraceptives (ethinyl estradiol and norethindrone), which are predominantly metabolized by CYP3A4.

Gemfibrozil: Concomitant administration of gemfibrozil (600 mg twice daily), an inhibitor of CYP2C8, and rosiglitazone (4 mg once daily) for 7 days increased rosiglitazone AUC by 127%, compared with the administration of rosiglitazone (4 mg once daily) alone. Given the potential for dose-related adverse events with rosiglitazone, a decrease in the dose of rosiglitazone may be needed when gemfibrozil is introduced [see Drug Interactions (7.1)].

Rifampin: Rifampin administration (600 mg once a day), an inducer of CYP2C8, for 6 days is reported to decrease rosiglitazone AUC by 66%, compared with the administration of rosiglitazone (8 mg) alone [see Drug Interactions (7.1)].[1]

Glyburide: Rosiglitazone (2 mg twice daily) taken concomitantly with glyburide (3.75 to 10 mg/day) for 7 days did not

Table 7. Glycemic Parameters in a 28-Week Trial of AVANDARYL in Patients With Type 2 Diabetes Mellitus Inadequately Controlled on Diet and Exercise

Parameter	Glimepiride	Rosiglitazone	AVANDARYL 4 mg/4 mg	AVANDARYL 8 mg/4 mg
Mean Final Dose	3.5 mg	7.5 mg	4.0 mg/3.2 mg	6.8 mg/2.9 mg
N	221	227	221	214
FPG (mg/dL) [mean (SD)]				
• Baseline	211 (70)	212 (66)	207 (58)	214 (61)
• Change from baseline	-42 (66)	-57 (58)	-70 (57)	-80 (57)
• Treatment difference between				
• – AVANDARYL and glimepiride	—	—	-30[a]	-37[a]
• – AVANDARYL and rosiglitazone	—	—	-16[a]	-23[a]
• % of patients with ≥ 30 mg/dL decrease from baseline	56%	64%	77%	85%
HbA1c (%) [mean (SD)]				
• Baseline	9.0 (1.3)	9.1 (1.3)	9.0 (1.3)	9.2 (1.4)
• Change from baseline	-1.7 (1.4)	-1.8 (1.5)	-2.4 (1.4)	-2.5 (1.4)
• Treatment difference between				
• – AVANDARYL and glimepiride	—	—	-0.6[a]	-0.7[a]
• – AVANDARYL and rosiglitazone	—	—	-0.7[a]	-0.8[a]
• % of patients with ≥ 0.7% decrease from baseline	82%	76%	93%	93%
• % of patients at HbA1c Target <7.0%[b]	49%	46%	75%	72%

[a] Least squared means, P <0.0001 compared with monotherapy.
[b] Response is related to baseline HbA1c

alter the mean steady-state 24-hour plasma glucose concentrations in diabetic patients stabilized on glyburide therapy. Repeat doses of rosiglitazone (8 mg once daily) for 8 days in healthy adult Caucasian subjects caused a decrease in glyburide AUC and C_{max} of approximately 30%. In Japanese subjects, glyburide AUC and C_{max} slightly increased following coadministration of rosiglitazone.

Digoxin: Repeat oral dosing of rosiglitazone (8 mg once daily) for 14 days did not alter the steady-state pharmacokinetics of digoxin (0.375 mg once daily) in healthy volunteers.

Warfarin: Repeat dosing with rosiglitazone had no clinically relevant effect on the steady-state pharmacokinetics of warfarin enantiomers.

Additional pharmacokinetic trials demonstrated no clinically relevant effect of acarbose, ranitidine, or metformin on the pharmacokinetics of rosiglitazone.

Glimepiride: The hypoglycemic action of sulfonylureas may be potentiated by certain drugs, including nonsteroidal anti-inflammatory drugs (NSAIDs) and other drugs that are highly protein bound, such as salicylates, sulfonamides, chloramphenicol, coumarins, probenecid, monoamine oxidase inhibitors, and beta-adrenergic blocking agents. When these drugs are administered to a patient receiving glimepiride, the patient should be observed closely for hypoglycemia. When these drugs are withdrawn from a patient receiving glimepiride, the patient should be observed closely for loss of glycemic control.

Certain drugs tend to produce hyperglycemia and may lead to loss of control. These drugs include the thiazides and other diuretics, corticosteroids, phenothiazines, thyroid products, estrogens, oral contraceptives, phenytoin, nicotinic acid, sympathomimetics, and isoniazid. When these drugs are administered to a patient receiving glimepiride, the patient should be closely observed for loss of control. When these drugs are withdrawn from a patient receiving glimepiride, the patient should be observed closely for hypoglycemia.

Drugs Metabolized by Cytochrome P450: A potential interaction between oral miconazole and oral hypoglycemic agents leading to severe hypoglycemia has been reported. Whether this interaction also occurs with the IV, topical, or vaginal preparations of miconazole is not known. There is a potential interaction of glimepiride with inhibitors (e.g., fluconazole) and inducers (e.g., rifampicin) of cytochrome P450 2C9.

Aspirin: Coadministration of aspirin (1 g three times daily) and glimepiride led to a 34% decrease in the mean glimepiride AUC and, therefore, a 34% increase in the mean CL/F. The mean C_{max} had a decrease of 4%. Blood glucose and serum C-peptide concentrations were unaffected and no hypoglycemic symptoms were reported.

H_2-receptor Antagonists: Coadministration of either cimetidine (800 mg once daily) or ranitidine (150 mg twice daily) with a single 4-mg oral dose of glimepiride did not significantly alter the absorption and disposition of glimepiride, and no differences were seen in hypoglycemic symptomatology.

Beta-Blockers: Concomitant administration of propranolol (40 mg three times daily) and glimepiride significantly increased C_{max}, AUC, and $t_{1/2}$ of glimepiride by 23%, 22%, and 15%, respectively, and it decreased CL/F by 18%. The recovery of M1 and M2 from urine, however, did not change. The pharmacodynamic responses to glimepiride were nearly identical in normal subjects receiving propranolol and placebo. Pooled data from clinical trials in patients with type 2 diabetes showed no evidence of clinically significant adverse interactions with uncontrolled concurrent administration of beta-blockers. However, if beta-blockers are used, caution should be exercised and patients should be warned about the potential for hypoglycemia.

Warfarin: Concomitant administration of glimepiride tablets (4 mg once daily) did not alter the pharmacokinetic characteristics of R- and S-warfarin enantiomers following administration of a single dose (25 mg) of racemic warfarin to healthy subjects. No changes were observed in warfarin plasma protein binding. Glimepiride treatment did result in a slight, but statistically significant, decrease in the pharmacodynamic response to warfarin. The reductions in mean area under the prothrombin time (PT) curve and maximum PT values during glimepiride treatment were very small (3.3% and 9.9%, respectively) and are unlikely to be clinically important.

ACE Inhibitors: The responses of serum glucose, insulin, C-peptide, and plasma glucagon to 2 mg glimepiride were unaffected by coadministration of ramipril (an ACE inhibitor) 5 mg once daily in normal subjects. No hypoglycemic symptoms were reported.

Other: Although no specific interaction trials were performed, pooled data from clinical trials showed no evidence of clinically significant adverse interactions with uncontrolled concurrent administration of aspirin and other salicylates, H_2-receptor antagonists, ACE inhibitors, calcium-channel blockers, estrogens, fibrates, NSAIDs, HMG CoA reductase inhibitors, sulfonamides, or thyroid hormone.

13 NONCLINICAL TOXICOLOGY

13.1 Carcinogenesis, Mutagenesis, Impairment of Fertility

No animal studies have been conducted with AVANDARYL. The following data are based on findings in studies performed with rosiglitazone or glimepiride alone.

Rosiglitazone: *Carcinogenesis:* A 2-year carcinogenicity study was conducted in Charles River CD-1 mice at doses of 0.4, 1.5, and 6 mg/kg/day in the diet (highest dose equiva-

lent to approximately 12 times human AUC at the maximum recommended human daily dose). Sprague-Dawley rats were dosed for 2 years by oral gavage at doses of 0.05 mg/kg/day, 0.3 mg/kg/day, and 2 mg/kg/day (highest dose equivalent to approximately 10 and 20 times human AUC at the maximum recommended human daily dose for male and female rats, respectively).

Rosiglitazone was not carcinogenic in the mouse. There was an increase in incidence of adipose hyperplasia in the mouse at doses ≥1.5 mg/kg/day (approximately 2 times human AUC at the maximum recommended human daily dose). In rats, there was a significant increase in the incidence of benign adipose tissue tumors (lipomas) at doses ≥0.3 mg/kg/day (approximately 2 times human AUC at the maximum recommended human daily dose). These proliferative changes in both species are considered due to the persistent pharmacological overstimulation of adipose tissue.

Mutagenesis: Rosiglitazone was not mutagenic or clastogenic in the in vitro bacterial assays for gene mutation, the in vitro chromosome aberration test in human lymphocytes, the in vivo mouse micronucleus test, and the in vivo/in vitro rat UDS assay. There was a small (about 2-fold) increase in mutation in the in vitro mouse lymphoma assay in the presence of metabolic activation.

Impairment of Fertility: Rosiglitazone had no effects on mating or fertility of male rats given up to 40 mg/kg/day (approximately 116 times human AUC at the maximum recommended human daily dose). Rosiglitazone altered estrous cyclicity (2 mg/kg/day) and reduced fertility (40 mg/kg/day) of female rats in association with lower plasma levels of progesterone and estradiol (approximately 20 and 200 times human AUC at the maximum recommended human daily dose, respectively). No such effects were noted at 0.2 mg/kg/day (approximately 3 times human AUC at the maximum recommended human daily dose). In juvenile rats dosed from 27 days of age through to sexual maturity (at up to 40 mg/kg/day), there was no effect on male reproductive performance, or on estrous cyclicity, mating performance or pregnancy incidence in females (approximately 68 times human AUC at the maximum recommended daily dose). In monkeys, rosiglitazone (0.6 and 4.6 mg/kg/day; approximately 3 and 15 times human AUC at the maximum recommended human daily dose, respectively) diminished the follicular phase rise in serum estradiol with consequential reduction in the luteinizing hormone surge, lower luteal phase progesterone levels, and amenorrhea. The mechanism for these effects appears to be direct inhibition of ovarian steroidogenesis.

Glimepiride: *Carcinogenesis:* Studies in rats at doses of up to 5,000 parts per million (ppm) in complete feed (approximately 340 times the maximum recommended human dose, based on surface area) for 30 months showed no evidence of carcinogenesis. In mice, administration of glimepiride for 24 months resulted in an increase in benign pancreatic adenoma formation which was dose-related and is thought to be the result of chronic pancreatic stimulation. The no-effect dose for adenoma formation in mice in this study was 320 ppm in complete feed, or 46 to 54 mg/kg body weight/day. This is about 35 times the maximum human recommended dose based on surface area.

Mutagenesis: Glimepiride was non-mutagenic in a battery of in vitro and in vivo mutagenicity studies (Ames test, somatic cell mutation, chromosomal aberration, unscheduled DNA synthesis, mouse micronucleus test).

Impairment of Fertility: There was no effect of glimepiride on male mouse fertility in animals exposed up to 2,500 mg/kg body weight (>1,700 times the maximum recommended human dose based on surface area). Glimepiride had no effect on the fertility of male and female rats administered up to 4,000 mg/kg body weight (approximately 4,000 times the maximum recommended human dose based on surface area).

13.2 Animal Toxicology and/or Pharmacology

Rosiglitazone: Heart weights were increased in mice (3 mg/kg/day), rats (5 mg/kg/day), and dogs (2 mg/kg/day) with rosiglitazone treatments (approximately 5, 22, and 2 times human AUC at the maximum recommended human daily dose, respectively). Effects in juvenile rats were consistent with those seen in adults. Morphometric measurement indicated that there was hypertrophy in cardiac ventricular tissues, which may be due to increased heart work as a result of plasma volume expansion.

Glimepiride: Reduced serum glucose values and degranulation of the pancreatic beta cells were observed in beagle dogs exposed to glimepiride 320 mg/kg/day for 12 months (approximately 1,000 times the recommended human dose based on surface area). No evidence of tumor formation was observed in any organ. One female and one male dog developed bilateral subcapsular cataracts. Non-GLP studies indicated that glimepiride was unlikely to exacerbate cataract formation. Evaluation of the co-cataractogenic potential of glimepiride in several diabetic and cataract rat models was negative and there was no adverse effect of glimepiride on bovine ocular lens metabolism in organ culture [see Adverse Reactions (6.1)].

14 CLINICAL STUDIES

14.1 Patients Inadequately Controlled on Diet and Exercise

In a 28-week, randomized, double-blind, clinical trial, 901 patients with type 2 diabetes inadequately controlled on diet and exercise alone (baseline mean fasting plasma glucose [FPG] 211 mg/dL and baseline mean HbA1c 9.1%) were started on AVANDARYL 4 mg/1 mg, rosiglitazone 4 mg, or glimepiride 1 mg. Doses could be increased at 4-week intervals to reach a target mean daily glucose of ≤110 mg/dL. Patients who received AVANDARYL were randomized to 1 of 2 titration schemes differing in the maximum total daily dose (4 mg/4 mg or 8 mg/4 mg). The maximum total daily dose was 8 mg for rosiglitazone monotherapy and 4 mg for glimepiride monotherapy. All treatments were administered as a once-daily regimen. Improvements in FPG and HbA1c were observed in patients treated with AVANDARYL compared with either rosiglitazone or glimepiride alone (see Table 7).

[See table 7 at top of previous page]

Treatment with AVANDARYL resulted in statistically significant improvements in FPG and HbA1c compared with each of the monotherapies. However, when considering choice of therapy for drug-naïve patients, the risk-benefit of initiating monotherapy or dual therapy should be considered. In particular, the risk of hypoglycemia and weight gain with dual therapy should be taken into account. [See Warnings and Precautions (5.4, 5.6), Adverse Reactions (6.1).]

14.2 Patients Previously Treated With Sulfonylureas

The safety and efficacy of rosiglitazone added to a sulfonylurea have been studied in clinical trials in patients with type 2 diabetes inadequately controlled on sulfonylureas alone. No clinical trials have been conducted with the fixed-dose combination of AVANDARYL in patients inadequately controlled on a sulfonylurea or who have initially responded to rosiglitazone alone and require additional glycemic control.

A total of 3,457 patients with type 2 diabetes participated in ten 24- 26-week randomized, double-blind, placebo/active-controlled trials and one 2-year double-blind, active-controlled trial in elderly patients designed to assess the efficacy and safety of rosiglitazone in combination with a sulfonylurea. Rosiglitazone 2 mg, 4 mg, or 8 mg daily, was administered either once daily (3 trials) or in divided doses twice daily (7 trials), to patients inadequately controlled on a submaximal or maximal dose of sulfonylurea.

In these trials, the combination of rosiglitazone 4 mg or 8 mg daily (administered as single- or twice-daily divided doses) and a sulfonylurea significantly reduced FPG and HbA1c compared with placebo plus sulfonylurea or further up-titration of the sulfonylurea. Table 8 shows pooled data for 8 trials in which rosiglitazone added to sulfonylurea was compared with placebo plus sulfonylurea.

[See table 8 above]

One of the 24- to 26-week trials included patients who were inadequately controlled on maximal doses of glyburide and switched to 4 mg of rosiglitazone daily as monotherapy; in this group, loss of glycemic control was demonstrated, as evidenced by increases in FPG and HbA1c.

In a 2-year double-blind trial, elderly patients (aged 59 to 89 years) on half-maximal sulfonylurea (glipizide 10 mg twice daily) were randomized to the addition of rosiglitazone (N = 115, 4 mg once daily to 8 mg as needed) or to continued up-titration of glipizide (N = 110), to a maximum of 20 mg twice daily. Mean baseline FPG and HbA1c were 157 mg/dL and 7.72%, respectively, for the rosiglitazone plus glipizide arm and 159 mg/dL and 7.65%, respectively, for the glipizide up-titration arm. Loss of glycemic control (FPG ≥180 mg/dL) occurred in a significantly lower proportion of patients (2%) on rosiglitazone plus glipizide compared with patients in the glipizide up-titration arm (28.7%). About 78% of the patients on combination therapy completed the 2 years of therapy while only 51% completed on glipizide monotherapy. The effect of combination therapy on FPG and HbA1c was durable over the 2-year trial period, with patients achieving a mean of 132 mg/dL for FPG and a mean of 6.98% for HbA1c compared with no change on the glipizide arm.

15 REFERENCES

1. Park JY, Kim KA, Kang MH, et al. Effect of rifampin on the pharmacokinetics of rosiglitazone in healthy subjects. *Clin Pharmacol Ther* 2004;75:157-162.

16 HOW SUPPLIED/STORAGE AND HANDLING

Each rounded triangular tablet contains rosiglitazone as the maleate and glimepiride as follows:
4 mg/1 mg – yellow, gsk debossed on one side and 4/1 on the other.
4 mg/2 mg – orange, gsk debossed on one side and 4/2 on the other.
4 mg/4 mg – pink, gsk debossed on one side and 4/4 on the other.

8 mg/2 mg – pale pink, gsk debossed on one side and 8/2 on the other.
8 mg/4 mg – red, gsk debossed on one side and 8/4 on the other.

4 mg/1 mg bottles of 30:	NDC 0173-0841-13
4 mg/2 mg bottles of 30:	NDC 0173-0842-13
4 mg/4 mg bottles of 30:	NDC 0173-0843-13
8 mg/2 mg bottles of 30:	NDC 0173-0844-13
8 mg/4 mg bottles of 30:	NDC 0173-0845-13

Store at 25°C (77°F); excursions permitted to 15° to 30°C (59° to 86°F). Dispense in a tight, light-resistant container.

17 PATIENT COUNSELING INFORMATION

Advise the patient to read the FDA-approved patient labeling (Medication Guide).

There are multiple medications available to treat type 2 diabetes. The benefits and risks of each available diabetes medication should be taken into account when choosing a particular diabetes medication for a given patient.

Patients should be informed of the following:

- AVANDARYL is not recommended in patients with symptomatic heart failure.
- A meta-analysis of mostly short-term trials suggested an increased risk for myocardial infarction with rosiglitazone compared with placebo. Data from long-term clinical trials of rosiglitazone versus other antidiabetes agents (metformin or sulfonylureas), including a cardiovascular outcome trial (RECORD), observed no difference in overall mortality or in major adverse cardiovascular events (MACE) and its components.
- AVANDARYL is not recommended for patients who are taking insulin.
- **Management of type 2 diabetes should include diet control. Caloric restriction, weight loss, and exercise are essential for the proper treatment of the diabetic patient because they help improve insulin sensitivity. This is im-**portant not only in the primary treatment of type 2 diabetes, but also in maintaining the efficacy of drug therapy.
- It is important to adhere to dietary instructions and to regularly have blood glucose and glycosylated hemoglobin (HbA1c) tested. It can take 2 weeks to see a reduction in blood glucose and 2 to 3 months to see the full effect of AVANDARYL.
- The risks of hypoglycemia, its symptoms and treatment, and conditions that predispose to its development should be explained to patients and their family members.
- Blood will be drawn to check their liver function prior to the start of therapy and periodically thereafter per the clinical judgment of the healthcare professional. Patients with unexplained symptoms of nausea, vomiting, abdominal pain, fatigue, anorexia, or dark urine should immediately report these symptoms to their physician.
- Patients who experience an unusually rapid increase in weight or edema or who develop shortness of breath or other symptoms of heart failure while on AVANDARYL should immediately report these symptoms to their physician.
- AVANDARYL should be taken with the first meal of the day.
- Therapy with rosiglitazone, like other thiazolidinediones, may result in ovulation in some premenopausal anovulatory women. As a result, these patients may be at an increased risk for pregnancy while taking AVANDARYL. Thus, adequate contraception in premenopausal women should be recommended. This possible effect has not been specifically investigated in clinical trials so the frequency of this occurrence is not known.

AVANDARYL is a registered trademark of the GSK group of companies.
GlaxoSmithKline
Research Triangle Park, NC 27709
©2014, the GSK group of companies. All rights reserved.
AVR:14PI

Table 8. Glycemic Parameters in 24- to 26-Week Combination Trials of Rosiglitazone Plus Sulfonylurea

Twice-Daily Divided Dosing (5 Trials)	Sulfonylurea	Rosiglitazone 2 mg Twice Daily + Sulfonylurea	Sulfonylurea	Rosiglitazone 4 mg Twice Daily + Sulfonylurea
N	397	497	248	346
FPG (mg/dL)				
• Baseline (mean)	204	198	188	187
• Change from baseline (mean)	11	-29	8	-43
• Difference from sulfonylurea alone (adjusted mean)	—	-42[a]	—	-53[a]
• % of patients with ≥30 mg/dL decrease from baseline	17%	49%	15%	61%
HbA1c (%)				
• Baseline (mean)	9.4	9.5	9.3	9.6
• Change from baseline (mean)	0.2	-1.0	0.0	-1.6
• Difference from sulfonylurea alone (adjusted mean)		-1.1[a]		-1.4[a]
• % of patients with ≥0.7% decrease from baseline	21%	60%	23%	75%

Once-Daily Dosing (3 Trials)	Sulfonylurea	Rosiglitazone 4 mg Once Daily + Sulfonylurea	Sulfonylurea	Rosiglitazone 8 mg Once Daily + Sulfonylurea
N	172	172	173	176
FPG (mg/dL)				
• Baseline (mean)	198	206	188	192
• Change from baseline (mean)	17	-25	17	-43
• Difference from sulfonylurea alone (adjusted mean)	—	-47[a]	—	-66[a]
• % of patients with ≥30 mg/dL decrease from baseline	17%	48%	19%	55%
HbA1c (%)				
• Baseline (mean)	8.6	8.8	8.9	8.9
• Change from baseline (mean)	0.4	-0.5	0.1	-1.2
• Difference from sulfonylurea alone (adjusted mean)	-	-0.9[a]	-	-1.4[a]
• % of patients with ≥0.7% decrease from baseline	11%	36%	20%	68%

[a] $P < 0.0001$ compared with sulfonylurea alone.

MEDICATION GUIDE
AVANDARYL® (ah-VAN-duh-ril)
(rosiglitazone maleate and glimepiride) tablets

Read this Medication Guide carefully before you start taking AVANDARYL and each time you get a refill. There may be new information. This information does not take the place of talking with your doctor about your medical condition or your treatment. If you have any questions about AVANDARYL, ask your doctor or pharmacist.

What is the most important information I should know about AVANDARYL?

AVANDARYL may cause serious side effects, including:
New or worse heart failure
- The risk of heart failure may be higher in people who take AVANDARYL with insulin. Most people who take insulin should not also take AVANDARYL.
- Rosiglitazone, one of the two drugs that make up AVANDARYL, can cause your body to keep extra fluid (fluid retention), which leads to swelling (edema) and weight gain. Extra body fluid can make some heart problems worse or lead to heart failure. Heart failure means your heart does not pump blood well enough.
- If you have severe heart failure, you cannot start AVANDARYL.
- If you have heart failure with symptoms (such as shortness of breath or swelling), even if these symptoms are not severe, AVANDARYL may not be right for you.

Call your doctor right away if you have any of the following:
- swelling or fluid retention, especially in the ankles or legs
- shortness of breath or trouble breathing, especially when you lie down
- an unusually fast increase in weight
- unusual tiredness

AVANDARYL can have other serious side effects. Be sure to read the section "What are possible side effects of AVANDARYL?"

What is AVANDARYL?
AVANDARYL contains 2 prescription medicines to treat diabetes, rosiglitazone maleate (AVANDIA®) and glimepiride. AVANDARYL is used with diet and exercise to treat adults with type 2 ("adult-onset" or "non-insulin dependent") diabetes mellitus ("high blood sugar").
Glimepiride can help your body release more of its own insulin. Rosiglitazone can help your body respond better to the insulin made in your body and does not cause your body to make more insulin. These medicines can work together to help control your blood sugar.
AVANDARYL is not for people with type 1 diabetes mellitus or to treat a condition called diabetic ketoacidosis.
It is not known if AVANDARYL is safe and effective in children younger than 18 years old.

Who should not take AVANDARYL?
Many people with heart failure should not start taking AVANDARYL. See "What should I tell my doctor before taking AVANDARYL?"
Do not take AVANDARYL if you are allergic to rosiglitazone or any of the ingredients in AVANDARYL. See the end of this leaflet for a complete list of ingredients in AVANDARYL.
Symptoms of a severe allergic reaction with AVANDARYL may include:
- swelling of your face, lips, tongue, or throat
- problems with breathing or swallowing
- skin rash or itching
- raised red areas on your skin (hives)
- blisters on your skin or in your mouth, nose, or eyes
- peeling of your skin
- fainting or feeling dizzy
- very rapid heartbeat

What should I tell my doctor before taking AVANDARYL?
Before starting AVANDARYL, ask your doctor about what the choices are for diabetes medicines and what the expected benefits and possible risks are for you in particular. Before taking AVANDARYL, tell your doctor about all of your medical conditions, including if you:
- **have heart problems or heart failure.**
- **have type 1 ("juvenile") diabetes or had diabetic ketoacidosis.** These conditions should be treated with insulin and should not be treated with AVANDARYL.
- **have a type of diabetic eye disease called macular edema** (swelling of the back of the eye).
- **have liver problems.** Your doctor should do blood tests to check your liver before you start taking AVANDARYL and during treatment as needed.
- **had liver problems while taking REZULIN™ (troglitazone),** another medicine for diabetes.
- **have kidney problems.** If people with kidney problems use AVANDARYL, they may need a lower dose of the medication.
- **have glucose 6-phosphate dehydrogenase (G6PD) deficiency.** This condition runs in families. People with G6PD deficiency who take glimepiride (one of the medicines in AVANDARYL) may develop hemolytic anemia (fast breakdown of red blood cells).

- **are pregnant or plan to become pregnant.** It is not known if AVANDARYL can harm your unborn baby. You and your doctor should talk about the best way to control your diabetes during pregnancy. If you are a premenopausal woman (before the "change of life") who does not have regular monthly periods, AVANDARYL may increase your chances of becoming pregnant. Talk to your doctor about birth control choices while taking AVANDARYL. Tell your doctor right away if you become pregnant while taking AVANDARYL.
- **are breastfeeding or planning to breastfeed.** It is not known if AVANDARYL passes into breast milk. You and your doctor should decide if you will take AVANDARYL or breastfeed. You should not do both.

Tell your doctor about all of the medicines you take including prescription and non-prescription medicines, vitamins or herbal supplements. AVANDARYL and certain other medicines can affect each other and may lead to serious side effects including high or low blood sugar, or heart problems. Especially tell your doctor if you take:
- insulin.
- **any medicines for high blood pressure, high cholesterol or heart failure, or for prevention of heart disease or stroke.**

Know the medicines you take. Keep a list of all your medicines and show it to your doctor and pharmacist before you start a new medicine. They will tell you if it is alright to take AVANDARYL with other medicines.

How should I take AVANDARYL?
- Take AVANDARYL exactly as prescribed. Your doctor may need to change your dose until your blood sugar is better controlled.
- Take AVANDARYL by mouth one time each day with your first main meal.
- It usually takes a few days for AVANDARYL to start lowering your blood sugar. It may take 2 to 3 months to see the full effect on your blood sugar level.
- If you miss a dose of AVANDARYL, take it as soon as you remember unless it is time to take your next dose. Take your next dose at the usual time. Do not take double doses to make up for a missed dose.
- If you take too much AVANDARYL, call your doctor or poison control center right away.
- Test your blood sugar regularly as your doctor tells you.
- Your doctor should do blood tests to check your liver before you start AVANDARYL and during treatment as needed. Your doctor should also do regular blood sugar tests (for example, "A1c") to monitor your response to AVANDARYL.
- Call your doctor if you get sick, get injured, get an infection, or have surgery. AVANDARYL may not control your blood sugar levels during these times. Your doctor may need to stop AVANDARYL for a short time and give you insulin to control your blood sugar level.
- Diet and exercise can help your body use its blood sugar better. It is important to stay on your recommended diet, lose extra weight, and get regular exercise while taking AVANDARYL.

What are possible side effects of AVANDARYL?
AVANDARYL may cause serious side effects, including:
- **New or worse heart failure.** See "What is the most important information I should know about AVANDARYL?"
- **Heart attack.** AVANDARYL may increase the risk of a heart attack. Talk to your doctor about what this means to you.

Symptoms of a heart attack can include the following:
- chest discomfort in the center of your chest that lasts for more than a few minutes, or that goes away or comes back
- chest discomfort that feels like uncomfortable pressure, squeezing, fullness, or pain
- pain or discomfort in your arms, back, neck, jaw, or stomach
- shortness of breath with or without chest discomfort
- breaking out in a cold sweat
- nausea or vomiting
- feeling lightheaded
- **Call your doctor or go to the nearest hospital emergency room right away if you think you are having a heart attack.**
- **Swelling (edema).** AVANDARYL can cause swelling due to fluid retention. See "What is the most important information I should know about AVANDARYL?"
- **Low blood sugar (hypoglycemia).** Lightheadedness, dizziness, shakiness, or hunger may mean that your blood sugar is too low. This can happen if you skip meals, drink alcohol, use another medicine that lowers blood sugar, exercise (particularly hard or long), or if you have certain medical problems. Call your doctor if low blood sugar levels are a problem for you.
- **Weight gain.** Rosiglitazone, one of the medicines in AVANDARYL, can cause weight gain that may be due to fluid retention or extra body fat. Weight gain can be a serious problem for people with certain conditions including heart problems. See "What is the most important information I should know about AVANDARYL?"

- **Liver problems.** It is important for your liver to be working normally when you take AVANDARYL. Your doctor should do blood tests to check your liver before you start taking AVANDARYL and during treatment as needed. Call your doctor right away if you have unexplained symptoms such as:
- nausea or vomiting
- stomach pain
- unusual or unexplained tiredness
- loss of appetite
- dark urine
- yellowing of your skin or the whites of your eyes.
- **Macular edema** (a diabetic eye disease with swelling in the back of the eye). Tell your doctor right away if you have any changes in your vision. Your doctor should check your eyes regularly. Very rarely, some people have had vision changes due to swelling in the back of the eye while taking rosiglitazone, one of the medicines in AVANDARYL.
- **Fractures (broken bones),** usually in the hand, upper arm, or foot. Talk to your doctor for advice on how to keep your bones healthy.
- **Low red blood cell count (anemia).**
- **Ovulation** (release of egg from an ovary in women) leading to pregnancy. Ovulation may happen in premenopausal women who do not have regular monthly periods. This can increase the chance of pregnancy. See "What should I tell my doctor before taking AVANDARYL?"

The most common side effects with AVANDARYL include cold-like symptoms and headache.
Call your doctor for medical advice about side effects. You may report side effects to FDA at 1-800-FDA-1088.

How should I store AVANDARYL?
- Store AVANDARYL at room temperature, 59°F to 86°F (15°C to 30°C). Keep AVANDARYL in the container it comes in. Keep the container closed tightly.
- Safely, throw away AVANDARYL that is out of date or no longer needed.

Keep AVANDARYL and all medicines out of the reach of children.

General information about AVANDARYL
Medicines are sometimes prescribed for purposes other than those listed in a Medication Guide. Do not use AVANDARYL for a condition for which it was not prescribed. Do not give AVANDARYL to other people, even if they have the same symptoms you have. It may harm them.
This Medication Guide summarizes important information about AVANDARYL. If you would like more information, talk with your doctor. You can ask your doctor or pharmacist for information about AVANDARYL that is written for healthcare professionals. You can also find out more about AVANDARYL by calling 1-888-825-5249.

What are the ingredients in AVANDARYL?
Active Ingredients: rosiglitazone maleate and glimepiride.
Inactive Ingredients: hypromellose 2910, lactose monohydrate, macrogol (polyethylene glycol), magnesium stearate, microcrystalline cellulose, sodium starch glycolate, titanium dioxide, triacetin, and 1 or more of the following: yellow, red, or black iron oxides.
Always check to make sure that the medicine you are taking is the correct one. AVANDARYL tablets are triangles with rounded corners and look like this:
4 mg/1 mg – yellow with "gsk" on one side and "4/1" on the other.
4 mg/2 mg – orange with "gsk" on one side and "4/2" on the other.
4 mg/4 mg – pink with "gsk" on one side and "4/4" on the other.
8 mg/2 mg – pale pink with "gsk" on one side and "8/2" on the other.
8 mg/4 mg – red with "gsk" on one side and "8/4" on the other.

AVANDARYL and AVANDIA are registered trademarks of the GSK group of companies.
REZULIN is a trademark of its respective owner and is not a trademark of the GSK group of companies. The maker of this brand is not affiliated with and does not endorse the GSK group of companies or its products.
This Medication Guide has been approved by the U.S. Food and Drug Administration.
GlaxoSmithKline
Research Triangle Park, NC 27709
©2014, the GSK group of companies. All rights reserved.
May 2014
AVR:5MG

AVANDIA
[ə-van′dē-ə]
(rosiglitazone maleate)
tablets

HIGHLIGHTS OF PRESCRIBING INFORMATION
These highlights do not include all the information needed to use AVANDIA safely and effectively. See full prescribing information for AVANDIA.
AVANDIA (rosiglitazone maleate) tablets
Initial U.S. Approval: 1999

℞

WARNING: CONGESTIVE HEART FAILURE
See full prescribing information for complete boxed warning.

- Thiazolidinediones, including rosiglitazone, cause or exacerbate congestive heart failure in some patients (5.1). After initiation of AVANDIA, and after dose increases, observe patients carefully for signs and symptoms of heart failure (including excessive, rapid weight gain, dyspnea, and/or edema). If these signs and symptoms develop, the heart failure should be managed according to current standards of care. Furthermore, discontinuation or dose reduction of AVANDIA must be considered.
- AVANDIA is not recommended in patients with symptomatic heart failure. Initiation of AVANDIA in patients with established NYHA Class III or IV heart failure is contraindicated. (4, 5.1)

———————RECENT MAJOR CHANGES———————

Boxed Warning, AVANDIA-Rosiglitazone Medicines Access Program removal	05/2014
Indications and Usage, patient population restrictions removal (1)	05/2014
Contraindications (4)	05/2014
Warnings and Precautions, Cardiac Failure (5.1)	05/2014
Warnings and Precautions, Major Adverse Cardiovascular Events (5.2)	05/2014
Warnings and Precautions, Rosiglitazone REMS (Risk Evaluation and Mitigation Strategy) Program removal (formerly 5.3)	05/2014

———————INDICATIONS AND USAGE———————

AVANDIA is a thiazolidinedione antidiabetic agent indicated as an adjunct to diet and exercise to improve glycemic control in adults with type 2 diabetes mellitus. (1)
Important Limitations of Use:
- AVANDIA should not be used in patients with type 1 diabetes mellitus or for the treatment of diabetic ketoacidosis. (1)
- Coadministration of AVANDIA and insulin is not recommended. (1, 5.1, 5.2)

———————DOSAGE AND ADMINISTRATION———————

- Start at 4 mg daily in single or divided doses; do not exceed 8 mg daily. (2)
- Dose increases should be accompanied by careful monitoring for adverse events related to fluid retention. (2)
- Do not initiate AVANDIA if the patient exhibits clinical evidence of active liver disease or increased serum transaminase levels. (2.1)

———————DOSAGE FORMS AND STRENGTHS———————

Pentagonal, film-coated tablets in the following strengths: 2 mg, 4 mg, and 8 mg (3)

———————CONTRAINDICATIONS———————

- Initiation in patients with established NYHA Class III or IV heart failure. (4)
- Hypersensitivity to rosiglitazone or any of the product's ingredients. (4)

———————WARNINGS AND PRECAUTIONS———————

- Fluid retention, which may exacerbate or lead to heart failure, may occur. Combination use with insulin and use in congestive heart failure NYHA Class I and II may increase risk of other cardiovascular effects. (5.1)
- Meta-analysis of 52 mostly short-term trials suggested a potential risk of ischemic cardiovascular (CV) events relative to placebo, not confirmed in a long-term CV outcome trial versus metformin or sulfonylurea. (5.2)
- Dose-related edema (5.3), weight gain (5.4), and anemia (5.8) may occur.
- Macular edema has been reported. (5.6)
- Increased incidence of bone fracture. (5.7)

———————ADVERSE REACTIONS———————

Common adverse reactions (>5%) reported in clinical trials without regard to causality were upper respiratory tract infection, injury, and headache. (6.1)
To report SUSPECTED ADVERSE REACTIONS, contact GlaxoSmithKline at 1-888-825-5249 or FDA at 1-800-FDA-1088 or www.fda.gov/medwatch.

———————DRUG INTERACTIONS———————

Inhibitors of CYP2C8 (e.g., gemfibrozil) may increase rosiglitazone levels; inducers of CYP2C8 (e.g., rifampin) may decrease rosiglitazone levels. (7.1)

———————USE IN SPECIFIC POPULATIONS———————

- Pregnancy: No adequate and well-controlled studies in pregnant women. Use during pregnancy only if the potential benefit justifies the potential risk to the fetus. (8.1)

- Nursing Mothers: Discontinue drug or nursing. (8.3)
- Safety and effectiveness in children younger than 18 years have not been established. (8.4)

See 17 for PATIENT COUNSELING INFORMATION and Medication Guide

Revised: 05/2014

FULL PRESCRIBING INFORMATION: CONTENTS*

FULL PRESCRIBING INFORMATION

WARNING: CONGESTIVE HEART FAILURE
- Thiazolidinediones, including rosiglitazone, cause or exacerbate congestive heart failure in some patients *[see Warnings and Precautions (5.1)]*. After initiation of AVANDIA®, and after dose increases, observe patients carefully for signs and symptoms of heart failure (including excessive, rapid weight gain, dyspnea, and/or edema). If these signs and symptoms develop, the heart failure should be managed according to current standards of care. Furthermore, discontinuation or dose reduction of AVANDIA must be considered.
- AVANDIA is not recommended in patients with symptomatic heart failure. Initiation of AVANDIA in patients with established NYHA Class III or IV heart failure is contraindicated. *[See Contraindications (4), Warnings and Precautions (5.1)]*

---

1   INDICATIONS AND USAGE

AVANDIA is a thiazolidinedione antidiabetic agent indicated as an adjunct to diet and exercise to improve glycemic control in adults with type 2 diabetes mellitus.
Important Limitations of Use:
- Due to its mechanism of action, AVANDIA is active only in the presence of endogenous insulin. Therefore, AVANDIA should not be used in patients with type 1 diabetes mellitus or for the treatment of diabetic ketoacidosis.
- The coadministration of AVANDIA and insulin is not recommended *[see Warnings and Precautions (5.1)]*.

2   DOSAGE AND ADMINISTRATION

AVANDIA may be administered at a starting dose of 4 mg either as a single daily dose or in 2 divided doses. For pa-

---

tients who respond inadequately following 8 to 12 weeks of treatment, as determined by reduction in fasting plasma glucose (FPG), the dose may be increased to 8 mg daily. Increases in the dose of AVANDIA should be accompanied by careful monitoring for adverse events related to fluid retention *[see Boxed Warning, Warnings and Precautions (5.1)]*. AVANDIA may be taken with or without food.
The total daily dose of AVANDIA should not exceed 8 mg. Patients receiving AVANDIA in combination with other hypoglycemic agents may be at risk for hypoglycemia, and a reduction in the dose of the concomitant agent may be necessary.

2.1   Specific Patient Populations
Renal Impairment: No dosage adjustment is necessary when AVANDIA is used as monotherapy in patients with renal impairment. Since metformin is contraindicated in such patients, concomitant administration of metformin and AVANDIA is also contraindicated in patients with renal impairment.
Hepatic Impairment: Liver enzymes should be measured prior to initiating treatment with AVANDIA. Therapy with AVANDIA should not be initiated if the patient exhibits clinical evidence of active liver disease or increased serum transaminase levels (ALT >2.5× upper limit of normal at start of therapy). After initiation of AVANDIA, liver enzymes should be monitored periodically per the clinical judgment of the healthcare professional. *[See Warnings and Precautions (5.5), Clinical Pharmacology (12.3).]*
Pediatric: Data are insufficient to recommend pediatric use of AVANDIA *[see Use in Specific Populations (8.4)]*.

3   DOSAGE FORMS AND STRENGTHS

Pentagonal film-coated TILTAB® tablet contains rosiglitazone as the maleate as follows:
- 2 mg – pink, debossed with GSK on one side and 2 on the other
- 4 mg – orange, debossed with GSK on one side and 4 on the other
- 8 mg – red-brown, debossed with GSK on one side and 8 on the other

4   CONTRAINDICATIONS

- Initiation of AVANDIA in patients with established New York Heart Association (NYHA) Class III or IV heart failure is contraindicated *[see Boxed Warning]*.
- Use in patients with a history of a hypersensitivity reaction to rosiglitazone or any of the product's ingredients.

5   WARNINGS AND PRECAUTIONS
5.1   Cardiac Failure
AVANDIA, like other thiazolidinediones, alone or in combination with other antidiabetic agents, can cause fluid retention, which may exacerbate or lead to heart failure. Patients should be observed for signs and symptoms of heart failure. If these signs and symptoms develop, the heart failure should be managed according to current standards of care. Furthermore, discontinuation or dose reduction of rosiglitazone must be considered *[see Boxed Warning]*.
Patients with congestive heart failure (CHF) NYHA Class I and II treated with AVANDIA have an increased risk of cardiovascular events. A 52-week, double-blind, placebo-controlled, echocardiographic trial was conducted in 224 patients with type 2 diabetes mellitus and NYHA Class I or II CHF (ejection fraction ≤45%) on background antidiabetic and CHF therapy. An independent committee conducted a blinded evaluation of fluid-related events (including congestive heart failure) and cardiovascular hospitalizations according to predefined criteria (adjudication). Separate from the adjudication, other cardiovascular adverse events were reported by investigators. Although no treatment difference in change from baseline of ejection fractions was observed, more cardiovascular adverse events were observed following treatment with AVANDIA compared with placebo during the 52-week trial. (See Table 1.)

Table 1. Emergent Cardiovascular Adverse Events in Patients With Congestive Heart Failure (NYHA Class I and II) Treated With AVANDIA or Placebo (in Addition to Background Antidiabetic and CHF Therapy)

Events	AVANDIA N = 110 n (%)	Placebo N = 114 n (%)
Adjudicated		
Cardiovascular deaths	5 (5%)	4 (4%)
CHF worsening	7 (6%)	4 (4%)
– with overnight hospitalization	5 (5%)	4 (4%)
– without overnight hospitalization	2 (2%)	0 (0%)
New or worsening edema	28 (25%)	10 (9%)
New or worsening dyspnea	29 (26%)	19 (17%)

Figure 1. Hazard Ratios for the Risk of MACE, Myocardial Infarction, and Total Mortality With AVANDIA Compared With a Control Group in Long-term Trials

Study	N	MACE n (%)	Myocardial Infarction * n (%)	Total Mortality n (%)
RECORD				
RSG+SU or MET	2220	154 (6.9%)	72 (3.2%)	136 (6.1%)
vs SU+MET	2227	165 (7.4%)	68 (3.1%)	157 (7.0%)
ADOPT				
RSG	1456	35 (2.4%)	20 (1.4%)	12 (0.8%)
vs. SU	1441	28 (1.9%)	15 (1.0%)	21 (1.5%)
vs. MET	1454	36 (2.5%)	17 (1.2%)	15 (1.0%)
DREAM				
RSG	1325	15 (1.1%)	5 (0.4%)	15 (1.1%)
vs. Placebo	1321	14 (1.1%)	7 (0.5%)	17 (1.3%)
RSG+RAM	1310	18 (1.4%)	12 (0.9%)	15 (1.1%)
vs. RAM	1313	9 (0.7%)	5 (0.4%)	16 (1.2%)
OVERALL				
RSG	6311	222 (3.5%)	109 (1.7%)	178 (2.8%)
vs control	7756	252 (3.3%)	112 (1.4%)	226 (2.9%)

RSG = rosiglitazone; SU = sulfonylurea; MET = metformin; RAM = ramipril
* Myocardial infarction includes fatal and non-fatal MI plus sudden death

Increases in CHF medication	36 (33%)	20 (18%)
Cardiovascular hospitalization[a]	21 (19%)	15 (13%)
Investigator-reported, non-adjudicated		
Ischemic adverse events	10 (9%)	5 (4%)
– Myocardial infarction	5 (5%)	2 (2%)
– Angina	6 (5%)	3 (3%)

[a] Includes hospitalization for any cardiovascular reason.

In a long-term, cardiovascular outcome trial (RECORD) in patients with type 2 diabetes *[see Adverse Reactions (6.1)]*, the incidence of heart failure was higher in patients treated with AVANDIA [2.7% (61/2,220) compared with active control 1.3% (29/2,227), HR 2.10 (95% CI: 1.35, 3.27)].
Initiation of AVANDIA in patients with established NYHA Class III or IV heart failure is contraindicated. AVANDIA is not recommended in patients with symptomatic heart failure. *[See Boxed Warning.]*
Patients experiencing acute coronary syndromes have not been studied in controlled clinical trials. In view of the potential for development of heart failure in patients having an acute coronary event, initiation of AVANDIA is not recommended for patients experiencing an acute coronary event, and discontinuation of AVANDIA during this acute phase should be considered.
Patients with NYHA Class III and IV cardiac status (with or without CHF) have not been studied in controlled clinical trials. AVANDIA is not recommended in patients with NYHA Class III and IV cardiac status.
Congestive Heart Failure During Coadministration of AVANDIA With Insulin: In trials in which AVANDIA was added to insulin, AVANDIA increased the risk of congestive heart failure. Coadministration of AVANDIA and insulin is not recommended. *[See Indications and Usage (1), Warnings and Precautions (5.2).]*
In 7 controlled, randomized, double-blind trials which had durations from 16 to 26 weeks and which were included in a meta-analysis *[see Warnings and Precautions (5.2)]*, patients with type 2 diabetes mellitus were randomized to coadministration of AVANDIA and insulin (N = 1,018) or insulin (N = 815). In these 7 trials, AVANDIA was added to insulin. These trials included patients with long-standing diabetes (median duration of 12 years) and a high prevalence of pre-existing medical conditions, including peripheral neuropathy, retinopathy, ischemic heart disease, vascular disease, and congestive heart failure. The total number of patients with emergent congestive heart failure was 23 (2.3%) and 8 (1.0%) in the group receiving AVANDIA plus insulin and the insulin group, respectively.
Heart Failure in Observational Studies of Elderly Diabetic Patients Comparing AVANDIA to Pioglitazone: Three observational studies in elderly diabetic patients (age 65 years and older) found that AVANDIA statistically significantly increased the risk of hospitalized heart failure compared to use of pioglitazone. One other observational study in patients with a mean age of 54 years, which also included an analysis in a subpopulation of patients >65 years of age, found no statistically significant increase in emergency department visits or hospitalization for heart failure in patients treated with AVANDIA compared to pioglitazone in the older subgroup.

5.2 Major Adverse Cardiovascular Events
Data from long-term, prospective, randomized, controlled clinical trials of AVANDIA versus metformin or sulfonylureas, particularly a cardiovascular outcome trial (RECORD), observed no difference in overall mortality or in major adverse cardiovascular events (MACE) and its components. A meta-analysis of mostly short-term trials suggested an increased risk for myocardial infarction with AVANDIA compared with placebo.
Cardiovascular Events in Large, Long-term, Prospective, Randomized, Controlled Trials of AVANDIA: RECORD, a prospectively designed cardiovascular outcome trial (mean follow-up 5.5 years; 4,447 patients), compared the addition of AVANDIA to metformin or a sulfonylurea (N = 2,220) with a control group of metformin plus sulfonylurea (N = 2,227) in patients with type 2 diabetes *[see Adverse Reactions (6.1)]*. Non-inferiority was demonstrated for the primary endpoint, cardiovascular hospitalization or cardiovascular death, for AVANDIA compared with control [HR 0.99 (95% CI: 0.85, 1.16)] demonstrating no overall increased risk in cardiovascular morbidity or mortality. The hazard ratios for total mortality and MACE were consistent with the primary endpoint and the 95% CI similarly excluded a 20% increase in risk for AVANDIA. The hazard ratios for the components of MACE were 0.72 (95% CI: 0.49, 1.06) for stroke, 1.14 (95% CI: 0.80, 1.63) for myocardial infarction, and 0.84 (95% CI: 0.59, 1.18) for cardiovascular death.
The results of RECORD are consistent with the findings of 2 earlier long-term, prospective, randomized, controlled clinical trials (each trial >3 years' duration; total of 9,620 patients) (see Figure 1). In patients with impaired glucose tolerance (DREAM trial), although the incidence of cardiovascular events was higher among subjects who were randomized to AVANDIA in combination with ramipril than among subjects randomized to ramipril alone, no statistically significant differences were observed for MACE and its components between AVANDIA and placebo. In type 2 diabetes patients who were initiating oral agent monotherapy (ADOPT trial), no statistically significant differences were observed for MACE and its components between AVANDIA and metformin or a sulfonylurea.
[See figure 1 above]
Cardiovascular Events in a Group of 52 Clinical Trials: In a meta-analysis of 52 double-blind, randomized, controlled clinical trials designed to assess glucose-lowering efficacy in type 2 diabetes (mean duration 6 months), a statistically significant increased risk of myocardial infarction with AVANDIA versus pooled comparators was observed [0.4% versus 0.3%; OR 1.8, (95% CI: 1.03, 3.25)]. A statistically non-significant increased risk of MACE was observed with AVANDIA versus pooled comparators (OR 1.44, 95% CI: 0.95, 2.20). In the placebo-controlled trials, a statistically significant increased risk of myocardial infarction [0.4% versus 0.2%, OR 2.23 (95% CI: 1.14, 4.64)] and statistically non-significant increased risk of MACE [0.7% versus 0.5%, OR 1.53 (95% CI: 0.94, 2.54)] with AVANDIA were observed. In the active-controlled trials, there was no increased risk of myocardial infarction or MACE.
Mortality in Observational Studies of AVANDIA Compared to Pioglitazone: Three observational studies in elderly diabetic patients (age 65 years and older) found that AVANDIA statistically significantly increased the risk of all-cause mortality compared to use of pioglitazone. One observational study in patients with a mean age of 54 years found no difference in all-cause mortality between patients treated with AVANDIA compared to pioglitazone and reported similar results in the subpopulation of patients >65 years of age. One additional small, prospective, observational study found no statistically significant differences for CV mortality and all-cause mortality in patients treated with AVANDIA compared to pioglitazone.

5.3 Edema
AVANDIA should be used with caution in patients with edema. In a clinical trial in healthy volunteers who received 8 mg of AVANDIA once daily for 8 weeks, there was a statistically significant increase in median plasma volume compared with placebo.
Since thiazolidinediones, including rosiglitazone, can cause fluid retention, which can exacerbate or lead to congestive heart failure, AVANDIA should be used with caution in patients at risk for heart failure. Patients should be monitored for signs and symptoms of heart failure *[see Boxed Warning, Warnings and Precautions (5.1), Patient Counseling Information (17)]*.
In controlled clinical trials of patients with type 2 diabetes, mild to moderate edema was reported in patients treated with AVANDIA, and may be dose related. Patients with ongoing edema were more likely to have adverse events associated with edema if started on combination therapy with insulin and AVANDIA *[see Adverse Reactions (6.1)]*.

5.4 Weight Gain
Dose-related weight gain was seen with AVANDIA alone and in combination with other hypoglycemic agents (Table 2). The mechanism of weight gain is unclear but probably involves a combination of fluid retention and fat accumulation.
In postmarketing experience, there have been reports of unusually rapid increases in weight and increases in excess of that generally observed in clinical trials. Patients who experience such increases should be assessed for fluid accumulation and volume-related events such as excessive edema and congestive heart failure *[see Boxed Warning]*.
[See table 2 at top of next page]
In a 4- to 6-year, monotherapy, comparative trial (ADOPT) in patients recently diagnosed with type 2 diabetes not previously treated with antidiabetic medication *[see Clinical Studies (14.1)]*, the median weight change (25th, 75th percentiles) from baseline at 4 years was 3.5 kg (0.0, 8.1) for AVANDIA, 2.0 kg (-1.0, 4.8) for glyburide, and -2.4 kg (-5.4, 0.5) for metformin.
In a 24-week trial in pediatric patients aged 10 to 17 years treated with AVANDIA 4 to 8 mg daily, a median weight gain of 2.8 kg (25th, 75th percentiles: 0.0, 5.8) was reported.

5.5 Hepatic Effects
Liver enzymes should be measured prior to the initiation of therapy with AVANDIA in all patients and periodically thereafter per the clinical judgment of the healthcare professional. Therapy with AVANDIA should not be initiated in patients with increased baseline liver enzyme levels (ALT >2.5× upper limit of normal). Patients with mildly elevated liver enzymes (ALT levels ≤2.5× upper limit of normal) at baseline or during therapy with AVANDIA should be evaluated to determine the cause of the liver enzyme elevation. Initiation of, or continuation of, therapy with AVANDIA in patients with mild liver enzyme elevations should proceed with caution and include close clinical follow-up, including liver enzyme monitoring, to determine if the liver enzyme elevations resolve or worsen. If at any time ALT levels increase to >3× the upper limit of normal in patients on therapy with AVANDIA, liver enzyme levels should be rechecked as soon as possible. If ALT levels remain >3× the upper limit of normal, therapy with AVANDIA should be discontinued.
If any patient develops symptoms suggesting hepatic dysfunction, which may include unexplained nausea, vomiting, abdominal pain, fatigue, anorexia and/or dark urine, liver enzymes should be checked. The decision whether to continue the patient on therapy with AVANDIA should be

guided by clinical judgment pending laboratory evaluations. If jaundice is observed, drug therapy should be discontinued. *[See Adverse Reactions (6.2, 6.3).]*

5.6 Macular Edema

Macular edema has been reported in postmarketing experience in some diabetic patients who were taking AVANDIA or another thiazolidinedione. Some patients presented with blurred vision or decreased visual acuity, but some patients appear to have been diagnosed on routine ophthalmologic examination. Most patients had peripheral edema at the time macular edema was diagnosed. Some patients had improvement in their macular edema after discontinuation of their thiazolidinedione. Patients with diabetes should have regular eye exams by an ophthalmologist, per the Standards of Care of the American Diabetes Association. Additionally, any diabetic who reports any kind of visual symptom should be promptly referred to an ophthalmologist, regardless of the patient's underlying medications or other physical findings. *[see Adverse Reactions (6.1).]*

5.7 Fractures

Long-term trials (ADOPT and RECORD) show an increased incidence of bone fracture in patients, particularly female patients, taking AVANDIA *[see Adverse Reactions (6.1)]*. This increased incidence was noted after the first year of treatment and persisted during the course of the trial. The majority of the fractures in the women who received AVANDIA occurred in the upper arm, hand, and foot. These sites of fracture are different from those usually associated with postmenopausal osteoporosis (e.g., hip or spine). Other trials suggest that this risk may also apply to men, although the risk of fracture among women appears higher than that among men. The risk of fracture should be considered in the care of patients treated with AVANDIA, and attention given to assessing and maintaining bone health according to current standards of care.

5.8 Hematologic Effects

Decreases in mean hemoglobin and hematocrit occurred in a dose-related fashion in adult patients treated with AVANDIA *[see Adverse Reactions (6.2)]*. The observed changes may be related to the increased plasma volume observed with treatment with AVANDIA.

5.9 Diabetes and Blood Glucose Control

Patients receiving AVANDIA in combination with other hypoglycemic agents may be at risk for hypoglycemia, and a reduction in the dose of the concomitant agent may be necessary.

Periodic fasting blood glucose and HbA1c measurements should be performed to monitor therapeutic response.

5.10 Ovulation

Therapy with AVANDIA, like other thiazolidinediones, may result in ovulation in some premenopausal anovulatory women. As a result, these patients may be at an increased risk for pregnancy while taking AVANDIA *[see Use in Specific Populations (8.1)]*. Thus, adequate contraception in premenopausal women should be recommended. This possible effect has not been specifically investigated in clinical trials; therefore, the frequency of this occurrence is not known. Although hormonal imbalance has been seen in preclinical studies *[see Nonclinical Toxicology (13.1)]*, the clinical significance of this finding is not known. If unexpected menstrual dysfunction occurs, the benefits of continued therapy with AVANDIA should be reviewed.

6 ADVERSE REACTIONS

The following adverse reactions are discussed in more detail elsewhere in the labeling:

- Cardiac Failure *[see Warnings and Precautions (5.1)]*
- Major Adverse Cardiovascular Events *[see Warnings and Precautions (5.2)]*
- Edema *[see Warnings and Precautions (5.3)]*
- Weight Gain *[see Warnings and Precautions (5.4)]*
- Hepatic Effects *[see Warnings and Precautions (5.5)]*
- Macular Edema *[see Warnings and Precautions (5.6)]*
- Fractures *[see Warnings and Precautions (5.7)]*
- Hematologic Effects *[see Warnings and Precautions (5.8)]*
- Ovulation *[see Warnings and Precautions (5.10)]*

6.1 Clinical Trial Experience

Because clinical trials are conducted under widely varying conditions, adverse reaction rates observed in the clinical trials of a drug cannot be directly compared with rates in the clinical trials of another drug and may not reflect the rates observed in practice.

Adult: In clinical trials, approximately 9,900 patients with type 2 diabetes have been treated with AVANDIA.

Short-term Trials of AVANDIA as Monotherapy and in Combination With Other Hypoglycemic Agents: The incidence and types of adverse events reported in short-term clinical trials of AVANDIA as monotherapy are shown in Table 3.

[See table 3 above]

Overall, the types of adverse reactions without regard to causality reported when AVANDIA was used in combination with a sulfonylurea or metformin were similar to those during monotherapy with AVANDIA.

Table 2. Weight Changes (kg) From Baseline at Endpoint During Clinical Trials

Monotherapy	Duration		Control Group Median (25th, 75th percentiles)	AVANDIA 4 mg Median (25th, 75th percentiles)	AVANDIA 8 mg Median (25th, 75th percentiles)
	26 weeks	placebo	-0.9 (-2.8, 0.9) N = 210	1.0 (-0.9, 3.6) N = 436	3.1 (1.1, 5.8) N = 439
	52 weeks	sulfonylurea	2.0 (0, 4.0) N = 173	2.0 (-0.6, 4.0) N = 150	2.6 (0, 5.3) N = 157
Combination Therapy					
Sulfonylurea	24-26 weeks	sulfonylurea	0 (-1.0, 1.3) N = 1,155	2.2 (0.5, 4.0) N = 613	3.5 (1.4, 5.9) N = 841
Metformin	26 weeks	metformin	-1.4 (-3.2, 0.2) N = 175	0.8 (-1.0, 2.6) N = 100	2.1 (0, 4.3) N = 184
Insulin	26 weeks	insulin	0.9 (-0.5, 2.7) N = 162	4.1 (1.4, 6.3) N = 164	5.4 (3.4, 7.3) N = 150
Sulfonylurea + metformin	26 weeks	sulfonylurea + metformin	0.2 (-1.2, 1.6) N = 272	2.5 (0.8, 4.6) N = 275	4.5 (2.4, 7.3) N = 276

Table 3. Adverse Events (≥5% in any Treatment Group) Reported by Patients in Short-term[a] Double-blind Clinical Trials With AVANDIA as Monotherapy

Preferred Term	AVANDIA Monotherapy N = 2,526 %	Placebo N = 601 %	Metformin N = 225 %	Sulfonylureas[b] N = 626 %
Upper respiratory tract infection	9.9	8.7	8.9	7.3
Injury	7.6	4.3	7.6	6.1
Headache	5.9	5.0	8.9	5.4
Back pain	4.0	3.8	4.0	5.0
Hyperglycemia	3.9	5.7	4.4	8.1
Fatigue	3.6	5.0	4.0	1.9
Sinusitis	3.2	4.5	5.3	3.0
Diarrhea	2.3	3.3	15.6	3.0
Hypoglycemia	0.6	0.2	1.3	5.9

[a] Short-term trials ranged from 8 weeks to 1 year.
[b] Includes patients receiving glyburide (N = 514), gliclazide (N = 91), or glipizide (N = 21).

Events of anemia and edema tended to be reported more frequently at higher doses, and were generally mild to moderate in severity and usually did not require discontinuation of treatment with AVANDIA.

In double-blind trials, anemia was reported in 1.9% of patients receiving AVANDIA as monotherapy compared with 0.7% on placebo, 0.6% on sulfonylureas, and 2.2% on metformin. Reports of anemia were greater in patients treated with a combination of AVANDIA and metformin (7.1%) and with a combination of AVANDIA and a sulfonylurea plus metformin (6.7%) compared with monotherapy with AVANDIA or in combination with a sulfonylurea (2.3%). Lower pre-treatment hemoglobin/hematocrit levels in patients enrolled in the metformin combination clinical trials may have contributed to the higher reporting rate of anemia in these trials *[see Adverse Reactions (6.2)]*.

In clinical trials, edema was reported in 4.8% of patients receiving AVANDIA as monotherapy compared with 1.3% on placebo, 1.0% on sulfonylureas, and 2.2% on metformin. The reporting rate of edema was higher for AVANDIA 8 mg in sulfonylurea combinations (12.4%) compared with other combinations, with the exception of insulin. Edema was reported in 14.7% of patients receiving AVANDIA in the insulin combination trials compared with 5.4% on insulin alone. Reports of new onset or exacerbation of congestive heart failure occurred at rates of 1% for insulin alone, and 2% (4 mg) and 3% (8 mg) for insulin in combination with AVANDIA *[see Boxed Warning, Warnings and Precautions (5.1)]*.

In controlled combination therapy trials with sulfonylureas, mild to moderate hypoglycemic symptoms, which appear to be dose related, were reported. Few patients were withdrawn for hypoglycemia (<1%) and few episodes of hypoglycemia were considered to be severe (<1%). Hypoglycemia was the most frequently reported adverse event in the fixed-dose insulin combination trials, although few patients withdrew for hypoglycemia (4 of 408 for AVANDIA plus insulin and 1 of 203 for insulin alone). Rates of hypoglycemia, confirmed by capillary blood glucose concentration ≤50 mg/dL, were 6% for insulin alone and 12% (4 mg) and 14% (8 mg) for insulin in combination with AVANDIA. *[See Warnings and Precautions (5.9).]*

Long-term Trial of AVANDIA as Monotherapy: A 4- to 6-year trial (ADOPT) compared the use of AVANDIA (n = 1,456), glyburide (n = 1,441), and metformin (n = 1,454) as monotherapy in patients recently diagnosed with type 2 diabetes who were not previously treated with antidiabetic medication. Table 4 presents adverse reactions without regard to causality; rates are expressed per 100 patient-years (PY) exposure to account for the differences in exposure to trial medication across the 3 treatment groups.

In ADOPT, fractures were reported in a greater number of women treated with AVANDIA (9.3%, 2.7/100 patient-years) compared with glyburide (3.5%, 1.3/100 patient-years) or metformin (5.1%, 1.5/100 patient-years). The majority of the fractures in the women who received rosiglitazone were reported in the upper arm, hand, and foot. *[See Warnings and Precautions (5.7).]* The observed incidence of fractures for male patients was similar among the 3 treatment groups.

Table 4. On-therapy Adverse Events [≥5 Events/100 Patient-Years (PY)] in any Treatment Group Reported in a 4- to 6-Year Clinical Trial of AVANDIA as Monotherapy (ADOPT)

Preferred Term	AVANDIA N = 1,456 PY = 4,954	Glyburide N = 1,441 PY = 4,244	Metformin N = 1,454 PY = 4,906
Nasopharyngitis	6.3	6.9	6.6
Back pain	5.1	4.9	5.3

Table 5. Cardiovascular (CV) Outcomes for the RECORD Trial

Primary Endpoint	AVANDIA N = 2,220	Active Control N = 2,227	Hazard Ratio	95% CI
CV death or CV hospitalization	321	323	0.99	0.85-1.16
Secondary Endpoint				
All-cause death	136	157	0.86	0.68-1.08
CV death	60	71	0.84	0.59-1.18
Myocardial infarction	64	56	1.14	0.80-1.63
Stroke	46	63	0.72	0.49-1.06
CV death, myocardial infarction, or stroke	154	165	0.93	0.74-1.15
Heart failure	61	29	2.10	1.35-3.27

Arthralgia	5.0	4.8	4.2
Hypertension	4.4	6.0	6.1
Upper respiratory tract infection	4.3	5.0	4.7
Hypoglycemia	2.9	13.0	3.4
Diarrhea	2.5	3.2	6.8

Long-term Trial of AVANDIA as Combination Therapy (RECORD): RECORD (Rosiglitazone Evaluated for Cardiac Outcomes and Regulation of Glycemia in Diabetes) was a multicenter, randomized, open-label, non-inferiority trial in subjects with type 2 diabetes inadequately controlled on maximum doses of metformin or sulfonylurea (glyburide, gliclazide, or glimepiride) to compare the time to reach the combined cardiovascular endpoint of cardiovascular death or cardiovascular hospitalization between patients randomized to the addition of AVANDIA versus metformin or sulfonylurea. The trial included patients who have failed metformin or sulfonylurea monotherapy; those who failed metformin (n = 2,222) were randomized to receive either AVANDIA as add-on therapy (n = 1,117) or add-on sulfonylurea (n = 1,105), and those who failed sulfonylurea (n = 2,225) were randomized to receive either AVANDIA as add-on therapy (n = 1,103) or add-on metformin (n = 1,122). Patients were treated to target HbA1c ≤7% throughout the trial.

The mean age of patients in this trial was 58 years, 52% were male, and the mean duration of follow-up was 5.5 years. AVANDIA demonstrated non-inferiority to active control for the primary endpoint of cardiovascular hospitalization or cardiovascular death (HR 0.99, 95% CI: 0.85-1.16). There were no significant differences between groups for secondary endpoints with the exception of congestive heart failure (see Table 5). The incidence of congestive heart failure was significantly greater among patients randomized to AVANDIA.

[See table 5 above]

There was an increased incidence of bone fracture for subjects randomized to AVANDIA in addition to metformin or sulfonylurea compared with those randomized to metformin plus sulfonylurea (8.3% versus 5.3%) *[see Warnings and Precautions (5.7)]*. The majority of fractures were reported in the upper limbs and distal lower limbs. The risk of fracture appeared to be higher in females relative to control (11.5% versus 6.3%), than in males relative to control (5.3% versus 4.3%). Additional data are necessary to determine whether there is an increased risk of fracture in males after a longer period of follow-up.

Pediatric: AVANDIA has been evaluated for safety in a single, active-controlled trial of pediatric patients with type 2 diabetes in which 99 were treated with AVANDIA and 101 were treated with metformin. The most common adverse reactions (>10%) without regard to causality for either AVANDIA or metformin were headache (17% versus 14%), nausea (4% versus 11%), nasopharyngitis (3% versus 12%), and diarrhea (1% versus 13%). In this trial, one case of diabetic ketoacidosis was reported in the metformin group. In addition, there were 3 patients in the rosiglitazone group who had FPG of approximately 300 mg/dL, 2+ ketonuria, and an elevated anion gap.

6.2 Laboratory Abnormalities
Hematologic: Decreases in mean hemoglobin and hematocrit occurred in a dose-related fashion in adult patients treated with AVANDIA (mean decreases in individual trials as much as 1.0 g/dL hemoglobin and as much as 3.3% hematocrit). The changes occurred primarily during the first 3 months following initiation of therapy with AVANDIA or following a dose increase in AVANDIA. The time course and magnitude of decreases were similar in patients treated with a combination of AVANDIA and other hypoglycemic agents or monotherapy with AVANDIA. Pre-treatment levels of hemoglobin and hematocrit were lower in patients in metformin combination trials and may have contributed to the higher reporting rate of anemia. In a single trial in pediatric patients, decreases in hemoglobin and hematocrit (mean decreases of 0.29 g/dL and 0.95%, respectively) were reported. Small decreases in hemoglobin and hematocrit have also been reported in pediatric patients treated with AVANDIA. White blood cell counts also decreased slightly in adult patients treated with AVANDIA. Decreases in hematologic parameters may be related to increased plasma volume observed with treatment with AVANDIA.

Lipids: Changes in serum lipids have been observed following treatment with AVANDIA in adults *[see Clinical Pharmacology (12.2)]*. Small changes in serum lipid parameters were reported in children treated with AVANDIA for 24 weeks.

Serum Transaminase Levels: In pre-approval clinical trials in 4,598 patients treated with AVANDIA (3,600 patient-years of exposure) and in a long-term 4- to 6-year trial in 1,456 patients treated with AVANDIA (4,954 patient-years exposure), there was no evidence of drug-induced hepatotoxicity.

In pre-approval controlled trials, 0.2% of patients treated with AVANDIA had elevations in ALT >3× the upper limit of normal compared with 0.2% on placebo and 0.5% on active comparators. The ALT elevations in patients treated with AVANDIA were reversible. Hyperbilirubinemia was found in 0.3% of patients treated with AVANDIA compared with 0.9% treated with placebo and 1% in patients treated with active comparators. In pre-approval clinical trials, there were no cases of idiosyncratic drug reactions leading to hepatic failure. *[See Warnings and Precautions (5.5).]*

In the 4- to 6-year ADOPT trial, patients treated with AVANDIA (4,954 patient-years exposure), glyburide (4,244 patient-years exposure), or metformin (4,906 patient-years exposure), as monotherapy, had the same rate of ALT increase to >3× upper limit of normal (0.3 per 100 patient-years exposure).

In the RECORD trial, patients randomized to AVANDIA in addition to metformin or sulfonylurea (10,849 patient-years exposure) and to metformin plus sulfonylurea (10,209 patient-years exposure) had a rate of ALT increase to ≥3× upper limit of normal of approximately 0.2 and 0.3 per 100 patient-years exposure, respectively.

6.3 Postmarketing Experience
In addition to adverse reactions reported from clinical trials, the events described below have been identified during post-approval use of AVANDIA. Because these events are reported voluntarily from a population of unknown size, it is not possible to reliably estimate their frequency or to always establish a causal relationship to drug exposure.

In patients receiving thiazolidinedione therapy, serious adverse events with or without a fatal outcome, potentially related to volume expansion (e.g., congestive heart failure, pulmonary edema, and pleural effusions) have been reported *[see Boxed Warning, Warnings and Precautions (5.1)]*.

There are postmarketing reports with AVANDIA of hepatitis, hepatic enzyme elevations to 3 or more times the upper limit of normal, and hepatic failure with and without fatal outcome, although causality has not been established.

There are postmarketing reports with AVANDIA of rash, pruritus, urticaria, angioedema, anaphylactic reaction, Stevens-Johnson syndrome *[see Contraindications (4)]*, and new onset or worsening diabetic macular edema with decreased visual acuity *[see Warnings and Precautions (5.6)]*.

7 DRUG INTERACTIONS
7.1 CYP2C8 Inhibitors and Inducers
An inhibitor of CYP2C8 (e.g., gemfibrozil) may increase the AUC of rosiglitazone and an inducer of CYP2C8 (e.g., rifam-pin) may decrease the AUC of rosiglitazone. Therefore, if an inhibitor or an inducer of CYP2C8 is started or stopped during treatment with rosiglitazone, changes in diabetes treatment may be needed based upon clinical response. *[See Clinical Pharmacology (12.4).]*

8 USE IN SPECIFIC POPULATIONS
8.1 Pregnancy
Pregnancy Category C.
All pregnancies have a background risk of birth defects, loss, or other adverse outcome regardless of drug exposure. This background risk is increased in pregnancies complicated by hyperglycemia and may be decreased with good metabolic control. It is essential for patients with diabetes or history of gestational diabetes to maintain good metabolic control before conception and throughout pregnancy. Careful monitoring of glucose control is essential in such patients. Most experts recommend that insulin monotherapy be used during pregnancy to maintain blood glucose levels as close to normal as possible.
Human Data: Rosiglitazone has been reported to cross the human placenta and be detectable in fetal tissue. The clinical significance of these findings is unknown. There are no adequate and well-controlled trials in pregnant women. AVANDIA should be used during pregnancy only if the potential benefit justifies the potential risk to the fetus.
Animal Studies: There was no effect on implantation or the embryo with rosiglitazone treatment during early pregnancy in rats, but treatment during mid-late gestation was associated with fetal death and growth retardation in both rats and rabbits. Teratogenicity was not observed at doses up to 3 mg/kg in rats and 100 mg/kg in rabbits (approximately 20 and 75 times human AUC at the maximum recommended human daily dose, respectively). Rosiglitazone caused placental pathology in rats (3 mg/kg/day). Treatment of rats during gestation through lactation reduced litter size, neonatal viability, and postnatal growth, with growth retardation reversible after puberty. For effects on the placenta, embryo/fetus, and offspring, the no-effect dose was 0.2 mg/kg in rats and 15 mg/kg/day in rabbits. These no-effect levels are approximately 4 times human AUC at the maximum recommended human daily dose. Rosiglitazone reduced the number of uterine implantations and live offspring when juvenile female rats were treated at 40 mg/kg/day from 27 days of age through to sexual maturity (approximately 68 times human AUC at the maximum recommended daily dose). The no-effect level was 2 mg/kg/day (approximately 4 times human AUC at the maximum recommended daily dose). There was no effect on pre- or post-natal survival or growth.

8.2 Labor and Delivery
The effect of rosiglitazone on labor and delivery in humans is not known.

8.3 Nursing Mothers
Drug-related material was detected in milk from lactating rats. It is not known whether AVANDIA is excreted in human milk. Because many drugs are excreted in human milk, a decision should be made whether to discontinue nursing or to discontinue AVANDIA, taking into account the importance of the drug to the mother.

8.4 Pediatric Use
After placebo run-in including diet counseling, children with type 2 diabetes mellitus, aged 10 to 17 years and with a baseline mean body mass index (BMI) of 33 kg/m², were randomized to treatment with 2 mg twice daily of AVANDIA (n = 99) or 500 mg twice daily of metformin (n = 101) in a 24-week, double-blind clinical trial. As expected, FPG decreased in patients naïve to diabetes medication (n = 104) and increased in patients withdrawn from prior medication (usually metformin) (n = 90) during the run-in period. After at least 8 weeks of treatment, 49% of patients treated with AVANDIA and 55% of metformin-treated patients had their dose doubled if FPG >126 mg/dL. For the overall intent-to-treat population, at Week 24, the mean change from baseline in HbA1c was -0.14% with AVANDIA and -0.49% with metformin. There was an insufficient number of patients in this trial to establish statistically whether these observed mean treatment effects were similar or different. Treatment effects differed for patients naïve to therapy with antidiabetic drugs and for patients previously treated with antidiabetic therapy (Table 6).
[See table 6 on next page]
Treatment differences depended on baseline BMI or weight such that the effects of AVANDIA and metformin appeared more closely comparable among heavier patients. The median weight gain was 2.8 kg with rosiglitazone and 0.2 kg with metformin *[see Warnings and Precautions (5.4)]*. Fifty-four percent of patients treated with rosiglitazone and 32% of patients treated with metformin gained ≥2 kg, and 33% of patients treated with rosiglitazone and 7% of patients treated with metformin gained ≥5 kg on trial.

Adverse events observed in this trial are described in *Adverse Reactions (6.1)*.

Figure 2. Mean HbA1c Over Time in a 24-Week Trial of AVANDIA and Metformin in Pediatric Patients — Drug-naïve Subgroup

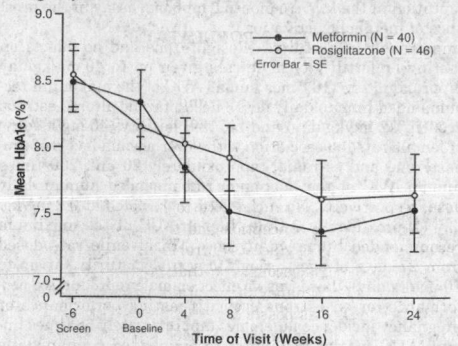

8.5 Geriatric Use

Results of the population pharmacokinetic analysis showed that age does not significantly affect the pharmacokinetics of rosiglitazone *[see Clinical Pharmacology (12.3)]*. Therefore, no dosage adjustments are required for the elderly. In controlled clinical trials, no overall differences in safety and effectiveness between older (≥65 years) and younger (<65 years) patients were observed.

10 OVERDOSAGE

Limited data are available with regard to overdosage in humans. In clinical trials in volunteers, AVANDIA has been administered at single oral doses of up to 20 mg and was well tolerated. In the event of an overdose, appropriate supportive treatment should be initiated as dictated by the patient's clinical status.

11 DESCRIPTION

AVANDIA (rosiglitazone maleate) is an oral antidiabetic agent which acts primarily by increasing insulin sensitivity. AVANDIA improves glycemic control while reducing circulating insulin levels.

Rosiglitazone maleate is not chemically or functionally related to the sulfonylureas, the biguanides, or the alpha-glucosidase inhibitors.

Chemically, rosiglitazone maleate is (±)-5-[[4-[2-(methyl-2-pyridinylamino)ethoxy]phenyl]methyl]-2,4-thiazolidinedione, (Z)-2-butenedioate (1:1) with a molecular weight of 473.52 (357.44 free base). The molecule has a single chiral center and is present as a racemate. Due to rapid interconversion, the enantiomers are functionally indistinguishable. The structural formula of rosiglitazone maleate is:

The molecular formula is $C_{18}H_{19}N_3O_3S \bullet C_4H_4O_4$. Rosiglitazone maleate is a white to off-white solid with a melting point range of 122° to 123°C. The pKa values of rosiglitazone maleate are 6.8 and 6.1. It is readily soluble in ethanol and a buffered aqueous solution with pH of 2.3; solubility decreases with increasing pH in the physiological range.

Each pentagonal film-coated TILTAB tablet contains rosiglitazone maleate equivalent to rosiglitazone, 2 mg, 4 mg, or 8 mg, for oral administration. Inactive ingredients are: hypromellose 2910, lactose monohydrate, magnesium stearate, microcrystalline cellulose, polyethylene glycol 3000, sodium starch glycolate, titanium dioxide, triacetin, and 1 or more of the following: synthetic red and yellow iron oxides and talc.

12 CLINICAL PHARMACOLOGY

12.1 Mechanism of Action

Rosiglitazone, a member of the thiazolidinedione class of antidiabetic agents, improves glycemic control by improving insulin sensitivity. Rosiglitazone is a highly selective and potent agonist for the peroxisome proliferator-activated receptor-gamma (PPARγ). In humans, PPAR receptors are found in key target tissues for insulin action such as adipose tissue, skeletal muscle, and liver. Activation of PPARγ nuclear receptors regulates the transcription of insulin-responsive genes involved in the control of glucose production, transport, and utilization. In addition, PPARγ-responsive genes also participate in the regulation of fatty acid metabolism.

Insulin resistance is a common feature characterizing the pathogenesis of type 2 diabetes. The antidiabetic activity of rosiglitazone has been demonstrated in animal models of type 2 diabetes in which hyperglycemia and/or impaired glucose tolerance is a consequence of insulin resistance in target tissues. Rosiglitazone reduces blood glucose concentrations and reduces hyperinsulinemia in the ob/ob obese mouse, db/db diabetic mouse, and fa/fa fatty Zucker rat.

In animal models, the antidiabetic activity of rosiglitazone was shown to be mediated by increased sensitivity to insulin's action in the liver, muscle, and adipose tissues. Pharmacological studies in animal models indicate that rosiglitazone inhibits hepatic gluconeogenesis. The expression of the insulin-regulated glucose transporter GLUT-4 was increased in adipose tissue. Rosiglitazone did not induce hypoglycemia in animal models of type 2 diabetes and/or impaired glucose tolerance.

12.2 Pharmacodynamics

Patients with lipid abnormalities were not excluded from clinical trials of AVANDIA. In all 26-week controlled trials, across the recommended dose range, AVANDIA as monotherapy was associated with increases in total cholesterol, LDL, and HDL and decreases in free fatty acids. These changes were statistically significantly different from placebo or glyburide controls (Table 7).

Increases in LDL occurred primarily during the first 1 to 2 months of therapy with AVANDIA and LDL levels remained elevated above baseline throughout the trials. In contrast, HDL continued to rise over time. As a result, the LDL/HDL ratio peaked after 2 months of therapy and then appeared to decrease over time. Because of the temporal nature of lipid changes, the 52-week, glyburide-controlled trial is most pertinent to assess long-term effects on lipids. At baseline, Week 26, and Week 52, mean LDL/HDL ratios were 3.1, 3.2, and 3.0, respectively, for AVANDIA 4 mg twice daily. The corresponding values for glyburide were 3.2, 3.1, and 2.9. The differences in change from baseline between AVANDIA and glyburide at Week 52 were statistically significant.

The pattern of LDL and HDL changes following therapy with AVANDIA in combination with other hypoglycemic agents were generally similar to those seen with AVANDIA in monotherapy.

The changes in triglycerides during therapy with AVANDIA were variable and were generally not statistically different from placebo or glyburide controls.

[See table 7 above]

12.3 Pharmacokinetics

Maximum plasma concentration (C_{max}) and the area under the curve (AUC) of rosiglitazone increase in a dose-proportional manner over the therapeutic dose range (Table 8). The elimination half-life is 3 to 4 hours and is independent of dose.

Table 6. Week 24 FPG and HbA1c Change From Baseline Last-observation—carried Forward in Children With Baseline HbA1c >6.5%

Parameter	Naïve Patients		Previously-treated Patients	
	Metformin	Rosiglitazone	Metformin	Rosiglitazone
	N = 40	N = 45	N = 43	N = 32
FPG (mg/dL)				
Baseline (mean)	170	165	221	205
Change from baseline (mean)	-21	-11	-33	-5
Adjusted treatment difference[a] (rosiglitazone–metformin)[b] (95% CI)		8 (-15, 30)		21 (-9, 51)
% of patients with ≥ 30 mg/dL decrease from baseline	43%	27%	44%	28%
HbA1c (%)				
Baseline (mean)	8.3	8.2	8.8	8.5
Change from baseline (mean)	-0.7	-0.5	-0.4	0.1
Adjusted treatment difference[a] (rosiglitazone–metformin)[b] (95% CI)		0.2 (-0.6, 0.9)		0.5 (-0.2, 1.3)
% of patients with ≥ 0.7% decrease from baseline	63%	52%	54%	31%

[a] Change from baseline means are least squares means adjusting for baseline HbA1c, gender, and region.
[b] Positive values for the difference favor metformin.

Table 7. Summary of Mean Lipid Changes in 26-Week, Placebo-controlled and 52-Week, Glyburide-controlled Monotherapy Trials

Parameter	Placebo-controlled Trials Week 26			Glyburide-controlled Trial Week 26 and Week 52			
	Placebo	AVANDIA		Glyburide Titration		AVANDIA 8 mg	
		4 mg Daily[a]	8 mg Daily[a]	Week 26	Week 52	Week 26	Week 52
Free fatty acids							
N	207	428	436	181	168	166	145
Baseline (mean)	18.1	17.5	17.9	26.4	26.4	26.9	26.6
% Change from baseline (mean)	+0.2%	-7.8%	-14.7%	-2.4%	-4.7%	-20.8%	-21.5%
LDL							
N	190	400	374	175	160	161	133
Baseline (mean)	123.7	126.8	125.3	142.7	141.9	142.1	142.1
% Change from baseline (mean)	+4.8%	+14.1%	+18.6%	-0.9%	-0.5%	+11.9%	+12.1%
HDL							
N	208	429	436	184	170	170	145
Baseline (mean)	44.1	44.4	43.0	47.2	47.7	48.4	48.3
% Change from baseline (mean)	+8.0%	+11.4%	+14.2%	+4.3%	+8.7%	+14.0%	+18.5%

[a] Once-daily and twice-daily dosing groups were combined

Table 8. Mean (SD) Pharmacokinetic Parameters for Rosiglitazone Following Single Oral Doses (N = 32)

Parameter	1 mg Fasting	2 mg Fasting	8 mg Fasting	8 mg Fed
AUC_{0-inf} (ng.h/mL)	358 (112)	733 (184)	2,971 (730)	2,890 (795)
C_{max} (ng/mL)	76 (13)	156 (42)	598 (117)	432 (92)
$T\frac{1}{2}$ (h)	3.16 (0.72)	3.15 (0.39)	3.37 (0.63)	3.59 (0.70)

CL/F (L/h)	3.03 (0.87)	2.89 (0.71)	2.85 (0.69)	2.97 (0.81)

AUC = area under the curve; C_{max} = maximum concentration; $T_{1/2}$ = terminal half-life; CL/F = Oral clearance.

Absorption: The absolute bioavailability of rosiglitazone is 99%. Peak plasma concentrations are observed about 1 hour after dosing. Administration of rosiglitazone with food resulted in no change in overall exposure (AUC), but there was an approximately 28% decrease in C_{max} and a delay in T_{max} (1.75 hours). These changes are not likely to be clinically significant; therefore, AVANDIA may be administered with or without food.

Distribution: The mean (CV%) oral volume of distribution (Vss/F) of rosiglitazone is approximately 17.6 (30%) liters, based on a population pharmacokinetic analysis. Rosiglitazone is approximately 99.8% bound to plasma proteins, primarily albumin.

Metabolism: Rosiglitazone is extensively metabolized with no unchanged drug excreted in the urine. The major routes of metabolism were N-demethylation and hydroxylation, followed by conjugation with sulfate and glucuronic acid. All the circulating metabolites are considerably less potent than parent and, therefore, are not expected to contribute to the insulin-sensitizing activity of rosiglitazone.

In vitro data demonstrate that rosiglitazone is predominantly metabolized by Cytochrome P450 (CYP) isoenzyme 2C8, with CYP2C9 contributing as a minor pathway.

Excretion: Following oral or intravenous administration of [^{14}C]rosiglitazone maleate, approximately 64% and 23% of the dose was eliminated in the urine and in the feces, respectively. The plasma half-life of [^{14}C]related material ranged from 103 to 158 hours.

Population Pharmacokinetics in Patients With Type 2 Diabetes: Population pharmacokinetic analyses from 3 large clinical trials including 642 men and 405 women with type 2 diabetes (aged 35 to 80 years) showed that the pharmacokinetics of rosiglitazone are not influenced by age, race, smoking, or alcohol consumption. Both oral clearance (CL/F) and oral steady-state volume of distribution (Vss/F) were shown to increase with increases in body weight. Over the weight range observed in these analyses (50 to 150 kg), the range of predicted CL/F and Vss/F values varied by <1.7-fold and <2.3-fold, respectively. Additionally, rosiglitazone CL/F was shown to be influenced by both weight and gender, being lower (about 15%) in female patients.

Special Populations: *Geriatric:* Results of the population pharmacokinetic analysis (n = 716 <65 years; n = 331 ≥65 years) showed that age does not significantly affect the pharmacokinetics of rosiglitazone.

Gender: Results of the population pharmacokinetics analysis showed that the mean oral clearance of rosiglitazone in female patients (n = 405) was approximately 6% lower compared with male patients of the same body weight (n = 642). As monotherapy and in combination with metformin, AVANDIA improved glycemic control in both males and females. In metformin combination trials, efficacy was demonstrated with no gender differences in glycemic response. In monotherapy trials, a greater therapeutic response was observed in females; however, in more obese patients, gender differences were less evident. For a given body mass index (BMI), females tend to have a greater fat mass than males. Since the molecular target PPARγ is expressed in adipose tissues, this differentiating characteristic may account, at least in part, for the greater response to AVANDIA in females. Since therapy should be individualized, no dose adjustments are necessary based on gender alone.

Hepatic Impairment: Unbound oral clearance of rosiglitazone was significantly lower in patients with moderate to severe liver disease (Child-Pugh Class B/C) compared with healthy subjects. As a result, unbound C_{max} and AUC_{0-inf} were increased 2- and 3-fold, respectively. Elimination half-life for rosiglitazone was about 2 hours longer in patients with liver disease, compared with healthy subjects. Therapy with AVANDIA should not be initiated if the patient exhibits clinical evidence of active liver disease or increased serum transaminase levels (ALT >2.5× upper limit of normal) at baseline [see Warnings and Precautions (5.5)].

Pediatric: Pharmacokinetic parameters of rosiglitazone in pediatric patients were established using a population pharmacokinetic analysis with sparse data from 96 pediatric patients in a single pediatric clinical trial including 33 males and 63 females with ages ranging from 10 to 17 years (weights ranging from 35 to 178.3 kg). Population mean CL/F and V/F of rosiglitazone were 3.15 L/h and 13.5 L, respectively. These estimates of CL/F and V/F were consistent with the typical parameter estimates from a prior adult population analysis.

Renal Impairment: There are no clinically relevant differences in the pharmacokinetics of rosiglitazone in patients with mild to severe renal impairment or in hemodialysis-dependent patients compared with subjects with normal renal function. No dosage adjustment is therefore required in such patients receiving AVANDIA. Since metformin is contraindicated in patients with renal impairment, coadministration of metformin with AVANDIA is contraindicated in these patients.

Race: Results of a population pharmacokinetic analysis including subjects of Caucasian, black, and other ethnic origins indicate that race has no influence on the pharmacokinetics of rosiglitazone.

12.4 Drug-drug Interactions

Drugs That Inhibit, Induce, or are Metabolized by Cytochrome P450: In vitro drug metabolism studies suggest that rosiglitazone does not inhibit any of the major P450 enzymes at clinically relevant concentrations. In vitro data demonstrate that rosiglitazone is predominantly metabolized by CYP2C8, and to a lesser extent, 2C9. AVANDIA (4 mg twice daily) was shown to have no clinically relevant effect on the pharmacokinetics of nifedipine and oral contraceptives (ethinyl estradiol and norethindrone), which are predominantly metabolized by CYP3A4.

Gemfibrozil: Concomitant administration of gemfibrozil (600 mg twice daily), an inhibitor of CYP2C8, and rosiglitazone (4 mg once daily) for 7 days increased rosiglitazone AUC by 127%, compared with the administration of rosiglitazone (4 mg once daily) alone. Given the potential for dose-related adverse events with rosiglitazone, a decrease in the dose of rosiglitazone may be needed when gemfibrozil is introduced [see Drug Interactions (7.1)].

Rifampin: Rifampin administration (600 mg once a day), an inducer of CYP2C8, for 6 days is reported to decrease rosiglitazone AUC by 66%, compared with the administration of rosiglitazone (8 mg) alone [see Drug Interactions (7.1)].[1]

Glyburide: AVANDIA (2 mg twice daily) taken concomitantly with glyburide (3.75 to 10 mg/day) for 7 days did not alter the mean steady-state 24-hour plasma glucose concentrations in diabetic patients stabilized on glyburide therapy. Repeat doses of AVANDIA (8 mg once daily) for 8 days in healthy adult Caucasian subjects caused a decrease in glyburide AUC and C_{max} of approximately 30%. In Japanese subjects, glyburide AUC and C_{max} slightly increased following coadministration of AVANDIA.

Glimepiride: Single oral doses of glimepiride in 14 healthy adult subjects had no clinically significant effect on the steady-state pharmacokinetics of AVANDIA. No clinically significant reductions in glimepiride AUC and C_{max} were observed after repeat doses of AVANDIA (8 mg once daily) for 8 days in healthy adult subjects.

Metformin: Concurrent administration of AVANDIA (2 mg twice daily) and metformin (500 mg twice daily) in healthy volunteers for 4 days had no effect on the steady-state pharmacokinetics of either metformin or rosiglitazone.

Acarbose: Coadministration of acarbose (100 mg three times daily) for 7 days in healthy volunteers had no clinically relevant effect on the pharmacokinetics of a single oral dose of AVANDIA.

Digoxin: Repeat oral dosing of AVANDIA (8 mg once daily) for 14 days did not alter the steady-state pharmacokinetics of digoxin (0.375 mg once daily) in healthy volunteers.

Warfarin: Repeat dosing with AVANDIA had no clinically relevant effect on the steady-state pharmacokinetics of warfarin enantiomers.

Ethanol: A single administration of a moderate amount of alcohol did not increase the risk of acute hypoglycemia in type 2 diabetes mellitus patients treated with AVANDIA.

Ranitidine: Pre-treatment with ranitidine (150 mg twice daily for 4 days) did not alter the pharmacokinetics of either single oral or intravenous doses of rosiglitazone in healthy volunteers. These results suggest that the absorption of oral rosiglitazone is not altered in conditions accompanied by increases in gastrointestinal pH.

13 NONCLINICAL TOXICOLOGY

13.1 Carcinogenesis, Mutagenesis, Impairment of Fertility

Carcinogenesis: A 2-year carcinogenicity study was conducted in Charles River CD-1 mice at doses of 0.4, 1.5, and 6 mg/kg/day in the diet (highest dose equivalent to approximately 12 times human AUC at the maximum recommended human daily dose). Sprague-Dawley rats were dosed for 2 years by oral gavage at doses of 0.05, 0.3, and 2 mg/kg/day (highest dose equivalent to approximately 10 and 20 times human AUC at the maximum recommended human daily dose for male and female rats, respectively). Rosiglitazone was not carcinogenic in the mouse. There was an increase in incidence of adipose hyperplasia in the mouse at doses ≥1.5 mg/kg/day (approximately 2 times human AUC at the maximum recommended human daily dose). In rats, there was a significant increase in the incidence of benign adipose tissue tumors (lipomas) at doses ≥0.3 mg/kg/day (approximately 2 times human AUC at the maximum recommended human daily dose). These proliferative changes in both species are considered due to the persistent pharmacological overstimulation of adipose tissue.

Mutagenesis: Rosiglitazone was not mutagenic or clastogenic in the in vitro bacterial assays for gene mutation, the in vitro chromosome aberration test in human lymphocytes, the in vivo mouse micronucleus test, and the in vivo/in vitro rat UDS assay. There was a small (about 2-fold) increase in mutation in the in vitro mouse lymphoma assay in the presence of metabolic activation.

Impairment of Fertility: Rosiglitazone had no effects on mating or fertility of male rats given up to 40 mg/kg/day (approximately 116 times human AUC at the maximum recommended human daily dose). Rosiglitazone altered estrous cyclicity (2 mg/kg/day) and reduced fertility (40 mg/kg/day) of female rats in association with lower plasma levels of progesterone and estradiol (approximately 20 and 200 times human AUC at the maximum recommended human daily dose, respectively). No such effects were noted at 0.2 mg/kg/day (approximately 3 times human AUC at the maximum recommended human daily dose). In juvenile rats dosed from 27 days of age through to sexual maturity (at up to 40 mg/kg/day), there was no effect on male reproductive performance, or on estrous cyclicity, mating performance or pregnancy incidence in females (approximately 68 times human AUC at the maximum recommended human daily dose). In monkeys, rosiglitazone (0.6 and 4.6 mg/kg/day; approximately 3 and 15 times human AUC at the maximum recommended human daily dose, respectively) diminished the follicular phase rise in serum estradiol with consequential reduction in the luteinizing hormone surge, lower luteal phase progesterone levels, and amenorrhea. The mechanism for these effects appears to be direct inhibition of ovarian steroidogenesis.

13.2 Animal Toxicology

Heart weights were increased in mice (3 mg/kg/day), rats (5 mg/kg/day), and dogs (2 mg/kg/day) with rosiglitazone treatments (approximately 5, 22, and 2 times human AUC at the maximum recommended human daily dose, respectively). Effects in juvenile rats were consistent with those seen in adults. Morphometric measurement indicated that there was hypertrophy in cardiac ventricular tissues, which may be due to increased heart work as a result of plasma volume expansion.

14 CLINICAL STUDIES

Monotherapy

In clinical trials, treatment with AVANDIA resulted in an improvement in glycemic control, as measured by FPG and HbA1c, with a concurrent reduction in insulin and C-peptide. Postprandial glucose and insulin were also reduced. This is consistent with the mechanism of action of AVANDIA as an insulin sensitizer.

The maximum recommended daily dose is 8 mg. Dose-ranging trials suggested that no additional benefit was obtained with a total daily dose of 12 mg.

Short-term Clinical Trials: A total of 2,315 patients with type 2 diabetes, previously treated with diet alone or antidiabetic medication(s), were treated with AVANDIA as monotherapy in 6 double-blind trials, which included two 26-week, placebo-controlled trials; one 52-week, glyburide-controlled trial; and 3 placebo-controlled, dose-ranging trials of 8 to 12 weeks' duration. Previous antidiabetic medication(s) were withdrawn and patients entered a 2- to 4-week placebo run-in period prior to randomization.

Two 26-week, double-blind, placebo-controlled trials, in patients with type 2 diabetes (n = 1,401) with inadequate glycemic control [mean baseline FPG approximately 228 mg/dL (101 to 425 mg/dL) and mean baseline HbA1c 8.9% (5.2% to 16.2%)], were conducted. Treatment with AVANDIA produced statistically significant improvements in FPG and HbA1c compared with baseline and relative to placebo. Data from one of these trials are summarized in Table 9.

[See table 9 at top of next page]

When administered at the same total daily dose, AVANDIA was generally more effective in reducing FPG and HbA1c when administered in divided doses twice daily compared with once-daily doses. However, for HbA1c, the difference between the 4 mg once-daily and 2 mg twice-daily doses was not statistically significant.

Long-term Clinical Trials: Long-term maintenance of effect was evaluated in a 52-week, double-blind, glyburide-controlled trial in patients with type 2 diabetes. Patients were randomized to treatment with AVANDIA 2 mg twice daily (N = 195) or AVANDIA 4 mg twice daily (N = 189) or glyburide (N = 202) for 52 weeks. Patients receiving glyburide were given an initial dosage of either 2.5 mg/day or 5.0 mg/day. The dosage was then titrated in 2.5-mg/day increments over the next 12 weeks, to a maximum dosage of 15.0 mg/day in order to optimize glycemic control. Thereafter, the glyburide dose was kept constant.

The median titrated dose of glyburide was 7.5 mg. All treatments resulted in a statistically significant improvement in glycemic control from baseline (Figure 3 and Figure 4). At the end of Week 52, the reduction from baseline in FPG and HbA1c was -40.8 mg/dL and -0.53% with AVANDIA 4 mg twice daily; -25.4 mg/dL and -0.27% with AVANDIA 2 mg twice daily; and -30.0 mg/dL and -0.72% with glyburide. For HbA1c, the difference between AVANDIA 4 mg twice daily and glyburide was not statistically significant at Week 52. The initial fall in FPG with glyburide was greater than with AVANDIA; however, this effect was less durable over time. The improvement in glycemic control seen with AVANDIA 4 mg twice daily at Week 26 was maintained through Week 52 of the trial.

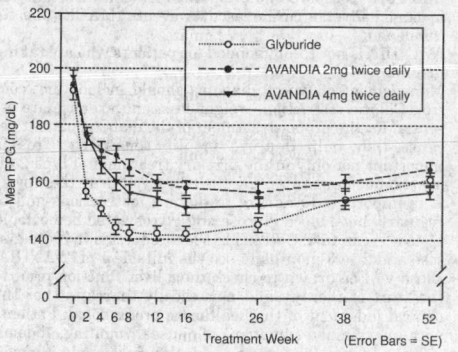

Figure 3. Mean FPG Over Time in a 52-Week, Glyburide-controlled Trial

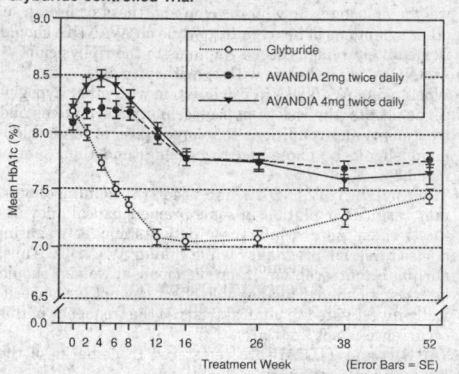

Figure 4. Mean HbA1c Over Time in a 52-Week, Glyburide-controlled Trial

Hypoglycemia was reported in 12.1% of glyburide-treated patients versus 0.5% (2 mg twice daily) and 1.6% (4 mg twice daily) of patients treated with AVANDIA. The improvements in glycemic control were associated with a mean weight gain of 1.75 kg and 2.95 kg for patients treated with 2 mg and 4 mg twice daily of AVANDIA, respectively, versus 1.9 kg in glyburide-treated patients. In patients treated with AVANDIA, C-peptide, insulin, pro-insulin, and pro-insulin split products were significantly reduced in a dose-ordered fashion, compared with an increase in the glyburide-treated patients.

A Diabetes Outcome Progression Trial (ADOPT) was a multicenter, double-blind, controlled trial (N = 4,351) conducted over 4 to 6 years to compare the safety and efficacy of AVANDIA, metformin, and glyburide monotherapy in patients recently diagnosed with type 2 diabetes mellitus (≤3 years) inadequately controlled with diet and exercise. The mean age of patients in this trial was 57 years and the majority of patients (83%) had no known history of cardiovascular disease. The mean baseline FPG and HbA1c were 152 mg/dL and 7.4%, respectively. Patients were randomized to receive either AVANDIA 4 mg once daily, glyburide 2.5 mg once daily, or metformin 500 mg once daily, and doses were titrated to optimal glycemic control up to a maximum of 4 mg twice daily for AVANDIA, 7.5 mg twice daily for glyburide, and 1,000 mg twice daily for metformin. The primary efficacy outcome was time to consecutive FPG >180 mg/dL after at least 6 weeks of treatment at the maximum tolerated dose of study medication or time to inadequate glycemic control, as determined by an independent adjudication committee.

The cumulative incidence of the primary efficacy outcome at 5 years was 15% with AVANDIA, 21% with metformin, and 34% with glyburide (HR 0.68 [95% CI: 0.55, 0.85] versus metformin, HR 0.37 [95% CI: 0.30, 0.45] versus glyburide). Cardiovascular and adverse event data (including effects on body weight and bone fracture) from ADOPT for AVANDIA, metformin, and glyburide are described in *Warnings and Precautions (5.2, 5.4, and 5.7)* and *Adverse Reactions (6.1)*, respectively. As with all medications, efficacy results must be considered together with safety information to assess the potential benefit and risk for an individual patient.

14.2 Combination With Metformin or Sulfonylurea

The addition of AVANDIA to either metformin or sulfonylurea resulted in significant reductions in hyperglycemia compared with either of these agents alone. These results are consistent with an additive effect on glycemic control when AVANDIA is used as combination therapy.

Combination With Metformin: A total of 670 patients with type 2 diabetes participated in two 26-week, randomized, double-blind, placebo/active-controlled trials designed to assess the efficacy of AVANDIA in combination with metformin. AVANDIA, administered in either once-daily or twice-daily dosing regimens, was added to the therapy of patients who were inadequately controlled on a maximum dose (2.5 grams/day) of metformin.

In one trial, patients inadequately controlled on 2.5 grams/day of metformin (mean baseline FPG 216 mg/dL and mean baseline HbA1c 8.8%) were randomized to receive 4 mg of AVANDIA once daily, 8 mg of AVANDIA once daily, or placebo in addition to metformin. A statistically significant improvement in FPG and HbA1c was observed in patients treated with the combinations of metformin and 4 mg of AVANDIA once daily and 8 mg of AVANDIA once daily, versus patients continued on metformin alone (Table 10).
[See table 10 above]

In a second 26-week trial, patients with type 2 diabetes inadequately controlled on 2.5 grams/day of metformin who were randomized to receive the combination of AVANDIA 4 mg twice daily and metformin (N = 105) showed a statistically significant improvement in glycemic control with a mean treatment effect for FPG of -56 mg/dL and a mean treatment effect for HbA1c of -0.8% over metformin alone. The combination of metformin and AVANDIA resulted in lower levels of FPG and HbA1c than either agent alone. Patients who were inadequately controlled on a maximum dose (2.5 grams/day) of metformin and who were switched to monotherapy with AVANDIA demonstrated loss of glycemic control, as evidenced by increases in FPG and HbA1c. In this group, increases in LDL and VLDL were also seen.

Combination With a Sulfonylurea: A total of 3,457 patients with type 2 diabetes participated in ten 24- to 26-week randomized, double-blind, placebo/active-controlled trials and one 2-year double-blind, active-controlled trial in elderly patients designed to assess the efficacy and safety of AVANDIA in combination with a sulfonylurea. AVANDIA 2 mg, 4 mg, or 8 mg daily was administered, either once

daily (3 trials) or in divided doses twice daily (7 trials), to patients inadequately controlled on a submaximal or maximal dose of sulfonylurea.

In these trials, the combination of AVANDIA 4 mg or 8 mg daily (administered as single- or twice-daily divided doses) and a sulfonylurea significantly reduced FPG and HbA1c compared with placebo plus sulfonylurea or further up-titration of the sulfonylurea. Table 11 shows pooled data for 8 trials in which AVANDIA added to sulfonylurea was compared with placebo plus sulfonylurea.
[See table 11 at top of next page]

One of the 24- to 26-week trials included patients who were inadequately controlled on maximal doses of glyburide and switched to 4 mg of AVANDIA daily as monotherapy; in this group, loss of glycemic control was demonstrated, as evidenced by increases in FPG and HbA1c.

In a 2-year, double-blind trial, elderly patients (aged 59 to 89 years) on half-maximal sulfonylurea (glipizide 10 mg twice daily) were randomized to the addition of AVANDIA (n = 115, 4 mg once daily to 8 mg as needed) or to continued up-titration of glipizide (n = 110), to a maximum of 20 mg twice daily. Mean baseline FPG and HbA1c were 157 mg/dL and 7.72%, respectively, for the arm receiving AVANDIA plus glipizide and 159 mg/dL and 7.65%, respectively, for the glipizide up-titration arm. Loss of glycemic control (FPG ≥180 mg/dL) occurred in a significantly lower proportion of patients (2%) on AVANDIA plus glipizide compared with patients in the glipizide up-titration arm (28.7%). About 78% of the patients on combination therapy completed the 2 years of therapy while only 51% completed on glipizide monotherapy. The effect of combination therapy on FPG and HbA1c was durable over the 2-year trial period, with patients achieving a mean of 132 mg/dL for FPG and a mean of 6.98% for HbA1c compared with no change on the glipizide arm.

14.3 Combination With Sulfonylurea Plus Metformin

In two 24- to 26-week, double-blind, placebo-controlled trials designed to assess the efficacy and safety of AVANDIA in combination with sulfonylurea plus metformin, AVANDIA 4 mg or 8 mg daily, was administered in divided doses twice daily, to patients inadequately controlled on submaximal (10 mg) and maximal (20 mg) doses of glyburide and maximal dose of metformin (2 g/day). A statistically significant improvement in FPG and HbA1c was observed in patients treated with the combinations of sulfonylurea plus met-

Table 9. Glycemic Parameters in a 26-Week, Placebo-controlled Trial

Parameter	Placebo	AVANDIA		AVANDIA	
		4 mg Once Daily	2 mg Twice Daily	8 mg Once Daily	4 mg Twice Daily
	N = 173	N = 180	N = 186	N = 181	N = 187
FPG (mg/dL)					
Baseline (mean)	225	229	225	228	228
Change from baseline (mean)	8	-25	-35	-42	-55
Difference from placebo (adjusted mean)	–	-31[a]	-43[a]	-49[a]	-62[a]
% of patients with ≥ 30 mg/dL decrease from baseline	19%	45%	54%	58%	70%
HbA1c (%)					
Baseline (mean)	8.9	8.9	8.9	8.9	9.0
Change from baseline (mean)	0.8	0.0	-0.1	-0.3	-0.7
Difference from placebo (adjusted mean)	–	-0.8[a]	-0.9[a]	-1.1[a]	-1.5[a]
% of patients with ≥ 0.7% decrease from baseline	9%	28%	29%	39%	54%

[a] $P < 0.0001$ compared with placebo.

Table 10. Glycemic Parameters in a 26-Week Combination Trial of AVANDIA Plus Metformin

Parameter	Metformin N = 113	AVANDIA 4 mg Once Daily + Metformin N = 116	AVANDIA 8 mg Once Daily + Metformin N = 110
FPG (mg/dL)			
Baseline (mean)	214	215	220
Change from baseline (mean)	6	-33	-48
Difference from metformin alone (adjusted mean)	–	-40[a]	-53[a]
% of patients with ≥ 30 mg/dL decrease from baseline	20%	45%	61%
HbA1c (%)			
Baseline (mean)	8.6	8.9	8.9
Change from baseline (mean)	0.5	-0.6	-0.8
Difference from metformin alone (adjusted mean)	–	-1.0[a]	-1.2[a]
% of patients with ≥ 0.7% decrease from baseline	11%	45%	52%

[a] $P < 0.0001$ compared with metformin.

Table 11. Glycemic Parameters in 24- to 26-Week Combination Trials of AVANDIA Plus Sulfonylurea

Twice-Daily Divided Dosing (5 Trials)	Sulfonylurea	AVANDIA 2 mg Twice Daily + Sulfonylurea	Sulfonylurea	AVANDIA 4 mg Twice Daily + Sulfonylurea
	N = 397	N = 497	N = 248	N = 346
FPG (mg/dL)				
Baseline (mean)	204	198	188	187
Change from baseline (mean)	11	-29	8	-43
Difference from sulfonylurea alone (adjusted mean)	–	-42[a]	–	-53[a]
% of patients with ≥ 30 mg/dL decrease from baseline	17%	49%	15%	61%
HbA1c (%)				
Baseline (mean)	9.4	9.5	9.3	9.6
Change from baseline (mean)	0.2	-1.0	0.0	-1.6
Difference from sulfonylurea alone (adjusted mean)	–	-1.1[a]	–	-1.4[a]
% of patients with ≥ 0.7% decrease from baseline	21%	60%	23%	75%
Once-Daily Dosing (3 Trials)	Sulfonylurea	AVANDIA 4 mg Once Daily + Sulfonylurea	Sulfonylurea	AVANDIA 8 mg Once Daily + Sulfonylurea
	N = 172	N = 172	N = 173	N = 176
FPG (mg/dL)				
Baseline (mean)	198	206	188	192
Change from baseline (mean)	17	-25	17	-43
Difference from sulfonylurea alone (adjusted mean)	–	-47[a]	–	-66[a]
% of patients with ≥ 30 mg/dL decrease from baseline	17%	48%	19%	55%
HbA1c (%)				
Baseline (mean)	8.6	8.8	8.9	8.9
Change from baseline (mean)	0.4	-0.5	0.1	-1.2
Difference from sulfonylurea alone (adjusted mean)	–	-0.9[a]	–	-1.4[a]
% of patients with ≥ 0.7% decrease from baseline	11%	36%	20%	68%

[a] *P* <0.0001 compared with sulfonylurea alone.

Table 12. Glycemic Parameters in a 26-Week Combination Trial of AVANDIA Plus Sulfonylurea and Metformin

Parameter	Sulfonylurea + Metformin	AVANDIA 2 mg Twice Daily + Sulfonylurea + Metformin	AVANDIA 4 mg Twice Daily + Sulfonylurea + Metformin
	N = 273	N = 276	N = 277
FPG (mg/dL)			
Baseline (mean)	189	190	192
Change from baseline (mean)	14	-19	-40
Difference from sulfonylurea plus metformin (adjusted mean)	–	-30[a]	-52[a]
% of patients with ≥30 mg/dL decrease from baseline	16%	46%	62%
HbA1c (%)			
Baseline (mean)	8.7	8.6	8.7
Change from baseline (mean)	0.2	-0.4	-0.9
Difference from sulfonylurea plus metformin (adjusted mean)	–	-0.6[a]	-1.1[a]
% of patients with ≥0.7% decrease from baseline	16%	39%	63%

[a] *P* <0.0001 compared with placebo.

formin and 4 mg of AVANDIA and 8 mg of AVANDIA versus patients continued on sulfonylurea plus metformin, as shown in Table 12.
[See table 12 above]

15   REFERENCES
1. Park JY, Kim KA, Kang MH, et al. Effect of rifampin on the pharmacokinetics of rosiglitazone in healthy subjects. *Clin Pharmacol Ther* 2004;75:157-162.

16   HOW SUPPLIED/STORAGE AND HANDLING
Each pentagonal film-coated TILTAB tablet contains rosiglitazone as the maleate as follows: 2 mg–pink, de-

bossed with GSK on one side and 2 on the other; 4 mg–orange, debossed with GSK on one side and 4 on the other; 8 mg–red-brown, debossed with GSK on one side and 8 on the other.
2 mg bottles of 60:   NDC 0173-0861-18
4 mg bottles of 30:   NDC 0173-0863-13
8 mg bottles of 30:   NDC 0173-0864-13
Store at 25°C (77°F); excursions 15° to 30°C (59° to 86°F). Dispense in a tight, light-resistant container.

17   PATIENT COUNSELING INFORMATION
Advise the patient to read the FDA-approved patient labeling (Medication Guide).

There are multiple medications available to treat type 2 diabetes. The benefits and risks of each available diabetes medication should be taken into account when choosing a particular diabetes medication for a given patient. Patients should be informed of the following:
• AVANDIA is not recommended for patients with symptomatic heart failure.
• A meta-analysis of mostly short-term trials suggested an increased risk for myocardial infarction with AVANDIA compared with placebo. Data from long-term clinical trials of AVANDIA versus other antidiabetes agents (metformin or sulfonylureas), including a cardiovascular outcome trial (RECORD), observed no difference in overall mortality or in major adverse cardiovascular events (MACE) and its components.
• AVANDIA is not recommended for patients who are taking insulin.
• Management of type 2 diabetes should include diet control. Caloric restriction, weight loss, and exercise are essential for the proper treatment of the diabetic patient because they help improve insulin sensitivity. This is important not only in the primary treatment of type 2 diabetes, but in maintaining the efficacy of drug therapy.
• It is important to adhere to dietary instructions and to regularly have blood glucose and glycosylated hemoglobin tested. It can take 2 weeks to see a reduction in blood glucose and 2 to 3 months to see the full effect of AVANDIA.
• Blood will be drawn to check their liver function prior to the start of therapy and periodically thereafter per the clinical judgment of the healthcare professional. Patients with unexplained symptoms of nausea, vomiting, abdominal pain, fatigue, anorexia, or dark urine should immediately report these symptoms to their physician.
• Patients who experience an unusually rapid increase in weight or edema or who develop shortness of breath or other symptoms of heart failure while on AVANDIA should immediately report these symptoms to their physician.
• AVANDIA can be taken with or without meals.
• When using AVANDIA in combination with other hypoglycemic agents, the risk of hypoglycemia, its symptoms and treatment, and conditions that predispose to its development should be explained to patients and their family members.
• Therapy with AVANDIA, like other thiazolidinediones, may result in ovulation in some premenopausal anovulatory women. As a result, these patients may be at an increased risk for pregnancy while taking AVANDIA. Thus, adequate contraception in premenopausal women should be recommended. This possible effect has not been specifically investigated in clinical trials so the frequency of this occurrence is not known.

AVANDIA and TILTAB are registered trademarks of the GSK group of companies.
GlaxoSmithKline
Research Triangle Park, NC 27709
©2014, the GSK group of companies. All rights reserved.
AVD:32PI

MEDICATION GUIDE
AVANDIA® (ah-VAN-dee-a)
(rosiglitazone maleate) tablets
Read this Medication Guide carefully before you start taking AVANDIA and each time you get a refill. There may be new information. This information does not take the place of talking with your doctor about your medical condition or your treatment. If you have any questions about AVANDIA, ask your doctor or pharmacist.
What is the most important information I should know about AVANDIA?
AVANDIA may cause serious side effects, including:
New or worse heart failure
• The risk of heart failure may be higher in people who take AVANDIA with insulin. Most people who take insulin should not also take AVANDIA.
• AVANDIA can cause your body to keep extra fluid (fluid retention), which leads to swelling (edema) and weight gain. Extra body fluid can make some heart problems worse or lead to heart failure. Heart failure means your heart does not pump blood well enough.
• If you have severe heart failure, you cannot start AVANDIA.
• If you have heart failure with symptoms (such as shortness of breath or swelling), even if these symptoms are not severe, AVANDIA may not be right for you.
Call your doctor right away if you have any of the following:
• swelling or fluid retention, especially in the ankles or legs
• shortness of breath or trouble breathing, especially when you lie down
• an unusually fast increase in weight
• unusual tiredness
AVANDIA can have other serious side effects. Be sure to read the section below "What are possible side effects of AVANDIA?"
What is AVANDIA?
AVANDIA is a prescription medicine used with diet and exercise to treat adults with type 2 ("adult-onset" or "non-insulin dependent") diabetes mellitus ("high blood sugar"),

AVANDIA helps to control high blood sugar. AVANDIA may be used alone or with other diabetes medicines. AVANDIA can help your body respond better to insulin made in your body. AVANDIA does not cause your body to make more insulin.

AVANDIA is not for people with type 1 diabetes mellitus or to treat a condition called diabetic ketoacidosis.

It is not known if AVANDIA is safe and effective in children younger than 18 years old.

Who should not take AVANDIA?

Many people with heart failure should not start taking AVANDIA. See "What should I tell my doctor before taking AVANDIA?"

Do not take AVANDIA if you are allergic to rosiglitazone or any of the ingredients in AVANDIA. See the end of this leaflet for a complete list of ingredients in AVANDIA.

Symptoms of a severe allergic reaction with AVANDIA may include:

• swelling of your face, lips, tongue, or throat
• problems with breathing or swallowing
• skin rash or itching
• raised red areas on your skin (hives)
• blisters on your skin or in your mouth, nose, or eyes
• peeling of your skin
• fainting or feeling dizzy
• very rapid heartbeat

What should I tell my doctor before taking AVANDIA?

Before starting AVANDIA, ask your doctor about what the choices are for diabetes medicines, and what the expected benefits and possible risks are for you in particular.

Before taking AVANDIA, tell your doctor about all of your medical conditions, including if you:

• **have heart problems or heart failure.**
• **have type 1 ("juvenile") diabetes or had diabetic ketoacidosis.** These conditions should be treated with insulin.
• **have a type of diabetic eye disease called macular edema** (swelling of the back of the eye).
• **have liver problems.** Your doctor should do blood tests to check your liver before you start taking AVANDIA and during treatment as needed.
• **had liver problems while taking REZULIN™ (troglitazone), another medicine for diabetes.**
• **are pregnant or plan to become pregnant.** It is not known if AVANDIA can harm your unborn baby. You and your doctor should talk about the best way to control your diabetes during pregnancy. If you are a premenopausal woman (before the "change of life") who does not have regular monthly periods, AVANDIA may increase your chances of becoming pregnant. Talk to your doctor about birth control choices while taking AVANDIA. Tell your doctor right away if you become pregnant while taking AVANDIA.
• **are breastfeeding or planning to breastfeed.** It is not known if AVANDIA passes into breast milk. You and your doctor should decide if you will take AVANDIA or breastfeed. You should not do both.

Tell your doctor about all of the medicines you take including prescription and non-prescription medicines, vitamins or herbal supplements. AVANDIA and certain other medicines can affect each other and may lead to serious side effects including high or low blood sugar, or heart problems. Especially tell your doctor if you take:

• insulin
• **any medicines for high blood pressure, high cholesterol or heart failure, or for prevention of heart disease or stroke.**

Know the medicines you take. Keep a list of your medicines and show it to your doctor and pharmacist before you start a new medicine. They will tell you if it is alright to take AVANDIA with other medicines.

How should I take AVANDIA?

• Take AVANDIA exactly as prescribed. Your doctor will tell you how many tablets to take and how often. The usual daily starting dose is 4 mg a day taken one time each day or 2 mg taken two times each day. Your doctor may need to adjust your dose until your blood sugar is better controlled.
• AVANDIA may be prescribed alone or with other diabetes medicines. This will depend on how well your blood sugar is controlled.
• Take AVANDIA with or without food.
• It can take 2 weeks for AVANDIA to start lowering blood sugar. It may take 2 to 3 months to see the full effect on your blood sugar level.
• If you miss a dose of AVANDIA, take it as soon as you remember, unless it is time to take your next dose. Take your next dose at the usual time. Do not take double doses to make up for a missed dose.
• If you take too much AVANDIA, call your doctor or poison control center right away.
• Test your blood sugar regularly as your doctor tells you.
• Diet and exercise can help your body use its blood sugar better. It is important to stay on your recommended diet, lose extra weight, and get regular exercise while taking AVANDIA.

• Your doctor should do blood tests to check your liver before you start AVANDIA and during treatment as needed. Your doctor should also do regular blood sugar tests (for example, "A1C") to monitor your response to AVANDIA.

What are possible side effects of AVANDIA?

AVANDIA may cause serious side effects including:

• **New or worse heart failure.** See "What is the most important information I should know about AVANDIA?"
• **Heart attack.** AVANDIA may increase the risk of a heart attack. Talk to your doctor about what this means to you.
  Symptoms of a heart attack can include the following:
  ○ chest discomfort in the center of your chest that lasts for more than a few minutes, or that goes away or comes back
  ○ chest discomfort that feels like uncomfortable pressure, squeezing, fullness, or pain
  ○ pain or discomfort in your arms, back, neck, jaw, or stomach
  ○ shortness of breath with or without chest discomfort
  ○ breaking out in a cold sweat
  ○ nausea or vomiting
  ○ feeling lightheaded
  Call your doctor or go to the nearest hospital emergency room right away if you think you are having a heart attack.
• **Swelling (edema).** AVANDIA can cause swelling due to fluid retention. See "What is the most important information I should know about AVANDIA?"
• **Weight gain.** AVANDIA can cause weight gain that may be due to fluid retention or extra body fat. Weight gain can be a serious problem for people with certain conditions including heart problems. See "What is the most important information I should know about AVANDIA?"
• **Liver problems.** It is important for your liver to be working normally when you take AVANDIA. Your doctor should do blood tests to check your liver before you start taking AVANDIA and during treatment as needed. Call your doctor right away if you have unexplained symptoms such as:
  ○ nausea or vomiting
  ○ stomach pain
  ○ unusual or unexplained tiredness
  ○ loss of appetite
  ○ dark urine
  ○ yellowing of your skin or the whites of your eyes.
• **Macular edema** (a diabetic eye disease with swelling in the back of the eye). Tell your doctor right away if you have any changes in your vision. Your doctor should check your eyes regularly. Very rarely, some people have had vision changes due to swelling in the back of the eye while taking AVANDIA.
• **Fractures (broken bones)**, usually in the hand, upper arm, or foot. Talk to your doctor for advice on how to keep your bones healthy.
• **Low red blood cell count (anemia).**
• **Low blood sugar (hypoglycemia).** Lightheadedness, dizziness, shakiness or hunger may mean that your blood sugar is too low. This can happen if you skip meals, if you use another medicine that lowers blood sugar, or if you have certain medical problems. Call your doctor if low blood sugar levels are a problem for you.
• **Ovulation** (release of egg from an ovary in a woman) leading to pregnancy. Ovulation may happen in premenopausal women who do not have regular monthly periods. This can increase the chance of pregnancy. See "What should I tell my doctor before taking AVANDIA?"

The most common side effects of AVANDIA reported in clinical trials included cold-like symptoms and headache.

Call your doctor for medical advice about side effects. You may report side effects to FDA at 1-800-FDA-1088.

How should I store AVANDIA?

• Store AVANDIA at room temperature, 59°F to 86°F (15°C to 30°C). Keep AVANDIA in the container it comes in.
• Safely throw away AVANDIA that is out of date or no longer needed.
• Keep AVANDIA and all medicines out of the reach of children.

General information about AVANDIA

Medicines are sometimes prescribed for purposes other than those listed in a Medication Guide. Do not use AVANDIA for a condition for which it was not prescribed. Do not give AVANDIA to other people, even if they have the same symptoms you have. It may harm them.

This Medication Guide summarizes important information about AVANDIA. If you would like more information, talk with your doctor. You can ask your doctor or pharmacist for information about AVANDIA that is written for healthcare professionals. You can also find out more about AVANDIA by calling 1-888-825-5249.

What are the ingredients in AVANDIA?

Active Ingredient: rosiglitazone maleate.

Inactive Ingredients: hypromellose 2910, lactose monohydrate, magnesium stearate, microcrystalline cellulose, polyethylene glycol 3000, sodium starch glycolate, titanium dioxide, triacetin, and 1 or more of the following: synthetic red and yellow iron oxides and talc.

Always check to make sure that the medicine you are taking is the correct one. AVANDIA tablets are triangles with rounded corners and look like this:

2 mg – pink with "GSK" on one side and "2" on the other.
4 mg – orange with "GSK" on one side and "4" on the other.
8 mg – red-brown with "GSK" on one side and "8" on the other.

AVANDIA is a registered trademark of the GSK group of companies.

REZULIN is a trademark of its respective owner and is not a trademark of the GSK group of companies. The maker of this brand is not affiliated with and does not endorse the GSK group of companies or its products.

This Medication Guide has been approved by the U.S. Food and Drug Administration.

GlaxoSmithKline
Research Triangle Park, NC 27709
©2014, the GSK group of companies. All rights reserved.
May 2014
AVD:8MG

AVODART ℞

[av'ō dart]
(dutasteride)
Soft Gelatin Capsules

HIGHLIGHTS OF PRESCRIBING INFORMATION
These highlights do not include all the information needed to use AVODART safely and effectively. See full prescribing information for AVODART.
AVODART (dutasteride) Soft Gelatin Capsules
Initial U.S. Approval: 2001

————RECENT MAJOR CHANGES————

Warnings and Precautions, Evaluation for Other Urological Diseases (5.3) 03/2012

————INDICATIONS AND USAGE————

AVODART is a 5 alpha-reductase inhibitor indicated for the treatment of symptomatic benign prostatic hyperplasia (BPH) in men with an enlarged prostate to: (1.1)
• improve symptoms,
• reduce the risk of acute urinary retention, and
• reduce the risk of the need for BPH-related surgery.
AVODART in combination with the alpha adrenergic antagonist, tamsulosin, is indicated for the treatment of symptomatic BPH in men with an enlarged prostate. (1.2)
Limitations of Use: AVODART is not approved for the prevention of prostate cancer. (1.3)

————DOSAGE AND ADMINISTRATION————

Monotherapy: 0.5 mg once daily. (2.1)
Combination with tamsulosin: 0.5 mg once daily and tamsulosin 0.4 mg once daily. (2.2)
Dosing considerations: Swallow whole. May take with or without food. (2)

————DOSAGE FORMS AND STRENGTHS————

0.5-mg soft gelatin capsules (3)

————CONTRAINDICATIONS————

• Pregnancy and women of childbearing potential. (4, 5.4, 8.1)
• Pediatric patients. (4)
• Patients with previously demonstrated, clinically significant hypersensitivity (e.g., serious skin reactions, angioedema) to AVODART or other 5 alpha-reductase inhibitors. (4)

————WARNINGS AND PRECAUTIONS————

• AVODART reduces serum prostate-specific antigen (PSA) concentration by approximately 50%. However, any confirmed increase in PSA while on AVODART may signal the presence of prostate cancer and should be evaluated, even if those values are still within the normal range for untreated men. (5.1)
• AVODART may increase the risk of high-grade prostate cancer. (5.2, 6.1)
• Prior to initiating treatment with AVODART, consideration should be given to other urological conditions that may cause similar symptoms. (5.3)
• Women who are pregnant or could become pregnant should not handle AVODART Capsules due to potential risk to a male fetus. (5.4, 8.1)
• Patients should not donate blood until 6 months after their last dose of AVODART. (5.5)

————ADVERSE REACTIONS————

The most common adverse reactions, reported in ≥1% of subjects treated with AVODART and more commonly than in subjects treated with placebo, are impotence, decreased libido, ejaculation disorders, and breast disorders. (6.1)
To report SUSPECTED ADVERSE REACTIONS, contact GlaxoSmithKline at 1-888-825-5249 or FDA at 1-800-FDA-1088 or www.fda.gov/medwatch.

DRUG INTERACTIONS

Use with caution in patients taking potent, chronic CYP3A4 enzyme inhibitors (e.g., ritonavir). (7)

See 17 for PATIENT COUNSELING INFORMATION and FDA-approved patient labeling

Revised: 10/2012

FULL PRESCRIBING INFORMATION

1   INDICATIONS AND USAGE

1.1   Monotherapy

AVODART® (dutasteride) Soft Gelatin Capsules are indicated for the treatment of symptomatic benign prostatic hyperplasia (BPH) in men with an enlarged prostate to:
• improve symptoms,
• reduce the risk of acute urinary retention (AUR), and
• reduce the risk of the need for BPH-related surgery.

1.2   Combination With Alpha Adrenergic Antagonist

AVODART in combination with the alpha adrenergic antagonist, tamsulosin, is indicated for the treatment of symptomatic BPH in men with an enlarged prostate.

1.3   Limitations of Use

AVODART is not approved for the prevention of prostate cancer.

2   DOSAGE AND ADMINISTRATION

The capsules should be swallowed whole and not chewed or opened, as contact with the capsule contents may result in irritation of the oropharyngeal mucosa. AVODART may be administered with or without food.

2.1   Monotherapy

The recommended dose of AVODART is 1 capsule (0.5 mg) taken once daily.

2.2   Combination With Alpha Adrenergic Antagonist

The recommended dose of AVODART is 1 capsule (0.5 mg) taken once daily and tamsulosin 0.4 mg taken once daily.

3   DOSAGE FORMS AND STRENGTHS

0.5-mg, opaque, dull yellow, gelatin capsules imprinted with "GX CE2" in red ink on one side.

4   CONTRAINDICATIONS

AVODART is contraindicated for use in:
• Pregnancy. In animal reproduction and developmental toxicity studies, dutasteride inhibited development of male fetus external genitalia. Therefore, AVODART may cause fetal harm when administered to a pregnant woman. If AVODART is used during pregnancy or if the patient becomes pregnant while taking AVODART, the patient should be apprised of the potential hazard to the fetus [see Warnings and Precautions (5.4), Use in Specific Populations (8.1)].
• Women of childbearing potential [see Warnings and Precautions (5.4), Use in Specific Populations (8.1)].
• Pediatric patients [see Use in Specific Populations (8.4)].
• Patients with previously demonstrated, clinically significant hypersensitivity (e.g., serious skin reactions, angioedema) to AVODART or other 5 alpha-reductase inhibitors [see Adverse Reactions (6.2)].

5   WARNINGS AND PRECAUTIONS

5.1   Effects on Prostate-Specific Antigen (PSA) and the Use of PSA in Prostate Cancer Detection

In clinical trials, AVODART reduced serum PSA concentration by approximately 50% within 3 to 6 months of treatment. This decrease was predictable over the entire range of PSA values in subjects with symptomatic BPH, although it may vary in individuals. AVODART may also cause decreases in serum PSA in the presence of prostate cancer. To interpret serial PSAs in men taking AVODART, a new PSA baseline should be established at least 3 months after starting treatment and PSA monitored periodically thereafter. Any confirmed increase from the lowest PSA value while on AVODART may signal the presence of prostate cancer and should be evaluated, even if PSA levels are still within the normal range for men not taking a 5 alpha-reductase inhibitor. Noncompliance with AVODART may also affect PSA test results.

To interpret an isolated PSA value in a man treated with AVODART for 3 months or more, the PSA value should be doubled for comparison with normal values in untreated men. The free-to-total PSA ratio (percent free PSA) remains constant, even under the influence of AVODART. If clinicians elect to use percent free PSA as an aid in the detection of prostate cancer in men receiving AVODART, no adjustment to its value appears necessary.

Coadministration of dutasteride and tamsulosin resulted in similar changes to serum PSA as dutasteride monotherapy.

5.2   Increased Risk of High-Grade Prostate Cancer

In men aged 50 to 75 years with a prior negative biopsy for prostate cancer and a baseline PSA between 2.5 ng/mL and 10.0 ng/mL taking AVODART in the 4-year Reduction by Dutasteride of Prostate Cancer Events (REDUCE) trial, there was an increased incidence of Gleason score 8-10 prostate cancer compared with men taking placebo (AVODART 1.0% versus placebo 0.5%) [see Indications and Usage (1.3), Adverse Reactions (6.1)]. In a 7-year placebo-controlled clinical trial with another 5 alpha-reductase inhibitor (finasteride 5 mg, PROSCAR), similar results for Gleason score 8-10 prostate cancer were observed (finasteride 1.8% versus placebo 1.1%).

5 alpha-reductase inhibitors may increase the risk of development of high-grade prostate cancer. Whether the effect of 5 alpha-reductase inhibitors to reduce prostate volume, or trial-related factors, impacted the results of these trials has not been established.

5.3   Evaluation for Other Urological Diseases

Prior to initiating treatment with AVODART, consideration should be given to other urological conditions that may cause similar symptoms. In addition, BPH and prostate cancer may coexist.

5.4   Exposure of Women—Risk to Male Fetus

AVODART Capsules should not be handled by a woman who is pregnant or who could become pregnant. Dutasteride is absorbed through the skin and could result in unintended fetal exposure. If a woman who is pregnant or who could become pregnant comes in contact with leaking dutasteride capsules, the contact area should be washed immediately with soap and water [see Use in Specific Populations (8.1)].

5.5   Blood Donation

Men being treated with AVODART should not donate blood until at least 6 months have passed following their last dose. The purpose of this deferred period is to prevent administration of dutasteride to a pregnant female transfusion recipient.

5.6   Effect on Semen Characteristics

The effects of dutasteride 0.5 mg/day on semen characteristics were evaluated in normal volunteers aged 18 to 52

(n = 27 dutasteride, n = 23 placebo) throughout 52 weeks of treatment and 24 weeks of post-treatment follow-up. At 52 weeks, the mean percent reductions from baseline in total sperm count, semen volume, and sperm motility were 23%, 26%, and 18%, respectively, in the dutasteride group when adjusted for changes from baseline in the placebo group. Sperm concentration and sperm morphology were unaffected. After 24 weeks of follow-up, the mean percent change in total sperm count in the dutasteride group remained 23% lower than baseline. While mean values for all semen parameters at all time-points remained within the normal ranges and did not meet predefined criteria for a clinically significant change (30%), 2 subjects in the dutasteride group had decreases in sperm count of greater than 90% from baseline at 52 weeks, with partial recovery at the 24-week follow-up. The clinical significance of dutasteride's effect on semen characteristics for an individual patient's fertility is not known.

6   ADVERSE REACTIONS

6.1   Clinical Trials Experience

Because clinical trials are conducted under widely varying conditions, adverse reaction rates observed in the clinical trials of a drug cannot be directly compared with rates in the clinical trial of another drug and may not reflect the rates observed in practice.

From clinical trials with AVODART as monotherapy or in combination with tamsulosin:
• The most common adverse reactions reported in subjects receiving AVODART were impotence, decreased libido, breast disorders (including breast enlargement and tenderness), and ejaculation disorders. The most common adverse reactions reported in subjects receiving combination therapy (AVODART plus tamsulosin) were impotence, decreased libido, breast disorders (including breast enlargement and tenderness), ejaculation disorders, and dizziness. Ejaculation disorders occurred significantly more in subjects receiving combination therapy (11%) compared with those receiving AVODART (2%) or tamsulosin (4%) as monotherapy.
• Trial withdrawal due to adverse reactions occurred in 4% of subjects receiving AVODART, and 3% of subjects receiving placebo in placebo-controlled trials with AVODART. The most common adverse reaction leading to trial withdrawal was impotence (1%).
• In the clinical trial evaluating the combination therapy, trial withdrawal due to adverse reactions occurred in 6% of subjects receiving combination therapy (AVODART plus tamsulosin) and 4% of subjects receiving AVODART or tamsulosin as monotherapy. The most common adverse reaction in all treatment arms leading to trial withdrawal was erectile dysfunction (1% to 1.5%).

Monotherapy: Over 4,300 male subjects with BPH were randomly assigned to receive placebo or 0.5-mg daily doses of AVODART in 3 identical 2-year, placebo-controlled, double-blind, Phase 3 treatment trials, each followed by a 2-year open-label extension. During the double-blind treatment period, 2,167 male subjects were exposed to AVODART, including 1,772 exposed for 1 year and 1,510 exposed for 2 years. When including the open-label extensions, 1,009 male subjects were exposed to AVODART for 3 years and 812 were exposed for 4 years. The population was aged 47 to 94 years (mean age: 66 years) and greater than 90% were Caucasian. Table 1 summarizes clinical adverse reactions reported in at least 1% of subjects receiving AVODART and at a higher incidence than subjects receiving placebo.

[See table 1 at top of next page]

Long-Term Treatment (Up to 4 Years): *High-Grade Prostate Cancer:* The REDUCE trial was a randomized, double-blind, placebo-controlled trial that enrolled 8,231 men aged 50 to 75 years with a serum PSA of 2.5 ng/mL to 10 ng/mL and a negative prostate biopsy within the previous 6 months. Subjects were randomized to receive placebo (N = 4,126) or 0.5-mg daily doses of AVODART (N = 4,105) for up to 4 years. The mean age was 63 years and 91% were Caucasian. Subjects underwent protocol-mandated scheduled prostate biopsies at 2 and 4 years of treatment or had "for-cause biopsies" at non-scheduled times if clinically indicated. There was a higher incidence of Gleason score 8-10 prostate cancer in men receiving AVODART (1.0%) compared with men on placebo (0.5%) [see Indications and Usage (1.3), Warnings and Precautions (5.2)]. In a 7-year placebo-controlled clinical trial with another 5 alpha-reductase inhibitor (finasteride 5 mg, PROSCAR), similar results for Gleason score 8-10 prostate cancer were observed (finasteride 1.8% versus placebo 1.1%).

No clinical benefit has been demonstrated in patients with prostate cancer treated with AVODART.

Reproductive and Breast Disorders: In the 3 pivotal placebo-controlled BPH trials with AVODART, each 4 years in duration, there was no evidence of increased sexual adverse reactions (impotence, decreased libido, and ejaculation disorder) or breast disorders with increased duration of treatment. Among these 3 trials, there was 1 case of breast cancer in the dutasteride group and 1 case in the placebo group. No cases of breast cancer were reported in any treatment group in the 4-year CombAT trial or the 4-year REDUCE trial.

The relationship between long-term use of dutasteride and male breast neoplasia is currently unknown.

Combination With Alpha-Blocker Therapy (CombAT): Over 4,800 male subjects with BPH were randomly assigned to receive 0.5-mg AVODART, 0.4-mg tamsulosin, or combination therapy (0.5-mg AVODART plus 0.4-mg tamsulosin) administered once daily in a 4-year double-blind trial. Overall, 1,623 subjects received monotherapy with AVODART; 1,611 subjects received monotherapy with tamsulosin; and 1,610 subjects received combination therapy. The population was aged 49 to 88 years (mean age: 66 years) and 88% were Caucasian. Table 2 summarizes adverse reactions reported in at least 1% of subjects in the combination group and at a higher incidence than subjects receiving monotherapy with AVODART or tamsulosin. [See table 2]

Cardiac Failure: In CombAT, after 4 years of treatment, the incidence of the composite term cardiac failure in the combination therapy group (12/1,610; 0.7%) was higher than in either monotherapy group: AVODART, 2/1,623 (0.1%) and tamsulosin, 9/1,611 (0.6%). Composite cardiac failure was also examined in a separate 4-year placebo-controlled trial evaluating AVODART in men at risk for development of prostate cancer. The incidence of cardiac failure in subjects taking AVODART was 0.6% (26/4,105) compared with 0.4% (15/4,126) in subjects on placebo. A majority of subjects with cardiac failure in both trials had co-morbidities associated with an increased risk of cardiac failure. Therefore, the clinical significance of the numerical imbalances in cardiac failure is unknown. No causal relationship between AVODART, alone or in combination with tamsulosin, and cardiac failure has been established. No imbalance was observed in the incidence of overall cardiovascular adverse events in either trial.

6.2 Postmarketing Experience

The following adverse reactions have been identified during post-approval use of AVODART. Because these reactions are reported voluntarily from a population of uncertain size, it is not always possible to reliably estimate their frequency or establish a causal relationship to drug exposure. These reactions have been chosen for inclusion due to a combination of their seriousness, frequency of reporting, or potential causal connection to AVODART.

Immune System Disorders: Hypersensitivity reactions, including rash, pruritus, urticaria, localized edema, serious skin reactions, and angioedema.

Neoplasms: Male breast cancer.

Psychiatric Disorders: Depressed mood.

Reproductive System and Breast Disorders: Testicular pain and testicular swelling.

7 DRUG INTERACTIONS

7.1 Cytochrome P450 3A Inhibitors

Dutasteride is extensively metabolized in humans by the CYP3A4 and CYP3A5 isoenzymes. The effect of potent CYP3A4 inhibitors on dutasteride has not been studied. Because of the potential for drug-drug interactions, use caution when prescribing AVODART to patients taking potent, chronic CYP3A4 enzyme inhibitors (e.g., ritonavir) *[see Clinical Pharmacology (12.3)]*.

7.2 Alpha Adrenergic Antagonists

The administration of AVODART in combination with tamsulosin or terazosin has no effect on the steady-state pharmacokinetics of either alpha adrenergic antagonist. The effect of administration of tamsulosin or terazosin on dutasteride pharmacokinetic parameters has not been evaluated.

7.3 Calcium Channel Antagonists

Coadministration of verapamil or diltiazem decreases dutasteride clearance and leads to increased exposure to dutasteride. The change in dutasteride exposure is not considered to be clinically significant. No dose adjustment is recommended *[see Clinical Pharmacology (12.3)]*.

7.4 Cholestyramine

Administration of a single 5-mg dose of AVODART followed 1 hour later by 12 g of cholestyramine does not affect the relative bioavailability of dutasteride *[see Clinical Pharmacology (12.3)]*.

7.5 Digoxin

AVODART does not alter the steady-state pharmacokinetics of digoxin when administered concomitantly at a dose of 0.5 mg/day for 3 weeks *[see Clinical Pharmacology (12.3)]*.

7.6 Warfarin

Concomitant administration of AVODART 0.5 mg/day for 3 weeks with warfarin does not alter the steady-state pharmacokinetics of the S- or R-warfarin isomers or alter the effect of warfarin on prothrombin time *[see Clinical Pharmacology (12.3)]*.

Table 1. Adverse Reactions Reported in ≥1% of Subjects Over a 24-Month Period and More Frequently in the Group Receiving AVODART Than the Placebo Group (Randomized, Double-Blind, Placebo-Controlled Trials Pooled) by Time of Onset

Adverse Reaction	Adverse Reaction Time of Onset			
	Months 0–6	Months 7–12	Months 13–18	Months 19–24
AVODART (n)	(n = 2,167)	(n = 1,901)	(n = 1,725)	(n = 1,605)
Placebo (n)	(n = 2,158)	(n = 1,922)	(n = 1,714)	(n = 1,555)
Impotence[a]				
AVODART	4.7%	1.4%	1.0%	0.8%
Placebo	1.7%	1.5%	0.5%	0.9%
Decreased libido[a]				
AVODART	3.0%	0.7%	0.3%	0.3%
Placebo	1.4%	0.6%	0.2%	0.1%
Ejaculation disorders[a]				
AVODART	1.4%	0.5%	0.5%	0.1%
Placebo	0.5%	0.3%	0.1%	0.0%
Breast disorders[b]				
AVODART	0.5%	0.8%	1.1%	0.6%
Placebo	0.2%	0.3%	0.3%	0.1%

[a]These sexual adverse reactions are associated with dutasteride treatment (including monotherapy and combination with tamsulosin). These adverse reactions may persist after treatment discontinuation. The role of dutasteride in this persistence is unknown.
[b]Includes breast tenderness and breast enlargement.

Table 2. Adverse Reactions Reported Over a 48-Month Period in ≥1% of Subjects and More Frequently in the Coadministration Therapy Group Than the Groups Receiving Monotherapy With AVODART or Tamsulosin (CombAT) by Time of Onset

Adverse Reaction	Adverse Reaction Time of Onset				
	Year 1		Year 2	Year 3	Year 4
	Months 0–6	Months 7–12			
Combination[a]	(n = 1,610)	(n = 1,527)	(n = 1,428)	(n = 1,283)	(n = 1,200)
AVODART	(n = 1,623)	(n = 1,548)	(n = 1,464)	(n = 1,325)	(n = 1,200)
Tamsulosin	(n = 1,611)	(n = 1,545)	(n = 1,468)	(n = 1,281)	(n = 1,112)
Ejaculation disorders[b,c]					
Combination	7.8%	1.6%	1.0%	0.5%	<0.1%
AVODART	1.0%	0.5%	0.5%	0.2%	0.3%
Tamsulosin	2.2%	0.5%	0.5%	0.2%	0.3%
Impotence[c,d]					
Combination	5.4%	1.1%	1.8%	0.9%	0.4%
AVODART	4.0%	1.1%	1.6%	0.6%	0.3%
Tamsulosin	2.6%	0.8%	1.0%	0.6%	1.1%
Decreased libido[c,e]					
Combination	4.5%	0.9%	0.8%	0.2%	0.0%
AVODART	3.1%	0.7%	1.0%	0.2%	0.0%
Tamsulosin	2.0%	0.6%	0.7%	0.2%	<0.1%
Breast disorders[f]					
Combination	1.1%	1.1%	0.8%	0.9%	0.6%
AVODART	0.9%	0.9%	1.2%	0.5%	0.7%
Tamsulosin	0.4%	0.4%	0.4%	0.2%	0.0%
Dizziness					
Combination	1.1%	0.4%	0.1%	<0.1%	0.2%
AVODART	0.5%	0.3%	0.1%	<0.1%	<0.1%
Tamsulosin	0.9%	0.5%	0.4%	<0.1%	0.0%

[a]Combination = AVODART 0.5 mg once daily plus tamsulosin 0.4 mg once daily.
[b]Includes anorgasmia, retrograde ejaculation, semen volume decreased, orgasmic sensation decreased, orgasm abnormal, ejaculation delayed, ejaculation disorder, ejaculation failure, and premature ejaculation.
[c]These sexual adverse reactions are associated with dutasteride treatment (including monotherapy and combination with tamsulosin). These adverse reactions may persist after treatment discontinuation. The role of dutasteride in this persistence is unknown.
[d]Includes erectile dysfunction and disturbance in sexual arousal.
[e]Includes libido decreased, libido disorder, loss of libido, sexual dysfunction, and male sexual dysfunction.
[f]Includes breast enlargement, gynecomastia, breast swelling, breast pain, breast tenderness, nipple pain, and nipple swelling.

8 USE IN SPECIFIC POPULATIONS

8.1 Pregnancy

Pregnancy Category X. AVODART is contraindicated for use in women of childbearing potential and during pregnancy. AVODART is a 5 alpha-reductase inhibitor that prevents conversion of testosterone to dihydrotestosterone (DHT), a hormone necessary for normal development of male genitalia. In animal reproduction and developmental toxicity studies, dutasteride inhibited normal development of external genitalia in male fetuses. Therefore, AVODART may cause fetal harm when administered to a pregnant woman. If AVODART is used during pregnancy or if the patient becomes pregnant while taking AVODART, the patient should be apprised of the potential hazard to the fetus.

Abnormalities in the genitalia of male fetuses is an expected physiological consequence of inhibition of the conversion of testosterone to DHT by 5 alpha-reductase inhibitors. These results are similar to observations in male infants with genetic 5 alpha-reductase deficiency. Dutasteride is absorbed through the skin. To avoid potential fetal exposure, women who are pregnant or could become pregnant should not handle AVODART Soft Gelatin Capsules. If contact is made with leaking capsules, the contact area should be washed immediately with soap and water [see Warnings and Precautions (5.4)]. Dutasteride is secreted into semen. The highest measured semen concentration of dutasteride in treated men was 14 ng/mL. Assuming exposure of a 50-kg woman to 5 mL of semen and 100% absorption, the woman's dutasteride concentration would be about 0.0175 ng/mL. This concentration is more than 100 times less than concentrations producing abnormalities of male genitalia in animal studies. Dutasteride is highly protein bound in human semen (greater than 96%), which may reduce the amount of dutasteride available for vaginal absorption.

In an embryo-fetal development study in female rats, oral administration of dutasteride at doses 10 times less than the maximum recommended human dose (MRHD) of 0.5 mg daily resulted in abnormalities of male genitalia in the fetus (decreased anogenital distance at 0.05 mg/kg/day, nipple development, hypospadias, and distended preputial glands in male offspring (at all doses of 0.05, 2.5, 12.5, and 30 mg/kg/day). An increase in stillborn pups was observed at 111 times the MRHD, and reduced fetal body weight was observed at doses of about 15 times the MRHD (animal dose of 2.5 mg/kg/day). Increased incidences of skeletal variations considered to be delays in ossification associated with reduced body weight were observed at doses about 56 times the MRHD (animal dose of 12.5 mg/kg/day).

In a rabbit embryo-fetal study, doses 28- to 93-fold the MRHD (animal doses of 30, 100, and 200 mg/kg/day) were administered orally during the period of major organogenesis (gestation days 7 to 29) to encompass the late period of external genitalia development. Histological evaluation of the genital papilla of fetuses revealed evidence of feminization of the male fetus at all doses. A second embryo-fetal study in rabbits at 0.3- to 53-fold the expected clinical exposure (animal doses of 0.05, 0.4, 3.0, and 30 mg/kg/day) also produced evidence of feminization of the genitalia in male fetuses at all doses.

In an oral pre- and post-natal development study in rats, dutasteride doses of 0.05, 2.5, 12.5, or 30 mg/kg/day were administered. Unequivocal evidence of feminization of the genitalia (i.e., decreased anogenital distance, increased incidence of hypospadias, nipple development) of male offspring occurred at 14- to 90-fold the MRHD (animal doses of 2.5 mg/kg/day or greater). At 0.05-fold the expected clinical exposure (animal dose of 0.05 mg/kg/day), evidence of feminization was limited to a small, but statistically significant, decrease in anogenital distance. Animal doses of 2.5 to 30 mg/kg/day resulted in prolonged gestation in the parental females and a decrease in time to vaginal patency for female offspring and a decrease in prostate and seminal vesicle weights in male offspring. Effects on newborn startle response were noted at doses greater than or equal to 12.5 mg/kg/day. Increased stillbirths were noted at 30 mg/kg/day.

In an embryo-fetal development study, pregnant rhesus monkeys were exposed intravenously to a dutasteride blood level comparable to the dutasteride concentration found in human semen. Dutasteride was administered on gestation days 20 to 100 at doses of 400, 780, 1,325, or 2,010 ng/day (12 monkeys/group). The development of male external genitalia of monkey offspring was not adversely affected. Reduction of fetal adrenal weights, reduction in fetal prostate weights, and increases in fetal ovarian and testis weights were observed at the highest dose tested in monkeys. Based on the highest measured semen concentration of dutasteride in treated men (14 ng/mL), these doses represent 0.8 to 16 times the potential maximum exposure of a 50-kg human female to 5 mL semen daily from a dutasteride-treated man, assuming 100% absorption. (These calculations are based on blood levels of parent drug which are achieved at 32 to 186 times the daily doses administered to pregnant monkeys on a ng/kg basis). Dutasteride is highly bound to proteins in human semen (greater than 96%), potentially reducing the amount of dutasteride available for vaginal absorption. It is not known whether rabbits or rhesus monkeys produce any of the major human metabolites.

Estimates of exposure multiples comparing animal studies to the MRHD for dutasteride are based on clinical serum concentration at steady state.

8.3 Nursing Mothers
AVODART is contraindicated for use in women of childbearing potential, including nursing women. It is not known whether dutasteride is excreted in human milk.

8.4 Pediatric Use
AVODART is contraindicated for use in pediatric patients. Safety and effectiveness in pediatric patients have not been established.

8.5 Geriatric Use
Of 2,167 male subjects treated with AVODART in 3 clinical trials, 60% were aged 65 years and older and 15% were aged 75 years and older. No overall differences in safety or efficacy were observed between these subjects and younger subjects. Other reported clinical experience has not identified differences in responses between the elderly and

younger patients, but greater sensitivity of some older individuals cannot be ruled out [see Clinical Pharmacology (12.3)].

8.6 Renal Impairment
No dose adjustment is necessary for AVODART in patients with renal impairment [see Clinical Pharmacology (12.3)].

8.7 Hepatic Impairment
The effect of hepatic impairment on dutasteride pharmacokinetics has not been studied. Because dutasteride is extensively metabolized, exposure could be higher in hepatically impaired patients. However, in a clinical trial where 60 subjects received 5 mg (10 times the therapeutic dose) daily for 24 weeks, no additional adverse events were observed compared with those observed at the therapeutic dose of 0.5 mg [see Clinical Pharmacology (12.3)].

10 OVERDOSAGE
In volunteer trials, single doses of dutasteride up to 40 mg (80 times the therapeutic dose) for 7 days have been administered without significant safety concerns. In a clinical trial, daily doses of 5 mg (10 times the therapeutic dose) were administered to 60 subjects for 6 months with no additional adverse effects to those seen at therapeutic doses of 0.5 mg.

There is no specific antidote for dutasteride. Therefore, in cases of suspected overdosage symptomatic and supportive treatment should be given as appropriate, taking the long half-life of dutasteride into consideration.

11 DESCRIPTION
AVODART is a synthetic 4-azasteroid compound that is a selective inhibitor of both the type 1 and type 2 isoforms of steroid 5 alpha-reductase, an intracellular enzyme that converts testosterone to DHT.

Dutasteride is chemically designated as $(5\alpha,17\beta)$-N-{2,5 bis(trifluoromethyl)phenyl}-3-oxo-4-azaandrost-1-ene-17-carboxamide. The empirical formula of dutasteride is $C_{27}H_{30}F_6N_2O_2$, representing a molecular weight of 528.5 with the following structural formula:

Dutasteride is a white to pale yellow powder with a melting point of 242° to 250°C. It is soluble in ethanol (44 mg/mL), methanol (64 mg/mL), and polyethylene glycol 400 (3 mg/mL), but it is insoluble in water.

Each AVODART Soft Gelatin Capsule, administered orally, contains 0.5 mg of dutasteride dissolved in a mixture of mono-di-glycerides of caprylic/capric acid and butylated hydroxytoluene. The inactive excipients in the capsule shell are ferric oxide (yellow), gelatin (from certified BSE-free bovine sources), glycerin, and titanium dioxide. The soft gelatin capsules are printed with edible red ink.

12 CLINICAL PHARMACOLOGY
12.1 Mechanism of Action
Dutasteride inhibits the conversion of testosterone to dihydrotestosterone (DHT). DHT is the androgen primarily responsible for the initial development and subsequent enlargement of the prostate gland. Testosterone is converted to DHT by the enzyme 5 alpha-reductase, which exists as 2 isoforms, type 1 and type 2. The type 2 isoenzyme is primarily active in the reproductive tissues, while the type 1 isoenzyme is also responsible for testosterone conversion in the skin and liver.

Dutasteride is a competitive and specific inhibitor of both type 1 and type 2 5 alpha-reductase isoenzymes, with which it forms a stable enzyme complex. Dissociation from this complex has been evaluated under in vitro and in vivo conditions and is extremely slow. Dutasteride does not bind to the human androgen receptor.

12.2 Pharmacodynamics
Effect on 5 Alpha-Dihydrotestosterone and Testosterone: The maximum effect of daily doses of dutasteride on the reduction of DHT is dose dependent and is observed within 1 to 2 weeks. After 1 and 2 weeks of daily dosing with dutasteride 0.5 mg, median serum DHT concentrations were reduced by 85% and 90%, respectively. In patients with BPH treated with dutasteride 0.5 mg/day for 4 years, the median decrease in serum DHT was 94% at 1 year, 93% at 2 years, and 95% at both 3 and 4 years. The median increase in serum testosterone was 19% at both 1 and 2 years, 26% at 3 years, and 22% at 4 years, but the mean and median levels remained within the physiologic range.

In patients with BPH treated with 5 mg/day of dutasteride or placebo for up to 12 weeks prior to transurethral resection of the prostate, mean DHT concentrations in prostatic

tissue were significantly lower in the dutasteride group compared with placebo (784 and 5,793 pg/g, respectively, $P<0.001$). Mean prostatic tissue concentrations of testosterone were significantly higher in the dutasteride group compared with placebo (2,073 and 93 pg/g, respectively, $P<0.001$).

Adult males with genetically inherited type 2 5 alpha-reductase deficiency also have decreased DHT levels. These 5 alpha-reductase deficient males have a small prostate gland throughout life and do not develop BPH. Except for the associated urogenital defects present at birth, no other clinical abnormalities related to 5 alpha-reductase-deficiency have been observed in these individuals.

Effects on Other Hormones: In healthy volunteers, 52 weeks of treatment with dutasteride 0.5 mg/day (n = 26) resulted in no clinically significant change compared with placebo (n = 23) in sex hormone-binding globulin, estradiol, luteinizing hormone, follicle-stimulating hormone, thyroxine (free T4), and dehydroepiandrosterone. Statistically significant, baseline-adjusted mean increases compared with placebo were observed for total testosterone at 8 weeks (97.1 ng/dL, $P<0.003$) and thyroid-stimulating hormone at 52 weeks (0.4 mcIU/mL, $P<0.05$). The median percentage changes from baseline within the dutasteride group were 17.9% for testosterone at 8 weeks and 12.4% for thyroid-stimulating hormone at 52 weeks. After stopping dutasteride for 24 weeks, the mean levels of testosterone and thyroid-stimulating hormone had returned to baseline in the group of subjects with available data at the visit. In subjects with BPH treated with dutasteride in a large randomized, double-blind, placebo-controlled trial, there was a median percent increase in luteinizing hormone of 12% at 6 months and 19% at both 12 and 24 months.

Other Effects: Plasma lipid panel and bone mineral density were evaluated following 52 weeks of dutasteride 0.5 mg once daily in healthy volunteers. There was no change in bone mineral density as measured by dual energy x-ray absorptiometry compared with either placebo or baseline. In addition, the plasma lipid profile (i.e., total cholesterol, low density lipoproteins, high density lipoproteins, and triglycerides) was unaffected by dutasteride. No clinically significant changes in adrenal hormone responses to adrenocorticotropic hormone (ACTH) stimulation were observed in a subset population (n = 13) of the 1-year healthy volunteer trial.

12.3 Pharmacokinetics
Absorption: Following administration of a single 0.5-mg dose of a soft gelatin capsule, time to peak serum concentrations (T_{max}) of dutasteride occurs within 2 to 3 hours. Absolute bioavailability in 5 healthy subjects is approximately 60% (range: 40% to 94%). When the drug is administered with food, the maximum serum concentrations were reduced by 10% to 15%. This reduction is of no clinical significance.

Distribution: Pharmacokinetic data following single and repeat oral doses show that dutasteride has a large volume of distribution (300 to 500 L). Dutasteride is highly bound to plasma albumin (99.0%) and alpha-1 acid glycoprotein (96.6%).

In a trial of healthy subjects (n = 26) receiving dutasteride 0.5 mg/day for 12 months, semen dutasteride concentrations averaged 3.4 ng/mL (range: 0.4 to 14 ng/mL) at 12 months and, similar to serum, achieved steady-state concentrations at 6 months. On average, at 12 months 11.5% of serum dutasteride concentrations partitioned into semen.

Metabolism and Elimination: Dutasteride is extensively metabolized in humans. In vitro studies showed that dutasteride is metabolized by the CYP3A4 and CYP3A5 isoenzymes. Both of these isoenzymes produced the 4'-hydroxydutasteride, 6-hydroxydutasteride, and the 6,4'-dihydroxydutasteride metabolites. In addition, the 15-hydroxydutasteride metabolite was formed by CYP3A4. Dutasteride is not metabolized in vitro by human cytochrome P450 isoenzymes CYP1A2, CYP2A6, CYP2B6, CYP2C8, CYP2C9, CYP2C19, CYP2D6, and CYP2E1. In human serum following dosing to steady state, unchanged dutasteride, 3 major metabolites (4'-hydroxydutasteride, 1,2-dihydrodutasteride, and 6-hydroxydutasteride), and 2 minor metabolites (6,4'-dihydroxydutasteride and 15-hydroxydutasteride), as assessed by mass spectrometric response, have been detected. The absolute stereochemistry of the hydroxyl additions in the 6 and 15 positions is not known. In vitro, the 4'-hydroxydutasteride and 1,2-dihydrodutasteride metabolites are much less potent than dutasteride against both isoforms of human 5 alpha-reductase. The activity of 6β-hydroxydutasteride is comparable to that of dutasteride.

Dutasteride and its metabolites were excreted mainly in feces. As a percent of dose, there was approximately 5% unchanged dutasteride (~1% to ~15%) and 40% as dutasteride-related metabolites (~2% to ~90%). Only trace amounts of unchanged dutasteride were found in urine (<1%). Therefore, on average, the dose unaccounted for approximated 55% (range, 5% to 97%).

The terminal elimination half-life of dutasteride is approximately 5 weeks at steady state. The average steady-state serum dutasteride concentration was 40 ng/mL following 0.5 mg/day for 1 year. Following daily dosing, dutasteride serum concentrations achieve 65% of steady-state concentration after 1 month and approximately 90% after 3 months. Due to the long half-life of dutasteride, serum concentrations remain detectable (greater than 0.1 ng/mL) for up to 4 to 6 months after discontinuation of treatment.

Specific Populations: *Pediatric:* Dutasteride pharmacokinetics have not been investigated in subjects younger than 18 years.

Geriatric: No dose adjustment is necessary in the elderly. The pharmacokinetics and pharmacodynamics of dutasteride were evaluated in 36 healthy male subjects aged between 24 and 87 years following administration of a single 5-mg dose of dutasteride. In this single-dose trial, dutasteride half-life increased with age (approximately 170 hours in men aged 20 to 49 years, approximately 260 hours in men aged 50 to 69 years, and approximately 300 hours in men older than 70 years). Of 2,167 men treated with dutasteride in the 3 pivotal trials, 60% were age 65 and over and 15% were age 75 and over. No overall differences in safety or efficacy were observed between these patients and younger patients.

Gender: AVODART is contraindicated in pregnancy and women of childbearing potential and is not indicated for use in other women *[see Contraindications (4), Warnings and Precautions (5.1)].* The pharmacokinetics of dutasteride in women have not been studied.

Race: The effect of race on dutasteride pharmacokinetics has not been studied.

Renal Impairment: The effect of renal impairment on dutasteride pharmacokinetics has not been studied. However, less than 0.1% of a steady-state 0.5-mg dose of dutasteride is recovered in human urine, so no adjustment in dosage is anticipated for patients with renal impairment.

Hepatic Impairment: The effect of hepatic impairment on dutasteride pharmacokinetics has not been studied. Because dutasteride is extensively metabolized, exposure could be higher in hepatically impaired patients.

Drug Interactions:
Cytochrome P450 Inhibitors: No clinical drug interaction trials have been performed to evaluate the impact of CYP3A enzyme inhibitors on dutasteride pharmacokinetics. However, based on in vitro data, blood concentrations of dutasteride may increase in the presence of inhibitors of CYP3A4/5 such as ritonavir, ketoconazole, verapamil, diltiazem, cimetidine, troleandomycin, and ciprofloxacin.

Dutasteride does not inhibit the in vitro metabolism of model substrates for the major human cytochrome P450 isoenzymes (CYP1A2, CYP2C9, CYP2C19, CYP2D6, and CYP3A4) at a concentration of 1,000 ng/mL, 25 times greater than steady-state serum concentrations in humans.

Alpha Adrenergic Antagonists: In a single-sequence, crossover trial in healthy volunteers, the administration of tamsulosin or terazosin in combination with AVODART had no effect on the steady-state pharmacokinetics of either alpha-adrenergic antagonist. Although the effect of administration of tamsulosin or terazosin on dutasteride pharmacokinetic parameters was not evaluated, the percent change in DHT concentrations was similar for AVODART alone compared with the combination treatment.

Calcium Channel Antagonists: In a population pharmacokinetics analysis, a decrease in clearance of dutasteride was noted when coadministered with the CYP3A4 inhibitors verapamil (-37%, n = 6) and diltiazem (-44%, n = 5). In contrast, no decrease in clearance was seen when amlodipine, another calcium channel antagonist that is not a CYP3A4 inhibitor, was coadministered with dutasteride (+7%, n = 4).

The decrease in clearance and subsequent increase in exposure to dutasteride in the presence of verapamil and diltiazem is not considered to be clinically significant. No dose adjustment is recommended.

Cholestyramine: Administration of a single 5-mg dose of AVODART followed 1 hour later by 12 g cholestyramine did not affect the relative bioavailability of dutasteride in 12 normal volunteers.

Digoxin: In a trial of 20 healthy volunteers, AVODART did not alter the steady-state pharmacokinetics of digoxin when administered concomitantly at a dose of 0.5 mg/day for 3 weeks.

Warfarin: In a trial of 23 healthy volunteers, 3 weeks of treatment with AVODART 0.5 mg/day did not alter the steady-state pharmacokinetics of the S- or R-warfarin isomers or alter the effect of warfarin on prothrombin time when administered with warfarin.

Other Concomitant Therapy: Although specific interaction trials were not performed with other compounds, approximately 90% of the subjects in the 3 randomized, double-blind, placebo-controlled safety and efficacy trials receiving AVODART were taking other medications concomitantly. No clinically significant adverse interactions could be attributed to the combination of AVODART and concurrent therapy when AVODART was coadministered with anti-hyperlipidemics, angiotensin-converting enzyme (ACE) inhibitors, beta-adrenergic blocking agents, calcium channel blockers, corticosteroids, diuretics, nonsteroidal anti-inflammatory drugs (NSAIDs), phosphodiesterase Type V inhibitors, and quinolone antibiotics.

13 NONCLINICAL TOXICOLOGY

13.1 Carcinogenesis, Mutagenesis, Impairment of Fertility

Carcinogenesis: A 2-year carcinogenicity study was conducted in B6C3F1 mice at doses of 3, 35, 250, and 500 mg/kg/day for males and 3, 35, and 250 mg/kg/day for females; an increased incidence of benign hepatocellular adenomas was noted at 250 mg/kg/day (290-fold the MRHD of a 0.5-mg daily dose) in female mice only. Two of the 3 major human metabolites have been detected in mice. The exposure to these metabolites in mice is either lower than in humans or is not known.

In a 2-year carcinogenicity study in Han Wistar rats, at doses of 1.5, 7.5, and 53 mg/kg/day in males and 0.8, 6.3, and 15 mg/kg/day in females, there was an increase in Leydig cell adenomas in the testes at 135-fold the MRHD (53 mg/kg/day and greater). An increased incidence of Leydig cell hyperplasia was present at 52-fold the MRHD (rat doses of 7.5 mg/kg/day and greater). A positive correlation between proliferative changes in the Leydig cells and an increase in circulating luteinizing hormone levels has been demonstrated with 5 alpha-reductase inhibitors and is consistent with an effect on the hypothalamic-pituitary-testicular axis following 5 alpha-reductase inhibition. At tumorigenic doses, luteinizing hormone levels in rats were increased by 167%. In this study, the major human metabolites were tested for carcinogenicity at approximately 1 to 3 times the expected clinical exposure.

Mutagenesis: Dutasteride was tested for genotoxicity in a bacterial mutagenesis assay (Ames test), a chromosomal aberration assay in CHO cells, and a micronucleus assay in rats. The results did not indicate any genotoxic potential of the parent drug. Two major human metabolites were also negative in either the Ames test or an abbreviated Ames test.

Impairment of Fertility: Treatment of sexually mature male rats with dutasteride at 0.1- to 110-fold the MRHD (animal doses of 0.05, 10, 50, and 500 mg/kg/day for up to 31 weeks) resulted in dose- and time-dependent decreases in fertility; reduced cauda epididymal (absolute) sperm counts but not sperm concentration (at 50 and 500 mg/kg/day); reduced weights of the epididymis, prostate, and seminal vesicles; and microscopic changes in the male reproductive organs. The fertility effects were reversed by recovery week 6 at all doses, and sperm counts were normal at the end of a 14-week recovery period. The 5 alpha-reductase–related changes consisted of cytoplasmic vacuolation of tubular epithelium in the epididymides and decreased cytoplasmic content of epithelium, consistent with decreased secretory activity in the prostate and seminal vesicles. The microscopic changes were no longer present at recovery week 14 in the low-dose group and were partly recovered in the remaining treatment groups. Low levels of dutasteride (0.6 to 17 ng/mL) were detected in the serum of untreated female rats mated to males dosed at 10, 50, or 500 mg/kg/day for 29 to 30 weeks.

In a fertility study in female rats, oral administration of dutasteride at doses of 0.05, 2.5, 12.5, and 30 mg/kg/day resulted in reduced litter size, increased embryo resorption, and feminization of male fetuses (decreased anogenital distance) at 2- to 10-fold the MRHD (animal doses of 2.5 mg/kg/day or greater). Fetal body weights were also reduced at less than 0.02-fold the MRHD in rats (0.5 mg/kg/day).

13.2 Animal Toxicology and/or Pharmacology

Central Nervous System Toxicology Studies: In rats and dogs, repeated oral administration of dutasteride resulted in some animals showing signs of non-specific, reversible, centrally-mediated toxicity without associated histopathological changes at exposures 425- and 315-fold the expected clinical exposure (of parent drug), respectively.

14 CLINICAL STUDIES

14.1 Monotherapy

AVODART 0.5 mg/day (n = 2,167) or placebo (n = 2,158) was evaluated in male subjects with BPH in three 2-year multi-center, placebo-controlled, double-blind trials, each with 2-year open-label extensions (n = 2,340). More than 90% of the trial population was Caucasian. Subjects were at least 50 years of age with a serum PSA ≥1.5 ng/mL and <10 ng/mL and BPH diagnosed by medical history and physical examination, including enlarged prostate (≥30 cc) and BPH symptoms that were moderate to severe according to the American Urological Association Symptom Index (AUA-SI). Most of the 4,325 subjects randomly assigned to receive either dutasteride or placebo completed 2 years of double-blind treatment (70% and 67%, respectively). Most of the 2,340 subjects in the trial extensions completed 2 additional years of open-label treatment (71%).

Effect on Symptom Scores: Symptoms were quantified using the AUA-SI, a questionnaire that evaluates urinary symptoms (incomplete emptying, frequency, intermittency, urgency, weak stream, straining, and nocturia) by rating on a 0 to 5 scale for a total possible score of 35, with higher numerical total symptom scores representing greater severity of symptoms. The baseline AUA-SI score across the 3 trials was approximately 17 units in both treatment groups. Subjects receiving dutasteride achieved statistically significant improvement in symptoms versus placebo by Month 3 in 1 trial and by Month 12 in the other 2 pivotal trials. At Month 12, the mean decrease from baseline in AUA-SI total symptom scores across the 3 trials pooled was -3.3 units for dutasteride and -2.0 units for placebo with a mean difference between the 2 treatment groups of -1.3 (range: -1.1 to -1.5 units in each of the 3 trials, $P<0.001$) and was consistent across the 3 trials. At Month 24, the mean decrease from baseline was -3.8 units for dutasteride and -1.7 units for placebo with a mean difference of -2.1 (range: -1.9 to -2.2 units in each of the 3 trials, $P<0.001$). See Figure 1. The improvement in BPH symptoms seen during the first 2 years of double-blind treatment was maintained throughout an additional 2 years of open-label extension trials.

These trials were prospectively designed to evaluate effects on symptoms based on prostate size at baseline. In men with prostate volumes ≥40 cc, the mean decrease was -3.8 units for dutasteride and -1.6 units for placebo with a mean difference between the 2 treatment groups of -2.2 at Month 24. In men with prostate volumes <40 cc, the mean decrease was -3.7 units for dutasteride and -2.2 units for placebo, with a mean difference between the 2 treatment groups of -1.5 at Month 24.

Figure 1. AUA-SI Score[a] Change From Baseline (Randomized, Double-Blind, Placebo-Controlled Trials Pooled)

■ Placebo	n = 2,122	n = 2,123	n = 2,123	n = 2,123
O Dutasteride	n = 2,122	n = 2,122	n = 2,122	n = 2,122

[a] AUA-SI score ranges from 0 to 35.

Effect on Acute Urinary Retention and the Need for BPH-Related Surgery: Efficacy was also assessed after 2 years of treatment by the incidence of AUR requiring catheterization and BPH-related urological surgical intervention. Compared with placebo, AVODART was associated with a statistically significantly lower incidence of AUR (1.8% for AVODART versus 4.2% for placebo, $P<0.001$; 57% reduction in risk, [95% CI: 38% to 71%]) and with a statistically significantly lower incidence of surgery (2.2% for AVODART versus 4.1% for placebo, $P<0.001$; 48% reduction in risk, [95% CI: 26% to 63%]). See Figures 2 and 3.

Figure 2. Percent of Subjects Developing Acute Urinary Retention Over a 24-Month Period (Randomized, Double-Blind, Placebo-Controlled Trials Pooled)

--- Placebo Group				
No. of events, cumulative	28	49	70	90
No. at risk	2,158	2,039	1,919	1,793
— Dutasteride Group				
No. of events, cumulative	19	27	31	39
No. at risk	2,167	2,052	1,928	1,827

Figure 3. Percent of Subjects Having Surgery for Benign Prostatic Hyperplasia Over a 24-Month Period (Randomized, Double-Blind, Placebo-Controlled Trials Pooled)

Placebo Group				
No. of events, cumulative	13	40	59	89
No. at risk	2,158	2,057	1,944	1,823
Dutasteride Group				
No. of events, cumulative	12	25	39	47
No. at risk	2,167	2,064	1,944	1,846

Effect on Prostate Volume: A prostate volume of at least 30 cc measured by transrectal ultrasound was required for trial entry. The mean prostate volume at trial entry was approximately 54 cc.

Statistically significant differences (AVODART versus placebo) were noted at the earliest post-treatment prostate volume measurement in each trial (Month 1, Month 3, or Month 6) and continued through Month 24. At Month 12, the mean percent change in prostate volume across the 3 trials pooled was -24.7% for dutasteride and -3.4% for placebo; the mean difference (dutasteride minus placebo) was -21.3% (range: -21.0% to -21.6% in each of the 3 trials, $P<0.001$). At Month 24, the mean percent change in prostate volume across the 3 trials pooled was -26.7% for dutasteride and -2.2% for placebo with a mean difference of -24.5% (range: -24.0% to -25.1% in each of the 3 trials, $P<0.001$). See Figure 4. The reduction in prostate volume seen during the first 2 years of double-blind treatment was maintained throughout an additional 2 years of open-label extension trials.

Figure 4. Prostate Volume Percent Change From Baseline (Randomized, Double-Blind, Placebo-Controlled Trials Pooled)

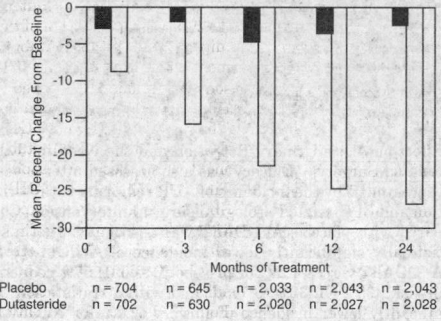

Placebo	n = 704	n = 645	n = 2,033	n = 2,043	n = 2,043
Dutasteride	n = 702	n = 630	n = 2,020	n = 2,027	n = 2,028

Effect on Maximum Urine Flow Rate: A mean peak urine flow rate (Q_{max}) of ≤15 mL/sec was required for trial entry. Q_{max} was approximately 10 mL/sec at baseline across the 3 pivotal trials.

Differences between the 2 groups were statistically significant from baseline at Month 3 in all 3 trials and were maintained through Month 12. At Month 12, the mean increase in Q_{max} across the 3 trials pooled was 1.6 mL/sec for AVODART and 0.7 mL/sec for placebo; the mean difference (dutasteride minus placebo) was 0.8 mL/sec (range: 0.7 to 1.0 mL/sec in each of the 3 trials, $P<0.001$). At Month 24, the mean increase in Q_{max} was 1.8 mL/sec for dutasteride and 0.7 mL/sec for placebo, with a mean difference of 1.1 mL/sec (range: 1.0 to 1.2 mL/sec in each of the 3 trials $P<0.001$). See Figure 5. The increase in maximum urine flow rate seen during the first 2 years of double-blind treatment was maintained throughout an additional 2 years of open-label extension trials.

[See figure 5 at top of next column]

Summary of Clinical Trials: Data from 3 large, well-controlled efficacy trials demonstrate that treatment with AVODART (0.5 mg once daily) reduces the risk of both AUR and BPH-related surgical intervention relative to placebo, improves BPH-related symptoms, decreases prostate volume, and increases maximum urinary flow rates. These data suggest that AVODART arrests the disease process of BPH in men with an enlarged prostate.

Figure 5. Q_{max} Change From Baseline (Randomized, Double-Blind, Placebo-Controlled Trials Pooled)

Placebo	n = 2,101	n = 2,105	n = 2,105	n = 2,105	
Dutasteride	n = 2,103	n = 2,104	n = 2,104	n = 2,104	

14.2 Combination With Alpha-Blocker Therapy (CombAT)

The efficacy of combination therapy (AVODART 0.5 mg/day plus tamsulosin 0.4 mg/day, n = 1,610) was compared with AVODART alone (n = 1,623) or tamsulosin alone (n = 1,611) in a 4-year multicenter, randomized, double-blind trial. Trial entry criteria were similar to the double-blind, placebo-controlled monotherapy efficacy trials described above in section 14.1. Eighty-eight percent (88%) of the enrolled trial population was Caucasian. Approximately 52% of subjects had previous exposure to 5 alpha-reductase inhibitor or alpha adrenergic antagonist treatment. Of the 4,844 subjects randomly assigned to receive treatment, 69% of subjects in the combination group, 67% in the group receiving AVODART, and 61% in the tamsulosin group completed 4 years of double-blind treatment.

Effect on Symptom Score: Symptoms were quantified using the first 7 questions of the International Prostate Symptom Score (IPSS) (identical to the AUA-SI). The baseline score was approximately 16.4 units for each treatment group. Combination therapy was statistically superior to each of the monotherapy treatments in decreasing symptom score at Month 24, the primary time point for this endpoint. At Month 24 the mean changes from baseline (±SD) in IPSS total symptom scores were -6.2 (±7.14) for combination, -4.9 (±6.81) for AVODART, and -4.3 (±7.01) for tamsulosin, with a mean difference between combination and AVODART of -1.3 units ($P<0.001$; [95% CI: -1.69, -0.86]), and between combination and tamsulosin of -1.8 units ($P<0.001$; [95% CI: -2.23, -1.40]). A significant difference was seen by Month 9 and continued through Month 48. At Month 48 the mean changes from baseline (±SD) in IPSS total symptom scores were -6.3 (±7.40) for combination, -5.3 (±7.14) for AVODART, and -3.8 (±7.74) for tamsulosin, with a mean difference between combination and AVODART of -0.96 units ($P<0.001$; [95% CI: -1.40, -0.52]), and between combination and tamsulosin of -2.5 units ($P<0.001$; [95% CI: -2.96, -2.07]). See Figure 6.

Figure 6. International Prostate Symptom Score Change From Baseline Over a 48-Month Period (Randomized, Double-Blind, Parallel Group Trial [CombAT Trial])

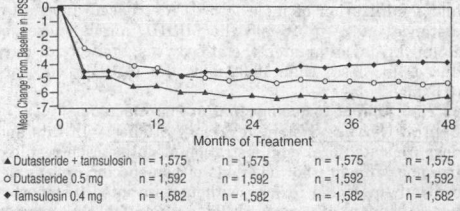

Dutasteride + tamsulosin	n = 1,575	n = 1,575	n = 1,575	n = 1,575
Dutasteride 0.5 mg	n = 1,592	n = 1,592	n = 1,592	n = 1,592
Tamsulosin 0.4 mg	n = 1,582	n = 1,582	n = 1,582	n = 1,582

Effect on Acute Urinary Retention or the Need for BPH-Related Surgery: After 4 years of treatment, combination therapy with AVODART and tamsulosin did not provide benefit over monotherapy with AVODART in reducing the incidence of AUR or BPH-related surgery.

Effect on Maximum Urine Flow Rate: The baseline Q_{max} was approximately 10.7 mL/sec for each treatment group. Combination therapy was statistically superior to each of the monotherapy treatments in increasing Q_{max} at Month 24, the primary time point for this endpoint. At Month 24, the mean increases from baseline (±SD) in Q_{max} were 2.4 (±5.26) mL/sec for combination, 1.9 (±5.10) mL/sec for AVODART, and 0.9 (±4.57) mL/sec for tamsulosin, with a mean difference between combination and AVODART of 0.5 mL/sec ($P = 0.003$; [95% CI: 0.17, 0.84]), and between combination and tamsulosin of 1.5 mL/sec ($P<0.001$; [95% CI: 1.19, 1.86]). This difference was seen by Month 6 and continued through Month 24. See Figure 7.

The additional improvement in Q_{max} of combination therapy over monotherapy with AVODART was no longer statistically significant at Month 48.

Figure 7. Q_{max} Change From Baseline Over a 24-Month Period (Randomized, Double-Blind, Parallel Group Trial [CombAT Trial])

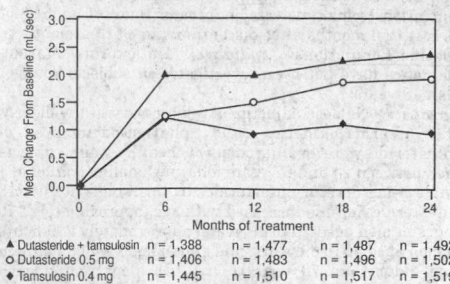

Dutasteride + tamsulosin	n = 1,388	n = 1,477	n = 1,487	n = 1,492
Dutasteride 0.5 mg	n = 1,406	n = 1,483	n = 1,496	n = 1,502
Tamsulosin 0.4 mg	n = 1,445	n = 1,510	n = 1,517	n = 1,519

Effect on Prostate Volume: The mean prostate volume at trial entry was approximately 55 cc. At Month 24, the primary time point for this endpoint, the mean percent changes from baseline (±SD) in prostate volume were -26.9% (±22.57) for combination therapy, -28.0% (±24.88) for AVODART, and 0% (±31.14) for tamsulosin, with a mean difference between combination and AVODART of 1.1% ($P =$ NS; [95% CI: -0.6, 2.8]), and between combination and tamsulosin of -26.9% ($P<0.001$; [95% CI: -28.9, -24.9]). Similar changes were seen at Month 48: -27.3% (±24.91) for combination therapy, -28.0% (±25.74) for AVODART, and +4.6% (±35.45) for tamsulosin.

16 HOW SUPPLIED/STORAGE AND HANDLING

AVODART Soft Gelatin Capsules 0.5 mg are oblong, opaque, dull yellow, gelatin capsules imprinted with "GX CE2" with red edible ink on one side packaged in bottles of 30 (NDC 0173-0712-15) and 90 (NDC 0173-0712-04) with child-resistant closures.

Store at 25°C (77°F); excursions permitted to 15-30°C (59-86°F) [see USP Controlled Room Temperature].

Dutasteride is absorbed through the skin. AVODART Capsules should not be handled by women who are pregnant or who could become pregnant because of the potential for absorption of dutasteride and the subsequent potential risk to a developing male fetus [see Warnings and Precautions (5.4)].

17 PATIENT COUNSELING INFORMATION

See FDA-approved patient labeling (Patient Information).

17.1 PSA Monitoring

Physicians should inform patients that AVODART reduces serum PSA levels by approximately 50% within 3 to 6 months of therapy, although it may vary for each individual. For patients undergoing PSA screening, increases in PSA levels while on treatment with AVODART may signal the presence of prostate cancer and should be evaluated by a healthcare provider [see Warnings and Precautions (5.1)].

17.2 Increased Risk of High-Grade Prostate Cancer

Physicians should inform patients that there was an increase in high-grade prostate cancer in men treated with 5 alpha-reductase inhibitors (which are indicated for BPH treatment), including AVODART, compared with those treated with placebo in trials looking at the use of these drugs to reduce the risk of prostate cancer [see Indications and Usage (1.3), Warnings and Precautions (5.2), Adverse Reactions (6.1)].

17.3 Exposure of Women—Risk to Male Fetus

Physicians should inform patients that AVODART Capsules should not be handled by a woman who is pregnant or who could become pregnant because of the potential for absorption of dutasteride and the subsequent potential risk to a developing male fetus. Dutasteride is absorbed through the skin and could result in unintended fetal exposure. If a pregnant woman or woman of childbearing potential comes in contact with leaking AVODART Capsules, the contact area should be washed immediately with soap and water [see Warnings and Precautions (5.4), Use in Specific Populations (8.1)].

17.4 Blood Donation

Physicians should inform men treated with AVODART that they should not donate blood until at least 6 months following their last dose to prevent pregnant women from receiving dutasteride through blood transfusion [see Warnings and Precautions (5.5)]. Serum levels of dutasteride are detectable for 4 to 6 months after treatment ends [see Clinical Pharmacology (12.3)].

GlaxoSmithKline
Research Triangle Park, NC 27709
Manufactured by Catalent Pharma Solutions
Somerset, NJ 08873 for
GlaxoSmithKline, Research Triangle Park, NC 27709
©2012, GlaxoSmithKline. All rights reserved.
AVT:11PI

PHARMACIST-DETACH HERE AND GIVE INSTRUCTIONS TO PATIENT

PATIENT INFORMATION
AVODART® (av' ō dart)
(dutasteride) Capsules
AVODART is for use by men only.

Read this patient information before you start taking AVODART and each time you get a refill. There may be new information. This information does not take the place of talking with your healthcare provider about your medical condition or your treatment.

What is AVODART?
AVODART is a prescription medicine that contains dutasteride. AVODART is used to treat the symptoms of benign prostatic hyperplasia (BPH) in men with an enlarged prostate to:
• improve symptoms
• reduce the risk of acute urinary retention (a complete blockage of urine flow)
• reduce the risk of the need for BPH-related surgery

Who should NOT take AVODART?
Do Not Take AVODART if you are:
• pregnant or could become pregnant. AVODART may harm your unborn baby. Pregnant women should not touch AVODART Capsules. If a woman who is pregnant with a male baby gets enough AVODART in her body by swallowing or touching AVODART, the male baby may be born with sex organs that are not normal. If a pregnant woman or woman of childbearing potential comes in contact with leaking AVODART Capsules, the contact area should be washed immediately with soap and water.
• a child or a teenager.
• allergic to dutasteride or any of the ingredients in AVODART. See the end of this leaflet for a complete list of ingredients in AVODART.
• allergic to other 5 alpha-reductase inhibitors, for example, PROSCAR (finasteride) Tablets.

What should I tell my healthcare provider before taking AVODART?
Before you take AVODART, tell your healthcare provider if you:
• have liver problems
Tell your healthcare provider about all the medicines you take, including prescription and non-prescription medicines, vitamins, and herbal supplements. AVODART and other medicines may affect each other, causing side effects. AVODART may affect the way other medicines work, and other medicines may affect how AVODART works.
Know the medicines you take. Keep a list of them to show your healthcare provider and pharmacist when you get a new medicine.

How should I take AVODART?
• Take 1 AVODART capsule once a day.
• Swallow AVODART capsules whole. Do not crush, chew, or open AVODART capsules because the contents of the capsule may irritate your lips, mouth, or throat.
• You can take AVODART with or without food.
• If you miss a dose, you may take it later that day. Do not make up the missed dose by taking 2 doses the next day.

What should I avoid while taking AVODART?
• You should not donate blood while taking AVODART or for 6 months after you have stopped AVODART. This is important to prevent pregnant women from receiving AVODART through blood transfusions.

What are the possible side effects of AVODART?
AVODART may cause serious side effects, including:
• **Rare and serious allergic reactions, including:**
  ○ swelling of your face, tongue, or throat
  ○ serious skin reactions, such as skin peeling
Get medical help right away if you have these serious allergic reactions.
• **Higher chance of a more serious form of prostate cancer.**

The most common side effects of AVODART include:
• trouble getting or keeping an erection (impotence) [1]
• a decrease in sex drive (libido) [1]
• ejaculation problems [1]
• enlarged or painful breasts. If you notice breast lumps or nipple discharge, you should talk to your healthcare provider.

Depressed mood has been reported in patients receiving AVODART.

AVODART has been shown to reduce sperm count, semen volume, and sperm movement. However, the effect of AVODART on male fertility is not known.

Prostate-Specific Antigen (PSA) Test: Your healthcare provider may check you for other prostate problems, including prostate cancer before you start and while you take AVODART. A blood test called PSA (prostate-specific antigen) is sometimes used to see if you might have prostate cancer. AVODART will reduce the amount of PSA measured in your blood. Your healthcare provider is aware of this effect and can still use PSA to see if you might have prostate

cancer. Increases in your PSA levels while on treatment with AVODART (even if the PSA levels are in the normal range) should be evaluated by your healthcare provider.
Tell your healthcare provider if you have any side effect that bothers you or that does not go away.
These are not all the possible side effects with AVODART. For more information, ask you healthcare provider or pharmacist.
Call your doctor for medical advice about side effects. You may report side effects to FDA at 1-800-FDA-1088.

[1]Some of these events may continue after you stop taking AVODART.

How should I store AVODART?
• Store AVODART Capsules at room temperature (59°F to 86°F or 15°C to 30°C).
• AVODART Capsules may become deformed and/or discolored if kept at high temperatures.
• Do not use AVODART if your capsules are deformed, discolored, or leaking.
• Safely throw away medicine that is no longer needed.
Keep AVODART and all medicines out of the reach of children.
Medicines are sometimes prescribed for purposes other than those listed in a patient leaflet. Do not use AVODART for a condition for which it was not prescribed. Do not give AVODART to other people, even if they have the same symptoms that you have. It may harm them.
This patient information leaflet summarizes the most important information about AVODART. If you would like more information, talk with your healthcare provider. You can ask your pharmacist or healthcare provider for information about AVODART that is written for health professionals.
For more information, go to www.AVODART.com or call 1-888-825-5249.

What are the ingredients in AVODART?
Active ingredient: dutasteride.
Inactive ingredients: butylated hydroxytoluene, ferric oxide (yellow), gelatin (from certified BSE-free bovine sources), glycerin, mono-di-glycerides of caprylic/capric acid, titanium dioxide, and edible red ink.

How does AVODART work?
Prostate growth is caused by a hormone in the blood called dihydrotestosterone (DHT). AVODART lowers DHT production in the body, leading to shrinkage of the enlarged prostate in most men. While some men have fewer problems and symptoms after 3 months of treatment with AVODART, a treatment of period of at least 6 months is usually necessary to see if AVODART will work for you.

GlaxoSmithKline
Research Triangle Park, NC 27709
Manufactured by Catalent Pharma Solutions
Somerset, NJ 08873 for
GlaxoSmithKline
Research Triangle Park, NC 27709
©2012, GlaxoSmithKline. All rights reserved.
October 2012
AVT:8PIL

BECONASE AQ® ℞
[be'kō-nāz]
(beclomethasone dipropionate, monohydrate)
Nasal Spray, 42 mcg
For Intranasal Use Only.
SHAKE WELL BEFORE USE.

DESCRIPTION
Beclomethasone dipropionate, monohydrate, the active component of BECONASE AQ Nasal Spray, is an anti-inflammatory steroid having the chemical name 9-chloro-11β,17,21-trihydroxy-16β-methylpregna-1,4-diene-3,20-dione 17,21-dipropionate, monohydrate and the following chemical structure:

Beclomethasone 17,21-dipropionate is a diester of beclomethasone, a synthetic halogenated corticosteroid. Beclomethasone dipropionate, monohydrate is a white to creamy-white, odorless powder with a molecular weight of 539.06. It is very slightly soluble in water, very soluble in chloroform, and freely soluble in acetone and in ethanol.
BECONASE AQ Nasal Spray is a metered-dose, manual pump spray unit containing a microcrystalline suspension of beclomethasone dipropionate, monohydrate equivalent to 42 mcg of beclomethasone dipropionate, calculated on the

dried basis, in an aqueous medium containing microcrystalline cellulose, carboxymethylcellulose sodium, dextrose, benzalkonium chloride, polysorbate 80, and 0.25% v/w phenylethyl alcohol. The pH through expiry is 5.0 to 6.8.
After initial priming (6 actuations), each actuation of the pump delivers from the nasal adapter 100 mg of suspension containing beclomethasone dipropionate, monohydrate equivalent to 42 mcg of beclomethasone dipropionate. If the pump is not used for 7 days, it should be primed until a fine spray appears. Each 25-g bottle of BECONASE AQ Nasal Spray provides 180 metered sprays.

CLINICAL PHARMACOLOGY
Mechanism of Action
Following topical administration, beclomethasone dipropionate produces anti-inflammatory and vasoconstrictor effects. The mechanisms responsible for the anti-inflammatory action of beclomethasone dipropionate are unknown. Corticosteroids have been shown to have a wide range of effects on multiple cell types (e.g., mast cells, eosinophils, neutrophils, macrophages, and lymphocytes) and mediators (e.g., histamine, eicosanoids, leukotrienes, and cytokines) involved in inflammation. The direct relationship of these findings to the effects of beclomethasone dipropionate on allergic rhinitis symptoms is not known.
Biopsies of nasal mucosa obtained during clinical studies showed no histopathologic changes when beclomethasone dipropionate was administered intranasally.
Beclomethasone dipropionate is a pro-drug with weak glucocorticoid receptor binding affinity. It is hydrolyzed via esterase enzymes to its active metabolite beclomethasone-17-monopropionate (B-17-MP), which has high topical anti-inflammatory activity.

Pharmacokinetics
Absorption: Beclomethasone dipropionate is sparingly soluble in water. When given by nasal inhalation in the form of an aqueous or aerosolized suspension, the drug is deposited primarily in the nasal passages. The majority of the drug is eventually swallowed. Following intranasal administration of aqueous beclomethasone dipropionate, the systemic absorption was assessed by measuring the plasma concentrations of its active metabolite B-17-MP, for which the absolute bioavailability following intranasal administration is 44% (43% of the administered dose came from the swallowed portion and only 1% of the total dose was bioavailable from the nose). The absorption of unchanged beclomethasone dipropionate following oral and intranasal dosing was undetectable (plasma concentrations <50 pg/mL).
Distribution: The tissue distribution at steady state for beclomethasone dipropionate is moderate (20 L) but more extensive for B-17-MP (424 L). There is no evidence of tissue storage of beclomethasone dipropionate or its metabolites. Plasma protein binding is moderately high (87%).
Metabolism: Beclomethasone dipropionate is cleared very rapidly from the systemic circulation by metabolism mediated via esterase enzymes that are found in most tissues. The main product of metabolism is the active metabolite (B-17-MP). Minor inactive metabolites, beclomethasone-21-monopropionate (B-21-MP) and beclomethasone (BOH), are also formed, but these contribute little to systemic exposure.
Elimination: The elimination of beclomethasone dipropionate and B-17-MP after intravenous administration are characterized by high plasma clearance (150 and 120 L/hour) with corresponding terminal elimination half-lives of 0.5 and 2.7 hours. Following oral administration of tritiated beclomethasone dipropionate, approximately 60% of the dose was excreted in the feces within 96 hours, mainly as free and conjugated polar metabolites. Approximately 12% of the dose was excreted as free and conjugated polar metabolites in the urine. The renal clearance of beclomethasone dipropionate and its metabolites is negligible.

Pharmacodynamics
The effects of beclomethasone dipropionate on hypothalamic-pituitary-adrenal (HPA) function have been evaluated in adult volunteers by other routes of administration. Studies with beclomethasone dipropionate by the intranasal route may demonstrate that there is more or that there is less absorption by this route of administration. There was no suppression of early morning plasma cortisol concentrations when beclomethasone dipropionate was administered in a dose of 1,000 mcg/day for 1 month as an oral aerosol or for 3 days by intramuscular injection. However, partial suppression of plasma cortisol concentrations was observed when beclomethasone dipropionate was administered in doses of 2,000 mcg/day either by oral aerosol or intramuscular injection. Immediate suppression of plasma cortisol concentrations was observed after single doses of 4,000 mcg of beclomethasone dipropionate. Suppression of HPA function (reduction of early morning plasma cortisol levels) has been reported in adult patients who received 1,600-mcg daily doses of oral beclomethasone dipropionate for 1 month. In clinical studies using beclomethasone

dipropionate aerosol intranasally, there was no evidence of adrenal insufficiency. The effect of BECONASE AQ Nasal Spray on HPA function was not evaluated but would not be expected to differ from intranasal beclomethasone dipropionate aerosol.

In 1 study in children with asthma, the administration of inhaled beclomethasone at recommended daily doses for at least 1 year was associated with a reduction in nocturnal cortisol secretion. The clinical significance of this finding is not clear. It reinforces other evidence, however, that topical beclomethasone may be absorbed in amounts that can have systemic effects and that physicians should be alert for evidence of systemic effects, especially in chronically treated patients (see PRECAUTIONS).

INDICATIONS AND USAGE

BECONASE AQ Nasal Spray is indicated for the relief of the symptoms of seasonal or perennial allergic and nonallergic (vasomotor) rhinitis.

Results from 2 clinical trials have shown that significant symptomatic relief was obtained within 3 days. However, symptomatic relief may not occur in some patients for as long as 2 weeks. BECONASE AQ Nasal Spray should not be continued beyond 3 weeks in the absence of significant symptomatic improvement. BECONASE AQ Nasal Spray should not be used in the presence of untreated localized infection involving the nasal mucosa.

BECONASE AQ Nasal Spray is also indicated for the prevention of recurrence of nasal polyps following surgical removal.

Clinical studies have shown that treatment of the symptoms associated with nasal polyps may have to be continued for several weeks or more before a therapeutic result can be fully assessed. Recurrence of symptoms due to polyps can occur after stopping treatment, depending on the severity of the disease.

CONTRAINDICATIONS

Hypersensitivity to any of the ingredients of this preparation contraindicates its use.

WARNINGS

The replacement of a systemic corticosteroid with BECONASE AQ Nasal Spray can be accompanied by signs of adrenal insufficiency.

Careful attention must be given when patients previously treated for prolonged periods with systemic corticosteroids are transferred to BECONASE AQ Nasal Spray. This is particularly important in those patients who have associated asthma or other clinical conditions where too rapid a decrease in systemic corticosteroids may cause a severe exacerbation of their symptoms.

If recommended doses of intranasal beclomethasone are exceeded or if individuals are particularly sensitive or predisposed by virtue of recent systemic steroid therapy, symptoms of hypercorticism may occur, including very rare cases of menstrual irregularities, acneiform lesions, cataracts, and cushingoid features. If such changes occur, BECONASE AQ Nasal Spray should be discontinued slowly consistent with accepted procedures for discontinuing oral steroid therapy.

Persons who are using drugs that suppress the immune system are more susceptible to infections than healthy individuals. Chickenpox and measles, for example, can have a more serious or even fatal course in susceptible children or adults using corticosteroids. In children or adults who have not had these diseases or been properly immunized, particular care should be taken to avoid exposure. How the dose, route, and duration of corticosteroid administration affect the risk of developing a disseminated infection is not known. The contribution of the underlying disease and/or prior corticosteroid treatment to the risk is also not known. If exposed to chickenpox, prophylaxis with varicella zoster immune globulin (VZIG) may be indicated. If exposed to measles, prophylaxis with pooled intramuscular immunoglobulin (IG) may be indicated. (See the respective package inserts for complete VZIG and IG prescribing information.) If chickenpox develops, treatment with antiviral agents may be considered.

Avoid spraying in eyes.

PRECAUTIONS

General

Intranasal corticosteroids may cause a reduction in growth velocity when administered to pediatric patients (see PRECAUTIONS: Pediatric Use).

During withdrawal from oral corticosteroids, some patients may experience symptoms of withdrawal, e.g., joint and/or muscular pain, lassitude, and depression.

Rarely, immediate hypersensitivity reactions may occur after the intranasal administration of beclomethasone (see ADVERSE REACTIONS).

Rare instances of nasal septum perforation have been spontaneously reported.

Rare instances of wheezing, cataracts, glaucoma, and increased intraocular pressure have been reported following the intranasal use of beclomethasone dipropionate.

In clinical studies with beclomethasone dipropionate administered intranasally, the development of localized infections of the nose and pharynx with *Candida albicans* has occurred only rarely. When such an infection develops, it may require treatment with appropriate local therapy and discontinuation of treatment with BECONASE AQ Nasal Spray.

If persistent nasopharyngeal irritation occurs, it may be an indication for stopping BECONASE AQ Nasal Spray.

Beclomethasone dipropionate is absorbed into the circulation. Use of excessive doses of BECONASE AQ Nasal Spray may suppress HPA function.

Intranasal corticosteroids should be used with caution, if at all, in patients with active or quiescent tuberculous infections of the respiratory tract, untreated local or systemic fungal or bacterial infections, systemic viral or parasitic infections, or ocular herpes simplex.

For BECONASE AQ Nasal Spray to be effective in the treatment of nasal polyps, the spray must be able to enter the nose. Therefore, treatment of nasal polyps with BECONASE AQ Nasal Spray should be considered adjunctive therapy to surgical removal and/or the use of other medications that will permit effective penetration of BECONASE AQ Nasal Spray into the nose. Nasal polyps may recur after any form of treatment.

As with any long-term treatment, patients using BECONASE AQ Nasal Spray over several months or longer should be examined periodically for possible changes in the nasal mucosa.

Because of the inhibitory effect of corticosteroids on wound healing, patients who have experienced recent nasal septal ulcers, nasal surgery, or nasal trauma should not use a nasal corticosteroid until healing has occurred.

Although systemic effects have been minimal with recommended doses, this potential increases with excessive doses. Therefore, larger than recommended doses should be avoided.

Information for Patients

Patients being treated with BECONASE AQ Nasal Spray should receive the following information and instructions. This information is intended to aid them in the safe and effective use of this medication. It is not a disclosure of all possible adverse or intended effects.

Patients should use BECONASE AQ Nasal Spray at regular intervals since its effectiveness depends on its regular use. The patient should take the medication as directed. It is not acutely effective, and the prescribed dosage should not be increased. Instead, nasal vasoconstrictors or oral antihistamines may be needed until the effects of BECONASE AQ Nasal Spray are fully manifested. One to 2 weeks may pass before full relief is obtained. The patient should contact the physician if symptoms do not improve, if the condition worsens, or if sneezing or nasal irritation occurs.

For the proper use of BECONASE AQ Nasal Spray and to attain maximum improvement, the patient should read and follow carefully the patient's instructions accompanying the product.

Persons who are using immunosuppressant doses of corticosteroids should be warned to avoid exposure to chickenpox or measles. Patients should also be advised that if they are exposed, medical advice should be sought without delay.

Carcinogenesis, Mutagenesis, Impairment of Fertility

The carcinogenicity of beclomethasone dipropionate was evaluated in rats that were exposed for a total of 95 weeks, 13 weeks at inhalation doses up to 0.4 mg/kg and the remaining 82 weeks at combined oral and inhalation doses up to 2.4 mg/kg. There was no evidence of carcinogenicity in this study at the highest dose, approximately 60 times the maximum recommended daily intranasal dose in adults on a mg/m^2 basis or approximately 35 times the maximum recommended daily intranasal dose in children on a mg/m^2 basis.

Beclomethasone dipropionate did not induce gene mutation in bacterial cells or mammalian Chinese hamster ovary (CHO) cells in vitro. No significant clastogenic effect was seen in cultured CHO cells in vitro or in the mouse micronucleus test in vivo.

In rats, beclomethasone dipropionate caused decreased conception rates at an oral dose of 16 mg/kg (approximately 390 times the maximum recommended daily intranasal dose in adults on a mg/m^2 basis). There was no significant effect of beclomethasone dipropionate on fertility in rats at oral doses of 1.6 mg/kg (approximately 40 times the maximum recommended daily intranasal dose in adults on a mg/m^2 basis). Inhibition of the estrous cycle in dogs was observed following oral dosing at 0.5 mg/kg (approximately 40 times the maximum recommended daily intranasal dose in adults on a mg/m^2 basis). No inhibition of the estrous cycle in dogs was seen following 12 months' exposure at an estimated in-

halation dose of 0.33 mg/kg (approximately 25 times the maximum recommended daily intranasal dose in adults on a mg/m^2 basis).

Pregnancy

Teratogenic Effects: Pregnancy Category C. Like other corticosteroids, beclomethasone dipropionate was teratogenic and embryocidal in the mouse and rabbit at a subcutaneous dose of 0.1 mg/kg in mice or 0.025 mg/kg in rabbits (approximately equal to the maximum recommended daily intranasal dose in adults on a mg/m^2 basis). No teratogenicity or embryocidal effects were seen in rats when exposed to an inhalation dose of 0.1 mg/kg plus oral doses of up to 10 mg/kg per day for a combined dose of 10.1 mg/kg (approximately 240 times the maximum recommended daily intranasal dose in adults on a mg/m^2 basis).

There are no adequate and well-controlled studies in pregnant women. Beclomethasone dipropionate should be used during pregnancy only if the potential benefit justifies the potential risk to the fetus.

Nonteratogenic Effects: Hypoadrenalism may occur in infants born of mothers receiving corticosteroids during pregnancy. Such infants should be carefully observed.

Nursing Mothers

It is not known whether beclomethasone dipropionate is excreted in human milk. Because other corticosteroids are excreted in human milk, caution should be exercised when BECONASE AQ Nasal Spray is administered to a nursing woman.

Pediatric Use

The safety and effectiveness of BECONASE AQ Nasal Spray have been established in children aged 6 years and above through evidence from extensive clinical use in adult and pediatric patients. The safety and effectiveness of BECONASE AQ Nasal Spray in children below 6 years of age have not been established.

Controlled clinical studies have shown that intranasal corticosteroids may cause a reduction in growth velocity in pediatric patients. This effect has been observed in the absence of laboratory evidence of HPA axis suppression, suggesting that growth velocity is a more sensitive indicator of systemic corticosteroid exposure in pediatric patients than some commonly used tests of HPA axis function. The long-term effects of this reduction in growth velocity associated with intranasal corticosteroids, including the impact on final adult height, are unknown. The potential for "catch-up" growth following discontinuation of treatment with intranasal corticosteroids has not been adequately studied. The growth of pediatric patients receiving intranasal corticosteroids, including BECONASE AQ Nasal Spray, should be monitored routinely (e.g., via stadiometry). The potential growth effects of prolonged treatment should be weighed against the clinical benefits obtained and the risks/benefits of treatment alternatives. To minimize the systemic effects of intranasal corticosteroids, including BECONASE AQ Nasal Spray, each patient should be titrated to the lowest dose that effectively controls his/her symptoms.

In a double-blind, controlled trial, 100 children between the ages of 6 and 9½ years with allergic rhinitis were randomized to receive aqueous intranasal beclomethasone dipropionate 168 mcg twice daily or placebo for 1 year. As measured by stadiometry, children who received beclomethasone dipropionate grew more slowly than those who received placebo. A difference in mean change in height was observed within 1 month of drug initiation. At the end of 12 months, the beclomethasone dipropionate-treated group had a growth velocity on average of 4.75 cm/year compared to 6.20 cm/year in the placebo group (p<0.01). While the placebo group had an expected distribution of growth velocity, approximately 50% of the beclomethasone dipropionate-treated children grew below the 10th percentile.

In children 7.3 years of age, the mean age of children in this study, the range for expected growth velocity is: boys – 3rd percentile = 4.1 cm/year, 50th percentile = 5.8 cm/year, and 97th percentile = 7.5 cm/year; girls – 3rd percentile = 4.3 cm/year, 50th percentile = 5.9 cm/year, and 97th percentile = 7.5 cm/year. The potential reversibility of the reduction in growth velocity was not studied. No significant differences were observed between the 2 groups for mean basal plasma cortisol or ACTH-stimulated plasma cortisol levels.

Geriatric Use

Clinical studies of BECONASE AQ Nasal Spray did not include sufficient numbers of subjects aged 65 and over to determine whether they respond differently from younger subjects. Other reported clinical experience has not identified differences in responses between the elderly and younger patients. In general, dose selection for an elderly patient should be cautious, starting at the low end of the dosing range, reflecting the greater frequency of decreased hepatic, renal, or cardiac function, and of concomitant disease or other drug therapy.

ADVERSE REACTIONS

In general, side effects in clinical studies have been primarily associated with irritation of the nasal mucous membranes.

Adverse reactions reported in controlled clinical trials and open studies in patients treated with BECONASE AQ Nasal Spray are described below.

Mild nasopharyngeal irritation following the use of beclomethasone aqueous nasal spray has been reported in up to 24% of patients treated, including occasional sneezing attacks (about 4%) occurring immediately following use of the spray. In patients experiencing these symptoms, none had to discontinue treatment. The incidence of transient irritation and sneezing was approximately the same in the group of patients who received placebo in these studies, implying that these complaints may be related to vehicle components of the formulation.

Fewer than 5 per 100 patients reported headache, nausea, or lightheadedness following the use of BECONASE AQ Nasal Spray. Fewer than 3 per 100 patients reported nasal stuffiness, nosebleeds, rhinorrhea, or tearing eyes.

Rare cases of ulceration of the nasal mucosa and instances of nasal septum perforation have been spontaneously reported (see PRECAUTIONS).

Reports of dryness and irritation of the nose and throat and unpleasant taste and smell have been received. There are rare reports of loss of taste and smell.

Rare instances of wheezing, cataracts, glaucoma, and increased intraocular pressure have been reported following the use of intranasal beclomethasone dipropionate (see PRECAUTIONS).

Rare cases of immediate and delayed hypersensitivity reactions, including anaphylactoid/anaphylactic reactions, urticaria, angioedema, rash, and bronchospasm, have been reported following the oral and intranasal inhalation of beclomethasone dipropionate.

Cases of growth suppression have been reported for intranasal corticosteroids, including BECONASE AQ (see PRECAUTIONS: Pediatric Use).

OVERDOSAGE

When used at excessive doses, systemic corticosteroid effects such as hypercorticism and adrenal suppression may appear. If such changes occur, BECONASE AQ Nasal Spray should be discontinued slowly consistent with accepted procedures for discontinuing oral steroid therapy. No deaths occurred when beclomethasone dipropionate was given as single oral doses of 3,000 mg/kg to mice (approximately 36,000 times the maximum recommended daily intranasal dose in adults on a mg/m^2 basis, or approximately 21,000 times the maximum recommended daily intranasal dose in children on a mg/m^2 basis) and 2,000 mg/kg to rats (approximately 48,000 times the maximum recommended daily intranasal dose in adults or approximately 29,000 times the maximum recommended daily intranasal dose in children on a mg/m^2 basis). One bottle of BECONASE AQ Nasal Spray contains beclomethasone dipropionate, monohydrate equivalent to 10.5 mg of beclomethasone dipropionate; therefore, acute overdosage is unlikely.

DOSAGE AND ADMINISTRATION
Adults and Children 12 Years of Age and Older
The usual dosage is 1 or 2 nasal inhalations (42 to 84 mcg) in each nostril twice a day (total dose, 168 to 336 mcg/day).
Children 6 to 12 Years of Age
Patients should be started with 1 nasal inhalation in each nostril twice daily; patients not adequately responding to 168 mcg or those with more severe symptoms may use 336 mcg (2 inhalations in each nostril). Once adequate control is achieved, the dosage should be decreased to 84 mcg (1 spray in each nostril) twice daily. BECONASE AQ Nasal Spray is *not* recommended for children below 6 years of age. The maximum total daily dosage should not exceed 2 sprays in each nostril twice daily (336 mcg/day).

In patients who respond to BECONASE AQ Nasal Spray, an improvement of the symptoms of seasonal or perennial rhinitis usually becomes apparent within a few days after the start of therapy with BECONASE AQ Nasal Spray. However, symptomatic relief may not occur in some patients for as long as 2 weeks. BECONASE AQ Nasal Spray should not be continued beyond 3 weeks in the absence of significant symptomatic improvement.

The therapeutic effects of corticosteroids, unlike those of decongestants, are not immediate. This should be explained to the patient in advance in order to ensure cooperation and continuation of treatment with the prescribed dosage regimen.

In the presence of excessive nasal mucous secretion or edema of the nasal mucosa, the drug may fail to reach the site of intended action. In such cases it is advisable to use a nasal vasoconstrictor during the first 2 to 3 days of therapy with BECONASE AQ Nasal Spray.
Directions for Use
Illustrated Patient's Instructions for Use accompany each package of BECONASE AQ Nasal Spray.

HOW SUPPLIED
BECONASE AQ Nasal Spray, 42 mcg is supplied in an amber glass bottle fitted with a metering atomizing pump and nasal adapter in a box of 1 (NDC 0173-0388-79) with patient's instructions for use. Each bottle contains 25 g of suspension and will provide 180 metered sprays.

The correct amount of medication in each spray cannot be assured after 180 sprays even though the bottle is not completely empty. The bottle should be discarded when the labeled number of actuations has been used.

Store between 15° and 30°C (59° and 86°F).

GlaxoSmithKline
Research Triangle Park, NC 27709
April 2005 RL-2182

Patient's Instructions for Use

PHARMACIST—DETACH HERE AND GIVE INSTRUCTIONS TO PATIENT

BECONASE AQ®
(beclomethasone dipropionate, monohydrate)
Nasal Spray, 42 mcg
For Intranasal Use Only. SHAKE WELL BEFORE USE.
Patient's Instructions for Use
Shake the suspension spray bottle well before using it. Read complete instructions carefully and use only as directed.
To Use:
1. Remove the safety clip and the plastic dust cap from the nasal applicator (Figure 1).

Figure 1
2. The very first time the spray is used, prime the pump into the air by pressing downward on the white collar, using your forefinger and middle finger while supporting the base of the bottle with your thumb. When you prime the pump for the first time, press down and release the pump 6 times or until a fine spray appears (Figure 2).
The pump is now ready for use. If the pump is not used for 7 days, prime until a fine spray appears.

Figure 2
3. Gently blow your nose to clear your nostrils. Close 1 nostril. Tilt your head forward slightly and, keeping the bottle upright, carefully insert the nasal applicator into the other nostril (Figure 3).

Figure 3
4. For each spray, press firmly downward once on the white collar, using your forefinger and middle finger while supporting the base of the bottle with your thumb. Avoid spraying in eyes. Breathe gently inward through the nostril.
5. Breathe out through your mouth.
6. Repeat steps 5 through 7 in the other nostril.
7. Replace the plastic dust cap and safety clip.
8. DISCARD THE BOTTLE AFTER the date calculated by your doctor or pharmacist. The correct amount of medication in each spray cannot be assured after 180 sprays even though the bottle is not completely empty. Discard the bottle after 180 sprays. Before the discard date you should consult your doctor to see if a refill is needed. Do not take extra doses or stop taking BECONASE AQ Nasal Spray without consulting your doctor.
Cleansing: To clean the nasal applicator, remove the plastic dust cap and safety clip and then press gently upward on the white collar to free the nasal applicator. Wash the applicator and dust cap with cold water. Dry and replace with the plastic dust cap and safety clip back in position.
If the nasal applicator becomes blocked, remove the dust cap, unscrew the complete pump mechanism, and soak the pump in warm water for a few minutes. Rinse with cold water, dry, refit to bottle, and reprime the pump.

Caution: BECONASE AQ Nasal Spray is not intended to give rapid relief of your nasal symptoms. BECONASE AQ Nasal Spray controls the underlying disorders responsible for your attacks, so it is important that you use it regularly at the times recommended by your doctor. The full benefit of BECONASE AQ Nasal Spray may take a few days to develop.
Storage: Store between 15° and 30°C (59° and 86°F).
GlaxoSmithKline
Research Triangle Park, NC 27709
April 2005 RL-2182

BENLYSTA®
(belimumab)
for injection, for intravenous use only   ℞

HIGHLIGHTS OF PRESCRIBING INFORMATION
These highlights do not include all the information needed to use BENLYSTA safely and effectively. See full prescribing information for BENLYSTA.
BENLYSTA® (belimumab)
for injection, for intravenous use only
Initial U.S. Approval: 2011

——RECENT MAJOR CHANGES——
Warnings and Precautions, Serious Infections (5.2)   04/2014
Warnings and Precautions, Hypersensitivity Reactions, Including Anaphylaxis (5.4)   12/2013

——INDICATIONS AND USAGE——
BENLYSTA is a B-lymphocyte stimulator (BLyS)-specific inhibitor indicated for the treatment of adult patients with active, autoantibody-positive, systemic lupus erythematosus who are receiving standard therapy. (1, 14)
Limitations of Use: The efficacy of BENLYSTA has not been evaluated in patients with severe active lupus nephritis or severe active central nervous system lupus (1). BENLYSTA has not been studied in combination with other biologics or intravenous cyclophosphamide (1). Use of BENLYSTA is not recommended in these situations.

——DOSAGE AND ADMINISTRATION——
• Recommended dosage regimen is 10 mg/kg at 2-week intervals for the first 3 doses and at 4-week intervals thereafter. Reconstitute, dilute and administer as an intravenous infusion only, over a period of 1 hour. (2.1)
• Consider administering premedication for prophylaxis against infusion reactions and hypersensitivity reactions. (2.2)

——DOSAGE FORMS AND STRENGTHS——
Single-use vials of belimumab lyophilized powder:
• 120 mg per vial (3)
• 400 mg per vial (3)

——CONTRAINDICATIONS——
Previous anaphylaxis to belimumab. (4)

——WARNINGS AND PRECAUTIONS——
• Mortality: There were more deaths reported with BENLYSTA than with placebo during the controlled period of clinical trials. (5.1)
• Serious Infections: Serious and sometimes fatal infections have been reported in patients receiving immunosuppressive agents, including BENLYSTA. Use with caution in patients with chronic infections. Consider interrupting therapy with BENLYSTA if patients develop a new infection during treatment with BENLYSTA. (5.2)
• Progressive Multifocal Leukoencephalopathy (PML): Patients presenting with new-onset or deteriorating neurological signs and symptoms should be evaluated for PML by an appropriate specialist. If PML is confirmed, consider discontinuation of immunosuppressant therapy, including BENLYSTA. (5.2)
• Hypersensitivity Reactions, Including Anaphylaxis: Serious and fatal reactions have been reported. BENLYSTA should be administered by healthcare providers prepared to manage anaphylaxis. Monitor patients during and for an appropriate period of time after administration of BENLYSTA. (2.2, 5.4)
• Depression: Depression and suicidality have been reported in trials with BENLYSTA. Patients should be instructed to contact their healthcare provider if they experience new or worsening depression, suicidal thoughts or other mood changes. (5.6)
• Immunization: Live vaccines should not be given concurrently with BENLYSTA. (5.7)

——ADVERSE REACTIONS——
Common adverse reactions (≥5%) in clinical trials were: nausea, diarrhea, pyrexia, nasopharyngitis, bronchitis, insomnia, pain in extremity, depression, migraine, and pharyngitis. (6.1)

To report SUSPECTED ADVERSE REACTIONS, contact GlaxoSmithKline at 1-877-423-6597 or FDA at 1-800-FDA-1088 or www.fda.gov/medwatch.

See 17 for PATIENT COUNSELING INFORMATION and Medication Guide

Revised: 04/2014

FULL PRESCRIBING INFORMATION: CONTENTS*
RECENT MAJOR CHANGES

FULL PRESCRIBING INFORMATION

1 INDICATIONS AND USAGE

BENLYSTA® (belimumab) is indicated for the treatment of adult patients with active, autoantibody-positive, systemic lupus erythematosus (SLE) who are receiving standard therapy.

Limitations of Use: The efficacy of BENLYSTA has not been evaluated in patients with severe active lupus nephritis or severe active central nervous system lupus. BENLYSTA has not been studied in combination with other biologics or intravenous cyclophosphamide. Use of BENLYSTA is not recommended in these situations.

2 DOSAGE AND ADMINISTRATION
2.1 Dosage Schedule

BENLYSTA is for intravenous infusion **only** and must be reconstituted and diluted prior to administration [see Dosage and Administration (2.3)]. Do not administer as an intravenous push or bolus.

The recommended dosage regimen is 10 mg/kg at 2-week intervals for the first 3 doses and at 4-week intervals thereafter. Reconstitute, dilute, and administer as an intravenous infusion only, over a period of 1 hour. The infusion rate may be slowed or interrupted if the patient develops an infusion reaction. The infusion must be discontinued immediately if the patient experiences a serious hypersensitivity reaction [see Contraindications (4), Warnings and Precautions (5.4)].

2.2 Premedication Recommendations

Prior to dosing with BENLYSTA, consider administering premedication for prophylaxis against infusion reactions and hypersensitivity reactions. [see Warnings and Precautions (5.4, 5.5), Adverse Reactions (6.1)].

2.3 Preparation of Solutions

BENLYSTA is provided as a lyophilized powder in a single-use vial for intravenous infusion only and should be reconstituted and diluted by a healthcare professional using aseptic technique as follows:

Reconstitution Instructions

1. Remove BENLYSTA from the refrigerator and allow to stand 10 to 15 minutes for the vial to reach room temperature.
2. Reconstitute the BENLYSTA powder with Sterile Water for Injection, USP, as follows: The reconstituted solution will contain a concentration of 80 mg/mL belimumab.
• Reconstitute the 120-mg vial with 1.5 mL Sterile Water for Injection, USP.
• Reconstitute the 400-mg vial with 4.8 mL Sterile Water for Injection, USP.
3. The stream of sterile water should be directed toward the side of the vial to minimize foaming. Gently swirl the vial for 60 seconds. Allow the vial to sit at room temperature during reconstitution, gently swirling the vial for 60 seconds every 5 minutes until the powder is dissolved. *Do not shake.* Reconstitution is typically complete within 10 to 15 minutes after the sterile water has been added, but it may take up to 30 minutes. Protect the reconstituted solution from sunlight.
4. If a mechanical reconstitution device (swirler) is used to reconstitute BENLYSTA, it should not exceed 500 rpm and the vial swirled for no longer than 30 minutes.
5. Once reconstitution is complete, the solution should be opalescent and colorless to pale yellow, and without particles. Small air bubbles, however, are expected and acceptable.

Dilution Instructions

6. Dextrose intravenous solutions are incompatible with BENLYSTA. BENLYSTA should only be diluted in 0.9% Sodium Chloride Injection, USP. Dilute the reconstituted product to 250 mL in 0.9% Sodium Chloride Injection, USP (normal saline) for intravenous infusion. From a 250-mL infusion bag or bottle of normal saline, withdraw and discard a volume equal to the volume of the reconstituted solution of BENLYSTA required for the patient's dose. Then add the required volume of the reconstituted solution of BENLYSTA into the infusion bag or bottle. Gently invert the bag or bottle to mix the solution. Any unused solution in the vials must be discarded.
7. Parenteral drug products should be inspected visually for particulate matter and discoloration prior to administration, whenever solution and container permit. Discard the solution if any particulate matter or discoloration is observed.
8. The reconstituted solution of BENLYSTA, if not used immediately, should be stored protected from direct sunlight and refrigerated at 2° to 8°C (36° to 46°F). Solutions of BENLYSTA diluted in normal saline may be stored at 2° to 8°C (36° to 46°F) or room temperature. The total time from reconstitution of BENLYSTA to completion of infusion should not exceed 8 hours.
9. No incompatibilities between BENLYSTA and polyvinylchloride or polyolefin bags have been observed.

2.4 Administration Instructions

1. The diluted solution of BENLYSTA should be administered by intravenous infusion only, over a period of 1 hour.
2. BENLYSTA should be administered by healthcare providers prepared to manage anaphylaxis [Warnings and Precautions (5.4)].
3. BENLYSTA should not be infused concomitantly in the same intravenous line with other agents. No physical or biochemical compatibility studies have been conducted to evaluate the coadministration of BENLYSTA with other agents.

3 DOSAGE FORMS AND STRENGTHS

Single-use vials of belimumab lyophilized powder for injection:
• 120 mg per vial
• 400 mg per vial

4 CONTRAINDICATIONS

BENLYSTA is contraindicated in patients who have had anaphylaxis with belimumab.

5 WARNINGS AND PRECAUTIONS
5.1 Mortality

There were more deaths reported with BENLYSTA than with placebo during the controlled period of the clinical trials. Out of 2,133 patients in 3 clinical trials, a total of 14 deaths occurred during the placebo-controlled, double-blind treatment periods: 3/675 (0.4%), 5/673 (0.7%), 0/111 (0%), and 6/674 (0.9%) deaths in the groups receiving placebo, BENLYSTA 1 mg/kg, BENLYSTA 4 mg/kg, and BENLYSTA 10 mg/kg, respectively. No single cause of death predominated. Etiologies included infection, cardiovascular disease, and suicide.

5.2 Serious Infections

Serious and sometimes fatal infections have been reported in patients receiving immunosuppressive agents, including BENLYSTA. Physicians should exercise caution when considering the use of BENLYSTA in patients with chronic infections. Patients receiving any therapy for chronic infection should not begin therapy with BENLYSTA. Consider interrupting therapy with BENLYSTA in patients who develop a new infection while undergoing treatment with BENLYSTA and monitor these patients closely.

In the controlled clinical trials, the overall incidence of infections was 71% in patients treated with BENLYSTA compared with 67% in patients who received placebo. The most frequent infections (>5% of patients receiving BENLYSTA) were upper respiratory tract infection, urinary tract infection, nasopharyngitis, sinusitis, bronchitis, and influenza. Serious infections occurred in 6.0% of patients treated with BENLYSTA and in 5.2% of patients who received placebo. The most frequent serious infections included pneumonia, urinary tract infection, cellulitis, and bronchitis. Infections leading to discontinuation of treatment occurred in 0.7% of patients receiving BENLYSTA and 1.0% of patients receiving placebo. Infections resulting in death occurred in 0.3% (4/1,458) of patients treated with BENLYSTA and in 0.1% (1/675) of patients receiving placebo.

Progressive Multifocal Leukoencephalopathy (PML): Cases of JC virus-associated PML resulting in neurological deficits, including fatal cases, have been reported in patients with SLE receiving immunosuppressants, including BENLYSTA. Risk factors for PML include treatment with immunosuppressant therapies and impairment of immune function. Consider the diagnosis of PML in any patient presenting with new-onset or deteriorating neurological signs and symptoms and consult with a neurologist or other appropriate specialist as clinically indicated. In patients with confirmed PML, consider stopping immunosuppressant therapy, including BENLYSTA.

5.3 Malignancy

The impact of treatment with BENLYSTA on the development of malignancies is not known. In the controlled clinical trials, malignancies (including non-melanoma skin cancers) were reported in 0.4% of patients receiving BENLYSTA and 0.4% of patients receiving placebo. In the controlled clinical trials, malignancies, excluding non-melanoma skin cancers, were observed in 0.2% (3/1,458) and 0.3% (2/675) of patients receiving BENLYSTA and placebo, respectively. The mechanism of action of BENLYSTA could increase the risk for the development of malignancies.

5.4 Hypersensitivity Reactions, Including Anaphylaxis

Acute hypersensitivity reactions, including anaphylaxis and death, have been reported in association with BENLYSTA. These events generally occurred within hours of the infusion; however, they may occur later. Non-acute hypersensitivity reactions including rash, nausea, fatigue, myalgia, headache, and facial edema, have been reported and typically occurred up to a week following the most recent infusion. Hypersensitivity, including serious reactions, has occurred in patients who have previously tolerated infusions of BENLYSTA. Limited data suggest that patients with a history of multiple drug allergies or significant hypersensitivity may be at increased risk. In the controlled clinical trials, hypersensitivity reactions (occurring on the same day of infusion) were reported in 13% (191/1,458) of patients receiving BENLYSTA and 11% (76/675) of patients receiving placebo. Anaphylaxis was observed in 0.6% (9/1,458) of patients receiving BENLYSTA and 0.4% (3/675) of patients receiving placebo. Manifestations included hypotension, angioedema, urticaria or other rash, pruritus, and dyspnea. Due to overlap in signs and symptoms, it was not possible to distinguish between hypersensitivity reactions and infusion reactions in all cases [see Warnings and Precautions (5.5)]. Some patients (13%) received premedication, which may have mitigated or masked a hypersensitivity response; however, there is insufficient evidence to determine whether premedication diminishes the frequency or severity of hypersensitivity reactions.

BENLYSTA should be administered by healthcare providers prepared to manage anaphylaxis. In the event of a serious reaction, administration of BENLYSTA must be discontinued immediately and appropriate medical therapy administered. Patients should be monitored during and for an appropriate period of time after administration of BENLYSTA. Patients should be informed of the signs and symptoms of an acute hypersensitivity reaction and be instructed to seek immediate medical care should a reaction occur.

5.5 Infusion Reactions

In the controlled clinical trials, adverse events associated with the infusion (occurring on the same day of the infusion) were reported in 17% (251/1,458) of patients receiving BENLYSTA and 15% (99/675) of patients receiving placebo. Serious infusion reactions (excluding hypersensitivity reactions) were reported in 0.5% of patients receiving BENLYSTA and 0.4% of patients receiving placebo and included bradycardia, myalgia, headache, rash, urticaria, and hypotension. The most common infusion reactions (≥3% of patients receiving BENLYSTA) were headache, nausea, and skin reactions. Due to overlap in signs and symptoms, it was not possible to distinguish between hypersensitivity reactions and infusion reactions in all cases [see Warnings and Precautions (5.4)]. Some patients (13%) received premedication, which may have mitigated or masked an infusion reaction; however, there is insufficient evidence to determine whether premedication diminishes the frequency or severity of infusion reactions [see Adverse Reactions (6.1)].

BENLYSTA should be administered by healthcare providers prepared to manage infusion reactions. The infusion rate may be slowed or interrupted if the patient develops an infusion reaction. Healthcare providers should be aware of the risk of hypersensitivity reactions, which may present as infusion reactions, and monitor patients closely.

5.6 Depression

In the controlled clinical trials, psychiatric events were reported more frequently with BENLYSTA (16%) than with placebo (12%), related primarily to depression-related events (6.3% BENLYSTA and 4.7% placebo), insomnia (6.0% BENLYSTA and 5.3% placebo), and anxiety (3.9% BENLYSTA and 2.8% placebo). Serious psychiatric events were reported in 0.8% of patients receiving BENLYSTA (0.6% and 1.2% with 1 and 10 mg/kg, respectively) and 0.4% of patients receiving placebo. Serious depression was reported in 0.4% (6/1,458) of patients receiving BENLYSTA and 0.1% (1/675) of patients receiving placebo. Two suicides (0.1%) were reported in patients receiving BENLYSTA. The majority of patients who reported serious depression or suicidal behavior had a history of depression or other serious psychiatric disorders and most were receiving psychoactive medications. It is unknown if treatment with BENLYSTA is associated with increased risk for these events.

Patients receiving BENLYSTA should be instructed to contact their healthcare provider if they experience new or worsening depression, suicidal thoughts, or other mood changes.

5.7 Immunization

Live vaccines should not be given for 30 days before or concurrently with BENLYSTA as clinical safety has not been established. No data are available on the secondary transmission of infection from persons receiving live vaccines to patients receiving BENLYSTA or the effect of BENLYSTA on new immunizations. Because of its mechanism of action, BENLYSTA may interfere with the response to immunizations.

5.8 Concomitant Use With Other Biologic Therapies or Intravenous Cyclophosphamide

BENLYSTA has not been studied in combination with other biologic therapies, including B-cell targeted therapies, or intravenous cyclophosphamide. Therefore, use of BENLYSTA is not recommended in combination with biologic therapies or intravenous cyclophosphamide.

6 ADVERSE REACTIONS

Because clinical trials are conducted under widely varying conditions, adverse reaction rates observed in the clinical trials of a drug cannot be directly compared with rates in the clinical trials of another drug and may not reflect the rates observed in practice.

The following have been observed with BENLYSTA and are discussed in detail in the Warnings and Precautions section:
- Mortality [see Warnings and Precautions (5.1)]
- Serious Infections [see Warnings and Precautions (5.2)]
- Malignancy [see Warnings and Precautions (5.3)]
- Hypersensitivity Reactions, Including Anaphylaxis [see Warnings and Precautions (5.4)]
- Infusion Reactions [see Warnings and Precautions (5.5)]
- Depression [see Warnings and Precautions (5.6)]

6.1 Clinical Trials Experience

The data described below reflect exposure to BENLYSTA plus standard of care compared with placebo plus standard of care in 2,133 patients in 3 controlled trials. Patients received BENLYSTA at doses of 1 mg/kg (N = 673), 4 mg/kg (N = 111; Trial 1 only), or 10 mg/kg (N = 674) or placebo (N = 675) intravenously over a 1-hour period on Days 0, 14, 28, and then every 28 days. In 2 of the trials (Trial 1 and Trial 3), treatment was given for 48 weeks, while in the other trial (Trial 2) treatment was given for 72 weeks [see Clinical Studies (14)]. Because there was no apparent dose-related increase in the majority of adverse events observed with BENLYSTA, the safety data summarized below are presented for the 3 doses pooled, unless otherwise indicated; the adverse reaction table displays the results for the recommended dose of 10 mg/kg compared with placebo.

The population had a mean age of 39 (range: 18 to 75), 94% were female, and 52% were Caucasian. In these trials, 93% of patients treated with BENLYSTA reported an adverse reaction compared with 92% treated with placebo.

The most common serious adverse reactions were serious infections (6.0% and 5.2% in the groups receiving BENLYSTA and placebo, respectively) [see Warnings and Precautions (5.2)].

The most commonly-reported adverse reactions, occurring in ≥5% of patients in clinical trials were nausea, diarrhea, pyrexia, nasopharyngitis, bronchitis, insomnia, pain in extremity, depression, migraine, and pharyngitis.

The proportion of patients who discontinued treatment due to any adverse reaction during the controlled clinical trials

was 6.2% for patients receiving BENLYSTA and 7.1% for patients receiving placebo. The most common adverse reactions resulting in discontinuation of treatment (≥1% of patients receiving BENLYSTA or placebo) were infusion reactions (1.6% BENLYSTA and 0.9% placebo), lupus nephritis (0.7% BENLYSTA and 1.2% placebo), and infections (0.7% BENLYSTA and 1.0% placebo).

Table 1 lists adverse reactions, regardless of causality, occurring in at least 3% of patients with SLE who received BENLYSTA 10 mg/kg and at an incidence at least 1% greater than that observed with placebo in the 3 controlled studies.

Table 1. Incidence of Adverse Reactions Occurring in at Least 3% of Patients Treated With BENLYSTA 10 mg/kg Plus Standard of Care and at Least 1% More Frequently Than in Patients Receiving Placebo Plus Standard of Care in 3 Controlled SLE Studies

Preferred Term	BENLYSTA 10 mg/kg + Standard of Care (n = 674) %	Placebo + Standard of Care (n = 675) %
Nausea	15	12
Diarrhea	12	9
Pyrexia	10	8
Nasopharyngitis	9	7
Bronchitis	9	5
Insomnia	7	5
Pain in extremity	6	4
Depression	5	4
Migraine	5	4
Pharyngitis	5	3
Cystitis	4	3
Leukopenia	4	2
Gastroenteritis viral	3	1

6.2 Immunogenicity

In Trials 2 and 3, anti-belimumab antibodies were detected in 4 of 563 (0.7%) patients receiving BENLYSTA 10 mg/kg and in 27 of 559 (4.8%) patients receiving BENLYSTA 1 mg/kg. The reported frequency for the group receiving 10 mg/kg may underestimate the actual frequency due to lower assay sensitivity in the presence of high drug concentrations. Neutralizing antibodies were detected in 3 patients receiving BENLYSTA 1 mg/kg. Three patients with anti-belimumab antibodies experienced mild infusion reactions of nausea, erythematous rash, pruritus, eyelid edema, headache, and dyspnea; none of the reactions was life-threatening. The clinical relevance of the presence of anti-belimumab antibodies is not known.

The data reflect the percentage of patients whose test results were positive for antibodies to belimumab in specific assays. The observed incidence of antibody positivity in an assay is highly dependent on several factors, including assay sensitivity and specificity, assay methodology, sample handling, timing of sample collection, concomitant medications, and underlying disease. For these reasons, comparison of the incidence of antibodies to belimumab with the incidence of antibodies to other products may be misleading.

6.3 Postmarketing Experience

The following adverse reactions have been identified during postapproval use of BENLYSTA. Because these reactions are reported voluntarily from a population of uncertain size, it is not always possible to reliably estimate their frequency or establish a causal relationship to drug exposure.
- Fatal anaphylaxis [see Warnings and Precautions (5.4)].

7 DRUG INTERACTIONS

Formal drug interaction studies have not been performed with BENLYSTA. In clinical trials of patients with SLE, BENLYSTA was administered concomitantly with other drugs, including corticosteroids, antimalarials, immunomodulatory and immunosuppressive agents (including azathioprine, methotrexate, and mycophenolate), angiotensin pathway antihypertensives, HMG-CoA reductase inhibitors (statins), and NSAIDs without evidence of a clinically meaningful effect of these concomitant medications on belimumab pharmacokinetics. The effect of belimumab on the pharmacokinetics of other drugs has not been evaluated [see Clinical Pharmacology (12.3)].

8 USE IN SPECIFIC POPULATIONS

8.1 Pregnancy

Pregnancy Category C. There are no adequate and well-controlled clinical studies using BENLYSTA in pregnant women. Immunoglobulin G (IgG) antibodies, including BENLYSTA, can cross the placenta. Because animal reproduction studies are not always predictive of human response, BENLYSTA should be used during pregnancy only if the potential benefit to the mother justifies the potential risk to the fetus. Women of childbearing potential should use adequate contraception during treatment with BENLYSTA and for at least 4 months after the final treatment.

Nonclinical reproductive studies have been performed in pregnant cynomolgus monkeys receiving belimumab at doses of 0, 5, and 150 mg/kg by intravenous infusion (the high dose was approximately 9 times the anticipated maximum human exposure) every 2 weeks from gestation day 20 to 150. Belimumab was shown to cross the placenta. Belimumab was not associated with direct or indirect teratogenicity under the conditions tested. Fetal deaths were observed in 14%, 24%, and 15% of pregnant females in the 0, 5 and 150 mg/kg groups, respectively. Infant deaths occurred with an incidence of 0%, 8%, and 5%. The cause of fetal and infant deaths is not known. The relevance of these findings to humans is not known. Other treatment-related findings were limited to the expected reversible reduction of B cells in both dams and infants and reversible reduction of immunoglobulin M (IgM) in infant monkeys. B-cell numbers recovered after the cessation of belimumab treatment by about 1 year post-partum in adult monkeys and by 3 months of age in infant monkeys. IgM levels in infants exposed to belimumab in utero recovered by 6 months of age.

Pregnancy Registry: To monitor maternal-fetal outcomes of pregnant women exposed to BENLYSTA, a pregnancy registry has been established. Healthcare professionals are encouraged to register patients and pregnant women are encouraged to enroll themselves by calling 1-877-681-6296.

8.3 Nursing Mothers

It is not known whether BENLYSTA is excreted in human milk or absorbed systemically after ingestion. However, belimumab was excreted into the milk of cynomolgus monkeys. Because maternal antibodies are excreted in human breast milk, a decision should be made whether to discontinue breastfeeding or to discontinue the drug, taking into account the importance of breastfeeding to the infant and the importance of the drug to the mother.

8.4 Pediatric Use

Safety and effectiveness of BENLYSTA have not been established in children.

8.5 Geriatric Use

Clinical studies of BENLYSTA did not include sufficient numbers of subjects aged 65 or over to determine whether they respond differently from younger subjects. Use with caution in elderly patients.

8.6 Race

In Trial 2 and Trial 3, response rates for the primary endpoint were lower for black subjects receiving BENLYSTA relative to black subjects receiving placebo [see Clinical Studies (14)]. Use with caution in black/African-American patients.

10 OVERDOSAGE

There is no clinical experience with overdosage of BENLYSTA. Two doses of up to 20 mg/kg have been given by intravenous infusion to humans with no increase in incidence or severity of adverse reactions compared with doses of 1, 4, or 10 mg/kg.

11 DESCRIPTION

BENLYSTA (belimumab) is a human IgG1λ monoclonal antibody specific for soluble human B lymphocyte stimulator protein (BLyS, also referred to as BAFF and TNFSF13B). Belimumab has a molecular weight of approximately 147 kDa. Belimumab is produced by recombinant DNA technology in a mammalian cell expression system.

BENLYSTA is supplied as a sterile, white to off-white, preservative-free, lyophilized powder for intravenous infusion. Upon reconstitution with Sterile Water for Injection, USP [see Dosage and Administration (2.3)], each single-use vial delivers 80 mg/mL belimumab in 0.16 mg/mL citric acid, 0.4 mg/mL polysorbate 80, 2.7 mg/mL sodium citrate, and 80 mg/mL sucrose, with a pH of 6.5.

12 CLINICAL PHARMACOLOGY

12.1 Mechanism of Action

BENLYSTA is a BLyS-specific inhibitor that blocks the binding of soluble BLyS, a B-cell survival factor, to its receptors on B cells. BENLYSTA does not bind B cells directly, but by binding BLyS, BENLYSTA inhibits the survival of B cells, including autoreactive B cells, and reduces the differentiation of B cells into immunoglobulin-producing plasma cells.

12.2 Pharmacodynamics

In Trial 1 and Trial 2 in which B cells were measured, treatment with BENLYSTA significantly reduced circulating

Table 3. Clinical Response Rate in Patients With SLE After 52 Weeks of Treatment

	Trial 2			Trial 3		
Response[a]	Placebo + Standard of Care (n = 275)	BENLYSTA 1 mg/kg + Standard of Care[b] (n = 271)	BENLYSTA 10 mg/kg + Standard of Care (n = 273)	Placebo + Standard of Care (n = 287)	BENLYSTA 1 mg/kg + Standard of Care[b] (n = 288)	BENLYSTA 10 mg/kg + Standard of Care (n = 290)
SLE Responder Index	34%	41% (P= 0.104)	43% (P= 0.021)	44%	51% (P= 0.013)	58% (P<0.001)
Odds Ratio (95% CI) vs. placebo		1.3 (0.9, 1.9)	1.5 (1.1, 2.2)		1.6 (1.1, 2.2)	1.8 (1.3, 2.6)
Components of SLE Responder Index						
Percent of patients with reduction in SELENA-SLEDAI ≥4	36%	43%	47%	46%	53%	58%
Percent of patients with no worsening by BILAG index	65%	75%	69%	73%	79%	81%
Percent of patients with no worsening by PGA	63%	73%	69%	69%	79%	80%

CD19+, CD20+, naïve, and activated B cells, plasmacytoid cells, and the SLE B-cell subset at Week 52. Reductions in naïve and the SLE B-cell subset were observed as early as Week 8 and were sustained to Week 52. Memory cells increased initially and slowly declined toward baseline levels by Week 52. The clinical relevance of these effects on B cells has not been established.

Treatment with BENLYSTA led to reductions in IgG and anti-dsDNA, and increases in complement (C3 and C4). These changes were observed as early as Week 8 and were sustained through Week 52. The clinical relevance of normalizing these biomarkers has not been definitively established.

12.3   Pharmacokinetics
The pharmacokinetic parameters displayed in Table 2 are based on population parameter estimates which are specific to the 563 patients who received BENLYSTA 10 mg/kg in Trials 2 and 3 [see Clinical Studies (14)].

Table 2. Population Pharmacokinetic Parameters in Patients With SLE After Intravenous Infusion of BENLYSTA 10 mg/kg[a]

Pharmacokinetic Parameter	Population Estimates (n = 563)
Peak concentration (C$_{max,}$ mcg/mL)	313
Area under the curve (AUC$_{0-\infty}$, day•mcg/mL)	3,083
Distribution half-life (t$_{½}$, days)	1.75
Terminal half-life (t$_{½}$, days)	19.4
Systemic clearance (CL, mL/day)	215
Volume of distribution (Vss, L)	5.29

[a] Intravenous infusions were administered at 2-week intervals for the first 3 doses and at 4-week intervals thereafter.
Drug Interactions: No formal drug interaction studies have been conducted with BENLYSTA. Concomitant use of mycophenolate, azathioprine, methotrexate, antimalarials, NSAIDs, aspirin, and HMG-CoA reductase inhibitors did not significantly influence belimumab pharmacokinetics. Coadministration of steroids and angiotensin-converting enzyme (ACE) inhibitors resulted in an increase of systemic clearance of belimumab that was not clinically significant because the magnitude was well within the range of normal variability of clearance. The effect of belimumab on the pharmacokinetics of other drugs has not been evaluated.
Special Populations: The following information is based on the population pharmacokinetic analysis.
Age: Age did not significantly influence belimumab pharmacokinetics in the trial population, where the majority of subjects (70%) were aged between 18 and 45 years. No pharmacokinetic data are available in pediatric patients. Lim-

ited pharmacokinetic data are available for elderly patients as only 1.4% of the subjects included in the pharmacokinetic analysis were aged 65 years or older [see Use in Specific Populations (8.5)].
Gender: Gender did not significantly influence belimumab pharmacokinetics in the largely (94%) female trial population.
Race: Race did not significantly influence belimumab pharmacokinetics. The racial distribution was 53% white/Caucasian, 16% Asian, 16% Alaska native/American Indian, and 14% black/African-American.
Renal Impairment: No formal trials were conducted to examine the effects of renal impairment on the pharmacokinetics of belimumab. BENLYSTA has been studied in a limited number of patients with SLE and renal impairment (261 subjects with moderate renal impairment, creatinine clearance ≥30 and <60 mL/min; 14 subjects with severe renal impairment, creatinine clearance ≥15 and <30 mL/min). Although increases in creatinine clearance and proteinuria (>2 g/day) increased belimumab clearance, these effects were within the expected range of variability. Therefore, dosage adjustment in patients with renal impairment is not recommended.
Hepatic Impairment: No formal trials were conducted to examine the effects of hepatic impairment on the pharmacokinetics of belimumab. Baseline ALT and AST levels did not significantly influence belimumab pharmacokinetics.

13   NONCLINICAL TOXICOLOGY
13.1   Carcinogenesis, Mutagenesis, Impairment of Fertility
Long-term animal studies have not been performed to evaluate the carcinogenic potential of belimumab. The mutagenic potential of belimumab was not evaluated.
Effects on male and female fertility have not been directly evaluated in animal studies.

14   CLINICAL STUDIES
The safety and effectiveness of BENLYSTA were evaluated in 3 randomized, double-blind, placebo-controlled trials involving 2,133 patients with SLE according to the American College of Rheumatology criteria (Trial 1, 2, and 3). Patients with severe active lupus nephritis and severe active CNS lupus were excluded. Patients were on a stable standard of care SLE treatment regimen comprising any of the following (alone or in combination): corticosteroids, antimalarials, NSAIDs, and immunosuppressives. Use of other biologics and intravenous cyclophosphamide were not permitted.
Trial 1:   BENLYSTA 1 mg/kg, 4 mg/kg, 10 mg/kg
Trial 1 enrolled 449 patients and evaluated doses of 1, 4, and 10 mg/kg BENLYSTA plus standard of care compared with placebo plus standard of care over 52 weeks in patients with SLE. Patients had to have a SELENA-SLEDAI score ≥4 at baseline and a history of autoantibodies (anti-nuclear antibody [ANA] and/or anti-double-stranded DNA [anti-dsDNA]), but 28% of the population was autoantibody negative at baseline. The co-primary endpoints were percent change in SELENA-SLEDAI score at Week 24 and time to first flare over 52 weeks. No significant differences between

any of the groups receiving BENLYSTA and the group receiving placebo were observed. Exploratory analysis of this trial identified a subgroup of patients (72%), who were autoantibody positive, in whom BENLYSTA appeared to offer benefit. The results of this trial informed the design of Trials 2 and 3 and led to the selection of a target population and indication that is limited to autoantibody-positive SLE patients.
Trials 2 and 3:   BENLYSTA 1 mg/kg and 10 mg/kg
Trials 2 and 3 were randomized, double-blind, placebo-controlled trials in patients with SLE that were similar in design except duration - Trial 2 was 76 weeks duration and Trial 3 was 52 weeks duration. Eligible patients had active SLE disease, defined as a SELENA-SLEDAI score ≥6, and positive autoantibody test results at screening. Patients were excluded from the trial if they had ever received treatment with a B-cell targeted agent or if they were currently receiving other biologic agents. Intravenous cyclophosphamide was not permitted within the previous 6 months or during the trial. Trial 2 was conducted primarily in North America and Europe. Trial 3 was conducted in South America, Eastern Europe, Asia, and Australia.
Baseline concomitant medications included corticosteroids (Trial 2: 76%, Trial 3: 96%), immunosuppressives (Trial 2: 56%, Trial 3: 42%; including azathioprine, methotrexate and mycophenolate), and antimalarials (Trial 2: 63%, Trial 3: 67%). Most patients (>70%) were receiving 2 or more classes of SLE medications.
In Trial 2 and Trial 3, more than 50% of patients had 3 or more active organ systems at baseline. The most common active organ systems at baseline based on SELENA-SLEDAI were mucocutaneous (82% in both trials); immune (Trial 2: 74%, Trial 3: 85%); and musculoskeletal (Trial 2: 73%, Trial 3: 59%). Less than 16% of patients had some degree of renal activity and less than 7% of patients had activity in the vascular, cardio-respiratory, or CNS systems.
At screening, patients were stratified by disease severity based on their SELENA-SLEDAI score (≤9 vs. ≥10), proteinuria level (<2 g/24 hr vs. ≥2 g/24 hr), and race (African or Indigenous-American descent vs. other), and then randomly assigned to receive BENLYSTA 1 mg/kg, BENLYSTA 10 mg/kg, or placebo in addition to standard of care. The patients were administered trial medication intravenously over a 1-hour period on Days 0, 14, 28, and then every 28 days for 48 weeks in Trial 3 and for 72 weeks in Trial 2.
The primary efficacy endpoint was a composite endpoint (SLE Responder Index or SRI) that defined response as meeting each of the following criteria at Week 52 compared with baseline:
• ≥4-point reduction in the SELENA-SLEDAI score, and
• no new British Isles Lupus Assessment Group (BILAG) A organ domain score or 2 new BILAG B organ domain scores, and
• no worsening (<0.30-point increase) in Physician's Global Assessment (PGA) score.
The SRI uses the SELENA-SLEDAI score as an objective measure of reduction in global disease activity; the BILAG index to ensure no significant worsening in any specific organ system; and the PGA to ensure that improvements in disease activity are not accompanied by worsening of the patient's condition overall.
In both Trials 2 and 3, the proportion of SLE patients achieving an SRI response, as defined for the primary endpoint, was significantly higher in the group receiving BENLYSTA 10 mg/kg than in the group receiving placebo. The effect on the SRI was not consistently significantly different for patients receiving BENLYSTA 1 mg/kg relative to placebo in both trials. The 1 mg/kg dose is not recommended. The trends in comparisons between the treatment groups for the rates of response for the individual components of the endpoint were generally consistent with that of the SRI (Table 3). At Week 76 in Trial 2, the SRI response rate with BENLYSTA 10 mg/kg was not significantly different from that of placebo (39% and 32%, respectively).
[See table 3 above]
[a]Patients dropping out of the trial early or experiencing certain increases in background medication were considered as failures in these analyses. In both trials, a higher proportion of placebo patients were considered as failures for this reason as compared with the groups receiving BENLYSTA.
[b] The 1-mg/kg dose is not recommended.
The reduction in disease activity seen in the SRI was related primarily to improvement in the most commonly involved organ systems namely, mucocutaneous, musculoskeletal, and immune.
Effect in Black/African-American Patients: Exploratory sub-group analyses of SRI response rate in patients of black race were performed. In Trial 2 and Trial 3 combined, the SRI response rate in black patients (N = 148) in groups receiving placebo (22/50 or 44% for placebo, 15/48 or 31% for BENLYSTA 1 mg/kg, and 18/50 or 36% for BENLYSTA 10 mg/kg). In Trial 1, black patients (N = 106) in the groups receiving BENLYSTA did not appear to have a different re-

sponse than the rest of the trial population. Although no definitive conclusions can be drawn from these subgroup analyses, caution should be used when considering treatment with BENLYSTA in black/African-American SLE patients.
Effect on Concomitant Steroid Treatment: In Trial 2 and Trial 3, 46% and 69% of patients, respectively, were receiving prednisone at doses >7.5 mg/day at baseline. The proportion of patients able to reduce their average prednisone dose by at least 25% to ≤7.5 mg/day during Weeks 40 through 52 was not consistently significantly different for BENLYSTA relative to placebo in both trials. In Trial 2, 17% of patients receiving BENLYSTA 10 mg/kg and 19% of patients receiving BENLYSTA 1 mg/kg achieved this level of steroid reduction compared with 13% of patients receiving placebo. In Trial 3, 19%, 21%, and 12% of patients receiving BENLYSTA 10 mg/kg, BENLYSTA 1 mg/kg, and placebo, respectively, achieved this level of steroid reduction.
Effect on Severe SLE Flares: The probability of experiencing a severe SLE flare, as defined by a modification of the SELENA Trial flare criteria which excluded severe flares triggered only by an increase of the SELENA-SLEDAI score to >12, was calculated for both Trials 2 and 3. The proportion of patients having at least 1 severe flare over 52 weeks was not consistently significantly different for BENLYSTA relative to placebo in both trials. In Trial 2, 18% of patients receiving BENLYSTA 10 mg/kg and 16% of patients receiving BENLYSTA 1 mg/kg had a severe flare compared with 24% of patients receiving placebo. In Trial 3, 14%, 18%, and 23% of patients receiving BENLYSTA 10 mg/kg, BENLYSTA 1 mg/kg and placebo, respectively, had a severe flare.

16 HOW SUPPLIED/STORAGE AND HANDLING

BENLYSTA is a sterile, preservative-free, lyophilized powder for reconstitution, dilution, and intravenous infusion provided in single-use glass vials with a rubber stopper (not made with natural rubber latex) and a flip-off seal. Each 5-mL vial contains 120 mg of belimumab. Each 20-mL vial contains 400 mg of belimumab.
BENLYSTA is supplied as follows:

| 120 mg belimumab in a 5-mL single-use vial | NDC 49401-101-01 |
| 400 mg belimumab in a 20-mL single-use vial | NDC 49401-102-01 |

Store vials of BENLYSTA refrigerated between 2° to 8°C (36° to 46°F). Vials should be protected from light and stored in the original carton until use. *Do not freeze.* Avoid exposure to heat. Do not use beyond the expiration date.

17 PATIENT COUNSELING INFORMATION

See the FDA-approved patient labeling (Medication Guide).
17.1 Advice for the Patient
Give patients the Medication Guide for BENLYSTA and provide them an opportunity to read it prior to each treatment session. It is important that the patient's overall health be assessed at each infusion visit and any questions resulting from the patient's reading of the Medication Guide be discussed.
Mortality: Advise patients that more patients receiving BENLYSTA in the main clinical trials died than did patients receiving placebo treatment *[see Warnings and Precautions (5.1)]*.
Serious Infections: Advise patients that BENLYSTA may decrease their ability to fight infections. Ask patients if they have a history of chronic infections and if they are currently on any therapy for an infection *[see Warnings and Precautions (5.2)]*. Instruct patients to tell their healthcare provider if they develop signs or symptoms of an infection.
Progressive Multifocal Leukoencephalopathy (PML): Advise patients to contact their healthcare professional if they experience new or worsening neurological symptoms such as memory loss, confusion, dizziness or loss of balance, difficulty talking or walking, or vision problems *[see Warnings and Precautions (5.2)]*.
Hypersensitivity/Anaphylactic and Infusion Reactions: Educate patients on the signs and symptoms of hypersensitivity and infusion reactions, including wheezing, difficulty breathing, angioedema, rash, hypotension, bradycardia, and headache. Instruct patients to immediately tell their healthcare provider if they experience symptoms of an allergic reaction during or after the administration of BENLYSTA. Inform patients to tell their healthcare provider about possible reactions that may include a combination of symptoms such as rash, nausea, fatigue, muscle aches, headache, and/or facial swelling and may occur after administration of BENLYSTA *[see Warnings and Precautions (5.4, 5.5)]*.
Depression: Instruct patients to contact their healthcare provider if they experience new or worsening depression, suicidal thoughts or other mood changes *[see Warnings and Precautions (5.6)]*.

Immunizations: Inform patients that they should not receive live vaccines while taking BENLYSTA. Response to vaccinations could be impaired by BENLYSTA *[see Warnings and Precautions (5.7)]*.
Pregnancy and Nursing Mothers: Inform patients that BENLYSTA has not been studied in pregnant women or nursing mothers so the effects of BENLYSTA on pregnant women or nursing infants are not known. Instruct patients to tell their healthcare provider if they are pregnant, become pregnant, or are thinking about becoming pregnant *[see Use in Specific Populations (8.1)]*. Encourage pregnant patients to enroll in the pregnancy registry for BENLYSTA *[see Use in Specific Populations (8.1)]*. Instruct patients to tell their healthcare provider if they plan to breastfeed their infant *[see Use in Specific Populations (8.3)]*.
BENLYSTA is a registered trademark of the GlaxoSmithKline group of companies.
Manufactured by:
Human Genome Sciences, Inc.
Rockville, Maryland 20850
US License No. 1820
Marketed by:
GlaxoSmithKline
Research Triangle Park, NC 27709
©2014, GlaxoSmithKline group of companies. All rights reserved.
BNL:2PI
MEDICATION GUIDE
BENLYSTA® (ben-LIST-ah)
(belimumab)
Injection for intravenous use
Read this Medication Guide before you start receiving BENLYSTA and before each treatment. There may be new information. This information does not take the place of talking with your healthcare provider about your medical condition or your treatment.
What is the most important information I should know about BENLYSTA?
BENLYSTA can cause serious side effects. Some of these side effects may cause death. It is not known if BENLYSTA causes these serious side effects. Tell your healthcare provider right away if you have any of the symptoms listed below while receiving BENLYSTA.
1. Infections. Symptoms of an infection can include:
• fever
• chills
• pain or burning with urination
• urinating often
• bloody diarrhea
• coughing up mucus
2. Heart Problems. Symptoms of heart problems can include:
• chest discomfort or pain
• shortness of breath
• cold sweats
• nausea
• dizziness
• discomfort in other areas of the upper body
3. Mental health problems and suicide. Symptoms of mental health problems can include:
• thoughts of suicide or dying
• attempt to commit suicide
• trouble sleeping (insomnia)
• new or worse anxiety
• new or worse depression
• acting on dangerous impulses
• other unusual changes in your behavior or mood
• thoughts of hurting yourself or others
What is BENLYSTA?
BENLYSTA is a prescription medicine used to treat adults with active systemic lupus erythematosus (SLE or lupus) who are receiving other lupus medicines.
BENLYSTA contains belimumab which is in a group of medicines called monoclonal antibodies. Lupus is a disease of the immune system (the body system that fights infection). People with active lupus often have high levels of a certain protein in their blood. BENLYSTA binds to and limits the activity of the protein. When given together with other medicines for lupus, BENLYSTA decreases lupus disease activity more than other lupus medicines alone.
• It is not known if BENLYSTA is safe and effective in people with severe active lupus nephritis or severe active central nervous system lupus.
• It is not known if BENLYSTA is safe and effective in children.
Who should not receive BENLYSTA?
Do not receive BENLYSTA if you:
• are allergic to belimumab or any of the ingredients in BENLYSTA. See the end of this Medication Guide for a complete list of ingredients in BENLYSTA.
What should I tell my healthcare provider before receiving BENLYSTA?
Before you receive BENLYSTA, tell your healthcare provider if you:

• think you have an infection or have infections that keep coming back. You should not receive BENLYSTA if you have an infection unless your healthcare provider tells you to. See "What is the most important information I should know about BENLYSTA?"
• have or have had mental health problems such as depression or thoughts of suicide
• have recently received a vaccination or if you think you may need a vaccination. If you are receiving BENLYSTA, you should not receive live vaccines.
• are allergic to other medicines
• are receiving other biologic medicines, monoclonal antibodies or IV infusions of cyclophosphamide (Cytoxan®)
• have or have had any type of cancer
• have any other medical conditions
• are pregnant or plan to become pregnant. It is not known if BENLYSTA will harm your unborn baby. Tell your healthcare provider if you become pregnant during your treatment with BENLYSTA.
• If you become pregnant while receiving BENLYSTA, talk to your healthcare provider about enrolling in the BENLYSTA Pregnancy Registry. You can enroll in this registry by calling 1-877-681-6296. The purpose of this registry is to monitor the health of you and your baby.
• are breastfeeding or plan to breastfeed. It is not known if BENLYSTA passes into your breast milk. You and your healthcare provider should decide if you will receive BENLYSTA or breastfeed. You should not do both.
Tell your healthcare provider about all the medicines you take, including prescription and non-prescription medicines, vitamins, and herbal supplements.
Know the medicines you take. Keep a list of your medicines with you to show to your healthcare provider and pharmacist when you get a new medicine.
How will I receive BENLYSTA?
• You will be given BENLYSTA by a healthcare provider through a needle placed in a vein (IV infusion). It takes about 1 hour to give you the full dose of BENLYSTA.
• Your healthcare provider will tell you how often you should receive BENLYSTA.
• Your healthcare provider may give you medicines before you receive BENLYSTA to help reduce your chance of having a reaction. A healthcare provider will watch you closely while you are receiving BENLYSTA and after your infusion for signs of a reaction.
What are the possible side effects of BENLYSTA?
BENLYSTA can cause serious side effects.
• See "What is the most important information I should know about BENLYSTA?"
• **Cancer.** BENLYSTA may reduce the activity of your immune system. Medicines that affect the immune system may increase your risk of certain cancers.
• **Allergic (hypersensitivity) and infusion reactions.** Serious allergic or infusion reactions can happen on the day of or days after receiving BENLYSTA and may cause death. Your healthcare provider will watch you closely while you are receiving BENLYSTA and after your infusion for signs of a reaction. Allergic reactions can sometimes be delayed; tell your healthcare provider right away if you have any of the following symptoms of an allergic or infusion reaction:
• itching
• swelling of the face, lips, mouth, tongue, or throat
• trouble breathing
• anxiousness
• low blood pressure
• dizziness or fainting
• headache
• nausea
• skin rash, redness, or swelling
• **Progressive multifocal leukoencephalopathy (PML).** PML is a serious and life-threatening brain infection. Your chance of getting PML may be higher if you are treated with medicines that weaken your immune system, including BENLYSTA. PML can result in death or severe disability. If you notice any new or worsening medical problems such as those below, tell your healthcare provider right away:
• memory loss
• trouble thinking
• dizziness or loss of balance
• difficulty talking or walking
• loss of vision
The most common side effects of BENLYSTA include:
• nausea
• diarrhea
• fever
• stuffy or runny nose
• sore throat
• cough (bronchitis)
• trouble sleeping
• leg or arm pain
• depression
• headache (migraine)
• urinary tract infection

- decreased white blood cell count (leukopenia)
- vomiting
- stomach pain

Tell your healthcare provider if you have any side effect that bothers you or that does not go away.

These are not all the possible side effects of BENLYSTA. For more information, ask your healthcare provider.

Call your doctor for medical advice about side effects. You may report side effects to FDA at 1-800-FDA-1088.

General information about the safe and effective use of BENLYSTA

Medicines are sometimes prescribed for purposes other than those listed in a Medication Guide. Do not use BENLYSTA for a condition for which it was not prescribed.

This Medication Guide summarizes the most important information about BENLYSTA. For more information about BENLYSTA, talk with your healthcare provider.

You can ask your healthcare provider or pharmacist for information about BENLYSTA that is written for healthcare professionals.

For more information about BENLYSTA, go to www.BENLYSTA.com or call 1-877-423-6597.

What are the ingredients in BENLYSTA?

Active ingredient: belimumab.

Inactive ingredients: citric acid, polysorbate 80, sodium citrate, sucrose.

BENLYSTA is a registered trademark of the GlaxoSmithKline group of companies.

Manufactured by
Human Genome Sciences, Inc.
Rockville, Maryland 20850
US License No. 1820
Marketed by
GlaxoSmithKline
Research Triangle Park, NC 27709

This Medication Guide has been approved by the U.S. Food and Drug Administration.

©2014, GlaxoSmithKline group of companies. All rights reserved.

April 2014
BNL:2MG

BOOSTRIX ℞

[boos' trix]
(Tetanus Toxoid, Reduced Diphtheria Toxoid and Acellular Pertussis Vaccine, Adsorbed)
Suspension for Intramuscular Injection

HIGHLIGHTS OF PRESCRIBING INFORMATION

These highlights do not include all the information needed to use BOOSTRIX safely and effectively. See full prescribing information for BOOSTRIX.

BOOSTRIX (Tetanus Toxoid, Reduced Diphtheria Toxoid and Acellular Pertussis Vaccine, Adsorbed)
Suspension for Intramuscular Injection
Initial U.S. Approval: 2005

————INDICATIONS AND USAGE————

BOOSTRIX is a vaccine indicated for active booster immunization against tetanus, diphtheria, and pertussis. BOOSTRIX is approved for use as a single dose in individuals 10 years of age and older. (1)

————DOSAGE AND ADMINISTRATION————

A single intramuscular injection (0.5 mL). (2.2)

————DOSAGE FORMS AND STRENGTHS————

Single-dose vials and prefilled syringes containing a 0.5-mL suspension for injection. (3)

————CONTRAINDICATIONS————

- Severe allergic reaction (e.g., anaphylaxis) after a previous dose of any tetanus toxoid-, diphtheria toxoid-, or pertussis antigen-containing vaccine or to any component of BOOSTRIX. (4.1)
- Encephalopathy (e.g., coma, decreased level of consciousness, prolonged seizures) within 7 days of administration of a previous pertussis antigen-containing vaccine. (4.2)

————WARNINGS AND PRECAUTIONS————

- The tip caps of the prefilled syringes may contain natural rubber latex which may cause allergic reactions in latex-sensitive individuals. (5.1)
- If Guillain-Barré syndrome occurred within 6 weeks of receipt of a prior vaccine containing tetanus toxoid, the risk of Guillain-Barré syndrome may be increased following a subsequent dose of tetanus toxoid-containing vaccine, including BOOSTRIX. (5.2)
- Syncope (fainting) can occur in association with administration of injectable vaccines, including BOOSTRIX. Procedures should be in place to avoid falling injury and to restore cerebral perfusion following syncope. (5.3)

- Progressive or unstable neurologic conditions are reasons to defer vaccination with a pertussis-containing vaccine, including BOOSTRIX. (5.4)
- Persons who experienced an Arthus-type hypersensitivity reaction following a prior dose of a tetanus toxoid-containing vaccine should not receive BOOSTRIX unless at least 10 years have elapsed since the last dose of a tetanus toxoid-containing vaccine. (5.5)

————ADVERSE REACTIONS————

- Common solicited adverse events (≥15%) in adolescents (10 to 18 years of age) were pain, redness, and swelling at the injection site, increase in arm circumference of injected arm, headache, fatigue, and gastrointestinal symptoms. (6.1)
- Common solicited adverse events (≥15%) in adults (19 to 64 years of age) were pain, redness, and swelling at the injection site, headache, fatigue, and gastrointestinal symptoms. (6.1)
- The most common solicited adverse event (≥15%) in the elderly (65 years of age and older) was pain at the injection site. (6.1)

To report SUSPECTED ADVERSE REACTIONS, contact GlaxoSmithKline at 1-888-825-5249 or VAERS at 1-800-822-7967 or www.vaers.hhs.gov.

————DRUG INTERACTIONS————

- In subjects 11 to 18 years of age, lower levels for antibodies to pertactin were observed when BOOSTRIX was administered concomitantly with meningococcal conjugate vaccine (serogroups A, C, Y, and W-135) as compared to BOOSTRIX administered first. (7.1)
- In subjects 19 to 64 years of age, lower levels for antibodies to FHA and pertactin were observed when BOOSTRIX was administered concomitantly with an inactivated influenza vaccine as compared to BOOSTRIX alone. (7.1)
- Do not mix BOOSTRIX with any other vaccine in the same syringe or vial. (7.1)

————USE IN SPECIFIC POPULATIONS————

- Safety and effectiveness of BOOSTRIX have not been established in pregnant women. (8.1)
- Register women who receive BOOSTRIX while pregnant in the pregnancy registry by calling 1-888-452-9622. (8.1)

See 17 for PATIENT COUNSELING INFORMATION
Revised: 11/2013

FULL PRESCRIBING INFORMATION

1   INDICATIONS AND USAGE

BOOSTRIX® is indicated for active booster immunization against tetanus, diphtheria, and pertussis. *BOOSTRIX is approved for use as a single dose in individuals 10 years of age and older.*

2   DOSAGE AND ADMINISTRATION
2.1   Preparation for Administration

Shake vigorously to obtain a homogeneous, turbid, white suspension before administration. Do not use if resuspension does not occur with vigorous shaking. Parenteral drug products should be inspected visually for particulate matter and discoloration prior to administration, whenever solution and container permit. If either of these conditions exists, the vaccine should not be administered.

For the prefilled syringes, attach a sterile needle and administer intramuscularly.

For the vials, use a sterile needle and sterile syringe to withdraw the 0.5-mL dose and administer intramuscularly. Changing needles between drawing vaccine from a vial and injecting it into a recipient is not necessary unless the needle has been damaged or contaminated. Use a separate sterile needle and syringe for each individual.

Do not administer this product intravenously, intradermally, or subcutaneously.

2.2   Dose and Schedule

BOOSTRIX is administered as a single 0.5-mL intramuscular injection into the deltoid muscle of the upper arm.

There are no data to support repeat administration of BOOSTRIX.

Five years should elapse between the last dose of the recommended series of Diphtheria and Tetanus Toxoids and Acellular Pertussis Vaccine Adsorbed (DTaP) and/or Tetanus and Diphtheria Toxoids Adsorbed For Adult Use (Td) vaccine and the administration of BOOSTRIX.

2.3   Additional Dosing Information

Primary Series: The use of BOOSTRIX as a primary series or to complete the primary series for diphtheria, tetanus, or pertussis has not been studied.

Wound Management: If tetanus prophylaxis is needed for wound management, BOOSTRIX may be given if no previous dose of any Tetanus Toxoid, Reduced Diphtheria Toxoid and Acellular Pertussis Vaccine, Adsorbed (Tdap) has been administered.

3   DOSAGE FORMS AND STRENGTHS

BOOSTRIX is a suspension for injection available in 0.5-mL single-dose vials and prefilled TIP-LOK® syringes.

4   CONTRAINDICATIONS
4.1   Hypersensitivity

A severe allergic reaction (e.g., anaphylaxis) after a previous dose of any tetanus toxoid-, diphtheria toxoid-, or pertussis antigen-containing vaccine or any component of this vaccine is a contraindication to administration of BOOSTRIX *[see Description (11)].* Because of the uncertainty as to which component of the vaccine might be responsible, none of the components should be administered. Alternatively, such individuals may be referred to an allergist for evaluation if immunization with any of these components is considered.

4.2   Encephalopathy

Encephalopathy (e.g., coma, decreased level of consciousness, prolonged seizures) within 7 days of administration of a previous dose of a pertussis antigen-containing vaccine that is not attributable to another identifiable cause is a contraindication to administration of any pertussis antigen-containing vaccine, including BOOSTRIX.

5   WARNINGS AND PRECAUTIONS
5.1   Latex

The tip caps of the prefilled syringes may contain natural rubber latex which may cause allergic reactions in latex-sensitive individuals.

5.2   Guillain-Barré Syndrome and Brachial Neuritis

If Guillain-Barré syndrome occurred within 6 weeks of receipt of a prior vaccine containing tetanus toxoid, the risk of Guillain-Barré syndrome may be increased following a subsequent dose of tetanus toxoid-containing vaccine, including BOOSTRIX. A review by the Institute of Medicine (IOM) found evidence for a causal relationship between receipt of tetanus toxoid and both brachial neuritis and Guillain-Barré syndrome.[1]

5.3   Syncope

Syncope (fainting) can occur in association with administration of injectable vaccines, including BOOSTRIX. Syncope can be accompanied by transient neurological signs such as visual disturbance, paresthesia, and tonic-clonic limb movements. Procedures should be in place to avoid falling injury and to restore cerebral perfusion following syncope.

5.4   Progressive or Unstable Neurologic Disorders

Progressive or unstable neurologic conditions (e.g., cerebrovascular events and acute encephalopathic conditions) are reasons to defer vaccination with a pertussis-containing vaccine, including BOOSTRIX. It is not known whether administration of BOOSTRIX to persons with an unstable or progressive neurologic disorder might hasten manifestations of the disorder or affect the prognosis. Administration of BOOSTRIX to persons with an unstable or progressive neurologic disorder may result in diagnostic confusion between manifestations of the underlying illness and possible adverse effects of vaccination.

5.5 Arthus-Type Hypersensitivity

Persons who experienced an Arthus-type hypersensitivity reaction following a prior dose of a tetanus toxoid-containing vaccine usually have a high serum tetanus antitoxin level and should not receive BOOSTRIX or other tetanus toxoid-containing vaccines unless at least 10 years have elapsed since the last dose of tetanus toxoid-containing vaccine.

5.6 Altered Immunocompetence

As with any vaccine, if administered to immunosuppressed persons, including individuals receiving immunosuppressive therapy, the expected immune response may not be obtained.

5.7 Prevention and Management of Acute Allergic Reactions

Prior to administration, the healthcare provider should review the immunization history for possible vaccine sensitivity and previous vaccination-related adverse reactions to allow an assessment of benefits and risks. Epinephrine and other appropriate agents used for the control of immediate allergic reactions must be immediately available should an acute anaphylactic reaction occur.

6 ADVERSE REACTIONS

6.1 Clinical Trials Experience

Because clinical trials are conducted under widely varying conditions, adverse reaction rates observed in the clinical trials of a vaccine cannot be directly compared to rates in the clinical trials of another vaccine, and may not reflect the rates observed in practice. As with any vaccine, there is the possibility that broad use of BOOSTRIX could reveal adverse reactions not observed in clinical trials.

In clinical studies, 4,949 adolescents (10 to 18 years of age) and 4,076 adults (19 years of age and older) were vaccinated with a single dose of BOOSTRIX. Of these adolescents, 1,341 were vaccinated with BOOSTRIX in a coadministration study with meningococcal conjugate vaccine *[see Drug Interactions (7.1) and Clinical Studies (14.5)]*. Of these adults, 1,104 were 65 years of age and older *[see Clinical Studies (14.4)]*. A total of 860 adults 19 years of age and older received concomitant vaccination with BOOSTRIX and influenza vaccines in a coadministration study *[see Drug Interactions (7.1) and Clinical Studies (14.5)]*. An additional 1,092 adolescents 10 to 18 years of age received a non-US formulation of BOOSTRIX (formulated to contain 0.5 mg aluminum per dose) in non-US clinical studies.

In a randomized, observer-blinded, controlled study in the US, 3,080 adolescents 10 to 18 years of age received a single dose of BOOSTRIX and 1,034 received the comparator Td vaccine, manufactured by MassBioLogics. There were no substantive differences in demographic characteristics between the vaccine groups. Among BOOSTRIX and comparator vaccine recipients, approximately 75% were 10 to 14 years of age and approximately 25% were 15 to 18 years of age. Approximately 98% of participants in this study had received the recommended series of 4 or 5 doses of either Diphtheria and Tetanus Toxoids and Pertussis Vaccine Adsorbed (DTwP) or a combination of DTwP and DTaP in childhood. Subjects were monitored for solicited adverse events using standardized diary cards (day 0-14). Unsolicited adverse events were monitored for the 31-day period following vaccination (day 0-30). Subjects were also monitored for 6 months post-vaccination for non-routine medical visits, visits to an emergency room, onset of new chronic illness, and serious adverse events. Information regarding late onset adverse events was obtained via a telephone call 6 months following vaccination. At least 97% of subjects completed the 6-month follow-up evaluation.

In a study conducted in Germany, BOOSTRIX was administered to 319 children 10 to 12 years of age previously vaccinated with 5 doses of acellular pertussis antigen-containing vaccines; 193 of these subjects had previously received 5 doses of INFANRIX® (Diphtheria and Tetanus Toxoids and Acellular Pertussis Vaccine Adsorbed). Adverse events were recorded on diary cards during the 15 days following vaccination. Unsolicited adverse events that occurred within 31 days of vaccination (day 0-30) were recorded on the diary card or verbally reported to the investigator. Subjects were monitored for 6 months post-vaccination for physician office visits, emergency room visits, onset of new chronic illness, and serious adverse events. The 6-month follow-up evaluation, conducted via telephone interview, was completed by 90% of subjects.

The US adult (19 to 64 years of age) study, a randomized, observer-blinded study, evaluated the safety of BOOSTRIX (N = 1,522) compared with ADACEL® (Tetanus Toxoid, Reduced Diphtheria Toxoid and Acellular Pertussis Vaccine Adsorbed) (N = 762), a Tdap vaccine manufactured by

Sanofi Pasteur SA. Vaccines were administered as a single dose. There were no substantive differences in demographic characteristics between the vaccine groups. Subjects were monitored for solicited adverse events using standardized diary cards (day 0-14). Unsolicited adverse events were monitored for the 31-day period following vaccination (day 0-30). Subjects were also monitored for 6 months post-vaccination for serious adverse events, visits to an emergency room, hospitalizations, and onset of new chronic illness. Approximately 95% of subjects completed the 6-month follow-up evaluation.

The US elderly (65 years of age and older) study, a randomized, observer-blinded study, evaluated the safety of BOOSTRIX (N = 887) compared with DECAVAC® (Tetanus and Diphtheria Toxoids Adsorbed) (N = 445), a US-licensed Td vaccine, manufactured by Sanofi Pasteur SA. Vaccines were administered as a single dose. Among all vaccine recipients, the mean age was approximately 72 years; 54% were female and 95% were white. Subjects were monitored for solicited adverse events using standardized diary cards (day 0-3). Unsolicited adverse events were monitored for the 31-day period following vaccination (day 0-30). Subjects were also monitored for 6 months post-vaccination for serious adverse events. Approximately 99% of subjects completed the 6-month follow-up evaluation.

Solicited Adverse Events in the US Adolescent Study: Table 1 presents the solicited local adverse reactions and general adverse events within 15 days of vaccination with BOOSTRIX or Td vaccine for the total vaccinated cohort.

The primary safety endpoint was the incidence of grade 3 pain (spontaneously painful and/or prevented normal activity) at the injection site within 15 days of vaccination. Grade 3 pain was reported in 4.6% of those who received BOOSTRIX compared with 4.0% of those who received the Td vaccine. The difference in rate of grade 3 pain was within the pre-defined clinical limit for non-inferiority (upper limit of the 95% CI for the difference [BOOSTRIX minus Td] ≤4%).

Table 1. Rates of Solicited Local Adverse Reactions or General Adverse Events Within the 15-day[a] Post-Vaccination Period in Adolescents 10 to 18 Years of Age (Total Vaccinated Cohort)

	BOOSTRIX (N = 3,032) %	Td (N = 1,013) %
Local		
Pain, any[b]	75.3	71.7
Pain, grade 2 or 3[b]	51.2	42.5
Pain, grade 3[c]	4.6	4.0
Redness, any	22.5	19.8
Redness, >20 mm	4.1	3.9
Redness, ≥50 mm	1.7	1.6
Swelling, any	21.1	20.1
Swelling, >20 mm	5.3	4.9
Swelling, ≥50 mm	2.5	3.2
Arm circumference increase, >5 mm[d]	28.3	29.5
Arm circumference increase, >20 mm[d]	2.0	2.2
Arm circumference increase, >40 mm[d]	0.5	0.3
General		
Headache, any	43.1	41.5
Headache, grade 2 or 3[b]	15.7	12.7
Headache, grade 3	3.7	2.7
Fatigue, any	37.0	36.7
Fatigue, grade 2 or 3	14.4	12.9
Fatigue, grade 3	3.7	3.2
Gastrointestinal symptoms, any[e]	26.0	25.8
Gastrointestinal symptoms, grade 2 or 3[e]	9.8	9.7
Gastrointestinal symptoms, grade 3[e]	3.0	3.2
Fever, ≥99.5°F (37.5°C)[f]	13.5	13.1
Fever, >100.4°F (38.0°C)[f]	5.0	4.7
Fever, >102.2°F (39.0°C)[f]	1.4	1.0

Td = Tetanus and Diphtheria Toxoids Adsorbed For Adult Use manufactured by MassBioLogics.
N = Number of subjects in the total vaccinated cohort with local/general symptoms sheets completed.
Grade 2 = Local: painful when limb moved; General: interfered with normal activity.

Grade 3 = Local: spontaneously painful and/or prevented normal activity; General: prevented normal activity.
[a] Day of vaccination and the next 14 days.
[b] Statistically significantly higher (*P* <0.05) following BOOSTRIX as compared to Td vaccine.
[c] Grade 3 injection site pain following BOOSTRIX was not inferior to Td vaccine (upper limit of two-sided 95% CI for the difference [BOOSTRIX minus Td] in the percentage of subjects ≤4%).
[d] Mid-upper region of the vaccinated arm.
[e] Gastrointestinal symptoms included nausea, vomiting, diarrhea, and/or abdominal pain.
[f] Oral temperatures or axillary temperatures.

Unsolicited Adverse Events in the US Adolescent Study: The incidence of unsolicited adverse events reported in the 31 days after vaccination was comparable between the 2 groups (25.4% and 24.5% for BOOSTRIX and Td vaccine, respectively).

Solicited Adverse Events in the German Adolescent Study: Table 2 presents the rates of solicited local adverse reactions and fever within 15 days of vaccination for those subjects who had previously been vaccinated with 5 doses of INFANRIX. No cases of whole arm swelling were reported. Two individuals (2/193) reported large injection site swelling (range 110 to 200 mm diameter), in one case associated with grade 3 pain. Neither individual sought medical attention. These episodes were reported to resolve without sequelae within 5 days.

Table 2. Rates of Solicited Adverse Events Reported Within the 15-day[a] Post-Vaccination Period Following Administration of BOOSTRIX in Adolescents 10 to 12 Years of Age Who Had Previously Received 5 Doses of INFANRIX

	BOOSTRIX (N = 193) %
Pain, any	62.2
Pain, grade 2 or 3	33.2
Pain, grade 3	5.7
Redness, any	47.7
Redness, >20 mm	15.0
Redness, ≥50 mm	10.9
Swelling, any	38.9
Swelling, >20 mm	17.6
Swelling, ≥50 mm	14.0
Fever, ≥99.5°F (37.5°C)[b]	8.8
Fever, >100.4°F (38.0°C)[b]	4.1
Fever, >102.2°F (39.0°C)[b]	1.0

N = Number of subjects with local/general symptoms sheets completed.
Grade 2 = Painful when limb moved.
Grade 3 = Spontaneously painful and/or prevented normal activity.
[a] Day of vaccination and the next 14 days.
[b] Oral temperatures or axillary temperatures.

Solicited Adverse Events in the US Adult (19 to 64 Years of Age) Study: Table 3 presents solicited local adverse reactions and general adverse events within 15 days of vaccination with BOOSTRIX or the comparator Tdap vaccine for the total vaccinated cohort.

Table 3. Rates of Solicited Local Adverse Reactions or General Adverse Events Within the 15-day[a] Post-Vaccination Period in Adults 19 to 64 Years of Age (Total Vaccinated Cohort)

	BOOSTRIX (N = 1,480) %	Tdap (N = 741) %
Local		
Pain, any	61.0	69.2
Pain, grade 2 or 3	35.1	44.4
Pain, grade 3	1.6	2.3
Redness, any	21.1	27.1
Redness, >20 mm	4.0	6.2

Redness, ≥50 mm	1.6	2.3
Swelling, any	17.6	25.6
Swelling, >20 mm	3.9	6.3
Swelling, ≥50 mm	1.4	2.8
General		
Headache, any	30.1	31.0
Headache, grade 2 or 3	11.1	10.5
Headache, grade 3	2.2	1.5
Fatigue, any	28.1	28.9
Fatigue, grade 2 or 3	9.1	9.4
Fatigue, grade 3	2.5	1.2
Gastrointestinal symptoms, any[b]	15.9	17.5
Gastrointestinal symptoms, grade 2 or 3[b]	4.3	5.7
Gastrointestinal symptoms, grade 3[b]	1.2	1.3
Fever, ≥99.5°F (37.5°C)[c]	5.5	8.0
Fever, >100.4°F (38.0°C)[c]	1.0	1.5
Fever, >102.2°F (39.0°C)[c]	0.1	0.4

Tdap = Tetanus Toxoid, Reduced Diphtheria Toxoid and Acellular Pertussis Vaccine Adsorbed, a Tdap vaccine manufactured by Sanofi Pasteur SA.

N = Number of subjects in the total vaccinated cohort with local/general symptoms sheets completed.

Grade 2 = Local: painful when limb moved; General: interfered with normal activity.

Grade 3 = Local/General: prevented normal activity.

[a] Day of vaccination and the next 14 days.

[b] Gastrointestinal symptoms included nausea, vomiting, diarrhea, and/or abdominal pain.

[c] Oral temperatures.

Unsolicited Adverse Events in the US Adult (19 to 64 Years of Age) Study: The incidence of unsolicited adverse events reported in the 31 days after vaccination was comparable between the 2 groups (17.8% and 22.2% for BOOSTRIX and Tdap vaccine, respectively).

Solicited Adverse Events in the US Elderly (65 Years of Age and Older) Study: Table 4 presents solicited local adverse reactions and general adverse events within 4 days of vaccination with BOOSTRIX or the comparator Td vaccine for the total vaccinated cohort.

Table 4. Rates of Solicited Local Adverse Reactions or General Adverse Events Within 4 Days[a] of Vaccination in the Elderly 65 Years of Age and Older (Total Vaccinated Cohort)

	BOOSTRIX %	Td %
Local	(N = 882)	(N = 444)
Pain, any	21.5	27.7
Pain, grade 2 or 3	7.5	10.1
Pain, grade 3	0.2	0.7
Redness, any	10.8	12.6
Redness, >20 mm	1.4	2.5
Redness, ≥50 mm	0.6	0.9
Swelling, any	7.5	11.7
Swelling, >20 mm	2.2	3.4
Swelling, ≥50 mm	0.7	0.7
General	(N = 882)	(N = 445)
Fatigue, any	12.5	14.8
Fatigue, grade 2 or 3	2.5	2.9
Fatigue, grade 3	0.7	0.7
Headache, any	11.5	11.7
Headache, grade 2 or 3	1.9	2.2
Headache, grade 3	0.6	0.0
Gastrointestinal symptoms, any[b]	7.6	9.2
Gastrointestinal symptoms, grade 2 or 3[b]	1.7	1.8
Gastrointestinal symptoms, grade 3[b]	0.3	0.4
Fever, ≥99.5°F (37.5°C)[c]	2.0	2.5
Fever, >100.4°F (38.0°C)[c]	0.2	0.2

Table 5. Rates of Solicited Local Adverse Reactions or General Adverse Events Reported Within the 4-day Post-Vaccination Period following Administration of BOOSTRIX in Individuals 11 to 18 Years of Age (Total Vaccinated Cohort)

	BOOSTRIX+MCV4[a] (N = 441) %	BOOSTRIX→MCV4[b] (N = 432-433) %	MCV4→BOOSTRIX[c] (N = 441) %
Local (at injection site for BOOSTRIX)			
Pain, any	70.1	70.4	47.8
Redness, any	22.7	25.7	17.9
Swelling, any	17.7	18.1	12.0
General (following administration of BOOSTRIX)			
Fatigue	34.0	32.1	20.4
Headache	34.0	30.7	17.0
Gastrointestinal symptoms[d]	15.2	14.5	7.7
Fever, ≥99.5°F (37.5°C)[e]	5.2	3.5	2.3

MCV4 = MENACTRA (Meningococcal (Groups A, C, Y, and W-135) Polysaccharide Diphtheria Toxoid Conjugate Vaccine), Sanofi Pasteur SA.

N = number of subjects in the total vaccinated cohort with local/general symptoms sheets completed.

[a] BOOSTRIX+MCV4 = concomitant vaccination with BOOSTRIX and MENACTRA.

[b] BOOSTRIX→MCV4 = BOOSTRIX followed by MCV4 1 month later.

[c] MCV4→BOOSTRIX = MCV4 followed by BOOSTRIX 1 month later.

[d] Gastrointestinal symptoms included nausea, vomiting, diarrhea, and/or abdominal pain.

[e] Oral temperatures.

Fever, >102.2°F (39.0°C)[c]	0.0	0.0

Td = Tetanus and Diphtheria Toxoids Adsorbed, a US-licensed Td vaccine, manufactured by Sanofi Pasteur SA.

N = Number of subjects with a documented dose.

Grade 2 = Local: painful when limb moved; General: interfered with normal activity.

Grade 3 = Local/General: prevented normal activity.

[a] Day of vaccination and the next 3 days.

[b] Gastrointestinal symptoms included nausea, vomiting, diarrhea, and/or abdominal pain.

[c] Oral temperatures.

Unsolicited Adverse Events in the US Elderly (65 Years of Age and Older) Study: The incidence of unsolicited adverse events reported in the 31 days after vaccination was comparable between the 2 groups (17.1% and 14.4% for BOOSTRIX and Td vaccine, respectively).

Serious Adverse Events (SAEs): In the US and German adolescent safety studies, no serious adverse events were reported to occur within 31 days of vaccination. During the 6-month extended safety evaluation period, no serious adverse events that were of potential autoimmune origin or new onset and chronic in nature were reported to occur. In non-US adolescent studies in which serious adverse events were monitored for up to 37 days, one subject was diagnosed with insulin-dependent diabetes 20 days following administration of BOOSTRIX. No other serious adverse events of potential autoimmune origin or that were new onset and chronic in nature were reported to occur in these studies. In the US adult (19 to 64 years of age) study, serious adverse events were reported to occur during the entire study period (0-6 months) by 1.4% and 1.7% of subjects who received BOOSTRIX and the comparator Tdap vaccine, respectively. During the 6-month extended safety evaluation period, no serious adverse events of a neuroinflammatory nature or with information suggesting an autoimmune etiology were reported in subjects who received BOOSTRIX. In the US elderly (65 years of age and older) study, serious adverse events were reported to occur by 0.7% and 0.9% of subjects who received BOOSTRIX and the comparator Td vaccine, respectively, during the 31-day period after vaccination. Serious adverse events were reported to occur by 4.2% and 2.2% of subjects who received BOOSTRIX and the comparator Td vaccine, respectively, during the 6-month period after vaccination.

Concomitant Vaccination With Meningococcal Conjugate Vaccine in Adolescents: In a randomized study in the US, 1,341 adolescents (11 to 18 years of age) received either BOOSTRIX administered concomitantly with MENACTRA® (Meningococcal (Groups A, C, Y, and W-135) Polysaccharide Diphtheria Toxoid Conjugate Vaccine), (Sanofi Pasteur SA), or each vaccine administered separately 1 month apart [see Drug Interactions (7.1) and Clinical Studies (14.5)]. Safety was evaluated in 446 subjects who received BOOSTRIX administered concomitantly with meningococcal conjugate vaccine at different injection sites, 446 subjects who received BOOSTRIX followed by meningococcal conjugate vaccine 1 month later, and 449 subjects who received meningococcal conjugate vaccine followed by BOOSTRIX 1 month later. Solicited local adverse reactions and general adverse events were recorded on diary cards for 4 days (day 0-3) following each vaccination. Unsolicited adverse events were monitored for the 31-day period following each vaccination (day 0-30). Table 5 presents the percentages of subjects experiencing local reactions at the injection site for BOOSTRIX and solicited general events following BOOSTRIX. The incidence of unsolicited adverse events reported in the 31 days after any vaccination was similar following each dose of BOOSTRIX in all cohorts.

[See table 5 above]

6.2 Postmarketing Experience

In addition to reports in clinical trials, worldwide voluntary reports of adverse events received for BOOSTRIX in persons 10 years of age and older since market introduction of this vaccine are listed below. This list includes serious events or events which have causal connection to components of this or other vaccines or drugs. Because these events are reported voluntarily from a population of uncertain size, it is not possible to reliably estimate their frequency or establish a causal relationship to the vaccine.

Blood and Lymphatic System Disorders: Lymphadenitis, lymphadenopathy.

Immune System Disorders: Allergic reactions, including anaphylactic and anaphylactoid reactions.

Cardiac Disorders: Myocarditis.

General Disorders and Administration Site Conditions: Extensive swelling of the injected limb, injection site induration, injection site inflammation, injection site mass, injection site pruritus, injection site nodule, injection site warmth, injection site reaction.

Musculoskeletal and Connective Tissue Disorders: Arthralgia, back pain, myalgia.

Nervous System Disorders: Convulsions (with and without fever), encephalitis, facial palsy, loss of consciousness, paraesthesia, syncope.

Skin and Subcutaneous Tissue Disorders: Angioedema, exanthem, Henoch-Schönlein purpura, rash, urticaria.

7 DRUG INTERACTIONS

7.1 Concomitant Vaccine Administration

BOOSTRIX was administered concomitantly with MENACTRA in a clinical study of subjects 11 to 18 years of age [see Clinical Studies (14.5)]. Post-vaccination geometric mean antibody concentrations (GMCs) to pertactin were lower following BOOSTRIX administered concomitantly with meningococcal conjugate vaccine compared to BOOSTRIX administered first. It is not known if the efficacy of BOOSTRIX is affected by the reduced response to pertactin.

BOOSTRIX was administered concomitantly with FLUARIX® (Influenza Virus Vaccine) in a clinical study of subjects 19 to 64 years of age [see Clinical Studies (14.5)]. Lower GMCs for antibodies to the pertussis antigens filamentous hemagglutinin (FHA) and pertactin were observed when BOOSTRIX was administered concomitantly with FLUARIX as compared with BOOSTRIX alone. It is not known if the efficacy of BOOSTRIX is affected by the reduced response to FHA and pertactin.

When BOOSTRIX is administered concomitantly with other injectable vaccines or Tetanus Immune Globulin, they should be given with separate syringes and at different injection sites. BOOSTRIX should not be mixed with any other vaccine in the same syringe or vial.

7.2 Immunosuppressive Therapies

Immunosuppressive therapies, including irradiation, antimetabolites, alkylating agents, cytotoxic drugs, and corticosteroids (used in greater than physiologic doses), may reduce the immune response to BOOSTRIX.

8 USE IN SPECIFIC POPULATIONS

8.1 Pregnancy

Pregnancy Category B

A developmental toxicity study has been performed in female rats at a dose approximately 40 times the human dose (on a mL/kg basis) and revealed no evidence of harm to the fetus due to BOOSTRIX. Animal fertility studies have not been conducted with BOOSTRIX. There are no adequate and well-controlled studies in pregnant women. Because animal reproduction studies are not always predictive of human response, BOOSTRIX should be given to a pregnant woman only if clearly needed.

In a developmental toxicity study, the effect of BOOSTRIX on embryo-fetal and pre-weaning development was evaluated in pregnant rats. Animals were administered INFANRIX by intramuscular injection once prior to gestation and BOOSTRIX by intramuscular injection during the period of organogenesis (gestation days 6, 8, 11, and 15), 0.1 mL/rat/occasion (approximately 40-fold excess relative to the projected human dose of BOOSTRIX on a body weight basis). The antigens in INFANRIX are the same as those in BOOSTRIX, but INFANRIX is formulated with higher quantities of these antigens. No adverse effects on pregnancy, parturition, lactation parameters, and embryo-fetal or pre-weaning development were observed. There were no vaccine-related fetal malformations or other evidence of teratogenesis.

Pregnancy Registry: GlaxoSmithKline maintains a surveillance registry to collect data on pregnancy outcomes and newborn health status outcomes following vaccination with BOOSTRIX during pregnancy. Women who receive BOOSTRIX during pregnancy should be encouraged to contact GlaxoSmithKline directly or their healthcare provider should contact GlaxoSmithKline by calling 1-888-452-9622.

8.3 Nursing Mothers

It is not known whether BOOSTRIX is excreted in human milk. Because many drugs are excreted in human milk, caution should be exercised when BOOSTRIX is administered to a nursing woman.

8.4 Pediatric Use

BOOSTRIX is not indicated for use in children younger than 10 years of age. Safety and effectiveness of BOOSTRIX in this age group have not been established.

8.5 Geriatric Use

In clinical trials, 1,104 subjects 65 years of age and older received BOOSTRIX; of these subjects, 299 were 75 years of age and older. In the US elderly (65 years and older) study, immune responses to tetanus and diphtheria toxoids following BOOSTRIX were non-inferior to the comparator Td vaccine. Antibody responses to pertussis antigens following a single dose of BOOSTRIX in the elderly were non-inferior to those observed with INFANRIX administered as a 3-dose series in infants *[see Clinical Studies (14.4)]*. Solicited adverse events following BOOSTRIX were similar in frequency to those reported with the comparator Td vaccine *[see Adverse Reactions (6.1)]*.

11 DESCRIPTION

BOOSTRIX (Tetanus Toxoid, Reduced Diphtheria Toxoid and Acellular Pertussis Vaccine, Adsorbed) is a noninfectious, sterile, vaccine for intramuscular administration. It contains tetanus toxoid, diphtheria toxoid, and pertussis antigens (inactivated pertussis toxin [PT] and formaldehyde-treated filamentous hemagglutinin [FHA] and pertactin). The antigens are the same as those in INFANRIX, but BOOSTRIX is formulated with reduced quantities of these antigens.

Tetanus toxin is produced by growing *Clostridium tetani* in a modified Latham medium derived from bovine casein. The diphtheria toxin is produced by growing *Corynebacterium diphtheriae* in Fenton medium containing a bovine extract. The bovine materials used in these extracts are sourced from countries which the United States Department of Agriculture (USDA) has determined neither have nor are at risk of bovine spongiform encephalopathy (BSE). Both toxins are detoxified with formaldehyde, concentrated by ultrafiltration, and purified by precipitation, dialysis, and sterile filtration.

The acellular pertussis antigens (PT, FHA, and pertactin) are isolated from *Bordetella pertussis* culture grown in modified Stainer-Scholte liquid medium. PT and FHA are isolated from the fermentation broth; pertactin is extracted from the cells by heat treatment and flocculation. The anti-

Table 6. Antibody Responses to Tetanus and Diphtheria Toxoids Following BOOSTRIX Compared With Td Vaccine in Adolescents 10 to 18 Years of Age (ATP Cohort for Immunogenicity)

	N	% ≥0.1 IU/mL[a] (95% CI)	% ≥1.0 IU/mL[a] (95% CI)	% Booster Response[b] (95% CI)
Anti-Tetanus				
BOOSTRIX	2,469-2,516			
Pre-vaccination		97.7 (97.1, 98.3)	36.8 (34.9, 38.7)	–
Post-vaccination		100 (99.8, 100)[c]	99.5 (99.1, 99.7)[d]	89.7 (88.4, 90.8)[c]
Td	817-834			
Pre-vaccination		96.8 (95.4, 97.9)	39.9 (36.5, 43.4)	–
Post-vaccination		100 (99.6, 100)	99.8 (99.1, 100)	92.5 (90.5, 94.2)
Anti-Diphtheria				
BOOSTRIX	2,463-2,515			
Pre-vaccination		85.8 (84.3, 87.1)	17.1 (15.6, 18.6)	–
Post-vaccination		99.9 (99.7, 100)[c]	97.3 (96.6, 97.9)[d]	90.6 (89.4, 91.7)[c]
Td	814-834			
Pre-vaccination		84.8 (82.1, 87.2)	19.5 (16.9, 22.4)	–
Post-vaccination		99.9 (99.3, 100)	99.3 (98.4, 99.7)	95.9 (94.4, 97.2)

Td manufactured by MassBioLogics.
ATP = according-to-protocol; CI = Confidence Interval.
[a]Measured by ELISA.
[b]Booster response: In subjects with pre-vaccination <0.1 IU/mL, post-vaccination concentration ≥0.4 IU/mL. In subjects with pre-vaccination concentration ≥0.1 IU/mL, an increase of at least 4 times the pre-vaccination concentration.
[c]Seroprotection rate or booster response rate to BOOSTRIX was non-inferior to Td (upper limit of two-sided 95% CI on the difference for Td minus BOOSTRIX ≤10%).
[d]Non-inferiority criteria not prospectively defined for this endpoint.

gens are purified in successive chromatographic and precipitation steps. PT is detoxified using glutaraldehyde and formaldehyde. FHA and pertactin are treated with formaldehyde.

Each antigen is individually adsorbed onto aluminum hydroxide. Each 0.5-mL dose is formulated to contain 5 Lf of tetanus toxoid, 2.5 Lf of diphtheria toxoid, 8 mcg of inactivated PT, 8 mcg of FHA, and 2.5 mcg of pertactin (69 kiloDalton outer membrane protein).

Tetanus and diphtheria toxoid potency is determined by measuring the amount of neutralizing antitoxin in previously immunized guinea pigs. The potency of the acellular pertussis components (inactivated PT and formaldehyde-treated FHA and pertactin) is determined by enzyme-linked immunosorbent assay (ELISA) on sera from previously immunized mice.

Each 0.5-mL dose contains aluminum hydroxide as adjuvant (not more than 0.39 mg aluminum by assay), 4.5 mg of sodium chloride, ≤100 mcg of residual formaldehyde, and ≤100 mcg of polysorbate 80 (Tween 80).

BOOSTRIX is available in vials and prefilled syringes. The tip caps of the prefilled syringes may contain natural rubber latex; the plungers are not made with natural rubber latex. The vial stoppers are not made with natural rubber latex.

12 CLINICAL PHARMACOLOGY

12.1 Mechanism of Action

Tetanus: Tetanus is a condition manifested primarily by neuromuscular dysfunction caused by a potent exotoxin released by *C. tetani*. Protection against disease is due to the development of neutralizing antibodies to the tetanus toxin. A serum tetanus antitoxin level of at least 0.01 IU/mL, measured by neutralization assays, is considered the minimum protective level.[2] A level ≥0.1 IU/mL by ELISA has been considered as protective.

Diphtheria: Diphtheria is an acute toxin-mediated infectious disease caused by toxigenic strains of *C. diphtheriae*. Protection against disease is due to the development of neutralizing antibodies to the diphtheria toxin. A serum diphtheria antitoxin level of 0.01 IU/mL, measured by neutralization assays, is the lowest level giving some degree of protection; a level of 0.1 IU/mL by ELISA is regarded as protective.[3] Diphtheria antitoxin levels ≥1.0 IU/mL by ELISA have been associated with long-term protection.[3]

Pertussis: Pertussis (whooping cough) is a disease of the respiratory tract caused by *B. pertussis*. The role of the different components produced by *B. pertussis* in either the pathogenesis of, or the immunity to, pertussis is not well understood.

13 NONCLINICAL TOXICOLOGY

13.1 Carcinogenesis, Mutagenesis, Impairment of Fertility

BOOSTRIX has not been evaluated for carcinogenic or mutagenic potential, or for impairment of fertility.

14 CLINICAL STUDIES

The efficacy of the tetanus and diphtheria toxoid components of BOOSTRIX is based on the immunogenicity of the individual antigens compared to US-licensed vaccines using

established serologic correlates of protection. The efficacy of the pertussis components of BOOSTRIX was evaluated by comparison of the immune response of adolescents and adults following a single dose of BOOSTRIX to the immune response of infants following a 3-dose primary series of INFANRIX. In addition, the ability of BOOSTRIX to induce a booster response to each of the antigens was evaluated.

14.1 Efficacy of INFANRIX

The efficacy of a 3-dose primary series of INFANRIX in infants has been assessed in 2 clinical studies: A prospective efficacy trial conducted in Germany employing a household contact study design and a double-blind, randomized, active Diphtheria and Tetanus Toxoids (DT)-controlled trial conducted in Italy sponsored by the National Institutes of Health (NIH) (for details see INFANRIX prescribing information). Serological data from a subset of infants immunized with INFANRIX in the household contact study were compared with the sera of adolescents and adults immunized with BOOSTRIX *[see Clinical Studies (14.2, 14.3)]*. In the household contact study, the protective efficacy of INFANRIX, in infants, against WHO-defined pertussis (21 days or more of paroxysmal cough with infection confirmed by culture and/or serologic testing) was calculated to be 89% (95% CI: 77%, 95%). When the definition of pertussis was expanded to include clinically milder disease, with infection confirmed by culture and/or serologic testing, the efficacy of INFANRIX against ≥7 days of any cough was 67% (95% CI: 52%, 78%) and against ≥7 days of paroxysmal cough was 81% (95% CI: 68%, 89%) (for details see INFANRIX prescribing information).

14.2 Immunological Evaluation in Adolescents

In a multicenter, randomized, controlled study conducted in the United States, the immune responses to each of the antigens contained in BOOSTRIX were evaluated in sera obtained approximately 1 month after administration of a single dose of vaccine to adolescent subjects (10 to 18 years of age). Of the subjects enrolled in this study, approximately 76% were 10 to 14 years of age and 24% were 15 to 18 years of age. Approximately 98% of participants in this study had received the recommended series of 4 or 5 doses of either DTwP or a combination of DTwP and DTaP in childhood. The racial/ethnic demographics were as follows: white 85.8%, black 5.7%, Hispanic 5.6%, Oriental 0.8%, and other 2.1%.

Response to Tetanus and Diphtheria Toxoids: The antibody responses to the tetanus and diphtheria toxoids of BOOSTRIX compared with Td vaccine are shown in Table 6. One month after a single dose, anti-tetanus and anti-diphtheria seroprotective rates (≥0.1 IU/mL by ELISA) and booster response rates were comparable between BOOSTRIX and the comparator Td vaccine.

[See table 6 above]

Response to Pertussis Antigens: The booster response rates of adolescents to the pertussis antigens are shown in Table 7. For each of the pertussis antigens the lower limit of the two-sided 95% CI for the percentage of subjects with a booster response exceeded the pre-defined lower limit of 80% for demonstration of an acceptable booster response.

Table 9. Antibody Responses to Tetanus and Diphtheria Toxoids Following One Dose of BOOSTRIX Compared With the Comparator Tdap Vaccine in Adults 19 to 64 Years of Age (ATP Cohort for Immunogenicity)

	N	% ≥0.1 IU/mL[a] (95% CI)	% ≥1.0 IU/mL[a] (95% CI)
Anti-Tetanus			
BOOSTRIX	1,445-1,447		
Pre-vaccination		95.9 (94.8, 96.9)	71.9 (69.5, 74.2)
Post-vaccination		99.6 (99.1, 99.8)[b]	98.3 (97.5, 98.9)[b]
Tdap	727-728		
Pre-vaccination		97.2 (95.8, 98.3)	74.7 (71.4, 77.8)
Post-vaccination		100 (95.5, 100)	99.3 (98.4, 99.8)
Anti-Diphtheria			
BOOSTRIX	1,440-1,444		
Pre-vaccination		85.2 (83.3, 87.0)	23.7 (21.5, 26.0)
Post-vaccination		98.2 (97.4, 98.8)[b]	87.9 (86.1, 89.5)[c]
Tdap	720-727		
Pre-vaccination		89.2 (86.7, 91.3)	26.5 (23.3, 29.9)
Post-vaccination		98.6 (97.5, 99.3)	92.0 (89.8, 93.9)

Tdap = Tetanus Toxoid, Reduced Diphtheria Toxoid and Acellular Pertussis Vaccine, Adsorbed manufactured by Sanofi Pasteur SA.
ATP = according-to-protocol; CI = Confidence Interval.
[a]Measured by ELISA.
[b]Seroprotection rates for BOOSTRIX were non-inferior to the comparator Tdap vaccine (lower limit of 95% CI on the difference of BOOSTRIX minus Tdap ≥-10%).
[c]Non-inferiority criteria not prospectively defined for this endpoint.

Table 7. Booster Responses to the Pertussis Antigens Following BOOSTRIX in Adolescents 10 to 18 Years of Age (ATP Cohort for Immunogenicity)

	N	BOOSTRIX % Booster Response[a] (95% CI)
Anti-PT	2,677	84.5 (83.0, 85.9)
Anti-FHA	2,744	95.1 (94.2, 95.9)
Anti-pertactin	2,752	95.4 (94.5, 96.1)

ATP = according-to-protocol; CI = Confidence Interval.

[a]Booster response: In initially seronegative subjects (<5 EL.U./mL), post-vaccination antibody concentrations ≥20 EL.U./mL. In initially seropositive subjects with pre-vaccination antibody concentrations ≥5 EL.U./mL and <20 EL.U./mL, an increase of at least 4 times the pre-vaccination antibody concentration. In initially seropositive subjects with pre-vaccination antibody concentrations ≥20 EL.U./mL, an increase of at least 2 times the pre-vaccination antibody concentration.

The GMCs to each of the pertussis antigens 1 month following a single dose of BOOSTRIX in the US adolescent study (N = 2,941-2,979) were compared with the GMCs observed in infants following a 3-dose primary series of INFANRIX administered at 3, 4, and 5 months of age (N = 631-2,884). Table 8 presents the results for the total immunogenicity cohort in both studies (vaccinated subjects with serology data available for at least one pertussis antigen; the majority of subjects in the study of INFANRIX had anti-PT serology data only). These infants were a subset of those who formed the cohort for the German household contact study in which the efficacy of INFANRIX was demonstrated [see Clinical Studies (14.1)]. Although a serologic correlate of protection for pertussis has not been established, anti-PT, anti-FHA, and anti-pertactin antibody concentrations observed in adolescents 1 month after a single dose of BOOSTRIX were non-inferior to those observed in infants following a primary vaccination series with INFANRIX.

Table 8. Ratio of GMCs to Pertussis Antigens Following One Dose of BOOSTRIX in Adolescents 10 to 18 Years of Age Compared With 3 Doses of INFANRIX in Infants (Total Immunogenicity Cohort)

	GMC Ratio: BOOSTRIX/INFANRIX (95% CI)
Anti-PT	1.90 (1.82, 1.99)[a]
Anti-FHA	7.35 (6.85, 7.89)[a]
Anti-pertactin	4.19 (3.73, 4.71)[a]

GMC = geometric mean antibody concentration, measured in ELISA units; CI = Confidence Interval.
Number of subjects for BOOSTRIX GMC evaluation: Anti-PT = 2,941, anti-FHA = 2,979, and anti-pertactin = 2,978.
Number of subjects for INFANRIX GMC evaluation: Anti-PT = 2,884, anti-FHA = 685, and anti-pertactin = 631.
[a]GMC following BOOSTRIX was non-inferior to GMC following INFANRIX (lower limit of 95% CI for the GMC ratio of BOOSTRIX/INFANRIX >0.67).

14.3 Immunological Evaluation in Adults (19 to 64 Years of Age)

A multicenter, randomized, observer-blinded study, conducted in the United States, evaluated the immunogenicity of BOOSTRIX compared with the licensed comparator Tdap vaccine (Sanofi Pasteur SA). Vaccines were administered as a single dose to subjects (N = 2,284) who had not received a tetanus-diphtheria booster within 5 years. The immune responses to each of the antigens contained in BOOSTRIX were evaluated in sera obtained approximately 1 month after administration. Approximately 33% of patients were 19 to 29 years of age, 33% were 30 to 49 years of age and 34% were 50 to 64 years of age. Among subjects in the combined vaccine groups, 62% were female; 84% of subjects were white, 8% black, 1% Asian, and 7% were of other racial/ethnic groups.

Response to Tetanus and Diphtheria Toxoids: The antibody responses to the tetanus and diphtheria toxoids of BOOSTRIX compared with the comparator Tdap vaccine are shown in Table 9. One month after a single dose, anti-tetanus and anti-diphtheria seroprotective rates (≥0.1 IU/mL by ELISA) were comparable between BOOSTRIX and the comparator Tdap vaccine.
[See table 9 above]

Response to Pertussis Antigens: Booster response rates to the pertussis antigens are shown in Table 10. For the FHA and pertactin antigens, the lower limit of the 95% CI for the booster responses exceeded the pre-defined limit of 80% demonstrating an acceptable booster response following BOOSTRIX. The PT antigen booster response lower limit of the 95% CI (74.9%) did not exceed the pre-defined limit of 80%.

Table 10. Booster Responses to the Pertussis Antigens Following One Dose of BOOSTRIX in Adults 19 to 64 Years of Age (ATP Cohort for Immunogenicity)

	N	BOOSTRIX % Booster Response[a] (95% CI)
Anti-PT	1,419	77.2 (74.9, 79.3)[b]
Anti-FHA	1,433	96.9 (95.8, 97.7)[c]
Anti-pertactin	1,441	93.2 (91.8, 94.4)[c]

ATP = according-to-protocol; CI = Confidence Interval.
[a]Booster response: In initially seronegative subjects (<5 EL.U./mL), post-vaccination antibody concentrations ≥20 EL.U./mL. In initially seropositive subjects with pre-vaccination antibody concentrations ≥5 EL.U./mL and <20 EL.U./mL, an increase of at least 4 times the pre-vaccination antibody concentration. In initially seropositive subjects with pre-vaccination antibody concentrations ≥20 EL.U./mL, an increase of at least 2 times the pre-vaccination antibody concentration.
[b]The PT antigen booster response lower limit of the 95% CI did not exceed the pre-defined limit of 80%.
[c]The FHA and pertactin antigens booster response lower limit of the 95% CI exceeded the pre-defined limit of 80%.

The GMCs to each of the pertussis antigens 1 month following a single dose of BOOSTRIX in the US adult (19 to 64 years of age) study were compared with the GMCs observed in infants following a 3-dose primary series of INFANRIX administered at 3, 4, and 5 months of age. Table 11 presents the results for the total immunogenicity cohort in both studies (vaccinated subjects with serology data available for at least one pertussis antigen). These infants were a subset of those who formed the cohort for the German household contact study in which the efficacy of INFANRIX was demonstrated [see Clinical Studies (14.1)]. Although a serologic correlate of protection for pertussis has not been established, anti-PT, anti-FHA, and anti-pertactin antibody concentrations observed in adults 1 month after a single dose of BOOSTRIX were non-inferior to those observed in infants following a primary vaccination series with INFANRIX.

Table 11. Ratio of GMCs to Pertussis Antigens Following One Dose of BOOSTRIX in Adults 19 to 64 Years of Age Compared With 3 Doses of INFANRIX in Infants (Total Immunogenicity Cohort)

	GMC Ratio: BOOSTRIX/INFANRIX (95% CI)
Anti-PT	1.39 (1.32, 1.47)[a]
Anti-FHA	7.46 (6.86, 8.12)[a]
Anti-pertactin	3.56 (3.10, 4.08)[a]

GMC = geometric mean antibody concentration; CI = Confidence Interval.
Number of subjects for BOOSTRIX GMC evaluation: Anti-PT = 1,460, anti-FHA = 1,472, and anti-pertactin = 1,473.
Number of subjects for INFANRIX GMC evaluation: Anti-PT = 2,884, anti-FHA = 685, and anti-pertactin = 631.
[a]BOOSTRIX was non-inferior to INFANRIX (lower limit of 95% CI for the GMC ratio of BOOSTRIX/INFANRIX ≥0.67).

14.4 Immunological Evaluation in the Elderly (65 Years of Age and Older)

The US elderly (65 years of age and older) study, a randomized, observer-blinded study, evaluated the immunogenicity of BOOSTRIX (N = 887) compared with a US-licensed comparator Td vaccine (N = 445) (Sanofi Pasteur SA). Vaccines were administered as a single dose to subjects who had not received a tetanus-diphtheria booster within 5 years. Among all vaccine recipients, the mean age was approximately 72 years of age; 54% were female and 95% were white. The immune responses to each of the antigens contained in BOOSTRIX were evaluated in sera obtained approximately 1 month after administration.

Response to Tetanus and Diphtheria Toxoids and Pertussis Antigens: Immune responses to tetanus and diphtheria toxoids and pertussis antigens were measured 1 month after administration of a single dose of BOOSTRIX or a comparator Td vaccine. Anti-tetanus and anti-diphtheria seroprotective rates (≥0.1 IU/mL) were comparable between BOOSTRIX and the comparator Td vaccine (Table 12).

Table 12. Immune Responses to Tetanus and Diphtheria Toxoids Following BOOSTRIX or Comparator Td Vaccine in the Elderly 65 Years of Age and Older (ATP Cohort for Immunogenicity)

	BOOSTRIX (N = 844-864)	Td (N = 430-439)
Anti-T		
% ≥0.1 IU/mL (95% CI)	96.8 (95.4, 97.8)[a]	97.5 (95.6, 98.7)
% ≥1.0 IU/mL (95% CI)	88.8 (86.5, 90.8)[a]	90.0 (86.8, 92.6)

Anti-D		
% ≥0.1 IU/mL (95% CI)	84.9 (82.3, 87.2)[a]	86.6 (83.0, 89.6)
% ≥1.0 IU/mL (95% CI)	52.0 (48.6, 55.4)[b]	51.2 (46.3, 56.0)

Td = Tetanus and Diphtheria Toxoids Adsorbed, a US-licensed Td vaccine, manufactured by Sanofi Pasteur SA.

ATP = according-to-protocol; CI = Confidence Interval.

[a]Seroprotection rates for BOOSTRIX were non-inferior to the comparator Td vaccine (lower limit of 95% CI on the difference of BOOSTRIX minus Td ≥-10%).

[b]Non-inferiority criteria not prospectively defined for this endpoint.

The GMCs to each of the pertussis antigens 1 month following a single dose of BOOSTRIX were compared with the GMCs of infants following a 3-dose primary series of INFANRIX administered at 3, 4, and 5 months of age. Table 13 presents the results for the total immunogenicity cohort in both studies (vaccinated subjects with serology data available for at least one pertussis antigen). These infants were a subset of those who formed the cohort for the German household contact study in which the efficacy of INFANRIX was demonstrated [see Clinical Studies (14.1)]. Although a serologic correlate of protection for pertussis has not been established, anti-PT, anti-FHA, and anti-pertactin antibody concentrations in the elderly (65 years of age and older) 1 month after a single dose of BOOSTRIX were non-inferior to those of infants following a primary vaccination series with INFANRIX.

Table 13. Ratio of GMCs to Pertussis Antigens Following One Dose of BOOSTRIX in the Elderly 65 Years of Age and Older Compared With 3 Doses of INFANRIX in Infants (Total Immunogenicity Cohort)

	GMC Ratio: BOOSTRIX/INFANRIX (95% CI)
Anti-PT	1.07 (1.00, 1.15)[a]
Anti-FHA	8.24 (7.45, 9.12)[a]
Anti-pertactin	0.93 (0.79, 1.10)[a]

GMC = geometric mean antibody concentration; CI = Confidence Interval.

Number of subjects for BOOSTRIX GMC evaluation: Anti-PT = 865, anti-FHA = 847, and anti-pertactin = 878. Number of subjects for INFANRIX GMC evaluation: Anti-PT = 2,884, anti-FHA = 685, and anti-pertactin = 631.

[a]BOOSTRIX was non-inferior to INFANRIX (lower limit of 95% CI for the GMC ratio of BOOSTRIX/INFANRIX ≥0.67).

14.5 Concomitant Vaccine Administration

Concomitant Administration With Meningococcal Conjugate Vaccine: The concomitant use of BOOSTRIX and a tetravalent meningococcal (groups A, C, Y, and W-135) conjugate vaccine (Sanofi Pasteur SA) was evaluated in a randomized study in healthy adolescents 11 to 18 years of age. A total of 1,341 adolescents were vaccinated with BOOSTRIX. Of these, 446 subjects received BOOSTRIX administered concomitantly with meningococcal conjugate vaccine at different injection sites, 446 subjects received BOOSTRIX followed by meningococcal conjugate vaccine 1 month later, and 449 subjects received meningococcal conjugate vaccine followed by BOOSTRIX 1 month later. Immune responses to diphtheria and tetanus toxoids (% of subjects with anti-tetanus and anti-diphtheria antibodies ≥1.0 IU/mL by ELISA), pertussis antigens (booster responses and GMCs), and meningococcal antigens (vaccine responses) were measured 1 month (range 30 to 48 days) after concomitant or separate administration of BOOSTRIX and meningococcal conjugate vaccine. For BOOSTRIX given concomitantly with meningococcal conjugate vaccine compared to BOOSTRIX administered first, non-inferiority was demonstrated for all antigens, with the exception of the anti-pertactin GMC. The lower limit of the 95% CI for the GMC ratio was 0.54 for anti-pertactin (pre-specified limit ≥0.67). For the anti-pertactin booster response, non-inferiority was demonstrated. It is not known if the efficacy of BOOSTRIX is affected by the reduced response to pertactin.

There was no evidence that BOOSTRIX interfered with the antibody responses to the meningococcal antigens when measured by serum bactericidal assays (rSBA) when given concomitantly or sequentially (meningococcal conjugate vaccine followed by BOOSTRIX or BOOSTRIX followed by meningococcal conjugate vaccine.

Concomitant Administration With FLUARIX (Influenza Virus Vaccine): The concomitant use of BOOSTRIX and

FLUARIX was evaluated in a multicenter, open-label, randomized, controlled study of 1,497 adults 19 to 64 years of age. In one group, subjects received BOOSTRIX and FLUARIX concurrently (n = 748). The other group received FLUARIX at the first visit, then 1 month later received BOOSTRIX (n = 749). Sera was obtained prior to and 1 month following concomitant or separate administration of BOOSTRIX and/or FLUARIX, as well as 1 month after the separate administration of FLUARIX.

Immune responses following concurrent administration of BOOSTRIX and FLUARIX were non-inferior to separate administration for diphtheria (seroprotection defined as ≥0.1 IU/mL), tetanus (seroprotection defined as ≥0.1 IU/mL and based on concentrations ≥1.0 IU/mL), pertussis toxin (PT) antigen (anti-PT GMC) and influenza antigens (percent of subjects with hemagglutination-inhibition [HI] antibody titer ≥1:40 and ≥4-fold rise in HI titer). Non-inferiority criteria were not met for the anti-pertussis antigens FHA and pertactin. The lower limit of the 95% CI of the GMC ratio was 0.64 for anti-FHA and 0.60 for anti-pertactin and the pre-specified limit was ≥0.67. It is not known if the efficacy of BOOSTRIX is affected by the reduced response to FHA and pertactin.

15 REFERENCES

1. Institute of Medicine (IOM). Stratton KR, Howe CJ, Johnston RB, eds. *Adverse events associated with childhood vaccines. Evidence bearing on causality.* Washington, DC: National Academy Press; 1994.
2. Wassilak SGF, Roper MH, Kretsinger K, and Orenstein WA. Tetanus Toxoid. In: Plotkin SA, Orenstein WA, and Offit PA, eds. *Vaccines.* 5th ed. Saunders; 2008:805-839.
3. Vitek CR and Wharton M. Diphtheria Toxoid. In: Plotkin SA, Orenstein WA, and Offit PA, eds. *Vaccines.* 5th ed. Saunders; 2008:139-156.

16 HOW SUPPLIED/STORAGE AND HANDLING

BOOSTRIX is available in 0.5-mL single-dose vials and disposable prefilled TIP-LOK syringes (packaged without needles):

NDC 58160-842-01 Vial in Package of 10: NDC 58160-842-11

NDC 58160-842-05 Syringe in Package of 1: NDC 58160-842-34

NDC 58160-842-43 Syringe in Package of 10: NDC 58160-842-52

Store refrigerated between 2° and 8°C (36° and 46°F). Do not freeze. Discard if the vaccine has been frozen.

17 PATIENT COUNSELING INFORMATION

The patient, parent, or guardian should be:
- informed of the potential benefits and risks of immunization with BOOSTRIX.
- informed about the potential for adverse reactions that have been temporally associated with administration of BOOSTRIX or other vaccines containing similar components.
- instructed to report any adverse events to their healthcare provider.
- informed that safety and efficacy have not been established in pregnant women. Register women who receive BOOSTRIX while pregnant in the pregnancy registry by calling 1-888-452-9622.
- given the Vaccine Information Statements, which are required by the National Childhood Vaccine Injury Act of 1986 to be given prior to immunization. These materials are available free of charge at the Centers for Disease Control and Prevention (CDC) website (www.cdc.gov/vaccines).

BOOSTRIX, FLUARIX, INFANRIX, and TIP-LOK are registered trademarks of the GlaxoSmithKline group of companies. The following are registered trademarks of their respective owners: ADACEL and DECAVAC/Sanofi Pasteur Limited; MENACTRA/Connaught Technology Corporation.

Manufactured by **GlaxoSmithKline Biologicals**
Rixensart, Belgium, US License 1617, and
Novartis Vaccines and Diagnostics GmbH
Marburg, Germany, US License 1754
Distributed by **GlaxoSmithKline**
Research Triangle Park, NC 27709
©2013, GlaxoSmithKline group of companies. All rights reserved.
BTX:26PI

BREO ELLIPTA   ℞
(fluticasone furoate and vilanterol inhalation powder)
FOR ORAL INHALATION USE

HIGHLIGHTS OF PRESCRIBING INFORMATION
These highlights do not include all the information needed to use BREO ELLIPTA safely and effectively. See full prescribing information for BREO ELLIPTA.

BREO ELLIPTA (fluticasone furoate and vilanterol inhalation powder)
FOR ORAL INHALATION USE
Initial U.S. Approval: 2013

> **WARNING: ASTHMA-RELATED DEATH**
> *See full prescribing information for complete boxed warning.*
> - Long-acting beta$_2$-adrenergic agonists (LABA), such as vilanterol, one of the active ingredients in BREO ELLIPTA, increase the risk of asthma-related death. A placebo-controlled trial with another LABA (salmeterol) showed an increase in asthma-related deaths in subjects receiving salmeterol. This finding with salmeterol is considered a class effect of all LABA, including vilanterol. (5.1)
> - The safety and efficacy of BREO ELLIPTA in patients with asthma have not been established. BREO ELLIPTA is not indicated for the treatment of asthma. (5.1)

INDICATIONS AND USAGE

BREO ELLIPTA is a combination of fluticasone furoate, an inhaled corticosteroid (ICS), and vilanterol, a long-acting beta$_2$–adrenergic agonist (LABA), indicated for long-term, once-daily, maintenance treatment of airflow obstruction and for reducing exacerbations in patients with chronic obstructive pulmonary disease (COPD). (1)
Important limitations: Not indicated for relief of acute bronchospasm or for treatment of asthma. (1, 5.2)

DOSAGE AND ADMINISTRATION

- For oral inhalation only. (2)
- Maintenance treatment of COPD: 1 inhalation of BREO ELLIPTA 100 mcg/25 mcg once daily. (2)

DOSAGE FORMS AND STRENGTHS

Inhalation Powder. Inhaler containing 2 double-foil blister strips of powder formulation for oral inhalation. One strip contains fluticasone furoate 100 mcg per blister and the other contains vilanterol 25 mcg per blister. (3)

CONTRAINDICATIONS

Severe hypersensitivity to milk proteins or any ingredients. (4)

WARNINGS AND PRECAUTIONS

- LABA increase the risk of asthma-related death. (5.1)
- Do not initiate in acutely deteriorating COPD or to treat acute symptoms. (5.2)
- Do not use in combination with an additional medicine containing LABA because of risk of overdose. (5.3)
- *Candida albicans* infection of the mouth and pharynx may occur. Monitor patients periodically. Advise the patient to rinse his/her mouth without swallowing after inhalation to help reduce the risk. (5.4)
- Increased risk of pneumonia in patients with COPD taking BREO ELLIPTA. Monitor patients for signs and symptoms of pneumonia. (5.5)
- Potential worsening of infections (e.g., existing tuberculosis; fungal, bacterial, viral, or parasitic infection; ocular herpes simplex). Use with caution in patients with these infections. More serious or even fatal course of chickenpox or measles can occur in susceptible patients. (5.6)
- Risk of impaired adrenal function when transferring from systemic corticosteroids. Taper patients slowly from systemic corticosteroids if transferring to BREO ELLIPTA. (5.7)
- Hypercorticism and adrenal suppression may occur with very high dosages or at the regular dosage in susceptible individuals. If such changes occur, discontinue BREO ELLIPTA slowly. (5.8)
- If paradoxical bronchospasm occurs, discontinue BREO ELLIPTA and institute alternative therapy. (5.10)
- Use with caution in patients with cardiovascular disorders because of beta-adrenergic stimulation. (5.12)
- Assess for decrease in bone mineral density initially and periodically thereafter. (5.13)
- Close monitoring for glaucoma and cataracts is warranted. (5.14)
- Use with caution in patients with convulsive disorders, thyrotoxicosis, diabetes mellitus, and ketoacidosis. (5.15)
- Be alert to hypokalemia and hyperglycemia. (5.16)

ADVERSE REACTIONS

Most common adverse reactions (incidence ≥3%) are nasopharyngitis, upper respiratory tract infection, headache, and oral candidiasis. (6.1)
To report SUSPECTED ADVERSE REACTIONS, contact GlaxoSmithKline at 1-888-825-5249 or FDA at 1-800-FDA-1088 or www.fda.gov/medwatch.

DRUG INTERACTIONS

- Strong cytochrome P450 3A4 inhibitors (e.g., ketoconazole): Use with caution. May cause systemic corticosteroid and cardiovascular effects. (7.1)

- Monoamine oxidase inhibitors and tricyclic antidepressants: Use with extreme caution. May potentiate effect of vilanterol on vascular system. (7.2)
- Beta-blockers: Use with caution. May block bronchodilatory effects of beta-agonists and produce severe bronchospasm. (7.3)
- Diuretics: Use with caution. Electrocardiographic changes and/or hypokalemia associated with non–potassium-sparing diuretics may worsen with concomitant beta-agonists. (7.4)

USE IN SPECIFIC POPULATIONS

Hepatic impairment: Fluticasone furoate exposure may increase in patients with moderate or severe impairment. Monitor for systemic corticosteroid effects. (8.6, 12.3)

See 17 for PATIENT COUNSELING INFORMATION and Medication Guide

Revised: 04/2014

FULL PRESCRIBING INFORMATION: CONTENTS*

* Sections or subsections omitted from the full prescribing information are not listed

FULL PRESCRIBING INFORMATION

WARNING: ASTHMA-RELATED DEATH

Long-acting beta₂-adrenergic agonists (LABA) increase the risk of asthma-related death. Data from a large placebo-controlled US trial that compared the safety of another LABA (salmeterol) with placebo added to usual asthma therapy showed an increase in asthma-related deaths in subjects receiving salmeterol. This finding with salmeterol is considered a class effect of LABA, including vilanterol, an active ingredient in BREO® ELLIPTA® *[see Warnings and Precautions (5.1)]*.

The safety and efficacy of BREO ELLIPTA in patients with asthma have not been established. BREO ELLIPTA is not indicated for the treatment of asthma.

1 INDICATIONS AND USAGE

BREO ELLIPTA is a combination inhaled corticosteroid/long-acting beta₂-adrenergic agonist (ICS/LABA) indicated for the long-term, once-daily, maintenance treatment of airflow obstruction in patients with chronic obstructive pulmonary disease (COPD), including chronic bronchitis and/or emphysema. BREO ELLIPTA is also indicated to reduce exacerbations of COPD in patients with a history of exacerbations.

Important Limitations of Use: BREO ELLIPTA is NOT indicated for the relief of acute bronchospasm or for the treatment of asthma.

2 DOSAGE AND ADMINISTRATION

BREO ELLIPTA 100 mcg/25 mcg should be administered as 1 inhalation once daily by the orally inhaled route only. After inhalation, the patient should rinse his/her mouth with water without swallowing to help reduce the risk of oropharyngeal candidiasis.

BREO ELLIPTA should be taken at the same time every day. Do not use BREO ELLIPTA more than 1 time every 24 hours.

No dosage adjustment is required for geriatric patients, patients with hepatic impairment, or renally impaired patients *[see Clinical Pharmacology (12.3)]*.

3 DOSAGE FORMS AND STRENGTHS

Inhalation Powder. Disposable light grey and pale blue plastic inhaler containing 2 double-foil blister strips, each with 30 blisters containing powder intended for oral inhalation only. One strip contains fluticasone furoate (100 mcg per blister), and the other strip contains vilanterol (25 mcg per blister). An institutional pack containing 14 blisters per strip is also available.

4 CONTRAINDICATIONS

The use of BREO ELLIPTA is contraindicated in patients with severe hypersensitivity to milk proteins or who have demonstrated hypersensitivity to either fluticasone furoate, vilanterol, or any of the excipients *[see Warnings and Precautions (5.11), Description (11)]*.

5 WARNINGS AND PRECAUTIONS

5.1 Asthma-Related Death

- Data from a large placebo-controlled trial in subjects with asthma showed that LABA may increase the risk of asthma-related death. Data are not available to determine whether the rate of death in patients with COPD is increased by LABA.
- A 28-week, placebo-controlled, US trial comparing the safety of another LABA (salmeterol) with placebo, each added to usual asthma therapy, showed an increase in asthma-related deaths in subjects receiving salmeterol (13/13,176 in subjects treated with salmeterol vs 3/13,179 in subjects treated with placebo; relative risk: 4.37 [95% CI: 1.25, 15.34]). The increased risk of asthma-related death is considered a class effect of LABA, including vilanterol, one of the active ingredients in BREO ELLIPTA.
- No study adequate to determine whether the rate of asthma-related death is increased in subjects treated with BREO ELLIPTA has been conducted. The safety and efficacy of BREO ELLIPTA in patients with asthma have not been established. BREO ELLIPTA is not indicated for the treatment of asthma.

5.2 Deterioration of Disease and Acute Episodes

BREO ELLIPTA should not be initiated in patients during rapidly deteriorating or potentially life-threatening episodes of COPD. BREO ELLIPTA has not been studied in patients with acutely deteriorating COPD. The initiation of BREO ELLIPTA in this setting is not appropriate.

BREO ELLIPTA should not be used for the relief of acute symptoms, i.e., as rescue therapy for the treatment of acute episodes of bronchospasm. BREO ELLIPTA has not been studied in the relief of acute symptoms and extra doses should not be used for that purpose. Acute symptoms should be treated with an inhaled, short-acting beta₂-agonist.

When beginning treatment with BREO ELLIPTA, patients who have been taking oral or inhaled, short-acting beta₂-agonists on a regular basis (e.g., 4 times a day) should be instructed to discontinue the regular use of these drugs and to use them only for symptomatic relief of acute respiratory symptoms. When prescribing BREO ELLIPTA, the healthcare provider should also prescribe an inhaled, short-acting beta₂-agonist and instruct the patient on how it should be used. Increasing inhaled, short-acting beta₂-agonist use is a signal of deteriorating disease for which prompt medical attention is indicated.

COPD may deteriorate acutely over a period of hours or chronically over several days or longer. If BREO ELLIPTA no longer controls symptoms of bronchoconstriction; the patient's inhaled, short-acting, beta₂-agonist becomes less effective; or the patient needs more short-acting beta₂-agonist than usual, these may be markers of deterioration of disease. In this setting a re-evaluation of the patient and the COPD treatment regimen should be undertaken at once. Increasing the daily dose of BREO ELLIPTA beyond the recommended dose is not appropriate in this situation.

5.3 Excessive Use of BREO ELLIPTA and Use With Other Long-Acting Beta₂-Agonists

BREO ELLIPTA should not be used more often than recommended, at higher doses than recommended, or in conjunction with other medicines containing LABA, as an overdose may result. Clinically significant cardiovascular effects and fatalities have been reported in association with excessive use of inhaled sympathomimetic drugs. Patients using BREO ELLIPTA should not use another medicine containing a LABA (e.g., salmeterol, formoterol fumarate, arformoterol tartrate, indacaterol) for any reason.

5.4 Local Effects of Inhaled Corticosteroids

In clinical trials, the development of localized infections of the mouth and pharynx with *Candida albicans* has occurred in subjects treated with BREO ELLIPTA. When such an infection develops, it should be treated with appropriate local or systemic (i.e., oral) antifungal therapy while treatment with BREO ELLIPTA continues, but at times therapy with BREO ELLIPTA may need to be interrupted. Advise the patient to rinse his/her mouth without swallowing following inhalation to help reduce the risk of oropharyngeal candidiasis.

5.5 Pneumonia

An increase in the incidence of pneumonia has been observed in subjects with COPD receiving the fluticasone furoate/vilanterol combination, including BREO ELLIPTA 100 mcg/25 mcg, in clinical trials. There was also an increased incidence of pneumonias resulting in hospitalization. In some incidences these pneumonia events were fatal. Physicians should remain vigilant for the possible development of pneumonia in patients with COPD as the clinical features of such infections overlap with the symptoms of COPD exacerbations.

In replicate 12-month trials in 3,255 subjects with COPD who had experienced a COPD exacerbation in the previous year, there was a higher incidence of pneumonia reported in subjects receiving the fluticasone furoate/vilanterol combination (50 mcg/25 mcg: 6% [48 of 820 subjects]; 100 mcg/25 mcg: 6% [51 of 806 subjects]; or 200 mcg/25 mcg: 7% [55 of 811 subjects]) than in subjects receiving vilanterol 25 mcg (3% [27 of 818 subjects]). There was no fatal pneumonia in subjects receiving vilanterol or fluticasone furoate/vilanterol 50 mcg/25 mcg. There was fatal pneumonia in 1 subject receiving fluticasone furoate/vilanterol 100 mcg/25 mcg and in 7 subjects receiving fluticasone furoate/vilanterol 200 mcg/25 mcg (less than 1% for each treatment group).

5.6 Immunosuppression

Persons who are using drugs that suppress the immune system are more susceptible to infections than healthy individuals. Chickenpox and measles, for example, can have a more serious or even fatal course in susceptible children or adults using corticosteroids. In such children or adults who have not had these diseases or been properly immunized, particular care should be taken to avoid exposure. How the dose, route, and duration of corticosteroid administration affect the risk of developing a disseminated infection is not known. The contribution of the underlying disease and/or prior corticosteroid treatment to the risk is also not known. If a patient is exposed to chickenpox, prophylaxis with varicella zoster immune globulin (VZIG) may be indicated. If a patient is exposed to measles, prophylaxis with pooled intramuscular immunoglobulin (IG) may be indicated. (See the respective package inserts for complete VZIG and IG prescribing information.) If chickenpox develops, treatment with antiviral agents may be considered.

Inhaled corticosteroids should be used with caution, if at all, in patients with active or quiescent tuberculosis infections of the respiratory tract; systemic fungal, bacterial, viral, or parasitic infections; or ocular herpes simplex.

5.7 Transferring Patients From Systemic Corticosteroid Therapy

Particular care is needed for patients who have been transferred from systemically active corticosteroids to inhaled corticosteroids because deaths due to adrenal insufficiency have occurred in patients with asthma during and after transfer from systemic corticosteroids to less systemically available inhaled corticosteroids. After withdrawal from systemic corticosteroids, a number of months are required for recovery of hypothalamic-pituitary-adrenal (HPA) function.

Patients who have been previously maintained on 20 mg or more of prednisone (or its equivalent) may be most susceptible, particularly when their systemic corticosteroids have been almost completely withdrawn. During this period of HPA suppression, patients may exhibit signs and symptoms of adrenal insufficiency when exposed to trauma, surgery, or infection (particularly gastroenteritis) or other conditions associated with severe electrolyte loss. Although BREO ELLIPTA may control COPD symptoms during these episodes, in recommended doses it supplies less than normal physiological amount of glucocorticoid systemically and does NOT provide the mineralocorticoid activity that is necessary for coping with these emergencies.

During periods of stress or a severe COPD exacerbation, patients who have been withdrawn from systemic corticosteroids should be instructed to resume oral corticosteroids (in large doses) immediately and to contact their physicians for further instruction. These patients should also be instructed to carry a warning card indicating that they may need supplementary systemic corticosteroids during periods of stress or severe COPD exacerbation.

Patients requiring oral corticosteroids should be weaned slowly from systemic corticosteroid use after transferring to BREO ELLIPTA. Prednisone reduction can be accomplished by reducing the daily prednisone dose by 2.5 mg on a weekly basis during therapy with BREO ELLIPTA. Lung function (mean forced expiratory volume in 1 second [FEV$_1$]), beta-agonist use, and COPD symptoms should be carefully monitored during withdrawal of oral corticosteroids. In addition, patients should be observed for signs and symptoms of adrenal insufficiency, such as fatigue, lassitude, weakness, nausea and vomiting, and hypotension.

Transfer of patients from systemic corticosteroid therapy to BREO ELLIPTA may unmask allergic conditions previously suppressed by the systemic corticosteroid therapy (e.g., rhinitis, conjunctivitis, eczema, arthritis, eosinophilic conditions).

During withdrawal from oral corticosteroids, some patients may experience symptoms of systemically active corticosteroid withdrawal (e.g., joint and/or muscular pain, lassitude, depression) despite maintenance or even improvement of respiratory function.

5.8   Hypercorticism and Adrenal Suppression
Inhaled fluticasone furoate is absorbed into the circulation and can be systemically active. Effects of fluticasone furoate on the HPA axis are not observed with the therapeutic dose of BREO ELLIPTA. However, exceeding the recommended dosage or coadministration with a strong cytochrome P450 3A4 (CYP3A4) inhibitor may result in HPA dysfunction *[see Warnings and Precautions (5.9), Drug Interactions (7.1)].*

Because of the possibility of significant systemic absorption of inhaled corticosteroids in sensitive patients, patients treated with BREO ELLIPTA should be observed carefully for any evidence of systemic corticosteroid effects. Particular care should be taken in observing patients postoperatively or during periods of stress for evidence of inadequate adrenal response.

It is possible that systemic corticosteroid effects such as hypercorticism and adrenal suppression (including adrenal crisis) may appear in a small number of patients who are sensitive to these effects. If such effects occur, BREO ELLIPTA should be reduced slowly, consistent with accepted procedures for reducing systemic corticosteroids, and other treatments for management of COPD symptoms should be considered.

5.9   Drug Interactions With Strong Cytochrome P450 3A4 Inhibitors
Caution should be exercised when considering the coadministration of BREO ELLIPTA with long-term ketoconazole and other known strong CYP3A4 inhibitors (e.g., ritonavir, clarithromycin, conivaptan, indinavir, itraconazole, lopinavir, nefazodone, nelfinavir, saquinavir, telithromycin, troleandomycin, voriconazole) because increased systemic corticosteroid and increased cardiovascular adverse effects may occur *[see Drug Interactions (7.1), Clinical Pharmacology (12.3)].*

5.10   Paradoxical Bronchospasm
As with other inhaled medicines, BREO ELLIPTA can produce paradoxical bronchospasm, which may be life threatening. If paradoxical bronchospasm occurs following dosing with BREO ELLIPTA, it should be treated immediately with an inhaled, short-acting bronchodilator; BREO ELLIPTA should be discontinued immediately; and alternative therapy should be instituted.

5.11   Hypersensitivity Reactions
Hypersensitivity reactions may occur after administration of BREO ELLIPTA. There have been reports of anaphylactic reactions in patients with severe milk protein allergy after inhalation of other powder products containing lactose; therefore, patients with severe milk protein allergy should not use BREO ELLIPTA *[see Contraindications (4)].*

Table 1. Adverse Reactions With ≥3% Incidence and More Common Than Placebo With BREO ELLIPTA in Subjects With Chronic Obstructive Pulmonary Disease

Adverse Event	BREO ELLIPTA 100 mcg/25 mcg (n = 410) %	Vilanterol 25 mcg (n = 408) %	Fluticasone Furoate 100 mcg (n = 410) %	Placebo (n = 412) %
Infections and infestations				
Nasopharyngitis	9	10	8	8
Upper respiratory tract infection	7	5	4	3
Oropharyngeal candidiasis[a]	5	2	3	2
Nervous system disorders				
Headache	7	9	7	5

[a] Includes terms oral candidiasis, oropharyngeal candidiasis, candidiasis, and oropharyngitis fungal.

5.12   Cardiovascular Effects
Vilanterol, like other beta$_2$-agonists, can produce a clinically significant cardiovascular effect in some patients as measured by increases in pulse rate, systolic or diastolic blood pressure, and also cardiac arrhythmias, such as supraventricular tachycardia and extrasystoles. If such effects occur, BREO ELLIPTA may need to be discontinued. In addition, beta-agonists have been reported to produce electrocardiographic changes, such as flattening of the T wave, prolongation of the QTc interval, and ST segment depression, although the clinical significance of these findings is unknown. In healthy subjects, large doses of inhaled fluticasone furoate/vilanterol (4 times the recommended dose of vilanterol, representing a 12-fold higher systemic exposure than seen in patients with COPD) have been associated with clinically significant prolongation of the QTc interval, which has the potential for producing ventricular arrhythmias. Therefore, BREO ELLIPTA, like other sympathomimetic amines, should be used with caution in patients with cardiovascular disorders, especially coronary insufficiency, cardiac arrhythmias, and hypertension.

5.13   Reduction in Bone Mineral Density
Decreases in bone mineral density (BMD) have been observed with long-term administration of products containing inhaled corticosteroids. The clinical significance of small changes in BMD with regard to long-term consequences such as fracture is unknown. Patients with major risk factors for decreased bone mineral content, such as prolonged immobilization, family history of osteoporosis, postmenopausal status, tobacco use, advanced age, poor nutrition, or chronic use of drugs that can reduce bone mass (e.g., anticonvulsants, oral corticosteroids) should be monitored and treated with established standards of care. Since patients with COPD often have multiple risk factors for reduced BMD, assessment of BMD is recommended prior to initiating BREO ELLIPTA and periodically thereafter. If significant reductions in BMD are seen and BREO ELLIPTA is still considered medically important for that patient's COPD therapy, use of medicine to treat or prevent osteoporosis should be strongly considered.

In replicate 12-month trials in 3,255 subjects with COPD, bone fractures were reported by 2% of subjects receiving the fluticasone furoate/vilanterol combination (50 mcg/25 mcg: 2% [14 of 820 subjects]; 100 mcg/25 mcg: 2% [19 of 806 subjects]; or 200 mcg/25 mcg: 2% [14 of 811 subjects]) than in subjects receiving vilanterol 25 mcg alone (less than 1% [8 of 818 subjects]).

5.14   Glaucoma and Cataracts
Glaucoma, increased intraocular pressure, and cataracts have been reported in patients with COPD following the long-term administration of inhaled corticosteroids. Therefore, close monitoring is warranted in patients with a change in vision or with a history of increased intraocular pressure, glaucoma, and/or cataracts.

In replicate 12-month trials in 3,255 subjects with COPD, similar incidences of ocular effects (including glaucoma and cataracts) were reported in subjects receiving the fluticasone furoate/vilanterol combination (50 mcg/25 mcg: less than 1% [7 of 820 subjects]; 100 mcg/25 mcg: 1% [12 of 806 subjects]; 200 mcg/25 mcg: less than 1% [7 of 811 subjects]) as those receiving vilanterol 25 mcg alone (1% [9 of 818 subjects]).

5.15   Coexisting Conditions
BREO ELLIPTA, like all medicines containing sympathomimetic amines, should be used with caution in patients with convulsive disorders or thyrotoxicosis and in those who are unusually responsive to sympathomimetic amines. Doses of the related beta$_2$-adrenoceptor agonist albuterol, when administered intravenously, have been reported to aggravate preexisting diabetes mellitus and ketoacidosis.

5.16   Hypokalemia and Hyperglycemia
Beta-adrenergic agonist medicines may produce significant hypokalemia in some patients, possibly through intracellular shunting, which has the potential to produce adverse cardiovascular effects. The decrease in serum potassium is usually transient, not requiring supplementation. Beta-agonist medications may produce transient hyperglycemia in some patients. In 4 clinical trials of 6- and 12-month duration evaluating BREO ELLIPTA in subjects with COPD, there was no evidence of a treatment effect on serum glucose or potassium.

6   ADVERSE REACTIONS
LABA, such as vilanterol, one of the active ingredients in BREO ELLIPTA, increase the risk of asthma-related death. BREO ELLIPTA is not indicated for the treatment of asthma. *[See Boxed Warnings and Warnings and Precautions (5.1).]*

Systemic and local corticosteroid use may result in the following:
- Increased risk of pneumonia in COPD *[see Warnings and Precautions (5.5)]*
- Increased risk for decrease in bone mineral density *[see Warnings and Precautions (5.13)]*

6.1   Clinical Trials Experience
Because clinical trials are conducted under widely varying conditions, adverse reaction rates observed in the clinical trials of a drug cannot be directly compared with rates in the clinical trials of another drug and may not reflect the rates observed in practice.

The clinical program for BREO ELLIPTA included 7,700 subjects with COPD in two 6-month lung function trials, two 12-month exacerbation trials, and 6 other trials of shorter duration. A total of 2,034 subjects have received at least 1 dose of BREO ELLIPTA 100 mcg/25 mcg, and 1,087 subjects have received higher doses of fluticasone furoate/vilanterol. The safety data described below are based on the confirmatory 6-month and 12-month trials. Adverse reactions observed in the other trials were similar to those observed in the confirmatory trials.

6-Month Trials: The incidence of adverse reactions associated with BREO ELLIPTA in Table 1 is based on 2 placebo-controlled, 6-month clinical trials (Trials 1 and 2; n = 1,224 and n = 1,030, respectively). Of the 2,254 subjects, 70% were male and 84% were Caucasian. They had a mean age of 62 years and an average smoking history of 44 pack years, with 54% identified as current smokers. At screening, the mean postbronchodilator percent predicted FEV$_1$ was 48% (range: 14% to 87%), the mean postbronchodilator FEV$_1$/forced vital capacity (FVC) ratio was 47% (range: 17% to 88%), and the mean percent reversibility was 14% (range: -41% to 152%).

Subjects received 1 inhalation once daily of the following: BREO ELLIPTA 100 mcg/25 mcg, fluticasone furoate/vilanterol 50 mcg/25 mcg, fluticasone furoate/vilanterol 200 mcg/25 mcg, fluticasone furoate 100 mcg, fluticasone furoate 200 mcg, vilanterol 25 mcg, or placebo. [See table 1 above]

12-Month Trials: Long-term safety data is based on two 12-month trials (Trials 3 and 4; n = 1,633 and n = 1,622, respectively). Trials 3 and 4 included 3,255 subjects, of which 57% were male and 85% were Caucasian. They had a mean age of 64 years and an average smoking history of 46 pack years, with 44% identified as current smokers. At screening, the mean postbronchodilator percent predicted FEV$_1$ was 45% (range: 12% to 91%), and the mean postbronchodilator FEV$_1$/FVC ratio was 46% (range: 17% to 81%), indicating that the subject population had moderate to very severely impaired airflow obstruction. Subjects received 1 inhalation once daily of the following: BREO ELLIPTA 100 mcg/25 mcg, fluticasone furoate/vilanterol 50 mcg/ 25 mcg, fluticasone furoate/vilanterol 200 mcg/25 mcg, or vilanterol 25 mcg. In addition to the events shown in Table 1, adverse reactions occurring in greater than or equal to 3% of the subjects treated with BREO ELLIPTA (N = 806) for 12 months included COPD, back pain, pneumonia *[see Warnings and Precautions (5.5)],* bronchitis, sinusitis, cough, oropharyngeal pain, arthralgia, hypertension, influenza, pharyngitis, diarrhea, peripheral edema, and pyrexia.

7   DRUG INTERACTIONS
7.1   Inhibitors of Cytochrome P450 3A4
Fluticasone furoate and vilanterol, the individual components of BREO ELLIPTA, are both substrates of CYP3A4.

Concomitant administration of the potent CYP3A4 inhibitor ketoconazole increases the systemic exposure to fluticasone furoate and vilanterol. Caution should be exercised when considering the coadministration of BREO ELLIPTA with long-term ketoconazole and other known strong CYP3A4 inhibitors (e.g., ritonavir, clarithromycin, conivaptan, indinavir, itraconazole, lopinavir, nefazodone, nelfinavir, saquinavir, telithromycin, troleandomycin, voriconazole) [see Warnings and Precautions (5.9) and Clinical Pharmacology (12.3)].

7.2 Monoamine Oxidase Inhibitors and Tricyclic Antidepressants

Vilanterol, like other beta$_2$-agonists, should be administered with extreme caution to patients being treated with monoamine oxidase inhibitors, tricyclic antidepressants, or drugs known to prolong the QTc interval or within 2 weeks of discontinuation of such agents, because the effect of adrenergic agonists on the cardiovascular system may be potentiated by these agents. Drugs that are known to prolong the QTc interval have an increased risk of ventricular arrhythmias.

7.3 Beta-Adrenergic Receptor Blocking Agents

Beta-blockers not only block the pulmonary effect of beta-agonists, such as vilanterol, a component of BREO ELLIPTA, but may produce severe bronchospasm in patients with reversible obstructive airways disease. Therefore, patients with COPD should not normally be treated with beta-blockers. However, under certain circumstances, there may be no acceptable alternatives to the use of beta-adrenergic blocking agents for these patients; cardioselective beta-blockers could be considered, although they should be administered with caution.

7.4 Non–Potassium-Sparing Diuretics

The electrocardiographic changes and/or hypokalemia that may result from the administration of non–potassium-sparing diuretics (such as loop or thiazide diuretics) can be acutely worsened by beta-agonists, especially when the recommended dose of the beta-agonist is exceeded. Although the clinical significance of these effects is not known, caution is advised in the coadministration of beta-agonists with non–potassium-sparing diuretics.

8 USE IN SPECIFIC POPULATIONS

8.1 Pregnancy

Teratogenic Effects: Pregnancy Category C. There are no adequate and well-controlled trials with BREO ELLIPTA in pregnant women. Corticosteroids and beta$_2$-agonists have been shown to be teratogenic in laboratory animals when administered systemically at relatively low dosage levels. Because animal studies are not always predictive of human response, BREO ELLIPTA should be used during pregnancy only if the potential benefit justifies the potential risk to the fetus. Women should be advised to contact their physicians if they become pregnant while taking BREO ELLIPTA.

Fluticasone Furoate and Vilanterol: There was no evidence of teratogenic interactions between fluticasone furoate and vilanterol in rats at approximately 9 and 40 times, respectively, the maximum recommended human daily inhalation dose (MRHDID) in adults (on a mcg/m^2 basis at maternal inhaled doses of fluticasone furoate and vilanterol, alone or in combination, up to approximately 95 mcg/kg/day).

Fluticasone Furoate: There were no teratogenic effects in rats and rabbits at approximately 9 and 2 times, respectively, the MRHDID in adults (on a mcg/m^2 basis at maternal inhaled doses up to 91 and 8 mcg/kg/day in rats and rabbits, respectively). There were no effects on perinatal and postnatal development in rats at approximately 3 times the MRHDID in adults (on a mcg/m^2 basis at maternal doses up to 27 mcg/kg/day).

Vilanterol: There were no teratogenic effects in rats and rabbits at approximately 13,000 and 160 times, respectively, the MRHDID in adults (on a mcg/m^2 basis at maternal inhaled doses up to 33,700 mcg/kg/day in rats and on an AUC basis at maternal inhaled doses up to 591 mcg/kg/day in rabbits). However, fetal skeletal variations were observed in rabbits at approximately 1,000 times the MRHDID in adults (on an AUC basis at maternal inhaled or subcutaneous doses of 5,740 or 300 mcg/kg/day, respectively). The skeletal variations included decreased or absent ossification in cervical vertebral centrum and metacarpals. There were no effects on perinatal and postnatal development in rats at approximately 3,900 times the MRHDID in adults (on a mcg/m^2 basis at maternal oral doses up to 10,000 mcg/kg/day).

Nonteratogenic Effects: Hypoadrenalism may occur in infants born of mothers receiving corticosteroids during pregnancy. Such infants should be carefully monitored.

8.2 Labor and Delivery

There are no adequate and well-controlled human trials that have investigated the effects of BREO ELLIPTA during labor and delivery.

Because beta-agonists may potentially interfere with uterine contractility, BREO ELLIPTA should be used during labor only if the potential benefit justifies the potential risk.

8.3 Nursing Mothers

It is not known whether fluticasone furoate or vilanterol are excreted in human breast milk. However, other corticosteroids and beta$_2$-agonists have been detected in human milk. Since there are no data from controlled trials on the use of BREO ELLIPTA by nursing mothers, caution should be exercised when it is administered to a nursing woman.

8.4 Pediatric Use

BREO ELLIPTA is not indicated for use in children. The safety and efficacy in pediatric patients have not been established.

8.5 Geriatric Use

Based on available data, no adjustment of the dosage of BREO ELLIPTA in geriatric patients is necessary, but greater sensitivity in some older individuals cannot be ruled out.

Clinical trials of BREO ELLIPTA for COPD included 2,508 subjects aged 65 and older and 564 subjects aged 75 and older. No overall differences in safety or effectiveness were observed between these subjects and younger subjects, and other reported clinical experience has not identified differences in responses between the elderly and younger subjects.

8.6 Hepatic Impairment

Fluticasone furoate systemic exposure increased by up to 3-fold in subjects with hepatic impairment compared with healthy subjects. Hepatic impairment had no effect on vilanterol systemic exposure. Use BREO ELLIPTA with caution in patients with moderate or severe hepatic impairment. Monitor patients for corticosteroid-related side effects [see Clinical Pharmacology (12.3)].

8.7 Renal Impairment

There were no significant increases in either fluticasone furoate or vilanterol exposure in subjects with severe renal impairment (CrCl<30 mL/min) compared with healthy subjects. No dosage adjustment is required in patients with renal impairment [see Clinical Pharmacology (12.3)].

10 OVERDOSAGE

No human overdosage data has been reported for BREO ELLIPTA.

BREO ELLIPTA contains both fluticasone furoate and vilanterol; therefore, the risks associated with overdosage for the individual components described below apply to BREO ELLIPTA.

10.1 Fluticasone Furoate

Because of low systemic bioavailability (15.2%) and an absence of acute drug-related systemic findings in clinical trials, overdosage of fluticasone furoate is unlikely to require any treatment other than observation. If used at excessive doses for prolonged periods, systemic effects such as hypercorticism may occur [see Warnings and Precautions (5.8)].

Single- and repeat-dose trials of fluticasone furoate at doses of 50 to 4,000 mcg have been studied in human subjects. Decreases in mean serum cortisol were observed at dosages of 500 mcg or higher given once daily for 14 days.

10.2 Vilanterol

The expected signs and symptoms with overdosage of vilanterol are those of excessive beta-adrenergic stimulation and/or occurrence or exaggeration of any of the signs and symptoms of beta-adrenergic stimulation (e.g., angina, hypertension or hypotension, tachycardia with rates up to 200 beats/min, arrhythmias, nervousness, headache, tremor, seizures, muscle cramps, dry mouth, palpitation, nausea, dizziness, fatigue, malaise, insomnia, hyperglycemia, hypokalemia, metabolic acidosis). As with all inhaled sympathomimetic medicines, cardiac arrest and even death may be associated with an overdose of vilanterol.

Treatment of overdosage consists of discontinuation of BREO ELLIPTA together with institution of appropriate symptomatic and/or supportive therapy. The judicious use of a cardioselective beta-receptor blocker may be considered, bearing in mind that such medicine can produce bronchospasm. Cardiac monitoring is recommended in cases of overdosage.

11 DESCRIPTION

BREO ELLIPTA is a combination of fluticasone furoate (an ICS) and vilanterol (a LABA).

One active component of BREO ELLIPTA is fluticasone furoate, a synthetic trifluorinated corticosteroid having the chemical name (6α,11β,16α,17α)-6,9-difluoro-17-[[(fluoromethyl)thio]carbonyl]-11-hydroxy-16-methyl-3-oxoandrosta-1,4-dien-17-yl 2-furancarboxylate and the following chemical structure:

Fluticasone furoate is a white powder with a molecular weight of 538.6, and the empirical formula is $C_{27}H_{29}F_3O_6S$. It is practically insoluble in water.

The other active component of BREO ELLIPTA is vilanterol trifenatate, a LABA with the chemical name triphenylacetic acid-4-[(1R)-2-[(6-{2-[(2,6-dichlorobenzyl)oxy]ethoxy}hexyl)amino]-1-hydroxyethyl]-2-(hydroxymethyl)phenol (1:1) and the following chemical structure:

Vilanterol trifenatate is a white powder with a molecular weight of 774.8, and the empirical formula is $C_{24}H_{33}Cl_2NO_5 \cdot C_{20}H_{16}O_2$. It is practically insoluble in water.

BREO ELLIPTA is a light grey and pale blue plastic inhaler containing 2 double-foil blister strips. Each blister on one strip contains a white powder mix of micronized fluticasone furoate (100 mcg) and lactose monohydrate (12.4 mg), and each blister on the other strip contains a white powder mix of micronized vilanterol trifenatate (40 mcg equivalent to 25 mcg of vilanterol), magnesium stearate (125 mcg), and lactose monohydrate (12.34 mg). The lactose monohydrate contains milk proteins. After the inhaler is activated, the powder within both blisters is exposed and ready for dispersion into the airstream created by the patient inhaling through the mouthpiece.

Under standardized in vitro test conditions, BREO ELLIPTA delivers 92 mcg of fluticasone furoate and 22 mcg of vilanterol per blister when tested at a flow rate of 60 L/min for 4 seconds.

In adult subjects with obstructive lung disease and severely compromised lung function (COPD with FEV$_1$/FVC less than 70% and FEV$_1$ less than 30% predicted or FEV$_1$ less than 50% predicted plus chronic respiratory failure), mean peak inspiratory flow through the ELLIPTA inhaler was 66.5 L/min (range: 43.5 to 81.0 L/min).

The actual amount of drug delivered to the lung will depend on patient factors, such as inspiratory flow profile.

12 CLINICAL PHARMACOLOGY

12.1 Mechanism of Action

BREO ELLIPTA: Since BREO ELLIPTA contains both fluticasone furoate and vilanterol, the mechanisms of action described below for the individual components apply to BREO ELLIPTA. These drugs represent 2 different classes of medications (a synthetic corticosteroid and a LABA) that have different effects on clinical and physiological indices.

Fluticasone Furoate: Fluticasone furoate is a synthetic trifluorinated corticosteroid with anti-inflammatory activity. Fluticasone furoate has been shown in vitro to exhibit a binding affinity for the human glucocorticoid receptor that is approximately 29.9 times that of dexamethasone and 1.7 times that of fluticasone propionate. The clinical relevance of these in vitro findings is unknown. The precise mechanism through which fluticasone furoate affects COPD symptoms is not known. Corticosteroids have been shown to have a wide range of actions on multiple cell types (e.g., mast cells, eosinophils, neutrophils, macrophages, lymphocytes) and mediators (e.g., histamine, eicosanoids, leukotrienes, cytokines) involved in inflammation. Specific effects of fluticasone furoate demonstrated in in vitro and in vivo models included activation of the glucocorticoid response element, inhibition of pro-inflammatory transcription factors such as NFkB, and inhibition of antigen-induced lung eosinophilia in sensitized rats.

Vilanterol: Vilanterol is a LABA. In vitro tests have shown the functional selectivity of vilanterol was similar to salmeterol. The clinical relevance of this in vitro finding is unknown.

Although beta$_2$-receptors are the predominant adrenergic receptors in bronchial smooth muscle and beta$_1$-receptors are the predominant receptors in the heart, there are also beta$_2$-receptors in the human heart comprising 10% to 50% of the total beta-adrenergic receptors. The precise function of these receptors has not been established, but they raise the possibility that even highly selective beta$_2$-agonists may have cardiac effects.

The pharmacologic effects of beta$_2$-adrenoceptor agonist drugs, including vilanterol, are at least in part attributable to stimulation of intracellular adenyl cyclase, the enzyme that catalyzes the conversion of adenosine triphosphate (ATP) to cyclic-3',5'-adenosine monophosphate (cyclic AMP). Increased cyclic AMP levels cause relaxation of bronchial smooth muscle and inhibition of release of mediators of immediate hypersensitivity from cells, especially from mast cells.

12.2 Pharmacodynamics

Cardiovascular Effects: Healthy Subjects: QTc interval prolongation was studied in a double-blind, multiple dose, placebo- and positive-controlled crossover study in 85 healthy volunteers. The maximum mean (95% upper confidence bound) difference in QTcF from placebo after baseline-correction was 4.9 (7.5) milliseconds and 9.6 (12.2) milliseconds seen 30 minutes after dosing for fluticasone furoate /vilanterol 200mcg/25 mcg and fluticasone furoate/vilanterol 800 mcg/100 mcg, respectively.

A dose-dependent increase in heart rate was also observed. The maximum mean (95% upper confidence bound) difference in heart rate from placebo after baseline-correction was 7.8 (9.4) beats/min and 17.1 (18.7) beats/min seen 10 minutes after dosing for fluticasone furoate/vilanterol 200 mcg/25 mcg and fluticasone furoate/vilanterol 800 mcg/100 mcg, respectively.

Chronic Obstructive Pulmonary Disease: In 4 clinical trials of 6- and 12-month duration, there was no evidence of a treatment effect on heart rate, QTcF, or blood pressure in subjects with COPD given combination doses of fluticasone furoate (50, 100, or 200 mcg)/vilanterol 25 mcg, the individual components of fluticasone furoate or vilanterol alone, or placebo [see Clinical Studies (14)].

HPA Axis Effects: Healthy Subjects: Inhaled fluticasone furoate at repeat doses up to 400 mcg was not associated with statistically significant decreases in serum or urinary cortisol in healthy subjects. Decreases in serum and urine cortisol levels were observed at fluticasone furoate exposures several-fold higher than exposures observed at the therapeutic dose.

Chronic Obstructive Pulmonary Disease: In a trial with subjects with COPD, treatment with fluticasone furoate/vilanterol (50 mcg/25 mcg, 100 mcg/25 mcg, and 200 mcg/25 mcg), vilanterol 25 mcg, and fluticasone furoate (100 and 200 mcg) for 6 months did not affect 24-hour urinary cortisol excretion. A separate trial with subjects with COPD demonstrated no effects on serum cortisol after 28 days of treatment with fluticasone furoate/vilanterol (50 mcg/25 mcg, 100 mcg/25 mcg, and 200 mcg/25 mcg).

12.3 Pharmacokinetics

Linear pharmacokinetics was observed for fluticasone furoate (200 to 800 mcg) and vilanterol (25 to 100 mcg). On repeated once-daily inhalation administration, steady state of fluticasone furoate and vilanterol plasma concentrations was achieved after 6 days, and the accumulation was up to 2.6-fold for fluticasone furoate and 2.4-fold for vilanterol as compared with single dose.

Absorption: Fluticasone Furoate: Fluticasone furoate plasma levels may not predict therapeutic effect. Peak plasma concentrations are reached within 0.5 to 1 hour. Absolute bioavailability of fluticasone furoate when administrated by inhalation was 15.2%, primarily due to absorption of the inhaled portion of the dose delivered to the lung. Oral bioavailability from the swallowed portion of the dose is low (approximately 1.3%) due to extensive first-pass metabolism. Systemic exposure (AUC) in subjects with COPD was 46% lower than observed in healthy subjects.

Vilanterol: Vilanterol plasma levels may not predict therapeutic effect. Peak plasma concentrations are reached within 10 minutes following inhalation. Absolute bioavailability of vilanterol when administrated by inhalation was 27.3%, primarily due to absorption of the inhaled portion of the dose delivered to the lung. Oral bioavailability from the swallowed portion of the dose of vilanterol is low (less than 2%) due to extensive first-pass metabolism. Systemic exposure in subjects with COPD was 24% higher than observed in healthy subjects.

Distribution: Fluticasone Furoate: Following intravenous administration to healthy subjects, the mean volume of distribution at steady state was 661 L. Binding of fluticasone furoate to human plasma proteins was high (99.6%).

Vilanterol: Following intravenous administration to healthy subjects, the mean volume of distribution at steady state was 165 L. Binding of vilanterol to human plasma proteins was 93.9%.

Metabolism: Fluticasone Furoate: Fluticasone furoate is cleared from systemic circulation principally by hepatic metabolism via CYP3A4 to metabolites with significantly reduced corticosteroid activity. There was no in vivo evidence for cleavage of the furoate moiety resulting in the formation of fluticasone.

Vilanterol: Vilanterol is mainly metabolized, principally via CYP3A4, to a range of metabolites with significantly reduced β_1- and β_2-agonist activity.

Elimination: Fluticasone Furoate: Fluticasone furoate and its metabolites are eliminated primarily in the feces, accounting for approximately 101% and 90% of the orally and intravenously administered dose, respectively. Urinary excretion accounted for approximately 1% and 2% of the orally and intravenously administered doses, respectively. Following repeat-dose inhaled administration, the plasma elimination phase half-life averaged 24 hours.

Vilanterol: Following oral administration, vilanterol was eliminated mainly by metabolism followed by excretion of metabolites in urine and feces (approximately 70% and 30% of the recovered radioactive dose, respectively). The effec-

tive half-life for accumulation of vilanterol, as determined from inhalation administration of multiple doses of vilanterol 25 mcg, is 21.3 hours in subjects with COPD.

Special Populations: The effect of renal and hepatic impairment and other intrinsic factors on the pharmacokinetics of fluticasone furoate and vilanterol is shown in Figure 1.

Figure 1. Impact of Intrinsic Factors on the Pharmacokinetics (PK) of Fluticasone Furoate and Vilanterol Following Administration as Fluticasone Furoate/Vilanterol Combination

[a]Age, gender, and ethnicity comparison for BREO ELLIPTA (fluticasone furoate/vilanterol 100 mcg/25 mcg) in subjects with COPD.

[b]Renal groups (fluticasone furoate/vilanterol 200 mcg/25 mcg) and hepatic groups (fluticasone furoate/vilanterol 200 mcg/25 mcg or fluticasone furoate/vilanterol 100 mcg/12.5 mcg) compared with healthy control group.

Race: Systemic exposure (AUC(0-24)) to inhaled fluticasone furoate 200 mcg was 27% to 49% higher in healthy subjects of Japanese, Korean, and Chinese heritage compared with Caucasian subjects. Similar differences were observed for subjects with COPD (Figure 1). However, there is no evidence that this higher exposure to fluticasone furoate results in clinically relevant effects on urinary cortisol excretion or on efficacy in these racial groups.

There was no effect of race on the pharmacokinetics of vilanterol in subjects with COPD.

Hepatic Impairment: Fluticasone Furoate: Following repeat dosing of fluticasone furoate/vilanterol 200 mcg/25 mcg (100 mcg/12.5 mcg in the severe impairment group) for 7 days, there was an increase of 34%, 83%, and 75% in fluticasone furoate systemic exposure (AUC) in subjects with mild, moderate, and severe hepatic impairment, respectively, compared with healthy subjects (see Figure 1).

In subjects with moderate hepatic impairment receiving fluticasone furoate/vilanterol 200 mcg/25 mcg, mean serum cortisol (0 to 24 hours) was reduced by 34% (95% CI: 11%, 51%) compared with healthy subjects. In subjects with severe hepatic impairment receiving fluticasone furoate/vilanterol 100 mcg/12.5 mcg, mean serum cortisol (0 to 24 hours) was increased by 14% (95% CI: -16%, 55%) compared with healthy subjects. Patients with moderate to severe hepatic disease should be closely monitored.

Vilanterol: Hepatic impairment had no effect on vilanterol systemic exposure (C_{max} and AUC(0-24) on Day 7) following repeat-dose administration of fluticasone furoate/vilanterol 200 mcg/25 mcg (100 mcg/12.5 mcg in the severe impairment group) for 7 days (see Figure 1).

There were no additional clinically relevant effects of the fluticasone furoate/vilanterol combinations on heart rate or serum potassium in subjects with mild or moderate hepatic impairment (vilanterol 25 mcg combination) or with severe hepatic impairment (vilanterol 12.5 mcg combination) compared with healthy subjects.

Renal Impairment: Fluticasone Furoate: Fluticasone furoate systemic exposure was not increased and vilanterol systemic exposure (AUC(0-24)) was 56% higher in subjects with severe renal impairment compared with healthy subjects (see Figure 1). There was no evidence of greater corticosteroid or beta-agonist class-related systemic effects (assessed by serum cortisol, heart rate, and serum potassium) in subjects with severe renal impairment compared with healthy subjects.

Drug Interactions: There were no clinically relevant differences in the pharmacokinetics or pharmacodynamics of either fluticasone furoate or vilanterol when administered in combination compared with administration alone. The potential for fluticasone furoate and vilanterol to inhibit or induce metabolic enzymes and transporter systems is negligible at low inhalation doses.

Inhibitors of Cytochrome P450 3A4: The exposure (AUC) of fluticasone furoate and vilanterol were 36% and 65% higher, respectively, when coadministered with ketoconazole 400 mg compared with placebo (see Figure 2). The increase in fluticasone furoate exposure was associated with a 27% reduction in weighted mean serum cortisol (0 to 24

hours). The increase in vilanterol exposure was not associated with an increase in beta-agonist–related systemic effects on heart rate or blood potassium.

Figure 2. Impact of Coadministered Drugs[a] on the Pharmacokinetics (PK) of Fluticasone Furoate and Vilanterol Following Administration as Fluticasone Furoate/Vilanterol Combination or Vilanterol Coadministered With a Long-Acting Muscarinic Antagonist

[a] Compared with placebo group.

Inhibitors of P-glycoprotein: Fluticasone furoate and vilanterol are both substrates of P-glycoprotein (P-gp). Co-administration of repeat-dose (240 mg once daily) verapamil (a potent P-gp inhibitor and moderate CYP3A4 inhibitor) did not affect the vilanterol C_{max} or AUC in healthy subjects (see Figure 2). Drug interaction trials with a specific P-gp inhibitor and fluticasone furoate have not been conducted.

13 NONCLINICAL TOXICOLOGY

13.1 Carcinogenesis, Mutagenesis, Impairment of Fertility

BREO ELLIPTA: No studies of carcinogenicity, mutagenicity, or impairment of fertility were conducted with BREO ELLIPTA; however, studies are available for the individual components, fluticasone furoate and vilanterol, as described below.

Fluticasone Furoate: Fluticasone furoate produced no treatment-related increases in the incidence of tumors in 2-year inhalation studies in rats and mice at inhaled doses up to 9 and 19 mcg/kg/day, respectively (approximately equal to the MRHDID in adults on a mcg/m[2] basis).

Fluticasone furoate did not induce gene mutation in bacteria or chromosomal damage in a mammalian cell mutation test in mouse lymphoma L5178Y cells in vitro. There was also no evidence of genotoxicity in the in vivo micronucleus test in rats.

No evidence of impairment of fertility was observed in male and female rats at inhaled fluticasone furoate doses up to 29 and 91 mcg/kg/day, respectively (approximately 3 and 9 times, respectively, the MRHDID in adults on a mcg/m[2]basis).

Vilanterol: In a 2-year carcinogenicity study in mice, vilanterol caused a statistically significant increase in ovarian tubulostromal adenomas in females at an inhalation dose of 29,500 mcg/kg/day (approximately 8,750 times the MRHDID in adults on an AUC basis). No increase in tumors was seen at an inhalation dose of 615 mcg/kg/day (approximately 530 times the MRHDID in adults on an AUC basis). In a 2-year carcinogenicity study in rats, vilanterol caused statistically significant increases in mesovarian leiomyomas in females and shortening of the latency of pituitary tumors at inhalation doses greater than or equal to 84.4 mcg/kg/day (greater than or equal to approximately 45 times the MRHDID in adults on an AUC basis). No tumors were seen at an inhalation dose of 10.5 mcg/kg/day (approximately 2 times the MRHDID in adults on an AUC basis).

These tumor findings in rodents are similar to those reported previously for other beta-adrenergic agonist drugs. The relevance of these findings to human use is unknown. Vilanterol tested negative in the following genotoxicity assays: the in vitro Ames assay, in vivo rat bone marrow micronucleus assay, in vivo rat unscheduled DNA synthesis (UDS) assay, and in vitro Syrian hamster embryo (SHE) cell assay. Vilanterol tested equivocal in the in vitro mouse lymphoma assay.

No evidence of impairment of fertility was observed in reproductive studies conducted in male and female rats at inhaled vilanterol doses up to 31,500 and 37,100 mcg/kg/day, respectively (approximately 12,000 and 14,000 times, respectively, the MRHDID in adults on a mcg/m[2] basis).

14 CLINICAL STUDIES

The safety and efficacy of BREO ELLIPTA were evaluated in 7,700 subjects with COPD. The development program included 4 confirmatory trials of 6- and 12-months' duration, three 12-week active comparator trials, and dose-ranging trials of shorter duration. The efficacy of BREO ELLIPTA is based primarily on the dose-ranging trials and the 4 confirmatory trials described below.

14.1 Dose-Ranging Trials

Dose selection for BREO ELLIPTA for COPD was based on dose-ranging trials for the individual components,

Table 2. Least Squares Mean Change From Baseline in Weighted Mean FEV₁ (0-4 h) and Trough FEV₁ at 6 Months

Treatment	N	Weighted Mean FEV_1 (0-4 h)[a] (mL)			Trough FEV_1[b] (mL)	
			Difference from			Difference from
		Placebo (95% CI)	Fluticasone Furoate 100 mcg (95% CI)	Fluticasone Furoate 200 mcg (95% CI)	Placebo (95% CI)	Vilanterol 25 mcg (95% CI)
Trial 1						
BREO ELLIPTA 100 mcg/25 mcg	204	214 (161, 266)	168 (116, 220)	—	144 (91, 197)	45 (-8, 97)
Fluticasone furoate/ vilanterol 200 mcg/25 mcg	205	209 (157, 261)	—	168 (117, 219)	131 (80, 183)	32 (-19, 83)
Trial 2						
BREO ELLIPTA 100 mcg/25 mcg	206	173 (123, 224)	120 (70, 170)	—	115 (60, 169)	48 (-6, 102)

[a] At Day 168.
[b] At Day 169.

vilanterol and fluticasone furoate, in patients with COPD and asthma. **BREO ELLIPTA 100 mcg/25 mcg is not indicated for asthma.**

Vilanterol: Dose selection for vilanterol in COPD was supported by a 28-day, randomized, double-blind, placebo-controlled, parallel-group trial evaluating 5 doses of vilanterol (3 to 50 mcg) or placebo dosed in the morning in 602 patients with COPD. Results demonstrated dose-related increases in FEV₁ compared with placebo at Day 1 and Day 28 (Figure 3).

Figure 3. Least Squares (LS) Mean Difference From Placebo in Post-Dose Serial FEV₁ (0-24 h, mL) on Days 1 and 28

The differences in trough FEV₁ on Day 28 from placebo for the 3-, 6.25-, 12.5-, 25-, and 50-mcg doses were 92 mL (95% CI: 39, 144), 98 mL (95% CI: 46, 150), 110 mL (95% CI: 57, 162), 137 mL (95% CI: 85, 190), and 165 mL (95% CI: 112, 217), respectively. These results supported the evaluation of vilanterol 25 mcg in the confirmatory COPD trials.

Dose-ranging trials in subjects with asthma evaluated doses from 3 to 50 mcg and 12.5 mcg once-daily versus 6.25 mcg twice-daily dosing frequency. The results supported the selection of the vilanterol 25 mcg once-daily dose for further evaluation in the confirmatory COPD trials.

Fluticasone Furoate: Eight doses of fluticasone furoate ranging from 25 to 800 mcg once daily were evaluated in 3 randomized, double-blind, placebo-controlled, 8-week trials in subjects with asthma. A dose-related increase in trough FEV₁ at Week 8 was seen for doses from 25 to 200 mcg with no consistent additional benefit for doses above 200 mcg. To

evaluate dosing frequency, a separate trial compared fluticasone furoate 200 mcg once-daily, fluticasone furoate 100 mcg twice-daily, fluticasone propionate 100 mcg twice-daily, and fluticasone propionate 200 mcg once-daily. The results supported the selection of the once-daily dosing frequency.

Based on the dose-ranging trials in asthma and COPD, once-daily doses of fluticasone furoate/vilanterol 50 mcg/ 25 mcg, 100 mcg/25 mcg, and 200 mcg/25 mcg were evaluated in the confirmatory COPD trials.

14.2 Confirmatory Trials

The clinical development program for BREO ELLIPTA included 4 confirmatory trials in subjects with COPD designed to evaluate the efficacy of BREO ELLIPTA on lung function (Trials 1 and 2) and exacerbations (Trials 3 and 4).

Lung Function: Trials 1 and 2 were 24-week, randomized, double-blind, placebo-controlled trials designed to evaluate the efficacy of BREO ELLIPTA on lung function in subjects with COPD. In Trial 1, subjects were randomized to BREO ELLIPTA 100 mcg/25 mcg, fluticasone furoate/vilanterol 200 mcg/25 mcg, fluticasone furoate 100 mcg, fluticasone furoate 200 mcg, vilanterol 25 mcg, and placebo. In Trial 2, subjects were randomized to BREO ELLIPTA 100 mcg/ 25 mcg, fluticasone furoate/vilanterol 50 mcg/25 mcg, fluticasone furoate 100 mcg, vilanterol 25 mcg, and placebo. All treatments were administered as 1 inhalation once daily.

Of the 2,254 patients, 70% were male and 84% were Caucasian. They had a mean age of 62 years and an average smoking history of 44 pack years, with 54% identified as current smokers. At screening, the mean postbronchodilator percent predicted FEV₁ was 48% (range: 14% to 87%), mean postbronchodilator FEV₁/FVC ratio was 47% (range: 17% to 88%), and the mean percent reversibility was 14% (range: -41% to 152%).

The co-primary efficacy variables in both trials were weighted mean FEV₁ (0 to 4 hours) postdose on Day 168 and change from baseline in trough FEV₁ on Day 169 (the mean of the FEV₁ values obtained 23 and 24 hours after the final dose on Day 168). The weighted mean comparison of the fluticasone furoate/vilanterol combination with fluticasone furoate was assessed to evaluate the contribution of vilanterol to BREO ELLIPTA. The trough FEV₁ comparison of the fluticasone furoate/vilanterol combination with vilanterol was assessed to evaluate the contribution of fluticasone furoate to BREO ELLIPTA.

BREO ELLIPTA 100 mcg/25 mcg demonstrated a larger increase in the weighted mean FEV₁ (0 to 4 hours) relative to placebo and fluticasone furoate 100 mcg at Day 168 (Table 2).

[See table 2 above]

Serial spirometric evaluations were performed pre-dose and up to 4 hours after dosing. Results from Trial 1 at Day 1 and Day 168 are shown in Figure 4. Similar results were seen in Trial 2 (not shown).

[See figure 4 at top of next column]

The second co-primary variable was change from baseline in trough FEV₁ following the final treatment day. At Day 169, both Trials 1 and 2 demonstrated significant increases in trough FEV₁ for all strengths of the fluticasone furoate/vilanterol combination compared with placebo (Table 2). The comparison of BREO ELLIPTA 100 mcg/25 mcg with vilanterol did not achieve statistical significance (Table 2). Trials 1 and 2 evaluated FEV₁ as a secondary endpoint. Peak FEV₁ was defined as the maximum postdose FEV₁ recorded within 4 hours after the first dose of trial medicine

Figure 4. Raw Mean Change From Baseline in Post-Dose Serial FEV1 (0-4 h, mL) on Days 1 and 168

on Day 1 (measurements recorded at 5, 15, and 30 minutes and 1, 2, and 4 hours). In both trials, differences in mean change from baseline in peak FEV₁ were observed for the groups receiving fluticasone furoate/vilanterol 100 mcg/ 25 mcg compared with placebo (152 and 139 mL, respectively). The median time to onset, defined as a 100-mL increase from baseline in FEV₁, was 16 minutes in subjects receiving fluticasone furoate/vilanterol 100 mcg/25 mcg.

Exacerbations: Trials 3 and 4 were randomized, double-blind, 52-week trials designed to evaluate the effect of BREO ELLIPTA on the rate of moderate and severe COPD exacerbations. All patients were treated with fluticasone propionate/salmeterol 250 mcg/50 mcg twice daily during a 4-week run-in period prior to being randomly assigned to 1 of the following treatment groups: BREO ELLIPTA 100 mcg/25 mcg, fluticasone furoate/vilanterol 50 mcg/ 25 mcg, fluticasone furoate/vilanterol 200 mcg/25 mcg, or vilanterol 25 mcg.

The primary efficacy variable in both trials was the annual rate of moderate/severe exacerbations. The comparison of the fluticasone furoate/vilanterol combination with vilanterol was assessed to evaluate the contribution of fluticasone furoate to BREO ELLIPTA. In these 2 trials, exacerbations were defined as worsening of 2 or more major symptoms (dyspnea, sputum volume, and sputum purulence) or worsening of any 1 major symptom together with any 1 of the following minor symptoms: sore throat, colds (nasal discharge and/or nasal congestion), fever without other cause, and increased cough or wheeze for at least 2 consecutive days. COPD exacerbations were considered to be of moderate severity if treatment with systemic corticosteroids and/or antibiotics was required and were considered to be severe if hospitalization was required.

Trials 3 and 4 included 3,255 subjects, of which 57% were male and 85% were Caucasian. They had a mean age of 64 years and an average smoking history of 46 pack years, with 44% identified as current smokers. At screening, the mean postbronchodilator percent predicted FEV₁ was 45% (range: 12% to 91%), and mean postbronchodilator FEV₁/ FVC ratio was 46% (range: 17% to 81%), indicating that the subject population had moderate to very severely impaired airflow obstruction. The mean percent reversibility was 15% (range: -65% to 313%).

Patients treated with BREO ELLIPTA 100 mcg/25 mcg had a lower annual rate of moderate/severe COPD exacerbations compared with vilanterol in both trials (Table 3).

[See table 3 at top of next page]

16 HOW SUPPLIED/STORAGE AND HANDLING

BREO ELLIPTA is supplied as a disposable light grey and pale blue plastic inhaler containing 2 double-foil strips, each with 30 blisters. The inhaler is packaged within a moisture-protective foil tray with a desiccant and a peelable lid (NDC 0173-0859-10).

BREO ELLIPTA is also supplied in an institutional pack as a disposable light grey and pale blue plastic inhaler containing 2 double-foil strips, each with 14 blisters. It is packaged within a moisture-protective foil tray with a desiccant and a peelable lid (NDC 0173-0859-14).

Store at room temperature between 68°F and 77°F (20°C and 25°C); excursions permitted from 59° to 86°F (15° to 30°C) [See USP Controlled Room Temperature]. Store in a dry place away from direct heat or sunlight. Keep out of reach of children.

BREO ELLIPTA should be stored inside the unopened moisture-protective foil tray and only removed from the tray immediately before initial use. Discard BREO ELLIPTA 6 weeks after opening the foil tray or when the counter reads "0" (after all blisters have been used), whichever comes first. The inhaler is not reusable. Do not attempt to take the inhaler apart.

17   PATIENT COUNSELING INFORMATION

Advise the patient to read the FDA-approved patient labeling (Medication Guide and Instructions for Use).

17.1   Asthma-Related Death

Patients should be informed that LABA, such as vilanterol, one of the active ingredients in BREO ELLIPTA, increase the risk of asthma-related death. BREO ELLIPTA is not indicated for the treatment of asthma.

17.2   Not for Acute Symptoms

BREO ELLIPTA is not meant to relieve acute symptoms of COPD and extra doses should not be used for that purpose. Acute symptoms should be treated with a rescue inhaler such as albuterol. The physician should provide the patient with such medicine and instruct the patient in how it should be used.

Patients should be instructed to notify their physicians immediately if they experience any of the following:
- Symptoms get worse
- Need for more inhalations than usual of their rescue inhaler
- Significant decrease in lung function as outlined by the physician

Patients should not stop therapy with BREO ELLIPTA without physician/provider guidance since symptoms may recur after discontinuation.

17.3   Do Not Use Additional Long-Acting Beta₂-Agonists

When patients are prescribed BREO ELLIPTA, other medicines containing a LABA should not be used.

17.4   Risks Associated With Corticosteroid Therapy

Local Effects: Patients should be advised that localized infections with *Candida albicans* occurred in the mouth and pharynx in some patients. If oropharyngeal candidiasis develops, it should be treated with appropriate local or systemic (i.e., oral) antifungal therapy while still continuing therapy with BREO ELLIPTA, but at times therapy with BREO ELLIPTA may need to be temporarily interrupted under close medical supervision. Rinsing the mouth without swallowing after inhalation is advised to help reduce the risk of thrush.

Pneumonia: Patients with COPD who have received BREO ELLIPTA have a higher risk of pneumonia and should be instructed to contact their healthcare providers if they develop symptoms of pneumonia (e.g., fever, chills, change in sputum color, increase in breathing problems).

Immunosuppression: Patients who are on immunosuppressant doses of corticosteroids should be warned to avoid exposure to chickenpox or measles and, if exposed, to consult their physicians without delay. Patients should be informed of potential worsening of existing tuberculosis, fungal, bacterial, viral, or parasitic infections, or ocular herpes simplex.

Hypercorticism and Adrenal Suppression: Patients should be advised that BREO ELLIPTA may cause systemic corticosteroid effects of hypercorticism and adrenal suppression. Additionally, patients should be instructed that deaths due to adrenal insufficiency have occurred during and after transfer from systemic corticosteroids.

Reduction in Bone Mineral Density: Patients who are at an increased risk for decreased BMD should be advised that the use of corticosteroids may pose an additional risk.

Ocular Effects: Long-term use of inhaled corticosteroids may increase the risk of some eye problems (cataracts or glaucoma); regular eye examinations should be considered.

17.5   Risks Associated With Beta-Agonist Therapy

Patients should be informed of adverse effects associated with beta₂-agonists, such as palpitations, chest pain, rapid heart rate, tremor, or nervousness.

BREO and ELLIPTA are registered trademarks of the GSK group of companies.

BREO ELLIPTA was developed in collaboration with Theravance.

GlaxoSmithKline
Research Triangle Park, NC 27709
©2014, the GSK group of companies. All rights reserved.
BRE:2PI

MEDICATION GUIDE

BREO® ELLIPTA® (*BREE-oh ee-LIP-ta*)
(fluticasone furoate and vilanterol inhalation powder)

Read the Medication Guide that comes with BREO ELLIPTA before you start using it and each time you get a

Table 3. Moderate and Severe Chronic Obstructive Pulmonary Disease Exacerbations

Treatment	N	Mean Annual Rate (exacerbations/year)	Ratio vs Vilanterol	95% CI
Trial 3				
Fluticasone furoate/vilanterol 200 mcg/25 mcg	409	0.79	0.69	(0.56, 0.85)
BREO ELLIPTA 100 mcg/25 mcg	403	0.90	0.79	(0.64, 0.97)
Fluticasone furoate/vilanterol 50 mcg/25 mcg	412	0.92	0.81	(0.66, 0.99)
Vilanterol 25 mcg	409	1.14	—	—
Trial 4				
Fluticasone furoate/vilanterol 200 mcg/25 mcg	402	0.90	0.85	(0.70, 1.04)
BREO ELLIPTA 100 mcg/25 mcg	403	0.70	0.66	(0.54, 0.81)
Fluticasone furoate/vilanterol 50 mcg/25 mcg	408	0.92	0.87	(0.72, 1.06)
Vilanterol 25 mcg	409	1.05	—	—

refill. There may be new information. This Medication Guide does not take the place of talking to your healthcare provider about your medical condition or treatment.

What is the most important information I should know about BREO ELLIPTA?

BREO ELLIPTA is only approved for use in chronic obstructive pulmonary disease (COPD). BREO ELLIPTA is NOT approved for use in asthma.

BREO ELLIPTA can cause serious side effects, including:
- **People with asthma who take long-acting beta₂-adrenergic agonist (LABA) medicines, such as vilanterol (one of the medicines in BREO ELLIPTA), have an increased risk of death from asthma problems.** It is not known whether fluticasone furoate, the other medicine in BREO ELLIPTA, reduces the risk of death from asthma problems seen with LABA medicines.
- **It is not known if LABA medicines, such as vilanterol (one of the medicines in BREO ELLIPTA), increase the risk of death in people with COPD.**
- **Call your healthcare provider if breathing problems worsen over time while using BREO ELLIPTA.** You may need different treatment.
- **Get emergency medical care if:**
  - your breathing problems worsen quickly
  - you use your rescue inhaler, but it does not relieve your breathing problems.

What is BREO ELLIPTA?
BREO ELLIPTA combines an inhaled corticosteroid (ICS) medicine, fluticasone furoate, and a LABA medicine, vilanterol.
- ICS medicines, such as fluticasone furoate (one of the medicines in BREO ELLIPTA), help to decrease inflammation in the lungs. Inflammation in the lungs can lead to breathing problems.
- LABA medicines, such as vilanterol (one of the medicines in BREO ELLIPTA), help the muscles around the airways in your lungs stay relaxed to prevent symptoms such as wheezing, cough, chest tightness, and shortness of breath. These symptoms can happen when the muscles around the airways tighten. This makes it hard to breathe.

BREO ELLIPTA is used for COPD. COPD is a chronic lung disease that includes chronic bronchitis, emphysema, or both. BREO ELLIPTA is a prescription medicine that is used long term as 1 inhalation 1 time each day to improve symptoms of COPD for better breathing and to reduce the number of flare-ups (the worsening of your COPD symptoms for several days).
- **BREO ELLIPTA is not for use to treat sudden symptoms of COPD.** Always have a rescue inhaler (an inhaled, short-acting bronchodilator) with you to treat sudden symptoms. If you do not have a rescue inhaler, contact your healthcare provider to have one prescribed for you.
- **BREO ELLIPTA is not for the treatment of asthma. It is not known if BREO ELLIPTA is safe and effective in people with asthma.**
- BREO ELLIPTA should not be used in children. It is not known if BREO ELLIPTA is safe and effective in children.

Who should not use BREO ELLIPTA?
Do not use BREO ELLIPTA if you:
- have a severe allergy to milk proteins. Ask your healthcare provider if you are not sure.
- are allergic to fluticasone furoate, vilanterol, or any of the ingredients in BREO ELLIPTA. See "What are the ingredients in BREO ELLIPTA?" below for a complete list of ingredients.

What should I tell my healthcare provider before using BREO ELLIPTA?

Tell your healthcare provider about all of your health conditions, including if you:
- have heart problems
- have high blood pressure
- have seizures
- have thyroid problems
- have diabetes
- have liver problems
- have weak bones (osteoporosis)
- have an immune system problem
- have eye problems such as glaucoma or cataracts
- are allergic to any of the ingredients in BREO ELLIPTA, any other medicines, or food products. See "What are the ingredients in BREO ELLIPTA?" below for a complete list of ingredients.
- have any type of viral, bacterial, or fungal infection
- are exposed to chickenpox or measles or been around anyone who has chickenpox or measles
- have any other medical conditions
- are pregnant or planning to become pregnant. It is not known if BREO ELLIPTA may harm your unborn baby.
- are breastfeeding. It is not known if the medicines in BREO ELLIPTA pass into your milk and if they can harm your baby.

Tell your healthcare provider about all the medicines you take, including prescription and non-prescription medicines, vitamins, and herbal supplements. BREO ELLIPTA and certain other medicines may interact with each other. This may cause serious side effects. Especially, tell your healthcare provider if you take antifungal or anti-HIV medicines.

Know the medicines you take. Keep a list of them to show your healthcare provider and pharmacist when you get a new medicine.

How should I use BREO ELLIPTA?
Read the step-by-step instructions for using BREO ELLIPTA at the end of this Medication Guide.
- **Do not** use BREO ELLIPTA unless your healthcare provider has taught you how to use the inhaler and you understand how to use it correctly.
- Use BREO ELLIPTA exactly as prescribed. **Do not** use BREO ELLIPTA more often than prescribed.
- Use 1 inhalation of BREO ELLIPTA 1 time each day. Use BREO ELLIPTA at the same time each day.
- If you miss a dose of BREO ELLIPTA, take it as soon as you remember. Do not take more than 1 inhalation per day. Take your next dose at your usual time. Do not take 2 doses at one time.
- If you take too much BREO ELLIPTA, call your healthcare provider and get medical help right away if you have any unusual symptoms, such as worsening shortness of breath, chest pain, increased heart rate, or shakiness.
- **Do not use other medicines that contain a LABA for any reason.** Ask your healthcare provider or pharmacist if any of your other medicines are LABA medicines.
- Do not stop using BREO ELLIPTA unless told to do so by your healthcare provider because your symptoms might get worse. Your healthcare provider will change your medicines as needed.
- **BREO ELLIPTA does not relieve sudden symptoms.** Always have a rescue inhaler with you to treat sudden symptoms. If you do not have a rescue inhaler, call your healthcare provider to have one prescribed for you.

- Call your healthcare provider or get medical care right away if:
  - your breathing problems get worse
  - you need to use your rescue inhaler more often than usual
  - your rescue inhaler does not work as well to relieve your symptoms
  - you need to use 4 or more inhalations of your rescue inhaler in 24 hours for 2 or more days in a row
  - you use 1 whole canister of your rescue inhaler in 8 weeks

What are the possible side effects with BREO ELLIPTA?
BREO ELLIPTA can cause serious side effects, including:
- See "What is the most important information I should know about BREO ELLIPTA?"
- **pneumonia.** People with COPD have a higher chance of getting pneumonia. BREO ELLIPTA may increase the chance of getting pneumonia. Call your healthcare provider if you notice any of the following symptoms:
  - increase in mucus (sputum) production
  - change in mucus color
  - fever
  - chills
  - increased cough
  - increased breathing problems
- **thrush (fungal infection) in mouth and throat.** You may develop a yeast infection (*Candida albicans*) in your mouth or throat. Rinse your mouth with water without swallowing after using BREO ELLIPTA to help prevent thrush in your mouth and throat.
- **serious allergic reactions.** Call your healthcare provider or get emergency medical care if you get any of the following symptoms of a serious allergic reaction:
  - rash
  - hives
  - swelling of the face, mouth, and tongue
  - breathing problems
- **sudden breathing problems immediately after inhaling your medicine**
- **effects on heart**
  - increased blood pressure
  - a fast and/or irregular heartbeat
  - chest pain
- **effects on nervous system**
  - tremor
  - nervousness
- **reduced adrenal function (adrenal insufficiency).** Adrenal insufficiency is a condition in which the adrenal glands do not make enough steroid hormones. This can happen when you stop taking oral corticosteroid medicines (such as prednisone) and start taking a medicine containing an inhaled corticosteroid (such as BREO ELLIPTA). When your body is under stress from fever, trauma (such as a car accident), infection, surgery, or worse COPD symptoms, adrenal insufficiency can get worse and may cause death. Symptoms of adrenal insufficiency include:
  - feeling tired (fatigue)
  - lack of energy
  - weakness
  - nausea and vomiting
  - low blood pressure
- **changes in laboratory blood values (sugar, potassium)**
- **weakened immune system and increased chance of getting infections (immunosuppression)**
- **bone thinning or weakness (osteoporosis)**
- **eye problems including glaucoma and cataracts.** You should have regular eye exams while using BREO ELLIPTA.

Common side effects of BREO ELLIPTA include:
- runny nose and sore throat
- upper respiratory tract infection
- headache
- thrush in the mouth and/or throat. Rinse your mouth without swallowing after use to help prevent this.

Tell your healthcare provider about any side effect that bothers you or that does not go away.
These are not all the side effects with BREO ELLIPTA. Ask your healthcare provider or pharmacist for more information.
Call your doctor for medical advice about side effects. You may report side effects to FDA at 1-800-FDA-1088.

How do I store BREO ELLIPTA?
- Store BREO ELLIPTA at room temperature between 68°F and 77°F (20°C and 25°C). Keep in a dry place away from heat and sunlight.
- Store BREO ELLIPTA in the unopened foil tray and only open when ready for use.
- Safely throw away BREO ELLIPTA in the trash 6 weeks after you open the foil tray or when the counter reads "0", whichever comes first. Write the date you open the tray on the label on the inhaler.
- **Keep BREO ELLIPTA and all medicines out of the reach of children.**

General Information about BREO ELLIPTA
Medicines are sometimes prescribed for purposes not mentioned in a Medication Guide. Do not use BREO ELLIPTA for a condition for which it was not prescribed. Do not give your BREO ELLIPTA to other people, even if they have the same condition that you have. It may harm them.
This Medication Guide summarizes the most important information about BREO ELLIPTA. If you would like more information, talk with your healthcare provider or pharmacist. You can ask your healthcare provider or pharmacist for information about BREO ELLIPTA that was written for healthcare professionals.
For more information about BREO ELLIPTA, call 1-888-825-5249 or visit our website at www.myBREO.com.

What are the ingredients in BREO ELLIPTA?
Active ingredients: fluticasone furoate, vilanterol
Inactive ingredients: lactose monohydrate (contains milk proteins), magnesium stearate

Instructions for Use
For Oral Inhalation Only.
Read this before you start:
- **If you open and close the cover without inhaling the medicine, you will lose the dose.**
- **The lost dose will be securely held inside the inhaler, but it will no longer be available to be inhaled.**
- **It is not possible to accidentally take a double dose or an extra dose in one inhalation.**

Your BREO ELLIPTA inhaler

Figure labels: Tray Lid, Inhaler, Desiccant, Tray, Carton, Medication Guide

How to use your inhaler
- BREO ELLIPTA comes in a foil tray.
- Peel back the lid to open the tray. See Figure A.
- The tray contains a desiccant to reduce moisture. Do not eat or inhale. Throw it away in the household trash out of reach of children and pets. See Figure B.

Figure A

Figure B

Important Notes:
- Your inhaler contains 30 doses (14 doses if you have a sample or institutional pack).
- Each time you open the cover of the inhaler fully (you will hear a clicking sound), a dose is ready to be inhaled. This is shown by a decrease in the number on the counter.
- If you open and close the cover without inhaling the medicine, you will lose the dose. The lost dose will be held in the inhaler, but it will no longer be available to be inhaled. It is not possible to accidentally take a double dose or an extra dose in one inhalation.
- **Do not** open the cover of the inhaler until you are ready to use it. To avoid wasting doses after the inhaler is ready, **do not** close the cover until after you have inhaled the medicine.
- Write the "Tray opened" and "Discard" dates on the inhaler label. The "Discard" date is 6 weeks from the date you open the tray.

Check the counter. See Figure C.

Figure labels: Cover, 30, Counter

Figure C

- Before the inhaler is used for the first time, the counter should show the number 30 (14 if you have a sample or institutional pack). This is the number of doses in the inhaler.
- Each time you open the cover, you prepare 1 dose of medicine.
- The counter counts down by 1 each time you open the cover.

Prepare your dose:
Wait to open the cover until you are ready to take your dose.

Figure labels: Mouthpiece, Counter, 29, Air vent, Cover, "Click"

Figure D

Step 1. Open the cover of the inhaler. See Figure D.
- Slide the cover down to expose the mouthpiece. You should hear a "click." The counter will count down by 1 number. You do not need to shake this kind of inhaler. **Your inhaler is now ready to use.**
- If the counter does not count down as you hear the click, the inhaler will not deliver the medicine. Call your healthcare provider or pharmacist if this happens.

Figure E

Step 2. Breathe out. See Figure E.
- While holding the inhaler away from your mouth, breathe out (exhale) fully. Do not breathe out into the mouthpiece.

Figure F

Step 3. Inhale your medicine. See Figure F.
- Put the mouthpiece between your lips, and close your lips firmly around it. Your lips should fit over the curved shape of the mouthpiece.
- Take one long, steady, deep breath in through your mouth. **Do not** breathe in through your nose.

Figure label: Do not block the air vent with your fingers.

Figure G

- Do not block the air vent with your fingers. **See Figure G.**

Figure H

- **Remove the inhaler from your mouth and hold your breath for about 3 to 4 seconds** (or as long as comfortable for you). **See Figure H.**

Figure I

Step 4. Breathe out slowly and gently. See Figure I.
- You may not taste or feel the medicine, even when you are using the inhaler correctly.
- **Do not** take another dose from the inhaler even if you do not feel or taste the medicine.

Figure J

Step 5. Close the inhaler. See Figure J.
- You can clean the mouthpiece if needed, using a dry tissue, before you close the cover. Routine cleaning is not required.
- Slide the cover up and over the mouthpiece as far as it will go.

Figure K

Step 6. Rinse your mouth. See Figure K.
- Rinse your mouth with water after you have used the inhaler and spit the water out. **Do not** swallow the water.
Important Note: When should you get a refill?

Figure L

- When you have less than 10 doses remaining in your inhaler, the left half of the counter shows red as a reminder to get a refill. **See Figure L.**
- After you have inhaled the last dose, the counter will show "0" and will be empty.
- Throw the empty inhaler away in your household trash out of reach of children and pets.
If you have questions about BREO ELLIPTA or how to use your inhaler, call GlaxoSmithKline (GSK) at 1-888-825-5249 or visit www.myBREO.com.
This Medication Guide has been approved by the U.S. Food and Drug Administration.
BREO and ELLIPTA are registered trademarks of the GSK group of companies.
BREO ELLIPTA was developed in collaboration with Theravance.
GlaxoSmithKline
Research Triangle Park, NC 27709
©2014, the GSK group of companies. All rights reserved.
April 2014
BRE:2MG

CEFTIN® Tablets ℞
[sĕf´tin]
(cefuroxime axetil tablets)

CEFTIN® for Oral Suspension ℞
(cefuroxime axetil powder for oral suspension)

To reduce the development of drug-resistant bacteria and maintain the effectiveness of CEFTIN and other antibacterial drugs, CEFTIN should be used only to treat or prevent infections that are proven or strongly suspected to be caused by bacteria.

DESCRIPTION
CEFTIN Tablets and CEFTIN for Oral Suspension contain cefuroxime as cefuroxime axetil. CEFTIN is a semisynthetic, broad-spectrum cephalosporin antibiotic for oral administration.
Chemically, cefuroxime axetil, the 1-(acetyloxy) ethyl ester of cefuroxime, is (RS)-1-hydroxyethyl (6R ,7R)-7-[2-(2-furyl)glyoxyl-amido]-3-(hydroxymethyl)-8-oxo-5-thia-1-azabicyclo[4.2.0]-oct-2-ene-2-carboxylate, 7^2-(Z)-(O -methyl-oxime), 1-acetate 3-carbamate. Its molecular formula is $C_{20}H_{22}N_4O_{10}S$, and it has a molecular weight of 510.48.
Cefuroxime axetil is in the amorphous form and has the following structural formula:

CEFTIN Tablets are film-coated and contain the equivalent of 250 or 500 mg of cefuroxime as cefuroxime axetil. CEFTIN Tablets contain the inactive ingredients colloidal silicon dioxide, croscarmellose sodium, hydrogenated vegetable oil, hypromellose, methylparaben, microcrystalline cellulose, propylene glycol, propylparaben, sodium benzoate, sodium lauryl sulfate, and titanium dioxide.
CEFTIN for Oral Suspension, when reconstituted with water, provides the equivalent of 125 mg or 250 mg of cefuroxime (as cefuroxime axetil) per 5 mL of suspension. CEFTIN for Oral Suspension contains the inactive ingredients acesulfame potassium, aspartame, povidone K30, stearic acid, sucrose, tutti-frutti flavoring, and xanthan gum.

CLINICAL PHARMACOLOGY
Absorption and Metabolism
After oral administration, cefuroxime axetil is absorbed from the gastrointestinal tract and rapidly hydrolyzed by nonspecific esterases in the intestinal mucosa and blood to cefuroxime. Cefuroxime is subsequently distributed throughout the extracellular fluids. The axetil moiety is metabolized to acetaldehyde and acetic acid.
Pharmacokinetics
Approximately 50% of serum cefuroxime is bound to protein. Serum pharmacokinetic parameters for CEFTIN Tablets and CEFTIN for Oral Suspension are shown in Tables 1 and 2.
[See table 1 below]
[See table 2 at top of next page]
Comparative Pharmacokinetic Properties
A 250 mg/5 mL-dose of CEFTIN Suspension is bioequivalent to 2 times 125 mg/5 mL-dose of CEFTIN Suspension when administered with food (see Table 3). **CEFTIN for Oral Suspension was not bioequivalent to CEFTIN Tablets when tested in healthy adults. The tablet and powder for oral suspension formulations are NOT substitutable on a milligram-per-milligram basis.** The area under the curve for the suspension averaged 91% of that for the tablet, and the peak plasma concentration for the suspension averaged 71% of the peak plasma concentration of the tablets. There-

fore, the safety and effectiveness of both the tablet and oral suspension formulations had to be established in separate clinical trials.
[See table 3 at top of next page]
Food Effect on Pharmacokinetics
Absorption of the tablet is greater when taken after food (absolute bioavailability of CEFTIN Tablets increases from 37% to 52%). Despite this difference in absorption, the clinical and bacteriologic responses of patients were independent of food intake at the time of tablet administration in 2 studies where this was assessed.
All pharmacokinetic and clinical effectiveness and safety studies in pediatric patients using the suspension formulation were conducted in the fed state. No data are available on the absorption kinetics of the suspension formulation when administered to fasted pediatric patients.
Renal Excretion
Cefuroxime is excreted unchanged in the urine; in adults, approximately 50% of the administered dose is recovered in the urine within 12 hours. The pharmacokinetics of cefuroxime in the urine of pediatric patients have not been studied at this time. Until further data are available, the renal pharmacokinetic properties of cefuroxime axetil established in adults should not be extrapolated to pediatric patients.
Because cefuroxime is renally excreted, the serum half-life is prolonged in patients with reduced renal function. In a study of 20 elderly patients (mean age = 83.9 years) having a mean creatinine clearance of 34.9 mL/min, the mean serum elimination half-life was 3.5 hours. Despite the lower elimination of cefuroxime in geriatric patients, dosage adjustment based on age is not necessary (see PRECAUTIONS: Geriatric Use).
Microbiology
The in vivo bactericidal activity of cefuroxime axetil is due to cefuroxime's binding to essential target proteins and the resultant inhibition of cell-wall synthesis.
Cefuroxime has bactericidal activity against a wide range of common pathogens, including many beta-lactamase-producing strains. Cefuroxime is stable to many bacterial beta-lactamases, especially plasmid-mediated enzymes that are commonly found in enterobacteriaceae.
Cefuroxime has been demonstrated to be active against most strains of the following microorganisms both in vitro and in clinical infections as described in the INDICATIONS AND USAGE (see INDICATIONS AND USAGE).
Aerobic Gram-Positive Microorganisms
Staphylococcus aureus (including beta-lactamase-producing strains)
Streptococcus pneumoniae
Streptococcus pyogenes
Aerobic Gram-Negative Microorganisms
Escherichia coli
Haemophilus influenzae (including beta-lactamase-producing strains)
Haemophilus parainfluenzae
Klebsiella pneumoniae
Moraxella catarrhalis (including beta-lactamase-producing strains)
Neisseria gonorrhoeae (including beta-lactamase-producing strains)
Spirochetes
Borrelia burgdorferi
Cefuroxime has been shown to be active in vitro against most strains of the following microorganisms; however, the clinical significance of these findings is unknown.
Cefuroxime exhibits in vitro minimum inhibitory concentrations (MICs) of 4.0 mcg/mL or less (systemic susceptible breakpoint) against most (≥90%) strains of the following microorganisms; however, the safety and effectiveness of cefuroxime in treating clinical infections due to these microorganisms have not been established in adequate and well-controlled trials.

Table 1. Postprandial Pharmacokinetics of Cefuroxime Administered as CEFTIN Tablets to Adults[a]				
Dose[b] (Cefuroxime Equivalent)	Peak Plasma Concentration (mcg/mL)	Time of Peak Plasma Concentration (hr)	Mean Elimination Half-life (hr)	AUC (mcg•hr/mL)
125 mg	2.1	2.2	1.2	6.7
250 mg	4.1	2.5	1.2	12.9
500 mg	7.0	3.0	1.2	27.4
1,000 mg	13.6	2.5	1.3	50.0

[a]Mean values of 12 healthy adult volunteers.
[b]Drug administered immediately after a meal.

Table 2. Postprandial Pharmacokinetics of Cefuroxime Administered as CEFTIN for Oral Suspension to Pediatric Patients[a]

Dose[b] (Cefuroxime Equivalent)	n	Peak Plasma Concentration (mcg/mL)	Time of Peak Plasma Concentration (hr)	Mean Elimination Half-life (hr)	AUC (mcg•hr/mL)
10 mg/kg	8	3.3	3.6	1.4	12.4
15 mg/kg	12	5.1	2.7	1.9	22.5
20 mg/kg	8	7.0	3.1	1.9	32.8

[a]Mean age = 23 months.
[b]Drug administered with milk or milk products.

Table 3. Pharmacokinetics of Cefuroxime Administered as 250 mg/5 mL or 2 × 125 mg/5 mL CEFTIN for Oral Suspension to Adults[a] With Food

Dose (Cefuroxime Equivalent)	Peak Plasma Concentration (mcg/mL)	Time of Peak Plasma Concentration (hr)	Mean Elimination Half-life (hr)	AUC (mcg•hr/mL)
250 mg/5 mL	2.23	3	1.40	8.92
2 × 125 mg/5 mL	2.37	3	1.44	9.75

[a]Mean values of 18 healthy adult volunteers.

Aerobic Gram-Positive Microorganisms
Staphylococcus epidermidis
Staphylococcus saprophyticus
Streptococcus agalactiae
NOTE: *Listeria monocytogenes* and certain strains of enterococci, e.g., *Enterococcus faecalis* (formerly *Streptococcus faecalis*), are resistant to cefuroxime. Methicillin-resistant staphylococci are resistant to cefuroxime.
Aerobic Gram-Negative Microorganisms
Morganella morganii
Proteus inconstans
Proteus mirabilis
Providencia rettgeri
NOTE: *Pseudomonas* spp., *Campylobacter* spp., *Acinetobacter calcoaceticu* , *Legionella* spp., and most strains of *Serratia* spp. and *Proteus vulgaris* are resistant to most first- and second-generation cephalosporins. Some strains of *Morganella morganii*, *Enterobacter cloacae*, and *Citrobacter* spp. have been shown by in vitro tests to be resistant to cefuroxime and other cephalosporins.
Anaerobic Microorganisms
Peptococcus niger
NOTE: Most strains of *Clostridium difficile* and *Bacteroides fragilis* are resistant to cefuroxime.
Susceptibility Tests
Dilution Techniques
Quantitative methods that are used to determine MICs provide reproducible estimates of the susceptibility of bacteria to antimicrobial compounds. One such standardized procedure uses a standardized dilution method[1] (broth, agar, or microdilution) or equivalent with cefuroxime powder. The MIC values obtained should be interpreted according to the following criteria:

MIC (mcg/mL)	Interpretation
≤4	(S) Susceptible
8-16	(I) Intermediate
≥32	(R) Resistant

A report of "Susceptible" indicates that the pathogen, if in the blood, is likely to be inhibited by usually achievable concentrations of the antimicrobial compound in blood. A report of "Intermediate" indicates that inhibitory concentrations of the antibiotic may be achieved if high dosage is used or if the infection is confined to tissues or fluids in which high antibiotic concentrations are attained. This category also provides a buffer zone that prevents small, uncontrolled technical factors from causing major discrepancies in interpretation. A report of "Resistant" indicates that usually achievable concentrations of the antimicrobial compound in the blood are unlikely to be inhibitory and that other therapy should be selected.
Standardized susceptibility test procedures require the use of laboratory control microorganisms. Standard cefuroxime powder should give the following MIC values:

Microorganism	MIC (mcg/mL)
Escherichia coli ATCC 25922	2-8
Staphylococcus aureus ATCC 29213	0.5-2

Diffusion Techniques
Quantitative methods that require measurement of zone diameters provide estimates of the susceptibility of bacteria to antimicrobial compounds. One such standardized procedure[2] that has been recommended (for use with disks) to test the susceptibility of microorganisms to cefuroxime uses the 30-mcg cefuroxime disk. Interpretation involves correlation of the diameter obtained in the disk test with the MIC for cefuroxime.
Reports from the laboratory providing results of the standard single-disk susceptibility test with a 30-mcg cefuroxime disk should be interpreted according to the following criteria:

Zone Diameter (mm)	Interpretation
≥23	(S) Susceptible
15-22	(I) Intermediate
≤14	(R) Resistant

Interpretation should be as stated above for results using dilution techniques.
As with standard dilution techniques, diffusion methods require the use of laboratory control microorganisms. The 30-mcg cefuroxime disk provides the following zone diameters in these laboratory test quality control strains:

Microorganism	Zone Diameter (mm)
Escherichia coli ATCC 25922	20-26
Staphylococcus aureus ATCC 25923	27-35

INDICATIONS AND USAGE

NOTE: CEFTIN TABLETS AND CEFTIN FOR ORAL SUSPENSION ARE NOT BIOEQUIVALENT AND ARE NOT SUBSTITUTABLE ON A MILLIGRAM-PER-MILLIGRAM BASIS (SEE CLINICAL PHARMACOLOGY).
CEFTIN Tablets
CEFTIN Tablets are indicated for the treatment of patients with mild to moderate infections caused by susceptible strains of the designated microorganisms in the conditions listed below:
1. **Pharyngitis/Tonsillitis** caused by *Streptococcus pyogenes*.
   NOTE: The usual drug of choice in the treatment and prevention of streptococcal infections, including the prophylaxis of rheumatic fever, is penicillin given by the intramuscular route. CEFTIN Tablets are generally effective in the eradication of streptococci from the nasopharynx; however, substantial data establishing the efficacy of cefuroxime in the subsequent prevention of rheumatic fever are not available. Please also note that in all clinical trials, all isolates had to be sensitive to both penicillin and cefuroxime. There are no data from adequate and well-controlled trials to demonstrate the effectiveness of cefuroxime in the treatment of penicillin-resistant strains of *Streptococcus pyogenes*.

2. **Acute Bacterial Otitis Media** caused by *Streptococcus pneumoniae*, *Haemophilus influenzae* (including beta-lactamase-producing strains), *Moraxella catarrhalis* (including beta-lactamase-producing strains), or *Streptococcus pyogenes*.
3. **Acute Bacterial Maxillary Sinusitis** caused by *Streptococcus pneumoniae* or *Haemophilus influenzae* (non-beta-lactamase-producing strains only) *(see CLINICAL STUDIES)*.
   NOTE: In view of the insufficient numbers of isolates of beta-lactamase-producing strains of *Haemophilus influenzae* and *Moraxella catarrhalis* that were obtained from clinical trials with CEFTIN Tablets for patients with acute bacterial maxillary sinusitis, it was not possible to adequately evaluate the effectiveness of CEFTIN Tablets for sinus infections known, suspected, or considered potentially to be caused by beta-lactamase-producing *Haemophilus influenzae* or *Moraxella catarrhalis*.
4. **Acute Bacterial Exacerbations of Chronic Bronchitis and Secondary Bacterial Infections of Acute Bronchitis** caused by *Streptococcus pneumoniae*, *Haemophilus influenzae* (beta-lactamase negative strains), or *Haemophilus parainfluenzae* (beta-lactamase negative strains) *(see DOSAGE AND ADMINISTRATION and CLINICAL STUDIES)*.
5. **Uncomplicated Skin and Skin-Structure Infections** caused by *Staphylococcus aureus* (including beta-lactamase-producing strains) or *Streptococcus pyogenes*.
6. **Uncomplicated Urinary Tract Infections** caused by *Escherichia coli* or *Klebsiella pneumoniae*.
7. **Uncomplicated Gonorrhea**, urethral and endocervical, caused by penicillinase-producing and non-penicillinase-producing strains of *Neisseria gonorrhoeae* and uncomplicated gonorrhea, rectal, in females, caused by non-penicillinase-producing strains of *Neisseria gonorrhoeae*.
8. **Early Lyme Disease (erythema migrans)** caused by *Borrelia burgdorferi*.
CEFTIN for Oral Suspension
CEFTIN for Oral Suspension is indicated for the treatment of pediatric patients 3 months to 12 years of age with mild to moderate infections caused by susceptible strains of the designated microorganisms in the conditions listed below. The safety and effectiveness of CEFTIN for Oral Suspension in the treatment of infections other than those specifically listed below have not been established either by adequate and well-controlled trials or by pharmacokinetic data with which to determine an effective and safe dosing regimen.
1. **Pharyngitis/Tonsillitis** caused by *Streptococcus pyogenes*.
   NOTE: The usual drug of choice in the treatment and prevention of streptococcal infections, including the prophylaxis of rheumatic fever, is penicillin given by the intramuscular route. CEFTIN for Oral Suspension is generally effective in the eradication of streptococci from the nasopharynx; however, substantial data establishing the efficacy of cefuroxime in the subsequent prevention of rheumatic fever are not available. Please also note that in all clinical trials, all isolates had to be sensitive to both penicillin and cefuroxime. There are no data from adequate and well-controlled trials to demonstrate the effectiveness of cefuroxime in the treatment of penicillin-resistant strains of *Streptococcus pyogenes*.
2. **Acute Bacterial Otitis Media** caused by *Streptococcus pneumoniae*, *Haemophilus influenzae* (including beta-lactamase-producing strains), *Moraxella catarrhalis* (including beta-lactamase-producing strains), or *Streptococcus pyogenes*.
3. **Impetigo** caused by *Staphylococcus aureus* (including beta-lactamase-producing strains) or *Streptococcus pyogenes*.
To reduce the development of drug-resistant bacteria and maintain the effectiveness of CEFTIN and other antibacterial drugs, CEFTIN should be used only to treat or prevent infections that are proven or strongly suspected to be caused by susceptible bacteria. When culture and susceptibility information are available, they should be considered in selecting or modifying antibacterial therapy. In the absence of such data, local epidemiology and susceptibility patterns may contribute to the empiric selection of therapy.

CONTRAINDICATIONS

CEFTIN products are contraindicated in patients with known allergy to the cephalosporin group of antibiotics.

WARNINGS

CEFTIN TABLETS AND CEFTIN FOR ORAL SUSPENSION ARE NOT BIOEQUIVALENT AND ARE THEREFORE NOT SUBSTITUTABLE ON A MILLIGRAM-PER-MILLIGRAM BASIS (SEE CLINICAL PHARMACOLOGY).
BEFORE THERAPY WITH CEFTIN PRODUCTS IS INSTITUTED, CAREFUL INQUIRY SHOULD BE MADE TO DETER-

MINE WHETHER THE PATIENT HAS HAD PREVIOUS HYPERSENSITIVITY REACTIONS TO CEFTIN PRODUCTS, OTHER CEPHALOSPORINS, PENICILLINS, OR OTHER DRUGS. IF THIS PRODUCT IS TO BE GIVEN TO PENICILLIN-SENSITIVE PATIENTS, CAUTION SHOULD BE EXERCISED BECAUSE CROSS-HYPERSENSITIVITY AMONG BETA-LACTAM ANTIBIOTICS HAS BEEN CLEARLY DOCUMENTED AND MAY OCCUR IN UP TO 10% OF PATIENTS WITH A HISTORY OF PENICILLIN ALLERGY. IF A CLINICALLY SIGNIFICANT ALLERGIC REACTION TO CEFTIN PRODUCTS OCCURS, DISCONTINUE THE DRUG AND INSTITUTE APPROPRIATE THERAPY. SERIOUS ACUTE HYPERSENSITIVITY REACTIONS MAY REQUIRE TREATMENT WITH EPINEPHRINE AND OTHER EMERGENCY MEASURES, INCLUDING OXYGEN, INTRAVENOUS FLUIDS, INTRAVENOUS ANTIHISTAMINES, CORTICOSTEROIDS, PRESSOR AMINES, AND AIRWAY MANAGEMENT, AS CLINICALLY INDICATED.

Clostridium difficile associated diarrhea (CDAD) has been reported with use of nearly all antibacterial agents, including CEFTIN, and may range in severity from mild diarrhea to fatal colitis. Treatment with antibacterial agents alters the normal flora of the colon leading to overgrowth of *C. difficile*.

C. difficile produces toxins A and B which contribute to the development of CDAD. Hypertoxin producing strains of *C. difficile* cause increased morbidity and mortality, as these infections can be refractory to antimicrobial therapy and may require colectomy. CDAD must be considered in all patients who present with diarrhea following antibiotic use. Careful medical history is necessary since CDAD has been reported to occur over 2o months after the administration of antibacterial agents.

If CDAD is suspected or confirmed, ongoing antibiotic use not directed against *C. difficile* may need to be discontinued. Appropriate fluid and electrolyte management, protein supplementation, antibiotic treatment of *C. difficile*, and surgical evaluation should be instituted as clinically indicated.

PRECAUTIONS
General
As with other broad-spectrum antibiotics, prolonged administration of cefuroxime axetil may result in overgrowth of nonsusceptible microorganisms. If superinfection occurs during therapy, appropriate measures should be taken.

Cephalosporins, including cefuroxime axetil, should be given with caution to patients receiving concurrent treatment with potent diuretics because these diuretics are suspected of adversely affecting renal function.

Cefuroxime axetil, as with other broad-spectrum antibiotics, should be prescribed with caution in individuals with a history of colitis. The safety and effectiveness of cefuroxime axetil have not been established in patients with gastrointestinal malabsorption. Patients with gastrointestinal malabsorption were excluded from participating in clinical trials of cefuroxime axetil.

Cephalosporins may be associated with a fall in prothrombin activity. Those at risk include patients with renal or hepatic impairment or poor nutritional state, as well as patients receiving a protracted course of antimicrobial therapy, and patients previously stabilized on anticoagulant therapy. Prothrombin time should be monitored in patients at risk and exogenous Vitamin K administered as indicated. Prescribing CEFTIN in the absence of a proven or strongly suspected bacterial infection or a prophylactic indication is unlikely to provide benefit to the patient and increases the risk of the development of drug-resistant bacteria.

Diarrhea is a common problem caused by antibiotics which usually ends when the antibiotic is discontinued. Sometimes after starting treatment with antibiotics, patients can develop watery and bloody stools (with or without stomach cramps and fever) even as late as 2 or more months after having taken the last dose of the antibiotic. If this occurs, patients should contact their physician as soon as possible.

Information for Patients/Caregivers (Pediatric)
Phenylketonurics
CEFTIN for Oral Suspension 125 mg/5 mL contains phenylalanine 11.8 mg per 5 mL (1 teaspoonful) constituted suspension. CEFTIN for Oral Suspension 250 mg/5 mL contains phenylalanine 25.2 mg per 5 mL (1 teaspoonful) constituted suspension.

1. During clinical trials, the tablet was tolerated by pediatric patients old enough to swallow the cefuroxime axetil tablet whole. The crushed tablet has a strong, persistent, bitter taste and should not be administered to pediatric patients in this manner. Pediatric patients who cannot swallow the tablet whole should receive the oral suspension.
2. Discontinuation of therapy due to taste and/or problems of administering this drug occurred in 1.4% of pediatric patients given the oral suspension. Complaints about taste (which may impair compliance) occurred in 5% of pediatric patients.

3. Patients should be counseled that antibacterial drugs, including CEFTIN, should only be used to treat bacterial infections. They do not treat viral infections (e.g., the common cold). When CEFTIN is prescribed to treat a bacterial infection, patients should be told that although it is common to feel better early in the course of therapy, the medication should be taken exactly as directed. Skipping doses or not completing the full course of therapy may: (1) decrease the effectiveness of the immediate treatment, and (2) increase the likelihood that bacteria will develop resistance and will not be treatable by CEFTIN or other antibacterial drugs in the future.

Drug/Laboratory Test Interactions
A false-positive reaction for glucose in the urine may occur with copper reduction tests (Benedict's or Fehling's solution or with CLINITEST® tablets), but not with enzyme-based tests for glycosuria (e.g., CLINISTIX®). As a false-negative result may occur in the ferricyanide test, it is recommended that either the glucose oxidase or hexokinase method be used to determine blood/plasma glucose levels in patients receiving cefuroxime axetil. The presence of cefuroxime does not interfere with the assay of serum and urine creatinine by the alkaline picrate method.

Drug/Drug Interactions
Concomitant administration of probenecid with cefuroxime axetil tablets increases the area under the serum concentration versus time curve by 50%. The peak serum cefuroxime concentration after a 1.5-g single dose is greater when taken with 1 g of probenecid (mean = 14.8 mcg/mL) than without probenecid (mean = 12.2 mcg/mL).

Drugs that reduce gastric acidity may result in a lower bioavailability of CEFTIN compared with that of fasting state and tend to cancel the effect of postprandial absorption.

In common with other antibiotics, cefuroxime axetil may affect the gut flora, leading to lower estrogen reabsorption and reduced efficacy of combined oral estrogen/progesterone contraceptives.

Carcinogenesis, Mutagenesis, Impairment of Fertility
Although lifetime studies in animals have not been performed to evaluate carcinogenic potential, no mutagenic activity was found for cefuroxime axetil in a battery of bacterial mutation tests. Positive results were obtained in an in vitro chromosome aberration assay; however, negative results were found in an in vivo micronucleus test at doses up to 1.5 g/kg. Reproduction studies in rats at doses up to 1,000 mg/kg/day (9 times the recommended maximum human dose based on mg/m²) have revealed no impairment of fertility.

Pregnancy
Teratogenic Effects
Pregnancy Category B. Reproduction studies have been performed in mice at doses up to 3,200 mg/kg/day (14 times the recommended maximum human dose based on mg/m²) and in rats at doses up to 1,000 mg/kg/day (9 times the recommended maximum human dose based on mg/m²) and have revealed no evidence of impaired fertility or harm to the fetus due to cefuroxime axetil. There are, however, no adequate and well-controlled studies in pregnant women. Because animal reproduction studies are not always predictive of human response, this drug should be used during pregnancy only if clearly needed.

Labor and Delivery
Cefuroxime axetil has not been studied for use during labor and delivery.

Nursing Mothers
Because cefuroxime is excreted in human milk, consideration should be given to discontinuing nursing temporarily during treatment with cefuroxime axetil.

Pediatric Use
The safety and effectiveness of CEFTIN have been established for pediatric patients aged 3 months to 12 years for acute bacterial maxillary sinusitis based upon its approval in adults. Use of CEFTIN in pediatric patients is supported by pharmacokinetic and safety data in adults and pediatric patients, and by clinical and microbiological data from adequate and well-controlled studies of the treatment of acute bacterial maxillary sinusitis in adults and of acute otitis media with effusion in pediatric patients. It is also supported by postmarketing adverse events surveillance *(see CLINICAL PHARMACOLOGY, INDICATIONS AND USAGE, ADVERSE REACTIONS, DOSAGE AND ADMINISTRATION, and CLINICAL STUDIES).*

Geriatric Use
Of the total number of subjects who received cefuroxime axetil in 20 clinical studies of CEFTIN, 375 were 65 and older while 151 were 75 and older. No overall differences in safety or effectiveness were observed between these subjects and younger adult subjects. The geriatric patients reported somewhat fewer gastrointestinal events and less frequent vaginal candidiasis compared with patients aged 12 to 64 years old; however, no clinically significant differences were

reported between the elderly and younger adult patients. Other reported clinical experience has not identified differences in responses between the elderly and younger adult patients.

ADVERSE REACTIONS
CEFTIN TABLETS IN CLINICAL TRIALS
Multiple-Dose Dosing Regimens
7 to 10 Days Dosing
Using multiple doses of cefuroxime axetil tablets, 912 patients were treated with cefuroxime axetil (125 to 500 mg twice daily). There were no deaths or permanent disabilities thought related to drug toxicity. Twenty (2.2%) patients discontinued medication due to adverse events thought by the investigators to be possibly, probably, or almost certainly related to drug toxicity. Seventeen (85%) of the 20 patients who discontinued therapy did so because of gastrointestinal disturbances, including diarrhea, nausea, vomiting, and abdominal pain. The percentage of cefuroxime axetil tablet-treated patients who discontinued study drug because of adverse events was very similar at daily doses of 1,000, 500, and 250 mg (2.3%, 2.1%, and 2.2%, respectively). However, the incidence of gastrointestinal adverse events increased with the higher recommended doses.

The following adverse events were thought by the investigators to be possibly, probably, or almost certainly related to cefuroxime axetil tablets in multiple-dose clinical trials (n = 912 cefuroxime axetil-treated patients).

Table 4. Adverse Reactions--CEFTIN Tablets

Multiple-Dose Dosing Regimens--Clinical Trials

Incidence ≥1%	Diarrhea/loose stools 3.7% Nausea/vomiting 3.0% Transient elevation in AST 2.0% Transient elevation in ALT 1.6% Eosinophilia 1.1% Transient elevation in LDH 1.0%
Incidence <1% but >0.1%	Abdominal pain Abdominal cramps Flatulence Indigestion Headache Vaginitis Vulvar itch Rash Hives Itch Dysuria Chills Chest pain Shortness of breath Mouth ulcers Swollen tongue Sleepiness Thirst Anorexia Positive Coombs test

5-Day Experience (see CLINICAL STUDIES)
In clinical trials using CEFTIN in a dose of 250 mg twice daily in the treatment of secondary bacterial infections of acute bronchitis, 399 patients were treated for 5 days and 402 patients were treated for 10 days. No difference in the occurrence of adverse events was found between the 2 regimens.

In Clinical Trials for Early Lyme Disease With 20 Days Dosing
Two multicenter trials assessed cefuroxime axetil tablets 500 mg twice a day for 20 days. The most common drug-related adverse experiences were diarrhea (10.6% of patients), Jarisch-Herxheimer reaction (5.6%), and vaginitis (5.4%). Other adverse experiences occurred with frequencies comparable to those reported with 7 to 10 days dosing.

Single-Dose Regimen for Uncomplicated Gonorrhea
In clinical trials using a single dose of cefuroxime axetil tablets, 1,061 patients were treated with the recommended dosage of cefuroxime axetil (1,000 mg) for the treatment of uncomplicated gonorrhea. There were no deaths or permanent disabilities thought related to drug toxicity in these studies.

The following adverse events were thought by the investigators to be possibly, probably, or almost certainly related to cefuroxime axetil in 1,000-mg single-dose clinical trials of cefuroxime axetil tablets in the treatment of uncomplicated gonorrhea conducted in the United States.

Table 5. Adverse Reactions--CEFTIN Tablets

1-g Single-Dose Regimen for Uncomplicated Gonorrhea— Clinical Trials

Incidence ≥1%	Nausea/vomiting 6.8%
	Diarrhea 4.2%
Incidence <1% but >0.1%	Abdominal pain
	Dyspepsia
	Erythema
	Rash
	Pruritus
	Vaginal candidiasis
	Vaginal itch
	Vaginal discharge
	Headache
	Dizziness
	Somnolence
	Muscle cramps
	Muscle stiffness
	Muscle spasm of neck
	Tightness/pain in chest
	Bleeding/pain in urethra
	Kidney pain
	Tachycardia
	Lockjaw-type reaction

CEFTIN FOR ORAL SUSPENSION IN CLINICAL TRIALS

In clinical trials using multiple doses of cefuroxime axetil powder for oral suspension, pediatric patients (96.7% of whom were younger than 12 years of age) were treated with the recommended dosages of cefuroxime axetil (20 to 30 mg/kg/day divided twice a day up to a maximum dose of 500 or 1,000 mg/day, respectively). There were no deaths or permanent disabilities in any of the patients in these studies. Eleven US patients (1.2%) discontinued medication due to adverse events thought by the investigators to be possibly, probably, or almost certainly related to drug toxicity. The discontinuations were primarily for gastrointestinal disturbances, usually diarrhea or vomiting. During clinical trials, discontinuation of therapy due to the taste and/or problems with administering this drug occurred in 13 (1.4%) pediatric patients enrolled at centers in the United States.
The following adverse events were thought by the investigators to be possibly, probably, or almost certainly related to cefuroxime axetil for oral suspension in multiple-dose clinical trials (n = 931 cefuroxime axetil-treated US patients).

Table 6. Adverse Reactions—CEFTIN for Oral Suspension

Multiple-Dose Dosing Regimens—Clinical Trials

Incidence ≥1%	Diarrhea/loose stools 8.6%
	Dislike of taste 5.0%
	Diaper rash 3.4%
	Nausea/vomiting 2.6%
Incidence <1% but >0.1%	Abdominal pain
	Flatulence
	Gastrointestinal infection
	Candidiasis
	Vaginal irritation
	Rash
	Hyperactivity
	Irritable behavior
	Eosinophilia
	Positive direct Coombs test
	Elevated liver enzymes
	Viral illness
	Upper respiratory infection
	Sinusitis
	Cough
	Urinary tract infection
	Joint swelling
	Arthralgia
	Fever
	Ptyalism

POSTMARKETING EXPERIENCE WITH CEFTIS

In addition to adverse events reported during clinical trials, the following events have been identified during clinical practice in patients treated with CEFTIN Tablets or CEFTIN for Oral Suspension and were reported spontaneously. Data are generally insufficient to allow an estimate of incidence or to establish causation.

General
The following hypersensitivity reactions have been reported: Anaphylaxis, angioedema, pruritus, rash, serum sickness-like reaction, urticaria.

Gastrointestinal
Pseudomembranous colitis (*see WARNINGS*).
Hematologic
Hemolytic anemia, leukopenia, pancytopenia, thrombocytopenia, and increased prothrombin time.
Hepatic
Hepatic impairment including hepatitis and cholestasis, jaundice.
Neurologic
Seizure.
Skin
Erythema multiforme, Stevens-Johnson syndrome, toxic epidermal necrolysis.
Urologic
Renal dysfunction.

CEPHALOSPORIN-CLASS ADVERSE REACTIONS

In addition to the adverse reactions listed above that have been observed in patients treated with cefuroxime axetil, the following adverse reactions and altered laboratory tests have been reported for cephalosporin-class antibiotics: Toxic nephropathy, aplastic anemia, hemorrhage, increased BUN, increased creatinine, false-positive test for urinary glucose, increased alkaline phosphatase, neutropenia, elevated bilirubin, and agranulocytosis.
Several cephalosporins have been implicated in triggering seizures, particularly in patients with renal impairment when the dosage was not reduced (*see DOSAGE AND ADMINISTRATION and OVERDOSAGE*). If seizures associated with drug therapy occur, the drug should be discontinued. Anticonvulsant therapy can be given if clinically indicated.

OVERDOSAGE

Overdosage of cephalosporins can cause cerebral irritation leading to convulsions. Serum levels of cefuroxime can be reduced by hemodialysis and peritoneal dialysis.

DOSAGE AND ADMINISTRATION

NOTE: CEFTIN TABLETS AND CEFTIN FOR ORAL SUSPENSION ARE NOT BIOEQUIVALENT AND ARE NOT SUBSTITUTABLE ON A MILLIGRAM-PER-MILLIGRAM BASIS (*SEE CLINICAL PHARMACOLOGY*).

Table 7. CEFTIN Tablets

(May be administered without regard to meals.)

Population/Infection	Dosage	Duration (days)
Adolescents and Adults (13 years and older)		
Pharyngitis/tonsillitis	250 mg b.i.d.	10
Acute bacterial maxillary sinusitis	250 mg b.i.d.	10
Acute bacterial exacerbations of chronic bronchitis	250 or 500 mg b.i.d.	10[a]
Secondary bacterial infections of acute bronchitis	250 or 500 mg b.i.d.	5-10
Uncomplicated skin and skin-structure infections	250 or 500 mg b.i.d.	10
Uncomplicated urinary tract infections	250 mg b.i.d.	7-10
Uncomplicated gonorrhea	1,000 mg once	single dose
Early Lyme disease	500 mg b.i.d.	20
Pediatric Patients (who can swallow tablets whole)		
Acute otitis media	250 mg b.i.d.	10
Acute bacterial maxillary sinusitis	250 mg b.i.d.	10

[a]The safety and effectiveness of CEFTIN administered for less than 10 days in patients with acute exacerbations of chronic bronchitis have not been established.

CEFTIN for Oral Suspension
CEFTIN for Oral Suspension may be administered to pediatric patients ranging in age from 3 months to 12 years, according to dosages in Table 8:

Table 8. CEFTIN for Oral Suspension

(Must be administered with food. Shake well each time before using.)

Population/Infection	Dosage	Daily Maximum Dose	Duration (days)
Pediatric Patients (3 months to 12 years)			
Pharyngitis/tonsillitis	20 mg/kg/day divided b.i.d.	500 mg	10
Acute otitis media	30 mg/kg/day divided b.i.d.	1,000 mg	10
Acute bacterial maxillary sinusitis	30 mg/kg/day divided b.i.d.	1,000 mg	10
Impetigo	30 mg/kg/day divided b.i.d.	1,000 mg	10

Patients With Renal Failure
The safety and efficacy of cefuroxime axetil in patients with renal failure have not been established. Since cefuroxime is renally eliminated, its half-life will be prolonged in patients with renal failure.

Directions for Mixing CEFTIN for Oral Suspension
Prepare a suspension at the time of dispensing as follows:
1. Shake the bottle to loosen the powder.
2. Remove the cap.
3. Add the total amount of water for reconstitution (see Table 9) and replace the cap.
4. Invert the bottle and vigorously rock the bottle from side to side so that water rises through the powder.
5. Once the sound of the powder against the bottle disappears, turn the bottle upright and vigorously shake it in a diagonal direction.

Table 9. Amount of Water Required for Reconstitution of Labeled Volumes of CEFTIN for Oral Suspension

CEFTIN for Oral Suspension	Labeled Volume After Reconstitution	Amount of Water Required for Reconstitution
125 mg/5 mL	100 mL	37 mL
250 mg/5 mL	50 mL	19 mL
	100 mL	35 mL

NOTE: SHAKE THE ORAL SUSPENSION WELL BEFORE EACH USE. Replace cap securely after each opening. Store the reconstituted suspension between 2° and 8°C (36° and 46°F) (in a refrigerator). DISCARD AFTER 10 DAYS.

HOW SUPPLIED
CEFTIN Tablets
CEFTIN Tablets, 250 mg of cefuroxime (as cefuroxime axetil), are white, capsule-shaped, film-coated tablets engraved with "GX ES7" on one side and blank on the other side as follows:
20 Tablets/Bottle NDC 0173-0387-00
CEFTIN Tablets, 500 mg of cefuroxime (as cefuroxime axetil), are white, capsule-shaped, film-coated tablets engraved with "GX EG2" on one side and blank on the other side as follows:
20 Tablets/Bottle NDC 0173-0394-00
Store the tablets between 15° and 30°C (59° and 86°F). Replace cap securely after each opening.
CEFTIN for Oral Suspension
CEFTIN for Oral Suspension is provided as dry, white to off-white, tutti-frutti-flavored powder. When reconstituted as directed, CEFTIN for Oral Suspension provides the equivalent of 125 mg or 250 mg of cefuroxime (as cefuroxime axetil) per 5 mL of suspension. It is supplied in amber glass bottles as follows:
125 mg/5 mL:
100-mL Suspension NDC 0173-0740-00
250 mg/5 mL:
50-mL Suspension NDC 0173-0741-10
100-mL Suspension NDC 0173-0741-00
Before reconstitution, store dry powder between 2° and 30°C (36° and 86°F).
After reconstitution, immediately store suspension between 2° and 8°C (36° and 46°F), in a refrigerator. DISCARD AFTER 10 DAYS.

CLINICAL STUDIES

Ceftin Tablets

Acute Bacterial Maxillary Sinusitis

One adequate and well-controlled study was performed in patients with acute bacterial maxillary sinusitis. In this study each patient had a maxillary sinus aspirate collected by sinus puncture before treatment was initiated for presumptive acute bacterial sinusitis. All patients had to have radiographic and clinical evidence of acute maxillary sinusitis. As shown in the following summary of the study, the general clinical effectiveness of CEFTIN Tablets was comparable to an oral antimicrobial agent that contained a specific beta-lactamase inhibitor in treating acute maxillary sinusitis. However, sufficient microbiology data were obtained to demonstrate the effectiveness of CEFTIN Tablets in treating acute bacterial maxillary sinusitis due only to *Streptococcus pneumoniae* or non-beta-lactamase-producing *Haemophilus influenzae*. An insufficient number of beta-lactamase-producing *Haemophilus influenzae* and *Moraxella catarrhalis* isolates were obtained in this trial to adequately evaluate the effectiveness of CEFTIN Tablets in the treatment of acute bacterial maxillary sinusitis due to these 2 organisms.

This study enrolled 317 adult patients, 132 patients in the United States and 185 patients in South America. Patients were randomized in a 1:1 ratio to cefuroxime axetil 250 mg twice daily or an oral antimicrobial agent that contained a specific beta-lactamase inhibitor. An intent-to-treat analysis of the submitted clinical data yielded the following results:

[See table 10 above]

In this trial and in a supporting maxillary puncture trial, 15 evaluable patients had non-beta-lactamase-producing *Haemophilus influenzae* as the identified pathogen. Ten (10) of these 15 patients (67%) had their pathogen (non-beta-lactamase-producing *Haemophilus influenzae*) eradicated. Eighteen (18) evaluable patients had *Streptococcus pneumoniae* as the identified pathogen. Fifteen (15) of these 18 patients (83%) had their pathogen (*Streptococcus pneumoniae*) eradicated.

Safety

The incidence of drug-related gastrointestinal adverse events was statistically significantly higher in the control arm (an oral antimicrobial agent that contained a specific beta-lactamase inhibitor) versus the cefuroxime axetil (12% versus 1%, respectively; $P<.001$), particularly drug-related diarrhea (8% versus 1%, respectively; $P = .001$).

Early Lyme Disease

Two adequate and well-controlled studies were performed in patients with early Lyme disease. In these studies all patients had to present with physician-documented erythema migrans, with or without systemic manifestations of infection. Patients were randomized in a 1:1 ratio to a 20-day course of treatment with cefuroxime axetil 500 mg twice daily or doxycycline 100 mg 3 times daily. Patients were assessed at 1 month posttreatment for success in treating early Lyme disease (Part I) and at 1 year posttreatment for success in preventing the progression to the sequelae of late Lyme disease (Part II).

A total of 355 adult patients (181 treated with cefuroxime axetil and 174 treated with doxycycline) were enrolled in the 2 studies. In order to objectively validate the clinical diagnosis of early Lyme disease in these patients, 2 approaches were used: 1) blinded expert reading of photographs, when available, of the pretreatment erythema migrans skin lesion; and 2) serologic confirmation (using enzyme-linked immunosorbent assay [ELISA] and immunoblot assay ["Western" blot]) of the presence of antibodies specific to *Borrelia burgdorferi*, the etiologic agent of Lyme disease. By these procedures, it was possible to confirm the physician diagnosis of early Lyme disease in 281 (79%) of the 355 study patients. The efficacy data summarized below are specific to this "validated" patient subset, while the safety data summarized below reflect the entire patient population for the 2 studies.

Analysis of the submitted clinical data for evaluable patients in the "validated" patient subset yielded the following results:

[See table 11 above]

CEFTIN and doxycycline were effective in prevention of the development of sequelae of late Lyme disease.

Safety

Drug-related adverse events affecting the skin were reported significantly more frequently by patients treated with doxycycline than by patients treated with cefuroxime axetil (12% versus 3%, respectively; $P = .002$), primarily reflecting the statistically significantly higher incidence of drug-related photosensitivity reactions in the doxycycline arm versus the cefuroxime axetil arm (9% versus 0%, respectively; $P<.001$). While the incidence of drug-related gastrointestinal adverse events was similar in the 2 treatment groups (cefuroxime axetil - 13%; doxycycline - 11%), the incidence of drug-related diarrhea was statistically significantly higher in the cefuroxime axetil arm versus the doxycycline arm (11% versus 3%, respectively; $P = .005$).

Table 10. Clinical Effectiveness of CEFTIN Tablets Compared to Beta-Lactamase Inhibitor-Containing Control Drug in the Treatment of Acute Bacterial Maxillary Sinusitis

	US Patients[a]		South American Patients[b]	
	CEFTIN (n = 49)	Control (n = 43)	CEFTIN (n = 87)	Control (n = 89)
Clinical success (cure + improvement)	65%	53%	77%	74%
Clinical cure	53%	44%	72%	64%
Clinical improvement	12%	9%	5%	10%

[a] 95% Confidence interval around the success difference [-0.08, +0.32].
[b] 95% Confidence interval around the success difference [-0.10, +0.16].

Table 11. Clinical Effectiveness of CEFTIN Tablets Compared to Doxycycline in the Treatment of Early Lyme Disease

	Part I (1 Month Posttreatment)[a]		Part II (1 Year Posttreatment)[b]	
	CEFTIN (n = 125)	Doxycycline (n = 108)	CEFTIN (n = 105[c])	Doxycycline (n = 83[c])
Satisfactory clinical outcome[d]	91%	93%	84%	87%
Clinical cure/success	72%	73%	73%	73%
Clinical improvement	19%	19%	10%	13%

[a] 95% confidence interval around the satisfactory difference for Part I (-0.08, +0.05).
[b] 95% confidence interval around the satisfactory difference for Part II (-0.13, +0.07).
[c] n's include patients assessed as unsatisfactory clinical outcomes (failure + recurrence) in Part I (CEFTIN - 11 [5 failure, 6 recurrence]; doxycycline - 8 [6 failure, 2 recurrence]).
[d] Satisfactory clinical outcome includes cure + improvement (Part I) and success + improvement (Part II).

Table 12. Clinical Effectiveness of CEFTIN Tablets 250 mg Twice Daily in Secondary Bacterial Infections of Acute Bronchitis: Comparison of 5 Versus 10 Days' Treatment Duration

	CAE-516 and CAE-517[a]		CAEA4001 and CAEA4002[b]	
	5 Day (n = 127)	10 Day (n = 139)	5 Day (n = 173)	10 Day (n = 192)
Clinical success (cure + improvement)	80%	87%	84%	82%
Clinical cure	61%	70%	73%	72%
Clinical improvement	19%	17%	11%	10%

[a] 95% Confidence interval around the success difference [-0.164, +0.029].
[b] 95% Confidence interval around the success difference [-0.061, +0.103].

Secondary Bacterial Infections of Acute Bronchitis

Four randomized, controlled clinical studies were performed comparing 5 days versus 10 days of CEFTIN for the treatment of patients with secondary bacterial infections of acute bronchitis. These studies enrolled a total of 1,253 patients (CAE-516 n = 360; CAE-517 n = 177; CAEA4001 n = 362; CAEA4002 n = 354). The protocols for CAE-516 and CAE-517 were identical and compared CEFTIN 250 mg twice daily for 5 days, CEFTIN 250 mg twice daily for 10 days, and AUGMENTIN® 500 mg 3 times daily for 10 days. These 2 studies were conducted simultaneously. CAEA4001 and CAEA4002 compared CEFTIN 250 mg twice daily for 5 days, CEFTIN 250 mg twice daily for 10 days, and CECLOR® 250 mg 3 times daily for 10 days. They were otherwise identical to CAE-516 and CAE-517 and were conducted over the following 2 years. Patients were required to have polymorphonuclear cells present on the Gram stain of their screening sputum specimen, but isolation of a bacterial pathogen from the sputum culture was not required for inclusion. The following table demonstrates the results of the clinical outcome analysis of the pooled studies CAE-516/CAE-517 and CAEA4001/CAEA4002, respectively:

[See table 12 above]

The response rates for patients who were both clinically and bacteriologically evaluable were consistent with those reported for the clinically evaluable patients.

Safety

In these clinical trials, 399 patients were treated with CEFTIN for 5 days and 402 patients with CEFTIN for 10 days. No difference in the occurrence of adverse events was observed between the 2 regimens.

REFERENCES

1. National Committee for Clinical Laboratory Standards. *Methods for Dilution Antimicrobial Susceptibility Tests for Bacteria that Grow Aerobically*. 3rd ed. Approved Standard NCCLS Document M7-A3, Vol. 13, No. 25. Villanova, Pa: NCCLS; 1993.

2. National Committee for Clinical Laboratory Standards. *Performance Standards for Antimicrobial Disk Susceptibility Tests*. 4th ed. Approved Standard NCCLS Document M2-A4, Vol. 10, No. 7. Villanova, Pa: NCCLS; 1990.

CEFTIN and AUGMENTIN are registered trademarks of GlaxoSmithKline.

CLINITEST and CLINISTIX are registered trademarks of Ames Division, Miles Laboratories, Inc.

GlaxoSmithKline
Research Triangle Park, NC 27709
©2009, GlaxoSmithKline
All rights reserved.
January 2010 CFT:1PI

CERVARIX   ℞

[serv'-ah-rix]
[Human Papillomavirus Bivalent (Types 16 and 18) Vaccine, Recombinant]
Suspension for Intramuscular Injection

HIGHLIGHTS OF PRESCRIBING INFORMATION

These highlights do not include all the information needed to use CERVARIX safely and effectively. See full prescribing information for CERVARIX.

CERVARIX [Human Papillomavirus Bivalent (Types 16 and 18) Vaccine, Recombinant]
Suspension for Intramuscular Injection
Initial U.S. Approval: 2009

——————INDICATIONS AND USAGE——————

CERVARIX is a vaccine indicated for the prevention of the following diseases caused by oncogenic human papillomavirus (HPV) types 16 and 18:
• cervical cancer,
• cervical intraepithelial neoplasia (CIN) grade 2 or worse and adenocarcinoma *in situ*, and
• cervical intraepithelial neoplasia (CIN) grade 1. (1.1)

Help Patients Save on Rx Drugs: PDR.net/PharmacyDiscountCard

CERVARIX is approved for use in females 9 through 25 years of age.
Limitations of Use and Effectiveness (1.2)
• CERVARIX does not provide protection against disease due to all HPV types. (14.3)
• CERVARIX has not been demonstrated to provide protection against disease from vaccine and non-vaccine HPV types to which a woman has previously been exposed through sexual activity. (14.2)

———DOSAGE AND ADMINISTRATION———
Three doses (0.5-mL each) by intramuscular injection according to the following schedule: 0, 1, and 6 months. (2.2)

———DOSAGE FORMS AND STRENGTHS———
Single-dose prefilled syringes containing a 0.5-mL suspension for injection. (3)

———CONTRAINDICATIONS———
Severe allergic reactions (e.g., anaphylaxis) to any component of CERVARIX. (4)

———WARNINGS AND PRECAUTIONS———
• Because vaccinees may develop syncope, sometimes resulting in falling with injury, observation for 15 minutes after administration is recommended. Syncope, sometimes associated with tonic-clonic movements and other seizure-like activity, has been reported following vaccination with CERVARIX. When syncope is associated with tonic-clonic movements, the activity is usually transient and typically responds to restoring cerebral perfusion by maintaining a supine or Trendelenburg position. (5.1)
• The tip caps of the prefilled syringes may contain natural rubber latex which may cause allergic reactions in latex-sensitive individuals. (5.2)

———ADVERSE REACTIONS———
• Most common local adverse reactions in ≥20% of subjects were pain, redness, and swelling at the injection site. (6.1)
• Most common general adverse events in ≥20% of subjects were fatigue, headache, myalgia, gastrointestinal symptoms, and arthralgia. (6.1)
To report SUSPECTED ADVERSE REACTIONS, contact GlaxoSmithKline at 1-888-825-5249 or VAERS at 1-800-822-7967 or www.vaers.hhs.gov

———DRUG INTERACTIONS———
Do not mix CERVARIX with any other vaccine in the same syringe or vial. (7.1)

———USE IN SPECIFIC POPULATIONS———
• Safety has not been established in pregnant women. Register women who receive CERVARIX while pregnant in the pregnancy registry by calling 1-888-452-9622. (8.1)
• Immunocompromised individuals may have a reduced immune response to CERVARIX. (8.6)
See 17 for PATIENT COUNSELING INFORMATION and FDA-approved patient labeling

Revised: 07/2014

FULL PRESCRIBING INFORMATION: CONTENTS*

Table 1. Rates of Solicited Local Adverse Reactions and General Adverse Events in Females 9 Through 25 Years of Age Within 7 Days of Vaccination (Total Vaccinated Cohort[a])

	CERVARIX (9-25 years) %	HAV 720[b] (15-25 years) %	HAV 360[c] (10-14 years) %	Al(OH)$_3$ Control[d] (15-25 years) %
Local Adverse Reaction	N = 6,669	N = 3,079	N = 1,027	N = 549
Pain	91.9	78.0	64.2	87.2
Redness	48.4	27.6	25.2	24.4
Swelling	44.3	19.8	17.3	21.3
General Adverse Event	N = 6,670	N = 3,079	N = 1,027	N = 549
Fatigue	54.6	53.7	42.3	53.6
Headache	53.4	51.3	45.2	61.4
GI[e]	27.9	27.3	24.6	32.8
Fever (≥99.5°F)	12.9	10.9	16.0	13.5
Rash	9.5	8.4	6.7	10.0
	N = 6,119	N = 3,079	N = 1,027	—
Myalgia[f]	48.8	44.9	33.1	—
Arthralgia[f]	20.7	17.9	19.9	—
Urticaria[f]	7.2	7.9	5.4	—

[a]Total vaccinated cohort included subjects with at least one documented dose (N).
[b]HAV 720 = Hepatitis A Vaccine control group [720 EL.U. of antigen and 500 mcg Al(OH)$_3$].
[c]HAV 360 = Hepatitis A Vaccine control group [360 EL.U. of antigen and 250 mcg of Al(OH)$_3$].
[d]Al(OH)$_3$ Control = control containing 500 mcg Al(OH)$_3$.
[e]GI = Gastrointestinal symptoms, including nausea, vomiting, diarrhea, and/or abdominal pain.
[f]Adverse events solicited in a subset of subjects.

FULL PRESCRIBING INFORMATION

1   INDICATIONS AND USAGE
1.1   Indications
CERVARIX® is indicated for the prevention of the following diseases caused by oncogenic human papillomavirus (HPV) types 16 and 18 [see Clinical Studies (14)]:
• cervical cancer,
• cervical intraepithelial neoplasia (CIN) grade 2 or worse and adenocarcinoma in situ, and
• cervical intraepithelial neoplasia (CIN) grade 1.
CERVARIX is approved for use in females 9 through 25 years of age.
1.2   Limitations of Use and Effectiveness
CERVARIX does not provide protection against disease due to all HPV types [see Clinical Studies (14.3)].
CERVARIX has not been demonstrated to provide protection against disease from vaccine and non-vaccine HPV types to which a woman has previously been exposed through sexual activity [see Clinical Studies (14.2)].
Females should continue to adhere to recommended cervical cancer screening procedures [see Patient Counseling Information (17)].
Vaccination with CERVARIX may not result in protection in all vaccine recipients.

2   DOSAGE AND ADMINISTRATION
2.1   Preparation for Administration
Shake syringe well before withdrawal and use. Parenteral drug products should be inspected visually for particulate matter and discoloration prior to administration, whenever solution and container permit. If either of these conditions exists, the vaccine should not be administered. With thorough agitation, CERVARIX is a homogeneous, turbid, white suspension. Do not administer if it appears otherwise. Attach a sterile needle and administer intramuscularly.

Do not administer this product intravenously, intradermally, or subcutaneously.
2.2   Dose and Schedule
Immunization with CERVARIX consists of 3 doses of 0.5-mL each, by intramuscular injection according to the following schedule: 0, 1, and 6 months. The preferred site of administration is the deltoid region of the upper arm.

3   DOSAGE FORMS AND STRENGTHS
CERVARIX is a suspension for intramuscular injection available in 0.5-mL single-dose prefilled TIP-LOK® syringes.

4   CONTRAINDICATIONS
Severe allergic reactions (e.g., anaphylaxis) to any component of CERVARIX [see Description (11)].

5   WARNINGS AND PRECAUTIONS
5.1   Syncope
Because vaccinees may develop syncope, sometimes resulting in falling with injury, observation for 15 minutes after administration is recommended. Syncope, sometimes associated with tonic-clonic movements and other seizure-like activity, has been reported following vaccination with CERVARIX. When syncope is associated with tonic-clonic movements, the activity is usually transient and typically responds to restoring cerebral perfusion by maintaining a supine or Trendelenburg position.
5.2   Latex
The tip caps of the prefilled syringes may contain natural rubber latex which may cause allergic reactions in latex-sensitive individuals.
5.3   Preventing and Managing Allergic Vaccine Reactions
Prior to administration, the healthcare provider should review the immunization history for possible vaccine hypersensitivity and previous vaccination-related adverse reactions to allow an assessment of benefits and risks. Appropriate medical treatment and supervision should be readily available in case of anaphylactic reactions following administration of CERVARIX.

6   ADVERSE REACTIONS
The most common local adverse reactions (≥20% of subjects) were pain, redness, and swelling at the injection site.
The most common general adverse events (≥20% of subjects) were fatigue, headache, myalgia, gastrointestinal symptoms, and arthralgia.
6.1   Clinical Studies Experience
Because clinical trials are conducted under widely varying conditions, adverse reaction rates observed in the clinical

Table 2. Rates of Solicited Local Adverse Reactions in Females 9 Through 25 Years of Age by Dose Within 7 Days of Vaccination (Total Vaccinated Cohort[a])

	CERVARIX (9-25 years) %			HAV 720[b] (15-25 years) %			HAV 360[c] (10-14 years) %			Al(OH)$_3$ Control[d] (15-25 years) %		
	Post-Dose			Post-Dose			Post-Dose			Post-Dose		
	1	2	3	1	2	3	1	2	3	1	2	3
N	6,653	6,428	6,168	3,070	2,919	2,758	1,027	1,021	1,011	546	521	500
Pain	87.0	76.4	78.5	65.6	54.4	56.1	48.5	38.5	36.9	79.1	66.8	72.4
Pain, Grade 3[e]	7.5	5.6	7.7	2.0	1.4	2.0	0.8	0.2	1.6	9.0	6.0	8.6
Redness	28.4	30.1	35.7	16.6	15.2	16.1	15.6	13.3	12.1	11.5	11.5	15.6
Redness, >50 mm	0.2	0.5	1.0	0.1	0.1	0.0	0.1	0.2	0.1	0.2	0.0	0.0
Swelling	22.8	25.5	32.7	10.5	9.4	10.5	9.4	8.6	7.6	10.3	10.4	12.0
Swelling, >50 mm	1.1	1.0	1.3	0.2	0.2	0.2	0.4	0.3	0.0	0.0	0.0	0.0

[a]Total vaccinated cohort included subjects with at least one documented dose (N).
[b]HAV 720 = Hepatitis A Vaccine control group [720 EL.U. of antigen and 500 mcg Al(OH)$_3$].
[c]HAV 360 = Hepatitis A Vaccine control group [360 EL.U. of antigen and 250 mcg of Al(OH)$_3$].
[d]Al(OH)$_3$ Control = control containing 500 mcg Al(OH)$_3$.
[e]Defined as spontaneously painful or pain that prevented normal daily activities.

trials of a vaccine cannot be directly compared with rates in the clinical trials of another vaccine, and may not reflect the rates observed in practice. There is the possibility that broad use of CERVARIX could reveal adverse reactions not observed in clinical trials.

Studies in Females 9 Through 25 Years of Age: The safety of CERVARIX was evaluated by pooling data from controlled and uncontrolled clinical trials involving 23,952 females 9 through 25 years of age in the pre-licensure clinical development program. In these studies, 13,024 females (9 through 25 years of age) received at least one dose of CERVARIX and 10,928 females received at least one dose of a control [Hepatitis A Vaccine containing 360 EL.U. (10 through 14 years of age), Hepatitis A Vaccine containing 720 EL.U. (15 through 25 years of age), or Al(OH)$_3$ (500 mcg, 15 through 25 years of age)].

Data on solicited local and general adverse events were collected by subjects or parents using standardized diary cards for 7 consecutive days following each vaccine dose (i.e., day of vaccination and the next 6 days). Unsolicited adverse events were recorded with diary cards for 30 days following each vaccination (day of vaccination and 29 subsequent days). Parents and/or subjects were also asked at each study visit about the occurrence of any adverse events and instructed to immediately report serious adverse events throughout the study period. These studies were conducted in North America, Latin America, Europe, Asia, and Australia. Overall, the majority of subjects were white (59.5%), followed by Asian (25.9%), Hispanic (8.5%), black (3.4%), and other racial/ethnic groups (2.7%).

Solicited Adverse Events: The reported frequencies of solicited local injection site reactions (pain, redness, and swelling) and general adverse events (fatigue, fever, gastrointestinal symptoms, headache, arthralgia, myalgia, and urticaria) within 7 days after vaccination in females 9 through 25 years of age are presented in Table 1. An analysis of solicited local injection site reactions by dose is presented in Table 2. Local reactions were reported more frequently with CERVARIX when compared with the control groups; in ≥76% of recipients of CERVARIX, these local reactions were mild to moderate in intensity. Compared with dose 1, pain was reported less frequently after doses 2 and 3 of CERVARIX, in contrast to redness and swelling where there was a small increased incidence. There was no increase in the frequency of general adverse events with successive doses.

[See table 1 at top of previous page]
[See table 2 above]

The pattern of solicited local adverse reactions and general adverse events following administration of CERVARIX was similar between the age cohorts (9 through 14 years and 15 through 25 years).

Unsolicited Adverse Events: The frequency of unsolicited adverse events that occurred within 30 days of vaccination (≥1% for CERVARIX and greater than any of the control groups) in females 9 through 25 years of age are presented in Table 3.

[See table 3 below]

New Onset Autoimmune Diseases (NOADs): The pooled safety database, which included controlled and uncontrolled trials which enrolled females 9 through 25 years of age, was searched for new medical conditions indicative of potential new onset autoimmune diseases. Overall, the incidence of

potential NOADs, as well as NOADs, in the group receiving CERVARIX was 0.8% (96/12,772) and comparable to the pooled control group (0.8%, 87/10,730) during the 4.3 years of follow-up (Table 4).

In the largest randomized, controlled trial (Study 2) which enrolled females 15 through 25 years of age and which included active surveillance for potential NOADs, the incidence of potential NOADs and NOADs was 0.8% among subjects who received CERVARIX (78/9,319) and 0.8% among subjects who received Hepatitis A Vaccine [720 EL.U. of antigen and 500 mcg Al(OH)$_3$] control (77/9,325).

[See table 4 at top of next page]

Serious Adverse Events: In the pooled safety database, inclusive of controlled and uncontrolled studies, which enrolled females 9 through 72 years of age, 5.3% (864/16,381) of subjects who received CERVARIX and 5.9% (814/13,811) of subjects who received control reported at least one serious adverse event, without regard to causality, during the entire follow-up period (up to 7.4 years).

Among females 9 through 25 years of age enrolled in these clinical studies, 6.3% of subjects who received CERVARIX

and 7.2% of subjects who received the control reported at least one serious adverse event during the entire follow-up period (up to 7.4 years).

Deaths: In completed and ongoing studies which enrolled 57,323 females 9 through 72 years of age, 37 deaths were reported during the 7.4 years of follow-up: 20 in subjects who received CERVARIX (0.06%, 20/33,623) and 17 in subjects who received control (0.07%, 17/23,700). Causes of death among subjects were consistent with those reported in adolescent and adult female populations. The most common causes of death were motor vehicle accident (5 subjects who received CERVARIX; 5 subjects who received control) and suicide (2 subjects who received CERVARIX; 5 subjects who received control), followed by neoplasm (3 subjects who received CERVARIX; 2 subjects who received control), autoimmune disease (3 subjects who received CERVARIX; 1 subject who received control), infectious disease (3 subjects who received CERVARIX; 1 subject who received control), homicide (2 subjects who received CERVARIX; 1 subject who received control), cardiovascular disorders (2 subjects who received CERVARIX), and death of unknown cause (2 subjects who received control). Among females 10 through 25 years

Table 3. Rates of Unsolicited Adverse Events in Females 9 Through 25 Years of Age Within 30 Days of Vaccination (≥1% For CERVARIX and Greater Than HAV 720, HAV 360, or Al(OH)$_3$ Control) (Total Vaccinated Cohort[a])

	CERVARIX % N = 6,893	HAV 720[b] % N = 3,186	HAV 360[c] % N = 1,032	Al(OH)$_3$ Control[d] % N = 581
Headache	5.2	7.6	3.3	9.3
Nasopharyngitis	3.7	3.4	5.9	3.3
Influenza	3.1	5.6	1.3	1.9
Pharyngolaryngeal pain	2.9	2.7	2.2	2.2
Dizziness	2.2	2.6	1.5	3.1
Upper respiratory infection	2.0	1.3	6.7	1.5
Chlamydia infection	1.9	4.4	0.0	0.0
Dysmenorrhea	1.9	2.3	1.9	4.0
Pharyngitis	1.4	1.8	2.2	0.5
Injection site bruising	1.4	1.8	0.7	1.5
Vaginal infection	1.3	2.2	0.1	0.9
Injection site pruritus	1.3	0.5	0.6	0.2
Back pain	1.1	1.3	0.7	3.1
Urinary tract infection	1.0	1.4	0.3	1.2

[a]Total vaccinated cohort included subjects with at least one dose administered (N).
[b]HAV 720 = Hepatitis A Vaccine control group [720 EL.U. of antigen and 500 mcg Al(OH)$_3$].
[c]HAV 360 = Hepatitis A Vaccine control group [360 EL.U. of antigen and 250 mcg of Al(OH)$_3$].
[d]Al(OH)$_3$ Control = control containing 500 mcg Al(OH)$_3$.

Table 4. Incidence of New Medical Conditions Indicative of Potential New Onset Autoimmune Disease and New Onset Autoimmune Disease Throughout the Follow-up Period Regardless of Causality in Females 9 Through 25 Years of Age (Total Vaccinated Cohort[a])

	CERVARIX N = 12,772	Pooled Control Group[b] N = 10,730
	n (%)[c]	n (%)[c]
Total Number of Subjects With at Least One Medical Condition	96 (0.8)	87 (0.8)
Arthritis[d]	9 (0.1)	4 (0.0)
Celiac disease	2 (0.0)	5 (0.0)
Dermatomyositis	0 (0.0)	1 (0.0)
Diabetes mellitus insulin-dependent (Type 1 or unspecified)	5 (0.0)	5 (0.0)
Erythema nodosum	3 (0.0)	0 (0.0)
Hyperthyroidism[e]	15 (0.1)	15 (0.1)
Hypothyroidism[f]	30 (0.2)	28 (0.3)
Inflammatory bowel disease[g]	8 (0.1)	4 (0.0)
Multiple sclerosis	4 (0.0)	1 (0.0)
Myelitis transverse	1 (0.0)	0 (0.0)
Optic neuritis/Optic neuritis retrobulbar	3 (0.0)	1 (0.0)
Psoriasis[h]	8 (0.1)	11 (0.1)
Raynaud's phenomenon	0 (0.0)	1 (0.0)
Rheumatoid arthritis	4 (0.0)	3 (0.0)
Systemic lupus erythematosus[i]	2 (0.0)	3 (0.0)
Thrombocytopenia[j]	1 (0.0)	1 (0.0)
Vasculitis[k]	1 (0.0)	3 (0.0)
Vitiligo	2 (0.0)	2 (0.0)

[a]Total vaccinated cohort included subjects with at least one documented dose (N).
[b]Pooled Control Group = Hepatitis A Vaccine control group [720 EL.U. of antigen and 500 mcg Al(OH)$_3$], Hepatitis A Vaccine control group [360 EL.U. of antigen and 250 mcg of Al(OH)$_3$], and a control containing 500 mcg Al(OH)$_3$.
[c]n (%): number and percentage of subjects with medical condition.
[d]Term includes reactive arthritis and arthritis.
[e]Term includes Basedow's disease, goiter, and hyperthyroidism.
[f]Term includes thyroiditis, autoimmune thyroiditis, and hypothyroidism.
[g]Term includes colitis ulcerative, Crohn's disease, proctitis ulcerative, and inflammatory bowel disease.
[h]Term includes psoriatic arthropathy, nail psoriasis, guttate psoriasis, and psoriasis.
[i]Term includes systemic lupus erythematosus and cutaneous lupus erythematosus.
[j]Term includes idiopathic thrombocytopenic purpura and thrombocytopenia.
[k]Term includes leukocytoclastic vasculitis and vasculitis.

of age, 31 deaths were reported (0.05%, 16/29,467 of subjects who received CERVARIX and 0.07%, 15/20,192 of subjects who received control).

6.2   Postmarketing Experience
In addition to reports in clinical trials, worldwide voluntary reports of adverse events received for CERVARIX since market introduction (2007) are listed below. This list includes serious events or events which have suspected causal association to CERVARIX. Because these events are reported voluntarily from a population of uncertain size, it is not always possible to reliably estimate their frequency or establish a causal relationship to vaccination.
Blood and Lymphatic System Disorders: Lymphadenopathy.
Immune System Disorders: Allergic reactions (including anaphylactic and anaphylactoid reactions), angioedema, erythema multiforme.
Nervous System Disorders: Syncope or vasovagal responses to injection (sometimes accompanied by tonic-clonic movements).

7   DRUG INTERACTIONS
7.1   Concomitant Vaccine Administration
There are no data to assess the concomitant use of CERVARIX with other vaccines.
Do not mix CERVARIX with any other vaccine in the same syringe or vial.
7.2   Hormonal Contraceptives
Among 7,693 subjects 15 through 25 years of age in Study 2 (CERVARIX, N = 3,821 or Hepatitis A Vaccine 720 EL.U., N = 3,872) who used hormonal contraceptives for a mean of 2.8 years, the observed efficacy of CERVARIX was similar to that observed among subjects who did not report use of hormonal contraceptives.

7.3   Immunosuppressive Therapies
Immunosuppressive therapies, including irradiation, antimetabolites, alkylating agents, cytotoxic drugs, and corticosteroids (used in greater than physiologic doses), may reduce the immune response to CERVARIX [see Use in Specific Populations (8.6)].

8   USE IN SPECIFIC POPULATIONS
8.1   Pregnancy
Pregnancy Category B
Reproduction studies have been performed in rats at a dose approximately 47 times the human dose (on a mg/kg basis) and revealed no evidence of impaired fertility or harm to the fetus due to CERVARIX. There are, however, no adequate and well-controlled studies in pregnant women. Because animal reproduction studies are not always predictive of human response, this drug should be used during pregnancy only if clearly needed.
Non-Clinical Studies: An evaluation of the effect of CERVARIX on embryo-fetal, pre- and post-natal development was conducted using rats. One group of rats was administered CERVARIX 30 days prior to gestation and during the period of organogenesis (gestation days 6, 8, 11, and 15). A second group of rats was administered saline at 30 days prior to gestation followed by CERVARIX on days 6, 8, 11, and 15 of gestation. Two additional groups of rats received either saline or adjuvant following the same dosing regimen. CERVARIX was administered at 0.1 mL/rat/occasion (approximately 47-fold excess relative to the projected human dose on a mg/kg basis) by intramuscular injection. No adverse effects on mating, fertility, pregnancy, parturition, lactation, or embryo-fetal, pre- and post-natal development were observed. There were no vaccine-related fetal malformations or other evidence of teratogenesis.

Clinical Studies: Overall Outcomes: In clinical studies, pregnancy testing was performed prior to each vaccine administration and vaccination was discontinued if a subject had a positive pregnancy test. In all clinical trials, subjects were instructed to take precautions to avoid pregnancy until 2 months after the last vaccination. During pre-licensure clinical development, a total of 7,276 pregnancies were reported among 3,696 females receiving CERVARIX and 3,580 females receiving a control (Hepatitis A Vaccine 360 EL.U., Hepatitis A Vaccine 720 EL.U., or 500 mcg Al(OH)$_3$). The overall proportions of pregnancy outcomes were similar between treatment groups. The majority of women gave birth to normal infants (62.2% and 62.6% of recipients of CERVARIX and control, respectively). Other outcomes included spontaneous abortion (11.0% and 10.8% of recipients of CERVARIX and control, respectively), elective termination (5.8% and 6.1% of recipients of CERVARIX and control, respectively), abnormal infant other than congenital anomaly (2.8% and 3.2% of recipients of CERVARIX and control, respectively), and premature birth (2.0% and 1.7% of recipients of CERVARIX and control, respectively). Other outcomes (congenital anomaly, stillbirth, ectopic pregnancy, and therapeutic abortion) were reported less frequently in 0.1% to 0.8% of pregnancies in both groups.
Outcomes Around Time of Vaccination: Sub-analyses were conducted to describe pregnancy outcomes in 761 women [N = 396 for CERVARIX and N = 365 pooled control, HAV 360 EL.U., HAV 720 EL.U., and 500 mcg Al(OH)$_3$] who had their last menstrual period within 30 days prior to, or 45 days after a vaccine dose and for whom pregnancy outcome was known. The majority of women gave birth to normal infants (65.2% and 69.3% of recipients of CERVARIX and control, respectively). Spontaneous abortion was reported in a total of 11.7% of subjects (13.6% of recipients of CERVARIX and 9.6% of control recipients) and elective termination was reported in a total of 9.7% of subjects (9.9% of recipients of CERVARIX and 9.6% of control recipients). Abnormal infant other than congenital anomaly was reported in a total of 4.9% of subjects (5.1% of recipients of CERVARIX and 4.7% of control recipients) and premature birth was reported in a total of 2.5% of subjects (2.5% of both groups). Other outcomes (congenital anomaly, stillbirth, ectopic pregnancy, and therapeutic abortion) were reported in 0.3% to 1.8% of pregnancies among recipients of CERVARIX and in 0.3% to 1.4% of pregnancies among control recipients.
It is not known whether the observed numerical imbalance in spontaneous abortions in pregnancies which occurred around the time of vaccination is due to a vaccine-related effect.
Pregnancy Registry: GlaxoSmithKline maintains a surveillance registry to collect data on pregnancy outcomes and newborn health status outcomes following vaccination with CERVARIX during pregnancy. Women who receive CERVARIX during pregnancy should be encouraged to contact GlaxoSmithKline directly or their healthcare provider should contact GlaxoSmithKline by calling 1-888-452-9622.
8.3   Nursing Mothers
In non-clinical studies in rats, serological data suggest a transfer of anti-HPV-16 and anti-HPV-18 antibodies via milk during lactation in rats. Excretion of vaccine-induced antibodies in human milk has not been studied for CERVARIX. Because many drugs are excreted in human milk, caution should be exercised when CERVARIX is administered to a nursing woman.
8.4   Pediatric Use
Safety and effectiveness in pediatric patients younger than 9 years of age have not been established. The safety and effectiveness of CERVARIX have been evaluated in 1,275 subjects 9 through 14 years of age and 6,362 subjects 15 through 17 years of age. [See Adverse Reactions (6.1) and Clinical Studies (14.5).]
8.5   Geriatric Use
Clinical studies of CERVARIX did not include sufficient numbers of subjects 65 years of age and older to determine whether they respond differently from younger subjects. CERVARIX is not approved for use in subjects 65 years of age and older.
8.6   Immunocompromised Individuals
The immune response to CERVARIX may be diminished in immunocompromised individuals [see Drug Interactions (7.3)].

11   DESCRIPTION
CERVARIX [Human Papillomavirus Bivalent (Types 16 and 18) Vaccine, Recombinant] is a non-infectious recombinant, AS04-adjuvanted vaccine that contains recombinant L1 protein, the major antigenic protein of the capsid, of oncogenic HPV types 16 and 18. The L1 proteins are produced in separate bioreactors using the recombinant Baculovirus expression vector system in a serum-free culture media composed of chemically-defined lipids, vitamins, amino acids, and mineral salts. Following replication of the L1 encoding recombinant Baculovirus in Trichoplusia ni insect cells, the L1 protein accumulates in the cytoplasm of the cells. The L1

Table 5. Efficacy of CERVARIX Against Histopathological Lesions Associated With HPV-16 or HPV-18 in Females 15 Through 25 Years of Age (According to Protocol Cohort[a]) (Study 2)

	Final Analysis					End of Study Analysis				
	CERVARIX		Control[b]		% Efficacy (96.1% CI)[c]	CERVARIX		Control[b]		% Efficacy (95% CI)
	N	n	N	n		N	n	N	n	
CIN2/3 or AIS	7,344	4	7,312	56	92.9 (79.9, 98.3)	7,338	5	7,305	97	94.9 (87.7, 98.4)
CIN1/2/3 or AIS	7,344	8	7,312	96	91.7 (82.4, 96.7)	7,338	12	7,305	165	92.8 (87.1, 96.4)

CI = Confidence Interval; n = number of cases.
[a]Subjects (including women who had normal cytology, ASC-US, or LSIL at baseline) who received 3 doses of vaccine and were HPV DNA negative and seronegative at baseline and HPV DNA negative at month 6 for the corresponding HPV type (N).
[b]Hepatitis A Vaccine control group [720 EL.U. of antigen and 500 mcg Al(OH)$_3$].
[c]The 96.1% confidence interval reflected in the final analysis results from statistical adjustment for the previously conducted interim analysis.

Table 6. Efficacy of CERVARIX Against Disease Associated With HPV-16 or HPV-18 in Females 15 Through 25 Years of Age, Regardless of Current or Prior Exposure to Vaccine HPV Types (Study 2)

	Final Analysis					End of Study Analysis				
	CERVARIX		Control[a]		% Efficacy (96.1% CI)[b]	CERVARIX		Control[a]		% Efficacy (95% CI)
	N	n	N	n		N	n	N	n	
CIN1/2/3 or AIS										
Prophylactic Efficacy[c]	5,449	3	5,436	85	96.5 (89.0, 99.4)	5,466	5	5,452	141	96.5 (91.6, 98.9)
HPV-16 or 18 DNA Positive at Baseline[d]	641	90	592	92	--	642	99	593	101	--
Regardless of Baseline Status[e]	8,667	107	8,682	240	55.5[f] (43.2, 65.3)	8,694	121	8,708	324	62.9[f] (54.1, 70.1)
CIN2/3 or AIS										
Prophylactic Efficacy[c]	5,449	1	5,436	63	98.4 (90.4, 100)	5,466	1	5,452	97	99.0 (94.2, 100)
HPV-16 or 18 DNA Positive at Baseline[d]	641	74	592	73	--	642	80	593	82	--
Regardless of Baseline Status[e]	8,667	82	8,682	174	52.8[f] (37.5, 64.7)	8,694	90	8,708	228	60.7[f] (49.6, 69.5)
CIN3 or AIS										
Prophylactic Efficacy[c]	5,449	0	5,436	13	100 (64.7, 100)	5,466	0	5,452	27	100 (85.5, 100)
HPV-16 or 18 DNA Positive at Baseline[d]	641	41	592	38	--	642	48	593	47	--
Regardless of Baseline Status[e]	8,667	43	8,682	65	33.6[f] (-1.1, 56.9)	8,694	51	8,708	94	45.7[f] (22.9, 62.2)

CI = Confidence Interval; n = number of histopathological cases associated with HPV-16 and/or HPV-18.
Table does not include disease due to non-vaccine HPV types.
[a]Hepatitis A Vaccine control group [720 EL.U. of antigen and 500 mcg Al(OH)$_3$].
[b]The 96.1% confidence interval reflected in the final analysis results from statistical adjustment for the previously conducted interim analysis.
[c]TVC naïve: includes all vaccinated subjects (who received at least one dose of vaccine) who had normal cytology, were HPV DNA negative for 14 oncogenic HPV types, and seronegative for HPV-16 and HPV-18 at baseline (N). Case counting started on day 1 after the first dose.
[d]TVC subset: includes all vaccinated subjects (who received at least one dose of vaccine) who were HPV DNA positive for HPV-16 or HPV-18 irrespective of serostatus at baseline (N). Case counting started on day 1 after the first dose.
[e]TVC: includes all vaccinated subjects (who received at least one dose of vaccine) irrespective of HPV DNA status and serostatus at baseline (N). Case counting started on day 1 after the first dose.
[f]Observed vaccine efficacy includes the prophylactic efficacy of CERVARIX and the impact of CERVARIX on the course of infections present at first vaccination.

proteins are released by cell disruption and purified by a series of chromatographic and filtration methods. Assembly of the L1 proteins into virus-like particles (VLPs) occurs at the end of the purification process. The purified, non-infectious VLPs are then adsorbed on to aluminum (as hydroxide salt). The adjuvant system, AS04, is composed of 3-O-desacyl-4'-monophosphoryl lipid A (MPL) adsorbed on to aluminum (as hydroxide salt).

CERVARIX is prepared by combining the adsorbed VLPs of each HPV type together with the AS04 adjuvant system in sodium chloride, sodium dihydrogen phosphate dihydrate, and Water for Injection.

CERVARIX is a sterile suspension for intramuscular injection. Each 0.5-mL dose is formulated to contain 20 mcg of HPV type 16 L1 protein, 20 mcg of HPV type 18 L1 protein, 50 mcg of the 3-O-desacyl-4'-monophosphoryl lipid A (MPL), and 0.5 mg of aluminum hydroxide. Each dose also contains 4.4 mg of sodium chloride and 0.624 mg of sodium dihydrogen phosphate dihydrate. Each dose may also contain residual amounts of insect cell and viral protein (<40 ng) and bacterial cell protein (<150 ng) from the manufacturing process. CERVARIX does not contain a preservative.

The tip caps may contain natural rubber latex; the plungers are not made with natural rubber latex.

12 CLINICAL PHARMACOLOGY

12.1 Mechanism of Action

Animal studies suggest that the efficacy of L1 VLP vaccines may be mediated by the development of IgG neutralizing antibodies directed against HPV-L1 capsid proteins generated as a result of vaccination.

13 NONCLINICAL TOXICOLOGY

13.1 Carcinogenesis, Mutagenesis, Impairment of Fertility

CERVARIX has not been evaluated for its carcinogenic or mutagenic potential. Vaccination of female rats with CERVARIX, at doses shown to be significantly immunogenic in the rat, had no effect on fertility.

14 CLINICAL STUDIES

Cervical intraepithelial neoplasia (CIN) grade 2 and 3 lesions or cervical adenocarcinoma in situ (AIS) are the immediate and necessary precursors of squamous cell carcinoma and adenocarcinoma of the cervix, respectively. Their detection and removal has been shown to prevent cancer. Therefore, CIN2/3 and AIS (precancerous lesions) serve as surrogate markers for the prevention of cervical cancer. In

Table 7. Efficacy of CERVARIX in Prevention of CIN or AIS Irrespective of Any HPV Type in Females 15 Through 25 Years of Age, Regardless of Current or Prior Infection with Vaccine or Non-Vaccine Types (Study 2)

	Final Analysis					End of Study Analysis				
	CERVARIX		Control[a]		% Efficacy (96.1% CI)[b]	CERVARIX		Control[a]		% Efficacy (95% CI)
	N	n	N	n		N	n	N	n	
CIN1/2/3 or AIS										
Prophylactic Efficacy[c]	5,449	106	5,436	211	50.1 (35.9, 61.4)	5,466	174	5,452	346	50.3 (40.2, 58.8)
Irrespective of HPV DNA at Baseline[d]	8,667	451	8,682	577	21.7 (10.7, 31.4)	8,694	579	8,708	798	27.7 (19.5, 35.2)
CIN2/3 or AIS										
Prophylactic Efficacy[c]	5,449	33	5,436	110	70.2 (54.7, 80.9)	5,466	61	5,452	172	64.9 (52.7, 74.2)
Irrespective of HPV DNA at Baseline[d]	8,667	224	8,682	322	30.4 (16.4, 42.1)	8,694	287	8,708	428	33.1 (22.2, 42.6)
CIN3 or AIS										
Prophylactic Efficacy[c]	5,449	3	5,436	23	87.0 (54.9, 97.7)	5,466	3	5,452	44	93.2 (78.9, 98.7)
Irrespective of HPV DNA at Baseline[d]	8,667	77	8,682	116	33.4 (9.1, 51.5)	8,694	86	8,708	158	45.6 (28.8, 58.7)

CI = Confidence Interval; n = number of cases.
[a]Hepatitis A Vaccine control group [720 EL.U. of antigen and 500 mcg Al(OH)$_3$].
[b]The 96.1% confidence interval reflected in the final analysis results from statistical adjustment for the previously conducted interim analysis.
[c]TVC naïve: includes all vaccinated subjects (who received at least one dose of vaccine) who had normal cytology, were HPV DNA negative for 14 oncogenic HPV types (including HPV-16 and HPV-18), and seronegative for HPV-16 and HPV-18 at baseline (N). Case counting started on day 1 after the first dose.
[d]TVC: includes all vaccinated subjects (who received at least one dose of vaccine) irrespective of HPV DNA status and serostatus at baseline (N). Case counting started on day 1 after the first dose.

clinical studies to evaluate the efficacy of CERVARIX, the endpoints were cases of CIN2/3 and AIS associated with HPV-16, HPV-18, and other oncogenic HPV types. Persistent infection with HPV-16 and HPV-18 that lasts for 12 months was also an endpoint.

The efficacy of CERVARIX to prevent histopathologically-confirmed CIN2/3 or AIS was assessed in 2 double-blind, randomized, controlled clinical studies that enrolled a total of 19,778 females 15 through 25 years of age.

Study 1 (HPV 001) enrolled women who were negative for oncogenic HPV DNA (HPV types 16, 18, 31, 33, 35, 39, 45, 51, 52, 56, 58, 59, 66, and 68) in cervical samples, seronegative for HPV-16 and HPV-18 antibodies and had normal cytology. This represents a population presumed "naïve" without current HPV infection at the time of vaccination and without prior exposure to either HPV-16 or HPV-18. Subjects were enrolled in an extended follow-up study (Study 1 extension [HPV 007]) to evaluate the long-term efficacy, immunogenicity, and safety. These subjects have been followed for up to 6.4 years.

In Study 2 (HPV 008), women were vaccinated regardless of baseline HPV DNA status, serostatus or cytology. This study reflects a population of women naïve (without current infection and without prior exposure) or non-naïve (with current infection and/or prior exposure) to HPV. Before vaccination, cervical samples were assessed for oncogenic HPV DNA (HPV types 16, 18, 31, 33, 35, 39, 45, 51, 52, 56, 58, 59, 66, and 68) and serostatus of HPV-16 and HPV-18 antibodies.

In both studies, testing for oncogenic HPV types was conducted using SPF$_{10}$-LiPA$_{25}$ PCR to detect HPV DNA in archived biopsy samples.

14.1 Prophylactic Efficacy Against HPV Types 16 and 18

Study 2: A randomized, double-blind, controlled clinical trial was conducted in which 18,665 healthy females 15 through 25 years of age received CERVARIX or Hepatitis A Vaccine control on a 0-, 1-, and 6-month schedule. Among subjects, 54.8% of subjects were white, 31.5% Asian, 7.1% Hispanic, 3.7% black, and 2.9% were of other racial/ethnic groups.

In this study, women were randomized and vaccinated regardless of baseline HPV DNA status, serostatus or cytology. Women with HPV-16 or HPV-18 DNA present in baseline cervical samples (HPV DNA positive) at study entry were considered currently infected with that specific HPV type. If HPV DNA was not detected by PCR, women were considered HPV DNA negative. Additionally, cervical samples were assessed for cytologic abnormalities and serologic testing was performed for anti-HPV-16 and anti-HPV-18 serum antibodies at baseline. Women with anti-

HPV serum antibodies present were considered to have prior exposure to HPV and characterized as seropositive. Women seropositive for HPV-16 or HPV-18 but DNA negative for that specific serotype were considered as having cleared a previous natural infection. Women without antibodies to HPV-16 and HPV-18 were characterized as seronegative. Before vaccination, 73.6% of subjects were naïve (without current infection [DNA negative] and without prior exposure [seronegative]) to HPV-16 and/or HPV-18.

Efficacy endpoints included histological evaluation of precancerous and dysplastic lesions (CIN grade 1, grade 2, or grade 3), and AIS. Virological endpoints (HPV DNA in cervical samples detected by PCR) included 12-month persistent infection (defined as at least 2 positive specimens for the same HPV type over a minimum interval of 10 months). The according to protocol (ATP) cohort for efficacy analyses for HPV-16 and/or HPV-18 included all subjects who received 3 doses of vaccine, for whom efficacy endpoint measures were available and who were HPV-16 and/or HPV-18 DNA negative and seronegative at baseline and HPV-16 and/or HPV-18 DNA negative at month 6 for the HPV type considered in the analysis. Case counting for the ATP cohort started on day 1 after the third dose of vaccine. This cohort included women who had normal or low-grade cytology (cytological abnormalities including atypical squamous cells of undetermined significance [ASC-US] or low grade squamous intraepithelial lesions [LSIL]) at baseline and excluded women with high-grade cytology.

The total vaccinated cohort (TVC) for each efficacy analysis included all subjects who received at least one dose of the vaccine, for whom efficacy endpoint measures were available, irrespective of their HPV DNA status, cytology, and serostatus at baseline. This cohort included women with or without current HPV infection and/or prior exposure. Case counting for the TVC started on day 1 after the first dose. The TVC naïve is a subset of the TVC that had normal cytology, and were HPV DNA negative for 14 oncogenic HPV types and seronegative for HPV-16 and HPV-18 at baseline. The pre-defined final analysis was event-triggered, i.e., performed when at least 36 CIN2/3 or AIS cases associated with HPV-16 or HPV-18 were accrued in the ATP cohort. The mean follow-up after the first dose was approximately 39 months and included approximately 3,300 women who completed the month 48 visit.

The pre-defined end of study analysis was performed at the end of the 4-year follow-up period (i.e., after all subjects completed the month 48 visit) and included all subjects from the TVC. The mean follow-up after the first dose was approximately 44 months and included approximately 15,600 women who completed the month 48 visit.

CERVARIX was efficacious in the prevention of precancerous lesions or AIS associated with HPV-16 or HPV-18 (Table 5).

[See table 5 at top of previous page]

Since CIN3 or AIS represents a more immediate precursor to cervical cancer, cases of CIN3 or AIS associated with HPV-16 or HPV-18 were evaluated. In the ATP cohort, CERVARIX was efficacious in the prevention of CIN3 or AIS associated with HPV-16 or HPV-18 in the final analysis (80.0% [96.1% CI: 0.3, 98.1]); these results were confirmed in the end of study analysis (91.7% [95% CI: 66.6, 99.1]).

Subjects who were already infected with one vaccine HPV type (16 or 18) prior to vaccination were protected from precancerous lesions or AIS and infection caused by the other vaccine HPV type.

Efficacy of CERVARIX against 12-month persistent infection with HPV-16 or HPV-18 was also evaluated. In the ATP cohort, CERVARIX reduced the incidence of 12-month persistent infection with HPV-16 and/or HPV-18 by 91.4% (96.1% CI: 86.1, 95.0) in the final analysis; these results were confirmed in the end of study analysis (92.9% [95% CI: 89.4, 95.4]).

Immune response following natural infection does not reliably confer protection against future infections. Among subjects who received 3 doses of CERVARIX and who were seropositive at baseline and DNA negative for HPV-16 or HPV-18 at baseline and month 6, CERVARIX reduced the incidence of 12-month persistent infection by 95.8% (96.1% CI: 72.4, 99.9) in the final analysis; these results were confirmed in the end of study analysis (94.0% [95% CI: 76.7, 99.3]). However, the number of cases of CIN2/3 or AIS was too few in these analyses to determine efficacy against histopathological endpoints in this population.

Study 1 and Study 1 Extension: In a second double-blind, randomized, controlled study (Study 1), the efficacy of CERVARIX in the prevention of HPV-16 or HPV-18 incident and persistent infections was compared with aluminum hydroxide control in 1,113 females 15 through 25 years of age. The population was naïve to current oncogenic HPV infection or prior exposure to HPV-16 and HPV-18 at the time of vaccination (total cohort). A total of 776 subjects were enrolled in the extended follow-up study (Study 1 Extension) to evaluate the long-term efficacy, immunogenicity, and safety of CERVARIX. These subjects have been followed for up to 6.4 years.

In Study 1 and Study 1 Extension, with up to 6.4 years of follow-up (mean 5.9 years), in naïve females 15 through 25 years of age, efficacy against CIN2/3 or AIS associated with HPV-16 or HPV-18 was 100% (98.67% CI: 28.4, 100). Efficacy against 12-month persistent infection with HPV-16 or

HPV-18 was 100% (98.67% CI: 74.4, 100). The confidence interval reflected in this final analysis results from statistical adjustment for analyses previously conducted.

14.2 Efficacy Against HPV Types 16 and 18, Regardless of Current Infection or Prior Exposure to HPV-16 or HPV-18

Study 2: The study included women regardless of HPV DNA status (current infection) and serostatus (prior exposure) to vaccine types, HPV-16 or HPV-18 at baseline. Efficacy analyses included lesions arising among women regardless of baseline DNA status and serostatus, including HPV infections present at first vaccination and those from infections acquired after dose 1. In this population which includes naïve (without current infection and prior exposure) and non-naïve women, CERVARIX was efficacious in the prevention of precancerous lesions or AIS associated with HPV-16 or HPV-18 (Table 6).

However, among women HPV DNA positive regardless of serostatus at baseline, there was no clear evidence of efficacy against precancerous lesions or AIS associated with HPV-16 or HPV-18 (Table 6).

[See table 6 at top of page 961]

14.3 Efficacy Against Cervical Disease Irrespective of HPV Type, Regardless of Current or Prior Infection with Vaccine or Non-Vaccine HPV Types

Study 2: The impact of CERVARIX against the overall burden of HPV-related cervical disease results from a combination of prophylactic efficacy against, and disease contribution of, HPV-16, HPV-18, and non-vaccine HPV types.

In the population naïve to oncogenic HPV (TVC naïve), CERVARIX reduced the overall incidence of CIN1/2/3 or AIS, CIN2/3 or AIS, and CIN3 or AIS regardless of the HPV DNA type in the lesion (Table 7). In the population of women naïve and non-naïve (TVC), vaccine efficacy against CIN1/2/3 or AIS, CIN2/3 or AIS, and CIN3 or AIS was demonstrated in all women regardless of HPV DNA type in the lesion (Table 7).

[See table 7 at top of previous page]

In exploratory end of study analyses, CERVARIX reduced definitive cervical therapy procedures (includes loop electrosurgical excision procedure [LEEP], cold-knife Cone, and laser procedures) by 33.2% (95% CI: 20.8, 43.7) in the TVC and by 70.2% (95% CI: 57.8, 79.3) in the TVC naïve.

To assess reductions in disease caused by non-vaccine HPV types, analyses were conducted combining 12 non-vaccine oncogenic HPV types, including and excluding lesions in which HPV-16 or HPV-18 were also detected. Among females who received 3 doses of CERVARIX and were DNA negative for the specific HPV type at baseline and month 6, CERVARIX reduced the incidence of CIN2/3 or AIS in the final analysis by 54.0% (96.1% CI: 34.0, 68.4) and 37.4% (96.1% CI: 7.4, 58.2), respectively. In the end of study analysis, CERVARIX reduced the incidence of CIN2/3 or AIS by 46.8% (95% CI: 30.7, 59.4) and 24.1% (95% CI: -1.5, 43.5), respectively.

End of study analyses were conducted to assess the impact of CERVARIX on CIN2/3 or AIS due to specific non-vaccine HPV types. The ATP cohort for these analyses included all subjects irrespective of serostatus who received 3 doses of CERVARIX and were DNA negative for the specific HPV type at baseline and month 6. These analyses were also conducted in the TVC naïve population.

In analyses including lesions in which HPV-16 or HPV-18 were also detected, vaccine efficacy in prevention of CIN2/3 or AIS associated with HPV-31 was 87.5% (95% CI: 68.3, 96.1) and 89.4% (95% CI: 65.5, 97.9), respectively. In analyses excluding lesions in which HPV-16 or HPV-18 were detected, vaccine efficacy in prevention of CIN2/3 or AIS associated with HPV-31 was 84.3% (95% CI: 59.5, 95.2) and 83.4% (95% CI: 43.3, 96.9), respectively.

14.4 Immunogenicity

The minimum anti-HPV titer that confers protective efficacy has not been determined.

The antibody response to HPV-16 and HPV-18 was measured using a type-specific binding ELISA (developed by GlaxoSmithKline) and a pseudovirion-based neutralization assay (PBNA). In a subset of subjects tested for HPV-16 and HPV-18, the ELISA has been shown to correlate with the PBNA. The scales for these assays are unique to each HPV type and each assay, thus, comparison between HPV types or assays is not appropriate.

Duration of Immune Response: The duration of immunity following a complete schedule of immunization with CERVARIX has not been established. In Study 1 and Study 1 Extension, the immune response against HPV-16 and HPV-18 was evaluated for up to 76 months post-dose 1, in females 15 through 25 years of age. Vaccine-induced geometric mean titers (GMTs) for both HPV-16 and HPV-18 peaked at month 7 and thereafter reached a plateau that was sustained from month 18 up to month 76. At all timepoints, >98% of subjects were seropositive for both HPV-16 (≥8 EL.U./mL, the limit of detection) and HPV-18 (≥7 EL.U./mL, the limit of detection) by ELISA.

In Study 2, immunogenicity was measured by seropositivity rates and GMTs for ELISA and PBNA (Table 8). The ATP

cohort for immunogenicity included all evaluable subjects for whom data concerning immunogenicity endpoint measures were available. These included subjects for whom assay results were available for antibodies against at least one vaccine type. Subjects who acquired either HPV-16 or HPV-18 infection during the trial were excluded.

[See table 8 above]

14.5 Bridging of Efficacy from Women to Adolescent Girls

The immunogenicity of CERVARIX was evaluated in 3 clinical studies involving 1,275 girls 9 through 14 years of age who received at least one dose of CERVARIX.

Study 3 (HPV 013) was a double-blind, randomized, controlled study in which 1,035 subjects received CERVARIX and 1,032 subjects received a Hepatitis A Vaccine 360 EL.U. as the control vaccine with a subset of subjects evaluated for immunogenicity. All initially seronegative subjects in the group who received CERVARIX were seropositive after vaccination, i.e., had levels of antibody greater than the limit of detection of the assay to both HPV-16 (≥8 EL.U./mL) and HPV-18 (≥7 EL.U./mL) antigens. The GMTs for anti-HPV-16 and anti-HPV-18 antibodies in initially seronegative subjects are presented in Table 9.

[See table 9 above]

In Study 4 (HPV 012), the immunogenicity of CERVARIX administered to girls 10 through 14 years of age was compared with that in females 15 through 25 years of age. The immune response in girls 10 through 14 years of age measured one month post-dose 3 was non-inferior to that seen in females 15 through 25 years of age for both HPV-16 and HPV-18 antigens (Table 10).

[See table 10 at top of next page]

In Study 5, a post-hoc analysis compared the immunogenicity of CERVARIX administered to girls 9 through 14 years of age (n = 68) with that in females 15 through 25 years of age (n = 114). In these initially seronegative subjects, the im-

Table 8. Persistence of Anti-HPV Geometric Mean Titers (GMTs) and Seropositivity Rates for HPV-16 and HPV-18 for Initially Seronegative Females 15 Through 25 Years of Age (According to Protocol Cohort for Immunogenicity[a]) (Study 2)

Time Point	N	% Seropositive (95% CI)	GMT (95% CI)
Anti-HPV-16 ELISA[b] (EL.U./mL)			
Month 7	816	99.5	9,120.0 (8,504.9, 9,779.7)
Month 12	793	99.7	3,266.3 (3,043.3, 3,505.6)
Month 24	755	99.9	1,587.7 (1,484.8, 1,697.7)
Month 36	759	100	1,281.7 (1,198.3, 1,370.9)
Month 48	746	100	1,174.3 (1,096.1, 1,258.0)
Anti-HPV-18 ELISA[b] (EL.U./mL)			
Month 7	879	99.4	4,682.9 (4,388.8, 4,996.7)
Month 12	853	100	1,514.7 (1,422.3, 1,613.0)
Month 24	810	99.9	702.2 (655.2, 752.6)
Month 36	817	100	538.1 (502.0, 576.8)
Month 48	806	99.8	476.2 (443.2, 511.6)
Anti-HPV-16 PBNA[c] (ED50)			
Month 7	46	100	26,457.0 (19,167.5, 36,518.6)
Month 12	45	100	7,885.5 (5,500.4, 11,304.8)
Month 24	46	100	3,396.4 (2,388.0, 4,830.6)
Month 36	41	100	2,245.1 (1,616.6, 3,117.9)
Month 48	41	97.6	1,931.1 (1,294.4, 2,880.8)
Anti-HPV-18 PBNA[c] (ED50)			
Month 7	46	100	8,413.9 (6,394.7, 1,1070.7)
Month 12	45	97.8	1,748.2 (1,223.6, 2,497.7)
Month 24	46	100	1,552.5 (1,112.9, 2,165.5)
Month 36	41	100	1,326.9 (948.0, 1,857.3)
Month 48	41	95.1	1,078.1 (714.9, 1,625.6)

[a]Subjects who received 3 doses of vaccine for whom assay results were available for at least one post-vaccination antibody measurement (N). Subjects who acquired either HPV-16 or HPV-18 infection during the study were excluded.
[b]Enzyme linked immunosorbent assay (assay cut-off 8 EL.U./mL for anti-HPV-16 antibody and 7 EL.U./mL for anti-HPV-18 antibody).
[c]Pseudovirion-based neutralization assay (assay cut-off 40 ED50 for both anti-HPV-16 antibody and anti-HPV-18 antibody).

Table 9. Geometric Mean Titers (GMTs) at Months 7 and 18 for Initially Seronegative Females 10 Through 14 Years of Age (According To Protocol Cohort for Immunogenicity[a]) (Study 3)

Age Group	Anti-HPV-16 Antibodies GMT EL.U./mL (95% CI)			Anti-HPV-18 Antibodies GMT EL.U./mL (95% CI)		
	N	Month 7	Month 18	N	Month 7	Month 18
10-14 years of age	556-619	19,882.0 (18,626.7, 21,221.9)	3,888.8 (3,605.0, 4,195.0)	562-628	8,262.0 (7,725.0, 8,836.2)	1,539.4 (1,418.8, 1,670.3)

[a]Subjects who received 3 doses of vaccine for whom assay results were available for at least one post-vaccination antibody measurement (N).

Table 10. Geometric Mean Titers (GMTs) and Seropositivity Rates at Month 7 for Initially Seronegative Females 10 Through 14 Years of Age Compared With Females 15 Through 25 Years of Age (According To Protocol Cohort for Immunogenicity[a]) (Study 4)

Antibody Assay	10-14 Years of Age			15-25 Years of Age		
	N	GMT[b] EL.U./mL (95% CI)	SeropositivityRate[c] %	N	GMT[b] EL.U./mL (95% CI)	SeropositivityRate[c] %
Anti-HPV-16	143	17,272.5 (15,117.9, 19,734.1)	100	118	7,438.9 (6,324.6, 8,749.6)	100
Anti-HPV-18	141	6,863.8 (5,976.3, 7,883.0)	100	116	3,070.1 (2,600.0, 3,625.4)	100

[a]Subjects who received 3 doses of vaccine for whom assay results were available for at least one post-vaccination antibody measurement (N).

[b]Non-inferiority based on the upper limit of the 2-sided 95% CI for the GMT ratio (15-25 year olds/10-14 year olds) was <2.

[c]Non-inferiority based on the upper limit of the 2-sided 95% CI for the difference between the seropositivity rates for 10-14 year olds and 15-25 year olds was <10%.

mune response in girls 9 through 14 years of age measured one month post-dose 3 was non-inferior to that observed in females 15 through 25 years of age for both HPV-16 and HPV-18 antigens [lower limit of the 2-sided 95% CI for the GMT ratio (9-14 year olds/15-25 year olds) was >0.5]. The GMTs for anti-HPV-16 and anti-HPV-18 antibodies at month 7 were 22,261.3 EL.U./mL and 7,398.8 EL.U./mL, respectively, in girls 9 through 14 years of age and 10,322.0 EL.U./mL and 4,261.5 EL.U./mL, respectively, in females 15 through 25 years of age.

Based on these immunogenicity data, the efficacy of CERVARIX is inferred in girls 9 through 14 years of age.

16 HOW SUPPLIED/STORAGE AND HANDLING

CERVARIX is available in 0.5-mL single-dose disposable prefilled TIP-LOK syringes (packaged without needles): NDC 58160-830-05 Syringe in Package of 1: NDC 58160-830-34

NDC 58160-830-43 Syringe in Package of 10: NDC 58160-830-52

Store refrigerated between 2° and 8°C (36° and 46°F). Do not freeze. Discard if the vaccine has been frozen. Upon storage, a fine, white deposit with a clear, colorless supernatant may be observed. This does not constitute a sign of deterioration.

17 PATIENT COUNSELING INFORMATION

Advise the patient to read the FDA-approved patient labeling (Patient Information). Patient labeling is provided as a tear-off leaflet at the end of this Full Prescribing Information.

Provide the Vaccine Information Statements prior to immunization. These are required by the National Childhood Vaccine Injury Act of 1986 and are available free of charge at the Centers for Disease Control and Prevention (CDC) website (www.cdc.gov/vaccines).

Inform the patient, parent, or guardian:
- Vaccination does not substitute for routine cervical cancer screening. Women who receive CERVARIX should continue to undergo cervical cancer screening per standard of care.
- CERVARIX does not protect against disease from HPV types to which a woman has previously been exposed through sexual activity.
- Since syncope has been reported following vaccination in young females, sometimes resulting in falling with injury, observation for 15 minutes after administration is recommended.
- Safety has not been established in pregnant women. CERVARIX is not recommended for use in pregnant women or women planning to become pregnant during the vaccination course. Register women who receive CERVARIX while pregnant in the pregnancy registry by calling 1-888-452-9622.

CERVARIX and TIP-LOK are registered trademarks of the GSK group of companies.

Manufactured by **GlaxoSmithKline Biologicals**
Rixensart, Belgium, US License 1617
Distributed by **GlaxoSmithKline**
Research Triangle Park, NC 27709
©2014, the GSK group of companies. All rights reserved.
CRX:10PI
PATIENT INFORMATION
CERVARIX®(SERV-ah-rix)
[Human Papillomavirus Bivalent (Types 16 and 18) Vaccine, Recombinant]
Read this Patient Information carefully before getting CERVARIX. You (the person getting CERVARIX) will need 3 doses of the vaccine. Read this information before each dose of CERVARIX. This information does not take the place of talking with your healthcare provider about CERVARIX.

What is CERVARIX?
CERVARIX is a vaccine given by injection (shot) to girls and women 9 through 25 years of age.
- CERVARIX helps protect against cervical cancer and pre-cancers caused by human papillomavirus (HPV) types 16 and 18.
- There are many types of HPV but only certain types cause cervical cancer. HPV types 16 and 18 are the 2 most common types of HPV that lead to cervical cancer and precancers.
- Abnormal Pap smear results can indicate the presence of precancers. Some precancers can lead to cervical cancer.
- CERVARIX is not a treatment for HPV.
- You can not get HPV diseases from CERVARIX.

What important information should I know about CERVARIX?
- You should continue to get routine cervical cancer screening (such as a Pap smear).
- CERVARIX may not fully protect everyone who gets the vaccine.
- Not all cervical cancers are caused by the HPV types CERVARIX protects against. CERVARIX will not protect against diseases from all HPV types.
- CERVARIX will not protect against HPV types that you already have.

Who should not get CERVARIX?
You should not get CERVARIX if you have or have had:
- an allergic reaction to a previous dose of CERVARIX.
- an allergy to any of the ingredients in CERVARIX (listed below).

What should I tell my healthcare provider before getting CERVARIX?
Tell your healthcare provider about all your health conditions, including if you:
- have had an allergic reaction after a previous dose of CERVARIX.
- have an allergy to latex.
- have a weakened immune system.
- are taking any other medicine or have recently gotten any other vaccine.
- have a fever over 100°F (37.8°C).
- are pregnant or are planning to get pregnant during the time period of the 3 shots. CERVARIX is not recommended for use in pregnant women.

Pregnancy Registry: If you are vaccinated during pregnancy, there is a registry. The purpose of the registry is to collect safety information about the health of you and your baby. Contact the registry as soon as you become aware of the pregnancy or ask your healthcare provider to contact the registry for you. You or your healthcare provider can get information and enroll in the registry by calling 1-888-452-9622.

Your healthcare provider will decide if you should get CERVARIX.

How is CERVARIX given?
CERVARIX is given as an injection (shot) in a muscle in your arm.
You will need a total of 3 shots as follows:
- First dose: given at a time decided by you and your healthcare provider
- Second dose: given 1 month after the first dose
- Third dose: given 6 months after the first dose
Fainting may occur, sometimes resulting in falling with injury, especially in young females. Your healthcare provider may ask you to sit or lie down for 15 minutes after you get CERVARIX. Some people who faint may shake or become stiff. If this happens, it may require evaluation or treatment by your healthcare provider.
Make sure you get all 3 shots on time for the best protection. If you miss a scheduled dose, talk to your healthcare provider.

What are the possible side effects of CERVARIX?
The most common side effects of CERVARIX are:
- pain, redness, and swelling where you got the shot
- feeling tired
- headache
- muscle aches
- nausea, vomiting, diarrhea, and stomach pain
- joint aches
Other possible side effects include:
- swollen glands (neck, armpit, or groin).
Call your healthcare provider or seek medical treatment immediately if you develop hives, difficulty breathing, or swelling of the throat, because these may be signs of a severe allergic reaction.
Tell your healthcare provider about these or any other side effects that concern you. For a more complete list of side effects, ask your healthcare provider.

What are the ingredients in CERVARIX?
CERVARIX contains proteins of HPV types 16 and 18. The vaccine also contains 3-*O*-desacyl-4'-monophosphoryl lipid A (MPL), aluminum hydroxide, sodium chloride, and sodium dihydrogen phosphate dehydrate.
CERVARIX contains no preservatives.
This is a summary of information about CERVARIX. If you would like more information, please talk with your healthcare provider or visit www.cervarix.com.
CERVARIX is a registered trademark of the GSK group of companies.
Manufactured by **GlaxoSmithKline Biologicals**
Rixensart, Belgium, US License 1617
Distributed by **GlaxoSmithKline**
Research Triangle Park, NC 27709
©2014, the GSK group of companies. All rights reserved.
July 2014
CRX:4PIL

COREG®   ℞
[kor' eg]
(carvedilol)
tablets

HIGHLIGHTS OF PRESCRIBING INFORMATION
These highlights do not include all the information needed to use COREG safely and effectively. See full prescribing information for COREG.
COREG (carvedilol) tablets
Initial U.S. Approval: 1995

———INDICATIONS AND USAGE———
COREG is an alpha/beta-adrenergic blocking agent indicated for the treatment of:
- Mild to severe chronic heart failure (1.1)
- Left ventricular dysfunction following myocardial infarction in clinically stable patients (1.2)
- Hypertension (1.3)

———DOSAGE AND ADMINISTRATION———
Take with food. Individualize dosage and monitor during up-titration. (2)
- Heart failure: Start at 3.125 mg twice daily and increase to 6.25, 12.5, and then 25 mg twice daily over intervals of at least 2 weeks. Maintain lower doses if higher doses are not tolerated. (2.1)
- Left ventricular dysfunction following myocardial infarction: Start at 6.25 mg twice daily and increase to 12.5 mg then 25 mg twice daily after intervals of 3 to 10 days. A lower starting dose or slower titration may be used. (2.2)
- Hypertension: Start at 6.25 mg twice daily and increase if needed for blood pressure control to 12.5 mg then 25 mg twice daily over intervals of 1 to 2 weeks. (2.3)

———DOSAGE FORMS AND STRENGTHS———
Tablets: 3.125 mg, 6.25 mg, 12.5 mg, 25 mg (3)

———CONTRAINDICATIONS———
- Bronchial asthma or related bronchospastic conditions. (4)
- Second- or third-degree AV block. (4)
- Sick sinus syndrome. (4)
- Severe bradycardia (unless permanent pacemaker in place). (4)
- Patients in cardiogenic shock or decompensated heart failure requiring the use of IV inotropic therapy. (4)
- Severe hepatic impairment (2.4, 4).
- History of serious hypersensitivity reaction (e.g., Stevens-Johnson syndrome, anaphylactic reaction, angioedema) to any component of this medication or other medications containing carvedilol. (4)

———WARNINGS AND PRECAUTIONS———
- Acute exacerbation of coronary artery disease upon cessation of therapy: Do not abruptly discontinue. (5.1)

- Bradycardia, hypotension, worsening heart failure/fluid retention may occur. Reduce the dose as needed. (5.2, 5.3, 5.4)
- Non-allergic bronchospasm (e.g., chronic bronchitis and emphysema): Avoid β-blockers. (4) However, if deemed necessary, use with caution and at lowest effective dose. (5.5)
- Diabetes: Monitor glucose as β-blockers may mask symptoms of hypoglycemia or worsen hyperglycemia. (5.6)

————————ADVERSE REACTIONS————————

Most common adverse events (6.1):
- Heart failure and left ventricular dysfunction following myocardial infarction (≥10%): Dizziness, fatigue, hypotension, diarrhea, hyperglycemia, asthenia, bradycardia, weight increase
- Hypertension (≥5%): Dizziness

To report SUSPECTED ADVERSE REACTIONS, contact GlaxoSmithKline at 1-888-825-5249 or FDA at 1-800-FDA-1088 or www.fda.gov/medwatch.

————————DRUG INTERACTIONS————————

- CYP P450 2D6 enzyme inhibitors may increase and rifampin may decrease carvedilol levels. (7.1, 7.5)
- Hypotensive agents (e.g., reserpine, MAO inhibitors, clonidine) may increase the risk of hypotension and/or severe bradycardia. (7.2)
- Cyclosporine or digoxin levels may increase. (7.3, 7.4)
- Both digitalis glycosides and β-blockers slow atrioventricular conduction and decrease heart rate. Concomitant use can increase the risk of bradycardia. (7.4)
- Amiodarone may increase carvedilol levels resulting in further slowing of the heart rate or cardiac conduction. (7.6)
- Verapamil- or diltiazem-type calcium channel blockers may affect ECG and/or blood pressure. (7.7)
- Insulin and oral hypoglycemics action may be enhanced. (7.8)

See 17 for PATIENT COUNSELING INFORMATION and FDA-approved patient labeling

Revised: 08/2013

FULL PRESCRIBING INFORMATION: CONTENTS*

* Sections or subsections omitted from the full prescribing information are not listed

FULL PRESCRIBING INFORMATION

1   INDICATIONS AND USAGE

1.1   Heart Failure

COREG® is indicated for the treatment of mild-to-severe chronic heart failure of ischemic or cardiomyopathic origin, usually in addition to diuretics, ACE inhibitors, and digitalis, to increase survival and, also, to reduce the risk of hospitalization *[see Drug Interactions (7.4) and Clinical Studies (14.1)]*.

1.2   Left Ventricular Dysfunction Following Myocardial Infarction

COREG is indicated to reduce cardiovascular mortality in clinically stable patients who have survived the acute phase of a myocardial infarction and have a left ventricular ejection fraction of ≤40% (with or without symptomatic heart failure) *[see Clinical Studies (14.2)]*.

1.3   Hypertension

COREG is indicated for the management of essential hypertension *[see Clinical Studies (14.3, 14.4)]*. It can be used alone or in combination with other antihypertensive agents, especially thiazide-type diuretics *[see Drug Interactions (7.2)]*.

2   DOSAGE AND ADMINISTRATION

COREG should be taken with food to slow the rate of absorption and reduce the incidence of orthostatic effects.

2.1   Heart Failure

DOSAGE MUST BE INDIVIDUALIZED AND CLOSELY MONITORED BY A PHYSICIAN DURING UP-TITRATION. Prior to initiation of COREG, it is recommended that fluid retention be minimized. The recommended starting dose of COREG is 3.125 mg twice daily for 2 weeks. If tolerated, patients may have their dose increased to 6.25, 12.5, and 25 mg twice daily over successive intervals of at least 2 weeks. Patients should be maintained on lower doses if higher doses are not tolerated. A maximum dose of 50 mg twice daily has been administered to patients with mild-to-moderate heart failure weighing over 85 kg (187 lbs).

Patients should be advised that initiation of treatment and (to a lesser extent) dosage increases may be associated with transient symptoms of dizziness or lightheadedness (and rarely syncope) within the first hour after dosing. During these periods, patients should avoid situations such as driving or hazardous tasks, where symptoms could result in injury. Vasodilatory symptoms often do not require treatment, but it may be useful to separate the time of dosing of COREG from that of the ACE inhibitor or to reduce temporarily the dose of the ACE inhibitor. The dose of COREG should not be increased until symptoms of worsening heart failure or vasodilation have been stabilized.

Fluid retention (with or without transient worsening heart failure symptoms) should be treated by an increase in the dose of diuretics.

The dose of COREG should be reduced if patients experience bradycardia (heart rate <55 beats/minute).

Episodes of dizziness or fluid retention during initiation of COREG can generally be managed without discontinuation of treatment and do not preclude subsequent successful titration of, or a favorable response to, carvedilol.

2.2   Left Ventricular Dysfunction Following Myocardial Infarction

DOSAGE MUST BE INDIVIDUALIZED AND MONITORED DURING UP-TITRATION. Treatment with COREG may be started as an inpatient or outpatient and should be started after the patient is hemodynamically stable and fluid retention has been minimized. It is recommended that COREG be started at 6.25 mg twice daily and increased after 3 to 10 days, based on tolerability, to 12.5 mg twice daily, then again to the target dose of 25 mg twice daily. A lower starting dose may be used (3.125 mg twice daily) and/or the rate of up-titration may be slowed if clinically indicated (e.g., due to low blood pressure or heart rate, or fluid retention). Patients should be maintained on lower doses if higher doses are not tolerated. The recommended dosing regimen need not be altered in patients who received treatment with an IV or oral β-blocker during the acute phase of the myocardial infarction.

2.3   Hypertension

DOSAGE MUST BE INDIVIDUALIZED. The recommended starting dose of COREG is 6.25 mg twice daily. If this dose is tolerated, using standing systolic pressure measured about 1 hour after dosing as a guide, the dose should be maintained for 7 to 14 days, and then increased to 12.5 mg twice daily if needed, based on trough blood pressure, again using standing systolic pressure one hour after dosing as a guide for tolerance. This dose should also be maintained for 7 to 14 days and can then be adjusted upward to 25 mg twice daily if tolerated and needed. The full antihypertensive effect of COREG is seen within 7 to 14 days. Total daily dose should not exceed 50 mg. Concomitant administration with a diuretic can be expected to produce additive effects and exaggerate the orthostatic component of carvedilol action.

2.4   Hepatic Impairment

COREG should not be given to patients with severe hepatic impairment *[see Contraindications (4)]*.

3   DOSAGE FORMS AND STRENGTHS

The white, oval, film-coated tablets are available in the following strengths: 3.125 mg – engraved with 39 and SB, 6.25 mg – engraved with 4140 and SB, 12.5 mg – engraved with 4141 and SB, and 25 mg – engraved with 4142 and SB.

4   CONTRAINDICATIONS

COREG is contraindicated in the following conditions:
- Bronchial asthma or related bronchospastic conditions. Deaths from status asthmaticus have been reported following single doses of COREG.
- Second- or third-degree AV block.
- Sick sinus syndrome.
- Severe bradycardia (unless a permanent pacemaker is in place).
- Patients with cardiogenic shock or who have decompensated heart failure requiring the use of intravenous inotropic therapy. Such patients should first be weaned from intravenous therapy before initiating COREG.
- Patients with severe hepatic impairment.
- Patients with a history of a serious hypersensitivity reaction (e.g., Stevens-Johnson syndrome, anaphylactic reaction, angioedema) to any component of this medication or other medications containing carvedilol.

5   WARNINGS AND PRECAUTIONS

5.1   Cessation of Therapy

Patients with coronary artery disease, who are being treated with COREG, should be advised against abrupt discontinuation of therapy. Severe exacerbation of angina and the occurrence of myocardial infarction and ventricular arrhythmias have been reported in angina patients following the abrupt discontinuation of therapy with β-blockers. The last 2 complications may occur with or without preceding exacerbation of the angina pectoris. As with other β-blockers, when discontinuation of COREG is planned, the patients should be carefully observed and advised to limit physical activity to a minimum. COREG should be discontinued over 1 to 2 weeks whenever possible. If the angina worsens or acute coronary insufficiency develops, it is recommended that COREG be promptly reinstituted, at least temporarily. Because coronary artery disease is common and may be unrecognized, it may be prudent not to discontinue therapy with COREG abruptly even in patients treated only for hypertension or heart failure.

5.2   Bradycardia

In clinical trials, COREG caused bradycardia in about 2% of hypertensive subjects, 9% of heart failure subjects, and 6.5% of myocardial infarction subjects with left ventricular dysfunction. If pulse rate drops below 55 beats/minute, the dosage should be reduced.

5.3   Hypotension

In clinical trials of primarily mild-to-moderate heart failure, hypotension and postural hypotension occurred in 9.7% and syncope in 3.4% of subjects receiving COREG compared with 3.6% and 2.5% of placebo subjects, respectively. The risk for these events was highest during the first 30 days of dosing, corresponding to the up-titration period and was a cause for discontinuation of therapy in 0.7% of subjects receiving COREG, compared with 0.4% of placebo subjects. In a long-term, placebo-controlled trial in severe heart failure (COPERNICUS), hypotension and postural hypotension occurred in 15.1% and syncope in 2.9% of heart failure subjects receiving COREG compared with 8.7% and 2.3% of placebo subjects, respectively. These events were a cause for discontinuation of therapy in 1.1% of subjects receiving COREG, compared with 0.8% of placebo subjects.

Postural hypotension occurred in 1.8% and syncope in 0.1% of hypertensive subjects, primarily following the initial dose or at the time of dose increase and was a cause for discontinuation of therapy in 1% of subjects.

Table 1. Adverse Events (%) Occurring More Frequently With COREG Than With Placebo in Subjects With Mild-to-Moderate Heart Failure (HF) Enrolled in US Heart Failure Trials or in Subjects With Severe Heart Failure in the COPERNICUS Trial (Incidence >3% in Subjects Treated With Carvedilol, Regardless of Causality)

Body System/ Adverse Event	Mild-to-Moderate HF		Severe HF	
	COREG	Placebo	COREG	Placebo
	(n = 765)	(n = 437)	(n = 1,156)	(n = 1,133)
Body as a Whole				
Asthenia	7	7	11	9
Fatigue	24	22	—	—
Digoxin level increased	5	4	2	1
Edema generalized	5	3	6	5
Edema dependent	4	2	—	—
Cardiovascular				
Bradycardia	9	1	10	3
Hypotension	9	3	14	8
Syncope	3	3	8	5
Angina pectoris	2	3	6	4
Central Nervous System				
Dizziness	32	19	24	17
Headache	8	7	5	3
Gastrointestinal				
Diarrhea	12	6	5	3
Nausea	9	5	4	3
Vomiting	6	4	1	2
Metabolic				
Hyperglycemia	12	8	5	3
Weight increase	10	7	12	11
BUN increased	6	5	—	—
NPN increased	6	5	—	—
Hypercholesterolemia	4	3	1	1
Edema peripheral	2	1	7	6
Musculoskeletal				
Arthralgia	6	5	1	1
Respiratory				
Cough increased	8	9	5	4
Rales	4	4	4	2
Vision				
Vision abnormal	5	2	—	—

In the CAPRICORN trial of survivors of an acute myocardial infarction, hypotension or postural hypotension occurred in 20.2% of subjects receiving COREG compared with 12.6% of placebo subjects. Syncope was reported in 3.9% and 1.9% of subjects, respectively. These events were a cause for discontinuation of therapy in 2.5% of subjects receiving COREG, compared with 0.2% of placebo subjects. Starting with a low dose, administration with food, and gradual up-titration should decrease the likelihood of syncope or excessive hypotension [see Dosage and Administration (2.1, 2.2, 2.3)]. During initiation of therapy, the patient should be cautioned to avoid situations such as driving or hazardous tasks, where injury could result should syncope occur.

5.4　Heart Failure/Fluid Retention
Worsening heart failure or fluid retention may occur during up-titration of carvedilol. If such symptoms occur, diuretics should be increased and the carvedilol dose should not be advanced until clinical stability resumes [see Dosage and Administration (2)]. Occasionally it is necessary to lower the carvedilol dose or temporarily discontinue it. Such episodes do not preclude subsequent successful titration of, or a favorable response to, carvedilol. In a placebo-controlled trial of subjects with severe heart failure, worsening heart failure during the first 3 months was reported to a similar degree with carvedilol and with placebo. When treatment was maintained beyond 3 months, worsening heart failure was reported less frequently in subjects treated with carvedilol than with placebo. Worsening heart failure observed during long-term therapy is more likely to be related to the patients' underlying disease than to treatment with carvedilol.

5.5　Non-allergic Bronchospasm
Patients with bronchospastic disease (e.g., chronic bronchitis and emphysema) should, in general, not receive β-blockers. COREG may be used with caution, however, in patients who do not respond to, or cannot tolerate, other antihypertensive agents. It is prudent, if COREG is used, to use the smallest effective dose, so that inhibition of endogenous or exogenous β-agonists is minimized.
In clinical trials of subjects with heart failure, subjects with bronchospastic disease were enrolled if they did not require oral or inhaled medication to treat their bronchospastic disease. In such patients, it is recommended that carvedilol be used with caution. The dosing recommendations should be followed closely and the dose should be lowered if any evidence of bronchospasm is observed during up-titration.

5.6　Glycemic Control in Type 2 Diabetes
In general, β-blockers may mask some of the manifestations of hypoglycemia, particularly tachycardia. Nonselective β-blockers may potentiate insulin-induced hypoglycemia and delay recovery of serum glucose levels. Patients subject to spontaneous hypoglycemia, or diabetic patients receiving insulin or oral hypoglycemic agents, should be cautioned about these possibilities.
In heart failure patients with diabetes, carvedilol therapy may lead to worsening hyperglycemia, which responds to intensification of hypoglycemic therapy. It is recommended that blood glucose be monitored when carvedilol dosing is initiated, adjusted, or discontinued. Trials designed to examine the effects of carvedilol on glycemic control in patients with diabetes and heart failure have not been conducted.
In a trial designed to examine the effects of carvedilol on glycemic control in a population with mild-to-moderate hypertension and well-controlled type 2 diabetes mellitus, carvedilol had no adverse effect on glycemic control, based on HbA1c measurements [see Clinical Studies (14.4)].

5.7　Peripheral Vascular Disease
β-blockers can precipitate or aggravate symptoms of arterial insufficiency in patients with peripheral vascular disease. Caution should be exercised in such individuals.

5.8　Deterioration of Renal Function
Rarely, use of carvedilol in patients with heart failure has resulted in deterioration of renal function. Patients at risk appear to be those with low blood pressure (systolic blood pressure <100 mm Hg), ischemic heart disease and diffuse vascular disease, and/or underlying renal insufficiency. Renal function has returned to baseline when carvedilol was stopped. In patients with these risk factors it is recommended that renal function be monitored during up-titration of carvedilol and the drug discontinued or dosage reduced if worsening of renal function occurs.

5.9　Major Surgery
Chronically administered beta-blocking therapy should not be routinely withdrawn prior to major surgery; however, the impaired ability of the heart to respond to reflex adrenergic stimuli may augment the risks of general anesthesia and surgical procedures.

5.10　Thyrotoxicosis
β-adrenergic blockade may mask clinical signs of hyperthyroidism, such as tachycardia. Abrupt withdrawal of β-blockade may be followed by an exacerbation of the symptoms of hyperthyroidism or may precipitate thyroid storm.

5.11　Pheochromocytoma
In patients with pheochromocytoma, an α-blocking agent should be initiated prior to the use of any β-blocking agent. Although carvedilol has both α- and β-blocking pharmacologic activities, there has been no experience with its use in this condition. Therefore, caution should be taken in the administration of carvedilol to patients suspected of having pheochromocytoma.

5.12　Prinzmetal's Variant Angina
Agents with non-selective β-blocking activity may provoke chest pain in patients with Prinzmetal's variant angina. There has been no clinical experience with carvedilol in these patients although the α-blocking activity may prevent such symptoms. However, caution should be taken in the administration of carvedilol to patients suspected of having Prinzmetal's variant angina.

5.13　Risk of Anaphylactic Reaction
While taking β-blockers, patients with a history of severe anaphylactic reaction to a variety of allergens may be more reactive to repeated challenge, either accidental, diagnostic, or therapeutic. Such patients may be unresponsive to the usual doses of epinephrine used to treat allergic reaction.

5.14　Intraoperative Floppy Iris Syndrome
Intraoperative Floppy Iris Syndrome (IFIS) has been observed during cataract surgery in some patients treated with alpha-1 blockers (COREG is an alpha/beta blocker). This variant of small pupil syndrome is characterized by the combination of a flaccid iris that billows in response to intraoperative irrigation currents, progressive intraoperative miosis despite preoperative dilation with standard mydriatic drugs, and potential prolapse of the iris toward the phacoemulsification incisions. The patient's ophthalmologist should be prepared for possible modifications to the surgical technique, such as utilization of iris hooks, iris dilator rings, or viscoelastic substances. There does not appear to be a benefit of stopping alpha-1 blocker therapy prior to cataract surgery.

6　ADVERSE REACTIONS
6.1　Clinical Studies Experience
COREG has been evaluated for safety in subjects with heart failure (mild, moderate, and severe), in subjects with left ventricular dysfunction following myocardial infarction and in hypertensive subjects The observed adverse event profile was consistent with the pharmacology of the drug and the health status of the subjects in the clinical trials. Adverse events reported for each of these patient populations are provided below. Excluded are adverse events considered too general to be informative, and those not reasonably associated with the use of the drug because they were associated with the condition being treated or are very common in the treated population. Rates of adverse events were generally similar across demographic subsets (men and women, elderly and non-elderly, blacks and non-blacks).
Heart Failure
COREG has been evaluated for safety in heart failure in more than 4,500 subjects worldwide of whom more than 2,100 participated in placebo-controlled clinical trials. Approximately 60% of the total treated population in placebo-controlled clinical trials received COREG for at least 6 months and 30% received COREG for at least 12 months. In the COMET trial, 1,511 subjects with mild-to-moderate heart failure were treated with COREG for up to 5.9 years (mean: 4.8 years). Both in US clinical trials in mild-to-moderate heart failure that compared COREG in daily doses up to 100 mg (n = 765) with placebo (n = 437), and in a multinational clinical trial in severe heart failure (COPERNICUS) that compared COREG in daily doses up to 50 mg (n = 1,156) with placebo (n = 1,133), discontinuation rates for adverse experiences were similar in carvedilol and placebo subjects. In placebo-controlled clinical trials, the only cause of discontinuation >1%, and occurring more often on carvedilol was dizziness (1.3% on carvedilol, 0.6% on placebo in the COPERNICUS trial).
Table 1 shows adverse events reported in subjects with mild-to-moderate heart failure enrolled in US placebo-controlled clinical trials, and with severe heart failure enrolled in the COPERNICUS trial. Shown are adverse events that occurred more frequently in drug-treated subjects than placebo-treated subjects with an incidence of >3% in subjects treated with carvedilol regardless of causality. Median trial medication exposure was 6.3 months for both carvedilol and placebo subjects in the trials of mild-to-moderate heart failure, and 10.4 months in the trial of severe heart failure subjects. The adverse event profile of COREG observed in the long-term COMET trial was generally similar to that observed in the US Heart Failure Trials. [See table 1 above]
Cardiac failure and dyspnea were also reported in these trials, but the rates were equal or greater in subjects who received placebo.

The following adverse events were reported with a frequency of >1% but ≤3% and more frequently with COREG in either the US placebo-controlled trials in subjects with mild-to-moderate heart failure, or in subjects with severe heart failure in the COPERNICUS trial.

Incidence >1% to ≤3%

Body as a Whole: Allergy, malaise, hypovolemia, fever, leg edema.

Cardiovascular: Fluid overload, postural hypotension, aggravated angina pectoris, AV block, palpitation, hypertension.

Central and Peripheral Nervous System: Hypesthesia, vertigo, paresthesia.

Gastrointestinal: Melena, periodontitis.

Liver and Biliary System: SGPT increased, SGOT increased.

Metabolic and Nutritional: Hyperuricemia, hypoglycemia, hyponatremia, increased alkaline phosphatase, glycosuria, hypervolemia, diabetes mellitus, GGT increased, weight loss, hyperkalemia, creatinine increased.

Musculoskeletal: Muscle cramps.

Platelet, Bleeding and Clotting: Prothrombin decreased, purpura, thrombocytopenia.

Psychiatric: Somnolence.

Reproductive, male: Impotence.

Special Senses: Blurred vision.

Urinary System: Renal insufficiency, albuminuria, hematuria.

Left Ventricular Dysfunction Following Myocardial Infarction

COREG has been evaluated for safety in survivors of an acute myocardial infarction with left ventricular dysfunction in the CAPRICORN trial which involved 969 subjects who received COREG and 980 who received placebo. Approximately 75% of the subjects received COREG for at least 6 months and 53% received COREG for at least 12 months. Subjects were treated for an average of 12.9 months and 12.8 months with COREG and placebo, respectively.

The most common adverse events reported with COREG in the CAPRICORN trial were consistent with the profile of the drug in the US heart failure trials and the COPERNICUS trial. The only additional adverse events reported in CAPRICORN in >3% of the subjects and more commonly on carvedilol were dyspnea, anemia, and lung edema. The following adverse events were reported with a frequency of >1% but ≤3% and more frequently with COREG:flu syndrome, cerebrovascular accident, peripheral vascular disorder, hypotonia, depression, gastrointestinal pain, arthritis, and gout. The overall rates of discontinuations due to adverse events were similar in both groups of subjects. In this database, the only cause of discontinuation >1%, and occurring more often on carvedilol was hypotension (1.5% on carvedilol, 0.2% on placebo).

Hypertension

COREG has been evaluated for safety in hypertension in more than 2,193 subjects in US clinical trials and in 2,976 subjects in international clinical trials. Approximately 36% of the total treated population received COREG for at least 6 months. Most adverse events reported during therapy with COREG were of mild to moderate severity. In US controlled clinical trials directly comparing COREG in doses up to 50 mg (n = 1,142) with placebo (n = 462), 4.9% of subjects receiving COREG discontinued for adverse events versus 5.2% of placebo subjects. Although there was no overall difference in discontinuation rates, discontinuations were more common in the carvedilol group for postural hypotension (1% versus 0). The overall incidence of adverse events in US placebo-controlled trials increased with increasing dose of COREG. For individual adverse events this could only be distinguished for dizziness, which increased in frequency from 2% to 5% as total daily dose increased from 6.25 mg to 50 mg.

Table 2 shows adverse events in US placebo-controlled clinical trials for hypertension that occurred with an incidence of ≥1% regardless of causality, and that were more frequent in drug-treated subjects than placebo-treated subjects.

Table 2. Adverse Events (%) Occurring in US Placebo-Controlled Hypertension Trials (Incidence ≥1%, Regardless of Causality)[a]

Body System/ Adverse Event	COREG (n = 1,142)	Placebo (n = 462)
Cardiovascular		
Bradycardia	2	—
Postural hypotension	2	—
Peripheral edema	1	—
Central Nervous System		
Dizziness	6	5
Insomnia	2	1
Gastrointestinal		
Diarrhea	2	1
Hematologic		
Thrombocytopenia	1	—
Metabolic		
Hypertriglyceridemia	1	—

[a] Shown are events with rate >1% rounded to nearest integer.

Dyspnea and fatigue were also reported in these trials, but the rates were equal or greater in subjects who received placebo.

The following adverse events not described above were reported as possibly or probably related to COREG in worldwide open or controlled trials with COREG in subjects with hypertension or heart failure.

Incidence >0.1% to ≤1%

Cardiovascular: Peripheral ischemia, tachycardia.

Central and Peripheral Nervous System: Hypokinesia.

Gastrointestinal: Bilirubinemia, increased hepatic enzymes (0.2% of hypertension patients and 0.4% of heart failure patients were discontinued from therapy because of increases in hepatic enzymes) *[see Adverse Reactions (6.2)]*.

Psychiatric: Nervousness, sleep disorder, aggravated depression, impaired concentration, abnormal thinking, paroniria, emotional lability.

Respiratory System: Asthma *[see Contraindications (4)]*.

Reproductive, male: Decreased libido.

Skin and Appendages: Pruritus, rash erythematous, rash maculopapular, rash psoriaform, photosensitivity reaction.

Special Senses: Tinnitus.

Urinary System: Micturition frequency increased.

Autonomic Nervous System: Dry mouth, sweating increased.

Metabolic and Nutritional: Hypokalemia, hypertriglyceridemia.

Hematologic: Anemia, leukopenia.

The following events were reported in ≤0.1% of subjects and are potentially important: complete AV block, bundle branch block, myocardial ischemia, cerebrovascular disorder, convulsions, migraine, neuralgia, paresis, anaphylactoid reaction, alopecia, exfoliative dermatitis, amnesia, GI hemorrhage, bronchospasm, pulmonary edema, decreased hearing, respiratory alkalosis, increased BUN, decreased HDL, pancytopenia, and atypical lymphocytes.

6.2   Laboratory Abnormalities

Reversible elevations in serum transaminases (ALT or AST) have been observed during treatment with COREG. Rates of transaminase elevations 2 to 3 times the upper limit of normal) observed during controlled clinical trials have generally been similar between subjects treated with COREG and those treated with placebo. However, transaminase elevations, confirmed by rechallenge, have been observed with COREG. In a long-term, placebo-controlled trial in severe heart failure, subjects treated with COREG had lower values for hepatic transaminases than subjects treated with placebo, possibly because improvements in cardiac function induced by COREG led to less hepatic congestion and/or improved hepatic blood flow.

COREG has not been associated with clinically significant changes in serum potassium, total triglycerides, total cholesterol, HDL cholesterol, uric acid, blood urea nitrogen, or creatinine. No clinically relevant changes were noted in fasting serum glucose in hypertensive patients; fasting serum glucose was not evaluated in the heart failure clinical trials.

6.3   Postmarketing Experience

The following adverse reactions have been identified during post-approval use of COREG. Because these reactions are reported voluntarily from a population of uncertain size, it is not always possible to reliably estimate their frequency or establish a causal relationship to drug exposure.

Blood and Lymphatic System Disorders: Aplastic anemia.

Immune System Disorders: Hypersensitivity (e.g., anaphylactic reactions, angioedema, urticaria).

Renal and Urinary Disorders: Urinary incontinence.

Respiratory, Thoracic and Mediastinal Disorders: Interstitial pneumonitis.

Skin and Subcutaneous Tissue Disorders: Stevens-Johnson syndrome, toxic epidermal necrolysis, erythema multiforme.

7   DRUG INTERACTIONS

7.1   CYP2D6 Inhibitors and Poor Metabolizers

Interactions of carvedilol with potent inhibitors of CYP2D6 isoenzyme (such as quinidine, fluoxetine, paroxetine, and propafenone) have not been studied, but these drugs would be expected to increase blood levels of the R(+) enantiomer of carvedilol *[see Clinical Pharmacology (12.3)]*. Retrospective analysis of side effects in clinical trials showed that poor 2D6 metabolizers had a higher rate of dizziness during up-titration, presumably resulting from vasodilating effects of the higher concentrations of the α-blocking R(+) enantiomer.

7.2   Hypotensive Agents

Patients taking both agents with β-blocking properties and a drug that can deplete catecholamines (e.g., reserpine and monoamine oxidase inhibitors) should be observed closely for signs of hypotension and/or severe bradycardia.

Concomitant administration of clonidine with agents with β-blocking properties may potentiate blood-pressure- and heart-rate-lowering effects. When concomitant treatment with agents with β-blocking properties and clonidine is to be terminated, the β-blocking agent should be discontinued first. Clonidine therapy can then be discontinued several days later by gradually decreasing the dosage.

7.3   Cyclosporine

Modest increases in mean trough cyclosporine concentrations were observed following initiation of carvedilol treatment in 21 renal transplant subjects suffering from chronic vascular rejection. In about 30% of subjects, the dose of cyclosporine had to be reduced in order to maintain cyclosporine concentrations within the therapeutic range, while in the remainder no adjustment was needed. On the average for the group, the dose of cyclosporine was reduced about 20% in these subjects. Due to wide interindividual variability in the dose adjustment required, it is recommended that cyclosporine concentrations be monitored closely after initiation of carvedilol therapy and that the dose of cyclosporine be adjusted as appropriate.

7.4   Digitalis Glycosides

Both digitalis glycosides and β-blockers slow atrioventricular conduction and decrease heart rate. Concomitant use can increase the risk of bradycardia. Digoxin concentrations are increased by about 15% when digoxin and carvedilol are administered concomitantly. Therefore, increased monitoring of digoxin is recommended when initiating, adjusting, or discontinuing COREG *[see Clinical Pharmacology (12.5)]*.

7.5   Inducers/Inhibitors of Hepatic Metabolism

Rifampin reduced plasma concentrations of carvedilol by about 70% *[see Clinical Pharmacology (12.5)]*. Cimetidine increased AUC by about 30% but caused no change in C_{max} *[see Clinical Pharmacology (12.5)]*.

7.6   Amiodarone

Amiodarone, and its metabolite desethyl amiodarone, inhibitors of CYP2C9 and P-glycoprotein, increased concentrations of the S(-)-enantiomer of carvedilol by at least 2-fold *[see Clinical Pharmacology (12.5)]*. The concomitant administration of amiodarone or other CYP2C9 inhibitors such as fluconazole with COREG may enhance the β-blocking properties of carvedilol resulting in further slowing of the heart rate or cardiac conduction. Patients should be observed for signs of bradycardia or heart block, particularly when one agent is added to pre-existing treatment with the other.

7.7   Calcium Channel Blockers

Conduction disturbance (rarely with hemodynamic compromise) has been observed when COREG is co-administered with diltiazem. As with other agents with β-blocking properties, if COREG is to be administered with calcium channel blockers of the verapamil or diltiazem type, it is recommended that ECG and blood pressure be monitored.

7.8   Insulin or Oral Hypoglycemics

Agents with β-blocking properties may enhance the blood-sugar-reducing effect of insulin and oral hypoglycemics. Therefore, in patients taking insulin or oral hypoglycemics, regular monitoring of blood glucose is recommended *[see Warnings and Precautions (5.6)]*.

7.9   Anesthesia

If treatment with COREG is to be continued perioperatively, particular care should be taken when anesthetic agents which depress myocardial function, such as ether, cyclopropane, and trichloroethylene, are used *[see Overdosage (10)]*.

8   USE IN SPECIFIC POPULATIONS

8.1   Pregnancy

Pregnancy Category C. Studies performed in pregnant rats and rabbits given carvedilol revealed increased postimplantation loss in rats at doses of 300 mg/kg/day (50 times the maximum recommended human dose [MRHD] as mg/m[2]) and in rabbits at doses of 75 mg/kg/day (25 times the MRHD as mg/m[2]). In the rats, there was also a decrease in fetal body weight at the maternally toxic dose of 300 mg/kg/day (50 times the MRHD as mg/m[2]), which was accompanied by an elevation in the frequency of fetuses with delayed skeletal development (missing or stunted 13th rib). In rats the no-observed-effect level for developmental toxicity was 60 mg/kg/day (10 times the MRHD as mg/m[2]); in rabbits it was 15 mg/kg/day (5 times the MRHD as mg/m[2]). There are no adequate and well-controlled studies in pregnant women. COREG should be used during pregnancy only if the potential benefit justifies the potential risk to the fetus.

8.3 Nursing Mothers

It is not known whether this drug is excreted in human milk. Studies in rats have shown that carvedilol and/or its metabolites (as well as other β-blockers) cross the placental barrier and are excreted in breast milk. There was increased mortality at one week post-partum in neonates from rats treated with 60 mg/kg/day (10 times the MRHD as mg/m²) and above during the last trimester through day 22 of lactation. Because many drugs are excreted in human milk and because of the potential for serious adverse reactions in nursing infants from β-blockers, especially bradycardia, a decision should be made whether to discontinue nursing or to discontinue the drug, taking into account the importance of the drug to the mother. The effects of other α- and β-blocking agents have included perinatal and neonatal distress.

8.4 Pediatric Use

Effectiveness of COREG in patients younger than 18 years has not been established.

In a double-blind trial, 161 children (mean age: 6 years, range: 2 months to 17 years; 45% younger than 2 years) with chronic heart failure [NYHA class II-IV, left ventricular ejection fraction <40% for children with a systemic left ventricle (LV), and moderate-severe ventricular dysfunction qualitatively by echo for those with a systemic ventricle that was not an LV] who were receiving standard background treatment were randomized to placebo or to 2 dose levels of carvedilol. These dose levels produced placebo-corrected heart rate reduction of 4 to 6 heart beats per minute, indicative of β -blockade activity. Exposure appeared to be lower in pediatric subjects than adults. After 8 months of follow-up, there was no significant effect of treatment on clinical outcomes. Adverse reactions in this trial that occurred in greater than 10% of subjects treated with COREG and at twice the rate of placebo-treated subjects included chest pain (17% versus 6%), dizziness (13% versus 2%), and dyspnea (11% versus 4%).

8.5 Geriatric Use

Of the 765 subjects with heart failure randomized to COREG in US clinical trials, 31% (235) were 65 years of age or older, and 7.3% (56) were 75 years of age or older. Of the 1,156 subjects randomized to COREG in a long-term, placebo-controlled trial in severe heart failure, 47% (547) were 65 years of age or older, and 15% (174) were 75 years of age or older. Of 3,025 subjects receiving COREG in heart failure trials worldwide, 42% were 65 years of age or older. Of the 975 myocardial infarction subjects randomized to COREG in the CAPRICORN trial, 48% (468) were 65 years of age or older, and 11% (111) were 75 years of age or older. Of the 2,065 hypertensive subjects in US clinical trials of efficacy or safety who were treated with COREG, 21% (436) were 65 years of age or older. Of 3,722 subjects receiving COREG in hypertension clinical trials conducted worldwide, 24% were 65 years of age or older.

With the exception of dizziness in hypertensive subjects (incidence 8.8% in the elderly versus 6% in younger subjects), no overall differences in the safety or effectiveness (see Figures 2 and 4) were observed between the older subjects and younger subjects in each of these populations. Similarly, other reported clinical experience has not identified differences in responses between the elderly and younger subjects, but greater sensitivity of some older individuals cannot be ruled out.

10   OVERDOSAGE

Overdosage may cause severe hypotension, bradycardia, cardiac insufficiency, cardiogenic shock, and cardiac arrest. Respiratory problems, bronchospasms, vomiting, lapses of consciousness, and generalized seizures may also occur.

The patient should be placed in a supine position and, where necessary, kept under observation and treated under intensive-care conditions. Gastric lavage or pharmacologically induced emesis may be used shortly after ingestion. The following agents may be administered:

For excessive bradycardia: Atropine, 2 mg IV.

To support cardiovascular function: Glucagon, 5 to 10 mg IV rapidly over 30 seconds, followed by a continuous infusion of 5 mg/hour; sympathomimetics (dobutamine, isoprenaline, adrenaline) at doses according to body weight and effect.

If peripheral vasodilation dominates, it may be necessary to administer adrenaline or noradrenaline with continuous monitoring of circulatory conditions. For therapy-resistant bradycardia, pacemaker therapy should be performed. For bronchospasm, β-sympathomimetics (as aerosol or IV) or aminophylline IV should be given. In the event of seizures, slow IV injection of diazepam or clonazepam is recommended.

NOTE: In the event of severe intoxication where there are symptoms of shock, treatment with antidotes must be continued for a sufficiently long period of time consistent with the 7- to 10-hour half-life of carvedilol.

Cases of overdosage with COREG alone or in combination with other drugs have been reported. Quantities ingested in some cases exceeded 1,000 milligrams. Symptoms experienced included low blood pressure and heart rate. Standard supportive treatment was provided and individuals recovered.

11   DESCRIPTION

Carvedilol is a nonselective β-adrenergic blocking agent with $α_1$-blocking activity. It is (±)-1-(Carbazol-4-yloxy)-3-[[2-(o-methoxyphenoxy)ethyl]amino]-2-propanol. Carvedilol is a racemic mixture with the following structure:

COREG is a white, oval, film-coated tablet containing 3.125 mg, 6.25 mg, 12.5 mg, or 25 mg of carvedilol. The 6.25-mg, 12.5-mg, and 25-mg tablets are TILTAB® tablets. Inactive ingredients consist of colloidal silicon dioxide, crospovidone, hypromellose, lactose, magnesium stearate, polyethylene glycol, polysorbate 80, povidone, sucrose, and titanium dioxide.

Carvedilol is a white to off-white powder with a molecular weight of 406.5 and a molecular formula of $C_{24}H_{26}N_2O_4$. It is freely soluble in dimethylsulfoxide; soluble in methylene chloride and methanol; sparingly soluble in 95% ethanol and isopropanol; slightly soluble in ethyl ether; and practically insoluble in water, gastric fluid (simulated, TS, pH 1.1), and intestinal fluid (simulated, TS without pancreatin, pH 7.5).

12   CLINICAL PHARMACOLOGY

12.1   Mechanism of Action

COREG is a racemic mixture in which nonselective β-adrenoreceptor blocking activity is present in the S(-) enantiomer and $α_1$-adrenergic blocking activity is present in both R(+) and S(-) enantiomers at equal potency. COREG has no intrinsic sympathomimetic activity.

12.2   Pharmacodynamics

Heart Failure

The basis for the beneficial effects of COREG in heart failure is not established.

Two placebo-controlled trials compared the acute hemodynamic effects of COREG with baseline measurements in 59 and 49 subjects with NYHA class II-IV heart failure receiving diuretics, ACE inhibitors, and digitalis. There were significant reductions in systemic blood pressure, pulmonary artery pressure, pulmonary capillary wedge pressure, and heart rate. Initial effects on cardiac output, stroke volume index, and systemic vascular resistance were small and variable.

These trials measured hemodynamic effects again at 12 to 14 weeks. COREG significantly reduced systemic blood pressure, pulmonary artery pressure, right atrial pressure, systemic vascular resistance, and heart rate, while stroke volume index was increased.

Among 839 subjects with NYHA class II-III heart failure treated for 26 to 52 weeks in 4 US placebo-controlled trials, average left ventricular ejection fraction (EF) measured by radionuclide ventriculography increased by 9 EF units (%) in subjects receiving COREG and by 2 EF units in placebo subjects at a target dose of 25 to 50 mg twice daily. The effects of carvedilol on ejection fraction were related to dose. Doses of 6.25 mg twice daily, 12.5 mg twice daily, and 25 mg twice daily were associated with placebo-corrected increases in EF of 5 EF units, 6 EF units, and 8 EF units, respectively; each of these effects were nominally statistically significant.

Left Ventricular Dysfunction Following Myocardial Infarction

The basis for the beneficial effects of COREG in patients with left ventricular dysfunction following an acute myocardial infarction is not established.

Hypertension

The mechanism by which β-blockade produces an antihypertensive effect has not been established.

β-adrenoreceptor blocking activity has been demonstrated in animal and human studies showing that carvedilol (1) reduces cardiac output in normal subjects; (2) reduces exercise- and/or isoproterenol-induced tachycardia; and (3) reduces reflex orthostatic tachycardia. Significant β-adrenoreceptor blocking effect is usually seen within 1 hour of drug administration.

$α_1$-adrenoreceptor blocking activity has been demonstrated in human and animal studies, showing that carvedilol (1) attenuates the pressor effects of phenylephrine; (2) causes vasodilation; and (3) reduces peripheral vascular resistance. These effects contribute to the reduction of blood pressure and usually are seen within 30 minutes of drug administration.

Due to the $α_1$-receptor blocking activity of carvedilol, blood pressure is lowered more in the standing than in the supine position, and symptoms of postural hypotension (1.8%), including rare instances of syncope, can occur. Following oral administration, when postural hypotension has occurred, it has been transient and is uncommon when COREG is administered with food at the recommended starting dose and titration increments are closely followed *[see Dosage and Administration (2)].*

In hypertensive patients with normal renal function, therapeutic doses of COREG decreased renal vascular resistance with no change in glomerular filtration rate or renal plasma flow. Changes in excretion of sodium, potassium, uric acid, and phosphorus in hypertensive patients with normal renal function were similar after COREG and placebo.

COREG has little effect on plasma catecholamines, plasma aldosterone, or electrolyte levels, but it does significantly reduce plasma renin activity when given for at least 4 weeks. It also increases levels of atrial natriuretic peptide.

12.3   Pharmacokinetics

COREG is rapidly and extensively absorbed following oral administration, with absolute bioavailability of approximately 25% to 35% due to a significant degree of first-pass metabolism. Following oral administration, the apparent mean terminal elimination half-life of carvedilol generally ranges from 7 to 10 hours. Plasma concentrations achieved are proportional to the oral dose administered. When administered with food, the rate of absorption is slowed, as evidenced by a delay in the time to reach peak plasma levels, with no significant difference in extent of bioavailability. Taking COREG with food should minimize the risk of orthostatic hypotension.

Carvedilol is extensively metabolized. Following oral administration of radiolabelled carvedilol to healthy volunteers, carvedilol accounted for only about 7% of the total radioactivity in plasma as measured by area under the curve (AUC). Less than 2% of the dose was excreted unchanged in the urine. Carvedilol is metabolized primarily by aromatic ring oxidation and glucuronidation. The oxidative metabolites are further metabolized by conjugation via glucuronidation and sulfation. The metabolites of carvedilol are excreted primarily via the bile into the feces. Demethylation and hydroxylation at the phenol ring produce 3 active metabolites with β-receptor blocking activity. Based on preclinical studies, the 4'-hydroxyphenyl metabolite is approximately 13 times more potent than carvedilol for β-blockade. Compared with carvedilol, the 3 active metabolites exhibit weak vasodilating activity. Plasma concentrations of the active metabolites are about one-tenth of those observed for carvedilol and have pharmacokinetics similar to the parent. Carvedilol undergoes stereoselective first-pass metabolism with plasma levels of R(+)-carvedilol approximately 2 to 3 times higher than S(-)-carvedilol following oral administration in healthy subjects. The mean apparent terminal elimination half-lives for R(+)-carvedilol range from 5 to 9 hours compared with 7 to 11 hours for the S(-)-enantiomer.

The primary P450 enzymes responsible for the metabolism of both R(+) and S(-)-carvedilol in human liver microsomes were CYP2D6 and CYP2C9 and to a lesser extent CYP3A4, 2C19, 1A2, and 2E1. CYP2D6 is thought to be the major enzyme in the 4'- and 5'-hydroxylation of carvedilol, with a potential contribution from 3A4. CYP2C9 is thought to be of primary importance in the O-methylation pathway of S(-)-carvedilol.

Carvedilol is subject to the effects of genetic polymorphism with poor metabolizers of debrisoquin (a marker for cytochrome P450 2D6) exhibiting 2- to 3-fold higher plasma concentrations of R(+)-carvedilol compared with extensive metabolizers. In contrast, plasma levels of S(-)-carvedilol are increased only about 20% to 25% in poor metabolizers, indicating this enantiomer is metabolized to a lesser extent by cytochrome P450 2D6 than R(+)-carvedilol. The pharmacokinetics of carvedilol do not appear to be different in poor metabolizers of S-mephenytoin (patients deficient in cytochrome P450 2C19).

Carvedilol is more than 98% bound to plasma proteins, primarily with albumin. The plasma-protein binding is independent of concentration over the therapeutic range. Carvedilol is a basic, lipophilic compound with a steady-state volume of distribution of approximately 115 L, indicating substantial distribution into extravascular tissues. Plasma clearance ranges from 500 to 700 mL/min.

12.4   Specific Populations

Heart Failure

Steady-state plasma concentrations of carvedilol and its enantiomers increased proportionally over the 6.25 to 50 mg dose range in subjects with heart failure. Compared with healthy subjects, heart failure subjects had increased mean AUC and C_{max} values for carvedilol and its enantiomers, with up to 50% to 100% higher values observed in 6 subjects with NYHA class IV heart failure. The mean apparent terminal elimination half-life for carvedilol was similar to that observed in healthy subjects.

Geriatric

Plasma levels of carvedilol average about 50% higher in the elderly compared with young subjects.

Hepatic Impairment

Compared with healthy subjects, patients with severe liver impairment (cirrhosis) exhibit a 4- to 7-fold increase in carvedilol levels. Carvedilol is contraindicated in patients with severe liver impairment.

Renal Impairment

Although carvedilol is metabolized primarily by the liver, plasma concentrations of carvedilol have been reported to be increased in patients with renal impairment. Based on mean AUC data, approximately 40% to 50% higher plasma concentrations of carvedilol were observed in hypertensive subjects with moderate to severe renal impairment compared to a control group of hypertensive subjects with normal renal function. However, the ranges of AUC values were similar for both groups. Changes in mean peak plasma levels were less pronounced, approximately 12% to 26% higher in subjects with impaired renal function.

Consistent with its high degree of plasma protein-binding, carvedilol does not appear to be cleared significantly by hemodialysis.

12.5   Drug-Drug Interactions

Since carvedilol undergoes substantial oxidative metabolism, the metabolism and pharmacokinetics of carvedilol may be affected by induction or inhibition of cytochrome P450 enzymes.

Amiodarone

In a pharmacokinetic trial conducted in 106 Japanese subjects with heart failure, coadministration of small loading and maintenance doses of amiodarone with carvedilol resulted in at least a 2-fold increase in the steady-state trough concentrations of S(-)-carvedilol *[see Drug Interactions (7.6)]*.

Cimetidine

In a pharmacokinetic trial conducted in 10 healthy male subjects, cimetidine (1,000 mg/day) increased the steady-state AUC of carvedilol by 30% with no change in C_{max} *[see Drug Interactions (7.5)]*.

Digoxin

Following concomitant administration of carvedilol (25 mg once daily) and digoxin (0.25 mg once daily) for 14 days, steady-state AUC and trough concentrations of digoxin were increased by 14% and 16%, respectively, in 12 hypertensive subjects *[see Drug Interactions (7.4)]*.

Glyburide

In 12 healthy subjects, combined administration of carvedilol (25 mg once daily) and a single dose of glyburide did not result in a clinically relevant pharmacokinetic interaction for either compound.

Hydrochlorothiazide

A single oral dose of carvedilol 25 mg did not alter the pharmacokinetics of a single oral dose of hydrochlorothiazide 25 mg in 12 subjects with hypertension. Likewise, hydrochlorothiazide had no effect on the pharmacokinetics of carvedilol.

Rifampin

In a pharmacokinetic trial conducted in 8 healthy male subjects, rifampin (600 mg daily for 12 days) decreased the AUC and C_{max} of carvedilol by about 70% *[see Drug Interactions (7.5)]*.

Torsemide

In a trial of 12 healthy subjects, combined oral administration of carvedilol 25 mg once daily and torsemide 5 mg once daily for 5 days did not result in any significant differences in their pharmacokinetics compared with administration of the drugs alone.

Warfarin

Carvedilol (12.5 mg twice daily) did not have an effect on the steady-state prothrombin time ratios and did not alter the pharmacokinetics of R(+)- and S(-)-warfarin following concomitant administration with warfarin in 9 healthy volunteers.

13   NONCLINICAL TOXICOLOGY

13.1   Carcinogenesis, Mutagenesis, Impairment of Fertility

In 2-year studies conducted in rats given carvedilol at doses up to 75 mg/kg/day (12 times the MRHD when compared on a mg/m² basis) or in mice given up to 200 mg/kg/day (16 times the MRHD on a mg/m² basis), carvedilol had no carcinogenic effect.

Carvedilol was negative when tested in a battery of genotoxicity assays, including the Ames and the CHO/HGPRT assays for mutagenicity and the in vitro hamster micronucleus and in vivo human lymphocyte cell tests for clastogenicity.

At doses ≥200 mg/kg/day (≥32 times the MRHD as mg/m²) carvedilol was toxic to adult rats (sedation, reduced weight gain) and was associated with a reduced number of successful matings, prolonged mating time, significantly fewer corpora lutea and implants per dam, and complete resorption of 18% of the litters. The no-observed-effect dose level for overt toxicity and impairment of fertility was 60 mg/kg/day (10 times the MRHD as mg/m²).

Table 3. Results of COMET

End point	Carvedilol N = 1,511	Metoprolol N = 1,518	Hazard ratio	(95% CI)
All-cause mortality	34%	40%	0.83	0.74 – 0.93
Mortality + all hospitalization	74%	76%	0.94	0.86 – 1.02
Cardiovascular death	30%	35%	0.80	0.70 – 0.90
Sudden death	14%	17%	0.81	0.68 – 0.97
Death due to circulatory failure	11%	13%	0.83	0.67 – 1.02
Death due to stroke	0.9%	2.5%	0.33	0.18 – 0.62

Table 4. Results of COPERNICUS Trial in Subjects With Severe Heart Failure

End point	Placebo (N = 1,133)	Carvedilol (N = 1,156)	Hazard ratio (95% CI)	% Reduction	Nominal P value
Mortality	190	130	0.65 (0.52 – 0.81)	35	0.00013
Mortality + all hospitalization	507	425	0.76 (0.67 – 0.87)	24	0.00004
Mortality + CV hospitalization	395	314	0.73 (0.63 – 0.84)	27	0.00002
Mortality + HF hospitalization	357	271	0.69 (0.59 – 0.81)	31	0.000004

Cardiovascular = CV; Heart failure = HF.

14   CLINICAL STUDIES

14.1   Heart Failure

A total of 6,975 subjects with mild to severe heart failure were evaluated in placebo-controlled trials of carvedilol.

Mild-to-Moderate Heart Failure

Carvedilol was studied in 5 multicenter, placebo-controlled trials, and in 1 active-controlled trial (COMET trial) involving subjects with mild-to-moderate heart failure.

Four US multicenter, double-blind, placebo-controlled trials enrolled 1,094 subjects (696 randomized to carvedilol) with NYHA class II-III heart failure and ejection fraction ≤0.35. The vast majority were on digitalis, diuretics, and an ACE inhibitor at trial entry. Patients were assigned to the trials based upon exercise ability. An Australia-New Zealand double-blind, placebo-controlled trial enrolled 415 subjects (half randomized to carvedilol) with less severe heart failure. All protocols excluded subjects expected to undergo cardiac transplantation during the 7.5 to 15 months of double-blind follow-up. All randomized subjects had tolerated a 2-week course on carvedilol 6.25 mg twice daily.

In each trial, there was a primary end point, either progression of heart failure (1 US trial) or exercise tolerance (2 US trials meeting enrollment goals and the Australia-New Zealand trial). There were many secondary end points specified in these trials, including NYHA classification, patient and physician global assessments, and cardiovascular hospitalization. Other analyses not prospectively planned included the sum of deaths and total cardiovascular hospitalizations. In situations where the primary end points of a trial do not show a significant benefit of treatment, assignment of significance values to the other results is complex, and such values need to be interpreted cautiously.

The results of the US and Australia-New Zealand trials were as follows:

Slowing Progression of Heart Failure: One US multicenter trial (366 subjects) had as its primary end point the sum of cardiovascular mortality, cardiovascular hospitalization, and sustained increase in heart failure medications. Heart failure progression was reduced, during an average follow-up of 7 months, by 48% (P = 0.008).

In the Australia-New Zealand trial, death and total hospitalizations were reduced by about 25% over 18 to 24 months. In the 3 largest US trials, death and total hospitalizations were reduced by 19%, 39%, and 49%, nominally statistically significant in the last 2 trials. The Australia-New Zealand results were statistically borderline.

Functional Measures: None of the multicenter trials had NYHA classification as a primary end point, but all such trials had it as a secondary end point. There was at least a trend toward improvement in NYHA class in all trials. Exercise tolerance was the primary end point in 3 trials; in none was a statistically significant effect found.

Subjective Measures: Health-related quality of life, as measured with a standard questionnaire (a primary end point in 1 trials), was unaffected by carvedilol. However, patients' and investigators' global assessments showed significant improvement in most trials.

Mortality: Death was not a pre-specified end point in any trial, but was analyzed in all trials. Overall, in these 4 US trials, mortality was reduced, nominally significantly so in 2 trials.

COMET Trial

In this double-blind trial, 3,029 subjects with NYHA class II-IV heart failure (left ventricular ejection fraction ≤35%) were randomized to receive either carvedilol (target dose: 25 mg twice daily) or immediate-release metoprolol tartrate (target dose: 50 mg twice daily). The mean age of the subjects was approximately 62 years, 80% were males, and the mean left ventricular ejection fraction at baseline was 26%. Approximately 96% of the subjects had NYHA class II or III heart failure. Concomitant treatment included diuretics (99%), ACE inhibitors (91%), digitalis (59%), aldosterone antagonists (11%), and "statin" lipid-lowering agents (21%). The mean duration of follow-up was 4.8 years. The mean dose of carvedilol was 42 mg per day.

The trial had 2 primary end points: all-cause mortality and the composite of death plus hospitalization for any reason. The results of COMET are presented in Table 3 below. All-cause mortality carried most of the statistical weight and was the primary determinant of the trial size. All-cause mortality was 34% in the subjects treated with carvedilol and was 40% in the immediate-release metoprolol group (P = 0.0017; hazard ratio = 0.83, 95%CI: 0.74 to 0.93). The effect on mortality was primarily due to a reduction in cardiovascular death. The difference between the 2 groups with respect to the composite end point was not significant (P = 0.122). The estimated mean survival was 8.0 years with carvedilol and 6.6 years with immediate-release metoprolol.

[See table 3 above]

It is not known whether this formulation of metoprolol at any dose or this low dose of metoprolol in any formulation has any effect on survival or hospitalization in patients with heart failure. Thus, this trial extends the time over which carvedilol manifests benefits on survival in heart failure, but it is not evidence that carvedilol improves outcome over the formulation of metoprolol (TOPROL-XL®) with benefits in heart failure.

Severe Heart Failure (COPERNICUS)

In a double-blind trial (COPERNICUS), 2,289 subjects with heart failure at rest or with minimal exertion and left ventricular ejection fraction <25% (mean 20%), despite digitalis (66%), diuretics (99%), and ACE inhibitors (89%) were randomized to placebo or carvedilol. Carvedilol was titrated from a starting dose of 3.125 mg twice daily to the maximum tolerated dose or up to 25 mg twice daily over a minimum of 6 weeks. Most subjects achieved the target dose of 25 mg. The trial was conducted in Eastern and Western Europe, the United States, Israel, and Canada. Similar numbers of subjects per group (about 100) withdrew during the titration period.

The primary end point of the trial was all-cause mortality, but cause-specific mortality and the risk of death or hospitalization (total, cardiovascular [CV], or heart failure [HF])

Help Patients Save on Rx Drugs: PDR.net/PharmacyDiscountCard

were also examined. The developing trial data were followed by a data monitoring committee, and mortality analyses were adjusted for these multiple looks. The trial was stopped after a median follow-up of 10 months because of an observed 35% reduction in mortality (from 19.7% per patient-year on placebo to 12.8% on carvedilol, hazard ratio 0.65, 95% CI: 0.52 to 0.81, P = 0.0014, adjusted) (see Figure 1). The results of COPERNICUS are shown in Table 4. [See table 4 at top of previous page]

Figure 1. Survival Analysis for COPERNICUS (Intent-to-Treat)

The effect on mortality was principally the result of a reduction in the rate of sudden death among subjects without worsening heart failure.

Patients' global assessments, in which carvedilol-treated subjects were compared with placebo, were based on prespecified, periodic patient self-assessments regarding whether clinical status post-treatment showed improvement, worsening or no change compared with baseline. Subjects treated with carvedilol showed significant improvements in global assessments compared with those treated with placebo in COPERNICUS.

The protocol also specified that hospitalizations would be assessed. Fewer subjects on COREG than on placebo were hospitalized for any reason (372 versus 432, P = 0.0029), for cardiovascular reasons (246 versus 314, P = 0.0003), or for worsening heart failure (198 versus 268, P = 0.0001). COREG had a consistent and beneficial effect on all-cause mortality as well as the combined end points of all-cause mortality plus hospitalization (total, CV, or for heart failure) in the overall trial population and in all subgroups examined, including men and women, elderly and non-elderly, blacks and non-blacks, and diabetics and non-diabetics (see Figure 2).

Figure 2. Effects on Mortality for Subgroups in COPERNICUS

14.2 Left Ventricular Dysfunction Following Myocardial Infarction

CAPRICORN was a double-blind trial comparing carvedilol and placebo in 1,959 subjects with a recent myocardial infarction (within 21 days) and left ventricular ejection fraction of ≤40%, with (47%) or without symptoms of heart failure. Subjects given carvedilol received 6.25 mg twice daily, titrated as tolerated to 25 mg twice daily. Subjects had to have a systolic blood pressure >90 mm Hg, a sitting heart rate >60 beats/minute, and no contraindication to β-blocker use. Treatment of the index infarction included aspirin (85%), IV or oral β-blockers (37%), nitrates (73%), heparin (64%), thrombolytics (40%), and acute angioplasty (12%). Background treatment included ACE inhibitors or angiotensin receptor blockers (97%), anticoagulants (20%), lipid-lowering agents (23%), and diuretics (34%). Baseline population characteristics included an average age of 63 years, 74% male, 95% Caucasian, mean blood pressure 121/74 mm Hg, 22% with diabetes, and 54% with a history of hypertension. Mean dosage achieved of carvedilol was 20 mg twice daily; mean duration of follow-up was 15 months.

All-cause mortality was 15% in the placebo group and 12% in the carvedilol group, indicating a 23% risk reduction in

Figure 4. Effects on Mortality for Subgroups in CAPRICORN

subjects treated with carvedilol (95% CI: 2% to 40%, P = 0.03), as shown in Figure 3. The effects on mortality in various subgroups are shown in Figure 4. Nearly all deaths were cardiovascular (which were reduced by 25% by carvedilol), and most of these deaths were sudden or related to pump failure (both types of death were reduced by carvedilol). Another trial end point, total mortality and all-cause hospitalization, did not show a significant improvement.

There was also a significant 40% reduction in fatal or non-fatal myocardial infarction observed in the group treated with carvedilol (95% CI: 11% to 60%, P = 0.01). A similar reduction in the risk of myocardial infarction was also observed in a meta-analysis of placebo-controlled trials of carvedilol in heart failure.

Figure 3. Survival Analysis for CAPRICORN (Intent-to-Treat)

[See figure 4 above]

14.3 Hypertension

COREG was studied in 2 placebo-controlled trials that utilized twice-daily dosing, at total daily doses of 12.5 to 50 mg. In these and other trials, the starting dose did not exceed 12.5 mg. At 50 mg/day, COREG reduced sitting trough (12-hour) blood pressure by about 9/5.5 mm Hg; at 25 mg/day the effect was about 7.5/3.5 mm Hg. Comparisons of trough to peak blood pressure showed a trough to peak ratio for blood pressure response of about 65%. Heart rate fell by about 7.5 beats/minute at 50 mg/day. In general, as is true for other β-blockers, responses were smaller in black than non-black subjects. There were no age- or gender-related differences in response.

The peak antihypertensive effect occurred 1 to 2 hours after a dose. The dose-related blood pressure response was accompanied by a dose-related increase in adverse effects [see Adverse Reactions (6)].

14.4 Hypertension With Type 2 Diabetes Mellitus

In a double-blind trial (GEMINI), COREG, added to an ACE inhibitor or angiotensin receptor blocker, was evaluated in a population with mild-to-moderate hypertension and well-controlled type 2 diabetes mellitus. The mean HbA1c at baseline was 7.2%. COREG was titrated to a mean dose of 17.5 mg twice daily and maintained for 5 months. COREG had no adverse effect on glycemic control, based on HbA1c measurements (mean change from baseline of 0.02%, 95% CI: -0.06 to 0.10, P = NS) [see Warnings and Precautions (5.6)].

16 HOW SUPPLIED/STORAGE AND HANDLING

The white, oval, film-coated tablets are available in the following strengths: 3.125 mg – engraved with 39 and SB, in bottles of 100; 6.25 mg – engraved with 4140 and SB, in bottles of 100; 12.5 mg – engraved with 4141 and SB, in bottles of 100; 25 mg – engraved with 4142 and SB, in bottles of 100. The 6.25-mg, 12.5-mg, and 25-mg tablets are TILTAB tablets.

3.125 mg 100's: NDC 0007-4139-20
- 6.25 mg 100's: NDC 0007-4140-20
- 12.5 mg 100's: NDC 0007-4141-20
- 25 mg 100's: NDC 0007-4142-20

Store below 30°C (86°F). Protect from moisture. Dispense in a tight, light-resistant container.

17 PATIENT COUNSELING INFORMATION

See FDA-Approved Patient Labeling (Patient Information)

17.1 Patient Advice

Patients taking COREG should be advised of the following:
- Patients should take COREG with food.
- Patients should not interrupt or discontinue using COREG without a physician's advice.
- Patients with heart failure should consult their physician if they experience signs or symptoms of worsening heart failure such as weight gain or increasing shortness of breath.
- Patients may experience a drop in blood pressure when standing, resulting in dizziness and, rarely, fainting. Patients should sit or lie down when these symptoms of lowered blood pressure occur.
- If experiencing dizziness or fatigue, patients should avoid driving or hazardous tasks.
- Patients should consult a physician if they experience dizziness or faintness, in case the dosage should be adjusted.
- Diabetic patients should report any changes in blood sugar levels to their physician.
- Contact lens wearers may experience decreased lacrimation.

COREG, COREG CR, and TILTAB are registered trademarks of GlaxoSmithKline.

TOPROL-XL is a registered trademark of the AstraZeneca group of companies.

Manufactured for

GlaxoSmithKline

Research Triangle Park, NC 27709

©2013, GlaxoSmithKline. All rights reserved.

CRG:23PI

PHARMACIST-DETACH HERE AND GIVE INSTRUCTIONS TO PATIENT

PATIENT INFORMATION

COREG® (Co-REG)

Carvedilol Tablets

Read the Patient Information that comes with COREG before you start taking it and each time you get a refill. There may be new information. This information does not take the place of talking with your doctor about your medical condition or your treatment. If you have any questions about COREG, ask your doctor or pharmacist.

What is COREG?

COREG is a prescription medicine that belongs to a group of medicines called "beta-blockers". COREG is used, often with other medicines, for the following conditions:

- to treat patients with certain types of heart failure
- to treat patients who had a heart attack that worsened how well the heart pumps
- to treat patients with high blood pressure (hypertension)

COREG is not approved for use in children under 18 years of age.

Who should not take COREG?

Do not take COREG if you:

- have severe heart failure and are hospitalized in the intensive care unit or require certain intravenous medications that help support circulation (inotropic medications).
- are prone to asthma or other breathing problems.
- have a slow heartbeat or a heart that skips a beat (irregular heartbeat).
- have liver problems.
- are allergic to any of the ingredients in COREG. The active ingredient is carvedilol. See the end of this leaflet for a list of all the ingredients in COREG.

What should I tell my doctor before taking COREG?

Tell your doctor about all of your medical conditions, including if you:

- have asthma or other lung problems (such as bronchitis or emphysema).
- have problems with blood flow in your feet and legs (peripheral vascular disease). COREG can make some of your symptoms worse.
- have diabetes.
- have thyroid problems.
- have a condition called pheochromocytoma.
- have had severe allergic reactions.
- are pregnant or trying to become pregnant. It is not known if COREG is safe for your unborn baby. You and your doctor should talk about the best way to control your high blood pressure during pregnancy.
- are breastfeeding. It is not known if COREG passes into your breast milk. You should not breastfeed while using COREG.
- are scheduled for surgery and will be given anesthetic agents.
- are scheduled for cataract surgery and have taken or are currently taking COREG.
- are taking prescription or non-prescription medicines, vitamins, and herbal supplements. COREG and certain other medicines can affect each other and cause serious side effects. COREG may affect the way other medicines work. Also, other medicines may affect how well COREG works.

Keep a list of all the medicines you take. Show this list to your doctor and pharmacist before you start a new medicine.

How should I take COREG?

It is important for you to take your medicine every day as directed by your doctor. If you stop taking COREG suddenly, you could have chest pain and/or a heart attack. If your doctor decides that you should stop taking COREG, your doctor may slowly lower your dose over a period of time before stopping it completely.

- Take COREG exactly as prescribed. Your doctor will tell you how many tablets to take and how often. In order to minimize possible side effects, your doctor might begin with a low dose and then slowly increase the dose.
- **Do not stop taking COREG and do not change the amount of COREG you take without talking to your doctor.**
- Tell your doctor if you gain weight or have trouble breathing while taking COREG.
- Take COREG with food.
- If you miss a dose of COREG, take your dose as soon as you remember, unless it is time to take your next dose. Take your next dose at the usual time. Do not take 2 doses at the same time.
- If you take too much COREG, call your doctor or poison control center right away.

What should I avoid while taking COREG?

- COREG can cause you to feel dizzy, tired, or faint. Do not drive a car, use machinery, or do anything that needs you to be alert if you have these symptoms.

What are possible side effects of COREG?

- **Low blood pressure (which may cause dizziness or fainting when you stand up).** If these happen, sit or lie down right away and tell your doctor.
- **Tiredness.** If you feel tired or dizzy you should not drive, use machinery, or do anything that needs you to be alert.
- **Slow heartbeat.**
- **Changes in your blood sugar. If you have diabetes, tell your doctor if you have any changes in your blood sugar levels.**
- COREG may hide some of the symptoms of low blood sugar, especially a fast heartbeat.
- COREG may mask the symptoms of hyperthyroidism (overactive thyroid).
- **Worsening of severe allergic reactions.**
- **Rare but serious allergic reactions** (including hives or swelling of the face, lips, tongue, and/or throat that may

cause difficulty in breathing or swallowing) have happened in patients who were on COREG. These reactions can be life-threatening.

Other side effects of COREG include shortness of breath, weight gain, diarrhea, and fewer tears or dry eyes that become bothersome if you wear contact lenses.

Call your doctor if you have any side effects that bother you or don't go away.

Call your doctor for medical advice about side effects. You may report side effects to FDA at 1-800-FDA-1088.

How should I store COREG?

- Store COREG at less than 86°F (30°C). Keep the tablets dry.
- Safely, throw away COREG that is out of date or no longer needed.
- Keep COREG and all medicines out of the reach of children.

General Information about COREG

Medicines are sometimes prescribed for conditions other than those described in patient information leaflets. Do not use COREG for a condition for which it was not prescribed. Do not give COREG to other people, even if they have the same symptoms you have. It may harm them.

This leaflet summarizes the most important information about COREG. If you would like more information, talk with your doctor. You can ask your doctor or pharmacist for information about COREG that is written for healthcare professionals. You can also find out more about COREG by visiting the website www.COREG.com or calling 1-888-825-5249. This call is free.

What are the ingredients in COREG?

Active Ingredient: carvedilol.

Inactive Ingredients: colloidal silicon dioxide, crospovidone, hypromellose, lactose, magnesium stearate, polyethylene glycol, polysorbate 80, povidone, sucrose, and titanium dioxide.

Carvedilol tablets come in the following strengths: 3.125 mg, 6.25 mg, 12.5 mg, 25 mg.

What is high blood pressure (hypertension)?

Blood pressure is the force of blood in your blood vessels when your heart beats and when your heart rests. You have high blood pressure when the force is too much. High blood pressure makes the heart work harder to pump blood through the body and causes damage to blood vessels. COREG can help your blood vessels relax so your blood pressure is lower. Medicines that lower blood pressure may lower your chance of having a stroke or heart attack.

COREG is a registered trademark of GlaxoSmithKline.

Manufactured for

GlaxoSmithKline

Research Triangle Park, NC 27709

©2013, GlaxoSmithKline. All rights reserved.

August 2013

CRG:5PIL

COREG CR®   ℞

[kor′ eg]

(carvedilol phosphate)

Extended-release Capsules

HIGHLIGHTS OF PRESCRIBING INFORMATION

These highlights do not include all the information needed to use COREG CR safely and effectively. See full prescribing information for COREG CR.

COREG CR (carvedilol phosphate) Extended-release Capsules

Initial U.S. Approval: 1995

──────INDICATIONS AND USAGE──────

COREG CR is an alpha-/beta-adrenergic blocking agent indicated for the treatment of:

- mild to severe chronic heart failure. (1.1)
- left ventricular dysfunction following myocardial infarction in clinically stable patients. (1.2)
- hypertension. (1.3)

──────DOSAGE AND ADMINISTRATION──────

Take with food. Do not crush or chew capsules. Individualize dosage and monitor during up-titration. (2)

- Heart failure: Start at 10 mg once daily and increase to 20, 40, and then 80 mg once daily over intervals of at least 2 weeks. Maintain lower doses if higher doses are not tolerated. (2.1)
- Left ventricular dysfunction following myocardial infarction: Start at 20 mg once daily and increase to 40 mg then 80 mg once daily after intervals of 3 to 10 days. A lower starting dose or slower titration may be used. (2.2)
- Hypertension: Start at 20 mg once daily and increase if needed for blood pressure control to 40 mg then 80 mg once daily over intervals of 1 to 2 weeks. (2.3)
- Elderly patients (>65 years of age): When switching from higher doses of immediate-release carvedilol to COREG CR, a lower starting dose should be considered to reduce the risk of hypotension and syncope. (2.5)

──────DOSAGE FORMS AND STRENGTHS──────

Capsules: 10 mg, 20 mg, 40 mg, 80 mg (3)

──────CONTRAINDICATIONS──────

- Bronchial asthma or related bronchospastic conditions. (4)
- Second- or third-degree AV block. (4)
- Sick sinus syndrome. (4)
- Severe bradycardia (unless permanent pacemaker in place). (4)
- Patients in cardiogenic shock or decompensated heart failure requiring the use of IV inotropic therapy. (4)
- Severe hepatic impairment. (2.4, 4)
- History of serious hypersensitivity reaction (e.g., Stevens-Johnson syndrome, anaphylactic reaction, angioedema) to carvedilol or any of the components of COREG CR. (4)

──────WARNINGS AND PRECAUTIONS──────

- Acute exacerbation of coronary artery disease upon cessation of therapy: Do not abruptly discontinue. (5.1)
- Bradycardia, hypotension, worsening heart failure/fluid retention may occur. Reduce the dose as needed. (5.2, 5.3, 5.4)
- Non-allergic bronchospasm (e.g., chronic bronchitis and emphysema): Avoid β-blockers. (4) However, if deemed necessary, use with caution and at lowest effective dose. (5.5)
- Diabetes: Monitor glucose as β-blockers may mask symptoms of hypoglycemia or worsen hyperglycemia. (5.6)

──────ADVERSE REACTIONS──────

The safety profile of COREG CR was similar to that observed for immediate-release carvedilol. Most common adverse events seen with immediate-release carvedilol (6.1):

- Heart failure and left ventricular dysfunction following myocardial infarction (≥10%): Dizziness, fatigue, hypotension, diarrhea, hyperglycemia, asthenia, bradycardia, weight increase.
- Hypertension (≥5%): Dizziness.

To report SUSPECTED ADVERSE REACTIONS, contact GlaxoSmithKline at 1-888-825-5249 or FDA at 1-800-FDA-1088 or www.fda.gov/medwatch.

──────DRUG INTERACTIONS──────

- CYP P450 2D6 enzyme inhibitors may increase and rifampin may decrease carvedilol levels. (7.1, 7.5)
- Hypotensive agents (e.g., reserpine, MAO inhibitors, clonidine) may increase the risk of hypotension and/or severe bradycardia. (7.2)
- Cyclosporine or digoxin levels may increase. (7.3, 7.4)
- Both digitalis glycosides and β-blockers slow atrioventricular conduction and decrease heart rate. Concomitant use can increase the risk of bradycardia. (7.4)
- Amiodarone may increase carvedilol levels resulting in further slowing of the heart rate or cardiac conduction. (7.6)
- Verapamil- or diltiazem-type calcium channel blockers may affect ECG and/or blood pressure. (7.7)
- Insulin and oral hypoglycemics action may be enhanced. (7.8)

See 17 for PATIENT COUNSELING INFORMATION and FDA-approved patient labeling

Revised: 05/2014

FULL PRESCRIBING INFORMATION: CONTENTS*

FULL PRESCRIBING INFORMATION

1   INDICATIONS AND USAGE

1.1   Heart Failure
COREG CR® is indicated for the treatment of mild-to-severe chronic heart failure of ischemic or cardiomyopathic origin, usually in addition to diuretics, ACE inhibitors, and digitalis, to increase survival and, also, to reduce the risk of hospitalization *[see Clinical Studies (14.1)]*.

1.2   Left Ventricular Dysfunction Following Myocardial Infarction
COREG CR is indicated to reduce cardiovascular mortality in clinically stable patients who have survived the acute phase of a myocardial infarction and have a left ventricular ejection fraction of ≤40% (with or without symptomatic heart failure) *[see Clinical Studies (14.2)]*.

1.3   Hypertension
COREG CR is indicated for the management of essential hypertension *[see Clinical Studies (14.3, 14.4)]*. It can be used alone or in combination with other antihypertensive agents, especially thiazide–type diuretics *[see Drug Interactions (7.2)]*.

2   DOSAGE AND ADMINISTRATION
COREG CR is an extended-release capsule intended for once–daily administration. Patients controlled with immediate–release carvedilol tablets alone or in combination with other medications may be switched to COREG CR extended–release capsules based on the total daily doses shown in Table 1.

Table 1. Dosing Conversion

Daily Dose of Immediate-Release Carvedilol Tablets	Daily Dose of COREG CR Capsules[a]
6.25 mg (3.125 mg twice daily)	10 mg once daily
12.5 mg (6.25 mg twice daily)	20 mg once daily
25 mg (12.5 mg twice daily)	40 mg once daily
50 mg (25 mg twice daily)	80 mg once daily

[a] When switching from carvedilol 12.5 mg or 25 mg twice daily, a starting dose of COREG CR 20 mg or 40 mg once daily, respectively, may be warranted for elderly patients or those at increased risk of hypotension, dizziness, or syncope. Subsequent titration to higher doses should, as appropriate, be made after an interval of at least 2 weeks.

COREG CR should be taken once daily in the morning with food. COREG CR should be swallowed as a whole capsule. COREG CR and/or its contents should not be crushed, chewed, or taken in divided doses.

Alternative Administration: The capsules may be carefully opened and the beads sprinkled over a spoonful of applesauce. The applesauce should not be warm because it could affect the modified-release properties of this formulation. The mixture of drug and applesauce should be consumed immediately in its entirety. The drug and applesauce mixture should not be stored for future use. Absorption of the beads sprinkled on other foods has not been tested.

2.1   Heart Failure
DOSAGE MUST BE INDIVIDUALIZED AND CLOSELY MONITORED BY A PHYSICIAN DURING UP–TITRATION. Prior to initiation of COREG CR, it is recommended that fluid retention be minimized. The recommended starting dose of COREG CR is 10 mg once daily for 2 weeks. Patients who tolerate a dose of 10 mg once daily may have their dose increased to 20, 40, and 80 mg over successive intervals of at least 2 weeks. Patients should be maintained on lower doses if higher doses are not tolerated.

Patients should be advised that initiation of treatment and (to a lesser extent) dosage increases may be associated with transient symptoms of dizziness or lightheadedness (and rarely syncope) within the first hour after dosing. Thus, during these periods, they should avoid situations such as driving or hazardous tasks, where symptoms could result in injury. Vasodilatory symptoms often do not require treatment, but it may be useful to separate the time of dosing of COREG CR from that of the ACE inhibitor or to reduce temporarily the dose of the ACE inhibitor. The dose of COREG CR should not be increased until symptoms of worsening heart failure or vasodilation have been stabilized.

Fluid retention (with or without transient worsening heart failure symptoms) should be treated by an increase in the dose of diuretics.

The dose of COREG CR should be reduced if patients experience bradycardia (heart rate <55 beats/minute).

Episodes of dizziness or fluid retention during initiation of COREG CR can generally be managed without discontinuation of treatment and do not preclude subsequent successful titration of, or a favorable response to, COREG CR.

2.2   Left Ventricular Dysfunction Following Myocardial Infarction
DOSAGE MUST BE INDIVIDUALIZED AND MONITORED DURING UP–TITRATION. Treatment with COREG CR may be started as an inpatient or outpatient and should be started after the patient is hemodynamically stable and fluid retention has been minimized. It is recommended that COREG CR be started at 20 mg once daily and increased after 3 to 10 days, based on tolerability, to 40 mg once daily, then again to the target dose of 80 mg once daily. A lower starting dose may be used (10 mg once daily) and/or the rate of up–titration may be slowed if clinically indicated (e.g., due to low blood pressure or heart rate, or fluid retention). Patients should be maintained on lower doses if higher doses are not tolerated. The recommended dosing regimen need not be altered in patients who received treatment with an IV or oral β–blocker during the acute phase of the myocardial infarction.

2.3   Hypertension
DOSAGE MUST BE INDIVIDUALIZED. The recommended starting dose of COREG CR is 20 mg once daily. If this dose is tolerated, using standing systolic pressure measured about 1 hour after dosing as a guide, the dose should be maintained for 7 to 14 days, and then increased to 40 mg once daily if needed, based on trough blood pressure, again using standing systolic pressure 1 hour after dosing as a guide for tolerance. This dose should also be maintained for 7 to 14 days and can then be adjusted upward to 80 mg once daily if tolerated and needed. Although not specifically studied, it is anticipated the full antihypertensive effect of COREG CR would be seen within 7 to 14 days as had been demonstrated with immediate–release carvedilol. Total daily dose should not exceed 80 mg.

Concomitant administration with a diuretic can be expected to produce additive effects and exaggerate the orthostatic component of carvedilol action.

2.4   Hepatic Impairment
COREG CR should not be given to patients with severe hepatic impairment *[see Contraindications (4)]*.

2.5   Geriatric Use
When switching elderly patients (65 years of age or older) who are taking the higher doses of immediate-release carvedilol tablets (25 mg twice daily) to COREG CR, a lower starting dose (40 mg) of COREG CR is recommended to minimize the potential for dizziness, syncope, or hypotension *[see Dosage and Administration (2)]*. Patients who have switched and who tolerate COREG CR should, as appropriate, have their dose increased after an interval of at least 2 weeks *[see Use in Specific Populations (8.5)]*.

3   DOSAGE FORMS AND STRENGTHS
The hard gelatin capsules are filled with white to off-white microparticles and are available in the following strengths:
- 10 mg – white and green capsule shell printed with "GSK COREG CR" and "10 mg"
- 20 mg – white and yellow capsule shell printed with "GSK COREG CR" and "20 mg"
- 40 mg – yellow and green capsule shell printed with "GSK COREG CR" and "40 mg"
- 80 mg – white capsule shell printed with "GSK COREG CR" and "80 mg"

4   CONTRAINDICATIONS
COREG CR is contraindicated in the following conditions:
- Bronchial asthma or related bronchospastic conditions. Deaths from status asthmaticus have been reported following single doses of immediate-release carvedilol.
- Second– or third–degree AV block.
- Sick sinus syndrome.
- Severe bradycardia (unless a permanent pacemaker is in place).
- Patients with cardiogenic shock or who have decompensated heart failure requiring the use of intravenous inotropic therapy. Such patients should first be weaned from intravenous therapy before initiating COREG CR.
- Patients with severe hepatic impairment.
- Patients with a history of a serious hypersensitivity reaction (e.g., Stevens-Johnson syndrome, anaphylactic reaction, angioedema) to carvedilol or any of the components of COREG CR.

5   WARNINGS AND PRECAUTIONS
In clinical trials of COREG CR in subjects with hypertension (338 subjects) and in subjects with left ventricular dysfunction following a myocardial infarction or heart failure (187 subjects), the profile of adverse events observed with carvedilol phosphate was generally similar to that observed with the administration of immediate–release carvedilol. Therefore, the information included within this section is based on data from controlled clinical trials with COREG CR as well as immediate–release carvedilol.

5.1   Cessation of Therapy
Patients with coronary artery disease, who are being treated with COREG CR, should be advised against abrupt discontinuation of therapy. Severe exacerbation of angina and the occurrence of myocardial infarction and ventricular arrhythmias have been reported in angina patients following the abrupt discontinuation of therapy with β–blockers. The last 2 complications may occur with or without preceding exacerbation of the angina pectoris. As with other β–blockers, when discontinuation of COREG CR is planned, the patients should be carefully observed and advised to limit physical activity to a minimum. COREG CR should be discontinued over 1 to 2 weeks whenever possible. If the angina worsens or acute coronary insufficiency develops, it is recommended that COREG CR be promptly reinstituted, at least temporarily. Because coronary artery disease is common and may be unrecognized, it may be prudent not to discontinue therapy with COREG CR abruptly even in patients treated only for hypertension or heart failure.

5.2   Bradycardia
In clinical trials with immediate–release carvedilol, bradycardia was reported in about 2% of hypertensive subjects, 9% of heart failure subjects, and 6.5% of myocardial infarction subjects with left ventricular dysfunction. Bradycardia was reported in 0.5% of subjects receiving COREG CR in a trial of heart failure subjects and myocardial infarction subjects with left ventricular dysfunction. There were no reports of bradycardia in the clinical trial of COREG CR in hypertension. However, if pulse rate drops below 55 beats/minute, the dosage of COREG CR should be reduced.

5.3   Hypotension
In clinical trials of primarily mild–to–moderate heart failure with immediate–release carvedilol, hypotension and postural hypotension occurred in 9.7% and syncope in 3.4% of subjects receiving carvedilol compared with 3.6% and 2.5% of placebo subjects, respectively. The risk for these events was highest during the first 30 days of dosing, corresponding to the up–titration period and was a cause for discontinuation of therapy in 0.7% of carvedilol subjects, compared with 0.4% of placebo subjects. In a long–term, placebo–controlled trial in severe heart failure (COPERNICUS), hypotension and postural hypotension occurred in 15.1% and syncope in 2.9% of subjects with heart failure receiving carvedilol compared with 8.7% and 2.3% of placebo subjects, respectively. These events were a cause for discontinuation of therapy in 1.1% of carvedilol subjects, compared with 0.8% of placebo subjects.

In a trial comparing subjects with heart failure switched to COREG CR or maintained on immediate-release carvedilol, there was a 2-fold increase in the combined incidence of hypotension, syncope, or dizziness in elderly subjects (>65 years) switched from the highest dose of carvedilol (25 mg twice daily) to COREG CR 80 mg once daily *[see Dosage and Administration (2), Use in Specific Populations (8.5)]*.

In the clinical trial of COREG CR in hypertensive subjects, syncope was reported in 0.3% of subjects receiving COREG CR compared with 0% of subjects receiving placebo. There were no reports of postural hypotension in this trial. Postural hypotension occurred in 1.8% and syncope in 0.1% of hypertensive subjects receiving immediate–release carvedilol, primarily following the initial dose or at the time of dose increase and was a cause for discontinuation of therapy in 1% of subjects.

In the CAPRICORN trial of survivors of an acute myocardial infarction with left ventricular dysfunction, hypotension or postural hypotension occurred in 20.2% of subjects receiving carvedilol compared with 12.6% of placebo subjects. Syncope was reported in 3.9% and 1.9% of subjects, respectively. These events were a cause for discontinuation of therapy in 2.5% of subjects receiving carvedilol, compared with 0.2% of placebo subjects.

Starting with a low dose, administration with food, and gradual up-titration should decrease the likelihood of syncope or excessive hypotension [see Dosage and Administration (2.1, 2.2, 2.3)]. During initiation of therapy, the patient should be cautioned to avoid situations such as driving or hazardous tasks, where injury could result should syncope occur.

5.4 Heart Failure/Fluid Retention

Worsening heart failure or fluid retention may occur during up–titration of carvedilol. If such symptoms occur, diuretics should be increased and the dose of COREG CR should not be advanced until clinical stability resumes [see Dosage and Administration (2)]. Occasionally it is necessary to lower the dose of COREG CR or temporarily discontinue it. Such episodes do not preclude subsequent successful titration of, or a favorable response to, COREG CR. In a placebo–controlled trial of subjects with severe heart failure, worsening heart failure during the first 3 months was reported to a similar degree with immediate-release carvedilol and with placebo. When treatment was maintained beyond 3 months, worsening heart failure was reported less frequently in subjects treated with carvedilol than with placebo. Worsening heart failure observed during long–term therapy is more likely to be related to the patients' underlying disease than to treatment with carvedilol.

5.5 Non-allergic Bronchospasm

Patients with bronchospastic disease (e.g., chronic bronchitis and emphysema) should, in general, not receive β–blockers. COREG CR may be used with caution, however, in patients who do not respond to, or cannot tolerate, other antihypertensive agents. It is prudent, if COREG CR is used, to use the smallest effective dose, so that inhibition of endogenous or exogenous β–agonists is minimized.

In clinical trials of subjects with heart failure, subjects with bronchospastic disease were enrolled if they did not require oral or inhaled medication to treat their bronchospastic disease. In such patients, it is recommended that COREG CR be used with caution. The dosing recommendations should be followed closely and the dose should be lowered if any evidence of bronchospasm is observed during up–titration.

5.6 Glycemic Control in Type 2 Diabetes

In general, β–blockers may mask some of the manifestations of hypoglycemia, particularly tachycardia. Nonselective β–blockers may potentiate insulin–induced hypoglycemia and delay recovery of serum glucose levels. Patients subject to spontaneous hypoglycemia, or diabetic patients receiving insulin or oral hypoglycemic agents, should be cautioned about these possibilities.

In heart failure patients with diabetes, carvedilol therapy may lead to worsening hyperglycemia, which responds to intensification of hypoglycemic therapy. It is recommended that blood glucose be monitored when dosing with COREG CR is initiated, adjusted, or discontinued. Trials designed to examine the effects of carvedilol on glycemic control in patients with diabetes and heart failure have not been conducted.

In a trial designed to examine the effects of immediate–release carvedilol on glycemic control in a population with mild–to–moderate hypertension and well-controlled type 2 diabetes mellitus, carvedilol had no adverse effect on glycemic control, based on HbA1c measurements [see Clinical Studies (14.4)].

5.7 Peripheral Vascular Disease

β–blockers can precipitate or aggravate symptoms of arterial insufficiency in patients with peripheral vascular disease. Caution should be exercised in such individuals.

5.8 Deterioration of Renal Function

Rarely, use of carvedilol in patients with heart failure has resulted in deterioration of renal function. Patients at risk appear to be those with low blood pressure (systolic blood pressure <100 mm Hg), ischemic heart disease and diffuse vascular disease, and/or underlying renal insufficiency. Renal function has returned to baseline when carvedilol was stopped. In patients with these risk factors it is recommended that renal function be monitored during up–titration of COREG CR and the drug discontinued or dosage reduced if worsening of renal function occurs.

5.9 Major Surgery

Chronically administered beta-blocking therapy should not be routinely withdrawn prior to major surgery; however, the impaired ability of the heart to respond to reflex adrenergic stimuli may augment the risks of general anesthesia and surgical procedures.

5.10 Thyrotoxicosis

β–adrenergic blockade may mask clinical signs of hyperthyroidism, such as tachycardia. Abrupt withdrawal of β–blockade may be followed by an exacerbation of the symptoms of hyperthyroidism or may precipitate thyroid storm.

5.11 Pheochromocytoma

In patients with pheochromocytoma, an α–blocking agent should be initiated prior to the use of any β–blocking agent. Although carvedilol has both α– and β–blocking pharmacologic activities, there has been no experience with its use in this condition. Therefore, caution should be taken in the administration of carvedilol to patients suspected of having pheochromocytoma.

5.12 Prinzmetal's Variant Angina

Agents with non–selective β–blocking activity may provoke chest pain in patients with Prinzmetal's variant angina. There has been no clinical experience with carvedilol in these patients although the α–blocking activity may prevent such symptoms. However, caution should be taken in the administration of COREG CR to patients suspected of having Prinzmetal's variant angina.

5.13 Risk of Anaphylactic Reaction

While taking β–blockers, patients with a history of severe anaphylactic reaction to a variety of allergens may be more reactive to repeated challenge, either accidental, diagnostic, or therapeutic. Such patients may be unresponsive to the usual doses of epinephrine used to treat allergic reaction.

5.14 Intraoperative Floppy Iris Syndrome

Intraoperative Floppy Iris Syndrome (IFIS) has been observed during cataract surgery in some patients treated with alpha-1 blockers (COREG CR is an alpha/beta blocker). This variant of small pupil syndrome is characterized by the combination of a flaccid iris that billows in response to intraoperative irrigation currents, progressive intraoperative miosis despite preoperative dilation with standard mydriatic drugs, and potential prolapse of the iris toward the phacoemulsification incisions. The patient's ophthalmologist should be prepared for possible modifications to the surgical technique, such as utilization of iris hooks,

Table 2. Adverse Events (%) Occurring More Frequently With Immediate-Release Carvedilol Than With Placebo in Subjects With Mild-to-Moderate Heart Failure (HF) Enrolled in US Heart Failure Trials or in Subjects With Severe Heart Failure in the COPERNICUS Trial (Incidence >3% in Subjects Treated With Carvedilol, Regardless of Causality)

Body System/ Adverse Event	Mild-to-Moderate HF		Severe HF	
	Carvedilol (n = 765)	Placebo (n = 437)	Carvedilol (n = 1,156)	Placebo (n = 1,133)
Body as a Whole				
Asthenia	7	7	11	9
Fatigue	24	22	—	—
Digoxin level increased	5	4	2	1
Edema generalized	5	3	6	5
Edema dependent	4	2	—	—
Cardiovascular				
Bradycardia	9	1	10	3
Hypotension	9	3	14	8
Syncope	3	3	8	5
Angina pectoris	2	3	6	4
Central Nervous System				
Dizziness	32	19	24	17
Headache	8	7	5	3
Gastrointestinal				
Diarrhea	12	6	5	3
Nausea	9	5	4	3
Vomiting	6	4	1	2
Metabolic				
Hyperglycemia	12	8	5	3
Weight increase	10	7	12	11
BUN increased	6	5	—	—
NPN increased	6	5	—	—
Hypercholesterolemia	4	3	1	1
Edema peripheral	2	1	7	6
Musculoskeletal				
Arthralgia	6	5	1	1
Respiratory				
Cough increased	8	9	5	4
Rales	4	4	4	2
Vision				
Vision abnormal	5	2		

iris dilator rings, or viscoelastic substances. There does not appear to be a benefit of stopping alpha-1 blocker therapy prior to cataract surgery.

6   ADVERSE REACTIONS
6.1   Clinical Trials Experience
Carvedilol has been evaluated for safety in subjects with heart failure (mild, moderate, and severe), in subjects with left ventricular dysfunction following myocardial infarction, and in hypertensive subjects. The observed adverse event profile was consistent with the pharmacology of the drug and the health status of the subjects in the clinical trials. Adverse events reported for each of these populations reflecting the use of either COREG CR or immediate-release carvedilol are provided below. Excluded are adverse events considered too general to be informative, and those not reasonably associated with the use of the drug because they were associated with the condition being treated or are very common in the treated population. Rates of adverse events were generally similar across demographic subsets (men and women, elderly and non–elderly, blacks and non–blacks). COREG CR has been evaluated for safety in a 4-week (2 weeks of immediate-release carvedilol and 2 weeks of COREG CR) clinical trial (n = 187) which included 157 subjects with stable mild, moderate, or severe chronic heart failure and 30 subjects with left ventricular dysfunction following acute myocardial infarction. The profile of adverse events observed with COREG CR in this small, short-term trial was generally similar to that observed with immediate-release carvedilol. Differences in safety would not be expected based on the similarity in plasma levels for COREG CR and immediate-release carvedilol.

Heart Failure
The following information describes the safety experience in heart failure with immediate-release carvedilol.

Carvedilol has been evaluated for safety in heart failure in more than 4,500 subjects worldwide of whom more than 2,100 participated in placebo–controlled clinical trials. Approximately 60% of the total treated population in placebo–controlled clinical trials received carvedilol for at least 6 months and 30% received carvedilol for at least 12 months. In the COMET trial, 1,511 subjects with mild–to–moderate heart failure were treated with carvedilol for up to 5.9 years (mean: 4.8 years). Both in US clinical trials in mild–to–moderate heart failure that compared carvedilol in daily doses up to 100 mg (n = 765) with placebo (n = 437), and in a multinational clinical trial in severe heart failure (COPERNICUS) that compared carvedilol in daily doses up to 50 mg (n = 1,156) with placebo (n = 1,133), discontinuation rates for adverse experiences were similar in carvedilol and placebo subjects. In placebo–controlled clinical trials, the only cause of discontinuation >1%, and occurring more often on carvedilol was dizziness (1.3% on carvedilol, 0.6% on placebo in the COPERNICUS trial).

Table 2 shows adverse events reported in subjects with mild–to–moderate heart failure enrolled in US placebo–controlled clinical trials, and with severe heart failure enrolled in the COPERNICUS trial. Shown are adverse events that occurred more frequently in drug–treated subjects than placebo–treated subjects with an incidence of >3% in subjects treated with carvedilol regardless of causality. Median trial medication exposure was 6.3 months for both carvedilol and placebo subjects in the trials of mild–to–moderate heart failure, and 10.4 months in the trial of subjects with severe heart failure. The adverse event profile of carvedilol observed in the long-term COMET trial was generally similar to that observed in the US Heart Failure Trials.

[See table 2 at top of previous page]

Cardiac failure and dyspnea were also reported in these trials, but the rates were equal or greater in subjects who received placebo.

The following adverse events were reported with a frequency of >1% but ≤3% and more frequently with carvedilol in either the US placebo-controlled trials in subjects with mild-to-moderate heart failure, or in subjects with severe heart failure in the COPERNICUS trial.

Incidence >1% to ≤3%
Body as a Whole: Allergy, malaise, hypovolemia, fever, leg edema.
Cardiovascular: Fluid overload, postural hypotension, aggravated angina pectoris, AV block, palpitation, hypertension.
Central and Peripheral Nervous System: Hypesthesia, vertigo, paresthesia.
Gastrointestinal: Melena, periodontitis.
Liver and Biliary System: SGPT increased, SGOT increased.
Metabolic and Nutritional: Hyperuricemia, hypoglycemia, hyponatremia, increased alkaline phosphatase, glycosuria, hypervolemia, diabetes mellitus, GGT increased, weight loss, hyperkalemia, creatinine increased.
Musculoskeletal: Muscle cramps.

Platelet, Bleeding, and Clotting: Prothrombin decreased, purpura, thrombocytopenia.
Psychiatric: Somnolence.
Reproductive, male: Impotence.
Special Senses: Blurred vision.
Urinary System: Renal insufficiency, albuminuria, hematuria.

Left Ventricular Dysfunction Following Myocardial Infarction
The following information describes the safety experience in left ventricular dysfunction following acute myocardial infarction with immediate-release carvedilol.

Carvedilol has been evaluated for safety in survivors of an acute myocardial infarction with left ventricular dysfunction in the CAPRICORN trial which involved 969 subjects who received carvedilol and 980 who received placebo. Approximately 75% of the subjects received carvedilol for at least 6 months and 53% received carvedilol for at least 12 months. Subjects were treated for an average of 12.9 months and 12.8 months with carvedilol and placebo, respectively.

The most common adverse events reported with carvedilol in the CAPRICORN trial were consistent with the profile of the drug in the US heart failure trials and the COPERNICUS trial. The only additional adverse events reported in CAPRICORN in >3% of the subjects and more commonly on carvedilol were dyspnea, anemia, and lung edema. The following adverse events were reported with a frequency of >1% but ≤3% and more frequently with carvedilol: flu syndrome, cerebrovascular accident, peripheral vascular disorder, hypotonia, depression, gastrointestinal pain, arthritis, and gout. The overall rates of discontinuations due to adverse events were similar in both groups of subjects. In this database, the only cause of discontinuation >1%, and occurring more often on carvedilol was hypotension (1.5% on carvedilol, 0.2% on placebo).

Hypertension
COREG CR was evaluated for safety in an 8-week double-blind trial in 337 subjects with essential hypertension. The profile of adverse events observed with COREG CR was generally similar to that observed with immediate-release carvedilol. The overall rates of discontinuations due to adverse events were similar between COREG CR and placebo.

Table 3. Adverse Events (%) Occurring More Frequently With COREG CR Than With Placebo in Subjects With Hypertension (Incidence ≥1% in Subjects Treated With Carvedilol, Regardless of Causality)

Adverse Event	COREG CR (n = 253)	Placebo (n = 84)
Nasopharyngitis	4	0
Dizziness	2	1
Nausea	2	0
Edema peripheral	2	1
Nasal congestion	1	0
Paresthesia	1	0
Sinus congestion	1	0
Diarrhea	1	0
Insomnia	1	0

The following information describes the safety experience in hypertension with immediate-release carvedilol.

Carvedilol has been evaluated for safety in hypertension in more than 2,193 subjects in US clinical trials and in 2,976 subjects in international clinical trials. Approximately 36% of the total treated population received carvedilol for at least 6 months. In general, carvedilol was well tolerated at doses up to 50 mg daily. Most adverse events reported during carvedilol therapy were of mild to moderate severity. In US controlled clinical trials directly comparing carvedilol monotherapy in doses up to 50 mg (n = 1,142) with placebo (n = 462), 4.9% of carvedilol subjects discontinued for adverse events versus 5.2% of placebo subjects. Although there was no overall difference in discontinuation rates, discontinuations were more common in the carvedilol group for postural hypotension (1% versus 0). The overall incidence of adverse events in US placebo–controlled trials was found to increase with increasing dose of carvedilol. For individual adverse events this could only be distinguished for dizziness, which increased in frequency from 2% to 5% as total daily dose increased from 6.25 mg to 50 mg as single or divided doses.

Table 4 shows adverse events in US placebo–controlled clinical trials for hypertension that occurred with an incidence of ≥1%, regardless of causality, and that were more frequent in drug–treated subjects than placebo–treated subjects.

Table 4. Adverse Events (% Occurrence) in US Placebo-Controlled Hypertension Trials With Immediate-Release Carvedilol (Incidence ≥1% in Subjects Treated With Carvedilol, Regardless of Causality)*

Adverse Event	Carvedilol (n = 1,142)	Placebo (n = 462)
Cardiovascular		
Bradycardia	2	—
Postural hypotension	2	—
Peripheral edema	1	—
Central Nervous System		
Dizziness	6	5
Insomnia	2	1
Gastrointestinal		
Diarrhea	2	1
Hematologic		
Thrombocytopenia	1	—
Metabolic		
Hypertriglyceridemia	1	—

* Shown are events with rate >1% rounded to nearest integer.

Dyspnea and fatigue were also reported in these trials, but the rates were equal or greater in subjects who received placebo.

The following adverse events not described above were reported as possibly or probably related to carvedilol in worldwide open or controlled trials with carvedilol in subjects with hypertension or heart failure.

Incidence >0.1% to ≤1%
Cardiovascular: Peripheral ischemia, tachycardia.
Central and Peripheral Nervous System: Hypokinesia.
Gastrointestinal: Bilirubinemia, increased hepatic enzymes (0.2% of hypertension patients and 0.4% of heart failure patients were discontinued from therapy because of increases in hepatic enzymes) [see Adverse Reactions (6.2)].
Psychiatric: Nervousness, sleep disorder, aggravated depression, impaired concentration, abnormal thinking, paroniria, emotional lability.
Respiratory System: Asthma [see Contraindications (4)].
Reproductive, male: Decreased libido.
Skin and Appendages: Pruritus, rash erythematous, rash maculopapular, rash psoriaform, photosensitivity reaction.
Special Senses: Tinnitus.
Urinary System: Micturition frequency increased.
Autonomic Nervous System: Dry mouth, sweating increased.
Metabolic and Nutritional: Hypokalemia, hypertriglyceridemia.
Hematologic: Anemia, leukopenia.
The following events were reported in ≤0.1% of subjects and are potentially important: complete AV block, bundle branch block, myocardial ischemia, cerebrovascular disorder, convulsions, migraine, neuralgia, paresis, anaphylactoid reaction, alopecia, exfoliative dermatitis, amnesia, GI hemorrhage, bronchospasm, pulmonary edema, decreased hearing, respiratory alkalosis, increased BUN, decreased HDL, pancytopenia, and atypical lymphocytes.

6.2   Laboratory Abnormalities
Reversible elevations in serum transaminases (ALT or AST) have been observed during treatment with carvedilol. Rates of transaminase elevations (2 to 3 times the upper limit of normal) observed during controlled clinical trials have generally been similar between subjects treated with carvedilol and those treated with placebo. However, transaminase elevations, confirmed by rechallenge, have been observed with carvedilol. In a long-term, placebo-controlled trial in severe heart failure, subjects treated with carvedilol had lower values for hepatic transaminases than subjects treated with placebo, possibly because carvedilol-induced improvements in cardiac function led to less hepatic congestion and/or improved hepatic blood flow.

Carvedilol therapy has not been associated with clinically significant changes in serum potassium, total triglycerides, total cholesterol, HDL cholesterol, uric acid, blood urea nitrogen, or creatinine. No clinically relevant changes were noted in fasting serum glucose in hypertensive subjects; fasting serum glucose was not evaluated in the heart failure clinical trials.

6.3   Postmarketing Experience
The following adverse reactions have been identified during post-approval use of COREG® or COREG CR. Because these reactions are reported voluntarily from a population of uncertain size, it is not always possible to reliably estimate their frequency or establish a causal relationship to drug exposure.

Blood and Lymphatic System Disorders: Aplastic anemia. *Immune System Disorders:* Hypersensitivity (e.g., anaphylactic reactions, angioedema, urticaria).
Renal and Urinary Disorders: Urinary incontinence.
Respiratory, Thoracic and Mediastinal Disorders: Interstitial pneumonitis.
Skin and Subcutaneous Tissue Disorders: Stevens-Johnson syndrome, toxic epidermal necrolysis, erythema multiforme.

7 DRUG INTERACTIONS

7.1 CYP2D6 Inhibitors and Poor Metabolizers

Interactions of carvedilol with potent inhibitors of CYP2D6 isoenzyme (such as quinidine, fluoxetine, paroxetine, and propafenone) have not been studied, but these drugs would be expected to increase blood levels of the R(+) enantiomer of carvedilol *[see Clinical Pharmacology (12.3)]*. Retrospective analysis of side effects in clinical trials showed that poor 2D6 metabolizers had a higher rate of dizziness during up-titration, presumably resulting from vasodilating effects of the higher concentrations of the α–blocking R(+) enantiomer.

7.2 Hypotensive Agents

Patients taking both agents with β–blocking properties and a drug that can deplete catecholamines (e.g., reserpine and monoamine oxidase inhibitors) should be observed closely for signs of hypotension and/or severe bradycardia.
Concomitant administration of clonidine with agents with β–blocking properties may potentiate blood–pressure– and heart–rate–lowering effects. When concomitant treatment with agents with β–blocking properties and clonidine is to be terminated, the β–blocking agent should be discontinued first. Clonidine therapy can then be discontinued several days later by gradually decreasing the dosage.

7.3 Cyclosporine

Modest increases in mean trough cyclosporine concentrations were observed following initiation of carvedilol treatment in 21 renal transplant subjects suffering from chronic vascular rejection. In about 30% of subjects, the dose of cyclosporine had to be reduced in order to maintain cyclosporine concentrations within the therapeutic range, while in the remainder no adjustment was needed. On the average for the group, the dose of cyclosporine was reduced about 20% in these subjects. Due to wide interindividual variability in the dose adjustment required, it is recommended that cyclosporine concentrations be monitored closely after initiation of carvedilol therapy and that the dose of cyclosporine be adjusted as appropriate.

7.4 Digitalis Glycosides

Both digitalis glycosides and β–blockers slow atrioventricular conduction and decrease heart rate. Concomitant use can increase the risk of bradycardia. Digoxin concentrations are increased by about 15% when digoxin and carvedilol are administered concomitantly. Therefore, increased monitoring of digoxin is recommended when initiating, adjusting, or discontinuing COREG CR *[see Clinical Pharmacology (12.5)]*.

7.5 Inducers/Inhibitors of Hepatic Metabolism

Rifampin reduced plasma concentrations of carvedilol by about 70% *[see Clinical Pharmacology (12.5)]*. Cimetidine increased area under the curve (AUC) by about 30% but caused no change in C_{max} *[see Clinical Pharmacology (12.5)]*.

7.6 Amiodarone

Amiodarone, and its metabolite desethyl amiodarone, inhibitors of CYP2C9 and P-glycoprotein, increased concentrations of the S(-) enantiomer of carvedilol by at least 2-fold *[see Clinical Pharmacology (12.5)]*. The concomitant administration of amiodarone or other CYP2C9 inhibitors such as fluconazole with COREG CR may enhance the β–blocking properties of carvedilol resulting in further slowing of the heart rate or cardiac conduction. Patients should be observed for signs of bradycardia or heart block, particularly when one agent is added to pre-existing treatment with the other.

7.7 Calcium Channel Blockers

Conduction disturbance (rarely with hemodynamic compromise) has been observed when carvedilol is coadministered with diltiazem. As with other agents with β–blocking properties, if COREG CR is to be administered orally with calcium channel blockers of the verapamil or diltiazem type, it is recommended that ECG and blood pressure be monitored.

7.8 Insulin or Oral Hypoglycemics

Agents with β–blocking properties may enhance the blood–sugar–reducing effect of insulin and oral hypoglycemics. Therefore, in patients taking insulin or oral hypoglycemics, regular monitoring of blood glucose is recommended *[see Warnings and Precautions (5.6)]*.

7.9 Proton Pump Inhibitors

There is no clinically meaningful increase in AUC and C_{max} with concomitant administration of carvedilol extended-release capsules with pantoprazole.

7.10 Anesthesia

If treatment with COREG CR is to be continued perioperatively, particular care should be taken when anesthetic agents which depress myocardial function, such as ether, cyclopropane, and trichloroethylene, are used *[see Overdosage (10)]*.

8 USE IN SPECIFIC POPULATIONS

8.1 Pregnancy

Pregnancy Category C. Studies performed in pregnant rats and rabbits given carvedilol revealed increased post-implantation loss in rats at doses of 300 mg/kg/day (50 times the maximum recommended human dose [MRHD] as mg/m²) and in rabbits at doses of 75 mg/kg/day (25 times the MRHD as mg/m²). In the rats, there was also a decrease in fetal body weight at the maternally toxic dose of 300 mg/kg/day (50 times the MRHD as mg/m²), which was accompanied by an elevation in the frequency of fetuses with delayed skeletal development (missing or stunted 13th rib). In rats the no–observed–effect level for developmental toxicity was 60 mg/kg/day (10 times the MRHD as mg/m²); in rabbits it was 15 mg/kg/day (5 times the MRHD as mg/m²). There are no adequate and well-controlled studies in pregnant women. COREG CR should be used during pregnancy only if the potential benefit justifies the potential risk to the fetus.

8.3 Nursing Mothers

It is not known whether this drug is excreted in human milk. Studies in rats have shown that carvedilol and/or its metabolites (as well as other β–blockers) cross the placental barrier and are excreted in breast milk. There was increased mortality at 1 week post partum in neonates from rats treated with 60 mg/kg/day (10 times the MRHD as mg/m²) and above during the last trimester through day 22 of lactation. Because many drugs are excreted in human milk and because of the potential for serious adverse reactions in nursing infants from β–blockers, especially bradycardia, a decision should be made whether to discontinue nursing or to discontinue the drug, taking into account the importance of the drug to the mother. The effects of other α– and β–blocking agents have included perinatal and neonatal distress.

8.4 Pediatric Use

Effectiveness of carvedilol in patients younger than 18 years has not been established.
In a double-blind trial, 161 children (mean age: 6 years; range: 2 months to 17 years; 45% younger than 2 years) with chronic heart failure [NYHA class II-IV, left ventricular ejection fraction <40% for children with a systemic left ventricle (LV), and moderate-severe ventricular dysfunction qualitatively by echo for those with a systemic ventricle that was not an LV] who were receiving standard background treatment were randomized to placebo or to 2 dose levels of carvedilol. These dose levels produced placebo-corrected heart rate reduction of 4 to 6 heart beats per minute, indicative of β–blockade activity. Exposure appeared to be lower in pediatric subjects than adults. After 8 months of follow-up, there was no significant effect of treatment on clinical outcomes. Adverse reactions in this trial that occurred in greater than 10% of subjects treated with immediate-release carvedilol and at twice the rate of placebo-treated subjects included chest pain (17% versus 6%), dizziness (13% versus 2%), and dyspnea (11% versus 0%).

8.5 Geriatric Use

The initial clinical trials of COREG CR in subjects with hypertension, heart failure, and left ventricular dysfunction following myocardial infarction did not include sufficient numbers of subjects 65 years of age or older to determine whether they respond differently from younger patients.
A randomized trial (n = 405) comparing subjects with mild to severe heart failure switched to COREG CR or maintained on immediate-release carvedilol included 220 subjects who were 65 years of age or older. In this elderly subgroup, the combined incidence of dizziness, hypotension, or syncope was 24% (18/75) in subjects switched from the highest dose of immediate-release carvedilol (25 mg twice daily) to the highest dose of COREG CR (80 mg once daily) compared with 11% (4/36) in subjects maintained on immediate-release carvedilol (25 mg twice daily). When switching from the higher doses of immediate-release carvedilol to COREG CR, a lower starting dose is recommended for elderly patients *[see Dosage and Administration (2.5)]*.
The following information is available for trials with immediate-release carvedilol. Of the 765 subjects with heart failure randomized to carvedilol in US clinical trials, 31% (235) were 65 years of age or older, and 7.3% (56) were 75 years of age or older. Of the 1,156 subjects randomized to carvedilol in a long–term, placebo–controlled trial in severe heart failure, 47% (547) were 65 years of age or older, and 15% (174) were 75 years of age or older. Of 3,025 subjects receiving carvedilol in heart failure trials worldwide, 42% were 65 years of age or older. Of the 975 subjects with myocardial infarction randomized to carvedilol in the CAPRICORN trial, 48% (468) were 65 years of age or older, and 11% (111) were 75 years of age or older. Of the 2,065 hypertensive subjects in US clinical trials of efficacy or safety who were treated with carvedilol, 21% (436) were 65 years of age or older. Of 3,722 subjects receiving immediate-release carvedilol in hypertension clinical trials conducted worldwide, 24% were 65 years of age or older.
With the exception of dizziness in hypertensive subjects (incidence 8.8% in the elderly versus 6% in younger subjects), no overall differences in the safety or effectiveness (see Figures 2 and 4) were observed between the older subjects and younger subjects in each of these populations. Similarly, other reported clinical experience has not identified differences in responses between the elderly and younger subjects, but greater sensitivity of some older individuals cannot be ruled out.

10 OVERDOSAGE

Overdosage may cause severe hypotension, bradycardia, cardiac insufficiency, cardiogenic shock, and cardiac arrest. Respiratory problems, bronchospasms, vomiting, lapses of consciousness, and generalized seizures may also occur.
The patient should be placed in a supine position and, where necessary, kept under observation and treated under intensive-care conditions. Gastric lavage or pharmacologically induced emesis may be used shortly after ingestion. The following agents may be administered:
For excessive bradycardia: atropine, 2 mg IV.
To support cardiovascular function: glucagon, 5 to 10 mg IV rapidly over 30 seconds, followed by a continuous infusion of 5 mg/hour; sympathomimetics (dobutamine, isoprenaline, adrenaline) at doses according to body weight and effect.
If peripheral vasodilation dominates, it may be necessary to administer adrenaline or noradrenaline with continuous monitoring of circulatory conditions. For therapy-resistant bradycardia, pacemaker therapy should be performed. For bronchospasm, β–sympathomimetics (as aerosol or IV) or aminophylline IV should be given. In the event of seizures, slow IV injection of diazepam or clonazepam is recommended.
NOTE: In the event of severe intoxication where there are symptoms of shock, treatment with antidotes must be continued for a sufficiently long period of time consistent with the 7- to 10-hour half-life of carvedilol.
There is no experience of overdosage with COREG CR. Cases of overdosage with carvedilol alone or in combination with other drugs have been reported. Quantities ingested in some cases exceeded 1,000 milligrams. Symptoms experienced included low blood pressure and heart rate. Standard supportive treatment was provided and individuals recovered.

11 DESCRIPTION

Carvedilol phosphate is a nonselective β–adrenergic blocking agent with α₁-blocking activity. It is (2RS)-1-(9H-Carbazol-4-yloxy)-3-[[2-(2-methoxyphenoxy)ethyl]amino]propan-2-ol phosphate salt (1:1) hemihydrate. It is a racemic mixture with the following structure:

Carvedilol phosphate is a white to almost white solid with a molecular weight of 513.5 (406.5 carvedilol free base) and a molecular formula of $C_{24}H_{26}N_2O_4 \cdot H_3PO_4 \cdot 1/2\ H_2O$.
COREG CR is available for once-a-day administration as controlled-release oral capsules containing 10, 20, 40, or 80 mg carvedilol phosphate. COREG CR hard gelatin capsules are filled with carvedilol phosphate immediate-release and controlled-release microparticles that are drug-layered and then coated with methacrylic acid copolymers. Inactive ingredients include crospovidone, hydrogenated castor oil, hydrogenated vegetable oil, magnesium stearate, methacrylic acid copolymers, microcrystalline cellulose, and povidone.

12 CLINICAL PHARMACOLOGY

12.1 Mechanism of Action

Carvedilol is a racemic mixture in which nonselective β–adrenoreceptor blocking activity is present in the S(-) enantiomer and α₁–adrenergic blocking activity is present in both R(+) and S(-) enantiomers at equal potency. Carvedilol has no intrinsic sympathomimetic activity.

12.2 Pharmacodynamics

Heart Failure and Left Ventricular Dysfunction Following Myocardial Infarction
The basis for the beneficial effects of carvedilol in patients with heart failure and in patients with left ventricular dysfunction following an acute myocardial infarction is not known. The concentration-response relationship for β₁–blockade following administration of COREG CR is equivalent (±20%) to immediate-release carvedilol tablets.

Hypertension

The mechanism by which β–blockade produces an antihypertensive effect has not been established.

β–adrenoreceptor blocking activity has been demonstrated in animal and human studies showing that carvedilol (1) reduces cardiac output in normal subjects; (2) reduces exercise- and/or isoproterenol-induced tachycardia; and (3) reduces reflex orthostatic tachycardia. Significant β–adrenoreceptor blocking effect is usually seen within 1 hour of drug administration.

α_1–adrenoreceptor blocking activity has been demonstrated in human and animal studies, showing that carvedilol (1) attenuates the pressor effects of phenylephrine; (2) causes vasodilation; and (3) reduces peripheral vascular resistance. These effects contribute to the reduction of blood pressure and usually are seen within 30 minutes of drug administration.

Due to the α_1–receptor blocking activity of carvedilol, blood pressure is lowered more in the standing than in the supine position, and symptoms of postural hypotension (1.8%), including rare instances of syncope, can occur. Following oral administration, when postural hypotension has occurred, it has been transient and is uncommon when immediate-release carvedilol is administered with food at the recommended starting dose and titration increments are closely followed [see Dosage and Administration (2)].

In a randomized, double-blind, placebo-controlled trial, the β_1–blocking effect of COREG CR, as measured by heart rate response to submaximal bicycle ergometry, was shown to be equivalent to that observed with immediate-release carvedilol at steady state in adult subjects with essential hypertension.

In hypertensive subjects with normal renal function, therapeutic doses of carvedilol decreased renal vascular resistance with no change in glomerular filtration rate or renal plasma flow. Changes in excretion of sodium, potassium, uric acid, and phosphorus in hypertensive patients with normal renal function were similar after carvedilol and placebo.

Carvedilol has little effect on plasma catecholamines, plasma aldosterone, or electrolyte levels, but it does significantly reduce plasma renin activity when given for at least 4 weeks. It also increases levels of atrial natriuretic peptide.

12.3 Pharmacokinetics

Absorption

Carvedilol is rapidly and extensively absorbed following oral administration of immediate-release carvedilol tablets, with an absolute bioavailability of approximately 25% to 35% due to a significant degree of first-pass metabolism. COREG CR extended-release capsules have approximately 85% of the bioavailability of immediate-release carvedilol tablets. For corresponding dosages [see Dosage and Administration (2)], the exposure (AUC, C_{max}, trough concentration) of carvedilol as COREG CR extended-release capsules is equivalent to those of immediate-release carvedilol tablets when both are administered with food. The absorption of carvedilol from COREG CR is slower and more prolonged compared with the immediate-release carvedilol tablet with peak concentrations achieved approximately 5 hours after administration. Plasma concentrations of carvedilol increase in a dose-proportional manner over the dosage range of COREG CR 10 to 80 mg. Within-subject and between-subject variability for AUC and C_{max} is similar for COREG CR and immediate-release carvedilol.

Effect of Food

Administration of COREG CR with a high-fat meal resulted in increases (~20%) in AUC and C_{max} compared with COREG CR administered with a standard meal. Decreases in AUC (27%) and C_{max} (43%) were observed when COREG CR was administered in the fasted state compared with administration after a standard meal. COREG CR should be taken with food.

In a trial with adult subjects, sprinkling the contents of the COREG CR capsule on applesauce did not appear to have a significant effect on overall exposure (AUC) compared with administration of the intact capsule following a standard meal but did result in a decrease in C_{max} (18%).

Distribution

Carvedilol is more than 98% bound to plasma proteins, primarily with albumin. The plasma-protein binding is independent of concentration over the therapeutic range. Carvedilol is a basic, lipophilic compound with a steady-state volume of distribution of approximately 115 L, indicating substantial distribution into extravascular tissues.

Metabolism and Excretion

Carvedilol is extensively metabolized. Following oral administration of radiolabelled carvedilol to healthy volunteers, carvedilol accounted for only about 7% of the total radioactivity in plasma as measured by AUC. Less than 2% of the dose was excreted unchanged in the urine. Carvedilol is metabolized primarily by aromatic ring oxidation and glucuronidation. The oxidative metabolites are further metabolized by conjugation via glucuronidation and sulfation. The metabolites of carvedilol are excreted primarily via the bile

into the feces. Demethylation and hydroxylation at the phenol ring produce 3 active metabolites with β–receptor blocking activity. Based on preclinical studies, the 4'-hydroxyphenyl metabolite is approximately 13 times more potent than carvedilol for β–blockade.

Compared with carvedilol, the 3 active metabolites exhibit weak vasodilating activity. Plasma concentrations of the active metabolites are about one-tenth of those observed for carvedilol and have pharmacokinetics similar to the parent. Carvedilol undergoes stereoselective first-pass metabolism with plasma levels of R(+)-carvedilol approximately 2 to 3 times higher than S(-)-carvedilol following oral administration of COREG CR in healthy subjects. Apparent clearance is 90 L/h and 213 L/h for R(+)- and S(-)-carvedilol, respectively.

The primary P450 enzymes responsible for the metabolism of both R(+) and S(-)-carvedilol in human liver microsomes were CYP2D6 and CYP2C9 and to a lesser extent CYP3A4, 2C19, 1A2, and 2E1. CYP2D6 is thought to be the major enzyme in the 4'- and 5'-hydroxylation of carvedilol, with a potential contribution from 3A4. CYP2C9 is thought to be of primary importance in the O-methylation pathway of S(-)-carvedilol.

Carvedilol is subject to the effects of genetic polymorphism with poor metabolizers of debrisoquin (a marker for cytochrome P450 2D6) exhibiting 2- to 3-fold higher plasma concentrations of R(+)-carvedilol compared with extensive metabolizers. In contrast, plasma levels of S(-)-carvedilol are increased only about 20% to 25% in poor metabolizers, indicating this enantiomer is metabolized to a lesser extent by cytochrome P450 2D6 than R(+)-carvedilol. The pharmacokinetics of carvedilol do not appear to be different in poor metabolizers of S-mephenytoin (patients deficient in cytochrome P450 2C19).

12.4 Specific Populations

Heart Failure

Following administration of immediate-release carvedilol tablets, steady–state plasma concentrations of carvedilol and its enantiomers increased proportionally over the dose range in subjects with heart failure. Compared with healthy subjects, subjects with heart failure had increased mean AUC and C_{max} values for carvedilol and its enantiomers, with up to 50% to 100% higher values observed in 6 subjects with NYHA class IV heart failure. The mean apparent terminal elimination half–life for carvedilol was similar to that observed in healthy subjects.

For corresponding dose levels [see Dosage and Administration (2)], the steady-state pharmacokinetics of carvedilol (AUC, C_{max}, trough concentrations) observed after administration of COREG CR to subjects with chronic heart failure (mild, moderate, and severe) were similar to those observed after administration of immediate-release carvedilol tablets.

Hypertension

For corresponding dose levels [see Dosage and Administration (2)], the pharmacokinetics (AUC, C_{max}, and trough concentrations) observed with administration of COREG CR were equivalent (±20%) to those observed with immediate-release carvedilol tablets following repeat dosing in subjects with essential hypertension.

Geriatric

Plasma levels of carvedilol average about 50% higher in the elderly compared with young subjects after administration of immediate-release carvedilol.

Hepatic Impairment

No trials have been performed with COREG CR in subjects with hepatic impairment. Compared with healthy subjects, subjects with severe liver impairment (cirrhosis) exhibit a 4- to 7-fold increase in carvedilol levels. Carvedilol is contraindicated in patients with severe liver impairment.

Renal Impairment

No trials have been performed with COREG CR in subjects with renal impairment. Although carvedilol is metabolized primarily by the liver, plasma concentrations of carvedilol have been reported to be increased in patients with renal impairment after dosing with immediate-release carvedilol. Based on mean AUC data, approximately 40% to 50% higher plasma concentrations of carvedilol were observed in hypertensive subjects with moderate to severe renal impairment compared with a control group of hypertensive subjects with normal renal function. However, the ranges of AUC values were similar for both groups. Changes in mean peak plasma levels were less pronounced, approximately 12% to 26% higher in subjects with impaired renal function. Consistent with its high degree of plasma protein binding, carvedilol does not appear to be cleared significantly by hemodialysis.

12.5 Drug-Drug Interactions

Since carvedilol undergoes substantial oxidative metabolism, the metabolism and pharmacokinetics of carvedilol may be affected by induction or inhibition of cytochrome P450 enzymes.

The following drug interaction trials were performed with immediate-release carvedilol tablets.

Amiodarone

In a pharmacokinetic trial conducted in 106 Japanese subjects with heart failure, coadministration of small loading and maintenance doses of amiodarone with carvedilol resulted in at least a 2-fold increase in the steady-state trough concentrations of S(-)-carvedilol [see Drug Interactions (7.6)].

Cimetidine

In a pharmacokinetic trial conducted in 10 healthy male subjects, cimetidine (1,000 mg/day) increased the steady-state AUC of carvedilol by 30% with no change in C_{max} [see Drug Interactions (7.5)].

Digoxin

Following concomitant administration of carvedilol (25 mg once daily) and digoxin (0.25 mg once daily) for 14 days, steady-state AUC and trough concentrations of digoxin were increased by 14% and 16%, respectively, in 12 hypertensive subjects [see Drug Interactions (7.4)].

Glyburide

In 12 healthy subjects, combined administration of carvedilol (25 mg once daily) and a single dose of glyburide did not result in a clinically relevant pharmacokinetic interaction for either compound.

Hydrochlorothiazide

A single oral dose of carvedilol 25 mg did not alter the pharmacokinetics of a single oral dose of hydrochlorothiazide 25 mg in 12 subjects with hypertension. Likewise, hydrochlorothiazide had no effect on the pharmacokinetics of carvedilol.

Rifampin

In a pharmacokinetic trial conducted in 8 healthy male subjects, rifampin (600 mg daily for 12 days) decreased the AUC and C_{max} of carvedilol by about 70% [see Drug Interactions (7.5)].

Torsemide

In a trial of 12 healthy subjects, combined oral administration of carvedilol 25 mg once daily and torsemide 5 mg once daily for 5 days did not result in any significant differences in their pharmacokinetics compared with administration of the drugs alone.

Warfarin

Carvedilol (12.5 mg twice daily) did not have an effect on the steady-state prothrombin time ratios and did not alter the pharmacokinetics of R(+)- and S(-)-warfarin following concomitant administration with warfarin in 9 healthy volunteers.

13 NONCLINICAL TOXICOLOGY

13.1 Carcinogenesis, Mutagenesis, Impairment of Fertility

In 2-year studies conducted in rats given carvedilol at doses up to 75 mg/kg/day (12 times the MRHD when compared on a mg/m² basis) or in mice given up to 200 mg/kg/day (16 times the MRHD on a mg/m² basis), carvedilol had no carcinogenic effect.

Carvedilol was negative when tested in a battery of genotoxicity assays, including the Ames and the CHO/HGPRT assays for mutagenicity and the in vitro hamster micronucleus and in vivo human lymphocyte cell tests for clastogenicity.

At doses ≥200 mg/kg/day (≥32 times the MRHD as mg/m²) carvedilol was toxic to adult rats (sedation, reduced weight gain) and was associated with a reduced number of successful matings, prolonged mating time, significantly fewer corpora lutea and implants per dam, and complete resorption of 18% of the litters. The no-observed-effect dose level for overt toxicity and impairment of fertility was 60 mg/kg/day (10 times the MRHD as mg/m²).

14 CLINICAL STUDIES

Support for the use of COREG CR extended-release capsules for the treatment of mild-to-severe heart failure and for patients with left ventricular dysfunction following myocardial infarction is based on the equivalence of pharmacokinetic and pharmacodynamic (β_1–blockade) parameters between COREG CR and immediate-release carvedilol [see Clinical Pharmacology (12.2, 12.3)].

The clinical trials performed with immediate-release carvedilol in heart failure and left ventricular dysfunction following myocardial infarction are presented below.

14.1 Heart Failure

A total of 6,975 subjects with mild-to-severe heart failure were evaluated in placebo-controlled and active-controlled trials of immediate-release carvedilol.

Mild-to-Moderate Heart Failure

Carvedilol was studied in 5 multicenter, placebo–controlled trials, and in 1 active-controlled trial (COMET trial) involving subjects with mild-to-moderate heart failure.

Four US multicenter, double–blind, placebo–controlled trials enrolled 1,094 subjects (696 randomized to carvedilol) with NYHA class II–III heart failure and ejection fraction ≤0.35. The vast majority were on digitalis, diuretics, and an ACE inhibitor at trial entry. Subjects were assigned to the trials based upon exercise ability. An Australia–New

Zealand double–blind, placebo–controlled trial enrolled 415 subjects (half randomized to immediate–release carvedilol) with less severe heart failure. All protocols excluded subjects expected to undergo cardiac transplantation during the 7.5 to 15 months of double–blind follow–up. All randomized subjects had tolerated a 2–week course on immediate–release carvedilol 6.25 mg twice daily.

In each trial, there was a primary end point, either progression of heart failure (1 US trial) or exercise tolerance (2 US trials meeting enrollment goals and the Australia–New Zealand trial). There were many secondary end points specified in these trials, including NYHA classification, patient and physician global assessments, and cardiovascular hospitalization. Other analyses not prospectively planned included the sum of deaths and total cardiovascular hospitalizations. In situations where the primary end points of a trial do not show a significant benefit of treatment, assignment of significance values to the other results is complex, and such values need to be interpreted cautiously.

The results of the US and Australia–New Zealand trials were as follows:

Slowing Progression of Heart Failure: One US multicenter trial (366 subjects) had as its primary end point the sum of cardiovascular mortality, cardiovascular hospitalization, and sustained increase in heart failure medications. Heart failure progression was reduced, during an average follow–up of 7 months, by 48% ($P = 0.008$).

In the Australia–New Zealand trial, death and total hospitalizations were reduced by about 25% over 18 to 24 months. In the 3 largest US trials, death and total hospitalizations were reduced by 19%, 39%, and 49%, nominally statistically significant in the last 2 trials. The Australia–New Zealand results were statistically borderline.

Functional Measures: None of the multicenter trials had NYHA classification as a primary end point, but all such trials had it as a secondary end point. There was at least a trend toward improvement in NYHA class in all trials. Exercise tolerance was the primary end point in 3 trials; in none was a statistically significant effect found.

Subjective Measures: Health-related quality of life, as measured with a standard questionnaire (a primary end point in 1 trial), was unaffected by carvedilol. However, patients' and investigators' global assessments showed significant improvement in most trials.

Mortality: Death was not a pre-specified end point in any trial, but was analyzed in all trials. Overall, in these 4 US trials, mortality was reduced, nominally significantly so in 2 trials.

The COMET Trial

In this double-blind trial, 3,029 subjects with NYHA class II-IV heart failure (left ventricular ejection fraction ≤35%) were randomized to receive either carvedilol (target dose: 25 mg twice daily) or immediate-release metoprolol tartrate (target dose: 50 mg twice daily). The mean age of the subjects was approximately 62 years, 80% were males, and the mean left ventricular ejection fraction at baseline was 26%. Approximately 96% of the subjects had NYHA class II or III heart failure. Concomitant treatment included diuretics (99%), ACE inhibitors (91%), digitalis (59%), aldosterone antagonists (11%), and "statin" lipid-lowering agents (21%). The mean duration of follow-up was 4.8 years. The mean dose of carvedilol was 42 mg per day.

The trial had 2 primary end points: all-cause mortality and the composite of death plus hospitalization for any reason. The results of COMET are presented in Table 5 below. All-cause mortality carried most of the statistical weight and was the primary determinant of the trial size. All-cause mortality was 34% in the subjects treated with carvedilol and was 40% in the immediate-release metoprolol group ($P = 0.0017$; hazard ratio = 0.83, 95% CI: 0.74 to 0.93). The effect on mortality was primarily due to a reduction in cardiovascular death. The difference between the 2 groups with respect to the composite end point was not significant ($P = 0.122$). The estimated mean survival was 8.0 years with carvedilol and 6.6 years with immediate-release metoprolol.

[See table 5 above]

It is not known whether this formulation of metoprolol at any dose or this low dose of metoprolol in any formulation has any effect on survival or hospitalization in patients with heart failure. Thus, this trial extends the time over which carvedilol manifests benefits on survival in heart failure, but it is not evidence that carvedilol improves outcome over the formulation of metoprolol (TOPROL-XL®) with benefits in heart failure.

Severe Heart Failure (COPERNICUS)

In a double-blind trial, 2,289 subjects with heart failure at rest or with minimal exertion and left ventricular ejection fraction <25% (mean 20%), despite digitalis (66%), diuretics (99%), and ACE inhibitors (89%) were randomized to placebo or carvedilol. Carvedilol was titrated from a starting dose of 3.125 mg twice daily to the maximum tolerated dose or up to 25 mg twice daily over a minimum of 6 weeks. Most subjects achieved the target dose of 25 mg. The trial was

Table 5. Results of COMET				
End point	Carvedilol N = 1,511	Metoprolol N = 1,518	Hazard ratio	(95% CI)
All-cause mortality	34%	40%	0.83	0.74 – 0.93
Mortality + all hospitalization	74%	76%	0.94	0.86 – 1.02
Cardiovascular death	30%	35%	0.80	0.70 – 0.90
Sudden death	14%	17%	0.81	0.68 – 0.97
Death due to circulatory failure	11%	13%	0.83	0.67 – 1.02
Death due to stroke	0.9%	2.5%	0.33	0.18 – 0.62

Table 6. Results of COPERNICUS Trial in Subjects With Severe Heart Failure					
End point	Placebo (N = 1,133)	Carvedilol (N = 1,156)	Hazard ratio (95% CI)	% Reduction	Nominal P value
Mortality	190	130	0.65 (0.52 – 0.81)	35	0.00013
Mortality + all hospitalization	507	425	0.76 (0.67 – 0.87)	24	0.00004
Mortality + CV hospitalization	395	314	0.73 (0.63 – 0.84)	27	0.00002
Mortality + HF hospitalization	357	271	0.69 (0.59 – 0.81)	31	0.000004

Cardiovascular = CV; Heart failure = HF

conducted in Eastern and Western Europe, the United States, Israel, and Canada. Similar numbers of subjects per group (about 100) withdrew during the titration period.

The primary end point of the trial was all-cause mortality, but cause–specific mortality and the risk of death or hospitalization (total, cardiovascular [CV], or heart failure [HF]) were also examined. The developing trial data were followed by a data monitoring committee, and mortality analyses were adjusted for these multiple looks. The trial was stopped after a median follow–up of 10 months because of an observed 35% reduction in mortality (from 19.7% per patient-year on placebo to 12.8% on carvedilol, hazard ratio 0.65, 95% CI: 0.52 to 0.81, $P = 0.0014$, adjusted) (see Figure 1). The results of COPERNICUS are shown in Table 6.

[See table 6 above]

Figure 1. Survival Analysis for COPERNICUS (Intent-to-Treat)

The effect on mortality was principally the result of a reduction in the rate of sudden death among subjects without worsening heart failure.

Patients' global assessments, in which carvedilol–treated subjects were compared with placebo, were based on pre-specified, periodic patient self-assessments regarding whether clinical status post-treatment showed improvement, worsening, or no change compared with baseline. Subjects treated with carvedilol showed significant improvements in global assessments compared with those treated with placebo in COPERNICUS.

The protocol also specified that hospitalizations would be assessed. Fewer subjects on immediate–release carvedilol than on placebo were hospitalized for any reason (372 versus 432, $P = 0.0029$), for cardiovascular reasons (246 versus 314, $P = 0.0003$), or for worsening heart failure (198 versus 268, $P = 0.0001$).

Immediate–release carvedilol had a consistent and beneficial effect on all–cause mortality as well as the combined end points of all–cause mortality plus hospitalization (total, CV, or for heart failure) in the overall trial population and in all subgroups examined, including men and women, elderly and non–elderly, blacks and non–blacks, and diabetics and non-diabetics (see Figure 2).

Figure 2. Effects on Mortality for Subgroups in COPERNICUS

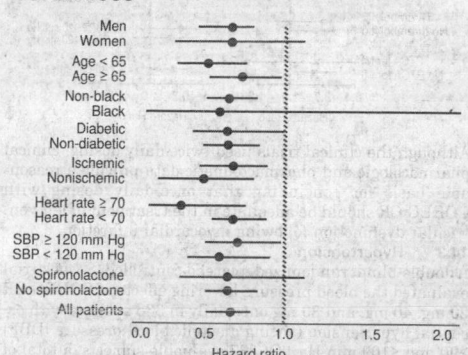

Although the clinical trials used twice-daily dosing, clinical pharmacologic and pharmacokinetic data provide a reasonable basis for concluding that once-daily dosing with COREG CR should be adequate in the treatment of heart failure.

14.2 Left Ventricular Dysfunction Following Myocardial Infarction

CAPRICORN was a double–blind trial comparing carvedilol and placebo in 1,959 subjects with a recent myocardial infarction (within 21 days) and left ventricular ejection fraction of ≤40%, with (47%) or without symptoms of heart failure. Subjects given carvedilol received 6.25 mg twice daily, titrated as tolerated to 25 mg twice daily. Subjects had to have a systolic blood pressure >90 mm Hg, a sitting heart rate >60 beats/minute, and no contraindication to β–blocker use. Treatment of the index infarction included aspirin (85%), IV or oral β–blockers (37%), nitrates (73%), heparin (64%), thrombolytics (40%), and acute angioplasty (12%). Background treatment included ACE inhibitors or angiotensin receptor blockers (97%), anticoagulants (20%), lipid-lowering agents (23%), and diuretics (34%). Baseline population characteristics included an average age of 63 years, 74% male, 95% Caucasian, mean blood pressure 121/74 mm Hg, 22% with diabetes, and 54% with a history of hypertension. Mean dosage achieved of carvedilol was 20 mg twice daily; mean duration of follow–up was 15 months.

All–cause mortality was 15% in the placebo group and 12% in the carvedilol group, indicating a 23% risk reduction in subjects treated with carvedilol (95% CI: 2% to 40%, $P = 0.03$), as shown in Figure 3. The effects on mortality in various subgroups are shown in Figure 4. Nearly all deaths were cardiovascular (which were reduced by 25% by carvedilol), and most of these deaths were sudden or related to pump failure (both types of death were reduced by carvedilol). Another trial end point, total mortality and all-cause hospitalization, did not show a significant improvement.

There was also a significant 40% reduction in fatal or non-fatal myocardial infarction observed in the group treated with carvedilol (95% CI: 11% to 60%, $P = 0.01$). A similar reduction in the risk of myocardial infarction was also observed in a meta-analysis of placebo-controlled trials of carvedilol in heart failure.

Figure 3. Survival Analysis for CAPRICORN (Intent-to-Treat)

Figure 4. Effects on Mortality for Subgroups in CAPRICORN

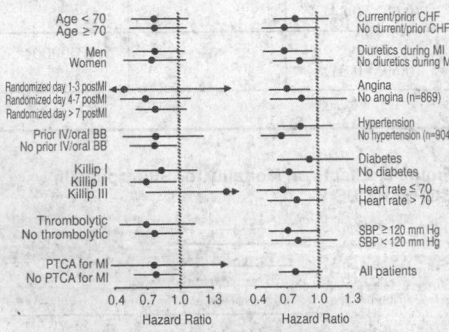

Although the clinical trials used twice-daily dosing, clinical pharmacologic and pharmacokinetic data provide a reasonable basis for concluding that once-daily dosing with COREG CR should be adequate in the treatment of left ventricular dysfunction following myocardial infarction.

14.3 Hypertension

A double-blind, randomized, placebo-controlled, 8-week trial evaluated the blood pressure lowering effects of COREG CR 20 mg, 40 mg, and 80 mg once daily in 338 subjects with essential hypertension (sitting diastolic blood pressure [DBP] ≥90 and ≤109 mm Hg). Of 337 evaluable subjects, a total of 273 subjects (81%) completed the trial. Of the 64 (19%) subjects withdrawn from the trial, 10 (3%) were due to adverse events, 10 (3%) were due to lack of efficacy; the remaining 44 (13%) withdrew for other reasons. The mean age of the subjects was approximately 53 years, 66% were male, and the mean sitting systolic blood pressure (SBP) and DBP at baseline were 150 mm Hg and 99 mm Hg, respectively. Dose titration occurred at 2-week intervals.

Statistically significant reductions in blood pressure as measured by 24-hour ambulatory blood pressure monitoring (ABPM) were observed with each dose of COREG CR compared with placebo. Placebo-subtracted mean changes from baseline in mean SBP/DBP were −6.1/−4.0 mm Hg, −9.4/−7.6 mm Hg, and −11.8/−9.2 mm Hg for COREG CR 20 mg, 40 mg, and 80 mg, respectively. Placebo-subtracted mean changes from baseline in mean trough (average of hours 20 to 24) SBP/DBP were −3.3/−2.8 mm Hg, −4.9/−5.2 mm Hg, and −8.4/−7.4 mm Hg for COREG CR 20 mg, 40 mg, and 80 mg, respectively. The placebo-corrected trough to peak (3 to 7 h) ratio was approximately 0.6 for COREG CR 80 mg. In this trial, assessments of 24-hour ABPM monitoring demonstrated statistically significant blood pressure reductions with COREG CR throughout the dosing period (Figure 5).

[See figure 5 at top of next column]

Immediate-release carvedilol was studied in 2 placebo-controlled trials that utilized twice-daily dosing, at total daily doses of 12.5 to 50 mg. In these and other trials, the starting dose did not exceed 12.5 mg. At 50 mg/day, COREG reduced sitting trough (12-hour) blood pressure by about 9/5.5 mm Hg; at 25 mg/day the effect was about 7.5/3.5 mm Hg. Comparisons of trough-to-peak blood pressure showed a trough-to-peak ratio for blood pressure response of about 65%. Heart rate fell by about 7.5 beats/minute at 50 mg/day. In general, as is true for other β-blockers, responses were smaller in black than non-black subjects. There were no age- or gender-related differences in response. The dose-related blood pressure response was accompanied by a dose-related increase in adverse effects [see Adverse Reactions (6)].

14.4 Hypertension With Type 2 Diabetes Mellitus

In a double-blind trial (GEMINI), carvedilol, added to an ACE inhibitor or angiotensin receptor blocker, was evaluated in a population with mild-to-moderate hypertension and well-controlled type 2 diabetes mellitus. The mean HbA1c at baseline was 7.2%. COREG was titrated to a mean dose of 17.5 mg twice daily and maintained for 5 months. COREG had no adverse effect on glycemic control, based on HbA1c measurements (mean change from baseline of 0.02%, 95% CI: −0.06 to 0.10, P = NS) [see Warnings and Precautions (5.6)].

Figure 5. Changes from Baseline in Systolic Blood Pressure and Diastolic Blood Pressure Measured by 24-Hour ABPM

Lines smoothed using locally weighted regression smoothing methodology.

16   HOW SUPPLIED/STORAGE AND HANDLING

The hard gelatin capsules are available in the following strengths:

- 10 mg – white and green capsule shell printed with "GSK COREG CR" and "10 mg"
- 20 mg – white and yellow capsule shell printed with "GSK COREG CR" and "20 mg"
- 40 mg – yellow and green capsule shell printed with "GSK COREG CR" and "40 mg"
- 80 mg – white capsule shell printed with "GSK COREG CR" and "80 mg"
- 10 mg 30's: NDC 0007-3370-13
- 20 mg 30's: NDC 0007-3371-13
- 40 mg 30's: NDC 0007-3372-13
- 80 mg 30's: NDC 0007-3373-13

Store at 25°C (77°F); excursions 15° to 30°C (59° to 86°F). Dispense in a tight, light-resistant container.

17   PATIENT COUNSELING INFORMATION

Advise the patient to read the FDA-approved patient labeling (Patient Information)

Patients taking COREG CR should be advised of the following:

- Patients should not interrupt or discontinue using COREG CR without a physician's advice.
- Patients with heart failure should consult their physician if they experience signs or symptoms of worsening heart failure such as weight gain or increasing shortness of breath.
- Patients may experience a drop in blood pressure when standing, resulting in dizziness and, rarely, fainting. Patients should sit or lie down when these symptoms of lowered blood pressure occur.
- If experiencing dizziness or fatigue, patients should avoid driving or hazardous tasks.
- Patients should consult a physician if they experience dizziness or faintness, in case the dosage should be adjusted.
- Patients should not crush or chew COREG CR capsules.
- Patients should take COREG CR with food.
- Diabetic patients should report any changes in blood sugar levels to their physician.
- Contact lens wearers may experience decreased lacrimation.

COREG CR and COREG are registered trademarks of the GSK group of companies.

TOPROL-XL is a trademark of its respective owner and is not a trademark of the GSK group of companies. The maker of this brand is not affiliated with and does not endorse the GSK group of companies or its products.

GlaxoSmithKline
Research Triangle Park, NC 27709
©2014, the GSK group of companies. All rights reserved.
May 2014
CCR:17PI

PHARMACIST—DETACH HERE AND GIVE INSTRUCTIONS TO PATIENT

PATIENT INFORMATION LEAFLET
COREG CR® (Co-REG)
(carvedilol phosphate)
Extended-release Capsules

Read the Patient Information that comes with COREG CR before you start taking it and each time you get a refill. There may be new information. This information does not take the place of talking with your doctor about your medical condition or your treatment. If you have any questions about COREG CR, ask your doctor or pharmacist.

What is the most important information I should know about COREG CR?

It is important for you to take your medicine every day as directed by your doctor. If you stop taking COREG CR suddenly, you could have chest pain and a heart attack. If your doctor decides that you should stop taking COREG CR, your doctor may slowly lower your dose over time before stopping it completely.

What is COREG CR?

COREG CR is a prescription medicine that belongs to a group of medicines called "beta-blockers". COREG CR is used, often with other medicines, for the following conditions:

- to treat patients with certain types of heart failure
- to treat patients who had a heart attack that worsened how well the heart pumps
- to treat patients with high blood pressure (hypertension)

COREG CR is not approved for use in children under 18 years of age.

Who should not take COREG CR?

Do not take COREG CR if you:

- have severe heart failure and require certain intravenous medicines that help support circulation.
- have asthma or other breathing problems.
- have a slow heartbeat or certain conditions that cause your heart to skip a beat (irregular heartbeat).
- have liver problems.
- are allergic to any of the ingredients in COREG CR. See *"What are the ingredients in COREG CR?"*

What should I tell my doctor before taking COREG CR?

Tell your doctor about all of your medical conditions, including if you:

- have asthma or other lung problems (such as bronchitis or emphysema).
- have problems with blood flow in your feet and legs (peripheral vascular disease). COREG CR can make some of your symptoms worse.
- have diabetes.
- have thyroid problems.
- have a condition called pheochromocytoma.
- have had severe allergic reactions.
- are scheduled for surgery and will be given anesthetic agents.
- are scheduled for cataract surgery and have taken or are currently taking COREG CR.
- are pregnant or trying to become pregnant. It is not known if COREG CR is safe for your unborn baby. You and your doctor should talk about the best way to control your high blood pressure during pregnancy.
- are breastfeeding. It is not known if COREG CR passes into your breast milk. You should not breastfeed while using COREG CR.

Tell your doctor about all of the medicines you take including prescription and non-prescription medicines, vitamins, and herbal supplements. COREG CR and certain other medicines can affect each other and cause serious side effects. COREG CR may affect the way other medicines work. Also, other medicines may affect how well COREG CR works.

Know the medicines you take. Keep a list of your medicines and show it to your doctor and pharmacist before you start a new medicine.

How should I take COREG CR?

- Take COREG CR exactly as prescribed. Take COREG CR **one** time each day with food. **It is important that you take COREG CR only one time each day.** To lessen possible side effects, your doctor might begin with a low dose and then slowly increase the dose.
- Swallow COREG CR capsules whole. Do not chew or crush COREG CR capsules.
- If you have trouble swallowing COREG CR whole:
  - The capsule may be carefully opened and the beads sprinkled over a spoonful of applesauce which should be eaten right away. The applesauce should not be warm.
  - Do not sprinkle beads on foods other than applesauce.
- **Do not stop taking COREG CR and do not change the amount of COREG CR you take without talking to your doctor.**
- If you miss a dose of COREG CR, take your dose as soon as you remember, unless it is time to take your next dose. Take your next dose at the usual time. Do not take 2 doses at the same time.

- If you take too much COREG CR, call your doctor or poison control center right away.

What should I avoid while taking COREG CR?
COREG CR can cause you to feel dizzy, tired, or faint. Do not drive a car, use machinery, or do anything that needs you to be alert if you have these symptoms.

What are possible side effects of COREG CR?
Serious side effects of COREG CR include:

- **chest pain and heart attack if you suddenly stop taking COREG CR.** See "What is the most important information I should know about COREG CR?"
- **slow heart beat.**
- **low blood pressure (which may cause dizziness or fainting when you stand up).** If these happen, sit or lie down, and tell your doctor right away.
- **worsening heart failure.** Tell your doctor right away if you have signs and symptoms that your heart failure may be worse, such as weight gain or increased shortness of breath.
- **changes in your blood sugar. If you have diabetes, tell your doctor if you have any changes in your blood sugar levels.**
- masking (hiding) the symptoms of low blood sugar, especially a fast heartbeat.
- **new or worsening symptoms of peripheral vascular disease.**
  - leg pain that happens when you walk, but goes away when you rest
  - no feeling (numbness) in your legs or feet while you are resting
  - cold legs or feet
- masking the symptoms of hyperthyroidism (overactive thyroid), such as a fast heartbeat.
- **worsening of severe allergic reactions.** Medicines to treat a severe allergic reaction may not work as well while you are taking COREG CR.
- **rare but serious allergic reactions** (including hives or swelling of the face, lips, tongue, and/or throat that may cause difficulty in breathing or swallowing) have happened in patients who were on COREG or COREG CR. These reactions can be life-threatening. In some cases, these reactions happened in patients who had been on COREG before taking COREG CR.

Common side effects of COREG CR include shortness of breath, weight gain, diarrhea, and tiredness. If you wear contact lenses, you may have fewer tears or dry eyes that can become bothersome.
Call your doctor if you have any side effects that bother you or don't go away.
Call your doctor for medical advice about side effects. You may report side effects to FDA at 1-800-FDA-1088.

How should I store COREG CR?
Store COREG CR at less than 86°F (30°C).
Safely throw away COREG CR that is out of date or no longer needed.
Keep COREG CR and all medicines out of the reach of children.

General information about COREG CR
Medicines are sometimes prescribed for conditions other than those described in patient information leaflets. Do not use COREG CR for a condition for which it was not prescribed. Do not give COREG CR to other people, even if they have the same symptoms you have. It may harm them.
This leaflet summarizes the most important information about COREG CR. If you would like more information, talk with your doctor. You can ask your doctor or pharmacist for information about COREG CR that is written for healthcare professionals. You can also find out more about COREG CR by visiting the website www.COREGCR.com or calling 1-888-825-5249. This call is free.

What are the ingredients in COREG CR?
Active ingredient: carvedilol phosphate
Inactive ingredients: crospovidone, hydrogenated castor oil, hydrogenated vegetable oil, magnesium stearate, methacrylic acid copolymers, microcrystalline cellulose, and povidone
COREG CR capsules come in the following strengths: 10 mg, 20 mg, 40 mg, and 80 mg.

What is high blood pressure (hypertension)? Blood pressure is the force of blood in your blood vessels when your heart beats and when your heart rests. You have high blood pressure when the force is too much. High blood pressure makes the heart work harder to pump blood through the body and causes damage to blood vessels. COREG CR can help your blood vessels relax so your blood pressure is lower. Medicines that lower blood pressure may lower your chance of having a stroke or heart attack.
COREG CR and COREG are registered trademarks of the GSK group of companies.
GlaxoSmithKline
Research Triangle Park, NC 27709
©2014, the GSK group of companies. All rights reserved.
May 2014
CCR:6PIL

DYAZIDE® ℞
[dī'ə-zīd]
(hydrochlorothiazide/triamterene) Capsules

DESCRIPTION
Each capsule of DYAZIDE (hydrochlorothiazide and triamterene) for oral use, with opaque red cap and opaque white body, contains hydrochlorothiazide 25 mg and triamterene 37.5 mg, and is imprinted with the product name DYAZIDE and SB. Hydrochlorothiazide is a diuretic/antihypertensive agent and triamterene is an antikaliuretic agent.
Hydrochlorothiazide is slightly soluble in water. It is soluble in dilute ammonia, dilute aqueous sodium hydroxide, and dimethylformamide. It is sparingly soluble in methanol.
Hydrochlorothiazide is 6-chloro-3,4-dihydro-2$\underline{H}$-1, 2, 4-benzothiadiazine-7-sulfonamide 1,1-dioxide, and its structural formula is:

At 50°C, triamterene is practically insoluble in water (less than 0.1%). It is soluble in formic acid, sparingly soluble in methoxyethanol, and very slightly soluble in alcohol.
Triamterene is 2, 4, 7-triamino-6-phenylpteridine and its structural formula is:

Inactive ingredients consist of benzyl alcohol, cetylpyridinium chloride, D&C Red No. 33, D&C Yellow No. 6, gelatin, glycine, lactose, magnesium stearate, microcrystalline cellulose, povidone, polysorbate 80, sodium starch glycolate, titanium dioxide, and trace amounts of other inactive ingredients.
Capsules of DYAZIDE meet Drug Release Test 3 as published in the current USP monograph for Triamterene and Hydrochlorothiazide Capsules.

CLINICAL PHARMACOLOGY
DYAZIDE is a diuretic/antihypertensive drug product that combines natriuretic and antikaliuretic effects. Each component complements the action of the other. The hydrochlorothiazide component blocks the reabsorption of sodium and chloride ions, and thereby increases the quantity of sodium traversing the distal tubule and the volume of water excreted. A portion of the additional sodium presented to the distal tubule is exchanged there for potassium and hydrogen ions. With continued use of hydrochlorothiazide and depletion of sodium, compensatory mechanisms tend to increase this exchange and may produce excessive loss of potassium, hydrogen, and chloride ions. Hydrochlorothiazide also decreases the excretion of calcium and uric acid, may increase the excretion of iodide, and may reduce glomerular filtration rate. The exact mechanism of the antihypertensive effect of hydrochlorothiazide is not known.
The triamterene component of DYAZIDE exerts its diuretic effect on the distal renal tubule to inhibit the reabsorption of sodium in exchange for potassium and hydrogen ions. Its natriuretic activity is limited by the amount of sodium reaching its site of action. Although it blocks the increase in this exchange that is stimulated by mineralocorticoids (chiefly aldosterone), it is not a competitive antagonist of aldosterone and its activity can be demonstrated in adrenalectomized rats and patients with Addison's disease. As a result, the dose of triamterene required is not proportionally related to the level of mineralocorticoid activity, but is dictated by the response of the individual patients, and the kaliuretic effect of concomitantly administered drugs. By inhibiting the distal tubular exchange mechanism, triamterene maintains or increases the sodium excretion and reduces the excess loss of potassium, hydrogen and chloride ions induced by hydrochlorothiazide. As with hy-

drochlorothiazide, triamterene may reduce glomerular filtration and renal plasma flow. Via this mechanism it may reduce uric acid excretion although it has no tubular effect on uric acid reabsorption or secretion. Triamterene does not affect calcium excretion. No predictable antihypertensive effect has been demonstrated for triamterene.
Duration of diuretic activity and effective dosage range of the hydrochlorothiazide and triamterene components of DYAZIDE are similar. Onset of diuresis with DYAZIDE takes place within 1 hour, peaks at 2 to 3 hours and tapers off during the subsequent 7 to 9 hours.
DYAZIDE is well absorbed.
Upon administration of a single oral dose to fasted normal male volunteers, the following mean pharmacokinetic parameters were determined:
[See table below]
where $AUC_{(0-48)}$, C_{max}, T_{max} and Ae represent area under the plasma concentration versus time plot, maximum plasma concentration, time to reach C_{max}, and amount excreted in urine over 48 hours.
A capsule of DYAZIDE is bioequivalent to a single-entity 25 mg hydrochlorothiazide tablet and 37.5 mg triamterene capsule used in the double-blind clinical trial below (see Clinical Trials).
In a limited study involving 12 subjects, coadministration of DYAZIDE with a high-fat meal resulted in: (1) an increase in the mean bioavailability of triamterene by about 67% (90% confidence interval = 0.99, 1.90), p-hydroxytriamterene sulfate by about 50% (90% confidence interval = 1.06, 1.77), hydrochlorothiazide by about 17% (90% confidence interval = 0.90, 1.34); (2) increases in the peak concentrations of triamterene and p-hydroxytriamterene; and (3) a delay of up to 2 hours in the absorption of the active constituents.

CLINICAL TRIALS
A placebo-controlled, double-blind trial was conducted to evaluate the efficacy of DYAZIDE. This trial demonstrated that DYAZIDE (25 mg hydrochlorothiazide/37.5 mg triamterene) was effective in controlling blood pressure while reducing the incidence of hydrochlorothiazide-induced hypokalemia. This trial involved 636 patients with mild to moderate hypertension controlled by hydrochlorothiazide 25 mg daily and who had hypokalemia (serum potassium <3.5 mEq/L) secondary to the hydrochlorothiazide. Patients were randomly assigned to 4 weeks' treatment with once-daily regimens of 25 mg hydrochlorothiazide plus placebo, or 25 mg hydrochlorothiazide combined with one of the following doses of triamterene: 25 mg, 37.5 mg, 50 mg, or 75 mg.
Blood pressure and serum potassium were monitored at baseline and throughout the trial. All five treatment groups had similar mean blood pressure and serum potassium concentrations at baseline (mean systolic blood pressure range: 137±14 mmHg to 140±16 mmHg; mean diastolic blood pressure range: 86±9 mmHg to 88±8 mmHg; mean serum potassium range: 2.3 to 3.4 mEq/L with the majority of patients having values between 3.1 and 3.4 mEq/L).
While all triamterene regimens reversed hypokalemia, at week 4 the 37.5 mg regimen proved optimal compared with the other tested regimens. On this regimen, 81% of the patients had a significant (p<0.05) reversal of hypokalemia vs. 59% of patients on the placebo/hydrochlorothiazide regimen. The mean serum potassium concentration on 37.5 mg triamterene went from 3.2±0.2 mEq/L at baseline to 3.7±0.3 mEq/L at week 4, a significantly greater (p<0.05) improvement than that achieved with placebo/hydrochlorothiazide (i.e., 3.2±0.2 mEq/L at baseline and 3.5±0.4 mEq/L at week 4). Also, 51% of patients in the 37.5 mg triamterene group had an increase in serum potassium of ≥0.5 mEq/L at week 4 vs. 33% in the placebo group. The 37.5 mg triamterene/25 mg hydrochlorothiazide regimen also maintained control of blood pressure; mean supine systolic blood pressure at week 4 was 138±21 mmHg while mean supine diastolic blood pressure was 87±13 mmHg.

INDICATIONS AND USAGE
This fixed combination drug is not indicated for the initial therapy of edema or hypertension except in individuals in whom the development of hypokalemia cannot be risked.
DYAZIDE is indicated for the treatment of hypertension or edema in patients who develop hypokalemia on hydrochlorothiazide alone.

	$AUC_{(0-48)}$ ng*hrs/mL (± SD)	C_{max} ng/mL (± SD)	Median T_{max} Hrs	Ae Mg (± SD)
Triamterene	148.7 (87.9)	46.4 (29.4)	1.1	2.7 (1.4)
hydroxytriamterene sulfate	1,865 (471)	720 (364)	1.3	19.7 (6.1)
hydrochlorothiazide	834 (177)	135.1 (35.7)	2.0	14.3 (3.8)

DYAZIDE is also indicated for those patients who require a thiazide diuretic and in whom the development of hypokalemia cannot be risked.

DYAZIDE may be used alone or as an adjunct to other antihypertensive drugs, such as beta-blockers. Since DYAZIDE may enhance the action of these agents, dosage adjustments may be necessary.

Usage in Pregnancy

The routine use of diuretics in an otherwise healthy woman is inappropriate and exposes mother and fetus to unnecessary hazard. Diuretics do not prevent development of toxemia of pregnancy, and there is no satisfactory evidence that they are useful in the treatment of developed toxemia. Edema during pregnancy may arise from pathological causes or from the physiologic and mechanical consequences of pregnancy. Diuretics are indicated in pregnancy when edema is due to pathologic causes, just as they are in the absence of pregnancy. Dependent edema in pregnancy resulting from restriction of venous return by the expanded uterus is properly treated through elevation of the lower extremities and use of support hose; use of diuretics to lower intravascular volume in this case is illogical and unnecessary. There is hypervolemia during normal pregnancy which is harmful to neither the fetus nor the mother (in the absence of cardiovascular disease), but which is associated with edema, including generalized edema in the majority of pregnant women. If this edema produces discomfort, increased recumbency will often provide relief. In rare instances this edema may cause extreme discomfort which is not relieved by rest. In these cases a short course of diuretics may provide relief and may be appropriate.

CONTRAINDICATIONS

Antikaliuretic Therapy and Potassium Supplementation

DYAZIDE should not be given to patients receiving other potassium-sparing agents such as spironolactone, amiloride, or other formulations containing triamterene. Concomitant potassium-containing salt substitutes should also not be used.

Potassium supplementation should not be used with DYAZIDE except in severe cases of hypokalemia. Such concomitant therapy can be associated with rapid increases in serum potassium levels. If potassium supplementation is used, careful monitoring of the serum potassium level is necessary.

Impaired Renal Function

DYAZIDE is contraindicated in patients with anuria, acute and chronic renal insufficiency or significant renal impairment.

Hypersensitivity

Hypersensitivity to either drug in the preparation or to other sulfonamide-derived drugs is a contraindication.

Hyperkalemia

DYAZIDE should not be used in patients with preexisting elevated serum potassium.

WARNINGS

> **Hyperkalemia:** Abnormal elevation of serum potassium levels (greater than or equal to 5.5 mEq/liter) can occur with all potassium-sparing diuretic combinations, including DYAZIDE. Hyperkalemia is more likely to occur in patients with renal impairment and diabetes (even without evidence of renal impairment), and in the elderly or severely ill. Since uncorrected hyperkalemia may be fatal, serum potassium levels must be monitored at frequent intervals especially in patients first receiving DYAZIDE, when dosages are changed or with any illness that may influence renal function.

If hyperkalemia is suspected (warning signs include paresthesias, muscular weakness, fatigue, flaccid paralysis of the extremities, bradycardia, and shock), an electrocardiogram (ECG) should be obtained. However, it is important to monitor serum potassium levels because hyperkalemia may not be associated with ECG changes.

If hyperkalemia is present, DYAZIDE should be discontinued immediately and a thiazide alone should be substituted. If the serum potassium exceeds 6.5 mEq/liter more vigorous therapy is required. The clinical situation dictates the procedures to be employed. These include the intravenous administration of calcium chloride solution, sodium bicarbonate solution, and/or the oral or parenteral administration of glucose with a rapid-acting insulin preparation. Cationic exchange resins such as sodium polystyrene sulfonate may be orally or rectally administered. Persistent hyperkalemia may require dialysis.

The development of hyperkalemia associated with potassium-sparing diuretics is accentuated in the presence of renal impairment (see CONTRAINDICATIONS section). Patients with mild renal functional impairment should not receive this drug without frequent and continuing monitoring of serum electrolytes. Cumulative drug effects may be observed in patients with impaired renal function. The renal clearances of hydrochlorothiazide and the pharmacologically active metabolite of triamterene, the sulfate ester of hydroxytriamterene, have been shown to be reduced and the plasma levels increased following administration of DYAZIDE to elderly patients and patients with impaired renal function.

Hyperkalemia has been reported in diabetic patients with the use of potassium-sparing agents even in the absence of apparent renal impairment. Accordingly, serum electrolytes must be frequently monitored if DYAZIDE is used in diabetic patients.

Metabolic or Respiratory Acidosis

Potassium-sparing therapy should also be avoided in severely ill patients in whom respiratory or metabolic acidosis may occur. Acidosis may be associated with rapid elevations in serum potassium levels. If DYAZIDE is employed, frequent evaluations of acid/base balance and serum electrolytes are necessary.

Acute Myopia and Secondary Angle-Closure Glaucoma

Hydrochlorothiazide, a sulfonamide, can cause an idiosyncratic reaction, resulting in acute transient myopia and acute angle-closure glaucoma. Symptoms include acute onset of decreased visual acuity or ocular pain and typically occur within hours to weeks of drug initiation. Untreated acute angle-closure glaucoma can lead to permanent vision loss. The primary treatment is to discontinue hydrochlorothiazide as rapidly as possible. Prompt medical or surgical treatments may need to be considered if the intraocular pressure remains uncontrolled. Risk factors for developing acute angle-closure glaucoma may include a history of sulfonamide or penicillin allergy.

PRECAUTIONS

Diabetes

Caution should be exercised when administering DYAZIDE to patients with diabetes, since thiazides may cause hyperglycemia, glycosuria, and alter insulin requirements in diabetes. Also, diabetes mellitus may become manifest during thiazide administration.

Impaired Hepatic Function

Thiazides should be used with caution in patients with impaired hepatic function. They can precipitate hepatic coma in patients with severe liver disease. Potassium depletion induced by the thiazide may be important in this connection. Administer DYAZIDE cautiously and be alert for such early signs of impending coma as confusion, drowsiness, and tremor; if mental confusion increases discontinue DYAZIDE for a few days. Attention must be given to other factors that may precipitate hepatic coma, such as blood in the gastrointestinal tract or preexisting potassium depletion.

Hypokalemia

Hypokalemia is uncommon with DYAZIDE; but, should it develop, corrective measures should be taken such as potassium supplementation or increased intake of potassium-rich foods. Institute such measures cautiously with frequent determinations of serum potassium levels, especially in patients receiving digitalis or with a history of cardiac arrhythmias. If serious hypokalemia (serum potassium less than 3.0 mEq/L) is demonstrated by repeat serum potassium determinations, DYAZIDE should be discontinued and potassium chloride supplementation initiated. Less serious hypokalemia should be evaluated with regard to other coexisting conditions and treated accordingly.

Electrolyte Imbalance

Electrolyte imbalance, often encountered in such conditions as heart failure, renal disease or cirrhosis of the liver, may also be aggravated by diuretics and should be considered during therapy with DYAZIDE when using high doses for prolonged periods or in patients on a salt-restricted diet. Serum determinations of electrolytes should be performed, and are particularly important if the patient is vomiting excessively or receiving fluids parenterally. Possible fluid and electrolyte imbalance may be indicated by such warning signs as: dry mouth, thirst, weakness, lethargy, drowsiness, restlessness, muscle pain or cramps, muscular fatigue, hypotension, oliguria, tachycardia, and gastrointestinal symptoms.

Hypochloremia

Although any chloride deficit is generally mild and usually does not require specific treatment except under extraordinary circumstances (as in liver disease or renal disease), chloride replacement may be required in the treatment of metabolic alkalosis. Dilutional hyponatremia may occur in edematous patients in hot weather; appropriate therapy is water restriction, rather than administration of salt, except in rare instances when the hyponatremia is life threatening. In actual salt depletion, appropriate replacement is the therapy of choice.

Renal Stones

Triamterene has been found in renal stones in association with the other usual calculus components. DYAZIDE should be used with caution in patients with a history of renal stones.

Laboratory Tests

Serum Potassium

The normal adult range of serum potassium is 3.5 to 5.0 mEq per liter with 4.5 mEq often being used for a reference point. If hypokalemia should develop, corrective measures should be taken such as potassium supplementation or increased dietary intake of potassium-rich foods.

Institute such measures cautiously with frequent determinations of serum potassium levels. Potassium levels persistently above 6 mEq per liter require careful observation and treatment. Serum potassium levels do not necessarily indicate true body potassium concentration. A rise in plasma pH may cause a decrease in plasma potassium concentration and an increase in the intracellular potassium concentration. Discontinue corrective measures for hyperkalemia immediately if laboratory determinations reveal an abnormal elevation of serum potassium.

Discontinue DYAZIDE and substitute a thiazide diuretic alone until potassium levels return to normal.

Serum Creatinine and BUN

DYAZIDE may produce an elevated blood urea nitrogen level, creatinine level or both. This apparently is secondary to a reversible reduction of glomerular filtration rate or a depletion of intravascular fluid volume (prerenal azotemia) rather than renal toxicity; levels usually return to normal when DYAZIDE is discontinued. If azotemia increases, discontinue DYAZIDE. Periodic BUN or serum creatinine determinations should be made, especially in elderly patients and in patients with suspected or confirmed renal insufficiency.

Serum PBI

Thiazide may decrease serum PBI levels without sign of thyroid disturbance.

Parathyroid Function

Thiazides should be discontinued before carrying out tests for parathyroid function. Calcium excretion is decreased by thiazides.

Pathologic changes in the parathyroid glands with hypercalcemia and hypophosphatemia have been observed in a few patients on prolonged thiazide therapy. The common complications of hyperparathyroidism such as bone resorption and peptic ulceration have not been seen.

Drug Interactions

Angiotensin-converting Enzyme Inhibitors

Potassium-sparing agents should be used with caution in conjunction with angiotensin-converting enzyme (ACE) inhibitors due to an increased risk of hyperkalemia.

Oral Hypoglycemic Drugs

Concurrent use with chlorpropamide may increase the risk of severe hyponatremia.

Nonsteroidal Anti-inflammatory Drugs

A possible interaction resulting in acute renal failure has been reported in a few patients on DYAZIDE when treated with indomethacin, a nonsteroidal anti-inflammatory agent. Caution is advised in administering nonsteroidal anti-inflammatory agents with DYAZIDE.

Lithium

Lithium generally should not be given with diuretics because they reduce its renal clearance and increase the risk of lithium toxicity. Read circulars for lithium preparations before use of such concomitant therapy with DYAZIDE.

Surgical Considerations

Thiazides have been shown to decrease arterial responsiveness to norepinephrine (an effect attributed to loss of sodium). This diminution is not sufficient to preclude effectiveness of the pressor agent for therapeutic use. Thiazides have also been shown to increase the paralyzing effect of nondepolarizing muscle relaxants such as tubocurarine (an effect attributed to potassium loss); consequently caution should be observed in patients undergoing surgery.

Other Considerations

Concurrent use of hydrochlorothiazide with amphotericin B or corticosteroids or corticotropin (ACTH) may intensify electrolyte imbalance, particularly hypokalemia, although the presence of triamterene minimizes the hypokalemic effect.

Thiazides may add to or potentiate the action of other antihypertensive drugs. See INDICATIONS AND USAGE for concomitant use with other antihypertensive drugs.

The effect of oral anticoagulants may be decreased when used concurrently with hydrochlorothiazide; dosage adjustments may be necessary.

DYAZIDE may raise the level of blood uric acid; dosage adjustments of antigout medication may be necessary to control hyperuricemia and gout.

The following agents given together with triamterene may promote serum potassium accumulation and possibly result in hyperkalemia because of the potassium-sparing nature of triamterene, especially in patients with renal insufficiency: blood from blood bank (may contain up to 30 mEq of potassium per liter of plasma or up to 65 mEq per liter of whole blood when stored for more than 10 days); low-salt milk (may contain up to 60 mEq of potassium per liter);

potassium-containing medications (such as parenteral penicillin G potassium); salt substitutes (most contain substantial amounts of potassium).

Exchange resins, such as sodium polystyrene sulfonate, whether administered orally or rectally, reduce serum potassium levels by sodium replacement of the potassium; fluid retention may occur in some patients because of the increased sodium intake.

Chronic or overuse of laxatives may reduce serum potassium levels by promoting excessive potassium loss from the intestinal tract; laxatives may interfere with the potassium-retaining effects of triamterene.

The effectiveness of methenamine may be decreased when used concurrently with hydrochlorothiazide because of alkalinization of the urine.

Drug/Laboratory Test Interactions

Triamterene and quinidine have similar fluorescence spectra; thus, DYAZIDE will interfere with the fluorescent measurement of quinidine.

Carcinogenesis, Mutagenesis, Impairment of Fertility

Carcinogenesis

Long-term studies have not been conducted with DYAZIDE (the triamterene/hydrochlorothiazide combination), or with triamterene alone.

Hydrochlorothiazide

Two-year feeding studies in mice and rats, conducted under the auspices of the National Toxicology Program (NTP), treated mice and rats with doses of hydrochlorothiazide up to 600 and 100 mg/kg/day, respectively. On a body-weight basis, these doses are 600 times (in mice) and 100 times (in rats) the Maximum Recommended Human Dose (MRHD) for the hydrochlorothiazide component of DYAZIDE at 50 mg/day (or 1.0 mg/kg/day based on 50 kg individuals). On the basis of body-surface area, these doses are 56 times (in mice) and 21 times (in rats) the MRHD. These studies uncovered no evidence of carcinogenic potential of hydrochlorothiazide in rats or female mice, but there was equivocal evidence of hepatocarcinogenicity in male mice.

Mutagenesis

Studies of the mutagenic potential of DYAZIDE (the triamterene/hydrochlorothiazide combination), or of triamterene alone have not been performed.

Hydrochlorothiazide

Hydrochlorothiazide was not genotoxic in in vitro assays using strains TA 98, TA 100, TA 1535, TA 1537 and TA 1538 of *Salmonella typhimurium* (the Ames test); in the Chinese Hamster Ovary (CHO) test for chromosomal aberrations; or in in vivo assays using mouse germinal cell chromosomes, Chinese hamster bone marrow chromosomes, and the *Drosophila* sex-linked recessive lethal trait gene. Positive test results were obtained in the in vitro CHO Sister Chromatid Exchange (clastogenicity) test, and in the mouse Lymphoma Cell (mutagenicity) assays, using concentrations of hydrochlorothiazide of 43 to 1300 mcg/mL. Positive test results were also obtained in the *Aspergillus nidulans* nondisjunction assay, using an unspecified concentration of hydrochlorothiazide.

Impairment of Fertility

Studies of the effects of DYAZIDE (the triamterene/hydrochlorothiazide combination), or of triamterene alone on animal reproductive function have not been conducted.

Hydrochlorothiazide

Hydrochlorothiazide had no adverse effects on the fertility of mice and rats of either sex in studies wherein these species were exposed, via their diet, to doses of up to 100 and 4 mg/kg/day, respectively, prior to mating and throughout gestation. Corresponding multiples of the MRHD are 100 (mice) and 4 (rats) on the basis of body-weight and 9.4 (mice) and 0.8 (rats) on the basis of body-surface area.

Pregnancy: Category C

Teratogenic Effects

DYAZIDE

Animal reproduction studies to determine the potential for fetal harm by DYAZIDE have not been conducted. However, a One Generation Study in the rat approximated composition of DYAZIDE by using a 1:1 ratio of triamterene to hydrochlorothiazide (30:30 mg/kg/day); there was no evidence of teratogenicity at those doses which were, on a body-weight basis, 15 and 30 times, respectively, the MRHD, and on the basis of body-surface area, 3.1 and 6.2 times, respectively, the MRHD.

The safe use of DYAZIDE in pregnancy has not been established since there are no adequate and well-controlled studies with DYAZIDE in pregnant women. DYAZIDE should be used during pregnancy only if the potential benefit justifies the risk to the fetus.

Triamterene

Reproduction studies have been performed in rats at doses as high as 20 times the MRHD on the basis of body-weight, and 6 times the human dose on the basis of body-surface area without evidence of harm to the fetus due to triamterene.

Because animal reproduction studies are not always predictive of human response, this drug should be used during pregnancy only if clearly needed.

Hydrochlorothiazide

Hydrochlorothiazide was orally administered to pregnant mice and rats during respective periods of major organogenesis at doses up to 3,000 and 1,000 mg/kg/day, respectively. At these doses, which are multiples of the MRHD equal to 3,000 for mice and 1,000 for rats, based on body-weight, and equal to 282 for mice and 206 for rats, based on body-surface area, there was no evidence of harm to the fetus.

There are, however, no adequate and well-controlled studies in pregnant women. Because animal reproduction studies are not always predictive of human response, this drug should be used during pregnancy only if clearly needed.

Nonteratogenic Effects

Thiazides and triamterene have been shown to cross the placental barrier and appear in cord blood. The use of thiazides and triamterene in pregnant women requires that the anticipated benefit be weighed against possible hazards to the fetus. These hazards include fetal or neonatal jaundice, pancreatitis, thrombocytopenia, and possible other adverse reactions which have occurred in the adult.

Nursing Mothers

Thiazides and triamterene in combination have not been studied in nursing mothers. Triamterene appears in animal milk; this may occur in humans. Thiazides are excreted in human breast milk. If use of the combination drug product is deemed essential, the patient should stop nursing.

Pediatric Use

Safety and effectiveness in pediatric patients have not been established.

ADVERSE REACTIONS

Adverse effects are listed in decreasing order of severity.

Hypersensitivity

Anaphylaxis, rash, urticaria, subacute cutaneous lupus erythematosus-like reactions, photosensitivity.

Cardiovascular

Arrhythmia, postural hypotension.

Metabolic

Diabetes mellitus, hyperkalemia, hypokalemia, hyponatremia, acidosis, hypercalcemia, hyperglycemia, glycosuria, hyperuricemia, hypochloremia.

Gastrointestinal

Jaundice and/or liver enzyme abnormalities, pancreatitis, nausea and vomiting, diarrhea, constipation, abdominal pain.

Renal

Acute renal failure (one case of irreversible renal failure has been reported), interstitial nephritis, renal stones composed primarily of triamterene, elevated BUN, and serum creatinine, abnormal urinary sediment.

Hematologic

Leukopenia, thrombocytopenia and purpura, megaloblastic anemia.

Musculoskeletal

Muscle cramps.

Central Nervous System

Weakness, fatigue, dizziness, headache, dry mouth.

Miscellaneous

Impotence, sialadenitis.

Thiazides alone have been shown to cause the following additional adverse reactions:

Central Nervous System

Paresthesias, vertigo.

Ophthalmic

Xanthopsia, transient blurred vision.

Respiratory

Allergic pneumonitis, pulmonary edema, respiratory distress.

Other

Necrotizing vasculitis, exacerbation of lupus.

Hematologic

Aplastic anemia, agranulocytosis, hemolytic anemia.

Neonate and infancy

Thrombocytopenia and pancreatitis–rarely, in newborns whose mothers have received thiazides during pregnancy.

Skin

Erythema multiforme including Stevens-Johnson syndrome, exfoliative dermatitis including toxic epidermal necrolysis.

DOSAGE AND ADMINISTRATION

The usual dose of DYAZIDE is one or two capsules given once daily, with appropriate monitoring of serum potassium and of the clinical effect (see WARNINGS, Hyperkalemia).

OVERDOSAGE

Electrolyte imbalance is the major concern (see WARNINGS section). Symptoms reported include: polyuria, nausea, vomiting, weakness, lassitude, fever, flushed face, and hyperactive deep tendon reflexes. If hypotension occurs, it may be treated with pressor agents such as levarterenol to maintain blood pressure. Carefully evaluate the electrolyte pattern and fluid balance. Induce immediate evacuation of the stomach through emesis or gastric lavage. There is no specific antidote.

Reversible acute renal failure following ingestion of 50 tablets of a product containing a combination of 50 mg triamterene and 25 mg hydrochlorothiazide has been reported. Although triamterene is largely protein-bound (approximately 67%), there may be some benefit to dialysis in cases of overdosage.

HOW SUPPLIED

Capsules containing 25 mg hydrochlorothiazide and 37.5 mg triamterene, in bottles of 1,000 capsules; in Patient-Pak™ unit-of-use bottles of 100.

They are supplied as follows:

NDC 0007-3650-22–in Patient-Pak™ unit-of-use bottles of 100.

NDC 0007-3650-30–bottles of 1,000.

Store at controlled room temperature 20° to 25°C (68° to 77°F); excursions permitted to 15° to 30°C (59° to 86°F). Protect from light. Dispense in a tight, light-resistant container.

GlaxoSmithKline
Research Triangle Park, NC 27709
DYAZIDE is a registered trademark of GlaxoSmithKline.
©2011, GlaxoSmithKline. All rights reserved.
February 2011
DYZ:74PI

ENGERIX-B   ℞

[in' jə-rix]

[Hepatitis B Vaccine (Recombinant)]
Suspension for Intramuscular Injection

HIGHLIGHTS OF PRESCRIBING INFORMATION

These highlights do not include all the information needed to use ENGERIX-B safely and effectively. See full prescribing information for ENGERIX-B.

ENGERIX-B [Hepatitis B Vaccine (Recombinant)]
Suspension for Intramuscular Injection
Initial U.S. Approval: 1989

INDICATIONS AND USAGE

ENGERIX-B is a vaccine indicated for immunization against infection caused by all known subtypes of hepatitis B virus. (1)

DOSAGE AND ADMINISTRATION

- ENGERIX-B is administered by intramuscular injection. (2.2)
- Persons from birth through 19 years of age: A series of 3 doses (0.5 mL each) given on a 0-, 1-, 6-month schedule. (2.3)
- Persons 20 years of age and older: A series of 3 doses (1 mL each) given on a 0-, 1-, 6-month schedule. (2.3)
- Adults on hemodialysis: A series of 4 doses (2 mL each) given as a single 2-mL dose or as two 1-mL doses on a 0-, 1-, 2-, 6-month schedule. (2.3)

DOSAGE FORMS AND STRENGTHS

- ENGERIX-B is a sterile suspension available in the following presentations:
- 0.5-mL (10 mcg) single-dose vials and prefilled syringes (3)
- 1-mL (20 mcg) single-dose vials and prefilled syringes (3)

CONTRAINDICATIONS

Severe allergic reaction (e.g., anaphylaxis) after a previous dose of any hepatitis B-containing vaccine, or to any component of ENGERIX-B, including yeast. (4)

WARNINGS AND PRECAUTIONS

- The tip caps of the prefilled syringes may contain natural rubber latex which may cause allergic reactions in latex-sensitive individuals. (5.1)
- Syncope (fainting) can occur in association with administration of injectable vaccines, including ENGERIX-B. Procedures should be in place to avoid falling injury and to restore cerebral perfusion following syncope. (5.2)
- Apnea following intramuscular vaccination has been observed in some infants born prematurely. Decisions about when to administer an intramuscular vaccine, including ENGERIX-B, to infants born prematurely should be based on consideration of the infant's medical status, and the potential benefits and possible risks of vaccination. (5.4)

ADVERSE REACTIONS

The most common solicited adverse events were injection-site soreness (22%) and fatigue (14%). (6.1)

To report SUSPECTED ADVERSE REACTIONS, contact GlaxoSmithKline at 1-888-825-5249 or VAERS at 1-800-822-7967 or www.vaers.hhs.gov.

DRUG INTERACTIONS

Do not mix ENGERIX-B with any other vaccine or product in the same syringe or vial. (7.1)

USE IN SPECIFIC POPULATIONS

- Safety and effectiveness of ENGERIX-B have not been established in pregnant women and nursing mothers. ENGERIX-B should only be given to a pregnant woman if clearly needed. (8.1, 8.3)
- Antibody responses are lower in persons older than 60 years of age than in younger adults. (8.5)

See 17 for PATIENT COUNSELING INFORMATION
                                    Revised: 12/2013

FULL PRESCRIBING INFORMATION

1   INDICATIONS AND USAGE

ENGERIX-B® is indicated for immunization against infection caused by all known subtypes of hepatitis B virus.

2   DOSAGE AND ADMINISTRATION

2.1   Preparation for Administration

Shake well before use. With thorough agitation, ENGERIX-B is a homogeneous, turbid white suspension. Do not administer if it appears otherwise. Parenteral drug products should be inspected visually for particulate matter and discoloration prior to administration, whenever solution and container permit. If either of these conditions exists, the vaccine should not be administered.

For the prefilled syringes, attach a sterile needle and administer intramuscularly.

For the vials, use a sterile needle and sterile syringe to withdraw the vaccine dose and administer intramuscularly. Changing needles between drawing vaccine from a vial and injecting it into a recipient is not necessary unless the needle has been damaged or contaminated. Use a separate sterile needle and syringe for each individual.

2.2   Administration

ENGERIX-B should be administered by intramuscular injection. The preferred administration site is the antero-

lateral aspect of the thigh for infants younger than 1 year and the deltoid muscle in older children (whose deltoid is large enough for an intramuscular injection) and adults. ENGERIX-B should not be administered in the gluteal region; such injections may result in suboptimal response. ENGERIX-B may be administered subcutaneously to persons at risk of hemorrhage (e.g., hemophiliacs). However, hepatitis B vaccines administered subcutaneously are known to result in a lower antibody response. Additionally, when other aluminum-adsorbed vaccines have been administered subcutaneously, an increased incidence of local reactions including subcutaneous nodules has been observed. Therefore, subcutaneous administration should be used only in persons who are at risk of hemorrhage with intramuscular injections.

Do not administer this product intravenously or intradermally.

2.3   Recommended Dose and Schedule

Persons From Birth Through 19 Years of Age: Primary immunization for infants (born of hepatitis B surface antigen [HBsAg]-negative or HBsAg-positive mothers), children (birth through 10 years of age), and adolescents (11 through 19 years of age) consists of a series of 3 doses (0.5 mL each) given on a 0-, 1-, and 6-month schedule.

Persons 20 Years of Age and Older: Primary immunization for persons 20 years of age and older consists of a series of 3 doses (1 mL each) given on a 0-, 1-, and 6-month schedule.

Adults on Hemodialysis: Primary immunization consists of a series of 4 doses (2 mL each) given as a single 2-mL dose or two 1-mL doses on a 0-, 1-, 2-, and 6-month schedule. In hemodialysis patients, antibody response is lower than in healthy persons and protection may persist only as long as antibody levels remain above 10 mIU/mL. Therefore, the need for booster doses should be assessed by annual antibody testing. A 2-mL booster dose (as a single 2-mL dose or two 1-mL doses) should be given when antibody levels decline below 10 mIU/mL.[1] [See Clinical Studies (14.2).]

Table 1. Recommended Dosage and Administration Schedules

Group	Dose[a]	Schedules
Infants born of:		
HBsAg-negative mothers	0.5 mL	0, 1, 6 months
HBsAg-positive mothers[b]	0.5 mL	0, 1, 6 months
Children: Birth through 10 years of age	0.5 mL	0, 1, 6 months
Adolescents: 11 through 19 years of age	0.5 mL	0, 1, 6 months
Adults: 20 years of age and older	1 mL	0, 1, 6 months
Adults on hemodialysis	2 mL[c]	0, 1, 2, 6 months

HBsAg = Hepatitis B surface antigen
[a] 0.5 mL (10 mcg); 1 mL (20 mcg).
[b] Infants born to HBsAg-positive mothers should also receive hepatitis B immune globulin (HBIG) [see Dosage and Administration (2.6)].
[c] Given as a single 2-mL dose or as two 1-mL doses.

2.4   Alternate Dosing Schedules

There are alternate dosing and administration schedules which may be used for specific populations (e.g., neonates born of hepatitis B–infected mothers, persons who have or might have been recently exposed to the virus, and travelers to high-risk areas) (Table 2). For some of these alternate schedules, an additional dose at 12 months is recommended for prolonged maintenance of protective titers.

Table 2. Alternate Dosage and Administration Schedules

Group	Dose[a]	Schedules
Infants born of: HBsAg-positive mothers[b]	0.5 mL	0, 1, 2, 12 months
Children Birth through 10 years of age	0.5 mL	0, 1, 2, 12 months
5 through 10 years of age	0.5 mL	0, 12, 24 months[c]
Adolescents: 11 through 16 years of age	0.5 mL	0, 12, 24 months[c]
11 through 19 years of age	1 mL	0, 1, 6 months
11 through 19 years of age	1 mL	0, 1, 2, 12 months

| Adults: 20 years of age and older | 1 mL | 0, 1, 2, 12 months |

HBsAg = Hepatitis B surface antigen
[a] 0.5 mL (10 mcg); 1 mL (20 mcg).
[b] Infants born to HBsAg-positive mothers should also receive hepatitis B immune globulin (HBIG) [see Dosage and Administration (2.6)].
[c] For children and adolescents for whom an extended administration schedule is acceptable based on risk of exposure.

2.5   Booster Vaccinations

Whenever administration of a booster dose is appropriate, the dose of ENGERIX-B is 0.5 mL for children 10 years of age and younger and 1 mL for persons 11 years of age and older. Studies have demonstrated a substantial increase in antibody titers after booster vaccination with ENGERIX-B. See Section 2.3 for information on booster vaccination for adults on hemodialysis.

2.6   Known or Presumed Exposure to Hepatitis B Virus

Persons with known or presumed exposure to the hepatitis B virus (e.g., neonates born of infected mothers, persons who experienced percutaneous or permucosal exposure to the virus) should be given hepatitis B immune globulin (HBIG) in addition to ENGERIX-B in accordance with Advisory Committee on Immunization Practices recommendations and with the package insert for HBIG. ENGERIX-B can be given on either dosing schedule (0, 1, and 6 months or 0, 1, 2, and 12 months).

3   DOSAGE FORMS AND STRENGTHS

ENGERIX-B is a sterile suspension available in the following presentations:
- 0.5-mL (10 mcg) single-dose vials and prefilled TIP-LOK® syringes
- 1-mL (20 mcg) single-dose vials and prefilled TIP-LOK syringes

[See Description (11) and How Supplied/Storage and Handling (16).]

4   CONTRAINDICATIONS

Severe allergic reaction (e.g., anaphylaxis) after a previous dose of any hepatitis B-containing vaccine, or to any component of ENGERIX-B, including yeast, is a contraindication to administration of ENGERIX-B [see Description (11)].

5   WARNINGS AND PRECAUTIONS

5.1   Latex

The tip caps of the prefilled syringes may contain natural rubber latex which may cause allergic reactions in latex-sensitive individuals.

5.2   Syncope

Syncope (fainting) can occur in association with administration of injectable vaccines, including ENGERIX-B. Syncope can be accompanied by transient neurological signs such as visual disturbance, paresthesia, and tonic-clonic limb movements. Procedures should be in place to avoid falling injury and to restore cerebral perfusion following syncope.

5.3   Infants Weighing Less Than 2,000 g

Hepatitis B vaccine should be deferred for infants weighing <2,000 g if the mother is documented to be HBsAg negative at the time of the infant's birth. Vaccination can commence at chronological age 1 month or hospital discharge. Infants weighing <2,000 g born to HBsAg-positive mothers or mothers of unknown HBsAg status should receive vaccine and hepatitis B immune globulin (HBIG) within 12 hours if HBsAg status cannot be determined; the birth dose should not be counted as the first dose in the vaccine series and it should be followed with a full 3-dose standard regimen (total of 4 doses).[2] [See Dosage and Administration (2).]

5.4   Apnea in Premature Infants

Apnea following intramuscular vaccination has been observed in some infants born prematurely. Decisions about when to administer an intramuscular vaccine, including ENGERIX-B, to infants born prematurely should be based on consideration of the infant's medical status, and the potential benefits and possible risks of vaccination. For ENGERIX-B, this assessment should include consideration of the mother's hepatitis B antigen status and the high probability of maternal transmission of hepatitis B virus to infants born of mothers who are HBsAg positive if vaccination is delayed.

5.5   Preventing and Managing Allergic Vaccine Reactions

Prior to immunization, the healthcare provider should review the immunization history for possible vaccine sensitivity and previous vaccination-related adverse reactions to allow an assessment of benefits and risks. Epinephrine and other appropriate agents used for the control of immediate allergic reactions must be immediately available should an acute anaphylactic reaction occur. [See Contraindications (4).]

5.6 Moderate or Severe Acute Illness

To avoid diagnostic confusion between manifestations of an acute illness and possible vaccine adverse effects, vaccination with ENGERIX-B should be postponed in persons with moderate or severe acute febrile illness unless they are at immediate risk of hepatitis B infection (e.g., infants born of HBsAg-positive mothers).

5.7 Altered Immunocompetence

Immunocompromised persons may have a diminished immune response to ENGERIX-B, including individuals receiving immunosuppressant therapy.

5.8 Multiple Sclerosis

Results from 2 clinical studies indicate that there is no association between hepatitis B vaccination and the development of multiple sclerosis,[3] and that vaccination with hepatitis B vaccine does not appear to increase the short–term risk of relapse in multiple sclerosis.[4]

5.9 Limitations of Vaccine Effectiveness

Hepatitis B has a long incubation period. ENGERIX-B may not prevent hepatitis B infection in individuals who had an unrecognized hepatitis B infection at the time of vaccine administration. Additionally, it may not prevent infection in individuals who do not achieve protective antibody titers.

6 ADVERSE REACTIONS

6.1 Clinical Trials Experience

Because clinical trials are conducted under widely varying conditions, adverse reaction rates observed in the clinical trials of a vaccine cannot be directly compared to rates in the clinical trials of another vaccine and may not reflect the rates observed in practice.

The most common solicited adverse events were injection site soreness (22%) and fatigue (14%).

In 36 clinical studies, a total of 13,495 doses of ENGERIX-B were administered to 5,071 healthy adults and children who were initially seronegative for hepatitis B markers, and healthy neonates. All subjects were monitored for 4 days post-administration. Frequency of adverse events tended to decrease with successive doses of ENGERIX-B.

Using a symptom checklist, the most frequently reported adverse events were injection site soreness (22%) and fatigue (14%). Other events are listed below. Parent or guardian completed forms for children and neonates. Neonatal checklist did not include headache, fatigue, or dizziness.

Incidence 1% to 10% of Injections: Nervous System Disorders: Dizziness, headache.

General Disorders and Administration Site Conditions: Fever (>37.5°C), injection site erythema, injection site induration, injection site swelling.

Incidence <1% of Injections: Infections and Infestations: Upper respiratory tract illnesses.

Blood and Lymphatic System Disorders: Lymphadenopathy.

Metabolism and Nutrition Disorders: Anorexia.

Psychiatric Disorders: Agitation, insomnia.

Nervous System Disorders: Somnolence, tingling.

Vascular Disorders: Flushing, hypotension.

Gastrointestinal Disorders: Abdominal pain/cramps, constipation, diarrhea, nausea, vomiting.

Skin and Subcutaneous Tissue Disorders: Erythema, petechiae, pruritus, rash, sweating, urticaria.

Musculoskeletal and Connective Tissue Disorders: Arthralgia, back pain, myalgia, pain/stiffness in arm, shoulder, or neck.

General Disorders and Administration Site Conditions: Chills, influenza-like symptoms, injection site ecchymosis, injection site pain, injection site pruritus, irritability, malaise, weakness.

6.2 Postmarketing Experience

In addition to reports in clinical trials, worldwide voluntary reports of adverse events received for ENGERIX-B since market introduction (1990) are listed below. This list includes serious adverse events or events which have a suspected causal connection to components of ENGERIX-B.

The following adverse events have been identified during postapproval use of ENGERIX-B. Because these events are reported voluntarily from a population of unknown size, it is not always possible to reliably estimate their frequency or establish a causal relationship to the vaccine.

Infections and Infestations: Herpes zoster, meningitis.

Blood and Lymphatic System Disorders: Thrombocytopenia.

Immune System Disorders: Allergic reaction, anaphylactoid reaction, anaphylaxis. An apparent hypersensitivity syndrome (serum sickness-like) of delayed onset has been reported days to weeks after vaccination, including: arthralgia/arthritis (usually transient), fever, and dermatologic reactions such as urticaria, erythema multiforme, ecchymoses, and erythema nodosum.

Nervous System Disorders: Encephalitis, encephalopathy, migraine, multiple sclerosis, neuritis, neuropathy including hypoesthesia, paresthesia, Guillain-Barré syndrome and Bell's palsy, optic neuritis, paralysis, paresis, seizures, syncope, transverse myelitis.

Eye Disorders: Conjunctivitis, keratitis, visual disturbances.

Ear and Labyrinth Disorders: Earache, tinnitus, vertigo.

Cardiac Disorders: Palpitations, tachycardia.

Vascular Disorders: Vasculitis.

Respiratory, Thoracic and Mediastinal Disorders: Apnea, bronchospasm including asthma-like symptoms.

Gastrointestinal Disorders: Dyspepsia.

Skin and Subcutaneous Tissue Disorders: Alopecia, angioedema, eczema, erythema multiforme including Stevens-Johnson syndrome, erythema nodosum, lichen planus, purpura.

Musculoskeletal and Connective Tissue Disorders: Arthritis, muscular weakness.

General Disorders and Administration Site Conditions: Injection site reaction.

Investigations: Abnormal liver function tests.

7 DRUG INTERACTIONS

7.1 Concomitant Administration With Vaccines and Immune Globulin

ENGERIX-B may be administered concomitantly with immune globulin.

When concomitant administration of other vaccines or immune globulin is required, they should be given with different syringes and at different injection sites. Do not mix ENGERIX-B with any other vaccine or product in the same syringe or vial.

8 USE IN SPECIFIC POPULATIONS

8.1 Pregnancy

Pregnancy Category C

Animal reproduction studies have not been conducted with ENGERIX-B. It is also not known whether ENGERIX-B can cause fetal harm when administered to a pregnant woman or can affect reproduction capacity. ENGERIX-B should be given to a pregnant woman only if clearly needed.

8.3 Nursing Mothers

It is not known whether ENGERIX-B is excreted in human milk. Because many drugs are excreted in human milk, caution should be exercised when ENGERIX-B is administered to a nursing woman.

8.4 Pediatric Use

Safety and effectiveness of ENGERIX-B have been established in all pediatric age groups. Maternally transferred antibodies do not interfere with the active immune response to the vaccine. *[See Adverse Reactions (6) and Clinical Studies (14.1, 14.3, 14.4).]*

8.5 Geriatric Use

Clinical studies of ENGERIX-B used for licensure did not include sufficient numbers of subjects 65 years of age and older to determine whether they respond differently from younger subjects. However, in later studies it has been shown that a diminished antibody response and seroprotective levels can be expected in persons older than 60 years of age.[5]

11 DESCRIPTION

ENGERIX-B [Hepatitis B Vaccine (Recombinant)] is a sterile suspension of noninfectious hepatitis B virus surface antigen (HBsAg) for intramuscular administration. It contains purified surface antigen of the virus obtained by culturing genetically engineered *Saccharomyces cerevisiae* cells, which carry the surface antigen gene of the hepatitis B virus. The HBsAg expressed in the cells is purified by several physicochemical steps and formulated as a suspension of the antigen adsorbed on aluminum hydroxide. The procedures used to manufacture ENGERIX-B result in a product that contains no more than 5% yeast protein.

Each 0.5-mL pediatric/adolescent dose contains 10 mcg of HBsAg adsorbed on 0.25 mg aluminum as aluminum hydroxide.

Each 1-mL adult dose contains 20 mcg of HBsAg adsorbed on 0.5 mg aluminum as aluminum hydroxide.

ENGERIX-B contains the following excipients: Sodium chloride (9 mg/mL) and phosphate buffers (disodium phosphate dihydrate, 0.98 mg/mL; sodium dihydrogen phosphate dihydrate, 0.71 mg/mL).

ENGERIX-B is available in vials and prefilled syringes. The tip caps of the prefilled syringes may contain natural rubber latex; the plungers are not made with natural rubber latex. The vial stoppers are not made with natural rubber latex. ENGERIX-B is formulated without preservatives.

12 CLINICAL PHARMACOLOGY

12.1 Mechanism of Action

Infection with hepatitis B virus can have serious consequences including acute massive hepatic necrosis and chronic active hepatitis. Chronically infected persons are at increased risk for cirrhosis and hepatocellular carcinoma.

Antibody concentrations ≥10 mIU/mL against HBsAg are recognized as conferring protection against hepatitis B virus infection.[1] Seroconversion is defined as antibody titers ≥1 mIU/mL.

13 NONCLINICAL TOXICOLOGY

13.1 Carcinogenesis, Mutagenesis, Impairment of Fertility

ENGERIX-B has not been evaluated for carcinogenic or mutagenic potential, or for impairment of fertility.

14 CLINICAL STUDIES

14.1 Efficacy in Neonates

Protective efficacy with ENGERIX-B has been demonstrated in a clinical trial in neonates at high risk of hepatitis B infection.[6,7] Fifty-eight neonates born of mothers who were both HBsAg-positive and hepatitis B "e" antigen (HBeAg)-positive were given ENGERIX-B (10 mcg/0.5 mL) at 0, 1, and 2 months, without concomitant hepatitis B immune globulin (HBIG). Two infants became chronic carriers in the 12-month follow-up period after initial inoculation. Assuming an expected carrier rate of 70%, the protective efficacy rate against the chronic carrier state during the first 12 months of life was 95%.

14.2 Efficacy and Immunogenicity in Specific Populations

Homosexual Men: ENGERIX-B (20 mcg/1 mL) given at 0, 1, and 6 months was evaluated in homosexual men 16 to 59 years of age. Four of 244 subjects became infected with hepatitis B during the period prior to completion of the 3-dose immunization schedule. No additional subjects became infected during the 18-month follow-up period after completion of the immunization course.

Adults with Chronic Hepatitis C: In a clinical trial of 67 adults 25 to 67 years of age with chronic hepatitis C, ENGERIX-B (20 mcg/1 mL) was given at 0, 1, and 6 months. Of the subjects assessed at month 7 (N = 31), 100% responded with seroprotective titers. The geometric mean antibody titer (GMT) was 1,260 mIU/mL (95% Confidence Interval [CI]: 709, 2,237).

Adults on Hemodialysis: Hemodialysis patients given hepatitis B vaccines respond with lower titers, which remain at protective levels for shorter durations than in normal subjects. In a clinical trial of 56 adults who had been on hemodialysis for a mean period of 56 months, ENGERIX-B (40 mcg/2 mL given as two 1-mL doses) was given at 0, 1, 2, and 6 months. Two months after the fourth dose, 67% (29/43) of patients had seroprotective antibody levels (≥10 mIU/mL) and the GMT among seroconverters was 93 mIU/mL.

14.3 Immunogenicity in Neonates

In clinical studies, neonates were given ENGERIX-B (10 mcg/0.5 mL) at 0, 1, and 6 months or at 0, 1, and 2 months of age. The immune response to vaccination was evaluated in sera obtained one month after the third dose of ENGERIX-B.

Among infants administered ENGERIX-B at 0, 1, and 6 months, 100% of evaluable subjects (N = 52) seroconverted by month 7. The GMT was 713 mIU/mL. Of these, 97% had seroprotective levels (≥10 mIU/mL).

Among infants enrolled (N = 381) to receive ENGERIX-B at 0, 1, and 2 months of age, 96% had seroprotective levels (≥10 mIU/mL) by month 4. The GMT among seroconverters (N = 311) (antibody titer ≥1 mIU/mL) was 210 mIU/mL. A subset of these children received a fourth dose of ENGERIX-B at 12 months of age. One month following this dose, seroconverters (N = 126) had a GMT of 2,941 mIU/mL.

14.4 Immunogenicity in Children and Adults

Persons 6 Months Through 10 Years of Age: In clinical trials, children (N = 242) 6 months through 10 years of age were given ENGERIX-B (10 mcg/0.5 mL) at 0, 1, and 6 months. One to 2 months after the third dose, the seroprotection rate was 98% and the GMT of seroconverters was 4,023 mIU/mL.

Persons 5 Through 16 Years of Age: In a separate clinical trial including both children and adolescents 5 through 16 years of age, ENGERIX-B (10 mcg/0.5 mL) was administered at 0, 1, and 6 months (N = 181) or 0, 12, and 24 months (N = 161). Immediately before the third dose of vaccine, seroprotection was achieved in 92.3% of subjects vaccinated on the 0-, 1-, and 6-month schedule and 88.8% of subjects on the 0-, 12-, and 24-month schedule (GMT: 117.9 mIU/mL versus 162.1 mIU/mL, respectively, P = 0.18). One month following the third dose, seroprotection was achieved in 99.5% of children vaccinated on the 0-, 1-, and 6-month schedule compared to 98.1% of those on the 0-, 12-, and 24-month schedule. GMTs were higher (P = 0.02) for children receiving vaccine on the 0-, 1-, and 6-month schedule compared to those on the 0-, 12-, and 24-month schedule (5,687.4 mIU/mL versus 3,158.7 mIU/mL, respectively).

Persons 11 Through 19 Years of Age: In clinical trials with healthy adolescent subjects 11 through 19 years of age, ENGERIX-B (10 mcg/0.5 mL) given at 0, 1, and 6 months produced a seroprotection rate of 97% at month 8 (N = 119) with a GMT of 1,989 mIU/mL (N = 118, 95% CI: 1,318, 3,020). Immunization with ENGERIX-B (20 mcg/1 mL) at 0, 1, and 6 months produced a seroprotection rate of 99% at month 8 (N = 122) with a GMT of 7,672 mIU/mL (N = 122, 95% CI: 5,248, 10,965).

Persons 16 Through 65 Years of Age: Clinical trials in healthy adult and adolescent subjects (16 through 65 years of age) have shown that following a course of 3 doses of ENGERIX-B (20 mcg/1 mL) given at 0, 1, and 6 months, the seroprotection (antibody titers ≥10 mIU/mL) rate for all individuals was 79% at month 6 (5 months after second dose) and 96% at month 7 (1 month after third dose); the GMT for seroconverters was 2,204 mIU/mL at month 7 (N = 110). An alternate 3-dose schedule (20 mcg/1 mL given at 0, 1, and 2 months) designed for certain populations (e.g., individuals who have or might have been recently exposed to the virus and travelers to high-risk areas) was also evaluated. At month 3 (1 month after third dose), 99% of all individuals were seroprotected and remained protected through month 12. On the alternate schedule, a fourth dose of ENGERIX-B (20 mcg/1 mL) at 12 months produced a GMT of 9,163 mIU/mL at month 13 (1 month after fourth dose) (N = 373).

Persons 40 Years of Age and Older: Among subjects 40 years of age and older given ENGERIX-B (20 mcg/1 mL) at 0, 1, and 6 months, the seroprotection rate 1 month after the third dose was 88% and the GMT for seroconverters was 610 mIU/mL (N = 50). In adults older than 40 years of age, ENGERIX-B produced anti-HBsAg antibody titers that were lower than those in younger adults.

14.5 Interchangeability With Other Hepatitis B Vaccines
A controlled study (N = 48) demonstrated that completion of a course of immunization with 1 dose of ENGERIX-B (20 mcg/1 mL) at month 6 following 2 doses of RECOMBIVAX HB® (10 mcg) at months 0 and 1 produced a similar GMT (4,077 mIU/mL) to immunization with 3 doses of RECOMBIVAX HB (10 mcg) at months 0, 1, and 6 (GMT: 2,654 mIU/mL). Thus, ENGERIX-B can be used to complete a vaccination course initiated with RECOMBIVAX HB.[8]

15   REFERENCES

1. Centers for Disease Control and Prevention. Hepatitis B. In: Atkinson W, Wolfe C, Humiston S, Nelson R, eds. *Epidemiology and Prevention of Vaccine-Preventable Diseases.* 6th ed. Atlanta, GA: Public Health Foundation; 2000:207-229.
2. Centers for Disease Control and Prevention. A Comprehensive Immunization Strategy to Eliminate Transmission of Hepatitis B Virus Infection in the United States. Recommendations of the Advisory Committee on Immunization Practices (ACIP). Part 1: Immunization of Infants, Children, and Adolescents, MMWR 2005;54(RR-16);1-23.
3. Ascherio A, Zhang SM, Hernán MA, et al. Hepatitis B vaccination and the risk of multiple sclerosis. *N Engl J Med.* 2001;344(5):327-332.
4. Confavreux C, Suissa S, Saddier P, et al. Vaccination and the risk of relapse in multiple sclerosis. *N Engl J Med.* 2001-344(5):319-326.
5. Centers for Disease Control and Prevention. A Comprehensive Immunization Strategy to Eliminate Transmission of Hepatitis B Virus Infection in the United States. Recommendations of the Advisory Committee on Immunization Practices (ACIP). Part 2: Immunization of Adults, MMWR 2006;55(RR-16);1-25.
6. André FE, Safary A. Clinical experience with a yeast-derived hepatitis B vaccine. In: Zuckerman AJ, ed. *Viral Hepatitis and Liver Disease.* New York, NY: Alan R Liss, Inc.; 1988:1025-1030.
7. Poovorawan Y, Sanpavat S, Pongpunlert W, et al. Protective efficacy of a recombinant DNA hepatitis B vaccine in neonates of HBe antigen-positive mothers. *JAMA.* 1989;261(22):3278-3281.
8. Bush LM, Moonsammy GI, Boscia JA. Evaluation of initiating a hepatitis B vaccination schedule with one vaccine and completing it with another. *Vaccine.* 1991;9(11):807-809.

16   HOW SUPPLIED/STORAGE AND HANDLING

ENGERIX-B is available in single-dose vials and prefilled disposable TIP-LOK syringes (packaged without needles) (Preservative Free Formulation):
10 mcg/0.5 mL Pediatric/Adolescent Dose
NDC 58160-820-01 Vial in Package of 10: NDC 58160-820-11
NDC 58160-820-43 Syringe in Package of 10: NDC 58160-820-52
20 mcg/mL Adult Dose
NDC 58160-821-01 Vial in Package of 10: NDC 58160-821-11
NDC 58160-821-05 Syringe in Package of 1: NDC 58160-821-34
NDC 58160-821-43 Syringe in Package of 10: NDC 58160-821-52
Store refrigerated between 2° and 8° C (36° and 46° F). Do not freeze; discard if product has been frozen. Do not dilute to administer.

17   PATIENT COUNSELING INFORMATION

- Inform vaccine recipients and parents or guardians of the potential benefits and risks of immunization with ENGERIX-B.

- Emphasize, when educating vaccine recipients and parents or guardians regarding potential side effects, that ENGERIX-B contains non-infectious purified HBsAg and cannot cause hepatitis B infection.
- Instruct vaccine recipients and parents or guardians to report any adverse events to their healthcare provider.
- Give vaccine recipients and parents or guardians the Vaccine Information Statements, which are required by the National Childhood Vaccine Injury Act of 1986 to be given prior to immunization. These materials are available free of charge at the Centers for Disease Control and Prevention (CDC) website (www.cdc.gov/vaccines).

ENGERIX-B and TIP-LOK are registered trademarks of the GlaxoSmithKline group of companies. RECOMBIVAX HB is a registered trademark of Merck & Co.
Manufactured by **GlaxoSmithKline Biologicals**
Rixensart, Belgium, US License No. 1617
Distributed by **GlaxoSmithKline**
Research Triangle Park, NC 27709
©2013, GlaxoSmithKline group of companies. All rights reserved.
ENG:53PI

EPIVIR-HBV   ℞
[ĕp′ə-vir]
(lamivudine)
tablets for oral use

EPIVIR-HBV
(lamivudine)
oral solution

HIGHLIGHTS OF PRESCRIBING INFORMATION
These highlights do not include all the information needed to use EPIVIR-HBV safely and effectively. See full prescribing information for EPIVIR-HBV.
EPIVIR-HBV (lamivudine) tablets for oral use
EPIVIR-HBV (lamivudine) oral solution
Initial U.S. Approval: 1995

> **WARNING: RISK OF LACTIC ACIDOSIS, EXACERBATIONS OF HEPATITIS B UPON DISCONTINUATION OF EPIVIR-HBV, AND RISK OF HIV-1 RESISTANCE IF EPIVIR-HBV IS USED IN PATIENTS WITH UNRECOGNIZED OR UNTREATED HIV-1 INFECTION.**
>
> *See full prescribing information for complete Boxed Warning.*
>
> - Lactic acidosis and severe hepatomegaly with steatosis, including fatal cases, have been reported with the use of nucleoside analogues. Suspend treatment if clinical or laboratory findings suggestive of lactic acidosis or pronounced hepatotoxicity occur. (5.1)
> - Severe acute exacerbations of hepatitis B have been reported in patients who have discontinued anti-hepatitis B therapy (including EPIVIR-HBV). Monitor hepatic function closely in these patients and, if appropriate, initiate anti-hepatitis B treatment. (5.2)
> - EPIVIR-HBV tablets and oral solution contain a lower dose of the same active ingredient (lamivudine) as EPIVIR tablets and oral Solution used to treat HIV-1 infection. HIV-1 resistance may emerge in chronic hepatitis B patients with unrecognized or untreated HIV-1 infection because the lamivudine dosage in EPIVIR-HBV is subtherapeutic and monotherapy is inappropriate for the treatment of HIV-1 infection. HIV counseling and testing should be offered to all patients before beginning treatment with EPIVIR-HBV and periodically during treatment. (5.3)

INDICATIONS AND USAGE
- EPIVIR-HBV is a nucleoside analogue reverse transcriptase inhibitor indicated for the treatment of chronic hepatitis B virus infection associated with evidence of hepatitis B viral replication and active liver inflammation. (1)

DOSAGE AND ADMINISTRATION
- Adult patients: 100 mg, once daily. (2.2)
- Pediatric patients aged 2 to 17 years: 3 mg per kg once daily up to 100 mg once daily. Prescribe oral solution for pediatric patients requiring less than 100 mg once daily. (2.3)
- Patients with renal impairment: Doses of EPIVIR-HBV must be adjusted in accordance with renal function. (2.4)
- EPIVIR-HBV should not be used with other medications that contain lamivudine or emtricitabine. (2.5)

DOSAGE FORMS AND STRENGTHS
- Tablets: 100 mg (3)
- Oral Solution: 5 mg per mL (3)

CONTRAINDICATIONS
Patients with previously demonstrated clinically significant hypersensitivity (e.g., anaphylaxis) to any of the components of the products. (4)

WARNINGS AND PRECAUTIONS
- EPIVIR-HBV should not be used with other medications that contain lamivudine or with medications that contain emtricitabine. (5.4)
- Emergence of Resistance-Associated HBV Substitutions: Monitor ALT and HBV DNA levels during lamivudine treatment to aid in treatment decisions if emergence of viral mutants or loss of therapeutic response is suspected. (2.6, 5.5)

ADVERSE REACTIONS
- The most common reported adverse reactions in those receiving EPIVIR-HBV (incidence greater than or equal to 10% and reported at a rate greater than placebo) were ear, nose and throat infections, sore throat, and diarrhea. (6.1)
To report SUSPECTED ADVERSE REACTIONS, contact GlaxoSmithKline at 1-888-825-5249 at 1-877-844-8872 or FDA at 1-800-FDA-1088 or www.fda.gov/medwatch.
See 17 for PATIENT COUNSELING INFORMATION and FDA-approved patient labeling

Revised: 12/2013

FULL PRESCRIBING INFORMATION: CONTENTS*
WARNING: RISK OF LACTIC ACIDOSIS, EXACERBATIONS OF HEPATITIS B UPON DISCONTINUATION OF EPIVIR-HBV®, AND RISK OF HIV-1 RESISTANCE IF EPIVIR-HBV IS USED IN PATIENTS WITH UNRECOGNIZED OR UNTREATED HIV-1 INFECTION.

FULL PRESCRIBING INFORMATION

> **WARNING: RISK OF LACTIC ACIDOSIS, EXACERBATIONS OF HEPATITIS B UPON DISCONTINUATION OF EPIVIR-HBV®, AND RISK OF HIV-1 RESISTANCE IF EPIVIR-HBV IS USED IN PATIENTS WITH UNRECOGNIZED OR UNTREATED HIV-1 INFECTION.**
>
> **Lactic Acidosis and Severe Hepatomegaly:** Lactic acidosis and severe hepatomegaly with steatosis, in-

cluding fatal cases, have been reported with the use of nucleoside analogues alone or in combination, including EPIVIR-HBV. Suspend treatment if clinical or laboratory findings suggestive of lactic acidosis or pronounced hepatotoxicity occur *[see Warnings and Precautions (5.1)]*.

Exacerbations of Hepatitis B Upon Discontinuation of EPIVIR-HBV: Severe acute exacerbations of hepatitis B have been reported in patients who have discontinued anti-hepatitis B therapy (including EPIVIR-HBV). Hepatic function should be monitored closely with both clinical and laboratory follow-up for at least several months in patients who discontinue anti-hepatitis B therapy. If appropriate, initiation of anti-hepatitis B therapy may be warranted *[see Warnings and Precautions (5.2)]*.

Risk of HIV-1 Resistance if EPIVIR-HBV Is Used in Patients With Unrecognized or Untreated HIV-1 Infection: EPIVIR-HBV is not approved for the treatment of HIV-1 infection because the lamivudine dosage in EPIVIR-HBV is subtherapeutic and monotherapy is inappropriate for the treatment of HIV-1 infection. HIV-1 resistance may emerge in chronic hepatitis B-infected patients with unrecognized or untreated HIV-1 infection. Counseling and testing should be offered to all patients before beginning treatment with EPIVIR-HBV and periodically during treatment *[see Warnings and Precautions (5.3)]*.

1 INDICATIONS AND USAGE

EPIVIR-HBV is indicated for the treatment of chronic hepatitis B virus (HBV) infection associated with evidence of hepatitis B viral replication and active liver inflammation *[see Clinical Studies (14.1, 14.2)]*.

The following points should be considered when initiating therapy with EPIVIR-HBV:

- Due to high rates of resistance development in treated patients, initiation of treatment with EPIVIR-HBV should only be considered when the use of an alternative antiviral agent with a higher genetic barrier to resistance is not available or appropriate.
- EPIVIR-HBV has not been evaluated in patients co-infected with HIV, hepatitis C virus (HCV), or hepatitis delta virus.
- EPIVIR-HBV has not been evaluated in liver transplant recipients or in patients with chronic hepatitis B virus infection with decompensated liver disease.
- EPIVIR-HBV has not been evaluated in pediatric patients younger than 2 years of age with chronic HBV infection.

2 DOSAGE AND ADMINISTRATION

2.1 HIV Counseling and Testing

HIV counseling and testing should be offered to all patients before beginning treatment with EPIVIR-HBV and periodically during treatment because of the risk of emergence of resistant-HIV-1 and limitation of treatment options if EPIVIR-HBV is prescribed to treat chronic hepatitis B infection in a patient who has unrecognized HIV-1 infection or acquires HIV-1 infection during treatment *[see Warnings and Precautions (5.3)]*.

2.2 Dosage in Adult Patients

The recommended oral dosage of EPIVIR-HBV is 100 mg once daily.

2.3 Dosage in Pediatric Patients

The recommended oral dosage of EPIVIR-HBV for pediatric patients aged 2 to 17 years is 3 mg per kg once daily up to a maximum daily dosage of 100 mg. The oral solution formulation should be prescribed for patients requiring a dosage less than 100 mg or if unable to swallow tablets.

2.4 Dosage Adjustment in Adult Patients With Renal Impairment

Dosage recommendations for adult patients with reduced renal function are provided in Table 1 *[see Clinical Pharmacology (12.3)]*.

Table 1. Dosage of EPIVIR-HBV in Adult Patients With Renal Impairment

Creatinine Clearance (mL/min)	Recommended Dosage of EPIVIR-HBV
≥50	100 mg once daily
30-49	100 mg first dose, then 50 mg once daily
15-29	100 mg first dose, then 25 mg once daily
5-14	35 mg first dose, then 15 mg once daily
<5	35 mg first dose, then 10 mg once daily

Following correction of the dosage for renal impairment, no additional dosage modification of EPIVIR-HBV is required after routine (4-hour) hemodialysis or peritoneal dialysis *[see Clinical Pharmacology (12.3)]*.

There are insufficient data to recommend a specific dosage of EPIVIR-HBV in pediatric patients with renal impairment.

2.5 Important Administration Instructions

- EPIVIR-HBV tablets and oral solution may be administered with or without food.
- The tablets and oral solution may be used interchangeably *[see Clinical Pharmacology (12.3)]*.
- The oral solution should be used for doses less than 100 mg.
- EPIVIR-HBV should not be used with other medications that contain lamivudine or medications that contain emtricitabine *[see Warnings and Precautions (5.4)]*.

2.6 Assessing Patients During Treatment

Patients should be monitored regularly during treatment by a physician experienced in the management of chronic hepatitis B. During treatment, combinations of such events such as return of persistently elevated ALT, increasing levels of HBV DNA over time after an initial decline below assay limit, progression of clinical signs or symptoms of hepatic disease, and/or worsening of hepatic necroinflammatory findings may be considered as potentially reflecting loss of therapeutic response. Such observations should be taken into consideration when determining the advisability of continuing therapy with EPIVIR-HBV.

The optimal duration of treatment, the durability of HBeAg seroconversions occurring during treatment, and the relationship between treatment response and long-term outcomes such as hepatocellular carcinoma or decompensated cirrhosis are not known.

3 DOSAGE FORMS AND STRENGTHS

- EPIVIR-HBV tablets: 100 mg, butterscotch-colored, film-coated, biconvex, capsule-shaped tablets imprinted with "GX CG5" on one side.
- EPIVIR-HBV oral solution: A clear, colorless to pale yellow, strawberry-banana-flavored liquid, containing 5 mg of lamivudine per 1 mL.

4 CONTRAINDICATIONS

EPIVIR-HBV is contraindicated in patients who have experienced a previous hypersensitivity reaction (e.g., anaphylaxis) to lamivudine or to any component of the tablets or oral solution.

5 WARNINGS AND PRECAUTIONS

5.1 Lactic Acidosis and Severe Hepatomegaly With Steatosis

Lactic acidosis and severe hepatomegaly with steatosis, including fatal cases, have been reported with the use of nucleoside analogues alone or in combination, including EPIVIR-HBV and other antiretrovirals. A majority of these cases have been in women. Obesity and prolonged nucleoside exposure may be risk factors. Most of these reports have described patients receiving nucleoside analogues for treatment of HIV infection, but there have been reports of lactic acidosis in patients receiving lamivudine for hepatitis B. Particular caution should be exercised when administering EPIVIR-HBV to any patient with known risk factors for liver disease; however, cases have also been reported in patients with no known risk factors. Treatment with EPIVIR-HBV should be suspended in any patient who develops clinical or laboratory findings suggestive of lactic acidosis or pronounced hepatotoxicity (which may include hepatomegaly and steatosis even in the absence of marked transaminase elevations).

5.2 Exacerbation of Hepatitis After Discontinuation of Treatment

Clinical and laboratory evidence of exacerbations of hepatitis have occurred after discontinuation of EPIVIR-HBV (these have been primarily detected by serum ALT elevations, in addition to the re-emergence of HBV DNA commonly observed after stopping treatment; see Table 4 for more information regarding frequency of posttreatment ALT elevations) *[see Adverse Reactions (6.1)]*. Although most events appear to have been self-limited, fatalities have been reported in some cases. The causal relationship of hepatitis exacerbation after discontinuation of EPIVIR-HBV has not been clearly established. Patients should be closely monitored with both clinical and laboratory follow-up for at least several months after stopping treatment with EPIVIR-HBV. There is insufficient evidence to determine whether reinitiation of EPIVIR-HBV alters the course of posttreatment exacerbations of hepatitis.

5.3 Risk of HIV-1 Resistance if EPIVIR-HBV Is Used in Patients With Unrecognized or Untreated HIV-1 Infection

EPIVIR-HBV tablets and oral solution contain a lower lamivudine dose than the lamivudine dose in the following drugs used to treat HIV-1 infection:

- EPIVIR® tablets and oral solution,
- COMBIVIR® (lamivudine/zidovudine) tablets,
- EPZICOM® (abacavir sulfate and lamivudine) tablets, and
- TRIZIVIR® (abacavir, lamivudine, and zidovudine) tablets

The formulation and dosage of lamivudine in EPIVIR-HBV are not approved for patients co-infected with HBV and

HIV. If a decision is made to administer lamivudine to such patients, the higher dosage indicated for HIV therapy should be used as part of an appropriate combination regimen, and the prescribing information for EPIVIR, COMBIVIR, EPZICOM, or TRIZIVIR as well as for EPIVIR-HBV should be consulted. HIV counseling and testing should be offered to all patients before beginning EPIVIR-HBV and periodically during treatment because of the risk of rapid emergence of resistant HIV and limitation of treatment options if EPIVIR-HBV is prescribed to treat chronic hepatitis B in a patient who has unrecognized or untreated HIV-1 infection or acquires HIV-1 infection during treatment.

5.4 Coadministration With Other Medications Containing Lamivudine or Emtricitabine

Do not coadminister EPIVIR-HBV with other lamivudine-containing products including EPIVIR (lamivudine), COMBIVIR (lamivudine/zidovudine), EPZICOM (abacavir/lamivudine), or TRIZIVIR (abacavir/lamivudine/zidovudine).

Do not coadminister EPIVIR-HBV with emtricitabine-containing products including ATRIPLA® (efavirenz/emtricitabine/tenofovir disoproxil fumarate), COMPLERA® (rilpivirine/emtricitabine/tenofovir disoproxil fumarate), EMTRIVA® (emtricitabine), STRIBILD® (elvitegravir/cobicistat/emtricitabine/tenofovir disoproxil fumarate), or TRUVADA® (emtricitabine/tenofovir disoproxil fumarate).

5.5 Emergence of Resistance-Associated HBV Substitutions

In controlled clinical trials, YMDD-mutant HBV was detected in subjects with on-EPIVIR-HBV re-appearance of HBV DNA after an initial decline below the solution-hybridization assay limit *[see Microbiology (12.4)]*. Subjects treated with EPIVIR-HBV (adults and children) with YMDD-mutant HBV at 52 weeks showed diminished treatment responses in comparison with subjects treated with EPIVIR-HBV without evidence of YMDD substitutions, including the following: lower rates of HBeAg seroconversion and HBeAg loss (no greater than placebo recipients), more frequent return of positive HBV DNA, and more frequent ALT elevations. In the controlled trials, when subjects developed YMDD-mutant HBV, they had a rise in HBV DNA and ALT from their own previous on-treatment levels. Progression of hepatitis B, including death, has been reported in some subjects with YMDD-mutant HBV, including subjects from the liver transplant setting and from other clinical trials. In clinical practice, monitoring of ALT and HBV DNA levels during treatment with EPIVIR-HBV may aid in treatment decisions if emergence of viral mutants is suspected.

6 ADVERSE REACTIONS

The following adverse reactions are discussed in greater detail in other sections of the labeling:

- Lactic acidosis and severe hepatomegaly with steatosis *[see Warnings and Precautions (5.1)]*.
- Exacerbation of hepatitis B after discontinuation of treatment *[see Warnings and Precautions (5.2)]*.
- Risk of emergence of resistant HIV-1 infection *[see Warnings and Precautions (5.3)]*.
- Risk of emergence of resistant HBV infection *[see Warnings and Precautions (5.4)]*.

6.1 Clinical Trials Experience

Because clinical trials are conducted under widely varying conditions, adverse reaction rates observed in the clinical trials of a drug cannot be directly compared with rates in the clinical trials of another drug and may not reflect the rates observed in practice.

Adverse Reactions in Clinical Trials of Adults With Chronic Hepatitis B Virus Infection: Clinical adverse reactions (regardless of investigator's causality assessment) reported in greater or equal to 10% of subjects who received EPIVIR-HBV and reported at a rate greater than placebo are listed in Table 2.

Table 2. Clinical Adverse Reactions[a] Reported in ≥10% of Subjects who Received EPIVIR-HBV for 52 to 68 Weeks and at an Incidence Greater than Placebo (Trials 1-3)

Adverse Event	EPIVIR-HBV (n = 332)	Placebo (n = 200)
Ear, Nose, and Throat		
Ear, nose, and throat infections	25%	21%
Sore throat	13%	8%
Gastrointestinal		
Diarrhea	14%	12%

[a]Includes adverse events regardless of severity and causality assessment.

Specified laboratory abnormalities reported in subjects who received EPIVIR-HBV and reported at a rate greater than in subjects who received placebo are listed in Table 3.

Table 3. Frequencies of Specified Laboratory Abnormalities Reported During Treatment at a Greater Frequency in Subjects Treated with EPIVIR-HBV Than With Placebo (Trials 1–3)[a]

Test (Abnormal Level)	Subjects With Abnormality/ Subjects With Observations	
	EPIVIR-HBV	Placebo
Serum Lipase ≥2.5 × ULN[b]	10%	7%
CPK ≥7 × baseline	9%	5%
Platelets <50,000/mm³	4%	3%

[a] Includes subjects treated for 52 to 68 weeks.
[b] Includes observations during and after treatment in the 2 placebo-controlled trials that collected this information.
ULN = Upper limit of normal.

In subjects followed for up to 16 weeks after discontinuation of treatment, posttreatment ALT elevations were observed more frequently in subjects who had received EPIVIR-HBV than in subjects who had received placebo. A comparison of ALT elevations between Weeks 52 and 68 in subjects who discontinued EPIVIR-HBV at Week 52 and subjects in the same trials who received placebo throughout the treatment course is shown in Table 4.

Table 4. Posttreatment ALT Elevations With No-Active-Treatment Follow-up (Trails 1 and 3)

Abnormal Value	Subjects With ALT Elevation/ Subjects With Observations[a]	
	EPIVIR-HBV[b]	Placebo[b]
ALT ≥2 × baseline value	27%	19%
ALT ≥3 × baseline value[c]	21%	8%
ALT ≥2 × baseline value and absolute ALT >500 IU/L	15%	7%
ALT ≥2 × baseline value; and bilirubin >2 × ULN and ≥2 × baseline value	0.7%	0.9%

[a] Each subject may be represented in one or more category.
[b] During treatment phase.
[c] Comparable to a Grade 3 toxicity in accordance with modified WHO criteria.
ULN = Upper limit of normal.

Adverse Reactions in Clinical Trials of Pediatric Subjects With Chronic Hepatitis B Virus Infection: Most commonly observed adverse reactions in the pediatric trials were similar to those in adult trials. Posttreatment transaminase elevations were observed in some subjects followed after cessation of EPIVIR-HBV.

6.2 Postmarketing Experience
In addition to adverse reactions reported from clinical trials, the following adverse reactions have been reported during postmarketing use of EPIVIR-HBV. Because these reactions are reported voluntarily from a population of unknown size, it is not always possible to reliably estimate the frequency or establish a causal relationship to drug exposure. These reactions have been chosen for inclusion due to a combination of their seriousness, frequency of reporting, or potential causal connection to lamivudine.
Blood and Lympatic System Disorders: Thrombocytopenia.
Digestive: Stomatitis.
Endocrine and Metabolic: Hyperglycemia.
General: Weakness.
Blood and Lymphatic: Anemia (including pure red cell aplasia and severe anemias progressing on therapy), lymphadenopathy, splenomegaly.
Hepatic and Pancreatic: Lactic acidosis and steatosis, posttreatment exacerbation of hepatitis [see Boxed Warning], pancreatitis.
Hypersensitivity: Anaphylaxis, urticaria.
Musculoskeletal: Cramps, rhabdomyolysis.
Nervous: Paresthesia, peripheral neuropathy.
Respiratory: Abnormal breath sounds/wheezing.
Skin: Alopecia, pruritus, rash.

7 DRUG INTERACTIONS
Lamivudine is predominantly eliminated in the urine by active organic cationic secretion. The possibility of interactions with other drugs administered concurrently should be considered, particularly when their main route of elimination is active renal secretion via the organic cationic transport system (e.g., trimethoprim). No data are available regarding interactions with other drugs that have renal clearance mechanisms similar to that of lamivudine.

8 USE IN SPECIFIC POPULATIONS
8.1 Pregnancy
Pregnancy Category C.
There are no adequate and well-controlled trials of EPIVIR-HBV in pregnant women. Because animal reproduction studies are not always predictive of human response, EPIVIR-HBV should be used during pregnancy only if the potential benefits outweigh the potential risks to the fetus.
Antiretroviral Pregnancy Registry: To monitor maternal-fetal outcomes of pregnant women exposed to lamivudine, a Pregnancy Registry has been established. Healthcare providers are encouraged to register patients by calling 1-800-258-4263.
Animal Data: Animal reproduction studies in rats and rabbits revealed no evidence of teratogenicity. Reproduction studies have been performed in rats and rabbits at orally administered doses up to 4,000 mg/kg/day and 1,000 mg/kg/day, respectively, producing plasma levels up to approximately 60 times that for the adult HBV dose. Evidence of early embryolethality was seen in the rabbit at exposure levels similar to those observed in humans, but there was no indication of this effect in the rat at exposure levels up to 60 times those in humans.
Studies in pregnant rats and rabbits showed that lamivudine is transferred to the fetus through the placenta.

8.3 Nursing Mothers
Lamivudine is excreted in human milk. Samples of breast milk obtained from 20 mothers receiving lamivudine monotherapy (300 mg twice daily, 6 times the recommended dosage for hepatitis B infection) or combination therapy (150 mg lamivudine twice daily [3 times the recommended dosage for hepatitis B infection] and 300 mg zidovudine twice daily) had measurable concentrations of lamivudine. Because of the potential for serious adverse reactions in nursing infants, a decision should be made to discontinue EPIVIR-HBV taking into consideration the importance of continued hepatitis B therapy to the mother and the known benefits of breastfeeding.

8.4 Pediatric Use
EPIVIR-HBV is indicated for the treatment of chronic hepatitis B virus infection in pediatric patients aged 2 to 17 years [see Indications and Usage (1), Clinical Pharmacology (12.3), Clinical Studies (14.2)]. The safety and efficacy of EPIVIR-HBV in pediatric patients younger than 2 years have not been established.

8.5 Geriatric Use
Clinical trials of EPIVIR-HBV did not include sufficient numbers of subjects aged 65 and over to determine whether they respond differently from younger subjects. In general, dose selection for an elderly patient should be cautious, reflecting the greater frequency of decreased hepatic, renal, or cardiac function, and of concomitant disease or other drug therapy. In particular, because lamivudine is substantially excreted by the kidney and elderly patients are more likely to have decreased renal function, renal function should be monitored and dosage adjustments should be made accordingly [see Dosage and Administration (2.4), Clinical Pharmacology (12.4)].

8.6 Patients With Impaired Renal Function
Reduction of the dosage of EPIVIR-HBV is recommended for patients with impaired renal function [see Dosage and Administration (2.4), Clinical Pharmacology (12.3)].

8.7 Patients With Impaired Liver Function
No dose adjustment for lamivudine is required for patients with impaired hepatic function.

10 OVERDOSAGE
There is no known antidote for EPIVIR-HBV. If overdose occurs, the patient should be monitored, and standard supportive treatment utilized, as required.
Because a negligible amount of lamivudine was removed via (4-hour) hemodialysis, continuous ambulatory peritoneal dialysis, and automated peritoneal dialysis, it is not known if continuous hemodialysis would provide clinical benefit in a lamivudine overdose event.

11 DESCRIPTION
EPIVIR-HBV is a synthetic nucleoside analogue with activity against HBV. The chemical name of lamivudine is (2R,cis)-4-amino-1-(2-hydroxymethyl-1,3-oxathiolan-5-yl)-(1H)-pyrimidin-2-one. Lamivudine is the (-)enantiomer of a dideoxy analogue of cytidine. Lamivudine has also been referred to as (-)2′,3′-dideoxy, 3′-thiacytidine. It has a molecular formula of $C_8H_{11}N_3O_3S$ and a molecular weight of 229.3. It has the following structural formula:

Lamivudine is a white to off-white crystalline solid with a solubility of approximately 70 mg per mL in water at 20°C. EPIVIR-HBV tablets are for oral administration. Each tablet contains 100 mg of lamivudine and the inactive ingredients hypromellose, macrogol 400, magnesium stearate, microcrystalline cellulose, polysorbate 80, red iron oxide, sodium starch glycolate, titanium dioxide, and yellow iron oxide.
EPIVIR-HBV oral solution is for oral administration. One milliliter (1 mL) of EPIVIR-HBV oral solution contains 5 mg of lamivudine (5 mg per mL) in an aqueous solution and the inactive ingredients artificial strawberry and banana flavors, citric acid (anhydrous), methylparaben, propylene glycol, propylparaben, sodium citrate (dihydrate), and sucrose (200 mg).

12 CLINICAL PHARMACOLOGY
12.1 Mechanism of Action
Lamivudine is an antiviral agent [see Microbiology (12.4)].
12.3 Pharmacokinetics
Pharmacokinetics in Adults: The pharmacokinetic properties of lamivudine have been studied as single and multiple oral doses ranging from 5 mg to 600 mg per day administered to HBV-infected patients.
Absorption and Bioavailability: Following single oral doses of 100 mg, the peak serum lamivudine concentration (C_{max}) in HBV-infected patients (steady state) and healthy subjects (single dose) was 1.28 ± 0.56 mcg per mL and 1.05 ± 0.32 mcg per mL (mean ± SD), respectively, which occurred between 0.5 and 2 hours after administration. The area under the plasma concentration versus time curve ($AUC_{[0-24\ h]}$) following 100 mg lamivudine oral single and repeated daily doses to steady state was 4.3 ± 1.4 (mean ± SD) and 4.7 ± 1.7 mcg•hour per mL, respectively. The relative bioavailability of the tablet and oral solution were demonstrated in healthy subjects. Although the solution demonstrated a slightly higher peak serum concentration (C_{max}), there was no significant difference in systemic exposure (AUC) between the oral solution and the tablet. Therefore, the oral solution and the tablet may be used interchangeably.
After oral administration of lamivudine once daily to HBV-infected adults, the AUC and C_{max} increased in proportion to dose over the range from 5 mg to 600 mg once daily.
Absolute bioavailability in 12 adult subjects was 86% ± 16% (mean ± SD) for the 150-mg tablet and 87% ± 13% for the 10-mg per mL oral solution.
Effects of Food on Oral Absorption: The 100-mg tablet was administered orally to 24 healthy subjects on 2 occasions, once in the fasted state and once with food (standard meal: 967 kcal; 67 grams fat, 33 grams protein, 58 grams carbohydrate). There was no significant difference in systemic exposure (AUC) in the fed and fasted states.
Distribution: The apparent volume of distribution after IV administration of lamivudine to 20 asymptomatic HIV-1-infected subjects was 1.3 ± 0.4 L per kg, suggesting that lamivudine distributes into extravascular spaces. Volume of distribution was independent of dose and did not correlate with body weight.
Binding of lamivudine to human plasma proteins is less than 36% and independent of dose. In vitro studies showed that over the concentration range of 0.1 to 100 mcg per mL, the amount of lamivudine associated with erythrocytes ranged from 53% to 57% and was independent of concentration.
Metabolism: Metabolism of lamivudine is a minor route of elimination. In humans, the only known metabolite of lamivudine is the trans-sulfoxide metabolite. In 9 healthy subjects receiving 300 mg of lamivudine as single oral doses, a total of 4.2% (range 1.5% to 7.5%) of the dose was excreted as the trans-sulfoxide metabolite in the urine, the majority of which was excreted in the first 12 hours. Serum concentrations of the trans-sulfoxide metabolite have not been determined.
Elimination: The majority of lamivudine is eliminated unchanged in urine by active organic cationic secretion. In 9 healthy subjects given a single 300-mg oral dose of lamivudine, renal clearance was 199.7 ± 56.9 mL per min (mean ± SD). In 20 HIV-1-infected subjects given a single IV dose, renal clearance was 280.4 ± 75.2 mL per min (mean ± SD), representing 71% ± 16% (mean ± SD) of total clearance of lamivudine.
In most single-dose trials in HIV-1-infected subjects, HBV-infected subjects, or healthy subjects with serum sampling for 24 hours after dosing, the observed mean elimination half-life ($t_{1/2}$) ranged from 5 to 7 hours. In HIV-1-infected subjects, total clearance was 398.5 ± 69.1 mL per min (mean

± SD). Oral clearance and elimination half-life were independent of dose and body weight over an oral dosing range of 0.25 to 10 mg per kg.

Special Populations: Adults With Renal Impairment: The pharmacokinetic properties of lamivudine have been determined in healthy subjects and in subjects with impaired renal function, with and without hemodialysis (Table 5).

[See table 5 above]

Exposure (AUC), C_{max}, and half-life increased with diminishing renal function (as expressed by creatinine clearance). Apparent total oral clearance (Cl/F) of lamivudine decreased as creatinine clearance decreased. T_{max} was not significantly affected by renal function. Based on these observations, it is recommended that the dosage of lamivudine be modified in patients with renal impairment *[see Dosage and Administration (2.4)].*

Hemodialysis increases lamivudine clearance from a mean of 64 to 88 mL per min; however, the length of time of hemodialysis (4 hours) was insufficient to significantly alter mean lamivudine exposure after a single-dose administration. Continuous ambulatory peritoneal dialysis and automated peritoneal dialysis have negligible effects on lamivudine clearance. Therefore, it is recommended, following correction of dose for creatinine clearance, that no additional dose modification be made after routine hemodialysis or peritoneal dialysis.

It is not known whether lamivudine can be removed by continuous (24-hour) hemodialysis.

Pediatric Patients With Renal Impairment: The effect of renal impairment on lamivudine pharmacokinetics in pediatric patients with chronic hepatitis B is not known.

Adults With Hepatic Impairment: The pharmacokinetic properties of lamivudine in adults with hepatic impairment are shown in Table 6. Subjects were stratified by severity of hepatic impairment.

[See table 6 above]

Pharmacokinetic parameters were not altered by diminishing hepatic impairment. Therefore, no dose adjustment for lamivudine is required for patients with impaired hepatic function. Safety and efficacy of EPIVIR-HBV have not been established in the presence of decompensated liver disease *[see Indications and Usage (1)].*

Adults Post-Hepatic Transplant: Fourteen HBV-infected subjects received liver transplant following lamivudine therapy and completed pharmacokinetic assessments at enrollment, 2 weeks after 100-mg once-daily dosing (pretransplant), and 3 months following transplant; there were no significant differences in pharmacokinetic parameters. The overall exposure of lamivudine is primarily affected by renal impairment; consequently, transplant patients with renal impairment had generally higher exposure than patients with normal renal function. Safety and efficacy of EPIVIR-HBV have not been established in this population *[see Indications and Usage (1)].*

Pediatric Subjects: Lamivudine pharmacokinetics were evaluated in a 28-day dose-ranging trial in 53 pediatric subjects with chronic hepatitis B. Subjects aged 2 to 12 years were randomized to receive lamivudine 0.35 mg per kg twice daily, 3 mg per kg once daily, 1.5 mg per kg twice daily, or 4 mg per kg twice daily. Subjects aged 13 to 17 years received lamivudine 100 mg once daily. Lamivudine T_{max} was 0.5 to 1 hour. In general, both C_{max} and exposure (AUC) showed dose proportionality in the dosing range studied. Weight-corrected oral clearance was highest at age 2 and declined from 2 to 12 years, where values were then similar to those seen in adults. A dose of 3 mg per kg once daily produced a steady-state lamivudine AUC (mean 5,953 ng•hour per mL ± 1,562 SD) similar to that associated with a dose of 100 mg per day in adults.

Gender: There are no significant gender differences in lamivudine pharmacokinetics.

Race: There are no significant racial differences in lamivudine pharmacokinetics.

Drug Interactions: Interferon Alfa: Multiple doses of lamivudine and a single dose of interferon were coadministered to 19 healthy male subjects in a pharmacokinetics study. Results indicated a 10% reduction in lamivudine AUC, but no change in interferon pharmacokinetic parameters when the 2 drugs were given in combination. All other pharmacokinetic parameters (C_{max}, T_{max}, and $t_{1/2}$) were unchanged. There was no significant pharmacokinetic interaction between lamivudine and interferon alfa in this trial.

Ribavirin: In vitro data indicate ribavirin reduces phosphorylation of lamivudine, stavudine, and zidovudine. However, no pharmacokinetic (e.g., plasma concentrations or intracellular triphosphorylated active metabolite concentrations) or pharmacodynamic (e.g., loss of HIV-1/HCV virologic suppression) interaction was observed when ribavirin and lamivudine (n = 18), stavudine (n = 10), or zidovudine (n = 6) were coadministered as part of a multidrug regimen in HIV–1/HCV co-infected subjects.

Trimethoprim/Sulfamethoxazole: Lamivudine and trimethoprim/sulfamethoxazole (TMP/SMX) were coadminis-

tered to 14 HIV-positive subjects in a single-center, open-label, randomized, crossover trial. Each subject received treatment with a single 300-mg dose of lamivudine and TMP 160 mg/SMX 800 mg once a day for 5 days with concomitant administration of lamivudine 300 mg with the fifth dose in a crossover design. Coadministration of TMP/SMX with lamivudine resulted in an increase of 44% ± 23% (mean ± SD) in lamivudine AUC, a decrease of 29% ± 13% in lamivudine oral clearance, and a decrease of 30% ± 36% in lamivudine renal clearance. The pharmacokinetic properties of TMP and SMX were not altered by coadministration with lamivudine.

Zidovudine: Lamivudine and zidovudine were coadministered to 12 asymptomatic HIV-positive adult subjects in a single-center, open-label, randomized, crossover trial. No significant differences were observed in AUC or total clearance for lamivudine or zidovudine when the 2 drugs were administered together. Coadministration of lamivudine with zidovudine resulted in an increase of 39% ± 62% (mean ± SD) in C_{max} of zidovudine.

12.4 Microbiology

Mechanism of Action: Lamivudine is a synthetic nucleoside analogue. Intracellularly, lamivudine is phosphorylated to its active 5'-triphosphate metabolite, lamivudine triphosphate, 3TC-TP. The principal mode of action of 3TC-TP is the inhibition of the RNA- and DNA- dependent polymerase activities of HBV reverse transcriptase (rt) via DNA chain termination after incorporation of the nucleotide analogue into viral DNA. 3TC-TP is a weak inhibitor of mammalian α, β, and γ-DNA polymerases.

Antiviral Activity: Activity of lamivudine against HBV in cell culture was assessed in HBV DNA-transfected 2.2.15 cells, HB611 cells, and infected human primary hepatocytes. EC_{50} values (the concentration of drug needed to reduce the level of extracellular HBV DNA by 50%) varied from 0.01 μM (2.3 ng per mL) to 5.6 μM (1.3 mcg per mL) depending upon the duration of exposure of cells to lamivudine, the cell model system, and the protocol used. See the EPIVIR prescribing information for information regarding activity of lamivudine against HIV

Resistance: Lamivudine-resistant isolates were identified in subjects with virologic breakthrough, defined when using solution hybridization assay as the detection of HBV DNA in serum on 2 or more occasions after failing to detect HBV DNA on 2 or more occasions and defined when using PCR assay as a greater than 1 $\log_{10}$ (10-fold) increase in serum HBV DNA from nadir during treatment in a subject who had an initial virologic response.

Lamivudine-resistant HBV isolates develop rtM204V/I substitutions in the YMDD motif of the catalytic domain of the viral reverse transcriptase. rtM204V/I substitutions are frequently accompanied by other substitutions (rtV173L, rtL180M) which enhance the level of lamivudine resistance

or act as compensatory substitutions improving replication efficiency. Other substitutions detected in lamivudine-resistant HBV isolates include rtL80I and rtA181T.

In 4 controlled clinical trials in adults with HBeAg-positive chronic hepatitis B virus infection (CHB), YMDD-mutant HBV was detected in 81 of 335 subjects receiving EPIVIR-HBV 100 mg once daily for 52 weeks. The prevalence of YMDD substitutions was less than 10% in each of these trials for subjects studied at 24 weeks and increased to an average of 24% (range in 4 trials: 16% to 32%) at 52 weeks. In limited data from a long-term follow-up trial in subjects who continued 100 mg per day EPIVIR-HBV after one of these trials, YMDD substitutions further increased from 18% (10 of 57) at 1 year to 41% (20 of 49), 53% (27 of 51), and 69% (31 of 45) after 2, 3, and 4 years of treatment, respectively. Over the 5-year treatment period, the proportion of subjects who developed YMDD-mutant HBV at any time was 69% (40 of 58).

In a controlled trial, treatment-naive subjects with HBeAg-positive CHB were treated with EPIVIR-HBV or EPIVIR-HBV plus adefovir dipivoxil combination therapy. Following 104 weeks of therapy, YMDD-mutant HBV was detected in 7 of 40 (18%) subjects receiving combination therapy compared with 15 of 35 (43%) subjects receiving therapy with only EPIVIR-HBV. In another controlled trial, combination therapy was evaluated in adult subjects with HBeAg-positive CHB who had YMDD-mutant HBV and diminished clinical and virologic response to EPIVIR-HBV. Following 52 weeks of EPIVIR-HBV plus adefovir dipivoxil combination therapy (n = 46) or therapy with only EPIVIR-HBV (n = 49), YMDD–mutant HBV was detected less frequently in subjects receiving combination therapy, 62% versus 96%.

A published trial suggested that the rates of lamivudine resistance in subjects treated for HBeAg-negative CHB appear to be more variable (0% to 27% at 1 year and 10% to 56% at 2 years).

Pediatric Subjects: In a controlled trial in pediatric subjects, YMDD-mutant HBV was detected in 31 of 166 (19%) subjects receiving EPIVIR-HBV for 52 weeks. For a subgroup that remained on therapy with EPIVIR-HBV in a follow-up trial, YMDD substitutions increased from 24% (29 of 121) at 12 months to 59% (68 of 115) at 24 months and 64% (66 of 103) at 36 months of treatment with EPIVIR-HBV.

Cross-Resistance: HBV containing lamivudine resistance-associated substitutions (rtL180M, rtM204I, rtM204V, rtL180M and rtM204V, rtV173L and rtL180M and rtM204V) retain susceptibility to adefovir dipivoxil but have reduced susceptibility to entecavir (30 fold) and telbivudine (greater than 100 fold). The lamivudine resistance-associated substitution rtA181T results in diminished response to adefovir and telbivudine. Similarly, HBV with en-

Table 5. Pharmacokinetic Parameters (Mean ± SD) Dose-Normalized to a Single 100-mg Oral Dose of Lamivudine in Subjects With Varying Degrees of Renal Function

Parameter	Creatinine Clearance Criterion (Number of Subjects)		
	≥80 mL/min (n = 9)	20-59 mL/min (n = 8)	<20 mL/min (n = 6)
Creatinine clearance (mL/min)	97 (range 82-117)	39 (range 25-49)	15 (range 13-19)
C_{max} (mcg/mL)	1.31 ± 0.35	1.85 ± 0.40	1.55 ± 0.31
AUC (mcg•h/mL)	5.28 ± 1.01	14.67 ± 3.74	27.33 ± 6.56
Cl/F (mL/min)	326.4 ± 63.8	120.1 ± 29.5	64.5 ± 18.3

Table 6. Pharmacokinetic Parameters (Mean ± SD) Dose-Normalized to a Single 100-mg Dose of Lamivudine in Subjects With Normal or Impaired Hepatic Function

Parameter	Normal (n = 8)	Impairment[a]	
		Moderate (n = 8)	Severe (n = 8)
C_{max} (mcg/mL)	0.92 ± 0.31	1.06 ± 0.58	1.08 ± 0.27
AUC (mcg•h/mL)	3.96 ± 0.58	3.97 ± 1.36	4.30 ± 0.63
T_{max}(h)	1.3 ± 0.8	1.4 ± 0.8	1.4 ± 1.2
Cl/F (mL/min)	424.7 ± 61.9	456.9 ± 129.8	395.2 ± 51.8
Clr (mL/min)	279.2 ± 79.2	323.5 ± 100.9	216.1 ± 58.0

[a]Hepatic impairment assessed by aminopyrine breath test.

Table 7. Histologic Response at Week 52 Among Adult Subjects Receiving EPIVIR-HBV 100 mg Once Daily or Placebo

Assessment	Trial 1		Trial 2		Trial 3	
	EPIVIR-HBV (n = 62)	Placebo (n = 63)	EPIVIR-HBV (n = 131)	Placebo (n = 68)	EPIVIR-HBV (n = 110)	Placebo (n = 54)
Improvement[a]	55%	25%	56%	26%	56%	26%
No Improvement	27%	59%	36%	62%	25%	54%
Missing Data	18%	16%	8%	12%	19%	20%

[a]Improvement was defined as a greater than or equal to 2-point decrease in the Knodell Histologic Activity Index (HAI) at Week 52 compared with pretreatment HAI. Subjects with missing data at baseline were excluded.

Table 8. HBeAg Seroconverters[a] at Week 52 Among Adult Subjects Receiving EPIVIR-HBV 100 mg Once Daily or Placebo

Seroconversion	Trial 1		Trial 2		Trial 3	
	EPIVIR-HBV (n = 63)	Placebo (n = 69)	EPIVIR-HBV (n = 140)	Placebo (n = 70)	EPIVIR-HBV (n = 108)	Placebo (n = 53)
Seroconverters	17%	6%	16%	4%	15%	13%

[a] Three-component seroconversion was defined as Week 52 values showing loss of HBeAg, gain of HBeAb, and reduction of HBV DNA to below the solution-hybridization assay limit. Subjects with negative baseline HBeAg or HBV DNA assay were excluded from the analysis.

tecavir resistance-associated substitutions (I169T/M250V and T184G/S202I) have greater than 1,000-fold reductions in susceptibility to lamivudine.

13 NONCLINICAL TOXICOLOGY

13.1 Carcinogenesis, Mutagenesis, Impairment of Fertility

Carcinogenesis: Long-term carcinogenicity studies with lamivudine in mice and rats showed no evidence of carcinogenic potential at exposures up to 34 times (mice) and 200 times (rats) those observed in humans at the recommended therapeutic dose for chronic hepatitis B.

Mutagenesis: Lamivudine was not active in a microbial mutagenicity screen or an in vitro cell transformation assay, but showed weak in vitro mutagenic activity in a cytogenetic assay using cultured human lymphocytes and in the mouse lymphoma assay. However, lamivudine showed no evidence of in vivo genotoxic activity in the rat at oral doses of up to 2,000 mg per kg producing plasma levels of 60 to 70 times those in humans at the recommended dose for chronic hepatitis B.

Impairment of Fertility: In a study of reproductive performance, lamivudine administered to rats at doses up to 4,000 mg per kg per day, producing plasma levels 80 to 120 times those in humans, revealed no evidence of impaired fertility and no effect on the survival, growth, and development to weaning of the offspring.

14 CLINICAL STUDIES

14.1 Clinical Studies of EPIVIR-HBV in Adult Patients

The safety and efficacy of EPIVIR-HBV 100 mg once daily versus placebo were evaluated in 3 controlled trials in subjects with compensated chronic hepatitis B virus infection. All subjects were aged 16 years or older and had chronic hepatitis B virus infection (serum HBsAg-positive for at least 6 months) accompanied by evidence of HBV replication (serum HBeAg-positive and positive for serum HBV DNA) and persistently elevated ALT levels and/or chronic inflammation on liver biopsy compatible with a diagnosis of chronic viral hepatitis. The results of these trials are summarized below.

- Trial 1 was a randomized, double-blind trial of EPIVIR-HBV 100 mg once daily versus placebo for 52 weeks followed by a 16-week no-treatment period in 141 treatment-naive US subjects.
- Trial 2 was a randomized, double-blind, 3-arm trial that compared EPIVIR-HBV 25 mg once daily versus EPIVIR-HBV 100 mg once daily versus placebo for 52 weeks in 358 Asian subjects.
- Trial 3 was a randomized, partially-blind trial conducted primarily in North America and Europe in 238 subjects who had ongoing evidence of active chronic hepatitis B despite previous treatment with interferon alfa. The trial compared EPIVIR-HBV 100 mg once daily for 52 weeks, followed by either EPIVIR-HBV 100 mg or matching placebo once daily for 16 weeks (Arm 1), versus placebo once daily for 68 weeks (Arm 2).

Principal endpoint comparisons for the histologic and serologic outcomes in subjects receiving EPIVIR-HBV (100 mg daily) or placebo in these trials are shown in the following tables.

[See table 7 above]
[See table 8 above]

Normalization of serum ALT levels was more frequent with EPIVIR-HBV treatment compared with placebo in Trials 1-3.

The majority of subjects treated with EPIVIR-HBV showed a decrease of HBV DNA to below the assay limit early in the course of therapy. However, reappearance of assay-detectable HBV DNA during treatment with EPIVIR-HBV was observed in approximately one-third of subjects after this initial response.

14.2 Clinical Studies of EPIVIR-HBV in Pediatric Subjects

The safety and efficacy of EPIVIR-HBV were evaluated in a double-blind clinical trial in 286 subjects aged from 2 to 17 years, who were randomized (2:1) to receive 52 weeks of EPIVIR-HBV (3 mg per kg once daily to a maximum of 100 mg once daily) or placebo. All subjects had compensated chronic hepatitis B accompanied by evidence of hepatitis B virus replication (positive serum HBeAg and positive for serum HBV DNA by a research branched-chain DNA assay) and persistently elevated serum ALT levels. The combination of loss of HBeAg and reduction of HBV DNA to below the assay limit of the research assay, evaluated at Week 52, was observed in 23% of subjects treated with EPIVIR-HBV and 13% of placebo-treated subjects. Normalization of serum ALT was achieved and maintained to Week 52 more frequently in subjects treated with EPIVIR-HBV compared with placebo (55% versus 13%). As in the adult controlled trials, most subjects treated with EPIVIR-HBV had decreases in HBV DNA below the assay limit early in treatment, but about one third of subjects with this initial response had reappearance of assay-detectable HBV DNA during treatment. Adolescents (aged 13 to 17 years) showed less evidence of treatment effect than younger pediatric subjects.

16 HOW SUPPLIED/STORAGE AND HANDLING

EPIVIR-HBV tablets, 100 mg, are butterscotch-colored, film-coated, biconvex, capsule-shaped tablets imprinted with "GX CG5" on one side.

Bottles of 60 tablets (NDC 0173-0662-00) with child-resistant closures.

Store at 25°C (77°F), excursions permitted to 15° to 30°C (59° to 86°F) [see USP Controlled Room Temperature].

EPIVIR-HBV oral solution, a clear, colorless to pale yellow, strawberry-banana-flavored liquid, contains 5 mg of lamivudine in each 1 mL in plastic bottles of 240 mL. Bottles of 240 mL (NDC 0173-0663-00) with child-resistant closures. This product does not require reconstitution.

Store at controlled room temperature of 20° to 25°C (68° to 77°F) (see USP) in tightly closed bottles.

17 PATIENT COUNSELING INFORMATION

Advise the patient to read the FDA-approved patient labeling (Patient Information).

Advice for the Patient

- Advise patients to remain under the care of a physician while taking EPIVIR-HBV and discuss any new symptoms or concurrent medications with their physician.
- Advise patients that EPIVIR-HBV is not a cure for hepatitis B, that the long-term treatment benefits of EPIVIR-HBV are unknown at this time, and, in particular, that the relationship of initial treatment response to

outcomes such as hepatocellular carcinoma and decompensated cirrhosis is unknown [see Dosage and Administration (2.6)].

- Inform patients that deterioration of liver disease has occurred in some cases when treatment was discontinued. Instruct patients to discuss any changes in regimen with their physician [see Warnings and Precautions (5.2)].
- Inform patients that emergence of resistant hepatitis B virus and worsening of disease can occur during treatment, and they should promptly report any new symptoms to their physician [see Warnings and Precautions (5.5)].
- Counsel patients on the importance of testing for HIV to avoid inappropriate therapy and development of resistant HIV. HIV counseling and testing should be offered before starting EPIVIR-HBV and periodically during therapy.
- Advise patients that EPIVIR-HBV tablets and EPIVIR-HBV oral solution contain a lower dose of the same active ingredient (lamivudine) as EPIVIR tablets, EPIVIR oral solution, COMBIVIR tablets, EPZICOM tablets, and TRIZIVIR tablets. EPIVIR-HBV should not be taken concurrently with EPIVIR, COMBIVIR, EPZICOM, or TRIZIVIR [see Dosage and Administration (2.1), Warnings and Precautions (5.3, 5.4)].
- Advise patients not to take EPIVIR-HBV with emtricitabine-containing medicines, such as ATRIPLA, COMPLERA, EMTRIVA, STRIBILD, or TRUVADA [see Warnings and Precautions (5.4)].
- Advise patients that treatment with EPIVIR-HBV has not been shown to reduce the risk of transmission of HBV to others through sexual contact or blood contamination [see Use in Specific Populations (8.1)].
- Instruct patients to avoid doing things that can spread HBV infection to others.
  ◦ **Do not share needles or other injection equipment.**
  ◦ **Do not share personal items that can have blood or body fluids on them, like toothbrushes and razor blades.**
  ◦ **Do not have any kind of sex without protection.** Always practice safe sex by using a latex or polyurethane condom to lower the chance of sexual contact with semen, vaginal secretions, or blood.
- Advise diabetic patients that each 20-mL dose of EPIVIR-HBV oral solution contains 4 grams of sucrose [see Description (11)].

EPIVIR-HBV is a registered trademark of the GlaxoSmithKline group of companies.

EPIVIR, COMBIVIR, EPZICOM, and TRIZIVIR are registered trademarks of the ViiV Healthcare group of companies.

The other brands listed are trademarks of their respective owners and are not trademarks of the GlaxoSmithKline group of companies. The makers of these brands are not affiliated with and do not endorse the GlaxoSmithKline group of companies or its products.

GlaxoSmithKline
Research Triangle Park, NC 27709
Manufactured under agreement from
Shire Pharmaceuticals Group plc
Basingstoke, UK
©2013, GlaxoSmithKline group of companies. All rights reserved.
EPV:3PI

PATIENT INFORMATION

EPIVIR HBV® (EP-i-veer h-b-v)
(lamivudine)
tablets
EPIVIR HBV® (EP-i-veer h-b-v)
(lamivudine)
oral solution

Read this Patient Information before you start taking EPIVIR-HBV and each time you get a refill. There may be new information. This information does not take the place of talking with your healthcare provider about your medical condition or treatment.

What is the most important information I should know about EPIVIR-HBV?

EPIVIR-HBV can cause serious side effects, including:

Build-up of an acid in your blood (lactic acidosis). Lactic acidosis can happen in some people who take EPIVIR-HBV or similar (nucleoside analogs) medicines. Lactic acidosis is a serious medical emergency that can lead to death.

Lactic acidosis can be hard to identify early because the symptoms could seem like symptoms of other health problems. **Call your healthcare provider right away if you get any of the following symptoms that could be signs of lactic acidosis:**

- feel very weak or tired
- unusual (not normal) muscle pain
- trouble breathing
- stomach pain with nausea and vomiting
- feel cold, especially in your arms and legs
- feel dizzy or light-headed
- have a fast or irregular heartbeat

Severe liver problems. Severe liver problems can happen in people who take EPIVIR-HBV or similar medicines. In some cases these liver problems can lead to death. Your liver may become large (hepatomegaly) and you may develop fat in your liver (steatosis) when you take EPIVIR-HBV. **Call your healthcare provider right away if you get any of the following signs of liver problems:**

• your skin or the white part of your eyes turns yellow (jaundice)
• dark "tea-colored" urine
• light-colored bowel movements (stools)
• loss of appetite for several days or longer
• nausea
• stomach pain

You may be more likely to get lactic acidosis or severe liver problems if you are female, very overweight, or have been taking nucleoside analogue medicines for a long time.

Worsening liver disease. Your hepatitis B infection may become worse after stopping treatment with EPIVIR-HBV. Worsening liver disease can be serious and may lead to death. If you stop treatment with EPIVIR-HBV, your healthcare provider will need to check your health and do blood tests to check your liver for at least several months after you stop taking EPIVIR-HBV.

Risk of HIV-1 resistance in people with unknown HIV-1 infection or in people with untreated HIV-1 infection. If you have or get HIV that is not being treated with medicines while taking EPIVIR-HBV, the HIV virus may develop resistance to certain HIV medicines and become harder to treat.

• Your healthcare provider should offer you counseling and testing for HIV-1 infection before you start treatment for hepatitis B with EPIVIR-HBV and during treatment.
• EPIVIR-HBV tablets and EPIVIR–HBV oral solution contain a lower dose of lamivudine than other medicines that contain lamivudine and are used to treat HIV-1 infection. See **"What should I tell my healthcare provider?"** for a list of medicines you should not take with EPIVIR-HBV.

Resistant Hepatitis B Virus (HBV). The hepatitis B virus can change (mutate) during your treatment with EPIVIR-HBV and become harder to treat (resistant). If this happens, your liver disease can become worse and may lead to death. Tell your healthcare provider right away if you have any new symptoms.

What is EPIVIR-HBV?

EPIVIR-HBV is a prescription medicine used to treat long-term (chronic) hepatitis B virus (HBV) when the disease is progressing and there is liver swelling (inflammation).
• EPIVIR-HBV will not cure HBV.
• EPIVIR-HBV may lower the amount of HBV in your body.
• EPIVIR-HBV may lower the ability of HBV to multiply and infect new liver cells.
• EPIVIR-HBV may improve the condition of your liver.
• The long-term benefits of taking EPIVIR-HBV for treatment of chronic hepatitis B infection are not known.

It is not known if EPIVIR-HBV is safe and effective in:
• people with chronic HBV who have a severely damaged liver that is unable to work properly (decompensated liver disease)
• people with hepatitis C virus or hepatitis D (delta) virus
• people who have had a liver transplant
• children with chronic HBV less than 2 years of age

EPIVIR-HBV does not stop you from spreading HBV to others by sex, sharing needles, or being exposed to your blood. Avoid doing things that can spread HBV infection to others.

• Do not share or re-use needles or other injection equipment.
• Do not share personal items that can have blood or body fluids on them, like toothbrushes and razor blades.
• Do not have any kind of sex without protection. Always practice safer sex by using a latex or polyurethane condom to lower the chance of sexual contact with semen, vaginal secretions, or blood.

A vaccine is available to protect people at risk for becoming infected with HBV. You can ask your healthcare provider for information about this vaccine.

Who should not take EPIVIR-HBV?

Do not take EPIVIR-HBV if you are allergic to lamivudine or any of the ingredients in EPIVIR-HBV. See the end of this leaflet for a complete list of ingredients in EPIVIR-HBV.

What should I tell my healthcare provider before taking EPIVIR-HBV?

Before you take EPIVIR-HBV, tell your healthcare provider if you:
• have HIV-1 infection.
• have kidney problems
• have diabetes. Each 20-mL dose (100 mg) of EPIVIR-HBV oral solution contains 4 grams of sucrose.
• have any other medical condition
• are pregnant or plan to become pregnant. It is not known if EPIVIR-HBV will harm your unborn baby.

Pregnancy Registry. There is a pregnancy registry for women who take antiviral medicines during pregnancy.

The purpose of this registry is to collect information about the health of you and your baby. Talk to your healthcare provider about how you can take part in this registry.
• are breastfeeding or plan to breastfeed. EPIVIR-HBV can pass into your breast milk and may harm your baby. You and your healthcare provider should decide if you will take EPIVIR-HBV or breastfeed.

Tell your healthcare provider about all the medicines you take, including prescription and over-the-counter medicines, vitamins,and herbal supplements.

Do not take EPIVIR-HBV if you also take:
• other medicines that contain lamivudine (COMBIVIR®, EPIVIR®, EPZICOM®, TRIZIVIR®)
• medicines that contain emtricitabine (ATRIPLA®, COMPLERA®, EMTRIVA®, STRIBILD®, TRUVADA®)

How should I take EPIVIR-HBV?
• Take EPIVIR-HBV exactly as your healthcare provider tells you to take it.
• Do not change your dose or stop taking EPIVIR-HBV without talking with your healthcare provider.
• EPIVIR-HBV is taken 1 time each day.
• Your healthcare provider may prescribe a lower dose if you have problems with your kidneys.
• For children 2 to 17 years of age, your healthcare provider will prescribe the right dose of EPIVIR-HBV based on your child's body weight.
• Take EPIVIR-HBV by mouth, with or without food.
• Tell your healthcare provider if you have trouble swallowing tablets. EPIVIR-HBV also comes as a liquid (oral solution).
• If you take too much EPIVIR-HBV, call your healthcare provider or go to the nearest hospital emergency room right away.
• It is important to stay under your healthcare provider's care while taking EPIVIR-HBV. Tell your healthcare provider about any new symptoms that you have.

What are the possible side effects of EPIVIR-HBV?
EPIVIR-HBV may cause serious side effects, including:
See **"What is the most important information I should know about EPIVIR-HBV?".**
The most common side effects of EPIVIR-HBV include:
• ear, nose, and throat infections
• sore throat
• diarrhea
Tell your healthcare provider if you have any side effect that bothers you or that does not go away.
These are not all the possible side effects of EPIVIR-HBV. For more information, ask your healthcare provider or pharmacist.
Call your doctor for medical advice about side effects. You may report side effects to FDA at 1-800-FDA-1088.

How should I store EPIVIR-HBV?
• Store EPIVIR–HBV tablets and oral solution at room temperature between 68°F to 77°F (20°C to 25°C).
• Keep bottles of EPIVIR-HBV oral solution tightly closed.
Keep EPIVIR-HBV and all medicines out of the reach of children.

General information about the safe and effective use of EPIVIR-HBV
Medicines are sometimes prescribed for purposes other than those listed in a Patient Information leaflet. Do not use EPIVIR-HBV for a condition for which it was not prescribed. Do not give EPIVIR-HBV to other people, even if they have the same symptoms that you have. It may harm them.
If you would like more information, talk with your healthcare provider. You can ask your pharmacist or healthcare provider for information about EPIVIR-HBV that is written for health professionals.
For more information, go to www.gsk.com or call 1-800-25-5249.

What are the ingredients in EPIVIR-HBV?
Active ingredient: lamivudine.
Inactive ingredients:
EPIVIR-HBVtablets: hypromellose, macrogol 400, magnesium stearate, microcrystalline cellulose, polysorbate 80, red iron oxide, sodium starch glycolate, titanium dioxide, and yellow iron oxide.
EPIVIR-HBV oral solution: artificial strawberry and banana flavors, citric acid (anhydrous), methylparaben, propylene glycol, propylparaben, sodium citrate (dihydrate), and sucrose (200 mg per mL).
This Patient Information has been approved by the U.S. Food and Drug Administration.
EPIVIR-HBV is a registered trademark of the GlaxoSmithKline group of companies.
EPIVIR, COMBIVIR, EPZICOM, and TRIZIVIR are registered trademarks of the ViiV Healthcare group of companies.
The other brands listed are trademarks of their respective owners and are not trademarks of the GlaxoSmithKline group of companies. The makers of these brands are not affiliated with and do not endorse the GlaxoSmithKline group of companies or its products.

GlaxoSmithKline
Research Triangle Park, NC 27709
Manufactured under agreement from
Shire Pharmaceuticals Group plc
Basingstoke, UK
©2013, GlaxoSmithKline group of companies. All rights reserved.
Revised: December 2013
EPH:3PIL

FLOLAN®   ℞

[flō′lan]
(epoprostenol sodium)
for Injection

DESCRIPTION

FLOLAN (epoprostenol sodium) for Injection is a sterile sodium salt formulated for intravenous (IV) administration. Each vial of FLOLAN contains epoprostenol sodium equivalent to either 0.5 mg (500,000 ng) or 1.5 mg (1,500,000 ng) epoprostenol, 3.76 mg glycine, 2.93 mg sodium chloride, and 50 mg mannitol. Sodium hydroxide may have been added to adjust pH.

Epoprostenol (PGI$_2$, PGX, prostacyclin), a metabolite of arachidonic acid, is a naturally occurring prostaglandin with potent vasodilatory activity and inhibitory activity of platelet aggregation.

Epoprostenol is $(5Z,9\alpha,11\alpha,13E,15S)$-6,9-epoxy-11,15-dihydroxyprosta-5,13-dien-1-oic acid.

Epoprostenol sodium has a molecular weight of 374.45 and a molecular formula of $C_{20}H_{31}NaO_5$. The structural formula is:

FLOLAN is a white to off-white powder that must be reconstituted with STERILE DILUENT for FLOLAN. STERILE DILUENT for FLOLAN is supplied in glass vials containing 50 mL of 94 mg glycine, 73.3 mg sodium chloride, sodium hydroxide (added to adjust pH), and Water for Injection, USP.

The reconstituted solution of FLOLAN has a pH of 10.2 to 10.8 and is increasingly unstable at a lower pH.

CLINICAL PHARMACOLOGY
General

Epoprostenol has 2 major pharmacological actions: (1) direct vasodilation of pulmonary and systemic arterial vascular beds, and (2) inhibition of platelet aggregation. In animals, the vasodilatory effects reduce right- and left-ventricular afterload and increase cardiac output and stroke volume. The effect of epoprostenol on heart rate in animals varies with dose. At low doses, there is vagally mediated bradycardia, but at higher doses, epoprostenol causes reflex tachycardia in response to direct vasodilation and hypotension. No major effects on cardiac conduction have been observed. Additional pharmacologic effects of epoprostenol in animals include bronchodilation, inhibition of gastric acid secretion, and decreased gastric emptying.

Pharmacokinetics

Epoprostenol is rapidly hydrolyzed at neutral pH in blood and is also subject to enzymatic degradation. Animal studies using tritium-labeled epoprostenol have indicated a high clearance (93 mL/kg/min), small volume of distribution (357 mL/kg), and a short half-life (2.7 minutes). During infusions in animals, steady-state plasma concentrations of tritium-labeled epoprostenol were reached within 15 minutes and were proportional to infusion rates.

No available chemical assay is sufficiently sensitive and specific to assess the in vivo human pharmacokinetics of epoprostenol. The in vitro half-life of epoprostenol in human blood at 37°C and pH 7.4 is approximately 6 minutes; therefore, the in vivo half-life of epoprostenol in humans is expected to be no greater than 6 minutes. The in vitro pharmacologic half-life of epoprostenol in human plasma, based on inhibition of platelet aggregation, was similar for males (n = 954) and females (n = 1,024).

Tritium-labeled epoprostenol has been administered to humans in order to identify the metabolic products of epoprostenol. Epoprostenol is metabolized to 2 primary metabolites: 6-keto-PGF$_{1\alpha}$ (formed by spontaneous degradation) and 6,15-diketo-13,14-dihydro-PGF$_{1\alpha}$ (enzymatically formed), both of which have pharmacological activity orders of magnitude less than epoprostenol in animal test systems. The recovery of radioactivity in urine and feces over a

Table 1. Hemodynamics During Chronic Administration of FLOLAN in Patients With Idiopathic or Heritable PAH

Hemodynamic Parameter	Baseline		Mean Change from Baseline at End of Treatment Period[*]	
	FLOLAN (N = 52)	Standard Therapy (N = 54)	FLOLAN (N = 48)	Standard Therapy (N = 41)
CI (L/min/m²)	2.0	2.0	0.3[†]	-0.1
PAPm (mm Hg)	60	60	-5[†]	1
PVR (Wood U)	16	17	-4[†]	1
SAPm (mm Hg)	89	91	-4	-3
SV (mL/beat)	44	43	6[†]	-1
TPR (Wood U)	20	21	-5[†]	1

[*] At 8 weeks: FLOLAN N = 10, conventional therapy N = 11 (N is the number of patients with hemodynamic data).
At 12 weeks: FLOLAN N = 38, conventional therapy N = 30 (N is the number of patients with hemodynamic data).
[†] Denotes statistically significant difference between FLOLAN and conventional therapy groups.
CI = cardiac index, PAPm = mean pulmonary arterial pressure, PVR = pulmonary vascular resistance, SAPm = mean systemic arterial pressure, SV = stroke volume, TPR = total pulmonary resistance.

Table 2. Hemodynamics During Chronic Administration of FLOLAN in Patients With PAH/SSD

Hemodynamic Parameter	Baseline		Mean Change from Baseline at 12 Weeks	
	FLOLAN (N = 56)	Conventional Therapy (N = 55)	FLOLAN (N = 50)	Conventional Therapy (N = 48)
CI (L/min/m²)	1.9	2.2	0.5[*]	-0.1
PAPm (mm Hg)	51	49	-5[*]	1
RAPm (mm Hg)	13	11	-1[*]	1
PVR (Wood U)	14	11	-5[*]	1
SAPm (mm Hg)	93	89	-8[*]	-1

[*] Denotes statistically significant difference between FLOLAN and conventional therapy groups (N is the number of patients with hemodynamic data).
CI = cardiac index, PAPm = mean pulmonary arterial pressure, RAPm = mean right arterial pressure, PVR = pulmonary vascular resistance, SAPm = mean systemic arterial pressure.

1-week period was 82% and 4% of the administered dose, respectively. Fourteen additional minor metabolites have been isolated from urine, indicating that epoprostenol is extensively metabolized in humans.

CLINICAL TRIALS IN PULMONARY ARTERIAL HYPERTENSION (PAH)

Acute Hemodynamic Effects

Acute intravenous infusions of FLOLAN for up to 15 minutes in patients with idiopathic or heritable PAH or PAH associated with scleroderma spectrum of diseases (PAH/SSD) produce dose-related increases in cardiac index (CI) and stroke volume (SV) and dose-related decreases in pulmonary vascular resistance (PVR), total pulmonary resistance (TPR), and mean systemic arterial pressure (SAPm). The effects of FLOLAN on mean pulmonary artery pressure (PAPm) are variable and minor.

Chronic Infusion in Idiopathic or Heritable PAH

Hemodynamic Effects

Chronic continuous infusions of FLOLAN in patients with idiopathic or heritable PAH were studied in 2 prospective, open, randomized trials of 8 and 12 weeks' duration comparing FLOLAN plus conventional therapy to conventional therapy alone. Dosage of FLOLAN was determined as described in DOSAGE AND ADMINISTRATION and averaged 9.2 ng/kg/min at study's end. Conventional therapy varied among patients and included some or all of the following: anticoagulants in essentially all patients; oral vasodilators, diuretics, and digoxin in one half to two thirds of patients; and supplemental oxygen in about half the patients. Except for 2 New York Heart Association (NYHA) functional Class II patients, all patients were either functional Class III or Class IV. As results were similar in the 2 studies, the pooled results are described. Chronic hemodynamic effects were generally similar to acute effects. Increases in CI, SV, and arterial oxygen saturation and decreases in PAPm, mean right atrial pressure (RAPm), TPR, and systemic vascular resistance (SVR) were observed in patients who received FLOLAN chronically compared to those who did not. Table 1 illustrates the treatment-related hemodynamic changes in these patients after 8 or 12 weeks of treatment.

[See table 1 above]

These hemodynamic improvements appeared to persist when FLOLAN was administered for at least 36 months in an open, nonrandomized study.

Clinical Effects

Statistically significant improvement was observed in exercise capacity, as measured by the 6-minute walk test in patients receiving continuous intravenous FLOLAN plus conventional therapy (N = 52) for 8 or 12 weeks compared to those receiving conventional therapy alone (N = 54). Improvements were apparent as early as the first week of therapy. Increases in exercise capacity were accompanied by statistically significant improvement in dyspnea and fatigue, as measured by the Chronic Heart Failure Questionnaire and the Dyspnea Fatigue Index.

Survival was improved in NYHA functional Class III and Class IV patients with idiopathic or heritable PAH treated with FLOLAN for 12 weeks in a multicenter, open, randomized, parallel study. At the end of the treatment period, 8 of 40 (20%) patients receiving conventional therapy alone died, whereas none of the 41 patients receiving FLOLAN died (p = 0.003).

Chronic Infusion in PAH/Scleroderma Spectrum of Diseases (SSD)

Hemodynamic Effects

Chronic continuous infusions of FLOLAN in patients with PAH/SSD were studied in a prospective, open, randomized trial of 12 weeks' duration comparing FLOLAN plus conventional therapy (N = 56) to conventional therapy alone (N = 55). Except for 5 NYHA functional Class II patients, all patients were either functional Class III or Class IV. Dosage of FLOLAN was determined as described in DOSAGE AND ADMINISTRATION and averaged 11.2 ng/kg/min at study's end. Conventional therapy varied among patients and included some or all of the following: anticoagulants in essentially all patients, supplemental oxygen and diuretics in two thirds of the patients, oral vasodilators in 40% of the patients, and digoxin in a third of the patients. A statistically significant increase in CI, and statistically significant decreases in PAPm, RAPm, PVR, and SAPm after 12 weeks of treatment were observed in patients who received FLOLAN chronically compared to those who did not. Table 2 illustrates the treatment-related hemodynamic changes in these patients after 12 weeks of treatment.

[See table 2 above]

Clinical Effects

Statistically significant improvement was observed in exercise capacity, as measured by the 6-minute walk, in patients receiving continuous intravenous FLOLAN plus conventional therapy for 12 weeks compared to those receiving conventional therapy alone. Improvements were apparent in some patients at the end of the first week of therapy. Increases in exercise capacity were accompanied by statistically significant improvements in dyspnea and fatigue, as measured by the Borg Dyspnea Index and Dyspnea Fatigue Index. At week 12, NYHA functional class improved in 21 of 51 (41%) patients treated with FLOLAN compared to none of the 48 patients treated with conventional therapy alone. However, more patients in both treatment groups (28/51 [55%] with FLOLAN and 35/48 [73%] with conventional therapy alone) showed no change in functional class, and 2/51 (4%) with FLOLAN and 13/48 (27%) with conventional therapy alone worsened. Of the patients randomized, NYHA functional class data at 12 weeks were not available for 5 patients treated with FLOLAN and 7 patients treated with conventional therapy alone.

No statistical difference in survival over 12 weeks was observed in PAH/SSD patients treated with FLOLAN as compared to those receiving conventional therapy alone. At the end of the treatment period, 4 of 56 (7%) patients receiving FLOLAN died, whereas 5 of 55 (9%) patients receiving conventional therapy alone died.

No controlled clinical trials with FLOLAN have been performed in patients with pulmonary hypertension associated with other diseases.

INDICATIONS AND USAGE

FLOLAN is indicated for the treatment of pulmonary arterial hypertension (WHO Group I) to improve exercise capacity. Studies establishing effectiveness included predominantly patients with NYHA Functional Class III-IV symptoms and etiologies of idiopathic or heritable PAH or PAH associated with connective tissue diseases.

CONTRAINDICATIONS

A large study evaluating the effect of FLOLAN on survival in NYHA Class III and IV patients with congestive heart failure due to severe left ventricular systolic dysfunction was terminated after an interim analysis of 471 patients revealed a higher mortality in patients receiving FLOLAN plus conventional therapy than in those receiving conventional therapy alone. The chronic use of FLOLAN in patients with congestive heart failure due to severe left ventricular systolic dysfunction is therefore contraindicated.

Some patients with pulmonary hypertension have developed pulmonary edema during dose initiation, which may be associated with pulmonary veno-occlusive disease. FLOLAN should not be used chronically in patients who develop pulmonary edema during dose initiation.

FLOLAN is also contraindicated in patients with known hypersensitivity to the drug or to structurally related compounds.

WARNINGS

FLOLAN must be reconstituted only as directed using STERILE DILUENT for FLOLAN. FLOLAN must not be reconstituted or mixed with any other parenteral medications or solutions prior to or during administration.

Abrupt Withdrawal

Abrupt withdrawal (including interruptions in drug delivery) or sudden large reductions in dosage of FLOLAN may result in symptoms associated with rebound pulmonary hypertension, including dyspnea, dizziness, and asthenia. In clinical trials, one Class III patient's death was judged attributable to the interruption of FLOLAN. Avoid abrupt withdrawal.

Sepsis
See ADVERSE REACTIONS: Adverse Events Attributable to the Drug Delivery System.

PRECAUTIONS

General
FLOLAN should be used only by clinicians experienced in the diagnosis and treatment of pulmonary hypertension. Carefully establish the diagnosis of idiopathic or heritable PAH or PAH/CTD.

FLOLAN is a potent pulmonary and systemic vasodilator. Initiate FLOLAN in a setting with adequate personnel and equipment for physiologic monitoring and emergency care. Dose initiation has been performed during right heart catheterization and without cardiac catheterization. During dose initiation, asymptomatic increases in pulmonary artery pressure coincident with increases in cardiac output occurred rarely. In such cases, consider dose reduction, but such an increase does not imply that chronic treatment is contraindicated.

FLOLAN is a potent inhibitor of platelet aggregation. Therefore, expect an increased risk for hemorrhagic complications, particularly for patients with other risk factors for bleeding (see PRECAUTIONS: Drug Interactions).

During chronic use, deliver FLOLAN continuously on an ambulatory basis through a permanent indwelling central venous catheter. Unless contraindicated, administer anticoagulant therapy to patients receiving FLOLAN to reduce the risk of pulmonary thromboembolism or systemic embolism through a patent foramen ovale. To reduce the risk of infection, use aseptic technique in the reconstitution and administration of FLOLAN and in routine catheter care. Because FLOLAN is metabolized rapidly, even brief interruptions in the delivery of FLOLAN may result in symptoms associated with rebound pulmonary hypertension including dyspnea, dizziness, and asthenia. Intravenous therapy with FLOLAN will likely be needed for prolonged periods, possibly years, so consider the patient's ability to accept and care for a permanent intravenous catheter and infusion pump.

Based on clinical trials, the acute hemodynamic response to FLOLAN did not correlate well with improvement in exercise tolerance or survival during chronic use of FLOLAN. Adjust dosage of FLOLAN during chronic use at the first sign of recurrence or worsening of symptoms attributable to pulmonary hypertension or the occurrence of adverse events associated with FLOLAN (see DOSAGE AND ADMINISTRATION). Following dosage adjustments, monitor standing and supine blood pressure and heart rate closely for several hours.

Information for Patients
Patients receiving FLOLAN should receive the following information. **FLOLAN must be reconstituted only with STERILE DILUENT for FLOLAN.** FLOLAN is infused continuously through a permanent indwelling central venous catheter via a small, portable infusion pump. Thus, therapy with FLOLAN requires commitment by the patient to drug reconstitution, drug administration, and care of the permanent central venous catheter. Patients must adhere to sterile technique in preparing the drug and in the care of the catheter, and even brief interruptions in the delivery of FLOLAN may result in rapid symptomatic deterioration. A patient's decision to receive FLOLAN should be based upon the understanding that there is a high likelihood that therapy with FLOLAN will be needed for prolonged periods, possibly years. The patient's ability to accept and care for a permanent intravenous catheter and infusion pump should also be carefully considered.

Drug Interactions
Additional reductions in blood pressure may occur when FLOLAN is administered with diuretics, antihypertensive agents, or other vasodilators. When other antiplatelet agents or anticoagulants are used concomitantly, there is the potential for FLOLAN to increase the risk of bleeding. However, patients receiving infusions of FLOLAN in clinical trials were maintained on anticoagulants without evidence of increased bleeding. In clinical trials, FLOLAN was used with digoxin, diuretics, anticoagulants, oral vasodilators, and supplemental oxygen.

In a pharmacokinetic substudy in patients with congestive heart failure receiving furosemide or digoxin in whom therapy with FLOLAN was initiated, apparent oral clearance values for furosemide (n = 23) and digoxin (n = 30) were decreased by 13% and 15%, respectively, on the second day of therapy and had returned to baseline values by day 87. The change in furosemide clearance value is not likely to be clinically significant. However, patients on digoxin may show elevations of digoxin concentrations after initiation of therapy with FLOLAN, which may be clinically significant in patients prone to digoxin toxicity.

Carcinogenesis, Mutagenesis, Impairment of Fertility
Long-term studies in animals have not been performed to evaluate carcinogenic potential. A micronucleus test in rats revealed no evidence of mutagenicity. The Ames test and DNA elution tests were also negative, although the instability of epoprostenol makes the significance of these tests uncertain. Fertility was not impaired in rats given FLOLAN by subcutaneous injection at doses up to 100 mcg/kg/day (600 mcg/m²/day), 2.5 times the recommended human dose [4.6 ng/kg/min or 245.1 mcg/m²/day, IV] based on body surface area).

Pregnancy
Pregnancy Category B. Reproductive studies have been performed in pregnant rats and rabbits at doses up to 100 mcg/kg/day (600 mcg/m²/day in rats, 2.5 times the recommended human dose, and 1,180 mcg/m²/day in rabbits, 4.8 times the recommended human dose based on body surface area) and have revealed no evidence of impaired fertility or harm to the fetus due to FLOLAN. There are, however, no adequate and well-controlled studies in pregnant women. Because animal reproduction studies are not always predictive of human response, this drug should be used during pregnancy only if clearly needed.

Labor and Delivery
The use of FLOLAN during labor, vaginal delivery, or cesarean section has not been adequately studied in humans.

Nursing Mothers
It is not known whether this drug is excreted in human milk. Because many drugs are excreted in human milk, caution should be exercised when FLOLAN is administered to a nursing woman.

Pediatric Use
Safety and effectiveness in pediatric patients have not been established.

Geriatric Use
Clinical studies of FLOLAN in pulmonary hypertension did not include sufficient numbers of subjects aged 65 and over to determine whether they respond differently from younger patients. Other reported clinical experience has not identified differences in responses between the elderly and younger patients. In general, dose selection for an elderly patient should be cautious, usually starting at the low end of the dosing range, reflecting the greater frequency of decreased hepatic, renal, or cardiac function and of concomitant disease or other drug therapy.

ADVERSE REACTIONS

During clinical trials, adverse events were classified as follows: (1) adverse events during dose initiation and escalation, (2) adverse events during chronic dosing, and (3) adverse events associated with the drug delivery system.

Adverse Events During Dose Initiation and Escalation
During early clinical trials, FLOLAN was increased in 2-ng/kg/min increments until the patients developed symptomatic intolerance. The most common adverse events and the adverse events that limited further increases in dose were generally related to vasodilation, the major pharmacologic effect of FLOLAN. The most common dose-limiting adverse events (occurring in ≥1% of patients) were nausea, vomiting, headache, hypotension, and flushing, but also include chest pain, anxiety, dizziness, bradycardia, dyspnea, abdominal pain, musculoskeletal pain, and tachycardia. Table 3 lists the adverse events reported during dose initiation and escalation in decreasing order of frequency.

Table 3. Adverse Events During Dose Initiation and Escalation

Adverse Events Occurring in ≥1% of Patients	FLOLAN (n = 391)
Flushing	58%
Headache	49%
Nausea/vomiting	32%
Hypotension	16%
Anxiety, nervousness, agitation	11%
Chest pain	11%
Dizziness	8%
Bradycardia	5%
Abdominal pain	5%
Musculoskeletal pain	3%
Dyspnea	2%
Back pain	2%
Sweating	1%
Dyspepsia	1%
Hypesthesia/paresthesia	1%
Tachycardia	1%

Adverse Events During Chronic Administration
Interpretation of adverse events is complicated by the clinical features of PAH, which are similar to some of the pharmacologic effects of FLOLAN (e.g., dizziness, syncope). Adverse events which may be related to the underlying disease include dyspnea, fatigue, chest pain, edema, hypoxia, right ventricular failure, and pallor. Several adverse events, on the other hand, can clearly be attributed to FLOLAN. These include hypotension, bradycardia, tachycardia, pulmonary edema, bleeding at various sites, thrombocytopenia, headache, abdominal pain, pain (unspecified), sweating, rash, arthralgia, jaw pain, flushing, diarrhea, nausea and vomiting, flu-like symptoms, anxiety/nervousness, and agitation. In addition, chest pain, fatigue, and pallor have been reported during FLOLAN therapy, and a role for the drug in these events cannot be excluded.

Adverse Events During Chronic Administration for Idiopathic or Heritable PAH
In an effort to separate the adverse effects of the drug from the adverse effects of the underlying disease, Table 4 lists adverse events that occurred at a rate at least 10% greater on FLOLAN in controlled trials.

Table 4. Adverse Events Regardless of Attribution Occurring in Patients With Idiopathic or Heritable PAH With ≥10% Difference Between FLOLAN and Conventional Therapy Alone

Adverse Event	FLOLAN (n = 52)	Conventional Therapy (n = 54)
Occurrence More Common With FLOLAN		
General		
Chills/fever/sepsis/flu-like symptoms	25%	11%
Cardiovascular		
Tachycardia	35%	24%
Flushing	42%	2%
Gastrointestinal		
Diarrhea	37%	6%
Nausea/vomiting	67%	48%
Musculoskeletal		
Jaw pain	54%	0%
Myalgia	44%	31%
Nonspecific musculoskeletal pain	35%	15%
Neurological		
Anxiety/nervousness/tremor	21%	9%
Dizziness	83%	70%
Headache	83%	33%
Hypesthesia, hyperesthesia, paresthesia	12%	2%

Thrombocytopenia has been reported during uncontrolled clinical trials in patients receiving FLOLAN.

Adverse Events During Chronic Administration for PAH/SSD
In an effort to separate the adverse effects of the drug from the adverse effects of the underlying disease, Table 5 lists adverse events that occurred at a rate at least 10% greater on FLOLAN in the controlled trial.

Table 5. Adverse Events Regardless of Attribution Occurring in Patients with PAH/SSD With ≥10% Difference Between FLOLAN and Conventional Therapy Alone

Adverse Event	FLOLAN (n = 56)	Conventional Therapy (n = 55)
Occurrence More Common With FLOLAN		
Cardiovascular		
Flushing	23%	0%
Hypotension	13%	0%
Gastrointestinal		
Anorexia	66%	47%
Nausea/vomiting	41%	16%
Diarrhea	50%	5%
Musculoskeletal		
Jaw pain	75%	0%
Pain/neck pain/arthralgia	84%	65%
Neurological		
Headache	46%	5%
Skin and Appendages		
Skin ulcer	39%	24%
Eczema/rash/urticaria	25%	4%

Although the relationship to FLOLAN administration has not been established, pulmonary embolism has been reported in several patients taking FLOLAN and there have been reports of hepatic failure.

Adverse Events Attributable to the Drug Delivery System
Chronic infusions of FLOLAN are delivered using a small, portable infusion pump through an indwelling central venous catheter. During controlled PAH trials of up to 12 weeks' duration, the local infection rate was about 18%, and the rate for pain was about 11%. During long-term follow-up, sepsis was reported at a rate of 0.3 infections/patient per year in patients treated with FLOLAN. This rate was higher than reported in patients using chronic indwelling

central venous catheters to administer parenteral nutrition, but lower than reported in oncology patients using these catheters. Malfunctions in the delivery system resulting in an inadvertent bolus of or a reduction in FLOLAN were associated with symptoms related to excess or insufficient FLOLAN, respectively (see ADVERSE REACTIONS: Adverse Events During Chronic Administration).

Observed During Clinical Practice

In addition to adverse reactions reported from clinical trials, the following events have been identified during post-approval use of FLOLAN. Because they are reported voluntarily from a population of unknown size, estimates of frequency cannot be made. These events have been chosen for inclusion due to a combination of their seriousness, frequency of reporting, or potential causal connection to FLOLAN.

Blood and Lymphatic

Anemia, hypersplenism, pancytopenia, splenomegaly.

Endocrine and Metabolic

Hyperthyroidism.

OVERDOSAGE

Signs and symptoms of excessive doses of FLOLAN during clinical trials are the expected dose-limiting pharmacologic effects of FLOLAN, including flushing, headache, hypotension, tachycardia, nausea, vomiting, and diarrhea. Treatment will ordinarily require dose reduction of FLOLAN.

One patient with PAH/CTD accidentally received 50 mL of an unspecified concentration of FLOLAN. The patient vomited and became unconscious with an initially unrecordable blood pressure. FLOLAN was discontinued and the patient regained consciousness within seconds. In clinical practice, fatal occurrences of hypoxemia, hypotension, and respiratory arrest have been reported following overdosage of FLOLAN.

Single intravenous doses of FLOLAN at 10 and 50 mg/kg (2,703 and 27,027 times the recommended acute phase human dose based on body surface area) were lethal to mice and rats, respectively. Symptoms of acute toxicity were hypoactivity, ataxia, loss of righting reflex, deep slow breathing, and hypothermia.

DOSAGE AND ADMINISTRATION

Important Note

FLOLAN must be reconstituted only with STERILE DILUENT for FLOLAN. Do not dilute reconstituted solutions of FLOLAN or administer with other parenteral solutions or medications (see WARNINGS).

Dosage

Administer continuous chronic infusion of FLOLAN through a central venous catheter. Temporary peripheral intravenous infusion may be used until central access is established. Initiate chronic infusion of FLOLAN at 2 ng/kg/min and increase in increments of 2 ng/kg/min every 15 minutes or longer until dose-limiting pharmacologic effects are elicited or until a tolerance limit to the drug is established or further increases in the infusion rate are not clinically warranted (see Dosage Adjustments). If dose-limiting pharmacologic effects occur, then decrease the infusion rate until tolerance is established. In clinical trials, the most common dose-limiting adverse events were nausea, vomiting, hypotension, sepsis, headache, abdominal pain, or respiratory disorder (most treatment-limiting adverse events were not serious). If the initial infusion rate of 2 ng/kg/min is not tolerated, identify a lower dose that is tolerated by the patient.

In the controlled 12-week trial in PAH/SSD, for example, the dose increased from a mean starting dose of 2.2 ng/kg/min. During the first 7 days of treatment, the dose was increased daily to a mean dose of 4.1 ng/kg/min on day 7 of treatment. At the end of week 12, the mean dose was 11.2 ng/kg/min. The mean incremental increase was 2 to 3 ng/kg/min every 3 weeks.

Dosage Adjustments

Base changes in the chronic infusion rate on persistence, recurrence, or worsening of the patient's symptoms of pulmonary hypertension and the occurrence of adverse events due to excessive doses of FLOLAN. In general, expect increases in dose from the initial chronic dose.

Consider increments in dose if symptoms of PAH persist or recur Increase the infusion by 1- to 2-ng/kg/min increments at intervals sufficient to allow assessment of clinical response; these intervals should be at least 15 minutes. In clinical trials, incremental increases in dose occurred at intervals of 24 to 48 hours or longer. Following establishment of a new chronic infusion rate, observe the patient, and monitor standing and supine blood pressure and heart rate for several hours to ensure that the new dose is tolerated. During chronic infusion, the occurrence of dose-limiting pharmacological events may necessitate a decrease in infusion rate, but the adverse event may occasionally resolve without dosage adjustment. Make dosage decreases gradually in 2-ng/kg/min decrements every 15 minutes or longer until the dose-limiting effects resolve. Avoid abrupt withdrawal of FLOLAN or sudden large reductions in infusion rates. Except in life-threatening situations (e.g., unconsciousness, collapse, etc.), adjust infusion rates of FLOLAN only under the direction of a physician.

In patients receiving lung transplants, doses of FLOLAN were tapered after the initiation of cardiopulmonary bypass.

Administration

FLOLAN is administered by continuous intravenous infusion via a central venous catheter using an ambulatory infusion pump. During initiation of treatment, FLOLAN may be administered peripherally.

The ambulatory infusion pump used to administer FLOLAN should: (1) be small and lightweight, (2) be able to adjust infusion rates in 2-ng/kg/min increments, (3) have occlusion, end-of-infusion, and low-battery alarms, (4) be accurate to ±6% of the programmed rate, and (5) be positive pressure-driven (continuous or pulsatile) with intervals between pulses not exceeding 3 minutes at infusion rates used to deliver FLOLAN. The reservoir should be made of polyvinyl chloride, polypropylene, or glass. The infusion pump used in the most recent clinical trials was the CADD-1 HFX 5100 (SIMS Deltec). A 60-inch microbore non-DEHP extension set with proximal antisyphon valve, low priming volume (0.9 mL), and in-line 0.22 micron filter was used during clinical trials.

To avoid interruptions in drug delivery, the patient should have access to a backup infusion pump and intravenous infusion sets. Consider a multi-lumen catheter if other intravenous therapies are routinely administered.

To facilitate extended use at ambient temperatures exceeding 25°C (77°F), a cold pouch with frozen gel packs was used in clinical trials (see DOSAGE AND ADMINISTRATION: Storage and Stability). The cold pouches and gel packs used in clinical trials were obtained from Palco Labs, Palo Alto, California. Any cold pouch used must be capable of maintaining the temperature of reconstituted FLOLAN between 2° and 8°C for 12 hours.

Reconstitution

FLOLAN is stable only when reconstituted with STERILE DILUENT for FLOLAN. FLOLAN must not be reconstituted or mixed with any other parenteral medications or solutions prior to or during administration.

Select a concentration for the solution of FLOLAN that is compatible with the infusion pump being used with respect to minimum and maximum flow rates, reservoir capacity, and the infusion pump criteria listed above. When administered chronically, prepare FLOLAN in a drug delivery reservoir appropriate for the infusion pump with a total reservoir volume of at least 100 mL, using 2 vials of STERILE DILUENT for FLOLAN for use during a 24-hour period. Table 6 gives directions for preparing several different concentrations of FLOLAN.

Table 7. Infusion Rates for FLOLAN at a Concentration of 3,000 ng/mL

Patient Weight (kg)	Dose or Drug Delivery Rate (ng/kg/min)							
	2	4	6	8	10	12	14	16
	Infusion Delivery Rate (mL/h)							
10	---	---	1.2	1.6	2.0	2.4	2.8	3.2
20	---	1.6	2.4	3.2	4.0	4.8	5.6	6.4
30	1.2	2.4	3.6	4.8	6.0	7.2	8.4	9.6
40	1.6	3.2	4.8	6.4	8.0	9.6	11.2	12.8
50	2.0	4.0	6.0	8.0	10.0	12.0	14.0	16.0
60	2.4	4.8	7.2	9.6	12.0	14.4	16.8	19.2
70	2.8	5.6	8.4	11.2	14.0	16.8	19.6	22.4
80	3.2	6.4	9.6	12.8	16.0	19.2	22.4	25.6
90	3.6	7.2	10.8	14.4	18.0	21.6	25.2	28.8
100	4.0	8.0	12.0	16.0	20.0	24.0	28.0	32.0

Table 8. Infusion Rates for FLOLAN at a Concentration of 5,000 ng/mL

Patient Weight (kg)	Dose or Drug Delivery Rate (ng/kg/min)							
	2	4	6	8	10	12	14	16
	Infusion Delivery Rate (mL/h)							
10	---	---	---	1.0	1.2	1.4	1.7	1.9
20	---	1.0	1.4	1.9	2.4	2.9	3.4	3.8
30	---	1.4	2.2	2.9	3.6	4.3	5.0	5.8
40	1.0	1.9	2.9	3.8	4.8	5.8	6.7	7.7
50	1.2	2.4	3.6	4.8	6.0	7.2	8.4	9.6
60	1.4	2.9	4.3	5.8	7.2	8.6	10.1	11.5
70	1.7	3.4	5.0	6.7	8.4	10.1	11.8	13.4
80	1.9	3.8	5.8	7.7	9.6	11.5	13.4	15.4
90	2.2	4.3	6.5	8.6	10.8	13.0	15.1	17.3
100	2.4	4.8	7.2	9.6	12.0	14.4	16.8	19.2

Table 6. Reconstitution and Dilution Instructions

To make 100 mL of solution with Final Concentration (ng/mL) of:	Directions:
3,000 ng/mL	Dissolve contents of one 0.5-mg vial with 5 mL of STERILE DILUENT for FLOLAN. Withdraw 3 mL and add to sufficient STERILE DILUENT for FLOLAN to make a total of 100 mL.
5,000 ng/mL	Dissolve contents of one 0.5-mg vial with 5 mL of STERILE DILUENT for FLOLAN. Withdraw entire vial contents and add sufficient STERILE DILUENT for FLOLAN to make a total of 100 mL.
10,000 ng/mL	Dissolve contents of two 0.5-mg vials each with 5 mL of STERILE DILUENT for FLOLAN. Withdraw entire vial contents and add sufficient STERILE DILUENT for FLOLAN to make a total of 100 mL.
15,000 ng/mL*	Dissolve contents of one 1.5-mg vial with 5 mL of STERILE DILUENT for FLOLAN. Withdraw entire vial contents and add sufficient STERILE DILUENT for FLOLAN to make a total of 100 mL.

* Higher concentrations may be required for patients who receive FLOLAN long-term.

Generally, 3,000 ng/mL and 10,000 ng/mL are satisfactory concentrations to deliver between 2 to 16 ng/kg/min in adults. Infusion rates may be calculated using the following formula:

Infusion Rate (mL/hr) = [Dose (ng/kg/min) × Weight (kg) × 60 min/hr]

Final Concentration (ng/mL)

Tables 7 through 10 provide infusion delivery rates for doses up to 16 ng/kg/min based upon patient weight, drug delivery rate, and concentration of the solution of FLOLAN to be used. These tables may be used to select the most appropriate concentration of FLOLAN that will result in an infusion rate between the minimum and maximum flow rates of the infusion pump and that will allow the desired duration of infusion from a given reservoir volume. Higher infusion rates, and therefore, more concentrated solutions may be necessary with long-term administration of FLOLAN.

[See table 7 above]
[See table 8 above]
[See table 9 at top of next page]
[See table 10 at top of next page]

Table 9. Infusion Rates for FLOLAN at a Concentration of 10,000 ng/mL

Patient Weight (kg)	Dose or Drug Delivery Rate (ng/kg/min)						
	4	6	8	10	12	14	16
	Infusion Delivery Rate (mL/h)						
20	---	---	1.0	1.2	1.4	1.7	1.9
30	---	1.1	1.4	1.8	2.2	2.5	2.9
40	1.0	1.4	1.9	2.4	2.9	3.4	3.8
50	1.2	1.8	2.4	3.0	3.6	4.2	4.8
60	1.4	2.2	2.9	3.6	4.3	5.0	5.8
70	1.7	2.5	3.4	4.2	5.0	5.9	6.7
80	1.9	2.9	3.8	4.8	5.8	6.7	7.7
90	2.2	3.2	4.3	5.4	6.5	7.6	8.6
100	2.4	3.6	4.8	6.0	7.2	8.4	9.6

Table 10. Infusion Rates for FLOLAN at a Concentration of 15,000 ng/mL

Patient Weight (kg)	Dose or Drug Delivery Rate (ng/kg/min)						
	4	6	8	10	12	14	16
	Infusion Delivery Rate (mL/h)						
30	---	---	1.0	1.2	1.4	1.7	1.9
40	---	1.0	1.3	1.6	1.9	2.2	2.6
50	---	1.2	1.6	2.0	2.4	2.8	3.2
60	1.0	1.4	1.9	2.4	2.9	3.4	3.8
70	1.1	1.7	2.2	2.8	3.4	3.9	4.5
80	1.3	1.9	2.6	3.2	3.8	4.5	5.1
90	1.4	2.2	2.9	3.6	4.3	5.0	5.8
100	1.6	2.4	3.2	4.0	4.8	5.6	6.4

Storage and Stability

Unopened vials of FLOLAN are stable until the date indicated on the package when stored at 15° to 25°C (59° to 77°F) and protected from light in the carton. Unopened vials of STERILE DILUENT for FLOLAN are stable until the date indicated on the package when stored at 15° to 25°C (59° to 77°F).

Prior to use, reconstituted solutions of FLOLAN must be protected from light and must be refrigerated at 2° to 8°C (36° to 46°F) if not used immediately. **Do not freeze reconstituted solutions of FLOLAN. Discard any reconstituted solution that has been frozen. Discard any reconstituted solution if it has been refrigerated for more than 48 hours.** During use, a single reservoir of reconstituted solution of FLOLAN can be administered at room temperature for a total duration of 8 hours, or it can be used with a cold pouch and administered up to 24 hours with the use of 2 frozen 6-oz gel packs in a cold pouch. When stored or in use, insulate reconstituted FLOLAN from temperatures greater than 25°C (77°F) and less than 0°C (32°F), and do not expose to direct sunlight.

Use at Room Temperature

Prior to use at room temperature, 15° to 25°C (59° to 77°F), reconstituted solutions of FLOLAN may be stored refrigerated at 2° to 8°C (36° to 46°F) for no longer than 40 hours. When administered at room temperature, reconstituted solutions may be used for no longer than 8 hours. This 48-hour period allows the patient to reconstitute a 2-day supply (200 mL) of FLOLAN. Each 100-mL daily supply may be divided into 3 equal portions. Two of the portions are stored refrigerated at 2° to 8°C (36° to 46°F) until they are used.

Use with a Cold Pouch

Prior to infusion with the use of a cold pouch, solutions may be stored refrigerated at 2° to 8°C (36° to 46°F) for up to 24 hours. When a cold pouch is employed during the infusion, reconstituted solutions of FLOLAN may be used for no longer than 24 hours. Change gel packs every 12 hours. Reconstituted solutions may be kept at 2° to 8°C (36° to 46°F), either in refrigerated storage or in a cold pouch or a combination of the two, for no more than 48 hours.

Inspect parenteral drug products for particulate matter and discoloration prior to administration whenever solution and container permit. If either occurs, do not administer.

HOW SUPPLIED

FLOLAN for Injection is supplied as a sterile freeze-dried powder in 17-mL flint glass vials with gray butyl rubber closures, individually packaged in a carton.

17-mL vial containing epoprostenol sodium equivalent to 0.5 mg (500,000 ng), carton of 1 (NDC 0173-0517-00).

17-mL vial containing epoprostenol sodium equivalent to 1.5 mg (1,500,000 ng), carton of 1 (NDC 0173-0519-00).

Store the vials of FLOLAN at 15° to 25°C (59° to 77°F). Protect from light.

The STERILE DILUENT for FLOLAN is supplied in flint glass vials containing 50-mL diluent with fluororesin-faced butyl rubber closures.

50-mL of STERILE DILUENT for FLOLAN, tray of 2 vials (NDC 0173-0518-01).

Store the vials of STERILE DILUENT for FLOLAN at 15° to 25°C (59° to 77°F). DO NOT FREEZE.

GlaxoSmithKline
Research Triangle Park, NC 27709
©2011, GlaxoSmithKline. All rights reserved.
March 2011
FLL:2PI

FLONASE® ℞

[flō'nāz]

(fluticasone propionate)
Nasal Spray, 50 mcg
For Intranasal Use Only. SHAKE GENTLY BEFORE USE.

DESCRIPTION

Fluticasone propionate, the active component of FLONASE Nasal Spray, is a synthetic corticosteroid having the chemical name S-(fluoromethyl)6α,9-difluoro-11β-17-dihydroxy-16α-methyl-3-oxoandrosta-1,4-diene-17β-carbothioate, 17-propionate and the following chemical structure:

Fluticasone propionate is a white powder with a molecular weight of 500.6, and the empirical formula is $C_{25}H_{31}F_3O_5S$. It is practically insoluble in water, freely soluble in dimethyl sulfoxide and dimethylformamide, and slightly soluble in methanol and 95% ethanol.

FLONASE Nasal Spray, 50 mcg is an aqueous suspension of microfine fluticasone propionate for topical administration to the nasal mucosa by means of a metering, atomizing spray pump. FLONASE Nasal Spray also contains microcrystalline cellulose and carboxymethylcellulose sodium, dextrose, 0.02% w/w benzalkonium chloride, polysorbate 80, and 0.25% w/w phenylethyl alcohol, and has a pH between 5 and 7.

It is necessary to prime the pump before first use or after a period of non-use (1 week or more). After initial priming (6 actuations), each actuation delivers 50 mcg of fluticasone propionate in 100 mg of formulation through the nasal adapter. Each 16-g bottle of FLONASE Nasal Spray provides 120 metered sprays. After 120 metered sprays, the amount of fluticasone propionate delivered per actuation may not be consistent and the unit should be discarded.

CLINICAL PHARMACOLOGY

Mechanism of Action

Fluticasone propionate is a synthetic trifluorinated corticosteroid with anti-inflammatory activity. In vitro dose response studies on a cloned human glucocorticoid receptor system involving binding and gene expression afforded 50% responses at 1.25 and 0.17 nM concentrations, respectively. Fluticasone propionate was 3-fold to 5-fold more potent than dexamethasone in these assays. Data from the McKenzie vasoconstrictor assay in man also support its potent glucocorticoid activity.

In preclinical studies, fluticasone propionate revealed progesterone-like activity similar to the natural hormone. However, the clinical significance of these findings in relation to the low plasma levels (see Pharmacokinetics) is not known.

The precise mechanism through which fluticasone propionate affects allergic rhinitis symptoms is not known. Corticosteroids have been shown to have a wide range of effects on multiple cell types (e.g., mast cells, eosinophils, neutrophils, macrophages, and lymphocytes) and mediators (e.g., histamine, eicosanoids, leukotrienes, and cytokines) involved in inflammation. In 7 trials in adults, FLONASE Nasal Spray has decreased nasal mucosal eosinophils in 66% (35% for placebo) of patients and basophils in 39% (28% for placebo) of patients. The direct relationship of these findings to long-term symptom relief is not known.

FLONASE Nasal Spray, like other corticosteroids, is an agent that does not have an immediate effect on allergic symptoms. A decrease in nasal symptoms has been noted in some patients 12 hours after initial treatment with FLONASE Nasal Spray. Maximum benefit may not be reached for several days. Similarly, when corticosteroids are discontinued, symptoms may not return for several days.

Pharmacokinetics

Absorption: The activity of FLONASE Nasal Spray is due to the parent drug, fluticasone propionate. Indirect calculations indicate that fluticasone propionate delivered by the intranasal route has an absolute bioavailability averaging less than 2%. After intranasal treatment of patients with allergic rhinitis for 3 weeks, fluticasone propionate plasma concentrations were above the level of detection (50 pg/mL) only when recommended doses were exceeded and then only in occasional samples at low plasma levels. Due to the low bioavailability by the intranasal route, the majority of the pharmacokinetic data was obtained via other routes of administration. Studies using oral dosing of radiolabeled drug have demonstrated that fluticasone propionate is highly extracted from plasma and absorption is low. Oral bioavailability is negligible, and the majority of the circulating radioactivity is due to an inactive metabolite.

Distribution: Following intravenous administration, the initial disposition phase for fluticasone propionate was rapid and consistent with its high lipid solubility and tissue binding. The volume of distribution averaged 4.2 L/kg.

The percentage of fluticasone propionate bound to human plasma proteins averaged 91% with no obvious concentration relationship. Fluticasone propionate is weakly and reversibly bound to erythrocytes and freely equilibrates between erythrocytes and plasma. Fluticasone propionate is not significantly bound to human transcortin.

Metabolism: The total blood clearance of fluticasone propionate is high (average, 1,093 mL/min), with renal clearance accounting for less than 0.02% of the total. The only circulating metabolite detected in man is the 17β-carboxylic acid derivative of fluticasone propionate, which is formed through the cytochrome P450 3A4 pathway. This inactive metabolite had less affinity (approximately 1/2,000) than the parent drug for the glucocorticoid receptor of human lung cytosol in vitro and negligible pharmacological activity in animal studies. Other metabolites detected in vitro using cultured human hepatoma cells have not been detected in man.

Elimination: Following intravenous dosing, fluticasone propionate showed polyexponential kinetics and had a terminal elimination half-life of approximately 7.8 hours. Less than 5% of a radiolabeled oral dose was excreted in the urine as metabolites, with the remainder excreted in the feces as parent drug and metabolites.

Special Populations

Fluticasone propionate nasal spray was not studied in any special populations, and no gender-specific pharmacokinetic data have been obtained.

Drug Interactions

Fluticasone propionate is a substrate of cytochrome P450 3A4. Coadministration of fluticasone propionate and the highly potent cytochrome P450 3A4 inhibitor ritonavir is not recommended based upon a multiple-dose, crossover drug interaction study in 18 healthy subjects. Fluticasone propionate aqueous nasal spray (200 mcg once daily) was coadministered for 7 days with ritonavir (100 mg twice daily). Plasma fluticasone propionate concentrations following fluticasone propionate aqueous nasal spray alone were undetectable (<10 pg/mL) in most subjects, and when concentrations were detectable, peak levels (C_{max}) averaged 11.9 pg/mL (range, 10.8 to 14.1 pg/mL) and $AUC_{(0-\tau)}$ averaged 8.43 pg•hr/mL (range, 4.2 to 18.8 pg•hr/mL). Fluticasone propionate C_{max} and $AUC_{(0-\tau)}$ increased to 318 pg/mL (range, 110 to 648 pg/mL) and 3,102.6 pg•hr/mL (range, 1,207.1 to 5,662.0 pg•hr/mL), respectively, after coadministration of ritonavir with fluticasone propionate aqueous nasal spray. This significant increase in plasma fluticasone propionate exposure resulted in a significant decrease (86%) in plasma cortisol area under the plasma concentration versus time curve (AUC).

Caution should be exercised when other potent cytochrome P450 3A4 inhibitors are coadministered with fluticasone propionate. In a drug interaction study, coadministration of orally inhaled fluticasone propionate (1,000 mcg) and keto-conazole (200 mg once daily) resulted in increased fluticasone propionate exposure and reduced plasma corti-sol AUC, but had no effect on urinary excretion of cortisol. In another multiple-dose drug interaction study, coadminis-tration of orally inhaled fluticasone propionate (500 mcg twice daily) and erythromycin (333 mg 3 times daily) did not affect fluticasone propionate pharmacokinetics.

Pharmacodynamics

In a trial to evaluate the potential systemic and topical ef-fects of FLONASE Nasal Spray on allergic rhinitis symp-toms, the benefits of comparable drug blood levels produced by FLONASE Nasal Spray and oral fluticasone propionate were compared. The dosages used were 200 mcg of FLONASE Nasal Spray, the nasal spray vehicle (plus oral placebo), and 5 and 10 mg of oral fluticasone propionate (plus nasal spray vehicle) per day for 14 days. Plasma levels were undetectable in the majority of patients after intrana-sal dosing, but present at low levels in the majority after oral dosing. FLONASE Nasal Spray was significantly more effective in reducing symptoms of allergic rhinitis than ei-ther the oral fluticasone propionate or the nasal vehicle. This trial demonstrated that the therapeutic effect of FLONASE Nasal Spray can be attributed to the topical ef-fects of fluticasone propionate.

In another trial, the potential systemic effects of FLONASE Nasal Spray on the hypothalamic-pituitary-adrenal (HPA) axis were also studied in allergic patients. FLONASE Nasal Spray given as 200 mcg once daily or 400 mcg twice daily was compared with placebo or oral prednisone 7.5 or 15 mg given in the morning. FLONASE Nasal Spray at either dos-age for 4 weeks did not affect the adrenal response to 6-hour cosyntropin stimulation, while both dosages of oral predni-sone significantly reduced the response to cosyntropin.

CLINICAL TRIALS

A total of 13 randomized, double-blind, parallel-group, mul-ticenter, vehicle placebo-controlled clinical trials were con-ducted in the United States in adults and pediatric patients (4 years of age and older) to investigate regular use of FLONASE Nasal Spray in patients with seasonal or peren-nial allergic rhinitis. The trials included 2,633 adults (1,439 men and 1,194 women) with a mean age of 37 (range, 18 to 79 years). A total of 440 adolescents (405 boys and 35 girls), mean age of 14 (range, 12 to 17 years), and 500 children (325 boys and 175 girls), mean age of 9 (range, 4 to 11 years) were also studied. The overall racial distribution was 89% white, 4% black, and 7% other. These trials evaluated the total nasal symptom scores (TNSS) that included rhinor-rhea, nasal obstruction, sneezing, and nasal itching in known allergic patients who were treated for 2 to 24 weeks. Subjects treated with FLONASE Nasal Spray exhibited sig-nificantly greater decreases in TNSS than vehicle placebo-treated patients. Nasal mucosal basophils and eosinophils were also reduced at the end of treatment in adult studies; however, the clinical significance of this decrease is not known.

There were no significant differences between fluticasone propionate regimens whether administered as a single daily dose of 200 mcg (two 50-mcg sprays in each nostril) or as 100 mcg (one 50-mcg spray in each nostril) twice daily in 6 clinical trials. A clear dose response could not be identified in clinical trials. In 1 trial, 200 mcg/day was slightly more effective than 50 mcg/day during the first few days of treat-ment; thereafter, no difference was seen.

Two randomized, double-blind, parallel-group, multicenter, vehicle placebo-controlled 28-day trials were conducted in the United States in 732 patients (243 given FLONASE) 12 years of age and older to investigate "as-needed" use of FLONASE Nasal Spray (200 mcg) in patients with seasonal allergic rhinitis. Patients were instructed to take the study medication only on days when they thought they needed the medication for symptom control, not to exceed 2 sprays per nostril on any day, and not more than once daily. "As-needed" use was prospectively defined as average use of study medication no more than 75% of study days. Average use of study medications was 57% to 70% of days for all treatment arms. The studies demonstrated significantly greater reduction in TNSS (sum of nasal congestion, rhinor-rhea, sneezing, and nasal itching) with FLONASE Nasal Spray 200 mcg compared to placebo. The relative difference in efficacy with as-needed use as compared to regularly ad-ministered doses was not studied.

Three randomized, double-blind, parallel-group, vehicle placebo-controlled trials were conducted in 1,191 patients to investigate regular use of FLONASE Nasal Spray in pa-tients with perennial nonallergic rhinitis. These trials eval-uated the patient-rated TNSS (nasal obstruction, postnasal drip, rhinorrhea) in patients treated for 28 days of double-blind therapy and in 1 of the 3 trials for 6 months of open-label treatment. Two of these trials demonstrated that pa-tients treated with FLONASE Nasal Spray at a dosage of 100 mcg twice daily exhibited statistically significant de-creases in TNSS compared with patients treated with vehi-cle.

Individualization of Dosage

Patients should use FLONASE Nasal Spray at regular in-tervals for optimal effect.

Adult patients may be started on a 200-mcg once-daily reg-imen (two 50-mcg sprays in each nostril once daily). An al-ternative 200-mcg/day dosage regimen can be given as 100 mcg twice daily (one 50-mcg spray in each nostril twice daily).

Individual patients will experience a variable time to onset and different degree of symptom relief. In 4 randomized, double-blind, vehicle placebo-controlled, parallel-group al-lergic rhinitis studies and 2 studies of patients in an outdoor "park" setting (park studies), a decrease in nasal symptoms in treated subjects compared to placebo was shown to occur as soon as 12 hours after treatment with a 200-mcg dose of FLONASE Nasal Spray. Maximum effect may take several days. Regular-use patients who have responded may be able to be maintained (after 4 to 7 days) on 100 mcg/day (1 spray in each nostril once daily).

Some patients (12 years of age and older) with seasonal al-lergic rhinitis may find as-needed use of FLONASE Nasal Spray (not to exceed 200 mcg daily) effective for symptom control (see CLINICAL TRIALS). Greater symptom control may be achieved with scheduled regular use. Efficacy of as-needed use of FLONASE Nasal Spray has not been studied in pediatric patients under 12 years of age with seasonal allergic rhinitis, or patients with perennial allergic or non-allergic rhinitis.

Pediatric patients (4 years of age and older) should be started with 100 mcg (1 spray in each nostril once daily). Treatment with 200 mcg (2 sprays in each nostril once daily or 1 spray in each nostril twice daily) should be reserved for pediatric patients not adequately responding to 100 mcg daily. Once adequate control is achieved, the dosage should be decreased to 100 mcg (1 spray in each nostril) daily.

Maximum total daily doses should not exceed 2 sprays in each nostril (total dose, 200 mcg/day). There is no evidence that exceeding the recommended dose is more effective.

INDICATIONS AND USAGE

FLONASE Nasal Spray is indicated for the management of the nasal symptoms of seasonal and perennial allergic and nonallergic rhinitis in adults and pediatric patients 4 years of age and older.

Safety and effectiveness of FLONASE Nasal Spray in chil-dren below 4 years of age have not been adequately estab-lished.

CONTRAINDICATIONS

FLONASE Nasal Spray is contraindicated in patients with a hypersensitivity to any of its ingredients.

WARNINGS

The replacement of a systemic corticosteroid with a topical corticosteroid can be accompanied by signs of adrenal insuf-ficiency, and in addition some patients may experience symptoms of withdrawal, e.g., joint and/or muscular pain, lassitude, and depression. Patients previously treated for prolonged periods with systemic corticosteroids and trans-ferred to topical corticosteroids should be carefully moni-tored for acute adrenal insufficiency in response to stress. In those patients who have asthma or other clinical conditions requiring long-term systemic corticosteroid treatment, too rapid a decrease in systemic corticosteroids may cause a se-vere exacerbation of their symptoms.

The concomitant use of intranasal corticosteroids with other inhaled corticosteroids could increase the risk of signs or symptoms of hypercorticism and/or suppression of the HPA axis.

A drug interaction study in healthy subjects has shown that ritonavir (a highly potent cytochrome P450 3A4 inhibitor) can significantly increase plasma fluticasone propionate ex-posure, resulting in significantly reduced serum cortisol concentrations (see CLINICAL PHARMACOLOGY: Drug Interactions and PRECAUTIONS: Drug Interactions). Dur-ing postmarketing use, there have been reports of clinically significant drug interactions in patients receiving fluticasone propionate and ritonavir, resulting in systemic corticosteroid effects including Cushing syndrome and adre-nal suppression. Therefore, coadministration of fluticasone propionate and ritonavir is not recommended unless the po-tential benefit to the patient outweighs the risk of systemic corticosteroid side effects.

Persons who are using drugs that suppress the immune sys-tem are more susceptible to infections than healthy indi-viduals. Chickenpox and measles, for example, can have a more serious or even fatal course in susceptible children or adults using corticosteroids. In children or adults who have not had these diseases or been properly immunized, partic-ular care should be taken to avoid exposure. How the dose, route, and duration of corticosteroid administration affect the risk of developing a disseminated infection is not known. The contribution of the underlying disease and/or prior corticosteroid treatment to the risk is also not known. If exposed to chickenpox, prophylaxis with varicella zoster

immune globulin (VZIG) may be indicated. If exposed to measles, prophylaxis with pooled intramuscular immuno-globulin (IG) may be indicated. (See the respective package inserts for complete VZIG and IG prescribing information.) If chickenpox develops, treatment with antiviral agents may be considered.

Avoid spraying in eyes.

PRECAUTIONS

General

Intranasal corticosteroids may cause a reduction in growth velocity when administered to pediatric patients (see PRE-CAUTIONS: Pediatric Use).

Rarely, immediate hypersensitivity reactions or contact der-matitis may occur after the administration of FLONASE Nasal Spray. Rare instances of wheezing, nasal septum per-foration, cataracts, glaucoma, and increased intraocular pressure have been reported following the intranasal appli-cation of corticosteroids, including fluticasone propionate.

Use of excessive doses of corticosteroids may lead to signs or symptoms of hypercorticism and/or suppression of HPA function.

Although systemic effects have been minimal with recom-mended doses of FLONASE Nasal Spray, potential risk in-creases with larger doses. Therefore, larger than recom-mended doses of FLONASE Nasal Spray should be avoided. When used at higher than recommended doses or in rare individuals at recommended doses, systemic corticosteroid effects such as hypercorticism and adrenal suppression may appear. If such changes occur, the dosage of FLONASE Nasal Spray should be discontinued slowly consistent with accepted procedures for discontinuing oral corticosteroid therapy.

In clinical studies with fluticasone propionate administered intranasally, the development of localized infections of the nose and pharynx with *Candida albicans* has occurred only rarely. When such an infection develops, it may require treatment with appropriate local therapy and discontinua-tion of treatment with FLONASE Nasal Spray. Patients us-ing FLONASE Nasal Spray over several months or longer should be examined periodically for evidence of *Candida* in-fection or other signs of adverse effects on the nasal mucosa. Intranasal corticosteroids should be used with caution, if at all, in patients with active or quiescent tuberculous infec-tions of the respiratory tract; untreated local or systemic fungal or bacterial infections; systemic viral or parasitic in-fections; or ocular herpes simplex.

Because of the inhibitory effect of corticosteroids on wound healing, patients who have experienced recent nasal septal ulcers, nasal surgery, or nasal trauma should not use a na-sal corticosteroid until healing has occurred.

Information for Patients

Patients being treated with FLONASE Nasal Spray should receive the following information and instructions. This in-formation is intended to aid them in the safe and effective use of this medication. It is not a disclosure of all possible adverse or intended effects.

Patients should be warned to avoid exposure to chickenpox or measles and, if exposed, to consult their physician with-out delay.

Patients should use FLONASE Nasal Spray at regular in-tervals for optimal effect. Some patients (12 years of age and older) with seasonal allergic rhinitis may find as-needed use of 200 mcg once daily effective for symptom control (see CLINICAL TRIALS).

A decrease in nasal symptoms may occur as soon as 12 hours after starting therapy with FLONASE Nasal Spray. Results in several clinical trials indicate statistically signif-icant improvement within the first day or two of treatment; however, the full benefit of FLONASE Nasal Spray may not be achieved until treatment has been administered for sev-eral days. The patient should not increase the prescribed dosage but should contact the physician if symptoms do not improve or if the condition worsens.

For the proper use of FLONASE Nasal Spray and to attain maximum improvement, the patient should read and follow carefully the patient's instructions accompanying the prod-uct.

Drug Interactions

Fluticasone propionate is a substrate of cytochrome P450 3A4. A drug interaction study with fluticasone propionate aqueous nasal spray in healthy subjects has shown that ritonavir (a highly potent cytochrome P450 3A4 inhibitor) can significantly increase plasma fluticasone propionate ex-posure, resulting in significantly reduced serum cortisol concentrations (see CLINICAL PHARMACOLOGY: Drug Interactions). During postmarketing use, there have been reports of clinically significant drug interactions in patients receiving fluticasone propionate and ritonavir, resulting in systemic corticosteroid effects including Cushing syndrome and adrenal suppression. Therefore, coadministration of fluticasone propionate and ritonavir is not recommended unless the potential benefit to the patient outweighs the risk of systemic corticosteroid side effects.

In a placebo-controlled crossover study in 8 healthy volunteers, coadministration of a single dose of orally inhaled fluticasone propionate (1,000 mcg; 5 times the maximum daily intranasal dose) with multiple doses of ketoconazole (200 mg) to steady state resulted in increased plasma fluticasone propionate exposure, a reduction in plasma cortisol AUC, and no effect on urinary excretion of cortisol. Caution should be exercised when FLONASE Nasal Spray is coadministered with ketoconazole and other known potent cytochrome P450 3A4 inhibitors.

Carcinogenesis, Mutagenesis, Impairment of Fertility
Fluticasone propionate demonstrated no tumorigenic potential in mice at oral doses up to 1,000 mcg/kg (approximately 20 times the maximum recommended daily intranasal dose in adults and approximately 10 times the maximum recommended daily intranasal dose in children on a mcg/m^2 basis) for 78 weeks or in rats at inhalation doses up to 57 mcg/kg (approximately 2 times the maximum recommended daily intranasal dose in adults and approximately equivalent to the maximum recommended daily intranasal dose in children on a mcg/m^2 basis) for 104 weeks.

Fluticasone propionate did not induce gene mutation in prokaryotic or eukaryotic cells in vitro. No significant clastogenic effect was seen in cultured human peripheral lymphocytes in vitro or in the mouse micronucleus test.

No evidence of impairment of fertility was observed in reproductive studies conducted in male and female rats at subcutaneous doses up to 50 mcg/kg (approximately 2 times the maximum recommended daily intranasal dose in adults on a mcg/m^2 basis). Prostate weight was significantly reduced at a subcutaneous dose of 50 mcg/kg.

Pregnancy
Teratogenic Effects: Pregnancy Category C. Subcutaneous studies in the mouse and rat at 45 and 100 mcg/kg, respectively (approximately equivalent to and 4 times, respectively, the maximum recommended daily intranasal dose in adults on a mcg/m^2 basis), revealed fetal toxicity characteristic of potent corticosteroid compounds, including embryonic growth retardation, omphalocele, cleft palate, and retarded cranial ossification.

In the rabbit, fetal weight reduction and cleft palate were observed at a subcutaneous dose of 4 mcg/kg (less than the maximum recommended daily intranasal dose in adults on a mcg/m^2 basis). However, no teratogenic effects were reported at oral doses up to 300 mcg/kg (approximately 25 times the maximum recommended daily intranasal dose in adults on a mcg/m^2 basis) of fluticasone propionate to the rabbit. No fluticasone propionate was detected in the plasma in this study, consistent with the established low bioavailability following oral administration (see CLINICAL PHARMACOLOGY).

Fluticasone propionate crossed the placenta following oral administration of 100 mcg/kg to rats and 300 mcg/kg to rabbits (approximately 4 and 25 times, respectively, the maximum recommended daily intranasal dose in adults on a mcg/m^2 basis).

There are no adequate and well-controlled studies in pregnant women. Fluticasone propionate should be used during pregnancy only if the potential benefit justifies the potential risk to the fetus.

Experience with oral corticosteroids since their introduction in pharmacologic, as opposed to physiologic, doses suggests that rodents are more prone to teratogenic effects from corticosteroids than humans. In addition, because there is a natural increase in corticosteroid production during pregnancy, most women will require a lower exogenous corticosteroid dose and many will not need corticosteroid treatment during pregnancy.

Nursing Mothers
It is not known whether fluticasone propionate is excreted in human breast milk. However, other corticosteroids have been detected in human milk. Subcutaneous administration to lactating rats of 10 mcg/kg of tritiated fluticasone propionate (less than the maximum recommended daily intranasal dose in adults on a mcg/m^2 basis) resulted in measurable radioactivity in the milk. Since there are no data from controlled trials on the use of intranasal fluticasone propionate by nursing mothers, caution should be exercised when FLONASE Nasal Spray is administered to a nursing woman.

Pediatric Use
Six hundred fifty (650) patients aged 4 to 11 years and 440 patients aged 12 to 17 years were studied in US clinical trials with fluticasone propionate nasal spray. The safety and effectiveness of FLONASE Nasal Spray in children below 4 years of age have not been established.

Controlled clinical studies have shown that intranasal corticosteroids may cause a reduction in growth velocity in pediatric patients. This effect has been observed in the absence of laboratory evidence of HPA axis suppression, suggesting that growth velocity is a more sensitive indicator of systemic corticosteroid exposure in pediatric patients than some commonly used tests of HPA axis function. The long-term effects of this reduction in growth velocity associated with intranasal corticosteroids, including the impact on final adult height, are unknown. The potential for "catch-up" growth following discontinuation of treatment with intranasal corticosteroids has not been adequately studied. The growth of pediatric patients receiving intranasal corticosteroids, including FLONASE Nasal Spray, should be monitored routinely (e.g., via stadiometry). The potential growth effects of prolonged treatment should be weighed against the clinical benefits obtained and the risks/benefits of treatment alternatives. To minimize the systemic effects of intranasal corticosteroids, including FLONASE Nasal Spray, each patient should be titrated to the lowest dose that effectively controls his/her symptoms.

A 1-year placebo-controlled clinical growth study was conducted in 150 pediatric patients (ages 3 to 9 years) to assess the effect of FLONASE Nasal Spray (single daily dose of 200 mcg, the maximum approved dose) on growth velocity. From the primary population of 56 patients receiving FLONASE Nasal Spray and 52 receiving placebo, the point estimate for growth velocity with FLONASE Nasal Spray was 0.14 cm/year lower than that noted with placebo (95% confidence interval ranging from 0.54 cm/year lower than placebo to 0.27 cm/year higher than placebo). Thus, no statistically significant effect on growth was noted compared to placebo. No evidence of clinically relevant changes in HPA axis function or bone mineral density was observed as assessed by 12-hour urinary cortisol excretion and dual-energy x-ray absorptiometry, respectively.

The potential for FLONASE Nasal Spray to cause growth suppression in susceptible patients or when given at higher doses cannot be ruled out.

Geriatric Use
A limited number of patients 65 years of age and older (n = 129) or 75 years of age and older (n = 11) have been treated with FLONASE Nasal Spray in US and non-US clinical trials. While the number of patients is too small to permit separate analysis of efficacy and safety, the adverse reactions reported in this population were similar to those reported by younger patients.

ADVERSE REACTIONS

In controlled US studies, more than 3,300 patients with seasonal allergic, perennial allergic, or perennial nonallergic rhinitis received treatment with intranasal fluticasone propionate. In general, adverse reactions in clinical studies have been primarily associated with irritation of the nasal mucous membranes, and the adverse reactions were reported with approximately the same frequency by patients treated with the vehicle itself. The complaints did not usually interfere with treatment. Less than 2% of patients in clinical trials discontinued because of adverse events; this rate was similar for vehicle placebo and active comparators. Systemic corticosteroid side effects were not reported during controlled clinical studies up to 6 months' duration with FLONASE Nasal Spray. If recommended doses are exceeded, however, or if individuals are particularly sensitive or taking FLONASE Nasal Spray in conjunction with administration of other corticosteroids, symptoms of hypercorticism, e.g., Cushing syndrome, could occur.

The following incidence of common adverse reactions (>3%, where incidence in fluticasone propionate-treated subjects exceeded placebo) is based upon 7 controlled clinical trials in which 536 patients (57 girls and 108 boys aged 4 to 11 years, 137 female and 234 male adolescents and adults) were treated with FLONASE Nasal Spray 200 mcg once daily over 2 to 4 weeks and 2 controlled clinical trials in which 246 patients (119 female and 127 male adolescents and adults) were treated with FLONASE Nasal Spray 200 mcg once daily over 6 months. Also included in the table are adverse reactions from 2 studies in which 167 children (45 girls and 122 boys aged 4 to 11 years) were treated with FLONASE Nasal Spray 100 mcg once daily for 2 to 4 weeks. [See table above]

Other adverse events that occurred in ≤3% but ≥1% of patients and that were more common with fluticasone propionate (with uncertain relationship to treatment) included: blood in nasal mucus, runny nose, abdominal pain, diarrhea, fever, flu-like symptoms, aches and pains, dizziness, bronchitis.

Observed During Clinical Practice
In addition to adverse events reported from clinical trials, the following events have been identified during postapproval use of intranasal fluticasone propionate in clinical practice. Because they are reported voluntarily from a population of unknown size, estimates of frequency cannot be made. These events have been chosen for inclusion due to either their seriousness, frequency of reporting, or causal connection to fluticasone propionate or a combination of these factors.

General: Hypersensitivity reactions, including angioedema, skin rash, edema of the face and tongue, pruritus, urticaria, bronchospasm, wheezing, dyspnea, and anaphylaxis/anaphylactoid reactions, which in rare instances were severe.

Ear, Nose, and Throat: Alteration or loss of sense of taste and/or smell and, rarely, nasal septal perforation, nasal ulcer, sore throat, throat irritation and dryness, cough, hoarseness, and voice changes.

Eye: Dryness and irritation, conjunctivitis, blurred vision, glaucoma, increased intraocular pressure, and cataracts.

Cases of growth suppression have been reported for intranasal corticosteroids, including FLONASE (see PRECAUTIONS: Pediatric Use).

OVERDOSAGE

Chronic overdosage may result in signs/symptoms of hypercorticism (see PRECAUTIONS). Intranasal administration of 2 mg (10 times the recommended dose) of fluticasone propionate twice daily for 7 days to healthy human volunteers was well tolerated. Single oral doses up to 16 mg have been studied in human volunteers with no acute toxic effects reported. Repeat oral doses up to 80 mg daily for 10 days in volunteers and repeat oral doses up to 10 mg daily for 14 days in patients were well tolerated. Adverse reactions were of mild or moderate severity, and incidences were similar in active and placebo treatment groups. Acute overdosage with this dosage form is unlikely since 1 bottle of FLONASE Nasal Spray contains approximately 8 mg of fluticasone propionate.

The oral and subcutaneous median lethal doses in mice and rats were >1,000 mg/kg (>20,000 and >41,000 times, respectively, the maximum recommended daily intranasal dose in adults and >10,000 and >20,000 times, respectively, the maximum recommended daily intranasal dose in children on a mg/m^2 basis).

DOSAGE AND ADMINISTRATION

Patients should use FLONASE Nasal Spray at regular intervals for optimal effect.

Adults
The recommended starting dosage in **adults** is 2 sprays (50 mcg of fluticasone propionate each) in each nostril once daily (total daily dose, 200 mcg). The same dosage divided into 100 mcg given twice daily (e.g., 8 a.m. and 8 p.m.) is also effective. After the first few days, patients may be able to reduce their dosage to 100 mcg (1 spray in each nostril) once daily for maintenance therapy. Some patients (12 years of age and older) with seasonal allergic rhinitis may find as-needed use of 200 mcg once daily effective for symptom control (see CLINICAL TRIALS). Greater symptom control may be achieved with scheduled regular use.

Adolescents and Children (4 Years of Age and Older)
Patients should be started with 100 mcg (1 spray in each nostril once daily). Patients not adequately responding to 100 mcg may use 200 mcg (2 sprays in each nostril). Once adequate control is achieved, the dosage should be decreased to 100 mcg (1 spray in each nostril) daily.

The maximum total daily dosage should not exceed 2 sprays in each nostril (200 mcg/day) (see CLINICAL TRIALS: Individualization of Dosage)

FLONASE Nasal Spray is not recommended for children under 4 years of age.

Overall Adverse Experiences With >3% Incidence on Fluticasone Propionate in Controlled Clinical Trials With FLONASE Nasal Spray in Patients ≥4 Years With Seasonal or Perennial Allergic Rhinitis			
Adverse Experience	Vehicle Placebo (n = 758) %	FLONASE 100 mcg Once Daily (n = 167) %	FLONASE 200 mcg Once Daily (n = 782) %
Headache	14.6	6.6	16.1
Pharyngitis	7.2	6.0	7.8
Epistaxis	5.4	6.0	6.9
Nasal burning/nasal irritation	2.6	2.4	3.2
Nausea/vomiting	2.0	4.8	2.6
Asthma symptoms	2.9	7.2	3.3
Cough	2.8	3.6	3.8

Directions for Use
Illustrated patient's instructions for proper use accompany each package of FLONASE Nasal Spray.

HOW SUPPLIED
FLONASE Nasal Spray, 50 mcg is supplied in an amber glass bottle fitted with a white metering atomizing pump, white nasal adapter, and green dust cover in a box of 1 (NDC 0173-0453-01) with patient's instructions for use. Each bottle contains a net fill weight of 16 g and will provide 120 actuations. Each actuation delivers 50 mcg of fluticasone propionate in 100 mg of formulation through the nasal adapter. The correct amount of medication in each spray cannot be assured after 120 sprays even though the bottle is not completely empty. The bottle should be discarded when the labeled number of actuations has been used.

Store between 4° and 30°C (39° and 86°F).
GlaxoSmithKline
Research Triangle Park, NC 27709
©2007, GlaxoSmithKline. All rights reserved.
August 2007 FLN:1PI

Flonase®
(fluticasone propionate)
Nasal Spray, 50 mcg
Please read this leaflet carefully before you start to take your medicine. It provides a summary of information on your medicine.
For further information ask your doctor or pharmacist.
WHAT YOU SHOULD KNOW ABOUT RHINITIS
Rhinitis is a word that means inflammation of the lining of the nose. If you suffer from rhinitis, your nose becomes stuffy and runny. Rhinitis can also make your nose itchy, and you may sneeze a lot. Rhinitis can be caused by allergies to pollen, animals, molds, or other materials—or it may have a nonallergic cause.
WHAT YOU SHOULD KNOW ABOUT FLONASE NASAL SPRAY
Your doctor has prescribed FLONASE Nasal Spray, a medicine that can help treat your rhinitis. FLONASE Nasal Spray contains fluticasone propionate, which is a synthetic corticosteroid. Corticosteroids are natural substances found in the body that help fight inflammation. When you spray FLONASE into your nose, it helps to reduce the symptoms of allergic reactions and the stuffiness, runniness, itching, and sneezing that can bother you.
THINGS TO REMEMBER ABOUT FLONASE NASAL SPRAY
1. Shake gently before using.
2. Use your nasal spray as directed by your doctor. The directions are on the pharmacy label.
3. Keep your nasal spray **out of the reach of children.**
BEFORE USING YOUR NASAL SPRAY
• If you are pregnant (or intending to become pregnant),
• If you are breastfeeding a baby,
• If you are allergic to FLONASE Nasal Spray or any other nasal corticosteroid,
• If you are taking a medicine containing ritonavir (commonly used to treat HIV infection or AIDS),
TELL YOUR DOCTOR BEFORE STARTING TO TAKE THIS MEDICINE. In some circumstances, this medicine may not be suitable and your doctor may wish to give you a different medicine. Make sure that your doctor knows what other medicines you are taking.
USING YOUR NASAL SPRAY
• Follow the instructions shown in the rest of this leaflet. If you have any problems, tell your doctor or pharmacist.
• It is important that you use it as directed by your doctor. The pharmacist's label will usually tell you what dose to take and how often. If it doesn't, or you are not sure, ask your doctor or pharmacist.
DOSAGE
• For **ADULTS**, the usual starting dosage is *2 sprays in each nostril once daily.* Sometimes your doctor may recommend using 1 spray in each nostril twice a day (morning and evening). You should not use more than a total of 2 sprays in each nostril daily. After you have begun to feel better, 1 spray in each nostril daily may be adequate for you.
For **ADOLESCENTS and CHILDREN** (4 years of age and older), the usual starting dosage is *1 spray in each nostril once daily.* Sometimes your doctor may recommend using 2 sprays in each nostril daily. Then, after you have begun to feel better, 1 spray in each nostril daily may be adequate for you.

• DO NOT use more of your medicine or take it more often than your doctor advises.
• FLONASE may begin to work within 12 hours of the first dose, but it takes several days of regular use to reach its greatest effect. It is important that you use FLONASE Nasal Spray as prescribed by your doctor. Best results will be obtained by using the spray on a regular basis. If symptoms disappear, contact your doctor for further instructions.
• If you also have itchy, watery eyes, you should tell your doctor. You may be given an additional medicine to treat your eyes. Be careful not to confuse them, particularly if the second medicine is an eye drop.
• If you miss a dose, just take your regularly scheduled next dose when it is due. DO NOT DOUBLE the dose.
HOW TO USE YOUR NASAL SPRAY
Read the complete instructions carefully and use only as directed.
BEFORE USING
1. Shake the bottle gently and then remove the dust cover (Figure 1).

Figure 1

2. It is necessary to prime the pump into the air the first time it is used, or when you have not used it for a week or more. To prime the pump, hold the bottle as shown with the nasal applicator pointing away from you and with your forefinger and middle finger on either side of the nasal applicator and your thumb underneath the bottle. When you prime the pump for the first time, press down and release the pump 6 times (Figure 2). The pump is now ready for use. If the pump is not used for 7 days, prime until a fine spray appears.

Figure 2

USING THE SPRAY
3. Blow your nose to clear your nostrils.
4. Close one nostril. Tilt your head forward slightly and, keeping the bottle upright, carefully insert the nasal applicator into the other nostril (Figure 3).

Figure 3

5. Start to breathe in through your nose, and WHILE BREATHING IN press firmly and quickly down once on the applicator to release the spray. To get a full actuation, use your forefinger and middle finger to spray while supporting the base of the bottle with your thumb. Avoid spraying in eyes. Breathe gently inwards through the nostril (Figure 4).

Figure 4

6. Breathe out through your mouth.
7. If a second spray is required in that nostril, repeat steps 4 through 6.

8. Repeat steps 4 through 7 in the other nostril.
9. Wipe the nasal applicator with a clean tissue and replace the dust cover (Figure 5).

Figure 5

10. Do not use this bottle for more than the labeled number of sprays even though the bottle is not completely empty. Before you throw the bottle away, you should consult your doctor to see if a refill is needed. Do not take extra doses or stop taking FLONASE Nasal Spray without consulting your doctor.
CLEANING
Your nasal spray should be cleaned at least once a week. To do this:
1. Remove the dust cover and then gently pull upwards to free the nasal applicator.
2. Wash the applicator and dust cover under warm tap water. Allow to dry at room temperature, then place the applicator and dust cover back on the bottle.
3. If the nasal applicator becomes blocked, it can be removed as above and left to soak in warm water. Rinse with cold tap water, dry, and refit. **Do not try to unblock the nasal applicator by inserting a pin or other sharp object.**
STORING YOUR NASAL SPRAY
• Keep your FLONASE Nasal Spray **out of the reach of children.**
• Avoid spraying in eyes.
• Store between 4° and 30°C (39° and 86°F).
• Do not use your FLONASE Nasal Spray after the date shown as "EXP" on the label or box.
REMEMBER: This medicine has been prescribed for you by your doctor. DO NOT give this medicine to anyone else.
FURTHER INFORMATION
This leaflet does not contain the complete information about your medicine. *If you have any questions, or are not sure about something, then you should ask your doctor or pharmacist.*
You may want to read this leaflet again. Please DO NOT THROW IT AWAY until you have finished your medicine.
GlaxoSmithKline
Research Triangle Park, NC 27709
©2003, GlaxoSmithKline. All rights reserved.
July 2003 RL-2019

FLOVENT DISKUS 50 mcg ℞
[flō′vent]
(fluticasone propionate inhalation powder, 50 mcg)
FLOVENT DISKUS 100 mcg ℞
(fluticasone propionate inhalation powder, 100 mcg)
FLOVENT DISKUS 250 mcg ℞
(fluticasone propionate inhalation powder, 250 mcg)
FOR ORAL INHALATION

HIGHLIGHTS OF PRESCRIBING INFORMATION
These highlights do not include all the information needed to use FLOVENT DISKUS safely and effectively. See full prescribing information for FLOVENT DISKUS.
FLOVENT DISKUS 50 mcg
(fluticasone propionate inhalation powder, 50 mcg)
FLOVENT DISKUS 100 mcg
(fluticasone propionate inhalation powder, 100 mcg)
FLOVENT DISKUS 250 mcg
(fluticasone propionate inhalation powder, 250 mcg)
FOR ORAL INHALATION
USEInitial U.S. Approval: 1994

——INDICATIONS AND USAGE——
FLOVENT DISKUS is an inhaled corticosteroid indicated for:
• Maintenance treatment of asthma as prophylactic therapy in patients aged 4 years and older. (1)
• Treatment of asthma in patients requiring oral corticosteroid therapy. (1)
Important limitation:
• Not indicated for the relief of acute bronchospasm. (1)

——DOSAGE AND ADMINISTRATION——
For oral inhalation only. Dosing is based on prior asthma therapy. (2)

Previous Therapy	Recommended Starting Dosage	Highest Recommended Dosage
Patients aged 12 years and older		
Bronchodilators alone	100 mcg twice daily	500 mcg twice daily
Inhaled corticosteroids	100-250 mcg twice daily	500 mcg twice daily
Oral corticosteroids	500-1,000 mcg twice daily	1,000 mcg twice daily
Patients aged 4-11 years	50 mcg twice daily	100 mcg twice daily

DOSAGE FORMS AND STRENGTHS

Inhalation Powder. Inhaler containing fluticasone propionate (50, 100, or 250 mcg) as a powder formulation for oral inhalation. (3)

CONTRAINDICATIONS

- Primary treatment of status asthmaticus or acute episodes of asthma requiring intensive measures. (4)
- Severe hypersensitivity to milk proteins. (4)

WARNINGS AND PRECAUTIONS

- *Candida albicans* infection of the mouth and pharynx may occur. Monitor patients periodically. Advise the patient to rinse his/her mouth with water without swallowing after inhalation to help reduce the risk. (5.1)
- Potential worsening of infections (e.g., existing tuberculosis; fungal, bacterial, viral, or parasitic infection; ocular herpes simplex). Use with caution in patients with these infections.More serious or even fatal course of chickenpox or measles can occur in susceptible patients. (5.3)
- Risk of impaired adrenal function when transferring from systemic corticosteroids. Taper patients slowly from systemic corticosteroids if transferring to FLOVENT DISKUS. (5.4)
- Hypercorticism and adrenal suppression may occur with very high dosages or at the regular dosage in susceptible individuals. If such changes occur, discontinue FLOVENT DISKUS slowly. (5.5)
- Assess for decrease in bone mineral density initially and periodically thereafter. (5.7)
- Monitor growth of pediatric patients. (5.8)
- Close monitoring for glaucoma and cataracts is warranted. (5.9)

ADVERSE REACTIONS

Most common adverse reactions (incidence >3%) include upper respiratory tract infection or inflammation, throat irritation, sinusitis, rhinitis, oral candidiasis, nausea and vomiting, gastrointestinal discomfort, fever, cough, bronchitis, and headache. (6.1)

To report SUSPECTED ADVERSE REACTIONS, contact GlaxoSmithKline at 1-888-825-5249 or FDA at 1-800-FDA-1088 or www.fda.gov/medwatch.

DRUG INTERACTIONS

Strong cytochrome P450 3A4 inhibitors (e.g., ritonavir, ketoconazole): Use not recommended. May increase risk of systemic corticosteroid effects (7.1)

USE IN SPECIFIC POPULATIONS

Hepatic impairment: Monitor patients for signs of increased drug exposure. (8.6)

See 17 for PATIENT COUNSELING INFORMATION and FDA-approved patient labeling

Revised: 05/2014

FULL PRESCRIBING INFORMATION

1   INDICATIONS AND USAGE

FLOVENT® DISKUS® is indicated for the maintenance treatment of asthma as prophylactic therapy in patients aged 4 years and older. It is also indicated for patients requiring oral corticosteroid therapy for asthma. Many of these patients may be able to reduce or eliminate their requirement for oral corticosteroids over time.

Important Limitation of Use: FLOVENT DISKUS is NOT indicated for the relief of acute bronchospasm.

2   DOSAGE AND ADMINISTRATION

Flovent DISKUS should be administered by the orally inhaled route only in patients aged 4 years and older. After inhalation, the patient should rinse his/her mouth with water without swallowing to help reduce the risk of oropharyngeal candidiasis.

Individual patients will experience a variable time to onset and degree of symptom relief. Maximum benefit may not be achieved for 1 to 2 weeks or longer after starting treatment. After asthma stability has been achieved, it is always desirable to titrate to the lowest effective dosage to reduce the possibility of side effects. For patients who do not respond adequately to the starting dosage after 2 weeks of therapy, higher dosages may provide additional asthma control. The safety and efficacy of FLOVENT DISKUS when administered in excess of recommended dosages have not been established.

The recommended starting dosage and the highest recommended dosage of FLOVENT DISKUS, based on prior asthma therapy, are listed in Table 1.

Table 1. Recommended Dosages of FLOVENT DISKUS

NOTE: In all patients, it is desirable to titrate to the lowest effective dosage once asthma stability is achieved.

Previous Therapy	Recommended Starting Dosage	Highest Recommended Dosage
Adult and adolescent patients (aged 12 years and older)		
Bronchodilators alone	100 mcg twice daily	500 mcg twice daily
Inhaled corticosteroids	100-250 mcg twice daily[a]	500 mcg twice daily
Oral corticosteroids[b]	500-1,000 mcg twice daily[c]	1,000 mcg twice daily
Pediatric patients (aged 4-11 years)[d]	50 mcg twice daily[a]	100 mcg twice daily

[a]Starting dosages above 100 mcg twice daily for adult and adolescent patients and 50 mcg twice daily for pediatric patients aged 4 to 11 years may be considered for patients with poorer asthma control or those who have previously required doses of inhaled corticosteroids that are in the higher range for the specific agent.

[b]For patients currently receiving chronic oral corticosteroid therapy, prednisone should be reduced no faster than 2.5 to 5 mg/day on a weekly basis beginning after at least 1 week of therapy with FLOVENT DISKUS. Patients should be carefully monitored for signs of asthma instability, including serial objective measures of airflow, and for signs of adrenal insufficiency [see Warnings and Precautions (5.4)]. Once prednisone reduction is complete, the dosage of FLOVENT DISKUS should be reduced to the lowest effective dosage.

[c]The choice of starting dosage should be made on the basis of individual patient assessment. A controlled clinical trial of 111 oral corticosteroid-dependent subjects with asthma showed few significant differences between the 2 doses of FLOVENT DISKUS on safety and efficacy endpoints. However, inability to decrease the dose of oral corticosteroids further during corticosteroid reduction may be indicative of the need to increase the dose of fluticasone propionate up to the maximum of 1,000 mcg twice daily.

[d]Because individual responses may vary, pediatric patients previously maintained on other inhaled corticosteroids may require dosage adjustments upon transfer to FLOVENT DISKUS.

3   DOSAGE FORMS AND STRENGTHS

Inhalation Powder. Inhaler containing a foil blister strip of powder formulation for oral inhalation. The strip contains fluticasone propionate 50, 100, or 250 mcg per blister.

4   CONTRAINDICATIONS

The use of FLOVENT DISKUS is contraindicated in the following conditions:

- Primary treatment of status asthmaticus or other acute episodes of asthma where intensive measures are required *[see Warnings and Precautions (5.2)]*
- Severe hypersensitivity to milk proteins *[see Warnings and Precautions (5.6), Adverse Reactions (6.2), Description (11)]*

5   WARNINGS AND PRECAUTIONS

5.1   Local Effects of Inhaled Corticosteroids

In clinical trials, the development of localized infections of the mouth and pharynx with *Candida albicans* has occurred in subjects treated with FLOVENT DISKUS. When such an infection develops, it should be treated with appropriate local or systemic (i.e., oral) antifungal therapy while treatment with FLOVENT DISKUS continues, but at times therapy with FLOVENT DISKUS may need to be interrupted. Advise the patient to rinse his/her mouth with water without swallowing following inhalation to help reduce the risk of oropharyngeal candidiasis.

5.2   Acute Asthma Episodes

FLOVENT DISKUS is not to be regarded as a bronchodilator and is not indicated for rapid relief of bronchospasm. Patients should be instructed to contact their physicians immediately when episodes of asthma that are not responsive to bronchodilators occur during the course of treatment with FLOVENT DISKUS. During such episodes, patients may require therapy with oral corticosteroids.

5.3   Immunosuppression

Persons who are using drugs that suppress the immune system are more susceptible to infections than healthy individuals. Chickenpox and measles, for example, can have a more serious or even fatal course in susceptible children or adults using corticosteroids. In such children or adults who have not had these diseases or been properly immunized, particular care should be taken to avoid exposure. How the dose, route, and duration of corticosteroid administration affect the risk of developing a disseminated infection is not known. The contribution of the underlying disease and/or prior corticosteroid treatment to the risk is also not known. If a patient is exposed to chickenpox, prophylaxis with varicella zoster immune globulin (VZIG) may be indicated. If a patient is exposed to measles, prophylaxis with pooled intramuscular immunoglobulin (IG) may be indicated. (See the respective package inserts for complete VZIG and IG prescribing information.) If chickenpox develops, treatment with antiviral agents may be considered.

Inhaled corticosteroids should be used with caution, if at all, in patients with active or quiescent tuberculosis infections of the respiratory tract; systemic fungal, bacterial, viral or parasitic infections; or ocular herpes simplex.

5.4   Transferring Patients From Systemic Corticosteroid Therapy

Particular care is needed for patients who have been transferred from systemically active corticosteroids to inhaled corticosteroids because deaths due to adrenal insufficiency have occurred in patients with asthma during and after transfer from systemic corticosteroids to less systemically available inhaled corticosteroids. After withdrawal from systemic corticosteroids, a number of months are required for recovery of hypothalamic-pituitary-adrenal (HPA) function.

Table 2. Adverse Reactions With FLOVENT DISKUS With >3% Incidence and More Common Than Placebo in Subjects With Asthma

Adverse Event	FLOVENT DISKUS 50 mcg Twice Daily (n = 178) %	FLOVENT DISKUS 100 mcg Twice Daily (n = 305) %	FLOVENT DISKUS 250 mcg Twice Daily (n = 86) %	FLOVENT DISKUS 500 mcg Twice Daily (n = 64) %	Placebo (n = 543) %
Ear, nose, and throat					
Upper respiratory tract infection	20	18	21	14	16
Throat irritation	13	13	3	22	8
Sinusitis/sinus infection	9	10	6	6	6
Upper respiratory inflammation	5	5	0	5	3
Rhinitis	4	3	1	2	2
Oral candidiasis	<1	9	6	5	7
Gastrointestinal					
Nausea and vomiting	8	4	1	2	4
Gastrointestinal discomfort and pain	4	3	2	2	3
Viral gastrointestinal infection	4	3	3	5	1
Non-site specific					
Fever	7	7	1	2	4
Viral infection	2	2	0	5	2
Lower respiratory					
Viral respiratory infection	4	5	1	2	4
Cough	3	5	1	5	4
Bronchitis	2	3	0	8	1
Neurological					
Headache	12	12	3	14	7
Musculoskeletal and trauma					
Muscle injury	2	0	1	5	1
Musculoskeletal pain	4	3	2	5	2
Injury	2	<1	0	5	<1

Patients who have been previously maintained on 20 mg or more of prednisone (or its equivalent) may be most susceptible, particularly when their systemic corticosteroids have been almost completely withdrawn. During this period of HPA suppression, patients may exhibit signs and symptoms of adrenal insufficiency when exposed to trauma, surgery, or infection (particularly gastroenteritis) or other conditions associated with severe electrolyte loss. Although FLOVENT DISKUS may control asthma symptoms during these episodes, in recommended doses it supplies less than normal physiological amounts of glucocorticoid systemically and does NOT provide the mineralocorticoid activity that is necessary for coping with these emergencies.

During periods of stress or a severe asthma attack, patients who have been withdrawn from systemic corticosteroids should be instructed to resume oral corticosteroids (in large doses) immediately and to contact their physicians for further instruction. These patients should also be instructed to carry a warning card indicating that they may need supplementary systemic corticosteroids during periods of stress or a severe asthma attack.

Patients requiring oral corticosteroids should be weaned slowly from systemic corticosteroid use after transferring to FLOVENT DISKUS. Prednisone reduction can be accomplished by reducing the daily prednisone dose by 2.5 mg on a weekly basis during therapy with FLOVENT DISKUS. Lung function (mean forced expiratory volume in 1 second [FEV$_1$] or morning peak expiratory flow [AM PEF]), beta-agonist use, and asthma symptoms should be carefully monitored during withdrawal of oral corticosteroids. In addition, patients should be observed for signs and symptoms of adrenal insufficiency, such as fatigue, lassitude, weakness, nausea and vomiting, and hypotension.

Transfer of patients from systemic corticosteroid therapy to FLOVENT DISKUS may unmask allergic conditions previously suppressed by the systemic corticosteroid therapy (e.g., rhinitis, conjunctivitis, eczema, arthritis, eosinophilic conditions).

During withdrawal from oral corticosteroids, some patients may experience symptoms of systemically active corticosteroid withdrawal (e.g., joint and/or muscular pain, lassitude, depression) despite maintenance or even improvement of respiratory function.

5.5   Hypercorticism and Adrenal Suppression
Fluticasone propionate will often help control asthma symptoms with less suppression of HPA function than therapeutically equivalent oral doses of prednisone. Since fluticasone propionate is absorbed into the circulation and can be systemically active at higher doses, the beneficial effects of FLOVENT DISKUS in minimizing HPA dysfunction may be expected only when recommended dosages are not exceeded and individual patients are titrated to the lowest effective

dose. A relationship between plasma levels of fluticasone propionate and inhibitory effects on stimulated cortisol production has been shown after 4 weeks of treatment with fluticasone propionate inhalation aerosol. Since individual sensitivity to effects on cortisol production exists, physicians should consider this information when prescribing FLOVENT DISKUS.

Because of the possibility of significant systemic absorption of inhaled corticosteroids in sensitive patients, patients treated with FLOVENT DISKUS should be observed carefully for any evidence of systemic corticosteroid effects. Particular care should be taken in observing patients postoperatively or during periods of stress for evidence of inadequate adrenal response.

It is possible that systemic corticosteroid effects such as hypercorticism and adrenal suppression (including adrenal crisis) may appear in a small number of patients who are sensitive to these effects. If such effects occur, FLOVENT DISKUS should be reduced slowly, consistent with accepted procedures for reducing systemic corticosteroids, and other treatments for management of asthma symptoms should be considered.

5.6   Immediate Hypersensitivity Reactions
Immediate hypersensitivity reactions (e.g., urticaria, angioedema, rash, bronchospasm, hypotension), including anaphylaxis, may occur after administration of FLOVENT DISKUS. There have been reports of anaphylactic reactions in patients with severe milk protein allergy after inhalation of powder products containing lactose; therefore, patients with severe milk protein allergy should not use FLOVENT DISKUS [see Contraindications (4)].

5.7   Reduction in Bone Mineral Density
Decreases in bone mineral density (BMD) have been observed with long-term administration of products containing inhaled corticosteroids. The clinical significance of small changes in BMD with regard to long-term consequences such as fracture is unknown. Patients with major risk factors for decreased bone mineral content, such as prolonged immobilization, family history of osteoporosis, postmenopausal status, tobacco use, advanced age, poor nutrition, or chronic use of drugs that can reduce bone mass (e.g., anticonvulsants, oral corticosteroids) should be monitored and treated with established standards of care.

A 2-year trial in 160 subjects (females aged 18 to 40 years, males 18 to 50) with asthma receiving CFC-propelled fluticasone propionate inhalation aerosol 88 or 440 mcg twice daily demonstrated no statistically significant changes in BMD at any time point (24, 52, 76, and 104 weeks of double-blind treatment) as assessed by dual-energy x-ray absorptiometry at lumbar regions L1 through L4.

5.8   Effect on Growth
Orally inhaled corticosteroids may cause a reduction in growth velocity when administered to pediatric patients.

Monitor the growth of pediatric patients receiving FLOVENT DISKUS routinely (e.g., via stadiometry). To minimize the systemic effects of orally inhaled corticosteroids, including FLOVENT DISKUS, titrate each patient's dosage to the lowest dosage that effectively controls his/her symptoms [see Dosage and Administration (2), Use in Specific Populations (8.4)].

5.9   Glaucoma and Cataracts
Glaucoma, increased intraocular pressure, and cataracts have been reported in patients following the long-term administration of inhaled corticosteroids, including fluticasone propionate. Therefore, close monitoring is warranted in patients with a change in vision or with a history of increased intraocular pressure, glaucoma, and/or cataracts.

5.10   Paradoxical Bronchospasm
As with other inhaled medicines, bronchospasm may occur with an immediate increase in wheezing after dosing. If bronchospasm occurs following dosing with FLOVENT DISKUS, it should be treated immediately with an inhaled, short-acting bronchodilator; FLOVENT DISKUS should be discontinued immediately; and alternative therapy should be instituted.

5.11   Drug Interactions With Strong Cytochrome P450 3A4 Inhibitors
The use of strong cytochrome P450 3A4 (CYP3A4) inhibitors (e.g., ritonavir, atazanavir, clarithromycin, indinavir, itraconazole, nefazodone, nelfinavir, saquinavir, ketoconazole, telithromycin) with FLOVENT DISKUS is not recommended because increased systemic corticosteroid adverse effects may occur [see Drug Interactions (7.1), Clinical Pharmacology (12.3)].

5.12   Eosinophilic Conditions and Churg-Strauss Syndrome
In rare cases, patients on inhaled fluticasone propionate may present with systemic eosinophilic conditions. Some of these patients have clinical features of vasculitis consistent with Churg-Strauss syndrome, a condition that is often treated with systemic corticosteroid therapy. These events usually, but not always, have been associated with the reduction and/or withdrawal of oral corticosteroid therapy following the introduction of fluticasone propionate. Cases of serious eosinophilic conditions have also been reported with other inhaled corticosteroids in this clinical setting. Physicians should be alert to eosinophilia, vasculitic rash, worsening pulmonary symptoms, cardiac complications, and/or neuropathy presenting in their patients. A causal relationship between fluticasone propionate and these underlying conditions has not been established.

6   ADVERSE REACTIONS

Systemic and local corticosteroid use may result in the following:

- Candida albicans infection [see Warnings and Precautions (5.1)]
- Immunosuppression [see Warnings and Precautions (5.3)]
- Hypercorticism and adrenal suppression [see Warnings and Precautions (5.5)]
- Reduction in bone mineral density [see Warnings and Precautions (5.7)]
- Growth effects [see Warnings and Precautions (5.8)]
- Glaucoma and cataracts [see Warnings and Precautions (5.9)]

6.1   Clinical Trials Experience
Because clinical trials are conducted under widely varying conditions, adverse reaction rates observed in the clinical trials of a drug cannot be directly compared with rates in the clinical trials of another drug and may not reflect the rates observed in practice.

The incidence of common adverse reactions in Table 2 is based upon 7 placebo-controlled US clinical trials in which 1,176 pediatric, adolescent, and adult subjects (466 females and 710 males) previously treated with as-needed bronchodilators and/or inhaled corticosteroids were treated twice daily for up to 12 weeks with FLOVENT DISKUS (doses of 50 to 500 mcg) or placebo.

[See table 2 above]

Table 2 includes all events (whether considered drug-related or nondrug-related by the investigator) that occurred at a rate of over 3% in any of the groups treated with FLOVENT DISKUS and were more common than in the placebo group. Less than 2% of subjects discontinued from the trials because of adverse reactions. The average duration of exposure was 73 to 79 days in the active treatment groups compared with 56 days in the placebo group.
Additional Adverse Reactions: Other adverse reactions not previously listed, whether considered drug-related or not by the investigators, that were reported more frequently by subjects with asthma treated with FLOVENT DISKUS compared with subjects treated with placebo include the following: palpitations; soft tissue injuries; contusions and hematomas; wounds and lacerations; burns; poisoning and toxicity; pressure-induced disorders; hoarseness/dysphonia; epistaxis; ear, nose, throat, and tonsil signs and symptoms; ear, nose, and throat polyps; allergic ear, nose, and throat

disorders; throat constriction; fluid disturbances; weight gain; appetite disturbances; keratitis and conjunctivitis; blepharoconjunctivitis; gastrointestinal signs and symptoms; oral ulcerations; dental discomfort and pain; oral erythema and rashes; mouth and tongue disorders; oral discomfort and pain; tooth decay; cholecystitis; arthralgia and articular rheumatism; muscle cramps and spasms; musculoskeletal inflammation; dizziness; sleep disorders; migraines; paralysis of cranial nerves; edema and swelling; bacterial infections; fungal infections; mobility disorders; mood disorders; bacterial reproductive infections; photodermatitis; dermatitis and dermatosis; viral skin infections; eczema; pruritus; acne and folliculitis; urinary infections.

Three (3) of the 7 placebo-controlled US clinical trials were pediatric trials. A total of 592 subjects aged 4 to 11 years were treated with FLOVENT DISKUS (dosages of 50 or 100 mcg twice daily) or placebo; an additional 174 subjects aged 4 to 11 years received FLOVENT® ROTADISK® (fluticasone propionate inhalation powder) at the same doses. There were no clinically relevant differences in the pattern or severity of adverse events in children compared with those reported in adults.

In the first 16 weeks of a 52-week clinical trial in adult subjects with asthma who previously required oral corticosteroids (daily doses of 5 to 40 mg oral prednisone), the effects of FLOVENT DISKUS 500 mcg twice daily (n = 41) and 1,000 mcg twice daily (n = 36) were compared with placebo (n = 34) for the frequency of reported adverse events. The average duration of exposure for subjects taking FLOVENT DISKUS was 105 days compared with 75 days for placebo. Adverse events, whether or not considered drug related by the investigators, reported in more than 5 subjects in the group taking FLOVENT DISKUS and that occurred more frequently with FLOVENT DISKUS than with placebo are shown below (percent FLOVENT DISKUS and percent placebo).

Ear, Nose, and Throat: Hoarseness/dysphonia (9% and 0%), nasal congestion/blockage (16% and 0%), oral candidiasis (31% and 21%), rhinitis (13% and 9%), sinusitis/sinus infection (33% and 12%), throat irritation (10% and 9%), and upper respiratory tract infection (31% and 24%).

Gastrointestinal: Nausea and vomiting (9% and 0%).

Lower Respiratory: Cough (9% and 3%) and viral respiratory infections (9% and 6%).

Musculoskeletal: Arthralgia and articular rheumatism (17% and 3%) and muscle pain (12% and 0%).

Non-Site Specific: Malaise and fatigue (16% and 9%) and pain (10% and 3%).

Skin: Pruritus (6% and 0%) and skin rashes (8% and 3%).

6.2 Postmarketing Experience

In addition to adverse reactions reported from clinical trials, the following adverse reactions have been identified during postapproval use of fluticasone propionate. Because these reactions are reported voluntarily from a population of uncertain size, it is not always possible to reliably estimate their frequency or establish a causal relationship to drug exposure. These events have been chosen for inclusion due to either their seriousness, frequency of reporting, or causal connection to fluticasone propionate or a combination of these factors.

Ear, Nose, and Throat: Aphonia, facial and oropharyngeal edema, and throat soreness.

Endocrine and Metabolic: Cushingoid features, growth velocity reduction in children/adolescents, hyperglycemia, and osteoporosis.

Eye: Cataracts.

Immune System Disorders: Immediate and delayed hypersensitivity reactions, including anaphylaxis, rash, angioedema, and bronchospasm, have been reported. Anaphylactic reactions in patients with severe milk protein allergy have been reported.

Infections and Infestations: Esophageal candidiasis

Psychiatry: Agitation, aggression, anxiety, depression, and restlessness. Behavioral changes, including hyperactivity and irritability, have been reported very rarely and primarily in children.

Respiratory: Asthma exacerbation, bronchospasm, chest tightness, dyspnea, immediate bronchospasm, pneumonia, and wheeze.

Skin: Contusions and ecchymoses.

7 DRUG INTERACTIONS

7.1 Inhibitors of Cytochrome P450 3A4

Fluticasone propionate is a substrate of CYP3A4. The use of strong CYP3A4 inhibitors (e.g., ritonavir, atazanavir, clarithromycin, indinavir, itraconazole, nefazodone, nelfinavir, saquinavir, ketoconazole, telithromycin) with FLOVENT DISKUS is not recommended because increased systemic corticosteroid adverse effects may occur.

Ritonavir: A drug interaction trial with fluticasone propionate aqueous nasal spray in healthy subjects has shown that ritonavir (a strong CYP3A4 inhibitor) can significantly increase plasma fluticasone propionate exposure, resulting in significantly reduced serum cortisol concentra-

tions [see Clinical Pharmacology (12.3)]. During postmarketing use, there have been reports of clinically significant drug interactions in patients receiving fluticasone propionate and ritonavir, resulting in systemic corticosteroid effects including Cushing's syndrome and adrenal suppression.

Ketoconazole: Coadministration of orally inhaled fluticasone propionate (1,000 mcg) and ketoconazole (200 mg once daily) resulted in a 1.9-fold increase in plasma fluticasone propionate exposure and a 45% decrease in plasma cortisol area under the curve (AUC), but had no effect on urinary excretion of cortisol.

8 USE IN SPECIFIC POPULATIONS

8.1 Pregnancy

Teratogenic Effects: Pregnancy Category C. There are no adequate and well-controlled trials with FLOVENT DISKUS in pregnant women. Corticosteroids have been shown to be teratogenic in laboratory animals when administered systemically at relatively low dosage levels. Because animal reproduction studies are not always predictive of human response, FLOVENT DISKUS should be used during pregnancy only if the potential benefit justifies the potential risk to the fetus. Women should be advised to contact their physicians if they become pregnant while taking FLOVENT DISKUS.

Mice and rats at fluticasone propionate doses approximately 0.1 and 0.4 times, respectively, the maximum recommended human daily inhalation dose (MRHDID) for adults (on a mg/m² basis at maternal subcutaneous doses of 45 and 100 mcg/kg/day, respectively) showed fetal toxicity characteristic of potent corticosteroid compounds, including embryonic growth retardation, omphalocele, cleft palate, and retarded cranial ossification. No teratogenicity was seen in rats at doses up to 0.3 times the MRHDID (on a mg/m² basis at maternal inhaled doses up to 68.7 mg/kg/day).

In rabbits, fetal weight reduction and cleft palate were observed at a fluticasone propionate dose approximately 0.03 times the MRHDID for adults (on a mg/m² basis at a maternal subcutaneous dose of 4 mcg/kg/day). However, no teratogenic effects were reported at fluticasone propionate doses up to approximately 2 times the MRHDID for adults (on a mg/m² basis at a maternal oral dose up to 300 mcg/kg/day). No fluticasone propionate was detected in the plasma in this study, consistent with the established low bioavailability following oral administration [see Clinical Pharmacology (12.3)].

Fluticasone propionate crossed the placenta following subcutaneous administration to mice and rats and oral administration to rabbits.

Experience with oral corticosteroids since their introduction in pharmacologic, as opposed to physiologic, doses suggests that rodents are more prone to teratogenic effects from corticosteroids than humans. In addition, because there is a natural increase in corticosteroid production during pregnancy, most women will require a lower exogenous corticosteroid dose and many will not need corticosteroid treatment during pregnancy.

Nonteratogenic Effects: Hypoadrenalism may occur in infants born of mothers receiving corticosteroids during pregnancy. Such infants should be carefully monitored.

8.3 Nursing Mothers

It is not known whether fluticasone propionate is excreted in human breast milk. However, other corticosteroids have been detected in human milk. Subcutaneous administration to lactating rats of tritiated fluticasone propionate at a dose approximately 0.04 times the MRHDID for adults on a mg/m² basis resulted in measurable radioactivity in milk.

Since there are no data from controlled trials on the use of FLOVENT DISKUS by nursing mothers, caution should be exercised when FLOVENT DISKUS is administered to a nursing woman.

8.4 Pediatric Use

The safety and effectiveness of FLOVENT DISKUS in children aged 4 years and older have been established [see Adverse Reactions (6.1), Clinical Pharmacology (12.3), Clinical Studies (14.2)]. The safety and effectiveness of FLOVENT DISKUS in children younger than 4 years have not been established.

Effects on Growth: Orally inhaled corticosteroids may cause a reduction in growth velocity when administered to pediatric patients. A reduction of growth velocity in children or teenagers may occur as a result of poorly controlled asthma or from use of corticosteroids, including inhaled corticosteroids. The effects of long-term treatment of children and adolescents with inhaled corticosteroids, including fluticasone propionate, on final adult height are not known. Controlled clinical trials have shown that inhaled corticosteroids may cause a reduction in growth in pediatric patients. In these trials, the mean reduction in growth velocity was approximately 1 cm/year (range: 0.3 to 1.8 cm/year) and appeared to depend upon dose and duration of exposure. This effect was observed in the absence of laboratory evidence of HPA axis suppression, suggesting that growth ve-

locity is a more sensitive indicator of systemic corticosteroid exposure in pediatric patients than some commonly used tests of HPA axis function. The long-term effects of this reduction in growth velocity associated with orally inhaled corticosteroids, including the impact on final adult height, are unknown. The potential for "catch-up" growth following discontinuation of treatment with orally inhaled corticosteroids has not been adequately studied. The effects on growth velocity of treatment with orally inhaled corticosteroids for over 1 year, including the impact on final adult height, are unknown. The growth of children and adolescents receiving orally inhaled corticosteroids, including FLOVENT DISKUS, should be monitored routinely (e.g., via stadiometry). The potential growth effects of prolonged treatment should be weighed against the clinical benefits obtained and the risks associated with alternative therapies. To minimize the systemic effects of orally inhaled corticosteroids, including FLOVENT DISKUS, each patient should be titrated to the lowest dose that effectively controls his/her symptoms. A 52-week placebo-controlled trial to assess the potential growth effects of fluticasone propionate inhalation powder (FLOVENT ROTADISK) at 50 and 100 mcg twice daily was conducted in the US in 325 prepubescent children (244 males and 81 females) aged 4 to 11 years. The mean growth velocities at 52 weeks observed in the intent-to-treat population were 6.32 cm/year in the placebo group (n = 76), 6.07 cm/year in the 50-mcg group (n = 98), and 5.66 cm/year in the 100-mcg group (n = 89). An imbalance in the proportion of children entering puberty between groups and a higher dropout rate in the placebo group due to poorly controlled asthma may be confounding factors in interpreting these data. A separate subset analysis of children who remained prepubertal during the trial revealed growth rates at 52 weeks of 6.10 cm/year in the placebo group (n = 57), 5.91 cm/year in the 50-mcg group (n = 74), and 5.67 cm/year in the 100-mcg group (n = 79). In children aged 8.5 years, the mean age of children in this trial, the range for expected growth velocity is: boys – 3rd percentile = 3.8 cm/year, 50th percentile = 5.4 cm/year, and 97th percentile = 7.0 cm/year; girls – 3rd percentile = 4.2 cm/year, 50th percentile = 5.7 cm/year, and 97th percentile = 7.3 cm/year. The clinical relevance of these growth data is not certain.

8.5 Geriatric Use

Safety data have been collected on 280 subjects (FLOVENT DISKUS n = 83, FLOVENT Rotadisk n = 197) aged 65 years and older and 33 subjects (FLOVENT DISKUS n = 14, FLOVENT ROTADISK n = 19) aged 75 years and older who have been treated with fluticasone propionate inhalation powder in US and non-US clinical trials. No overall differences in safety or effectiveness were observed between these subjects and younger subjects, and other reported clinical experience has not identified differences in responses between the elderly and younger subjects, but greater sensitivity of some older individuals cannot be ruled out.

8.6 Hepatic Impairment

Formal pharmacokinetic studies using FLOVENT DISKUS have not been conducted in patients with hepatic impairment. Since fluticasone propionate is predominantly cleared by hepatic metabolism, impairment of liver function may lead to accumulation of fluticasone propionate in plasma. Therefore, patients with hepatic disease should be closely monitored.

8.7 Renal Impairment

Formal pharmacokinetic studies using FLOVENT DISKUS have not been conducted in patients with renal impairment.

10 OVERDOSAGE

Chronic overdosage may result in signs/symptoms of hypercorticism [see Warnings and Precautions (5.5)]. Inhalation by healthy volunteers of a single dose of 4,000 mcg of fluticasone propionate inhalation powder or single doses of 1,760 or 3,520 mcg of fluticasone propionate CFC inhalation aerosol was well tolerated. Fluticasone propionate given by inhalation aerosol at dosages of 1,320 mcg twice daily for 7 to 15 days to healthy human volunteers was also well tolerated. Repeat oral doses up to 80 mg daily for 10 days in healthy volunteers and repeat oral doses up to 20 mg daily for 42 days in subjects were well tolerated. Adverse reactions were of mild or moderate severity, and incidences were similar in active and placebo treatment groups.

11 DESCRIPTION

The active component of FLOVENT DISKUS 50 mcg, FLOVENT DISKUS 100 mcg, and FLOVENT DISKUS 250 mcg is fluticasone propionate, a corticosteroid having the chemical name S-(fluoromethyl) 6α,9-difluoro-11β,17-dihydroxy-16α-methyl-3-oxoandrosta-1,4-diene-17β-carbothioate, 17-propionate and the following chemical structure: [See chemical structure at top of next column]

Fluticasone propionate is a white powder with a molecular weight of 500.6, and the empirical formula is $C_{25}H_{31}F_3O_5S$. It is practically insoluble in water, freely soluble in dimethyl sulfoxide and dimethylformamide, and slightly soluble in methanol and 95% ethanol.

FLOVENT DISKUS is an orange plastic inhaler containing a foil blister strip. Each blister on the strip contains a white powder mix of micronized fluticasone propionate (50, 100, or 250 mcg) in 12.5 mg of formulation containing lactose monohydrate (which contains milk proteins). After the inhaler is activated, the powder is dispersed into the airstream created by the patient inhaling through the mouthpiece.

Under standardized in vitro test conditions, FLOVENT DISKUS delivers 46, 94, and 229 mcg of fluticasone propionate from FLOVENT DISKUS 50 mcg, FLOVENT DISKUS 100 mcg, and FLOVENT DISKUS 250 mcg, respectively, when tested at a flow rate of 60 L/min for 2 seconds.

In adult subjects with obstructive lung disease and severely compromised lung function (mean FEV_1 20% to 30% of predicted), mean peak inspiratory flow (PIF) through the DISKUS® inhaler was 82.4 L/min (range: 46.1 to 115.3 L/min). In children with asthma aged 4 and 8 years, mean PIF through FLOVENT DISKUS was 70 and 104 L/min, respectively (range: 48 to 123 L/min).

The actual amount of drug delivered to the lung will depend on patient factors, such as inspiratory flow profile.

12   CLINICAL PHARMACOLOGY
12.1   Mechanism of Action

Fluticasone propionate is a synthetic trifluorinated corticosteroid with anti-inflammatory activity. Fluticasone propionate has been shown in vitro to exhibit a binding affinity for the human glucocorticoid receptor that is 18 times that of dexamethasone, almost twice that of beclomethasone-17-monopropionate (BMP), the active metabolite of beclomethasone dipropionate, and over 3 times that of budesonide. Data from the McKenzie vasoconstrictor assay in man are consistent with these results. The clinical significance of these findings is unknown.

Inflammation is an important component in the pathogenesis of asthma. Corticosteroids have been shown to have a wide range of actions on multiple cell types (e.g., mast cells, eosinophils, neutrophils, macrophages, lymphocytes) and mediators (e.g., histamine, eicosanoids, leukotrienes, cytokines) involved in inflammation. These anti–inflammatory actions of corticosteroids contribute to their efficacy in asthma.

Though effective for the treatment of asthma, corticosteroids do not affect asthma symptoms immediately. Individual patients will experience a variable time to onset and degree of symptom relief. Maximum benefit may not be achieved for 1 to 2 weeks or longer after starting treatment. When corticosteroids are discontinued, asthma stability may persist for several days or longer.

Trials in subjects with asthma have shown a favorable ratio between topical anti-inflammatory activity and systemic corticosteroid effects with recommended doses of orally inhaled fluticasone propionate. This is explained by a combination of a relatively high local anti-inflammatory effect, negligible oral systemic bioavailability (<1%), and the minimal pharmacological activity of the only metabolite detected in man.

12.2   Pharmacodynamics

In clinical trials with fluticasone propionate inhalation powder using dosages up to and including 250 mcg twice daily, occasional abnormal short cosyntropin tests (peak serum cortisol <18 mcg/dL assessed by radioimmunoassay) were noted both in subjects receiving fluticasone propionate and in subjects receiving placebo. The incidence of abnormal tests at 500 mcg twice daily was greater than placebo. In a 2-year trial carried out with the DISKHALER® inhalation device in 64 subjects with mild, persistent asthma (mean FEV_1 91% of predicted) randomized to fluticasone propionate 500 mcg twice daily or placebo, no subject receiving fluticasone propionate had an abnormal response to 6-hour cosyntropin infusion (peak serum cortisol <18 mcg/dL). With a peak cortisol threshold of <35 mcg/dL, 1 subject receiving fluticasone propionate (4%) had an abnormal response at 1 year; repeat testing at 18 months and 2 years was normal. Another subject receiving fluticasone propionate (5%) had an abnormal response at 2 years. No subject on placebo had an abnormal response at 1 or 2 years.

In a placebo-controlled clinical trial conducted in subjects aged 4 to 11 years, a 30-minute cosyntropin stimulation test was performed in 41 subjects after 12 weeks of dosing with 50 or 100 mcg twice daily of fluticasone propionate via the DISKUS inhaler. One subject receiving fluticasone propionate via the DISKUS inhaler had a prestimulation

plasma cortisol concentration <5 mcg/dL, and 2 subjects had a rise in cortisol of <7 mcg/dL. However, all poststimulation values were >18 mcg/dL.

The potential systemic effects of inhaled fluticasone propionate on the HPA axis were also studied in subjects with asthma. Fluticasone propionate given by inhalation aerosol at dosages of 220, 440, 660, or 880 mcg twice daily was compared with placebo or oral prednisone 10 mg given once daily for 4 weeks. For most subjects, the ability to increase cortisol production in response to stress, as assessed by 6-hour cosyntropin stimulation, remained intact with inhaled fluticasone propionate treatment. No subject had an abnormal response (peak serum cortisol <18 mcg/dL) after dosing with placebo or fluticasone propionate 220 mcg twice daily. For subjects treated with 440, 660, and 880 mcg twice daily, 10%, 16%, and 12%, respectively, had an abnormal response as compared with 29% of subjects treated with prednisone.

12.3   Pharmacokinetics

Absorption: Fluticasone propionate acts locally in the lung; therefore, plasma levels do not predict therapeutic effect. Trials using oral dosing of labeled and unlabeled drug have demonstrated that the oral systemic bioavailability of fluticasone propionate is negligible (<1%), primarily due to incomplete absorption and presystemic metabolism in the gut and liver. In contrast, the majority of the fluticasone propionate delivered to the lung is systemically absorbed. The absolute bioavailability of fluticasone propionate from the DISKUS inhaler in healthy volunteers averages 7.8%. Peak steady-state fluticasone propionate plasma concentrations in adult subjects with asthma (N = 11) ranged from undetectable to 266 pg/mL after a 500-mcg twice-daily dose of fluticasone propionate inhalation powder using the DISKUS inhaler. The mean fluticasone propionate plasma concentration was 110 pg/mL.

Distribution: Following intravenous administration, the initial disposition phase for fluticasone propionate was rapid and consistent with its high lipid solubility and tissue binding. The volume of distribution averaged 4.2 L/kg.

The percentage of fluticasone propionate bound to human plasma proteins averages 99%. Fluticasone propionate is weakly and reversibly bound to erythrocytes and is not significantly bound to human transcortin.

Metabolism: The total clearance of fluticasone propionate is high (average, 1,093 mL/min), with renal clearance accounting for less than 0.02% of the total. The only circulating metabolite detected in man is the 17β-carboxylic acid derivative of fluticasone propionate, which is formed through the CYP3A4 pathway. This metabolite had less affinity (approximately 1/2,000) than the parent drug for the glucocorticoid receptor of human lung cytosol in vitro and negligible pharmacological activity in animal studies. Other metabolites detected in vitro using cultured human hepatoma cells have not been detected in man.

Elimination: Following intravenous dosing, fluticasone propionate showed polyexponential kinetics and had a terminal elimination half-life of approximately 7.8 hours. Less than 5% of a radiolabeled oral dose was excreted in the urine as metabolites, with the remainder excreted in the feces as parent drug and metabolites.

Special Populations: Gender: Full pharmacokinetic profiles were obtained from 9 female and 16 male subjects given 500 mcg twice daily. No overall differences in fluticasone propionate pharmacokinetics were observed.

Pediatrics: In a clinical trial conducted in subjects aged 4 to 11 years with mild to moderate asthma, fluticasone propionate concentrations were obtained in 61 subjects at 20 and 40 minutes after dosing with 50 and 100 mcg twice daily of fluticasone propionate inhalation powder using the DISKUS. Plasma concentrations were low and ranged from undetectable (about 80% of the plasma samples) to 88 pg/mL. Mean peak fluticasone propionate plasma concentrations at the 50- and 100-mcg dose levels were 5 and 8 pg/mL, respectively.

Hepatic and Renal Impairment: Formal pharmacokinetic studies using FLOVENT DISKUS have not been conducted in patients with hepatic or renal impairment. However, since fluticasone propionate is predominantly cleared by hepatic metabolism, impairment of liver function may lead to accumulation of fluticasone propionate in plasma. Therefore, patients with hepatic disease should be closely monitored.

Drug Interactions: Inhibitors of Cytochrome P450 3A4: Ritonavir: Fluticasone propionate is a substrate of CYP3A4. Coadministration of fluticasone propionate and the strong CYP3A4 inhibitor ritonavir is not recommended based upon a multiple-dose, crossover drug interaction trial in 18 healthy subjects. Fluticasone propionate aqueous nasal spray (200 mcg once daily) was coadministered for 7 days with ritonavir (100 mg twice daily). Plasma fluticasone propionate concentrations following fluticasone propionate aqueous nasal spray alone were undetectable (<10 pg/mL) in most subjects, and when concentrations were detectable, peak levels (C_{max}) averaged 11.9 pg/mL (range: 10.8 to

14.1 pg/mL) and $AUC_{(0-\tau)}$ averaged 8.43 pg•h/mL (range: 4.2 to 18.8 pg•h/mL). Fluticasone propionate C_{max} and $AUC_{(0-\tau)}$ increased to 318 pg/mL (range: 110 to 648 pg/mL) and 3,102.6 pg•h/mL (range: 1,207.1 to 5,662.0 pg•h/mL), respectively, after coadministration of ritonavir with fluticasone propionate aqueous nasal spray. This significant increase in plasma fluticasone propionate exposure resulted in a significant decrease (86%) in serum cortisol AUC.

Ketoconazole: In a placebo-controlled, crossover trial in 8 healthy adult volunteers, coadministration of a single dose of orally inhaled fluticasone propionate (1,000 mcg) with multiple doses of ketoconazole (200 mg) to steady state resulted in increased plasma fluticasone propionate exposure, a reduction in plasma cortisol AUC, and no effect on urinary excretion of cortisol.

Following orally inhaled fluticasone propionate alone, $AUC_{(2-last)}$ averaged 1.559 ng•h/mL (range: 0.555 to 2.906 ng•h/mL) and $AUC_{(2-\infty)}$ averaged 2.269 ng•h/mL (range: 0.836 to 3.707 ng•h/mL). Fluticasone propionate $AUC_{(2-last)}$ and $AUC_{(2-\infty)}$ increased to 2.781 ng•h/mL (range: 2.489 to 8.486 ng•h/mL) and 4.317 ng•h/mL (range: 3.256 to 9.408 ng•h/mL), respectively, after coadministration of ketoconazole with orally inhaled fluticasone propionate. This increase in plasma fluticasone propionate concentration resulted in a decrease (45%) in serum cortisol AUC.

Erythromycin: In a multiple-dose drug interaction trial, coadministration of orally inhaled fluticasone propionate (500 mcg twice daily) and erythromycin (333 mg 3 times daily) did not affect fluticasone propionate pharmacokinetics.

13   NONCLINICAL TOXICOLOGY
13.1   Carcinogenesis, Mutagenesis, Impairment of Fertility

Fluticasone propionate demonstrated no tumorigenic potential in mice at oral doses up to 1,000 mcg/kg (approximately 2 and 10 times the MRHDID for adults and children aged 4 to 11 years, respectively, on a mg/m^2 basis) for 78 weeks or in rats at inhalation doses up to 57 mcg/kg (approximately 0.2 times and approximately equivalent to the MRHDID for adults and children aged 4 to 11 years, respectively, on a mg/m^2 basis) for 104 weeks.

Fluticasone propionate did not induce gene mutation in prokaryotic or eukaryotic cells in vitro. No significant clastogenic effect was seen in cultured human peripheral lymphocytes in vitro or in the in vivo mouse micronucleus test.

No evidence of impairment of fertility was observed in male and female rats at subcutaneous doses up to 50 mcg/kg (approximately 0.2 times the MRHDID for adults on a mg/m^2 basis). Prostate weight was significantly reduced.

14   CLINICAL STUDIES
14.1   Adult and Adolescent Subjects Aged 12 Years and Older

Four randomized, double-blind, parallel-group, placebo-controlled, US clinical trials were conducted in 1,036 adult and adolescent subjects (aged 12 years and older) with asthma to assess the efficacy and safety of FLOVENT DISKUS in the treatment of asthma. Fixed dosages of 100, 250, and 500 mcg twice daily were compared with placebo to provide information about appropriate dosing to cover a range of asthma severity. Subjects in these trials included those inadequately controlled with bronchodilators alone and those already maintained on daily inhaled corticosteroids. All doses were delivered by inhalation of the contents of 1 or 2 blisters from FLOVENT DISKUS twice daily.

Figures 1 through 4 display results of pulmonary function tests (mean percent change from baseline in FEV_1 prior to AM dose) for 3 recommended dosages of FLOVENT DISKUS (100, 250, and 500 mcg twice daily) and placebo from the four 12-week trials in adolescents and adults. These trials used predetermined criteria for lack of efficacy (indicators of worsening asthma), resulting in withdrawal of more patients in the placebo group. Therefore, pulmonary function results at Endpoint (the last evaluable FEV_1 result, including most patients' lung function data) are also displayed. Pulmonary function, as determined by percent change from baseline in FEV_1 at recommended dosages of FLOVENT DISKUS improved significantly compared with placebo by the first week of treatment, and improvement was maintained for up to 1 year or more.

[See figure 1 at top of next column]
[See figure 2 at top of next column]
[See figure 3 at top of next column]
[See figure 4 at top of next column]

In all 4 efficacy trials, measures of pulmonary function (FEV_1) were statistically significantly improved as compared with placebo at all twice-daily doses. Subjects on all dosages of FLOVENT DISKUS were also less likely to discontinue study participation due to asthma deterioration (as defined by predetermined criteria for lack of efficacy including lung function and subject-recorded variables such as AM PEF, albuterol use, and nighttime awakenings due to asthma) compared with placebo.

In a clinical trial of 111 subjects with severe asthma requiring chronic oral corticosteroid therapy (average baseline daily prednisone dose was 14 mg), fluticasone propionate given by inhalation powder at doses of 500 and 1,000 mcg twice daily

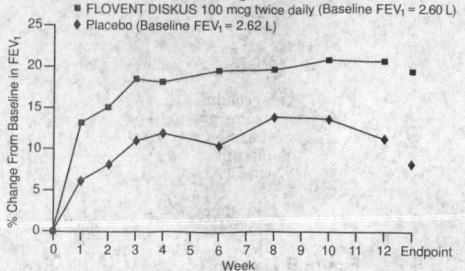

Figure 1. A 12-Week Clinical Trial Evaluating FLOVENT DISKUS 100 mcg Twice Daily in Adults and Adolescents Receiving Bronchodilators Alone

Figure 2. A 12-Week Clinical Trial Evaluating FLOVENT DISKUS 100 mcg Twice Daily in Adults and Adolescents Receiving Inhaled Corticosteroids

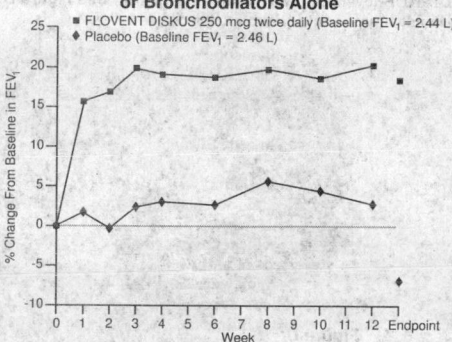

Figure 3. A 12-Week Clinical Trial Evaluating FLOVENT DISKUS 250 mcg Twice Daily in Adults and Adolescents Receiving Inhaled Corticosteroids or Bronchodilators Alone

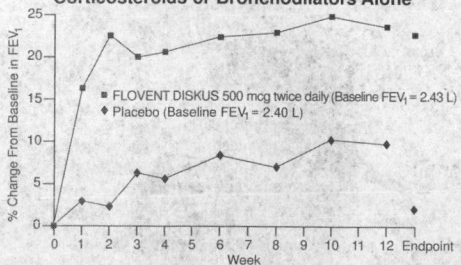

Figure 4. A 12-Week Clinical Trial Evaluating FLOVENT DISKUS 500 mcg Twice Daily in Adults and Adolescents Receiving Inhaled Corticosteroids or Bronchodilators Alone

was evaluated. Both doses enabled a statistically significantly larger percentage of subjects to wean from oral prednisone as compared with placebo (75% of the subjects on 500 mcg twice daily and 89% of the subjects on 1,000 mcg twice daily as compared with 9% of subjects on placebo). Accompanying the reduction in oral corticosteroid use, subjects treated with fluticasone propionate had significantly improved lung function and fewer asthma symptoms as compared with the placebo group.

14.2   Pediatric Subjects Aged 4 to 11 Years
A 12-week, placebo-controlled clinical trial was conducted in 437 pediatric subjects (177 received FLOVENT DISKUS), approximately half of whom were receiving inhaled corticosteroids at baseline. In this trial, doses of fluticasone propionate inhalation powder 50 and 100 mcg twice daily significantly improved FEV_1 (15% and 18% change from baseline at Endpoint, respectively) compared with placebo

(7% change). AM PEF was also significantly improved with doses of fluticasone propionate 50 and 100 mcg twice daily (26% and 27% change from baseline at Endpoint, respectively) compared with placebo (14% change). In this trial, subjects on active treatment were significantly less likely to discontinue treatment due to asthma deterioration (as defined by predetermined criteria for lack of efficacy including lung function and subject-recorded variables such as AM PEF, albuterol use, and nighttime awakenings due to asthma).

Two other 12-week placebo-controlled clinical trials were conducted in 504 pediatric subjects with asthma, approximately half of whom were receiving inhaled corticosteroids at baseline. In these trials, FLOVENT DISKUS was efficacious at doses of 50 and 100 mcg twice daily when compared with placebo on major endpoints including lung function and symptom scores. Pulmonary function improved significantly compared with placebo by the first week of treatment, and subjects treated with FLOVENT DISKUS were also less likely to discontinue trial participation due to asthma deterioration. One hundred ninety-two (192) subjects received FLOVENT DISKUS for up to 1 year during an open-label extension. Data from this open-label extension suggested that lung function improvements could be maintained up to 1 year.

16   HOW SUPPLIED/STORAGE AND HANDLING

FLOVENT DISKUS 50 mcg is supplied as a disposable orange plastic inhaler containing a foil blister strip with 60 blisters. The inhaler is packaged in a plastic-coated, moisture-protective foil pouch (NDC 0173-0600-02).

FLOVENT DISKUS 100 mcg is supplied as a disposable orange plastic inhaler containing a foil blister strip with 60 blisters. The inhaler is packaged in a plastic-coated, moisture-protective foil pouch (NDC 0173-0602-02). FLOVENT DISKUS 100 mcg is also supplied in an institutional pack containing 28 blisters (NDC 0173-0602-00).

FLOVENT DISKUS 250 mcg is supplied as a disposable orange plastic inhaler containing a foil blister strip with 60 blisters. The inhaler is packaged in a plastic-coated, moisture-protective foil pouch (NDC 0173-0601-02). FLOVENT DISKUS 250 mcg is also supplied in an institutional pack containing 28 blisters (NDC 0173-0601-00).

Store at room temperature between 68°F and 77°F (20°C and 25°C); excursions permitted from 59°F to 86°F (15°C to 30°C) [See USP Controlled Room Temperature]. Store in a dry place away from direct heat or sunlight. Keep out of reach of children.

FLOVENT DISKUS should be stored inside the unopened moisture-protective foil pouch and only removed from the pouch immediately before initial use. Discard FLOVENT DISKUS 6 weeks (50-mcg strength) or 2 months (100- and 250-mcg strengths) after opening the foil pouch or when the counter reads "0" (after all blisters have been used), whichever comes first. The inhaler is not reusable. Do not attempt to take the inhaler apart.

17   PATIENT COUNSELING INFORMATION

Advise the patient to read the FDA-approved patient labeling (Patient Information and Instructions for Use).

Local Effects: Inform patients that localized infections with *Candida albicans* occurred in the mouth and pharynx in some patients. If oropharyngeal candidiasis develops, treat it with appropriate local or systemic (i.e., oral) antifungal therapy while still continuing therapy with FLOVENT DISKUS, but at times therapy with FLOVENT DISKUS may need to be temporarily interrupted under close medical supervision. Rinsing the mouth with water without swallowing after inhalation is advised to help reduce the risk of thrush.

Status Asthmaticus and Acute Asthma Symptoms: Inform patients that FLOVENT DISKUS is not a bronchodilator and is not intended for use as rescue medicine for acute asthma exacerbations. Advise patients to treat acute asthma symptoms with an inhaled, short-acting beta$_2$-agonist such as albuterol. Instruct patients to contact their physicians immediately if there is deterioration of their asthma.

Immunosuppression: Warn patients who are on immunosuppressant doses of corticosteroids to avoid exposure to chickenpox or measles and, if exposed, to consult their physicians without delay. Inform patients of potential worsening of existing tuberculosis; fungal, bacterial, viral, or parasitic infections; or ocular herpes simplex.

Hypercorticism and Adrenal Suppression: Advise patients that FLOVENT DISKUS may cause systemic corticosteroid effects of hypercorticism and adrenal suppression. Additionally, inform patients that deaths due to adrenal insufficiency have occurred during and after transfer from systemic corticosteroids. Patients should taper slowly from systemic corticosteroids if transferring to FLOVENT DISKUS.

Immediate Hypersensitivity Reactions: Advise patients that immediate hypersensitivity reactions (e.g., urticaria,

angioedema, rash, bronchospasm, hypotension), including anaphylaxis, may occur after administration of FLOVENT DISKUS. Patients should discontinue FLOVENT DISKUS if such reactions occur. There have been reports of anaphylactic reactions in patients with severe milk protein allergy after inhalation of powder products containing lactose; therefore, patients with severe milk protein allergy should not take FLOVENT DISKUS.

Reduction in Bone Mineral Density: Advise patients who are at an increased risk for decreased BMD that the use of corticosteroids may pose an additional risk.

Reduced Growth Velocity: Inform patients that orally inhaled corticosteroids, including FLOVENT DISKUS, may cause a reduction in growth velocity when administered to pediatric patients. Physicians should closely follow the growth of children and adolescents taking corticosteroids by any route.

Ocular Effects: Long-term use of inhaled corticosteroids may increase the risk of some eye problems (cataracts or glaucoma); consider regular eye examinations.

Use Daily for Best Effect: Patients should use Flovent DISKUS at regular intervals as directed. Individual patients will experience a variable time to onset and degree of symptom relief and the full benefit may not be achieved until treatment has been administered for 1 to 2 weeks or longer. Patients should not increase the prescribed dosage but should contact their physicians if symptoms do not improve or if the condition worsens. Instruct patients not to stop use of FLOVENT DISKUS abruptly. Patients should contact their physicians immediately if they discontinue use of FLOVENT DISKUS.

DISKHALER, DISKUS, FLOVENT, and ROTADISK are registered trademarks of the GSK group of companies.
GlaxoSmithKline
Research Triangle Park, NC 27709
©2014, the GSK group of companies. All rights reserved.
FLD:8PI

Patient Information
FLOVENT® DISKUS *[flō′ ventdisk′ us]* **50 mcg**
(fluticasone propionate inhalation powder, 50 mcg)
FLOVENT® DISKUS® 100 mcg
(fluticasone propionate inhalation powder, 100 mcg)
FLOVENT® DISKUS® 250 mcg
(fluticasone propionate inhalation powder, 250 mcg)
Read the Patient Information that comes with FLOVENT DISKUS before you start using it and each time you get a refill. There may be new information. This Patient Information does not take the place of talking to your healthcare provider about your medical condition or treatment.

What is FLOVENT DISKUS?
FLOVENT DISKUS is a prescription inhaled corticosteroid (ICS) medicine for the long-term treatment of asthma in people aged 4 years and older.
• ICS medicines such as fluticasone propionate help to decrease inflammation in the lungs. Inflammation in the lungs can lead to breathing problems.
• FLOVENT DISKUS is not used to relieve sudden breathing problems.
• It is not known if FLOVENT DISKUS is safe and effective in children younger than 4 years of age.

Who should not use FLOVENT DISKUS?
Do not use FLOVENT DISKUS if you:
• have a severe allergy to milk proteins. Ask your healthcare provider if you are not sure.
• are allergic to fluticasone propionate or any of the ingredients in FLOVENT DISKUS. See "What are the ingredients in FLOVENT DISKUS?" below for a complete list of ingredients.

What should I tell my healthcare provider before using FLOVENT DISKUS?
Tell your healthcare provider about all of your health conditions, including if you:
• have liver problems.
• have weak bones (osteoporosis).
• have an immune system problem.
• have eye problems such as glaucoma or cataracts.
• are allergic to any of the ingredients in FLOVENT DISKUS, any other medicines, or food products. See "What are the ingredients in FLOVENT DISKUS?" below for a complete list of ingredients.
• have any type of viral, bacterial, or fungal infection.
• are exposed to chickenpox or measles.
• have any other medical conditions.
• are pregnant or planning to become pregnant. It is not known if FLOVENT DISKUS may harm your unborn baby.
• are breastfeeding. It is not known if the medicine in FLOVENT DISKUS passes into your milk and if it can harm your baby.

Tell your healthcare provider about all the medicines you take, including prescription and over-the-counter medicines, vitamins, and herbal supplements. FLOVENT DISKUS and certain other medicines may interact with each other. This may cause serious side effects. Especially, tell your health-care provider if you take antifungal or anti-HIV medicines. Know the medicines you take. Keep a list of them to show your healthcare provider and pharmacist when you get a new medicine.

How should I use FLOVENT DISKUS?
Read the step-by-step instructions for using FLOVENT DISKUS at the end of this Patient Information.
• **Do not** use FLOVENT DISKUS unless your healthcare provider has taught you how to use the inhaler and you understand how to use it correctly.
• Children should use FLOVENT DISKUS with an adult's help, as instructed by the child's healthcare provider.
• Flovent DISKUS comes in 3 different strengths. Your healthcare provider prescribed the strength that is best for you.
• Use FLOVENT DISKUS exactly as your healthcare provider tells you to use it. **Do not** use FLOVENT DISKUS more often than prescribed.
• It may take 1 to 2 weeks or longer after you start FLOVENT DISKUS for your asthma symptoms to get better. You must use FLOVENT DISKUS regularly.
• **Do not** stop using FLOVENT DISKUS, even if you are feeling better, unless your healthcare provider tells you to.
• If you miss a dose of FLOVENT DISKUS, just skip that dose. Take your next dose at your usual time. Do not take 2 doses at 1 time.
• **FLOVENT DISKUS does not relieve sudden symptoms.** Always have a rescue inhaler with you to treat sudden symptoms. If you do not have a rescue inhaler, call your healthcare provider to have one prescribed for you.
• Call your healthcare provider or get medical care right away if:
  • your breathing problems get worse.
  • you need to use your rescue inhaler more often than usual.
  • your rescue inhaler does not work as well to relieve your symptoms.
  • you need to use 4 or more inhalations of your rescue inhaler in 24 hours for 2 or more days in a row.
  • you use 1 whole canister of your rescue inhaler in 8 weeks.
  • your peak flow meter results decrease. Your healthcare provider will tell you the numbers that are right for you.

What are the possible side effects with FLOVENT DISKUS?
FLOVENT DISKUS can cause serious side effects, including:
• **fungal infection in your mouth or throat (thrush).** Rinse your mouth with water without swallowing after using FLOVENT DISKUS to help reduce your chance of getting thrush.
• **weakened immune system and increased chance of getting infections (immunosuppression)**
• **reduced adrenal function (adrenal insufficiency).** Adrenal insufficiency is a condition where the adrenal glands do not make enough steroid hormones. This can happen when you stop taking oral corticosteroid medicines (such as prednisone) and start taking a medicine containing an inhaled steroid (such as FLOVENT DISKUS). When your body is under stress such as from fever, trauma (such as a car accident), infection, or surgery, adrenal insufficiency can get worse and may cause death.
Symptoms of adrenal insufficiency include:
  • feeling tired
  • lack of energy
  • weakness
  • nausea and vomiting
  • low blood pressure
• **serious allergic reactions.** Call your healthcare provider or get emergency medical care if you get any of the following symptoms of a serious allergic reaction:
  • rash
  • hives
  • swelling of your face, mouth, and tongue
  • breathing problems
• **bone thinning or weakness (osteoporosis)**
• **slowed growth in children. A child's growth should be checked often.**
• **eye problems including glaucoma and cataracts.** You should have regular eye exams while using FLOVENT DISKUS.
• **increased wheezing (bronchospasm).** Increased wheezing can happen right away after using FLOVENT DISKUS. Always have a rescue inhaler with you to treat sudden wheezing.
Common side effects of FLOVENT DISKUS include:
• upper respiratory tract infection
• throat irritation
• nausea and vomiting
• fever
• headache
Tell your healthcare provider about any side effect that bothers you or that does not go away.
These are not all the side effects with FLOVENT DISKUS. Ask your healthcare provider or pharmacist for more information.

Call your doctor for medical advice about side effects. You may report side effects to FDA at 1-800-FDA-1088.
How should I store FLOVENT DISKUS?
• Store FLOVENT DISKUS at room temperature between 68°F and 77°F (20°C and 25°C). Keep in a dry place away from heat and sunlight.
• Store FLOVENT DISKUS in the unopened foil pouch and only open when ready for use.
• Safely throw away FLOVENT DISKUS 50 mcg in the trash **6 weeks** after you open the foil pouch or when the counter reads **0**, whichever comes first.
• Safely throw away FLOVENT DISKUS 100 mcg and FLOVENT DISKUS 250 mcg in the trash **2 months** after you open the foil pouch or when the counter reads **0**, whichever comes first.
• **Keep FLOVENT DISKUS and all medicines out of the reach of children.**
  General information about FLOVENT DISKUS
Medicines are sometimes prescribed for purposes not mentioned in a Patient Information leaflet. Do not use FLOVENT DISKUS for a condition for which it was not prescribed. Do not give your FLOVENT DISKUS to other people, even if they have the same condition that you have. It may harm them.
This Patient Information leaflet summarizes the most important information about FLOVENT DISKUS. If you would like more information, talk with your healthcare provider or pharmacist. You can ask your healthcare provider or pharmacist for information about FLOVENT DISKUS that was written for healthcare professionals.
For more information about FLOVENT DISKUS, call 1-888-825-5249 or visit our website at www.floventdiskus.com.
What are the ingredients in FLOVENT DISKUS?
Active ingredient: fluticasone propionate
Inactive ingredient: lactose monohydrate (contains milk proteins)
Instructions for Use
For Oral Inhalation Only
Your FLOVENT DISKUS inhaler

Figure A

Read this information before you start using your FLOVENT DISKUS inhaler:
• Take FLOVENT DISKUS out of the foil pouch just before you use it for the first time. Safely throw away the pouch. The DISKUS will be in the closed position.
• Write the date you opened the foil pouch in the first blank line on the label. **See Figure A.**
• Write the "use by" date in the second blank line on the label. **See Figure A.** If you are using FLOVENT DISKUS 50 mcg, that date is 6 weeks after the date you wrote in the first line. If you are using FLOVENT DISKUS 100 mcg or 250 mcg, that date is 2 months after the date you wrote in the first line.
• The counter should read **60**. If you have a sample (with "Sample" on the back label) or institutional (with "INSTITUTIONAL PACK" on the foil pouch) pack, the counter should read **28**.
How to use your FLOVENT DISKUS inhaler
Follow these steps every time you use FLOVENT DISKUS.
Step 1. Open your FLOVENT DISKUS.
• Hold the DISKUS in your left hand and place the thumb of your right hand in the thumb grip. Push the thumb grip away from you as far as it will go until the mouthpiece shows and snaps into place. **See Figure B.**
[See figure B at top of next column]
Step 2. Slide the lever until you hear it click.
• Hold the Diskus in a level, flat position with the mouthpiece towards you. Slide the lever away from the mouthpiece as far as it will go until it **clicks. See Figure C.**
[See figure C at top of next column]
• The number on the counter will count down by 1. The DISKUS is now ready to use.
Follow the instructions below so you will not accidentally waste a dose:
  Do not close the DISKUS.
• **Do not** close the DISKUS.
• **Do not** tilt the DISKUS.
• **Do not** move the lever on the DISKUS.

Figure B

Figure C

Step 3. Inhale your medicine.
• Before you breathe in your dose from the DISKUS, breathe out (exhale) as long as you can while you hold the DISKUS level and away from your mouth. **See Figure D.** Do not breathe into the mouthpiece.

Figure D

• Put the mouthpiece to your lips. **See Figure E.** Breathe in quickly and deeply through the DISKUS. Do not breathe in through your nose.

Figure E

• Remove the DISKUS from your mouth and **hold your breath for about 10 seconds,** or for as long as is comfortable for you.
• **Breathe out slowly as long as you can. See Figure D.**
• If your healthcare provider has told you to take more than 1 inhalation of FLOVENT DISKUS, repeat Steps 2 and 3.
• The DISKUS delivers your dose of medicine as a very fine powder that you may or may not taste or feel. **Do not** take an extra dose from the DISKUS even if you do not taste or feel the medicine.
Step 4. Close the DISKUS.
• Place your thumb in the thumb grip and slide it back towards you as far as it will go. **See Figure F.** Make sure the DISKUS clicks shut and you cannot see the mouthpiece.

Figure F

- The DISKUS is now ready for you to take your next scheduled dose in about 12 hours. **When you are ready to take your next dose, repeat Steps 1 through 4.**

Step 5. Rinse your mouth.

- **Rinse your mouth with water after breathing in the medicine.** Spit out the water. Do not swallow it. **See Figure G.**

Figure G

When should you get a refill?

The counter on top of the DISKUS shows you how many doses are left. After you have taken 55 doses (23 doses from the sample or institutional pack), the numbers 5 to 0 will show in red. **See Figure H.** These numbers warn you there are only a few doses left and are a reminder to get a refill.

Figure H

For correct use of the DISKUS, remember:

- Always use the DISKUS in a level, flat position.
- Make sure the lever firmly clicks into place.
- Hold your breath for about 10 seconds after inhaling. Then breathe out fully.
- After each dose, rinse your mouth with water and spit it out. Do not swallow the water.
- **Do not** take an extra dose, even if you did not taste or feel the powder.
- **Do not** take the DISKUS apart.
- **Do not** wash the DISKUS.
- Always keep the DISKUS in a dry place.
- **Do not** use the DISKUS with a spacer device.

If you have questions about FLOVENT DISKUS or how to use your inhaler, call GlaxoSmithKline (GSK) at 1-888-825-5249 or visit www.floventdiskus.com.

This Patient Information and Instructions for Use have been approved by the U.S. Food and Drug Administration.

FLOVENT and DISKUS are registered trademarks of the GSK group of companies.

GlaxoSmithKline

Research Triangle Park, NC 27709

©2014, the GSK group of companies. All rights reserved.

April 2014

FLD:6PIL

Patient Information

FLOVENT® DISKUS® *[flō′ ventdisk′ us]* 50 mcg

(fluticasone propionate inhalation powder, 50 mcg)

FLOVENT® DISKUS® 100 mcg

(fluticasone propionate inhalation powder, 100 mcg)

FLOVENT® DISKUS® 250 mcg

(fluticasone propionate inhalation powder, 250 mcg)

Read the Patient Information that comes with FLOVENT DISKUS before you start using it and each time you get a refill. There may be new information. This Patient Information does not take the place of talking to your healthcare provider about your medical condition or treatment.

What is FLOVENT DISKUS?

FLOVENT DISKUS is a prescription inhaled corticosteroid (ICS) medicine for the long-term treatment of asthma in people aged 4 years and older.

- ICS medicines such as fluticasone propionate help to decrease inflammation in the lungs. Inflammation in the lungs can lead to breathing problems.
- FLOVENT DISKUS is not used to relieve sudden breathing problems.
- It is not known if FLOVENT DISKUS is safe and effective in children younger than 4 years of age.

Who should not use FLOVENT DISKUS?

Do not use FLOVENT DISKUS if you:

- have a severe allergy to milk proteins. Ask your healthcare provider if you are not sure.
- are allergic to fluticasone propionate or any of the ingredients in FLOVENT DISKUS. See "What are the ingredients in FLOVENT DISKUS?" below for a complete list of ingredients.

What should I tell my healthcare provider before using FLOVENT DISKUS?

Tell your healthcare provider about all of your health conditions, including if you:

- have liver problems.
- have weak bones (osteoporosis).
- have an immune system problem.
- have eye problems such as glaucoma or cataracts.
- are allergic to any of the ingredients in FLOVENT DISKUS, any other medicines, or food products. See "What are the ingredients in FLOVENT DISKUS?" below for a complete list of ingredients.
- have any type of viral, bacterial, or fungal infection.
- are exposed to chickenpox or measles.
- have any other medical conditions.
- are pregnant or planning to become pregnant. It is not known if FLOVENT DISKUS may harm your unborn baby.
- are breastfeeding. It is not known if the medicine in FLOVENT DISKUS passes into your milk and if it can harm your baby.

Tell your healthcare provider about all the medicines you take, including prescription and over-the-counter medicines, vitamins, and herbal supplements. FLOVENT DISKUS and certain other medicines may interact with each other. This may cause serious side effects. Especially, tell your healthcare provider if you take antifungal or anti-HIV medicines.

Know the medicines you take. Keep a list of them to show your healthcare provider and pharmacist when you get a new medicine.

How should I use FLOVENT DISKUS?

Read the step-by-step instructions for using FLOVENT DISKUS at the end of this Patient Information.

- Do not use FLOVENT DISKUS unless your healthcare provider has taught you how to use the inhaler and you understand how to use it correctly.
- Children should use FLOVENT DISKUS with an adult's help, as instructed by the child's healthcare provider.
- Flovent DISKUS comes in 3 different strengths. Your healthcare provider prescribed the strength that is best for you.
- Use FLOVENT DISKUS exactly as your healthcare provider tells you to use it. **Do not** use FLOVENT DISKUS more often than prescribed.
- It may take 1 to 2 weeks or longer after you start FLOVENT DISKUS for your asthma symptoms to get better. You must use FLOVENT DISKUS regularly.
- **Do not** stop using FLOVENT DISKUS, even if you are feeling better, unless your healthcare provider tells you to.
- If you miss a dose of FLOVENT DISKUS, just skip that dose. Take your next dose at your usual time. Do not take 2 doses at 1 time.
- **FLOVENT DISKUS does not relieve sudden symptoms.** Always have a rescue inhaler with you to treat sudden symptoms. If you do not have a rescue inhaler, call your healthcare provider to have one prescribed for you.
- Call your healthcare provider or get medical care right away if:
- your breathing problems get worse.
- you need to use your rescue inhaler more often than usual.
- your rescue inhaler does not work as well to relieve your symptoms.
- you need to use 4 or more inhalations of your rescue inhaler in 24 hours for 2 or more days in a row.
- you use 1 whole canister of your rescue inhaler in 8 weeks.

- your peak flow meter results decrease. Your healthcare provider will tell you the numbers that are right for you.

What are the possible side effects with FLOVENT DISKUS?

FLOVENT DISKUS can cause serious side effects, including:

- **fungal infection in your mouth or throat (thrush).** Rinse your mouth with water without swallowing after using FLOVENT DISKUS to help reduce your chance of getting thrush.
- **weakened immune system and increased chance of getting infections (immunosuppression)**
- **reduced adrenal function (adrenal insufficiency).** Adrenal insufficiency is a condition where the adrenal glands do not make enough steroid hormones. This can happen when you stop taking oral corticosteroid medicines (such as prednisone) and start taking a medicine containing an inhaled steroid (such as FLOVENT DISKUS). When your body is under stress such as from fever, trauma (such as a car accident), infection, or surgery, adrenal insufficiency can get worse and may cause death.

Symptoms of adrenal insufficiency include:

- feeling tired
- lack of energy
- weakness
- nausea and vomiting
- low blood pressure

- **serious allergic reactions.** Call your healthcare provider or get emergency medical care if you get any of the following symptoms of a serious allergic reaction:
- rash
- hives
- swelling of your face, mouth, and tongue
- breathing problems
- **bone thinning or weakness (osteoporosis)**
- **slowed growth in children.** A child's growth should be checked often.
- **eye problems including glaucoma and cataracts.** You should have regular eye exams while using FLOVENT DISKUS.
- **increased wheezing (bronchospasm).** Increased wheezing can happen right away after using FLOVENT DISKUS. Always have a rescue inhaler with you to treat sudden wheezing.

Common side effects of FLOVENT DISKUS include:

upper respiratory tract infection

- upper respiratory tract infection
- throat irritation
- nausea and vomiting
- fever
- headache

Tell your healthcare provider about any side effect that bothers you or that does not go away.

These are not all the side effects with FLOVENT DISKUS. Ask your healthcare provider or pharmacist for more information.

Call your doctor for medical advice about side effects. You may report side effects to FDA at 1-800-FDA-1088.

How should I store FLOVENT DISKUS?

- Store FLOVENT DISKUS at room temperature between 68°F and 77°F (20°C and 25°C). Keep in a dry place away from heat and sunlight.
- Store FLOVENT DISKUS in the unopened foil pouch and only open when ready for use.
- Safely throw away FLOVENT DISKUS 50 mcg in the trash **6 weeks** after you open the foil pouch or when the counter reads **0**, whichever comes first.
- Safely throw away FLOVENT DISKUS 100 mcg and FLOVENT DISKUS 250 mcg in the trash **2 months** after you open the foil pouch or when the counter reads **0**, whichever comes first.
- **Keep FLOVENT DISKUS and all medicines out of the reach of children.**

General information about FLOVENT DISKUS

Medicines are sometimes prescribed for purposes not mentioned in a Patient Information leaflet. Do not use FLOVENT DISKUS for a condition for which it was not prescribed. Do not give your FLOVENT DISKUS to other people, even if they have the same condition that you have. It may harm them.

This Patient Information leaflet summarizes the most important information about FLOVENT DISKUS. If you would like more information, talk with your healthcare provider or pharmacist. You can ask your healthcare provider or pharmacist for information about FLOVENT DISKUS that was written for healthcare professionals.

For more information about FLOVENT DISKUS, call 1-888-825-5249 or visit our website at www.floventdiskus.com.

What are the ingredients in FLOVENT DISKUS?

Active ingredient: fluticasone propionate

Inactive ingredient: lactose monohydrate (contains milk proteins)

Help Patients Save on Rx Drugs: PDR.net/PharmacyDiscountCard

Instructions for Use
For Oral Inhalation Only
Your FLOVENT DISKUS inhaler

Figure A

Read this information before you start using your FLOVENT DISKUS inhaler:

• Take FLOVENT DISKUS out of the foil pouch just before you use it for the first time. Safely throw away the pouch. The DISKUS will be in the closed position.
• Write the date you opened the foil pouch in the first blank line on the label. **See Figure A.**
• Write the "use by" date in the second blank line on the label. **See Figure A.** If you are using FLOVENT DISKUS 50 mcg, that date is 6 weeks after the date you wrote on the first line. If you are using FLOVENT DISKUS 100 mcg or 250 mcg, that date is 2 months after the date you wrote on the first line.
• The counter should read **60**. If you have a sample (with "Sample" on the back label) or institutional (with "INSTITUTIONAL PACK" on the foil pouch) pack, the counter should read **28**.

How to use your FLOVENT DISKUS inhaler
Follow these steps every time you use FLOVENT DISKUS.
Step 1. Open your FLOVENT DISKUS.
• Hold the DISKUS in your left hand and place the thumb of your right hand in the thumb grip. Push the thumb grip away from you as far as it will go until the mouthpiece shows and snaps into place. **See Figure B.**

Figure B

Step 2. Slide the lever until you hear it click.
• Hold the Diskus in a level, **flat position** with the mouthpiece towards you. Slide the lever away from the mouthpiece as far as it will go until it **clicks. See Figure C.**

Figure C

• The number on the counter will count down by 1. The DISKUS is now ready to use.
Follow the instructions below so you will not accidentally waste a dose:
Do not close the DISKUS.
• **Do not** close the DISKUS.
• **Do not** tilt the DISKUS.
• **Do not** move the lever on the DISKUS.
Step 3. Inhale your medicine.
• Before you breathe in your dose from the DISKUS, breathe out (exhale) as long as you can while you hold the DISKUS level and away from your mouth. **See Figure D.** Do not breathe into the mouthpiece.

Figure D

• Put the mouthpiece to your lips. **See Figure E.** Breathe in quickly and deeply through the DISKUS. Do not breathe in through your nose.

Figure E

• Remove the DISKUS from your mouth and **hold your breath for about 10 seconds**, or for as long as is comfortable for you.
• Breathe out slowly as long as you can. **See Figure D.**
• If your healthcare provider has told you to take more than 1 inhalation of FLOVENT DISKUS, repeat steps 2 and 3.
• The DISKUS delivers your dose of medicine as a very fine powder that you may or may not taste or feel. **Do not** take an extra dose from the DISKUS even if you do not taste or feel the medicine.

Step 4. Close the DISKUS.
• Place your thumb in the thumb grip and slide it back towards you as far as it will go. **See Figure F.** Make sure the DISKUS clicks shut and you cannot see the mouthpiece.

Figure F

• The DISKUS is now ready for you to take your next scheduled dose in about 12 hours. **When you are ready to take your next dose, repeat steps 1 through 4.**
Step 5. Rinse your mouth.
• **Rinse your mouth with water after breathing in the medicine.** Spit out the water. Do not swallow it. **See Figure G.**

Figure G

When should you get a refill?
The counter on top of the DISKUS shows you how many doses are left. After you have taken **55** doses (**23** doses from the sample or institutional pack), the numbers **5** to **0** will show in red. **See Figure H.** These numbers warn you there are only a few doses left and are a reminder to get a refill.

Figure H

For correct use of the DISKUS, remember:
• Always use the DISKUS in a level, flat position.
• Make sure the lever firmly clicks into place.
• Hold your breath for about 10 seconds after inhaling. Then breathe out fully.
• After each dose, rinse your mouth with water and spit it out. Do not swallow the water.
• **Do not** take an extra dose, even if you did not taste or feel the powder.
• **Do not** take the DISKUS apart.
• **Do not** wash the DISKUS.
• Always keep the DISKUS in a dry place.
• **Do not** use the DISKUS with a spacer device.
If you have questions about FLOVENT DISKUS or how to use your inhaler, call GlaxoSmithKline (GSK) at 1-888-825-5249 or visit www.floventdiskus.com.
This Patient Information and Instructions for Use have been approved by the U.S. Food and Drug Administration.
FLOVENT and DISKUS are registered trademarks of the GSK group of companies.
GlaxoSmithKline
Research Triangle Park, NC 27709
©2014, the GSK group of companies. All rights reserved.
April 2014
FLD:6PIL

FLOVENT HFA 44 mcg   Rx
[flō' vent]
(fluticasone propionate 44 mcg)
Inhalation Aerosol
FLOVENT HFA 110 mcg   Rx
(fluticasone propionate 110 mcg)
Inhalation Aerosol
FLOVENT HFA 220 mcg   Rx
(fluticasone propionate 220 mcg)
Inhalation Aerosol
For Oral Inhalation Only

HIGHLIGHTS OF PRESCRIBING INFORMATION
These highlights do not include all the information needed to use FLOVENT HFA safely and effectively. See full prescribing information for FLOVENT HFA.
FLOVENT HFA 44 mcg (fluticasone propionate 44 mcg) Inhalation Aerosol
FLOVENT HFA 110 mcg (fluticasone propionate 110 mcg) Inhalation Aerosol
FLOVENT HFA 220 mcg (fluticasone propionate 220 mcg) Inhalation Aerosol
FOR ORAL INHALATION ONLY
Initial U.S. Approval: 1994

─────────INDICATIONS AND USAGE─────────
FLOVENT HFA is an inhaled corticosteroid indicated for:
• Maintenance treatment of asthma as prophylactic therapy in patients aged 4 years and older. (1)
• Treatment of asthma in patients requiring oral corticosteroid therapy. (1)
FLOVENT HFA is NOT indicated for the relief of acute bronchospasm. (1)

──────DOSAGE AND ADMINISTRATION──────
For oral inhalation only. Dosing is based on prior asthma therapy. (2)

Previous Therapy	Recommended Starting Dosage	Highest Recommended Dosage
Patients aged 12 years and older		
Bronchodilators alone	88 mcg twice daily	440 mcg twice daily
Inhaled corticosteroids	88-220 mcg twice daily	440 mcg twice daily
Oral corticosteroids	440 mcg twice daily	880 mcg twice daily
Patients aged 4-11 years	88 mcg twice daily	88 mcg twice daily

──────DOSAGE FORMS AND STRENGTHS──────
Inhalation aerosol with 44, 110, or 220 mcg per actuation. (3)

CONTRAINDICATIONS

- Primary treatment of status asthmaticus or acute episodes of asthma requiring intensive measures. (4)
- Hypersensitivity to any ingredient. (4)

WARNINGS AND PRECAUTIONS

- Localized infections: *Candida albicans* infection of the mouth and pharynx. Monitor patients periodically for signs of adverse effects on the oral cavity. Advise patients to rinse mouth following inhalation. (5.1)
- Immunosuppression: Potential worsening of existing tuberculosis; fungal, bacterial, viral, or parasitic infection; or ocular herpes simplex. More serious or even fatal course of chickenpox or measles in susceptible patients. Use caution in patients with above because of the potential for worsening of these infections. (5.3)
- Transferring patients from systemic corticosteroids: Risk of impaired adrenal function when transferring from oral steroids. Taper patients slowly from systemic corticosteroids if transferring to FLOVENT HFA. (5.4)
- Hypercorticism and adrenal suppression: May occur with very high dosages or at the regular dosage in susceptible individuals. If such changes occur, discontinue FLOVENT HFA slowly. (5.5)
- Hypersensitivity reactions, including anaphylaxis, may occur after administration of FLOVENT HFA. Discontinue FLOVENT HFA if such reactions occur. (4, 5.6)
- Decreases in bone mineral density: Assess bone mineral density initially and periodically thereafter in patients at risk. (5.7)
- Effect on growth: Monitor growth of pediatric patients. (5.8)
- Glaucoma and cataracts: Close monitoring is warranted. (5.9)

ADVERSE REACTIONS

Most common adverse reactions (incidence >3%) include upper respiratory tract infection or inflammation, throat irritation, sinusitis, dysphonia, candidiasis, cough, bronchitis, and headache. (6.1)

To report SUSPECTED ADVERSE REACTIONS, contact GlaxoSmithKline at 1-888-825-5249 or FDA at 1-800-FDA-1088 or www.fda.gov/medwatch

DRUG INTERACTIONS

Use with strong cytochrome P450 3A4 inhibitors such as ritonavir and ketoconazole is not recommended. Systemic corticosteroid effects may occur. (7.1)

USE IN SPECIFIC POPULATIONS

Hepatic impairment: Monitor patients for signs of increased drug exposure. (8.6)

See 17 for PATIENT COUNSELING INFORMATION and FDA-approved patient labeling

Revised: 05/2014

FULL PRESCRIBING INFORMATION

1   INDICATIONS AND USAGE

FLOVENT® HFA Inhalation Aerosol is indicated for the maintenance treatment of asthma as prophylactic therapy in patients aged 4 years and older. It is also indicated for patients requiring oral corticosteroid therapy for asthma. Many of these patients may be able to reduce or eliminate their requirement for oral corticosteroids over time.

FLOVENT HFA Inhalation Aerosol is NOT indicated for the relief of acute bronchospasm.

2   DOSAGE AND ADMINISTRATION

FLOVENT HFA should be administered by the orally inhaled route only in patients aged 4 years and older. Individual patients will experience a variable time to onset and degree of symptom relief. Maximum benefit may not be achieved for 1 to 2 weeks or longer after starting treatment. After asthma stability has been achieved, it is always desirable to titrate to the lowest effective dosage to reduce the possibility of side effects. For patients who do not respond adequately to the starting dosage after 2 weeks of therapy, higher dosages may provide additional asthma control. The safety and efficacy of FLOVENT HFA when administered in excess of recommended dosages have not been established. The recommended starting dosage and the highest recommended dosage of FLOVENT HFA, based on prior asthma therapy, are listed in Table 1.

Table 1. Recommended Dosages of FLOVENT HFA Inhalation Aerosol

NOTE: In all patients, it is desirable to titrate to the lowest effective dosage once asthma stability is achieved.

Previous Therapy	Recommended Starting Dosage	Highest Recommended Dosage
Adult and adolescent patients (aged 12 years and older)		
Bronchodilators alone	88 mcg twice daily	440 mcg twice daily
Inhaled corticosteroids	88-220 mcg twice daily[a]	440 mcg twice daily
Oral corticosteroids[b]	440 mcg twice daily	880 mcg twice daily
Pediatric patients (aged 4-11 years)[c]	88 mcg twice daily	88 mcg twice daily

[a] Starting dosages above 88 mcg twice daily may be considered for patients with poorer asthma control or those who have previously required doses of inhaled corticosteroids that are in the higher range for the specific agent.

[b] For patients currently receiving chronic oral corticosteroid therapy, prednisone should be reduced no faster than 2.5 to 5 mg/day on a weekly basis beginning after at least 1 week of therapy with FLOVENT HFA. Patients should be carefully monitored for signs of asthma instability, including serial objective measures of airflow, and for signs of adrenal insufficiency [see Warnings and Precautions (5.4)]. Once prednisone reduction is complete, the dosage of FLOVENT HFA should be reduced to the lowest effective dosage.

[c] Recommended pediatric dosage is 88 mcg twice daily regardless of prior therapy. A valved holding chamber and mask may be used to deliver FLOVENT HFA to young patients.

FLOVENT HFA should be primed before using for the first time by releasing 4 test sprays into the air away from the face, shaking well for 5 seconds before each spray. In cases where the inhaler has not been used for more than 7 days or when it has been dropped, prime the inhaler again by shaking well for 5 seconds and releasing 1 test spray into the air away from the face.

3   DOSAGE FORMS AND STRENGTHS

FLOVENT HFA is an inhalation aerosol. Each actuation delivers 44, 110, or 220 mcg of fluticasone propionate from the actuator. FLOVENT HFA 44 mcg is supplied in 10.6-g pressurized aluminum canisters, and FLOVENT HFA 110 mcg and FLOVENT HFA 220 mcg are supplied in 12-g pressurized aluminum canisters. Each canister contains 120 metered inhalations and is fitted with a counter and a dark orange oral actuator with a peach strapcap.

4   CONTRAINDICATIONS

The use of FLOVENT HFA is contraindicated in the following conditions:
- Primary treatment of status asthmaticus or other acute episodes of asthma where intensive measures are required [see Warnings and Precautions (5.2)]
- Hypersensitivity to any of the ingredients of FLOVENT HFA contraindicates their use [see Warnings and Precautions (5.6), Adverse Reactions (6.2), Description (11)]

5   WARNINGS AND PRECAUTIONS

5.1   Local Effects

In clinical studies, the development of localized infections of the mouth and pharynx with *Candida albicans* has occurred in patients treated with FLOVENT HFA. When such an infection develops, it should be treated with appropriate local or systemic (i.e., oral antifungal) therapy while treatment with FLOVENT HFA continues, but at times therapy with FLOVENT HFA may need to be interrupted. Patients should rinse the mouth after inhalation of FLOVENT HFA [see Adverse Reactions (6.1)].

5.2   Acute Asthma Episodes

FLOVENT HFA is not to be regarded as a bronchodilator and is not indicated for rapid relief of bronchospasm. Patients should be instructed to contact their physicians immediately when episodes of asthma that are not responsive to bronchodilators occur during the course of treatment with FLOVENT HFA. During such episodes, patients may require therapy with oral corticosteroids.

5.3   Immunosuppression

Persons who are using drugs that suppress the immune system are more susceptible to infections than healthy individuals. Chickenpox and measles, for example, can have a more serious or even fatal course in susceptible children or adults using corticosteroids. In such children or adults who have not had these diseases or been properly immunized, particular care should be taken to avoid exposure. How the dose, route, and duration of corticosteroid administration affect the risk of developing a disseminated infection is not known. The contribution of the underlying disease and/or prior corticosteroid treatment to the risk is also not known. If a patient is exposed to chickenpox, prophylaxis with varicella zoster immune globulin (VZIG) may be indicated. If a patient is exposed to measles, prophylaxis with pooled intramuscular immunoglobulin (IG) may be indicated. (See the respective package inserts for complete VZIG and IG prescribing information.) If chickenpox develops, treatment with antiviral agents may be considered.

Because of the potential for worsening infections, inhaled corticosteroids should be used with caution, if at all, in patients with active or quiescent tuberculosis infection of the respiratory tract; untreated systemic fungal, bacterial, viral, or parasitic infections; or ocular herpes simplex.

5.4   Transferring Patients From Systemic Corticosteroid Therapy

Particular care is needed for patients who have been transferred from systemically active corticosteroids to inhaled corticosteroids because deaths due to adrenal insufficiency have occurred in patients with asthma during and after transfer from systemic corticosteroids to less systemically available inhaled corticosteroids. After withdrawal from systemic corticosteroids, a number of months are required for recovery of hypothalamic-pituitary-adrenal (HPA) function.

Patients requiring oral corticosteroids should be weaned slowly from systemic corticosteroid use after transferring to FLOVENT HFA. In a clinical trial of 168 patients, prednisone reduction was successfully accomplished by reducing the daily prednisone dose on a weekly basis following initiation of treatment with FLOVENT HFA. Successive reduction of prednisone dose was allowed only when lung function, symptoms, and as-needed short-acting beta-agonist use were better than or comparable to that seen before initiation of prednisone dose reduction. Lung function (forced expiratory volume in 1 second [FEV$_1$] or morning peak expiratory flow [AM PEF]), beta-agonist use, and asthma

Table 2. Adverse Reactions With >3% Incidence in US Controlled Clinical Trials With FLOVENT HFA in Patients Aged 12 Years and Older With Asthma Previously Receiving Bronchodilators and/or Inhaled Corticosteroids

Adverse Event	FLOVENT HFA 88 mcg Twice Daily (n = 203) %	FLOVENT HFA 220 mcg Twice Daily (n = 204) %	FLOVENT HFA 440 mcg Twice Daily (n = 202) %	Placebo (n = 203) %
Ear, nose, and throat				
Upper respiratory tract infection	18	16	16	14
Throat irritation	8	8	10	5
Upper respiratory inflammation	2	5	5	1
Sinusitis/sinus infection	6	7	4	3
Hoarseness/dysphonia	2	3	6	<1
Gastrointestinal				
Candidiasis mouth/throat and non-site specific	4	2	5	<1
Lower respiratory				
Cough	4	6	4	5
Bronchitis	2	2	6	5
Neurological				
Headache	11	7	5	6

symptoms should be carefully monitored during withdrawal of oral corticosteroids. In addition to monitoring asthma signs and symptoms, patients should be observed for signs and symptoms of adrenal insufficiency such as fatigue, lassitude, weakness, nausea and vomiting, and hypotension. Patients who have been previously maintained on 20 mg or more per day of prednisone (or its equivalent) may be most susceptible, particularly when their systemic corticosteroids have been almost completely withdrawn. During this period of HPA suppression, patients may exhibit signs and symptoms of adrenal insufficiency when exposed to trauma, surgery, or infection (particularly gastroenteritis) or other conditions associated with severe electrolyte loss. Although inhaled corticosteroids may provide control of asthma symptoms during these episodes, in recommended doses they supply less than normal physiological amounts of glucocorticoid (cortisol) systemically and do NOT provide the mineralocorticoid activity that is necessary for coping with these emergencies.

During periods of stress or a severe asthma attack, patients who have been withdrawn from systemic corticosteroids should be instructed to resume oral corticosteroids immediately and to contact their physicians for further instruction. These patients should also be instructed to carry a warning card indicating that they may need supplementary systemic corticosteroids during periods of stress or a severe asthma attack.

Transfer of patients from systemic corticosteroid therapy to FLOVENT HFA may unmask conditions previously suppressed by the systemic corticosteroid therapy (e.g., rhinitis, conjunctivitis, eczema, arthritis, eosinophilic conditions). Some patients may experience symptoms of systemically active corticosteroid withdrawal (e.g., joint and/or muscular pain, lassitude, and depression, despite maintenance or even improvement of respiratory function).

5.5   Hypercorticism and Adrenal Suppression
Fluticasone propionate will often help control asthma symptoms with less suppression of HPA function than therapeutically equivalent oral doses of prednisone. Since fluticasone propionate is absorbed into the circulation and can be systemically active at higher doses, the beneficial effects of FLOVENT HFA in minimizing HPA dysfunction may be expected only when recommended dosages are not exceeded and individual patients are titrated to the lowest effective dose. A relationship between plasma levels of fluticasone propionate and inhibitory effects on stimulated cortisol production has been shown after 4 weeks of treatment with fluticasone propionate. Since individual sensitivity to effects on cortisol production exists, physicians should consider this information when prescribing FLOVENT HFA.
Because of the possibility of systemic absorption of inhaled corticosteroids, patients treated with FLOVENT HFA should be observed carefully for any evidence of systemic corticosteroid effects. Particular care should be taken in observing patients postoperatively or during periods of stress for evidence of inadequate adrenal response.
It is possible that systemic corticosteroid effects such as hypercorticism and adrenal suppression (including adrenal crisis) may appear in a small number of patients, particularly when FLOVENT HFA is administered at higher than recommended doses over prolonged periods of time. If such effects occur, the dosage of FLOVENT HFA should be reduced slowly, consistent with accepted procedures for reducing systemic corticosteroids and for management of asthma.

5.6   Hypersensitivity Reactions, Including Anaphylaxis
Hypersensitivity reactions, including anaphylaxis, angioedema, urticaria, and bronchospasm, may occur after administration of FLOVENT HFA *[see Contraindications (4)].*
5.7   Reduction in Bone Mineral Density
Decreases in bone mineral density (BMD) have been observed with long-term administration of products containing inhaled corticosteroids. The clinical significance of small changes in BMD with regard to long-term outcomes is unknown. Patients with major risk factors for decreased bone mineral content, such as prolonged immobilization, family history of osteoporosis, postmenopausal status, tobacco use, advanced age, poor nutrition, or chronic use of drugs that can reduce bone mass (e.g., anticonvulsants, oral corticosteroids), should be monitored and treated with established standards of care.
5.8   Effect on Growth
Orally inhaled corticosteroids may cause a reduction in growth velocity when administered to pediatric patients *[see Use in Specific Populations (8.4)].* Monitor the growth of pediatric patients receiving FLOVENT HFA routinely (e.g., via stadiometry). To minimize the systemic effects of orally inhaled corticosteroids, including FLOVENT HFA, titrate each patient's dosage to the lowest dosage that effectively controls his/her symptoms *[see Dosage and Administration (2)].*
5.9   Glaucoma and Cataracts
Glaucoma, increased intraocular pressure, and cataracts have been reported in patients following the long-term administration of inhaled corticosteroids, including fluticasone propionate. Therefore, close monitoring is warranted in patients with a change in vision or with a history of increased intraocular pressure, glaucoma, and/or cataracts.
5.10   Paradoxical Bronchospasm
As with other inhaled medications, bronchospasm may occur with an immediate increase in wheezing after dosing. If bronchospasm occurs following dosing with FLOVENT HFA, it should be treated immediately with a fast-acting inhaled bronchodilator. Treatment with FLOVENT HFA should be discontinued immediately and alternative therapy instituted.
5.11   Drug Interactions With Strong Cytochrome P450 3A4 Inhibitors
The use of strong cytochrome P450 3A4 (CYP3A4) inhibitors (e.g., ritonavir, atazanavir, clarithromycin, indinavir, itraconazole, nefazodone, nelfinavir, saquinavir, ketoconazole, telithromycin) with FLOVENT HFA is not recommended because increased systemic corticosteroid adverse effects may occur *[see Drug Interactions (7.1), Clinical Pharmacology (12.3)].*
5.12   Eosinophilic Conditions and Churg-Strauss Syndrome
In rare cases, patients on inhaled fluticasone propionate may present with systemic eosinophilic conditions. Some of these patients have clinical features of vasculitis consistent with Churg-Strauss syndrome, a condition that is often treated with systemic corticosteroid therapy. These events usually, but not always, have been associated with the reduction and/or withdrawal of oral corticosteroid therapy following the introduction of fluticasone propionate. Cases of serious eosinophilic conditions have also been reported with other inhaled corticosteroids in this clinical setting. Physicians should be alert to eosinophilia, vasculitic rash, worsening pulmonary symptoms, cardiac complications, and/or

neuropathy presenting in their patients. A causal relationship between fluticasone propionate and these underlying conditions has not been established.

6   ADVERSE REACTIONS
Systemic and local corticosteroid use may result in the following:
• *Candida albicans* infection *[see Warnings and Precautions (5.1)]*
• Immunosuppression *[see Warnings and Precautions (5.3)]*
• Hypercorticism and adrenal suppression *[see Warnings and Precautions (5.5)]*
• Reduction in bone mineral density *[see Warnings and Precautions (5.7)]*
• Growth effects *[see Warnings and Precautions (5.8)]*
• Glaucoma and cataracts *[see Warnings and Precautions (5.9)]*
6.1   Clinical Trials Experience
Because clinical trials are conducted under widely varying conditions, adverse reaction rates observed in the clinical trials of a drug cannot be directly compared with rates in the clinical trials of another drug and may not reflect the rates observed in practice.
The incidence of common adverse reactions in Table 2 is based upon 2 placebo-controlled US clinical trials in which 812 adult and adolescent patients (457 females and 355 males) previously treated with as-needed bronchodilators and/or inhaled corticosteroids were treated twice daily for up to 12 weeks with 2 inhalations of FLOVENT HFA 44 mcg Inhalation Aerosol, FLOVENT HFA 110 mcg Inhalation Aerosol, FLOVENT HFA 220 mcg Inhalation Aerosol (dosages of 88, 220, or 440 mcg twice daily), or placebo.
[See table 2 above]
Table 2 includes all events (whether considered drug-related or nondrug-related by the investigator) that occurred at a rate of over 3% in any of the groups treated with FLOVENT HFA and were more common than in the placebo group. Less than 2% of patients discontinued from the studies because of adverse reactions. The average duration of exposure was 73 to 76 days in the active treatment groups compared with 60 days in the placebo group.
Additional Adverse Reactions: Other adverse reactions not previously listed, whether considered drug-related or not by the investigators, that were reported more frequently by patients with asthma treated with FLOVENT HFA compared with patients treated with placebo include the following: rhinitis, rhinorrhea/post-nasal drip, nasal sinus disorders, laryngitis, diarrhea, viral gastrointestinal infections, dyspeptic symptoms, gastrointestinal discomfort and pain, hyposalivation, musculoskeletal pain, muscle pain, muscle stiffness/tightness/rigidity, dizziness, migraines, fever, viral infections, pain, chest symptoms, viral skin infections, muscle injuries, soft tissue injuries, urinary infections.
Fluticasone propionate inhalation aerosol (440 or 880 mcg twice daily) was administered for 16 weeks to 168 patients with asthma requiring oral corticosteroids (Study 3). Adverse reactions not included above, but reported by more than 3 patients in either group treated with FLOVENT HFA and more commonly than in the placebo group included nausea and vomiting, arthralgia and articular rheumatism, and malaise and fatigue.
In 2 long-term studies (26 and 52 weeks), the pattern of adverse reactions in patients treated with FLOVENT HFA at dosages up to 440 mcg twice daily was similar to that observed in the 12-week studies. There were no new and/or unexpected adverse reactions with long-term treatment.
Pediatric Patients Aged 4 to 11 Years: FLOVENT HFA has been evaluated for safety in 56 pediatric patients who received 88 mcg twice daily for 4 weeks. Types of adverse reactions in these pediatric patients were generally similar to those observed in adults and adolescents.
6.2   Postmarketing Experience
In addition to adverse reactions reported from clinical trials, the following adverse reactions have been identified during postmarketing use of fluticasone propionate. Because these reactions are reported voluntarily from a population of uncertain size, it is not always possible to reliably estimate their frequency or establish a causal relationship to drug exposure. These events have been chosen for inclusion due to either their seriousness, frequency of reporting, or causal connection to fluticasone propionate or a combination of these factors.
Ear, Nose, and Throat: Aphonia, facial and oropharyngeal edema, and throat soreness and irritation.
Endocrine and Metabolic: Cushingoid features, growth velocity reduction in children/adolescents, hyperglycemia, osteoporosis, and weight gain.
Eye: Cataracts.
Gastrointestinal Disorders: Dental caries and tooth discoloration.
Immune System Disorders: Immediate and delayed hypersensitivity reactions, including urticaria, anaphylaxis, rash, and angioedema and bronchospasm, have been reported.

Infections and Infestations: Esophageal candidiasis.

Psychiatry: Agitation, aggression, anxiety, depression, and restlessness. Behavioral changes, including hyperactivity and irritability, have been reported very rarely and primarily in children.

Respiratory: Asthma exacerbation, chest tightness, cough, dyspnea, immediate and delayed bronchospasm, paradoxical bronchospasm, pneumonia, and wheeze.

Skin: Contusions, cutaneous hypersensitivity reactions, ecchymoses, and pruritus.

Eosinophilic Conditions: In rare cases, patients on inhaled fluticasone propionate may present with systemic eosinophilic conditions, with some patients presenting with clinical features of vasculitis consistent with Churg-Strauss syndrome, a condition that is often treated with systemic corticosteroid therapy. These events usually, but not always, have been associated with the reduction and/or withdrawal of oral corticosteroid therapy following the introduction of fluticasone propionate [see Warnings and Precautions (5.12)].

7 DRUG INTERACTIONS

7.1 Strong Cytochrome P450 3A4 Inhibitors

Fluticasone propionate is a substrate of CYP3A4. The use of strong CYP3A4 inhibitors (e.g., ritonavir, atazanavir, clarithromycin, indinavir, itraconazole, nefazodone, nelfinavir, saquinavir, ketoconazole, telithromycin) with FLOVENT HFA is not recommended because increased systemic corticosteroid adverse effects may occur.

A drug interaction study with fluticasone propionate aqueous nasal spray in healthy subjects has shown that ritonavir (a strong CYP3A4 inhibitor) can significantly increase plasma fluticasone propionate concentration, resulting in significantly reduced serum cortisol concentrations [see Clinical Pharmacology (12.3)]. During postmarketing use, there have been reports of clinically significant drug interactions in patients receiving fluticasone propionate and ritonavir, resulting in systemic corticosteroid effects including Cushing's syndrome and adrenal suppression. Therefore, coadministration of fluticasone propionate and ritonavir is not recommended unless the potential benefit to the patient outweighs the risk of systemic corticosteroid side effects.

Coadministration of orally inhaled fluticasone propionate (1,000 mcg) and ketoconazole (200 mg once daily) resulted in a 1.9-fold increase in plasma fluticasone propionate exposure and a 45% decrease in plasma cortisol area under the curve (AUC), but had no effect on urinary excretion of cortisol. Coadministration of fluticasone propionate and ketoconazole is not recommended unless the potential benefit to the patient outweighs the risk of systemic corticosteroid side effects.

8 USE IN SPECIFIC POPULATIONS

8.1 Pregnancy

Pregnancy Category C. There are no adequate and well-controlled studies with FLOVENT HFA in pregnant women. FLOVENT HFA should be used during pregnancy only if the potential benefit justifies the potential risk to the fetus.

Teratogenic Effects: Subcutaneous studies in mice at a dose approximately 0.1 times the maximum recommended human daily inhalation dose (MRHD) for adults on a mg/m^2 basis and in the rat at a dose approximately 0.5 times the MRHD in adults on a mg/m^2 basis revealed fetal toxicity characteristic of potent corticosteroid compounds, including embryonic growth retardation, omphalocele, cleft palate, and retarded cranial ossification.

In rabbits, fetal weight reduction and cleft palate were observed at a subcutaneous dose approximately 0.04 times the MRHD for adults on a mg/m^2 basis. However, no teratogenic effects were reported at oral doses up to approximately 3 times the MRHD for adults on a mg/m^2 basis. No fluticasone propionate was detected in the plasma in this study, consistent with the established low bioavailability following oral administration [see Clinical Pharmacology (12.3)].

Experience with oral corticosteroids since their introduction in pharmacologic, as opposed to physiologic, doses suggests that rodents are more prone to teratogenic effects from corticosteroids than humans. In addition, because there is a natural increase in corticosteroid production during pregnancy, most women will require a lower exogenous corticosteroid dose and many will not need corticosteroid treatment during pregnancy.

8.3 Nursing Mothers

It is not known whether fluticasone propionate is excreted in human breast milk. However, other corticosteroids have been detected in human milk. Subcutaneous administration to lactating rats of tritiated fluticasone propionate (approximately 0.05 times the MRHD in adults on a mg/m^2 basis) resulted in measurable radioactivity in milk.

Since there are no data from controlled trials on the use of FLOVENT HFA by nursing mothers, caution should be exercised when FLOVENT HFA is administered to a nursing woman.

8.4 Pediatric Use

The safety and effectiveness of FLOVENT HFA in children aged 4 years and older have been established [see Adverse Reactions (6.1), Clinical Pharmacology (12.3), Clinical Studies (14.2)]. The safety and effectiveness of FLOVENT HFA in children younger than 4 years have not been established. Use of FLOVENT HFA in patients aged 4 to 11 years is supported by evidence from adequate and well-controlled studies in adults and adolescents aged 12 years and older, pharmacokinetic studies in patients aged 4 to 11 years, established efficacy of fluticasone propionate formulated as FLOVENT® DISKUS® (fluticasone propionate inhalation powder) and FLOVENT® ROTADISK® (fluticasone propionate inhalation powder) in patients aged 4 to 11 years, and supportive findings with FLOVENT HFA in a study conducted in patients aged 4 to 11 years.

Effects on Growth: Orally inhaled corticosteroids may cause a reduction in growth velocity when administered to pediatric patients. A reduction of growth velocity in children or teenagers may occur as a result of poorly controlled asthma or from use of corticosteroids including inhaled corticosteroids. The effects of long-term treatment of children and adolescents with inhaled corticosteroids, including fluticasone propionate, on final adult height are not known. Controlled clinical studies have shown that inhaled corticosteroids may cause a reduction in growth in pediatric patients. In these studies, the mean reduction in growth velocity was approximately 1 cm/year (range: 0.3 to 1.8 cm/year) and appeared to depend upon dose and duration of exposure. This effect was observed in the absence of laboratory evidence of HPA axis suppression, suggesting that growth velocity is a more sensitive indicator of systemic corticosteroid exposure in pediatric patients than some commonly used tests of HPA axis function. The longterm effects of this reduction in growth velocity associated with orally inhaled corticosteroids, including the impact on final adult height, are unknown. The potential for "catch-up" growth following discontinuation of treatment with orally inhaled corticosteroids has not been adequately studied. The effects on growth velocity of treatment with orally inhaled corticosteroids for over 1 year, including the impact on final adult height, are unknown. The growth of children and adolescents receiving orally inhaled corticosteroids, including FLOVENT HFA, should be monitored routinely (e.g., via stadiometry). The potential growth effects of prolonged treatment should be weighed against the clinical benefits obtained and the risks associated with alternative therapies. To minimize the systemic effects of orally inhaled corticosteroids, including FLOVENT HFA, each patient should be titrated to the lowest dose that effectively controls his/her symptoms.

Since a cross study comparison in adult and adolescent patients (aged 12 years and older) indicated that systemic exposure of inhaled fluticasone propionate from FLOVENT HFA would be higher than exposure from FLOVENT ROTADISK, results from a study to assess the potential growth effects of FLOVENT ROTADISK in pediatric patients (aged 4 to 11 years) are provided.

A 52-week placebo-controlled study to assess the potential growth effects of fluticasone propionate inhalation powder (FLOVENT ROTADISK) at 50 and 100 mcg twice daily was conducted in the US in 325 prepubescent children (244 males and 81 females) aged 4 to 11 years. The mean growth velocities at 52 weeks observed in the intent-to-treat population were 6.32 cm/year in the placebo group (n = 76), 6.07 cm/year in the 50-mcg group (n = 98), and 5.66 cm/year in the 100-mcg group (n = 89). An imbalance in the proportion of children entering puberty between groups and a higher dropout rate in the placebo group due to poorly controlled asthma may be confounding factors in interpreting these data. A separate subset analysis of children who remained prepubertal during the study revealed growth rates at 52 weeks of 6.10 cm/year in the placebo group (n = 57), 5.91 cm/year in the 50-mcg group (n = 74), and 5.67 cm/year in the 100-mcg group (n = 79). In children aged 8.5 years, the mean age of children in this study, the range for expected growth velocity is: boys – 3rd percentile = 3.8 cm/year, 50th percentile = 5.4 cm/year, and 97th percentile = 7.0 cm/year; girls – 3rd percentile = 4.2 cm/year, 50th percentile = 5.7 cm/year, and 97th percentile = 7.3 cm/year. The clinical significance of these growth data is not certain. Physicians should closely follow the growth of children and adolescents taking corticosteroids by any route, and weigh the benefits of corticosteroid therapy against the possibility of growth suppression if growth appears slowed. Patients should be maintained on the lowest dose of inhaled corticosteroid that effectively controls their asthma.

Children Younger Than 4 Years: Pharmacokinetics: [see Clinical Pharmacology (12.3)].

Pharmacodynamics: A 12-week, double-blind, placebo-controlled, parallel-group study was conducted in children with asthma aged 1 to younger than 4 years. Twelve-hour overnight urinary cortisol excretion after a 12-week treatment period with 88 mcg of FLOVENT HFA twice daily (n =

73) and with placebo (n = 42) were calculated. The mean and median change from baseline in urine cortisol over 12 hours were -0.7 and 0.0 mcg for FLOVENT HFA and 0.3 and -0.2 mcg for placebo, respectively.

In a 1-way crossover study in children aged 6 to younger than 12 months with reactive airways disease (N = 21), serum cortisol was measured over a 12-hour dosing period. Patients received placebo treatment for a 2-week period followed by a 4-week treatment period with 88 mcg of FLOVENT HFA twice daily with an AeroChamber Plus® Valved Holding Chamber (VHC) with mask. The geometric mean ratio of serum cortisol over 12 hours ($AUC_{0-12\,h}$) following FLOVENT HFA (n = 16) versus placebo (n = 18) was 0.95 (95% CI: 0.72, 1.27).

Safety: FLOVENT HFA administered as 88 mcg twice daily has been evaluated for safety in 239 pediatric patients aged 1 to younger than 4 years in a 12-week, double-blind, placebo-controlled study. Treatments were administered with an AeroChamber Plus VHC with mask. In pediatric patients aged 1 to younger than 4 years receiving FLOVENT HFA, the following events occurred with a frequency greater than 3% and more frequently than in pediatric patients who received placebo, regardless of causality assessment: pyrexia, nasopharyngitis, upper respiratory tract infection, vomiting, otitis media, diarrhea, bronchitis, pharyngitis, and viral infection.

FLOVENT HFA administered as 88 mcg twice daily has also been evaluated for safety in 23 pediatric patients aged 6 to 12 months in an open-label placebo-controlled study. Treatments were administered with an AeroChamber Plus VHC with mask for 2 weeks with placebo followed by 4 weeks with active drug. There was no discernable difference in the types of adverse events reported between patients receiving placebo compared to the active drug.

In Vitro Testing of Dose Delivery With Holding Chambers: In vitro dose characterization studies were performed to evaluate the delivery of FLOVENT HFA via holding chambers with attached masks. The studies were conducted with 2 different holding chambers (AeroChamber Plus VHC and AeroChamber Z-STAT Plus™ VHC) with masks (small and medium size) at inspiratory flow rates of 4.9, 8.0, and 12.0 L/min in combination with holding times of 0, 2, 5, and 10 seconds. The flow rates were selected to be representative of inspiratory flow rates of children aged 6 to 12 months, 2 to 5 years, and over 5 years, respectively. The mean delivered dose of fluticasone propionate through the holding chambers with masks was lower than the 44 mcg of fluticasone propionate delivered directly from the actuator mouthpiece. The results were similar through both holding chambers (see Table 3 for data for the AeroChamber Plus VHC). The fine particle fraction (approximately 1 to 5 μm) across the flow rates used in these studies was 70% to 84% of the delivered dose, consistent with the removal of the coarser fraction by the holding chamber. In contrast, the fine particle fraction for FLOVENT HFA delivered without a holding chamber typically represents 42% to 55% of the delivered dose measured at the standard flow rate of 28.3 L/min. These data suggest that, on a per kilogram basis, young children receive a comparable dose of fluticasone propionate when delivered via a holding chamber and mask as adults do without their use.

[See Table 3 at top of next page]

8.5 Geriatric Use

Of the total number of patients treated with FLOVENT HFA in US and non-US clinical trials, 173 were aged 65 years or older, 19 of which were 75 years or older. No overall differences in safety or effectiveness were observed between these patients and younger patients, and other reported clinical experience has not identified differences in responses between the elderly and younger patients, but greater sensitivity of some older individuals cannot be ruled out.

8.6 Hepatic Impairment

Formal pharmacokinetic studies using FLOVENT HFA have not been conducted in patients with hepatic impairment. Since fluticasone propionate is predominantly cleared by hepatic metabolism, impairment of liver function may lead to accumulation of fluticasone propionate in plasma. Therefore, patients with hepatic disease should be closely monitored.

8.7 Renal Impairment

Formal pharmacokinetic studies using FLOVENT HFA have not been conducted in patients with renal impairment.

10 OVERDOSAGE

Chronic overdosage may result in signs/symptoms of hypercorticism [see Warnings and Precautions (5.5)]. Inhalation by healthy volunteers of a single dose of 1,760 or 3,520 mcg of fluticasone propionate CFC inhalation aerosol was well tolerated. Doses of 1,320 mcg administered to healthy human volunteers twice daily for 7 to 15 days were also well tolerated. Repeat oral doses up to 80 mg daily for 10 days in healthy volunteers and repeat oral doses up to 20 mg daily for 42 days in patients were well tolerated. Adverse reactions were of mild or moderate severity, and incidences were similar in active and placebo treatment groups.

Table 3. In Vitro Medication Delivery Through AeroChamber Plus Valved Holding Chamber With a Mask

Age	Mask	Flow Rate (L/min)	Holding Time (seconds)	Mean Medication Delivery Through AeroChamber Plus VHC (mcg/actuation)	Body Weight 50th Percentile (kg)[a]	Medication Delivered per Actuation (mcg/kg)[b]
6 to 12 Months	Small	4.9	0	8.3	7.5-9.9	0.8-1.1
			2	6.7		0.7-0.9
			5	7.5		0.8-1.0
			10	7.5		0.8-1.0
2 to 5 Years	Small	8.0	0	7.3	12.3-18.0	0.4-0.6
			2	6.8		0.4-0.6
			5	6.7		0.4-0.5
			10	7.7		0.4-0.6
2 to 5 Years	Medium	8.0	0	7.8	12.3-18.0	0.4-0.6
			2	7.7		0.4-0.6
			5	8.1		0.5-0.7
			10	9.0		0.5-0.7
>5 Years	Medium	12.0	0	12.3	18.0	0.7
			2	11.8		0.7
			5	12.0		0.7
			10	10.1		0.6

[a] Centers for Disease Control growth charts, developed by the National Center for Health Statistics in collaboration with the National Center for Chronic Disease Prevention and Health Promotion (2000). Ranges correspond to the average of the 50th percentile weight for boys and girls at the ages indicated.
[b] A single inhalation of FLOVENT HFA in a 70-kg adult without use of a valved holding chamber and mask delivers approximately 44 mcg, or 0.6 mcg/kg.

No deaths were seen in mice given an oral dose of 1,000 mg/kg (approximately 2,300 and 11,000 times the MRHD for adults and children aged 4 to 11 years, respectively, on a mg/m^2 basis). No deaths were seen in rats given an oral dose of 1,000 mg/kg (approximately 4,600 and 22,000 times the MRHD in adults and children aged 4 to 11 years, respectively, on a mg/m^2 basis).

11 DESCRIPTION

The active component of FLOVENT HFA 44 mcg Inhalation Aerosol, FLOVENT HFA 110 mcg Inhalation Aerosol, and FLOVENT HFA 220 mcg Inhalation Aerosol is fluticasone propionate, a corticosteroid having the chemical name S-(fluoromethyl) 6α,9-difluoro-11β,17-dihydroxy-16α-methyl-3-oxoandrosta-1,4-diene-17β-carbothioate, 17-propionate and the following chemical structure:

Fluticasone propionate is a white powder with a molecular weight of 500.6, and the empirical formula is $C_{25}H_{31}F_3O_5S$. It is practically insoluble in water, freely soluble in dimethyl sulfoxide and dimethylformamide, and slightly soluble in methanol and 95% ethanol.

FLOVENT HFA 44 mcg Inhalation Aerosol, FLOVENT HFA 110 mcg Inhalation Aerosol, and FLOVENT HFA 220 mcg Inhalation Aerosol are pressurized metered-dose aerosol units fitted with a counter. FLOVENT HFA is intended for oral inhalation only. Each unit contains a microcrystalline suspension of fluticasone propionate (micronized) in propellant HFA-134a (1,1,1,2-tetrafluoroethane). It contains no other excipients.

After priming, each actuation of the inhaler delivers 50, 125, or 250 mcg of fluticasone propionate in 60 mg of suspension (for the 44-mcg product) or in 75 mg of suspension (for the 110- and 220-mcg products) from the valve. Each actuation delivers 44, 110, or 220 mcg of fluticasone propionate from the actuator. The actual amount of drug delivered to the lung may depend on patient factors, such as the coordination between the actuation of the device and inspiration through the delivery system.

Each 10.6-g canister (44 mcg) and each 12-g canister (110 and 220 mcg) provides 120 inhalations.

FLOVENT HFA should be primed before using for the first time by releasing 4 test sprays into the air away from the face, shaking well for 5 seconds before each spray. In cases where the inhaler has not been used for more than 7 days or when it has been dropped, prime the inhaler again by shaking well for 5 seconds and releasing 1 test spray into the air away from the face.

This product does not contain any chlorofluorocarbon (CFC) as the propellant.

12 CLINICAL PHARMACOLOGY

12.1 Mechanism of Action

Fluticasone propionate is a synthetic trifluorinated corticosteroid with potent anti-inflammatory activity. In vitro assays using human lung cytosol preparations have established fluticasone propionate as a human glucocorticoid receptor agonist with an affinity 18 times greater than dexamethasone, almost twice that of beclomethasone–17–monopropionate (BMP), the active metabolite of beclomethasone dipropionate, and over 3 times that of budesonide. Data from the McKenzie vasoconstrictor assay in man are consistent with these results. The clinical significance of these findings is unknown.

Inflammation is an important component in the pathogenesis of asthma. Corticosteroids have been shown to inhibit multiple cell types (e.g., mast cells, eosinophils, basophils, lymphocytes, macrophages, neutrophils) and mediator production or secretion (e.g., histamine, eicosanoids, leukotrienes, cytokines) involved in the asthmatic response. These anti-inflammatory actions of corticosteroids contribute to their efficacy in asthma.

Though effective for the treatment of asthma, corticosteroids do not affect asthma symptoms immediately. Individual patients will experience a variable time to onset and degree of symptom relief. Maximum benefit may not be achieved for 1 to 2 weeks or longer after starting treatment. When corticosteroids are discontinued, asthma stability may persist for several days or longer.

Studies in patients with asthma have shown a favorable ratio between topical anti-inflammatory activity and systemic corticosteroid effects with recommended doses of orally inhaled fluticasone propionate. This is explained by a combination of a relatively high local anti-inflammatory effect, negligible oral systemic bioavailability (less than 1%), and the minimal pharmacological activity of the only metabolite detected in man.

12.2 Pharmacodynamics

Serum cortisol concentrations, urinary excretion of cortisol, and urine 6-β-hydroxycortisol excretion collected over 24 hours in 24 healthy subjects following 8 inhalations of fluticasone propionate HFA 44, 110, and 220 mcg decreased with increasing dose. However, in patients with asthma treated with 2 inhalations of fluticasone propionate HFA 44, 110, and 220 mcg twice daily for at least 4 weeks, differences in serum cortisol $AUC_{(0-12\ h)}$ (n = 65) and 24-hour urinary excretion of cortisol (n = 47) compared with placebo were not related to dose and generally not significant. In the study with healthy volunteers, the effect of propellant was also evaluated by comparing results following the 220-mcg strength inhaler containing HFA 134a propellant with the same strength of inhaler containing CFC 11/12 propellant. A lesser effect on the HPA axis with the HFA formulation was observed for serum cortisol, but not urine cortisol and 6-betahydroxy cortisol excretion. In addition, in a crossover study of children with asthma aged 4 to 11 years (N = 40),

24-hour urinary excretion of cortisol was not affected after a 4-week treatment period with 88 mcg of fluticasone propionate HFA twice daily compared with urinary excretion after the 2-week placebo period. The ratio (95% CI) of urinary excretion of cortisol over 24 hours following fluticasone propionate HFA versus placebo was 0.987 (0.796, 1.223).

The potential systemic effects of fluticasone propionate HFA on the HPA axis were also studied in patients with asthma. Fluticasone propionate given by inhalation aerosol at dosages of 440 or 880 mcg twice daily was compared with placebo in oral corticosteroid-dependent patients with asthma (range of mean dose of prednisone at baseline: 13 to 14 mg/day) in a 16-week study. Consistent with maintenance treatment with oral corticosteroids, abnormal plasma cortisol responses to short cosyntropin stimulation (peak plasma cortisol less than 18 mcg/dL) were present at baseline in the majority of patients participating in this study (69% of patients later randomized to placebo and 72% to 78% of patients later randomized to fluticasone propionate HFA). At week 16, 8 patients (73%) on placebo compared with 14 (54%) and 13 (68%) patients receiving fluticasone propionate HFA (440 and 880 mcg twice daily, respectively) had post-stimulation cortisol levels of less than 18 mcg/dL.

12.3 Pharmacokinetics

Absorption: Fluticasone propionate acts locally in the lung; therefore, plasma levels do not predict therapeutic effect. Studies using oral dosing of labeled and unlabeled drug have demonstrated that the oral systemic bioavailability of fluticasone propionate is negligible (less than 1%), primarily due to incomplete absorption and presystemic metabolism in the gut and liver. In contrast, the majority of the fluticasone propionate delivered to the lung is systemically absorbed.

Distribution: Following intravenous administration, the initial disposition phase for fluticasone propionate was rapid and consistent with its high lipid solubility and tissue binding. The volume of distribution averaged 4.2 L/kg.

The percentage of fluticasone propionate bound to human plasma proteins averages 99%. Fluticasone propionate is weakly and reversibly bound to erythrocytes and is not significantly bound to human transcortin.

Metabolism: The total clearance of fluticasone propionate is high (average, 1,093 mL/min), with renal clearance accounting for less than 0.02% of the total. The only circulating metabolite detected in man is the 17β-carboxylic acid derivative of fluticasone propionate, which is formed through the CYP 3A4 pathway. This metabolite had less affinity (approximately 1/2,000) than the parent drug for the corticosteroid receptor of human lung cytosol in vitro and negligible pharmacological activity in animal studies. Other metabolites detected in vitro using cultured human hepatoma cells have not been detected in man.

Elimination: Following intravenous dosing, fluticasone propionate showed polyexponential kinetics and had a terminal elimination half-life of approximately 7.8 hours. Less than 5% of a radiolabeled oral dose was excreted in the urine as metabolites, with the remainder excreted in the feces as parent drug and metabolites.

Special Populations: *Gender:* No significant difference in clearance (CL/F) of fluticasone propionate was observed.

Pediatrics: A population pharmacokinetic analysis was performed for FLOVENT HFA using steady-state data from 4 controlled clinical trials and single-dose data from 1 controlled clinical trial. The combined cohort for analysis included 269 patients (161 males and 108 females) with asthma aged 6 months to 66 years who received treatment with FLOVENT HFA. Most of these subjects (n = 215) were treated with FLOVENT HFA 44 mcg given as 88 mcg twice daily. FLOVENT HFA was delivered using an AeroChamber Plus VHC with a mask to patients aged younger than 4 years. Data from adult patients with asthma following FLOVENT HFA 110 mcg given as 220 mcg twice daily (n = 15) and following FLOVENT HFA 220 mcg given as 440 mcg twice daily (n = 17) at steady state were also included. Data for 22 patients came from a single-dose crossover study of 264 mcg (6 doses of FLOVENT HFA 44 mcg) with and without AeroChamber Plus VHC in children with asthma aged 4 to 11 years.

Stratification of exposure data following FLOVENT HFA 88 mcg by age and study indicated that systemic exposure to fluticasone propionate at steady state was similar in children aged 6 to younger than 12 months, children aged 1 to younger than 4 years, and adults and adolescents aged 12 years and older. Exposure was lower in children aged 4 to 11 years, who did not use a VHC, as shown in Table 4.

[See table 4 at top of next page]

The lower exposure to fluticasone propionate in children aged 4 to 11 years who did not use a VHC may reflect the inability to coordinate actuation and inhalation of the metered-dose inhaler. The impact of the use of a VHC on exposure to fluticasone propionate in patients aged 4 to 11 years was evaluated in a single-dose crossover study with FLOVENT HFA 44 mcg given as 264 mcg. In this study, use of a VHC increased systemic exposure to fluticasone propionate (Table 5), possibly correcting for the inability to coordinate actuation and inhalation.

[See table 5 above]

There was a dose-related increase in systemic exposure in patients aged 12 years and older receiving higher doses of fluticasone propionate (220 and 440 mcg twice daily). The $AUC_{(0-\tau)}$ in pg•h/mL was 358 (95% CI: 272, 473) and 640 (95% CI: 477, 858), and C_{max} in pg/mL was 47.3 (95% CI: 37, 61) and 87 (95% CI: 68, 112) following fluticasone propionate 220 and 440 mcg, respectively.

Hepatic and Renal Impairment: Formal pharmacokinetic studies using FLOVENT HFA have not been conducted in patients with hepatic or renal impairment. However, since fluticasone propionate is predominantly cleared by hepatic metabolism, impairment of liver function may lead to accumulation of fluticasone propionate in plasma. Therefore, patients with hepatic disease should be closely monitored.

Race: No significant difference in clearance (CL/F) of fluticasone propionate in Caucasian, African-American, Asian, or Hispanic populations was observed.

Drug Interactions: Ritonavir: Fluticasone propionate is a substrate of CYP3A4. Coadministration of fluticasone propionate and the strong CYP3A4 inhibitor ritonavir is not recommended based upon a multiple-dose, crossover drug interaction study in 18 healthy subjects. Fluticasone propionate aqueous nasal spray (200 mcg once daily) was coadministered for 7 days with ritonavir (100 mg twice daily). Plasma fluticasone propionate concentrations following fluticasone propionate aqueous nasal spray alone were undetectable (less than 10 pg/mL) in most subjects, and when concentrations were detectable, peak levels (C_{max}) averaged 11.9 pg/mL (range: 10.8 to 14.1 pg/mL) and $AUC_{(0-\tau)}$ averaged 8.43 pg•h/mL (range: 4.2 to 18.8 pg•h/mL). Fluticasone propionate C_{max} and $AUC_{(0-\tau)}$ increased to 318 pg/mL (range: 110 to 648 pg/mL) and 3,102.6 pg•h/mL (range: 1,207.1 to 5,662.0 pg•h/mL), respectively, after coadministration of ritonavir with fluticasone propionate aqueous nasal spray. This significant increase in plasma fluticasone propionate exposure resulted in a significant decrease (86%) in serum cortisol AUC.

Ketoconazole: In a placebo-controlled crossover study in 8 healthy adult volunteers, coadministration of a single dose of orally inhaled fluticasone propionate (1,000 mcg) with multiple doses of ketoconazole (200 mg) to steady state resulted in increased plasma fluticasone propionate exposure, a reduction in plasma cortisol AUC, and no effect on urinary excretion of cortisol.

Following orally inhaled fluticasone propionate alone, $AUC_{(2-last)}$ averaged 1.559 ng•h/mL (range: 0.555 to 2.906 ng•h/mL) and $AUC_{(2-\infty)}$ averaged 2.269 ng•h/mL (range: 0.836 to 3.707 ng•h/mL). Fluticasone propionate $AUC_{(2-last)}$ and $AUC_{(2-\infty)}$ increased to 2.781 ng•h/mL (range: 2.489 to 8.486 ng•h/mL) and 4.317 ng•h/mL (range: 3.256 to 9.408 ng•h/mL), respectively, after coadministration of ketoconazole with orally inhaled fluticasone propionate. This increase in plasma fluticasone propionate concentration resulted in a decrease (45%) in serum cortisol AUC.

Erythromycin: In a multiple-dose drug interaction study, coadministration of orally inhaled fluticasone propionate (500 mcg twice daily) and erythromycin (333 mg 3 times daily) did not affect fluticasone propionate pharmacokinetics.

13 NONCLINICAL TOXICOLOGY

13.1 Carcinogenesis, Mutagenesis, Impairment of Fertility

Fluticasone propionate demonstrated no tumorigenic potential in mice at oral doses up to 1,000 mcg/kg (approximately 2 and 10 times the MRHD for adults and children aged 4 to 11 years, respectively, on a mg/m² basis) for 78 weeks or in rats at inhalation doses up to 57 mcg/kg (approximately 0.3 times and approximately equivalent to the MRHD for adults and children aged 4 to 11 years, respectively, on a mg/m² basis) for 104 weeks.

Fluticasone propionate did not induce gene mutation in prokaryotic or eukaryotic cells in vitro. No significant clastogenic effect was seen in cultured human peripheral lymphocytes in vitro or in the in vivo mouse micronucleus test.

No evidence of impairment of fertility was observed in reproductive studies conducted in male and female rats at subcutaneous doses up to 50 mcg/kg (approximately 0.2 times the MRHD for adults on a mg/m² basis). Prostate weight was significantly reduced at a subcutaneous dose of 50 mcg/kg.

13.2 Animal Toxicology and/or Pharmacology

Reproductive Toxicology: Subcutaneous studies in mice and rats at 45 and 100 mcg/kg (approximately 0.1 and 0.5 times the MRHD for adults on a mg/m² basis, respectively)

revealed fetal toxicity characteristic of potent corticosteroid compounds, including embryonic growth retardation, omphalocele, cleft palate, and retarded cranial ossification.

In rabbits, fetal weight reduction and cleft palate were observed at a subcutaneous dose of 4 mcg/kg (approximately 0.04 times the MRHD for adults on a mg/m² basis). However, no teratogenic effects were reported at oral doses up to 300 mcg/kg (approximately 3 times the MRHD for adults on a mg/m² basis) of fluticasone propionate. No fluticasone propionate was detected in the plasma in this study, consistent with the established low bioavailability following oral administration [see Clinical Pharmacology (12.3)].

Fluticasone propionate crossed the placenta following subcutaneous administration to mice and rats and oral administration to rabbits.

In animals and humans, propellant HFA-134a was found to be rapidly absorbed and rapidly eliminated, with an elimination half-life of 3 to 27 minutes in animals and 5 to 7 minutes in humans. Time to maximum plasma concentration (T_{max}) and mean residence time are both extremely short, leading to a transient appearance of HFA-134a in the blood with no evidence of accumulation.

Propellant HFA-134a is devoid of pharmacological activity except at very high doses in animals (i.e., 380 to 1,300 times the maximum human exposure based on comparisons of AUC values), primarily producing ataxia, tremors, dyspnea, or salivation. These events are similar to effects produced by the structurally related CFCs, which have been used extensively in metered-dose inhalers.

14 CLINICAL STUDIES

14.1 Adult and Adolescent Patients Aged 12 Years and Older

Three randomized, double-blind, parallel-group, placebo-controlled, US clinical trials were conducted in 980 adult and adolescent patients (aged 12 years and older) with asthma to assess the efficacy and safety of FLOVENT HFA in the treatment of asthma. Fixed dosages of 88, 220, and 440 mcg twice daily (each dose administered as 2 inhalations of the 44-, 110-, and 220-mcg strengths, respectively) and 880 mcg twice daily (administered as 4 inhalations of the 220-mcg strength) were compared with placebo to provide information about appropriate dosing to cover a range of asthma severity. Patients in these studies included those inadequately controlled with bronchodilators alone (Study 1), those already receiving inhaled corticosteroids (Study 2), and those requiring oral corticosteroid therapy (Study 3). In all 3 studies, patients (including placebo-treated patients) were allowed to use VENTOLIN® (albuterol, USP) Inhalation Aerosol as needed for relief of acute asthma symptoms. In Studies 1 and 2, other maintenance asthma therapies were discontinued.

Study 1 enrolled 397 patients with asthma inadequately controlled on bronchodilators alone. FLOVENT HFA was evaluated at dosages of 88, 220, and 440 mcg twice daily for 12 weeks. Baseline FEV_1 values were similar across groups (mean 67% of predicted normal). All 3 dosages of FLOVENT HFA demonstrated a statistically significant improvement in lung function as measured by improvement in AM pre-dose FEV_1 compared with placebo. This improvement was observed after the first week of treatment, and was maintained over the 12-week treatment period.

At Endpoint (last observation), mean change from baseline in AM pre-dose percent predicted FEV_1 was greater in all 3 groups treated with FLOVENT HFA (9.0% to 11.2%) compared with the placebo group (3.4%). The mean differences between the groups treated with FLOVENT HFA 88, 220, and 440 mcg and the placebo group were statistically significant, and the corresponding 95% confidence intervals were (2.2%, 9.2%), (2.8%, 9.9%), and (4.3%, 11.3%), respectively.

Figure 1 displays results of pulmonary function tests (mean percent change from baseline in FEV_1 prior to AM dose) for the recommended starting dosage of FLOVENT HFA (88 mcg twice daily) and placebo from Study 1. This trial used predetermined criteria for lack of efficacy (indicators of worsening asthma), resulting in withdrawal of more patients in the placebo group. Therefore, pulmonary function results at Endpoint (the last evaluable FEV_1 result, including most patients' lung function data) are also displayed.

Figure 1. A 12-Week Clinical Trial in Patients Aged 12 Years and Older Inadequately Controlled on Bronchodilators Alone: Mean Percent Change From Baseline in FEV1 Prior to AM Dose (Study 1)

In Study 2, FLOVENT HFA at dosages of 88, 220, and 440 mcg twice daily was evaluated over 12 weeks of treatment in 415 patients with asthma who were already receiving an inhaled corticosteroid at a daily dose within its recommended dose range in addition to as-needed albuterol. Baseline FEV_1 values were similar across groups (mean 65% to 66% of predicted normal). All 3 dosages of FLOVENT HFA demonstrated a statistically significant improvement in lung function, as measured by improvement in FEV_1, compared with placebo. This improvement was observed after the first week of treatment and was maintained over the 12-week treatment period. Discontinuations from the study for lack of efficacy (defined by a pre-specified decrease in FEV_1 or PEF, or an increase in use of VENTOLIN or nighttime awakenings requiring treatment with VENTOLIN) were lower in the groups treated with FLOVENT HFA (6% to 11%) compared with placebo (50%).

At Endpoint (last observation), mean change from baseline in AM pre-dose percent predicted FEV_1 was greater in all 3 groups treated with FLOVENT HFA (2.2% to 4.6%) compared with the placebo group (-8.3%). The mean differences between the groups treated with FLOVENT HFA 88, 220, and 440 mcg and the placebo group were statistically significant, and the corresponding 95% confidence intervals were (7.1%, 13.8%), (8.2%, 14.9%), and (9.6%, 16.4%), respectively.

Figure 2 displays the mean percent change from baseline in FEV_1 from Week 1 through Week 12. This study also used predetermined criteria for lack of efficacy, resulting in withdrawal of more patients in the placebo group; therefore, pulmonary function results at Endpoint are also displayed.

[See figure 2 at top of next column]

In both studies, use of VENTOLIN, AM and PM PEF, and asthma symptom scores showed numerical improvement with FLOVENT HFA compared with placebo.

Study 3 enrolled 168 patients with asthma requiring oral prednisone therapy (average baseline daily prednisone dose ranged from 13 to 14 mg). FLOVENT HFA at dosages of 440 and 880 mcg twice daily was evaluated over a 16-week treatment period. Baseline FEV_1 values were similar across groups (mean 59% to 62% of predicted normal). Over the course of the study, patients treated with either dosage of FLOVENT HFA required a statistically significantly lower mean daily oral prednisone dose (6 mg) compared with placebo-treated patients (15 mg). Both dosages of

Table 4. Systemic Exposure to Fluticasone Propionate Following FLOVENT HFA 88 mcg Twice Daily

Age	Valved Holding Chamber	N	$AUC_{0-\tau}$, pg•h/mL (95% CI)	C_{max}, pg/mL (95% CI)
6 to <12 Months	Yes	17	141 (88, 227)	19 (13, 29)
1 to <4 Years	Yes	164	143 (131, 157)	20 (18, 21)
4 to 11 Years	No	14	68 (48, 97)	11 (8, 16)
≥12 Years	No	20	149 (106, 210)	20 (15, 27)

Table 5. Systemic Exposure to Fluticasone Propionate Following a Single Dose of FLOVENT HFA 264 mcg

Age	Valved Holding Chamber	N	$AUC_{(0-\infty)}$, pg•h/mL (95% CI)	C_{max}, pg/mL (95% CI)
4 to 11 Years	Yes	22	373 (297, 468)	61 (51, 73)
4 to 11 Years	No	21	141 (111, 178)	23 (19, 28)

Figure 2. A 12-Week Clinical Trial in Patients Aged 12 Years and Older Already Receiving Daily Inhaled Corticosteroids: Mean Percent Change From Baseline in FEV1 Prior to AM Dose (Study 2)

FLOVENT HFA enabled a larger percentage of patients (59% and 56% in the groups treated with FLOVENT HFA 440 and 880 mcg, respectively, twice daily) to eliminate oral prednisone as compared with placebo (13%) (see Figure 3). There was no efficacy advantage of FLOVENT HFA 880 mcg twice daily compared with 440 mcg twice daily. Accompanying the reduction in oral corticosteroid use, patients treated with either dosage of FLOVENT HFA had statistically significantly improved lung function, fewer asthma symptoms, and less use of VENTOLIN Inhalation Aerosol compared with the placebo-treated patients.

Figure 3. A 16-Week Clinical Trial in Patients Aged 12 Years and Older Requiring Chronic Oral Prednisone Therapy: Change in Maintenance Prednisone Dose

Two long-term safety studies (Study 4 and Study 5) of ≥6 months' duration were conducted in 507 adult and adolescent patients with asthma. Study 4 was designed to monitor the safety of 2 doses of FLOVENT HFA, while Study 5 compared fluticasone propionate HFA with fluticasone propionate CFC. Study 4 enrolled 182 patients who were treated daily with low to high doses of inhaled corticosteroids, beta-agonists (short-acting [as needed or regularly scheduled] or long-acting), theophylline, inhaled cromolyn or nedocromil sodium, leukotriene receptor antagonists, or 5-lipoxygenase inhibitors at baseline. FLOVENT HFA at dosages of 220 and 440 mcg twice daily was evaluated over a 26-week treatment period in 89 and 93 patients, respectively. Study 5 enrolled 325 patients who were treated daily with moderate to high doses of inhaled corticosteroids, with or without concurrent use of salmeterol or albuterol, at baseline. Fluticasone propionate HFA at a dosage of 440 mcg twice daily and fluticasone propionate CFC at a dosage of 440 mcg twice daily were evaluated over a 52-week treatment period in 163 and 162 patients, respectively. Baseline FEV_1 values were similar across groups (mean 81% to 84% of predicted normal). Throughout the 52-week treatment period, asthma control was maintained with both formulations of fluticasone propionate compared with baseline. In both studies, none of the patients were withdrawn due to lack of efficacy.

14.2   Pediatric Patients Aged 4 to 11 Years
A 12-week clinical trial conducted in 241 pediatric patients with asthma was supportive of efficacy but inconclusive due to measurable levels of fluticasone propionate in 6/48 (13%) of the plasma samples from patients randomized to placebo. Efficacy in patients aged 4 to 11 years is extrapolated from adult data with FLOVENT HFA and other supporting data [see Use in Specific Populations (8.4)].

16   HOW SUPPLIED/STORAGE AND HANDLING
Flovent HFA 44 mcg Inhalation Aerosol is supplied in 10.6-g pressurized aluminum canisters containing 120 metered inhalations in boxes of 1 with patient instructions (NDC 0173-0718-20).
Flovent HFA 110 mcg Inhalation Aerosol is supplied in 12-g pressurized aluminum canisters containing 120 metered inhalations in boxes of 1 with patient instructions (NDC 0173-0719-20).

Flovent HFA 220 mcg Inhalation Aerosol is supplied in 12-g pressurized aluminum canisters containing 120 metered inhalations in boxes of 1 with patient instructions (NDC 0173-0720-20).
Each canister is fitted with a counter and a dark orange oral actuator with a peach strapcap. The dark orange actuator supplied with FLOVENT HFA should not be used with any other product canisters, and actuators from other products should not be used with a FLOVENT HFA canister.
The correct amount of medication in each inhalation cannot be assured after the counter reads 000, even though the canister is not completely empty and will continue to operate. The inhaler should be discarded when the counter reads 000.
Keep out of reach of children. Avoid spraying in eyes.
Contents Under Pressure: Do not puncture. Do not use or store near heat or open flame. Exposure to temperatures above 120°F may cause bursting. Never throw into fire or incinerator.
Store at 25°C (77°F); excursions permitted from 15° to 30°C (59° to 86°F). Store the inhaler with the mouthpiece down. For best results, the inhaler should be at room temperature before use. SHAKE WELL BEFORE USING.
FLOVENT HFA does not contain CFCs as the propellant.

17   PATIENT COUNSELING INFORMATION
See FDA-approved patient labeling (Patient Information and Instructions for Use).
17.1   Oral Candidiasis
Patients should be advised that localized infections with *Candida albicans* have occurred in the mouth and pharynx in some patients. If oropharyngeal candidiasis develops, it should be treated with appropriate local or systemic (i.e., oral antifungal) therapy while still continuing therapy with FLOVENT HFA, but at times therapy with FLOVENT HFA may need to be temporarily interrupted under close medical supervision. Rinsing the mouth after inhalation is advised.
17.2   Status Asthmaticus and Acute Asthma Symptoms
Patients should be advised that FLOVENT HFA is not a bronchodilator and is not intended for use as rescue medication for acute asthma exacerbations. Acute asthma symptoms should be treated with an inhaled, short-acting beta₂-agonist such as albuterol. Patients should be instructed to contact their physicians immediately if there is deterioration of their asthma.
17.3   Immunosuppression
Patients who are on immunosuppressant doses of corticosteroids should be warned to avoid exposure to chickenpox or measles and if they are exposed to consult their physicians without delay. Patients should be informed of potential worsening of existing tuberculosis, fungal, bacterial, viral, or parasitic infections, or ocular herpes simplex.
17.4   Hypercorticism and Adrenal Suppression
Patients should be advised that FLOVENT HFA may cause systemic corticosteroid effects of hypercorticism and adrenal suppression. Additionally, patients should be instructed that deaths due to adrenal insufficiency have occurred during and after transfer from systemic corticosteroids. Patients should taper slowly from systemic corticosteroids if transferring to FLOVENT HFA.
17.5   Hypersensitivity Reactions, Including Anaphylaxis
Patients should be advised that hypersensitivity reactions including anaphylaxis, angioedema, urticaria, and bronchospasm may occur after administration of FLOVENT HFA. Patients should discontinue FLOVENT HFA if such reactions occur.
17.6   Reduction in Bone Mineral Density
Patients who are at an increased risk for decreased BMD should be advised that the use of corticosteroids may pose an additional risk.
17.7   Reduced Growth Velocity
Patients should be informed that orally inhaled corticosteroids, including FLOVENT HFA, may cause a reduction in growth velocity when administered to pediatric patients. Physicians should closely follow the growth of children and adolescents taking corticosteroids by any route.
17.8   Ocular Effects
Long-term use of inhaled corticosteroids may increase the risk of some eye problems (cataracts or glaucoma); regular eye examinations should be considered.
17.9   Use Daily for Best Effect
Patients should use FLOVENT HFA at regular intervals as directed. Individual patients will experience a variable time to onset and degree of symptom relief and the full benefit may not be achieved until treatment has been administered for 1 to 2 weeks or longer. Patients should not increase the prescribed dosage but should contact their physicians if symptoms do not improve or if the condition worsens. Patients should be instructed not to stop use of FLOVENT HFA abruptly. Patients should contact their physicians immediately if they discontinue use of FLOVENT HFA.
DISKUS, FLOVENT, ROTADISK, and VENTOLIN are registered trademarks of the GSK group of companies. The other brands listed are trademarks of their respective own-

ers and are not trademarks of the GSK group of companies. The makers of these brands are not affiliated with and do not endorse GlaxoSmithKline or its products.
GlaxoSmithKline
Research Triangle Park, NC 27709
©2014, the GSK group of companies. All rights reserved.
FLH:6PI

PHARMACIST—DETACH HERE AND GIVE LEAFLET TO PATIENT
Patient Information
FLOVENT® *[flō' vent]* **HFA 44 mcg**
(fluticasone propionate 44 mcg)
Inhalation Aerosol
FLOVENT® HFA 110 mcg
(fluticasone propionate 110 mcg)
Inhalation Aerosol
FLOVENT® HFA 220 mcg
(fluticasone propionate 220 mcg)
Inhalation Aerosol
FOR ORAL INHALATION ONLY
Read this leaflet carefully before you start to use FLOVENT HFA Inhalation Aerosol.
Keep this leaflet because it has important summary information about FLOVENT HFA. This leaflet does not contain all the information about your medicine. If you have any questions or are not sure about something, you should ask your doctor or pharmacist.
Read the new leaflet that comes with each refill of your prescription because there may be new information.
What is FLOVENT HFA?
FLOVENT HFA contains a medicine called fluticasone propionate, which is a synthetic corticosteroid. Corticosteroids are natural substances found in the body that help fight inflammation. Corticosteroids are used to treat asthma because they reduce airway inflammation.
FLOVENT HFA is used to treat asthma in patients 4 years and older. When inhaled regularly, FLOVENT HFA also helps to prevent symptoms of asthma.
FLOVENT HFA comes in 3 strengths. Your doctor has prescribed the one that is best for your condition.
Who should not use FLOVENT HFA?
Do not use FLOVENT HFA if you:
• are allergic to any of the ingredients in FLOVENT HFA or other inhaled corticosteroids. See "What are the ingredients in FLOVENT HFA?" below.
• have an acute asthma attack or status asthmaticus.
FLOVENT HFA is not a bronchodilator and should not be used to give you fast relief from your breathing problems during an asthma attack. Always use a short-acting bronchodilator (rescue medicine), such as albuterol inhaler, during a sudden asthma attack. You must take FLOVENT HFA at regular times as recommended by your doctor, and not as an emergency medicine.
What should I tell my doctor before taking FLOVENT HFA?
Tell your doctor if you:
• have liver problems.
• have been exposed to chickenpox or measles.
• have any other medical conditions.
• are pregnant or planning to become pregnant. It is not known if FLOVENT HFA will harm your unborn baby.
• are breastfeeding a baby. It is not known if FLOVENT HFA passes into your breast milk.
Tell your doctor about all the medicines you take including prescription and non-prescription medicines, vitamins, and herbal supplements. FLOVENT HFA may affect the way other medicines work, and other medicines may affect how FLOVENT HFA works. Especially, tell your doctor if you take:
• a medicine containing ritonavir (commonly used to treat HIV infection or AIDS). The anti-HIV medicines NORVIR® (ritonavir capsules) Soft Gelatin, NORVIR (ritonavir oral solution), and KALETRA® (lopinavir/ritonavir) tablets contain ritonavir.
• any other corticosteroid medicines.
• ketoconazole (NIZORAL®), an antifungal medicine.
How should I use FLOVENT HFA?
1. It is important that you inhale each dose as your doctor has prescribed. The prescription label provided by your pharmacist will usually tell you what dose to take and how often. If it doesn't or if you aren't sure, ask your doctor or pharmacist. DO NOT inhale more doses or use your FLOVENT HFA more often than your doctor has prescribed.
2. It may take 1 to 2 weeks or longer for this medicine to work, and it is very important that you use it regularly. **Do not stop taking FLOVENT HFA, even if you are feeling better, unless your doctor tells you to.**
3. If you miss a dose, just take your next scheduled dose when it is due. **Do not double the dose.**
4. Your doctor may prescribe additional medicine (such as fast-acting bronchodilators) for emergency relief if a sudden asthma attack occurs. Contact your doctor if:
• an asthma attack does not respond to the additional medicine or
• you need more of the additional medicine than usual.

5. If you also use another medicine by inhalation, you should ask your doctor for instructions on when to use it while you are also using FLOVENT HFA.

6. Children should use FLOVENT HFA with an adult's help, as instructed by the child's healthcare provider. A valved holding chamber (a kind of spacer) and mask may be used to deliver FLOVENT HFA to young patients.

What should I avoid while taking FLOVENT HFA?

If you have not had or not been vaccinated against chickenpox, measles, or active tuberculosis, you should stay away from people who are infected.

What are the possible side effects of FLOVENT HFA?

FLOVENT HFA can cause serious side effects, including:

- **fungal infections (thrush) in your mouth and throat.** Tell your doctor if you have any redness or white-colored coating in your mouth.
- **decreased ability to fight infections.** Symptoms of infection may include: fever, pain, aches, chills, feeling tired, nausea and vomiting. Tell your doctor about any signs of infection while you use FLOVENT HFA.
- **decreased adrenal function (adrenal insufficiency).** Symptoms of decreased adrenal function include tiredness, weakness, nausea and vomiting, and low blood pressure. Decreased adrenal function can lead to death.
- **allergic reaction (anaphylaxis).** Call your doctor and stop FLOVENT HFA right away if you have any symptoms of an allergic reaction:
  - swelling of the face, throat and tongue
  - hives
  - rash
  - breathing problems
- **lower bone mineral density.** This may be a problem for people who already have a higher chance of low bone density (osteoporosis).
- **slow growth in children.** The growth of children using FLOVENT HFA should be checked regularly.
- **eye problems including glaucoma and cataracts.** Tell your doctor about any vision changes while using FLOVENT HFA. Your doctor may tell you to have your eyes checked.
- **increased wheezing (bronchospasm).** Increased wheezing can happen right away after using FLOVENT HFA. Always have a rescue inhaler with you to treat sudden wheezing.

Tell your doctor right away if you have any of the serious side effects listed above or if you have worsening lung symptoms.

The most common side effects of FLOVENT HFA include:
- a cold or upper respiratory tract infection
- throat irritation
- headache
- fever
- diarrhea
- ear infection

Tell your doctor if you have any side effects that bother you or that do not go away. These are not all the possible side effects of FLOVENT HFA. For more information ask your doctor or pharmacist.

Call your doctor for medical advice about side effects. You may report side effects to FDA at 1-800-FDA-1088 or 1-800-332-1088.

How should I store FLOVENT HFA?

Store FLOVENT HFA at room temperature between 59°and 86°F (15°-30°C). Store the inhaler with the mouthpiece down. For best results, the inhaler should be at room temperature before use.

Keep FLOVENT HFA and all medicines out of the reach of children.

This Patient Information leaflet summarizes the most important information about FLOVENT HFA. If you would like more information, talk with your healthcare provider. You can ask your pharmacist or doctor for information about FLOVENT HFA that is written for health professionals. You can also contact the company that makes FLOVENT HFA (toll free) at 1-888-825-5249.

What are the ingredients in FLOVENT HFA?

Active ingredient: fluticasone propionate (micronized)
Inactive ingredient: propellant HFA-134a

Instructions for Use

The parts of your FLOVENT HFA

There are 2 main parts to your FLOVENT HFA inhaler—the metal canister that holds the medicine and the dark orange plastic actuator that sprays the medicine from the canister (see Figure 1).

[See figure 1 at top of next column]

The canister has a counter to show how many sprays of medicine you have left. The number shows through a window in the back of the actuator. The counter starts at 124. The number will count down by 1 each time you spray the inhaler. The counter will stop counting at 000:

Never try to change the numbers or take the counter off the metal canister. The counter cannot be reset, and it is permanently attached to the canister.

The mouthpiece of the actuator is covered by a cap. A strap on this cap keeps it attached to the actuator.

Metal Canister
Counter
Plastic Actuator
Strap
Mouthpiece
Cap

Figure 1

Do not use the actuator with a canister of medicine from any other inhaler. And do not use a FLOVENT HFA canister with an actuator from any other inhaler.

Using your FLOVENT HFA

- The inhaler should be at room temperature before you use it.
- **Priming the inhaler:**

  Before you use FLOVENT HFA for the first time, you must prime the inhaler so that you will get the right amount of medicine when you use it. To prime the inhaler, take the cap off the mouthpiece and shake the inhaler well for 5 seconds. Then spray the inhaler into the air away from your face. **Avoid spraying in eyes.** Shake and spray the inhaler like this 3 more times to finish priming it. The counter should now read 120.

  You must prime the inhaler again if you have not used it in more than 7 days or if you drop it. Take the cap off the mouthpiece and shake the inhaler well for 5 seconds. Then spray it 1 time into the air away from your face.

- If a child needs help using the inhaler, an adult should help the child use the inhaler with or without a valved holding chamber, which may also be attached to a mask. The adult should follow the instructions that came with the valved holding chamber. An adult should watch a child use the inhaler to be sure it is used correctly.

Read the following 7 steps before using FLOVENT HFA and follow them at each use. If you have any questions, ask your doctor or pharmacist.

1. **Take the cap off the mouthpiece of the actuator** (see Figure 2).

   Look inside the mouthpiece for foreign objects, and take out any you see.

   Make sure the canister fits firmly in the actuator.

   Shake the inhaler well for 5 seconds.

2. Hold the inhaler with the mouthpiece down (see Figure 2). **Breathe out through your mouth** and push as much air from your lungs as you can. Put the mouthpiece in your mouth and close your lips around it.

Mouthpiece-Down Position

Mouthpiece
Strap
Cap

Figure 2

3. Push the top of the canister all the way down while you breathe in deeply and slowly through your mouth (see Figure 3).

Right after the spray comes out, take your finger off the canister. After you have breathed in all the way, take the inhaler out of your mouth and close your mouth.

Push down and breathe in.

Figure 3

4. **Hold your breath as long as you can,** up to 10 seconds. Then breathe normally.

5. **Wait about 30 seconds and shake the inhaler well** for 5 seconds. Repeat steps 2 through 4.

   After you finish taking this medicine, rinse your mouth with water. Spit out the water. Do not swallow it.

6. Put the cap back on the mouthpiece after each time you use the inhaler. Make sure it snaps firmly into place.

Cleaning your FLOVENT HFA

Clean the inhaler at least once a week after your evening dose. It is important to keep the canister and plastic actuator clean so the medicine will not build-up and block the spray.

Figure 4

1. Take the cap off the mouthpiece. The strap on the cap will stay attached to the actuator. Do not take the canister out of the plastic actuator.

2. Use a clean cotton swab dampened with water to clean the small circular opening where the medicine sprays out of the canister. Gently twist the swab in a circular motion to take off any medicine (see Figure 4). Repeat with a new swab dampened with water to take off any medicine still at the opening.

3. Wipe the inside of the mouthpiece with a clean tissue dampened with water. Let the actuator air-dry overnight.

4. Put the cap back on the mouthpiece after the actuator has dried.

Replacing your FLOVENT HFA

- **When the counter reads 020,** you should refill your prescription or ask your doctor if you need a refill of your prescription.

- **When the counter reads 000,** throw the inhaler away. You should not keep using the inhaler because you will not receive the right amount of medicine.

- **Do not use the inhaler** after the expiration date, which is on the packaging it comes in.

This Patient Information and Instructions for Use have been approved by the U.S. Food and Drug Administration.

FLOVENT is a registered trademark of the GSK group of companies. The other brands listed are trademarks of their respective owners and are not trademarks of the GSK group of companies. The makers of these brands are not affiliated with and do not endorse GlaxoSmithKline or its products.

GlaxoSmithKline
Research Triangle Park, NC 27709
©2014, the GSK group of companies. All rights reserved.
May 2014
FLH:4PIL

FLUARIX QUADRIVALENT   ℞
(Influenza Vaccine)
Suspension for Intramuscular Injection
2014-2015 Formula

HIGHLIGHTS OF PRESCRIBING INFORMATION
These highlights do not include all the information needed to use FLUARIX QUADRIVALENT safely and effectively. See full prescribing information for FLUARIX QUADRIVALENT.
FLUARIX QUADRIVALENT (Influenza Vaccine)
Suspension for Intramuscular Injection
2014-2015 Formula
Initial U.S. Approval: 2012

—————RECENT MAJOR CHANGES—————

Warning and Precautions, Latex (removal)   05/2014

—————INDICATIONS AND USAGE—————

FLUARIX QUADRIVALENT is a vaccine indicated for active immunization for the prevention of disease caused by influenza A subtype viruses and type B viruses contained in the vaccine. FLUARIX QUADRIVALENT is approved for use in persons 3 years of age and older. (1)

—————DOSAGE AND ADMINISTRATION—————

For intramuscular injection only. (2)

Age	Vaccination Status	Dose and Schedule
3 through 8 years of age	Not previously vaccinated with influenza vaccine	Two doses (0.5–mL each) at least 4 weeks apart (2.1)
	Vaccinated with influenza vaccine in a previous season	One or two doses[a] (0.5–mL each) (2.1)
9 years of age and older	Not applicable	One 0.5–mL dose (2.1)

[a] One dose or two doses (0.5-mL each) depending on vaccination history as per the annual Advisory Committee on Immunization Practices (ACIP) recommendation on prevention and control of influenza with vaccines. If two doses, administer each 0.5–mL dose at least 4 weeks apart. (2.1)

—————DOSAGE FORMS AND STRENGTHS—————

Suspension for injection supplied in 0.5–mL single-dose prefilled syringes. (3)

—————CONTRAINDICATIONS—————

History of severe allergic reactions (e.g., anaphylaxis) to any component of the vaccine, including egg protein, or following a previous dose of any influenza vaccine. (4, 11)

—————WARNINGS AND PRECAUTIONS—————

• If Guillain-Barré syndrome has occurred within 6 weeks of receipt of a prior influenza vaccine, the decision to give FLUARIX QUADRIVALENT should be based on careful consideration of potential benefits and risks. (5.1)
• Syncope (fainting) can occur in association with administration of injectable vaccines, including FLUARIX QUADRIVALENT. Procedures should be in place to avoid falling injury and to restore cerebral perfusion following syncope. (5.2)

—————ADVERSE REACTIONS—————

• In adults, the most common (≥10%) injection site adverse reaction was pain (36%); the most common systemic adverse events were muscle aches (16%), headache (16%), and fatigue (16%). (6.1)
• In children 3 through 17 years of age, the injection site adverse reactions were pain (44%), redness (23%), and swelling (19%). (6.1)
• In children 3 through 5 years of age, the most common (≥10%) systemic adverse events were drowsiness (17%), irritability (17%), and loss of appetite (16%); in children 6 through 17 years of age, the most common systemic adverse events were fatigue (20%), muscle aches (18%), headache (16%), arthralgia (10%), and gastrointestinal symptoms (10%). (6.1)

To report SUSPECTED ADVERSE REACTIONS, contact GlaxoSmithKline at 1-888-825-5249 or VAERS at 1-800-822-7967 or www.vaers.hhs.gov.

Table 2. FLUARIX QUADRIVALENT: Incidence of Solicited Local Adverse Reactions and Systemic Adverse Events Within 7 Days[a] of Vaccination in Adults[b] (Total Vaccinated Cohort)

	FLUARIX QUADRIVALENT[c] N = 3,011-3,015 %	Trivalent Influenza Vaccine (TIV)	
		TIV-1 (B Victoria)[d] N = 1,003 %	TIV-2 (B Yamagata)[e] N = 607 %
Local			
Pain	36	37	31
Redness	2	2	2
Swelling	2	2	1
Systemic			
Muscle aches	16	19	16
Headache	16	16	13
Fatigue	16	18	15
Arthralgia	8	10	9
Gastrointestinal symptoms[f]	7	7	6
Shivering	4	5	4
Fever ≥99.5°F (37.5°C)	2	1	2

Total vaccinated cohort for safety included all vaccinated subjects for whom safety data were available.
[a] 7 days included day of vaccination and the subsequent 6 days.
[b] Study 1: NCT01204671.
[c] Contained the same composition as FLUARIX (trivalent formulation) manufactured for the 2010-2011 season and an additional influenza type B virus of Yamagata lineage.
[d] Contained the same composition as FLUARIX manufactured for the 2010-2011 season (2 influenza A subtype viruses and an influenza type B virus of Victoria lineage).
[e] Contained the same 2 influenza A subtype viruses as FLUARIX manufactured for the 2010-2011 season and an influenza type B virus of Yamagata lineage.
[f] Gastrointestinal symptoms included nausea, vomiting, diarrhea, and/or abdominal pain.

—————USE IN SPECIFIC POPULATIONS—————

• Safety and effectiveness of FLUARIX QUADRIVALENT have not been established in pregnant women or nursing mothers. (8.1, 8.3)
• Register women who receive FLUARIX QUADRIVALENT while pregnant in the pregnancy registry by calling 1-888-452-9622. (8.1)
• Geriatric Use: Antibody responses were lower in geriatric subjects who received FLUARIX QUADRIVALENT than in younger subjects. (8.5)

See 17 for PATIENT COUNSELING INFORMATION
Revised: 06/2014

FULL PRESCRIBING INFORMATION: CONTENTS*

1   INDICATIONS AND USAGE
2   DOSAGE AND ADMINISTRATION
   2.1   Dosage and Schedule
   2.2   Administration Instructions
3   DOSAGE FORMS AND STRENGTHS
4   CONTRAINDICATIONS
5   WARNINGS AND PRECAUTIONS
   5.1   Guillain-Barré Syndrome
   5.2   Syncope
   5.3   Preventing and Managing Allergic Vaccine Reactions
   5.4   Altered Immunocompetence
   5.5   Limitations of Vaccine Effectiveness
   5.6   Persons at Risk of Bleeding
6   ADVERSE REACTIONS
   6.1   Clinical Trials Experience
   6.2   Postmarketing Experience
7   DRUG INTERACTIONS
   7.1   Concomitant Vaccine Administration
   7.2   Immunosuppressive Therapies
8   USE IN SPECIFIC POPULATIONS
   8.1   Pregnancy
   8.3   Nursing Mothers
   8.4   Pediatric Use
   8.5   Geriatric Use
11   DESCRIPTION
12   CLINICAL PHARMACOLOGY
   12.1   Mechanism of Action
13   NONCLINICAL TOXICOLOGY
   13.1   Carcinogenesis, Mutagenesis, Impairment of Fertility
14   CLINICAL STUDIES
   14.1   Efficacy Against Culture-Confirmed Influenza
   14.2   Immunological Evaluation of FLUARIX QUADRIVALENT in Adults
   14.3   Immunological Evaluation of FLUARIX QUADRIVALENT in Children
15   REFERENCES
16   HOW SUPPLIED/STORAGE AND HANDLING
17   PATIENT COUNSELING INFORMATION
* Sections or subsections omitted from the full prescribing information are not listed

FULL PRESCRIBING INFORMATION

1   INDICATIONS AND USAGE

FLUARIX® QUADRIVALENT is indicated for active immunization for the prevention of disease caused by influenza A subtype viruses and type B viruses contained in the vaccine [see Description (11)]. FLUARIX QUADRIVALENT is approved for use in persons 3 years of age and older.

2   DOSAGE AND ADMINISTRATION

For intramuscular injection only.
2.1   Dosage and Schedule
The dose and schedule for FLUARIX QUADRIVALENT are presented in Table 1.

Table 1. FLUARIX QUADRIVALENT: Dosing

Age	Vaccination Status	Dose and Schedule
3 through 8 years of age	Not previously vaccinated with influenza vaccine	Two doses (0.5–mL each) at least 4 weeks apart
	Vaccinated with influenza vaccine in a previous season	One or two doses[a] (0.5–mL each)
9 years of age and older	Not applicable	One 0.5–mL dose

[a] One dose or two doses (0.5-mL each) depending on vaccination history as per the annual Advisory Committee on Immunization Practices (ACIP) recommendation on prevention and control of influenza with vaccines. If two doses, administer each 0.5–mL dose at least 4 weeks apart.

2.2   Administration Instructions
Shake well before administration. Parenteral drug products should be inspected visually for particulate matter and dis-

coloration prior to administration, whenever solution and container permit. If either of these conditions exists, the vaccine should not be administered.

Attach a sterile needle to the prefilled syringe and administer intramuscularly.

The preferred site for intramuscular injection is the deltoid muscle of the upper arm. Do not inject in the gluteal area or areas where there may be a major nerve trunk.

Do not administer this product intravenously, intradermally, or subcutaneously.

3 DOSAGE FORMS AND STRENGTHS

FLUARIX QUADRIVALENT is a suspension for injection. Each 0.5–mL dose is supplied in single-dose prefilled TIP–LOK® syringes.

4 CONTRAINDICATIONS

Do not administer FLUARIX QUADRIVALENT to anyone with a history of severe allergic reactions (e.g., anaphylaxis) to any component of the vaccine, including egg protein, or following a previous administration of any influenza vaccine [see Description (11)].

5 WARNINGS AND PRECAUTIONS

5.1 Guillain-Barré Syndrome

If Guillain–Barré syndrome (GBS) has occurred within 6 weeks of receipt of a prior influenza vaccine, the decision to give FLUARIX QUADRIVALENT should be based on careful consideration of the potential benefits and risks.

The 1976 swine influenza vaccine was associated with an increased frequency of GBS. Evidence for a causal relation of GBS with subsequent vaccines prepared from other influenza viruses is inconclusive. If influenza vaccine does pose a risk, it is probably slightly more than one additional case/one million persons vaccinated.

5.2 Syncope

Syncope (fainting) can occur in association with administration of injectable vaccines, including FLUARIX QUADRIVALENT. Syncope can be accompanied by transient neurological signs such as visual disturbance, paresthesia, and tonic-clonic limb movements. Procedures should be in place to avoid falling injury and to restore cerebral perfusion following syncope.

5.3 Preventing and Managing Allergic Vaccine Reactions

Prior to administration, the healthcare provider should review the immunization history for possible vaccine sensitivity and previous vaccination–related adverse reactions. Appropriate medical treatment and supervision must be available to manage possible anaphylactic reactions following administration of FLUARIX QUADRIVALENT.

5.4 Altered Immunocompetence

If FLUARIX QUADRIVALENT is administered to immunosuppressed persons, including individuals receiving immunosuppressive therapy, the immune response may be lower than in immunocompetent persons.

5.5 Limitations of Vaccine Effectiveness

Vaccination with FLUARIX QUADRIVALENT may not protect all susceptible individuals.

5.6 Persons at Risk of Bleeding

As with other intramuscular injections, FLUARIX QUADRIVALENT should be given with caution in individuals with bleeding disorders such as hemophilia or on anticoagulant therapy, to avoid the risk of hematoma following the injection.

6 ADVERSE REACTIONS

The safety experience with FLUARIX (trivalent influenza vaccine) is relevant to FLUARIX QUADRIVALENT because both vaccines are manufactured using the same process and have overlapping compositions [see Description (11)].

6.1 Clinical Trials Experience

In adults who received FLUARIX QUADRIVALENT, the most common (≥10%) injection site adverse reaction was pain (36%). The most common (≥10%) systemic adverse events were muscle aches (16%), headache (16%), and fatigue (16%).

In children 3 through 17 years of age who received FLUARIX QUADRIVALENT, injection site adverse reactions were pain (44%), redness (23%), and swelling (19%). In children 3 through 5 years of age, the most common (≥10%) systemic adverse events were drowsiness (17%), irritability (17%), and loss of appetite (16%); in children 6 through 17 years of age, the most common systemic adverse events were fatigue (20%), muscle aches (18%), headache (16%), arthralgia (10%) and gastrointestinal symptoms (10%).

Because clinical trials are conducted under widely varying conditions, adverse reaction rates observed in the clinical trials of a vaccine cannot be directly compared to rates in the clinical trials of another vaccine, and may not reflect the rates observed in practice. There is the possibility that broad use of FLUARIX QUADRIVALENT could reveal adverse reactions not observed in clinical trials.

FLUARIX QUADRIVALENT in Adults: Study 1 was a randomized, double-blind (2 arms) and open-label

Table 3. FLUARIX QUADRIVALENT: Incidence of Solicited Local Adverse Reactions and Systemic Adverse Events Within 7 Days[a] After First Vaccination in Children 3 Through 17 Years of Age[b] (Total Vaccinated Cohort)

	FLUARIX QUADRIVALENT[c] %	Trivalent Influenza Vaccine (TIV)	
		TIV-1 (B Victoria)[d] %	TIV-2 (B Yamagata)[e] %
3 Through 17 Years of Age			
Local	N = 903	N = 901	N = 905
Pain[f]	44	42	40
Redness	23	21	21
Swelling	19	17	15
3 Through 5 Years of Age			
Systemic	N = 291	N = 314	N = 279
Drowsiness	17	12	14
Irritability	17	13	14
Loss of appetite	16	8	10
Fever ≥99.5°F (37.5°C)	9	9	8
6 Through 17 Years of Age			
Systemic	N = 613	N = 588	N = 626
Fatigue	20	19	16
Muscle aches	18	16	16
Headache	16	19	15
Arthralgia	10	9	7
Gastrointestinal symptoms[g]	10	10	7
Shivering	6	4	5
Fever ≥99.5°F (37.5°C)	6	9	6

Total vaccinated cohort for safety included all vaccinated subjects for whom safety data were available.
[a] 7 days included day of vaccination and the subsequent 6 days.
[b] Study 2: NCT01196988.
[c] Contained the same composition as FLUARIX (trivalent formulation) manufactured for the 2010-2011 season and an additional influenza type B virus of Yamagata lineage.
[d] Contained the same composition as FLUARIX manufactured for the 2010-2011 season (2 influenza A subtype viruses and an influenza type B virus of Victoria lineage).
[e] Contained the same 2 influenza A subtype viruses as FLUARIX manufactured for the 2010-2011 season and an influenza type B virus of Yamagata lineage.
[f] Percentage of subjects with pain by age subgroup: 39%, 38%, and 37% for FLUARIX QUADRIVALENT, TIV-1, and TIV-2, respectively, in children 3 through 8 years of age and 52%, 50%, and 46% for FLUARIX QUADRIVALENT, TIV-1, and TIV-2, respectively, in children 9 through 17 years of age.
[g] Gastrointestinal symptoms included nausea, vomiting, diarrhea, and/or abdominal pain.

(one arm), active-controlled, safety, and immunogenicity study. In this study, subjects received FLUARIX QUADRIVALENT (N = 3,036) or one of two formulations of comparator trivalent influenza vaccine (FLUARIX, TIV-1, N = 1,010 or TIV-2, N = 610), each containing an influenza type B virus that corresponded to one of the two type B viruses in FLUARIX QUADRIVALENT (a type B virus of the Victoria lineage or a type B virus of the Yamagata lineage). The population was 18 years of age and older (mean age 58 years) and 57% were female; 69% were white, 27% were Asian, and 4% were of other racial/ethnic groups. Solicited events were collected for 7 days (day of vaccination and the next 6 days). The frequencies of solicited adverse events are shown in Table 2.

[See table 2 at top of previous page]

Unsolicited events occurring within 21 days of vaccination (day 0-20) were reported in 13%, 14%, and 15% of subjects who received FLUARIX QUADRIVALENT, TIV-1, or TIV-2, respectively. The unsolicited adverse reactions that occurred most frequently (≥0.1% for FLUARIX QUADRIVALENT) included dizziness, injection site hematoma, injection site pruritus, and rash. Serious adverse events occurring within 21 days of vaccination were reported in 0.5%, 0.6%, and 0.2% of subjects who received FLUARIX QUADRIVALENT, TIV-1, or TIV-2, respectively.

FLUARIX QUADRIVALENT in Children: Study 2 was a randomized, double-blind, active-controlled, safety, and immunogenicity study. In this study, subjects received FLUARIX QUADRIVALENT (N = 915) or one of two formulations of comparator trivalent influenza vaccine (FLUARIX, TIV-1, N = 912 or TIV-2, N = 911), each contain-

ing an influenza type B virus that corresponded to one of the two type B viruses in FLUARIX QUADRIVALENT (a type B virus of the Victoria lineage or a type B virus of the Yamagata lineage). Subjects were 3 through 17 years of age and 52% were male; 56% were white, 29% were Asian, 12% were black, and 3% were of other racial/ethnic groups. Children 3 through 8 years of age with no history of influenza vaccination received 2 doses approximately 28 days apart. Children 3 through 8 years of age with a history of influenza vaccination and children 9 years of age and older received one dose. Solicited local adverse reactions and systemic adverse events were collected using diary cards for 7 days (day of vaccination and the next 6 days). The frequencies of solicited adverse events are shown in Table 3.

[See table 3 above]

In children who received a second dose of FLUARIX QUADRIVALENT, TIV-1, or TIV-2, the incidences of adverse events following the second dose were generally lower than those observed after the first dose.

Unsolicited adverse events occurring within 28 days of any vaccination were reported in 31%, 33%, and 34% of subjects who received FLUARIX QUADRIVALENT, TIV-1, or TIV-2, respectively. The unsolicited adverse reactions that occurred most frequently (≥0.1% for FLUARIX QUADRIVALENT) included injection site pruritus and rash. Serious adverse events occurring within 28 days of any vaccination were reported in 0.1%, 0.1%, and 0.1% of subjects who received FLUARIX QUADRIVALENT, TIV-1, or TIV-2, respectively.

FLUARIX (Trivalent Formulation): FLUARIX has been administered to 10,317 adults 18 through 64 years of age,

Table 4. FLUARIX (Trivalent Formulation): Incidence of Solicited Local Adverse Reactions and Systemic Adverse Events Within 4 Days[a] of Vaccination in Adults (Total Vaccinated Cohort)

	Study 3[b]		Study 4[c]	
	18 Through 64 Years of Age		65 Years of Age and Older	
	FLUARIX N = 760 %	Placebo N = 192 %	FLUARIX N = 601-602 %	Comparator N = 596 %
Local				
Pain	55	12	19	18
Redness	18	10	11	13
Swelling	9	6	6	9
Systemic				
Muscle aches	23	12	7	7
Fatigue	20	18	9	10
Headache	19	21	8	8
Arthralgia	6	6	6	5
Shivering	3	3	2	2
Fever ≥100.4°F (38.0°C)	2	2	–	–
Fever ≥99.5°F (37.5°C)	–	–	2	1

Total vaccinated cohort for safety included all vaccinated subjects for whom safety data were available.
[a] 4 days included day of vaccination and the subsequent 3 days.
[b] Study 3 was a randomized, double-blind, placebo-controlled, safety, and immunogenicity study (NCT00100399).
[c] Study 4 was a randomized, single-blind, active-controlled, safety, and immunogenicity study (NCT00197288). The active control was Fluzone, a US-licensed trivalent, inactivated influenza vaccine (Sanofi Pasteur SA).

Table 5. FLUARIX (Trivalent Formulation): Incidence of Solicited Local Adverse Reactions and Systemic Adverse Events Within 4 Days[a] of First Vaccination in Children 3 Through 17 Years of Age[b] (Total Vaccinated Cohort)

	3 Through 4 Years of Age		5 Through 17 Years of Age	
	FLUARIX N = 350 %	Comparator N = 341 %	FLUARIX N = 1,348 %	Comparator N = 451 %
Local				
Pain	35	38	56	56
Redness	23	20	18	16
Swelling	14	13	14	13
Systemic				
Irritability	21	22	–	–
Loss of appetite	13	15	–	–
Drowsiness	13	20	–	–
Fever ≥99.5°F (37.5°C)	7	8	4	3
Muscle aches	–	–	29	29
Fatigue	–	–	20	19
Headache	–	–	15	16
Arthralgia	–	–	6	6
Shivering	–	–	3	4

Total vaccinated cohort for safety included all vaccinated subjects for whom safety data were available.
[a] 4 days included day of vaccination and the subsequent 3 days.
[b] Study 6 was a single-blind, active-controlled, safety, and immunogenicity US study (NCT00383123). The active control was Fluzone, a US-licensed trivalent, inactivated influenza vaccine (Sanofi Pasteur SA).

606 subjects 65 years of age and older, and 2,115 children 6 months through 17 years of age in clinical trials. The incidence of solicited adverse events in each age group is shown in Tables 4 and 5.
[See table 4 above]
[See table 5 above]
In children who received a second dose of FLUARIX or the comparator vaccine, the incidences of adverse events following the second dose were similar to those observed after the first dose.

Serious Adverse Events: In the 4 clinical trials in adults (N = 10,923), there was a single case of anaphylaxis within one day following administration of FLUARIX (<0.01%).

6.2   Postmarketing Experience
Beyond those events reported above in the clinical trials for FLUARIX QUADRIVALENT or FLUARIX, the following adverse events have been spontaneously reported during postapproval use of FLUARIX (trivalent influenza vaccine). This list includes serious events or events which have causal connection to FLUARIX. Because these events are re-ported voluntarily from a population of uncertain size, it is not always possible to reliably estimate their frequency or establish a causal relationship to the vaccine.

Blood and Lymphatic System Disorders: Lymphadenopathy.
Cardiac Disorders: Tachycardia.
Ear and Labyrinth Disorders: Vertigo.
Eye Disorders: Conjunctivitis, eye irritation, eye pain, eye redness, eye swelling, eyelid swelling.
Gastrointestinal Disorders: Abdominal pain or discomfort, swelling of the mouth, throat, and/or tongue.
General Disorders and Administration Site Conditions: Asthenia, chest pain, feeling hot, injection site mass, injection site reaction, injection site warmth, body aches.
Immune System Disorders: Anaphylactic reaction including shock, anaphylactoid reaction, hypersensitivity, serum sickness.
Infections and Infestations: Injection site abscess, injection site cellulitis, pharyngitis, rhinitis, tonsillitis.
Nervous System Disorders: Convulsion, encephalomyelitis, facial palsy, facial paresis, Guillain-Barré syndrome, hypoesthesia, myelitis, neuritis, neuropathy, paresthesia, syncope.
Respiratory, Thoracic, and Mediastinal Disorders: Asthma, bronchospasm, dyspnea, respiratory distress, stridor.
Skin and Subcutaneous Tissue Disorders: Angioedema, erythema, erythema multiforme, facial swelling, pruritus, Stevens-Johnson syndrome, sweating, urticaria.
Vascular Disorders: Henoch-Schönlein purpura, vasculitis.

7   DRUG INTERACTIONS
7.1   Concomitant Vaccine Administration
FLUARIX QUADRIVALENT should not be mixed with any other vaccine in the same syringe or vial.
There are insufficient data to assess the concurrent administration of FLUARIX QUADRIVALENT with other vaccines. When concomitant administration of other vaccines is required, the vaccines should be administered at different injection sites.
7.2   Immunosuppressive Therapies
Immunosuppressive therapies, including irradiation, antimetabolites, alkylating agents, cytotoxic drugs, and corticosteroids (used in greater than physiologic doses), may reduce the immune response to FLUARIX QUADRIVALENT.

8   USE IN SPECIFIC POPULATIONS
8.1   Pregnancy
Pregnancy Category B
A reproductive and developmental toxicity study has been performed in female rats at doses approximately 80 times the human dose (on a mg/kg basis) and revealed no evidence of impaired female fertility or harm to the fetus due to FLUARIX QUADRIVALENT. There are, however, no adequate and well-controlled studies in pregnant women. Because animal reproduction studies are not always predictive of human response, FLUARIX QUADRIVALENT should be given to a pregnant woman only if clearly needed.
In a reproductive and developmental toxicity study, the effect of FLUARIX QUADRIVALENT on embryo-fetal and pre-weaning development was evaluated in rats. Animals were administered FLUARIX QUADRIVALENT by intramuscular injection twice prior to gestation, during the period of organogenesis (gestation days 3, 8, 11, and 15), and during lactation (day 7), 0.2 mL/rat/occasion (approximately 80-fold excess relative to the projected human dose on a body weight basis). No adverse effects on mating, female fertility, pregnancy, parturition, lactation parameters, and embryo-fetal or pre-weaning development were observed. There were no vaccine-related fetal malformations or other evidence of teratogenesis.
Pregnancy Registry: GlaxoSmithKline maintains a surveillance registry to collect data on pregnancy outcomes and newborn health status outcomes following vaccination with FLUARIX QUADRIVALENT during pregnancy. Women who receive FLUARIX QUADRIVALENT during pregnancy should be encouraged to contact GlaxoSmithKline directly or their healthcare provider should contact GlaxoSmithKline by calling 1-888-452-9622.
8.3   Nursing Mothers
It is not known whether FLUARIX QUADRIVALENT is excreted in human milk. Because many drugs are excreted in human milk, caution should be exercised when FLUARIX QUADRIVALENT is administered to a nursing woman.
8.4   Pediatric Use
Safety and effectiveness of FLUARIX QUADRIVALENT in children younger than 3 years of age have not been established.
Safety and immunogenicity of FLUARIX QUADRIVALENT in children 3 through 17 years of age have been evaluated [see Adverse Reactions (6.1) and Clinical Studies (14.3)].

8.5   Geriatric Use

In a randomized, double-blind (2 arms) and open-label (one arm), active-controlled study, immunogenicity and safety were evaluated in a cohort of subjects 65 years of age and older who received FLUARIX QUADRIVALENT (N = 1,517); 469 of these subjects were 75 years of age and older. In subjects 65 years of age and older, the geometric mean antibody titers post-vaccination and seroconversion rates were lower than in younger subjects (18 through 64 years of age) and the frequencies of solicited and unsolicited adverse events were generally lower than in younger subjects.

11   DESCRIPTION

FLUARIX QUADRIVALENT, Influenza Vaccine, for intramuscular injection, is a sterile colorless and slightly opalescent suspension. FLUARIX QUADRIVALENT is prepared from influenza viruses propagated in embryonated chicken eggs. Each of the influenza viruses is produced and purified separately. After harvesting the virus-containing fluids, each influenza virus is concentrated and purified by zonal centrifugation using a linear sucrose density gradient solution containing detergent to disrupt the viruses. Following dilution, the vaccine is further purified by diafiltration. Each influenza virus solution is inactivated by the consecutive effects of sodium deoxycholate and formaldehyde leading to the production of a "split virus." Each split inactivated virus is then suspended in sodium phosphate-buffered isotonic sodium chloride solution. Each vaccine is formulated from the split inactivated virus solutions.

FLUARIX QUADRIVALENT has been standardized according to USPHS requirements for the 2014–2015 influenza season and is formulated to contain 60 micrograms (mcg) hemagglutinin (HA) per 0.5–mL dose, in the recommended ratio of 15 mcg HA of each of the following 4 influenza virus strains: A/Christchurch/16/2010 NIB-74XP (H1N1) (an A/California/7/2009-like virus), A/Texas/50/2012 NYMC X-223A (H3N2), B/Massachusetts/2/2012 NYMC BX-51B, and B/Brisbane/60/2008.

FLUARIX QUADRIVALENT is formulated without preservatives. FLUARIX QUADRIVALENT does not contain thimerosal. Each 0.5–mL dose also contains octoxynol-10 (TRITON® X-100) ≤0.115 mg, α-tocopheryl hydrogen succinate ≤0.135 mg, and polysorbate 80 (Tween 80) ≤0.550 mg. Each dose may also contain residual amounts of hydrocortisone ≤0.0016 mcg, gentamicin sulfate ≤0.15 mcg, ovalbumin ≤0.05 mcg, formaldehyde ≤5 mcg, and sodium deoxycholate ≤65 mcg from the manufacturing process.

The tip caps and plungers of the prefilled syringes of FLUARIX QUADRIVALENT are not made with natural rubber latex.

12   CLINICAL PHARMACOLOGY

12.1   Mechanism of Action

Influenza illness and its complications follow infection with influenza viruses. Global surveillance of influenza identifies yearly antigenic variants. Since 1977, antigenic variants of influenza A (H1N1 and H3N2) viruses and influenza B viruses have been in global circulation.

Public health authorities give annual influenza vaccine composition recommendations. Inactivated influenza vaccines are standardized to contain the hemagglutinins of influenza viruses representing the virus types or subtypes likely to circulate in the United States during the influenza season. Two influenza type B virus lineages (Victoria and Yamagata) are of public health importance because they have co-circulated since 2001. FLUARIX (trivalent influenza vaccine) contains 2 influenza A subtype viruses and one influenza type B virus.

Specific levels of hemagglutination-inhibition (HI) antibody titer post-vaccination with inactivated influenza virus vaccines have not been correlated with protection from influenza illness but the HI antibody titers have been used as a measure of vaccine activity. In some human challenge studies, HI antibody titers of ≥1:40 have been associated with protection from influenza illness in up to 50% of subjects.[1,2] Antibody against one influenza virus type or subtype confers little or no protection against another virus. Furthermore, antibody to one antigenic variant of influenza virus might not protect against a new antigenic variant of the same type or subtype. Frequent development of antigenic variants through antigenic drift is the virological basis for seasonal epidemics and the reason for the usual replacement of one or more influenza viruses in each year's influenza vaccine.

Annual revaccination is recommended because immunity declines during the year after vaccination, and because circulating strains of influenza virus change from year to year.[3]

13   NONCLINICAL TOXICOLOGY

13.1   Carcinogenesis, Mutagenesis, Impairment of Fertility

FLUARIX QUADRIVALENT has not been evaluated for carcinogenic or mutagenic potential. Vaccination of female rats with FLUARIX QUADRIVALENT, at doses shown to be immunogenic in the rat, had no effect on fertility.

Table 6. FLUARIX (Trivalent Formulation): Attack Rates and Vaccine Efficacy Against Culture-Confirmed Influenza A and/or B in Adults (Total Vaccinated Cohort)

		Attack Rates (n/N)		Vaccine Efficacy		
	N	N	%	%	LL	UL
Antigenically Matched Strains[a]						
FLUARIX	5,103	49	1.0	66.9[b]	51.9	77.4
Placebo	2,549	74	2.9	–	–	–
All Culture-Confirmed Influenza (Matched, Unmatched, and Untyped)[c]						
FLUARIX	5,103	63	1.2	61.6[b]	46.0	72.8
Placebo	2,549	82	3.2	–	–	–

[a] There were no vaccine matched culture-confirmed cases of A/New Caledonia/20/1999 (H1N1) or B/Malaysia/2506/2004 influenza virus strains with FLUARIX or placebo.
[b] Vaccine efficacy for FLUARIX exceeded a pre-defined threshold of 35% for the lower limit of the 2-sided 95% CI.
[c] Of the 22 additional cases, 18 were unmatched and 4 were untyped; 15 of the 22 cases were A (H3N2) (11 cases with FLUARIX and 4 cases with placebo).

Table 7. FLUARIX QUADRIVALENT: Immune Responses to Each Antigen 21 Days After Vaccination in Adults (ATP Cohort for Immunogenicity)

	FLUARIX QUADRIVALENT[a]	Trivalent Influenza Vaccine (TIV)	
		TIV-1 (B Victoria)[b]	TIV-2 (B Yamagata)[c]
GMTs	N = 1,809 (95% CI)	N = 608 (95% CI)	N = 534 (95% CI)
A/California/7/2009 (H1N1)	201.1 (188.1, 215.1)	218.4 (194.2, 245.6)	213.0 (187.6, 241.9)
A/Victoria/210/2009 (H3N2)	314.7 (296.8, 333.6)	298.2 (268.4, 331.3)	340.4 (304.3, 380.9)
B/Brisbane/60/2008 (Victoria lineage)	404.6 (386.6, 423.4)	393.8 (362.7, 427.6)	258.5 (234.6, 284.8)
B/Brisbane/3/2007 (Yamagata lineage)	601.8 (573.3, 631.6)	386.6 (351.5, 425.3)	582.5 (534.6, 634.7)
Seroconversion[d]	N = 1,801 % (95% CI)	N = 605 % (95% CI)	N = 530 % (95% CI)
A/California/7/2009 (H1N1)	77.5 (75.5, 79.4)	77.2 (73.6, 80.5)	80.2 (76.5, 83.5)
A/Victoria/210/2009 (H3N2)	71.5 (69.3, 73.5)	65.8 (61.9, 69.6)	70.0 (65.9, 73.9)
B/Brisbane/60/2008 (Victoria lineage)	58.1 (55.8, 60.4)	55.4 (51.3, 59.4)	47.5 (43.2, 51.9)
B/Brisbane/3/2007 (Yamagata lineage)	61.7 (59.5, 64.0)	45.6 (41.6, 49.7)	59.1 (54.7, 63.3)

ATP = according–to–protocol; GMT = geometric mean antibody titer; CI = Confidence Interval.
ATP cohort for immunogenicity included subjects for whom assay results were available after vaccination for at least one study vaccine antigen.
[a] Contained the same composition as FLUARIX (trivalent formulation) manufactured for the 2010-2011 season and an additional influenza type B virus of Yamagata lineage.
[b] Contained the same composition as FLUARIX manufactured for the 2010-2011 season (2 influenza A subtype viruses and an influenza type B virus of Victoria lineage).
[c] Contained the same 2 influenza A subtype viruses as FLUARIX manufactured for the 2010-2011 season and an influenza type B virus of Yamagata lineage.
[d] Seroconversion defined as a pre-vaccination HI titer of <1:10 with a post-vaccination titer ≥1:40 or at least a 4-fold increase in serum titers of HI antibodies to ≥1:40.

14   CLINICAL STUDIES

14.1   Efficacy Against Culture-Confirmed Influenza

The efficacy experience with FLUARIX is relevant to FLUARIX QUADRIVALENT because both vaccines are manufactured using the same process and have overlapping compositions [see Description (11)].

The efficacy of FLUARIX was evaluated in a randomized, double-blind, placebo-controlled study conducted in 2 European countries during the 2006-2007 influenza season. Efficacy of FLUARIX, containing A/New Caledonia/20/1999 (H1N1), A/Wisconsin/67/2005 (H3N2), and B/Malaysia/2506/2004 influenza virus strains, was defined as the prevention of culture-confirmed influenza A and/or B cases, for vaccine antigenically matched strains, compared with placebo. Healthy subjects 18 through 64 years of age (mean age 40 years) were randomized (2:1) to receive FLUARIX (N = 5,103) or placebo (N = 2,549) and monitored for influenza-like illnesses (ILI) starting 2 weeks post-vaccination and lasting for approximately 7 months. In the overall population, 60% of subjects were female and 99.9% were white. Culture-confirmed influenza was assessed by active and passive surveillance of ILI. Influenza-like illness was defined as at least one general symptom (fever ≥100°F and/or myalgia) and at least one respiratory symptom (cough and/or sore throat). After an episode of ILI, nose and throat swab samples were collected for analysis; attack rates and vaccine efficacy were calculated (Table 6).
[See table 6 above]

In a post-hoc, exploratory analysis by age, vaccine efficacy (against culture-confirmed influenza A and/or B cases, for vaccine antigenically matched strains) in subjects 18 through 49 years of age was 73.4% (95% CI: 59.3, 82.8) [number of influenza cases: FLUARIX (n = 35/3,602) and placebo (n = 66/1,810)]. In subjects 50 through 64 years of age, vaccine efficacy was 13.8% (95% CI: −137.0, 66.3) [number of influenza cases: FLUARIX (n = 14/1,501) and placebo (n = 8/739)]. As the study lacked statistical power to evaluate efficacy within age subgroups, the clinical significance of these results is unknown.

Table 8. FLUARIX QUADRIVALENT: Immune Responses to Each Antigen 28 Days After Last Vaccination in Children 3 Through 17 Years of Age (ATP Cohort for Immunogenicity)

| | FLUARIX QUADRIVALENT[a] | Trivalent Influenza Vaccine (TIV) | |
		TIV-1 (B Victoria)[b]	TIV-2 (B Yamagata)[c]
GMTs	N = 791 (95% CI)	N = 818 (95% CI)	N = 801 (95% CI)
A/California/7/2009 (H1N1)	386.2 (357.3, 417.4)	433.2 (401.0, 468.0)	422.3 (390.5, 456.5)
A/Victoria/210/2009 (H3N2)	228.8 (215.0, 243.4)	227.3 (213.3, 242.3)	234.0 (219.1, 249.9)
B/Brisbane/60/2008 (Victoria lineage)	244.2 (227.5, 262.1)	245.6 (229.2, 263.2)	88.4 (81.5, 95.8)
B/Brisbane/3/2007 (Yamagata lineage)	569.6 (533.6, 608.1)	224.7 (207.9, 242.9)	643.3 (603.2, 686.1)
Seroconversion[d]	N = 790 % (95% CI)	N = 818 % (95% CI)	N = 800 % (95% CI)
A/California/7/2009 (H1N1)	91.4 (89.2, 93.3)	89.9 (87.6, 91.8)	91.6 (89.5, 93.5)
A/Victoria/210/2009 (H3N2)	72.3 (69.0, 75.4)	70.7 (67.4, 73.8)	71.9 (68.6, 75.0)
B/Brisbane/60/2008 (Victoria lineage)	70.0 (66.7, 73.2)	68.5 (65.2, 71.6)	29.6 (26.5, 32.9)
B/Brisbane/3/2007 (Yamagata lineage)	72.5 (69.3, 75.6)	37.0 (33.7, 40.5)	70.8 (67.5, 73.9)

ATP = according–to–protocol; GMT = geometric mean antibody titer; CI = Confidence Interval.
ATP cohort for immunogenicity included subjects for whom assay results were available after vaccination for at least one study vaccine antigen.
[a] Contained the same composition as FLUARIX (trivalent formulation) manufactured for the 2010-2011 season and an additional influenza type B virus of Yamagata lineage.
[b] Contained the same composition as FLUARIX manufactured for the 2010-2011 season (2 influenza A subtype viruses and an influenza type B virus of Victoria lineage).
[c] Contained the same 2 influenza A subtype viruses as FLUARIX manufactured for the 2010-2011 season and an influenza B virus of Yamagata lineage.
[d] Seroconversion defined as a pre-vaccination HI titer of <1:10 with a post-vaccination titer ≥1:40 or at least a 4-fold increase in serum titers of HI antibodies to ≥1:40.

14.2 Immunological Evaluation of FLUARIX QUADRIVALENT in Adults
Study 1 was a randomized, double-blind (2 arms) and open-label (one arm), active-controlled, safety, immunogenicity, and non-inferiority study. In this study, subjects received FLUARIX QUADRIVALENT (N = 1,809) or one of two formulations of comparator trivalent influenza vaccine (FLUARIX, TIV-1, N = 608 or TIV-2, N = 534), each containing an influenza type B virus that corresponded to one of the two type B viruses in FLUARIX QUADRIVALENT (a type B virus of the Victoria lineage or a type B virus of the Yamagata lineage). Subjects 18 years of age and older (mean age 58 years) were evaluated for immune responses to each of the vaccine antigens 21 days following vaccination. In the overall population, 57% of subjects were female; 69% were white, 27% were Asian, and 4% were of other racial/ethnic groups.
The immunogenicity endpoints were geometric mean antibody titers (GMTs) of serum hemagglutination-inhibition (HI) antibodies adjusted for baseline, and the percentage of subjects who achieved seroconversion, defined as a pre-vaccination HI titer of <1:10 with a post-vaccination titer ≥1:40 or at least a 4–fold increase in serum HI antibody titer over baseline to ≥1:40 following vaccination, performed on the According-to-Protocol (ATP) cohort for whom immunogenicity assay results were available after vaccination. FLUARIX QUADRIVALENT was non–inferior to both TIVs based on adjusted GMTs (upper limit of the 2–sided 95% CI for the GMT ratio [TIV/FLUARIX QUADRIVALENT] ≤1.5) and seroconversion rates (upper limit of the 2–sided 95% CI on difference of the TIV minus FLUARIX QUADRIVALENT ≤10%). The antibody response to influenza B strains contained in FLUARIX QUADRIVALENT was higher than the antibody response after vaccination with a TIV containing an influenza B strain from a different lineage. There was no evidence that the addition of the second B strain resulted in immune interference to other strains included in the vaccine (Table 7).
[See table 7 at top of previous page]
14.3 Immunological Evaluation of FLUARIX QUADRIVALENT in Children
Study 2 was a randomized, double-blind, active-controlled, safety, immunogenicity, and non-inferiority study. In this study, subjects received FLUARIX QUADRIVALENT

(N = 791) or one of two formulations of comparator trivalent influenza vaccine (FLUARIX, TIV-1, N = 819 or TIV-2, N = 801), each containing an influenza type B virus that corresponded to one of the two type B viruses in FLUARIX QUADRIVALENT (a type B virus of the Victoria lineage or a type B virus of the Yamagata lineage). In children 3 through 17 years of age, immune responses to each of the vaccine antigens were evaluated in sera 28 days following 1 or 2 doses. In the overall population, 52% of subjects were male; 56% were white, 29% were Asian, 12% were black, and 3% were of other racial/ethnic groups.
The immunogenicity endpoints were geometric mean antibody titers (GMTs) adjusted for baseline, and the percentage of subjects who achieved seroconversion, defined as a pre-vaccination HI titer of <1:10 with a post-vaccination titer ≥1:40 or at least a 4–fold increase in serum HI titer over baseline to ≥1:40, following vaccination, performed on the According–to–Protocol (ATP) cohort for whom immunogenicity assay results were available after vaccination. FLUARIX QUADRIVALENT was non-inferior to both TIVs based on adjusted GMTs (upper limit of the 2–sided 95% CI for the GMT ratio [TIV/FLUARIX QUADRIVALENT] ≤1.5) and seroconversion rates (upper limit of the 2–sided 95% CI on difference of the TIV minus FLUARIX QUADRIVALENT ≤10%). The antibody response to influenza B strains contained in FLUARIX QUADRIVALENT was higher than the antibody response after vaccination with a TIV containing an influenza B strain from a different lineage. There was no evidence that the addition of the second B strain resulted in immune interference to other strains included in the vaccine (Table 8).
[See table 8 above]

15 REFERENCES
1. Hannoun C, Megas F, Piercy J. Immunogenicity and protective efficacy of influenza vaccination. *Virus Res.* 2004;103:133-138.
2. Hobson D, Curry RL, Beare AS, et al. The role of serum haemagglutination-inhibiting antibody in protection against challenge infection with influenza A2 and B viruses. *J Hyg Camb.* 1972;70:767-777.
3. Centers for Disease Control and Prevention. Prevention and Control of Influenza with Vaccines: Recommendations of the Advisory Committee on Immunization Practices (ACIP). *MMWR* 2010;59(RR-8):1-62.

16 HOW SUPPLIED/STORAGE AND HANDLING
NDC 58160-901-41 Syringe in Package of 10: NDC 58160-901-52
Store refrigerated between 2° and 8°C (36° and 46°F). Do not freeze. Discard if the vaccine has been frozen. Store in the original package to protect from light.

17 PATIENT COUNSELING INFORMATION
Provide the following information to the vaccine recipient or guardian:
• Inform of the potential benefits and risks of immunization with FLUARIX QUADRIVALENT.
• Educate regarding potential side effects, emphasizing that: (1) FLUARIX QUADRIVALENT contain non–infectious killed viruses and cannot cause influenza and (2) FLUARIX QUADRIVALENT are intended to provide protection against illness due to influenza viruses only, and cannot provide protection against all respiratory illness.
• Inform that safety and efficacy have not been established in pregnant women. Register women who receive FLUARIX QUADRIVALENT while pregnant in the pregnancy registry by calling 1-888-452-9622.
• Give the Vaccine Information Statements, which are required by the National Childhood Vaccine Injury Act of 1986 prior to each immunization. These materials are available free of charge at the Centers for Disease Control and Prevention (CDC) website (www.cdc.gov/vaccines).
• Instruct that annual revaccination is recommended.
FLUARIX and TIP–LOK are registered trademarks of the GSK group of companies. FLUZONE is a registered trademark of Sanofi Pasteur Limited. TRITON is a registered trademark of Union Carbide Chemicals & Plastics Technology Corp.
Manufactured by **GlaxoSmithKline Biologicals**, Dresden, Germany,
a branch of **SmithKline Beecham Pharma GmbH & Co. KG**, Munich, Germany
Licensed by **GlaxoSmithKline Biologicals**, Rixensart, Belgium, US License 1617
Distributed by **GlaxoSmithKline**, Research Triangle Park, NC 27709
©2014, the GSK group of companies. All rights reserved.
FLQ:4PI

FLULAVAL   ℞
[flū' la-val]
(Influenza Vaccine)
Suspension for Intramuscular Injection
2014-2015 Formula

HIGHLIGHTS OF PRESCRIBING INFORMATION
These highlights do not include all the information needed to use FLULAVAL safely and effectively. See full prescribing information for FLULAVAL.
FLULAVAL (Influenza Vaccine)
Suspension for Intramuscular Injection
2014-2015 Formula
Initial U.S. Approval: 2006

———————RECENT MAJOR CHANGES———————

Indications and Usage (1)   08/2013
Dosage and Administration (2.1)   08/2013

———————INDICATIONS AND USAGE———————

FLULAVAL is a vaccine indicated for active immunization for the prevention of disease caused by influenza A subtype viruses and type B virus contained in the vaccine. FLULAVAL is approved for use in persons 3 years of age and older. (1)

———————DOSAGE AND ADMINISTRATION———————

For intramuscular injection only. (2)

Age	Vaccination Status	Dose and Schedule
3 through 8 years of age	Not previously vaccinated with influenza vaccine	Two doses (0.5-mL each) at least 4 weeks apart (2.1)
	Vaccinated with influenza vaccine in a previous season	One or two doses[a] (0.5-mL each) (2.1)
9 years of age and older	Not applicable	One 0.5-mL dose (2.1)

[a] One dose or two doses (0.5-mL each) depending on vaccination history as per the annual Advisory Committee on Immunization Practices (ACIP) recommendation on prevention and control of influenza with vaccines. If two doses, administer each 0.5 mL dose at least 4 weeks apart. (2.1)

---DOSAGE FORMS AND STRENGTHS---

Suspension for injection in 0.5-mL single-dose prefilled syringes and 5-mL multi-dose vials containing 10 doses (each dose is 0.5 mL). (3)

---CONTRAINDICATIONS---

History of severe allergic reactions (e.g., anaphylaxis) to any component of the vaccine, including egg protein, or following a previous dose of any influenza vaccine. (4, 11)

---WARNINGS AND PRECAUTIONS---

• If Guillain-Barré syndrome has occurred within 6 weeks of receipt of a prior influenza vaccine, the decision to give FLULAVAL should be based on careful consideration of the potential benefits and risks. (5.1)
• Syncope (fainting) can occur in association with administration of injectable vaccines, including FLULAVAL. Procedures should be in place to avoid falling injury and to restore cerebral perfusion following syncope. (5.2)

---ADVERSE REACTIONS---

• In adults, the most common (≥10%) solicited local adverse reactions were pain (51%), redness (13%), and/or swelling (11%); the most common solicited systemic adverse events were fatigue (20%), headache (18%), and muscle aches/arthralgia (18%). (6.1)
• In children 3 through 17 years of age, the most common (≥10%) solicited local adverse reaction was pain (56%). (6.1)
• In children 3 through 4 years of age, the most common (≥10%) solicited systemic adverse events were irritability (25%), drowsiness (19%), and loss of appetite (16%). (6.1)
• In children 5 through 17 years of age, the most common (≥10%) solicited systemic adverse events were muscle aches (24%), headache (17%), and fatigue (17%). (6.1)

To report SUSPECTED ADVERSE REACTIONS, contact GlaxoSmithKline at 1-888-825-5249 or VAERS at 1-800-822-7967 or www.vaers.hhs.gov.

---USE IN SPECIFIC POPULATIONS---

• Safety and effectiveness of FLULAVAL have not been established in pregnant women or nursing mothers. (8.1, 8.3)
• Register women who receive FLULAVAL while pregnant in the pregnancy registry by calling 1-888-452-9622. (8.1)
• Geriatric Use: Antibody responses were lower in geriatric subjects who received FLULAVAL than in younger subjects. (8.5)

See 17 for PATIENT COUNSELING INFORMATION
Revised: 06/2014

FULL PRESCRIBING INFORMATION

1   INDICATIONS AND USAGE

FLULAVAL® is indicated for active immunization for the prevention of disease caused by influenza A subtype viruses and type B virus contained in the vaccine. FLULAVAL is approved for use in persons 3 years of age and older.

2   DOSAGE AND ADMINISTRATION

For intramuscular injection only.
2.1   Dosage and Schedule
The dose and schedule for FLULAVAL are presented in Table 1.

Table 1. FLULAVAL: Dosing

Age	Vaccination Status	Dose and Schedule
3 through 8 years of age	Not previously vaccinated with influenza vaccine	Two doses (0.5–mL each) at least 4 weeks apart
	Vaccinated with influenza vaccine in a previous season	One or two doses[a] (0.5–mL each)
9 years of age and older	Not applicable	One 0.5–mL dose

[a] One dose or two doses (0.5–mL each) depending on vaccination history as per the annual Advisory Committee on Immunization Practices (ACIP) recommendation on prevention and control of influenza with vaccines. If two doses, administer each 0.5–mL dose at least 4 weeks apart.

2.2   Administration Instructions
Shake well before administration. Parenteral drug products should be inspected visually for particulate matter and discoloration prior to administration, whenever solution and container permit. If either of these conditions exists, the vaccine should not be administered.
Attach a sterile needle to the prefilled syringe and administer intramuscularly.
For the multi-dose vial, use a sterile needle and sterile syringe to withdraw the 0.5–mL dose from the multi-dose vial and administer intramuscularly. A sterile syringe with a needle bore no larger than 23 gauge is recommended for administration. It is recommended that small syringes (0.5-mL or 1-mL) be used to minimize any product loss. Use a separate sterile needle and syringe for each dose withdrawn from the multi-dose vial.
Between uses, return the multi-dose vial to the recommended storage conditions, between 2° and 8°C (36° and 46°F). Do not freeze. Discard if the vaccine has been frozen. Once entered, a multi-dose vial, and any residual contents, should be discarded after 28 days.
The preferred site for intramuscular injection is the deltoid muscle of the upper arm. Do not inject in the gluteal area or areas where there may be a major nerve trunk.
Do not administer this product intravenously, intradermally, or subcutaneously.

3   DOSAGE FORMS AND STRENGTHS

FLULAVAL is a suspension for injection available in 0.5-mL prefilled TIP–LOK® syringes and 5-mL multi-dose vials containing 10 doses (each dose is 0.5 mL).

4   CONTRAINDICATIONS

Do not administer FLULAVAL to anyone with a history of severe allergic reactions (e.g., anaphylaxis) to any component of the vaccine, including egg protein, or following a previous dose of any influenza vaccine [see Description (11)].

5   WARNINGS AND PRECAUTIONS

5.1   Guillain-Barré Syndrome
If Guillain-Barré syndrome (GBS) has occurred within 6 weeks of receipt of a prior influenza vaccine, the decision to give FLULAVAL should be based on careful consideration of the potential benefits and risks.
The 1976 swine influenza vaccine was associated with an elevated risk of GBS. Evidence for a causal relation of GBS with other influenza vaccines is inconclusive; if an excess risk exists, it is probably slightly more than one additional case/one million persons vaccinated.
5.2   Syncope
Syncope (fainting) can occur in association with administration of injectable vaccines, including FLULAVAL. Syncope can be accompanied by transient neurological signs such as visual disturbance, paresthesia, and tonic-clonic limb movements. Procedures should be in place to avoid falling injury and to restore cerebral perfusion following syncope.
5.3   Preventing and Managing Allergic Vaccine Reactions
Prior to administration, the healthcare provider should review the immunization history for possible vaccine sensitivity and previous vaccination-related adverse reactions. Appropriate medical treatment and supervision must be available to manage possible anaphylactic reactions following administration of FLULAVAL.
5.4   Altered Immunocompetence
If FLULAVAL is administered to immunosuppressed persons, including individuals receiving immunosuppressive therapy, the immune response may be lower than in immunocompetent persons.
5.5   Limitations of Vaccine Effectiveness
Vaccination with FLULAVAL may not protect all susceptible individuals.
5.6   Persons at Risk of Bleeding
As with other intramuscular injections, FLULAVAL should be given with caution in individuals with bleeding disorders such as hemophilia or on anticoagulant therapy to avoid the risk of hematoma following the injection.

6   ADVERSE REACTIONS

6.1   Clinical Trials Experience
In adults who received FLULAVAL, the most common (≥10%) solicited local adverse reactions were pain (51%), redness (13%), and swelling (11%); the most common (≥10%) solicited systemic adverse events were fatigue (20%), headache (18%), and muscle aches/arthralgia (18%).
In children 3 through 17 years of age who received FLULAVAL, the most common (≥10%) solicited local adverse reaction was pain (56%). In children 3 through 4 years of age, the most common (≥10%) solicited systemic adverse events were irritability (25%), drowsiness (19%), and loss of appetite (16%). In children 5 through 17 years of age, the most common (≥10%) systemic adverse events were muscle aches (24%), headache (17%), and fatigue (17%).
Because clinical trials are conducted under widely varying conditions, adverse reaction rates observed in the clinical trials of a vaccine cannot be directly compared to rates in the clinical trials of another vaccine, and may not reflect the rates observed in practice. There is the possibility that broad use of FLULAVAL could reveal adverse reactions not observed in clinical trials.
FLULAVAL in Adults: Safety data was obtained from 3 randomized, controlled trials, one of which was a placebo-controlled efficacy study. In these trials, 9,836 subjects were randomized to receive either FLULAVAL (5,114 subjects in the safety analysis), FLUZONE, a US-licensed trivalent, inactivated influenza vaccine, manufactured by Sanofi Pasteur SA (894 subjects in the safety analysis), or placebo (3,828 subjects in the safety analysis), intramuscularly. In these studies, solicited events were collected for 4 days (i.e., 30 minutes post-vaccination through the next 3 days). Unsolicited adverse events that occurred within 22 days of vaccination (day 0–21) were recorded based on spontaneous reports or in response to queries about changes in health status.
Study 1 (Immunogenicity): Safety information was collected in a randomized, controlled US study. This study included 1,000 adults 18 through 64 years of age who were randomized to receive FLULAVAL (N = 721) or a US-licensed trivalent, inactivated influenza vaccine (N = 279). Among recipients of FLULAVAL, 57% were female; 91% of subjects were white and 9% were of other racial/ethnic groups. The mean age of subjects was 38 years; 80% were 18 through 49 years of age and 20% were 50 through 64 years of age.
Study 2 (Immunogenicity Non-Inferiority): Safety information was collected in a randomized, double-blind, active-controlled US study. The study included 1,225 adults ≥50 years of age randomized to receive FLULAVAL (N = 610) or a US-licensed trivalent, inactivated influenza vaccine (N = 615). In the total population, 57% were female; 95% of subjects were white and 5% were of other racial/ethnic groups. The mean age of subjects was 66 years; 46% were 50 through 64 years of age, 41% were 65 through 79 years of age, and 13% were ≥80 years of age.
Study 3 (Efficacy): Safety information was collected in a double-blind, placebo-controlled US study. The study included 7,658 adults 18 through 49 years of age randomized to receive FLULAVAL (N = 3,807) or placebo (N = 3,851). In the total population, 61% were female; 84% of subjects were white, 10% black, 2% Asian, and 4% were of other racial/ethnic groups. The mean age of subjects was 33 years.
Solicited Adverse Events: Solicited local adverse reactions and systemic adverse events collected for 4 days (day of vaccination and the next 3 days) are presented in Table 2.
[See table 2 at top of next page]
Unsolicited Adverse Events: The incidence of unsolicited adverse events in the 21 days post-vaccination was comparable for FLULAVAL and the active comparator in Study 1 (16% and 15%, respectively) and in Study 2 (18% and 21%, respectively). In Study 3, the incidence of unsolicited adverse events was comparable for the groups (21% for FLULAVAL and 19% for placebo).
Unsolicited adverse events defined as reported with FLULAVAL in >1.0% of subjects are described as fol-

Table 2. FLULAVAL: Incidence of Solicited Local Adverse Reactions and Systemic Adverse Events Within 4 Days[a] of Vaccination in Adults (Total Vaccinated Cohort)

	Percentage of Subjects Reporting Event					
	Study 1[b] 18 Through 64 Years of Age		Study 2[b] 50 Years of Age and Older		Study 3[b] 18 Through 49 Years of Age	
	FLULAVAL N = 721	Comparator[c] N = 279	FLULAVAL N = 610	Comparator[c] N = 615	FLULAVAL N = 3,783	Placebo N = 3,828
Local Adverse Reactions						
Pain	24	31	25	32	51	14
Redness	11	10	10	11	13	6
Swelling	10	10	7	9	11	3
Systemic Adverse Events						
Headache	18	17	11	12	18	19
Fatigue	17	15	12	13	20	18
Muscle aches[d]	13	16	11	10	18	10
Fever (≥99.5°F (37.5°C)	11	10	1	1	3	1
Malaise	10	10	6	7	9	6
Sore throat	9	9	5	6	9	9
Reddened eyes	6	5	4	7	7	6
Cough	6	7	5	6	8	7
Chills	5	2	3	6	4	4
Chest tightness	3	1	2	2	3	3
Facial swelling	1	1	1	2	1	1

Total vaccinated cohort for safety included all vaccinated subjects for whom safety data were available.
[a] 4 days included day of vaccination and the subsequent 3 days.
[b] Study 1: NCT01389479; Study 2: NCT00232947; Study 3: NCT00216242.
[c] US-licensed trivalent, inactivated influenza vaccine (manufactured by Sanofi Pasteur SA).
[d] For Study 2 and Study 3, includes muscle aches and arthralgia.

lows: Study 1: Cough, headache, and pharyngolaryngeal pain; Study 2: Diarrhea, headache, and nasopharyngitis; and Study 3: Pharyngolaryngeal pain, headache, fatigue, cough, injection site pain, upper respiratory tract infection, musculoskeletal pain, nasopharyngitis, injection site erythema and discomfort.

Serious Adverse Events (SAEs): In Study 1, no SAEs were reported. In Study 2, 3% of subjects receiving FLULAVAL and 3% of subjects receiving the active comparator reported SAEs. In Study 3, 1% of subjects receiving FLULAVAL and 1% of subjects receiving placebo reported SAEs. In the 3 clinical trials, the rates of SAEs were comparable between groups and none of the SAEs were considered related to vaccination.

FLULAVAL in Children: *Study 4 (Immunogenicity Non-Inferiority):* An observer-blind, active-controlled US study evaluated subjects 3 through 17 years of age who received FLULAVAL (N = 1,055) or FLUZONE (N = 1,061), a US-licensed trivalent, inactivated influenza vaccine, manufactured by Sanofi Pasteur SA. In the overall population, 53% were male; 78% of subjects were white, 12% were black, 2% were Asian, and 8% were of other racial/ethnic groups. The mean age of subjects was 8 years. Children 3 through 8 years of age with no history of influenza vaccination received 2 doses approximately 28 days apart. Children 3 through 8 years of age with a history of influenza vaccination and children 9 years of age and older received one dose. Solicited local adverse reactions and systemic adverse events were collected for 4 days (day of vaccination and the next 3 days) (Table 3).

Table 3. FLULAVAL: Incidence of Solicited Local Adverse Reactions and Systemic Adverse Events Within 4 Days[a] of First Vaccination in Children 3 Through 17 Years of Age[b] (Total Vaccinated Cohort)

	FLULAVAL %	Active Comparator[c] %
	3 Through 17 Years of Age	
Local Adverse Reactions	N = 1,042	N = 1,026
Pain	56	53
Redness	4	5
Swelling	4	5
	3 Through 4 Years of Age	
Systemic Adverse Events	N = 293	N = 279
Irritability	25	27
Drowsiness	19	19
Loss of appetite	16	13
Fever ≥100.4°F (38.0°C)	5	3
	5 Through 17 Years of Age	
Systemic Adverse Events	N = 750	N = 747
Muscle aches	24	23
Headache	17	15
Fatigue	17	17
Arthralgia	8	10
Shivering	6	5
Fever ≥100.4°F (38.0°C)	5	4

Total vaccinated cohort for safety included all vaccinated subjects for whom safety data were available.
[a] 4 days included day of vaccination and the subsequent 3 days.
[b] Study 4: NCT00980005.
[c] US-licensed trivalent, inactivated influenza vaccine (manufactured by Sanofi Pasteur SA).

In children who received a second dose of FLULAVAL or the comparator vaccine, the incidences of adverse events following the second dose were generally lower than those observed after the first dose.

The incidence of unsolicited adverse events that occurred within 28 days (day 0-27) of any vaccination reported in subjects who received FLULAVAL (N = 1,055) or FLUZONE (N = 1,061) was 40% and 37%, respectively. The unsolicited adverse events that occurred most frequently (≥0.1% of subjects for FLULAVAL) and considered possibly related to vaccination included diarrhea, influenza-like illness, injection site hematoma, injection site rash, injection site warmth, rash, upper abdominal pain, and vomiting. The rates of SAEs were comparable between groups (0.9% and 0.6% for FLULAVAL and the comparator, respectively); none of the SAEs were considered related to vaccination.

6.2 Postmarketing Experience
In addition to reports in clinical trials, the following adverse events have been identified during postapproval use of FLULAVAL. Because these events are reported voluntarily from a population of uncertain size, it is not always possible to reliably estimate their incidence rate or establish a causal relationship to the vaccine. Adverse events described here are included because: a) they represent reactions which are known to occur following immunizations generally or influenza immunizations specifically; b) they are potentially serious; or c) the frequency of reporting.

Blood and Lymphatic System Disorders: Lymphadenopathy.
Eye Disorders: Eye pain, photophobia.
Gastrointestinal Disorders: Dysphagia.
General Disorders and Administration Site Conditions: Chest pain, injection site inflammation, asthenia, injection site rash, abnormal gait, injection site bruising, injection site sterile abscess.
Immune System Disorders: Allergic reactions including anaphylaxis, angioedema.
Infections and Infestations: Rhinitis, laryngitis, cellulitis.
Musculoskeletal and Connective Tissue Disorders: Muscle weakness, arthritis.
Nervous System Disorders: Dizziness, paresthesia, hypoesthesia, hypokinesia, tremor, somnolence, syncope, Guillain-Barré syndrome, convulsions/seizures, facial or cranial nerve paralysis, encephalopathy, limb paralysis.
Psychiatric Disorders: Insomnia.
Respiratory, Thoracic, and Mediastinal Disorders: Dyspnea, dysphonia, bronchospasm, throat tightness.
Skin and Subcutaneous Tissue Disorders: Urticaria, pruritus, sweating.
Vascular Disorders: Flushing, pallor.

7 DRUG INTERACTIONS
7.1 Concomitant Administration With Other Vaccines
FLULAVAL should not be mixed with any other vaccine in the same syringe or vial.
There are insufficient data to assess the concomitant administration of FLULAVAL with other vaccines. When concomitant administration of other vaccines is required, the vaccines should be administered at different injection sites.
7.2 Immunosuppressive Therapies
Immunosuppressive therapies, including irradiation, antimetabolites, alkylating agents, cytotoxic drugs, and corticosteroids (used in greater than physiologic doses), may reduce the immune response to FLULAVAL.

8 USE IN SPECIFIC POPULATIONS
8.1 Pregnancy
Pregnancy Category B
A reproductive and developmental toxicity study has been performed in female rats at a dose 40-fold the human dose (on a mg/kg basis) and showed no evidence of impaired female fertility or harm to the fetus due to FLULAVAL. There are, however, no adequate and well-controlled studies in pregnant women. Because animal reproduction studies are not always predictive of human response, FLULAVAL should be given to a pregnant woman only if clearly needed. In a reproductive and developmental toxicity study, the effect of FLULAVAL on embryo-fetal and pre-weaning development was evaluated in rats. Animals were administered FLULAVAL by intramuscular injection once prior to gestation, and during the period of organogenesis (gestation days 6, 8, 11, and 15), 0.1 mL/dose/rat (approximately 40-fold higher than the projected human dose on a body weight basis). No adverse effects on mating, female fertility, pregnancy, parturition, lactation parameters, and embryo-fetal or pre-weaning development were observed. There were no vaccine-related fetal malformations or other evidence of teratogenesis.
Pregnancy Registry: GlaxoSmithKline maintains a surveillance registry to collect data on pregnancy outcomes and newborn health status outcomes following vaccination with FLULAVAL during pregnancy. Women who receive FLULAVAL during pregnancy should be encouraged to contact GlaxoSmithKline directly or their healthcare provider should contact GlaxoSmithKline by calling 1-888-452-9622.
8.3 Nursing Mothers
It is not known whether FLULAVAL is excreted in human milk. Because many drugs are excreted in human milk, caution should be exercised when FLULAVAL is administered to a nursing woman.
8.4 Pediatric Use
Safety and effectiveness of FLULAVAL in children younger than 3 years of age have not been established.
Safety and immunogenicity of FLULAVAL in children 3 through 17 years of age have been evaluated *[see Adverse Reactions (6.1) and Clinical Studies (14)]*.
8.5 Geriatric Use
In clinical trials, there were 330 subjects 65 years of age and older who received FLULAVAL; 142 of these subjects were 75 years of age and older. Hemagglutination inhibition antibody responses were lower in geriatric subjects than younger subjects after administration of FLULAVAL. *[See Clinical Studies (14.2).]* Solicited adverse events were similar in frequency to those reported in younger subjects *[see Adverse Reactions (6.1)]*.

11 DESCRIPTION
FLULAVAL, Influenza Vaccine, for intramuscular injection, is a trivalent, split-virion, inactivated influenza virus

vaccine prepared from virus propagated in the allantoic cavity of embryonated hens' eggs. Each of the influenza viruses is produced and purified separately. The virus is inactivated with ultraviolet light treatment followed by formaldehyde treatment, purified by centrifugation, and disrupted with sodium deoxycholate.

FLULAVAL is a sterile, opalescent, translucent to off-white suspension in a phosphate-buffered saline solution that may sediment slightly. The sediment resuspends upon shaking to form a homogeneous suspension.

FLULAVAL has been standardized according to USPHS requirements for the 2014–2015 influenza season and is formulated to contain 45 micrograms (mcg) hemagglutinin (HA) per 0.5-mL dose in the recommended ratio of 15 mcg HA of each of the following 3 strains: A/California/7/2009 NYMC X–179A (H1N1), A/Texas/50/2012 NYMC X–223A (H3N2), and B/Massachusetts/2/2012 NYMC BX-51B.

The prefilled syringe is formulated without preservatives and does not contain thimerosal. Each 0.5-mL dose from the multi-dose vial contains 50 mcg thimerosal (<25 mcg mercury); thimerosal, a mercury derivative, is added as a preservative.

Each 0.5-mL dose of either presentation may also contain residual amounts of ovalbumin (≤0.3 mcg), formaldehyde (≤25 mcg), sodium deoxycholate (≤50 mcg), α-tocopheryl hydrogen succinate (≤240 mcg), and polysorbate 80 (≤665 mcg) from the manufacturing process. Antibiotics are not used in the manufacture of this vaccine.

The tip caps and plungers of the prefilled syringes are not made with natural rubber latex. The vial stoppers are not made with natural rubber latex.

12 CLINICAL PHARMACOLOGY

12.1 Mechanism of Action

Influenza illness and its complications follow infection with influenza viruses. Global surveillance of influenza identifies yearly antigenic variants. Since 1977, antigenic variants of influenza A (H1N1 and H3N2) viruses and influenza B viruses have been in global circulation.

Specific levels of hemagglutination inhibition (HI) antibody titer post-vaccination with inactivated influenza virus vaccines have not been correlated with protection from influenza illness but the antibody titers have been used as a measure of vaccine activity. In some human challenge studies, antibody titers of ≥1:40 have been associated with protection from influenza illness in up to 50% of subjects.[1,2] Antibody against one influenza virus type or subtype confers little or no protection against another virus. Furthermore, antibody to one antigenic variant of influenza virus might not protect against a new antigenic variant of the same type or subtype. Frequent development of antigenic variants through antigenic drift is the virological basis for seasonal epidemics and the reason for the usual change of one or more new strains in each year's influenza vaccine. Therefore, inactivated influenza vaccines are standardized to contain the hemagglutinins of strains (i.e., typically 2 type A and 1 type B), representing the influenza viruses likely to circulate in the United States in the upcoming winter.

Annual revaccination is recommended because immunity declines during the year after vaccination, and because circulating strains of influenza virus change from year to year.[3]

13 NONCLINICAL TOXICOLOGY

13.1 Carcinogenesis, Mutagenesis, Impairment of Fertility

FLULAVAL has not been evaluated for carcinogenic or mutagenic potential. Vaccination of female rats with FLULAVAL, at doses shown to be immunogenic in the rat, had no effect on fertility.

14 CLINICAL STUDIES

The effectiveness of FLULAVAL was demonstrated based on clinical endpoint efficacy data for FLULAVAL QUADRIVALENT (Influenza Vaccine), clinical endpoint efficacy data for FLULAVAL, and on an evaluation of serum HI antibody responses to FLULAVAL. FLULAVAL QUADRIVALENT, an inactivated influenza vaccine that contains the hemagglutinins of two influenza A subtype viruses and two influenza type B viruses, is manufactured according to the same process as FLULAVAL.

14.1 Efficacy Against Influenza

Efficacy Trial in Children: The efficacy of FLULAVAL QUADRIVALENT was evaluated in Study 5, a randomized, observer-blind, non-influenza vaccine-controlled study conducted in 3 countries in Asia, 3 in Latin America, and 2 in the Middle East/Europe during the 2010-2011 influenza season. Healthy subjects 3 through 8 years of age were randomized (1:1) to receive FLULAVAL QUADRIVALENT (N = 2,584), containing A/California/7/2009 (H1N1), A/Victoria/210/2009 (H3N2), B/Brisbane/60/2008 (Victoria lineage), and B/Florida/4/2006 (Yamagata lineage) influenza strains, or HAVRIX® (Hepatitis A Vaccine) (N = 2,584), as a control vaccine. Children with no history of influenza vaccination received 2 doses of FLULAVAL QUADRIVALENT or

HAVRIX approximately 28 days apart. Children with a history of influenza vaccination received one dose of FLULAVAL QUADRIVALENT or HAVRIX. In the overall population, 52% were male; 60% were Asian, 5% were white, and 35% were of other racial/ethnic groups. The mean age of subjects was 5 years.

Efficacy of FLULAVAL QUADRIVALENT was assessed for the prevention of reverse transcriptase polymerase chain reaction (RT-PCR)-positive influenza A and/or B disease presenting as influenza-like illness (ILI). ILI was defined as a temperature ≥100°F in the presence of at least one of the following symptoms on the same day: cough, sore throat, runny nose, or nasal congestion. Subjects with ILI (monitored by passive and active surveillance for approximately 6 months) had nasal and throat swabs collected and tested for influenza A and/or B by RT-PCR. All RT-PCR-positive specimens were further tested in cell culture. Vaccine efficacy was calculated based on the ATP cohort for efficacy (Table 4).

[See table 4 above]

Table 4. FLULAVAL QUADRIVALENT: Influenza Attack Rates and Vaccine Efficacy Against Influenza A and/or B in Children 3 Through 8 Years of Age[a] (According to Protocol Cohort for Efficacy)

	N[b]	n[c]	Influenza Attack Rate % (n/N)	Vaccine Efficacy % (CI)
All RT-PCR-Positive Influenza				
FLULAVAL QUADRIVALENT	2,379	58	2.4	55.4[d] (95% CI: 39.1, 67.3)
HAVRIX[e]	2,398	128	5.3	–
All Culture-Confirmed Influenza[f]				
FLULAVAL QUADRIVALENT	2,379	50	2.1	55.9 (97.5% CI: 35.4, 69.9)
HAVRIX[e]	2,398	112	4.7	–
Antigenically Matched Culture-Confirmed Influenza				
FLULAVAL QUADRIVALENT	2,379	31	1.3	45.1[g] (97.5% CI: 9.3, 66.8)
HAVRIX[e]	2,398	56	2.3	

CI = Confidence Interval; RT-PCR = reverse transcriptase polymerase chain reaction.
[a] Study 5: NCT01218308.
[b] According to protocol cohort for efficacy included subjects who met all eligibility criteria, were successfully contacted at least once post-vaccination, and complied with the protocol-specified efficacy criteria.
[c] Number of influenza cases.
[d] Vaccine efficacy for FLULAVAL QUADRIVALENT met the pre-defined criterion of >30% for the lower limit of the 2-sided 95% CI.
[e] Hepatitis A Vaccine used as a control vaccine.
[f] Of 162 culture-confirmed influenza cases, 108 (67%) were antigenically typed (87 matched; 21 unmatched); 54 (33%) could not be antigenically typed [but were typed by RT-PCR and nucleic acid sequence analysis: 5 cases A (H1N1) (5 with HAVRIX), 47 cases A (H3N2) (10 with FLULAVAL QUADRIVALENT; 37 with HAVRIX), and 2 cases B Victoria (2 with HAVRIX)].
[g] Since only 67% of cases could be typed, the clinical significance of this result is unknown.

Table 5. FLULAVAL QUADRIVALENT: Incidence of Adverse Outcomes Associated With RT-PCR-Positive Influenza in Children 3 Through 8 Years of Age[a] (Total Vaccinated Cohort)[b]

Adverse Outcome[d]	FLULAVAL QUADRIVALENT N = 2,584			HAVRIX[c] N = 2,584		
	Number of Events	Number of Subjects[e]	%	Number of Events	Number of Subjects[e]	%
Fever >102.2°F/39.0°C	16[f]	15	0.6	51[f]	50	1.9
Shortness of breath	0	0	0	5	5	0.2
Pneumonia	0	0	0	3	3	0.1
Wheezing	1	1	0	1	1	0
Bronchitis	1	1	0	1	1	0
Pulmonary congestion	0	0	0	1	1	0
Acute otitis media	0	0	0	1	1	0
Bronchiolitis	0	0	0	0	0	0
Croup	0	0	0	0	0	0
Encephalitis	0	0	0	0	0	0
Myocarditis	0	0	0	0	0	0
Myositis	0	0	0	0	0	0
Seizure	0	0	0	0	0	0

[a] Study NCT01218308.
[b] Total vaccinated cohort included all vaccinated subjects for whom data were available.
[c] Hepatitis A Vaccine used as a control vaccine.
[d] In subjects who presented with more than one adverse outcome, each outcome was counted in the respective category.
[e] Number of subjects presenting with at least one event in each group.
[f] One subject in each group had sequential influenza due to influenza type A and type B viruses.

In an exploratory analysis by age, vaccine efficacy against RT-PCR-positive influenza A and/or B disease presenting as ILI was evaluated in subjects 3 through 4 years of age and 5 through 8 years of age; vaccine efficacy was 35.3% (95% CI: –1.3, 58.6) and 67.7% (95% CI: 49.7, 79.2), respectively. As the study lacked statistical power to evaluate efficacy within age subgroups, the clinical significance of these results is unknown.

As a secondary objective in the study, subjects with RT-PCR-positive influenza A and/or B were prospectively classified based on the presence of adverse outcomes that have been associated with influenza infection (defined as fever >102.2°F/39.0°C, physician-verified shortness of breath, pneumonia, wheezing, bronchitis, bronchiolitis, pulmonary congestion, croup and/or acute otitis media, and/or physician-diagnosed serious extra-pulmonary complications, including myositis, encephalitis, seizure and/or myocarditis).

The risk reduction of fever >102.2°F/39.0°C associated with RT-PCR-positive influenza was 71.0% (95% CI: 44.8, 84.8) based on the ATP cohort for efficacy [FLULAVAL QUADRIVALENT (n = 12/2,379); HAVRIX (n = 41/2,398)]. The other pre-specified adverse outcomes had too few cases to calculate a risk reduction. The incidence of these adverse outcomes is presented in Table 5.
[See table 5 at top of previous page]

Efficacy Trial in Adults: The efficacy of FLULAVAL was evaluated in a randomized, double-blind, placebo-controlled study conducted in the United States during the 2005-2006 and 2006-2007 influenza seasons (Study 3). Efficacy of FLULAVAL was defined as the prevention of culture-confirmed influenza A and/or B cases, for vaccine antigenically matched strains, compared with placebo. Healthy subjects 18 through 49 years of age were randomized (1:1); a total of 3,783 subjects received FLULAVAL and 3,828 subjects received placebo [see Adverse Reactions (6.1)]. Subjects were monitored for influenza-like illnesses (ILI) starting 2 weeks post-vaccination and for duration of approximately 7 months thereafter. Culture-confirmed influenza was assessed by active and passive surveillance of ILI. Influenza-like illness was defined as illness sufficiently severe to limit daily activity and including cough, and at least one of the following: Fever >99.9°F, nasal congestion or runny nose, sore throat, muscle aches or arthralgia, headache, feverishness or chills. After an episode of ILI, nose and throat swab samples were collected for analysis; attack rates and vaccine efficacy were calculated using the per protocol cohort (Table 6). Of note, the 1.2% attack rate in the placebo group for culture-confirmed, antigenically matched strains was lower than expected, contributing to a wide confidence interval for the estimate of vaccine efficacy.

Table 6. FLULAVAL: Influenza Attack Rates and Vaccine Efficacy Against Culture-Confirmed Influenza in Adults 18 Through 49 Years of Age[a] (Per Protocol Cohort)

	N[b]	n[c]	Influenza Attack Rates % (n/N)	Vaccine Efficacy %	Vaccine Efficacy 97.5% CI Lower Limit
Antigenically Matched Strains					
FLULAVAL	3,714	23	0.6	46.3	9.8[d]
Placebo	3,768	45	1.2	–	–
All Culture-Confirmed Influenza (Matched, Unmatched, and Untyped)					
FLULAVAL	3,714	30	0.8	49.3	20.3
Placebo	3,768	60	1.6	–	–

CI = Confidence Interval.
[a] Study 3: NCT00216242.
[b] Per Protocol Cohort for efficacy included subjects with no protocol deviations considered to compromise efficacy data.
[c] Number of influenza cases.
[d] Lower limit of the one-sided 97.5% CI for vaccine efficacy against influenza due to antigenically matched strains was less than the pre-defined success criterion of ≥35%.

14.2 Immunological Evaluation

Adults: Study 1 was a randomized, blinded, active-controlled US study performed in healthy adults 18 through 64 years of age (N = 1,000). A total of 721 subjects received FLULAVAL, and 279 received a US-licensed trivalent, inactivated influenza vaccine, FLUZONE (manufactured by Sanofi Pasteur SA), intramuscularly; 959 subjects had complete serological data and no major protocol deviations [see Adverse Reactions (6.1)].

Analyses of immunogenicity (Table 7) were performed for each hemagglutinin (HA) antigen contained in the vaccine: 1) assessment of the lower bounds of 2-sided 95% confidence intervals for the proportion of subjects with HI antibody titers of ≥1:40 after vaccination, and 2) assessment of the lower bounds of 2-sided 95% confidence intervals for rates of seroconversion (defined as a 4-fold increase in post-vaccination HI antibody titer from pre-vaccination titer ≥1:10, or an increase in titer from <1:10 to ≥1:40). The pre-specified success criteria for HI titer ≥1:40 was 70% and for seroconversion rate was 40%. The lower limit of the 2-sided 95% CI for the percentage of subjects who achieved an HI titer of ≥1:40 exceeded the pre-defined criteria for the A strains. The lower limit of the 2-sided 95% CI for the percentage of subjects who achieved seroconversion exceeded the pre-defined criteria for all 3 strains.

Table 7. Immune Responses to Each Antigen 21 Days After Vaccination With FLULAVAL[a] in Adults 18 Through 64 Years of Age (Per Protocol Cohort)[b]

	FLULAVAL N = 692 % of Subjects (95% CI)	
HI titers ≥1:40	**Pre-vaccination**	**Post-vaccination**
A/New Caledonia/20/99 (H1N1)	24.6	96.5 (94.9, 97.8)
A/Wyoming/03/03 (H3N2)	58.7	98.7 (97.6, 99.4)
B/Jiangsu/10/03	5.4	62.9 (59.1, 66.5)
Seroconversion[c] to:		
A/New Caledonia/20/99 (H1N1)	85.6 (82.7, 88.1)	
A/Wyoming/03/03 (H3N2)	79.3 (76.1, 82.3)	
B/Jiangsu/10/03	58.4 (54.6, 62.1)	

HI – hemagglutination inhibition; CI = Confidence Interval.
[a] Results obtained following vaccination with FLULAVAL manufactured for the 2004–2005 season.
[b] Per Protocol Cohort for immunogenicity included subjects with complete pre- and post-dose HI titer data and no major protocol deviations.
[c] Seroconversion defined as a 4-fold increase in post-vaccination HI antibody titers from pre-vaccination titer ≥1:10, or an increase in titer from <1:10 to ≥1:40.

Study 2 (Immunogenicity Non-Inferiority): In a randomized, double-blind, active-controlled US study, immunological non-inferiority of FLULAVAL was compared with a US-licensed trivalent, inactivated influenza vaccine, FLUZONE, manufactured by Sanofi Pasteur SA. A total of 1,225 adults ≥50 years of age and older in stable health were randomized to receive FLULAVAL or the comparator vaccine intramuscularly [see Adverse Reactions (6.1)].

Analyses of immunogenicity were performed for each HA antigen contained in the vaccines: 1) assessment of the lower bounds of 2-sided 95% confidence intervals for the geometric mean antibody titer (GMT) ratio (FLULAVAL/comparator), and 2) assessment of the lower bounds of 2-sided 95% confidence intervals for seroconversion rates (defined as a 4-fold increase in post-vaccination HI antibody titer from pre-vaccination titer ≥1:10, or an increase in titer from <1:10 to ≥1:40). Non-inferiority of FLULAVAL to the comparator vaccine was established for all 6 co-primary endpoints (Table 8). Within each age stratum, immunogenicity results were similar between the groups.
[See table 8 below]

Children: In Study 4, the immune response of FLULAVAL (N = 987) was compared to FLUZONE, a US-licensed trivalent, inactivated influenza vaccine (N = 979), manufactured by Sanofi Pasteur SA, in an observer-blind, randomized study in children 3 through 17 years of age. The immune responses to each of the antigens contained in FLULAVAL formulated for the 2009-2010 season were evaluated in sera obtained after one or 2 doses of FLULAVAL and were compared to those following the comparator influenza vaccine [see Adverse Reactions (6.1)].

The non-inferiority endpoints were geometric mean antibody titers (GMTs) adjusted for baseline, and the percentage of subjects who achieved seroconversion, defined as at least a 4-fold increase in serum HI titer over baseline to ≥1:40, following vaccination, performed on the According-to-Protocol (ATP) cohort. FLULAVAL was non-inferior to the comparator influenza for all strains based on adjusted GMTs and seroconversion rates (Table 9).

Table 8. Immune Responses to Each Antigen 21 Days After Vaccination With FLULAVAL Versus Comparator Influenza Vaccine in Adults 50 Years of Age and Older[a] (Per Protocol Cohort)[b]

GMTs Against	FLULAVAL N = 592 GMT (95% CI)	Active Comparator[c] N = 595 GMT (95% CI)	GMT Ratio[d] (95% CI)
A/New Caledonia/20/99 (H1N1)	113.4 (104.7, 122.8)	110.2 (101.8, 119.3)	1.03 (0.92, 1.15)
A/New York/55/04 (H3N2)	223.9 (199.5, 251.3)	214.6 (191.3, 240.7)	1.04 (0.89, 1.23)
B/Jiangsu/10/03	82.3 (74.7, 90.6)	97.1 (88.2, 106.8)	0.85 (0.74, 0.97)
Seroconversion[e] to:	**% of Subjects (95% CI)**	**% of Subjects (95% CI)**	**Difference in Seroconversion Rates[f] (95% CI)**
A/New Caledonia/20/99 (H1N1)	34 (30.0, 37.6)	32 (28.3, 35.9)	2 (-3.7, 7.0)
A/New York/55/04 (H3N2)	83 (80.3, 86.3)	82 (78.4, 84.6)	1 (-2.6, 6.1)
B/Jiangsu/10/03	53 (49.0, 57.1)	56 (51.6, 59.6)	-3 (-8.3, 3.1)

GMT = geometric mean antibody titer; CI = Confidence Interval.
[a] Results obtained following vaccination with influenza vaccines manufactured for the 2005–2006 season.
[b] Per Protocol Cohort for immunogenicity included subjects with complete pre- and post-dose HI titer data and no major protocol deviations.
[c] US-licensed trivalent, inactivated influenza vaccine (manufactured by Sanofi Pasteur SA).
[d] FLULAVAL met non-inferiority criteria based on GMTs (lower limit of 2-sided 95% CI for GMT ratio [FLULAVAL/comparator vaccine] ≥0.67).
[e] Seroconversion defined as a 4-fold increase in post-vaccination HI antibody titer from pre-vaccination titer ≥1:10, or an increase in titer from <1:10 to ≥1:40.
[f] FLULAVAL met non-inferiority criteria based on seroconversion rates (lower limit of 2-sided 95% CI for difference of FLULAVAL minus the comparator vaccine ≥–10%).

Table 9. Immune Responses to Each Antigen 28 Days After Last Vaccination With FLULAVAL Versus Comparator Influenza Vaccine in Children 3 Through 17 Years of Age[a] (According to Protocol Cohort for Immunogenicity)[b]

GMTs Against	FLULAVAL N = 987 (95% CI)	Active Comparator[c] N = 979 (95% CI)	GMT Ratio[d] (95% CI)
A/Brisbane (H1N1)	320.9 (298.3, 345.2)	329.4 (306.8, 353.7)	1.03 (0.94, 1.13)
A/Uruguay (H3N2)	414.7 (386.5, 444.9)	451.9 (423.8, 481.8)	1.05 (0.96, 1.13)
B/Brisbane	213.7 (198.5, 230.1)	200.2 (186.1, 215.3)	0.93 (0.85, 1.02)
Seroconversion[e] to:	N = 987 % (95% CI)	N = 978 % (95% CI)	Difference in Seroconversion Rate[f] (95% CI)
A/Brisbane (H1N1)	59.8 (56.6, 62.9)	58.2 (55.0, 61.3)	-1.6 (-5.9, 2.8)
A/Uruguay (H3N2)	68.2 (65.2, 71.1)	66.2 (63.1, 69.1)	-2.0 (-6.1, 2.1)
B/Brisbane	81.1 (78.5, 83.5)	78.6 (75.9, 81.2)	-2.4 (-6.0, 1.1)

GMT = geometric mean antibody titer; CI = Confidence Interval.
[a] Results obtained following vaccination with influenza vaccines formulated for the 2009-2010 season.
[b] According to protocol cohort for immunogenicity included all evaluable subjects for whom assay results were available after vaccination for at least one study vaccine antigen.
[c] US-licensed trivalent, inactivated influenza vaccine (Sanofi Pasteur SA).
[d] FLULAVAL met non–inferiority criteria based on GMTs (upper limit of 2–sided 95% CI for GMT ratio [comparator vaccine/FLULAVAL] ≤1.5).
[e] Seroconversion defined as a 4–fold increase in post-vaccination HI antibody titer from pre-vaccination titer ≥1:10, or an increase in titer from <1:10 to ≥1:40.
[f] FLULAVAL met non–inferiority criteria based on seroconversion rates (upper limit of 2–sided 95% CI for difference of the comparator vaccine minus FLULAVAL ≤10%).

[See table 9 above]

15   REFERENCES
1. Hannoun C, Megas F, Piercy J. Immunogenicity and protective efficacy of influenza vaccination. *Virus Res* 2004;103:133-138.
2. Hobson D, Curry RL, Beare AS, et al. The role of serum haemagglutination-inhibiting antibody in protection against challenge infection with influenza A2 and B viruses. *J Hyg Camb* 1972;70:767-777.
3. Centers for Disease Control and Prevention. Prevention and control of influenza with vaccines: Recommendations of the Advisory Committee on Immunization Practices (ACIP). *MMWR* 2010;59(RR-8):1-62.

16   HOW SUPPLIED/STORAGE AND HANDLING
FLULAVAL is available in 0.5-mL single-dose disposable prefilled TIP-LOK syringes (packaged without needles) and in 5-mL multi-dose vials containing 10 doses (0.5-mL each). NDC 19515-892-41 Syringe in Package of 10: NDC 19515-892-52
NDC 19515-893-02 Multi-Dose Vial (containing 10 doses) in Package of 1: NDC 19515-893-07
Store refrigerated between 2° and 8°C (36° and 46°F). Do not freeze. Discard if the vaccine has been frozen. Store in the original package to protect from light. Once entered, a multi-dose vial should be discarded after 28 days.

17   PATIENT COUNSELING INFORMATION
Provide the following information to the vaccine recipient or guardian:
• Inform of the potential benefits and risks of immunization with FLULAVAL.
• Educate regarding potential side effects, emphasizing that: (1) FLULAVAL contains non-infectious killed viruses and cannot cause influenza, and (2) FLULAVAL is intended to provide protection against illness due to influenza viruses only, and cannot provide protection against all respiratory illness.
• Inform that safety and efficacy have not been established in pregnant women. Register women who receive FLULAVAL while pregnant in the pregnancy registry by calling 1-888-452-9622.
• Give the Vaccine Information Statements, which are required by the National Childhood Vaccine Injury Act of 1986 prior to each immunization. These materials are available free of charge at the Centers for Disease Control and Prevention (CDC) website (www.cdc.gov/vaccines).
• Instruct that annual revaccination is recommended.
FLULAVAL, TIP-LOK and HAVRIX are registered trademarks of the GSK group of companies. FLUZONE is a registered trademark of Sanofi Pasteur Limited.

Manufactured by **ID Biomedical Corporation of Quebec**
Quebec City, QC, Canada, US License 1739
Distributed by **GlaxoSmithKline**
Research Triangle Park, NC 27709
©2014, the GSK group of companies. All rights reserved.
FLV:13PI

FLULAVAL QUADRIVALENT   ℞
(Influenza Virus Vaccine)
Suspension for Intramuscular Injection
2014-2015 Formula

HIGHLIGHTS OF PRESCRIBING INFORMATION
These highlights do not include all the information needed to use FLULAVAL QUADRIVALENT safely and effectively. See full prescribing information for FLULAVAL QUADRIVALENT.
FLULAVAL QUADRIVALENT (Influenza Vaccine)
Suspension for Intramuscular Injection
2014-2015 Formula
Initial U.S. Approval: 2013

INDICATIONS AND USAGE
FLULAVAL QUADRIVALENT is a vaccine indicated for active immunization for the prevention of disease caused by influenza A subtype viruses and type B viruses contained in the vaccine. FLULAVAL QUADRIVALENT is approved for use in persons 3 years of age and older. (1)

DOSAGE AND ADMINISTRATION
For intramuscular injection only. (2)

Age	Vaccination Status	Dose and Schedule
3 through 8 years of age	Not previously vaccinated with influenza vaccine	Two doses (0.5-mL each) at least 4 weeks apart (2.1)
	Vaccinated with influenza vaccine in a previous season	One or two doses[a] (0.5-mL each) (2.1)
9 years of age and older	Not applicable	One 0.5-mL dose (2.1)

[a] One dose or two doses (0.5-mL each) depending on vaccination history as per the annual Advisory Committee on Immunization Practices (ACIP) recommendation on prevention and control of influenza with vaccines. If two doses, administer each 0.5-mL dose at least 4 weeks apart. (2.1)

DOSAGE FORMS AND STRENGTHS
Suspension for injection in 0.5-mL single-dose prefilled syringes and 5-mL multi-dose vials containing 10 doses (each dose is 0.5 mL). (3)

CONTRAINDICATIONS
History of severe allergic reactions (e.g., anaphylaxis) to any component of the vaccine, including egg protein, or following a previous dose of any influenza vaccine. (4, 11)

WARNINGS AND PRECAUTIONS
• If Guillain-Barré syndrome has occurred within 6 weeks of receipt of a prior influenza vaccine, the decision to give FLULAVAL QUADRIVALENT should be based on careful consideration of the potential benefits and risks. (5.1)
• Syncope (fainting) can occur in association with administration of injectable vaccines, including FLULAVAL QUADRIVALENT. Procedures should be in place to avoid falling injury and to restore cerebral perfusion following syncope. (5.2)

ADVERSE REACTIONS
• In adults, the most common (≥10%) solicited local adverse reaction was pain (60%); most common solicited systemic adverse events were muscle aches (26%), headache (22%), fatigue (22%), and arthralgia (15%). (6.1)
• In children 3 through 17 years of age, the most common (≥10%) solicited local adverse reaction was pain (65%). (6.1)
• In children 3 through 4 years of age, the most common (≥10%) solicited systemic adverse events were irritability (26%), drowsiness (21%), and loss of appetite (17%). (6.1)
• In children 5 through 17 years of age, the most common (≥10%) solicited systemic adverse events were muscle aches (29%), fatigue (22%), headache (22%), arthralgia (13%), and gastrointestinal symptoms (10%). (6.1)
To report SUSPECTED ADVERSE REACTIONS, contact GlaxoSmithKline at 1-888-825-5249 or VAERS at 1-800-822-7967 or www.vaers.hhs.gov

USE IN SPECIFIC POPULATIONS
• Safety and effectiveness of FLULAVAL QUADRIVALENT have not been established in pregnant women or nursing mothers. (8.1, 8.3)
• Register women who receive FLULAVAL QUADRIVALENT while pregnant in the pregnancy registry by calling 1-888-452-9622. (8.1)
• Geriatric Use: Antibody responses were lower in geriatric subjects who received FLULAVAL QUADRIVALENT than in younger subjects. (8.5)
See 17 for PATIENT COUNSELING INFORMATION
Revised: 05/2014

FULL PRESCRIBING INFORMATION

1 INDICATIONS AND USAGE

FLULAVAL® QUADRIVALENT is indicated for active immunization for the prevention of disease caused by influenza A subtype viruses and type B viruses contained in the vaccine. FLULAVAL QUADRIVALENT is approved for use in persons 3 years of age and older.

2 DOSAGE AND ADMINISTRATION

For intramuscular injection only.

2.1 Dosage and Schedule

The dose and schedule for FLULAVAL QUADRIVALENT are presented in Table 1.

Table 1. FLULAVAL QUADRIVALENT: Dosing

Age	Vaccination Status	Dose and Schedule
3 through 8 years of age	Not previously vaccinated with influenza vaccine	Two doses (0.5-mL each) at least 4 weeks apart
	Vaccinated with influenza vaccine in a previous season	One or two doses[a] (0.5-mL each)
9 years of age and older	Not applicable	One 0.5-mL dose

[a] One dose or two doses (0.5-mL each) depending on vaccination history as per the annual Advisory Committee on Immunization Practices (ACIP) recommendation on prevention and control of influenza with vaccines. If two doses, administer each 0.5-mL dose at least 4 weeks apart.

2.2 Administration Instructions

Shake well before administration. Parenteral drug products should be inspected visually for particulate matter and discoloration prior to administration, whenever solution and container permit. If either of these conditions exists, the vaccine should not be administered.

Attach a sterile needle to the prefilled syringe and administer intramuscularly.

For the multi-dose vial, use a sterile needle and sterile syringe to withdraw the 0.5-mL dose from the multi-dose vial and administer intramuscularly. A sterile syringe with a needle bore no larger than 23 gauge is recommended for administration. It is recommended that small syringes (0.5-mL or 1-mL) be used to minimize any product loss. Use a separate sterile needle and syringe for each dose withdrawn from the multi-dose vial.

Between uses, return the multi-dose vial to the recommended storage conditions, between 2° and 8°C (36° and 46°F). Do not freeze. Discard if the vaccine has been frozen. Once entered, a multi-dose vial, and any residual contents, should be discarded after 28 days.

The preferred site for intramuscular injection is the deltoid muscle of the upper arm. Do not inject in the gluteal area or areas where there may be a major nerve trunk.

Do not administer this product intravenously, intradermally, or subcutaneously.

3 DOSAGE FORMS AND STRENGTHS

FLULAVAL QUADRIVALENT is a suspension for injection available in 0.5-mL prefilled TIP-LOK® syringes and 5-mL multi-dose vials containing 10 doses (each dose is 0.5 mL).

4 CONTRAINDICATIONS

Do not administer FLULAVAL QUADRIVALENT to anyone with a history of severe allergic reactions (e.g., anaphylaxis) to any component of the vaccine, including egg protein, or following a previous dose of any influenza vaccine [see Description (11)].

5 WARNINGS AND PRECAUTIONS

5.1 Guillain-Barré Syndrome

If Guillain-Barré syndrome (GBS) has occurred within 6 weeks of receipt of a prior influenza vaccine, the decision to give FLULAVAL QUADRIVALENT should be based on careful consideration of the potential benefits and risks.

The 1976 swine influenza vaccine was associated with an elevated risk of GBS. Evidence for a causal relation of GBS with other influenza vaccines is inconclusive; if an excess risk exists, it is probably slightly more than one additional case/one million persons vaccinated.

5.2 Syncope

Syncope (fainting) can occur in association with administration of injectable vaccines, including FLULAVAL QUADRIVALENT. Syncope can be accompanied by transient neurological signs such as visual disturbance, paresthesia, and tonic-clonic limb movements. Procedures should be in place to avoid falling injury and to restore cerebral perfusion following syncope.

5.3 Preventing and Managing Allergic Vaccine Reactions

Prior to administration, the healthcare provider should review the immunization history for possible vaccine sensitivity and previous vaccination-related adverse reactions. Appropriate medical treatment and supervision must be available to manage possible anaphylactic reactions following administration of FLULAVAL QUADRIVALENT.

5.4 Altered Immunocompetence

If FLULAVAL QUADRIVALENT is administered to immunosuppressed persons, including individuals receiving immunosuppressive therapy, the immune response may be lower than in immunocompetent persons.

5.5 Limitations of Vaccine Effectiveness

Vaccination with FLULAVAL QUADRIVALENT may not protect all susceptible individuals.

5.6 Persons at Risk of Bleeding

As with other intramuscular injections, FLULAVAL QUADRIVALENT should be given with caution in individuals with bleeding disorders such as hemophilia or on anticoagulant therapy to avoid the risk of hematoma following the injection.

6 ADVERSE REACTIONS

6.1 Clinical Trials Experience

In adults who received FLULAVAL QUADRIVALENT, the most common (≥10%) solicited local adverse reaction was pain (60%); the most common (≥10%) solicited systemic adverse events were muscle aches (26%), headache (22%), fatigue (22%), and arthralgia (15%).

In children 3 through 17 years of age who received FLULAVAL QUADRIVALENT, the most common (≥10%) solicited local adverse reaction was pain (65%). In children 3 through 4 years of age, the most common (≥10%) solicited systemic adverse events were irritability (26%), drowsiness (21%), and loss of appetite (17%). In children 5 through 17 years of age, the most common (≥10%) systemic adverse events were muscle aches (29%), fatigue (22%), headache (22%), arthralgia (13%), and gastrointestinal symptoms (10%).

Because clinical trials are conducted under widely varying conditions, adverse reaction rates observed in the clinical trials of a vaccine cannot be directly compared to rates in the clinical trials of another vaccine, and may not reflect the rates observed in practice. There is the possibility that broad use of FLULAVAL QUADRIVALENT could reveal adverse reactions not observed in clinical trials.

FLULAVAL QUADRIVALENT has been administered to 1,384 adults 18 years of age and older and 3,516 pediatric subjects 3 through 17 years of age in 4 clinical trials.

FLULAVAL QUADRIVALENT in Adults: Study 1 was a randomized, double-blind, active-controlled, safety and immunogenicity study. In this study, subjects received FLULAVAL QUADRIVALENT (N = 1,272), or one of two formulations of a comparator trivalent influenza vaccine (FLULAVAL, TIV-1, N = 213 or TIV-2, N = 218), each containing an influenza type B virus that corresponded to one of the two B viruses in FLULAVAL QUADRIVALENT (a type B virus of the Victoria lineage or a type B virus of the Yamagata lineage). The population was 18 years of age and older (mean age 50 years) and 61% were female; 61% of subjects were white, 3% were black, 1% were Asian, and 35% were of other racial/ethnic groups. Solicited adverse events were collected for 7 days (day of vaccination and the next 6 days). The incidence of local adverse reactions and systemic adverse events occurring within 7 days of vaccination in adults are shown in Table 2.

[See table 2 below]

Unsolicited adverse events occurring within 21 days of vaccination were reported in 19%, 23%, and 23% of subjects who received FLULAVAL QUADRIVALENT (N = 1,272), TIV-1 (B Victoria) (N = 213), or TIV-2 (B Yamagata) (N = 218), respectively. The unsolicited adverse events that occurred most frequently (≥1% for FLULAVAL QUADRIVALENT) included nasopharyngitis, upper respiratory tract infection, headache, cough and oropharyngeal pain. Serious adverse events occurring within 21 days of vaccination were reported in 0.4%, 0%, and 0% of subjects who received FLULAVAL QUADRIVALENT, TIV-1 (B Victoria), or TIV-2 (B Yamagata), respectively.

FLULAVAL QUADRIVALENT in Children: Study 2 was a randomized, double-blind, active-controlled study. In this study, subjects received FLULAVAL QUADRIVALENT (N = 932), or one of two formulations of a comparator trivalent influenza vaccine [FLUARIX® (Influenza Vaccine), TIV-1, N = 929 or TIV-2, N = 932], each containing an influenza type B virus that corresponded to one of the two B viruses in FLULAVAL QUADRIVALENT (a type B virus of the Victoria lineage or a type B virus of the Yamagata lineage). The population was 3 through 17 years of age (mean age 9 years) and 53% were male; 65% were white, 13% were Asian, 9% were black, and 13% were of other racial/ethnic groups. Children 3 through 8 years of age with no history of influenza vaccination received 2 doses approximately 28 days apart. Children 3 through 8 years of age with a history of influenza vaccination and children 9 years of age and older received one dose. Solicited local adverse reactions and systemic adverse events were collected for 7 days (day

Table 2. FLULAVAL QUADRIVALENT: Incidence of Solicited Local Adverse Reactions and Systemic Adverse Events Within 7 Days[a] of Vaccination in Adults 18 Years of Age and Older[b] (Total Vaccinated Cohort)

	FLULAVAL QUADRIVALENT[c] N = 1,260 %	Trivalent Influenza Vaccine (TIV)	
		TIV-1 (B Victoria)[d] N = 208 %	TIV-2 (B Yamagata)[e] N = 216 %
Local Adverse Reactions			
Pain	60	45	41
Swelling	3	1	4
Redness	2	3	1
Systemic Adverse Events			
Muscle aches	26	25	19
Headache	22	20	23
Fatigue	22	22	17
Arthralgia	15	17	15
Gastrointestinal symptoms[f]	9	10	7
Shivering	9	8	6
Fever ≥100.4°F (38.0°C)	2	1	1

Total vaccinated cohort for safety included all vaccinated subjects for whom safety data were available.
[a] 7 days included day of vaccination and the subsequent 6 days.
[b] Study 1: NCT01196975.
[c] Contained two A strains and two B strains, one of Victoria lineage and one of Yamagata lineage.
[d] Contained two A strains and a B strain of Victoria lineage.
[e] Contained the same two A strains as FLULAVAL and a B strain of Yamagata lineage.
[f] Gastrointestinal symptoms included nausea, vomiting, diarrhea, and/or abdominal pain.

Table 3. FLULAVAL QUADRIVALENT: Incidence of Solicited Local Adverse Reactions and Systemic Adverse Events Within 7 Days[a] of First Vaccination in Children 3 Through 17 Years of Age[b] (Total Vaccinated Cohort)

| | FLULAVAL QUADRIVALENT[c] % | Trivalent Influenza Vaccine (TIV) | |
		TIV-1 (B Victoria)[d] %	TIV-2 (B Yamagata)[e] %
3 Through 17 Years of Age			
Local Adverse Reactions	N = 913	N = 911	N = 915
Pain	65	55	56
Swelling	6	3	4
Redness	5	3	4
3 Through 4 Years of Age			
Systemic Adverse Events	N = 185	N = 187	N = 189
Irritability	26	17	22
Drowsiness	21	20	23
Loss of appetite	17	16	13
Fever ≥100.4°F (38.0°C)	5	6	4
5 Through 17 Years of Age			
Systemic Adverse Events	N = 727	N = 724	N = 725
Muscle aches	29	25	25
Fatigue	22	24	23
Headache	22	22	20
Arthralgia	13	12	11
Gastrointestinal symptoms[f]	10	10	9
Shivering	7	7	7
Fever ≥100.4°F (38.0°C)	2	4	3

Total vaccinated cohort for safety included all vaccinated subjects for whom safety data were available.
[a] 7 days included day of vaccination and the subsequent 6 days.
[b] Study 2: NCT01198756.
[c] Contained two A strains and two B strains, one of Victoria lineage and one of Yamagata lineage.
[d] Contained two A strains and a B strain of Victoria lineage.
[e] Contained the same two A strains as FLUARIX and a B strain of Yamagata lineage.
[f] Gastrointestinal symptoms included nausea, vomiting, diarrhea, and/or abdominal pain.

of vaccination and the next 6 days). The incidence of local adverse reactions and systemic adverse events occurring within 7 days of vaccination in children are shown in Table 3.
[See table 3 above]
In children who received a second dose of FLULAVAL QUADRIVALENT, FLUARIX TIV-1 (B Victoria), or TIV-2 (B Yamagata), the incidences of adverse events following the second dose were generally lower than those observed after the first dose.
Unsolicited adverse events occurring within 28 days of vaccination were reported in 30%, 31% and 30% of subjects who received FLULAVAL QUADRIVALENT (N = 932), FLUARIX TIV-1 (B Victoria) (N = 929), or TIV-2 (B Yamagata) (N = 932), respectively. The unsolicited adverse events that occurred most frequently (≥1% for FLULAVAL QUADRIVALENT) included vomiting, pyrexia, bronchitis, nasopharyngitis, pharyngitis, upper respiratory tract infection, headache, cough, oropharyngeal pain, and rhinorrhea. Serious adverse events occurring within 28 days of any vaccination were reported in 0.1%, 0.2%, and 0.2% of subjects who received FLULAVAL QUADRIVALENT, FLUARIX TIV-1 (B Victoria), or TIV-2 (B Yamagata), respectively.
Study 3 was a randomized, observer-blind, non-influenza vaccine-controlled study evaluating the efficacy of FLULAVAL QUADRIVALENT. The study included subjects 3 through 8 years of age who received FLULAVAL QUADRIVALENT (N = 2,584) or HAVRIX® (Hepatitis A Vaccine) (N = 2,584), as a control vaccine. Children with no history of influenza vaccination received 2 doses of FLULAVAL QUADRIVALENT or HAVRIX approximately 28 days apart. Children with a history of influenza vaccination received one dose of FLULAVAL QUADRIVALENT or HAVRIX. In the overall population, 52% were male; 60% were Asian, 5% were white, and 35% were of other racial/ethnic groups. The mean age of subjects was 5 years. Solic-

ited local adverse reactions and systemic adverse events were collected for 7 days (day of vaccination and the next 6 days). The incidence of local adverse reactions and systemic adverse events occurring within 7 days of vaccination in children are shown in Table 4.

Table 4. FLULAVAL QUADRIVALENT: Incidence of Solicited Local Adverse Reactions and Systemic Adverse Events Within 7 Days[a] of First Vaccination in Children 3 Through 8 Years of Age[b] (Total Vaccinated Cohort)

	FLULAVAL QUADRIVALENT %	HAVRIX[c] %
3 Through 8 Years of Age		
Local Adverse Reactions	N = 2,546	N = 2,551
Pain	39	28
Swelling	1	0.3
Redness	0.4	0.2
3 Through 4 Years of Age		
Systemic Adverse Events	N = 898	N = 895
Loss of appetite	9	8
Irritability	8	8
Drowsiness	8	7
Fever ≥100.4°F (38.0°C)	4	4

| | 5 Through 8 Years of Age | |
Systemic Adverse Events	N = 1,648	N = 1,654
Muscle aches	12	10
Headache	11	11
Fatigue	8	7
Arthralgia	6	5
Gastrointestinal symptoms[d]	6	6
Shivering	3	3
Fever ≥100.4°F (38.0°C)	3	3

Total vaccinated cohort for safety included all vaccinated subjects for whom safety data were available.
[a] 7 days included day of vaccination and the subsequent 6 days.
[b] Study 3: NCT01218308.
[c] Hepatitis A Vaccine used as a control vaccine.
[d] Gastrointestinal symptoms included nausea, vomiting, diarrhea, and/or abdominal pain.

In children who received a second dose of FLULAVAL QUADRIVALENT or HAVRIX, the incidences of adverse events following the second dose were generally lower than those observed after the first dose.
The frequency of unsolicited adverse events occurring within 28 days of vaccination was similar in both groups (33% for both FLULAVAL QUADRIVALENT and HAVRIX). The unsolicited adverse events that occurred most frequently (≥1% for FLULAVAL QUADRIVALENT) included diarrhea, pyrexia, gastroenteritis, nasopharyngitis, upper respiratory tract infection, varicella, cough, and rhinorrhea. Serious adverse events occurring within 28 days of any vaccination were reported in 0.7% of subjects who received FLULAVAL QUADRIVALENT and in 0.2% of subjects who received HAVRIX.

6.2 Postmarketing Experience
There are no postmarketing data available for FLULAVAL QUADRIVALENT. The following adverse events have been spontaneously reported during postapproval use of FLULAVAL (trivalent influenza vaccine). Because these events are reported voluntarily from a population of uncertain size, it is not always possible to reliably estimate their incidence rate or establish a causal relationship to the vaccine. Adverse events described here are included because: a) they represent reactions which are known to occur following immunizations generally or influenza immunizations specifically; b) they are potentially serious; or c) the frequency of reporting.
Blood and Lymphatic System Disorders: Lymphadenopathy.
Eye Disorders: Eye pain, photophobia.
Gastrointestinal Disorders: Dysphagia, vomiting.
General Disorders and Administration Site Conditions: Chest pain, injection site inflammation, asthenia, injection site rash, influenza-like symptoms, abnormal gait, injection site bruising, injection site sterile abscess.
Immune System Disorders: Allergic reactions including anaphylaxis, angioedema.
Infections and Infestations: Rhinitis, laryngitis, cellulitis.
Musculoskeletal and Connective Tissue Disorders: Muscle weakness, arthritis.
Nervous System Disorders: Dizziness, paresthesia, hypoesthesia, hypokinesia, tremor, somnolence, syncope, Guillain-Barré syndrome, convulsions/seizures, facial or cranial nerve paralysis, encephalopathy, limb paralysis.
Psychiatric Disorders: Insomnia.
Respiratory, Thoracic, and Mediastinal Disorders: Dyspnea, dysphonia, bronchospasm, throat tightness.
Skin and Subcutaneous Tissue Disorders: Urticaria, localized or generalized rash, pruritus, sweating.
Vascular Disorders: Flushing, pallor.

7 DRUG INTERACTIONS
7.1 Concomitant Administration With Other Vaccines
FLULAVAL QUADRIVALENT should not be mixed with any other vaccine in the same syringe or vial.
There are insufficient data to assess the concomitant administration of FLULAVAL QUADRIVALENT with other vaccines. When concomitant administration of other vaccines is required, the vaccines should be administered at different injection sites.
7.2 Immunosuppressive Therapies
Immunosuppressive therapies, including irradiation, antimetabolites, alkylating agents, cytotoxic drugs, and corticosteroids (used in greater than physiologic doses), may reduce the immune response to FLULAVAL QUADRIVALENT.

Table 5. FLULAVAL QUADRIVALENT: Influenza Attack Rates and Vaccine Efficacy Against Influenza A and/or B in Children 3 Through 8 Years of Age[a] (According to Protocol Cohort for Efficacy)

	N[b]	n[c]	Influenza Attack Rate % (n/N)	Vaccine Efficacy % (CI)
All RT-PCR-Positive Influenza				
FLULAVAL QUADRIVALENT	2,379	58	2.4	55.4[d] (95% CI: 39.1, 67.3)
HAVRIX[e]	2,398	128	5.3	-
All Culture-Confirmed Influenza[f]				
FLULAVAL QUADRIVALENT	2,379	50	2.1	55.9 (97.5% CI: 35.4, 69.9)
HAVRIX[e]	2,398	112	4.7	-
Antigenically Matched Culture-Confirmed Influenza				
FLULAVAL QUADRIVALENT	2,379	31	1.3	45.1[g] (97.5% CI: 9.3, 66.8)
HAVRIX[e]	2,398	56	2.3	-

CI = Confidence Interval; RT-PCR = reverse transcriptase polymerase chain reaction.
[a] Study 3: NCT01218308.
[b] According to protocol cohort for efficacy included subjects who met all eligibility criteria, were successfully contacted at least once post-vaccination, and complied with the protocol-specified efficacy criteria.
[c] Number of influenza cases.
[d] Vaccine efficacy for FLULAVAL QUADRIVALENT met the pre-defined criterion of >30% for the lower limit of the 2-sided 95% CI.
[e] Hepatitis A Vaccine used as a control vaccine.
[f] Of 162 culture-confirmed influenza cases, 108 (67%) were antigenically typed (87 matched; 21 unmatched); 54 (33%) could not be antigenically typed [but were typed by RT-PCR and nucleic acid sequence analysis: 5 cases A (H1N1) (5 with HAVRIX), 47 cases A (H3N2) (10 with FLULAVAL QUADRIVALENT; 37 with HAVRIX), and 2 cases B Victoria (2 with HAVRIX)].
[g] Since only 67% of cases could be typed, the clinical significance of this result is unknown.

Table 6. FLULAVAL QUADRIVALENT: Incidence of Adverse Outcomes Associated With RT-PCR-Positive Influenza in Children 3 Through 8 Years of Age[a] (Total Vaccinated Cohort)[b]

Adverse Outcome[d]	FLULAVAL QUADRIVALENT N = 2,584			HAVRIX[c] N = 2,584		
	Number of Events	Number of Subjects[e]	%	Number of Events	Number of Subjects[e]	%
Fever >102.2°F/39.0°C	16[f]	15	0.6	51[f]	50	1.9
Shortness of breath	0	0	0	5	5	0.2
Pneumonia	0	0	0	3	3	0.1
Wheezing	1	1	0	1	1	0
Bronchitis	1	1	0	1	1	0
Pulmonary congestion	0	0	0	1	1	0
Acute otitis media	0	0	0	1	1	0
Bronchiolitis	0	0	0	0	0	0
Croup	0	0	0	0	0	0
Encephalitis	0	0	0	0	0	0
Myocarditis	0	0	0	0	0	0
Myositis	0	0	0	0	0	0
Seizure	0	0	0	0	0	0

[a] Study 3: NCT01218308.
[b] Total vaccinated cohort included all vaccinated subjects for whom data were available.
[c] Hepatitis A Vaccine used as a control vaccine.
[d] In subjects who presented with more than one adverse outcome, each outcome was counted in the respective category.
[e] Number of subjects presenting with at least one event in each group.
[f] One subject in each group had sequential influenza due to influenza type A and type B viruses.

8　USE IN SPECIFIC POPULATIONS

8.1　Pregnancy

Pregnancy Category B

A reproductive and developmental toxicity study has been performed in female rats at a dose 80-fold the human dose (on a mg/kg basis) and showed no evidence of impaired female fertility or harm to the fetus due to FLULAVAL QUADRIVALENT. There are, however, no adequate and well-controlled studies in pregnant women. Because animal reproduction studies are not always predictive of human response, FLULAVAL QUADRIVALENT should be given to a pregnant woman only if clearly needed.

In a reproductive and developmental toxicity study, the effect of FLULAVAL QUADRIVALENT on embryo-fetal and pre-weaning development was evaluated in rats. Animals were administered FLULAVAL QUADRIVALENT by intramuscular injection twice prior to gestation, during the period of organogenesis (gestation days 3, 8, 11, and 15), and during lactation (day 7), 0.2 mL/dose/rat (80-fold higher than the projected human dose on a body weight basis). No adverse effects on mating, female fertility, pregnancy, parturition, lactation parameters, and embryo-fetal or pre-weaning development were observed. There were no vaccine-related fetal malformations or other evidence of teratogenesis.

Pregnancy Registry:
GlaxoSmithKline maintains a surveillance registry to collect data on pregnancy outcomes and newborn health status outcomes following vaccination with FLULAVAL QUADRIVALENT during pregnancy. Women who receive FLULAVAL QUADRIVALENT during pregnancy should be encouraged to contact GlaxoSmithKline directly or their healthcare provider should contact GlaxoSmithKline by calling 1-888-452-9622.

8.3　Nursing Mothers

It is not known whether FLULAVAL QUADRIVALENT is excreted in human milk. Because many drugs are excreted in human milk, caution should be exercised when FLULAVAL QUADRIVALENT is administered to a nursing woman.

8.4　Pediatric Use

Safety and effectiveness of FLULAVAL QUADRIVALENT in children younger than 3 years of age have not been established.

Safety and immunogenicity of FLULAVAL QUADRIVALENT in children 3 through 17 years of age have been evaluated [see Adverse Reactions (6.1) and Clinical Studies (14.2)].

8.5　Geriatric Use

In a randomized, double-blind, active-controlled study, immunogenicity and safety were evaluated in a cohort of subjects 65 years of age and older who received FLULAVAL QUADRIVALENT (N = 397); approximately one-third of these subjects were 75 years of age and older. In subjects 65 years of age and older, the geometric mean antibody titers post-vaccination and seroconversion rates were lower than in younger subjects (18 to 64 years of age) and the frequencies of solicited and unsolicited adverse events were generally lower than in younger subjects [see Adverse Reactions (6.1) and Clinical Studies (14.2)].

11　DESCRIPTION

FLULAVAL QUADRIVALENT, Influenza Vaccine, for intramuscular injection, is a quadrivalent, split-virion, inactivated influenza virus vaccine prepared from virus propagated in the allantoic cavity of embryonated hens' eggs. Each of the influenza viruses is produced and purified separately. The virus is inactivated with ultraviolet light treatment followed by formaldehyde treatment, purified by centrifugation, and disrupted with sodium deoxycholate.

FLULAVAL QUADRIVALENT is a sterile, opalescent, translucent to off-white suspension in a phosphate-buffered saline solution that may sediment slightly. The sediment resuspends upon shaking to form a homogeneous suspension.

FLULAVAL QUADRIVALENT has been standardized according to USPHS requirements for the 2014-2015 influenza season and is formulated to contain 60 micrograms (mcg) hemagglutinin (HA) per 0.5-mL dose in the recommended ratio of 15 mcg HA of each of the following 4 viruses (two A strains and two B strains): A/California/7/2009 NYMC X-179A (H1N1), A/Texas/50/2012 NYMC X-223A (H3N2), B/Massachusetts/2/2012 NYMC BX-51B, and B/Brisbane/60/2008.

The prefilled syringe is formulated without preservatives and does not contain thimerosal. Each 0.5-mL dose from the multi-dose vial contains 50 mcg thimerosal (<25 mcg mercury); thimerosal, a mercury derivative, is added as a preservative.

Each 0.5-mL dose of either presentation may also contain residual amounts of ovalbumin (≤0.3 mcg), formaldehyde (≤25 mcg), sodium deoxycholate (≤50 mcg), α-tocopheryl hydrogen succinate (≤320 mcg) and polysorbate 80 (≤887 mcg) from the manufacturing process. Antibiotics are not used in the manufacture of this vaccine.

The tip caps and plungers of the prefilled syringes are not made with natural rubber latex. The vial stoppers are not made with natural rubber latex.

12　CLINICAL PHARMACOLOGY

12.1　Mechanism of Action

Influenza illness and its complications follow infection with influenza viruses. Global surveillance of influenza identifies yearly antigenic variants. Since 1977, antigenic variants of influenza A (H1N1 and H3N2) viruses and influenza B viruses have been in global circulation.

Public health authorities recommend influenza vaccine strains annually. Inactivated influenza vaccines are standardized to contain the hemagglutinins of strains representing the influenza viruses likely to circulate in the United States during the influenza season. Two B strain lineages (Victoria and Yamagata) are of public health importance because they have co-circulated since 2001. FLULAVAL (trivalent influenza vaccine) contains only two influenza A subtype viruses and one influenza type B virus. In 6 of the last 11 seasons, the most predominant circulating influenza B lineage was not included in the annual trivalent vaccine. Quadrivalent vaccines, such as FLULAVAL QUADRIVALENT, contain two influenza A subtype viruses and two influenza type B viruses (one of the Victoria lineage and one of the Yamagata lineage).

Specific levels of hemagglutination inhibition (HI) antibody titer post-vaccination with inactivated influenza virus vaccines have not been correlated with protection from influenza illness but the antibody titers have been used as a measure of vaccine activity. In some human challenge studies, antibody titers of ≥1:40 have been associated with protection from influenza illness in up to 50% of subjects.[1,2] Antibody against one influenza virus type or subtype confers little or no protection against another virus. Furthermore, antibody to one antigenic variant of influenza virus might not protect against a new antigenic variant of the same type or subtype. Frequent development of antigenic variants through antigenic drift is the virological basis for seasonal epidemics and the reason for the usual change of one or more new strains in each year's influenza vaccine. Annual revaccination is recommended because immunity declines during the year after vaccination, and because circulating strains of influenza virus change from year to year.[3]

13   NONCLINICAL TOXICOLOGY
13.1   Carcinogenesis, Mutagenesis, Impairment of Fertility
FLULAVAL QUADRIVALENT has not been evaluated for carcinogenic or mutagenic potential. Vaccination of female rats with FLULAVAL QUADRIVALENT, at doses shown to be immunogenic in the rat, had no effect on fertility.

14   CLINICAL STUDIES
14.1   Efficacy Against Influenza
The efficacy of FLULAVAL QUADRIVALENT was evaluated in Study 3, a randomized, observer-blind, non-influenza vaccine-controlled study conducted in 3 countries in Asia, 3 in Latin America, and 2 in the Middle East/Europe during the 2010-2011 influenza season. Healthy subjects 3 through 8 years of age were randomized (1:1) to receive FLULAVAL QUADRIVALENT (N = 2,584), containing A/California/7/2009 (H1N1), A/Victoria/210/2009 (H3N2), B/Brisbane/60/2008 (Victoria lineage), and B/Florida/4/2006 (Yamagata lineage) influenza strains, or HAVRIX (N = 2,584), as a control vaccine. Children with no history of influenza vaccination received 2 doses of FLULAVAL QUADRIVALENT or HAVRIX approximately 28 days apart. Children with a history of influenza vaccination received one dose of FLULAVAL QUADRIVALENT or HAVRIX [see Adverse Reactions (6.1)].
Efficacy of FLULAVAL QUADRIVALENT was assessed for the prevention of reverse transcriptase polymerase chain reaction (RT-PCR)-positive influenza A and/or B disease presenting as influenza-like illness (ILI). ILI was defined as a temperature ≥100°F in the presence of at least one of the following symptoms on the same day: cough, sore throat, runny nose, or nasal congestion. Subjects with ILI (monitored by passive and active surveillance for approximately 6 months) had nasal and throat swabs collected and tested for influenza A and/or B by RT-PCR. All RT-PCR-positive specimens were further tested in cell culture. Vaccine efficacy was calculated based on the ATP cohort for efficacy (Table 5).
[See table 5 at top of previous page]
In an exploratory analysis by age, vaccine efficacy against RT-PCR-positive influenza A and/or B disease presenting as ILI was evaluated in subjects 3 through 4 years of age and 5 through 8 years of age; vaccine efficacy was 35.3% (95% CI: -1.3, 58.6) and 67.7% (95% CI: 49.7, 79.2), respectively. As the study lacked statistical power to evaluate efficacy within age subgroups, the clinical significance of these results is unknown.
As a secondary objective in the study, subjects with RT-PCR-positive influenza A and/or B were prospectively classified based on the presence of adverse outcomes that have been associated with influenza infection (defined as fever >102.2°F/39.0°C, physician-verified shortness of breath, pneumonia, wheezing, bronchitis, bronchiolitis, pulmonary congestion, croup and/or acute otitis media, and/or physician-diagnosed serious extra-pulmonary complications, including myositis, encephalitis, seizure and/or myocarditis).
The risk reduction of fever >102.2°F/39.0°C associated with RT-PCR-positive influenza was 71.0% (95% CI: 44.8, 84.8) based on the ATP cohort for efficacy [FLULAVAL QUADRIVALENT (n = 12/2,379); HAVRIX (n = 41/2,398)]. The other pre-specified adverse outcomes had too few cases to calculate a risk reduction. The incidence of these adverse outcomes is presented in Table 6.

Table 7. Non-inferiority of FLULAVAL QUADRIVALENT Relative to Trivalent Influenza Vaccine (TIV) 21 Days Post-Vaccination in Adults 18 Years of Age and Older[a] (According to Protocol Cohort for Immunogenicity)[b]

Geometric Mean Titers Against	FLULAVAL QUADRIVALENT[c]	TIV-1 (B Victoria)[d]	TIV-2 (B Yamagata)[e]
	N = 1,245-1,246 (95% CI)	N = 204 (95% CI)	N = 210-211 (95% CI)
A/California/7/2009 (H1N1)	204.6[f] (190.4, 219.9)	176.0 (149.1, 207.7)	149.0 (122.9, 180.7)
A/Victoria/210/2009 (H3N2)	125.4[f] (117.4, 133.9)	147.5 (124.1, 175.2)	141.0 (118.1, 168.3)
B/Brisbane/60/2008 (Victoria lineage)	177.7[f] (167.8, 188.1)	135.9 (118.1, 156.5)	71.9 (61.3, 84.2)
B/Florida/4/2006 (Yamagata lineage)	399.7[f] (378.1, 422.6)	176.9 (153.8, 203.5)	306.6 (266.2, 353.3)

CI = Confidence Interval.
[a] Study 1:   NCT01196975.
[b] According to protocol cohort for immunogenicity included all evaluable subjects for whom assay results were available after vaccination for at least one study vaccine antigen.
[c] Containing A/California/07/2009 (H1N1), A/Victoria/210/2009 (H3N2), B/Florida/04/2006 (Yamagata lineage), and B/Brisbane/60/2008 (Victoria lineage)
[d] Containing A/California/07/2009 (H1N1), A/Victoria/210/2009 (H3N2), and B/Brisbane/60/2008 (Victoria lineage)
[e] Containing A/California/07/2009 (H1N1), A/Victoria/210/2009 (H3N2), and B/Florida/04/2006 (Yamagata lineage)
[f] Non-inferior to both TIVs based on adjusted GMTs [upper limit of the 2-sided 95% CI for the GMT ratio (TIV/FLULAVAL QUADRIVALENT) ≤1.5]; superior to TIV-1 (B Victoria) with respect to the B strain of Yamagata lineage and to TIV-2 (B Yamagata) with respect to the B strain of Victoria lineage based on adjusted GMTs [lower limit of the 2-sided 95% CI for the GMT ratio (FLULAVAL QUADRIVALENT/TIV) >1.5].

Table 8. Non-inferiority of FLULAVAL QUADRIVALENT Relative to Trivalent Influenza Vaccine (TIV) at 28 Days Post-Vaccination in Children 3 Through 17 Years of Age[a] (According to Protocol Cohort for Immunogenicity)[b]

Geometric Mean Titers Against	FLULAVAL QUADRIVALENT[c]	TIV-1 (B Victoria)[d]	TIV-2 (B Yamagata)[e]
	N = 878 (95% CI)	N = 871 (95% CI)	N = 877-878 (95% CI)
A/California/7/2009 (H1N1)	362.7[f] (335.3, 392.3)	429.1 (396.5, 464.3)	420.2 (388.8, 454.0)
A/Victoria/210/2009 (H3N2)	143.7[f] (134.2, 153.9)	139.6 (130.5, 149.3)	151.0 (141.0, 161.6)
B/Brisbane/60/2008 (Victoria lineage)	250.5[f] (230.8, 272.0)	245.4 (226.9, 265.4)	68.1 (61.9, 74.9)
B/Florida/4/2006 (Yamagata lineage)	512.5[f] (477.6, 549.9)	197.0 (180.7, 214.8)	579.0 (541.2, 619.3)
Seroconversion[g] to:	N = 876 % (95% CI)	N = 870 % (95% CI)	N = 876-877 % (95% CI)
A/California/7/2009 (H1N1)	84.4[f] (81.8, 86.7)	86.8 (84.3, 89.0)	85.5 (83.0, 87.8)
A/Victoria/210/2009 (H3N2)	70.1[f] (66.9, 73.1)	67.8 (64.6, 70.9)	69.6 (66.5, 72.7)
B/Brisbane/60/2008 (Victoria lineage)	74.5[f] (71.5, 77.4)	71.5 (68.4, 74.5)	29.9 (26.9, 33.1)
B/Florida/4/2006 (Yamagata lineage)	75.2[f] (72.2, 78.1)	41.3 (38.0, 44.6)	73.4 (70.4, 76.3)

CI = Confidence Interval.
[a] Study 2: NCT01198756.
[b] According to protocol cohort for immunogenicity included all evaluable subjects for whom assay results were available after vaccination for at least one study vaccine antigen.
[c] Containing A/California/07/2009 (H1N1), A/Victoria/210/2009 (H3N2), B/Florida/04/2006 (Yamagata lineage), and B/Brisbane/60/2008 (Victoria lineage).
[d] Containing A/California/07/2009 (H1N1), A/Victoria/210/2009 (H3N2), and B/Brisbane/60/2008 (Victoria lineage).
[e] Containing A/California/07/2009 (H1N1), A/Victoria/210/2009 (H3N2), and B/Florida/04/2006 (Yamagata lineage).
[f] Non-inferior to both TIVs based on adjusted GMTs [upper limit of the 2-sided 95% CI for the GMT ratio (TIV/FLULAVAL QUADRIVALENT) ≤1.5] and seroconversion rates (upper limit of the 2-sided 95% CI on difference of the TIV minus FLULAVAL QUADRIVALENT ≤10%); superior to TIV-1 (B Victoria) with respect to the B strain of Yamagata lineage and to TIV-2 (B Yamagata) with respect to the B strain of Victoria lineage based on adjusted GMTs [lower limit of the 2-sided 95% CI for the GMT ratio (FLULAVAL QUADRIVALENT/TIV) >1.5] and seroconversion rates (lower limit of the 2-sided 95% CI on difference of FLULAVAL QUADRIVALENT minus the TIV >10%).
[g] Seroconversion defined as a 4-fold increase in post-vaccination antibody titer from pre-vaccination titer ≥1:10, or an increase in titer from <1:10 to ≥1:40.

[See table 6 at top of previous page]
14.2   Immunological Evaluation
Adults: Study 1 was a randomized, double-blind, active-controlled, safety and immunogenicity study conducted in subjects 18 years of age and older. In this study, subjects received FLULAVAL QUADRIVALENT (N = 1,246), or one of two formulations of a comparator trivalent influenza vaccine (FLULAVAL, TIV-1, N = 204 or TIV-2, N = 211), each containing an influenza type B virus that corresponded to one of the two B viruses in FLULAVAL QUADRIVALENT (a type B virus of the Victoria lineage or a type B virus of the Yamagata lineage) [see Adverse Reactions (6.1)].

Immune responses, specifically hemagglutination inhibition (HI) antibody titers to each virus strain in the vaccine, were evaluated in sera obtained 21 days after administration of FLULAVAL QUADRIVALENT or the comparators. The immunogenicity endpoint was geometric mean antibody titers (GMTs) adjusted for baseline, performed on the According-to-Protocol (ATP) cohort for whom immunogenicity assay results were available after vaccination. FLULAVAL QUADRIVALENT was non-inferior to both TIVs based on adjusted GMTs (Table 7). The antibody response to influenza B strains contained in FLULAVAL QUADRIVALENT was higher than the antibody response after vaccination with a TIV containing an influenza B strain from a different lineage. There was no evidence that the addition of the second B strain resulted in immune interference to other strains included in the vaccine (Table 7). [See table 7 at top of previous page]

Children: Study 2 was a randomized, double-blind, active-controlled study conducted in children 3 through 17 years of age. In this study, subjects received FLULAVAL QUADRIVALENT (N = 878), or one of two formulations of a comparator trivalent influenza vaccine (FLUARIX, TIV-1, N = 871 or TIV-2 N = 878), each containing an influenza type B virus that corresponded to one of the two B viruses in FLULAVAL QUADRIVALENT (a type B virus of the Victoria lineage or a type B virus of the Yamagata lineage) [see Adverse Reactions (6.1)].

Immune responses, specifically HI antibody titers to each virus strain in the vaccine, were evaluated in sera obtained 28 days following one or 2 doses of FLULAVAL QUADRIVALENT or the comparators. The immunogenicity endpoints were GMTs adjusted for baseline, and the percentage of subjects who achieved seroconversion, defined as at least a 4-fold increase in serum HI titer over baseline to ≥1:40, following vaccination, performed on the ATP cohort. FLULAVAL QUADRIVALENT was non-inferior to both TIVs based on adjusted GMTs and seroconversion rates (Table 8). The antibody response to influenza B strains contained in FLULAVAL QUADRIVALENT was higher than the antibody response after vaccination with a TIV containing an influenza B strain from a different lineage. There was no evidence that the addition of the second B strain resulted in immune interference to other strains included in the vaccine (Table 8). [See table 8 at top of previous page]

15 REFERENCES

1. Hannoun C, Megas F, Piercy J. Immunogenicity and protective efficacy of influenza vaccination. Virus Res 2004;103:133-138.
2. Hobson D, Curry RL, Beare AS, et al. The role of serum haemagglutination-inhibiting antibody in protection against challenge infection with influenza A2 and B viruses. J Hyg Camb 1972;70:767-777.
3. Centers for Disease Control and Prevention. Prevention and control of influenza with vaccines: Recommendations of the Advisory Committee on Immunization Practices (ACIP). MMWR 2010;59(RR-8):1-62.

16 HOW SUPPLIED/STORAGE AND HANDLING

FLULAVAL QUADRIVALENT is available in 0.5-mL single-dose disposable prefilled TIP-LOK syringes (packaged without needles) and in 5-mL multi-dose vials containing 10 doses (0.5 mL each).

NDC 19515-894-41 Syringe in Package of 10: NDC 19515-894-52

NDC 19515-891-01 Multi-Dose Vial (containing 10 doses) in Package of 1: NDC 19515-891-11

Store refrigerated between 2° and 8°C (36° and 46°F). Do not freeze. Discard if the vaccine has been frozen. Store in the original package to protect from light. Once entered, a multi-dose vial should be discarded after 28 days.

17 PATIENT COUNSELING INFORMATION

Provide the following information to the vaccine recipient or guardian:
- Inform of the potential benefits and risks of immunization with FLULAVAL QUADRIVALENT.
- Educate regarding potential side effects, emphasizing that (1) FLULAVAL QUADRIVALENT contains non-infectious killed viruses and cannot cause influenza, and (2) FLULAVAL QUADRIVALENT is intended to provide protection against illness due to influenza viruses only, and cannot provide protection against all respiratory illness.
- Inform that safety and efficacy have not been established in pregnant women. Register women who receive FLULAVAL QUADRIVALENT while pregnant in the pregnancy registry by calling 1-888-452-9622.
- Give the Vaccine Information Statements, which are required by the National Childhood Vaccine Injury Act of 1986 prior to each immunization. These materials are available free of charge at the Centers for Disease Control and Prevention (CDC) website (www.cdc.gov/vaccines).
- Instruct that annual revaccination is recommended.

FLUARIX, FLULAVAL, HAVRIX and TIP-LOK are registered trademarks of the GSK group of companies.
Manufactured by **ID Biomedical Corporation of Quebec** Quebec City, QC, Canada, US License 1739
Distributed by **GlaxoSmithKline** Research Triangle Park, NC 27709
©2014, the GSK group of companies. All rights reserved.
FVQ:2PI

HAVRIX   ℞
[hav' rix]
(Hepatitis A Vaccine)
Suspension for Intramuscular Injection

HIGHLIGHTS OF PRESCRIBING INFORMATION
These highlights do not include all the information needed to use HAVRIX safely and effectively. See full prescribing information for HAVRIX.
HAVRIX (Hepatitis A Vaccine)
Suspension for Intramuscular Injection
Initial U.S. Approval: 1995

——INDICATIONS AND USAGE——

HAVRIX is a vaccine indicated for active immunization against disease caused by hepatitis A virus (HAV). HAVRIX is approved for use in persons 12 months of age and older. Primary immunization should be administered at least 2 weeks prior to expected exposure to HAV. (1)

——DOSAGE AND ADMINISTRATION——

- HAVRIX is administered by intramuscular injection. (2.2)
- Children and adolescents: A single 0.5-mL dose and a 0.5-mL booster dose administered between 6 to 12 months later. (2.3)
- Adults: A single 1-mL dose and a 1-mL booster dose administered between 6 to 12 months later. (2.3)

——DOSAGE FORMS AND STRENGTHS——

- Suspension for injection available in the following presentations:
- 0.5-mL single-dose vials and prefilled syringes. (3)
- 1-mL single-dose vials and prefilled syringes. (3)

——CONTRAINDICATIONS——

Severe allergic reaction (e.g., anaphylaxis) after a previous dose of any hepatitis A-containing vaccine, or to any component of HAVRIX, including neomycin. (4)

——WARNINGS AND PRECAUTIONS——

- The tip caps of the prefilled syringes may contain natural rubber latex which may cause allergic reactions in latex-sensitive individuals. (5.1)
- Syncope (fainting) can occur in association with administration of injectable vaccines, including HAVRIX. Procedures should be in place to avoid falling injury and to restore cerebral perfusion following syncope. (5.2)

——ADVERSE REACTIONS——

- In studies of adults and children 2 years of age and older, the most common solicited adverse events were injection-site soreness (56% of adults and 21% of children) and headache (14% of adults and less than 9% of children). (6.1)
- In studies of children 11 to 25 months of age, the most frequently reported solicited local reactions were pain (32%) and redness (29%). Common solicited general adverse events were irritability (42%), drowsiness (28%), and loss of appetite (28%). (6.1)

To report SUSPECTED ADVERSE REACTIONS, contact GlaxoSmithKline at 1-888-825-5249 or VAERS at 1-800-822-7967 or www.vaers.hhs.gov.

——DRUG INTERACTIONS——

Do not mix HAVRIX with any other vaccine or product in the same syringe or vial. (7.1)

——USE IN SPECIFIC POPULATIONS——

Safety and effectiveness of HAVRIX have not been established in pregnant women and nursing mothers. (8.1)
See 17 for PATIENT COUNSELING INFORMATION
Revised: 07/2014

FULL PRESCRIBING INFORMATION: CONTENTS*

FULL PRESCRIBING INFORMATION

1 INDICATIONS AND USAGE

HAVRIX® is indicated for active immunization against disease caused by hepatitis A virus (HAV). HAVRIX is approved for use in persons 12 months of age and older. Primary immunization should be administered at least 2 weeks prior to expected exposure to HAV.

2 DOSAGE AND ADMINISTRATION

2.1 Preparation for Administration

Shake well before use. With thorough agitation, HAVRIX is a homogeneous, turbid, white suspension. Do not administer if it appears otherwise. Parenteral drug products should be inspected visually for particulate matter and discoloration prior to administration, whenever solution and container permit. If either of these conditions exists, the vaccine should not be administered.

For the prefilled syringes, attach a sterile needle and administer intramuscularly.

For the vials, use a sterile needle and sterile syringe to withdraw the vaccine dose and administer intramuscularly. Changing needles between drawing vaccine from a vial and injecting it into a recipient is not necessary unless the needle has been damaged or contaminated. Use a separate sterile needle and syringe for each individual.

2.2 Administration

HAVRIX should be administered by intramuscular injection only. HAVRIX should not be administered in the gluteal region; such injections may result in suboptimal response.

Do not administer this product intravenously, intradermally, or subcutaneously.

2.3 Recommended Dose and Schedule

Children and Adolescents: Primary immunization for children and adolescents (12 months through 18 years of age) consists of a single 0.5-mL dose and a 0.5-mL booster dose administered anytime between 6 and 12 months later. The preferred sites for intramuscular injections are the anterolateral aspect of the thigh in young children or the deltoid muscle of the upper arm in older children.

Adults: Primary immunization for adults consists of a single 1-mL dose and a 1-mL booster dose administered anytime between 6 and 12 months later. In adults, the injection should be given in the deltoid region.

3 DOSAGE FORMS AND STRENGTHS

Suspension for injection available in the following presentations:
- 0.5-mL single-dose vials and prefilled TIP-LOK® syringes.
- 1-mL single-dose vials and prefilled TIP-LOK syringes.
[See How Supplied/Storage and Handling (16).]

4 CONTRAINDICATIONS

Severe allergic reaction (e.g., anaphylaxis) after a previous dose of any hepatitis A-containing vaccine, or to any component of HAVRIX, including neomycin, is a contraindication to administration of HAVRIX [see Description (11)].

5 WARNINGS AND PRECAUTIONS

5.1 Latex

The tip caps of the prefilled syringes may contain natural rubber latex which may cause allergic reactions in latex-sensitive individuals.

5.2 Syncope

Syncope (fainting) can occur in association with administration of injectable vaccines, including HAVRIX. Syncope can be accompanied by transient neurological signs such as visual disturbance, paresthesia, and tonic-clonic limb movements. Procedures should be in place to avoid falling injury and to restore cerebral perfusion following syncope.

5.3 Preventing and Managing Allergic Vaccine Reactions

Appropriate medical treatment and supervision must be available to manage possible anaphylactic reactions following administration of the vaccine [see Contraindications (4)].

5.4 Altered Immunocompetence

Immunocompromised persons may have a diminished immune response to HAVRIX, including individuals receiving immunosuppressant therapy.

5.5 Limitations of Vaccine Effectiveness

Hepatitis A virus has a relatively long incubation period (15 to 50 days). HAVRIX may not prevent hepatitis A infection in individuals who have an unrecognized hepatitis A infection at the time of vaccination. Additionally, vaccination with HAVRIX may not protect all individuals.

6 ADVERSE REACTIONS

6.1 Clinical Trials Experience

Because clinical trials are conducted under widely varying conditions, adverse reaction rates observed in the clinical trials of a vaccine cannot be directly compared to rates in the clinical trials of another vaccine, and may not reflect the rates observed in practice.

The safety of HAVRIX has been evaluated in 61 clinical trials involving approximately 37,000 individuals receiving doses of 360 EL.U. (n = 21,928 in 3- or 4-dose schedule), 720 EL.U. (n = 12,274 in 2- or 3-dose schedule), or 1440 EL.U. (n = 2,782 in 2- or 3-dose schedule).

Of solicited adverse events in clinical trials of adults, who received HAVRIX 1440 EL.U., and children (2 years of age and older), who received either HAVRIX 360 EL.U. or 720 EL.U., the most frequently reported was injection-site soreness (56% of adults and 21% of children); less than 0.5% of soreness was reported as severe. Headache was reported by 14% of adults and less than 9% of children. Other solicited and unsolicited events occurring during clinical trials are listed below.

Incidence 1% to 10% of Injections: *Metabolism and Nutrition Disorders:* Anorexia.

Gastrointestinal Disorders: Nausea.

General Disorders and Administration Site Conditions: Fatigue, fever >99.5°F (37.5°C), induration, redness, and swelling of the injection site; malaise.

Incidence <1% of Injections: *Infections and Infestations:* Pharyngitis, upper respiratory tract infections.

Blood and Lymphatic System Disorders: Lymphadenopathy.

Psychiatric Disorders: Insomnia.

Nervous System Disorders: Dysgeusia, hypertonia.

Eye Disorders: Photophobia.

Ear and Labyrinth Disorders: Vertigo.

Gastrointestinal Disorders: Abdominal pain, diarrhea, vomiting.

Skin and Subcutaneous Tissue Disorders: Pruritus, rash, urticaria.

Musculoskeletal and Connective Tissue Disorders: Arthralgia, myalgia.

General Disorders and Administration Site Conditions: Injection site hematoma.

Investigations: Creatine phosphokinase increased.

Coadministration Studies of HAVRIX in Children 11 to 25 Months of Age: In 4 studies, 3,152 children 11 to 25 months of age received at least one dose of HAVRIX 720 EL.U. administered alone or concomitantly with other routine childhood vaccinations [see Clinical Studies (14.2, 14.5)]. The studies included HAV 210 (N = 1,084), HAV 232 (N = 394), HAV 220 (N = 433), and HAV 231 (N = 1,241). In the largest of these studies (HAV 231) conducted in the US, 1,241 children 15 months of age were randomized to receive: Group 1) HAVRIX alone; Group 2) HAVRIX concomitantly with measles, mumps, and rubella (MMR) vaccine (manufactured by Merck and Co.) and varicella vaccine (manufactured by Merck and Co.); or Group 3) MMR and varicella vaccines. Subjects in Group 3 who received MMR and varicella vaccines received the first dose of HAVRIX 42 days later. A second dose of HAVRIX was administered to all subjects 6 to 9 months after the first dose of HAVRIX. Solicited local adverse reactions and general events were recorded by parents/guardians on diary cards for 4 days (days 0 to 3) after vaccination. Unsolicited adverse events were recorded on the diary card for 31 days after vaccination. Telephone follow-up was conducted 6 months after the last vaccination to inquire about serious adverse events, new onset chronic illnesses and medically significant events. A total of 1,035 children completed the 6-month follow-up.

Table 1. Solicited Local Adverse Reactions and General Adverse Events Occurring Within 4 Days of Vaccination[a] in Children 15 to 24 Months of Age With HAVRIX Administered Alone or Concomitantly With MMR and Varicella Vaccines (TVC)

	Group 1 HAVRIX Dose 1 %	Group 2 HAVRIX+ MMR+V[b] Dose 1 %	Group 1 HAVRIX Dose 2 %	Group 2 HAVRIX Dose 2 %
Local (at injection site for HAVRIX)				
N	298	411	272	373
Pain, any	23.8	23.6	24.3	30.3
Redness, any	20.1	20.0	22.8	23.9
Swelling, any	8.7	10.2	9.6	9.9
General				
N	300	417	271	375
Irritability, any	33.3	43.9	31.0	27.2
Irritability, grade 3	0.3	1.9	1.5	0.3
Drowsiness, any	22.3	35.3	21.0	20.8
Drowsiness, grade 3	1.0	2.2	1.1	0.0
Loss of appetite, any	18.3	26.1	19.9	20.5
Loss of appetite, grade 3	1.0	1.4	0.4	0.3
Fever ≥100.6°F (38.1°C)	3.0	4.8	3.3	2.7
Fever ≥101.5°F (38.6°C)	2.0	2.6	1.8	1.6
Fever ≥102.4°F (39.1°C)	0.7	0.7	0.4	1.1

Total vaccinated cohort (TVC) = all subjects who received at least one dose of vaccine.
N = number of subjects who received at least one dose of vaccine and for whom diary card information was available.
Grade 3: drowsiness defined as prevented normal daily activities; irritability/fussiness defined as crying that could not be comforted/prevented normal daily activities; loss of appetite defined as no eating at all.
[a] Within 4 days of vaccination defined as day of vaccination and the next 3 days.
[b] MMR = measles, mumps, and rubella vaccine; V = varicella vaccine.

Among subjects in all groups combined, 53% were male; 69% of subjects were white, 16% were Hispanic, 9% were black and 6% were other racial/ethnic groups.

Percentages of subjects with solicited local adverse reactions and general adverse events following HAVRIX administered alone (Group 1) or concomitantly with MMR and varicella vaccines (Group 2) are presented in Table 1. The solicited adverse events from the 3 additional coadministration studies conducted with HAVRIX were comparable to those from Study HAV 231.

[See table 1 above]

Serious Adverse Events in Children 11 to 25 Months of Age: Among these 4 studies, 0.9% (29/3,152) of subjects reported a serious adverse event within the 31-day period following vaccination with HAVRIX. Among subjects administered HAVRIX alone 1.0% (13/1,332) reported a serious adverse event. Among subjects who received HAVRIX concomitantly with other childhood vaccines, 0.9% (8/909) reported a serious adverse event. In these 4 studies, there were 4 reports of seizure within 31 days post-vaccination: these occurred 2, 9, and 27 days following the first dose of HAVRIX administered alone and 12 days following the second dose of HAVRIX. In one subject who received INFANRIX and Hib conjugate vaccine followed by HAVRIX 6 weeks later, bronchial hyperreactivity and respiratory distress were reported on the day of administration of HAVRIX alone.

6.2 Postmarketing Experience

In addition to reports in clinical trials, worldwide voluntary reports of adverse events received for HAVRIX since market introduction of this vaccine are listed below. This list includes serious adverse events or events which have a suspected causal connection to components of HAVRIX or other vaccines or drugs. Because these events are reported voluntarily from a population of uncertain size, it is not always possible to reliably estimate their frequency or establish a causal relationship to the vaccine.

Infections and Infestations: Rhinitis.

Blood and Lymphatic System Disorders: Thrombocytopenia.

Immune System Disorders: Anaphylactic reaction, anaphylactoid reaction, serum sickness–like syndrome.

Nervous System Disorders: Convulsion, dizziness, encephalopathy, Guillain-Barré syndrome, hypoesthesia, multiple sclerosis, myelitis, neuropathy, paresthesia, somnolence, syncope.

Vascular Disorders: Vasculitis.

Respiratory, Thoracic, and Mediastinal Disorders: Dyspnea.

Hepatobiliary Disorders: Hepatitis, jaundice.

Skin and Subcutaneous Tissue Disorders: Angioedema, erythema multiforme, hyperhidrosis.

Congenital, Familial, and Genetic Disorders: Congenital anomaly.

Musculoskeletal and Connective Tissue Disorders: Musculoskeletal stiffness.

General Disorders and Administration Site Conditions: Chills, influenza-like symptoms, injection site reaction, local swelling.

7 DRUG INTERACTIONS

7.1 Concomitant Administration With Vaccines and Immune Globulin

In clinical studies HAVRIX was administered concomitantly with the following vaccines [see Adverse Reactions (6.1) and Clinical Studies (14.5)]:
• INFANRIX (DTaP);
• Hib conjugate vaccine;
• pneumococcal 7-valent conjugate vaccine;
• MMR vaccine;
• varicella vaccine.

HAVRIX may be administered concomitantly with immune globulin.

When concomitant administration of other vaccines or immune globulin is required, they should be given with different syringes and at different injection sites. Do not mix HAVRIX with any other vaccine or product in the same syringe or vial.

7.2 Immunosuppressive Therapies

Immunosuppressive therapies, including irradiation, antimetabolites, alkylating agents, cytotoxic drugs, and corticosteroids (used in greater than physiologic doses), may reduce the immune response to HAVRIX.

8 USE IN SPECIFIC POPULATIONS

8.1 Pregnancy

Pregnancy Category C

Animal reproduction studies have not been conducted with HAVRIX. It is also not known whether HAVRIX can cause fetal harm when administered to a pregnant woman or can affect reproduction capacity. HAVRIX should be given to a pregnant woman only if clearly needed.

8.3 Nursing Mothers

It is not known whether HAVRIX is excreted in human milk. Because many drugs are excreted in human milk, caution should be exercised when HAVRIX is administered to a nursing woman.

8.4 Pediatric Use

The safety and effectiveness of HAVRIX, doses of 360 EL.U. or 720 EL.U., have been evaluated in more than 22,000 subjects 1 year to 18 years of age.

The safety and effectiveness of HAVRIX have not been established in subjects younger than 12 months of age.

8.5 Geriatric Use

Clinical studies of HAVRIX did not include sufficient numbers of subjects 65 years of age and older to determine whether they respond differently from younger subjects. Other reported clinical experience has not identified differences in overall safety between these subjects and younger adult subjects.

8.6 Hepatic Impairment

Subjects with chronic liver disease had a lower antibody response to HAVRIX than healthy subjects [see Clinical Studies (14.3)].

11 DESCRIPTION

HAVRIX (Hepatitis A Vaccine) is a sterile suspension of inactivated virus for intramuscular administration. The virus (strain HM175) is propagated in MRC-5 human diploid cells. After removal of the cell culture medium, the cells are lysed to form a suspension. This suspension is purified through ultrafiltration and gel permeation chromatography procedures. Treatment of this lysate with formalin ensures viral inactivation. Viral antigen activity is referenced to a standard using an enzyme linked immunosorbent assay (ELISA), and is therefore expressed in terms of ELISA Units (EL.U.).

Each 1-mL adult dose of vaccine contains 1440 EL.U. of viral antigen, adsorbed on 0.5 mg of aluminum as aluminum hydroxide.

Each 0.5-mL pediatric dose of vaccine contains 720 EL.U. of viral antigen, adsorbed onto 0.25 mg of aluminum as aluminum hydroxide.

HAVRIX contains the following excipients: Amino acid supplement (0.3% w/v) in a phosphate-buffered saline solution and polysorbate 20 (0.05 mg/mL). From the manufacturing process, HAVRIX also contains residual MRC-5 cellular proteins (not more than 5 mcg/mL), formalin (not more than 0.1 mg/mL), and neomycin sulfate (not more than 40 ng/mL), an aminoglycoside antibiotic included in the cell growth media.

HAVRIX is formulated without preservatives.

HAVRIX is available in vials and prefilled syringes. The tip caps of the prefilled syringes may contain natural rubber latex; the plungers are not made with natural rubber latex. The vial stoppers are not made with natural rubber latex.

12 CLINICAL PHARMACOLOGY

12.1 Mechanism of Action

The hepatitis A virus belongs to the picornavirus family. It is one of several hepatitis viruses that cause systemic disease with pathology in the liver.

The incubation period for hepatitis A averages 28 days (range: 15 to 50 days).[1] The course of hepatitis A infection is extremely variable, ranging from asymptomatic infection to icteric hepatitis and death.

The presence of antibodies to HAV confers protection against hepatitis A infection. However, the lowest titer needed to confer protection has not been determined.

13 NONCLINICAL TOXICOLOGY

13.1 Carcinogenesis, Mutagenesis, Impairment of Fertility

HAVRIX has not been evaluated for its carcinogenic potential, mutagenic potential, or potential for impairment of fertility.

14 CLINICAL STUDIES

14.1 Pediatric Effectiveness Studies

Protective efficacy with HAVRIX has been demonstrated in a double-blind, randomized controlled study in school children (age 1 to 16 years) in Thailand who were at high risk of HAV infection. A total of 40,119 children were randomized to be vaccinated with either HAVRIX 360 EL.U. or ENGERIX-B 10 mcg at 0, 1, and 12 months. Of these, 19,037 children received 2 doses of HAVRIX (0 and 1 months) and 19,120 children received 2 doses of control vaccine, ENGERIX-B (0 and 1 months). A total of 38,157 children entered surveillance at day 138 and were observed for an additional 8 months. Using the protocol-defined endpoint (≥2 days absence from school, ALT level >45 U/mL, and a positive result in the HAVAB-M test), 32 cases of clinical hepatitis A occurred in the control group. In the HAVRIX group, 2 cases were identified. These 2 cases were mild in terms of both biochemical and clinical indices of hepatitis A disease. Thus the calculated efficacy rate for prevention of clinical hepatitis A was 94% (95% Confidence Interval [CI]: 74, 98).

In outbreak investigations occurring in the trial, 26 clinical cases of hepatitis A (of a total of 34 occurring in the trial) occurred. No cases occurred in vaccinees who received HAVRIX.

Using additional virological and serological analyses post hoc, the efficacy of HAVRIX was confirmed. Up to 3 additional cases of mild clinical illness may have occurred in vaccinees. Using available testing, these illnesses could neither be proven nor disproven to have been caused by HAV. By including these as cases, the calculated efficacy rate for prevention of clinical hepatitis A would be 84% (95% CI: 60, 94).

14.2 Immunogenicity in Children and Adolescents

Immune Response to HAVRIX 720 EL.U./0.5 mL at 11 to 25 Months of Age (Study HAV 210): In this prospective, open-label, multicenter study, 1,084 children were administered study vaccine in one of 5 groups:
(1) Children 11 to 13 months of age who received HAVRIX on a 0- and 6-month schedule;
(2) Children 15 to 18 months of age who received HAVRIX on a 0- and 6-month schedule;
(3) Children 15 to 18 months of age who received HAVRIX coadministered with INFANRIX and Haemophilus b (Hib) conjugate vaccine (no longer US-licensed) at month 0 and HAVRIX at month 6;
(4) Children 15 to 18 months of age who received INFANRIX coadministered with Hib conjugate vaccine at month 0 and HAVRIX at months 1 and 7;
(5) Children 23 to 25 months of age who received HAVRIX on a 0- and 6-month schedule.

Among subjects in all groups, 52% were male; 61% of subjects were white, 9% were black, 3% were Asian, and 27% were other racial/ethnic groups. The anti-hepatitis A antibody vaccine responses and GMTs, calculated on responders for groups 1, 2, and 5 are presented in Table 2. Vaccine response rates were similar among the 3 age groups that received HAVRIX. One month after the second dose of HAVRIX, the GMT in each of the younger age groups (11 to 13 and 15 to 18 months of age) was shown to be similar to that achieved in the 23 to 25 months of age group.

Table 2. Anti-Hepatitis A Immune Response Following 2 Doses of HAVRIX 720 EL.U./0.5 mL Administered 6 Months Apart in Children Given the First Dose of HAVRIX at 11 to 13 Months of Age, 15 to 18 Months of Age, or 23 to 25 Months of Age

Age group	N	Vaccine Response		GMT (mIU/mL)
		%	95% CI	
11-13 months (Group 1)	218	99	97, 100	1,461[a]
15-18 months (Group 2)	200	100	98, 100	1,635[a]
23-25 months (Group 5)	211	100	98, 100	1,911

Vaccine response = Seroconversion (anti-HAV ≥15 mIU/mL [lower limit of antibody measurement by assay]) in children initially seronegative or at least the maintenance of the pre-vaccination anti-HAV concentration in initially seropositive children.

CI = Confidence Interval; GMT = Geometric mean antibody titer.

[a] Calculated on vaccine responders one month post-dose 2. GMTs in children 11 to 13 months of age and 15 to 18 months of age were non-inferior (similar) to the GMT in children 23 to 25 months of age (i.e., the lower limit of the two-sided 95% CI on the GMT ratio for Group 1/Group 5 and for Group 2/Group 5 were both ≥0.5).

In 3 additional clinical studies (HAV 232, HAV 220, and HAV 231), children received either 2 doses of HAVRIX alone or the first dose of HAVRIX concomitantly administered with other routinely recommended US-licensed vaccines followed by a second dose of HAVRIX. After the second dose of HAVRIX, there was no evidence for interference with the anti-HAV response in the children who received concomitantly administered vaccines compared to those who received HAVRIX alone. [See Adverse Reactions (6.1) and Clinical Studies (14.5).]

Immune Response to HAVRIX 360 EL.U. Among Individuals 2 to 18 Years of Age: In 6 clinical studies, 762 subjects 2 to 18 years of age received 2 doses of HAVRIX (360 EL.U.) given 1 month apart (GMT ranged from 197 to 660 mIU/mL). Ninety-nine percent of subjects seroconverted following 2 doses. When a third dose of HAVRIX 360 EL.U. was administered 6 months following the initial dose, all subjects were seropositive (anti-HAV ≥20 mIU/mL) 1 month following the third dose, with GMTs rising to a range of 3,388 to 4,643 mIU/mL. In 1 study in which children were followed for an additional 6 months, all subjects remained seropositive.

Immune Response to HAVRIX 720 EL.U./0.5 mL Among Individuals 2 to 19 Years of Age: In 4 clinical studies, 314 children and adolescents ranging from 2 to 19 years of age were immunized with 2 doses of HAVRIX 720 EL.U./0.5 mL given 6 months apart. One month after the first dose, seroconversion (anti-HAV ≥20 mIU/mL [lower limit of antibody measurement by assay]) ranged from 96.8% to 100%, with GMTs of 194 mIU/mL to 305 mIU/mL. In studies in which sera were obtained 2 weeks following the initial dose, seroconversion ranged from 91.6% to 96.1%. One month following the booster dose at month 6, all subjects were seropositive, with GMTs ranging from 2,495 mIU/mL to 3,644 mIU/mL.

In an additional study in which the booster dose was delayed until 1 year following the initial dose, 95.2% of the subjects were seropositive just prior to administration of the booster dose. One month later, all subjects were seropositive, with a GMT of 2,657 mIU/mL.

14.3 Immunogenicity in Adults

More than 400 healthy adults 18 to 50 years of age in 3 clinical studies were given a single 1440 EL.U. dose of HAVRIX. All subjects were seronegative for hepatitis A antibodies at baseline. Specific humoral antibodies against HAV were elicited in more than 96% of subjects when measured 1 month after vaccination. By day 15, 80% to 98% of vaccinees had already seroconverted (anti-HAV ≥20 mIU/mL [lower limit of antibody measurement by assay]). GMTs of seroconverters ranged from 264 to 339 mIU/mL at day 15 and increased to a range of 335 to 637 mIU/mL by 1 month following vaccination.

The GMTs obtained following a single dose of HAVRIX are at least several times higher than that expected following receipt of immune globulin.

In a clinical study using 2.5 to 5 times the standard dose of immune globulin (standard dose = 0.02 to 0.06 mL/kg), the GMT in recipients was 146 mIU/mL at 5 days post-administration, 77 mIU/mL at month 1, and 63 mIU/mL at month 2.

In 2 clinical trials in which a booster dose of 1440 EL.U. was given 6 months following the initial dose, 100% of vaccinees (n = 269) were seropositive 1 month after the booster dose, with GMTs ranging from 3,318 mIU/mL to 5,925 mIU/mL. The titers obtained from this additional dose approximate those observed several years after natural infection.

In a subset of vaccinees (n = 89), a single dose of HAVRIX 1440 EL.U. elicited specific anti-HAV neutralizing antibodies in more than 94% of vaccinees when measured 1 month after vaccination. These neutralizing antibodies persisted until month 6. One hundred percent of vaccinees had neutralizing antibodies when measured 1 month after a booster dose given at month 6.

Immunogenicity of HAVRIX was studied in subjects with chronic liver disease of various etiologies. 189 healthy adults and 220 adults with either chronic hepatitis B (n = 46), chronic hepatitis C (n = 104), or moderate chronic liver disease of other etiology (n = 70) were vaccinated with HAVRIX 1440 EL.U. on a 0- and 6-month schedule. The last group consisted of alcoholic cirrhosis (n = 17), autoimmune hepatitis (n = 10), chronic hepatitis/cryptogenic cirrhosis (n = 9), hemochromatosis (n = 2), primary biliary cirrhosis (n = 15), primary sclerosing cholangitis (n = 4), and unspecified (n = 13). At each time point, geometric mean antibody titers (GMTs) were lower for subjects with chronic liver disease than for healthy subjects. At month 7, the GMTs ranged from 478 mIU/mL (chronic hepatitis C) to 1,245 mIU/mL (healthy). One month after the first dose, seroconversion rates in adults with chronic liver disease were lower than in healthy adults. However, 1 month after the booster dose at month 6, seroconversion rates were similar in all groups; rates ranged from 94.7% to 98.1%. The relevance of these data to the duration of protection afforded by HAVRIX is unknown.

In subjects with chronic liver disease, local injection site reactions with HAVRIX were similar among all 4 groups, and no serious adverse events attributed to the vaccine were reported in subjects with chronic liver disease.

14.4 Duration of Immunity

The duration of immunity following a complete schedule of immunization with HAVRIX has not been established.

14.5 Immune Response to Concomitantly Administered Vaccines

In 3 clinical studies HAVRIX was administered concomitantly with other routinely recommended US-licensed vaccines: Study HAV 232: Diphtheria and tetanus toxoids and acellular pertussis vaccine adsorbed (INFANRIX, DTaP) and Haemophilus b (Hib) conjugate vaccine (tetanus toxoid conjugate) (manufactured by sanofi pasteur SA); Study HAV 220: Pneumococcal 7-valent conjugate vaccine (PCV-7) (manufactured by Pfizer), and Study HAV 231: MMR and varicella vaccines. [See Adverse Reactions (6.1).]

Concomitant Administration With DTaP and Hib Conjugate Vaccine (Study HAV 232): In this US multicenter study, 468 subjects, children 15 months of age were randomized to receive: Group 1) HAVRIX coadministered with INFANRIX and Hib conjugate vaccine (n = 127); Group 2) INFANRIX and Hib conjugate vaccine alone followed by a first dose of HAVRIX one month later (n = 132); or Group 3) HAVRIX alone (n = 135). All subjects received a second dose of HAVRIX alone 6 to 9 months following the first dose. Among subjects in all groups combined, 53% were male; 64% of subjects were white, 12% were black, 6% were Hispanic, and 18% were other racial/ethnic groups.

There was no evidence for reduced antibody response to diphtheria and tetanus toxoids (percentage of subjects with antibody levels ≥0.1 mIU/mL to each antigen), pertussis antigens (percentage of subjects with seroresponse, antibody concentrations ≥5 EL.U./mL in seronegative subjects or post-vaccination antibody concentration ≥2 times the pre-vaccination antibody concentration in seropositive subjects, and GMTs), or Hib (percentage of subjects with antibody levels ≥1 mcg/mL to polyribosyl-ribitol phosphate, PRP) when HAVRIX was administered concomitantly with INFANRIX and Hib conjugate vaccine (Group 1) relative to INFANRIX and Hib conjugate vaccine administered together (Group 2).

Concomitant Administration With Pneumococcal 7-Valent Conjugate Vaccine (Study HAV 220): In this US multicenter study, 433 children 15 months of age were randomized to receive: Group 1) HAVRIX coadministered with PCV-7 vaccine (n = 137); Group 2) HAVRIX administered alone (n = 147); or Group 3) PCV-7 vaccine administered alone (n = 149) followed by a first dose of HAVRIX one month later. All subjects received a second dose of HAVRIX 6 to 9 months after the first dose. Among subjects in all groups combined, 53% were female; 61% of subjects were white, 16% were Hispanic, 15% were black, and 8% were other racial/ethnic groups.

There was no evidence for reduced antibody response to PCV-7 (GMC to each serotype) when HAVRIX was administered concomitantly with PCV-7 vaccine (Group 1) relative to PCV-7 administered alone (Group 3).

Concomitant Administration With MMR and Varicella Vaccines (Study HAV 231): In a US multicenter study, there was no evidence for interference in the immune response to MMR and varicella vaccines (the percentage of subjects with pre-specified seroconversion/seroresponse levels) administered at 15 months of age concomitantly with HAVRIX relative to the response when MMR and varicella vaccines are administered without HAVRIX. *[See Adverse Reactions (6.1).]*

15 REFERENCES

1. Centers for Disease Control and Prevention. Prevention of hepatitis A through active or passive immunization: Recommendations of the Immunization Practices Advisory Committee (ACIP). *MMWR* 2006;55(RR-7):1-23.

16 HOW SUPPLIED/STORAGE AND HANDLING

HAVRIX is available in single-dose vials and prefilled disposable TIP-LOK syringes (packaged without needles) (Preservative Free Formulation):

720 EL.U./0.5 mL

NDC 58160-825-01 Vial in Package of 10: NDC 58160-825-11

NDC 58160-825-43 Syringe in Package of 10: NDC 58160-825-52

1440 EL.U./mL

NDC 58160-826-01 Vial in Package of 10: NDC 58160-826-11

NDC 58160-826-05 Syringe in Package of 1: NDC 58160-826-34

NDC 58160-826-43 Syringe in Package of 10: NDC 58160-826-52

Store refrigerated between 2° and 8°C (36° and 46°F). Do not freeze. Discard if the vaccine has been frozen. Do not dilute to administer.

17 PATIENT COUNSELING INFORMATION

- Inform vaccine recipients and parents or guardians of the potential benefits and risks of immunization with HAVRIX.
- Emphasize, when educating vaccine recipients and parents or guardians regarding potential side effects, that HAVRIX contains non-infectious killed viruses and cannot cause hepatitis A infection.
- Instruct vaccine recipients and parents or guardians to report any adverse events to their healthcare provider.
- Give vaccine recipients and parents or guardians the Vaccine Information Statements, which are required by the National Childhood Vaccine Injury Act of 1986 to be given prior to immunization. These materials are available free of charge at the Centers for Disease Control and Prevention (CDC) website (www.cdc.gov/vaccines).

HAVRIX, ENGERIX-B, INFANRIX, and TIP-LOK are registered trademarks of the GSK group of companies.

Manufactured by GlaxoSmithKline Biologicals
Rixensart, Belgium, US License No. 1617
Distributed by GlaxoSmithKline
Research Triangle Park, NC 27709

©2014, the GSK group of companies. All rights reserved.
HVX:42PI

HYCAMTIN ℞
[hī-kam' tin]
(topotecan)
capsules, for oral use

HIGHLIGHTS OF PRESCRIBING INFORMATION
These highlights do not include all the information needed to use HYCAMTIN capsules safely and effectively. See full prescribing information for HYCAMTIN capsules.
HYCAMTIN (topotecan) capsules, for oral use
Initial U.S. Approval: 1996

> **WARNING: BONE MARROW SUPPRESSION**
> *See full prescribing information for complete boxed warning*
> HYCAMTIN can cause severe myelosuppression. Administer only to patients with baseline neutrophil counts of ≥1,500 cells/mm³ and a platelet count ≥100,000 cells/mm³. Monitor blood cell counts (5.1).

---RECENT MAJOR CHANGES---

Boxed Warning	06/2014
Dosage and Administration, Dose Modification Guidelines (2.2)	06/2014
Contraindications, Severe Bone Marrow Depression (4)	Removed 06/2014
Warnings and Precautions, Embryofetal Toxicity (5.4)	06/2014
Warnings and Precautions, Drug Interactions (5.5)	Removed 06/2014

---INDICATIONS AND USAGE---

HYCAMTIN is a topoisomerase inhibitor. HYCAMTIN capsules are indicated for treatment of patients with relapsed small cell lung cancer. (1)

---DOSAGE AND ADMINISTRATION---

- 2.3 mg/m²/day orally once daily for 5 consecutive days repeated every 21 days. (2)
- Renal impairment: Adjust the dose of HYCAMTIN in patients with renal impairment. (2.2)

---DOSAGE FORMS AND STRENGTHS---

0.25-mg and 1-mg capsules. (3)

---CONTRAINDICATIONS---

- History of severe hypersensitivity reactions to topotecan. (4)

---WARNINGS AND PRECAUTIONS---

- Bone marrow suppression: Administer HYCAMTIN only to patients with adequate bone marrow reserves. Monitor peripheral blood counts. (5.1) Adjust dose as needed. (2.2)
- Diarrhea: Severe diarrhea can occur and may require hospitalization. (5.2) Withhold for severe diarrhea. Reduce dose upon recovery. (2.2)
- Interstitial lung disease (ILD): Fatal cases have occurred. Permanently discontinue for confirmed ILD. (5.3)
- Embryofetal toxicity: Can cause fetal harm. Advise women of potential risk to the fetus. (5.4, 8.1)

---ADVERSE REACTIONS---

The most common Grade 3 or 4 hematologic adverse reactions with HYCAMTIN capsules were neutropenia (56%), anemia (25%), and thrombocytopenia (35%). The most common (≥10%) non-hematologic adverse reactions (all grades) were nausea (33%), diarrhea (22%), vomiting (21%), alopecia (20%), and fatigue (19%). (6.1)

To report SUSPECTED ADVERSE REACTIONS, contact GlaxoSmithKline at 1-888-825-5249 or FDA at 1-800-FDA-1088 or www.fda.gov/medwatch.

---DRUG INTERACTIONS---

- Avoid concomitant use of P-gp and BCRP inhibitors with HYCAMTIN. (7, 12.3)

---USE IN SPECIFIC POPULATIONS---

- Geriatric use: Diarrhea was more frequent in patients aged ≥65 years (28%) compared with those younger than 65 years (19%). (5.2, 6.1, 8.5)
- Nursing mothers: Discontinue nursing or discontinue HYCAMTIN. (8.3)

See 17 for PATIENT COUNSELING INFORMATION and FDA-approved patient labeling

Revised: 06/2014

FULL PRESCRIBING INFORMATION: CONTENTS*
WARNING: BONE MARROW SUPPRESSION

* Sections or subsections omitted from the full prescribing information are not listed

---

FULL PRESCRIBING INFORMATION

> **WARNING: BONE MARROW SUPPRESSION**
> HYCAMTIN® can cause severe myelosuppression. Administer only to patients with neutrophil counts of ≥1,500 cells/mm³ and platelet counts ≥100,000 cells/mm³. Monitor blood cell counts.

1 INDICATIONS AND USAGE

HYCAMTIN capsules are indicated for the treatment of relapsed small cell lung cancer in patients with a prior complete or partial response and who are at least 45 days from the end of first-line chemotherapy.

2 DOSAGE AND ADMINISTRATION

2.1 Recommended Dosing

The recommended dose of HYCAMTIN capsules is 2.3 mg/m²/day orally once daily for 5 consecutive days repeated every 21 days. Round the dose to the nearest 0.25 mg, and prescribe the minimum number of 1-mg and 0.25-mg capsules. Prescribe the same number of capsules for each of the 5 dosing days.

Take HYCAMTIN capsules with or without food. Swallow capsules whole. Do not chew, crush, or divide the capsules. Do not prescribe a replacement dose for emesis.

Diarrhea:
Do not administer HYCAMTIN capsules to patients with Grade 3 or 4 diarrhea. After recovery to Grade 1 or less, reduce the dose of HYCAMTIN by 0.4 mg/m²/day for subsequent courses *[see Warnings and Precautions (5.2)].*

2.2 Dose Modification Guidelines

Hematologic Toxicities:
Do not administer subsequent courses of HYCAMTIN capsules until neutrophils recover to greater than 1,000 cells/mm3, platelets recover to greater than 100,000 cells/mm3, hemoglobin levels recover to greater than or equal to 9.0 g/dL (with transfusion if necessary).

Renal Impairment:
The recommended starting doses of HYCAMTIN capsules in patients with moderate and severe renal impairment are as follows:

- Dose reduce HYCAMTIN capsules by 0.4 mg/m2/day for:
  ◦ neutrophil counts of less than 500 cells/mm3 associated with fever or infection or lasting for 7 days or more;
  ◦ neutrophil counts of 500 to 1,000 cells/mm3 lasting beyond day 21 of the treatment course;
  ◦ platelet counts less than 25,000 cells/mm3.

Renal Impairment:
The recommended starting doses of HYCAMTIN capsules in patients with moderate and severe renal impairment are as follows:

Table 1. Dose Reduction Guidelines for Renal Impairment

Degree of Renal Impairment	Creatinine Clearance[a] (mL/min)	Dose (mg/m2)/day
Moderate	30 – 49	1.5b
Severe	<30	0.6b

a Calculated with the Cockroft-Gault method using ideal body weight.
b Dose can be increased after the first course by 0.4 mg/m2/day if no severe hematologic or gastrointestinal toxicities occur.

3 DOSAGE FORMS AND STRENGTHS

HYCAMTIN capsules contain topotecan hydrochloride expressed as topotecan free base. The 0.25-mg capsules are opaque white to yellowish-white and imprinted with HYCAMTIN and 0.25 mg. The 1-mg capsules are opaque pink and imprinted with HYCAMTIN and 1 mg.

4 CONTRAINDICATIONS

HYCAMTIN is contraindicated in patients who have a history of severe hypersensitivity reactions to topotecan.

5 WARNINGS AND PRECAUTIONS
5.1 Bone Marrow Suppression

Bone marrow suppression (primarily neutropenia) is a dose-limiting toxicity of HYCAMTIN. Neutropenia is not cumulative over time. The following data on myelosuppression are based on an integrated safety database from 4 thoracic malignancy trials (N = 682) using HYCAMTIN capsules at 2.3 mg/m^2/day for 5 consecutive days. The median day for neutrophil and platelet nadirs occurred on Day 15.
Neutropenia:
Grade 4 neutropenia (<500 cells/mm^3) occurred in 32% of patients with a median duration of 7 days and was most common during Course 1 of treatment (20% of patients). Clinical sequelae of neutropenia included infection (17%), febrile neutropenia (4%), sepsis (2%), and septic death (1%). Pancytopenia has been reported.
Topotecan can cause fatal typhlitis (neutropenic enterocolitis). Consider the possibility of typhlitis in patients presenting with fever, neutropenia, and abdominal pain [see Dosage and Administration (2.2)].
Thrombocytopenia:
Grade 4 thrombocytopenia (<10,000 cells/mm^3) occurred in 6% of patients, with a median duration of 3 days.
Anemia:
Grade 3 or 4 anemia (<8 g/dL) occurred in 25% of patients. Administer the first course of HYCAMTIN only to patients with a neutrophil count of ≥1,500 cells/mm^3 and a platelet count ≥100,000 cells/mm^3. Monitor peripheral blood cell counts frequently during treatment with HYCAMTIN. Refer to Section 2.2 for dose modification guidelines for hematological toxicities in subsequent courses.
5.2 Diarrhea
Diarrhea, including severe and life-threatening diarrhea requiring hospitalization, can occur during treatment with HYCAMTIN capsules. Diarrhea caused by HYCAMTIN capsules can occur at the same time as drug-induced neutropenia and its sequelae. In the 682 patients who received HYCAMTIN capsules in the 4 lung cancer trials, the incidence of diarrhea caused by HYCAMTIN capsules was 22%, with 4% Grade 3 and 0.4% Grade 4.The incidence of Grade 3 or 4 diarrhea proximate (within 5 days) to Grade 3 or 4 neutropenia events in the group receiving HYCAMTIN capsules was 5%. The median time to onset of Grade 2 or worse diarrhea was 9 days in the group receiving HYCAMTIN capsules. Manage diarrhea caused by HYCAMTIN capsules aggressively. Do not administer HYCAMTIN capsules to patients with Grade 3 or 4 diarrhea. Reduce the dose of HYCAMTIN after recovery to Grade 1 or less [see Dosage and Administration (2.2)].
5.3 Interstitial Lung Disease
Interstitial lung disease (ILD), including fatalities, has occurred with HYCAMTIN. Underlying risk factors include history of ILD, pulmonary fibrosis, lung cancer, thoracic radiation, and use of pneumotoxic drugs and/or colony stimulating factors. Monitor patients for pulmonary symptoms indicative of interstitial lung disease (e.g., cough, fever, dyspnea, and/or hypoxia), and discontinue HYCAMTIN if a new diagnosis of ILD is confirmed.
5.4 Embryofetal Toxicity
HYCAMTIN can cause fetal harm when administered to a pregnant woman. Topotecan caused embryolethality, fetotoxicity, and teratogenicity in rats and rabbits when administered during organogenesis. If this drug is used during pregnancy, or if a patient becomes pregnant while taking this drug, the patient should be apprised of the potential hazard to a fetus [see Use in Specific Populations (8.1)].
Advise females of reproductive potential to use highly effective contraception during treatment and for at least 1 month after the last dose of HYCAMTIN. Advise patients to contact their healthcare provider if they become pregnant, or if pregnancy is suspected, while taking HYCAMTIN [see Use in Specific Populations (8.1, 8.7)].

6 ADVERSE REACTIONS
The following serious adverse reactions are described below and elsewhere in the labeling:
• Bone Marrow Suppression [see Warnings and Precautions (5.1)]
• Diarrhea [see Warnings and Precautions (5.2)]
• Interstitial Lung Disease [see Warnings and Precautions (5.3)]
6.1 Clinical Trials Experience
Because clinical trials are conducted under widely varying conditions, adverse reaction rates observed in the clinical trials of a drug cannot be directly compared with rates in the clinical trials of another drug and may not reflect the rates observed in practice.
The safety of HYCAMTIN capsules was evaluated in 682 patients with lung cancer (3 recurrent small cell lung cancer [SCLC] trials and 1 recurrent non-small cell lung cancer [NSCLC] trial) who received at least one dose of HYCAMTIN capsules. Patients in all four trials had advanced lung malignancies and received prior chemotherapy in the first-line setting. The dose regimen for HYCAMTIN capsules was 2.3 mg/m^2/day for five consecutive days every 21 days. The median number of courses was 3 (range: 1 to 20) in these four trials. Table 2 describes the hematologic and non-hematologic adverse reactions in recurrent SCLC patients treated with HYCAMTIN capsules in the overall lung cancer patient population.
[See table 2 below]
Adverse reactions were graded using NCI Common Toxicity Criteria Version 2.0.
On-Study Death Due to Toxicity of HYCAMTIN:
In the 682 patients who received HYCAMTIN capsules in the four lung cancer trials, 39 deaths (6%) occurred within 30 days after the last dose for a reason other than progressive disease: 13 due to hematologic toxicity, 5 due to non-hematologic toxicity (2 from diarrhea), and 21 due to other causes.

7 DRUG INTERACTIONS

Topotecan is a substrate for both P-glycoprotein (P-gp) and breast cancer resistance protein (BCRP). Inhibitors of these transporters increase the systemic exposure to oral topotecan. Avoid concomitant use of P-gp inhibitors (e.g., amiodarone, azithromycin, captopril, carvedilol, clarithromycin, conivaptan, cyclosporine, diltiazem, dronedarone, erythromycin, felodipine, itraconazole, ketoconazole, lopinavir, ritonavir, quercetin, quinidine, ranolazine, ticagrelor, verapamil) and BCRP inhibitors (e.g., cyclosporine, eltrombopag) with HYCAMTIN capsules [see Clinical Pharmacology (12.3)].

8 USE IN SPECIFIC POPULATIONS
8.1 Pregnancy
Pregnancy Category D.
Risk Summary:
HYCAMTIN can cause fetal harm when administered to a pregnant woman. Topotecan caused embryolethality, fetotoxicity, and teratogenicity in rats and rabbits when administered during organogenesis. If this drug is used during pregnancy, or if the patient becomes pregnant while taking this drug, inform the patient of the potential hazard to a fetus.
Animal Data:
In rabbits, an IV dose of 0.10 mg/kg/day (about equal to the clinical IV dose on a mg/m^2 basis) given on days 6 through 20 of gestation caused maternal toxicity, embryolethality, and reduced fetal body weight. In the rat, an IV dose of 0.23 mg/kg/day (about equal to the clinical IV dose on a mg/m^2 basis) given for 14 days before mating through gestation day 6 caused fetal resorption, microphthalmia, pre-implant loss, and mild maternal toxicity. Administration of an IV dose of 0.10 mg/kg/day (about half the clinical IV dose on a mg/m^2 basis) to rats on days 6 through 17 of gestation caused an increase in post-implantation mortality. This dose also caused an increase in total fetal malformations. The most frequent malformations were of the eye (microphthalmia, anophthalmia, rosette formation of the retina, coloboma of the retina, ectopic orbit), brain (dilated lateral and third ventricles), skull, and vertebrae.
8.3 Nursing Mothers
It is not known whether topotecan is present in human milk. Lactating rats excrete high concentrations of topotecan into milk. Female rats given 4.72 mg/m^2 IV (about twice the clinical dose on a mg/m^2 basis) excreted topotecan into milk at concentrations up to 48-fold higher than those in plasma. Because many drugs are present in human milk, and because of the potential for serious adverse reactions in nursing infants from HYCAMTIN, a decision should be made whether to discontinue nursing or to discontinue the drug, taking into account the importance of the drug to the mother.
8.4 Pediatric Use
Safety and effectiveness in pediatric patients have not been established.
8.5 Geriatric Use
Of the 682 patients with thoracic cancer in 4 clinical trials who received HYCAMTIN capsules, 33% (n = 225) were aged 65 years and older, while 4.8% (n = 33) were aged 75 years and older. Treatment-related diarrhea was more frequent in patients aged ≥65 years (28%) compared with those younger than 65 years (19%). [See Warnings and Precautions (5.2), Adverse Reactions (6.1).]
No overall differences in effectiveness were observed between patients 65 years and older and younger patients.

Table 2. Incidence (≥5%) of Adverse Reactions in Small Cell Lung Cancer Patients Treated With HYCAMTIN Capsules Plus BSC and in Four Lung Cancer Trials

Adverse Reaction	HYCAMTIN Capsules + BSC (N = 70)			HYCAMTIN Capsules Lung Cancer Population (N = 682)		
	All Grades (%)	Grade 3 (%)	Grade 4 (%)	All Grades (%)	Grade 3 (%)	Grade 4 (%)
Hematologic						
Anemia	94	15	10	98	18	7
Neutropenia	91	28	33	83	24	32
Thrombocytopenia	81	30	7	81	29	6
Non-hematologic						
Nausea	27	1	0	33	3	0
Diarrhea	14	4	1	22	4	0.4
Vomiting	19	1	0	21	3	0.4
Alopecia	10	0	0	20	0.1	0
Fatigue	11	0	0	19	4	0.1
Anorexia	7	0	0	14	2	0
Asthenia	3	0	0	7	2	0
Pyrexia	7	1	0	5	1	1

BSC = Best Supportive Care.
N = Total number of patients treated.

8.6 Renal Impairment

The systemic exposure to both topotecan lactone and total topotecan increased in patients with renal impairment compared with that in patients with normal renal function. No dosage adjustment is recommended for patients with mild renal impairment (CLcr = 50-79 mL/min). Adjust the dose of HYCAMTIN capsules in patients with moderate (CLcr = 30-49 mL/min) and severe (CLcr <30 mL/min) renal impairment [see Dosage and Administration (2.2), Clinical Pharmacology (12.3)].

8.7 Females and Males of Reproductive Potential

Contraception:
Females: Counsel patients on pregnancy planning and prevention. Advise female patients of reproductive potential to use highly effective contraception during and for 1 month following treatment with HYCAMTIN. Advise patients to contact their healthcare provider if they become pregnant, or if pregnancy is suspected, while taking HYCAMTIN [see Use in Specific Populations (8.1)].
Males: HYCAMTIN may damage spermatozoa, resulting in possible genetic and fetal abnormalities. Advise males with a female sexual partner of reproductive potential to use effective contraception during and for 3 months after treatment with HYCAMTIN [see Nonclinical Toxicology (13.1)].
Infertility:
Females: In females of reproductive potential, HYCAMTIN may have both acute and long-term effects on fertility [see Nonclinical Toxicology (13.1)].
Males: Effects on spermatogenesis have been observed in animals administered HYCAMTIN. Advise males of the potential risk for impaired fertility and to seek counseling on fertility and family planning options prior to starting treatment.

10 OVERDOSAGE

Overdoses (up to 5-fold of the prescribed dose) occurred in patients treated with HYCAMTIN capsules. The primary complication of overdosage is bone marrow suppression. The observed signs and symptoms of overdose are consistent with the known adverse reactions associated with HYCAMTIN for oral use [see Adverse Reactions (6.1)]. Mucositis has also been reported in association with overdose. There is no known antidote for overdosage with HYCAMTIN. If an overdose is suspected, monitor the patient closely for bone marrow suppression, and institute supportive-care measures (such as the prophylactic use of G-CSF and/or antibiotic therapy) as appropriate.

11 DESCRIPTION

Topotecan hydrochloride is a semi-synthetic derivative of camptothecin and is an anti-tumor drug with topoisomerase I-inhibitory activity.
The chemical name for topotecan hydrochloride is (S)-10-[(dimethylamino)methyl]-4-ethyl-4,9-dihydroxy-1H-pyrano-[3',4':6,7] indolizino [1,2-b]quinoline-3,14-(4H,12H)-dione monohydrochloride. It has the molecular formula $C_{23}H_{23}N_3O_5\bullet HCl$ and a molecular weight of 457.9. It is soluble in water and melts with decomposition at 213° to 218°C.
Topotecan hydrochloride has the following structural formula:

HYCAMTIN capsules for oral use contain topotecan hydrochloride, the content of which is expressed as topotecan free base. The excipients are gelatin, glyceryl monostearate, hydrogenated vegetable oil, and titanium dioxide. The capsules are imprinted with edible black ink. The 1-mg capsules also contain red iron oxide.

12 CLINICAL PHARMACOLOGY

12.1 Mechanism of Action

Topoisomerase I relieves torsional strain in DNA by inducing reversible single-strand breaks. Topotecan binds to the topoisomerase I-DNA complex and prevents re-ligation of these single strand breaks. The cytotoxicity of topotecan is thought to be due to double-strand DNA damage produced during DNA synthesis, when replication enzymes interact with the ternary complex formed by topotecan, topoisomerase I, and DNA. Mammalian cells cannot efficiently repair these double-strand breaks.

12.3 Pharmacokinetics

Following administration of HYCAMTIN capsules at doses of 1.2 to 3.1 mg/m² administered daily for 5 days in cancer patients, topotecan exhibited biexponential pharmacokinet-

Table 3. Renal Function Groups With Initial Doses of HYCAMTIN Received

Renal Function Group	Creatinine Clearance (CLcr) (mL/min)	N	Dose (mg/m²) Once Daily for 5 Days
Normal (without prior P-B CT)[a]	>80	6	2.3
Normal (with prior P-B CT)	>80	12	2.3
Mild renal impairment	50-79	19	1.9 or 2.3
Moderate renal impairment	30-49	14	1.2, 1.5 or 1.8
Severe renal impairment	<30	8	0.6, 0.8 or 1.2

[a] P-B CT = Platinum-based chemotherapy.

ics with a mean terminal half-life of 3 to 6 hours. Total exposure (AUC) increased approximately proportionally to dose.
Absorption:
Topotecan is rapidly absorbed with peak plasma concentrations occurring between 1 to 2 hours following oral administration. The oral bioavailability of topotecan is approximately 40%. Following a high-fat meal, the extent of exposure was similar in the fed and fasted states, while T_{max} was delayed from 1.5 to 3 hours for topotecan lactone and from 3 to 4 hours for total topotecan. HYCAMTIN capsules can be given without regard to food.
Distribution:
Binding of topotecan to plasma proteins is approximately 35%.
Metabolism:
Topotecan undergoes a reversible pH-dependent hydrolysis of its lactone moiety; it is the lactone form that is pharmacologically active. At pH ≤4, the lactone is exclusively present, whereas the ring-opened hydroxy-acid form predominates at physiologic pH. The mean metabolite:parent AUC ratio was <10% for total topotecan and topotecan lactone.
Excretion:
In a mass balance study in 4 patients with advanced solid tumors, the overall recovery of drug-related material following 5 daily doses of topotecan was 57% of the administered oral dose. In the urine, 20% of the orally administered dose was excreted as total topotecan and 2% was excreted as N-desmethyl topotecan [see Use in Specific Populations (8.6)].
Fecal elimination of total topotecan accounted for 33%, while fecal elimination of N-desmethyl topotecan was 1.5%. Overall, the N-desmethyl metabolite contributed a mean of <6% (range: 4% to 8%) of the total drug-related material accounted for in the urine and feces. O-glucuronides of both topotecan and N-desmethyl topotecan have been identified in the urine.
Specific Populations:
Age and Gender: A cross-study analysis in 217 patients with advanced solid tumors indicated that age and gender did not significantly affect the pharmacokinetics of oral topotecan.
Race: In patients with normal renal function, the exposures (geometric mean dose-normalized AUC_{inf}) to topotecan lactone and total topotecan each were approximately 30% higher in Asian patients (n = 7) compared with Caucasian patients (n = 11).
In patients with mild renal impairment, the exposure was 30% higher for topotecan lactone in Asian (n = 7) compared with Caucasian (n = 12) patients, but the exposure to total topotecan was similar.
In patients with moderate renal impairment, the exposure was 60% higher for both topotecan lactone and total topotecan in Asian (n = 8) compared with Caucasian patients (n = 6).
In patients with severe renal impairment, the exposure was 112% higher for topotecan lactone and 70% higher for total topotecan in Asian (n = 3) compared with Caucasian patients (n = 4).
Renal Impairment: A trial was conducted in 59 patients with advanced cancer who were grouped based on the degree of their renal function and received HYCAMTIN capsules as shown in the table below.
[See table 3 above]
The exposure (geometric mean dose-normalized AUC_{inf}) for topotecan lactone increased by 34%, 80%, and 114% in Caucasian patients with mild, moderate, and severe renal impairment, respectively, compared with that in Caucasian patients with normal renal function. The corresponding values for total topotecan in Caucasian patients were 70%, 108%, and 227%, respectively. Asian patients with mild, moderate, and severe renal impairment had a 34%, 121%, and 247% higher exposure to topotecan lactone, respectively, than Asian patients with normal renal function. The corresponding values for total topotecan in Asian patients

are 26%, 153%, and 331%, respectively. Prior platinum-based chemotherapy (P-B CT) had no effect on the systemic exposure to both total topotecan and topotecan lactone in patients with normal renal function.
No dosage adjustment is recommended for patients with mild renal impairment. Adjust the dosage of HYCAMTIN capsules in patients with moderate and severe renal impairment [see Dosage and Administration (2.2), Use in Specific Populations (8.6)].
Hepatic Impairment: In a population pharmacokinetic analysis involving oral topotecan administered at doses of 0.15 to 2.7 mg/m2/day to 118 cancer patients, the pharmacokinetics of total topotecan did not differ significantly based on patient serum bilirubin, ALT, or AST.
Drug Interactions:
Effects of Topotecan on Drug-Metabolizing Enzymes: In vitro inhibition studies using marker substrates known to be metabolized by human cytochromes P450 (CYP1A2, CYP2A6, CYP2C8/9, CYP2C19, CYP2D6, CYP2E, CYP3A, or CYP4A) or dihydropyrimidine dehydrogenase indicate that the activities of these enzymes were not altered by topotecan. Enzyme inhibition by topotecan has not been evaluated in vivo.
Drugs That Inhibit Drug Efflux Transporters: Following coadministration of escalating doses of a dual inhibitor of BCRP and P-gp with oral topotecan, the AUC_{inf} of topotecan lactone and total topotecan increased approximately 2.5-fold compared with control [see Drug Interactions (7.1)]. Administration of oral cyclosporine A (15 mg/kg), an inhibitor of P-gp, multidrug-resistance-associated protein (MRP-1), and cytochrome P450 3A4 (CYP3A4) within 4 hours of oral topotecan increased the dose-normalized AUC_{0-24h} of topotecan lactone and total topotecan 2.0- to 3.0-fold compared with control [see Drug Interactions (7.1)].
Effect of pH-Elevating Agents: The pharmacokinetics of oral topotecan were unchanged when coadministered with ranitidine.

13 NONCLINICAL TOXICOLOGY

13.1 Carcinogenesis, Mutagenesis, Impairment of Fertility

Carcinogenicity testing of topotecan has not been done. Nevertheless, topotecan is known to be genotoxic to mammalian cells and is a probable carcinogen. Topotecan was mutagenic to L5178Y mouse lymphoma cells and clastogenic to cultured human lymphocytes with and without metabolic activation. It was also clastogenic to mouse bone marrow. Topotecan did not cause mutations in bacterial cells.
Topotecan given to female rats prior to mating at a dose of 1.4 mg/m² IV (about 0.6 times the oral clinical dose on a mg/m² basis) caused superovulation possibly related to inhibition of follicular atresia. This dose given to pregnant female rats also caused increased pre-implantation loss. Studies in dogs given 0.4 mg/m² IV (about 0.2 times the oral clinical dose on a mg/m² basis) of topotecan daily for a month suggest that treatment may cause an increase in the incidence of multinucleated spermatogonial giant cells in the testes. Topotecan may impair fertility in women and men.

14 CLINICAL STUDIES

14.1 Small Cell Lung Cancer

The efficacy of HYCAMTIN capsules was studied in 141 patients with relapsed SCLC in a randomized, controlled, open-label trial. The patients were prior responders (complete or partial) to first-line chemotherapy, were not considered candidates for standard intravenous chemotherapy, and had relapsed at least 45 days from the end of first-line chemotherapy. Seventy-one patients were randomized to HYCAMTIN capsules (2.3 mg/m²/day administered for 5 consecutive days repeated every 21 days) and Best Supportive Care (BSC) and 70 patients were randomized to BSC alone. The primary objective was to compare the overall survival between the treatment arms. Patients in the arm receiving HYCAMTIN capsules plus BSC received a median of 4 courses (range: 1 to 10) and maintained a median dose intensity of 3.77 mg/m²/week. The median patient age in the arm receiving HYCAMTIN capsules plus BSC and the BSC-alone treatment arm was 60 years and 58 years while the percentage of patients aged ≥65 years was 34% and 29%, respectively. The majority of patients were Caucasian (99.3%) and male (73%). Eighty percent of patients receiving HYCAMTIN capsules plus BSC previously received carboplatin or cisplatin, and 77% of patients in the BSC-alone arm received prior carboplatin or cisplatin. The arm receiving HYCAMTIN capsules plus BSC included 68% of patients with extensive disease and 28% with liver metastasis. In the BSC- alone arm, 61% of patients had extensive disease and 20% had liver metastases. Both treatment arms recruited 73% males. In the arm receiving HYCAMTIN capsules plus BSC, 18% of patients had prior carboplatin and 62% had prior cisplatin. In the BSC-alone arm, 26% of patients had prior carboplatin and 51% had prior cisplatin. The arm receiving HYCAMTIN capsules plus BSC showed a statistically significant improvement in overall survival compared with the BSC-alone arm (Log-rank *P* = 0.0104). Survival results are shown in Table 4 and Figure 1.

Table 4. Overall Survival in Patients With Small Cell Lung Cancer With HYCAMTIN Capsules Plus BSC Compared With BSC Alone

	Treatment Group	
	HYCAMTIN Capsules + BSC (N = 71)	BSC (N = 70)
Median (months) (95% CI)	6.0 (4.2, 7.3)	3.2 (2.6, 4.3)
Hazard ratio (95% CI) Log-rank *P*-value	0.64 (0.45, 0.90) 0.0104	

BSC = Best Supportive Care.
N = Total number of patients randomized.
CI = Confidence interval.

Figure 1. Kaplan-Meier Estimates for Survival

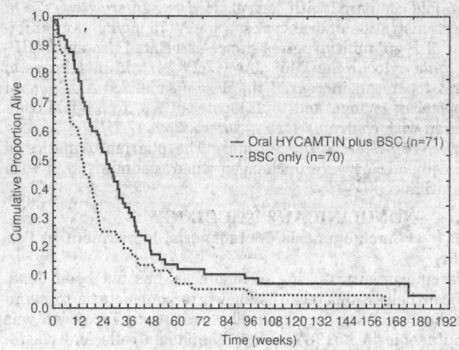

— Oral HYCAMTIN plus BSC (n=71)
··· BSC only (n=70)

BSC = Best Supportive Care

15 REFERENCES

• "OSHA Hazardous Drugs." OSHA. http://www.osha.gov/SLTC/hazardousdrugs/index.html.

16 HOW SUPPLIED/STORAGE AND HANDLING

The 0.25-mg HYCAMTIN capsules are opaque white to yellowish-white imprinted with HYCAMTIN and 0.25 mg and are available in bottles of 10: NDC 0007-4205-11.
The 1-mg HYCAMTIN capsules are opaque pink imprinted with HYCAMTIN and 1 mg and are available in bottles of 10: NDC 0007-4207-11.
Store refrigerated 2°C to 8°C (36°F to 46°F). Store the bottles protected from light in the original outer cartons. HYCAMTIN is a cytotoxic drug. Follow applicable special handling and disposable procedures.[1]

17 PATIENT COUNSELING INFORMATION

Advise the patient to read the FDA-approved patient labeling (Patient Information)
• **Bone Marrow Suppression**
Inform patients that HYCAMTIN decreases blood cell counts such as white blood cells, platelets, and red blood cells. Instruct patients to notify their healthcare provider promptly for fever or other signs of infection such as chills, cough, or burning pain on urination. Advise patients that frequent blood tests will be performed while taking HYCAMTIN to monitor for bone marrow suppression *[see Warnings and Precautions (5.1)].*

• **Embryofetal Toxicity**
Advise patients on pregnancy planning and prevention. Advise females of reproductive potential to use highly effective contraception during treatment and for 1 month following treatment with HYCAMTIN *[see Warnings and Precautions (5.6), Use in Specific Populations (8.1, 8.7)].*
Advise males with a female sexual partner of reproductive potential to use effective contraception during and for 3 months after treatment *[see Nonclinical Toxicology (13.1)].*
• **Nursing Mothers**
Advise patients to discontinue nursing during treatment with HYCAMTIN *[see Use in Specific Populations 8.1, 8.7)].*
• **Infertility**
Advise male and female patients of the potential risk for impaired fertility and possible family planning options.
• **Diarrhea**
Inform patients that HYCAMTIN capsules cause diarrhea which may be severe and life-threatening. Instruct patients how to manage and/or prevent diarrhea and to inform their physician if severe diarrhea occurs during treatment with HYCAMTIN capsules *[see Warnings and Precautions (5.2)].*
HYCAMTIN is a registered trademark of the GSK group of companies.
GlaxoSmithKline
Research Triangle Park, NC 27709
©2014, the GSK group of companies. All rights reserved.
HYC:6PI
PATIENT INFORMATION
HYCAMTIN® (hi-CAM-tin)
(topotecan) capsules
What is the most important information I should know about HYCAMTIN capsules?
HYCAMTIN capsules can cause serious side effects, including:
Decreased blood counts. HYCAMTIN capsules affects your bone marrow and can cause a severe decrease in your blood cell counts (bone marrow suppression) including neutrophils (a type of white blood cell important in fighting bacterial infections), red blood cells (blood cells that carry oxygen to the tissues), and platelets (important for clotting and control of bleeding).
• You should have blood tests regularly to check your blood counts. A decrease in neutrophils (neutropenia) may affect how your body fights infection.
• Your healthcare provider will tell you if your blood counts are too low before you begin treatment with HYCAMTIN.
• Your dose of HYCAMTIN may need to be changed or stopped until your blood counts recover enough after each cycle of treatment.
• Call your healthcare provider right away if you get any of the following signs of infection:
  ∘ fever (temperature of 100.5°F or greater)
  ∘ chills
  ∘ cough
  ∘ burning or pain on urination
• Tell your healthcare provider about any abnormal bleeding or bruising.
Diarrhea. HYCAMTIN capsules can cause severe and life-threatening diarrhea that may need to be treated in hospital. Tell your healthcare provider right away if you have:
• diarrhea with fever
• diarrhea 3 or more times a day
• diarrhea with stomach-area pain or cramps
See "What are the possible side effects of HYCAMTIN capsules?" for more information about side effects.
What are HYCAMTIN capsules?
HYCAMTIN capsules is a prescription medicine used to treat small cell lung cancer that has come back (relapsed). HYCAMTIN capsules may be right for you if:
• your cancer responded to your first chemotherapy, and
• it has been at least 45 days after you finished your last dose of chemotherapy
It is not known if HYCAMTIN is safe and effective in children.
Who should not take HYCAMTIN capsules?
Do not take HYCAMTIN if:
• you are allergic to topotecan. See the end of this leaflet for a complete list of ingredients in HYCAMTIN capsules.
What should I tell my healthcare provider before taking HYCAMTIN capsules?
Before you take HYCAMTIN capsules, tell your healthcare provider if you:
• have kidney problems
• are pregnant or plan to become pregnant. HYCAMTIN capsules can harm your unborn baby. You should not become pregnant while you are taking HYCAMTIN capsules.
  ∘ Females who can become pregnant should use effective birth control (contraception) during treatment with HYCAMTIN and for 1 month after treatment.
  ∘ If you are a male and your female sexual partner is able to become pregnant, you should use effective birth control during treatment with HYCAMTIN and for 3 months after treatment.

  ∘ Talk to your healthcare provider about birth control options to prevent pregnancy while you are taking HYCAMTIN.
  ∘ Tell your healthcare provider right away if you or your female partner becomes pregnant while taking HYCAMTIN.
• are breastfeeding or plan to breastfeed. It is not known if HYCAMTIN passes into your breast milk. You and your healthcare provider should decide if you will take HYCAMTIN or breastfeed. You should not do both.
Tell your healthcare provider about all the medicines you take, including prescription and over-the-counter medicines, vitamins, and herbal supplements. Know the medicines you take. Keep a list of them to show your healthcare provider and pharmacist when you get a new medicine.
How should I take HYCAMTIN capsules?
• Take HYCAMTIN capsules exactly as your healthcare provider tells you to take it.
• Your healthcare provider will tell you how many HYCAMTIN capsules to take and when to take them.
• Your healthcare provider may change your dose if needed.
• Your healthcare provider may want you to take both 1-mg and 0.25-mg capsules together to make up your complete dose. You must be able to tell the difference between the capsules. The 1-mg capsule is a pink color and the 0.25-mg capsule is a white to yellowish-white color.
• Take HYCAMTIN one time a day for 5 days in a row. This treatment will normally be repeated every 3 weeks (a treatment cycle). Your healthcare provider will decide how long you will take HYCAMTIN capsules.
• Swallow HYCAMTIN capsules whole. Do not open, chew, or crush HYCAMTIN capsules.
• Take HYCAMTIN with or without food.
• If any of the HYCAMTIN capsules are broken or leaking, do not touch them with your bare hands. Carefully throw away (dispose of) the capsules, and then wash your hands well with soap and water.
• If you get any of the contents of HYCAMTIN capsules on your skin or in your eyes, do the following:
  ∘ Wash the area of skin well with soap and water right away.
  ∘ Wash your eyes right away with gently flowing water for at least 15 minutes.
  ∘ Call your healthcare provider if you get a skin reaction or get HYCAMTIN in your eyes.
• If you take too much HYCAMTIN, call your healthcare provider right away.
• If you vomit after taking your HYCAMTIN, just take the next scheduled dose. Do not take another dose on the same day.
What are the possible side effects of HYCAMTIN capsules?
HYCAMTIN can cause serious side effects including:
• See "What is the most important information I should know about HYCAMTIN capsules?"
• **Lung problems that can cause death.** Tell your healthcare provider right away if you have **new or worse** symptoms of coughing, fever, shortness of breath, or problems breathing. Your healthcare provider may tell you to stop taking HYCAMTIN capsules.
The most common side effects of HYCAMTIN include:
• nausea
• diarrhea
• vomiting
• hair loss
• tiredness
HYCAMTIN may cause short-term and long-term fertility problems in females. This could affect your ability to become pregnant.
HYCAMTIN may cause lower sperm count problems in men. This could affect your ability to father a child and cause birth defects. Talk to your healthcare provider about family planning options that might be right for you.
Tell your healthcare provider if you have any side effect that bothers you or does not go away.
These are not all of the possible side effects of HYCAMTIN capsules. For more information, ask your healthcare provider or pharmacist.
Call your doctor for medical advice about side effects. You may report side effects to FDA at 1-800-FDA-1088.
How should I store HYCAMTIN capsules?
• Store HYCAMTIN capsules in a refrigerator between 36°F to 46°F (2°C to 8°C).
• Keep the bottle of HYCAMTIN capsules in the carton that it comes in to protect it from light.
• Ask your healthcare provider or pharmacist how to safely throw away any unused or expired HYCAMTIN.
Keep HYCAMTIN capsules and all medicines out of the reach of children.
General information about HYCAMTIN capsules
Medicines are sometimes prescribed for purposes other than those listed in a Patient Information leaflet. Do not use HYCAMTIN for a condition for which it was not prescribed. Do not give HYCAMTIN to other people, even if they have the same symptoms that you have. It may harm them.

You can ask your pharmacist or healthcare provider for information about HYCAMTIN that is written for health professionals.

For more information go to www.gsk.com or call 1-888-825-5249.

What are the ingredients in HYCAMTIN capsules?
Active ingredient: topotecan hydrochloride
Inactive ingredients: gelatin, glyceryl monostearate, hydrogenated vegetable oil, and titanium oxide. The 1-mg capsules also contain red iron oxide. The capsules are imprinted with edible black ink.

This Patient Information has been approved by the U.S. Food and Drug Administration.

HYCAMTIN is a registered trademark of the GSK group of companies.

GlaxoSmithKline
Research Triangle Park, NC 27709
©2014, the GSK group of companies. All rights reserved.
Revised June 2014
HYC:6PIL

HYCAMTIN ℞
[hī-kam′tin]
(topotecan hydrochloride)
for Injection

HIGHLIGHTS OF PRESCRIBING INFORMATION
These highlights do not include all the information needed to use HYCAMTIN safely and effectively. See full prescribing information for HYCAMTIN.
HYCAMTIN (topotecan hydrochloride) for Injection
Initial U.S. Approval: 1996

WARNING: BONE MARROW SUPPRESSION
See full prescribing information for complete boxed warning
Do not give HYCAMTIN to patients with baseline neutrophil counts less than 1,500 cells/mm³. In order to monitor the occurrence of bone marrow suppression, primarily neutropenia, which may be severe and result in infection and death, monitor peripheral blood cell counts frequently on all patients receiving HYCAMTIN (5.1).

-----RECENT MAJOR CHANGES-----
Dosage and Administration (2). 02/2014

-----INDICATIONS AND USAGE-----
HYCAMTIN for Injection is a topoisomerase inhibitor indicated for:
• metastatic carcinoma of the ovary after failure of initial or subsequent chemotherapy. (1)
• small cell lung cancer sensitive disease after failure of first-line chemotherapy. (1)
• combination therapy with cisplatin for Stage IV-B, recurrent, or persistent carcinoma of the cervix which is not amenable to curative treatment with surgery and/or radiation therapy. (1)

-----DOSAGE AND ADMINISTRATION-----
• Ovarian cancer and small cell lung cancer: 1.5 mg/m² by intravenous infusion over 30 minutes daily for 5 consecutive days, starting on day one of a 21-day course. (2.1)
• Cervical cancer: 0.75 mg/m² by intravenous infusion over 30 minutes on days 1, 2, and 3 followed by cisplatin 50 mg/m² by intravenous infusion on day 1 repeated every 21 days. (2.2)
See Dosage Modification Guidelines for patients with neutropenia or reduced platelets. (2.1, 2.2)
See Dosage Adjustment in Renal Impairment. (2.3)

-----DOSAGE FORMS AND STRENGTHS-----
4-mg (free base) single-dose vial. (3)

-----CONTRAINDICATIONS-----
• History of severe hypersensitivity reactions (e.g., anaphylactoid reactions) to topotecan or any of its ingredients (4)
• Severe bone marrow depression (4)

-----WARNINGS AND PRECAUTIONS-----
• Bone marrow suppression: Administer HYCAMTIN only to patients with adequate bone marrow reserves. Monitor peripheral blood counts and adjust the dose if needed. (5.1)
• Topotecan-induced neutropenia can lead to neutropenic colitis. (5.2)
• Interstitial lung disease: HYCAMTIN has been associated with reports of interstitial lung disease. Monitor patients for symptoms and discontinue HYCAMTIN if the diagnosis is confirmed. (5.3)
• Pregnancy: Can cause fetal harm. Advise women of potential risk to the fetus. (5.4, 8.1)

-----ADVERSE REACTIONS-----
Ovarian and small cell lung cancer:
• The most common hematologic adverse reactions were: neutropenia (97%), leukopenia (97%), anemia (89%), and thrombocytopenia (69%). (6.1)
• The most common (>25%) non-hematologic adverse reactions (all grades) were: nausea, alopecia, vomiting, sepsis or pyrexia/infection with neutropenia, diarrhea, constipation, fatigue, and pyrexia. (6.1)
Cervical cancer (HYCAMTIN plus cisplatin):
• The most common hematologic adverse reactions (all grades) were: anemia (94%), leukopenia (91%), neutropenia (89%), and thrombocytopenia (74%). (6.1)
• The most common (>25%) non-hematologic adverse reactions (all grades) were: pain, nausea, vomiting, and infection/febrile neutropenia. (6.1)
To report SUSPECTED ADVERSE REACTIONS, contact GlaxoSmithKline at 1-888-825-5249 or FDA at 1-800-FDA-1088 or www.fda.gov/medwatch.

-----DRUG INTERACTIONS-----
• Do not initiate G-CSF until 24 hours after completion of treatment with HYCAMTIN. Concomitant administration can prolong duration of neutropenia. (7)
• Greater myelosuppression is likely to be seen when used in combination with other cytotoxic agents. (7)

-----USE IN SPECIFIC POPULATIONS-----
• Nursing Mothers: Discontinue nursing when receiving HYCAMTIN. (8.3)
See 17 for PATIENT COUNSELING INFORMATION
Revised: 03/2014

FULL PRESCRIBING INFORMATION: CONTENTS*
WARNING: BONE MARROW SUPPRESSION
* Sections or subsections omitted from the full prescribing information are not listed

FULL PRESCRIBING INFORMATION

WARNING: BONE MARROW SUPPRESSION
Do not give HYCAMTIN® to patients with baseline neutrophil counts less than 1,500 cells/mm³. In order to monitor the occurrence of bone marrow suppression, primarily neutropenia, which may be severe and result in infection and death, monitor peripheral blood counts frequently on all patients receiving HYCAMTIN *[see Warnings and Precautions (5.1)].*

---

1   INDICATIONS AND USAGE
HYCAMTIN is indicated for the treatment of:
• metastatic carcinoma of the ovary after failure of initial or subsequent chemotherapy.
• small cell lung cancer sensitive disease after failure of first-line chemotherapy. In clinical studies submitted to support approval, sensitive disease was defined as disease responding to chemotherapy but subsequently progressing at least 60 days (in the Phase 3 study) or at least 90 days (in the Phase 2 studies) after chemotherapy *[see Clinical Studies (14)].*
HYCAMTIN in combination with cisplatin is indicated for the treatment of:
• Stage IV-B, recurrent, or persistent carcinoma of the cervix which is not amenable to curative treatment with surgery and/or radiation therapy.

2   DOSAGE AND ADMINISTRATION
Verify dose using body surface area prior to dispensing. Recommended dosage should generally not exceed 4 mg intravenously [see Overdosage (10)].
Prior to administration of the first course of HYCAMTIN, patients must have a baseline neutrophil count of >1,500 cells/mm³ and a platelet count of >100,000 cells/mm³.
2.1   Ovarian Cancer and Small Cell Lung Cancer
Recommended Dosage:
• The recommended dose of HYCAMTIN is 1.5 mg/m² by intravenous infusion over 30 minutes daily for 5 consecutive days, starting on day 1 of a 21-day course.
• In the absence of tumor progression, a minimum of 4 courses is recommended because tumor response may be delayed. The median time to response in 3 ovarian clinical trials was 9 to 12 weeks, and median time to response in 4 small cell lung cancer trials was 5 to 7 weeks.
Dosage Modification Guidelines:
• In the event of severe neutropenia (defined as <500 cells/mm³) during any course, reduce the dose by 0.25 mg/m² (to 1.25 mg/m²) for subsequent courses.
• Alternatively, in the event of severe neutropenia, administer G-CSF (granulocyte-colony stimulating factor) following the subsequent course (before resorting to dose reduction) starting from day 6 of the course (24 hours after completion of topotecan administration).
• In the event the platelet count falls below 25,000 cells/mm³, reduce doses by 0.25 mg/m² (to 1.25 mg/m²) for subsequent courses.
2.2   Cervical Cancer
Recommended Dosage:
The recommended dose of HYCAMTIN is 0.75 mg/m² by intravenous infusion over 30 minutes daily on days 1, 2, and 3; followed by cisplatin 50 mg/m² by intravenous infusion on day 1 repeated every 21 days (a 21-day course).
Dosage Modification Guidelines:
Dosage adjustments for subsequent courses of HYCAMTIN in combination with cisplatin are specific for each drug. See manufacturer's prescribing information for cisplatin administration and hydration guidelines and for cisplatin dosage adjustment in the event of hematologic toxicity.
• In the event of severe febrile neutropenia (defined as <1,000 cells/mm³ with temperature of 38.0°C or 100.4°F), reduce the dose of HYCAMTIN to 0.60 mg/m² for subsequent courses.
• Alternatively, in the event of severe febrile neutropenia, administer G-CSF following the subsequent course (before resorting to dose reduction) starting from day 4 of the course (24 hours after completion of administration of HYCAMTIN).
• If febrile neutropenia occurs despite the use of G-CSF, reduce the dose of HYCAMTIN to 0.45 mg/m² for subsequent courses.
• In the event the platelet count falls below 25,000 cells/mm³, reduce doses to 0.60 mg/m² for subsequent courses.
2.3   Dosage Adjustment in Specific Populations
Renal Impairment:
No dosage adjustment of HYCAMTIN appears to be required for patients with mild renal impairment (Clcr 40 to 60 mL/min). Dosage adjustment of HYCAMTIN to 0.75 mg/m² is recommended for patients with moderate renal impairment (20 to 39 mL/min). Insufficient data are available in patients with severe renal impairment to provide a dosage recommendation for HYCAMTIN *[see Use in Specific Populations (8.6) and Clinical Pharmacology (12.3)].*
HYCAMTIN in combination with cisplatin for the treatment of cervical cancer should only be initiated in patients with serum creatinine ≤1.5 mg/dL. In the clinical trial, cisplatin was discontinued for a serum creatinine >1.5 mg/dL. Insufficient data are available regarding continuing monotherapy with HYCAMTIN after cisplatin discontinuation in patients with cervical cancer.
2.4   Instructions for Handling, Preparation, and Intravenous Administration
Handling:
HYCAMTIN is a cytotoxic anticancer drug. Prepare HYCAMTIN under a vertical laminar flow hood while wear-

ing gloves and protective clothing. If HYCAMTIN solution contacts the skin, wash the skin immediately and thoroughly with soap and water. If HYCAMTIN contacts mucous membranes, flush thoroughly with water.

Use procedures for proper handling and disposal of anticancer drugs. Several guidelines on this subject have been published.[1-4]

Preparation and Administration:
Each 4-mg vial of HYCAMTIN is reconstituted with 4 mL Sterile Water for Injection. Then the appropriate volume of the reconstituted solution is diluted in either 0.9% Sodium Chloride Intravenous Infusion or 5% Dextrose Intravenous Infusion prior to administration.

Stability:
Unopened vials of HYCAMTIN are stable until the date indicated on the package when stored between 20° and 25°C (68° and 77°F) [see USP] and protected from light in the original package. Because the vials contain no preservative, contents should be used immediately after reconstitution. Reconstituted vials of HYCAMTIN diluted for infusion are stable at approximately 20° to 25°C (68° to 77°F) and ambient lighting conditions for 24 hours.

3 DOSAGE FORMS AND STRENGTHS

4-mg (free base) single-dose vial; light yellow to greenish powder.

4 CONTRAINDICATIONS

HYCAMTIN is contraindicated in patients who have a history of severe hypersensitivity reactions (e.g., anaphylactoid reactions) to topotecan or to any of its ingredients. HYCAMTIN should not be used in patients with severe bone marrow depression.

5 WARNINGS AND PRECAUTIONS

5.1 Bone Marrow Suppression

Bone marrow suppression (primarily neutropenia) is the dose-limiting toxicity of HYCAMTIN. Neutropenia is not cumulative over time. In ovarian cancer, the overall treatment-related death rate was 1%. In the comparative trial in small cell lung cancer, however, the treatment-related death rates were 5% for HYCAMTIN and 4% for CAV (cyclophosphamide-doxorubicin-vincristine).

Neutropenia:
- Ovarian and small cell lung cancer experience: Grade 4 neutropenia (<500 cells/mm^3) was most common during course 1 of treatment (60% of patients) and occurred in 39% of all courses, with a median duration of 7 days. The nadir neutrophil count occurred at a median of 12 days. Therapy-related sepsis or febrile neutropenia occurred in 23% of patients, and sepsis was fatal in 1%. Pancytopenia has been reported.
- Cervical cancer experience: Grade 3 and Grade 4 neutropenia affected 26% and 48% of patients, respectively.

Thrombocytopenia:
- Ovarian and small cell lung cancer experience: Grade 4 thrombocytopenia (<25,000/mm^3) occurred in 27% of patients and in 9% of courses, with a median duration of 5 days and platelet nadir at a median of 15 days. Platelet transfusions were given to 15% of patients in 4% of courses.
- Cervical cancer experience: Grade 3 and Grade 4 thrombocytopenia affected 26% and 7% of patients, respectively.

Anemia:
- Ovarian and small cell lung cancer experience: Grade 3/4 anemia (<8 g/dL) occurred in 37% of patients and in 14% of courses. Median nadir was at day 15. Transfusions were needed in 52% of patients in 22% of courses.
- Cervical cancer experience: Grade 3 and Grade 4 anemia affected 34% and 6% of patients, respectively.

Monitoring of Bone Marrow Function:
Administer HYCAMTIN only in patients with adequate bone marrow reserves, including baseline neutrophil count of at least 1,500 cells/mm^3 and platelet count at least 100,000/mm^3. Monitor peripheral blood counts frequently during treatment with HYCAMTIN. Do not treat patients with subsequent courses of HYCAMTIN until neutrophils recover to >1,000 cells/mm^3, platelets recover to >100,000 cells/mm^3, and hemoglobin levels recover to 9.0 g/dL (with transfusion if necessary). Severe myelotoxicity has been reported when HYCAMTIN is used in combination with cisplatin [see Drug Interactions (7)].

5.2 Neutropenic Colitis

Topotecan-induced neutropenia can lead to neutropenic colitis. Fatalities due to neutropenic colitis have been reported in clinical trials with HYCAMTIN. In patients presenting with fever, neutropenia, and a compatible pattern of abdominal pain, consider the possibility of neutropenic colitis.

5.3 Interstitial Lung Disease

HYCAMTIN has been associated with reports of interstitial lung disease (ILD), some of which have been fatal [see Adverse Reactions (6.2)]. Underlying risk factors include history of ILD, pulmonary fibrosis, lung cancer, thoracic exposure to radiation, and use of pneumotoxic drugs and/or colony stimulating factors. Monitor patients for pulmo-

nary symptoms indicative of interstitial lung disease (e.g., cough, fever, dyspnea, and/or hypoxia), and discontinue HYCAMTIN if a new diagnosis of ILD is confirmed.

5.4 Pregnancy

Pregnancy Category D.
HYCAMTIN can cause fetal harm when administered to a pregnant woman.

Topotecan caused embryolethality, fetotoxicity, and teratogenicity in rats and rabbits when administered during organogenesis. There are no adequate and well-controlled studies of HYCAMTIN in pregnant women. If this drug is used during pregnancy, or if a patient becomes pregnant while receiving HYCAMTIN, the patient should be apprised of the potential hazard to the fetus [see Use in Specific Populations (8.1)].

5.5 Inadvertent Extravasation

Inadvertent extravasation with HYCAMTIN has been observed; most reactions have been mild, but severe cases have been reported.

6 ADVERSE REACTIONS

6.1 Clinical Trials Experience

Because clinical trials are conducted under widely varying conditions, adverse reaction rates observed in the clinical trials of a drug cannot be directly compared with rates in the clinical trials of another drug and may not reflect the rates observed in practice.

Ovarian Cancer and Small Cell Lung Cancer:
Data in the following section are based on the combined experience of 453 patients with metastatic ovarian carcinoma, and 426 patients with small cell lung cancer treated with HYCAMTIN. Table 1 lists the principal hematologic adverse reactions and Table 2 lists non-hematologic adverse reactions occurring in at least 15% of patients.

Table 1. Hematologic Adverse Reactions Experienced in ≥15% Ovarian Cancer and Small Cell Lung Cancer Patients Receiving HYCAMTIN

Hematologic Adverse Reaction	Patients (n = 879) % Incidence
Neutropenia <1,500 cells/mm^3 <500 cells/mm^3	97 78
Leukopenia <3,000 cells/mm^3 <1,000 cells/mm^3	97 32
Thrombocytopenia <75,000/mm^3 <25,000/mm^3	69 27
Anemia <10 g/dL <8 g/dL	89 37

Table 2. Non-hematologic Adverse Reactions Experienced by ≥15% of Ovarian Cancer and Small Cell Lung Cancer Patients Receiving HYCAMTIN

Non-hematologic Adverse Reaction	Percentage of Patients With Adverse Reaction (879 Patients)		
	All Grades	Grade 3	Grade 4
Infections and infestations Sepsis or pyrexia/ infection with neutropenia [a]	43	NR	23
Metabolism and nutrition disorders Anorexia	19	2	<1
Nervous system disorders Headache	18	1	<1
Respiratory, thoracic, and mediastinal disorders Dyspnea Coughing	22 15	5 1	3 0
Gastrointestinal disorders Nausea Vomiting Diarrhea	64 45 32	7 4 3	1 1 1
Constipation	29	2	1
Abdominal pain	22	2	2
Stomatitis	18	1	<1
Skin and subcutaneous tissue disorders Alopecia Rash[b]	49 16	NA 1	NA 0
General disorders and administrative site conditions Fatigue Pyrexia Pain[c] Asthenia	29 28 23 25	5 1 2 4	0 <1 1 2

NA = Not applicable.

NR = Not reported separately.

[a] Does not include Grade 1 sepsis or pyrexia.

[b] Rash also includes pruritus, rash erythematous, urticaria, dermatitis, bullous eruption, and maculopapular rash.

[c] Pain includes body pain, back pain, and skeletal pain.

Nervous System Disorders:
Paresthesia occurred in 7% of patients but was generally Grade 1.

Hepatobiliary Disorders:
Grade 1 transient elevations in hepatic enzymes occurred in 8% of patients. Greater elevations, Grade 3/4, occurred in 4%. Grade 3/4 elevated bilirubin occurred in <2% of patients.

Table 3 shows the Grade 3/4 hematologic and major non-hematologic adverse reactions in the topotecan/paclitaxel comparator trial in ovarian cancer.

Table 3. Adverse Reactions Experienced by ≥5% of Ovarian Cancer Patients Randomized to Receive HYCAMTIN or Paclitaxel

Adverse Reaction	HYCAMTIN (n = 112)	Paclitaxel (n = 114)
Hematologic Grade 3/4	%	%
Grade 4 neutropenia (<500 cells/mm^3)	80	21
Grade 3/4 anemia (Hgb <8 g/dL)	41	6
Grade 4 thrombocytopenia (<25,000 plts/mm^3)	27	3
Pyrexia/Grade 4 neutropenia	23	4
Non-hematologic Grade 3/4	%	%
Infections and infestations Documented sepsis[a]	5	2
Respiratory, thoracic, and mediastinal disorders Dyspnea	6	5
Gastrointestinal disorders Abdominal pain Constipation Diarrhea Intestinal obstruction Nausea Vomiting	5 5 6 5 10 10	4 0 1 4 2 3
General disorders and administrative site conditions Fatigue Asthenia Pain[b]	7 5 5	6 3 7

[a] Death related to sepsis occurred in 2% of patients receiving HYCAMTIN and 0% of patients receiving paclitaxel.
[b] Pain includes body pain, skeletal pain, and back pain.

Table 4 shows the Grade 3/4 hematologic and major non-hematologic adverse reactions in the topotecan/CAV (cyclophosphamide–doxorubicin–vincristine) comparator trial in small cell lung cancer.

Table 4. Adverse Reactions Experienced by ≥5% of Small Cell Lung Cancer Patients Randomized to Receive HYCAMTIN or CAV

Adverse Reaction	HYCAMTIN (n = 107)	CAV (n = 104)
Hematologic Grade 3/4	%	%
Grade 4 neutropenia (<500 cells/mm³)	70	72
Grade 3/4 anemia (Hgb <8 g/dL)	42	20
Grade 4 thrombocytopenia (<25,000 plts/mm³)	29	5
Pyrexia/Grade 4 neutropenia	28	26
Non-hematologic Grade 3/4	%	%
Infections and infestations Documented sepsis[a]	5	5
Respiratory, thoracic, and mediastinal disorders Dyspnea	9	14
Pneumonia	8	6
Gastrointestinal disorders Abdominal pain	6	4
Nausea	8	6
General disorders and administrative site conditions Fatigue	6	10
Asthenia	9	7
Pain[b]	5	7

[a] Death related to sepsis occurred in 3% of patients receiving HYCAMTIN, and 1% of patients receiving CAV.
[b] Pain includes body pain, skeletal pain, and back pain.

Cervical Cancer:
In the comparative trial with HYCAMTIN plus cisplatin versus cisplatin in patients with cervical cancer, the most common dose-limiting adverse reaction was myelosuppression. Table 5 shows the hematologic adverse reactions and Table 6 shows the non-hematologic adverse reactions in patients with cervical cancer.

Table 5. Hematologic Adverse Reactions in Patients with Cervical Cancer Treated with HYCAMTIN Plus Cisplatin or Cisplatin Monotherapy[a]

Hematologic Adverse Reaction	HYCAMTIN Plus Cisplatin (n = 140)	Cisplatin (n = 144)
Anemia		
All Grades (Hgb <12 g/dL)	131 (94%)	130 (90%)
Grade 3 (Hgb <8-6.5 g/dL)	47 (34%)	28 (19%)
Grade 4 (Hgb <6.5 g/dL)	9 (6%)	5 (3%)
Leukopenia		
All Grades (<3,800 cells/mm3)	128 (91%)	43 (30%)
Grade 3 (<2,000-1,000 cells/mm3)	58 (41%)	1 (1%)
Grade 4 (<1,000 cells/mm3)	35 (25%)	0 (0%)
Neutropenia		
All Grades (<2,000 cells/mm3)	125 (89%)	28 (19%)
Grade 3 (<1,000-500 cells/mm3)	36 (26%)	1 (1%)
Grade 4 (<500 cells/mm3)	67 (48%)	1 (1%)
Thrombocytopenia		
All Grades (<130,000 cells/mm3)	104 (74%)	21 (15%)
Grade 3 (<50,000-10,000 cells/mm3)	36 (26%)	5 (3%)
Grade 4 (<10,000 cells/mm3)	10 (7%)	0 (0%)

[a] Includes patients who were eligible and treated.

[See table 6 above]

6.2 Postmarketing Experience
In addition to adverse reactions reported from clinical trials or listed in other sections of the prescribing information, the following reactions have been identified during postmarketing use of HYCAMTIN. Because they are reported voluntarily from a population of unknown size, estimates of frequency cannot be made. These reactions have been chosen for inclusion due to a combination of their seriousness, frequency of reporting, or potential causal connection to HYCAMTIN.
Blood and Lymphatic System Disorders:
Severe bleeding (in association with thrombocytopenia) [see Warnings and Precautions (5.1)].
Immune System Disorders:
Allergic manifestations, anaphylactoid reactions.
Gastrointestinal Disorders:
Abdominal pain potentially associated with neutropenic colitis [see Warnings and Precautions (5.2)].
Pulmonary Disorders:
Interstitial lung disease [see Warnings and Precautions (5.3)].
Skin and Subcutaneous Tissue Disorders:
Angioedema, severe dermatitis, severe pruritus.
General Disorders and Administration Site Conditions:
Inadvertent extravasation [see Warnings and Precautions (5.5)].

7 DRUG INTERACTIONS

G-CSF: Concomitant administration of G–CSF can prolong the duration of neutropenia, so if G–CSF is to be used, do not initiate it until day 6 of the course of therapy, 24 hours after completion of treatment with HYCAMTIN.
Platinum and Other Cytotoxic Agents: Myelosuppression was more severe when HYCAMTIN, at a dose of 1.25 mg/m²/day for 5 days, was given in combination with cisplatin at a dose of 50 mg/m² in Phase 1 trials. In one trial, 1 of 3 patients had severe neutropenia for 12 days and a second patient died with neutropenic sepsis.
Greater myelosuppression is also likely to be seen when HYCAMTIN is used in combination with other cytotoxic agents, thereby necessitating a dose reduction. However, when combining HYCAMTIN with platinum agents (e.g., cisplatin or carboplatin), a distinct sequence-dependent interaction on myelosuppression has been reported. Coadministration of a platinum agent on day 1 of dosing with HYCAMTIN required lower doses of each agent compared to coadministration on day 5 of the dosing schedule for HYCAMTIN.
For information on the pharmacokinetics, efficacy, safety, and dosing of HYCAMTIN at a dose of 0.75 mg/m²/day on days 1, 2, and 3 in combination with cisplatin 50 mg/m² on day 1 for cervical cancer, see Dosage and Administration (2), Adverse Reactions (6), Clinical Pharmacology (12.3), and Clinical Studies (14).

8 USE IN SPECIFIC POPULATIONS
8.1 Pregnancy
Pregnancy Category D [see Warnings and Precautions (5.4)]. HYCAMTIN can cause fetal harm when administered to a pregnant woman. In rabbits, a dose of 0.10 mg/kg/day (about equal to the clinical dose on a mg/m² basis) given on days 6 through 20 of gestation caused maternal toxicity, embryolethality, and reduced fetal body weight. In the rat, a dose of 0.23 mg/kg/day (about equal to the clinical dose on a

Table 6. Non-hematologic Adverse Reactions Experienced by ≥5% of Patients with Cervical Cancer Treated with HYCAMTIN Plus Cisplatin or Cisplatin Monotherapy[a]

Adverse Reaction	HYCAMTIN Plus Cisplatin (n = 140)			Cisplatin (n = 144)		
	All Grades[b]	Grade 3	Grade 4	All Grades[b]	Grade 3	Grade 4
General disorders and administrative site conditions						
Constitutional[c]	96 (69%)	11 (8%)	0	89 (62%)	17 (12%)	0
Pain[d]	82 (59%)	28 (20%)	3 (2%)	72 (50%)	18 (13%)	5 (3%)
Gastrointestinal disorders						
Vomiting	56 (40%)	20 (14%)	2 (1%)	53 (37%)	13 (9%)	0
Nausea	77 (55%)	18 (13%)	2 (1%)	79 (55%)	13 (9%)	0
Stomatitis-pharyngitis	8 (6%)	1 (<1%)	0	0	0	0
Other	88 (63%)	16 (11%)	4 (3%)	80 (56%)	12 (8%)	3 (2%)
Dermatology	67 (48%)	1 (<1%)	0	29 (20%)	0	0
Metabolic-Laboratory	55 (39%)	13 (9%)	7 (5%)	44 (31%)	14 (10%)	1 (<1%)
Genitourinary	51 (36%)	9 (6%)	9 (6%)	49 (34%)	7 (5%)	7 (5%)
Nervous system disorders						
Neuropathy	4 (3%)	1 (<1%)	0	3 (2%)	1 (<1%)	0
Other	49 (35%)	3 (2%)	1 (<1%)	43 (30%)	7 (5%)	2 (1%)
Infection-febrile neutropenia	39 (28%)	21 (15%)	5 (4%)	26 (18%)	11 (8%)	0
Cardiovascular	35 (25%)	7 (5%)	6 (4%)	22 (15%)	8 (6%)	3 (2%)
Hepatic	34 (24%)	5 (4%)	2 (1%)	23 (16%)	2 (1%)	0
Pulmonary	24 (17%)	4 (3%)	0	23 (16%)	5 (3%)	3 (2%)
Vascular disorders						
Hemorrhage	21 (15%)	8 (6%)	1 (<1%)	20 (14%)	3 (2%)	1 (<1%)
Coagulation	8 (6%)	4 (3%)	3 (2%)	10 (7%)	7 (5%)	0
Musculoskeletal	19 (14%)	3 (2%)	0	7 (5%)	1 (<1%)	1 (<1%)
Allergy-Immunology	8 (6%)	2 (1%)	1 (<1%)	4 (3%)	0	1 (<1%)
Endocrine	8 (6%)	0	0	4 (3%)	2 (1%)	0
Sexual reproduction function	7 (5%)	0	0	10 (7%)	1 (<1%)	0
Ocular-visual	7 (5%)	0	0	7 (5%)	1 (<1%)	0

Data were collected using NCI Common Toxicity Criteria, v. 2.0.
[a] Includes patients who were eligible and treated.
[b] Grades 1 through 4 only. There were 3 patients who experienced Grade 5 deaths with investigator-designated attribution. One was a Grade 5 hemorrhage in which the drug-related thrombocytopenia aggravated the event. A second patient experienced bowel obstruction, cardiac arrest, pleural effusion and respiratory failure which were not treatment related but probably aggravated by treatment. A third patient experienced a pulmonary embolism and adult respiratory distress syndrome; the latter was indirectly treatment-related.
[c] Constitutional includes fatigue (lethargy, malaise, asthenia), fever (in the absence of neutropenia), rigors, chills, sweating, and weight gain or loss.
[d] Pain includes abdominal pain or cramping, arthralgia, bone pain, chest pain (non-cardiac and non-pleuritic), dysmenorrhea, dyspareunia, earache, headache, hepatic pain, myalgia, neuropathic pain, pain due to radiation, pelvic pain, pleuritic pain, rectal or perirectal pain, and tumor pain.

mg/m^2 basis) given for 14 days before mating through gestation day 6 caused fetal resorption, microphthalmia, pre-implant loss, and mild maternal toxicity. A dose of 0.10 mg/kg/day (about half the clinical dose on a mg/m^2 basis) given to rats on days 6 through 17 of gestation caused an increase in post-implantation mortality. This dose also caused an increase in total fetal malformations. The most frequent malformations were of the eye (microphthalmia, anophthalmia, rosette formation of the retina, coloboma of the retina, ectopic orbit), brain (dilated lateral and third ventricles), skull, and vertebrae.

There are no adequate and well-controlled studies of HYCAMTIN in pregnant women. If this drug is used during pregnancy, or if a patient becomes pregnant while receiving HYCAMTIN, the patient should be apprised of the potential hazard to the fetus [see Warnings and Precautions (5.4)].

8.3 Nursing Mothers
Rats excrete high concentrations of topotecan into milk. Lactating female rats given 4.72 mg/m^2 IV (about twice the clinical dose on a mg/m^2 basis) excreted topotecan into milk at concentrations up to 48-fold higher than those in plasma. It is not known whether the drug is excreted in human milk. Because many drugs are excreted in human milk and because of the potential for serious adverse reactions in nursing infants from HYCAMTIN, discontinue breastfeeding when women are receiving HYCAMTIN.

8.4 Pediatric Use
Safety and effectiveness in pediatric patients have not been established.

8.5 Geriatric Use
Of the 879 patients with metastatic ovarian cancer or small cell lung cancer in clinical trials of HYCAMTIN, 32% (n = 281) were 65 years of age and older, while 3.8% (n = 33) were 75 years of age and older. Of the 140 patients with Stage IV-B, relapsed, or refractory cervical cancer in clinical trials of HYCAMTIN who received HYCAMTIN plus cisplatin in the randomized clinical trial, 6% (n = 9) were 65 years of age and older, while 3% (n = 4) were 75 years of age and older. No overall differences in effectiveness or safety were observed between these patients and younger adult patients, and other reported clinical experience has not identified differences in responses between the elderly and younger adult patients, but greater sensitivity of some older individuals cannot be ruled out.

There were no apparent differences in the pharmacokinetics of topotecan in elderly patients, once the age-related decrease in renal function was considered [see Clinical Pharmacology (12.3)].

This drug is known to be substantially excreted by the kidney, and the risk of toxic reactions to this drug may be greater in patients with impaired renal function. Because elderly patients are more likely to have decreased renal function, care should be taken in dose selection, and it may be useful to monitor renal function [see Dosage and Administration (2.3)].

8.6 Renal Impairment
No dosage adjustment of HYCAMTIN appears to be required for patients with mild renal impairment (Clcr 40 to 60 mL/min). Dosage reduction is recommended for patients with moderate renal impairment (Clcr 20 to 39 mL/min). Insufficient data are available in patients with severe renal impairment to provide a dosage recommendation for HYCAMTIN [see Dosage and Administration (2.3) and Clinical Pharmacology (12.3)].

10 OVERDOSAGE
Overdoses (up to 10-fold of the prescribed dose) occurred in patients treated with intravenous topotecan. The primary complication of overdosage is bone marrow suppression. The observed signs and symptoms of overdose are consistent with the known adverse reactions associated with HYCAMTIN for intravenous use [see Adverse Reactions (6.1, 6.2)]. In addition, elevated hepatic enzymes and mucositis have been reported following overdose. One patient received a single dose of 40 mg/m^2 of intravenous topotecan and developed gastrointestinal toxicity, skin toxicity, and myelosuppression leading to septic shock. Another patient received a single dose of 35 mg/m^2 and experienced severe, reversible neutropenia.

There is no known antidote for overdosage with HYCAMTIN. If an overdose is suspected, monitor the patient for bone marrow suppression and institute supportive-care measures (such as prophylactic G-CSF and antibiotic therapy) as appropriate.

11 DESCRIPTION
HYCAMTIN (topotecan hydrochloride) is a semi-synthetic derivative of camptothecin and is an anti-tumor drug with topoisomerase I-inhibitory activity.

HYCAMTIN for Injection is supplied as a sterile, lyophilized, buffered, light yellow to greenish powder available in single-dose vials. Each vial contains topotecan hydrochloride equivalent to 4 mg of topotecan as free base. The reconstituted solution ranges in color from yellow to yellow-green and is intended for administration by intravenous infusion.

Inactive ingredients are mannitol, 48 mg, and tartaric acid, 20 mg. Hydrochloric acid and sodium hydroxide may be used to adjust the pH. The solution pH ranges from 2.5 to 3.5.

The chemical name for topotecan hydrochloride is (S)-10-[(dimethylamino)methyl]-4-ethyl-4,9-dihydroxy-1H-pyrano[3',4':6,7] indolizino [1,2-b]quinoline-3,14-(4H,12H)-dione monohydrochloride. It has the molecular formula $C_{23}H_{23}N_3O_5 \cdot HCl$ and a molecular weight of 457.9.

Topotecan hydrochloride has the following structural formula:

It is soluble in water and melts with decomposition at 213° to 218°C.

12 CLINICAL PHARMACOLOGY
12.1 Mechanism of Action
Topoisomerase I relieves torsional strain in DNA by inducing reversible single-strand breaks. Topotecan binds to the topoisomerase I-DNA complex and prevents religation of these single-strand breaks. The cytotoxicity of topotecan is thought to be due to double-strand DNA damage produced during DNA synthesis, when replication enzymes interact with the ternary complex formed by topotecan, topoisomerase I, and DNA. Mammalian cells cannot efficiently repair these double strand breaks.

12.2 Pharmacodynamics
The dose-limiting toxicity of topotecan is leukopenia. White blood cell count decreases with increasing topotecan dose or topotecan AUC. When topotecan is administered at a dose of 1.5 mg/m^2/day for 5 days, an 80% to 90% decrease in white blood cell count at nadir is typically observed after the first cycle of therapy.

12.3 Pharmacokinetics
The pharmacokinetics of topotecan have been evaluated in cancer patients following doses of 0.5 to 1.5 mg/m^2 administered as a 30-minute infusion. Topotecan exhibits multiexponential pharmacokinetics with a terminal half-life of 2 to 3 hours. Total exposure (AUC) is approximately dose-proportional.

Distribution:
Binding of topotecan to plasma proteins is about 35%.
Metabolism:
Topotecan undergoes a reversible pH-dependent hydrolysis of its lactone moiety; it is the lactone form that is pharmacologically active. At pH ≤4, the lactone is exclusively present, whereas the ring-opened hydroxy-acid form predominates at physiologic pH. In vitro studies in human liver microsomes indicate topotecan is metabolized to an N-demethylated metabolite. The mean metabolite:parent AUC ratio was about 3% for total topotecan and topotecan lactone following IV administration.
Excretion:
Renal clearance is an important determinant of topotecan elimination.
In a mass balance/excretion trial in 4 patients with solid tumors, the overall recovery of total topotecan and its N-desmethyl metabolite in urine and feces over 9 days averaged 73.4% ± 2.3% of the administered IV dose. Mean values of 50.8% ± 2.9% as total topotecan and 3.1% ± 1.0% as N-desmethyl topotecan were excreted in the urine following IV administration. Fecal elimination of total topotecan accounted for 17.9% ± 3.6% while fecal elimination of N-desmethyl topotecan was 1.7% ± 0.6%. An O-glucuronidation metabolite of topotecan and N-desmethyl topotecan has been identified in the urine alone. These metabolites, topotecan-O-glucuronide and N-desmethyl topotecan-O-glucuronide, were less than 2% of the administered dose.
Effect of Gender:
The overall mean topotecan plasma clearance in male patients was approximately 24% higher than that in female patients, largely reflecting difference in body size.
Effect of Age:
Topotecan pharmacokinetics have not been specifically studied in an elderly population, but population pharmacokinetic analysis in female patients did not identify age as a significant factor. Decreased renal clearance, which is common in the elderly, is a more important determinant of topotecan clearance [see Dosage and Administration (2.3) and Use in Specific Populations (8.5)].
Effect of Race:
The effect of race on topotecan pharmacokinetics has not been studied.

Effect of Renal Impairment:
In patients with mild renal impairment (creatinine clearance of 40 to 60 mL/min), topotecan plasma clearance was decreased to about 67% of the value in patients with normal renal function. In patients with moderate renal impairment (Clcr of 20 to 39 mL/min), topotecan plasma clearance was reduced to about 34% of the value in control patients, with an increase in half-life. Mean half-life, estimated in 3 patients with renal impairment, was about 5.0 hours. Dosage adjustment is recommended for these patients [see Dosage and Administration (2.3)].
Effect of Hepatic Impairment:
Plasma clearance in patients with hepatic impairment (serum bilirubin levels between 1.7 and 15.0 mg/dL) was decreased to about 67% of the value in patients without hepatic impairment. Topotecan half-life increased slightly, from 2.0 hours to 2.5 hours, but these patients with hepatic impairment tolerated the usual recommended topotecan dosage regimen.
Drug Interactions:
Pharmacokinetic trials of the interaction of topotecan with concomitantly administered medications have not been formally investigated.
In vitro inhibition studies using marker substrates known to be metabolized by human P450 CYP1A2, CYP2A6, CYP2C8/9, CYP2C19, CYP2D6, CYP2E, CYP3A, or CYP4A or dihydropyrimidine dehydrogenase indicate that the activities of these enzymes were not altered by topotecan. Enzyme inhibition by topotecan has not been evaluated in vivo.
Cisplatin:
Administration of cisplatin (60 or 75 mg/m^2 on day 1) before topotecan (0.75 mg/m^2/day on days 1 to 5) in 9 patients with ovarian cancer had no significant effect on the C_{max} and AUC of total topotecan.
Topotecan had no effect on the pharmacokinetics of free platinum in 15 patients with ovarian cancer who were administered cisplatin 50 mg/m^2 (n = 9) or 75 mg/m^2 (n = 6) on day 2 after paclitaxel 110 mg/m^2 on day 1 before topotecan 0.3 mg/m^2 IV daily on days 2 to 6. Topotecan had no effect on dose-normalized (60 mg/m^2) C_{max} values of free platinum in 13 patients with ovarian cancer who were administered 60 mg/m^2 (n = 10) or 75 mg/m^2 (n = 3) cisplatin on day 1 before topotecan 0.75 mg/m^2 IV daily on days 1 to 5.
No pharmacokinetic data are available following topotecan (0.75 mg/m^2/day for 3 consecutive days) and cisplatin (50 mg/m^2/day on day 1) in patients with cervical cancer. Myelosuppression was more severe when HYCAMTIN was given in combination with cisplatin. [see Drug Interactions (7)].

13 NONCLINICAL TOXICOLOGY
13.1 Carcinogenesis, Mutagenesis, Impairment of Fertility
Carcinogenicity testing of topotecan has not been performed. Topotecan is known to be genotoxic to mammalian cells and is a probable carcinogen. Topotecan was mutagenic to L5178Y mouse lymphoma cells and clastogenic to cultured human lymphocytes with and without metabolic activation. It was also clastogenic to mouse bone marrow. Topotecan did not cause mutations in bacterial cells.
Topotecan given to female rats prior to mating at a dose of 1.4 mg/m^2 IV (about equal to the clinical dose on a mg/m^2 basis) caused superovulation possibly related to inhibition of follicular atresia. This dose given to pregnant female rats also caused increased pre-implantation loss. Studies in dogs given 0.4 mg/m^2 IV (about 1/4th the clinical dose on a mg/m^2 basis) of topotecan daily for a month suggest that treatment may cause an increase in the incidence of multinucleated spermatogonial giant cells in the testes. Topotecan may impair fertility in women and men.

14 CLINICAL STUDIES
14.1 Ovarian Cancer
HYCAMTIN was studied in 2 clinical trials of 223 patients given topotecan with metastatic ovarian carcinoma. All patients had disease that had recurred on, or was unresponsive to, a platinum-containing regimen. Patients in these 2 trials received an initial dose of 1.5 mg/m^2 given by intravenous infusion over 30 minutes for 5 consecutive days, starting on day 1 of a 21-day course.
One trial was a randomized trial of 112 patients treated with HYCAMTIN (1.5 mg/m^2/day × 5 days starting on day 1 of a 21-day course) and 114 patients treated with paclitaxel (175 mg/m^2 over 3 hours on day 1 of a 21-day course). All patients had recurrent ovarian cancer after a platinum-containing regimen or had not responded to at least 1 prior platinum-containing regimen. Patients who did not respond to the trial therapy, or who progressed, could be given the alternative therapy.
Response rates, response duration, and time to progression are shown in Table 7.

Table 7. Efficacy of HYCAMTIN Versus Paclitaxel in Ovarian Cancer

Parameter	HYCAMTIN (n = 112)	Paclitaxel (n = 114)
Complete response rate	5%	3%
Partial response rate	16%	11%
Overall response rate	21%	14%
95% Confidence interval	13 to 28%	8 to 20%
(P-value)	(0.20)	
Response duration[a] (weeks)	n = 23	n = 16
Median	25.9	21.6
95% Confidence interval	22.1 to 32.9	16.0 to 34.0
Hazard-ratio (HYCAMTIN:paclitaxel)	0.78	
(P-value)	(0.48)	
Time to progression (weeks)		
Median	18.9	14.7
95% Confidence interval	12.1 to 23.6	11.9 to 18.3
Hazard-ratio (HYCAMTIN:paclitaxel)	0.76	
(P-value)	(0.07)	
Survival (weeks)		
Median	63.0	53.0
95% Confidence interval	46.6 to 71.9	42.3 to 68.7
Hazard-ratio (HYCAMTIN:paclitaxel)	0.97	
(P-value)	(0.87)	

[a] The calculation for duration of response was based on the interval between first response and time to progression.

The median time to response was 7.6 weeks (range: 3.1 to 21.7) with HYCAMTIN compared with 6.0 weeks (range: 2.4 to 18.1) with paclitaxel. Consequently, the efficacy of HYCAMTIN may not be achieved if patients are withdrawn from treatment prematurely.

In the crossover phase, 8 of 61 (13%) patients who received HYCAMTIN after paclitaxel had a partial response and 5 of 49 (10%) patients who received paclitaxel after HYCAMTIN had a response (2 complete responses).

HYCAMTIN was active in ovarian cancer patients who had developed resistance to platinum-containing therapy, defined as tumor progression while on, or tumor relapse within 6 months after completion of, a platinum-containing regimen. One complete and 6 partial responses were seen in 60 patients, for a response rate of 12%. In the same trial, there were no complete responders and 4 partial responders on the paclitaxel arm, for a response rate of 7%.

HYCAMTIN was also studied in an open-label, non-comparative trial in 111 patients with recurrent ovarian cancer after treatment with a platinum-containing regimen, or who had not responded to 1 prior platinum-containing regimen. The response rate was 14% (95% CI: 7% to 20%). The median duration of response was 22 weeks (range: 4.6 to 41.9 weeks). The time to progression was 11.3 weeks (range: 0.7 to 72.1 weeks). The median survival was 67.9 weeks (range: 1.4 to 112.9 weeks).

14.2 Small Cell Lung Cancer

HYCAMTIN was studied in 426 patients with recurrent or progressive small cell lung cancer in 1 randomized, comparative trial and in 3 single-arm trials.

Randomized Comparative Trial:

In a randomized, comparative, Phase 3 trial, 107 patients were treated with HYCAMTIN (1.5 mg/m²/day × 5 days starting on day 1 of a 21-day course) and 104 patients were treated with CAV (1,000 mg/m² cyclophosphamide, 45 mg/m² doxorubicin, 2 mg vincristine administered sequentially on day 1 of a 21-day course). All patients were considered sensitive to first-line chemotherapy (responders who then subsequently progressed ≥60 days after completion of first-line therapy). A total of 77% of patients treated with HYCAMTIN and 79% of patients treated with CAV received platinum/etoposide with or without other agents as first-line chemotherapy.

Response rates, response duration, time to progression, and survival are shown in Table 8.

Table 8. Efficacy of HYCAMTIN Versus CAV (cyclophosphamide-doxorubicin-vincristine) in Small Cell Lung Cancer Patients Sensitive to First-Line Chemotherapy

Parameter	HYCAMTIN (n = 107)	CAV (n = 104)
Complete response rate	0%	1%
Partial response rate	24%	17%

Table 9. Percentage of Patients With Symptom Improvement[a]: HYCAMTIN Versus CAV in Patients With Small Cell Lung Cancer

Symptom	HYCAMTIN (n = 107) n[b]	HYCAMTIN (%)	CAV (n = 104) n[b]	CAV (%)
Shortness of breath	68	(28)	61	(7)
Interference with daily activity	67	(27)	63	(11)
Fatigue	70	(23)	65	(9)
Hoarseness	40	(33)	38	(13)
Cough	69	(25)	61	(15)
Insomnia	57	(33)	53	(19)
Anorexia	56	(32)	57	(16)
Chest pain	44	(25)	41	(17)
Hemoptysis	15	(27)	12	(33)

[a] Defined as improvement sustained over at least 2 courses compared with baseline.
[b] Number of patients with baseline and at least 1 post-baseline assessment.

Overall response rate	24%	18%
Difference in overall response rates	6%	
95% Confidence interval of the difference	(–6 to 18%)	
Response duration[a] (weeks)	n = 26	n = 19
Median	14.4	15.3
95% Confidence interval	13.1 to 18.0	13.1 to 23.1
Hazard-ratio (HYCAMTIN:CAV) (95% CI)	1.42 (0.73 to 2.76)	
(P-value)	(0.30)	
Time to progression (weeks)		
Median	13.3	12.3
95% Confidence interval	11.4 to 16.4	11.0 to 14.1
Hazard-ratio (HYCAMTIN:CAV) (95% CI)	0.92 (0.69 to 1.22)	
(P-value)	(0.55)	
Survival (weeks)		
Median	25.0	24.7
95% Confidence interval	20.6 to 29.6	21.7 to 30.3
Hazard-ratio (HYCAMTIN:CAV) (95% CI)	1.04 (0.78 to 1.39)	
(P-value)	(0.80)	

[a] The calculation for duration of response was based on the interval between first response and time to progression.

The time to response was similar in both arms: HYCAMTIN median of 6 weeks (range: 2.4 to 15.7) versus CAV median 6 weeks (range: 5.1 to 18.1).

Changes on a disease-related symptom scale in patients who received HYCAMTIN or who received CAV are presented in Table 9. It should be noted that not all patients had all symptoms, nor did all patients respond to all questions. Each symptom was rated on a 4-category scale with an improvement defined as a change in 1 category from baseline sustained over 2 courses. Limitations in interpretation of the rating scale and responses preclude formal statistical analysis.

[See table 9 above]

Single-Arm Trials:

HYCAMTIN was also studied in 3 open-label, non-comparative trials in a total of 319 patients with recurrent or progressive small cell lung cancer after treatment with first-line chemotherapy. In all 3 trials, patients were stratified as either sensitive (responders who then subsequently progressed ≥90 days after completion of first-line therapy) or refractory (no response to first-line chemotherapy or who responded to first-line therapy and then progressed within 90 days of completing first-line therapy). Response rates ranged from 11% to 31% for sensitive patients and 2% to 7% for refractory patients. Median time to progression and median survival were similar in all 3 trials and the comparative trial.

14.3 Cervical Cancer

In a comparative trial, 147 eligible women were randomized to HYCAMTIN (0.75 mg/m²/day IV over 30 minutes × 3 consecutive days starting on day 1 of a 21-day course) plus cisplatin (50 mg/m² on day 1) and 146 eligible women were randomized to cisplatin (50 mg/m² IV on day 1 of a 21-day course). All patients had histologically confirmed Stage IV-B, recurrent, or persistent carcinoma of the cervix considered not amenable to curative treatment with surgery and/or radiation. Fifty-six percent (56%) of patients treated with HYCAMTIN plus cisplatin and 56% of patients treated with cisplatin had received prior cisplatin with or without other agents as first-line chemotherapy.

Median survival of eligible patients receiving HYCAMTIN plus cisplatin was 9.4 months (95% CI: 7.9 to 11.9) compared with 6.5 months (95% CI: 5.8 to 8.8) among patients randomized to cisplatin alone with a log rank P-value of 0.033 (significance level was 0.044 after adjusting for the interim analysis). The unadjusted hazard ratio for overall survival was 0.76 (95% CI: 0.59 to 0.98).

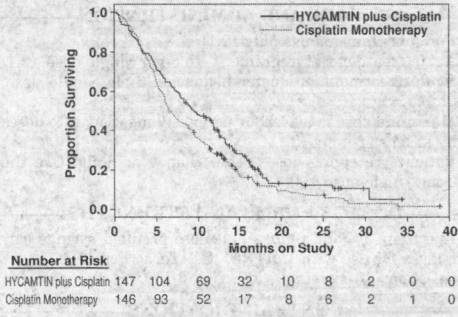

Figure 1. Overall Survival Curves Comparing HYCAMTIN plus Cisplatin versus Cisplatin Monotherapy in Cervical Cancer Patients

15 REFERENCES

1. Preventing Occupational Exposures to Antineoplastic and Other Hazardous Drugs in Health Care Settings. NIOSH Alert 2004-165.
2. OSHA Technical Manual, TED 1-0.15A, Section VI: Chapter 2. Controlling Occupational Exposure to Hazardous Drugs. OSHA, 1999. http://www.osha.gov/dts/osta/otm/otm_vi/otm_vi_2.html
3. American Society of Health-System Pharmacists. ASHP Guidelines on Handling Hazardous Drugs. Am J Health-Syst Pharm. 2006;63:1172-1193.
4. Polovich M, White JM, Kelleher LO (eds.) 2005. Chemotherapy and Biotherapy Guidelines and Recommendations for Practice. (2nd ed) Pittsburgh, PA: Oncology Nursing Society.

16 HOW SUPPLIED/STORAGE AND HANDLING

HYCAMTIN for Injection is supplied in 4-mg (free base) single-dose vials.

NDC 0007-4201-01 (package of 1)

Storage: Store the vials protected from light in the original cartons at controlled room temperature between 20° and 25°C (68° and 77°F) [see USP].

17 PATIENT COUNSELING INFORMATION

17.1 Bone Marrow Suppression

Inform patients that HYCAMTIN decreases blood cell counts such as white blood cells, platelets, and red blood cells. Patients who develop fever, other signs of infection (e.g., chills, cough, or burning pain on urination), or bleeding while on therapy should notify their physician promptly. Inform patients that frequent blood tests will be performed while taking HYCAMTIN to monitor for the occurrence of bone marrow suppression.

17.2 Pregnancy and Breastfeeding

Advise patients to use effective contraceptive measures to prevent pregnancy and to avoid breastfeeding during treatment with HYCAMTIN.

17.3 Asthenia and Fatigue

Inform patients that HYCAMTIN may cause asthenia or fatigue. If these symptoms occur, caution should be observed when driving or operating machinery.

HYCAMTIN is a registered trademark of the GSK group of companies.

GlaxoSmithKline
Research Triangle Park, NC 27709
©2014, the GSK group of companies. All rights reserved.
HYJ:22PI

IMITREX   ℞

[ĭm′ĭ-trĕx]
(sumatriptan succinate)
Injection
For Subcutaneous Use

HIGHLIGHTS OF PRESCRIBING INFORMATION

These highlights do not include all the information needed to use IMITREX safely and effectively. See full prescribing information for IMITREX.

IMITREX (sumatriptan succinate) Injection
For Subcutaneous Use
Initial U.S. Approval: 1992

——————INDICATIONS AND USAGE——————

IMITREX is a serotonin (5-HT$_{1B/1D}$) receptor agonist (triptan) indicated for:
- Acute treatment of migraine with or without aura in adults (1)
- Acute treatment of cluster headache in adults (1)

Limitations of Use:
- Use only if a clear diagnosis of migraine or cluster headache has been established. (1)
- Not indicated for the prevention of migraine attacks. (1)

——————DOSAGE AND ADMINISTRATION——————

- For subcutaneous use only. (2.1)
- Acute treatment of migraine: 1- to 6-mg Single dose. (2.1)
- Acute treatment of cluster headache: 6-mg Single dose. (2.1)
- Maximum dose in a 24-hour period: 12 mg, Separate doses by at least 1 hour. (2.1)
- Patients receiving doses other than 4 or 6 mg: Use the 6-mg single-dose vial. (2.3)

——————DOSAGE FORMS AND STRENGTHS——————

- Injection: 4- and 6-mg single-dose prefilled syringe cartridges for use with IMITREX STATdose Pen (3)
- Injection: 6-mg single-dose vial (3)

——————CONTRAINDICATIONS——————

- Coronary artery disease or coronary vasospasm (4)
- Wolff-Parkinson-White syndrome or other cardiac accessory conduction pathway disorders (4)
- History of stroke, transient ischemic attack, or hemiplegic or basilar migraine (4)
- Peripheral vascular disease (4)
- Ischemic bowel disease (4)
- Uncontrolled hypertension (4)
- Recent (within 24 hours) use of another 5-HT$_1$ agonist (e.g., another triptan) or of an ergotamine-containing medication (4)
- Concurrent or recent (past 2 weeks) use of monoamine oxidase-A inhibitor (4)
- Known hypersensitivity to sumatriptan (4)
- Severe hepatic impairment (4)

——————WARNINGS AND PRECAUTIONS——————

- Myocardial ischemia/infarction and Prinzmetal's angina: Perform cardiac evaluation in patients with multiple cardiovascular risk factors. (5.1)
- Arrhythmias: Discontinue IMITREX if occurs. (5.2)
- Chest/throat/neck/jaw pain, tightness, pressure, or heaviness: Generally not associated with myocardial ischemia; evaluate for coronary artery disease in patients at high risk. (5.3)
- Cerebral hemorrhage, subarachnoid hemorrhage, and stroke: Discontinue IMITREX if occurs. (5.4)
- Gastrointestinal ischemia and infarction events, peripheral vasospastic reactions: Discontinue IMITREX if occurs. (5.5)
- Medication overuse headache: Detoxification may be necessary. (5.6)
- Serotonin syndrome: Discontinue IMITREX if occurs. (5.7)
- Increase in blood pressure: Monitor blood pressure. (5.8)
- Anaphylactic/anaphylactoid reactions: Discontinue IMITREX if occurs. (5.9)
- Seizures: Use with caution in patients with epilepsy or a lowered seizure threshold. (5.10)

——————ADVERSE REACTIONS——————

Most common adverse reactions (≥5% and > placebo) were injection site reactions, tingling, dizziness/vertigo, warm/

hot sensation, burning sensation, feeling of heaviness, pressure sensation, flushing, feeling of tightness, and numbness. (6.1)

To report SUSPECTED ADVERSE REACTIONS, contact GlaxoSmithKline at 1-888-825-5249 or FDA at 1-800-FDA-1088 or www.fda.gov/medwatch.

——————USE IN SPECIFIC POPULATIONS——————

- Pregnancy: Based on animal data, may cause fetal harm (8.1)
- Geriatric use: A cardiovascular evaluation is recommended in those who have other cardiovascular risk factors prior to receiving IMITREX. (8.5)

See 17 for PATIENT COUNSELING INFORMATION and FDA-approved patient labeling

Revised: 10/2012

FULL PRESCRIBING INFORMATION: CONTENTS*

FULL PRESCRIBING INFORMATION

1 INDICATIONS AND USAGE

IMITREX® Injection is indicated in adults for (1) the acute treatment of migraine, with or without aura, and (2) the acute treatment of cluster headache.

Limitations of Use:
- Use only if a clear diagnosis of migraine or cluster headache has been established.
- If a patient has no response to the first migraine attack treated with IMITREX, reconsider the diagnosis of migraine before IMITREX is administered to treat any subsequent attacks.

- IMITREX is not indicated for the prevention of migraine attacks.

2 DOSAGE AND ADMINISTRATION

2.1 Dosing Information

The maximum single recommended adult dose of IMITREX Injection for the acute treatment of migraine or cluster headache is 6 mg injected subcutaneously. For the treatment of migraine, if side effects are dose limiting, lower doses (1 to 5 mg) may be used [see Clinical Studies (14.1)]. For the treatment of cluster headache, the efficacy of lower doses has not been established.

The maximum cumulative dose that may be given in 24 hours is 12 mg, two 6-mg injections separated by at least 1 hour. A second 6-mg dose should only be considered if some response to a first injection was observed.

2.2 Administration Using the IMITREX STATdose Pen®

An autoinjector device (IMITREX STATdose Pen) is available for use with 4- and 6-mg prefilled syringe cartridges. With this device, the needle penetrates approximately 1/4 inch (5 to 6 mm). The injection is intended to be given subcutaneously, and intramuscular or intravascular delivery must be avoided. Instruct patients on the proper use of IMITREX STATdose Pen and direct them to use injection sites with an adequate skin and subcutaneous thickness to accommodate the length of the needle.

2.3 Administration of Doses of IMITREX Other Than 4 or 6 mg

In patients receiving doses other than 4 or 6 mg, use the 6-mg single-dose vial; do not use the IMITREX STATdose Pen. Visually inspect the vial for particulate matter and discoloration before administration. Do not use if particulates and discolorations are noted.

3 DOSAGE FORMS AND STRENGTHS

- Injection: 4- and 6-mg single-dose prefilled syringe cartridges for use with the IMITREX STATdose Pen
- Injection: 6-mg single-dose vial

4 CONTRAINDICATIONS

IMITREX Injection is contraindicated in patients with:
- Ischemic coronary artery disease (CAD) (angina pectoris, history of myocardial infarction, or documented silent ischemia) or coronary artery vasospasm, including Prinzmetal's angina [see Warnings and Precautions (5.1)].
- Wolff-Parkinson-White syndrome or arrhythmias associated with other cardiac accessory conduction pathway disorders [see Warnings and Precautions (5.2)].
- History of stroke or transient ischemic attack (TIA) because these patients are at a higher risk of stroke [see Warnings and Precautions (5.4)].
- History of hemiplegic or basilar migraine.
- Peripheral vascular disease [see Warnings and Precautions (5.5)].
- Ischemic bowel disease [see Warnings and Precautions (5.5)].
- Uncontrolled hypertension [see Warnings and Precautions (5.8)].
- Recent (i.e., within 24 hours) use of ergotamine-containing medication, ergot-type medication (such as dihydroergotamine or methysergide), or another 5-hydroxytryptamine$_1$ (5-HT$_1$) agonist [see Drug Interactions (7.1, 7.3)].
- Concurrent administration of an MAO-A inhibitor or recent (within 2 weeks) use of an MAO-A inhibitor [see Drug Interactions (7.2) and Clinical Pharmacology (12.3)].
- Known hypersensitivity to sumatriptan [see Warnings and Precautions (5.9) and Adverse Reactions (6.2)].
- Severe hepatic impairment [see Clinical Pharmacology (12.3)].

5 WARNINGS AND PRECAUTIONS

5.1 Myocardial Ischemia, Myocardial Infarction, and Prinzmetal's Angina

The use of IMITREX Injection is contraindicated in patients with ischemic or vasospastic CAD. There have been rare reports of serious cardiac adverse reactions, including acute myocardial infarction, occurring within a few hours following administration of IMITREX Injection. Some of these reactions occurred in patients without known CAD. 5-HT$_1$ agonists, including IMITREX Injection, may cause coronary artery vasospasm (Prinzmetal's angina), even in patients without a history of CAD.

Perform a cardiovascular evaluation in triptan-naive patients who have multiple cardiovascular risk factors (e.g., increased age, diabetes, hypertension, smoking, obesity, strong family history of CAD) prior to receiving IMITREX Injection. If there is evidence of CAD or coronary artery vasospasm, IMITREX Injection is contraindicated. For patients with multiple cardiovascular risk factors who have a negative cardiovascular evaluation, consider administering the first dose of IMITREX Injection in a medically supervised setting and performing an electrocardiogram (ECG) immediately following IMITREX Injection. For such patients, consider periodic cardiovascular evaluation in intermittent long-term users of IMITREX Injection.

Evaluate patients with signs or symptoms suggestive of angina following IMITREX Injection for the presence of CAD or Prinzmetal's angina before receiving additional doses of IMITREX Injection.

5.2 Arrhythmias

Life-threatening disturbances of cardiac rhythm, including ventricular tachycardia and ventricular fibrillation leading to death, have been reported within a few hours following the administration of 5-HT$_1$ agonists. Discontinue IMITREX Injection if these disturbances occur. IMITREX Injection is contraindicated in patients with Wolff-Parkinson-White syndrome or arrhythmias associated with other cardiac accessory conduction pathway disorders.

5.3 Chest, Throat, Neck, and/or Jaw Pain/Tightness/Pressure

As with other 5-HT$_1$ agonists, sensations of tightness, pain, pressure, and heaviness in the precordium, throat, neck, and jaw commonly occur after treatment with IMITREX Injection and are usually non-cardiac in origin. However, perform a cardiac evaluation if these patients are at high cardiac risk. The use of IMITREX Injection is contraindicated in patients shown to have CAD and those with Prinzmetal's variant angina.

5.4 Cerebrovascular Events

Cerebral hemorrhage, subarachnoid hemorrhage, and stroke have occurred in patients treated with 5-HT$_1$ agonists, and some have resulted in fatalities. In a number of cases, it appears possible that the cerebrovascular events were primary, the 5-HT$_1$ agonist having been administered in the incorrect belief that the symptoms experienced were a consequence of migraine when they were not. Also, patients with migraine may be at increased risk of certain cerebrovascular events (e.g., stroke, hemorrhage, TIA). Discontinue IMITREX Injection if a cerebrovascular event occurs.

As with other acute migraine therapies, before treating headaches in patients not previously diagnosed as migraineurs, and in migraineurs who present with atypical symptoms, exclude other potentially serious neurological conditions. IMITREX Injection is contraindicated in patients with a history of stroke or TIA.

5.5 Other Vasospasm Reactions

5-HT$_1$ agonists, including IMITREX Injection, may cause non-coronary vasospastic reactions, such as peripheral vascular ischemia, gastrointestinal vascular ischemia and infarction (presenting with abdominal pain and bloody diarrhea), splenic infarction, and Raynaud's syndrome. Until further evaluation, IMITREX Injection is contraindicated in patients who experience symptoms or signs suggestive of non-coronary vasospasm reaction following the use of any 5-HT$_1$ agonist.

Reports of transient and permanent blindness and significant partial vision loss have been reported with the use of 5-HT$_1$ agonists. Since visual disorders may be part of a migraine attack, a causal relationship between these events and the use of 5-HT$_1$ agonists have not been clearly established.

5.6 Medication Overuse Headache

Overuse of acute migraine drugs (e.g., ergotamine, triptans, opioids, combination of drugs for 10 or more days per month) may lead to exacerbation of headache (medication overuse headache). Medication overuse headache may present as migraine-like daily headaches, or as a marked increase in frequency of migraine attacks. Detoxification of patients, including withdrawal of the overused drugs, and treatment of withdrawal symptoms (which often includes a transient worsening of headache) may be necessary.

5.7 Serotonin Syndrome

Serotonin syndrome may occur with triptans, including IMITREX Injection, particularly during coadministration with selective serotonin reuptake inhibitors (SSRIs), serotonin norepinephrine reuptake inhibitors (SNRIs), tricyclic antidepressants (TCAs) and MAO inhibitors [see Drug Interactions (7.4)]. Serotonin syndrome symptoms may include mental status changes (e.g., agitation, hallucinations, coma), autonomic instability (e.g., tachycardia, labile blood pressure, hyperthermia), neuromuscular aberrations (e.g., hyperreflexia, incoordination), and/or gastrointestinal symptoms (e.g., nausea, vomiting, diarrhea). The onset of symptoms usually occurs within minutes to hours of receiving a new or a greater dose of a serotonergic medication. Discontinue IMITREX Injection if serotonin syndrome is suspected.

5.8 Increase in Blood Pressure

Significant elevation in blood pressure, including hypertensive crisis with acute impairment of organ systems, has been reported on rare occasions in patients treated with 5-HT$_1$ agonists, including patients without a history of hypertension. Monitor blood pressure in patients treated with IMITREX. IMITREX Injection is contraindicated in patients with uncontrolled hypertension.

5.9 Anaphylactic/Anaphylactoid Reactions

Anaphylactic/anaphylactoid reactions have occurred in patients receiving sumatriptan. Such reactions can be life threatening or fatal. In general, anaphylactic reactions to drugs are more likely to occur in individuals with a history of sensitivity to multiple allergens. IMITREX Injection is contraindicated in patients with prior serious anaphylactic reaction.

5.10 Seizures

Seizures have been reported following administration of sumatriptan. Some have occurred in patients with either a history of seizures or concurrent conditions predisposing to seizures. There are also reports in patients where no such predisposing factors are apparent. IMITREX Injection should be used with caution in patients with a history of epilepsy or conditions associated with a lowered seizure threshold.

6 ADVERSE REACTIONS

The following adverse reactions are discussed in more detail in other sections of the labeling:
- Myocardial ischemia, myocardial infarction, and Prinzmetal's angina [see Warnings and Precautions (5.1)]
- Arrhythmias [see Warnings and Precautions (5.2)]
- Chest, throat, neck, and/or jaw pain/tightness/pressure [see Warnings and Precautions (5.3)]
- Cerebrovascular events [see Warnings and Precautions (5.4)]
- Other vasospasm reactions [see Warnings and Precautions (5.5)]
- Medication overuse headache [see Warnings and Precautions (5.6)]
- Serotonin syndrome [see Warnings and Precautions (5.7)]
- Increase in blood pressure [see Warnings and Precautions (5.8)]
- Anaphylactic/anaphylactoid reactions [see Warnings and Precautions (5.9)]
- Seizures [see Warnings and Precautions (5.10)]

6.1 Clinical Trials Experience

Because clinical trials are conducted under widely varying conditions, adverse reaction rates observed in the clinical trials of a drug cannot be directly compared with rates in the clinical trials of another drug and may not reflect the rates observed in practice.

Migraine Headache: Table 1 lists adverse reactions that occurred in 2 US placebo-controlled clinical trials in migraine subjects [Studies 2 and 3, see Clinical Studies (14.1)] following either a single 6-mg dose of IMITREX Injection or placebo. Only reactions that occurred at a frequency of 2% or more in groups treated with IMITREX Injection 6 mg and that occurred at a frequency greater than the placebo group are included in Table 1.

Table 1. Adverse Reactions Reported by at Least 2% of Subjects and at a Greater Frequency Than Placebo in 2 Placebo-Controlled Migraine Clinical Trials (Studies 2 and 3)[a]

Adverse Reaction	Percent of Subjects Reporting	
	IMITREX Injection 6 mg Subcutaneous (n = 547)	Placebo (n = 370)
Atypical sensations	42	9
Tingling	14	3
Warm/hot sensation	11	4
Burning sensation	7	<1
Feeling of heaviness	7	1
Pressure sensation	7	2
Feeling of tightness	5	<1
Numbness	5	2
Feeling strange	2	<1
Tight feeling in head	2	<1
Cardiovascular		
Flushing	7	2
Chest discomfort	5	1
Tightness in chest	3	<1
Pressure in chest	2	<1
Ear, nose, and throat		
Throat discomfort	3	<1
Discomfort: nasal cavity/sinuses	2	<1
Injection site reaction[b]	59	24
Miscellaneous		
Jaw discomfort	2	0
Musculoskeletal		
Weakness	5	<1
Neck pain/stiffness	5	<1
Myalgia	2	<1
Neurological		
Dizziness/vertigo	12	4
Drowsiness/sedation	3	2
Headache	2	<1
Skin		
Sweating	2	1

[a] The sum of the percentages cited is greater than 100% because subjects may have experienced more than 1 type of adverse reaction. Only reactions that occurred at a frequency of 2% or more in groups treated with IMITREX Injection and occurred at a frequency greater than the placebo groups are included.
[b] Includes injection site pain, stinging/burning, swelling, erythema, bruising, bleeding.

The incidence of adverse reactions in controlled clinical trials was not affected by gender or age of the subjects. There were insufficient data to assess the impact of race on the incidence of adverse reactions.

Cluster Headache: In the controlled clinical trials assessing the efficacy of IMITREX Injection as a treatment for cluster headache [Studies 4 and 5, see Clinical Studies (14.2)], no new significant adverse reactions were detected that had not already been identified in trials of IMITREX in subjects with migraine.

Overall, the frequency of adverse reactions reported in the trials of cluster headache was generally lower than in the migraine trials. Exceptions include reports of paresthesia (5% IMITREX, 0% placebo), nausea and vomiting (4% IMITREX, 0% placebo), and bronchospasm (1% IMITREX, 0% placebo).

Other Adverse Reactions: In the paragraphs that follow, the frequencies of less commonly reported adverse reactions are presented. Reaction frequencies were calculated as the number of subjects reporting a reaction divided by the total number of subjects (N = 6,218) exposed to subcutaneous IMITREX Injection. All reported reactions are included except those already listed in the previous table. Reactions are further classified within body system categories and enumerated in order of decreasing frequency using the following definitions: frequent are defined as those occurring in at least 1/100 subjects, infrequent are those occurring in 1/100 to 1/1,000 subjects, and rare are those occurring in fewer than 1/1,000 subjects.

Cardiovascular: Infrequent were hypertension, hypotension, bradycardia, tachycardia, palpitations, and syncope. Rare was arrhythmia.

Gastrointestinal: Frequent was abdominal discomfort.

Musculoskeletal: Frequent were muscle cramps.

Neurological: Frequent was anxiety. Infrequent were mental confusion, euphoria, agitation, tremor. Rare were myoclonia, sleep disturbance, and dystonia.

Respiratory: Infrequent was dyspnea.

Skin: Infrequent were erythema, pruritus, and skin rashes.

Miscellaneous: Infrequent was "serotonin agonist effect".

Adverse Events Observed With Other Formulations of IMITREX: The following adverse events occurred in clinical trials with IMITREX® Tablets and IMITREX® Nasal Spray. Because the reports include events observed in open and uncontrolled trials, the role of IMITREX in their causation cannot be reliably determined. All reported events are included except those already listed, those too general to be informative, and those not reasonably associated with the use of the drug.

Cardiovascular: Angina, cerebrovascular lesion, heart block, peripheral cyanosis, phlebitis, thrombosis.

Gastrointestinal: Abdominal distention and colitis.

Neurological: Convulsions, hallucinations, syncope, suicide, and twitching.

Miscellaneous: Edema, hypersensitivity, swelling of extremities, and swelling of face.

6.2 Postmarketing Experience

The following adverse reactions have been identified during postapproval use of IMITREX Tablets, IMITREX Nasal Spray, and IMITREX Injection. Because these reactions are reported voluntarily from a population of uncertain size, it is not always possible to reliably estimate their frequency or establish a causal relationship to drug exposure. These reactions have been chosen for inclusion due to either their seriousness, frequency of reporting, or causal connection to IMITREX or a combination of these factors.

Blood: Hemolytic anemia, pancytopenia, thrombocytopenia.

Ear, Nose, and Throat: Deafness.

Eye: Ischemic optic neuropathy, retinal artery occlusion, retinal vein thrombosis.

Neurological: Central nervous system vasculitis, cerebrovascular accident, serotonin syndrome, subarachnoid hemorrhage.

Non-Site Specific: Angioedema, cyanosis, temporal arteritis.

Skin: Exacerbation of sunburn, hypersensitivity reactions (allergic vasculitis, erythema, pruritus, rash, shortness of breath, urticaria), photosensitivity. Following subcutaneous administration of IMITREX, pain, redness, stinging, induration, swelling, contusion, subcutaneous bleeding, and, on rare occasions, lipoatrophy (depression in the skin) or lipohypertrophy (enlargement or thickening of tissue) have been reported.

Urogenital: Acute renal failure.

7 DRUG INTERACTIONS

7.1 Ergot-Containing Drugs
Ergot-containing drugs have been reported to cause prolonged vasospastic reactions. Because these effects may be additive, use of ergotamine-containing or ergot-type medications (like dihydroergotamine or methysergide) and IMITREX Injection within 24 hours of each other is contraindicated.

7.2 Monoamine Oxidase-A Inhibitors
MAO-A inhibitors increase systemic exposure by 2-fold. Therefore, the use of IMITREX Injection in patients receiving MAO-A inhibitors is contraindicated [see Clinical Pharmacology (12.3)].

7.3 Other 5-HT$_1$ Agonists
Because their vasospastic effects may be additive, coadministration of IMITREX Injection and other 5-HT$_1$ agonists (e.g., triptans) within 24 hours of each other is contraindicated.

7.4 Selective Serotonin Reuptake Inhibitors/Serotonin Norepinephrine Reuptake Inhibitors and Serotonin Syndrome
Cases of serotonin syndrome have been reported during coadministration of triptans and SSRIs, or SNRIs, TCAs, and MAO inhibitors [see Warnings and Precautions (5.7)].

8 USE IN SPECIFIC POPULATIONS

8.1 Pregnancy
Pregnancy Category C: There are no adequate and well-controlled trials of IMITREX Injection in pregnant women. IMITREX Injection should be used during pregnancy only if the potential benefit justifies the potential risk to the fetus. When sumatriptan was administered intravenously to pregnant rabbits daily throughout the period of organogenesis, embryolethality was observed at doses at or close to those producing maternal toxicity. These doses were less than the maximum recommended human dose (MRHD) of 12 mg/day on a mg/m^2 basis. Oral administration of sumatriptan to rabbits during organogenesis was associated with increased incidences of fetal vascular and skeletal abnormalities. The highest no-effect dose for these effects was 15 mg/kg/day. The intravenous administration of sumatriptan to pregnant rats throughout organogenesis at doses that are approximately 10 times the MRHD on a mg/m^2 basis, did not produce evidence of embryolethality. The subcutaneous administration of sumatriptan to pregnant rats prior to and throughout pregnancy did not produce evidence of embryolethality or teratogenicity.

8.3 Nursing Mothers
It is not known whether sumatriptan is excreted in human breast milk following subcutaneous administration. Because many drugs are excreted in human milk, and because of the potential for serious adverse reactions in nursing infants from IMITREX, a decision should be made whether to discontinue nursing or to discontinue the drug, taking into account the importance of the drug to the mother.

8.4 Pediatric Use
Safety and effectiveness of IMITREX Injection in pediatric patients under 18 years of age have not been established; therefore, IMITREX Injection is not recommended for use in patients under 18 years of age.

Two controlled clinical trials evaluated IMITREX Nasal Spray (5 to 20 mg) in 1,248 adolescent migraineurs aged 12 to 17 years who treated a single attack. The trials did not establish the efficacy of IMITREX Nasal Spray compared with placebo in the treatment of migraine in adolescents. Adverse reactions observed in these clinical trials were similar in nature to those reported in clinical trials in adults. Five controlled clinical trials (2 single-attack trials, 3 multiple-attack trials) evaluating oral IMITREX (25 to 100 mg) in pediatric subjects aged 12 to 17 years enrolled a total of 701 adolescent migraineurs. These trials did not establish the efficacy of oral IMITREX compared with placebo in the treatment of migraine in adolescents. Adverse reactions observed in these clinical trials were similar in nature to those reported in clinical trials in adults. The frequency of all adverse reactions in these subjects appeared to be both dose- and age-dependent, with younger subjects reporting reactions more commonly than older adolescents. Postmarketing experience documents that serious adverse reactions have occurred in the pediatric population after use of subcutaneous, oral, and/or intranasal IMITREX. These reports include reactions similar in nature to those reported rarely in adults, including stroke, visual loss, and death. A

myocardial infarction has been reported in a 14-year-old male following the use of oral IMITREX; clinical signs occurred within 1 day of drug administration. Since clinical data to determine the frequency of serious adverse reactions in pediatric patients who might receive subcutaneous, oral, or intranasal IMITREX are not presently available, the use of IMITREX in patients under 18 years of age is not recommended.

8.5 Geriatric Use
Clinical trials of IMITREX Injection did not include sufficient numbers of subjects aged 65 and over to determine whether they respond differently from younger subjects. Other reported clinical experience has not identified differences in responses between the elderly and younger subjects. In general, dose selection for an elderly patient should be cautious, usually starting at the low end of the dosing range, reflecting the greater frequency of decreased hepatic, renal, or cardiac function and of concomitant disease or other drug therapy.

A cardiovascular evaluation is recommended for geriatric patients who have other cardiovascular risk factors (e.g., diabetes, hypertension, smoking, obesity, strong family history of CAD) prior to receiving IMITREX Injection [see Warnings and Precautions (5.1)].

10 OVERDOSAGE
No gross overdoses in clinical practice have been reported. Coronary vasospasm was observed after intravenous administration of IMITREX Injection [see Contraindications (4)]. Overdoses would be expected from animal data (dogs at 0.1 g/kg, rats at 2 g/kg) to possibly cause convulsions, tremor, inactivity, erythema of the extremities, reduced respiratory rate, cyanosis, ataxia, mydriasis, injection site reactions (desquamation, hair loss, and scab formation), and paralysis.

The elimination half-life of sumatriptan is about 2 hours [see Clinical Pharmacology (12.3)], and therefore monitoring of patients after overdose with IMITREX Injection should continue for at least 10 hours or while symptoms or signs persist.

It is unknown what effect hemodialysis or peritoneal dialysis has on the serum concentrations of sumatriptan.

11 DESCRIPTION
IMITREX Injection contains sumatriptan succinate, a selective 5-HT$_{1B/1D}$ receptor agonist. Sumatriptan succinate is chemically designated as 3-[2-(dimethylamino)ethyl]-N-methyl-indole-5-methanesulfonamide succinate (1:1), and it has the following structure:

The empirical formula is $C_{14}H_{21}N_3O_2S•C_4H_6O_4$, representing a molecular weight of 413.5. Sumatriptan succinate is a white to off-white powder that is readily soluble in water and in saline.

IMITREX Injection is a clear, colorless to pale yellow, sterile, nonpyrogenic solution for subcutaneous injection. Each 0.5 mL of IMITREX Injection 8 mg/mL solution contains 4 mg of sumatriptan (base) as the succinate salt and 3.8 mg of sodium chloride, USP in Water for Injection, USP. Each 0.5 mL of IMITREX Injection 12 mg/mL solution contains 6 mg of sumatriptan (base) as the succinate salt and 3.5 mg of sodium chloride, USP in Water for Injection, USP. The pH range of both solutions is approximately 4.2 to 5.3. The osmolality of both injections is 291 mOsmol.

12 CLINICAL PHARMACOLOGY

12.1 Mechanism of Action
Sumatriptan binds with high affinity to human cloned 5-HT$_{1B/1D}$ receptors. IMITREX presumably exerts its therapeutic effects in the treatment of migraine headache by binding to 5-HT$_{1B/1D}$ receptors located on intracranial blood vessels and sensory nerves of the trigeminal system.

Current theories proposed to explain the etiology of migraine headache suggest that symptoms are due to local cranial vasodilatation and/or to the release of sensory neuropeptides (including substance P and calcitonin gene-related peptide) through nerve endings in the trigeminal system. The therapeutic activity of IMITREX for the treatment of migraine and cluster headaches is thought to be due to the agonist effects at the 5-HT$_{1B/1D}$ receptors on intracranial blood vessels (including the arterio-venous anastomoses) and sensory nerves of the trigeminal system, which result in cranial vessel constriction and inhibition of proinflammatory neuropeptide release.

12.2 Pharmacodynamics
Blood Pressure: Significant elevation in blood pressure, including hypertensive crisis, has been reported in patients with and without a history of hypertension [see Warnings and Precautions (5.8)].

Peripheral (Small) Arteries: In healthy volunteers (N = 18), a trial evaluating the effects of sumatriptan on peripheral (small vessel) arterial reactivity failed to detect a clinically significant increase in peripheral resistance.

Heart Rate: Transient increases in blood pressure observed in some subjects in clinical trials carried out during sumatriptan's development as a treatment for migraine were not accompanied by any clinically significant changes in heart rate.

12.3 Pharmacokinetics
Absorption and Bioavailability: The bioavailability of sumatriptan via subcutaneous site injection to 18 healthy male subjects was 97% ± 16% of that obtained following intravenous injection.

After a single 6-mg subcutaneous manual injection into the deltoid area of the arm in 18 healthy males (age: 24 ± 6 years, weight: 70 kg), the maximum serum concentration (C$_{max}$) of sumatriptan was (mean ± standard deviation) 74 ± 15 ng/mL and the time to peak concentration (T$_{max}$) was 12 minutes after injection (range: 5 to 20 minutes). In this trial, the same dose injected subcutaneously in the thigh gave a C$_{max}$ of 61 ± 15 ng/mL by manual injection versus 52 ± 15 ng/mL by autoinjector techniques. The T$_{max}$ or amount absorbed was not significantly altered by either the site or technique of injection.

Distribution: Protein binding, determined by equilibrium dialysis over the concentration range of 10 to 1,000 ng/mL, is low, approximately 14% to 21%. The effect of sumatriptan on the protein binding of other drugs has not been evaluated.

Following a 6-mg subcutaneous injection into the deltoid area of the arm in 9 males (mean age: 33 years, mean weight: 77 kg) the volume of distribution central compartment of sumatriptan was 50 ± 8 liters and the distribution half-life was 15 ± 2 minutes.

Metabolism: In vitro studies with human microsomes suggest that sumatriptan is metabolized by MAO, predominantly the A isoenzyme. Most of a radiolabeled dose of sumatriptan excreted in the urine is the major metabolite indole acetic acid (IAA) or the IAA glucuronide, both of which are inactive.

Elimination: After a single 6-mg subcutaneous dose, 22% ± 4% was excreted in the urine as unchanged sumatriptan and 38% ± 7% as the IAA metabolite.

Following a 6-mg subcutaneous injection into the deltoid area of the arm, the systemic clearance of sumatriptan was 1,194 ± 149 mL/min and the terminal half-life was 115 ± 19 minutes.

Special Populations: Age: The pharmacokinetics of sumatriptan in the elderly (mean age: 72 years, 2 males and 4 females) and in subjects with migraine (mean age: 38 years, 25 males and 155 females) were similar to that in healthy male subjects (mean age: 30 years).

Renal Impairment: The effect of renal impairment on the pharmacokinetics of sumatriptan has not been examined.

Hepatic Impairment: The effect of mild to moderate hepatic disease on the pharmacokinetics of subcutaneously administered sumatriptan has been evaluated. There were no significant differences in the pharmacokinetics of subcutaneously administered sumatriptan in moderately hepatically impaired subjects compared with healthy controls. The pharmacokinetics of subcutaneously administered sumatriptan in patients with severe hepatic impairment has not been studied. The use of IMITREX Injection in this population is contraindicated [see Contraindications (4)].

Race: The systemic clearance and C$_{max}$ of sumatriptan were similar in black (n = 34) and Caucasian (n = 38) healthy male subjects.

Drug Interaction Studies: Monoamine Oxidase-A Inhibitors: In a trial of 14 healthy females, pretreatment with an MAO-A inhibitor decreased the clearance of sumatriptan, resulting in a 2-fold increase in the area under the sumatriptan plasma concentration-time curve (AUC), corresponding to a 40% increase in elimination half-life.

13 NONCLINICAL TOXICOLOGY

13.1 Carcinogenesis, Mutagenesis, Impairment of Fertility
Carcinogenesis: In carcinogenicity studies, rats and mice were given sumatriptan by oral gavage. Mice were dosed for 78 weeks and rats were dosed for 104 weeks. Average exposures achieved in mice receiving the highest dose were approximately 110 times the exposure attained in humans after the maximum recommended single dose of 6 mg. The highest dose to rats was approximately 260 times the maximum single dose of 6 mg on a mg/m2 basis. There was no evidence of an increase in tumors in either species related to sumatriptan administration.

Mutagenesis: Sumatriptan was not mutagenic in the presence or absence of metabolic activation when tested in 2 gene mutation assays (the Ames test and the in vitro mammalian Chinese hamster V79/HGPRT assay). It was not clastogenic in 2 cytogenetics assays (the in vitro human lymphocyte assay and the in vivo rat micronucleus assay).

Impairment of Fertility: A fertility study (Segment I) by the subcutaneous route, during which male and female rats were dosed daily with sumatriptan prior to and throughout the mating period, has shown no evidence of impaired fertility at doses equivalent to approximately 100 times the maximum recommended single human dose of 6 mg on a mg/m^2 basis. However, following oral administration, a treatment-related decrease in fertility, secondary to a decrease in mating, was seen for rats treated with 50 and 500 mg/kg/day. The no-effect dose for this finding was approximately 8 times the maximum recommended single human dose of 6 mg on a mg/m^2 basis. It is not clear whether the problem is associated with the treatment of males or females or both.

13.2 Animal Toxicology and/or Pharmacology

Corneal Opacities: Dogs receiving oral sumatriptan developed corneal opacities and defects in the corneal epithelium. Corneal opacities were seen at the lowest dosage tested, 2 mg/kg/day, and were present after 1 month of treatment. Defects in the corneal epithelium were noted in a 60-week study. Earlier examinations for these toxicities were not conducted and no-effect doses were not established; however, the relative exposure at the lowest dose tested was approximately 5 times the human exposure after a 100-mg oral dose or 3 times the human exposure after a 6-mg subcutaneous dose.

Melanin Binding: In rats with a single subcutaneous dose (0.5 mg/kg) of radiolabeled sumatriptan, the elimination half-life of radioactivity from the eye was 15 days, suggesting that sumatriptan and its metabolites bind to the melanin of the eye. The clinical significance of this binding is unknown.

14 CLINICAL STUDIES

14.1 Migraine

In controlled clinical trials enrolling more than 1,000 subjects during migraine attacks who were experiencing moderate or severe pain and 1 or more of the symptoms enumerated in Table 3, onset of relief began as early as 10 minutes following a 6-mg IMITREX Injection. Lower doses of IMITREX Injection may also prove effective, although the proportion of subjects obtaining adequate relief was decreased and the latency to that relief is greater with lower doses.

In Study 1, 6 different doses of IMITREX Injection (n = 30 each group) were compared with placebo (n = 62), in a single-attack, parallel-group design, the dose response relationship was found to be as shown in Table 2.

[See table 2 above]

In 2 randomized, placebo-controlled clinical trials of IMITREX Injection 6 mg in 1,104 subjects with moderate or severe migraine pain (Studies 2 and 3), the onset of relief was less than 10 minutes. Headache relief, as defined by a reduction in pain from severe or moderately severe to mild or no headache, was achieved in 70% of the subjects within 1 hour of a single 6-mg subcutaneous dose of IMITREX Injection. Approximately 82% and 65% of subjects treated with IMITREX 6 mg had headache relief and were pain free within 2 hours, respectively.

Table 3 shows the 1- and 2-hour efficacy results for IMITREX Injection 6 mg in Studies 2 and 3.

[See table 3 above]

IMITREX Injection also relieved photophobia, phonophobia (sound sensitivity), nausea, and vomiting associated with migraine attacks. Similar efficacy was seen when subjects self-administered IMITREX Injection using the IMITREX STATdose Pen.

The efficacy of IMITREX Injection was unaffected by whether or not the migraine was associated with aura, duration of attack, gender or age of the subject, or concomitant use of common migraine prophylactic drugs (e.g., betablockers).

14.2 Cluster Headache

The efficacy of IMITREX Injection in the acute treatment of cluster headache was demonstrated in 2 randomized, double-blind, placebo-controlled, 2-period crossover trials (Studies 4 and 5). Subjects aged 21 to 65 years were enrolled and were instructed to treat a moderate to very severe headache within 10 minutes of onset. Headache relief was defined as a reduction in headache severity to mild or no pain. In both trials, the proportion of individuals gaining relief at 10 or 15 minutes was significantly greater among subjects receiving 6 mg of IMITREX Injection compared with those who received placebo (see Table 4).

[See table 4 above]

An estimate of the cumulative probability of a subject with a cluster headache obtaining relief after being treated with either IMITREX Injection or placebo is presented in Figure 1.

[See figure 1 at top of next column]

The plot was constructed with data from subjects who either experienced relief or did not require (request) rescue medication within a period of 2 hours following treatment. As a consequence, the data in the plot are derived from only a subset of the 258 headaches treated (rescue medication was required in 52 of the 127 placebo-treated headaches and 18 of the 131 headaches treated with IMITREX Injection).

Other data suggest that treatment with IMITREX Injection is not associated with an increase in early recurrence of headache and has little effect on the incidence of later-occurring headaches (i.e., those occurring after 2, but before 18 or 24 hours).

Table 2. Proportion of Subjects With Migraine Relief and Incidence of Adverse Events by Time and by IMITREX Dose in Study 1

Dose of IMITREX Injection	Percent Subjects With Relief[a]				Adverse Events Incidence (%)
	at 10 Minutes	at 30 Minutes	at 1 Hour	at 2 Hours	
Placebo	5	15	24	21	55
1 mg	10	40	43	40	63
2 mg	7	23	57	43	63
3 mg	17	47	57	60	77
4 mg	13	37	50	57	80
6 mg	10	63	73	70	83
8 mg	23	57	80	83	93

[a] Relief is defined as the reduction of moderate or severe pain to no or mild pain after dosing without use of rescue medication.

Table 3. Proportion of Subjects With Pain Relief and Relief of Migraine Symptoms After 1 and 2 Hours of Treatment in Studies 2 and 3

1-Hour Data	Study 2		Study 3	
	Placebo (n = 190)	IMITREX 6 mg (n = 384)	Placebo (n = 180)	IMITREX 6 mg (n = 350)
Subjects with pain relief (grade 0/1)	18%	70%[a]	26%	70%[a]
Subjects with no pain	5%	48%[a]	13%	49%[a]
Subjects without nausea	48%	73%[a]	50%	73%[a]
Subjects without photophobia	23%	56%[a]	25%	58%[a]
Subjects with little or no clinical disability[b]	34%	76%[a]	34%	76%[a]

2-Hour Data	Study 2		Study 3	
	Placebo[c]	IMITREX 6 mg[d]	Placebo[c]	IMITREX 6 mg[d]
Subjects with pain relief (grade 0/1)	31%	81%[a]	39%	82%[a]
Subjects with no pain	11%	63%[a]	19%	65%[a]
Subjects without nausea	56%	82%[a]	63%	81%[a]
Subjects without photophobia	31%	72%[a]	35%	71%[a]
Subjects with little or no clinical disability[b]	42%	85%[a]	49%	84%[a]

[a] P <0.05 versus placebo.
[b] A successful outcome in terms of clinical disability was defined prospectively as ability to work mildly impaired or ability to work and function normally.
[c] Includes subjects that may have received an additional placebo injection 1 hour after the initial injection.
[d] Includes subjects that may have received an additional 6 mg of IMITREX Injection 1 hour after the initial injection.

Table 4. Proportion of Subjects With Cluster Headache Relief by Time in Studies 4 and 5

	Study 4		Study 5	
	Placebo (n = 39)	IMITREX 6 mg (n = 39)	Placebo (n = 88)	IMITREX 6 mg (n = 92)
Subjects with pain relief (no/mild)				
5 Minutes post-injection	8%	21%	7%	23%[a]
10 Minutes post-injection	10%	49%[a]	25%	49%[a]
15 minutes post-injection	26%	74%[a]	35%	75%[a]

[a] P <0.05.
(n = Number of headaches treated.)

Figure 1. Time to Relief of Cluster Headache from Time of Injection[a]

■ Placebo (N = 127)
● Sumatriptan (N = 131)

[a] The figure uses Kaplan-Meier (product limit) Survivorship Plot. Subjects taking rescue medication were censored at 15 minutes.

16 HOW SUPPLIED/STORAGE AND HANDLING

IMITREX Injection contains sumatriptan (base) as the succinate salt and is supplied as a clear, colorless to pale yellow, sterile, nonpyrogenic solution as follows:

Prefilled Syringe and/or Autoinjector Pen: Each pack contains a Patient Information and Patients Instructions for Use leaflet.

- IMITREX STATdose System®, 4 mg, containing 1 IMITREX STATdose Pen, 2 prefilled single-dose syringe cartridges, and 1 carrying case (NDC 0173-0739-00).
- IMITREX STATdose System, 6 mg, containing 1 IMITREX STATdose Pen, 2 prefilled single-dose syringe cartridges, and 1 carrying case (NDC 0173-0479-00).
- Two 4-mg single-dose prefilled syringe cartridges for use with IMITREX STATdose System (NDC 0173-0739-02).
- Two 6-mg single-dose prefilled syringe cartridges for use with IMITREX STATdose System (NDC 0173-0478-00).

Single-Dose Vial:

- IMITREX Injection single-dose vial (6 mg/0.5 mL) in cartons containing 5 vials (NDC 0173-0449-02).

Store between 2° and 30°C (36° and 86°F). Protect from light.

17 PATIENT COUNSELING INFORMATION

See FDA-approved patient labeling (Patient Information and Instructions for Use).

17.1 Risk of Myocardial Ischemia and/or Infarction, Prinzmetal's Angina, Other Vasospasm-Related Events, Arrhythmias, and Cerebrovascular Events

Inform patients that IMITREX Injection may cause serious cardiovascular side effects such as myocardial infarction or stroke. Although serious cardiovascular events can occur without warning symptoms, patients should be alert for the signs and symptoms of chest pain, shortness of breath, irregular heartbeat, significant rise in blood pressure, weakness, and slurring of speech and should ask for medical advice when observing any indicative sign or symptoms. Patients should be apprised of the importance of this follow-up *[see Warnings and Precautions (5.1, 5.2, 5.4, 5.5, 5.8)]*.

17.2 Anaphylactic/Anaphylactoid Reactions

Inform patients that anaphylactic/anaphylactoid reactions have occurred in patients receiving IMITREX Injection. Such reactions can be life threatening or fatal. In general, anaphylactic reactions to drugs are more likely to occur in individuals with a history of sensitivity to multiple allergens *[see Warnings and Precautions (5.9)]*.

17.3 Medication Overuse Headache

Inform patients that use of acute migraine drugs for 10 or more days per month may lead to an exacerbation of headache and encourage patients to record headache frequency and drug use (e.g., by keeping a headache diary) *[see Warnings and Precautions (5.6)]*.

17.4 Pregnancy

Inform patients that IMITREX Injection should not be used during pregnancy unless the potential benefit justifies the potential risk to the fetus *[see Use in Specific Populations (8.1)]*.

17.5 Nursing Mothers

Advise patients to notify their healthcare provider if they are breastfeeding or plan to breastfeed *[see Use in Specific Populations (8.3)]*.

17.6 Ability To Perform Complex Tasks

Since migraines or treatment with IMITREX Injection may cause somnolence and dizziness, instruct patients to evaluate their ability to perform complex tasks during migraine attacks and after administration of IMITREX Injection.

17.7 Serotonin Syndrome

Patients should be cautioned about the risk of serotonin syndrome with the use of IMITREX Injection or other triptans, particularly during combined use with SSRIs, SNRIs, TCAs, and MAO inhibitors *[see Warnings and Precautions (5.7) and Drug Interactions (7.4)]*.

17.8 How to Use IMITREX Injection

Provide patients instruction on the proper use of IMITREX Injection if they are able to self-administer IMITREX Injection in medically unsupervised situation.

Inform patients that the needle in the IMITREX STATdose Pen penetrates approximately 1/4 of an inch (5 to 6 mm). Inform patients that the injection is intended to be given subcutaneously and intramuscular or intravascular delivery should be avoided. Instruct patients to use injection sites with an adequate skin and subcutaneous thickness to accommodate the length of the needle.

IMITREX, IMITREX STATdose Pen, and IMITREX STATdose System are registered trademarks of GlaxoSmithKline.

GlaxoSmithKline

Research Triangle Park, NC 27709

©2012, GlaxoSmithKline. All rights reserved.

IMJ:4PI

Patient Information

IMITREX® (IM-i-trex)

(sumatriptan succinate)

Injection

Read this Patient Information before you start taking IMITREX and each time you get a refill. There may be new information. This information does not take the place of talking with your healthcare provider about your medical condition or treatment.

What is the most important information I should know about IMITREX?

IMITREX can cause serious side effects, including:

Heart attack and other heart problems. Heart problems may lead to death.

Stop taking IMITREX and get emergency medical help right away if you have any of the following symptoms of a heart attack:

- discomfort in the center of your chest that lasts for more than a few minutes, or that goes away and comes back
- severe tightness, pain, pressure, or heaviness in your chest, throat, neck, or jaw
- pain or discomfort in your arms, back, neck, jaw, or stomach
- shortness of breath with or without chest discomfort
- breaking out in a cold sweat

- nausea or vomiting
- feeling lightheaded

IMITREX is not for people with risk factors for heart disease unless a heart exam is done and shows no problem. You have a higher risk for heart disease if you:

- have high blood pressure
- have high cholesterol levels
- smoke
- are overweight
- have diabetes
- have a family history of heart disease

What is IMITREX?

IMITREX is a prescription medicine used to treat acute migraine headaches with or without aura and acute cluster headaches in adults who have been diagnosed with migraine or cluster headaches.

IMITREX is not used to treat other types of headaches such as hemiplegic (that make you unable to move on one side of your body) or basilar (rare form of migraine with aura) migraines.

IMITREX is not used to prevent or decrease the number of migraine or cluster headaches you have.

It is not known if IMITREX is safe and effective in children under 18 years of age.

Who should not take IMITREX?

Do not take IMITREX if you have:

- heart problems or a history of heart problems
- narrowing of blood vessels to your legs, arms, stomach, or kidney (peripheral vascular disease)
- uncontrolled high blood pressure
- hemiplegic migraines or basilar migraines. If you are not sure if you have these types of migraines, ask your healthcare provider.
- had a stroke, transient ischemic attacks (TIAs), or problems with your blood circulation
- taken any of the following medicines in the last 24 hours:
  - almotriptan (AXERT®)
  - eletriptan (RELPAX®)
  - frovatriptan (FROVA®)
  - naratriptan (AMERGE®)
  - rizatriptan (MAXALT®, MAXALT-MLT®)
  - sumatriptan and naproxen (TREXIMET®)
  - ergotamines (CAFERGOT®, ERGOMAR®, MIGERGOT®)
  - dihydroergotamine (D.H.E. 45®, MIGRANAL®)
  Ask your healthcare provider if you are not sure if your medicine is listed above.
- an allergy to sumatriptan or any of the ingredients in IMITREX. See the end of this leaflet for a complete list of ingredients in IMITREX.

What should I tell my healthcare provider before taking IMITREX?

Before you take IMITREX, tell your healthcare provider about all of your medical conditions, including if you:

- have high blood pressure
- have high cholesterol
- have diabetes
- smoke
- are overweight
- have heart problems or family history of heart problems or stroke
- have liver problems
- have had epilepsy or seizures
- are not using effective birth control
- become pregnant while taking IMITREX
- are breastfeeding or plan to breastfeed. IMITREX passes into your breast milk and may harm your baby. Talk with your healthcare provider about the best way to feed your baby if you take IMITREX.

Tell your healthcare provider about all the medicines you take, including prescription and nonprescription medicines, vitamins, and herbal supplements.

Using IMITREX with certain other medicines can affect each other, causing serious side effects.

Especially tell your healthcare provider if you take antidepressant medicines called:

- selective serotonin reuptake inhibitors (SSRIs)
- serotonin norepinephrine reuptake inhibitors (SNRIs)
- tricyclic antidepressants (TCAs)
- monoamine oxidase inhibitors (MAOIs)

Ask your healthcare provider or pharmacist for a list of these medicines if you are not sure.

Know the medicines you take. Keep a list of them to show your healthcare provider or pharmacist when you get a new medicine.

How should I take IMITREX?

- Certain people should take their first dose of IMITREX in their healthcare provider's office or in another medical setting. Ask your healthcare provider if you should take your first dose in a medical setting.
- Use IMITREX exactly as your healthcare provider tells you to use it.

- Your healthcare provider may change your dose. Do not change your dose without first talking with your healthcare provider.
- For adults, the usual dose is a single injection given just below the skin.
- You should give an injection as soon as the symptoms of your headache start, but it may be given at any time during a migraine attack.
- If you did not get any relief after the first injection, do not give a second injection without first talking with your healthcare provider.
- You can take a second injection 1 hour after the first injection, but not sooner, if your headache came back after your first injection.
- Do not take more than 12 mg in a 24-hour period.
- If you use too much IMITREX, call your healthcare provider or go to the nearest hospital emergency room right away.
- You should write down when you have headaches and when you take IMITREX so you can talk with your healthcare provider about how IMITREX is working for you.

What should I avoid while taking IMITREX?

IMITREX can cause dizziness, weakness, or drowsiness. If you have these symptoms, do not drive a car, use machinery, or do anything where you need to be alert.

What are the possible side effects of IMITREX?

IMITREX may cause serious side effects. See "What is the most important information I should know about IMITREX?"

These serious side effects include:

- changes in color or sensation in your fingers and toes (Raynaud's syndrome)
- stomach and intestinal problems (gastrointestinal and colonic ischemic events). Symptoms of gastrointestinal and colonic ischemic events include:
  - sudden or severe stomach pain
  - stomach pain after meals
  - weight loss
  - nausea or vomiting
  - constipation or diarrhea
  - bloody diarrhea
  - fever
- problems with blood circulation to your legs and feet (peripheral vascular ischemia). Symptoms of peripheral vascular ischemia include:
  - cramping and pain in your legs or hips
  - feeling of heaviness or tightness in your leg muscles
  - burning or aching pain in your feet or toes while resting
  - numbness, tingling, or weakness in your legs
  - cold feeling or color changes in 1 or both legs or feet
- medication overuse headaches. Some people who use too many IMITREX injections may have worse headaches (medication overuse headache). If your headaches get worse, your healthcare provider may decide to stop your treatment with IMITREX.
- serotonin syndrome. Serotonin syndrome is a rare but serious problem that can happen in people using IMITREX, especially if IMITREX is used with anti-depressant medicines called SSRIs or SNRIs.

Call your healthcare provider right away if you have any of the following symptoms of serotonin syndrome:

- mental changes such as seeing things that are not there (hallucinations), agitation, or coma
- fast heartbeat
- changes in blood pressure
- high body temperature
- tight muscles
- trouble walking
- seizures. Seizures have happened in people taking IMITREX who have never had seizures before. Talk with your healthcare provider about your chance of having seizures while you take IMITREX.

The most common side effects of IMITREX include:

- pain or redness at your injection site
- tingling or numbness in your fingers or toes
- dizziness
- warm, hot, burning feeling to your face (flushing)
- discomfort or stiffness in your neck
- feeling weak, drowsy, or tired

Tell your healthcare provider if you have any side effect that bothers you or that does not go away.

These are not all the possible side effects of IMITREX. For more information, ask your healthcare provider or pharmacist.

Call your doctor for medical advice about side effects. You may report side effects to FDA at 1-800-FDA-1088.

How should I store IMITREX Injection?

- Store IMITREX between 36°F to 86°F (2°C to 30°C).
- Store your medicine away from light.
- Keep your medicine in the packaging or carrying case provided with it.

Keep IMITREX and all medicines out of the reach of children.

General information about the safe and effective use of IMITREX

Medicines are sometimes prescribed for purposes other than those listed in Patient Information leaflets. Do not use

IMITREX for a condition for which it was not prescribed. Do not give IMITREX to other people, even if they have the same symptoms you have. It may harm them.

This Patient Information leaflet summarizes the most important information about IMITREX. If you would like more information, talk with your healthcare provider. You can ask your healthcare provider or pharmacist for information about IMITREX that is written for healthcare professionals. For more information, go to www.gsk.com or call 1-888-825-5249.

What are the ingredients in IMITREX Injection?

Active ingredient: sumatriptan succinate

Inactive ingredients: sodium chloride, water for injection

This Patient Information and Instructions for Use has been approved by the U.S. Food and Drug Administration.

IMITREX, AMERGE, TREXIMET are registered trademarks of GlaxoSmithKline. The other brands listed are trademarks of their respective owners and are not trademarks of GlaxoSmithKline. The makers of these brands are not affiliated with and do not endorse GlaxoSmithKline or its products.

GlaxoSmithKline

Research Triangle Park, NC 27709

©2012, GlaxoSmithKline. All rights reserved.

October 2012

IMJ:3PPI

Patient Instructions for Use
IMITREX STATdose System®

Read this Patient Instructions for Use before you start to use the IMITREX STATdose System. There may be new information. This information does not take the place of talking with your healthcare provider about your medical condition or treatment. You and your healthcare provider should talk about IMITREX Injection when you start taking it and at regular checkups.

Keep the IMITREX STATdose System out of the reach of children.

Before you use the IMITREX STATdose System

When you first open the IMITREX STATdose System box, the Cartridge Pack and the IMITREX STATdose Pen® are already in the Carrying Case for your convenience.

The grey and blue **Carrying Case** is used for storing the unloaded Pen and the Cartridge Pack when they are not being used.

The **Cartridge Pack** holds 2 individually sealed **Syringe Cartridges**. Each Syringe Cartridge holds 1 dose of IMITREX® (sumatriptan succinate) Injection. The Cartridge Pack for the 4-mg strength of this medicine is yellow, and the Cartridge Pack for the 6-mg strength is blue (as shown). Refill Cartridge Packs are available.

The grey and blue **Pen** is used to automatically inject 1 dose of medicine from a Syringe Cartridge. Do not touch the **Blue Button** until you have pressed the Pen against your skin to give a dose. If you press it at any other time, you might lose a dose. The **Safety Catch** keeps the Pen from accidentally firing until you are ready. The Pen will only work when you slide the grey part of the barrel down to the blue part. Always check to make sure that the white Priming Rod is not sticking out from the end of the Pen (as shown in Figure B) before you load a new Syringe Cartridge. If it is sticking out, you will lose that dose.

How to load the IMITREX STATdose Pen

Do not load the Pen until you are ready to give yourself an injection.

Do not touch the Blue Button on top of the Pen (see Figure A) while you are loading the Pen.

1. Open the lid of the Carrying Case. The tamper-evident seals over the 2 Syringe Cartridges are labeled "A" and "B" **(see Figure A inset)**.

Always use the Syringe Cartridge marked "A" before the one marked "B" to help you keep track of your doses. **Do not use if either seal is broken or missing when you first open the Carrying Case.**

Figure A

2. Tear off one of the tamper-evident seals **(see Figure A)**. Throw away the seal. Open the lid over the Syringe Cartridge.

3. Hold the Pen by the ridges at the top. Take the Pen out of the Carrying Case **(see Figure B)**.

Check to make sure the white Priming Rod is not sticking out from the lower end of the Pen **(see Figure B inset)**. If it is sticking out, put the Pen back into the Carrying Case and press down firmly until you feel it click. Take the Pen out of the Carrying Case.

Figure B

4. Put the Pen in the Cartridge Pack. Turn it to the right (clockwise) until it will not turn any more (about half a turn) **(see Figure C)**.

Figure C

5. Hold the loaded Pen by the ridges and pull it **straight out (see Figure D)**. You may need to pull hard on the Pen, but this is normal. **Do not** press the Blue Button yet.

[See figure D at top of next column]

The Pen is now ready to use. **Do not** put the loaded Pen back into the Carrying Case because that will damage the needle.

How to use the IMITREX STATdose Pen to take your medicine

Before injecting your medicine, choose an area with a fatty tissue layer (see Figure E or Figure F). Ask your healthcare provider if you have a question about where to inject your medicine.

To prepare the area of skin where IMITREX is to be injected, wipe the injection site with an alcohol swab. Do not touch this area again before giving the injection.

[See figure E at top of next column]
[See figure F at top of next column]

Syringe Cartridge

Figure D

Figure E

Figure F

6. Without pushing the Blue Button, press the loaded Pen firmly against the skin so that the grey barrel slides down toward the blue section that holds the Syringe Cartridge **(see Figure D)**. (This releases the Safety Catch that keeps the Pen from firing by mistake until you are ready.)

7. Push the Blue Button. Hold the Pen still for **at least 5 seconds**. If the Pen is taken away from the skin too soon, not all the medicine will come out.

8. **After 5 seconds**, carefully take the Pen away from your skin. The needle will be showing **(see Figure G)**. **Do not touch the needle.**

Figure G

How to unload the IMITREX STATdose Pen after taking your medicine

Right after you take a dose with the Pen, you need to return the used Syringe Cartridge to the Cartridge Pack.

9. Push the Pen down into the empty side of the Cartridge Pack as far as it will go **(see Figure H)**.

[See figure H at top of next column]

10. Turn the Pen to the left (counterclockwise) about half a turn until it is released from the Syringe Cartridge **(see Figure I)**.

[See figure I at top of next column]

Figure H

Figure I

11. Pull the empty Pen out of the Cartridge Pack (see Figure J).
Because the Pen has now been used, the white Priming Rod will stick out from the lower end of the Pen (see Figure J).

Figure J

12. Close the Cartridge Pack lid over the used Syringe Cartridge. When the used Syringe Cartridges are inserted correctly, the Cartridge Pack is a disposable, protective case to help you avoid needle sticks and use the syringes correctly.
13. Put the Pen back into the Carrying Case and press it down firmly until you feel it click. Close the Carrying Case lid. This gets the Pen ready for the next use.
If the lid will not close, push the Pen down until you feel it click. Then close the lid.

How to take out a used Cartridge Pack
After both Syringe Cartridges have been used, take the Cartridge Pack out of the Carrying Case. **Never reuse or recycle a Syringe Cartridge.**
14. Open the Carrying Case lid.
15. Hold the Carrying Case with one hand and press the 2 buttons on either side of the Carrying Case (see Figure K).

Figure K

16. Gently pull out the Cartridge Pack with the other hand (see Figure L).
[See figure L at top of next column]
17. Throw away the Cartridge Pack or dispose of it as instructed by your healthcare provider. There may be special state and local laws for disposing of used needles and syringes. Always keep out of the reach of children.

Figure L

How to insert a new Cartridge Pack
18. Take the new Cartridge Pack out of its box. **Do not take off the tamper– evident seals (see Figure M).**

Figure M

19. Put the Cartridge Pack in the Carrying Case. Slide it down smoothly (see Figure N).

Figure N

20. The Cartridge Pack will click into place when the 2 buttons show through the holes in the Carrying Case (see Figure O). Close the lid.

Figure O

This Patient Information and Instructions for Use has been approved by the U.S. Food and Drug Administration.
AMERGE, IMITREX, IMITREX STATdose System, IMITREX STATdose Pen, and TREXIMET are registered trademarks of GlaxoSmithKline. The other brands listed are trademarks of their respective owners and are not trademarks of GlaxoSmithKline. The makers of these brands are not affiliated with and do not endorse GlaxoSmithKline or its products.
GlaxoSmithKline
Research Triangle Park, NC 27709
©2012, GlaxoSmithKline. All rights reserved.
October 2012
IMJ:3PIL

IMITREX
[ĭm'ĭ-trĕx]
(sumatriptan)
Nasal Spray ℞

HIGHLIGHTS OF PRESCRIBING INFORMATION
These highlights do not include all the information needed to use IMITREX safely and effectively. See full prescribing information for IMITREX.
IMITREX (sumatriptan) Nasal Spray
Initial U.S. Approval: 1992

―――――**INDICATIONS AND USAGE**―――――
IMITREX is a serotonin ($5\text{-HT}_{1B/1D}$) receptor agonist (triptan) indicated for acute treatment of migraine with or without aura in adults. (1)
Limitations of Use:
• Use only if a clear diagnosis of migraine headache has been established. (1)
• Not indicated for the prophylactic therapy of migraine attacks. (1)
• Not indicated for the treatment of cluster headache. (1)

―――**DOSAGE AND ADMINISTRATION**―――
• Single dose of 5 mg, 10 mg, or 20 mg of nasal spray. (2)
• A second dose should only be considered if some response to the first dose was observed. Separate doses by at least 2 hours. (2)
• Maximum dose in a 24-hour period: 40 mg. (2)

―――**DOSAGE FORMS AND STRENGTHS**―――
Nasal spray: 5 mg and 20 mg (3, 16)

―――――**CONTRAINDICATIONS**―――――
• History of coronary artery disease or coronary artery vasospasm. (4)
• Wolff-Parkinson-White syndrome or other cardiac accessory conduction pathway disorders. (4)
• History of stroke, transient ischemic attack, or hemiplegic or basilar migraine. (4)
• Peripheral vascular disease. (4)
• Ischemic bowel disease. (4)
• Uncontrolled hypertension. (4)
• Recent (within 24 hours) use of another 5-HT1 agonist (e.g., another triptan) or of an ergotamine-containing medication. (4)
• Concurrent or recent (past 2 weeks) use of monoamine oxidase-A inhibitor. (4)
• Hypersensitivity to IMITREX (angioedema and anaphylaxis seen). (4)
• Severe hepatic impairment. (4)

―――**WARNINGS AND PRECAUTIONS**―――
• Myocardial ischemia/infarction and Prinzmetal's angina: Perform cardiac evaluation in patients with multiple cardiovascular risk factors. (5.1)
• Arrhythmias: Discontinue IMITREX if occurs. (5.2)
• Chest/throat/neck/jaw pain, tightness, pressure, or heaviness: Generally not associated with myocardial ischemia; evaluate for coronary artery disease in patients at high risk. (5.3)
• Cerebral hemorrhage, subarachnoid hemorrhage, and stroke: Discontinue IMITREX if occurs. (5.4)
• Gastrointestinal ischemic reactions and peripheral vasospastic reactions: Discontinue IMITREX if occurs. (5.5)
• Medication overuse headache: Detoxification may be necessary. (5.6)
• Serotonin syndrome: Discontinue IMITREX if occurs. (5.7)
• Seizures: Use with caution in patients with epilepsy or a lowered seizure threshold. (5.11)

―――――**ADVERSE REACTIONS**―――――
Most common adverse reactions (≥1% and >placebo) were burning sensation, disorder/discomfort of nasal cavity/sinuses, throat discomfort, nausea and/or vomiting, bad/unusual taste, and dizziness/vertigo. (6.1)
To report SUSPECTED ADVERSE REACTIONS, contact GlaxoSmithKline at 1-888-825-5249 or FDA at 1-800-FDA-1088 or www.fda.gov/medwatch.

―――**USE IN SPECIFIC POPULATIONS**―――
Pregnancy: Based on animal data, may cause fetal harm. (8.1)
See 17 for PATIENT COUNSELING INFORMATION and FDA-approved patient labeling

Revised: 11/2013

FULL PRESCRIBING INFORMATION

1 INDICATIONS AND USAGE

IMITREX® Nasal Spray is indicated for the acute treatment of migraine with or without aura in adults.

Limitations of Use:
• Use only if a clear diagnosis of migraine headache has been established. If a patient has no response to the first migraine attack treated with IMITREX, reconsider the diagnosis of migraine before IMITREX is administered to treat any subsequent attacks.
• IMITREX is not indicated for the prevention of migraine attacks.
• Safety and effectiveness of IMITREX Nasal Spray have not been established for cluster headache.

2 DOSAGE AND ADMINISTRATION

The recommended adult dose of IMITREX Nasal Spray for the acute treatment of migraine is 5 mg, 10 mg, or 20 mg. The 20-mg dose may provide a greater effect than the 5-mg and 10-mg doses, but may have a greater risk of adverse reactions [see Clinical Studies (14)].

The 5-mg and 20-mg doses are given as a single spray in 1 nostril. The 10-mg dose may be achieved by the administration of a single 5-mg dose in each nostril.

If the migraine has not resolved by 2 hours after taking IMITREX Nasal Spray, or returns after a transient improvement, 1 additional dose may be administered at least 2 hours after the first dose. The maximum daily dose is 40 mg in a 24-hour period.

The safety of treating an average of more than 4 headaches in a 30–day period has not been established.

3 DOSAGE FORMS AND STRENGTHS

Unit dose nasal spray devices containing 5 mg or 20 mg sumatriptan.

4 CONTRAINDICATIONS

IMITREX Nasal Spray is contraindicated in patients with:
• Ischemic coronary artery disease (CAD) (angina pectoris, history of myocardial infarction, or documented silent ischemia) or coronary artery vasospasm, including Prinzmetal's angina [see Warnings and Precautions (5.1)]
• Wolff-Parkinson-White syndrome or arrhythmias associated with other cardiac accessory conduction pathway disorders [see Warnings and Precautions (5.2)]
• History of stroke, transient ischemic attack (TIA), or history of hemiplegic or basilar migraine because these patients are at a higher risk of stroke [see Warnings and Precautions (5.4)]
• Peripheral vascular disease [see Warnings and Precautions (5.5)]
• Ischemic bowel disease [see Warnings and Precautions (5.5)]
• Uncontrolled hypertension [see Warnings and Precautions (5.8)]
• Recent use (i.e., within 24 hours) of ergotamine-containing medication, ergot-type medication (such as dihydroergotamine or methysergide), or another 5-hydroxytryptamine$_1$ (5-HT$_1$) agonist [see Drug Interactions (7.1, 7.3)]
• Concurrent administration of a monoamine oxidase (MAO)-A inhibitor or recent (within 2 weeks) use of an MAO-A inhibitor [see Drug Interactions (7.2) and Clinical Pharmacology (12.3)]
• Hypersensitivity to IMITREX (angioedema and anaphylaxis seen) [see Warnings and Precautions (5.10)]
• Severe hepatic impairment [see Clinical Pharmacology (12.3)]

5 WARNINGS AND PRECAUTIONS

5.1 Myocardial Ischemia, Myocardial Infarction, and Prinzmetal's Angina

The use of IMITREX Nasal Spray is contraindicated in patients with ischemic or vasospastic CAD. There have been rare reports of serious cardiac adverse reactions, including acute myocardial infarction, occurring within a few hours following administration of IMITREX Nasal Spray. Some of these reactions occurred in patients without known CAD. IMITREX Nasal Spray may cause coronary artery vasospasm (Prinzmetal's angina), even in patients without a history of CAD.

Perform a cardiovascular evaluation in triptan-naive patients who have multiple cardiovascular risk factors (e.g., increased age, diabetes, hypertension, smoking, obesity, strong family history of CAD) prior to receiving IMITREX Nasal Spray. If there is evidence of CAD or coronary artery vasospasm, IMITREX Nasal Spray is contraindicated. For patients with multiple cardiovascular risk factors who have a negative cardiovascular evaluation, consider administering the first dose of IMITREX Nasal Spray in a medically supervised setting and performing an electrocardiogram (ECG) immediately following administration of IMITREX Nasal Spray. For such patients, consider periodic cardiovascular evaluation in intermittent long-term users of IMITREX Nasal Spray.

5.2 Arrhythmias

Life-threatening disturbances of cardiac rhythm, including ventricular tachycardia and ventricular fibrillation leading to death, have been reported within a few hours following the administration of 5-HT$_1$ agonists. Discontinue IMITREX Nasal Spray if these disturbances occur. IMITREX Nasal Spray is contraindicated in patients with Wolff-Parkinson-White syndrome or arrhythmias associated with other cardiac accessory conduction pathway disorders.

5.3 Chest, Throat, Neck, and/or Jaw Pain/Tightness/Pressure

Sensations of tightness, pain, pressure, and heaviness in the precordium, throat, neck, and jaw may occur after treatment with IMITREX Nasal Spray and are usually noncardiac in origin. However, perform a cardiac evaluation if these patients are at high cardiac risk. The use of IMITREX Nasal Spray is contraindicated in patients with CAD and those with Prinzmetal's variant angina.

5.4 Cerebrovascular Events

Cerebral hemorrhage, subarachnoid hemorrhage, and stroke have occurred in patients treated with 5-HT$_1$ agonists, and some have resulted in fatalities. In a number of cases, it appears possible that the cerebrovascular events were primary, the 5-HT$_1$ agonist having been administered in the incorrect belief that the symptoms experienced were a consequence of migraine when they were not. Also, patients with migraine may be at increased risk of certain cerebrovascular events (e.g., stroke, hemorrhage, TIA). Discontinue IMITREX Nasal Spray if a cerebrovascular event occurs.

Before treating headaches in patients not previously diagnosed as migraineurs, and in migraineurs who present with atypical symptoms, exclude other potentially serious neurological conditions. IMITREX Nasal Spray is contraindicated in patients with a history of stroke or TIA.

5.5 Other Vasospasm Reactions

IMITREX Nasal Spray may cause non-coronary vasospastic reactions, such as peripheral vascular ischemia, gastrointestinal vascular ischemia and infarction (presenting with abdominal pain and bloody diarrhea), splenic infarction, and Raynaud's syndrome. In patients who experience symptoms or signs suggestive of non-coronary vasospasm reaction following the use of any 5-HT$_1$ agonist, rule out a vasospastic reaction before using additional IMITREX Nasal Spray.

Reports of transient and permanent blindness and significant partial vision loss have been reported with the use of 5-HT$_1$ agonists. Since visual disorders may be part of a migraine attack, a causal relationship between these events and the use of 5-HT$_1$ agonists have not been clearly established.

5.6 Medication Overuse Headache

Overuse of acute migraine drugs (e.g., ergotamine, triptans, opioids, or combination of these drugs for 10 or more days per month) may lead to exacerbation of headache (medication overuse headache). Medication overuse headache may present as migraine-like daily headaches or as a marked increase in frequency of migraine attacks. Detoxification of patients, including withdrawal of the overused drugs, and treatment of withdrawal symptoms (which often includes a transient worsening of headache) may be necessary.

5.7 Serotonin Syndrome

Serotonin syndrome may occur with IMITREX Nasal Spray, particularly during co-administration with selective serotonin reuptake inhibitors (SSRIs), serotonin norepinephrine reuptake inhibitors (SNRIs), tricyclic antidepressants (TCAs), and MAO inhibitors [see Drug Interactions (7.4)]. Serotonin syndrome symptoms may include mental status changes (e.g., agitation, hallucinations, coma), autonomic instability (e.g., tachycardia, labile blood pressure, hyperthermia), neuromuscular aberrations (e.g., hyperreflexia, incoordination), and/or gastrointestinal symptoms (e.g., nausea, vomiting, diarrhea). The onset of symptoms usually occurs within minutes to hours of receiving a new or a greater dose of a serotonergic medication. Discontinue IMITREX Nasal Spray if serotonin syndrome is suspected.

5.8 Increase in Blood Pressure

Significant elevation in blood pressure, including hypertensive crisis with acute impairment of organ systems, has been reported on rare occasions in patients treated with 5-HT$_1$ agonists, including patients without a history of hypertension. Monitor blood pressure in patients treated with IMITREX. IMITREX Nasal Spray is contraindicated in patients with uncontrolled hypertension.

5.9 Local Irritation

Local irritative symptoms such as burning, numbness, paresthesia, discharge, and pain or soreness were reported in approximately 5% of patients in controlled clinical trials and were noted to be severe in about 1%. The symptoms were transient and generally resolved in less than 2 hours. Limited examinations of the nose and throat did not reveal any clinically noticeable injury in these patients. The consequences of extended and repeated use of Imitrex Nasal Spray on the nasal and/or respiratory mucosa have not been systematically evaluated in patients.

5.10 Anaphylactic/Anaphylactoid Reactions

Anaphylactic/anaphylactoid reactions have occurred in patients receiving IMITREX. Such reactions can be life threatening or fatal. In general, anaphylactic reactions to drugs are more likely to occur in individuals with a history of sensitivity to multiple allergens. IMITREX Nasal Spray is contraindicated in patients with a history of hypersensitivity reaction to IMITREX.

5.11 Seizures

Seizures have been reported following administration of IMITREX. Some have occurred in patients with either a history of seizures or concurrent conditions predisposing to seizures. There are also reports in patients where no such predisposing factors are apparent. IMITREX Nasal Spray should be used with caution in patients with a history of epilepsy or conditions associated with a lowered seizure threshold.

6 ADVERSE REACTIONS

The following adverse reactions are discussed in more detail in other sections of the prescribing information:
• Myocardial ischemia, myocardial infarction, and Prinzmetal's angina [see Warnings and Precautions (5.1)]
• Arrhythmias [see Warnings and Precautions (5.2)]
• Chest, throat, neck, and/or jaw pain/tightness/pressure [see Warnings and Precautions (5.3)]
• Cerebrovascular events [see Warnings and Precautions (5.4)]
• Other vasospasm reactions [see Warnings and Precautions (5.5)]
• Medication overuse headache [see Warnings and Precautions (5.6)]
• Serotonin syndrome [see Warnings and Precautions (5.7)]
• Increase in blood pressure [see Warnings and Precautions (5.8)]
• Local irritation [see Warnings and Precautions (5.9)]
• Hypersensitivity reactions [see Contraindications (4) and Warnings and Precautions (5.10)]
• Seizures [see Warnings and Precautions (5.11)]

6.1 Clinical Trials Experience

Because clinical trials are conducted under widely varying conditions, adverse reaction rates observed in the clinical trials of a drug cannot be directly compared with rates in the clinical trials of another drug and may not reflect the rates observed in practice.

Table 1 lists adverse reactions that occurred in worldwide placebo-controlled clinical trials in 3,419 patients with migraine. Only treatment-emergent adverse reactions that occurred at a frequency of 1% or more in the group treated with IMITREX Nasal Spray 20 mg and that occurred at a frequency greater than the placebo group are included in Table 1.

Table 1. Adverse Reactions Reported by at Least 1% of Patients and at a Greater Frequency Than Placebo in Controlled Migraine Clinical Trials

Adverse Reaction	Percent of Patients Reporting			
	IMITREX Nasal Spray 5 mg (n = 496)	IMITREX Nasal Spray 10 mg (n = 1,007)	IMITREX Nasal Spray 20 mg (n = 1,212)	Placebo (n = 704)
Atypical sensations				
Burning sensation	0.4	0.6	1.4	0.1
Ear, nose, and throat				
Disorder/discomfort of nasal cavity/sinuses	2.8	2.5	3.8	2.4
Throat discomfort	0.8	1.8	2.4	0.9
Gastrointestinal				
Nausea and/or vomiting	12.2	11.0	13.5	11.3
Neurological				
Bad/unusual taste	13.5	19.3	24.5	1.7
Dizziness/vertigo	1.0	1.7	1.4	0.9

[See table 1 above]
The incidence of adverse reactions in controlled clinical trials was not affected by gender, weight, or age of the patients; use of prophylactic medications; or presence of aura. There were insufficient data to assess the impact of race on the incidence of adverse reactions.

6.2   Postmarketing Experience
The following adverse reactions have been identified during postapproval use of IMITREX Tablets, IMITREX Nasal Spray, and IMITREX Injection. Because these reactions are reported voluntarily from a population of uncertain size, it is not always possible to reliably estimate their frequency or establish a causal relationship to drug exposure. These reactions have been chosen for inclusion due to either their seriousness, frequency of reporting, or causal connection to IMITREX or a combination of these factors.
Cardiovascular: Hypotension, palpitations.
Neurological: Dystonia, tremor.

7   DRUG INTERACTIONS
7.1   Ergot-Containing Drugs
Ergot-containing drugs have been reported to cause prolonged vasospastic reactions. Because these effects may be additive, use of ergotamine-containing or ergot-type medications (like dihydroergotamine or methysergide) and IMITREX Nasal Spray within 24 hours of each other is contraindicated.
7.2   Monoamine Oxidase-A Inhibitors
MAO-A inhibitors increase systemic exposure by up to 7-fold. Therefore, the use of IMITREX Nasal Spray in patients receiving MAO-A inhibitors is contraindicated [see Clinical Pharmacology (12.3)].
7.3   Other 5-HT₁ Agonists
Because their vasospastic effects may be additive, co-administration of IMITREX Nasal Spray and other 5-HT₁ agonists (e.g., triptans) within 24 hours of each other is contraindicated.
7.4   Selective Serotonin Reuptake Inhibitors/Serotonin Norepinephrine Reuptake Inhibitors and Serotonin Syndrome
Cases of serotonin syndrome have been reported during coadministration of triptans and SSRIs, SNRIs, TCAs, and MAO inhibitors [see Warnings and Precautions (5.7)].

8   USE IN SPECIFIC POPULATIONS
8.1   Pregnancy
Pregnancy Category C: There are no adequate and well-controlled trials in pregnant women. In developmental toxicity studies in rats and rabbits, oral administration of sumatriptan to pregnant animals was associated with embryolethality, fetal abnormalities, and pup mortality. When administered by the intravenous route to pregnant rabbits, sumatriptan was embryolethal. Developmental toxicity studies of sumatriptan by the intranasal route have not been conducted. IMITREX Nasal Spray should be used during pregnancy only if the potential benefit justifies the potential risk to the fetus.
Oral administration of sumatriptan to pregnant rats during the period of organogenesis resulted in an increased incidence of fetal blood vessel (cervicothoracic and umbilical) abnormalities. The highest no-effect dose for embryofetal developmental toxicity in rats was 60 mg/kg/day. Oral administration of sumatriptan to pregnant rabbits during the period of organogenesis resulted in increased incidences of embryolethality and fetal cervicothoracic vascular and skeletal abnormalities. Intravenous administration of sumatriptan to pregnant rabbits during the period of organogenesis resulted in an increased incidence of embryolethal-

ity. The highest oral and intravenous no-effect doses for developmental toxicity in rabbits were 15 and 0.75 mg/kg/day, respectively.
Oral administration of sumatriptan to rats prior to and throughout gestation resulted in embryofetal toxicity (decreased body weight, decreased ossification, increased incidence of skeletal abnormalities). The highest no-effect dose was 50 mg/kg/day. In offspring of pregnant rats treated orally with sumatriptan during organogenesis, there was a decrease in pup survival. The highest no-effect dose for this effect was 60 mg/kg/day. Oral treatment of pregnant rats with sumatriptan during the latter part of gestation and throughout lactation resulted in a decrease in pup survival. The highest no-effect dose for this finding was 100 mg/kg/day.
8.3   Nursing Mothers
Sumatriptan is excreted in human milk following subcutaneous administration. Infant exposure to sumatriptan can be minimized by avoiding breastfeeding for 12 hours after treatment with IMITREX Nasal Spray.
8.4   Pediatric Use
Safety and effectiveness in pediatric patients have not been established. IMITREX Nasal Spray is not recommended for use in patients younger than 18 years of age.
Two controlled clinical trials evaluated IMITREX Nasal Spray (5 to 20 mg) in 1,248 adolescent migraineurs aged 12 to 17 years who treated a single attack. The trials did not establish the efficacy of IMITREX Nasal Spray compared with placebo in the treatment of migraine in adolescents. Adverse reactions observed in these clinical trials were similar in nature to those reported in clinical trials in adults.
Five controlled clinical trials (2 single-attack trials, 3 multiple-attack trials) evaluating oral IMITREX (25 to 100 mg) in pediatric patients aged 12 to 17 years enrolled a total of 701 adolescent migraineurs. These trials did not establish the efficacy of oral IMITREX compared with placebo in the treatment of migraine in adolescents. Adverse reactions observed in these clinical trials were similar in nature to those reported in clinical trials in adults. The frequency of all adverse reactions in these patients appeared to be both dose- and age-dependent, with younger patients reporting reactions more commonly than older adolescents.
Postmarketing experience documents that serious adverse reactions have occurred in the pediatric population after use of subcutaneous, oral, and/or intranasal IMITREX. These reports include reactions similar in nature to those reported rarely in adults, including stroke, visual loss, and death. A myocardial infarction has been reported in a 14–year–old male following the use of oral IMITREX; clinical signs occurred within 1 day of drug administration. Clinical data to determine the frequency of serious adverse reactions in pediatric patients who might receive subcutaneous, oral, or intranasal IMITREX are not presently available.
8.5   Geriatric Use
Clinical trials of IMITREX Nasal Spray did not include sufficient numbers of patients aged 65 and older to determine whether they respond differently from younger patients. Other reported clinical experience has not identified differences in responses between the elderly and younger patients. In general, dose selection for an elderly patient should be cautious, usually starting at the low end of the dosing range, reflecting the greater frequency of decreased hepatic, renal, or cardiac function and of concomitant disease or other drug therapy.
A cardiovascular evaluation is recommended for geriatric patients who have other cardiovascular risk factors (e.g., diabetes, hypertension, smoking, obesity, strong family history of CAD) prior to receiving IMITREX Nasal Spray [see Warnings and Precautions (5.1)].

10   OVERDOSAGE
In clinical trials, the highest single doses of IMITREX Nasal Spray administered without significant reactions were 40 mg to 12 volunteers and 40 mg to 85 subjects with migraine, which is twice the highest single recommended dose. In addition, 12 volunteers were administered a total daily dose of 60 mg (20 mg 3 times daily) for 3.5 days without significant adverse reactions.
Overdose in animals has been fatal and has been heralded by convulsions, tremor, paralysis, inactivity, ptosis, erythema of the extremities, abnormal respiration, cyanosis, ataxia, mydriasis, salivation, and lacrimation.
The elimination half–life of sumatriptan is approximately 2 hours [see Clinical Pharmacology (12.3)], and therefore monitoring of patients after overdose with IMITREX Nasal Spray should continue for at least 10 hours or while symptoms or signs persist.
It is unknown what effect hemodialysis or peritoneal dialysis has on the serum concentrations of sumatriptan.

11   DESCRIPTION
IMITREX Nasal Spray contains sumatriptan, a selective 5-HT$_{1B/1D}$ receptor agonist. Sumatriptan is chemically designated as 3-[2-(dimethylamino)ethyl]-N-methyl-indole-5-methanesulfonamide, and it has the following structure:

The empirical formula is $C_{14}H_{21}N_3O_2S$, representing a molecular weight of 295.4. Sumatriptan is a white to off-white powder that is readily soluble in water and in saline.
Each IMITREX Nasal Spray contains 5 or 20 mg of sumatriptan in a 100-µL unit dose aqueous buffered solution containing monobasic potassium phosphate NF, anhydrous dibasic sodium phosphate USP, sulfuric acid NF, sodium hydroxide NF, and purified water USP. The pH of the solution is approximately 5.5. The osmolality of the solution is 372 or 742 mOsmol for the 5- and 20-mg IMITREX Nasal Spray, respectively.

12   CLINICAL PHARMACOLOGY
12.1   Mechanism of Action
Sumatriptan binds with high affinity to human cloned 5-HT$_{1B/1D}$ receptors. Sumatriptan presumably exerts its therapeutic effects in the treatment of migraine headache through agonist effects at the 5–HT$_{1B/1D}$ receptors on intracranial blood vessels and sensory nerves of the trigeminal system, which result in cranial vessel constriction and inhibition of pro-inflammatory neuropeptide release..
12.2   Pharmacodynamics
Blood Pressure: Significant elevation in blood pressure, including hypertensive crisis, has been reported in patients with and without a history of hypertension [see Warnings and Precautions (5.8)].
Peripheral (Small) Arteries: In healthy volunteers (N = 18), a trial evaluating the effects of sumatriptan on peripheral (small vessel) arterial reactivity failed to detect a clinically significant increase in peripheral resistance.
Heart Rate: Transient increases in blood pressure observed in some patients in clinical trials carried out during sumatriptan's development as a treatment for migraine were not accompanied by any clinically significant changes in heart rate.
12.3   Pharmacokinetics
Absorption and Bioavailability: In a trial of 20 female volunteers, the mean maximum concentration following a 5- and 20-mg intranasal dose was 5 and 16 ng/mL, respectively. The mean C$_{max}$ following a 6–mg subcutaneous injection is 71 ng/mL (range: 49 to 110 ng/mL). The mean C$_{max}$ is 18 ng/mL (range: 7 to 47 ng/mL) following oral dosing with 25 mg and 51 ng/mL (range: 28 to 100 ng/mL) following oral dosing with 100 mg of sumatriptan. In a trial of 24 male volunteers, the bioavailability relative to subcutaneous injection was low, approximately 17%, primarily due to presystemic metabolism and partly due to incomplete absorption.
Clinical and pharmacokinetic data indicate that administration of two 5-mg doses, 1 dose in each nostril, is equivalent to administration of a single 10-mg dose in 1 nostril.
Distribution: Protein binding, determined by equilibrium dialysis over the concentration range of 10 to 1,000 ng/mL, is low, approximately 14% to 21%. The effect of sumatriptan on the protein binding of other drugs has not been evaluated. The apparent volume of distribution is 2.7 L/kg.
Metabolism: In vitro studies with human microsomes suggest that sumatriptan is metabolized by MAO, predominantly the A isoenzyme. Most of a radiolabeled dose of sumatriptan excreted in the urine is the major metabolite indole acetic acid (IAA) or the IAA glucuronide, both of which are inactive.
Elimination: The elimination half-life of sumatriptan administered as a nasal spray is approximately 2 hours, sim-

ilar to the half-life seen after subcutaneous injection. Only 3% of the dose is excreted in the urine as unchanged sumatriptan; 42% of the dose is excreted as the major metabolite, the indole acetic acid analogue of sumatriptan. The total plasma clearance is approximately 1,200 mL/min.

Special Populations: *Age:* The pharmacokinetics of sumatriptan in the elderly (mean age: 72 years, 2 males and 4 females) and in subjects with migraine (mean age: 38 years, 25 males and 155 females) were similar to that in healthy male subjects (mean age: 30 years). Intranasal sumatriptan has not been evaluated for age differences.

Renal Impairment: The effect of renal impairment on the pharmacokinetics of sumatriptan has not been examined.

Hepatic Impairment: The effect of mild to moderate hepatic disease on the pharmacokinetics of the intranasal formulation of sumatriptan has not been evaluated. Sumatriptan bioavailability following intranasal administration is 17%, similar to that after oral administration (15%). Following oral administration, an approximately 70% increase in C_{max} and AUC was observed in one small trial of patients with moderate liver impairment (n = 8) matched for sex, age and weight with healthy subjects (n = 8). Similar changes can be expected following intranasal administration.

The pharmacokinetics of sumatriptan in patients with severe hepatic impairment has not been studied. The use of IMITREX Nasal Spray in patients with severe hepatic impairment is contraindicated *[see Contraindications (4)]*.

Race: The systemic clearance and C_{max} of subcutaneous sumatriptan were similar in black (n = 34) and Caucasian (n = 38) healthy male subjects. Intranasal sumatriptan has not been evaluated for race differences.

Drug Interaction Studies: *Monoamine Oxidase-A Inhibitors:* Treatment with MAO-A inhibitors generally leads to an increase of sumatriptan plasma levels *[see Contraindications (4) and Drug Interactions (7.2)]*. MAO inhibitors interaction studies have not been performed with intranasal sumatriptan.

Due to gut and hepatic metabolic first-pass effects, the increase of systemic exposure after co-administration of an MAO-A inhibitor with oral sumatriptan is greater than after co-administration of the MAO inhibitors with subcutaneous sumatriptan. The effects of an MAO inhibitor on systemic exposure after intranasal sumatriptan would be expected to be greater than the effect after subcutaneous sumatriptan but smaller than the effect after oral sumatriptan because only swallowed drug would be subject to first-pass effects.

In a trial of 14 healthy females, pretreatment with an MAO-A inhibitor decreased the clearance of subcutaneous sumatriptan, resulting in a 2-fold increase in the area under the sumatriptan plasma concentration-time curve (AUC), corresponding to a 40% increase in elimination half-life.

A small trial evaluating the effect of pretreatment with an MAO-A inhibitor on the bioavailability from a 25-mg oral sumatriptan tablet resulted in an approximately 7-fold increase in systemic exposure.

Xylometazoline: An in vivo drug interaction trial indicated that 3 drops of xylometazoline (0.1% w/v), a decongestant, administered 15 minutes prior to a 20-mg nasal dose of sumatriptan did not alter the pharmacokinetics of sumatriptan.

13 NONCLINICAL TOXICOLOGY

13.1 Carcinogenesis, Mutagenesis, Impairment of Fertility

Carcinogenesis: In carcinogenicity studies in mouse and rat in which sumatriptan was administered orally for 78 and 104 weeks, respectively, there was no evidence in either species of an increase in tumors related to sumatriptan administration.

Carcinogenicity studies of sumatriptan using the nasal route have not been conducted.

Mutagenesis: Sumatriptan was negative in in vitro(bacterial reverse mutation [Ames], gene cell mutation in Chinese hamster V79/HGPRT, chromosomal aberration in human lymphocytes) and in vivo (rat micronucleus) assays.

Impairment of Fertility: When sumatriptan was administered by subcutaneous injection to male and female rats prior to and throughout the mating period, there was no evidence of impaired fertility at doses up to 60 mg/kg/day. When sumatriptan (5, 50, or 500 mg/kg/day) was administered orally to male and female rats prior to and throughout the mating period, there was a treatment-related decrease in fertility secondary to a decrease in mating in animals treated with doses greater than 5 mg/kg/day. It is not clear whether this finding was due to an effect on males or females or both.

Fertility studies of sumatriptan using the intranasal route have not been conducted.

13.2 Animal Toxicology and/or Pharmacology

Corneal Opacities: Dogs receiving oral sumatriptan developed corneal opacities and defects in the corneal epithelium. Corneal opacities were seen at the lowest dose tested,

2 mg/kg/day, and were present after 1 month of treatment. Defects in the corneal epithelium were noted in a 60–week study. Earlier examinations for these toxicities were not conducted and no-effect doses were not established.

14 CLINICAL STUDIES

The efficacy of Imitrex Nasal Spray in the acute treatment of migraine headaches was demonstrated in 8, randomized, double-blind, placebo-controlled trials, of which 5 used the recommended dosing regimen and used the marketed formulation. Patients enrolled in these 5 trials were predominately female (86%) and Caucasian (95%), with a mean age of 41 years (range of 18 to 65 years). Patients were instructed to treat a moderate to severe headache. Headache response, defined as a reduction in headache severity from moderate or severe pain to mild or no pain, was assessed up to 2 hours after dosing. Associated symptoms such as nausea, photophobia, and phonophobia were also assessed. Maintenance of response was assessed for up to 24 hours postdose. A second dose of IMITREX Nasal Spray or other medication was allowed 2 to 24 hours after the initial treatment for recurrent headache. The frequency and time to use of these additional treatments were also determined. In all trials, doses of 10 and 20 mg were compared with placebo in the treatment of 1 to 3 migraine attacks. Patients received doses as a single spray into 1 nostril. In 2 trials, a 5-mg dose was also evaluated.

In all 5 trials utilizing the market formulation and recommended dosage regimen, the percentage of patients achieving headache response 2 hours after treatment was significantly greater among patients receiving Imitrex Nasal Spray at all doses (with one exception) compared with those who received placebo. In 4 of the 5 trials, there was a statistically significant greater percentage of patients with headache response at 2 hours in the 20-mg group when compared with the lower dose groups (5 and 10 mg). There were no statistically significant differences between the 5- and 10-mg dose groups in any trial. The results from the 5 controlled clinical trials are summarized in Table 2. Note that, in general, comparisons of results obtained in trials conducted under different conditions by different investigators with different samples of patients are ordinarily unreliable for purposes of quantitative comparison

[See table 2 above]

The estimated probability of achieving an initial headache response over the 2 hours following treatment is depicted in Figure 1.

[See figure 1 at top of next column]

For patients with migraine-associated nausea, photophobia, and phonophobia at baseline, there was a lower incidence of these symptoms at 2 hours following administration of IMITREX Nasal Spray compared with placebo.

Two to 24 hours following the initial dose of study treatment, patients were allowed to use additional treatment for pain relief in the form of a second dose of study treatment or other medication. The estimated probability of patients taking a second dose or other medication for migraine over the 24 hours following the initial dose of study treatment is summarized in Figure 2.

[See figure 2 at top of next column]

There is evidence that doses above 20 mg do not provide a greater effect than 20 mg. There was no evidence to suggest that treatment with sumatriptan was associated with an increase in the severity of recurrent headaches. The efficacy of IMITREX Nasal Spray was unaffected by presence of aura; duration of headache prior to treatment; gender, age, or weight of the subject; or concomitant use of common mi-

Table 2. Percentage of Patients With Headache Response (No or Mild Pain) 2 Hours Following Treatment

	IMITREX Nasal Spray 5 mg	IMITREX Nasal Spray 10 mg	IMITREX Nasal Spray 20 mg	Placebo
Trial 1	49%[a] (n = 121)	46%[a] (n = 112)	64%[a,b,c] (n = 118)	25% (n = 63)
Trial 2	Not applicable	44%[a] (n = 273)	55%[a,b] (n = 277)	25% (n = 138)
Trial 3	Not applicable	54%[a] (n = 106)	63%[a] (n = 202)	35% (n = 100)
Trial 4	Not applicable	43% (n = 106)	62%[a,b] (n = 215)	29% (n = 112)
Trial 5[d]	45%[a] (n = 296)	53%[a] (n = 291)	60%[a,c] (n = 286)	36% (n = 198)

[a]$P<0.05$ in comparison with placebo.
[b]$P<0.05$ in comparison with 10 mg.
[c]$P<0.05$ in comparison with 5 mg.
[d]Data are for attack 1 only of multi-attack trial for comparison.

Figure 1. Estimated Probability of Achieving Initial Headache Response Within 120 Minutes[a]

[a]The figure shows the probability over time of obtaining headache response (no or mild pain) following treatment with intranasal sumatriptan. The averages displayed are based on pooled data from the 5 clinical controlled trials providing evidence of efficacy. Kaplan-Meier plot with patients not achieving response within 120 minutes censored to 120 minutes.

Figure 2. The Estimated Probability of Patients Taking a Second Dose or Other Medication for Migraine Over the 24 Hours Following the Initial Dose of Study Treatment[a]

[a]Kaplan-Meier plot based on data obtained in the 3 clinical controlled trials providing evidence of efficacy with patients not using additional treatments censored to 24 hours. Plot also includes patients who had no response to the initial dose. No remediation was allowed within 2 hours postdose.

graine prophylactic drugs (e.g., beta-blockers, calcium channel blockers, tricyclic antidepressants). There were insufficient data to assess the impact of race on efficacy.

16 HOW SUPPLIED/STORAGE AND HANDLING

IMITREX Nasal Spray 5 mg (NDC 0173-0524-00) and 20 mg (NDC 0173-0523-00) are each supplied in boxes of 6 nasal spray devices. Each unit dose spray supplies 5 mg and 20 mg, respectively, of sumatriptan.

Store between 2°C and 30°C (36°F and 86°F). Protect from light.

17 PATIENT COUNSELING INFORMATION

Advise the patient to read the FDA-approved patient labeling (Patient Information).

Risk of Myocardial Ischemia and/or Infarction, Prinzmetal's Angina, Other Vasospasm-Related Events, Arrhythmias, and Cerebrovascular Events: Inform patients that IMITREX Nasal Spray may cause serious cardiovascular side effects such as myocardial infarction or stroke. Although serious cardiovascular events can occur without warning symptoms, patients should be alert for the signs and symptoms of chest pain, shortness of breath, irregular heartbeat, significant rise in blood pressure, weakness, and slurring of speech and should ask for medical advice if any indicative sign or symptoms are observed. Apprise patients of the importance of this follow-up [see Warnings and Precautions (5.1, 5.2, 5.4, 5.5, 5.8)].

Anaphylactic/Anaphylactoid Reactions: Inform patients that anaphylactic/anaphylactoid reactions have occurred in patients receiving IMITREX Nasal Spray. Such reactions can be life threatening or fatal. In general, anaphylactic reactions to drugs are more likely to occur in individuals with a history of sensitivity to multiple allergens [see Contraindications (4) and Warnings and Precautions (5.10)].

Concomitant Use With Other Triptans or Ergot Medications: Inform patients that use of IMITREX Nasal Spray within 24 hours of another triptan or an ergot-type medication (including dihydroergotamine or methysergide) is contraindicated [see Contraindications (4) and Drug Interactions (7.1, 7.3)].

Serotonin Syndrome: Caution patients about the risk of serotonin syndrome with the use of IMITREX Nasal Spray or other triptans, particularly during combined use with SSRIs, SNRIs, TCAs, and MAO inhibitors [see Warnings and Precautions (5.7) and Drug Interactions (7.4)].

Medication Overuse Headache: Inform patients that use of acute migraine drugs for 10 or more days per month may lead to an exacerbation of headache and encourage patients to record headache frequency and drug use (e.g., by keeping a headache diary) [see Warnings and Precautions (5.6)].

Pregnancy: Inform patients that IMITREX Nasal Spray should not be used during pregnancy unless the potential benefit justifies the potential risk to the fetus [see Use in Specific Populations (8.1)].

Nursing Mothers: Advise patients to notify their healthcare provider if they are breastfeeding or plan to breastfeed [see Use in Specific Populations (8.3)].

Ability to Perform Complex Tasks: Treatment with IMITREX Nasal Spray may cause somnolence and dizziness; instruct patients to evaluate their ability to perform complex tasks after administration of IMITREX Nasal Spray.

Local Irritation: Inform patients that they may experience local irritation of their nose and throat. The symptoms will generally resolve in less than 2 hours.

How to Use IMITREX Nasal Spray: Provide patients instruction on the proper use of IMITREX Nasal Spray. Caution patients to avoid spraying the contents of the device in their eyes.

Imitrex is a registered trademark of the GlaxoSmithKline group of companies.

GlaxoSmithKline
Research Triangle Park, NC 27709
©2013, GlaxoSmithKline group of companies. All rights reserved.

IMN:4PI

Patient Information
IMITREX® (IM-i-trex)
(sumatriptan)
Nasal Spray

Read this Patient Information before you start using IMITREX and each time you get a refill. There may be new information. This information does not take the place of talking with your healthcare provider about your medical condition or treatment.

What is the most important information I should know about IMITREX?
IMITREX can cause serious side effects, including:
Heart attack and other heart problems. Heart problems may lead to death.
Stop taking IMITREX and get emergency medical help right away if you have any of the following symptoms of a heart attack:
• discomfort in the center of your chest that lasts for more than a few minutes, or that goes away and comes back
• severe tightness, pain, pressure, or heaviness in your chest, throat, neck, or jaw
• pain or discomfort in your arms, back, neck, jaw, or stomach
• shortness of breath with or without chest discomfort
• breaking out in a cold sweat
• nausea or vomiting
• feeling lightheaded
IMITREX is not for people with risk factors for heart disease unless a heart exam is done and shows no problem. You have a higher risk for heart disease if you:
• have high blood pressure
• have high cholesterol levels
• smoke
• are overweight
• have diabetes
• have a family history of heart disease

What is IMITREX?
IMITREX is a prescription medicine used to treat acute migraine headaches with or without aura in adults.
IMITREX is not used to treat other types of headaches, such as hemiplegic (that make you unable to move on one side of your body) or basilar (rare form of migraine with aura) migraines.
IMITREX is not used to prevent or decrease the number of migraine headaches you have.
It is not known if IMITREX is safe and effective to treat cluster headaches.
It is not known if IMITREX is safe and effective in children under 18 years of age.
Who should not use IMITREX?
Do not use IMITREX if you have:
• heart problems or a history of heart problems
• narrowing of blood vessels to your legs, arms, stomach, or kidneys (peripheral vascular disease)
• uncontrolled high blood pressure
• severe liver problems
• hemiplegic migraines or basilar migraines. If you are not sure if you have these types of migraines, ask your healthcare provider.
• had a stroke, transient ischemic attacks (TIAs), or problems with your blood circulation
• taken any of the following medicines in the last 24 hours:
  ◦ almotriptan (AXERT®)
  ◦ eletriptan (RELPAX®)
  ◦ frovatriptan (FROVA®)
  ◦ naratriptan (AMERGE®)
  ◦ rizatriptan (MAXALT®, MAXALT-MLT®)
  ◦ sumatriptan and naproxen (TREXIMET®)
  ◦ ergotamines (CAFERGOT®, ERGOMAR®, MIGERGOT®)
  ◦ dihydroergotamine (D.H.E. 45®, MIGRANAL®)
  Ask your healthcare provider if you are not sure if your medicine is listed above.
• an allergy to sumatriptan or any of the ingredients in IMITREX. See below for a complete list of ingredients in IMITREX.
What should I tell my healthcare provider before using IMITREX?
Before you use IMITREX, tell your healthcare provider about all of your medical conditions, including if you:
• have high blood pressure
• have high cholesterol
• have diabetes
• smoke
• are overweight
• have heart problems or family history of heart problems or stroke
• have kidney problems
• have liver problems
• have had epilepsy or seizures
• are not using effective birth control
• become pregnant while taking IMITREX
• are breastfeeding or plan to breastfeed. IMITREX passes into your breast milk and may harm your baby. Talk with your healthcare provider about the best way to feed your baby if you use IMITREX.
Tell your healthcare provider about all the medicines you take, including prescription and nonprescription medicines, vitamins, and herbal supplements.
IMITREX and certain other medicines can affect each other, causing serious side effects.
Especially tell your healthcare provider if you take anti-depressant medicines called:
• selective serotonin reuptake inhibitors (SSRIs)
• serotonin norepinephrine reuptake inhibitors (SNRIs)
• tricyclic antidepressants (TCAs)
• monoamine oxidase inhibitors (MAOIs)
Ask your healthcare provider or pharmacist for a list of these medicines if you are not sure.
Know the medicines you take. Keep a list of them to show your healthcare provider or pharmacist when you get a new medicine.
How should I use IMITREX?
• Certain people should use their first dose of IMITREX in their healthcare provider's office or in another medical setting. Ask your healthcare provider if you should use your first dose in a medical setting.
• Use IMITREX exactly as your healthcare provider tells you to use it.
• Your healthcare provider may change your dose. Do not change your dose without first talking with your healthcare provider.
• If you do not get any relief after your first nasal spray, do not use a second nasal spray without first talking with your healthcare provider.
• If your headache comes back after the first nasal spray or you only get some relief from your headache, you can use a second nasal spray 2 hours after the first nasal spray.
• Do not use more than 40 mg of IMITREX Nasal Spray in a 24–hour period.

• It is not known how using IMITREX Nasal Spray for a long time affects the nose and throat.
• If you use too much IMITREX, call your healthcare provider or go to the nearest hospital emergency room right away.
• You should write down when you have headaches and when you use IMITREX so you can talk with your healthcare provider about how IMITREX is working for you.
What should I avoid while using IMITREX?
IMITREX can cause dizziness, weakness, or drowsiness. If you have these symptoms, do not drive a car, use machinery, or do anything where you need to be alert.
What are the possible side effects of IMITREX?
IMITREX may cause serious side effects. See "What is the most important information I should know about IMITREX?"
These serious side effects include:
• changes in color or sensation in your fingers and toes (Raynaud's syndrome)
• stomach and intestinal problems (gastrointestinal and colonic ischemic events). Symptoms of gastrointestinal and colonic ischemic events include:
  ◦ sudden or severe stomach pain
  ◦ stomach pain after meals
  ◦ weight loss
  ◦ nausea or vomiting
  ◦ constipation or diarrhea
  ◦ bloody diarrhea
  ◦ fever
• problems with blood circulation to your legs and feet (peripheral vascular ischemia). Symptoms of peripheral vascular ischemia include:
  ◦ cramping and pain in your legs or hips
  ◦ feeling of heaviness or tightness in your leg muscles
  ◦ burning or aching pain in your feet or toes while resting
  ◦ numbness, tingling, or weakness in your legs
  ◦ cold feeling or color changes in 1 or both legs or feet
• hives (itchy bumps); swelling of your tongue, mouth, or throat
• medication overuse headaches. Some people who use too many IMITREX nasal sprays may have worse headaches (medication overuse headache). If your headaches get worse, your healthcare provider may decide to stop your treatment with IMITREX.
• serotonin syndrome. Serotonin syndrome is a rare but serious problem that can happen in people using IMITREX, especially if IMITREX is used with anti-depressant medicines called SSRIs or SNRIs.
Call your healthcare provider right away if you have any of the following symptoms of serotonin syndrome:
  ◦ mental changes such as seeing things that are not there (hallucinations), agitation, or coma
  ◦ fast heartbeat
  ◦ changes in blood pressure
  ◦ high body temperature
  ◦ tight muscles
  ◦ trouble walking
• seizures. Seizures have happened in people taking IMITREX who have never had seizures before. Talk with your healthcare provider about your chance of having seizures while you take IMITREX.
The most common side effects of IMITREX Nasal Spray include:
• unusual or bad taste in your mouth
• nausea and/or vomiting
• discomfort of your throat or nose
• dizziness
• warm, hot, burning feeling
Tell your healthcare provider if you have any side effect that bothers you or that does not go away.
These are not all the possible side effects of IMITREX. For more information, ask your healthcare provider or pharmacist.
Call your doctor for medical advice about side effects. You may report side effects to FDA at 1-800-FDA-1088.
How should I store IMITREX Nasal Spray?
• Store IMITREX between 36°F to 86°F (2°C to 30°C).
• Store your medicine away from light.
Keep IMITREX and all medicines out of the reach of children.
General information about the safe and effective use of IMITREX.
Medicines are sometimes prescribed for purposes other than those listed in Patient Information leaflets. Do not use IMITREX for a condition for which it was not prescribed. Do not give IMITREX to other people, even if they have the same symptoms you have. It may harm them.
This Patient Information leaflet summarizes the most important information about IMITREX. If you would like more information, talk with your healthcare provider. You can ask your healthcare provider or pharmacist for information about IMITREX that is written for healthcare professionals.
For more information, go to www.gsk.com or call 1-888-825-5249.

What are the ingredients in IMITREX Nasal Spray?

Active ingredient: sumatriptan

Inactive ingredients: monobasic potassium phosphate NF, anhydrous dibasic sodium phosphate USP, sulfuric acid NF, sodium hydroxide NF, and purified water USP.

This Patient Information has been approved by the U.S. Food and Drug Administration.

IMITREX, AMERGE, and TREXIMET are registered trademarks of the GlaxoSmithKline group of companies. The other brands listed are trademarks of their respective owners and are not trademarks of GlaxoSmithKline. The makers of these brands are not affiliated with and do not endorse GlaxoSmithKline or its products.

GlaxoSmithKline

Research Triangle Park, NC 27709

©2013, GlaxoSmithKline group of companies. All rights reserved.

November 2013

IMN:4PPI

Instructions for Use

IMITREX® (IM-i-trex)

(sumatriptan)

Nasal Spray

For use in the nose only. Do not spray in your eyes.

Step 1. Remove the IMITREX Nasal Spray unit from the plastic pack **(see Figure A)**. Do not remove the unit until you are ready to use. The unit contains only 1 spray. **Do not test before use.**

Figure A

Step 2. While sitting down, gently blow your nose to clear your nasal passages **(see Figure B).**

Figure B

Step 3. Keeping your head in an upright position, gently close 1 nostril with your index finger and breathe out gently through your mouth **(see Figure C).**

Figure C

Step 4. With your other hand, hold the container with your thumb supporting the container at the bottom, and your index and middle fingers on either side of the nozzle **(see Figure D).** Insert the nozzle into your open nostril about ½ inch. **Do not press the blue plunger yet.**

Figure D

Step 5. Keep your head upright and close your mouth. While gently taking a breath in through your nose, press the blue plunger firmly to release the dose of IMITREX Nasal Spray **(see Figure E).**

Figure E

Step 6. Keep your head level and remove the nozzle from your nostril. While holding your head level, gently breathe in through your nose and out through your mouth for 10 to 20 seconds **(see Figure F). Do not breathe in deeply.**

Figure F

IIMITREX, AMERGE, and TREXIMET are registered trademarks of the GlaxoSmithKline group of companies. The other brands listed are trademarks of their respective owners and are not trademarks of the GlaxoSmithKline

group of companies. The makers of these brands are not affiliated with and do not endorse the GlaxoSmithKline group of companies or its products.

This Patient Information and Instructions for Use have been approved by the U.S. Food and Drug Administration.

GlaxoSmithKline

Research Triangle Park, NC 27709

©2013, GlaxoSmithKline group of companies. All rights reserved.

November 2013

IMN:4PIL

IMITREX®

[Ĭm'ĭ-trĕx]

(sumatriptan succinate)

Tablets

℞

HIGHLIGHTS OF PRESCRIBING INFORMATION

These highlights do not include all the information needed to use IMITREX safely and effectively. See full prescribing information for IMITREX.

IMITREX (sumatriptan succinate) Tablets

Initial U.S. Approval: 1992

——INDICATIONS AND USAGE——

IMITREX is a serotonin (5-HT1B/1D) receptor agonist (triptan) indicated for acute treatment of migraine with or without aura in adults. (1)

Limitations of Use:

- Use only if a clear diagnosis of migraine headache has been established. (1)
- Not indicated for the prophylactic therapy of migraine attacks. (1)
- Not indicated for the treatment of cluster headache. (1)

——DOSAGE AND ADMINISTRATION——

- Single dose of 25- mg, 50-mg, or 100-mg tablet. (2.1)
- A second dose should only be considered if some response to the first dose was observed. Separate doses by at least 2 hours. (2.1)
- Maximum dose in a 24-hour period: 200 mg. (2.1)
- Maximum single dose should not exceed 50 mg in patients with mild to moderate hepatic impairment. (2.2)

——DOSAGE FORMS AND STRENGTHS——

Tablets: 25 mg, 50 mg, and 100 mg (3)

——CONTRAINDICATIONS——

- History of coronary artery disease or coronary artery vasospasm. (4)
- Wolff-Parkinson-White syndrome or other cardiac accessory conduction pathway disorders. (4)
- History of stroke, transient ischemic attack, or hemiplegic or basilar migraine. (4)
- Peripheral vascular disease. (4)
- Ischemic bowel disease. (4)
- Uncontrolled hypertension. (4)
- Recent (within 24 hours) use of another 5-HT₁ agonist (e.g., another triptan) or of an ergotamine-containing medication. (4)
- Concurrent or recent (past 2 weeks) use of monoamine oxidase-A inhibitor. (4)
- Hypersensitivity to IMITREX (angioedema and anaphylaxis seen). (4)
- Severe hepatic impairment. (4)

——WARNINGS AND PRECAUTIONS——

- Myocardial ischemia/infarction and Prinzmetal's angina: Perform cardiac evaluation in patients with multiple cardiovascular risk factors. (5.1)
- Arrhythmias: Discontinue IMITREX if occurs. (5.2)
- Chest/throat/neck/jaw pain, tightness, pressure, or heaviness: Generally not associated with myocardial ischemia; evaluate for coronary artery disease in patients at high risk. (5.3)
- Cerebral hemorrhage, subarachnoid hemorrhage, and stroke: Discontinue IMITREX if occurs. (5.4)
- Gastrointestinal ischemic reactions and peripheral vasospastic reactions: Discontinue IMITREX if occurs. (5.5)
- Medication overuse headache: Detoxification may be necessary. (5.6)
- Serotonin syndrome: Discontinue IMITREX if occurs. (5.7)
- Seizures: Use with caution in patients with epilepsy or a lowered seizure threshold. (5.10)

——ADVERSE REACTIONS——

Most common adverse reactions (≥2% and >placebo) were paresthesia, warm/cold sensation, chest pain/tightness/pressure and/or heaviness, neck/throat/jaw pain/tightness/pressure, other sensations of pain/pressure/tightness/heaviness, vertigo, and malaise/fatigue. (6.1)

To report SUSPECTED ADVERSE REACTIONS, contact GlaxoSmithKline at 1-888-825-5249 or FDA at 1-800-FDA-1088 or www.fda.gov/medwatch

——USE IN SPECIFIC POPULATIONS——

Pregnancy: Based on animal data, may cause fetal harm. (8.1)

See 17 for PATIENT COUNSELING INFORMATION and FDA-approved patient labeling

Revised: 11/2013

FULL PRESCRIBING INFORMATION

1 INDICATIONS AND USAGE

IMITREX® Tablets are indicated for the acute treatment of migraine with or without aura in adults.

Limitations of Use:

- Use only if a clear diagnosis of migraine headache has been established. If a patient has no response to the first migraine attack treated with IMITREX, reconsider the diagnosis of migraine before IMITREX is administered to treat any subsequent attacks.
- IMITREX is not indicated for the prevention of migraine attacks.
- Safety and effectiveness of IMITREX Tablets have not been established for cluster headache.

2 DOSAGE AND ADMINISTRATION

2.1 Dosing Information

The recommended dose of IMITREX Tablets is 25 mg, 50 mg, or 100 mg. Doses of 50 mg and 100 mg may provide a greater effect than the 25-mg dose, but doses of 100 mg may not provide a greater effect than the 50-mg dose. Higher doses may have a greater risk of adverse reactions [see Clinical Studies (14)].

If the migraine has not resolved by 2 hours after taking IMITREX Tablets, or returns after a transient improvement, a second dose may be administered at least 2 hours after the first dose. The maximum daily dose is 200 mg in a 24-hour period.

Use after IMITREX Injection: If the migraine returns following an initial treatment with IMITREX (sumatriptan succinate) Injection, additional IMITREX Tablets (up to 100 mg/day) may be given with an interval of at least 2 hours between tablet doses.

The safety of treating an average of more than 4 headaches in a 30-day period has not been established.

Table 1. Adverse Reactions Reported by at Least 2% of Patients Treated With IMITREX Tablets and at a Greater Frequency Than Placebo

Adverse Reaction	Percent of Patients Reporting			
	IMITREX Tablets 25 mg (n = 417)	IMITREX Tablets 50 mg (n = 771)	IMITREX Tablets 100 mg (n = 437)	Placebo (n = 309)
Atypical sensations	5	6	6	4
Paresthesia (all types)	3	5	3	2
Sensation warm/cold	3	2	3	2
Pain and other pressure sensations	6	6	8	4
Chest - pain/tightness/pressure and/or heaviness	1	2	2	1
Neck/throat/jaw - pain/tightness/pressure	<1	2	3	<1
Pain - location specified	2	1	1	1
Other - pressure/tightness/heaviness	1	2	3	2
Neurological				
Vertigo	<1	<1	2	<1
Other				
Malaise/fatigue	2	2	3	<1

2.2 Dosing in Patients With Hepatic Impairment
If treatment is deemed advisable in the presence of mild to moderate hepatic impairment, the maximum single dose should not exceed 50 mg [see Use in Specific Populations (8.6) and Clinical Pharmacology (12.3)].

3 DOSAGE FORMS AND STRENGTHS
25 mg Tablets: White, triangular-shaped, film-coated, and debossed with "I" on one side and "25" on the other.
50 mg Tablets: White, triangular-shaped, film-coated, and debossed with "IMITREX 50" on one side and a chevron shape (^) on the other.
100 mg Tablets: Pink, triangular-shaped, film-coated, and debossed with "IMITREX 100" on one side and a chevron shape (^) on the other.

4 CONTRAINDICATIONS
IMITREX Tablets are contraindicated in patients with:
- Ischemic coronary artery disease (CAD) (angina pectoris, history of myocardial infarction, or documented silent ischemia) or coronary artery vasospasm, including Prinzmetal's angina [see Warnings and Precautions (5.1)]
- Wolff-Parkinson-White syndrome or arrhythmias associated with other cardiac accessory conduction pathway disorders [see Warnings and Precautions (5.2)]
- History of stroke or transient ischemic attack (TIA) or history of hemiplegic or basilar migraine because these patients are at a higher risk of stroke [see Warnings and Precautions (5.4)]
- Peripheral vascular disease [see Warnings and Precautions (5.5)]
- Ischemic bowel disease [see Warnings and Precautions (5.5)]
- Uncontrolled hypertension [see Warnings and Precautions (5.8)]
- Recent use (i.e., within 24 hours) of ergotamine-containing medication, ergot-type medication (such as dihydroergotamine or methysergide), or another 5-hydroxytryptamine₁ (5-HT₁) agonist [see Drug Interactions (7.1, 7.3)]
- Concurrent administration of a monoamine oxidase (MAO)-A inhibitor or recent (within 2 weeks) use of an MAO-A inhibitor [see Drug Interactions (7.2) and Clinical Pharmacology (12.3)]
- Hypersensitivity to IMITREX (angioedema and anaphylaxis seen) [see Warnings and Precautions (5.9)]
- Severe hepatic impairment [see Use in Specific Populations (8.6) and Clinical Pharmacology (12.3)]

5 WARNINGS AND PRECAUTIONS
5.1 Myocardial Ischemia, Myocardial Infarction, and Prinzmetal's Angina
The use of IMITREX Tablets is contraindicated in patients with ischemic or vasospastic CAD. There have been rare reports of serious cardiac adverse reactions, including acute myocardial infarction, occurring within a few hours following administration of IMITREX Tablets. Some of these reactions occurred in patients without known CAD. IMITREX Tablets may cause coronary artery vasospasm (Prinzmetal's angina), even in patients without a history of CAD.
Perform a cardiovascular evaluation in triptan-naive patients who have multiple cardiovascular risk factors (e.g., increased age, diabetes, hypertension, smoking, obesity, strong family history of CAD) prior to receiving IMITREX Tablets. If there is evidence of CAD or coronary artery vasospasm, IMITREX Tablets are contraindicated. For patients with multiple cardiovascular risk factors who have a nega-

tive cardiovascular evaluation, consider administering the first dose of IMITREX Tablets in a medically supervised setting and performing an electrocardiogram (ECG) immediately following administration of IMITREX Tablets. For such patients, consider periodic cardiovascular evaluation in intermittent long-term users of IMITREX Tablets.
5.2 Arrhythmias
Life-threatening disturbances of cardiac rhythm, including ventricular tachycardia and ventricular fibrillation leading to death, have been reported within a few hours following the administration of 5-HT₁ agonists. Discontinue IMITREX Tablets if these disturbances occur. IMITREX Tablets are contraindicated in patients with Wolff-Parkinson-White syndrome or arrhythmias associated with other cardiac accessory conduction pathway disorders.
5.3 Chest, Throat, Neck, and/or Jaw Pain/Tightness/Pressure
Sensations of tightness, pain, pressure, and heaviness in the precordium, throat, neck, and jaw commonly occur after treatment with IMITREX Tablets and are usually noncardiac in origin. However, perform a cardiac evaluation if these patients are at high cardiac risk. The use of IMITREX Tablets is contraindicated in patients with CAD and those with Prinzmetal's variant angina.
5.4 Cerebrovascular Events
Cerebral hemorrhage, subarachnoid hemorrhage, and stroke have occurred in patients treated with 5-HT₁ agonists, and some have resulted in fatalities. In a number of cases, it appears possible that the cerebrovascular events were primary, the 5-HT₁ agonist having been administered in the incorrect belief that the symptoms experienced were a consequence of migraine when they were not. Also, patients with migraine may be at increased risk of certain cerebrovascular events (e.g., stroke, hemorrhage, TIA). Discontinue IMITREX Tablets if a cerebrovascular event occurs.
Before treating headaches in patients not previously diagnosed as migraineurs, and in migraineurs who present with atypical symptoms, exclude other potentially serious neurological conditions. IMITREX Tablets are contraindicated in patients with a history of stroke or TIA.
5.5 Other Vasospasm Reactions
IMITREX Tablets may cause non-coronary vasospastic reactions, such as peripheral vascular ischemia, gastrointestinal vascular ischemia and infarction (presenting with abdominal pain and bloody diarrhea), splenic infarction, and Raynaud's syndrome. In patients who experience symptoms or signs suggestive of non-coronary vasospasm reaction following the use of any 5-HT₁ agonist, rule out a vasospastic reaction before receiving additional IMITREX Tablets.
Reports of transient and permanent blindness and significant partial vision loss have been reported with the use of 5-HT₁ agonists. Since visual disorders may be part of a migraine attack, a causal relationship between these events and the use of 5-HT₁ agonists have not been clearly established.
5.6 Medication Overuse Headache
Overuse of acute migraine drugs (e.g., ergotamine, triptans, opioids, or combination of these drugs for 10 or more days per month) may lead to exacerbation of headache (medication overuse headache). Medication overuse headache may present as migraine-like daily headaches or as a marked increase in frequency of migraine attacks. Detoxification of patients, including withdrawal of the overused drugs, and treatment of withdrawal symptoms (which often includes a transient worsening of headache) may be necessary.

5.7 Serotonin Syndrome
Serotonin syndrome may occur with IMITREX Tablets, particularly during co-administration with selective serotonin reuptake inhibitors (SSRIs), serotonin norepinephrine reuptake inhibitors (SNRIs), tricyclic antidepressants (TCAs), and MAO inhibitors [see Drug Interactions (7.4)]. Serotonin syndrome symptoms may include mental status changes (e.g., agitation, hallucinations, coma), autonomic instability (e.g., tachycardia, labile blood pressure, hyperthermia), neuromuscular aberrations (e.g., hyperreflexia, incoordination), and/or gastrointestinal symptoms (e.g., nausea, vomiting, diarrhea). The onset of symptoms usually occurs within minutes to hours of receiving a new or a greater dose of a serotonergic medication. Discontinue IMITREX Tablets if serotonin syndrome is suspected.
5.8 Increase in Blood Pressure
Significant elevation in blood pressure, including hypertensive crisis with acute impairment of organ systems, has been reported on rare occasions in patients treated with 5-HT1 agonists, including patients without a history of hypertension. Monitor blood pressure in patients treated with IMITREX. IMITREX Tablets are contraindicated in patients with uncontrolled hypertension.
5.9 Anaphylactic/Anaphylactoid Reactions
Anaphylactic/anaphylactoid reactions have occurred in patients receiving IMITREX. Such reactions can be life threatening or fatal. In general, anaphylactic reactions to drugs are more likely to occur in individuals with a history of sensitivity to multiple allergens. IMITREX Tablets are contraindicated in patients with a history of hypersensitivity reaction to IMITREX.
5.10 Seizures
Seizures have been reported following administration of IMITREX. Some have occurred in patients with either a history of seizures or concurrent conditions predisposing to seizures. There are also reports in patients where no such predisposing factors are apparent. IMITREX Tablets should be used with caution in patients with a history of epilepsy or conditions associated with a lowered seizure threshold.

6 ADVERSE REACTIONS
The following adverse reactions are discussed in more detail in other sections of the prescribing information:
- Myocardial ischemia, myocardial infarction, and Prinzmetal's angina [see Warnings and Precautions (5.1)]
- Arrhythmias [see Warnings and Precautions (5.2)]
- Chest, throat, neck, and/or jaw pain/tightness/pressure [see Warnings and Precautions (5.3)]
- Cerebrovascular events [see Warnings and Precautions (5.4)]
- Other vasospasm reactions [see Warnings and Precautions (5.5)]
- Medication overuse headache [see Warnings and Precautions (5.6)]
- Serotonin syndrome [see Warnings and Precautions (5.7)]
- Increase in blood pressure [see Warnings and Precautions (5.8)]
- Hypersensitivity reactions [see Contraindications (4) and Warnings and Precautions (5.9)]
- Seizures [see Warnings and Precautions (5.10)]
6.1 Clinical Trials Experience
Because clinical trials are conducted under widely varying conditions, adverse reaction rates observed in the clinical trials of a drug cannot be directly compared with rates in the clinical trials of another drug and may not reflect the rates observed in practice.
Table 1 lists adverse reactions that occurred in placebo-controlled clinical trials in patients who took at least 1 dose of study drug. Only treatment-emergent adverse reactions that occurred at a frequency of 2% or more in any group treated with IMITREX Tablets and that occurred at a frequency greater than the placebo group are included in Table 1.
[See table 1 above]
The incidence of adverse reactions in controlled clinical trials was not affected by gender or age of the patients. There were insufficient data to assess the impact of race on the incidence of adverse reactions.
6.2 Postmarketing Experience
The following adverse reactions have been identified during postapproval use of IMITREX Tablets, IMITREX Nasal Spray, and IMITREX Injection. Because these reactions are reported voluntarily from a population of uncertain size, it is not always possible to reliably estimate their frequency or establish a causal relationship to drug exposure. These reactions have been chosen for inclusion due to either their seriousness, frequency of reporting, or causal connection to IMITREX or a combination of these factors.
Cardiovascular: Hypotension, palpitations.
Neurological: Dystonia, tremor.

7 DRUG INTERACTIONS
7.1 Ergot-Containing Drugs
Ergot-containing drugs have been reported to cause prolonged vasospastic reactions. Because these effects may be

additive, use of ergotamine-containing or ergot-type medications (like dihydroergotamine or methysergide) and IMITREX Tablets within 24 hours of each other is contraindicated.

7.2 Monoamine Oxidase-A Inhibitors
MAO–A inhibitors increase systemic exposure by 7-fold. Therefore, the use of IMITREX Tablets in patients receiving MAO–A inhibitors is contraindicated *[see Clinical Pharmacology (12.3)]*.

7.3 Other 5-HT₁ Agonists
Because their vasospastic effects may be additive, co-administration of IMITREX Tablets and other 5–HT₁ agonists (e.g., triptans) within 24 hours of each other is contraindicated.

7.4 Selective Serotonin Reuptake Inhibitors/Serotonin Norepinephrine Reuptake Inhibitors and Serotonin Syndrome
Cases of serotonin syndrome have been reported during co-administration of triptans and SSRIs, SNRIs, TCAs, and MAO inhibitors *[see Warnings and Precautions (5.7)]*.

8 USE IN SPECIFIC POPULATIONS
8.1 Pregnancy
Pregnancy Category C: There are no adequate and well-controlled trials in pregnant women. In developmental toxicity studies in rats and rabbits, oral administration of sumatriptan to pregnant animals was associated with embryolethality, fetal abnormalities, and pup mortality. When administered by the intravenous route to pregnant rabbits, sumatriptan was embryolethal. IMITREX Tablets should be used during pregnancy only if the potential benefit justifies the potential risk to the fetus.

Oral administration of sumatriptan to pregnant rats during the period of organogenesis resulted in an increased incidence of fetal blood vessel (cervicothoracic and umbilical) abnormalities. The highest no-effect dose for embryofetal developmental toxicity in rats was 60 mg/kg/day, or approximately 3 times the maximum recommended human dose (MRHD) of 200 mg/day on a mg/m² basis. Oral administration of sumatriptan to pregnant rabbits during the period of organogenesis resulted in increased incidences of embryolethality and fetal cervicothoracic vascular and skeletal abnormalities. Intravenous administration of sumatriptan to pregnant rabbits during the period of organogenesis resulted in an increased incidence of embryolethality. The highest oral and intravenous no-effect doses for developmental toxicity in rabbits were 15 (approximately 2 times the MRHD on a mg/m² basis) and 0.75 mg/kg/day, respectively.

Oral administration of sumatriptan to rats prior to and throughout gestation resulted in embryofetal toxicity (decreased body weight, decreased ossification, increased incidence of skeletal abnormalities). The highest no-effect dose was 50 mg/kg/day, or approximately 2 times the MRHD on a mg/m² basis. In offspring of pregnant rats treated orally with sumatriptan during organogenesis, there was a decrease in pup survival. The highest no-effect dose for this effect was 60 mg/kg/day, or approximately 3 times the MRHD on a mg/m² basis. Oral treatment of pregnant rats with sumatriptan during the latter part of gestation and throughout lactation resulted in a decrease in pup survival. The highest no-effect dose for this finding was 100 mg/kg/day, or approximately 5 times the MRHD on a mg/m² basis.

8.3 Nursing Mothers
Sumatriptan is excreted in human milk following subcutaneous administration. Infant exposure to sumatriptan can be minimized by avoiding breastfeeding for 12 hours after treatment with IMITREX Tablets.

8.4 Pediatric Use
Safety and effectiveness in pediatric patients have not been established. IMITREX Tablets are not recommended for use in patients younger than 18 years of age.

Two controlled clinical trials evaluated IMITREX Nasal Spray (5 to 20 mg) in 1,248 adolescent migraineurs aged 12 to 17 years who treated a single attack. The trials did not establish the efficacy of IMITREX Nasal Spray compared with placebo in the treatment of migraine in adolescents. Adverse reactions observed in these clinical trials were similar in nature to those reported in clinical trials in adults.

Five controlled clinical trials (2 single-attack trials, 3 multiple-attack trials) evaluating oral IMITREX (25 to 100 mg) in pediatric patients aged 12 to 17 years enrolled a total of 701 adolescent migraineurs. These trials did not establish the efficacy of oral IMITREX compared with placebo in the treatment of migraine in adolescents. Adverse reactions observed in these clinical trials were similar in nature to those reported in clinical trials in adults. The frequency of all adverse reactions in these patients appeared to be both dose- and age- dependent, with younger patients reporting reactions more commonly than older adolescents.

Postmarketing experience documents that serious adverse reactions have occurred in the pediatric population after use of subcutaneous, oral, and/or intranasal IMITREX. These reports include reactions similar in nature to those reported rarely in adults, including stroke, visual loss, and death. A myocardial infarction has been reported in a 14–year–old male following the use of oral IMITREX; clinical signs occurred within 1 day of drug administration. Clinical data to determine the frequency of serious adverse reactions in pediatric patients who might receive subcutaneous, oral, or intranasal IMITREX are not presently available.

8.5 Geriatric Use
Clinical trials of IMITREX Tablets did not include sufficient numbers of patients aged 65 and older to determine whether they respond differently from younger patients. Other reported clinical experience has not identified differences in responses between the elderly and younger patients. In general, dose selection for an elderly patient should be cautious, usually starting at the low end of the dosing range, reflecting the greater frequency of decreased hepatic, renal, or cardiac function and of concomitant disease or other drug therapy.

A cardiovascular evaluation is recommended for geriatric patients who have other cardiovascular risk factors (e.g., diabetes, hypertension, smoking, obesity, strong family history of CAD) prior to receiving IMITREX Tablets *[see Warnings and Precautions (5.1)]*.

8.6 Hepatic Impairment
The maximum single dose in patients with mild to moderate hepatic impairment should not exceed 50 mg. IMITREX Tablets are contraindicated in patients with severe hepatic impairment *[see Clinical Pharmacology (12.3)]*.

10 OVERDOSAGE
Patients in clinical trials (N = 670) received single oral doses of 140 to 300 mg without significant adverse reactions. Volunteers (N = 174) received single oral doses of 140 to 400 mg without serious adverse reactions.

Overdose in animals has been fatal and has been heralded by convulsions, tremor, paralysis, inactivity, ptosis, erythema of the extremities, abnormal respiration, cyanosis, ataxia, mydriasis, salivation, and lacrimation.

The elimination half-life of sumatriptan is approximately 2.5 hours *[see Clinical Pharmacology (12.3)]*, and therefore monitoring of patients after overdose with IMITREX Tablets should continue for at least 12 hours or while symptoms or signs persist.

It is unknown what effect hemodialysis or peritoneal dialysis has on the serum concentrations of sumatriptan.

11 DESCRIPTION
IMITREX Tablets contain sumatriptan succinate, a selective 5–HT₁B/1D receptor agonist. Sumatriptan succinate is chemically designated as 3-[2-(dimethylamino)ethyl]-N-methyl-indole-5-methanesulfonamide succinate (1:1), and it has the following structure:

The empirical formula is $C_{14}H_{21}N_3O_2S \bullet C_4H_6O_4$, representing a molecular weight of 413.5. Sumatriptan succinate is a white to off–white powder that is readily soluble in water and in saline.

Each IMITREX Tablet for oral administration contains 35, 70, or 140 mg of sumatriptan succinate equivalent to 25, 50, or 100 mg of sumatriptan, respectively. Each tablet also contains the inactive ingredients croscarmellose sodium, dibasic calcium phosphate, magnesium stearate, microcrystalline cellulose, and sodium bicarbonate. Each 100-mg tablet also contains hypromellose, iron oxide, titanium dioxide, and triacetin.

12 CLINICAL PHARMACOLOGY
12.1 Mechanism of Action
Sumatriptan binds with high affinity to human cloned 5–HT₁B/1D receptors. Sumatriptan presumably exerts its therapeutic effects in the treatment of migraine headache through agonist effects at the 5–HT₁B/1D receptors on intracranial blood vessels and sensory nerves of the trigeminal system, which result in cranial vessel constriction and inhibition of pro–inflammatory neuropeptide release.

12.2 Pharmacodynamics
Blood Pressure: Significant elevation in blood pressure, including hypertensive crisis, has been reported in patients with and without a history of hypertension *[see Warnings and Precautions (5.8)]*.

Peripheral (Small) Arteries: In healthy volunteers (N = 18), a trial evaluating the effects of sumatriptan on peripheral (small vessel) arterial reactivity failed to detect a clinically significant increase in peripheral resistance.

Heart Rate: Transient increases in blood pressure observed in some patients in clinical trials carried out during sumatriptan's development as a treatment for migraine were not accompanied by any clinically significant changes in heart rate.

12.3 Pharmacokinetics
Absorption and Bioavailability: The mean maximum concentration following oral dosing with 25 mg is 18 ng/mL (range: 7 to 47 ng/mL) and 51 ng/mL (range: 28 to 100 ng/mL) following oral dosing with 100 mg of sumatriptan. This compares with a C_{max} of 5 and 16 ng/mL following dosing with a 5- and 20–mg intranasal dose, respectively. The mean C_{max} following a 6–mg subcutaneous injection is 71 ng/mL (range: 49 to 110 ng/mL). The bioavailability is approximately 15%, primarily due to presystemic metabolism and partly due to incomplete absorption. The C_{max} is similar during a migraine attack and during a migraine–free period, but the T_{max} is slightly later during the attack, approximately 2.5 hours compared with 2.0 hours. When given as a single dose, sumatriptan displays dose proportionality in its extent of absorption (area under the curve [AUC]) over the dose range of 25 to 200 mg, but the C_{max} after 100 mg is approximately 25% less than expected (based on the 25–mg dose).

A food effect trial involving administration of IMITREX Tablets 100 mg to healthy volunteers under fasting conditions and with a high– fat meal indicated that the C_{max} and AUC were increased by 15% and 12%, respectively, when administered in the fed state.

Distribution: Protein binding, determined by equilibrium dialysis over the concentration range of 10 to 1,000 ng/mL is low, approximately 14% to 21%. The effect of sumatriptan on the protein binding of other drugs has not been evaluated. The apparent volume of distribution is 2.7 L/kg.

Metabolism: In vitro studies with human microsomes suggest that sumatriptan is metabolized by MAO, predominantly the A isoenzyme. Most of a radiolabeled dose of sumatriptan excreted in the urine is the major metabolite indole acetic acid (IAA) or the IAA glucuronide, both of which are inactive.

Elimination: The elimination half-life of sumatriptan is approximately 2.5 hours. Radiolabeled ¹⁴C-sumatriptan administered orally is largely renally excreted (about 60%) with about 40% found in the feces. Most of the radiolabeled compound excreted in the urine is the major metabolite, indole acetic acid (IAA), which is inactive, or the IAA glucuronide. Only 3% of the dose can be recovered as unchanged sumatriptan.

Special Populations: *Age:* The pharmacokinetics of sumatriptan in the elderly (mean age: 72 years, 2 males and 4 females) and in subjects with migraine (mean age: 38 years, 25 males and 155 females) were similar to that in healthy male subjects (mean age: 30 years).

Renal Impairment: The effect of renal impairment on the pharmacokinetics of sumatriptan has not been examined.

Hepatic Impairment: The liver plays an important role in the presystemic clearance of orally administered sumatriptan. Accordingly, the bioavailability of sumatriptan following oral administration may be markedly increased in patients with liver disease. In one small trial of patients with moderate liver impairment (n = 8) matched for sex, age, and weight with healthy subjects (n = 8), the hepatically-impaired patients had an approximately 70% increase in AUC and C_{max} and a T_{max} 40 minutes earlier compared to the healthy subjects.

The pharmacokinetics of sumatriptan in patients with severe hepatic impairment has not been studied. The use of IMITREX Tablets in this population is contraindicated *[see Contraindications (4) and Use in Specific Populations (8.6)]*.

Gender: In a trial comparing females to males, no pharmacokinetic differences were observed between genders for AUC, C_{max}, T_{max}, and half–life.

Race: The systemic clearance and C_{max} of subcutaneous sumatriptan were similar in black (n = 34) and Caucasian (n = 38) healthy male subjects. Oral sumatriptan has not been evaluated for race differences.

Drug Interaction Studies: Monoamine Oxidase-A Inhibitors: Treatment with MAO-A inhibitors generally leads to an increase of sumatriptan plasma levels *[see Contraindications (4) and Drug Interactions (7.2)]* .

Due to gut and hepatic metabolic first-pass effects, the increase of systemic exposure after co-administration of an MAO-A inhibitor with oral sumatriptan is greater than after co-administration of the MAO inhibitors with subcutaneous sumatriptan.

In a trial of 14 healthy females, pretreatment with an MAO-A inhibitor decreased the clearance of subcutaneous sumatriptan, resulting in a 2-fold increase in the area under the sumatriptan plasma concentration-time curve (AUC), corresponding to a 40% increase in elimination half-life.

A small trial evaluating the effect of pretreatment with an MAO-A inhibitor on the bioavailability from a 25-mg oral sumatriptan tablet resulted in an approximately 7-fold increase in systemic exposure.

Table 2. Percentage of Patients With Headache Response (Mild or No Headache) 2 and 4 Hours Following Treatment

	IMITREX Tablets 25 mg		IMITREX Tablets 50 mg		IMITREX Tablets 100 mg		Placebo	
	2 hr	4 hr	2 hr	4 hr	2 hr	4 hr	2 hr	4 hr
Trial 1	52%[a]	67%[a]	61%[a,b]	78%[a,b]	62%[a,b]	79%[a,b]	27%	38%
	(n = 298)		(n = 296)		(n = 296)		(n = 94)	
Trial 2	52%[a]	70%[a]	50%[a]	68%[a]	56%[a]	71%[a]	26%	38%
	(n = 66)		(n = 62)		(n = 66)		(n = 65)	
Trial 3	52%[a]	65%[a]	54%[a]	72%[a]	57%[a]	78%[a]	17%	19%
	(n = 48)		(n = 46)		(n = 46)		(n = 47)	

[a] $P<0.05$ in comparison with placebo.
[b] $P<0.05$ in comparison with 25 mg.

Alcohol: Alcohol consumed 30 minutes prior to sumatriptan ingestion had no effect on the pharmacokinetics of sumatriptan.

13 NONCLINICAL TOXICOLOGY

13.1 Carcinogenesis, Mutagenesis, Impairment of Fertility

Carcinogenesis: In carcinogenicity studies in mouse and rat, sumatriptan was administered orally for 78 and 104 weeks, respectively, at doses up to 160 mg/kg/day (the high dose in rat was reduced from 360 mg/kg/day during week 21). There was no evidence in either species of an increase in tumors related to sumatriptan administration. Plasma exposures (AUC) at the highest doses tested were 20 and 8 times that in humans at the maximum recommended human dose (MRHD) of 200 mg/day.

Mutagenesis: Sumatriptan was negative in in vitro (bacterial reverse mutation [Ames], gene cell mutation in Chinese hamster V79/HGPRT, chromosomal aberration in human lymphocytes) and in vivo (rat micronucleus) assays.

Impairment of Fertility: When sumatriptan (5, 50, 500 mg/kg/day) was administered orally to male and female rats prior to and throughout the mating period, there was a treatment-related decrease in fertility secondary to a decrease in mating in animals treated with doses greater than 5 mg/kg/day (less than the MRHD on a mg/m² basis). It is not clear whether this finding was due to an effect on males or females or both..

13.2 Animal Toxicology and/or Pharmacology

Corneal Opacities: Dogs receiving oral sumatriptan developed corneal opacities and defects in the corneal epithelium. Corneal opacities were seen at the lowest dose tested, 2 mg/kg/day, and were present after 1 month of treatment. Defects in the corneal epithelium were noted in a 60-week study. Earlier examinations for these toxicities were not conducted and no-effect doses were not established. Plasma exposure at the lowest dose tested was approximately 2 times that in humans at the MRHD.

14 CLINICAL STUDIES

The efficacy of IMITREX Tablets in the acute treatment of migraine headaches was demonstrated in 3, randomized, double-blind, placebo-controlled trials. Patients enrolled in these 3 trials were predominately female (87%) and Caucasian (97%), with a mean age of 40 years (range of 18 to 65 years). Patients were instructed to treat a moderate to severe headache. Headache response, defined as a reduction in headache severity from moderate or severe pain to mild or no pain, was assessed up to 4 hours after dosing. Associated symptoms such as nausea, photophobia, and phonophobia were also assessed. Maintenance of response was assessed for up to 24 hours postdose. A second dose of IMITREX Tablets or other medication was allowed 4 to 24 hours after the initial treatment for recurrent headache. Acetaminophen was offered to patients in Trials 2 and 3 beginning at 2 hours after initial treatment if the migraine pain had not improved or worsened. Additional medications were allowed 4 to 24 hours after the initial treatment for recurrent headache or as rescue in all 3 trials. The frequency and time to use of these additional treatments were also determined. In all trials, doses of 25, 50, and 100 mg were compared with placebo in the treatment of migraine attacks. In 1 trial, doses of 25, 50, and 100 mg were also compared with each other.

In all 3 trials, the percentage of patients achieving headache response 2 and 4 hours after treatment was significantly greater among patients receiving IMITREX Tablets at all doses compared with those who received placebo. In 1 of the 3 trials, there was a statistically significant greater percentage of patients with headache response at 2 and 4 hours in the 50-mg or 100-mg group when compared with the 25-mg dose groups. There were no statistically significant differences between the 50-mg and 100-mg dose groups in any trial. The results from the 3 controlled clinical trials are summarized in Table 2.
[See table 2 above]

The estimated probability of achieving an initial headache response over the 4 hours following treatment in pooled Trials 1, 2, and 3 is depicted in Figure 1.

Figure 1. Estimated Probability of Achieving Initial Headache Response Within 4 Hours of Treatment in Pooled Trials 1, 2, and 3[a]

[a] The figure shows the probability over time of obtaining headache response (no or mild pain) following treatment with oral sumatriptan. The averages displayed are based on pooled data from the 3 clinical controlled trials providing evidence of efficacy. Kaplan–Meier plot with patients not achieving response and/or taking rescue within 240 minutes censored to 240 minutes.

For patients with migraine-associated nausea, photophobia, and/or phonophobia at baseline, there was a lower incidence of these symptoms at 2 hours (Trial 1) and at 4 hours (Trials 1, 2, and 3) following administration of IMITREX Tablets compared with placebo.

As early as 2 hours in Trials 2 and 3, or as early as 4 hours in Trial 1, through 24 hours following the initial dose of study treatment, patients were allowed to use additional treatment for pain relief in the form of a second dose of study treatment or other medication. The estimated probability of patients taking a second dose or other medication for migraine over the 24 hours following the initial dose of study treatment is summarized in Figure 2.

Figure 2. The Estimated Probability of Patients Taking a Second Dose of IMITREX Tablets or Other Medication to Treat Migraine Over the 24 Hours Following the Initial Dose of Study Treatment in Pooled Trials 1, 2, and 3[a]

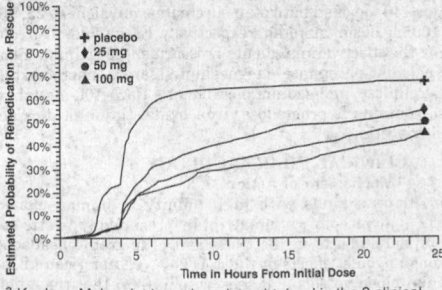

[a] Kaplan–Meier plot based on data obtained in the 3 clinical controlled trials providing evidence of efficacy with patients not using additional treatments censored to 24 hours. Plot also includes patients who had no response to the initial dose. No remediation was allowed within 2 hours postdose.

There is evidence that doses above 50 mg do not provide a greater effect than 50 mg. There was no evidence to suggest that treatment with IMITREX Tablets was associated with an increase in the severity of recurrent headaches. The efficacy of IMITREX Tablets was unaffected by presence of aura; duration of headache prior to treatment; gender, age, or weight of the subject; relationship to menses; or concomitant use of common migraine prophylactic drugs (e.g., beta-blockers, calcium channel blockers, tricyclic antidepressants). There were insufficient data to assess the impact of race on efficacy.

16 HOW SUPPLIED/STORAGE AND HANDLING

IMITREX Tablets, 25 mg, 50 mg, and 100 mg of sumatriptan (base) as the succinate.

IMITREX Tablets, 25 mg, are white, triangular–shaped, film–coated tablets debossed with "I" on one side and "25" on the other in blister packs of 9 tablets (NDC 0173-0735-00).

IMITREX Tablets, 50 mg, are white, triangular–shaped, film–coated tablets debossed with "IMITREX 50" on one side and a chevron shape (^) on the other in blister packs of 9 tablets (NDC 0173-0736-01).

IMITREX Tablets, 100 mg, are pink, triangular–shaped, film–coated tablets debossed with "IMITREX 100" on one side and a chevron shape (^) on the other in blister packs of 9 tablets (NDC 0173-0737-01).

Store between 2°C and 30°C (36°F and 86°F).

17 PATIENT COUNSELING INFORMATION

Advise the patient to read the FDA-approved patient labeling (Patient Information).

Risk of Myocardial Ischemia and/or Infarction, Prinzmetal's Angina, Other Vasospasm-Related Events, Arrhythmias, and Cerebrovascular Events: Inform patients that IMITREX Tablets may cause serious cardiovascular side effects such as myocardial infarction or stroke. Although serious cardiovascular events can occur without warning symptoms, patients should be alert for the signs and symptoms of chest pain, shortness of breath, irregular heartbeat, significant rise in blood pressure, weakness, and slurring of speech, and should ask for medical advice if any indicative sign or symptoms are observed. Apprise patients of the importance of this follow-up [see Warnings and Precautions (5.1, 5.2, 5.4, 5.5, 5.8)].

Anaphylactic/Anaphylactoid Reactions: Inform patients that anaphylactic/anaphylactoid reactions have occurred in patients receiving IMITREX Tablets. Such reactions can be life threatening or fatal. In general, anaphylactic reactions to drugs are more likely to occur in individuals with a history of sensitivity to multiple allergens [see Contraindications (4) and Warnings and Precautions (5.9)].

Concomitant Use With Other Triptans or Ergot Medications: Inform patients that use of IMITREX Tablets within 24 hours of another triptan or an ergot-type medication (including dihydroergotamine or methysergide) is contraindicated [see Contraindications (4), Drug Interactions (7.1, 7.3)].

Serotonin Syndrome: Caution patients about the risk of serotonin syndrome with the use of IMITREX Tablets and other triptans, particularly during combined use with SSRIs, SNRIs, TCAs, and MAO inhibitors [see Warnings and Precautions (5.7), Drug Interactions (7.4)].

Medication Overuse Headache: Inform patients that use of acute migraine drugs for 10 or more days per month may lead to an exacerbation of headache and encourage patients to record headache frequency and drug use (e.g., by keeping a headache diary) [see Warnings and Precautions (5.6)].

Pregnancy: Inform patients that IMITREX Tablets should not be used during pregnancy unless the potential benefit justifies the potential risk to the fetus [see Use in Specific Populations (8.1)].

Nursing Mothers: Advise patients to notify their healthcare provider if they are breastfeeding or plan to breastfeed [see Use in Specific Populations (8.3)].

Ability to Perform Complex Tasks: Treatment with IMITREX Tablets may cause somnolence and dizziness; instruct patients to evaluate their ability to perform complex tasks after administration of IMITREX Tablets.

IMITREX is a registered trademark of the GlaxoSmithKline group of companies.

GlaxoSmithKline
Research Triangle Park, NC 27709
©2013, GlaxoSmithKline group of companies. All rights reserved.
IMT:4PI

Patient Information
IMITREX® (IM-i-trex)
(sumatriptan succinate)
Tablets

Read this Patient Information before you start taking IMITREX and each time you get a refill. There may be new information. This information does not take the place of talking with your healthcare provider about your medical condition or treatment.

What is the most important information I should know about IMITREX?

IMITREX can cause serious side effects, including:

Heart attack and other heart problems. Heart problems may lead to death.

Stop taking IMITREX and get emergency medical help right away if you have any of the following symptoms of a heart attack:

- discomfort in the center of your chest that lasts for more than a few minutes, or that goes away and comes back
- severe tightness, pain, pressure, or heaviness in your chest, throat, neck, or jaw
- pain or discomfort in your arms, back, neck, jaw, or stomach
- shortness of breath with or without chest discomfort
- breaking out in a cold sweat
- nausea or vomiting
- feeling lightheaded

IMITREX is not for people with risk factors for heart disease unless a heart exam is done and shows no problem. You have a higher risk for heart disease if you:

- have high blood pressure
- have high cholesterol levels
- smoke
- are overweight
- have diabetes
- have a family history of heart disease

What is IMITREX?

IMITREX is a prescription medicine used to treat acute migraine headaches with or without aura in adults.

IMITREX is not used to treat other types of headaches such as hemiplegic (that make you unable to move on one side of your body) or basilar (rare form of migraine with aura) migraines.

IMITREX is not used to prevent or decrease the number of migraine headaches you have.

It is not known if IMITREX is safe and effective to treat cluster headaches.

It is not known if IMITREX is safe and effective in children under 18 years of age.

Who should not take IMITREX?

Do not take IMITREX if you have:

- heart problems or a history of heart problems
- narrowing of blood vessels to your legs, arms, stomach, or kidneys (peripheral vascular disease)
- uncontrolled high blood pressure
- severe liver problems
- hemiplegic migraines or basilar migraines. If you are not sure if you have these types of migraines, ask your healthcare provider.
- had a stroke, transient ischemic attacks (TIAs), or problems with your blood circulation
- taken any of the following medicines in the last 24 hours:
  ◦ almotriptan (AXERT®)
  ◦ eletriptan (RELPAX®)
  ◦ frovatriptan (FROVA®)
  ◦ naratriptan (AMERGE®)
  ◦ rizatriptan (MAXALT®), MAXALT-MLT®)
  ◦ sumatriptan and naproxen (TREXIMET®)
  ◦ ergotamines (CAFERGOT®, ERGOMAR®, MIGERGOT®)
  ◦ dihydroergotamine (D.H.E. 45®, MIGRANAL®)

Ask your healthcare provider if you are not sure if your medicine is listed above.

- an allergy to sumatriptan or any of the ingredients in IMITREX. See the end of this leaflet for a complete list of ingredients in IMITREX.

What should I tell my healthcare provider before taking IMITREX?

Before you take IMITREX, tell your healthcare provider about all of your medical conditions, including if you:

- have high blood pressure
- have high cholesterol
- have diabetes
- smoke
- are overweight
- have heart problems or family history of heart problems or stroke
- have kidney problems
- have liver problems
- have had epilepsy or seizures
- are not using effective birth control
- become pregnant while taking IMITREX.
- are breastfeeding or plan to breastfeed. IMITREX passes into your breast milk and may harm your baby. Talk with your healthcare provider about the best way to feed your baby if you take IMITREX.

Tell your healthcare provider about all the medicines you take, including prescription and nonprescription medicines, vitamins, and herbal supplements.

IMITREX and certain other medicines can affect each other, causing serious side effects.

Especially tell your healthcare provider if you take antidepressant medicines called:

- selective serotonin reuptake inhibitors (SSRIs)
- serotonin norepinephrine reuptake inhibitors (SNRIs)
- tricyclic antidepressants (TCAs)
- monoamine oxidase inhibitors (MAOIs)

Ask your healthcare provider or pharmacist for a list of these medicines if you are not sure.

Know the medicines you take. Keep a list of them to show your healthcare provider or pharmacist when you get a new medicine.

How should I take IMITREX?

- Certain people should take their first dose of IMITREX in their healthcare provider's office or in another medical setting. Ask your healthcare provider if you should take your first dose in a medical setting.
- Take IMITREX exactly as your healthcare provider tells you to take it.
- Your healthcare provider may change your dose. Do not change your dose without first talking to your healthcare provider.
- Take IMITREX Tablets whole with water or other liquids.
- If you do not get any relief after your first tablet, do not take a second tablet without first talking with your healthcare provider.
- If your headache comes back or you only get some relief from your headache, you can take a second tablet 2 hours after the first tablet.
- Do not take more than 200 mg of IMITREX Tablets in a 24–hour period.
- If you take too much IMITREX, call your healthcare provider or go to the nearest hospital emergency room right away.
- You should write down when you have headaches and when you take IMITREX so you can talk with your healthcare provider about how IMITREX is working for you.

What should I avoid while taking IMITREX?

IMITREX can cause dizziness, weakness, or drowsiness. If you have these symptoms, do not drive a car, use machinery, or do anything where you need to be alert.

What are the possible side effects of IMITREX?

IMITREX may cause serious side effects. See "What is the most important information I should know about IMITREX?"

These serious side effects include:

- changes in color or sensation in your fingers and toes (Raynaud's syndrome)
- stomach and intestinal problems (gastrointestinal and colonic ischemic events). Symptoms of gastrointestinal and colonic ischemic events include:
  ◦ sudden or severe stomach pain
  ◦ stomach pain after meals
  ◦ weight loss
  ◦ nausea or vomiting
  ◦ constipation or diarrhea
  ◦ bloody diarrhea
  ◦ fever
- problems with blood circulation to your legs and feet (peripheral vascular ischemia). Symptoms of peripheral vascular ischemia include:
  ◦ cramping and pain in your legs or hips
  ◦ feeling of heaviness or tightness in your leg muscles
  ◦ burning or aching pain in your feet or toes while resting
  ◦ numbness, tingling, or weakness in your legs
  ◦ cold feeling or color changes in 1 or both legs or feet
- hives (itchy bumps); swelling of your tongue, mouth, or throat
- medication overuse headaches. Some people who use too many IMITREX tablets may have worse headaches (medication overuse headache). If your headaches get worse, your healthcare provider may decide to stop your treatment with IMITREX.
- serotonin syndrome. Serotonin syndrome is a rare but serious problem that can happen in people using IMITREX, especially if IMITREX is used with anti–depressant medicines called SSRIs or SNRIs.

Call your healthcare provider right away if you have any of the following symptoms of serotonin syndrome:

  ◦ mental changes such as seeing things that are not there (hallucinations), agitation, or coma
  ◦ fast heartbeat
  ◦ changes in blood pressure
  ◦ high body temperature
  ◦ tight muscles
  ◦ trouble walking

- seizures. Seizures have happened in people taking IMITREX who have never had seizures before. Talk with your healthcare provider about your chance of having seizures while you take IMITREX.

The most common side effects of IMITREX Tablets include:

- tingling or numbness in your fingers or toes
- warm or cold feeling
- feeling weak, drowsy, or tired
- pain, discomfort, or stiffness in your neck, throat, jaw, or chest
- dizziness

Tell your healthcare provider if you have any side effect that bothers you or that does not go away.

These are not all the possible side effects of IMITREX. For more information, ask your healthcare provider or pharmacist.

Call your doctor for medical advice about side effects. You may report side effects to FDA at 1-800-FDA-1088.

How should I store IMITREX Tablets?

Store IMITREX between 36°F to 86°F (2°C to 30°C).

Keep IMITREX and all medicines out of the reach of children.

General information about the safe and effective use of IMITREX.

Medicines are sometimes prescribed for purposes other than those listed in Patient Information leaflets. Do not use IMITREX for a condition for which it was not prescribed. Do not give IMITREX to other people, even if they have the same symptoms you have. It may harm them.

This Patient Information leaflet summarizes the most important information about IMITREX. If you would like more information, talk with your healthcare provider. You can ask your healthcare provider or pharmacist for information about IMITREX that is written for healthcare professionals. For more information, go to www.gsk.com or call 1-888-825-5249.

What are the ingredients in IMITREX Tablets?

Active ingredient: sumatriptan succinate

Inactive ingredients: croscarmellose sodium, dibasic calcium phosphate, magnesium stearate, microcrystalline cellulose, and sodium bicarbonate

100–mg tablets also contain hypromellose, iron oxide, titanium dioxide, and triacetin.

This Patient Information has been approved by the U.S. Food and Drug Administration.

IMITREX, AMERGE, and TREXIMET are registered trademarks of the GlaxoSmithKline group of companies. The other brands listed are trademarks of their respective owners and are not trademarks of the GlaxoSmithKline group. The makers of these brands are not affiliated with and do not endorse GlaxoSmithKline or its products.

GlaxoSmithKline

Research Triangle Park, NC 27709

©2013, GlaxoSmithKline group of companies. All rights reserved.

November 2013

IMT:4PIL

INCRUSE ELLIPTA   ℞

[IN-cruise e-LIP-ta]
(umeclidinium)
inhalation powder

HIGHLIGHTS OF PRESCRIBING INFORMATION
These highlights do not include all the information needed to use INCRUSE ELLIPTA safely and effectively. See full prescribing information for INCRUSE ELLIPTA.
INCRUSE ELLIPTA (umeclidinium inhalation powder)
FOR ORAL INHALATION USE
Initial U.S. Approval: 2013

────────INDICATIONS AND USAGE────────

INCRUSE ELLIPTA is an anticholinergic indicated for the long-term, once-daily, maintenance treatment of airflow obstruction in patients with chronic obstructive pulmonary disease (COPD). (1)

──────DOSAGE AND ADMINISTRATION──────

- For oral inhalation only. (2)
- Maintenance treatment of COPD: 1 inhalation of INCRUSE ELLIPTA once daily. (2)

──────DOSAGE FORMS AND STRENGTHS──────

Inhalation Powder. Inhaler containing a double-foil blister strip of powder formulation for oral inhalation. Each blister contains umeclidinium 62.5 mcg. (3)

────────────CONTRAINDICATIONS────────────

- Severe hypersensitivity to milk proteins. (4)
- Hypersensitivity to any ingredient. (4)

──────WARNINGS AND PRECAUTIONS──────

- Do not initiate in acutely deteriorating COPD or to treat acute symptoms. (5.1)
- If paradoxical bronchospasm occurs, discontinue INCRUSE ELLIPTA and institute alternative therapy. (5.2)
- Worsening of narrow-angle glaucoma may occur. Use with caution in patients with narrow-angle glaucoma and instruct patients to contact a physician immediately if symptoms occur. (5.4)
- Worsening of urinary retention may occur. Use with caution in patients with prostatic hyperplasia or bladder-neck obstruction and instruct patients to contact a physician immediately if symptoms occur. (5.5)

────────────ADVERSE REACTIONS────────────

Most common adverse reactions (incidence ≥2% and more common than placebo) were nasopharyngitis, upper respiratory tract infection, cough, arthralgia. (6.1)

To report SUSPECTED ADVERSE REACTIONS, contact GlaxoSmithKline at 1-888-825-5249 or FDA at 1-800-FDA-1088 or www.fda.gov/medwatch.

DRUG INTERACTIONS

Anticholinergics: May interact additively with concomitantly used anticholinergic medications. Avoid administration of INCRUSE ELLIPTA with other anticholinergic-containing drugs. (7.1)

See 17 for PATIENT COUNSELING INFORMATION and FDA-approved patient labeling

Revised: 06/2014

FULL PRESCRIBING INFORMATION: CONTENTS*

FULL PRESCRIBING INFORMATION

1   INDICATIONS AND USAGE

INCRUSE® ELLIPTA® is an anticholinergic indicated for the long-term, once-daily, maintenance treatment of airflow obstruction in patients with chronic obstructive pulmonary disease (COPD), including chronic bronchitis and/or emphysema.

2   DOSAGE AND ADMINISTRATION

INCRUSE ELLIPTA (umeclidinium 62.5 mcg) should be administered as 1 inhalation once daily by the orally inhaled route only.

INCRUSE ELLIPTA should be taken at the same time every day. Do not use INCRUSE ELLIPTA more than 1 time every 24 hours.

No dosage adjustment is required for geriatric patients, patients with renal impairment, or patients with moderate hepatic impairment [see Clinical Pharmacology (12.3)].

3   DOSAGE FORMS AND STRENGTHS

Inhalation Powder. Disposable light grey and light green plastic inhaler containing a double-foil blister strip with 30 blisters containing powder intended for oral inhalation only. Each blister contains umeclidinium 62.5 mcg. An institutional pack containing a blister strip with 7 blisters is also available.

4   CONTRAINDICATIONS

The use of INCRUSE ELLIPTA is contraindicated in the following conditions:
• Severe hypersensitivity to milk proteins [see Warnings and Precautions (5.3)]
• Hypersensitivity to umeclidinium or any of the excipients [see Warnings and Precautions (5.3), Description (11)]

5   WARNINGS AND PRECAUTIONS

5.1   Deterioration of Disease and Acute Episodes

INCRUSE ELLIPTA should not be initiated in patients during rapidly deteriorating or potentially life-threatening episodes of COPD. INCRUSE ELLIPTA has not been studied in subjects with acutely deteriorating COPD. The initiation of INCRUSE ELLIPTA in this setting is not appropriate. INCRUSE ELLIPTA should not be used for the relief of acute symptoms, i.e., as rescue therapy for the treatment of acute episodes of bronchospasm. INCRUSE ELLIPTA has not been studied in the relief of acute symptoms and extra doses should not be used for that purpose. Acute symptoms should be treated with an inhaled, short-acting beta₂-agonist.

COPD may deteriorate acutely over a period of hours or chronically over several days or longer. If INCRUSE ELLIPTA no longer controls symptoms of bronchoconstriction; the patient's inhaled, short-acting beta₂-agonist becomes less effective; or the patient needs more short-acting beta₂-agonist than usual, these may be markers of deterioration of disease. In this setting a re-evaluation of the patient and the COPD treatment regimen should be undertaken at once. Increasing the daily dose of INCRUSE ELLIPTA beyond the recommended dose is not appropriate in this situation.

5.2   Paradoxical Bronchospasm

As with other inhaled medicines, INCRUSE ELLIPTA can produce paradoxical bronchospasm, which may be life threatening. If paradoxical bronchospasm occurs following dosing with INCRUSE ELLIPTA, it should be treated immediately with an inhaled, short-acting bronchodilator; INCRUSE ELLIPTA should be discontinued immediately; and alternative therapy should be instituted.

5.3   Hypersensitivity Reactions

Hypersensitivity reactions may occur after administration of INCRUSE ELLIPTA. There have been reports of anaphylactic reactions in patients with severe milk protein allergy after inhalation of other powder products containing lactose; therefore, patients with severe milk protein allergy should not use INCRUSE ELLIPTA [see Contraindications (4)].

5.4   Worsening of Narrow-Angle Glaucoma

INCRUSE ELLIPTA should be used with caution in patients with narrow-angle glaucoma. Prescribers and patients should be alert for signs and symptoms of acute narrow-angle glaucoma (e.g., eye pain or discomfort, blurred vision, visual halos or colored images in association with red eyes from conjunctival congestion and corneal edema). Instruct patients to consult a physician immediately if any of these signs or symptoms develops.

5.5   Worsening of Urinary Retention

INCRUSE ELLIPTA should be used with caution in patients with urinary retention. Prescribers and patients should be alert for signs and symptoms of urinary retention (e.g., difficulty passing urine, painful urination), especially in patients with prostatic hyperplasia or bladder-neck obstruction. Instruct patients to consult a physician immediately if any of these signs or symptoms develops.

6   ADVERSE REACTIONS

The following adverse reactions are described in greater detail in other sections:
• Paradoxical bronchospasm [see Warnings and Precautions (5.2)]
• Worsening of narrow-angle glaucoma [see Warnings and Precautions (5.4)]
• Worsening of urinary retention [see Warnings and Precautions (5.5)]

6.1   Clinical Trials Experience

Because clinical trials are conducted under widely varying conditions, adverse reaction rates observed in the clinical trials of a drug cannot be directly compared with rates in the clinical trials of another drug and may not reflect the rates observed in practice.

A total of 1,663 subjects with COPD across 8 clinical trials (mean age: 62.7 years; 89% white; 65% male across all treatments, including placebo) received at least 1 inhalation dose of umeclidinium at doses of 62.5 or 125 mcg. In the 4 randomized, double-blind, placebo- or active-controlled, efficacy clinical trials, 1,185 subjects received umeclidinium for up to 24 weeks, of which 487 subjects received the recommended dose of umeclidinium 62.5 mcg. In a 12-month, randomized, double-blind, placebo-controlled, long-term safety trial, 227 subjects received umeclidinium 125 mcg for up to 52 weeks [see Clinical Studies (14)].

The incidence of adverse reactions associated with INCRUSE ELLIPTA in Table 1 is based upon 2 placebo-controlled efficacy trials: one 12-week trial and one 24-week trial.

Table 1. Adverse Reactions With INCRUSE ELLIPTA With ≥1% Incidence and More Common Than With Placebo in Subjects With Chronic Obstructive Pulmonary Disease

Adverse Reaction	INCRUSE ELLIPTA (n = 487) %	Placebo (n = 348) %
Infections and infestations		
Nasopharyngitis	8%	7%
Upper respiratory tract infection	5%	4%
Pharyngitis	1%	<1%
Viral upper respiratory tract infection	1%	<1%
Respiratory, thoracic, and mediastinal disorders		
Cough	3%	2%
Musculoskeletal and connective tissue disorders		
Arthralgia	2%	1%
Myalgia	1%	<1%
Gastrointestinal disorders		
Abdominal pain upper	1%	<1%
Toothache	1%	<1%
Injury, poisoning, and procedural complications		
Contusion	1%	<1%
Cardiac disorders		
Tachycardia	1%	<1%

Other adverse reactions with INCRUSE ELLIPTA observed with an incidence less than 1% but more common than placebo included atrial fibrillation.

In a long-term safety trial, 336 subjects (n = 227 umeclidinium 125 mcg, n = 109 placebo) were treated for up to 52 weeks with umeclidinium 125 mcg or placebo. The demographic and baseline characteristics of the long-term safety trial were similar to those of the efficacy trials described above. Adverse reactions that occurred with a frequency greater than or equal to 1% in subjects receiving umeclidinium 125 mcg that exceeded that in placebo in this trial were: nasopharyngitis, upper respiratory tract infection, urinary tract infection, pharyngitis, pneumonia, lower respiratory tract infection, rhinitis, supraventricular tachycardia, supraventricular extrasystoles, sinus tachycardia, idioventricular rhythm, headache, dizziness, sinus headache, cough, back pain, arthralgia, pain in extremity, neck pain, myalgia, nausea, dyspepsia, diarrhea, rash, depression, and vertigo.

7   DRUG INTERACTIONS

7.1   Anticholinergics

There is potential for an additive interaction with concomitantly used anticholinergic medicines. Therefore, avoid co-administration of INCRUSE ELLIPTA with other anticholinergic-containing drugs as this may lead to an increase in anticholinergic adverse effects [see Warnings and Precautions (5.4, 5.5), Adverse Reactions (6)].

8   USE IN SPECIFIC POPULATIONS

8.1   Pregnancy

Teratogenic Effects: Pregnancy Category C. There are no adequate and well-controlled trials with INCRUSE ELLIPTA in pregnant women. Because animal reproduction studies are not always predictive of human response, INCRUSE ELLIPTA should be used during pregnancy only if the potential benefit justifies the potential risk to the fetus. Women should be advised to contact their physicians if they become pregnant while taking INCRUSE ELLIPTA.

There was no evidence of teratogenic effects in rats and rabbits at approximately 50 and 200 times, respectively, the MRHDID (maximum recommended human daily inhaled dose) in adults (on an AUC basis at maternal inhaled doses up to 278 mcg/kg/day in rats and maternal subcutaneous doses up to 180 mcg/kg/day in rabbits).

Nonteratogenic Effects: There were no effects on perinatal and postnatal developments in rats at approximately 80 times the MRHDID in adults (on an AUC basis at maternal subcutaneous doses up to 180 mcg/kg/day).

8.2   Labor and Delivery

There are no adequate and well-controlled human trials that have investigated the effects of INCRUSE ELLIPTA during labor and delivery. INCRUSE ELLIPTA should be used during labor only if the potential benefit justifies the potential risk.

8.3   Nursing Mothers

It is not known whether INCRUSE ELLIPTA is excreted in human breast milk. Because many drugs are excreted in human milk, caution should be exercised when INCRUSE ELLIPTA is administered to a nursing woman. Since there are no data from well-controlled human studies on the use of INCRUSE ELLIPTA by nursing mothers, a decision should be made whether to discontinue nursing or to discontinue INCRUSE ELLIPTA, taking into account the importance of INCRUSE ELLIPTA to the mother.

Subcutaneous administration of umeclidinium to lactating rats at approximately 25 times the MRHDID in adults resulted in a quantifiable level of umeclidinium in 2 pups, which may indicate transfer of umeclidinium in milk.

8.4 Pediatric Use

INCRUSE ELLIPTA is not indicated for use in children. The safety and efficacy in pediatric patients have not been established.

8.5 Geriatric Use

Based on available data, no adjustment of the dosage of INCRUSE ELLIPTA in geriatric patients is necessary, but greater sensitivity in some older individuals cannot be ruled out.

Clinical trials of INCRUSE ELLIPTA included 810 subjects aged 65 years and older, and, of those, 183 subjects were aged 75 years and older. No overall differences in safety or effectiveness were observed between these subjects and younger subjects, and other reported clinical experience has not identified differences in responses between the elderly and younger subjects.

8.6 Hepatic Impairment

Patients with moderate hepatic impairment (Child-Pugh score of 7-9) showed no relevant increases in C_{max} or AUC, nor did protein binding differ between subjects with moderate hepatic impairment and their healthy controls. Studies in subjects with severe hepatic impairment have not been performed [see Clinical Pharmacology (12.3)].

8.7 Renal Impairment

Patients with severe renal impairment (creatinine clearance less than 30 mL/min) showed no relevant increases in C_{max} or AUC, nor did protein binding differ between subjects with severe renal impairment and their healthy controls. No dosage adjustment is required in patients with renal impairment [see Clinical Pharmacology (12.3)].

10 OVERDOSAGE

No case of overdose has been reported with INCRUSE ELLIPTA.

High doses of umeclidinium may lead to anticholinergic signs and symptoms. However, there were no systemic anticholinergic adverse effects following a once-daily inhaled dose of up to 1,000 mcg umeclidinium (16 times the maximum recommended daily dose) for 14 days in subjects with COPD.

Treatment of overdosage consists of discontinuation of INCRUSE ELLIPTA together with institution of appropriate symptomatic and/or supportive therapy.

11 DESCRIPTION

INCRUSE ELLIPTA contains the active ingredient umeclidinium, an anticholinergic.

Umeclidinium bromide has the chemical name 1-[2-(benzyloxy)ethyl]-4-(hydroxydiphenylmethyl)-1-azoniabicyclo-[2.2.2]octane bromide and the following chemical structure:

Umeclidinium bromide is a white powder with a molecular weight of 508.5, and the empirical formula is $C_{29}H_{34}NO_2 \cdot Br$ (as a quaternary ammonium bromide compound). It is slightly soluble in water.

INCRUSE ELLIPTA is a light grey and light green plastic inhaler containing a double-foil blister strip. Each blister on the strip contains a white powder mix of micronized umeclidinium bromide (74.2 mcg equivalent to 62.5 mcg of umeclidinium), magnesium stearate (75 mcg), and lactose monohydrate (to 12.5 mg). The lactose monohydrate contains milk proteins. After the inhaler is activated, the powder within the blister is exposed and ready for dispersion into the airstream created by the patient inhaling through the mouthpiece.

Under standardized in vitro test conditions, INCRUSE ELLIPTA delivers 55 mcg of umeclidinium per dose when tested at a flow rate of 60 L/min for 4 seconds.

In adult subjects with obstructive lung disease and severely compromised lung function (COPD with forced expiratory volume in 1 second/forced vital capacity [FEV₁/FVC] less than 70% and FEV₁ less than 30% predicted or FEV₁ less than 50% predicted plus chronic respiratory failure), mean peak inspiratory flow through the ELLIPTA inhaler was 67.5 L/min (range: 41.6 to 83.3 L/min).

The actual amount of drug delivered to the lung will depend on patient factors, such as inspiratory flow profile.

12 CLINICAL PHARMACOLOGY

12.1 Mechanism of Action

Umeclidinium is a long-acting, antimuscarinic agent, which is often referred to as an anticholinergic. It has similar affinity to the subtypes of muscarinic receptors M1 to M5. In the airways, it exhibits pharmacological effects through the inhibition of M3 receptor at the smooth muscle leading to bronchodilation. The competitive and reversible nature of antagonism was shown with human and animal origin re-

Figure 1. Impact of Intrinsic and Extrinsic Factors on the Systemic Exposure of Umeclidinium

Impact of Factors on Umeclidinium PK

Population Description:	PK	Fold Change and 90% CI	Recommendation
Gender:			
Male	AUC		No dose adjustment
	Cmax		
Age:			
>65 Years	AUC		No dose adjustment
	Cmax		
Severe Renal Impairment	AUC		No dose adjustment
	Cmax		
Moderate Hepatic Impairment	AUC		No dose adjustment
	Cmax		
CYP2D6 Inhibitor:			
Poor Metabolizer	AUC		No dose adjustment
	Cmax		
P-gp Transport Inhibitor:			
Verapamil	AUC		No dose adjustment
	Cmax		

Change relative to reference (x-axis: 0.0, 0.5, 1.0, 1.5, 2.0)

ceptors and isolated organ preparations. In preclinical in vitro as well as in vivo studies, prevention of methacholine and acetylcholine-induced bronchoconstrictive effects was dose-dependent and lasted longer than 24 hours. The clinical relevance of these findings is unknown. The bronchodilation following inhalation of umeclidinium is predominantly a site-specific effect.

12.2 Pharmacodynamics

Cardiac Electrophysiology: QTc interval prolongation was studied in a double-blind, multiple dose, placebo- and positive-controlled, crossover trial in 86 healthy subjects. Following repeat doses of umeclidinium 500 mcg once daily (8 times the recommended dosage) for 10 days, umeclidinium does not prolong QTc to any clinically relevant extent.

12.3 Pharmacokinetics

Linear pharmacokinetics was observed for umeclidinium (62.5 to 500 mcg).

Absorption: Umeclidinium plasma levels may not predict therapeutic effect. Following inhaled administration of umeclidinium in healthy subjects, C_{max} occurred at 5 to 15 minutes. Umeclidinium is mostly absorbed from the lung after inhaled doses with minimum contribution from oral absorption. Following repeat dosing of inhaled INCRUSE ELLIPTA, steady state was achieved within 14 days with 1.8-fold accumulation.

Distribution: Following intravenous administration to healthy subjects, the mean volume of distribution was 86 L. In vitro plasma protein binding in human plasma was on average 89%.

Metabolism: In vitro data showed that umeclidinium is primarily metabolized by the enzyme cytochrome P450 2D6 (CYP2D6) and is a substrate for the P-glycoprotein (P-gp) transporter. The primary metabolic routes for umeclidinium are oxidative (hydroxylation, O-dealkylation) followed by conjugation (e.g., glucuronidation), resulting in a range of metabolites with either reduced pharmacological activity or for which the pharmacological activity has not been established. Systemic exposure to the metabolites is low.

Elimination: Following intravenous dosing with radiolabeled umeclidinium, mass balance showed 58% of the radiolabel in the feces and 22% in the urine. The excretion of the drug-related material in the feces following intravenous dosing indicated elimination in the bile. Following oral dosing to healthy male subjects, radiolabel recovered in feces was 92% of the total dose and that in urine was less than 1% of the total dose, suggesting negligible oral absorption. The effective half-life after once daily dosing is 11 hours.

Special Populations: Population pharmacokinetic analysis showed no evidence of a clinically significant effect of age (40 to 93 years) (see Figure 1), gender (69% male) (see Figure 1), inhaled corticosteroid use (48%), or weight (34 to 161 kg) on systemic exposure of umeclidinium. In addition, there was no evidence of a clinically significant effect of race.

Hepatic Impairment: The impact of hepatic impairment on the pharmacokinetics of INCRUSE ELLIPTA has been evaluated in subjects with moderate hepatic impairment (Child-Pugh score of 7-9). There was no evidence of an increase in systemic exposure to umeclidinium (C_{max} and AUC) (see Figure 1). There was no evidence of altered protein binding in subjects with moderate hepatic impairment compared with healthy subjects. INCRUSE ELLIPTA has not been evaluated in subjects with severe hepatic impairment.

Renal Impairment: The pharmacokinetics of INCRUSE ELLIPTA has been evaluated in subjects with severe renal impairment (creatinine clearance less than 30 mL/min). There was no evidence of an increase in systemic exposure to umeclidinium (C_{max} and AUC) (see Figure 1). There was no evidence of altered protein binding in subjects with severe renal impairment compared with healthy subjects.
[See figure above]

Drug Interactions: Umeclidinium and P-glycoprotein Transporter: Umeclidinium is a substrate of P-gp. The effect of the moderate P-gp transporter inhibitor verapamil (240 mg once daily) on the steady-state pharmacokinetics of umeclidinium was assessed in healthy subjects. No effect on umeclidinium C_{max} was observed; however, an approximately 1.4-fold increase in umeclidinium AUC was observed (see Figure 1).

Umeclidinium and Cytochrome P450 2D6: In vitro metabolism of umeclidinium is mediated primarily by CYP2D6. However, no clinically meaningful difference in systemic exposure to umeclidinium (500 mcg) (8 times the approved dose) was observed following repeat daily inhaled dosing to normal (ultrarapid, extensive, and intermediate metabolizers) and CYP2D6 poor metabolizer subjects (see Figure 1).

13 NONCLINICAL TOXICOLOGY

13.1 Carcinogenesis, Mutagenesis, Impairment of Fertility

Umeclidinium produced no treatment-related increases in the incidence of tumors in 2-year inhalation studies in rats and mice at inhaled doses up to 137 and 295/200 mcg/kg/day (male/female), respectively (approximately 20 and 25/20 times the MRHDID in adults on an AUC basis, respectively).

Umeclidinium tested negative in the following genotoxicity assays: the in vitro Ames assay, in vitro mouse lymphoma assay, and in vivo rat bone marrow micronucleus assay.

No evidence of impairment of fertility was observed in male and female rats at subcutaneous doses up to 180 mcg/kg/day and inhaled doses up to 294 mcg/kg/day, respectively (approximately 100 and 50 times, respectively, the MRHDID in adults on an AUC basis).

14 CLINICAL STUDIES

The safety and efficacy of umeclidinium 62.5 mcg were evaluated in 3 dose-ranging trials, 2 placebo-controlled clinical trials (one 12-week trial and one 24-week trial), and a 12-month long-term safety trial. The efficacy of INCRUSE ELLIPTA is based primarily on the dose-ranging trials in 624 subjects with COPD and the 2 placebo-controlled confirmatory trials in 1,738 subjects with COPD.

Figure 2. Adjusted Mean Change From Baseline in Post-Dose Serial FEV$_1$ (mL) on Days 1 and 7

Day 1

Day 7

Placebo ◆◆◆   Umeclidinium 31.25 mcg ★★★   Umeclidinium 125 mcg ◆◆◆
Umeclidinium 15.6 mcg ●●●   Umeclidinium 62.5 mcg ■■■

14.1   Dose-Ranging Trials

Dose selection for umeclidinium in COPD was supported by a 7-day, randomized, double-blind, placebo-controlled, cross-over trial evaluating 4 doses of umeclidinium (15.6 to 125 mcg) or placebo dosed once daily in the morning in 163 subjects with COPD. A dose ordering was observed, with the 62.5- and 125-mcg doses demonstrating larger improvements in FEV$_1$ over 24 hours compared with the lower doses of 15.6 and 31.25 mcg (Figure 2).

The differences in trough FEV$_1$ from baseline after 7 days for placebo and the 15.6-, 31.25-, 62.5-, and 125-mcg doses were -74 mL (95% CI: -118, -31), 38 mL (95% CI: -6, 83), 27 mL (95% CI: -18, 72), 49 mL (95% CI: 6, 93), and 109 mL (95% CI: 65, 152), respectively. Two additional dose-ranging trials in subjects with COPD demonstrated minimal additional benefit at doses above 125 mcg. The dose-ranging results supported the evaluation of 2 doses of umeclidinium, 62.5 and 125 mcg, in the confirmatory COPD trials to further assess dose response.

Evaluations of dosing interval by comparing once- and twice-daily dosing supported selection of a once-daily dosing interval for further evaluation in the confirmatory COPD trials.

[See figure above]

14.2   Confirmatory Trials

The clinical development program for INCRUSE ELLIPTA included 2 randomized, double-blind, placebo-controlled, parallel-group trials in subjects with COPD designed to evaluate the efficacy of INCRUSE ELLIPTA on lung function. Trial 1 was a 24-week placebo-controlled trial, and Trial 2 was a 12-week placebo-controlled trial. These trials treated subjects that had a clinical diagnosis of COPD, were 40 years of age or older, had a history of smoking greater than or equal to 10 pack-years, had a post-albuterol FEV$_1$ less than or equal to 70% of predicted normal values, had a ratio of FEV$_1$/FVC of less than 0.7, and had a Modified Medical Research Council (mMRC) score greater than or equal to 2. Subjects in Trial 1 had a mean age of 63 years and an average smoking history of 46 pack-years, with 50% identified as current smokers. At screening, the mean post-

bronchodilator percent predicted FEV$_1$ was 47% (range: 13% to 74%), the mean post-bronchodilator FEV$_1$/FVC ratio was 0.47 (range: 0.20 to 0.74), and the mean percent reversibility was 15% (range: -35% to 109%). Baseline demographics and lung function for subjects in Trial 2 were similar to those in Trial 1.

Trial 1 evaluated umeclidinium 62.5 mcg and placebo. The primary endpoint was change from baseline in trough (predose) FEV$_1$ at Day 169 (defined as the mean of the FEV$_1$ values obtained at 23 and 24 hours after the previous dose on Day 168) compared with placebo. INCRUSE ELLIPTA 62.5 mcg demonstrated a larger increase in mean change from baseline in trough (predose) FEV$_1$ relative to placebo (see Table 2). Similar results were obtained from Trial 2.

Table 2. Least Squares (LS) Mean Change From Baseline in Trough FEV$_1$ (mL) at Day 169 in the Intent-to-Treat Population (Trial 1)

Treatment	n	Trough FEV$_1$ (mL) at Day 169
		Difference From Placebo (95% CI) n = 280
INCRUSE ELLIPTA	n = 418	115 (76, 155)

n = Number in intent-to-treat population.

Serial spirometric evaluations throughout the 24-hour dosing interval were performed in a subset of subjects (n = 54, umeclidinium 62.5 mcg; n = 36, placebo) at Days 1, 84, and 168 in Trial 1, and for all patients at Days 1 and 84 in Trial 2. Results from Trial 1 at Day 1 and Day 168 are shown in Figure 3.

[See figure 2 at top of next page]

In Trial 1, the mean peak FEV$_1$ (over the first 6 hours relative to baseline) at Day 1 and at Day 168 for the group receiving umeclidinium 62.5 mcg compared with placebo was 126 and 130 mL, respectively.

Health-related quality of life was measured using St. George's Respiratory Questionnaire (SGRQ). Umeclidinium demonstrated an improvement in mean SGRQ total score compared with placebo treatment at Day 168: -4.69 (95% CI: -7.07,-2.31). The proportion of patients with a clinically meaningful decrease (defined as a decrease of at least 4 units from baseline) at Week 24 was greater for INCRUSE ELLIPTA 62.5 mcg (42%; 172/410) compared with placebo (31%; 86/274).

16   HOW SUPPLIED/STORAGE AND HANDLING

INCRUSE ELLIPTA is supplied as a disposable light grey and light green plastic inhaler containing a double-foil blister strip with 30 blisters. The inhaler is packaged in a moisture-protective foil tray with a desiccant and a peelable lid (NDC 0173-0873-10).

INCRUSE ELLIPTA is also supplied in an institutional pack of a disposable light grey and light green plastic inhaler containing a double-foil blister strip with 7 blisters. The inhaler is packaged in a moisture-protective foil tray with a desiccant and a peelable lid (NDC 0173-0873-06).

Store at room temperature between 68°F and 77°F (20°C and 25°C); excursions permitted from 59°F to 86°F (15°C to 30°C) [See USP Controlled Room Temperature]. Store in a dry place away from direct heat or sunlight. Keep out of reach of children.

INCRUSE ELLIPTA should be stored inside the unopened moisture-protective foil tray and only removed from the tray immediately before initial use. Discard INCRUSE ELLIPTA 6 weeks after opening the foil tray or when the counter reads "0" (after all blisters have been used), whichever comes first. The inhaler is not reusable. Do not attempt to take the inhaler apart.

17   PATIENT COUNSELING INFORMATION

Advise the patient to read the FDA-approved patient labeling (Patient Information and Instructions for Use).

Not for Acute Symptoms: Inform patients that INCRUSE ELLIPTA is not meant to relieve acute symptoms of COPD and extra doses should not be used for that purpose. Advise them to treat acute symptoms with a rescue inhaler such as albuterol. Provide patients with such medicine and instruct them in how it should be used.

Instruct patients to seek medical attention immediately if they experience any of the following:
• Symptoms get worse
• Need for more inhalations than usual of their rescue inhaler

Patients should not stop therapy with INCRUSE ELLIPTA without physician/provider guidance since symptoms may recur after discontinuation.

Paradoxical Bronchospasm: As with other inhaled medicines, INCRUSE ELLIPTA can cause paradoxical bronchospasm. If paradoxical bronchospasm occurs, instruct patients to discontinue INCRUSE ELLIPTA.

Worsening of Narrow-Angle Glaucoma: Instruct patients to be alert for signs and symptoms of acute narrow-angle glaucoma (e.g., eye pain or discomfort, blurred vision, visual halos or colored images in association with red eyes from conjunctival congestion and corneal edema). Instruct patients to consult a physician immediately if any of these signs or symptoms develops.

Worsening of Urinary Retention: Instruct patients to be alert for signs and symptoms of urinary retention (e.g., difficulty passing urine, painful urination). Instruct patients to consult a physician immediately if any of these signs or symptoms develops.

INCRUSE and ELLIPTA are registered trademarks of the GSK group of companies.

GlaxoSmithKline

Research Triangle Park, NC 27709

©2014, the GSK group of companies. All rights reserved.

INC:3PI

Patient Information

INCRUSE® ELLIPTA® *[IN-cruse e-LIP-ta]*
(umeclidinium inhalation powder)

Read the Patient Information that comes with INCRUSE ELLIPTA before you start using it and each time you get a refill. There may be new information. This Patient Information does not take the place of talking to your healthcare provider about your medical condition or treatment.

What is INCRUSE ELLIPTA?

INCRUSE ELLIPTA is an anticholinergic medicine. Anticholinergic medicines help the muscles around the airways in your lungs stay relaxed to prevent symptoms such as wheezing, cough, chest tightness, and shortness of breath. These symptoms can happen when the muscles around the airways tighten. This makes it hard to breathe.

INCRUSE ELLIPTA is a prescription medicine used to treat COPD. COPD is a chronic lung disease that includes chronic bronchitis, emphysema, or both. INCRUSE ELLIPTA is used long term as 1 inhalation, 1 time each day, to improve symptoms of COPD for better breathing.

Figure 3. Least Squares (LS) Mean Change From Baseline in FEV_1 (mL) Over Time (0-24 hr) on Days 1 and 168 (Trial 1 Subset Population)

Day 1

Day 168

- rash
- hives
- swelling of the face, mouth, and tongue
- breathing problems
- **new or worsened eye problems including acute narrow-angle glaucoma.** Acute narrow-angle glaucoma can cause permanent loss of vision if not treated. Symptoms of acute narrow-angle glaucoma may include:
  - eye pain or discomfort
  - nausea or vomiting
  - blurred vision
  - seeing halos or bright colors around lights
  - red eyes
  If you have these symptoms, call your doctor right away before taking another dose.
- **urinary retention.** People who take INCRUSE ELLIPTA may develop new or worse urinary retention. Symptoms of urinary retention may include:
  - difficulty urinating
  - painful urination
  - urinating frequently
  - urination in a weak stream or drips
  If you have these symptoms of urinary retention, stop taking INCRUSE ELLIPTA, and call your doctor right away before taking another dose.

Common side effects of INCRUSE ELLIPTA include:
- upper respiratory infection
- stuffy or runny nose
- cough
- sore throat
- joint pain
- muscle pain
- tooth pain
- stomach pain
- bruising or dark areas of skin
- fast or irregular heartbeat

Tell your healthcare provider about any side effect that bothers you or that does not go away.

These are not all the side effects with INCRUSE ELLIPTA. Ask your healthcare provider or pharmacist for more information.

Call your doctor for medical advice about side effects. You may report side effects to FDA at 1-800-FDA-1088.

How do I store INCRUSE ELLIPTA?
- Store INCRUSE ELLIPTA at room temperature between 68°F and 77°F (20°C and 25°C). Keep in a dry place away from heat and sunlight.
- Store INCRUSE ELLIPTA in the unopened foil tray and only open when ready for use.
- Safely throw away INCRUSE ELLIPTA in the trash 6 weeks after you open the foil tray or when the counter reads "0," whichever comes first. Write the date you open the tray on the label on the inhaler.
- **Keep INCRUSE ELLIPTA and all medicines out of the reach of children.**

General information about INCRUSE ELLIPTA
Medicines are sometimes prescribed for purposes not mentioned in a Patient Information leaflet. Do not use INCRUSE ELLIPTA for a condition for which it was not prescribed. Do not give your INCRUSE ELLIPTA to other people, even if they have the same condition that you have. It may harm them.

This Patient Information leaflet summarizes the most important information about INCRUSE ELLIPTA. If you would like more information, talk with your healthcare provider or pharmacist. You can ask your healthcare provider or pharmacist for information about INCRUSE ELLIPTA that was written for healthcare professionals.

For more information about INCRUSE ELLIPTA, call 1-888-825-5249 or visit our website at www.INCRUSE.com.

What are the ingredients in INCRUSE ELLIPTA?
Active ingredients: umeclidinium
Inactive ingredients: lactose monohydrate (contains milk proteins), magnesium stearate

Instructions for Use
For Oral Inhalation Only.
Read this before you start:
- **If you open and close the cover without inhaling the medicine, you will lose the dose.**
- **The lost dose will be securely held inside the inhaler, but it will no longer be available to be inhaled.**
- **It is not possible to accidentally take a double dose or an extra dose in one inhalation.**

Your INCRUSE ELLIPTA inhaler
[See figure at top of next column]
How to use your inhaler
- INCRUSE ELLIPTA comes in a foil tray.
- Peel back the lid to open the tray. See Figure A.

- **INCRUSE ELLIPTA is not for use to treat sudden symptoms of COPD.** Always have a rescue inhaler (an inhaled, short-acting bronchodilator) with you to treat sudden symptoms. If you do not have a rescue inhaler, contact your healthcare provider to have one prescribed for you.
- INCRUSE ELLIPTA should not be used in children. It is not known if INCRUSE ELLIPTA is safe and effective in children.

Who should not use INCRUSE ELLIPTA?
Do not use INCRUSE ELLIPTA if you:
- have a severe allergy to milk proteins. Ask your healthcare provider if you are not sure.
- are allergic to umeclidinium or any of the ingredients in INCRUSE ELLIPTA. See "What are the ingredients in INCRUSE ELLIPTA?" below for a complete list of ingredients.

What should I tell my healthcare provider before using INCRUSE ELLIPTA?
Tell your healthcare provider about all of your health conditions, including if you:
- have heart problems.
- have eye problems such as glaucoma. INCRUSE ELLIPTA may make your glaucoma worse.
- have prostate or bladder problems, or problems passing urine. INCRUSE ELLIPTA may make these problems worse.
- are allergic to any of the ingredients in INCRUSE ELLIPTA, any other medicines, or food products. See "What are the ingredients in INCRUSE ELLIPTA?" below for a complete list of ingredients.
- have any other medical conditions.
- are pregnant or planning to become pregnant. It is not known if INCRUSE ELLIPTA may harm your unborn baby.
- are breastfeeding. It is not known if the medicine in INCRUSE ELLIPTA passes into your milk and if it can harm your baby.

Tell your healthcare provider about all the medicines you take, including prescription and over-the-counter medicines, vitamins, and herbal supplements. INCRUSE ELLIPTA and certain other medicines may interact with each other. This may cause serious side effects.

Especially tell your healthcare provider if you take:
- anticholinergics (including tiotropium, ipratropium, aclidinium)
- atropine

Know the medicines you take. Keep a list of them to show your healthcare provider and pharmacist when you get a new medicine.

How should I use INCRUSE ELLIPTA?
Read the step-by-step instructions for using INCRUSE ELLIPTA at the end of this Patient Information.
- **Do not** use INCRUSE ELLIPTA unless your healthcare provider has taught you how to use the inhaler and you understand how to use it correctly.
- Use INCRUSE ELLIPTA exactly as your healthcare provider tells you to use it. **Do not** use INCRUSE ELLIPTA more often than prescribed.
- Use 1 inhalation of INCRUSE ELLIPTA 1 time each day. Use INCRUSE ELLIPTA at the same time each day.
- If you miss a dose of INCRUSE ELLIPTA, take it as soon as you remember. Do not take more than 1 inhalation each day. Take your next dose at your usual time. Do not take 2 doses at one time.
- If you take too much INCRUSE ELLIPTA, call your healthcare provider or go to the nearest hospital emergency room right away if you have any unusual symptoms, such as worsening shortness of breath, chest pain, increased heart rate, or shakiness.
- **Do not use other medicines that contain an anticholinergic for any reason.** Ask your healthcare provider or pharmacist if any of your other medicines are anticholinergic medicines.
- Do not stop using INCRUSE ELLIPTA unless told to do so by your healthcare provider because your symptoms might get worse. Your healthcare provider will change your medicines as needed.
- **INCRUSE ELLIPTA does not relieve sudden symptoms.** Always have a rescue inhaler with you to treat sudden symptoms. If you do not have a rescue inhaler, call your healthcare provider to have one prescribed for you.
- Call your healthcare provider or get medical care right away if:
  - your breathing problems get worse
  - you need to use your rescue inhaler more often than usual
  - your rescue inhaler does not work as well to relieve your symptoms

What are the possible side effects with INCRUSE ELLIPTA?
INCRUSE ELLIPTA can cause serious side effects, including:
- **sudden breathing problems immediately after inhaling your medicine.** If you have sudden breathing problems immediately after inhaling your medicine, stop taking INCRUSE ELLIPTA and call your doctor right away.
- **serious allergic reactions.** Call your healthcare provider or get emergency medical care if you get any of the following symptoms of a serious allergic reaction:

Figure A

- The tray contains a desiccant to reduce moisture. Do not eat or inhale. Throw it away in the household trash out of reach of children and pets. See Figure B.

Figure A

Figure B

Important Notes:
- Your inhaler contains 30 doses (7 doses if you have a sample or institutional pack).
- Each time you fully open the cover of the inhaler (you will hear a clicking sound), a dose is ready to be inhaled. This is shown by a decrease in the number on the counter.
- If you open and close the cover without inhaling the medicine, you will lose the dose. The lost dose will be held in the inhaler, but it will no longer be available to be inhaled. It is not possible to accidentally take a double dose or an extra dose in one inhalation.
- **Do not** open the cover of the inhaler until you are ready to use it. To avoid wasting doses after the inhaler is ready, **do not** close the cover until after you have inhaled the medicine.
- Write the "Tray opened" and "Discard" dates on the inhaler label. The "Discard" date is 6 weeks from the date you open the tray.

Check the counter. See Figure C.

Figure C

- Before the inhaler is used for the first time, the counter should show the number 30 (7 if you have a sample or institutional pack). This is the number of doses in the inhaler.
- Each time you open the cover, you prepare 1 dose of medicine.
- The counter counts down by 1 each time you open the cover.

Prepare your dose:
Wait to open the cover until you are ready to take your dose.
Step 1. Open the cover of the inhaler. See Figure D.

Figure D

- Slide the cover down to expose the mouthpiece. You should hear a "click." The counter will count down by 1 number. You do not need to shake this kind of inhaler. **Your inhaler is now ready to use.**
- If the counter does not count down as you hear the click, the inhaler will not deliver the medicine. Call your healthcare provider or pharmacist if this happens.

Step 2. Breathe out. See Figure E.

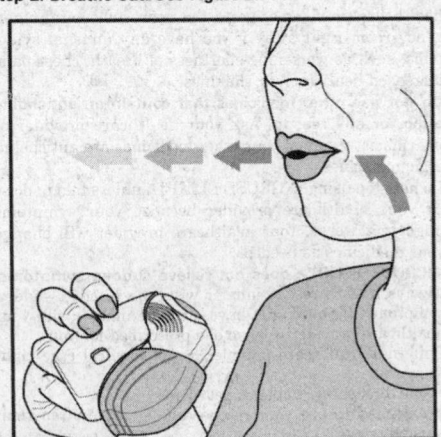

Figure E

- While holding the inhaler away from your mouth, breathe out (exhale) fully. Do not breathe out into the mouthpiece.

Step 3. Inhale your medicine. See Figure F.
[See figure F at top of next column]
- Put the mouthpiece between your lips, and close your lips firmly around it. Your lips should fit over the curved shape of the mouthpiece.
- Take one long, steady, deep breath in through your mouth. **Do not** breathe in through your nose.

Figure F

- Do not block the air vent with your fingers. **See Figure G.**

Do not block the air vent with your fingers.

Figure G

- **Remove the inhaler from your mouth and hold your breath for about 3 to 4 seconds** (or as long as comfortable for you). **See Figure H.**

Figure H

Step 4. Breathe out slowly and gently. See Figure I.
[See figure I at top of next column]
- You may not taste or feel the medicine, even when you are using the inhaler correctly.
- **Do not** take another dose from the inhaler even if you do not feel or taste the medicine.

Step 5. Close the inhaler. See Figure J.
[See figure J at top of next column]
- You can clean the mouthpiece if needed, using a dry tissue, before you close the cover. Routine cleaning is not required.
- Slide the cover up and over the mouthpiece as far as it will go.

Important Note: When should you get a refill?
- **When you have less than 10 doses remaining** in your inhaler, the left half of the counter shows red as a reminder to get a refill. **See Figure K.**
[See figure K at top of next column]

Figure I

Figure J

Figure K

- After you have inhaled the last dose, the counter will show "0" and will be empty.
- Throw the empty inhaler away in your household trash out of reach of children and pets.

If you have questions about INCRUSE ELLIPTA or how to use your inhaler, call GlaxoSmithKline (GSK) at 1-888-825-5249 or visit www.INCRUSE.com.

This Patient Information and Instructions for Use have been approved by the U.S. Food and Drug Administration.
INCRUSE and ELLIPTA are registered trademarks of the GSK group of companies.

GlaxoSmithKline
Research Triangle Park, NC 27709
©2014, the GSK group of companies. All rights reserved.
June 2014
INC:2PIL

INFANRIX
[in' fan-rix]   ℞
(Diphtheria and Tetanus Toxoids
and Acellular Pertussis Vaccine Adsorbed)
Suspension for Intramuscular Injection

HIGHLIGHTS OF PRESCRIBING INFORMATION
These highlights do not include all the information needed to use INFANRIX safely and effectively. See full prescribing information for INFANRIX.

INFANRIX (Diphtheria and Tetanus Toxoids and Acellular Pertussis Vaccine Adsorbed)
Suspension for Intramuscular Injection
Initial U.S. Approval: 1997

————INDICATIONS AND USAGE————
INFANRIX is a vaccine indicated for active immunization against diphtheria, tetanus, and pertussis as a 5-dose series in infants and children 6 weeks to 7 years of age. (1)

————DOSAGE AND ADMINISTRATION————
A 0.5-mL intramuscular injection given as a 5-dose series: (2.2)
- One dose each at 2, 4, and 6 months of age.
- One booster dose at 15 to 20 months of age and another booster dose at 4 to 6 years of age.

————DOSAGE FORMS AND STRENGTHS————
Single-dose vials and prefilled syringes containing a 0.5-mL suspension for injection. (3)

————CONTRAINDICATIONS————
- Severe allergic reaction (e.g., anaphylaxis) after a previous dose of any diphtheria toxoid, tetanus toxoid, or pertussis-containing vaccine, or to any component of INFANRIX. (4.1)
- Encephalopathy within 7 days of administration of a previous pertussis-containing vaccine. (4.2)
- Progressive neurologic disorders. (4.3)

————WARNINGS AND PRECAUTIONS————
- If Guillain-Barré syndrome occurs within 6 weeks of receipt of a prior vaccine containing tetanus toxoid, the decision to give INFANRIX should be based on potential benefits and risks. (5.1)
- The tip caps of the prefilled syringes may contain natural rubber latex which may cause allergic reactions in latex-sensitive individuals. (5.2)
- Syncope (fainting) can occur in association with administration of injectable vaccines, including INFANRIX. Procedures should be in place to avoid falling injury and to restore cerebral perfusion following syncope. (5.3)
- If temperature ≥105°F, collapse or shock-like state, or persistent, inconsolable crying lasting ≥3 hours have occurred within 48 hours after receipt of a pertussis-containing vaccine, or if seizures have occurred within 3 days after receipt of a pertussis-containing vaccine, the decision to give INFANRIX should be based on potential benefits and risks. (5.4)
- For children at higher risk for seizures, an antipyretic may be administered at the time of vaccination with INFANRIX. (5.5)
- Apnea following intramuscular vaccination has been observed in some infants born prematurely. Decisions about when to administer an intramuscular vaccine, including INFANRIX, to infants born prematurely should be based on consideration of the individual infant's medical status, and the potential benefits and possible risks of vaccination. (5.6)

————ADVERSE REACTIONS————
Rates of injection site reactions (pain, redness, swelling) ranged from 10% to 53%, depending on reaction and dose number, and were highest following doses 4 and 5. Fever was common (20% to 30%) following doses 1-3. Other common solicited adverse events were drowsiness, irritability/fussiness, and loss of appetite, reported in approximately 15% to 60% of subjects, depending on event and dose number. (6.1)

To report SUSPECTED ADVERSE REACTIONS, contact GlaxoSmithKline at 1-888-825-5249 or VAERS at 1-800-822-7967 or www.vaers.hhs.gov.

————DRUG INTERACTIONS————
Do not mix INFANRIX with any other vaccine in the same syringe or vial. (7.1)

See 17 for PATIENT COUNSELING INFORMATION
Revised: 11/2013

FULL PRESCRIBING INFORMATION

1   INDICATIONS AND USAGE
INFANRIX® is indicated for active immunization against diphtheria, tetanus, and pertussis as a 5-dose series in infants and children 6 weeks to 7 years of age (prior to seventh birthday).

2   DOSAGE AND ADMINISTRATION
2.1   Preparation for Administration
Shake vigorously to obtain a homogeneous, turbid, white suspension. Do not use if resuspension does not occur with vigorous shaking. Parenteral drug products should be inspected visually for particulate matter and discoloration prior to administration, whenever solution and container permit. If either of these conditions exists, the vaccine should not be administered.
For the prefilled syringes, attach a sterile needle and administer intramuscularly.
For the vials, use a sterile needle and sterile syringe to withdraw the 0.5-mL dose and administer intramuscularly. Changing needles between drawing vaccine from a vial and injecting it into a recipient is not necessary unless the needle has been damaged or contaminated. Use a separate sterile needle and syringe for each individual.
Do not administer this product intravenously, intradermally, or subcutaneously.
2.2   Dose and Schedule
A 0.5-mL dose of INFANRIX is approved for intramuscular administration in infants and children 6 weeks to 7 years of age (prior to the seventh birthday) as a 5-dose series. The series consists of a primary immunization course of 3 doses administered at 2, 4, and 6 months of age (at intervals of 4 to 8 weeks), followed by 2 booster doses, administered at 15 to 20 months of age and at 4 to 6 years of age. The first dose may be given as early as 6 weeks of age.
The preferred administration site is the anterolateral aspect of the thigh for most infants younger than 12 months of age and the deltoid muscle of the upper arm for most children 12 months of age to 7 years of age.
2.3   Use of INFANRIX With Other DTaP Vaccines
Sufficient data are not available on the safety and effectiveness of interchanging INFANRIX and Diphtheria and Tetanus Toxoids and Acellular Pertussis (DTaP) vaccines from different manufacturers for successive doses of the DTaP vaccination series. Because the pertussis antigen components of INFANRIX and PEDIARIX® [Diphtheria and Tetanus Toxoids and Acellular Pertussis Adsorbed, Hepatitis B (Recombinant) and Inactivated Poliovirus Vaccine] are the same, INFANRIX may be used to complete a DTaP vaccination series initiated with PEDIARIX.
2.4   Additional Dosing Information
If any recommended dose of pertussis vaccine cannot be given [see Contraindications (4.2, 4.3) and Warnings and Precautions (5.5)], Diphtheria and Tetanus Toxoids Adsorbed (DT) For Pediatric Use should be given according to its prescribing information.

3   DOSAGE FORMS AND STRENGTHS
INFANRIX is a suspension for injection available in 0.5-mL single-dose vials and prefilled TIP-LOK® syringes.

4   CONTRAINDICATIONS
4.1   Hypersensitivity
Severe allergic reaction (e.g., anaphylaxis) after a previous dose of any diphtheria toxoid, tetanus toxoid, or pertussis-

containing vaccine, or to any component of INFANRIX is a contraindication [see Description (11)]. Because of the uncertainty as to which component of the vaccine might be responsible, no further vaccination with any of these components should be given. Alternatively, such individuals may be referred to an allergist for evaluation if immunization with any of these components is being considered.

4.2 Encephalopathy

Encephalopathy (e.g., coma, decreased level of consciousness, prolonged seizures) within 7 days of administration of a previous dose of a pertussis-containing vaccine that is not attributable to another identifiable cause is a contraindication to administration of any pertussis-containing vaccine, including INFANRIX.

4.3 Progressive Neurologic Disorder

Progressive neurologic disorder, including infantile spasms, uncontrolled epilepsy, or progressive encephalopathy is a contraindication to administration of any pertussis-containing vaccine, including INFANRIX. Pertussis vaccine should not be administered to individuals with these conditions until a treatment regimen has been established and the condition has stabilized.

5 WARNINGS AND PRECAUTIONS

5.1 Guillain-Barré Syndrome

If Guillain-Barré syndrome occurs within 6 weeks of receipt of a prior vaccine containing tetanus toxoid, the decision to give any tetanus toxoid-containing vaccine, including INFANRIX, should be based on careful consideration of the potential benefits and possible risks. When a decision is made to withhold tetanus toxoid, other available vaccines should be given, as indicated.

5.2 Latex

The tip caps of the prefilled syringes may contain natural rubber latex which may cause allergic reactions in latex-sensitive individuals.

5.3 Syncope

Syncope (fainting) can occur in association with administration of injectable vaccines, including INFANRIX. Syncope can be accompanied by transient neurological signs such as visual disturbance, paresthesia, and tonic-clonic limb movements. Procedures should be in place to avoid falling injury and to restore cerebral perfusion following syncope.

5.4 Adverse Events Following Prior Pertussis Vaccination

If any of the following events occur in temporal relation to receipt of a pertussis-containing vaccine, the decision to give any pertussis-containing vaccine, including INFANRIX, should be based on careful consideration of the potential benefits and possible risks:

- Temperature of ≥40.5°C (105°F) within 48 hours not due to another identifiable cause;
- Collapse or shock-like state (hypotonic-hyporesponsive episode) within 48 hours;
- Persistent, inconsolable crying lasting ≥3 hours, occurring within 48 hours;
- Seizures with or without fever occurring within 3 days.

5.5 Children at Risk for Seizures

For children at higher risk for seizures than the general population, an appropriate antipyretic may be administered at the time of vaccination with a pertussis-containing vaccine, including INFANRIX, and for the ensuing 24 hours to reduce the possibility of post-vaccination fever.

5.6 Apnea in Premature Infants

Apnea following intramuscular vaccination has been observed in some infants born prematurely. Decisions about when to administer an intramuscular vaccine, including INFANRIX, to infants born prematurely should be based on consideration of the individual infant's medical status, and the potential benefits and possible risks of vaccination.

5.7 Preventing and Managing Allergic Vaccine Reactions

Prior to administration, the healthcare provider should review the patient's immunization history for possible vaccine hypersensitivity. Epinephrine and other appropriate agents used for the control of immediate allergic reactions must be immediately available should an acute anaphylactic reaction occur.

6 ADVERSE REACTIONS

6.1 Clinical Trials Experience

Because clinical trials are conducted under widely varying conditions, adverse reaction rates observed in the clinical trials of a vaccine cannot be directly compared to rates in the clinical trials of another vaccine and may not reflect the rates observed in practice. There is the possibility that broad use of INFANRIX could reveal adverse reactions not observed in clinical trials.

Approximately 95,000 doses of INFANRIX have been administered in clinical studies. In these studies, 29,243 infants have received INFANRIX in primary series studies,

6,081 children have received a fourth consecutive dose of INFANRIX, 1,764 children have received a fifth consecutive dose of INFANRIX, and 559 children have received a dose of INFANRIX following 3 doses of PEDIARIX.

Solicited Adverse Events: In a US study, 335 infants received INFANRIX, ENGERIX-B® [Hepatitis B Vaccine (Recombinant)], inactivated poliovirus vaccine (IPV, Sanofi Pasteur SA), Haemophilus b (Hib) conjugate vaccine (Wyeth Pharmaceuticals Inc.), and pneumococcal 7-valent conjugate (PCV7) vaccine (Wyeth Pharmaceuticals Inc.) concomitantly at separate sites. All vaccines were administered at 2, 4, and 6 months of age. Data on solicited local reactions and general adverse events were collected by parents using standardized diary cards for 4 consecutive days following each vaccine dose (i.e., day of vaccination and the next 3 days) (Table 1). Among subjects, 69% were White, 16% were Hispanic, 8% were Black, 4% were Asian, and 2% were of other racial/ethnic groups.

Table 1. Solicited Local Reactions and General Adverse Events (%) Occurring Within 4 Days of Vaccination[a] With Separate Concomitant Administration of INFANRIX, ENGERIX-B, IPV, Haemophilus b (Hib) Conjugate Vaccine, and Pneumococcal Conjugate Vaccine (PCV7) (Modified Intent To Treat Cohort)

	INFANRIX, ENGERIX-B, IPV, Hib Vaccine, & PCV7		
	Dose 1	Dose 2	Dose 3
Local[b]			
N	335	323	315
Pain, any	31.9	30.0	29.8
Pain, grade 2 or 3	9.0	8.7	8.9
Pain, grade 3	2.7	1.5	1.3
Redness, any	18.2	32.8	39.0
Redness, >20 mm	0.3	0.0	1.9
Swelling, any	9.6	20.4	24.8
Swelling, >20 mm	0.6	0.0	1.3
General			
N	333	321	311
Fever[c] (≥100.4°F)	19.8	30.2	23.8
Fever[c] (>101.3°F)	4.5	9.7	5.8
Fever[c] (>102.2°F)	0.3	3.1	2.3
Fever[c] (>103.1°F)	0.0	0.3	0.3
N	335	323	315
Drowsiness, any	54.0	48.3	38.4
Drowsiness, grade 2 or 3	17.6	12.4	11.1
Drowsiness, grade 3	3.6	0.6	1.9
Irritability/ Fussiness, any	61.5	61.6	56.5
Irritability/ Fussiness, grade 2 or 3	19.4	21.1	19.4
Irritability/ Fussiness, grade 3	3.9	3.4	3.2
Loss of appetite, any	27.8	26.6	23.8
Loss of appetite, grade 2 or 3	5.1	3.4	5.4
Loss of appetite, grade 3	0.6	0.3	0.0

Hib conjugate vaccine and PCV7 manufactured by Wyeth Pharmaceuticals Inc. IPV manufactured by Sanofi Pasteur SA.
Modified intent to treat cohort = all vaccinated subjects for whom safety data were available.

N = number of infants for whom at least one symptom sheet was completed; for fever, numbers exclude missing temperature recordings or tympanic measurements.
Grade 2: pain defined as cried/protested on touch; drowsiness defined as interfered with normal daily activities; irritability/fussiness defined as crying more than usual/interfered with normal daily activities; loss of appetite defined as eating less than usual/interfered with normal daily activities.
Grade 3: pain defined as cried when limb was moved/spontaneously painful; drowsiness defined as prevented normal daily activities; irritability/fussiness defined as crying that could not be comforted/prevented normal daily activities; loss of appetite defined as no eating at all.
[a] Within 4 days of vaccination defined as day of vaccination and the next 3 days.
[b] Local reactions at the injection site for INFANRIX.
[c] Axillary temperatures increased by 1°C and oral temperatures increased by 0.5°C to derive equivalent rectal temperature.

In a US study, the safety of a booster dose of INFANRIX was evaluated in children 15 to 18 months of age whose previous 3 DTaP doses were with INFANRIX (N = 251) or PEDIARIX (N = 559). Vaccines administered concurrently with the fourth dose of INFANRIX included measles, mumps, and rubella (MMR) vaccine (Merck & Co., Inc.), varicella vaccine (Merck & Co., Inc.), pneumococcal 7-valent conjugate (PCV7) vaccine (Wyeth Pharmaceuticals Inc.), and any US-licensed Hib conjugate vaccine; these were given concomitantly in 13.2%, 6.3%, 37.4%, and 41.2% of subjects, respectively. Data on solicited adverse events were collected by parents using standardized diary cards for 4 consecutive days following each vaccine dose (i.e., day of vaccination and the next 3 days) (Table 2). Among subjects, 85% were White, 6% were Hispanic, 6% were Black, 1% were Asian, and 2% were of other racial/ethnic groups.

Table 2. Solicited Local Reactions and General Adverse Events (%) Occurring Within 4 Days of Vaccination[a] With INFANRIX Administered as the Fourth Dose Following 3 Previous Doses of INFANRIX or PEDIARIX (Total Vaccinated Cohort)

	Group Primed With INFANRIX[b] N = 247	Group Primed With PEDIARIX[c] N = 553
Local[d]		
Pain, any	44.5	48.3
Pain, grade 2 or 3	19.0	18.6
Pain, grade 3	3.6	3.4
Redness, any	48.2	49.9
Redness, >20 mm	6.1	6.0
Swelling, any	32.8	32.7
Swelling, >20 mm	3.6	5.2
Increase in mid-thigh circumference, any	33.2	26.2
Increase in mid-thigh circumference, >40 mm	0.0	1.3
General		
Fever[e] (>99.5°F)	8.9	15.4
Fever[e] (>100.4°F)	4.5	6.7
Fever[e] (>101.3°F)	2.0	2.0
Drowsiness, any	35.6	31.3
Drowsiness, grade 2 or 3	9.3	6.7
Drowsiness, grade 3	2.4	1.3
Irritability, any	52.2	53.9
Irritability, grade 2 or 3	18.2	19.7
Irritability, grade 3	3.2	1.4
Loss of appetite, any	24.7	23.3

Loss of appetite, grade 2 or 3	5.3	4.9
Loss of appetite, grade 3	2.4	0.5

Total Vaccinated Cohort = all subjects who received a dose of study vaccine.

N = number of subjects for whom at least one symptom sheet was completed.

Grade 2: pain defined as cried/protested on touch; drowsiness defined as interfered with normal daily activities; irritability defined as crying more than usual/interfered with normal daily activities; loss of appetite defined as eating less than usual/no effect on normal daily activities.

Grade 3: pain defined as cried when limb was moved/spontaneously painful; drowsiness defined as prevented normal daily activities; irritability defined as crying that could not be comforted/prevented normal daily activities; loss of appetite defined as eating less than usual/interfered with normal daily activities.

[a]Within 4 days of vaccination defined as day of vaccination and the next 3 days.

[b]Received INFANRIX, ENGERIX-B, IPV (Sanofi Pasteur SA), PCV7 vaccine (Wyeth Pharmaceuticals Inc.), and Hib conjugate vaccine (Wyeth Pharmaceuticals Inc.) at 2, 4, and 6 months of age.

[c]Received PEDIARIX, PCV7 vaccine (Wyeth Pharmaceuticals Inc.), and Hib conjugate vaccine (Wyeth Pharmaceuticals Inc.) at 2, 4, and 6 months of age or PCV7 vaccine 2 weeks later.

[d] Local reactions at the injection site for INFANRIX.

[e]Axillary temperatures.

In a US study, the safety of a fifth consecutive dose of INFANRIX coadministered at separate sites with a fourth dose of IPV (Sanofi Pasteur SA) and a second dose of MMR vaccine (Merck & Co., Inc.) was evaluated in 1,053 children 4 to 6 years of age. Data on solicited adverse events were collected by parents using standardized diary cards for 4 consecutive days following each vaccine dose (i.e., day of vaccination and the next 3 days) (Table 3). Among subjects, 43% were White, 18% Hispanic, 15% Asian, 7% Black, and 17% were of other racial/ethnic groups.

Table 3. Solicited Local Reactions and General Adverse Events (%) Occurring Within 4 Days of Vaccination[a] With a Fifth Consecutive Dose of INFANRIX When Coadministered With IPV and MMR Vaccine (Total Vaccinated Cohort)

Local[b]	N = 1,039-1,043
Pain, any	53.3
Pain, grade 2 or 3[c]	12.0
Pain, grade 3[c]	0.6
Redness, any	36.6
Redness, ≥50 mm	20.0
Redness, ≥110 mm	4.1
Arm circumference increase, any	37.8
Arm circumference increase, >20 mm	7.4
Arm circumference increase, >30 mm	3.2
Swelling, any	27.0
Swelling, ≥50 mm	11.5
Swelling, ≥110 mm	1.8
General	**N = 993-1,036**
Drowsiness, any	17.5
Drowsiness, grade 3[d]	0.8
Fever, ≥99.5°F	14.8
Fever, >100.4°F	4.4
Fever, >102.2°F	1.1
Fever, >104°F	0.0

Table 4. Selected Adverse Events Occurring Within 48 Hours Following Vaccination With INFANRIX or Whole-Cell DTP in Italian Infants at 2, 4, or 6 Months of Age

Event	INFANRIX (N = 13,761 Doses)		Whole-Cell DTP Vaccine (N = 13,520 Doses)	
	Number	Rate/1,000 Doses	Number	Rate/1,000 Doses
Fever (≥104°F)[a][b]	5	0.36	32	2.4
Hypotonic-hyporesponsive episode[c]	0	0	9	0.67
Persistent crying ≥3 hours[a]	6	0.44	54	4.0
Seizures[d]	1[e]	0.07	3[f]	0.22

[a]P <0.001.
[b]Rectal temperatures.
[c]P = 0.002.
[d]Not statistically significant at P <0.05.
[e]Maximum rectal temperature within 72 hours of vaccination = 103.1°F.
[f]Maximum rectal temperature within 72 hours of vaccination = 99.5°F, 101.3°F, and 102.2°F.

Loss of appetite, any	16.0
Loss of appetite, grade 3[e]	0.6

IPV manufactured by Sanofi Pasteur SA. MMR vaccine manufactured by Merck & Co., Inc.

Total Vaccinated Cohort = all vaccinated subjects for whom safety data were available.

N = number of children with evaluable data for the events listed.

[a] Within 4 days of vaccination defined as day of vaccination and the next 3 days.

[b]Local reactions at the injection site for INFANRIX.

[c]Grade 2 defined as painful when the limb was moved; Grade 3 defined as preventing normal daily activities.

[d]Grade 3 defined as preventing normal daily activities.

[e] Grade 3 defined as not eating at all.

In the US booster immunization studies in which INFANRIX was administered as the fourth or fifth dose in the DTaP series following previous doses with INFANRIX or PEDIARIX, large swelling reactions of the limb injected with INFANRIX were assessed.

In the fourth dose study, a large swelling reaction was defined as injection site swelling with a diameter of >50 mm, a >50 mm increase in the mid-thigh circumference compared to the pre-vaccination measurement, and/or any diffuse swelling that interfered with or prevented daily activities. The overall incidence of large swelling reactions occurring within 4 days (Day 0-Day 3) following INFANRIX was 2.3%. In the fifth dose study, a large swelling reaction was defined as swelling that involved >50% of the injected upper arm length and that was associated with a >30 mm increase in mid-upper arm circumference within 4 days following vaccination. The incidence of large swelling reactions following the fifth consecutive dose of INFANRIX was 1.0%.

Less Common and Serious General Adverse Events: Selected adverse events reported from a double-blind, randomized Italian clinical efficacy trial involving 4,696 children administered INFANRIX or 4,678 children administered whole-cell DTP vaccine (DTwP) (manufactured by Connaught Laboratories, Inc.) as a 3-dose primary series are shown in Table 4. The incidence of rectal temperature ≥104°F, hypotonic-hyporesponsive episodes and persistent crying ≥3 hours following administration of INFANRIX was significantly less than that following administration of whole-cell DTP vaccine.

[See table 4 above]

In a German safety study that enrolled 22,505 infants (66,867 doses of INFANRIX administered as a 3-dose primary series at 3, 4, and 5 months of age), all subjects were monitored for unsolicited adverse events that occurred within 28 days following vaccination using report cards. In a subset of subjects (N = 2,457), these cards were standardized diaries which solicited specific adverse events that occurred within 8 days of each vaccination in addition to unsolicited adverse events which occurred from enrollment until approximately 30 days following the third vaccination. Cards from the whole cohort were returned at subsequent visits and were supplemented by spontaneous reporting by parents and a medical history after the first and second doses of vaccine. In the subset of 2,457, adverse events following the third dose of vaccine were reported via standardized diaries and spontaneous reporting at a follow-up visit. Adverse events in the remainder of the cohort were reported via report cards which were returned by mail approximately 28 days after the third dose of vaccine. Adverse events (rates per 1,000 doses) occurring within 7 days following any of the first 3 doses included: unusual crying (0.09), febrile seizure (0.0), afebrile seizure (0.13), and hypotonic-hyporesponsive episodes (0.01).

6.2   Postmarketing Experience
In addition to reports in clinical trials, worldwide voluntary reports of adverse events received for INFANRIX since market introduction are listed below. This list includes serious events and events which have a plausible causal connection to INFANRIX. These adverse events were reported voluntarily from a population of uncertain size; therefore, it is not always possible to reliably estimate their frequency or establish a causal relationship to INFANRIX.
Infections and Infestations: Bronchitis, cellulitis, respiratory tract infection.
Blood and Lymphatic System Disorders: Lymphadenopathy, thrombocytopenia.
Immune System Disorders: Anaphylactic reaction, hypersensitivity.
Nervous System Disorders: Encephalopathy, headache, hypotonia, syncope.
Ear and Labyrinth Disorders: Ear pain.
Cardiac Disorders: Cyanosis.
Respiratory, Thoracic, and Mediastinal Disorders: Apnea, cough.
Skin and Subcutaneous Tissue Disorders: Angioedema, erythema, pruritus, rash, urticaria.
General Disorders and Administration Site Conditions: Fatigue, injection site induration, injection site reaction, Sudden Infant Death Syndrome.

7   DRUG INTERACTIONS
7.1   Concomitant Vaccine Administration
In clinical trials, INFANRIX was given concomitantly with Hib conjugate vaccine, pneumococcal 7-valent conjugate vaccine, hepatitis B vaccine, IPV, and the second dose of MMR vaccine [see Adverse Reactions (6.1) and Clinical Studies (14.3)].
When INFANRIX is administered concomitantly with other injectable vaccines, they should be given with separate syringes. INFANRIX should not be mixed with any other vaccine in the same syringe or vial.
7.2   Immunosuppressive Therapies
Immunosuppressive therapies, including irradiation, antimetabolites, alkylating agents, cytotoxic drugs, and corticosteroids (used in greater than physiologic doses), may reduce the immune response to INFANRIX.

8   USE IN SPECIFIC POPULATIONS
8.1   Pregnancy
Pregnancy Category C
Animal reproduction studies have not been conducted with INFANRIX. It is also not known whether INFANRIX can cause fetal harm when administered to a pregnant woman or can affect reproduction capacity.
8.4   Pediatric Use
Safety and effectiveness of INFANRIX in infants younger than 6 weeks of age and children 7 to 16 years of age have not been established. INFANRIX is not approved for use in these age groups.

11   DESCRIPTION
INFANRIX (Diphtheria and Tetanus Toxoids and Acellular Pertussis Vaccine Adsorbed) is a noninfectious, sterile vaccine for intramuscular administration. Each 0.5-mL dose is formulated to contain 25 Lf of diphtheria toxoid, 10 Lf of tetanus toxoid, 25 mcg of inactivated pertussis toxin (PT), 25 mcg of filamentous hemagglutinin (FHA), and 8 mcg of pertactin (69 kiloDalton outer membrane protein).
The diphtheria toxin is produced by growing Corynebacterium diphtheriae in Fenton medium containing a bovine extract. Tetanus toxin is produced by growing Clostridium tetani in a modified Latham medium derived from bovine casein. The bovine materials used in these extracts are sourced from countries which the United States

Department of Agriculture (USDA) has determined neither have nor present an undue risk for bovine spongiform encephalopathy (BSE). Both toxins are detoxified with formaldehyde, concentrated by ultrafiltration, and purified by precipitation, dialysis, and sterile filtration.

The acellular pertussis antigens (PT, FHA, and pertactin) are isolated from *Bordetella pertussis* culture grown in modified Stainer-Scholte liquid medium. PT and FHA are isolated from the fermentation broth; pertactin is extracted from the cells by heat treatment and flocculation. The antigens are purified in successive chromatographic and precipitation steps. PT is detoxified using glutaraldehyde and formaldehyde. FHA and pertactin are treated with formaldehyde.

Diphtheria and tetanus toxoids and pertussis antigens (PT, FHA, and pertactin) are individually adsorbed onto aluminum hydroxide.

Diphtheria and tetanus toxoid potency is determined by measuring the amount of neutralizing antitoxin in previously immunized guinea pigs. The potency of the acellular pertussis components (PT, FHA, and pertactin) is determined by enzyme-linked immunosorbent assay (ELISA) on sera from previously immunized mice.

Each 0.5-mL dose contains aluminum hydroxide as adjuvant (not more than 0.625 mg aluminum by assay) and 4.5 mg of sodium chloride. Each dose also contains ≤100 mcg of residual formaldehyde and ≤100 mcg of polysorbate 80 (Tween 80).

INFANRIX is available in vials and prefilled syringes. The tip caps of the prefilled syringes may contain natural rubber latex; the plungers are not made with natural rubber latex. The vial stoppers are not made with natural rubber latex. INFANRIX is formulated without preservatives.

12 CLINICAL PHARMACOLOGY

12.1 Mechanism of Action

<u>Diphtheria</u>: Diphtheria is an acute toxin-mediated infectious disease caused by toxigenic strains of *C. diphtheriae*. Protection against disease is due to the development of neutralizing antibodies to the diphtheria toxin. A serum diphtheria antitoxin level of 0.01 IU/mL is the lowest level giving some degree of protection; a level of 0.1 IU/mL is regarded as protective.[1]

<u>Tetanus</u>: Tetanus is an acute toxin-mediated infectious disease caused by a potent exotoxin released by *C. tetani*. Protection against disease is due to the development of neutralizing antibodies to the tetanus toxin. A serum tetanus antitoxin level of at least 0.01 IU/mL, measured by neutralization assays, is considered the minimum protective level.[2,3] A level of 0.1 IU/mL is considered protective.[4]

<u>Pertussis</u>: Pertussis (whooping cough) is a disease of the respiratory tract caused by *B. pertussis*. The role of the different components produced by *B. pertussis* in either the pathogenesis of, or the immunity to, pertussis is not well understood. There is no well established serological correlate of protection for pertussis.

13 NONCLINICAL TOXICOLOGY

13.1 Carcinogenesis, Mutagenesis, Impairment of Fertility

INFANRIX has not been evaluated for carcinogenic or mutagenic potential, or for impairment of fertility.

14 CLINICAL STUDIES

14.1 Diphtheria and Tetanus

Efficacy of diphtheria toxoid used in INFANRIX was determined on the basis of immunogenicity studies. A VERO cell toxin neutralizing test confirmed the ability of infant sera (N = 45), obtained one month after a 3-dose primary series, to neutralize diphtheria toxin. Levels of diphtheria antitoxin ≥0.01 IU/mL were achieved in 100% of the sera tested. Efficacy of tetanus toxoid used in INFANRIX was determined on the basis of immunogenicity studies. An in vivo mouse neutralization assay confirmed the ability of infant sera (N = 45), obtained one month after a 3-dose primary series, to neutralize tetanus toxin. Levels of tetanus antitoxin ≥0.01 IU/mL were achieved in 100% of the sera tested.

14.2 Pertussis

Efficacy of a 3-dose primary series of INFANRIX has been assessed in 2 clinical studies.

A double-blind, randomized, active Diphtheria and Tetanus Toxoids (DT)-controlled trial conducted in Italy assessed the absolute protective efficacy of INFANRIX when administered at 2, 4, and 6 months of age. The population used in the primary analysis of the efficacy of INFANRIX included 4,481 infants vaccinated with INFANRIX and 1,470 DT vaccinees. The mean length of follow-up was 17 months, beginning 30 days after the third dose of vaccine. After 3 doses, the absolute protective efficacy of INFANRIX against WHO-defined typical pertussis (21 days or more of paroxysmal cough with infection confirmed by culture and/or serologic testing) was 84% (95% CI: 76, 89). When the definition of pertussis was expanded to include clinically milder disease with respect to type and duration of cough, with infection confirmed by culture and/or serologic testing, the efficacy of

INFANRIX was calculated to be 71% (95% CI: 60, 78) against >7 days of any cough and 73% (95% CI: 63, 80) against ≥14 days of any cough. Vaccine efficacy after 3 doses and with no booster dose in the second year of life was assessed in 2 subsequent follow-up periods. A follow-up period from 24 months to a mean age of 33 months was conducted in a partially unblinded cohort (children who received DT were offered pertussis vaccine and those who declined were retained in the study cohort). During this period, the efficacy of INFANRIX against WHO-defined pertussis was 78% (95% CI: 62, 87). During the third follow-up period which was conducted in an unblinded manner among children from 3 to 6 years of age, the efficacy of INFANRIX against WHO-defined pertussis was 86% (95% CI: 79, 91). Thus, protection against pertussis in children administered 3 doses of INFANRIX in infancy was sustained to 6 years of age.

A prospective efficacy trial was also conducted in Germany employing a household contact study design. In preparation for this study, 3 doses of INFANRIX were administered at 3, 4, and 5 months of age to more than 22,000 children living in 6 areas of Germany in a safety and immunogenicity study. Infants who did not participate in the safety and immunogenicity study could have received a DTwP vaccine or DT vaccine. Index cases were identified by spontaneous presentation to a physician. Households with at least one other member (i.e., besides index case) aged 6 through 47 months were enrolled. Household contacts of index cases were monitored for incidence of pertussis by a physician who was blinded to the vaccination status of the household. Calculation of vaccine efficacy was based on attack rates of pertussis in household contacts classified by vaccination status. Of the 173 household contacts who had not received a pertussis vaccine, 96 developed WHO-defined pertussis, as compared with 7 of 112 contacts vaccinated with INFANRIX. The protective efficacy of INFANRIX was calculated to be 89% (95% CI: 77, 95), with no indication of waning of protection up until the time of the booster vaccination. The average age of infants vaccinated with INFANRIX at the end of follow-up in this trial was 13 months (range 6 to 25 months). When the definition of pertussis was expanded to include clinically milder disease, with infection confirmed by culture and/or serologic testing, the efficacy of INFANRIX against ≥7 days of any cough was 67% (95% CI: 52, 78) and against ≥7 days of paroxysmal cough was 81% (95% CI: 68, 89). The corresponding efficacy of INFANRIX against ≥14 days of any cough or paroxysmal cough were 73% (95% CI: 59, 82) and 84% (95% CI: 71, 91), respectively.

<u>Pertussis Immune Response to INFANRIX Administered as a 3-Dose Primary Series</u>: The immune responses to each of the 3 pertussis antigens contained in INFANRIX were evaluated in sera obtained 1 month after the third dose of vaccine in each of 3 studies (schedule of administration: 2, 4, and 6 months of age in the Italian efficacy study and one US study; 3, 4, and 5 months of age in the German efficacy study). One month after the third dose of INFANRIX, the response rates to each pertussis antigen were similar in all 3 studies. Thus, although a serologic correlate of protection for pertussis has not been established, the antibody responses to these 3 pertussis antigens (PT, FHA, and pertactin) in a US population were similar to those achieved in 2 populations in which efficacy of INFANRIX was demonstrated.

14.3 Immune Response to Concomitantly Administered Vaccines

In a US study, INFANRIX was given concomitantly, at separate sites, with Hib conjugate vaccine (Sanofi Pasteur SA) at 2, 4, and 6 months of age. Subjects also received ENGERIX-B and oral poliovirus vaccine (OPV). One month after the third dose of Hib conjugate vaccine, 90% of 72 infants had anti-PRP (polyribosyl-ribitol-phosphate) ≥1.0 mcg/mL.

In a US study, INFANRIX was given concomitantly, at separate sites, with ENGERIX-B, IPV (Sanofi Pasteur SA), pneumococcal 7-valent conjugate (PCV7), and Hib conjugate vaccines (Wyeth Pharmaceuticals Inc.) at 2, 4, and 6 months of age. Immune responses were measured in sera obtained approximately one month after the third dose of vaccines. Among 121 subjects who had not received a birth dose of hepatitis B vaccine, 99.2% had anti-HBsAg (hepatitis B surface antigen) ≥10 mIU/mL following the third dose of ENGERIX-B. Among 153 subjects, 100% had anti-poliovirus 1, 2, and 3, ≥1:8 following the third dose of IPV. Although serological correlates for protection have not been established for the pneumococcal serotypes, a threshold level of ≥0.3 mcg/mL was evaluated. Following the third dose of PCV7 vaccine, 91.8% to 99.4% of subjects (N = 146-156) had anti-pneumococcal polysaccharide ≥0.3 mcg/mL for serotypes 4, 9V, 14, 18C, 19F, and 23F, and 73.0% had a level ≥0.3 mcg/mL for serotype 6B.

15 REFERENCES

1. Vitek CR and Wharton M. Diphtheria Toxoid. In: Plotkin SA, Orenstein WA, and Offit PA, eds. *Vaccines*. 5th ed. Saunders; 2008:139-156.

2. Wassilak SGF, Roper MH, Kretsinger K, and Orenstein WA. Tetanus Toxoid. In: Plotkin SA, Orenstein WA, and Offit PA, eds. *Vaccines*. 5th ed. Saunders; 2008:805-839.
3. Department of Health and Human Services, Food and Drug Administration. Biological products; Bacterial vaccines and toxoids; Implementation of efficacy review; Proposed rule. *Federal Register* December 13, 1985;50(240):51002-51117.
4. Centers for Disease Control and Prevention. General Recommendations on Immunization. Recommendations of the Advisory Committee on Immunization Practices (ACIP). *MMWR* 2006;55(RR-15):1-48.

16 HOW SUPPLIED/STORAGE AND HANDLING

INFANRIX is available in 0.5-mL single-dose vials and disposable prefilled TIP-LOK syringes (packaged without needles):

NDC 58160-810-01 Vial in Package of 10: NDC 58160-810-11

NDC 58160-810-43 Syringe in Package of 10: NDC 58160-810-52

Store refrigerated between 2° and 8°C (36° and 46°F). Do not freeze. Discard if the vaccine has been frozen.

17 PATIENT COUNSELING INFORMATION

The parent or guardian should be:

- informed of the potential benefits and risks of immunization with INFANRIX, and of the importance of completing the immunization series.
- informed about the potential for adverse reactions that have been temporally associated with administration of INFANRIX or other vaccines containing similar components.
- instructed to report any adverse events to their healthcare provider.
- given the Vaccine Information Statements, which are required by the National Childhood Vaccine Injury Act of 1986 to be given prior to immunization. These materials are available free of charge at the Centers for Disease Control and Prevention (CDC) website (www.cdc.gov/vaccines).

ENGERIX-B, INFANRIX, PEDIARIX, and TIP-LOK are registered trademarks of the GlaxoSmithKline group of companies.

Manufactured by **GlaxoSmithKline Biologicals**
Rixensart, Belgium, US License 1617
Novartis Vaccines and Diagnostics GmbH
Marburg, Germany, US License 1754
Distributed by **GlaxoSmithKline**
Research Triangle Park, NC 27709
©2013, GlaxoSmithKline group of companies. All rights reserved.
INF:25PI

JALYN   ℞
[*JAY-LIN*]
(dutasteride and tamsulosin hydrochloride)
Capsules

HIGHLIGHTS OF PRESCRIBING INFORMATION
These highlights do not include all the information needed to use JALYN safely and effectively. See full prescribing information for JALYN.
JALYN (dutasteride and tamsulosin hydrochloride) Capsules
Initial U.S. Approval: 2010

―――――INDICATIONS AND USAGE―――――

JALYN is a combination of dutasteride, a 5 alpha-reductase inhibitor, and tamsulosin, an alpha adrenergic antagonist, indicated for the treatment of symptomatic benign prostatic hyperplasia (BPH) in men with an enlarged prostate. (1.1) Limitations of Use: Dutasteride-containing products, including JALYN, are not approved for the prevention of prostate cancer. (1.2)

―――――DOSAGE AND ADMINISTRATION―――――

- Take one capsule daily approximately 30 minutes after the same meal each day. (2)
- Swallow capsule whole. (2)

―――――DOSAGE FORMS AND STRENGTHS―――――

0.5 mg dutasteride and 0.4 mg tamsulosin hydrochloride. (3)

―――――CONTRAINDICATIONS―――――

- Pregnancy and women of childbearing potential. (4, 5.6, 8.1)
- Pediatric patients. (4)
- Patients with previously demonstrated, clinically significant hypersensitivity (e.g., serious skin reactions, angioedema, urticaria, pruritus, respiratory symptoms) to dutasteride, other 5 alpha-reductase inhibitors, tamsulosin, or any component of JALYN. (4)

WARNINGS AND PRECAUTIONS

- Orthostatic hypotension and/or syncope can occur. Advise patients of symptoms related to postural hypotension and to avoid situations where injury could result if syncope occurs. (5.1)
- Do not use JALYN with other alpha adrenergic antagonists, as this may increase the risk of hypotension. (5.2)
- JALYN reduces serum prostate-specific antigen (PSA) concentration by approximately 50%. However, any confirmed increase in PSA while on JALYN may signal the presence of prostate cancer and should be evaluated, even if those values are still within the normal range for untreated men. (5.3)
- Do not use JALYN with strong inhibitors of cytochrome P450 (CYP) 3A4 (e.g., ketoconazole). Use caution in combination with moderate CYP3A4 inhibitors (e.g., erythromycin) or strong (e.g., paroxetine) or moderate CYP2D6 inhibitors, or known poor metabolizers of CYP2D6. Concomitant use with known inhibitors can cause a marked increase in drug exposure. (5.2, 7.1, 12.3)
- Exercise caution with concomitant use of PDE-5 inhibitors, as this may increase the risk of hypotension. (5.2)
- Drugs that contain dutasteride, including JALYN, may increase the risk of high-grade prostate cancer. (5.4, 6.1)
- Prior to initiating treatment with JALYN, consideration should be given to other urological conditions that may cause similar symptoms. (5.5)
- Women who are pregnant or could become pregnant should not handle JALYN Capsules due to potential risk to a male fetus. (5.6, 8.1)
- Advise patients about the possibility and seriousness of priapism. (5.7)
- Patients should not donate blood until 6 months after their last dose of JALYN. (5.8)
- Intraoperative Floppy Iris Syndrome has been observed during cataract surgery after alpha adrenergic antagonist exposure. Advise patients considering cataract surgery to tell their ophthalmologist that they take or have taken JALYN Capsules. (5.9)
- Exercise caution with concomitant use of warfarin. (5.2, 7.2, 12.3)

ADVERSE REACTIONS

The most common adverse reactions, reported in ≥1% of subjects treated with coadministered dutasteride and tamsulosin are ejaculation disorders, impotence, decreased libido, dizziness, and breast disorders. (6.1)

To report SUSPECTED ADVERSE REACTIONS, contact GlaxoSmithKline at 1-888-825-5249 or FDA at 1-800-FDA-1088 or www.fda.gov/medwatch.

See 17 for PATIENT COUNSELING INFORMATION and FDA-approved patient labeling

Revised: 06/2014

FULL PRESCRIBING INFORMATION

1 INDICATIONS AND USAGE

1.1 Benign Prostatic Hyperplasia (BPH) Treatment
JALYN® (dutasteride and tamsulosin hydrochloride) Capsules are indicated for the treatment of symptomatic BPH in men with an enlarged prostate.

1.2 Limitations of Use
Dutasteride-containing products, including JALYN, are not approved for the prevention of prostate cancer.

2 DOSAGE AND ADMINISTRATION

The recommended dosage of JALYN is 1 capsule (0.5 mg dutasteride and 0.4 mg tamsulosin hydrochloride) taken once daily approximately 30 minutes after the same meal each day.
The capsules should be swallowed whole and not chewed or opened. Contact with the contents of the JALYN capsule may result in irritation of the oropharyngeal mucosa.

3 DOSAGE FORMS AND STRENGTHS

JALYN Capsules, containing 0.5 mg dutasteride and 0.4 mg tamsulosin hydrochloride, are oblong, hard-shell capsules with a brown body and an orange cap imprinted with "GS 7CZ" in black ink.

4 CONTRAINDICATIONS

JALYN is contraindicated for use in:
- Pregnancy. In animal reproduction and developmental toxicity studies, dutasteride inhibited development of male fetus external genitalia. Therefore, JALYN may cause fetal harm when administered to a pregnant woman. If JALYN is used during pregnancy, or if the patient becomes pregnant while taking JALYN, the patient should be apprised of the potential hazard to the fetus [see Warnings and Precautions (5.6), Use in Specific Populations (8.1)].
- Women of childbearing potential [see Warnings and Precautions (5.6), Use in Specific Populations (8.1)].
- Pediatric patients [see Use in Specific Populations (8.4)].
- Patients with previously demonstrated, clinically significant hypersensitivity (e.g., serious skin reactions, angioedema, urticaria, pruritus, respiratory symptoms) to dutasteride, other 5 alpha-reductase inhibitors, tamsulosin, or any other component of JALYN [see Adverse Reactions (6.2)].

5 WARNINGS AND PRECAUTIONS

5.1 Orthostatic Hypotension
As with other alpha adrenergic antagonists, orthostatic hypotension (postural hypotension, dizziness, and vertigo) may occur in patients treated with tamsulosin-containing products, including JALYN, and can result in syncope. Patients starting treatment with JALYN should be cautioned to avoid situations where syncope could result in an injury [see Adverse Reactions (6.1)].

5.2 Drug-Drug Interactions
Strong Inhibitors of CYP3A4: Tamsulosin-containing products, including JALYN, should not be coadministered with strong CYP3A4 inhibitors (e.g., ketoconazole) as this can significantly increase tamsulosin exposure [see Drug Interactions (7.1), Clinical Pharmacology (12.3)].
Inhibitors of CYP2D6 and Moderate Inhibitors of CYP3A4: Tamsulosin-containing products, including JALYN, should be used with caution when coadministered with moderate inhibitors of CYP3A4 (e.g., erythromycin), strong (e.g., paroxetine) or moderate (e.g., terbinafine) inhibitors of CYP2D6, or in patients known to be poor metabolizers of CYP2D6, as there is a potential for significant increase in tamsulosin exposure [see Drug Interactions (7.1), Clinical Pharmacology (12.3)].
Cimetidine: Caution is advised when tamsulosin-containing products, including JALYN, are coadministered with cimetidine [see Drug Interactions (7.1), Clinical Pharmacology (12.3)].
Other Alpha Adrenergic Antagonists: Tamsulosin-containing products, including JALYN, should not be coadministered with other alpha adrenergic antagonists because of the increased risk of symptomatic hypotension.

Phosphodiesterase-5 Inhibitors (PDE-5 Inhibitors): Caution is advised when alpha adrenergic antagonist-containing products, including JALYN, are coadministered with PDE-5 inhibitors. Alpha adrenergic antagonists and PDE-5 inhibitors are both vasodilators that can lower blood pressure. Concomitant use of these 2 drug classes can potentially cause symptomatic hypotension.
Warfarin: Caution should be exercised with concomitant administration of warfarin and tamsulosin-containing products, including JALYN [see Drug Interactions (7.2), Clinical Pharmacology (12.3)].

5.3 Effects on Prostate-Specific Antigen (PSA) and the Use of PSA in Prostate Cancer Detection
Coadministration of dutasteride with tamsulosin resulted in similar changes to serum PSA as with dutasteride monotherapy.
In clinical trials, dutasteride reduced serum PSA concentration by approximately 50% within 3 to 6 months of treatment. This decrease was predictable over the entire range of PSA values in patients with symptomatic BPH, although it may vary in individuals. Dutasteride-containing treatment, including JALYN, may also cause decreases in serum PSA in the presence of prostate cancer. To interpret serial PSAs in men treated with a dutasteride-containing product, including JALYN, a new baseline PSA should be established at least 3 months after starting treatment and PSA monitored periodically thereafter. Any confirmed increase from the lowest PSA value while on a dutasteride-containing treatment, including JALYN, may signal the presence of prostate cancer and should be evaluated, even if PSA levels are still within the normal range for men not taking a 5 alpha-reductase inhibitor. Noncompliance with JALYN may also affect PSA test results.
To interpret an isolated PSA value in a man treated with JALYN, for 3 months or more, the PSA value should be doubled for comparison with normal values in untreated men. The free-to-total PSA ratio (percent free PSA) remains constant, even under the influence of dutasteride. If clinicians elect to use percent free PSA as an aid in the detection of prostate cancer in men receiving JALYN, no adjustment to its value appears necessary.

5.4 Increased Risk of High-Grade Prostate Cancer
In men aged 50 to 75 years with a prior negative biopsy for prostate cancer and a baseline PSA between 2.5 ng/mL and 10.0 ng/mL taking dutasteride in the 4-year Reduction by Dutasteride of Prostate Cancer Events (REDUCE) trial, there was an increased incidence of Gleason score 8-10 prostate cancer compared with men taking placebo (dutasteride 1.0% versus placebo 0.5%) [see Indications and Usage (1.2), Adverse Reactions (6.1)]. In a 7-year placebo-controlled clinical trial with another 5 alpha-reductase inhibitor (finasteride 5 mg, PROSCAR®), similar results for Gleason score 8-10 prostate cancer were observed (finasteride 1.8% versus placebo 1.1%).
5 alpha-reductase inhibitors may increase the risk of development of high-grade prostate cancer. Whether the effect of 5 alpha-reductase inhibitors to reduce prostate volume or trial-related factors impacted the results of these trials has not been established.

5.5 Evaluation for Other Urological Diseases
Prior to initiating treatment with JALYN, consideration should be given to other urological conditions that may cause similar symptoms. In addition, BPH and prostate cancer may coexist.

5.6 Exposure of Women—Risk to Male Fetus
JALYN Capsules should not be handled by a woman who is pregnant or who could become pregnant. Dutasteride is absorbed through the skin and could result in unintended fetal exposure. If a woman who is pregnant or could become pregnant comes in contact with a leaking capsule, the contact area should be washed immediately with soap and water [see Use in Specific Populations (8.1)].

5.7 Priapism
Priapism (persistent painful penile erection unrelated to sexual activity) has been associated (probably less than 1 in 50,000) with the use of alpha-adrenergic antagonists, including tamsulosin, which is a component of JALYN. Because this condition can lead to permanent impotence if not properly treated, patients should be advised about the seriousness of the condition.

5.8 Blood Donation
Men being treated with a dutasteride-containing product, including JALYN, should not donate blood until at least 6 months have passed following their last dose. The purpose of this deferred period is to prevent administration of dutasteride to a pregnant female transfusion recipient.

5.9 Intraoperative Floppy Iris Syndrome
Intraoperative Floppy Iris Syndrome (IFIS) has been observed during cataract surgery in some patients on or previously treated with alpha adrenergic antagonists, including tamsulosin, which is a component of JALYN.
Most reports were in patients taking the alpha adrenergic antagonist when IFIS occurred, but in some cases, the alpha adrenergic antagonist had been stopped prior to surgery. In

Table 1. Adverse Reactions Reported Over a 48-Month Period in ≥1% of Subjects and More Frequently in the Coadministration Therapy Group Than the Dutasteride or Tamsulosin Monotherapy Group (CombAT) by Time of Onset

Adverse Reaction	Adverse Reaction Time of Onset				
	Year 1		Year 2	Year 3	Year 4
	Months 0–6	Months 7–12			
Coadministration[a]	(n = 1,610)	(n = 1,527)	(n = 1,428)	(n = 1,283)	(n = 1,200)
Dutasteride	(n = 1,623)	(n = 1,548)	(n = 1,464)	(n = 1,325)	(n = 1,200)
Tamsulosin	(n = 1,611)	(n = 1,545)	(n = 1,468)	(n = 1,281)	(n = 1,112)
Ejaculation disorders[b,c]					
Coadministration	7.8%	1.6%	1.0%	0.5%	<0.1%
Dutasteride	1.0%	0.5%	0.5%	0.2%	0.3%
Tamsulosin	2.2%	0.5%	0.5%	0.2%	0.3%
Impotence[c,d]					
Coadministration	5.4%	1.1%	1.8%	0.9%	0.4%
Dutasteride	4.0%	1.1%	1.6%	0.6%	0.3%
Tamsulosin	2.6%	0.8%	1.0%	0.6%	1.1%
Decreased libido[c,e]					
Coadministration	4.5%	0.9%	0.8%	0.2%	0.0%
Dutasteride	3.1%	0.7%	1.0%	0.2%	0.0%
Tamsulosin	2.0%	0.6%	0.7%	0.2%	<0.1%
Breast disorders[f]					
Coadministration	1.1%	1.1%	0.8%	0.9%	0.6%
Dutasteride	0.9%	0.9%	1.2%	0.5%	0.7%
Tamsulosin	0.4%	0.4%	0.4%	0.2%	0.0%
Dizziness					
Coadministration	1.1%	0.4%	0.1%	<0.1%	0.2%
Dutasteride	0.5%	0.3%	0.1%	<0.1%	<0.1%
Tamsulosin	0.9%	0.5%	0.4%	<0.1%	0.0%

[a]Coadministration = AVODART® 0.5 mg once daily plus tamsulosin 0.4 mg once daily.
[b]Includes anorgasmia, retrograde ejaculation, semen volume decreased, orgasmic sensation decreased, orgasm abnormal, ejaculation delayed, ejaculation disorder, ejaculation failure, and premature ejaculation.
[c]These sexual adverse reactions are associated with dutasteride treatment (including monotherapy and combination with tamsulosin). These adverse reactions may persist after treatment discontinuation. The role of dutasteride in this persistence is unknown.
[d]Includes erectile dysfunction and disturbance in sexual arousal.
[e]Includes libido decreased, libido disorder, loss of libido, sexual dysfunction, and male sexual dysfunction.
[f]Includes breast enlargement, gynecomastia, breast swelling, breast pain, breast tenderness, nipple pain, and nipple swelling.

most of these cases, the alpha adrenergic antagonist had been stopped recently prior to surgery (2 to 14 days), but in a few cases, IFIS was reported after the patients had been off the alpha adrenergic antagonist for a longer period (5 weeks to 9 months). IFIS is a variant of small pupil syndrome and is characterized by the combination of a flaccid iris that billows in response to intraoperative irrigation currents, progressive intraoperative miosis despite preoperative dilation with standard mydriatic drugs, and potential prolapse of the iris toward the phacoemulsification incisions. The patient's ophthalmologist should be prepared for possible modifications to their surgical technique, such as the utilization of iris hooks, iris dilator rings, or viscoelastic substances.

IFIS may increase the risk of eye complications during and after the operation. The benefit of stopping alpha adrenergic antagonist therapy prior to cataract surgery has not been established. The initiation of therapy with tamsulosin in patients for whom cataract surgery is scheduled is not recommended.

5.10   Sulfa Allergy
In patients with sulfa allergy, allergic reaction to tamsulosin has been rarely reported. If a patient reports a serious or life-threatening sulfa allergy, caution is warranted when administering tamsulosin-containing products, including JALYN.

5.11   Effect on Semen Characteristics
Dutasteride: The effects of dutasteride 0.5 mg/day on semen characteristics were evaluated in normal volunteers aged 18 to 52 (n = 27 dutasteride, n = 23 placebo) throughout 52 weeks of treatment and 24 weeks of post-treatment follow-up. At 52 weeks, the mean percent reductions from baseline in total sperm count, semen volume, and sperm motility were 23%, 26%, and 18%, respectively, in the dutasteride group when adjusted for changes from baseline in the placebo group. Sperm concentration and sperm morphology were unaffected. After 24 weeks of follow-up, the mean percent change in total sperm count in the dutasteride group remained 23% lower than baseline. While mean values for all semen parameters at all time-points remained within the normal ranges and did not meet predefined criteria for a clinically significant change (30%), 2 subjects in the dutasteride group had decreases in sperm count of greater than 90% from baseline at 52 weeks, with

partial recovery at the 24-week follow-up. The clinical significance of dutasteride's effect on semen characteristics for an individual patient's fertility is not known.
Tamsulosin: The effects of tamsulosin hydrochloride on sperm counts or sperm function have not been evaluated.

6   ADVERSE REACTIONS
6.1   Clinical Trials Experience
There have been no clinical trials conducted with JALYN; however, the clinical efficacy and safety of coadministered dutasteride and tamsulosin, which are individual components of JALYN, have been evaluated in a multicenter, randomized, double-blind, parallel group trial (the Combination with Alpha-Blocker Therapy, or CombAT, trial). Because clinical trials are conducted under widely varying conditions, adverse reaction rates observed in the clinical trials of a drug cannot be directly compared with rates in the clinical trial of another drug and may not reflect the rates observed in practice.
- The most common adverse reactions reported in subjects receiving coadministered dutasteride and tamsulosin were impotence, decreased libido, breast disorders (including breast enlargement and tenderness), ejaculation disorders, and dizziness. Ejaculation disorders occurred significantly more in subjects receiving coadministration therapy (11%) compared with those receiving dutasteride (2%) or tamsulosin (4%) as monotherapy.
- Trial withdrawal due to adverse reactions occurred in 6% of subjects receiving coadministered dutasteride and tamsulosin, and in 4% of subjects receiving dutasteride or tamsulosin as monotherapy. The most common adverse reaction in all treatment arms leading to trial withdrawal was erectile dysfunction (1% to 1.5%).

In the CombAT trial, over 4,800 male subjects with BPH were randomly assigned to receive 0.5 mg dutasteride, 0.4 mg tamsulosin hydrochloride, or coadministration therapy (0.5 mg dutasteride and 0.4 mg tamsulosin hydrochloride) administered once daily in a 4-year double-blind trial. Overall, 1,623 subjects received monotherapy with dutasteride; 1,611 subjects received monotherapy with tamsulosin; and 1,610 subjects received coadministration therapy. The population was aged 49 to 88 years (mean age: 66 years) and 88% were Caucasian. Table 1 summarizes adverse reactions reported in at least 1% of subjects receiving coadministration therapy and at a higher incidence than subjects receiving either dutasteride or tamsulosin as monotherapy.

[See table 1 above]
Cardiac Failure: In CombAT, after 4 years of treatment, the incidence of the composite term cardiac failure in the coadministration group (12/1,610; 0.7%) was higher than in either monotherapy group: dutasteride, 2/1,623 (0.1%) and tamsulosin, 9/1,611 (0.6%). Composite cardiac failure was also examined in a separate 4-year placebo-controlled trial evaluating dutasteride in men at risk for development of prostate cancer. The incidence of cardiac failure in subjects taking dutasteride was 0.6% (26/4,105) compared with 0.4% (15/4,126) in subjects on placebo. A majority of subjects with cardiac failure in both trials had comorbidities associated with an increased risk of cardiac failure. Therefore, the clinical significance of the numerical imbalances in cardiac failure is unknown. No causal relationship between dutasteride, alone or coadministered with tamsulosin, and cardiac failure has been established. No imbalance was observed in the incidence of overall cardiovascular adverse events in either trial.
Additional information regarding adverse reactions in placebo-controlled trials with dutasteride or tamsulosin monotherapy follows:
Dutasteride:
Long-Term Treatment (Up to 4 Years):   High-Grade Prostate Cancer: The REDUCE trial was a randomized, double-blind, placebo-controlled trial that enrolled 8,231 men aged 50 to 75 years with a serum PSA of 2.5 ng/mL to 10 ng/mL and a negative prostate biopsy within the previous 6 months. Subjects were randomized to receive placebo (N = 4,126) or 0.5-mg daily doses of dutasteride (N = 4,105) for up to 4 years. The mean age was 63 years and 91% were Caucasian. Subjects underwent protocol-mandated scheduled prostate biopsies at 2 and 4 years of treatment or had "for-cause biopsies" at non-scheduled times if clinically indicated. There was a higher incidence of Gleason score 8-10 prostate cancer in men receiving dutasteride (1.0%) compared with men on placebo (0.5%) [see Indications and Usage (1.2), Warnings and Precautions (5.4)]. In a 7-year placebo-controlled clinical trial with another 5 alpha-reductase inhibitor (finasteride 5 mg, PROSCAR), similar results for Gleason score 8-10 prostate cancer were observed (finasteride 1.8% versus placebo 1.1%).
No clinical benefit has been demonstrated in patients with prostate cancer treated with dutasteride.
Reproductive and Breast Disorders: In the 3 pivotal placebo-controlled BPH trials with dutasteride, each 4 years in duration, there was no evidence of increased sexual adverse reactions (impotence, decreased libido, and ejaculation disorder) or breast disorders with increased duration of treatment. Among these 3 trials, there was 1 case of breast cancer in the dutasteride group and 1 case in the placebo group. No cases of breast cancer were reported in any treatment group in the 4-year CombAT trial or the 4-year REDUCE trial.
The relationship between long-term use of dutasteride and male breast neoplasia is currently unknown.
Tamsulosin: According to the tamsulosin prescribing information, in two 13-week treatment trials with tamsulosin monotherapy, adverse reactions occurring in at least 2% of subjects receiving 0.4 mg tamsulosin hydrochloride and at an incidence higher than in subjects receiving placebo were: infection, asthenia, back pain, chest pain, somnolence, insomnia, rhinitis, pharyngitis, cough increased, sinusitis, and diarrhea.
Signs and Symptoms of Orthostasis: According to the tamsulosin prescribing information, in clinical trials with tamsulosin monotherapy, a positive orthostatic test result was observed in 16% (81/502) of subjects receiving 0.4 mg tamsulosin hydrochloride versus 11% (54/493) of subjects receiving placebo. Because orthostasis was detected more frequently in the tamsulosin-treated subjects than in placebo recipients, there is a potential risk of syncope [see Warnings and Precaution (5.1)].
6.2   Postmarketing Experience
The following adverse reactions have been identified during post-approval use of the individual components of JALYN. Because these reactions are reported voluntarily from a population of uncertain size, it is not always possible to reliably estimate their frequency or establish a causal relationship to drug exposure. These reactions have been chosen for inclusion due to a combination of their seriousness, frequency of reporting, or potential causal connection to drug exposure.
Dutasteride:
Immune System Disorders: Hypersensitivity reactions, including rash, pruritus, urticaria, localized edema, serious skin reactions, and angioedema.
Neoplasms: Male breast cancer.
Psychiatric Disorders: Depressed mood.
Reproductive System and Breast Disorders: Testicular pain and testicular swelling.

Tamsulosin:

Immune System Disorders: Hypersensitivity reactions, including rash, urticaria, pruritus, angioedema, and respiratory problems have been reported with positive rechallenge in some cases.

Cardiac Disorders: Palpitations, dyspnea, atrial fibrillation, arrhythmia, and tachycardia.

Skin Disorders: Skin desquamation, including Stevens–Johnson syndrome.

Gastrointestinal Disorders: Constipation, vomiting.

Reproductive System and Breast Disorders: Priapism.

Vascular Disorders: Hypotension.

Ophthalmologic Disorders: During cataract surgery, a variant of small pupil syndrome known as Intraoperative floppy iris syndrome (IFIS) associated with alpha adrenergic antagonist therapy *[see Warnings and Precautions (5.9)]*.

7 DRUG INTERACTIONS

There have been no drug interaction trials using JALYN. The following sections reflect information available for the individual components.

7.1 Cytochrome P450 3A Inhibitors

Dutasteride: Dutasteride is extensively metabolized in humans by the CYP3A4 and CYP3A5 isoenzymes. The effect of potent CYP3A4 inhibitors on dutasteride has not been studied. Because of the potential for drug-drug interactions, use caution when prescribing a dutasteride-containing product, including JALYN, to patients taking potent, chronic CYP3A4 enzyme inhibitors (e.g., ritonavir) *[see Clinical Pharmacology (12.3)]*.

Tamsulosin: *Strong and Moderate Inhibitors of CYP3A4 or CYP2D6:* Tamsulosin is extensively metabolized, mainly by CYP3A4 or CYP2D6.

Concomitant treatment with ketoconazole (a strong inhibitor of CYP3A4) resulted in increases in the C_{max} and AUC of tamsulosin by factors of 2.2 and 2.8, respectively. Concomitant treatment with paroxetine (a strong inhibitor of CYP2D6) resulted in increases in the C_{max} and AUC of tamsulosin by factors of 1.3 and 1.6, respectively. A similar increase in exposure is expected in poor metabolizers (PM) of CYP2D6 as compared to extensive metabolizers (EM). Since CYP2D6 PMs cannot be readily identified and the potential for significant increase in tamsulosin exposure exists when tamsulosin 0.4 mg is coadministered with strong CYP3A4 inhibitors in CYP2D6 PMs, tamsulosin 0.4 mg capsules should not be used in combination with strong inhibitors of CYP3A4 (e.g., ketoconazole). The effects of coadministration of both a CYP3A4 and a CYP2D6 inhibitor with tamsulosin have not been evaluated. However, there is a potential for significant increase in tamsulosin exposure when tamsulosin 0.4 mg is coadministered with a combination of both CYP3A4 and CYP2D6 inhibitors *[see Warnings and Precautions (5.2), Clinical Pharmacology (12.3)]*.

Cimetidine: Treatment with cimetidine resulted in a moderate increase in tamsulosin hydrochloride AUC (44%) *[see Warnings and Precautions (5.2), Clinical Pharmacology (12.3)]*.

7.2 Warfarin

Dutasteride: Concomitant administration of dutasteride 0.5 mg/day for 3 weeks with warfarin does not alter the steady-state pharmacokinetics of the S- or R-warfarin isomers or alter the effect of warfarin on prothrombin time *[see Clinical Pharmacology (12.3)]*.

Tamsulosin: A definitive drug-drug interaction trial between tamsulosin hydrochloride and warfarin was not conducted. Results from limited in vitro and in vivo studies are inconclusive. Caution should be exercised with concomitant administration of warfarin and tamsulosin-containing products, including JALYN *[see Warnings and Precautions (5.2), Clinical Pharmacology (12.3)]*.

7.3 Nifedipine, Atenolol, Enalapril

Tamsulosin: Dosage adjustments are not necessary when tamsulosin is administered concomitantly with nifedipine, atenolol, or enalapril *[see Clinical Pharmacology (12.3)]*.

7.4 Digoxin and Theophylline

Dutasteride: Dutasteride does not alter the steady-state pharmacokinetics of digoxin when administered concomitantly at a dose of 0.5 mg/day for 3 weeks *[see Clinical Pharmacology (12.3)]*.

Tamsulosin: Dosage adjustments are not necessary when tamsulosin is administered concomitantly with digoxin or theophylline *[see Clinical Pharmacology (12.3)]*.

7.5 Furosemide

Tamsulosin: Tamsulosin had no effect on the pharmacodynamics (excretion of electrolytes) of furosemide. While furosemide produced an 11% to 12% reduction in tamsulosin hydrochloride C_{max} and AUC, these changes are expected to be clinically insignificant and do not require adjustment of the dose of tamsulosin *[see Clinical Pharmacology (12.3)]*.

7.6 Calcium Channel Antagonists

Dutasteride: Coadministration of verapamil or diltiazem decreases dutasteride clearance and leads to increased exposure to dutasteride. The change in dutasteride exposure is not considered to be clinically significant. No dosage adjustment of dutasteride is recommended *[see Clinical Pharmacology (12.3)]*.

7.7 Cholestyramine

Dutasteride: Administration of a single 5-mg dose of dutasteride followed 1 hour later by a 12-g dose of cholestyramine does not affect the relative bioavailability of dutasteride *[see Clinical Pharmacology (12.3)]*.

8 USE IN SPECIFIC POPULATIONS

8.1 Pregnancy

Pregnancy Category X. There are no adequate and well-controlled studies in pregnant women with JALYN or its individual components.

Dutasteride: Dutasteride is contraindicated for use in women of childbearing potential and during pregnancy. Dutasteride is a 5 alpha-reductase inhibitor that prevents conversion of testosterone to dihydrotestosterone (DHT), a hormone necessary for normal development of male genitalia. In animal reproduction and developmental toxicity studies, dutasteride inhibited normal development of external genitalia in male fetuses. Therefore, dutasteride may cause fetal harm when administered to a pregnant woman. If dutasteride is used during pregnancy or if the patient becomes pregnant while taking dutasteride, the patient should be apprised of the potential hazard to the fetus.

Abnormalities in the genitalia of male fetuses is an expected physiological consequence of inhibition of the conversion of testosterone to DHT by 5 alpha-reductase inhibitors. These results are similar to observations in male infants with genetic 5 alpha-reductase deficiency. Dutasteride is absorbed through the skin. To avoid potential fetal exposure, women who are pregnant or could become pregnant should not handle dutasteride-containing capsules, including JALYN Capsules. If contact is made with leaking capsules, the contact area should be washed immediately with soap and water *[see Warnings and Precautions (5.6)]*. Dutasteride is secreted into semen. The highest measured semen concentration of dutasteride in treated men was 14 ng/mL. Assuming exposure of a 50-kg woman to 5 mL of semen and 100% absorption, the woman's dutasteride concentration would be about 0.0175 ng/mL. This concentration is more than 100 times less than concentrations producing abnormalities of male genitalia in animal studies. Dutasteride is highly protein bound in human semen (greater than 96%), which may reduce the amount of dutasteride available for vaginal absorption.

In an embryo-fetal development study in female rats, oral administration of dutasteride at doses 10 times less than the maximum recommended human dose (MRHD) of 0.5 mg daily resulted in abnormalities of male genitalia in the fetus (decreased anogenital distance at 0.05 mg/kg/day), nipple development, hypospadias, and distended preputial glands in male offspring (at all doses of 0.05, 2.5, 12.5, and 30 mg/kg/day). An increase in stillborn pups was observed at 111 times the MRHD, and reduced fetal body weight was observed at doses of about 15 times the MRHD (animal dose of 2.5 mg/kg/day). Increased incidences of skeletal variations considered to be delays in ossification associated with reduced body weight were observed at doses at about 56 times the MRHD (animal dose of 12.5 mg/kg/day).

In a rabbit embryo-fetal study, doses 28- to 93-fold the MRHD (animal doses of 30, 100, and 200 mg/kg/day) were administered orally during the period of major organogenesis (gestation days 7 to 29) to encompass the late period of external genitalia development. Histological evaluation of the genital papilla of fetuses revealed evidence of feminization of the male fetus at all doses. A second embryo-fetal study in rabbits at 0.3- to 53-fold the expected clinical exposure (animal doses of 0.05, 0.4, 3.0, and 30 mg/kg/day) also produced evidence of feminization of the genitalia in male fetuses at all doses.

In an oral pre- and post-natal development study in rats, dutasteride doses of 0.05, 2.5, 12.5, or 30 mg/kg/day were administered. Unequivocal evidence of feminization of the genitalia (i.e., decreased anogenital distance, increased incidence of hypospadias, nipple development) of male offspring occurred at 14- to 90-fold the MRHD (animal doses of 2.5 mg/kg/day or greater). At 0.05-fold the expected clinical exposure (animal dose of 0.05 mg/kg/day), evidence of feminization was limited to a small, but statistically significant, decrease in anogenital distance. Animal doses of 2.5 to 30 mg/kg/day resulted in prolonged gestation in the parental females and a decrease in time to vaginal patency for female offspring and a decrease in prostate and seminal vesicle weights in male offspring. Effects on newborn startle response were noted at doses greater than or equal to 12.5 mg/kg/day. Increased stillbirths were noted at 30 mg/kg/day.

In an embryo-fetal development study, pregnant rhesus monkeys were exposed intravenously to a dutasteride blood level comparable to the dutasteride concentration found in human semen. Dutasteride was administered on gestation days 20 to 100 at doses of 400, 780, 1,325, or 2,010 ng/day (12 monkeys/group). The development of male external genitalia of monkey offspring was not adversely affected. Reduction of fetal adrenal weights, reduction in fetal prostate weights, and increases in fetal ovarian and testis weights were observed at the highest dose tested in monkeys. Based on the highest measured semen concentration of dutasteride in treated men (14 ng/mL), these doses represent 0.8 to 16 times the potential maximum exposure of a 50-kg human female to 5 mL semen daily from a dutasteride-treated man, assuming 100% absorption. (These calculations are based on blood levels of parent drug which are achieved at 32 to 186 times the daily doses administered to pregnant monkeys on a ng/kg basis). Dutasteride is highly bound to proteins in human semen (greater than 96%), potentially reducing the amount of dutasteride available for vaginal absorption. It is not known whether rabbits or rhesus monkeys produce any of the major human metabolites.

Estimates of exposure multiples comparing animal studies to the MRHD for dutasteride are based on clinical serum concentration at steady state.

Tamsulosin: Administration of tamsulosin to pregnant female rats at dose levels up to approximately 50 times the human therapeutic AUC exposure (animal dose of 300 mg/kg/day) revealed no evidence of harm to the fetus. Administration of tamsulosin hydrochloride to pregnant rabbits at dose levels up to 50 mg/kg/day produced no evidence of fetal harm. However, because of the effect of dutasteride on the fetus, JALYN is contraindicated for use in pregnant women. Estimates of exposure multiples comparing animal studies to the MRHD for tamsulosin are based on AUC.

8.3 Nursing Mothers

JALYN is contraindicated for use in women of childbearing potential, including nursing women. It is not known whether dutasteride or tamsulosin is excreted in human milk.

8.4 Pediatric Use

JALYN is contraindicated for use in pediatric patients. Safety and effectiveness of JALYN in pediatric patients have not been established.

8.5 Geriatric Use

Of 1,610 male subjects treated with coadministered dutasteride and tamsulosin in the CombAT trial, 58% of enrolled subjects were aged 65 years and older and 13% of enrolled subjects were aged 75 years and older. No overall differences in safety or efficacy were observed between these subjects and younger subjects but greater sensitivity of some older individuals cannot be ruled out *[see Clinical Pharmacology (12.3)]*.

8.6 Renal Impairment

The effect of renal impairment on dutasteride and tamsulosin pharmacokinetics has not been studied using JALYN. Because no dosage adjustment is necessary for dutasteride or tamsulosin in patients with moderate-to-severe renal impairment ($10 \leq CL_{cr} < 30$ mL/min/1.73 m^2), no dosage adjustment is necessary for JALYN in patients with moderate-to-severe renal impairment. However, patients with end-stage renal disease ($CL_{cr} < 10$ mL/min/1.73 m^2) have not been studied *[see Clinical Pharmacology (12.3)]*.

8.7 Hepatic Impairment

The effect of hepatic impairment on dutasteride and tamsulosin pharmacokinetics has not been studied using JALYN. The following text reflects information available for the individual components.

Dutasteride: The effect of hepatic impairment on dutasteride pharmacokinetics has not been studied. Because dutasteride is extensively metabolized, exposure could be higher in hepatically impaired patients. However, in a clinical trial where 60 subjects received 5 mg (10 times the therapeutic dose) daily for 24 weeks, no additional adverse events were observed compared with those observed at the therapeutic dose of 0.5 mg *[see Clinical Pharmacology (12.3)]*.

Tamsulosin: Patients with moderate hepatic impairment do not require an adjustment in tamsulosin dosage. Tamsulosin has not been studied in patients with severe hepatic impairment *[see Clinical Pharmacology (12.3)]*.

10 OVERDOSAGE

No data are available with regard to overdosage with JALYN. The following text reflects information available for the individual components.

Dutasteride: In volunteer trials, single doses of dutasteride up to 40 mg (80 times the therapeutic dose) for 7 days have been administered without significant safety concerns. In a clinical trial, daily doses of 5 mg (10 times the therapeutic dose) were administered to 60 subjects for 6 months with no additional adverse effects to those seen at therapeutic doses of 0.5 mg.

There is no specific antidote for dutasteride. Therefore, in cases of suspected overdosage symptomatic and supportive treatment should be given as appropriate, taking the long half-life of dutasteride into consideration.

Table 2. Arithmetic Means (SD) of Serum Dutasteride and Tamsulosin in Single-Dose Pharmacokinetic Parameters Under Fed Conditions

Component	N	$AUC_{(0-t)}$ (ng h/mL)	C_{max} (ng/mL)	T_{max} (h)[a]	$t_{\frac{1}{2}}$ (h)
Dutasteride	92	39.6 (23.1)	2.14 (0.77)	3.00 (1.00-10.00)	
Tamsulosin	92	187.2 (95.7)	11.3 (4.44)	6.00 (2.00-24.00)	13.5 (3.92)[b]

[a] Median (range).
[b] N = 91.

Tamsulosin: Should overdosage of tamsulosin lead to hypotension [see Warnings and Precautions (5.1), Adverse Reactions (6.1)], support of the cardiovascular system is of first importance. Restoration of blood pressure and normalization of heart rate may be accomplished by keeping the patient in the supine position. If this measure is inadequate, then administration of intravenous fluids should be considered. If necessary, vasopressors should then be used and renal function should be monitored and supported as needed. Laboratory data indicate that tamsulosin is 94% to 99% protein bound; therefore, dialysis is unlikely to be of benefit.

11 DESCRIPTION

JALYN (dutasteride and tamsulosin hydrochloride) Capsules contain dutasteride (a selective inhibitor of both the type 1 and type 2 isoforms of steroid 5 alpha-reductase, an intracellular enzyme that converts testosterone to DHT) and tamsulosin (an antagonist of alpha$_{1A}$-adrenoreceptors in the prostate). Each JALYN Capsule contains the following:
- One dutasteride oblong, opaque, dull-yellow soft gelatin capsule, containing 0.5 mg of dutasteride dissolved in a mixture of butylated hydroxytoluene and mono-diglycerides of caprylic/capric acid. The inactive ingredients in the soft-gelatin capsule shell are ferric oxide (yellow), gelatin (from certified BSE-free bovine sources), glycerin, and titanium dioxide.
- Tamsulosin hydrochloride white to off-white pellets, containing 0.4 mg tamsulosin hydrochloride and the inactive ingredients: methacrylic acid copolymer dispersion, microcrystalline cellulose, talc, and triethyl citrate.

The above components are encapsulated in a hard-shell capsule made with the inactive ingredients of carrageenan, FD&C yellow 6, hypromellose, iron oxide red, potassium chloride, titanium dioxide, and imprinted with "GS 7CZ" in black ink.

Dutasteride: Dutasteride is a synthetic 4-azasteroid compound chemically designated as (5α,17β)-N-{2,5 bis(trifluoromethyl)phenyl}-3-oxo-4-azaandrost-1-ene-17-carboxamide. The empirical formula of dutasteride is $C_{27}H_{30}F_6N_2O_2$, representing a molecular weight of 528.5 with the following structural formula:

Dutasteride is a white to pale yellow powder with a melting point of 242° to 250°C. It is soluble in ethanol (44 mg/mL), methanol (64 mg/mL), and polyethylene glycol 400 (3 mg/mL), but it is insoluble in water.

Tamsulosin: Tamsulosin hydrochloride is a synthetic compound chemically designated as (-)-(R)-5-[2-[[2-(o-Ethoxyphenoxy)ethyl]amino]propyl]-2-methoxybenzenesulfonamide, monohydrochloride.

The empirical formula of tamsulosin hydrochloride is $C_{20}H_{28}N_2O_5S•HCl$. The molecular weight of tamsulosin hydrochloride is 444.97. Its structural formula is:

Tamsulosin hydrochloride is a white or almost white crystalline powder that melts with decomposition at approximately 234°C. It is sparingly soluble in water and slightly soluble in methanol, ethanol, acetone, and ethyl acetate.

12 CLINICAL PHARMACOLOGY

12.1 Mechanism of Action

JALYN is a combination of 2 drugs with different mechanisms of action to improve symptoms in patients with BPH: dutasteride, a 5 alpha-reductase inhibitor, and tamsulosin, an antagonist of alpha$_{1A}$-adrenoreceptors.

Dutasteride: Dutasteride inhibits the conversion of testosterone to DHT. DHT is the androgen primarily responsible for the initial development and subsequent enlargement of the prostate gland. Testosterone is converted to DHT by the enzyme 5 alpha-reductase, which exists as 2 isoforms, type 1 and type 2. The type 2 isoenzyme is primarily active in the reproductive tissues, while the type 1 isoenzyme is also responsible for testosterone conversion in the skin and liver. Dutasteride is a competitive and specific inhibitor of both type 1 and type 2 5 alpha-reductase isoenzymes, with which it forms a stable enzyme complex. Dissociation from this complex has been evaluated under in vitro and in vivo conditions and is extremely slow. Dutasteride does not bind to the human androgen receptor.

Tamsulosin: Smooth muscle tone is mediated by the sympathetic nervous stimulation of alpha$_1$-adrenoceptors, which are abundant in the prostate, prostatic capsule, prostatic urethra, and bladder neck. Blockade of these adrenoceptors can cause smooth muscles in the bladder neck and prostate to relax, resulting in an improvement in urine flow rate and a reduction in symptoms of BPH.

Tamsulosin, an alpha$_1$-adrenoceptor blocking agent, exhibits selectivity for alpha$_1$-receptors in the human prostate. At least 3 discrete alpha$_1$-adrenoceptor subtypes have been identified: alpha$_{1A}$, alpha$_{1B}$, and alpha$_{1D}$; their distribution differs between human organs and tissue. Approximately 70% of the alpha$_1$-receptors in human prostate are of the alpha$_{1A}$ subtype. Tamsulosin is not intended for use as an antihypertensive.

12.2 Pharmacodynamics

Dutasteride: *Effect on 5 Alpha-Dihydrotestosterone and Testosterone:* The maximum effect of daily doses of dutasteride on the reduction of DHT is dose-dependent and is observed within 1 to 2 weeks. After 1 and 2 weeks of daily dosing with dutasteride 0.5 mg, median serum DHT concentrations were reduced by 85% and 90%, respectively. In patients with BPH treated with dutasteride 0.5 mg/day for 4 years, the median decrease in serum DHT was 94% at 1 year, 93% at 2 years, and 95% at both 3 and 4 years. The median increase in serum testosterone was 19% at both 1 and 2 years, 26% at 3 years, and 22% at 4 years, but the mean and median levels remained within the physiologic range.

In patients with BPH treated with 5 mg/day of dutasteride or placebo for up to 12 weeks prior to transurethral resection of the prostate, mean DHT concentrations in prostatic tissue were significantly lower in the dutasteride group compared with placebo (784 and 5,793 pg/g, respectively, P<0.001). Mean prostatic tissue concentrations of testosterone were significantly higher in the dutasteride group compared with placebo (2,073 and 93 pg/g, respectively, P<0.001).

Adult males with genetically inherited type 2 5 alpha-reductase deficiency also have decreased DHT levels. These 5 alpha-reductase-deficient males have a small prostate gland throughout life and do not develop BPH. Except for the associated urogenital defects present at birth, no other clinical abnormalities related to 5 alpha-reductase deficiency have been observed in these individuals.

Effects on Other Hormones: In healthy volunteers, 52 weeks of treatment with dutasteride 0.5 mg/day (n = 26) resulted in no clinically significant change compared with placebo (n = 23) in sex hormone-binding globulin, estradiol, luteinizing hormone, follicle-stimulating hormone, thyroxine (free T4), and dehydroepiandrosterone. Statistically significant, baseline-adjusted mean increases compared with placebo were observed for total testosterone at 8 weeks (97.1 ng/dL, P<0.003) and thyroid-stimulating hormone at 52 weeks (0.4 mcIU/mL, P<0.05). The median percentage changes from baseline within the dutasteride group were 17.9% for testosterone at 8 weeks and 12.4% for thyroid-stimulating hormone at 52 weeks. After stopping dutasteride for 24 weeks, the mean levels of testosterone and thyroid-stimulating hormone had returned to baseline in the group of subjects with available data at the visit. In subjects with BPH treated with dutasteride in a large randomized, double-blind, placebo-controlled trial, there was a median percent increase in luteinizing hormone of 12% at 6 months and 19% at both 12 and 24 months.

Other Effects: Plasma lipid panel and bone mineral density were evaluated following 52 weeks of dutasteride

0.5 mg once daily in healthy volunteers. There was no change in bone mineral density as measured by dual energy x-ray absorptiometry compared with either placebo or baseline. In addition, the plasma lipid profile (i.e., total cholesterol, low density lipoproteins, high density lipoproteins, and triglycerides) was unaffected by dutasteride. No clinically significant changes in adrenal hormone responses to adrenocorticotropic hormone (ACTH) stimulation were observed in a subset population (n = 13) of the 1-year healthy volunteer trial.

12.3 Pharmacokinetics

The pharmacokinetics of dutasteride and tamsulosin from JALYN are comparable to the pharmacokinetics of dutasteride and tamsulosin when administered separately.

Absorption: The pharmacokinetic parameters of dutasteride and tamsulosin observed after administration of JALYN in a single dose, randomized, 3-period partial, cross-over trial are summarized in Table 2 below.
[See table 2 above]

Dutasteride: Following administration of a single 0.5-mg dose of a soft gelatin capsule, time to peak absolute bioavailability in 5 healthy subjects is approximately 60% (range: 40% to 94%).

Tamsulosin: Absorption of tamsulosin is essentially complete (>90%) following oral administration of 0.4-mg tamsulosin hydrochloride capsules under fasting conditions. Tamsulosin exhibits linear kinetics following single and multiple dosing, with achievement of steady-state concentrations by the fifth day of once-daily dosing.

Effect of Food: Food does not affect the pharmacokinetics of dutasteride following administration of JALYN. However, a mean 30% decrease in tamsulosin C_{max} was observed when JALYN was administered with food, similar to that seen when tamsulosin monotherapy was administered under fed versus fasting conditions.

Distribution: *Dutasteride:* Pharmacokinetic data following single and repeat oral doses show that dutasteride has a large volume of distribution (300 to 500 L). Dutasteride is highly bound to plasma albumin (99.0%) and alpha-1 acid glycoprotein (96.6%).

In a trial of healthy subjects (n = 26) receiving dutasteride 0.5 mg/day for 12 months, semen dutasteride concentrations averaged 3.4 ng/mL (range: 0.4 to 14 ng/mL) at 12 months and, similar to serum, achieved steady-state concentrations at 6 months. On average, at 12 months 11.5% of serum dutasteride concentrations partitioned into semen.

Tamsulosin: The mean steady-state apparent volume of distribution of tamsulosin after intravenous administration to 10 healthy male adults was 16 L, which is suggestive of distribution into extracellular fluids in the body. Tamsulosin is extensively bound to human plasma proteins (94% to 99%), primarily alpha-1 acid glycoprotein (AAG), with linear binding over a wide concentration range (20 to 600 ng/mL). The results of 2-way in vitro studies indicate that the binding of tamsulosin to human plasma proteins is not affected by amitriptyline, diclofenac, glyburide, simvastatin plus simvastatin-hydroxy acid metabolite, warfarin, diazepam, or propranolol. Likewise, tamsulosin had no effect on the extent of binding of these drugs.

Metabolism: *Dutasteride:* Dutasteride is extensively metabolized in humans. In vitro studies showed that dutasteride is metabolized by the CYP3A4 and CYP3A5 isoenzymes. Both of these isoenzymes produced the 4'-hydroxydutasteride, 6-hydroxydutasteride, and the 6,4'-dihydroxydutasteride metabolites. In addition, the 15-hydroxydutasteride metabolite was formed by CYP3A4. Dutasteride is not metabolized in vitro by human cytochrome P450 isoenzymes CYP1A2, CYP2A6, CYP2B6, CYP2C8, CYP2C9, CYP2C19, CYP2D6, and CYP2E1. In human serum following dosing to steady state, unchanged dutasteride, 3 major metabolites (4'-hydroxydutasteride, 1,2-dihydrodutasteride, and 6-hydroxydutasteride), and 2 minor metabolites (6,4'-dihydroxydutasteride and 15-hydroxydutasteride), as assessed by mass spectrometric response, have been detected. The absolute stereochemistry of the hydroxyl additions in the 6 and 15 positions is not known. In vitro, the 4'-hydroxydutasteride and 1,2-dihydrodutasteride metabolites are much less potent than dutasteride against both isoforms of human 5α-reductase. The activity of 6β-hydroxydutasteride is comparable to that of dutasteride.

Tamsulosin: There is no enantiomeric bioconversion from tamsulosin [R(-) isomer] to the S(+) isomer in humans. Tamsulosin is extensively metabolized by cytochrome P450 enzymes in the liver and less than 10% of the dose is excreted in urine unchanged. However, the pharmacokinetic profile of the metabolites in humans has not been established. In vitro studies indicate that CYP3A4 and CYP2D6 are involved in metabolism of tamsulosin as well as some minor participation of other CYP isoenzymes. Inhibition of hepatic drug-metabolizing enzymes may lead to increased exposure to tamsulosin [see Drug Interactions (7.1)]. The metabolites of tamsulosin undergo extensive conjugation to glucuronide or sulfate prior to renal excretion.

Incubations with human liver microsomes showed no evidence of clinically significant metabolic interactions between tamsulosin and amitriptyline, albuterol, glyburide, and finasteride. However, results of the in vitro testing of the tamsulosin interaction with diclofenac and warfarin were equivocal.

Excretion: *Dutasteride:* Dutasteride and its metabolites were excreted mainly in feces. As a percent of dose, there was approximately 5% unchanged dutasteride (approximately 1% to approximately 15%) and 40% as dutasteride-related metabolites (approximately 2% to approximately 90%). Only trace amounts of unchanged dutasteride were found in urine (<1%). Therefore, on average, the dose unaccounted for approximated 55% (range: 5% to 97%). The terminal elimination half-life of dutasteride is approximately 5 weeks at steady state. The average steady-state serum dutasteride concentration was 40 ng/mL following 0.5 mg/day for 1 year. Following daily dosing, dutasteride serum concentrations achieve 65% of steady-state concentration after 1 month and approximately 90% after 3 months. Due to the long half-life of dutasteride, serum concentrations remain detectable (greater than 0.1 ng/mL) for up to 4 to 6 months after discontinuation of treatment.

Tamsulosin: On administration of the radiolabeled dose of tamsulosin to 4 healthy volunteers, 97% of the administered radioactivity was recovered, with urine (76%) representing the primary route of excretion compared with feces (21%) over 168 hours.

Following intravenous or oral administration of an immediate-release formulation, the elimination half-life of tamsulosin in plasma ranges from 5 to 7 hours. Because of absorption rate-controlled pharmacokinetics with tamsulosin hydrochloride capsules, the apparent half-life of tamsulosin is approximately 9 to 13 hours in healthy volunteers and 14 to 15 hours in the target population.

Tamsulosin undergoes restrictive clearance in humans, with a relatively low systemic clearance (2.88 L/h).

Specific Populations: *Pediatric:* The pharmacokinetics of dutasteride and tamsulosin administered together have not been investigated in subjects younger than 18 years.

Geriatric: Dutasteride and tamsulosin pharmacokinetics using JALYN have not been studied in geriatric patients. The following text reflects information for the individual components.

Dutasteride: No dosage adjustment is necessary in the elderly. The pharmacokinetics and pharmacodynamics of dutasteride were evaluated in 36 healthy male subjects aged between 24 and 87 years following administration of a single 5-mg dose of dutasteride. In this single-dose trial, dutasteride half-life increased with age (approximately 170 hours in men aged 20 to 49 years, approximately 260 hours in men aged 50 to 69 years, and approximately 300 hours in men older than 70 years).

Tamsulosin: Cross-study comparison of tamsulosin overall exposure (AUC) and half-life indicate that the pharmacokinetic disposition of tamsulosin may be slightly prolonged in geriatric males compared with young, healthy male volunteers. Intrinsic clearance is independent of tamsulosin binding to AAG, but diminishes with age, resulting in a 40% overall higher exposure (AUC) in subjects aged 55 to 75 years compared with subjects aged 20 to 32 years.

Gender: *Dutasteride:* Dutasteride is contraindicated in pregnancy and women of childbearing potential and is not indicated for use in other women [see Contraindications (4), Warnings and Precautions (5.6)]. The pharmacokinetics of dutasteride in women have not been studied.

Tamsulosin: Tamsulosin is not indicated for use in women. No information is available on the pharmacokinetics of tamsulosin in women.

Race: The effect of race on pharmacokinetics of dutasteride and tamsulosin administered together or separately has not been studied.

Renal Impairment: The effect of renal impairment on dutasteride and tamsulosin pharmacokinetics has not been studied using JALYN. The following text reflects information for the individual components.

Dutasteride: The effect of renal impairment on dutasteride pharmacokinetics has not been studied. However, less than 0.1% of a steady-state 0.5-mg dose of dutasteride is recovered in human urine, so no adjustment in dosage is anticipated for patients with renal impairment.

Tamsulosin: The pharmacokinetics of tamsulosin have been compared in 6 subjects with mild-moderate (30≤ CL_{cr} <70 mL/min/1.73 m^2) or moderate-severe (10≤ CL_{cr} <30 mL/min/1.73 m^2) renal impairment and 6 normal subjects (CL_{cr} >90 mL/min/1.73 m^2). While a change in the overall plasma concentration of tamsulosin was observed as the result of altered binding to AAG, the unbound (active) concentration of tamsulosin, as well as the intrinsic clearance, remained relatively constant. Therefore, patients with renal impairment do not require an adjustment in tamsulosin dosing. However, patients with end-stage renal disease (CL_{cr} <10 mL/min/1.73 m^2) have not been studied.

Hepatic Impairment: The effect of hepatic impairment on dutasteride and tamsulosin pharmacokinetics has not been studied using JALYN. The following text reflects information available for the individual components.

Dutasteride: The effect of hepatic impairment on dutasteride pharmacokinetics has not been studied. Because dutasteride is extensively metabolized, exposure could be higher in hepatically impaired patients.

Tamsulosin: The pharmacokinetics of tamsulosin have been compared in 8 subjects with moderate hepatic impairment (Child-Pugh classification: Grades A and B) and 8 normal subjects. While a change in the overall plasma concentration of tamsulosin was observed as the result of altered binding to AAG, the unbound (active) concentration of tamsulosin does not change significantly with only a modest (32%) change in intrinsic clearance of unbound tamsulosin. Therefore, patients with moderate hepatic impairment do not require an adjustment in tamsulosin dosage. Tamsulosin has not been studied in patients with severe hepatic impairment.

Drug Interactions: There have been no drug interaction studies using JALYN. The following text reflects information available for the individual components.

Cytochrome P450 Inhibitors: Dutasteride: No clinical drug interaction trials have been performed to evaluate the impact of CYP3A enzyme inhibitors on dutasteride pharmacokinetics. However, based on in vitro data, blood concentrations of dutasteride may increase in the presence of inhibitors of CYP3A4/5 such as ritonavir, ketoconazole, verapamil, diltiazem, cimetidine, troleandomycin, and ciprofloxacin.

Dutasteride does not inhibit the in vitro metabolism of model substrates for the major human cytochrome P450 isoenzymes (CYP1A2, CYP2C9, CYP2C19, CYP2D6, and CYP3A4) at a concentration of 1,000 ng/mL, 25 times greater than steady-state serum concentrations in humans.

Tamsulosin: Strong and Moderate Inhibitors of CYP3A4 or CYP2D6: The effects of ketoconazole (a strong inhibitor of CYP3A4) at 400 mg once daily for 5 days on the pharmacokinetics of a single tamsulosin hydrochloride capsule 0.4-mg dose was investigated in 24 healthy volunteers (age range: 23 to 47 years). Concomitant treatment with ketoconazole resulted in increases in the C_{max} and AUC of tamsulosin by factors of 2.2 and 2.8, respectively. The effects of concomitant administration of a moderate CYP3A4 inhibitor (e.g., erythromycin) on the pharmacokinetics of tamsulosin have not been evaluated.

The effects of paroxetine (a strong inhibitor of CYP2D6) at 20 mg once daily for 9 days on the pharmacokinetics of a single tamsulosin capsule 0.4-mg dose was investigated in 24 healthy volunteers (age range: 23 to 47 years). Concomitant treatment with paroxetine resulted in increases in the C_{max} and AUC of tamsulosin by factors of 1.3 and 1.6, respectively. A similar increase in exposure is expected in poor metabolizers (PM) of CYP2D6 as compared with extensive metabolizers (EM). A fraction of the population (about 7% of Caucasians and 2% of African-Americans) are CYP2D6 PMs. Since CYP2D6 PMs cannot be readily identified and the potential for significant increase in tamsulosin exposure exists when tamsulosin 0.4 mg is coadministered with strong CYP3A4 inhibitors in CYP2D6 PMs, tamsulosin 0.4-mg capsules should not be used in combination with strong inhibitors of CYP3A4 (e.g., ketoconazole).

The effects of concomitant administration of a moderate CYP2D6 inhibitor (e.g., terbinafine) on the pharmacokinetics of tamsulosin have not been evaluated.

The effects of coadministration of both a CYP3A4 and a CYP2D6 inhibitor with tamsulosin capsules have not been evaluated. However, there is a potential for significant increase in tamsulosin exposure when tamsulosin 0.4 mg is coadministered with a combination of both CYP3A4 and CYP2D6 inhibitors.

Cimetidine: The effects of cimetidine at the highest recommended dose (400 mg every 6 hours for 6 days) on the pharmacokinetics of a single tamsulosin capsule 0.4 mg dose was investigated in 10 healthy volunteers (age range: 21 to 38 years). Treatment with cimetidine resulted in a significant decrease (26%) in the clearance of tamsulosin hydrochloride, which resulted in a moderate increase in tamsulosin hydrochloride AUC (44%).

Alpha Adrenergic Antagonists: Dutasteride: In a single-sequence, crossover trial in healthy volunteers, the administration of tamsulosin or terazosin in combination with dutasteride had no effect on the steady-state pharmacokinetics of either alpha-adrenergic antagonist. Although the effect of administration of tamsulosin or terazosin on dutasteride pharmacokinetic parameters was not evaluated, the percent change in DHT concentrations was similar for dutasteride, alone or in combination with tamsulosin or terazosin.

Warfarin: Dutasteride: In a trial of 23 healthy volunteers, 3 weeks of treatment with dutasteride 0.5 mg/day did not alter the steady-state pharmacokinetics of the S- or R-warfarin isomers or alter the effect of warfarin on prothrombin time when administered with warfarin.

Tamsulosin: A definitive drug-drug interaction trial between tamsulosin and warfarin was not conducted. Results

from limited in vitro and in vivo studies are inconclusive. Therefore, caution should be exercised with concomitant administration of warfarin and tamsulosin.

Nifedipine, Atenolol, Enalapril: Tamsulosin: In 3 trials in hypertensive subjects (age range: 47 to 79 years) whose blood pressure was controlled with stable doses of nifedipine extended-release, atenolol, or enalapril for at least 3 months, tamsulosin hydrochloride capsules 0.4 mg for 7 days followed by tamsulosin hydrochloride capsules 0.8 mg for another 7 days (n = 8 per trial) resulted in no clinically significant effects on blood pressure and pulse rate compared with placebo (n = 4 per trial). Therefore, dosage adjustments are not necessary when tamsulosin is administered concomitantly with nifedipine extended-release, atenolol, or enalapril.

Digoxin and Theophylline: Dutasteride: In a trial of 20 healthy volunteers, dutasteride did not alter the steady-state pharmacokinetics of digoxin when administered concomitantly at a dose of 0.5 mg/day for 3 weeks.

Tamsulosin: In 2 trials in healthy volunteers (n = 10 per trial; age range: 19 to 39 years) receiving tamsulosin capsules 0.4 mg/day for 2 days, followed by tamsulosin capsules 0.8 mg/day for 5 to 8 days, single intravenous doses of digoxin 0.5 mg or theophylline 5 mg/kg resulted in no change in the pharmacokinetics of digoxin or theophylline. Therefore, dosage adjustments are not necessary when a tamsulosin capsule is administered concomitantly with digoxin or theophylline.

Furosemide: Tamsulosin: The pharmacokinetic and pharmacodynamic interaction between tamsulosin hydrochloride capsules 0.8 mg/day (steady-state) and furosemide 20 mg intravenously (single dose) was evaluated in 10 healthy volunteers (age range: 21 to 40 years). Tamsulosin had no effect on the pharmacodynamics (excretion of electrolytes) of furosemide. While furosemide produced an 11% to 12% reduction in tamsulosin C_{max} and AUC, these changes are expected to be clinically insignificant and do not require dose adjustment for tamsulosin.

Calcium Channel Antagonists: Dutasteride: In a population pharmacokinetics analysis, a decrease in clearance of dutasteride was noted when coadministered with the CYP3A4 inhibitors verapamil (-37%, n = 6) and diltiazem (-44%, n = 5). In contrast, no decrease in clearance was seen when amlodipine, another calcium channel antagonist that is not a CYP3A4 inhibitor, was coadministered with dutasteride (+7%, n = 4). The decrease in clearance and subsequent increase in exposure to dutasteride in the presence of verapamil and diltiazem is not considered to be clinically significant. No dosage adjustment is recommended.

Cholestyramine: Dutasteride: Administration of a single 5-mg dose of dutasteride followed 1 hour later by 12 g cholestyramine did not affect the relative bioavailability of dutasteride in 12 normal volunteers.

13 NONCLINICAL TOXICOLOGY

13.1 Carcinogenesis, Mutagenesis, Impairment of Fertility

No non-clinical studies have been conducted with JALYN. The following information is based on studies performed with dutasteride or tamsulosin.

Carcinogenesis:

Dutasteride: A 2-year carcinogenicity study was conducted in B6C3F1 mice at doses of 3, 35, 250, and 500 mg/kg/day for males and 3, 35, 250 mg/kg/day for females; an increased incidence of benign hepatocellular adenomas was noted at 250 mg/kg/day (290-fold the MRHD of a 0.5-mg daily dose) in female mice only. Two of the 3 major human metabolites have been detected in mice. The exposure to these metabolites in mice is either lower than in humans or is not known.

In a 2-year carcinogenicity study in Han Wistar rats, at doses of 1.5, 7.5, and 53 mg/kg/day in males and 0.8, 6.3, and 15 mg/kg/day in females, there was an increase in Leydig cell adenomas in the testes at 135-fold the MRHD (53 mg/kg/day and greater). An increased incidence of Leydig cell hyperplasia was present at 52-fold the MRHD (male rat doses of 7.5 mg/kg/day and greater). A positive correlation between proliferative changes in the Leydig cells and an increase in circulating luteinizing hormone levels has been demonstrated with 5 alpha-reductase inhibitors and is consistent with an effect on the hypothalamic-pituitary-testicular axis following 5 alpha-reductase inhibition. At tumorigenic doses, luteinizing hormone levels in rats were increased by 167%. In this study, the major human metabolites were tested for carcinogenicity at approximately 1 to 3 times the expected clinical exposure.

Tamsulosin: In a rat carcinogenicity assay, no increases in tumor incidence was observed in rats administered up to 3 times the MRHD of 0.8 mg/day (based on AUC of animal doses up to 43 mg/kg/day in males and up to 52 mg/kg/day in females), with the exception of a modest increase in the frequency of mammary gland fibroadenomas in female rats receiving doses of 5.4 mg/kg or greater.

In a carcinogenicity assay, mice were administered up to 8 times the MRHD of tamsulosin (oral doses up to

127 mg/kg/day in males and 158 mg/kg/day in females). There were no significant tumor findings in male mice. Female mice treated for 2 years with the 2 highest doses of 45 and 158 mg/kg/day had statistically significant increases in the incidence of mammary gland fibroadenomas (P<0.0001) and adenocarcinomas.

The increased incidences of mammary gland neoplasms in female rats and mice were considered secondary to tamsulosin-induced hyperprolactinemia. It is not known if tamsulosin elevates prolactin in humans. The relevance for human risk of the findings of prolactin-mediated endocrine tumors in rodents is not known.

Mutagenesis:
Dutasteride: Dutasteride was tested for genotoxicity in a bacterial mutagenesis assay (Ames test), a chromosomal aberration assay in CHO cells, and a micronucleus assay in rats. The results did not indicate any genotoxic potential of the parent drug. Two major human metabolites were also negative in either the Ames test or an abbreviated Ames test.

Tamsulosin: Tamsulosin produced no evidence of mutagenic potential in vitro in the Ames reverse mutation test, mouse lymphoma thymidine kinase assay, unscheduled DNA repair synthesis assay, and chromosomal aberration assays in CHO cells or human lymphocytes. There were no mutagenic effects in the in vivo sister chromatid exchange and mouse micronucleus assay.

Impairment of Fertility:
Dutasteride: Treatment of sexually mature male rats with dutasteride at 0.1- to 110-fold the MRHD (animal doses of 0.05, 10, 50, and 500 mg/kg/day for up to 31 weeks) resulted in dose- and time-dependent decreases in fertility; reduced cauda epididymal (absolute) sperm counts but not sperm concentration (at 50 and 500 mg/kg/day); reduced weights of the epididymis, prostate, and seminal vesicles; and microscopic changes in the male reproductive organs. The fertility effects were reversed by recovery week 6 at all doses, and sperm counts were normal at the end of a 14-week recovery period. The 5 alpha-reductase–related changes consisted of cytoplasmic vacuolation of tubular epithelium in the epididymides and decreased cytoplasmic content of epithelium, consistent with decreased secretory activity in the prostate and seminal vesicles. The microscopic changes were no longer present at recovery week 14 in the low-dose group and were partly recovered in the remaining treatment groups. Low levels of dutasteride (0.6 to 17 ng/mL) were detected in the serum of untreated female rats mated to males dosed at 10, 50, or 500 mg/kg/day for 29 to 30 weeks.

In a fertility study in female rats, oral administration of dutasteride at doses of 0.05, 2.5, 12.5, and 30 mg/kg/day resulted in reduced litter size, increased embryo resorption and feminization of male fetuses (decreased anogenital distance) at 2- to 10-fold the MRHD (animal doses of 2.5 mg/kg/day or greater). Fetal body weights were also reduced at less than 0.02-fold the MRHD in rats (0.5 mg/kg/day).

Tamsulosin: Studies in rats revealed significantly reduced fertility in males at approximately 50 times the MRHD based on AUC (single or multiple daily doses of 300 mg/kg/day of tamsulosin hydrochloride). The mechanism of decreased fertility in male rats is considered to be an effect of the compound on the vaginal plug formation possibly due to changes of semen content or impairment of ejaculation. The effects on fertility were reversible showing improvement by 3 days after a single dose and 4 weeks after multiple dosing. Effects on fertility in males were completely reversed within nine weeks of discontinuation of multiple dosing. Multiple doses of 0.2 and 16 times the MRHD (animal doses of 10 and 100 mg/kg/day tamsulosin hydrochloride) did not significantly alter fertility in male rats. Effects of tamsulosin on sperm counts or sperm function have not been evaluated.

Studies in female rats revealed significant reductions in fertility after single or multiple dosing with 300 mg/kg/day of the R-isomer or racemic mixture of tamsulosin hydrochloride, respectively. In female rats, the reductions in fertility after single doses were considered to be associated with impairments in fertilization. Multiple dosing with 10 or 100 mg/kg/day of the racemic mixture did not significantly alter fertility in female rats.

Estimates of exposure multiples comparing animal studies to the MRHD for dutasteride are based on clinical serum concentration at steady state.

Estimates of exposure multiples comparing animal studies to the MRHD for tamsulosin are based on AUC.

13.2   Animal Toxicology and/or Pharmacology
Central Nervous System Toxicology Studies: *Dutasteride:* In rats and dogs, repeated oral administration of dutasteride resulted in some animals showing signs of non-specific, reversible, centrally-mediated toxicity without associated histopathological changes at exposures 425- and 315-fold the expected clinical exposure (of parent drug), respectively.

14   CLINICAL STUDIES

The trial supporting the efficacy of JALYN was a 4-year multicenter, randomized, double-blind, parallel-group trial (CombAT trial) investigating the efficacy of the coadministration of dutasteride 0.5 mg/day and tamsulosin hydrochloride 0.4 mg/day (n = 1,610) compared with dutasteride alone (n = 1,623) or tamsulosin alone (n = 1,611). Subjects were at least 50 years of age with a serum PSA ≥1.5 ng/mL and <10 ng/mL and BPH diagnosed by medical history and physical examination, including enlarged prostate (≥30 cc) and BPH symptoms that were moderate to severe according to the International Prostate Symptom Score (IPSS). Eighty-eight percent (88%) of the enrolled trial population was Caucasian. Approximately 52% of subjects had previous exposure to 5 alpha-reductase inhibitor or alpha adrenergic antagonist treatment. Of the 4,844 subjects randomly assigned to receive treatment, 69% of subjects in the coadministration group, 67% in the dutasteride group, and 61% in the tamsulosin group completed 4 years of double-blind treatment.

Effect on Symptom Score: Symptoms were quantified using the first 7 questions of the International Prostate Symptom Score (IPSS). The baseline score was approximately 16.4 units for each treatment group. Coadministration therapy was statistically superior to each of the monotherapy treatments in decreasing symptom score at Month 24, the primary time point for this endpoint. At Month 24, the mean changes from baseline (±SD) in IPSS total symptom scores were -6.2 (±7.14) for the coadministration group, -4.9 (±6.81) for dutasteride, and -4.3 (±7.01) for tamsulosin, with a mean difference between coadministration and dutasteride of -1.3 units (P<0.001; [95% CI: -1.69, -0.86]), and between coadministration and tamsulosin of -1.8 units (P<0.001; [95% CI: -2.23, -1.40]). A significant difference was seen by Month 9 and continued through Month 48. At Month 48 the mean changes from baseline (±SD) in IPSS total symptom scores were -6.3 (±7.40) for coadministration, -5.3 (±7.14) for dutasteride, and -3.8 (±7.74) for tamsulosin, with a mean difference between coadministration and dutasteride of -0.96 units (P<0.001; [95% CI: -1.40, -0.52]), and between coadministration and tamsulosin of -2.5 units (P<0.001; [95% CI: -2.96, -2.07]). See Figure 1.

Figure 1. International Prostate Symptom Score Change From Baseline Over a 48-Month Period (Randomized, Double-Blind, Parallel-Group Trial [CombAT Trial])

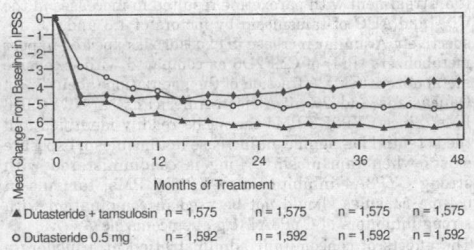

▲ Dutasteride + tamsulosin	n = 1,575	n = 1,575	n = 1,575	n = 1,575
○ Dutasteride 0.5 mg	n = 1,592	n = 1,592	n = 1,592	n = 1,592
◆ Tamsulosin 0.4 mg	n = 1,582	n = 1,582	n = 1,582	n = 1,582

Effect on Acute Urinary Retention or the Need for BPH-Related Surgery: After 4 years of treatment, coadministration therapy with dutasteride and tamsulosin did not provide benefit over dutasteride monotherapy in reducing the incidence of AUR or BPH-related surgery.

In separate 2-year randomized, double-blind trials, compared with placebo, dutasteride monotherapy was associated with a statistically significantly lower incidence of AUR (1.8% for dutasteride versus 4.2% for placebo; 57% reduction in risk) and with a statistically significantly lower incidence of BPH-related surgery (2.2% for dutasteride versus. 4.1% for placebo; 48% reduction in risk).

Effect on Maximum Urine Flow Rate: The baseline Q_{max} was approximately 10.7 mL/sec for each treatment group. Coadministration therapy was statistically superior to each of the monotherapy treatments in increasing Q_{max} at Month 24, the primary time point for this endpoint. At Month 24, the mean increases from baseline (±SD) in Q_{max} were 2.4 (±5.26) mL/sec for coadministration group, 1.9 (±5.10) mL/sec for dutasteride, and 0.9 (±4.57) mL/sec for tamsulosin, with a mean difference between coadministration and dutasteride of 0.5 mL/sec (P = 0.003; [95% CI: 0.17, 0.84]), and between coadministration and tamsulosin of 1.5 mL/sec (P<0.001; [95% CI: 1.19, 1.86]). This difference was seen by Month 6 and continued through Month 24. See Figure 2. The additional improvement in Q_{max} of coadministration therapy over dutasteride monotherapy was no longer statistically significant at Month 48.

[See figure 2 at top of next column]

Effect on Prostate Volume: The mean prostate volume at trial entry was approximately 55 cc. At Month 24, the primary time point for this endpoint, the mean percent

Figure 2. Q_{max} Change From Baseline Over a 24-Month Period (Randomized, Double-Blind, Parallel-Group Trial [CombAT Trial])

▲ Dutasteride + tamsulosin	n = 1,388	n = 1,477	n = 1,487	n = 1,492
○ Dutasteride 0.5 mg	n = 1,406	n = 1,483	n = 1,496	n = 1,502
◆ Tamsulosin 0.4 mg	n = 1,445	n = 1,510	n = 1,517	n = 1,519

changes from baseline (±SD) in prostate volume were -26.9% (±22.57) for coadministration therapy, -28.0% (±24.88) for dutasteride, and 0% (±31.14) for tamsulosin, with a mean difference between coadministration and dutasteride of 1.1% (P = NS; [95% CI: -0.6, 2.8]), and between coadministration and tamsulosin of -26.9% (P<0.001; [95% CI: -28.9, -24.9]). Similar changes were seen at Month 48: -27.3% (±24.91) for coadministration therapy, -28.0% (±25.74) for dutasteride, and +4.6% (±35.45) for tamsulosin.

16   HOW SUPPLIED/STORAGE AND HANDLING

JALYN Capsules, containing 0.5 mg dutasteride and 0.4 mg tamsulosin hydrochloride, are oblong hard-shell capsules with a brown body and an orange cap imprinted with "GS 7CZ" in black ink. They are available in bottles with child-resistant closures as follows:
Bottle of 30 (NDC 0173-0809-13).
Bottle of 90 (NDC 0173-0809-59).
Store at 25°C (77°F); excursions permitted 15° to 30°C (59° to 86°F) [see USP Controlled Room Temperature]. Capsules may become deformed and/or discolored if kept at high temperatures.
Dutasteride is absorbed through the skin. JALYN Capsules should not be handled by women who are pregnant or who could become pregnant because of the potential for absorption of dutasteride and the subsequent potential risk to a developing male fetus [see Warnings and Precautions (5.6)]

17   PATIENT COUNSELING INFORMATION

Advise the patient to read the FDA-approved patient labeling (Patient Information)
Orthostatic Hypotension: Inform patients about the possible occurrence of symptoms related to orthostatic hypotension, such as dizziness and vertigo, and the potential risk of syncope when taking JALYN. Caution patients starting treatment with JALYN to avoid situations where injury could result should syncope occur (e.g., driving, operating machinery, performing hazardous tasks). Advise patients to sit or lie down at the first signs of orthostatic hypotension [see Warnings and Precautions (5.1)].
PSA Monitoring: Inform patients that JALYN reduces serum PSA levels by approximately 50% within 3 to 6 months of therapy, although it may vary for each individual. For patients undergoing PSA screening, increases in PSA levels while on treatment with JALYN may signal the presence of prostate cancer and should be evaluated by a healthcare provider [see Warnings and Precautions (5.3)].
Risk of High-Grade Prostate Cancer: Inform patients that there was an increase in high-grade prostate cancer in men treated with 5 alpha-reductase inhibitors (which are indicated for BPH treatment), including dutasteride, which is a component of JALYN, compared with those treated with placebo in trials looking at the use of these drugs to reduce the risk of prostate cancer [see Indications and Usage (1.2), Warnings and Precautions (5.4), Adverse Reactions (6.1)].
Exposure of Women—Risk to Male Fetus: Inform patients that JALYN Capsules should not be handled by a woman who is pregnant or who could become pregnant because of the potential for absorption of dutasteride and the subsequent potential risk to a developing male fetus. Dutasteride is absorbed through the skin and could result in unintended fetal exposure. If a pregnant woman or woman of childbearing potential comes in contact with leaking JALYN Capsules, the contact area should be washed immediately with soap and water [see Warnings and Precautions (5.6), Use in Specific Populations (8.1)].
Instructions for Use: JALYN Capsules should be swallowed whole and not chewed, crushed, or opened. JALYN Capsules may become deformed and/or discolored if kept at high temperatures. If this occurs, capsules should not be used.
Priapism: Inform patients about the possibility of priapism as a result of treatment with JALYN or other alpha adrenergic antagonist-containing medications. Inform pa-

tients that this reaction is extremely rare, but can lead to permanent erectile dysfunction if not brought to immediate medical attention [see Warnings and Precautions (5.7)].

Blood Donation: Inform men treated with JALYN that they should not donate blood until at least 6 months following their last dose to prevent pregnant women from receiving dutasteride through blood transfusion [see Warnings and Precautions (5.8)]. Serum levels of dutasteride are detectable for 4 to 6 months after treatment ends [see Clinical Pharmacology (12.3)].

Intraoperative Floppy Iris Syndrome (IFIS): Advise patients considering cataract surgery to tell their ophthalmologist that they take or have taken JALYN, an alpha adrenergic antagonist-containing product [see Warnings and Precautions (5.9)].

JALYN and AVODART are trademarks of the GSK group of companies.

The other brands listed are trademarks of their respective owners and are not trademarks of the GSK group of companies. The makers of these brands are not affiliated with and do not endorse the GSK group of companies or its products.

Manufactured for:
GlaxoSmithKline
Research Triangle Park, NC 27709
©2014, the GSK group of companies. All rights reserved.
JLN:9PI

PATIENT INFORMATION
JALYN® [JAY-lin]
(dutasteride and tamsulosin hydrochloride)
Capsules
JALYN is for use by men only.

Read this patient information before you start taking JALYN and each time you get a refill. There may be new information. This information does not take the place of talking with your healthcare provider about your medical condition or your treatment.

What is JALYN?

JALYN is a prescription medicine that contains 2 medicines: dutasteride and tamsulosin. JALYN is used to treat the symptoms of benign prostatic hyperplasia (BPH) in men with an enlarged prostate.

Who should not take JALYN?
Do Not Take JALYN if you are:

- pregnant or could become pregnant. JALYN may harm your unborn baby. Pregnant women should not touch JALYN Capsules. If a woman who is pregnant with a male baby gets enough JALYN in her body by swallowing or touching JALYN, the male baby may be born with sex organs that are not normal. If a pregnant woman or woman of childbearing potential comes in contact with leaking JALYN Capsules, the contact area should be washed immediately with soap and water.
- a child or teenager.
- allergic to dutasteride, tamsulosin, or any of the ingredients in JALYN. See the end of this leaflet for a complete list of ingredients in JALYN.
- taking another medicine that contains an alpha-blocker.
- allergic to other 5 alpha-reductase inhibitors, for example, PROSCAR® (finasteride) Tablets.

What should I tell my healthcare provider before taking JALYN?
Before you take JALYN, tell your healthcare provider if you:

- have a history of low blood pressure
- take medicines to treat high blood pressure
- plan to have cataract surgery
- have liver problems
- are allergic to sulfa medications
- have any other medical conditions

Tell your healthcare provider about all the medicines you take, including prescription and non-prescription medicines, vitamins, and herbal supplements. JALYN and other medicines may affect each other, causing side effects. JALYN may affect the way other medicines work, and other medicines may affect how JALYN works.

Know the medicines you take. Keep a list of them to show your healthcare provider and pharmacist when you get a new medicine.

How should I take JALYN?

- Take JALYN exactly as your healthcare provider tells you to take it.
- Swallow JALYN Capsules whole. Do not crush, chew, or open JALYN Capsules because the contents of the capsule may irritate your lips, mouth, or throat.
- Take your JALYN 1 time each day, about 30 minutes after the same meal every day. For example, you may take JALYN 30 minutes after dinner every day.
- If you miss a dose, you can take it later that same day, 30 minutes after a meal. Do not take 2 JALYN capsules in the same day. If you stop or forget to take JALYN for several days, talk with your healthcare provider before starting again.
- If you take too much JALYN, call your healthcare provider or go to the nearest hospital emergency room right away.

What should I avoid while taking JALYN?

- Avoid driving, operating machinery, or other dangerous activities when starting treatment with JALYN until you know how JALYN affects you. JALYN can cause a sudden drop in your blood pressure, especially at the start of treatment. A sudden drop in blood pressure may cause you to faint, feel dizzy or lightheaded.
- You should not donate blood while taking JALYN or for 6 months after you have stopped JALYN. This is important to prevent pregnant women from receiving JALYN through blood transfusions.

What are the possible side effects of JALYN?
JALYN may cause serious side effects, including:

- **Decreased blood pressure.** JALYN may cause a sudden drop in your blood pressure upon standing from a sitting or lying position, especially at the start of treatment. Symptoms of low blood pressure may include:
- fainting
- dizziness
- feeling lightheaded
- **Rare and serious allergic reactions, including:**
- swelling of your face, tongue, or throat
- difficulty breathing
- serious skin reactions, such as skin peeling

Get medical help right away if you have these serious allergic reactions.

- **Higher chance of a more serious form of prostate cancer.**
- **Eye problems during cataract surgery.** During cataract surgery, a condition called intraoperative floppy iris syndrome (IFIS) can happen if you take or have taken JALYN in the past. If you need to have cataract surgery, tell your surgeon if you take or have taken JALYN.
- **A painful erection that will not go away.** Rarely, JALYN can cause a painful erection (priapism), which cannot be relieved by having sex. If this happens, get medical help right away. If priapism is not treated, there could be lasting damage to your penis, including not being able to have an erection.

The most common side effects of JALYN include:

- ejaculation problems[1]
- trouble getting or keeping an erection (impotence)[1]
- a decrease in sex drive (libido)[1]
- dizziness
- enlarged or painful breasts. If you notice breast lumps or nipple discharge, you should talk to your healthcare provider.
- runny nose

[1]Some of these events may continue after you stop taking JALYN.

Depressed mood has been reported in patients receiving dutasteride, an ingredient of JALYN.

Dutasteride, an ingredient of JALYN, has been shown to reduce sperm count, semen volume, and sperm movement. However, the effect of JALYN on male fertility is not known.

Prostate-Specific Antigen (PSA) Test: Your healthcare provider may check you for other prostate problems, including prostate cancer before you start and while you take JALYN. A blood test called PSA (prostate-specific antigen) is sometimes used to see if you might have prostate cancer. JALYN will reduce the amount of PSA measured in your blood. Your healthcare provider is aware of this effect and can still use PSA to see if you might have prostate cancer. Increases in your PSA levels while on treatment with JALYN (even if the PSA levels are in the normal range) should be evaluated by your healthcare provider.

Tell your healthcare provider if you have any side effect that bothers you or that does not go away.

These are not all the possible side effects with JALYN. For more information, ask your healthcare provider or pharmacist.

Call your doctor for medical advice about side effects. You may report side effects to FDA at 1-800-FDA-1088.

How should I store JALYN?

- Store JALYN Capsules at room temperature (59° to 86°F or 15° to 30°C).
- JALYN Capsules may become deformed and/or discolored if kept at high temperatures.
- Do not use or touch JALYN if your capsules are deformed, discolored, or leaking.
- Safely throw away medicine that is no longer needed.

Keep JALYN and all medicines out of the reach of children.

Medicines are sometimes prescribed for purposes other than those listed in a patient leaflet. Do not use JALYN for a condition for which it was not prescribed. Do not give JALYN to other people, even if they have the same symptoms that you have. It may harm them.

This patient information leaflet summarizes the most important information about JALYN. If you would like more information, talk with your healthcare provider. You can ask your pharmacist or healthcare provider for information about JALYN that is written for health professionals.

For more information, go to www.JALYN.com or call 1-888-825-5249.

What are the ingredients in JALYN?
Active ingredients: dutasteride and tamsulosin hydrochloride

Inactive ingredients: black ink, butylated hydroxytoluene, carrageenan, FD&C yellow 6, ferric oxide (yellow), gelatin (from certified BSE-free bovine sources), glycerin, hypromellose, iron oxide red, methacrylic acid copolymer dispersion, microcrystalline cellulose, mono-di-glycerides of caprylic/capric acid, potassium chloride, talc, titanium dioxide, and triethyl citrate.

How does JALYN work?

JALYN contains 2 medications, dutasteride and tamsulosin. These 2 medications work in different ways to improve symptoms of BPH. Dutasteride shrinks the enlarged prostate and tamsulosin relaxes muscles in the prostate and neck of the bladder. These 2 medications, when used together, can improve symptoms of BPH better than either medication when used alone.

JALYN is a registered trademark of the GSK group of companies.

The other brands listed are trademarks of their respective owners and are not trademarks of the GSK group of companies. The makers of these brands are not affiliated with and do not endorse the GSK group of companies or its products.

Manufactured for:
GlaxoSmithKline
Research Triangle Park, NC 27709
©2014, the GSK group of companies. All rights reserved.
June 2014
JLN:8PIL

KINRIX   ℞
[kin' rix]
(Diphtheria and Tetanus Toxoids and Acellular Pertussis Adsorbed and Inactivated Poliovirus Vaccine)
Suspension for Intramuscular Injection

HIGHLIGHTS OF PRESCRIBING INFORMATION
These highlights do not include all the information needed to use KINRIX safely and effectively. See full prescribing information for KINRIX.
KINRIX (Diphtheria and Tetanus Toxoids and Acellular Pertussis Adsorbed and Inactivated Poliovirus Vaccine)
Suspension for Intramuscular Injection
Initial U.S. Approval: 2008

————INDICATIONS AND USAGE————

A single dose of KINRIX is indicated for active immunization against diphtheria, tetanus, pertussis, and poliomyelitis as the fifth dose in the diphtheria, tetanus, and acellular pertussis (DTaP) vaccine series and the fourth dose in the inactivated poliovirus (IPV) series in children 4 through 6 years of age whose previous DTaP vaccine doses have been with INFANRIX and/or PEDIARIX for the first three doses and INFANRIX for the fourth dose. (1)

————DOSAGE AND ADMINISTRATION————

A single intramuscular injection (0.5 mL). (2.2)

————DOSAGE FORMS AND STRENGTHS————

Single-dose vials and prefilled syringes containing a 0.5-mL suspension for injection. (3)

————CONTRAINDICATIONS————

- Severe allergic reaction (e.g., anaphylaxis) after a previous dose of any diphtheria toxoid, tetanus toxoid, pertussis- or poliovirus-containing vaccine, or to any component of KINRIX, including neomycin and polymyxin B. (4.1)
- Encephalopathy within 7 days of administration of a previous pertussis-containing vaccine. (4.2)
- Progressive neurologic disorders. (4.3)

————WARNINGS AND PRECAUTIONS————

- If Guillain-Barré syndrome occurs within 6 weeks of receipt of a prior vaccine containing tetanus toxoid, the decision to give KINRIX should be based on potential benefits and risks. (5.1)
- The tip caps of the prefilled syringes may contain natural rubber latex which may cause allergic reactions in latex-sensitive individuals. (5.2)
- Syncope (fainting) can occur in association with administration of injectable vaccines, including KINRIX. Procedures should be in place to avoid falling injury and to restore cerebral perfusion following syncope. (5.3)
- If adverse events (i.e., temperature ≥105°F, collapse or shock-like state, persistent, inconsolable crying lasting ≥3 hours, occurring within 48 hours of vaccination; seizures within 3 days of vaccination) have occurred in temporal relation to receipt of a pertussis-containing vaccine, the decision to give KINRIX should be based on potential benefits and risks. (5.4)
- For children at higher risk for seizures, an antipyretic may be administered at the time of vaccination with KINRIX. (5.5)

---ADVERSE REACTIONS---
- The most frequently reported solicited local reaction (>50%) was injection site pain. Other common solicited local reactions (≥25%) were redness, increase in arm circumference, and swelling. (6.1)
- Common solicited general adverse events (≥15%) were drowsiness, fever (≥99.5°F), and loss of appetite. (6.1)

To report SUSPECTED ADVERSE REACTIONS, contact GlaxoSmithKline at 1-888-825-5249 or VAERS at 1-800-822-7967 or www.vaers.hhs.gov.

---DRUG INTERACTIONS---
Do not mix KINRIX with any other vaccine in the same syringe or vial. (7.1)

See 17 for PATIENT COUNSELING INFORMATION
                                        Revised: 11/2013

FULL PRESCRIBING INFORMATION: CONTENTS*

FULL PRESCRIBING INFORMATION

1 INDICATIONS AND USAGE

A single dose of KINRIX® is indicated for active immunization against diphtheria, tetanus, pertussis, and poliomyelitis as the fifth dose in the diphtheria, tetanus, and acellular pertussis (DTaP) vaccine series and the fourth dose in the inactivated poliovirus vaccine (IPV) series in children 4 through 6 years of age whose previous DTaP vaccine doses have been with INFANRIX® (Diphtheria and Tetanus Toxoids and Acellular Pertussis Vaccine Adsorbed) and/or PEDIARIX® [Diphtheria and Tetanus Toxoids and Acellular Pertussis Adsorbed, Hepatitis B (Recombinant) and Inactivated Poliovirus Vaccine] for the first three doses and INFANRIX for the fourth dose.

2 DOSAGE AND ADMINISTRATION

2.1 Preparation for Administration

Shake vigorously to obtain a homogeneous, turbid, white suspension. Do not use if resuspension does not occur with vigorous shaking. Parenteral drug products should be inspected visually for particulate matter and discoloration prior to administration, whenever solution and container permit. If either of these conditions exists, the vaccine should not be administered.

For the prefilled syringes, attach a sterile needle and administer intramuscularly.

For the vials, use a sterile needle and sterile syringe to withdraw the 0.5-mL dose and administer intramuscularly. Changing needles between drawing vaccine from a vial and injecting it into a recipient is not necessary unless the needle has been damaged or contaminated. Use a separate sterile needle and syringe for each individual.

Do not administer this product intravenously, intradermally, or subcutaneously.

2.2 Recommended Dose and Schedule

KINRIX is to be administered as a 0.5-mL dose by intramuscular injection. The preferred site of administration is the deltoid muscle of the upper arm.

KINRIX may be used for the fifth dose in the DTaP immunization series and the fourth dose in the IPV immunization series in children 4 through 6 years of age (prior to the seventh birthday) whose previous DTaP vaccine doses have been with INFANRIX and/or PEDIARIX for the first three doses and INFANRIX for the fourth dose [see Indications and Usage (1)].

3 DOSAGE FORMS AND STRENGTHS

KINRIX is a suspension for injection available in 0.5-mL single-dose vials and prefilled TIP-LOK® syringes.

4 CONTRAINDICATIONS

4.1 Hypersensitivity

Severe allergic reaction (e.g., anaphylaxis) after a previous dose of any diphtheria toxoid, tetanus toxoid, pertussis- or poliovirus-containing vaccine, or to any component of KINRIX, including neomycin and polymyxin B, is a contraindication to administration of KINRIX [see Description (11)]. Because of the uncertainty as to which component of the vaccine might be responsible, no further vaccination with any of these components should be given. Alternatively, such individuals may be referred to an allergist for evaluation if immunization with any of these components is considered.

4.2 Encephalopathy

Encephalopathy (e.g., coma, decreased level of consciousness, prolonged seizures) within 7 days of administration of a previous dose of a pertussis-containing vaccine that is not attributable to another identifiable cause is a contraindication to administration of any pertussis-containing vaccine, including KINRIX.

4.3 Progressive Neurologic Disorder

Progressive neurologic disorder, including infantile spasms, uncontrolled epilepsy, or progressive encephalopathy is a contraindication to administration of any pertussis-containing vaccine, including KINRIX. Pertussis vaccine should not be administered to individuals with such conditions until a treatment regimen has been established and the condition has stabilized.

5 WARNINGS AND PRECAUTIONS

5.1 Guillain-Barré Syndrome

If Guillain-Barré syndrome occurs within 6 weeks of receipt of a prior vaccine containing tetanus toxoid, the decision to give any tetanus toxoid-containing vaccine, including KINRIX, should be based on careful consideration of the potential benefits and possible risks. When a decision is made to withhold tetanus toxoid, other available vaccines should be given, as indicated.

5.2 Latex

The tip caps of the prefilled syringes may contain natural rubber latex which may cause allergic reactions in latex-sensitive individuals.

5.3 Syncope

Syncope (fainting) can occur in association with administration of injectable vaccines, including KINRIX. Syncope can be accompanied by transient neurological signs such as visual disturbance, paresthesia, and tonic-clonic limb movements. Procedures should be in place to avoid falling injury and to restore cerebral perfusion following syncope.

5.4 Adverse Events Following Prior Pertussis Vaccination

If any of the following events occur in temporal relation to receipt of a pertussis-containing vaccine, the decision to give any pertussis-containing vaccine, including KINRIX, should be based on careful consideration of the potential benefits and possible risks:
- Temperature of ≥40.5oC (105oF) within 48 hours not due to another identifiable cause;
- Collapse or shock-like state (hypotonic-hyporesponsive episode) within 48 hours;
- Persistent, inconsolable crying lasting ≥3 hours, occurring within 48 hours;
- Seizures with or without fever occurring within 3 days.

When a decision is made to withhold pertussis vaccination, other available vaccines should be given, as indicated.

5.5 Children at Risk for Seizures

For children at higher risk for seizures than the general population, an appropriate antipyretic may be administered at the time of vaccination with a pertussis-containing vaccine, including KINRIX, and for the ensuing 24 hours to reduce the possibility of post-vaccination fever.

5.6 Preventing and Managing Allergic Vaccine Reactions

Prior to administration, the healthcare provider should review the patient's immunization history for possible vaccine sensitivity and previous vaccination-related adverse reactions to allow an assessment of benefits and risks. Epinephrine and other appropriate agents used for the control of immediate allergic reactions must be immediately available should an acute anaphylactic reaction occur.

6 ADVERSE REACTIONS

6.1 Clinical Trials Experience

Because clinical trials are conducted under widely varying conditions, adverse reaction rates observed in the clinical trials of a vaccine cannot be directly compared with rates in the clinical trials of another vaccine, and may not reflect the rates observed in practice.

A total of 3,537 children were vaccinated with a single dose of KINRIX in 3 clinical trials. Of these, 381 children received a non-US formulation of KINRIX (containing ≤2.5 mg 2-phenoxyethanol per dose as preservative). The primary study (Study 048), conducted in the United States, was a randomized, controlled clinical trial in which children 4 to 6 years of age were vaccinated with KINRIX (N = 3,156) or control vaccines (INFANRIX and IPOL® vaccine [IPV, Sanofi Pasteur SA]; N = 1,053) as a fifth DTaP vaccine dose following 4 doses of INFANRIX and as a fourth IPV dose following 3 doses of IPOL. Subjects also received the second dose of US-licensed measles, mumps, and rubella (MMR) vaccine (Merck & Co., Inc.) administered concomitantly, at separate sites.

Data on adverse events were collected by parents/guardians using standardized forms for 4 consecutive days following vaccination with KINRIX or control vaccines (i.e., day of vaccination and the next 3 days). The reported frequencies of solicited local reactions and general adverse events in Study 048 are presented in Table 1.

In 3 studies (Study 046, 047, and 048), children were monitored for unsolicited adverse events, including serious adverse events, that occurred in the 31-day period following vaccination and in 2 studies (Study 047 and 048), parents/guardians were actively queried about changes in the child's health status, including the occurrence of serious adverse events, through 6 months post-vaccination.

Table 1. Percentage of Children 4 to 6 Years of Age Reporting Solicited Local Reactions or General Adverse Events Within 4 Days of Vaccination[a] With KINRIX or Separate Concomitant Administration of INFANRIX and IPV When Coadministered With MMR Vaccine (Study 048) (Total Vaccinated Cohort)

	KINRIX	INFANRIX + IPV
Local[b]	N = 3,121-3,128	N = 1,039-1,043
Pain, any	57.0[c]	53.3
Pain, grade 2 or 3[d]	13.7	12.0
Pain, grade 3[d]	1.6[c]	0.6
Redness, any	36.6	36.6
Redness, ≥50 mm	17.6	20.0
Redness, ≥110 mm	2.9	4.1
Arm circumference increase, any	36.0	37.8
Arm circumference increase, >20 mm	6.9	7.4
Arm circumference increase, >30 mm	2.4	3.2
Swelling, any	26.0	27.0
Swelling, ≥50 mm	10.2	11.5
Swelling, ≥110 mm	1.4	1.8
General	N = 3,037-3,120	N = 993-1,036
Drowsiness, any	19.1	17.5
Drowsiness, grade 3[e]	0.8	0.8
Fever, ≥99.5°F	16.0	14.8
Fever, >100.4°F	6.5[c]	4.4
Fever, >102.2°F	1.1	1.1
Fever, >104°F	0.1	0.0
Loss of appetite, any	15.5	16.0
Loss of appetite, grade 3[f]	0.8	0.6

IPV manufactured by Sanofi Pasteur SA. MMR vaccine manufactured by Merck & Co., Inc.
Total Vaccinated Cohort = all vaccinated subjects for whom safety data were available.
N = number of children with evaluable data for the events listed.
[a] Within 4 days of vaccination defined as day of vaccination and the next 3 days.
[b] Local reactions at the injection site for KINRIX or INFANRIX.
[c] Statistically higher than comparator group (P <0.05).
[d] Grade 2 defined as painful when the limb was moved; Grade 3 defined as preventing normal daily activities.
[e] Grade 3 defined as preventing normal daily activities.
[f] Grade 3 defined as not eating at all.

In Study 048, KINRIX was non-inferior to INFANRIX with regard to swelling that involved >50% of the injected upper arm length and that was associated with a >30 mm increase in mid-upper arm circumference within 4 days following vaccination (upper limit of two-sided 95% Confidence Interval for difference in percentage of KINRIX [0.6%, n = 20] minus INFANRIX [1.0%, n = 11] ≤2%).

Serious Adverse Events: Within the 31-day period following study vaccination in 3 studies (Study 046, 047, and 048), in which all subjects received concomitant MMR vaccine (US-licensed MMR vaccine [Merck & Co., Inc.] in Study 047 and 048; non-US-licensed MMR vaccine in Study 046), 3 subjects (0.1% [3/3,537]) who received KINRIX reported serious adverse events (dehydration and hypernatremia; cerebrovascular accident; dehydration and gastroenteritis) and 4 subjects (0.3% [4/1,434]) who received INFANRIX and IPV (Sanofi Pasteur SA) reported serious adverse events (cellulitis; constipation; foreign body trauma; fever without identified etiology).

6.2 Postmarketing Experience

In addition to reports in clinical trials, the following adverse events, for which a causal relationship to components of KINRIX is plausible, have been reported since market introduction of DTaP-IPV manufactured by GlaxoSmithKline outside the U.S. Because these events are reported voluntarily from a population of uncertain size, it is not always possible to reliably estimate their frequency or establish a causal relationship to vaccination.

General Disorders and Administration Site Conditions: Injection site vesicles.

Nervous System Disorders: Syncope.

Skin and Subcutaneous Tissue Disorders: Pruritus.

Additional adverse events reported following postmarketing use of INFANRIX, for which a causal relationship to vaccination is plausible, are: Allergic reactions, including anaphylactoid reactions, anaphylaxis, angioedema, and urticaria, apnea, collapse or shock-like state (hypotonic-hyporesponsive episode), convulsions (with or without fever), lymphadenopathy, and thrombocytopenia.

7 DRUG INTERACTIONS

7.1 Concomitant Vaccine Administration

In clinical trials, KINRIX was administered concomitantly with the second dose of MMR vaccine *[see Clinical Studies (14)]*.

Data are not available on concomitant use of KINRIX and varicella vaccine.

When KINRIX is administered concomitantly with other injectable vaccines, they should be given with separate syringes. KINRIX should not be mixed with any other vaccine in the same syringe or vial.

7.2 Immunosuppressive Therapies

Immunosuppressive therapies, including irradiation, antimetabolites, alkylating agents, cytotoxic drugs, and corticosteroids (used in greater than physiologic doses), may reduce the immune response to KINRIX.

8 USE IN SPECIFIC POPULATIONS

8.1 Pregnancy

Pregnancy Category C

Animal reproduction studies have not been conducted with KINRIX. It is also not known whether KINRIX can cause fetal harm when administered to a pregnant woman or can affect reproduction capacity.

8.4 Pediatric Use

Safety and effectiveness of KINRIX in children younger than 4 years of age and children 7 to 16 years of age have not been evaluated. KINRIX is not approved for use in persons in these age groups.

11 DESCRIPTION

KINRIX (Diphtheria and Tetanus Toxoids and Acellular Pertussis Adsorbed and Inactivated Poliovirus Vaccine) is a noninfectious, sterile vaccine for intramuscular administration. Each 0.5-mL dose is formulated to contain 25 Lf of diphtheria toxoid, 10 Lf of tetanus toxoid, 25 mcg of inactivated pertussis toxin (PT), 25 mcg of filamentous hemagglutinin (FHA), 8 mcg of pertactin (69 kiloDalton outer membrane protein), 40 D-antigen Units (DU) of Type 1 poliovirus (Mahoney), 8 DU of Type 2 poliovirus (MEF-1), and 32 DU of Type 3 poliovirus (Saukett). The diphtheria, tetanus, and pertussis components of KINRIX are the same as those in INFANRIX and PEDIARIX and the poliovirus component is the same as that in PEDIARIX.

The diphtheria toxin is produced by growing *Corynebacterium diphtheriae* in Fenton medium containing a bovine extract. Tetanus toxin is produced by growing *Clostridium tetani* in a modified Latham medium derived from bovine casein. The bovine materials used in these extracts are sourced from countries which the United States Department of Agriculture (USDA) has determined neither have nor are at risk of bovine spongiform encephalopathy (BSE). Both toxins are detoxified with formaldehyde, concentrated by ultrafiltration, and purified by precipitation, dialysis, and sterile filtration.

Table 2. Pre-Vaccination Antibody Levels and Post-Vaccination[a] Antibody Responses Following KINRIX Compared With Separate Concomitant Administration of INFANRIX and IPV in Children 4 to 6 Years of Age When Coadministered With MMR Vaccine (Study 048) (ATP Cohort for Immunogenicity)

	KINRIX	INFANRIX + IPV
	N = 787-851	N = 237-262
Anti-Diphtheria Toxoid		
Pre-vaccination % ≥0.1 IU/mL (95% CI)[b]	87.7 (85.3, 89.9)	85.5 (80.6, 89.5)
Post-vaccination % ≥0.1 IU/mL (95% CI)[b]	100 (99.6, 100)	100 (98.6, 100)
% Booster Response (95% CI)[c]	99.5 (98.8, 99.9)[d]	100 (98.6, 100)
Anti-Tetanus Toxoid		
Pre-vaccination % ≥0.1 IU/mL (95% CI)[b]	87.8 (85.4, 90.0)	88.2 (83.6, 91.8)
Post-vaccination % ≥0.1 IU/mL (95% CI)[b]	100 (99.6, 100)	100 (98.6, 100)
% Booster Response (95% CI)[c]	96.7 (95.2, 97.8)[d]	93.9 (90.2, 96.5)
Anti-PT		
% Booster Response (95% CI)[e]	92.2 (90.2, 94.0)[d]	92.6 (88.7, 95.5)
Anti-FHA		
% Booster Response (95% CI)[e]	95.4 (93.7, 96.7)[d]	96.2 (93.1, 98.1)
Anti-Pertactin		
% Booster Response (95% CI)[e]	97.8 (96.5, 98.6)[d]	96.9 (94.1, 98.7)
Anti-Poliovirus 1		
Pre-vaccination % ≥1:8 (95% CI)[b]	88.3 (85.9, 90.4)	85.1 (80.1, 89.2)
Post-vaccination % ≥1:8 (95% CI)[b]	99.9 (99.3, 100)	100 (98.5, 100)
Post-vaccination GMT (95% CI)	2,127 (1,976, 2,290)[f]	1,685 (1,475, 1,925)
Anti-Poliovirus 2		
Pre-vaccination % ≥1:8 (95% CI)[b]	91.8 (89.7, 93.6)	87.0 (82.3, 90.8)
Post-vaccination % ≥1:8 (95% CI)[b]	100 (99.6, 100)	100 (98.5, 100)
Post-vaccination GMT (95% CI)	2,265 (2,114, 2,427)[f]	1,818 (1,606, 2,057)
Anti-Poliovirus 3		
Pre-vaccination % ≥1:8 (95% CI)[b]	84.7 (82.0, 87.0)	85.0 (80.1, 89.1)
Post-vaccination % ≥1:8 (95% CI)[b]	100 (99.5, 100)	100 (98.5, 100)
Post-vaccination GMT (95% CI)	3,588 (3,345, 3,849)[f]	3,365 (2,961, 3,824)

IPV manufactured by Sanofi Pasteur SA. MMR vaccine manufactured by Merck & Co., Inc.

ATP = according-to-protocol; CI = Confidence Interval; GMT = geometric mean antibody titer

N = number of subjects with available results.

[a] One month blood sampling, range 31 to 48 days.

[b] Seroprotection defined as anti-diphtheria toxoid and anti-tetanus toxoid antibody concentrations ≥0.1 IU/mL by ELISA and as anti-poliovirus Type 1, Type 2, and Type 3 antibody titer ≥1:8 by micro-neutralization assay for poliovirus.

[c] Booster response: In subjects with pre-vaccination <0.1 IU/mL, post-vaccination concentration ≥0.4 IU/mL. In subjects with pre-vaccination concentration ≥0.1 IU/mL, an increase of at least 4 times the pre-vaccination concentration.

[d] KINRIX was non-inferior to INFANRIX + IPV based on booster response rates (upper limit of two-sided 95% CI on the difference of INFANRIX + IPV minus KINRIX ≤10%).

[e] Booster response: In subjects with pre-vaccination <5 EL.U./mL, post-vaccination concentration ≥20 EL.U./mL. In subjects with pre-vaccination ≥5 EL.U./mL and <20 EL.U./mL, an increase of at least 4 times the pre-vaccination concentration. In subjects with pre-vaccination ≥20 EL.U./mL, an increase of at least 2 times the pre-vaccination concentration.

[f] KINRIX was non-inferior to INFANRIX + IPV based on post-vaccination anti-poliovirus antibody GMTs adjusted for baseline titer (upper limit of two-sided 95% CI for the GMT ratio [INFANRIX + IPV:KINRIX] ≤1.5).

The acellular pertussis antigens (PT, FHA, and pertactin) are isolated from *Bordetella pertussis* culture grown in modified Stainer-Scholte liquid medium. PT and FHA are isolated from the fermentation broth; pertactin is extracted from the cells by heat treatment and flocculation. The antigens are purified in successive chromatographic and precipitation steps. PT is detoxified using glutaraldehyde and formaldehyde. FHA and pertactin are treated with formaldehyde.

Diphtheria and tetanus toxoids and pertussis antigens (inactivated PT, FHA, and pertactin) are individually adsorbed onto aluminum hydroxide.

The inactivated poliovirus component of KINRIX is an enhanced potency component. Each of the 3 strains of poliovirus is individually grown in VERO cells, a continuous line of monkey kidney cells, cultivated on microcarriers. Calf serum and lactalbumin hydrolysate are used during VERO cell culture and/or virus culture. Calf serum is sourced from countries the USDA has determined neither have nor are at risk of BSE. After clarification, each viral suspension is purified by ultrafiltration, diafiltration, and successive chromatographic steps, and inactivated with formaldehyde. The 3 purified viral strains are then pooled to form a trivalent concentrate.

Diphtheria and tetanus toxoid potency is determined by measuring the amount of neutralizing antitoxin in previously immunized guinea pigs. The potency of the acellular pertussis components (inactivated PT, FHA, and pertactin) is determined by enzyme-linked immunosorbent assay (ELISA) on sera from previously immunized mice. The potency of the inactivated poliovirus component is determined by using the D-antigen ELISA and by a poliovirus neutralizing cell culture assay on sera from previously immunized rats.

Each 0.5-mL dose contains aluminum hydroxide as adjuvant (not more than 0.6 mg aluminum by assay) and 4.5 mg of sodium chloride. Each dose also contains ≤100 mcg of residual formaldehyde and ≤100 mcg of polysorbate 80 (Tween 80). Neomycin sulfate and polymyxin B are used in the poliovirus vaccine manufacturing process and may be present in the final vaccine at ≤0.05 ng neomycin and ≤0.01 ng polymyxin B per dose.

The tip caps of the prefilled syringes may contain natural rubber latex; the plungers are not made with natural rubber latex. The vial stoppers are not made with natural rubber latex.

KINRIX does not contain a preservative.

12 CLINICAL PHARMACOLOGY

12.1 Mechanism of Action

Diphtheria: Diphtheria is an acute toxin-mediated infectious disease caused by toxigenic strains of *C. diphtheriae*. Protection against disease is due to the development of neutralizing antibodies to the diphtheria toxin. A serum diphtheria antitoxin level of 0.01 IU/mL is the lowest level giving some degree of protection; a level of 0.1 IU/mL is regarded as protective.[1]

Tetanus: Tetanus is an acute toxin-mediated disease caused by a potent exotoxin released by *C. tetani*. Protection against disease is due to the development of neutralizing antibodies to the tetanus toxin. A serum tetanus antitoxin level of at least 0.01 IU/mL, measured by neutralization assays, is considered the minimum protective level.[2,3] A level of ≥0.1 IU/mL is considered protective.[4]

Pertussis: Pertussis (whooping cough) is a disease of the respiratory tract caused by *B. pertussis*. The role of the different components produced by *B. pertussis* in either the pathogenesis of, or the immunity to, pertussis is not well understood. There is no well established serological correlate of protection for pertussis. The efficacy of the pertussis component of KINRIX was determined in clinical trials of INFANRIX administered as a 3-dose series in infants (see INFANRIX prescribing information).

Poliomyelitis: Poliovirus is an enterovirus that belongs to the picornavirus family. Three serotypes of poliovirus have been identified (Types 1, 2, and 3). Neutralizing antibodies against the 3 poliovirus serotypes are recognized as conferring protection against poliomyelitis disease.[5]

13 NONCLINICAL TOXICOLOGY

13.1 Carcinogenesis, Mutagenesis, Impairment of Fertility

KINRIX has not been evaluated for carcinogenic or mutagenic potential, or for impairment of fertility.

14 CLINICAL STUDIES

14.1 Immunological Evaluation

In a US multicenter study (Study 048), 4,209 children were randomized in a 3:1 ratio to receive either KINRIX or INFANRIX and IPV (Sanofi Pasteur SA) administered concomitantly at separate sites. Subjects also received MMR vaccine (Merck & Co., Inc.) administered concomitantly at a separate site. Subjects were children 4 through 6 years of age who previously received 4 doses of INFANRIX, 3 doses of IPV, and 1 dose of MMR vaccine. Among subjects in both vaccine groups combined, 49.6% were female; 45.6% of subjects were White, 18.8% Hispanic, 13.6% Asian, 7.0% Black, and 15.0% were of other racial/ethnic groups.

Levels of antibodies to the diphtheria, tetanus, pertussis (PT, FHA, and pertactin), and poliovirus antigens were measured in sera obtained immediately prior to vaccination and 1 month (range 31 to 48 days) after vaccination (Table 2). The co-primary immunogenicity endpoints were anti-diphtheria toxoid, anti-tetanus toxoid, anti-PT, anti-FHA, and anti-pertactin booster responses, and anti-poliovirus Type 1, Type 2, and Type 3 geometric mean antibody titers (GMTs) 1 month after vaccination. KINRIX was shown to be non-inferior to INFANRIX and IPV administered separately, in terms of booster responses to DTaP antigens and post-vaccination GMTs for anti-poliovirus antibodies (Table 2).

[See table 2 at top of previous page]

14.2 Concomitant Vaccine Administration

In a US study (Study 047), among recipients of DTaP-IPV (same formulation as KINRIX but not containing 2-phenoxyethanol) and the second dose of MMR vaccine (Merck & Co., Inc.) who had pre-vaccination sera tested for antibodies to measles, mumps, and rubella (N = 175-181), 99% of subjects were seropositive for antibodies to measles, mumps, and rubella prior to vaccination.

15 REFERENCES

1. Vitek CR and Wharton M. Diphtheria Toxoid. In: Plotkin SA, Orenstein WA, and Offit PA, eds. *Vaccines*. 5th ed. Saunders; 2008:139-156.
2. Wassilak SGF, Roper MH, Kretsinger K, and Orenstein WA. Tetanus Toxoid. In: Plotkin SA, Orenstein WA, and Offit PA, eds. *Vaccines*. 5th ed. Saunders; 2008:805-839.
3. Department of Health and Human Services, Food and Drug Administration. Biological products; Bacterial vaccines and toxoids; Implementation of efficacy review; Proposed rule. *Federal Register* December 13, 1985;50(240):51002-51117.
4. Centers for Disease Control and Prevention. General Recommendations on Immunization. Recommendations of the Advisory Committee on Immunization Practices (ACIP). *MMWR* 2006;55(RR-15):1-48.
5. Sutter RW, Pallansch MA, Sawyer LA, et al. Defining surrogate serologic tests with respect to predicting protective vaccine efficacy: Poliovirus vaccination. In: Williams JC, Goldenthal KL, Burns DL, Lewis Jr BP, eds. Combined vaccines and simultaneous administration. Current issues and perspectives. New York, NY: The New York Academy of Sciences; 1995:289-299.

16 HOW SUPPLIED/STORAGE AND HANDLING

KINRIX is available in 0.5-mL single-dose vials and disposable prefilled TIP-LOK syringes (packaged without needles):
NDC 58160-812-01 Vial in Package of 10: NDC 58160-812-11
NDC 58160-812-43 Syringe in Package of 10: NDC 58160-812-52
Store refrigerated between 2° and 8°C (36° and 46°F). Do not freeze. Discard if the vaccine has been frozen.

17 PATIENT COUNSELING INFORMATION

Parents or guardians should be:
- informed of the potential benefits and risks of immunization with KINRIX.
- informed about the potential for adverse reactions that have been temporally associated with administration of KINRIX or other vaccines containing similar components.

- instructed to report any adverse events to their healthcare provider.
- given the Vaccine Information Statements, which are required by the National Childhood Vaccine Injury Act of 1986 to be given prior to immunization. These materials are available free of charge at the Centers for Disease Control and Prevention (CDC) website (www.cdc.gov/vaccines).

INFANRIX, KINRIX, PEDIARIX, and TIP-LOK are registered trademarks of the GlaxoSmithKline group of companies. IPOL is a registered trademark of Sanofi Pasteur Limited.

Manufactured by **GlaxoSmithKline Biologicals**
Rixensart, Belgium, US License 1617, and
Novartis Vaccines and Diagnostics GmbH
Marburg, Germany, US License 1754
Distributed by **GlaxoSmithKline**
Research Triangle Park, NC 27709
©2013, GlaxoSmithKline group of companies. All rights reserved.
KNX:10PI

LAMICTAL ℞
[*la-mǐk' tal*]
(lamotrigine)
Tablets
LAMICTAL ℞
(lamotrigine)
Chewable Dispersible Tablets
LAMICTAL ODT ℞
(lamotrigine)
Orally Disintegrating Tablets

HIGHLIGHTS OF PRESCRIBING INFORMATION

These highlights do not include all the information needed to use LAMICTAL safely and effectively. See full prescribing information for LAMICTAL.
LAMICTAL (lamotrigine) Tablets
LAMICTAL (lamotrigine) Chewable Dispersible Tablets
LAMICTAL ODT (lamotrigine) Orally Disintegrating Tablets
Initial U.S. Approval: 1994

> **WARNING: SERIOUS SKIN RASHES**
> *See full prescribing information for complete boxed warning.*
> **Cases of life-threatening serious rashes, including Stevens-Johnson syndrome, toxic epidermal necrolysis, and/or rash-related death, have been caused by LAMICTAL. The rate of serious rash is greater in pediatric patients than in adults. Additional factors that may increase the risk of rash include (5.1):**
> - **coadministration with valproate**
> - **exceeding recommended initial dose of LAMICTAL**
> - **exceeding recommended dose escalation of LAMICTAL**
> **Benign rashes are also caused by LAMICTAL; however, it is not possible to predict which rashes will prove to be serious or life threatening. LAMICTAL should be discontinued at the first sign of rash, unless the rash is clearly not drug related. (5.1)**

INDICATIONS AND USAGE

LAMICTAL is an antiepileptic drug (AED) indicated for:
Epilepsy—adjunctive therapy in patients ≥2 years of age: (1.1)
- partial seizures
- primary generalized tonic-clonic seizures
- generalized seizures of Lennox-Gastaut syndrome

Epilepsy—monotherapy in patients ≥16 years of age: conversion to monotherapy in patients with partial seizures who are receiving treatment with carbamazepine, phenobarbital, phenytoin, primidone, or valproate as the single AED. (1.1)
Bipolar Disorder in patients ≥18 years of age: maintenance treatment of Bipolar I Disorder to delay the time to occurrence of mood episodes in patients treated for acute mood episodes with standard therapy. (1.2)

DOSAGE AND ADMINISTRATION

- Dosing is based on concomitant medications, indication, and patient age. (2.2, 2.4)
- To avoid an increased risk of rash, the recommended initial dose and subsequent dose escalations should not be exceeded. LAMICTAL Starter Kits and LAMICTAL ODT Patient Titration Kits are available for the first 5 weeks of treatment. (2.1, 16)
- Do not restart LAMICTAL in patients who discontinued due to rash unless the potential benefits clearly outweigh the risks. (2.1)
- Adjustments to maintenance doses will in most cases be required in patients starting or stopping estrogen-containing oral contraceptives. (2.1, 5.8)

- LAMICTAL should be discontinued over a period of at least 2 weeks (approximately 50% reduction per week). (2.1, 5.9)
Epilepsy
- Adjunctive therapy—See Table 1 for patients >12 years of age and Tables 2 and 3 for patients 2 to 12 years. (2.2)
- Conversion to monotherapy—See Table 4. (2.3)
Bipolar Disorder: See Tables 5 and 6. (2.4)

DOSAGE FORMS AND STRENGTHS

Tablets: 25 mg, 100 mg, 150 mg, and 200 mg scored. (3.1, 16)
Chewable Dispersible Tablets: 2 mg, 5 mg, and 25 mg. (3.2, 16)
Orally Disintegrating Tablets: 25 mg, 50 mg, 100 mg, and 200 mg. (3.3, 16)

CONTRAINDICATIONS

Hypersensitivity to the drug or its ingredients. (Boxed Warning, 4)

WARNINGS AND PRECAUTIONS

- Life-threatening serious rash and/or rash-related death may result. (Boxed Warning, 5.1)
- Fatal or life-threatening hypersensitivity reaction: Multiorgan hypersensitivity reactions, also known as Drug Reaction with Eosinophilia and Systemic Symptoms (DRESS), may be fatal or life threatening. Early signs may include rash, fever, and lymphadenopathy. These reactions may be associated with other organ involvement, such as hepatitis, hepatic failure, blood dyscrasias, or acute multiorgan failure. LAMICTAL should be discontinued if alternate etiology for this reaction is not found. (5.2)
- Blood dyscrasias (e.g., neutropenia, thrombocytopenia, pancytopenia): May occur, either with or without an associated hypersensitivity syndrome. (5.3)
- Suicidal behavior and ideation. (5.4)
- Clinical worsening, emergence of new symptoms, and suicidal ideation/behaviors may be associated with treatment of bipolar disorder. Patients should be closely monitored, particularly early in treatment or during dosage changes. (5.5)
- Aseptic meningitis reported in pediatric and adult patients. (5.6)
- Medication errors involving LAMICTAL have occurred. In particular the names LAMICTAL or lamotrigine can be confused with names of other commonly used medications. Medication errors may also occur between the different formulations of LAMICTAL. (3.4, 5.7, 16, 17.10)

ADVERSE REACTIONS

- Most common adverse reactions (incidence ≥10%) in adult epilepsy clinical studies were dizziness, headache, diplopia, ataxia, nausea, blurred vision, somnolence, rhinitis, and rash. Additional adverse reactions (incidence ≥10%) reported in children in epilepsy clinical studies included vomiting, infection, fever, accidental injury, pharyngitis, abdominal pain, and tremor. (6.1)
- Most common adverse reactions (incidence >5%) in adult bipolar clinical studies were nausea, insomnia, somnolence, back pain, fatigue, rash, rhinitis, abdominal pain, and xerostomia. (6.1)

To report SUSPECTED ADVERSE REACTIONS, contact GlaxoSmithKline at 1-888-825-5249 or FDA at 1-800-FDA-1088 or www.fda.gov/medwatch.

DRUG INTERACTIONS

- Valproate increases lamotrigine concentrations more than 2-fold. (7, 12.3)
- Carbamazepine, phenytoin, phenobarbital, and primidone decrease lamotrigine concentrations by approximately 40%. (7, 12.3)
- Oral estrogen-containing contraceptives and rifampin also decrease lamotrigine concentrations by approximately 50%. (7, 12.3)

USE IN SPECIFIC POPULATIONS

- Hepatic impairment: Dosage adjustments required. (2.1)
- Healthcare professionals can enroll patients in the Lamotrigine Pregnancy Registry (1-800-336-2176). Patients can enroll themselves in the North American Antiepileptic Drug Pregnancy Registry (1-888-233-2334). (8.1)
- Efficacy of LAMICTAL, used as adjunctive treatment for partial seizures, was not demonstrated in a small, randomized, double-blind, placebo-controlled study in very young pediatric patients (1 to 24 months). (8.4)

See 17 for PATIENT COUNSELING INFORMATION and Medication Guide

Revised: 06/2014

FULL PRESCRIBING INFORMATION: CONTENTS*
WARNING: SERIOUS SKIN RASHES
1 INDICATIONS AND USAGE
 1.1 Epilepsy
 1.2 Bipolar Disorder

FULL PRESCRIBING INFORMATION

WARNING: SERIOUS SKIN RASHES

LAMICTAL® can cause serious rashes requiring hospitalization and discontinuation of treatment. The incidence of these rashes, which have included Stevens-Johnson syndrome, is approximately 0.8% (8 per 1,000) in pediatric patients (2 to 16 years of age) receiving LAMICTAL as adjunctive therapy for epilepsy and 0.3% (3 per 1,000) in adults on adjunctive therapy for epilepsy. In clinical trials of bipolar and other mood disorders, the rate of serious rash was 0.08% (0.8 per 1,000) in adult patients receiving LAMICTAL as initial monotherapy and 0.13% (1.3 per 1,000) in adult patients receiving LAMICTAL as adjunctive therapy. In a prospectively followed cohort of 1,983 pediatric patients (2 to 16 years of age) with epilepsy taking adjunctive LAMICTAL, there was 1 rash-related death. In worldwide postmarketing experience, rare cases of toxic epidermal necrolysis and/or rash-related death have been reported in adult and pediatric patients, but their numbers are too few to permit a precise estimate of the rate.

Other than age, there are as yet no factors identified that are known to predict the risk of occurrence or the severity of rash caused by LAMICTAL. There are suggestions, yet to be proven, that the risk of rash may also be increased by (1) coadministration of LAMICTAL with valproate (includes valproic acid and divalproex sodium), (2) exceeding the recommended initial dose of LAMICTAL, or (3) exceeding the recommended dose escalation for LAMICTAL. However, cases have occurred in the absence of these factors.

Nearly all cases of life-threatening rashes caused by LAMICTAL have occurred within 2 to 8 weeks of treatment initiation. However, isolated cases have occurred after prolonged treatment (e.g., 6 months). Accordingly, duration of therapy cannot be relied upon as means to predict the potential risk heralded by the first appearance of a rash.

Although benign rashes are also caused by LAMICTAL, it is not possible to predict reliably which rashes will prove to be serious or life threatening. Accordingly, LAMICTAL should ordinarily be discontinued at the first sign of rash, unless the rash is clearly not drug related. Discontinuation of treatment may not prevent a rash from becoming life threatening or permanently disabling or disfiguring [see Warnings and Precautions (5.1)].

1   INDICATIONS AND USAGE

1.1   Epilepsy

Adjunctive Therapy: LAMICTAL is indicated as adjunctive therapy for the following seizure types in patients ≥2 years of age:

- partial seizures
- primary generalized tonic-clonic seizures
- generalized seizures of Lennox-Gastaut syndrome

Monotherapy: LAMICTAL is indicated for conversion to monotherapy in adults (≥16 years of age) with partial seizures who are receiving treatment with carbamazepine, phenytoin, phenobarbital, primidone, or valproate as the single antiepileptic drug (AED).

Safety and effectiveness of LAMICTAL have not been established (1) as initial monotherapy; (2) for conversion to monotherapy from AEDs other than carbamazepine, phenytoin, phenobarbital, primidone, or valproate; or (3) for simultaneous conversion to monotherapy from 2 or more concomitant AEDs.

1.2   Bipolar Disorder

LAMICTAL is indicated for the maintenance treatment of Bipolar I Disorder to delay the time to occurrence of mood episodes (depression, mania, hypomania, mixed episodes) in adults (≥18 years of age) treated for acute mood episodes with standard therapy. The effectiveness of LAMICTAL in the acute treatment of mood episodes has not been established.

The effectiveness of LAMICTAL as maintenance treatment was established in 2 placebo-controlled trials in patients with Bipolar I Disorder as defined by DSM-IV [see Clinical Studies (14.2)]. The physician who elects to prescribe LAMICTAL for periods extending beyond 16 weeks should periodically re-evaluate the long-term usefulness of the drug for the individual patient.

2   DOSAGE AND ADMINISTRATION

2.1   General Dosing Considerations

Rash: There are suggestions, yet to be proven, that the risk of severe, potentially life-threatening rash may be increased by (1) coadministration of LAMICTAL with valproate, (2) exceeding the recommended initial dose of LAMICTAL, or (3) exceeding the recommended dose escalation for LAMICTAL. However, cases have occurred in the absence of these factors [see Boxed Warning]. Therefore, it is important that the dosing recommendations be followed closely.

The risk of nonserious rash may be increased when the recommended initial dose and/or the rate of dose escalation of LAMICTAL is exceeded and in patients with a history of allergy or rash to other AEDs.

LAMICTAL Starter Kits and LAMICTAL ODT® Patient Titration Kits provide LAMICTAL at doses consistent with the recommended titration schedule for the first 5 weeks of treatment, based upon concomitant medications, for patients with epilepsy (>12 years of age) and Bipolar I Disorder (≥18 years of age) and are intended to help reduce the potential for rash. The use of LAMICTAL Starter Kits and LAMICTAL ODT Patient Titration Kits is recommended for appropriate patients who are starting or restarting LAMICTAL [see How Supplied/Storage and Handling (16)]. It is recommended that LAMICTAL not be restarted in patients who discontinued due to rash associated with prior treatment with lamotrigine, unless the potential benefits clearly outweigh the risks. If the decision is made to restart a patient who has discontinued lamotrigine, the need to restart with the initial dosing recommendations should be assessed. The greater the interval of time since the previous dose, the greater consideration should be given to restarting with the initial dosing recommendations. If a patient has discontinued lamotrigine for a period of more than 5 half-lives, it is recommended that initial dosing recommendations and guidelines be followed. The half-life of lamotrigine is affected by other concomitant medications [see Clinical Pharmacology (12.3)].

LAMICTAL Added to Drugs Known to Induce or Inhibit Glucuronidation: Drugs other than those listed in the Clinical Pharmacology section [see Clinical Pharmacology (12.3)] have not been systematically evaluated in combination with lamotrigine. Because lamotrigine is metabolized predominantly by glucuronic acid conjugation, drugs that are known to induce or inhibit glucuronidation may affect the apparent clearance of lamotrigine and doses of LAMICTAL may require adjustment based on clinical response.

Target Plasma Levels for Patients With Epilepsy or Bipolar Disorder: A therapeutic plasma concentration range has not been established for lamotrigine. Dosing of LAMICTAL should be based on therapeutic response [see Clinical Pharmacology (12.3)].

Women Taking Estrogen-Containing Oral Contraceptives:
Starting LAMICTAL in Women Taking Estrogen-Containing Oral Contraceptives: Although estrogen-containing oral contraceptives have been shown to increase the clearance of lamotrigine [see Clinical Pharmacology (12.3)], no adjustments to the recommended dose-escalation guidelines for LAMICTAL should be necessary solely based on the use of estrogen-containing oral contraceptives. Therefore, dose escalation should follow the recommended guidelines for initiating adjunctive therapy with LAMICTAL based on the concomitant AED or other concomitant medications (see Table 1 or Table 5). See below for adjustments to maintenance doses of LAMICTAL in women taking estrogen-containing oral contraceptives.

Adjustments to the Maintenance Dose of LAMICTAL in Women Taking Estrogen-Containing Oral Contraceptives:
(1) Taking Estrogen-Containing Oral Contraceptives: For women not taking carbamazepine, phenytoin, phenobarbital, primidone, or other drugs such as rifampin that induce lamotrigine glucuronidation [see Drug Interactions (7), Clinical Pharmacology (12.3)], the maintenance dose of LAMICTAL will in most cases need to be increased by as much as 2-fold over the recommended target maintenance dose to maintain a consistent lamotrigine plasma level [see Clinical Pharmacology (12.3)].
(2) Starting Estrogen-Containing Oral Contraceptives: In women taking a stable dose of LAMICTAL and not taking carbamazepine, phenytoin, phenobarbital, primidone, or other drugs such as rifampin that induce lamotrigine glucuronidation [see Drug Interactions (7), Clinical Pharmacology (12.3)], the maintenance dose will in most cases need to be increased by as much as 2-fold to maintain a consistent lamotrigine plasma level. The dose increases should begin at the same time that the oral contraceptive is introduced and continue, based on clinical response, no more rapidly than 50 to 100 mg/day every week. Dose increases should not exceed the recommended rate (see Table 1 or Table 5) unless lamotrigine plasma levels or clinical response support larger increases. Gradual transient increases in lamotrigine plasma levels may occur during the week of inactive hormonal preparation ("pill-free" week), and these increases will be greater if dose increases are made in the days before or during the week of inactive hormonal preparation. Increased lamotrigine plasma levels could result in additional adverse reactions, such as dizziness, ataxia, and diplopia. If adverse reactions attributable to LAMICTAL consistently occur during the "pill-free" week, dose adjustments to the overall maintenance dose may be necessary. Dose adjustments limited to the "pill-free" week are not recommended. For women taking LAMICTAL in addition to carbamazepine, phenytoin, phenobarbital, primidone, or other drugs such as rifampin that induce lamotrigine glucuronidation [see Drug Interactions (7), Clinical Pharmacology (12.3)], no adjustment to the dose of LAMICTAL should be necessary.
(3) Stopping Estrogen-Containing Oral Contraceptives: For women not taking carbamazepine, phenytoin, phenobarbital, primidone, or other drugs such as rifampin that induce lamotrigine glucuronidation [see Drug Interactions (7), Clinical Pharmacology (12.3)], the maintenance dose of LAMICTAL will in most cases need to be decreased by as much as 50% in order to maintain a consistent lamotrigine plasma level. The decrease in dose of

Table 1. Escalation Regimen for LAMICTAL in Patients Over 12 Years of Age With Epilepsy

	For Patients TAKING Valproate[a]	For Patients NOT TAKING Carbamazepine, Phenytoin, Phenobarbital, Primidone,[b] or Valproate[a]	For Patients TAKING Carbamazepine, Phenytoin, Phenobarbital, or Primidone[b] and NOT TAKING Valproate[a]
Weeks 1 and 2	25 mg every *other* day	25 mg every day	50 mg/day
Weeks 3 and 4	25 mg every day	50 mg/day	100 mg/day (in 2 divided doses)
Week 5 onwards to maintenance	Increase by 25 to 50 mg/day every 1 to 2 weeks	Increase by 50 mg/day every 1 to 2 weeks	Increase by 100 mg/day every 1 to 2 weeks.
Usual maintenance dose	100 to 200 mg/day with valproate alone 100 to 400 mg/day with valproate and other drugs that induce glucuronidation (in 1 or 2 divided doses)	225 to 375 mg/day (in 2 divided doses)	300 to 500 mg/day (in 2 divided doses)

[a]Valproate has been shown to inhibit glucuronidation and decrease the apparent clearance of lamotrigine [see *Drug Interactions (7), Clinical Pharmacology (12.3)*].
[b]These drugs induce lamotrigine glucuronidation and increase clearance [see *Drug Interactions (7), Clinical Pharmacology (12.3)*]. Other drugs that have similar effects include estrogen-containing oral contraceptives [see *Drug Interactions (7), Clinical Pharmacology (12.3)*]. Dosing recommendations for oral contraceptives can be found in General Dosing Considerations [see *Dosage and Administration (2.1)*]. Patients on rifampin, or other drugs that induce lamotrigine glucuronidation and increase clearance, should follow the same dosing titration/maintenance regimen as that used with anticonvulsants that have this effect.

Table 2. Escalation Regimen for LAMICTAL in Patients 2 to 12 Years of Age With Epilepsy

	For Patients TAKING Valproate[a]	For Patients NOT TAKING Carbamazepine, Phenytoin, Phenobarbital, Primidone,[b] or Valproate[a]	For Patients TAKING Carbamazepine, Phenytoin, Phenobarbital, or Primidone[b] and NOT TAKING Valproate[a]
Weeks 1 and 2	0.15 mg/kg/day in 1 or 2 divided doses, rounded down to the nearest whole tablet (see Table 3 for weight-based dosing guide)	0.3 mg/kg/day in 1 or 2 divided doses, rounded down to the nearest whole tablet	0.6 mg/kg/day in 2 divided doses, rounded down to the nearest whole tablet
Weeks 3 and 4	0.3 mg/kg/day in 1 or 2 divided doses, rounded down to the nearest whole tablet (see Table 3 for weight-based dosing guide)	0.6 mg/kg/day in 2 divided doses, rounded down to the nearest whole tablet	1.2 mg/kg/day in 2 divided doses, rounded down to the nearest whole tablet
Week 5 onwards to maintenance	The dose should be increased every 1 to 2 weeks as follows: calculate 0.3 mg/kg/day, round this amount down to the nearest whole tablet, and add this amount to the previously administered daily dose	The dose should be increased every 1 to 2 weeks as follows: calculate 0.6 mg/kg/day, round this amount down to the nearest whole tablet, and add this amount to the previously administered daily dose	The dose should be increased every 1 to 2 weeks as follows: calculate 1.2 mg/kg/day, round this amount down to the nearest whole tablet, and add this amount to the previously administered daily dose
Usual maintenance dose	1 to 5 mg/kg/day (maximum 200 mg/day in 1 or 2 divided doses) 1 to 3 mg/kg/day with valproate alone	4.5 to 7.5 mg/kg/day (maximum 300 mg/day in 2 divided doses)	5 to 15 mg/kg/day (maximum 400 mg/day in 2 divided doses)
Maintenance dose in patients less than 30 kg	May need to be increased by as much as 50%, based on clinical response	May need to be increased by as much as 50%, based on clinical response	May need to be increased by as much as 50%, based on clinical response

Note: Only whole tablets should be used for dosing.
[a]Valproate has been shown to inhibit glucuronidation and decrease the apparent clearance of lamotrigine [see *Drug Interactions (7), Clinical Pharmacology (12.3)*].
[b]These drugs induce lamotrigine glucuronidation and increase clearance [see *Drug Interactions (7), Clinical Pharmacology (12.3)*]. Other drugs that have similar effects include estrogen-containing oral contraceptives [see *Drug Interactions (7), Clinical Pharmacology (12.3)*]. Dosing recommendations for oral contraceptives can be found in General Dosing Considerations [see *Dosage and Administration (2.1)*]. Patients on rifampin, or other drugs that induce lamotrigine glucuronidation and increase clearance, should follow the same dosing titration/maintenance regimen as that used with anticonvulsants that have this effect.

LAMICTAL should not exceed 25% of the total daily dose per week over a 2-week period, unless clinical response or lamotrigine plasma levels indicate otherwise [see *Clinical Pharmacology (12.3)*]. For women taking LAMICTAL in addition to carbamazepine, phenytoin, phenobarbital, primidone, or other drugs such as rifampin that induce lamotrigine glucuronidation [see *Drug Interactions (7), Clinical Pharmacology (12.3)*], no adjustment to the dose of LAMICTAL would be necessary.
Women and Other Hormonal Contraceptive Preparations or Hormone Replacement Therapy: The effect of other hormonal contraceptive preparations or hormone replacement therapy on the pharmacokinetics of lamotrigine has not been systematically evaluated. It has been reported that ethinylestradiol, not progestogens, increased the clearance of lamotrigine up to 2-fold, and the progestin-only pills had no effect on lamotrigine plasma levels. Therefore, adjustments to the dosage of LAMICTAL in the presence of progestogens alone will likely not be needed.
Patients With Hepatic Impairment: Experience in patients with hepatic impairment is limited. Based on a clinical pharmacology study in 24 patients with mild, moderate,

and severe liver impairment [see *Use in Specific Populations (8.6), Clinical Pharmacology (12.3)*], the following general recommendations can be made. No dosage adjustment is needed in patients with mild liver impairment. Initial, escalation, and maintenance doses should generally be reduced by approximately 25% in patients with moderate and severe liver impairment without ascites and 50% in patients with severe liver impairment with ascites. Escalation and maintenance doses may be adjusted according to clinical response.
Patients With Renal Impairment: Initial doses of LAMICTAL should be based on patients' concomitant medications (see Tables 1-3 or Table 5); reduced maintenance doses may be effective for patients with significant renal impairment [see *Use in Specific Populations (8.7), Clinical Pharmacology (12.3)*]. Few patients with severe renal impairment have been evaluated during chronic treatment with LAMICTAL. Because there is inadequate experience in this population, LAMICTAL should be used with caution in these patients.
Discontinuation Strategy: *Epilepsy:* For patients receiving LAMICTAL in combination with other AEDs, a re-evaluation of all AEDs in the regimen should be considered if a change in seizure control or an appearance or worsening of adverse reactions is observed.
If a decision is made to discontinue therapy with LAMICTAL, a step-wise reduction of dose over at least 2 weeks (approximately 50% per week) is recommended unless safety concerns require a more rapid withdrawal [see *Warnings and Precautions (5.9)*].
Discontinuing carbamazepine, phenytoin, phenobarbital, primidone, or other drugs such as rifampin that induce lamotrigine glucuronidation should prolong the half-life of lamotrigine; discontinuing valproate should shorten the half-life of lamotrigine.
Bipolar Disorder: In the controlled clinical trials, there was no increase in the incidence, type, or severity of adverse reactions following abrupt termination of LAMICTAL. In clinical trials in patients with Bipolar Disorder, 2 patients experienced seizures shortly after abrupt withdrawal of LAMICTAL. However, there were confounding factors that may have contributed to the occurrence of seizures in these bipolar patients. Discontinuation of LAMICTAL should involve a step-wise reduction of dose over at least 2 weeks (approximately 50% per week) unless safety concerns require a more rapid withdrawal [see *Warnings and Precautions (5.9)*].
2.2 Epilepsy – Adjunctive Therapy
This section provides specific dosing recommendations for patients greater than 12 years of age and patients 2 to 12 years of age. Within each of these age-groups, specific dosing recommendations are provided depending upon concomitant AED or other concomitant medications (Table 1 for patients greater than 12 years of age and Table 2 for patients 2 to 12 years of age). A weight-based dosing guide for patients 2 to 12 years of age on concomitant valproate is provided in Table 3.
Patients Over 12 Years of Age: Recommended dosing guidelines are summarized in Table 1.
[See table 1 above]
Patients 2 to 12 Years of Age: Recommended dosing guidelines are summarized in Table 2.
Smaller starting doses and slower dose escalations than those used in clinical trials are recommended because of the suggestion that the risk of rash may be decreased by smaller starting doses and slower dose escalations. Therefore, maintenance doses will take longer to reach in clinical practice than in clinical trials. It may take several weeks to months to achieve an individualized maintenance dose. Maintenance doses in patients weighing less than 30 kg, regardless of age or concomitant AED, may need to be increased by as much as 50%, based on clinical response.
The smallest available strength of LAMICTAL Chewable Dispersible Tablets is 2 mg, and only whole tablets should be administered. If the calculated dose cannot be achieved using whole tablets, the dose should be rounded down to the nearest whole tablet [see *How Supplied/Storage and Handling (16)* and *Medication Guide*].
[See table 2 above]

Table 3. The Initial Weight-Based Dosing Guide for Patients 2 to 12 Years of Age Taking Valproate (Weeks 1 to 4) With Epilepsy

If the patient's weight is		Give this daily dose, using the most appropriate combination of LAMICTAL 2-mg and 5-mg tablets	
Greater than	And less than	Weeks 1 and 2	Weeks 3 and 4
6.7 kg	14 kg	2 mg every *other* day	2 mg every day
14.1 kg	27 kg	2 mg every day	4 mg every day

Table 4. Conversion From Adjunctive Therapy With Valproate to Monotherapy With LAMICTAL in Patients ≥16 Years of Age With Epilepsy

	LAMICTAL	Valproate
Step 1	Achieve a dose of 200 mg/day according to guidelines in Table 1 (if not already on 200 mg/day).	Maintain previous stable dose.
Step 2	Maintain at 200 mg/day.	Decrease to 500 mg/day by decrements no greater than 500 mg/day/week and then maintain the dose of 500 mg/day for 1 week.
Step 3	Increase to 300 mg/day and maintain for 1 week.	Simultaneously decrease to 250 mg/day and maintain for 1 week.
Step 4	Increase by 100 mg/day every week to achieve maintenance dose of 500 mg/day.	Discontinue.

Table 5. Escalation Regimen for LAMICTAL for Patients With Bipolar Disorder

	For Patients TAKING Valproate[a]	For Patients NOT TAKING Carbamazepine, Phenytoin, Phenobarbital, Primidone,[b] or Valproate[a]	For Patients TAKING Carbamazepine, Phenytoin, Phenobarbital, or Primidone[b] and NOT TAKING Valproate[a]
Weeks 1 and 2	25 mg every *other* day	25 mg daily	50 mg daily
Weeks 3 and 4	25 mg daily	50 mg daily	100 mg daily, in divided doses
Week 5	50 mg daily	100 mg daily	200 mg daily, in divided doses
Week 6	100 mg daily	200 mg daily	300 mg daily, in divided doses
Week 7	100 mg daily	200 mg daily	up to 400 mg daily, in divided doses

[a]Valproate has been shown to inhibit glucuronidation and decrease the apparent clearance of lamotrigine [see Drug Interactions (7), Clinical Pharmacology (12.3)].

[b]These drugs induce lamotrigine glucuronidation and increase clearance [see Drug Interactions (7), Clinical Pharmacology (12.3)]. Other drugs that have similar effects include estrogen-containing oral contraceptives [see Drug Interactions (7), Clinical Pharmacology (12.3)]. Dosing recommendations for oral contraceptives can be found in General Dosing Considerations [see Dosage and Administration (2.1)]. Patients on rifampin, or other drugs that induce lamotrigine glucuronidation and increase clearance, should follow the same dosing titration/maintenance regimen as that used with anticonvulsants that have this effect.

27.1 kg	34 kg	4 mg every day	8 mg every day
34.1 kg	40 kg	5 mg every day	10 mg every day

Usual Adjunctive Maintenance Dose for Epilepsy: The usual maintenance doses identified in Tables 1 and 2 are derived from dosing regimens employed in the placebo-controlled adjunctive studies in which the efficacy of LAMICTAL was established. In patients receiving multidrug regimens employing carbamazepine, phenytoin, phenobarbital, or primidone **without valproate**, maintenance doses of adjunctive LAMICTAL as high as 700 mg/day have been used. In patients receiving **valproate alone**, maintenance doses of adjunctive LAMICTAL as high as 200 mg/day have been used. The advantage of using doses above those recommended in Tables 1 through 4 has not been established in controlled trials.

2.3   Epilepsy – Conversion From Adjunctive Therapy to Monotherapy
The goal of the transition regimen is to effect the conversion to monotherapy with LAMICTAL under conditions that ensure adequate seizure control while mitigating the risk of serious rash associated with the rapid titration of LAMICTAL.
The recommended maintenance dose of LAMICTAL as monotherapy is 500 mg/day given in 2 divided doses.
To avoid an increased risk of rash, the recommended initial dose and subsequent dose escalations of LAMICTAL should not be exceeded [see Boxed Warning].
Conversion From Adjunctive Therapy With Carbamazepine, Phenytoin, Phenobarbital, or Primidone to Monotherapy With LAMICTAL: After achieving a dose of 500 mg/day of LAMICTAL according to the guidelines in Table 1, the concomitant AED should be withdrawn by 20% decrements each week over a 4-week period. The regimen for the withdrawal of the concomitant AED is based on experience gained in the controlled monotherapy clinical trial.
Conversion From Adjunctive Therapy With Valproate to Monotherapy With LAMICTAL: The conversion regimen involves 4 steps outlined in Table 4.
[See table 4 above]
Conversion From Adjunctive Therapy With Antiepileptic Drugs Other Than Carbamazepine, Phenytoin, Phenobarbital, Primidone, or Valproate to Monotherapy With LAMICTAL: No specific dosing guidelines can be

provided for conversion to monotherapy with LAMICTAL with AEDs other than carbamazepine, phenobarbital, phenytoin, primidone, or valproate.
2.4   Bipolar Disorder
The goal of maintenance treatment with LAMICTAL is to delay the time to occurrence of mood episodes (depression, mania, hypomania, mixed episodes) in patients treated for acute mood episodes with standard therapy. The target dose of LAMICTAL is 200 mg/day (100 mg/day in patients taking valproate, which decreases the apparent clearance of lamotrigine, and 400 mg/day in patients not taking valproate and taking either carbamazepine, phenytoin, phenobarbital, primidone, or other drugs such as rifampin that increase the apparent clearance of lamotrigine). In the clinical trials, doses up to 400 mg/day as monotherapy were evaluated; however, no additional benefit was seen at 400 mg/day compared with 200 mg/day [see Clinical Studies (14.2)]. Accordingly, doses above 200 mg/day are not recommended. Treatment with LAMICTAL is introduced, based on concurrent medications, according to the regimen outlined in Table 5. If other psychotropic medications are withdrawn following stabilization, the dose of LAMICTAL should be adjusted. For patients discontinuing valproate, the dose of LAMICTAL should be doubled over a 2-week period in equal weekly increments (see Table 6). For patients discontinuing carbamazepine, phenytoin, phenobarbital, primidone, or other drugs such as rifampin that induce lamotrigine glucuronidation, the dose of LAMICTAL should remain constant for the first week and then should be decreased by half over a 2-week period in equal weekly decrements (see Table 6). The dose of LAMICTAL may then be further adjusted to the target dose (200 mg) as clinically indicated.
If other drugs are subsequently introduced, the dose of LAMICTAL may need to be adjusted. In particular, the introduction of valproate requires reduction in the dose of LAMICTAL [see Drug Interactions (7), Clinical Pharmacology (12.3)].
To avoid an increased risk of rash, the recommended initial dose and subsequent dose escalations of LAMICTAL should not be exceeded [see Boxed Warning].
[See table 5 above]
[See table 6 at top of next page]
The benefit of continuing treatment in patients who had been stabilized in an 8- to 16-week open-label phase with

LAMICTAL was established in 2 randomized, placebo-controlled clinical maintenance trials [see Clinical Studies (14.2)]. However, the optimal duration of treatment with LAMICTAL has not been established. Thus, patients should be periodically reassessed to determine the need for maintenance treatment.
2.5   Administration of LAMICTAL Chewable Dispersible Tablets
LAMICTAL Chewable Dispersible Tablets may be swallowed whole, chewed, or dispersed in water or diluted fruit juice. If the tablets are chewed, consume a small amount of water or diluted fruit juice to aid in swallowing.
To disperse LAMICTAL Chewable Dispersible Tablets, add the tablets to a small amount of liquid (1 teaspoon, or enough to cover the medication). Approximately 1 minute later, when the tablets are completely dispersed, swirl the solution and consume the entire quantity immediately. *No attempt should be made to administer partial quantities of the dispersed tablets.*
2.6   Administration of LAMICTAL ODT Orally Disintegrating Tablets
LAMICTAL ODT Orally Disintegrating Tablets should be placed onto the tongue and moved around in the mouth. The tablet will disintegrate rapidly, can be swallowed with or without water, and can be taken with or without food.
3   DOSAGE FORMS AND STRENGTHS
3.1   Tablets
25 mg, white, scored, shield-shaped tablets debossed with "LAMICTAL" and "25."
100 mg, peach, scored, shield-shaped tablets debossed with "LAMICTAL" and "100."
150 mg, cream, scored, shield-shaped tablets debossed with "LAMICTAL" and "150."
200 mg, blue, scored, shield-shaped tablets debossed with "LAMICTAL" and "200."
3.2   Chewable Dispersible Tablets
2 mg, white to off-white, round tablets debossed with "LTG" over "2."
5 mg, white to off-white, caplet-shaped tablets debossed with "GX CL2."
25 mg, white, super elliptical-shaped tablets debossed with "GX CL5."
3.3   Orally Disintegrating Tablets
25 mg, white to off-white, round, flat-faced, radius edge, tablets debossed with "LMT" on one side and "25" on the other side.
50 mg, white to off-white, round, flat-faced, radius edge, tablets debossed with "LMT" on one side and "50" on the other side.
100 mg, white to off-white, round, flat-faced, radius edge, tablets debossed with "LAMICTAL" on one side and "100" on the other side.
200 mg, white to off-white, round, flat-faced, radius edge, tablets debossed with "LAMICTAL" on one side and "200" on the other side.
3.4   Potential Medication Errors
Patients should be strongly advised to visually inspect their tablets to verify that they are receiving LAMICTAL as well as the correct formulation of LAMICTAL each time they fill their prescription. Depictions of the LAMICTAL Tablets, Chewable Dispersible Tablets, and Orally Disintegrating Tablets can be found in the Medication Guide that accompanies the product.
4   CONTRAINDICATIONS
LAMICTAL is contraindicated in patients who have demonstrated hypersensitivity to the drug or its ingredients [see Boxed Warning, Warnings and Precautions (5.1, 5.2)].
5   WARNINGS AND PRECAUTIONS
5.1   Serious Skin Rashes [see Boxed Warning]
Pediatric Population: The incidence of serious rash associated with hospitalization and discontinuation of LAMICTAL in a prospectively followed cohort of pediatric patients (2 to 16 years of age) with epilepsy receiving adjunctive therapy was approximately 0.8% (16 of 1,983). When 14 of these cases were reviewed by 3 expert dermatologists, there was considerable disagreement as to their proper classification. To illustrate, one dermatologist considered none of the cases to be Stevens-Johnson syndrome; another assigned 7 of the 14 to this diagnosis. There was 1 rash-related death in this 1,983-patient cohort. Additionally, there have been rare cases of toxic epidermal necrolysis with and without permanent sequelae and/or death in US and foreign postmarketing experience.
There is evidence that the inclusion of valproate in a multidrug regimen increases the risk of serious, potentially life-threatening rash in pediatric patients. In pediatric patients who used valproate concomitantly, 1.2% (6 of 482) experienced a serious rash compared with 0.6% (6 of 952) patients not taking valproate.
Adult Population: Serious rash associated with hospitalization and discontinuation of LAMICTAL occurred in 0.3% (11 of 3,348) of adult patients who received LAMICTAL in premarketing clinical trials of epilepsy. In the bipolar and

Table 6. Dosage Adjustments to LAMICTAL for Patients With Bipolar Disorder Following Discontinuation of Psychotropic Medications

Discontinuation of Psychotropic Drugs (excluding Carbamazepine, Phenytoin, Phenobarbital, Primidone,[b] or Valproate[a])	After Discontinuation of Valproate[a] Current dose of LAMICTAL (mg/day) 100	After Discontinuation of Carbamazepine, Phenytoin, Phenobarbital, or Primidone[b] Current dose of LAMICTAL (mg/day) 400
Week 1	Maintain current dose of LAMICTAL	150	400
Week 2	Maintain current dose of LAMICTAL	200	300
Week 3 onward	Maintain current dose of LAMICTAL	200	200

[a]Valproate has been shown to inhibit glucuronidation and decrease the apparent clearance of lamotrigine [see Drug Interactions (7), Clinical Pharmacology (12.3)].
[b]These drugs induce lamotrigine glucuronidation and increase clearance [see Drug Interactions (7), Clinical Pharmacology (12.3)]. Other drugs that have similar effects include estrogen-containing oral contraceptives [see Drug Interactions (7), Clinical Pharmacology (12.3)]. Dosing recommendations for oral contraceptives can be found in General Dosing Considerations [see Dosage and Administration (2.1)]. Patients on rifampin, or other drugs that induce lamotrigine glucuronidation and increase clearance, should follow the same dosing titration/maintenance regimen as that used with anticonvulsants that have this effect.

Table 7. Risk by Indication for Antiepileptic Drugs in the Pooled Analysis

Indication	Placebo Patients With Events Per 1,000 Patients	Drug Patients With Events Per 1,000 Patients	Relative Risk: Incidence of Events in Drug Patients/ Incidence in Placebo Patients	Risk Difference: Additional Drug Patients With Events Per 1,000 Patients
Epilepsy	1.0	3.4	3.5	2.4
Psychiatric	5.7	8.5	1.5	2.9
Other	1.0	1.8	1.9	0.9
Total	2.4	4.3	1.8	1.9

other mood disorders clinical trials, the rate of serious rash was 0.08% (1 of 1,233) of adult patients who received LAMICTAL as initial monotherapy and 0.13% (2 of 1,538) of adult patients who received LAMICTAL as adjunctive therapy. No fatalities occurred among these individuals. However, in worldwide postmarketing experience, rare cases of rash-related death have been reported, but their numbers are too few to permit a precise estimate of the rate.
Among the rashes leading to hospitalization were Stevens-Johnson syndrome, toxic epidermal necrolysis, angioedema, and those associated with multiorgan hypersensitivity [see Warnings and Precautions (5.2)].
There is evidence that the inclusion of valproate in a multidrug regimen increases the risk of serious, potentially life-threatening rash in adults. Specifically, of 584 patients administered LAMICTAL with valproate in epilepsy clinical trials, 6 (1%) were hospitalized in association with rash; in contrast, 4 (0.16%) of 2,398 clinical trial patients and volunteers administered LAMICTAL in the absence of valproate were hospitalized.
Patients With History of Allergy or Rash to Other Antiepileptic Drugs: The risk of nonserious rash may be increased when the recommended initial dose and/or the rate of dose escalation of LAMICTAL is exceeded and in patients with a history of allergy or rash to other AEDs.

5.2 Multiorgan Hypersensitivity Reactions and Organ Failure
Multiorgan hypersensitivity reactions, also known as Drug Reaction with Eosinophilia and Systemic Symptoms (DRESS), have occurred in LAMICTAL. Some have been fatal or life threatening. DRESS typically, although not exclusively, presents with fever, rash, and/or lymphadenopathy in association with other organ system involvement, such as hepatitis, nephritis, hematologic abnormalities, myocarditis, or myositis, sometimes resembling an acute viral infection. Eosinophilia is often present. This disorder is variable in its expression, and other organ systems not noted here may be involved.
Fatalities associated with acute multiorgan failure and various degrees of hepatic failure have been reported in 2 of 3,796 adult patients and 4 of 2,435 pediatric patients who received LAMICTAL in epilepsy clinical trials. Rare fatalities from multiorgan failure have also been reported in postmarketing use.
Isolated liver failure without rash or involvement of other organs has also been reported with LAMICTAL.
It is important to note that early manifestations of hypersensitivity (e.g., fever, lymphadenopathy) may be present even though a rash is not evident. If such signs or symptoms are present, the patient should be evaluated immediately. LAMICTAL should be discontinued if an alternative etiology for the signs or symptoms cannot be established.
Prior to initiation of treatment with LAMICTAL, the patient should be instructed that a rash or other signs or symptoms of hypersensitivity (e.g., fever, lymphadenopathy) may herald a serious medical event and that the patient should report any such occurrence to a physician immediately.

5.3 Blood Dyscrasias
There have been reports of blood dyscrasias that may or may not be associated with multiorgan hypersensitivity (also known as DRESS) [see Warnings and Precautions (5.2)]. These have included neutropenia, leukopenia, anemia, thrombocytopenia, pancytopenia, and, rarely, aplastic anemia and pure red cell aplasia.

5.4 Suicidal Behavior and Ideation
AEDs, including LAMICTAL, increase the risk of suicidal thoughts or behavior in patients taking these drugs for any indication. Patients treated with any AED for any indication should be monitored for the emergence or worsening of depression, suicidal thoughts or behavior, and/or any unusual changes in mood or behavior.
Pooled analyses of 199 placebo-controlled clinical trials (monotherapy and adjunctive therapy) of 11 different AEDs showed that patients randomized to 1 of the AEDs had approximately twice the risk (adjusted Relative Risk 1.8, 95% CI:1.2, 2.7) of suicidal thinking or behavior compared to patients randomized to placebo. In these trials, which had a median treatment duration of 12 weeks, the estimated incidence of suicidal behavior or ideation among 27,863 AED-treated patients was 0.43%, compared to 0.24% among 16,029 placebo-treated patients, representing an increase of approximately 1 case of suicidal thinking or behavior for every 530 patients treated. There were 4 suicides in drug-treated patients in the trials and none in placebo-treated patients, but the number of events is too small to allow any conclusion about drug effect on suicide.
The increased risk of suicidal thoughts or behavior with AEDs was observed as early as 1 week after starting treatment with AEDs and persisted for the duration of treatment assessed. Because most trials included in the analysis did not extend beyond 24 weeks, the risk of suicidal thoughts or behavior beyond 24 weeks could not be assessed.
The risk of suicidal thoughts or behavior was generally consistent among drugs in the data analyzed. The finding of increased risk with AEDs of varying mechanism of action and across a range of indications suggests that the risk applies to all AEDs used for any indication. The risk did not vary substantially by age (5 to 100 years) in the clinical trials analyzed.
Table 7 shows absolute and relative risk by indication for all evaluated AEDs.
[See table above]
The relative risk for suicidal thoughts or behavior was higher in clinical trials for epilepsy than in clinical trials for psychiatric or other conditions, but the absolute risk differences were similar for the epilepsy and psychiatric indications.
Anyone considering prescribing LAMICTAL or any other AED must balance the risk of suicidal thoughts or behavior with the risk of untreated illness. Epilepsy and many other illnesses for which AEDs are prescribed are themselves associated with morbidity and mortality and an increased risk of suicidal thoughts and behavior. Should suicidal thoughts and behavior emerge during treatment, the prescriber needs to consider whether the emergence of these symptoms in any given patient may be related to the illness being treated.
Patients, their caregivers, and families should be informed that AEDs increase the risk of suicidal thoughts and behavior and should be advised of the need to be alert for the emergence or worsening of the signs and symptoms of depression, any unusual changes in mood or behavior, or the emergence of suicidal thoughts, behavior, or thoughts about self-harm. Behaviors of concern should be reported immediately to healthcare providers.

5.5 Use in Patients With Bipolar Disorder
Acute Treatment of Mood Episodes: Safety and effectiveness of LAMICTAL in the acute treatment of mood episodes have not been established.
Children and Adolescents (less than 18 years of age): Safety and effectiveness of LAMICTAL in patients below the age of 18 years with mood disorders have not been established [see Suicidal Behavior and Ideation (5.4)].
Clinical Worsening and Suicide Risk Associated With Bipolar Disorder: Patients with bipolar disorder may experience worsening of their depressive symptoms and/or the emergence of suicidal ideation and behaviors (suicidality) whether or not they are taking medications for bipolar disorder. Patients should be closely monitored for clinical worsening (including development of new symptoms) and suicidality, especially at the beginning of a course of treatment or at the time of dose changes.
In addition, patients with a history of suicidal behavior or thoughts, those patients exhibiting a significant degree of suicidal ideation prior to commencement of treatment, and young adults are at an increased risk of suicidal thoughts or suicide attempts and should receive careful monitoring during treatment [see Suicidal Behavior and Ideation (5.4)].
Consideration should be given to changing the therapeutic regimen, including possibly discontinuing the medication, in patients who experience clinical worsening (including development of new symptoms) and/or the emergence of suicidal ideation/behavior especially if these symptoms are severe, abrupt in onset, or were not part of the patient's presenting symptoms.
Prescriptions for LAMICTAL should be written for the smallest quantity of tablets consistent with good patient management in order to reduce the risk of overdose. Overdoses have been reported for LAMICTAL, some of which have been fatal [see Overdosage (10.1)].

5.6 Aseptic Meningitis
Therapy with LAMICTAL increases the risk of developing aseptic meningitis. Because of the potential for serious outcomes of untreated meningitis due to other causes, patients should also be evaluated for other causes of meningitis and treated as appropriate.
Postmarketing cases of aseptic meningitis have been reported in pediatric and adult patients taking LAMICTAL for various indications. Symptoms upon presentation have included headache, fever, nausea, vomiting, and nuchal rigidity. Rash, photophobia, myalgia, chills, altered consciousness, and somnolence were also noted in some cases. Symptoms have been reported to occur within 1 day to one and a half months following the initiation of treatment. In most cases, symptoms were reported to resolve after discontinuation of LAMICTAL. Re-exposure resulted in a rapid return of symptoms (from within 30 minutes to 1 day following re-initiation of treatment) that were frequently more severe. Some of the patients treated with LAMICTAL who developed aseptic meningitis had underlying diagnoses of systemic lupus erythematosus or other autoimmune diseases. Cerebrospinal fluid (CSF) analyzed at the time of clinical presentation in reported cases was characterized by a mild to moderate pleocytosis, normal glucose levels, and mild to moderate increase in protein. CSF white blood cell count differentials showed a predominance of neutrophils in a majority of the cases, although a predominance of lymphocytes was reported in approximately one third of the cases. Some patients also had new onset of signs and symptoms of involvement of other organs (predominantly hepatic and renal involvement), which may suggest that in these cases the aseptic meningitis observed was part of a hypersensitivity reaction [see Warnings and Precautions (5.2)].

5.7 Potential Medication Errors

Medication errors involving LAMICTAL have occurred. In particular, the names LAMICTAL or lamotrigine can be confused with the names of other commonly used medications. Medication errors may also occur between the different formulations of LAMICTAL. To reduce the potential of medication errors, write and say LAMICTAL clearly. Depictions of the LAMICTAL Tablets, Chewable Dispersible Tablets, and Orally Disintegrating Tablets can be found in the Medication Guide that accompanies the product to highlight the distinctive markings, colors, and shapes that serve to identify the different presentations of the drug and thus may help reduce the risk of medication errors. To avoid the medication error of using the wrong drug or formulation, patients should be strongly advised to visually inspect their tablets to verify that they are LAMICTAL, as well as the correct formulation of LAMICTAL, each time they fill their prescription.

5.8 Concomitant Use With Oral Contraceptives

Some estrogen-containing oral contraceptives have been shown to decrease serum concentrations of lamotrigine [see Clinical Pharmacology (12.3)]. Dosage adjustments will be necessary in most patients who start or stop estrogen-containing oral contraceptives while taking LAMICTAL [see Dosage and Administration (2.1)]. During the week of inactive hormone preparation ("pill-free" week) of oral contraceptive therapy, plasma lamotrigine levels are expected to rise, as much as doubling at the end of the week. Adverse reactions consistent with elevated levels of lamotrigine, such as dizziness, ataxia, and diplopia, could occur.

5.9 Withdrawal Seizures

As with other AEDs, LAMICTAL should not be abruptly discontinued. In patients with epilepsy there is a possibility of increasing seizure frequency. In clinical trials in patients with Bipolar Disorder, 2 patients experienced seizures shortly after abrupt withdrawal of LAMICTAL; however, there were confounding factors that may have contributed to the occurrence of seizures in these bipolar patients. Unless safety concerns require a more rapid withdrawal, the dose of LAMICTAL should be tapered over a period of at least 2 weeks (approximately 50% reduction per week) [see Dosage and Administration (2.1)].

5.10 Status Epilepticus

Valid estimates of the incidence of treatment-emergent status epilepticus among patients treated with LAMICTAL are difficult to obtain because reporters participating in clinical trials did not all employ identical rules for identifying cases. At a minimum, 7 of 2,343 adult patients had episodes that could unequivocally be described as status epilepticus. In addition, a number of reports of variably defined episodes of seizure exacerbation (e.g., seizure clusters, seizure flurries) were made.

5.11 Sudden Unexplained Death in Epilepsy (SUDEP)

During the premarketing development of LAMICTAL, 20 sudden and unexplained deaths were recorded among a cohort of 4,700 patients with epilepsy (5,747 patient-years of exposure).

Some of these could represent seizure-related deaths in which the seizure was not observed, e.g., at night. This represents an incidence of 0.0035 deaths per patient-year. Although this rate exceeds that expected in a healthy population matched for age and sex, it is within the range of estimates for the incidence of sudden unexplained deaths in patients with epilepsy not receiving LAMICTAL (ranging from 0.0005 for the general population of patients with epilepsy, to 0.004 for a recently studied clinical trial population similar to that in the clinical development program for LAMICTAL, to 0.005 for patients with refractory epilepsy). Consequently, whether these figures are reassuring or suggest concern depends on the comparability of the populations reported upon to the cohort receiving LAMICTAL and the accuracy of the estimates provided. Probably most reassuring is the similarity of estimated SUDEP rates in patients receiving LAMICTAL and those receiving other AEDs, chemically unrelated to each other, that underwent clinical testing in similar populations. Importantly, that drug is chemically unrelated to LAMICTAL. This evidence suggests, although it certainly does not prove, that the high SUDEP rates reflect population rates, not a drug effect.

5.12 Addition of LAMICTAL to a Multidrug Regimen That Includes Valproate

Because valproate reduces the clearance of lamotrigine, the dosage of lamotrigine in the presence of valproate is less than half of that required in its absence.

5.13 Binding in the Eye and Other Melanin-Containing Tissues

Because lamotrigine binds to melanin, it could accumulate in melanin-rich tissues over time. This raises the possibility that lamotrigine may cause toxicity in these tissues after extended use. Although ophthalmological testing was performed in 1 controlled clinical trial, the testing was inadequate to exclude subtle effects or injury occurring after long-term exposure. Moreover, the capacity of available tests to detect potentially adverse consequences, if any, of lamotrigine's binding to melanin is unknown [see Clinical Pharmacology (12.2)].

Accordingly, although there are no specific recommendations for periodic ophthalmological monitoring, prescribers should be aware of the possibility of long-term ophthalmologic effects.

5.14 Laboratory Tests

The value of monitoring plasma concentrations of lamotrigine in patients treated with LAMICTAL has not been established. Because of the possible pharmacokinetic interactions between lamotrigine and other drugs including AEDs (see Table 15), monitoring of the plasma levels of lamotrigine and concomitant drugs may be indicated, particularly during dosage adjustments. In general, clinical judgment should be exercised regarding monitoring of plasma levels of lamotrigine and other drugs and whether or not dosage adjustments are necessary.

6 ADVERSE REACTIONS

The following adverse reactions are described in more detail in the Warnings and Precautions section of the label:
- Serious skin rashes [see Warnings and Precautions (5.1)]
- Multiorgan hypersensitivity reactions and organ failure [see Warnings and Precautions (5.2)]
- Blood dyscrasias [see Warnings and Precautions (5.3)]
- Suicidal behavior and ideation [see Warnings and Precautions (5.4)]
- Aseptic meningitis [see Warnings and Precautions (5.6)]
- Withdrawal seizures [see Warnings and Precautions (5.9)]
- Status epilepticus [see Warnings and Precautions (5.10)]
- Sudden unexplained death in epilepsy [see Warnings and Precautions (5.11)]

6.1 Clinical Trials

Because clinical trials are conducted under widely varying conditions, adverse reaction rates observed in the clinical trials of a drug cannot be directly compared with rates in the clinical trials of another drug and may not reflect the rates observed in practice.

LAMICTAL has been evaluated for safety in patients with epilepsy and in patients with Bipolar I Disorder. Adverse reactions reported for each of these patient populations are provided below. Excluded are adverse reactions considered too general to be informative and those not reasonably attributable to the use of the drug.

Epilepsy: *Most Common Adverse Reactions in All Clinical Studies: Adjunctive Therapy in Adults With Epilepsy:* The most commonly observed (≥5% for LAMICTAL and more common on drug than placebo) adverse reactions seen in association with LAMICTAL during adjunctive therapy in adults and not seen at an equivalent frequency among placebo-treated patients were: dizziness, ataxia, somnolence, headache, diplopia, blurred vision, nausea, vomiting, and rash. Dizziness, diplopia, ataxia, blurred vision, nausea, and vomiting were dose-related. Dizziness, diplopia, ataxia, and blurred vision occurred more commonly in patients receiving carbamazepine with LAMICTAL than in patients receiving other AEDs with LAMICTAL. Clinical data suggest a higher incidence of rash, including serious rash, in patients receiving concomitant valproate than in patients not receiving valproate [see Warnings and Precautions (5.1)].

Approximately 11% of the 3,378 adult patients who received LAMICTAL as adjunctive therapy in premarketing clinical trials discontinued treatment because of an adverse reaction. The adverse reactions most commonly associated with discontinuation were rash (3.0%), dizziness (2.8%), and headache (2.5%).

In a dose-response study in adults, the rate of discontinuation of LAMICTAL for dizziness, ataxia, diplopia, blurred vision, nausea, and vomiting was dose-related.

Monotherapy in Adults With Epilepsy: The most commonly observed (≥5% for LAMICTAL and more common on drug than placebo) adverse reactions seen in association with the use of LAMICTAL during the monotherapy phase of the controlled trial in adults not seen at an equivalent rate in the control group were vomiting, coordination abnormality, dyspepsia, nausea, dizziness, rhinitis, anxiety, insomnia, infection, pain, weight decrease, chest pain, and dysmenorrhea. The most commonly observed (≥5% for LAMICTAL and more common on drug than placebo) adverse reactions associated with the use of LAMICTAL during the conversion to monotherapy (add-on) period, not seen at an equivalent frequency among low-dose valproate-treated patients, were dizziness, headache, nausea, asthenia, coordination abnormality, vomiting, rash, somnolence, diplopia, ataxia, accidental injury, tremor, blurred vision, insomnia, nystagmus, diarrhea, lymphadenopathy, pruritus, and sinusitis.

Approximately 10% of the 420 adult patients who received LAMICTAL as monotherapy in premarketing clinical trials discontinued treatment because of an adverse reaction. The adverse reactions most commonly associated with discontinuation were rash (4.5%), headache (3.1%), and asthenia (2.4%).

Adjunctive Therapy in Pediatric Patients With Epilepsy: The most commonly observed (≥5% for LAMICTAL and more common on drug than placebo) adverse reactions seen in association with the use of LAMICTAL as adjunctive treatment in pediatric patients 2 to 16 years of age and not seen at an equivalent rate in the control group were infection, vomiting, rash, fever, somnolence, accidental injury, dizziness, diarrhea, abdominal pain, nausea, ataxia, tremor, asthenia, bronchitis, flu syndrome, and diplopia.

In 339 patients 2 to 16 years of age with partial seizures or generalized seizures of Lennox-Gastaut syndrome, 4.2% of patients on LAMICTAL and 2.9% of patients on placebo discontinued due to adverse reactions. The most commonly reported adverse reaction that led to discontinuation of LAMICTAL was rash.

Approximately 11.5% of the 1,081 pediatric patients 2 to 16 years of age who received LAMICTAL as adjunctive therapy in premarketing clinical trials discontinued treatment because of an adverse reaction. The adverse reactions most commonly associated with discontinuation were rash (4.4%), reaction aggravated (1.7%), and ataxia (0.6%).

Controlled Adjunctive Clinical Studies in Adults With Epilepsy: Table 8 lists treatment-emergent adverse reactions that occurred in at least 2% of adult patients with epilepsy treated with LAMICTAL in placebo-controlled trials and were numerically more common in the patients treated with LAMICTAL. In these studies, either LAMICTAL or placebo was added to the patient's current AED therapy. Adverse reactions were usually mild to moderate in intensity.

Table 8. Treatment-Emergent Adverse Reaction Incidence in Placebo-Controlled Adjunctive Trials in Adult Patients With Epilepsy[a] (Adverse reactions in at least 2% of patients treated with LAMICTAL and numerically more frequent than in the placebo group.)

Body System/Adverse Reaction	Percent of Patients Receiving Adjunctive LAMICTAL (n = 711)	Percent of Patients Receiving Adjunctive Placebo (n = 419)
Body as a whole		
Headache	29	19
Flu syndrome	7	6
Fever	6	4
Abdominal pain	5	4
Neck pain	2	1
Reaction aggravated (seizure exacerbation)	2	1
Digestive		
Nausea	19	10
Vomiting	9	4
Diarrhea	6	4
Dyspepsia	5	2
Constipation	4	3
Anorexia	2	1
Musculoskeletal		
Arthralgia	2	0
Nervous		
Dizziness	38	13
Ataxia	22	6
Somnolence	14	7
Incoordination	6	2
Insomnia	6	2
Tremor	4	1
Depression	4	3
Anxiety	4	3
Convulsion	3	1
Irritability	3	2
Speech disorder	3	0
Concentration disturbance	2	1
Respiratory		
Rhinitis	14	9
Pharyngitis	10	9
Cough increased	8	6
Skin and appendages		
Rash	10	5
Pruritus	3	2
Special senses		
Diplopia	28	7
Blurred vision	16	5
Vision abnormality	3	1
Urogenital		
Female patients only	(n = 365)	(n = 207)
Dysmenorrhea	7	6

Vaginitis	4	1
Amenorrhea	2	1

[a]Patients in these adjunctive studies were receiving 1 to 3 of the following concomitant AEDs (carbamazepine, phenytoin, phenobarbital, or primidone) in addition to LAMICTAL or placebo. Patients may have reported multiple adverse reactions during the study or at discontinuation; thus, patients may be included in more than one category.

In a randomized, parallel study comparing placebo and 300 and 500 mg/day of LAMICTAL, some of the more common drug-related adverse reactions were dose-related (see Table 9).

Table 9. Dose-Related Adverse Reactions From a Randomized, Placebo-Controlled Adjunctive Trial in Adults With Epilepsy

	Percent of Patients Experiencing Adverse Reactions		
Adverse Reaction	Placebo (n = 73)	LAMICTAL 300 mg (n = 71)	LAMICTAL 500 mg (n = 72)
Ataxia	10	10	28[ab]
Blurred vision	10	11	25[ab]
Diplopia	8	24[a]	49[ab]
Dizziness	27	31	54[ab]
Nausea	11	18	25[a]
Vomiting	4	11	18[a]

[a]Significantly greater than placebo group (*P*<0.05).
[b]Significantly greater than group receiving LAMICTAL 300 mg (*P*<0.05).

The overall adverse reaction profile for LAMICTAL was similar between females and males, and was independent of age. Because the largest non-Caucasian racial subgroup was only 6% of patients exposed to LAMICTAL in placebo-controlled trials, there are insufficient data to support a statement regarding the distribution of adverse reaction reports by race. Generally, females receiving either LAMICTAL as adjunctive therapy or placebo were more likely to report adverse reactions than males. The only adverse reaction for which the reports on LAMICTAL were greater than 10% more frequent in females than males (without a corresponding difference by gender on placebo) was dizziness (difference = 16.5%). There was little difference between females and males in the rates of discontinuation of LAMICTAL for individual adverse reactions.

Controlled Monotherapy Trial in Adults With Partial Seizures: Table 10 lists treatment-emergent adverse reactions that occurred in at least 5% of patients with epilepsy treated with monotherapy with LAMICTAL in a double-blind trial following discontinuation of either concomitant carbamazepine or phenytoin not seen at an equivalent frequency in the control group.
[See table 10 below]
Adverse reactions that occurred with a frequency of less than 5% and greater than 2% of patients receiving LAMICTAL and numerically more frequent than placebo were:
Body as a Whole: Asthenia, fever.
Digestive: Anorexia, dry mouth, rectal hemorrhage, peptic ulcer.
Metabolic and Nutritional: Peripheral edema.
Nervous System: Amnesia, ataxia, depression, hypesthesia, libido increase, decreased reflexes, increased reflexes, nystagmus, irritability, suicidal ideation.
Respiratory: Epistaxis, bronchitis, dyspnea.
Skin and Appendages: Contact dermatitis, dry skin, sweating.
Special Senses: Vision abnormality.
Incidence in Controlled Adjunctive Trials in Pediatric Patients With Epilepsy: Table 11 lists adverse reactions that occurred in at least 2% of 339 pediatric patients with partial seizures or generalized seizures of Lennox-Gastaut syndrome, who received LAMICTAL up to 15 mg/kg/day or a maximum of 750 mg/day. Reported adverse reactions were classified using COSTART terminology.

Table 11. Treatment-Emergent Adverse Reaction Incidence in Placebo-Controlled Adjunctive Trials in Pediatric Patients With Epilepsy (Adverse reactions in at least 2% of patients treated with LAMICTAL and numerically more frequent than in the placebo group.)

Body System/ Adverse Reaction	Percent of Patients Receiving LAMICTAL (n = 168)	Percent of Patients Receiving Placebo (n = 171)
Body as a whole		
Infection	20	17
Fever	15	14
Accidental injury	14	12
Abdominal pain	10	5
Asthenia	8	4
Flu syndrome	7	6
Pain	5	4
Facial edema	2	1
Photosensitivity	2	0

Body System/ Adverse Reaction	LAMICTAL	Placebo
Cardiovascular		
Hemorrhage	2	1
Digestive		
Vomiting	20	16
Diarrhea	11	9
Nausea	10	2
Constipation	4	2
Dyspepsia	2	1
Hemic and lymphatic		
Lymphadenopathy	2	1
Metabolic and nutritional		
Edema	2	0
Nervous system		
Somnolence	17	15
Dizziness	14	4
Ataxia	11	3
Tremor	10	1
Emotional lability	4	2
Gait abnormality	4	2
Thinking abnormality	3	2
Convulsions	2	1
Nervousness	2	1
Vertigo	2	1
Respiratory		
Pharyngitis	14	11
Bronchitis	7	5
Increased cough	7	6
Sinusitis	2	1
Bronchospasm	2	1
Skin		
Rash	14	12
Eczema	2	1
Pruritus	2	1
Special senses		
Diplopia	5	1
Blurred vision	4	1
Visual abnormality	2	0
Urogenital		
Male and female patients		
Urinary tract infection	3	0

Bipolar Disorder: The most commonly observed (≥5%) treatment-emergent adverse reactions seen in association with the use of LAMICTAL as monotherapy (100 to 400 mg/day) in adult patients (≥18 years of age) with Bipolar Disorder in the 2 double-blind, placebo-controlled trials of 18 months' duration, and numerically more frequent than in placebo-treated patients are included in Table 12. Adverse reactions that occurred in at least 5% of patients and were numerically more common during the dose-escalation phase of LAMICTAL in these trials (when patients may have been receiving concomitant medications) compared with the monotherapy phase were: headache (25%), rash (11%), dizziness (10%), diarrhea (8%), dream abnormality (6%), and pruritus (6%).
During the monotherapy phase of the double-blind, placebo-controlled trials of 18 months' duration, 13% of 227 patients who received LAMICTAL (100 to 400 mg/day), 16% of 190 patients who received placebo, and 23% of 166 patients who received lithium discontinued therapy because of an adverse reaction. The adverse reactions which most commonly led to discontinuation of LAMICTAL were rash (3%) and mania/hypomania/mixed mood adverse reactions (2%). Approximately 16% of 2,401 patients who received LAMICTAL (50 to 500 mg/day) for Bipolar Disorder in premarketing trials discontinued therapy because of an adverse reaction, most commonly due to rash (5%) and mania/hypomania/mixed mood adverse reactions (2%).
The overall adverse reaction profile for LAMICTAL was similar between females and males, between elderly and nonelderly patients, and among racial groups.

Table 12. Treatment-Emergent Adverse Reaction Incidence in 2 Placebo-Controlled Trials in Adults With Bipolar I Disorder[a] (Adverse reactions in at least 5% of patients treated with LAMICTAL as monotherapy and numerically more frequent than in the placebo group.)

Body System/ Adverse Reaction	Percent of Patients Receiving LAMICTAL (n = 227)	Percent of Patients Receiving Placebo (n = 190)
General		
Back pain	8	6

Table 10. Treatment-Emergent Adverse Reaction Incidence in Adults With Partial Seizures in a Controlled Monotherapy Trial[a] (Adverse reactions in at least 5% of patients treated with LAMICTAL and numerically more frequent than in the valproate group.)

Body System/ Adverse Reaction	Percent of Patients Receiving LAMICTAL as Monotherapy[b] (n = 43)	Percent of Patients Receiving Low-Dose Valproate[c] Monotherapy (n = 44)
Body as a whole		
Pain	5	0
Infection	5	2
Chest pain	5	2
Digestive		
Vomiting	9	0
Dyspepsia	7	2
Nausea	7	2
Metabolic and nutritional		
Weight decrease	5	2
Nervous		
Coordination abnormality	7	0
Dizziness	7	0
Anxiety	5	0
Insomnia	5	2
Respiratory		
Rhinitis	7	2
Urogenital (female patients only)	(n = 21)	(n = 28)
Dysmenorrhea	5	0

[a]Patients in these studies were converted to LAMICTAL or valproate monotherapy from adjunctive therapy with carbamazepine or phenytoin. Patients may have reported multiple adverse reactions during the study; thus, patients may be included in more than one category.
[b]Up to 500 mg/day.
[c]1,000 mg/day.

Fatigue	8	5
Abdominal pain	6	3
Digestive		
Nausea	14	11
Constipation	5	2
Vomiting	5	2
Nervous System		
Insomnia	10	6
Somnolence	9	7
Xerostomia (dry mouth)	6	4
Respiratory		
Rhinitis	7	4
Exacerbation of cough	5	3
Pharyngitis	5	4
Skin		
Rash (nonserious)[b]	7	5

[a]Patients in these studies were converted to LAMICTAL (100 to 400 mg/day) or placebo monotherapy from add-on therapy with other psychotropic medications. Patients may have reported multiple adverse reactions during the study; thus, patients may be included in more than one category.

[b]In the overall bipolar and other mood disorders clinical trials, the rate of serious rash was 0.08% (1 of 1,233) of adult patients who received LAMICTAL as initial monotherapy and 0.13% (2 of 1,538) of adult patients who received LAMICTAL as adjunctive therapy [see Warnings and Precautions (5.1)].

These adverse reactions were usually mild to moderate in intensity. Other reactions that occurred in 5% or more patients but equally or more frequently in the placebo group included: dizziness, mania, headache, infection, influenza, pain, accidental injury, diarrhea, and dyspepsia.

Adverse reactions that occurred with a frequency of less than 5% and greater than 1% of patients receiving LAMICTAL and numerically more frequent than placebo were:

General: Fever, neck pain.
Cardiovascular: Migraine.
Digestive: Flatulence.
Metabolic and Nutritional: Weight gain, edema.
Musculoskeletal: Arthralgia, myalgia.
Nervous System: Amnesia, depression, agitation, emotional lability, dyspraxia, abnormal thoughts, dream abnormality, hypoesthesia.
Respiratory: Sinusitis.
Urogenital: Urinary frequency.
Adverse Reactions Following Abrupt Discontinuation: In the 2 maintenance trials, there was no increase in the incidence, severity, or type of adverse reactions in Bipolar Disorder patients after abruptly terminating therapy with LAMICTAL. In clinical trials in patients with Bipolar Disorder, 2 patients experienced seizures shortly after abrupt withdrawal of LAMICTAL. However, there were confounding factors that may have contributed to the occurrence of seizures in these bipolar patients [see Warnings and Precautions (5.9)].
Mania/Hypomania/Mixed Episodes: During the double-blind, placebo-controlled clinical trials in Bipolar I Disorder in which patients were converted to monotherapy with LAMICTAL (100 to 400 mg/day) from other psychotropic medications and followed for up to 18 months, the rates of manic or hypomanic or mixed mood episodes reported as adverse reactions were 5% for patients treated with LAMICTAL (n = 227), 4% for patients treated with lithium (n = 166), and 7% for patients treated with placebo (n = 190). In all bipolar controlled trials combined, adverse reactions of mania (including hypomania and mixed mood episodes) were reported in 5% of patients treated with LAMICTAL (n = 956), 3% of patients treated with lithium (n = 280), and 4% of patients treated with placebo (n = 803).

6.2   Other Adverse Reactions Observed in All Clinical Trials

LAMICTAL has been administered to 6,694 individuals for whom complete adverse reaction data was captured during all clinical trials, only some of which were placebo controlled. During these trials, all adverse reactions were recorded by the clinical investigators using terminology of their own choosing. To provide a meaningful estimate of the proportion of individuals having adverse reactions, similar types of adverse reactions were grouped into a smaller number of standardized categories using modified COSTART dictionary terminology. The frequencies presented represent the proportion of the 6,694 individuals exposed to LAMICTAL who experienced an event of the type cited on at least one occasion while receiving LAMICTAL. All reported adverse reactions are included except those already listed in the previous tables or elsewhere in the labeling, those too general to be informative, and those not reasonably associated with the use of the drug.

Adverse reactions are further classified within body system categories and enumerated in order of decreasing frequency using the following definitions: *frequent* adverse reactions are defined as those occurring in at least 1/100 patients; *infrequent* adverse reactions are those occurring in 1/100 to 1/1,000 patients; *rare* adverse reactions are those occurring in fewer than 1/1,000 patients.

Body as a Whole: *Infrequent:* Allergic reaction, chills, and malaise.
Cardiovascular System: *Infrequent:* Flushing, hot flashes, hypertension, palpitations, postural hypotension, syncope, tachycardia, and vasodilation.
Dermatological: *Infrequent:* Acne, alopecia, hirsutism, maculopapular rash, skin discoloration, and urticaria. *Rare:* Angioedema, erythema, exfoliative dermatitis, fungal dermatitis, herpes zoster, leukoderma, multiforme erythema, petechial rash, pustular rash, Stevens-Johnson syndrome, and vesiculobullous rash.
Digestive System: *Infrequent:* Dysphagia, eructation, gastritis, gingivitis, increased appetite, increased salivation, liver function tests abnormal, and mouth ulceration. *Rare:* Gastrointestinal hemorrhage, glossitis, gum hemorrhage, gum hyperplasia, hematemesis, hemorrhagic colitis, hepatitis, melena, stomach ulcer, stomatitis, and tongue edema.
Endocrine System: *Rare:* Goiter and hypothyroidism.
Hematologic and Lymphatic System: *Infrequent:* Ecchymosis and leukopenia. *Rare:* Anemia, eosinophilia, fibrin decrease, fibrinogen decrease, iron deficiency anemia, leukocytosis, lymphocytosis, macrocytic anemia, petechia, and thrombocytopenia.
Metabolic and Nutritional Disorders: *Infrequent:* Aspartate transaminase increased. *Rare:* Alcohol intolerance, alkaline phosphatase increase, alanine transaminase increase, bilirubinemia, general edema, gamma glutamyl transpeptidase increase, and hyperglycemia.
Musculoskeletal System: *Infrequent:* Arthritis, leg cramps, myasthenia, and twitching. *Rare:* Bursitis, muscle atrophy, pathological fracture, and tendinous contracture.
Nervous System: *Frequent:* Confusion and paresthesia. *Infrequent:* Akathisia, apathy, aphasia, central nervous system (CNS) depression, depersonalization, dysarthria, dyskinesia, euphoria, hallucinations, hostility, hyperkinesia, hypertonia, libido decreased, memory decrease, mind racing, movement disorder, myoclonus, panic attack, paranoid reaction, personality disorder, psychosis, sleep disorder, stupor, and suicidal ideation. *Rare:* Choreoathetosis, delirium, delusions, dysphoria, dystonia, extrapyramidal syndrome, faintness, grand mal convulsions, hemiplegia, hyperalgesia, hyperesthesia, hypokinesia, hypotonia, manic depression reaction, muscle spasm, neuralgia, neurosis, paralysis, and peripheral neuritis.

Respiratory System: *Infrequent:* Yawn. *Rare:* Hiccup and hyperventilation.
Special Senses: *Frequent:* Amblyopia. *Infrequent:* Abnormality of accommodation, conjunctivitis, dry eyes, ear pain, photophobia, taste perversion, and tinnitus. *Rare:* Deafness, lacrimation disorder, oscillopsia, parosmia, ptosis, strabismus, taste loss, uveitis, and visual field defect.
Urogenital System: *Infrequent:* Abnormal ejaculation, hematuria, impotence, menorrhagia, polyuria, and urinary incontinence. *Rare:* Acute kidney failure, anorgasmia, breast abscess, breast neoplasm, creatinine increase, cystitis, dysuria, epididymitis, female lactation, kidney failure, kidney pain, nocturia, urinary retention, and urinary urgency.

6.3   Postmarketing Experience
The following adverse events (not listed above in clinical trials or other sections of the prescribing information) have been identified during postapproval use of LAMICTAL. Because these events are reported voluntarily from a population of uncertain size, it is not always possible to reliably estimate their frequency or establish a causal relationship to drug exposure.

Blood and Lymphatic: Agranulocytosis, hemolytic anemia, lymphadenopathy not associated with hypersensitivity disorder.
Gastrointestinal: Esophagitis.
Hepatobiliary Tract and Pancreas: Pancreatitis.
Immunologic: Lupus-like reaction, vasculitis.
Lower Respiratory: Apnea.
Musculoskeletal: Rhabdomyolysis has been observed in patients experiencing hypersensitivity reactions.
Neurology: Exacerbation of Parkinsonian symptoms in patients with pre-existing Parkinson's disease, tics.
Non-site Specific: Progressive immunosuppression.

7   DRUG INTERACTIONS
Significant drug interactions with lamotrigine are summarized in Table 13. Additional details of these drug interaction studies are provided in the Clinical Pharmacology section [see Clinical Pharmacology (12.3)].
[See table 13 above]

8   USE IN SPECIFIC POPULATIONS
8.1   Pregnancy
Teratogenic Effects: Pregnancy Category C. No evidence of teratogenicity was found in mice, rats, or rabbits when lamotrigine was orally administered to pregnant animals during the period of organogenesis at doses up to 1.2, 0.5, and 1.1 times, respectively, on a mg/m^2 basis, the highest usual human maintenance dose (i.e., 500 mg/day). However, maternal toxicity and secondary fetal toxicity producing reduced fetal weight and/or delayed ossification were seen in mice and rats, but not in rabbits at these doses. Teratology studies were also conducted using bolus intravenous administration of the isethionate salt of lamotrigine in rats and rabbits. In rat dams administered an intravenous dose at

Table 13. Established and Other Potentially Significant Drug Interactions

Concomitant Drug	Effect on Concentration of Lamotrigine or Concomitant Drug	Clinical Comment
Estrogen-containing oral contraceptive preparations containing 30 mcg ethinylestradiol and 150 mcg levonorgestrel	↓ lamotrigine	Decreased lamotrigine levels approximately 50%.
	↓ levonorgestrel	Decrease in levonorgestrel component by 19%.
Carbamazepine (CBZ) and CBZ epoxide	↓ lamotrigine	Addition of carbamazepine decreases lamotrigine concentration approximately 40%.
	? CBZ epoxide	May increase CBZ epoxide levels
Phenobarbital/primidone	↓ lamotrigine	Decreased lamotrigine concentration approximately 40%.
Phenytoin (PHT)	↓ lamotrigine	Decreased lamotrigine concentration approximately 40%.
Rifampin	↓ lamotrigine	Decreased lamotrigine AUC approximately 40%.
Valproate	↑ lamotrigine	Increased lamotrigine concentrations slightly more than 2-fold.
	? valproate	Decreased valproate concentrations an average of 25% over a 3-week period then stabilized in healthy volunteers; no change in controlled clinical trials in epilepsy patients.

↓= Decreased (induces lamotrigine glucuronidation).
↑= Increased (inhibits lamotrigine glucuronidation).
? = Conflicting data.

0.6 times the highest usual human maintenance dose, the incidence of intrauterine death without signs of teratogenicity was increased.

A behavioral teratology study was conducted in rats dosed during the period of organogenesis. At day 21 postpartum, offspring of dams receiving 5 mg/kg/day or higher displayed a significantly longer latent period for open field exploration and a lower frequency of rearing. In a swimming maze test performed on days 39 to 44 postpartum, time to completion was increased in offspring of dams receiving 25 mg/kg/day. These doses represent 0.1 and 0.5 times the clinical dose on a mg/m^2 basis, respectively.

Lamotrigine did not affect fertility, teratogenesis, or postnatal development when rats were dosed prior to and during mating, and throughout gestation and lactation at doses equivalent to 0.4 times the highest usual human maintenance dose on a mg/m^2 basis.

When pregnant rats were orally dosed at 0.1, 0.14, or 0.3 times the highest human maintenance dose (on a mg/m^2 basis) during the latter part of gestation (days 15 to 20), maternal toxicity and fetal death were seen. In dams, food consumption and weight gain were reduced, and the gestation period was slightly prolonged (22.6 vs. 22.0 days in the control group). Stillborn pups were found in all 3 drug-treated groups with the highest number in the high-dose group. Postnatal death was also seen, but only in the 2 highest doses, and occurred between days 1 and 20. Some of these deaths appear to be drug-related and not secondary to the maternal toxicity. A no-observed-effect level (NOEL) could not be determined for this study.

Although lamotrigine was not found to be teratogenic in the above studies, lamotrigine decreases fetal folate concentrations in rats, an effect known to be associated with teratogenesis in animals and humans. There are no adequate and well-controlled studies in pregnant women. Because animal reproduction studies are not always predictive of human response, this drug should be used during pregnancy only if the potential benefit justifies the potential risk to the fetus.

Non-Teratogenic Effects: As with other AEDs, physiological changes during pregnancy may affect lamotrigine concentrations and/or therapeutic effect. There have been reports of decreased lamotrigine concentrations during pregnancy and restoration of pre-partum concentrations after delivery. Dosage adjustments may be necessary to maintain clinical response.

Pregnancy Exposure Registry: To provide information regarding the effects of in utero exposure to LAMICTAL, physicians are advised to recommend that pregnant patients taking LAMICTAL enroll in the North American Antiepileptic Drug (NAAED) Pregnancy Registry. This can be done by calling the toll-free number 1-888-233-2334, and must be done by patients themselves. Information on the registry can also be found at the website http://www.aedpregnancyregistry.org/.

Physicians are also encouraged to register patients in the Lamotrigine Pregnancy Registry; enrollment in this registry must be done prior to any prenatal diagnostic tests and before fetal outcome is known. Physicians can obtain information by calling the Lamotrigine Pregnancy Registry at 1-800-336-2176 (toll-free).

8.2 Labor and Delivery
The effect of LAMICTAL on labor and delivery in humans is unknown.

8.3 Nursing Mothers
Lamotrigine is present in milk from lactating women taking LAMICTAL. Data from multiple small studies indicate that lamotrigine plasma levels in human milk-fed infants have been reported to be as high as 50% of the maternal serum levels. Neonates and young infants are at risk for high serum levels because maternal serum and milk levels can rise to high levels postpartum if lamotrigine dosage has been increased during pregnancy but not later reduced to the pre-pregnancy dosage. Lamotrigine exposure is further increased due to the immaturity of the infant glucuronidation capacity needed for drug clearance. Events including apnea, drowsiness, and poor sucking have been reported in infants who have been human milk-fed by mothers using lamotrigine; whether or not these events were caused by lamotrigine is unknown. Human milk-fed infants should be closely monitored for adverse events resulting from lamotrigine. Measurement of infant serum levels should be performed to rule out toxicity if concerns arise. Human milk-feeding should be discontinued in infants with lamotrigine toxicity. Caution should be exercised when LAMICTAL is administered to a nursing woman.

8.4 Pediatric Use
LAMICTAL is indicated for adjunctive therapy in patients ≥2 years of age for partial seizures, the generalized seizures of Lennox-Gastaut syndrome, and primary generalized tonic-clonic seizures.

Safety and efficacy of LAMICTAL, used as adjunctive treatment for partial seizures, were not demonstrated in a small randomized, double-blind, placebo-controlled, withdrawal study in very young pediatric patients (1 to 24 months of age). LAMICTAL was associated with an increased risk for infectious adverse reactions (LAMICTAL 37%, placebo 5%), and respiratory adverse reactions (LAMICTAL 26%, placebo 5%). Infectious adverse reactions included bronchiolitis, bronchitis, ear infection, eye infection, otitis externa, pharyngitis, urinary tract infection, and viral infection. Respiratory adverse reactions included nasal congestion, cough, and apnea.

Safety and effectiveness in patients below the age of 18 years with Bipolar Disorder have not been established.

8.5 Geriatric Use
Clinical studies of LAMICTAL for epilepsy and in Bipolar Disorder did not include sufficient numbers of subjects 65 years of age and over to determine whether they respond differently from younger subjects or exhibit a different safety profile than that of younger patients. In general, dose selection for an elderly patient should be cautious, usually starting at the low end of the dosing range, reflecting the greater frequency of decreased hepatic, renal, or cardiac function, and of concomitant disease or other drug therapy.

8.6 Patients With Hepatic Impairment
Experience in patients with hepatic impairment is limited. Based on a clinical pharmacology study in 24 patients with mild, moderate, and severe liver impairment [see Clinical Pharmacology (12.3)], the following general recommendations can be made. No dosage adjustment is needed in patients with mild liver impairment. Initial, escalation, and maintenance doses should generally be reduced by approximately 25% in patients with moderate and severe liver impairment without ascites and 50% in patients with severe liver impairment with ascites. Escalation and maintenance doses may be adjusted according to clinical response [see Dosage and Administration (2.1)].

8.7 Patients With Renal Impairment
Lamotrigine is metabolized mainly by glucuronic acid conjugation, with the majority of the metabolites being recovered in the urine. In a small study comparing a single dose of lamotrigine in patients with varying degrees of renal impairment with healthy volunteers, the plasma half-life of lamotrigine was significantly longer in the patients with renal impairment [see Clinical Pharmacology (12.3)].

Initial doses of LAMICTAL should be based on patients' AED regimens; reduced maintenance doses may be effective for patients with significant renal impairment. Few patients with severe renal impairment have been evaluated during chronic treatment with LAMICTAL. Because there is inadequate experience in this population, LAMICTAL should be used with caution in these patients [see Dosage and Administration (2.1)].

10 OVERDOSAGE
10.1 Human Overdose Experience
Overdoses involving quantities up to 15 g have been reported for LAMICTAL, some of which have been fatal. Overdose has resulted in ataxia, nystagmus, seizures (including tonic-clonic seizures), decreased level of consciousness, coma, and intraventricular conduction delay.

10.2 Management of Overdose
There are no specific antidotes for lamotrigine. Following a suspected overdose, hospitalization of the patient is advised. General supportive care is indicated, including frequent monitoring of vital signs and close observation of the patient. If indicated, emesis should be induced; usual precautions should be taken to protect the airway. It should be kept in mind that lamotrigine is rapidly absorbed [see Clinical Pharmacology (12.3)]. It is uncertain whether hemodialysis is an effective means of removing lamotrigine from the blood. In 6 renal failure patients, about 20% of the amount of lamotrigine in the body was removed by hemodialysis during a 4-hour session. A Poison Control Center should be contacted for information on the management of overdosage of LAMICTAL.

11 DESCRIPTION
LAMICTAL (lamotrigine), an AED of the phenyltriazine class, is chemically unrelated to existing AEDs. Its chemical name is 3,5-diamino-6-(2,3-dichlorophenyl)-as-triazine, its molecular formula is $C_9H_7N_5Cl_2$, and its molecular weight is 256.09. Lamotrigine is a white to pale cream-colored powder and has a pK$_a$ of 5.7. Lamotrigine is very slightly soluble in water (0.17 mg/mL at 25°C) and slightly soluble in 0.1 M HCl (4.1 mg/mL at 25°C). The structural formula is:

LAMICTAL Tablets are supplied for oral administration as 25 mg (white), 100 mg (peach), 150 mg (cream), and 200 mg (blue) tablets. Each tablet contains the labeled amount of lamotrigine and the following inactive ingredients: lactose; magnesium stearate; microcrystalline cellulose; povidone; sodium starch glycolate; FD&C Yellow No. 6 Lake (100-mg tablet only); ferric oxide, yellow (150-mg tablet only); and FD&C Blue No. 2 Lake (200-mg tablet only).

LAMICTAL Chewable Dispersible Tablets are supplied for oral administration. The tablets contain 2 mg (white), 5 mg (white), or 25 mg (white) of lamotrigine and the following inactive ingredients: blackcurrant flavor, calcium carbonate, low-substituted hydroxypropylcellulose, magnesium aluminum silicate, magnesium stearate, povidone, saccharin sodium, and sodium starch glycolate.

LAMICTAL ODT Orally Disintegrating Tablets are supplied for oral administration. The tablets contain 25 mg (white to off-white), 50 mg (white to off-white), 100 mg (white to off-white), or 200 mg (white to off-white) of lamotrigine and the following inactive ingredients: artificial cherry flavor, crospovidone, ethylcellulose, magnesium stearate, mannitol, polyethylene, and sucralose.

LAMICTAL ODT Orally Disintegrating Tablets are formulated using technologies (Microcaps® and AdvaTab®) designed to mask the bitter taste of lamotrigine and achieve a rapid dissolution profile. Tablet characteristics including flavor, mouth-feel, after-taste, and ease of use were rated as favorable in a study of 108 healthy volunteers.

12 CLINICAL PHARMACOLOGY
12.1 Mechanism of Action
The precise mechanism(s) by which lamotrigine exerts its anticonvulsant action are unknown. In animal models designed to detect anticonvulsant activity, lamotrigine was effective in preventing seizure spread in the maximum electroshock (MES) and pentylenetetrazol (scMet) tests, and prevented seizures in the visually and electrically evoked after-discharge (EEAD) tests for antiepileptic activity. Lamotrigine also displayed inhibitory properties in the kindling model in rats both during kindling development and in the fully kindled state. The relevance of these models to human epilepsy, however, is not known.

One proposed mechanism of action of lamotrigine, the relevance of which remains to be established in humans, involves an effect on sodium channels. In vitro pharmacological studies suggest that lamotrigine inhibits voltage-sensitive sodium channels, thereby stabilizing neuronal membranes and consequently modulating presynaptic transmitter release of excitatory amino acids (e.g., glutamate and aspartate).

Although the relevance for human use is unknown, the following data characterize the performance of lamotrigine in receptor binding assays. Lamotrigine had a weak inhibitory effect on the serotonin 5-HT$_3$ receptor (IC$_{50}$ = 18 μM). It does not exhibit high affinity binding (IC$_{50}$>100 μM) to the following neurotransmitter receptors: adenosine A$_1$ and A$_2$; adrenergic α$_1$, α$_2$, and β; dopamine D$_1$ and D$_2$; γ-aminobutyric acid (GABA) A and B; histamine H$_1$; kappa opioid; muscarinic acetylcholine; and serotonin 5-HT$_2$. Studies have failed to detect an effect of lamotrigine on dihydropyridine-sensitive calcium channels. It had weak effects at sigma opioid receptors (IC$_{50}$ = 145 μM). Lamotrigine did not inhibit the uptake of norepinephrine, dopamine, or serotonin (IC$_{50}$>200 μM) when tested in rat synaptosomes and/or human platelets in vitro.

Effect of Lamotrigine on N-Methyl d-Aspartate-Receptor Mediated Activity: Lamotrigine did not inhibit N-methyl d-aspartate (NMDA)-induced depolarizations in rat cortical slices or NMDA-induced cyclic GMP formation in immature rat cerebellum, nor did lamotrigine displace compounds that are either competitive or noncompetitive ligands at this glutamate receptor complex (CNQX, CGS, TCHP). The IC$_{50}$ for lamotrigine effects on NMDA-induced currents (in the presence of 3 μM of glycine) in cultured hippocampal neurons exceeded 100 μM.

The mechanisms by which lamotrigine exerts its therapeutic action in Bipolar Disorder have not been established.

12.2 Pharmacodynamics
Folate Metabolism: In vitro, lamotrigine inhibited dihydrofolate reductase, the enzyme that catalyzes the reduction of dihydrofolate to tetrahydrofolate. Inhibition of this enzyme may interfere with the biosynthesis of nucleic acids and proteins. When oral daily doses of lamotrigine were given to pregnant rats during organogenesis, fetal, placental, and maternal folate concentrations were reduced. Significantly reduced concentrations of folate are associated with teratogenesis [see Use in Specific Populations (8.1)]. Folate concentrations were also reduced in male rats given repeated oral doses of lamotrigine. Reduced concentrations were partially returned to normal when supplemented with folinic acid.

Accumulation in Kidneys: Lamotrigine accumulated in the kidney of the male rat, causing chronic progressive nephrosis, necrosis, and mineralization. These findings are attributed to α-2 microglobulin, a species- and sex-specific protein that has not been detected in humans or other animal species.

Melanin Binding: Lamotrigine binds to melanin-containing tissues, e.g., in the eye and pigmented skin. It has been found in the uveal tract up to 52 weeks after a single dose in rodents.

Table 14. Mean[a] Pharmacokinetic Parameters in Healthy Volunteers and Adult Patients With Epilepsy

Adult Study Population	Number of Subjects	T_{max}: Time of Maximum Plasma Concentration (hr)	$t_{1/2}$: Elimination Half-life (hr)	Cl/F: Apparent Plasma Clearance (mL/min/kg)
Healthy volunteers taking no other medications:				
Single-dose LAMICTAL	179	2.2 (0.25-12.0)	32.8 (14.0-103.0)	0.44 (0.12-1.10)
Multiple-dose LAMICTAL	36	1.7 (0.5-4.0)	25.4 (11.6-61.6)	0.58 (0.24-1.15)
Healthy volunteers taking valproate:				
Single-dose LAMICTAL	6	1.8 (1.0-4.0)	48.3 (31.5-88.6)	0.30 (0.14-0.42)
Multiple-dose LAMICTAL	18	1.9 (0.5-3.5)	70.3 (41.9-113.5)	0.18 (0.12-0.33)
Patients with epilepsy taking valproate only:				
Single-dose LAMICTAL	4	4.8 (1.8-8.4)	58.8 (30.5-88.8)	0.28 (0.16-0.40)
Patients with epilepsy taking carbamazepine, phenytoin, phenobarbital, or primidone[b] plus valproate:				
Single-dose LAMICTAL	25	3.8 (1.0-10.0)	27.2 (11.2-51.6)	0.53 (0.27-1.04)
Patients with epilepsy taking carbamazepine, phenytoin, phenobarbital, or primidone:[b]				
Single-dose LAMICTAL	24	2.3 (0.5-5.0)	14.4 (6.4-30.4)	1.10 (0.51-2.22)
Multiple-dose LAMICTAL	17	2.0 (0.75-5.93)	12.6 (7.5-23.1)	1.21 (0.66-1.82)

[a]The majority of parameter means determined in each study had coefficients of variation between 20% and 40% for half-life and Cl/F and between 30% and 70% for T_{max}. The overall mean values were calculated from individual study means that were weighted based on the number of volunteers/patients in each study. The numbers in parentheses below each parameter mean represent the range of individual volunteer/patient values across studies.
[b]Carbamazepine, phenobarbital, phenytoin, and primidone have been shown to increase the apparent clearance of lamotrigine. Estrogen-containing oral contraceptives and other drugs such as rifampin that induce lamotrigine glucuronidation have also been shown to increase the apparent clearance of lamotrigine [see Drug Interactions (7)].

Cardiovascular: In dogs, lamotrigine is extensively metabolized to a 2-N-methyl metabolite. This metabolite causes dose-dependent prolongations of the PR interval, widening of the QRS complex, and, at higher doses, complete AV conduction block. Similar cardiovascular effects are not anticipated in humans because only trace amounts of the 2-N-methyl metabolite (<0.6% of lamotrigine dose) have been found in human urine [see Clinical Pharmacology (12.3)]. However, it is conceivable that plasma concentrations of this metabolite could be increased in patients with a reduced capacity to glucuronidate lamotrigine (e.g., in patients with liver disease).

12.3 Pharmacokinetics
The pharmacokinetics of lamotrigine have been studied in patients with epilepsy, healthy young and elderly volunteers, and volunteers with chronic renal failure. Lamotrigine pharmacokinetic parameters for adult and pediatric patients and healthy normal volunteers are summarized in Table 14 and 16.
[See table 14 above]

Absorption: Lamotrigine is rapidly and completely absorbed after oral administration with negligible first-pass metabolism (absolute bioavailability is 98%). The bioavailability is not affected by food. Peak plasma concentrations occur anywhere from 1.4 to 4.8 hours following drug administration. The lamotrigine chewable/dispersible tablets were found to be equivalent, whether they were administered as dispersed in water, chewed and swallowed, or swallowed as whole, to the lamotrigine compressed tablets in terms of rate and extent of absorption. In terms of rate and extent of absorption, lamotrigine orally disintegrating tablets whether disintegrated in the mouth or swallowed whole with water were equivalent to the lamotrigine compressed tablets swallowed with water.

Dose Proportionality: In healthy volunteers not receiving any other medications and given single doses, the plasma concentrations of lamotrigine increased in direct proportion to the dose administered over the range of 50 to 400 mg. In 2 small studies (n = 7 and 8) of patients with epilepsy who were maintained on other AEDs, there also was a linear relationship between dose and lamotrigine plasma concentrations at steady state following doses of 50 to 350 mg twice daily.

Distribution: Estimates of the mean apparent volume of distribution (Vd/F) of lamotrigine following oral administration ranged from 0.9 to 1.3 L/kg. Vd/F is independent of dose and is similar following single and multiple doses in both patients with epilepsy and in healthy volunteers.

Protein Binding: Data from in vitro studies indicate that lamotrigine is approximately 55% bound to human plasma proteins at plasma lamotrigine concentrations from 1 to 10 mcg/mL (10 mcg/mL is 4 to 6 times the trough plasma concentration observed in the controlled efficacy trials). Because lamotrigine is not highly bound to plasma proteins, clinically significant interactions with other drugs through competition for protein binding sites are unlikely. The binding of lamotrigine to plasma proteins did not change in the presence of therapeutic concentrations of phenytoin, phenobarbital, or valproate. Lamotrigine did not displace other AEDs (carbamazepine, phenytoin, phenobarbital) from protein-binding sites.

Metabolism: Lamotrigine is metabolized predominantly by glucuronic acid conjugation; the major metabolite is an inactive 2-N-glucuronide conjugate. After oral administration of 240 mg of ^{14}C-lamotrigine (15 μCi) to 6 healthy volunteers, 94% was recovered in the urine and 2% was recovered in the feces. The radioactivity in the urine consisted of unchanged lamotrigine (10%), the 2-N-glucuronide (76%), a 5-N-glucuronide (10%), a 2-N-methyl metabolite (0.14%), and other unidentified minor metabolites (4%).

Enzyme Induction: The effects of lamotrigine on the induction of specific families of mixed-function oxidase isozymes have not been systematically evaluated. Following multiple administrations (150 mg twice daily) to normal volunteers taking no other medications, lamotrigine induced its own metabolism, resulting in a 25% decrease in $t_{1/2}$ and a 37% increase in Cl/F at steady state compared with values obtained in the same volunteers following a single dose. Evidence gathered from other sources suggests that self-induction by lamotrigine may not occur when lamotrigine is given as adjunctive therapy in patients receiving enzyme-inducing drugs such as carbamazepine, phenytoin, phenobarbital, primidone, or drugs such as rifampin that induce lamotrigine glucuronidation [see Drug Interactions (7)].

Elimination: The elimination half-life and apparent clearance of lamotrigine following administration of LAMICTAL

to adult patients with epilepsy and healthy volunteers is summarized in Table 14. Half-life and apparent oral clearance vary depending on concomitant AEDs.

Drug Interactions: The apparent clearance of lamotrigine is affected by the coadministration of certain medications [see Warnings and Precautions (5.8, 5.12), Drug Interactions (7)].
The net effects of drug interactions with LAMICTAL are summarized in Tables 13 and 15, followed by details of the drug interaction studies below.

Table 15. Summary of Drug Interactions With LAMICTAL

Drug	Drug Plasma Concentration With Adjunctive LAMICTAL[a]	Lamotrigine Plasma Concentration With Adjunctive Drugs[b]
Oral contraceptives (e.g., ethinylestradiol/levonorgestrel)[c]	↔[d]	↓
Bupropion	Not assessed	↔
Carbamazepine (CBZ)	↔	↓
CBZ epoxide[e]	?	
Felbamate	Not assessed	↔
Gabapentin	Not assessed	↔
Levetiracetam	↔	↔
Lithium	↔	Not assessed
Olanzapine	↔	↔[f]
Oxcarbazepine	↔	↔
10-monohydroxy oxcarbazepine metabolite[g]	↔	
Phenobarbital/primidone	↔	↓
Phenytoin (PHT)	↔	↓
Pregabalin	↔	↔
Rifampin	Not assessed	↓
Topiramate	↔[h]	↔
Valproate	↓	↑
Valproate + PHT and/or CBZ	Not assessed	↔
Zonisamide	Not assessed	↔

[a]From adjunctive clinical trials and volunteer studies.
[b]Net effects were estimated by comparing the mean clearance values obtained in adjunctive clinical trials and volunteer studies.
[c]The effect of other hormonal contraceptive preparations or hormone replacement therapy on the pharmacokinetics of lamotrigine has not been systematically evaluated in clinical trials, although the effect may be similar to that seen with the ethinylestradiol/levonorgestrel combinations.
[d]Modest decrease in levonorgestrel.
[e]Not administered, but an active metabolite of carbamazepine.
[f]Slight decrease, not expected to be clinically relevant.
[g] Not administered, but an active metabolite of oxcarbazepine.
[h]Slight increase, not expected to be clinically relevant.
↔ = No significant effect.
? = Conflicting data.

Estrogen-Containing Oral Contraceptives: In 16 female volunteers, an oral contraceptive preparation containing 30 mcg ethinylestradiol and 150 mcg levonorgestrel increased the apparent clearance of lamotrigine (300 mg/day) by approximately 2-fold with mean decreases in AUC of 52% and in C_{max} of 39%. In this study, trough serum lamotrigine concentrations gradually increased and were approximately 2-fold higher on average at the end of the week of the inactive hormone preparation compared with trough lamotrigine concentrations at the end of the active hormone cycle.
Gradual transient increases in lamotrigine plasma levels (approximate 2-fold increase) occurred during the week of inactive hormone preparation ("pill-free" week) for women not also taking a drug that increased the clearance of lamotrigine (carbamazepine, phenytoin, phenobarbital, primidone, or other drugs such as rifampin that induce lamotrigine glucuronidation [see Drug Interactions (7)]). The increase in lamotrigine plasma levels will be greater if the dose of LAMICTAL is increased in the few days before or during the "pill-free" week. Increases in lamotrigine plasma levels could result in dose-dependent adverse reactions.
In the same study, coadministration of LAMICTAL (300 mg/day) in 16 female volunteers did not affect the pharmacokinetics of the ethinylestradiol component of the oral contraceptive preparation. There were mean decreases in the AUC

Table 16. Mean Pharmacokinetic Parameters in Pediatric Patients With Epilepsy

Pediatric Study Population	Number of Subjects	T_{max} (hr)	$t\frac{1}{2}$ (hr)	Cl/F (mL/min/kg)
Ages 10 months-5.3 years				
Patients taking carbamazepine, phenytoin, phenobarbital, or primidone[a]	10	3.0 (1.0-5.9)	7.7 (5.7-11.4)	3.62 (2.44-5.28)
Patients taking AEDs with no known effect on the apparent clearance of lamotrigine	7	5.2 (2.9-6.1)	19.0 (12.9-27.1)	1.2 (0.75-2.42)
Patients taking valproate only	8	2.9 (1.0-6.0)	44.9 (29.5-52.5)	0.47 (0.23-0.77)
Ages 5-11 years				
Patients taking carbamazepine, phenytoin, phenobarbital, or primidone[a]	7	1.6 (1.0-3.0)	7.0 (3.8-9.8)	2.54 (1.35-5.58)
Patients taking carbamazepine, phenytoin, phenobarbital, or primidone[a] plus valproate	8	3.3 (1.0-6.4)	19.1 (7.0-31.2)	0.89 (0.39-1.93)
Patients taking valproate only[b]	3	4.5 (3.0-6.0)	65.8 (50.7-73.7)	0.24 (0.21-0.26)
Ages 13-18 years				
Patients taking carbamazepine, phenytoin, phenobarbital, or primidone[a]	11	c	c	1.3
Patients taking carbamazepine, phenytoin, phenobarbital, or primidone[a] plus valproate	8	c	c	0.5
Patients taking valproate only	4	c	c	0.3

[a]Carbamazepine, phenobarbital, phenytoin, and primidone have been shown to increase the apparent clearance of lamotrigine. Estrogen-containing oral contraceptives and rifampin have also been shown to increase the apparent clearance of lamotrigine [see Drug Interactions (7)].
[b]Two subjects were included in the calculation for mean T_{max}.
[c]Parameter not estimated.

and C_{max} of the levonorgestrel component of 19% and 12%, respectively. Measurement of serum progesterone indicated that there was no hormonal evidence of ovulation in any of the 16 volunteers, although measurement of serum FSH, LH, and estradiol indicated that there was some loss of suppression of the hypothalamic-pituitary-ovarian axis.
The effects of doses of LAMICTAL other than 300 mg/day have not been systematically evaluated in controlled clinical trials.
The clinical significance of the observed hormonal changes on ovulatory activity is unknown. However, the possibility of decreased contraceptive efficacy in some patients cannot be excluded. Therefore, patients should be instructed to promptly report changes in their menstrual pattern (e.g., break-through bleeding).
Dosage adjustments may be necessary for women receiving estrogen-containing oral contraceptive preparations [see Dosage and Administration (2.1)].
Other Hormonal Contraceptives or Hormone Replacement Therapy: The effect of other hormonal contraceptive preparations or hormone replacement therapy on the pharmacokinetics of lamotrigine has not been systematically evaluated. It has been reported that ethinylestradiol, not progestogens, increased the clearance of lamotrigine up to 2-fold, and the progestin-only pills had no effect on lamotrigine plasma levels. Therefore, adjustments to the dosage of LAMICTAL in the presence of progestogens alone will likely not be needed.
Bupropion: The pharmacokinetics of a 100-mg single dose of LAMICTAL in healthy volunteers (n = 12) were not changed by coadministration of bupropion sustained-release formulation (150 mg twice daily) starting 11 days before LAMICTAL.
Carbamazepine: LAMICTAL has no appreciable effect on steady-state carbamazepine plasma concentration. Limited clinical data suggest there is a higher incidence of dizziness, diplopia, ataxia, and blurred vision in patients receiving carbamazepine with lamotrigine than in patients receiving other AEDs with lamotrigine [see Adverse Reactions (6.1)]. The mechanism of this interaction is unclear. The effect of lamotrigine on plasma concentrations of carbamazepine-epoxide is unclear. In a small subset of patients (n = 7) studied in a placebo-controlled trial, lamotrigine had no effect on carbamazepine-epoxide plasma concentrations, but in a small, uncontrolled study (n = 9), carbamazepine-epoxide levels increased.
The addition of carbamazepine decreases lamotrigine steady-state concentrations by approximately 40%.
Felbamate: In a study of 21 healthy volunteers, coadministration of felbamate (1,200 mg twice daily) with lamotrigine (100 mg twice daily for 10 days) appeared to have no clinically relevant effects on the pharmacokinetics of lamotrigine.
Folate Inhibitors: Lamotrigine is a weak inhibitor of dihydrofolate reductase. Prescribers should be aware of this action when prescribing other medications that inhibit folate metabolism.

Gabapentin: Based on a retrospective analysis of plasma levels in 34 patients who received lamotrigine both with and without gabapentin, gabapentin does not appear to change the apparent clearance of lamotrigine.
Levetiracetam: Potential drug interactions between levetiracetam and lamotrigine were assessed by evaluating serum concentrations of both agents during placebo-controlled clinical trials. These data indicate that lamotrigine does not influence the pharmacokinetics of levetiracetam and that levetiracetam does not influence the pharmacokinetics of lamotrigine.
Lithium: The pharmacokinetics of lithium were not altered in healthy subjects (n = 20) by coadministration of lamotrigine (100 mg/day) for 6 days.
Olanzapine: The AUC and C_{max} of olanzapine were similar following the addition of olanzapine (15 mg once daily) to lamotrigine (200 mg once daily) in healthy male volunteers (n = 16) compared with the AUC and C_{max} in healthy male volunteers receiving olanzapine alone (n = 16).
In the same study, the AUC and C_{max} of lamotrigine were reduced on average by 24% and 20%, respectively, following the addition of olanzapine to lamotrigine in healthy male volunteers compared with those receiving lamotrigine alone. This reduction in lamotrigine plasma concentrations is not expected to be clinically relevant.
Oxcarbazepine: The AUC and C_{max} of oxcarbazepine and its active 10-monohydroxy oxcarbazepine metabolite were not significantly different following the addition of oxcarbazepine (600 mg twice daily) to lamotrigine (200 mg once daily) in healthy male volunteers (n = 13) compared with healthy male volunteers receiving oxcarbazepine alone (n = 13).
In the same study, the AUC and C_{max} of lamotrigine were similar following the addition of oxcarbazepine (600 mg twice daily) to LAMICTAL in healthy male volunteers compared with those receiving LAMICTAL alone. Limited clinical data suggest a higher incidence of headache, dizziness, nausea, and somnolence with coadministration of lamotrigine and oxcarbazepine compared with lamotrigine alone or oxcarbazepine alone.
Phenobarbital, Primidone: The addition of phenobarbital or primidone decreases lamotrigine steady-state concentrations by approximately 40%.
Phenytoin: Lamotrigine has no appreciable effect on steady-state phenytoin plasma concentrations in patients with epilepsy. The addition of phenytoin decreases lamotrigine steady-state concentrations by approximately 40%.
Pregabalin: Steady-state trough plasma concentrations of lamotrigine were not affected by concomitant pregabalin (200 mg 3 times daily) administration. There are no pharmacokinetic interactions between lamotrigine and pregabalin.
Rifampin: In 10 male volunteers, rifampin (600 mg/day for 5 days) significantly increased the apparent clearance of a single 25-mg dose of lamotrigine by approximately 2-fold (AUC decreased by approximately 40%).

Topiramate: Topiramate resulted in no change in plasma concentrations of lamotrigine. Administration of lamotrigine resulted in a 15% increase in topiramate concentrations.
Valproate: When lamotrigine was administered to healthy volunteers (n = 18) receiving valproate, the trough steady-state valproate plasma concentrations decreased by an average of 25% over a 3-week period, and then stabilized. However, adding lamotrigine to the existing therapy did not cause a change in valproate plasma concentrations in either adult or pediatric patients in controlled clinical trials.
The addition of valproate increased lamotrigine steady-state concentrations in normal volunteers by slightly more than 2-fold. In one study, maximal inhibition of lamotrigine clearance was reached at valproate doses between 250 and 500 mg/day and did not increase as the valproate dose was further increased.
Zonisamide: In a study of 18 patients with epilepsy, coadministration of zonisamide (200 to 400 mg/day) with lamotrigine (150 to 500 mg/day for 35 days) had no significant effect on the pharmacokinetics of lamotrigine.
Known Inducers or Inhibitors of Glucuronidation: Drugs other than those listed above have not been systematically evaluated in combination with lamotrigine. Since lamotrigine is metabolized predominantly by glucuronic acid conjugation, drugs that are known to induce or inhibit glucuronidation may affect the apparent clearance of lamotrigine and doses of lamotrigine may require adjustment based on clinical response.
Other: Results of in vitro experiments suggest that clearance of lamotrigine is unlikely to be reduced by concomitant administration of amitriptyline, clonazepam, clozapine, fluoxetine, haloperidol, lorazepam, phenelzine, risperidone, sertraline, or trazodone.
Results of in vitro experiments suggest that lamotrigine does not reduce the clearance of drugs eliminated predominantly by CYP2D6.
Special Populations: *Patients With Renal Impairment:* Twelve volunteers with chronic renal failure (mean creatinine clearance: 13 mL/min, range: 6 to 23) and another 6 individuals undergoing hemodialysis were each given a single 100-mg dose of lamotrigine. The mean plasma half-lives determined in the study were 42.9 hours (chronic renal failure), 13.0 hours (during hemodialysis), and 57.4 hours (between hemodialysis) compared with 26.2 hours in healthy volunteers. On average, approximately 20% (range: 5.6 to 35.1) of the amount of lamotrigine present in the body was eliminated by hemodialysis during a 4-hour session [see Dosage and Administration (2.1)].
Hepatic Disease: The pharmacokinetics of lamotrigine following a single 100-mg dose of lamotrigine were evaluated in 24 subjects with mild, moderate, and severe hepatic impairment (Child-Pugh Classification system) and compared with 12 subjects without hepatic impairment. The patients with severe hepatic impairment were without ascites (n = 2) or with ascites (n = 5). The mean apparent clearances of lamotrigine in patients with mild (n = 12), moderate (n = 5), severe without ascites (n = 2), and severe with ascites (n = 5) liver impairment were 0.30 ± 0.09, 0.24 ± 0.1, 0.21 ± 0.04, and 0.15 ± 0.09 mL/min/kg, respectively, as compared with 0.37 ± 0.1 mL/min/kg in the healthy controls. Mean half-lives of lamotrigine in patients with mild, moderate, severe without ascites, and severe with ascites hepatic impairment were 46 ± 20, 72 ± 44, 67 ± 11, and 100 ± 48 hours, respectively, as compared with 33 ± 7 hours in healthy controls [see Dosage and Administration (2.1)].
Age: Pediatric Patients: The pharmacokinetics of lamotrigine following a single 2-mg/kg dose were evaluated in 2 studies of pediatric patients (n = 29 for patients 10 months to 5.9 years of age and n = 26 for patients 5 to 11 years of age). Forty-three patients received concomitant therapy with other AEDs and 12 patients received lamotrigine as monotherapy. Lamotrigine pharmacokinetic parameters for pediatric patients are summarized in Table 16.
Population pharmacokinetic analyses involving patients 2 to 18 years of age demonstrated that lamotrigine clearance was influenced predominantly by total body weight and concurrent AED therapy. The oral clearance of lamotrigine was higher, on a body weight basis, in pediatric patients than in adults. Weight-normalized lamotrigine clearance was higher in those subjects weighing less than 30 kg, compared with those weighing greater than 30 kg. Accordingly, patients weighing less than 30 kg may need an increase of as much as 50% in maintenance doses, based on clinical response, as compared with subjects weighing more than 30 kg being administered the same AEDs [see Dosage and Administration (2.2)]. These analyses also revealed that, after accounting for body weight, lamotrigine clearance was not significantly influenced by age. Thus, the same weight-adjusted doses should be administered to children irrespective of differences in age. Concomitant AEDs which influence lamotrigine clearance in adults were found to have similar effects in children.
[See table 16 above]

Elderly: The pharmacokinetics of lamotrigine following a single 150-mg dose of LAMICTAL were evaluated in 12 elderly volunteers between the ages of 65 and 76 years (mean creatinine clearance = 61 mL/min, range: 33 to 108 mL/min). The mean half-life of lamotrigine in these subjects was 31.2 hours (range: 24.5 to 43.4 hours), and the mean clearance was 0.40 mL/min/kg (range: 0.26 to 0.48 mL/min/kg).

Gender: The clearance of lamotrigine is not affected by gender. However, during dose escalation of LAMICTAL in one clinical trial in patients with epilepsy on a stable dose of valproate (n = 77), mean trough lamotrigine concentrations, unadjusted for weight, were 24% to 45% higher (0.3 to 1.7 mcg/mL) in females than in males.

Race: The apparent oral clearance of lamotrigine was 25% lower in non-Caucasians than Caucasians.

13 NONCLINICAL TOXICOLOGY

13.1 Carcinogenesis, Mutagenesis, Impairment of Fertility

No evidence of carcinogenicity was seen in 1 mouse study or 2 rat studies following oral administration of lamotrigine for up to 2 years at maximum tolerated doses (30 mg/kg/day for mice and 10 to 15 mg/kg/day for rats, doses that are equivalent to 90 mg/m^2 and 60 to 90 mg/m^2, respectively). Steady-state plasma concentrations ranged from 1 to 4 mcg/mL in the mouse study and 1 to 10 mcg/mL in the rat study. Plasma concentrations associated with the recommended human doses of 300 to 500 mg/day are generally in the range of 2 to 5 mcg/mL, but concentrations as high as 19 mcg/mL have been recorded.

Lamotrigine was not mutagenic in the presence or absence of metabolic activation when tested in 2 gene mutation assays (the Ames test and the in vitro mammalian mouse lymphoma assay). In 2 cytogenetic assays (the in vitro human lymphocyte assay and the in vivo rat bone marrow assay), lamotrigine did not increase the incidence of structural or numerical chromosomal abnormalities.

No evidence of impairment of fertility was detected in rats given oral doses of lamotrigine up to 2.4 times the highest usual human maintenance dose of 8.33 mg/kg/day or 0.4 times the human dose on a mg/m^2 basis. The effect of lamotrigine on human fertility is unknown.

14 CLINICAL STUDIES

14.1 Epilepsy

Monotherapy With LAMICTAL in Adults With Partial Seizures Already Receiving Treatment With Carbamazepine, Phenytoin, Phenobarbital, or Primidone as the Single Antiepileptic Drug: The effectiveness of monotherapy with LAMICTAL was established in a multicenter, double-blind clinical trial enrolling 156 adult outpatients with partial seizures. The patients experienced at least 4 simple partial, complex partial, and/or secondarily generalized seizures during each of 2 consecutive 4-week periods while receiving carbamazepine or phenytoin monotherapy during baseline. LAMICTAL (target dose of 500 mg/day) or valproate (1,000 mg/day) was added to either carbamazepine or phenytoin monotherapy over a 4-week period. Patients were then converted to monotherapy with LAMICTAL or valproate during the next 4 weeks, then continued on monotherapy for an additional 12-week period.

Study endpoints were completion of all weeks of study treatment or meeting an escape criterion. Criteria for escape relative to baseline were: (1) doubling of average monthly seizure count, (2) doubling of highest consecutive 2-day seizure frequency, (3) emergence of a new seizure type (defined as a seizure that did not occur during the 8-week baseline) that is more severe than seizure types that occur during study treatment, or (4) clinically significant prolongation of generalized tonic-clonic seizures. The primary efficacy variable was the proportion of patients in each treatment group who met escape criteria.

The percentages of patients who met escape criteria were 42% (32/76) in the group receiving LAMICTAL and 69% (55/80) in the valproate group. The difference in the percentage of patients meeting escape criteria was statistically significant (P = 0.0012) in favor of LAMICTAL. No differences in efficacy based on age, sex, or race were detected.

Patients in the control group were intentionally treated with a relatively low dose of valproate; as such, the sole objective of this study was to demonstrate the effectiveness and safety of monotherapy with LAMICTAL, and cannot be interpreted to imply the superiority of LAMICTAL to an adequate dose of valproate.

Adjunctive Therapy With LAMICTAL in Adults With Partial Seizures: The effectiveness of LAMICTAL as adjunctive therapy (added to other AEDs) was established in 3 multicenter, placebo-controlled, double-blind clinical trials in 355 adults with refractory partial seizures. The patients had a history of at least 4 partial seizures per month in spite of receiving one or more AEDs at therapeutic concentrations and, in 2 of the studies, were observed on their established AED regimen during baselines that varied be-

tween 8 to 12 weeks. In the third, patients were not observed in a prospective baseline. In patients continuing to have at least 4 seizures per month during the baseline, LAMICTAL or placebo was then added to the existing therapy. In all 3 studies, change from baseline in seizure frequency was the primary measure of effectiveness. The results given below are for all partial seizures in the intent-to-treat population (all patients who received at least one dose of treatment) in each study, unless otherwise indicated. The median seizure frequency at baseline was 3 per week while the mean at baseline was 6.6 per week for all patients enrolled in efficacy studies.

One study (n = 216) was a double-blind, placebo-controlled, parallel trial consisting of a 24-week treatment period. Patients could not be on more than 2 other anticonvulsants and valproate was not allowed. Patients were randomized to receive placebo, a target dose of 300 mg/day of LAMICTAL, or a target dose of 500 mg/day of LAMICTAL. The median reductions in the frequency of all partial seizures relative to baseline were 8% in patients receiving placebo, 20% in patients receiving 300 mg/day of LAMICTAL, and 36% in patients receiving 500 mg/day of LAMICTAL. The seizure frequency reduction was statistically significant in the 500-mg/day group compared with the placebo group, but not in the 300-mg/day group.

A second study (n = 98) was a double-blind, placebo-controlled, randomized, crossover trial consisting of two 14-week treatment periods (the last 2 weeks of which consisted of dose tapering) separated by a 4-week washout period. Patients could not be on more than 2 other anticonvulsants and valproate was not allowed. The target dose of LAMICTAL was 400 mg/day. When the first 12 weeks of the treatment periods were analyzed, the median change in seizure frequency was a 25% reduction on LAMICTAL compared with placebo (P<0.001).

The third study (n = 41) was a double-blind, placebo-controlled, crossover trial consisting of two 12-week treatment periods separated by a 4-week washout period. Patients could not be on more than 2 other anticonvulsants. Thirteen patients were on concomitant valproate; these patients received 150 mg/day of LAMICTAL. The 28 other patients had a target dose of 300 mg/day of LAMICTAL. The median change in seizure frequency was a 26% reduction on LAMICTAL compared with placebo (P<0.01).

No differences in efficacy based on age, sex, or race, as measured by change in seizure frequency, were detected.

Adjunctive Therapy With LAMICTAL in Pediatric Patients With Partial Seizures: The effectiveness of LAMICTAL as adjunctive therapy in pediatric patients with partial seizures was established in a multicenter, double-blind, placebo-controlled trial in 199 patients 2 to 16 years of age (n = 98 on LAMICTAL, n = 101 on placebo). Following an 8-week baseline phase, patients were randomized to 18 weeks of treatment with LAMICTAL or placebo added to their current AED regimen of up to 2 drugs. Patients were dosed based on body weight and valproate use. Target doses were designed to approximate 5 mg/kg/day for patients taking valproate (maximum dose: 250 mg/day) and 15 mg/kg/day for the patients not taking valproate (maximum dose: 750 mg/day). The primary efficacy endpoint was percentage change from baseline in all partial seizures. For the intent-to-treat population, the median reduction of all partial seizures was 36% in patients treated with LAMICTAL and 7% on placebo, a difference that was statistically significant (P<0.01).

Adjunctive Therapy With LAMICTAL in Pediatric and Adult Patients With Lennox-Gastaut Syndrome: The effectiveness of LAMICTAL as adjunctive therapy in patients with Lennox-Gastaut syndrome was established in a multicenter, double-blind, placebo-controlled trial in 169 patients 3 to 25 years of age (n = 79 on LAMICTAL, n = 90 on placebo). Following a 4-week single-blind, placebo phase, patients were randomized to 16 weeks of treatment with LAMICTAL or placebo added to their current AED regimen of up to 3 drugs. Patients were dosed on a fixed-dose regimen based on body weight and valproate use. Target doses were designed to approximate 5 mg/kg/day for patients taking valproate (maximum dose: 200 mg/day) and 15 mg/kg/day for patients not taking valproate (maximum dose: 400 mg/day). The primary efficacy endpoint was percentage change from baseline in major motor seizures (atonic, tonic, major myoclonic, and tonic-clonic seizures). For the intent-to-treat population, the median reduction of major motor seizures was 32% in patients treated with LAMICTAL and 9% on placebo, a difference that was statistically significant (P<0.05). Drop attacks were significantly reduced by LAMICTAL (34%) compared with placebo (9%), as were tonic-clonic seizures (36% reduction versus 10% increase for LAMICTAL and placebo, respectively).

Adjunctive Therapy With LAMICTAL in Pediatric and Adult Patients With Primary Generalized Tonic-Clonic Seizures: The effectiveness of LAMICTAL as adjunctive therapy in patients with primary generalized tonic-clonic seizures was established in a multicenter, double-blind,

placebo-controlled trial in 117 pediatric and adult patients ≥2 years (n = 58 on LAMICTAL, n = 59 on placebo). Patients with at least 3 primary generalized tonic-clonic seizures during an 8-week baseline phase were randomized to 19 to 24 weeks of treatment with LAMICTAL or placebo added to their current AED regimen of up to 2 drugs. Patients were dosed on a fixed-dose regimen, with target doses ranging from 3 mg/kg/day to 12 mg/kg/day for pediatric patients and from 200 mg/day to 400 mg/day for adult patients based on concomitant AED.

The primary efficacy endpoint was percentage change from baseline in primary generalized tonic-clonic seizures. For the intent-to-treat population, the median percent reduction of primary generalized tonic-clonic seizures was 66% in patients treated with LAMICTAL and 34% on placebo, a difference that was statistically significant (P = 0.006).

14.2 Bipolar Disorder

The effectiveness of LAMICTAL in the maintenance treatment of Bipolar I Disorder was established in 2 multicenter, double-blind, placebo-controlled studies in adult patients who met DSM-IV criteria for Bipolar I Disorder. Study 1 enrolled patients with a current or recent (within 60 days) depressive episode as defined by DSM-IV and Study 2 included patients with a current or recent (within 60 days) episode of mania or hypomania as defined by DSM-IV. Both studies included a cohort of patients (30% of 404 patients in Study 1 and 28% of 171 patients in Study 2) with rapid cycling Bipolar Disorder (4 to 6 episodes per year).

In both studies, patients were titrated to a target dose of 200 mg of LAMICTAL, as add-on therapy or as monotherapy, with gradual withdrawal of any psychotropic medications during an 8- to 16-week open-label period. Overall 81% of 1,305 patients participating in the open-label period were receiving 1 or more other psychotropic medications, including benzodiazepines, selective serotonin reuptake inhibitors (SSRIs), atypical antipsychotics (including olanzapine), valproate, or lithium, during titration of LAMICTAL. Patients with a CGI-severity score of 3 or less maintained for at least 4 continuous weeks, including at least the final week on monotherapy with LAMICTAL, were randomized to a placebo-controlled, double-blind treatment period for up to 18 months. The primary endpoint was TIME (time to intervention for a mood episode or one that was emerging, time to discontinuation for either an adverse event that was judged to be related to Bipolar Disorder, or for lack of efficacy). The mood episode could be depression, mania, hypomania, or a mixed episode.

In Study 1, patients received double-blind monotherapy with LAMICTAL 50 mg/day (n = 50), LAMICTAL 200 mg/day (n = 124), LAMICTAL 400 mg/day (n = 47), or placebo (n = 121). LAMICTAL (200- and 400-mg/day treatment groups combined) was superior to placebo in delaying the time to occurrence of a mood episode. Separate analyses of the 200- and 400-mg/day dose groups revealed no added benefit from the higher dose.

In Study 2, patients received double-blind monotherapy with LAMICTAL (100 to 400 mg/day, n = 59), or placebo (n = 70). LAMICTAL was superior to placebo in delaying time to occurrence of a mood episode. The mean dose of LAMICTAL was about 211 mg/day.

Although these studies were not designed to separately evaluate time to the occurrence of depression or mania, a combined analysis for the 2 studies revealed a statistically significant benefit for LAMICTAL over placebo in delaying the time to occurrence of both depression and mania, although the finding was more robust for depression.

16 HOW SUPPLIED/STORAGE AND HANDLING

LAMICTAL (lamotrigine) Tablets
25 mg, white, scored, shield-shaped tablets debossed with "LAMICTAL" and "25", bottles of 100 (NDC 0173-0633-02). Store at 25°C (77°F); excursions permitted to 15-30°C (59-86°F) [see USP Controlled Room Temperature] in a dry place.
100 mg, peach, scored, shield-shaped tablets debossed with "LAMICTAL" and "100", bottles of 100 (NDC 0173-0642-55).
150 mg, cream, scored, shield-shaped tablets debossed with "LAMICTAL" and "150", bottles of 60 (NDC 0173-0643-60).
200 mg, blue, scored, shield-shaped tablets debossed with "LAMICTAL" and "200", bottles of 60 (NDC 0173-0644-60).
Store at 25°C (77°F); excursions permitted to 15-30°C (59-86°F) [see USP Controlled Room Temperature] in a dry place and protect from light.

LAMICTAL (lamotrigine) Starter Kit for Patients Taking Valproate (Blue Kit)
25 mg, white, scored, shield-shaped tablets debossed with "LAMICTAL" and "25", blisterpack of 35 tablets (NDC 0173-0633-10).
Store at 25°C (77°F); excursions permitted to 15-30°C (59-86°F) [see USP Controlled Room Temperature] in a dry place.

LAMICTAL (lamotrigine) Starter Kit for Patients Taking Carbamazepine, Phenytoin, Phenobarbital, or Primidone and Not Taking Valproate (Green Kit)

25 mg, white, scored, shield-shaped tablets debossed with "LAMICTAL" and "25" and 100 mg, peach, scored, shield-shaped tablets debossed with "LAMICTAL" and "100", blister-pack of 98 tablets (84/25-mg tablets and 14/100-mg tablets) (NDC 0173-0817-28).

Store at 25°C (77°F); excursions permitted to 15-30°C (59-86°F) [see USP Controlled Room Temperature] in a dry place and protect from light.

LAMICTAL (lamotrigine) Starter Kit for Patients Not Taking Carbamazepine, Phenytoin, Phenobarbital, Primidone, or Valproate (Orange Kit)

25 mg, white, scored, shield-shaped tablets debossed with "LAMICTAL" and "25" and 100 mg, peach, scored, shield-shaped tablets debossed with "LAMICTAL" and "100", blister-pack of 49 tablets (42/25-mg tablets and 7/100-mg tablets) (NDC 0173-0594-02).

Store at 25°C (77°F); excursions permitted to 15-30°C (59-86°F) [see USP Controlled Room Temperature] in a dry place and protect from light.

LAMICTAL (lamotrigine) Chewable Dispersible Tablets

2 mg, white to off-white, round tablets debossed with "LTG" over "2", bottles of 30 (NDC 0173-0699-00). ORDER DIRECTLY FROM GlaxoSmithKline 1-800-334-4153.

5 mg, white to off-white, caplet-shaped tablets debossed with "GX CL2", bottles of 100 (NDC 0173-0526-00).

25 mg, white, super elliptical-shaped tablets debossed with "GX CL5", bottles of 100 (NDC 0173-0527-00).

Store at 25°C (77°F); excursions permitted to 15-30°C (59-86°F) [see USP Controlled Room Temperature] in a dry place.

LAMICTAL ODT (lamotrigine) Orally Disintegrating Tablets

25 mg, white to off-white, round, flat-faced, radius edge, tablets debossed with "LMT" on one side and "25" on the other, Maintenance Packs of 30 (NDC 0173-0772-02).

50 mg, white to off-white, round, flat-faced, radius edge, tablets debossed with "LMT" on one side and "50" on the other, Maintenance Packs of 30 (NDC 0173-0774-02).

100 mg, white to off-white, round, flat-faced, radius edge, tablets debossed with "LAMICTAL" on one side and "100" on the other, Maintenance Packs of 30 (NDC 0173-0776-02).

200 mg, white to off-white, round, flat-faced, radius edge, tablets debossed with "LAMICTAL" on one side and "200" on the other, Maintenance Packs of 30 (NDC 0173-0777-02).

Store between 20°C to 25°C (68°F to 77°F); with excursions permitted between 15°C and 30°C (59°F and 86°F).

LAMICTAL ODT (lamotrigine) Patient Titration Kit for Patients Taking Valproate (Blue ODT Kit)

25 mg, white to off-white, round, flat-faced, radius edge, tablets debossed with "LMT" on one side and "25" on the other, and 50 mg, white to off-white, round, flat-faced, radius edge, tablets debossed with "LMT" on one side and "50" on the other, blisterpack of 28 tablets (21/25-mg tablets and 7/50-mg tablets) (NDC 0173-0779-00).

LAMICTAL ODT (lamotrigine) Patient Titration Kit for Patients Taking Carbamazepine, Phenytoin, Phenobarbital, or Primidone and Not Taking Valproate (Green ODT Kit)

50 mg, white to off-white, round, flat-faced, radius edge, tablets debossed with "LMT" on one side and "50" on the other, and 100 mg, white to off-white, round, flat-faced, radius edge, tablets debossed with "LAMICTAL" on one side and "100" on the other, blisterpack of 56 tablets (42/50-mg tablets and 14/100-mg tablets) (NDC 0173-0780-00).

LAMICTAL ODT (lamotrigine) Patient Titration Kit for Patients Not Taking Carbamazepine, Phenytoin, Phenobarbital, Primidone, or Valproate (Orange ODT Kit)

25 mg, white to off-white, round, flat-faced, radius edge, tablets debossed with "LMT" on one side and "25" on the other, 50 mg, white to off-white, round, flat-faced, radius edge, tablets debossed with "LMT" on one side and "50" on the other, and 100 mg, white to off-white, round, flat-faced, radius edge, tablets debossed with "LAMICTAL" on one side and "100" on the other, blisterpack of 35 (14/25-mg tablets, 14/50-mg tablets, and 7/100-mg tablets) (NDC 0173-0778-00).

Store between 20°C to 25°C (68°F to 77°F); with excursions permitted between 15°C and 30°C (59°F and 86°F).

Blisterpacks: If the product is dispensed in a blisterpack, the patient should be advised to examine the blisterpack before use and not use if blisters are torn, broken, or missing.

17 PATIENT COUNSELING INFORMATION

See FDA-approved patient labeling (Medication Guide).

17.1 Rash

Prior to initiation of treatment with LAMICTAL, the patient should be instructed that a rash or other signs or symptoms of hypersensitivity (e.g., fever, lymphadenopathy) may herald a serious medical event and that the patient should report any such occurrence to a physician immediately.

17.2 Multiorgan Hypersensitivity Reactions, Blood Dyscrasias, and Organ Failure

Patients should be instructed that multiorgan hypersensitivity reactions and acute multiorgan failure may occur with LAMICTAL. Isolated organ failure or isolated blood dyscrasias without evidence of multiorgan hypersensitivity may also occur. Patients should contact their physician immediately if they experience any signs or symptoms of these conditions [see Warnings and Precautions (5.2, 5.3)].

17.3 Suicidal Thinking and Behavior

Patients, their caregivers, and families should be counseled that AEDs, including LAMICTAL, may increase the risk of suicidal thoughts and behavior and should be advised of the need to be alert for the emergence or worsening of symptoms of depression, any unusual changes in mood or behavior, or the emergence of suicidal thoughts, behavior, or thoughts about self-harm. Behaviors of concern should be reported immediately to healthcare providers.

17.4 Worsening of Seizures

Patients should be advised to notify their physician if worsening of seizure control occurs.

17.5 Central Nervous System Adverse Effects

Patients should be advised that LAMICTAL may cause dizziness, somnolence, and other symptoms and signs of CNS depression. Accordingly, they should be advised neither to drive a car nor to operate other complex machinery until they have gained sufficient experience on LAMICTAL to gauge whether or not it adversely affects their mental and/or motor performance.

17.6 Pregnancy and Nursing

Patients should be advised to notify their physicians if they become pregnant or intend to become pregnant during therapy. Patients should be advised to notify their physicians if they intend to breastfeed or are breastfeeding an infant.

Patients should also be encouraged to enroll in the NAAED Pregnancy Registry if they become pregnant. This registry is collecting information about the safety of antiepileptic drugs during pregnancy. To enroll, patients can call the toll-free number 1-888-233-2334 [see Use in Specific Populations (8.1)].

Patients who intend to breastfeed should be informed that LAMICTAL is present in breast milk and that they should monitor their child for potential adverse effects of this drug. Benefits and risks of continuing breastfeeding should be discussed with the patient.

17.7 Oral Contraceptive Use

Women should be advised to notify their physician if they plan to start or stop use of oral contraceptives or other female hormonal preparations. Starting estrogen-containing oral contraceptives may significantly decrease lamotrigine plasma levels and stopping estrogen-containing oral contraceptives (including the "pill-free" week) may significantly increase lamotrigine plasma levels [see Warnings and Precautions (5.8), Clinical Pharmacology (12.3)]. Women should also be advised to promptly notify their physician if they experience adverse reactions or changes in menstrual pattern (e.g., break-through bleeding) while receiving LAMICTAL in combination with these medications.

17.8 Discontinuing LAMICTAL

Patients should be advised to notify their physician if they stop taking LAMICTAL for any reason and not to resume LAMICTAL without consulting their physician.

17.9 Aseptic Meningitis

Patients should be advised that LAMICTAL may cause aseptic meningitis. Patients should be advised to notify their physician immediately if they develop signs and symptoms of meningitis such as headache, fever, nausea, vomiting, stiff neck, rash, abnormal sensitivity to light, myalgia, chills, confusion, or drowsiness while taking LAMICTAL.

17.10 Potential Medication Errors

Medication errors involving LAMICTAL have occurred. In particular the names LAMICTAL or lamotrigine can be confused with the names of other commonly used medications. Medication errors may also occur between the different formulations of LAMICTAL. To reduce the potential of medication errors, write and say LAMICTAL clearly. Depictions of the LAMICTAL Tablets, Chewable Dispersible Tablets, and Orally Disintegrating Tablets can be found in the Medication Guide that accompanies the product to highlight the distinctive markings, colors, and shapes that serve to identify the different presentations of the drug and thus may help reduce the risk of medication errors. **To avoid a medication error of using the wrong drug or formulation, patients should be strongly advised to visually inspect their tablets to verify that they are LAMICTAL, as well as the correct formulation of LAMICTAL, each time they fill their prescription** [see Dosage Forms and Strengths (3.1, 3.2, 3.3), How Supplied/Storage and Handling (16)].

LAMICTAL and LAMICTAL ODT are registered trademarks of the GSK group of companies.

Microcaps and AdvaTab are registered trademarks of Eurand, Inc.

GlaxoSmithKline
Research Triangle Park, NC 27709

LAMICTAL Tablets and Chewable Dispersible Tablets are manufactured by
DSM Pharmaceuticals, Inc., Greenville, NC 27834 or GlaxoSmithKline, Research Triangle Park, NC 27709

LAMICTAL Orally Disintegrating Tablets are manufactured by
Eurand, Inc., Vandalia, OH 45377

©2014, the GSK group of companies. All rights reserved.

LMT:10PI

MEDICATION GUIDE

LAMICTAL® (la-MIK-tal) (lamotrigine) **Tablets and Chewable Dispersible Tablets**
LAMICTAL ODT® (lamotrigine) **Orally Disintegrating Tablets**

Read this Medication Guide before you start taking LAMICTAL and each time you get a refill. There may be new information. This information does not take the place of talking with your healthcare provider about your medical condition or treatment. If you have questions about LAMICTAL, ask your healthcare provider or pharmacist.

What is the most important information I should know about LAMICTAL?

1. LAMICTAL may cause a serious skin rash that may cause you to be hospitalized or to stop LAMICTAL; it may rarely cause death.

There is no way to tell if a mild rash will develop into a more serious reaction. These serious skin reactions are more likely to happen when you begin taking LAMICTAL, within the first 2 to 8 weeks of treatment. But it can happen in people who have taken LAMICTAL for any period of time. Children between 2 to 16 years of age have a higher chance of getting this serious skin reaction while taking LAMICTAL.

The risk of getting a rash is higher if you:
• take LAMICTAL while taking valproate [DEPAKENE (valproic acid) or DEPAKOTE (divalproex sodium)].
• take a higher starting dose of LAMICTAL than your healthcare provider prescribed
• increase your dose of LAMICTAL faster than prescribed.

LAMICTAL can also cause other types of allergic reactions or serious problems which may affect organs and other parts of your body like the liver or blood cells. You may or may not have a rash with these types of reactions.

Call your healthcare provider right away if you have any of the following:
• a skin rash
• hives
• fever
• swollen lymph glands
• painful sores in the mouth or around your eyes
• swelling of your lips or tongue
• yellowing of your skin or eyes
• unusual bruising or bleeding
• severe fatigue or weakness
• severe muscle pain
• frequent infections

These symptoms may be the first signs of a serious reaction. A healthcare provider should examine you to decide if you should continue taking LAMICTAL.

2. Like other antiepileptic drugs, LAMICTAL may cause suicidal thoughts or actions in a very small number of people, about 1 in 500.

Call a healthcare provider right away if you have any of these symptoms, especially if they are new, worse, or worry you:
• thoughts about suicide or dying
• attempt to commit suicide
• new or worse depression
• new or worse anxiety
• feeling agitated or restless
• panic attacks
• trouble sleeping (insomnia)
• new or worse irritability
• acting aggressive, being angry, or violent
• acting on dangerous impulses
• an extreme increase in activity and talking (mania)
• other unusual changes in behavior or mood

Do not stop LAMICTAL without first talking to a healthcare provider.
• Stopping LAMICTAL suddenly can cause serious problems.
• Suicidal thoughts or actions can be caused by things other than medicines. If you have suicidal thoughts or actions, your healthcare provider may check for other causes.

How can I watch for early symptoms of suicidal thoughts and actions?
• Pay attention to any changes, especially sudden changes, in mood, behaviors, thoughts, or feelings.
• Keep all follow-up visits with your healthcare provider as scheduled.
• Call your healthcare provider between visits as needed, especially if you are worried about symptoms.

3. LAMICTAL may rarely cause aseptic meningitis, a serious inflammation of the protective membrane that covers the brain and spinal cord.

Call your healthcare provider right away if you have any of the following symptoms:
• Headache
• Fever

- Nausea
- Vomiting
- Stiff neck
- Rash
- Unusual sensitivity to light
- Muscle pains
- Chills
- Confusion
- Drowsiness

Meningitis has many causes other than LAMICTAL, which your doctor would check for if you developed meningitis while taking LAMICTAL.

LAMICTAL can have other serious side effects. For more information ask your healthcare provider or pharmacist. Tell your healthcare provider if you have any side effect that bothers you. Be sure to read the section below entitled "What are the possible side effects of LAMICTAL?"

4. Patients prescribed LAMICTAL have sometimes been given the wrong medicine because many medicines have names similar to LAMICTAL, so always check that you receive LAMICTAL.

Taking the wrong medication can cause serious health problems. When your healthcare provider gives you a prescription for LAMICTAL:

- Make sure you can read it clearly.
- Talk to your pharmacist to check that you are given the correct medicine.
- Each time you fill your prescription, check the tablets you receive against the pictures of the tablets below.
- These pictures show the distinct wording, colors, and shapes of the tablets that help to identify the right strength of LAMICTAL Tablets, Chewable Dispersible Tablets, and Orally Disintegrating Tablets. Immediately call your pharmacist if you receive a LAMICTAL tablet that does not look like one of the tablets shown below, as you may have received the wrong medication.

[See table above]

What is LAMICTAL?

LAMICTAL is a prescription medicine used:

1. together with other medicines to treat certain types of seizures (partial seizures, primary generalized tonic-clonic seizures, generalized seizures of Lennox-Gastaut syndrome) in people 2 years or older.
2. alone when changing from other medicines used to treat partial seizures in people 16 years or older.
3. for the long-term treatment of Bipolar I Disorder to lengthen the time between mood episodes in people 18 years or older who have been treated for mood episodes with other medicine.

It is not known if LAMICTAL is safe or effective in children or teenagers under the age of 18 with mood disorders such as bipolar disorder or depression.

It is not known if LAMICTAL is safe or effective when used alone as the first treatment of seizures in adults.

Who should not take LAMICTAL?

You should not take LAMICTAL if you have had an allergic reaction to lamotrigine or to any of the inactive ingredients in LAMICTAL. See the end of this leaflet for a complete list of ingredients in LAMICTAL.

What should I tell my healthcare provider before taking LAMICTAL?

Before taking LAMICTAL, tell your healthcare provider about all of your medical conditions, including if you:

- have had a rash or allergic reaction to another antiseizure medicine.
- have or have had depression, mood problems, or suicidal thoughts or behavior.
- are taking oral contraceptives (birth control pills) or other female hormonal medicines. Do not start or stop taking birth control pills or other female hormonal medicine until you have talked with your healthcare provider. Tell your healthcare provider if you have any changes in your menstrual pattern such as breakthrough bleeding. Stopping or starting these medicines may cause side effects (such as dizziness, lack of coordination, or double vision) or lessen how well LAMICTAL works.
- are pregnant or plan to become pregnant. It is not known if LAMICTAL will harm your unborn baby. If you become pregnant while taking LAMICTAL, talk to your healthcare provider about registering with the North American Antiepileptic Drug Pregnancy Registry. You can enroll in this registry by calling 1-888-233-2334. The purpose of this registry is to collect information about the safety of antiepileptic drugs during pregnancy.
- are breastfeeding. LAMICTAL passes into breast milk and may cause side effects in a breastfed baby. If you breastfeed while taking LAMICTAL, watch your baby closely for trouble breathing, episodes of temporarily stopping breathing, sleepiness, or poor sucking. Call your baby's

---

LAMICTAL (lamotrigine) Tablets

25 mg, white
Imprinted with
LAMICTAL 25

100 mg, peach
Imprinted with
LAMICTAL 100

150 mg, cream
Imprinted with
LAMICTAL 150

200 mg, blue
Imprinted with
LAMICTAL 200

LAMICTAL (lamotrigine) Chewable Dispersible Tablets

2 mg, white
Imprinted with
LTG 2

5 mg, white
Imprinted with
GX CL2

25 mg, white
Imprinted with
GX CL5

LAMICTAL ODT (lamotrigine) Orally Disintegrating Tablets

25 mg, white to off-white
Imprinted with LMT on one side
25 on the other

50 mg, white to off-white
Imprinted with LMT on one side
50 on the other

100 mg, white to off-white
Imprinted with LAMICTAL on one side
100 on the other

200 mg, white to off-white
Imprinted with LAMICTAL on one side
200 on the other

---

healthcare provider right away if you see any of these problems. Talk to your healthcare provider about the best way to feed your baby if you take LAMICTAL.

Tell your healthcare provider about all the medicines you take or if you are planning to take a new medicine, including prescription and non-prescription medicines, vitamins, and herbal supplements. Using LAMICTAL with certain other medicines can affect each other, causing side effects.

How should I take LAMICTAL?

- Take LAMICTAL exactly as prescribed.
- Your healthcare provider may change your dose. Do not change your dose without talking to your healthcare provider.
- Do not stop taking LAMICTAL without talking to your healthcare provider. Stopping LAMICTAL suddenly may cause serious problems. For example, if you have epilepsy and you stop taking LAMICTAL suddenly, you may get seizures that do not stop. Talk with your healthcare provider about how to stop LAMICTAL slowly.
- If you miss a dose of LAMICTAL, take it as soon as you remember. If it is almost time for your next dose, just skip the missed dose. Take the next dose at your regular time. **Do not take two doses at the same time.**
- If you take too much LAMICTAL, call your healthcare provider or your local Poison Control Center or go to the nearest hospital emergency room right away.
- You may not feel the full effect of LAMICTAL for several weeks.
- If you have epilepsy, tell your healthcare provider if your seizures get worse or if you have any new types of seizures.
- Swallow LAMICTAL tablets whole.
- If you have trouble swallowing LAMICTAL Tablets, there may be another form of LAMICTAL you can take.
- LAMICTAL ODT should be placed on the tongue and moved around the mouth. The tablet will rapidly disintegrate, can be swallowed with or without water, and can be taken with or without food.
- LAMICTAL Chewable Dispersible tablets may be swallowed whole, chewed, or mixed in water or diluted fruit juice. If the tablets are chewed, drink a small amount of water or diluted fruit juice to help in swallowing. To break up LAMICTAL Chewable Dispersible tablets, add the tablets to a small amount of liquid (1 teaspoon, or enough to cover the medicine) in a glass or spoon. Wait at least 1 minute or until the tablets are completely broken up, mix the solution together and take the whole amount right away.
- If you receive LAMICTAL in a blisterpack, examine the blisterpack before use. Do not use if blisters are torn, broken, or missing.

What should I avoid while taking LAMICTAL?

- Do not drive a car or operate complex, hazardous machinery until you know how LAMICTAL affects you.

What are possible side effects of LAMICTAL?

- See "What is the most important information I should know about LAMICTAL?"

Common side effects of LAMICTAL include:

dizziness	tremor
headache	rash
blurred or double vision	fever
lack of coordination	abdominal pain
sleepiness	back pain
nausea, vomiting	tiredness
insomnia	dry mouth

Tell your healthcare provider about any side effect that bothers you or that does not go away.

These are not all the possible side effects of LAMICTAL. For more information, ask your healthcare provider or pharmacist.

Call your doctor for medical advice about side effects. You may report side effects to FDA at 1-800-FDA-1088.

How should I store LAMICTAL?

- Store LAMICTAL at room temperature between 68°F to 77°F (20°C to 25°C).
- **Keep LAMICTAL and all medicines out of the reach of children.**

General information about LAMICTAL

Medicines are sometimes prescribed for purposes other than those listed in a Medication Guide. Do not use LAMICTAL for a condition for which it was not prescribed. Do not give LAMICTAL to other people, even if they have the same symptoms you have. It may harm them.

This Medication Guide summarizes the most important information about LAMICTAL. If you would like more information, talk with your healthcare provider. You can ask your healthcare provider or pharmacist for information about LAMICTAL that is written for healthcare professionals.

For more information, go to www.lamictal.com or call 1-888-825-5249.

What are the ingredients in LAMICTAL?

LAMICTAL Tablets

Active ingredient: lamotrigine.

Inactive ingredients: lactose; magnesium stearate, microcrystalline cellulose, povidone, sodium starch glycolate, FD&C Yellow No. 6 Lake (100 mg tablet only), ferric oxide, yellow (150 mg tablet only), and FD&C Blue No. 2 Lake (200 mg tablet only).

LAMICTAL Chewable Dispersible Tablets

Active ingredient: lamotrigine.

Inactive ingredients: blackcurrant flavor, calcium carbonate, low-substituted hydroxypropylcellulose, magnesium aluminum silicate, magnesium stearate, povidone, saccharin sodium, and sodium starch glycolate.

LAMICTAL ODT Orally Disintegrating Tablets

Active ingredient: lamotrigine

Inactive ingredients: artificial cherry flavor, crospovidone, ethylcellulose, magnesium stearate, mannitol, polyethylene, and sucralose.

This Medication Guide has been approved by the U.S. Food and Drug Administration.

LAMICTAL and LAMICTAL ODT are registered trademarks of the GSK group of companies.

DEPAKENE and DEPAKOTE are registered trademarks of Abbott Laboratories.

GlaxoSmithKline
Research Triangle Park, NC 27709
LAMICTAL Tablets and Chewable Dispersible Tablets are manufactured by
DSM Pharmaceuticals, Inc.,
Greenville, NC 27834 or
GlaxoSmithKline
Research Triangle Park, NC 27709
LAMICTAL Orally Disintegrating Tablets are manufactured by
Eurand, Inc., Vandalia, OH 45377
©2014, the GSK group of companies. All rights reserved.
June 2014
LMT:9MG

LAMICTAL XR   ℞
[la-mik' tal]
(lamotrigine)
Extended-Release Tablets

HIGHLIGHTS OF PRESCRIBING INFORMATION
These highlights do not include all the information needed to use LAMICTAL XR safely and effectively. See full prescribing information for LAMICTAL XR.
LAMICTAL XR (lamotrigine) Extended-Release Tablets
Initial U.S. Approval: 1994

WARNING: SERIOUS SKIN RASHES
See full prescribing information for complete boxed warning.
Cases of life-threatening serious rashes, including Stevens-Johnson syndrome and toxic epidermal necrolysis, and/or rash-related death have been caused by lamotrigine. The rate of serious rash is greater in pediatric patients than in adults. Additional factors that may increase the risk of rash include (5.1):
• **coadministration with valproate**
• **exceeding recommended initial dose of LAMICTAL XR**
• **exceeding recommended dose escalation for LAMICTAL XR**
Benign rashes are also caused by lamotrigine; however, it is not possible to predict which rashes will prove to be serious or life threatening. LAMICTAL XR should be discontinued at the first sign of rash, unless the rash is clearly not drug related. (5.1)

INDICATIONS AND USAGE
LAMICTAL XR is an antiepileptic drug (AED) indicated for:
• adjunctive therapy for primary generalized tonic-clonic (PGTC) seizures and partial onset seizures with or without secondary generalization in patients ≥13 years of age (1.1)
• conversion to monotherapy in patients ≥13 years of age with partial seizures who are receiving treatment with a single AED (1.2)
• Limitation of use: Safety and effectiveness in patients less than 13 years of age have not been established. (1.3)

DOSAGE AND ADMINISTRATION
• Do not exceed the recommended initial dosage and subsequent dose escalation. (2.1)
• Initiation of adjunctive therapy and conversion to monotherapy requires slow titration dependent on concomitant AEDs; the prescriber must refer to the appropriate algorithm in Dosage and Administration (2.2, 2.3)
  ◦ Adjunct therapy target therapeutic dose range is 200 to 600 mg daily and is dependent on concomitant AEDs. (2.2)
  ◦ Conversion to monotherapy: Target therapeutic dosage range is 250 to 300 mg daily. (2.3)
• Conversion from immediate-release lamotrigine to LAMICTAL XR: The initial dose of LAMICTAL XR should match the total daily dose of the immediate-release lamotrigine. Patients should be closely monitored for seizure control after conversion. (2.4)
• Do not restart LAMICTAL XR in patients who discontinued due to rash unless the potential benefits clearly outweigh the risks. (2.1, 5.1)

• Adjustments to maintenance doses are likely in patients starting or stopping estrogen-containing oral contraceptives. (2.1, 5.7)
• Discontinuation: Taper over a period of at least 2 weeks (approximately 50% dose reduction per week). (2.1, 5.8)

DOSAGE FORMS AND STRENGTHS
Extended-Release Tablets: 25 mg, 50 mg, 100 mg, 200 mg, 250 mg, and 300 mg. (3.1, 16)

CONTRAINDICATIONS
Hypersensitivity to the drug or its ingredients. (Boxed Warning, 4)

WARNINGS AND PRECAUTIONS
• Life-threatening serious rash and/or rash-related death: Discontinue at the first sign of rash, unless the rash is clearly not drug related. (Boxed Warning, 5.1)
• Fatal or life-threatening hypersensitivity reaction: Multiorgan hypersensitivity reactions, also known as Drug Reaction with Eosinophilia and Systemic Symptoms (DRESS), may be fatal or life threatening. Early signs may include rash, fever, and lymphadenopathy. These reactions may be associated with other organ involvement, such as hepatitis, hepatic failure, blood dyscrasias, or acute multiorgan failure. LAMICTAL XR should be discontinued if alternate etiology for this reaction is not found. (5.2)
• Blood dyscrasias (e.g., neutropenia, thrombocytopenia, pancytopenia): May occur, either with or without an associated hypersensitivity syndrome. Monitor for signs of anemia, unexpected infection, or bleeding. (5.3)
• Suicidal behavior and ideation: Monitor for suicidal thoughts or behaviors. (5.4)
• Aseptic meningitis: Monitor for signs of meningitis. (5.5)
• Medication errors due to product name confusion: Strongly advise patients to visually inspect tablets to verify the received drug is correct. (3.2, 5.6, 16, 17.10)

ADVERSE REACTIONS
• Most common adverse reactions with use as adjunctive therapy (treatment difference between LAMICTAL XR and placebo ≥4%) are dizziness, tremor/intention tremor, vomiting, and diplopia. (6.1)
• Most common adverse reactions with use as monotherapy were similar to those seen with previous studies conducted with immediate-release lamotrigine and LAMICTAL XR. (6.1)

To report SUSPECTED ADVERSE REACTIONS, contact GlaxoSmithKline at 1-888-825-5249 or FDA at 1-800-FDA-1088 or www.fda.gov/medwatch.

DRUG INTERACTIONS
• Valproate increases lamotrigine concentrations more than 2-fold. (7, 12.3)
• Carbamazepine, phenytoin, phenobarbital, and primidone decrease lamotrigine concentrations by approximately 40%. (7, 12.3)
• Estrogen-containing oral contraceptives and rifampin also decrease lamotrigine concentrations by approximately 50%. (7, 12.3)

USE IN SPECIFIC POPULATIONS
• Pregnancy: Based on animal data may cause fetal harm. Pregnancy registry available. (8.1)
• Hepatic impairment: Dosage adjustments required in patients with moderate and severe liver impairment. (2.1, 8.6)
• Renal impairment: Reduced maintenance doses may be effective for patients with significant renal impairment. (2.1, 8.7)
See 17 for PATIENT COUNSELING INFORMATION and Medication Guide

Revised: 06/2014

FULL PRESCRIBING INFORMATION: CONTENTS*
WARNING: SERIOUS SKIN RASHES

FULL PRESCRIBING INFORMATION

WARNING: SERIOUS SKIN RASHES

LAMICTAL® XR™ can cause serious rashes requiring hospitalization and discontinuation of treatment. The incidence of these rashes, which have included Stevens-Johnson syndrome, is approximately 0.8% (8 per 1,000) in pediatric patients (aged 2 to 16 years) receiving immediate-release lamotrigine as adjunctive therapy for epilepsy and 0.3% (3 per 1,000) in adults on adjunctive therapy for epilepsy. In a prospectively followed cohort of 1,983 pediatric patients (aged 2 to 16 years) with epilepsy taking adjunctive immediate-release lamotrigine, there was 1 rash-related death. LAMICTAL XR is not approved for patients less than 13 years of age. In worldwide postmarketing experience, rare cases of toxic epidermal necrolysis and/or rash-related death have been reported in adult and pediatric patients, but their numbers are too few to permit a precise estimate of the rate.

The risk of serious rash caused by treatment with LAMICTAL XR is not expected to differ from that with immediate-release lamotrigine. However, the relatively limited treatment experience with LAMICTAL XR makes it difficult to characterize the frequency and risk of serious rashes caused by treatment with LAMICTAL XR.

Other than age, there are as yet no factors identified that are known to predict the risk of occurrence or the severity of rash caused by LAMICTAL XR. There are suggestions, yet to be proven, that the risk of rash may also be increased by (1) coadministration of LAMICTAL XR with valproate (includes valproic acid and divalproex sodium), (2) exceeding the recommended initial dose of LAMICTAL XR, or (3) exceeding the recommended dose escalation for LAMICTAL XR. However, cases have occurred in the absence of these factors.

Nearly all cases of life-threatening rashes caused by immediate-release lamotrigine have occurred within 2 to 8 weeks of treatment initiation. However, isolated cases have occurred after prolonged treatment (e.g., 6 months). Accordingly, duration of therapy cannot be relied upon as means to predict the potential risk heralded by the first appearance of a rash.

Although benign rashes are also caused by LAMICTAL XR, it is not possible to predict reliably which rashes will prove to be serious or life threatening. Accordingly, LAMICTAL XR should ordinarily be discontinued at the first sign of rash, unless the rash is clearly not drug related. Discontinuation of treatment may not prevent a rash from becoming life threatening or permanently disabling or disfiguring *[see Warnings and Precautions (5.1)]*.

1 INDICATIONS AND USAGE

1.1 Adjunctive Therapy

LAMICTAL XR is indicated as adjunctive therapy for primary generalized tonic-clonic (PGTC) seizures and partial onset seizures with or without secondary generalization in patients ≥13 years of age.

1.2 Monotherapy

LAMICTAL XR is indicated for conversion to monotherapy in patients ≥13 years of age with partial seizures who are receiving treatment with a single antiepileptic drug (AED). Safety and effectiveness of LAMICTAL XR have not been established (1) as initial monotherapy or (2) for simultaneous conversion to monotherapy from two or more concomitant AEDs.

1.3 Limitation of Use

Safety and effectiveness of LAMICTAL XR for use in patients less than 13 years of age have not been established.

2 DOSAGE AND ADMINISTRATION

LAMICTAL XR Extended-Release Tablets are taken once daily, with or without food. Tablets must be swallowed whole and must not be chewed, crushed, or divided.

2.1 General Dosing Considerations

Rash: There are suggestions, yet to be proven, that the risk of severe, potentially life-threatening rash may be increased by (1) coadministration of LAMICTAL XR with valproate, (2) exceeding the recommended initial dose of LAMICTAL XR, or (3) exceeding the recommended dose escalation for LAMICTAL XR. However, cases have occurred in the absence of these factors *[see Boxed Warning]*. Therefore, it is important that the dosing recommendations be followed closely.

The risk of nonserious rash may be increased when the recommended initial dose and/or the rate of dose escalation for LAMICTAL XR is exceeded and in patients with a history of allergy or rash to other AEDs.

LAMICTAL XR Patient Titration Kits provide LAMICTAL XR at doses consistent with the recommended titration schedule for the first 5 weeks of treatment, based upon concomitant medications, for patients with partial onset seizures and are intended to help reduce the potential for rash. The use of LAMICTAL XR Patient Titration Kits is recommended for appropriate patients who are starting or restarting LAMICTAL XR *[see How Supplied/Storage and Handling (16)]*.

It is recommended that LAMICTAL XR not be restarted in patients who discontinued due to rash associated with prior treatment with lamotrigine, unless the potential benefits clearly outweigh the risks. If the decision is made to restart a patient who has discontinued LAMICTAL XR, the need to restart with the initial dosing recommendations should be assessed. The greater the interval of time since the previous dose, the greater consideration should be given to restarting with the initial dosing recommendations. If a patient has discontinued lamotrigine for a period of more than 5 half-lives, it is recommended that initial dosing recommendations and guidelines be followed. The half-life of lamotrigine is affected by other concomitant medications *[see Clinical Pharmacology (12.3)]*.

LAMICTAL XR Added to Drugs Known to Induce or Inhibit Glucuronidation: Drugs other than those listed in the Clinical Pharmacology section *[see Clinical Pharmacology (12.3)]* have not been systematically evaluated in combination with lamotrigine. Because lamotrigine is metabolized predominantly by glucuronic acid conjugation, drugs that are known to induce or inhibit glucuronidation may affect the apparent clearance of lamotrigine and doses of LAMICTAL XR may require adjustment based on clinical response.

Target Plasma Levels: A therapeutic plasma concentration range has not been established for lamotrigine. Dosing of LAMICTAL XR should be based on therapeutic response *[see Clinical Pharmacology (12.3)]*.

Women Taking Estrogen-Containing Oral Contraceptives:
Starting LAMICTAL XR in Women Taking Estrogen-Containing Oral Contraceptives: Although estrogen-containing oral contraceptives have been shown to increase the clearance of lamotrigine *[see Clinical Pharmacology (12.3)]*, no adjustments to the recommended dose-escalation guidelines for LAMICTAL XR should be necessary solely based on the use of estrogen-containing oral contraceptives. Therefore, dose escalation should follow the recommended guidelines for initiating adjunctive therapy with LAMICTAL XR based on the concomitant AED or other concomitant medications (see Table 1). See below for adjustments to maintenance doses of LAMICTAL XR in women taking estrogen-containing oral contraceptives.

Adjustments to the Maintenance Dose of LAMICTAL XR in Women Taking Estrogen-Containing Oral Contraceptives:
(1) Taking Estrogen-Containing Oral Contraceptives: For women not taking carbamazepine, phenytoin, phenobarbital, primidone, or other drugs such as rifampin that induce lamotrigine glucuronidation *[see Drug Interactions (7), Clinical Pharmacology (12.3)]*, the maintenance dose of LAMICTAL XR will in most cases need to be increased by as much as 2-fold over the recommended target maintenance dose to maintain a consistent lamotrigine plasma level *[see Clinical Pharmacology (12.3)]*.

(2) Starting Estrogen-Containing Oral Contraceptives: In women taking a stable dose of LAMICTAL XR and not taking carbamazepine, phenytoin, phenobarbital, primidone, or other drugs such as rifampin that induce lamotrigine glucuronidation *[see Drug Interactions (7), Clinical Pharmacology (12.3)]*, the maintenance dose will in most cases need to be increased by as much as 2-fold to maintain a consistent lamotrigine plasma level. The dose increases should begin at the same time that the oral contraceptive is introduced and continue, based on clinical response, no more rapidly than 50 to 100 mg/day every week. Dose increases should not exceed the recommended rate (see Table 1) unless lamotrigine plasma levels or clinical response support larger increases. Gradual transient increases in lamotrigine plasma levels may occur during the week of inactive hormonal preparation (pill-free week), and these increases will be greater if dose increases are made in the days before or during the week of inactive hormonal preparation. Increased lamotrigine plasma levels could result in additional adverse reactions, such as dizziness, ataxia, and diplopia. If adverse reactions attributable to LAMICTAL XR consistently occur during the pill-free week, dose adjustments to the overall maintenance dose may be necessary. Dose adjustments limited to the pill-free week are not recommended. For women taking LAMICTAL XR in addition to carbamazepine, phenytoin, phenobarbital, primidone, or other drugs such as rifampin that induce lamotrigine glucuronidation *[see Drug Interactions (7), Clinical Pharmacology (12.3)]*, no adjustment to the dose of LAMICTAL XR should be necessary.

(3) Stopping Estrogen-Containing Oral Contraceptives: For women not taking carbamazepine, phenytoin, phenobarbital, primidone, or other drugs such as rifampin that induce lamotrigine glucuronidation *[see Drug Interactions (7), Clinical Pharmacology (12.3)]*, the maintenance dose of LAMICTAL XR will in most cases need to be decreased by as much as 50% in order to maintain a consistent lamotrigine plasma level. The decrease in dose of LAMICTAL XR should not exceed 25% of the total daily dose per week over a 2-week period, unless clinical response or lamotrigine plasma levels indicate otherwise *[see Clinical Pharmacology (12.3)]*. For women taking LAMICTAL XR in addition to carbamazepine, phenytoin, phenobarbital, primidone, or other drugs such as rifampin that induce lamotrigine glucuronidation *[see Drug Interactions (7), Clinical Pharmacology (12.3)]*, no adjustment to the dose of LAMICTAL XR should be necessary.

Women and Other Hormonal Contraceptive Preparations or Hormone Replacement Therapy: The effect of other hormonal contraceptive preparations or hormone replacement therapy on the pharmacokinetics of lamotrigine has not been systematically evaluated. It has been reported that ethinylestradiol, not progestogens, increased the clearance of lamotrigine up to 2-fold, and the progestin-only pills had no effect on lamotrigine plasma levels. Therefore, adjustments to the dosage of LAMICTAL XR in the presence of progestogens alone will likely not be needed.

Patients With Hepatic Impairment: Experience in patients with hepatic impairment is limited. Based on a clinical pharmacology study in 24 patients with mild, moderate, and severe liver impairment *[see Use in Specific Populations (8.6), Clinical Pharmacology (12.3)]*, the following general recommendations can be made. No dosage adjustment is needed in patients with mild liver impairment. Initial, escalation, and maintenance doses should generally be reduced by approximately 25% in patients with moderate and severe liver impairment without ascites and 50% in patients with severe liver impairment with ascites. Escalation and maintenance doses may be adjusted according to clinical response.

Patients With Renal Impairment: Initial doses of LAMICTAL XR should be based on patients' concomitant medications (see Table 1); reduced maintenance doses may be effective for patients with significant renal impairment *[see Use in Specific Populations (8.7), Clinical Pharmacology (12.3)]*. Few patients with severe renal impairment have been evaluated during chronic treatment with immediate-release lamotrigine. Because there is inadequate experience in this population, LAMICTAL XR should be used with caution in these patients.

Discontinuation Strategy: For patients receiving LAMICTAL XR in combination with other AEDs, a re-evaluation of all AEDs in the regimen should be considered if a change in seizure control or an appearance or worsening of adverse reactions is observed.

If a decision is made to discontinue therapy with LAMICTAL XR, a step-wise reduction of dose over at least 2

Table 1. Escalation Regimen for LAMICTAL XR in Patients ≥13 Years of Age

	For Patients TAKING Valproate[a]	For Patients NOT TAKING Carbamazepine, Phenytoin, Phenobarbital, Primidone,[b] or Valproate[a]	For Patients TAKING Carbamazepine, Phenytoin, Phenobarbital, or Primidone[b] and NOT TAKING Valproate[a]
Weeks 1 and 2	25 mg every *other* day	25 mg every day	50 mg every day
Weeks 3 and 4	25 mg every day	50 mg every day	100 mg every day
Week 5	50 mg every day	100 mg every day	200 mg every day
Week 6	100 mg every day	150 mg every day	300 mg every day
Week 7	150 mg every day	200 mg every day	400 mg every day
Maintenance range (week 8 and onward)	200 to 250 mg every day[c]	300 to 400 mg every day[c]	400 to 600 mg every day[c]

[a]Valproate has been shown to inhibit glucuronidation and decrease the apparent clearance of lamotrigine *[see Drug Interactions (7), Clinical Pharmacology (12.3)]*.

[b]These drugs induce lamotrigine glucuronidation and increase clearance *[see Drug Interactions (7), Clinical Pharmacology (12.3)]*. Other drugs that have similar effects include estrogen-containing oral contraceptives *[see Drug Interactions (7), Clinical Pharmacology (12.3)]*. Dosing recommendations for oral contraceptives can be found in General Dosing Considerations *[see Dosage and Administration (2.1)]*. Patients on rifampin, or other drugs that induce lamotrigine glucuronidation and increase clearance, should follow the same dosing titration/maintenance regimen as that used with anticonvulsants that have this effect.

[c]Dose increases at week 8 or later should not exceed 100 mg daily at weekly intervals.

weeks (approximately 50% per week) is recommended unless safety concerns require a more rapid withdrawal *[see Warnings and Precautions (5.8)]*.

Discontinuing carbamazepine, phenytoin, phenobarbital, primidone, or other drugs such as rifampin that induce lamotrigine glucuronidation should prolong the half-life of lamotrigine; discontinuing valproate should shorten the half-life of lamotrigine.

2.2 Adjunctive Therapy for Primary Generalized Tonic-Clonic and Partial Onset Seizures

This section provides specific dosing recommendations for patients ≥13 years of age. Specific dosing recommendations are provided depending upon concomitant AED or other concomitant medications.

[See table 1 at top of previous page]

2.3 Conversion From Adjunctive Therapy to Monotherapy

The goal of the transition regimen is to attempt to maintain seizure control while mitigating the risk of serious rash associated with the rapid titration of LAMICTAL XR.

The recommended maintenance dosage range of LAMICTAL XR as monotherapy is 250 to 300 mg given once daily.

The recommended initial dose and subsequent dose escalations for LAMICTAL XR should not be exceeded *[see Boxed Warning]*.

Conversion From Adjunctive Therapy With Carbamazepine, Phenytoin, Phenobarbital, or Primidone to Monotherapy With LAMICTAL XR: After achieving a dosage of 500 mg/day of LAMICTAL XR using the guidelines in Table 1, the concomitant enzyme-inducing AED should be withdrawn by 20% decrements each week over a 4-week period. Two weeks after completion of withdrawal of the enzyme-inducing AED, the dosage of LAMICTAL XR may be decreased no faster than 100 mg/day each week to achieve the monotherapy maintenance dosage range of 250 to 300 mg/day.

The regimen for the withdrawal of the concomitant AED is based on experience gained in the controlled monotherapy clinical trial using immediate-release lamotrigine.

Conversion From Adjunctive Therapy With Valproate to Monotherapy With LAMICTAL XR: The conversion regimen involves the 4 steps outlined in Table 2.

Table 2. Conversion From Adjunctive Therapy With Valproate to Monotherapy With LAMICTAL XR in Patients ≥13 Years of Age With Epilepsy

	LAMICTAL XR	Valproate
Step 1	Achieve a dosage of 150 mg/day according to guidelines in Table 1.	Maintain established stable dose.
Step 2	Maintain at 150 mg/day.	Decrease dosage by decrements no greater than 500 mg/day/week to 500 mg/day and then maintain for 1 week.
Step 3	Increase to 200 mg/day.	Simultaneously decrease to 250 mg/day and maintain for 1 week.
Step 4	Increase to 250 or 300 mg/day.	Discontinue.

Conversion From Adjunctive Therapy With Antiepileptic Drugs Other Than Carbamazepine, Phenytoin, Phenobarbital, Primidone, or Valproate to Monotherapy With LAMICTAL XR: After achieving a dosage of 250 to 300 mg/day of LAMICTAL XR using the guidelines in Table 1, the concomitant AED should be withdrawn by 20% decrements each week over a 4-week period. No adjustment to the monotherapy dose of LAMICTAL XR is needed.

2.4 Conversion From Immediate-Release Lamotrigine Tablets to LAMICTAL XR

Patients may be converted directly from immediate-release lamotrigine to LAMICTAL XR Extended-Release Tablets. The initial dose of LAMICTAL XR should match the total daily dose of immediate-release lamotrigine. However, some subjects on concomitant enzyme-inducing agents may have lower plasma levels of lamotrigine on conversion and should be monitored *[see Clinical Pharmacology (12.3)]*.

Following conversion to LAMICTAL XR, all patients (but especially those on drugs that induce lamotrigine glucuronidation) should be closely monitored for seizure control *[see Drug Interactions (7)]*. Depending on the therapeutic response after conversion, the total daily dose may need to be adjusted within the recommended dosing instructions (Table 1).

3 DOSAGE FORMS AND STRENGTHS

3.1 Extended-Release Tablets

25 mg, yellow with white center, round, biconvex, film-coated tablets printed with "LAMICTAL" and "XR 25."

50 mg, green with white center, round, biconvex, film-coated tablets printed with "LAMICTAL" and "XR 50."

100 mg, orange with white center, round, biconvex, film-coated tablets printed with "LAMICTAL" and "XR 100."

200 mg, blue with white center, round, biconvex, film-coated tablets printed with "LAMICTAL" and "XR 200."

250 mg, purple with white center, caplet-shaped, film-coated tablets printed with "LAMICTAL" and "XR 250."

300 mg, gray with white center, caplet-shaped, film-coated tablets printed with "LAMICTAL" and "XR 300."

3.2 Potential Medication Errors

Patients should be strongly advised to visually inspect their tablets to verify that they are receiving LAMICTAL XR, as opposed to other medications, and that they are receiving the correct formulation of lamotrigine each time they fill their prescription. Depictions of the LAMICTAL XR tablets can be found in the Medication Guide.

4 CONTRAINDICATIONS

LAMICTAL XR is contraindicated in patients who have demonstrated hypersensitivity (e.g., rash, angioedema, acute urticaria, extensive pruritus, mucosal ulceration) to the drug or its ingredients *[see Boxed Warning, Warnings and Precautions (5.1, 5.2)]*.

5 WARNINGS AND PRECAUTIONS

5.1 Serious Skin Rashes

The risk of serious rash caused by treatment with LAMICTAL XR is not expected to differ from that with immediate-release lamotrigine *[see Boxed Warning]*. However, the relatively limited treatment experience with LAMICTAL XR makes it difficult to characterize the frequency and risk of serious rashes caused by treatment with LAMICTAL XR.

Pediatric Population: The incidence of serious rash associated with hospitalization and discontinuation of immediate-release lamotrigine in a prospectively followed cohort of pediatric patients (aged 2 to 16 years) with epilepsy receiving adjunctive therapy with immediate-release lamotrigine was approximately 0.8% (16 of 1,983). When 14 of these cases were reviewed by 3 expert dermatologists, there was considerable disagreement as to their proper classification. To illustrate, one dermatologist considered none of the cases to be Stevens-Johnson syndrome; another assigned 7 of the 14 to this diagnosis. There was 1 rash-related death in this 1,983-patient cohort. Additionally, there have been rare cases of toxic epidermal necrolysis with and without permanent sequelae and/or death in US and foreign postmarketing experience.

There is evidence that the inclusion of valproate in a multidrug regimen increases the risk of serious, potentially life-threatening rash in pediatric patients. In pediatric patients who used valproate concomitantly, 1.2% (6 of 482) experienced a serious rash compared with 0.6% (6 of 952) patients not taking valproate.

LAMICTAL XR is not approved in patients less than 13 years of age.

Adult Population: Serious rash associated with hospitalization and discontinuation of immediate-release lamotrigine occurred in 0.3% (11 of 3,348) of adult patients who received immediate-release lamotrigine in premarketing clinical trials of epilepsy. In worldwide postmarketing experience, rare cases of rash-related death have been reported, but their numbers are too few to permit a precise estimate of the rate.

Among the rashes leading to hospitalization were Stevens-Johnson syndrome, toxic epidermal necrolysis, angioedema, and those associated with multiorgan hypersensitivity *[see Warnings and Precautions (5.2)]*.

There is evidence that the inclusion of valproate in a multidrug regimen increases the risk of serious, potentially life-threatening rash in adults. Specifically, of 584 patients administered immediate-release lamotrigine with valproate in epilepsy clinical trials, 6 (1%) were hospitalized in association with rash; in contrast, 4 (0.16%) of 2,398 clinical trial patients and volunteers administered immediate-release lamotrigine in the absence of valproate were hospitalized.

Patients With History of Allergy or Rash to Other Antiepileptic Drugs: The risk of nonserious rash may be increased when the recommended initial dose and/or the rate of dose escalation for LAMICTAL XR is exceeded and in patients with a history of allergy or rash to other AEDs.

5.2 Multiorgan Hypersensitivity Reactions and Organ Failure

Multiorgan hypersensitivity reactions, also known as Drug Reaction with Eosinophilia and Systemic Symptoms (DRESS), have occurred with LAMICTAL. Some have been fatal or life threatening. DRESS typically, although not exclusively, presents with fever, rash, and/or lymphadenopathy in association with other organ system involvement, such as hepatitis, nephritis, hematologic abnormalities, myocarditis, or myositis, sometimes resembling an acute viral infection. Eosinophilia is often present. This disorder is variable in its expression and other organ systems not noted here may be involved.

Fatalities associated with acute multiorgan failure and various degrees of hepatic failure have been reported in 2 of 3,796 adult patients and 4 of 2,435 pediatric patients who received LAMICTAL in epilepsy clinical trials. Rare fatalities from multiorgan failure have also been reported in postmarketing use.

Isolated liver failure without rash or involvement of other organs has also been reported with LAMICTAL.

It is important to note that early manifestations of hypersensitivity (e.g., fever, lymphadenopathy) may be present even though a rash is not evident. If such signs or symptoms are present, the patient should be evaluated immediately. LAMICTAL XR should be discontinued if an alternative etiology for the signs or symptoms cannot be established.

Prior to initiation of treatment with LAMICTAL XR, the patient should be instructed that a rash or other signs or symptoms of hypersensitivity (e.g., fever, lymphadenopathy) may herald a serious medical event and that the patient should report any such occurrence to a physician immediately.

5.3 Blood Dyscrasias

There have been reports of blood dyscrasias with immediate-release lamotrigine that may or may not be associated with multiorgan hypersensitivity (also known as DRESS) *[see Warnings and Precautions (5.2)]*. These have included neutropenia, leukopenia, anemia, thrombocytopenia, pancytopenia, and, rarely, aplastic anemia and pure red cell aplasia.

5.4 Suicidal Behavior and Ideation

AEDs, including LAMICTAL XR, increase the risk of suicidal thoughts or behavior in patients taking these drugs for any indication. Patients treated with any AED for any indication should be monitored for the emergence or worsening of depression, suicidal thoughts or behavior, and/or any unusual changes in mood or behavior.

Pooled analyses of 199 placebo-controlled clinical trials (monotherapy and adjunctive therapy) of 11 different AEDs showed that patients randomized to 1 of the AEDs had approximately twice the risk (adjusted Relative Risk 1.8, 95% CI: 1.2, 2.7) of suicidal thinking or behavior compared to patients randomized to placebo. In these trials, which had a median treatment duration of 12 weeks, the estimated incidence of suicidal behavior or ideation among 27,863 AED-treated patients was 0.43%, compared to 0.24% among 16,029 placebo-treated patients, representing an increase of approximately 1 case of suicidal thinking or behavior for every 530 patients treated. There were 4 suicides in drug-treated patients in the trials and none in placebo-treated patients, but the number of events is too small to allow any conclusion about drug effect on suicide.

The increased risk of suicidal thoughts or behavior with AEDs was observed as early as 1 week after starting treatment with AEDs and persisted for the duration of treatment assessed. Because most trials included in the analysis did not extend beyond 24 weeks, the risk of suicidal thoughts or behavior beyond 24 weeks could not be assessed.

The risk of suicidal thoughts or behavior was generally consistent among drugs in the data analyzed. The finding of increased risk with AEDs of varying mechanism of action and across a range of indications suggests that the risk applies to all AEDs used for any indication. The risk did not vary substantially by age (5 to 100 years) in the clinical trials analyzed.

Table 3 shows absolute and relative risk by indication for all evaluated AEDs.

[See table 3 at top of next page]

The relative risk for suicidal thoughts or behavior was higher in clinical trials for epilepsy than in clinical trials for psychiatric or other conditions, but the absolute risk differences were similar for the epilepsy and psychiatric indications.

Anyone considering prescribing LAMICTAL XR or any other AED must balance the risk of suicidal thoughts or behavior with the risk of untreated illness. Epilepsy and many other illnesses for which AEDs are prescribed are themselves associated with morbidity and mortality and an increased risk of suicidal thoughts and behavior. Should suicidal thoughts and behavior emerge during treatment, the prescriber needs to consider whether the emergence of these symptoms in any given patient may be related to the illness being treated.

Patients, their caregivers, and families should be informed that AEDs increase the risk of suicidal thoughts and behavior and should be advised of the need to be alert for the emergence or worsening of the signs and symptoms of depression; any unusual changes in mood or behavior; or the emergence of suicidal thoughts, behavior, or thoughts about self-harm. Behaviors of concern should be reported immediately to healthcare providers.

5.5 Aseptic Meningitis

Therapy with lamotrigine increases the risk of developing aseptic meningitis. Because of the potential for serious outcomes of untreated meningitis due to other causes, patients should also be evaluated for other causes of meningitis and treated as appropriate.

Table 3. Risk by Indication for Antiepileptic Drugs in the Pooled Analysis

Indication	Placebo Patients With Events per 1,000 Patients	Drug Patients With Events per 1,000 Patients	Relative Risk: Incidence of Events in Drug Patients/Incidence in Placebo Patients	Risk Difference: Additional Drug Patients With Events per 1,000 Patients
Epilepsy	1.0	3.4	3.5	2.4
Psychiatric	5.7	8.5	1.5	2.9
Other	1.0	1.8	1.9	0.9
Total	2.4	4.3	1.8	1.9

Postmarketing cases of aseptic meningitis have been reported in pediatric and adult patients taking lamotrigine for various indications. Symptoms upon presentation have included headache, fever, nausea, vomiting, and nuchal rigidity. Rash, photophobia, myalgia, chills, altered consciousness, and somnolence were also noted in some cases. Symptoms have been reported to occur within 1 day to one and a half months following the initiation of treatment. In most cases, symptoms were reported to resolve after discontinuation of lamotrigine. Re-exposure resulted in a rapid return of symptoms (from within 30 minutes to 1 day following re-initiation of treatment) that were frequently more severe. Some of the patients treated with LAMICTAL who developed aseptic meningitis had underlying diagnoses of systemic lupus erythematosus or other autoimmune diseases.

Cerebrospinal fluid (CSF) analyzed at the time of clinical presentation in reported cases was characterized by a mild to moderate pleocytosis, normal glucose levels, and mild to moderate increase in protein. CSF white blood cell count differentials showed a predominance of neutrophils in a majority of the cases, although a predominance of lymphocytes was reported in approximately one third of the cases. Some patients also had new onset of signs and symptoms of involvement of other organs (predominantly hepatic and renal involvement), which may suggest that in these cases the aseptic meningitis observed was part of a hypersensitivity reaction [see Warnings and Precautions (5.2)].

5.6   Potential Medication Errors
Medication errors involving LAMICTAL have occurred. In particular, the names LAMICTAL or lamotrigine can be confused with the names of other commonly used medications. Medication errors may also occur between the different formulations of LAMICTAL. To reduce the potential of medication errors, write and say LAMICTAL XR clearly. Depictions of the LAMICTAL XR Extended-Release Tablets can be found in the Medication Guide. Each LAMICTAL XR tablet has a distinct color and white center, and is printed with "LAMICTAL XR" and the tablet strength. These distinctive features serve to identify the different presentations of the drug and thus may help reduce the risk of medication errors. LAMICTAL XR is supplied in round, unit-of-use bottles with orange caps containing 30 tablets. The label on the bottle includes a depiction of the tablets that further communicates to patients and pharmacists that the medication is LAMICTAL XR and the specific tablet strength included in the bottle. The unit-of-use bottle with a distinctive orange cap and distinctive bottle label features serves to identify the different presentations of the drug and thus may help to reduce the risk of medication errors. To avoid the medication error of using the wrong drug or formulation, patients should be strongly advised to visually inspect their tablets to verify that they are LAMICTAL XR each time they fill their prescription.

5.7   Concomitant Use With Oral Contraceptives
Some estrogen-containing oral contraceptives have been shown to decrease serum concentrations of lamotrigine [see Clinical Pharmacology (12.3)]. **Dosage adjustments will be necessary in most patients who start or stop estrogen-containing oral contraceptives while taking LAMICTAL XR** [see Dosage and Administration (2.1)]. During the week of inactive hormone preparation (pill-free week) of oral contraceptive therapy, plasma lamotrigine levels are expected to rise, as much as doubling at the end of the week. Adverse reactions consistent with elevated levels of lamotrigine, such as dizziness, ataxia, and diplopia, could occur.

5.8   Withdrawal Seizures
As with other AEDs, LAMICTAL XR should not be abruptly discontinued. In patients with epilepsy there is a possibility of increasing seizure frequency. Unless safety concerns require a more rapid withdrawal, the dose of LAMICTAL XR should be tapered over a period of at least 2 weeks (approximately 50% reduction per week) [see Dosage and Administration (2.1)].

5.9   Status Epilepticus
Valid estimates of the incidence of treatment-emergent status epilepticus among patients treated with immediate-release lamotrigine are difficult to obtain because reporters participating in clinical trials did not all employ identical rules for identifying cases. At a minimum, 7 of 2,343 adult patients had episodes that could unequivocally be described as status epilepticus. In addition, a number of reports of variably defined episodes of seizure exacerbation (e.g., seizure clusters, seizure flurries) were made.

5.10   Sudden Unexplained Death in Epilepsy
During the premarketing development of immediate-release lamotrigine, 20 sudden and unexplained deaths were recorded among a cohort of 4,700 patients with epilepsy (5,747 patient-years of exposure).

Some of these could represent seizure-related deaths in which the seizure was not observed, e.g., at night. This represents an incidence of 0.0035 deaths per patient-year. Although this rate exceeds that expected in a healthy population matched for age and sex, it is within the range of estimates for the incidence of sudden unexplained death in patients with epilepsy not receiving lamotrigine (ranging from 0.0005 for the general population of patients with epilepsy, to 0.004 for a recently studied clinical trial population similar to that in the clinical development program for immediate-release lamotrigine, to 0.005 for patients with refractory epilepsy). Consequently, whether these figures are reassuring or suggest concern depends on the comparability of the populations reported upon to the cohort receiving immediate-release lamotrigine and the accuracy of the estimates provided. Probably most reassuring is the similarity of estimated sudden unexplained death in epilepsy (SUDEP) rates in patients receiving immediate-release lamotrigine and those receiving other AEDs, chemically unrelated to each other, that underwent clinical testing in similar populations. Importantly, that drug is chemically unrelated to lamotrigine. This evidence suggests, although it certainly does not prove, that the high SUDEP rates reflect population rates, not a drug effect.

5.11   Addition of LAMICTAL XR to a Multidrug Regimen That Includes Valproate
Because valproate reduces the clearance of lamotrigine, the dosage of lamotrigine in the presence of valproate is less than half of that required in its absence [see Dosage and Administration (2.1, 2.2), Drug Interactions (7)].

5.12   Binding in the Eye and Other Melanin-Containing Tissues
Because lamotrigine binds to melanin, it could accumulate in melanin-rich tissues over time. This raises the possibility that lamotrigine may cause toxicity in these tissues after extended use. Although ophthalmological testing was performed in 1 controlled clinical trial, the testing was inadequate to exclude subtle effects or injury occurring after longterm exposure. Moreover, the capacity of available tests to detect potentially adverse consequences, if any, of lamotrigine binding to melanin is unknown [see Clinical Pharmacology (12.2)].

Accordingly, although there are no specific recommendations for periodic ophthalmological monitoring, prescribers should be aware of the possibility of long-term ophthalmologic effects.

5.13   Laboratory Tests
Plasma Concentrations of Lamotrigine: The value of monitoring plasma concentrations of lamotrigine in patients treated with LAMICTAL XR has not been established. Because of the possible pharmacokinetic interactions between lamotrigine and other drugs, including AEDs (see Table 6), monitoring of the plasma levels of lamotrigine and concomitant drugs may be indicated, particularly during dosage adjustments. In general, clinical judgment should be exercised regarding monitoring of plasma levels of lamotrigine and other drugs and whether or not dosage adjustments are necessary.

Effect on Leukocytes: Treatment with LAMICTAL XR caused an increased incidence of subnormal (below the reference range) values in some hematology analytes (e.g., total white blood cells, monocytes). The treatment effect (LAMICTAL XR % - Placebo %) incidence of subnormal counts was 3% for total white blood cells and 4% for monocytes.

6   ADVERSE REACTIONS

The following adverse reactions are described in more detail in the Warnings and Precautions section of the label:
- Serious skin rashes [see Warnings and Precautions (5.1)]
- Multiorgan hypersensitivity reactions and organ failure [see Warnings and Precautions (5.2)]
- Blood dyscrasias [see Warnings and Precautions (5.3)]
- Suicidal behavior and ideation [see Warnings and Precautions (5.4)]
- Aseptic meningitis [see Warnings and Precautions (5.5)]
- Withdrawal seizures [see Warnings and Precautions (5.8)]
- Status epilepticus [see Warnings and Precautions (5.9)]
- Sudden unexplained death in epilepsy [see Warnings and Precautions (5.10)]

6.1   Clinical Trial Experience With LAMICTAL XR for Treatment of Primary Generalized Tonic-Clonic and Partial Onset Seizures
Most Common Adverse Reactions in Clinical Studies: Adjunctive Therapy in Patients With Epilepsy: Because clinical trials are conducted under widely varying conditions, adverse reaction rates observed in the clinical trials of a drug cannot be directly compared with rates in the clinical trials of another drug and may not reflect the rates observed in practice.

LAMICTAL XR has been evaluated for safety in patients ≥13 years of age with PGTC and partial onset seizures. The most commonly observed adverse reactions in these 2 double-blind, placebo-controlled trials of adjunctive therapy with LAMICTAL XR were, in order of decreasing incidence (treatment difference between LAMICTAL XR and placebo ≥4%): dizziness, tremor/intention tremor, vomiting, and diplopia.

In these 2 trials, adverse reactions led to withdrawal of 4 (2%) patients in the group receiving placebo and 10 (5%) patients in the group receiving LAMICTAL XR. Dizziness was the most common reason for withdrawal in the group receiving LAMICTAL XR (5 patients [3%]). The next common adverse reactions leading to withdrawal in 2 patients each (1%) were rash, headache, nausea, and nystagmus.

Table 4 displays the incidence of adverse reactions in these two 19-week, double-blind, placebo-controlled studies of patients with PGTC and partial onset seizures.

Table 4. Adverse Reaction Incidence in Double-Blind, Placebo-Controlled Adjunctive Trials of Patients With Epilepsy (Adverse Reactions ≥2% of Patients Treated With LAMICTAL XR and Numerically More Frequent Than in the Placebo Group)

Body System/Adverse Reaction	LAMICTAL XR (n = 190) %	Placebo (n = 195) %
Ear and labyrinth disorders		
Vertigo	3	<1
Eye disorders		
Diplopia	5	<1
Vision blurred	3	2
Gastrointestinal disorders		
Nausea	7	4
Vomiting	6	3
Diarrhea	5	3
Constipation	2	<1
Dry mouth	2	1
General disorders and administration site conditions		
Asthenia and fatigue	6	4
Infections and infestations		
Sinusitis	2	1
Metabolic and nutritional disorders		
Anorexia	3	2
Musculoskeletal and connective tissue disorder		
Myalgia	2	0
Nervous system		
Dizziness	14	6
Tremor and intention tremor	6	1
Somnolence	5	3
Cerebellar coordination and balance disorder	3	0
Nystagmus	2	<1
Psychiatric disorders		
Depression	3	<1
Anxiety	3	0

Respiratory, thoracic, and mediastinal disorders		
Pharyngolaryngeal pain	3	2
Vascular disorder		
Hot flush	2	0

Note: In these trials the incidence of nonserious rash was 2% for LAMICTAL XR and 3% for placebo. In clinical trials evaluating immediate-release lamotrigine, the rate of serious rash was 0.3% in adults on adjunctive therapy for epilepsy [see Boxed Warning].

Adverse reactions were also analyzed to assess the incidence of the onset of an event in the titration period, and in the maintenance period, and if adverse reactions occurring in the titration phase persisted in the maintenance phase. The incidence for many adverse reactions caused by treatment with LAMICTAL XR was increased relative to placebo (i.e., treatment difference between LAMICTAL XR and placebo ≥2%) in either the titration or maintenance phases of the study. During the titration phase, an increased incidence (shown in descending order of % treatment difference) was observed for diarrhea, nausea, vomiting, somnolence, vertigo, myalgia, hot flush, and anxiety. During the maintenance phase, an increased incidence was observed for dizziness, tremor, and diplopia. Some adverse reactions developing in the titration phase were notable for persisting (>7 days) into the maintenance phase. These "persistent" adverse reactions included somnolence and dizziness.

There were inadequate data to evaluate the effect of dose and/or concentration on the incidence of adverse reactions because, although patients were randomized to different target doses based upon concomitant AED, the plasma exposure was expected to be generally similar among all patients receiving different doses. However, in a randomized, parallel study comparing placebo and 300 and 500 mg/day of immediate-release lamotrigine, the incidence of the most common adverse reactions (≥5%) such as ataxia, blurred vision, diplopia, and dizziness were dose related. Less common adverse reactions (<5%) were not assessed for dose-response relationships.

Monotherapy in Patients With Epilepsy: Adverse reactions observed in this study were generally similar to those observed and attributed to drug in adjunctive and monotherapy immediate-release lamotrigine and adjunctive LAMICTAL XR placebo-controlled studies. Only 2 adverse events, nasopharyngitis and upper respiratory tract infection, were observed at a rate of ≥3% and not reported at a similar rate in previous studies. Because this study did not include a placebo control group, causality could not be established [see Clinical Studies (14.3)].

6.2   Other Adverse Reactions Observed During the Clinical Development of Immediate-Release Lamotrigine
All reported reactions are included except those already listed in the previous tables or elsewhere in the labeling, those too general to be informative, and those not reasonably associated with the use of the drug.

Adjunctive Therapy in Adults With Epilepsy: In addition to the adverse reactions reported above from the development of LAMICTAL XR, the following adverse reactions with an uncertain relationship to lamotrigine were reported during the clinical development of immediate-release lamotrigine for treatment of epilepsy in adults. These reactions occurred in ≥2% of patients receiving immediate-release lamotrigine and more frequently than in the placebo group.
Body as a Whole: Headache, flu syndrome, fever, neck pain.
Musculoskeletal: Arthralgia.
Nervous: Insomnia, convulsion, irritability, speech disorder, concentration disturbance.
Respiratory: Pharyngitis, cough increased.
Skin and Appendages: Rash, pruritus.
Urogenital (female patients only): Vaginitis, amenorrhea, dysmenorrhea.
Monotherapy in Adults With Epilepsy: In addition to the adverse reactions reported above from the development of LAMICTAL XR, the following adverse reactions with an uncertain relationship to lamotrigine were reported during the clinical development of immediate-release lamotrigine for treatment of epilepsy in adults. These reactions occurred in >2% of patients receiving immediate-release lamotrigine and more frequently than in the placebo group.
Body as a Whole: Chest pain.
Digestive: Rectal hemorrhage, peptic ulcer.
Metabolic and Nutritional: Weight decrease, peripheral edema.
Nervous: Hypesthesia, libido increase, decreased reflexes.
Respiratory: Epistaxis, dyspnea.
Skin and Appendages: Contact dermatitis, dry skin, sweating.
Special Senses: Vision abnormality.
Urogenital (female patients only): Dysmenorrhea.
Other Clinical Trial Experience: Immediate-release lamotrigine has been administered to 6,694 individuals for whom complete adverse reaction data was captured during all clinical trials, only some of which were placebo controlled.

Adverse reactions are further classified within body system categories and enumerated in order of decreasing frequency using the following definitions: *frequent* adverse reactions are defined as those occurring in at least 1/100 patients; *in-*

frequent adverse reactions are those occurring in 1/100 to 1/1,000 patients; *rare* adverse reactions are those occurring in fewer than 1/1,000 patients.
Cardiovascular System: Infrequent: Hypertension, palpitations, postural hypotension, syncope, tachycardia, vasodilation.
Dermatological: Infrequent: Acne, alopecia, hirsutism, maculopapular rash, urticaria. *Rare:* Leukoderma, multiforme erythema, petechial rash, pustular rash.
Digestive System: Infrequent: Dysphagia, liver function tests abnormal, mouth ulceration. *Rare:* Gastrointestinal hemorrhage, hemorrhagic colitis, hepatitis, melena and stomach ulcer.
Endocrine System: Rare: Goiter, hypothyroidism.
Hematologic and Lymphatic System: Infrequent: Ecchymosis, leukopenia. *Rare:* Anemia, eosinophilia, fibrin decrease, fibrinogen decrease, iron deficiency anemia, leukocytosis, lymphocytosis, macrocytic anemia, petechia, thrombocytopenia.
Metabolic and Nutritional Disorders: Infrequent: Aspartate transaminase increased. *Rare:* Alcohol intolerance, alkaline phosphatase increase, alanine transaminase increase, bilirubinemia, gamma glutamyl transpeptidase increase, hyperglycemia.
Musculoskeletal System: Rare: Muscle atrophy, pathological fracture, tendinous contracture.
Nervous System: Frequent: Confusion. *Infrequent:* Akathisia, apathy, aphasia, depersonalization, dysarthria, dyskinesia, euphoria, hallucinations, hostility, hyperkinesia, hypertonia, libido decreased, memory decrease, mind racing, movement disorder, myoclonus, panic attack, paranoid reaction, personality disorder, psychosis, stupor. *Rare:* Choreoathetosis, delirium, delusions, dysphoria, dystonia, extrapyramidal syndrome, hemiplegia, hyperalgesia, hyperesthesia, hypokinesia, hypotonia, manic depression reaction, neuralgia, paralysis, peripheral neuritis.
Respiratory System: Rare: Hiccup, hyperventilation.
Special Senses: Frequent: Amblyopia. *Infrequent:* Abnormality of accommodation, conjunctivitis, dry eyes, ear pain, photophobia, taste perversion, tinnitus. *Rare:* Deafness, lacrimation disorder, oscillopsia, parosmia, ptosis, strabismus, taste loss, uveitis, visual field defect.
Urogenital System: Infrequent: Abnormal ejaculation, hematuria, impotence, menorrhagia, polyuria, urinary incontinence. *Rare:* Acute kidney failure, breast neoplasm, creatinine increase, female lactation, kidney failure, kidney pain, nocturia, urinary retention, urinary urgency.

6.3   Postmarketing Experience With Immediate-Release Lamotrigine
The following adverse events (not listed above in clinical trials or other sections of the prescribing information) have been identified during postapproval use of immediate-release lamotrigine. Because these events are reported voluntarily from a population of uncertain size, it is not always possible to reliably estimate their frequency or establish a causal relationship to drug exposure.
Blood and Lymphatic: Agranulocytosis, hemolytic anemia, lymphadenopathy not associated with hypersensitivity disorder.
Gastrointestinal: Esophagitis.
Hepatobiliary Tract and Pancreas: Pancreatitis.
Immunologic: Lupus-like reaction, vasculitis.
Lower Respiratory: Apnea.
Musculoskeletal: Rhabdomyolysis has been observed in patients experiencing hypersensitivity reactions.
Neurology: Exacerbation of Parkinsonian symptoms in patients with pre-existing Parkinson's disease, tics.
Non-site Specific: Progressive immunosuppression.

7   DRUG INTERACTIONS
Significant drug interactions with lamotrigine are summarized in Table 5. Additional details of these drug interaction studies, which were conducted using immediate-release lamotrigine, are provided in the Clinical Pharmacology section [see Clinical Pharmacology (12.3)].
[See table 5 below]

8   USE IN SPECIFIC POPULATIONS
8.1   Pregnancy
As with other AEDs, physiological changes during pregnancy may affect lamotrigine concentrations and/or therapeutic effect. There have been reports of decreased lamotrigine concentrations during pregnancy and restoration of pre-partum concentrations after delivery. Dosage adjustments may be necessary to maintain clinical response. Pregnancy Category C.
There are no adequate and well-controlled studies in pregnant women. In animal studies, lamotrigine was developmentally toxic at doses lower than those administered clinically. LAMICTAL XR should be used during pregnancy only if the potential benefit justifies the potential risk to the fetus.
When lamotrigine was administered to pregnant mice, rats, or rabbits during the period of organogenesis (oral doses of

Table 5. Established and Other Potentially Significant Drug Interactions

Concomitant Drug	Effect on Concentration of Lamotrigine or Concomitant Drug	Clinical Comment
Estrogen-containing oral contraceptive preparations containing 30 mcg ethinylestradiol and 150 mcg levonorgestrel	↓ lamotrigine	Decreased lamotrigine levels approximately 50%.
	↓ levonorgestrel	Decrease in levonorgestrel component by 19%.
Carbamazepine and carbamazepine epoxide	↓ lamotrigine	Addition of carbamazepine decreases lamotrigine concentration approximately 40%.
	? CBZ epoxide	May increase carbamazepine epoxide levels.
Phenobarbital/primidone	↓ lamotrigine	Decreased lamotrigine concentration approximately 40%.
Phenytoin	↓ lamotrigine	Decreased lamotrigine concentration approximately 40%.
Rifampin	↓ lamotrigine	Decreased lamotrigine AUC approximately 40%.
Valproate	↑ lamotrigine	Increased lamotrigine concentrations slightly more than 2-fold.
	? valproate	Decreased valproate concentrations an average of 25% over a 3-week period then stabilized in healthy volunteers; no change in controlled clinical trials in epilepsy patients.

↓ = Decreased (induces lamotrigine glucuronidation).
↑ = Increased (inhibits lamotrigine glucuronidation).
? = Conflicting data.

up to 125, 25, and 30 mg/kg, respectively), reduced fetal body weight and increased incidences of fetal skeletal variations were seen in mice and rats at doses that were also maternally toxic. The no-effect doses for embryo-fetal developmental toxicity in mice, rats, and rabbits (75, 6.25, 30 mg/kg, respectively) are similar to (mice and rabbits) or less than the human dose of 400 mg/day on a body surface area (mg/m^2) basis.

In a study in which pregnant rats were administered lamotrigine (oral doses of 5 or 25 mg/kg) during the period of organogenesis and offspring were evaluated postnatally, behavioral abnormalities were observed in exposed offspring at both doses. The lowest effect dose for developmental neurotoxicity in rats is less than the human dose of 400 mg/day on a mg/m^2 basis. Maternal toxicity was observed at the higher dose tested.

When pregnant rats were administered lamotrigine (oral doses of 5, 10, or 20 mg/kg) during the latter part of gestation, increased offspring mortality (including stillbirths) was seen at all doses. The lowest effect dose for peri/postnatal developmental toxicity in rats is less than the human dose of 400 mg/day on a mg/m^2 basis. Maternal toxicity was observed at the 2 highest doses tested.

Lamotrigine decreases fetal folate concentrations in rat, an effect known to be associated with adverse pregnancy outcomes in animals and humans.

Pregnancy Registry: To provide information regarding the effects of in utero exposure to LAMICTAL XR, physicians are advised to recommend that pregnant patients taking LAMICTAL XR enroll in the North American Antiepileptic Drug (NAAED) Pregnancy Registry. This can be done by calling the toll-free number 1-888-233-2334, and must be done by patients themselves. Information on the registry can also be found at the website http://www.aedpregnancyregistry.org.

8.2 Labor and Delivery
The effect of LAMICTAL XR on labor and delivery in humans is unknown.

8.3 Nursing Mothers
Lamotrigine is present in milk from lactating women taking LAMICTAL XR. Data from multiple small studies indicate that lamotrigine plasma levels in human milk-fed infants have been reported to be as high as 50% of the maternal serum levels. Neonates and young infants are at risk for high serum levels because maternal serum and milk levels can rise to high levels postpartum if lamotrigine dosage has been increased during pregnancy but not later reduced to the pre-pregnancy dosage. Lamotrigine exposure is further increased due to the immaturity of the infant glucuronidation capacity needed for drug clearance. Events including apnea, drowsiness, and poor sucking have been reported in infants who have been human milk-fed by mothers using lamotrigine; whether or not these events were caused by lamotrigine is unknown. Human milk-fed infants should be closely monitored for adverse events resulting from lamotrigine. Measurement of infant serum levels should be performed to rule out toxicity if concerns arise. Human milk-feeding should be discontinued in infants with lamotrigine toxicity. Caution should be exercised when LAMICTAL XR is administered to a nursing woman.

8.4 Pediatric Use
LAMICTAL XR is indicated as adjunctive therapy for PGTC and partial onset seizures with or without secondary generalization in patients ≥13 years of age. Safety and effectiveness of LAMICTAL XR for any use in patients less than 13 years of age have not been established.

Immediate-release lamotrigine is indicated for adjunctive therapy in patients ≥2 years of age for partial seizures, the generalized seizures of Lennox-Gastaut syndrome, and PGTC seizures.

Safety and efficacy of immediate-release lamotrigine, used as adjunctive treatment for partial seizures, were not demonstrated in a small, randomized, double-blind, placebo-controlled withdrawal study in very young pediatric patients (aged 1 to 24 months). Immediate-release lamotrigine was associated with an increased risk for infectious adverse reactions (lamotrigine 37%, placebo 5%), and respiratory adverse reactions (lamotrigine 26%, placebo 5%). Infectious adverse reactions included bronchiolitis, bronchitis, ear infection, eye infection, otitis externa, pharyngitis, urinary tract infection, and viral infection. Respiratory adverse reactions included nasal congestion, cough, and apnea.

In a juvenile animal study in which lamotrigine (oral doses of 5, 15, or 30 mg/kg) was administered to young rats (postnatal days 7 to 62), decreased viability and growth were seen at the highest dose tested and long-term behavioral abnormalities (decreased locomotor activity, increased reactivity, and learning deficits in animals tested as adults) were observed at the 2 highest doses. The no-effect dose for adverse effects on neurobehavioral development is less than the human dose of 400 mg/day on a mg/m^2 basis.

8.5 Geriatric Use
Clinical studies of LAMICTAL XR for epilepsy did not include sufficient numbers of subjects aged 65 years and over

to determine whether they respond differently from younger subjects or exhibit a different safety profile than that of younger patients. In general, dose selection for an elderly patient should be cautious, usually starting at the low end of the dosing range, reflecting the greater frequency of decreased hepatic, renal, or cardiac function and of concomitant disease or other drug therapy.

8.6 Patients With Hepatic Impairment
Experience in patients with hepatic impairment is limited. Based on a clinical pharmacology study with immediate-release lamotrigine in 24 patients with mild, moderate, and severe liver impairment [see Clinical Pharmacology (12.3)], the following general recommendations can be made. No dosage adjustment is needed in patients with mild liver impairment. Initial, escalation, and maintenance doses should generally be reduced by approximately 25% in patients with moderate and severe liver impairment without ascites and 50% in patients with severe liver impairment with ascites. Escalation and maintenance doses may be adjusted according to clinical response [see Dosage and Administration (2.1)].

8.7 Patients With Renal Impairment
Lamotrigine is metabolized mainly by glucuronic acid conjugation, with the majority of the metabolites being recovered in the urine. In a small study comparing a single dose of immediate-release lamotrigine in patients with varying degrees of renal impairment with healthy volunteers, the plasma half-life of lamotrigine was approximately twice as long in the patients with significant renal impairment [see Clinical Pharmacology (12.3)].

Initial doses of LAMICTAL XR should be based on patients' AED regimens; reduced maintenance doses may be effective for patients with significant renal impairment. Few patients with severe renal impairment have been evaluated during chronic treatment with lamotrigine. Because there is inadequate experience in this population, LAMICTAL XR should be used with caution in these patients [see Dosage and Administration (2.1)].

10 OVERDOSAGE
10.1 Human Overdose Experience
Overdoses involving quantities up to 15 g have been reported for immediate-release lamotrigine, some of which have been fatal. Overdose has resulted in ataxia, nystagmus, seizures (including tonic-clonic seizures), decreased level of consciousness, coma, and intraventricular conduction delay.

10.2 Management of Overdose
There are no specific antidotes for lamotrigine. Following a suspected overdose, hospitalization of the patient is advised. General supportive care is indicated, including frequent monitoring of vital signs and close observation of the patient. If indicated, emesis should be induced; usual precautions should be taken to protect the airway. It is uncertain whether hemodialysis is an effective means of removing lamotrigine from the blood. In 6 renal failure patients, about 20% of the amount of lamotrigine in the body was removed by hemodialysis during a 4-hour session. A Poison Control Center should be contacted for information on the management of overdosage of LAMICTAL XR.

11 DESCRIPTION
LAMICTAL XR (lamotrigine), an AED of the phenyltriazine class, is chemically unrelated to existing AEDs. Its chemical name is 3,5-diamino-6-(2,3-dichlorophenyl)-as-triazine, its molecular formula is $C_9H_7N_5Cl_2$, and its molecular weight is 256.09. Lamotrigine is a white to pale cream-colored powder and has a pK$_a$ of 5.7. Lamotrigine is very slightly soluble in water (0.17 mg/mL at 25°C) and slightly soluble in 0.1 M HCl (4.1 mg/mL at 25°C). The structural formula is:

LAMICTAL XR Extended-Release Tablets are supplied for oral administration as 25-mg (yellow with white center), 50-mg (green with white center), 100-mg (orange with white center), 200-mg (blue with white center), 250-mg (purple with white center), and 300-mg (gray with white center) tablets. Each tablet contains the labeled amount of lamotrigine and the following inactive ingredients: glycerol monostearate; hypromellose, lactose monohydrate; magnesium stearate; methacrylic acid copolymer dispersion, polyethylene glycol 400, polysorbate 80, silicon dioxide (25- and 50-mg tablets only), titanium dioxide, triethyl citrate, carmine (250-mg tablet only), iron oxide black (50-, 250-, and 300-mg tablets only), iron oxide yellow (25-, 50-, and 100-mg tablets only), iron oxide red (100-mg tablet only), FD&C Blue No. 2 Aluminum Lake (200- and 250-mg tablets only). Tablets are printed with edible black ink.

LAMICTAL XR Extended-Release Tablets contain a modified-release eroding formulation as the core. The tablets are coated with a clear enteric coat and have an aperture drilled through the coats on both faces of the tablet (DiffCORE™) to enable a controlled release of drug in the acidic environment of the stomach. The combination of this and the modified-release core are designed to control the dissolution rate of lamotrigine over a period of approximately 12 to 15 hours, leading to a gradual increase in serum lamotrigine levels.

12 CLINICAL PHARMACOLOGY
12.1 Mechanism of Action
The precise mechanism(s) by which lamotrigine exerts its anticonvulsant action is unknown. In animal models designed to detect anticonvulsant activity, lamotrigine was effective in preventing seizure spread in the maximum electroshock and pentylenetetrazol tests, and prevented seizures in the visually and electrically evoked after-discharge tests for antiepileptic activity. Lamotrigine also displayed inhibitory properties in a kindling model in rats both during kindling development and in the fully kindled state. The relevance of these models to human epilepsy, however, is not known.

One proposed mechanism of action of lamotrigine, the relevance of which remains to be established in humans, involves an effect on sodium channels. In vitro pharmacological studies suggest that lamotrigine inhibits voltage-sensitive sodium channels, thereby stabilizing neuronal membranes and consequently modulating presynaptic transmitter release of excitatory amino acids (e.g., glutamate and aspartate).

Effect of Lamotrigine on N-Methyl d-Aspartate-Receptor Mediated Activity: Lamotrigine did not inhibit N-methyl d-aspartate (NMDA)-induced depolarizations in rat cortical slices or NMDA-induced cyclic GMP formation in immature rat cerebellum, nor did lamotrigine displace compounds that are either competitive or noncompetitive ligands at this glutamate receptor complex (CNQX, CGS, TCHP). The IC$_{50}$ for lamotrigine effects on NMDA-induced currents (in the presence of 3 µM of glycine) in cultured hippocampal neurons exceeded 100 µM.

12.2 Pharmacodynamics
Folate Metabolism: In vitro, lamotrigine inhibited dihydrofolate reductase, the enzyme that catalyzes the reduction of dihydrofolate to tetrahydrofolate. Inhibition of this enzyme may interfere with the biosynthesis of nucleic acids and proteins. When oral daily doses of lamotrigine were given to pregnant rats during organogenesis, fetal, placental, and maternal folate concentrations were reduced. Significantly reduced concentrations of folate are associated with teratogenesis [see Use in Specific Populations (8.1)]. Folate concentrations were also reduced in male rats given repeated oral doses of lamotrigine. Reduced concentrations were partially returned to normal when supplemented with folinic acid.

Cardiovascular: In dogs, lamotrigine is extensively metabolized to a 2-N-methyl metabolite. This metabolite causes dose-dependent prolongation of the PR interval, widening of the QRS complex, and, at higher doses, complete AV conduction block. Similar cardiovascular effects are not anticipated in humans because only trace amounts of the 2-N-methyl metabolite (<0.6% of lamotrigine dose) have been found in human urine [see Clinical Pharmacology (12.3)]. However, it is conceivable that plasma concentrations of this metabolite could be increased in patients with a reduced capacity to glucuronidate lamotrigine (e.g., in patients with liver disease, patients taking concomitant medications that inhibit glucuronidation).

12.3 Pharmacokinetics
In comparison to immediate-release lamotrigine, the plasma lamotrigine levels following administration of LAMICTAL XR are not associated with any significant changes in trough plasma concentrations, and are characterized by lower peaks, longer time to peaks, and lower peak-to-trough fluctuation, as described in detail below.

Absorption: Lamotrigine is absorbed after oral administration with negligible first-pass metabolism. The bioavailability of lamotrigine is not affected by food.

In an open-label, crossover study of 44 subjects with epilepsy receiving concomitant AEDs, the steady-state pharmacokinetics of lamotrigine were compared following administration of equivalent total doses of LAMICTAL XR given once daily with those of lamotrigine immediate-release given twice daily. In this study, the median time to peak concentration (T_{max}) following administration of LAMICTAL XR was 4 to 6 hours in patients taking carbamazepine, phenytoin, phenobarbital, or primidone; 9 to 11 hours in patients taking valproate; and 6 to 10 hours in patients taking AEDs other than carbamazepine, phenytoin, phenobarbital, primidone, or valproate. In comparison, the median T_{max} following administration of immediate-release lamotrigine was between 1 and 1.5 hours.

The steady-state trough concentrations for extended-release lamotrigine were similar to or higher than those of immediate-release lamotrigine depending on concomitant AED (Table 6). A mean reduction in the lamotrigine C_{max} by 11% to 29% was observed for LAMICTAL XR compared to immediate-release lamotrigine, resulting in a decrease in the peak-to-trough fluctuation in serum lamotrigine concentrations. However, in some subjects receiving enzyme-inducing AEDs, a reduction in C_{max} of 44% to 77% was observed. The degree of fluctuation was reduced by 17% in patients taking enzyme-inducing AEDs; 34% in patients taking valproate; and 37% in patients taking AEDs other than carbamazepine, phenytoin, phenobarbital, primidone, or valproate. LAMICTAL XR and immediate-release lamotrigine regimens were similar with respect to area under the curve (AUC, a measure of the extent of bioavailability) for patients receiving AEDs other than those known to induce the metabolism of lamotrigine. The relative bioavailability of extended-release lamotrigine was approximately 21% lower than immediate-release lamotrigine in subjects receiving enzyme-inducing AEDs. However, a reduction in exposure of up to 70% was observed in some subjects in this group when they switched to LAMICTAL XR. Therefore, doses may need to be adjusted in some subjects based on therapeutic response.

Table 6. Steady-State Bioavailability of LAMICTAL XR Relative to Immediate-Release Lamotrigine at Equivalent Daily Doses (Ratio of Extended-Release to Immediate-Release 90% CI)

Concomitant Antiepileptic Drug	AUC(0-24ss)	C_{max}	C_{min}
Enzyme-inducing antiepileptic drugs[a]	0.79 (0.69, 0.90)	0.71 (0.61, 0.82)	0.99 (0.89, 1.09)
Valproate	0.94 (0.81, 1.08)	0.88 (0.75, 1.03)	0.99 (0.88, 1.10)
Antiepileptic drugs other than enzyme-inducing antiepileptic drugs[a] or valproate	1.00 (0.88, 1.14)	0.89 (0.78, 1.03)	1.14 (1.03, 1.25)

[a] Enzyme-inducing antiepileptic drugs include carbamazepine, phenytoin, phenobarbital, and primidone.

Dose Proportionality: In healthy volunteers not receiving any other medications and given LAMICTAL XR once daily, the systemic exposure to lamotrigine increased in direct proportion to the dose administered over the range of 50 to 200 mg. At doses between 25 and 50 mg, the increase was less than dose proportional, with a 2-fold increase in dose resulting in an approximately 1.6-fold increase in systemic exposure.

Distribution: Estimates of the mean apparent volume of distribution (Vd/F) of lamotrigine following oral administration ranged from 0.9 to 1.3 L/kg. Vd/F is independent of dose and is similar following single and multiple doses in both patients with epilepsy and in healthy volunteers.

Protein Binding: Data from in vitro studies indicate that lamotrigine is approximately 55% bound to human plasma proteins at plasma lamotrigine concentrations from 1 to 10 mcg/mL (10 mcg/mL is 4 to 6 times the trough plasma concentration observed in the controlled efficacy trials). Because lamotrigine is not highly bound to plasma proteins, clinically significant interactions with other drugs through competition for protein binding sites are unlikely. The binding of lamotrigine to plasma proteins did not change in the presence of therapeutic concentrations of phenytoin, phenobarbital, or valproate. Lamotrigine did not displace other AEDs (carbamazepine, phenytoin, phenobarbital) from protein-binding sites.

Metabolism: Lamotrigine is metabolized predominantly by glucuronic acid conjugation; the major metabolite is an inactive 2-N-glucuronide conjugate. After oral administration of 240 mg of ^{14}C-lamotrigine (15 μCi) to 6 healthy volunteers, 94% was recovered in the urine and 2% was recovered in the feces. The radioactivity in the urine consisted of unchanged lamotrigine (10%), the 2-N-glucuronide (76%), a 5-N-glucuronide (10%), a 2-N-methyl metabolite (0.14%), and other unidentified minor metabolites (4%).

Enzyme Induction: The effects of lamotrigine on the induction of specific families of mixed-function oxidase isozymes have not been systematically evaluated. Following multiple administrations (150 mg twice daily) to normal volunteers taking no other medications, lamotrigine induced its own metabolism, resulting in a 25% decrease in $t_{1/2}$ and a 37% increase in CL/F at steady state compared with values obtained in the same volunteers following a single dose. Evidence gathered from other sources suggests that self-induction by lamotrigine may not occur when lamotrigine is given as adjunctive therapy in patients receiving enzyme-inducing drugs such as carbamazepine, phenytoin, phenobarbital, primidone, or other drugs such as rifampin that induce lamotrigine glucuronidation [see Drug Interactions (7)].

Elimination: The elimination half-life and apparent clearance of lamotrigine following oral administration of immediate-release lamotrigine to adult patients with epilepsy and healthy volunteers is summarized in Table 7. Half-life and apparent clearance vary depending on concomitant AEDs.

Since the half-life of lamotrigine following administration of single doses of immediate-release lamotrigine is comparable to that observed following administration of LAMICTAL XR, similar changes in the half-life of lamotrigine would be expected for LAMICTAL XR.
[See table 7 below]

Drug Interactions: The apparent clearance of lamotrigine is affected by the coadministration of certain medications [see Warnings and Precautions (5.7, 5.11), Drug Interactions (7)].

The net effects of drug interactions with lamotrigine are summarized in Table 8. Details of the drug interaction studies, which were done using immediate-release lamotrigine, are provided in Table 8.
[See table 8 at top of next page]

Estrogen-Containing Oral Contraceptives: In 16 female volunteers, an oral contraceptive preparation containing 30 mcg ethinylestradiol and 150 mcg levonorgestrel increased the apparent clearance of lamotrigine (300 mg/day) by approximately 2-fold with mean decreases in AUC of 52% and in C_{max} of 39%. In this study, trough serum lamotrigine concentrations gradually increased and were approximately 2-fold higher on average at the end of the week of the inactive hormone preparation compared with trough lamotrigine concentrations at the end of the active hormone cycle.

Gradual transient increases in lamotrigine plasma levels (approximate 2-fold increase) occurred during the week of inactive hormone preparation (pill-free week) for women not also taking a drug that increased the clearance of lamotrigine (carbamazepine, phenytoin, phenobarbital, primidone, or other drugs such as rifampin that induce lamotrigine glucuronidation) [see Drug Interactions (7)]. The increase in lamotrigine plasma levels will be greater if the dose of LAMICTAL XR is increased in the few days before or during the pill-free week. Increases in lamotrigine plasma levels could result in dose-dependent adverse reactions.

In the same study, coadministration of lamotrigine (300 mg/day) in 16 female volunteers did not affect the pharmacokinetics of the ethinylestradiol component of the oral contraceptive preparation. There were mean decreases in the AUC and C_{max} of the levonorgestrel component of 19% and 12%, respectively. Measurement of serum progesterone indicated that there was no hormonal evidence of ovulation in any of the 16 volunteers, although measurement of serum FSH, LH, and estradiol indicated that there was some loss of suppression of the hypothalamic-pituitary-ovarian axis.

The effects of doses of lamotrigine other than 300 mg/day have not been systematically evaluated in controlled clinical trials.

The clinical significance of the observed hormonal changes on ovulatory activity is unknown. However, the possibility of decreased contraceptive efficacy in some patients cannot be excluded. Therefore, patients should be instructed to promptly report changes in their menstrual pattern (e.g., break-through bleeding).

Dosage adjustments may be necessary for women receiving estrogen-containing oral contraceptive preparations [see Dosage and Administration (2.1)].

Other Hormonal Contraceptives or Hormone Replacement Therapy: The effect of other hormonal contraceptive preparations or hormone replacement therapy on the pharmacokinetics of lamotrigine has not been systematically evaluated. It has been reported that ethinylestradiol, not progestogens, increased the clearance of lamotrigine up to 2-fold, and the progestin-only pills had no effect on lamotrigine plasma levels. Therefore, adjustments to the dosage of LAMICTAL XR in the presence of progestogens alone will likely not be needed.

Bupropion: The pharmacokinetics of a 100-mg single dose of lamotrigine in healthy volunteers (n = 12) were not changed by coadministration of bupropion sustained-release formulation (150 mg twice daily) starting 11 days before lamotrigine.

Carbamazepine: Lamotrigine has no appreciable effect on steady-state carbamazepine plasma concentration. Limited clinical data suggest there is a higher incidence of dizziness, diplopia, ataxia, and blurred vision in patients receiving carbamazepine with lamotrigine than in patients receiving other AEDs with lamotrigine [see Adverse Reactions (6.1)]. The mechanism of this interaction is unclear. The effect of lamotrigine on plasma concentrations of carbamazepine-epoxide is unclear. In a small subset of patients (n = 7) studied in a placebo-controlled trial, lamotrigine had no effect on carbamazepine-epoxide plasma concentrations, but in a small, uncontrolled study (n = 9), carbamazepine-epoxide levels increased.

Table 7. Mean[a] Pharmacokinetic Parameters of Immediate-Release Lamotrigine in Healthy Volunteers and Adult Patients With Epilepsy

Adult Study Population	Number of Subjects	t½: Elimination Half-life (hr)	CL/F: Apparent Plasma Clearance (mL/min/kg)
Healthy volunteers taking no other medications:			
Single-dose lamotrigine	179	32.8 (14.0-103.0)	0.44 (0.12-1.10)
Multiple-dose lamotrigine	36	25.4 (11.6-61.6)	0.58 (0.24-1.15)
Healthy volunteers taking valproate:			
Single-dose lamotrigine	6	48.3 (31.5-88.6)	0.30 (0.14-0.42)
Multiple-dose lamotrigine	18	70.3 (41.9-113.5)	0.18 (0.12-0.33)
Patients with epilepsy taking valproate only:			
Single-dose lamotrigine	4	58.8 (30.5-88.8)	0.28 (0.16-0.40)
Patients with epilepsy taking carbamazepine, phenytoin, phenobarbital, or primidone[b] plus valproate:			
Single-dose lamotrigine	25	27.2 (11.2-51.6)	0.53 (0.27-1.04)
Patients with epilepsy taking carbamazepine, phenytoin, phenobarbital, or primidone:[b]			
Single-dose lamotrigine	24	14.4 (6.4-30.4)	1.10 (0.51-2.22)
Multiple-dose lamotrigine	17	12.6 (7.5-23.1)	1.21 (0.66-1.82)

[a]The majority of parameter means determined in each study had coefficients of variation between 20% and 40% for half-life and CL/F and between 30% and 70% for T_{max}. The overall mean values were calculated from individual study means that were weighted based on the number of volunteers/patients in each study. The numbers in parentheses below each parameter mean represent the range of individual volunteer/patient values across studies.

[b]Carbamazepine, phenobarbital, phenytoin, and primidone have been shown to increase the apparent clearance of lamotrigine. Estrogen-containing oral contraceptives and other drugs such as rifampin that induce lamotrigine glucuronidation have also been shown to increase the apparent clearance of lamotrigine [see Drug Interactions (7)].

The addition of carbamazepine decreases lamotrigine steady-state concentrations by approximately 40%.

Esomeprazole: In a study of 30 subjects, coadministration of LAMICTAL XR with esomeprazole resulted in no significant change in lamotrigine levels and a small decrease in T_{max}. The levels of gastric pH were not altered compared with pre-lamotrigine dosing.

Felbamate: In a study of 21 healthy volunteers, coadministration of felbamate (1,200 mg twice daily) with lamotrigine (100 mg twice daily for 10 days) appeared to have no clinically relevant effects on the pharmacokinetics of lamotrigine.

Folate Inhibitors: Lamotrigine is a weak inhibitor of dihydrofolate reductase. Prescribers should be aware of this action when prescribing other medications that inhibit folate metabolism.

Gabapentin: Based on a retrospective analysis of plasma levels in 34 patients who received lamotrigine both with and without gabapentin, gabapentin does not appear to change the apparent clearance of lamotrigine.

Levetiracetam: Potential drug interactions between levetiracetam and lamotrigine were assessed by evaluating serum concentrations of both agents during placebo-controlled clinical trials. These data indicate that lamotrigine does not influence the pharmacokinetics of levetiracetam and that levetiracetam does not influence the pharmacokinetics of lamotrigine.

Lithium: The pharmacokinetics of lithium were not altered in healthy subjects (n = 20) by coadministration of lamotrigine (100 mg/day) for 6 days.

Olanzapine: The AUC and C_{max} of olanzapine were similar following the addition of olanzapine (15 mg once daily) to lamotrigine (200 mg once daily) in healthy male volunteers (n = 16) compared with the AUC and C_{max} in healthy male volunteers receiving olanzapine alone (n = 16).

In the same study, the AUC and C_{max} of lamotrigine were reduced on average by 24% and 20%, respectively, following the addition of olanzapine to lamotrigine in healthy male volunteers compared with those receiving lamotrigine alone. This reduction in lamotrigine plasma concentrations is not expected to be clinically relevant.

Oxcarbazepine: The AUC and C_{max} of oxcarbazepine and its active 10-monohydroxy oxcarbazepine metabolite were not significantly different following the addition of oxcarbazepine (600 mg twice daily) to lamotrigine (200 mg once daily) in healthy male volunteers (n = 13) compared with healthy male volunteers receiving oxcarbazepine alone (n = 13).

In the same study, the AUC and C_{max} of lamotrigine were similar following the addition of oxcarbazepine (600 mg twice daily) to lamotrigine in healthy male volunteers compared with those receiving lamotrigine alone. Limited clinical data suggest a higher incidence of headache, dizziness, nausea, and somnolence with coadministration of lamotrigine and oxcarbazepine compared with lamotrigine alone or oxcarbazepine alone.

Phenobarbital, Primidone: The addition of phenobarbital or primidone decreases lamotrigine steady-state concentrations by approximately 40%.

Phenytoin: Lamotrigine has no appreciable effect on steady-state phenytoin plasma concentrations in patients with epilepsy. The addition of phenytoin decreases lamotrigine steady-state concentrations by approximately 40%.

Pregabalin: Steady-state trough plasma concentrations of lamotrigine were not affected by concomitant pregabalin (200 mg 3 times daily) administration. There are no pharmacokinetic interactions between lamotrigine and pregabalin.

Rifampin: In 10 male volunteers, rifampin (600 mg/day for 5 days) significantly increased the apparent clearance of a single 25-mg dose of lamotrigine by approximately 2-fold (AUC decreased by approximately 40%).

Topiramate: Topiramate resulted in no change in plasma concentrations of lamotrigine. Administration of lamotrigine resulted in a 15% increase in topiramate concentrations.

Valproate: When lamotrigine was administered to healthy volunteers (n = 18) receiving valproate, the trough steady-state valproate plasma concentrations decreased by an average of 25% over a 3-week period, and then stabilized. However, adding lamotrigine to the existing therapy did not cause a change in valproate plasma concentrations in either adult or pediatric patients in controlled clinical trials.

The addition of valproate increased lamotrigine steady-state concentrations in normal volunteers by slightly more than 2-fold. In one study, maximal inhibition of lamotrigine clearance was reached at valproate doses between 250 and 500 mg/day and did not increase as the valproate dose was further increased.

Zonisamide: In a study of 18 patients with epilepsy, coadministration of zonisamide (200 to 400 mg/day) with lamotrigine (150 to 500 mg/day for 35 days) had no significant effect on the pharmacokinetics of lamotrigine.

Table 8. Summary of Drug Interactions With Lamotrigine

Drug	Drug Plasma Concentration With Adjunctive Lamotrigine[a]	Lamotrigine Plasma Concentration With Adjunctive Drugs[b]
Oral contraceptives (e.g., ethinylestradiol/levonorgestrel[c])	↔[d]	↓
Bupropion	Not assessed	↔
Carbamazepine	↔	↓
Carbamazepine epoxide[e]	?	
Felbamate	Not assessed	↔
Gabapentin	Not assessed	↔
Levetiracetam	↔	↔
Lithium	↔	Not assessed
Olanzapine	↔	↔[f]
Oxcarbazepine	↔	↔
10-monohydroxy oxcarbazepine metabolite[g]	↔	
Phenobarbital/primidone	↔	↓
Phenytoin	↔	↓
Pregabalin	↔	↔
Rifampin	Not assessed	↓
Topiramate	↔[h]	↔
Valproate	↓	↑
Valproate + phenytoin and/or carbamazepine	Not assessed	↔
Zonisamide	Not assessed	↔

[a]From adjunctive clinical trials and volunteer studies.
[b]Net effects were estimated by comparing the mean clearance values obtained in adjunctive clinical trials and volunteer studies.
[c]The effect of other hormonal contraceptive preparations or hormone replacement therapy on the pharmacokinetics of lamotrigine has not been systematically evaluated in clinical trials, although the effect may be similar to that seen with the ethinylestradiol/levonorgestrel combinations.
[d]Modest decrease in levonorgestrel.
[e]Not administered, but an active metabolite of carbamazepine.
[f]Slight decrease, not expected to be clinically relevant.
[g]Not administered, but an active metabolite of oxcarbazepine.
[h]Slight increase, not expected to be clinically relevant.
↔ = No significant effect.
? = Conflicting data.

Known Inducers or Inhibitors of Glucuronidation: Drugs other than those listed above have not been systematically evaluated in combination with lamotrigine. Since lamotrigine is metabolized predominately by glucuronic acid conjugation, drugs that are known to induce or inhibit glucuronidation may affect the apparent clearance of lamotrigine, and doses of LAMICTAL XR may require adjustment based on clinical response.

Other: Results of in vitro experiments suggest that clearance of lamotrigine is unlikely to be reduced by concomitant administration of amitriptyline, clonazepam, clozapine, fluoxetine, haloperidol, lorazepam, phenelzine, risperidone, sertraline, or trazodone.

Results of in vitro experiments suggest that lamotrigine does not reduce the clearance of drugs eliminated predominantly by CYP2D6.

Special Populations: *Patients With Renal Impairment:* Twelve volunteers with chronic renal failure (mean creatinine clearance: 13 mL/min, range: 6 to 23) and another 6 individuals undergoing hemodialysis were each given a single 100 mg dose of immediate-release lamotrigine. The mean plasma half-lives determined in the study were 42.9 hours (chronic renal failure), 13.0 hours (during hemodialysis), and 57.4 hours (between hemodialysis) compared with 26.2 hours in healthy volunteers. On average, approximately 20% (range: 5.6 to 35.1) of the amount of lamotrigine present in the body was eliminated by hemodialysis during a 4-hour session *[see Dosage and Administration (2.1)]*.

Hepatic Disease: The pharmacokinetics of lamotrigine following a single 100-mg dose of immediate-release lamotrigine were evaluated in 24 subjects with mild, moderate, and severe hepatic impairment (Child-Pugh Classification system) and compared with 12 subjects without hepatic impairment. The patients with severe hepatic impairment were without ascites (n = 2) or with ascites (n = 5). The mean apparent clearances of lamotrigine in patients with mild (n = 12), moderate (n = 5), severe without ascites (n = 2), and severe with ascites (n = 5) liver impairment were 0.30 ± 0.09, 0.24 ± 0.1, 0.21 ± 0.04, and 0.15 ± 0.09 mL/min/kg, respectively, as compared with 0.37 ± 0.1 mL/min/kg in the healthy controls. Mean half-lives of lamotrigine in patients with mild, moderate, severe without ascites, and severe with ascites hepatic impairment were 46 ± 20, 72 ± 44, 67 ± 11, and 100 ± 48 hours, respectively, as compared with 33 ± 7 hours in healthy controls *[see Dosage and Administration (2.1)]*.

Elderly: The pharmacokinetics of lamotrigine following a single 150-mg dose of immediate-release lamotrigine were evaluated in 12 elderly volunteers between the ages of 65 and 76 years (mean creatinine clearance: 61 mL/min, range: 33 to 108 mL/min). The mean half-life of lamotrigine in these subjects was 31.2 hours (range: 24.5 to 43.4 hours), and the mean clearance was 0.40 mL/min/kg (range: 0.26 to 0.48 mL/min/kg).

Gender: The clearance of lamotrigine is not affected by gender. However, during dose escalation of immediate-release lamotrigine in one clinical trial in patients with epilepsy on a stable dose of valproate (n = 77), mean trough lamotrigine concentrations, unadjusted for weight, were 24% to 45% higher (0.3 to 1.7 mcg/mL) in females than in males.

Race: The apparent oral clearance of lamotrigine was 25% lower in non-Caucasians than Caucasians.

Pediatric Patients: Safety and effectiveness of LAMICTAL XR for use in patients less than 13 years of age have not been established.

13 NONCLINICAL TOXICOLOGY

13.1 Carcinogenesis, Mutagenesis, Impairment of Fertility

No evidence of carcinogenicity was seen in mouse or rat following oral administration of lamotrigine for up to 2 years at doses up to 30 mg/kg/day and 10 to 15 mg/kg/day in mouse and rat, respectively. The highest doses tested are less than the human dose of 400 mg/day on a body surface area (mg/m^2) basis.

Lamotrigine was negative in in vitro gene mutation (Ames and mouse lymphoma *tk*) assays and in clastogenicity (in vitro human lymphocyte and in vivo rat bone marrow) assays.

No evidence of impaired fertility was detected in rats given oral doses of lamotrigine up to 20 mg/kg/day. The highest dose tested is less than the human dose of 400 mg/day on a mg/m^2 basis.

14 CLINICAL STUDIES

14.1 Adjunctive Therapy for Primary Generalized Tonic-Clonic Seizures

The effectiveness of LAMICTAL XR as adjunctive therapy was established in PGTC seizures in a 19-week, international, multicenter, double-blind, randomized, placebo-controlled study in 143 patients 13 years of age and older (n = 70 on LAMICTAL XR and n = 73 on placebo). Patients with at least 3 PGTC seizures during an 8-week baseline phase were randomized to 19 weeks of treatment with LAMICTAL XR or placebo added to their current AED regimen of up to 2 drugs. Patients were dosed on a fixed-dose regimen, with target doses ranging from 200 to 500 mg/day of LAMICTAL XR based on concomitant AED(s) (target dose = 200 mg for valproate, 300 mg for AEDs not altering plasma lamotrigine levels, and 500 mg for enzyme-inducing AEDs).

The primary efficacy endpoint was percent change from baseline in PGTC seizure frequency during the double-blind treatment phase. For the intent-to-treat population, the median percent reduction in PGTC seizure frequency was 75%

Help Patients Save on Rx Drugs: PDR.net/PharmacyDiscountCard

in patients treated with LAMICTAL XR and 32% in patients treated with placebo, a difference that was statistically significant, defined as a 2-sided P value ≥0.05.

Figure 1 presents the percentage of patients (X-axis) with a percent reduction in PGTC seizure frequency (responder rate) from baseline through the entire treatment period at least as great as that represented on the Y-axis. A positive value on the Y-axis indicates an improvement from baseline (i.e., a decrease in seizure frequency), while a negative value indicates a worsening from baseline (i.e., an increase in seizure frequency). Thus, in a display of this type, a curve for an effective treatment is shifted to the left of the curve for placebo. The proportion of patients achieving any particular level of reduction in PGTC seizure frequency was consistently higher for the group treated with LAMICTAL XR compared with the placebo group. For example, 70% of patients randomized to LAMICTAL XR experienced a 50% or greater reduction in PGTC seizure frequency, compared with 32% of patients randomized to placebo. Patients with an increase in seizure frequency >100% are represented on the Y-axis as equal to or greater than -100%.

Figure 1. Proportion of Patients by Responder Rate for LAMICTAL XR and Placebo Group (Primary Generalized Tonic-Clonic Seizures Study)

14.2   Adjunctive Therapy for Partial Onset Seizures
The effectiveness of immediate-release lamotrigine as adjunctive therapy was initially established in 3 pivotal, multicenter, placebo-controlled, double-blind clinical trials in 355 adults with refractory partial onset seizures.

The effectiveness of LAMICTAL XR as adjunctive therapy in partial onset seizures, with or without secondary generalization, was established in a 19-week, multicenter, double-blind, placebo-controlled trial in 236 patients 13 years of age and older (approximately 93% of patients were aged 16 to 65 years). Approximately 36% were from the U.S. and approximately 64% were from other countries including Argentina, Brazil, Chile, Germany, India, Korea, Russian Federation, and Ukraine. Patients with at least 8 partial onset seizures during an 8-week prospective baseline phase (or 4-week prospective baseline coupled with a 4-week historical baseline documented with seizure diary data) were randomized to treatment with LAMICTAL XR (n = 116) or placebo (n = 120) added to their current regimen of 1 or 2 AEDs. Approximately half of the patients were taking 2 concomitant AEDs at baseline. Target doses ranged from 200 to 500 mg/day of LAMICTAL XR based on concomitant AED (target dose = 200 mg for valproate, 300 mg for AEDs not altering plasma lamotrigine, and 500 mg for enzyme-inducing AEDs). The median partial seizure frequency per week at baseline was 2.3 for LAMICTAL XR and 2.1 for placebo.

The primary endpoint was the median percent change from baseline in partial onset seizure frequency during the entire double-blind treatment phase. The median percent reductions in weekly partial onset seizures were 47% in patients treated with LAMICTAL XR and 25% on placebo, a difference that was statistically significant, defined as a 2-sided P value ≤0.05.

Figure 2 presents the percentage of patients (X-axis) with a percent reduction in partial seizure frequency (responder rate) from baseline through the entire treatment period at least as great as that represented on the Y-axis. The proportion of patients achieving any particular level of reduction in partial seizure frequency was consistently higher for the group treated with LAMICTAL XR compared with the placebo group. For example, 44% of patients randomized to LAMICTAL XR experienced a 50% or greater reduction in partial seizure frequency compared with 21% of patients randomized to placebo.

[See figure 2 at top of next column]

14.3   Conversion to Monotherapy for Partial Onset Seizures
The effectiveness of LAMICTAL XR as monotherapy for partial onset seizures was established in a historical-control trial in 223 adults with partial seizures. The historical control methodology is described in a publication by French, et

Figure 2. Proportion of Patients by Responder Rate for LAMICTAL XR and Placebo Group (Partial Onset Seizure Study)

al. [see References (15)]. Briefly, in this study, patients were randomized to ultimately receive either LAMICTAL XR 300 mg or 250 mg once a day, and their responses were compared to those of a historical control group. The historical control consisted of a pooled analysis of the control groups from 8 studies of similar design, which utilized a subtherapeutic dose of an AED as a comparator. Statistical superiority to the historical control was considered to be demonstrated if the upper 95% confidence interval for the proportion of patients meeting escape criteria in patients receiving LAMICTAL XR remained below the lower 95% prediction interval of 65.3% derived from the historical control data.

In this study, patients ≥13 years of age experienced at least 4 partial seizures during an 8-week baseline period with at least 2 seizures occurring during each of 2 consecutive 4-week periods while receiving valproate or a non–enzyme-inducing AED. LAMICTAL XR was added to either valproate or a non–enzyme-inducing AED over a 6- to 7-week period followed by the gradual withdrawal of the background AED. Patients were then continued on monotherapy with LAMICTAL XR for 12 weeks. The escape criteria were one or more of the following: (1) doubling of average monthly seizure count during any 28 consecutive days, (2) doubling of highest consecutive 2-day seizure frequency during the entire treatment phase, (3) emergence of a new seizure type compared to baseline (4) clinically significant prolongation of generalized tonic-clonic seizures or worsening of seizure considered by the investigator to require intervention. These criteria were similar to those in the 8 controlled trials from which the historical control group was constituted.

The upper 95% confidence limits of the proportion of subjects meeting escape criteria (40.2% at 300 mg/day and 44.5% at 250 mg/day) were below the threshold of 65.3% derived from the historical control data.

Although the study population was not fully comparable to the historical controlled population and the study was not fully blinded, numerous sensitivity analyses supported the primary results. Efficacy was further supported by the established effectiveness of the immediate-release formulation as monotherapy.

15   REFERENCES
1. French JA, Wang S, Warnock B, Temkin N. Historical control monotherapy design in the treatment of epilepsy. *Epilepsia.* 2010; 51(10):1936-1943.

16   HOW SUPPLIED/STORAGE AND HANDLING
LAMICTAL XR (lamotrigine) Extended-Release Tablets
25 mg, yellow with a white center, round, biconvex, film-coated tablets printed on one face in black ink with "LAMICTAL" and "XR 25", unit-of-use bottles of 30 with orange caps (NDC 0173-0754-00).

50 mg, green with a white center, round, biconvex, film-coated tablets printed on one face in black ink with "LAMICTAL" and "XR 50", unit-of-use bottles of 30 with orange caps (NDC 0173-0755-00).

100 mg, orange with a white center, round, biconvex, film-coated tablets printed on one face in black ink with "LAMICTAL" and "XR 100", unit-of-use bottles of 30 with orange caps (NDC 0173-0756-00).

200 mg, blue with a white center, round, biconvex, film-coated tablets printed on one face in black ink with "LAMICTAL" and "XR 200", unit-of-use bottles of 30 with orange caps (NDC 0173-0757-00).

250 mg, purple with a white center, caplet-shaped, film-coated tablets printed on one face in black ink with "LAMICTAL" and "XR 250", unit-of-use bottles of 30 with orange caps (NDC 0173-0781-00).

300 mg, gray with a white center, caplet-shaped, film-coated tablets printed on one face in black ink with "LAMICTAL" and "XR 300", unit-of-use bottles of 30 with orange caps (NDC 0173-0761-00).

LAMICTAL XR (lamotrigine) Patient Titration Kit for Patients Taking Valproate (Blue XR Kit)
25 mg, yellow with a white center, round, biconvex, film-coated tablets printed on one face in black ink with "LAMICTAL" and "XR 25" and 50 mg, green with a white center, round, biconvex, film-coated tablets printed on one face in black ink with "LAMICTAL" and "XR 50"; blister-pack of 21/25-mg tablets and 7/50-mg tablets (NDC 0173-0758-00).

LAMICTAL XR (lamotrigine) Patient Titration Kit for Patients Taking Carbamazepine, Phenytoin, Phenobarbital, or Primidone, and Not Taking Valproate (Green XR Kit)
50 mg, green with a white center, round, biconvex, film-coated tablets printed on one face in black ink with "LAMICTAL" and "XR 50"; 100 mg, orange with a white center, round, biconvex, film-coated tablets printed on one face in black ink with "LAMICTAL" and "XR 100"; and 200 mg, blue with a white center, round, biconvex, film-coated tablets printed on one face in black ink with "LAMICTAL" and "XR 200"; blisterpack of 14/50-mg tablets, 14/100-mg tablets, and 7/200-mg tablets (NDC 0173-0759-00).

LAMICTAL XR (lamotrigine) Patient Titration Kit for Patients Not Taking Carbamazepine, Phenytoin, Phenobarbital, Primidone, or Valproate (Orange XR Kit) 25 mg, yellow with a white center, round, biconvex, film-coated tablets printed on one face in black ink with "LAMICTAL" and "XR 25"; 50 mg, green with a white center, round, biconvex, film-coated tablets printed on one face in black ink with "LAMICTAL" and "XR 50"; and 100 mg, orange with a white center, round, biconvex, film-coated tablets printed on one face in black ink with "LAMICTAL" and "XR 100"; blisterpack of 14/25-mg tablets, 14/50-mg tablets, and 7/100-mg tablets (NDC 0173-0760-00).

Storage: Store at 25°C (77°F); excursions permitted to 15-30°C (59-86°F) [see USP Controlled Room Temperature].

17   PATIENT COUNSELING INFORMATION
See FDA-approved patient labeling (Medication Guide).
17.1   Rash
Prior to initiation of treatment with LAMICTAL XR, the patient should be instructed that a rash or other signs or symptoms of hypersensitivity (e.g., fever, lymphadenopathy) may herald a serious medical event and that the patient should report any such occurrence to a physician immediately.
17.2   Multiorgan Hypersensitivity Reactions, Blood Dyscrasias, and Organ Failure
Patients should be instructed that multiorgan hypersensitivity reactions and acute multiorgan failure may occur with LAMICTAL. Isolated organ failure or isolated blood dyscrasias without evidence of multiorgan hypersensitivity may also occur. Patients should contact their physician immediately if they experience any signs or symptoms of these conditions [see Warnings and Precautions (5.2, 5.3)].
17.3   Suicidal Thinking and Behavior
Patients, their caregivers, and families should be counseled that AEDs, including LAMICTAL XR, may increase the risk of suicidal thoughts and behavior and should be advised of the need to be alert for the emergence or worsening of symptoms of depression; any unusual changes in mood or behavior; or the emergence of suicidal thoughts, behavior, or thoughts about self-harm. Behaviors of concern should be reported immediately to healthcare providers.
17.4   Worsening of Seizures
Patients should be advised to notify their physicians if worsening of seizure control occurs.
17.5   Central Nervous System Adverse Effects
Patients should be advised that LAMICTAL XR may cause dizziness, somnolence, and other symptoms and signs of central nervous system depression. Accordingly, they should be advised neither to drive a car nor to operate other complex machinery until they have gained sufficient experience on LAMICTAL XR to gauge whether or not it adversely affects their mental and/or motor performance.
17.6   Pregnancy and Nursing
Patients should be advised to notify their physicians if they become pregnant or intend to become pregnant during therapy. Patients should be advised to notify their physicians if they intend to breastfeed or are breastfeeding an infant.
Patients should also be encouraged to enroll in the NAAED Pregnancy Registry if they become pregnant. This registry is collecting information about the safety of antiepileptic drugs during pregnancy. To enroll, patients can call the toll-free number 1-888-233-2334 [see Use in Specific Populations (8.1)].
Patients who intend to breastfeed should be informed that LAMICTAL XR is present in breast milk and that they should monitor their child for potential adverse effects of this drug. Benefits and risks of continuing breastfeeding should be discussed with the patient.
17.7   Oral Contraceptive Use
Women should be advised to notify their physicians if they plan to start or stop use of oral contraceptives or other female hormonal preparations. Starting estrogen-containing oral contraceptives may significantly decrease lamotrigine

plasma levels and stopping estrogen-containing oral contraceptives (including the pill-free week) may significantly increase lamotrigine plasma levels [see Warnings and Precautions (5.7), Clinical Pharmacology (12.3)]. Women should also be advised to promptly notify their physicians if they experience adverse reactions or changes in menstrual pattern (e.g., break-through bleeding) while receiving LAMICTAL XR in combination with these medications.

17.8 Discontinuing LAMICTAL XR

Patients should be advised to notify their physicians if they stop taking LAMICTAL XR for any reason and not to resume LAMICTAL XR without consulting their physicians.

17.9 Aseptic Meningitis

Patients should be advised that LAMICTAL XR may cause aseptic meningitis. Patients should be advised to notify their physicians immediately if they develop signs and symptoms of meningitis such as headache, fever, nausea, vomiting, stiff neck, rash, abnormal sensitivity to light, myalgia, chills, confusion, or drowsiness while taking LAMICTAL XR.

17.10 Potential Medication Errors

Medication errors involving LAMICTAL have occurred. In particular the names LAMICTAL or lamotrigine can be confused with the names of other commonly used medications. Medication errors may also occur between the different formulations of LAMICTAL. To reduce the potential of medication errors, write and say LAMICTAL XR clearly. Depictions of the LAMICTAL XR Extended-Release Tablets can be found in the Medication Guide. Each LAMICTAL XR tablet has a distinct color and white center, and is printed with "LAMICTAL XR" and the tablet strength. These distinctive features serve to identify the different presentations of the drug and thus may help reduce the risk of medication errors. LAMICTAL XR is supplied in round, unit-of-use bottles with orange caps containing 30 tablets. The label on the bottle includes a depiction of the tablets that further communicates to patients and pharmacists that the medication is LAMICTAL XR and the specific tablet strength included in the bottle. The unit-of-use bottle with a distinctive orange cap and distinctive bottle label features serves to identify the different presentations of the drug and thus may help to reduce the risk of medication errors. **To avoid a medication error of using the wrong drug or formulation, patients should be strongly advised to visually inspect their tablets to verify that they are LAMICTAL XR each time they fill their prescription and to immediately talk to their doctor/pharmacist if they receive a LAMICTAL XR tablet without a white center and without "LAMICTAL XR" and the strength printed on the tablet as they may have received the wrong medication** [see Dosage Forms and Strengths (3), How Supplied/Storage and Handling (16)].

LAMICTAL XR and DiffCORE are trademarks of the GSK group of companies.

GlaxoSmithKline
Research Triangle Park, NC 27709
©2014, the GSK group of companies. All rights reserved.
LXR:15PI

MEDICATION GUIDE
LAMICTAL® (la-MIK-tal) XR™ (lamotrigine) Extended-Release Tablets

Read this Medication Guide before you start taking LAMICTAL XR and each time you get a refill. There may be new information. This information does not take the place of talking with your healthcare provider about your medical condition or treatment. If you have questions about LAMICTAL XR, ask your healthcare provider or pharmacist.

What is the most important information I should know about LAMICTAL XR?

1. LAMICTAL XR may cause a serious skin rash that may cause you to be hospitalized or to stop LAMICTAL XR; it may rarely cause death.

There is no way to tell if a mild rash will develop into a more serious reaction. These serious skin reactions are more likely to happen when you begin taking LAMICTAL XR, within the first 2 to 8 weeks of treatment. But it can happen in people who have taken LAMICTAL XR for any period of time. Children between 2 to 16 years of age have a higher chance of getting this serious skin reaction while taking lamotrigine. LAMICTAL XR is not approved for use in children less than 13 years of age.

The risk of getting a rash is higher if you:
- take LAMICTAL XR while taking valproate [DEPAKENE (valproic acid) or DEPAKOTE (divalproex sodium)].
- take a higher starting dose of LAMICTAL XR than your healthcare provider prescribed.
- increase your dose of LAMICTAL XR faster than prescribed.

LAMICTAL XR can also cause other types of allergic reactions or serious problems that may affect organs and other parts of your body like the liver or blood cells. You may or may not have a rash with these types of reactions.

Call your healthcare provider right away if you have any of the following:
- a skin rash
- hives
- fever
- swollen lymph glands
- painful sores in the mouth or around your eyes
- swelling of your lips or tongue
- yellowing of your skin or eyes
- unusual bruising or bleeding
- severe fatigue or weakness
- severe muscle pain
- frequent infections

These symptoms may be the first signs of a serious reaction. A healthcare provider should examine you to decide if you should continue taking LAMICTAL XR.

2. Like other antiepileptic drugs, LAMICTAL XR may cause suicidal thoughts or actions in a very small number of people, about 1 in 500.

Call a healthcare provider right away if you have any of these symptoms, especially if they are new, worse, or worry you:
- thoughts about suicide or dying
- attempt to commit suicide
- new or worse depression
- new or worse anxiety
- feeling agitated or restless
- panic attacks
- trouble sleeping (insomnia)
- new or worse irritability
- acting aggressive, being angry, or violent
- acting on dangerous impulses
- an extreme increase in activity and talking (mania)
- other unusual changes in behavior or mood

Do not stop LAMICTAL XR without first talking to a healthcare provider.
- Stopping LAMICTAL XR suddenly can cause serious problems.
- Suicidal thoughts or actions can be caused by things other than medicines. If you have suicidal thoughts or actions, your healthcare provider may check for other causes.

How can I watch for early symptoms of suicidal thoughts and actions?
- Pay attention to any changes, especially sudden changes, in mood, behaviors, thoughts, or feelings.
- Keep all follow-up visits with your healthcare provider as scheduled.
- Call your healthcare provider between visits as needed, especially if you are worried about symptoms.

3. LAMICTAL XR may rarely cause aseptic meningitis, a serious inflammation of the protective membrane that covers the brain and spinal cord.

Call your healthcare provider right away if you have any of the following symptoms:
- Headache
- Fever
- Nausea
- Vomiting
- Stiff neck
- Rash
- Unusual sensitivity to light
- Muscle pains
- Chills
- Confusion
- Drowsiness

Meningitis has many causes other than LAMICTAL XR, which your doctor would check for if you developed meningitis while taking LAMICTAL XR.

LAMICTAL XR can have other serious side effects. For more information ask your healthcare provider or pharmacist. Tell your healthcare provider if you have any side effect that bothers you. Be sure to read the section below entitled "What are the possible side effects of LAMICTAL XR?"

4. Patients prescribed LAMICTAL have sometimes been given the wrong medicine because many medicines have names similar to LAMICTAL, so always check that you receive LAMICTAL XR.

Taking the wrong medication can cause serious health problems. When your healthcare provider gives you a prescription for LAMICTAL XR:
- Make sure you can read it clearly.
- Talk to your pharmacist to check that you are given the correct medicine.
- Each time you fill your prescription, check the tablets you receive against the pictures of the tablets below.

These pictures show the distinct wording, colors, and shapes of the tablets that help to identify the right strength of LAMICTAL XR. Immediately call your pharmacist if you receive a LAMICTAL XR tablet that does not look like one of the tablets shown below, as you may have received the wrong medication.

LAMICTAL XR (lamotrigine) Extended-Release Tablets

25 mg, yellow with white center Imprinted with LAMICTAL XR 25

50 mg, green with white center Imprinted with LAMICTAL XR 50

100 mg, orange with white center Imprinted with LAMICTAL XR 100

200 mg, blue with white center Imprinted with LAMICTAL XR 200

250 mg, purple with white center Imprinted with LAMICTAL XR 250

300 mg, gray with white center Imprinted with LAMICTAL XR 300

What is LAMICTAL XR?
LAMICTAL XR is a prescription medicine used:
- together with other medicines to treat primary generalized tonic-clonic seizures and partial onset seizures in people 13 years of age and older.
- alone to treat partial seizures when changing from certain other medicines used in people 13 years and older.

It is not known if LAMICTAL XR is safe or effective in children less than 13 years of age. Other forms of lamotrigine can be used in children aged 2 to 12 years.

Who should not take LAMICTAL XR?
You should not take LAMICTAL XR if you have had an allergic reaction to lamotrigine or to any of the inactive ingredients in LAMICTAL XR. See the end of this leaflet for a complete list of ingredients in LAMICTAL XR.

What should I tell my healthcare provider before taking LAMICTAL XR?
Before taking LAMICTAL XR, tell your healthcare provider about all of your medical conditions, including if you:
- have had a rash or allergic reaction to another antiseizure medicine.
- have or have had depression, mood problems, or suicidal thoughts or behavior.
- are taking oral contraceptives (birth control pills) or other female hormonal medicines. Do not start or stop taking birth control pills or other female hormonal medicine until you have talked with your healthcare provider. Tell your healthcare provider if you have any changes in your menstrual pattern such as breakthrough bleeding. Stopping these medicines may cause side effects (such as dizziness, lack of coordination, or double vision). Starting these medicines may lessen how well LAMICTAL XR works.
- are pregnant or plan to become pregnant. It is not known if LAMICTAL XR will harm your unborn baby. If you become pregnant while taking LAMICTAL XR, talk to your healthcare provider about registering with the North American Antiepileptic Drug Pregnancy Registry. You can enroll in this registry by calling 1-888-233-2334. The purpose of this registry is to collect information about the safety of antiepileptic drugs during pregnancy.
- are breastfeeding. LAMICTAL XR passes into breast milk and may cause side effects in a breastfed baby. If you breastfeed while taking LAMICTAL XR, watch your baby closely for trouble breathing, episodes of temporarily stopping breathing, sleepiness, or poor sucking. Call your baby's healthcare provider right away if you see any of these problems. Talk to your healthcare provider about the best way to feed your baby if you take LAMICTAL XR.

Tell your healthcare provider about all the medicines you take or if you are planning to take a new medicine, including prescription and non-prescription medicines, vitamins, and herbal supplements. Using LAMICTAL XR with certain other medicines can affect each other, causing side effects.

How should I take LAMICTAL XR?
- Take LAMICTAL XR exactly as prescribed.
- Your healthcare provider may change your dose. Do not change your dose without talking to your healthcare provider.
- Do not stop taking LAMICTAL XR without talking to your healthcare provider. Stopping LAMICTAL XR suddenly may cause serious problems. For example, if you have epilepsy and you stop taking LAMICTAL XR suddenly, you may get seizures that do not stop. Talk with your healthcare provider about how to stop LAMICTAL XR slowly.

- If you miss a dose of LAMICTAL XR, take it as soon as you remember. If it is almost time for your next dose, just skip the missed dose. Take the next dose at your regular time. **Do not take 2 doses at the same time.**
- If you take too much LAMICTAL XR, call your healthcare provider or your local Poison Control Center or go to the nearest hospital emergency room right away.
- You may not feel the full effect of LAMICTAL XR for several weeks.
- If you have epilepsy, tell your healthcare provider if your seizures get worse or if you have any new types of seizures.
- LAMICTAL XR can be taken with or without food.
- Do not chew, crush, or divide LAMICTAL XR.
- Swallow LAMICTAL XR tablets whole.
- If you have trouble swallowing LAMICTAL XR Tablets, tell your healthcare provider because there may be another form of lamotrigine you can take.
- If you receive LAMICTAL XR in a blisterpack, examine the blisterpack before use. Do not use if blisters are torn, broken, or missing.

What should I avoid while taking LAMICTAL XR?
Do not drive a car or operate complex, hazardous machinery until you know how LAMICTAL XR affects you.

What are possible side effects of LAMICTAL XR?
- See "What is the most important information I should know about LAMICTAL XR?" Common side effects of LAMICTAL XR include:
- Dizziness
- Tremor
- Double vision
- Nausea
- Vomiting
- Trouble with balance and coordination
- Anxiety

Other common side effects that have been reported with another form of lamotrigine include headache, sleepiness, blurred vision, runny nose, and rash.
Tell your healthcare provider about any side effect that bothers you or that does not go away.
These are not all the possible side effects of LAMICTAL XR. For more information, ask your healthcare provider or pharmacist.
Call your doctor for medical advice about side effects. You may report side effects to FDA at 1-800-FDA-1088.

How should I store LAMICTAL XR?
- Store LAMICTAL XR at room temperature between 59°F to 86°F (15°C to 30°C).
- **Keep LAMICTAL XR and all medicines out of the reach of children.**

General information about LAMICTAL XR
Medicines are sometimes prescribed for purposes other than those listed in a Medication Guide. Do not use LAMICTAL XR for a condition for which it was not prescribed. Do not give LAMICTAL XR to other people, even if they have the same symptoms you have. It may harm them.
This Medication Guide summarizes the most important information about LAMICTAL XR. If you would like more information, talk with your healthcare provider. You can ask your healthcare provider or pharmacist for information about LAMICTAL XR that is written for healthcare professionals.
For more information, go to www.lamictalxr.com or call 1-888-825-5249.

What are the ingredients in LAMICTAL XR?
Active ingredient: Lamotrigine.
Inactive ingredients: glycerol monostearate, hypromellose, lactose monohydrate, magnesium stearate, methacrylic acid copolymer dispersion, polyethylene glycol 400, polysorbate 80, silicon dioxide (25- and 50-mg tablets only), titanium dioxide, triethyl citrate, carmine (250 mg tablet only), iron oxide black (50-, 250-, and 300-mg tablets only), iron oxide yellow (25-, 50-, and 100-mg tablets only), iron oxide red (100 mg tablet only), FD&C Blue No. 2 Aluminum Lake (200- and 250-mg tablets only). Tablets are printed with edible black ink.
This Medication Guide has been approved by the U.S. Food and Drug Administration.
LAMICTAL XR is a trademark of the GSK group of companies.
DEPAKENE and DEPAKOTE are registered trademarks of Abbott Laboratories.
GlaxoSmithKline
Research Triangle Park, NC 27709
©2014, the GSK group of companies. All rights reserved.
June 2014
LXR:12MG

LOVAZA®
[lō-vă′ ză]
(omega-3-acid ethyl esters)
Capsules, for oral use

HIGHLIGHTS OF PRESCRIBING INFORMATION
These highlights do not include all the information needed to use LOVAZA safely and effectively. See full prescribing information for LOVAZA.

R℥

LOVAZA®(omega-3-acid ethyl esters) Capsules, for oral use
Initial U.S. Approval: 2004

---RECENT MAJOR CHANGES---

Indications and Usage, Limitations of Use (1)   05/2014

---INDICATIONS AND USAGE---
LOVAZA is a combination of ethyl esters of omega 3 fatty acids, principally EPA and DHA, indicated as an adjunct to diet to reduce triglyceride (TG) levels in adult patients with severe (≥500 mg/dL) hypertriglyceridemia (HTG). (1)
Limitations of Use:
- The effect of LOVAZA on the risk for pancreatitis has not been determined. (1)
- The effect of LOVAZA on cardiovascular mortality and morbidity has not been determined. (1)

---DOSAGE AND ADMINISTRATION---
- The daily dose of LOVAZA is 4 grams per day taken as a single 4-gram dose (4 capsules) or as two 2-gram doses (2 capsules given twice daily). (2)
- Patients should be advised to swallow LOVAZA capsules whole. Do not break open, crush, dissolve, or chew LOVAZA. (2)

---DOSAGE FORMS AND STRENGTHS---
Capsules: 1-gram (3)

---CONTRAINDICATIONS---
LOVAZA is contraindicated in patients with known hypersensitivity (e.g., anaphylactic reaction) to LOVAZA or any of its components. (4)

---WARNINGS AND PRECAUTIONS---
- In patients with hepatic impairment, monitor ALT and AST levels periodically during therapy. (5.1)
- LOVAZA may increase levels of LDL. Monitor LDL levels periodically during therapy. (5.1)
- Use with caution in patients with known hypersensitivity to fish and/or shellfish. (5.2)
- There is a possible association between LOVAZA and more frequent recurrences of symptomatic atrial fibrillation or flutter in patients with paroxysmal or persistent atrial fibrillation, particularly within the first months of initiating therapy. (5.3)

---ADVERSE REACTIONS---
The most common adverse reactions (incidence >3% and greater than placebo) were eructation, dyspepsia, and taste perversion. (6)
To report SUSPECTED ADVERSE REACTIONS, contact GlaxoSmithKline at 1-888-825-5249 or FDA at 1-800-FDA-1088 or www.fda.gov/medwatch

---DRUG INTERACTIONS---
Omega-3-acids may prolong bleeding time. Patients taking LOVAZA and an anticoagulant or other drug affecting coagulation (e.g., anti-platelet agents) should be monitored periodically. (7.1)

---USE IN SPECIFIC POPULATIONS---
- Pregnancy: Use during pregnancy only if the potential benefit justifies the potential risk to the fetus. (8.1)
See 17 for PATIENT COUNSELING INFORMATION and FDA-approved patient labeling

Revised: 05/2014

FULL PRESCRIBING INFORMATION

1   INDICATIONS AND USAGE
LOVAZA® (omega-3-acid ethyl esters) is indicated as an adjunct to diet to reduce triglyceride (TG) levels in adult patients with severe (≥500 mg/dL) hypertriglyceridemia (HTG).
Usage Considerations: Patients should be placed on an appropriate lipid-lowering diet before receiving LOVAZA and should continue this diet during treatment with LOVAZA.
Laboratory studies should be done to ascertain that the lipid levels are consistently abnormal before instituting therapy with LOVAZA. Every attempt should be made to control serum lipids with appropriate diet, exercise, weight loss in obese patients, and control of any medical problems such as diabetes mellitus and hypothyroidism that are contributing to the lipid abnormalities. Medications known to exacerbate hypertriglyceridemia (such as beta blockers, thiazides, estrogens) should be discontinued or changed if possible prior to consideration of triglyceride-lowering drug therapy.
Limitations of Use:
The effect of LOVAZA on the risk for pancreatitis has not been determined.
The effect of LOVAZA on cardiovascular mortality and morbidity has not been determined.

2   DOSAGE AND ADMINISTRATION
- Assess triglyceride levels carefully before initiating therapy. Identify other causes (e.g., diabetes mellitus, hypothyroidism, medications) of high triglyceride levels and manage as appropriate *[see Indications and Usage (1)]*.
- Patients should be placed on an appropriate lipid-lowering diet before receiving LOVAZA, and should continue this diet during treatment with LOVAZA. In clinical studies, LOVAZA was administered with meals.
The daily dose of LOVAZA is 4 grams per day. The daily dose may be taken as a single 4-gram dose (4 capsules) or as two 2-gram doses (2 capsules given twice daily).
Patients should be advised to swallow LOVAZA capsules whole. Do not break open, crush, dissolve, or chew LOVAZA.

3   DOSAGE FORMS AND STRENGTHS
LOVAZA (omega-3-acid ethyl esters) capsules are supplied as 1-gram transparent, soft-gelatin capsules filled with light-yellow oil and bearing the designation LOVAZA.

4   CONTRAINDICATIONS
LOVAZA is contraindicated in patients with known hypersensitivity (e.g., anaphylactic reaction) to LOVAZA or any of its components.

5   WARNINGS AND PRECAUTIONS
5.1   Monitoring: Laboratory Tests
In patients with hepatic impairment, alanine aminotransferase (ALT) and aspartate aminotransferase (AST) levels should be monitored periodically during therapy with LOVAZA. In some patients, increases in ALT levels without a concurrent increase in AST levels were observed.
In some patients, LOVAZA increases LDL-C levels. LDL-C levels should be monitored periodically during therapy with LOVAZA.
Laboratory studies should be performed periodically to measure the patient's TG levels during therapy with LOVAZA.
5.2   Fish Allergy
LOVAZA contains ethyl esters of omega-3 fatty acids (EPA and DHA) obtained from the oil of several fish sources. It is not known whether patients with allergies to fish and/or shellfish, are at increased risk of an allergic reaction to LOVAZA. LOVAZA should be used with caution in patients with known hypersensitivity to fish and/or shellfish.
5.3   Recurrent Atrial Fibrillation (AF) or Flutter
In a double-blind, placebo-controlled trial of 663 subjects with symptomatic paroxysmal AF (n = 542) or persistent AF (n = 121), recurrent AF or flutter was observed in subjects randomized to LOVAZA who received 8 grams/day for 7 days and 4 grams/day thereafter for 23 weeks at a higher rate relative to placebo. Subjects in this trial had median baseline triglycerides of 127 mg/dL, had no substantial structural heart disease, were taking no anti-arrhythmic therapy (rate control permitted), and were in normal sinus rhythm at baseline.
At 24 weeks, in the paroxysmal AF stratum, there were 129 (47%) first recurrent symptomatic AF or flutter events on

placebo and 141 (53%) on LOVAZA [primary endpoint, HR 1.19; 95% CI: 0.93, 1.35]. In the persistent AF stratum, there were 19 (35%) events on placebo and 34 (52%) events on LOVAZA [HR 1.63; 95% CI: 0.91, 2.18]. For both strata combined, the HR was 1.25; 95% CI: 1.00, 1.40. Although the clinical significance of these results is uncertain, there is a possible association between LOVAZA and more frequent recurrences of symptomatic atrial fibrillation or flutter in patients with paroxysmal or persistent atrial fibrillation, particularly within the first 2 to 3 months of initiating therapy.

LOVAZA is not indicated for the treatment of AF or flutter.

6 ADVERSE REACTIONS
6.1 Clinical Trials Experience
Because clinical trials are conducted under widely varying conditions, adverse reaction rates observed in the clinical trials of a drug cannot be directly compared with rates in the clinical trials of another drug and may not reflect the rates observed in practice.

Adverse reactions reported in at least 3% and at a greater rate than placebo for subjects treated with LOVAZA based on pooled data across 23 clinical trials are listed in Table 1.

Table 1. Adverse Reactions Occurring at Incidence ≥3% and Greater than Placebo in Clinical Trials of LOVAZA

Adverse Reaction[a]	LOVAZA (N = 655)		Placebo (N = 370)	
	n	%	n	%
Eructation	29	4	5	1
Dyspepsia	22	3	6	2
Taste perversion	27	4	1	<1

[a] Trials included subjects with HTG and severe HTG.

Additional adverse reactions from clinical trials are listed below:

Digestive System: Constipation, gastrointestinal disorder and vomiting.
Metabolic and Nutritional Disorders: Increased ALT and increased AST.
Skin: Pruritus and rash.

6.2 Postmarketing Experience
In addition to adverse reactions reported from clinical trials, the events described below have been identified during post-approval use of LOVAZA. Because these events are reported voluntarily from a population of unknown size, it is not possible to reliably estimate their frequency or to always establish a causal relationship to drug exposure.

The following events have been reported: anaphylactic reaction, hemorrhagic diathesis.

7 DRUG INTERACTIONS
7.1 Anticoagulants or Other Drugs Affecting Coagulation
Some trials with omega-3-acids demonstrated prolongation of bleeding time. The prolongation of bleeding time reported in these trials has not exceeded normal limits and did not produce clinically significant bleeding episodes. Clinical trials have not been done to thoroughly examine the effect of LOVAZA and concomitant anticoagulants. Patients receiving treatment with LOVAZA and an anticoagulant or other drug affecting coagulation (e.g., anti-platelet agents) should be monitored periodically.

8 USE IN SPECIFIC POPULATIONS
8.1 Pregnancy
Pregnancy Category C: There are no adequate and well-controlled studies in pregnant women. It is unknown whether LOVAZA can cause fetal harm when administered to a pregnant woman or can affect reproductive capacity. LOVAZA should be used during pregnancy only if the potential benefit to the patient justifies the potential risk to the fetus.

Animal Data:
Omega-3-acid ethyl esters have been shown to have an embryocidal effect in pregnant rats when given in doses resulting in exposures 7 times the recommended human dose of 4 grams/day based on a body surface area comparison.

In female rats given oral gavage doses of 100, 600, and 2,000 mg/kg/day beginning 2 weeks prior to mating and continuing through gestation and lactation, no adverse effects were observed in the high-dose group (5 times human systemic exposure following an oral dose of 4 grams/day based on body surface area comparison).

In pregnant rats given oral gavage doses of 1,000, 3,000, and 6,000 mg/kg/day from gestation day 6 through 15, no adverse effects were observed (14 times human systemic exposure following an oral dose of 4 grams/day based on a body surface area comparison).

In pregnant rats given oral gavage doses of 100, 600, and 2,000 mg/kg/day from gestation day 14 through lactation

Table 2. Median Baseline and Percent Change From Baseline in Lipid Parameters in Patients with Very High TG Levels (≥500 mg/dL)

Parameter	LOVAZA N = 42		Placebo N = 42		Difference
	BL	% Change	BL	% Change	
TG	816	-44.9	788	+6.7	-51.6
Non-HDL-C	271	-13.8	292	-3.6	-10.2
TC	296	-9.7	314	-1.7	-8.0
VLDL-C	175	-41.7	175	-0.9	-40.8
HDL-C	22	+9.1	24	0.0	+9.1
LDL-C	89	+44.5	108	-4.8	+49.3

BL = Baseline (mg/dL); % Change = Median Percent Change from Baseline; Difference = LOVAZA Median % Change – Placebo Median % Change

day 21, no adverse effects were seen at 2,000 mg/kg/day (5 times the human systemic exposure following an oral dose of 4 grams/day based on a body surface area comparison). However, decreased live births (20% reduction) and decreased survival to postnatal day 4 (40% reduction) were observed in a dose-ranging study using higher doses of 3,000 mg/kg/day (7 times the human systemic exposure following an oral dose of 4 grams/day based on a body surface area comparison).

In pregnant rabbits given oral gavage doses of 375, 750, and 1,500 mg/kg/day from gestation day 7 through 19, no findings were observed in the fetuses in groups given 375 mg/kg/day (2 times human systemic exposure following an oral dose of 4 grams/day based on a body surface area comparison). However, at higher doses, evidence of maternal toxicity was observed (4 times human systemic exposure following an oral dose of 4 grams/day based on a body surface area comparison).

8.3 Nursing Mothers
Studies with omega-3-acid ethyl esters have demonstrated excretion in human milk. The effect of this excretion on the infant of a nursing mother is unknown; caution should be exercised when LOVAZA is administered to a nursing mother. An animal study in lactating rats given oral gavage ^{14}C-ethyl EPA demonstrated that drug levels were 6 to 14 times higher in milk than in plasma.

8.4 Pediatric Use
Safety and effectiveness in pediatric patients have not been established.

8.5 Geriatric Use
A limited number of subjects older than 65 years were enrolled in the clinical trials of LOVAZA. Safety and efficacy findings in subjects older than 60 years did not appear to differ from those of subjects younger than 60 years.

9 DRUG ABUSE AND DEPENDENCE
LOVAZA does not have any known drug abuse or withdrawal effects.

11 DESCRIPTION
LOVAZA, a lipid-regulating agent, is supplied as a liquid-filled gel capsule for oral administration. Each 1-gram capsule of LOVAZA contains at least 900 mg of the ethyl esters of omega-3 fatty acids sourced from fish oils. These are predominantly a combination of ethyl esters of eicosapentaenoic acid (EPA - approximately 465 mg) and docosahexaenoic acid (DHA - approximately 375 mg).

The empirical formula of EPA ethyl ester is $C_{22}H_{34}O_2$, and the molecular weight of EPA ethyl ester is 330.51. The structural formula of EPA ethyl ester is:

The empirical formula of DHA ethyl ester is $C_{24}H_{36}O_2$, and the molecular weight of DHA ethyl ester is 356.55. The structural formula of DHA ethyl ester is:

LOVAZA capsules also contain the following inactive ingredients: 4 mg α-tocopherol (in a carrier of soybean oil), and gelatin, glycerol, and purified water (components of the capsule shell).

12 CLINICAL PHARMACOLOGY
12.1 Mechanism of Action
The mechanism of action of LOVAZA is not completely understood. Potential mechanisms of action include inhibition

of acyl-CoA:1,2-diacylglycerol acyltransferase, increased mitochondrial and peroxisomal β-oxidation in the liver, decreased lipogenesis in the liver, and increased plasma lipoprotein lipase activity. LOVAZA may reduce the synthesis of triglycerides in the liver because EPA and DHA are poor substrates for the enzymes responsible for TG synthesis, and EPA and DHA inhibit esterification of other fatty acids.

12.3 Pharmacokinetics
In healthy volunteers and in subjects with hypertriglyceridemia, EPA and DHA were absorbed when administered as ethyl esters orally. Omega-3-acids administered as ethyl esters (LOVAZA) induced significant, dose-dependent increases in serum phospholipid EPA content, though increases in DHA content were less marked and not dose-dependent when administered as ethyl esters.

Specific Populations:
Age:
Uptake of EPA and DHA into serum phospholipids in subjects treated with LOVAZA was independent of age (<49 years versus ≥49 years).

Gender:
Females tended to have more uptake of EPA into serum phospholipids than males. The clinical significance of this is unknown.

Pediatric:
Pharmacokinetics of LOVAZA have not been studied.

Renal or Hepatic Impairment:
LOVAZA has not been studied in patients with renal or hepatic impairment.

Drug-Drug Interactions:
Simvastatin:
In a 14-day trial of 24 healthy adult subjects, daily coadministration of simvastatin 80 mg with LOVAZA 4 grams did not affect the extent (AUC) or rate (C_{max}) of exposure to simvastatin or the major active metabolite, beta-hydroxy simvastatin at steady state.

Atorvastatin:
In a 14-day trial of 50 healthy adult subjects, daily coadministration of atorvastatin 80 mg with LOVAZA 4 grams did not affect AUC or C_{max} of exposure to atorvastatin, 2-hydroxyatorvastatin, or 4-hydroxyatorvastatin at steady state.

Rosuvastatin:
In a 14-day trial of 48 healthy adult subjects, daily coadministration of rosuvastatin 40 mg with LOVAZA 4 grams did not affect AUC or C_{max} of exposure to rosuvastatin at steady state.

In vitro studies using human liver microsomes indicated that clinically significant cytochrome P450-mediated inhibition by EPA/DHA combinations are not expected in humans.

13 NONCLINICAL TOXICOLOGY
13.1 Carcinogenesis, Mutagenesis, impairment of Fertility
In a rat carcinogenicity study with oral gavage doses of 100, 600, and 2,000 mg/kg/day, males were treated with omega-3-acid ethyl esters for 101 weeks and females for 89 weeks without an increased incidence of tumors (up to 5 times human systemic exposures following an oral dose of 4 grams/day based on a body surface area comparison). Standard lifetime carcinogenicity bioassays were not conducted in mice.

Omega-3-acid ethyl esters were not mutagenic or clastogenic with or without metabolic activation in the bacterial mutagenesis (Ames) test with *Salmonella typhimurium* and *Escherichia coli* or in the chromosomal aberration assay in Chinese hamster V79 lung cells or human lymphocytes. Omega-3-acid ethyl esters were negative in the in vivo mouse micronucleus assay.

In a rat fertility study with oral gavage doses of 100, 600, and 2,000 mg/kg/day, males were treated for 10 weeks prior to mating and females were treated for 2 weeks prior to and throughout mating, gestation, and lactation. No adverse effect on fertility was observed at 2,000 mg/kg/day (5 times human systemic exposure following an oral dose of 4 grams/day based on a body surface area comparison).

14 CLINICAL STUDIES

14.1 Severe Hypertriglyceridemia

The effects of LOVAZA 4 grams per day were assessed in 2 randomized, placebo-controlled, double-blind, parallel-group trials of 84 adult subjects (42 on LOVAZA, 42 on placebo) with very high triglyceride levels. Subjects whose baseline triglyceride levels were between 500 and 2,000 mg/dL were enrolled in these 2 trials of 6 and 16 weeks' duration. The median triglyceride and LDL-C levels in these subjects were 792 mg/dL and 100 mg/dL, respectively. Median HDL-C level was 23.0 mg/dL.

The changes in the major lipoprotein lipid parameters for the groups receiving LOVAZA or placebo are shown in Table 2.

[See table 2 at top of previous page]

LOVAZA 4 grams per day reduced median TG, VLDL-C, and non-HDL-C levels and increased median HDL-C from baseline relative to placebo. Treatment with LOVAZA to reduce very high TG levels may result in elevations in LDL-C and non-HDL-C in some individuals. Patients should be monitored to ensure that the LDL-C level does not increase excessively.

The effect of LOVAZA on the risk of pancreatitis has not been determined.

The effect of LOVAZA on cardiovascular mortality and morbidity has not been determined.

16 HOW SUPPLIED/STORAGE AND HANDLING

LOVAZA (omega-3-acid ethyl esters) capsules are supplied as 1-gram, transparent, soft-gelatin capsules filled with light-yellow oil and bearing the designation LOVAZA.

Bottles of 120: NDC 0173-0783-02.

Store at 25°C (77°F); excursions permitted to 15° to 30°C (59° to 86°F) [see USP Controlled Room Temperature]. Do not freeze. Keep out of reach of children.

17 PATIENT COUNSELING INFORMATION

Advise the patient to read the FDA-approved patient labeling (Patient Information).

Information for Patients:

- LOVAZA should be used with caution in patients with known sensitivity or allergy to fish and/or shellfish *[see Warnings and Precautions (5.2)]*.
- Advise patients that use of lipid-regulating agents does not reduce the importance of adhering to diet *[see Dosage and Administration (2)]*.
- Advise patients not to alter LOVAZA capsules in any way and to ingest intact capsules only *[see Dosage and Administration (2)]*.
- Instruct patients to take LOVAZA as prescribed. If a dose is missed, advise patients to take it as soon as they remember. However, if they miss one day of LOVAZA, they should not double the dose when they take it.

Manufactured for:

GlaxoSmithKline

Research Triangle Park, NC 27709

LOVAZA is a registered trademark of the GSK group of companies.

©2014, the GSK group of companies. All rights reserved.

LVZ:12PI

PHARMACIST-DETACH HERE AND GIVE INSTRUCTIONS TO PATIENT

PATIENT INFORMATION

LOVAZA® (lō-vä-zä)

(omega-3-acid ethyl esters)

Capsules

Read this Patient Information before you start taking LOVAZA, and each time you get a refill. There may be new information. This information does not take the place of talking with your doctor about your medical condition or your treatment.

What is LOVAZA?

LOVAZA is a prescription medicine used along with a low fat and low cholesterol diet to lower very high triglyceride (fat) levels in adults.

It is not known if LOVAZA changes your risk of having inflammation of your pancreas (pancreatitis).

It is not known if LOVAZA prevents you from having a heart attack or stroke.

It is not known if LOVAZA is safe and effective in children.

Who should not take LOVAZA?

Do not take LOVAZA if you are allergic to omega-3-acid ethyl esters or any of the ingredients in LOVAZA. See the end of this leaflet for a complete list of ingredients in LOVAZA.

What should I tell my doctor before taking LOVAZA?

Before you take LOVAZA, tell your doctor if you:

- have diabetes.
- have a low thyroid problem (hypothyroidism).
- have a liver problem.
- have a pancreas problem.
- have a certain heart rhythm problem called atrial fibrillation or flutter.
- are allergic to fish or shellfish. It is not known if people who are allergic to fish or shellfish are also allergic to LOVAZA.
- are pregnant or plan to become pregnant. It is not known if LOVAZA will harm your unborn baby.
- are breastfeeding or plan to breastfeed. LOVAZA can pass into your breast milk. You and your doctor should decide if you will take LOVAZA or breastfeed.

Tell your doctor about all the medicines you take, including prescription and non-prescription medicine, vitamins, and herbal supplements.

LOVAZA can interact with certain other medicines that you are taking. Using LOVAZA with medicines that affect blood clotting (anticoagulants or blood thinners) may cause serious side effects.

Know the medicines you take. Keep a list of them to show your doctor and pharmacist when you get a new medicine.

How should I take LOVAZA?

- Take LOVAZA exactly as your doctor tells you to take it.
- You should not take more than 4 capsules of LOVAZA each day. Either take all 4 capsules at one time, or 2 capsules two times a day.
- Do not change your dose or stop LOVAZA without talking to your doctor.
- Take LOVAZA with or without food.
- Take LOVAZA capsules whole. Do not break, crush, dissolve, or chew LOVAZA capsules before swallowing. If you cannot swallow LOVAZA capsules whole, tell your doctor. You may need a different medicine.
- Your doctor may start you on a diet that is low in saturated fat, cholesterol, carbohydrates, and low in added sugars before giving you LOVAZA. Stay on this diet while taking LOVAZA.
- Your doctor should do blood tests to check your triglyceride, bad cholesterol and liver function levels while you take LOVAZA.

What are the possible side effects of LOVAZA?

LOVAZA may cause serious side effects, including:

- increases in the results of blood tests used to check your liver function (ALT and AST) and your bad cholesterol levels (LDL-C).
- increases in the frequency of a heart rhythm problem (atrial fibrillation or flutter) may especially happen in the first few months of taking LOVAZA if you already have that problem.

The most common side effects of LOVAZA include:

- burping
- upset stomach
- a change in your sense of taste.

Talk to your doctor if you have a side effect that bothers you or does not go away.

These are not all the possible side effects of LOVAZA. For more information, ask your doctor or pharmacist.

Call your doctor for medical advice about side effects. You may report side effects to FDA at 1-800-FDA-1088.

How should I store LOVAZA?

- Store LOVAZA at room temperature between 68°F to 77°F (20°C to 25°C).
- Do not freeze LOVAZA.
- Safely throw away medicine that is out of date or no longer needed.

Keep LOVAZA and all medicines out of the reach of children.

General information about the safe and effective use of LOVAZA

Medicines are sometimes prescribed for purposes other than those listed in a Patient Information leaflet. Do not use LOVAZA for a condition for which it was not prescribed. Do not give LOVAZA to other people, even if they have the same symptoms you have. It may harm them.

This Patient Information Leaflet summarizes the most important information about LOVAZA. If you would like more information, talk with your doctor. You can ask your doctor or pharmacist for information about LOVAZA that is written for health professionals.

For more information go to www.LOVAZA.com or call 1-888-825-5249.

What are the ingredients in LOVAZA?

Active Ingredient: omega-3-acid ethyl esters, mostly EPA and DHA

Inactive Ingredients: alpha-tocopherol (in soybean oil), gelatin, glycerol, purified water.

This patient labeling has been approved by the U.S. Food and Drug Administration.

Manufactured for:

GlaxoSmithKline

Research Triangle Park, NC 27709

LOVAZA is a registered trademark of the GSK group of companies.

©2014, the GSK group of companies. All rights reserved.

May 2014

LVZ:10PIL

MALARONE   ℞

[mal'ə-rōn]

(atovaquone and proguanil hydrochloride)

Tablets

MALARONE   ℞

(atovaquone and proguanil hydrochloride)

Pediatric Tablets

HIGHLIGHTS OF PRESCRIBING INFORMATION

These highlights do not include all the information needed to use MALARONE safely and effectively. See full prescribing information for MALARONE.

MALARONE (atovaquone and proguanil hydrochloride) Tablets

MALARONE (atovaquone and proguanil hydrochloride) Pediatric Tablets

Initial U.S. Approval: 2000

——————INDICATIONS AND USAGE——————

MALARONE is an antimalarial indicated for:

- prophylaxis of *Plasmodium falciparum* malaria, including in areas where chloroquine resistance has been reported. (1.1)
- treatment of acute, uncomplicated *P. falciparum* malaria. (1.2)

————DOSAGE AND ADMINISTRATION————

- MALARONE should be taken with food or a milky drink.

Prophylaxis (2.1):

- Start prophylaxis 1 or 2 days before entering a malaria-endemic area and continue daily during the stay and for 7 days after return.
- Adults: One adult strength tablet per day.
- Pediatric Patients: Dosage based on body weight (see Table 1).

Treatment (2.2):

- Adults: Four adult strength tablets as a single daily dose for 3 days.
- Pediatric Patients: Dosage based on body weight (see Table 2).

Renal Impairment (2.3):

- Do not use for prophylaxis of malaria in patients with severe renal impairment.
- Use with caution for treatment of malaria in patients with severe renal impairment.

————DOSAGE FORMS AND STRENGTHS————

- Tablets (adult strength): 250 mg atovaquone and 100 mg proguanil hydrochloride. (3)
- Pediatric Tablets: 62.5 mg atovaquone and 25 mg proguanil hydrochloride. (3)

——————CONTRAINDICATIONS——————

- Known serious hypersensitivity reactions to atovaquone or proguanil hydrochloride or any component of the formulation. (4.1)
- Prophylaxis of *P. falciparum* malaria in patients with severe renal impairment (creatinine clearance <30 mL/min). (4.2)

————WARNINGS AND PRECAUTIONS————

- Atovaquone absorption may be reduced in patients with diarrhea or vomiting. If used in patients who are vomiting, parasitemia should be closely monitored and the use of an antiemetic considered. In patients with severe or persistent diarrhea or vomiting, alternative antimalarial therapy may be required. (5.1)
- In mixed *P. falciparum* and *Plasmodium vivax* infection, *P. vivax* relapse occurred commonly when patients were treated with MALARONE alone. (5.2)
- In the event of recrudescent *P. falciparum* infections after treatment or prophylaxis failure, patients should be treated with a different blood schizonticide. (5.2)
- Elevated liver laboratory tests and cases of hepatitis and hepatic failure requiring liver transplantation have been reported with prophylactic use. (5.3)
- MALARONE has not been evaluated for the treatment of cerebral malaria or other severe manifestations of complicated malaria. Patients with severe malaria are not candidates for oral therapy. (5.4)

——————ADVERSE REACTIONS——————

- Prophylaxis: common adverse reactions (4%) in adults were diarrhea, dreams, oral ulcers, and headache; these events occurred in a similar or lower proportion of subjects receiving MALARONE than an active comparator. Common adverse reactions (5%) in pediatric patients included abdominal pain, headache, cough, and vomiting. (6.1)

• Treatment: common adverse reactions (5%) in adolescents and adults were abdominal pain, nausea, vomiting, headache, diarrhea, asthenia, anorexia, and dizziness. Common adverse reactions (6%) in pediatric patients included vomiting, pruritus, and diarrhea. (6.1)

To report SUSPECTED ADVERSE REACTIONS, contact GlaxoSmithKline at 1-888-825-5249 or FDA at 1-800-FDA-1088 or www.fda.gov/medwatch

─────────DRUG INTERACTIONS─────────

• Administration with rifampin or rifabutin is known to reduce atovaquone concentrations; concomitant use with MALARONE is not recommended. (7.1)
• Proguanil may potentiate anticoagulant effect of warfarin and other coumarin-based anticoagulants. Caution advised when initiating or withdrawing MALARONE in patients on anticoagulants; coagulation tests should be closely monitored. (7.2)
• Tetracycline may reduce atovaquone concentrations; parasitemia should be closely monitored. (7.3)

──────USE IN SPECIFIC POPULATIONS──────

• Caution should be exercised when administered to a nursing woman as proguanil is excreted into human milk. (8.3)
• Renal impairment: contraindicated for prophylaxis of *P. falciparum* malaria in patients with severe renal impairment (8.6).

See 17 for PATIENT COUNSELING INFORMATION
                                    Revised: 06/2013

FULL PRESCRIBING INFORMATION: CONTENTS*

FULL PRESCRIBING INFORMATION

1   INDICATIONS AND USAGE
1.1   Prevention of Malaria
MALARONE® is indicated for the prophylaxis of *Plasmodium falciparum* malaria, including in areas where chloroquine resistance has been reported.
1.2   Treatment of Malaria
MALARONE is indicated for the treatment of acute, uncomplicated *P. falciparum* malaria. MALARONE has been shown to be effective in regions where the drugs chloro-

quine, halofantrine, mefloquine, and amodiaquine may have unacceptable failure rates, presumably due to drug resistance.

2   DOSAGE AND ADMINISTRATION
The daily dose should be taken at the same time each day with food or a milky drink. In the event of vomiting within 1 hour after dosing, a repeat dose should be taken.
MALARONE may be crushed and mixed with condensed milk just prior to administration to patients who may have difficulty swallowing tablets.
2.1   Prevention of Malaria
Start prophylactic treatment with MALARONE 1 or 2 days before entering a malaria-endemic area and continue daily during the stay and for 7 days after return.
Adults: One MALARONE Tablet (adult strength = 250 mg atovaquone/100 mg proguanil hydrochloride) per day.
Pediatric Patients: The dosage for prevention of malaria in pediatric patients is based upon body weight (Table 1).

Table 1. Dosage for Prevention of Malaria in Pediatric Patients

Weight (kg)	Atovaquone/Proguanil HCl Total Daily Dose	Dosage Regimen
11-20	62.5 mg/ 25 mg	1 MALARONE Pediatric Tablet daily
21-30	125 mg/ 50 mg	2 MALARONE Pediatric Tablets as a single daily dose
31-40	187.5 mg/ 75 mg	3 MALARONE Pediatric Tablets as a single daily dose
>40	250 mg/ 100 mg	1 MALARONE Tablet (adult strength) as a single daily dose

2.2   Treatment of Acute Malaria
Adults: Four MALARONE Tablets (adult strength; total daily dose 1 g atovaquone/400 mg proguanil hydrochloride) as a single daily dose for 3 consecutive days.
Pediatric Patients: The dosage for treatment of acute malaria in pediatric patients is based upon body weight (Table 2).

Table 2. Dosage for Treatment of Acute Malaria in Pediatric Patients

Weight (kg)	Atovaquone/Proguanil HCl Total Daily Dose	Dosage Regimen
5-8	125 mg/ 50 mg	2 MALARONE Pediatric Tablets daily for 3 consecutive days
9-10	187.5 mg/ 75 mg	3 MALARONE Pediatric Tablets daily for 3 consecutive days
11-20	250 mg/ 100 mg	1 MALARONE Tablet (adult strength) daily for 3 consecutive days
21-30	500 mg/ 200 mg	2 MALARONE Tablets (adult strength) as a single daily dose for 3 consecutive days
31-40	750 mg/ 300 mg	3 MALARONE Tablets (adult strength) as a single daily dose for 3 consecutive days
>40	1 g/ 400 mg	4 MALARONE Tablets (adult strength) as a single daily dose for 3 consecutive days

2.3   Renal Impairment
Do not use MALARONE for malaria prophylaxis in patients with severe renal impairment (creatinine clearance <30 mL/min) *[see Contraindications (4.2)]*. Use with caution for the treatment of malaria in patients with severe renal impairment, only if the benefits of the 3-day treatment regimen outweigh the potential risks associated with increased drug exposure. No dosage adjustments are needed in patients with mild (creatinine clearance 50 to 80 mL/min) or moderate (creatinine clearance 30 to 50 mL/min) renal impairment. *[See Clinical Pharmacology (12.3).]*

3   DOSAGE FORMS AND STRENGTHS
Each MALARONE Tablet (adult strength) contains 250 mg atovaquone and 100 mg proguanil hydrochloride. MALARONE Tablets are pink, film-coated, round, biconvex tablets engraved with "GX CM3" on one side.

Each MALARONE Pediatric Tablet contains 62.5 mg atovaquone and 25 mg proguanil hydrochloride. MALARONE Pediatric Tablets are pink, film-coated, round, biconvex tablets engraved with "GX CG7" on one side.

4   CONTRAINDICATIONS
4.1   Hypersensitivity
MALARONE is contraindicated in individuals with known hypersensitivity reactions (e.g., anaphylaxis, erythema multiforme or Stevens-Johnson syndrome, angioedema, vasculitis) to atovaquone or proguanil hydrochloride or any component of the formulation.
4.2   Severe Renal Impairment
MALARONE is contraindicated for prophylaxis of *P. falciparum* malaria in patients with severe renal impairment (creatinine clearance <30 mL/min) because of pancytopenia in patients with severe renal impairment treated with proguanil *[see Use in Specific Populations (8.6), and Clinical Pharmacology (12.3)].*

5   WARNINGS AND PRECAUTIONS
5.1   Vomiting and Diarrhea
Absorption of atovaquone may be reduced in patients with diarrhea or vomiting. If MALARONE is used in patients who are vomiting, parasitemia should be closely monitored and the use of an antiemetic considered. *[See Dosage and Administration (2).]* Vomiting occurred in up to 19% of pediatric patients given treatment doses of MALARONE. In the controlled clinical trials, 15.3% of adults received an antiemetic when they received atovaquone/proguanil and 98.3% of these patients were successfully treated. In patients with severe or persistent diarrhea or vomiting, alternative antimalarial therapy may be required.
5.2   Relapse of Infection
In mixed *P. falciparum* and *Plasmodium vivax* infections, *P. vivax* parasite relapse occurred commonly when patients were treated with MALARONE alone.
In the event of recrudescent *P. falciparum* infections after treatment with MALARONE or failure of chemoprophylaxis with MALARONE, patients should be treated with a different blood schizonticide.
5.3   Hepatotoxicity
Elevated liver laboratory tests and cases of hepatitis and hepatic failure requiring liver transplantation have been reported with prophylactic use of MALARONE.
5.4   Severe or Complicated Malaria
MALARONE has not been evaluated for the treatment of cerebral malaria or other severe manifestations of complicated malaria, including hyperparasitemia, pulmonary edema, or renal failure. Patients with severe malaria are not candidates for oral therapy.

6   ADVERSE REACTIONS
6.1   Clinical Trials Experience
Because clinical trials are conducted under widely varying conditions, adverse reaction rates observed in the clinical trials of a drug cannot be directly compared to rates in the clinical trials of another drug and may not reflect the rates observed in practice.
Because MALARONE contains atovaquone and proguanil hydrochloride, the type and severity of adverse reactions associated with each of the compounds may be expected. The lower prophylactic doses of MALARONE were better tolerated than the higher treatment doses.
Prophylaxis of *P. falciparum* Malaria: In 3 clinical trials (2 of which were placebo-controlled) 381 adults (mean age 31 years) received MALARONE for the prophylaxis of malaria; the majority of adults were black (90%) and 79% were male. In a clinical trial for the prophylaxis of malaria, 125 pediatric patients (mean age 9 years) received MALARONE; all subjects were black and 52% were male. Adverse experiences reported in adults and pediatric patients, considered attributable to therapy, occurred in similar proportions of subjects receiving MALARONE or placebo in all studies. Prophylaxis with MALARONE was discontinued prematurely due to a treatment-related adverse experience in 3 of 381 (0.8%) adults and 0 of 125 pediatric patients.
In a placebo-controlled study of malaria prophylaxis with MALARONE involving 330 pediatric patients (aged 4 to 14 years) in Gabon, a malaria-endemic area, the safety profile of MALARONE was consistent with that observed in the earlier prophylactic studies in adults and pediatric patients. The most common treatment-emergent adverse events with MALARONE were abdominal pain (13%), headache (13%), and cough (10%). Abdominal pain (13% vs. 8%) and vomiting (5% vs. 3%) were reported more often with MALARONE than with placebo. No patient withdrew from the study due to an adverse experience with MALARONE. No routine laboratory data were obtained during this study.
Non-immune travelers visiting a malaria-endemic area received MALARONE (n = 1,004) for prophylaxis of malaria in 2 active-controlled clinical trials. In one study (n = 493), the mean age of subjects was 33 years and 53% were male; 90% of subjects were white, 6% of subjects were black and the remaining were of other racial/ethnic groups. In the

Table 3. Adverse Experiences in Active-Controlled Clinical Trials of MALARONE for Prophylaxis of P. falciparum Malaria

	Percent of Subjects With Adverse Experiences[a] (Percent of Subjects With Adverse Experiences Attributable to Therapy)							
	Study 1				Study 2			
	MALARONE n = 493 (28 days)[b]		Mefloquine n = 483 (53 days)[b]		MALARONE n = 511 (26 days)[b]		Chloroquine plus Proguanil n = 511 (49 days)[b]	
Diarrhea	38	(8)	36	(7)	34	(5)	39	(7)
Nausea	14	(3)	20	(8)	11	(2)	18	(7)
Abdominal pain	17	(5)	16	(5)	14	(3)	22	(6)
Headache	12	(4)	17	(7)	12	(4)	14	(4)
Dreams	7	(7)	16	(14)	6	(4)	7	(3)
Insomnia	5	(3)	16	(13)	4	(2)	5	(2)
Fever	9	(<1)	11	(1)	8	(<1)	8	(<1)
Dizziness	5	(2)	14	(9)	7	(3)	8	(4)
Vomiting	8	(1)	10	(2)	8	(0)	14	(2)
Oral ulcers	9	(6)	6	(4)	5	(4)	7	(5)
Pruritus	4	(2)	5	(2)	3	(1)	2	(<1)
Visual difficulties	2	(2)	5	(3)	3	(2)	3	(2)
Depression	<1	(<1)	5	(4)	<1	(<1)	1	(<1)
Anxiety	1	(<1)	5	(4)	<1	(<1)	1	(<1)
Any adverse experience	64	(30)	69	(42)	58	(22)	66	(28)
Any neuropsychiatric event	20	(14)	37	(29)	16	(10)	20	(10)
Any GI event	49	(16)	50	(19)	43	(12)	54	(20)

[a] Adverse experiences that started while receiving active study drug.
[b] Mean duration of dosing based on recommended dosing regimens.

other study (n = 511), the mean age of subjects was 36 years and 51% were female; the majority of subjects (97%) were white. Adverse experiences occurred in a similar or lower proportion of subjects receiving MALARONE than an active comparator (Table 3). Fewer neuropsychiatric adverse experiences occurred in subjects who received MALARONE than mefloquine. Fewer gastrointestinal adverse experiences occurred in subjects receiving MALARONE than chloroquine/proguanil. Compared with active comparator drugs, subjects receiving MALARONE had fewer adverse experiences overall that were attributed to prophylactic therapy (Table 3). Prophylaxis with MALARONE was discontinued prematurely due to a treatment-related adverse experience in 7 of 1,004 travelers.
[See table 3 above]
In a third active-controlled study, MALARONE (n = 110) was compared with chloroquine/proguanil (n = 111) for the prophylaxis of malaria in 221 non-immune pediatric patients (2 to 17 years of age). The mean duration of exposure was 23 days for MALARONE, 46 days for chloroquine, and 43 days for proguanil, reflecting the different recommended dosage regimens for these products. Fewer patients treated with MALARONE reported abdominal pain (2% vs. 7%) or nausea (<1% vs. 7%) than children who received chloroquine/proguanil. Oral ulceration (2% vs. 2%), vivid dreams (2% vs. <1%), and blurred vision (0% vs. 2%) occurred in similar proportions of patients receiving either MALARONE or chloroquine/proguanil, respectively. Two patients discontinued prophylaxis with chloroquine/proguanil due to adverse events, while none of those receiving MALARONE discontinued due to adverse events.
Treatment of Acute, Uncomplicated *P. falciparum* Malaria: In 7 controlled trials, 436 adolescents and adults received MALARONE for treatment of acute, uncomplicated *P. falciparum* malaria. The range of mean ages of subjects was 26 to 29 years; 79% of subjects were male. In these studies, 48% of subjects were classified as other racial/ethnic groups, primarily Asian; 42% of subjects were black and the remaining subjects were white. Attributable adverse experiences that occurred in ≥5% of subjects were abdominal pain (17%), nausea (12%), vomiting (12%), headache (10%), diarrhea (8%), asthenia (8%), anorexia (5%), and dizziness (5%). Treatment was discontinued prematurely due to an adverse experience in 4 of 436 (0.9%) adolescents and adults treated with MALARONE.
In 2 controlled trials, 116 pediatric patients (weighing 11 to 40 kg) (mean age 7 years) received MALARONE for the

treatment of malaria. The majority of subjects were black (72%); 28% were of other racial/ethnic groups, primarily Asian. Attributable adverse experiences that occurred in ≥5% of patients were vomiting (10%) and pruritus (6%). Vomiting occurred in 43 of 319 (13%) pediatric patients who did not have symptomatic malaria but were given treatment doses of MALARONE for 3 days in a clinical trial. The design of this clinical trial required that any patient who vomited be withdrawn from the trial. Among pediatric patients with symptomatic malaria treated with MALARONE, treatment was discontinued prematurely due to an adverse experience in 1 of 116 (0.9%).
In a study of 100 pediatric patients (5 to <11 kg body weight) who received MALARONE for the treatment of uncomplicated *P. falciparum* malaria, only diarrhea (6%) occurred in ≥5% of patients as an adverse experience attributable to MALARONE. In 3 patients (3%), treatment was discontinued prematurely due to an adverse experience.
Abnormalities in laboratory tests reported in clinical trials were limited to elevations of transaminases in malaria patients being treated with MALARONE. The frequency of these abnormalities varied substantially across trials of treatment and were not observed in the randomized portions of the prophylaxis trials.
One active-controlled trial evaluated the treatment of malaria in Thai adults (n = 182); the mean age of subjects was 26 years (range 15 to 63 years); 80% of subjects were male. Early elevations of ALT and AST occurred more frequently in patients treated with MALARONE (n = 91) compared to patients treated with an active control, mefloquine (n = 91). On Day 7, rates of elevated ALT and AST with MALARONE and mefloquine (for patients who had normal baseline levels of these clinical laboratory parameters) were ALT 26.7% vs. 15.6%; AST 16.9% vs. 8.6%, respectively. By Day 14 of this 28-day study, the frequency of transaminase elevations equalized across the 2 groups.
6.2   Postmarketing Experience
In addition to adverse events reported from clinical trials, the following events have been identified during postmarketing use of MALARONE. Because they are reported voluntarily from a population of unknown size, estimates of frequency cannot be made. These events have been chosen for inclusion due to a combination of their seriousness, frequency of reporting, or potential causal connection to MALARONE.
Blood and Lymphatic System Disorders: Neutropenia and anemia. Pancytopenia in patients with severe renal impairment treated with proguanil [see Contraindications (4.2)].

Immune System Disorders: Allergic reactions including anaphylaxis, angioedema, and urticaria, and vasculitis.
Nervous System Disorders: Seizures and psychotic events (such as hallucinations); however, a causal relationship has not been established.
Gastrointestinal Disorders: Stomatitis.
Hepatobiliary Disorders: Elevated liver laboratory tests, hepatitis, cholestasis; hepatic failure requiring transplant has been reported.
Skin and Subcutaneous Tissue Disorders: Photosensitivity, rash, erythema multiforme, and Stevens-Johnson syndrome.

7   DRUG INTERACTIONS
7.1   Rifampin/Rifabutin
Concomitant administration of rifampin or rifabutin is known to reduce atovaquone concentrations [see Clinical Pharmacology (12.3)]. The concomitant administration of MALARONE and rifampin or rifabutin is not recommended.
7.2   Anticoagulants
Proguanil may potentiate the anticoagulant effect of warfarin and other coumarin-based anticoagulants. The mechanism of this potential drug interaction has not been established. Caution is advised when initiating or withdrawing malaria prophylaxis or treatment with MALARONE in patients on continuous treatment with coumarin-based anticoagulants. When these products are administered concomitantly, coagulation tests should be closely monitored.
7.3   Tetracycline
Concomitant treatment with tetracycline has been associated with a reduction in plasma concentrations of atovaquone [see Clinical Pharmacology (12.3)]. Parasitemia should be closely monitored in patients receiving tetracycline.
7.4   Metoclopramide
While antiemetics may be indicated for patients receiving MALARONE, metoclopramide may reduce the bioavailability of atovaquone and should be used only if other antiemetics are not available [see Clinical Pharmacology (12.3)].
7.5   Indinavir
Concomitant administration of atovaquone and indinavir did not result in any change in the steady-state AUC and C_{max} of indinavir but resulted in a decrease in the C_{trough} of indinavir [see Clinical Pharmacology (12.3)]. Caution should be exercised when prescribing atovaquone with indinavir due to the decrease in trough concentrations of indinavir.

8   USE IN SPECIFIC POPULATIONS
8.1   Pregnancy
Pregnancy Category C
Atovaquone: Atovaquone was not teratogenic and did not cause reproductive toxicity in rats at doses up to 1,000 mg/kg/day corresponding to maternal plasma concentrations up to 7.3 times the estimated human exposure during treatment of malaria based on AUC. In rabbits, atovaquone caused adverse fetal effects and maternal toxicity at a dose of 1,200 mg/kg/day corresponding to plasma concentrations that were approximately 1.3 times the estimated human exposure during treatment of malaria based on AUC. Adverse fetal effects in rabbits, including decreased fetal body lengths and increased early resorptions and post-implantation losses, were observed only in the presence of maternal toxicity.
In a pre- and post-natal study in rats, atovaquone did not produce adverse effects in offspring at doses up to 1,000 mg/kg/day corresponding to AUC exposures of approximately 7.3 times the estimated human exposure during treatment of malaria.
Proguanil: A pre- and post-natal study in Sprague-Dawley rats revealed no adverse effects at doses up to 16 mg/kg/day of proguanil hydrochloride (up to 0.04-times the average human exposure based on AUC). Pre- and post-natal studies of proguanil in animals at exposures similar to or greater than those observed in humans have not been conducted.
Atovaquone and Proguanil: The combination of atovaquone and proguanil hydrochloride was not teratogenic in pregnant rats at atovaquone:proguanil hydrochloride (50:20 mg/kg/day) corresponding to plasma concentrations up to 1.7 and 0.1 times, respectively, the estimated human exposure during treatment of malaria based on AUC. In pregnant rabbits, the combination of atovaquone and proguanil hydrochloride was not teratogenic or embryotoxic to rabbit fetuses at atovaquone:proguanil hydrochloride (100:40 mg/kg/day) corresponding to plasma concentrations of approximately 0.3 and 0.5 times, respectively, the estimated human exposure during treatment of malaria based on AUC.
There are no adequate and well-controlled studies of atovaquone and/or proguanil hydrochloride in pregnant women. MALARONE should be used during pregnancy only if the potential benefit justifies the potential risk to the fetus.
Falciparum malaria carries a higher risk of morbidity and mortality in pregnant women than in the general population. Maternal death and fetal loss are both known complications of falciparum malaria in pregnancy. In pregnant

women who must travel to malaria-endemic areas, personal protection against mosquito bites should always be employed in addition to antimalarials. *[See Patient Counseling Information (17).]*

The proguanil component of MALARONE acts by inhibiting the parasitic dihydrofolate reductase *[see Clinical Pharmacology (12.1)].* However, there are no clinical data indicating that folate supplementation diminishes drug efficacy. For women of childbearing age receiving folate supplements to prevent neural tube birth defects, such supplements may be continued while taking MALARONE.

8.3 Nursing Mothers

It is not known whether atovaquone is excreted into human milk. In a rat study, atovaquone concentrations in the milk were 30% of the concurrent atovaquone concentrations in the maternal plasma.

Proguanil is excreted into human milk in small quantities. Caution should be exercised when MALARONE is administered to a nursing woman.

8.4 Pediatric Use

Prophylaxis of Malaria: Safety and effectiveness have not been established in pediatric patients who weigh less than 11 kg. The efficacy and safety of MALARONE have been established for the prophylaxis of malaria in controlled trials involving pediatric patients weighing 11 kg or more *[see Clinical Studies (14.1)].*

Treatment of Malaria: Safety and effectiveness have not been established in pediatric patients who weigh less than 5 kg. The efficacy and safety of MALARONE for the treatment of malaria have been established in controlled trials involving pediatric patients weighing 5 kg or more *[see Clinical Studies (14.2)].*

8.5 Geriatric Use

Clinical trials of MALARONE did not include sufficient numbers of subjects aged 65 years and older to determine whether they respond differently from younger subjects. In general, dose selection for an elderly patient should be cautious, reflecting the greater frequency of decreased hepatic, renal, or cardiac function, the higher systemic exposure to cycloguanil, and the greater frequency of concomitant disease or other drug therapy. *[See Clinical Pharmacology (12.3).]*

8.6 Renal Impairment

Do not use MALARONE for malaria prophylaxis in patients with severe renal impairment (creatinine clearance <30 mL/min). Use with caution for the treatment of malaria in patients with severe renal impairment, only if the benefits of the 3-day treatment regimen outweigh the potential risks associated with increased drug exposure. No dosage adjustments are needed in patients with mild (creatinine clearance 50 to 80 mL/min) or moderate (creatinine clearance 30 to 50 mL/min) renal impairment. *[See Clinical Pharmacology (12.3).]*

8.7 Hepatic Impairment

No dosage adjustments are needed in patients with mild or moderate hepatic impairment *[see Clinical Pharmacology (12.3)].* No trials have been conducted in patients with severe hepatic impairment.

10 OVERDOSAGE

There is no information on overdoses of MALARONE substantially higher than the doses recommended for treatment.

There is no known antidote for atovaquone, and it is currently unknown if atovaquone is dialyzable. Overdoses up to 31,500 mg of atovaquone have been reported. In one such patient who also took an unspecified dose of dapsone, methemoglobinemia occurred. Rash has also been reported after overdose.

Overdoses of proguanil hydrochloride as large as 1,500 mg have been followed by complete recovery, and doses as high as 700 mg twice daily have been taken for over 2 weeks without serious toxicity. Adverse experiences occasionally associated with proguanil hydrochloride doses of 100 to 200 mg/day, such as epigastric discomfort and vomiting, would be likely to occur with overdose. There are also reports of reversible hair loss and scaling of the skin on the palms and/or soles, reversible aphthous ulceration, and hematologic side effects.

11 DESCRIPTION

MALARONE (atovaquone and proguanil hydrochloride) Tablets (adult strength) and MALARONE (atovaquone and proguanil hydrochloride) Pediatric Tablets, for oral administration, contain a fixed-dose combination of the antimalarial agents atovaquone and proguanil hydrochloride.

The chemical name of atovaquone is *trans*-2-[4-(4-chlorophenyl)cyclohexyl]-3-hydroxy-1,4-naphthalenedione. Atovaquone is a yellow crystalline solid that is practically insoluble in water. It has a molecular weight of 366.84 and the molecular formula $C_{22}H_{19}ClO_3$. The compound has the following structural formula:

Table 4. Apparent Clearance for Atovaquone and Proguanil in Patients as a Function of Body Weight

Body Weight	Atovaquone		Proguanil	
	N	CL/F (L/hr) Mean ± SD[a] (range)	N	CL/F (L/hr) Mean ± SD[a] (range)
11-20 kg	159	1.34 ± 0.63 (0.52-4.26)	146	29.5 ± 6.5 (10.3-48.3)
21-30 kg	117	1.87 ± 0.81 (0.52-5.38)	113	40.0 ± 7.5 (15.9-62.7)
31-40 kg	95	2.76 ± 2.07 (0.97-12.5)	91	49.5 ± 8.30 (25.8-71.5)
>40 kg	368	6.61 ± 3.92 (1.32-20.3)	282	67.9 ± 19.9 (14.0-145)

[a] SD = standard deviation.

The chemical name of proguanil hydrochloride is 1-(4-chlorophenyl)-5-isopropyl-biguanide hydrochloride. Proguanil hydrochloride is a white crystalline solid that is sparingly soluble in water. It has a molecular weight of 290.22 and the molecular formula $C_{11}H_{16}ClN_5 \cdot HCl$. The compound has the following structural formula:

Each MALARONE Tablet (adult strength) contains 250 mg of atovaquone and 100 mg of proguanil hydrochloride and each MALARONE Pediatric Tablet contains 62.5 mg of atovaquone and 25 mg of proguanil hydrochloride. The inactive ingredients in both tablets are low-substituted hydroxypropyl cellulose, magnesium stearate, microcrystalline cellulose, poloxamer 188, povidone K30, and sodium starch glycolate. The tablet coating contains hypromellose, polyethylene glycol 400, polyethylene glycol 8000, red iron oxide, and titanium dioxide.

12 CLINICAL PHARMACOLOGY

12.1 Mechanism of Action

The constituents of MALARONE, atovaquone and proguanil hydrochloride, interfere with 2 different pathways involved in the biosynthesis of pyrimidines required for nucleic acid replication. Atovaquone is a selective inhibitor of parasite mitochondrial electron transport. Proguanil hydrochloride primarily exerts its effect by means of the metabolite cycloguanil, a dihydrofolate reductase inhibitor. Inhibition of dihydrofolate reductase in the malaria parasite disrupts deoxythymidylate synthesis.

12.2 Pharmacodynamics

No trials of the pharmacodynamics of MALARONE have been conducted.

12.3 Pharmacokinetics

Absorption: Atovaquone is a highly lipophilic compound with low aqueous solubility. The bioavailability of atovaquone shows considerable inter-individual variability. Dietary fat taken with atovaquone increases the rate and extent of absorption, increasing AUC 2 to 3 times and C_{max} 5 times over fasting. The absolute bioavailability of the tablet formulation of atovaquone when taken with food is 23%. MALARONE Tablets should be taken with food or a milky drink.

Distribution: Atovaquone is highly protein bound (>99%) over the concentration range of 1 to 90 mcg/mL. A population pharmacokinetic analysis demonstrated that the apparent volume of distribution of atovaquone (V/F) in adult and pediatric patients after oral administration is approximately 8.8 L/kg.

Proguanil is 75% protein bound. A population pharmacokinetic analysis demonstrated that the apparent V/F of proguanil in adult and pediatric patients >15 years of age with body weights from 31 to 110 kg ranged from 1,617 to 2,502 L. In pediatric patients ≤15 years of age with body weights from 11 to 56 kg, the V/F of proguanil ranged from 462 to 966 L.

In human plasma, the binding of atovaquone and proguanil was unaffected by the presence of the other.

Metabolism: In a study where ^{14}C-labeled atovaquone was administered to healthy volunteers, greater than 94% of the dose was recovered as unchanged atovaquone in the feces over 21 days. There was little or no excretion of atovaquone in the urine (less than 0.6%). There is indirect evidence that atovaquone may undergo limited metabolism; however, a specific metabolite has not been identified. Between 40% to 60% of proguanil is excreted by the kidneys. Proguanil is metabolized to cycloguanil (primarily via CYP2C19) and 4-chlorophenylbiguanide. The main routes of elimination are hepatic biotransformation and renal excretion.

Elimination: The elimination half-life of atovaquone is about 2 to 3 days in adult patients.

The elimination half-life of proguanil is 12 to 21 hours in both adult patients and pediatric patients, but may be longer in individuals who are slow metabolizers.

A population pharmacokinetic analysis in adult and pediatric patients showed that the apparent clearance (CL/F) of both atovaquone and proguanil are related to the body weight. The values CL/F for both atovaquone and proguanil in subjects with body weight ≥11 kg are shown in Table 4. [See table 4 above]

The pharmacokinetics of atovaquone and proguanil in patients with body weight below 11 kg have not been adequately characterized.

Pediatrics: The pharmacokinetics of proguanil and cycloguanil are similar in adult and pediatric patients. However, the elimination half-life of atovaquone is shorter in pediatric patients (1 to 2 days) than in adult patients (2 to 3 days). In clinical trials, plasma trough concentrations of atovaquone and proguanil in pediatric patients weighing 5 to 40 kg were within the range observed in adults after dosing by body weight.

Geriatrics: In a single-dose study, the pharmacokinetics of atovaquone, proguanil, and cycloguanil were compared in 13 elderly subjects (age 65 to 79 years) to 13 younger subjects (age 30 to 45 years). In the elderly subjects, the extent of systemic exposure (AUC) of cycloguanil was increased (point estimate = 2.36, 90% CI = 1.70, 3.28). T_{max} was longer in elderly subjects (median 8 hours) compared with younger subjects (median 4 hours) and average elimination half-life was longer in elderly subjects (mean 14.9 hours) compared with younger subjects (mean 8.3 hours).

Renal Impairment: In patients with mild renal impairment (creatinine clearance 50 to 80 mL/min), oral clearance and/or AUC data for atovaquone, proguanil, and cycloguanil are within the range of values observed in patients with normal renal function (creatinine clearance >80 mL/min). In patients with moderate renal impairment (creatinine clearance 30 to 50 mL/min), mean oral clearance for proguanil was reduced by approximately 35% compared with patients with normal renal function (creatinine clearance >80 mL/min) and the oral clearance of atovaquone was comparable between patients with normal renal function and mild renal impairment. No data exist on the use of MALARONE for long-term prophylaxis (over 2 months) in individuals with moderate renal failure. In patients with severe renal impairment (creatinine clearance <30 mL/min), atovaquone C_{max} and AUC are reduced but the elimination half-lives for proguanil and cycloguanil are prolonged, with corresponding increases in AUC, resulting in the potential of drug accumulation and toxicity with repeated dosing *[see Contraindications (4.2)].*

Hepatic Impairment: In a single-dose study, the pharmacokinetics of atovaquone, proguanil, and cycloguanil were compared in 13 subjects with hepatic impairment (9 mild, 4 moderate, as indicated by the Child-Pugh method) to 13 subjects with normal hepatic function. In subjects with mild or moderate hepatic impairment as compared to healthy subjects, there were no marked differences (<50%) in the

Table 5. Point Estimates (90% CI) for Proguanil and Cycloguanil Parameters in Subjects With Mild and Moderate Hepatic Impairment Compared to Healthy Volunteers

Parameter	Comparison	Proguanil	Cycloguanil
$AUC_{(0-inf)}$[a]	mild:healthy	1.96 (1.51, 2.54)	0.32 (0.22, 0.45)
C_{max}[a]	mild:healthy	1.41 (1.16, 1.71)	0.35 (0.24, 0.50)
$t_{1/2}$[b]	mild:healthy	1.21 (0.92, 1.60)	0.86 (0.49, 1.48)
$AUC_{(0-inf)}$[a]	moderate:healthy	1.64 (1.14, 2.34)	ND
C_{max}[a]	moderate:healthy	0.97 (0.69, 1.36)	ND
$t_{1/2}$[b]	moderate:healthy	1.46 (1.05, 2.05)	ND

ND = not determined due to lack of quantifiable data.
[a] Ratio of geometric means.
[b] Mean difference.

Table 7. Prevention of Parasitemia[a] in Active-Controlled Clinical Trials of MALARONE for Prophylaxis of P. falciparum Malaria in Non-Immune Travelers

	MALARONE	Mefloquine	Chloroquine plus Proguanil
Total number of randomized patients who received study drug	1,004	483	511
Failed to complete study	14	6	4
Developed parasitemia (P. falciparum)	0	0	3

[a] Free of parasitemia during the period of prophylactic therapy.

rate or extent of systemic exposure of atovaquone. However, in subjects with moderate hepatic impairment, the elimination half-life of atovaquone was increased (point estimate = 1.28, 90% CI = 1.00 to 1.63). Proguanil AUC, C_{max}, and its elimination half-life increased in subjects with mild hepatic impairment when compared to healthy subjects (Table 5). Also, the proguanil AUC and its elimination half-life increased in subjects with moderate hepatic impairment when compared to healthy subjects. Consistent with the increase in proguanil AUC, there were marked decreases in the systemic exposure of cycloguanil (C_{max} and AUC) and an increase in its elimination half-life in subjects with mild hepatic impairment when compared to healthy volunteers (Table 5). There were few measurable cycloguanil concentrations in subjects with moderate hepatic impairment. The pharmacokinetics of atovaquone, proguanil, and cycloguanil after administration of MALARONE have not been studied in patients with severe hepatic impairment.
[See table 5 above]
Drug Interactions: There are no pharmacokinetic interactions between atovaquone and proguanil at the recommended dose.
Atovaquone is highly protein bound (>99%) but does not displace other highly protein-bound drugs in vitro.
Proguanil is metabolized primarily by CYP2C19. Potential pharmacokinetic interactions between proguanil or cycloguanil and other drugs that are CYP2C19 substrates or inhibitors are unknown.
Rifampin/Rifabutin: Concomitant administration of rifampin or rifabutin is known to reduce atovaquone concentrations by approximately 50% and 34%, respectively. The mechanisms of these interactions are unknown.
Tetracycline: Concomitant treatment with tetracycline has been associated with approximately a 40% reduction in plasma concentrations of atovaquone.
Metoclopramide: Concomitant treatment with metoclopramide has been associated with decreased bioavailability of atovaquone.
Indinavir: Concomitant administration of atovaquone (750 mg twice daily with food for 14 days) and indinavir (800 mg three times daily without food for 14 days) did not result in any change in the steady-state AUC and C_{max} of indinavir but resulted in a decrease in the C_{trough} of indinavir (23% decrease [90% CI = 8%, 35%]).

12.4 Microbiology
Activity *In Vitro* and *In Vivo:* Atovaquone and cycloguanil (an active metabolite of proguanil) are active against the erythrocytic and exoerythrocytic stages of *Plasmodium* spp. Enhanced efficacy of the combination compared to either atovaquone or proguanil hydrochloride alone was demonstrated in clinical trials in both immune and non-immune patients *[see Clinical Studies (14.1, 14.2)]*.
Drug Resistance: Strains of *P. falciparum* with decreased susceptibility to atovaquone or proguanil/cycloguanil alone can be selected in vitro or in vivo. The combination of

atovaquone and proguanil hydrochloride may not be effective for treatment of recrudescent malaria that develops after prior therapy with the combination.

13 NONCLINICAL TOXICOLOGY
13.1 Carcinogenesis, Mutagenesis, Impairment of Fertility
Genotoxicity studies have not been performed with atovaquone in combination with proguanil. Effects of MALARONE on male and female reproductive performance are unknown.
Atovaquone: A 24-month carcinogenicity study in CD rats was negative for neoplasms at doses up to 500 mg/kg/day corresponding to approximately 54 times the average steady-state plasma concentrations in humans during prophylaxis of malaria. In CD-1 mice, a 24-month study showed treatment-related increases in incidence of hepatocellular adenoma and hepatocellular carcinoma at all doses tested (50, 100, and 200 mg/kg/day) which correlated with at least 15 times the average steady-state plasma concentrations in humans during prophylaxis of malaria.
Atovaquone was negative with or without metabolic activation in the Ames *Salmonella* mutagenicity assay, the Mouse Lymphoma mutagenesis assay, and the Cultured Human Lymphocyte cytogenetic assay. No evidence of genotoxicity was observed in the in vivo Mouse Micronucleus assay.
Atovaquone did not impair fertility in male and female rats at doses up to 1,000 mg/kg/day corresponding to plasma exposures of approximately 7.3 times the estimated human exposure during treatment of malaria based on AUC.
Proguanil: No evidence of a carcinogenic effect was observed in 24-month studies conducted in CD-1 mice at doses up to 16 mg/kg/day corresponding to 1.5 times the average human plasma exposure during prophylaxis of malaria based on AUC, and in Wistar Hannover rats at doses up to 20 mg/kg/day corresponding to 1.1 times the average human plasma exposure during prophylaxis of malaria based on AUC.
Proguanil was negative with or without metabolic activation in the Ames *Salmonella* mutagenicity assay and the Mouse Lymphoma mutagenesis assay. No evidence of genotoxicity was observed in the in vivo Mouse Micronucleus assay.
Cycloguanil, the active metabolite of proguanil, was also negative in the Ames test, but was positive in the Mouse Lymphoma assay and the Mouse Micronucleus assay. These positive effects with cycloguanil, a dihydrofolate reductase inhibitor, were significantly reduced or abolished with folinic acid supplementation.
A fertility study in Sprague-Dawley rats revealed no adverse effects at doses up to 16 mg/kg/day of proguanil hydrochloride (up to 0.04-times the average human exposure during treatment of malaria based on AUC). Fertility studies of proguanil in animals at exposures similar to or greater than those observed in humans have not been conducted.

13.2 Animal Toxicology and/or Pharmacology
Fibrovascular proliferation in the right atrium, pyelonephritis, bone marrow hypocellularity, lymphoid atrophy, and gastritis/enteritis were observed in dogs treated with proguanil hydrochloride for 6 months at a dose of 12 mg/kg/day (approximately 3.9 times the recommended daily human dose for malaria prophylaxis on a mg/m² basis). Bile duct hyperplasia, gall bladder mucosal atrophy, and interstitial pneumonia were observed in dogs treated with proguanil hydrochloride for 6 months at a dose of 4 mg/kg/day (approximately 1.3 times the recommended daily human dose for malaria prophylaxis on a mg/m² basis). Mucosal hyperplasia of the cecum and renal tubular basophilia were observed in rats treated with proguanil hydrochloride for 6 months at a dose of 20 mg/kg/day (approximately 1.6 times the recommended daily human dose for malaria prophylaxis on a mg/m² basis). Adverse heart, lung, liver, and gall bladder effects observed in dogs and kidney effects observed in rats were not shown to be reversible.

14 CLINICAL STUDIES
14.1 Prevention of P. falciparum Malaria
MALARONE was evaluated for prophylaxis of *P. falciparum* malaria in 5 clinical trials in malaria-endemic areas and in 3 active-controlled trials in non-immune travelers to malaria-endemic areas.
Three placebo-controlled trials of 10 to 12 weeks' duration were conducted among residents of malaria-endemic areas in Kenya, Zambia, and Gabon. The mean age of subjects was 30 (range 17-55), 32 (range 16-64), and 10 (range 5-16) years, respectively. Of a total of 669 randomized patients (including 264 pediatric patients 5 to 16 years of age), 103 were withdrawn for reasons other than falciparum malaria or drug-related adverse events (55% of these were lost to follow-up and 45% were withdrawn for protocol violations). The results are listed in Table 6.

Table 6. Prevention of Parasitemia[a] in Placebo Controlled Clinical Trials of MALARONE for Prophylaxis of P. falciparum Malaria in Residents of Malaria Endemic Areas

	MALARONE	Placebo
Total number of patients randomized	326	343
Failed to complete study	57	46
Developed parasitemia (P. falciparum)	2	92

[a] Free of parasitemia during the 10 to 12-week period of prophylactic therapy.

In another study, 330 Gabonese pediatric patients (weighing 13 to 40 kg, and aged 4 to 14 years) who had received successful open-label radical cure treatment with artesunate, were randomized to receive either MALARONE (dosage based on body weight) or placebo in a double-blind fashion for 12 weeks. Blood smears were obtained weekly and any time malaria was suspected. Nineteen of the 165 children given MALARONE and 18 of 165 patients given placebo withdrew from the study for reasons other than parasitemia (primary reason was lost to follow-up). One out of 150 evaluable patients (<1%) who received MALARONE developed *P. falciparum* parasitemia while receiving prophylaxis with MALARONE compared with 31 (22%) of the 144 evaluable placebo recipients.
In a 10-week study in 175 South African subjects who moved into malaria-endemic areas and were given prophylaxis with 1 MALARONE Tablet daily, parasitemia developed in 1 subject who missed several doses of medication. Since no placebo control was included, the incidence of malaria in this study was not known.
Two active-controlled trials were conducted in non-immune travelers who visited a malaria-endemic area. The mean duration of travel was 18 days (range 2 to 38 days). Of a total of 1,998 randomized patients who received MALARONE or controlled drug, 24 discontinued from the study before follow-up evaluation 60 days after leaving the endemic area. Nine of these were lost to follow-up, 2 withdrew because of an adverse experience, and 13 were discontinued for other reasons. These trials were not large enough to allow for statements of comparative efficacy. In addition, the true exposure rate to *P. falciparum* malaria in both trials is unknown. The results are listed in Table 7.
[See table 7 above]
A third randomized, open-label study was conducted which included 221 otherwise healthy pediatric patients (weighing ≥11 kg and 2 to 17 years of age) who were at risk of contracting malaria by traveling to an endemic area. The mean duration of travel was 15 days (range 1 to 30 days). Prophylaxis with MALARONE (n = 110, dosage based on body weight) began 1 or 2 days before entering the endemic area

Table 8. Parasitological Response in 8 Clinical Trials of MALARONE for Treatment of P. falciparum Malaria

| Study Site | MALARONE[a] | | Comparator | | |
	Evaluable Patients (n)	% Sensitive Response[b]	Drug(s)	Evaluable Patients (n)	% Sensitive Response[b]
Brazil	74	98.6%	Quinine and tetracycline	76	100.0%
Thailand	79	100.0%	Mefloquine	79	86.1%
France[c]	21	100.0%	Halofantrine	18	100.0%
Kenya[c,d]	81	93.8%	Halofantrine	83	90.4%
Zambia	80	100.0%	Pyrimethamine/sulfadoxine (P/S)	80	98.8%
Gabon[c]	63	98.4%	Amodiaquine	63	81.0%
Philippines	54	100.0%	Chloroquine (Cq) Cq and P/S	23 32	30.4% 87.5%
Peru	19	100.0%	Chloroquine P/S	13 7	7.7% 100.0%

[a] MALARONE = 1,000 mg atovaquone and 400 mg proguanil hydrochloride (or equivalent based on body weight for patients weighing ≤ 40 kg) once daily for 3 days.
[b] Elimination of parasitemia with no recurrent parasitemia during follow-up for 28 days.
[c] Patients hospitalized only for acute care. Follow-up conducted in outpatients
[d] Study in pediatric patients 3 to 12 years of age.

and lasted until 7 days after leaving the area. A control group (n = 111) received prophylaxis with chloroquine/proguanil dosed according to WHO guidelines. No cases of malaria occurred in either group of children. However, the study was not large enough to allow for statements of comparative efficacy. In addition, the true exposure rate to *P. falciparum* malaria in this study is unknown.

Causal Prophylaxis: In separate trials with small numbers of volunteers, atovaquone and proguanil hydrochloride were independently shown to have causal prophylactic activity directed against liver-stage parasites of *P. falciparum*. Six patients given a single dose of atovaquone 250 mg 24 hours prior to malaria challenge were protected from developing malaria, whereas all 4 placebo-treated patients developed malaria.

During the 4 weeks following cessation of prophylaxis in clinical trial participants who remained in malaria-endemic areas and were available for evaluation, malaria developed in 24 of 211 (11.4%) subjects who took placebo and 9 of 328 (2.7%) who took MALARONE. While new infections could not be distinguished from recrudescent infections, all but 1 of the infections in patients treated with MALARONE occurred more than 15 days after stopping therapy. The single case occurring on day 8 following cessation of therapy with MALARONE probably represents a failure of prophylaxis with MALARONE.

The possibility that delayed cases of *P. falciparum* malaria may occur some time after stopping prophylaxis with MALARONE cannot be ruled out. Hence, returning travelers developing febrile illnesses should be investigated for malaria.

14.2 Treatment of Acute, Uncomplicated P. falciparum Malaria Infections

In 3 phase II clinical trials, atovaquone alone, proguanil hydrochloride alone, and the combination of atovaquone and proguanil hydrochloride were evaluated for the treatment of acute, uncomplicated malaria caused by *P. falciparum*. Among 156 evaluable patients, the parasitological cure rate (elimination of parasitemia with no recurrent parasitemia during follow-up for 28 days) was 59/89 (66%) with atovaquone alone, 1/17 (6%) with proguanil hydrochloride alone, and 50/50 (100%) with the combination of atovaquone and proguanil hydrochloride.

MALARONE was evaluated for treatment of acute, uncomplicated malaria caused by *P. falciparum* in 8 phase III randomized, open-label, controlled clinical trials (N = 1,030 enrolled in both treatment groups). The mean age of subjects was 27 years and 16% were children ≤12 years of age; 74% of subjects were male. Evaluable patients included those whose outcome at 28 days was known. Among 471 evaluable patients treated with the equivalent of 4 MALARONE Tablets once daily for 3 days, 464 had a sensitive response (elimination of parasitemia with no recurrent parasitemia during follow-up for 28 days) (Table 8). Seven patients had a response of RI resistance (elimination of parasitemia but with recurrent parasitemia between 7 and 28 days after starting treatment). In these trials, the response to treatment with MALARONE was similar to treatment with the comparator drug in 4 trials. [See table above]

When these 8 trials were pooled and 2 additional trials evaluating MALARONE alone (without a comparator arm) were added to the analysis, the overall efficacy (elimination of parasitemia with no recurrent parasitemia during follow-up for 28 days) in 521 evaluable patients was 98.7%.

The efficacy of MALARONE in the treatment of the erythrocytic phase of nonfalciparum malaria was assessed in a small number of patients. Of the 23 patients in Thailand infected with *P. vivax* and treated with atovaquone/proguanil hydrochloride 1,000 mg/400 mg daily for 3 days, parasitemia cleared in 21 (91.3%) at 7 days. Parasite relapse occurred commonly when *P. vivax* malaria was treated with MALARONE alone. Relapsing malarias including *P. vivax* and *P. ovale* require additional treatment to prevent relapse.

The efficacy of MALARONE in treating acute uncomplicated *P. falciparum* malaria in children weighing ≥5 and <11 kg was examined in an open-label, randomized trial conducted in Gabon. Patients received either MALARONE (2 or 3 MALARONE Pediatric Tablets once daily depending upon body weight) for 3 days (n = 100) or amodiaquine (10 mg/kg/day) for 3 days (n = 100). In this study, the MALARONE Tablets were crushed and mixed with condensed milk just prior to administration. An adequate clinical response (elimination of parasitemia with no recurrent parasitemia during follow-up for 28 days) was obtained in 95% (87/92) of the evaluable pediatric patients who received MALARONE and in 53% (41/78) of those evaluable who received amodiaquine. A response of RI resistance (elimination of parasitemia but with recurrent parasitemia between 7 and 28 days after starting treatment) was noted in 3% and 40% of the patients, respectively. Two cases of RIII resistance (rising parasite count despite therapy) were reported in the patients receiving MALARONE. There were 4 cases of RIII in the amodiaquine arm.

16 HOW SUPPLIED/STORAGE AND HANDLING

MALARONE Tablets, containing 250 mg atovaquone and 100 mg proguanil hydrochloride.
• Bottle of 100 tablets with child-resistant closure (NDC 0173-0675-01).
• Unit Dose Pack of 24 (NDC 0173-0675-02).
MALARONE Pediatric Tablets, containing 62.5 mg atovaquone and 25 mg proguanil hydrochloride.
• Bottle of 100 tablets with child-resistant closure (NDC 0173-0676-01).
Storage Conditions: Store at 25°C (77°F). Temperature excursions are permitted to 15° to 30°C (59° to 86°F) (see USP Controlled Room Temperature).

17 PATIENT COUNSELING INFORMATION

Patients should be instructed:
• to take MALARONE at the same time each day with food or a milky drink.
• to take a repeat dose of MALARONE if vomiting occurs within 1 hour after dosing.
• to take a dose as soon as possible if a dose is missed, then return to their normal dosing schedule. However, if a dose is skipped, the patient should not double the next dose.
• that rare serious adverse events such as hepatitis, severe skin reactions, neurological, and hematological events have been reported when MALARONE was used for the prophylaxis or treatment of malaria.

• to consult a healthcare professional regarding alternative forms of prophylaxis if prophylaxis with MALARONE is prematurely discontinued for any reason.
• that protective clothing, insect repellents, and bednets are important components of malaria prophylaxis.
• that no chemoprophylactic regimen is 100% effective; therefore, patients should seek medical attention for any febrile illness that occurs during or after return from a malaria-endemic area and inform their healthcare professional that they may have been exposed to malaria.
• that falciparum malaria carries a higher risk of death and serious complications in pregnant women than in the general population. Pregnant women anticipating travel to malarious areas should discuss the risks and benefits of such travel with their physicians.

GlaxoSmithKline
Research Triangle Park, NC 27709
©2013, GlaxoSmithKline. All rights reserved.
MLR:6PI

MEKINIST ℞
(trametinib)
tablets, for oral use

HIGHLIGHTS OF PRESCRIBING INFORMATION
These highlights do not include all the information needed to use MEKINIST safely and effectively. See full prescribing information for MEKINIST.
MEKINIST (trametinib) tablets, for oral use
Initial U.S. Approval: 2013

———RECENT MAJOR CHANGES———

Indications and Usage (1)	01/2014
Dosage and Administration (2.2-2.3)	01/2014
Warnings and Precautions (5-5.10)	01/2014

———INDICATIONS AND USAGE———

MEKINIST is a kinase inhibitor indicated as a single agent and in combination with dabrafenib for the treatment of patients with unresectable or metastatic melanoma with BRAF V600E or V600K mutations as detected by an FDA-approved test. The use in combination is based on the demonstration of durable response rate. Improvement in disease-related symptoms or overall survival has not been demonstrated for MEKINIST in combination with dabrafenib. (1, 14.1)
Limitation of use: MEKINIST as a single agent is not indicated for treatment of patients who have received prior BRAF-inhibitor therapy. (1)

———DOSAGE AND ADMINISTRATION———

• Confirm the presence of BRAF V600E or V600K mutation in tumor specimens prior to initiation of treatment with MEKINIST. (2.1)
• The recommended dosage regimens of MEKINIST are 2 mg orally once daily as a single agent or in combination with dabrafenib 150 mg orally twice daily. Take MEKINIST at least 1 hour before or at least 2 hours after a meal. (2.2)

———DOSAGE FORMS AND STRENGTHS———

Tablets: 0.5 mg, 1 mg, and 2 mg. (3)

———CONTRAINDICATIONS———

None. (4)

———WARNINGS AND PRECAUTIONS———

• New primary malignancies, cutaneous and noncutaneous, can occur when MEKINIST is used in combination with dabrafenib. Monitor patients for new malignancies prior to initiation of therapy while on therapy, and following discontinuation of the combination treatment. (5.1, 2.3)
• Hemorrhage: Major hemorrhagic events can occur in patients receiving MEKINIST in combination with dabrafenib. Monitor for signs and symptoms of bleeding (5.2, 2.3)
• Venous Thromboembolism: Deep vein thrombosis and pulmonary embolism can occur in patients receiving MEKINIST in combination with dabrafenib. (5.3, 2.3)
• Cardiomyopathy: Assess LVEF before treatment, after one month of treatment, then every 2 to 3 months thereafter. (5.4, 2.3)
• Ocular Toxicities: Perform ophthalmologic evaluation for any visual disturbances. For Retinal Vein Occlusion (RVO), permanently discontinue MEKINIST. (5.5, 2.3)
• Interstitial Lung Disease (ILD): Withhold MEKINIST for new or progressive unexplained pulmonary symptoms. Permanently discontinue MEKINIST for treatment-related ILD or pneumonitis. (5.6, 2.3)
• Serious Febrile Reactions can occur when MEKINIST is used in combination with dabrafenib. (5.7, 2.3)

- **Serious Skin Toxicity:** Monitor for skin toxicities and for secondary infections. Discontinue for intolerable Grade 2, or Grade 3 or 4 rash not improving within 3 weeks despite interruption of MEKINIST. (5.8, 2.3)
- **Hyperglycemia:** Monitor serum glucose levels in patients with pre-existing diabetes or hyperglycemia. (5.9, 2.3)
- **Embryofetal Toxicity:** Can cause fetal harm. Advise females of reproductive potential of potential risk to the fetus. (5.10, 8.1, 8.6)

————————ADVERSE REACTIONS————————

- Most common adverse reactions (≥20%) for MEKINIST as a single agent include rash, diarrhea, and lymphedema. (6.1)
- Most common adverse reactions (≥20%) for MEKINIST in combination with dabrafenib include pyrexia, chills, fatigue, rash, nausea, vomiting, diarrhea, abdominal pain, peripheral edema, cough, headache, arthralgia, night sweats, decreased appetite, constipation, and myalgia. (6.1)

To report SUSPECTED ADVERSE REACTIONS, contact GlaxoSmithKline at 1-888-825-5249 or FDA at 1-800-FDA-1088 or www.fda.gov/medwatch.

————————DRUG INTERACTIONS————————

- Avoid concurrent administration of strong inhibitors of CYP3A4 or CYP2C8 when MEKINIST is used in combination with dabrafenib. (7.1)
- Avoid concurrent administration of strong inducers of CYP3A4 or CYP2C8 when MEKINIST is used in combination with dabrafenib. (7.1)
- Concomitant use with agents that are sensitive substrates of CYP3A4, CYP2C8, CYP2C9, CYP2C19, or CYP2B6 may result in loss of efficacy of these agents when MEKINIST is used in combination with dabrafenib. (7.1)

————————USE IN SPECIFIC POPULATIONS————————

- **Nursing Mothers:** Discontinue drug or nursing. (8.3)
- **Females and Males of Reproductive Potential:** Counsel female patients on pregnancy planning and prevention. May impair fertility. (8.6)

See 17 for PATIENT COUNSELING INFORMATION and FDA-approved patient labeling

Revised: 01/2014

FULL PRESCRIBING INFORMATION: CONTENTS*

FULL PRESCRIBING INFORMATION

1 INDICATIONS AND USAGE

MEKINIST® as a single agent is indicated for the treatment of patients with unresectable or metastatic melanoma with BRAF V600E or V600K mutations, as detected by an FDA-approved test [see Clinical Studies (14.1)].

MEKINIST, in combination with dabrafenib, is indicated for the treatment of patients with unresectable or metastatic melanoma with BRAF V600E or V600K mutations, as detected by an FDA-approved test. This indication is based on the demonstration of durable response rate [see Clinical Studies (14.1)]. Improvement in disease-related symptoms or overall survival has not been demonstrated for MEKINIST in combination with dabrafenib.

Limitation of use: MEKINIST as a single agent is not indicated for treatment of patients who have received prior BRAF-inhibitor therapy [see Clinical Studies (14.2)].

2 DOSAGE AND ADMINISTRATION

2.1 Patient Selection

Select patients for treatment of unresectable or metastatic melanoma with MEKINIST based on presence of BRAF V600E or V600K mutation in tumor specimens [see Clinical Studies (14.1)]. Information on FDA-approved tests for the detection of BRAF V600 mutations in melanoma is available at: http://www.fda.gov/CompanionDiagnostics.

2.2 Recommended Dosing

The recommended dosage regimens of MEKINIST are:
- 2 mg orally taken once daily as a single agent
- 2 mg orally taken once daily in combination with dabrafenib 150 mg orally taken twice daily

Continue treatment until disease progression or unacceptable toxicity occurs. Take MEKINIST as a single agent, or MEKINIST in combination with dabrafenib, at least 1 hour before or 2 hours after a meal [see Clinical Pharmacology (12.3)]. Do not take a missed dose of MEKINIST within 12 hours of the next dose of MEKINIST. When administered in combination with dabrafenib, take the once daily dose of MEKINIST at the same time each day with either the morning dose or the evening dose of dabrafenib.

2.3 Dose Modifications

For New Primary Cutaneous Malignancies: No dose modifications are required.

For New Primary Non-Cutaneous Malignancies: No dose modifications are required for MEKINIST. If used in combination with dabrafenib, permanently discontinue dabrafenib in patients who develop RAS mutation-positive noncutaneous malignancies.

Table 1. Recommended Dose Reductions

Dose Reductions for MEKINIST When Administered as a Single Agent or in Combination With Dabrafenib

First Dose Reduction	1.5 mg orally once daily
Second Dose Reduction	1 mg orally once daily
Subsequent Modification	Permanently discontinue if unable to tolerate MEKINIST 1 mg orally once daily

Dose Reductions for Dabrafenib When Administered in Combination With MEKINIST

First Dose Reduction	100 mg orally twice daily
Second Dose Reduction	75 mg orally twice daily
Third Dose Reduction	50 mg orally twice daily
Subsequent Modification	Permanently discontinue dabrafenib if unable to tolerate 50 mg orally twice daily

[See table 2 on next page]

3 DOSAGE FORMS AND STRENGTHS

0.5-mg Tablets: Yellow, modified oval, biconvex, film-coated tablets with 'GS' debossed on one face and 'TFC' on the opposing face.

1-mg Tablets: White, round, biconvex, film-coated tablets with 'GS' debossed on one face and 'LHE' on the opposing face.

2-mg Tablets: Pink, round, biconvex, film-coated tablets with 'GS' debossed on one face and 'HMJ' on the opposing face.

4 CONTRAINDICATIONS

None.

5 WARNINGS AND PRECAUTIONS

Review the Full Prescribing Information for dabrafenib prior to initiation of MEKINIST in combination with dabrafenib. The following serious adverse reactions of dabrafenib as a single agent, which may occur when MEKINIST is used in combination with dabrafenib, are not described in the Full Prescribing Information for MEKINIST:

- Tumor promotion in patients with BRAF wild-type melanoma
- Hemolytic anemia in patients with glucose-6-phosphate dehydrogenase deficiency

5.1 New Primary Malignancies

New primary malignancies, cutaneous and non-cutaneous, can occur when MEKINIST is used in combination with dabrafenib and with dabrafenib as a single agent [refer to Full Prescribing Information for dabrafenib].

Cutaneous Malignancies:

In Trial 2, the incidence of basal cell carcinoma was increased in patients receiving MEKINIST in combination with dabrafenib, with an incidence of 9% (5/55) in patients receiving MEKINIST in combination with dabrafenib compared with 2% (1/53) in patients receiving dabrafenib as a single agent. The range of time to diagnosis of basal cell carcinoma was 28 to 249 days in patients receiving MEKINIST in combination with dabrafenib and was 197 days for the patient receiving dabrafenib as a single agent. Cutaneous squamous cell carcinoma (SCC), including keratoacanthoma, occurred in 7% of patients receiving MEKINIST in combination with dabrafenib and 19% of patients receiving dabrafenib as a single agent. The range of time to diagnosis of cuSCC was 136 to 197 days in the combination arm and was 9 to 197 days in the arm receiving dabrafenib as a single agent.

New primary melanoma occurred in 2% (1/53) of patients receiving dabrafenib and in none of the 55 patients receiving MEKINIST in combination with dabrafenib.

Perform dermatologic evaluations prior to initiation of MEKINIST in combination with dabrafenib, every 2 months while on therapy, and for up to 6 months following discontinuation of the combination. No dose modifications of MEKINIST or dabrafenib are recommended in patients who develop new primary cutaneous malignancies.

Non-Cutaneous Malignancies:

Based on its mechanism of action, dabrafenib may promote growth and development of malignancies with activation of RAS through mutation or other mechanisms [refer to the Full Prescribing Information for dabrafenib]. In patients receiving MEKINIST in combination with dabrafenib, four cases of non-cutaneous malignancies were identified: KRAS mutation-positive pancreatic adenocarcinoma (n = 1), recurrent NRAS mutation-positive colorectal carcinoma (n = 1), head and neck carcinoma (n = 1), and glioblastoma (n = 1). Monitor patients receiving the combination closely for signs or symptoms of non-cutaneous malignancies. If used in combination with dabrafenib, no dose modification is required for MEKINIST in patients who develop non-cutaneous malignancies. Permanently discontinue dabrafenib in patients who develop RAS mutation-positive noncutaneous malignancies.

5.2 Hemorrhage

Hemorrhages, including major hemorrhages defined as symptomatic bleeding in a critical area or organ, can occur when MEKINIST is used in combination with dabrafenib.

In Trial 2, treatment with MEKINIST in combination with dabrafenib resulted in an increased incidence and severity of any hemorrhagic event: 16% (9/55) of patients treated with MEKINIST in combination with dabrafenib compared with 2% (1/53) of patients treated with dabrafenib as a single agent. The major hemorrhagic events of intracranial or gastric hemorrhage occurred in 5% (3/55) of patients treated with MEKINIST in combination with dabrafenib compared with none of the 53 patients treated with dabrafenib as a single agent. Intracranial hemorrhage was fatal in two (4%) patients receiving the combination of MEKINIST and dabrafenib.

Permanently discontinue MEKINIST, and also permanently discontinue dabrafenib if administered in combination, for all Grade 4 hemorrhagic events and for any Grade 3 hemorrhagic events that do not improve. Withhold MEKINIST for up to 3 weeks for Grade 3 hemorrhagic events; if improved resume at a lower dose level. Withhold dabrafenib for Grade 3 hemorrhagic events; if improved resume at a lower dose level.

5.3 Venous Thromboembolism

Venous thromboembolism can occur when MEKINIST is used in combination with dabrafenib.

In Trial 2, treatment with MEKINIST in combination with dabrafenib resulted in an increased incidence of deep venous thrombosis (DVT) and pulmonary embolism (PE): 7% (4/55) of patients treated with MEKINIST in combination with dabrafenib compared with none of the 53 patients treated with dabrafenib as a single agent. Pulmonary embolism was fatal in one (2%) patient receiving the combination of MEKINIST and dabrafenib.

Advise patients to immediately seek medical care if they develop symptoms of DVT or PE, such as shortness of breath, chest pain, or arm or leg swelling. Permanently discontinue MEKINIST and dabrafenib for life threatening PE. Withhold MEKINIST for uncomplicated DVT and PE for up to 3 weeks; if improved, MEKINIST may be resumed at a lower dose level. Do not modify the dose of dabrafenib [see Dosage and Administration (2.3)].

5.4 Cardiomyopathy

Cardiomyopathy can occur when MEKINIST is administered as a single agent or when used in combination with dabrafenib.

In Trial 1, cardiomyopathy (defined as cardiac failure, left ventricular dysfunction, or decreased left ventricular ejection fraction [LVEF]) occurred in 7% (14/211) of patients treated with MEKINIST; no chemotherapy-treated patients in Trial 1 developed cardiomyopathy. In Trial 2, cardiomyopathy occurred in 9% (5/55) of patients treated with MEKINIST in combination with dabrafenib and in none of patients treated with dabrafenib as a single agent. The median time to onset of cardiomyopathy in patients treated with MEKINIST was 63 days (range: 16 to 156 days) for Trial 1 and 86 days (range: 27 to 253 days) for Trial 2. Cardiomyopathy was identified within the first month of treatment with MEKINIST in 5 of 14 patients in Trial 1 and in 2 of 5 patients in Trial 2. Development of cardiomyopathy resulted in dose reduction (7/211) and/or discontinuation (4/211) of study drug in Trial 1, and resulted in dose reduction (4/55) and/or dose interruption (1/55) in Trial 2. Cardiomyopathy resolved in 10 of 14 (71%) patients in Trial 1 and in all 5 patients in Trial 2.

Across clinical trials of MEKINIST administered either as a single agent (N = 329), or in combination with dabrafenib (N = 202), 11% and 8% of patients, respectively, developed evidence of cardiomyopathy (decrease in LVEF below institutional lower limits of normal with an absolute decrease in LVEF ≥10% below baseline). Five percent and 2% in single-agent and in combination trials, respectively, demonstrated a decrease in LVEF below institutional lower limits of normal with an absolute decrease in LVEF of ≥20% below baseline.

Assess LVEF by echocardiogram or multigated acquisition (MUGA) scan before initiation of MEKINIST as a single agent and in combination with dabrafenib, one month after initiation, and then at 2- to 3-month intervals while on treatment. Withhold treatment with MEKINIST for up to 4 weeks if absolute LVEF value decreases by 10% from pretreatment values and is less than the lower limit of normal. For symptomatic cardiomyopathy or persistent, asymptomatic LV dysfunction that does not resolve within 4 weeks, permanently discontinue MEKINIST and withhold dabrafenib. Resume dabrafenib at the same dose upon recovery of cardiac function [see Dosage and Administration (2.3)].

5.5 Ocular Toxicities

Retinal Vein Occlusion (RVO):
Across all clinical trials of MEKINIST, the incidence of RVO was 0.2% (4/1,749). RVO may lead to macular edema, decreased visual function, neovascularization, and glaucoma. Urgently (within 24 hours) perform ophthalmological evaluation for patient-reported loss of vision or other visual disturbances. Permanently discontinue MEKINIST in patients with documented RVO. If MEKINIST is used in combination with dabrafenib, do not modify dabrafenib dose [see Dosage and Administration (2.3)].

Retinal Pigment Epithelial Detachment (RPED):
Retinal pigment epithelial detachment (RPED) can occur when MEKINIST is administered as a single agent or when used in combination with dabrafenib.

In Trial 1 and Trial 2, ophthalmologic examinations including retinal evaluation were performed pretreatment and at regular intervals during treatment.

In Trial 1, one patient (0.5%) receiving MEKINIST developed RPED and no cases of RPED were identified in chemotherapy-treated patients. Across all clinical trials of MEKINIST, the incidence of RPED was 0.8% (14/1,749). Retinal detachments were often bilateral and multifocal, occurring in the macular region of the retina. RPED led to reduction in visual acuity that resolved after a median of 11.5 days (range: 3 to 71 days) following the interruption of dosing with MEKINIST, although Ocular Coherence Tomography (OCT) abnormalities persisted beyond a month in at least several cases.

In Trial 2, one patient (2%) receiving MEKINIST in combination with dabrafenib developed RPED.

Perform ophthalmological evaluation at any time a patient reports visual disturbances and compare with baseline, if available. Withhold MEKINIST if RPED is diagnosed. If resolution of the RPED is documented on repeat ophthalmological evaluation within 3 weeks, resume MEKINIST at a

Table 2. Recommended Dose Modifications for MEKINIST as a Single Agent and for MEKINIST and Dabrafenib Administered in Combination

Severity of Adverse Reaction[a]	MEKINIST[b]	Dabrafenib (When Used in Combination)[b,c]
Febrile drug reaction		
• Fever of 101.3°F to 104°F	Do not modify the dose of MEKINIST.	Withhold dabrafenib until fever resolves. Then resume at same or lower dose level.
• Fever higher than 104°F • Fever complicated by rigors, hypotension, dehydration, or renal failure	Withhold MEKINIST until fever resolves. Then resume MEKINIST at same or lower dose level.	• Withhold dabrafenib until fever resolves. Then resume at a lower dose level. Or • Permanently discontinue dabrafenib.
Cutaneous		
• Intolerable Grade 2 skin toxicity • Grade 3 or 4 skin toxicity	Withhold MEKINIST for up to 3 weeks. • If improved, resume at a lower dose level. • If not improved, permanently discontinue.	Withhold dabrafenib for up to 3 weeks. • If improved, resume at a lower dose level. • If not improved, permanently discontinue.
Cardiac		
• Asymptomatic, absolute decrease in LVEF of 10% or greater from baseline and is below institutional lower limits of normal (LLN) from pretreatment value	Withhold MEKINIST for up to 4 weeks. • If improved to normal LVEF value, resume at a lower dose level. • If not improved to normal LVEF value, permanently discontinue.	Do not modify the dose of dabrafenib.
• Symptomatic congestive heart failure • Absolute decrease in LVEF of greater than 20% from baseline that is below LLN	Permanently discontinue MEKINIST.	Withhold dabrafenib, if improved, then resume at the same dose.
Venous Thromboembolism		
• Uncomplicated DVT or PE	Withhold MEKINIST for up to 3 weeks. • If improved to Grade 0-1, resume at a lower dose level. • If not improved, permanently discontinue.	Do not modify the dose of dabrafenib.
• Life Threatening PE	Permanently discontinue MEKINIST.	Permanently discontinue dabrafenib.
Ocular Toxicities		
• Grade 2-3 retinal pigment epithelial detachments (RPED)	Withhold MEKINIST for up to 3 weeks. • If improved to Grade 0-1, resume at a lower dose level. • If not improved, permanently discontinue.	Do not modify the dose of dabrafenib.
• Retinal vein occlusion	Permanently discontinue MEKINIST.	Do not modify the dose of dabrafenib.
• Uveitis and Iritis	Do not modify the dose of MEKINIST.	Withhold dabrafenib for up to 6 weeks. • If improved to Grade 0-1, then resume at the same dose. • If not improved, permanently discontinue.
Pulmonary		
• Interstitial lung disease/pneumonitis	Permanently discontinue MEKINIST.	Do not modify the dose of dabrafenib.
Other		
• Intolerable Grade 2 adverse reactions • Any Grade 3 adverse reactions	Withhold MEKINIST for up to 3 weeks. • If improved to Grade 0-1, resume at a lower dose level. • If not improved, permanently discontinue.	Withhold dabrafenib • If improved to Grade 0-1, resume at a lower dose level. • If not improved, permanently discontinue.
• First occurrence of any Grade 4 adverse reaction	• Withhold MEKINIST until adverse reaction improves to Grade 0-1. Then resume at a lower dose level. Or • Permanently discontinue.	• Withhold dabrafenib until adverse reaction improves to Grade 0-1. Then resume at a lower dose level. Or • Permanently discontinue.
• Recurrent Grade 4 adverse reaction	Permanently discontinue MEKINIST.	Permanently discontinue dabrafenib.

[a]National Cancer Institute Common Terminology Criteria for Adverse Events (CTCAE) version 4.0.
[b]See Table 1 for recommended dose reductions of MEKINIST and dabrafenib.
[c]Refer to Full Prescribing Information for dabrafenib.

Table 3. Selected Adverse Reactions Occurring in ≥10% of Patients Receiving MEKINIST and at a Higher Incidence (≥5%) Than in the Chemotherapy Arm or ≥2% (Grades 3 or 4) Adverse Reactions

Adverse Reactions	MEKINIST N = 211		Chemotherapy N = 99	
	All Grades[a]	Grades 3 and 4[b]	All Grades[a]	Grades 3 and 4[b]
Skin and subcutaneous tissue disorders				
Rash	57	8	10	0
Dermatitis acneiform	19	<1	1	0
Dry skin	11	0	0	0
Pruritus	10	2	1	0
Paronychia	10	0	1	0
Gastrointestinal disorders				
Diarrhea	43	0	16	2
Stomatitis[c]	15	2	2	0
Abdominal pain[d]	13	1	5	1
Vascular disorders				
Lymphedema[e]	32	1	4	0
Hypertension	15	12	7	3
Hemorrhage[f]	13	<1	0	0

[a]National Cancer Institute Common Terminology Criteria for Adverse Events, version 4.0.
[b]Grade 4 adverse reactions limited to rash (n = 1) in trametinib arm and diarrhea (n = 1) in chemotherapy arm.
[c]Includes the following terms: stomatitis, aphthous stomatitis, mouth ulceration, and mucosal inflammation.
[d]Includes the following terms: abdominal pain, abdominal pain lower, abdominal pain upper, and abdominal tenderness.
[e]Includes the following terms: lymphedema, edema, and peripheral edema.
[f]Includes the following terms: epistaxis, gingival bleeding, hematochezia, rectal hemorrhage, melena, vaginal hemorrhage, hemorrhoidal hemorrhage, hematuria, and conjunctival hemorrhage.

Table 4. Percent-Patient Incidence of Laboratory Abnormalities Occurring at a Higher Incidence in Patients Treated With MEKINIST in Trial 1 (Between-Arm Difference of ≥5% [All Grades] or ≥2% [Grades 3 or 4][a])

Test	MEKINIST N = 211		Chemotherapy N = 99	
	All Grades	Grades 3 and 4	All Grades	Grades 3 and 4
Increased aspartate aminotransferase (AST)	60	2	16	1
Increased alanine aminotransferase (ALT)	39	3	20	3
Hypoalbuminemia	42	2	23	1
Anemia	38	2	26	3
Increased alkaline phosphatase	24	2	18	3

[a]No Grade 4 events were reported in either treatment arm.

lower dose level. Discontinue MEKINIST if no improvement after 3 weeks. If MEKINIST is used in combination with dabrafenib, do not modify the dose of dabrafenib [see Dosage and Administration (2.3)].
Uveitis and Iritis:
Uveitis and iritis can occur when MEKINIST is used in combination with dabrafenib and with dabrafenib as a single agent [refer to Full Prescribing Information for dabrafenib].
Uveitis occurred in 1% (2/202) of patients treated with MEKINIST in combination with dabrafenib.
Symptomatic treatment employed in clinical trials included steroid and mydriatic ophthalmic drops. Monitor patients for visual signs and symptoms of uveitis (e.g., change in vision, photophobia, eye pain). If diagnosed, withhold dabrafenib for up to 6 weeks until uveitis/iritis resolves to Grade 0-1. If not improved, permanently discontinue dabrafenib. If MEKINIST is used in combination with dabrafenib, do not modify the dose of MEKINIST [see Dosage and Administration (2.3)].

5.6 Interstitial Lung Disease
In clinical trials of MEKINIST (N = 329) as a single agent, ILD or pneumonitis occurred in 2% of patients. In Trial 1, 2% (5/211) of patients treated with MEKINIST developed ILD or pneumonitis; all five patients required hospitalization. The median time to first presentation of ILD or pneumonitis was 160 days (range: 60 to 172 days).

Withhold MEKINIST in patients presenting with new or progressive pulmonary symptoms and findings including cough, dyspnea, hypoxia, pleural effusion, or infiltrates, pending clinical investigations. Permanently discontinue MEKINIST for patients diagnosed with treatment-related ILD or pneumonitis. If MEKINIST is used in combination with dabrafenib, do not modify the dose of dabrafenib [see Dosage and Administration (2.3)].

5.7 Serious Febrile Reactions
Serious febrile reactions and fever of any severity accompanied by hypotension, rigors or chills, dehydration, or renal failure, can occur when MEKINIST is used in combination with dabrafenib and with dabrafenib as a single agent [refer to Full Prescribing Information for dabrafenib].
The incidence and severity of pyrexia are increased when MEKINIST is used in combination with dabrafenib compared with dabrafenib as a single agent [see Adverse Reactions (6.1)].
In Trial 2, the incidence of fever (serious and non-serious) was 71% (39/55) in patients treated with MEKINIST in combination with dabrafenib and 26% (14/53) in patients treated with dabrafenib as a single agent. Serious febrile reactions and fever of any severity accompanied by hypotension, rigors, or chills occurred in 25% (14/55) of patients treated with MEKINIST in combination with dabrafenib compared with 2% (1/53) of patients treated with dabrafenib as a single agent. Fever was complicated with chills/rigors

in 51% (28/55), dehydration in 9% (5/55), renal failure in 4% (2/55), and syncope in 4% (2/55) of patients in Trial 2. In patients treated with MEKINIST in combination with dabrafenib, the median time to initial onset of fever was 30 days compared with 19 days in patients treated with dabrafenib as a single agent; the median duration of fever was 6 days with the combination compared with 4 days with dabrafenib as a single agent.
Across clinical trials of MEKINIST administered in combination with dabrafenib (N = 202), the incidence of pyrexia was 57% (116/202).
Withhold dabrafenib for fever of 101.3°F or higher. Withhold MEKINIST for fever higher than 104°F. Withhold dabrafenib and MEKINIST for any serious febrile reaction or fever accompanied by hypotension, rigors or chills, dehydration, or renal failure, and evaluate for signs and symptoms of infection. Refer to Table 2 for recommended dose modifications for adverse reactions [see Dosage and Administration (2.3)]. Prophylaxis with antipyretics may be required when resuming MEKINIST or dabrafenib.

5.8 Serious Skin Toxicity
Serious skin toxicity can occur when MEKINIST is administered as a single agent or when used in combination with dabrafenib. Serious skin toxicity can also occur with dabrafenib as a single agent [refer to Full Prescribing Information for dabrafenib].
In Trial 1, the overall incidence of any skin toxicity, the most common of which were rash, dermatitis acneiform rash, palmar-plantar erythrodysesthesia syndrome, and erythema, was 87% in patients treated with MEKINIST and 13% in chemotherapy-treated patients. Severe skin toxicity occurred in 12% of patients treated with MEKINIST. Skin toxicity requiring hospitalization occurred in 6% of patients treated with MEKINIST, most commonly for secondary infections of the skin requiring intravenous antibiotics or severe skin toxicity without secondary infection. In comparison, no patients treated with chemotherapy required hospitalization for severe skin toxicity or infections of the skin. The median time to onset of skin toxicity in patients treated with MEKINIST was 15 days (range: 1 to 221 days) and median time to resolution of skin toxicity was 48 days (range: 1 to 282 days). Reductions in the dose of MEKINIST were required in 12% and permanent discontinuation of MEKINIST was required in 1% of patients with skin toxicity.
In Trial 2, the incidence of any skin toxicity was similar for patients receiving MEKINIST in combination with dabrafenib (65% [36/55] compared with patients receiving dabrafenib as a single agent (68% [36/53]). The median time to onset of skin toxicity in patients treated with MEKINIST in combination with dabrafenib was 37 days (range: 1 to 225 days) and median time to resolution of skin toxicity was 33 days (range: 3 to 421 days). No patient required dose reduction or permanent discontinuation of MEKINIST or dabrafenib for skin toxicity.
Across clinical trials of MEKINIST administered in combination with dabrafenib (n = 202), severe skin toxicity and secondary infection of the skin requiring hospitalization occurred in 2.5% (5/202) of patients treated with MEKINIST in combination with dabrafenib.
Withhold MEKINIST, and dabrafenib if used in combination, for intolerable or severe skin toxicity. MEKINIST and dabrafenib may be resumed at lower dose levels in patients with improvement or recovery from skin toxicity within 3 weeks [see Dosage and Administration (2.3)].

5.9 Hyperglycemia
Hyperglycemia can occur when MEKINIST is used in combination with dabrafenib and with dabrafenib as a single agent. Hyperglycemia requiring an increase in the dose of, or initiation of insulin or oral hypoglycemic agent therapy occurred with dabrafenib as a single agent [refer to Full Prescribing Information for dabrafenib].
In Trial 2, the incidence of Grade 3 hyperglycemia based on laboratory values was 5% (3/55) in patients treated with MEKINIST in combination with dabrafenib compared with 2% (1/53) in patients treated with dabrafenib as a single agent.
Monitor serum glucose levels as clinically appropriate during treatment with MEKINIST in combination with dabrafenib in patients with pre-existing diabetes or hyperglycemia. Advise patients to report symptoms of severe hyperglycemia.

5.10 Embryofetal Toxicity
Based on its mechanism of action, MEKINIST can cause fetal harm when administered to a pregnant woman. MEKINIST was embryotoxic and abortifacient in rabbits at doses greater than or equal to those resulting in exposures approximately 0.3 times the human exposure at the recommended clinical dose. If this drug is used during pregnancy, or if the patient becomes pregnant while taking this drug, the patient should be apprised of the potential hazard to a fetus [see Use in Specific Populations (8.1)].
Advise female patients of reproductive potential to use highly effective contraception during treatment with

MEKINIST and for 4 months after treatment. Advise patients to use a highly effective non-hormonal method of contraception when MEKINIST is administered in combination with dabrafenib, since dabrafenib can render hormonal contraceptives ineffective. Advise patients to contact their healthcare provider if they become pregnant, or if pregnancy is suspected, while taking MEKINIST [see Use in Specific Populations (8.1, 8.6)].

6 ADVERSE REACTIONS

The following adverse reactions are discussed in greater detail in another section of the label:
• New Primary Malignancies [see Warnings and Precautions (5.1)]
• Hemorrhage [see Warnings and Precautions (5.2)]
• Venous Thromboembolism [see Warnings and Precautions (5.3)]
• Cardiomyopathy [see Warnings and Precautions (5.4)]
• Ocular Toxicities [see Warnings and Precautions (5.5)]
• Interstitial Lung Disease [see Warnings and Precautions (5.6)]
• Serious Febrile Reactions [see Warnings and Precautions (5.7)]
• Serious Skin Toxicity [see Warnings and Precautions (5.8)]
• Hyperglycemia [see Warnings and Precautions (5.9)]

6.1 Clinical Trials Experience

Because clinical trials are conducted under widely varying conditions, adverse reaction rates observed in the clinical trials of a drug cannot be directly compared with rates in the clinical trials of another drug and may not reflect the rates observed in practice.

The data described in the Warnings and Precautions section and below reflect exposure to MEKINIST as a single agent and in combination with dabrafenib. MEKINIST as a single agent was evaluated in 329 patients including 107 (33%) exposed for greater than or equal to 6 months and 30 (9%) exposed for greater than or equal to one year. MEKINIST as a single agent was studied in open-label, single-arm trials (N = 118) or in an open-label, randomized, active-controlled trial (N = 211). The median age was 54 years, 60% were male, >99% were white, and all patients had metastatic melanoma. All patients received 2 mg once-daily doses of MEKINIST. The incidence of RPED and RVO are obtained from the 1,749 patients from all clinical trials with MEKINIST.

The safety of MEKINIST in combination with dabrafenib was evaluated in Trial 2 and other trials consisting of 202 patients with BRAF V600 mutation-positive unresectable or metastatic melanoma who received MEKINIST 2 mg orally once daily in combination with dabrafenib 150 mg orally twice daily until disease progression or unacceptable toxicity. Among these 202 patients, 68 (34%) were exposed to MEKINIST and 66 (33%) were exposed to dabrafenib for greater than 6 to 12 months while 36 (18%) were exposed to MEKINIST and 40 (20%) were exposed to dabrafenib for greater than one year. The median age was 54 years, 57% were male and >99% were white.

Table 3 presents adverse reactions identified from analyses of Trial 1, a randomized, open-label trial of patients with BRAF V600E or V600K mutation-positive melanoma receiving MEKINIST (N = 211) 2 mg orally once daily or chemotherapy (N = 99) (either dacarbazine 1,000 mg/m² every 3 weeks or paclitaxel 175 mg/m² every 3 weeks) [see Clinical Studies (14.1)]. Patients with abnormal LVEF, history of acute coronary syndrome within 6 months, or current evidence of Class II or greater congestive heart failure (New York Heart Association) were excluded from Trial 1. The median duration of treatment with MEKINIST was 4.3 months. In Trial 1, 9% of patients receiving MEKINIST experienced adverse reactions resulting in permanent discontinuation of trial medication. The most common adverse reactions resulting in permanent discontinuation of MEKINIST were decreased left ventricular ejection fraction (LVEF), pneumonitis, renal failure, diarrhea, and rash. Adverse reactions led to dose reductions in 27% of patients treated with MEKINIST. Rash and decreased LVEF were the most common reasons cited for dose reductions of MEKINIST.

[See table 3 at top of previous page]
Other clinically important adverse reactions observed in ≤10% of patients (N = 329) treated with MEKINIST were:
Cardiac Disorders: Bradycardia.
Gastrointestinal Disorders: Xerostomia.
Infections and Infestations: Folliculitis, rash pustular, cellulitis.
Musculoskeletal and Connective Tissue Disorders: Rhabdomyolysis.
Nervous System Disorders: Dizziness, dysgeusia.
Ocular Disorders: Vision blurred, dry eye.
[See table 4 on previous page]
Table 5 presents adverse reactions from Trial 2, a multicenter, open-label, randomized trial of 162 patients with BRAF V600E or V600K mutation-positive melanoma receiving MEKINIST 2 mg once daily in combination with dab-

rafenib 150 mg twice daily (N = 55), MEKINIST 1 mg once daily in combination with dabrafenib 150 mg twice daily (N = 54), and dabrafenib as a single agent 150 mg twice daily (N = 53) [see Clinical Studies (14.1)]. Patients with abnormal LVEF, history of acute coronary syndrome within 6 months, current evidence of Class II or greater congestive heart failure (New York Heart Association), history of RVO, or RPED, QTc interval ≥480 msec, treatment refractory hypertension, uncontrolled arrhythmias, history of pneumonitis or interstitial lung disease, or a known history of G6PD deficiency were excluded. The median duration of treatment was 10.9 months for both MEKINIST (2-mg once-daily treatment group) and dabrafenib when used in combination, 10.6 months for both MEKINIST (1-mg once-daily treatment group) and dabrafenib when used in combination, and 6.1 months for dabrafenib as a single agent.
In Trial 2, 13% of patients receiving MEKINIST in combination with dabrafenib at the recommended dose experienced adverse reactions resulting in permanent discontinu-

ation of trial medication(s). The most common adverse reaction resulting in permanent discontinuation was pyrexia (4%). Adverse reactions led to dose reductions in 49% and dose interruptions in 67% of patients treated with MEKINIST in combination with dabrafenib. Pyrexia, chills, and nausea were the most common reasons cited for dose reductions, and pyrexia, chills, and decreased ejection fraction were the most common reasons cited for dose interruptions of MEKINIST and dabrafenib when used in combination.
[See table 5 above and on next page]
Other clinically important adverse reactions (N = 202) observed in <10% of patients treated with MEKINIST in combination with dabrafenib were:
Eye Disorders: Vision blurred, transient blindness.
Gastrointestinal Disorders: Stomatitis, pancreatitis.
General Disorders and Administration Site Conditions: Asthenia.
Infections and Infestations: Cellulitis, folliculitis, paronychia, rash pustular.

Table 5. Common Adverse Drug Reactions Occurring in >10% (All Grades) or ≥5% (Grades 3 or 4) of Patients Treated With MEKINIST in Combination With Dabrafenib in Trial 2

Adverse Reactions	MEKINIST 2 mg plus Dabrafenib N = 55		MEKINIST 1 mg plus Dabrafenib N = 54		Dabrafenib N = 53	
	All Grades[a]	Grades 3 and 4	All Grades[a]	Grades 3 and 4	All Grades[a]	Grades 3 and 4
General disorders and administrative site conditions						
Pyrexia	71	5	69	9	26	0
Chills	58	2	50	2	17	0
Fatigue	53	4	57	2	40	6
Edema peripheral[b]	31	0	28	0	17	0
Skin and subcutaneous tissue disorders						
Rash[c]	45	0	43	0	53	0
Night sweats	24	0	15	0	6	0
Dry skin	18	0	9	0	6	0
Dermatitis acneiform	16	0	11	0	4	0
Actinic keratosis	15	0	7	0	9	0
Erythema	15	0	6	0	2	0
Pruritus	11	0	11	0	13	0
Gastrointestinal disorders						
Nausea	44	2	46	6	21	0
Vomiting	40	2	43	4	15	0
Diarrhea	36	2	26	0	28	0
Abdominal pain[d]	33	2	24	2	21	2
Constipation	22	0	17	2	11	0
Dry mouth	11	0	11	0	6	0
Nervous system disorders						
Headache	29	0	37	2	28	0
Dizziness	16	0	13	0	9	0
Respiratory, thoracic, and mediastinal disorders						
Cough	29	0	11	0	21	0
Oropharyngeal pain	13	0	7	0	0	0
Musculoskeletal, connective tissue, and bone disorders						
Arthralgia	27	0	44	0	34	0
Myalgia	22	2	24	0	23	2
Back pain	18	5	11	0	11	2
Muscle spasms	16	0	2	0	4	0
Pain in extremity	16	0	11	2	19	0

(Table continued on next page)

Table 5 (cont.). Common Adverse Drug Reactions Occurring in >10% (All Grades) or ≥5% (Grades 3 or 4) of Patients Treated With MEKINIST in Combination With Dabrafenib in Trial 2

Adverse Reactions	MEKINIST 2 mg plus Dabrafenib N = 55		MEKINIST 1 mg plus Dabrafenib N = 54		Dabrafenib N = 53	
	All Grades[a]	Grades 3 and 4	All Grades[a]	Grades 3 and 4	All Grades[a]	Grades 3 and 4
Metabolism and nutritional disorders						
Decreased appetite	22	0	30	0	19	0
Dehydration	11	0	6	2	2	0
Psychiatric disorders						
Insomnia	18	0	11	0	8	2
Vascular disorders						
Hemorrhage[e]	16	5	11	0	2	0
Infections and infestations						
Urinary tract infection	13	2	6	0	9	2
Renal and urinary disorders						
Renal failure[f]	7	7	2	0	0	0

[a]National Cancer Institute Common Terminology Criteria for Adverse Events, version 4.
[b]Includes the following terms: peripheral edema, edema, and lymphedema.
[c]Includes the following terms: rash, rash generalized, rash pruritic, rash erythematous, rash papular, rash vesicular, rash macular, and rash maculo-papular.
[d]Includes the following terms: abdominal pain, abdominal pain upper, abdominal pain lower, and abdominal discomfort.
[e]Includes the following terms: brain stem hemorrhage, cerebral hemorrhage, gastric hemorrhage, epistaxis, gingival hemorrhage, hematuria, vaginal hemorrhage, hemorrhage intracranial, eye hemorrhage, and vitreous hemorrhage.
[f]Includes the following terms: renal failure and renal failure acute.

Neoplasms Benign, Malignant, and Unspecified (including cysts and polyps): Skin papilloma.
Skin and Subcutaneous Tissue Disorders: Palmar-plantar erythrodysesthesia syndrome, hyperkeratosis, hyperhidrosis.
Vascular Disorders: Hypertension.
[See table at top of next page]
QT Prolongation: In Trial 2, QTcF prolongation to >500 msec occurred in 4% (2/55) of patients treated with MEKINIST in combination with dabrafenib and in 2% (1/53) of patients treated with dabrafenib as a single agent. The QTcF was increased more than 60 msec from baseline in 13% (7/55) of patients treated with MEKINIST in combination with dabrafenib and 2% (1/53) of patients treated with dabrafenib as a single agent.

7 DRUG INTERACTIONS

No formal clinical trials have been conducted to evaluate human cytochrome P450 (CYP) enzyme-mediated drug interactions with trametinib [see Clinical Pharmacology (12.3)].

7.1 Dabrafenib

Coadministration of MEKINIST 2 mg once daily and dabrafenib 150 mg twice daily resulted in no clinically relevant pharmacokinetic drug interactions [see Clinical Pharmacology (12.3)].
Refer to the Full Prescribing Information for dabrafenib for further details on the drug interaction potential of dabrafenib. Avoid concurrent administration of strong inhibitors or strong inducers of CYP3A4 or CYP2C8 with dabrafenib. If concomitant use of strong inhibitors or strong inducers of CYP3A4 or CYP2C8 is unavoidable, monitor patients closely for adverse reactions when taking strong inhibitors or loss of efficacy when taking strong inducers. Concomitant use of dabrafenib with agents that are sensitive substrates of CYP3A4, CYP2C8, CYP2C9, CYP2C19, or CYP2B6 may result in loss of efficacy of these agents. Substitute for these medications or monitor patients for loss of efficacy if use of these medications is unavoidable.

8 USE IN SPECIFIC POPULATIONS

8.1 Pregnancy

Pregnancy Category D
Risk Summary: MEKINIST can cause fetal harm when administered to a pregnant woman. Trametinib was embryotoxic and abortifacient in rabbits at doses greater than or equal to those resulting in exposures approximately 0.3 times the human exposure at the recommended clinical dose. If this drug is used during pregnancy, or if the patient becomes pregnant while taking this drug, the patient should be apprised of the potential hazard to the fetus [see Warnings and Precautions (5.10)].

Animal Data: In reproductive toxicity studies, administration of trametinib to rats during the period of organogenesis resulted in decreased fetal weights at doses greater than or equal to 0.031 mg/kg/day (approximately 0.3 times the human exposure based on AUC at the recommended dose). In rats, at a dose resulting in exposures 1.8-fold higher than the human exposure at the recommended dose, there was maternal toxicity and an increase in post-implantation loss. In pregnant rabbits, administration of trametinib during the period of organogenesis resulted in decreased fetal body weight and increased incidence of variations in ossification at doses greater than or equal to 0.039 mg/kg/day (approximately 0.08 times the human exposure at the recommended dose based on AUC). In rabbits administered trametinib at 0.15 mg/kg/day (approximately 0.3 times the human exposure at the recommended dose based on AUC) there was an increase in post-implantation loss, including total loss of pregnancy, compared with control animals.

8.3 Nursing Mothers

It is not known whether this drug is present in human milk. Because many drugs are present in human milk and because of the potential for serious adverse reactions in nursing infants from MEKINIST, a decision should be made whether to discontinue nursing or to discontinue the drug taking into account the importance of the drug to the mother.

8.4 Pediatric Use

The safety and effectiveness of MEKINIST as a single agent or in combination with dabrafenib have not been established in pediatric patients.
Adequate juvenile animal studies using trametinib have not been completed. In a repeat-dose toxicity study in juvenile rats, an increased incidence of kidney cysts and tubular deposits were noted at doses as low as 0.2 times the human exposure at the recommended adult dose of dabrafenib based on AUC. Additionally, forestomach hyperplasia, decreased bone length, and early vaginal opening were noted at doses as low as 0.8 times the human exposure at the recommended adult dose based on AUC.

8.5 Geriatric Use

Clinical trials of MEKINIST as a single agent did not include sufficient numbers of subjects aged 65 and over to determine whether they respond differently from younger subjects. In Trial 1, 49 patients (23%) were 65 years of age and older, and 9 patients (4%) were 75 years of age and older. Across all clinical trials of MEKINIST administered in combination with dabrafenib, there was an insufficient number of patients aged 65 years and over to determine whether they respond differently from younger patients. In Trial 2, 11 patients (20%) were 65 years of age and older, and 2 patients (4%) were 75 years of age and older.

8.6 Females and Males of Reproductive Potential

Contraception:
Females: MEKINIST can cause fetal harm when administered during pregnancy. Advise female patients of reproductive potential to use highly effective contraception during treatment and for 4 months after the last dose of MEKINIST. When MEKINIST is used in combination with dabrafenib, counsel patients to use a non-hormonal method of contraception since dabrafenib can render hormonal contraceptives ineffective. Advise patients to contact their healthcare provider if they become pregnant, or if pregnancy is suspected, while taking MEKINIST [see Use in Specific Populations (8.1)].
Infertility:
Females: MEKINIST may impair fertility in female patients [see Nonclinical Toxicology (13.1)].
Males: Effects on spermatogenesis have been observed in animals treated with dabrafenib. Advise male patients of the potential risk for impaired spermatogenesis, and to seek counseling on fertility and family planning options prior to starting treatment with MEKINIST in combination with dabrafenib.

8.7 Hepatic Impairment

No formal clinical trial has been conducted to evaluate the effect of hepatic impairment on the pharmacokinetics of trametinib. No dose adjustment is recommended in patients with mild hepatic impairment based on a population pharmacokinetic analysis [see Clinical Pharmacology (12.3)].
The appropriate dose of MEKINIST has not been established in patients with moderate or severe hepatic impairment.

8.8 Renal Impairment

No formal clinical trial has been conducted to evaluate the effect of renal impairment on the pharmacokinetics of trametinib. No dose adjustment is recommended in patients with mild or moderate renal impairment based on a population pharmacokinetic analysis [see Clinical Pharmacology (12.3)]. The appropriate dose of MEKINIST has not been established in patients with severe renal impairment.

10 OVERDOSAGE

There were no reported cases of overdosage with MEKINIST. The highest doses of MEKINIST evaluated in clinical trials were 4 mg orally once daily and 10 mg administered orally once daily on 2 consecutive days followed by 3 mg once daily. In seven patients treated on one of these two schedules, there were two cases of retinal pigment epithelial detachments for an incidence of 28%. Since trametinib is highly bound to plasma proteins, hemodialysis is likely to be ineffective in the treatment of overdose with MEKINIST.

11 DESCRIPTION

Trametinib dimethyl sulfoxide is a kinase inhibitor. The chemical name is acetamide, N-[3-[3-cyclopropyl-5-[(2-fluoro-4-iodophenyl)amino]-3,4,6,7-tetrahydro-6,8-dimethyl- 2,4,7-trioxopyrido[4,3-d]pyrimidin-1(2H)-yl]phenyl]-, compound with 1,1'-sulfinylbis[methane] (1:1). It has a molecular formula $C_{26}H_{23}FIN_5O_4 \cdot C_2H_6OS$ with a molecular mass of 693.53. Trametinib dimethyl sulfoxide has the following chemical structure:

Trametinib dimethyl sulfoxide is a white to almost white powder. It is practically insoluble in the pH range of 2 to 8 in aqueous media.
MEKINIST (trametinib) tablets are supplied as 0.5-mg, 1-mg, and 2-mg tablets for oral administration. Each 0.5-mg tablet contains 0.5635 mg trametinib dimethyl sulfoxide equivalent to 0.5 mg of trametinib non-solvated parent. Each 1-mg tablet contains 1.127 mg trametinib dimethyl sulfoxide equivalent to 1 mg of trametinib non-solvated parent. Each 2-mg tablet contains 2.254 mg trametinib dimethyl sulfoxide equivalent to 2 mg of trametinib non-solvated parent.
The inactive ingredients of MEKINIST tablets are: **Tablet Core:** colloidal silicon dioxide, croscarmellose sodium, hypromellose, magnesium stearate (vegetable source), mannitol, microcrystalline cellulose, sodium lauryl sulfate. **Coating:** hypromellose, iron oxide red (2-mg tablets), iron oxide yellow (0.5-mg tablets), polyethylene glycol, polysorbate 80 (2-mg tablets), titanium dioxide.

12 CLINICAL PHARMACOLOGY

12.1 Mechanism of Action

Trametinib is a reversible inhibitor of mitogen-activated extracellular signal regulated kinase 1 (MEK1) and MEK2 activation and of MEK1 and MEK2 kinase activity. MEK proteins are upstream regulators of the extracellular signal-related kinase (ERK) pathway, which promotes cellular proliferation. BRAF V600E mutations result in constitutive activation of the BRAF pathway which includes MEK1 and MEK2. Trametinib inhibits BRAF V600 mutation-positive melanoma cell growth in vitro and in vivo.

Trametinib and dabrafenib target two different tyrosine kinases in the RAS/RAF/MEK/ERK pathway. Use of trametinib and dabrafenib in combination resulted in greater growth inhibition of BRAF V600 mutation-positive melanoma cell lines in vitro and prolonged inhibition of tumor growth in BRAF V600 mutation positive melanoma xenografts compared with either drug alone.

12.2 Pharmacodynamics

Administration of 1 mg and 2 mg trametinib to patients with BRAF V600 mutation-positive melanoma resulted in dose-dependent changes in tumor biomarkers including inhibition of phosphorylated ERK, inhibition of Ki67 (a marker of cell proliferation), and increases in p27 (a marker of apoptosis).

12.3 Pharmacokinetics

The pharmacokinetics (PK) of trametinib were characterized following single- and repeat-oral administration in patients with solid tumors and BRAF V600 mutation-positive metastatic melanoma.

Absorption: After oral administration, the median time to achieve peak plasma concentrations (T_{max}) is 1.5 hours post-dose. The mean absolute bioavailability of a single 2-mg oral dose of trametinib tablet is 72%. The increase in C_{max} was dose proportional after a single dose of 0.125 to 10 mg while the increase in AUC was greater than dose proportional. After repeat doses of 0.125 to 4 mg daily, both C_{max} and AUC increase proportionally with dose. Inter-subject variability in AUC and C_{max} at steady state is 22% and 28%, respectively.

Administration of a single dose of trametinib with a high-fat, high-calorie meal decreased AUC by 24%, C_{max} by 70%, and delayed T_{max} by approximately 4 hours as compared with fasted conditions [see Dosage and Administration (2.2)].

Distribution: Trametinib is 97.4% bound to human plasma proteins. The apparent volume of distribution (V_c/F) is 214 L.

Metabolism: Trametinib is metabolized predominantly via deacetylation alone or with mono-oxygenation or in combination with glucuronidation biotransformation pathways in vitro. Deacetylation is likely mediated by hydrolytic enzymes, such as carboxyl-esterases or amidases.

Following a single dose of [^{14}C]-trametinib, approximately 50% of circulating radioactivity is represented as the parent compound. However, based on metabolite profiling after repeat dosing of trametinib, ≥75% of drug-related material in plasma is the parent compound.

Elimination: The estimated elimination half-life based on the population PK model is 3.9 to 4.8 days. The apparent clearance is 4.9 L/h.

Following oral administration of [^{14}C]-trametinib, >80% of excreted radioactivity was recovered in the feces while <20% of excreted radioactivity was recovered in the urine with <0.1% of the excreted dose as parent.

Specific Populations:

Based on a population pharmacokinetic analysis, age, gender, and body weight do not have a clinically important effect on the exposure of trametinib. There are insufficient data to evaluate potential differences in the exposure of trametinib by race or ethnicity.

Hepatic Impairment: Based on a population pharmacokinetic analysis in 64 patients with mild hepatic impairment (total bilirubin ≤ULN and AST >ULN or total bilirubin >1.0 to 1.5 × ULN and any AST), mild hepatic impairment has no clinically important effect on the systemic exposure of trametinib. The pharmacokinetics of trametinib have not been studied in patients with moderate or severe hepatic impairment [see Use in Specific Populations (8.7)].

Renal Impairment: As renal excretion of trametinib is low (<20%), renal impairment is unlikely to have a clinically important effect on the exposure of trametinib. Based on a population PK analysis in 223 patients with mild renal impairment (GFR 60 to 89 mL/min/1.73 m^2) and 35 patients with moderate renal impairment (GFR 30 to 59 mL/min/1.73 m^2), mild and moderate renal impairment have no clinically important effects on the systemic exposure of trametinib. The pharmacokinetics of trametinib have not been studied in patients with severe renal impairment [see Use in Specific Populations (8.8)].

Pediatrics: No trials have been conducted to evaluate the pharmacokinetics of trametinib in pediatric patients.

Table 6. Treatment-Emergent Laboratory Abnormalities Occurring at ≥10% (All Grades) or ≥2% (Grades 3 or 4) of Patients Treated With MEKINIST in Combination With Dabrafenib in Trial 2

Test	MEKINIST 2 mg plus Dabrafenib N = 55		MEKINIST 1 mg plus Dabrafenib N = 54		Dabrafenib N = 53	
	All Grades	Grades 3 and 4	All Grades	Grades 3 and 4	All Grades	Grades 3 and 4[a]
Hematology						
Leukopenia	62	5	46	4	21	0
Lymphopenia	55	22	59	19	40	6
Neutropenia	55	13	37	2	9	2
Anemia	55	4	46	7	28	0
Thrombocytopenia	31	4	31	2	8	0
Liver Function Tests						
Increased AST	60	5	54	0	15	0
Increased alkaline phosphatase	60	2	67	6	26	2
Increased ALT	42	4	35	4	11	0
Hyperbilirubinemia	15	0	7	4	0	0
Chemistry						
Hyperglycemia	58	5	67	6	49	2
Increased GGT	56	11	54	17	38	2
Hyponatremia	55	11	48	15	36	2
Hypoalbuminemia	53	0	43	2	23	0
Hypophosphatemia	47	5	41	11	40	0
Hypokalemia	29	2	15	0	23	6
Increased creatinine	24	5	20	2	9	0
Hypomagnesemia	18	2	2	0	6	0
Hyperkalemia	18	0	22	0	15	4
Hypercalcemia	15	0	19	2	4	0
Hypocalcemia	13	0	20	0	0	0

[a] No Grade 4 events were reported in dabrafenib arm.
ALT = Alanine aminotransferase; AST = Aspartate aminotransferase; GGT = Gamma glutamyltransferase.

Drug Interactions:

Trametinib is not a substrate of CYP enzymes or efflux transporters human P-glycoprotein (P-gp) or breast cancer resistance protein (BCRP) in vitro.

Based on in vitro studies, trametinib is not an inhibitor of CYP450 including CYP1A2, CYP2A6, CYP2B6, CYP2C9, CYP2C19, CYP2D6, and CYP3A4, or of transporters including human organic anion transporting polypeptide (OATP1B1, OATP1B3), P-gp, and BCRP at a clinically relevant systemic concentration of 0.04 μM. Trametinib is an inhibitor of CYP2C8 in vitro.

Trametinib is an inducer of CYP3A4 in vitro. Based on cross-study comparisons, oral administration of trametinib 2 mg once daily with everolimus (sensitive CYP3A4 substrate) 5 mg once daily, had no clinically important effect on the AUC and C_{max} of everolimus.

Coadministration of trametinib 2 mg daily with dabrafenib 150 mg twice daily resulted in a 23% increase in AUC of dabrafenib, a 33% increase in AUC of desmethyl-dabrafenib, and no change in AUC of trametinib or hydroxy-dabrafenib as compared with administration of either drug alone.

13 NONCLINICAL TOXICOLOGY

13.1 Carcinogenesis, Mutagenesis, Impairment of Fertility

Carcinogenicity studies with trametinib have not been conducted. Trametinib was not genotoxic in studies evaluating reverse mutations in bacteria, chromosomal aberrations in mammalian cells, and micronuclei in the bone marrow of rats.

Trametinib may impair fertility in humans. In female rats given trametinib for up to 13 weeks, increased follicular cysts and decreased corpora lutea were observed at doses ≥0.016 mg/kg/day (approximately 0.3 times the human exposure at the recommended dose based on AUC). In rat and dog toxicity studies up to 13 weeks in duration, there were no treatment effects observed on male reproductive tissues [see Use in Specific Populations (8.6)].

14 CLINICAL STUDIES

14.1 BRAF V600E or V600K Mutation-Positive Unresectable or Metastatic Melanoma

The safety and efficacy of MEKINIST were evaluated in two clinical trials. Trial 1 was an international, multicenter, randomized (2:1), open-label, active-controlled trial in 322 patients with BRAF V600E or V600K mutation-positive, unresectable or metastatic melanoma. Trial 2 was a multicenter, randomized (1:1:1), open-label, dose-ranging trial designed to evaluate the clinical activity and safety of MEKINIST (at two different doses) in combination with dabrafenib and to compare the safety with dabrafenib as a single agent in 162 patients with BRAF V600E or V600K mutation-positive, unresectable or metastatic melanoma.

In Trial 1, patients were not permitted to have more than one prior chemotherapy regimen for advanced or metastatic disease; prior treatment with a BRAF inhibitor or MEK inhibitor was not permitted. The primary efficacy outcome measure was progression-free survival (PFS). Patients were randomized to receive MEKINIST 2 mg orally once daily (N = 214) or chemotherapy (N = 108) consisting of either dacarbazine 1,000 mg/m^2 intravenously every 3 weeks or paclitaxel 175 mg/m^2 intravenously every 3 weeks. Treatment continued until disease progression or unacceptable toxicity. Randomization was stratified according to prior use of chemotherapy for advanced or metastatic disease (yes versus no) and lactate dehydrogenase level (normal versus greater than upper limit of normal). Tumor tissue was evaluated for BRAF mutations at a central testing site using a clinical trial assay. Tumor samples from 289 patients (196 patients treated with MEKINIST and 93 chemotherapy-treated patients) were also tested retrospectively using an FDA-approved companion diagnostic test, THxID™-BRAF assay.

The median age for randomized patients was 54 years, 54% were male, >99% were white, and all patients had baseline ECOG performance status of 0 or 1. Most patients had metastatic disease (94%), were Stage M1c (64%), had elevated LDH (36%), no history of brain metastasis (97%), and received no prior chemotherapy for advanced or metastatic disease (66%). The distribution of BRAF V600 mutations was BRAF V600E (87%), V600K (12%), or both (<1%). The median durations of follow-up prior to initiation of alternative treatment were 4.9 months for patients treated with MEKINIST and 3.1 months for patients treated with chemotherapy. Fifty-one (47%) patients crossed over from the chemotherapy arm at the time of disease progression to receive MEKINIST.

Trial 1 demonstrated a statistically significant increase in progression-free survival in the patients treated with MEKINIST. Table 7 and Figure 1 summarize the PFS results.

Table 7. Investigator-Assessed Progression-Free Survival and Confirmed Objective Response Results in Trial 1

	MEKINIST N = 214	Chemotherapy N = 108
PFS		
Number of Events (%)	117 (55%)	77 (71%)
Progressive Disease	107 (50%)	70 (65%)
Death	10 (5%)	7 (6%)
Median, months (95% CI)	4.8 (4.3, 4.9)	1.5 (1.4, 2.7)
HR[a] (95% CI)	0.47 (0.34, 0.65)	
P value (log-rank test)	P<0.0001	
Confirmed Tumor Responses		
Objective Response Rate	22%	8%
(95% CI)	(17, 28)	(4, 15)
CR, n (%)	4 (2%)	0
PR, n (%)	43 (20%)	9 (8%)
Duration of Response		
Median, months (95% CI)	5.5 (4.1, 5.9)	NR (3.5, NR)

[a] Pike estimator.
CI = Confidence interval; CR = Complete response; HR = Hazard ratio; NR = Not reached, PFS = Progression-free survival; PR = Partial response.

Figure 1. Kaplan-Meier Curves of Investigator-Assessed Progression-Free Survival (ITT population) in Trial 1

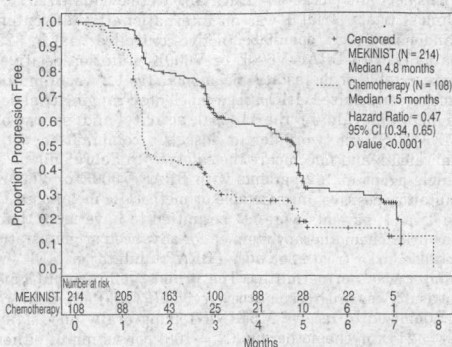

In supportive analyses based on independent radiologic review committee (IRRC) assessment, the PFS results were consistent with those of the primary efficacy analysis.

Trial 2 randomized (1:1:1) patients to MEKINIST (at two different doses) in combination with dabrafenib compared with dabrafenib as a single agent in 162 patients with BRAF V600E or V600K mutation-positive, unresectable or metastatic melanoma. Patients were permitted to have had one prior chemotherapy regimen and prior aldesleukin; patients with prior exposure to BRAF or MEK inhibitors were ineligible. Patients were randomized to receive MEKINIST 2 mg orally once daily with dabrafenib 150 mg orally twice daily (n = 54), MEKINIST 1 mg orally once daily with dabrafenib 150 mg orally twice daily (n = 54), or dabrafenib 150 mg orally twice daily (n = 54). Treatment continued until disease progression or unacceptable toxicity. Patients randomized to receive dabrafenib as a single agent were offered MEKINIST 2 mg orally once daily with dabrafenib 150 mg orally twice daily at the time of investigator-assessed disease progression. The major efficacy outcome measure was investigator-assessed overall response rate (ORR). Additional efficacy outcome measures were investigator-assessed duration of response, independent radiology review committee (IRRC)-assessed ORR, and IRRC-assessed duration of response.

The median age of patients in Trial 2 was 53 years, 57% were male, >99% were white, 66% of patients had a pretreatment ECOG performance status of 0, 67% had M1c disease, 54% had a normal LDH at baseline, and 8% had a history of brain metastases. Most patients (81%) had not received prior anti-cancer therapy for unresectable or metastatic disease. All patients had tumor containing BRAF V600E or V600K mutations as determined by local laboratory or centralized testing, 85% with BRAF V600E mutations and 15% with BRAF V600K mutations.

The median duration of follow-up was 14 months. Efficacy outcomes for the arm receiving MEKINIST 2 mg daily in combination with dabrafenib and the arm receiving dabrafenib as a single agent are summarized in Table 8.

Table 8. Investigator-Assessed and Independent Review Committee-Assessed Response Rates and Response Durations in Trial 2

Endpoints	MEKINIST plus Dabrafenib N = 54	Dabrafenib N = 54
Investigator Assessment		
Responders (ORR%) (95% CI)	41 (76%) (62%, 87%)	29 (54%) (40%, 67%)
Complete response	9%	4%
Partial response	67%	50%
Duration of Response (months)		
Median (95% CI)	10.5 (7, 15)	5.6 (5, 7)
Independent Radiology Review Committee Assessment		
Responders (ORR%) (95% CI)	31 (57%) (43%, 71%)	25 (46%) (33%, 60%)
Complete response	9%	7%
Partial response	48%	39%
Duration of Response (months)		
Median (95% CI)	7.6 (7, NR)	7.6 (6, NR)

CI = Confidence interval; ORR = Confirmed overall response rate; NR = Not reported.

The ORR results were similar in subgroups defined by BRAF mutation subtype, i.e., in the 85% of patients with V600E mutation-positive melanoma and in the 15% of patients with V600K mutation-positive melanoma. In exploratory subgroup analyses of the patients with retrospectively confirmed BRAF V600E or V600K mutation-positive melanoma using the THxID™-BRAF assay, the ORR results were also similar to the intent-to-treat analysis.

14.2   Lack of Clinical Activity in Metastatic Melanoma Following BRAF-Inhibitor Therapy
The clinical activity of MEKINIST as a single agent was evaluated in a single-arm, multicenter, international trial (Trial 3) in 40 patients with BRAF V600E or V600K mutation-positive, unresectable or metastatic melanoma who had received prior treatment with a BRAF inhibitor. All patients received MEKINIST at a dose of 2 mg orally once daily until disease progression or unacceptable toxicity. The median age was 58 years, 63% were male, all were white, 98% had baseline ECOG PS of 0 or 1, and the distribution of BRAF V600 mutations was V600E (83%), V600K (10%), and the remaining patients had multiple V600 mutations (5%), or unknown mutational status (2%). No patient in Trial 3 achieved a confirmed partial or complete response as determined by the clinical investigators.

16   HOW SUPPLIED/STORAGE AND HANDLING
0.5-mg Tablets: Yellow, modified oval, biconvex, film-coated tablets with 'GS' debossed on one face and 'TFC' on the opposing face and are available in bottles of 30 (NDC 0173-0849-13).
1-mg Tablets: White, round, biconvex, film-coated tablets with 'GS' debossed on one face and 'LHE' on the opposing face and are available in bottles of 30 (NDC 0173-0858-13).
2-mg Tablets: Pink, round, biconvex, film-coated tablets with 'GS' debossed on one face and 'HMJ' on the opposing face and are available in bottles of 30 (NDC 0173-0848-13).
Store refrigerated at 2° to 8°C (36° to 46°F). Do not freeze. Dispense in original bottle. Do not remove desiccant. Protect from moisture and light. Do not place medication in pill boxes.

17   PATIENT COUNSELING INFORMATION
See FDA-approved patient labeling (Patient Information). Inform patients of the following:
- Evidence of BRAF V600E or V600K mutation within the tumor specimen is necessary to identify patients for whom treatment with MEKINIST is indicated [see Dosage and Administration (2.1)].
- MEKINIST administered in combination with dabrafenib can result in the development of new primary cutaneous and non-cutaneous malignancies. Advise patients to contact their doctor immediately for any new lesions, changes to existing lesions on their skin, or other signs and symptoms of malignancies [see Warnings and Precautions (5.1)].
- MEKINIST administered in combination with dabrafenib increases the risk of intracranial and gastrointestinal hemorrhage. Advise patients to contact their healthcare provider to seek immediate medical attention for signs or symptoms of unusual bleeding or hemorrhage [see Warnings and Precautions (5.2)].
- MEKINIST administered in combination with dabrafenib increases the risks of pulmonary embolism and deep venous thrombosis. Advise patients to seek immediate medical attention for sudden onset of difficulty breathing, leg pain, or swelling [see Warnings and Precautions (5.3)].
- MEKINIST can cause cardiomyopathy. Advise patients to immediately report any signs or symptoms of heart failure to their healthcare provider [see Warnings and Precautions (5.4)].
- MEKINIST can cause severe visual disturbances that can lead to blindness. Advise patients to contact their healthcare provider if they experience any changes in their vision [see Warnings and Precautions (5.5)].
- MEKINIST can cause interstitial lung disease (or pneumonitis). Advise patients to contact their healthcare provider as soon as possible if they experience signs such as cough or dyspnea [see Warnings and Precautions (5.6)].
- MEKINIST used in combination with dabrafenib can cause serious febrile reactions. Instruct patients to contact their healthcare provider if they develop fever while taking MEKINIST with dabrafenib [see Warnings and Precautions (5.7)].
- MEKINIST can cause skin toxicities which may require hospitalization. Advise patients to contact their healthcare provider for progressive or intolerable rash [see Warnings and Precautions (5.8)].
- MEKINIST causes hypertension. Advise patients that they need to undergo blood pressure monitoring and to contact their healthcare provider if they develop symptoms of hypertension such as severe headache, blurry vision, or dizziness.
- MEKINIST often causes diarrhea which may be severe in some cases. Inform patients of the need to contact their healthcare provider if severe diarrhea occurs during treatment.
- MEKINIST should be taken at least 1 hour before or at least 2 hours after a meal.
- MEKINIST can cause fetal harm if taken during pregnancy. Instruct female patients to use highly effective contraception during treatment and for 4 months after treatment. Advise patients to use a highly effective non-hormonal method of contraception when MEKINIST is administered in combination with dabrafenib. Advise patients to contact their healthcare provider if they become pregnant, or if pregnancy is suspected, while taking MEKINIST [see Use in Specific Populations (8.1, 8.6)].
- Nursing infants may experience serious adverse reactions if the mother is taking MEKINIST. Advise lactating mothers to discontinue nursing while taking MEKINIST [see Use in Specific Populations (8.3)].

MEKINIST is a registered trademark of the GlaxoSmithKline group of companies.
THxID BRAF™ assay is a trademark of bioMerieux.
GlaxoSmithKline
Research Triangle Park, NC 27709

©2014, GlaxoSmithKline group of companies. All rights reserved.
MKN:3PI

Patient Information
MEKINIST® (MEK-in-ist)
(trametinib)
tablets
If your healthcare provider prescribes MEKINIST for you in combination with dabrafenib, also read the Medication Guide that comes with dabrafenib.

What is MEKINIST?
MEKINIST is a prescription medicine used by itself or in combination with dabrafenib to treat people with a type of skin cancer called melanoma:
- that has spread to other parts of the body or cannot be removed by surgery, and
- that has a certain type of abnormal "BRAF" gene.
MEKINIST should not be used alone to treat people who already have received a BRAF inhibitor for treatment of their melanoma.
Your healthcare provider will perform a test to make sure that MEKINIST is right for you.
It is not known if MEKINIST is safe and effective in children.

What should I tell my healthcare provider before taking MEKINIST?
Before you take MEKINIST, tell your healthcare provider if you:
- have had bleeding problems or blood clots
- have heart problems
- have eye problems
- have lung or breathing problems
- have high blood pressure (hypertension)
- have liver or kidney problems
- have any other medical conditions
- are pregnant or plan to become pregnant. MEKINIST can harm your unborn baby.
  - Females who are able to become pregnant should use effective birth control (contraception) during treatment with MEKINIST and for 4 months after stopping treatment.
  - Birth control using hormones (such as birth control pills, injections, or patches) may not work as well while you are taking MEKINIST in combination with dabrafenib. You should use another effective method of birth control while taking MEKINIST in combination with dabrafenib.
  - Talk to your healthcare provider about birth control methods that may be right for you during this time.
  - Tell your healthcare provider right away if you become pregnant during treatment with MEKINIST.
- are breastfeeding or plan to breastfeed. It is not known if MEKINIST passes into your breast milk. You and your healthcare provider should decide if you will take MEKINIST or breastfeed. You should not do both.
Tell your healthcare provider about all the medicines you take, including prescription and over-the-counter medicines, vitamins, and herbal supplements.
Know the medicines you take. Keep a list of them to show your healthcare provider and pharmacist when you get a new medicine.

How should I take MEKINIST?
- Take MEKINIST exactly as your healthcare provider tells you to take it. Do not change your dose or stop MEKINIST unless your healthcare provider tells you.
- Take MEKINIST one time a day. If you are taking MEKINIST in combination with dabrafenib, you can take it at the same time as one of your doses of dabrafenib.
- Take MEKINIST at least 1 hour before or 2 hours after a meal.
- If you miss a dose, take it as soon as you remember. If it is within 12 hours of your next scheduled dose, skip the missed dose. Just take the next dose at your regular time.
- If you take too much MEKINIST, call your healthcare provider or go to the nearest hospital emergency room right away.

What are the possible side effects of MEKINIST?
MEKINIST may cause serious side effects, including:
- **bleeding problems.** MEKINIST, when taken in combination with dabrafenib, can cause serious bleeding problems, especially in your brain or stomach, and can lead to death. Call your healthcare provider and get medical help right away if you have any unusual signs of bleeding, including:
  - headaches, dizziness, or feeling weak
  - cough up blood or blood clots
  - vomit blood or your vomit looks like "coffee grounds"
  - red or black stools that look like tar
- **blood clots.** MEKINIST, when taken in combination with dabrafenib, can cause blood clots in your arms or legs, which can travel to your lungs and can lead to death. Get medical help right away if you have the following symptoms:
  - chest pain
  - sudden shortness of breath or trouble breathing

- pain in your legs with or without swelling
- swelling in your arms or legs
- a cool or pale arm or leg
- **heart problems, including heart failure.** Your healthcare provider should check your heart function before you start taking MEKINIST by itself or in combination with dabrafenib, and during treatment. Call your healthcare provider right away if you have any of the following signs and symptoms of a heart problem:
  - feeling like your heart is pounding or racing
  - shortness of breath
  - swelling of your ankles and feet
  - feeling lightheaded
- **eye problems.** MEKINIST can cause severe eye problems that might lead to blindness. Call your healthcare provider right away if you get these symptoms of eye problems:
  - blurred vision, loss of vision, or other vision changes
  - see color dots
  - halo (seeing blurred outline around objects)
  - eye pain, swelling, or redness
- **lung or breathing problems.** Tell your healthcare provider if you have any new or worsening symptoms of lung or breathing problems, including:
  - shortness of breath
  - cough
- **skin reactions.** Rash is a common side effect of MEKINIST. MEKINIST can also cause other skin reactions. In some cases these rashes and other skin reactions can be severe, and may need to be treated in a hospital. Call your healthcare provider if you get any of the following symptoms:
  - skin rash that bothers you or does not go away
  - acne
  - redness, swelling, peeling, or tenderness of hands or feet
  - skin redness
- **fever.** MEKINIST in combination with dabrafenib can cause fever, which may be serious. In some cases, chills or shaking chills, too much fluid loss (dehydration), low blood pressure, dizziness, or kidney problems may happen with the fever. Call your healthcare provider right away if you get a fever while taking MEKINIST.
- **increased blood sugar (hyperglycemia).** Some people may develop high blood sugar or worsening diabetes during treatment with MEKINIST in combination with dabrafenib. If you are diabetic, your healthcare provider should check your blood sugar levels closely during treatment with MEKINIST in combination with dabrafenib. Your diabetes medicine may need to be changed. Tell your healthcare provider if you have any of the following symptoms of severe high blood sugar:
  - increased thirst
  - urinating more often than normal or urinating an increased amount of urine
The most common side effects of MEKINIST when used alone include:
- diarrhea. Call your healthcare provider if you get severe diarrhea.
- swelling of the face, arms, or legs
Other common side effects of MEKINIST when used in combination with dabrafenib include:
- tiredness
- nausea or vomiting
- stomach-area (abdominal) pain
- diarrhea
- cough
- swelling of the face, arms, or legs
- headache
- night sweats
- decreased appetite
- constipation
- muscle or joint aches
MEKINIST can cause new or worsening high blood pressure (hypertension). Your healthcare provider should check your blood pressure during treatment with MEKINIST. Call your healthcare provider right away if you develop high blood pressure, your blood pressure worsens, or you have severe headache, lightheadedness, or dizziness.
MEKINIST may cause fertility problems in females. This could affect your ability to become pregnant. Talk to your healthcare provider if this is a concern for you.
Tell your healthcare provider if you have any side effect that bothers you or that does not go away.
These are not all the possible side effects of MEKINIST. For more information, ask your healthcare provider or pharmacist.
Call your doctor for medical advice about side effects. You may report side effects to FDA at 1-800-FDA-1088.

How should I store MEKINIST?
- Store MEKINIST in the refrigerator between 36°F to 46°F (2°C to 8°C). Do not freeze.
- Keep MEKINIST dry and away from moisture and light.
- The bottle of MEKINIST contains a desiccant packet to help keep your medicine dry. Do not throw away the desiccant packet.

- Keep MEKINIST in its original bottle. Do not place tablets in a pill box.
- Safely throw away MEKINIST that is out of date or no longer needed.
Keep MEKINIST and all medicine out of the reach of children.

General information about MEKINIST
Medicines are sometimes prescribed for purposes other than those listed in a Patient Information leaflet. Do not use MEKINIST for a condition for which it was not prescribed. Do not give MEKINIST to other people, even if they have the same symptoms that you have. It may harm them.
You can ask your healthcare provider or pharmacist for information about MEKINIST that is written for health professionals.
For more information, go to www.MEKINIST.com or call 1-888-825-5249.

What are the ingredients in MEKINIST?
Active ingredient: trametinib
Inactive ingredients:
Tablet Core: colloidal silicon dioxide, croscarmellose sodium, hypromellose, magnesium stearate (vegetable source), mannitol, microcrystalline cellulose, sodium lauryl sulfate.
Tablet Coating: hypromellose, iron oxide red (2-mg tablets), iron oxide yellow (0.5-mg tablets), polyethylene glycol, polysorbate 80 (2-mg tablets), titanium dioxide.
This Patient Information has been approved by the U.S. Food and Drug Administration.
GlaxoSmithKline
Research Triangle Park, NC 27709
Revised: January 2014
MEKINIST is a registered trademark of the GlaxoSmithKline group of companies.
©2014, GlaxoSmithKline group of companies. All rights reserved.
MKN:3PIL

MENHIBRIX   R
(Meningococcal Groups C and Y and Haemophilus b Tetanus Toxoid Conjugate Vaccine)
Solution for Intramuscular Injection

HIGHLIGHTS OF PRESCRIBING INFORMATION
These highlights do not include all the information needed to use MENHIBRIX safely and effectively. See full prescribing information for MENHIBRIX.
MENHIBRIX (Meningococcal Groups C and Y and Haemophilus b Tetanus Toxoid Conjugate Vaccine)
Solution for Intramuscular Injection
Initial U.S. Approval: 2012

————————INDICATIONS AND USAGE————————
MENHIBRIX is a vaccine indicated for active immunization to prevent invasive disease caused by *Neisseria meningitidis* serogroups C and Y and *Haemophilus influenzae* type b. MENHIBRIX is approved for use in children 6 weeks of age through 18 months of age. (1)

————————DOSAGE AND ADMINISTRATION————————
Four doses (0.5 mL each) by intramuscular injection at 2, 4, 6, and 12 through 15 months of age. The first dose may be given as early as 6 weeks of age. The fourth dose may be given as late as 18 months of age. (2.3)

————————DOSAGE FORMS AND STRENGTHS————————
Solution for injection supplied as a single-dose vial of lyophilized vaccine to be reconstituted with the accompanying vial of saline diluent. A single dose after reconstitution is 0.5 mL. (3)

————————CONTRAINDICATIONS————————
Severe allergic reaction (e.g., anaphylaxis) after a previous dose of any meningococcal-, *H. influenzae* type b-, or tetanus toxoid-containing vaccine or any component of MENHIBRIX. (4)

————————WARNINGS AND PRECAUTIONS————————
- If Guillain-Barré syndrome has occurred within 6 weeks of receipt of a prior vaccine containing tetanus toxoid, the decision to give any tetanus toxoid-containing vaccine, including MENHIBRIX, should be based on consideration of the potential benefits and possible risks. (5.1)
- Syncope (fainting) can occur in association with administration of injectable vaccines, including MENHIBRIX. Procedures should be in place to avoid falling injury and to restore cerebral perfusion following syncope. (5.2)
- Apnea following intramuscular vaccination has been observed in some infants born prematurely. Decisions about when to administer an intramuscular vaccine, including MENHIBRIX, to infants born prematurely should be based on consideration of the individual infant's medical status, and the potential benefits and possible risks of vaccination. (5.3)

Figure 1. Cleanse both vial stoppers. Withdraw 0.6 mL of saline from diluent vial.

Figure 2. Transfer saline diluent into the lyophilized vaccine vial.

Figure 3. Shake the vial well.

Figure 4. After reconstitution, withdraw 0.5 mL of reconstituted vaccine and administer **intramuscularly.**

ADVERSE REACTIONS

Rates of local injection site pain, redness, and swelling ranged from 15% to 46% depending on reaction and specific dose in schedule. Commonly reported systemic events included irritability (62% to 71%), drowsiness (49% to 63%), loss of appetite (30% to 34%), and fever (11% to 26%) (specific rate depended on the event and dose in the schedule). (6.1)

To report SUSPECTED ADVERSE REACTIONS, contact GlaxoSmithKline at 1-888-825-5249 or VAERS at 1-800-822-7967 or www.vaers.hhs.gov.

DRUG INTERACTIONS

Do not mix MENHIBRIX with any other vaccine in the same syringe or vial. (7.1)
See 17 for PATIENT COUNSELING INFORMATION
Revised: 11/2013

FULL PRESCRIBING INFORMATION: CONTENTS*

FULL PRESCRIBING INFORMATION

1 INDICATIONS AND USAGE

MENHIBRIX® is indicated for active immunization to prevent invasive disease caused by *Neisseria meningitidis* serogroups C and Y and *Haemophilus influenzae* type b. MENHIBRIX is approved for use in children 6 weeks of age through 18 months of age.

2 DOSAGE AND ADMINISTRATION

2.1 Reconstitution

MENHIBRIX is to be reconstituted only with the accompanying saline diluent. The reconstituted vaccine should be a clear and colorless solution. Parenteral drug products should be inspected visually for particulate matter and discoloration prior to administration, whenever solution and container permit. If either of these conditions exists, the vaccine should not be administered.
[See table above]

2.2 Administration

For intramuscular use only. Do not administer this product intravenously, intradermally, or subcutaneously.
After reconstitution, administer MENHIBRIX immediately. Use a separate sterile needle and sterile syringe for each individual. The preferred administration site is the anterolateral aspect of the thigh for most infants younger than 1 year of age. In older children, the deltoid muscle is usually large enough for an intramuscular injection.

2.3 Dose and Schedule

A 4-dose series, with each 0.5-mL dose given by intramuscular injection at 2, 4, 6, and 12 through 15 months of age. The first dose may be given as early as 6 weeks of age. The fourth dose may be given as late as 18 months of age.

3 DOSAGE FORMS AND STRENGTHS

MENHIBRIX is a solution for injection supplied as a single-dose vial of lyophilized vaccine to be reconstituted with the accompanying vial of saline diluent. A single dose after reconstitution is 0.5 mL.

4 CONTRAINDICATIONS

Severe allergic reaction (e.g., anaphylaxis) after a previous dose of any meningococcal-, *H. influenzae* type b-, or tetanus toxoid-containing vaccine or any component of this vaccine is a contraindication to administration of MENHIBRIX *[see Description (11)]*.

5 WARNINGS AND PRECAUTIONS

5.1 Guillain-Barré Syndrome

If Guillain-Barré syndrome has occurred within 6 weeks of receipt of a prior vaccine containing tetanus toxoid, the decision to give any tetanus toxoid-containing vaccine, including MENHIBRIX, should be based on consideration of the potential benefits and possible risks.

5.2 Syncope

Syncope (fainting) can occur in association with administration of injectable vaccines, including MENHIBRIX. Syncope can be accompanied by transient neurological signs such as visual disturbance, paresthesia, and tonic-clonic limb movements. Procedures should be in place to avoid falling injury and to restore cerebral perfusion following syncope.

5.3 Apnea in Premature Infants

Apnea following intramuscular vaccination has been observed in some infants born prematurely. Decisions about when to administer an intramuscular vaccine, including MENHIBRIX, to infants born prematurely should be based on consideration of the individual infant's medical status, and the potential benefits and possible risks of vaccination.

5.4 Preventing and Managing Allergic Vaccine Reactions

Prior to administration, the healthcare provider should review the patient's immunization history for possible vaccine hypersensitivity. Epinephrine and other appropriate agents used for the control of immediate allergic reactions must be immediately available should an acute anaphylactic reaction occur.

5.5 Altered Immunocompetence

Safety and effectiveness of MENHIBRIX in immunosuppressed children have not been evaluated. If MENHIBRIX is administered to immunosuppressed children, including children receiving immunosuppressive therapy, the expected immune response may not be obtained.

5.6 Tetanus Immunization

Immunization with MENHIBRIX does not substitute for routine tetanus immunization.

6 ADVERSE REACTIONS

6.1 Clinical Trials Experience

Because clinical trials are conducted under widely varying conditions, adverse reaction rates observed in the clinical trials of a vaccine cannot be directly compared with rates in the clinical trials of another vaccine, and may not reflect the rates observed in practice. There is the possibility that broad use of MENHIBRIX could reveal adverse reactions not observed in clinical trials.

A total of 7,521 infants received at least one dose of MENHIBRIX in 6 clinical studies.[1-6] In 5 of these studies, 6,686 children received 4 consecutive doses of MENHIBRIX.[2-6] Across all studies, approximately half of participants were female; 50% were white, 41% were Hispanic, 4% were black, 1% were Asian and 4% were of other racial/ethnic groups.

Two randomized, controlled, pivotal trials enrolled participants to receive 4 doses of MENHIBRIX or a monovalent Haemophilus b Conjugate (Hib) vaccine, administered at 2, 4, 6, and 12 to 15 months of age (Study 009/010[5] and Study 011/012[6]). Together, these trials evaluated safety in 8,571 infants who received at least one dose of MENHIBRIX (N = 6,414) or Hib vaccine (N = 2,157).[5,6]

In Study 009/010[5], conducted in the United States, Australia, and Mexico, 4,180 infants were randomized 3:1 to receive MENHIBRIX or a control US-licensed Hib vaccine. Safety data are available for 3,136 infants who received MENHIBRIX and 1,044 infants who received a control Haemophilus b Conjugate Vaccine (Tetanus Toxoid Conjugate) (PRP-T, manufactured by Sanofi Pasteur SA) at 2, 4, and 6 months of age. For dose 4 administered at 12 to 15 months of age, safety data are available for 2,769 toddlers who received MENHIBRIX and 923 toddlers who received a control Haemophilus b Conjugate Vaccine (Meningococcal Protein Conjugate) (PRP-OMP, manufactured by Merck and Co., Inc.). With doses 1, 2, and 3 of MENHIBRIX or PRP-T, infants concomitantly received PEDIARIX® [Diphtheria and Tetanus Toxoids and Acellular Pertussis Adsorbed, Hepatitis B (Recombinant) and Inactivated Poliovirus Vaccine] and Pneumococcal 7-valent Conjugate Vaccine (Diphtheria CRM$_{197}$ Protein) (PCV7, manufactured by Wyeth Pharmaceuticals, Inc.). With dose 4 of MENHIBRIX or PRP-OMP, toddlers concomitantly received PCV7, Measles, Mumps, and Rubella Virus Vaccine Live (MMR, manufactured by Merck & Co., Inc.), and Varicella Virus Vaccine Live (manufactured by Merck & Co., Inc.).

Data on solicited adverse events were collected by parents/guardians using standardized forms for 4 consecutive days following vaccination with MENHIBRIX or control Hib vaccine (i.e., day of vaccination and the next 3 days).[5] Children were monitored for unsolicited adverse events that occurred in the 31-day period following vaccination and were monitored for serious adverse events, new onset chronic disease, rash, and conditions prompting emergency department visits or physician office visits during the entire study period (6 months following the last vaccine administered). Among participants in both groups, 66% were from the United States, 19% were from Mexico, and 14% were from Australia. Forty-eight percent of participants were female; 64% were white, 22% were Hispanic, 6% were black, 1% were Asian, and 7% were of other racial/ethnic groups.

In the second pivotal study (Study 011/012[6]), conducted in the United States and Mexico and evaluating the same vaccines and vaccination schedule, participants were monitored for serious adverse events, new onset chronic disease, rash, and conditions prompting emergency department visits during the entire study period (6 months following the last vaccine administered). Among participants in both groups, 30% were from the United States and 70% were from Mexico.

In addition to the pivotal studies, safety data are available from 4 studies which either did not include a fourth dose of MENHIBRIX[1], used a dosing regimen not approved in the United States[2,3], or incorporated a comparator vaccine which was not licensed in the United States.[4] In these studies, participants were monitored for unsolicited adverse events and serious adverse events occurring in the 31-day period following vaccination. In 2 of these studies[3,4], participants were monitored for serious adverse events, new onset chronic disease, rash, and conditions prompting emergency department visits or physician office visits through 6 months after the last vaccination.

Solicited Adverse Events: The reported frequencies of solicited local and systemic adverse events from US participants in Study 009/010 are presented in Table 1.[5] Because of differences in reported rates of solicited adverse events between US and non-US participants, only the solicited adverse event data in US participants are presented. Among the US participants included in Table 1, 48% were female; 76% were white, 10% were black, 4% were Hispanic, 2% were Asian, and 8% were of other racial/ethnic groups.
[See table 1 at top of next page]

The reported rates of some solicited adverse events in participants from Australia and Mexico varied from those in the United States.[5] For example, in Australia, pain after dose 1 was reported in 28.4% of participants who received MENHIBRIX and 33.3% of control participants, while in Mexico pain after dose 1 was reported in 73.7% of participants who received MENHIBRIX and 79.4% of control participants. Fever after dose 1 was reported in 10.4% of participants who received MENHIBRIX and 10.7% of control participants in Australia, while it was reported in 44.0% of participants who received MENHIBRIX and 35.7% of control participants in Mexico. The reported incidences of pain and fever in US participants after dose 1 are provided in Table 1.

Unsolicited Adverse Events: Among participants who received MENHIBRIX or Hib control vaccine co-administered with US-licensed vaccines at 2, 4, 6 and 12 to 15 months of age[1,3-5], the incidence of unsolicited adverse events reported within the 31-day period following study vaccination (doses 1, 2, and 3) was comparable between MENHIBRIX (61.9%; 2,578/4,166) and PRP-T (62.5%; 1,042/1,666). The incidence of unsolicited adverse events reported within the 31-day period following dose 4 was also comparable between MENHIBRIX (42.5%; 1,541/3,630) and PRP-OMP (41.4%; 520/1,257).

Serious Adverse Events: Following doses 1, 2, and 3[1,3-6], 1.8% (137/7,444) of participants who received MENHIBRIX and 2.1% (59/2,779) of participants who received PRP-T reported at least one serious adverse event within the 31-day period. Up to 6 months following the last vaccine administered (doses 1, 2, and 3) or until administration of dose 4[3-6], 4.8% (365/7,362) of participants who received MENHIBRIX and 5.0% (134/2,697) of participants in the PRP-T group reported at least one serious adverse event.

Following dose 4[3-6], 0.5% (35/6,640) of participants who received MENHIBRIX and 0.5% (12/2,267) of participants who received PRP-OMP reported at least one serious adverse event within the 31-day period. Up to 6 months following the last vaccine administered (dose 4), 2.5% (165/6,640) of participants who received MENHIBRIX and 2.0% (46/2,267) of participants who received PRP-OMP reported at least one serious adverse event.

6.2 Postmarketing Experience

The following adverse events have been spontaneously reported during post-approval use of HIBERIX® (Haemophilus b Conjugate Vaccine [Tetanus Toxoid Conjugate]) in the United States and other countries. These events are relevant because the Haemophilus b capsular polysaccharide tetanus toxoid conjugate is included as a component antigen in both MENHIBRIX and HIBERIX. Because these events are reported voluntarily from a population of uncertain size, it is not possible to reliably estimate their frequency or to establish a causal relationship to vaccine exposure.

The following adverse events were included based on one or more of the following factors: seriousness, frequency of reporting, or strength of evidence for a causal relationship to HIBERIX.

General Disorders and Administration Site Conditions: Extensive swelling of the vaccinated limb, injection site induration.

Immune System Disorders: Allergic reactions (including anaphylactic and anaphylactoid reactions), angioedema.

Nervous System Disorders: Convulsions (with or without fever), hypotonic-hyporesponsive episode, somnolence, syncope or vasovagal responses to injection.

Respiratory, Thoracic, and Mediastinal Disorders: Apnea.

Skin and Subcutaneous Tissue Disorders: Rash, urticaria.

7 DRUG INTERACTIONS

7.1 Concomitant Vaccine Administration

In clinical studies, MENHIBRIX was administered concomitantly with routinely recommended pediatric US-licensed vaccines [see Adverse Reactions (6.1) and Clinical Studies (14.2)].

If MENHIBRIX is administered concomitantly with other injectable vaccines, they should be given with separate syringes and at different injection sites. MENHIBRIX should not be mixed with any other vaccine in the same syringe or vial.

7.2 Interference With Laboratory Tests

Haemophilus b capsular polysaccharide derived from Haemophilus b Conjugate Vaccines has been detected in the urine of some vaccinees.[7] Urine antigen detection may not have a diagnostic value in suspected disease due to H. influenzae type b within 1 to 2 weeks after receipt of a H. influenzae type b-containing vaccine, including MENHIBRIX.

7.3 Immunosuppressive Therapies

Immunosuppressive therapies, including irradiation, antimetabolites, alkylating agents, cytotoxic drugs, and corticosteroids (used in greater than physiologic doses), may reduce the immune response to MENHIBRIX.

Table 1. Percentage of US Children from Study 009/010 With Solicited Local and General Adverse Events within 4 Days of Vaccination[a] With MENHIBRIX or Haemophilus b Conjugate Vaccine (Total Vaccinated Cohort)

	MENHIBRIX[b]				Haemophilus b Conjugate Vaccine[b,c]			
	Dose 1	Dose 2	Dose 3	Dose 4	Dose 1	Dose 2	Dose 3	Dose 4
Local[d]								
N	2,009	1,874	1,725	1,533	659	612	569	492
Pain, any	46.2	44.6	41.4	42.1	61.6	52.8	49.9	50.4
Pain, grade 3[e]	3.7	3.3	2.3	1.6	11.4	5.1	3.0	5.3
Redness, any	20.6	31.0	35.5	34.6	27.9	33.7	42.2	46.7
Redness, >30 mm	0.1	0.3	0.1	0.7	1.8	0.3	0.4	1.2
Swelling, any	14.7	20.4	23.8	25.4	20.5	20.8	28.6	31.7
Swelling, >30 mm	0.5	0.3	0.3	0.6	1.5	0.2	0.4	0.8
Systemic								
N	2,008-2,009	1,871	1,723	1,535-1,536	659	609-610	569	493-494
Irritability	67.5	70.8	65.8	62.1	76.9	75.1	65.4	66.1
Irritability, grade 3[f]	3.7	4.8	3.3	2.5	7.4	5.6	4.2	4.3
Drowsiness, any	62.8	57.7	49.5	48.7	66.9	61.8	52.4	48.5
Drowsiness, grade 3[g]	2.7	3.2	1.7	2.1	2.7	2.6	1.4	2.0
Loss of appetite, any	33.8	32.1	30.1	32.1	37.6	33.6	30.2	32.5
Loss of appetite, grade 3[h]	0.5	0.7	0.5	1.1	0.3	0.7	1.1	2.2
Fever, ≥100.4°F[i]	18.9	25.9	23.0	11.0	21.4	28.2	23.7	12.6
Fever, ≥102.2°F[i]	1.1	1.9	3.2	1.5	0.9	2.6	2.8	2.0
Fever, >104°F[i]	0.0	0.0	0.3	0.3	0.0	0.0	0.4	0.2

Total Vaccinated Cohort = all participants who received at least one dose of either vaccine.
N = number of participants who completed the symptom sheet for a given symptom at the specified dose.
[a] Within 4 days of vaccination defined as day of vaccination and the next 3 days.
[b] Co-administered with PEDIARIX and PCV7 at doses 1, 2, 3 and PCV7, MMR and varicella vaccines at dose 4.
[c] US-licensed monovalent Haemophilus b Conjugate Vaccine manufactured by Sanofi Pasteur SA for doses 1, 2, and 3 (PRP-T) and by Merck & Co., Inc for dose 4 (PRP-OMP).
[d] Local reactions at the injection site for MENHIBRIX or Haemophilus b Conjugate Vaccine.
[e] Cried when limb was moved/spontaneously painful.
[f] Crying that could not be comforted/prevented normal daily activities.
[g] Prevented normal daily activities.
[h] Not eating at all.
[i] Across both treatment groups, 54%, 56%, and 59% of participants had temperatures measured rectally following doses 1, 2, and 3, respectively; 45%, 44%, and 40% of participants had temperatures measured by the axillary route for doses 1, 2, and 3, respectively. For dose 4, >90% of participants had temperatures measured via the axillary route.

8 USE IN SPECIFIC POPULATIONS

8.1 Pregnancy

Pregnancy Category C

Animal reproduction studies have not been conducted with MENHIBRIX. It is also not known whether MENHIBRIX can cause fetal harm when administered to a pregnant woman or can affect reproduction capacity.

8.4 Pediatric Use

Safety and effectiveness of MENHIBRIX in children younger than 6 weeks of age and in children 19 months to 16 years of age have not been established.

11 DESCRIPTION

MENHIBRIX (Meningococcal Groups C and Y and Haemophilus b Tetanus Toxoid Conjugate Vaccine), for intramuscular injection, is supplied as a sterile, lyophilized powder which is reconstituted at the time of use with the accompanying saline diluent. MENHIBRIX contains Neisseria meningitidis serogroup C and Y capsular polysaccharide antigens and Haemophilus b capsular polysaccharide (polyribosyl-ribitol-phosphate [PRP]). The Neisseria meningitidis C strain and Y strain are grown in semi-synthetic media and undergo heat inactivation and purification. The PRP is a high molecular weight polymer prepared from the Haemophilus influenzae type b strain 20,752 grown in a synthetic medium that undergoes heat inactivation and purification. The tetanus toxin, prepared from Clostridium tetani grown in a semi-synthetic medium, is detoxified with formaldehyde and purified. Each capsular polysaccharide is individually covalently bound to the inactivated tetanus toxoid. After purification, the conjugate is lyophilized in the presence of sucrose as a stabilizer. The diluent for MENHIBRIX is a sterile saline solution (0.9% sodium chloride) supplied in vials.

When MENHIBRIX is reconstituted with the accompanying vial of saline diluent, each 0.5-mL dose is formulated to contain 5 mcg of purified Neisseria meningitidis C capsular polysaccharide conjugated to approximately 5 mcg of tetanus toxoid, 5 mcg of purified Neisseria meningitidis Y capsular polysaccharide conjugated to approximately 6.5 mcg of tetanus toxoid, and 2.5 mcg of purified Haemophilus b capsular polysaccharide conjugated to approximately 6.25 mcg of tetanus toxoid. Each dose also contains 96.8 mcg of Tris (trometamol)-HCl, 12.6 mg of sucrose, and ≤0.72 mcg of residual formaldehyde. MENHIBRIX does not contain preservatives. The lyophilized vaccine and saline diluent vial stoppers are not made with natural rubber latex.

12 CLINICAL PHARMACOLOGY

12.1 Mechanism of Action

Neisseria meningitidis: The presence of bactericidal anticapsular meningococcal antibodies has been associated with protection from invasive meningococcal disease.[8] MENHIBRIX induces production of bactericidal antibodies specific to the capsular polysaccharides of serogroups C and Y.

Haemophilus influenzae type b: Specific levels of antibodies to PRP (anti-PRP) have been shown to correlate with protection against invasive disease due to H. influenzae type b. Based on data from passive antibody studies[9] and a clinical efficacy study with unconjugated Haemophilus b polysaccharide vaccine[10], an anti-PRP concentration of 0.15 mcg/mL has been accepted as a minimal protective level. Data from an efficacy study with unconjugated Haemophilus b polysaccharide vaccine indicate that an anti-PRP concentration of ≥1.0 mcg/mL predicts protection through at least a 1-year period.[11,12] These antibody levels have been used to evaluate the effectiveness of H. influenzae type b-containing vaccines, including MENHIBRIX.

13 NONCLINICAL TOXICOLOGY

13.1 Carcinogenesis, Mutagenesis, Impairment of Fertility

MENHIBRIX has not been evaluated for carcinogenic or mutagenic potential, or for impairment of fertility.

14 CLINICAL STUDIES

14.1 Immunological Evaluation

In Study 009/010[5] the immune response to MENHIBRIX and control vaccines was evaluated in a subset of US participants. In this clinical study, MENHIBRIX and Hib control vaccines were administered concomitantly with routinely recommended US-licensed vaccines [see Adverse Reactions (6.1)]. Among participants in the ATP immunogenicity cohort for both vaccine groups combined, 47% were

Table 3. Comparison of anti-PRP Responses Following MENHIBRIX or Haemophilus b Conjugate Vaccine[a] (One Month After Dose 3 and 6 Weeks After Dose 4) in US Children Vaccinated at 2, 4, 6, and 12 to 15 Months of Age (ATP Cohort for Immunogenicity)

	Post-Dose 3		Post-Dose 4	
	MENHIBRIX	PRP-T	MENHIBRIX	PRP-OMP
Anti-PRP	N = 518	N = 171	N = 361	N = 126
% ≥0.15 mcg/mL	100	98.2	100	100
95% CI	99.3, 100	95.0, 99.6	99.0, 100	97.1, 100
% ≥1.0 mcg/mL	96.3[b]	91.2	99.2[b]	99.2
95% CI	94.3, 97.8	85.9, 95.0	97.6, 99.8	95.7, 100
GMC (mcg/mL)	11.0	6.5	34.9	20.2
95% CI	10.0, 12.1	5.3, 7.9	30.7, 39.6	16.4, 24.9

ATP = according to protocol; anti-PRP = antibody concentrations to *H. influenzae* capsular polysaccharide; CI = confidence interval; GMC = geometric mean antibody concentration.
N = number of US children eligible for inclusion in the ATP immunogenicity cohort for whom serological results were available for the post-dose 3 and post-dose 4 immunological evaluations.
[a] US-licensed monovalent Haemophilus b Conjugate Vaccine for doses 1, 2, and 3 (PRP-T) and for dose 4 (PRP-OMP).
[b] Non-inferiority was demonstrated (lower limit of 95% CI on the group difference of MENHIBRIX minus Haemophilus b Conjugate Vaccine ≥-10%).

female; 81% of participants were white, 8% were black, 4% were Hispanic, 1% were Asian, and 6% were of other racial/ethnic groups.

Study objectives included evaluation of *N. meningitidis* serogroups C (MenC) and Y (MenY) as measured by serum bactericidal assay using human complement (hSBA) and antibodies to PRP as measured by enzyme-linked immunosorbent assay (ELISA) in sera obtained approximately one month (range 21 to 48 days) after dose 3 of MENHIBRIX or PRP-T and approximately 6 weeks (range 35 to 56 days) after dose 4 of MENHIBRIX or PRP-OMP. The hSBA-MenC and hSBA-MenY geometric mean antibody titers (GMTs) and the percentage of participants with hSBA-MenC and hSBA-MenY levels ≥1:8 are presented in Table 2. Anti-PRP geometric mean antibody concentrations (GMCs) and the percentage of participants with anti-PRP levels ≥0.15 mcg/mL and ≥1.0 mcg/mL are presented in Table 3.

Table 2. Bactericidal Antibody Responses Following MENHIBRIX (One Month After Dose 3 and 6 Weeks After Dose 4) in US Children Vaccinated at 2, 4, 6, and 12 to 15 Months of Age (ATP Cohort for Immunogenicity)

	MENHIBRIX Post-Dose 3	MENHIBRIX Post-Dose 4
hSBA-MenC	N = 491	N = 331
% ≥1:8	98.8	98.5[a]
95% CI	97.4, 99.6	96.5, 99.5
GMT	968	2040
95% CI	864, 1084	1746, 2383
hSBA-MenY	N = 481	N = 342
% ≥1:8	95.8	98.8[a]
95% CI	93.7, 97.4	97.0, 99.7
GMT	237	1390
95% CI	206, 272	1205, 1602

ATP = according to protocol; CI = confidence interval; GMT = geometric mean antibody titer.
N = number of US children eligible for inclusion in the ATP immunogenicity cohort for whom serological results were available for the post-dose 3 and post-dose 4 immunological evaluations.
[a] Acceptance criteria were met (lower limit of 95% CI for the percentage of participants with hSBA-MenC and hSBA-MenY titers ≥1:8 ≥90% following 4 doses).

[See table 3 above]

14.2   Concomitant Vaccine Administration
In participants who received MENHIBRIX concomitantly with PEDIARIX and PCV7 at 2, 4, and 6 months of age, there was no evidence for reduced antibody response to pertussis antigens (GMC to pertussis toxin, filamentous hemagglutinin, and pertactin), diphtheria toxoid (antibody levels ≥0.1 IU/mL), tetanus toxoid (antibody levels ≥0.1 IU/mL), poliovirus types 1, 2, and 3 (neutralizing antibody levels ≥1:8 to each virus), hepatitis B (anti-hepatitis B surface antigen ≥10 mIU/mL) or PCV7 (antibody levels ≥0.2 mcg/mL and GMC to each serotype) relative to the response in control participants administered PRP-T concom-

itantly with PEDIARIX and PCV7. The immune responses to PEDIARIX[3,5] and PCV7[3] were evaluated one month following dose 3.

There was no evidence for interference in the immune response to MMR and varicella vaccines (initially seronegative participants with anti-measles ≥200 mIU/mL, anti-mumps ≥51 ED$_{50}$, anti-rubella ≥10 IU/mL, and anti-varicella ≥1:40) administered at 12 to 15 months of age concomitantly with MENHIBRIX and PCV7 relative to these vaccines administered concomitantly with PRP-OMP and PCV7.[4,5] The immune responses to MMR and varicella vaccines were evaluated 6 weeks post-vaccination. Data are insufficient to evaluate potential interference when a fourth PCV7 dose is administered concomitantly with MENHIBRIX at 12 to 15 months of age.

15   REFERENCES
All NCT numbers are as noted in the National Library of Medicine clinical trial database (see www.clinicaltrials.gov).

1. NCT00127855 (001).
2. NCT00129116 (003/004).
3. NCT00129129 (005/006).
4. NCT00134719 (007/008).
5. NCT00289783 (009/010).
6. NCT00345579/NCT00345683 (011/012).
7. Rothstein EP, Madore DV, Girone JAC, et al. Comparison of antigenuria after immunization with three *Haemophilus influenzae* type b conjugate vaccines. *Pediatr Infect Dis J* 1991;10:311-314.
8. Goldschneider I, Gotschlich EC, Artenstein MS. Human immunity to the meningococcus. I. The role of humoral antibodies. *J Exp Med* 1969;129:1307-1326.
9. Robbins JB, Parke JC, Schneerson R, et al. Quantitative measurement of "natural" and immunization-induced *Haemophilus influenzae* type b capsular polysaccharide antibodies. *Pediatr Res* 1973;7:103-110.
10. Peltola H, Käythy H, Sivonen A, et al. *Haemophilus influenzae* type b capsular polysaccharide vaccine in children: A double-blind field study of 100,000 vaccinees 3 months to 5 years of age in Finland. *Pediatrics* 1977;60:730-737.
11. Käythy H, Peltola H, Karanko V, et al. The protective level of serum antibodies to the capsular polysaccharide of *Haemophilus influenzae* type b. *J Infect Dis* 1983;147:1100.
12. Anderson P. The protective level of serum antibodies to the capsular polysaccharide of *Haemophilus influenzae* type b. *J Infect Dis* 1984;149:1034.

16   HOW SUPPLIED/STORAGE AND HANDLING
MENHIBRIX is available in single-dose vials of lyophilized vaccine, accompanied by vials containing 0.85 mL of saline diluent (packaged without syringes or needles).
Supplied as package of 10 doses (NDC 58160-801-11):
NDC 58160-809-01 Vial of lyophilized vaccine in Package of 10: NDC 58160-809-05
NDC 58160-813-01 Vial of saline diluent in Package of 10: NDC 58160-813-05

16.1   Storage Before Reconstitution
Lyophilized vaccine vials: Store refrigerated between 2° and 8°C (36° and 46°F). Protect vials from light.
Diluent: Store refrigerated or at controlled room temperature between 2° and 25°C (36° and 77°F). Do not freeze. Discard if the diluent has been frozen.

16.2   Storage After Reconstitution
After reconstitution, administer MENHIBRIX immediately. Do not freeze. Discard if the vaccine has been frozen.

17   PATIENT COUNSELING INFORMATION
- Inform parents or guardians of the potential benefits and risks of immunization with MENHIBRIX, and of the importance of completing the immunization series.
- Inform parents or guardians about the potential for adverse reactions that have been temporally associated with administration of MENHIBRIX or other vaccines containing similar components.
- Instruct parents or guardians to report any adverse events to their healthcare provider.
- Give parents or guardians the Vaccine Information Statements, which are required by the National Childhood Vaccine Injury Act of 1986 to be given prior to immunization. These materials are available free of charge at the Centers for Disease Control and Prevention (CDC) website (www.cdc.gov/vaccines).

HIBERIX, MENHIBRIX, and PEDIARIX are registered trademarks of the GlaxoSmithKline group of companies.
Manufactured by **GlaxoSmithKline Biologicals**
Rixensart, Belgium, US License 1617, and
Distributed by **GlaxoSmithKline**
Research Triangle Park, NC 27709
©2013, GlaxoSmithKline group of companies. All rights reserved.
MNX:2PI

MEPRON®
(atovaquone)
Suspension   ℞

DESCRIPTION
MEPRON (atovaquone) is an antiprotozoal agent. The chemical name of atovaquone is *trans*-2-[4-(4-chlorophenyl)cyclohexyl]-3-hydroxy-1,4-naphthalenedione. Atovaquone is a yellow crystalline solid that is practically insoluble in water. It has a molecular weight of 366.84 and the molecular formula $C_{22}H_{19}ClO_3$. The compound has the following structural formula:

MEPRON Suspension is a formulation of micro-fine particles of atovaquone. The atovaquone particles, reduced in size to facilitate absorption, are significantly smaller than those in the previously marketed tablet formulation. MEPRON Suspension is for oral administration and is bright yellow with a citrus flavor. Each teaspoonful (5 mL) contains 750 mg of atovaquone and the inactive ingredients benzyl alcohol, flavor, poloxamer 188, purified water, saccharin sodium, and xanthan gum.

MICROBIOLOGY
Mechanism of Action
Atovaquone is a hydroxy-1,4-naphthoquinone, an analog of ubiquinone, with antipneumocystis activity. The mechanism of action against *Pneumocystis jiroveci* has not been fully elucidated. In *Plasmodium* species, the site of action appears to be the cytochrome bc_1 complex (Complex III). Several metabolic enzymes are linked to the mitochondrial electron transport chain via ubiquinone. Inhibition of electron transport by atovaquone will result in indirect inhibition of these enzymes. The ultimate metabolic effects of such blockade may include inhibition of nucleic acid and ATP synthesis.

Activity In Vitro
Several laboratories, using different in vitro methodologies, have shown the IC_{50} (50% inhibitory concentration) of atovaquone against rat *P. jiroveci* to be in the range of 0.1 to 3.0 mcg/mL.

Drug Resistance
Phenotypic resistance to atovaquone in vitro has not been demonstrated for *P. jiroveci*. However, in 2 patients who developed *Pneumocystis carinii* pneumonia (PCP) after prophylaxis with atovaquone, DNA sequence analysis identified mutations in the predicted amino acid sequence of *P. jiroveci* cytochrome b (a likely target site for atovaquone). The clinical significance of this is unknown.

CLINICAL PHARMACOLOGY
Pharmacokinetics
Absorption
Atovaquone is a highly lipophilic compound with low aqueous solubility. The bioavailability of atovaquone is highly dependent on formulation and diet. The suspension formu-

lation provides an approximately 2-fold increase in atovaquone bioavailability in the fasting or fed state compared to the previously marketed tablet formulation. The absolute bioavailability of a 750-mg dose of MEPRON Suspension administered under fed conditions in 9 HIV-infected (CD4 >100 cells/mm³) volunteers was 47% ± 15%. In the same study, the bioavailability of a 750-mg dose of the previously marketed tablet formulation was 23% ± 11%. Administering atovaquone with food enhances its absorption by approximately 2 fold. In one study, 16 healthy volunteers received a single dose of 750 mg MEPRON Suspension after an overnight fast and following a standard breakfast (23 g fat: 610 kCal). The mean (±SD) area under the concentration-time curve (AUC) values were 324 ± 115 and 801 ± 320 hr•mcg/mL under fasting and fed conditions, respectively, representing a 2.6 ± 1.0-fold increase. The effect of food (23 g fat: 400 kCal) on plasma atovaquone concentrations was also evaluated in a multiple-dose, randomized, crossover study in 19 HIV-infected volunteers (CD4 <200 cells/mm³) receiving daily doses of 500 mg MEPRON Suspension. AUC was 280 ± 114 hr•mcg/mL when atovaquone was administered with food as compared to 169 ± 77 hr•mcg/mL under fasting conditions. Maximum plasma atovaquone concentration (C_{max}) was 15.1 ± 6.1 and 8.8 ± 3.7 mcg/mL when atovaquone was administered with food and under fasting conditions, respectively.

Dose Proportionality

Plasma atovaquone concentrations do not increase proportionally with dose. When MEPRON Suspension was administered with food at dosage regimens of 500 mg once daily, 750 mg once daily, and 1,000 mg once daily, average steady-state plasma atovaquone concentrations were 11.7 ± 4.8, 12.5 ± 5.8, and 13.5 ± 5.1 mcg/mL, respectively. The corresponding C_{max} concentrations were 15.1 ± 6.1, 15.3 ± 7.6, and 16.8 ± 6.4 mcg/mL. When MEPRON Suspension was administered to 5 HIV-infected volunteers at a dose of 750 mg twice daily, the average steady-state plasma atovaquone concentration was 21.0 ± 4.9 mcg/mL and C_{max} was 24.0 ± 5.7 mcg/mL. The minimum plasma atovaquone concentration (C_{min}) associated with the 750-mg twice-daily regimen was 16.7 ± 4.6 mcg/mL.

Distribution

Following the intravenous administration of atovaquone, the volume of distribution at steady state (Vd_{ss}) was 0.60 ± 0.17 L/kg (n = 9). Atovaquone is extensively bound to plasma proteins (99.9%) over the concentration range of 1 to 90 mcg/mL. In 3 HIV-infected children who received 750 mg atovaquone as the tablet formulation 4 times daily for 2 weeks, the cerebrospinal fluid concentrations of atovaquone were 0.04, 0.14, and 0.26 mcg/mL, representing less than 1% of the plasma concentration.

Elimination

The plasma clearance of atovaquone following intravenous (IV) administration in 9 HIV-infected volunteers was 10.4 ± 5.5 mL/min (0.15 ± 0.09 mL/min/kg). The half-life of atovaquone was 62.5 ± 35.3 hours after IV administration and ranged from 67.0 ± 33.4 to 77.6 ± 23.1 hours across studies following administration of MEPRON Suspension. The half-life of atovaquone is long due to presumed enterohepatic cycling and eventual fecal elimination. In a study where ¹⁴C-labelled atovaquone was administered to healthy volunteers, greater than 94% of the dose was recovered as unchanged atovaquone in the feces over 21 days. There was little or no excretion of atovaquone in the urine (less than 0.6%). There is indirect evidence that atovaquone may undergo limited metabolism; however, a specific metabolite has not been identified.

Special Populations

Pediatrics

In a study of MEPRON Suspension in 27 HIV-infected, asymptomatic infants and children between 1 month and 13 years of age, the pharmacokinetics of atovaquone were age dependent. These patients were dosed once daily with food for 12 days. The average steady-state plasma atovaquone concentrations in the 24 patients with available concentration data are shown in Table 1.

Table 1. Average Steady-State Plasma Atovaquone Concentrations in Pediatric Patients

Age	Dose of MEPRON Suspension		
	10 mg/kg	30 mg/kg	45 mg/kg
	Average C_{ss} in mcg/mL (mean ± SD)		
1-3 months	5.9 (n = 1)	27.8 ± 5.8 (n = 4)	____
>3-24 months	5.7 ± 5.1 (n = 4)	9.8 ± 3.2 (n = 4)	15.4 ± 6.6 (n = 4)
>2-13 years	16.8 ± 6.4 (n = 4)	37.1 ± 10.9 (n = 3)	

Hepatic/Renal Impairment

The pharmacokinetics of atovaquone have not been studied in patients with hepatic or renal impairment.

Drug Interactions

Rifampin

In a study with 13 HIV-infected volunteers, the oral administration of rifampin 600 mg every 24 hours with MEPRON Suspension 750 mg every 12 hours resulted in a 52% ± 13% decrease in the average steady-state plasma atovaquone concentration and a 37% ± 42% increase in the average steady-state plasma rifampin concentration. The half-life of atovaquone decreased from 82 ± 36 hours when administered without rifampin to 50 ± 16 hours with rifampin. Rifabutin, another rifamycin, is structurally similar to rifampin and may possibly have some of the same drug interactions as rifampin. No interaction trials have been conducted with MEPRON and rifabutin.

Trimethoprim/Sulfamethoxazole (TMP-SMX)

The possible interaction between atovaquone and TMP-SMX was evaluated in 6 HIV-infected adult volunteers as part of a larger multiple-dose, dose-escalation, and chronic dosing study of MEPRON Suspension. In this crossover study, MEPRON Suspension 500 mg once daily, or TMP-SMX tablets (160 mg trimethoprim and 800 mg sulfamethoxazole) twice daily, or the combination were administered with food to achieve steady state. No difference was observed in the average steady-state plasma atovaquone concentration after coadministration with TMP-SMX. Coadministration of MEPRON with TMP-SMX resulted in a 17% and 8% decrease in average plasma steady-state concentrations of trimethoprim and sulfamethoxazole in plasma, respectively. This effect is minor and would not be expected to produce clinically significant events.

Zidovudine

Data from 14 HIV-infected volunteers who were given atovaquone tablets 750 mg every 12 hours with zidovudine 200 mg every 8 hours showed a 24% ± 12% decrease in zidovudine apparent oral clearance, leading to a 35% ± 23% increase in plasma zidovudine AUC. The glucuronide metabolite:parent ratio decreased from a mean of 4.5 when zidovudine was administered alone to 3.1 when zidovudine was administered with atovaquone tablets. This effect is minor and would not be expected to produce clinically significant events. Zidovudine had no effect on atovaquone pharmacokinetics.

Relationship Between Plasma Atovaquone Concentration and Clinical Outcome

In a comparative study of atovaquone tablets with TMP-SMX for oral treatment of mild-to-moderate *PCP* (see INDICATIONS AND USAGE), where AIDS patients received 750 mg atovaquone tablets 3 times daily for 21 days, the mean steady-state atovaquone concentration was 13.9 ± 6.9 mcg/mL (n = 133). Analysis of these data established a relationship between plasma atovaquone concentration and successful treatment. This is shown in Table 2.

Table 2. Relationship Between Plasma Atovaquone Concentration and Successful Treatment

Steady-State Plasma Atovaquone Concentrations (mcg/mL)	Successful Treatment[a] No. Successes/No. in Group (%)			
	Observed		Predicted[b]	
0 to <5	0/6	(0)	1.5/6	(25)
5 to <10	18/26	(69)	14.7/26	(57)
10 to <15	30/38	(79)	31.9/38	(84)
15 to <20	18/19	(95)	18.1/19	(95)
20 to <25	18/18	(100)	17.8/18	(99)
25+	6/6	(100)	6/6	(100)

[a] Successful treatment was defined as improvement in clinical and respiratory measures persisting at least 4 weeks after cessation of therapy. This was based on data from patients for which both outcome and steady-state plasma atovaquone concentration data are available.
[b] Based on logistic regression analysis.

A dosing regimen of MEPRON Suspension for the treatment of mild-to-moderate PCP has been selected to achieve average plasma atovaquone concentrations of approximately 20 mcg/mL, because this plasma concentration was previously shown to be well tolerated and associated with the highest treatment success rates (Table 2). In an open-label PCP treatment study with MEPRON Suspension, dosing regimens of 1,000 mg once daily, 750 mg twice daily, 1,500 mg once daily, and 1,000 mg twice daily were explored. The average steady-state plasma atovaquone concentration achieved at the 750-mg twice-daily dose given with meals was 22.0 ± 10.1 mcg/mL (n = 18).

INDICATIONS AND USAGE

MEPRON Suspension is indicated for the prevention of *Pneumocystis jiroveci* pneumonia in patients who are intolerant to trimethoprim-sulfamethoxazole (TMP-SMX).

MEPRON Suspension is also indicated for the acute oral treatment of mild-to-moderate PCP in patients who are intolerant to TMP-SMX.

Prevention of PCP

The indication for prevention of PCP is based on the results of 2 clinical trials comparing MEPRON Suspension to dapsone or aerosolized pentamidine in HIV-infected adult and adolescent patients at risk of PCP (CD4 count <200 cells/mm³ or a prior episode of PCP) and intolerant to TMP-SMX.

Dapsone Comparative Study

This randomized, open-label trial enrolled a total of 1,057 patients at 48 study centers. Patients were randomized to receive 1,500 mg MEPRON Suspension once daily (n = 536) or 100 mg dapsone once daily (n = 521). Median follow-up was 24 months. Patients randomized to the dapsone arm who were seropositive for *Toxoplasma gondii* and had a CD4 count <100 cells/mm³ also received pyrimethamine and folinic acid. PCP event rates are shown in Table 3. There was no significant difference in mortality rates between the groups.

Aerosolized Pentamidine Comparative Study

This randomized, open-label trial enrolled a total of 549 patients at 35 study centers. Patients were randomized to receive 1,500 mg MEPRON Suspension once daily (n = 175), 750 mg MEPRON Suspension once daily (n = 188), or 300 mg aerosolized pentamidine once monthly (n = 186). Median follow-up was 11.3 months. The results of the PCP event rates appear in Table 3. There were no significant differences in mortality rates among the groups.

[See table 3 at top of next page]

Treatment of PCP

The indication for treatment of mild-to-moderate PCP is based on the results of comparative pharmacokinetic studies of the suspension and tablet formulations (see CLINICAL PHARMACOLOGY) and clinical efficacy studies of the tablet formulation which established a relationship between plasma atovaquone concentration and successful treatment. The results of a randomized, double-blind trial comparing MEPRON to TMP-SMX in AIDS patients with mild-to-moderate PCP (defined in the study protocol as an alveolar-arterial oxygen diffusion gradient [(A-a)DO₂]≤45 mm Hg and PaO₂≥60 mm Hg on room air) and a randomized trial comparing MEPRON to IV pentamidine isethionate in patients with mild-to-moderate PCP intolerant to trimethoprim or sulfa-antimicrobials are summarized below:

TMP-SMX Comparative Study

This double-blind, randomized trial initiated in 1990 was designed to compare the safety and efficacy of MEPRON to that of TMP-SMX for the treatment of AIDS patients with histologically confirmed PCP. Only patients with mild-to-moderate PCP were eligible for enrollment.

A total of 408 patients were enrolled into the trial at 37 study centers. Eighty-six patients without histologic confirmation of PCP were excluded from the efficacy analyses. Of the 322 patients with histologically confirmed PCP, 160 were randomized to receive MEPRON and 162 to TMP-SMX.

Study participants randomized to treatment with MEPRON were to receive 750 mg MEPRON (three 250-mg tablets) 3 times daily for 21 days and those randomized to TMP-SMX were to receive 320 mg TMP plus 1,600 mg SMX 3 times daily for 21 days.

Therapy success was defined as improvement in clinical and respiratory measures persisting at least 4 weeks after cessation of therapy. Therapy failures included lack of response, treatment discontinuation due to an adverse experience, and unevaluable.

There was a significant difference (P = 0.03) in mortality rates between the treatment groups. Among the 322 patients with confirmed PCP, 13 of 160 (8%) patients treated with MEPRON and 4 of 162 (2.5%) patients receiving TMP-SMX died during the 21-day treatment course or 8-week follow-up period. In the intent-to-treat analysis for all 408 randomized patients, there were 16 (8%) deaths in the arm treated with MEPRON and 7 (3.4%) deaths in the TMP-SMX arm (P = 0.051). Of the 13 patients treated with MEPRON who died, 4 died of PCP and 5 died with a combination of bacterial infections and PCP; bacterial infections did not appear to be a factor in any of the 4 deaths among TMP-SMX-treated patients.

A correlation between plasma atovaquone concentrations and death was demonstrated; in general, patients with lower plasma concentrations were more likely to die. For those patients for whom day 4 plasma atovaquone concentration data are available, 5 (63%) of the 8 patients with concentrations <5 mcg/mL died during participation in the study. However, only 1 (2.0%) of the 49 patients with day 4 plasma atovaquone concentrations ≥5 mcg/mL died. Sixty-two percent of patients on MEPRON and 64% of patients on TMP-SMX were classified as protocol-defined therapy successes (Table 4).

Table 3. Confirmed or Presumed/Probable PCP Events (As-Treated Analysis)[a]

Assessment	Study 115-211		Study 115-213		
	Atovaquone 1,500 mg/day (n = 527)	Dapsone 100 mg/day (n = 510)	Atovaquone 750 mg/day (n = 188)	Atovaquone 1,500 mg/day (n = 172)	Aerosolized Pentamidine 300 mg/month (n = 169)
%	15	19	23	18	17
Relative Risk[b] (CI)[c]	0.77 (0.57, 1.04)		1.47 (0.86, 2.50)	1.14 (0.63, 2.06)	

[a]Those events occurring during or within 30 days of stopping assigned treatment.
[b]Relative risk <1 favors atovaquone and values >1 favor comparator. These trials were designed to show superiority of atovaquone to the comparator. This was not shown.
[c]The confidence level of the interval for the dapsone comparative study was 95% and for the pentamidine comparative study was 97.5%.
An analysis of all PCP events (intent-to-treat analysis) showed results similar to those above.

Table 4. Outcome of Treatment for PCP-Positive Patients Enrolled in the TMP-SMX Comparative Study

Outcome of Therapy[a]	Number of Patients (% of Total)				P Value
	MEPRON (n = 160)		TMP-SMX (n = 162)		
Therapy success	99	(62)	103	(64)	0.75
Therapy failure					
-Lack of response	28	(17)	10	(6)	<0.01
-Adverse experience	11	(7)	33	(20)	<0.01
-Unevaluable	22	(14)	16	(10)	0.28
Required alternate PCP therapy during study	55	(34)	55	(34)	0.95

[a] As defined by the protocol and described in study description above.

Table 5. Outcome of Treatment for PCP-Positive Patients Enrolled in the Pentamidine Comparative Study

Outcome of Therapy	Primary Treatment					Salvage Treatment				
	MEPRON (n = 56)		Pentamidine (n = 53)		P Value	MEPRON (n = 14)		Pentamidine (n = 11)		P Value
Therapy success	32	(57%)	21	(40%)	0.09	13	(93%)	7	(64%)	0.14
Therapy failure										
-Lack of response	16	(29%)	9	(17%)	0.18	0		0		—
-Adverse experience	2	(3.6%)	19	(36%)	<0.01	0		3	(27%)	0.07
-Unevaluable	6	(11%)	4	(8%)	0.75	1	(7%)	1	(9%)	1.00
Required alternate PCP therapy during study	19	(34%)	29	(55%)	0.04	0		4	(36%)	0.03

[See table 4 above]
The failure rate due to lack of response was significantly larger for patients receiving MEPRON while the failure rate due to adverse experiences was significantly larger for patients receiving TMP-SMX.

There were no significant differences in the effect of either treatment on additional indicators of response (i.e., arterial blood gas measurements, vital signs, serum LDH levels, clinical symptoms, and chest radiographs).

Pentamidine Comparative Study
This unblinded, randomized trial initiated in 1991 was designed to compare the safety and efficacy of MEPRON to that of pentamidine for the treatment of histologically confirmed mild or moderate PCP in AIDS patients. Approximately 80% of the patients either had a history of intolerance to trimethoprim or sulfa-antimicrobials (the primary therapy group) or were experiencing intolerance to TMP-SMX with treatment of an episode of PCP at the time of enrollment in the study (the salvage treatment group).

Patients randomized to MEPRON were to receive 750 mg atovaquone (three 250-mg tablets) 3 times daily for 21 days and those randomized to pentamidine isethionate were to receive a 3- to 4-mg/kg single IV infusion daily for 21 days.
A total of 174 patients were enrolled into the trial at 22 study centers. Thirty-nine patients without histologic confirmation of PCP were excluded from the efficacy analyses. Of the 135 patients with histologically confirmed PCP, 70 were randomized to receive MEPRON and 65 to pentamidine. One hundred and ten (110) of these were in the primary therapy group and 25 were in the salvage therapy

group. One patient in the primary therapy group randomized to receive pentamidine did not receive study medication.

There was no difference in mortality rates between the treatment groups. Among the 135 patients with confirmed PCP, 10 of 70 (14%) patients randomized to MEPRON and 9 of 65 (14%) patients randomized to pentamidine died during the 21-day treatment course or 8-week follow-up period. In the intent-to-treat analysis for all randomized patients, there were 11 (12.5%) deaths in the arm treated with MEPRON and 12 (14%) deaths in the pentamidine arm. For those patients for whom day 4 plasma atovaquone concentrations are available, 3 of 5 (60%) patients with concentrations <5 mcg/mL died during participation in the study. However, only 2 of 21 (9%) patients with day 4 plasma concentrations ≥5 mcg/mL died.

The therapeutic outcomes for the 134 patients who received study medication in this trial are presented in Table 5.
[See table 5 above]

CONTRAINDICATIONS

MEPRON Suspension is contraindicated for patients who develop or have a history of potentially life-threatening allergic reactions to any of the components of the formulation.

WARNINGS

Clinical experience with MEPRON for the treatment of PCP has been limited to patients with mild-to-moderate PCP ([(A-a)DO$_2$]^1 ≤45 mm Hg). Treatment of more severe episodes of PCP has not been systematically studied with this agent. Also, the efficacy of MEPRON in patients who are failing therapy with TMP-SMX has not been systematically studied.

PRECAUTIONS
General
Absorption of orally administered MEPRON is limited but can be significantly increased when the drug is taken with food. Plasma atovaquone concentrations have been shown to correlate with the likelihood of successful treatment and survival. Therefore, parenteral therapy with other agents should be considered for patients who have difficulty taking MEPRON with food (see CLINICAL PHARMACOLOGY). Gastrointestinal disorders may limit absorption of orally administered drugs. Patients with these disorders also may not achieve plasma concentrations of atovaquone associated with response to therapy in controlled trials.

Based upon the spectrum of in vitro antimicrobial activity, atovaquone is not effective therapy for concurrent pulmonary conditions such as bacterial, viral, or other fungal pneumonia or mycobacterial diseases. Clinical deterioration in patients may be due to infections with other pathogens, as well as progressive PCP. All patients with acute PCP should be carefully evaluated for other possible causes of pulmonary disease and treated with additional agents as appropriate.

Rare cases of hepatitis, elevated liver function tests and one case of fatal liver failure have been reported in patients treated with atovaquone. A causal relationship between atovaquone use and these events could not be established because of numerous confounding medical conditions and concomitant drug therapies. (See ADVERSE REACTIONS.) If it is necessary to treat patients with severe hepatic impairment, caution is advised and administration should be closely monitored.

Information for Patients
The importance of taking the prescribed dose of MEPRON should be stressed. Patients should be instructed to take their daily doses of MEPRON with meals, as the presence of food will significantly improve the absorption of the drug.

Drug Interactions
Atovaquone is highly bound to plasma protein (>99.9%). Therefore, caution should be used when administering MEPRON concurrently with other highly plasma protein-bound drugs with narrow therapeutic indices, as competition for binding sites may occur. The extent of plasma protein binding of atovaquone in human plasma is not affected by the presence of therapeutic concentrations of phenytoin (15 mcg/mL), nor is the binding of phenytoin affected by the presence of atovaquone.

Rifampin
Coadministration of rifampin and MEPRON Suspension results in a significant decrease in average steady-state plasma atovaquone concentrations (see CLINICAL PHARMACOLOGY: Drug Interactions). Alternatives to rifampin should be considered during the course of PCP treatment with MEPRON.

Rifabutin, another rifamycin, is structurally similar to rifampin and may possibly have some of the same drug interactions as rifampin. No interaction trials have been conducted with MEPRON and rifabutin.

Drug/Laboratory Test Interactions
It is not known if MEPRON interferes with clinical laboratory test or assay results.

Carcinogenesis, Mutagenesis, Impairment of Fertility
Carcinogenicity studies in rats were negative; 24-month studies in mice showed treatment-related increases in incidence of hepatocellular adenoma and hepatocellular carcinoma at all doses tested which ranged from 1.4 to 3.6 times the average steady-state plasma concentrations in humans during acute treatment of *PCP*. Atovaquone was negative with or without metabolic activation in the Ames *Salmonella* mutagenicity assay, the Mouse Lymphoma mutagenesis assay, and the Cultured Human Lymphocyte cytogenetic assay. No evidence of genotoxicity was observed in the in vivo Mouse Micronucleus assay.

Pregnancy
Pregnancy Category C. Atovaquone was not teratogenic and did not cause reproductive toxicity in rats at plasma concentrations up to 2 to 3 times the estimated human exposure. Atovaquone caused maternal toxicity in rabbits at plasma concentrations that were approximately one half the estimated human exposure. Mean fetal body lengths and weights were decreased and there were higher numbers of early resorption and post-implantation loss per dam. It is not clear whether these effects were caused by atovaquone directly or were secondary to maternal toxicity. Concentrations of atovaquone in rabbit fetuses averaged 30% of the concurrent maternal plasma concentrations. In a separate study in rats given a single ^{14}C-radiolabelled dose, concentrations of radiocarbon in rat fetuses were 18% (middle gestation) and 60% (late gestation) of concurrent maternal plasma concentrations. There are no adequate and well-controlled studies in pregnant women. MEPRON should be used during pregnancy only if the potential benefit justifies the potential risk to the fetus.

Nursing Mothers
It is not known whether atovaquone is excreted into human milk. Because many drugs are excreted into human milk,

caution should be exercised when MEPRON is administered to a nursing woman. In a rat study, atovaquone concentrations in the milk were 30% of the concurrent atovaquone concentrations in the maternal plasma.

Pediatric Use
Evidence of safety and effectiveness in pediatric patients has not been established. A relationship between plasma atovaquone concentrations and successful treatment of PCP has been established in adults (see Table 2). In a study of MEPRON Suspension in 27 HIV-infected, asymptomatic infants and children between 1 month and 13 years of age, the pharmacokinetics of atovaquone were age-dependent (see CLINICAL PHARMACOLOGY: Special Populations). No drug-related treatment-limiting adverse events were observed in the pharmacokinetic study.

Geriatric Use
Clinical studies of MEPRON did not include sufficient numbers of subjects aged 65 and over to determine whether they respond differently from younger subjects. Other reported clinical experience has not identified differences in responses between the elderly and younger patients. In general, dose selection for an elderly patient should be cautious, reflecting the greater frequency of decreased hepatic, renal, or cardiac function, and of concomitant disease or other drug therapy.

ADVERSE REACTIONS
Because many patients who participated in clinical trials with MEPRON had complications of advanced HIV disease, it was often difficult to distinguish adverse events caused by MEPRON from those caused by underlying medical conditions. There were no life-threatening or fatal adverse experiences caused by MEPRON.

PCP Prevention Studies
In the dapsone comparative study of MEPRON Suspension, adverse experience data were collected only for treatment-limiting events. Among the entire population (n = 1,057), treatment-limiting events occurred at similar frequencies in patients treated with MEPRON Suspension or dapsone (Table 6). Among patients who were taking neither dapsone nor atovaquone at enrollment (n = 487), treatment-limiting events occurred in 43% of patients treated with dapsone and 20% of patients treated with MEPRON Suspension (P <0.001). In both populations, the type of treatment-limiting events differed between the 2 treatment arms. Hypersensitivity reactions (rash, fever, allergic reaction) and anemia were more common in patients treated with dapsone, while gastrointestinal events (nausea, diarrhea, and vomiting) were more common in patients treated with MEPRON Suspension.

[See table 6 above]

Table 7 summarizes the clinical adverse experiences reported by ≥20% of patients in any group in the aerosolized pentamidine comparative study of MEPRON Suspension (n = 549), regardless of attribution. The incidence of adverse experiences at the recommended dose was similar to that seen with aerosolized pentamidine. Rash was the only individual adverse experience that occurred significantly more commonly in patients treated with both dosages of MEPRON Suspension (39% to 46%) than in patients treated with aerosolized pentamidine (28%). Among patients treated with MEPRON Suspension, there was no evidence of a dose-related increase in the incidence of adverse experiences. Treatment-limiting adverse experiences occurred less often in patients treated with aerosolized pentamidine (7%) than in patients treated with 1,500 mg MEPRON Suspension once daily (25%, P≤0.001) or 750 mg MEPRON Suspension once daily (16%, P = 0.004). The most common adverse experiences requiring discontinuation of dosing in the group receiving 1,500 mg MEPRON Suspension once daily were rash (6%), diarrhea (4%), and nausea (3%). The most common adverse experience requiring discontinuation of dosing in the group receiving aerosolized pentamidine was bronchospasm (2%).

[See table 7 above]

Other events occurring in ≥10% of the patients receiving the recommended dose of MEPRON included sweating, flu syndrome, pain, sinusitis, pruritus, insomnia, depression, and myalgia. Bronchospasm occurred more frequently in patients receiving aerosolized pentamidine (11%) than in patients receiving MEPRON 1,500 mg/day (4%) and MEPRON 750 mg/day (2%).

Neither MEPRON nor aerosolized pentamidine was associated with a substantial change from baseline values in any measured laboratory parameter, nor were there any significant differences in any measured laboratory parameter between MEPRON and aerosolized pentamidine. Some patients had laboratory abnormalities considered serious by the investigator or that contributed to discontinuation of therapy.

PCP Treatment Studies
Table 8 summarizes all the clinical adverse experiences reported by ≥5% of the study population during the TMP-SMX comparative study of MEPRON (n = 408), regardless of attribution. The incidence of adverse experiences with MEPRON Suspension at the recommended dose was similar to that seen with the tablet formulation of atovaquone.

Table 6. Treatment-Limiting Adverse Experiences in the Dapsone Comparative PCP Prevention Study

Treatment-Limiting Adverse Experience	Percentage of Patients with Treatment-Limiting Adverse Experience			
	All Patients		Patients Not Taking Either Drug at Enrollment	
	MEPRON 1,500 mg/day (n = 536)	Dapsone 100 mg/day (n = 521)	MEPRON 1,500 mg/day (n = 238)	Dapsone 100 mg/day (n = 249)
Any event	24.4	25.9	20.2	43.4
Rash	6.3	8.8	7.6	16.1
Nausea	4.1	0.6	2.5	0.8
Diarrhea	3.2	0.2	2.1	0.4
Vomiting	2.2	0.6	1.3	0.8
Allergic reaction	1.1	2.9	0.8	4.8
Fever	0.6	2.9	0	5.6
Anemia	0	1.5	0	2.0

Table 7. Treatment-Emergent Adverse Experiences in the Aerosolized Pentamidine Comparative PCP Prevention Study

Treatment-Emergent Adverse Experience	Percentage of Patients with Treatment-Emergent Adverse Experience		
	MEPRON 1,500 mg/day (n = 175)	MEPRON 750 mg/day (n = 188)	Aerosolized Pentamidine (n = 186)
Diarrhea	42	42	35
Rash	39	46	28
Headache	28	31	22
Nausea	26	32	23
Cough increased	25	25	31
Fever	25	31	18
Rhinitis	24	18	17
Asthenia	22	31	31
Infection	22	18	19
Abdominal pain	20	21	20
Dyspnea	15	21	16
Vomiting	15	22	11
Patients discontinuing therapy due to an adverse experience	25	16	7
Patients reporting at least 1 adverse experience	98	96	89

Table 8. Treatment-Emergent Adverse Experiences in the TMP-SMX Comparative PCP Treatment Study

Treatment-Emergent Adverse Experience	Percentage of Patients with Treatment-Emergent Adverse Experience	
	MEPRON (n = 203)	TMP-SMX (n = 205)
Rash (including maculopapular)	23	34
Nausea	21	44
Diarrhea	19	7
Headache	16	22
Vomiting	14	35
Fever	14	25
Insomnia	10	9
Asthenia	8	8
Pruritus	5	9
Monilia, oral	5	10
Abdominal pain	4	7
Constipation	3	17
Dizziness	3	8
Patients discontinuing therapy due to an adverse experience	9	24
Patients reporting at least 1 adverse experience	63	65

Although an equal percentage of patients receiving MEPRON and TMP-SMX reported at least 1 adverse experience, more patients receiving TMP-SMX required discontinuation of therapy due to an adverse event. Twenty-four percent of patients receiving TMP-SMX were prematurely discontinued from therapy due to an adverse experience versus 9% of patients receiving MEPRON. Four percent of patients receiving MEPRON had therapy discontinued due to development of rash. The majority of cases of rash among patients receiving MEPRON were mild and did not require the discontinuation of dosing. The only other clinical adverse experience that led to premature discontinuation of dosing of MEPRON by more than 1 patient was vomiting (<1%). The most common adverse experience requiring discontinuation of dosing in the TMP-SMX group was rash (8%).

Laboratory test abnormalities reported for ≥5% of the study population during the treatment period are summarized in Table 9. Two percent of patients treated with MEPRON and 7% of patients treated with TMP-SMX had therapy prematurely discontinued due to elevations in ALT/AST. In general, patients treated with MEPRON developed fewer abnormalities in measures of hepatocellular function (ALT, AST, alkaline phosphatase) or amylase values than patients treated with TMP-SMX.

Table 9. Treatment-Emergent Laboratory Test Abnormalities in the TMP-SMX Comparative PCP Treatment Study

Laboratory Test Abnormality	Percentage of Patients Developing a Laboratory Test Abnormality	
	MEPRON	TMP-SMX
Anemia (Hgb<8.0 g/dL)	6	7
Neutropenia (ANC<750 cells/mm³)	3	9
Elevated ALT (>5 × ULN)	6	16
Elevated AST (>5 × ULN)	4	14
Elevated alkaline phosphatase (>2.5 × ULN)	8	6
Elevated amylase (>1.5 × ULN)	7	12
Hyponatremia (<0.96 × LLN)	7	26

ULN = upper limit of normal range.
LLN = lower limit of normal range.

Table 10 summarizes the clinical adverse experiences reported by ≥5% of the primary therapy study population (n = 144) during the comparative trial of MEPRON and intravenous pentamidine, regardless of attribution. A slightly lower percentage of patients who received MEPRON reported occurrence of adverse events than did those who received pentamidine (63% vs 72%). However, only 7% of patients discontinued treatment with MEPRON due to adverse events, while 41% of patients who received pentamidine discontinued treatment for this reason (P<0.001). Of the 5 patients who discontinued therapy with MEPRON, 3 reported rash (4%). Rash was not severe in any patient. No other reason for discontinuation of MEPRON was cited more than once. The most frequently cited reasons for discontinuation of pentamidine therapy were hypoglycemia (11%) and vomiting (9%).

Table 10. Treatment-Emergent Adverse Experiences in the Pentamidine Comparative PCP Treatment Study (Primary Therapy Group)

Treatment-Emergent Adverse Experience	Percentage of Patients with Treatment-Emergent Adverse Experience	
	MEPRON (n = 73)	Pentamidine (n = 71)
Fever	40	25
Nausea	22	37
Rash	22	13
Diarrhea	21	31
Insomnia	19	14
Headache	18	28
Vomiting	14	17
Cough	14	1
Abdominal pain	10	11
Pain	10	10
Sweat	10	3
Monilia, oral	10	3
Asthenia	8	14
Dizziness	8	14
Anxiety	7	10
Anorexia	7	10
Sinusitis	7	6
Dyspepsia	5	10
Rhinitis	5	7
Taste perversion	3	13
Hypoglycemia	1	15
Hypotension	1	10
Patients discontinuing therapy due to an adverse experience	7	41
Patients reporting at least 1 adverse experience	63	72

Laboratory test abnormalities reported in ≥5% of patients in the pentamidine comparative study are presented in Table 11. Laboratory abnormality was reported as the reason for discontinuation of treatment in 2 of 73 patients who received MEPRON. One patient (1%) had elevated creatinine and BUN levels and 1 patient (1%) had elevated amylase levels. Laboratory abnormalities were the sole or contributing factor in 14 patients who prematurely discontinued pentamidine therapy. In the 71 patients who received pentamidine, laboratory parameters most frequently reported as reasons for discontinuation were hypoglycemia (11%), elevated creatinine levels (6%), and leukopenia (4%).

Table 11. Treatment-Emergent Laboratory Test Abnormalities in the Pentamidine Comparative PCP Treatment Study

Laboratory Test Abnormality	Percentage of Patients Developing a Laboratory Test Abnormality	
	MEPRON	Pentamidine
Anemia (Hgb<8.0 g/dL)	4	9
Neutropenia (ANC<750 cells/mm³)	5	9
Hyponatremia (<0.96 × LLN)	10	10
Hyperkalemia (>1.18 × ULN)	0	5
Alkaline phosphatase (>2.5 × ULN)	5	2
Hyperglycemia (>1.8 × ULN)	9	13
Elevated AST (>5 × ULN)	0	5
Elevated amylase (>1.5 × ULN)	8	4
Elevated creatinine (>1.5 × ULN)	0	7

ULN = upper limit of normal range.
LLN = lower limit of normal range.

Postmarketing Experience
In addition to adverse events reported from clinical trials, the following events have been identified during post-approval use of MEPRON. Because they are reported voluntarily from a population of unknown size, estimates of frequency cannot be made. These events have been chosen for inclusion due to a combination of their seriousness, frequency of reporting, or potential causal connection to MEPRON.

Blood and Lymphatic System Disorders:
Methemoglobinemia, thrombocytopenia.
Immune System Disorders:
Hypersensitivity reactions including angioedema, bronchospasm, throat tightness, and urticaria.
Eye Disorders:
Vortex keratopathy.
Gastrointestinal Disorders:
Pancreatitis.
Hepatobiliary Disorders:
Rare cases of hepatitis, and one case of fatal liver failure have been reported with atovaquone usage.
Skin and Subcutaneous Tissue Disorders:
Erythema multiforme, Stevens-Johnson syndrome, and skin desquamation have been reported in patients receiving multiple drug therapy including atovaquone.
Renal and Urinary Disorders:
Acute renal impairment.

OVERDOSAGE

There is no known antidote for atovaquone, and it is currently unknown if atovaquone is dialyzable. The median lethal oral dose is higher than the maximum oral dose tested in mice and rats (1,825 mg/kg/day). Overdoses up to 31,500 mg of atovaquone have been reported. In 1 such patient who also took an unspecified dose of dapsone, methemoglobinemia occurred. Rash has also been reported after overdose.

DOSAGE AND ADMINISTRATION

Dosage
Prevention of PCP: Adults and Adolescents (13 to 16 Years):
The recommended oral dose is 1,500 mg (10 mL) once daily administered with a meal.
Treatment of Mild-to-Moderate PCP: Adults and Adolescents (13 to 16 Years):
The recommended oral dose is 750 mg (5 mL) administered with meals twice daily for 21 days (total daily dose 1,500 mg).
Note: Failure to administer MEPRON Suspension with meals may result in lower plasma atovaquone concentrations and may limit response to therapy (see CLINICAL PHARMACOLOGY and PRECAUTIONS).
Administration
Foil Pouch
Open pouch by removing tab at perforation and tear at notch. Take entire contents by mouth. Can be discharged into a dosing spoon or cup or directly into the mouth.
Bottle
SHAKE BOTTLE GENTLY BEFORE USING.

HOW SUPPLIED

MEPRON Suspension (bright yellow, citrus flavored) containing 750 mg atovaquone in each teaspoonful (5 mL).
Bottle of 210 mL with child-resistant cap (NDC 0173-0665-18).
Store at 15° to 25°C (59° to 77°F). DO NOT FREEZE. Dispense in tight container as defined in USP.
5-mL child-resistant foil pouch - unit dose pack of 42 (NDC 0173-0547-00).
Store at 15° to 25°C (59° to 77°F). DO NOT FREEZE.
[1] (A-a)DO$_2$ = [(713 × FiO$_2$) – (PaCO$_2$/0.8)]– PaO$_2$ (mm Hg)
GlaxoSmithKline
Research Triangle Park, NC 27709
©2013, GlaxoSmithKline. All rights reserved.
March 2013
MPR:2PI

PEDIARIX ℞

[pēd'ē-ə-rix]
[Diphtheria and Tetanus Toxoids and Acellular Pertussis Adsorbed, Hepatitis B (Recombinant) and Inactivated Poliovirus Vaccine]
Suspension for Intramuscular Injection

HIGHLIGHTS OF PRESCRIBING INFORMATION
These highlights do not include all the information needed to use PEDIARIX safely and effectively. See full prescribing information for PEDIARIX.
PEDIARIX [Diphtheria and Tetanus Toxoids and Acellular Pertussis Adsorbed, Hepatitis B (Recombinant) and Inactivated Poliovirus Vaccine]
Suspension for Intramuscular Injection
Initial U.S. Approval: 2002

——————INDICATIONS AND USAGE——————
PEDIARIX is a vaccine indicated for active immunization against diphtheria, tetanus, pertussis, infection caused by all known subtypes of hepatitis B virus, and poliomyelitis. PEDIARIX is approved for use as a three-dose series in infants born of hepatitis B surface antigen (HBsAg)-negative mothers. PEDIARIX may be given as early as 6 weeks of age through 6 years of age (prior to the 7th birthday). (1)

————DOSAGE AND ADMINISTRATION————

Three doses (0.5 mL each) by intramuscular injection at 2, 4, and 6 months of age. (2.2)

————DOSAGE FORMS AND STRENGTHS————

Single-dose prefilled syringes containing a 0.5-mL suspension for injection. (3)

————CONTRAINDICATIONS————

- Severe allergic reaction (e.g., anaphylaxis) after a previous dose of any diphtheria toxoid, tetanus toxoid, pertussis, hepatitis B, or poliovirus-containing vaccine, or to any component of PEDIARIX. (4.1)
- Encephalopathy within 7 days of administration of a previous pertussis-containing vaccine. (4.2)
- Progressive neurologic disorders. (4.3)

————WARNINGS AND PRECAUTIONS————

- In clinical trials, PEDIARIX was associated with higher rates of fever, relative to separately administered vaccines. (5.1)
- If Guillain-Barré syndrome occurs within 6 weeks of receipt of a prior vaccine containing tetanus toxoid, the decision to give PEDIARIX should be based on potential benefits and risks. (5.2)
- The tip caps of the prefilled syringes may contain natural rubber latex which may cause allergic reactions in latex-sensitive individuals. (5.3)
- Syncope (fainting) can occur in association with administration of injectable vaccines, including PEDIARIX. Procedures should be in place to avoid falling injury and to restore cerebral perfusion following syncope. (5.4)
- If specified adverse events (i.e., temperature ≥105°F, collapse or shock-like state, or inconsolable crying lasting ≥3 hours, within 48 hours after vaccination; seizures within 3 days after vaccination) have occurred following a pertussis-containing vaccine, the decision to give PEDIARIX should be based on potential benefits and risks. (5.5)
- For children at higher risk for seizures, an antipyretic may be administered at the time of vaccination with PEDIARIX. (5.6)
- Apnea following intramuscular vaccination has been observed in some infants born prematurely. Decisions about when to administer an intramuscular vaccine, including PEDIARIX, to infants born prematurely should be based on consideration of the individual infant's medical status, and the potential benefits and possible risks of vaccination. (5.7)

————ADVERSE REACTIONS————

Common solicited adverse events following any dose (≥25%) included local injection site reactions (pain, redness, and swelling), fever (≥100.4°F), drowsiness, irritability/fussiness and loss of appetite. (6.1)

To report SUSPECTED ADVERSE REACTIONS, contact GlaxoSmithKline at 1-888-825-5249 or VAERS at 1-800-822-7967 or www.vaers.hhs.gov

————DRUG INTERACTIONS————

Do not mix PEDIARIX with any other vaccine in the same syringe or vial. (7.1)

See 17 for PATIENT COUNSELING INFORMATION

Revised: 11/2013

FULL PRESCRIBING INFORMATION

1   INDICATIONS AND USAGE

PEDIARIX® is indicated for active immunization against diphtheria, tetanus, pertussis, infection caused by all known subtypes of hepatitis B virus, and poliomyelitis. PEDIARIX is approved for use as a three-dose series in infants born of hepatitis B surface antigen (HBsAg)-negative mothers. PEDIARIX may be given as early as 6 weeks of age through 6 years of age (prior to the 7th birthday).

2   DOSAGE AND ADMINISTRATION

2.1   Preparation for Administration

Shake vigorously to obtain a homogeneous, turbid, white suspension. Do not use if resuspension does not occur with vigorous shaking. Parenteral drug products should be inspected visually for particulate matter and discoloration prior to administration, whenever solution and container permit. If either of these conditions exists, the vaccine should not be administered.

Attach a sterile needle and administer intramuscularly.

The preferred administration site is the anterolateral aspect of the thigh for children younger than 1 year. In older children, the deltoid muscle is usually large enough for an intramuscular injection. The vaccine should not be injected in the gluteal area or areas where there may be a major nerve trunk. Gluteal injections may result in suboptimal hepatitis B immune response.

Do not administer this product intravenously, intradermally, or subcutaneously.

2.2   Recommended Dose and Schedule

Immunization with PEDIARIX consists of 3 doses of 0.5 mL each, by intramuscular injection, at 2, 4, and 6 months of age (at intervals of 6 to 8 weeks, preferably 8 weeks). The first dose may be given as early as 6 weeks of age. Three doses of PEDIARIX constitute a primary immunization course for diphtheria, tetanus, pertussis, and poliomyelitis and the complete vaccination course for hepatitis B.

2.3   Modified Schedules in Previously Vaccinated Children

Children Previously Vaccinated With Diphtheria and Tetanus Toxoids and Acellular Pertussis Vaccine Adsorbed (DTaP): PEDIARIX may be used to complete the first 3 doses of the DTaP series in children who have received 1 or 2 doses of INFANRIX® (Diphtheria and Tetanus Toxoids and Acellular Pertussis Vaccine Adsorbed), manufactured by GlaxoSmithKline, identical to the DTaP component of PEDIARIX [see Description (11)] and are also scheduled to receive the other vaccine components of PEDIARIX. Data are not available on the safety and effectiveness of using PEDIARIX following one or more doses of a DTaP vaccine from a different manufacturer.

Children Previously Vaccinated With Hepatitis B Vaccine: PEDIARIX may be used to complete the hepatitis B vaccination series following 1 or 2 doses of another hepatitis B vaccine (monovalent or as part of a combination vaccine), including vaccines from other manufacturers, in children born of HBsAg-negative mothers who are also scheduled to receive the other vaccine components of PEDIARIX.

A 3-dose series of PEDIARIX may be administered to infants born of HBsAg-negative mothers and who received a dose of hepatitis B vaccine at or shortly after birth. However, data are limited regarding the safety of PEDIARIX in such infants [see Adverse Reactions (6.1)]. There are no data to support the use of a 3-dose series of PEDIARIX in infants who have previously received more than one dose of hepatitis B vaccine.

Children Previously Vaccinated With Inactivated Poliovirus Vaccine (IPV): PEDIARIX may be used to complete the first 3 doses of the IPV series in children who have received 1 or 2 doses of IPV from a different manufacturer and are also scheduled to receive the other vaccine components of PEDIARIX.

2.4   Booster Immunization Following PEDIARIX

Children who have received a 3-dose series with PEDIARIX should complete the DTaP and IPV series according to the recommended schedule.[1] Because the pertussis antigens contained in INFANRIX and KINRIX® (Diphtheria and Tetanus Toxoids and Acellular Pertussis Adsorbed and Inactivated Poliovirus Vaccine), manufactured by GlaxoSmithKline, are the same as those in PEDIARIX, these children should receive INFANRIX as their fourth dose of DTaP and either INFANRIX or KINRIX as their fifth dose of DTaP, according to the respective prescribing information for these vaccines. KINRIX or another manufacturer's IPV may be used to complete the 4-dose IPV series according to the respective prescribing information.

3   DOSAGE FORMS AND STRENGTHS

PEDIARIX is a suspension for injection available in 0.5-mL single-dose prefilled TIP-LOK® syringes.

4   CONTRAINDICATIONS

4.1   Hypersensitivity

A severe allergic reaction (e.g., anaphylaxis) after a previous dose of any diphtheria toxoid-, tetanus toxoid-, pertussis antigen-, hepatitis B-, or poliovirus-containing vaccine or any component of this vaccine, including yeast, neomycin, and polymyxin B, is a contraindication to administration of PEDIARIX [see Description (11)].

4.2   Encephalopathy

Encephalopathy (e.g., coma, decreased level of consciousness, prolonged seizures) within 7 days of administration of a previous dose of a pertussis-containing vaccine that is not attributable to another identifiable cause is a contraindication to administration of any pertussis-containing vaccine, including PEDIARIX.

4.3   Progressive Neurologic Disorder

Progressive neurologic disorder, including infantile spasms, uncontrolled epilepsy, or progressive encephalopathy is a contraindication to administration of any pertussis-containing vaccine, including PEDIARIX. PEDIARIX should not be administered to individuals with such conditions until the neurologic status is clarified and stabilized.

5   WARNINGS AND PRECAUTIONS

5.1   Fever

In clinical trials, administration of PEDIARIX in infants was associated with higher rates of fever, relative to separately administered vaccines [see Adverse Reactions (6.1)].

5.2   Guillain-Barré Syndrome

If Guillain-Barré syndrome occurs within 6 weeks of receipt of a prior vaccine containing tetanus toxoid, the decision to give PEDIARIX or any vaccine containing tetanus toxoid should be based on careful consideration of the potential benefits and possible risks.

5.3   Latex

The tip caps of the prefilled syringes may contain natural rubber latex which may cause allergic reactions in latex-sensitive individuals.

5.4   Syncope

Syncope (fainting) can occur in association with administration of injectable vaccines, including PEDIARIX. Syncope can be accompanied by transient neurological signs such as visual disturbance, paresthesia, and tonic-clonic limb movements. Procedures should be in place to avoid falling injury and to restore cerebral perfusion following syncope.

5.5   Adverse Events Following Prior Pertussis Vaccination

If any of the following events occur in temporal relation to receipt of a vaccine containing a pertussis component, the decision to give any pertussis-containing vaccine, including PEDIARIX, should be based on careful consideration of the potential benefits and possible risks:
- Temperature of ≥40.5oC (105oF) within 48 hours not due to another identifiable cause;
- Collapse or shock-like state (hypotonic-hyporesponsive episode) within 48 hours;
- Persistent, inconsolable crying lasting ≥3 hours, occurring within 48 hours;
- Seizures with or without fever occurring within 3 days.

5.6   Children at Risk for Seizures

For children at higher risk for seizures than the general population, an appropriate antipyretic may be administered at the time of vaccination with a vaccine containing a pertussis component, including PEDIARIX, and for the ensuing 24 hours to reduce the possibility of post-vaccination fever.

5.7   Apnea in Premature Infants

Apnea following intramuscular vaccination has been observed in some infants born prematurely. Decisions about when to administer an intramuscular vaccine, including PEDIARIX, to infants born prematurely should be based on consideration of the individual infant's medical status, and the potential benefits and possible risks of vaccination.

Table 1. Percentage of Infants With Solicited Local Reactions or General Adverse Events Within 4 Days of Vaccination[a] at 2, 4, and 6 Months of Age With PEDIARIX Administered Concomitantly With Hib Conjugate Vaccine and 7-valent Pneumococcal Conjugate Vaccine (PCV7) or With Separate Concomitant Administration of INFANRIX, ENGERIX-B, IPV, Hib Conjugate Vaccine, and PCV7 (Modified Intent To Treat Cohort)

	PEDIARIX, Hib Vaccine, & PCV7			INFANRIX, ENGERIX-B, IPV, Hib Vaccine, & PCV7		
	Dose 1	Dose 2	Dose 3	Dose 1	Dose 2	Dose 3
Local[b]						
N	671	653	648	335	323	315
Pain, any	36.1	36.1	31.2	31.9	30.0	29.8
Pain, grade 2 or 3	11.5	10.9	10.6	9.0	8.7	8.9
Pain, grade 3	2.4	2.5	1.7	2.7	1.5	1.3
Redness, any	24.9[c]	37.2	40.1	18.2	32.8	39.0
Redness, >5 mm	6.0[c]	9.6[c]	12.7[c]	1.8	5.9	7.3
Redness, >20 mm	0.9	1.2[c]	2.8	0.3	0.0	1.9
Swelling, any	17.3[c]	26.5[c]	28.7	9.6	20.4	24.8
Swelling, >5 mm	5.8[c]	9.6[c]	9.3[c]	1.8	5.0	4.1
Swelling, >20 mm	1.9	2.5[c]	3.1	0.6	0.0	1.3
General						
N	667	644	645	333	321	311
Fever[d], ≥100.4°F	27.9[c]	38.8[c]	33.5[c]	19.8	30.2	23.8
Fever[d], >101.3°F	7.0	14.1[c]	8.8	4.5	9.7	5.8
Fever[d], >102.2°F	2.2[c]	3.6	3.4	0.3	3.1	2.3
Fever[d], >103.1°F	0.4	1.4	1.1	0.0	0.3	0.3
Fever[d], M.A.	1.2[c]	0.2	0.8	0.0	0.6	0.0
N	671	653	648	335	323	315
Drowsiness, any	57.2	51.6	40.9	54.0	48.3	38.4
Drowsiness, grade 2 or 3	15.8	13.8	11.4	17.6	12.4	11.1
Drowsiness, grade 3	2.5	1.2	0.9	3.6	0.6	1.9
Irritability/Fussiness, any	60.5	64.9	61.1	61.5	61.6	56.5
Irritability/Fussiness, grade 2 or 3	19.8	27.9[c]	25.2[c]	19.4	21.1	19.4
Irritability/Fussiness, grade 3	3.4	4.4	3.5	3.9	3.4	3.2
Loss of appetite, any	30.4	30.6	26.2	27.8	26.6	23.8
Loss of appetite, grade 2 or 3	6.6	7.8[c]	5.9	5.1	3.4	5.4
Loss of appetite, grade 3	0.7	0.3	0.2	0.6	0.3	0.0

Hib conjugate vaccine (Wyeth Pharmaceuticals Inc.; no longer licensed in the US); PCV7 (Wyeth Pharmaceuticals Inc.); IPV (Sanofi Pasteur SA).
Modified intent to treat cohort = all vaccinated subjects for whom safety data were available.
N = number of infants for whom at least one symptom sheet was completed; for fever, numbers exclude missing temperature recordings or tympanic measurements.
M.A. = medically attended (a visit to or from medical personnel).
Grade 2 defined as sufficiently discomforting to interfere with daily activities.
Grade 3 defined as preventing normal daily activities.
[a] Within 4 days of vaccination defined as day of vaccination and the next 3 days.
[b] Local reactions at the injection site for PEDIARIX or INFANRIX.
[c] Rate significantly higher in the group that received PEDIARIX compared to separately administered vaccines [P value <0.05 (2-sided Fisher Exact test) or the 95% CI on the difference between groups (Separate minus PEDIARIX) does not include 0].
[d] Axillary temperatures increased by 1°C and oral temperatures increased by 0.5°C to derive equivalent rectal temperature.

5.8 Preventing and Managing Allergic Vaccine Reactions

Prior to administration, the healthcare provider should review the immunization history for possible vaccine sensitivity and previous vaccination-related adverse reactions to allow an assessment of benefits and risks. Epinephrine and other appropriate agents used for the control of immediate allergic reactions must be immediately available should an acute anaphylactic reaction occur.

6 ADVERSE REACTIONS
6.1 Clinical Trials Experience
Because clinical trials are conducted under widely varying conditions, adverse event rates observed in the clinical trials of a vaccine cannot be directly compared to rates in the clinical trials of another vaccine, and may not reflect the rates observed in practice.
A total of 23,849 doses of PEDIARIX have been administered to 8,088 infants who received one or more doses as part of the 3-dose series during 14 clinical studies. Common adverse events that occurred in ≥25% of subjects following any dose of PEDIARIX included local injection site reactions (pain, redness, and swelling), fever, drowsiness, irritability/fussiness, and loss of appetite. In comparative studies (including the German and US studies described below), administration of PEDIARIX was associated with higher rates of fever relative to separately administered vaccines [see *Warnings and Precautions (5.1)*]. The prevalence of fever

was highest on the day of vaccination and the day following vaccination. More than 96% of episodes of fever resolved within the 4-day period following vaccination (i.e., the period including the day of vaccination and the next 3 days). In the largest of the 14 studies, conducted in Germany, safety data were available for 4,666 infants who received PEDIARIX administered concomitantly at separate sites with 1 of 4 *Haemophilus influenzae* type b (Hib) conjugate vaccines (GlaxoSmithKline [licensed in the US only for booster immunization], Wyeth Pharmaceuticals Inc. [no longer licensed in the US], Sanofi Pasteur SA [US-licensed], or Merck & Co, Inc. [US-licensed]) at 3, 4, and 5 months of age and for 768 infants in the control group that received separate US-licensed vaccines (INFANRIX, Hib conjugate vaccine [Sanofi Pasteur SA], and oral poliovirus vaccine [OPV] [Wyeth Pharmaceuticals, Inc.; no longer licensed in the US]). In this study, information on adverse events that occurred within 30 days following vaccination was collected. More than 95% of study participants were white.
In a US study, the safety of PEDIARIX administered to 673 infants was compared to the safety of separately administered INFANRIX, ENGERIX-B® [Hepatitis B Vaccine (Recombinant)], and IPV (Sanofi Pasteur SA) in 335 infants. In both groups, infants received Hib conjugate vaccine (Wyeth Pharmaceuticals Inc.; no longer licensed in the US) and 7-valent pneumococcal conjugate vaccine (Wyeth Pharmaceuticals Inc.) concomitantly at separate sites. All vaccines were administered at 2, 4, and 6 months of age. Data

on solicited local reactions and general adverse events were collected by parents using standardized diary cards for 4 consecutive days following each vaccine dose (i.e., day of vaccination and the next 3 days). Telephone follow-up was conducted 1 month and 6 months after the third vaccination to inquire about serious adverse events. At the 6-month follow-up, information also was collected on new onset of chronic illnesses. A total of 638 subjects who received PEDIARIX and 313 subjects who received INFANRIX, ENGERIX-B, and IPV completed the 6-month follow-up. Among subjects in both study groups combined, 69% were white, 18% were Hispanic, 7% were black, 3% were Oriental, and 3% were of other racial/ethnic groups.
Solicited Adverse Events: Data on solicited local reactions and general adverse events from the US safety study are presented in Table 1. This study was powered to evaluate fever >101.3°F following dose 1. The rate of fever ≥100.4°F following each dose was significantly higher in the group that received PEDIARIX compared to separately administered vaccines. Other statistically significant differences between groups in rates of fever, as well as other solicited adverse events, are noted in Table 1. Medical attention (a visit to or from medical personnel) for fever within 4 days following vaccination was sought in the group who received PEDIARIX for 8 infants after the first dose (1.2%), 1 infant following the second dose (0.2%), and 5 infants following the third dose (0.8%) (Table 1). Following dose 2, medical attention for fever was sought for 2 infants (0.6%) who received separately administered vaccines (Table 1). Among infants who had a medical visit for fever within 4 days following vaccination, 9 of 14 who received PEDIARIX and 1 of 2 who received separately administered vaccines, had one or more diagnostic studies performed to evaluate the cause of fever. [See table 1 above]
Serious Adverse Events: Within 30 days following any dose of vaccine in the US safety study in which all subjects received concomitant Hib and pneumococcal conjugate vaccines, 7 serious adverse events were reported in 7 subjects (1% [7/673]) who received PEDIARIX (1 case each of pyrexia, gastroenteritis, and culture negative clinical sepsis and 4 cases of bronchiolitis) and 5 serious adverse events were reported in 4 subjects (1% [4/335]) who received INFANRIX, ENGERIX-B, and IPV (uteropelvic junction obstruction and testicular atrophy in one subject and 3 cases of bronchiolitis).
Deaths: In 14 clinical trials, 5 deaths were reported among 8,088 (0.06%) recipients of PEDIARIX and 1 death was reported among 2,287 (0.04%) recipients of comparator vaccines. Causes of death in the group that received PEDIARIX included 2 cases of Sudden Infant Death Syndrome (SIDS) and one case of each of the following: convulsive disorder, congenital immunodeficiency with sepsis, and neuroblastoma. One case of SIDS was reported in the comparator group. The rate of SIDS among all recipients of PEDIARIX across the 14 trials was 0.25/1,000. The rate of SIDS observed for recipients of PEDIARIX in the German safety study was 0.2/1,000 infants (reported rate of SIDS in Germany in the latter part of the 1990s was 0.7/1,000 newborns). The reported rate of SIDS in the United States from 1990 to 1994 was 1.2/1,000 live births. By chance alone, some cases of SIDS can be expected to follow receipt of pertussis-containing vaccines.
Onset of Chronic Illnesses: In the US safety study in which all subjects received concomitant Hib and pneumococcal conjugate vaccines, 21 subjects (3%) who received PEDIARIX and 14 subjects (4%) who received INFANRIX, ENGERIX-B, and IPV reported new onset of a chronic illness during the period from 1 to 6 months following the last dose of study vaccines. Among the chronic illnesses reported in the subjects who received PEDIARIX, there were 4 cases of asthma and 1 case each of diabetes mellitus and chronic neutropenia. There were 4 cases of asthma in subjects who received INFANRIX, ENGERIX-B, and IPV.
Seizures: In the German safety study over the entire study period, 6 subjects in the group that received PEDIARIX (N = 4,666) reported seizures. Two of these subjects had a febrile seizure, 1 of whom also developed afebrile seizures. The remaining 4 subjects had afebrile seizures, including 2 with infantile spasms. Two subjects reported seizures within 7 days following vaccination (1 subject had both febrile and afebrile seizures, and 1 subject had afebrile seizures), corresponding to a rate of 0.22 seizures per 1,000 doses (febrile seizures 0.07 per 1,000 doses, afebrile seizures 0.14 per 1,000 doses). No subject who received concomitant INFANRIX, Hib vaccine, and OPV (N = 768) reported seizures. In a separate German study that evaluated the safety of INFANRIX in 22,505 infants who received 66,867 doses of INFANRIX administered as a 3-dose primary series, the rate of seizures within 7 days of vaccination with INFANRIX was 0.13 per 1,000 doses (febrile seizures 0.0 per 1,000 doses, afebrile seizures 0.13 per 1,000 doses).
Over the entire study period in the US safety study in which all subjects received concomitant Hib and pneumococcal conjugate vaccines, 4 subjects in the group that received PEDIARIX (N = 673) reported seizures. Three of these subjects had a febrile seizure and 1 had an afebrile seizure.

Over the entire study period, 2 subjects in the group that received INFANRIX, ENGERIX-B, and IPV (N = 335) reported febrile seizures. There were no afebrile seizures in this group. No subject in either study group had seizures within 7 days following vaccination.

Other Neurological Events of Interest: No cases of hypotonic-hyporesponsiveness or encephalopathy were reported in either the German or US safety studies.

Safety of PEDIARIX After a Previous Dose of Hepatitis B Vaccine: Limited data are available on the safety of administering PEDIARIX after a previous dose of hepatitis B vaccine. In 2 separate studies, 160 Moldovan infants and 96 US infants, respectively, received 3 doses of PEDIARIX following 1 previous dose of hepatitis B vaccine. Neither study was designed to detect significant differences in rates of adverse events associated with PEDIARIX administered after a previous dose of hepatitis B vaccine compared to PEDIARIX administered without a previous dose of hepatitis B vaccine.

6.2 Postmarketing Safety Surveillance Study

In a safety surveillance study conducted at a health maintenance organization in the US, infants who received one or more doses of PEDIARIX from approximately mid-2003 through mid-2005 were compared to age-, gender-, and area-matched historical controls who received one or more doses of separately administered US-licensed DTaP vaccine from 2002 through approximately mid-2003. Only infants who received 7-valent pneumococcal conjugate vaccine (Wyeth Pharmaceuticals Inc.) concomitantly with PEDIARIX or DTaP vaccine were included in the cohorts. Other US-licensed vaccines were administered according to routine practices at the study sites, but concomitant administration with PEDIARIX or DTaP was not a criterion for inclusion in the cohorts. A birth dose of hepatitis B vaccine had been administered routinely to infants in the historical DTaP control cohort, but not to infants who received PEDIARIX. For each of Doses 1-3, a random sample of 40,000 infants who received PEDIARIX was compared to the historical DTaP control cohort for the incidence of seizures (with or without fever) during the 8-day period following vaccination. For each dose, random samples of 7,500 infants in each cohort were also compared for the incidence of medically-attended fever (fever ≥100.4°F that resulted in hospitalization, an emergency department visit, or an outpatient visit) during the 4-day period following vaccination. Possible seizures and medical visits plausibly related to fever were identified by searching automated inpatient and outpatient data files. Medical record reviews of identified events were conducted to verify the occurrence of seizures or medically-attended fever. The incidence of verified seizures and medically-attended fever from this study are presented in Table 2.

[See table 2 above]

6.3 Postmarketing Spontaneous Reports for PEDIARIX

In addition to reports in clinical trials, worldwide voluntary reports of adverse events received for PEDIARIX since market introduction of this vaccine are listed below. This list includes serious adverse events or events which have a suspected causal connection to components of PEDIARIX. Because these events are reported voluntarily from a population of uncertain size, it is not possible to reliably estimate their frequency or establish a causal relationship to vaccine exposure.

Cardiac Disorders: Cyanosis.

Gastrointestinal Disorders: Diarrhea, vomiting.

General Disorders and Administration Site Conditions: Fatigue, injection site cellulitis, injection site induration, injection site itching, injection site nodule/lump, injection site reaction, injection site vesicles, injection site warmth, limb pain, limb swelling.

Immune System Disorders: Anaphylactic reaction, anaphylactoid reaction, hypersensitivity.

Infections and Infestations: Upper respiratory tract infection.

Investigations: Abnormal liver function tests.

Nervous System Disorders: Bulging fontanelle, depressed level of consciousness, encephalitis, hypotonia, hypotonic-hyporesponsive episode, lethargy, somnolence, syncope.

Psychiatric Disorders: Crying, insomnia, nervousness, restlessness, screaming, unusual crying.

Respiratory, Thoracic, and Mediastinal Disorders: Apnea, cough, dyspnea.

Skin and Subcutaneous Tissue Disorders: Angioedema, erythema, rash, urticaria.

Vascular Disorders: Pallor, petechiae.

6.4 Postmarketing Spontaneous Reports for INFANRIX and/or ENGERIX-B

Worldwide voluntary reports of adverse events received for INFANRIX and/or ENGERIX-B in children younger than 7 years of age but not already reported for PEDIARIX are listed below. This list includes serious adverse events or events which have a suspected causal connection to components of INFANRIX and/or ENGERIX-B. Because these events are reported voluntarily from a population of uncertain size, it is not possible to reliably estimate their frequency or establish a causal relationship to vaccine exposure.

Blood and Lymphatic System Disorders: Idiopathic thrombocytopenic purpura[1,2], lymphadenopathy[1], thrombocytopenia[1,2].

Gastrointestinal Disorders: Abdominal pain[2], intussusception[1,2], nausea[2].

General Disorders and Administration Site Conditions: Asthenia[2], malaise[2].

Hepatobiliary Disorders: Jaundice[2].

Immune System Disorders: Anaphylactic shock[1], serum sickness–like disease[2].

Musculoskeletal and Connective Tissue Disorders: Arthralgia[2], arthritis[2], muscular weakness[2], myalgia[2].

Nervous System Disorders: Encephalopathy[1], headache[1], meningitis[2], neuritis[2], neuropathy[2], paralysis[2].

Skin and Subcutaneous Tissue Disorders: Alopecia[2], erythema multiforme[2], lichen planus[2], pruritus[1,2], Stevens Johnson syndrome[1].

Vascular Disorders: Vasculitis[2].

---

[1]Following INFANRIX (licensed in the United States in 1997).

[2]Following ENGERIX-B (licensed in the United States in 1989).

7 DRUG INTERACTIONS

7.1 Concomitant Vaccine Administration

Immune responses following concomitant administration of PEDIARIX, Hib conjugate vaccine (Wyeth Pharmaceuticals Inc.; no longer licensed in the US), and 7-valent pneumococcal conjugate vaccine (Wyeth Pharmaceuticals Inc.) were evaluated in a clinical trial [see Clinical Studies (14.3)].

When PEDIARIX is administered concomitantly with other injectable vaccines, they should be given with separate syringes and at different injection sites. PEDIARIX should not be mixed with any other vaccine in the same syringe or vial.

7.2 Immunosuppressive Therapies

Immunosuppressive therapies, including irradiation, antimetabolites, alkylating agents, cytotoxic drugs, and corticosteroids (used in greater than physiologic doses), may reduce the immune response to PEDIARIX.

8 USE IN SPECIFIC POPULATIONS

8.1 Pregnancy

Pregnancy Category C

Animal reproduction studies have not been conducted with PEDIARIX. It is not known whether PEDIARIX can cause fetal harm when administered to a pregnant woman or if PEDIARIX can affect reproduction capacity.

8.4 Pediatric Use

Safety and effectiveness of PEDIARIX were established in the age group 6 weeks through 6 months on the basis of clinical studies [see Adverse Reactions (6.1) and Clinical Studies (14.1, 14.2)]. Safety and effectiveness of PEDIARIX in the age group 7 months through 6 years are supported by evidence in infants 6 weeks through 6 months of age. Safety and effectiveness of PEDIARIX in infants younger than 6 weeks of age and children 7 to 16 years of age have not been evaluated.

11 DESCRIPTION

PEDIARIX [Diphtheria and Tetanus Toxoids and Acellular Pertussis Adsorbed, Hepatitis B (Recombinant) and Inactivated Poliovirus Vaccine] is a noninfectious, sterile vaccine for intramuscular administration. Each 0.5-mL dose is formulated to contain 25 Lf of diphtheria toxoid, 10 Lf of tetanus toxoid, 25 mcg of inactivated pertussis toxin (PT), 25 mcg of filamentous hemagglutinin (FHA), 8 mcg of pertactin (69 kiloDalton outer membrane protein), 10 mcg of HBsAg, 40 D-antigen Units (DU) of Type 1 poliovirus (Mahoney), 8 DU of Type 2 poliovirus (MEF-1), and 32 DU of Type 3 poliovirus (Saukett). The diphtheria, tetanus, and pertussis components are the same as those in INFANRIX and KINRIX. The hepatitis B surface antigen is the same as that in ENGERIX-B.

The diphtheria toxin is produced by growing Corynebacterium diphtheriae in Fenton medium containing a bovine extract. Tetanus toxin is produced by growing Clostridium tetani in a modified Latham medium derived from bovine casein. The bovine materials used in these extracts are sourced from countries which the United States Department of Agriculture (USDA) has determined neither have nor present an undue risk for bovine spongiform encephalopathy (BSE). Both toxins are detoxified with formaldehyde, concentrated by ultrafiltration, and purified by precipitation, dialysis, and sterile filtration.

The acellular pertussis antigens (PT, FHA, and pertactin) are isolated from Bordetella pertussis culture grown in modified Stainer-Scholte liquid medium. PT and FHA are isolated from the fermentation broth; pertactin is extracted from the cells by heat treatment and flocculation. The antigens are purified in successive chromatographic and precipitation steps. PT is detoxified using glutaraldehyde and formaldehyde. FHA and pertactin are treated with formaldehyde.

The hepatitis B surface antigen is obtained by culturing genetically engineered Saccharomycescerevisiae cells, which carry the surface antigen gene of the hepatitis B virus, in synthetic medium. The surface antigen expressed in the S. cerevisiae cells is purified by several physicochemical steps, which include precipitation, ion exchange chromatography, and ultrafiltration.

The inactivated poliovirus component is an enhanced potency component. Each of the 3 strains of poliovirus is individually grown in VERO cells, a continuous line of monkey

---

Table 2. Percentage of Infants With Seizures (With or Without Fever) Within 8 Days of Vaccination and Medically-Attended Fever Within 4 Days of Vaccination With PEDIARIX Compared With Historical Controls

	PEDIARIX			Historical DTaP Controls			Difference (PEDIARIX–DTaP Controls)
	N	n	% (95% CI)	N	n	% (95% CI)	% (95% CI)
All seizures (with or without fever)							
Dose 1, Days 0-7	40,000	7	0.02 (0.01, 0.04)	39,232	6	0.02 (0.01, 0.03)	0.00 (-0.02, 0.02)
Dose 2, Days 0-7	40,000	3	0.01 (0.00, 0.02)	37,405	4	0.01 (0.00, 0.03)	0.00 (-0.02, 0.01)
Dose 3, Days 0-7	40,000	6	0.02 (0.01, 0.03)	40,000	5	0.01 (0.00, 0.03)	0.00 (-0.01, 0.02)
Total doses	120,000	16	0.01 (0.01, 0.02)	116,637	15	0.01 (0.01, 0.02)	0.00 (-0.01, 0.01)
Medically-attended fever[a]							
Dose 1, Days 0-3	7,500	14	0.19 (0.11, 0.30)	7,500	14	0.19 (0.11, 0.30)	0.00 (-0.14, 0.14)
Dose 2, Days 0-3	7,500	25	0.33 (0.22, 0.48)	7,500	15	0.20 (0.11, 0.33)	0.13 (-0.03, 0.30)
Dose 3, Days 0-3	7,500	21	0.28 (0.17, 0.43)	7,500	19	0.25 (0.15, 0.39)	0.03 (-0.14, 0.19)
Total doses	22,500	60	0.27 (0.20, 0.34)	22,500	48	0.21 (0.16, 0.28)	0.05 (-0.01, 0.14)

DTaP – any US-licensed DTaP vaccine. Infants received 7-valent pneumococcal conjugate vaccine (Wyeth Pharmaceuticals Inc.) concomitantly with each dose of PEDIARIX or DTaP. Other US-licensed vaccines were administered according to routine practices at the study sites.
N = number of subjects in the given cohort.
n = number of subjects with events reported in the given cohort.
[a] Medically-attended fever defined as fever ≥100.4°F that resulted in hospitalization, an emergency department visit, or an outpatient visit.

kidney cells, cultivated on microcarriers. Calf serum and lactalbumin hydrolysate are used during VERO cell culture and/or virus culture. Calf serum is sourced from countries the USDA has determined neither have nor present an undue risk for BSE. After clarification, each viral suspension is purified by ultrafiltration, diafiltration, and successive chromatographic steps, and inactivated with formaldehyde. The 3 purified viral strains are then pooled to form a trivalent concentrate.

Diphtheria and tetanus toxoids and pertussis antigens (inactivated PT, FHA, and pertactin) are individually adsorbed onto aluminum hydroxide. The hepatitis B component is adsorbed onto aluminum phosphate.

Diphtheria and tetanus toxoid potency is determined by measuring the amount of neutralizing antitoxin in previously immunized guinea pigs. The potency of the acellular pertussis component (inactivated PT, FHA, and pertactin) is determined by enzyme-linked immunosorbent assay (ELISA) on sera from previously immunized mice. Potency of the hepatitis B component is established by HBsAg ELISA. The potency of the inactivated poliovirus component is determined by using the D-antigen ELISA and by a poliovirus neutralizing cell culture assay on sera from previously immunized rats.

Each 0.5-mL dose contains aluminum salts as adjuvant (not more than 0.85 mg aluminum by assay) and 4.5 mg of sodium chloride. Each dose also contains ≤100 mcg of residual formaldehyde and ≤100 mcg of polysorbate 80 (Tween 80). Neomycin sulfate and polymyxin B are used in the poliovirus vaccine manufacturing process and may be present in the final vaccine at ≤0.05 ng neomycin and ≤0.01 ng polymyxin B per dose. The procedures used to manufacture the HBsAg antigen result in a product that contains ≤5% yeast protein.

The tip caps of the prefilled syringes may contain natural rubber latex; the plungers are not made with natural rubber latex.

PEDIARIX is formulated without preservatives.

12 CLINICAL PHARMACOLOGY

12.1 Mechanism of Action

Diphtheria: Diphtheria is an acute toxin-mediated infectious disease caused by toxigenic strains of *C. diphtheriae*. Protection against disease is due to the development of neutralizing antibodies to the diphtheria toxin. A serum diphtheria antitoxin level of 0.01 IU/mL is the lowest level giving some degree of protection; a level of 0.1 IU/mL is regarded as protective.[2]

Tetanus: Tetanus is an acute toxin-mediated disease caused by a potent exotoxin released by *C. tetani*. Protection against disease is due to the development of neutralizing antibodies to the tetanus toxin. A serum tetanus antitoxin level of at least 0.01 IU/mL, measured by neutralization assays, is considered the minimum protective level.[3,4] A level ≥0.1 IU/mL is considered protective.[5]

Pertussis: Pertussis (whooping cough) is a disease of the respiratory tract caused by *B. pertussis*. The role of the different components produced by *B. pertussis* in either the pathogenesis of, or the immunity to, pertussis is not well understood. There is no established serological correlate of protection for pertussis.

Hepatitis B: Infection with hepatitis B virus can have serious consequences including acute massive hepatic necrosis and chronic active hepatitis. Chronically infected persons are at increased risk for cirrhosis and hepatocellular carcinoma.

Antibody concentrations ≥10 mIU/mL against HBsAg are recognized as conferring protection against hepatitis B virus infection.[6]

Poliomyelitis: Poliovirus is an enterovirus that belongs to the picornavirus family. Three serotypes of poliovirus have been identified (Types 1, 2, and 3). Poliovirus neutralizing antibodies confer protection against poliomyelitis disease.[7]

13 NONCLINICAL TOXICOLOGY

13.1 Carcinogenesis, Mutagenesis, Impairment of Fertility

PEDIARIX has not been evaluated for carcinogenic or mutagenic potential, or for impairment of fertility.

14 CLINICAL STUDIES

The efficacy of PEDIARIX is based on the immunogenicity of the individual antigens compared to licensed vaccines. Serological correlates of protection exist for the diphtheria, tetanus, hepatitis B, and poliovirus components. The efficacy of the pertussis component, which does not have a well established correlate of protection, was determined in clinical trials of INFANRIX.

14.1 Efficacy of INFANRIX

Efficacy of a 3-dose primary series of INFANRIX has been assessed in 2 clinical studies.

A double-blind, randomized, active Diphtheria and Tetanus Toxoids (DT)-controlled trial conducted in Italy, sponsored by the National Institutes of Health (NIH), assessed the absolute protective efficacy of INFANRIX when administered

at 2, 4, and 6 months of age. The population used in the primary analysis of the efficacy of INFANRIX included 4,481 infants vaccinated with INFANRIX and 1,470 DT vaccinees. After 3 doses, the absolute protective efficacy of INFANRIX against WHO-defined typical pertussis (21 days or more of paroxysmal cough with infection confirmed by culture and/or serologic testing) was 84% (95% CI: 76%, 89%). When the definition of pertussis was expanded to include clinically milder disease, with infection confirmed by culture and/or serologic testing, the efficacy of INFANRIX was 71% (95% CI: 60%, 78%) against >7 days of any cough and 73% (95% CI: 63%, 80%) against ≥14 days of any cough. A longer unblinded follow-up period showed that after 3 doses and with no booster dose in the second year of life, the efficacy of INFANRIX against WHO-defined pertussis was 86% (95% CI: 79%, 91%) among children followed to 6 years of age. For details see INFANRIX prescribing information. A prospective efficacy trial was also conducted in Germany employing a household contact study design. In this study, the protective efficacy of INFANRIX administered to infants at 3, 4, and 5 months of age, against WHO-defined pertussis was 89% (95% CI: 77%, 95%). When the definition of pertussis was expanded to include clinically milder disease, with infection confirmed by culture and/or serologic testing, the efficacy of INFANRIX against ≥7 days of any cough was 67% (95% CI: 52%, 78%) and against ≥7 days of paroxysmal cough was 81% (95% CI: 68%, 89%). For details see INFANRIX prescribing information.

14.2 Immunological Evaluation of PEDIARIX

In a US multicenter study, infants were randomized to 1 of 3 groups: (1) a combination vaccine group that received PEDIARIX concomitantly with Hib conjugate vaccine (Wyeth Pharmaceuticals Inc.; no longer licensed in the US) and US-licensed 7-valent pneumococcal conjugate vaccine (Wyeth Pharmaceuticals Inc.); (2) a separate vaccine group that received US-licensed INFANRIX, ENGERIX-B, and IPV (Sanofi Pasteur SA) concomitantly with the same Hib and pneumococcal conjugate vaccines; and (3) a staggered vaccine group that received PEDIARIX concomitantly with the same Hib conjugate vaccine but with the same pneumococcal conjugate vaccine administered 2 weeks later. The schedule of administration was 2, 4, and 6 months of age. Infants either did not receive a dose of hepatitis B vaccine prior to enrollment or were permitted to receive one dose of hepatitis B vaccine administered at least 30 days prior to enrollment. For the separate vaccine group, ENGERIX-B was not administered at 4 months of age to subjects who received a dose of hepatitis B vaccine prior to enrollment. Among subjects in all 3 vaccine groups combined, 84% were white, 7% were Hispanic, 6% were black, 0.7% were Oriental, and 2.4% were of other racial/ethnic groups.

The immune responses to the pertussis (PT, FHA, and pertactin), diphtheria, tetanus, poliovirus, and hepatitis B antigens were evaluated in sera obtained one month (range 20 to 60 days) after the third dose of PEDIARIX or INFANRIX. Geometric mean antibody concentrations (GMCs) adjusted for pre-vaccination values for PT, FHA, and pertactin and the seroprotection rates for diphtheria, tetanus, and the polioviruses among subjects who received PEDIARIX in the combination vaccine group were shown to be non-inferior to those achieved following separately administered vaccines (Table 3).

Because of differences in the hepatitis B vaccination schedule among subjects in the study, no clinical limit for non-inferiority was pre-defined for the hepatitis B immune response. However, in a previous US study, non-inferiority of PEDIARIX relative to separately administered INFANRIX, ENGERIX-B, and an oral poliovirus vaccine, with respect to the hepatitis B immune response was demonstrated.

Table 3. Antibody Responses Following PEDIARIX as Compared to Separate Concomitant Administration of INFANRIX, ENGERIX-B, and IPV (One Month[a] After Administration of Dose 3) in Infants Vaccinated at 2, 4, and 6 Months of Age When Administered Concomitantly With Hib Conjugate Vaccine and Pneumococcal Conjugate Vaccine (PCV7)

	PEDIARIX, Hib Vaccine, & PCV7	INFANRIX, ENGERIX-B, IPV, Hib Vaccine, & PCV7
	(N = 154-168)	(N = 141-155)
Anti-Diphtheria Toxoid % ≥0.1 IU/mL[b]	99.4	98.7
Anti-Tetanus Toxoid % ≥0.1 IU/mL[b]	100	98.1
Anti-PT % VR[c]	98.7	95.1
GMC[b]	48.1	28.6
Anti-FHA % VR[c]	98.7	96.5
GMC[b]	111.9	97.6
Anti-Pertactin % VR[c]	91.7	95.1
GMC[b]	95.3	80.6
Anti-Polio 1 % ≥1:8[b,d]	100	100
Anti-Polio 2 % ≥1:8[b,d]	100	100
Anti-Polio 3 % ≥1:8[b,d]	100	100
	(N = 114-128)	(N = 111-121)
Anti-HBsAg[e] % ≥10 mIU/mL[f]	97.7	99.2
GMC (mIU/mL)[f]	1032.1	614.5

Hib conjugate vaccine (Wyeth Pharmaceuticals Inc.; no longer licensed in the US); PCV7 (Wyeth Pharmaceuticals Inc.); IPV (Sanofi Pasteur SA).

Assay methods used: ELISA for anti-diphtheria, anti-tetanus, anti-PT, anti-FHA, anti-pertactin, and anti-HBsAg; micro-neutralization for anti-polio (1, 2, and 3).

VR = vaccine response: In initially seronegative infants, appearance of antibodies (concentration ≥5 EL.U./mL); in initially seropositive infants, at least maintenance of pre-vaccination concentration.

GMC = geometric mean antibody concentration. GMCs are adjusted for pre-vaccination levels.

a One month blood sampling, range 20 to 60 days.

b Seroprotection rate or GMC for PEDIARIX not inferior to separately administered vaccines [upper limit of 90% CI on GMC ratio (separate vaccine group/combination vaccine group) <1.5 for anti-PT, anti-FHA, and anti-pertactin, and upper limit of 95% CI for the difference in seroprotection rates (separate vaccine group minus combination vaccine group) <10% for diphtheria and tetanus and <5% for the 3 polioviruses]. GMCs are adjusted for pre-vaccination levels.

c The upper limit of 95% CI for differences in vaccine response rates (separate vaccine group minus combination group) was 0.31, 1.52, and 9.46 for PT, FHA, and pertactin, respectively. No clinical limit defined for non-inferiority.

d Poliovirus neutralizing antibody titer.

e Subjects who received a previous dose of hepatitis B vaccine were excluded from the analysis of hepatitis B seroprotection rates and GMCs presented in the table.

f No clinical limit defined for non-inferiority.

14.3 Concomitant Vaccine Administration

In a US multicenter study *[see Clinical Studies (14.2)]*, there was no evidence for interference with the immune responses to PEDIARIX when administered concomitantly with 7-valent pneumococcal conjugate vaccine (Wyeth Pharmaceuticals Inc.) relative to 2 weeks prior.

Anti-PRP (Hib polyribosyl-ribitol-phosphate) seroprotection rates and GMCs of pneumococcal antibodies one month (range 20 to 60 days) after the third dose of vaccines for the combination vaccine group and the separate vaccine group from the US multicenter study *[see Clinical Studies (14.2)]*, are presented in Table 4.

Table 4. Anti-PRP Seroprotection Rates and GMCs (mcg/mL) of Pneumococcal Antibodies One Month[a] Following the Third Dose of Hib Conjugate Vaccine and Pneumococcal Conjugate Vaccine (PCV7) Administered Concomitantly With PEDIARIX or With INFANRIX, ENGERIX-B, and IPV

	PEDIARIX, Hib Vaccine, & PCV7	INFANRIX, ENGERIX-B, IPV, Hib Vaccine, & PCV7
	(N = 161-168)	(N = 146-156)
	% (95% CI)	% (95% CI)
Anti-PRP ≥0.15 mcg/mL	100 (97.8, 100)	99.4 (96.5, 100)
Anti-PRP ≥1.0 mcg/mL	95.8 (91.6, 98.3)	91.0 (85.3, 95.0)

Pneumococcal Serotype	GMC (95% CI)	GMC (95% CI)
4	1.7 (1.5, 2.0)	2.1 (1.8, 2.4)
6B	0.8 (0.7, 1.0)	0.7 (0.5, 0.9)
9V	1.6 (1.4, 1.8)	1.6 (1.4, 1.9)
14	4.7 (4.0, 5.4)	6.3 (5.4, 7.4)
18C	2.6 (2.3, 3.0)	3.0 (2.5, 3.5)
19F	1.1 (1.0, 1.3)	1.1 (0.9, 1.2)
23F	1.5 (1.2, 1.8)	1.8 (1.5, 2.3)

Hib conjugate vaccine (Wyeth Pharmaceuticals Inc.; no longer licensed in the US); PCV7 (Wyeth Pharmaceuticals Inc.); IPV (Sanofi Pasteur SA).
Assay method used: ELISA for anti-PRP and 7 pneumococcal serotypes.
GMC = geometric mean antibody concentration.
[a] One month blood sampling, range 20 to 60 days.

15   REFERENCES

1. Centers for Disease and Control and Prevention. Recommended immunization schedules for persons aged 0-18 years—United States, 2010. *MMWR* 2010;58(51&52).
2. Vitek CR and Wharton M. Diphtheria Toxoid. In: Plotkin SA, Orenstein WA, and Offit PA, eds. *Vaccines*. 5th ed. Saunders;2008:139-156.
3. Wassilak SGF, Roper MH, Kretsinger K, and Orenstein WA. Tetanus Toxoid. In: Plotkin SA, Orenstein WA, and Offit PA, eds. *Vaccines*. 5th ed. Saunders;2008:805-839.
4. Department of Health and Human Services, Food and Drug Administration. Biological products; Bacterial vaccines and toxoids; Implementation of efficacy review; Proposed rule. *Federal Register* December 13, 1985;50(240):51002-51117.
5. Centers for Disease Control and Prevention. General Recommendations on Immunization. Recommendations of the Advisory Committee on Immunization Practices (ACIP). *MMWR* 2006;55(RR-15):1-48.
6. Ambrosch F, Frisch-Niggemeyer W, Kremsner P, et al. Persistence of vaccine-induced antibodies to hepatitis B surface antigen and the need for booster vaccination in adult subjects. *Postgrad Med J* 1987;63(Suppl. 2):129-135.
7. Sutter RW, Pallansch MA, Sawyer LA, et al. Defining surrogate serologic tests with respect to predicting protective vaccine efficacy: Poliovirus vaccination. In: Williams JC, Goldenthal KL, Burns DL, Lewis Jr BP, eds. Combined vaccines and simultaneous administration. Current issues and perspectives. New York, NY: The New York Academy of Sciences; 1995:289-299.

16   HOW SUPPLIED/STORAGE AND HANDLING

PEDIARIX is available in 0.5 mL single-dose disposable prefilled TIP-LOK syringes (packaged without needles): NDC 58160-811-43 Syringe in Package of 10: NDC 58160-811-52
Store refrigerated between 2° and 8°C (36° and 46°F). Do not freeze. Discard if the vaccine has been frozen.

17   PATIENT COUNSELING INFORMATION

The parent or guardian should be:
• informed of the potential benefits and risks of immunization with PEDIARIX, and of the importance of completing the immunization series.
• informed about the potential for adverse reactions that have been temporally associated with administration of PEDIARIX or other vaccines containing similar components.
• instructed to report any adverse events to their healthcare provider.
• given the Vaccine Information Statements, which are required by the National Childhood Vaccine Injury Act of 1986 to be given prior to immunization. These materials are available free of charge at the Centers for Disease Control and Prevention (CDC) website (www.cdc.gov/nip).
PEDIARIX, INFANRIX, KINRIX, TIP-LOK, and ENGERIX-B are registered trademarks of the GlaxoSmithKline group of companies.
Manufactured by **GlaxoSmithKline Biologicals**
Rixensart, Belgium, US License 1617, and
Novartis Vaccines and Diagnostics GmbH
Marburg, Germany, US License 1754
Distributed by **GlaxoSmithKline**
Research Triangle Park, NC 27709

©2013, GlaxoSmithKline group of companies. All rights reserved.
PDX:22PI

POTIGA
(ezogabine)
Tablets

HIGHLIGHTS OF PRESCRIBING INFORMATION
These highlights do not include all the information needed to use POTIGA safely and effectively. See full prescribing information for POTIGA.
POTIGA (ezogabine) Tablets, CV
Initial U.S. Approval: 2011

> **WARNING: RETINAL ABNORMALITIES AND POTENTIAL VISION LOSS**
> *See full prescribing information for complete boxed warning.*
> • POTIGA can cause retinal abnormalities with funduscopic features similar to those seen in retinal pigment dystrophies, which are known to result in damage to the photoreceptors and vision loss.
> • Some patients with retinal abnormalities have been found to have abnormal visual acuity. It is not possible to determine whether POTIGA caused this decreased visual acuity.
> • The rate of progression of retinal abnormalities and their reversibility are unknown.
> • Patients who fail to show substantial clinical benefit after adequate titration should be discontinued from POTIGA.
> • All patients taking POTIGA should have baseline and periodic (every 6 months) systematic visual monitoring by an ophthalmic professional. Testing should include visual acuity and dilated fundus photography.
> • If retinal pigmentary abnormalities or vision changes are detected, POTIGA should be discontinued unless no other suitable treatment options are available and the benefits of treatment outweigh the potential risk of vision loss.

———RECENT MAJOR CHANGES———

Boxed Warning, WARNING: RETINAL ABNORMALITIES AND POTENTIAL VISION LOSS	09/2013
Indications and Usage (1)	09/2013
Dosage and Administration (2)	09/2013
Warnings and Precautions, Retinal Abnormalities and Potential Vision Loss (5.1)	09/2013
Warnings and Precautions, Skin Discoloration (5.3)	09/2013

———INDICATIONS AND USAGE———
POTIGA is a potassium channel opener indicated as adjunctive treatment of partial-onset seizures in patients aged 18 years and older who have responded inadequately to several alternative treatments and for whom the benefits outweigh the risk of retinal abnormalities and potential decline in visual acuity. (1)

———DOSAGE AND ADMINISTRATION———
• Administer in 3 divided doses daily, with or without food. (2.1)
• The initial dosage should be 100 mg 3 times daily (300 mg per day) for 1 week. (2.1)
• Titrate to maintenance dosage by increasing the dosage at weekly intervals by no more than 150 mg per day. (2.1)
• Optimize effective dosage between 200 mg 3 times daily (600 mg per day) to 400 mg 3 times daily (1,200 mg per day). (2.1)
• In controlled clinical trials, 400 mg 3 times daily (1,200 mg per day) showed limited improvement compared to 300 mg 3 times daily (900 mg per day) with an increase in adverse reactions and discontinuations. (2.1)
• When discontinuing POTIGA, reduce the dosage gradually over a period of at least 3 weeks. (2.1, 5.8)
• POTIGA may cause retinal abnormalities with long-term use; therefore, treatment should be discontinued if patients fail to show substantial clinical benefit after adequate titration. (2.2)
• Testing of visual function should be done at baseline and every 6 months during therapy with POTIGA. (2.2)
• If retinal pigmentary abnormalities or vision changes are detected, POTIGA should be discontinued unless no other suitable treatment options are available and the benefits of treatment outweigh the potential risk of vision loss. (2.2)

• Dosing adjustments are required for geriatric patients and patients with moderate to severe renal or hepatic impairment. (2.3)

———DOSAGE FORMS AND STRENGTHS———
Tablets: 50 mg, 200 mg, 300 mg, and 400 mg. (3)

———CONTRAINDICATIONS———
None. (4)

———WARNINGS AND PRECAUTIONS———
• Urinary retention: Patients should be carefully monitored for urologic symptoms. (5.2)
• POTIGA can cause skin discoloration: If a patient develops skin discoloration, serious consideration should be given to an alternative treatment. (5.3)
• Neuropsychiatric symptoms: Monitor for confusional state, psychotic symptoms, and hallucinations. (5.4)
• Dizziness and somnolence: Monitor for dizziness and somnolence. (5.5)
• QT prolongation: QT interval should be monitored in patients taking concomitant medications known to increase the QT interval or with certain heart conditions. (5.6)
• Suicidal behavior and ideation: Monitor for suicidal thoughts or behaviors. (5.7)

———ADVERSE REACTIONS———
The most common adverse reactions (incidence ≥4% and approximately twice placebo) are dizziness, somnolence, fatigue, confusional state, vertigo, tremor, abnormal coordination, diplopia, disturbance in attention, memory impairment, asthenia, blurred vision, gait disturbance, aphasia, dysarthria, and balance disorder. (6.1)
To report SUSPECTED ADVERSE REACTIONS, contact GlaxoSmithKline at 1-888-825-5249 or FDA at 1-800-FDA-1088 or www.fda.gov/medwatch.

———DRUG INTERACTIONS———
• Ezogabine plasma levels may be reduced by concomitant administration of phenytoin or carbamazepine. An increase in dosage of POTIGA should be considered when adding phenytoin or carbamazepine. (7.1)
• N-acetyl metabolite of ezogabine may inhibit renal clearance of digoxin, a P-glycoprotein substrate. Monitor digoxin levels. (7.2)

———USE IN SPECIFIC POPULATIONS———
• Pregnancy: Based on animal data, may cause fetal harm. Pregnancy registry available. (8.1)
• Pediatric use: Safety and effectiveness in patients under 18 years of age have not been established. (8.4)
See 17 for PATIENT COUNSELING INFORMATION and Medication Guide

Revised: 09/2013

FULL PRESCRIBING INFORMATION: CONTENTS*
WARNING: RETINAL ABNORMALITIES AND POTENTIAL VISION LOSS

FULL PRESCRIBING INFORMATION

> **WARNING: RETINAL ABNORMALITIES AND POTENTIAL VISION LOSS**
> - POTIGA can cause retinal abnormalities with funduscopic features similar to those seen in retinal pigment dystrophies, which are known to result in damage to the photoreceptors and vision loss.
> - Some patients with retinal abnormalities have been found to have abnormal visual acuity. It is not possible to determine whether POTIGA caused this decreased visual acuity, as baseline assessments are not available for these patients.
> - Approximately one third of the patients who had eye examinations performed after approximately 4 years of treatment were found to have retinal pigmentary abnormalities. An earlier onset cannot be ruled out, and it is possible that retinal abnormalities were present earlier in the course of exposure to POTIGA. The rate of progression of retinal abnormalities and their reversibility are unknown.
> - POTIGA should only be used in patients who have responded inadequately to several alternative treatments and for whom the benefits outweigh the potential risk of vision loss. Patients who fail to show substantial clinical benefit after adequate titration should be discontinued from POTIGA.
> - All patients taking POTIGA should have baseline and periodic (every 6 months) systematic visual monitoring by an ophthalmic professional. Testing should include visual acuity and dilated fundus photography. Additional testing may include fluorescein angiograms (FA), ocular coherence tomography (OCT), perimetry, and electroretinograms (ERG).
> - If retinal pigmentary abnormalities or vision changes are detected, POTIGA should be discontinued unless no other suitable treatment options are available and the benefits of treatment outweigh the potential risk of vision loss.

1   INDICATIONS AND USAGE

POTIGA® is indicated as adjunctive treatment of partial-onset seizures in patients aged 18 years and older who have responded inadequately to several alternative treatments and for whom the benefits outweigh the risk of retinal abnormalities and potential decline in visual acuity [see Warnings and Precautions (5.1)].

2   DOSAGE AND ADMINISTRATION

2.1   Dosing Information

The initial dosage should be 100 mg 3 times daily (300 mg per day). The dosage should be increased gradually at weekly intervals by no more than 50 mg 3 times daily (increase in the daily dose of no more than 150 mg per day) up to a maintenance dosage of 200 mg to 400 mg 3 times daily (600 mg to 1,200 mg per day), based on individual patient response and tolerability. This information is summarized in Table 1 under Dosing in Specific Populations. In the controlled clinical trials, 400 mg 3 times daily showed limited evidence of additional improvement in seizure reduction, but an increase in adverse events and discontinuations, compared to the 300 mg 3 times daily dosage. The safety and efficacy of doses greater than 400 mg 3 times daily (1,200 mg per day) have not been examined in controlled trials.

POTIGA should be given orally in 3 equally divided doses daily, with or without food.

POTIGA Tablets should be swallowed whole.

If POTIGA is discontinued, the dosage should be gradually reduced over a period of at least 3 weeks, unless safety concerns require abrupt withdrawal.

2.2   Dosing Considerations to Mitigate the Risk of Visual Adverse Reactions

Because POTIGA may cause retinal abnormalities with long-term use, patients who fail to show substantial clinical benefit after adequate titration should be discontinued from POTIGA. Testing of visual function should be done at baseline and every 6 months during therapy with POTIGA. Patients who cannot be monitored should usually not be treated with POTIGA. If retinal pigmentary abnormalities or vision changes are detected, POTIGA should be discontinued unless no other suitable treatment options are available and the benefits of treatment outweigh the potential risk of vision loss [see Warnings and Precautions (5.1)].

2.3   Dosing in Specific Populations

No adjustment in dosage is required for patients with mild renal or hepatic impairment (see Table 1). Dosage adjustment is required in geriatric and patients with moderate and greater renal or hepatic impairment (see Table 1).

[See table 1 below]

3   DOSAGE FORMS AND STRENGTHS

50 mg, purple, round, film-coated tablets debossed with "RTG 50" on one side.

200 mg, yellow, oblong, film-coated tablets debossed with "RTG-200" on one side.

300 mg, green, oblong, film-coated tablets debossed with "RTG-300" on one side.

400 mg, purple, oblong, film-coated tablets debossed with "RTG-400" on one side.

4   CONTRAINDICATIONS

None.

5   WARNINGS AND PRECAUTIONS

5.1   Retinal Abnormalities and Potential Vision Loss

POTIGA can cause abnormalities of the retina. The abnormalities seen in patients treated with POTIGA have funduscopic features similar to those seen in retinal pigment dystrophies that are known to result in damage to photoreceptors and vision loss.

The retinal abnormalities observed with POTIGA have been reported in patients who were originally enrolled in clinical trials with POTIGA and who have generally taken the drug for a long period of time in 2 ongoing extension studies. Approximately one third of the patients who had eye examinations performed after approximately 4 years of treatment were found to have retinal pigmentary abnormalities. However, an earlier onset cannot be ruled out, and it is possible that retinal abnormalities were present earlier in the course of exposure to POTIGA. POTIGA causes skin, scleral, nail, and mucous membrane discoloration and it is not clear whether this discoloration is related to retinal abnormalities [see Warnings and Precautions (5.3)]. Approximately 15% of patients with retinal pigmentary abnormalities had no such discoloration.

Funduscopic abnormalities have most commonly been described as perivascular pigmentation (bone spicule pattern) in the retinal periphery and/or as areas of focal retinal pigment epithelium clumping. Although some of the patients with retinal abnormalities have been found to have abnormal visual acuity, it is not possible to assess whether POTIGA caused their decreased visual acuity, as baseline assessments are not available for these patients. Two patients with retinal abnormalities have had more extensive diagnostic retinal evaluations. The results of these evaluations were consistent with a retinal dystrophy, including abnormalities in the electroretinogram and electrooculogram of both patients, with abnormal fluorescein angiography and diminished sensitivity on visual field testing in one patient.

The rate of progression of retinal abnormalities and the reversibility after drug discontinuation are unknown.

Because of the observed ophthalmologic adverse reactions, POTIGA should only be used in patients who have responded inadequately to several alternative treatments and for whom the benefits outweigh the risk of retinal abnormalities and potential vision loss. Patients who fail to show substantial clinical benefit after adequate titration should be discontinued from POTIGA.

Patients should have baseline ophthalmologic testing by an ophthalmic professional and follow-up testing every 6 months. The best method of detection of these abnormalities and the optimal frequency of periodic ophthalmologic monitoring are unknown. Patients who cannot be monitored should usually not be treated with POTIGA. The ophthalmologic monitoring program should include visual acuity testing and dilated fundus photography. Additional testing may include fluorescein angiograms (FA), ocular coherence tomography (OCT), perimetry, and electroretinograms (ERG). If retinal pigmentary abnormalities or vision changes are detected, POTIGA should be discontinued unless no other suitable treatment options are available and the benefits of treatment outweigh the potential risk of vision loss.

5.2   Urinary Retention

POTIGA caused urinary retention in clinical trials. Urinary retention was generally reported within the first 6 months of treatment, but was also observed later. Urinary retention was reported as an adverse event in 29 of 1,365 (approximately 2%) patients treated with POTIGA in the open-label and placebo-controlled epilepsy database [see Clinical Studies (14)]. Of these 29 patients, 5 (17%) required catheterization, with post-voiding residuals of up to 1,500 mL. POTIGA was discontinued in 4 patients who required catheterization. Following discontinuation, these 4 patients were able to void spontaneously; however, 1 of the 4 patients continued intermittent self-catheterization. A fifth patient continued treatment with POTIGA and was able to void spontaneously after catheter removal. Hydronephrosis occurred in 2 patients, one of whom had associated renal function impairment that resolved upon discontinuation of POTIGA. Hydronephrosis was not reported in placebo patients.

In the placebo-controlled epilepsy trials, "urinary retention," "urinary hesitation," and "dysuria" were reported in 0.9%, 2.2%, and 2.3% of patients on POTIGA, respectively, and in 0.5%, 0.9%, and 0.7% of patients on placebo, respectively.

Because of the increased risk of urinary retention on POTIGA, urologic symptoms should be carefully monitored. Closer monitoring is recommended for patients who have other risk factors for urinary retention (e.g., benign prostatic hyperplasia [BPH]), patients who are unable to communicate clinical symptoms (e.g., cognitively impaired patients), or patients who use concomitant medications that may affect voiding (e.g., anticholinergics). In these patients, a comprehensive evaluation of urologic symptoms prior to and during treatment with POTIGA may be appropriate.

5.3   Skin Discoloration

POTIGA can cause skin discoloration. The skin discoloration is generally described as blue, but has also been described as grey-blue or brown. It is predominantly on or around the lips or in the nail beds of the fingers or toes, but more widespread involvement of the face and legs has also been reported. Discoloration of the palate, sclera, and conjunctiva has also been reported.

Table 1. Dosing in Specific Populations

Specific Population	Initial Dose	Titration	Maximum Dose
General Dosing			
General population (including patients with mild renal or hepatic impairment)	100 mg 3 times daily (300 mg per day)	Increase by no more than 50 mg 3 times daily, at weekly intervals	400 mg 3 times daily (1,200 mg per day)
Dosing in Specific Populations			
Geriatrics (patients >65 years)	50 mg 3 times daily (150 mg per day)	Increase by no more than 50 mg 3 times daily, at weekly intervals	250 mg 3 times daily (750 mg per day)
Renal impairment (patients with CrCL <50 mL per min or end-stage renal disease on dialysis)	50 mg 3 times daily (150 mg per day)		200 mg 3 times daily (600 mg per day)
Hepatic impairment (patients with Child-Pugh 7-9)	50 mg 3 times daily (150 mg per day)		250 mg 3 times daily (750 mg per day)
Hepatic impairment (patients with Child-Pugh >9)	50 mg 3 times daily (150 mg per day)		200 mg 3 times daily (600 mg per day)

Approximately 10% of patients in long-term clinical trials developed skin discoloration, generally after 2 or more years of treatment and at higher doses (900 mg or greater) of POTIGA. Among patients in whom the status of both skin, nail, lip, or mucous membrane discoloration and retinal pigmentary abnormalities are reported, approximately a quarter of those with skin, nail, lip, or mucous membrane discoloration had concurrent retinal pigmentary abnormalities *[see Warnings and Precautions (5.1)]*.

Information on the consequences, reversibility, time to onset, and pathophysiology of the skin abnormalities remains incomplete. The possibility of more extensive systemic involvement has not been excluded. If a patient develops skin discoloration, serious consideration should be given to changing to an alternate medication.

5.4 Neuro-Psychiatric Symptoms

Confusional state, psychotic symptoms, and hallucinations were reported more frequently as adverse reactions in patients treated with POTIGA than in those treated with placebo in placebo-controlled epilepsy trials (see Table 2). Discontinuations resulting from these reactions were more common in the drug-treated group (see Table 2). These effects were dose-related and generally appeared within the first 8 weeks of treatment. Half of the patients in the controlled trials who discontinued POTIGA due to hallucinations or psychosis required hospitalization. Approximately two-thirds of patients with psychosis in controlled trials had no prior psychiatric history. The psychiatric symptoms in the vast majority of patients in both controlled and open-label trials resolved within 7 days of discontinuation of POTIGA. Rapid titration at greater than the recommended doses appeared to increase the risk of psychosis and hallucinations.

[See table 2 above]

5.5 Dizziness and Somnolence

POTIGA causes dose-related increases in dizziness and somnolence *[see Adverse Reactions (6.1)]*. In placebo-controlled trials in patients with epilepsy, dizziness was reported in 23% of patients treated with POTIGA and 9% of patients treated with placebo. Somnolence was reported in 22% of patients treated with POTIGA and 12% of patients treated with placebo. In these trials 6% of patients on POTIGA and 1.2% on placebo discontinued treatment because of dizziness; 3% of patients on POTIGA and <1.0% on placebo discontinued because of somnolence.

Most of these adverse reactions were mild to moderate in intensity and occurred during the titration phase. For those patients continued on POTIGA, dizziness and somnolence appeared to diminish with continued use.

5.6 QT Interval Effect

A study of cardiac conduction showed that POTIGA produced a mean 7.7-msec QT prolongation in healthy volunteers titrated to 400 mg 3 times daily. The QT-prolonging effect occurred within 3 hours. The QT interval should be monitored when POTIGA is prescribed with medicines known to increase QT interval and in patients with known prolonged QT interval, congestive heart failure, ventricular hypertrophy, hypokalemia, or hypomagnesemia *[see Clinical Pharmacology (12.2)]*.

5.7 Suicidal Behavior and Ideation

Antiepileptic drugs (AEDs), including POTIGA, increase the risk of suicidal thoughts or behavior in patients taking these drugs for any indication. Patients treated with any AED for any indication should be monitored for the emergence or worsening of depression, suicidal thoughts or behavior, and/or any unusual changes in mood or behavior.

Pooled analyses of 199 placebo-controlled clinical trials (mono- and adjunctive-therapy) of 11 different AEDs showed that patients randomized to one of the AEDs had approximately twice the risk (adjusted relative risk 1.8, 95% confidence interval [CI]: 1.2, 2.7) of suicidal thinking or behavior compared to patients randomized to placebo. In these trials, which had a median treatment duration of 12 weeks, the estimated incidence of suicidal behavior or ideation among 27,863 AED-treated patients was 0.43% compared to 0.24% among 16,029 placebo-treated patients, representing an increase of approximately 1 case of suicidal thinking or behavior for every 530 patients treated. There were 4 suicides in drug-treated patients in the trials and none in placebo-treated patients, but the number is too small to allow any conclusion about drug effect on suicide.

The increased risk of suicidal thoughts or behavior with AEDs was observed as early as 1 week after starting treatment with AEDs and persisted for the duration of treatment assessed. Because most trials included in the analysis did not extend beyond 24 weeks, the risk of suicidal thoughts or behavior beyond 24 weeks could not be assessed.

The risk of suicidal thoughts or behavior was generally consistent among drugs in the data analyzed. The finding of increased risk with AEDs of varying mechanism of action and across a range of indications suggests that the risk applies to all AEDs used for any indication. The risk did not vary substantially by age (5 to 100 years) in the clinical trials analyzed.

Table 2. Major Neuro-Psychiatric Symptoms in Placebo-Controlled Epilepsy Trials

Adverse Reaction	Number (%) With Adverse Reaction		Number (%) Discontinuing	
	POTIGA (n = 813)	Placebo (n = 427)	POTIGA (n = 813)	Placebo (n = 427)
Confusional state	75 (9%)	11 (3%)	32 (4%)	4 (<1%)
Psychosis	9 (1%)	0	6 (<1%)	0
Hallucinations[a]	14 (2%)	2 (<1%)	6 (<1%)	0

[a]Hallucinations includes visual, auditory, and mixed hallucinations.

Table 3. Risk of Suicidal Thoughts or Behaviors by Indication for Antiepileptic Drugs in the Pooled Analysis

Indication	Placebo Patients With Events per 1,000 Patients	Drug Patients With Events per 1,000 Patients	Relative Risk: Incidence of Events in Drug Patients/ Incidence in Placebo Patients	Risk Difference: Additional Drug Patients With Events per 1,000 Patients
Epilepsy	1.0	3.4	3.5	2.4
Psychiatric	5.7	8.5	1.5	2.9
Other	1.0	1.8	1.9	0.9
Total	2.4	4.3	1.8	1.9

Table 3 shows absolute and relative risk by indication for all evaluated AEDs.

[See table 3 above]

The relative risk for suicidal thoughts or behavior was higher in clinical trials in patients with epilepsy than in clinical trials in patients with psychiatric or other conditions, but the absolute risk differences were similar for epilepsy and psychiatric indications.

Anyone considering prescribing POTIGA or any other AED must balance this risk with the risk of untreated illness. Epilepsy and many other illnesses for which AEDs are prescribed are themselves associated with morbidity and mortality and an increased risk of suicidal thoughts and behavior. Should suicidal thoughts and behavior emerge during treatment, the prescriber needs to consider whether the emergence of these symptoms in any given patient may be related to the illness being treated.

Patients, their caregivers, and families should be informed that AEDs increase the risk of suicidal thoughts and behavior and should be advised of the need to be alert for the emergence or worsening of the signs and symptoms of depression; any unusual changes in mood or behavior; or the emergence of suicidal thoughts, behavior, or thoughts about self-harm. Behaviors of concern should be reported immediately to healthcare providers.

5.8 Withdrawal Seizures

As with all AEDs, when POTIGA is discontinued, it should be withdrawn gradually when possible to minimize the potential of increased seizure frequency *[see Dosage and Administration (2)]*. The dosage of POTIGA should be reduced over a period of at least 3 weeks, unless safety concerns require abrupt withdrawal.

6 ADVERSE REACTIONS

The following adverse reactions are described in more detail in the *Warnings and Precautions* section of the label:

- Retinal abnormalities and potential vision loss *[see Warnings and Precautions (5.1)]*
- Urinary retention *[see Warnings and Precautions (5.2)]*
- Skin discoloration *[see Warnings and Precautions (5.3)]*
- Neuro-psychiatric symptoms *[see Warnings and Precautions (5.4)]*
- Dizziness and somnolence *[see Warnings and Precautions (5.5)]*
- QT interval effect *[see Warnings and Precautions (5.6)]*
- Suicidal behavior and ideation *[see Warnings and Precautions (5.7)]*
- Withdrawal seizures *[see Warnings and Precautions (5.8)]*

6.1 Clinical Trials Experience

Because clinical trials are conducted under widely varying conditions and for varying durations, adverse reaction frequencies observed in the clinical trials of a drug cannot be directly compared with frequencies in the clinical trials of another drug and may not reflect the frequencies observed in practice.

POTIGA was administered as adjunctive therapy to 1,365 patients with epilepsy in all controlled and uncontrolled clinical studies during the premarketing development. A total of 801 patients were treated for at least 6 months, 585 patients were treated for 1 year or longer, and 311 patients were treated for at least 2 years.

Adverse Reactions Leading to Discontinuation in All Controlled Clinical Studies: In the 3 randomized, double-blind, placebo-controlled studies, 199 of 813 patients (25%) receiving POTIGA and 45 of 427 patients (11%) receiving placebo discontinued treatment because of adverse reactions. The most common adverse reactions leading to withdrawal in patients receiving POTIGA were dizziness (6%), confusional state (4%), fatigue (3%), and somnolence (3%).

Common Adverse Reactions in All Controlled Clinical Studies: Overall, the most frequently reported adverse reactions in patients receiving POTIGA (≥4% and occurring approximately twice the placebo rate) were dizziness (23%), somnolence (22%), fatigue (15%), confusional state (9%), vertigo (8%), tremor (8%), abnormal coordination (7%), diplopia (7%), disturbance in attention (6%), memory impairment (6%), asthenia (5%), blurred vision (5%), gait disturbance (4%), aphasia (4%), dysarthria (4%), and balance disorder (4%). In most cases the reactions were of mild or moderate intensity.

[See table 4 at top of next page]

Other adverse reactions reported in these 3 studies in <2% of patients treated with POTIGA and numerically greater than placebo were increased appetite, hallucinations, myoclonus, peripheral edema, hypokinesia, dry mouth, dysphagia, hyperhydrosis, urinary retention, malaise, and increased liver enzymes.

Most of the adverse reactions appear to be dose related (especially those classified as psychiatric and nervous system symptoms), including dizziness, somnolence, confusional state, tremor, abnormal coordination, memory impairment, blurred vision, gait disturbance, aphasia, balance disorder, constipation, dysuria, and chromaturia.

POTIGA was associated with dose-related weight gain, with mean weight increasing by 0.2 kg, 1.2 kg, 1.6 kg, and 2.7 kg in the placebo, 600 mg per day, 900 mg per day, and 1,200 mg per day groups, respectively.

Additional Adverse Reactions Observed During All Phase 2 and 3 Clinical Trials: Following is a list of adverse reactions reported by patients treated with POTIGA during all clinical trials: rash, nystagmus, dyspnea, leukopenia, muscle spasms, alopecia, nephrolithiasis, syncope, neutropenia, thrombocytopenia, euphoric mood, renal colic, coma, encephalopathy.

Comparison of Gender, Age, and Race: The overall adverse reaction profile of POTIGA was similar for females and males.

There are insufficient data to support meaningful analyses of adverse reactions by age or race. Approximately 86% of the population studied was Caucasian, and 0.8% of the population was older than 65 years.

7 DRUG INTERACTIONS

7.1 Antiepileptic Drugs

The potentially significant interactions between POTIGA and concomitant AEDs are summarized in Table 5.

[See table 5 at top of next page]

7.2 Digoxin

Data from an *in vitro* study showed that the N-acetyl metabolite of ezogabine (NAMR) inhibited P-glycoprotein–mediated transport of digoxin in a concentration-dependent manner, indicating that NAMR may inhibit renal clearance of digoxin. Administration of POTIGA at therapeutic doses may increase digoxin serum concentrations. Serum levels of digoxin should be monitored *[see Clinical Pharmacology (12.3)]*.

Table 4. Adverse Reaction Incidence in Placebo-Controlled Adjunctive Trials in Adult Patients With Partial Onset Seizures (Adverse reactions in at least 2% of patients treated with POTIGA in any treatment group and numerically more frequent than in the placebo group.)

Body System/ Adverse Reaction	Placebo (N = 427) %	POTIGA 600 mg/day (N = 281) %	POTIGA 900 mg/day (N = 273) %	POTIGA 1,200 mg/day (N = 259) %	POTIGA All (N = 813) %
Eye					
Diplopia	2	8	6	7	7
Blurred vision	2	2	4	10	5
Gastrointestinal					
Nausea	5	6	6	9	7
Constipation	1	1	4	5	3
Dyspepsia	2	3	2	3	2
General					
Fatigue	6	16	15	13	15
Asthenia	2	4	6	4	5
Infections and infestations					
Influenza	2	4	1	5	3
Investigations					
Weight increased	1	2	3	3	3
Nervous system					
Dizziness	9	15	23	32	23
Somnolence	12	15	25	27	22
Memory impairment	3	3	6	9	6
Tremor	3	3	10	12	8
Vertigo	2	8	8	9	8
Abnormal coordination	3	5	5	12	7
Disturbance in attention	<1	6	6	7	6
Gait disturbance	1	2	5	6	4
Aphasia	<1	1	3	7	4
Dysarthria	<1	4	2	8	4
Balance disorder	<1	3	3	5	4
Paresthesia	2	3	2	5	3
Amnesia	<1	<1	3	3	2
Dysphasia	<1	1	1	3	2
Psychiatric					
Confusional state	3	4	8	16	9
Anxiety	2	3	2	5	3
Disorientation	<1	<1	<1	5	2
Psychotic disorder	0	0	<1	2	<1
Renal and urinary					
Dysuria	<1	1	2	4	2
Urinary hesitation	<1	2	1	4	2
Hematuria	<1	2	1	2	2
Chromaturia	<1	<1	2	3	2

Table 5. Significant Interactions Between POTIGA and Concomitant Antiepileptic Drugs

AED	Dose of AED (mg/day)	Dose of POTIGA (mg/day)	Influence of POTIGA on AED	Influence of AED on POTIGA	Dosage Adjustment
Carbamazepine[a,b]	600-2,400	300-1,200	None	31% decrease in AUC, 23% decrease in C_{max}	consider an increase in dosage of POTIGA when adding carbamazepine[c]
Phenytoin[a,b]	120-600	300-1,200	None	34% decrease in AUC, 18% decrease in C_{max}	consider an increase in dosage of POTIGA when adding phenytoin[c]

[a] Based on results of a Phase 2 study.
[b] Inducer for uridine 5'-diphosphate (UDP)-glucuronyltransferases (UGTs).
[c] A decrease in dosage of POTIGA should be considered when carbamazepine or phenytoin is discontinued.
[See Clinical Pharmacology (12.3)]

7.3 Alcohol
Alcohol increased systemic exposure to POTIGA. Patients should be advised of possible worsening of ezogabine's general dose-related adverse reactions if they take POTIGA with alcohol [see Clinical Pharmacology (12.3)].

7.4 Laboratory Tests
Ezogabine has been shown to interfere with clinical laboratory assays of both serum and urine bilirubin, which can result in falsely elevated readings.

8 USE IN SPECIFIC POPULATIONS
8.1 Pregnancy
Pregnancy Category C. There are no adequate and well-controlled studies in pregnant women. POTIGA should be used during pregnancy only if the potential benefit justifies the potential risk to the fetus.

In animal studies, doses associated with maternal plasma exposures (AUC) to ezogabine and its major circulating metabolite, NAMR, similar to or below those expected in humans at the maximum recommended human dose (MRHD) of 1,200 mg per day produced developmental toxicity when administered to pregnant rats and rabbits. The maximum doses evaluated were limited by maternal toxicity (acute neurotoxicity).

Treatment of pregnant rats with ezogabine (oral doses of up to 46 mg/kg/day) throughout organogenesis increased the incidences of fetal skeletal variations. The no-effect dose for embryo-fetal toxicity in rats (21 mg/kg/day) was associated with maternal plasma exposures (AUC) to ezogabine and NAMR less than those in humans at the MRHD. Treatment of pregnant rabbits with ezogabine (oral doses of up to 60 mg/kg/day) throughout organogenesis resulted in de-

creased fetal body weights and increased incidences of fetal skeletal variations. The no-effect dose for embryo-fetal toxicity in rabbits (12 mg/kg/day) was associated with maternal plasma exposures to ezogabine and NAMR less than those in humans at the MRHD.

Administration of ezogabine (oral doses of up to 61.9 mg/kg/day) to rats throughout pregnancy and lactation resulted in increased pre- and postnatal mortality, decreased body weight gain, and delayed reflex development in the offspring. The no-effect dose for pre- and postnatal developmental effects in rats (17.8 mg/kg/day) was associated with maternal plasma exposures to ezogabine and NAMR less than those in humans at the MRHD.

Pregnancy Registry: To provide information regarding the effects of in utero exposure to POTIGA, physicians are advised to recommend that pregnant patients taking POTIGA enroll in the North American Antiepileptic Drug (NAAED) Pregnancy Registry. This can be done by calling the toll-free number 1-888-233-2334, and must be done by patients themselves. Information on the registry can also be found at the website www.aedpregnancyregistry.org.

8.2 Labor and Delivery
The effects of POTIGA on labor and delivery in humans are unknown.

8.3 Nursing Mothers
It is not known whether ezogabine is excreted in human milk. However, ezogabine and/or its metabolites are present in the milk of lactating rats. Because of the potential for serious adverse reactions in nursing infants from POTIGA, a decision should be made whether to discontinue nursing or to discontinue the drug, taking into account the importance of the drug to the mother.

8.4 Pediatric Use
The safety and effectiveness of POTIGA in patients under 18 years of age have not been established.

In juvenile animal studies, increased sensitivity to acute neurotoxicity and urinary bladder toxicity was observed in young rats compared to adults. In studies in which rats were dosed starting on postnatal day 7, ezogabine-related mortality, clinical signs of neurotoxicity, and renal and urinary tract toxicities were observed at doses ≥2 mg/kg/day. The no-effect level was associated with plasma ezogabine exposures (AUC) less than those expected in human adults at the MRHD of 1,200 mg per day. In studies in which dosing began on postnatal day 28, acute central nervous system effects, but no apparent renal or urinary tract effects, were observed at doses of up to 30 mg/kg/day. These doses were associated with plasma ezogabine exposures less than those achieved clinically at the MRHD.

8.5 Geriatric Use
There were insufficient numbers of elderly patients enrolled in partial-onset seizure controlled trials (n = 8 patients on ezogabine) to determine the safety and efficacy of POTIGA in this population. Dosage adjustment is recommended in patients aged 65 years and older [see Dosage and Administration (2), Clinical Pharmacology (12.3)].

POTIGA may cause urinary retention. Elderly men with symptomatic BPH may be at increased risk for urinary retention.

8.6 Patients With Renal Impairment
Dosage adjustment is recommended for patients with creatinine clearance <50 mL/min or patients with end-stage renal disease (ESRD) receiving dialysis treatments [see Dosage and Administration (2), Clinical Pharmacology (12.3)].

8.7 Patients With Hepatic Impairment
No dosage adjustment is required for patients with mild hepatic impairment.

In patients with moderate or severe hepatic impairment, the initial and maintenance dosage of POTIGA should be reduced [see Dosage and Administration (2), Clinical Pharmacology (12.3)].

9 DRUG ABUSE AND DEPENDENCE
9.1 Controlled Substance
POTIGA is a Schedule V controlled substance.

9.2 Abuse
A human abuse potential study was conducted in recreational sedative-hypnotic abusers (n = 36) in which single oral doses of ezogabine (300 mg [n = 33], 600 mg [n = 34], 900 mg [n = 6]), the sedative-hypnotic alprazolam (1.5 mg and 3.0 mg), and placebo were administered. Euphoria-type subjective responses to the 300-mg and 600-mg doses of ezogabine were statistically different from placebo but statistically indistinguishable from those produced by either dose of alprazolam. Adverse events reported following administration of single oral doses of 300 mg, 600 mg, and 900 mg ezogabine given without titration included euphoric mood (18%, 21%, and 33%, respectively; 8% from placebo), hallucination (0%, 0%, and 17%, respectively; 0% from placebo) and somnolence (18%, 15%, and 67%, respectively; 15% from placebo).

In Phase 1 clinical studies, healthy individuals who received oral doses of ezogabine (200 mg to 1,650 mg) reported euphoria (8.5%), feeling drunk (5.5%), hallucination (5.1%), disorientation (1.7%), and feeling abnormal (1.5%).

In the 3 randomized, double-blind, placebo-controlled Phase 2 and 3 clinical studies, patients with partial seizures who received oral ezogabine (300 mg to 1,200 mg) reported euphoric mood (0.5%) and feeling drunk (0.9%), while those who received placebo did not report either adverse event (0%).

9.3 Dependence

In a 28-day physical dependence study in which rats received daily ezogabine administration, abrupt drug discontinuation produced behavioral changes that included piloerection, increases in high step gait, and tremors, compared to vehicle-treated animals. These data show that ezogabine produces a withdrawal syndrome indicative of physical dependence.

10 OVERDOSAGE

10.1 Signs, Symptoms, and Laboratory Findings

There is limited experience of overdose with POTIGA. Total daily doses of POTIGA over 2,500 mg were reported during clinical trials. In addition to adverse reactions seen at therapeutic doses, symptoms reported with POTIGA overdose included agitation, aggressive behavior, and irritability. There were no reported sequelae.

In an abuse potential study, cardiac arrhythmia (asystole or ventricular tachycardia) occurred in 2 volunteers within 3 hours of receiving a single 900-mg dose of POTIGA. The arrhythmias spontaneously resolved and both volunteers recovered without sequelae.

10.2 Management of Overdose

There is no specific antidote for overdose with POTIGA. In the event of overdose, standard medical practice for the management of any overdose should be used. An adequate airway, oxygenation, and ventilation should be ensured; monitoring of cardiac rhythm and vital sign measurement is recommended. A certified poison control center should be contacted for updated information on the management of overdose with POTIGA.

11 DESCRIPTION

The chemical name of ezogabine is N-[2-amino-4-(4-fluorobenzylamino)-phenyl] carbamic acid ethyl ester, and it has the following structure:

The empirical formula is $C_{16}H_{18}FN_3O_2$, representing a molecular weight of 303.3. Ezogabine is a white to slightly colored, odorless, tasteless, crystalline powder. At room temperature, ezogabine is practically insoluble in aqueous media at pH values above 4, while the solubility is higher in polar organic solvents. At gastric pH, ezogabine is sparingly soluble in water (about 16 g/L). The pKa is approximately 3.7 (basic).

POTIGA is supplied for oral administration as 50-mg, 200-mg, 300-mg, and 400-mg film-coated immediate-release tablets. Each tablet contains the labeled amount of ezogabine and the following inactive ingredients: carmine (50-mg and 400-mg tablets), croscarmellose sodium, FD&C Blue No. 2 (50-mg, 300-mg, and 400-mg tablets), hypromellose, iron oxide yellow (200-mg and 300-mg tablets), lecithin, magnesium stearate, microcrystalline cellulose, polyvinyl alcohol, talc, titanium dioxide, and xanthan gum.

12 CLINICAL PHARMACOLOGY

12.1 Mechanism of Action

The mechanism by which ezogabine exerts its therapeutic effects has not been fully elucidated. *In vitro* studies indicate that ezogabine enhances transmembrane potassium currents mediated by the KCNQ (Kv7.2 to 7.5) family of ion channels. By activating KCNQ channels, ezogabine is thought to stabilize the resting membrane potential and reduce brain excitability. *In vitro* studies suggest that ezogabine may also exert therapeutic effects through augmentation of GABA-mediated currents.

12.2 Pharmacodynamics

The QTc prolongation risk of POTIGA was evaluated in healthy subjects. In a randomized, double-blind, active- and placebo-controlled parallel-group study, 120 healthy subjects (40 in each group) were administered POTIGA titrated up to the final dose of 400 mg 3 times daily, placebo, and placebo and moxifloxacin (on day 22). After 22 days of dosing, the maximum mean (upper 1-sided, 95% CI) increase of baseline- and placebo-adjusted QTc interval based on Fridericia correction method (QTcF) was 7.7 msec (11.9 msec) and was observed at 3 hours after dosing in subjects who achieved 1,200 mg per day. No effects on heart rate, PR, or QRS intervals were noted.

Patients who are prescribed POTIGA with medicines known to increase QT interval or who have known prolonged QT interval, congestive heart failure, ventricular hypertrophy, hypokalemia, or hypomagnesemia should be observed closely [see Warnings and Precautions (5.4)].

Table 6. Interactions Between POTIGA and Concomitant Antiepileptic Drugs

AED	Dose of AED (mg/day)	Dose of POTIGA (mg/day)	Influence of POTIGA on AED	Influence of AED on POTIGA	Dosage Adjustment
Carbamazepine[a,b]	600-2,400	300-1,200	None	31% decrease in AUC, 23% decrease in C_{max}, 28% increase in clearance	consider an increase in dosage of POTIGA when adding carbamazepine[c]
Phenytoin[a,b]	120-600	300-1,200	None	34% decrease in AUC, 18% decrease in C_{max}, 33% increase in clearance	consider an increase in dosage of POTIGA when adding phenytoin[c]
Topiramate[a]	250-1,200	300-1,200	None	None	None
Valproate[a]	750-2,250	300-1,200	None	None	None
Phenobarbital	90	600	None	None	None
Lamotrigine	200	600	18% decrease in AUC, 22% increase in clearance	None	None
Others[d]			None	None	None

[a]Based on results of a Phase 2 study.
[b]Inducer for uridine 5'-diphosphate (UDP)-glucuronyltransferases (UGTs).
[c]A decrease in dose of POTIGA should be considered when carbamazepine or phenytoin is discontinued.
[d]Zonisamide, valproic acid, clonazepam, gabapentin, levetiracetam, oxcarbazepine, phenobarbital, pregabalin, topiramate, clobazam, and lamotrigine, based on a population pharmacokinetic analysis using pooled data from Phase 3 clinical trials.

12.3 Pharmacokinetics

The pharmacokinetic profile is approximately linear in daily doses between 600 mg and 1,200 mg in patients with epilepsy, with no unexpected accumulation following repeated administration. The pharmacokinetics of ezogabine are similar in healthy volunteers and patients with epilepsy.

Absorption: After both single and multiple oral doses, ezogabine is rapidly absorbed with median time to maximum plasma concentration (T_{max}) values generally between 0.5 and 2 hours. Absolute oral bioavailability of ezogabine relative to an intravenous dose of ezogabine is approximately 60%. High-fat food does not affect the extent to which ezogabine is absorbed based on plasma AUC values, but it increases peak concentration (C_{max}) by approximately 38% and delays T_{max} by 0.75 hour.

POTIGA can be taken with or without food.

Distribution: Data from *in vitro* studies indicate that ezogabine and NAMR are approximately 80% and 45% bound to plasma protein, respectively. Clinically significant interactions with other drugs through displacement from proteins are not anticipated. The steady-state volume of distribution of ezogabine is 2 to 3 L/kg following intravenous dosing, suggesting that ezogabine is well distributed in the body.

Metabolism: Ezogabine is extensively metabolized primarily via glucuronidation and acetylation in humans. A substantial fraction of the ezogabine dose is converted to inactive N-glucuronides, the predominant circulating metabolites in humans. Ezogabine is also metabolized to NAMR that is also subsequently glucuronidated. NAMR has antiepileptic activity, but it is less potent than ezogabine in animal seizure models. Additional minor metabolites of ezogabine are an N-glucoside of ezogabine and a cyclized metabolite believed to be formed from NAMR. *In vitro* studies using human biomaterials showed that the N-acetylation of ezogabine was primarily carried out by NAT2, while glucuronidation was primarily carried out by UGT1A4, with contributions by UGT1A1, UGT1A3, and UGT1A9.

In vitro studies showed no evidence of oxidative metabolism of ezogabine or NAMR by cytochrome P450 enzymes. Coadministration of ezogabine with medications that are inhibitors or inducers of cytochrome P450 enzymes is therefore unlikely to affect the pharmacokinetics of ezogabine or NAMR.

Elimination: Results of a mass balance study suggest that renal excretion is the major route of elimination for ezogabine and NAMR. About 85% of the dose was recovered in the urine, with the unchanged parent drug and NAMR accounting for 36% and 18% of the administered dose, respectively, and the total N-glucuronides of ezogabine and NAMR accounting for 24% of the administered dose. Approximately 14% of the radioactivity was recovered in the feces, with unchanged ezogabine accounting for 3% of the total dose. Average total recovery in both urine and feces within 240 hours after dosing is approximately 98%.

Ezogabine and its N-acetyl metabolite have similar elimination half-lives ($t_{½}$) of 7 to 11 hours. The clearance of ezogabine following intravenous dosing was approximately 0.4 to 0.6 L/hr/kg. Ezogabine is actively secreted into the urine.

Specific Populations: *Race:* No study has been conducted to investigate the impact of race on pharmacokinetics of ezogabine. A population pharmacokinetic analysis comparing Caucasians and non-Caucasians (predominantly African American and Hispanic patients) showed no significant pharmacokinetic difference. No adjustment of the ezogabine dose for race is recommended.

Gender: The impact of gender on the pharmacokinetics of ezogabine was examined following a single dose of POTIGA to healthy young (aged 21 to 40 years) and elderly (aged 66 to 82 years) subjects. The AUC values were approximately 20% higher in young females compared to young males and approximately 30% higher in elderly females compared to elderly males. The C_{max} values were approximately 50% higher in young females compared to young males and approximately 100% higher in elderly females compared to elderly males. There was no gender difference in weight-normalized clearance. Overall, no adjustment of the dosage of POTIGA is recommended based on gender.

Pediatric Patients: The pharmacokinetics of ezogabine in pediatric patients have not been investigated.

Geriatric: The impact of age on the pharmacokinetics of ezogabine was examined following a single dose of ezogabine to healthy young (aged 21 to 40 years) and elderly (aged 66 to 82 years) subjects. Systemic exposure (AUC) of ezogabine was approximately 40% to 50% higher and terminal half-life was prolonged by approximately 30% in the elderly compared to the younger subjects. The peak concentration (C_{max}) was similar to that observed in younger subjects. A dosage reduction in the elderly is recommended [see Dosage and Administration (2), Use in Specific Populations (8.5)].

Renal Impairment: The pharmacokinetics of ezogabine were studied following a single 100-mg dose of POTIGA in subjects with normal (CrCL >80 ml/min), mild (CrCL ≥50 to <80 mL/min), moderate (CrCL ≥30 to <50 mL/min), or severe renal impairment (CrCL <30 mL/min) (n = 6 in each cohort) and in subjects with ESRD requiring hemodialysis (n = 6). The ezogabine AUC was increased by approximately 30% in patients with mild renal impairment and doubled in patients with moderate impairment to ESRD (CrCL <50 mL/min) relative to healthy subjects. Similar increases in NAMR exposure were observed in the various degrees of renal impairment. The effect of hemodialysis on ezogabine clearance has not been established. Dosage reduction is recommended for patients with creatinine clearance <50 mL/min and for patients with ESRD receiving dialysis [see Dosage and Administration (2), Use in Specific Populations (8.6)].

Hepatic Impairment: The pharmacokinetics of ezogabine were studied following a single 100-mg dose of POTIGA in subjects with normal, mild (Child-Pugh score 5 to 6), moderate (Child-Pugh score 7 to 9), or severe hepatic (Child-Pugh score >9) impairment (n = 6 in each cohort). Relative to healthy subjects, ezogabine AUC was not affected by mild

Figure 1. Median Percent Reduction From Baseline in Seizure Frequency per 28 Days by Dose

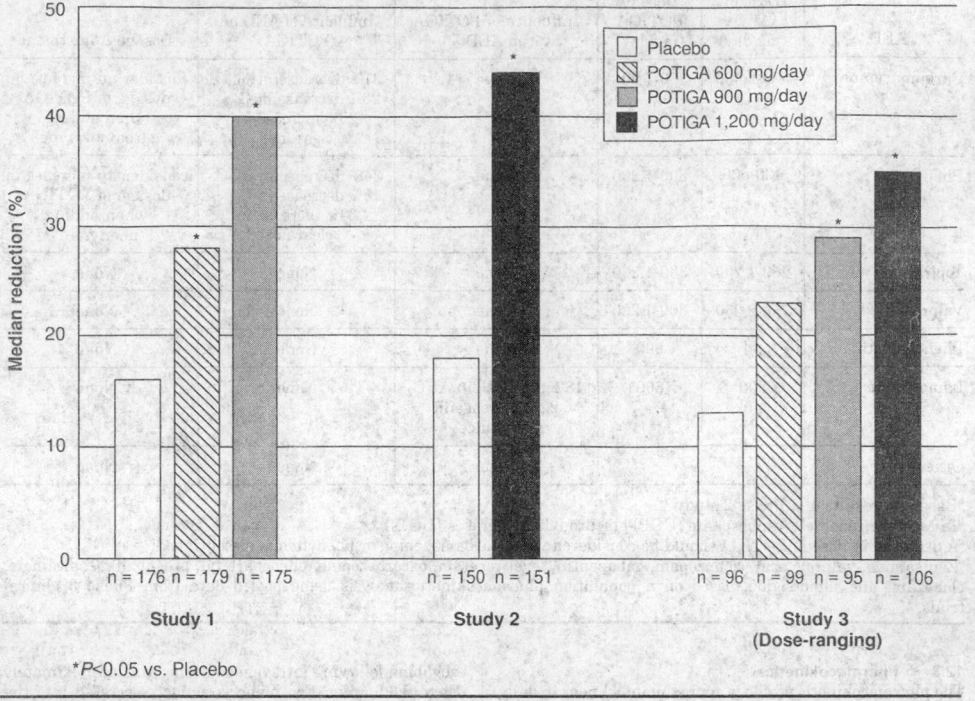

n = 176 n = 179 n = 175   n = 150 n = 151   n = 96 n = 99 n = 95 n = 106

Study 1   Study 2   Study 3 (Dose-ranging)

*P<0.05 vs. Placebo

Legend: Placebo, POTIGA 600 mg/day, POTIGA 900 mg/day, POTIGA 1,200 mg/day

Figure 2. Proportion of Patients by Category of Seizure Response for POTIGA and Placebo Across All Three Double-blind Trials

Legend: Placebo, Potiga 600 mg/day, Potiga 900 mg/day, Potiga 1,200 mg/day

Reduction in seizure frequency from baseline (%): Worse, 0 to <20, 20 to <40, 40 to <60, 60 to <80, 80 to 100

hepatic impairment, but was increased by approximately 50% in subjects with moderate hepatic impairment and doubled in subjects with severe hepatic impairment. There was an increase of approximately 30% in exposure to NAMR in patients with moderate to severe impairment. Dosage reduction is recommended for patients with moderate and severe hepatic impairment [see Dosage and Administration (2), Use in Specific Populations (8.7)].

Drug Interactions: In vitro studies using human liver microsomes indicated that ezogabine does not inhibit enzyme activity for CYP1A2, CYP2A6, CYP2C8, CYP2C9, CYP2C19, CYP2D6, CYP2E1, and CYP3A4/5. Inhibition of CYP2B6 by ezogabine has not been evaluated. In addition, in vitro studies in human primary hepatocytes showed that ezogabine and NAMR did not induce CYP1A2 or CYP3A4/5 activity. Therefore, ezogabine is unlikely to affect the pharmacokinetics of substrates of the major cytochrome P450 isoenzymes through inhibition or induction mechanisms.

Ezogabine is neither a substrate nor an inhibitor of P-glycoprotein, an efflux transporter. NAMR is a P-glycoprotein inhibitor. Data from an in vitro study showed that NAMR inhibited P-glycoprotein–mediated transport of digoxin in a concentration-dependent manner, indicating that NAMR may inhibit renal clearance of digoxin. Administration of POTIGA at therapeutic doses may increase digoxin serum concentrations [see Drug Interactions (7.2)].

Interactions with Antiepileptic Drugs: The interactions between POTIGA and concomitant AEDs are summarized in Table 6.

[See table 6 at top of previous page]

Oral Contraceptives: In one study examining the potential interaction between ezogabine (150 mg 3 times daily for 3 days) and the combination oral contraceptive norgestrel/ ethinyl estradiol (0.3 mg/0.03 mg) tablets in 20 healthy females, no significant alteration in the pharmacokinetics of either drug was observed.

In a second study examining the potential interaction of repeated ezogabine dosing (250 mg 3 times daily for 14 days) and the combination oral contraceptive norethindrone/ethinyl estradiol (1 mg/0.035 mg) tablets in 25 healthy females, no significant alteration in the pharmacokinetics of either drug was observed.

Alcohol: In a healthy volunteer study, the coadministration of ethanol 1g/kg (5 standard alcohol drinks) over 20 minutes and ezogabine (200 mg) resulted in an increase in the ezogabine C_{max} and AUC by 23% and 37%, respectively [see Drug Interactions (7.3)].

13   NONCLINICAL TOXICOLOGY

13.1   Carcinogenesis, Mutagenesis, Impairment of Fertility

Carcinogenesis: In a one-year neonatal mouse study of ezogabine (2 single-dose oral administrations of up to 96 mg/kg on postnatal days 8 and 15), a dose-related increase in the frequency of lung neoplasms (bronchioalveolar carcinoma and/or adenoma) was observed in treated males. No evidence of carcinogenicity was observed in rats following oral administration of ezogabine (oral gavage doses of up to 50 mg/kg/day) for 2 years. Plasma exposure (AUC) to ezogabine at the highest doses tested was less than that in humans at the maximum recommended human dose (MRHD) of 1,200 mg per day.

Mutagenesis: Highly purified ezogabine was negative in the in vitro Ames assay, the in vitro Chinese hamster ovary (CHO) Hprt gene mutation assay, and the in vivo mouse micronucleus assay. Ezogabine was positive in the in vitro chromosomal aberration assay in human lymphocytes. The major circulating metabolite of ezogabine, NAMR, was negative in the in vitro Ames assay, but positive in the in vitro chromosomal aberration assay in CHO cells.

Impairment of Fertility: Ezogabine had no effect on fertility, general reproductive performance, or early embryonic development when administered to male and female rats at doses of up to 46.4 mg/kg/day (associated with a plasma ezogabine exposure [AUC] less than that in humans at the MRHD) prior to and during mating, and continuing in females through gestation day 7.

14   CLINICAL STUDIES

The efficacy of POTIGA as adjunctive therapy in partial-onset seizures was established in 3 multicenter, randomized, double-blind, placebo-controlled studies in 1,239 adult patients. The primary endpoint consisted of the percent change in seizure frequency from baseline in the double-blind treatment phase.

Patients enrolled in the studies had partial onset seizures with or without secondary generalization and were not adequately controlled with 1 to 3 concomitant AEDs, with or without concomitant vagus nerve stimulation. More than 75% of patients were taking 2 or more concomitant AEDs. During an 8-week baseline period, patients experienced at least 4 partial onset seizures per 28 days on average with no seizure-free period exceeding 3 to 4 weeks. Patients had a mean duration of epilepsy of 22 years. Across the 3 studies, the median baseline seizure frequency ranged from 8 to 12 seizures per month. The criteria for statistical significance was $P<0.05$.

Patients were randomized to the total daily maintenance dosages of 600 mg per day, 900 mg per day, or 1,200 mg per day, each administered in 3 equally divided doses. During the titration phase of all 3 studies, treatment was initiated at 300 mg per day (100 mg 3 times per day) and increased in weekly increments of 150 mg per day to the target maintenance dosage.

Figure 1 shows the median percent reduction in 28-day seizure frequency (baseline to double-blind phase) as compared with placebo across all 3 studies. A statistically significant effect was observed with POTIGA at doses of 600 mg per day (Study 1), at 900 mg per day (Studies 1 and 3), and at 1,200 mg per day (Studies 2 and 3).

[See figure 1 above]

Figure 2 shows changes from baseline in the 28-day total partial seizure frequency by category for patients treated with POTIGA and placebo in an integrated analysis across the 3 clinical trials. Patients in whom the seizure frequency increased are shown at left as "worse." Patients in whom the seizure frequency decreased are shown in five categories.

[See figure 2 above]

16   HOW SUPPLIED/STORAGE AND HANDLING

POTIGA is supplied as film-coated immediate-release tablets for oral administration containing 50 mg, 200 mg, 300 mg, or 400 mg of ezogabine in the following packs:

50-mg Tablets: purple, round, film-coated tablets debossed with "RTG 50" on one side in bottles of 90 tablets with desiccant (NDC 0173-0810-59).

200-mg Tablets: yellow, oblong, film-coated tablets debossed with "RTG-200" on one side in bottles of 90 tablets with desiccant (NDC 0173-0812-59).

300-mg Tablets: green, oblong, film-coated tablets debossed with "RTG-300" on one side in bottles of 90 tablets with desiccant (NDC 0173-0813-59).

400-mg Tablets: purple, oblong, film-coated tablets debossed with "RTG-400" on one side in bottles of 90 tablets with desiccant (NDC 0173-0814-59).

Store at 25°C (77°F); excursions permitted to 15°-30°C (59°-86°F) [See USP Controlled Room Temperature.]

17 PATIENT COUNSELING INFORMATION

See FDA-approved patient labeling (Medication Guide).

17.1 Retinal Abnormalities and Potential Vision Loss

Inform patients of the risk of retinal abnormalities and possible risk of vision loss, which may be permanent *[see Warnings and Precautions 5.1]*. All patients taking POTIGA should participate in baseline and periodic ophthalmologic monitoring of vision by an ophthalmic professional. Inform patients that if they suspect any vision changes, they should notify their physician immediately.

17.2 Urinary Retention

Patients should be informed that POTIGA can cause urinary retention (including urinary hesitation and dysuria). If patients experience any symptoms of urinary retention, inability to urinate, and/or pain with urination, they should be instructed to seek immediate medical assistance *[see Warnings and Precautions (5.2)]*. For patients who cannot reliably report symptoms of urinary retention (for example, patients with cognitive impairment), urologic consultation may be helpful.

17.3 Skin Discoloration

Inform patients that POTIGA can cause discoloration of nails, lips, skin, palate, and parts of the eye and that it is not known if the discoloration is reversible upon drug discontinuation *[see Warnings and Precautions 5.3]*. Most skin discoloration has been reported after at least 2 years of treatment with POTIGA, but may happen earlier. Inform patients that the possibility of more extensive systemic involvement has not been excluded. Instruct patients to notify their physician if they develop skin discoloration.

17.4 Psychiatric Symptoms

Patients should be informed that POTIGA can cause psychiatric symptoms such as confusional state, disorientation, hallucinations, and other symptoms of psychosis. Patients and their caregivers should be instructed to notify their physicians if they experience psychotic symptoms *[see Warnings and Precautions (5.4)]*.

17.5 Central Nervous System Effects

Patients should be informed that POTIGA may cause dizziness, somnolence, memory impairment, abnormal coordination/balance, disturbance in attention, and ophthalmological effects such as diplopia or blurred vision. Patients taking POTIGA should be advised not to drive, operate complex machinery, or engage in other hazardous activities until they have become accustomed to any such effects associated with POTIGA *[see Warnings and Precautions (5.5)]*.

17.6 Suicidal Thinking and Behavior

Patients, their caregivers, and families should be informed that AEDs, including POTIGA, may increase the risk of suicidal thoughts and behavior and should be advised of the need to be alert for the emergence or worsening of symptoms of depression, any unusual changes in mood or behavior, or the emergence of suicidal thoughts, behavior, or thoughts about self-harm. Behaviors of concern should be reported immediately to healthcare providers *[see Warnings and Precautions (5.7)]*.

17.7 Pregnancy

Patients should be advised to notify their physicians if they become pregnant or intend to become pregnant during therapy. Patients should be advised to notify their physicians if they intend to breastfeed or are breastfeeding an infant. Patients should be encouraged to enroll in the NAAED Pregnancy Registry if they become pregnant. This registry collects information about the safety of AEDs during pregnancy. To enroll, patients can call the toll-free number 1-888-233-2334 *[see Use in Specific Populations (8.1)]*.

POTIGA is a trademark of Valeant Pharmaceuticals North America LLC.

GlaxoSmithKline

Research Triangle Park, NC 27709

©2013, GlaxoSmithKline. All rights reserved.

PTG:7PI

MEDICATION GUIDE

POTIGA® (po-TEE-ga) Tablets, CV (ezogabine)

Read this Medication Guide before you start taking POTIGA and each time you get a refill. There may be new information. This Medication Guide does not take the place of talking to your healthcare provider about your medical condition or treatment. If you have questions about POTIGA, ask your healthcare provider or pharmacist.

What is the most important information I should know about POTIGA?

Do not stop POTIGA without first talking to a healthcare provider. Stopping POTIGA suddenly can cause serious problems. Stopping POTIGA suddenly can cause you to have more seizures more often.

1. **POTIGA can cause changes to your retina, which is located in the back of your eye and is needed for vision. These types of changes can cause vision loss.**
- If a decrease in your vision happens, it is not known if it will get better.
- You and your healthcare provider should decide if the benefit of taking POTIGA is more important than the possible risk of vision loss.
- You should have a complete eye exam if you are currently taking POTIGA or before starting treatment, and then every 6 months while taking POTIGA.
- Tell your healthcare provider right away if you notice any changes in your vision.

2. **POTIGA can make it hard for you to urinate** (empty your bladder) and may cause you to be unable to urinate. Call your healthcare provider right away if you:
- are unable to start urinating
- have trouble emptying your bladder
- have a weak urine stream
- have pain with urination

3. **POTIGA can cause changes in the color of your skin, nails, lips, roof of your mouth, and whites of your eyes or insides of your eyelids.**
- The changes in color may be blue, grey-blue, or brown.
- Most changes in color have happened in people who have taken POTIGA for at least 2 years, but may happen earlier.
- It is not known if the changes in color go away after stopping POTIGA.
- Tell your healthcare provider if you notice any changes in color to your body.

4. **POTIGA can cause mental (psychiatric) problems, including:**
- confusion
- new or worse aggressive behavior, hostility, anger, or irritability
- new or worse psychosis (hearing or seeing things that are not real)
- being suspicious or distrustful (believing things that are not true)
- other unusual or extreme changes in behavior or mood
Tell your healthcare provider right away if you have any new or worsening mental problems while using POTIGA.

5. **Like other antiepileptic drugs, POTIGA may cause suicidal thoughts or actions in a very small number of people, about 1 in 500.**
Call a healthcare provider right away if you have any of these symptoms, especially if they are new, worse, or worry you:
- thoughts about suicide or dying
- attempt to commit suicide
- new or worse depression
- new or worse anxiety
- feeling agitated or restless
- panic attacks
- trouble sleeping (insomnia)
- new or worse irritability
- acting aggressive, being angry, or violent
- acting on dangerous impulses
- an extreme increase in activity and talking (mania)
- other unusual changes in behavior or mood
Suicidal thoughts or actions can be caused by things other than medicines. If you have suicidal thoughts or actions, your healthcare provider may check for other causes.

How can I watch for early symptoms of suicidal thoughts and actions?
- Pay attention to any changes, especially sudden changes, in mood, behaviors, thoughts, or feelings.
- Keep all follow-up visits with your healthcare provider as scheduled.
Call your healthcare provider between visits as needed, especially if you are worried about symptoms.

What is POTIGA?

POTIGA is a prescription medicine that is used with other medicines to treat partial-onset seizures in adults with epilepsy when several other medicines have not worked well. POTIGA is used when the benefit of taking it is more important than the possible risk of vision loss.

POTIGA is a controlled substance (CV) because it can be abused or lead to drug dependence. Keep your POTIGA in a safe place to protect it from theft. Never give your POTIGA to anyone else because it may harm them. Selling or giving away this medicine is against the law.

It is not known if POTIGA is safe and effective in children under 18 years of age.

What should I tell my healthcare provider before taking POTIGA?

Before you take POTIGA, tell your healthcare provider if you:
- have trouble urinating
- have an enlarged prostate
- have or have had depression, mood problems, or suicidal thoughts or behavior

- have heart problems, including a condition called long QT Syndrome, or have low potassium or magnesium in your blood
- have liver problems
- have kidney problems
- drink alcohol
- have any other medical conditions
- are pregnant or plan to become pregnant. It is not known if POTIGA will harm your unborn baby.
  - If you become pregnant while taking POTIGA, talk to your healthcare provider about registering with the North American Antiepileptic Drug Pregnancy Registry. The purpose of this registry is to collect information about the safety of medicines used to treat seizures during pregnancy. You can enroll in this registry by calling 1-888-233-2334.
- are breastfeeding or plan to breastfeed. It is not known if POTIGA passes into your breast milk. Talk to your healthcare provider about the best way to feed your baby if you take POTIGA. You and your healthcare provider should decide if you will take POTIGA or breastfeed. You should not do both.

Tell your healthcare provider about all the medicines you take, including prescription and over-the-counter medicines, vitamins, and herbal supplements.

Taking POTIGA with certain other medicines can affect each other, causing side effects.

Especially tell your healthcare provider if you take:
- digoxin (LANOXIN®)
- phenytoin (DILANTIN®, PHENYTEK®)
- carbamazepine (CARBATROL®, TEGRETOL®, TEGRETOL®-XR, EQUETRO®, EPITOL®)

Know the medicines you take. Keep a list of them to show your healthcare provider and pharmacist when you get a new medicine.

How should I take POTIGA?
- Take POTIGA exactly as your healthcare provider tells you to take it. Your healthcare provider will tell you how much POTIGA to take and when to take it.
- Your healthcare provider may change your dose of POTIGA. Do not change your dose without talking to your healthcare provider.
- POTIGA can be taken with or without food.
- Swallow POTIGA tablets whole. Do not break, crush, dissolve, or chew POTIGA tablets before swallowing.
- If you take too much POTIGA, call your local Poison Control Center or go to the nearest hospital emergency room right away.

What should I avoid while taking POTIGA?

Do not drive, operate machinery, or do other dangerous activities until you know how POTIGA affects you. POTIGA can cause dizziness, sleepiness, double-vision, and blurred vision.

What are the possible side effects of POTIGA?

POTIGA may cause serious side effects, including:
- See "What is the most important information I should know about POTIGA?"
- **Dizziness and sleepiness.** These symptoms can increase when your dose of POTIGA is increased. See "What should I avoid while taking POTIGA?"
- **Changes in your heart rhythm and the electrical activity of your heart.** Your healthcare provider should monitor your heart during treatment if you have a certain type of heart disease or take certain medications.
- Drinking alcohol during treatment with POTIGA may increase the side effects that you get with POTIGA.

The most common side effects of POTIGA include:
- dizziness
- somnolence
- sleepiness
- tiredness
- confusion
- spinning sensation (vertigo)
- tremor
- problems with balance and muscle coordination, including trouble with walking and moving
- blurred or double vision
- trouble concentrating
- memory problems
- weakness

Tell your healthcare provider about any side effect that bothers you or that does not go away.

These are not all the possible side effects of POTIGA. Ask your healthcare provider or pharmacist for more information.

Call your doctor for medical advice about side effects. You may report side effects to FDA at 1-800-FDA-1088.

How should I store POTIGA?
- Store POTIGA at room temperature between 68°F and 77°F (20°C and 25°C).
- Keep POTIGA and all medicines out of the reach of children.

General information about the safe and effective use of POTIGA.
Medicines are sometimes prescribed for purposes other than those listed in a Medication Guide. Do not use POTIGA for a condition for which it was not prescribed. Do not give POTIGA to other people, even if they have the same symptoms you have. It may harm them.
This Medication Guide summarizes the most important information about POTIGA. If you would like more information, talk with your healthcare provider. You can ask your healthcare provider or pharmacist for information about POTIGA that is written for healthcare professionals.
For more information, go to www.potiga.com or call 1-877-3POTIGA (1-877-376-8442).
What are the ingredients in POTIGA?
Active ingredient: ezogabine
Inactive ingredients in all strengths: croscarmellose sodium, hypromellose, lecithin, magnesium stearate, microcrystalline cellulose, polyvinyl alcohol, talc, titanium dioxide, and xanthan gum
50-mg and 400-mg tablets also contain: carmine
50-mg, 300-mg, and 400-mg tablets also contain: FD&C Blue No 2
200-mg and 300-mg tablets also contain: iron oxide yellow
POTIGA is a trademark of Valeant Pharmaceuticals North America LLC.
The other brands listed are trademarks of their respective owners and are not trademarks of GlaxoSmithKline. The makers of these brands are not affiliated with and do not endorse GlaxoSmithKline or its products.
GlaxoSmithKline
Research Triangle Park, NC 27709
This Medication Guide has been approved by the U.S. Food and Drug Administration.
©2013, GlaxoSmithKline. All rights reserved.
September 2013
PTG:5MG

PROMACTA   R

[pro-MAC-ta]
(eltrombopag)
tablets, for oral use

HIGHLIGHTS OF PRESCRIBING INFORMATION
These highlights do not include all the information needed to use PROMACTA safely and effectively. See full prescribing information for PROMACTA.
PROMACTA (eltrombopag) tablets, for oral use
Initial U.S. Approval: 2008

WARNING: RISK FOR HEPATIC DECOMPENSATION IN PATIENTS WITH CHRONIC HEPATITIS C
See full prescribing information for complete boxed warning.
In patients with chronic hepatitis C, PROMACTA in combination with interferon and ribavirin may increase the risk of hepatic decompensation. (5.1)

────────RECENT MAJOR CHANGES────────

Boxed Warning	02/2014
Indications and Usage (1.3)	04/2014
Warnings and Precautions, Hepatic Decompensation in Patients With Chronic Hepatitis C moved (5.1)	02/2014
Warnings and Precautions, Hepatotoxicity (5.2)	02/2014
Warnings and Precautions, Bone Marrow Reticulin Formation removal (formerly 5.3)	02/2014
Warnings and Precautions, Laboratory Monitoring removal (formerly 5.5)	02/2014

────────INDICATIONS AND USAGE────────

PROMACTA is a thrombopoietin receptor agonist indicated for the treatment of thrombocytopenia in patients with chronic immune (idiopathic) thrombocytopenia (ITP) who have had an insufficient response to corticosteroids, immunoglobulins, or splenectomy. (1.1)
PROMACTA is indicated for the treatment of thrombocytopenia in patients with chronic hepatitis C to allow the initiation and maintenance of interferon-based therapy. (1.2)
Limitations of Use:
• PROMACTA should not be used to normalize platelet counts. (1.3)
• PROMACTA should be used only in patients with ITP whose degree of thrombocytopenia and clinical condition increase the risk for bleeding. (1.3)
• PROMACTA should be used only in patients with chronic hepatitis C whose degree of thrombocytopenia prevents the initiation of interferon-based therapy or limits the ability to maintain interferon-based therapy. (1.3)

• Safety and efficacy have not been established in combination with direct-acting antiviral agents used without interferon for treatment of chronic hepatitis C infection. (1.3)

────────DOSAGE AND ADMINISTRATION────────

• Take on an empty stomach (1 hour before or 2 hours after a meal). (2.3)
• Allow a 4-hour interval between PROMACTA and other medications, foods, or supplements containing polyvalent cations (e.g., iron, calcium, aluminum, magnesium, selenium, and zinc). (2.3)
• **Chronic ITP:** Initiate PROMACTA at 50 mg once daily for most patients. Reduce the initial dose in patients with hepatic impairment and/or patients of East Asian ancestry. Adjust to maintain a platelet count ≥50 × 10^9/L. Do not exceed 75 mg per day. (2.1)
• **Chronic Hepatitis C-associated Thrombocytopenia:** Initiate PROMACTA at 25 mg once daily for all patients. Adjust to achieve a target platelet count required to initiate antiviral therapy. Do not exceed a daily dose of 100 mg. (2.2)

────────DOSAGE FORMS AND STRENGTHS────────

12.5 mg, 25 mg, 50 mg, 75 mg, and 100 mg tablets. (3)

────────CONTRAINDICATIONS────────

None. (4)

────────WARNINGS AND PRECAUTIONS────────

• Hepatic Decompensation in Patients With Chronic Hepatitis C. (5.1)
• Hepatotoxicity: Monitor liver function before and during therapy. (5.2)
• Thrombotic/Thromboembolic Complications: Portal vein thrombosis has been reported in patients with chronic liver disease receiving PROMACTA. Monitor platelet counts regularly. (5.3)

────────ADVERSE REACTIONS────────

• The most common adverse reactions in ITP patients (≥3% and greater than placebo) were: nausea, diarrhea, upper respiratory tract infection, vomiting, increased ALT, myalgia, urinary tract infection, oropharyngeal pain, increased AST, pharyngitis, back pain, influenza, paresthesia, and rash. (6.1)
• The most common adverse reactions in thrombocytopenic patients with chronic hepatitis C (≥10% and greater than placebo) were: anemia, pyrexia, fatigue, headache, nausea, diarrhea, decreased appetite, influenza-like illness, asthenia, insomnia, cough, pruritus, chills, myalgia, alopecia, and peripheral edema. (6.1)
To report SUSPECTED ADVERSE REACTIONS, contact GlaxoSmithKline at 1-888-825-5249 or FDA at 1-800-FDA-1088 or www.fda.gov/medwatch.

────────DRUG INTERACTIONS────────

PROMACTA must not be taken within 4 hours of any medications or products containing polyvalent cations such as antacids, dairy products, and mineral supplements. (7.1)

────────USE IN SPECIFIC POPULATIONS────────

• Pregnancy: Based on animal data, PROMACTA may cause fetal harm. (8.1)
• Nursing Mothers: A decision should be made to discontinue PROMACTA or nursing, taking into account the importance of PROMACTA to the mother. (8.3)
• Reduce the initial dose in chronic ITP patients with hepatic impairment. (8.6)
See 17 for PATIENT COUNSELING INFORMATION and Medication Guide

Revised: 04/2014

FULL PRESCRIBING INFORMATION: CONTENTS*
WARNING: RISK FOR HEPATIC DECOMPENSATION IN PATIENTS WITH CHRONIC HEPATITIS C

FULL PRESCRIBING INFORMATION

WARNING: RISK FOR HEPATIC DECOMPENSATION IN PATIENTS WITH CHRONIC HEPATITIS C
In patients with chronic hepatitis C, PROMACTA® in combination with interferon and ribavirin may increase the risk of hepatic decompensation [see Warnings and Precautions (5.1)].

---

1 INDICATIONS AND USAGE
1.1 Treatment of Thrombocytopenia in Patients With Chronic ITP
PROMACTA is indicated for the treatment of thrombocytopenia in patients with chronic immune (idiopathic) thrombocytopenia (ITP) who have had an insufficient response to corticosteroids, immunoglobulins, or splenectomy.
1.2 Treatment of Thrombocytopenia in Patients With Hepatitis C Infection
PROMACTA is indicated for the treatment of thrombocytopenia in patients with chronic hepatitis C to allow the initiation and maintenance of interferon-based therapy.
1.3 Limitations of Use
• PROMACTA should not be used to normalize platelet counts.
• PROMACTA should be used only in patients with ITP whose degree of thrombocytopenia and clinical condition increase the risk for bleeding.
• PROMACTA should be used only in patients with chronic hepatitis C whose degree of thrombocytopenia prevents the initiation of interferon-based therapy or limits the ability to maintain interferon-based therapy.
• Safety and efficacy have not been established in combination with direct-acting antiviral agents used without interferon for treatment of chronic hepatitis C infection.

2 DOSAGE AND ADMINISTRATION
2.1 Chronic Immune (Idiopathic) Thrombocytopenia
Use the lowest dose of PROMACTA to achieve and maintain a platelet count greater than or equal to 50 × 10^9/L as necessary to reduce the risk for bleeding. Dose adjustments are based upon the platelet count response. Do not use PROMACTA to normalize platelet counts [see Warnings and Precautions (5.3)]. In clinical trials, platelet counts generally increased within 1 to 2 weeks after starting PROMACTA and decreased within 1 to 2 weeks after discontinuing PROMACTA [see Clinical Studies (14.1)].
Initial Dose Regimen: Initiate PROMACTA at a dose of 50 mg once daily, except in patients who are of East Asian ancestry (such as Chinese, Japanese, Taiwanese, or Korean) or who have mild to severe hepatic impairment (Child-Pugh Class A, B, C).
For ITP patients of East Asian ancestry, initiate PROMACTA at a reduced dose of 25 mg once daily [see Use in Specific Populations (8.8) and Clinical Pharmacology (12.3)].
For ITP patients with mild, moderate, or severe hepatic impairment (Child-Pugh Class A, B, C), initiate PROMACTA at a reduced dose of 25 mg once daily [see Use in Specific Populations (8.6) and Clinical Pharmacology (12.3)].

For ITP patients of East Asian ancestry with hepatic impairment (Child-Pugh Class A, B, C), consider initiating PROMACTA at a reduced dose of 12.5 mg once daily [see Clinical Pharmacology (12.3)].

Monitoring and Dose Adjustment: After initiating PROMACTA, adjust the dose to achieve and maintain a platelet count greater than or equal to 50×10^9/L as necessary to reduce the risk for bleeding. Do not exceed a dose of 75 mg daily. Monitor clinical hematology and liver tests regularly throughout therapy with PROMACTA and modify the dosage regimen of PROMACTA based on platelet counts as outlined in Table 1. During therapy with PROMACTA, assess CBCs with differentials, including platelet counts, weekly until a stable platelet count has been achieved. Obtain CBCs with differentials, including platelet counts, monthly thereafter.

Table 1. Dose Adjustments of PROMACTA in Adults With Chronic Immune (Idiopathic) Thrombocytopenia

Platelet Count Result	Dose Adjustment or Response
$<50 \times 10^9$/L following at least 2 weeks of PROMACTA	Increase daily dose by 25 mg to a maximum of 75 mg/day. For patients taking 12.5 mg once daily, increase the dose to 25 mg daily before increasing the dose amount by 25 mg.
$\geq 200 \times 10^9$/L to $\leq 400 \times 10^9$/L at any time	Decrease the daily dose by 25 mg. Wait 2 weeks to assess the effects of this and any subsequent dose adjustments.
$>400 \times 10^9$/L	Stop PROMACTA; increase the frequency of platelet monitoring to twice weekly. Once the platelet count is $<150 \times 10^9$/L, reinitiate therapy at a daily dose reduced by 25 mg. For patients taking 25 mg once daily, reinitiate therapy at a daily dose of 12.5 mg.
$>400 \times 10^9$/L after 2 weeks of therapy at lowest dose of PROMACTA	Discontinue PROMACTA.

In ITP patients with hepatic impairment (Child-Pugh Class A, B, C), after initiating PROMACTA or after any subsequent dosing increase, wait 3 weeks before increasing the dose.

Modify the dosage regimen of concomitant ITP medications, as medically appropriate, to avoid excessive increases in platelet counts during therapy with PROMACTA. Do not administer more than one dose of PROMACTA within any 24-hour period.

Discontinuation: Discontinue PROMACTA if the platelet count does not increase to a level sufficient to avoid clinically important bleeding after 4 weeks of therapy with PROMACTA at the maximum daily dose of 75 mg. Excessive platelet count responses, as outlined in Table 1, or important liver test abnormalities also necessitate discontinuation of PROMACTA [see Warnings and Precautions (5.2)]. Obtain CBCs with differentials, including platelet counts, weekly for at least 4 weeks following discontinuation of PROMACTA.

2.2   Chronic Hepatitis C-Associated Thrombocytopenia
Use the lowest dose of PROMACTA to achieve and maintain a platelet count necessary to initiate and maintain antiviral therapy with pegylated interferon and ribavirin. Dose adjustments are based upon the platelet count response. Do not use PROMACTA to normalize platelet counts [see Warnings and Precautions (5.3)]. In clinical trials, platelet counts generally began to rise within the first week of treatment with PROMACTA [see Clinical Studies (14.2)].

Initial Dose Regimen: Initiate PROMACTA at a dose of 25 mg once daily.

Monitoring and Dose Adjustment: Adjust the dose of PROMACTA in 25 mg increments every 2 weeks as necessary to achieve the target platelet count required to initiate antiviral therapy. Monitor platelet counts every week prior to starting antiviral therapy.

During antiviral therapy, adjust the dose of PROMACTA to avoid dose reductions of peginterferon. Monitor CBCs with differentials, including platelet counts, weekly during antiviral therapy until a stable platelet count is achieved. Monitor platelet counts monthly thereafter. Do not exceed a dose of 100 mg daily. Monitor clinical hematology and liver tests regularly throughout therapy with PROMACTA.

For specific dosage instructions for peginterferon or ribavirin, refer to their respective prescribing information.

Table 2. Dose Adjustments of PROMACTA in Adults With Chronic Hepatitis C

Platelet Count Result	Dose Adjustment or Response
$<50 \times 10^9$/L following at least 2 weeks of PROMACTA	Increase daily dose by 25 mg to a maximum of 100 mg/day.
$\geq 200 \times 10^9$/L to $\leq 400 \times 10^9$/L at any time	Decrease the daily dose by 25 mg. Wait 2 weeks to assess the effects of this and any subsequent dose adjustments.
$>400 \times 10^9$/L	Stop PROMACTA; increase the frequency of platelet monitoring to twice weekly. Once the platelet count is $<150 \times 10^9$/L, reinitiate therapy at a daily dose reduced by 25 mg. For patients taking 25 mg once daily, reinitiate therapy at a daily dose of 12.5 mg.
$>400 \times 10^9$/L after 2 weeks of therapy at lowest dose of PROMACTA	Discontinue PROMACTA.

Discontinuation: The prescribing information for pegylated interferon and ribavirin include recommendations for antiviral treatment discontinuation for treatment futility. Refer to pegylated interferon and ribavirin prescribing information for discontinuation recommendations for antiviral treatment futility.

PROMACTA should be discontinued when antiviral therapy is discontinued. Excessive platelet count responses, as outlined in Table 2, or important liver test abnormalities also necessitate discontinuation of PROMACTA [see Warnings and Precautions (5.2)].

2.3   Administration
Take PROMACTA on an empty stomach (1 hour before or 2 hours after a meal) [see Clinical Pharmacology (12.3)].

Allow at least a 4-hour interval between PROMACTA and other medications (e.g., antacids), calcium-rich foods (e.g., dairy products and calcium fortified juices), or supplements containing polyvalent cations such as iron, calcium, aluminum, magnesium, selenium, and zinc [see Drug Interactions (7.1)].

3   DOSAGE FORMS AND STRENGTHS

- 12.5 mg tablets — round, biconvex, white, film-coated tablets debossed with GS MZ1 and 12.5 on one side. Each tablet, for oral administration, contains eltrombopag olamine, equivalent to 12.5 mg of eltrombopag free acid.
- 25 mg tablets — round, biconvex, orange, film-coated tablets debossed with GS NX3 and 25 on one side. Each tablet, for oral administration, contains eltrombopag olamine, equivalent to 25 mg of eltrombopag free acid.
- 50 mg tablets — round, biconvex, blue, film-coated tablets debossed with GS UFU and 50 on one side. Each tablet, for oral administration, contains eltrombopag olamine, equivalent to 50 mg of eltrombopag free acid.
- 75 mg tablets — round, biconvex, pink, film-coated tablets debossed with GS FFS and 75 on one side. Each tablet, for oral administration, contains eltrombopag olamine, equivalent to 75 mg of eltrombopag free acid.
- 100 mg tablets — round, biconvex, green, film-coated tablets debossed with GS 1L5. Each tablet, for oral administration, contains eltrombopag olamine, equivalent to 100 mg of eltrombopag free acid.

4   CONTRAINDICATIONS
None.

5   WARNINGS AND PRECAUTIONS
5.1   Hepatic Decompensation in Patients With Chronic Hepatitis C
In patients with chronic hepatitis C, PROMACTA in combination with interferon and ribavirin may increase the risk of hepatic decompensation. In two controlled clinical trials in patients with chronic hepatitis C and thrombocytopenia, ascites and encephalopathy occurred more frequently on the arm receiving PROMACTA plus antivirals treatment (7%) than the placebo plus antivirals arm (4%). Patients with low albumin levels (<3.5 g/dL) or Model for End-Stage Liver Disease (MELD) score ≥10 at baseline had a greater risk for hepatic decompensation on the arm receiving PROMACTA plus antivirals treatment. Discontinue PROMACTA if antiviral therapy is discontinued.

5.2   Hepatotoxicity
PROMACTA can cause liver enzyme elevations [see Adverse Reactions (6.1)]. Measure serum ALT, AST, and bilirubin prior to initiation of PROMACTA, every 2 weeks during the dose adjustment phase, and monthly following establishment of a stable dose. PROMACTA inhibits UGT1A1 and OATP1B1, which may lead to indirect hyperbilirubinemia. If bilirubin is elevated, perform fractionation. Evaluate abnormal serum liver tests with repeat testing within 3 to 5 days. If the abnormalities are confirmed, monitor serum liver tests weekly until resolved or stabilized. Discontinue PROMACTA if ALT levels increase to ≥3× ULN in patients with normal liver function or ≥3× baseline in patients with pre-treatment elevations in transaminases and are:

- progressively increasing, or
- persistent for ≥4 weeks, or
- accompanied by increased direct bilirubin, or
- accompanied by clinical symptoms of liver injury or evidence for hepatic decompensation.

If the potential benefit for reinitiating treatment with PROMACTA is considered to outweigh the risk for hepatotoxicity, then consider cautiously reintroducing PROMACTA and measure serum liver tests weekly during the dose adjustment phase. Hepatotoxicity may reoccur if PROMACTA is reinitiated. If liver tests abnormalities persist, worsen or recur, then permanently discontinue PROMACTA.

5.3   Thrombotic/Thromboembolic Complications
In 2 controlled clinical trials in patients with chronic hepatitis C and thrombocytopenia, 3% (31/955) treated with PROMACTA experienced a thrombotic event compared to 1% (5/484) on placebo. The majority of events were of the portal venous system (1% in patients treated with PROMACTA versus <1% for placebo).

Thrombotic/thromboembolic complications may result from increases in platelet counts with PROMACTA. Reported thrombotic/thromboembolic complications included both venous and arterial events and were observed at low and at normal platelet counts.

Consider the potential for an increased risk of thromboembolism when administering PROMACTA to patients with known risk factors for thromboembolism (e.g., Factor V Leiden, ATIII deficiency, antiphospholipid syndrome, chronic liver disease). To minimize the risk for thrombotic/thromboembolic complications, do not use PROMACTA in an attempt to normalize platelet counts. Follow the dose adjustment guidelines to achieve and maintain target platelet counts [see Dosage and Administration (2.1, 2.2)].

In a controlled trial in non-ITP thrombocytopenic patients with chronic liver disease undergoing elective invasive procedures (N = 292), the risk of thrombotic events was increased in patients treated with 75 mg PROMACTA once daily. Seven thrombotic complications (six patients) were reported in the group that received PROMACTA and three thrombotic complications were reported in the placebo group (two patients). All of the thrombotic complications reported in the group that received PROMACTA were portal vein thrombosis (PVT). Symptoms of PVT included abdominal pain, nausea, vomiting, and diarrhea. Five of the six patients in the group that received PROMACTA experienced a thrombotic complication within 30 days of completing treatment with PROMACTA and at a platelet count above 200×10^9/L. The risk of portal venous thrombosis was increased in thrombocytopenic patients with chronic liver disease treated with 75 mg PROMACTA once daily for 2 weeks in preparation for invasive procedures.

5.4   Cataracts
In the 3 controlled clinical trials in chronic ITP, cataracts developed or worsened in 15 (7%) patients who received 50 mg PROMACTA daily and 8 (7%) placebo-group patients. In the extension trial, cataracts developed or worsened in 4% of patients who underwent ocular examination prior to therapy with PROMACTA. In the 2 controlled clinical trials in patients with chronic hepatitis C and thrombocytopenia, cataracts developed or worsened in 8% patients treated with PROMACTA and 5% patients treated with placebo.

Cataracts were observed in toxicology studies of eltrombopag in rodents [see Nonclinical Toxicology (13.2)]. Perform a baseline ocular examination prior to administration of PROMACTA, and during therapy with PROMACTA, regularly monitor patients for signs and symptoms of cataracts.

6   ADVERSE REACTIONS
The following serious adverse reactions associated with PROMACTA are described in other sections.

- Hepatic Decompensation in Patients With Chronic Hepatitis C [see Warnings and Precautions (5.1)]
- Hepatotoxicity [see Warnings and Precautions (5.2)]
- Thrombotic/Thromboembolic Complications [see Warnings and Precautions (5.3)]
- Cataracts [see Warnings and Precautions (5.4)]

6.1   Clinical Trials Experience
Because clinical trials are conducted under widely varying conditions, adverse reaction rates observed in the clinical trials of a drug cannot be directly compared to rates in the clinical trials of another drug and may not reflect the rates observed in practice.

Chronic Immune (Idiopathic) Thrombocytopenia: In clinical trials, hemorrhage was the most common serious adverse reaction and most hemorrhagic reactions followed discontinuation of PROMACTA. Other serious adverse reactions included thrombotic/thromboembolic complications [see Warnings and Precautions (5.3)].

The data described below reflect exposure of PROMACTA to 446 patients with chronic ITP aged 18 to 85, of whom 65% were female across the ITP clinical development program including 3 placebo-controlled trials. PROMACTA was administered to 277 patients for at least 6 months and 202 patients for at least 1 year.

Table 3 presents the most common adverse drug reactions (experienced by ≥3% of patients receiving PROMACTA) from the 3 placebo-controlled trials, with a higher incidence in PROMACTA versus placebo.

Table 3. Adverse Reactions (≥3%) from Three Placebo-Controlled Trials in Adults With Chronic Immune (Idiopathic) Thrombocytopenia

Adverse Reaction	PROMACTA 50 mg n = 241 (%)	Placebo n = 128 (%)
Nausea	9	3
Diarrhea	9	7
Upper respiratory tract infection	7	6
Vomiting	6	<1
Increased ALT	5	3
Myalgia	5	2
Urinary tract infection	5	3
Oropharyngeal pain	4	3
Increased AST	4	2
Pharyngitis	4	2
Back pain	3	2
Influenza	3	2
Paresthesia	3	2
Rash	3	2

In the 3 controlled clinical chronic ITP trials, alopecia, musculoskeletal pain, blood alkaline phosphatase increased, and dry mouth were the adverse reactions reported in 2% of patients treated with PROMACTA and in no patients who received placebo.

Among 299 patients with chronic ITP who received PROMACTA in the single-arm extension trial, the adverse reactions occurred in a pattern similar to that seen in the placebo-controlled trials. Table 4 presents the most common treatment-related adverse reactions (experienced by ≥3% of patients receiving PROMACTA) from the extension trial.

Table 4. Treatment-Related Adverse Reactions (≥3%) from Extension Trial in Adults With Chronic Immune (Idiopathic) Thrombocytopenia

Adverse Reaction	PROMACTA 50 mg n = 299 (%)
Headache	10
Hyperbilirubinemia	6
ALT increased	6
Cataract	5
AST increased	4
Fatigue	4
Nausea	4

In the 3 controlled chronic ITP trials, serum liver test abnormalities (predominantly Grade 2 or less in severity) were reported in 11% and 7% of the PROMACTA and placebo groups, respectively. Four patients (1%) treated with PROMACTA and three patients in the placebo group (2%) discontinued treatment due to hepatobiliary laboratory abnormalities. Seven of the patients treated with PROMACTA in the controlled trials with hepatobiliary laboratory abnor-

malities were re-exposed to PROMACTA in the extension trial. Six of these patients again experienced liver test abnormalities (predominantly Grade 1) resulting in discontinuation of PROMACTA in one patient. In the extension chronic ITP trial, one additional patient had PROMACTA discontinued due to liver test abnormalities (≤Grade 3).

In a placebo-controlled trial of PROMACTA in non-ITP thrombocytopenic patients with chronic liver disease, six patients in the PROMACTA group and one patient in the placebo group developed portal vein thromboses [see Warnings and Precautions (5.3)].

Chronic Hepatitis C-Associated Thrombocytopenia: In the 2 placebo-controlled trials, 955 patients with chronic hepatitis C-associated thrombocytopenia received PROMACTA. Table 5 presents the most common adverse drug reactions (experienced by ≥10% of patients receiving PROMACTA compared to placebo).

Table 5. Adverse Reactions (≥10% and Greater than Placebo) from Two Placebo-Controlled Trials in Adults With Chronic Hepatitis C

Adverse Reaction	PROMACTA + Peginterferon/ Ribavirin n = 955 (%)	Placebo + Peginterferon/ Ribavirin n = 484 (%)
Anemia	40	35
Pyrexia	30	24
Fatigue	28	23
Headache	21	20
Nausea	19	14
Diarrhea	19	11
Decreased appetite	18	14
Influenza-like illness	18	16
Asthenia	16	13
Insomnia	16	15
Cough	15	12
Pruritus	15	13
Chills	14	9
Myalgia	12	10
Alopecia	10	6
Peripheral edema	10	5

In the 2 controlled clinical trials in patients with chronic hepatitis C, hyperbilirubinemia was reported in 8% of patients receiving PROMACTA compared to 3% for placebo. Total bilirubin ≥1.5 × ULN was reported in 76% and 50% of patients receiving PROMACTA and placebo, respectively. ALT or AST ≥3× ULN was reported in 34% and 38% of the PROMACTA and placebo groups, respectively.

7   DRUG INTERACTIONS

In vitro, CYP1A2, CYP2C8, UDP-glucuronosyltransferase (UGT)1A1 and UGT1A3 are involved in the metabolism of eltrombopag. In vitro, eltrombopag inhibits the following metabolic or transporter systems: CYP2C8, CYP2C9, UGT1A1, UGT1A3, UGT1A4, UGT1A6, UGT1A9, UGT2B7, UGT2B15, OATP1B1 and breast cancer resistance protein (BCRP) [see Clinical Pharmacology (12.3)].

7.1   Polyvalent Cations (Chelation)

Eltrombopag chelates polyvalent cations (such as iron, calcium, aluminum, magnesium, selenium, and zinc) in foods, mineral supplements, and antacids. In a clinical trial, administration of PROMACTA with a polyvalent cation-containing antacid decreased plasma eltrombopag systemic exposure by approximately 70% [see Clinical Pharmacology (12.3)].

PROMACTA must not be taken within 4 hours of any medications or products containing polyvalent cations such as antacids, dairy products, and mineral supplements to avoid significant reduction in PROMACTA absorption due to chelation [see Dosage and Administration (2.3)].

7.2   Transporters

Co-administration of PROMACTA with the OATP1B1 and BCRP substrate, rosuvastatin, to healthy adult subjects increased plasma rosuvastatin $AUC_{0-\infty}$ by 55% and C_{max} by 103% [see Clinical Pharmacology (12.3)].

Use caution when concomitantly administering PROMACTA and drugs that are substrates of OATP1B1 [e.g., atorvastatin, bosentan, ezetimibe, fluvastatin, glyburide, olmesartan, pitavastatin, pravastatin, rosuvastatin, repaglinide, rifampin, simvastatin acid, SN-38 (active metabolite of irinotecan), valsartan] or BCRP (e.g., imatinib, irinotecan, lapatinib, methotrexate, mitoxantrone, rosuvastatin, sulfasalazine, topotecan). Monitor patients closely for signs and symptoms of excessive exposure to the drugs that are substrates of OATP1B1 or BCRP and consider reduction of the dose of these drugs, if appropriate. In clinical trials with PROMACTA, a dose reduction of rosuvastatin by 50% was recommended.

7.3   Protease Inhibitors

HIV Protease Inhibitors: In a drug interaction trial, co-administration of PROMACTA with lopinavir/ritonavir (LPV/RTV) decreased plasma eltrombopag exposure by 17% [see Clinical Pharmacology (12.3)]. No dose adjustment is recommended when PROMACTA is co-administered with LPV/RTV. Drug interactions with other HIV protease inhibitors have not been evaluated.

Hepatitis C Virus (HCV) Protease Inhibitors: Coadministration of PROMACTA with either boceprevir or telaprevir did not affect eltrombopag or protease inhibitor exposure significantly [see Clinical Pharmacology (12.3)]. No dose adjustments are recommended. Drug interactions with other HCV protease inhibitors have not been evaluated.

7.4   Peginterferon Alfa 2a/b Therapy

Co-administration of peginterferon alfa 2a (PEGASYS®) or 2b (PEGINTRON®) did not affect eltrombopag exposure in 2 randomized, double-blind, placebo-controlled trials with adult patients with chronic hepatitis C [see Clinical Pharmacology (12.3)].

8   USE IN SPECIFIC POPULATIONS

8.1   Pregnancy

Pregnancy Category C

There are no adequate and well-controlled studies of eltrombopag use in pregnancy. In animal reproduction and developmental toxicity studies, there was evidence of embryolethality and reduced fetal weights at maternally toxic doses. PROMACTA should be used in pregnancy only if the potential benefit to the mother justifies the potential risk to the fetus.

Pregnancy Registry: A pregnancy registry has been established to collect information about the effects of PROMACTA during pregnancy. Physicians are encouraged to register pregnant patients, or pregnant women may enroll themselves in the PROMACTA pregnancy registry by calling 1-888-825-5249.

In an early embryonic development study, female rats received oral eltrombopag at doses of 10, 20, or 60 mg/kg/day (0.8, 2, and 6 times, respectively, the human clinical exposure based on AUC in ITP patients at 75 mg/day and 0.3, 1, and 3 times, respectively, the human clinical exposure based on AUC in chronic hepatitis C patients at 100 mg/day). Increased pre- and post-implantation loss and reduced fetal weight were observed at the highest dose which also caused maternal toxicity.

Eltrombopag was administered orally to pregnant rats at 10, 20, or 60 mg/kg/day (0.8, 2, and 6 times, respectively, the human clinical exposure based on AUC in ITP patients at 75 mg/day and 0.3, 1, and 3 times, respectively, the human clinical exposure based on AUC in chronic hepatitis C patients at 100 mg/day). Decreased fetal weights (6% to 7%) and a slight increase in the presence of cervical ribs were observed at the highest dose which also caused maternal toxicity. However, no evidence of major structural malformations was observed.

Pregnant rabbits were treated with oral eltrombopag doses of 30, 80, or 150 mg/kg/day (0.04, 0.3, and 0.5 times, respectively, the human clinical exposure based on AUC in ITP patients at 75 mg/day and 0.02, 0.1, and 0.3 times, respectively, the human clinical exposure based on AUC in chronic hepatitis C patients at 100 mg/day). No evidence of fetotoxicity, embryolethality, or teratogenicity was observed.

In a pre- and post-natal developmental toxicity study in pregnant rats (F0), no adverse effects on maternal reproductive function or on the development of the offspring (F1) were observed at doses up to 20 mg/kg/day (2 times the human clinical exposure based on AUC in ITP patients at 75 mg/day and similar to the human clinical exposure based on AUC in chronic hepatitis C patients at 100 mg/day). Eltrombopag was detected in the plasma of offspring (F1). The plasma concentrations in pups increased with dose following administration of drug to the F0 dams.

8.3   Nursing Mothers

It is not known whether eltrombopag is excreted in human milk. Because many drugs are excreted in human milk and because of the potential for serious adverse reactions in nursing infants from PROMACTA, a decision should be made whether to discontinue nursing or to discontinue PROMACTA taking into account the importance of PROMACTA to the mother.

8.4 Pediatric Use

The safety and efficacy of PROMACTA in pediatric patients have not been established.

8.5 Geriatric Use

Of the 106 patients in 2 randomized clinical trials of PROMACTA 50 mg in chronic ITP, 22% were 65 years of age and over, while 9% were 75 years of age and over. In the 2 randomized clinical trials of PROMACTA in patients with chronic hepatitis C and thrombocytopenia, 7% were 65 years of age and over, while fewer than 1% were 75 years of age and over. No overall differences in safety or effectiveness were observed between these patients and younger patients in the placebo-controlled trials, but greater sensitivity of some older individuals cannot be ruled out.

8.6 Hepatic Impairment

Hepatic impairment influences the exposure of PROMACTA [see Clinical Pharmacology (12.3)].

A reduction in the initial dose of PROMACTA in patients with chronic ITP is recommended for patients with hepatic impairment (Child-Pugh Class A, B, C) [see Dosage and Administration (2.1) and Warnings and Precautions (5.2)]. No dosage adjustment is necessary for HCV patients with hepatic impairment [see Clinical Pharmacology (12.3)].

8.7 Renal Impairment

No adjustment in the initial PROMACTA dose is needed for patients with renal impairment [see Clinical Pharmacology (12.3)]. Closely monitor patients with impaired renal function when administering PROMACTA.

8.8 Ethnicity

Patients of East Asian ethnicity (i.e., Japanese, Chinese, Taiwanese, and Korean) exhibit higher eltrombopag exposures. A reduction in the initial dose of PROMACTA is recommended for ITP patients of East Asian ancestry and patients of East Asian ancestry with hepatic impairment (Child-Pugh Class A, B, C) [see Dosage and Administration (2.1)]. No dose reduction is needed in patients of East Asian ethnicity with chronic hepatitis C [see Clinical Pharmacology (12.3)].

10 OVERDOSAGE

In the event of overdose, platelet counts may increase excessively and result in thrombotic/thromboembolic complications.

In one report, a subject who ingested 5,000 mg of PROMACTA had a platelet count increase to a maximum of 929×10^9/L at 13 days following the ingestion. The patient also experienced rash, bradycardia, ALT/AST elevations, and fatigue. The patient was treated with gastric lavage, oral lactulose, intravenous fluids, omeprazole, atropine, furosemide, calcium, dexamethasone, and plasmapheresis; however, the abnormal platelet count and liver test abnormalities persisted for 3 weeks. After 2 months follow-up, all events had resolved without sequelae.

In case of an overdose, consider oral administration of a metal cation-containing preparation, such as calcium, aluminum, or magnesium preparations to chelate eltrombopag and thus limit absorption. Closely monitor platelet counts. Reinitiate treatment with PROMACTA in accordance with dosing and administration recommendations [see Dosage and Administration (2.1, 2.2)].

11 DESCRIPTION

PROMACTA (eltrombopag) tablets contain eltrombopag olamine, a small molecule thrombopoietin (TPO) receptor agonist for oral administration. Eltrombopag interacts with the transmembrane domain of the TPO receptor (also known as cMpl) leading to increased platelet production. Each tablet contains eltrombopag olamine in the amount equivalent to 12.5 mg, 25 mg, 50 mg, 75 mg, or 100 mg of eltrombopag free acid.

Eltrombopag olamine is a biphenyl hydrazone. The chemical name for eltrombopag olamine is 3'-[(2Z)-2-[1-(3,4-dimethylphenyl)-3-methyl-5-oxo-1,5-dihydro-4H-pyrazol-4-ylidene]hydrazino]-2'-hydroxy-3-biphenylcarboxylic acid - 2-aminoethanol (1:2). It has the molecular formula $C_{25}H_{22}N_4O_4 \cdot 2(C_2H_7NO)$. The molecular weight is 564.65 for eltrombopag olamine and 442.5 for eltrombopag free acid. Eltrombopag olamine has the following structural formula:

[See chemical structure at top of next column]

Eltrombopag olamine is practically insoluble in aqueous buffer across a pH range of 1 to 7.4, and is sparingly soluble in water.

The inactive ingredients of PROMACTA are: **Tablet Core:** magnesium stearate, mannitol, microcrystalline cellulose, povidone, and sodium starch glycolate. **Coating:** hypromellose (12.5 mg, 25 mg, 50 mg, and 75 mg tablet) or polyvinyl alcohol and talc (100 mg tablet), polyethylene glycol 400, titanium dioxide, polysorbate 80 (12.5 mg tablet), FD&C Yellow No. 6 aluminum lake (25 mg tablet), FD&C Blue No. 2 aluminum lake (50 mg tablet), Iron Oxide Red and Iron Oxide Black (75 mg tablet), or Iron Oxide Yellow and Iron Oxide Black (100 mg tablet).

12 CLINICAL PHARMACOLOGY

12.1 Mechanism of Action

Eltrombopag is an orally bioavailable, small-molecule TPO-receptor agonist that interacts with the transmembrane domain of the human TPO-receptor and initiates signaling cascades that induce proliferation and differentiation of megakaryocytes from bone marrow progenitor cells.

12.3 Pharmacokinetics

Absorption: Eltrombopag is absorbed with a peak concentration occurring 2 to 6 hours after oral administration. Based on urinary excretion and biotransformation products eliminated in feces, the oral absorption of drug-related material following administration of a single 75 mg solution dose was estimated to be at least 52%.

An open-label, randomized, crossover trial was conducted to assess the effect of food on the bioavailability of eltrombopag. A standard high-fat breakfast significantly decreased plasma eltrombopag $AUC_{0-\infty}$ by approximately 59% and C_{max} by 65% and delayed t_{max} by 1 hour. The calcium content of this meal may have also contributed to this decrease in exposure.

Distribution: The concentration of eltrombopag in blood cells is approximately 50% to 79% of plasma concentrations based on a radiolabel study. In vitro studies suggest that eltrombopag is highly bound to human plasma proteins (>99%). Eltrombopag is a substrate of BCRP, but is not a substrate for P-glycoprotein (P-gp) or OATP1B1.

Metabolism: Absorbed eltrombopag is extensively metabolized, predominantly through pathways including cleavage, oxidation, and conjugation with glucuronic acid, glutathione, or cysteine. In vitro studies suggest that CYP1A2 and CYP2C8 are responsible for the oxidative metabolism of eltrombopag. UGT1A1 and UGT1A3 are responsible for the glucuronidation of eltrombopag.

Elimination: The predominant route of eltrombopag excretion is via feces (59%), and 31% of the dose is found in the urine. Unchanged eltrombopag in feces accounts for approximately 20% of the dose; unchanged eltrombopag is not detectable in urine. The plasma elimination half-life of eltrombopag is approximately 21 to 32 hours in healthy subjects and 26 to 35 hours in ITP patients.

Drug Interactions: Polyvalent Cation-containing Antacids: In a clinical trial, co-administration of 75 mg of PROMACTA with a polyvalent cation-containing antacid (1,524 mg aluminum hydroxide, 1,425 mg magnesium carbonate, and sodium alginate) to 26 healthy adult subjects decreased plasma eltrombopag $AUC_{0-\infty}$ and C_{max} by approximately 70%. The contribution of sodium alginate to this interaction is not known.

Cytochrome P450 Enzymes (CYPs): In a clinical trial, PROMACTA 75 mg once daily was administered for 7 days to 24 healthy male subjects did not show inhibition or induction of the metabolism of a combination of probe substrates for CYP1A2 (caffeine), CYP2C19 (omeprazole), CYP2C9 (flurbiprofen), or CYP3A4 (midazolam) in humans. Probe substrates for CYP2C8 were not evaluated in this trial.

Rosuvastatin: In a clinical trial, co-administration of 75 mg of PROMACTA once daily for 5 days with a single 10 mg dose of the OATP1B1 and BCRP substrate, rosuvastatin to 39 healthy adult subjects increased plasma rosuvastatin $AUC_{0-\infty}$ by 55% and C_{max} by 103%.

Protease Inhibitors: HIV Protease Inhibitors: In a clinical trial, co-administration of repeat dose lopinavir 400 mg/ritonavir 100 mg twice daily with a single dose of PROMACTA 100 mg to 40 healthy adult subjects decreased plasma eltrombopag $AUC_{0-\infty}$ by 17%.

HCV Protease Inhibitors: In a clinical trial, co-administration of repeat dose telaprevir 750 mg every 8 hours or boceprevir 800 mg every 8 hours with a single dose of PROMACTA 200 mg to healthy adult subjects did not alter plasma telaprevir, boceprevir, or eltrombopag $AUC_{0-\infty}$ or C_{max} to a significant extent.

Pegylated Interferon alfa-2a + Ribavirin and Pegylated Interferon alfa-2b + Ribavirin: The pharmacokinetics of eltrombopag in both the presence and absence of pegylated interferon alfa 2a and 2b therapy were evaluated using a population pharmacokinetic analysis in 635 patients with chronic hepatitis C. The population PK model estimates of clearance indicate no significant difference in eltrombopag clearance in the presence of pegylated interferon alfa plus ribavirin therapy.

In vitro Studies: Eltrombopag is an inhibitor of CYP2C8 and CYP2C9 in vitro. Eltrombopag is an inhibitor of UGT1A1, UGT1A3, UGT1A4, UGT1A6, UGT1A9, UGT2B7, and UGT2B15 in vitro. Eltrombopag is an inhibitor of the organic anion transporting polypeptide OATP1B1 and BCRP in vitro.

Specific Populations: Ethnicity: Based on two population PK analyses of eltrombopag concentrations in ITP and chronic hepatitis C patients, East Asian (i.e., Japanese, Chinese, Taiwanese, and Korean) subjects exhibited 50 to 55% higher eltrombopag plasma concentrations compared to non-East Asian subjects [see Dosage and Administration (2.1, 2.2)].

An approximately 40% higher systemic eltrombopag exposure in healthy African-American subjects was noted in at least one clinical pharmacology trial. The effect of African-American ethnicity on exposure and related safety and efficacy of eltrombopag has not been established.

Hepatic Impairment: In a pharmacokinetic trial, the disposition of a single 50 mg dose of PROMACTA in patients with mild, moderate, and severe hepatic impairment was compared to subjects with normal hepatic function. The degree of hepatic impairment was based on Child-Pugh score. Plasma eltrombopag $AUC_{0-\infty}$ was 41% higher in patients with mild hepatic impairment (Child-Pugh Class A) compared to subjects with normal hepatic function. Plasma eltrombopag $AUC_{0-\infty}$ was approximately 2-fold higher in patients with moderate (Child-Pugh Class B) and severe hepatic impairment (Child-Pugh Class C). The half-life of eltrombopag was prolonged 2-fold in these patients. This clinical trial did not evaluate protein binding effects.

Chronic Liver Disease: A population PK analysis in thrombocytopenic patients with chronic liver disease following repeat doses of eltrombopag demonstrated that mild hepatic impairment resulted in an 87% to 110% higher plasma eltrombopag $AUC_{(0-\tau)}$ and patients with moderate hepatic impairment had approximately 141% to 240% higher plasma eltrombopag $AUC_{(0-\tau)}$ values compared to patients with normal hepatic function. The half-life of eltrombopag was prolonged 3-fold in patients with mild hepatic impairment and 4-fold in patients with moderate hepatic impairment. This clinical trial did not evaluate protein binding effects.

Chronic Hepatitis C: A population PK in 28 healthy adults and 635 patients with chronic hepatitis C demonstrated that patients with chronic hepatitis C treated with PROMACTA had higher plasma $AUC_{(0-\tau)}$ values as compared to healthy subjects, and $AUC_{(0-\tau)}$ increased with increasing Child-Pugh score. Patients with chronic hepatitis C and mild hepatic impairment had approximately 100% to 144% higher plasma $AUC_{(0-\tau)}$ compared with healthy subjects. This clinical trial did not evaluate protein binding effects.

Renal Impairment: The disposition of a single 50 mg dose of PROMACTA in patients with mild (creatinine clearance (CrCl) of 50 to 80 mL/min), moderate (CrCl of 30 to 49 mL/min), and severe (CrCl less than 30 mL/min) renal impairment was compared to subjects with normal renal function. Average total plasma eltrombopag $AUC_{0-\infty}$ was 32% to 36% lower in subjects with mild to moderate renal impairment and 60% lower in subjects with severe renal impairment compared with healthy subjects. The effect of renal impairment on unbound (active) eltrombopag exposure has not been assessed.

12.6 Assessment of Risk of QT/QTc Prolongation

There is no indication of a QT/QTc prolonging effect of PROMACTA at doses up to 150 mg daily for 5 days. The effects of PROMACTA at doses up to 150 mg daily for 5 days (supratherapeutic doses) on the QT/QTc interval was evaluated in a double-blind, randomized, placebo- and positive-controlled (moxifloxacin 400 mg, single oral dose) crossover trial in healthy adult subjects. Assay sensitivity was confirmed by significant QTc prolongation by moxifloxacin.

13 NONCLINICAL TOXICOLOGY

13.1 Carcinogenesis, Mutagenesis, Impairment of Fertility

Eltrombopag does not stimulate platelet production in rats, mice, or dogs because of unique TPO receptor specificity. Data from these animals do not fully model effects in humans.

Eltrombopag was not carcinogenic in mice at doses up to 75 mg/kg/day or in rats at doses up to 40 mg/kg/day (exposures up to 4 times the human clinical exposure based on AUC in ITP patients at 75 mg/day and 2 times the human clinical exposure based on AUC in chronic hepatitis C patients at 100 mg/day).

Eltrombopag was not mutagenic or clastogenic in a bacterial mutation assay or in 2 in vivo assays in rats (micronucleus and unscheduled DNA synthesis, 10 times the human

Table 8. Trials 1 and 2 Sustained Virologic Response in Adults With Chronic Hepatitis C

	Trial 1[a]		Trial 2[b]	
Pre-antiviral Treatment Phase	N = 715		N = 805	
% Patients who achieved target platelet counts and initiated antiviral therapy[c]	95%		94%	
Antiviral Treatment Phase	PROMACTA N = 450 %	Placebo N = 232 %	PROMACTA N = 506 %	Placebo N = 253 %
Overall SVR[d]	23	14	19	13
HCV Genotype 2,3	35	24	34	25
HCV Genotype 1,4,6	18	10	13	7

[a] PROMACTA given in combination with peginterferon alfa-2a (180 mcg once weekly for 48 weeks for genotypes 1/4/6; 24 weeks for genotype 2 or 3) plus ribavirin (800 to 1,200 mg daily in 2 divided doses orally).
[b] PROMACTA given in combination with peginterferon alfa-2b (1.5 mcg/kg once weekly for 48 weeks for genotypes 1/4/6; 24 weeks for genotype 2 or 3) plus ribavirin (800 to 1,400 mg daily in 2 divided doses orally).
[c] Target platelet count was $\geq 90 \times 10^9$ /L for Trial 1 and $\geq 100 \times 10^9$ /L for Trial 2.
[d] P value <0.05 for PROMACTA versus placebo.

clinical exposure based on C_{max} in ITP patients at 75 mg/day and 7 times the human clinical exposure based on C_{max} in chronic hepatitis C patients at 100 mg/day). In the *in vitro* mouse lymphoma assay, eltrombopag was marginally positive (<3-fold increase in mutation frequency). Eltrombopag did not affect female fertility in rats at doses up to 20 mg/kg/day (2 times the human clinical exposure based on AUC in ITP patients at 75 mg/day and similar to the human clinical exposure based on AUC in chronic hepatitis C patients at 100 mg/day). Eltrombopag did not affect male fertility in rats at doses up to 40 mg/kg/day, the highest dose tested (3 times the human clinical exposure based on AUC in ITP patients at 75 mg/day and 2 times the human clinical exposure based on AUC in chronic hepatitis C patients at 100 mg/day).

13.2 Animal Pharmacology/Toxicology
Eltrombopag is phototoxic *in vitro*. There was no evidence of *in vivo* cutaneous or ocular phototoxicity in rodents.
Treatment-related cataracts were detected in rodents in a dose- and time-dependent manner. At ≥ 6 times the human clinical exposure based on AUC in ITP patients at 75 mg/day and 3 times the human clinical exposure based on AUC in chronic hepatitis C patients at 100 mg/day, cataracts were observed in mice after 6 weeks and in rats after 28 weeks of dosing. At ≥ 4 times the human clinical exposure based on AUC in ITP patients at 75 mg/day and 2 times the human clinical exposure based on AUC in chronic hepatitis C patients at 100 mg/day, cataracts were observed in mice after 13 weeks and in rats after 39 weeks of dosing *[see Warnings and Precautions (5.4)]*.
Renal tubular toxicity was observed in studies up to 14 days in duration in mice and rats at exposures that were generally associated with morbidity and mortality. Tubular toxicity was also observed in a 2-year oral carcinogenicity study in mice at doses of 25, 75, and 150 mg/kg/day. The exposure at the lowest dose was 1.2 times the human clinical exposure based on AUC in ITP patients at 75 mg/day and 0.6 times the human clinical exposure based on AUC in chronic hepatitis C patients at 100 mg/day. No similar effects were observed in mice after 13 weeks at exposures greater than those associated with renal changes in the 2-year study, suggesting that this effect is both dose- and time-dependent.

14 CLINICAL STUDIES
14.1 Chronic ITP
The efficacy and safety of PROMACTA in adult patients with chronic ITP were evaluated in 3 randomized, double-blind, placebo-controlled trials and in an open-label extension trial.
Trials 1 and 2: In trials 1 and 2, patients who had completed at least one prior ITP therapy and who had a platelet count $<30 \times 10^9$ /L were randomized to receive either PROMACTA or placebo daily for up to 6 weeks, followed by 6 weeks off therapy. During the trials, PROMACTA or placebo was discontinued if the platelet count exceeded 200×10^9 /L. The primary efficacy endpoint was response rate, defined as a shift from a baseline platelet count of $<30 \times 10^9$ /L to $\geq 50 \times 10^9$ /L at any time during the treatment period.
The median age of the patients was 50 years and 60% were female. Approximately 70% of the patients had received at least 2 prior ITP therapies (predominantly corticosteroids, immunoglobulins, rituximab, cytotoxic therapies, danazol, and azathioprine) and 40% of the patients had undergone splenectomy. The median baseline platelet counts (approximately 18×10^9 /L) were similar among all treatment groups.
Trial 1 randomized 114 patients (2:1) to PROMACTA 50 mg or placebo. Trial 2 randomized 117 patients (1:1:1:1) among placebo or 1 of 3 dose regimens of PROMACTA, 30 mg, 50 mg, or 75 mg each administered daily.

Table 6 shows for each trial the primary efficacy outcomes for the placebo groups and the patient groups who received the 50 mg daily regimen of PROMACTA.

Table 6. Trials 1 and 2 Platelet Count Response ($\geq 50 \times 10^9$/L) Rates in Adults With Chronic Immune (Idiopathic) Thrombocytopenia

Trial	PROMACTA 50 mg Daily	Placebo
1	43/73 (59%)[a]	6/37 (16%)
2	19/27 (70%)[a]	3/27 (11%)

[a] P value <0.001 for PROMACTA versus placebo.

The platelet count response to PROMACTA was similar among patients who had or had not undergone splenectomy. In general, increases in platelet counts were detected 1 week following initiation of PROMACTA and the maximum response was observed after 2 weeks of therapy. In the placebo and 50 mg dose groups of PROMACTA, the trial drug was discontinued due to an increase in platelet counts to $>200 \times 10^9$ /L in 3% and 27% of the patients, respectively. The median duration of treatment with the 50 mg dose of PROMACTA was 42 days in Trial 1 and 43 days in Trial 2. Of 7 patients who underwent hemostatic challenges, additional ITP medications were required in 3 of 3 placebo group patients and 0 of 4 patients treated with PROMACTA. Surgical procedures accounted for most of the hemostatic challenges. Hemorrhage requiring transfusion occurred in one placebo group patient and no patients treated with PROMACTA.
Trial 3: In this trial, 197 patients were randomized (2:1) to receive either PROMACTA 50 mg once daily (n = 135) or placebo (n = 62) for 6 months, during which time the dose of PROMACTA could be adjusted based on individual platelet counts. Patients were allowed to taper or discontinue concomitant ITP medications after being treated with PROMACTA for 6 weeks. Patients were permitted to receive rescue treatments at any time during the trial as clinically indicated. The primary endpoint was the odds of achieving a platelet count $\geq 50 \times 10^9$ /L and $\leq 400 \times 10^9$ /L for patients receiving PROMACTA relative to placebo and was based on patient response profiles throughout the 6-month treatment period.
The median age of the patients treated with PROMACTA and placebo was 47 years and 52.5 years, respectively. Approximately half of the patients treated with PROMACTA and placebo (47% and 50%, respectively) were receiving concomitant ITP medication (predominantly corticosteroids) at randomization and had baseline platelet counts 15×10^9 /L (50% and 48%, respectively). A similar percentage of patients treated with PROMACTA and placebo (37% and 34%, respectively) had a prior splenectomy.
In 134 patients who completed 26 weeks of treatment, a sustained platelet response (platelet count $\geq 50 \times 10^9$ /L and $\leq 400 \times 10^9$ /L for 6 out of the last 8 weeks of the 26-week treatment period in the absence of rescue medication at any time) was achieved by 60% of patients treated with PROMACTA, compared to 10% of patients treated with placebo (splenectomized patients: PROMACTA 51%, placebo 8%; non-splenectomized patients: PROMACTA 66%, placebo 11%). The proportion of responders in the PROMACTA treatment group was between 37% and 56% compared to 7% and 19% in the placebo treatment group for all on-therapy visits. Patients treated with PROMACTA were significantly more likely to achieve a platelet count between 50×10^9 /L and 400×10^9 /L during the entire 6-month treatment period compared to those patients treated with placebo.

Outcomes of treatment are presented in Table 7 for all patients enrolled in the trial.

Table 7. Outcomes of Treatment from Trial 3 in Adults With Chronic Immune (Idiopathic) Thrombocytopenia

Outcome	PROMACTA N = 135	Placebo N = 62
Mean number of weeks with platelet counts $\geq 50 \times 10^9$/L	11.3	2.4
Requiring rescue therapy, n (%)	24 (18)	25 (40)

Among 94 patients receiving other ITP therapy at baseline, 37 (59%) of 63 patients in the PROMACTA group and 10 (32%) of 31 patients in the placebo group discontinued concomitant therapy at some time during the trial.
Extension Trial: Patients who completed any prior clinical trial with PROMACTA were enrolled in an open-label, single-arm trial in which attempts were made to decrease the dose or eliminate the need for any concomitant ITP medications. PROMACTA was administered to 299 patients; 249 completed 6 months, 210 patients completed 12 months, and 138 patients completed 24 months of therapy. The median baseline platelet count was 19×10^9 /L prior to administration of PROMACTA.

14.2 Chronic Hepatitis C-Associated Thrombocytopenia
The efficacy and safety of PROMACTA for the treatment of thrombocytopenia in adult patients with chronic hepatitis C were evaluated in 2 randomized, double-blind, placebo-controlled trials. Trial 1 utilized peginterferon alfa-2a (PEGASYS®) plus ribavirin for antiviral treatment and Trial 2 utilized peginterferon alfa-2b (PEGINTRON®) plus ribavirin. In both trials, patients with a platelet count of $<75 \times 10^9$ /L were enrolled and stratified by platelet count, screening HCV RNA, and HCV genotype. Patients were excluded if they had evidence of decompensated liver disease with Child-Pugh score > 6 (class B and C), history of ascites, or hepatic encephalopathy. The median age of the patients in both trials was 52 years, 63% were male, and 74% were Caucasian. Sixty-nine percent of patients had HCV genotypes 1, 4, 6 with the remainder genotypes 2 and 3. Approximately 30% of patients had been previously treated with interferon and ribavirin. The majority of patients (90%) had bridging fibrosis and cirrhosis, as indicated by noninvasive testing. A similar proportion (95%) of patients in both treatment groups had Child-Pugh level A (score 5-6) at baseline. A similar proportion of patients (2%) in both treatment groups had baseline international normalized ratio (INR) > 1.7. Median baseline platelet counts (approximately 60×10^9 /L) were similar in both treatment groups. The trials consisted of two phases – a pre-antiviral treatment phase and an antiviral treatment phase. In the pre-antiviral treatment phase, patients received open-label PROMACTA to increase the platelet count to a threshold of $\geq 90 \times 10^9$ /L for Trial 1 and $\geq 100 \times 10^9$ /L for Trial 2. PROMACTA was administered at an initial dose of 25 mg once daily for 2 weeks and increased in 25 mg increments over 2 to 3 week periods to achieve the optimal platelet count to initiate antiviral therapy. The maximal time patients could receive open-label PROMACTA was 9 weeks. If threshold platelet counts were achieved, patients were randomized (2:1) to the same dose of PROMACTA at the end of the pre-treatment phase or to placebo. PROMACTA was administered in combination with pegylated interferon and ribavirin per their respective prescribing information for up to 48 weeks.
The primary efficacy endpoint for both trials was sustained virologic response (SVR) defined as the percentage of patients with undetectable HCV-RNA at 24 weeks after completion of antiviral treatment. The median time to achieve the target platelet count $\geq 90 \times 10^9$ /L was approximately 2 weeks. Ninety-five percent of patients were able to initiate antiviral therapy.
In both trials, a significantly greater proportion of patients treated with PROMACTA achieved SVR (see Table 8). The improvement in the proportion of patients who achieved SVR was consistent across subgroups based on baseline platelet count ($<50 \times 10^9$ /L versus $\geq 50 \times 10^9$ /L). In patients with high baseline viral loads ($\geq 800,000$), the SVR rate was 18% (82/452) for PROMACTA versus 8% (20/239) for placebo.
[See table 8 above]
The majority of patients treated with PROMACTA (76%) maintained a platelet count $\geq 50 \times 10^9$ /L compared to 19% for placebo. A greater proportion of patients on PROMACTA did not require any antiviral dose reduction as compared to placebo (45% versus 27%).

16 HOW SUPPLIED/STORAGE AND HANDLING
• The 12.5 mg tablets are round, biconvex, white, film-coated tablets debossed with GS MZ1 and 12.5 on one side and are available in bottles of 30: NDC 0007-4643-13.
• The 25 mg tablets are round, biconvex, orange, film-coated tablets debossed with GS NX3 and 25 on one side and are available in bottles of 30: NDC 0007-4640-13.

- The 50 mg tablets are round, biconvex, blue, film-coated tablets debossed with GS UFU and 50 on one side and are available in bottles of 30: NDC 0007-4641-13.
- The 75 mg tablets are round, biconvex, pink, film-coated tablets debossed with GS FFS and 75 on one side and are available in bottles of 30: NDC 0007-4642-13.
- The 100 mg tablets are round, biconvex, green, film-coated tablets debossed with GS 1L5 and are available in bottles of 30: NDC 0007-4646-13. This product contains a desiccant.

Store at room temperature between 20°C and 25°C (68°F to 77°F); excursions permitted to 15° to 30°C (59° to 86°F) [see USP Controlled Room Temperature]. Do not remove desiccant if present. Dispense in original bottle.

17   PATIENT COUNSELING INFORMATION

See FDA-approved patient labeling (Medication Guide). Prior to treatment, patients should fully understand and be informed of the following risks and considerations for PROMACTA:

- For patients with chronic ITP, therapy with PROMACTA is administered to achieve and maintain a platelet count $\geq 50 \times 10^9$/L as necessary to reduce the risk for bleeding.
- For patients with chronic hepatitis C, therapy with PROMACTA is administered to achieve and maintain a platelet count necessary to initiate and maintain antiviral therapy with pegylated interferon and ribavirin.
- Therapy with PROMACTA may be associated with hepatobiliary laboratory abnormalities.
- Advise patients with chronic hepatitis C and cirrhosis that they may be at risk for hepatic decompensation when receiving alfa interferon therapy.
- Advise patients that they should report any of the following signs and symptoms of liver problems to their healthcare provider right away.
  - yellowing of the skin or the whites of the eyes (jaundice)
  - unusual darkening of the urine
  - unusual tiredness
  - right upper stomach area pain
  - confusion
  - swelling of the stomach area (abdomen)
- Advise patients that thrombocytopenia and risk of bleeding may reoccur upon discontinuing PROMACTA, particularly if PROMACTA is discontinued while the patient is on anticoagulants or antiplatelet agents.
- Advise patients that too much PROMACTA may result in excessive platelet counts and a risk for thrombotic/thromboembolic complications.
- Advise patients that during therapy with PROMACTA, they should continue to avoid situations or medications that may increase the risk for bleeding.
- Advise patients to have a baseline ocular examination prior to administration of PROMACTA and be monitored for signs and symptoms of cataracts during therapy.
- Advise patients to keep at least a 4-hour interval between PROMACTA and foods, mineral supplements, and antacids which contain polyvalent cations such as iron, calcium, aluminum, magnesium, selenium, and zinc.

PROMACTA is a registered trademark of the GSK group of companies. The following are registered trademarks of their respective owners: PEGASYS/Hoffmann-La Roche Inc.; PEGINTRON/Schering Corporation.

GlaxoSmithKline
Research Triangle Park, NC 27709
©2014, the GSK group of companies. All rights reserved.
PRM:7PI

MEDICATION GUIDE

PROMACTA®(pro-MAC-ta)
(eltrombopag)
tablets

Read this Medication Guide before you start taking PROMACTA and each time you get a refill. There may be new information. This Medication Guide does not take the place of talking with your healthcare provider about your medical condition or treatment.

What is the most important information I should know about PROMACTA?
PROMACTA can cause serious side effects, including:
Liver problems. If you have chronic hepatitis C virus, and take PROMACTA with interferon and ribavirin treatment, PROMACTA may increase your risk of liver problems. Tell your healthcare provider right away if you have any of these signs and symptoms of liver problems:
- yellowing of the skin or the whites of the eyes (jaundice)
- unusual darkening of the urine
- unusual tiredness
- right upper stomach area pain
- confusion
- swelling of the stomach area (abdomen)

See "What are the possible side effects of PROMACTA?" for other side effects of PROMACTA.
What is PROMACTA?
PROMACTA is a prescription medicine used to treat low blood platelet counts in people with:

- chronic immune (idiopathic) thrombocytopenia (ITP), when other medicines to treat your ITP or surgery to remove the spleen have not worked well enough
- chronic hepatitis C virus (HCV) infection before and during treatment with interferon

PROMACTA is used to try to raise your platelet count in order to lower your risk for bleeding.
PROMACTA is not used to make your platelet count normal.
PROMACTA is for treatment of certain people with low platelet counts caused by chronic ITP or chronic HCV, not low platelet counts caused by other conditions or diseases. It is not known if PROMACTA is safe and effective when used with other antiviral medicines that are approved to treat chronic hepatitis C.
It is not known if PROMACTA is safe and effective in children.
What should I tell my healthcare provider before taking PROMACTA?
Before you take PROMACTA, tell your healthcare provider if you:
- have liver or kidney problems
- have or had a blood clot
- have a history of cataracts
- have had surgery to remove your spleen (splenectomy)
- have bleeding problems
- are Asian and you are of Chinese, Japanese, Taiwanese, or Korean ancestry. You may need a lower dose of PROMACTA.
- have any other medical conditions
- are pregnant or plan to become pregnant. It is not known if PROMACTA will harm an unborn baby.
  Pregnancy Registry: There is a registry for women who become pregnant during treatment with PROMACTA. If you become pregnant, consider this registry. The purpose of the registry is to collect safety information about the health of you and your baby. Contact the registry as soon as you become aware of the pregnancy, or ask your healthcare provider to contact the registry for you. You and your healthcare provider can get information and enroll in the registry by calling 1-888-825-5249.
- are breastfeeding or plan to breastfeed. It is not known if PROMACTA passes into your breast milk. You and your healthcare provider should decide whether you will take PROMACTA or breastfeed. You should not do both.

Tell your healthcare provider about all the medicines you take, including prescription and over-the-counter medicines, vitamins, and herbal supplements. PROMACTA may affect the way certain medicines work. Certain other medicines may affect the way PROMACTA works.
Especially tell your healthcare provider if you take:
- certain medicines used to treat high cholesterol, called "statins"
- a blood thinner medicine
Certain medicines may keep PROMACTA from working correctly. Take PROMACTA at least 4 hours before or 4 hours after taking these products:
- antacids used to treat stomach ulcers or heartburn
- multivitamins or products that contain iron, calcium, aluminum, magnesium, selenium, and zinc which may be found in mineral supplements
Ask your healthcare provider if you are not sure if your medicine is one that is listed above.
Know the medicines you take. Keep a list of them and show it to your healthcare provider and pharmacist when you get a new medicine.
How should I take PROMACTA?
- Take PROMACTA exactly as your healthcare provider tells you to take it. Do not stop taking PROMACTA without talking with your healthcare provider first. Do not change your dose or schedule for taking PROMACTA unless your healthcare provider tells you to change it.
- Take PROMACTA on an empty stomach, either 1 hour before or 2 hours after eating food.
- Take PROMACTA at least 4 hours before or 4 hours after eating dairy products and calcium fortified juices.
- If you miss a dose of PROMACTA, wait and take your next scheduled dose. Do not take more than one dose of PROMACTA in one day.
- If you take too much PROMACTA, you may have a higher risk of serious side effects. Call your healthcare provider right away.
- Your healthcare provider will check your platelet count during your treatment with PROMACTA and change your dose of PROMACTA as needed.
- Tell your healthcare provider about any bruising or bleeding that happens while you take and after you stop taking PROMACTA.

What should I avoid while taking PROMACTA?
Avoid situations and medicines that may increase your risk of bleeding.

What are the possible side effects of PROMACTA?
PROMACTA may cause serious side effects, including:
- See "What is the most important information I should know about PROMACTA?"
- **Abnormal liver function tests.** Your healthcare provider will order blood tests to check your liver before you start taking PROMACTA and during your treatment. In some cases treatment with PROMACTA may need to be stopped due to changes in your liver function tests.
- **High platelet counts and higher risk for blood clots.** Your risk of getting a blood clot is increased if your platelet count is too high during treatment with PROMACTA. Your risk of getting a blood clot may also be increased during treatment with PROMACTA if you have normal or low platelet counts. You may have severe problems or die from some forms of blood clots, such as clots that travel to the lungs or that cause heart attacks or strokes. Your healthcare provider will check your blood platelet counts, and change your dose or stop PROMACTA if your platelet counts get too high. Tell your healthcare provider right away if you have signs and symptoms of a blood clot in the leg, such as swelling, pain, or tenderness in your leg. People with chronic liver disease may be at risk for a type of blood clot in the stomach area. Tell your healthcare provider right away if you have stomach area pain that may be a symptom of this type of blood clot.
- **New or worsened cataracts (a clouding of the lens in the eye).** New or worsened cataracts have happened in people taking PROMACTA. Your healthcare provider will check your eyes before and during your treatment with PROMACTA. Tell your healthcare provider about any changes in your eyesight while taking PROMACTA.

The most common side effects of PROMACTA when used to treat chronic ITP are:
- nausea
- diarrhea
- upper respiratory tract infection. Symptoms may include runny nose, stuffy nose, and sneezing
- vomiting
- muscle aches
- urinary tract infection. Symptoms may include frequent or urgent need to urinate, low fever in some people, pain or burning with urination
- pain or swelling (inflammation) in your throat or mouth (oropharyngeal pain and pharyngitis)
- abnormal liver function tests
- back pain
- "flu" like symptoms (influenza) including fever, headache, tiredness, cough, sore throat, and body aches
- skin tingling, itching, or burning
- rash

The most common side effects when PROMACTA is used in combination with other medicines to treat chronic HCV are:
- low red blood cell count (anemia)
- fever
- tiredness
- headache
- nausea
- diarrhea
- decreased appetite
- "flu" like symptoms (influenza) including fever, headache, tiredness, cough, sore throat, and body aches
- feeling weak
- trouble sleeping
- cough
- itching
- chills
- muscle aches
- hair loss
- swelling in your ankles, feet, and legs
Tell your healthcare provider if you have any side effect that bothers you or that does not go away. These are not all the possible side effects of PROMACTA. For more information, ask your healthcare provider or pharmacist.
Call your doctor for medical advice about side effects. You may report side effects to FDA at 1-800-FDA-1088.
How should I store PROMACTA tablets?
- Store PROMACTA at room temperature between 68°F to 77°F (20°C to 25°C).
- Keep PROMACTA tightly closed in the bottle given to you.
- The PROMACTA bottle may contain a desiccant pack to help keep your medicine dry. Do not remove the desiccant pack from the bottle.
Keep PROMACTA and all medicines out of the reach of children.
General information about the safe and effective use of PROMACTA
Medicines are sometimes prescribed for purposes other than those listed in a Medication Guide. Do not use PROMACTA for a condition for which it was not prescribed. Do not give PROMACTA to other people even, if they have the same symptoms that you have. It may harm them.
This Medication Guide summarizes the most important information about PROMACTA. If you would like more information, talk with your healthcare provider. You can ask

your healthcare provider or pharmacist for information about PROMACTA that is written for health professionals. For more information about PROMACTA, go to www.PROMACTA.com or call 1-888-825-5249.

What are the ingredients in PROMACTA?
Active ingredient: eltrombopag olamine.
Inactive ingredients:
- **Tablet Core:** magnesium stearate, mannitol, microcrystalline cellulose, povidone, and sodium starch glycolate.
- **Coating:** hypromellose (12.5 mg, 25 mg, 50 mg, and 75 mg tablets) or polyvinyl alcohol and talc (100 mg tablet), polyethylene glycol 400, titanium dioxide, polysorbate 80 (12.5 mg tablet), and FD&C Yellow No. 6 aluminum lake (25 mg tablet), FD&C Blue No. 2 aluminum lake (50 mg tablet), Iron Oxide Red and Iron Oxide Black (75 mg tablet), or Iron Oxide Yellow and Iron Oxide Black (100 mg tablet).

This Medication Guide has been approved by the U.S. Food and Drug Administration.
PROMACTA is a registered trademark of the GSK group of companies.
GlaxoSmithKline
Research Triangle Park, NC 27709
©2014, the GSK group of companies. All rights reserved.
Revised: February 2014
PRM:7MG

RAXIBACUMAB INJECTION
for intravenous use   ℞

HIGHLIGHTS OF PRESCRIBING INFORMATION
These highlights do not include all the information needed to use RAXIBACUMAB safely and effectively. See full prescribing information for RAXIBACUMAB.
RAXIBACUMAB injection, for intravenous use
Initial U.S. Approval: 2012

INDICATIONS AND USAGE
Raxibacumab is indicated for the treatment of adult and pediatric patients with inhalational anthrax due to *Bacillus anthracis* in combination with appropriate antibacterial drugs, and for prophylaxis of inhalational anthrax when alternative therapies are not available or are not appropriate. (1)
Limitations of Use:
- The effectiveness of raxibacumab is based solely on efficacy studies in animal models of inhalational anthrax. (1.2, 14.1)
- There have been no studies of raxibacumab in the pediatric population. Dosing in pediatric patients was derived using a population PK approach. (1.2, 8.4)
- Raxibacumab does not cross the blood-brain barrier and does not prevent or treat meningitis. Raxibacumab should be used in combination with appropriate antibacterial drugs. (1.2)

DOSAGE AND ADMINISTRATION
- Premedicate with diphenhydramine. (5.1)
- Dilute and administer as an intravenous infusion over 2 hours and 15 minutes. (2.2)
  - Adults: 40 mg/kg raxibacumab. (2.1)
  - Pediatrics greater than 50 kg: 40 mg/kg raxibacumab. (2.2)

- Pediatrics greater than 15 kg to 50 kg: 60 mg/kg raxibacumab. (2.2)
- Pediatrics 15 kg or less: 80 mg/kg raxibacumab. (2.2)

DOSAGE FORMS AND STRENGTHS
Single-use vial contains 1,700 mg/34 mL (50 mg/mL) raxibacumab solution. (3)

CONTRAINDICATIONS
None. (4)

WARNINGS AND PRECAUTIONS
Infusion reactions may occur. Premedicate with diphenhydramine. Slow or interrupt infusion and administer treatment based on severity of the reaction. (5.1)

ADVERSE REACTIONS
Common adverse reactions in healthy adult subjects (≥1.5%) were: rash, pain in extremity, pruritus, and somnolence. (6.1)

To report SUSPECTED ADVERSE REACTIONS, contact GlaxoSmithKline at 1-888-825-5249 or FDA at 1-800-FDA-1088 or www.fda.gov/medwatch.

USE IN SPECIFIC POPULATIONS
- Nursing Mothers: Caution should be exercised when administered to a nursing woman. (8.3)
- Pediatric Use: Safety and effectiveness in children <16 years of age not studied. (8.4)
See 17 for PATIENT COUNSELING INFORMATION and FDA-approved patient labeling

Revised: 04/2014

FULL PRESCRIBING INFORMATION
1 INDICATIONS AND USAGE
1.1 Inhalational Anthrax
Raxibacumab is indicated for the treatment of adult and pediatric patients with inhalational anthrax due to *Bacillus anthracis* in combination with appropriate antibacterial drugs. Raxibacumab is also indicated for prophylaxis of inhalational anthrax when alternative therapies are not available or are not appropriate.
1.2 Limitations of Use
The effectiveness of raxibacumab is based solely on efficacy studies in animal models of inhalational anthrax. It is not ethical or feasible to conduct controlled clinical trials with intentional exposure of humans to anthrax. [See Clinical Studies (14.1).]
Safety and pharmacokinetics (PK) of raxibacumab have been studied in adult healthy volunteers. There have been no trials of safety or PK of raxibacumab in the pediatric population. A population PK approach was used to derive dosing regimens that are predicted to provide pediatric patients with exposure comparable to the observed exposure in adults. [See Use in Specific Populations (8.4).]
Raxibacumab binds to the protective antigen (PA) of *B. anthracis*; it does not have direct antibacterial activity. Raxibacumab does not cross the blood-brain barrier and does not prevent or treat meningitis. Raxibacumab should be used in combination with appropriate antibacterial drugs.

2 DOSAGE AND ADMINISTRATION
2.1 Dose and Schedule for Adults
Administer raxibacumab as a single dose of 40 mg/kg intravenously over 2 hours and 15 minutes after dilution in 0.9% Sodium Chloride Injection, USP (normal saline) to a final volume of 250 mL. Administer 25 to 50 mg diphenhydramine within 1 hour prior to raxibacumab infusion to reduce the risk of infusion reactions. Diphenhydramine route of administration (oral or IV) should be based on the temporal proximity to the start of raxibacumab infusion. [See Warnings and Precautions (5.1), Adverse Reactions (6.1).]
2.2 Dose and Schedule for Pediatric Patients
The recommended dose for pediatric patients is based on weight as shown in Table 1.

Table 1. Recommended Pediatric Dose

Pediatric Body Weight	Pediatric Dose
Greater than 50 kg	40 mg/kg
Greater than 15 kg to 50 kg	60 mg/kg
15 kg or less	80 mg/kg

Premedicate with diphenhydramine within 1 hour prior to raxibacumab infusion. Diphenhydramine route of administration (oral or IV) should be based on the temporal proximity to the start of raxibacumab infusion. Infuse raxibacumab over 2 hours and 15 minutes. No pediatric patients were studied during the development of raxibacumab. The dosing recommendations in Table 1 are derived from simulations designed to match the observed adult exposure to raxibacumab at a 40 mg/kg dose. [See Use in Specific Populations (8.4).]
2.3 Preparation for Administration
The recommended dose of raxibacumab is weight-based, given as an intravenous infusion after dilution in a compatible solution to a final volume of 250 mL (adults and children 50 kg or heavier) or to a volume indicated based on the child's weight (Table 2). Dilute raxibacumab using one of the following compatible solutions:
- 0.9% Sodium Chloride Injection, USP
- 0.45% Sodium Chloride Injection, USP
Keep vials in their cartons prior to preparation of an infusion solution to protect raxibacumab from light. Raxibacumab vials contain no preservative.
[See table 2 below]
Preparation: Follow the steps below to prepare the raxibacumab intravenous infusion solution.
1. Calculate the milligrams of raxibacumab injection by multiplying the recommended mg/kg dose in Table 2 by patient weight in kilograms.
2. Calculate the required volume in milliliters of raxibacumab injection needed for the dose by dividing the calculated dose in milligrams (step 1) by the concentration, 50 mg/mL. Each single-use vial allows delivery of 34 mL raxibacumab.

Table 2. Raxibacumab Dose, Diluents, Infusion Volume and Rate by Body Weight

Body Weight (kg)	Dose (mg/kg)	Total Infusion Volume (mL)	Type of Diluent	Infusion Rate (mL/h) First 20 Minutes	Infusion Rate (mL/h) Remaining Infusion
1 or less	80	7	0.45% or 0.9% NaCl	0.5	3.5
1.1 to 2		15		1	7
2.1 to 3		20		1.2	10
3.1 to 4.9		25		1.5	12
5 to 10		50		3	25
11 to 15		100		6	50
16 to 30	60	100	0.9% NaCl	6	50
31 to 40		250		15	125
41 to 50		250		15	125
Greater than 50 or adult	40	250		15	125

Based on the total infusion volume selected in Table 2, prepare either a syringe or infusion bag as appropriate following the steps below.

Syringe Preparation

3. Select an appropriate size syringe for the total volume of infusion to be administered, as described in Table 2.
4. Using the selected syringe, withdraw the volume of raxibacumab as calculated in step 2.
5. Withdraw an appropriate amount of compatible solution to prepare a total volume infusion syringe as specified in Table 2.
6. Gently mix the solution. Do not shake.
7. Discard any unused portion remaining in the raxibacumab vial(s).
8. The prepared solution is stable for 8 hours stored at room temperature.

Infusion Bag Preparation

3. Select appropriate size bag of compatible solution (see compatible solutions listed in Table 2), withdraw a volume of solution from the bag equal to the calculated volume in milliliters of raxibacumab in Table 2. Discard the solution that was withdrawn from the bag.
4. Withdraw the required volume of raxibacumab injection from the raxibacumab vial(s).
5. Transfer the required volume of raxibacumab injection to the selected infusion bag (step 3). Gently invert the bag to mix the solution. Do not shake.
6. Discard any unused portion remaining in the raxibacumab vial(s).
7. The prepared solution is stable for 8 hours stored at room temperature.

Parenteral drug products should be inspected visually for particulate matter and discoloration prior to administration, whenever solution and container permit. Discard the solution if particulate matter is present or color is abnormal. *[See Description (11).]*

Administration: Administer the infusion solution as described in Table 2. The rate of infusion may be slowed or interrupted if the patient develops any signs of adverse reactions, including infusion-associated symptoms.

3 DOSAGE FORMS AND STRENGTHS

Raxibacumab is available as a single-use vial which contains 1,700 mg/34 mL (50 mg/mL) raxibacumab injection *[see Description (11)]*.

4 CONTRAINDICATIONS

None.

5 WARNINGS AND PRECAUTIONS
5.1 Infusion Reactions

Infusion-related reactions were reported during administration of raxibacumab in clinical trials including reports of rash, urticaria, and pruritus. If these reactions occur, slow or interrupt raxibacumab infusion and administer appropriate treatment based on severity of the reaction.

Premedicate with diphenhydramine within 1 hour prior to administering raxibacumab to reduce the risk of infusion reactions *[see Dosage and Administration (2.1), Adverse Reactions (6.1)]*.

6 ADVERSE REACTIONS
6.1 Clinical Trials Experience

Because clinical trials are conducted under widely varying conditions, adverse reaction rates observed in the clinical trials of a drug cannot be directly compared with rates in the clinical trials of another drug and may not reflect the rates observed in practice. The safety of raxibacumab has been studied only in healthy volunteers. It has not been studied in patients with inhalational anthrax.

The safety of raxibacumab has been evaluated in 326 healthy subjects treated with a dose of 40 mg/kg in 3 clinical trials: a drug interaction trial with ciprofloxacin (Study 1), a repeat-dose trial of 20 subjects with the second raxibacumab dose administered ≥4 months after the first dose (Study 2), and a placebo-controlled trial evaluating single doses with a subset of subjects receiving 2 raxibacumab doses 14 days apart (Study 3). Raxibacumab was administered to 86 healthy subjects in Study 1. In Study 3, 240 healthy subjects received raxibacumab (217 received 1 dose and 23 received 2 doses) and 80 subjects received placebo. The overall safety of raxibacumab was evaluated as an integrated summary of these 3 clinical trials. Of 326 raxibacumab subjects, 283 received single doses, 23 received 2 doses 14 days apart, and 20 received 2 doses more than 4 months apart. The subjects were 18 to 88 years of age, 53% female, 74% white, 17% black/African American, 6% Asian, and 15% Hispanic.

Adverse Reactions Leading to Discontinuation of Raxibacumab Infusion

Four subjects (1.2%) had their infusion of raxibacumab discontinued for adverse reactions: 2 subjects (neither of whom received diphenhydramine premedication) due to urticaria (mild), and 1 subject each discontinued for clonus (mild) and dyspnea (moderate).

Table 3. Adverse Reactions Reported in ≥1.5% of Healthy Adult Subjects Exposed to Raxibacumab 40 mg/kg IV

Preferred Term	Placebo N = 80 (%)	Single-dose Raxibacumab N = 283 (%)	Double-dose Raxibacumab ≥4 Months Apart N = 20 (%)	Double-dose Raxibacumab 2 Weeks Apart N = 23 (%)	Total Raxibacumab Subjects N = 326 (%)
Rash/Rash erythematous/Rash papular	1 (1.3)	9 (3.2)	0	0	9 (2.8)
Pain in extremity	1 (1.3)	7 (2.5)	0	0	7 (2.1)
Pruritus	0	7 (2.5)	0	0	7 (2.1)
Somnolence	0	4 (1.4)	0	1 (4.3)	5 (1.5)

Most Frequently Reported Adverse Reactions

The most frequently reported adverse reactions were rash, pain in extremity, pruritus, and somnolence.

[See table 3 above]

Rashes

For all subjects exposed to raxibacumab in clinical trials, the rate of rash was 2.8% (9/326) compared with 1.3% (1/80) of placebo subjects. Mild to moderate infusion-related rashes were reported in 22.2% (6/27) of subjects who did not receive diphenhydramine premedication compared to 3.3% (2/61) of subjects who were premedicated with diphenhydramine in the ciprofloxacin/raxibacumab combination trial (Study 1). In the placebo-controlled raxibacumab study where all subjects received diphenhydramine (Study 3), the rate of rash was 2.5% in both placebo- and raxibacumab-treated subjects.

Less Common Adverse Reactions

Clinically significant adverse reactions that were reported in <1.5% of subjects exposed to raxibacumab and at rates higher than in placebo subjects are listed below:

- *Blood and lymphatic system*: anemia, leukopenia, lymphadenopathy
- *Cardiac disorders*: palpitations
- *Ear and labyrinth*: vertigo
- *General disorders and administration site*: fatigue, infusion site pain, peripheral edema
- *Investigations*: blood amylase increased, blood creatine phosphokinase increased, prothrombin time prolonged
- *Musculoskeletal and connective tissue*: back pain, muscle spasms
- *Nervous system*: syncope vasovagal
- *Psychiatric*: insomnia
- *Vascular*: flushing, hypertension

Immunogenicity

The development of anti-raxibacumab antibodies was evaluated in all subjects receiving single and double doses of raxibacumab in Studies 1, 2, and 3. Immunogenic responses against raxibacumab were not detected in any raxibacumab-treated human subjects following single or repeat doses of raxibacumab.

The incidence of antibody formation is highly dependent on the sensitivity and specificity of the immunogenicity assay. Additionally, the observed incidence of any antibody positivity in an assay is highly dependent on several factors, including assay sensitivity and specificity, assay methodology, sample handling, timing of sample collection, concomitant medications, and underlying disease. For these reasons, comparison of the incidence of antibodies to raxibacumab with the incidence of antibodies to other products may be misleading.

7 DRUG INTERACTIONS
7.1 Ciprofloxacin

Co-administration of 40 mg/kg raxibacumab IV with IV or oral ciprofloxacin in human subjects did not alter the PK of either ciprofloxacin or raxibacumab *[see Clinical Pharmacology (12.3)]*.

8 USE IN SPECIFIC POPULATIONS
8.1 Pregnancy

Pregnancy Category B

A single embryonic-fetal development study was conducted in pregnant, healthy New Zealand White rabbits administered 2 intravenous doses of raxibacumab up to 120 mg/kg (3 times the human dose on a mg/kg basis) on gestation days 7 and 14. No evidence of harm to the pregnant dam or the fetuses due to raxibacumab was observed. C_{max} values in rabbits after dosing with 120 mg/kg were 3,629 mcg/mL and 4,337 mcg/mL after the first and second dose of raxibacumab, respectively; these are more than 3 and 4 times the mean C_{max} values in humans. Estimates of exposure (AUC) were not generated in the embryo-fetal rabbit study. No adequate and well-controlled studies in pregnant women were conducted. Because animal reproduction studies are not always predictive of human response, raxibacumab should be used during pregnancy only if clearly needed.

8.3 Nursing Mothers

Raxibacumab has not been evaluated in nursing women. Although human immunoglobulins are excreted in human milk, published data suggest that neonatal consumption of human milk does not result in substantial absorption of these maternal immunoglobulins into circulation. Inform a nursing woman that the effects of local gastrointestinal and systemic exposure to raxibacumab on a nursing infant are unknown.

8.4 Pediatric Use

As in adults, the effectiveness of raxibacumab in pediatric patients is based solely on efficacy studies in animal models of inhalational anthrax. As exposure of healthy children to raxibacumab is not ethical, a population PK approach was used to derive dosing regimens that are predicted to provide pediatric patients with exposure comparable to the observed exposure in adults receiving 40 mg/kg. The dose for pediatric patients is based on weight. *[See Dosage and Administration (2.2).]*

Safety or PK of raxibacumab have not been studied in the pediatric population.

8.5 Geriatric Use

Clinical trials of raxibacumab did not include sufficient numbers of subjects aged 65 years and older to determine whether they respond differently from younger subjects. Of the total number of subjects in clinical trials of raxibacumab, 6.4% (21/326) were 65 years and older, while 1.5% (5/326) were 75 years and older. However, no alteration of dosing is needed for patients ≥65 years of age *[see Clinical Pharmacology (12.3)]*.

10 OVERDOSAGE

There is no clinical experience with overdosage of raxibacumab. In case of overdosage, monitor patients for any signs or symptoms of adverse effects.

11 DESCRIPTION

Raxibacumab is a human IgG1λ monoclonal antibody that binds the PA component of *B. anthracis* toxin. Raxibacumab has a molecular weight of approximately 146 kilodaltons. Raxibacumab is produced by recombinant DNA technology in a murine cell expression system.

Raxibacumab is supplied as a sterile, liquid formulation in single-dose vials for intravenous infusion. Each vial contains 50 mg/mL raxibacumab in citric acid (0.13 mg/mL), glycine (18 mg/mL), polysorbate 80 [0.2 mg/mL (w/v)], sodium citrate (2.8 mg/mL), and sucrose (10 mg/mL), with a pH of 6.5. Each vial contains a minimum of 35.1 mL filled into a 50 mL vial (to allow delivery of 1,700 mg/34 mL). Raxibacumab is a clear to opalescent, colorless to pale yellow, liquid.

12 CLINICAL PHARMACOLOGY
12.1 Mechanism of Action

Raxibacumab is a monoclonal antibody that binds the PA of *B. anthracis [see Clinical Pharmacology (12.4)]*.

12.3 Pharmacokinetics

The PK of raxibacumab are linear over the dose range of 1 to 40 mg/kg following single IV dosing in humans; raxibacumab was not tested at doses higher than 40 mg/kg in humans. Following single IV administration of raxibacumab 40 mg/kg in healthy, male and female human subjects, the mean C_{max} and AUC_{inf} were 1,020.3 ± 140.6 mcg/mL and 15,845.8 ± 4,333.5 mcg•day/mL, respectively. Mean raxibacumab steady-state volume of distribution was greater than plasma volume, suggesting some tissue distribution. Clearance values were much smaller than the glomerular filtration rate indicating that there is virtually no renal clearance of raxibacumab.

Because the effectiveness of raxibacumab cannot be tested in humans, a comparison of raxibacumab exposures achieved in healthy human subjects to those observed in animal models of inhalational anthrax in therapeutic efficacy studies is necessary to support the dosage regimen of 40 mg/kg IV as a single dose for the treatment of inhalational anthrax in humans. Humans achieve similar or greater systemic exposure (C_{max} and AUC_{inf}) to

Table 4. Survival Rates in NZW Rabbits in Combination Therapy Study, All Treated Animals

	NZW Rabbits (35 days)[a] Study 1		
	Number (%) Survivors	P value[b]	95% CI[c] Levofloxacin versus Levofloxacin + Raxibacumab
Levofloxacin alone	24/37 (65%)	-	-
Levofloxacin + Raxibacumab 40 mg/kg IV single dose	32/39 (82%)	0.0874	(-2.4, 36.7)

[a] Survival assessed 28 days after last dose of levofloxacin.
[b] P value based on a two-sided likelihood ratio chi-square test.
[c] 95% confidence interval based on normal approximation.

Table 5. Survival Rates in Animals Treated With Raxibacumab, All Treated Animals

	Cynomolgus Macaques at 28 days[a] Study 2			NZW Rabbits at 14 days[b] Study 3			NZW Rabbits at 28 days[a] Study 4		
	Number (%) Survivors	P value[c]	95% CI[d]	Number (%) Survivors	P value[c]	95% CI[d]	Number (%) Survivors	P value[c]	95% CI[d]
Placebo	0/12			0/17			0/24		
20 mg/kg raxibacumab	7/14 (50%)	0.0064	(19.3, 73.7)	5/18 (28%)	0.0455	(6.6, 52.5)	-		
40 mg/kg raxibacumab	9/14 (64%)	0.0007	(31.6, 84.7)	8/18 (44%)	0.0029	(21.3, 66.7)	11/24 (46%)	0.0002	(27.0, 66.1)

[a] Survival measured at 28 days after spore challenge.
[b] Survival measured at 14 days after spore challenge.
[c] P value based on two-sided Fisher's exact test for comparisons between raxibacumab and placebo.
[d] 95% CIs are exact confidence intervals for the difference between raxibacumab and placebo.

raxibacumab following a single 40 mg/kg IV dose compared with New Zealand White rabbits and cynomolgus macaques receiving the same dosage regimen.

Effects of Gender, Age, and Race
Raxibacumab PK were evaluated via a population PK analysis using serum samples from 322 healthy subjects who received a single 40 mg/kg IV dose across 3 clinical trials. Based on this analysis, gender (female versus male), race (non-white versus white), or age (elderly versus young) had no meaningful effects on the PK parameters for raxibacumab.
Raxibacumab PK have not been evaluated in children [see Dosage and Administration (2.2), Use in Specific Populations (8.4)].

Repeat Dosing
Although raxibacumab is intended for single dose administration, the PK of raxibacumab following a second administration of 40 mg/kg IV given 14 days after the first 40 mg/kg IV dose was assessed in 23 healthy subjects (Study 3). The mean raxibacumab concentration at 28 days after the second dose was approximately twice the mean raxibacumab concentration at 14 days following the first dose. In the human trial assessing the immunogenicity of raxibacumab (Study 2), 20 healthy subjects who had initially received a single dose of raxibacumab 40 mg/kg IV received a second 40 mg/kg IV dose at ≥4 months following their first dose. No statistically significant differences in mean estimates of AUC_{inf}, CL, or half-life of raxibacumab between the 2 doses administered ≥4 months apart were observed. The mean C_{max} following the second dose was 15% lower than the C_{max} following the first dose.

Ciprofloxacin Interaction Trial
In an open-label trial evaluating the effect of raxibacumab on ciprofloxacin PK in healthy adult male and female subjects (Study 1), the administration of 40 mg/kg raxibacumab IV following ciprofloxacin IV infusion or ciprofloxacin oral tablet ingestion did not alter the PK of ciprofloxacin administered orally and/or intravenously. Likewise, ciprofloxacin did not alter the PK of raxibacumab. [See Drug Interactions (7.1).]

12.4   Microbiology
Mechanism of Action
Raxibacumab is a monoclonal antibody that binds free PA with an affinity equilibrium dissociation constant (Kd) of 2.78 ± 0.9 nM. Raxibacumab inhibits the binding of PA to its cellular receptors, preventing the intracellular entry of the anthrax lethal factor and edema factor, the enzymatic toxin components responsible for the pathogenic effects of anthrax toxin.

Activity In Vitro and In Vivo
Raxibacumab binds in vitro to PA from the Ames, Vollum, and Sterne strains of B. anthracis. Raxibacumab binds to an epitope on PA that is conserved across reported strains of B. anthracis.
In vivo studies in rats suggest that raxibacumab neutralizes the toxicity due to lethal toxin, as animals slowly infused with lethal toxin (a combination of PA + lethal factor) survived 7 days following administration. The median time to death in control rats was 16 hours. Similar observations were noted in animal efficacy studies in rabbits and monkeys challenged with B. anthracis spores by the inhalational route. PA was detected in animals following exposure to B. anthracis spores. PA levels rose and then fell to undetectable levels in animals that responded to treatment and survived, whereas levels continued to rise in animals that failed treatment and died or were euthanized because of poor clinical condition. [See Clinical Studies (14.1).]

13   NONCLINICAL TOXICOLOGY
13.1   Carcinogenesis, Mutagenesis, Impairment of Fertility
Carcinogenicity, genotoxicity, and fertility studies have not been conducted with raxibacumab.

13.2   Animal Toxicology
Healthy cynomolgus macaques administered 3 intravenous doses or 3 subcutaneous doses of 40 mg/kg raxibacumab once every 12 days, or a single intramuscular dose (40 mg/kg) of raxibacumab, showed no adverse effects, including no effects up to 120 days post-dosing.
Studies with raxibacumab in rabbit, cynomolgus macaque, and human donor tissues showed no cross reactivity with brain.
Anthrax-infected rabbits and monkeys administered an intravenous injection of raxibacumab (40 mg/kg) at time of PA toxemia reproducibly showed greater severity of central nervous system (CNS) lesions (bacteria, inflammation, hemorrhage, and necrosis) in non-surviving animals compared to dead placebo control animals, with no difference in mean time to death from spore challenge. The raxibacumab monoclonal antibody appears unable to penetrate the CNS until compromise of the blood-brain barrier (BBB) during the later stages of anthrax infection. The most severe brain lesions in rabbits were associated with bacteria and raxibacumab tissue binding in a similar pattern as endogenous IgG antibody that leaked across the compromised BBB. No dose/exposure-response relationship for brain histopathology was identified. Surviving rabbits and monkeys at the end of the 28-day studies showed no microscopic evidence of CNS lesions. CNS toxicity was not observed in healthy monkeys administered raxibacumab (40 mg/kg) or in GLP combination treatment studies with antibacterials in rabbits (levofloxacin) or in monkeys (ciprofloxacin) at any time.

14   CLINICAL STUDIES
Because it is not feasible or ethical to conduct controlled clinical trials in humans with inhalational anthrax, the effectiveness of raxibacumab for therapeutic treatment of inhalational anthrax is based on efficacy studies in rabbits and monkeys. Raxibacumab effectiveness has not been studied in humans. Because the animal efficacy studies are conducted under widely varying conditions, the survival rates observed in the animal studies cannot be directly compared between studies and may not reflect the rates observed in clinical practice.
The efficacy of raxibacumab for treatment of inhalational anthrax was studied in a monkey model (study 2) and a rabbit model (studies 3 and 4) of inhalational anthrax disease. These 3 studies tested raxibacumab efficacy compared to placebo. Another study in a rabbit model (study 1) evaluated the efficacy of raxibacumab in combination with an antibacterial drug relative to the antibacterial drug alone. Studies were randomized and blinded.
The animals were challenged with aerosolized B. anthracis spores (Ames strain) at $200 \times LD_{50}$ to achieve 100% mortality if untreated. In rabbit study 1, treatment was delayed until 84 hours after spore challenge. In monkey study 2, study treatment commenced at the time of a positive serum electrochemiluminescence (ECL) assay for B. anthracis PA. The mean time between spore challenge and initiation of study treatment was 42 hours. In rabbit studies 3 and 4, sustained elevation of body temperature above baseline for 2 hours or a positive result on serum ECL assay for PA served as the trigger for initiation of study treatment. The mean time between spore challenge and initiation of study treatment was 28 hours post-exposure. Efficacy in all therapeutic studies in animals was determined based on survival at the end of the study. Most study animals (88% to 100%) were bacteremic and had a positive ECL assay for PA prior to treatment in all 4 studies.

14.1   Treatment of Inhalational Anthrax in Combination With Antibacterial Drug
The efficacy of raxibacumab administered with levofloxacin as treatment of animals with systemic anthrax disease (84 hours after spore challenge) was evaluated in New Zealand White rabbits (study 1). The dose of levofloxacin was chosen to yield a comparable exposure to that achieved by the recommended doses in humans. Levofloxacin and raxibacumab PK in this study were unaffected by product co-administration. Forty-two percent of challenged animals survived to treatment. Treatment with antibacterial drug plus raxibacumab resulted in 82% survival compared to 65% survival in rabbits treated with antibacterial drug alone, $P = 0.0874$ (Table 4).
[See table 4 above]

14.2   Post-exposure Prophylaxis/Early Treatment of Inhalational Anthrax
Monkey study 2 and rabbit studies 3 and 4 evaluated treatment with raxibacumab alone at an earlier time point after exposure than rabbit study 1. Treatment with raxibacumab alone resulted in a statistically significant dose-dependent improvement in survival relative to placebo when administered at the time of initial manifestations of anthrax disease in the rabbit and monkey infection models (Table 5). Raxibacumab at 40 mg/kg IV single dose was superior to placebo in the rabbit and monkey studies in the all treated and the bacteremic animal analysis populations. All surviving animals developed toxin-neutralizing antibodies.
[See table 5 above]
In other animal studies evaluating antibacterial drug alone and raxibacumab-antibacterial drug combination, the efficacy of an antibacterial drug alone (levofloxacin in rabbits and ciprofloxacin in monkeys) was very high (95-100%) when given at the initial manifestations of inhalational anthrax disease. The timing of treatment was similar to that reported for studies 2, 3, and 4 above.
In another study, rabbits were exposed to $100 \times LD_{50}$ B. anthracis spores and administered raxibacumab at a single dose of 40 mg/kg at the time of exposure, 12 hours, 24 hours, or 36 hours after exposure. Survival was 12/12 (100%) in animals treated at time of exposure or 12 hours, but decreased to 6/12 (50%) and 5/12 (42%) at 24 and 36 hours, respectively.

16   HOW SUPPLIED/STORAGE AND HANDLING
Raxibacumab is supplied in single-use vials containing 1,700 mg/34 mL (50 mg/mL) raxibacumab injection and is available in the following packaging configuration:
Single Unit Carton: Contains one (1) single-use vial of raxibacumab 1,700 mg/34 mL (deliverable) (NDC 49401-103-01).
Raxibacumab must be refrigerated at 2° to 8°C (36° to 46°F). DO NOT FREEZE. Protect the vial from exposure to

light, prior to use. Brief exposure to light, as with normal use, is acceptable. Store vial in original carton until time of use.

17 PATIENT COUNSELING INFORMATION

See FDA-approved patient labeling (Patient Information).

Efficacy Based on Animal Models: Inform patients that the efficacy of raxibacumab is based solely on efficacy studies demonstrating a survival benefit in animals and that the effectiveness of raxibacumab has not been tested in humans with anthrax. The safety of raxibacumab has been tested in healthy adults, but no safety data are available in children or pregnant women. Limited data are available in geriatric patients [See Use in Specific Populations (8.5).]

Pregnancy and Nursing Mothers: Inform patients that raxibacumab has not been studied in pregnant women or nursing mothers so the effects of raxibacumab on pregnant women or nursing infants are not known. Instruct patients to tell their healthcare professional if they are pregnant, become pregnant, or are thinking about becoming pregnant. Instruct patients to tell their healthcare professional if they plan to breastfeed their infant. [See Use in Specific Populations (8.1, 8.3).]

Infusion Reactions: Infusion-related reactions were reported during administration of raxibacumab in clinical trials, including reports of rash, urticaria, and pruritus. Prophylactic administration of diphenhydramine is recommended within 1 hour prior to administering raxibacumab. Diphenhydramine route of administration (oral or IV) should be based on the temporal proximity to the start of raxibacumab infusion.

Manufactured by
Human Genome Sciences, Inc.
(a subsidiary of GlaxoSmithKline)
Rockville, MD 20850
U.S. License No. 1820
Marketed by
GlaxoSmithKline
Research Triangle Park, NC 27709
©2014, the GSK group of companies. All rights reserved.
RXB:4PI

PATIENT INFORMATION

RAXIBACUMAB (rack-see-BACK-u-mab)
Injection Solution for IV use

What is RAXIBACUMAB?
- RAXIBACUMAB is a prescription medicine used along with antibiotic medicines to treat people with inhalational anthrax. Raxibacumab can also be used to prevent anthrax disease when there are no other treatment options.
- The effectiveness of RAXIBACUMAB has been studied only in animals with inhalational anthrax. There have been no studies in people who have inhalational anthrax.
- The safety of RAXIBACUMAB was studied in healthy adults. There have been no studies of raxibacumab in children 16 years of age and younger.
- RAXIBACUMAB is not used for prevention or treatment of anthrax meningitis.

Before you receive RAXIBACUMAB, tell your healthcare provider about all of your medical conditions, including if you are:
- allergic to any of the ingredients in raxibacumab. See the end of this leaflet for a list of the ingredients in RAXIBACUMAB.
- allergic to diphenhydramine (Benadryl®).
- pregnant or planning to become pregnant. It is not known if RAXIBACUMAB will harm your unborn baby.
- breastfeeding or plan to breastfeed. It is not known if RAXIBACUMAB passes into your breast milk. You and your healthcare provider should decide if you will receive RAXIBACUMAB or breastfeed.

Tell your healthcare provider about all the medicines you take, including prescription and non-prescription medicines, vitamins, and herbal supplements.

How will I receive RAXIBACUMAB?
- You will be given 1 dose of RAXIBACUMAB by a healthcare provider through a vein (IV or intravenous infusion). It takes about 2 hours to give you the full dose of medicine.
- Your healthcare provider will give you a medicine called diphenhydramine (Benadryl®) before you receive RAXIBACUMAB to help reduce your chances of developing a skin reaction from RAXIBACUMAB. Benadryl may be given to you to take by mouth or through a vein.
- Benadryl may make you sleepy, and you should use caution if you will be driving or operating equipment.

What are the possible side effects of RAXIBACUMAB?
RAXIBACUMAB may cause serious side effects, including:
- **infusion reactions.** Tell your healthcare provider right away if you have rash, hives, or itching while receiving RAXIBACUMAB.

The most common side effects of RAXIBACUMAB include rash, pain in your arms or legs, itchiness, and sleepiness.

Tell your healthcare provider if you have any side effect that bothers you or that does not go away. These are not all the possible side effects of RAXIBACUMAB. For more information, ask your healthcare provider.

Call your healthcare provider for medical advice about side effects. You may report side effects to FDA at 1-800-FDA-1088. **For more information go to** dailymed.nlm.nih.gov.

General information about the safe and effective use of RAXIBACUMAB.
- This patient information leaflet summarizes the most important information about RAXIBACUMAB. If you would like more information, talk to your healthcare provider. You can ask your pharmacist or healthcare provider for information about RAXIBACUMAB that is written for health professionals.

What are the ingredients in RAXIBACUMAB?
Active ingredient: RAXIBACUMAB
Inactive ingredients: citric acid, glycine, polysorbate 80, sodium citrate, and sucrose
Manufactured by: Human Genome Sciences, Inc. (a subsidiary of GlaxoSmithKline), Rockville, MD 20850
Marketed by: GlaxoSmithKline, Research Triangle Park, NC 27709
For more information, go to www.gsk.com or call 1-888-825-5249.
This Patient Information has been approved by the U.S. Food and Drug Administration.
Issued: December 2012
©2014, the GSK group of companies. All rights reserved.
April 2014
RXB:2PIL

RELENZA ℞
[rə-lin′zə]
(zanamivir)
Inhalation Powder, for oral inhalation

HIGHLIGHTS OF PRESCRIBING INFORMATION
These highlights do not include all the information needed to use RELENZA safely and effectively. See full prescribing information for RELENZA.

RELENZA (zanamivir) Inhalation Powder, for oral inhalation
Initial U.S. Approval: 1999

———INDICATIONS AND USAGE———
RELENZA, an influenza neuraminidase inhibitor, is indicated for:
Treatment of influenza in patients aged 7 years and older who have been symptomatic for no more than 2 days. (1.1)
Prophylaxis of influenza in patients aged 5 years and older. (1.2)
Important Limitations on Use of RELENZA:
Not recommended for treatment or prophylaxis of influenza in:
- Individuals with underlying airways disease. (5.1)
Not proven effective for:
- Treatment in individuals with underlying airways disease. (1.3)
- Prophylaxis in nursing home residents. (1.3)
Not a substitute for annual influenza vaccination. (1.3)
Consider available information on influenza drug susceptibility patterns and treatment effects when deciding whether to use RELENZA. (1.3)

———DOSAGE AND ADMINISTRATION———

Indication	Dose
Treatment of Influenza (2.2)	10 mg twice daily for 5 days
Prophylaxis: (2.3) Household Setting	10 mg once daily for 10 days
Community Outbreaks	10 mg once daily for 28 days

Note: The 10-mg dose is provided by 2 inhalations (one 5-mg blister per inhalation). (2.1)

———DOSAGE FORMS AND STRENGTHS———
Blister for oral inhalation: 5 mg. Four 5-mg blisters of powder on a ROTADISK for oral inhalation via DISKHALER. Packaged in carton containing 5 ROTADISKs (total of 10 doses) and 1 DISKHALER inhalation device. (3)

———CONTRAINDICATIONS———
Do not use in patients with history of allergic reaction to any ingredient of RELENZA, including milk proteins. (4)

———WARNINGS AND PRECAUTIONS———
- **Bronchospasm:** Serious, sometimes fatal, cases have occurred. Not recommended in individuals with underlying airways disease. Discontinue RELENZA if bronchospasm or decline in respiratory function develops. (5.1)
- **Allergic Reactions:** Discontinue RELENZA and initiate appropriate treatment if an allergic reaction occurs or is suspected. (5.2)
- **Neuropsychiatric Events:** Patients with influenza, particularly pediatric patients, may be at an increased risk of seizures, confusion, or abnormal behavior early in their illness. Monitor for signs of abnormal behavior. (5.3)
- **High-risk Underlying Medical Conditions:** Safety and effectiveness have not been demonstrated in these patients. (5.4)

———ADVERSE REACTIONS———
The most common adverse events reported in >1.5% of subjects treated with RELENZA and more commonly than in subjects treated with placebo are:
- Treatment Trials – sinusitis, dizziness.
- Prophylaxis Trials – fever and/or chills, arthralgia and articular rheumatism. (6.1)
To report SUSPECTED ADVERSE REACTIONS, contact GlaxoSmithKline at 1-888-825-5249 or FDA at 1-800-FDA-1088 or www.fda.gov/medwatch.

———DRUG INTERACTIONS———
Live attenuated influenza vaccine, intranasal (7):
- Do not administer until 48 hours following cessation of RELENZA.
- Do not administer RELENZA until 2 weeks following administration of the live attenuated influenza vaccine, unless medically indicated.

See 17 for PATIENT COUNSELING INFORMATION and FDA-approved patient labeling

Revised: 10/2013

FULL PRESCRIBING INFORMATION

1 INDICATIONS AND USAGE
1.1 Treatment of Influenza
RELENZA® (zanamivir) Inhalation Powder is indicated for treatment of uncomplicated acute illness due to influenza A and B virus in adults and pediatric patients aged 7 years and older who have been symptomatic for no more than 2 days.
1.2 Prophylaxis of Influenza
RELENZA is indicated for prophylaxis of influenza in adults and pediatric patients aged 5 years and older.

1.3 Important Limitations on Use of RELENZA

- RELENZA is not recommended for treatment or prophylaxis of influenza in individuals with underlying airways disease (such as asthma or chronic obstructive pulmonary disease) due to risk of serious bronchospasm [see Warnings and Precautions (5.1)].
- RELENZA has not been proven effective for treatment of influenza in individuals with underlying airways disease.
- RELENZA has not been proven effective for prophylaxis of influenza in the nursing home setting.
- RELENZA is not a substitute for early influenza vaccination on an annual basis as recommended by the Centers for Disease Control's Immunization Practices Advisory Committee.
- Influenza viruses change over time. Emergence of resistance mutations could decrease drug effectiveness. Other factors (for example, changes in viral virulence) might also diminish clinical benefit of antiviral drugs. Prescribers should consider available information on influenza drug susceptibility patterns and treatment effects when deciding whether to use RELENZA.
- There is no evidence for efficacy of zanamivir in any illness caused by agents other than influenza virus A and B.
- Patients should be advised that the use of RELENZA for treatment of influenza has not been shown to reduce the risk of transmission of influenza to others.

2 DOSAGE AND ADMINISTRATION

2.1 Dosing Considerations

- RELENZA is for administration to the respiratory tract by oral inhalation only, using the DISKHALER® device provided [see Warnings and Precautions (5.6)].
- The 10-mg dose is provided by 2 inhalations (one 5-mg blister per inhalation).
- Patients should be instructed in the use of the delivery system. Instructions should include a demonstration whenever possible. If RELENZA is prescribed for children, it should be used only under adult supervision and instruction, and the supervising adult should first be instructed by a healthcare professional [see Patient Counseling Information (17)].
- Patients scheduled to use an inhaled bronchodilator at the same time as RELENZA should use their bronchodilator before taking RELENZA [see Patient Counseling Information (17)].

2.2 Treatment of Influenza

- The recommended dose of RELENZA for treatment of influenza in adults and pediatric patients aged 7 years and older is 10 mg twice daily (approximately 12 hours apart) for 5 days.
- Two doses should be taken on the first day of treatment whenever possible provided there is at least 2 hours between doses.
- On subsequent days, doses should be about 12 hours apart (e.g., morning and evening) at approximately the same time each day.
- The safety and efficacy of repeated treatment courses have not been studied.

2.3 Prophylaxis of Influenza

Household Setting:
- The recommended dose of RELENZA for prophylaxis of influenza in adults and pediatric patients aged 5 years and older in a household setting is 10 mg once daily for 10 days.
- The dose should be administered at approximately the same time each day.
- There are no data on the effectiveness of prophylaxis with RELENZA in a household setting when initiated more than 1.5 days after the onset of signs or symptoms in the index case.

Community Outbreaks:
- The recommended dose of RELENZA for prophylaxis of influenza in adults and adolescents in a community setting is 10 mg once daily for 28 days.
- The dose should be administered at approximately the same time each day.
- There are no data on the effectiveness of prophylaxis with RELENZA in a community outbreak when initiated more than 5 days after the outbreak was identified in the community.
- The safety and effectiveness of prophylaxis with RELENZA have not been evaluated for longer than 28 days' duration.

3 DOSAGE FORMS AND STRENGTHS

Blister for oral inhalation: 5 mg. Four 5-mg blisters of powder on a ROTADISK® for oral inhalation via DISKHALER. Packaged in carton containing 5 ROTADISKs (total of 10 doses) and 1 DISKHALER inhalation device [see How Supplied/Storage and Handling (16)].

4 CONTRAINDICATIONS

Do not use in patients with history of allergic reaction to any ingredient of RELENZA including milk proteins [see Warnings and Precautions (5.2), Description (11)].

5 WARNINGS AND PRECAUTIONS

5.1 Bronchospasm

RELENZA is not recommended for treatment or prophylaxis of influenza in individuals with underlying airways disease (such as asthma or chronic obstructive pulmonary disease).

Serious cases of bronchospasm, including fatalities, have been reported during treatment with RELENZA in patients with and without underlying airways disease. Many of these cases were reported during postmarketing and causality was difficult to assess.

RELENZA should be discontinued in any patient who develops bronchospasm or decline in respiratory function; immediate treatment and hospitalization may be required.

Some patients without prior pulmonary disease may also have respiratory abnormalities from acute respiratory infection that could resemble adverse drug reactions or increase patient vulnerability to adverse drug reactions.

Bronchospasm was documented following administration of zanamivir in 1 of 13 subjects with mild or moderate asthma (but without acute influenza-like illness) in a Phase I trial. In a Phase III trial in subjects with acute influenza-like illness superimposed on underlying asthma or chronic obstructive pulmonary disease, 10% (24 of 244) of subjects on zanamivir and 9% (22 of 237) on placebo experienced a greater than 20% decline in FEV_1 following treatment for 5 days.

If use of RELENZA is considered for a patient with underlying airways disease, the potential risks and benefits should be carefully weighed. If a decision is made to prescribe RELENZA for such a patient, this should be done only under conditions of careful monitoring of respiratory function, close observation, and appropriate supportive care including availability of fast-acting bronchodilators.

5.2 Allergic Reactions

Allergic-like reactions, including oropharyngeal edema, serious skin rashes, and anaphylaxis have been reported in postmarketing experience with RELENZA. RELENZA should be stopped and appropriate treatment instituted if an allergic reaction occurs or is suspected.

5.3 Neuropsychiatric Events

Influenza can be associated with a variety of neurologic and behavioral symptoms which can include events such as seizures, hallucinations, delirium, and abnormal behavior, in some cases resulting in fatal outcomes. These events may occur in the setting of encephalitis or encephalopathy but can occur without obvious severe disease.

There have been postmarketing reports (mostly from Japan) of delirium and abnormal behavior leading to injury in patients with influenza who were receiving neuraminidase inhibitors, including RELENZA. Because these events were reported voluntarily during clinical practice, estimates of frequency cannot be made, but they appear to be uncommon based on usage data for RELENZA. These events were reported primarily among pediatric patients and often had an abrupt onset and rapid resolution. The contribution of RELENZA to these events has not been established. Patients with influenza should be closely monitored for signs of abnormal behavior. If neuropsychiatric symptoms occur, the risks and benefits of continuing treatment should be evaluated for each patient.

5.4 Limitations of Populations Studied

Safety and efficacy have not been demonstrated in patients with high-risk underlying medical conditions. No information is available regarding treatment of influenza in patients with any medical condition sufficiently severe or unstable to be considered at imminent risk of requiring inpatient management.

5.5 Bacterial Infections

Serious bacterial infections may begin with influenza-like symptoms or may coexist with or occur as complications during the course of influenza. RELENZA has not been shown to prevent such complications.

5.6 Importance of Proper Route of Administration

RELENZA Inhalation Powder must not be made into an extemporaneous solution for administration by nebulization or mechanical ventilation. There have been reports of hospitalized patients with influenza who received a solution made with RELENZA Inhalation Powder administered by nebulization or mechanical ventilation, including a fatal case where it was reported that the lactose in this formulation obstructed the proper functioning of the equipment. RELENZA Inhalation Powder must only be administered using the device provided [see Dosage and Administration (2.1)].

5.7 Importance of Proper Use of DISKHALER

Effective and safe use of RELENZA requires proper use of the DISKHALER to inhale the drug. Prescribers should carefully evaluate the ability of young children to use the delivery system if use of RELENZA is considered [see Use in Specific Populations (8.4)].

6 ADVERSE REACTIONS

See Warnings and Precautions for information about risk of serious adverse events such as bronchospasm (5.1) and allergic-like reactions (5.2), and for safety information in patients with underlying airways disease (5.1).

6.1 Clinical Trials Experience

Because clinical trials are conducted under widely varying conditions, adverse reaction rates observed in the clinical trials of a drug cannot be directly compared with rates in the clinical trials of another drug and may not reflect the rates observed in practice.

The placebo used in clinical trials consisted of inhaled lactose powder, which is also the vehicle for the active drug; therefore, some adverse events occurring at similar frequencies in different treatment groups could be related to lactose vehicle inhalation.

Treatment of Influenza: _Clinical Trials in Adults and Adolescents:_ Adverse events that occurred with an incidence ≥1.5% in treatment trials are listed in Table 1. This table shows adverse events occurring in subjects aged 12 years and older receiving RELENZA 10 mg inhaled twice daily, RELENZA in all inhalation regimens, and placebo inhaled twice daily (where placebo consisted of the same lactose vehicle used in RELENZA).

Table 1. Summary of Adverse Events ≥1.5% Incidence During Treatment in Adults and Adolescents

Adverse Event	RELENZA		Placebo (Lactose Vehicle) (n = 1,520)
	10 mg b.i.d. Inhaled (n = 1,132)	All Dosing Regimens[a] (n = 2,289)	
Body as a whole			
Headaches	2%	2%	3%
Digestive			
Diarrhea	3%	3%	4%
Nausea	3%	3%	3%
Vomiting	1%	1%	2%
Respiratory			
Nasal signs and symptoms	2%	3%	3%
Bronchitis	2%	2%	3%
Cough	2%	2%	3%
Sinusitis	3%	2%	2%
Ear, nose, and throat infections	2%	1%	2%
Nervous system			
Dizziness	2%	1%	<1%

[a] Includes trials where RELENZA was administered intranasally (6.4 mg 2 to 4 times per day in addition to inhaled preparation) and/or inhaled more frequently (q.i.d.) than the currently recommended dose.

Additional adverse reactions occurring in less than 1.5% of subjects receiving RELENZA included malaise, fatigue, fever, abdominal pain, myalgia, arthralgia, and urticaria.

The most frequent laboratory abnormalities in Phase III treatment trials included elevations of liver enzymes and CPK, lymphopenia, and neutropenia. These were reported in similar proportions of zanamivir and lactose vehicle placebo recipients with acute influenza-like illness.

Clinical Trials in Pediatric Subjects: Adverse events that occurred with an incidence ≥1.5% in children receiving treatment doses of RELENZA in 2 Phase III trials are listed in Table 2. This table shows adverse events occurring in pediatric subjects aged 5 to 12 years receiving RELENZA 10 mg inhaled twice daily and placebo inhaled twice daily (where placebo consisted of the same lactose vehicle used in RELENZA).

Table 2. Summary of Adverse Events ≥1.5% Incidence During Treatment in Pediatric Subjects[a]

Adverse Event	RELENZA 10 mg b.i.d. Inhaled (n = 291)	Placebo (Lactose Vehicle) (n = 318)
Respiratory		
Ear, nose, and throat infections	5%	5%
Ear, nose, and throat hemorrhage	<1%	2%
Asthma	<1%	2%
Cough	<1%	2%
Digestive		
Vomiting	2%	3%
Diarrhea	2%	2%
Nausea	<1%	2%

[a] Includes a subset of subjects receiving RELENZA for treatment of influenza in a prophylaxis trial.

In 1 of the 2 trials described in Table 2, some additional information is available from children (aged 5 to 12 years) without acute influenza-like illness who received an investigational prophylaxis regimen of RELENZA; 132 children received RELENZA and 145 children received placebo. Among these children, nasal signs and symptoms (zanamivir 20%, placebo 9%), cough (zanamivir 16%, placebo 8%), and throat/tonsil discomfort and pain (zanamivir 11%, placebo 6%) were reported more frequently with RELENZA than placebo. In a subset with chronic pulmonary disease, lower respiratory adverse events (described as asthma, cough, or viral respiratory infections which could include influenza-like symptoms) were reported in 7 of 7 zanamivir recipients and 5 of 12 placebo recipients.

Prophylaxis of Influenza: *Family/Household Prophylaxis Studies:* Adverse events that occurred with an incidence of ≥1.5% in the 2 prophylaxis trials are listed in Table 3. This table shows adverse events occurring in subjects aged 5 years and older receiving RELENZA 10 mg inhaled once daily for 10 days.

Table 3. Summary of Adverse Events ≥1.5% Incidence During 10-Day Prophylaxis Trials in Adults, Adolescents, and Children[a]

Adverse Event	Contact Cases	
	RELENZA (n = 1,068)	Placebo (n = 1,059)
Lower respiratory		
Viral respiratory infections	13%	19%
Cough	7%	9%
Neurologic		
Headaches	13%	14%
Ear, nose, and throat		
Nasal signs and symptoms	12%	12%
Throat and tonsil discomfort and pain	8%	9%
Nasal inflammation	1%	2%
Musculoskeletal		
Muscle pain	3%	3%
Endocrine and metabolic		
Feeding problems (decreased or increased appetite and anorexia)	2%	2%
Gastrointestinal		
Nausea and vomiting	1%	2%
Non-site specific		
Malaise and fatigue	5%	5%
Temperature regulation disturbances (fever and/or chills)	5%	4%

[a] In prophylaxis trials, symptoms associated with influenza-like illness were captured as adverse events; subjects were enrolled during a winter respiratory season during which time any symptoms that occurred were captured as adverse events.

Community Prophylaxis Trials: Adverse events that occurred with an incidence of ≥1.5% in 2 prophylaxis trials are listed in Table 4. This table shows adverse events occurring in subjects aged 5 years and older receiving RELENZA 10 mg inhaled once daily for 28 days.

Table 4. Summary of Adverse Events ≥1.5% Incidence During 28-Day Prophylaxis Trials in Adults, Adolescents, and Children[a]

Adverse Event	RELENZA (n = 2,231)	Placebo (n = 2,239)
Neurologic		
Headaches	24%	26%
Ear, nose, and throat		
Throat and tonsil discomfort and pain	19%	20%
Nasal signs and symptoms	12%	13%
Ear, nose, and throat infections	2%	2%
Lower respiratory		
Cough	17%	18%
Viral respiratory infections	3%	4%
Musculoskeletal		
Muscle pain	8%	8%
Musculoskeletal pain	6%	6%
Arthralgia and articular rheumatism	2%	<1%
Endocrine and metabolic		
Feeding problems (decreased or increased appetite and anorexia)	4%	4%
Gastrointestinal		
Nausea and vomiting	2%	3%
Diarrhea	2%	2%

(continued in next column)

Non-site specific		
Temperature regulation disturbances (fever and/or chills)	9%	10%
Malaise and fatigue	8%	8%

[a] In prophylaxis trials, symptoms associated with influenza-like illness were captured as adverse events; subjects were enrolled during a winter respiratory season during which time any symptoms that occurred were captured as adverse events.

6.2   Postmarketing Experience

In addition to adverse events reported from clinical trials, the following events have been identified during postmarketing use of zanamivir (RELENZA). Because they are reported voluntarily from a population of unknown size, estimates of frequency cannot be made. These events have been chosen for inclusion due to a combination of their seriousness, frequency of reporting, or potential causal connection to zanamivir (RELENZA).

Allergic Reactions: Allergic or allergic-like reaction, including oropharyngeal edema [see Warnings and Precautions (5.2)].

Psychiatric: Delirium, including symptoms such as altered level of consciousness, confusion, abnormal behavior, delusions, hallucinations, agitation, anxiety, nightmares[see Warnings and Precautions (5.3)].

Cardiac: Arrhythmias, syncope.

Neurologic: Seizures. Vasovagal-like episodes have been reported shortly following inhalation of zanamivir.

Respiratory: Bronchospasm, dyspnea [see Warnings and Precautions (5.1)].

Skin: Facial edema; rash, including serious cutaneous reactions (e.g., erythema multiforme, Stevens-Johnson syndrome, toxic epidermal necrolysis); urticaria [see Warnings and Precautions (5.2)].

7   DRUG INTERACTIONS

Zanamivir is not a substrate nor does it affect cytochrome P450 (CYP) isoenzymes (CYP1A1/2, 2A6, 2C9, 2C18, 2D6, 2E1, and 3A4) in human liver microsomes. No clinically significant pharmacokinetic drug interactions are predicted based on data from in vitro studies.

The concurrent use of RELENZA with live attenuated influenza vaccine (LAIV) intranasal has not been evaluated. However, because of potential interference between these products, LAIV should not be administered within 2 weeks before or 48 hours after administration of RELENZA, unless medically indicated. The concern about possible interference arises from the potential for antiviral drugs to inhibit replication of live vaccine virus.

Trivalent inactivated influenza vaccine can be administered at any time relative to use of RELENZA [see Clinical Pharmacology (12.4)].

8   USE IN SPECIFIC POPULATIONS

8.1   Pregnancy

Pregnancy Category C. There are no adequate and well-controlled studies of zanamivir in pregnant women. Zanamivir should be used during pregnancy only if the potential benefit justifies the potential risk to the fetus.

Embryo/fetal development studies were conducted in rats (dosed from days 6 to 15 of pregnancy) and rabbits (dosed from days 7 to 19 of pregnancy) using the same IV doses (1, 9, and 90 mg/kg/day). Pre- and post-natal developmental studies were performed in rats (dosed from day 16 of pregnancy until litter day 21 to 23). No malformations, maternal toxicity, or embryotoxicity were observed in pregnant rats or rabbits and their fetuses. Because of insufficient blood sampling timepoints in rat and rabbit reproductive toxicity studies, AUC values were not available. In a subchronic study in rats at the 90 mg/kg/day IV dose, the AUC values were greater than 300 times the human exposure at the proposed clinical dose.

An additional embryo/fetal study, in a different strain of rat, was conducted using subcutaneous administration of zanamivir, 3 times daily, at doses of 1, 9, or 80 mg/kg during days 7 to 17 of pregnancy. There was an increase in the incidence rates of a variety of minor skeleton alterations and variants in the exposed offspring in this study. Based on AUC measurements, the 80 mg/kg dose produced an exposure greater than 1,000 times the human exposure at the proposed clinical dose. However, in most instances, the individual incidence rate of each skeletal alteration or variant remained within the background rates of the historical occurrence in the strain studied.

Zanamivir has been shown to cross the placenta in rats and rabbits. In these animals, fetal blood concentrations of zanamivir were significantly lower than zanamivir concentrations in the maternal blood.

8.3   Nursing Mothers

Studies in rats have demonstrated that zanamivir is excreted in milk. However, nursing mothers should be instructed that it is not known whether zanamivir is excreted in human milk. Because many drugs are excreted in human milk, caution should be exercised when RELENZA is administered to a nursing mother.

8.4   Pediatric Use

Treatment of Influenza: Safety and effectiveness of RELENZA for treatment of influenza have not been assessed in pediatric patients younger than 7 years, but were studied in a Phase III treatment trial in pediatric subjects, where 471 children aged 5 to 12 years received zanamivir or placebo [see Clinical Studies (14.1)]. Adolescents were included in the 3 principal Phase III adult treatment trials. In these trials, 67 patients were aged 12 to 16 years. No definite differences in safety and efficacy were observed between these adolescent patients and young adults.

In a Phase I trial of 16 children aged 6 to 12 years with signs and symptoms of respiratory disease, 4 did not produce a measurable peak inspiratory flow rate (PIFR) through the DISKHALER (3 with no adequate inhalation on request, 1 with missing data), 9 had measurable PIFR on each of 2 inhalations, and 3 achieved measurable PIFR on only 1 of 2 inhalations. Neither of two 6-year-olds and one of two 7-year-olds produced measurable PIFR. Overall, 8 of the 16 children (including all those younger than 8 years) either did not produce measurable inspiratory flow through the DISKHALER or produced peak inspiratory flow rates below the 60 L/min considered optimal for the device under standardized in vitro testing; lack of measurable flow rate was related to low or undetectable serum concentrations [see Clinical Pharmacology (12.3), Clinical Studies (14.1)]. Prescribers should carefully evaluate the ability of young children to use the delivery system if prescription of RELENZA is considered.

Prophylaxis of Influenza: The safety and effectiveness of RELENZA for prophylaxis of influenza have been studied in 4 Phase III trials where 273 children aged 5 to 11 years and 239 adolescents aged 12 to 16 years received RELENZA. No differences in safety and effectiveness were observed between pediatric and adult subjects [see Clinical Studies (14.2)].

8.5   Geriatric Use

Of the total number of subjects in 6 clinical trials of RELENZA for treatment of influenza, 59 subjects were aged 65 years and older, while 24 subjects were aged 75 years and older. Of the total number of subjects in 4 clinical trials of RELENZA for prophylaxis of influenza in households and community settings, 954 subjects were aged 65 years and older, while 347 subjects were aged 75 years and older. No overall differences in safety or effectiveness were observed between these subjects and younger subjects, and other reported clinical experience has not identified differences in responses between the elderly and younger subjects, but greater sensitivity of some older individuals cannot be ruled out. Elderly patients may need assistance with use of the device.

In 2 additional trials of RELENZA for prophylaxis of influenza in the nursing home setting, efficacy was not demonstrated [see Indications and Usage (1.3)].

10   OVERDOSAGE

There have been no reports of overdosage from administration of RELENZA.

11   DESCRIPTION

The active component of RELENZA is zanamivir. The chemical name of zanamivir is 5-(acetylamino)-4-[(aminoiminomethyl)-amino]-2,6-anhydro-3,4,5-trideoxy-D-glycero-D-galacto-non-2-enonic acid. It has a molecular formula of $C_{12}H_{20}N_4O_7$ and a molecular weight of 332.3. It has the following structural formula:

Zanamivir is a white to off-white powder for oral inhalation with a solubility of approximately 18 mg/mL in water at 20°C.

RELENZA is for administration to the respiratory tract by oral inhalation only. Each RELENZA ROTADISK contains 4 regularly spaced double-foil blisters with each blister containing a powder mixture of 5 mg of zanamivir and 20 mg of lactose (which contains milk proteins). The contents of each blister are inhaled using a specially designed breath-activated plastic device for inhaling powder called the DISKHALER. After a RELENZA ROTADISK is loaded into the DISKHALER, a blister that contains medication is pierced and the zanamivir is dispersed into the air stream created when the patient inhales through the mouthpiece. The amount of drug delivered to the respiratory tract will depend on patient factors such as inspiratory flow. Under standardized in vitro testing, RELENZA ROTADISK delivers 4 mg of zanamivir from the DISKHALER device when tested at a pressure drop of 3 kPa (corresponding to a flow rate of about 62 to 65 L/min) for 3 seconds.

12 CLINICAL PHARMACOLOGY

12.1 Mechanism of Action
Zanamivir is an antiviral drug [see Clinical Pharmacology (12.4)].

12.3 Pharmacokinetics
Absorption and Bioavailability: Pharmacokinetic studies of orally inhaled zanamivir indicate that approximately 4% to 17% of the inhaled dose is systemically absorbed. The peak serum concentrations ranged from 17 to 142 ng/mL within 1 to 2 hours following a 10 mg dose. The area under the serum concentration versus time curve (AUC_∞) ranged from 111 to 1,364 ng•h/mL.

Distribution: Zanamivir has limited plasma protein binding (<10%).

Metabolism: Zanamivir is renally excreted as unchanged drug. No metabolites have been detected in humans.

Elimination: The serum half-life of zanamivir following administration by oral inhalation ranges from 2.5 to 5.1 hours. It is excreted unchanged in the urine with excretion of a single dose completed within 24 hours. Total clearance ranges from 2.5 to 10.9 L/h. Unabsorbed drug is excreted in the feces.

Impaired Hepatic Function: The pharmacokinetics of zanamivir have not been studied in patients with impaired hepatic function.

Impaired Renal Function: After a single intravenous dose of 4 mg or 2 mg of zanamivir in volunteers with mild/moderate or severe renal impairment, respectively, significant decreases in renal clearance (and hence total clearance: normals 5.3 L/h, mild/moderate 2.7 L/h, and severe 0.8 L/h; median values) and significant increases in half-life (normals 3.1 h, mild/moderate 4.7 h, and severe 18.5 h; median values) and systemic exposure were observed. Safety and efficacy have not been documented in the presence of severe renal insufficiency. Due to the low systemic bioavailability of zanamivir following oral inhalation, no dosage adjustments are necessary in patients with renal impairment. However, the potential for drug accumulation should be considered.

Pediatric Patients: The pharmacokinetics of zanamivir were evaluated in pediatric subjects with signs and symptoms of respiratory illness. Sixteen subjects, aged 6 to 12 years, received a single dose of 10 mg zanamivir dry powder via DISKHALER. Five subjects had either undetectable zanamivir serum concentrations or had low drug concentrations (8.32 to 10.38 ng/mL) that were not detectable after 1.5 hours. Eleven subjects had C_{max} median values of 43 ng/mL (range: 15 to 74) and AUC_∞ median values of 167 ng•h/mL (range: 58 to 279). Low or undetectable serum concentrations were related to lack of measurable PIFR in individual subjects [see Use in Specific Populations (8.4), Clinical Studies (14.1)].

Geriatric Patients: The pharmacokinetics of zanamivir have not been studied in subjects older than 65 years [see Use in Specific Populations (8.5)].

Gender, Race, and Weight: In a population pharmacokinetic analysis in patient trials, no clinically significant differences in serum concentrations and/or pharmacokinetic parameters (V/F, CL/F, ka, AUC_{0-3}, C_{max}, T_{max}, CLr, and % excreted in urine) were observed when demographic variables (gender, age, race, and weight) and indices of infection (laboratory evidence of infection, overall symptoms, symptoms of upper respiratory illness, and viral titers) were considered. There were no significant correlations between measures of systemic exposure and safety parameters.

12.4 Microbiology
Mechanism of Action: Zanamivir is an inhibitor of influenza virus neuraminidase affecting release of viral particles.

Antiviral Activity: The antiviral activity of zanamivir against laboratory and clinical isolates of influenza virus was determined in cell culture assays. The concentrations of zanamivir required for inhibition of influenza virus were highly variable depending on the assay method used and virus isolate tested. The 50% and 90% effective concentrations (EC_{50} and EC_{90}) of zanamivir were in the range of 0.005 to 16.0 µM and 0.05 to >100 µM, respectively (1 µM = 0.33 mcg/mL). The relationship between the cell culture inhibition of influenza virus by zanamivir and the inhibition of influenza virus replication in humans has not been established.

Resistance: Influenza viruses with reduced susceptibility to zanamivir have been selected in cell culture by multiple passages of the virus in the presence of increasing concentrations of the drug. Genetic analysis of these viruses showed that the reduced susceptibility in cell culture to zanamivir is associated with mutations that result in amino acid changes in the viral neuraminidase or viral hemagglutinin or both. Resistance mutations selected in cell culture

which result in neuraminidase amino acid substitutions include E119G/A/D and R292K. Mutations selected in cell culture in hemagglutinin include: K68R, G75E, E114K, N145S, S165N, S186F, N199S, and K222T.

In an immunocompromised patient infected with influenza B virus, a variant virus emerged after treatment with an investigational nebulized solution of zanamivir for 2 weeks. Analysis of this variant showed a hemagglutinin substitution (T198I) which resulted in a reduced affinity for human cell receptors, and a substitution in the neuraminidase active site (R152K) which reduced the enzyme's activity to zanamivir by 1,000-fold. Insufficient information is available to characterize the risk of emergence of zanamivir resistance in clinical use.

Cross-Resistance: Cross-resistance has been observed between some zanamivir-resistant and some oseltamivir-resistant influenza virus mutants generated in cell culture. However, some of the in cell culture zanamivir-induced resistance mutations, E119G/A/D and R292K, occurred at the same neuraminidase amino acid positions as in the clinical isolates resistant to oseltamivir, E119V and R292K. No trials have been performed to assess risk of emergence of cross-resistance during clinical use.

Influenza Vaccine Interaction Trial: An interaction trial (n = 138) was conducted to evaluate the effects of zanamivir (10 mg once daily) on the serological response to a single dose of trivalent inactivated influenza vaccine, as measured by hemagglutination inhibition titers. There was no difference in hemagglutination inhibition antibody titers at 2 weeks and 4 weeks after vaccine administration between zanamivir and placebo recipients.

Influenza Challenge Trials: Antiviral activity of zanamivir was supported for infection with influenza A virus, and to a more limited extent for infection with influenza B virus, by Phase I trials in volunteers who received intranasal inoculations of challenge strains of influenza virus, and received an intranasal formulation of zanamivir or placebo starting before or shortly after viral inoculation.

13 NONCLINICAL TOXICOLOGY

13.1 Carcinogenesis, Mutagenesis, Impairment of Fertility
Carcinogenesis: In 2-year carcinogenicity studies conducted in rats and mice using a powder formulation administered through inhalation, zanamivir induced no statistically significant increases in tumors over controls. The maximum daily exposures in rats and mice were approximately 23 to 25 and 20 to 22 times, respectively, greater than those in humans at the proposed clinical dose based on AUC comparisons.

Mutagenesis: Zanamivir was not mutagenic in in vitro and in vivo genotoxicity assays which included bacterial mutation assays in S. typhimurium and E. coli, mammalian mutation assays in mouse lymphoma, chromosomal aberration assays in human peripheral blood lymphocytes, and the in vivo mouse bone marrow micronucleus assay.

Impairment of Fertility: The effects of zanamivir on fertility and general reproductive performance were investigated in male (dosed for 10 weeks prior to mating, and throughout mating, gestation/lactation, and shortly after weaning) and female rats (dosed for 3 weeks prior to mating through Day 19 of pregnancy, or Day 21 post partum) at IV doses 1, 9, and 90 mg/kg/day. Zanamivir did not impair mating or fertility of male or female rats, and did not affect the sperm of treated male rats. The reproductive performance of the F1 generation born to female rats given zanamivir was not affected. Based on a subchronic study in rats at a 90 mg/kg/day IV dose, AUC values ranged between 142 and 199 mcg•h/mL (>300 times the human exposure at the proposed clinical dose).

14 CLINICAL STUDIES

14.1 Treatment of Influenza
Adults and Adolescents: The efficacy of RELENZA 10 mg inhaled twice daily for 5 days in the treatment of influenza has been evaluated in placebo-controlled trials conducted in North America, the Southern Hemisphere, and Europe during their respective influenza seasons. The magnitude of treatment effect varied between trials, with possible relationships to population-related factors including amount of symptomatic relief medication used.

Populations Studied: The principal Phase III trials enrolled 1,588 subjects aged 12 years and older (median age 34 years, 49% male, 91% Caucasian), with uncomplicated influenza-like illness within 2 days of symptom onset. Influenza was confirmed by culture, hemagglutination inhibition antibodies, or investigational direct tests. Of 1,164 subjects with confirmed influenza, 89% had influenza A and 11% had influenza B. These trials served as the principal basis for efficacy evaluation, with more limited Phase II studies providing supporting information where necessary. Following randomization to either zanamivir or placebo (inhaled lactose vehicle), all subjects received instruction and supervision by a healthcare professional for the initial dose.

Principal Results: The definition of time to improvement in major symptoms of influenza included no fever and self-assessment of "none" or "mild" for headache, myalgia, cough, and sore throat. A Phase II and a Phase III trial conducted in North America (total of over 600 influenza-positive subjects) suggested up to 1 day of shortening of median time to this defined improvement in symptoms in subjects receiving zanamivir compared with placebo, although statistical significance was not reached in either of these trials. In a trial conducted in the Southern Hemisphere (321 influenza-positive subjects), a 1.5-day difference in median time to symptom improvement was observed. Additional evidence of efficacy was provided by the European trial.

Other Findings: There was no consistent difference in treatment effect in subjects with influenza A compared with influenza B; however, these trials enrolled smaller numbers of subjects with influenza B and thus provided less evidence in support of efficacy in influenza B.

In general, subjects with lower temperature (e.g., 38.2°C or less) or investigator-rated as having less severe symptoms at entry derived less benefit from therapy.

No consistent treatment effect was demonstrated in subjects with underlying chronic medical conditions, including respiratory or cardiovascular disease [see Warnings and Precautions (5.4)].

No consistent differences in rate of development of complications were observed between treatment groups.

Some fluctuation of symptoms was observed after the primary trial endpoint in both treatment groups.

Pediatric Patients: The efficacy of RELENZA 10 mg inhaled twice daily for 5 days in the treatment of influenza in pediatric patients has been evaluated in a placebo-controlled trial conducted in North America and Europe, enrolling 471 subjects, aged 5 to 12 years (55% male, 90% Caucasian), within 36 hours of symptom onset. Of 346 subjects with confirmed influenza, 65% had influenza A and 35% had influenza B. The definition of time to improvement included no fever and parental assessment of no or mild cough and absent/minimal muscle and joint aches or pains, sore throat, chills/feverishness, and headache. Median time to symptom improvement was 1 day shorter in subjects receiving zanamivir compared with placebo. No consistent differences in rate of development of complications were observed between treatment groups. Some fluctuation of symptoms was observed after the primary trial endpoint in both treatment groups.

Although this trial was designed to enroll children aged 5 to 12 years, the product is indicated only for children aged 7 years and older. This evaluation is based on the combination of lower estimates of treatment effect in 5- and 6-year-olds compared with the overall trial population, and evidence of inadequate inhalation through the DISKHALER in a pharmacokinetic trial [see Use in Specific Populations (8.4), Clinical Pharmacology (12.3)].

14.2 Prophylaxis of Influenza
The efficacy of RELENZA in preventing naturally occurring influenza illness has been demonstrated in 2 post-exposure prophylaxis trials in households and 2 seasonal prophylaxis trials during community outbreaks of influenza. The primary efficacy endpoint in these trials was the incidence of symptomatic, laboratory-confirmed influenza, defined as the presence of 2 or more of the following symptoms: oral temperature ≥100°F/37.8°C or feverishness, cough, headache, sore throat, and myalgia; and laboratory confirmation of influenza A or B by culture, PCR, or seroconversion (defined as a 4-fold increase in convalescent antibody titer from baseline).

Household Prophylaxis Trials: Two trials assessed post-exposure prophylaxis in household contacts of an index case. Within 1.5 days of onset of symptoms in an index case, each household (including all family members aged 5 years and older) was randomized to RELENZA 10 mg inhaled once daily or placebo inhaled once daily for 10 days. In the first trial only, each index case was randomized to RELENZA 10 mg inhaled twice daily for 5 days or inhaled placebo twice daily for 5 days. In this trial, the proportion of households with at least 1 new case of symptomatic laboratory-confirmed influenza was reduced from 19.0% (32 of 168 households) for the placebo group to 4.1% (7 of 169 households) for the group receiving RELENZA.

In the second trial, index cases were not treated. The incidence of symptomatic laboratory-confirmed influenza was reduced from 19.0% (46 of 242 households) for the placebo group to 4.1% (10 of 245 households) for the group receiving RELENZA.

Seasonal Prophylaxis Trials: Two seasonal prophylaxis trials assessed RELENZA 10 mg inhaled once daily versus placebo inhaled once daily for 28 days during community outbreaks. The first trial enrolled subjects aged 18 years or older (mean age: 29 years) from 2 university communities. The majority of subjects were unvaccinated (86%). In this trial, the incidence of symptomatic laboratory-confirmed influenza was reduced from 6.1% (34 of 554) for the placebo group to 2.0% (11 of 553) for the group receiving RELENZA. The second seasonal prophylaxis trial enrolled subjects aged 12 to 94 years (mean age 60 years) with 56% of them older than 65 years. Sixty-seven percent of the subjects were vaccinated. In this trial, the incidence of symptomatic laboratory-confirmed influenza was reduced from 1.4% (23 of 1,685) for the placebo group to 0.2% (4 of 1,678) for the group receiving RELENZA.

16   HOW SUPPLIED/STORAGE AND HANDLING

RELENZA is supplied in a circular double-foil pack (a ROTADISK) containing 4 blisters of the drug. Five ROTADISKs are packaged in a white polypropylene tube. The tube is packaged in a carton with 1 blue and gray DISKHALER inhalation device (NDC 0173-0681-01).

Store at 25°C (77°F); excursions permitted to 15° to 30°C (59° to 86°F) (see USP Controlled Room Temperature). Keep out of reach of children. Do not puncture any RELENZA ROTADISK blister until taking a dose using the DISKHALER.

17   PATIENT COUNSELING INFORMATION

See FDA-approved patient labeling (Patient Information and Instructions for Use).

Bronchospasm: **Inform patients of the risk of bronchospasm, especially in the setting of underlying airways disease, and advise patients to stop RELENZA and contact their healthcare provider if they experience increased respiratory symptoms during treatment such as worsening wheezing, shortness of breath, or other signs or symptoms of bronchospasm*[see Warnings and Precautions (5.1)]*. If a decision is made to prescribe RELENZA for a patient with asthma or chronic obstructive pulmonary disease, the patient should be made aware of the risks and should have a fast-acting bronchodilator available.**

Concomitant Bronchodilator Use: Patients scheduled to take inhaled bronchodilators at the same time as RELENZA should be advised to use their bronchodilators before taking RELENZA.

Neuropsychiatric Events: Inform patients with influenza (the flu), particularly children and adolescents, they may be at an increased risk of seizures, confusion, or abnormal behavior early in their illness. These events may occur after beginning RELENZA or may occur when flu is not treated. These events are uncommon but may result in accidental injury to the patient. Therefore, patients should be observed for signs of unusual behavior and a healthcare professional should be contacted immediately if the patient shows any signs of unusual behavior *[see Warnings and Precautions (5.3)]*.

Instructions for Use: Instruct patients in use of the delivery system. Instructions should include a demonstration whenever possible. For the proper use of RELENZA, the patient should read and follow carefully the accompanying Instructions for Use.

If RELENZA is prescribed for children, it should be used only under adult supervision and instruction, and the supervising adult should first be instructed by a healthcare professional *[see Dosage and Administration (2.1)]*.

Risk of Influenza Transmission to Others: Inform patients that the use of RELENZA for treatment of influenza has not been shown to reduce the risk of transmission of influenza to others.

RELENZA, DISKHALER, and ROTADISK are registered trademarks of the GlaxoSmithKline group of companies.

GlaxoSmithKline
Research Triangle Park, NC 27709
©2013, GlaxoSmithKline group of companies. All rights reserved.

RLZ:10PI

Patient Information
RELENZA® (ruh-LENS-uh)
(zanamivir)
Inhalation Powder

This leaflet contains important patient information about RELENZA (zanamivir) Inhalation Powder, and should be read completely before beginning treatment. It does not, however, take the place of discussions with your healthcare provider about your medical condition or your treatment. This summary does not list all benefits and risks of RELENZA. The medication described here can only be prescribed and dispensed by a licensed healthcare provider, who has information about your medical condition and more information about the drug, including how to take it, what to expect, and potential side effects. If you have any questions about RELENZA, talk with your healthcare provider.

What is RELENZA?

RELENZA is a medicine for the treatment of influenza (flu, infection caused by influenza virus) and for reducing the chance of getting the flu in community and household settings. It belongs to a group of medicines called neuraminidase inhibitors. These medications attack the influenza vi-

rus and prevent it from spreading inside your body. RELENZA treats the cause of influenza at its source, rather than simply masking the symptoms.

Important Safety Information About RELENZA

Some patients have had bronchospasm (wheezing) or serious breathing problems when they used RELENZA. Many but not all of these patients had previous asthma or chronic obstructive pulmonary disease. RELENZA has not been shown to shorten the duration of influenza in people with these diseases. Because of the risk of side effects and because it has not been shown to help them, RELENZA is not recommended for people with chronic respiratory disease such as asthma or chronic obstructive pulmonary disease.

If you develop worsening respiratory symptoms such as wheezing or shortness of breath, stop using RELENZA and contact your healthcare provider right away.

If you have chronic respiratory disease such as asthma and chronic obstructive pulmonary disease and your healthcare provider has prescribed RELENZA, you should have a fast-acting, inhaled bronchodilator available for your use. If you are scheduled to use an inhaled bronchodilator at the same time as RELENZA, use the inhaled bronchodilator **before** using RELENZA.

Read the rest of this leaflet for more information about side effects and risks.

Other kinds of infections can appear like influenza or occur along with influenza, and need different kinds of treatment. Contact your healthcare provider if you feel worse or develop new symptoms during or after treatment, or if your influenza symptoms do not start to get better.

Who should not take RELENZA?

RELENZA is not recommended for people who have chronic lung disease such as asthma or chronic obstructive pulmonary disease. RELENZA has not been shown to shorten the duration of influenza in people with these diseases, and some people have had serious side effects of bronchospasm and worsening lung function. (See the section of this Patient Information entitled **"Important Safety Information About RELENZA."**)

You should not take RELENZA if you are allergic to zanamivir or any other ingredient of RELENZA. Also tell your healthcare provider if you have any type of chronic condition including lung or heart disease, if you are allergic to any other medicines, milk proteins or other food products, or if you are pregnant.

RELENZA was not effective in reducing the chance of getting the flu in 2 studies in nursing home patients.

RELENZA does not treat flu-like illness that is not caused by influenza virus.

Who should consider taking RELENZA?

Adult and pediatric patients at least 7 years of age who have influenza symptoms that appeared within the previous day or two. Typical symptoms of influenza include sudden onset of fever, cough, headache, fatigue, muscular weakness, and sore throat.

RELENZA can also help reduce the chance of getting the flu in adults and children at least 5 years of age who have a higher chance of getting the flu because they spend time with someone who has the flu. RELENZA can also reduce the chance of getting the flu if there is a flu outbreak in the community.

The use of RELENZA for the treatment of flu has not been shown to reduce the risk of spreading the virus to others.

Can I take other medications with RELENZA?

RELENZA has been shown to have an acceptable safety profile when used as labeled, with minimal risk of drug interactions. Your healthcare provider may recommend taking other medications, including over-the-counter medications, to reduce fever or other symptoms while you are taking RELENZA. Before starting treatment, make sure that your healthcare provider knows if you are taking other medicines. If you are scheduled to use an inhaled bronchodilator at the same time as RELENZA, you should use the inhaled bronchodilator **before** using RELENZA.

Before taking RELENZA, please let your healthcare provider know if you received live attenuated influenza vaccine (FLUMIST®) intranasal in the past 2 weeks.

How and when should I take RELENZA?

RELENZA is packaged in medicine disks called ROTADISKS® and is inhaled by mouth using a delivery device called a DISKHALER®. Each ROTADISK contains 4 blisters. Each blister contains 5 mg of active drug and 20 mg of lactose powder (which contains milk proteins).

You should receive a demonstration on how to use RELENZA in the DISKHALER from a healthcare provider. Before taking RELENZA, read the "Patient Instructions for Use." Make sure that you understand these instructions and talk to your healthcare provider if you have any questions. Children who use RELENZA should always be supervised by an adult who understands how to use RELENZA. Proper use of the DISKHALER to inhale the drug is necessary for safe and effective use of RELENZA.

If you have the flu the usual dose for treatment is 2 inhalations of RELENZA (1 blister per inhalation) twice daily (in

the morning and evening) for 5 days. It is important that you begin your treatment with RELENZA as soon as possible from the first appearance of your flu symptoms. Take 2 doses on the first day of treatment whenever possible if there are at least 2 hours between doses.

To reduce the chance of getting the flu, the usual dose is 2 inhalations of RELENZA (1 blister per inhalation) once daily for 10 or 28 days as prescribed by your healthcare provider.

Never share RELENZA with anyone, even if they have the same symptoms. If you feel worse or develop new symptoms during treatment with RELENZA, or if your flu symptoms do not start to get better, stop using the medicine and contact your healthcare provider.

What if I miss a dose?

If you forget to take your medicine at any time, take the missed dose as soon as you remember, except if it is near the next dose (within 2 hours). Then continue to take RELENZA at the usual times. You do not need to take a double dose. If you have missed several doses, inform your healthcare provider and follow the advice given to you.

What are important or common possible side effects of taking RELENZA?

Some patients have had breathing problems while taking RELENZA. This can be very serious and need treatment right away. Most of the patients who had this problem had asthma or chronic obstructive pulmonary disease, but some did not. If you have trouble breathing or have wheezing after your dose of RELENZA, stop taking RELENZA and get medical attention.

In studies, the most common side effects with RELENZA have been headaches; diarrhea; nausea; vomiting; nasal irritation; bronchitis; cough; sinusitis; ear, nose, and throat infections; and dizziness. Other side effects that have been reported, but were not as common, include rashes and allergic reactions, some of which were severe.

People with influenza (the flu), particularly children and adolescents, may be at an increased risk of seizures, confusion, or abnormal behavior early in their illness. These events may occur after beginning RELENZA or may occur when flu is not treated. These events are uncommon but may result in accidental injury to the patient. Therefore, patients should be observed for signs of unusual behavior and a healthcare professional should be contacted immediately if the patient shows any signs of unusual behavior.

If you are not feeling well when you take RELENZA, you may faint or become lightheaded after inhaling RELENZA. You should sit down in a relaxed position before inhaling the dose of RELENZA, and you should only hold your breath for as long as is comfortable after inhaling the dose.

If you are not feeling well, you are advised to have someone with you while you are inhaling the dose of RELENZA.

This list of side effects is not complete. Your healthcare provider or pharmacist can discuss with you a more complete list of possible side effects with RELENZA. Talk to your healthcare provider promptly about any side effects you have.

Call your healthcare provider for medical advice about side effects. You may report side effects to FDA at 1-800-FDA-1088.

Please refer to the section entitled **"Important Safety Information About RELENZA"** for additional information.

Should I get a flu shot?

RELENZA is not a substitute for a flu shot. You should receive an annual flu shot according to guidelines on immunization practices that your healthcare provider can share with you.

What if I am pregnant or nursing?

If you are pregnant or planning to become pregnant while taking RELENZA, talk to your healthcare provider before taking this medication. RELENZA is normally not recommended for use during pregnancy or nursing, as the effects on the unborn child or nursing infant are unknown.

How and where should I store RELENZA?

RELENZA should be stored at room temperature below 77°F (25°C). RELENZA is not in a childproof container. Keep RELENZA out of the reach of children. Discard the DISKHALER after finishing your treatment.

INSTRUCTIONS FOR USE

IMPORTANT: Read Step-by-Step Instructions before using the DISKHALER®.

Be sure to take the dose your healthcare provider has prescribed.

BEFORE YOU START:

Please read the entire Patient Information leaflet for important information about the effects of RELENZA including

the section "Important Safety Information About RELENZA" for information about the risk of breathing difficulties.

If RELENZA is prescribed for a child, dosing should be supervised by an adult who understands how to use RELENZA and has been instructed in its use by a healthcare provider.

Parts of the DISKHALER:

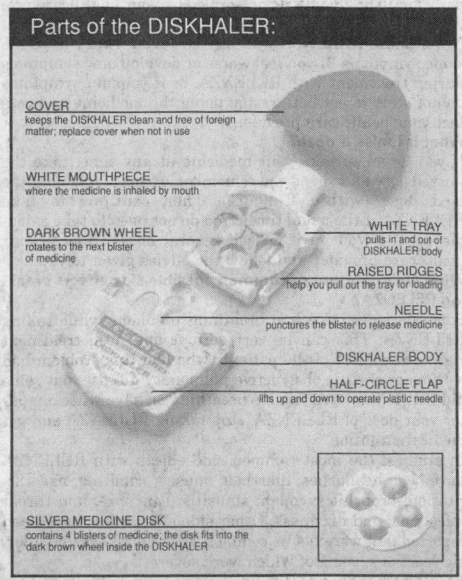

COVER
keeps the DISKHALER clean and free of foreign matter; replace cover when not in use

WHITE MOUTHPIECE
where the medicine is inhaled by mouth

DARK BROWN WHEEL
rotates to the next blister of medicine

WHITE TRAY
pulls in and out of DISKHALER body

RAISED RIDGES
help you pull out the tray for loading

NEEDLE
punctures the blister to release medicine

DISKHALER BODY

HALF-CIRCLE FLAP
lifts up and down to operate plastic needle

SILVER MEDICINE DISK
contains 4 blisters of medicine; the disk fits into the dark brown wheel inside the DISKHALER

Step-by-step instructions for using the DISKHALER®

Step A: Load the medicine into the DISKHALER

1. Start by pulling off the blue cover.
2. **Always check inside the mouthpiece to make sure it is clear before each use. If foreign objects are in the mouthpiece, they could be inhaled and cause serious harm.**
3. Pull the white mouthpiece by the edges to extend the white tray all the way.
4. Once the white tray is extended all the way, find the raised ridges on each side of it. Press in these ridges, both sides at the same time, and **pull the whole white tray out of the DISKHALER body.**
5. Place one silver medicine disk onto the dark brown wheel, flat side up. The four silver blisters on the underside of the medicine disk will drop neatly into the four holes in the wheel.
6. Push in the white tray as far as it will go. Now the DISKHALER is loaded with medicine.

Step B: Puncture the blister

Be sure to keep the DISKHALER level.

The DISKHALER punctures one blister of medicine at a time so you can inhale the right amount. It does not matter which blister you start with. Check to make sure that the silver foil is unbroken.

1. Be sure to keep the DISKHALER level so the medicine does not spill out.
2. Locate the half-circle flap with the name "RELENZA" on top of the DISKHALER.
3. Lift this flap from the outer edge until it cannot go any farther. Flap must be **straight up** for the plastic needle to puncture both the **top** and **bottom** of the silver medicine disk inside.

4. Keeping the DISKHALER level, click the flap down into place.

Step C: Inhale

1. Before putting the white mouthpiece into your mouth, breathe all the way out (exhale).
   Then put the white mouthpiece into your mouth. Be sure to keep the DISKHALER level so the medicine does not spill out.
2. Close your lips firmly around the mouthpiece. Be sure not to cover the small holes on either side of it.
3. Breathe in through your mouth steadily and as deeply as you can. Your breath pulls the medicine into your airways and lungs.
4. Hold your breath for a few seconds to help RELENZA stay in your lungs where it can work.

To take another inhalation, move to the next blister by following Step D below.

Once you've inhaled the number of blisters prescribed by your healthcare provider, replace the cover until your next dose.

Step D: Move the medicine disk to the next blister

1. **Pull** the mouthpiece to extend the white tray, without removing it.
2. Then **push** it back until it clicks. This pull-push motion rotates the medicine disk to the next blister.
3. To take your next inhalation, repeat Steps B and C.

If all 4 blisters in the medicine disk have been used, you are ready to start a new medicine disk (see Step A). Check to make sure that the silver foil is unbroken each time you are ready to puncture the next blister.

IMPORTANT INSTRUCTIONS

Read this entire leaflet before using RELENZA. Even if you have had a previous prescription for RELENZA, read this leaflet to see if any information has changed.

If you have the flu, the usual dose is 2 inhalations twice daily. To reduce the chance of getting the flu, the usual dose is 2 inhalations once daily. However, you must take the number of inhalations your healthcare provider has prescribed.

If you feel worse or develop new symptoms during or after treatment, or if your flu symptoms do not start to improve, stop using the medicine and contact your healthcare provider.

Keep out of reach of children.

Always check inside the mouthpiece to make sure it is clear before each use. If foreign objects are in the mouthpiece, they could be inhaled and cause serious harm.

Always replace the cover after each use.

Throw away the DISKHALER after treatment is completed.

This DISKHALER is for use only with RELENZA. Do not use the RELENZA DISKHALER device with FLOVENT® (fluticasone propionate) and do not use RELENZA with the FLOVENT DISKHALER device. Store at 25°C (77°F); excursions permitted to 15° to 30°C (59° to 86°F) (see USP Controlled Room Temperature).

REMEMBER: This medicine has been prescribed for you by your healthcare provider. DO NOT give this medicine to anyone else.

RELENZA, FLOVENT, ROTADISK, and DISKHALER are registered trademarks of the GlaxoSmithKline group of companies.
FLUMIST is a registered trademark of MedImmune, Inc.
GlaxoSmithKline
Research Triangle Park, NC 27709
©2013, GlaxoSmithKline group of companies. All rights reserved.
October 2013
RLZ:6PIL

REQUIP®

[rē'kwip]
(ropinirole tablets)
Patient Information Included

℞

DESCRIPTION

REQUIP (ropinirole) is an orally administered non-ergoline dopamine agonist. It is the hydrochloride salt of 4-[2-(dipropylamino)ethyl]-1,3-dihydro-2H-indol-2-one monohydrochloride and has an empirical formula of $C_{16}H_{24}N_2O \bullet HCl$. The molecular weight is 296.84 (260.38 as the free base).

The structural formula is:
Ropinirole hydrochloride is a white to yellow solid with a melting range of 243° to 250°C and a solubility of 133 mg/mL in water.

Each pentagonal film-coated TILTAB® tablet with beveled edges contains 0.29 mg, 0.57 mg, 1.14 mg, 2.28 mg, 3.42 mg, 4.56 mg, or 5.70 mg ropinirole hydrochloride equivalent to ropinirole, 0.25 mg, 0.5 mg, 1 mg, 2 mg, 3 mg, 4 mg, or 5 mg. Inactive ingredients consist of: croscarmellose sodium, hydrous lactose, magnesium stearate, microcrystalline cellulose, and one or more of the following: carmine, FD&C Blue No. 2 aluminum lake, FD&C Yellow No. 6 aluminum lake, hypromellose, iron oxides, polyethylene glycol, polysorbate 80, titanium dioxide.

CLINICAL PHARMACOLOGY

Mechanism of Action

REQUIP is a non-ergoline dopamine agonist with high relative in vitro specificity and full intrinsic activity at the D_2 and D_3 dopamine receptor subtypes, binding with higher affinity to D_3 than to D_2 or D_4 receptor subtypes.

Ropinirole has moderate in vitro affinity for opioid receptors. Ropinirole and its metabolites have negligible in vitro affinity for dopamine D_1, 5-HT$_1$, 5-HT$_2$, benzodiazepine, GABA, muscarinic, alpha$_1$-, alpha$_2$-, and beta-adrenoreceptors.

Parkinson's Disease: The precise mechanism of action of REQUIP as a treatment for Parkinson's disease is unknown, although it is believed to be due to stimulation of postsynaptic dopamine D_2-type receptors within the caudate-putamen in the brain. This conclusion is supported by studies that show that ropinirole improves motor function in various animal models of Parkinson's disease. In particular, ropinirole attenuates the motor deficits induced by lesioning the ascending nigrostriatal dopaminergic pathway with the neurotoxin 1-methyl-4-phenyl-1,2,3,6-tetrahydropyridine (MPTP) in primates. The relevance of D_3 receptor binding in Parkinson's disease is unknown.

Restless Legs Syndrome (RLS): The precise mechanism of action of REQUIP as a treatment for Restless Legs Syndrome (also known as Ekbom Syndrome) is unknown. Although the pathophysiology of RLS is largely unknown, neuropharmacological evidence suggests primary dopaminergic system involvement. Positron emission tomographic (PET) studies suggest that a mild striatal presynaptic dopaminergic dysfunction may be involved in the pathogenesis of RLS.

Clinical Pharmacology Studies

In healthy normotensive subjects, single oral doses of REQUIP in the range 0.01 to 2.5 mg had little or no effect on supine blood pressure and pulse rates. Upon standing, REQUIP caused decreases in systolic and diastolic blood pressure at doses above 0.25 mg. In some subjects, these changes were associated with the emergence of orthostatic symptoms, bradycardia, and, in one case, transient sinus arrest with syncope. With repeat dosing and slow titration up to 4 mg once daily in healthy volunteers, postural hypotension or hypotension-related adverse events were noted in 13% of subjects on REQUIP and none of the subjects on placebo.

The mechanism of postural hypotension induced by REQUIP is presumed to be due to a D_2-mediated blunting of the noradrenergic response to standing and subsequent decrease in peripheral vascular resistance. Nausea is a common concomitant symptom of orthostatic signs and symptoms.

At oral doses as low as 0.2 mg, REQUIP suppressed serum prolactin concentrations in healthy male volunteers.

REQUIP had no dose-related effect on ECG wave form and rhythm in young, healthy, male volunteers in the range of 0.01 to 2.5 mg.

REQUIP had no dose- or exposure-related effect on mean QT intervals in healthy male and female volunteers titrated to doses up to 4 mg/day. The effect of REQUIP on QT intervals at higher exposures achieved either due to drug interactions or at doses used in Parkinson's disease has not been systematically evaluated.

Pharmacokinetics

Absorption, Distribution, Metabolism, and Elimination:

The pharmacokinetics of ropinirole are similar in Parkinson's disease patients and patients with Restless Legs Syndrome. Ropinirole is rapidly absorbed after oral administration, reaching peak concentration in approximately 1-2 hours. In clinical studies, over 88% of a radiolabeled dose was recovered in urine and the absolute bioavailability was 55%, indicating a first-pass effect. Relative bioavailability from a tablet compared to an oral solution is 85%. Food does not affect the extent of absorption of ropinirole, although its T_{max} is increased by 2.5 hours and its C_{max} is decreased by approximately 25% when the drug is taken with a high-fat meal. The clearance of ropinirole after oral administration to patients is 47 L/hr (cv = 45%) and its elimination half-life is approximately 6 hours. Ropinirole is extensively metabolized by the liver to inactive metabolites and displays linear kinetics over the therapeutic dosing range of 1 to 8 mg 3 times daily. Steady-state concentrations are expected to be achieved within 2 days of dosing. Accumulation upon multiple dosing is predictive from single dosing.

Ropinirole is widely distributed throughout the body, with an apparent volume of distribution of 7.5 L/kg (cv = 32%). It is up to 40% bound to plasma proteins and has a blood-to-plasma ratio of 1:1.

The major metabolic pathways are N-despropylation and hydroxylation to form the inactive N-despropyl and hydroxy metabolites. In vitro studies indicate that the major cytochrome P_{450} isozyme involved in the metabolism of ropinirole is CYP1A2, an enzyme known to be stimulated by smoking and omeprazole, and inhibited by, for example, fluvoxamine, mexiletine, and the older fluoroquinolones such as ciprofloxacin and norfloxacin. The N-despropyl metabolite is converted to carbamyl glucuronide, carboxylic acid, and N-despropyl hydroxy metabolites. The hydroxy metabolite of ropinirole is rapidly glucuronidated. Less than 10% of the administered dose is excreted as unchanged drug in urine. N-despropyl ropinirole is the predominant metabolite found in urine (40%), followed by the carboxylic acid metabolite (10%), and the glucuronide of the hydroxy metabolite (10%).

P_{450} Interaction:

In vitro metabolism studies showed that CYP1A2 was the major enzyme responsible for the metabolism of ropinirole. Inhibitors or inducers of this enzyme have been shown to alter its clearance when coadministered with ropinirole. Therefore, if therapy with a drug known to be a potent inhibitor of CYP1A2 is stopped or started during treatment with REQUIP, adjustment of the dose of REQUIP may be required.

Population Subgroups

Because therapy with REQUIP is initiated at a low dose and gradually titrated upward according to clinical tolerability to obtain the optimum therapeutic effect, adjustment of the initial dose based on gender, weight, or age is not necessary.

Age:

Oral clearance of ropinirole is reduced by 15% in patients above 65 years of age compared to younger patients. Dosage adjustment is not necessary in the elderly (above 65 years), as the dose of ropinirole is to be individually titrated to clinical response.

Gender:

Female and male patients showed similar oral clearance.

Race:

The influence of race on the pharmacokinetics of ropinirole has not been evaluated.

Cigarette Smoking:

Smoking is expected to increase the clearance of ropinirole since CYP1A2 is known to be induced by smoking. In a study in patients with RLS, smokers (n = 7) had an approximate 30% lower C_{max} and a 38% lower AUC than did nonsmokers (n = 11), when those parameters were normalized for dose.

Renal Impairment:

Based on population pharmacokinetic analysis, no difference was observed in the pharmacokinetics of ropinirole in patients with moderate renal impairment (creatinine clearance between 30 to 50 mL/min.) compared to an age-matched population with creatinine clearance above 50 mL/min. Therefore, no dosage adjustment is necessary in moderately renally impaired patients. The use of REQUIP in patients with severe renal impairment has not been studied.

The effect of hemodialysis on drug removal is not known, but because of the relatively high apparent volume of distribution of ropinirole (525 L), the removal of the drug by hemodialysis is unlikely.

Hepatic Impairment:

The pharmacokinetics of ropinirole have not been studied in hepatically impaired patients. These patients may have higher plasma levels and lower clearance of the drug than patients with normal hepatic function. The drug should be titrated with caution in this population.

Other Diseases:

Population pharmacokinetic analysis revealed no change in the oral clearance of ropinirole in patients with concomitant diseases such as hypertension, depression, osteoporosis/arthritis, and insomnia compared to patients with Parkinson's disease only.

Clinical Trials

Parkinson's Disease:

The effectiveness of REQUIP in the treatment of Parkinson's disease was evaluated in a multinational drug development program consisting of 11 randomized, controlled trials. Four were conducted in patients with early Parkinson's disease and no concomitant levodopa (L-dopa), and 7 were conducted in patients with advanced Parkinson's disease with concomitant L-dopa.

Among these 11 studies, 3 placebo-controlled studies provide the most persuasive evidence of ropinirole's effectiveness in the management of patients with Parkinson's disease who were and were not receiving concomitant L-dopa. Two of these 3 trials enrolled patients with early Parkinson's disease (without L-dopa) and 1 enrolled patients receiving L-dopa.

In these studies a variety of measures were used to assess the effects of treatment (e.g., the Unified Parkinson's Disease Rating Scale [UPDRS], Clinical Global Impression [CGI] scores, patient diaries recording time "on" and "off," and tolerability of L-dopa dose reductions).

In both studies of early Parkinson's disease (without L-dopa) patients, the motor component (Part III) of the UPDRS was the primary outcome assessment. The UPDRS is a 4-part multi-item rating scale intended to evaluate mentation (Part I), activities of daily living (Part II), motor performance (Part III), and complications of therapy (Part IV). Part III of the UPDRS contains 14 items designed to assess the severity of the cardinal motor findings in patients with Parkinson's disease (e.g., tremor, rigidity, bradykinesia, postural instability, etc.) scored for different body regions and has a maximum (worst) score of 108. Responders were defined as patients with at least a 30% reduction in the Part III score.

In the study of advanced Parkinson's disease (with L-dopa) patients, both reduction in percent awake time spent "off" and the ability to reduce the daily use of L-dopa were assessed as a combined endpoint and individually.

Studies in Patients With Early Parkinson's Disease (Without L-dopa):

One early therapy study was a 12-week multicenter study in which 63 patients (41 on REQUIP) with idiopathic Parkinson's disease receiving concomitant anti-Parkinson medication (but not L-dopa) were randomized to either REQUIP or placebo. Patients had a mean disease duration of approximately 2 years. Patients were eligible for enrollment if they presented with bradykinesia and at least tremor, rigidity, or postural instability. In addition, they must have been classified as Hoehn & Yahr Stage I-IV. This scale, ranging from I = unilateral involvement with minimal impairment to V = confined to wheelchair or bed, is a standard instrument used for staging patients with Parkinson's disease. The primary outcome measure in this trial was the proportion of patients experiencing a decrease (compared to baseline) of at least 30% in the UPDRS motor score. Patients were titrated for up to 10 weeks, starting at 0.5 mg twice daily, with weekly increments of 0.5 mg twice daily to a maximum of 5 mg twice daily. Once patients reached their maximally tolerated dose (or 5 mg twice daily), they were maintained on that dose through 12 weeks. The mean dose achieved by patients at study endpoint was 7.4 mg/day. At the end of 12 weeks, 71% of patients treated with REQUIP were responders, compared with 41% of patients in the placebo group (p = 0.021).

Statistically significant differences between the percentage of responders on REQUIP compared to placebo were seen after 8 weeks of treatment.

In addition, the mean percentage improvement from baseline in the Total Motor Score was 43% in patients treated with REQUIP compared with 21% in patients treated with placebo (p = 0.018).

Statistically significant differences in UPDRS motor score between REQUIP and placebo were seen after 2 weeks of treatment.

The median daily dose at which a 30% reduction in UPDRS motor score was sustained was 4 mg.

The second trial in early Parkinson's disease (without L-dopa) patients was a double-blind, randomized, placebo-controlled, 6-month study. Patients were essentially similar to those in the study described above; concomitant use of selegiline was allowed, but patients were not permitted to

use anticholinergics or amantadine during the study. Patients had a mean disease duration of 2 years and limited (not more than a 6-week period) or no prior exposure to L-dopa. The starting dose of REQUIP in this trial was 0.25 mg 3 times daily. The dose was titrated at weekly intervals by increments of 0.25 mg 3 times daily to a dose of 1 mg 3 times daily. Further titrations at weekly intervals were at increments of 0.5 mg 3 times daily up to a dose of 3 mg 3 times daily, and then weekly at increments of 1 mg 3 times daily. Patients were to be titrated to a dose of at least 1.5 mg 3 times daily and then to their maximally tolerated dose, up to a maximum of 8 mg 3 times daily. The mean dose attained in patients at study endpoint was 15.7 mg/day.

The primary measure of effectiveness was the mean percent reduction (improvement) from baseline in the UPDRS Motor Score. In this study 241 patients were enrolled. At the end of the 6-month study, patients treated with REQUIP had 22% improvement in motor score, compared with a 4% worsening in the placebo group (p<0.001).

Statistically significant differences in UPDRS motor score improvement between REQUIP and placebo were seen after 12 weeks of treatment.

Study in Patients With Advanced Parkinson's Disease (With L-dopa):

This double-blind, randomized, placebo-controlled, 6-month trial evaluated 148 patients (Hoehn & Yahr II-IV) who were not adequately controlled on L-dopa. Patients in this study had a mean disease duration of approximately 9 years, had been exposed to L-dopa for approximately 7 years, and had experienced "on-off" periods with L-dopa therapy. Patients previously receiving stable doses of selegiline, amantadine, and/or anticholinergic agents could continue on these agents during the study. Patients were started at a dose of 0.25 mg 3 times daily of REQUIP and titrated upward by weekly intervals until an optimal therapeutic response was achieved. The maximum dose of study medication was 8 mg 3 times daily. All patients had to be titrated to at least a dose of 2.5 mg 3 times daily. Patients could then be maintained on this dose level or higher for the remainder of the study. Once a dose of 2.5 mg 3 times daily was achieved, patients underwent a mandatory reduction in their L-dopa dose, to be followed by additional mandatory reductions with continued escalation of the dose of REQUIP. Reductions in the dosage of L-dopa were also allowed if patients experienced adverse events that the investigator considered related to dopaminergic therapy. The mean dose attained at study endpoint was 16.3 mg/day. The primary outcome was the proportion of responders, defined as patients who were able both to achieve a decrease (compared to baseline) of at least 20% in their L-dopa dose and a decrease of at least 20% in the proportion of the time awake in the "off" condition (a period of time during the day when patients are particularly immobile), as determined by patient diary. In addition, the mean percent change from baseline in daily L-dopa dose was examined.

At the end of 6 months, 28% of patients treated with REQUIP were classified as responders (based on combined endpoint) while 11% of patients treated with placebo were responders (p = 0.02). Based on the protocol-mandated reductions in L-dopa dosage with escalating doses of REQUIP, patients treated with REQUIP had a 19.4% mean reduction in L-dopa dose while patients treated with placebo had a 3% reduction (p<0.001). L-dopa dosage reduction was also allowed during the study if dyskinesias or other dopaminergic effects occurred. Overall, reduction of L-dopa dose was sustained in 87% of patients treated with REQUIP and in 57% of patients on placebo. On average, the L-dopa dose was reduced by 31% in patients treated with REQUIP.

The mean number of "off" hours per day during baseline was 6.4 hours for patients treated with REQUIP and 7.3 hours for patients treated with placebo. At the end of the 6-month study, patients treated with REQUIP had a mean of 4.9 hours per day of "off" time, while placebo-treated patients had a mean of 6.4 hours per day of "off" time.

Restless Legs Syndrome (RLS):

The effectiveness of REQUIP in the treatment of RLS was demonstrated in randomized, double-blind, placebo-controlled studies in adults diagnosed with RLS using the International Restless Legs Syndrome Study Group diagnostic criteria (see INDICATIONS AND USAGE). Patients were required to have a history of a minimum of 15 RLS episodes/month during the previous month and a total score of ≥15 on the International RLS Rating Scale (IRLS scale) at baseline. Patients with RLS secondary to other conditions (e.g., pregnancy, renal failure, and anemia) were excluded. All studies employed flexible dosing, with patients initiating therapy at 0.25 mg REQUIP once daily. Patients were titrated based on clinical response and tolerability over 7 weeks to a maximum of 4 mg once daily. All doses were taken between 1 and 3 hours before bedtime.

A variety of measures were used to assess the effects of treatment, including the IRLS Scale and Clinical Global Impression-Global Improvement (CGI-I) scores. The IRLS Scale contains 10 items designed to assess the severity of sensory and motor symptoms, sleep disturbance, daytime

Table 1. Mean Change in IRLS Score and Percent Responders on CGI-I

	REQUIP	Placebo	p-value
Mean Change in IRLS score at Week 12			
US study	-13.5	-9.8	p<0.0001
Multinational study (excluding US)	-11.0	-8.0	p=0.0036
Multinational study (including US)	-11.2	-8.7	p=0.0197
Percent responders on CGI-I at Week 12			
US study	73.3%	56.5%	p=0.0006
Multinational study (excluding US)	53.4%	40.9%	p=0.0416
Multinational study (including US)	59.5%	39.6%	p=0.0010

somnolence, and impact on activities of daily living and mood associated with RLS. The range of scores is 0 to 40, with 0 being absence of RLS symptoms and 40 the most severe symptoms. Three of the controlled studies utilized the change from baseline in the IRLS Scale at the week 12 endpoint as the primary efficacy outcome.

Three hundred eighty patients were randomized to receive REQUIP (n = 187) or placebo (n = 193) in a US study; 284 were randomized to receive either REQUIP (n = 146) or placebo (n = 138) in a multinational study (excluding US); and 267 patients were randomized to REQUIP (n = 131) or placebo (n = 136) in a multinational study (including US). Across the 3 studies, the mean duration of RLS was 16 to 22 years (range of 0 to 65 years), mean age was approximately 54 years (range of 18 to 79 years), and approximately 61% were women. The mean dose at week 12 was approximately 2 mg/day for the 3 studies.

In all 3 studies, a statistically significant difference between the treatment group receiving REQUIP and the treatment group receiving placebo was observed at week 12 for both the mean change from baseline in the IRLS Scale total score and the percentage of patients rated as responders (much improved or very much improved) on the CGI-I (see Table 1).

[See table above]

Long-term maintenance of efficacy in the treatment of RLS was demonstrated in a 36-week study. Following a 24-week single-blind treatment phase (flexible doses of REQUIP of 0.25 to 4 mg once daily), patients who were responders (defined as a decrease of >6 points on the IRLS Scale total score relative to baseline) were randomized in double-blind fashion to placebo or continuation of REQUIP for an additional 12 weeks. Relapse was defined as an increase of at least 6 points on the IRLS Scale total score to a total score of at least 15, or withdrawal due to lack of efficacy. For patients who were responders at week 24, the mean dose of ropinirole was 2 mg (range 0.25 to 4 mg). Patients continued on REQUIP demonstrated a significantly lower relapse rate compared with patients randomized to placebo (32.6% vs 57.8%, p = 0.0156).

INDICATIONS AND USAGE
Parkinson's Disease
REQUIP is indicated for the treatment of the signs and symptoms of idiopathic Parkinson's disease.

The effectiveness of REQUIP was demonstrated in randomized, controlled trials in patients with early Parkinson's disease who were not receiving concomitant L-dopa therapy as well as in patients with advanced disease on concomitant L-dopa (see CLINICAL PHARMACOLOGY: Clinical Trials).

Restless Legs Syndrome
REQUIP is indicated for the treatment of moderate-to-severe primary Restless Legs Syndrome (RLS).

Key diagnostic criteria for RLS are: an urge to move the legs usually accompanied or caused by uncomfortable and unpleasant leg sensations; symptoms begin or worsen during periods of rest or inactivity such as lying or sitting; symptoms are partially or totally relieved by movement such as walking or stretching at least as long as the activity continues; and symptoms are worse or occur only in the evening or night. Difficulty falling asleep may frequently be associated with moderate-to-severe RLS.

CONTRAINDICATIONS
REQUIP is contraindicated for patients known to have hypersensitivity reaction (including urticaria, angioedema, rash, pruritus) to ropinirole or to any of the excipients.

WARNINGS
Falling Asleep During Activities of Daily Living
Patients treated with REQUIP have reported falling asleep while engaged in activities of daily living, including the operation of motor vehicles, which sometimes resulted in accidents. Although many of these patients reported somnolence while on REQUIP, some perceived that they had no warning signs such as excessive drowsiness, and believed that they were alert immediately prior to the event. Some of these events have been reported as late as 1 year after initiation of treatment.

In controlled clinical trials, somnolence was a common occurrence in patients receiving REQUIP and is more frequent in Parkinson's disease (up to 40% REQUIP, 6% placebo)

than in Restless Legs Syndrome (12% REQUIP, 6% placebo). Many clinical experts believe that falling asleep while engaged in activities of daily living always occurs in a setting of preexisting somnolence, although patients may not give such a history. For this reason, prescribers should continually reassess patients for drowsiness or sleepiness, especially since some of the events occur well after the start of treatment. Prescribers should also be aware that patients may not acknowledge drowsiness or sleepiness until directly questioned about drowsiness or sleepiness during specific activities.

Before initiating treatment with REQUIP, patients should be advised of the potential to develop drowsiness and specifically asked about factors that may increase the risk with REQUIP such as concomitant sedating medications, the presence of sleep disorders (other than Restless Legs Syndrome), and concomitant medications that increase ropinirole plasma levels (e.g., ciprofloxacin—see PRECAUTIONS: Drug Interactions). If a patient develops significant daytime sleepiness or episodes of falling asleep during activities that require active participation (e.g., conversations, eating, etc.), REQUIP should ordinarily be discontinued. (See DOSAGE AND ADMINISTRATION for guidance in discontinuing REQUIP.) If a decision is made to continue REQUIP, patients should be advised to not drive and to avoid other potentially dangerous activities. There is insufficient information to establish that dose reduction will eliminate episodes of falling asleep while engaged in activities of daily living.

Syncope
Syncope, sometimes associated with bradycardia, was observed in association with ropinirole in both Parkinson's disease patients and RLS patients. In the 2 double-blind, placebo-controlled studies of REQUIP in patients with Parkinson's disease who were not being treated with L-dopa, 11.5% (18 of 157) of patients on REQUIP had syncope compared to 1.4% (2 of 147) of patients on placebo. Most of these cases occurred more than 4 weeks after initiation of therapy with REQUIP, and were usually associated with a recent increase in dose.

Of 208 patients being treated with both L-dopa and REQUIP in placebo-controlled advanced Parkinson's disease trials, there were reports of syncope in 6 (2.9%) compared to 2 of 120 (1.7%) of placebo/L-dopa patients.

In patients with RLS, of 496 patients treated with REQUIP in 12-week placebo-controlled trials, there were reports of syncope in 5 (1.0%) compared with 1 of 500 (0.2%) patients treated with placebo.

Because the studies of REQUIP excluded patients with significant cardiovascular disease, it is not known to what extent the estimated incidence figures apply to either Parkinson's disease or RLS patients in clinical practice. Therefore, patients with severe cardiovascular disease should be treated with caution.

Two of 47 Parkinson's disease patient volunteers enrolled in phase 1 studies had syncope following a 1-mg dose. In 2 studies in RLS patients that used a forced titration regimen and orthostatic challenge with intensive blood pressure monitoring, 1 of 55 RLS patients treated with REQUIP compared with 0 of 27 patients receiving placebo reported syncope. In phase 1 studies including 110 healthy volunteers, 1 patient developed hypotension, bradycardia, and sinus arrest of 26 seconds accompanied by syncope; the patient recovered spontaneously without intervention. One other healthy volunteer reported syncope.

Symptomatic Hypotension
Dopamine agonists, in clinical studies and clinical experience, appear to impair the systemic regulation of blood pressure, with resulting postural hypotension, especially during dose escalation. Parkinson's disease patients, in addition, appear to have an impaired capacity to respond to a postural challenge. For these reasons, Parkinson's patients being treated with dopaminergic agonists ordinarily (1) require careful monitoring for signs and symptoms of postural hypotension, especially during dose escalation, and (2) should be informed of this risk (see PRECAUTIONS: Information for Patients).

Although the clinical trials were not designed to systematically monitor blood pressure, there were individual reported cases of postural hypotension in early Parkinson's

disease (without L-dopa) in patients treated with REQUIP. Most of these cases occurred more than 4 weeks after initiation of therapy with REQUIP and were usually associated with a recent increase in dose.

In 12-week placebo-controlled trials of patients with RLS, the adverse event orthostatic hypotension was reported by 4 of 496 patients (0.8%) treated with REQUIP compared with 2 of 500 patients (0.4%) receiving placebo.

In two phase 2 studies in patients with RLS that used a forced-titration regimen and orthostatic challenges with intensive blood pressure monitoring, 14 of 55 patients (25%) receiving REQUIP experienced an adverse event of hypotension or postural hypotension. As described above, one additional patient was noted to have an episode of vasovagal syncope (although no blood pressure recording was documented). None of the 27 patients receiving placebo had a similar adverse event. In these studies, 11 of the 55 patients (20%) receiving REQUIP and 3 of the 26 patients (12%) who had post-dose blood pressure assessments following placebo, experienced an orthostatic blood pressure decrease of at least 40 mm Hg systolic and/or at least 20 mm Hg diastolic; not all of these changes were associated with clinical symptoms. Except for its forced nature these studies used a similar titration schedule as those in the phase 3 efficacy trials. In phase 1 studies of REQUIP that included 110 healthy volunteers, 9 subjects had documented symptomatic postural hypotension. These episodes appeared mainly at doses above 0.8 mg and these doses are higher than the starting doses recommended for either Parkinson's disease patients or RLS patients. In 8 of these 9 individuals, the hypotension was accompanied by bradycardia, but did not develop into syncope (see Syncope subsection). None of these events resulted in death or hospitalization.

One of 47 Parkinson's disease patient volunteers enrolled in phase 1 studies had documented hypotension following a 2-mg dose on 2 occasions.

Hallucinations
In double-blind, placebo-controlled, early-therapy studies in patients with Parkinson's disease who were not treated with L-dopa, 5.2% (8 of 157) of patients treated with REQUIP reported hallucinations, compared to 1.4% of patients on placebo (2 of 147). Among those patients receiving both REQUIP and L-dopa in advanced Parkinson's disease (with L-dopa) studies, 10.1% (21 of 208) were reported to experience hallucinations, compared to 4.2% (5 of 120) of patients treated with placebo and L-dopa.

Hallucinations were of sufficient severity to cause discontinuation of treatment in 1.3% of the early Parkinson's disease (without L-dopa) patients and 1.9% of the advanced Parkinson's disease (with L-dopa) patients, compared to 0% and 1.7% of placebo patients, respectively.

In patients with RLS, hallucinations were reported by 0% of patients treated with REQUIP (0 of 496) compared with 0.2% of patients who received placebo (1 of 500) in the 12-week placebo-controlled trials; in premarketing long-term open-label studies, 0.5% of patients reported hallucinations during therapy with REQUIP (2 of 390) but did not discontinue treatment and symptoms resolved.

PRECAUTIONS
General
Dyskinesia: REQUIP may potentiate the dopaminergic side effects of L-dopa and may cause and/or exacerbate preexisting dyskinesia in patients treated with L-dopa for Parkinson's disease. Decreasing the dose of L-dopa may ameliorate this side effect.

Renal Impairment: No dosage adjustment is needed in patients with mild to moderate renal impairment (creatinine clearance of 30 to 50 mL/min). The use of REQUIP in patients with severe renal impairment has not been studied.

Hepatic Impairment: The pharmacokinetics of ropinirole have not been studied in patients with hepatic impairment. Since patients with hepatic impairment may have higher plasma levels and lower clearance, REQUIP should be titrated with caution in these patients.

Events Reported With Dopaminergic Therapy: *Withdrawal-Emergent Hyperpyrexia and Confusion:* Although not reported with REQUIP, a symptom complex resembling the neuroleptic malignant syndrome (characterized by elevated temperature, muscular rigidity, altered consciousness, and autonomic instability), with no other obvious etiology, has been reported in association with rapid dose reduction, withdrawal of, or changes in anti-Parkinsonian therapy.

Fibrotic Complications: Cases of retroperitoneal fibrosis, pulmonary infiltrates, pleural effusion, pleural thickening, pericarditis, and cardiac valvulopathy have been reported in some patients treated with ergot-derived dopaminergic agents. While these complications may resolve when the drug is discontinued, complete resolution does not always occur.

Although these adverse events are believed to be related to the ergoline structure of these compounds, whether other, nonergot-derived dopamine agonists can cause them is unknown.

A small number of reports have been received of possible fibrotic complications, including pleural effusion, pleural fibrosis, interstitial lung disease, and cardiac valvulopathy, in the development program and postmarketing experience for REQUIP. While the evidence is not sufficient to establish a causal relationship between REQUIP and these fibrotic complications, a contribution of REQUIP cannot be completely ruled out in rare cases.

Melanoma: Epidemiologic studies have shown that patients with Parkinson's disease have a higher risk (2- to approximately 6-fold higher) of developing melanoma than the general population. Whether the increased risk observed was due to Parkinson's disease or other factors, such as drugs used to treat Parkinson's disease, is unclear.

For the reasons stated above, patients and providers are advised to monitor for melanomas frequently and on a regular basis when using REQUIP for *any* indication. Ideally, periodic skin examinations should be performed by appropriately qualified individuals (e.g., dermatologists).

Augmentation and Rebound in RLS: Reports in the literature indicate treatment of RLS with dopaminergic medications can result in a worsening of symptoms in the early morning hours, referred to as rebound. Augmentation has also been described during therapy for RLS. Augmentation refers to the earlier onset of symptoms in the evening (or even the afternoon), increase in symptoms, and spread of symptoms to involve other extremities. The controlled trials of REQUIP in patients with RLS excluded patients with augmentation and rebound and were generally not of sufficient duration to capture these phenomena. The frequency of augmentation and/or rebound after longer use of REQUIP and the appropriate management of these events, have not been evaluated in controlled clinical trials.

Retinal Pathology: Albino Rats: Retinal degeneration was observed in albino rats in the 2-year carcinogenicity study at all doses tested (equivalent to 0.6 to 20 times the maximum recommended human dose on a mg/m² basis), but was statistically significant at the highest dose (50 mg/kg/day). Additional studies to further evaluate the specific pathology (e.g., loss of photoreceptor cells) have not been performed. Similar changes were not observed in a 2-year carcinogenicity study in albino mice or in rats or monkeys treated for 1 year. The potential significance of this effect in humans has not been established, but cannot be disregarded because disruption of a mechanism that is universally present in vertebrates (e.g., disk shedding) may be involved.

Human: In order to evaluate the effect of REQUIP in humans, ocular electroretinogram (ERG) assessments were conducted during a 2-year, double-blind, multicenter, flexible dose, L-dopa controlled clinical study of REQUIP in patients with Parkinson's disease. A total of 156 patients (78 on ropinirole, mean dose 11.9 mg/day and 78 on L-dopa, mean dose 555.2 mg/day) were evaluated for evidence of retinal dysfunction through electroretinograms. There was no clinically meaningful difference between the treatment groups in retinal function over the duration of the study.

Binding to Melanin: REQUIP binds to melanin-containing tissues (i.e., eyes, skin) in pigmented rats. After a single dose, long-term retention of drug was demonstrated, with a half-life in the eye of 20 days. It is not known if REQUIP accumulates in these tissues over time.

Information for Patients

Physicians should instruct their patients to read the Patient Information leaflet before starting therapy with REQUIP and to reread it upon prescription renewal for new information regarding the use of REQUIP.

Patients should be instructed to take REQUIP only as prescribed. If a dose is missed, patients should be advised not to double their next dose.

REQUIP can be taken with or without food. Patients may be advised that taking REQUIP with food may reduce the occurrence of nausea. However, this has not been established in controlled clinical trials.

Patients should be advised that they may develop postural (orthostatic) hypotension with or without symptoms such as dizziness, nausea, syncope, and sometimes sweating. Hypotension and/or orthostatic symptoms may occur more frequently during initial therapy or with an increase in dose at any time (cases have been seen after weeks of treatment). Accordingly, patients should be cautioned against rising rapidly after sitting or lying down, especially if they have been doing so for prolonged periods, and especially at the initiation of treatment with REQUIP.

Patients should be alerted to the potential sedating effects associated with REQUIP, including somnolence and the possibility of falling asleep while engaged in activities of daily living. Since somnolence is a frequent adverse event with potentially serious consequences, patients should neither drive a car nor engage in other potentially dangerous activities until they have gained sufficient experience with REQUIP to gauge whether or not it affects their mental and/or motor performance adversely. Patients should be advised that if increased somnolence or episodes of falling asleep during activities of daily living (e.g., watching television, passenger in a car, etc.) are experienced at any time during treatment, they should not drive or participate in potentially dangerous activities until they have contacted their physician.

Because of possible additive effects, caution should be advised when patients are taking other sedating medications or alcohol in combination with REQUIP and when taking concomitant medications that increase plasma levels of ropinirole (e.g., ciprofloxacin).

Because of the possible additive sedative effects, caution should also be used when patients are taking alcohol or other CNS depressants (e.g., benzodiazepines, antipsychotics, antidepressants, etc.) in combination with REQUIP. Patients should be informed they may experience hallucinations (unreal visions, sounds, or sensations) while taking REQUIP. These were uncommon in patients taking REQUIP for Restless Legs Syndrome. The risk is greater in patients with Parkinson's disease; the elderly are at greater risk than younger patients with Parkinson's disease; and the risk is greater in patients who are taking REQUIP with L-dopa, or taking higher doses of REQUIP.

Impulse Control Symptoms Including Compulsive Behaviors: There have been reports of patients experiencing intense urges to gamble, increased sexual urges, and other intense urges and the inability to control these urges while taking one or more of the medications that increase central dopaminergic tone, that are generally used for the treatment of Parkinson's disease or Restless Legs Syndrome, including REQUIP. Although it is not proven that the medications caused these events, these urges were reported to have stopped in some cases when the dose was reduced or the medication was stopped. Prescribers should ask patients about the development of new or increased gambling urges, sexual urges or other urges while being treated with REQUIP. Patients should inform their physician if they experience new or increased gambling urges, increased sexual urges or other intense urges while taking REQUIP. Physicians should consider dose reduction or stopping the medication if a patient develops such urges while taking REQUIP.

Because of the possibility that ropinirole may be excreted in breast milk, patients should be advised to notify their physicians if they intend to breastfeed or are breastfeeding an infant.

Because ropinirole has been shown to have adverse effects on embryo-fetal development, including teratogenic effects, in animals, and because experience in humans is limited, patients should be advised to notify their physician if they become pregnant or intend to become pregnant during therapy (see PRECAUTIONS: Pregnancy).

Drug Interactions

P450 Interaction: In vitro metabolism studies showed that CYP1A2 was the major enzyme responsible for the metabolism of ropinirole. There is thus the potential for substrates or inhibitors of this enzyme when coadministered with ropinirole to alter its clearance. Therefore, if therapy with a drug known to be a potent inhibitor of CYP1A2 is stopped or started during treatment with REQUIP, adjustment of the dose of REQUIP may be required.

L-dopa: Coadministration of carbidopa + l-dopa (SINEMET® 10/100 mg twice daily) with ropinirole (2 mg 3 times daily) had no effect on the steady-state pharmacokinetics of ropinirole (n = 28 patients). Oral administration of REQUIP 2 mg 3 times daily increased mean steady state C_{max} of l-dopa by 20%, but its AUC was unaffected (n = 23 patients).

Digoxin: Coadministration of REQUIP (2 mg 3 times daily) with digoxin (0.125 to 0.25 mg once daily) did not alter the steady-state pharmacokinetics of digoxin in 10 patients.

Theophylline: Administration of theophylline (300 mg twice daily, a substrate of CYP1A2) did not alter the steady-state pharmacokinetics of ropinirole (2 mg 3 times daily) in 12 patients with Parkinson's disease. Ropinirole (2 mg 3 times daily) did not alter the pharmacokinetics of theophylline (5 mg/kg IV) in 12 patients with Parkinson's disease.

Ciprofloxacin: Coadministration of ciprofloxacin (500 mg twice daily), an inhibitor of CYP1A2, with ropinirole (2 mg 3 times daily) increased ropinirole AUC by 84% on average and C_{max} by 60% (n = 12 patients).

Estrogens: Population pharmacokinetic analysis revealed that estrogens (mainly ethinylestradiol: intake 0.6 to 3 mg over 4-month to 23-year period) reduced the oral clearance of ropinirole by 36% in 16 patients. Dosage adjustment may not be needed for REQUIP in patients on estrogen therapy because patients must be carefully titrated with ropinirole to tolerance or adequate effect. However, if estrogen therapy is stopped or started during treatment with REQUIP, then adjustment of the dose of REQUIP may be required.

Dopamine Antagonists: Since ropinirole is a dopamine agonist, it is possible that dopamine antagonists such as neuroleptics (phenothiazines, butyrophenones, thioxanthenes) or metoclopramide may diminish the effectiveness of REQUIP. Patients with major psychotic disorders treated with neuroleptics should only be treated with dopamine agonists if the potential benefits outweigh the risks.

Population analysis showed that commonly administered drugs, e.g., selegiline, amantadine, tricyclic antidepressants, benzodiazepines, ibuprofen, thiazides, antihistamines, and anticholinergics, did not affect the oral clearance of ropinirole.

Carcinogenesis, Mutagenesis, Impairment of Fertility

Two-year carcinogenicity studies were conducted in Charles River CD-1 mice at doses of 5, 15, and 50 mg/kg/day and in Sprague-Dawley rats at doses of 1.5, 15, and 50 mg/kg/day (top doses equivalent to 10 and 20 times, respectively, the maximum recommended human dose (MRHD) of 24 mg/day on a mg/m² basis). In the male rat, there was a significant increase in testicular Leydig cell adenomas at all doses tested, i.e., ≥1.5 mg/kg (0.6 times the MRHD on a mg/m² basis). This finding is of questionable significance because the endocrine mechanisms believed to be involved in the production of Leydig cell hyperplasia and adenomas in rats are not relevant to humans. In the female mouse, there was an increase in benign uterine endometrial polyps at a dose of 50 mg/kg/day (10 times the MRHD on a mg/m² basis).

Ropinirole was not mutagenic or clastogenic in the in vitro Ames test, the in vitro chromosome aberration test in human lymphocytes, the in vitro mouse lymphoma (L1578Y cells) assay, and the in vivo mouse micronucleus test.

When administered to female rats prior to and during mating and throughout pregnancy, ropinirole caused disruption of implantation at doses of 20 mg/kg/day (8 times the MRHD on a mg/m² basis) or greater. This effect is thought to be due to the prolactin-lowering effect of ropinirole. In humans, chorionic gonadotropin, not prolactin, is essential for implantation. In rat studies using low doses (5 mg/kg) during the prolactin-dependent phase of early pregnancy (gestation days 0 to 8), ropinirole did not affect female fertility at dosages up to 100 mg/kg/day (40 times the MRHD on a mg/m² basis). No effect on male fertility was observed in rats at dosages up to 125 mg/kg/day (50 times the MRHD on a mg/m² basis).

Pregnancy

Pregnancy Category C. In animal reproduction studies, ropinirole has been shown to have adverse effects on embryo-fetal development, including teratogenic effects. Ropinirole given to pregnant rats during organogenesis (20 mg/kg on gestation days 6 and 7 followed by 20, 60, 90, 120, or 150 mg/kg on gestation days 8 through 15) resulted in decreased fetal body weight at 60 mg/kg/day, increased fetal death at 90 mg/kg/day, and digital malformations at 150 mg/kg/day (24, 36, and 60 times the MRHD on a mg/m² basis, respectively). The combined administration of ropinirole (10 mg/kg/day, 8 times the MRHD on a mg/m² basis) and L-dopa (250 mg/kg/day) to pregnant rabbits during organogenesis produced a greater incidence and severity of fetal malformations (primarily digit defects) than were seen in the offspring of rabbits treated with L-dopa alone. No indication of an effect on development of the conceptus was observed in rabbits when a maternally toxic dose of ropinirole was administered alone (20 mg/kg/day, 16 times the MRHD on a mg/m² basis). In a perinatal-postnatal study in rats, 10 mg/kg/day (4 times the MRHD on a mg/m² basis) of ropinirole impaired growth and development of nursing offspring and altered neurological development of female offspring.

There are no adequate and well-controlled studies using REQUIP in pregnant women. REQUIP should be used during pregnancy only if the potential benefit outweighs the potential risk to the fetus.

Nursing Mothers

REQUIP inhibits prolactin secretion in humans and could potentially inhibit lactation.

Studies in rats have shown that REQUIP and/or its metabolite(s) is excreted in breast milk. It is not known whether this drug is excreted in human milk. Because many drugs are excreted in human milk and because of the potential for serious adverse reactions in nursing infants from REQUIP, a decision should be made whether to discontinue nursing or to discontinue the drug, taking into account the importance of the drug to the mother.

Pediatric Use

Safety and effectiveness in the pediatric population have not been established.

ADVERSE REACTIONS

Parkinson's Disease

During the premarketing development of REQUIP, patients received REQUIP either without L-dopa (early Parkinson's disease studies) or as concomitant therapy with L-dopa (advanced Parkinson's disease studies). Because these 2 populations may have differential risks for various adverse events, this section will, in general, present adverse event data for these 2 populations separately.

Early Parkinson's Disease (Without L-dopa): The most commonly observed adverse events (>5%) in the double-blind, placebo-controlled early Parkinson's disease trials associated with the use of REQUIP (n = 157) not seen at an equivalent frequency among the placebo-treated patients (n = 147) were, in order of decreasing incidence: nausea, dizziness, somnolence, headache, vomiting, syncope, fatigue, dyspepsia, viral infection, constipation, pain, increased sweating, asthenia, dependent/leg edema, orthostatic symptoms, abdominal pain, pharyngitis, confusion, hallucinations, urinary tract infections, and abnormal vision.

Approximately 24% of 157 patients treated with REQUIP who participated in the double-blind, placebo-controlled early Parkinson's disease (without l-dopa) trials discontinued treatment due to adverse events compared to 13% of 147 patients who received placebo. The adverse events most commonly causing discontinuation of treatment by patients treated with REQUIP were: nausea (6.4%), dizziness (3.8%), aggravated Parkinson's disease (1.3%), hallucinations (1.3%), somnolence (1.3%), vomiting (1.3%), and headache (1.3%). Of these, hallucinations appear to be dose-related. While other adverse events leading to discontinuation may be dose-related, the titration design utilized in these trials precluded an adequate assessment of the dose response. For example, in the larger of the 2 trials described in CLINICAL PHARMACOLOGY: Clinical Trials, the difference in the rate of discontinuations emerged only after 10 weeks of treatment, suggesting, although not proving, that the effect could be related to dose.

Adverse Event Incidence in Controlled Clinical Studies: Table 2 lists treatment-emergent adverse events that occurred in ≥2% of patients with early Parkinson's disease (without l-dopa) treated with REQUIP participating in the double-blind, placebo-controlled studies and were numerically more common in the group treated with REQUIP. In these studies, either REQUIP or placebo was used as early therapy (i.e., without l-dopa).

The prescriber should be aware that these figures cannot be used to predict the incidence of adverse events in the course of usual medical practice where patient characteristics and other factors differ from those that prevailed in the clinical studies. Similarly, the cited frequencies cannot be compared with figures obtained from other clinical investigations involving different treatments, uses, and investigators. However, the cited figures do provide the prescribing physician with some basis for estimating the relative contribution of drug and non-drug factors to the adverse-events incidence rate in the population studied.

Table 2. Treatment-Emergent Adverse Event[*] Incidence in Double-Blind, Placebo-Controlled Early Parkinson's Disease (Without l-dopa) Trials (Events ≥2% of Patients Treated With REQUIP and Numerically More Frequent Than the Placebo Group)

Adverse Experience	REQUIP (n = 157) (%)	Placebo (n = 147) (%)
Autonomic nervous system		
Flushing	3	1
Dry mouth	5	3
Increased sweating	6	4
Body as a whole		
Asthenia	6	1
Chest pain	4	2
Dependent edema	6	3
Leg edema	7	1
Fatigue	11	4
Malaise	3	1
Pain	8	4
Cardiovascular general		
Hypertension	5	3
Hypotension	2	0
Orthostatic symptoms	6	5
Syncope	12	1
Central/peripheral nervous system		
Dizziness	40	22
Hyperkinesia	2	1
Hypesthesia	4	2
Vertigo	2	0
Gastrointestinal system		
Abdominal pain	6	3
Anorexia	4	1
Dyspepsia	10	5
Flatulence	3	1
Nausea	60	22
Vomiting	12	7
Heart rate/rhythm		
Extrasystoles	2	1
Atrial fibrillation	2	0
Palpitation	3	2
Tachycardia	2	0
Metabolic/nutritional		
Increased alkaline phosphatase	3	1
Psychiatric		
Amnesia	3	1
Impaired concentration	2	0
Confusion	5	1
Hallucination	5	1
Somnolence	40	6
Yawning	3	0
Reproductive male		
Impotence	3	1
Resistance mechanism		
Viral infection	11	3
Respiratory system		
Bronchitis	3	1
Dyspnea	3	0
Pharyngitis	6	4
Rhinitis	4	3
Sinusitis	4	3
Urinary system		
Urinary tract infection	5	4
Vascular extracardiac		
Peripheral ischemia	3	0
Vision		
Eye abnormality	3	1
Abnormal vision	6	3
Xerophthalmia	2	0

[*]Patients may have reported multiple adverse experiences during the study or at discontinuation; thus, patients may be included in more than one category.

Other events reported by 1% or more of early Parkinson's disease (without L-dopa) patients treated with REQUIP, but that were equally or more frequent in the placebo group, were: headache, upper respiratory infection, insomnia, arthralgia, tremor, back pain, anxiety, dyskinesias, aggravated Parkinsonism, depression, falls, myalgia, leg cramps, paresthesias, nervousness, diarrhea, arthritis, hot flushes, weight loss, rash, cough, hyperglycemia, muscle spasm, arthrosis, abnormal dreams, dystonia, increased salivation, bradycardia, gout, basal cell carcinoma, gingivitis, hematuria, and rigors.

Among the treatment-emergent adverse events in patients treated with REQUIP, hallucinations appear to be dose-related.

The incidence of adverse events was not materially different between women and men.

Advanced Parkinson's Disease (With L-dopa): The most commonly observed adverse events (>5%), in the double-blind, placebo-controlled advanced Parkinson's disease (with l-dopa) trials associated with the use of REQUIP (n = 208) as an adjunct to l-dopa not seen at an equivalent frequency among the placebo-treated patients (n = 120) were, in order of decreasing incidence: dyskinesias, nausea, dizziness, aggravated Parkinsonism, somnolence, headache, insomnia, injury, hallucinations, falls, abdominal pain, upper respiratory infection, confusion, increased sweating, vomiting, viral infection, increased drug level, arthralgia, tremor, anxiety, urinary tract infection, constipation, dry mouth, pain, hypokinesia, and paresthesia.

Approximately 24% of 208 patients who received REQUIP in the double-blind, placebo-controlled advanced Parkinson's disease (with l-dopa) trials discontinued treatment due to adverse events compared to 18% of 120 patients who received placebo. The events most commonly (≥1%) causing discontinuation of treatment by patients treated with REQUIP were: dizziness (2.9%), dyskinesias (2.4%), vomiting (2.4%), confusion (2.4%), nausea (1.9%), hallucinations (1.9%), anxiety (1.9%), and increased sweating (1.4%). Of these, hallucinations and dyskinesias appear to be dose-related.

Adverse Event Incidence in Controlled Clinical Studies: Table 3 lists treatment-emergent adverse events that occurred in ≥2% of patients with advanced Parkinson's disease (with l-dopa) treated with REQUIP who participated in the double-blind, placebo-controlled studies and were numerically more common in the group treated with REQUIP. In these studies, either REQUIP or placebo was used as an adjunct to l-dopa. Adverse events were usually mild or moderate in intensity.

The prescriber should be aware that these figures cannot be used to predict the incidence of adverse events in the course of usual medical practice where patient characteristics and other factors differ from those that prevailed in the clinical studies. Similarly, the cited frequencies cannot be compared with figures obtained from other clinical investigations involving different treatments, uses, and investigators. However, the cited figures do provide the prescribing physician with some basis for estimating the relative contribution of drug and non-drug factors to the adverse events incidence rate in the population studied.

Table 3. Treatment-Emergent Adverse Event[*] Incidence in Double-Blind, Placebo-Controlled Advanced Parkinson's Disease (With L-dopa) Trials (Events ≥2% of Patients Treated With REQUIP and Numerically More Frequent Than the Placebo Group)

Adverse Experience	REQUIP (n = 208) (%)	Placebo (n = 120) (%)
Autonomic nervous system		
Dry mouth	5	1
Increased sweating	7	2
Body as a whole		
Increased drug level	7	3
Pain	5	3
Cardiovascular general		
Hypotension	2	1
Syncope	3	2
Central/peripheral nervous system		
Dizziness	26	16
Dyskinesia	34	13
Falls	10	7
Headache	17	12
Hypokinesia	5	4
Paresis	3	0
Paresthesia	5	3
Tremor	6	3
Gastrointestinal system		
Abdominal pain	9	8
Constipation	6	3
Diarrhea	5	3
Dysphagia	2	1
Flatulence	2	1
Nausea	30	18
Increased saliva	2	1
Vomiting	7	4
Metabolic/nutritional		
Weight decrease	2	1
Musculoskeletal system		
Arthralgia	7	5
Arthritis	3	1
Psychiatric		
Amnesia	5	1
Anxiety	6	3
Confusion	9	2
Abnormal dreaming	3	2
Hallucinations	10	4
Nervousness	5	3
Somnolence	20	8
Red blood cell		
Anemia	2	0
Resistance mechanism		
Upper respiratory tract infection	9	8
Respiratory system		
Dyspnea	3	2
Urinary system		
Pyuria	2	1
Urinary incontinence	2	1
Urinary tract infection	6	3
Vision		
Diplopia	2	1

[*]Patients may have reported multiple adverse experiences during the study or at discontinuation; thus, patients may be included in more than one category.

Other events reported by 1% or more of patients treated with both REQUIP and L-dopa, but equally or more frequent in the placebo/L-dopa group, were: myocardial infarction, orthostatic symptoms, virus infections, asthenia, dyspepsia, myalgia, back pain, depression, leg cramps, fatigue, rhinitis, chest pain, hematuria, vertigo, tinnitus, leg edema, hot flushes, abnormal gait, hyperkinesia, and pharyngitis.

Among the treatment-emergent adverse events in patients treated with REQUIP, hallucinations and dyskinesias appear to be dose-related.

Restless Legs Syndrome

The most commonly observed adverse events (>5%) in the 12-week double-blind, placebo-controlled trials in the treatment of Restless Legs Syndrome with REQUIP (n = 496) and at least twice the rate for placebo-treated patients (n = 500) were, in order of decreasing incidence: nausea, somnolence, vomiting, dizziness, and fatigue (see Table 4). Occurrences of nausea in clinical trials were generally mild to moderate in intensity (see also DOSAGE AND ADMINISTRATION: General Dosing Considerations).

Approximately 5% of 496 patients treated with REQUIP who participated in the double-blind, placebo-controlled trials in the treatment of RLS discontinued treatment due to adverse events compared to 4% of 500 patients who received placebo. The adverse events most commonly causing discontinuation of treatment by patients treated with REQUIP were: nausea (1.6%), dizziness (0.8%), and headache (0.8%).

Adverse Event Incidence in Controlled Clinical Studies: Table 4 lists treatment-emergent adverse events that occurred in ≥2% of patients with RLS treated with REQUIP participating in the 12-week double-blind, placebo-controlled studies and were numerically more common in the group treated with REQUIP.

The prescriber should be aware that these figures cannot be used to predict the incidence of adverse events in the course of usual medical practice where patient characteristics and other factors differ from those that prevailed in the clinical studies. Similarly, the cited frequencies cannot be compared with figures obtained from other clinical investigations involving different treatments, uses, and investigators. However, the cited figures do provide the prescribing physician with some basis for estimating the relative contribution of drug and non-drug factors to the adverse-events incidence rate in the population studied.

Table 4. Treatment-Emergent Adverse Event Incidence in Double-Blind, Placebo-Controlled RLS Trials (Events ≥2% of Patients Treated With REQUIP and Numerically More Frequent Than the Placebo Group)

Adverse Experience	REQUIP (n = 496) (%)	Placebo (n = 500) (%)
Ear and labyrinth disorders		
Vertigo	2	1
Gastrointestinal disorders		
Nausea	40	8
Vomiting	11	2
Diarrhea	5	3
Dyspepsia	4	3
Dry mouth	3	2
Abdominal pain upper	3	1
General disorders and administration site conditions		
Fatigue	8	4
Edema peripheral	2	1
Infections and infestations		
Nasopharyngitis	9	8
Influenza	3	2
Musculoskeletal and connective tissue disorders		
Arthralgia	4	3
Muscle cramps	3	2
Pain in extremity	3	2
Nervous system disorders		
Somnolence	12	6
Dizziness	11	5
Paresthesia	3	1
Respiratory, thoracic, and mediastinal disorders		
Cough	3	2
Nasal congestion	2	1
Skin and subcutaneous tissue disorders		
Hyperhidrosis	3	1

Other events reported by 2% or more of patients treated with REQUIP, but equally or more frequent in the placebo group, were headache, insomnia, restless legs syndrome, upper respiratory tract infection, back pain, and sinusitis.

Other Adverse Events Observed During All Phase 2/3 Clinical Trials for Parkinson's Disease

REQUIP has been administered to 1,599 individuals in clinical trials. During these trials, all adverse events were recorded by the clinical investigators using terminology of their own choosing. To provide a meaningful estimate of the proportion of individuals having adverse events, similar types of events were grouped into a smaller number of standardized categories using modified WHOART dictionary terminology. These categories are used in the listing below. The frequencies presented represent the proportion of the 1,599 individuals exposed to REQUIP who experienced events of the type cited on at least 1 occasion while receiving REQUIP. All reported events that occurred at least twice (or once for serious or potentially serious events), except those already listed above, trivial events, and terms too vague to be meaningful, are included without regard to determination of a causal relationship to REQUIP, except that events very unlikely to be drug-related have been deleted.

Events are further classified within body system categories and enumerated in order of decreasing frequency using the following definitions: frequent adverse events are defined as those occurring in at least 1/100 patients and infrequent adverse events are those occurring in 1/100 to 1/1,000 patients and rare events are those occurring in fewer than 1/1,000 patients.

Body as a Whole: Infrequent: Cellulitis, peripheral edema, fever, influenza-like symptoms, enlarged abdomen, precordial chest pain, and generalized edema. *Rare:* Ascites.

Cardiovascular: Infrequent: Cardiac failure, bradycardia, tachycardia, supraventricular tachycardia, angina pectoris, bundle branch block, cardiac arrest, cardiomegaly, aneurysm, mitral insufficiency. *Rare:* Ventricular tachycardia.

Central/Peripheral Nervous System: Frequent: Neuralgia. *Infrequent:* Involuntary muscle contractions, hypertonia, dysphonia, abnormal coordination, extrapyramidal disorder, migraine, choreoathetosis, coma, stupor, aphasia, convulsions, hypotonia, peripheral neuropathy, paralysis. *Rare:* Grand mal convulsions, hemiparesis, hemiplegia.

Endocrine: Infrequent: Hypothyroidism, gynecomastia, hyperthyroidism. *Rare:* Goiter, SIADH.

Gastrointestinal: Infrequent: Increased hepatic enzymes, bilirubinemia, cholecystitis, cholelithiasis colitis, dysphagia, periodontitis, fecal incontinence, gastroesophageal reflux, hemorrhoids, toothache, eructation, gastritis, esophagitis, hiccups, diverticulitis, duodenal ulcer, gastric ulcer, melena, duodenitis, gastrointestinal hemorrhage, glossitis, rectal hemorrhage, pancreatitis, stomatitis and ulcerative stomatitis, tongue edema. *Rare:* Biliary pain, hemorrhagic gastritis, hematemesis, salivary duct obstruction.

Hematologic: Infrequent: Purpura, thrombocytopenia, hematoma, Vitamin B12 deficiency, hypochromic anemia, eosinophilia, leukocytosis, leukopenia, lymphocytosis, lymphopenia, lymphedema.

Metabolic/Nutritional: Frequent: Increased BUN. *Infrequent:* Hypoglycemia, increased alkaline phosphatase, increased LDH, weight increase, hyperphosphatemia, hyperuricemia, diabetes mellitus, glycosuria, hypokalemia, hypercholesterolemia, hyperkalemia, acidosis, hyponatremia, thirst, increased CPK, dehydration. *Rare:* Hypochloremia.

Musculoskeletal: Infrequent: Aggravated arthritis, tendonitis, osteoporosis, bursitis, polymyalgia rheumatica, muscle weakness, skeletal pain, torticollis. *Rare:* Dupuytren's contracture requiring surgery.

Neoplasm: Infrequent: Malignant breast neoplasm. *Rare:* Bladder carcinoma, benign brain neoplasm, esophageal carcinoma, malignant laryngeal neoplasm, lipoma, rectal carcinoma, uterine neoplasm.

Psychiatric: Infrequent: Increased libido, agitation, apathy, impaired concentration, depersonalization, paranoid reaction, personality disorder, euphoria, delirium, dementia, delusion, emotional lability, decreased libido, manic reaction, somnambulism, aggressive reaction, neurosis. *Rare:* Suicide attempt.

Genitourinary: Infrequent: Amenorrhea, vaginal hemorrhage, penile disorder, prostatic disorder, balanoposthitis, epididymitis, perineal pain, dysuria, micturition frequency, albuminuria, nocturia, polyuria, renal calculus. *Rare:* Breast enlargement, mastitis, uterine hemorrhage, ejaculation disorder, Peyronie's disease, pyelonephritis, acute renal failure, uremia.

Resistance Mechanism: Infrequent: Herpes zoster, otitis media, sepsis, abscess, herpes simplex, fungal infection, genital moniliasis.

Respiratory: Infrequent: Asthma, epistaxis, laryngitis, pleurisy, pulmonary edema.

Skin/Appendage: Infrequent: Pruritus, dermatitis, eczema, skin ulceration, alopecia, skin hypertrophy, skin discoloration, urticaria, fungal dermatitis, furunculosis, hyperkeratosis, photosensitivity reaction, psoriasis, maculopapular rash, psoriaform rash, seborrhea.

Special Senses: Infrequent: Tinnitus, earache, decreased hearing, abnormal lacrimation, conjunctivitis, blepharitis, glaucoma, abnormal accommodation, blepharospasm, eye pain, photophobia. *Rare:* Scotoma.

Vascular Extracardiac: Infrequent: Varicose veins, phlebitis, peripheral gangrene. *Rare:* Limb embolism, pulmonary embolism, gangrene, subarachnoid hemorrhage, deep thrombophlebitis, leg thrombophlebitis, thrombosis.

Falling Asleep During Activities of Daily Living:

Patients treated with REQUIP have reported falling asleep while engaged in activities of daily living, including operation of a motor vehicle which sometimes resulted in accidents (see bolded WARNING).

Other Adverse Events Observed During Phase 2/3 Clinical Trials for RLS

REQUIP has been administered to 911 individuals in clinical trials. During these trials, all adverse events were recorded by the clinical investigators using terminology of their own choosing. To provide a meaningful estimate of the proportion of individuals having adverse events, similar types of events were grouped into a smaller number of standardized categories using MedDRA dictionary terminology. These categories are used in the listing below. The frequencies presented represent the proportion of the 911 individuals exposed to REQUIP who experienced events of the type cited on at least one occasion while receiving REQUIP. All reported events that occurred at least twice (or once for serious or potentially serious events), except those already listed, trivial events, and terms too vague to be meaningful, are included without regard to determination of a causal relationship to REQUIP, except that events very unlikely to be drug-related have been deleted.

Events are further classified within body system categories and enumerated in order of decreasing frequency using the following definitions: frequent adverse events are defined as those occurring in at least 1/100 patients and infrequent adverse events are those occurring in 1/100 to 1/1,000 patients.

Blood and Lymphatic System Disorders: Infrequent: Anemia, lymphadenopathy.

Cardiac Disorders: Frequent: Palpitations. *Infrequent:* Acute coronary syndrome, angina pectoris, angina unstable, bradycardia, cardiac failure, cardiovascular disorder, coronary artery disease, myocardial infarction, sick sinus syndrome, tachycardia.

Congenital, Familial, and Genetic Disorders: Infrequent: Pigmented nevus.

Ear and Labyrinth Disorders: Infrequent: Ear pain, middle ear effusion, tinnitus.

Endocrine Disorders: Infrequent: Goiter, hypothyroidism.

Eye Disorders: Infrequent: Blepharitis, conjunctival hemorrhage, conjunctivitis, eye irritation, eye pain, keratoconjunctivitis sicca, vision blurred, visual acuity reduced, visual disturbance.

Gastrointestinal Disorders: Frequent: Abdominal pain, constipation, gastroesophageal reflux disease, stomach discomfort, toothache. *Infrequent:* Abdominal adhesions, abdominal discomfort, abdominal distension, abdominal pain lower, duodenal ulcer, dysphagia, eructation, flatulence, gastric disorder, gastric hemorrhage, gastric polyps, gastric ulcer, gastritis, gastrointestinal pain, hematemesis, hemorrhoids, hiatus hernia, intestinal obstruction, irritable bowel syndrome, loose stools, mouth ulceration, pancreatitis acute, peptic ulcer, rectal hemorrhage, reflux esophagitis.

General Disorders and Administration Site Conditions: Frequent: Asthenia, chest pain, influenza-like illness, rigors. *Infrequent:* Chest discomfort, feeling cold, feeling hot, hunger, lethargy, malaise, edema, pain, pyrexia.

Hepatobiliary Disorders: Infrequent: Cholecystitis, cholelithiasis, ischemic hepatitis.

Immune System Disorders: Infrequent: Hypersensitivity.

Infections and Infestations: Frequent: Bronchitis, gastroenteritis, gastroenteritis viral, lower respiratory tract infection, rhinitis, tooth abscess, urinary tract infection. *Infrequent:* Appendicitis, bacterial infection, bladder infection, bronchitis acute, candidiasis, cellulitis, cystitis, diarrhea infectious, diverticulitis, ear infection, folliculitis, fungal infection, gastrointestinal infection, herpes simplex, infected cyst, laryngitis, localized infection, mastitis, otitis externa, otitis media, pharyngitis, pneumonia, postoperative infection, respiratory tract infection, tonsillitis, tooth infection, vaginal candidiasis, vaginal infection, vaginal mycosis, viral infection, viral upper respiratory tract infection, wound infection.

Injury, Poisoning, and Procedural Complications: Infrequent: Concussion, lower limb fracture, post procedural hemorrhage, road traffic accident.

Investigations: Infrequent: Blood cholesterol increased, blood iron decreased, blood pressure increased, blood urine present, hemoglobin decreased, heart rate increased, protein urine present, weight decreased, weight increased.

Metabolism and Nutrition Disorders: Infrequent: Anorexia, decreased appetite, diabetes mellitus non-insulin-dependent, fluid retention, gout, hypercholesterolemia.

Musculoskeletal and Connective Tissue Disorders: Frequent: Muscle spasms, musculoskeletal stiffness, myalgia, neck pain, osteoarthritis, tendonitis. *Infrequent:* Arthritis, aseptic necrosis bone, bone pain, bone spur, bursitis, groin pain, intervertebral disc degeneration, intervertebral disc protrusion, joint stiffness, joint swelling, localized osteoarthritis, monoarthritis, muscle contracture, muscle tightness, muscle twitching, osteoporosis, rotator cuff syndrome, sacroiliitis, synovitis.

Neoplasms Benign, Malignant, and Unspecified: Infrequent: Anaplastic thyroid cancer, angiomyolipoma, basal cell carcinoma, breast cancer, gastric cancer, gastrointestinal stromal tumor, malignant melanoma, prostate cancer, skin papilloma, squamous cell carcinoma, uterine leiomyoma.

Nervous System Disorders: Frequent: Hypoesthesia, migraine. **Infrequent:** Amnesia, aphasia, ataxia, balance disorder, benign intracranial hypertension, burning sensation, carpal tunnel syndrome, disturbance in attention, dizziness postural, dysgeusia, dyskinesia, head discomfort, hyperesthesia, hypersomnia, lethargy, loss of consciousness, memory impairment, migraine with aura, migraine without aura, neuralgia, sciatica, sedation, sinus headache, sleep apnea syndrome, syncope vasovagal, tension headache, transient ischemic attack, tremor.

Psychiatric Disorders: Frequent: Anxiety, depression, irritability, sleep disorder. **Infrequent:** Abnormal dreams, agitation, bruxism, confusional state, depressed mood, disorientation, early morning awakening, libido decreased, loss of libido, mood swings, nervousness, nightmare, panic attack, stress symptoms, tension.

Renal and Urinary Disorders: Infrequent: Dysuria, hematuria, hypertonic bladder, micturition disorder, nephrolithiasis, nocturia, pollakiuria, proteinuria, urinary retention.

Reproductive System and Breast Disorders: Frequent: Erectile dysfunction. **Infrequent:** Breast cyst, dysmenorrhea, menorrhagia, pelvic peritoneal adhesions, postmenopausal hemorrhage, premenstrual syndrome, prostatitis.

Respiratory, Thoracic and Mediastinal Disorders: Frequent: Asthma, pharyngolaryngeal pain. **Infrequent:** Dry throat, dyspnea, epistaxis, hemoptysis, hoarseness, interstitial lung disease, nasal mucosal disorder, nasal polyps, respiratory tract congestion, rhinorrhea, sinus congestion, sneezing, wheezing, yawning.

Skin and Subcutaneous Tissue Disorders: Frequent: Night sweats, rash. **Infrequent:** Acne, actinic keratosis, alopecia, cold sweat, dermatitis, dermatitis allergic, dermatitis contact, eczema, exanthem, face edema, photosensitivity reaction, pruritus, psoriasis, rash pruritic, skin lesion, urticaria.

Vascular Disorders: Frequent: Hot flush, hypertension, hypotension. **Infrequent:** Atherosclerosis, circulatory collapse, flushing, hematoma, thrombosis, varicose vein.

Postmarketing Reports

The following adverse events (not listed above in clinical trials or other sections of the prescribing information) have been identified during postapproval use of ropinirole. Because these events are reported voluntarily from a population of uncertain size, it is not always possible to reliably estimate their frequency or establish a causal relationship to drug exposure.

Immune Systems Disorders: Hypersensitivity reactions (including urticaria, angioedema, rash, and pruritus).

Psychiatric Disorders: Impulse control symptoms, pathological gambling, increased libido including hypersexuality.

DRUG ABUSE AND DEPENDENCE
Controlled Substance Class
REQUIP is not a controlled substance.
Physical and Psychological Dependence
Animal studies and human clinical trials with REQUIP did not reveal any potential for drug-seeking behavior or physical dependence.

OVERDOSAGE
In the Parkinson's disease program, there have been patients who accidentally or intentionally took more than their prescribed dose of ropinirole. The largest overdose reported in the Parkinson's disease clinical trials was 435 mg taken over a 7-day period (62.1 mg/day). Of patients who received a dose greater than 24 mg/day, reported symptoms included adverse events commonly reported during dopaminergic therapy (nausea, dizziness), as well as visual hallucinations, hyperhidrosis, claustrophobia, chorea, palpitations, asthenia, and nightmares. Additional symptoms reported for doses of 24 mg or less or for overdoses of unknown amount included vomiting, increased coughing, fatigue, syncope, vasovagal syncope, dyskinesia, agitation, chest pain, orthostatic hypotension, somnolence, and confusional state.

Overdose Management
It is anticipated that the symptoms of overdose with REQUIP will be related to its dopaminergic activity. General supportive measures are recommended. Vital signs should be maintained, if necessary. Removal of any unabsorbed material (e.g., by gastric lavage) should be considered.

DOSAGE AND ADMINISTRATION
General Dosing Considerations for Parkinson's Disease and RLS
REQUIP can be taken with or without food. Patients may be advised that taking REQUIP with food may reduce the occurrence of nausea. However, this has not been established in controlled clinical trials.

If a significant interruption in therapy with REQUIP has occurred, retitration of therapy may be warranted.

Geriatric Use: Pharmacokinetic studies demonstrated a reduced clearance of ropinirole in the elderly (see CLINICAL PHARMACOLOGY). Dose adjustment is not necessary since the dose is individually titrated to clinical response.

Renal Impairment: The pharmacokinetics of ropinirole were not altered in patients with moderate renal impairment (see CLINICAL PHARMACOLOGY). Therefore, no dosage adjustment is necessary in patients with moderate renal impairment. The use of REQUIP in patients with severe renal impairment has not been studied.

Hepatic Impairment: The pharmacokinetics of ropinirole have not been studied in patients with hepatic impairment. Since patients with hepatic impairment may have higher plasma levels and lower clearance, REQUIP should be titrated with caution in these patients.

Dosing for Parkinson's Disease
In all clinical studies, dosage was initiated at a subtherapeutic level and gradually titrated to therapeutic response. The dosage should be increased to achieve a maximum therapeutic effect, balanced against the principal side effects of nausea, dizziness, somnolence, and dyskinesia.

The recommended starting dose for Parkinson's disease is 0.25 mg 3 times daily. Based on individual patient response, dosage should then be titrated with weekly increments as described in Table 5. After week 4, if necessary, daily dosage may be increased by 1.5 mg/day on a weekly basis up to a dose of 9 mg/day, and then by up to 3 mg/day weekly to a total dose of 24 mg/day. Doses greater than 24 mg/day have not been tested in clinical trials.

Table 5. Ascending-Dose Schedule of REQUIP for Parkinson's Disease

Week	Dosage	Total Daily Dose
1	0.25 mg 3 times daily	0.75 mg
2	0.5 mg 3 times daily	1.5 mg
3	0.75 mg 3 times daily	2.25 mg
4	1 mg 3 times daily	3 mg

When REQUIP is administered as adjunct therapy to L-dopa, the concurrent dose of L-dopa may be decreased gradually as tolerated. L-dopa dosage reduction was allowed during the advanced Parkinson's disease (with L-dopa) study if dyskinesias or other dopaminergic effects occurred. Overall, reduction of L-dopa dose was sustained in 87% of patients treated with REQUIP and in 57% of patients on placebo. On average the L-dopa dose was reduced by 31% in patients treated with REQUIP.

REQUIP for Parkinson's disease patients should be discontinued gradually over a 7-day period. The frequency of administration should be reduced from 3 times daily to twice daily for 4 days. For the remaining 3 days, the frequency should be reduced to once daily prior to complete withdrawal of REQUIP.

Dosing for Restless Legs Syndrome
In all clinical trials, the dose for REQUIP was initiated at 0.25 mg once daily, 1 to 3 hours before bedtime. Patients were titrated based on clinical response and tolerability.

The recommended adult starting dosage for RLS is 0.25 mg once daily, 1 to 3 hours before bedtime. After 2 days, the dosage can be increased to 0.5 mg once daily and to 1 mg once daily at the end of the first week of dosing, then as shown in Table 6 as needed to achieve efficacy. For RLS, the safety and effectiveness of doses greater than 4 mg once daily have not been established.

Table 6. Dose Titration Schedule for RLS

Day/Week	Dosage to be taken once daily, 1 to 3 hours before bedtime
Days 1 and 2	0.25 mg
Days 3-7	0.5 mg
Week 2	1 mg
Week 3	1.5 mg
Week 4	2 mg
Week 5	2.5 mg
Week 6	3 mg
Week 7	4 mg

In clinical trials of patients being treated for RLS with doses up to 4 mg once daily, REQUIP was discontinued without a taper.

HOW SUPPLIED
Tablets
Each pentagonal film-coated TILTAB® tablet with beveled edges contains ropinirole hydrochloride equivalent to the labeled amount of ropinirole as follows:
0.25 mg: white tablets imprinted with "SB" and "4890" in bottles of 100 (NDC 0007-4890-20).
0.5 mg: yellow tablets imprinted with "SB" and "4891" in bottles of 100 (NDC 0007-4891-20).
1 mg: green tablets imprinted with "SB" and "4892" in bottles of 100 (NDC 0007-4892-20).
2 mg: pale yellowish-pink tablets imprinted with "SB" and "4893" in bottles of 100 (NDC 0007-4893-20).
3 mg: pale to moderate reddish-purple tablets, imprinted with "SB" and"4895" in bottles of 100 (NDC 0007-4895-20).
4 mg: pale brown tablets imprinted with "SB" and "4896" in bottles of 100 (NDC 0007-4896-20).
5 mg: blue tablets imprinted with "SB" and "4894" in bottles of 100 (NDC 0007-4894-20).
STORAGE: Protect from light and moisture. Close container tightly after each use.
Store at controlled room temperature 20°-25°C (68°-77°F) [see USP].
GlaxoSmithKline
Research Triangle Park, NC 27709
REQUIP and TILTAB are registered trademarks of GlaxoSmithKline.
SINEMET is a registered trademark of Merck & Co., Inc.
©2009, GlaxoSmithKline. All rights reserved.
May 2009
REP:3PI
PHARMACIST DETACH HERE AND GIVE INSTRUCTIONS TO PATIENT
PATIENT INFORMATION
REQUIP® (ropinirole tablets)
If you have Restless Legs Syndrome (RLS, also known as Ekbom Syndrome), read this side
Read this information completely before you start taking REQUIP. Read the information each time you get more medicine. There may be new information. This leaflet provides a summary about REQUIP. It does not include everything there is to know about your medicine. This information should not take the place of discussions with your doctor about your medical condition or REQUIP.
What is REQUIP?
REQUIP is a prescription medicine to treat moderate-to-severe primary Restless Legs Syndrome. It is sometimes used to treat Parkinson's disease. Having one of these conditions does not mean you have or will develop the other.
What is the most important information I should know about REQUIP?
• Patients with RLS should take REQUIP differently than patients with Parkinson's disease (see **How should I take REQUIP for RLS?** for the recommended dosing for RLS). A lower dose of REQUIP is generally needed for patients with RLS, and is taken once daily before bedtime.
• There are known side effects of REQUIP. If you fall asleep or feel very sleepy while doing normal activities such as driving, faint, feel dizzy, nauseated, or sweaty when you stand up from sitting or lying down, you should talk with your doctor (see **What are the possible side effects of REQUIP?**).
• Before starting REQUIP, be sure to tell your doctor if you are taking any medicines that make you drowsy.
Unusual urges: Some patients taking REQUIP or REQUIP XL get urges to behave in a way unusual for them. Examples of this are an unusual urge to gamble or increased sexual urges and behaviors. If you notice or your family notices that you are developing any unusual behaviors, talk to your healthcare provider.
Who should not take REQUIP?
You should not take REQUIP if you are allergic to the active ingredient ropinirole or to any of the inactive ingredients. Your doctor and pharmacist have a list of the inactive ingredients.
What should I tell my doctor?
Be sure to tell your doctor if:
• you are pregnant or plan to become pregnant.
• you are breastfeeding.
• you have daytime sleepiness from a sleep disorder other than RLS or have unexpected sleepiness or periods of sleep while taking REQUIP.
• you are taking any other prescription or over-the-counter medicines. Some of these medicines may increase your chances of getting side effects while taking REQUIP.
• you start or stop taking other medicines while you are taking REQUIP. This may increase your chances of getting side effects.
• you start or stop smoking while you are taking REQUIP. Smoking may decrease the treatment effect of REQUIP.
• you feel dizzy, nauseated, sweaty, or faint when you stand up from sitting or lying down.

- you drink alcoholic beverages. This may increase your chances of becoming drowsy or sleepy while taking REQUIP.

How should I take REQUIP for RLS?

- Be sure to take REQUIP exactly as directed by your doctor or healthcare provider.
- The usual way to take REQUIP is once in the evening, 1 to 3 hours before bedtime.
- Your doctor will start you on a low dose of REQUIP. Your doctor may change the dose until you are taking the amount of medicine that is right for you to control your symptoms.
- **If you miss your dose, do not double your next dose.** Take only your usual dose 1 to 3 hours before your next bedtime.
- Contact your doctor, if you stop taking REQUIP for any reason. Do not restart without consulting your doctor.
- You can take REQUIP with or without food. Taking REQUIP with food may decrease the chances of feeling nauseated.

What are the possible side effects of REQUIP?

- Most people who take REQUIP tolerate it well. The most commonly reported side effects in people taking REQUIP for RLS are nausea, vomiting, dizziness, and drowsiness or sleepiness. You should be careful until you know if REQUIP affects your ability to remain alert while doing normal daily activities, and you should watch for the development of significant daytime sleepiness or episodes of falling asleep. It is possible that you could fall asleep while doing normal activities such as driving a car, doing physical tasks, or using hazardous machinery while taking REQUIP. Your chances of falling asleep while doing normal activities while taking REQUIP are greater if you are taking other medicines that cause drowsiness.
- When you start taking REQUIP or when you increase your dose, you may feel dizzy, nauseated, sweaty or faint, when first standing up from sitting or lying down. Therefore, do not stand up quickly after sitting or lying down, particularly if you have been sitting or lying down for a long period of time. Take a minute sitting on the edge of the bed or chair before you get up.
- Hallucinations (unreal sounds, visions, or sensations) have been reported in patients taking REQUIP. These were uncommon in patients taking REQUIP for RLS. The risk is greater in patients with Parkinson's disease who are elderly, taking REQUIP with L-dopa, or taking higher doses of REQUIP than recommended for RLS.

Some patients taking REQUIP get urges to behave in a way unusual for them. Examples of this are an unusual urge to gamble or increased sexual urges and behaviors. If you notice or your family notices that you are developing any unusual behaviors, talk to your healthcare provider.

This is not a complete list of side effects and should not take the place of discussions with your healthcare providers. Your doctor or pharmacist can give you a more complete list of possible side effects.

Call your healthcare provider for medical advice about side effects. You may report side effects to FDA at 1-800-FDA-1088.

Other Information about REQUIP

- Studies of people with Parkinson's disease show that they may be at an increased risk of developing melanoma, a form of skin cancer, when compared to people without Parkinson's disease. It is not known if this problem is associated with Parkinson's disease or the medicines used to treat Parkinson's disease. REQUIP is one of the medicines used to treat Parkinson's disease, therefore, patients being treated with REQUIP should have periodic skin examinations.
- Take REQUIP exactly as your doctor prescribes it.
- Do not share REQUIP with other people, even if they have the same symptoms you have.
- Keep REQUIP out of the reach of children.
- Store REQUIP at room temperature out of direct sunlight.
- Keep REQUIP in a tightly closed container.

This leaflet summarizes important information about REQUIP. Medicines are sometimes prescribed for purposes other than those listed in this leaflet. Do not take REQUIP for a condition for which it was not prescribed. For more information, talk with your doctor or pharmacist. They can give you information about REQUIP that is written for healthcare professionals.

PATIENT INFORMATION
REQUIP® (ropinirole tablets)
If you have Parkinson's disease, read this side
Read this information completely before you start taking REQUIP. Read the information each time you get more medicine. There may be new information. This leaflet provides a summary about REQUIP. It does not include everything there is to know about your medicine. This information should not take the place of discussions with your doctor about your medical condition or REQUIP.

What is REQUIP?
REQUIP is a prescription medicine used to treat Parkinson's disease. It is also used to treat moderate-to-severe primary Restless Legs Syndrome. Having one of these conditions does not mean you have or will develop the other.

What is the most important information I should know about REQUIP?

- Patients with Parkinson's disease should take REQUIP differently than patients with Restless Legs Syndrome (see **How should I take REQUIP for Parkinson's disease?**). For Parkinson's disease, a higher dose of REQUIP is generally needed, and is taken more frequently throughout the day.
- There are known side effects of REQUIP (see **What are the possible side effects of REQUIP?**).
- If you fall asleep or feel very sleepy while doing normal activities such as driving, faint, feel dizzy, nauseated, or sweaty when you stand up from sitting or lying down, you should talk with your doctor.
- Hallucinations (unreal visions, sounds, or sensations) have been reported in patients taking REQUIP. The risk is greater in patients with Parkinson's disease who are elderly, taking REQUIP with L-dopa or taking higher doses of REQUIP. If these occur, you should discuss them with your doctor.
- REQUIP may make some of the side effects of L-dopa worse. REQUIP may cause uncontrolled sudden movements or make such movements you already have worse or more frequent. You should notify your doctor in such a case as dosage adjustments to your anti-Parkinson's medications may be necessary.
- Before starting REQUIP, be sure to tell your doctor if you are taking any medicines that make you drowsy.

Unusual urges: Some patients taking REQUIP or REQUIP XL get urges to behave in a way unusual for them. Examples of this are an unusual urge to gamble or increased sexual urges and behaviors. If you notice or your family notices that you are developing any unusual behaviors, talk to your healthcare provider.

Who should not take REQUIP?
You should not take REQUIP if you are allergic to the active ingredient ropinirole or to any of the inactive ingredients. Your doctor and pharmacist have a list of the inactive ingredients.

What should I tell my doctor?
Be sure to tell your doctor if:

- you are pregnant or plan to become pregnant.
- you are breastfeeding.
- you have daytime sleepiness from a sleep disorder or have unexpected sleepiness or periods of sleep while taking REQUIP.
- you are taking any other prescription or over-the-counter medicines. Some of these medicines may increase your chances of getting side effects while taking REQUIP.
- you start or stop taking other medicines while you are taking REQUIP. This may increase your chances of getting side effects.
- you start or stop smoking while you are taking REQUIP. Smoking may decrease the treatment effect of REQUIP.
- you feel dizzy, nauseated, sweaty, or faint when you first stand up from sitting or lying down.
- you drink alcoholic beverages. This may increase your chances of becoming drowsy or sleepy while taking REQUIP.

How should I take REQUIP for Parkinson's disease?

- Be sure to take your REQUIP exactly as directed by your doctor or healthcare provider.
- Three times a day is the usual way to take REQUIP for Parkinson's disease.
- Your doctor will start you on a low dose of REQUIP. Your doctor will change the dose until you are taking the right amount of medicine to control your symptoms. It may take several weeks before you reach a dose that controls your symptoms.
- **If you miss a dose, do not double your next dose.**
- Contact your doctor, if you stop taking REQUIP for any reason. Do not restart without consulting your doctor.
- Your doctor may prescribe REQUIP alone or add REQUIP to medicine that you are already taking for Parkinson's disease.
- You can take REQUIP with or without food. Taking REQUIP with food may decrease the chances of feeling nauseated.

What are the possible side effects of REQUIP?

- Most people who take REQUIP tolerate it well. The most commonly reported side effects in people taking REQUIP are nausea, headache, dizziness, drowsiness or sleepiness.
- You should be careful until you know if REQUIP affects your ability to remain alert while doing normal daily activities, and you should watch for the development of significant daytime sleepiness or episodes of falling asleep. It is possible that you could fall asleep while doing normal activities such as driving a car, doing physical tasks, or using hazardous machinery while taking REQUIP. Your chances of falling asleep while doing normal activities while taking REQUIP are greater if you are taking other medicines that cause drowsiness.

- When you start taking REQUIP or when you increase your dose, you may feel dizzy, nauseated, sweaty or faint, when first standing up from sitting or lying down. Therefore, do not stand up quickly after sitting or lying down, particularly if you have been sitting or lying down for a long period of time. Take a minute sitting on the edge of the bed or chair before you get up.
- Hallucinations (unreal visions, sounds, or sensations) have been reported in patients taking REQUIP. The risk is greater in patients with Parkinson's disease who are elderly, taking REQUIP with L-dopa, or taking higher amounts of REQUIP.
- If you are taking L-dopa for Parkinson's disease, REQUIP may make some of the side effects of L-dopa worse. REQUIP may cause uncontrolled sudden movements or make such movements you already have worse or more frequent.

Some patients taking REQUIP get urges to behave in a way unusual for them. Examples of this are an unusual urge to gamble or increased sexual urges and behaviors. If you notice or your family notices that you are developing any unusual behaviors, talk to your healthcare provider.

This is not a complete list of side effects and should not take the place of discussions with your healthcare providers. Your doctor or pharmacist can give you a more complete list of possible side effects.

Call your healthcare provider for medical advice about side effects. You may report side effects to FDA at 1-800-FDA-1088.

Other Information about REQUIP

- Studies of people with Parkinson's disease show that they may be at an increased risk of developing melanoma, a form of skin cancer, when compared to people without Parkinson's disease. It is not known if this problem is associated with Parkinson's disease or the medicines used to treat Parkinson's disease, therefore, patients being treated with REQUIP should have periodic skin examinations.
- Take REQUIP exactly as your doctor prescribes it.
- Do not share REQUIP with other people, even if they have the same symptoms you have.
- Keep REQUIP out of the reach of children.
- Store REQUIP at room temperature out of direct sunlight.
- Keep REQUIP in a tightly closed container.

This leaflet summarizes important information about REQUIP. Medicines are sometimes prescribed for purposes other than those listed in this leaflet. Do not take REQUIP for a condition for which it was not prescribed. For more information, talk with your doctor or pharmacist. They can give you information about REQUIP that is written for healthcare professionals.

GlaxoSmithKline
Research Triangle Park, NC 27709
©2009, GlaxoSmithKline. All rights reserved.
April 2009
REP:2PIL

REQUIP XL   ℞
[rē' kwip]
(ropinirole extended-release tablets)

HIGHLIGHTS OF PRESCRIBING INFORMATION
These highlights do not include all the information needed to use REQUIP XL safely and effectively. See full prescribing information for REQUIP XL.
REQUIP XL (ropinirole extended-release tablets)
Initial U.S. Approval: 1997

————————INDICATIONS AND USAGE————————

REQUIP XL is an orally administered, non-ergoline dopamine agonist indicated for the treatment of signs and symptoms of idiopathic Parkinson's disease. (1.1)

————————DOSAGE AND ADMINISTRATION————————

- REQUIP XL tablets are taken once daily, with or without food. Tablets must be swallowed whole and must not be chewed, crushed, or divided. (2.1)
- The starting dose is 2 mg taken once daily for 1 to 2 weeks, followed by increases of 2 mg/day at 1 week or longer intervals as appropriate, depending on therapeutic response and tolerability, up to a maximally recommended dose of 24 mg/day. Patients should be assessed for therapeutic response and tolerability at a minimal interval of 1 week or longer after each dose increment. Caution should be exercised during dose titration because too rapid a rate of ti-

tration can lead to dose selection that does not provide additional benefit, but that increases the risk of adverse reactions. (2.2, 14.2)

• Patients may be switched directly from immediate-release ropinirole to REQUIP XL. The initial switching dose of REQUIP XL should most closely match the total daily dose of immediate-release ropinirole, see Table 1. (2.3)

• If REQUIP XL must be discontinued, it should be tapered gradually over a 7-day period. (2.2)

-----DOSAGE FORMS AND STRENGTHS-----

Tablets: 2 mg, 4 mg, 6 mg, 8 mg, and 12 mg (3)

-----CONTRAINDICATIONS-----

None (4)

-----WARNINGS AND PRECAUTIONS-----

• Falling asleep during activities of daily living may occur, including the operation of motor vehicles, which sometimes resulted in accidents. Sudden onset of sleep may occur without apparent warning or daytime drowsiness. Sedating medications (such as alcohol or CNS depressants), the presence of sleeping disorders, or other medications that increase plasma levels of ropinirole, may increase the risk of somnolence or falling asleep while engaged in activities of daily living. Before initiating treatment, patients should be advised of the potential of sudden onset of sleep or to develop drowsiness and asked about risk factors they may have. If a patient develops sudden onset of sleep during activities that require active participation (e.g., conversations, eating, etc.) and/or cannot avoid high-risk activities in the future, REQUIP XL should ordinarily be discontinued. (5.1)

• Syncope, sometimes associated with bradycardia, may occur. (5.2)

• Symptomatic hypotension (including postural/orthostatic hypotension) may occur, especially during dose escalation. (5.3)

• Elevation of blood pressure and changes in heart rate may occur. (5.4)

• Hallucination may occur. (5.5)

• Dyskinesia may be caused or exacerbated. Decreasing the L-dopa dose may lessen or eliminate this side effect. (5.6)

-----ADVERSE REACTIONS-----

• **Most common adverse reactions (incidence ≥5% and greater than placebo) in advanced Parkinson's disease with concomitant L-dopa were dyskinesia, nausea, dizziness, hallucination, somnolence, abdominal pain/discomfort, and orthostatic hypotension. (6.1)**

• **Most common adverse reactions (incidence ≥5%) in early Parkinson's disease without L-dopa were nausea, somnolence, abdominal pain/discomfort, dizziness, headache, and constipation. (6.1)**

To report SUSPECTED ADVERSE REACTIONS, contact GlaxoSmithKline at 1-888-825-5249 or FDA at 1-800-FDA-1088 or www.fda.gov/medwatch.

-----DRUG INTERACTIONS-----

• CYP1A2 is the major enzyme responsible for the metabolism of ropinirole. Thus inhibitors (e.g., ciprofloxacin, fluvoxamine) or inducers (e.g., omeprazole or smoking) of CYP1A2 may alter the clearance of ropinirole. Adjustment of dosage of REQUIP XL may be required. (7.1)

• Higher doses of estrogens, usually associated with hormone replacement therapy (HRT), reduced oral clearance of ropinirole. Starting or stopping HRT treatment may require adjustment of dosage of REQUIP XL. (7.3)

• Dopamine antagonists, such as neuroleptics (e.g., phenothiazines, butyrophenones, thioxanthenes) or metoclopramide, may diminish effectiveness of ropinirole. (7.4)

-----USE IN SPECIFIC POPULATIONS-----

Pregnancy: REQUIP XL should be used during pregnancy only if the potential benefit outweighs the potential risk to the fetus. (8.1)

See 17 for PATIENT COUNSELING INFORMATION and FDA-approved patient labeling

Revised: 12/2012

FULL PRESCRIBING INFORMATION: CONTENTS*

FULL PRESCRIBING INFORMATION

1   INDICATIONS AND USAGE
1.1   Parkinson's Disease
REQUIP XL® (ropinirole extended-release tablets) is indicated for the treatment of the signs and symptoms of idiopathic Parkinson's disease.

2   DOSAGE AND ADMINISTRATION
2.1   General Dosing Considerations
• REQUIP XL extended-release tablets are taken once daily, with or without food. Taking REQUIP XL with food may reduce the occurrence of nausea; this has not been established in controlled clinical trials [see Clinical Pharmacology (12.3)].
• Tablets must be swallowed whole and must not be chewed, crushed, or divided.
• If a significant interruption in therapy with REQUIP XL has occurred, retitration of therapy may be warranted.

2.2   Dosing for Parkinson's Disease
The starting dose is 2 mg taken once daily for 1 to 2 weeks, followed by increases of 2 mg/day at 1-week or longer intervals as appropriate, depending on therapeutic response and tolerability, up to a maximally recommended dose of 24 mg/day.
In clinical trials, dosage was initiated at 2 mg/day and gradually titrated based on individual therapeutic response and tolerability. Doses greater than 24 mg/day have not been studied in clinical trials. Patients should be assessed for therapeutic response and tolerability at a minimal interval of 1 week or longer after each dose increment. Caution should be exercised during dose titration because too rapid

a rate of titration may lead to dose selection that may not provide additional benefit, but that may increase the risk of adverse reactions [see Clinical Studies (14.2)]. Due to the flexible dosing design used in clinical studies, specific dose response information could not be determined.
When REQUIP XL is administered as adjunct therapy to L-dopa, the concurrent dose of L-dopa may be decreased gradually as tolerated. In the placebo-controlled advanced Parkinson's disease study, the L-dopa dose was reduced once patients reached a dose of REQUIP XL of 8 mg/day. Overall, L-dopa dose reduction was sustained in 93% of patients treated with REQUIP XL and in 72% of patients on placebo. On average the L-dopa dose was reduced by 34% in patients treated with REQUIP XL [see Clinical Studies (14)].
REQUIP XL should be discontinued gradually over a 7-day period.

2.3   Switching From Immediate-Release Ropinirole Tablets to REQUIP XL
Patients may be switched directly from immediate-release ropinirole to REQUIP XL tablets. The initial dose of REQUIP XL should most closely match the total daily dose of the immediate-release formulation of REQUIP, as shown in Table 1.

Table 1. Conversion from Immediate-Release REQUIP to REQUIP XL

Immediate-Release Ropinirole Tablets Total Daily Dose (mg)	REQUIP XL Tablets Total Daily Dose (mg)
0.75 to 2.25	2
3 to 4.5	4
6	6
7.5 to 9	8
12	12
15 to 18	16
21	20
24	24

Following conversion to REQUIP XL, the dose may be adjusted depending on therapeutic response and tolerability [see Dosage and Administration (2.2)].

3   DOSAGE FORMS AND STRENGTHS
• 2 mg, pink, biconvex, capsule-shaped, film-coated, tablets debossed with "GS" and "3V2"
• 4 mg, light brown, biconvex, capsule-shaped, film-coated, tablets debossed with "GS" and "WXG"
• 6 mg, white, biconvex, capsule-shaped, film-coated, tablets debossed with "GS" and "11F"
• 8 mg, red, biconvex, capsule-shaped, film-coated, tablets debossed with "GS" and "5CC"
• 12 mg, green, biconvex, capsule-shaped, film-coated, tablets debossed with "GS" and "YX7"

4   CONTRAINDICATIONS
None.

5   WARNINGS AND PRECAUTIONS
5.1   Falling Asleep During Activities of Daily Living
Patients treated with ropinirole have reported falling asleep while engaged in activities of daily living, including the operation of motor vehicles, which sometimes resulted in accidents. Although many of these patients reported somnolence while on ropinirole, some perceived that they had no warning signs such as excessive drowsiness, and believed that they were alert immediately prior to the event. Some of these events have been reported more than 1 year after initiation of treatment.
Among the 613 patients who received REQUIP XL in clinical trials, there were 5 cases of sudden onset of sleep and 2 cases of motor vehicle accident in which it is not known if falling asleep was a contributing factor.
During the 6-month trial in advanced Parkinson's disease, somnolence was reported in 7% (14 of 202) of patients receiving REQUIP XL compared with 4% (7 of 191) of patients receiving placebo. During the 36-week trial in early Parkinson's disease, somnolence was reported in 11% (16 of 140) of patients receiving REQUIP XL compared with 15% (22 of 149) of patients receiving the immediate-release formulation of REQUIP [see Adverse Reactions (6)]. However, because dose-response was not systematically studied with REQUIP XL, the occurrence of somnolence at the highest recommended doses may be higher than these reported frequencies [see Adverse Reactions (6)].

Many clinical experts believe that falling asleep while engaged in activities of daily living always occurs in a setting of preexisting somnolence, although patients may not give such a history. For this reason, prescribers should continually reassess patients for drowsiness or sleepiness, especially since some of the events occur well after the start of treatment. Prescribers should also be aware that patients may not acknowledge drowsiness or sleepiness until directly questioned about drowsiness or sleepiness during specific activities.

Before initiating treatment with REQUIP XL, patients should be advised of the potential to develop drowsiness and specifically asked about factors that may increase the risk with REQUIP XL such as concomitant sedating medications, the presence of sleep disorders, and concomitant medications that increase ropinirole plasma levels (e.g., ciprofloxacin) [see Drug Interactions (7.1)]. If a patient develops significant daytime sleepiness or episodes of falling asleep during activities that require active participation (e.g., driving a motor vehicle, conversations, eating, etc.), REQUIP XL should ordinarily be discontinued [see Dosage and Administration for guidance in discontinuing REQUIP XL (2.2)]. If a decision is made to continue REQUIP XL, patients should be advised to not drive and to avoid other potentially dangerous activities. There is insufficient information to establish that dose reduction will eliminate episodes of falling asleep while engaged in activities of daily living.

5.2 Syncope

Syncope, sometimes associated with bradycardia, was observed during treatment with ropinirole in Parkinson's disease patients.

In a placebo-controlled study involving patients with advanced Parkinson's disease, syncope occurred in 2 of the 202 patients (1%) who received REQUIP XL, and in none of the 191 patients who received placebo.

Because the study of REQUIP XL excluded patients with significant cardiovascular disease, it is not known to what extent the estimated incidence figure applies to patients with Parkinson's disease in clinical practice. Therefore, patients with significant cardiovascular disease should be treated with caution.

5.3 Hypotension

Dopamine agonists, in clinical studies and clinical experience, appear to impair the systemic regulation of blood pressure, with resulting postural hypotension, especially during dose escalation. In addition, patients with Parkinson's disease appear to have an impaired capacity to respond to a postural challenge. For these reasons, patients being treated with dopaminergic agonists ordinarily (1) require careful monitoring for signs and symptoms of postural hypotension, especially during dose escalation, and (2) should be informed of this risk [see Patient Counseling Information (17.2)].

In a placebo-controlled trial involving patients with advanced Parkinson's disease, hypotension was reported as an adverse event in 5 of 202 patients (2%) receiving REQUIP XL and in none of the 191 patients receiving placebo. Orthostatic hypotension was reported as an adverse event in 5% of patients receiving REQUIP XL, and in 1% of placebo recipients.

An analysis of the randomized, double-blinded, placebo-controlled study in advanced Parkinson's disease was conducted using a variety of adverse event terms possibly suggestive of hypotension, including hypotension, orthostatic hypotension, dizziness, vertigo, and blood pressure decreased. This analysis showed a higher incidence of these events with REQUIP XL (7%, 15 of 202) vs. placebo (3%, 6 of 191). This increased incidence was observed in a setting in which patients were very carefully titrated, and patients with clinically relevant cardiovascular disease or symptomatic orthostatic hypotension at baseline had been excluded from this study.

Orthostatic vital signs (semi-supine to standing) were monitored throughout the study in the advanced Parkinson's disease study and changes related to REQUIP XL (compared with placebo) from baseline were assessed.

The frequency of any orthostatic hypotension at any time during the study was 38% for REQUIP XL vs. 31% for placebo for mild to moderate systolic blood pressure decrements (≥20 mm Hg), 63% for REQUIP XL vs. 58% for placebo for mild to moderate diastolic blood pressure decrements (≥10 mm Hg), 10% for REQUIP XL vs. 7% for placebo for severe diastolic blood pressure decrements (≥20 mm Hg), and 23% for REQUIP XL vs. 19% for placebo for mild to moderate combined systolic and diastolic blood pressure decrements.

Significant decrements in blood pressure unrelated to standing were also reported in some patients taking REQUIP XL. In the semi-supine position, the frequency was 10% for REQUIP XL vs. 8% for placebo for severe systolic blood pressure decrease (≥40 mm Hg), and was 25% for REQUIP XL vs. 21% for placebo for severe diastolic blood pressure decrease (≥20 mm Hg).

The increased incidence for hypotension and/or orthostatic hypotension was observed in both the titration and maintenance phases and in some cases persisted into the maintenance period after developing in the titration phase.

5.4 Elevation of Blood Pressure and Changes in Heart Rate

In the placebo-controlled study in advanced Parkinson's disease, there were no clear effects of REQUIP XL on average changes in blood pressure or heart rate compared with placebo. However, there was an increased incidence of patients treated with REQUIP XL who met various outlier criteria, as described below.

In the semi-supine position, the frequency was 8% for REQUIP XL vs. 5% for placebo for severe systolic blood pressure increase (≥40 mm Hg). In the standing position, the frequency was 9% for REQUIP XL vs. 6% for placebo for severe systolic blood pressure increase (≥40 mm Hg).

In the semi-supine position, the frequency was 23% for REQUIP XL vs. 18% for placebo for moderate pulse increase (≥15 beats/minute), and 19% for REQUIP XL vs. 17% for placebo for moderate pulse decrease (≥15 beats/minute). In the standing position, the frequency was 2% for REQUIP XL vs. <1% for placebo for severe pulse increase (≥30 beats/minute), and 24% for REQUIP XL vs. 19% for placebo for moderate pulse decrease (≥15 beats/minute).

The increased incidence for various elevations of systolic and/or diastolic blood pressure and/or changes in pulse was observed in both the titration and maintenance phases as well as persisting into the maintenance period after developing in the titration phase.

Elevation of blood pressure and/or changes in heart rate in patients taking REQUIP XL should be considered when treating patients with cardiovascular disease.

5.5 Hallucination

In the double-blind, placebo-controlled, advanced Parkinson's disease trial 8% (17 of 202) of patients receiving REQUIP XL reported hallucination compared with 2% (4 of 191) patients receiving placebo. Hallucination led to discontinuation of treatment in 2% (4 of 202) of patients on REQUIP XL and 1% (2 of 191) of patients on placebo.

The incidence of hallucination is increased in patients over age 65. Coadministration of entacapone and L-dopa with ropinirole may also increase the risk of hallucination. In a placebo-controlled clinical trial, hallucination occurred in 0 of 43 patients taking entacapone plus L-dopa, in 9 of 155 patients taking REQUIP XL plus L-dopa (6%), and in 7 of 47 patients taking entacapone with REQUIP XL plus L-dopa (15%).

5.6 Dyskinesia

REQUIP XL may potentiate the dopaminergic side effects of L-dopa and may cause and/or exacerbate preexisting dyskinesia in patients treated with L-dopa for Parkinson's disease. Decreasing the dose of a dopaminergic drug may ameliorate this side effect.

5.7 Major Psychotic Disorders

Patients with a major psychotic disorder should ordinarily not be treated with REQUIP XL because of the risk of exacerbating the psychosis. In addition, many treatments for psychosis may decrease the effectiveness of REQUIP XL [see Drug Interactions (7.4)].

5.8 Events Reported With Dopaminergic Therapy

Withdrawal-Emergent Hyperpyrexia and Confusion: Although not reported during the clinical development of ropinirole, a symptom complex resembling the neuroleptic malignant syndrome (characterized by elevated temperature, muscular rigidity, altered consciousness, and autonomic instability), with no other obvious etiology, has been reported in association with rapid dose reduction, withdrawal of, or changes in dopaminergic therapy. Therefore, it is recommended that the dose be tapered at the end of treatment with REQUIP XL as a prophylactic measure [see Dosage and Administration (2.2)].

Fibrotic Complications: Cases of retroperitoneal fibrosis, pulmonary infiltrates, pleural effusion, pleural thickening, pericarditis, and cardiac valvulopathy have been reported in some patients treated with ergot-derived dopaminergic agents. While these complications may resolve when the drug is discontinued, complete resolution does not always occur.

Although these adverse reactions are believed to be related to the ergoline structure of these compounds, whether other, nonergot-derived dopamine agonists, such as REQUIP or REQUIP XL, can cause them is unknown.

A small number of reports have been received of possible fibrotic complications, including pleural infiltrates, pleural fibrosis, interstitial lung disease, and cardiac valvulopathy, in the development program and postmarketing experience for ropinirole. In the clinical development program (N = 613), 2 patients treated with REQUIP XL had pleural effusion. While the evidence is not sufficient to establish a causal relationship between ropinirole and these fibrotic complications, a contribution of ropinirole cannot be completely ruled out in rare cases.

Melanoma: Some epidemiologic studies have shown that patients with Parkinson's disease have a higher risk (perhaps 2- to 4-fold higher) of developing melanoma than the general population. Whether the observed increased risk was due to Parkinson's disease or other factors, such as drugs used to treat Parkinson's disease, was unclear. Ropinirole is one of the dopamine agonists used to treat Parkinson's disease. Although ropinirole has not been associated with an increased risk of melanoma specifically, its potential role as a risk factor has not been systematically studied. In the clinical development program (N = 613), one patient treated with REQUIP XL and also levodopa/carbidopa developed melanoma. Patients using REQUIP XL should be made aware of these results and undergo periodic dermatologic screening.

5.9 Retinal Pathology

Human: Because of observations made in albino rats (see below), ocular electroretinogram (ERG) assessments were conducted during a 2-year, double-blind, multicenter, flexible-dose, l-dopa controlled clinical study of immediate-release ropinirole in patients with Parkinson's disease. A total of 156 patients (78 on immediate-release ropinirole, mean dose 11.9 mg/day and 78 on l-dopa, mean dose 555.2 mg/day) were evaluated for evidence of retinal dysfunction through electroretinograms. There was no clinically meaningful difference between the treatment groups in retinal function over the duration of the study.

Albino Rats: Retinal degeneration was observed in albino rats in the 2-year carcinogenicity study at all doses tested (equivalent to 0.6 to 20 times the maximum recommended human dose (MRHD) of 24 mg/day on a mg/m^2 basis), but was statistically significant at the highest dose (50 mg/kg/day). Retinal degeneration was not observed in pigmented rats after 3 months in a 2-year carcinogenicity study in albino mice, or in 1-year studies in monkeys or albino rats. The potential significance of this effect for humans has not been established, but cannot be disregarded because disruption of a mechanism that is universally present in vertebrates (e.g., disk shedding) may be involved.

5.10 Binding to Melanin

Ropinirole binds to melanin-containing tissues (i.e., eyes, skin) in pigmented rats. After a single dose, long-term retention of drug was demonstrated, with a half-life in the eye of 20 days.

6 ADVERSE REACTIONS

The following adverse reactions are described in more detail in the Warnings and Precautions section of the label:
- Falling asleep during activities of daily living (5.1)
- Syncope (5.2)
- Symptomatic hypotension, hypotension, postural/orthostatic hypotension (5.3)
- Elevation of blood pressure and changes in heart rate (5.4)
- Hallucination (5.5)
- Dyskinesia (5.6)
- Major psychotic disorders (5.7)
- Events with dopaminergic therapy (5.8)
- Retinal pathology (5.9)

6.1 Clinical Trial Experience

Because clinical trials are conducted under widely varying conditions, adverse reaction rates observed in the clinical trials of a drug cannot be directly compared with rates in the clinical trials of another drug (or of another development program of a different formulation of the same drug) and may not reflect the rates observed in practice.

During the premarketing development of REQUIP XL, patients with advanced Parkinson's disease received REQUIP XL or placebo as adjunctive therapy in 1 clinical trial. In a second trial, patients with early Parkinson's disease were treated with REQUIP XL or the immediate-release formulation of REQUIP without L-dopa.

Advanced Parkinson's Disease (With L-dopa): The most commonly observed adverse reactions (≥5% and numerically greater than placebo) in the 24-week, double-blind, placebo-controlled trial for the treatment of advanced Parkinson's disease during treatment with REQUIP XL were, in order of decreasing incidence: dyskinesia, nausea, dizziness, hallucination, somnolence, abdominal pain/discomfort, and orthostatic hypotension.

Approximately 6% of 202 patients treated with REQUIP XL discontinued treatment due to adverse event(s) compared with 5% of 191 patients who received placebo. The adverse event most commonly causing discontinuation of treatment with REQUIP XL was hallucination (2%).

Table 2 lists adverse reactions that occurred with a frequency of at least 2% (and were numerically greater than placebo) in patients with advanced Parkinson's disease treated with REQUIP XL who participated in the 26-week, double-blind, placebo-controlled study. In this study, either REQUIP XL or placebo was used as an adjunct to L-dopa. Adverse reactions were generally mild or moderate in intensity.

Table 2. Treatment-Emergent Adverse Reaction Incidence in a Double-Blind, Placebo-Controlled Trial in Advanced Stage Parkinson's Disease (With L-dopa) (Events ≥2% of Patients Treated with REQUIP XL and >% with Placebo)

Body System/Adverse Reaction	REQUIP XL (n = 202) %	Placebo (n = 191) %
Ear and labyrinth disorders		
Vertigo	4	2
Gastrointestinal disorders		
Nausea	11	4
Constipation	4	2
Abdominal pain/discomfort	6	3
Diarrhea	3	2
Dry mouth	2	<1
General disorders		
Edema peripheral	4	1
Injury, poisoning, and procedural complications		
Fall*	2	1
Musculoskeletal and connective tissue disorders		
Back pain	3	2
Nervous system disorders		
Dyskinesia*	13	3
Dizziness	8	3
Somnolence	7	4
Psychiatric disorders		
Hallucination	8	2
Anxiety	2	1
Vascular disorders		
Orthostatic hypotension	5	1
Hypotension	2	0
Hypertension*	3	2

[a] Dose-related.

Although this study was not designed for optimally characterizing dose-related adverse reactions, there was a suggestion (based upon comparison of incidence of adverse reactions across dose ranges for REQUIP XL and placebo) that the incidence for dyskinesia, hypertension, and fall was dose-related to REQUIP XL.

The incidence for many adverse reactions with REQUIP XL treatment was increased relative to placebo (i.e., REQUIP XL % - Placebo % = treatment difference ≥2%) in either the titration or maintenance phases of the study. During the titration phase, an increased incidence (shown in descending order of % treatment difference) was observed for dyskinesia, nausea, abdominal pain/discomfort, orthostatic hypotension, dizziness, vertigo, hypertension, peripheral edema, and dry mouth. During the maintenance phase, an increased incidence was observed for dyskinesia, nausea, dizziness, hallucination, somnolence, fall, hypertension, abnormal dreams, constipation, chest pain, bronchitis, and nasopharyngitis. Some adverse reactions developing in the titration phase persisted (≥7 days) into the maintenance phase. These "persistent" adverse reactions included dyskinesia, hallucination, orthostatic hypotension, and dry mouth.

The incidence of adverse reactions was not clearly different between women and men.

Early Parkinson's Disease (Without L-dopa): The most commonly observed adverse reactions (≥5%) in the 36-week early Parkinson's disease trial during treatment with REQUIP XL were, in order of decreasing incidence: nausea (19%), somnolence (11%), abdominal pain/discomfort (7%), dizziness (6%), headache (6%), and constipation (5%). The type of adverse reactions and the frequency (i.e. incidence) with which they occurred were generally similar over the whole treatment period in this study of early Parkinson's disease patients who were initially treated with REQUIP XL or the immediate-release formulation of REQUIP and subsequently crossed over to treatment with the other formulation.

During the titration phase, an increased incidence with REQUIP XL compared with the immediate-release formulation of REQUIP (i.e., REQUIP XL % - REQUIP IR % = treatment difference ≥2%), shown in descending order of % treatment difference, was observed for: constipation, hallucination, vertigo, abdominal pain/discomfort, nausea, vomiting, fall, headache, diarrhea, pyrexia, and flatulence. During the maintenance phase, an increased incidence was observed for fall, myalgia, and sleep disorder. Several adverse reactions developing in the titration phase persisted

(≥7 days) into the maintenance phase. These "persistent" adverse reactions included: constipation, hallucination, muscle spasms, flatulence, insomnia, sleep disorder, abdominal pain/discomfort, cough, and nasopharyngitis.

6.2 Adverse Reactions Observed During the Clinical Development of the Immediate-Release Formulation of REQUIP for Parkinson's Disease (Advanced and Early)
Because clinical trials are conducted under widely varying conditions, adverse reaction rates observed in the clinical trials of a drug cannot be directly compared to rates in the clinical trials of another drug (or of another development program of a different formulation of the same drug) and may not reflect the rates observed in practice.

In patients with advanced Parkinson's disease who were treated with the immediate-release formulation of REQUIP, the most common adverse reactions (≥5% treatment difference from placebo; presented in order of decreasing treatment difference frequency) were dyskinesia (21%), somnolence (12%), nausea (12%), dizziness (10%), confusion (7%), hallucinations (6%), headache (5%), and increased sweating (5%). In patients with early Parkinson's disease who were treated with the immediate-release formulation of REQUIP, the most common adverse reactions (≥5% treatment difference from placebo; presented in order of decreasing treatment difference frequency) were nausea (38%), somnolence (34%), dizziness (18%), syncope (11%), viral infection (8%), fatigue (7%), leg edema (6%), asthenia (5%), and dyspepsia (5%).

7 DRUG INTERACTIONS
7.1 P450 Interaction
In vitro metabolism studies showed that CYP1A2 is the major enzyme responsible for the metabolism of ropinirole. There is thus the potential for inducers or inhibitors of this enzyme to alter the clearance of ropinirole. Therefore, if therapy with a drug known to be a potent inducer or inhibitor of CYP1A2 is stopped or started during treatment with ropinirole, adjustment of the dose of ropinirole may be required.
Coadministration of ciprofloxacin, an inhibitor of CYP1A2, with immediate-release ropinirole increased the AUC of ropinirole by 84% on average and C_{max} by 60% [see Clinical Pharmacology (12.3)].
Cigarette smoking is expected to increase the clearance of ropinirole since CYP1A2 is known to be induced by smoking. In one study in patients with Restless Legs Syndrome, cigarette smokers had an approximate 30% lower C_{max} and a 38% lower AUC than did nonsmokers, when those parameters were normalized for dose.
There is no evidence of interaction between ropinirole and other CYP1A2 substrates (e.g., theophylline).
Ropinirole and its circulating metabolites do not inhibit or induce P450 enzymes; therefore, ropinirole is unlikely to affect the pharmacokinetics of other drugs by a P450 mechanism [see Clinical Pharmacology (12.3)].
7.2 L-dopa
Coadministration of carbidopa + L-dopa (SINEMET®) with immediate-release ropinirole had no effect on the steady-state pharmacokinetics of ropinirole. Oral administration of immediate-release ropinirole increased mean steady-state C_{max} of L-dopa by 20%, but its AUC was unaffected [see Clinical Pharmacology (12.3)].
7.3 Estrogens
Population pharmacokinetic analysis revealed that higher doses of estrogens (usually associated with hormone replacement therapy [HRT]) reduced the oral clearance of ropinirole by approximately 35%. Dosage adjustment is not needed for initiating REQUIP XL in patients on estrogen therapy because patients are individually titrated with REQUIP XL to tolerance or adequate effect. If estrogen therapy is stopped or started during treatment with REQUIP XL, then adjustment of the dose of REQUIP XL may be required.
7.4 Dopamine Antagonists
Since ropinirole is a dopamine agonist, it is possible that dopamine antagonists such as neuroleptics (e.g., phenothiazines, butyrophenones, thioxanthenes) or metoclopramide may diminish the effectiveness of REQUIP XL. Patients with a history or presence of major psychotic disorders should be treated with dopamine agonists only if the potential benefits outweigh the risks.

8 USE IN SPECIFIC POPULATIONS
8.1 Pregnancy
Pregnancy Category C. There are no adequate and well-controlled studies using ropinirole in pregnant women. REQUIP XL should be used during pregnancy only if the potential benefit outweighs the potential risk to the fetus.
In animal reproduction studies, ropinirole has been shown to have adverse effects on embryo-fetal development, including teratogenic effects. Treatment of pregnant rats with ropinirole during organogenesis resulted in decreased fetal body weight, increased fetal death, and digital malformations at 24, 36, and 60 times the MRHD, respectively. The combined administration of ropinirole at 8 times the MRHD

and a clinically relevant dose of L-dopa to pregnant rabbits during organogenesis produced a greater incidence and severity of fetal malformations (primarily digit defects) than were seen in the offspring of rabbits treated with L-dopa alone. In a perinatal-postnatal study in rats, impaired growth and development of nursing offspring and altered neurological development of female offspring were observed when dams were treated with 4 times the MRHD.
8.3 Nursing Mothers
Ropinirole inhibits prolactin secretion in humans and could potentially inhibit lactation.
Ropinirole has been detected in the milk of lactating rats. Although many drugs are excreted in human milk, transfer of ropinirole into human milk has not been demonstrated. Due to the potential for serious adverse reactions in nursing infants, a decision should be made whether to discontinue nursing or to discontinue the drug, taking into account the importance of ropinirole to the mother.
8.4 Pediatric Use
Safety and effectiveness in the pediatric population have not been established.
8.5 Geriatric Use
Dosage adjustment is not necessary in the elderly (above 65 years), as the dose of REQUIP XL is to be individually titrated to clinical response [see Clinical Pharmacology (12.3)]. Pharmacokinetic studies conducted in patients demonstrated that oral clearance of ropinirole is reduced by 15% in patients above 65 years of age compared to younger patients.
Of the total number of patients who participated in clinical trials of REQUIP XL for Parkinson's disease, 387 patients were 65 and over and 107 patients were 75 and over. Among patients receiving REQUIP XL, hallucination was more common in elderly subjects (10%) compared with non-elderly subjects (2%). The incidence of overall adverse events increased with increasing age for both patients receiving REQUIP XL and placebo.
8.6 Renal Impairment
No dosage adjustment of ropinirole is needed in patients with moderate renal impairment (creatinine clearance of 30 to 50 mL/min). The use of ropinirole in patients with severe renal impairment has not been studied.
8.7 Hepatic Impairment
The pharmacokinetics of ropinirole have not been studied in patients with hepatic impairment. Since patients with hepatic impairment may have higher plasma levels and lower clearance, ropinirole should be titrated with caution in these patients.

9 DRUG ABUSE AND DEPENDENCE
9.1 Controlled Substance
Ropinirole is not a controlled substance.
9.3 Dependence
Animal studies and human clinical trials with ropinirole did not reveal any potential for drug-seeking behavior or physical dependence.

10 OVERDOSAGE
10.1 Human Overdose Experience
In the Parkinson's disease program, there have been patients who accidentally or intentionally took more than their prescribed dose of ropinirole. The largest overdose reported with immediate-release ropinirole in clinical trials was 435 mg taken over a 7-day period (62.1 mg/day). Of patients who received a dose greater than 24 mg/day, reported symptoms included adverse events commonly reported during dopaminergic therapy (nausea, dizziness), as well as visual hallucination, hyperhidrosis, claustrophobia, chorea, palpitations, asthenia, and nightmares. Additional symptoms reported for doses of 24 mg or less or for overdoses of unknown amount included vomiting, increased coughing, fatigue, syncope, vasovagal syncope, dyskinesia, agitation, chest pain, orthostatic hypotension, somnolence, and confusional state.
10.2 Overdose Management
The symptoms of overdose with ropinirole are generally related to its dopaminergic activity; these symptoms may be alleviated by appropriate treatment with dopamine antagonists such as neuroleptics or metoclopramide. General supportive measures are recommended. Vital signs should be maintained, if necessary. Removal of any unabsorbed material (e.g., by gastric lavage) may be considered.

11 DESCRIPTION
REQUIP (ropinirole) is an orally administered non-ergoline dopamine agonist. It is supplied as the hydrochloride salt of ropinirole 4-[2-(dipropylamino)ethyl]-1,3-dihydro-2H-indol-2-one and has an empirical formula of $C_{16}H_{24}N_2O\bullet HCl$. The molecular weight is 296.84 (260.38 as the free base).
The structural formula is:
[See chemical structure at top of next column]
Ropinirole hydrochloride is a white to yellow solid with a melting range of 243° to 250°C and a solubility of 133 mg/mL in water.
REQUIP XL extended-release tablets are formulated as a three-layered tablet with a central, active-containing, slow-

release layer, and 2 placebo outer layers acting as barrier layers which control the surface area available for drug release. Each biconvex, capsule-shaped tablet contains 2.28 mg, 4.56 mg, 6.84 mg, 9.12 mg, or 13.68 mg ropinirole hydrochloride equivalent to ropinirole 2 mg, 4 mg, 6 mg, 8 mg, or 12 mg, respectively. Inactive ingredients consist of carboxymethylcellulose sodium, colloidal silicon dioxide, glyceryl behenate, hydrogenated castor oil, hypromellose, lactose monohydrate, magnesium stearate, maltodextrin, mannitol, povidone, and one or more of the following: FD&C Yellow No. 6 aluminum lake, FD&C Blue No. 2 aluminum lake, ferric oxides (black, red, yellow), polyethylene glycol 400, titanium dioxide.

12 CLINICAL PHARMACOLOGY
12.1 Mechanism of Action
Ropinirole is a non-ergoline dopamine agonist with high relative in vitro specificity and full intrinsic activity at the D_2 and D_3 dopamine receptor subtypes, binding with higher affinity to D_3 than to D_2 or D_4 receptor subtypes.

Ropinirole has moderate in vitro affinity for opioid receptors. Ropinirole and its metabolites have negligible in vitro affinity for dopamine D_1, $5\text{-}HT_1$, $5\text{-}HT_2$, benzodiazepine, GABA, muscarinic, alpha$_1$-, alpha$_2$-, and beta-adrenoreceptors.

The precise mechanism of action of ropinirole as a treatment for Parkinson's disease is unknown, although it is believed to be due to stimulation of postsynaptic dopamine D_2-type receptors within the caudate-putamen in the brain. This conclusion is supported by studies that show that ropinirole improves motor function in various animal models of Parkinson's disease. In particular, ropinirole attenuates the motor deficits induced by lesioning the ascending nigrostriatal dopaminergic pathway with the neurotoxin 1-methyl-4-phenyl-1,2,3,6-tetrahydropyridine (MPTP) in primates. The relevance of D_3 receptor binding in Parkinson's disease is unknown.

12.2 Pharmacodynamics
Clinical experience with dopamine agonists, including ropinirole, suggests an association with impaired ability to regulate blood pressure with resulting postural hypotension, especially during dose escalation. In some subjects in clinical trials, blood pressure changes were associated with the emergence of orthostatic symptoms, bradycardia, and, in one case in a healthy volunteer, transient sinus arrest with syncope.

The mechanism of postural hypotension induced by ropinirole is presumed to be due to a D_2-mediated blunting of the noradrenergic response to standing and subsequent decrease in peripheral vascular resistance. Nausea is a common concomitant symptom of orthostatic signs and symptoms.

At oral doses as low as 0.2 mg, ropinirole suppressed serum prolactin concentrations in healthy male volunteers.

Immediate-release ropinirole had no dose-related effect on ECG wave form and rhythm in young, healthy, male volunteers in the range of 0.01 to 2.5 mg. Immediate-release ropinirole had no dose- or exposure-related effect on mean QT intervals in healthy male and female volunteers titrated to doses up to 4 mg/day. The effect of ropinirole on QTc intervals at higher exposures achieved either due to drug interactions, hepatic impairment, or at higher doses has not been systematically evaluated.

12.3 Pharmacokinetics
Absorption: In clinical studies with immediate-release ropinirole, over 88% of a radiolabeled dose was recovered in urine, and the absolute bioavailability was 45% to 55%, indicating approximately 50% first-pass effect.

Ropinirole displayed linear kinetics up to doses of 24 mg/day (8 mg immediate-release, 3 times a day). Increase in systemic exposure of ropinirole following oral administration of 2 to 12 mg of REQUIP XL was approximately dose-proportional. For REQUIP XL, steady-state concentrations of ropinirole are expected to be achieved within 4 days of dosing.

Relative bioavailability of REQUIP XL extended-release tablets compared with immediate-release tablets was approximately 100%. In a repeat-dose study in patients with Parkinson's disease using REQUIP XL 8 mg, the dose-normalized $AUC_{(0-24)}$ and C_{min} for REQUIP XL and immediate-release ropinirole were similar. Dose-normalized C_{max} was, on average, 12% lower for REQUIP XL than for the immediate-release formulation and the median time-to-peak concentration was 6 to 10 hours. In a single-dose study, administration of REQUIP XL to healthy volunteers with food (i.e., high-fat meal) increased oral AUC by approxi-

mately 30% and C_{max} by approximately 44%, compared with dosing under fasted conditions. In a repeat-dose study in patients with Parkinson's disease, food (i.e., high-fat meal) increased AUC by approximately 20% and C_{max} by approximately 44%; T_{max} was prolonged by 3 hours (median prolongation) compared with dosing under fasted conditions [see Dosage and Administration (2.1)].

Distribution: Ropinirole is widely distributed throughout the body, with an apparent volume of distribution of 7.5 L/kg (cv = 32%). It is up to 40% bound to plasma proteins and has a blood-to-plasma ratio of 1:1.

Metabolism: Ropinirole is extensively metabolized by the liver. The major metabolic pathways are N-despropylation and hydroxylation to form the inactive N-despropyl metabolite and hydroxy metabolites. The N-despropyl metabolite is converted to carbamyl glucuronide, carboxylic acid, and N-despropyl hydroxy metabolites. The hydroxy metabolite of ropinirole is rapidly glucuronidated.

In vitro studies indicate that the major cytochrome P450 isozyme involved in the metabolism of ropinirole is CYP1A2, an enzyme known to be induced by smoking and omeprazole, and inhibited by, for example, fluvoxamine, mexiletine, and the older fluoroquinolones such as ciprofloxacin and norfloxacin.

Elimination: The clearance of ropinirole after oral administration to patients is 47 L/hr (cv = 45%) and its elimination half-life is approximately 6 hours. Less than 10% of the administered dose is excreted as unchanged drug in urine. N-despropyl ropinirole is the predominant metabolite found in urine (40%), followed by the carboxylic acid metabolite (10%), and the glucuronide of the hydroxy metabolite (10%).

Drug Interactions: Ciprofloxacin: Coadministration of ciprofloxacin (500 mg twice daily), an inhibitor of CYP1A2, with immediate-release ropinirole (2 mg 3 times daily) increased ropinirole AUC by 84% on average and C_{max} by 60% (n = 12 patients).

Digoxin: Coadministration of immediate-release ropinirole (2 mg 3 times daily) with digoxin (0.125 to 0.25 mg once daily) did not alter the steady-state pharmacokinetics of digoxin in 10 patients.

Theophylline: Administration of theophylline (300 mg twice daily, a substrate of CYP1A2) did not alter the steady-state pharmacokinetics of immediate-release ropinirole (2 mg 3 times daily) in 12 patients with Parkinson's disease. Immediate-release ropinirole (2 mg 3 times daily) did not alter the pharmacokinetics of theophylline (5 mg/kg IV) in 12 patients with Parkinson's disease.

L-dopa: Coadministration of carbidopa + l-dopa (SINEMET 10/100 mg twice daily) with immediate-release ropinirole (2 mg 3 times daily) had no effect on the steady-state pharmacokinetics of ropinirole (n = 28 patients). Oral administration of immediate-release ropinirole 2 mg 3 times daily increased mean steady-state C_{max} of l-dopa by 20%, but its AUC was unaffected (n = 23 patients).

Estrogens: Population pharmacokinetic analysis revealed that higher doses of estrogens (usually associated with hormone replacement therapy [HRT]) reduced the oral clearance of ropinirole by approximately 35%.

Commonly Administered Drugs: Population analysis showed that commonly administered drugs, e.g., selegiline, amantadine, tricyclic antidepressants, benzodiazepines, ibuprofen, thiazides, antihistamines, and anticholinergics, did not affect the oral clearance of ropinirole.

Population Subgroups: Because therapy with REQUIP XL is initiated at a low dose and gradually titrated upward according to clinical tolerability to obtain the optimum therapeutic effect, adjustment of the initial dose based on gender, weight, or age is not necessary.

Age: Oral clearance of ropinirole is reduced by approximately 15% in patients above 65 years of age compared with younger patients. Dosage adjustment is not necessary in the elderly (above 65 years), as the dose of ropinirole is individually titrated to clinical response.

Gender: Female and male patients showed similar oral clearance.

Race: The influence of race on the pharmacokinetics of ropinirole has not been evaluated.

Renal Impairment: Based on population pharmacokinetic analysis, no difference was observed in the pharmacokinetics of ropinirole in patients with moderate renal impairment (creatinine clearance between 30 to 50 mL/min) compared with an age-matched population with creatinine clearance above 50 mL/min. Therefore, no dosage adjustment is necessary in patients with moderate renal impairment. The use of ropinirole in patients with severe renal impairment has not been studied.

The effect of hemodialysis on ropinirole clearance is not known, but because of the relatively high apparent volume of distribution of ropinirole (7.5 L/kg), significant removal of ropinirole by hemodialysis is unlikely.

Hepatic Impairment: The pharmacokinetics of ropinirole have not been studied in patients with hepatic impairment. These patients may have higher plasma levels and lower

clearance of ropinirole than patients with normal hepatic function. REQUIP XL should be titrated with caution in this population.

Other Diseases: Population pharmacokinetic analysis revealed no change in the oral clearance of ropinirole in patients with concomitant diseases such as hypertension, depression, osteoporosis/arthritis, and insomnia compared with patients who had Parkinson's disease only.

13 NONCLINICAL TOXICOLOGY
13.1 Carcinogenesis, Mutagenesis, Impairment of Fertility
Two-year carcinogenicity studies were conducted in Charles River CD-1 mice at doses of 5, 15, and 50 mg/kg/day and in Sprague-Dawley rats at doses of 1.5, 15, and 50 mg/kg/day (top doses which, based on mg/m^2, are equivalent to 10 and 20 times, respectively, the MRHD of 24 mg/day). In the male rat, there was a significant increase in testicular Leydig cell adenomas at all doses tested, i.e., ≥1.5 mg/kg (0.6 times the MRHD on a mg/m^2 basis). This finding is of questionable significance because the endocrine mechanisms believed to be involved in the production of Leydig cell hyperplasia and adenomas in rats are not relevant to humans. In the female mouse, there was an increase in benign uterine endometrial polyps at a dose of 50 mg/kg/day (10 times the MRHD on a mg/m^2 basis).

Ropinirole was not mutagenic or clastogenic in the in vitro Ames test, the in vitro chromosome aberration test in human lymphocytes, the in vitro mouse lymphoma (L5178Y cells) assay, and the in vivo mouse micronucleus test.

When administered to female rats prior to and during mating and throughout pregnancy, ropinirole caused disruption of implantation at doses of 20 mg/kg/day (8 times the MRHD on a mg/m^2 basis) or greater. This effect is thought to be due to the prolactin-lowering effect of ropinirole. In humans, chorionic gonadotropin, not prolactin, is essential for implantation. In rat studies using low doses (5 mg/kg) during the prolactin-dependent phase of early pregnancy (gestation days 0 to 8), ropinirole did not affect female fertility at dosages up to 100 mg/kg/day (40 times the MRHD on a mg/m^2 basis). No effect on male fertility was observed in rats at dosages up to 125 mg/kg/day (50 times the MRHD on a mg/m^2 basis).

14 CLINICAL STUDIES
The effectiveness of the immediate-release formulation of ropinirole (REQUIP tablets) in the treatment of early and advanced Parkinson's disease was initially established in 3 randomized, double-blind, placebo-controlled trials.

The effectiveness of REQUIP XL in the treatment of Parkinson's disease was supported by 2 randomized, double-blind, multicenter clinical trials and clinical pharmacokinetic considerations. One trial conducted in advanced Parkinson's disease patients compared REQUIP XL with placebo as adjunctive therapy to L-dopa. A second trial compared REQUIP XL with REQUIP tablets in early phase Parkinson's disease patients not receiving L-dopa.

In these studies a variety of measures were used to assess the effects of treatment (e.g., patient diaries recording time "on" and "off," tolerability of L-dopa dose reductions, and the Unified Parkinson's Disease Rating Scale [UPDRS] scores). The UPDRS is a multi-item rating scale evaluating mentation (Part I), activities of daily living (Part II), motor performance (Part III), and complications of therapy (Part IV). Part III of the UPDRS contains 14 items designed to assess the severity of the cardinal motor findings in patients with Parkinson's disease (e.g., tremor, rigidity, bradykinesia, postural instability, etc.) scored for different body regions and has a maximum (worst) score of 108.

14.1 Study in Patients With Advanced Parkinson's Disease (With L-dopa)
The effectiveness of REQUIP XL as adjunctive therapy to L-dopa in patients with Parkinson's disease was established in a randomized, double-blind, placebo-controlled, parallel group, 24-week clinical trial in 393 patients (Hoehn & Yahr criteria Stages II-IV) who were not adequately controlled by L-dopa therapy. Patients were allowed to be on concomitant selegiline, amantadine, anticholinergics, and catechol-O-methyltransferase (COMT) inhibitors provided the doses were stable for at least 4 weeks prior to screening and throughout the trial. The primary efficacy endpoint evaluated was the mean change from baseline in total awake time spent "off".

Patients in this study had a mean disease duration of 8.6 years, a mean duration of exposure to L-dopa of 6.5 years, had experienced a minimum of 3 hours awake time "off" with a baseline average of approximately 7 hours awake time "off", and had a mean baseline UPDRS motor score of approximately 30 points with similar mean data in each treatment group. The mean baseline dose of L-dopa in the group receiving REQUIP XL was 824 mg/day and 776 mg/day for the placebo group. Patients initiated treatment at 2 mg/day for 1 week followed by increases of 2 mg/day at weekly intervals to a minimum dose of

6 mg/day. The following week, the REQUIP XL total daily dose could be further increased (based upon therapeutic response and tolerability) to 8 mg/day. Once a daily dose of 8 mg/day was reached, the background L-dopa dosage was reduced. Thereafter, the daily dose could be increased by up to 4 mg/day approximately every 2 weeks until an optimal dose was achieved (based upon therapeutic response and tolerability). The mean dose of REQUIP XL at the end of Week 24 was 18.8 mg/day. Dose titrations were based upon the degree of symptom control, planned L-dopa dosage reduction, and/or tolerability. The maximal allowed daily dosage for REQUIP XL was 24 mg/day.

The primary efficacy endpoint was mean change from baseline in total awake time spent "off" at Week 24. At baseline the mean total awake time spent "off" was approximately 7 hours in each treatment group. At Week 24, the total awake time spent "off", on average, had decreased by approximately 2 hours in the group receiving REQUIP XL and by approximately half an hour in the placebo group. The adjusted mean difference in total awake time spent "off" between REQUIP XL and placebo was -1.7 hours, which was statistically significant (ANCOVA, p< 0.0001). Results for this endpoint showing the statistical superiority of REQUIP XL over Placebo are presented in Table 3.

Table 3. Change from Baseline in Total Awake Time Spent "Off" at Week 24

	REQUIP XL (n = 201)	Placebo (n = 190)
Mean "Off" time at Baseline (hours)	7.0	7.0
Mean Change from Baseline in "Off" time (hours)	-2.1	-0.4

The difference between groups in favor of REQUIP XL, with regard to a decrease in total "off" hours, was primarily related to an increase in total "on" hours without troublesome dyskinesia. Patients treated with REQUIP XL had a mean reduction in L-dopa dose of 278 mg/day (34%) while patients treated with placebo had a mean reduction of 164 mg/day (21%). In patients who reduced their L-dopa dose, reduction was sustained in 93% of patients treated with REQUIP XL and in 72% of patients treated with placebo (p<0.001).

14.2   Study in Patients With Early Parkinson's Disease (Without L-dopa)

A 36-week multicenter, double-blind, titration/3-period maintenance, cross-over study compared the efficacy of REQUIP XL with the immediate-release formulation of REQUIP (IR) in 161 patients with early phase Parkinson's disease (Hoehn & Yahr Stages I-III) with limited prior exposure to L-dopa or dopamine agonists. Eligible subjects were randomized (1:1:1:1) to 4 treatment sequences (2 were titrated on REQUIP IR and 2 on REQUIP XL). The REQUIP IR titration was slower in rate than that of the REQUIP XL. Patients were titrated, during the 12-week titration period, to their optimal dosage, based upon tolerance and therapeutic response. This was followed by 3 consecutive 8-week maintenance periods, during which patients were either maintained on the prior formulation or switched to the alternative formulation. All switches were performed overnight by using the approximately equivalent doses of ropinirole. The primary efficacy endpoint was the change of UPDRS motor score within each maintenance period.

Patients in all 4 groups started out with similar UPDRS motor scores (about 21) at baseline. All 4 groups exhibited similar improvement in UPDRS total motor scores from baseline until the completion of the titration phase, with a change in score of about -9 observed for the groups started on REQUIP IR and of about -10 for the groups started on REQUIP XL. No difference was observed between groups when switches were made between identical formulations or between different formulations. This suggests therapeutic dosage equivalence between REQUIP IR and REQUIP XL formulations.

The optimal daily dose at the end of the titration period for patients on REQUIP IR was substantially lower (mean 7 mg) compared to the dose at the end of the titration period for patients on REQUIP XL (mean 18 mg). In this study, the marked difference in the final optimal dosages suggests that the higher doses afforded no additional benefit when compared to the lower doses [see Dosage and Administration (2)].

16   HOW SUPPLIED/STORAGE AND HANDLING

Each biconvex, capsule-shaped, film-coated tablet contains ropinirole hydrochloride equivalent to the labeled amount of ropinirole as follows:
- 2 mg: pink tablets debossed with "GS" and "3V2", in bottles of 30 (NDC 0007-4885-13) and 90 (NDC 0007-4885-59).

- 4 mg: light brown tablets debossed with "GS" and "WXG", in bottles of 30 (NDC 0007-4887-13) and 90 (NDC 0007-4887-59).
- 6 mg: white tablets debossed with "GS" and "11F", in bottles of 30 (NDC 0007-4883-13)
- 8 mg: red tablets debossed with "GS" and "5CC", in bottles of 30 (NDC 0007-4888-13) and 90 (NDC 0007-4888-59).
- 12 mg: green tablets debossed with "GS" and "YX7", in bottles of 30 (NDC 0007-4882-13).

Storage: Store at 25°C (77°F); excursions permitted to 15-30°C (59-86°F) [see USP Controlled Room Temperature]. Dispense in a tight, light-resistant container as defined in the USP.

17   PATIENT COUNSELING INFORMATION

See FDA-approved patient labeling (Patient Information).
Physicians should instruct their patients to read the Patient Information leaflet before starting therapy with REQUIP XL and to reread it upon prescription renewal for new information regarding the use of REQUIP XL.

17.1   Dosing Instructions
- Patients should be instructed to take REQUIP XL only as prescribed. If a dose is missed, patients should be advised not to double their next dose.
- REQUIP XL can be taken with or without food. Taking REQUIP XL with food may reduce the occurrence of nausea [see Dosage and Administration (2.1)].
- REQUIP XL tablets should be swallowed whole. They should not be chewed, crushed, or divided [see Dosage and Administration (2.1)].
- Ropinirole is the active ingredient that is in both REQUIP XL and REQUIP tablets (the immediate-release formulation). Ask your patient if they are taking another medication containing ropinirole.

17.2   Postural (Orthostatic) Hypotension
Patients should be advised that they may develop postural (orthostatic) hypotension with or without symptoms such as dizziness, nausea, syncope, and sometimes sweating. Hypotension and/or orthostatic symptoms may occur more frequently during initial therapy with an increase in dose at any time (cases have been seen after weeks of treatment). Accordingly, patients should be cautioned against standing up rapidly after sitting or lying down, especially if they have been doing so for prolonged periods, and especially at the initiation of treatment with REQUIP XL [see Warnings and Precautions (5.2, 5.3)].

17.3   Elevation of Blood Pressure and Changes in Heart Rate
Patients should be alerted to the possibility of increases in blood pressure during treatment with REQUIP XL. Exacerbation of hypertension may occur. Medication dose adjustment may be necessary if elevation of blood pressure is sustained over multiple evaluations. Patients with cardiovascular disease, who may not tolerate marked changes in heart rate, should also be alerted to the possibility that they may experience significant increases or decreases in heart rate during treatment with REQUIP XL [see Warnings and Precautions (5.4)].

17.4   Sedating Effects
Patients should be alerted to the potential sedating effects caused by REQUIP XL, including somnolence and the possibility of falling asleep while engaged in activities of daily living. Since somnolence is a frequent adverse reaction with potentially serious consequences, patients should neither drive a car nor engage in other potentially dangerous activities until they have gained sufficient experience with REQUIP XL to gauge whether or not it affects their mental and/or motor performance adversely. Patients should be advised that if increased somnolence or episodes of falling asleep during activities of daily living (e.g., conversations, eating, driving a motor vehicle, etc.) are experienced at any time during treatment, they should not drive or participate in potentially dangerous activities until they have contacted their physician.
Because of possible additive effects, caution should be advised when patients are taking other sedating medications, alcohol, or other CNS depressants (e.g., benzodiazepines, antipsychotics, antidepressants, etc.) in combination with REQUIP XL or when taking concomitant medications that increase plasma levels of ropinirole (e.g., ciprofloxacin) [see Warnings and Precautions (5.1)].

17.5   Hallucination
Patients should be informed they may experience hallucinations (unreal visions, sounds, or sensations) while taking ropinirole. The elderly are at greater risk than younger patients with Parkinson's disease; and the risk is greater in patients who are taking ropinirole with L-dopa or taking higher doses of ropinirole, and may also be further increased in patients taking any other drugs that increase dopaminergic tone [see Warnings and Precautions (5.5)].

17.6   Impulse Control Symptoms, Including Compulsive Behaviors
There have been reports of patients experiencing intense urges to gamble, increased sexual urges, and other intense

urges and the inability to control these urges while taking one or more of the medications that increase central dopaminergic tone, that are generally used for the treatment of Parkinson's disease or Restless Legs Syndrome, including ropinirole. In the clinical development program (N = 613), 6 patients treated with REQUIP XL exhibited compulsive behaviors consisting of pathological gambling and/or hypersexuality. Although it is not proven that the medications caused these events, these urges were reported to have stopped in some cases when the dose was reduced or the medication was stopped. Prescribers should ask patients about the development of new or increased gambling urges, sexual urges or other urges while being treated with REQUIP XL. Patients should inform their physician if they experience new or increased gambling urges, increased sexual urges or other intense urges while taking REQUIP XL. Physicians should consider dose reduction or stopping the medication if a patient develops such urges while taking REQUIP XL.

17.7   Nursing Mothers
Because of the possibility that ropinirole may be excreted in breast milk, a decision should be made whether to discontinue nursing or to discontinue the drug, taking into account the importance of the drug to the mother [see Use in Specific Populations (8.3)].
Patients should be advised that ropinirole could inhibit lactation, as ropinirole inhibits prolactin secretion.

17.8   Pregnancy
Because ropinirole has been shown to have adverse effects on embryo-fetal development, including teratogenic effects, in animals, and because experience in humans is limited, patients should be advised to notify their physician if they become pregnant or intend to become pregnant during therapy [see Use in Specific Populations (8.1)].

REQUIP XL is a registered trademark of GlaxoSmithKline. SINEMET is a registered trademark of Merck & Co., Inc.
GlaxoSmithKline
Research Triangle Park, NC 27709
©2012, GlaxoSmithKline. All rights reserved.
RXL:5PI
PATIENT INFORMATION
REQUIP® (RE-qwip) (ropinirole tablets)
REQUIP XL® (RE-qwip)
(ropinirole extended-release tablets)
IF YOU HAVE PARKINSON'S DISEASE, READ THIS SIDE
IF YOU HAVE RESTLESS LEGS SYNDROME, READ THE OTHER SIDE

IMPORTANT NOTE: REQUIP XL has not been studied in Restless Legs Syndrome (RLS) and is not approved for the treatment of RLS. However, an immediate-release form of ropinirole (REQUIP) is approved for the treatment of RLS (see other side of this leaflet).

Read this information completely before you start taking REQUIP or REQUIP XL. Read the information each time you get more medicine. There may be new information. This leaflet provides a summary about REQUIP and REQUIP XL. It does not include everything there is to know about your medicine. This information should not take the place of discussions with your healthcare provider about your medical condition or treatment with REQUIP or REQUIP XL.
What are REQUIP and REQUIP XL?
REQUIP is a short-acting prescription medicine containing ropinirole (usually taken 3 times a day) used to treat Parkinson's disease. It is also used to treat a condition called Restless Legs Syndrome.
REQUIP XL is a long-acting prescription medicine containing ropinirole (taken once a day) used to treat Parkinson's disease.
You should not be taking more than one medicine containing ropinirole. Inform your physician if you are taking any other medicine containing ropinirole.
REQUIP and REQUIP XL have not been studied in children.
What is the most important information I should know about REQUIP and REQUIP XL?
REQUIP and REQUIP XL can cause serious side effects including:
- **Falling asleep during normal activities.** You may fall asleep while doing normal activities such as driving a car, doing physical tasks, or using hazardous machinery while taking REQUIP or REQUIP XL. You may suddenly fall asleep without being drowsy or without warning. This may result in having accidents. Your chances of falling asleep while doing normal activities while taking REQUIP or REQUIP XL are greater if you take other medicines that cause drowsiness. Tell your healthcare provider right away if this happens. Before starting REQUIP or REQUIP XL, be sure to tell your healthcare provider if you take any medicines that make you drowsy.

- **Changes in blood pressure.** REQUIP and REQUIP XL can decrease or increase your blood pressure. Lowering of your blood pressure is of special concern. If you faint, feel dizzy, nauseated, or sweaty when you stand up from sitting or lying down, this may mean that your blood pressure is decreased. If you notice this, you should contact your healthcare provider. Also, when changing position from lying down or sitting to standing up, you should do it carefully and slowly. Lowering of your blood pressure can happen especially when you start taking REQUIP or REQUIP XL or when your dose is increased.
- **Fainting.** Fainting can occur, and sometimes your heart rate may be decreased. This can happen especially when you start taking REQUIP or REQUIP XL or your dose is increased. Tell your healthcare provider if you faint or feel dizzy.
- **Hallucinations** (unreal visions, sounds, or sensations) can occur in patients taking REQUIP or REQUIP XL. The chances of having hallucinations are higher in patients with Parkinson's disease who are elderly, taking REQUIP or REQUIP XL with other Parkinson's disease drugs, or taking higher doses of REQUIP or REQUIP XL. If you have hallucinations, talk with your healthcare provider.
- **Uncontrolled sudden movements.** REQUIP or REQUIP XL may cause uncontrolled sudden movements or make such movements you already have worse or more frequent. Tell your healthcare provider if this happens. The doses of your anti-Parkinson's medicines may need to be changed.
Unusual urges. Some patients taking REQUIP or REQUIP XL get urges to behave in a way unusual for them. Examples of this are an unusual urge to gamble or increased sexual urges and behaviors. If you notice or your family notices that you are developing any unusual behaviors, talk to your healthcare provider.

See "What are the possible side effects of REQUIP and REQUIP XL?"

What should I tell my healthcare provider before taking REQUIP or REQUIP XL?
Be sure to tell your healthcare provider if you:
- have daytime sleepiness from a sleep disorder or have unexpected or unpredictable sleepiness or periods of sleep.
- are taking any other prescription or over-the-counter medicines. Some of these medicines may increase your chances of getting side effects while taking REQUIP or REQUIP XL.
- start or stop taking other medicines while you are taking REQUIP or REQUIP XL. This may increase your chances of getting side effects.
- start or stop smoking while you are taking REQUIP or REQUIP XL. Smoking may decrease the treatment effect of REQUIP or REQUIP XL.
- feel dizzy, nauseated, sweaty, or faint when you first stand up from sitting or lying down.
- drink alcoholic beverages. This may increase your chances of becoming drowsy or sleepy while taking REQUIP or REQUIP XL.
- have high or low blood pressure.
- are pregnant or plan to become pregnant. REQUIP and REQUIP XL should only be used during pregnancy if needed.
- are breastfeeding. It is not known if REQUIP or REQUIP XL passes into your breast milk. Talk to your healthcare provider to decide whether you will breastfeed or take REQUIP or REQUIP XL.
- are allergic to any of the ingredients in REQUIP or REQUIP XL. See the end of this Patient Information leaflet for a complete list of the ingredients in REQUIP and REQUIP XL.

How should I take REQUIP or REQUIP XL for Parkinson's disease?
- Take REQUIP or REQUIP XL exactly as directed by your healthcare provider.
- Do not suddenly stop taking REQUIP or REQUIP XL without talking to your healthcare provider. If you stop this medicine suddenly, you may develop fever, confusion, or severe muscle stiffness.
- Before starting REQUIP or REQUIP XL, you should talk to your healthcare provider about what to do if you miss a dose. If you have missed the previous dose and it is time for your next dose, **do not double the dose.**
- Your healthcare provider will start you on a low dose of REQUIP or REQUIP XL. Your healthcare provider will change the dose until you are taking the right amount of medicine to control your symptoms. **It may take several weeks before you reach a dose that controls your symptoms.**

If you are taking REQUIP:
- REQUIP tablets are usually taken 3 times each day for Parkinson's disease.

If you are taking REQUIP XL:
- Take REQUIP XL tablets 1 time each day for Parkinson's disease, preferably at or around the same time of day.
- Swallow REQUIP XL tablets whole. Do not chew, crush, or split REQUIP XL tablets.

If you are taking either REQUIP or REQUIP XL:
- Contact your healthcare provider if you stop taking REQUIP or REQUIP XL for any reason. Do not restart without talking with your healthcare provider.
- Your healthcare provider may prescribe REQUIP or REQUIP XL alone, or add REQUIP or REQUIP XL to medicine that you are already taking for Parkinson's disease.
- You should not substitute REQUIP for REQUIP XL or REQUIP XL for REQUIP without talking with your healthcare provider.
- You can take REQUIP or REQUIP XL with or without food. If you experience nausea you may try taking REQUIP or REQUIP XL with food.

What are the possible side effects of REQUIP and REQUIP XL?
Serious side effects in people taking REQUIP and REQUIP XL are described in the section "REQUIP and REQUIP XL can cause serious side effects including" and include:
- Falling asleep during normal activities
- Changes in blood pressure
- Fainting
- Hallucinations
- Uncontrolled sudden movements

Some patients taking REQUIP or REQUIP XL get urges to behave in a way unusual for them. Examples of this are an unusual urge to gamble or increased sexual urges and behaviors. If you notice or your family notices that you are developing any unusual behaviors, talk to your healthcare provider.

You should be careful until you know if REQUIP or REQUIP XL affects your ability to remain alert while doing normal daily activities, driving a car, operating machinery, or working at heights. You should also watch for the development of significant daytime sleepiness or episodes of falling asleep.

Common side effects in people taking REQUIP and REQUIP XL include:
- Fainting
- Sleepiness
- Hallucinations
- Dizziness
- Nausea or vomiting
- Uncontrolled sudden movements
- Leg swelling
- Fatigue
- Headache
- Upset stomach
- Increased sweating

This is not a complete list of side effects and should not take the place of discussions with your healthcare providers. Your healthcare provider or pharmacist can give you a more complete list of possible side effects.

Call your healthcare provider for medical advice about side effects. You may report side effects to FDA at 1-800-FDA-1088.

How should I store REQUIP and REQUIP XL?
- Store REQUIP tablets between 68°-77°F (20°-25°C).
- Store REQUIP XL tablets between 59°-86°F (15°-30°C).
- Store REQUIP or REQUIP XL at room temperature out of direct sunlight.
- Keep REQUIP or REQUIP XL in a tightly closed container.
- Keep REQUIP or REQUIP XL out of the reach of children.

Other Information about REQUIP and REQUIP XL:
- Do not share REQUIP or REQUIP XL with other people, even if they have the same symptoms you have.
- Studies of people with Parkinson's disease show that they may be at an increased risk of developing melanoma, a form of skin cancer, when compared to people without Parkinson's disease. It is not known if this problem is associated with Parkinson's disease or the medicines used to treat Parkinson's disease. REQUIP and REQUIP XL are two of the medicines used to treat Parkinson's disease; therefore, patients being treated with REQUIP or REQUIP XL should have periodic skin examinations.

This patient information leaflet summarizes the most important information about REQUIP and REQUIP XL for Parkinson's disease. Medicines are sometimes prescribed for purposes other than those listed in this leaflet. Do not take REQUIP or REQUIP XL for a condition for which it was not prescribed. For more information, talk with your healthcare provider or pharmacist. They can give you information about REQUIP and REQUIP XL that is written for healthcare professionals. For more information call 1-888-825-5249 (toll-free) or visit www.requipxl.com.

What are the ingredients in REQUIP and REQUIP XL?
The following ingredients are in REQUIP:
Active ingredient: ropinirole (as ropinirole hydrochloride)
Inactive ingredients: croscarmellose sodium, hydrous lactose, magnesium stearate, microcrystalline cellulose, and one or more of the following: carmine, FD&C Blue No. 2 aluminum lake, FD&C Yellow No. 6 aluminum lake, hypromellose, iron oxides, polyethylene glycol, polysorbate 80, titanium dioxide.

The following ingredients are in REQUIP XL:
Active ingredient: ropinirole (as ropinirole hydrochloride)
Inactive ingredients: carboxymethylcellulose sodium, colloidal silicon dioxide, glycerol behenate, hydrogenated castor oil, hypromellose, lactose monohydrate, magnesium stearate, maltodextrin, mannitol, povidone, and one or more of the following: FD&C Yellow No. 6 aluminum lake, FD&C Blue No. 2 aluminum lake, ferric oxides (black, red, yellow), polyethylene glycol 400, titanium dioxide.

PATIENT INFORMATION
REQUIP® (RE-qwip)
(ropinirole tablets)
IF YOU HAVE RESTLESS LEGS SYNDROME (RLS), READ THIS SIDE
IF YOU HAVE PARKINSON'S DISEASE, READ THE OTHER SIDE
Read this information completely before you start taking REQUIP. Read the information each time you get more medicine. There may be new information. This leaflet provides a summary about REQUIP. It does not include everything there is to know about your medicine. This information should not take the place of discussions with your healthcare provider about your medical condition or treatment with REQUIP.
Patients with RLS should take REQUIP differently than patients with Parkinson's disease (see **How should I take REQUIP for RLS?** for the recommended dosing for RLS). A lower dose of REQUIP is generally needed for patients with RLS, and is taken once daily before bedtime.

What is the most important information I should know about REQUIP?
REQUIP can cause serious side effects including:
- **Falling asleep during normal activities.** You may fall asleep while doing normal activities such as driving a car, doing physical tasks, or using hazardous machinery while taking REQUIP. You may suddenly fall asleep without being drowsy or without warning. This may result in having accidents. Your chances of falling asleep while doing normal activities while taking REQUIP are greater if you take other medicines that cause drowsiness. Tell your healthcare provider right away if this happens. Before starting REQUIP, be sure to tell your healthcare provider if you take any medicines that make you drowsy.
- **Decrease in blood pressure.** REQUIP can decrease your blood pressure. Lowering of your blood pressure is of special concern. If you faint, feel dizzy, nauseated, or sweaty when you stand up from sitting or lying down, this may mean that your blood pressure is decreased. If you notice this, you should contact your healthcare provider. Also, when changing position from lying down or sitting to standing up, you should do it carefully and slowly. Lowering of your blood pressure can happen especially when you start taking REQUIP or when your dose is increased.
- **Fainting.** Fainting can occur, and sometimes your heart rate may be decreased. This can happen especially when you start taking REQUIP or your dose is increased. Tell your healthcare provider if you faint or feel dizzy.
- **Hallucinations** (unreal visions, sounds, or sensations) can occur in patients taking REQUIP. If you have hallucinations, talk with your healthcare provider.
Unusual urges. Some patients taking REQUIP get urges to behave in a way unusual for them. Examples of this are an unusual urge to gamble or increased sexual urges and behaviors. If you notice or your family notices that you are developing any unusual behaviors, talk to your healthcare provider.

See "What are the possible side effects of REQUIP?"
What is REQUIP?
REQUIP is a prescription medicine containing ropinirole used to treat moderate-to-severe primary Restless Legs Syndrome. It is also used to treat Parkinson's disease. Having one of these conditions does not mean you have or will develop the other.
REQUIP has not been studied in children.

What should I tell my healthcare provider before taking REQUIP?
Be sure to tell your healthcare provider if you:
- have daytime sleepiness from a sleep disorder or have unexpected or unpredictable sleepiness or periods of sleep.
- are taking any other prescription or over-the-counter medicines. Some of these medicines may increase your chances of getting side effects while taking REQUIP.
- start or stop taking other medicines while you are taking REQUIP. This may increase your chances of getting side effects.
- start or stop smoking while you are taking REQUIP. Smoking may decrease the treatment effect of REQUIP.
- feel dizzy, nauseated, sweaty, or faint when you first stand up from sitting or lying down.
- drink alcoholic beverages. This may increase your chances of becoming drowsy or sleepy while taking REQUIP.
- have high or low blood pressure.
- are pregnant or plan to become pregnant. REQUIP should only be used during pregnancy if needed.

- are breastfeeding. It is not known if REQUIP passes into your breast milk. Talk to your healthcare provider to decide whether you will breastfeed or take REQUIP.
- are allergic to any of the ingredients in REQUIP. See the end of this Patient Information leaflet for a complete list of the ingredients in REQUIP.

How should I take REQUIP for RLS?

- Take REQUIP exactly as directed by your healthcare provider.
- The usual way to take REQUIP is once in the evening, 1 to 3 hours before bedtime.
- Your healthcare provider will start you on a low dose of REQUIP. Your healthcare provider may change the dose until you are taking the right amount of medicine to control your symptoms.
- **If you miss your dose, do not double your next dose.** Take only your usual dose 1 to 3 hours before your next bedtime.
- Contact your healthcare provider if you stop taking REQUIP for any reason. Do not restart without consulting your healthcare provider.
- You can take REQUIP with or without food. Taking REQUIP with food may decrease the chances of feeling nauseated.

What are the possible side effects of REQUIP?

Serious side effects in people taking REQUIP are described in the section "REQUIP can cause serious side effects including" and include:

- Falling asleep during normal activities
- Decrease in blood pressure
- Fainting
- Hallucinations

Some patients taking REQUIP get urges to behave in a way unusual for them. Examples of this are an unusual urge to gamble or increased sexual urges and behaviors. If you notice or your family notices that you are developing any unusual behaviors, talk to your healthcare provider.

You should be careful until you know if REQUIP affects your ability to remain alert while doing normal daily activities, driving a car, operating machinery, or working at heights. You should also watch for the development of significant daytime sleepiness or episodes of falling asleep.

Common side effects in people taking REQUIP include:

- Nausea or vomiting
- Sleepiness or drowsiness
- Dizziness
- Fatigue

This is not a complete list of side effects and should not take the place of discussions with your healthcare providers. Your healthcare provider or pharmacist can give you a more complete list of possible side effects.

Call your healthcare provider for medical advice about side effects. You may report side effects to FDA at 1-800-FDA-1088.

How should I store REQUIP?

- Store REQUIP tablets between 68°-77°F (20°-25°C).
- Store REQUIP at room temperature out of direct sunlight.
- Keep REQUIP in a tightly closed container.
- Keep REQUIP out of the reach of children.

Other Information about REQUIP

- Do not share REQUIP with other people, even if they have the same symptoms you have.
- Studies of people with Parkinson's disease show that they may be at an increased risk of developing melanoma, a form of skin cancer, when compared to people without Parkinson's disease. It is not known if this problem is associated with Parkinson's disease or the medicines used to treat Parkinson's disease. REQUIP is one of the medicines used to treat Parkinson's disease; therefore, patients being treated with REQUIP should have periodic skin examinations.

This patient information leaflet summarizes important information about REQUIP for Restless Legs Syndrome. Medicines are sometimes prescribed for purposes other than those listed in this leaflet. Do not take REQUIP for a condition for which it was not prescribed. For more information, talk with your healthcare provider or pharmacist. They can give you information about REQUIP that is written for healthcare providers. For more information call 1-888-825-5249 (toll-free) or visit www.requip.com.

What are the ingredients in REQUIP?

The following ingredients are in REQUIP:

Active ingredient: ropinirole (as ropinirole hydrochloride)

Inactive ingredients: croscarmellose sodium, hydrous lactose, magnesium stearate, microcrystalline cellulose, and one or more of these ingredients: carmine, FD&C Blue No. 2 aluminum lake, FD&C Yellow No. 6 aluminum lake, hypromellose, iron oxides, polyethylene glycol, polysorbate 80, titanium dioxide.

GlaxoSmithKline
Research Triangle Park, NC 27709
©2012, GlaxoSmithKline. All rights reserved.
RXL:3PIL
December 2012

ROTARIX ℞

[rōt'ə-rix]
(Rotavirus Vaccine, Live, Oral)
Oral Suspension

HIGHLIGHTS OF PRESCRIBING INFORMATION

These highlights do not include all the information needed to use ROTARIX safely and effectively. See full prescribing information for ROTARIX.

ROTARIX (Rotavirus Vaccine, Live, Oral)
Oral Suspension
Initial U.S. Approval: 2008

————RECENT MAJOR CHANGES————

Warnings and Precautions, 05/2014
Intussusception (5.5)

————INDICATIONS AND USAGE————

ROTARIX is a vaccine indicated for the prevention of rotavirus gastroenteritis caused by G1 and non-G1 types (G3, G4, and G9). ROTARIX is approved for use in infants 6 weeks to 24 weeks of age. (1)

————DOSAGE AND ADMINISTRATION————

FOR ORAL USE ONLY. (2.1)

- Each dose is 1-mL administered orally. (2.2)
- Administer first dose to infants beginning at 6 weeks of age. (2.2)
- Administer second dose after an interval of at least 4 weeks and prior to 24 weeks of age. (2.2)

————DOSAGE FORMS AND STRENGTHS————

- Vial of lyophilized vaccine to be reconstituted with a liquid diluent in a prefilled oral applicator. (3)
- Each 1-mL dose contains a suspension of at least $10^{6.0}$ median Cell Culture Infective Dose (CCID$_{50}$) of live, attenuated human G1P[8] rotavirus after reconstitution. (3)

————CONTRAINDICATIONS————

- A demonstrated history of hypersensitivity to the vaccine or any component of the vaccine. (4.1, 11)
- History of uncorrected congenital malformation of the gastrointestinal tract that would predispose the infant to intussusception. (4.2)
- History of intussusception. (4.3)
- History of Severe Combined Immunodeficiency Disease (SCID). (4.4, 4.3)

————WARNINGS AND PRECAUTIONS————

- The tip caps of the prefilled oral applicators of diluent may contain natural rubber latex which may cause allergic reactions in latex-sensitive individuals. (5.1)
- Administration of ROTARIX in infants suffering from acute diarrhea or vomiting should be delayed. Safety and effectiveness of ROTARIX in infants with chronic gastrointestinal disorders have not been evaluated. (5.2)
- Safety and effectiveness of ROTARIX in infants with known primary or secondary immunodeficiencies have not been established. (5.3)
- In a postmarketing study, cases of intussusception were observed in temporal association within 31 days following the first dose of ROTARIX, with a clustering of cases in the first 7 days. (5.5, 6.2)

————ADVERSE REACTIONS————

Common (≥5%) solicited adverse events included fussiness/irritability, cough/runny nose, fever, loss of appetite, and vomiting. (6.1)

To report SUSPECTED ADVERSE REACTIONS, contact GlaxoSmithKline at 1-888-825-5249 or VAERS at 1-800-822-7967 or www.vaers.hhs.gov.

See 17 for PATIENT COUNSELING INFORMATION and FDA-approved patient labeling

Revised: 05/2014

FULL PRESCRIBING INFORMATION

1 INDICATIONS AND USAGE

ROTARIX® is indicated for the prevention of rotavirus gastroenteritis caused by G1 and non-G1 types (G3, G4, and G9) when administered as a 2-dose series [see Clinical Studies (14.3)]. ROTARIX is approved for use in infants 6 weeks to 24 weeks of age.

2 DOSAGE AND ADMINISTRATION

2.1 Reconstitution Instructions for Oral Administration

For oral use only. Not for injection.

Reconstitute only with accompanying diluent. Do not mix ROTARIX with other vaccines or solutions.

[See table at top of next page]

2.2 Recommended Dose and Schedule

The vaccination series consists of two 1-mL doses administered **orally**. The first dose should be administered to infants beginning at 6 weeks of age. There should be an interval of at least 4 weeks between the first and second dose. The 2-dose series should be completed by 24 weeks of age. Safety and effectiveness have not been evaluated if ROTARIX were administered for the first dose and another rotavirus vaccine were administered for the second dose or vice versa.

In the event that the infant spits out or regurgitates most of the vaccine dose, a single replacement dose may be considered at the same vaccination visit.

2.3 Infant Feeding

Breast-feeding was permitted in clinical studies. There was no evidence to suggest that breast-feeding reduced the protection against rotavirus gastroenteritis afforded by ROTARIX. There are no restrictions on the infant's liquid consumption, including breast-milk, either before or after vaccination with ROTARIX.

3 DOSAGE FORMS AND STRENGTHS

ROTARIX is available as a vial of lyophilized vaccine to be reconstituted with a liquid diluent in a prefilled oral applicator.

Each 1-mL dose contains a suspension of at least $10^{6.0}$ median Cell Culture Infective Dose (CCID$_{50}$) of live, attenuated human G1P[8] rotavirus after reconstitution.

4 CONTRAINDICATIONS

4.1 Hypersensitivity

A demonstrated history of hypersensitivity to any component of the vaccine.

Infants who develop symptoms suggestive of hypersensitivity after receiving a dose of ROTARIX should not receive further doses of ROTARIX.

4.2 Gastrointestinal Tract Congenital Malformation

Infants with a history of uncorrected congenital malformation of the gastrointestinal tract (such as Meckel's diverticulum) that would predispose the infant for intussusception should not receive ROTARIX.

4.3 History of Intussusception

Infants with a history of intussusception should not receive ROTARIX [see Warnings and Precautions (5.5)]. In postmarketing experience, intussusception resulting in death following a second dose has been reported following a history of intussusception after the first dose [see Adverse Reactions (6.2)].

4.4 Severe Combined Immunodeficiency Disease

Infants with Severe Combined Immunodeficiency Disease (SCID) should not receive ROTARIX. Postmarketing reports of gastroenteritis, including severe diarrhea and prolonged shedding of vaccine virus, have been reported in infants who were administered live, oral rotavirus vaccines and later identified as having SCID [see Adverse Reactions (6.2)].

5 WARNINGS AND PRECAUTIONS

5.1 Latex

The tip caps of the prefilled oral applicators of diluent may contain natural rubber latex which may cause allergic reactions in latex-sensitive individuals.

5.2 Gastrointestinal Disorders

Administration of ROTARIX should be delayed in infants suffering from acute diarrhea or vomiting.

Safety and effectiveness of ROTARIX in infants with chronic gastrointestinal disorders have not been evaluated. [See Contraindications (4.2).]

5.3 Altered Immunocompetence

Safety and effectiveness of ROTARIX in infants with known primary or secondary immunodeficiencies, including infants with human immunodeficiency virus (HIV), infants on immunosuppressive therapy, or infants with malignant neoplasms affecting the bone marrow or lymphatic system have not been established.

5.4 Shedding and Transmission

Rotavirus shedding in stool occurs after vaccination with peak excretion occurring around day 7 after dose 1.

One clinical trial demonstrated that vaccinees transmit vaccine virus to healthy seronegative contacts [see Clinical Pharmacology (12.2)].

The potential for transmission of vaccine virus following vaccination should be weighed against the possibility of acquiring and transmitting natural rotavirus. Caution is advised when considering whether to administer ROTARIX to individuals with immunodeficient close contacts, such as individuals with malignancies, primary immunodeficiency or receiving immunosuppressive therapy.

5.5 Intussusception

Following administration of a previously licensed oral live rhesus rotavirus-based vaccine, an increased risk of intussusception was observed.[1] The risk of intussusception with ROTARIX was evaluated in a pre-licensure randomized, placebo-controlled safety study (including 63,225 infants) conducted in Latin America and Finland. No increased risk of intussusception was observed in this clinical trial following administration of ROTARIX when compared with placebo. [See Adverse Reactions (6.1).]

In a postmarketing, observational study conducted in Mexico, cases of intussusception were observed in temporal association within 31 days following the first dose of ROTARIX, with a clustering of cases in the first 7 days. [See Adverse Reactions (6.2).]

Other postmarketing observational studies conducted in Brazil and Australia also suggest an increased risk of intussusception within the first 7 days following the second dose of ROTARIX.[2,3] [See Adverse Reactions (6.2).]

In worldwide passive postmarketing surveillance, cases of intussusception have been reported in temporal association with ROTARIX [see Adverse Reactions (6.2)].

5.6 Post-Exposure Prophylaxis

Safety and effectiveness of ROTARIX when administered after exposure to rotavirus have not been evaluated.

6 ADVERSE REACTIONS

6.1 Clinical Trials Experience

Because clinical trials are conducted under widely varying conditions, adverse reaction rates observed in the clinical trials of a vaccine cannot be directly compared to rates in the clinical trials of another vaccine, and may not reflect the rates observed in practice. As with any vaccine, there is the possibility that broad use of ROTARIX could reveal adverse reactions not observed in clinical trials.

Solicited and unsolicited adverse events, serious adverse events and cases of intussusception were collected in 7 clinical studies. Cases of intussusception and serious adverse events were collected in an additional large safety study. These 8 clinical studies evaluated a total of 71,209 infants who received ROTARIX (N = 36,755) or placebo (N = 34,454). The racial distribution for these studies was as follows: Hispanic 73.4%, white 16.2%, black 1.0%, and other 9.4%; 51% were male.

Solicited Adverse Events: In 7 clinical studies, detailed safety information was collected by parents/guardians for 8 consecutive days following vaccination with ROTARIX (i.e., day of vaccination and the next 7 days). A diary card was completed to record fussiness/irritability, cough/runny nose, the infant's temperature, loss of appetite, vomiting, or diarrhea on a daily basis during the first week following each

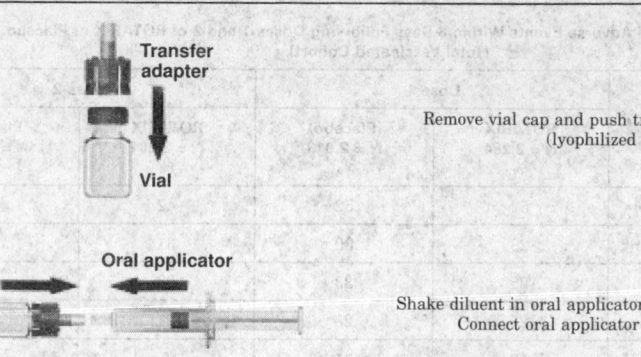

Remove vial cap and push transfer adapter onto vial (lyophilized vaccine).

Shake diluent in oral applicator (white, turbid suspension). Connect oral applicator to transfer adapter.

Push plunger of oral applicator to transfer diluent into vial. Suspension will appear white and turbid.

Withdraw vaccine into oral applicator.

Twist and remove the oral applicator.

Do not use a needle with ROTARIX. Not for injection.

Ready for **oral** administration.

dose of ROTARIX or placebo. Adverse events among recipients of ROTARIX and placebo occurred at similar rates (Table 1).

[See table 1 at top of next page]

Unsolicited Adverse Events: Infants were monitored for unsolicited serious and non-serious adverse events that occurred in the 31-day period following vaccination in 7 clinical studies. The following adverse events occurred at a statistically higher incidence (95% Confidence Interval [CI] of Relative Risk excluding 1) among recipients of ROTARIX (N = 5,082) as compared with placebo recipients (N = 2,902): irritability (ROTARIX 11.4%, placebo 8.7%) and flatulence (ROTARIX 2.2%, placebo 1.3%).

Serious Adverse Events (SAEs): Infants were monitored for serious adverse events that occurred in the 31-day period following vaccination in 8 clinical studies. Serious adverse events occurred in 1.7% of recipients of ROTARIX (N = 36,755) as compared with 1.9% of placebo recipients (N = 34,454). Among placebo recipients, diarrhea (placebo 0.07%, ROTARIX 0.02%), dehydration (placebo 0.06%, ROTARIX 0.02%), and gastroenteritis (placebo 0.3%, ROTARIX 0.2%) occurred at a statistically higher incidence (95% CI of Relative Risk excluding 1) as compared with recipients of ROTARIX.

Deaths: During the entire course of 8 clinical studies, there were 68 (0.19%) deaths following administration of

ROTARIX (N = 36,755) and 50 (0.15%) deaths following placebo administration (N = 34,454). The most commonly reported cause of death following vaccination was pneumonia, which was observed in 19 (0.05%) recipients of ROTARIX and 10 (0.03%) placebo recipients (Relative Risk: 1.74, 95% CI: 0.76, 4.23).

Intussusception: In a controlled safety study conducted in Latin America and Finland, the risk of intussusception was evaluated in 63,225 infants (31,673 received ROTARIX and 31,552 received placebo). Infants were monitored by active surveillance including independent, complementary methods (prospective hospital surveillance and parent reporting at scheduled study visits) to identify potential cases of intussusception within 31 days after vaccination and, in a subset of 20,169 infants (10,159 received ROTARIX and 10,010 received placebo), up to one year after the first dose. No increased risk of intussusception following administration of ROTARIX was observed within a 31-day period following any dose, and rates were comparable to the placebo group after a median of 100 days (Table 2). In a subset of 20,169 infants (10,159 received ROTARIX and 10,010 received placebo) followed up to one year after dose 1, there were 4 cases of intussusception with ROTARIX compared with 14 cases of intussusception with placebo [Relative Risk: 0.28 (95% CI: 0.10, 0.81)]. All of the infants who developed intussusception recovered without sequelae.

Table 1. Solicited Adverse Events Within 8 Days Following Doses 1 and 2 of ROTARIX or Placebo (Total Vaccinated Cohort)

	Dose 1		Dose 2	
	ROTARIX N = 3,284 %	Placebo N = 2,013 %	ROTARIX N = 3,201 %	Placebo N = 1,973 %
Fussiness/irritability[a]	52	52	42	42
Cough/runny nose[b]	28	30	31	33
Fever[c]	25	33	28	34
Loss of appetite[d]	25	25	21	21
Vomiting	13	11	8	8
Diarrhea	4	3	3	3

Total vaccinated cohort = all vaccinated infants for whom safety data were available.
N = number of infants for whom at least one symptom sheet was completed.
[a]Defined as crying more than usual.
[b]Data not collected in 1 of 7 studies; Dose 1: ROTARIX N = 2,583; placebo N = 1,897; Dose 2: ROTARIX N = 2,522; placebo N = 1,863.
[c]Defined as temperature ≥100.4°F (≥38.0°C) rectally or ≥99.5°F (≥37.5°C) orally.
[d]Defined as eating less than usual.

Table 3. Intussusception Cases by Day Range in Relation to Dose

Day Range	Dose 1		Dose 2		Any Dose	
	ROTARIX N = 31,673	Placebo N = 31,552	ROTARIX N = 29,616	Placebo N = 29,465	ROTARIX N = 31,673	Placebo N = 31,552
0-7	0	0	2	0	2	0
8-14	0	0	0	2	0	2
15-21	1	1	2	1	3	2
22-30	0	1	1	2	1	3
Total (0-30)	1	2	5	5	6	7

Table 2. Intussusception and Relative Risk With ROTARIX Compared With Placebo

Confirmed Cases of Intussusception	ROTARIX N = 31,673	Placebo N = 31,552
Within 31 days following diagnosis after any dose	6	7
Relative Risk (95% CI)	0.85 (0.30, 2.42)	
Within 100 days following dose 1[a]	9	16
Relative Risk (95% CI)	0.56 (0.25, 1.24)	

CI = Confidence Interval.
[a]Median duration after dose 1 (follow-up visit at 30 to 90 days after dose 2).

Among vaccine recipients, there were no confirmed cases of intussusception within the 0- to 14-day period after the first dose (Table 3), which was the period of highest risk for the previously licensed oral live rhesus rotavirus-based vaccine.[1]
[See tables 2 and 3 above]
Kawasaki Disease: Kawasaki disease has been reported in 18 (0.035%) recipients of ROTARIX and 9 (0.021%) placebo recipients from 16 completed or ongoing clinical trials. Of the 27 cases, 5 occurred following ROTARIX in clinical trials that were either not placebo-controlled or 1:1 randomized. In placebo-controlled trials, Kawasaki disease was reported in 17 recipients of ROTARIX and 9 placebo recipients [Relative Risk: 1.71 (95% CI: 0.71, 4.38)]. Three of the 27 cases were reported within 30 days post-vaccination: 2 cases (ROTARIX = 1, placebo = 1) were from placebo-controlled trials [Relative Risk: 1.00 (95% CI: 0.01, 78.35)] and one case following ROTARIX was from a non-placebo-controlled trial. Among recipients of ROTARIX, the time of onset after study dose ranged 3 days to 19 months.

6.2   Postmarketing Experience
The temporal association between vaccination with ROTARIX and intussusception was evaluated in a hospital-based active surveillance study that identified infants with intussusception at participating hospitals in Mexico. Using a self-controlled case series method,[4] the incidence of intus-

susception during the first 7 days after receipt of ROTARIX and during the 31-day period after receipt of ROTARIX was compared to a control period. The control period was from birth to one year, excluding the pre-defined risk period (first 7 days or first 31 days post-vaccination, respectively).
Over a 2-year period, the participating hospitals provided health services to approximately 1 million infants under 1 year of age. Among 750 infants with intussusception, the relative incidence of intussusception in the 31-day period after the first dose of ROTARIX compared to the control period was 1.96 (95.5% CI: 1.46, 2.63)]; the relative incidence of intussusception in the first 7 days after the first dose of ROTARIX compared to the control period was 6.07 (95.5% CI: 4.20, 8.63).
The Mexico study did not take into account all medical conditions that may predispose infants to intussusception. The results may not be generalizable to US infants who have a lower background rate of intussusception than Mexican infants. However, if a temporal increase in the risk for intussusception following ROTARIX similar in magnitude to that observed in the Mexico study does exist in US infants, it is estimated that approximately 1 to 3 additional cases of intussusception hospitalizations would occur per 100,000 vaccinated infants in the US within 7 days following the first dose of ROTARIX. In the first year of life, the background rate of intussusception hospitalizations in the US has been estimated to be approximately 34 per 100,000 infants.[5]
Other postmarketing observational studies conducted in Brazil and Australia also suggest an increased risk of intussusception within the first 7 days following the second dose of ROTARIX.[2,3]
Worldwide passive postmarketing surveillance data suggest that most cases of intussusception reported following ROTARIX occur in the 7-day period after the first dose.
The following adverse events have been reported since marketed introduction of ROTARIX. Because these events are reported voluntarily from a population of uncertain size, it is not always possible to reliably estimate their frequency or establish a causal relationship to vaccination with ROTARIX.
Gastrointestinal Disorders: Intussusception (including death), recurrent intussusception (including death), hematochezia, gastroenteritis with vaccine viral shedding in infants with Severe Combined Immunodeficiency Disease (SCID).
Blood and Lymphatic System Disorders: Idiopathic thrombocytopenic purpura.

Vascular Disorders: Kawasaki disease.
General Disorders and Administration Site Conditions: Maladministration.

7   DRUG INTERACTIONS
7.1   Concomitant Vaccine Administration
In clinical trials, ROTARIX was administered concomitantly with US-licensed and non-US-licensed vaccines. In a US coadministration study in 484 infants, there was no evidence of interference in the immune responses to any of the antigens when PEDIARIX® [Diphtheria and Tetanus Toxoids and Acellular Pertussis Adsorbed, Hepatitis B (Recombinant) and Inactivated Poliovirus Vaccine], a US-licensed 7-valent pneumococcal conjugate vaccine (Wyeth Pharmaceuticals Inc.), and a US-licensed Hib conjugate vaccine (Sanofi Pasteur SA) were coadministered with ROTARIX as compared with separate administration of ROTARIX.
7.2   Immunosuppressive Therapies
Immunosuppressive therapies, including irradiation, antimetabolites, alkylating agents, cytotoxic drugs, and corticosteroids (used in greater than physiologic doses), may reduce the immune response to ROTARIX. [See Warnings and Precautions (5.3).]

8   USE IN SPECIFIC POPULATIONS
8.1   Pregnancy
Pregnancy Category C
Animal reproduction studies have not been conducted with ROTARIX. It is also not known whether ROTARIX can cause fetal harm when administered to a pregnant woman or can affect reproduction capacity.
8.4   Pediatric Use
Safety and effectiveness of ROTARIX in infants younger than 6 weeks or older than 24 weeks of age have not been evaluated.
The effectiveness of ROTARIX in pre-term infants has not been established. Safety data are available in pre-term infants (ROTARIX = 134, placebo = 120) with a reported gestational age ≤36 weeks. These pre-term infants were followed for serious adverse events up to 30 to 90 days after dose 2. Serious adverse events were observed in 5.2% of recipients of ROTARIX as compared with 5.0% of placebo recipients. No deaths or cases of intussusception were reported in this population.

11   DESCRIPTION
ROTARIX (Rotavirus Vaccine, Live, Oral), for oral administration, is a live, attenuated rotavirus vaccine derived from the human 89-12 strain which belongs to G1P[8] type. The rotavirus strain is propagated on Vero cells. After reconstitution, the final formulation (1 mL) contains at least $10^{6.0}$ median Cell Culture Infective Dose ($CCID_{50}$) of live, attenuated rotavirus.
The lyophilized vaccine contains amino acids, dextran, Dulbecco's Modified Eagle Medium (DMEM), sorbitol, and sucrose. DMEM contains the following ingredients: sodium chloride, potassium chloride, magnesium sulfate, ferric (III) nitrate, sodium phosphate, sodium pyruvate, D-glucose, concentrated vitamin solution, L-cystine, L-tyrosine, amino acids solution, L-glutamine, calcium chloride, sodium hydrogenocarbonate, and phenol red.
In the manufacturing process, porcine-derived materials are used. Porcine circovirus type 1 (PCV-1) is present in ROTARIX. PCV-1 is not known to cause disease in humans. The liquid diluent contains calcium carbonate, sterile water, and xanthan. The diluent includes an antacid component (calcium carbonate) to protect the vaccine during passage through the stomach and prevent its inactivation due to the acidic environment of the stomach.
ROTARIX is available in single-dose vials of lyophilized vaccine, accompanied by a prefilled oral applicator of liquid diluent [see How Supplied/Storage and Handling (16)]. The tip caps of the prefilled oral applicators may contain natural rubber the vial stoppers are not made with natural rubber latex.
ROTARIX contains no preservatives.

12   CLINICAL PHARMACOLOGY
12.1   Mechanism of Action
Prior to rotavirus vaccination programs, rotavirus infected nearly all children by the time they were 5 years of age. Severe, dehydrating rotavirus gastroenteritis occurs primarily among children aged 3 to 35 months.[6] Among children up to 3 years of age, approximately 16% of cases before 6 months of age result in hospitalization.[7]
The exact immunologic mechanism by which ROTARIX protects against rotavirus gastroenteritis is unknown [see Clinical Pharmacology (12.2)]. ROTARIX contains a live, attenuated human rotavirus that replicates in the small intestine and induces immunity.
12.2   Pharmacodynamics
Immunogenicity: A relationship between antibody responses to rotavirus vaccination and protection against rotavirus gastroenteritis has not been established. Seroconversion was defined as the appearance of anti-rotavirus IgA

antibodies (concentration ≥20 U/mL) post-vaccination in the serum of infants previously negative for rotavirus. In 2 safety and efficacy studies, one to two months after a 2-dose series, 86.5% of 787 recipients of ROTARIX seroconverted compared with 6.7% of 420 placebo recipients and 76.8% of 393 recipients of ROTARIX seroconverted compared with 9.7% of 341 placebo recipients, respectively.

Shedding and Transmission: A prospective, randomized, double-blind, placebo-controlled study was performed in the Dominican Republic in twins within the same household to assess whether transmission of vaccine virus occurs from a vaccinated infant to a non-vaccinated infant. One hundred pairs of healthy twins 6 to 14 weeks of age (gestational age ≥32 weeks) were randomized with one twin to receive ROTARIX (N = 100) and the other twin to receive placebo (N = 100). Twenty subjects in each arm were excluded for reasons such as having rotavirus antibody at baseline. Stool samples were collected on the day of or 1 day prior to each dose, as well as 3 times weekly for 6 consecutive weeks after each dose of ROTARIX or placebo. Transmission was defined as presence of the vaccine virus strain in any stool sample from a twin receiving placebo.

Transmitted vaccine virus was identified in 15 of 80 twins receiving placebo (18.8% [95% CI: 10.9, 29.0]). Median duration of the rotavirus shedding was 10 days in twins who received ROTARIX as compared to 4 days in twins who received placebo in whom the vaccine virus was transmitted. In the 15 twins who received placebo, no gastrointestinal symptoms related to transmitted vaccine virus were observed.

13 NONCLINICAL TOXICOLOGY

13.1 Carcinogenesis, Mutagenesis, Impairment of Fertility

ROTARIX has not been evaluated for carcinogenic or mutagenic potential, or for impairment of fertility.

14 CLINICAL STUDIES

14.1 Efficacy Studies

The data demonstrating the efficacy of ROTARIX in preventing rotavirus gastroenteritis come from 24,163 infants randomized in two placebo-controlled studies conducted in 17 countries in Europe and Latin America. In these studies, oral polio vaccine (OPV) was not coadministered; however, other routine childhood vaccines could be concomitantly administered. Breast-feeding was permitted in both studies.

A randomized, double-blind, placebo-controlled study was conducted in 6 European countries. A total of 3,994 infants were enrolled to receive ROTARIX (n = 2,646) or placebo (n = 1,348). Vaccine or placebo was given to healthy infants as a 2-dose series with the first dose administered orally from 6 through 14 weeks of age followed by one additional dose administered at least 4 weeks after the first dose. The 2-dose series was completed by 24 weeks of age. For both vaccination groups, 98.3% of infants were white and 53% were male.

The clinical case definition of rotavirus gastroenteritis was an episode of diarrhea (passage of 3 or more loose or watery stools within a day), with or without vomiting, where rotavirus was identified in a stool sample. Severity of gastroenteritis was determined by a clinical scoring system, the Vesikari scale, assessing the duration and intensity of diarrhea and vomiting, the intensity of fever, use of rehydration therapy or hospitalization for each episode. Scores range from 0 to 20, where higher scores indicate greater severity. An episode of gastroenteritis with a score of 11 or greater was considered severe.[8]

The primary efficacy endpoint was prevention of any grade of severity of rotavirus gastroenteritis caused by naturally occurring rotavirus from 2 weeks after the second dose through one rotavirus season (according to protocol, ATP). Other efficacy evaluations included prevention of severe rotavirus gastroenteritis, as defined by the Vesikari scale, and reductions in hospitalizations due to rotavirus gastroenteritis and all cause gastroenteritis regardless of presumed etiology. Analyses were also done to evaluate the efficacy of ROTARIX against rotavirus gastroenteritis among infants who received at least one vaccination (total vaccinated cohort, TVC).

Efficacy of ROTARIX against any grade of severity of rotavirus gastroenteritis through one rotavirus season was 87.1% (95% CI: 79.6, 92.1); TVC efficacy was 87.3% (95% CI: 80.3, 92.0). Efficacy against severe rotavirus gastroenteritis through one rotavirus season was 95.8% (95% CI: 89.6, 98.7); TVC efficacy was 96.0% (95% CI: 90.2, 98.8) (Table 4). The protective effect of ROTARIX against any grade of severity of rotavirus gastroenteritis observed immediately following dose 1 administration and prior to dose 2 was 89.8% (95% CI: 8.9, 99.8).

Efficacy of ROTARIX in reducing hospitalizations for rotavirus gastroenteritis through one rotavirus season was 100% (95% CI: 81.8, 100); TVC efficacy was 100% (95% CI: 81.7, 100) (Table 4). ROTARIX reduced hospitalizations for all cause gastroenteritis regardless of presumed etiology by 74.7% (95% CI: 45.5, 88.9).

[See table 4 above]

A randomized, double-blind, placebo-controlled study was conducted in 11 countries in Latin America and Finland. A total of 63,225 infants received ROTARIX (n = 31,673) or placebo (n = 31,552). An efficacy subset of these infants consisting of 20,169 infants from Latin America received ROTARIX (n = 10,159) or placebo (n = 10,010). Vaccine or placebo was given to healthy infants as a 2-dose series with the first dose administered orally from 6 through 13 weeks of age followed by one additional dose administered at least 4 weeks after the first dose. The 2-dose series was completed by the age of 24 weeks of age. For both vaccination groups, the racial distribution of the efficacy subset was as follows: Hispanic 85.8%, white 7.9%, black 1.1%, and other 5.2%; 51% were male.

The clinical case definition of severe rotavirus gastroenteritis was an episode of diarrhea (passage of 3 or more loose or watery stools within a day), with or without vomiting, where rotavirus was identified in a stool sample, requiring hospitalization and/or rehydration therapy equivalent to World Health Organization (WHO) plan B (oral rehydration therapy) or plan C (intravenous rehydration therapy) in a medical facility.

The primary efficacy endpoint was prevention of severe rotavirus gastroenteritis caused by naturally occurring rotavirus from 2 weeks after the second dose through one year (ATP). Analyses were done to evaluate the efficacy of ROTARIX against severe rotavirus gastroenteritis among infants who received at least one vaccination (TVC). Reduction in hospitalizations due to rotavirus gastroenteritis was also evaluated (ATP).

Efficacy of ROTARIX against severe rotavirus gastroenteritis through one year was 84.7% (95% CI: 71.7, 92.4); TVC efficacy was 81.1% (95% CI: 68.5, 89.3) (Table 5). Efficacy of ROTARIX in reducing hospitalizations for rotavirus gastroenteritis through one year was 85.0% (95% CI: 69.6, 93.5); TVC efficacy was 80.8% (95% CI: 65.7, 90.0) (Table 5).

[See table 5 above]

14.2 Efficacy Through Two Rotavirus Seasons

The efficacy of ROTARIX persisting through two rotavirus seasons was evaluated in two studies.

In the European study, the efficacy of ROTARIX against any grade of severity of rotavirus gastroenteritis through two rotavirus seasons was 78.9% (95% CI: 72.7, 83.8). Efficacy in preventing any grade of severity of rotavirus gastroenteritis cases occurring only during the second season post-vaccination was 71.9% (95% CI: 61.2, 79.8). The efficacy of ROTARIX against severe rotavirus gastroenteritis through two rotavirus seasons was 90.4% (95% CI: 85.1, 94.1). Efficacy in preventing severe rotavirus gastroenteritis cases occurring only during the second season post-vaccination was 85.6% (95% CI: 75.8, 91.9).

The efficacy of ROTARIX in reducing hospitalizations for rotavirus gastroenteritis through two rotavirus seasons was 96.0% (95% CI: 83.8, 99.5).

In the Latin American study, the efficacy of ROTARIX against severe rotavirus gastroenteritis through two years was 80.5% (95% CI: 71.3, 87.1). Efficacy in preventing severe rotavirus gastroenteritis cases occurring only during the second year post-vaccination was 79.0% (95% CI: 66.4, 87.4). The efficacy of ROTARIX in reducing hospitalizations for rotavirus gastroenteritis through two years was 83.0% (95% CI: 73.1, 89.7).

The efficacy of ROTARIX beyond the second season post-vaccination was not evaluated.

14.3 Efficacy Against Specific Rotavirus Types

The type-specific efficacy against any grade of severity and severe rotavirus gastroenteritis caused by G1P[8], G3P[8], G4P[8], G9P[8], and combined non-G1 (G2, G3, G4, G9) types was statistically significant through one year. Additionally, type-specific efficacy against any grade of severity and severe rotavirus gastroenteritis caused by G1P[8], G2P[4], G3P[8], G4P[8], G9P[8], and combined non-G1 (G2, G3, G4, G9) types was statistically significant through two years (Table 6).

Table 4. Efficacy Evaluation of ROTARIX Through One Rotavirus Season

Infants in Cohort	According to Protocol[a]		Total Vaccinated Cohort[b]	
	ROTARIX N = 2,572	Placebo N = 1,302	ROTARIX N = 2,646	Placebo N = 1,348
Gastroenteritis cases				
Any severity	24	94	26	104
Severe[c]	5	60	5	64
Efficacy estimate against RV GE				
Any severity	87.1%[d]		87.3%[d]	
(95% CI)	(79.6, 92.1)		(80.3, 92.0)	
Severe[c]	95.8%[d]		96.0%[d]	
(95% CI)	(89.6, 98.7)		(90.2, 98.8)	
Cases of hospitalization due to RV GE	0	12	0	12
Efficacy in reducing hospitalizations due to RV GE	100%[d]		100%[d]	
(95% CI)	(81.8, 100)		(81.7, 100)	

RV GE = rotavirus gastroenteritis; CI = Confidence Interval.
[a]ATP analysis includes all infants in the efficacy cohort who received two doses of vaccine according to randomization.
[b]TVC analysis includes all infants in the efficacy cohort who received at least one dose of vaccine or placebo.
[c]Severe gastroenteritis defined as ≥11 on the Vesikari scale.
[d]Statistically significant vs. placebo (P <0.001).

Table 5. Efficacy Evaluation of ROTARIX Through One Year

Infants in Cohort	According to Protocol[a]		Total Vaccinated Cohort[b]	
	ROTARIX N = 9,009	Placebo N = 8,858	ROTARIX N = 10,159	Placebo N = 10,010
Gastroenteritis cases				
Severe	12	77	18	94
Efficacy estimate against RV GE				
Severe	84.7%[c]		81.1%[c]	
(95% CI)	(71.7, 92.4)		(68.5, 89.3)	
Cases of hospitalization due to RV GE	9	59	14	72
Efficacy in reducing hospitalizations due to RV GE	85.0%[c]		80.8%[c]	
(95% CI)	(69.6, 93.5)		(65.7, 90.0)	

RV GE = rotavirus gastroenteritis; CI = Confidence Interval.
[a]ATP analysis includes all infants in the efficacy cohort who received two doses of vaccine according to randomization.
[b]TVC analysis includes all infants in the efficacy cohort who received at least one dose of vaccine or placebo.
[c]Statistically significant vs. placebo (P <0.001).

Table 6. Type-Specific Efficacy of ROTARIX Against Any Grade of Severity and Severe Rotavirus Gastroenteritis (According to Protocol)

Type Identified[a]	Through One Rotavirus Season			Through Two Rotavirus Seasons		
	Number of Cases			Number of Cases		
	ROTARIX N = 2,572	Placebo N = 1,302	% Efficacy (95% CI)	ROTARIX N = 2,572	Placebo N = 1,302	% Efficacy (95% CI)
ANY GRADE OF SEVERITY						
G1P[8]	4	46	95.6%[b] (87.9, 98.8)	18	89[c,d]	89.8%[b] (82.9, 94.2)
G2P[4]	3	4[c]	NS	14	17[c]	58.3%[b] (10.1, 81.0)
G3P[8]	1	5	89.9%[b] (9.5, 99.8)	3	10	84.8%[b] (41.0, 97.3)
G4P[8]	3	13	88.3%[b] (57.5, 97.9)	6	18	83.1%[b] (55.6, 94.5)
G9P[8]	13	27	75.6%[b] (51.1, 88.5)	38	71[d]	72.9%[b] (59.3, 82.2)
Combined non-G1 (G2, G3, G4, G9, G12) types[e]	20	49	79.3%[b] (64.6, 88.4)	62	116	72.9%[b] (62.9, 80.5)
SEVERE						
G1P[8]	2	28	96.4%[b] (85.7, 99.6)	4	57	96.4%[b] (90.4, 99.1)
G2P[4]	1	2[c]	NS	2	7[c]	85.5%[b] (24.0, 98.5)
G3P[8]	0	5	100%[b] (44.8, 100)	1	8	93.7%[b] (52.8, 99.9)
G4P[8]	0	7	100%[b] (64.9, 100)	1	11	95.4%[b] (68.3, 99.9)
G9P[8]	2	19	94.7%[b] (77.9, 99.4)	13	44[d]	85.0%[b] (71.7, 92.6)
Combined non-G1 (G2, G3, G4, G9, G12) types[e]	3	33	95.4%[b] (85.3, 99.1)	17	70	87.7%[b] (78.9, 93.2)

CI = Confidence Interval; NS = Not significant.
[a]Statistical analyses done by G type; if more than one rotavirus type was detected from a rotavirus gastroenteritis episode, the episode was counted in each of the detected rotavirus type categories.
[b]Statistically significant vs. placebo (P <0.05).
[c]The P genotype was not typeable for one episode.
[d]P[8] genotype was not detected in one episode.
[e]Two cases of G12P[8] were isolated in the second season (one in each group).

[See table 6 above]

15 REFERENCES

1. Murphy TV, Gargiullo PM, Massoudi MS, et al. Intussusception among infants given an oral rotavirus vaccine. *N Engl J Med* 2001;344:564–572.
2. Carlin JB, Macartney KK, Lee KJ, et al. Intussusception Risk and Disease Prevention Associated with Rotavirus Vaccines in Australia's National Immunization Program. *CID* 2013;57(10):1427-1434.
3. Patel MM, López-Collada VR, Bulhões MM, et al. Intussusception Risk and Health Benefits of Rotavirus Vaccination in Mexico and Brazil. *N Engl J Med* 2011;364: 2283-2292.
4. Farrington CP, Whitaker HJ, Hocine MN, et al. Case series analysis for censored, perturbed, or curtailed post-event exposures. *Biostatistics* 2009;10(1):3–16.
5. Tate JE, Simonsen L, Viboud C, et al. Trends in intussusception hospitalizations among US infants, 1993–2004: implications for monitoring the safety of the new rotavirus vaccination program. *Pediatrics* 2008;121:e1125-e1132.
6. Centers for Disease Control and Prevention. Prevention of rotavirus gastroenteritis among infants and children. Recommendations of the Advisory Committee on Immunization Practices (ACIP). *MMWR* 2006;55(No. RR-12): 1-13.
7. Parashar UD, Holman RC, Clarke MJ, et al. Hospitalizations associated with rotavirus diarrhea in the United States, 1993 through 1995: surveillance based on the new ICD-9-CM rotavirus-specific diagnostic code. *J Infect Dis* 1998;177:13-17.
8. Ruuska T, Vesikari T. Rotavirus disease in Finnish children: use of numerical scores for severity of diarrheal episodes. *Scand J Infect Dis* 1990;22:259-267.

16 HOW SUPPLIED/STORAGE AND HANDLING

ROTARIX is available in single-dose vials of lyophilized vaccine, accompanied by a prefilled oral applicator of liquid diluent (1 mL) with a plunger stopper, and a transfer adapter for reconstitution.

Supplied as an outer package of 10 doses (NDC 58160-854-52) containing:

NDC 58160-851-01 vial of lyophilized vaccine in package of 10: NDC 58160-851-10

NDC 58160-853-02 oral applicator of diluent (10 applicators)

16.1 Storage Before Reconstitution

- Vials: Store the vials of lyophilized ROTARIX refrigerated at 2° to 8°C (36° to 46°F). **Protect vials from light.**
- Diluent: The diluent may be stored at a controlled room temperature 20° to 25°C (68° to 77°F). **Do not freeze. Discard if the diluent has been frozen.**

16.2 Storage After Reconstitution

ROTARIX should be administered within 24 hours of reconstitution. It may be stored refrigerated at 2° to 8°C (36° to 46°F) or at room temperature up to 25°C (77°F), after reconstitution. Discard the reconstituted vaccine if not used within 24 hours in biological waste container. **Do not freeze. Discard if the vaccine has been frozen.**

17 PATIENT COUNSELING INFORMATION

See FDA-approved patient labeling (Patient Information). Patient labeling is provided as a tear-off leaflet at the end of this full prescribing information.

- Parents or guardians should be informed by the healthcare provider of the potential benefits and risks of immunization with ROTARIX, and of the importance of completing the immunization series.
- The healthcare provider should inform the parents or guardians about the potential for adverse reactions that have been temporally associated with administration of ROTARIX or other vaccines containing similar components.
- The parent or guardian should immediately report any signs and/or symptoms of intussusception.
- The parent or guardian should be given the Vaccine Information Statements, which are required by the National Childhood Vaccine Injury Act of 1986 to be given prior to immunization. These materials are available free of charge at the Centers for Disease Control and Prevention (CDC) website (www.cdc.gov/vaccines).

ROTARIX and PEDIARIX are registered trademarks of the GSK group of companies.
Manufactured by GlaxoSmithKline Biologicals
Rixensart, Belgium, US License 1617
Distributed by **GlaxoSmithKline**
Research Triangle Park, NC 27709
©2014, the GSK group of companies. All rights reserved.
RTX:14PI

PATIENT INFORMATION
ROTARIX® (ROW-tah-rix)
Rotavirus Vaccine, Live, Oral
Read this Patient Information carefully before your baby gets ROTARIX and before your baby receives the next dose of ROTARIX. This leaflet is a summary of information about ROTARIX and does not take the place of talking with your baby's doctor.

What is ROTARIX?
ROTARIX is a vaccine that protects your baby from a kind of virus (called a rotavirus) that can cause bad diarrhea and vomiting. Rotavirus can cause diarrhea and vomiting that is so bad that your baby can lose too much body fluid and need to go to the hospital.
Rotavirus vaccine is a liquid that is given to your baby by mouth. It is not a shot.

Who should not take ROTARIX?
Your baby should not get ROTARIX if:
- He or she has had an allergic reaction after getting a dose of ROTARIX.
- He or she is allergic to any of the ingredients of this vaccine. A list of ingredients can be found at the end of this leaflet.
- A doctor has told you that your baby's digestive system has a defect (is not normal).
- He or she has a history of a serious problem called intussusception that happens when a part of the intestine gets blocked or twisted.
- He or she has Severe Combined Immunodeficiency Disease (SCID), a severe problem with his/her immune system.

Tell your doctor if your baby:
- Is allergic to latex.
- Has problems with his/her immune system.
- Has cancer.
- Will be in close contact with someone who has problems with his/her immune system or is getting treated for cancer as the spread of vaccine virus to non-vaccinated contacts could occur. Hand washing is recommended after diaper changes to help prevent the spread of vaccine virus. If your baby has been having diarrhea and vomiting, your doctor may want to wait before giving your baby a dose of ROTARIX.

What are possible side effects of ROTARIX?
The most common side effects of ROTARIX are:
- Crying
- Fussiness
- Cough
- Runny nose
- Fever
- Loss of appetite
- Vomiting.

Call your doctor right away or go to the emergency department if your baby has any of these problems after getting ROTARIX, even if it has been several weeks since the last vaccine dose because these may be signs of a serious problem called intussusception:
- Bad vomiting
- Bad diarrhea
- Bloody bowel movement
- High fever
- Severe stomach pain (if your baby brings his/her knees to his/her chest while crying or screaming).

Studies showed an increased risk of intussusception after the first and second dose of vaccine, especially in the first 7 days.
Since FDA approval, reports of infants with intussusception have been received by Vaccine Adverse Event Reporting System (VAERS). Intussusception occurred days and sometimes weeks after vaccination. Some infants needed hospitalization, surgery on their intestines, or a special enema to treat this problem. Death due to intussusception has occurred.
Other reported side effects include: Kawasaki disease (a serious condition that can affect the heart; symptoms may in-

clude fever, rash, red eyes, red mouth, swollen glands, swollen hands, and feet and, if not treated, death can occur). Talk to your baby's doctor if your baby has any problems that concern you.

How is ROTARIX given?
ROTARIX is a liquid that is dropped into your baby's mouth and swallowed.

Figure 1. Administration of ROTARIX

Your baby will get the first dose at around 6 weeks old. The second dose will be at least 4 weeks after the first dose (before 6 months old).
Be sure to plan the time for your baby's second dose with the doctor because it is important that your baby gets both doses of ROTARIX before your baby is 6 months old.
The doctor may decide to give your baby shots at the same time as ROTARIX.
Your baby can be fed normally after getting ROTARIX.

What are the ingredients in ROTARIX?
ROTARIX contains weakened human rotavirus.
ROTARIX also contains dextran, sorbitol, xanthan, and Dulbecco's Modified Eagle Medium (DMEM). The ingredients of DMEM are as follows: sodium chloride, potassium chloride, magnesium sulphate, ferric (III) nitrate, sodium phosphate, sodium pyruvate, D-glucose, concentrated vitamin solution, L-cystine, L-tyrosine, amino acids solution, L-glutamine, calcium chloride, sodium hydrogenocarbonate, and phenol red.
Porcine circovirus type 1 (PCV-1), a virus found in pigs, is present in ROTARIX. PCV-1 is not known to cause disease in humans.
ROTARIX contains no preservatives.
The dropper used to give your baby ROTARIX may contain latex.
ROTARIX is a registered trademark of the GSK group of companies.
Manufactured by GlaxoSmithKline Biologicals
Rixensart, Belgium, US License 1617
Distributed by GlaxoSmithKline
Research Triangle Park, NC 27709
©2014, the GSK group of companies. All rights reserved.
May 2014
RTX:11PIL

RYTHMOL℞

[rith'-mol]
(propafenone hydrochloride)
Tablets for oral use

HIGHLIGHTS OF PRESCRIBING INFORMATION
These highlights do not include all the information needed to use RYTHMOL safely and effectively. See full prescribing information for RYTHMOL.
RYTHMOL (propafenone hydrochloride) Tablets for oral use
Initial U.S. Approval: 1989

WARNING: MORTALITY
See full prescribing information for complete boxed warning.

- **An increased rate of death or reversed cardiac arrest rate was seen in subjects treated with encainide or flecainide (Class IC antiarrhythmics) compared with that seen in subjects assigned to placebo. At present it is prudent to consider any IC antiarrhythmic to have a significant risk of provoking proarrhythmic events in patients with structural heart disease.**
- **Given the lack of any evidence that these drugs improve survival, antiarrhythmic agents should generally be avoided in patients with non-life-threatening ventricular arrhythmias, even if the patients are experiencing unpleasant, but not life-threatening, symptoms or signs.**

——INDICATIONS AND USAGE——

RYTHMOL is an antiarrhythmic indicated to:
- prolong the time to recurrence of symptomatic atrial fibrillation (AF) in patients with episodic (most likely paroxysmal or persistent) AF who do not have structural heart disease. (1)

- prolong the time to recurrence of paroxysmal supraventricular tachycardia (PSVT) associated with disabling symptoms in patients who do not have structural heart disease. (1)
- treat documented life-threatening ventricular arrhythmias. (1)

Usage Considerations:
- Use in patients with permanent atrial fibrillation or with atrial flutter or PSVT has not been evaluated. Do not use to control ventricular rate during atrial fibrillation. (1)
- In patients with atrial fibrillation and atrial flutter, use RYTHMOL with drugs that increase the atrioventricular nodal refractory period. (1)
- Because of proarrhythmic effects, use with lesser ventricular arrhythmias is not recommended, even if patients are symptomatic. (1)
- The effect of propafenone on mortality has not been determined. (1)

——DOSAGE AND ADMINISTRATION——

- Initiate therapy with 150 mg given every 8 hours. (2)
- As needed, uptitrate in 3 to 4 days to 225 to 300 mg every 8 hours. (2)
- Consider reducing the dose in patients with hepatic impairment, significant widening of the QRS complex, or second- or third-degree AV block. (2)

——DOSAGE FORMS AND STRENGTHS——

Tablets: 150 mg, 225 mg. (3)

——CONTRAINDICATIONS——

- Heart failure, cardiogenic shock, or marked hypotension (4)
- Sinoatrial, atrioventricular, and intraventricular disorders of impulse generation or conduction in the absence of pacemaker (4)
- Known Brugada Syndrome (4)
- Bradycardia (4)
- Bronchospastic disorders and severe obstructive pulmonary disease (4)
- Marked electrolyte imbalance (4)

——WARNINGS AND PRECAUTIONS——

- May cause new or worsened arrhythmias. Evaluate patients via ECG prior to and during therapy. (5.1)
- RYTHMOL may unmask Brugada or Brugada-like Syndrome. (4, 5.2)
- Avoid use with other drugs that prolong the QT interval. (5.3)
- Avoid simultaneous use of propafenone with both a cytochrome P450 2D6 inhibitor and a 3A4 inhibitor. (5.4)
- May provoke overt heart failure. (5.5)
- May cause dose-related first-degree AV block or other conduction disturbances. Only use in patients with conduction disorders who have pacemakers. (5.6)
- May affect artificial pacemakers. Monitor pacemaker function. (5.7)
- Agranulocytosis: Patients should report signs of infection. (5.8)
- May exacerbate myasthenia gravis. (5.11)

——ADVERSE REACTIONS——

The most commonly reported adverse events with propafenone (>5%) included: unusual taste, nausea and/or vomiting, dizziness, constipation, headache, fatigue, first-degree AV block, and intraventricular conduction delay. (6.1)

To report SUSPECTED ADVERSE REACTIONS, contact GlaxoSmithKline at 1-888-825-5249 or FDA at 1-800-FDA-1088 or www.fda.gov/medwatch.

——DRUG INTERACTIONS——

- Inhibitors of CYP2D6, 1A2, and 3A4 increase propafenone exposure. (7.1)
- Propafenone may increase digoxin or warfarin levels. (7.2, 7.3)
- Orlistat may reduce propafenone exposure. Taper orlistat withdrawal. (7.4)
- Lidocaine may increase central nervous system side effects. (7.6)

See 17 for PATIENT COUNSELING INFORMATION and FDA-approved patient labeling

Revised: 03/2014

FULL PRESCRIBING INFORMATION

WARNING: MORTALITY

- **In the National Heart, Lung, and Blood Institute's Cardiac Arrhythmia Suppression Trial (CAST), a long-term, multi-center, randomized, double-blind trial in subjects with asymptomatic non-life-threatening ventricular arrhythmias who had a myocardial infarction more than 6 days but less than 2 years previously, an increased rate of death or reversed cardiac arrest rate (7.7%; 56/730) was seen in patients treated with encainide or flecainide (Class IC antiarrhythmics) compared with that seen in subjects assigned to placebo (3.0%; 22/725). The average duration of treatment with encainide or flecainide in this trial was 10 months.**
- **The applicability of the CAST results to other populations (e.g., those without recent myocardial infarction) or other antiarrhythmic drugs is uncertain, but at present, it is prudent to consider any IC antiarrhythmic to have a significant proarrhythmic risk in patients with structural heart disease. Given the lack of any evidence that these drugs improve survival, antiarrhythmic agents should generally be avoided in patients with non-life-threatening ventricular arrhythmias, even if the patients are experiencing unpleasant, but not life-threatening, symptoms or signs.**

---

1   INDICATIONS AND USAGE

RYTHMOL® is indicated to:
- prolong the time to recurrence of paroxysmal atrial fibrillation/flutter (PAF) associated with disabling symptoms in patients without structural heart disease.
- prolong the time to recurrence of paroxysmal supraventricular tachycardia (PSVT) associated with disabling symptoms in patients without structural heart disease.
- treat documented ventricular arrhythmias, such as sustained ventricular tachycardia that, in the judgment of the physician, are life-threatening. Initiate treatment in the hospital.

Usage Considerations:
- The use of RYTHMOL in patients with permanent atrial fibrillation (AF) or in patients exclusively with atrial flutter or PSVT has not been evaluated. Do not use RYTHMOL to control ventricular rate during AF.

- Some patients with atrial flutter treated with propafenone have developed 1:1 conduction, producing an increase in ventricular rate. Concomitant treatment with drugs that increase the functional atrioventricular (AV) nodal refractory period is recommended.
- The use of RYTHMOL in patients with chronic atrial fibrillation has not been evaluated.
- Because of the proarrhythmic effects of RYTHMOL, its use with lesser ventricular arrhythmias is not recommended, even if patients are symptomatic, and any use of the drug should be reserved for patients in whom, in the opinion of the physician, the potential benefits outweigh the risks.
- The effect of propafenone on mortality has not been determined [see Boxed Warning].

2 DOSAGE AND ADMINISTRATION

The dose of RYTHMOL must be individually titrated on the basis of response and tolerance. Initiate therapy with RYTHMOL 150 mg given every 8 hours (450 mg/day). Dosage may be increased at a minimum of 3 to 4 day intervals to 225 mg every 8 hours (675 mg/day). If additional therapeutic effect is needed, the dose of RYTHMOL may be increased to 300 mg every 8 hours (900 mg/day). The usefulness and safety of dosages exceeding 900 mg per day have not been established.

In patients with hepatic impairment or those with significant widening of the QRS complex or second- or third-degree AV block, consider reducing the dose.

As with other antiarrhythmic agents, in the elderly or in ventricular arrhythmia patients with marked previous myocardial damage, the dose of RYTHMOL should be increased more gradually during the initial phase of treatment.

The combination of CYP3A4 inhibition and either CYP2D6 deficiency or CYP2D6 inhibition with the simultaneous administration of propafenone may significantly increase the concentration of propafenone and thereby increase the risk of proarrhythmia and other adverse events. Therefore, avoid simultaneous use of RYTHMOL with both a CYP2D6 inhibitor and a CYP3A4 inhibitor [see Warnings and Precautions (5.4), Drug Interactions (7.1)].

3 DOSAGE FORMS AND STRENGTHS

150-mg and 225-mg scored, round, film-coated tablets.

4 CONTRAINDICATIONS

RYTHMOL is contraindicated in the following circumstances:
- Heart failure
- Cardiogenic shock
- Sinoatrial, atrioventricular, and intraventricular disorders of impulse generation or conduction (e.g., sick sinus node syndrome, AV block) in the absence of an artificial pacemaker
- Known Brugada Syndrome
- Bradycardia
- Marked hypotension
- Bronchospastic disorders or severe obstructive pulmonary disease
- Marked electrolyte imbalance

5 WARNINGS AND PRECAUTIONS

5.1 Proarrhythmic Effects

Propafenone has caused new or worsened arrhythmias. Such proarrhythmic effects include sudden death and life-threatening ventricular arrhythmias such as ventricular fibrillation, ventricular tachycardia, asystole, and torsade de pointes. It may also worsen premature ventricular contractions or supraventricular arrhythmias, and it may prolong the QT interval. It is therefore essential that each patient given RYTHMOL be evaluated electrocardiographically prior to and during therapy to determine whether the response to RYTHMOL supports continued treatment. Because propafenone prolongs the QRS interval in the electrocardiogram, changes in the QT interval are difficult to interpret [see Clinical Pharmacology (12.2)].

In a US uncontrolled, open-label, multicenter trial in subjects with symptomatic supraventricular tachycardia (SVT), 1.9% (9/474) of these subjects experienced ventricular tachycardia (VT) or ventricular fibrillation (VF) during the trial. However, in 4 of the 9 subjects, the ventricular tachycardia was of atrial origin. Six of the 9 subjects that developed ventricular arrhythmias did so within 14 days of onset of therapy. About 2.3% (11/474) of all subjects had a recurrence of SVT during the trial which could have been a change in the subjects' arrhythmia behavior or could represent a proarrhythmic event. Case reports in patients treated with propafenone for atrial fibrillation/flutter have included increased premature ventricular contractions (PVCs), VT, VF, torsade de pointes, asystole, and death.

Overall in clinical trials with RYTHMOL (which included subjects treated for ventricular arrhythmias, atrial fibrillation/flutter, and PSVT), 4.7% of all subjects had new or worsened ventricular arrhythmia possibly representing a proarrhythmic event (0.7% was an increase in PVCs; 4.0% a

worsening, or new appearance, of VT or VF). Of the subjects who had worsening of VT (4%), 92% had a history of VT and/or VT/VF, 71% had coronary artery disease, and 68% had a prior myocardial infarction. The incidence of proarrhythmia in subjects with less serious or benign arrhythmias, which include subjects with an increase in frequency of PVCs, was 1.6%. Although most proarrhythmic events occurred during the first week of therapy, late events also were seen and the CAST trial [see Boxed Warning: Mortality] suggests that an increased risk of proarrhythmia is present throughout treatment.

In a trial of sustained-release propafenone (RYTHMOL SR®), there were too few deaths to assess the long-term risk to patients. There were 5 deaths, 3 in the pooled group for RYTHMOL SR (0.8%) and 2 in the placebo group (1.6%). In the overall database of 8 trials of RYTHMOL SR and immediate-release RYTHMOL, the mortality rate was 2.5% per year on propafenone and 4.0% per year on placebo. Concurrent use of propafenone with other antiarrhythmic agents has not been well studied.

5.2 Unmasking Brugada Syndrome

Brugada Syndrome may be unmasked after exposure to RYTHMOL. Perform an ECG after initiation of RYTHMOL, and discontinue the drug if changes are suggestive of Brugada Syndrome [see Contraindications (4)].

5.3 Use With Drugs That Prolong the QT Interval and Antiarrhythmic Agents

The use of RYTHMOL in conjunction with other drugs that prolong the QT interval has not been extensively studied. Such drugs may include many antiarrhythmics, some phenothiazines, tricyclic antidepressants, and oral macrolides. Withhold Class IA and III antiarrhythmic agents for at least 5 half-lives prior to dosing with RYTHMOL. Avoid the use of propafenone with Class IA and III antiarrhythmic agents (including quinidine and amiodarone). There is only limited experience with the concomitant use of Class IB or IC antiarrhythmics.

5.4 Drug Interactions: Simultaneous Use With Inhibitors of Cytochrome P450 Isoenzymes 2D6 and 3A4

Propafenone is metabolized by CYP2D6, CYP3A4, and CYP1A2 isoenzymes. Approximately 6% of Caucasians in the US population are naturally deficient in CYP2D6 activity and to a somewhat lesser extent in other demographic groups. Drugs that inhibit these CYP pathways (such as desipramine, paroxetine, ritonavir, sertraline for CYP2D6; ketoconazole, erythromycin, saquinavir, and grapefruit juice for CYP3A4; and amiodarone and tobacco smoke for CYP1A2) can be expected to cause increased plasma levels of propafenone.

Increased exposure to propafenone may lead to cardiac arrhythmias and exaggerated beta-adrenergic blocking activity. Because of its metabolism, the combination of CYP3A4 inhibition and either CYP2D6 deficiency or CYP2D6 inhibition in users of propafenone is potentially hazardous. Therefore, avoid simultaneous use of RYTHMOL with both a CYP2D6 inhibitor and a CYP3A4 inhibitor.

5.5 Use in Patients With a History of Heart Failure

Propafenone exerts a negative inotropic activity on the myocardium as well as beta-blockade effects and may provoke overt heart failure.

In clinical trial experience with RYTHMOL, new or worsened congestive heart failure (CHF) has been reported in 3.7% of subjects with ventricular arrhythmia; of those 0.9% were considered probably or definitely related to propafenone HCl. Of the subjects with CHF probably related to propafenone, 80% had pre-existing heart failure and 85% had coronary artery disease. CHF attributable to propafenone HCl developed rarely (<0.2%) in ventricular arrhythmia subjects who had no previous history of CHF. CHF occurred in 1.9% of subjects studied with PAF or PSVT.

In a US trial of RYTHMOL SR in subjects with symptomatic AF, heart failure was reported in 4 (1.0%) subjects receiving RYTHMOL SR (all doses), compared with 1 (0.8%) subject receiving placebo.

5.6 Conduction Disturbances

Propafenone slows atrioventricular conduction and may also cause dose-related first-degree AV block. Average PR interval prolongation and increases in QRS duration are also dose-related. Do not give propafenone to patients with atrioventricular and intraventricular conduction defects in the absence of a pacemaker [see Contraindications (4), Clinical Pharmacology (12.2)].

The incidence of first-degree, second-degree, and third-degree AV block observed in 2,127 subjects with ventricular arrhythmia was 2.5%, 0.6%, and 0.2%, respectively. Development of second- or third-degree AV block requires a reduction in dosage or discontinuation of propafenone HCl. Bundle branch block (1.2%) and intraventricular conduction delay (1.1%) have been reported in subjects receiving propafenone. Bradycardia has also been reported (1.5%). Experience in patients with sick sinus node syndrome is limited and these patients should not be treated with propafenone.

In a US trial in 523 subjects with a history of symptomatic AF treated with RYTHMOL SR, sinus bradycardia (rate <50 beats/min) was reported with the same frequency with RYTHMOL SR and placebo.

5.7 Effects on Pacemaker Threshold

Propafenone may alter both pacing and sensing thresholds of implanted pacemakers and defibrillators. During and after therapy, monitor and re-program these devices accordingly.

5.8 Agranulocytosis

Agranulocytosis has been reported in patients receiving propafenone. Generally, the agranulocytosis occurred within the first 2 months of propafenone therapy and upon discontinuation of therapy; the white count usually normalized by 14 days. Unexplained fever or decrease in white cell count, particularly during the initial 3 months of therapy, warrant consideration of possible agranulocytosis or granulocytopenia. Instruct patients to report promptly any signs of infection such as fever, sore throat, or chills.

5.9 Use in Patients With Hepatic Dysfunction

Propafenone is highly metabolized by the liver. Severe liver dysfunction increases the bioavailability of propafenone to approximately 70% compared with 3% to 40% in patients with normal liver function. In 8 subjects with moderate to severe liver disease, the mean half-life was approximately 9 hours. Increased bioavailability of propafenone in these patients may result in excessive accumulation. Carefully monitor patients with impaired hepatic function for excessive pharmacological effects [see Overdosage (10)].

5.10 Use in Patients With Renal Dysfunction

Approximately 50% of propafenone metabolites are excreted in the urine following administration of RYTHMOL.

In patients with impaired renal function, monitor for signs of overdosage [see Overdosage (10)].

5.11 Use in Patients With Myasthenia Gravis

Exacerbation of myasthenia gravis has been reported during propafenone therapy.

5.12 Elevated ANA Titers

Positive ANA titers have been reported in patients receiving propafenone. They have been reversible upon cessation of treatment and may disappear even in the face of continued propafenone therapy. These laboratory findings were usually not associated with clinical symptoms, but there is one published case of drug-induced lupus erythematosis (positive rechallenge); it resolved completely upon discontinuation of therapy. Carefully evaluate patients who develop an abnormal ANA test and, if persistent or worsening elevation of ANA titers is detected, consider discontinuing therapy.

5.13 Impaired Spermatogenesis

Reversible disorders of spermatogenesis have been demonstrated in monkeys, dogs, and rabbits after high-dose intravenous administration of propafenone. Evaluation of the effects of short-term administration of RYTHMOL on spermatogenesis in 11 normal subjects suggested that propafenone produced a reversible, short-term drop (within normal range) in sperm count.

6 ADVERSE REACTIONS

6.1 Clinical Trials Experience

Because clinical trials are conducted under widely varying conditions, adverse reaction rates observed in the clinical trials of a drug cannot be directly compared with rates in the clinical trials of another drug and may not reflect the rates observed in practice.

Adverse reactions associated with RYTHMOL occur most frequently in the gastrointestinal, cardiovascular, and central nervous systems. About 20% of subjects treated with RYTHMOL have discontinued treatment because of adverse reactions.

Adverse reactions reported for > 1.5% of 474 subjects with SVT who received RYTHMOL in US clinical trials are presented in Table 1 by incidence and percent discontinuation, reported to the nearest percent.

Table 1. Adverse Reactions Reported for >1.5% of Subjects With SVT

	Incidence (N = 480)	% of Subjects Who Discontinued
Unusual taste	14%	1.3%
Nausea and/or vomiting	11%	2.9%
Dizziness	9%	1.7%
Constipation	8%	0.2%
Headache	6%	0.8%
Fatigue	6%	1.5%
Blurred Vision	3%	0.6%

Weakness	3%	1.3%
Dyspnea	2%	1.0%
Wide complex tachycardia	2%	1.9%
CHF	2%	0.6%
Bradycardia	2%	0.2%
Palpitations	2%	0.2%
Tremor	2%	0.4%
Anorexia	2%	0.2%
Diarrhea	2%	0.4%
Ataxia	2%	0.0%

In controlled trials in subjects with ventricular arrhythmia, the most common reactions reported for RYTHMOL and more frequent than on placebo were unusual taste, dizziness, first degree AV block, intraventricular conduction delay, nausea and/or vomiting, and constipation. Headache was relatively common also, but was not increased compared with placebo. Other reactions reported more frequently than on placebo or comparator and not already reported elsewhere included anxiety, angina, second-degree AV block, bundle branch block, loss of balance, congestive heart failure, and dyspepsia.

Adverse reactions reported for ≥1% of 2,127 subjects with ventricular arrhythmia who received propafenone in US clinical trials were evaluated by daily dose. The most common adverse reactions appeared dose-related (but note that most subjects spent more time at the larger doses), especially dizziness, nausea and/or vomiting, unusual taste, constipation, and blurred vision. Some less common reactions may also have been dose-related such as first-degree AV block, congestive heart failure, dyspepsia, and weakness. Other adverse reactions included rash, syncope, chest pain, abdominal pain, ataxia, and hypotension.

In addition, the following adverse reactions were reported less frequently than 1% either in clinical trials or in marketing experience. Causality and relationship to propafenone therapy cannot necessarily be judged from these events.

Cardiovascular System: Atrial flutter, AV dissociation, cardiac arrest, flushing, hot flashes, sick sinus syndrome, sinus pause or arrest, supraventricular tachycardia.

Nervous System: Abnormal dreams, abnormal speech, abnormal vision, confusion, depression, memory loss, numbness, paresthesias, psychosis/mania, seizures (0.3%), tinnitus, unusual smell sensation, vertigo.

Gastrointestinal: Cholestasis , elevated liver enzymes (alkaline phosphatase, serum transaminases), gastroenteritis, hepatitis .

Hematologic: Agranulocytosis, anemia, bruising, granulocytopenia, leukopenia, purpura, thrombocytopenia.

Other: Alopecia, eye irritation, impotence, increased glucose, positive ANA (0.7%), muscle cramps, muscle weakness, nephrotic syndrome, pain, pruritus.

6.2 Postmarketing Experience

The following adverse reactions have been identified during post-approval use of RYTHMOL. Because these reactions are reported voluntarily from a population of uncertain size, it is not always possible to reliably estimate their frequency or establish a causal relationship to drug exposure.

Gastrointestinal: A number of patients with liver abnormalities associated with propafenone therapy have been reported in postmarketing experience. Some appeared due to hepatocellular injury, some were cholestatic, and some showed a mixed picture. Some of these reports were simply discovered through clinical chemistries, others because of clinical symptoms including fulminant hepatitis and death. One case was rechallenged with a positive outcome.

Blood and Lymphatic System: Increased bleeding time.

Immune System: Lupus erythematosis.

Nervous System: Apnea, coma.

Renal and Urinary: Hyponatremia/inappropriate ADH secretion, kidney failure.

7 DRUG INTERACTIONS
7.1 CYP2D6 and CYP3A4 Inhibitors

Drugs that inhibit CYP2D6 (such as desipramine, paroxetine, ritonavir, or sertraline) and CYP3A4 (such as ketoconazole, ritonavir, saquinavir, erythromycin, or grapefruit juice) can be expected to cause increased plasma levels of propafenone. The combination of CYP3A4 inhibition and either CYP2D6 deficiency or CYP2D6 inhibition with administration of propafenone may increase the risk of adverse reactions, including proarrhythmia. Therefore, simultaneous use of RYTHMOL with both a CYP2D6 inhibitor and a CYP3A4 inhibitor should be avoided [see Warnings and Precautions (5.4), Dosage and Administration (2)].

Amiodarone: Concomitant administration of propafenone and amiodarone can affect conduction and repolarization and is not recommended.

Cimetidine: Concomitant administration of propafenone immediate-release tablets and cimetidine in 12 healthy subjects resulted in a 20% increase in steady-state plasma concentrations of propafenone.

Fluoxetine: Concomitant administration of propafenone and fluoxetine in extensive metabolizers increased the S-propafenone C_{max} and AUC by 39% and 50%, respectively, and the R propafenone C_{max} and AUC by 71% and 50%, respectively.

Quinidine: Small doses of quinidine completely inhibit the CYP2D6 hydroxylation metabolic pathway, making all patients, in effect, slow metabolizers [see Clinical Pharmacology (12)]. Concomitant administration of quinidine (50 mg 3 times daily) with 150 mg immediate-release propafenone 3 times daily decreased the clearance of propafenone by 60% in extensive metabolizers, making them slow metabolizers. Steady-state plasma concentrations more than doubled for propafenone, and decreased 50% for 5-OH-propafenone. A 100-mg dose of quinidine tripled steady-state concentrations of propafenone. Avoid concomitant use of propafenone and quinidine.

Rifampin: Concomitant administration of rifampin and propafenone in extensive metabolizers decreased the plasma concentrations of propafenone by 67% with a corresponding decrease of 5-OH-propafenone by 65%. The concentrations of norpropafenone increased by 30%. In slow metabolizers, there was a 50% decrease in propafenone plasma concentrations and an increase in the AUC and C_{max} of norpropafenone by 74% and 20%, respectively. Urinary excretion of propafenone and its metabolites decreased significantly. Similar results were noted in elderly patients: Both the AUC and C_{max} of propafenone decreased by 84%, with a corresponding decrease in AUC and C_{max} of 5-OH-propafenone by 69% and 57%, respectively.

7.2 Digoxin

Concomitant use of propafenone and digoxin increased steady-state serum digoxin exposure (AUC) in patients by 60% to 270%, and decreased the clearance of digoxin by 31% to 67%. Monitor plasma digoxin levels of patients receiving propafenone and adjust digoxin dosage as needed.

7.3 Warfarin

The concomitant administration of propafenone and warfarin increased warfarin plasma concentrations at steady state by 39% in healthy volunteers and prolonged the prothrombin time (PT) in patients taking warfarin. Adjust the warfarin dose as needed by monitoring INR (international normalized ratio).

7.4 Orlistat

Orlistat may limit the fraction of propafenone available for absorption. In postmarketing reports, abrupt cessation of orlistat in patients stabilized on propafenone has resulted in severe adverse events including convulsions, atrioventricular block, and acute circulatory failure.

7.5 Beta-Antagonists

Concomitant use of propafenone and propranolol in healthy subjects increased propranolol plasma concentrations at steady state by 113%. In 4 patients, administration of metoprolol with propafenone increased the metoprolol plasma concentrations at steady state by 100% to 400%. The pharmacokinetics of propafenone was not affected by the coadministration of either propranolol or metoprolol. In clinical trials using propafenone immediate-release tablets, subjects who were receiving beta-blockers concurrently did not experience an increased incidence of side effects.

7.6 Lidocaine

No significant effects on the pharmacokinetics of propafenone or lidocaine have been seen following their concomitant use in patients. However, concomitant use of propafenone and lidocaine has been reported to increase the risks of central nervous system side effects of lidocaine.

8 USE IN SPECIFIC POPULATIONS
8.1 Pregnancy

Pregnancy Category C. There are no adequate and well-controlled studies in pregnant women. RYTHMOL should be used during pregnancy only if the potential benefit justifies the potential risk to the fetus.

Animal Data: Teratogenic Effects: Propafenone has been shown to be embryotoxic (decreased survival) in rabbits and rats when given in oral maternally toxic doses of 150 mg/kg day (about 3 times the maximum recommended human dose [MRHD] on a mg/m² basis) and 600 mg/kg/day (about 6 times the MRHD on a mg/m² basis), respectively. Although maternally tolerated doses (up to 270 mg/kg/day, about 3 times the MRHD on a mg/m² basis) produced no evidence of embryotoxicity in rats; post-implantation loss was elevated in all rabbit treatment groups (doses as low as 15 mg/kg/ day, about 1/3 the MRHD on a mg/m² basis).

Non-teratogenic Effects: In a study in which female rats received daily oral doses of propafenone from mid-gestation through weaning of their offspring, doses as low as 90 mg/kg/day (equivalent to the MRHD on a mg/m² basis) produced increases in maternal deaths. Doses of 360 or more mg/kg/day (4 or more times the MRHD on a mg/m² basis) resulted in reductions in neonatal survival, body weight gain, and physiological development.

8.2 Labor and Delivery

It is not known whether the use of propafenone during labor or delivery has immediate or delayed adverse effects on the fetus, or whether it prolongs the duration of labor or increases the need for forceps delivery or other obstetrical intervention.

8.3 Nursing Mothers

Propafenone is excreted in human milk. Because of the potential for serious adverse reactions in nursing infants from propafenone, decide whether to discontinue nursing or to discontinue the drug, taking into account the importance of the drug to the mother.

8.4 Pediatric Use

The safety and effectiveness of propafenone in pediatric patients have not been established.

8.5 Geriatric Use

Clinical trials of RYTHMOL did not include sufficient numbers of subjects aged 65 and over to determine whether they respond differently from younger subjects. Other reported clinical experience has not identified differences in responses between the elderly and younger subjects. In general, dose selection for an elderly patient should be cautious, usually starting at the low end of the dosing range, reflecting the greater frequency of decreased hepatic, renal, or cardiac function, and of concomitant disease or other drug therapy.

10 OVERDOSAGE

The symptoms of overdosage may include hypotension, somnolence, bradycardia, intra-atrial and intraventricular conduction disturbances, and rarely, convulsions and high-grade ventricular arrhythmias. Defibrillation, as well as infusion of dopamine and isoproterenol have been effective in controlling abnormal rhythm and blood pressure. Convulsions have been alleviated with intravenous diazepam. General supportive measures such as mechanical respiratory assistance and external cardiac massage may be necessary. The hemodialysis of propafenone in patients with an overdose is expected to be of limited value in the removal of propafenone as a result of both its high protein binding (>95%) and large volume of distribution.

11 DESCRIPTION

RYTHMOL (propafenone hydrochloride) is an antiarrhythmic drug supplied in scored, film-coated tablets of 150 and 225 mg for oral administration. Propafenone has some structural similarities to beta-blocking agents.

Chemically, propafenone hydrochloride (HCl) is 2′-[2-hydroxy-3-(propylamino)-propoxy]-3-phenylpropiophenone hydrochloride, with a molecular weight of 377.92. The molecular formula is $C_{21}H_{27}NO_3 \cdot HCl$. The structural formula of propafenone HCl is given below:

Propafenone HCl occurs as colorless crystals or white crystalline powder with a very bitter taste. It is slightly soluble in water (20°C), chloroform and ethanol. The following inactive ingredients are contained in the tablet: corn starch, hypromellose, magnesium stearate, polyethylene glycol, polysorbate, povidone, propylene glycol, sodium starch glycolate, and titanium dioxide.

12 CLINICAL PHARMACOLOGY
12.1 Mechanism of Action

Propafenone is a Class 1C antiarrhythmic drug with local anesthetic effects, and a direct stabilizing action on myocardial membranes. The electrophysiological effect of propafenone manifests itself in a reduction of upstroke velocity (Phase 0) of the monophasic action potential. In Purkinje fibers, and to a lesser extent myocardial fibers, propafenone reduces the fast inward current carried by sodium ions. Diastolic excitability threshold is increased and effective refractory period prolonged. Propafenone reduces spontaneous automaticity and depresses triggered activity. Studies in anesthetized dogs and isolated organ preparations show that propafenone has beta-sympatholytic activity at about 1/50 the potency of propranolol. Clinical studies employing isoproterenol challenge and exercise testing after single doses of propafenone indicate a beta-adrenergic blocking potency (per mg) about 1/40 that of propranolol in man. In clinical trials, resting heart rate decreases of about 8% were noted at the higher end of the therapeutic plasma

Table 2. Mean Changes in Electrocardiogram Intervals [a]

	Total Daily Dose (mg)							
	337.5 mg		450 mg		675 mg		900 mg	
Interval	msec	%	msec	%	msec	%	msec	%
RR	-14.5	-1.8	30.6	3.8	31.5	3.9	41.7	5.1
PR	3.6	2.1	19.1	11.6	28.9	17.8	35.6	21.9
QRS	5.6	6.4	5.5	6.1	7.7	8.4	15.6	17.3
QTc	2.7	0.7	-7.5	-1.8	5.0	1.2	14.7	3.7

[a] Change and percent change based on mean baseline values for each treatment group.

Table 3. Reduction of Arrhythmias in Subjects with PAF or PSVT

	Trial 1		Trial 2	
	Propafenone	Placebo	Propafenone	Placebo
PAF	n = 30	n = 30	n = 9	n = 9
Percent attack free	53%	13%	67%	22%
Median time to first recurrence	>98 days	8 days	62 days	5 days
PSVT	n = 45	n = 45	n = 15	n = 15
Percent attack free	47%	16%	38%	7%
Median time to first recurrence	>98 days	12 days	31 days	8 days

concentration range. At very high concentrations in vitro, propafenone can inhibit the slow inward current carried by calcium, but this calcium antagonist effect probably does not contribute to antiarrhythmic efficacy. Moreover, propafenone inhibits a variety of cardiac potassium currents in in vitro studies (i.e., the transient outward, the delayed rectifier, and the inward rectifier current). Propafenone has local anesthetic activity approximately equal to procaine. Compared with propafenone, the main metabolite, 5-hydroxypropafenone, has similar sodium and calcium channel activity, but about 10 times less beta-blocking activity (N-depropylpropafenone has weaker sodium channel activity but equivalent affinity for beta-receptors).

12.2 Pharmacodynamics

Electrophysiology: Electrophysiology trials in subjects with ventricular tachycardia have shown that propafenone prolongs atrioventricular conduction while having little or no effect on sinus node function. Both atrioventricular nodal conduction time (AH interval) and His-Purkinje conduction time (HV interval) are prolonged. Propafenone has little or no effect on the atrial functional refractory period, but AV nodal functional and effective refractory periods are prolonged. In patients with Wolff-Parkinson-White syndrome, RYTHMOL reduces conduction and increases the effective refractory period of the accessory pathway in both directions.

Electrocardiograms: Propafenone slows prolongs the PR and QRS intervals. Prolongation of the QRS interval makes it difficult to interpret the effect of propafenone on the QT interval.

[See table 2 above]

In any individual patient, the above ECG changes cannot be readily used to predict either efficacy or plasma concentration.

RYTHMOL causes a dose-related and concentration-related decrease in the rate of single and multiple premature ventricular contractions (PVCs) and can suppress recurrence of ventricular tachycardia. Based on the percent of patients attaining substantial (80% to 90%) suppression of ventricular ectopic activity, it appears that trough plasma levels of 0.2 to 1.5 mcg/mL can provide good suppression, with higher concentrations giving a greater rate of good response.

When 600 mg/day propafenone was administered to subjects with paroxysmal atrial tachyarrhythmias, mean heart rate during arrhythmia decreased 14 beats/min and 37 beats/min for subjects with paroxysmal atrial fibrillation/flutter (PAF) and subjects with paroxysmal supraventricular tachycardia (PSVT), respectively.

Hemodynamics: Trials in humans have shown that propafenone HCl exerts a negative inotropic effect on the myocardium. Cardiac catheterization trials in subjects with moderately impaired ventricular function (mean C.I. = 2.61 L/min/m²) utilizing intravenous propafenone infusions (loading dose of 2 mg/kg over 10 min followed by 2 mg/min for 30 min) that gave mean plasma concentrations of 3.0 mcg/mL (a dose that produces plasma levels of propafenone greater than recommended oral dosing)

showed significant increases in pulmonary capillary wedge pressure, systemic and pulmonary vascular resistances, and depression of cardiac output and cardiac index.

12.3 Pharmacokinetics

Absorption/Bioavailability: Propafenone HCl is nearly completely absorbed after oral administration with peak plasma levels occurring approximately 3.5 hours after administration in most individuals. Propafenone exhibits extensive saturable presystemic biotransformation (first-pass effect) resulting in a dose dependent and dosage form dependent absolute bioavailability; e.g., a 150-mg tablet had absolute bioavailability of 3.4%, while a 300-mg tablet had absolute bioavailability of 10.6%. A 300-mg solution which was rapidly absorbed had absolute bioavailability of 21.4%. At still larger doses, above those recommended, bioavailability increases still further.

Propafenone HCl follows a nonlinear pharmacokinetic disposition presumably because of saturation of first-pass hepatic metabolism as the liver is exposed to higher concentrations of propafenone and shows a very high degree of interindividual variability. For example, for an increase in daily dose from 300 to 900 mg/day there is a 10-fold increase in steady-state plasma concentration. The top 25% of subjects given 337.5 mg/day, however, had a mean concentration of propafenone larger than the bottom 25%, and about equal to the second 25%, of subjects given a dose of 900 mg. Although food increased peak blood level and bioavailability in a single-dose trial, during multiple-dose administration of propafenone to healthy volunteers, food did not change bioavailability significantly.

Distribution: Following intravenous administration of propafenone, plasma levels decline in a bi-phasic manner consistent with a 2-compartment pharmacokinetic model. The average distribution half-life corresponding to the first phase was about 5 minutes. The volume of the central compartment was about 88 liters (1.1 L/kg) and the total volume of distribution about 252 liters.

In serum, propafenone is greater than 95% bound to proteins within the concentration range of 0.5 to 2 mcg/mL.

Metabolism: There are 2 genetically determined patterns of propafenone metabolism. In over 90% of patients, the drug is rapidly and extensively metabolized with an elimination half-life from 2 to 10 hours. These patients metabolize propafenone into 2 active metabolites: 5-hydroxypropafenone which is formed by CYP2D6 and N-depropylpropafenone (norpropafenone) which is formed by both CYP3A4 and CYP1A2.

In less than 10% of patients, metabolism of propafenone is slower because the 5-hydroxy metabolite is not formed or is minimally formed. In these patients, the estimated propafenone elimination half-life ranges from 10 to 32 hours. Decreased ability to form the 5-hydroxy metabolite of propafenone is associated with a diminished ability to metabolize debrisoquine and a variety of other drugs (such as encainide, metoprolol, and dextromethorphan) whose metabolism is mediated by the CYP2D6 isozyme. In these patients, the N-depropylpropafenone metabolite occurs in quantities comparable to the levels occurring in extensive metabolizers.

There are significant differences in plasma concentrations of propafenone in slow and extensive metabolizers, the former achieving concentrations 1.5 to 2.0 times those of the extensive metabolizers at daily doses of 675 to 900 mg/day. At low doses the differences are greater, with slow metabolizers attaining concentrations more than 5 times that of extensive metabolizers. Because the difference decreases at high doses and is mitigated by the lack of the active 5-hydroxy metabolite in the slow metabolizers, and because steady-state conditions are achieved after 4 to 5 days of dosing in all patients, the recommended dosing regimen is the same for all patients. The greater variability in blood levels require that the drug be titrated carefully in patients with close attention paid to clinical and ECG evidence of toxicity [see Dosage and Administration (2)].

Stereochemistry: RYTHMOL is a racemic mixture. The R- and S-enantiomers of propafenone display stereoselective disposition characteristics. In vitro and in vivo studies have shown that the R-isomer of propafenone is cleared faster than the S-isomer via the 5-hydroxylation pathway (CYP2D6). This results in a higher ratio of S-propafenone to R-propafenone at steady state. Both enantiomers have equivalent potency to block sodium channels; however, the S-enantiomer is a more potent beta-antagonist than the R-enantiomer. Following administration of RYTHMOL immediate-release tablets, the S/R ratio for the area under the plasma concentration-time curve was about 1.7. In addition, no difference in the average values of the S/R ratios is evident between genotypes or over time.

Special Populations: Hepatic Impairment: Decreased liver function increases the bioavailability of propafenone. Absolute bioavailability of RYTHMOL immediate-release tablets is inversely related to indocyanine green clearance, reaching 60% to 70% at clearances of 7 mL/min and below. Protein binding decreases to about 88% in patients with severe hepatic dysfunction. The clearance of propafenone is reduced and the elimination half-life increased in patients with significant hepatic dysfunction [see Warnings and Precautions (5,9)].

13 NONCLINICAL TOXICOLOGY

13.1 Carcinogenesis, Mutagenesis, Impairment of Fertility

Lifetime maximally tolerated oral dose studies in mice (up to 360 mg/kg/day, about twice the maximum recommended human oral daily dose [MRHD] on a mg/m² basis) and rats (up to 270 mg/kg/day, about 3 times the MRHD on a mg/m² basis) provided no evidence of a carcinogenic potential for propafenone HCl.

Propafenone HCl tested negative for mutagenicity in the Ames (salmonella) test and in the in vivo mouse dominant lethal test. It tested negative for clastogenicity in the human lymphocyte chromosome aberration assay in vitro and in rat and Chinese hamster micronucleus tests, and other in vivo tests for chromosomal aberrations in rat bone marrow and Chinese hamster bone marrow and spermatogonia.

Propafenone HCl, administered intravenously to rabbits, dogs, and monkeys, has been shown to decrease spermatogenesis. These effects were reversible, were not found following oral dosing of propafenone HCl, were seen at lethal or near lethal dose levels, and were not seen in rats treated either orally or intravenously [see Warnings and Precautions (5.13)]. Treatment of male rabbits for 10 weeks prior to mating at an oral dose of 120 mg/kg/day (about 2.4 times the MRHD on a mg/m² basis) or an intravenous dose of 3.5 mg/kg/day (a spermatogenesis-impairing dose) did not result in evidence of impaired fertility. Nor was there evidence of impaired fertility when propafenone HCl was administered orally to male and female rats at dose levels up to 270 mg/kg/day (about 3 times the MRHD on a mg/m² basis).

13.2 Animal Toxicology and/or Pharmacology

Renal changes have been observed in the rat following 6 months of oral administration of propafenone HCl at doses of 180 and 360 mg/kg/day (about 2 and 4 times, respectively, the MRHD on a mg/m² basis). Both inflammatory and non-inflammatory changes in the renal tubules, with accompanying interstitial nephritis, were observed. These changes were reversible, as they were not found in rats allowed to recover for 6 weeks. Fatty degenerative changes of the liver were found in rats following longer durations of administration of propafenone HCl at a dose of 270 mg/kg/day (about 3 times the MRHD on a mg/m² basis). There were no renal or hepatic changes at 90 mg/kg/day (equivalent to the MRHD on a mg/m² basis).

14 CLINICAL STUDIES

In 2 randomized, crossover, placebo-controlled, double-blind trials of 60 to 90 days' duration in subjects with paroxysmal supraventricular arrhythmias (paroxysmal atrial fibrillation/flutter [PAF], or paroxysmal supraventricular tachycardia [PSVT]), propafenone reduced the rate of both arrhythmias, as shown in Table 3.

[See table 3 above]

The patient population in the above trials was 50% male with a mean age of 57.3 years. Fifty percent of the subjects had a diagnosis of PAF and 50% had PSVT. Eighty percent of the subjects received 600 mg/day propafenone. No subject died in the above 2 trials.

In US long-term safety trials, 474 subjects (mean age: 57.4 ± 14.5 years) with supraventricular arrhythmias [195 with PAF, 274 with PSVT and 5 with both PAF and PSVT] were treated up to 5 years (mean: 14.4 months) with propafenone. Fourteen of the subjects died. When this mortality rate was compared with the rate in a similar patient population (n = 194 subjects; mean age: 43.0 ± 16.8 years) studied in an arrhythmia clinic, there was no age-adjusted difference in mortality. This comparison was not, however, a randomized trial and the 95% confidence interval around the comparison was large, such that neither a significant adverse or favorable effect could be ruled out.

16 HOW SUPPLIED/STORAGE AND HANDLING

RYTHMOL Tablets are supplied as white, biconvex, scored, round, film-coated tablets containing either 150 mg or 225 mg of propafenone hydrochloride and embossed (on the same side) with GS and TF5 for the 150-mg tablet, and GS and F1X for the 225-mg tablet, in the following package sizes:

150 mg - bottles of 100: NDC 0173-0792-20
225 mg - bottles of 100: NDC 0173-0794-20

Storage: Store at 25°C (77°F); excursions permitted to 15°C to 30°C (59°F to 86°F). Dispense in a tight, light-resistant container.

17 PATIENT COUNSELING INFORMATION

See FDA-approved patient labeling (Patient Information).

17.1 Information for Patients

- Patients should be instructed to notify their healthcare providers of any change in over-the-counter, prescription, and supplement use. The healthcare provider should assess the patients' medication history including all over-the-counter, prescription, and herbal/natural preparations for those that may affect the pharmacodynamics or kinetics of RYTHMOL [see Warnings and Precautions (5.4)].
- Patients should also check with their healthcare providers prior to taking a new over-the-counter medicine.
- If patients experience symptoms that may be associated with altered electrolyte balance, such as excessive or prolonged diarrhea, sweating, vomiting, or loss of appetite or thirst, these conditions should be immediately reported to their healthcare provider.
- Patients should be instructed NOT to double the next dose if a dose is missed. The next dose should be taken at the usual time.

RYTHMOL is a registered trademark of G. Petrik used under license by Abbott Laboratories.
Manufactured for:
GlaxoSmithKline
Research Triangle Park, NC 27709
©2014, the GSK group of companies. All rights reserved.
RML:6PI

PHARMACIST-DETACH HERE AND GIVE INSTRUCTIONS TO PATIENT

PATIENT INFORMATION
RYTHMOL® (RITH-Mall)
(propafenone hydrochloride) Tablets
What is RYTHMOL?
RYTHMOL is a prescription medicine that is used:
- in certain people who have ventricular heart rhythm disorders
- to increase the amount of time between having symptoms of heart rhythm disorders called atrial fibrillation (AF) or paroxysmal supraventricular tachycardia (PSVT)

It is not known if RYTHMOL is safe and effective in children.
Who should not take RYTHMOL?
Do not take RYTHMOL if you have:
- heart failure (weak heart)
- had a recent heart attack
- a heart rate that is too slow, and you do not have a pacemaker
- a heart condition called Brugada Syndrome
- very low blood pressure
- certain breathing problems that make you short of breath or wheeze
- certain abnormal body salt (electrolyte) levels in your blood

Talk to your doctor before taking RYTHMOL if you think you have any of the conditions listed above.
What should I tell my doctor before taking RYTHMOL?
Before you take RYTHMOL, tell your doctor if you:
- have liver or kidney problems
- have breathing problems
- have symptoms including diarrhea, sweating, vomiting, or loss of appetite or thirst that are severe. These symptoms may be a sign of abnormal electrolyte levels in your blood.

- have myasthenia gravis
- have lupus erythematosis
- have been told you have or had an abnormal blood test called Antinuclear Antibody Test or ANA Test
- have any other medical conditions
- are pregnant or plan to become pregnant. It is not known if RYTHMOL will harm your unborn baby.
- are breastfeeding or plan to breastfeed. RYTHMOL can pass into your milk and may harm your baby. You and your doctor should decide if you will breastfeed or take RYTHMOL. You should not do both.

Tell your doctor about all the medicines you take, including prescription and over-the-counter medicines, vitamins, and herbal supplements. RYTHMOL and certain other medicines can affect (interact) with each other and cause serious side effects. You can ask your pharmacist for a list of medicines that interact with RYTHMOL.
Know the medicines you take. Keep a list of them to show your doctor and pharmacist when you get a new medicine.
How should I take RYTHMOL?
- Take RYTHMOL exactly as prescribed. Your doctor will tell you how many tablets to take and how often to take them.
- To help reduce the chance of certain side effects, your doctor may start you with a low dose of RYTHMOL, and then slowly increase the dose.
- You should not drink grapefruit juice during treatment with RYTHMOL.
- If you miss a dose of RYTHMOL, take your next dose at the usual time. Do not take 2 doses at the same time.
- If you take too much RYTHMOL, call your doctor or go to the nearest hospital emergency room right away.
- Call your doctor if your heart problems get worse.
What are possible side effects of RYTHMOL?
RYTHMOL can cause serious side effects including:
- **New or worsened abnormal heart beats, that can cause sudden death or be life-threatening.** Your doctor may do an electrocardiogram (ECG or EKG) before and during treatment to check your heart for these problems.
- **New or worsened heart failure. Tell your doctor about any changes in your heart symptoms, including:**
  - any new or increased swelling in your arms or legs
  - trouble breathing
  - sudden weight gain
- **Effects on pacemaker function.** RYTHMOL may affect how an implanted pacemaker or defibrillator works. Your doctor should check how your pacemaker or defibrillator is working during and after treatment with RYTHMOL. They may need to be re-programmed.
- **Very low white blood cell levels in your blood (agranulocytosis).** Your bone marrow may not produce enough of a certain type of white blood cells called neutrophils. If this happens, you are more likely to get infections. Tell your doctor right away if you have any of these symptoms, especially during the first 3 months of treatment:
  - fever
  - sore throat
  - chills
- **Worsening of myasthenia gravis in people who already have this condition.** Tell your doctor about any change in your symptoms.
- **RYTHMOL may cause lower sperm counts in men.** This could affect the ability to father a child. Talk to your doctor if this is a concern for you.

Common side effects of RYTHMOL include:
1. unusual taste
2. nausea
3. vomiting
4. dizziness
5. constipation
6. headache
7. tiredness
8. irregular heart beats

Tell your doctor if you have any side effect that bothers you or that does not go away.
These are not all the possible side effects of RYTHMOL. For more information, ask your doctor or pharmacist.
Call your doctor for medical advice about side effects. You may report side effects to FDA at 1-800-FDA-1088.
How should I store RYTHMOL?
- Store RYTHMOL at room temperature between 68°F to 77°F (20°C to 25°C).
- Keep the bottle tightly closed.

Keep RYTHMOL and all medicines out of the reach of children.
General information about RYTHMOL
Medicines are sometimes prescribed for purposes other than those listed in a Patient Information Leaflet. Do not use RYTHMOL for a condition for which it was not prescribed. Do not give RYTHMOL to other people, even if they have the same symptoms you have. It may harm them.
If you would like more information, talk with your doctor. You can ask your doctor or pharmacist for information about

RYTHMOL that is written for health professionals. For more information about RYTHMOL, call 1-888-825-5249.
What are the ingredients in RYTHMOL?
Active ingredient: propafenone hydrochloride.
Inactive ingredients: corn starch, hypromellose, magnesium stearate, polyethylene glycol, polysorbate, povidone, propylene glycol, sodium starch glycolate, and titanium dioxide.
This Patient Information has been approved by the U.S. Food and Drug Administration.
RYTHMOL is a registered trademark of G. Petrik used under license by Abbott Laboratories.
Manufactured for:
GlaxoSmithKline
Research Triangle Park, NC 27709
©2014, the GSK group of companies. All rights reserved.
March 2014
RML:3PIL

RYTHMOL SR   ℞
[RITH-Mall]
(propafenone hydrochloride)
Extended-Release Capsules for oral use

HIGHLIGHTS OF PRESCRIBING INFORMATION
These highlights do not include all the information needed to use RYTHMOL SR safely and effectively. See full prescribing information for RYTHMOL SR.
RYTHMOL SR (propafenone hydrochloride) Extended-Release Capsules for oral use
Initial U.S. Approval: 1989

WARNING: MORTALITY
See full prescribing information for complete boxed warning
- **An increased rate of death or reversed cardiac arrest rate was seen in patients treated with encainide or flecainide (Class IC antiarrhythmics) compared with that seen in patients assigned to placebo. At present it is prudent to consider any IC antiarrhythmic to have a significant risk of provoking proarrhythmic events in patients with structural heart disease.**
- **Given the lack of any evidence that these drugs improve survival, antiarrhythmic agents should generally be avoided in patients with non-life-threatening ventricular arrhythmias, even if the patients are experiencing unpleasant, but not life-threatening, symptoms or signs.**

INDICATIONS AND USAGE
RYTHMOL SR is an antiarrhythmic indicated to prolong the time to recurrence of symptomatic atrial fibrillation (AF) in patients with episodic (most likely paroxysmal or persistent) AF who do not have structural heart disease. (1)
Usage Considerations:
- Use in patients with permanent atrial fibrillation or with atrial flutter or paroxysmal supraventricular tachycardia (PSVT) has not been evaluated. Do not use to control ventricular rate during atrial fibrillation. (1)
- In patients with atrial fibrillation and atrial flutter, use RYTHMOL SR with drugs that increase the atrioventricular nodal refractory period. (1)
- The effect of propafenone on mortality has not been determined. (1)

DOSAGE AND ADMINISTRATION
- Initiate therapy with 225 mg given every 12 hours. (2)
- Dosage may be increased at a minimum of 5-day intervals to 325 mg every 12 hours and, if necessary, to 425 mg every 12 hours. (2)
- Dose reduction should be considered in patients with hepatic impairment, significant widening of the QRS complex, or second-or third-degree AV block. (2)

DOSAGE FORMS AND STRENGTHS
Capsules: 225 mg, 325 mg, 425 mg. (3)

CONTRAINDICATIONS
- Heart failure (4)
- Cardiogenic shock (4)
- Sinoatrial, atrioventricular, and intraventricular disorders of impulse generation and/or conduction in the absence of pacemaker (4)
- Known Brugada Syndrome (4)
- Bradycardia (4)
- Marked hypotension (4)
- Bronchospastic disorders and severe obstructive pulmonary disease (4)
- Marked electrolyte imbalance (4)

WARNINGS AND PRECAUTIONS

- May cause new or worsened arrhythmias. Evaluate patients via ECG prior to and during therapy. (5.1)
- RYTHMOL SR may unmask Brugada or Brugada-like Syndrome. Evaluate patients via ECG after initiation of therapy. (4, 5.2)
- Avoid use with other antiarrhythmic agents or drugs that prolong the QT interval. (5.3)
- Avoid simultaneous use of propafenone with both a cytochrome P450 2D6 inhibitor and a 3A4 inhibitor. (5.4)
- May provoke overt heart failure. (5.5)
- May cause dose-related first-degree AV block or other conduction disturbances. Should not be given to patients with conduction defects in absence of a pacemaker. (5.6)
- May affect artificial pacemakers. Pacemakers should be monitored during therapy. (5.7)
- Agranulocytosis: Patients should report signs of infection. (5.8)
- Administer cautiously to patients with impaired hepatic and renal function. (5.9, 5.10)
- Exacerbation of myasthenia gravis has been reported. (5.11)

ADVERSE REACTIONS

The most commonly reported adverse events with propafenone (>5% and greater than placebo) excluding those not reasonably associated with the use of the drug included the following: dizziness, palpitations, chest pain, dyspnea, taste disturbance, nausea, fatigue, anxiety, constipation, upper respiratory tract infection, edema, and influenza. (6.1)

To report SUSPECTED ADVERSE REACTIONS, contact GlaxoSmithKline at 1-888-825-5249 or FDA at 1-800-FDA-1088 or www.fda.gov/medwatch.

DRUG INTERACTIONS

- Inhibitors of CYP2D6, 1A2, and 3A4 may increase propafenone levels which may lead to cardiac arrhythmias. Simultaneous use with both a CYP3A4 and CYP2D6 inhibitor (or in patients with CYP2D6 deficiency) should be avoided. (7.1)
- Propafenone may increase digoxin or warfarin levels. (7.2, 7.3)
- Orlistat may reduce propafenone concentrations. Abrupt cessation of orlistat in patients stable on RYTHMOL SR has resulted in convulsions, atrioventricular block, and circulatory failure. (7.4)
- Concomitant use of lidocaine may increase central nervous system side effects. (7.6)

See 17 for PATIENT COUNSELING INFORMATION and FDA-approved patient labeling

Revised: 02/2014

FULL PRESCRIBING INFORMATION: CONTENTS*

FULL PRESCRIBING INFORMATION

> **WARNING: MORTALITY**
> - In the National Heart, Lung, and Blood Institute's Cardiac Arrhythmia Suppression Trial (CAST), a long-term, multicenter, randomized, double-blind trial in patients with asymptomatic non-life-threatening ventricular arrhythmias who had a myocardial infarction more than 6 days but less than 2 years previously, an increased rate of death or reversed cardiac arrest rate (7.7%; 56/730) was seen in patients treated with encainide or flecainide (Class IC antiarrhythmics) compared with that seen in patients assigned to placebo (3.0%; 22/725). The average duration of treatment with encainide or flecainide in this trial was 10 months.
> - The applicability of the CAST results to other populations (e.g., those without recent myocardial infarction) or other antiarrhythmic drugs is uncertain, but at present, it is prudent to consider any IC antiarrhythmic to have a significant proarrhythmic risk in patients with structural heart disease. Given the lack of any evidence that these drugs improve survival, antiarrhythmic agents should generally be avoided in patients with non-life-threatening ventricular arrhythmias, even if the patients are experiencing unpleasant, but not life-threatening, symptoms or signs.

1 INDICATIONS AND USAGE

RYTHMOL SR® is indicated to prolong the time to recurrence of symptomatic atrial fibrillation (AF) in patients with episodic (most likely paroxysmal or persistent) AF who do not have structural heart disease.

Usage Considerations:
- The use of RYTHMOL SR in patients with permanent AF or in patients exclusively with atrial flutter or paroxysmal supraventricular tachycardia (PSVT) has not been evaluated. Do not use RYTHMOL SR to control ventricular rate during AF.
- Some patients with atrial flutter treated with propafenone have developed 1:1 conduction, producing an increase in ventricular rate. Concomitant treatment with drugs that increase the functional atrioventricular (AV) nodal refractory period is recommended.
- The effect of propafenone on mortality has not been determined [see Boxed Warning].

2 DOSAGE AND ADMINISTRATION

RYTHMOL SR can be taken with or without food. Do not crush or further divide the contents of the capsule.

The dose of RYTHMOL SR must be individually titrated on the basis of response and tolerance. Initiate therapy with RYTHMOL SR 225 mg given every 12 hours. Dosage may be increased at a minimum of 5-day intervals to 325 mg given every 12 hours. If additional therapeutic effect is needed, the dose of RYTHMOL SR may be increased to 425 mg given every 12 hours.

In patients with hepatic impairment or those with significant widening of the QRS complex or second-or third-degree AV block, consider reducing the dose.

The combination of CYP3A4 inhibition and either CYP2D6 deficiency or CYP2D6 inhibition with the simultaneous administration of propafenone may significantly increase the concentration of propafenone and thereby increase the risk of proarrhythmia and other adverse events. Therefore, avoid simultaneous use of RYTHMOL SR with both a CYP2D6 inhibitor and a CYP3A4 inhibitor [see Warnings and Precautions (5.4), Drug Interactions (7.1)].

3 DOSAGE FORMS AND STRENGTHS

RYTHMOL SR (propafenone HCl) Capsules are supplied as white, opaque, hard gelatin capsules containing either 225 mg, 325 mg, or 425 mg of propafenone HCl. The 225 mg strength is imprinted in red with GS EUG followed by 225. The 325-mg strength is imprinted in red with GS F1Y followed by 325, and also has a single red band around ¾ of the circumference of the body. The 425-mg strength is imprinted in red with GS UY2 followed by 425, and also has 3 red bands around ¾ of the circumference of the body.

4 CONTRAINDICATIONS

RYTHMOL SR is contraindicated in the following circumstances:
- Heart failure
- Cardiogenic shock
- Sinoatrial, atrioventricular, and intraventricular disorders of impulse generation or conduction (e.g., sick sinus node syndrome, AV block) in the absence of an artificial pacemaker
- Known Brugada Syndrome
- Bradycardia
- Marked hypotension
- Bronchospastic disorders or severe obstructive pulmonary disease
- Marked electrolyte imbalance

5 WARNINGS AND PRECAUTIONS

5.1 Proarrhythmic Effects

Propafenone has caused new or worsened arrhythmias. Such proarrhythmic effects include sudden death and life-threatening ventricular arrhythmias such as ventricular fibrillation, ventricular tachycardia, asystole, and torsade de pointes. It may also worsen premature ventricular contractions or supraventricular arrhythmias, and it may prolong the QT interval. It is therefore essential that each patient given RYTHMOL SR be evaluated electrocardiographically prior to and during therapy to determine whether the response to RYTHMOL SR supports continued treatment. Because propafenone prolongs the QRS interval in the electrocardiogram, changes in the QT interval are difficult to interpret [see Clinical Pharmacology (12.2)].

In the RAFT trial [see Clinical Studies (14)], there were too few deaths to assess the long-term risk to patients. There were 5 deaths, 3 in the pooled group for RYTHMOL SR (0.8%) and 2 in the placebo group (1.6%). In the overall database of 8 trials of RYTHMOL SR and immediate-release RYTHMOL, the mortality rate was 2.5% per year on propafenone and 4.0% per year on placebo. Concurrent use of propafenone with other antiarrhythmic agents has not been well studied.

In a US uncontrolled, open-label, multicenter trial using the immediate-release formulation in patients with symptomatic supraventricular tachycardia (SVT), 1.9% (9/474) of these patients experienced ventricular tachycardia (VT) or ventricular fibrillation (VF) during the trial. However, in 4 of the 9 patients, the ventricular tachycardia was of atrial origin. Six of the 9 patients that developed ventricular arrhythmias did so within 14 days of onset of therapy. About 2.3% (11/474) of all patients had recurrence of SVT during the trial which could have been a change in the patients' arrhythmia behavior or could represent a proarrhythmic event. Case reports in patients treated with propafenone for atrial fibrillation/flutter have included increased premature ventricular contractions (PVCs), VT, VF, torsades de pointes, asystole, and death.

Overall in clinical trials with RYTHMOL immediate-release (which included patients treated for ventricular arrhythmias, atrial fibrillation/flutter, and PSVT), 4.7% of all patients had new or worsened ventricular arrhythmia possibly representing a proarrhythmic event (0.7% was an increase in PVCs; 4.0% a worsening, or new appearance, of VT or VF). Of the patients who had worsening of VT (4%), 92% had a history of VT and/or VT/VF, 71% had coronary artery disease, and 68% had a prior myocardial infarction. The incidence of proarrhythmia in patients with less serious or benign arrhythmias, which include patients with an increase in frequency of PVCs, was 1.6%. Although most proarrhythmic events occurred during the first week of therapy, late events also were seen and the CAST trial [see Boxed Warning: Mortality] suggests that an increased risk of proarrhythmia is present throughout treatment.

5.2 Unmasking Brugada Syndrome

Brugada Syndrome may be unmasked after exposure to RYTHMOL SR. Perform an ECG after initiation of RYTHMOL SR and discontinue the drug if changes are suggestive of Brugada Syndrome [see Contraindications (4)].

5.3 Use With Drugs That Prolong the QT Interval and Antiarrhythmic Agents

The use of RYTHMOL SR in conjunction with other drugs that prolong the QT interval has not been extensively studied. Such drugs may include many antiarrhythmics, some phenothiazines, tricyclic antidepressants, and oral macrolides. Withhold Class IA and III antiarrhythmic agents for at least 5 half-lives prior to dosing with RYTHMOL SR. Avoid the use of propafenone with Class IA and III antiarrhythmic agents (including quinidine and amiodarone). There is only limited experience with the concomitant use of Class IB or IC antiarrhythmics.

5.4 Drug Interactions: Simultaneous Use With Inhibitors of Cytochrome P450 Isoenzymes 2D6 and 3A4

Propafenone is metabolized by CYP2D6, CYP3A4, and CYP1A2 isoenzymes. Approximately 6% of Caucasians in the US population are naturally deficient in CYP2D6 activity and to a somewhat lesser extent in other demographic groups. Drugs that inhibit these CYP pathways (such as desipramine, paroxetine, ritonavir, sertraline for CYP2D6; ketoconazole, erythromycin, saquinavir, and grapefruit juice for CYP3A4; and amiodarone and tobacco smoke for CYP1A2) can be expected to cause increased plasma levels of propafenone.

Increased exposure to propafenone may lead to cardiac arrhythmias and exaggerated beta-adrenergic blocking activity. Because of its metabolism, the combination of CYP3A4 inhibition and either CYP2D6 deficiency or CYP2D6 inhibition in users of propafenone is potentially hazardous. Therefore, avoid simultaneous use of RYTHMOL SR with both a CYP2D6 inhibitor and a CYP3A4 inhibitor.

5.5 Use in Patients With a History of Heart Failure

Propafenone exerts a negative inotropic activity on the myocardium as well as beta blockade effects and may provoke overt heart failure. In the US trial (RAFT) in patients with symptomatic AF, heart failure was reported in 4 (1.0%) patients receiving RYTHMOL SR (all doses), compared with 1 (0.8%) patient receiving placebo. Proarrhythmic effects more likely occur when propafenone is administered to patients with heart failure (NYHA III and IV) or severe myocardial ischemia [see Contraindications (4)].

In clinical trial experience with RYTHMOL immediate-release, new or worsened heart failure has been reported in 3.7% of patients with ventricular arrhythmia. These events were more likely in subjects with pre-existing heart failure and coronary artery disease. New onset of heart failure attributable to propafenone developed in <0.2% of patients with ventricular arrhythmia and in 1.9% of patients with paroxysmal AF or PSVT.

5.6 Conduction Disturbances

Propafenone slows atrioventricular conduction and may also cause dose-related first-degree AV block. Average PR interval prolongation and increases in QRS duration are also dose-related. Do not give propafenone to patients with atrioventricular and intraventricular conduction defects in the absence of a pacemaker [see Contraindications (4), Clinical Pharmacology (12.2)].

In a US trial (RAFT) in 523 patients with a history of symptomatic AF treated with RYTHMOL SR, sinus bradycardia (rate <50 beats/min) was reported with the same frequency with RYTHMOL SR and placebo.

5.7 Effects on Pacemaker Threshold

Propafenone may alter both pacing and sensing thresholds of implanted pacemakers and defibrillators. During and after therapy, monitor and re-program these devices accordingly.

5.8 Agranulocytosis

Agranulocytosis has been reported in patients receiving propafenone. Generally, the agranulocytosis occurred within the first 2 months of propafenone therapy and upon discontinuation of therapy; the white count usually normalized by 14 days. Unexplained fever or decrease in white cell count, particularly during the initial 3 months of therapy, warrant consideration of possible agranulocytosis or granulocytopenia. Instruct patients to report promptly any signs of infection such as fever, sore throat, or chills.

5.9 Use in Patients With Hepatic Dysfunction

Propafenone is highly metabolized by the liver. Severe liver dysfunction increases the bioavailability of propafenone to approximately 70% compared with 3% to 40% in patients with normal liver function when given RYTHMOL immediate-release tablets. In 8 patients with moderate to severe liver disease administered RYTHMOL immediate-release tablets, the mean half-life was approximately 9 hours. No trials have compared bioavailability of propafenone from RYTHMOL SR in patients with normal and impaired hepatic function. Increased bioavailability of propafenone in these patients may result in excessive accumulation. Carefully monitor patients with impaired hepatic function for excessive pharmacological effects [see Overdosage (10)].

5.10 Use in Patients With Renal Dysfunction

Approximately 50% of propafenone metabolites are excreted in the urine following administration of RYTHMOL immediate-release tablets. No trials have been performed to assess the percentage of metabolites eliminated in the urine following the administration of RYTHMOL SR Capsules.

In patients with impaired renal function monitor for signs of overdosage [see Overdosage (10)].

5.11 Use in Patients With Myasthenia Gravis

Exacerbation of myasthenia gravis has been reported during propafenone therapy.

5.12 Elevated ANA Titers

Positive ANA titers have been reported in patients receiving propafenone. They have been reversible upon cessation of treatment and may disappear even in the face of continued propafenone therapy. These laboratory findings were usually not associated with clinical symptoms, but there is one published case of drug-induced lupus erythematosus (positive rechallenge); it resolved completely upon discontinuation of therapy. Carefully evaluate patients who develop an abnormal ANA test and if persistent or worsening elevation of ANA titers is detected, consider discontinuing therapy.

5.13 Impaired Spermatogenesis

Reversible disorders of spermatogenesis have been demonstrated in monkeys, dogs, and rabbits after high-dose intravenous administration of propafenone. Evaluation of the effects of short-term administration of RYTHMOL on spermatogenesis in 11 normal subjects suggested that propafenone produced a reversible, short-term drop (within normal range) in sperm count.

6 ADVERSE REACTIONS

6.1 Clinical Trials Experience

Because clinical trials are conducted under widely varying conditions, adverse reaction rates observed in the clinical trials of a drug cannot be directly compared with rates in the clinical trials of another drug and may not reflect the rates observed in practice.

The data described below reflect exposure to RYTHMOL SR 225 mg twice daily in 126 patients, to RYTHMOL SR 325 mg twice daily in 135 patients, to RYTHMOL SR 425 mg twice daily in 136 patients, and to placebo in 126 patients for up to 39 weeks (mean 20 weeks) in a placebo-controlled trial (RAFT) conducted in the US. The most commonly reported adverse events with propafenone (>5% and greater than placebo) excluding those not reasonably associated with the use of the drug or because they were associated with the condition being treated, were dizziness, palpitations, chest pain, dyspnea, taste disturbance, nausea, fatigue, anxiety, constipation, upper respiratory tract infection, edema, and influenza. The frequency of discontinuation due to adverse events was 17%, and the rate was highest during the first 14 days of treatment.

Cardiac-related adverse events occurring in ≥ 2% of the patients in any of the RAFT propafenone SR treatment groups and more common with propafenone than with placebo, excluding those that are common in the population and those not plausibly related to drug therapy, included the following: angina pectoris, atrial flutter, AV block first-degree, bradycardia, congestive cardiac failure, cardiac murmur, edema, dyspnea, rales, wheezing, and cardioactive drug level above therapeutic.

Propafenone prolongs the PR and QRS intervals in patients with atrial and ventricular arrhythmias. Prolongation of the QRS interval makes it difficult to interpret the effect of propafenone on the QT interval [see Clinical Pharmacology (12.2)].

Non-cardiac related adverse events occurring in ≥2% of the patients in any of the RAFT propafenone SR treatment groups and more common with propafenone than with placebo, excluding those that are common in the population and those not plausibly related to drug therapy, included the following: blurred vision, constipation, diarrhea, dry mouth, flatulence, nausea, vomiting, fatigue, weakness, upper respiratory tract infection, blood alkaline phosphatase increased, hematuria, muscle weakness, dizziness (excluding vertigo), headache, taste disturbance, tremor, somnolence, anxiety, depression, ecchymosis.

No clinically important differences in incidence of adverse reactions were noted by age or gender. Too few non-Caucasian patients were enrolled to assess adverse events according to race.

Adverse events occurring in 2% or more of the patients in any of the ERAFT [see Clinical Studies (14)] propafenone SR treatment groups and not listed above include the following: bundle branch block left, bundle branch block right, conduction disorders, sinus bradycardia, and hypotension.

Other adverse events reported with propafenone clinical trials not already listed elsewhere in the prescribing information include the following adverse events by body system and preferred term.

Blood and Lymphatic System Disorders

Anemia, lymphadenopathy, spleen disorder, thrombocytopenia.

Cardiac Disorders

Unstable angina, atrial hypertrophy, cardiac arrest, coronary artery disease, extrasystoles, myocardial infarction, nodal arrhythmia, palpitations, pericarditis, sinoatrial block, sinus arrest, sinus arrhythmia, supraventricular extrasystoles, ventricular extrasystoles, ventricular hypertrophy.

Ear and Labyrinth Disorders

Hearing impaired, tinnitus, vertigo.

Eye Disorders

Eye hemorrhage, eye inflammation, eyelid ptosis, miosis, retinal disorder, visual acuity reduced.

Gastrointestinal Disorders

Abdominal distension, abdominal pain, duodenitis, dyspepsia, dysphagia, eructation, gastritis, gastroesophageal reflux disease, gingival bleeding, glossitis, glossodynia, gum pain, halitosis, intestinal obstruction, melena, mouth ulceration, pancreatitis, peptic ulcer, rectal bleeding, sore throat.

General Disorders and Administration Site Conditions

Chest pain, feeling hot, hemorrhage, malaise, pain, pyrexia.

Hepatobiliary Disorders

Hepatomegaly.

Investigations

Abnormal heart sounds, abnormal pulse, carotid bruit, decreased blood chloride, decreased blood pressure, decreased blood sodium, decreased hemoglobin, decreased neutrophil count, decreased platelet count, decreased prothrombin level, decreased red blood cell count, decreased weight, glycosuria present, increased alanine aminotransferase, increased aspartate aminotransferase, increased blood bilirubin, increased blood cholesterol, increased blood creatinine, increased blood glucose, increased blood lactate dehydrogenase, increased blood pressure, increased blood prolactin, increased blood triglycerides, increased blood urea, increased blood uric acid, increased eosinophil count, increased gamma-glutamyltransferase, increased monocyte count, increased prostatic specific antigen, increased prothrombin level, increased weight, increased white blood cell count, ketonuria present, proteinuria present.

Metabolism and Nutrition Disorders

Anorexia, dehydration, diabetes mellitus, gout, hypercholesterolemia, hyperglycemia, hyperlipidemia, hypokalemia.

Musculoskeletal, Connective Tissue and Bone Disorders

Arthritis, bursitis, collagen-vascular disease, costochondritis, joint disorder, muscle cramps, muscle spasms, myalgia, neck pain, pain in jaw, sciatica, tendonitis.

Nervous System Disorders

Amnesia, ataxia, balance impaired, brain damage, cerebrovascular accident, dementia, gait disorder, hypertonia, hypothesia, insomnia, paralysis, paresthesia, peripheral neuropathy, speech disorder, syncope, tongue hypoesthesia.

Psychiatric Disorders

Decreased libido, emotional disturbance, mental disorder, neurosis, nightmare, sleep disorder.

Renal and Urinary Disorder

Dysuria, nocturia, oliguria, pyuria, renal failure, urinary casts, urinary frequency, urinary incontinence, urinary retention, urine abnormal.

Reproductive System and Breast Disorders

Breast pain, impotence, prostatism.

Respiratory, Thoracic, and Mediastinal Disorders

Atelectasis, breath sounds decreased, chronic obstructive airways disease, cough, epistaxis, hemoptysis, lung disorder, pleural effusion, pulmonary congestion, rales, respiratory failure, rhinitis, throat tightness.

Skin and Subcutaneous Tissue Disorders

Alopecia, dermatitis, dry skin, erythema, nail abnormality, petechiae, pruritus, sweating increased, urticaria.

Vascular Disorders

Arterial embolism limb, deep limb venous thrombosis, flushing, hematoma, hypertension, hypertensive crisis, hypotension, labile blood pressure, pallor, peripheral coldness, peripheral vascular disease, thrombosis.

7 DRUG INTERACTIONS

7.1 CYP2D6 and CYP3A4 Inhibitors

Drugs that inhibit CYP2D6 (such as desipramine, paroxetine, ritonavir, sertraline) and CYP3A4 (such as ketoconazole, ritonavir, saquinavir, erythromycin, and grapefruit juice) can be expected to cause increased plasma levels of propafenone. The combination of CYP3A4 inhibition and either CYP2D6 deficiency or CYP2D6 inhibition with administration of propafenone may increase the risk of adverse reactions, including proarrhythmia. Therefore, simultaneous use of RYTHMOL SR with both a CYP2D6 inhibitor and a CYP3A4 inhibitor should be avoided [see Warnings and Precautions (5.4), Dosage and Administration (2)].

Amiodarone

Concomitant administration of propafenone and amiodarone can affect conduction and repolarization and is not recommended.

Cimetidine

Concomitant administration of propafenone immediate-release tablets and cimetidine in 12 healthy subjects resulted in a 20% increase in steady-state plasma concentrations of propafenone.

Fluoxetine

Concomitant administration of propafenone and fluoxetine in extensive metabolizers increased the S-propafenone C_{max} and AUC by 39% and 50%, respectively, and the R propafenone C_{max} and AUC by 71% and 50%, respectively.

Quinidine

Small doses of quinidine completely inhibit the CYP2D6 hydroxylation metabolic pathway, making all patients, in effect, slow metabolizers [see Clinical Pharmacology (12)]. Concomitant administration of quinidine (50 mg 3 times daily) with 150-mg immediate-release propafenone 3 times daily decreased the clearance of propafenone by 60% in extensive metabolizers, making them poor metabolizers. Steady-state plasma concentrations increased by more than 2 fold for propafenone, and decreased 50% for 5-OH-

Table 1. Mean Change ± SD in 12-Lead Electrocardiogram Results (RAFT)

	RYTHMOL SR Twice-Daily Dosing			
	225 mg	325 mg	425 mg	Placebo
	n = 126	n = 135	n = 136	n = 126
PR (ms)	9 ± 22	12 ± 23	21 ± 24	1 ± 16
QRS (ms)	4 ± 14	6 ± 15	6 ± 15	-2 ± 12
Heart rate	5 ± 24	7 ± 23	2 ± 22	8 ± 27
QTc[a] (ms)	2 ± 30	5 ± 36	6 ± 37	5 ± 35

[a] Calculated using Bazett's correction factor

Table 2. Number of Patients According to the Range of Maximum QTc Change Compared With Baseline Over the Trial in Each Dose Group (RAFT Trial).

Range Maximum QTc Change	RYTHMOL SR			
	225 mg Twice Daily N = 119 n (%)	325 mg Twice Daily N = 129 n (%)	425 mg Twice Daily N = 123 n (%)	Placebo N = 100 n (%)
>20%	1 (1)	6 (5)	3 (2)	5 (4)
10-20%	19 (16)	28 (22)	32 (26)	24 (20)
0 ≤10%	99 (83)	95 (74)	88 (72)	91 (76)

propafenone. A 100-mg dose of quinidine increased steady state concentrations of propafenone 3 fold. Avoid concomitant use of propafenone and quinidine.

Rifampin
Concomitant administration of rifampin and propafenone in extensive metabolizers decreased the plasma concentrations of propafenone by 67% with a corresponding decrease of 5-OH-propafenone by 65%. The concentrations of norpropafenone increased by 30%. In poor metabolizers, there was a 50% decrease in propafenone plasma concentrations and an increase in the AUC and C_{max} of norpropafenone by 74% and 20%, respectively. Urinary excretion of propafenone and its metabolites decreased significantly. Similar results were noted in elderly patients: Both the AUC and C_{max} propafenone decreased by 84%, with a corresponding decrease in AUC and C_{max} of 5-OH-propafenone by 69% and 57%, respectively.

7.2 Digoxin
Concomitant use of propafenone and digoxin increased steady-state serum digoxin exposure (AUC) in patients by 60% to 270%, and decreased the clearance of digoxin by 31% to 67%. Monitor plasma digoxin levels of patients receiving propafenone and adjust digoxin dosage as needed.

7.3 Warfarin
The concomitant administration of propafenone and warfarin increased warfarin plasma concentrations at steady state by 39% in healthy volunteers and prolonged the prothrombin time (PT) in patients taking warfarin. Adjust the warfarin dose as needed by monitoring INR (international normalized ratio).

7.4 Orlistat
Orlistat may limit the fraction of propafenone available for absorption. In postmarketing reports, abrupt cessation of orlistat in patients stabilized on propafenone has resulted in severe adverse events including convulsions, atrioventricular block, and acute circulatory failure.

7.5 Beta-Antagonists
Concomitant use of propafenone and propranolol in healthy subjects increased propranolol plasma concentrations at steady state by 113%. In 4 patients, administration of metoprolol with propafenone increased the metoprolol plasma concentrations at steady state by 100% to 400%. The pharmacokinetics of propafenone was not affected by the coadministration of either propranolol or metoprolol. In clinical trials using propafenone immediate-release tablets, patients who were receiving beta-blockers concurrently did not experience an increased incidence of side effects.

7.6 Lidocaine
No significant effects on the pharmacokinetics of propafenone or lidocaine have been seen following their concomitant use in patients. However, concomitant use of propafenone and lidocaine has been reported to increase the risks of central nervous system side effects of lidocaine.

8 USE IN SPECIFIC POPULATIONS
8.1 Pregnancy
Pregnancy Category C. There are no adequate and well-controlled studies in pregnant women. RYTHMOL SR should be used during pregnancy only if the potential benefit justifies the potential risk to the fetus.

Animal Data
Teratogenic Effects
Propafenone has been shown to be embryotoxic (decreased survival) in rabbits and rats when given in oral maternally toxic doses of 150 mg/kg/day (about 3 times the maximum recommended human dose [MRHD] on a mg/m² basis) and 600 mg/kg/day (about 6 times the MRHD on a mg/m² basis), respectively. Although maternally tolerated doses (up to 270 mg/kg/day, about 3 times the MRHD on a mg/m² basis) produced no evidence of embryotoxicity in rats, postimplantation loss was elevated in all rabbit treatment groups (doses as low as 15 mg/kg/day, about 1/3 the MRHD on a mg/m² basis).
Non-teratogenic Effects
In a study in which female rats received daily oral doses of propafenone from mid-gestation through weaning of their offspring, doses as low as 90 mg/kg/day (equivalent to the MRHD on a mg/m² basis) produced increases in maternal deaths. Doses of 360 or more mg/kg/day (4 or more times the MRHD on a mg/m² basis) resulted in reductions in neonatal survival, body weight gain, and physiological development.

8.2 Labor and Delivery
It is not known whether the use of propafenone during labor or delivery has immediate or delayed adverse effects on the fetus, or whether it prolongs the duration of labor or increases the need for forceps delivery or other obstetrical intervention.

8.3 Nursing Mothers
Propafenone is excreted in human milk. Because of the potential for serious adverse reactions in nursing infants from propafenone, decide whether to discontinue nursing or to discontinue the drug, taking into account the importance of the drug to the mother.

8.4 Pediatric Use
The safety and effectiveness of propafenone in pediatric patients have not been established.

8.5 Geriatric Use
Of the total number of patients in Phase 3 clinical trials of RYTHMOL SR (propafenone hydrochloride) 46% were 65 and over, while 16% were 75 and over. No overall differences in safety or effectiveness were observed between these patients and younger patients, but greater sensitivity of some older individuals at higher doses cannot be ruled out. The effect of age on the pharmacokinetics and pharmacodynamics of propafenone has not been studied.

10 OVERDOSAGE
The symptoms of overdosage may include hypotension, somnolence, bradycardia, intra-atrial and intraventricular conduction disturbances, and rarely convulsions and high grade ventricular arrhythmias. Defibrillation as well as infusion of dopamine and isoproterenol have been effective in controlling abnormal rhythm and blood pressure. Convulsions have been alleviated with intravenous diazepam. General supportive measures such as mechanical respiratory assistance and external cardiac massage may be necessary. The hemodialysis of propafenone in patients with an overdose is expected to be of limited value in the removal of propafenone as a result of both its high protein binding (>95%) and large volume of distribution.

11 DESCRIPTION
RYTHMOL SR (propafenone hydrochloride) is an antiarrhythmic drug supplied in extended-release capsules of 225, 325 and 425 mg for oral administration.
Chemically, propafenone hydrochloride is 2'-[2-Hydroxy-3-(propylamino)-propoxy]-3-phenylpropiophenone, with a molecular weight of 377.92. The molecular formula is $C_{21}H_{27}NO_3 \cdot HCl$.
Propafenone HCl has some structural similarities to beta-blocking agents. The structural formula of propafenone HCl is given below:

Propafenone HCl occurs as colorless crystals or white crystalline powder with a very bitter taste. It is slightly soluble in water (20°C), chloroform and ethanol. RYTHMOL SR capsules are filled with cylindrical-shaped 2 × 2 mm microtablets containing propafenone and the following inactive ingredients: antifoam, gelatin, hypromellose, magnesium stearate, red iron oxide, shellac, sodium dodecyl sulfate, sodium lauryl sulfate, soy lecithin, and titanium dioxide.

12 CLINICAL PHARMACOLOGY
12.1 Mechanism of Action
Propafenone is a Class 1C antiarrhythmic drug with local anesthetic effects, and a direct stabilizing action on myocardial membranes. The electrophysiological effect of propafenone manifests itself in a reduction of upstroke velocity (Phase 0) of the monophasic action potential. In Purkinje fibers, and to a lesser extent myocardial fibers, propafenone reduces the fast inward current carried by sodium ions. Diastolic excitability threshold is increased and effective refractory period prolonged. Propafenone reduces spontaneous automaticity and depresses triggered activity. Studies in anesthetized dogs and isolated organ preparations show that propafenone has beta-sympatholytic activity at about 1/50 the potency of propranolol. Clinical studies employing isoproterenol challenge and exercise testing after single doses of propafenone indicate a beta-adrenergic blocking potency (per mg) about 1/40 that of propranolol in man. In clinical trials with the immediate-release formulation, resting heart rate decreases of about 8% were noted at the higher end of the therapeutic plasma concentration range. At very high concentrations in vitro, propafenone can inhibit the slow inward current carried by calcium, but this calcium antagonist effect probably does not contribute to antiarrhythmic efficacy. Moreover, propafenone inhibits a variety of cardiac potassium currents in in vitro studies (i.e., the transient outward, the delayed rectifier, and the inward rectifier current). Propafenone has local anesthetic activity approximately equal to procaine. Compared with propafenone, the main metabolite, 5-hydroxypropafenone, has similar sodium and calcium channel activity, but about 10 times less beta-blocking activity (N-depropylpropafenone has weaker sodium channel activity but equivalent affinity for beta-receptors).

12.2 Pharmacodynamics
Electrophysiology
Electrophysiology trials in patients with ventricular tachycardia have shown that propafenone prolongs atrioventricular conduction while having little or no effect on sinus node function. Both atrioventricular nodal conduction time (AH interval) and His-Purkinje conduction time (HV interval) are prolonged. Propafenone has little or no effect on the atrial functional refractory period, but AV nodal functional and effective refractory periods are prolonged. In patients with Wolff-Parkinson-White syndrome, RYTHMOL immediate-release tablets reduce conduction and increase the effective refractory period of the accessory pathway in both directions.
Electrocardiograms
Propafenone prolongs the PR and QRS intervals. Prolongation of the QRS interval makes it difficult to interpret the effect of propafenone on the QT interval.
[See table 1 above]
In RAFT [see Clinical Studies (14)], the distribution of the maximum changes in QTc compared with baseline over the trial in each patient was similar in the groups receiving RYTHMOL SR 225 mg twice daily, 325 mg twice daily, and 425 mg twice daily, and placebo. Similar results were seen in the ERAFT trial.
[See table 2 above]
Hemodynamics
Trials in humans have shown that propafenone exerts a negative inotropic effect on the myocardium. Cardiac catheterization trials in patients with moderately impaired ventricular function (mean C.I. = 2.61 L/min/m²), utilizing intravenous propafenone infusions (loading dose of 2 mg/kg

over 10 min+ followed by 2 mg/min for 30 min) that gave mean plasma concentrations of 3.0 mcg/mL (a dose that produces plasma levels of propafenone greater than recommended oral dosing), showed significant increases in pulmonary capillary wedge pressure, systemic and pulmonary vascular resistances and depression of cardiac output and cardiac index.

12.3 Pharmacokinetics
Absorption/Bioavailability
Maximal plasma levels of propafenone are reached between 3 to 8 hours following the administration of RYTHMOL SR. Propafenone is known to undergo extensive and saturable presystemic biotransformation which results in a dose- and dosage-form-dependent absolute bioavailability; e.g., a 150-mg immediate-release tablet had an absolute bioavailability of 3.4%, while a 300-mg immediate-release tablet had an absolute bioavailability of 10.6%. Absorption from a 300-mg solution dose was rapid, with an absolute bioavailability of 21.4%. At still larger doses, above those recommended, bioavailability of propafenone from immediate-release tablets increased still further.

Relative bioavailability assessments have been performed between RYTHMOL SR capsules and RYTHMOL immediate-release tablets. In extensive metabolizers, the bioavailability of propafenone from the SR formulation was less than that of the immediate-release formulation as the more gradual release of propafenone from the prolonged-release preparations resulted in an increase of overall first-pass metabolism [see Metabolism]. As a result of the increased first-pass effect, higher daily doses of propafenone were required from the SR formulation relative to the immediate-release formulation, to obtain similar exposure to propafenone. The relative bioavailability of propafenone from the 325-mg twice daily regimens of RYTHMOL SR approximates that of RYTHMOL immediate-release 150-mg 3 times daily regimen. Mean exposure to 5-hydroxypropafenone was about 20% to 25% higher after SR capsule administration than after immediate-release tablet administration.

Food increased the exposure to propafenone 4-fold after single-dose administration of 425-mg of RYTHMOL SR. However, in the multiple-dose trial (425-mg dose twice daily), the difference between the fed and fasted state was not significant.

Distribution
Following intravenous administration of propafenone, plasma levels decline in a bi-phasic manner consistent with a 2-compartment pharmacokinetic model. The average distribution half-life corresponding to the first phase was about 5 minutes. The volume of the central compartment was about 88 liters (1.1 L/kg) and the total volume of distribution about 252 liters.

In serum, propafenone is greater than 95% bound to proteins within the concentration range of 0.5 to 2 mcg/mL.
Metabolism
There are 2 genetically determined patterns of propafenone metabolism. In over 90% of patients, the drug is rapidly and extensively metabolized with an elimination half-life from 2 to 10 hours. These patients metabolize propafenone into 2 active metabolites: 5-hydroxypropafenone which is formed by CYP2D6, and N-depropylpropafenone (norpropafenone) which is formed by both CYP3A4 and CYP1A2. In less than 10% of patients, metabolism of propafenone is slower because the 5-hydroxy metabolite is not formed or is minimally formed. In these patients, the estimated propafenone elimination half-life ranges from 10 to 32 hours. Decreased ability to form the 5-hydroxy metabolite of propafenone is associated with a diminished ability to metabolize debrisoquine and a variety of other drugs such as encainide, metoprolol, and dextromethorphan, whose metabolism is mediated by the CYP2D6 isozyme. In these patients, the N-depropylpropafenone metabolite occurs in quantities comparable to the levels occurring in extensive metabolizers.

As a consequence of the observed differences in metabolism, administration of RYTHMOL SR to slow and extensive metabolizers results in significant differences in plasma concentrations of propafenone, with slow metabolizers achieving concentrations about twice those of the extensive metabolizers at daily doses of 850 mg/day. At low doses the differences are greater, with slow metabolizers attaining concentrations about 3 to 4 times higher than extensive metabolizers. In extensive metabolizers, saturation of the hydroxylation pathway (CYP2D6) results in greater-than-linear increases in plasma levels following administration of RYTHMOL SR Capsules. In slow metabolizers, propafenone pharmacokinetics is linear. Because the difference decreases at high doses and is mitigated by the lack of the active 5-hydroxymetabolite in the slow metabolizers, and because steady-state conditions are achieved after 4 to 5 days of dosing in all patients, the recommended dosing regimen of RYTHMOL SR is the same for all patients. The larger inter-subject variability in blood levels require that the dose of the drug be titrated carefully in patients with close attention paid to clinical and ECG evidence of toxicity [see Dosage and Administration (2)].

Table 3. Analysis of Tachycardia-free Period (Days) from Day 1 of Randomization

Parameter	Dose of RYTHMOL SR			
	225 mg Twice Daily (N = 126) n (%)	325 mg Twice Daily (N = 135) n (%)	425 mg Twice Daily (N = 136) n (%)	Placebo (N = 126) n (%)
Patients completing with terminating event[a]	66 (52)	56 (41)	41 (30)	87 (69)
Comparison of tachycardia-free periods				
Kaplan-Meier Media	112	291	NA[b]	41
Range	0 - 285	0 - 293	0 - 300	0 – 289
p-Value (Log-rank test)	0.014	<0.0001	<0.0001	--
Hazard Ratio compared with placebo	0.67	0.43	0.35	--
95% CI for Hazard Ratio	(0.49, 0.93)	(0.31, 0.61)	(0.24, 0.51)	--

[a] Terminating events comprised 91% AF, 5% atrial flutter, and 4% PSVT.
[b] Not Applicable: Fewer than 50% of the patients had events. The median time is not calculable.

The 5-hydroxypropafenone and norpropafenone metabolites have electrophysiologic properties similar to propafenone in vitro. In man after administration of RYTHMOL SR, the 5-hydroxypropafenone metabolite is usually present in concentrations less than 40% of propafenone. The norpropafenone metabolite is usually present in concentrations less than 10% of propafenone.

Inter-Subject Variability
With propafenone, there is a considerable degree of inter-subject variability in pharmacokinetics which is due in large part to the first-pass hepatic effect and non-linear pharmacokinetics in extensive metabolizers. A higher degree of inter-subject variability in pharmacokinetic parameters of propafenone was observed following both single- and multiple-dose administration of RYTHMOL SR Capsules. Inter-subject variability appears to be substantially less in the poor metabolizer group than in the extensive metabolizer group, suggesting that a large portion of the variability is intrinsic to CYP2D6 polymorphism rather than to the formulation.

Stereochemistry
RYTHMOL is a racemic mixture. The R- and S-enantiomers of propafenone display stereoselective disposition characteristics. In vitro and in vivo studies have shown that the R-isomer of propafenone is cleared faster than the S-isomer via the 5-hydroxylation pathway (CYP2D6). This results in a higher ratio of S-propafenone to R-propafenone at steady state. Both enantiomers have equivalent potency to block sodium channels; however, the S-enantiomer is a more potent beta-antagonist than the R-enantiomer. Following administration of RYTHMOL immediate-release tablets or RYTHMOL SR Capsules, the S/R ratio for the area under the plasma concentration-time curve was about 1.7. The S/R ratios of propafenone obtained after administration of 225-, 325-, and 425-mg RYTHMOL SR are independent of dose. In addition, no difference in the average values of the S/R ratios is evident between genotypes or over time.

Special Populations
Hepatic Impairment
Decreased liver function increases the bioavailability of propafenone. Absolute bioavailability assessments have not been determined for the RYTHMOL SR capsule formulation. Absolute bioavailability of RYTHMOL immediate-release tablets is inversely related to indocyanine green clearance, reaching 60% to 70% at clearances of 7 mL/min and below. Protein binding decreases to about 88% in patients with severe hepatic dysfunction. The clearance of propafenone is reduced and the elimination half-life increased in patients with significant hepatic dysfunction [see Warnings and Precautions (5.9)].

13 NONCLINICAL TOXICOLOGY
13.1 Carcinogenesis, Mutagenesis, Impairment of Fertility
Lifetime maximally tolerated oral dose studies in mice (up to 360 mg/kg/day, about twice the maximum recommended human oral daily dose [MRHD] on a mg/m² basis) and rats (up to 270 mg/kg/day, about 3 times the MRHD on a mg/m² basis) provided no evidence of a carcinogenic potential for propafenone HCl.

Propafenone HCl tested negative for mutagenicity in the Ames (salmonella) test and in the in vivo mouse dominant lethal test. It tested negative for clastogenicity in the human lymphocyte chromosome aberration assay in vitro and in rat and Chinese hamster micronucleus tests, and other in vivo tests for chromosomal aberrations in rat bone marrow and Chinese hamster bone marrow and spermatogonia.

Propafenone HCl, administered intravenously to rabbits, dogs, and monkeys, has been shown to decrease spermatogenesis. These effects were reversible, were not found following oral dosing of propafenone HCl, were seen at lethal or near lethal dose levels, and were not seen in rats treated either orally or intravenously [see Warnings and Precautions (5.13)]. Treatment of male rabbits for 10 weeks prior to mating at an oral dose of 120 mg/kg/day (about 2.4 times the MRHD on a mg/m² basis) or an intravenous dose of 3.5 mg/kg/day (a spermatogenesis-impairing dose) did not result in evidence of impaired fertility. Nor was there evidence of impaired fertility when propafenone HCl was administered orally to male and female rats at dose levels up to 270 mg/kg/day (about 3 times the MRHD on a mg/m² basis).

13.2 Animal Toxicology and/or Pharmacology
Renal and Hepatic Toxicity in Animals
Renal changes have been observed in the rat following 6 months of oral administration of propafenone HCl at doses of 180 and 360 mg/kg/day (about 2 and 4 times, respectively, the MRHD on a mg/m² basis). Both inflammatory and non-inflammatory changes in the renal tubules, with accompanying interstitial nephritis, were observed. These changes were reversible, as they were not found in rats allowed to recover for 6 weeks. Fatty degenerative changes of the liver were found in rats following longer durations of administration of propafenone HCl at a dose of 270 mg/kg/day (about 3 times the MRHD on a mg/m² basis). There were no renal or hepatic changes at 90 mg/kg/day equivalent to the MRHD on a mg/m² basis).

14 CLINICAL STUDIES
RYTHMOL SR has been evaluated in patients with a history of electrocardiographically documented recurrent episodes of symptomatic AF in 2 randomized, double-blind, placebo-controlled trials.

RAFT: In one US multicenter trial (RYTHMOL SR Atrial Fibrillation Trial, RAFT), 3 doses of RYTHMOL SR (225 mg twice daily, 325 mg twice daily, and 425 mg twice daily) and placebo were compared in 523 patients with symptomatic, episodic AF. The patient population in this trial was 59% male with a mean age of 63 years, 91% white and 6% black. The patients had a median history of AF of 13 months, and documented symptomatic AF within 12 months of trial entry. Over 90% were NYHA Class I, and 21% had a prior electrical cardioversion. At baseline, 24% were treated with calcium channel blockers, 37% with beta blockers, and 38% with digoxin. Symptomatic arrhythmias after randomization were documented by transtelephonic electrocardiogram and centrally read and adjudicated by a blinded adverse event committee. RYTHMOL SR administered for up to 39 weeks was shown to prolong significantly the time to the first recurrence of symptomatic atrial arrhythmia, predominantly AF, from Day 1 of randomization (primary efficacy variable) compared with placebo, as shown in Table 3.
[See table 3 above]

There was a dose response for RYTHMOL SR for the tachycardia free period as shown in the proportional hazard analysis and the Kaplan-Meier curves presented in Figure 1.
[See figure 1 at top of next column]

In additional analyses, RYTHMOL SR (225 mg twice daily, 325 mg twice daily, and 425 mg twice daily) was also shown to prolong time to the first recurrence of symptomatic AF from Day 5 (steady-state pharmacokinetics were attained). The antiarrhythmic effect of RYTHMOL SR was not influenced by age, gender, history of cardioversion, duration of AF, frequency of AF, or use of medication that lowers heart

Figure 1. RAFT Kaplan-Meier Analysis for the Tachycardia-free Period From Day 1 of Randomization:

Days	0	25	50	75	100	125	150	175	200	225	250	275	300
Patients at Risk:													
Rythmol SR	397	220	191					166				76	
Placebo	126		50					25				7	

- Placebo
- △ Propafenone S R 325 mg bid
- □ Propafenone S R 225 mg bid
- ○ Propafenone S R 425 mg bid

p <0.001
p <0.001
p =0.014

Week 39

* Patient closeout started on Day 273 (week 39) and lasted until 300 days. On day 291, of the 2 patients that were left on 325 mg, 1 had an event, causing a 50% decline in the Kaplan-Meier curves

rate. Similarly, the antiarrhythmic effect of RYTHMOL SR was not influenced by the individual use of calcium channel blockers, beta-blockers, or digoxin. Too few non-white patients were enrolled to assess the influence of race on effects of RYTHMOL SR.

No difference in the average heart rate during the first recurrence of symptomatic arrhythmia between RYTHMOL SR and placebo was observed.

ERAFT: In a European multicenter trial [European Rythmonorm SR Atrial Fibrillation Trial (ERAFT)], 2 doses of RYTHMOL SR (325 mg twice daily and 425 mg twice daily) and placebo were compared in 293 patients with documented electrocardiographic evidence of symptomatic paroxysmal AF. The patient population in this trial was 61% male, 100% white with a mean age of 61 years. Patients had a median duration of AF of 3.3 years, and 61% were taking medications that lowered heart rate. At baseline, 15% of the patients were treated with calcium channel blockers (verapamil and diltiazem), 42% with beta-blockers, and 8% with digoxin. During a qualifying period of up to 28 days, patients had to have 1 ECG-documented incident of symptomatic AF. The double-blind treatment phase consisted of a 4-day loading period followed by a 91-day efficacy period. Symptomatic arrhythmias were documented by electrocardiogram monitoring.

In ERAFT, RYTHMOL SR was shown to prolong the time to the first recurrence of symptomatic atrial arrhythmia from Day 5 of randomization (primary efficacy analysis). The proportional hazard analysis revealed that both doses of RYTHMOL SR were superior to placebo. The antiarrhythmic effect of propafenone SR was not influenced by age, gender, duration of AF, frequency of AF or use of medication that lowers heart rate. It was also not influenced by the individual use of calcium channel blockers, beta-blockers, or digoxin. Too few non-white patients were enrolled to assess the influence of race on the effects of RYTHMOL SR. There was a slight increase in the incidence of centrally diagnosed asymptomatic AF or atrial flutter in each of the 2 treatment groups receiving RYTHMOL SR compared with placebo.

16 HOW SUPPLIED/STORAGE AND HANDLING

RYTHMOL SR (propafenone HCl) capsules are supplied as white, opaque, hard gelatin capsules containing either 225 mg, 325 mg, or 425 mg of propafenone HCl. The 225-mg strength is imprinted in red with GS EUG followed by 225. The 325-mg strength is imprinted in red with GS F1Y followed by 325, and also has a single red band around þ of the circumference of the body. The 425-mg strength is imprinted in red with GS UY2 followed by 425, and also has 3 red bands around þ of the circumference of the body.

Capsule Strength	60 count bottle NDC
225 mg	0173-0823-18
325 mg	0173-0824-18
425 mg	0173-0826-18

Storage: Store at 25°C (77°F); excursions permitted to 15°C to 30°C (59°F to 86°F). Dispense in a tight container.

17 PATIENT COUNSELING INFORMATION

See FDA-approved patient labeling (Patient Information).

17.1 Information for Patients

- Patients should be instructed to notify their health care providers of any change in over-the-counter, prescription, and supplement use. The health care provider should assess the patients' medication history including all over-the-counter, prescription, and herbal/natural preparations for those that may affect the pharmacodynamics or kinetics of RYTHMOL SR [see Warnings and Precautions (5.4)].
- Patients should also check with their healthcare providers prior to taking any new over-the-counter medicine.

- If patients experience symptoms that may be associated with altered electrolyte balance, such as excessive or prolonged diarrhea, sweating, vomiting, or loss of appetite or thirst, these conditions should be immediately reported to their healthcare provider.
- Patients should be instructed NOT to double the next dose if a dose is missed. The next dose should be taken at the usual time.

RYTHMOL SR is a registered trademark of G. Petrik used under license by Abbott Laboratories.

Manufactured for:
GlaxoSmithKline
Research Triangle Park, NC 27709
©2014, the GlaxoSmithKline group of companies. All rights reserved.
RMS:9PI

PATIENT INFORMATION
RYTHMOL SR® (RITH-Mall)
(propafenone hydrochloride) Extended-Release Capsules

Read this Patient Information Leaflet before you start taking RYTHMOL SR and each time you get a refill. There may be new information. This information does not take the place of talking with your doctor about your medical condition or your treatment.

What is RYTHMOL SR?

RYTHMOL SR is a prescription medicine that is used:
- in certain people who have a heart rhythm disorder called atrial fibrillation (AF)
- to increase the amount of time between having symptoms of AF

It is not known if RYTHMOL SR is safe and effective in children.

Who should not take RYTHMOL SR?

Do not take RYTHMOL SR if you have:
- heart failure (weak heart)
- had a recent heart attack
- have a heart condition called Brugada Syndrome
- a heart rate that is too slow, and you do not have a pacemaker
- very low blood pressure
- certain breathing problems that make you short of breath or wheeze
- certain abnormal body salt (electrolyte) levels in your blood

Talk to your doctor before taking RYTHMOL SR if you think you have any of the conditions listed above.

What should I tell my doctor before taking RYTHMOL SR?

Before you take RYTHMOL SR, tell your doctor if you:
- have liver or kidney problems
- have breathing problems
- have symptoms including diarrhea, sweating, vomiting, or loss of appetite or thirst that are severe. These symptoms may be a sign of abnormal electrolyte levels in your blood.
- have myasthenia gravis
- have lupus erythematosis
- have been told you have or had an abnormal blood test called Antinuclear Antibody Test or ANA Test
- are pregnant or plan to become pregnant. It is not known if RYTHMOL SR will harm your unborn baby.
- are breastfeeding or plan to breastfeed. RYTHMOL SR can pass into your milk and may harm your baby. You and your doctor should decide if you will breastfeed or take RYTHMOL SR. You should not do both.
- have any other medical conditions

Tell your doctor about all the medicines you take, including prescription and non-prescription medicines, vitamins, and herbal supplements. RYTHMOL SR and certain other medicines can affect each other and cause serious side effects. RYTHMOL SR may affect the way other medicines work, and other medicines may affect how RYTHMOL SR works.

Especially tell your doctor if you take:
- amiodarone or other medicines for your abnormal heart beats
- an antidepressant medicine
- a medicine to treat anxiety
- ritonavir (for example, KALETRA®, NORVIR®) or saquinavir (for example, INVIRASE®)
- an antibiotic medicine
- ketoconazole (for example, NIZORAL®)
- digoxin (LANOXIN®)
- warfarin sodium (for example, COUMADIN®, JANTOVEN®)

Know the medicines you take. Keep a list of them to show your doctor and pharmacist when you get a new medicine.

How should I take RYTHMOL SR?

- Take RYTHMOL SR exactly as prescribed. Your doctor will tell you how many capsules to take and how often to take them.
- To help reduce the chance of certain side effects, your doctor may start you with a low dose of RYTHMOL SR, and then slowly increase the dose.
- Do not open or crush the capsule.
- You may take RYTHMOL SR with or without food.

- You should not drink grapefruit juice during treatment with RYTHMOL SR.
- If you miss a dose of RYTHMOL SR, take your next dose at the usual time. Do not take 2 doses at the same time.
- If you take too much RYTHMOL SR, call your doctor or go to the nearest hospital emergency room right away.
- Call your doctor if your heart problems get worse.

What are possible side effects of RYTHMOL SR?

RYTHMOL SR can cause serious side effects including:
- **New or worsened abnormal heart beats, that can cause sudden death or be life-threatening.** Your doctor may do an electrocardiogram (ECG or EKG) before and during treatment to check your heart for these problems.
- **New or worsened heart failure. Tell your doctor about any changes in your heart symptoms, including:**
  ○ any new or increased swelling in your arms or legs
  ○ trouble breathing
  ○ sudden weight gain
- **Effects on pacemaker function.** RYTHMOL SR may affect how an implanted pacemaker or defibrillator works. Your doctor should check how your pacemaker or defibrillator is working during and after treatment with RYTHMOL SR. They may need to be re-programmed.
- **Very low white blood cell levels in your blood (agranulocytosis).** Your bone marrow may not produce enough of a certain type of white blood cells called neutrophils. If this happens, you are more likely to get infections. Tell your doctor right away if you have any of these symptoms, especially during the first 3 months of treatment:
  ○ fever
  ○ sore throat
  ○ chills
- **Worsening of myasthenia gravis in people who already have this condition.** Tell your doctor about any change in your symptoms.
- **RYTHMOL SR may cause lower sperm counts in men.** This could affect the ability to father a child. Talk to your doctor if this is a concern for you.

Common side effects of RYTHMOL SR include:
- dizziness
- fast or irregular heart beats
- chest pain
- trouble breathing
- taste changes
- nausea
- tiredness
- feeling anxious
- constipation
- upper respiratory infection or flu
- swelling

Tell your doctor if you have any side effect that bothers you or that does not go away.

These are not all the possible side effects of RYTHMOL SR. For more information, ask your doctor or pharmacist.

Call your doctor for medical advice about side effects. You may report side effects to FDA at 1-800-FDA-1088.

How should I store RYTHMOL SR?

- Store RYTHMOL SR at room temperature between 59°F to 86°F (15°C to 30°C).
- Keep the bottle tightly closed.

Keep RYTHMOL SR and all medicines out of the reach of children.

General information about RYTHMOL SR

Medicines are sometimes prescribed for conditions other than those described in patient information leaflets. Do not use RYTHMOL SR for a condition for which it was not prescribed by your doctor. Do not give RYTHMOL SR to other people, even if they have the same symptoms you have. It may harm them.

This leaflet summarizes the most important information about RYTHMOL SR. If you would like more information, talk with your doctor. You can ask your doctor or pharmacist for information about RYTHMOL SR that is written for healthcare professionals. For more information about RYTHMOL SR, call 1-888-825-5249.

What are the ingredients in RYTHMOL SR?

Active Ingredient: Propafenone hydrochloride
Inactive Ingredients: Antifoam, gelatin, hypromellose, magnesium stearate, red iron oxide, shellac, sodium dodecyl sulfate, sodium lauryl sulfate, soy lecithin and titanium dioxide.

RYTHMOL is a registered trademark of G. Petrik used under license by Abbott Laboratories. The other brands listed are trademarks of their respective owners and are not trademarks of the GlaxoSmithKline group of companies. The makers of these brands are not affiliated with and do not endorse the GlaxoSmithKline group of companies or its products.

Manufactured for:
GlaxoSmithKline
Research Triangle Park, NC 27709
©2014, the GlaxoSmithKline group of companies. All rights reserved.
February 2014
RMS:4PIL

SEREVENT DISKUS
[ser' ə-vent dĭsk' us]
(salmeterol xinafoate inhalation powder)
FOR ORAL INHALATION USE

HIGHLIGHTS OF PRESCRIBING INFORMATION
These highlights do not include all the information needed to use SEREVENT DISKUS safely and effectively. See full prescribing information for SEREVENT DISKUS.
SEREVENT DISKUS
(salmeterol xinafoate inhalation powder)
FOR ORAL INHALATION USE
Initial U.S. Approval: 1994

WARNING: ASTHMA-RELATED DEATH
See full prescribing information for complete boxed warning
- Long-acting beta$_2$-adrenergic agonists (LABA), such as salmeterol, the active ingredient in SEREVENT DISKUS, increase the risk of asthma-related death. A US trial showed an increase in asthma-related deaths in subjects receiving salmeterol (13 deaths out of 13,176 subjects treated for 28 weeks on salmeterol versus 3 out of 13,179 subjects on placebo). Currently available data are inadequate to determine whether concurrent use of inhaled corticosteroids or other long-term asthma control drugs mitigates the increased risk of asthma-related death from LABA. (5.1)
- Prescribe SEREVENT DISKUS only as additional therapy for patients with asthma who are currently taking but are inadequately controlled on a long-term asthma control medication, such as an inhaled corticosteroid. Once asthma control is achieved and maintained, assess the patient at regular intervals and step down therapy (e.g., discontinue SEREVENT DISKUS) if possible without loss of asthma control and maintain the patient on a long-term asthma control medication, such as an inhaled corticosteroid. Do not use SEREVENT DISKUS for patients whose asthma is adequately controlled on low- or medium-dose inhaled corticosteroids. (1.1, 5.1)
- Available data from controlled clinical trials suggest that LABA increase the risk of asthma-related hospitalization in pediatric and adolescent patients. (5.1)

INDICATIONS AND USAGE
SEREVENT DISKUS is a LABA indicated for:
- Treatment of asthma in patients aged 4 years and older. (1.1)
- Prevention of exercise-induced bronchospasm (EIB) in patients aged 4 years and older. (1.2)
- Maintenance treatment of bronchospasm associated with chronic obstructive pulmonary disease (COPD). (1.3)
Important limitation:
- Not indicated for the relief of acute bronchospasm. (1.1, 1.3)

DOSAGE AND ADMINISTRATION
For oral inhalation only.
- Treatment of asthma in patients aged 4 years and older: 1 inhalation twice daily in addition to concomitant treatment with an inhaled corticosteroid. (2.1)
- EIB: 1 inhalation at least 30 minutes before exercise. (2.2)
- Maintenance treatment of bronchospasm associated with COPD: 1 inhalation twice daily. (2.3)

DOSAGE FORMS AND STRENGTHS
Inhalation Powder. Inhaler containing salmeterol (50 mcg) as a powder formulation for oral inhalation. (3)

CONTRAINDICATIONS
- Asthma: Without concomitant use of a long-term asthma control medication such as an inhaled corticosteroid. (4)
- Primary treatment of status asthmaticus or acute episodes of asthma or COPD requiring intensive measures. (4)
- Severe hypersensitivity to milk proteins. (4)

WARNINGS AND PRECAUTIONS
- LABA increase the risk of asthma-related death and asthma-related hospitalizations. Prescribe for asthma only as concomitant therapy with an inhaled corticosteroid. (5.1)
- Do not initiate in acutely deteriorating asthma or COPD. Do not use to treat acute symptoms. (5.2)
- Not a substitute for corticosteroids. Patients with asthma must take a concomitant inhaled corticosteroid. (5.3)
- Do not use in combination with an additional medicine containing a LABA because of risk of overdose. (5.4)

- If paradoxical bronchospasm occurs, discontinue SEREVENT DISKUS and institute alternative therapy. (5.5)
- Use with caution in patients with cardiovascular or central nervous system disorders because of beta-adrenergic stimulation. (5.6)
- Use with caution in patients with convulsive disorders, thyrotoxicosis, diabetes mellitus, and ketoacidosis. (5.9)
- Be alert to hypokalemia and hyperglycemia. (5.10)

ADVERSE REACTIONS
Most common adverse reactions (incidence ≥5%) are:
- Asthma: Headache, influenza, nasal/sinus congestion, pharyngitis, rhinitis, tracheitis/bronchitis. (6.1)
- COPD: Cough, headache, musculoskeletal pain, throat irritation, viral respiratory infection. (6.2)

To report SUSPECTED ADVERSE REACTIONS, contact GlaxoSmithKline at 1-888-825-5249 or FDA at 1-800-FDA-1088 or www.fda.gov/medwatch

DRUG INTERACTIONS
- Strong cytochrome P450 3A4 inhibitors (e.g., ritonavir, ketoconazole): Use not recommended. May increase risk of cardiovascular effects. (7.1)
- Monoamine oxidase inhibitors and tricyclic antidepressants: Use with extreme caution. May potentiate effect of salmeterol on vascular system. (7.2)
- Beta-blockers: Use with caution. May block bronchodilatory effects of beta-agonists and produce severe bronchospasm. (7.3)
- Diuretics: Use with caution. Electrocardiographic changes and/or hypokalemia associated with non–potassium-sparing diuretics may worsen with concomitant beta-agonists. (7.4)

USE IN SPECIFIC POPULATIONS
Hepatic impairment: Monitor patients for signs of increased drug exposure. (8.6)
See 17 for PATIENT COUNSELING INFORMATION and Medication Guide

Revised: 04/2014

FULL PRESCRIBING INFORMATION: CONTENTS*

FULL PRESCRIBING INFORMATION

WARNING: ASTHMA-RELATED DEATH
Long-acting beta$_2$-adrenergic agonists (LABA), such as salmeterol, the active ingredient in SEREVENT® DISKUS®, increase the risk of asthma-related death. Data from a large placebo-controlled US trial that compared the safety of salmeterol with placebo added to usual asthma therapy showed an increase in asthma-related deaths in subjects receiving salmeterol (13 deaths out of 13,176 subjects treated for 28 weeks on salmeterol versus 3 deaths out of 13,179 subjects on placebo). Currently available data are inadequate to determine whether concurrent use of inhaled corticosteroids or other long-term asthma control drugs mitigates the increased risk of asthma-related death from LABA.
Because of this risk, use of SEREVENT DISKUS for the treatment of asthma without a concomitant long-term asthma control medication, such as an inhaled corticosteroid, is contraindicated. Use SEREVENT DISKUS only as additional therapy for patients with asthma who are currently taking but are inadequately controlled on a long-term asthma control medication, such as an inhaled corticosteroid. Once asthma control is achieved and maintained, assess the patient at regular intervals and step down therapy (e.g., discontinue SEREVENT DISKUS) if possible without loss of asthma control and maintain the patient on a long-term asthma control medication, such as an inhaled corticosteroid. Do not use SEREVENT DISKUS for patients whose asthma is adequately controlled on low- or medium-dose inhaled corticosteroids.
Pediatric and Adolescent Patients: Available data from controlled clinical trials suggest that LABA increase the risk of asthma-related hospitalization in pediatric and adolescent patients. For pediatric and adolescent patients with asthma who require addition of a LABA to an inhaled corticosteroid, a fixed-dose combination product containing both an inhaled corticosteroid and a LABA should ordinarily be used to ensure adherence with both drugs. In cases where use of a separate long-term asthma control medication (e.g., inhaled corticosteroid) and a LABA is clinically indicated, appropriate steps must be taken to ensure adherence with both treatment components. If adherence cannot be assured, a fixed-dose combination product containing both an inhaled corticosteroid and a LABA is recommended.

---

1   INDICATIONS AND USAGE
1.1   Treatment of Asthma
SEREVENT DISKUS is indicated for the treatment of asthma and in the prevention of bronchospasm only as concomitant therapy with a long-term asthma control medication, such as an inhaled corticosteroid, in patients aged 4 years and older with reversible obstructive airway disease, including patients with symptoms of nocturnal asthma. LABA, such as salmeterol, the active ingredient in SEREVENT DISKUS, increase the risk of asthma-related death *[see Warnings and Precautions (5.1)]*. Use of SEREVENT DISKUS for the treatment of asthma without concomitant use of a long-term asthma control medication, such as an inhaled corticosteroid, is contraindicated *[see Contraindications (4)]*. Use SEREVENT DISKUS only as additional therapy for patients with asthma who are currently taking but are inadequately controlled on a long-term asthma control medication, such as an inhaled corticosteroid. Once asthma control is achieved and maintained, assess the patient at regular intervals and step down therapy (e.g., discontinue SEREVENT DISKUS) if possible without loss of asthma control and maintain the patient on a long-term asthma control medication, such as an inhaled corticosteroid. Do not use SEREVENT DISKUS for patients whose asthma is adequately controlled on low- or medium-dose inhaled corticosteroids.
Pediatric and Adolescent Patients: Available data from controlled clinical trials suggest that LABA increase the

risk of asthma-related hospitalization in pediatric and adolescent patients. For pediatric and adolescent patients with asthma who require addition of a LABA to an inhaled corticosteroid, a fixed-dose combination product containing both an inhaled corticosteroid and a LABA should ordinarily be used to ensure adherence with both drugs. In cases where use of a separate long-term asthma control medication (e.g., inhaled corticosteroid) and a LABA is clinically indicated, appropriate steps must be taken to ensure adherence with both treatment components. If adherence cannot be assured, a fixed-dose combination product containing both an inhaled corticosteroid and a LABA is recommended.

Important Limitation of Use: SEREVENT DISKUS is NOT indicated for the relief of acute bronchospasm.

1.2   Prevention of Exercise-Induced Bronchospasm
SEREVENT DISKUS is also indicated for prevention of exercise-induced bronchospasm (EIB) in patients aged 4 years and older. Use of SEREVENT DISKUS as a single agent for the prevention of EIB may be clinically indicated in patients who do not have persistent asthma. In patients with persistent asthma, use of SEREVENT DISKUS for the prevention of EIB may be clinically indicated, but the treatment of asthma should include a long-term asthma control medication, such as an inhaled corticosteroid.

1.3   Maintenance Treatment of Chronic Obstructive Pulmonary Disease
SEREVENT DISKUS is indicated for the long-term twice-daily administration in the maintenance treatment of bronchospasm associated with chronic obstructive pulmonary disease (COPD) (including emphysema and chronic bronchitis).

Important Limitation of Use: SEREVENT DISKUS is NOT indicated for the relief of acute bronchospasm.

2   DOSAGE AND ADMINISTRATION
SEREVENT DISKUS should be administered by the orally inhaled route only.

More frequent administration or a greater number of inhalations (more than 1 inhalation twice daily) is not recommended as some patients are more likely to experience adverse effects. Patients using SEREVENT DISKUS should not use additional LABA for any reason. [See Warnings and Precautions (5.4, 5.6).]

2.1   Asthma
LABA, such as salmeterol, the active ingredient in SEREVENT DISKUS, increase the risk of asthma-related death [see Warnings and Precautions (5.1)].

Because of this risk, use of SEREVENT DISKUS for the treatment of asthma without concomitant use of a long-term asthma control medication, such as an inhaled corticosteroid is contraindicated. Use SEREVENT DISKUS only as additional therapy for patients with asthma who are currently taking but are inadequately controlled on a long-term asthma control medication, such as an inhaled corticosteroid. Once asthma control is achieved and maintained, assess the patient at regular intervals and step down therapy (e.g., discontinue SEREVENT DISKUS) if possible without loss of asthma control and maintain the patient on a long-term asthma control medication, such as an inhaled corticosteroid. Do not use SEREVENT DISKUS for patients whose asthma is adequately controlled on low- or medium-dose inhaled corticosteroids.

Pediatric and Adolescent Patients: Available data from controlled clinical trials suggest that LABA increase the risk of asthma-related hospitalization in pediatric and adolescent patients. For patients with asthma younger than 18 years who require addition of a LABA to an inhaled corticosteroid, a fixed-dose combination product containing both an inhaled corticosteroid and a LABA should ordinarily be used to ensure adherence with both drugs. In cases where use of a separate long-term asthma control medication (e.g., inhaled corticosteroid) and a LABA is clinically indicated, appropriate steps must be taken to ensure adherence with both treatment components. If adherence cannot be assured, a fixed-dose combination product containing both an inhaled corticosteroid and a LABA is recommended.

For bronchodilatation and prevention of symptoms of asthma, including the symptoms of nocturnal asthma, the usual dosage for adults and children aged 4 years and older is 1 inhalation (50 mcg) twice daily, approximately 12 hours apart. If a previously effective dosage regimen fails to provide the usual response, medical advice should be sought immediately as this is often a sign of destabilization of asthma. Under these circumstances, the therapeutic regimen should be reevaluated. If symptoms arise in the period between doses, an inhaled, short-acting beta$_2$-agonist should be taken for immediate relief.

2.2   Exercise-Induced Bronchospasm
Use of SEREVENT DISKUS as a single agent for the prevention of EIB may be clinically indicated in patients who do not have persistent asthma. In patients with persistent asthma, use of SEREVENT DISKUS for the prevention of EIB may be clinically indicated, but the treatment of

asthma should include a long-term asthma control medication, such as an inhaled corticosteroid. One inhalation of SEREVENT DISKUS at least 30 minutes before exercise has been shown to protect patients against EIB. When used intermittently as needed for prevention of EIB, this protection may last up to 9 hours in adults and adolescents and up to 12 hours in patients aged 4 to 11 years. Additional doses of SEREVENT should not be used for 12 hours after the administration of this drug. Patients who are receiving SEREVENT DISKUS twice daily should not use additional SEREVENT for prevention of EIB.

2.3   Chronic Obstructive Pulmonary Disease
For maintenance treatment of bronchospasm associated with COPD (including chronic bronchitis and emphysema), the dosage for adults is 1 inhalation (50 mcg) twice daily approximately 12 hours apart.

3   DOSAGE FORMS AND STRENGTHS
Inhalation Powder. Inhaler containing a foil blister strip of powder formulation for oral inhalation. The strip contains salmeterol 50 mcg per blister.

4   CONTRAINDICATIONS
Because of the risk of asthma-related death and hospitalization, use of SEREVENT DISKUS for the treatment of asthma without concomitant use of a long-term asthma control medication, such as an inhaled corticosteroid, is contraindicated [see Warnings and Precautions (5.1)].

The use of SEREVENT DISKUS is contraindicated in the following conditions:
- Primary treatment of status asthmaticus or other acute episodes of asthma or COPD where intensive measures are required [see Warnings and Precautions (5.2)].
- Severe hypersensitivity to milk proteins [see Warnings and Precautions (5.7), Adverse Reactions (6.3), Description (11)]

5   WARNINGS AND PRECAUTIONS
5.1   Asthma-Related Death
LABA, such as salmeterol, the active ingredient in SEREVENT DISKUS, increase the risk of asthma-related death. Currently available data are inadequate to determine whether concurrent use of inhaled corticosteroids or other long-term asthma control drugs mitigates the increased risk of asthma-related death from LABA.

Because of this risk, use of SEREVENT DISKUS for the treatment of asthma without concomitant use of a long-term asthma control medication, such as an inhaled corticosteroid, is contraindicated. Use SEREVENT DISKUS only as additional therapy for patients with asthma who are currently taking but are inadequately controlled on a long-term asthma control medication, such as an inhaled corticosteroid. Once asthma control is achieved and maintained, assess the patient at regular intervals and step down therapy (e.g., discontinue SEREVENT DISKUS) if possible without loss of asthma control and maintain the patient on a long-term asthma control medication, such as an inhaled corticosteroid. Do not use SEREVENT DISKUS for patients whose asthma is adequately controlled on low- or medium-dose inhaled corticosteroids.

Pediatric and Adolescent Patients: **Available data from controlled clinical trials suggest that LABA increase the risk of asthma-related hospitalization in pediatric and adolescent patients. For pediatric and adolescent patients with asthma who require addition of a LABA to an inhaled corticosteroid, a fixed-dose combination product containing both an inhaled corticosteroid and a LABA should ordinarily be used to ensure adherence with both drugs. In cases where use of a separate long-term asthma control medication (e.g., inhaled corticosteroid) and a LABA is clinically indicated, appropriate steps must be taken to ensure adherence with both treatment components. If adherence cannot be assured, a fixed-dose combination product containing both an inhaled corticosteroid and a LABA is recommended.**

The Salmeterol Multi-center Asthma Research Trial (SMART) was a large 28-week placebo-controlled US trial comparing the safety of salmeterol (SEREVENT® Inhalation Aerosol) with placebo, each added to usual asthma therapy, that showed an increase in asthma-related deaths in subjects receiving salmeterol [see Clinical Studies (14.1)]. Given the similar basic mechanisms of action of beta$_2$-agonists, the findings seen in the SMART trial are considered a class effect.

A 16-week clinical trial performed in the United Kingdom, the Salmeterol Nationwide Surveillance (SNS) trial, showed results similar to the SMART trial. In the SNS trial, the rate of asthma-related death was numerically, though not statistically significantly, greater in subjects with asthma treated with salmeterol (42 mcg twice daily) than those treated with albuterol (180 mcg 4 times daily) added to usual asthma therapy.

The SNS and SMART trials enrolled subjects with asthma. No trials have been conducted that were primarily designed to determine whether the rate of death in patients with COPD is increased by LABA.

5.2   Deterioration of Disease and Acute Episodes
SEREVENT DISKUS should not be initiated in patients during rapidly deteriorating or potentially life-threatening episodes of asthma or COPD. SEREVENT DISKUS has not been studied in subjects with acutely deteriorating asthma or COPD. The initiation of SEREVENT DISKUS in this setting is not appropriate.

Serious acute respiratory events, including fatalities, have been reported when salmeterol has been initiated in patients with significantly worsening or acutely deteriorating asthma. In most cases, these have occurred in patients with severe asthma (e.g., patients with a history of corticosteroid dependence, low pulmonary function, intubation, mechanical ventilation, frequent hospitalizations, previous life-threatening acute asthma exacerbations) and in some patients with acutely deteriorating asthma (e.g., patients with significantly increasing symptoms; increasing need for inhaled, short-acting beta$_2$-agonists; decreasing response to usual medications; increasing need for systemic corticosteroids; recent emergency room visits; deteriorating lung function). However, these events have occurred in a few patients with less severe asthma as well. It was not possible from these reports to determine whether salmeterol contributed to these events.

Increasing use of inhaled, short-acting beta$_2$-agonists is a marker of deteriorating asthma. In this situation, the patient requires immediate reevaluation with reassessment of the treatment regimen, giving special consideration to the possible need for adding additional inhaled corticosteroid or initiating systemic corticosteroids. Patients should not use more than 1 inhalation twice daily of SEREVENT DISKUS. SEREVENT DISKUS should not be used for the relief of acute symptoms, i.e., as rescue therapy for the treatment of acute episodes of bronchospasm. An inhaled, short-acting beta$_2$-agonist, not SEREVENT DISKUS, should be used to relieve acute symptoms such as shortness of breath. When prescribing SEREVENT DISKUS, the healthcare provider should also prescribe an inhaled, short-acting beta$_2$-agonist (e.g., albuterol) for treatment of acute symptoms.

When beginning treatment with SEREVENT DISKUS, patients who have been taking oral or inhaled, short-acting beta$_2$-agonists on a regular basis (e.g., 4 times a day) should be instructed to discontinue the regular use of these drugs.

5.3   SEREVENT DISKUS is Not a Substitute for Corticosteroids
There are no data demonstrating that SEREVENT DISKUS has a clinical anti-inflammatory effect such as that associated with corticosteroids. When initiating and throughout treatment with SEREVENT DISKUS in patients receiving oral or inhaled corticosteroids for treatment of asthma, patients must continue taking a suitable dosage of corticosteroids to maintain clinical stability even if they feel better as a result of initiating SEREVENT DISKUS. Any change in corticosteroid dosage should be made ONLY after clinical evaluation.

5.4   Excessive Use of SEREVENT DISKUS and Use With Other Long-Acting Beta$_2$-Agonists
SEREVENT DISKUS should not be used more often than recommended, at higher doses than recommended, or in conjunction with other medicines containing LABA, as an overdose may result. Clinically significant cardiovascular effects and fatalities have been reported in association with excessive use of inhaled sympathomimetic drugs. Patients using SEREVENT DISKUS should not use another medicine containing a LABA (e.g., formoterol fumarate, arformoterol tartrate, indacaterol) for any reason.

5.5   Paradoxical Bronchospasm and Upper Airway Symptoms
As with other inhaled medicines, SEREVENT DISKUS can produce paradoxical bronchospasm, which may be life threatening. If paradoxical bronchospasm occurs following dosing with SEREVENT DISKUS, it should be treated immediately with an inhaled, short-acting bronchodilator. SEREVENT DISKUS should be discontinued immediately, and alternative therapy should be instituted. Upper airway symptoms of laryngeal spasm, irritation, or swelling, such as stridor and choking, have been reported in patients receiving SEREVENT DISKUS.

5.6   Cardiovascular and Central Nervous System Effects
Excessive beta-adrenergic stimulation has been associated with seizures, angina, hypertension or hypotension, tachycardia with rates up to 200 beats/min, arrhythmias, nervousness, headache, tremor, palpitation, nausea, dizziness, fatigue, malaise, and insomnia [see Overdosage (10)]. Therefore, SEREVENT DISKUS, like all products containing sympathomimetic amines, should be used with caution in patients with cardiovascular disorders, especially coronary insufficiency, cardiac arrhythmias, and hypertension.

Salmeterol can produce a clinically significant cardiovascular effect in some patients as measured by pulse rate, blood pressure, and/or symptoms. Although such effects are uncommon after administration of salmeterol at recommended doses, if they occur, the drug may need to be discontinued. In addition, beta-agonists have been reported to produce electrocardiogram (ECG) changes, such as flattening of the T wave, prolongation of the QTc interval, and ST segment depression. The clinical significance of these findings is unknown. Large doses of inhaled or oral salmeterol (12 to 20 times the recommended dose) have been associated with clinically significant prolongation of the QTc interval, which has the potential for producing ventricular arrhythmias. Fatalities have been reported in association with excessive use of inhaled sympathomimetic drugs.

5.7   Immediate Hypersensitivity Reactions
Immediate hypersensitivity reactions (e.g., urticaria, angioedema, rash, bronchospasm, hypotension), including anaphylaxis, may occur after administration of SEREVENT DISKUS. There have been reports of anaphylactic reactions in patients with severe milk protein allergy after inhalation of powder products containing lactose; therefore, patients with severe milk protein allergy should not use SEREVENT DISKUS [see Contraindications (4)].

5.8   Drug Interactions With Strong Cytochrome P450 3A4 Inhibitors
The use of strong cytochrome P450 3A4 (CYP3A4) inhibitors (e.g., ritonavir, atazanavir, clarithromycin, indinavir, itraconazole, nefazodone, nelfinavir, saquinavir, ketoconazole, telithromycin) with SEREVENT DISKUS is not recommended because increased cardiovascular adverse effects may occur [see Drug Interactions (7.1), Clinical Pharmacology (12.3)].

5.9   Coexisting Conditions
SEREVENT DISKUS, like all medicines containing sympathomimetic amines, should be used with caution in patients with convulsive disorders or thyrotoxicosis and in those who are unusually responsive to sympathomimetic amines. Doses of the related beta$_2$-adrenoceptor agonist albuterol, when administered intravenously, have been reported to aggravate preexisting diabetes mellitus and ketoacidosis.

5.10   Hypokalemia and Hyperglycemia
Beta-adrenergic agonist medicines may produce significant hypokalemia in some patients, possibly through intracellular shunting, which has the potential to produce adverse cardiovascular effects [see Clinical Pharmacology (12.2)]. The decrease in serum potassium is usually transient, not requiring supplementation. Clinically significant and dose-related changes in blood glucose and/or serum potassium were seen infrequently during clinical trials with SEREVENT DISKUS at recommended doses.

6   ADVERSE REACTIONS
LABA, including salmeterol, the active ingredient in SEREVENT DISKUS, increase the risk of asthma-related death. Data from a large 28-week placebo-controlled US trial that compared the safety of salmeterol or placebo added to usual asthma therapy showed an increase in asthma-related deaths in subjects receiving salmeterol. Available data from controlled clinical trials suggest that LABA increase the risk of asthma-related hospitalization in pediatric and adolescent patients [see Warnings and Precautions (5.1), Clinical Studies (14.1)].

Because clinical trials are conducted under widely varying conditions, adverse reaction rates observed in the clinical trials of a drug cannot be directly compared with rates in the clinical trials of another drug and may not reflect the rates observed in practice.

6.1   Clinical Trials Experience in Asthma
Adult and Adolescent Subjects Aged 12 Years and Older: Two multicenter, 12-week, placebo-controlled clinical trials evaluated twice-daily doses of SEREVENT DISKUS in subjects aged 12 years and older with asthma. Table 1 reports the incidence of adverse reactions in these 2 trials.
[See table 1 above]
Table 1 includes all events (whether considered drug-related or nondrug-related by the investigator) that occurred at a rate of ≥3% in the group treated with SEREVENT DISKUS and were more common than in the placebo group.
Pharyngitis, sinusitis, upper respiratory tract infection, and cough occurred at ≥3% but were more common in the placebo group. However, throat irritation has been described at rates exceeding that of placebo in other controlled clinical trials.
Additional Adverse Reactions: Other adverse reactions not previously listed, whether considered drug-related or not by the investigators, that were reported more frequently by subjects with asthma treated with SEREVENT DISKUS compared with subjects treated with placebo include the following: contact dermatitis, eczema, localized aches and pains, nausea, oral mucosal abnormality, pain in joint, paresthesia, pyrexia of unknown origin, sinus headache, and sleep disturbance.
Pediatric Subjects Aged 4 to 11 Years: Two multicenter, 12-week, controlled trials have evaluated twice-daily doses of SEREVENT DISKUS in subjects aged 4 to 11 years with asthma. Table 2 includes all events (whether considered drug-related or nondrug-related by the investigator) that

Table 1. Adverse Reactions With SEREVENT DISKUS With ≥3 Incidence and More Common Than Placebo in Adult and Adolescent Subjects With Asthma

Adverse Event	Percent of Subjects		
	Placebo (n = 152)	SEREVENT DISKUS 50 mcg Twice Daily (n = 149)	Albuterol Inhalation Aerosol 180 mcg 4 Times Daily (n = 150)
Ear, nose, and throat			
Nasal/sinus congestion, pallor	6	9	8
Rhinitis	4	5	4
Neurological			
Headache	9	13	12
Respiratory			
Asthma	1	3	<1
Tracheitis/bronchitis	4	7	3
Influenza	2	5	5

Table 2. Adverse Reaction Incidence in Two 12-Week Pediatric Clinical Trials in Subjects With Asthma

Adverse Event	Percent of Subjects		
	Placebo (n = 215)	SEREVENT DISKUS 50 mcg Twice Daily (n = 211)	Albuterol Inhalation Aerosol 200 mcg 4 Times Daily (n = 115)
Ear, nose, and throat			
Ear signs and symptoms	3	4	9
Pharyngitis	3	6	5
Neurological			
Headache	14	17	20
Respiratory			
Asthma	2	4	<1
Skin			
Skin rashes	3	4	2
Urticaria	0	3	2

occurred at a rate of 3% or greater in the group receiving SEREVENT DISKUS and were more common than in the placebo group.
[See table 2 above]
The following events were reported at an incidence of >1% in the salmeterol group and with a higher incidence than in the albuterol and placebo groups: gastrointestinal signs and symptoms, lower respiratory signs and symptoms, photodermatitis, and arthralgia and articular rheumatism.
In clinical trials evaluating concurrent therapy of salmeterol with inhaled corticosteroids, adverse events were consistent with those previously reported for salmeterol, or with events that would be expected with the use of inhaled corticosteroids.
Laboratory Test Abnormalities: Elevation of hepatic enzymes was reported in ≥1% of subjects in clinical trials. The elevations were transient and did not lead to discontinuation from the trials. In addition, there were no clinically relevant changes noted in glucose or potassium.

6.2   Clinical Trials Experience in Chronic Obstructive Pulmonary Disease
Two multicenter, 24-week, placebo-controlled US trials evaluated twice-daily doses of SEREVENT DISKUS in subjects with COPD. For presentation (Table 3), the placebo data from a third trial, identical in design, subject entrance criteria, and overall conduct but comparing fluticasone propionate with placebo, were integrated with the placebo data from these 2 trials (total N = 341 for salmeterol and 576 for placebo).

Table 3. Adverse Reactions With SEREVENT DISKUS With ≥3% Incidence in US Controlled Clinical Trials in Subjects With Chronic Obstructive Pulmonary Disease[a]

Adverse Event	Percent of Subjects	
	Placebo (n = 576)	SEREVENT DISKUS 50 mcg Twice Daily (n = 341)
Cardiovascular		
Hypertension	2	4
Ear, nose, and throat		
Throat irritation	6	7
Nasal congestion/blockage	3	4
Sinusitis	2	4
Ear signs and symptoms	1	3
Gastrointestinal		
Nausea and vomiting	3	3
Lower respiratory		
Cough	4	5
Rhinitis	2	4
Viral respiratory infection	4	5
Musculoskeletal		
Musculoskeletal pain	10	12
Muscle cramps and spasms	1	3
Neurological		
Headache	11	14
Dizziness	2	4
Average duration of exposure (days)	128.9	138.5

[a]Table 3 includes all events (whether considered drug-related or nondrug-related by the investigator) that occurred at a rate of 3% or greater in the group receiving SEREVENT DISKUS and were more common than in the group receiving SEREVENT DISKUS than in the placebo group.

Additional Adverse Reactions: Other adverse reactions occurring in the group receiving SEREVENT DISKUS that occurred at a frequency of ≥1% and were more common than in the placebo group were as follows: anxiety; arthralgia and articular rheumatism; bone and skeletal pain; candidiasis mouth/throat; dental discomfort and pain; dyspeptic symptoms; edema and swelling; gastrointestinal infections; hyperglycemia; hyposalivation; keratitis and conjunctivitis; lower respiratory signs and symptoms; migraines; muscle pain; muscle stiffness, tightness, and rigidity; musculoskeletal inflammation; pain; and skin rashes.

Adverse reactions to salmeterol are similar in nature to those seen with other selective beta$_2$-adrenoceptor agonists, e.g., tachycardia; palpitations; immediate hypersensitivity reactions, including urticaria, angioedema, rash, bronchospasm; headache; tremor; nervousness; and paradoxical bronchospasm.

Laboratory Abnormalities: There were no clinically relevant changes in these trials. Specifically, no changes in potassium were noted.

6.3 Postmarketing Experience

In addition to adverse reactions reported from clinical trials, the following adverse reactions have been identified during postapproval use of salmeterol. Because these reactions are reported voluntarily from a population of uncertain size, it is not always possible to reliably estimate their frequency or establish a causal relationship to drug exposure. These events have been chosen for inclusion due to either their seriousness, frequency of reporting, or causal connection to salmeterol or a combination of these factors.

In extensive US and worldwide postmarketing experience with salmeterol, serious exacerbations of asthma, including some that have been fatal, have been reported. In most cases, these have occurred in patients with severe asthma and/or in some patients in whom asthma has been acutely deteriorating [see Warnings and Precautions (5.2)], but they have also occurred in a few patients with less severe asthma. It was not possible from these reports to determine whether salmeterol contributed to these events.

Cardiovascular: Arrhythmias (including atrial fibrillation, supraventricular tachycardia, extrasystoles) and anaphylaxis.

Non-Site Specific: Very rare anaphylactic reaction in patients with severe milk protein allergy.

Respiratory: Reports of upper airway symptoms of laryngeal spasm, irritation, or swelling such as stridor or choking; oropharyngeal irritation.

7 DRUG INTERACTIONS

7.1 Inhibitors of Cytochrome P450 3A4

Salmeterol is a substrate of CYP3A4. The use of strong CYP3A4 inhibitors (e.g., ritonavir, atazanavir, clarithromycin, indinavir, itraconazole, nefazodone, nelfinavir, saquinavir, ketoconazole, telithromycin) with SEREVENT DISKUS is not recommended because increased cardiovascular adverse effects may occur.

In a drug interaction trial in 20 healthy subjects, coadministration of inhaled salmeterol (50 mcg twice daily) and oral ketoconazole (400 mg once daily) for 7 days resulted in greater systemic exposure to salmeterol (AUC increased 16-fold and C_{max} increased 1.4-fold). Three (3) subjects were withdrawn due to beta$_2$-agonist side effects (2 with prolonged QTc and 1 with palpitations and sinus tachycardia). Although there was no statistical effect on the mean QTc, coadministration of salmeterol and ketoconazole was associated with more frequent increases in QTc duration compared with salmeterol and placebo administration.

7.2 Monoamine Oxidase Inhibitors and Tricyclic Antidepressants

SEREVENT DISKUS should be administered with extreme caution to patients being treated with monoamine oxidase inhibitors or tricyclic antidepressants, or within 2 weeks of discontinuation of such agents, because the action of salmeterol on the vascular system may be potentiated by these agents.

7.3 Beta-Adrenergic Receptor Blocking Agents

Beta-blockers not only block the pulmonary effect of beta-agonists, such as SEREVENT DISKUS, but may also produce severe bronchospasm in patients with asthma or COPD. Therefore, patients with asthma or COPD should not normally be treated with beta-blockers. However, under certain circumstances, there may be no acceptable alternatives to the use of beta-adrenergic blocking agents for these patients; cardioselective beta-blockers could be considered, although they should be administered with caution.

7.4 Non–Potassium-Sparing Diuretics

The ECG changes and/or hypokalemia that may result from the administration of non–potassium-sparing diuretics (such as loop or thiazide diuretics) can be acutely worsened by beta-agonists, especially when the recommended dose of the beta-agonist is exceeded. Although the clinical significance of these effects is not known, caution is advised in the coadministration of SEREVENT DISKUS with non–potassium-sparing diuretics.

8 USE IN SPECIFIC POPULATIONS

8.1 Pregnancy

Teratogenic Effects: Pregnancy Category C. There are no adequate and well-controlled trials with SEREVENT DISKUS in pregnant women. Beta$_2$-agonists have been shown to be teratogenic in laboratory animals when administered systemically at relatively low dosage levels. Because animal reproductive studies are not always predictive of human response, SEREVENT DISKUS should be used during pregnancy only if the potential benefit justifies the potential risk to the fetus. Women should be advised to contact their physicians if they become pregnant while taking SEREVENT DISKUS.

No teratogenic effects occurred in rats at salmeterol doses approximately 160 times the maximum recommended daily inhalation dose (MRHDID) (on a mg/m^2 basis at maternal oral doses up to 2 mg/kg/day). In pregnant Dutch rabbits administered oral doses approximately 50 times the MRHDID (on an AUC basis at maternal oral doses of 1 mg/kg/day and higher), fetal toxic effects were observed characteristically resulting from beta-adrenoceptor stimulation. These included precocious eyelid openings, cleft palate, sternebral fusion, limb and paw flexures, and delayed ossification of the frontal cranial bones. No such effects occurred at a salmeterol dose approximately 20 times the MRHDID (on an AUC basis at a maternal oral dose of 0.6 mg/kg/day). New Zealand White rabbits were less sensitive since only delayed ossification of the frontal cranial bones was seen at an oral dose approximately 1,600 times the MRHDID (on n mg/m^2 basis at a maternal oral dose of 10 mg/kg/day). Salmeterol crossed the placenta following oral administration to mice and rats.

8.2 Labor and Delivery

There are no well-controlled human trials that have investigated effects of salmeterol on preterm labor or labor at term. Because of the potential for beta-agonist interference with uterine contractility, use of SEREVENT DISKUS during labor should be restricted to those patients in whom the benefits clearly outweigh the risks.

8.3 Nursing Mothers

Plasma levels of salmeterol after inhaled therapeutic doses are very low. In rats, salmeterol xinafoate is excreted in the milk. Since there are no data from controlled trials on the use of SEREVENT DISKUS by nursing mothers, caution should be exercised when SEREVENT DISKUS is administered to a nursing woman.

8.4 Pediatric Use

Available data from controlled clinical trials suggest that LABA increase the risk of asthma-related hospitalization in pediatric and adolescent patients. For pediatric and adolescent patients with asthma who require addition of a LABA to an inhaled corticosteroid, a fixed-dose combination product containing both an inhaled corticosteroid and a LABA should ordinarily be used to ensure adherence with both drugs [see Indications and Usage (1.1), Warnings and Precautions (5.1)].

The safety and efficacy of SEREVENT DISKUS in adolescents (aged 12 years and older) have been established based on adequate and well-controlled trials conducted in adults and adolescents [see Clinical Studies (14.1)]. A large 28-week placebo-controlled US trial comparing salmeterol (SEREVENT Inhalation Aerosol) and placebo, each added to usual asthma therapy, showed an increase in asthma-related deaths in subjects receiving salmeterol [see Clinical Studies (14.1)]. Post-hoc analyses in pediatric subjects aged 12 to 18 years were also performed. Pediatric subjects accounted for approximately 12% of subjects in each treatment arm. Respiratory-related death or life-threatening experience occurred at a similar rate in the salmeterol group (0.12% [2/1,653) and the placebo group (0.12% [2/1,622]; relative risk: 1.0 [95% CI: 0.1, 7.2]). All-cause hospitalization, however, was increased in the salmeterol group (2% [35/1,653]) versus the placebo group (<1% [16/1,622]; relative risk: 2.1 [95% CI: 1.1, 3.7]).

The safety and efficacy of SEREVENT DISKUS have been evaluated in over 2,500 subjects aged 4 to 11 years with asthma, 346 of whom were administered SEREVENT DISKUS for 1 year. Based on available data, no adjustment of dosage of SEREVENT DISKUS in pediatric patients is warranted for either asthma or EIB.

In 2 randomized, double-blind, controlled clinical trials of 12 weeks' duration, SEREVENT DISKUS 50 mcg was administered to 211 pediatric subjects with asthma who did and who did not receive concurrent inhaled corticosteroids. The efficacy of SEREVENT DISKUS was demonstrated over the 12-week treatment period with respect to peak expiratory flow (PEF) and forced expiratory volume in 1 second (FEV$_1$). SEREVENT DISKUS was effective in demographic subgroups (gender and age) of the population.

In 2 randomized trials in children aged 4 to 11 years with asthma and EIB, a single 50-mcg dose of SEREVENT DISKUS prevented EIB when dosed 30 minutes prior to exercise, with protection lasting up to 11.5 hours in repeat testing following this single dose in many subjects.

8.5 Geriatric Use

Of the total number of adult and adolescent subjects with asthma who received SEREVENT DISKUS in chronic dosing clinical trials, 209 were aged 65 years and older. Of the total number of subjects with COPD who received SEREVENT DISKUS in chronic dosing clinical trials, 167 were aged 65 years and older and 45 were aged 75 years and older. No apparent differences in the safety of Serevent DISKUS were observed when geriatric subjects were compared with younger subjects in clinical trials. As with other beta$_2$-agonists, however, special caution should be observed when using Serevent DISKUS in geriatric patients who have concomitant cardiovascular disease that could be adversely affected by beta-agonists. Data from the trials in subjects with COPD suggested a greater effect on FEV$_1$ of SEREVENT DISKUS in subjects younger than 65 years, as compared with subjects aged 65 years and older. However, based on available data, no adjustment of dosage of SEREVENT DISKUS in geriatric patients is warranted.

8.6 Hepatic Impairment

Formal pharmacokinetic studies using SEREVENT DISKUS have not been conducted in patients with hepatic impairment. Since salmeterol is predominantly cleared by hepatic metabolism, impairment of liver function may lead to accumulation of salmeterol in plasma. Therefore, patients with hepatic disease should be closely monitored.

10 OVERDOSAGE

The expected signs and symptoms with overdosage of SEREVENT DISKUS are those of excessive beta-adrenergic stimulation and/or occurrence or exaggeration of any of the signs and symptoms of beta-adrenergic stimulation (e.g., seizures, angina, hypertension or hypotension, tachycardia with rates up to 200 beats/min, arrhythmias, nervousness, headache, tremor, muscle cramps, dry mouth, palpitation, nausea, dizziness, fatigue, malaise, insomnia, hyperglycemia, hypokalemia, metabolic acidosis). Overdosage with SEREVENT DISKUS can lead to clinically significant prolongation of the QTc interval, which can produce ventricular arrhythmias.

As with all inhaled sympathomimetic medicines, cardiac arrest and even death may be associated with an overdose of SEREVENT DISKUS.

Treatment consists of discontinuation of SEREVENT DISKUS together with appropriate symptomatic therapy. The judicious use of a cardioselective beta-receptor blocker may be considered, bearing in mind that such medication can produce bronchospasm. There is insufficient evidence to determine if dialysis is beneficial for overdosage of SEREVENT DISKUS. Cardiac monitoring is recommended in cases of overdosage.

11 DESCRIPTION

The active component of SEREVENT DISKUS is salmeterol xinafoate, a beta$_2$-adrenergic bronchodilator. Salmeterol xinafoate is the racemic form of the 1-hydroxy-2-naphthoic acid salt of salmeterol. It has the chemical name 4-hydroxy-α^1-[[[6-(4-phenylbutoxy)hexyl]amino]methyl]-1,3-benzenedimethanol, 1-hydroxy-2-naphthalenecarboxylate and the following chemical structure:

Salmeterol xinafoate is a white powder with a molecular weight of 603.8, and the empirical formula is $C_{25}H_{37}NO_4 \cdot C_{11}H_8O_3$. It is freely soluble in methanol; slightly soluble in ethanol, chloroform, and isopropanol; and sparingly soluble in water.

SEREVENT DISKUS is a teal green plastic inhaler containing a foil blister strip. Each blister on the strip contains a white powder mix of micronized salmeterol xinafoate salt (72.5 mcg, equivalent to 50 mcg of salmeterol base) in 12.5 mg of formulation containing lactose monohydrate (which contains milk proteins). After the inhaler is activated, the powder is dispersed into the airstream created by the patient inhaling through the mouthpiece.

Under standardized in vitro test conditions, SEREVENT DISKUS delivers 47 mcg of salmeterol base per blister when tested at a flow rate of 60 L/min for 2 seconds.

In adult subjects with obstructive lung disease and severely compromised lung function (mean FEV$_1$ 20% to 30% of predicted), mean peak inspiratory flow (PIF) through a DISKUS® inhaler was 82.4 L/min (range: 46.1 to 115.3 L/min).

The actual amount of drug delivered to the lung will depend on patient factors, such as inspiratory flow profile.

12 CLINICAL PHARMACOLOGY

12.1 Mechanism of Action

Salmeterol is a selective LABA. In vitro studies show salmeterol to be at least 50 times more selective for beta$_2$-adrenoceptors than albuterol. Although beta$_2$-adrenoceptors are the predominant adrenergic receptors in bronchial smooth muscle and beta$_1$-adrenoceptors are the predominant receptors in the heart, there are also beta$_2$-adrenoceptors in the human heart comprising 10% to 50% of the total beta-adrenoceptors. The precise function of these receptors has not been established, but their presence raises the possibility that even selective beta$_2$-agonists may have cardiac effects.

The pharmacologic effects of beta$_2$-adrenoceptor agonist drugs, including salmeterol, are at least in part attributable to stimulation of intracellular adenyl cyclase, the enzyme that catalyzes the conversion of adenosine triphosphate (ATP) to cyclic-3′,5′-adenosine monophosphate (cyclic AMP). Increased cyclic AMP levels cause relaxation of bronchial smooth muscle and inhibition of release of mediators of immediate hypersensitivity from cells, especially from mast cells.

In vitro tests show that salmeterol is a potent and long-lasting inhibitor of the release of mast cell mediators, such as histamine, leukotrienes, and prostaglandin D$_2$, from human lung. Salmeterol inhibits histamine-induced plasma protein extravasation and inhibits platelet-activating factor–induced eosinophil accumulation in the lungs of guinea pigs when administered by the inhaled route. In humans, single doses of salmeterol administered via inhalation aerosol attenuate allergen-induced bronchial hyperresponsiveness.

12.2 Pharmacodynamics

Inhaled salmeterol, like other beta-adrenergic agonist drugs, can produce dose-related cardiovascular effects and effects on blood glucose and/or serum potassium *[see Warnings and Precautions (5.6, 5.10)]*. The cardiovascular effects (heart rate, blood pressure) associated with salmeterol inhalation aerosol occur with similar frequency, and are of similar type and severity, as those noted following albuterol administration.

The effects of rising inhaled doses of salmeterol and standard inhaled doses of albuterol were studied in volunteers and in subjects with asthma. Salmeterol doses up to 84 mcg administered as inhalation aerosol resulted in heart rate increases of 3 to 16 beats/min, about the same as albuterol dosed at 180 mcg by inhalation aerosol (4 to 10 beats/min). Adult and adolescent subjects receiving 50-mcg doses of salmeterol inhalation powder (n = 60) underwent continuous electrocardiographic monitoring during two 12-hour periods after the first dose and after 1 month of therapy, and no clinically significant dysrhythmias were noted. Also, pediatric patients receiving 50-mcg doses of salmeterol inhalation powder (n = 67) underwent continuous electrocardiographic monitoring during two 12-hour periods after the first dose and after 3 months of therapy, and no clinically significant dysrhythmias were noted.

In 24-week clinical studies in patients with COPD, the incidence of clinically significant abnormalities on the predose ECGs at Weeks 12 and 24 in patients who received salmeterol 50 mcg was not different compared with placebo. No effect of treatment with salmeterol 50 mcg was observed on pulse rate and systolic and diastolic blood pressure in a subset of patients with COPD who underwent 12-hour serial vital sign measurements after the first dose (n = 91) and after 12 weeks of therapy (n = 74). Median changes from baseline in pulse rate and systolic and diastolic blood pressure were similar for patients receiving either salmeterol or placebo *[see Adverse Reactions (6.1)]*.

Concomitant Use of SEREVENT DISKUS With Other Respiratory Medications: *Short-Acting Beta$_2$-Agonists:* In two 12-week repetitive-dose clinical trials in adult and adolescent subjects with asthma (N = 149), the mean daily need for additional beta$_2$-agonist in subjects using SEREVENT DISKUS was approximately 1½ inhalations/day. Twenty-six percent (26%) of the subjects in these trials used between 8 and 24 inhalations of short-acting beta-agonist per day on 1 or more occasions. Nine percent (9%) of the subjects in these trials averaged over 4 inhalations/day over the course of the 12-week trials. No increase in frequency of cardiovascular events was observed among the 3 subjects who averaged 8 to 11 inhalations/day; however, the safety of concomitant use of more than 8 inhalations/day of short-acting beta$_2$-agonist with SEREVENT DISKUS has not been established. In 29 subjects who experienced worsening of asthma while receiving SEREVENT DISKUS during these trials, albuterol therapy administered via either nebulizer or inhalation aerosol (1 dose in most cases) led to improvement in FEV$_1$ and no increase in occurrence of cardiovascular adverse events.

In 2 clinical trials in subjects with COPD, the mean daily need for additional beta$_2$-agonist for subjects using SEREVENT DISKUS was approximately 4 inhalations/day. Twenty-four percent (24%) of subjects using SEREVENT DISKUS averaged 6 or more inhalations of albuterol per day over the course of the 24-week trials. No increase in frequency of cardiovascular adverse reactions was observed among subjects who averaged 6 or more inhalations per day.

Methylxanthines: The concurrent use of intravenously or orally administered methylxanthines (e.g., aminophylline, theophylline) by subjects receiving salmeterol has not been completely evaluated. In 1 clinical trial in subjects with asthma, 87 subjects receiving SEREVENT Inhalation Aerosol 42 mcg twice daily concurrently with a theophylline

product had adverse event rates similar to those in 71 subjects receiving SEREVENT Inhalation Aerosol without theophylline. Resting heart rates were slightly higher in the subjects on theophylline but were little affected by therapy with SEREVENT Inhalation Aerosol.

In 2 clinical trials in subjects with COPD, 39 subjects receiving SEREVENT DISKUS concurrently with a theophylline product had adverse event rates similar to those in 302 subjects receiving SEREVENT DISKUS without theophylline. Based on the available data, the concomitant administration of methylxanthines with SEREVENT DISKUS did not alter the observed adverse event profile.

Cromoglycate: In clinical trials, inhaled cromolyn sodium did not alter the safety profile of salmeterol when administered concurrently.

12.3 Pharmacokinetics

Salmeterol xinafoate, an ionic salt, dissociates in solution so that the salmeterol and 1-hydroxy-2-naphthoic acid (xinafoate) moieties are absorbed, distributed, metabolized, and eliminated independently. Salmeterol acts locally in the lung; therefore, plasma levels do not predict therapeutic effect.

Absorption: Because of the small therapeutic dose, systemic levels of salmeterol are low or undetectable after inhalation of recommended doses (50 mcg of salmeterol inhalation powder twice daily). Following chronic administration of an inhaled dose of 50 mcg of salmeterol inhalation powder twice daily, salmeterol was detected in plasma within 5 to 45 minutes in 7 subjects with asthma; plasma concentrations were very low, with mean peak concentrations of 167 pg/mL at 20 minutes and no accumulation with repeated doses.

Distribution: The percentage of salmeterol bound to human plasma proteins averages 96% in vitro over the concentration range of 8 to 7,722 ng of salmeterol base per milliliter, much higher concentrations than those achieved following therapeutic doses of salmeterol.

Metabolism: Salmeterol base is extensively metabolized by hydroxylation, with subsequent elimination predominantly in the feces. No significant amount of unchanged salmeterol base was detected in either urine or feces.

An in vitro study using human liver microsomes showed that salmeterol is extensively metabolized to α-hydroxysalmeterol (aliphatic oxidation) by CYP3A4. Ketoconazole, a strong inhibitor of CYP3A4, essentially completely inhibited the formation of α-hydroxysalmeterol in vitro.

Elimination: In 2 healthy adult subjects who received 1 mg of radiolabeled salmeterol (as salmeterol xinafoate) orally, approximately 25% and 60% of the radiolabeled salmeterol was eliminated in urine and feces, respectively, over a period of 7 days. The terminal elimination half-life was about 5.5 hours (1 volunteer only).

The xinafoate moiety has no apparent pharmacologic activity. The xinafoate moiety is highly protein bound (>99%) and has a long elimination half-life of 11 days.

Drug Interactions: *Inhibitors of Cytochrome P450 3A4: Ketoconazole:* In a placebo-controlled crossover drug interaction trial in 20 healthy male and female subjects, co-administration of salmeterol (50 mcg twice daily) and the strong CYP3A4 inhibitor ketoconazole (400 mg once daily) for 7 days resulted in a significant increase in plasma salmeterol exposure as determined by a 16-fold increase in AUC (ratio with and without ketoconazole 15.76 [90% CI: 10.66, 23.31]) mainly due to increased bioavailability of the swallowed portion of the dose. Peak plasma salmeterol con-

centrations were increased by 1.4-fold (90% CI: 1.23, 1.68). Three (3) out of 20 subjects (15%) were withdrawn from salmeterol and ketoconazole coadministration due to beta-agonist–mediated systemic effects (2 with QTc prolongation and 1 with palpitations and sinus tachycardia). Coadministration of salmeterol and ketoconazole did not result in a clinically significant effect on mean heart rate, mean blood potassium, or mean blood glucose. Although there was no statistical effect on the mean QTc, coadministration of salmeterol and ketoconazole was associated with more frequent increases in QTc duration compared with salmeterol and placebo administration.

Erythromycin: In a repeat-dose trial in 13 healthy subjects, concomitant administration of erythromycin (a moderate CYP3A4 inhibitor) and salmeterol inhalation aerosol resulted in a 40% increase in salmeterol C$_{max}$ at steady state (ratio with and without erythromycin 1.4 [90% CI: 0.96, 2.03], P = 0.12), a 3.6-beat/min increase in heart rate ([95% CI: 0.19, 7.03], P <0.04), a 5.8-msec increase in QTc interval ([95% CI: -6.14, 17.77], P = 0.34), and no change in plasma potassium.

13 NONCLINICAL TOXICOLOGY

13.1 Carcinogenesis, Mutagenesis, Impairment of Fertility

In an 18-month carcinogenicity study in CD-mice, salmeterol at oral doses of 1.4 mg/kg and above (approximately 20 times the MRHDID for adults and children based on comparison of the plasma AUCs) caused a dose-related increase in the incidence of smooth muscle hyperplasia, cystic glandular hyperplasia, leiomyomas of the uterus, and ovarian cysts. No tumors were seen at 0.2 mg/kg (approximately 3 times the MRHDID for adults and children based on comparison of the AUCs).

In a 24-month oral and inhalation carcinogenicity study in Sprague Dawley rats, salmeterol caused a dose-related increase in the incidence of mesovarian leiomyomas and ovarian cysts at doses of 0.68 mg/kg and above (approximately 55 and 25 times the MRHDID for adults and children, respectively, on a mg/m^2 basis). No tumors were seen at 0.21 mg/kg (approximately 15 and 8 times the MRHDID for adults and children, respectively, on a mg/m^2 basis). These findings in rodents are similar to those reported previously for other beta-adrenergic agonist drugs. The relevance of these findings to human use is unknown.

Salmeterol produced no detectable or reproducible increases in microbial and mammalian gene mutation in vitro. No clastogenic activity occurred in vitro in human lymphocytes or in vivo in a rat micronucleus test. No effects on fertility were identified in rats treated with salmeterol at oral doses up to 2 mg/kg (approximately 160 times the MRHDID for adults on a mg/m^2 basis).

13.2 Animal Toxicology and/or Pharmacology

Preclinical: Studies in laboratory animals (minipigs, rodents, and dogs) have demonstrated the occurrence of cardiac arrhythmias and sudden death (with histologic evidence of myocardial necrosis) when beta-agonists and methylxanthines are administered concurrently. The clinical relevance of these findings is unknown.

14 CLINICAL STUDIES

14.1 Asthma

The initial trials supporting the approval of SEREVENT DISKUS for the treatment of asthma did not require the regular use of inhaled corticosteroids. However, for the treatment of asthma, SEREVENT DISKUS is currently indicated only as concomitant therapy with an inhaled corticosteroid *[see Indications and Usage (1.1)]*.

Table 4. Daily Efficacy Measurements in Two 12-Week Clinical Trials (Combined Data)

Parameter	Time	Placebo	SEREVENT DISKUS	Albuterol Inhalation Aerosol
No. of randomized subjects		152	149	148
Mean AM peak expiratory flow (L/min)	Baseline 12 weeks	394	395	394
		396	427[a]	394
Mean % days with no asthma symptoms	Baseline 12 weeks	14	13	12
		20	33	21
Mean % nights with no awakenings	Baseline 12 weeks	70	63	68
		73	85[a]	71
Rescue medications (mean no. of inhalations per day)	Baseline 12 weeks	4.2	4.3	4.3
		3.3	1.6[b]	2.2
Asthma exacerbations (%)		14	15	16

[a]Statistically superior to placebo and albuterol ($P<0.001$).
[b]Statistically superior to placebo ($P<0.001$).

Table 5: Asthma-Related Deaths in the 28-Week Salmeterol Multi-center Asthma Research Trial (SMART)

	Salmeterol n (%[a])	Placebo n (%[a])	Relative Risk[b] (95% Confidence Interval)	Excess Deaths Expressed per 10,000 Subjects[c] (95% Confidence Interval)
Total Population[d]				
Salmeterol: n = 13,176	13 (0.10%)		4.37 (1.25, 15.34)	8 (3, 13)
Placebo: n = 13,179		3 (0.02%)		
Caucasian				
Salmeterol: n = 9,281	6 (0.07%)		5.82 (0.70, 48.37)	6 (1, 10)
Placebo: n = 9,361		1 (0.01%)		
African American				
Salmeterol: n = 2,366	7 (0.31%)		7.26 (0.89, 58.94)	27 (8, 46)
Placebo: n = 2,319		1 (0.04%)		

[a]Life-table 28-week estimate, adjusted according to the subjects' actual lengths of exposure to study treatment to account for early withdrawal of subjects from the study.
[b]Relative risk is the ratio of the rate of asthma-related death in the salmeterol group and the rate in the placebo group. The relative risk indicates how many more times likely an asthma-related death occurred in the salmeterol group than in the placebo group in a 28-week treatment period.
[c]Estimate of the number of additional asthma-related deaths in subjects treated with salmeterol in SMART, assuming 10,000 subjects received salmeterol for a 28-week treatment period. Estimate calculated as the difference between the salmeterol and placebo groups in the rates of asthma-related death multiplied by 10,000.
[d]The Total Population includes the following ethnic origins listed on the case report form: Caucasian, African American, Hispanic, Asian, and "Other." In addition, the Total Population includes those subjects whose ethnic origin was not reported. The results for Caucasian and African American subpopulations are shown above. No asthma-related deaths occurred in the Hispanic (salmeterol n = 996, placebo n = 999), Asian (salmeterol n = 173, placebo n = 149), or "Other" (salmeterol n = 230, placebo n = 224) subpopulations. One asthma-related death occurred in the placebo group in the subpopulation whose ethnic origin was not reported (salmeterol n = 130, placebo n = 127).

Adult and Adolescent Subjects Aged 12 Years and Older: In 2 randomized double-blind trials, SEREVENT DISKUS was compared with albuterol inhalation aerosol and placebo in adolescent and adult subjects with mild-to-moderate asthma (protocol defined as 50% to 80% predicted FEV$_1$, actual mean of 67.7% at baseline), including subjects who did and who did not receive concurrent inhaled corticosteroids. The efficacy of SEREVENT DISKUS was demonstrated over the 12-week period with no change in effectiveness over this time period (see Figure 1). There were no gender- or age-related differences in safety or efficacy. No development of tachyphylaxis to the bronchodilator effect was noted in these trials. FEV$_1$ measurements (mean change from baseline) from these two 12-week trials are shown in Figure 1 for both the first and last treatment days.

Figure 1. Serial 12-Hour FEV$_1$ From Two 12-Week Clinical Trials in Subjects With Asthma

First Treatment Day

Last Treatment Day (Week 12)

Table 4 shows the treatment effects seen during daily treatment with SEREVENT DISKUS for 12 weeks in adolescent and adult subjects with mild-to-moderate asthma.
[See table 4 at top of previous page]

Maintenance of efficacy for periods up to 1 year has been documented.

SEREVENT DISKUS and SEREVENT Inhalation Aerosol were compared with placebo in 2 additional randomized double-blind clinical trials in adolescent and adult subjects with mild-to-moderate asthma. SEREVENT DISKUS 50 mcg and SEREVENT Inhalation Aerosol 42 mcg, both administered twice daily, produced significant improvements in pulmonary function compared with placebo over the 12-week period. While no statistically significant differences were observed between the active treatments for any of the efficacy assessments or safety evaluations performed, there were some efficacy measures on which the metered-dose inhaler appeared to provide better results. Similar findings were noted in 2 randomized, single-dose, crossover comparisons of SEREVENT DISKUS and SEREVENT Inhalation Aerosol for the prevention of EIB. Therefore, while SEREVENT DISKUS was comparable to SEREVENT Inhalation Aerosol in clinical trials in mild-to-moderate subjects with asthma, it should not be assumed that they will produce clinically equivalent outcomes in all subjects.

Subjects on Concomitant Inhaled Corticosteroids: In 4 clinical trials in adult and adolescent subjects with asthma (N = 1,922), the effect of adding SEREVENT Inhalation Aerosol to inhaled corticosteroid therapy was evaluated over a 24-week treatment period. The trials compared the addition of salmeterol therapy to an increase (at least doubling) of the inhaled corticosteroid dose.

Two randomized, double-blind, controlled, parallel-group clinical trials (N = 997) enrolled subjects (aged 18 to 82 years) with persistent asthma who were previously maintained but not adequately controlled on inhaled corticosteroid therapy. During the 2-week run-in period, all subjects were switched to beclomethasone dipropionate (BDP) 168 mcg twice daily. Subjects still not adequately controlled were randomized to either the addition of SEREVENT Inhalation Aerosol 42 mcg twice daily or an increase of BDP to 336 mcg twice daily. As compared with the doubled dose of BDP, the addition of SEREVENT Inhalation Aerosol resulted in statistically significantly greater improvements in pulmonary function and asthma symptoms, and statistically significantly greater reduction in supplemental albuterol use. The percent of subjects who experienced asthma exacerbations overall was not different between groups (i.e., 16.2% in the group receiving SEREVENT Inhalation Aerosol versus 17.9% in the higher-dose beclomethasone dipropionate group).

Two randomized, double-blind, controlled, parallel-group clinical trials (N = 925) enrolled subjects (aged 12 to 78 years) with persistent asthma who were previously maintained but not adequately controlled on prior asthma therapy. During the 2- to 4-week run-in period, all subjects were switched to fluticasone propionate 88 mcg twice daily. Subjects still not adequately controlled were randomized to either the addition of SEREVENT Inhalation Aerosol 42 mcg twice daily or an increase of fluticasone propionate to 220 mcg twice daily. As compared with the increased (2.5 times) dose of fluticasone propionate, the addition of SEREVENT Inhalation Aerosol resulted in statistically significantly greater improvements in pulmonary function and

asthma symptoms, and statistically significantly greater reductions in supplemental albuterol use. Fewer subjects receiving SEREVENT Inhalation Aerosol experienced asthma exacerbations than those receiving the higher dose of fluticasone propionate (8.8% versus 13.8%).

Table 5 shows the treatment effects seen during daily treatment with SEREVENT Inhalation Aerosol for 24 weeks in adolescent and adult subjects with mild-to-moderate asthma.

Onset of Action: During the initial treatment day in several multiple-dose clinical trials with SEREVENT DISKUS in subjects with asthma, the median time to onset of clinically significant bronchodilatation (≥15% improvement in FEV$_1$) ranged from 30 to 48 minutes after a 50-mcg dose. One hour after a single dose of 50 mcg of SEREVENT DISKUS, the majority of subjects had ≥15% improvement in FEV$_1$. Maximum improvement in FEV$_1$ generally occurred within 180 minutes, and clinically significant improvement continued for 12 hours in most subjects.

Pediatric Subjects: In a randomized, double-blind, controlled trial (N = 449), 50 mcg of SEREVENT DISKUS was administered twice daily to pediatric subjects with asthma who did and who did not receive concurrent inhaled corticosteroids. The efficacy of salmeterol inhalation powder was demonstrated over the 12-week treatment period with respect to periodic serial PEF (36% to 39% postdose increase from baseline) and FEV$_1$ (32% to 33% postdose increase from baseline). Salmeterol was effective in demographic subgroup analyses (gender and age) and was effective when coadministered with other inhaled asthma medications such as short-acting bronchodilators and inhaled corticosteroids. A second randomized, double-blind, placebo-controlled trial (N = 207) with 50 mcg of salmeterol inhalation powder via an alternate device supported the findings of the trial with the DISKUS.

Salmeterol Multi-center Asthma Research Trial: The SMART trial was a randomized double-blind trial that enrolled LABA-naive subjects with asthma (average age of 39 years; 71% Caucasian, 18% African American, 8% Hispanic) to assess the safety of salmeterol (SEREVENT Inhalation Aerosol) 42 mcg twice daily over 28 weeks compared with placebo when added to usual asthma therapy.

A planned interim analysis was conducted when approximately half of the intended number of subjects had been enrolled (N = 26,355), which led to premature termination of the trial. The results of the interim analysis showed that subjects receiving salmeterol were at increased risk for fatal asthma events (see Table 5 and Figure 2). In the total population, a higher rate of asthma-related death occurred in subjects treated with salmeterol than those treated with placebo (0.10% versus 0.02%, relative risk: 4.37 [95% CI: 1.25, 15.34]).

Post-hoc subpopulation analyses were performed. In Caucasians, asthma-related death occurred at a higher rate in subjects treated with salmeterol than in subjects treated with placebo (0.07% versus 0.01%, relative risk: 5.82 [95% CI: 0.70, 48.37]). In African Americans also, asthma-related death occurred at a higher rate in subjects treated with salmeterol than those treated with placebo (0.31% versus 0.04%, relative risk: 7.26 [95% CI: 0.89, 58.94]). Although the relative risks of asthma-related death were similar in Caucasians and African Americans, the estimate of excess deaths in subjects treated with salmeterol was greater in African Americans because there was a higher overall rate of asthma-related death in African American subjects (see Table 5).

Post-hoc analyses in pediatric subjects aged 12 to 18 years were also performed. Pediatric subjects accounted for approximately 12% of subjects in each treatment arm. Respiratory-related death or life-threatening experience occurred at a similar rate in the salmeterol group (0.12% [2/1,653]) and the placebo group (0.12% [2/1,622]; relative risk: 1.0 [95% CI: 0.1, 7.2]). All-cause hospitalization, however, was increased in the salmeterol group (2% [35/1,653]) versus the placebo group (<1% [16/1,622]; relative risk: 2.1 [95% CI: 1.1, 3.7]).

The data from the SMART trial are not adequate to determine whether concurrent use of inhaled corticosteroids or other long-term asthma control therapy mitigates the risk of asthma-related death.

[See table 5 above]
[See figure 2 at top of next column]

14.2 Exercise-Induced Bronchospasm

In 2 randomized, single-dose, crossover trials in adolescents and adults with EIB (N = 52), 50 mcg of SEREVENT DISKUS prevented EIB when dosed 30 minutes prior to exercise. For some subjects, this protective effect against EIB was still apparent up to 8.5 hours following a single dose (see Table 6).

[See table 6 at top of next page]

In 2 randomized trials in children aged 4 to 11 years with asthma and EIB (N = 50), a single 50-mcg dose of SEREVENT DISKUS prevented EIB when dosed 30 min-

Figure 2. Cumulative Incidence of Asthma-Related Deaths in the 28-Week Salmeterol Multi-center Asthma Research Trial (SMART), by Duration of Treatment

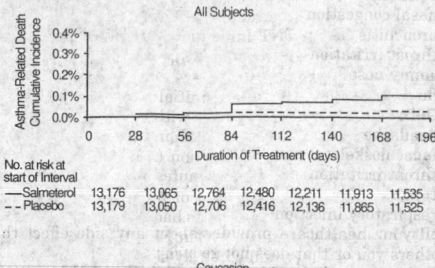

No. at risk at start of Interval

—Salmeterol	13,176	13,065	12,764	12,480	12,211	11,913	11,535
– – Placebo	13,179	13,050	12,706	12,416	12,136	11,865	11,525

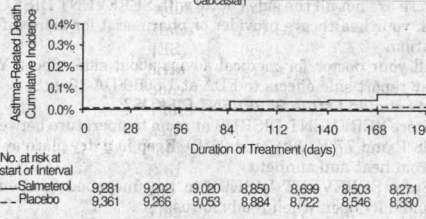

No. at risk at start of Interval

—Salmeterol	9,281	9,202	9,020	8,850	8,699	8,503	8,271
– – Placebo	9,361	9,266	9,053	8,884	8,722	8,546	8,330

No. at risk at start of Interval

—Salmeterol	2,366	2,351	2,271	2,201	2,114	2,048	1,972
– – Placebo	2,319	2,303	2,225	2,156	2,078	2,023	1,953

utes prior to exercise, with protection lasting up to 11.5 hours in repeat testing following this single dose in many subjects.

14.3 Chronic Obstructive Pulmonary Disease

In 2 clinical trials evaluating twice-daily treatment with SEREVENT DISKUS 50 mcg (n = 336) compared with placebo (n = 366) in subjects with chronic bronchitis with airflow limitation, with or without emphysema, improvements in pulmonary function endpoints were greater with salmeterol 50 mcg than with placebo. Treatment with SEREVENT DISKUS did not result in significant improvements in secondary endpoints assessing COPD symptoms in either clinical trial. Both trials were randomized, double-blind, parallel-group trials of 24 weeks' duration and were identical in design, subject entrance criteria, and overall conduct.

Figure 3 displays the integrated 2-hour postdose FEV_1 results from the 2 clinical trials. The percent change in FEV_1 refers to the change from baseline, defined as the predose value on Treatment Day 1. To account for subject withdrawals during the trial, Endpoint (last evaluable FEV_1) data are provided. Subjects receiving SEREVENT DISKUS 50 mcg had significantly greater improvements in 2-hour postdose FEV_1 at Endpoint (216 mL, 20%) compared with placebo (43 mL, 5%). Improvement was apparent on the first day of treatment and maintained throughout the 24 weeks of treatment.

Figure 3. Mean Percent Change From Baseline in Postdose FEV_1 Integrated Data From 2 Trials of Subjects With Chronic Bronchitis and Airflow Limitation

	Day 1	Week 12	Week 24	Endpoint
	N	N	N	N
SEREVENT DISKUS 50 mcg twice daily	335	265	222	326
Placebo	361	264	226	343

Table 6. Results of 2 Exercise-Induced Bronchospasm Trials in Adolescents and Adults

		Placebo (N = 52)		SEREVENT DISKUS (N = 52)	
		n	% Total	n	% Total
0.5-Hour postdose exercise challenge	% Fall in FEV_1				
	<10%	15	29	31	60
	≥10%, <20%	3	6	11	21
	≥20%	34	65	10	19
Mean maximal % fall in FEV_1 (SE)		-25% (1.8)		-11% (1.9)	
8.5-Hour postdose exercise challenge	% Fall in FEV_1				
	<10%	12	23	26	50
	≥10%, <20%	7	13	12	23
	≥20%	33	63	14	27
Mean maximal % fall in FEV_1 (SE)		-27% (1.5)		-16% (2.0)	

Onset of Action and Duration of Effect: The onset of action and duration of effect of SEREVENT DISKUS were evaluated in a subset of subjects (n = 87) from 1 of the 2 clinical trials discussed above. Following the first 50-mcg dose, significant improvement in pulmonary function (mean FEV_1 increase of 12% or more and at least 200 mL) occurred at 2 hours. The mean time to peak bronchodilator effect was 4.75 hours. As seen in Figure 4, evidence of bronchodilatation was seen throughout the 12-hour period. Figure 4 also demonstrates that the bronchodilating effect after 12 weeks of treatment was similar to that observed after the first dose. The mean time to peak bronchodilator effect after 12 weeks of treatment was 3.27 hours.

Figure 4. Serial 12-Hour FEV_1 on the First Day and at Week 12 of Treatment

Day 1 ● SEREVENT DISKUS 50 mcg twice daily (N = 87)
Day 1 ■ Placebo (N = 95)
Week 12 ○ SEREVENT DISKUS 50 mcg twice daily (N = 73)
Week 12 □ Placebo (N = 65)

16 HOW SUPPLIED/STORAGE AND HANDLING

SEREVENT DISKUS is supplied as a disposable teal green plastic inhaler containing a foil blister strip with 60 blisters. The inhaler is packaged in a plastic-coated, moisture-protective foil pouch (NDC 0173-0521-00).

Serevent Diskus is also supplied in an institutional pack containing 28 blisters (NDC 0173-0520-00).

Store at room temperature between 68°F and 77°F (20°C and 25°C); excursions permitted from 59°F to 86°F (15°C to 30°C) [See USP Controlled Room Temperature]. Store in a dry place away from direct heat or sunlight. Keep out of reach of children.

SEREVENT DISKUS should be stored inside the unopened moisture-protective foil pouch and only removed from the pouch immediately before initial use. Discard SEREVENT DISKUS 6 weeks after opening the foil pouch or when the counter reads "0" (after all blisters have been used), whichever comes first. The inhaler is not reusable. Do not attempt to take the inhaler apart.

17 PATIENT COUNSELING INFORMATION

Advise the patient to read the FDA-approved patient labeling (Medication Guide and Instructions for Use).

Asthma-Related Death: Inform patients that salmeterol increases the risk of asthma-related death and may increase the risk of asthma-related hospitalization in pediatric and adolescent patients. Inform patients that SEREVENT DISKUS should not be the only therapy for the treatment of asthma and must only be used as additional therapy when long-term asthma control medications (e.g., inhaled corticosteroids) do not adequately control asthma symptoms. Also inform them that currently available data are inadequate to determine whether concurrent use of inhaled corticosteroids or other long-term asthma control drugs mitigates the increased risk of asthma-related death from LABA. Inform patients that when SEREVENT DISKUS is added to their treatment regimen they must continue to use their long-term asthma control medication.

Not for Acute Symptoms: Inform patients that SEREVENT DISKUS is not meant to relieve acute asthma symptoms or exacerbations of COPD and extra doses should not be used for that purpose. Advise patients to treat acute symptoms with an inhaled, short-acting beta$_2$-agonist such as albuterol. Provide patients with such medication and instruct them in how it should be used.

Instruct patients to seek medical attention immediately if they experience any of the following:

• Decreasing effectiveness of inhaled, short-acting beta$_2$-agonists

• Need for more inhalations than usual of inhaled, short-acting beta$_2$-agonists

• Significant decrease in lung function as outlined by the physician

Tell patients they should not stop therapy with SEREVENT DISKUS without physician/provider guidance since symptoms may recur after discontinuation.

Not a Substitute for Corticosteroids: Advise all patients with asthma that they must also continue regular maintenance treatment with an inhaled corticosteroid if they are taking SEREVENT DISKUS.

SEREVENT DISKUS should not be used as a substitute for oral or inhaled corticosteroids. The dosage of these medications should not be changed and they should not be stopped without consulting the physician, even if the patient feels better after initiating treatment with SEREVENT DISKUS.

Do Not Use Additional Long-Acting Beta$_2$-Agonists: Instruct patients not to use other LABA.

Immediate Hypersensitivity Reactions: Advise patients that immediate hypersensitivity reactions (e.g., urticaria, angioedema, rash, bronchospasm, hypotension), including anaphylaxis, may occur after administration of SEREVENT DISKUS. Patients should discontinue SEREVENT DISKUS if such reactions occur. There have been reports of anaphylactic reactions in patients with severe milk protein allergy after inhalation of powder products containing lactose; therefore, patients with severe milk protein allergy should not take SEREVENT DISKUS.

Risks Associated With Beta-Agonist Therapy: Inform patients of adverse effects associated with beta$_2$-agonists, such as palpitations, chest pain, rapid heart rate, tremor, or nervousness.

Treatment of Exercise-Induced Bronchospasm: Patients using SEREVENT DISKUS for the treatment of EIB should not use additional doses for 12 hours. Patients who are receiving SEREVENT DISKUS twice daily should not use additional SEREVENT for prevention of EIB.

SEREVENT and DISKUS are registered trademarks of the GSK group of companies.

GlaxoSmithKline
Research Triangle Park, NC 27709
©2014, the GSK group of companies. All rights reserved.
SRD:10PI

MEDICATION GUIDE
SEREVENT® DISKUS® [ser′ uh-vent disk′ us]
(salmeterol xinafoate inhalation powder)
Read the Medication Guide that comes with SEREVENT DISKUS before you start using it and each time you get a refill. There may be new information. This Medication Guide does not take the place of talking to your healthcare provider about your medical condition or treatment.

What is the most important information I should know about SEREVENT DISKUS?
SEREVENT DISKUS can cause serious side effects, including:
- People with asthma who take long-acting beta$_2$-adrenergic agonist (LABA) medicines, such as salmeterol xinafoate (the medicine in SEREVENT DISKUS), have an increased risk of death from asthma problems.
- It is not known if LABA medicines such as salmeterol xinafoate increase the risk of death in people with COPD.
- Call your healthcare provider if breathing problems worsen over time while using SEREVENT DISKUS. You may need different treatment.
- Get emergency medical care if:
  ◦ your breathing problems worsen quickly.
  ◦ you use your rescue inhaler, but it does not relieve your breathing problems.
- Do not use SEREVENT DISKUS as your only asthma medicine. SEREVENT DISKUS must only be used with a long-term asthma control medicine, such as an inhaled corticosteroid.
- SEREVENT DISKUS should be used only if your healthcare provider decides that your asthma is not well controlled with a long-term asthma control medicine, such as an inhaled corticosteroid. When your asthma is well controlled, your healthcare provider may tell you to stop taking SEREVENT DISKUS. Your healthcare provider will decide if you can stop SEREVENT DISKUS without loss of asthma control. You will continue taking your long-term asthma control medicine, such as an inhaled corticosteroid.
- Children and adolescents who take LABA medicines may have an increased risk of being hospitalized for asthma problems.

What is SEREVENT DISKUS?
- SEREVENT DISKUS is a prescription inhaled LABA medicine. LABA medicines such as salmeterol xinafoate help the muscles around the airways in your lungs stay relaxed to prevent symptoms, such as wheezing, cough, chest tightness, and shortness of breath. These symptoms can happen when the muscles around the airways tighten. This makes it hard to breathe.
- SEREVENT DISKUS is not used to relieve sudden breathing problems.
- It is not known if SEREVENT DISKUS is safe and effective in children younger than 4 years.
- SEREVENT DISKUS is used for asthma, exercise-induced bronchospasm (EIB), and chronic obstructive pulmonary disease (COPD) as follows:

Asthma:
SEREVENT DISKUS is a prescription medicine used to control symptoms of asthma and to prevent symptoms such as wheezing in adults and children aged 4 years and older. SEREVENT DISKUS contains salmeterol xinafoate. LABA medicines such as salmeterol xinafoate increase the risk of death from asthma problems.
SEREVENT DISKUS is not for adults and children with asthma who are well controlled with an asthma control medicine, such as a low to medium dose of an inhaled corticosteroid medicine.

Exercise-Induced Bronchospasm (EIB):
SEREVENT DISKUS is used to prevent wheezing caused by exercise in adults and children aged 4 years and older.
- If you only have EIB, your healthcare provider may only prescribe SEREVENT DISKUS for your condition.
- If you have EIB and asthma, your healthcare provider should also prescribe an asthma control medicine, such as an inhaled corticosteroid.

Chronic Obstructive Pulmonary Disease (COPD):
COPD is a chronic lung disease that includes chronic bronchitis, emphysema, or both.
SEREVENT DISKUS is a prescription medicine used long term as 1 inhalation 2 times each day to improve symptoms of COPD for better breathing.

Who should not use SEREVENT DISKUS?
Do not use SEREVENT DISKUS:
- to treat your asthma without a long-term asthma control medicine, such as an inhaled corticosteroid.
- if you have a severe allergy to milk proteins. Ask your healthcare provider if you are not sure.
- if you are allergic to salmeterol xinafoate or any of the ingredients in SEREVENT DISKUS. See "What are the ingredients in SEREVENT DISKUS?" below for a complete list of ingredients.

What should I tell my healthcare provider before using SEREVENT DISKUS?
Tell your healthcare provider about all of your health conditions, including if you:
- have heart problems.
- have high blood pressure.
- have seizures.
- have thyroid problems.
- have diabetes.
- have liver problems.

- are allergic to any of the ingredients in SEREVENT DISKUS, any other medicines, or food products. See "What are the ingredients in SEREVENT DISKUS?" below for a complete list of ingredients.
- have any other medical conditions.
- are pregnant or planning to become pregnant. It is not known if SEREVENT DISKUS may harm your unborn baby.
- are breastfeeding. It is not known if the medicine in SEREVENT DISKUS passes into your milk and if it can harm your baby.

Tell your healthcare provider about all the medicines you take, including prescription and over-the-counter medicines, vitamins, and herbal supplements. SEREVENT DISKUS and certain other medicines may interact with each other. This may cause serious side effects. Especially, tell your healthcare provider if you take antifungal or anti-HIV medicines.
Know the medicines you take. Keep a list of them to show your healthcare provider and pharmacist when you get a new medicine.

How should I use SEREVENT DISKUS?
Read the step-by-step instructions for using SEREVENT DISKUS at the end of this Medication Guide.
- **Do not** use SEREVENT DISKUS unless your healthcare provider has taught you how to use the inhaler and you understand how to use it correctly.
- Children should use SEREVENT DISKUS with an adult's help, as instructed by the child's healthcare provider.
- Use SEREVENT DISKUS exactly as prescribed. **Do not** use SEREVENT DISKUS more often than prescribed.
- **For asthma and COPD,** the usual dose is 1 inhalation of SEREVENT DISKUS 2 times each day. Use SEREVENT DISKUS at the same time each day, about 12 hours apart.
- **For preventing exercise-induced bronchospasm,** the usual dose is 1 inhalation at least 30 minutes before exercise. Do not use SEREVENT DISKUS more often than every 12 hours. Do not use extra SEREVENT DISKUS before exercise if you already use it 2 times each day.
- If you miss a dose of SEREVENT DISKUS, just skip that dose. Take your next dose at your usual time. Do not take 2 doses at 1 time.
- If you take too much SEREVENT DISKUS, call your healthcare provider or go to the nearest hospital emergency room right away if you have any unusual symptoms, such as worsening shortness of breath, chest pain, increased heart rate, or shakiness.
- **Do not use other medicines that contain a LABA for any reason.** Ask your healthcare provider or pharmacist if any of your other medicines are LABA medicines.
- Do not stop using SEREVENT DISKUS unless told to do so by your healthcare provider because your symptoms might get worse. Your healthcare provider will change your medicines as needed.
- SEREVENT DISKUS does not relieve sudden symptoms. Always have a rescue inhaler with you to treat sudden symptoms. If you do not have a rescue inhaler, call your healthcare provider to have one prescribed for you.
- Call your healthcare provider or get medical care right away if:
  ◦ your breathing problems get worse.
  ◦ you need to use your rescue inhaler more often than usual.
  ◦ your rescue inhaler does not work as well to relieve your symptoms.
  ◦ you need to use 4 or more inhalations of your rescue inhaler in 24 hours for 2 or more days in a row.
  ◦ you use 1 whole canister of your rescue inhaler in 8 weeks.
  ◦ your peak flow meter results decrease. Your healthcare provider will tell you the numbers that are right for you.
  ◦ you have asthma and your symptoms do not improve after using SEREVENT DISKUS regularly for 1 week.

What are the possible side effects with SEREVENT DISKUS?
SEREVENT DISKUS can cause serious side effects, including:
- See "What is the most important information I should know about SEREVENT DISKUS?"
- **sudden breathing problems immediately after inhaling your medicine**
- **effects on heart**
  ◦ increased blood pressure
  ◦ a fast or irregular heartbeat
  ◦ chest pain
- **effects on nervous system**
  ◦ tremor
  ◦ nervousness
- **serious allergic reactions.** Call your healthcare provider or get emergency medical care if you get any of the following symptoms of a serious allergic reaction:
  ◦ rash
  ◦ hives
  ◦ swelling of your face, mouth, and tongue

◦ breathing problems.
- **changes in laboratory blood values (sugar, potassium)**
Common side effects of SEREVENT DISKUS include:
Asthma:
- headache
- nasal congestion
- bronchitis
- throat irritation
- runny nose
- flu
COPD:
- headache
- musculoskeletal pain
- throat irritation
- cough
- respiratory infection
Tell your healthcare provider about any side effect that bothers you or that does not go away.
These are not all the side effects with SEREVENT DISKUS. Ask your healthcare provider or pharmacist for more information.
Call your doctor for medical advice about side effects. You may report side effects to FDA at 1-800-FDA-1088.

How should I store SEREVENT DISKUS?
- Store SEREVENT DISKUS at room temperature between 68°F and 77°F (20°C and 25°C). Keep in a dry place away from heat and sunlight.
- Store SEREVENT DISKUS in the unopened foil pouch and only open when ready for use.
- Safely throw away SEREVENT DISKUS in the trash 6 weeks after you open the foil pouch or when the counter reads 0, whichever comes first.
- **Keep SEREVENT DISKUS and all medicines out of the reach of children.**

General information about SEREVENT DISKUS
Medicines are sometimes prescribed for purposes not mentioned in a Medication Guide. Do not use SEREVENT DISKUS for a condition for which it was not prescribed. Do not give your SEREVENT DISKUS to other people, even if they have the same condition that you have. It may harm them.
This Medication Guide summarizes the most important information about SEREVENT DISKUS. If you would like more information, talk with your healthcare provider or pharmacist. You can ask your healthcare provider or pharmacist for information about SEREVENT DISKUS that was written for healthcare professionals.
For more information about SEREVENT DISKUS, call 1-888-825-5249 or visit our website at www.serevent.com.

What are the ingredients in SEREVENT DISKUS?
Active ingredient: salmeterol xinafoate
Inactive ingredient: lactose monohydrate (contains milk proteins)

Instructions for Use
For Oral Inhalation Only
Your SEREVENT DISKUS inhaler

Figure A

Read this information before you start using your SEREVENT DISKUS inhaler:
- Take SEREVENT DISKUS out of the foil pouch just before you use it for the first time. Safely throw away the pouch. The DISKUS will be in the closed position.
- Write the date you opened the foil pouch in the first blank line on the label. **See Figure A.**
- Write the "use by" date in the second blank line on the label. **See Figure A.** That date is 6 weeks after the date you wrote in the first line.
- The counter should read **60**. If you have an institutional pack (with "INSTITUTIONAL PACK" on the foil pouch), the counter should read **28**.
How to use your SEREVENT DISKUS inhaler
Follow these steps every time you use SEREVENT DISKUS.
Step 1. Open your SEREVENT DISKUS.
- Hold the DISKUS in your left hand and place the thumb of your right hand in the thumb grip. Push the thumb grip away from you as far as it will go until the mouthpiece shows and snaps into place. **See Figure B.**

Figure B

Step 2. Slide the lever until you hear it click.
• **Hold the Diskus in a level, flat position** with the mouthpiece towards you. Slide the lever away from the mouthpiece as far as it will go until it **clicks**. **See Figure C.**

Figure C

• The number on the counter will count down by 1. The DISKUS is now ready to use.
Follow the instructions below so you will not accidentally waste a dose:
• **Do not** close the DISKUS.
• **Do not** tilt the DISKUS.
• **Do not** move the lever on the DISKUS.
Step 3. Inhale your medicine.
• Before you breathe in your dose from the DISKUS, breathe out (exhale) as long as you can while you hold the DISKUS level and away from your mouth. **See Figure D.** Do not breathe into the mouthpiece.

Figure D

• Put the mouthpiece to your lips. **See Figure E.** Breathe in quickly and deeply through the DISKUS. Do not breathe in through your nose.

Figure E

• Remove the DISKUS from your mouth and **hold your breath for about 10 seconds,** or for as long as is comfortable for you.
• **Breathe out slowly as long as you can. See Figure D.**
• The DISKUS delivers your dose of medicine as a very fine powder that you may or may not taste or feel. **Do not take an extra dose from the DISKUS even if you do not taste or feel the medicine.**

Step 4. Close the DISKUS.
• Place your thumb in the thumb grip and slide it back towards you as far as it will go. **See Figure F.** Make sure the DISKUS clicks shut and you cannot see the mouthpiece.
• The DISKUS is now ready for you to take your next scheduled dose in about 12 hours. **When you are ready to take your next dose, repeat Steps 1 through 4.**

Figure F

When should you get a refill?
The counter on top of the DISKUS shows you how many doses are left. After you have taken **55 doses** (**23 doses** from the institutional pack), the numbers **5 to 0** will show in red. **See Figure G.** These numbers warn you there are only a few doses left and are a reminder to get a refill.

Figure G

For correct use of the DISKUS, remember:
• Always use the DISKUS in a level, flat position.
• Make sure the lever firmly clicks into place.
• Hold your breath for about 10 seconds after inhaling. Then breathe out fully.
• **Do not** take an extra dose, even if you did not taste or feel the powder.
• **Do not** take the DISKUS apart.
• **Do not** wash the DISKUS.
• Always keep the DISKUS in a dry place.
• **Do not** use the DISKUS with a spacer device.
If you have questions about SEREVENT DISKUS or how to use your inhaler, call GlaxoSmithKline (GSK) at 1-888-825-5249 or visit www.serevent.com.
This Medication Guide and Instructions for Use have been approved by the U.S. Food and Drug Administration.
SEREVENT and DISKUS are registered trademarks of the GSK group of companies.
GlaxoSmithKline
Research Triangle Park, NC 27709
©2014, the GSK group of companies. All rights reserved.
April 2014
SRD:5MG

TAFINLAR ℞
(dabrafenib)
capsules, for oral use

HIGHLIGHTS OF PRESCRIBING INFORMATION
These highlights do not include all the information needed to use TAFINLAR safely and effectively. See full prescribing information for TAFINLAR.
TAFINLAR (dabrafenib) capsules, for oral use
Initial U.S. Approval: 2013

——————RECENT MAJOR CHANGES——————
Indications and Usage (1.2)	01/2014
Dosage and Administration (2.1-2.3)	01/2014
Warnings and Precautions (5-5.9, 5.11)	01/2014

——————INDICATIONS AND USAGE——————
• TAFINLAR is a kinase inhibitor indicated as a single agent for the treatment of patients with unresectable or metastatic melanoma with BRAF V600E mutation as detected by an FDA-approved test. (1.1, 2.1)
• TAFINLAR in combination with trametinib is indicated for the treatment of patients with unresectable or metastatic melanoma with BRAF V600E or V600K mutations as detected by an FDA-approved test. The use in combination is based on the demonstration of durable response rate. Improvement in disease-related symptoms or overall survival has not been demonstrated for TAFINLAR in combination with trametinib. (1.2, 2.1, 14.2)
Limitation of Use: TAFINLAR is not indicated for treatment of patients with wild-type BRAF melanoma. (1.3, 5.2)

——————DOSAGE AND ADMINISTRATION——————
• Confirm the presence of BRAF V600E mutation in tumor specimens prior to initiation of treatment with TAFINLAR as a single agent. Confirm the presence of BRAF V600E or V600K mutation in tumor specimens prior to initiation of treatment with TAFINLAR in combination with trametinib. (2.1)
• The recommended dose of TAFINLAR is 150 mg orally twice daily as a single agent or in combination with trametinib 2 mg orally once daily. Take TAFINLAR at least 1 hour before or at least 2 hours after a meal. (2.2)

——————DOSAGE FORMS AND STRENGTHS——————
Capsules: 50 mg, 75 mg. (3)

——————CONTRAINDICATIONS——————
None. (4)

——————WARNINGS AND PRECAUTIONS——————
• New primary malignancies, cutaneous and non-cutaneous, can occur when TAFINLAR is administered as a single agent or in combination with trametinib. Monitor patients for new malignancies prior to initiation of therapy, while on therapy, and following discontinuation of TAFINLAR or the combination therapy. (5.1, 2.3)
• Tumor Promotion in BRAF Wild-Type Melanoma: Increased cell proliferation can occur with BRAF inhibitors. (5.2)
• Hemorrhage: Major hemorrhagic events can occur in patients receiving TAFINLAR in combination with trametinib. Monitor for signs and symptoms of bleeding. (5.3)
• Venous Thromboembolism: Deep vein thrombosis and pulmonary embolism can occur in patients receiving TAFINLAR in combination with trametinib. (5.4, 2.3)
• Cardiomyopathy: Assess LVEF before treatment with TAFINLAR in combination with trametinib, after one month of treatment, then every 2 to 3 months thereafter. (5.5, 2.3)
• Ocular Toxicities: Perform ophthalmologic evaluation for any visual disturbances. (5.6, 2.3)
• Serious Febrile Reactions: Incidence and severity of pyrexia are increased with TAFINLAR in combination with trametinib. (5.7, 2.3)
• Serious Skin Toxicity: Monitor for skin toxicities and for secondary infections. Discontinue for intolerable Grade 2, or Grade 3 or 4 rash not improving within 3 weeks despite interruption of TAFINLAR. (5.8, 2.3)
• Hyperglycemia: Monitor serum glucose levels in patients with pre-existing diabetes or hyperglycemia. (5.9)
• Glucose-6-Phosphate Dehydrogenase Deficiency: Closely monitor for hemolytic anemia. (5.10)
• Embryofetal Toxicity: Can cause fetal harm. Advise females of reproductive potential of potential risk to a fetus. TAFINLAR may render hormonal contraceptives less effective and an alternative method of contraception should be used. (5.11, 8.1)

——————ADVERSE REACTIONS——————
• Most common adverse reactions (≥20%) for TAFINLAR as a single agent are hyperkeratosis, headache, pyrexia, arthralgia, papilloma, alopecia, and palmar-plantar erythrodysesthesia syndrome. (6.1)
• Most common adverse reactions (≥20%) for TAFINLAR in combination with trametinib are pyrexia, chills, fatigue, rash, nausea, vomiting, diarrhea, abdominal pain, peripheral edema, cough, headache, arthralgia, night sweats, decreased appetite, constipation, and myalgia. (6.1)
To report SUSPECTED ADVERSE REACTIONS, contact GlaxoSmithKline at 1-888-825-5249 or FDA at 1-800-FDA-1088 or www.fda.gov/medwatch.

——————DRUG INTERACTIONS——————
• Avoid concurrent administration of strong inhibitors of CYP3A4 or CYP2C8. (7.1)
• Avoid concurrent administration of strong inducers of CYP3A4 or CYP2C8. (7.1)
• Concomitant use with agents that are sensitive substrates of CYP3A4, CYP2C8, CYP2C9, CYP2C19, or CYP2B6 may result in loss of efficacy of these agents. (7.2)

——————USE IN SPECIFIC POPULATIONS——————
• Nursing Mothers: Discontinue drug or nursing. (8.3)
• Females and Males of Reproductive Potential: Advise females patients to use highly effective contraception during treatment and for 2 weeks following discontinuation of treatment. Advise male patients of potential risk for impaired spermatogenesis. (8.6)

See 17 for PATIENT COUNSELING INFORMATION and Medication Guide

Revised: 01/2014

FULL PRESCRIBING INFORMATION: CONTENTS*

FULL PRESCRIBING INFORMATION

1   INDICATIONS AND USAGE

1.1   BRAF V600E Mutation-Positive Unresectable or Metastatic Melanoma

TAFINLAR® as a single agent is indicated for the treatment of patients with unresectable or metastatic melanoma with BRAF V600E mutation as detected by an FDA-approved test.

1.2   BRAF V600E or V600K Mutation-Positive Unresectable or Metastatic Melanoma

TAFINLAR, in combination with trametinib, is indicated for the treatment of patients with unresectable or metastatic melanoma with BRAF V600E or V600K mutations, as detected by an FDA-approved test. This indication is based on the demonstration of durable response rate [see Clinical Studies (14.2)]. Improvement in disease-related symptoms or overall survival has not been demonstrated for TAFINLAR in combination with trametinib.

1.3   Limitation of Use

TAFINLAR is not indicated for treatment of patients with wild-type BRAF melanoma [see Warnings and Precautions (5.2)].

2   DOSAGE AND ADMINISTRATION

2.1   Patient Selection

Confirm the presence of BRAF V600E mutation in tumor specimens prior to initiation of treatment with TAFINLAR as a single agent [see Warnings and Precautions (5.2)]. Confirm the presence of BRAF V600E or V600K mutation in tu-mor specimens prior to initiation of treatment with TAFINLAR in combination with trametinib. Information on FDA-approved tests for the detection of BRAF V600 mutations in melanoma is available at: http://www.fda.gov/CompanionDiagnostics.

2.2   Recommended Dosing

The recommended dosage regimens of TAFINLAR are
• 150 mg orally taken twice daily, approximately 12 hours apart, as a single agent
• 150 mg orally taken twice daily, approximately 12 hours apart, in combination with trametinib 2 mg orally taken once daily

Continue treatment until disease progression or unacceptable toxicity occurs. Take TAFINLAR as a single agent, or TAFINLAR in combination with trametinib, at least 1 hour before or 2 hours after a meal [see Clinical Pharmacology (12.3)]. Do not take a missed dose of TAFINLAR within 6 hours of the next dose of TAFINLAR. Do not open, crush, or break TAFINLAR capsule.

When administered in combination with trametinib, take the once-daily dose of trametinib at the same time each day with either the morning dose or the evening dose of TAFINLAR.

2.3   Dose Modifications

For New Primary Cutaneous Malignancies: No dose modifications are required.

For New Primary Non-Cutaneous Malignancies: Permanently discontinue TAFINLAR in patients who develop RAS mutation-positive non-cutaneous malignancies. If used in combination with trametinib, no dose modifications are required for trametinib in patients who develop non-cutaneous malignancies.

Table 1. Recommended Dose Reductions

Dose Reductions for TAFINLAR When Administered as a Single Agent or in Combination With Trametinib	
First Dose Reduction	100 mg orally twice daily
Second Dose Reduction	75 mg orally twice daily
Third Dose Reduction	50 mg orally twice daily
Subsequent Modification	Permanently discontinue TAFINLAR if unable to tolerate 50 mg orally twice daily

Dose Reductions for Trametinib When Administered in Combination With TAFINLAR	
First Dose Reduction	1.5 mg orally once daily
Second Dose Reduction	1 mg orally once daily
Subsequent Modification	Permanently discontinue if unable to tolerate trametinib 1 mg orally once daily

[See table 2 on pages 1183 and 1184]

3   DOSAGE FORMS AND STRENGTHS

50 mg Capsules: Dark red capsule imprinted with 'GS TEW' and '50 mg'.
75 mg Capsules: Dark pink capsule imprinted with 'GS LHF' and '75 mg'.

4   CONTRAINDICATIONS

None.

5   WARNINGS AND PRECAUTIONS

Review the Full Prescribing Information for trametinib prior to initiation of TAFINLAR in combination with trametinib. The following serious adverse reactions of trametinib as a single agent, which may occur when TAFINLAR is used in combination with trametinib, are not described in the Full Prescribing Information for TAFINLAR:
• Retinal vein occlusion
• Interstitial lung disease

5.1   New Primary Malignancies

New primary malignancies, cutaneous and non-cutaneous, can occur when TAFINLAR is administered as a single agent or when used in combination with trametinib.

Cutaneous Malignancies:

TAFINLAR results in an increased incidence of cutaneous squamous cell carcinoma, keratoacanthoma, and melanoma. TAFINLAR when used in combination with trametinib results in an increased incidence of basal cell carcinoma.

In Trial 1, cutaneous squamous cell carcinomas and keratoacanthomas (cuSCC) occurred in 7% (14/187) of patients treated with TAFINLAR and in none of the patients treated with dacarbazine.

Across clinical trials of TAFINLAR (N = 586), the incidence of cuSCC was 11%. The median time to first cuSCC was 9 weeks (range: 1 to 53 weeks). Of those patients who developed new cuSCC, approximately 33% developed one or more cuSCC with continued administration of TAFINLAR. The median time between diagnosis of the first cuSCC and the second cuSCC was 6 weeks.

In Trial 1, the incidence of new primary malignant melanomas was 2% (3/187) for patients receiving TAFINLAR while no dacarbazine-treated patient was diagnosed with new primary malignant melanoma.

In Trial 2, the incidence of basal cell carcinoma was increased in patients receiving TAFINLAR in combination with trametinib: 9% (5/55) of patients receiving TAFINLAR in combination with trametinib compared with 2% (1/53) of patients receiving TAFINLAR as a single agent. The range of time to diagnosis of basal cell carcinoma was 28 to 249 days in patients receiving TAFINLAR in combination with trametinib and was 197 days for the patient receiving TAFINLAR as a single agent.

Cutaneous squamous cell carcinoma (SCC), including keratoacanthoma, occurred in 7% of patients receiving TAFINLAR in combination with trametinib and 19% of patients receiving TAFINLAR as a single agent. The range of time to diagnosis of cuSCC was 136 to197 days in the combination arm and was 9 to 197 days in the arm receiving TAFINLAR as a single agent.

New primary melanoma occurred in 2% (1/53) of patients receiving TAFINLAR as a single agent and in none of the 55 patients receiving TAFINLAR in combination with trametinib.

Perform dermatologic evaluations prior to initiation of TAFINLAR as a single agent or in combination with trametinib, every 2 months while on therapy, and for up to 6 months following discontinuation of TAFINLAR. No dose modifications of TAFINLAR or trametinib are required in patients who develop new primary cutaneous malignancies.

Non-cutaneous Malignancies:

Based on its mechanism of action, TAFINLAR may promote the growth and development of malignancies with activation of RAS through mutation or other mechanisms [see Warnings and Precautions (5.2)]. In patients receiving TAFINLAR in combination with trametinib four cases of non-cutaneous malignancies were identified: KRAS mutation-positive pancreatic adenocarcinoma (n = 1), recurrent NRAS mutation-positive colorectal carcinoma (n = 1), head and neck carcinoma (n = 1), and glioblastoma (n = 1). Monitor patients receiving the combination closely for signs or symptoms of non-cutaneous malignancies. Permanently discontinue TAFINLAR for RAS mutation-positive non-cutaneous malignancies. If used in combination with trametinib, no dose modification of trametinib is required for patients who develop non-cutaneous malignancies.

5.2   Tumor Promotion in BRAF Wild-Type Melanoma

In vitro experiments have demonstrated paradoxical activation of MAP-kinase signaling and increased cell proliferation in BRAF wild-type cells which are exposed to BRAF inhibitors. Confirm evidence of BRAF V600E or V600K mutation status prior to initiation of TAFINLAR as a single agent or combination therapy [see Indications and Usage (1), Dosage and Administration (2.1)].

5.3   Hemorrhage

Hemorrhages, including major hemorrhages defined as symptomatic bleeding in a critical area or organ, can occur when TAFINLAR is used in combination with trametinib.

In Trial 2, treatment with TAFINLAR in combination with trametinib resulted in an increased incidence and severity of any hemorrhagic event: 16% (9/55) of patients treated with TAFINLAR in combination with trametinib compared with 2% (1/53) of patients treated with TAFINLAR as a single agent. The major hemorrhagic events of intracranial or gastric hemorrhage occurred in 5% (3/55) of patients treated with TAFINLAR in combination with trametinib compared with none of the 53 patients treated with TAFINLAR as a single agent. Intracranial hemorrhage was fatal in 4% (2/55) of patients treated with TAFINLAR in combination with trametinib.

Permanently discontinue TAFINLAR and trametinib for all Grade 4 hemorrhagic events and for any Grade 3 hemorrhagic events that do not improve. Withhold TAFINLAR for Grade 3 hemorrhagic events; if improved resume at a lower dose level. Withhold trametinib for up to 3 weeks for Grade 3 hemorrhagic events; if improved, resume at a lower dose level.

5.4   Venous Thromboembolism

Venous thromboembolism can occur when TAFINLAR is used in combination with trametinib.

In Trial 2, treatment with TAFINLAR in combination with trametinib resulted in an increased incidence of deep venous thrombosis (DVT) and pulmonary embolism (PE): 7% (4/55) of patients treated with TAFINLAR in combination with trametinib compared with none of the 53 patients treated with TAFINLAR as a single agent. Pulmonary embolism was fatal in 2% (1/55) of patients receiving TAFINLAR in combination with trametinib.

Advise patients to immediately seek medical care if they develop symptoms of DVT or PE, such as shortness of breath, chest pain, or arm or leg swelling. Permanently discontinue TAFINLAR and trametinib for life-threatening PE. Withhold trametinib and continue TAFINLAR at the same dose for uncomplicated DVT or PE; if improved within 3 weeks, trametinib may be resumed at a lower dose level [see Dosage and Administration (2.3)].

5.5 Cardiomyopathy

Cardiomyopathy can occur when TAFINLAR is used in combination with trametinib and with trametinib as a single agent [refer to Full Prescribing Information for trametinib]. In Trial 2, cardiomyopathy occurred in 9% (5/55) of patients treated with TAFINLAR in combination with trametinib and in none of patients treated with TAFINLAR as a single agent. The median time to onset of cardiomyopathy in patients treated with TAFINLAR in combination with trametinib was 86 days (range: 27 to 253 days). Cardiomyopathy was identified within the first month of treatment with TAFINLAR in combination with trametinib in two of five patients. Development of cardiomyopathy resolved in all five patients following dose reduction (4/55) and/or dose interruption (1/55).

Across clinical trials of TAFINLAR administered in combination with trametinib (N = 202), 8% of patients developed evidence of cardiomyopathy (decrease in LVEF below institutional lower limits of normal with an absolute decrease in LVEF ≥10% below baseline). Two percent demonstrated a decrease in LVEF below institutional lower limits of normal with an absolute decrease in LVEF of ≥20% below baseline. Assess LVEF by echocardiogram or multigated acquisition (MUGA) scan before initiation of TAFINLAR in combination with trametinib, one month after initiation, and then at 2- to 3-month intervals while on treatment with the combination. Withhold treatment with trametinib and continue TAFINLAR at the same dose if absolute LVEF value decreases by 10% from pretreatment values and is less than the lower limit of normal. For symptomatic cardiomyopathy or persistent, asymptomatic LV dysfunction that does not resolve within 4 weeks, permanently discontinue trametinib and withhold TAFINLAR. Resume TAFINLAR at the same dose level upon recovery of cardiac function [see Dosage and Administration (2.3)].

5.6 Ocular Toxicities

Retinal Pigment Epithelial Detachment (RPED):
Retinal pigment epithelial detachments (RPED) can occur when TAFINLAR is used in combination with trametinib and with trametinib as a single agent [refer to Full Prescribing Information for trametinib]. Retinal detachments resulting from trametinib are often bilateral and multifocal, occurring in the macular region of the retina.

In Trial 2, ophthalmologic examinations including retinal evaluation were performed pretreatment and at regular intervals during treatment. RPED occurred in 2% (1/55) of patients receiving TAFINLAR in combination with trametinib. Across clinical trials of TAFINLAR administered in combination with trametinib (N = 202), the incidence of RPED was 1% (2/202).

Perform ophthalmological evaluation at any time a patient reports visual disturbances and compare with baseline, if available. If TAFINLAR is used in combination with trametinib, do not modify the dose of TAFINLAR. Withhold trametinib if RPED is diagnosed. If resolution of the RPED is documented on repeat ophthalmological evaluation within 3 weeks, resume trametinib at a lower dose level. Discontinue trametinib if no improvement after 3 weeks [see Dosage and Administration (2.3)].

Uveitis and Iritis:
Uveitis and iritis can occur when TAFINLAR is administered as a single agent or when used in combination with trametinib.

Uveitis (including iritis) occurred in 1% (6/586) of patients treated with TAFINLAR as a single agent and uveitis occurred in 1% (2/202) of patients treated with TAFINLAR in combination with trametinib. Symptomatic treatment employed in clinical trials included steroid and mydriatic ophthalmic drops. Monitor patients for visual signs and symptoms of uveitis (e.g., change in vision, photophobia, eye pain). If diagnosed, withhold TAFINLAR for up to 6 weeks until uveitis/iritis resolves to Grade 0-1. If TAFINLAR is used in combination with trametinib, do not modify the dose of trametinib.

5.7 Serious Febrile Reactions

Serious febrile reactions and fever of any severity complicated by hypotension, rigors or chills, dehydration, or renal failure, can occur when TAFINLAR is administered as a single agent or when used in combination with trametinib. The incidence and severity of pyrexia are increased when TAFINLAR is used in combination with trametinib compared with TAFINLAR as a single agent [see Adverse Reactions (6.1)].

In Trial 1, the incidence of fever (serious and non-serious) was 28% in patients treated with TAFINLAR and 10% in patients treated with dacarbazine. In patients treated with

Severity of Adverse Reaction[a]	TAFINLAR[b]	Trametinib (When Used in Combination)[b,c]
Febrile drug reaction		
• Fever of 101.3°F to 104°F	Withhold TAFINLAR until fever resolves. Then resume at same or lower dose level.	Do not modify the dose of trametinib.
• Fever higher than 104°F • Fever complicated by rigors, hypotension, dehydration, or renal failure	• Withhold TAFINLAR until fever resolves. Then resume at a lower dose level. Or • Permanently discontinue TAFINLAR.	Withhold trametinib until fever resolves. Then resume trametinib at same or lower dose level.
Cutaneous		
• Intolerable Grade 2 skin toxicity • Grade 3 or 4 skin toxicity	Withhold TAFINLAR for up to 3 weeks. • If improved, resume at a lower dose level. • If not improved, permanently discontinue.	Withhold trametinib for up to 3 weeks. • If improved, resume at a lower dose level. • If not improved, permanently discontinue.
Cardiac		
• Asymptomatic, absolute decrease in LVEF of 10% or greater from baseline and is below institutional lower limits of normal (LLN) from pretreatment value	Do not modify the dose of TAFINLAR.	Withhold trametinib for up to 4 weeks. • If improved to normal LVEF value, resume at a lower dose level. • If not improved to normal LVEF value, permanently discontinue.
• Symptomatic congestive heart failure • Absolute decrease in LVEF of greater than 20% from baseline that is below LLN	Withhold TAFINLAR, if improved, then resume at the same dose.	Permanently discontinue trametinib.
Venous Thromboembolism		
• Uncomplicated DVT or PE	Do not modify the dose of TAFINLAR.	Withhold trametinib for up to 3 weeks. • If improved to Grade 0-1, resume at a lower dose level. • If not improved, permanently discontinue.
• Life Threatening PE	Permanently discontinue TAFINLAR.	Permanently discontinue trametinib.
Ocular Toxicities		
• Grade 2-3 retinal pigment epithelial detachments (RPED)	Do not modify the dose of TAFINLAR.	Withhold trametinib for up to 3 weeks. • If improved to Grade 0-1, resume at a lower dose level. • If not improved, permanently discontinue.
• Retinal vein occlusion	Do not modify the dose of TAFINLAR.	Permanently discontinue trametinib.
• Uveitis and Iritis	Withhold TAFINLAR for up to 6 weeks. • If improved to Grade 0-1, then resume at the same dose. • If not improved, permanently discontinue.	Do not modify the dose of trametinib.
Pulmonary		
• Interstitial lung disease/pneumonitis	Do not modify the dose of TAFINLAR.	Permanently discontinue trametinib.

Table 2. Recommended Dose Modifications for TAFINLAR as a Single Agent and for TAFINLAR and Trametinib Administered in Combination

(Table continued on next page)

TAFINLAR, the median time to initial onset of fever (any severity) was 11 days (range: 1 to 202 days) and the median duration of fever was 3 days (range: 1 to 129 days). Serious febrile reactions and fever of any severity complicated by hypotension, rigors or chills occurred in 3.7% (7/187) of patients treated with TAFINLAR and in none of the 59 patients treated with dacarbazine.

In Trial 2, the incidence of fever (serious and non-serious) was 71% (39/55) in patients treated with TAFINLAR in combination with trametinib and 26% (14/53) in patients treated with TAFINLAR as a single agent. Serious febrile reactions and fever of any severity complicated by hypotension, rigors or chills occurred in 25% (14/55) of patients treated with TAFINLAR in combination with trametinib compared with 2% (1/53) of patients treated with

TAFINLAR as a single agent. Fever was complicated with chills/rigors in 51% (28/55), dehydration in 9% (5/55), renal failure in 4% (2/55), and syncope in 4% (2/55) of patients in Trial 2.

In patients treated with TAFINLAR in combination with trametinib, the median time to initial onset of fever was 30 days compared with 19 days in patients treated with TAFINLAR as a single agent; the median duration of fever was 6 days with the combination compared with 4 days with TAFINLAR as a single agent.

Across clinical trials of TAFINLAR administered in combination with trametinib (N = 202), the incidence of pyrexia was 57% (116/202).

Withhold TAFINLAR for fever of 101.3°F or higher. Withhold trametinib for any fever higher than 104°F. Withhold

Table 2 (cont.). Recommended Dose Modifications for TAFINLAR as a Single Agent and for TAFINLAR and Trametinib Administered in Combination

Severity of Adverse Reaction[a]	TAFINLAR[b]	Trametinib (When Used in Combination)[b,c]
Other		
• Intolerable Grade 2 adverse reactions • Any Grade 3 adverse reaction	Withhold TAFINLAR. • If improved to Grade 0-1, resume at a lower dose level. • If not improved, permanently discontinue.	Withhold trametinib for up to 3 weeks. • If improved to Grade 0-1, resume at a lower dose level. • If not improved, permanently discontinue.
• First occurrence of any Grade 4 adverse reaction	• Withhold TAFINLAR until adverse reaction improves to Grade 0-1. Then resume at a lower dose level. Or • Permanently discontinue TAFINLAR.	• Withhold trametinib until adverse reaction improves to Grade 0-1. Then resume at a lower dose level. Or • Permanently discontinue trametinib.
• Recurrent Grade 4 adverse reaction	Permanently discontinue TAFINLAR.	Permanently discontinue trametinib.

[a]National Cancer Institute Common Terminology Criteria for Adverse Events (CTCAE) version 4.0.
[b]See Table 1 for recommended dose reductions of TAFINLAR and trametinib.
[c]Refer to Full Prescribing Information for trametinib.

TAFINLAR, and trametinib if used in combination, for any serious febrile reaction or fever complicated by hypotension, rigors or chills, dehydration, or renal failure and evaluate for signs and symptoms of infection. Refer to Table 2 for recommended dose modifications for adverse reactions [see Dosage and Administration (2.3)]. Prophylaxis with antipyretics may be required when resuming TAFINLAR or trametinib.

5.8 Serious Skin Toxicity
Serious skin toxicity can occur when TAFINLAR is used in combination with trametinib and with trametinib as a single agent [refer to Full Prescribing Information for trametinib].
In Trial 2, the incidence of any skin toxicity was similar for patients receiving TAFINLAR in combination with trametinib (65% [36/55]) compared with patients receiving TAFINLAR as a single agent (68% [36/53]). The median time to onset of skin toxicity in patients treated with TAFINLAR in combination with trametinib was 37 days (range: 1 to 225 days) and median time to resolution of skin toxicity was 33 days (range: 3 to 421 days). No patient required dose reduction or permanent discontinuation of TAFINLAR or trametinib for skin toxicity.
Across clinical trials of TAFINLAR in combination with trametinib (N = 202), severe skin toxicity and secondary infections of the skin requiring hospitalization occurred in 2.5% (5/202) of patients treated with TAFINLAR in combination with trametinib.
Withhold TAFINLAR, and trametinib if used in combination, for intolerable or severe skin toxicity. TAFINLAR and trametinib may be resumed at lower dose levels in patients with improvement or recovery from skin toxicity within 3 weeks [see Dosage and Administration (2.3)].

5.9 Hyperglycemia
Hyperglycemia can occur when TAFINLAR is administered as a single agent or when used in combination with trametinib.
In Trial 1, 5 of 12 patients with a history of diabetes required more intensive hypoglycemic therapy while taking TAFINLAR. The incidence of Grade 3 hyperglycemia based on laboratory values was 6% (12/187) in patients treated with TAFINLAR compared with none of the dacarbazine-treated patients.
In Trial 2, the incidence of Grade 3 hyperglycemia based on laboratory values was 5% (3/55) in patients treated with TAFINLAR in combination with trametinib compared with 2% (1/53) in patients treated with TAFINLAR as a single agent.
Monitor serum glucose levels as clinically appropriate when TAFINLAR is administered as a single agent or when used in combination with trametinib in patients with pre-existing diabetes or hyperglycemia. Advise patients to report symptoms of severe hyperglycemia such as excessive thirst or any increase in the volume or frequency of urination.

5.10 Glucose-6-Phosphate Dehydrogenase Deficiency
TAFINLAR, which contains a sulfonamide moiety, confers a potential risk of hemolytic anemia in patients with glucose-6-phosphate dehydrogenase (G6PD) deficiency. Closely observe patients with G6PD deficiency for signs of hemolytic anemia.

5.11 Embryofetal Toxicity
Based on its mechanism of action, TAFINLAR can cause fetal harm when administered to a pregnant woman. Dabrafenib was teratogenic and embryotoxic in rats at doses three times greater than the human exposure at the recommended clinical dose. If this drug is used during pregnancy or if the patient becomes pregnant while taking this drug, the patient should be apprised of the potential hazard to a fetus [see Use in Specific Populations (8.1)].
Advise female patients of reproductive potential to use a highly effective non-hormonal method of contraception since TAFINLAR can render hormonal contraceptives ineffective, during treatment and for at least 2 weeks after treatment with TAFINLAR or for 4 months after treatment with TAFINLAR in combination with trametinib. Advise patients to contact their healthcare provider if they become pregnant, or if pregnancy is suspected, while taking TAFINLAR [see Drug Interactions (7.2), Use in Specific Populations (8.6)].

6 ADVERSE REACTIONS
The following adverse reactions are discussed in greater detail in another section of the label:
• New Primary Malignancies [see Warnings and Precautions (5.1)]
• Tumor Promotion in BRAF Wild-Type Melanoma [see Warnings and Precautions (5.2)]
• Hemorrhage [see Warnings and Precautions (5.3)]
• Venous Thromboembolism [see Warnings and Precautions (5.4)]
• Cardiomyopathy [see Warnings and Precautions (5.5)]
• Ocular Toxicities [see Warnings and Precautions (5.6)]
• Serious Febrile Reactions [see Warnings and Precautions (5.7)]
• Serious Skin Toxicity [see Warnings and Precautions (5.8)]
• Hyperglycemia [see Warnings and Precautions (5.9)]
• Glucose-6-Phosphate Dehydrogenase Deficiency [see Warnings and Precautions (5.10)]

6.1 Clinical Trials Experience
Because clinical trials are conducted under widely varying conditions, adverse reaction rates observed in the clinical trials of a drug cannot be directly compared to rates in the clinical trials of another drug and may not reflect the rates observed in practice.
The data described in the Warnings and Precautions section and below reflect exposure to TAFINLAR as a single agent and in combination with trametinib.
BRAF V600E Unresectable or Metastatic Melanoma:
The safety of TAFINLAR as a single agent was evaluated in 586 patients with BRAF V600 mutation-positive unresectable or metastatic melanoma, previously treated or untreated, who received TAFINLAR 150 mg orally twice daily until disease progression or unacceptable toxicity, including 181 patients treated for at least 6 months and 86 additional patients treated for more than 12 months. TAFINLAR was studied in open-label, single-arm trials and in an open-label, randomized, active-controlled trial. The median daily dose of TAFINLAR was 300 mg (range: 118 to 300 mg).
Table 3 and Table 4 present adverse drug reactions and laboratory abnormalities identified from analyses of Trial 1 [see Clinical Studies (14.1)]. Trial 1, a multicenter, international, open-label, randomized (3:1), controlled trial allo-

cated 250 patients with unresectable or metastatic BRAF V600E mutation-positive melanoma to receive TAFINLAR 150 mg orally twice daily (n = 187) or dacarbazine 1,000 mg/m^2 intravenously every 3 weeks (n = 63). The trial excluded patients with abnormal left ventricular ejection fraction or cardiac valve morphology (≥Grade 2), corrected QT interval ≥480 milliseconds on electrocardiogram, or a known history of glucose-6-phosphate dehydrogenase deficiency. The median duration on treatment was 4.9 months for patients treated with TAFINLAR and 2.8 months for dacarbazine-treated patients. The population exposed to TAFINLAR was 60% male, 99% white, and had a median age of 53 years.
The most commonly occurring adverse reactions (≥20%) in patients treated with TAFINLAR were, in order of decreasing frequency: hyperkeratosis, headache, pyrexia, arthralgia, papilloma, alopecia, and palmar-plantar erythrodysesthesia syndrome (PPES).
The incidence of adverse events resulting in permanent discontinuation of study medication in Trial 1 was 3% for patients treated with TAFINLAR and 3% for patients treated with dacarbazine. The most frequent (≥2%) adverse reactions leading to dose reduction of TAFINLAR were pyrexia (9%), PPES (3%), chills (3%), fatigue (2%), and headache (2%).
[See table 3 at top of next page]
[See table 4 at bottom of next page]
Other clinically important adverse reactions observed in <10% of patients (N = 586) treated with TAFINLAR were:
Gastrointestinal Disorders: Pancreatitis.
Immune System Disorders: Hypersensitivity manifesting as bullous rash.
Renal and Urinary Disorders: Interstitial nephritis.
BRAF V600E or V600K Unresectable or Metastatic Melanoma:
The safety of TAFINLAR in combination with trametinib was evaluated in Trial 2 and other trials consisting of a total of 202 patients with BRAF V600 mutation-positive unresectable or metastatic melanoma who received TAFINLAR 150 mg orally twice daily in combination with trametinib 2 mg orally once daily until disease progression or unacceptable toxicity. Among these 202 patients, 66 (33%) were exposed to TAFINLAR and 68 (34%) were exposed to trametinib for greater than 6 to 12 months while 40 (20%) were exposed to TAFINLAR and 36 (18%) were exposed to trametinib for greater than one year. The median age was 54 years, 57% were male, and >99% were white.
Table 5 presents adverse reactions from Trial 2, a multicenter, open-label, randomized trial of 162 patients with BRAF V600E or V600K mutation-positive melanoma receiving TAFINLAR 150 mg twice daily in combination with trametinib 2 mg orally once daily (n = 55), TAFINLAR 150 mg orally twice daily in combination with trametinib 1 mg once daily (n = 54), and TAFINLAR as a single agent 150 mg orally twice daily (n = 53) [see Clinical Studies (14.2)]. Patients with abnormal LVEF, history of acute coronary syndrome within 6 months, current evidence of Class II or greater congestive heart failure (New York Heart Association), history RVO or RPED, QTc interval ≥480 msec, treatment refractory hypertension, uncontrolled arrhythmias, history of pneumonitis or interstitial lung disease, or a known history of G6PD deficiency were excluded. The median duration of treatment was 10.9 months for both TAFINLAR and trametinib (2-mg orally once-daily treatment group) when used in combination, 10.6 months for both TAFINLAR and trametinib (1-mg orally once-daily treatment group) when used in combination, and 6.1 months for TAFINLAR as a single agent.
In Trial 2, 13% of patients receiving TAFINLAR in combination with trametinib experienced adverse reactions resulting in permanent discontinuation of trial medication(s). The most common adverse reaction resulting in permanent discontinuation was pyrexia (4%). Adverse reactions led to dose reductions in 49% and dose interruptions in 67% of patients treated with TAFINLAR in combination with trametinib. Pyrexia, chills, and nausea were the most common reasons cited for dose reductions and pyrexia, chills, and decreased ejection fraction were the most common reasons cited for dose interruptions of TAFINLAR and trametinib when used in combination.
[See table 5 on pages 1186 and 1887]
Other clinically important adverse reactions (N = 202) observed in <10% of patients treated with TAFINLAR in combination with trametinib were:
Eye Disorders: Vision blurred, transient blindness.
Gastrointestinal Disorders: Stomatitis, pancreatitis.
General Disorders and Administration Site Conditions: Asthenia.
Infections and Infestations: Cellulitis, folliculitis, paronychia, rash pustular.
Neoplasms Benign, Malignant, and Unspecified (including cysts and polyps): Skin papilloma.

Skin and Subcutaneous Tissue Disorders: Palmar-plantar erythrodysesthesia syndrome, hyperkeratosis, hyperhidrosis.

Vascular Disorders: Hypertension.

[See table at top of page 1187]

QT Prolongation: In Trial 2, QTcF prolongation to >500 msec occurred in 4% (2/55) of patients treated with TAFINLAR in combination with trametinib and in 2% (1/53) of patients treated with TAFINLAR as a single agent. The QTcF was increased more than 60 msec from baseline in 13% (7/55) of patients treated with TAFINLAR in combination with trametinib and 2% (1/53) of patients treated with TAFINLAR as a single agent.

7 DRUG INTERACTIONS

7.1 Effects of Other Drugs on Dabrafenib

Dabrafenib is primarily metabolized by CYP2C8 and CYP3A4. Strong inhibitors of CYP3A4 or CYP2C8 may increase concentrations of dabrafenib and strong inducers of CYP3A4 or CYP2C8 may decrease concentrations of dabrafenib *[see Clinical Pharmacology (12.3)]*. Substitution of strong inhibitors or strong inducers of CYP3A4 or CYP2C8 is recommended during treatment with TAFINLAR. If concomitant use of strong inhibitors (e.g., ketoconazole, nefazodone, clarithromycin, gemfibrozil) or strong inducers (e.g., rifampin, phenytoin, carbamazepine, phenobarbital, St John's wort) of CYP3A4 or CYP2C8 is unavoidable, monitor patients closely for adverse reactions when taking strong inhibitors or loss of efficacy when taking strong inducers.

7.2 Effects of Dabrafenib on Other Drugs

Dabrafenib induces CYP3A4 and CYP2C9. Dabrafenib decreased the systemic exposures of midazolam (a CYP3A4 substrate), S-warfarin (a CYP2C9 substrate), and R-warfarin (a CYP3A4/CYP1A2 substrate) *[see Clinical Pharmacology (12.3)]*. Monitor international normalized ratio (INR) levels more frequently in patients receiving warfarin during initiation or discontinuation of dabrafenib. Coadministration of TAFINLAR with other substrates of these enzymes, including dexamethasone or hormonal contraceptives, can result in decreased concentrations and loss of efficacy *[see Use in Specific Populations (8.1, 8.6)]*. Substitute for these medications or monitor patients for loss of efficacy if use of these medications is unavoidable.

7.3 Trametinib

Coadministration of TAFINLAR 150 mg twice daily and trametinib 2 mg once daily resulted in no clinically relevant pharmacokinetic drug interactions *[see Clinical Pharmacology (12.3)]*.

8 USE IN SPECIFIC POPULATIONS

8.1 Pregnancy

Pregnancy Category D

Risk Summary: Based on its mechanism of action, TAFINLAR can cause fetal harm when administered to a pregnant woman. Dabrafenib was teratogenic and embryotoxic in rats at doses three times greater than the human exposure at the recommended clinical dose of 150 mg twice daily based on AUC. If this drug is used during pregnancy or if the patient becomes pregnant while taking this drug, the patient should be apprised of the potential hazard to a fetus *[see Warnings and Precautions (5.11)]*.

Animal Data: In a combined female fertility and embryo-fetal development study in rats, developmental toxicity consisted of embryo-lethality, ventricular septal defects, and variation in thymic shape at a dabrafenib dose of 300 mg/kg/day (approximately three times the human exposure at the recommended dose based on AUC). At doses of 20 mg/kg/day or greater (equivalent to the human exposure at the recommended dose based on AUC), rats demonstrated delays in skeletal development and reduced fetal body weight.

8.3 Nursing Mothers

It is not known whether this drug is present in human milk. Because many drugs are present in human milk and because of the potential for serious adverse reactions from TAFINLAR in nursing infants, a decision should be made whether to discontinue nursing or discontinue the drug, taking into account the importance of the drug to the mother.

8.4 Pediatric Use

The safety and effectiveness of TAFINLAR have not been established in pediatric patients.

In a repeat-dose toxicity study in juvenile rats, an increased incidence of kidney cysts and tubular deposits were noted at doses as low as 0.2 times the human exposure at the recommended adult dose based on AUC. Additionally, forestomach hyperplasia, decreased bone length and early vaginal opening were noted at doses as low as 0.8 times the human exposure at the recommended adult dose based on AUC.

8.5 Geriatric Use

One hundred and twenty-six (22%) of 586 patients in clinical trials of TAFINLAR administered as a single agent and 40 (21%) of the 187 patients receiving TAFINLAR in Trial 1 were ≥65 years of age. No overall differences in the effectiveness or safety of TAFINLAR were observed in the elderly in Trial 1.

Table 3. Selected Common Adverse Reactions Occurring in ≥10% (All Grades) or ≥2% (Grades 3 or 4) of Patients Treated With TAFINLAR[a]

Primary System Organ Class Preferred Term	TAFINLAR N = 187		Dacarbazine N = 59	
	All Grades (%)	Grades 3 and 4[b] (%)	All Grades (%)	Grades 3 and 4 (%)
Skin and subcutaneous tissue disorders				
Hyperkeratosis	37	1	0	0
Alopecia	22	NA[f]	2	NA[f]
Palmar-plantar erythrodysesthesia syndrome	20	2	2	0
Rash	17	0	0	0
Nervous system disorders				
Headache	32	0	8	0
General disorders and administration site conditions				
Pyrexia	28	3	10	0
Musculoskeletal and connective tissue disorders				
Arthralgia	27	1	2	0
Back pain	12	3	7	0
Myalgia	11	0	0	0
Neoplasms benign, malignant, and unspecified (including cysts and polyps)				
Papilloma[c]	27	0	2	0
cuSCC[d, e]	7	4	0	0
Respiratory, thoracic, and mediastinal disorders				
Cough	12	0	5	0
Gastrointestinal disorders				
Constipation	11	2	14	0
Infections and infestations				
Nasopharyngitis	10	0	3	0

[a]Adverse drug reactions, reported using MedDRA and graded using CTCAE version 4.0 for assessment of toxicity.
[b]Grade 4 adverse reactions limited to hyperkeratosis (n = 1) and constipation (n = 1).
[c]Includes skin papilloma and papilloma.
[d]Includes squamous cell carcinoma of the skin and keratoacanthoma.
[e]Cases of cutaneous squamous cell carcinoma were required to be reported as Grade 3 per protocol.
[f]NA = not applicable.

Table 4. Incidence of Laboratory Abnormalities Increased From Baseline Occurring at a Higher Incidence in Patients Treated With TAFINLAR in Trial 1 [Between-Arm Difference of ≥5% (All Grades) or ≥2% (Grades 3 or 4)]

Test	TAFINLAR N = 187		DTIC N = 59	
	All Grades (%)	Grades 3 and 4 (%)	All Grades (%)	Grades 3 and 4 (%)
Hyperglycemia	50	6	43	0
Hypophosphatemia	37	6[a]	14	2
Increased alkaline phosphatase	19	0	14	2
Hyponatremia	8	2	3	0

[a]Grade 4 laboratory abnormality limited to hypophosphatemia (n = 1).

Across all clinical trials of TAFINLAR administered in combination with trametinib, there was an insufficient number of patients aged 65 years and over to determine whether they respond differently from younger patients. In Trial 2, 11 patients (20%) were 65 years of age and older, and 2 patients (4%) were 75 years of age and older.

8.6 Females and Males of Reproductive Potential

Contraception: *Females:* Advise female patients of reproductive potential to use highly effective contraception during treatment and for at least 2 weeks after the last dose of TAFINLAR or at least 4 months after the last dose of TAFINLAR taken in combination with trametinib. Counsel patients to use a non-hormonal method of contraception since TAFINLAR can render hormonal contraceptives ineffective. Advise patients to contact their healthcare provider if they become pregnant, or if pregnancy is suspected, while taking TAFINLAR *[see Warnings and Precautions (5.11), Drug Interactions (7.1), Use in Specific Populations (8.1)]*.

Infertility:

Females: Increased follicular cysts and decreased corpora lutea were observed in female rats treated with trametinib. Advise female patients of reproductive potential that TAFINLAR taken in combination with trametinib may impair fertility in female patients.

Table 5. Common Adverse Drug Reactions Occurring in ≥10% at (All Grades) or ≥5% (Grades 3 or 4) of Patients Treated With TAFINLAR in Combination With Trametinib in Trial 2

Adverse Reactions	TAFINLAR plus Trametinib 2 mg N = 55		TAFINLAR plus Trametinib 1 mg N = 54		TAFINLAR N = 53	
	All Grades[a]	Grades 3 and 4	All Grades[a]	Grades 3 and 4	All Grades[a]	Grades 3 and 4
General disorders and administrative site conditions						
Pyrexia	71	5	69	9	26	0
Chills	58	2	50	2	17	0
Fatigue	53	4	57	2	40	6
Edema peripheral[b]	31	0	28	0	17	0
Skin and subcutaneous tissue disorders						
Rash[c]	45	0	43	2	53	0
Night Sweats	24	0	15	0	6	0
Dry skin	18	0	9	0	6	0
Dermatitis acneiform	16	0	11	0	4	0
Actinic keratosis	15	0	7	0	9	0
Erythema	15	0	6	0	2	0
Pruritus	11	0	11	0	13	0
Gastrointestinal disorders						
Nausea	44	2	46	6	21	0
Vomiting	40	2	43	4	15	0
Diarrhea	36	2	26	0	28	0
Abdominal pain[d]	33	2	24	2	21	2
Constipation	22	0	17	2	11	0
Dry mouth	11	0	11	0	6	0
Nervous system disorders						
Headache	29	0	37	2	28	0
Dizziness	16	0	13	0	9	0
Respiratory, thoracic, and mediastinal disorders						
Cough	29	0	11	0	21	0
Oropharyngeal pain	13	0	7	0	0	0
Musculoskeletal, connective tissue, and bone disorders						
Arthralgia	27	0	44	0	34	0
Myalgia	22	2	24	0	23	2
Back pain	18	5	11	0	11	2
Muscle spasms	16	0	2	0	4	0
Pain in extremity	16	0	11	2	19	0
Metabolism and nutritional disorders						
Decreased appetite	22	0	30	0	19	0
Dehydration	11	0	6	2	2	0
Psychiatric Disorders						
Insomnia	18	0	11	0	8	2
Vascular disorders						
Hemorrhage[e]	16	5	11	0	2	0

(Table continued on next page)

Males: Effects on spermatogenesis have been observed in animals. Advise male patients of the potential risk for impaired spermatogenesis, and to seek counseling on fertility and family planning options prior to starting treatment with TAFINLAR [see *Nonclinical Toxicology (13.1)*].

8.7   Hepatic Impairment
No formal pharmacokinetic trial in patients with hepatic impairment has been conducted. Dose adjustment is not recommended for patients with mild hepatic impairment based on the results of the population pharmacokinetic analysis. As hepatic metabolism and biliary secretion are the primary routes of elimination of dabrafenib and its metabolites, patients with moderate to severe hepatic impairment may have increased exposure. An appropriate dose has not been established for patients with moderate to severe hepatic impairment [see *Clinical Pharmacology (12.3)*].

8.8   Renal Impairment
No formal pharmacokinetic trial in patients with renal impairment has been conducted. Dose adjustment is not recommended for patients with mild or moderate renal impairment based on the results of the population pharmacokinetic analysis. An appropriate dose has not been established for patients with severe renal impairment [see *Clinical Pharmacology (12.3)*].

10   OVERDOSAGE
There is no information on overdosage of TAFINLAR. Since dabrafenib is highly bound to plasma proteins, hemodialysis is likely to be ineffective in the treatment of overdose with TAFINLAR.

11   DESCRIPTION
Dabrafenib mesylate is a kinase inhibitor. The chemical name for dabrafenib mesylate is N-{3-[5-(2-Amino-4-pyrimidinyl)-2-(1,1-dimethylethyl)-1,3-thiazol-4-yl]-2-fluorophenyl}-2,6-difluorobenzene sulfonamide, methanesulfonate salt. It has the molecular formula $C_{23}H_{20}F_3N_5O_2S_2 \bullet CH_4O_3S$ and a molecular weight of 615.68. Dabrafenib mesylate has the following chemical structure.

Dabrafenib mesylate is a white to slightly colored solid with three pK_as: 6.6, 2.2, and -1.5. It is very slightly soluble at pH 1 and practically insoluble above pH 4 in aqueous media.
TAFINLAR (dabrafenib) capsules are supplied as 50-mg and 75-mg capsules for oral administration. Each 50-mg capsule contains 59.25 mg dabrafenib mesylate equivalent to 50 mg of dabrafenib free base. Each 75-mg capsule contains 88.88 mg dabrafenib mesylate equivalent to 75 mg of dabrafenib free base.
The inactive ingredients of TAFINLAR are colloidal silicon dioxide, magnesium stearate, and microcrystalline cellulose. Capsule shells contain hypromellose, red iron oxide (E172), and titanium dioxide (E171).

12   CLINICAL PHARMACOLOGY
12.1   Mechanism of Action
Dabrafenib is an inhibitor of some mutated forms of BRAF kinases with in vitro IC_{50} values of 0.65, 0.5, and 1.84 nM for BRAF V600E, BRAF V600K, and BRAF V600D enzymes, respectively. Dabrafenib also inhibits wild-type BRAF and CRAF kinases with IC_{50} values of 3.2 and 5.0 nM, respectively, and other kinases such as SIK1, NEK11, and LIMK1 at higher concentrations. Some mutations in the BRAF gene, including those that result in BRAF V600E, can result in constitutively activated BRAF kinases that may stimulate tumor cell growth [see *Indications and Usage (1)*]. Dabrafenib inhibits BRAF V600 mutation-positive melanoma cell growth in vitro and in vivo.
Dabrafenib and trametinib target two different tyrosine kinases in the RAS/RAF/MEK/ERK pathway. Use of dabrafenib and trametinib in combination resulted in greater growth inhibition of BRAF V600 mutation-positive melanoma cell lines in vitro and prolonged inhibition of tumor growth in BRAF V600 mutation positive melanoma xenograftscompared with either drug alone.

12.3   Pharmacokinetics
Absorption: After oral administration, median time to achieve peak plasma concentration (Tmax) is 2 hours. Mean absolute bioavailability of oral dabrafenib is 95%. Following a single dose, dabrafenib exposure (Cmax and AUC) increased in a dose-proportional manner across the dose range of 12 to 300 mg, but the increase was less than dose-

proportional after repeat twice-daily dosing. After repeat twice-daily dosing of 150 mg, the mean accumulation ratio was 0.73 and the inter-subject variability (CV%) of AUC at steady-state was 38%.

Administration of dabrafenib with a high-fat meal decreased C_{max} by 51%, decreased AUC by 31%, and delayed median T_{max} by 3.6 hours as compared with the fasted state [see Dosage and Administration (2.2)].

Distribution: Dabrafenib is 99.7% bound to human plasma proteins. The apparent volume of distribution (V_c/F) is 70.3 L.

Metabolism: The metabolism of dabrafenib is primarily mediated by CYP2C8 and CYP3A4 to form hydroxy-dabrafenib. Hydroxy-dabrafenib is further oxidized via CYP3A4 to form carboxy-dabrafenib and subsequently excreted in bile and urine. Carboxy-dabrafenib is decarboxylated to form desmethyl-dabrafenib; desmethyl-dabrafenib may be reabsorbed from the gut. Desmethyl-dabrafenib is further metabolized by CYP3A4 to oxidative metabolites. Hydroxy-dabrafenib terminal half-life (10 hours) parallels that of dabrafenib while the carboxy- and desmethyl-dabrafenib metabolites exhibited longer half-lives (21 to 22 hours). Mean metabolite-to-parent AUC ratios following repeat-dose administration are 0.9, 11, and 0.7 for hydroxy-, carboxy-, and desmethyl-dabrafenib, respectively. Based on systemic exposure, relative potency, and pharmacokinetic properties, both hydroxy- and desmethyl-dabrafenib are likely to contribute to the clinical activity of dabrafenib.

Elimination: The mean terminal half-life of dabrafenib is 8 hours after oral administration. The apparent clearance of dabrafenib is 17.0 L/h after single dosing and 34.4 L/h after 2 weeks of twice-daily dosing.

Fecal excretion is the major route of elimination accounting for 71% of radioactive dose while urinary excretion accounted for 23% of total radioactivity as metabolites only.

Specific Populations:

Age, Body Weight, and Gender: Based on the population pharmacokinetics analysis, age has no effect on dabrafenib pharmacokinetics. Pharmacokinetic differences based on gender and on weight are not clinically relevant.

Pediatric: Pharmacokinetics of dabrafenib has not been studied in pediatric patients.

Renal: No formal pharmacokinetic trial in patients with renal impairment has been conducted. The pharmacokinetics of dabrafenib were evaluated using a population analysis in 233 patients with mild renal impairment (GFR 60 to 89 mL/min/1.73 m^2) and 30 patients with moderate renal impairment (GFR 30 to 59 mL/min/1.73 m^2) enrolled in clinical trials. Mild or moderate renal impairment has no effect on systemic exposure to dabrafenib and its metabolites. No data are available in patients with severe renal impairment.

Hepatic: No formal pharmacokinetic trial in patients with hepatic impairment has been conducted. The pharmacokinetics of dabrafenib was evaluated using a population analysis in 65 patients with mild hepatic impairment enrolled in clinical trials. Mild hepatic impairment has no effect on systemic exposure to dabrafenib and its metabolites. No data are available in patients with moderate to severe hepatic impairment.

Drug Interactions:

In vitro studies show that dabrafenib is a substrate of CYP3A4 and CYP2C8 while hydroxy-dabrafenib and desmethyl-dabrafenib are CYP3A4 substrates. Coadministration of dabrafenib 75 mg twice daily and ketoconazole 400 mg once daily (a strong CYP3A4 inhibitor) for 4 days increased dabrafenib AUC by 71%, hydroxy-dabrafenib AUC by 82%, and desmethyl-dabrafenib AUC by 68%. Coadministration of dabrafenib 75 mg twice daily and gemfibrozil 600 mg twice daily (a strong CYP2C8 inhibitor) for 4 days increased dabrafenib AUC by 47%, with no change in the AUC of dabrafenib metabolites. Dabrafenib is a substrate of human P-glycoprotein (P-gp) and breast cancer resistance protein (BCRP) in vitro.

In vitro data demonstrate that dabrafenib is an inducer of CYP3A4 and CYP2B6 via activation of the pregnane X receptor (PXR) and constitutive androstane receptor (CAR) nuclear receptors. Dabrafenib may also induce CYP2C enzymes via the same mechanism. Coadministration of dabrafenib 150 mg twice daily for 15 days and a single dose of midazolam 3 mg (a CYP3A4 substrate) decreased midazolam AUC by 74%. Coadministration of dabrafenib 150 mg twice daily for 15 days and a single dose of warfarin 15 mg decreased the AUC of S-warfarin (a CYP2C9 substrate) by 37% and the AUC of R-warfarin (a CYP3A4/CYP1A2 substrate) by 33% [see Drug Interactions (7.2)].

Dabrafenib and its metabolites, hydroxy-dabrafenib, carboxy-dabrafenib, and desmethyl-dabrafenib, are inhibitors of human organic anion transporting polypeptide OATP1B1, OATP1B3 and organic anion transporter OAT1 and OAT3 in vitro. Dabrafenib and desmethyl-dabrafenib are inhibitors of BCRP in vitro.

Coadministration of trametinib 2 mg daily with dabrafenib 150 mg twice daily resulted in a 23% increase in AUC of dabrafenib, a 33% increase in AUC of desmethyl-dabrafenib, and no change in AUC of trametinib or hydroxy-dabrafenib as compared with administration of either drug alone.

Drugs that alter the pH of the upper GI tract (e.g., proton pump inhibitors, H$_2$-receptor antagonists, antacids) may alter the solubility of dabrafenib and reduce its bioavailability. However, no formal clinical trial has been conducted to evaluate the effect of gastric pH-altering agents on the systemic exposure of dabrafenib. When TAFINLAR is coadministered with a proton pump inhibitor, H$_2$-receptor antagonist, or antacid, systemic exposure of dabrafenib may be decreased and the effect on efficacy of TAFINLAR is unknown.

Table 5 (cont.). Common Adverse Drug Reactions Occurring in ≥10% at (All Grades) or ≥5% (Grades 3 or 4) of Patients Treated With TAFINLAR in Combination With Trametinib in Trial 2

Adverse Reactions	TAFINLAR plus Trametinib 2 mg N = 55		TAFINLAR plus Trametinib 1 mg N = 54		TAFINLAR N = 53	
	All Grades[a]	Grades 3 and 4	All Grades[a]	Grades 3 and 4	All Grades[a]	Grades 3 and 4
Infections and infestations						
Urinary tract infection	13	2	6	0	9	2
Renal and urinary disorders						
Renal failure[f]	7	7	2	0	0	0

[a]National Cancer Institute Common Terminology Criteria for Adverse Events, version 4.
[b]Includes the following terms: peripheral edema, edema, and lymphedema.
[c]Includes the following terms: rash, rash generalized, rash pruritic, rash erythematous, rash papular, rash vesicular, rash macular, and rash maculo-papular.
[d]Includes the following terms: abdominal pain, abdominal pain upper, abdominal pain lower, and abdominal discomfort.
[e]Includes the following terms: brain stem hemorrhage, cerebral hemorrhage, gastric hemorrhage, epistaxis, gingival hemorrhage, hematuria, vaginal hemorrhage, hemorrhage intracranial, eye hemorrhage, and vitreous hemorrhage.
[f]Includes the following terms: renal failure and renal failure acute.

Table 6. Treatment-Emergent Laboratory Abnormalities Occurring at ≥10% (All Grades) or ≥2% (Grades 3 or 4)] of Patients Treated With TAFINLAR in Combination With Trametinib in Trial 2

Tests	TAFINLAR plus Trametinib 2 mg N = 55		TAFINLAR plus Trametinib 1 mg N = 54		TAFINLAR N = 53	
	All Grades	Grades 3 and 4	All Grades	Grades 3 and 4	All Grades	Grades 3 and 4[a]
Hematology						
Leukopenia	62	5	46	4	21	0
Lymphopenia	55	22	59	19	40	6
Neutropenia	55	13	37	2	9	2
Anemia	55	4	46	7	28	0
Thrombocytopenia	31	4	31	2	8	0
Liver Function Tests						
Increased AST	60	5	54	0	15	0
Increased alkaline phosphatase	60	2	67	6	26	2
Increased ALT	42	4	35	4	11	0
Hyperbilirubinemia	15	0	7	4	0	0
Chemistry						
Hyperglycemia	58	5	67	6	49	2
Increased GGT	56	11	54	17	38	2
Hyponatremia	55	11	48	15	36	2
Hypoalbuminemia	53	0	43	2	23	0
Hypophosphatemia	47	5	41	11	40	0
Hypokalemia	29	2	15	2	23	6
Increased creatinine	24	0	20	2	9	0
Hypomagnesemia	18	2	2	0	6	0
Hyperkalemia	18	0	22	0	15	4
Hypercalcemia	15	0	19	2	4	0
Hypocalcemia	13	0	20	0	9	0

[a]No Grade 4 events were reported in patients receiving TAFINLAR as a single agent.
ALT = Alanine aminotransferase; AST = Aspartate aminotransferase; GGT = Gamma glutamyltransferase.

13 NONCLINICAL TOXICOLOGY

13.1 Carcinogenesis, Mutagenesis, Impairment of Fertility

Carcinogenicity studies with dabrafenib have not been conducted. TAFINLAR increased the risk of cutaneous squamous cell carcinomas in patients in clinical trials.

Dabrafenib was not mutagenic in vitro in the bacterial reverse mutation assay (Ames test) or the mouse lymphoma assay, and was not clastogenic in an in vivo rat bone marrow micronucleus test.

In a combined female fertility and embryofetal development study in rats, a reduction in fertility was noted at doses greater than or equal to 20 mg/kg/day (equivalent to the human exposure at the recommended dose based on AUC). A reduction in the number of ovarian corpora lutea was noted in pregnant females at 300 mg/kg/day (which is approximately three times the human exposure at the recommended dose based on AUC).

Male fertility studies with dabrafenib have not been conducted; however, in repeat-dose studies, testicular degeneration/depletion was seen in rats and dogs at doses equivalent to and three times the human exposure at the recommended dose based on AUC, respectively.

13.2 Animal Toxicology and/or Pharmacology

Adverse cardiovascular effects were noted in dogs at dabrafenib doses of 50 mg/kg/day (approximately five times the human exposure at the recommended dose based on AUC) or greater, when administered for up to 4 weeks. Adverse effects consisted of coronary arterial degeneration/necrosis and hemorrhage, as well as cardiac atrioventricular valve hypertrophy/hemorrhage.

14 CLINICAL STUDIES

14.1 BRAF V600E Mutation-Positive Unresectable or Metastatic Melanoma

In Trial 1, the safety and efficacy of TAFINLAR as a single agent were demonstrated in an international, multicenter, randomized (3:1), open-label, active-controlled trial conducted in 250 patients with previously untreated BRAF V600E mutation-positive, unresectable or metastatic melanoma. Patients with any prior use of BRAF inhibitors or MEK inhibitors were excluded. Patients were randomized to receive TAFINLAR 150 mg orally twice daily (n = 187) or dacarbazine 1,000 mg/m^2 intravenously every 3 weeks (n = 63). Randomization was stratified by disease stage at baseline [unresectable stage III (regional nodal or in-transit metastases), M1a (distant skin, subcutaneous, or nodal metastases), or M1b (lung metastases) versus M1c melanoma (all other visceral metastases or elevated serum LDH)]. The main efficacy outcome measure was progression-free survival (PFS) as assessed by the investigator. In addition, an independent radiology review committee (IRRC) assessed the following efficacy outcome measures in pre-specified supportive analyses: PFS, confirmed objective response rate (ORR), and duration of response.

The median age of patients in Trial 1 was 52 years. The majority of the trial population was male (60%), white (99%), had an ECOG performance status of 0 (67%), M1c disease (66%), and normal LDH (62%). All patients had tumor tissue with mutations in BRAF V600E as determined by a clinical trial assay at a centralized testing site. Tumor samples from 243 patients (97%) were tested retrospectively, using an FDA-approved companion diagnostic test, THxID™-BRAF assay.

The median durations of follow-up prior to initiation of alternative treatment in patients randomized to receive TAFINLAR was 5.1 months and in the dacarbazine arm was 3.5 months. Twenty-eight (44%) patients crossed over from the dacarbazine arm at the time of disease progression to receive TAFINLAR.

Trial 1 demonstrated a statistically significant increase in progression-free survival in the patients treated with TAFINLAR. Table 7 and Figure 1 summarize the PFS results.

Table 7. Investigator-Assessed Progression-Free Survival and Confirmed Objective Response Results in Trial 1

	TAFINLAR N = 187	Dacarbazine N = 63
Progression-free Survival		
Number of Events (%)	78 (42%)	41 (65%)
Progressive Disease	76	41
Death	2	0
Median, months (95% CI)	5.1 (4.9, 6.9)	2.7 (1.5, 3.2)
HR[a] (95% CI)	0.33 (0.20, 0.54)	
P-value[b]	P <0.0001	
Confirmed Tumor Responses		
Objective Response Rate	52%	17%

(95% CI)	(44, 59)	(9, 29)
CR, n (%)	6 (3%)	0
PR, n (%)	91 (48%)	11 (17%)
Duration of Response		
Median, months (95% CI)	5.6 (5.4, NR)	NR (5.0, NR)

[a]Pike estimator, stratified by disease state.
[b]Stratified log-rank test.
CI = Confidence interval; CR = Complete response; HR = Hazard ratio; NR = Not reached; PR = Partial response.

Figure 1. Kaplan-Meier Curves of Investigator-Assessed Progression-Free Survival

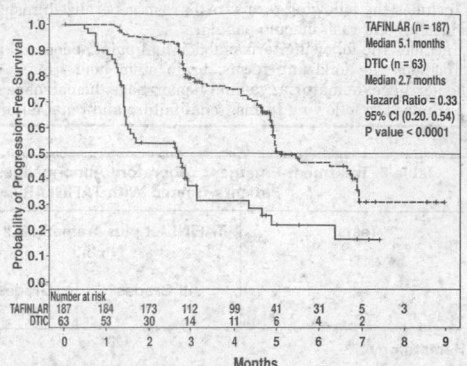

TAFINLAR (n = 187) Median 5.1 months
DTIC (n = 63) Median 2.7 months
Hazard Ratio = 0.33 95% CI (0.20. 0.54) P value < 0.0001

Number at risk

	TAFINLAR	DTIC
0	187	63
1	184	53
2	173	30
3	112	14
4	99	11
5	41	6
6	31	4
7	5	2
8	1	

In supportive analyses based on IRRC assessment and in an exploratory subgroup analysis of patients with retrospectively confirmed V600E mutation-positive melanoma with the THxID™-BRAF assay, the PFS results were consistent with those of the primary efficacy analysis.

The activity of TAFINLAR for the treatment of BRAF V600E mutation-positive melanoma, metastatic to the brain was evaluated in a single-arm, open-label, two-cohort multi-center trial (Trial 3). All patients received TAFINLAR 150 mg twice daily. Patients in Cohort A (n = 74) had received no prior local therapy for brain metastases, while patients in Cohort B (n = 65) had received at least one local therapy for brain metastases, including, but not limited to, surgical resection, whole brain radiotherapy, or stereotactic radiosurgery such as gamma knife, linear-accelerated-based radiosurgery, charged particles, or CyberKnife. In addition, patients in Cohort B were required to have evidence of disease progression in a previously treated lesion or an untreated lesion. Additional eligibility criteria were at least one measurable lesion of 0.5 cm or greater in largest diameter on contrast-enhanced MRI, stable or decreasing corticosteroid dose, and no more than two prior systemic regimens for treatment of metastatic disease. The primary outcome measure was estimation of the overall intracranial response rate (OIRR) in each cohort.

The median age of patients in Cohort A was 50 years, 72% were male, 100% were white, 59% had a pre-treatment ECOG performance status of 0, and 57% had an elevated LDH value at baseline. The median age of patients in Cohort B was 51 years, 63% were male, 98% were white, 66% had a pre-treatment ECOG performance status of 0, and 54% had an elevated LDH value at baseline. Efficacy results as determined by an independent radiology review committee, masked to investigator response assessments, are provided in Table 8.

Table 8. Efficacy Results in Patients With BRAF V600E Melanoma Brain Metastases (Trial 3)

Endpoint	IRRC Assessed Response	
	Cohort A N = 74	Cohort B N = 65
Overall Intracranial Response Rate (OIRR) % (95% CI)	18 (9.7, 28.2) (N = 13)	18 (9.9, 30.0) (N = 12)
Duration of OIRR Median, months (95% CI)	4.6 (2.8, NR)	4.6 (1.9, 4.6)

IRRC = Independent radiology review committee; CI = Confidence interval; NR = Not reached.

14.2 BRAF V600E or V600K Unresectable or Metastatic Melanoma

Trial 2 was a multicenter, open-label, randomized (1:1:1) dose-ranging trial designed to evaluate the clinical activity and safety of TAFINLAR in combination with trametinib (at two different doses) and to compare the safety with TAFINLAR as a single agent in 162 patients with BRAF V600E or V600K mutation-positive, unresectable or metastatic melanoma. Patients were permitted to have had one prior chemotherapy regimen and prior aldesleukin; patients with prior exposure to BRAF or MEK inhibitors were ineligible. Patients were randomized to receive TAFINLAR 150 mg orally twice daily with trametinib 2 mg orally once daily (n = 54), TAFINLAR 150 mg orally twice daily with trametinib 1 mg orally once daily (n = 54), or TAFINLAR 150 mg orally twice daily (n = 54). Treatment continued until disease progression or unacceptable toxicity. Patients randomized to TAFINLAR as a single agent were offered TAFINLAR 150 mg orally twice daily with trametinib 2 mg orally once daily at the time of investigator-assessed disease progression. The major efficacy outcome measure was investigator-assessed overall response rate (ORR). Additional efficacy outcome measures were investigator-assessed duration of response, independent radiology review committee (IRRC)-assessed ORR, and IRRC-assessed duration of response.

The median age of patients was 53 years, 57% were male, >99% were white, 66% of patients had a pre-treatment ECOG performance status of 0, 67% had M1c disease, 54% had a normal LDH at baseline, and 8% had history of brain metastases. Most patients (81%) had not received prior anti-cancer therapy for unresectable or metastatic disease. Based on local laboratory or centralized testing, 85% of patients' tumors had BRAF V600E mutations and 15% had BRAF V600K mutations.

The median duration of follow-up was 14 months. Efficacy outcomes for the trial arms receiving TAFINLAR in combination with trametinib 2 mg orally once daily and TAFINLAR as a single agent are summarized in Table 9.

Table 9. Investigator-Assessed and Independent Review Committee-Assessed Response Rates and Response Duration in Trial 2

Endpoints	TAFINLAR plus Trametinib N = 54	TAFINLAR N = 54
Investigator Assessment		
Responders (ORR%) (95% CI)	41 (76%) (62%, 87%)	29 (54%) (40%, 67%)
Complete response	9%	4%
Partial response	67%	50%
Duration of Response (months)		
Median (95% CI)	10.5 (7, 15)	5.6 (5, 7)
Independent Radiology Review Committee Assessment		
Responders (ORR%) (95% CI)	31 (57%) (43%, 71%)	25 (46%) (33%, 60%)
Complete response	9%	7%
Partial response	48%	39%
Duration of Response (months)		
Median (95% CI)	7.6 (7, NR)	7.6 (6, NR)

CI = Confidence interval; ORR = Confirmed overall response rate; NR = Not reported.

The ORR results were similar in subgroups defined by BRAF mutation subtype, i.e., in the 85% of patients with V600E mutation-positive melanoma and in the 15% of patients with V600K mutation-positive melanoma. In exploratory subgroup analyses of the patients with retrospectively confirmed BRAF V600E or V600K mutation-positive melanoma using the THxID™-BRAF assay, the ORR results were also similar to the intent-to-treat analysis.

16 HOW SUPPLIED/STORAGE AND HANDLING

50 mg Capsules: Dark red capsules imprinted with 'GS TEW' and '50 mg' available in bottles of 120 (NDC 0173-0846-08). Each bottle contains a silica gel desiccant.

75 mg Capsules: Dark pink capsule imprinted with 'GS LHF' and '75 mg' available in bottles of 120 (NDC 0173-0847-08). Each bottle contains a silica gel desiccant. Store at 25°C (77°F); excursions permitted to 15° to 30°C (59° to 86°F) [see USP Controlled Room Temperature].

17 PATIENT COUNSELING INFORMATION

See FDA-approved patient labeling (Medication Guide). Inform patients of the following:

- Evidence of BRAF V600E mutation in the tumor specimen is necessary to identify patients for whom treatment with TAFINLAR as a single agent is indicated and evidence of BRAF V600E or V600K mutation in tumor specimens is necessary to identify patients for whom treatment with TAFINLAR in combination with trametinib is indicated [see Dosage and Administration (2.1)].
- TAFINLAR increases the risk of developing new primary cutaneous and non-cutaneous malignancies. Advise patients to contact their doctor immediately for any new lesions, changes to existing lesions on their skin, or signs and symptoms of other malignancies [see Warnings and Precautions (5.1)].
- TAFINLAR administered in combination with trametinib increases the risk of intracranial and gastrointestinal hemorrhage. Advise patients to contact their healthcare provider to seek immediate medical attention for signs or symptoms of unusual bleeding or hemorrhage [see Warnings and Precautions (5.3)].
- TAFINLAR administered in combination with trametinib increases the risks of pulmonary embolism and deep venous thrombosis. Advise patients to seek immediate medical attention for sudden onset of difficulty breathing, leg pain, or swelling [see Warnings and Precautions (5.4)].
- TAFINLAR administered in combination with trametinib can cause cardiomyopathy. Advise patients to immediately report any signs or symptoms of heart failure to their healthcare provider [see Warnings and Precautions (5.5)].
- TAFINLAR can cause visual disturbances; TAFINLAR administered in combination with trametinib can lead to blindness. Advise patients to contact their healthcare provider if they experience any changes in their vision [see Warnings and Precautions (5.6)].
- TAFINLAR administered as a single agent and in combination with trametinib, can cause pyrexia including serious febrile reactions. Inform patients that the incidence and severity of pyrexia are increased when TAFINLAR is given in combination with trametinib. Instruct patients to contact their doctor if they develop fever while taking TAFINLAR [see Warnings and Precautions (5.7)].
- TAFINLAR in combination with trametinib can cause serious skin toxicities which may require hospitalization. Advise patients to contact their healthcare provider for progressive or intolerable rash [see Warnings and Precautions (5.8)].
- TAFINLAR can impair glucose control in diabetic patients resulting in the need for more intensive hypoglycemic treatment. Advise patients to contact their doctor to report symptoms of severe hyperglycemia [see Warnings and Precautions (5.9)].
- TAFINLAR may cause hemolytic anemia in patients with glucose-6-phosphate dehydrogenase (G6PD) deficiency. Advise patients with known G6PD deficiency to contact their doctor to report signs or symptoms of anemia or hemolysis [see Warnings and Precautions (5.10)].
- TAFINLAR can cause fetal harm if taken during pregnancy. Instruct female patients to use non-hormonal, highly effective contraception during treatment and for 2 weeks after discontinuation of treatment with TAFINLAR as a single agent, or for 4 months after discontinuation of treatment with TAFINLAR in combination with trametinib. Advise patients to contact their doctor if they become pregnant, or if pregnancy is suspected, while taking TAFINLAR [see Warnings and Precautions (5.11), Use in Specific Populations (8.1)].
- Nursing infants may experience serious adverse reactions if the mother is taking TAFINLAR during breastfeeding. Advise breastfeeding mothers to discontinue nursing while taking TAFINLAR [see Use in Specific Populations (8.3)].
- Male patients are at an increased risk for impaired spermatogenesis [see Use in Specific Populations (8.6)].
- TAFINLAR should be taken either at least 1 hour before or at least 2 hours after a meal [see Dosage and Administration (2.1)].

TAFINLAR is a registered trademark of the GlaxoSmithKline group of companies.
THxID™ is a trademark of bioMérieux.
GlaxoSmithKline
Research Triangle Park, NC 27709
©2014, GlaxoSmithKline group of companies. All rights reserved.
TFR:4PI

MEDICATION GUIDE
TAFINLAR® (TAFF-in-lar)
(dabrafenib)
capsules

If your healthcare provider prescribes TAFINLAR for you in combination with trametinib, also read the Patient Information leaflet that comes with trametinib.

What is the most important information I should know about TAFINLAR?

TAFINLAR may cause serious side effects, including the risk of new cancers:

- **TAFINLAR, when used alone or in combination with trametinib, may cause a type of skin cancer, called cutaneous squamous cell carcinoma (cuSCC). New melanoma lesions have also occurred in people who take TAFINLAR.**
- **TAFINLAR, in combination with trametinib, may cause new cancers including basal cell carcinoma.**

Talk with your healthcare provider about your risk for these cancers.

Check your skin and tell your healthcare provider right away about any skin changes including a:

- new wart
- skin sore or reddish bump that bleeds or does not heal
- change in size or color of a mole

Your healthcare provider should check your skin before you start taking TAFINLAR, and every two months while taking TAFINLAR to look for any new skin cancers. Your healthcare provider may continue to check your skin for six months after you stop taking TAFINLAR.

Your healthcare provider should also check for cancers that may not occur on the skin. Tell your healthcare provider about any new symptoms that have developed while taking TAFINLAR in combination with trametinib.

See "What are the possible side effects of TAFINLAR?" for more information about side effects.

What is TAFINLAR?

TAFINLAR is a prescription medicine used alone or in combination with trametinib to treat people with a type of skin cancer called melanoma:

- that has spread to other parts of the body or cannot be removed by surgery, and
- that has a certain type of abnormal "BRAF" gene.

Your healthcare provider will perform a test to make sure that TAFINLAR is right for you.

TAFINLAR (alone or in combination with trametinib) is not used to treat people with a type of skin cancer called wild-type BRAF melanoma.

It is not known if TAFINLAR is safe and effective in children.

What should I tell my healthcare provider before taking TAFINLAR?

Before you take TAFINLAR, tell your healthcare provider if you:

- have had bleeding problems or blood clots
- have heart problems
- have eye problems
- have liver or kidney problems
- have diabetes
- plan to have surgery, dental, or other medical procedures
- have a deficiency of the glucose-6-phosphate dehydrogenase (G6PD) enzyme
- have any other medical conditions
- are pregnant or plan to become pregnant. TAFINLAR can harm your unborn baby.
  ◦ Females who are able to become pregnant should use birth control (contraception) **during treatment** with TAFINLAR **and** for **2 weeks after stopping** treatment with **TAFINLAR alone, or for 4 months when taking TAFINLAR in combination with trametinib.**
  ◦ Birth control using hormones (such as birth control pills, injections, or patches) may not work as well while you are taking TAFINLAR alone or in combination with trametinib. You should use another effective method of birth control while taking TAFINLAR alone or in combination with trametinib.
  ◦ Talk to your healthcare provider about birth control methods that may be right for you during this time.
  ◦ Tell your healthcare provider right away if you become pregnant during treatment with TAFINLAR alone or in combination with trametinib.
- are breastfeeding or plan to breastfeed. It is not known if TAFINLAR passes into your breast milk. You and your healthcare provider should decide if you will take TAFINLAR or breastfeed. You should not do both.

Tell your healthcare provider about all the medicines you take, including prescription and over-the-counter medicines, vitamins, and herbal supplements. TAFINLAR and certain other medicines can affect each other, causing side effects. TAFINLAR may affect the way other medicines work, and other medicines may affect how TAFINLAR works. You can ask your pharmacist for a list of medicines that may interact with TAFINLAR.

Know the medicines you take. Keep a list of them to show your healthcare provider and pharmacist when you get a new medicine.

How should I take TAFINLAR?

- Take TAFINLAR exactly as your healthcare provider tells you. Do not change your dose or stop TAFINLAR unless your healthcare provider tells you.
- Take TAFINLAR 2 times a day, about 12 hours apart.
- If you take TAFINLAR in combination with trametinib, take the first dose of TAFINLAR in the morning, and take the second dose of TAFINLAR in the evening, about 12 hours apart. Take trametinib 1 time a day at the same time each day, either with the morning or the evening dose of TAFINLAR.
- Take TAFINLAR at least 1 hour before or 2 hours after a meal.
- Do not open, crush, or break TAFINLAR capsules.
- If you miss a dose of TAFINLAR, take it as soon as you remember. But, if it is within 6 hours of your next scheduled dose, just take your next dose at your regular time. Do not make up for the missed dose.
- If you are taking TAFINLAR in combination with trametinib and you miss a dose of trametinib, take it as soon as you remember. But, if it is within 12 hours of your next scheduled dose of trametinib, just take your next dose at your regular time. Do not make up for the missed dose.
- If you take too much TAFINLAR, call your healthcare provider or go to the nearest hospital emergency room right away.

What are the possible side effects of TAFINLAR?

TAFINLAR may cause serious side effects, including:

- See "What is the most important information I should know about TAFINLAR?"
- **bleeding problems.** TAFINLAR, in combination with trametinib, can cause serious bleeding problems, especially in your brain and stomach, and can lead to death. Call your healthcare provider and get medical help right away if you have any unusual signs of bleeding, including:
  ◦ headaches, dizziness, or feeling weak
  ◦ cough up blood or blood clots
  ◦ vomit blood or your vomit looks like "coffee grounds"
  ◦ red or black stools that look like tar
- **blood clots.** TAFINLAR, in combination with trametinib, can cause blood clots in your arms or legs, which can travel to your lungs and can lead to death. Get medical help right away if you have the following symptoms:
  ◦ chest pain
  ◦ sudden shortness of breath or trouble breathing
  ◦ pain in your legs with or without swelling
  ◦ swelling in your arms or legs
  ◦ a cool or pale arm or leg
- **heart problems, including heart failure.** Your healthcare provider should check your heart function before you start taking TAFINLAR in combination with trametinib and during treatment. Call your healthcare provider right away if you have any of the following signs and symptoms of a heart problem:
  ◦ feeling like your heart is pounding or racing
  ◦ shortness of breath
  ◦ swelling of your ankles and feet
  ◦ feeling lightheaded
- **eye problems.** TAFINLAR alone, or in combination with trametinib, can cause severe eye problems that can lead to blindness. Call your healthcare provider right away if you get these symptoms of eye problems:
  ◦ blurred vision, loss of vision, or other vision changes
  ◦ see color dots
  ◦ halo (seeing blurred outline around objects)
  ◦ eye pain, swelling, or redness
- **fever.** TAFINLAR alone or in combination with trametinib can cause fever which may be serious. When taking TAFINLAR, in combination with trametinib, fever may happen more often or may be more severe. In some cases, chills or shaking chills, too much fluid loss (dehydration), low blood pressure, dizziness, or kidney problems may happen with the fever. Call your healthcare provider right away if you get a fever while taking TAFINLAR.
- **skin reactions.** Rash is a common side effect of TAFINLAR alone, or when used in combination with trametinib. TAFINLAR alone, or in combination with trametinib, can also cause other skin reactions. In some cases these rashes and other skin reactions can be severe, and may need to be treated in a hospital. Call your healthcare provider if you get any of the following symptoms:
  ◦ skin rash that bothers you or does not go away
  ◦ acne
  ◦ redness, swelling, peeling, or tenderness of hands or feet
  ◦ skin redness
- **increased blood sugar (hyperglycemia).** Some people may develop high blood sugar or worsening diabetes during treatment with TAFINLAR, alone or in combination with trametinib. If you are diabetic, your healthcare provider should check your blood sugar levels closely during treatment with TAFINLAR alone or in combination with trametinib. Your diabetes medicine may need to be changed. Tell your healthcare provider if you have any of the following symptoms of severe high blood sugar:

○ increased thirst
○ urinating more often than normal, or urinating an increased amount of urine

- TAFINLAR may cause healthy red blood cells to break down too early in people with G6PD deficiency. This may lead to a type of anemia called hemolytic anemia where the body does not have enough healthy red blood cells. Tell your healthcare provider if you have any of the following signs or symptoms of anemia or breakdown of red blood cells:
  ○ yellow skin (jaundice)
  ○ weakness or dizziness
  ○ shortness of breath

The most common side effects of TAFINLAR when used alone include:
- thickening of the outer layers of the skin
- headache
- joint aches
- warts
- hair loss
- redness, swelling, peeling, or tenderness of hands or feet

Common side effects of TAFINLAR when used in combination with trametinib include:
- tiredness
- nausea or vomiting
- stomach-area (abdominal) pain
- diarrhea
- cough
- swelling of the face, arms, or legs
- headache
- night sweats
- decreased appetite
- constipation
- muscle or joint aches

TAFINLAR, in combination with trametinib, may cause fertility problems in females. This could affect your ability to become pregnant. Talk to your healthcare provider if this is a concern for you.

TAFINLAR may cause lower sperm counts in males. This could affect the ability to father a child. Talk to your healthcare provider if this is a concern for you.

Tell your healthcare provider if you have any side effect that bothers you or that does not go away.

These are not all of the possible side effects of TAFINLAR. For more information about side effects, ask your healthcare provider or pharmacist.

Call your doctor for medical advice about side effects. You may report side effects to FDA at 1-800-FDA-1088.

You may also report side effects to GlaxoSmithKline at 1-888-825-5249.

How should I store TAFINLAR?
Store TAFINLAR at room temperature, between 68°F to 77°F (20°C to 25°C).

Keep TAFINLAR and all medicine out of the reach of children.

General information about TAFINLAR
Medicines are sometimes prescribed for purposes other than those listed in a Medication Guide. Do not use TAFINLAR for a condition for which it was not prescribed. Do not give TAFINLAR to other people, even if they have the same symptoms that you have. It may harm them.

You can ask your healthcare provider or pharmacist for information about TAFINLAR that is written for health professionals.

For more information, call GlaxoSmithKline at 1-888-825-5249 or go to www.TAFINLAR.com.

What are the ingredients in TAFINLAR?
Active ingredient: dabrafenib
Inactive ingredients: colloidal silicon dioxide, magnesium stearate, microcrystalline cellulose

Capsule shells: hypromellose, red iron oxide (E172), titanium dioxide (E171).

This Medication Guide has been approved by the U.S. Food and Drug Administration.

GlaxoSmithKline
Research Triangle Park, NC 27709
Revised: January 2014
TAFINLAR is a registered trademark of the GlaxoSmithKline group of companies.
©2014, GlaxoSmithKline group of companies. All rights reserved.
TFR:3MG

TANZEUM   ℞
(albiglutide)
for injection, for subcutaneous use

HIGHLIGHTS OF PRESCRIBING INFORMATION
These highlights do not include all the information needed to use TANZEUM safely and effectively. See full prescribing information for TANZEUM.

TANZEUM (albiglutide) for injection, for subcutaneous use
Initial U.S. Approval: 2014

WARNING: RISK OF THYROID C-CELL TUMORS
See full prescribing information for complete boxed warning.

- Thyroid C-cell tumors have been observed in rodent studies with glucagon-like peptide-1 (GLP-1) receptor agonists at clinically relevant exposures. It is unknown whether TANZEUM causes thyroid C-cell tumors, including medullary thyroid carcinoma (MTC), in humans. (5.1)
- TANZEUM is contraindicated in patients with a personal or family history of MTC or in patients with Multiple Endocrine Neoplasia syndrome type 2 (MEN 2). (4, 5.1)

————INDICATIONS AND USAGE————

TANZEUM is a GLP-1 receptor agonist indicated as an adjunct to diet and exercise to improve glycemic control in adults with type 2 diabetes mellitus. (1)
Limitations of Use:
- Not recommended as first-line therapy for patients inadequately controlled on diet and exercise. (1, 5.1)
- Has not been studied in patients with a history of pancreatitis. Consider other antidiabetic therapies in patients with a history of pancreatitis. (1, 5.2)
- Not for treatment of type 1 diabetes mellitus or diabetic ketoacidosis. (1)
- Not for patients with pre-existing severe gastrointestinal disease. (1)
- Has not been studied in combination with prandial insulin. (1)

————DOSAGE AND ADMINISTRATION————

- Administer once weekly at any time of day, without regard to meals. (2.1)
- Inject subcutaneously in the abdomen, thigh, or upper arm. (2.1)
- Initiate at 30 mg subcutaneously once weekly. Dose can be increased to 50 mg once weekly in patients requiring additional glycemic control. (2.1)
- If a dose is missed, administer within 3 days of missed dose. (2.1)
- See Full Prescribing Information and Patient Instructions for Use for reconstitution of lyophilized powder and administration. (2.4, 2.5, 17)

————DOSAGE FORMS AND STRENGTHS————

- For injection: 30 mg or 50 mg in a single-dose Pen. (3)

————CONTRAINDICATIONS————

- Personal or family history of medullary thyroid carcinoma or in patients with Multiple Endocrine Neoplasia syndrome type 2. (4.1)
- History of serious hypersensitivity to albiglutide or any product components. (4.2, 5.4)

————WARNINGS AND PRECAUTIONS————

- Pancreatitis: Discontinue promptly if suspected. Do not restart if confirmed. Consider other antidiabetic therapies in patients with a history of pancreatitis. (5.2)
- Hypoglycemia: Can occur when used in combination with insulin secretagogues (e.g., sulfonylureas) or insulin. Consider lowering sulfonylurea or insulin dosage when starting TANZEUM. (5.3)
- Hypersensitivity Reactions: Discontinue TANZEUM if suspected. Monitor and treat promptly per standard of care until signs and symptoms resolve. (5.4)
- Renal Impairment: Monitor renal function in patients with renal impairment reporting severe adverse gastrointestinal reactions. (5.5)
- Macrovascular Outcomes: There have been no clinical trials establishing conclusive evidence of macrovascular risk reduction with TANZEUM or any other antidiabetic drug. (5.6)

————ADVERSE REACTIONS————

Adverse reactions, reported in ≥10% of patients treated with TANZEUM and more frequently than in patients on placebo, were upper respiratory tract infection, diarrhea, nausea, and injection site reaction. (6.1)
To report SUSPECTED ADVERSE REACTIONS, contact GlaxoSmithKline at 1-888-825-5249 or FDA at 1-800-FDA-1088 or www.fda.gov/medwatch

————DRUG INTERACTIONS————

TANZEUM delays gastric emptying. May impact absorption of concomitantly administered oral medications. (7)

————USE IN SPECIFIC POPULATIONS————

- Pregnancy: TANZEUM may cause fetal harm; only use if potential benefit justifies potential risk to fetus. (8.1)
- Nursing Mothers: Discontinue nursing or discontinue TANZEUM. (8.3)

- Renal Impairment: No dosage adjustment recommended. Monitor renal function in patients with renal impairment reporting severe adverse gastrointestinal reactions. (5.5, 8.6)

See 17 for PATIENT COUNSELING INFORMATION and Medication Guide

Revised: 06/2014

FULL PRESCRIBING INFORMATION: CONTENTS*
WARNING: RISK OF THYROID C-CELL TUMORS

FULL PRESCRIBING INFORMATION

> **WARNING: RISK OF THYROID C-CELL TUMORS**
> - Thyroid C-cell tumors have been observed in rodent studies with glucagon-like peptide-1 (GLP-1) receptor agonists at clinically relevant exposures. It is unknown whether TANZEUM™ causes thyroid C-cell tumors, including medullary thyroid carcinoma (MTC), in humans *[see Warnings and Precautions (5.1)]*.
> - TANZEUM is contraindicated in patients with a personal or family history of MTC or in patients with Multiple Endocrine Neoplasia syndrome type 2 (MEN 2). Routine serum calcitonin or thyroid ultrasound monitoring is of uncertain value in patients treated with TANZEUM. Patients should be counseled regarding the risk and symptoms of thyroid tumors *[see Contraindications (4.1), Warnings and Precautions (5.1)]*.

1   INDICATIONS AND USAGE

TANZEUM is indicated as an adjunct to diet and exercise to improve glycemic control in adults with type 2 diabetes mellitus *[see Clinical Studies (14)]*.
Limitations of Use:
- TANZEUM is not recommended as first-line therapy for patients inadequately controlled on diet and exercise *[see Warnings and Precautions (5.1)]*.
- TANZEUM has not been studied in patients with a history of pancreatitis *[see Warnings and Precautions (5.2)]*. Consider other antidiabetic therapies in patients with a history of pancreatitis.
- TANZEUM is not indicated in the treatment of patients with type 1 diabetes mellitus or for the treatment of patients with diabetic ketoacidosis. TANZEUM is not a substitute for insulin in these patients.

- TANZEUM has not been studied in patients with severe gastrointestinal disease, including severe gastroparesis. The use of TANZEUM is not recommended in patients with pre-existing severe gastrointestinal disease [see Adverse Reactions (6.1)].
- TANZEUM has not been studied in combination with prandial insulin.

2 DOSAGE AND ADMINISTRATION

2.1 Dosage

The recommended dosage of TANZEUM is 30 mg once weekly given as a subcutaneous injection in the abdomen, thigh, or upper arm region. The dosage may be increased to 50 mg once weekly if the glycemic response is inadequate. TANZEUM may be administered at any time of day without regard to meals. Instruct patients to administer TANZEUM once a week on the same day each week. The day of weekly administration may be changed if necessary as long as the last dose was administered 4 or more days before.

If a dose is missed, instruct patients to administer as soon as possible within 3 days after the missed dose. Thereafter, patients can resume dosing on their usual day of administration. If it is more than 3 days after the missed dose, instruct patients to wait until their next regularly scheduled weekly dose.

2.2 Concomitant Use with an Insulin Secretagogue (e.g., Sulfonylurea) or with Insulin

When initiating TANZEUM, consider reducing the dosage of concomitantly administered insulin secretagogues (e.g., sulfonylureas) or insulin to reduce the risk of hypoglycemia [see Warnings and Precautions (5.3)].

2.3 Dosage in Patients with Renal Impairment

No dose adjustment is needed in patients with mild, moderate, or severe renal impairment (eGFR 15 to 89 mL/min/1.73 m²). Use caution when initiating or escalating doses of TANZEUM in patients with renal impairment. Monitor renal function in patients with renal impairment reporting severe adverse gastrointestinal reactions [see Warnings and Precautions (5.5), Use in Specific Populations (8.6)].

2.4 Reconstitution of the Lyophilized Powder

The lyophilized powder contained within the Pen must be reconstituted prior to administration. See Patient Instructions for Use for complete administration instructions with illustrations. The instructions may also be found at www.TANZEUM.com. Instruct patients as follows:

Pen Reconstitution

a. Hold the Pen body with the clear cartridge pointing up to see the [1] in the number window.
b. To reconstitute the lyophilized powder with the diluent in the Pen, twist the clear cartridge on the Pen in the direction of the arrow until the Pen is felt/heard to "click" into place and the [2] is seen in the number window. This mixes the diluent with the lyophilized powder.
c. Slowly and gently rock the Pen side-to-side 5 times to mix the reconstituted solution of TANZEUM. Advise the patient to not shake the Pen hard to avoid foaming.
d. Wait 15 minutes for the 30-mg Pen and 30 minutes for the 50-mg Pen to ensure that the reconstituted solution is mixed.

Preparing Pen for Injection

e. Slowly and gently rock the Pen side-to-side 5 additional times to mix the reconstituted solution.
f. Visually inspect the reconstituted solution in the viewing window for particulate matter. The reconstituted solution will be yellow in color. After reconstitution, use TANZEUM within 8 hours.
g. Holding the Pen upright, attach the needle to the Pen. Gently tap the clear cartridge to bring large bubbles to the top.

See Dosage and Administration (2.5) for important administration instructions, including the injection procedure.

Alternate Method of Reconstitution (Healthcare Professional Use Only)

The Patient Instructions for Use provide directions for the patient to wait 15 minutes for the 30-mg Pen and 30 minutes for the 50-mg Pen after the lyophilized powder and diluent are mixed to ensure reconstitution.

Healthcare professionals may utilize the following alternate method of reconstitution. Because this method relies on appropriate swirling and visual inspection of the solution, it should only be performed by healthcare professionals.

a. Follow Step A (Inspect Your Pen and Mix Your Medication) in the Instructions for Use. Make sure you have:
  ○ Inspected the Pen for [1] in the number window and expiration date.
  ○ Twisted the clear cartridge until [2] appears in the number window and a "click" is heard. This combines the medicine powder and liquid in the clear cartridge.
b. Hold the Pen with the clear cartridge pointing up and maintain this orientation throughout the reconstitution.
c. Gently swirl the Pen in small circular motions for at least one minute. Avoid shaking as this can result in foaming, which may affect the dose.

d. Inspect the solution, and if needed, continue to gently swirl the Pen until all the powder is dissolved and you see a clear yellow solution that is free of particles. A small amount of foam, on top of the solution at the end of reconstitution, is normal.
  ○ For 30-mg Pen: Complete dissolution usually occurs within 2 minutes but may take up to 5 minutes, as confirmed by visual inspection for a clear yellow solution free of particles.
  ○ For 50-mg Pen: Complete dissolution usually occurs within 7 minutes but may take up to 10 minutes.
e. After reconstitution, continue to follow the steps in the Instructions for Use, starting at Step B: Attach the Needle.

2.5 Important Administration Instructions

Instruct patients as follows:
- The pen should be used within 8 hours of reconstitution prior to attaching the needle.
- After attaching the supplied needle, remove air bubbles by slowly twisting the Pen until you see the [3] in the number window. At the same time, the injection button will be automatically released from the bottom of the Pen.
- Use immediately after the needle is attached and primed. The product can clog the needle if allowed to dry in the primed needle.
- After subcutaneously inserting the needle into the skin in the abdomen, thigh, or upper arm region, press the injection button. Hold the injection button until you hear a "click" and then hold the button for 5 additional seconds to deliver the full dose.

When using TANZEUM with insulin, instruct patients to administer as separate injections and to never mix the products. It is acceptable to inject TANZEUM and insulin in the same body region but the injections should not be adjacent to each other.

When injecting in the same body region, advise patients to use a different injection site each week. TANZEUM must not be administered intravenously or intramuscularly.

3 DOSAGE FORMS AND STRENGTHS

TANZEUM is supplied as follows:
- For injection: 30-mg lyophilized powder in a single-dose Pen (pen injector) for reconstitution.
- For injection: 50-mg lyophilized powder in a single-dose Pen (pen injector) for reconstitution.

4 CONTRAINDICATIONS

4.1 Medullary Thyroid Carcinoma

TANZEUM is contraindicated in patients with a personal or family history of medullary thyroid carcinoma (MTC) or in patients with Multiple Endocrine Neoplasia syndrome type 2 (MEN 2) [see Warnings and Precautions (5.1)].

4.2 Hypersensitivity

TANZEUM is contraindicated in patients with a prior serious hypersensitivity reaction to albiglutide or to any of the product components [see Warnings and Precautions (5.4)].

5 WARNINGS AND PRECAUTIONS

5.1 Risk of Thyroid C-cell Tumors

Nonclinical studies in rodents of clinically relevant doses of GLP-1 receptor agonists showed dose-related and treatment-duration-dependent increases in the incidence of thyroid C-cell tumors (adenomas and carcinomas). Carcinogenicity studies could not be conducted with TANZEUM because drug-clearing, anti-drug antibodies develop in animals used for these types of studies [see Nonclinical Toxicology (13.1)]. It is unknown whether GLP-1 receptor agonists are associated with thyroid C-cell tumors, including MTC in humans [see Boxed Warning, Contraindications (4.1)].

Across 8 Phase III clinical trials [see Clinical Studies (14)], MTC was diagnosed in 1 patient receiving TANZEUM and 1 patient receiving placebo. Both patients had markedly elevated serum calcitonin levels at baseline.

TANZEUM is contraindicated in patients with a personal or family history of MTC or in patients with MEN 2. Counsel patients regarding the risk for MTC with the use of TANZEUM and inform them of symptoms of thyroid tumors (e.g., a mass in the neck, dysphagia, dyspnea, persistent hoarseness). The clinical value of routine monitoring of serum calcitonin to diagnose MTC in patients at risk for MTC has not been established.

Elevated serum calcitonin is a biological marker of MTC. Patients with MTC usually have calcitonin values >50 ng/L. Patients with thyroid nodules noted on physical examination or neck imaging should be referred to an endocrinologist for further evaluation. Routine monitoring of serum calcitonin or using thyroid ultrasound is of uncertain value for early detection of MTC in patients treated with TANZEUM. Such monitoring may increase the risk of unnecessary procedures, due to the low specificity of serum calcitonin testing for MTC and a high background incidence of thyroid disease. If serum calcitonin is measured and found to be elevated, the patient should be referred to an endocrinologist for further evaluation.

5.2 Acute Pancreatitis

In clinical trials, acute pancreatitis has been reported in association with TANZEUM.

Across 8 Phase III clinical trials [see Clinical Studies (14)], pancreatitis adjudicated as likely related to therapy occurred more frequently in patients receiving TANZEUM (6 of 2,365 [0.3%]) than in patients receiving placebo (0 of 468 [0%]) or active comparators (2 of 2,065 [0.1%]).

After initiation of TANZEUM, observe patients carefully for signs and symptoms of pancreatitis (including persistent severe abdominal pain, sometimes radiating to the back and which may or may not be accompanied by vomiting). If pancreatitis is suspected, promptly discontinue TANZEUM. If pancreatitis is confirmed, TANZEUM should not be restarted.

TANZEUM has not been studied in patients with a history of pancreatitis to determine whether these patients are at increased risk for pancreatitis. Consider other antidiabetic therapies in patients with a history of pancreatitis.

5.3 Hypoglycemia with Concomitant Use of Insulin Secretagogues or Insulin

The risk of hypoglycemia is increased when TANZEUM is used in combination with insulin secretagogues (e.g., sulfonylureas) or insulin. Therefore, patients may require a lower dose of sulfonylurea or insulin to reduce the risk of hypoglycemia in this setting [see Adverse Reactions (6.1)].

5.4 Hypersensitivity Reactions

Across 8 Phase III clinical trials [see Clinical Studies (14)], a serious hypersensitivity reaction with pruritus, rash, and dyspnea occurred in a patient treated with TANZEUM. If hypersensitivity reactions occur, discontinue use of TANZEUM; treat promptly per standard of care and monitor until signs and symptoms resolve [see Contraindications (4.2)].

5.5 Renal Impairment

In patients treated with GLP-1 receptor agonists, there have been postmarketing reports of acute renal failure and worsening of chronic renal failure, which may sometimes require hemodialysis. Some of these events were reported in patients without known underlying renal disease. A majority of reported events occurred in patients who had experienced nausea, vomiting, diarrhea, or dehydration. In a trial of TANZEUM in patients with renal impairment [see Clinical Studies (14.3)], the frequency of such gastrointestinal reactions increased as renal function declined [see Use in Specific Populations (8.6)]. Because these reactions may worsen renal function, use caution when initiating or escalating doses of TANZEUM in patients with renal impairment [see Dosage and Administration (2.3), Use in Specific Populations (8.6)].

5.6 Macrovascular Outcomes

There have been no clinical trials establishing conclusive evidence of macrovascular risk reduction with TANZEUM or any other antidiabetic drug.

6 ADVERSE REACTIONS

The following serious reactions are described below or elsewhere in the labeling:
- Risk of Thyroid C-cell Tumors [see Warnings and Precautions (5.1)]
- Acute Pancreatitis [see Warnings and Precautions (5.2)]
- Hypoglycemia with Concomitant Use of Insulin Secretagogues or Insulin [see Warnings and Precautions (5.3)]
- Hypersensitivity Reactions [see Warnings and Precautions (5.4)]
- Renal Impairment [see Warnings and Precautions (5.5)]

6.1 Clinical Trials Experience

Because clinical trials are conducted under widely varying conditions, adverse reaction rates observed in the clinical trials of a drug cannot be directly compared with rates in the clinical trials of another drug and may not reflect the rates observed in practice.

Pool of Placebo-Controlled Trials

The data in Table 1 are derived from 4 placebo-controlled trials. TANZEUM was used as monotherapy in 1 trial and as add-on therapy in 3 trials [see Clinical Studies (14)]. These data reflect exposure of 923 patients to TANZEUM and a mean duration of exposure to TANZEUM of 93 weeks. The mean age of participants was 55 years, 1% of participants were 75 years or older and 53% of participants were male. The population in these studies was 48% white, 13% African/African American, 7% Asian, and 29% Hispanic/Latino. At baseline, the population had diabetes for an average of 7 years and had a mean HbA1c of 8.1%. At baseline, 17% of the population in these studies reported peripheral neuropathy and 4% reported retinopathy. Baseline estimated renal function was normal or mildly impaired (eGFR >60 mL/min/1.73 m²) in 91% of the study population and moderately impaired (eGFR 30 to 60 mL/min/1.73 m²) in 9%.

Table 1 shows common adverse reactions excluding hypoglycemia associated with the use of TANZEUM in the pool of placebo-controlled trials. These adverse reactions were not present at baseline, occurred more commonly on TANZEUM than on placebo, and occurred in at least 5% of patients treated with TANZEUM.

Table 1. Adverse Reactions in Placebo-controlled Trials Reported in ≥5% of Patients Treated with TANZEUM[a]

Adverse Reaction	Placebo (N = 468) %	TANZEUM (N = 923) %
Upper respiratory tract infection	13.0	14.2
Diarrhea	10.5	13.1
Nausea	9.6	11.1
Injection site reaction[b]	2.1	10.5
Cough	6.2	6.9
Back pain	5.8	6.7
Arthralgia	6.4	6.6
Sinusitis	5.8	6.2
Influenza	3.2	5.2

[a] Adverse reactions reported includes adverse reactions occurring with the use of glycemic rescue medications which included metformin (17% for placebo and 10% for TANZEUM) and insulin (24% for placebo and 14% for TANZEUM).
[b] See below for other events of injection site reactions reported.

Gastrointestinal Adverse Reactions
In the pool of placebo-controlled trials, gastrointestinal complaints occurred more frequently among patients receiving TANZEUM (39%) than patients receiving placebo (33%). In addition to diarrhea and nausea (see Table 1), the following gastrointestinal adverse reactions also occurred more frequently in patients receiving TANZEUM: vomiting (2.6% versus 4.2% for placebo versus TANZEUM), gastro-esophageal reflux disease (1.9% versus 3.5% for placebo versus TANZEUM), and dyspepsia (2.8% versus 3.4% for placebo versus TANZEUM). Constipation also contributed to the frequently reported reactions. In the group treated with TANZEUM, investigators graded the severity of GI reactions as "mild" in 56% of cases, "moderate" in 37% of cases, and "severe" in 7% of cases. Discontinuation due to GI adverse reactions occurred in 2% of individuals on TANZEUM or placebo.

Injection Site Reactions
In the pool of placebo-controlled trials, injection site reactions occurred more frequently on TANZEUM (18%) than on placebo (8%). In addition to the term injection site reaction (see Table 1), the following other types of injection site reactions also occurred more frequently on TANZEUM: injection site hematoma (1.9% versus 2.1% for placebo versus TANZEUM), injection site erythema (0.4% versus 1.7% for placebo versus TANZEUM), injection site rash (0% versus 1.4% for placebo versus TANZEUM), injection site hypersensitivity (0% versus 0.8% for placebo versus TANZEUM), and injection site hemorrhage (0.6% versus 0.7% for placebo versus TANZEUM). Injection site pruritus also contributed to the frequently reported reactions. The majority of injection site reactions were judged as "mild" by investigators in both groups (73% for TANZEUM versus 94% for placebo). More patients on TANZEUM than on placebo: discontinued due to an injection site reaction (2% versus 0.2%), experienced more than 2 reactions (38% versus 20%), had a reaction judged by investigators to be "moderate" or "severe" (27% versus 6%) and required local or systemic treatment for the reactions (36% versus 11%).

Pool of Placebo- and Active-controlled Trials
The occurrence of adverse reactions was also evaluated in a larger pool of patients with type 2 diabetes participating in 7 placebo- and active-controlled trials. These trials evaluated the use of TANZEUM as monotherapy, and as add-on therapy to oral antidiabetic agents, and as add-on therapy to basal insulin [see Clinical Studies (14)]. In this pool, a total of 2,116 patients with type 2 diabetes were treated with TANZEUM for a mean duration of 75 weeks. The mean age of patients treated with TANZEUM was 55 years, 1.5% of the population in these studies was 75 years old or older and 51% of participants were male. Forty-eight percent of patients were white, 15% African/African American, 9% Asian, and 26% were Hispanic/Latino. At baseline, the population had diabetes for an average of 8 years and had a mean HbA1c of 8.2%. At baseline, 21% of the population reported peripheral neuropathy and 5% reported retinopathy. Baseline estimated renal function was normal or mildly impaired (eGFR >60 mL/min/1.73 m²) in 92% of the population and moderately impaired (eGFR 30 to 60 mL/min/1.73 m²) in 8% of the population.
In the pool of placebo- and active-controlled trials, the types and frequency of common adverse reactions excluding hypoglycemia were similar to those listed in Table 1.

Other Adverse Reactions
Hypoglycemia
The proportion of patients experiencing at least one documented symptomatic hypoglycemic episode on TANZEUM and the proportion of patients experiencing at least one severe hypoglycemic episode on TANZEUM in clinical trials [see Clinical Studies (14)] is shown in Table 2. Hypoglycemia was more frequent when TANZEUM was added to sulfonylurea or insulin [see Warnings and Precautions (5.3)].

Table 2. Incidence (%) of Hypoglycemia in Clinical Trials of TANZEUM[a]

	Placebo	TANZEUM 30 mg Weekly
Monotherapy[b] (52 Weeks)	Placebo N = 101	N = 101
Documented symptomatic[c]	2%	2%
Severe[d]	-	-
In Combination with Metformin Trial (104 Weeks)[e]	Placebo N = 101	TANZEUM N = 302
Documented symptomatic	4%	3%
Severe	-	-
In Combination with Pioglitazone ± Metformin (52 Weeks)	Placebo N = 151	TANZEUM N = 150
Documented symptomatic	1%	3%
Severe	-	1%
In Combination with Metformin and Sulfonylurea (52 Weeks)	Placebo N = 115	TANZEUM N = 271
Documented symptomatic	7%	13%
Severe	-	0.4%
In Combination with Insulin Glargine (26 Weeks)	Insulin Lispro N = 281	TANZEUM N = 285
Documented symptomatic	30%	16%
Severe	0.7%	-
In Combination with Metformin ± Sulfonylurea (52 Weeks)	Insulin Glargine N = 241	TANZEUM N = 504
Documented symptomatic	27%	17%
Severe	0.4%	0.4%
In Combination with OADs in Renal Impairment (26 Weeks)	Sitagliptin N = 246	TANZEUM N = 249
Documented symptomatic	6%	10%
Severe	0.8%	-

OAD = Oral antidiabetic agents.
[a] Data presented are to the primary endpoint and include only events occurring on-therapy with randomized medications and excludes events occurring after use of glycemic rescue medications (i.e., primarily metformin or insulin).
[b] In this trial, no documented symptomatic or severe hypoglycemia were reported for TANZEUM 50 mg and these data are omitted from the table.
[c] Plasma glucose concentration ≤70 mg/dL and presence of hypoglycemic symptoms.
[d] Event requiring another person to administer a resuscitative action.
[e] Rate of documented symptomatic hypoglycemia for active controls 18% (glimepiride) and 2% (sitagliptin).

Pneumonia
In the pool of 7 placebo- and active-controlled trials, the adverse reaction of pneumonia was reported more frequently in patients receiving TANZEUM (1.8%) than in patients in the all-comparators group (0.8%). More cases of pneumonia in the group receiving TANZEUM were serious (0.4% for TANZEUM versus 0.1% for all comparators).

Atrial Fibrillation/Flutter
In the pool of 7 placebo- and active-controlled trials, adverse reactions of atrial fibrillation (1.0%) and atrial flutter (0.2%) were reported more frequently for TANZEUM than for all comparators (0.5% and 0%, respectively). In both groups, patients with events were generally male, older, and had underlying renal impairment or cardiac disease (e.g., history of arrhythmia, palpitations, congestive heart failure, cardiomyopathy, etc.).

Appendicitis
In the pool of placebo- and active-controlled trials, serious events of appendicitis occurred in 0.3% of patients treated with TANZEUM compared with 0% among all comparators.
Immunogenicity
In the pool of 7 placebo- and active-controlled trials, 116 (5.5%) of 2,098 patients exposed to TANZEUM tested positive for anti-albiglutide antibodies at any time during the trials. None of these antibodies were shown to neutralize the activity of albiglutide in an in vitro bioassay. Presence of antibody did not correlate with reduced efficacy as measured by HbA1c and fasting plasma glucose or specific adverse reactions.
Consistent with the high homology of albiglutide with human GLP-1, the majority of patients (approximately 79%) with anti-albiglutide antibodies also tested positive for anti-GLP-1 antibodies; none were neutralizing. A minority of patients (approximately 17%) who tested positive for anti-albiglutide antibodies also transiently tested positive for antibodies to human albumin.
The detection of antibody formation is highly dependent on the sensitivity and specificity of the assay. Additionally, the observed incidence of antibody (including neutralizing antibody) positivity in an assay may be influenced by several factors including assay methodology, sample handling, timing of sample collection, concomitant medications, and underlying disease. For these reasons, the incidence of antibodies to albiglutide cannot be directly compared with the incidence of antibodies of other products.
Liver Enzyme Abnormalities
In the pool of placebo- and active-controlled trials, a similar proportion of patients experienced at least one event of alanine aminotransferase (ALT) increase of 3-fold or greater above the upper limit of normal (0.9% and 0.9% for all comparators versus TANZEUM). Three subjects on TANZEUM and one subject in the all-comparator group experienced at least one event of ALT increase of 10-fold or greater above the upper limit of normal. In one of the 3 cases an alternate etiology was identified to explain the rise in liver enzyme (acute viral hepatitis). In one case, insufficient information was obtained to establish or refute a drug-related causality. In the third case, elevation in ALT (10 times the upper limit of normal) was accompanied by an increase in total bilirubin (4 times the upper limit of normal) and occurred 8 days after the first dose of TANZEUM. The etiology of hepatocellular injury was possibly related to TANZEUM but direct attribution to TANZEUM was confounded by the presence of gallstone disease diagnosed on ultrasound 3 weeks after the event.
Gamma Glutamyltransferase (GGT) Increase
In the pool of placebo-controlled trials, the adverse event of increased GGT occurred more frequently in the group treated with TANZEUM (0.9% and 1.5% for placebo versus TANZEUM).
Heart Rate Increase
In the pool of placebo-controlled trials, mean heart rate in patients treated with TANZEUM was higher by an average of 1 to 2 bpm compared with mean heart rate in patients treated with placebo across study visits. The long-term clinical effects of the increase in heart rate have not been established [see Warnings and Precautions (5.6)].

7 DRUG INTERACTIONS

TANZEUM did not affect the absorption of orally administered medications tested in clinical pharmacology studies to any clinically relevant degree [see Clinical Pharmacology (12.3)]. However, TANZEUM causes a delay of gastric emptying, and thereby has the potential to impact the absorption of concomitantly administered oral medications. Caution should be exercised when oral medications are concomitantly administered with TANZEUM.

8 USE IN SPECIFIC POPULATIONS
8.1 Pregnancy
Pregnancy Category C
There are no adequate and well-controlled studies of TANZEUM in pregnant women. Nonclinical studies have shown reproductive toxicity, but not teratogenicity, in mice treated with albiglutide at up to 39 times human exposure resulting from the maximum recommended dose of 50 mg/week, based on AUC [see Nonclinical Toxicology (13.1, 13.3)]. TANZEUM should not be used during pregnancy unless the expected benefit outweighs the potential risks.
Due to the long washout period for TANZEUM, consider stopping TANZEUM at least 1 month before a planned pregnancy.
There are no data on the effects of TANZEUM on human fertility. Studies in mice showed no effects on fertility [see Nonclinical Toxicology (13.1)]. The potential risk to human fertility is unknown.
8.3 Nursing Mothers
There are no adequate data to support the use of TANZEUM during lactation in humans.

It is not known if TANZEUM is excreted into human milk during lactation. Given that TANZEUM is an albumin-based protein therapeutic, it is likely to be present in human milk. Decreased body weight in offspring was observed in mice treated with TANZEUM during gestation and lactation [see Nonclinical Toxicology (13.3)]. A decision should be made whether to discontinue nursing or to discontinue TANZEUM, taking into account the importance of the drug to the mother and the potential risks to the infant.

8.4   Pediatric Use
Safety and effectiveness of TANZEUM have not been established in pediatric patients (younger than 18 years).

8.5   Geriatric Use
Of the total number of patients (N = 2,365) in 8 Phase III clinical trials who received TANZEUM, 19% (N = 444) were 65 years and older, and <3% (N = 52) were 75 years and older. No overall differences in safety or effectiveness were observed between these patients and younger patients, but greater sensitivity of some older individuals cannot be ruled out.

8.6   Renal Impairment
Of the total number of patients (N = 2,365) in 8 Phase III clinical trials who received TANZEUM, 54% (N = 1,267) had mild renal impairment (eGFR 60 to 89 mL/min/1.73 m²), 12% (N = 275) had moderate renal impairment (eGFR 30 to 59 mL/min/1.73 m²) and 1% (N = 19) had severe renal impairment (eGFR 15 to <30 mL/min/1.73 m²).
No dosage adjustment is required in patients with mild (eGFR 60 to 89 mL/min/1.73 m²), moderate (eGFR 30 to 59 mL/min/1.73 m²), or severe (eGFR 15 to <30 mL/min/1.73 m²) renal impairment.
Efficacy of TANZEUM in patients with type 2 diabetes and renal impairment is described elsewhere [see Clinical Studies (14.3)]. There is limited clinical experience in patients with severe renal impairment (19 subjects). The frequency of GI events increased as renal function declined. For patients with mild, moderate, or severe impairment, the respective event rates were: diarrhea (6%, 13%, 21%), nausea (3%, 5%, 16%), and vomiting (1%, 2%, 5%). Therefore, caution is recommended when initiating or escalating doses of TANZEUM in patients with renal impairment [see Dosage and Administration (2.3), Warnings and Precautions (5.5), Clinical Pharmacology (12.3)].

10   OVERDOSAGE
No data are available with regard to overdosage in humans. Anticipated symptoms of an overdose may be severe nausea and vomiting.
In the event of an overdose, appropriate supportive treatment should be initiated as dictated by the patient's clinical signs and symptoms. A prolonged period of observation and treatment for these symptoms may be necessary, taking into account the half-life of TANZEUM (5 days).

11   DESCRIPTION
TANZEUM is a GLP-1 receptor agonist, a recombinant fusion protein comprised of 2 tandem copies of modified human GLP-1 genetically fused in tandem to human albumin. The human GLP-1 fragment sequence 7 – 36 has been modified with a glycine substituted for the naturally-occurring alanine at position 8 in order to confer resistance to dipeptidylpeptidase IV (DPP-IV) mediated proteolysis. The human albumin moiety of the recombinant fusion protein, together with the DPP-IV resistance, extends the half-life allowing once-weekly dosing. TANZEUM has a molecular weight of 72,970 Daltons.
TANZEUM is produced by a strain of Saccharomyces cerevisiae modified to express the therapeutic protein.
TANZEUM 30-mg Pen for injection (for subcutaneous use) contains 40.3 mg lyophilized albiglutide and 0.65 mL Water for Injection diluent designed to deliver a dose of 30 mg in a volume of 0.5 mL after reconstitution.
TANZEUM 50-mg Pen for injection (for subcutaneous use) contains 67 mg lyophilized albiglutide and 0.65 mL Water for Injection diluent designed to deliver a dose of 50 mg in a volume of 0.5 mL after reconstitution.
The lyophilized powder of both dose strengths is white to yellow in color and the solvent is a clear and colorless solution. The reconstituted solution is yellow in color.
Inactive ingredients include 153 mM mannitol, 0.01% (w/w) polysorbate 80, 10 mM sodium phosphate, and 117 mM trehalose dihydrate. TANZEUM does not contain a preservative.

12   CLINICAL PHARMACOLOGY
12.1   Mechanism of Action
TANZEUM is an agonist of the GLP-1 receptor and augments glucose-dependent insulin secretion. TANZEUM also slows gastric emptying.
12.2   Pharmacodynamics
TANZEUM lowers fasting glucose and reduces postprandial glucose excursions in patients with type 2 diabetes mellitus. The majority of the observed reduction in fasting plasma glucose occurs after a single dose, consistent with the pharmacokinetic profile of albiglutide. In a Phase II trial in Jap-

anese patients with type 2 diabetes mellitus who received TANZEUM 30 mg, a reduction (22%) in postprandial glucose $AUC_{(0-3\ h)}$ was observed at steady state (Week 16) compared with placebo following a mixed meal.
A single dose of TANZEUM 50 mg subcutaneous (SC) did not impair glucagon response to low glucose concentrations.
Gastric Motility
TANZEUM slowed gastric emptying compared with placebo for both solids and liquids when albiglutide 100 mg (2 times the maximum approved dosage) was administered as a single dose in healthy subjects.
Cardiac Electrophysiology
At doses up to the maximum recommended dose (50 mg), TANZEUM does not prolong QTc to any clinically relevant extent.
12.3   Pharmacokinetics
Absorption
Following SC administration of a single 30-mg dose to subjects with type 2 diabetes mellitus, maximum concentrations of albiglutide were reached at 3 to 5 days post-dosing. The mean peak concentration (C_{max}) and mean area under the time-concentration curve (AUC) of albiglutide were 1.74 mcg/mL and 465 mcg.h/mL, respectively, following a single dose of 30 mg albiglutide in type 2 diabetes mellitus subjects. Steady-state exposures are achieved following 4 to 5 weeks of once-weekly administration. Exposures at the 30-mg and 50-mg dose levels were consistent with a dose-proportional increase. Similar exposure is achieved with SC administration of albiglutide in the abdomen, thigh, or upper arm. The absolute bioavailability of albiglutide following SC administration has not been evaluated.
Distribution
The mean estimate of apparent volume of distribution of albiglutide following SC administration is 11 L. As albiglutide is an albumin fusion molecule, plasma protein binding has not been assessed.
Metabolism
Albiglutide is a protein for which the expected metabolic pathway is degradation to small peptides and individual amino acids by ubiquitous proteolytic enzymes. Classical biotransformation studies have not been performed. Because albiglutide is an albumin fusion protein, it likely follows a metabolic pathway similar to native human serum albumin which is catabolized primarily in the vascular endothelium.
Elimination
The mean apparent clearance of albiglutide is 67 mL/h with an elimination half-life of approximately 5 days, making albiglutide suitable for once-weekly administration.
Specific Patient Populations
Age, Gender, Race, and Body Weight: Based on the population pharmacokinetic analysis with data collected from 1,113 subjects, age, gender, race, and body weight had no clinically relevant effect on the pharmacokinetics of albiglutide.
Pediatric: No pharmacokinetic data are available in pediatric patients.

Renal: In a population pharmacokinetic analysis including a Phase III trial in patients with mild, moderate, and severe renal impairment, exposures were increased by approximately 30% to 40% in severe renal impairment compared with those observed in type 2 diabetic patients with normal renal function.
Hepatic: No clinical trials were conducted to examine the effects of mild, moderate, or severe hepatic impairment on the pharmacokinetics of albiglutide. Therapeutic proteins such as albiglutide are catabolized by widely distributed proteolytic enzymes, which are not restricted to hepatic tissue; therefore, changes in hepatic function are unlikely to have any effect on the elimination of albiglutide.
Drug Interactions
In multiple-dose, drug-drug interaction trials no significant change in systemic exposures of the co-administered drugs were observed, except simvastatin (see Table 3). When albiglutide was co-administered with simvastatin, C_{max} of simvastatin and its active metabolite simvastatin acid was increased by approximately 18% and 98%, respectively. In the same trial, AUC of simvastatin decreased by 40% and AUC of simvastatin acid increased by 36%. Clinical relevance of these changes has not been established (see Table 3).
Additionally, no clinically relevant pharmacodynamic effects on luteinizing hormone, follicle-stimulating hormone, or progesterone were observed when albiglutide and a combination oral contraceptive were co-administered. Albiglutide did not significantly alter the pharmacodynamic effects of warfarin as measured by the international normalized ratio (INR).
[See table 3 above]

13   NONCLINICAL TOXICOLOGY
13.1   Carcinogenesis, Mutagenesis, Impairment of Fertility
As albiglutide is a recombinant protein, no genotoxicity studies have been conducted.
Carcinogenicity studies have not been performed with albiglutide because such studies are not technically feasible due to the rapid development of drug-clearing, anti-drug antibodies in rodents. Thyroid C-cell tumors were observed in 2-year rodent carcinogenicity studies with some GLP-1 receptor agonists. The clinical relevance of rodent thyroid findings observed with GLP-1 receptor agonists is unknown. In a mouse fertility study, males were treated with SC doses of 5, 15, or 50 mg/kg/day for 7 days prior to cohabitation with females, and continuing through mating. In a separate fertility study, females were treated with SC doses of 5, 15, or 50 mg/kg/day for 7 days prior to cohabitation with males, and continuing through mating. Reductions in estrous cycles were observed at 50 mg/kg/day, a dose associated with maternal toxicity (body weight loss and reduced food consumption). There were no effects on mating or fertility in either sex at doses up to 50 mg/kg/day (up to 39 times clinical exposure based on AUC).
13.3   Reproductive and Developmental Toxicity
In order to minimize the impact of the drug-clearing, anti-drug antibody response, reproductive and developmental

Table 3. Effect of Albiglutide on Systemic Exposure of Co-administered Drugs

Co-administered Drug	Dose of Co-administered Drug[a]	Dose of TANZEUM	Geometric Mean Ratio (Ratio +/- Co-administered Drug) No Effect = 1		
			Analyte	AUC (90% CI)[b]	C_{max} (90% CI)
No dose adjustments of co-administered drug required for the following:					
Simvastatin	80 mg	50 mg QW for 5 weeks	Simvastatin	0.60 (0.52 – 0.69)	1.18 (1.02 – 1.38)
			Simvastatin acid	1.36 (1.19 – 1.55)	1.98 (1.75 – 2.25)
Digoxin	0.5 mg	50 mg QW for 5 weeks	Digoxin	1.09 (1.01 – 1.18)	1.11 (0.98 – 1.26)
Oral contraceptive[c]	0.035 mg ethinyl estradiol and 0.5 mg norethindrone	50 mg QW for 4 weeks	Norethindrone	1.00 (0.96 – 1.04)	1.04 (0.98 – 1.10)
			Levonorgestrel	1.09 (1.06 – 1.14)	1.20 (1.11 – 1.29)
Warfarin	25 mg	50 mg QW for 5 weeks	R-Warfarin	1.02 (0.98 – 1.07)	0.94 (0.89 – 0.99)
			S-Warfarin	0.99 (0.95 – 1.03)	0.93 (0.87 – 0.98)

QW = Once weekly.
[a] Single dose unless otherwise noted.
[b] AUC_{inf} for drugs given as a single dose and AUC24h for drugs given as multiple doses.
[c] Subjects received low-dose oral contraceptive for two 28-day treatment cycles (21 days active/7 days placebo).

Table 5. Results at Week 104 (LOCF[a]) in a Trial Comparing TANZEUM with Placebo as Add-on Therapy in Patients Inadequately Controlled on Metformin

	TANZEUM + Metformin	Placebo + Metformin	Sitagliptin + Metformin	Glimepiride + Metformin
ITT[a] (N)	297	100	300	302
HbA1c (%)				
Baseline (mean)	8.1	8.1	8.1	8.1
Change at Week 104[b]	-0.6	+0.3	-0.3	-0.4
Difference from placebo + metformin[b] (95% CI)	-0.9 (-1.16, -0.65)[c]			
Difference from sitagliptin + metformin[b] (95% CI)	-0.4 (-0.53, -0.17)[c]			
Difference from glimepiride + metformin[b] (95% CI)	-0.3 (-0.45, -0.09)[c]			
Proportion achieving HbA1c <7%	39	16	32	31
FPG (mg/dL)				
Baseline (mean)	165	162	165	168
Change at Week 104[b]	-18	+10	-2	-8
Difference from placebo + metformin[b] (95% CI)	-28 (-39, -16)[c]			
Difference from sitagliptin + metformin[b] (95% CI)	-16 (-24, -8)[c]			
Difference from glimepiride + metformin[b] (95% CI)	-10 (-18, -2)[c]			
Body Weight (kg)				
Baseline (mean)	90	92	90	92
Change at Week 104[b]	-1.2	-1.0	-0.9	+1.2
Difference from placebo + metformin[b] (95% CI)	-0.2 (-1.1, 0.7)			
Difference from sitagliptin + metformin[b] (95% CI)	-0.4 (-1.0, 0.3)			
Difference from glimepiride + metformin[b] (95% CI)	-2.4 (-3.0, -1.7)[c]			

[a] Intent-to-treat population. Last observation carried forward (LOCF) was used to impute missing data. Data post-onset of rescue therapy are treated as missing. At Week 104, primary efficacy data was imputed for 76%, 46%, 55%, and 51% of individuals randomized to placebo, TANZEUM, sitagliptin, and glimepiride, respectively.
[b] Least squares mean adjusted for baseline value and stratification factors.
[c] P <0.0137 for treatment difference.

toxicity assessments in the mouse were partitioned to limit the dosing period to no more than approximately 15 days in each study.

In pregnant mice given SC doses of 1, 5, or 50 mg/kg/day from gestation Day 1 to 6, there were no adverse effects on early embryonic development through implantation at 50 mg/kg/day (39 times clinical exposure based on AUC).

In pregnant mice given SC doses of 1, 5, or 50 mg/kg/day from gestation Day 6 through 15 (organogenesis), embryo-fetal lethality (post-implantation loss) and bent (wavy) ribs were observed at 50 mg/kg/day (39 times clinical exposure based on AUC), a dose associated with maternal toxicity (body weight loss and reduced food consumption).

Pregnant mice were given SC doses of 1, 5, or 50 mg/kg/day from gestation Day 6 to 17. Offspring of pregnant mice given 50 mg/kg/day (39 times clinical exposure based on AUC), a dose associated with maternal toxicity, had reduced body weight pre-weaning, dehydration and coldness, and a delay in balanopreputial separation.

Pregnant mice were given SC doses of 1, 5, or 50 mg/kg/day from gestation Day 15 to lactation Day 10. Increased mortality and morbidity were seen at all doses (≥1 mg/kg/day) in lactating females in mouse pre- and postnatal development studies. Mortalities have not been observed in previous toxicology studies in non-lactating or non-pregnant mice, nor in pregnant mice. These findings are consistent with lactational ileus syndrome which has been previously reported in mice. Since the relative stress of lactation energy demands is lower in humans than mice and humans have large energy reserves, the mortalities observed in lactating mice are of questionable relevance to humans. The offspring had decreased pre-weaning body weight which reversed post-weaning in males but not females at ≥5 mg/kg/day (2.2 times clinical exposure based on AUC) with no other effects on development. Low levels of albiglutide were detected in plasma of offspring.

Lactating mice were given SC doses of 1, 5, or 50 mg/kg/day from lactation Day 7 to 21 (weaning) under conditions that limit the impact of lactational ileus (increased caloric intake and culling of litters). Doses ≥1 mg/kg/day (exposures below clinical AUC) caused reduced weight gain in the pups during the treatment period.

14   CLINICAL STUDIES

TANZEUM has been studied as monotherapy and in combination with metformin, metformin and a sulfonylurea, a thiazolidinedione (with and without metformin), and insulin glargine (with or without oral anti-diabetic drugs). The efficacy of TANZEUM was compared with placebo, glimepiride, pioglitazone, liraglutide, sitagliptin, insulin lispro, and insulin glargine.

Trials evaluated the use of TANZEUM 30 mg and 50 mg. Five of the 8 trials allowed optional uptitration of TANZEUM from 30 mg to 50 mg if glycemic response with 30 mg was inadequate.

In patients with type 2 diabetes mellitus, TANZEUM produced clinically relevant reduction from baseline in HbA1c compared with placebo. No overall differences in glycemic effectiveness or body weight were observed across demographic subgroups (age, gender, race/ethnicity, duration of diabetes).

14.1   Monotherapy
The efficacy of TANZEUM as monotherapy was evaluated in a 52-week, randomized, double-blind, placebo-controlled, multicenter trial. In this trial, 296 patients with type 2 diabetes inadequately controlled on diet and exercise were randomized (1:1:1) to TANZEUM 30 mg SC once weekly, TANZEUM 30 mg SC once weekly uptitrated to 50 mg once weekly at Week 12, or placebo. The mean age of participants was 53 years, 55% of patients were men, the mean duration of diabetes was 4 years, and the mean baseline eGFR was 84 mL/min/1.73 m^2. Primary and secondary efficacy results are presented in Table 4. Figure 1 shows the mean adjusted changes in HbA1c from baseline across study visits.

Compared with placebo, treatment with TANZEUM 30 mg or 50 mg resulted in statistically significant reductions in HbA1c from baseline at Week 52 (see Table 4). The adjusted mean change in weight from baseline did not differ significantly between TANZEUM (-0.4 to -0.9 kg) and placebo (-0.7 kg) at Week 52.

Table 4. Results at Week 52 (LOCF[a]) in a Trial of TANZEUM as Monotherapy

	Placebo	TANZEUM 30 mg Weekly	TANZEUM 50 mg Weekly
ITT[a] (N)	99	100	97
HbA1c (%)			
Baseline (mean)	8.0	8.1	8.2
Change at Week 52[b]	+0.2	-0.7	-0.9
Difference from placebo[b] (95% CI)		-0.8 (-1.1, -0.6)[c]	-1.0 (-1.3, -0.8)[c]
Patients (%) achieving HbA1c <7%	21	49	40
FPG (mg/dL)			
Baseline (mean)	163	164	171
Change at Week 52[b]	+18	-16	-25
Difference from placebo[b] (95% CI)		-34 (-46, -22)[c]	-43 (-55, -31)[c]

[a] Intent-to-treat population. Last observation carried forward (LOCF) was used to impute missing data. Data post-onset of rescue therapy are treated as missing. At Week 52, primary efficacy data was imputed for 63%, 34%, and 41% of individuals randomized to placebo, TANZEUM 30 mg, and TANZEUM 50 mg.
[b] Least squares mean adjusted for baseline value and stratification factors.
[c] P <0.0001 for treatment difference.

Figure 1. Mean HbA1c Change from Baseline (ITT Population-LOCF) in a Trial of TANZEUM as Monotherapy

14.2   Combination Therapy
Add-on to Metformin
The efficacy of TANZEUM was evaluated in a 104-week randomized, double-blind, multicenter trial in 999 patients with type 2 diabetes mellitus inadequately controlled on background metformin therapy (≥1,500 mg daily). In this trial, TANZEUM 30 mg SC weekly (with optional uptitration to 50 mg weekly after a minimum of 4 weeks) was compared with placebo, sitagliptin 100 mg daily, or glimepiride 2 mg daily (with optional titration to 4 mg daily). The mean age of participants was 55 years, 48% of participants were men, the mean duration of type 2 diabetes was 6 years, and the mean baseline eGFR was 86 mL/min/1.73 m^2. Results of the primary and secondary analyses are presented in Table 5. Figure 2 shows the mean adjusted changes in HbA1c across study visits.

Reduction in HbA1c from baseline achieved with TANZEUM was significantly greater than HbA1c reduction achieved with placebo, sitagliptin, and glimepiride at Week 104 (see Table 5). The difference in body weight change from baseline between TANZEUM and glimepiride was significant at Week 104.
[See table 5 above]

Figure 2. Mean HbA1c Over Time (ITT Population-LOCF) in a Trial Comparing TANZEUM with Placebo as Add-on Therapy in Patients Inadequately Controlled on Metformin

Add-on to Pioglitazone
The efficacy of TANZEUM was evaluated in a 52-week randomized, double-blind, multicenter trial in 299 patients with type 2 diabetes mellitus inadequately controlled on pioglitazone ≥30 mg daily (with or without metformin ≥1,500 mg daily). Patients were randomized to receive TANZEUM 30 mg SC weekly or placebo. The mean age of participants was 55 years, 60% of patients were men, the mean duration of type 2 diabetes was 8 years, and the mean baseline eGFR was 83 mL/min/1.73 m^2. Results of the primary and secondary analyses are presented in Table 6. Compared with placebo, treatment with TANZEUM resulted in a statistically significant reduction in HbA1c from baseline at Week 52 (see Table 6). The adjusted mean change from baseline in weight did not differ significantly between TANZEUM (+0.3 kg) and placebo (+0.5 kg) at Week 52.

Table 6. Results at Week 52 (LOCF[a]) in a Trial Comparing TANZEUM with Placebo as Add-on Therapy in Patients Inadequately Controlled on Pioglitazone (with or without Metformin)

	TANZEUM + Pioglitazone (with or without Metformin)	Placebo + Pioglitazone (with or without Metformin)
ITT[a] (N)	150	149
HbA1c (%)		
Baseline (mean)	8.1	8.1
Change at Week 52[b]	-0.8	-0.1
Difference from placebo + pioglitazone[b] (95% CI)	-0.8 (-0.95, -0.56)[c]	
Proportion Achieving HbA1c <7%	44	15
FPG (mg/dL)		
Baseline (mean)	165	167
Change at Week 52[b]	-23	+6
Difference from placebo + pioglitazone[b] (95% CI)	-30 (-39, -20)[c]	

[a] Intent-to-treat population. Last observation carried forward (LOCF) was used to impute missing data. Data post-onset of rescue therapy are treated as missing. At Week 52, primary efficacy data was imputed for 58% and 32% of individuals randomized to placebo and TANZEUM, respectively.
[b] Least squares mean adjusted for baseline value and stratification factors.
[c] P <0.0001 for treatment difference.

Add-on to Metformin Plus Sulfonylurea

The efficacy of TANZEUM was evaluated in a 52-week randomized, double-blind, multicenter trial in 657 patients with type 2 diabetes mellitus inadequately controlled on metformin (≥1,500 mg daily) and glimepiride (4 mg daily). Patients were randomized to receive TANZEUM 30 mg SC weekly (with optional uptitration to 50 mg weekly after a minimum of 4 weeks), placebo, or pioglitazone 30 mg daily (with optional titration to 45 mg/day). The mean age of participants was 55 years, 53% of patients were men, the mean duration of type 2 diabetes was 9 years, and the mean baseline eGFR was 84 mL/min/1.73 m[2]. Results of the primary and main secondary analyses are presented in Table 7.

Treatment with TANZEUM resulted in statistically significant reductions in HbA1c from baseline compared with placebo (see Table 7). Treatment with TANZEUM did not meet the pre-specified, non-inferiority margin (0.3%) against pioglitazone. In this trial, TANZEUM provided less HbA1c reduction than pioglitazone and the treatment difference was statistically significant (see Table 7). The change from baseline in body weight for TANZEUM did not differ significantly from placebo but was significantly different compared with pioglitazone (see Table 7).
[See table 7 above]

Combination Therapy: Active-controlled Trial versus Liraglutide

The efficacy of TANZEUM was evaluated in a 32-week, randomized, open-label, liraglutide-controlled, non-inferiority trial in 805 patients with type 2 diabetes mellitus inadequately controlled on monotherapy or combination oral antidiabetic therapy (metformin, thiazolidinedione, sulfonylurea, or a combination of these). Patients were randomized to TANZEUM 30 mg SC weekly (with uptitration to 50 mg weekly at Week 6) or liraglutide 1.8 mg daily (titrated up from 0.6 mg at Week 1, and 1.2 mg at Week 1 to Week 2). The mean age of participants was 56 years, 50% of patients were men, the mean duration of type 2 diabetes was 8 years, and the mean baseline eGFR was 95 mL/min/1.73 m[2]. Results of the primary and main secondary analyses are presented in Table 8.

The between-treatment difference of 0.2% with 95% confidence interval (0.08, 0.34) between TANZEUM and liraglutide did not meet the pre-specified, non-inferiority margin (0.3%). In this trial, TANZEUM provided less HbA1c reduction than liraglutide and the treatment difference was statistically significant (see Table 8).

Table 7. Results at Week 52 (LOCF[a]) in a Trial Comparing TANZEUM with Placebo as Add-on Therapy in Patients Inadequately Controlled on Metformin Plus Sulfonylurea

	TANZEUM + Metformin + Glimepiride	Placebo + Metformin + Glimepiride	Pioglitazone + Metformin + Glimepiride
ITT[a] (N)	269	115	273
HbA1c (%)			
Baseline (mean)	8.2	8.3	8.3
Change at Week 52[b]	-0.6	+0.3	-0.8
Difference from placebo + met + glim[b] (95% CI)	-0.9 (-1.07, -0.68)[c]		
Difference from pioglitazone + met + glim[b] (95% CI)	0.25 (0.10, 0.40)[d]		
Proportion achieving HbA1c <7%	30	9	35
FPG (mg/dL)			
Baseline (mean)	171	174	177
Change at Week 52[b]	-12	+12	-31
Difference from placebo + met + glim[b] (95% CI)	-24 (-34, -14)[c]		
Difference from pioglitazone + met + glim[b] (95% CI)	19 (11, 27)[c]		
Body Weight (kg)			
Baseline (mean)	91	90	91
Change at Week 52[b]	-0.4	-0.4	+4.4
Difference from placebo + met + glim[b] (95% CI)	-0.0 (-0.9, 0.8)		
Difference from pioglitazone + met + glim[b] (95% CI)	-4.9 (-5.5, -4.2)[c]		

[a] Intent-to-treat population. Last observation carried forward (LOCF) was used to impute missing data. Data post-onset of rescue therapy are treated as missing. At Week 52, primary efficacy data was imputed for 70%, 35%, and 34% of individuals randomized to placebo, TANZEUM, and pioglitazone.
[b] Least squares mean adjusted for baseline value and stratification factors.
[c] P <0.0001 for treatment difference.
[d] Did not meet non-inferiority margin of 0.3%.

Table 8. Results of Controlled Trial of TANZEUM versus Liraglutide at Week 32 (LOCF[a])

	TANZEUM	Liraglutide
ITT[a] (N)	402	403
HbA1c (%)		
Baseline (mean)	8.2%	8.2%
Change at Week 32[b]	-0.8	-1.0
Difference from liraglutide[b] (95% CI)	0.2 (0.08, 0.34)[c]	
Proportion achieving HbA1c <7%	42%	52%
FPG (mg/dL)		
Baseline (mean)	169	167
Change at Week 32[b]	-22	-30
Difference from liraglutide[b] (95% CI)	8 (3, 14)[d]	
Body Weight (kg)		
Baseline (mean)	92	93
Change at Week 32[b]	-0.6	-2.2
Difference from liraglutide[b] (95% CI)	1.6 (1.1, 2.1)[d]	

[a] Intent-to-treat population. Last observation carried forward (LOCF) was used to impute missing data. Data post-onset of rescue therapy are treated as missing. At Week 32, primary efficacy data was imputed for 31% and 24% of individuals randomized to TANZEUM and liraglutide.
[b] Least squares mean adjusted for baseline value and stratification factors.
[c] Did not meet non-inferiority margin of 0.3%.
[d] P <0.005 for treatment difference in favor of liraglutide.

Combination Therapy: Active-controlled Trial versus Basal Insulin

The efficacy of TANZEUM was evaluated in a 52-week, randomized (2:1), open-label, insulin glargine-controlled, non-inferiority trial in 735 patients with type 2 diabetes mellitus inadequately controlled on metformin ≥1,500 mg daily (with or without sulfonylurea). Patients were randomized to receive TANZEUM 30 mg SC weekly (with optional uptitration to 50 mg weekly) or insulin glargine (started at 10 units and titrated weekly per prescribing information). The primary endpoint was change in HbA1c from baseline compared with insulin glargine. The starting total daily dose of insulin glargine ranged between 2 and 40 units (median daily dose of 10 units) and ranged between 3 and 230 units (median daily dose of 30 units) at Week 52. Seventy-seven percent of patients treated with TANZEUM were uptitrated to 50 mg SC weekly. The mean age of participants was 56 years, 56% of patients were men, the mean duration of type 2 diabetes was 9 years, and the mean baseline eGFR was 85 mL/min/1.73 m[2]. Results of the primary and main secondary analyses are presented in Table 9.

The between-treatment difference of 0.1% with 95% confidence interval (-0.04%, 0.27%) for TANZEUM and insulin glargine met the pre-specified, non-inferiority margin (0.3%). A mean decrease in body weight was observed for TANZEUM compared with a mean increase in body weight for insulin glargine, and the difference in weight change was statistically significant (see Table 9).
[See table 9 at top of next page]

Figure 3. Mean HbA1c Change from Baseline (Completers) in a Trial Comparing TANZEUM with Insulin Glargine as Add-on Therapy in Patients Inadequately Controlled on Metformin (with or without a Sulfonylurea)

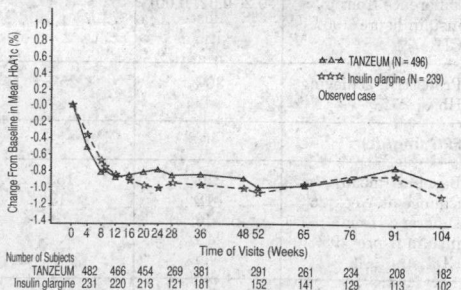

Combination Therapy: Active-controlled Trial versus Prandial Insulin

The efficacy of TANZEUM was evaluated in a 26-week, randomized, open-label, multicenter, non-inferiority trial in 563 patients with type 2 diabetes mellitus inadequately controlled on insulin glargine (started at 10 units and titrated to ≥20 units per day). Patients were randomized to receive TANZEUM 30 mg SC once weekly (with uptitration to 50 mg if inadequately controlled after Week 8) or insulin lispro (administered daily at meal times, started according to standard of care and titrated to effect). At Week 26, the mean daily dose of insulin glargine was 53 IU for TANZEUM and 51 IU for insulin lispro. The mean daily dose of insulin lispro at Week 26 was 31 IU, and 69% of patients treated with TANZEUM were on 50 mg weekly. The mean age of participants was 56 years, 47% of patients were men, the mean duration of type 2 diabetes was 11 years, and the mean baseline eGFR was 91 mL/min/1.73 m[2]. Results of

Table 9. Results at Week 52 (LOCF[a]) in a Trial Comparing TANZEUM with Insulin Glargine as Add-on Therapy in Patients Inadequately Controlled on Metformin ± Sulfonylurea

	TANZEUM + Metformin (with or without Sulfonylurea)	Insulin Glargine + Metformin (with or without Sulfonylurea)
ITT[a] (N)	496	239
HbA1c (%)		
Baseline (mean)	8.3	8.4
Change at Week 52[b]	-0.7	-0.8
Difference from insulin glargine[b] (95% CI)	0.1(-0.04, 0.27)[c]	
Proportion achieving HbA1c <7%	32	33
FPG (mg/dL)		
Baseline (mean)	169	175
Change at Week 52[b]	-16	-37
Difference from insulin glargine[b] (95% CI)	21 (14, 29)[d]	
Body Weight (kg)		
Baseline (mean)	95	95
Change at Week 52[b]	-1.1	1.6
Difference from insulin glargine[b] (95% CI)	-2.6 (-3.2, -2.0)[e]	

[a] Intent-to-treat population. Last observation carried forward (LOCF) was used to impute missing data. Data post-onset of rescue therapy are treated as missing. At Week 52, primary efficacy data was imputed for 41% and 36% of individuals randomized to TANZEUM and insulin glargine.
[b] Least squares mean adjusted for baseline value and stratification factors.
[c] Met non-inferiority margin of 0.3%.
[d] P <0.0001 in favor of insulin glargine.
[e] P <0.0001.

the primary and main secondary analyses are presented in Table 10. Figure 4 shows the mean adjusted changes in HbA1c from baseline across study visits.

The between-treatment difference of -0.2% with 95% confidence interval (-0.32%, 0.00%) between albiglutide and insulin lispro met the pre-specified non-inferiority margin (0.4%). Treatment with TANZEUM resulted in a mean weight loss for TANZEUM compared with a mean weight gain for insulin lispro, and the difference between treatment groups was statistically significant (see Table 10).

Table 10. Results at Week 26 (LOCF[a]) in a Trial Comparing TANZEUM with Insulin Lispro as Add-On Therapy in Patients Inadequately Controlled on Insulin Glargine

	TANZEUM + Insulin Glargine	Insulin Lispro + Insulin Glargine
ITT[a] (N)	282	281
HbA1c (%)		
Baseline (mean)	8.5	8.4
Change at Week 26[b]	-0.8	-0.7
Difference from insulin lispro[b] (95% CI)	-0.2(-0.32, 0.00)[c]	
Proportion achieving HbA1c <7%	30%	25%
FPG (mg/dL)		
Baseline (mean)	153	153
Change at Week 26[b]	-18	-13
Difference from insulin lispro[b] (95% CI)	-5 (-13, 3)	
Body Weight (kg)		
Baseline (mean)	93	92
Change at Week 26[b]	-0.7	+0.8
Difference from insulin lispro[b] (95% CI)	-1.5 (-2.1, -1.0)[d]	

[a] Intent-to-treat population. Last observation carried forward (LOCF) was used to impute missing data. Data post-onset of rescue therapy are treated as missing. At Week 26, primary efficacy data was imputed for 29% and 29% of individuals randomized to TANZEUM and insulin lispro.
[b] Least squares mean adjusted for baseline value and stratification factors.
[c] Rules out a non-inferiority margin of 0.4%.
[d] P <0.0001 for treatment difference.

Figure 4. Mean HbA1c Change from Baseline (ITT-LOCF population) in a Trial Comparing TANZEUM with Insulin Lispro as Add-on Therapy in Patients Inadequately Controlled on Insulin Glargine

TANZEUM (N = 279)
Insulin Lispro (N = 278)
* P <0.0001 for TANZEUM versus comparator

14.3 Type 2 Diabetes Mellitus Patients with Renal Impairment

The efficacy of TANZEUM was evaluated in a 26-week, randomized, double-blind, active-controlled trial in 486 patients with mild (n = 250), moderate (n = 200), and severe renal impairment (n = 36) inadequately controlled on a current regimen of diet and exercise or other antidiabetic therapy. Patients were randomized to receive TANZEUM 30 mg SC weekly (with uptitration to 50 mg weekly if needed as early as Week 4) or sitagliptin. Sitagliptin was dosed according to renal function (100 mg, 50 mg, and 25 mg daily in mild, moderate, and severe renal impairment, respectively). The mean age of participants was 63 years, 54% of patients were men, the mean duration of type 2 diabetes was 11 years, and the mean baseline eGFR was 60 mL/min/1.73 m². Results of the primary and main secondary analyses are presented in Table 11. Treatment with TANZEUM resulted in statistically significant reductions in HbA1c from baseline at Week 26 compared with sitagliptin (see Table 11).

Table 11. Results at Week 26 (LOCF[a]) in a Trial Comparing TANZEUM with Sitagliptin in Patients with Renal Impairment

	TANZEUM	Sitagliptin
ITT[a] (N)	246	240
HbA1c (%)		
Baseline (mean)	8.1	8.2
Change at Week 26[b]	-0.8	-0.5
Difference from sitagliptin[b] (95% CI)	-0.3 (-0.49, -0.15)[c]	
Proportion achieving HbA1c <7%	43%	31%
FPG (mg/dL)		
Baseline (mean)	166	165
Change at Week 26[b]	-26	-4
Difference from sitagliptin[b] (95% CI)	-22 (-31, -13)[c]	
Body Weight (kg)		
Baseline (mean)	84	83
Change at Week 26[b]	-0.8	-0.2
Difference from sitagliptin[b] (95% CI)	-0.6 (-1.1, -0.1)[d]	

[a] Intent-to-treat population. Last observation carried forward (LOCF) was used to impute missing data. Data post-onset of rescue therapy are treated as missing. At Week 26 primary efficacy data was imputed for 17% and 25% of individuals randomized to TANZEUM and sitagliptin.
[b] Least squares mean adjusted for baseline value and stratification factors.
[c] P <0.0003 for treatment difference.
[d] P = 0.0281 for treatment difference.

16 HOW SUPPLIED/STORAGE AND HANDLING

16.1 How Supplied

TANZEUM is available in the following strengths and package size:

30 mg single-dose Pen (NDC 0173-0866-01):
- carton of 4 (containing four 29-gauge, 5-mm, thinwall needles): NDC 0173-0866-35

50 mg single-dose Pen (NDC 0173-0867-01):
- carton of 4 (containing four 29-gauge, 5-mm, thinwall needles): NDC 0173-0867-35

16.2 Storage and Handling

- Prior to dispensing: Store Pens in the refrigerator at 36°F to 46°F (2°C to 8°C). Pens may be stored refrigerated until the expiration date.
- Following dispensing: Store Pens in the refrigerator at 36°F to 46°F (2°C to 8°C). Patients may store Pens at room temperature not to exceed 86°F (30°C) for up to 4 weeks prior to use. Store Pens in the original carton until use.
- Do not freeze.
- Do not use past the expiration date.
- Use within 8 hours after reconstitution.

17 PATIENT COUNSELING INFORMATION

See FDA-approved patient labeling (Medication Guide and Instructions for Use). The Medication Guide is contained in a separate leaflet that accompanies the product.

- Inform patients about self-management practices, including the importance of proper storage of TANZEUM, injection technique, timing of dosage of TANZEUM and concomitant oral drugs, and recognition and management of hypoglycemia.
- Inform patients that thyroid C-cell tumors have been observed in rodents treated with some GLP-1 receptor agonists, and the human relevance of this finding is unknown. Counsel patients to report symptoms of thyroid tumors to their physician [see Warnings and Precautions (5.1)].
- Advise patients that persistent, severe abdominal pain that may radiate to the back and which may (or may not) be accompanied by vomiting is the hallmark symptom of acute pancreatitis. Instruct patients to discontinue TANZEUM promptly and to contact their physician if persistent, severe abdominal pain occurs [see Warnings and Precautions (5.2)].
- The risk of hypoglycemia is increased when TANZEUM is used in combination with an agent that induces hypoglycemia, such as sulfonylurea or insulin. Instructions for hypoglycemia should be reviewed with patients and reinforced when initiating therapy with TANZEUM, particularly when concomitantly administered with a sulfonylurea or insulin [see Warnings and Precautions (5.3)].
- Advise patients on the symptoms of hypersensitivity reactions and instruct them to stop taking TANZEUM and seek medical advice promptly if such symptoms occur [see Warnings and Precautions (5.4)].
- Instruct patients to read the Instructions for Use before starting therapy. Instruct patients on proper use, storage, and disposal of the pen [see How Supplied/Storage and Handling (16.2), Patient Instructions for Use].
- Instruct patients to read the Medication Guide before starting TANZEUM and to read again each time the prescription is renewed. Instruct patients to inform their doctor or pharmacist if they develop any unusual symptom, or if any known symptom persists or worsens.
- Inform patients not to take an extra dose of TANZEUM to make up for a missed dose. If a dose is missed, instruct

patients to take a dose as soon as possible within 3 days after the missed dose. Instruct patients to then take their next dose at their usual weekly time. If it has been longer than 3 days after the missed dose, instruct patients to wait and take TANZEUM at the next usual weekly time. TANZEUM is a trademark of the GSK group of companies.
Manufactured by GlaxoSmithKline LLC
Wilmington, DE 19808
U.S. Lic. No. 1727
Marketed by GlaxoSmithKline
Research Triangle Park, NC 27709
©2014, the GSK group of companies. All rights reserved.
TNZ:3PI

Medication Guide
TANZEUM™ (TAN-zee-um)
(albiglutide)
for injection, for subcutaneous use

Read this Medication Guide before you start taking TANZEUM and each time you get a refill. There may be new information. This information does not take the place of talking to your healthcare provider about your medical condition or your treatment.

What is the most important information I should know about TANZEUM?
Serious side effects may happen in people who take TANZEUM, including:
- **Possible thyroid tumors, including cancer.** Tell your healthcare provider if you get a lump or swelling in your neck, hoarseness, trouble swallowing, or shortness of breath. These may be symptoms of thyroid cancer. In studies with rats and mice, medicines that work like TANZEUM caused thyroid tumors, including thyroid cancer. It is not known if TANZEUM will cause thyroid tumors or a type of thyroid cancer called medullary thyroid carcinoma in people.
- **Do not use TANZEUM if you** or your family have ever had a type of thyroid cancer called medullary thyroid carcinoma (MTC) or if you have an endocrine system cancer called Multiple Endocrine Neoplasia syndrome type 2 (MEN 2).

What is TANZEUM?
TANZEUM is an injectable prescription medicine that may improve blood sugar (glucose) in adults with type 2 diabetes mellitus, and should be used along with diet and exercise.
- TANZEUM is not recommended as the first choice of medicine for treating diabetes.
- It is not known if TANZEUM can be used in people who previously had pancreatitis.
- TANZEUM is not a substitute for insulin and is not for use in people with type 1 diabetes or people with diabetic ketoacidosis.
- TANZEUM is not recommended in people with severe stomach or intestinal problems.
- It is not known if TANZEUM can be used with short-acting or rapid-acting (mealtime) insulin.
- It is not known if TANZEUM is safe and effective in children under 18 years of age.

Who should not use TANZEUM?
Do not use TANZEUM if:
- you or your family have ever had a type of thyroid cancer called medullary thyroid carcinoma (MTC) or if you have an endocrine system cancer called Multiple Endocrine Neoplasia syndrome type 2 (MEN 2)
- you are allergic to albiglutide or any of the ingredients in TANZEUM.

Before using TANZEUM, tell your healthcare provider about your medical conditions including, if you:
- have or have had problems with your pancreas, kidneys, or liver
- have severe problems with your stomach, such as slowed emptying of your stomach (gastroparesis) or problems with digesting food
- are pregnant or plan to become pregnant. It is not known if TANZEUM will harm your unborn baby. Tell your healthcare provider if you become pregnant while using TANZEUM.
- are breastfeeding or plan to breastfeed. It is not known if TANZEUM passes into your breast milk. You and your healthcare provider should decide if you will use TANZEUM or breastfeed. You should not do both without talking with your healthcare provider first.
- are taking a new prescription or over-the-counter medicines, vitamins, or herbal supplements.

How should I use TANZEUM?
- Read the **Instructions for Use** that comes with TANZEUM.
- Use TANZEUM exactly as your healthcare provider tells you to.

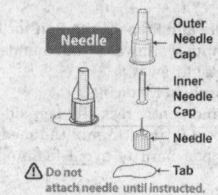

Needle — Outer Needle Cap
— Inner Needle Cap
— Needle
⚠ Do not attach needle until instructed. — Tab

Clean, Empty Cup

Clock Timer

Large Sharps Container
WARNING BIOHAZARD

- **Use TANZEUM 1 time each week on the same day each week at any time of the day.**
- You may change your day of the week as long as your last dose was given **4** or more days before.
- If you miss a dose of TANZEUM, take the missed dose of TANZEUM within **3** days after your usual scheduled day. If more than **3** days have gone by since your missed dose, wait until your next regularly scheduled weekly dose.
- TANZEUM may be taken with or without food.
- **Do not mix insulin and TANZEUM together in the same injection.**
- **Do not share your pen or needles with another person.** You may give another person an infection or get an infection from them.

What are the possible side effects of TANZEUM?
TANZEUM may cause serious side effects, including:
- **inflammation of your pancreas (pancreatitis).** Stop using TANZEUM and call your healthcare provider right away if you have severe pain in your stomach area (abdomen) that will not go away, with or without vomiting. You may feel pain that may go from your abdomen to your back.
- **low blood sugar (hypoglycemia).** Your risk is higher if you take TANZEUM with another medicine that can cause low blood sugar such as insulin or sulfonylurea. Signs and symptoms of low blood sugar may include:

• dizziness or light-headedness	• blurred vision	• anxiety, irritability, or mood changes
• sweating	• slurred speech	
• confusion	• shakiness	
• headache	• fast heart beat	• hunger
		• feeling jittery

- **allergic reactions.** Stop using TANZEUM and get medical help right away if you have any symptoms of an allergic reaction including itching, rash, or difficulty breathing.
- **kidney problems (kidney failure).** In people who have kidney problems, diarrhea, nausea, and vomiting may result in loss of fluids (dehydration) which may worsen kidney problems.

Common side effects of TANZEUM may include diarrhea, nausea, reactions at your injection site, cough, back pain, and cold or flu symptoms.
These are not all the possible side effects of TANZEUM. Call your doctor for medical advice about side effects. You may report side effects to FDA at 1-800-FDA-1088.

General information about the safe and effective use of TANZEUM.
Medicines are sometimes prescribed for purposes other than those listed in a Medication Guide. You can ask your pharmacist or healthcare provider for information about TANZEUM that is written for health professionals. Do not use TANZEUM for a condition for which it was not prescribed. Do not give TANZEUM to other people, even if they have the same symptoms that you have. It may harm them.

What are the ingredients in TANZEUM?
Active Ingredient: albiglutide
Inactive Ingredients: mannitol, polysorbate 80, sodium phosphate, and trehalose dihydrate. TANZEUM does not contain a preservative.
For more information, go to www.TANZEUM.com or call 1-888-825-5249.

This Medication Guide has been approved by the U.S. Food and Drug Administration. Approved: April 2014

Manufactured by
GlaxoSmithKline LLC
Wilmington, DE 19808
U.S. Lic No. 1727
Marketed by
GlaxoSmithKline
Research Triangle Park, NC 27709

TANZEUM is a trademark of the GSK group of companies.
©2014, the GSK group of companies. All rights reserved.
TNZ:1MG

INSTRUCTIONS FOR USE
TANZEUM™ (TAN-zee-um)
(albiglutide)
for injection, for subcutaneous use
TANZEUM (albiglutide) Pen 30 mg

Use 1 Time Each Week
Read all the instructions and follow the steps below to mix the medicine and prepare the pen for injection.
Failure to follow Steps A to C in the correct order may result in damage to your pen.
Information About This Pen
- This medicine is injected **1** time each week.
- The pen has medicine powder in 1 compartment and water in another compartment. You will need to mix them together by twisting the pen, then wait for **15** minutes for the medicine and water to fully mix.

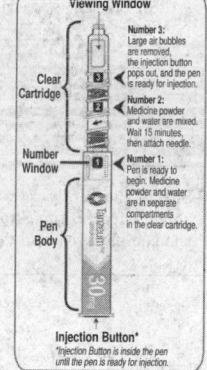

Viewing Window
Clear Cartridge
Number Window
Pen Body
Injection Button*

Number 3: Large air bubbles are removed, the injection button pops out, and the pen is ready for injection.
Number 2: Medicine powder and water are mixed. Wait 15 minutes, then attach needle.
Number 1: Pen is ready to begin. Medicine powder and water are in separate compartments in the clear cartridge.

*Injection Button is inside the pen until the pen is ready for injection.

⚠ **CAUTION:** Do not allow the pen to freeze. Throw away the pen if frozen.	If stored in refrigerator, allow to sit at room temperature for 15 minutes before starting Step A.	Dispose of the pen right away after injecting. Do not recap, remove, or reuse the needle.

Before you Begin: Wash Your Hands, Gather and Inspect Your Supplies
- Wash your hands.
- Take a pen and new needle out of the box and check the label on your pen to make sure it is your prescribed dose of medicine.
- Gather a **clean, empty cup** to hold the pen while the medicine mixes, a **clock timer** to measure the time while the medicine mixes, and a large **sharps container** for pen disposal. See "**Disposing of Your Used Pens and Needles**" at the end of these instructions.
[See table above]
Step A
Inspect Your Pen and Mix Your Medicine
Inspect Your Pen
- Make sure that you have all of the supplies listed above (pen, needle, cup, timer, sharps container).

- Check the expiration date on the pen. **Do not** use if expired.

Check expiration date.   Exp:

- Check that the pen has a **[1]** in the number window. **Do not** use if the **[1]** is not showing.

Twist Pen to Mix Your Medicine

- Hold the pen body with the clear cartridge pointing up so that you **see the [1] in the number window.**
- With your other hand, twist the clear cartridge several times in the direction of the arrow (clockwise) until you feel and hear the pen "click" into place and you **see the [2] in the number window.** This will mix the medicine powder and liquid in the clear cartridge.

"Click"

- Slowly and gently rock the pen side to side (like a windshield wiper) **5** times to mix the medicine. **Do not** shake the pen hard to avoid foaming; it may affect your dose.

5 Times

⚠ Do not shake the pen hard.

Wait for Medicine to Dissolve

- Place the pen into the clean, empty cup to keep the clear cartridge pointing up.
- **Set the clock timer for 15 minutes.**

You <u>must</u> wait 15 minutes for the medicine to dissolve before continuing to Step B.

Step B
Attach the Needle and Prepare the Pen for Injection

After the 15 minute wait, wash your hands and finish the rest of the steps right away.

Inspect Your Dissolved Medicine

- Again, slowly and gently rock the pen side to side (like a windshield wiper) **5** times to mix the medicine again. **Do not** shake the pen hard to avoid foaming; it may affect your dose.

Repeat rocking.

⚠ Do not shake the pen hard.

5 Times

- Look through the viewing window to check that the liquid in the cartridge is clear and free of solid particles.

Look for particles.

⚠ If you still see particles in the liquid, do not use the pen.

- The liquid will have a yellow color and there will be **large air bubbles** on top of the liquid.

Attach the Needle

- Peel the tab from the outer needle cap.

- Hold the pen with the clear cartridge pointing up and push the needle straight down onto the clear cartridge until you hear a "click" and feel the needle "snap" down into place. This means the needle is attached.

"Click"

Push down firmly.

⚠ Do not twist the needle or attach at an angle.

Tap for Air Bubbles

- With the needle point up, gently tap the clear cartridge **2 to 3** times to bring large air bubbles to the top.

Tap cartridge.

⚠ Keep pen upright.

Small bubbles are okay and do not need to rise to the top.

Twist Pen to Prime the Needle

- Twist the clear cartridge several times in the direction of the arrow (clockwise) until you feel and hear the pen "click" and you **see the [3] in the number window.** This removes the large air bubbles from the clear cartridge. The injection button will also pop out from the bottom of the pen.

"Click"

Step C
Remove Both Needle Caps and Inject Your Medicine
Remove Needle Caps

- Carefully remove the outer needle cap, then the inner needle cap. **A few drops of liquid may come out of the needle. This is normal.**

| Step 1: Remove Outer Needle Cap | → | Step 2: Remove Inner Needle Cap |

Inject the Medicine

- Insert the needle into the skin on your abdomen, thigh, or upper arm and inject as shown to you by your healthcare provider.

Injection Sites →

- With your thumb, press the injection button slowly and steadily to inject your medicine. The slower you press the button, the less pressure you will feel.

- Keep the injection button pressed down until you hear a "click". **After hearing the click, continue holding your thumb down on the button and then slowly count to 5 to deliver the full dose of the medicine.**

Then slowly count to 5.

"Click"

⚠ Inject slowly and steadily. After hearing the "click", count to 5 to deliver the full dose.

- After hearing the "click" and then slowly counting to **5**, pull the needle out of your skin.

Please make sure you are using the right dose. These instructions are for the 30 mg dose.

Disposing of Your Used Pens and Needles
- **Do not** recap the needle or remove needle from the pen.
- Put your used needles and pens in an FDA-cleared sharps disposal container right away after use. **Do not throw away (dispose of) loose needles and pens in your household trash.**

General Information About the Safe and Effective Use of TANZEUM
- Take **1** time each week. You can take your medicine at any time of day, with or without meals.
- Your healthcare provider will teach you how to mix and inject TANZEUM before you use it for the first time. If you have questions or do not understand the **Instructions for Use**, talk to your healthcare provider.
- Use TANZEUM exactly as your healthcare provider tells you. **Do not** change your dose or stop TANZEUM without talking to your healthcare provider.
- **Change (rotate) your injection site with each injection (weekly).**
- TANZEUM is injected under the skin (subcutaneously) in your stomach area (abdomen), upper leg (thigh), or upper arm.
- **Do not** inject TANZEUM into a vein or muscle.
- If you use TANZEUM with insulin, you should inject your TANZEUM and insulin separately. **Do not mix insulin and TANZEUM together.** You can inject TANZEUM and insulin in the same body area (for example, your stomach area), but you should not give the injections right next to each other.
- Keep pens and needles out of the reach of children.
- Always use a new needle for each injection.
- **Do not** share pens or needles.

Frequently Asked Questions
Medicine Dosing
What if i need to take my medicine on a different day of the week?
- You may take your next dose of medicine on a different day as long as it has been at least **4** days since your last dose.

What if I forget to take the medicine on the day I am supposed to?
- Take your missed dose of medicine within **3** days after your scheduled day, then return to your scheduled day for your next dose. If more than **3** days have passed since your usual scheduled day, wait until your next regularly scheduled day to take the injection of TANZEUM.

Storage
How should I store my medicine?
- Store your pens in the refrigerator between 36°F to 46°F (2°C to 8°C).
- You may store your pen in the box at room temperature below 86°F (30°C) for up to **4** weeks before you are ready to use the pen.
- Store pens in the carton they came in.
- **Do not** freeze pens. If the liquid in the pen is frozen, throw away the pen and use another pen.

Number Window
Are the Numbers 1, 2, and 3 used to select my dose of medicine?
- No, you do not have to select your dose. The numbers are to help you prepare and give your medicine.
Number 1: Pen is ready to begin. Medicine powder and water are in separate compartments in the clear cartridge. If you don't see a number **1** in the window, throw away the pen.
Number 2: Medicine powder and water are mixed and then gently rocked. Wait **15** minutes, then attach needle.
Number 3: Large air bubbles are removed, the injection button pops out, and the pen is ready for injection.
What if I do not hear the "click" when the 2 or 3 are moved into the Number Window?
- If you do not hear a "click" when **2** or **3** are moved into the number window, you may not have the number fully centered in the window. Twist the clear cartridge slightly in

the direction of the arrow to complete the "click" and center the number in the window. Do not turn the clear cartridge in the opposite direction from the arrows.

Step A: Inspect Your Pen and Mix Your Medicine
What if I do not wait 15 minutes after turning the pen to the Number 2?
- If you do not wait the full **15** minutes the medicine may not be mixed with the water the right way. This can result in particles floating in the clear cartridge, not getting your full dose, or a blocked needle. Waiting the full **15** minutes ensures that the medicine powder and water are mixed the right way, even though it may look like it is mixed sooner than that.

What if I leave my pen for more than 15 minutes after turning the pen to the Number 2 in Step A?
- As long as the needle has not been attached, the pen can be used for up to **8** hours from the time **Step A** was started. If it has been more than **8** hours since the medicine was mixed in **Step A**, throw away the pen and use another pen.
- If you have attached the needle, TANZEUM should be used right away.

Step B: Attach the Needle and Prepare Pen for Injection
What if I leave my pen with the needle attached at Step B, and come back later to finish Step C?
- This can cause your needle to block, you should continue from **Step B** to **Step C** right away.
What if I do not attach the needle at Step B?
- If the needle is attached at **Step A**, some of the medicine may be lost during mixing. Throw away the pen and use another pen.
- If the needle is not attached before turning the pen from Position **2 to 3** in **Step B**, this can damage the pen.

Step C: Remove Both Needle Caps and Inject Your Medicine
After I turn the pen to Number 3 (Step B), there are still some small air bubbles remaining. Can I still use the pen?
- Seeing small air bubbles remaining is normal and you can still use the pen.
After I give my medicine, there is some liquid still seen in the clear cartridge.
- This is normal. If you have heard and felt the injection button "click" and slowly counted to **5** before pulling the needle out of your skin, you should have received the full dose of your medicine.
How should I dispose of the pen?
- **Do not** recap the needle or remove needle from the pen.
- Put your used needles and pens in an FDA-cleared sharps disposal container right away after use. **Do not throw away (dispose of) loose needles and pens in your household trash.**
- If you do not have an FDA-cleared sharps disposal container, you may use a household container that is:
  ° made of a heavy-duty plastic,
  ° can be closed with a tight-fitting, puncture-resistant lid, without sharps being able to come out,
  ° upright and stable during use,
  ° leak-resistant, and
  ° properly labeled to warn of hazardous waste inside the container.
- When your sharps disposal container is almost full, you will need to follow your community guidelines for the right way to dispose of your sharps disposal container. There may be state or local laws about how you should throw away used needles and pens. For more information about safe sharps disposal, and for specific information about sharps disposal in the state that you live in, go to the FDA's website at: http://www.fda.gov/safesharpsdisposal.
- **Do not** dispose of your used sharps disposal container in your household trash unless your community guidelines permit this. **Do not** recycle your used sharps disposal container.

[See table above]

This Instructions for Use has been approved by the U.S. Food and Drug Administration.

Revised: June 2014

Manufactured by
GlaxoSmithKline LLC
Wilmington, DE 19808
U.S. Lic No. 1727
Marketed by
GlaxoSmithKline
Research Triangle
Park, NC 27709

TANZEUM is a trademark of the GSK group of companies. ©2014, the GSK group of companies. All rights reserved.
TNZ:2IFU-30

Instructions for Use
TANZEUM™ (TAN-zee-um) (albiglutide)
for injection, for subcutaneous use
TANZEUM (albiglutide) Pen 50 mg

Use 1 Time Each Week
Read all the instructions and follow the steps below to mix the medicine and prepare the pen for injection.
Failure to follow Steps A to C in the correct order may result in damage to your pen.
Information About This Pen
- This medicine is injected **1** time each week.
- The pen has medicine powder in 1 compartment and water in another compartment. You will need to mix them together by twisting the pen, then wait for **30** minutes for the medicine and water to fully mix.

CAUTION: Do not allow the pen to freeze. Throw away the pen if frozen.	If stored in refrigerator, allow to sit at room temperature for 15 minutes before starting Step A.	Dispose of the pen right away after injecting. Do not recap, remove, or reuse the needle.

Before you Begin: Wash Your Hands, Gather and Inspect Your Supplies
- Wash your hands.
- Take a pen and new needle out of the box and check the label on your pen to make sure it is your prescribed dose of medicine.
- Gather a **clean, empty cup** to hold the pen while the medicine mixes, a **clock timer** to measure the time while the medicine mixes, and a large **sharps container** for pen disposal. See "Disposing of Your Used Pens and Needles" at the end of these instructions.

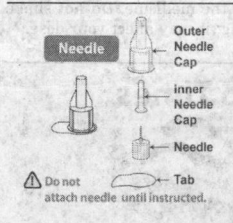

This TANZEUM 50 mg pen needs 30 minutes to let the medicine powder and water mix in Step A. This is different from the TANZEUM 30 mg pen you may have used before.

[See table at top of next page]
Step A
Inspect Your Pen and Mix Your Medicine
Inspect Your Pen
- Make sure that you have all of the supplies listed above (pen, needle, cup, timer, sharps container).
- Check the expiration date on the pen. **Do not** use if expired.

Check expiration date.

- Check that the pen has a **[1]** in the number window. **Do not** use if the **[1]** is not showing.

Clean, Empty Cup   Clock Timer   Large Sharps Container

Twist Pen to Mix Your Medicine
- Hold the pen body with the clear cartridge pointing up so that you **see the [1] in the number window**.
- With your other hand, twist the clear cartridge several times in the direction of the arrow (clockwise) until you feel and hear the pen "click" into place and you **see the [2] in the number window**. This will mix the medicine powder and liquid in the clear cartridge.

"Click"

- Slowly and gently rock the pen side to side (like a windshield wiper) **5 times** to mix the medicine. **Do not** shake the pen hard to avoid foaming; it may affect your dose.

5 Times

⚠ Do not shake the pen hard.

Wait for Medicine to Dissolve
- Place the pen into the clean, empty cup to keep the clear cartridge pointing up.
- **Set the clock timer for 30 minutes.**

Wait 30 minutes

You <u>must</u> wait 30 minutes for the medicine to dissolve before continuing to Step B.

Step B
Attach the Needle and Prepare the Pen for Injection
After the 30 minute wait, wash your hands and finish the rest of the steps right away.
Inspect Your Dissolved Medicine
- Again, slowly and gently rock the pen side to side (like a windshield wiper) **5 times** to mix the medicine again. **Do not** shake the pen hard to avoid foaming; it may affect your dose.

5 Times

Repeat rocking.

⚠ Do not shake the pen hard.

- Look through the viewing window to check that the liquid in the cartridge is clear and free of solid particles.

Look for particles.

⚠ If you still see particles in the liquid, do not use the pen.

- The liquid will have a yellow color and there will be **large air bubbles** on top of the liquid.
Attach the Needle
- Peel the tab from the outer needle cap.

- Hold the pen with the clear cartridge pointing up and push the needle straight down onto the clear cartridge until you hear a "click" and feel the needle "snap" down into place. This means the needle is attached.

"Click"

Push down firmly.

⚠ Do not twist the needle or attach at an angle.

Tap for Air Bubbles
- With the needle point up, gently tap the clear cartridge **2 to 3 times** to bring large air bubbles to the top.

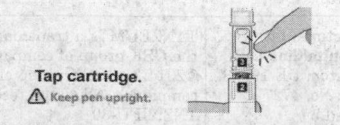

Tap cartridge.

⚠ Keep pen upright.

Small bubbles are okay and do not need to rise to the top.

Twist Pen to Prime the Needle
- Twist the clear cartridge several times in the direction of the arrow (clockwise) until you feel and hear the pen "click" and you **see the [3] in the number window**. This removes the large air bubbles from the clear cartridge. The injection button will also pop out from the bottom of the pen.

"Click"

Step C
Remove Both Needle Caps and Inject Your Medicine
Remove Needle Caps
- Carefully remove the outer needle cap, then the inner needle cap. **A few drops of liquid may come out of the needle. This is normal.**

Step 1: Remove Outer Needle Cap ➡ Step 2: Remove Inner Needle Cap

Inject the Medicine
- Insert the needle into the skin on your abdomen, thigh, or upper arm and inject as shown to you by your healthcare provider.

Injection Sites

- With your thumb, press the injection button slowly and steadily to inject your medicine. The slower you press the button, the less pressure you will feel.
- Keep the injection button pressed down until you hear a "click". **After hearing the click, continue holding your thumb down on the button and then slowly count to 5 to deliver the full dose of the medicine.**

"Click"   Then slowly count to 5.

⚠ Inject slowly and steadily. After hearing the "click", count to 5 to deliver the full dose.

- After hearing the "click" and then slowly counting to **5**, pull the needle out of your skin.

Please make sure you are using the right dose. These instructions are for the 50 mg dose.

Disposing of Your Used Pens and Needles
- **Do not** recap the needle or remove needle from the pen.
- Put your used needles and pens in an FDA-cleared sharps disposal container right away after use. **Do not throw away (dispose of) loose needles and pens in your household trash.**

General Information About the Safe and Effective Use of TANZEUM
- Take **1** time each week. You can take your medicine at any time of day, with or without meals.
- **Your healthcare provider will teach you how to mix and inject TANZEUM before you use it for the first time.** If you have questions or do not understand the **Instructions for Use**, talk to your healthcare provider.
- **Use TANZEUM exactly as your healthcare provider tells you. Do not** change your dose or stop TANZEUM without talking to your healthcare provider.
- **Change (rotate) your injection site with each injection (weekly).**
- TANZEUM is injected under the skin (subcutaneously) in your stomach area (abdomen), upper leg (thigh), or upper arm.
- **Do not** inject TANZEUM into a vein or muscle.
- If you use TANZEUM with insulin, you should inject your TANZEUM and insulin separately. **Do not mix insulin and TANZEUM together.** You can inject TANZEUM and insulin in the same body area (for example, your stomach area), but you should not give the injections right next to each other.
- Keep pens and needles out of the reach of children.
- Always use a new needle for each injection.
- Do not share pens or needles.

Frequently Asked Questions
Medicine Dosing
What if I need to take my medicine on a different day of the week?
- You may take your next dose of medicine on a different day as long as it has been at least **4** days since your last dose.

What if I forget to take the medicine on the day I am supposed to?
- Take your missed dose of medicine within **3** days after your scheduled day, then return to your scheduled day for your next dose. If more than **3** days have passed since your usual scheduled day, wait until your next regularly scheduled day to take the injection of TANZEUM.

Storage
How should I store my medicine?
- Store your pens in the refrigerator between 36°F to 46°F (2°C to 8°C).
- You may store your pen in the box at room temperature below 86°F (30°C) for up to **4** weeks before you are ready to use the pen.
- Store pens in the carton they came in.
- **Do not** freeze pens. If the liquid in the pen is frozen, throw away the pen and use another pen.

Number Window
Are the Numbers 1, 2, and 3 used to select my dose of medicine?
- No, you do not have to select your dose. The numbers are to help you prepare and give your medicine.
Number 1: Pen is ready to begin. Medicine powder and water are in separate compartments in the clear cartridge. If you don't see a number **1** in the window, throw away the pen.
Number 2: Medicine powder and water are mixed and then gently rocked. Wait **30** minutes, then attach needle.
Number 3: Large air bubbles are removed, the injection button pops out, and the pen is ready for injection.
What if I do not hear the "click" when the 2 or 3 are moved into the Number Window?
- If you do not hear a "click" when **2 or 3** are moved into the number window, you may not have the number fully centered in the window. Twist the clear cartridge slightly in

the direction of the arrow to complete the "click" and center the number in the window. Do not turn the clear cartridge in the opposite direction from the arrows.

Step A: Inspect Your Pen and Mix Your Medicine
What if I do not wait 30 minutes after turning the pen to the Number 2?
- If you do not wait the full **30** minutes the medicine may not be mixed with the water the right way. This can result in particles floating in the clear cartridge, not getting your full dose, or a blocked needle. Waiting the full **30** minutes ensures that the medicine powder and water are mixed the right way, even though it may look like it is mixed sooner than that.

What if I leave my pen for more than 30 minutes after turning the pen to the Number 2 in Step A?
- As long as the needle has not been attached, the pen can be used for up to **8** hours from the time **Step A** was started. If it has been more than **8** hours since the medicine was mixed in **Step A**, throw away the pen and use another pen.
- If you have attached the needle, TANZEUM should be used right away.

Step B: Attach the Needle and Prepare Pen for Injection
What if I leave my pen with the needle attached at Step B, and come back later to finish Step C?
- This can cause your needle to block, you should continue from **Step B** to **Step C** right away.

What if I do not attach the needle at Step B?
- If the needle is attached at **Step A**, some of the medicine may be lost during mixing. Throw away the pen and use another pen.
- If the needle is not attached before turning the pen from Position **2 to 3** in **Step B**, this can damage the pen.

Step C: Remove Both Needle Caps and Inject Your Medicine
After I turn the pen to Number 3 (Step B), there are still some small air bubbles remaining. Can I still use the pen?
- Seeing small air bubbles remaining is normal and you can still use the pen.

After I give my medicine, there is some liquid still seen in the clear cartridge.
- This is normal. If you have heard and felt the injection button "click" and slowly counted to **5** before pulling the needle out of your skin, you should have received the full dose of your medicine.

How should I dispose of the pen?
- **Do not** recap the needle or remove needle from the pen.
- Put your used needles and pens in an FDA-cleared sharps disposal container right away after use. **Do not throw away (dispose of) loose needles and pens in your household trash.**
- If you do not have an FDA-cleared sharps disposal container, you may use a household container that is:
  ○ made of a heavy-duty plastic,
  ○ can be closed with a tight-fitting, puncture-resistant lid, without sharps being able to come out,
  ○ upright and stable during use,
  ○ leak-resistant, and
  ○ properly labeled to warn of hazardous waste inside the container.
- When your sharps disposal container is almost full, you will need to follow your community guidelines for the right way to dispose of your sharps disposal container. There may be state or local laws about how you should throw away used needles and pens. For more information about safe sharps disposal, and for specific information about sharps disposal in the state that you live in, go to the FDA's website at: http://www.fda.gov/safesharpsdisposal.
- **Do not** dispose of your used sharps disposal container in your household trash unless your community guidelines permit this. **Do not** recycle your used sharps disposal container.

[See table above]
This Instructions for Use has been approved by the U.S. Food and Drug Administration.
Revised: June 2014

Manufactured by
GlaxoSmithKline LLC
Wilmington, DE 19808
U.S. Lic No. 1727
Marketed by
GlaxoSmithKline
Research Triangle
Park, NC 27709

TANZEUM is a trademark of the GSK group of companies. ©2014, the GSK group of companies. All rights reserved.
TNZ:2IFU-50

TIMENTIN
(ticarcillin disodium and clavulanate potassium)
for Injection
TIMENTIN
(ticarcillin disodium and clavulanate potassium)
for Injection: Pharmacy Bulk Package
TIMENTIN
(ticarcillin disodium and clavulanate potassium)
Injection: GALAXY Container
℞

HIGHLIGHTS OF PRESCRIBING INFORMATION
These highlights do not include all the information needed to use TIMENTIN safely and effectively. See full prescribing information for TIMENTIN.
TIMENTIN (ticarcillin disodium and clavulanate potassium) for Injection
TIMENTIN (ticarcillin disodium and clavulanate potassium) for Injection: Pharmacy Bulk Package
TIMENTIN (ticarcillin disodium and clavulanate potassium) Injection: GALAXY Container
Initial U.S. Approval: 1985

INDICATIONS AND USAGE
To reduce the development of drug-resistant bacteria and maintain the effectiveness of TIMENTIN and other antibacterial drugs, TIMENTIN should be used only to treat infections that are proven or strongly suspected to be caused by bacteria.
TIMENTIN is a combination of a β–lactam antibacterial and a β–lactamase inhibitor indicated for the treatment of the following infections due to designated susceptible bacteria:
- Septicemia (1.1)
- Lower respiratory infections (1.2)
- Bone and joint infections (1.3)
- Skin and skin structure infections (1.4)
- Urinary tract infections (1.5)
- Gynecologic infections (1.6)
- Intra–abdominal infections (1.7)

DOSAGE AND ADMINISTRATION
Administer TIMENTIN by intravenous infusion (30 minutes). (2)
Adults:
- Systemic and urinary tract infections: 3.1 g every 4 to 6 hours. (2.1)
- Gynecologic infections: 200 to 300 mg/kg/day in divided doses every 4 to 6 hours depending on severity of infection. (2.1)
Pediatric Patients:
- <60 kg: 200 to 300 mg/kg/day in divided doses every 4 to 6 hours depending on severity of infection. (2.2)
- ≥60 kg: 3.1 grams every 4 to 6 hours depending on severity of infection. (2.2)

DOSAGE FORMS AND STRENGTHS
- 3.1 gram vial of TIMENTIN for Injection containing ticarcillin disodium equivalent to 3 grams ticarcillin and clavulanate potassium equivalent to 0.1 gram clavulanic acid. (3)
- 31-gram Pharmacy Bulk Package of TIMENTIN for Injection containing ticarcillin disodium equivalent to 30 grams ticarcillin and clavulanate potassium equivalent to 1 gram clavulanic acid. (3)
- 100–mL single-dose GALAXY Container (PL 2040 Plastic) of TIMENTIN Injection containing ticarcillin disodium equivalent to 3.0 grams ticarcillin and clavulanate potassium equivalent to 0.1 gram clavulanic acid as a frozen solution. (3)

CONTRAINDICATIONS
History of a serious hypersensitivity reaction (anaphylaxis or Stevens-Johnson syndrome) to TIMENTIN or to other β–lactams (e.g., penicillins and cephalosporins). (4)

WARNINGS AND PRECAUTIONS
- Serious, including fatal, hypersensitivity (anaphylactic) reactions. Discontinue TIMENTIN and institute appropriate therapy. (5.1)
- *Clostridium difficile* associated diarrhea (CDAD). If diarrhea occurs, evaluate patients for CDAD. (5.2)
- Convulsions may occur when the recommended dose of TIMENTIN is exceeded, especially in the presence of impaired renal function. Institute supportive measures. (5.3)

ADVERSE REACTIONS
Most common adverse reactions (≥1%) are rash, nausea, diarrhea, and phlebitis at injection site. (6.1)

To report SUSPECTED ADVERSE REACTIONS, contact GlaxoSmithKline at 1-888-825-5249 or FDA at 1-800-FDA-1088 or www.fda.gov/medwatch.

---DRUG INTERACTIONS---

- Aminoglycosides: Mixing with TIMENTIN for parenteral administration can inactivate the aminoglycoside. (7.1)
- Probenecid: Interferes with renal tubular secretion of ticarcillin, therefore increases exposure to ticarcillin. (7.2)
- Oral Contraceptives: Effects on gut flora may lower estrogen reabsorption and reduce efficacy of oral contraceptives. (7.3)

---USE IN SPECIFIC POPULATIONS---

Renal Impairment: Adjust dose based on creatinine clearance and type of dialysis. (2.3, 8.6)
See 17 for PATIENT COUNSELING INFORMATION
Revised: 06/2014

FULL PRESCRIBING INFORMATION: CONTENTS*

FULL PRESCRIBING INFORMATION

1 INDICATIONS AND USAGE

TIMENTIN® is indicated in the treatment of infections caused by susceptible isolates of the designated bacteria in the conditions listed below:

1.1 Septicemia
Septicemia (including bacteremia) caused by β–lactamase–producing isolates of *Klebsiella* spp.*, *Escherichia coli*, *Staphylococcus aureus*, or *Pseudomonas aeruginosa** (or other *Pseudomonas* species*)

1.2 Lower Respiratory Infections
Lower respiratory infections caused by β–lactamase–producing isolates of *S. aureus*, *Haemophilus influenzae*, or *Klebsiella* spp.*

1.3 Bone and Joint Infections
Bone and joint infections caused by β–lactamase–producing isolates of *S. aureus*

1.4 Skin and Skin Structure Infections
Skin and skin structure infections caused by β–lactamase–producing isolates of *S. aureus*, *Klebsiella* spp.*, or *E. coli**

1.5 Urinary Tract Infections
Urinary tract infections (complicated and uncomplicated) caused by β–lactamase–producing isolates of *Klebsiella* spp.*, *P. aeruginosa** (or other *Pseudomonas* spp.*), *Citrobacter* spp.*, *Enterobacter cloacae**, *Serratia marcescens**, or *S. aureus**

1.6 Gynecologic Infections
Endometritis caused by β–lactamase–producing isolates of *Prevotella melaninogenicus**, *Enterobacter* spp. (including *E. cloacae**), *E. coli*, *Klebsiella pneumoniae**, *S. aureus*, or *Staphylococcus epidermidis*

1.7 Intra-abdominal Infections
Peritonitis caused by β–lactamase–producing isolates of *E. coli*, *K. pneumoniae*, or *Bacteroides fragilis** group

* Efficacy for this organism in this organ system was studied in fewer than 10 infections.

1.8 Usage
To reduce the development of drug–resistant bacteria and maintain the effectiveness of TIMENTIN and other antibacterial drugs, TIMENTIN should be used only to treat infections that are proven or strongly suspected to be caused by susceptible bacteria. When culture and susceptibility information are available, they should be considered in selecting or modifying antibacterial therapy. In the absence of such data, local epidemiology and susceptibility patterns may contribute to the empiric selection of therapy.

2 DOSAGE AND ADMINISTRATION

2.1 Adults
The usual recommended dosage for systemic and urinary tract infections for adults is 3.1 grams of TIMENTIN (3 grams ticarcillin and 100 mg clavulanic acid) given every 4 to 6 hours.
For gynecologic infections, TIMENTIN should be administered as follows (based on ticarcillin content): Moderate infections, 200 mg/kg/day in divided doses every 6 hours; severe infections, 300 mg/kg/day in divided doses every 4 hours.
For patients weighing less than 60 kg, the recommended dosage is 200 to 300 mg/kg/day given in divided doses every 4 to 6 hours.
The duration of therapy depends upon the severity of infection. The usual duration is 10 to 14 days; however, in difficult and complicated infections, more prolonged therapy may be required.

2.2 Pediatric Patients (≥3 Months of Age)
Patients <60 kg: Mild to moderate infections, 200 mg/kg/day based on ticarcillin content in divided doses every 6 hours; severe infections, 300 mg/kg/day in divided doses every 4 hours.
Patients ≥60 kg: Mild to moderate infections, 3.1 grams every 6 hours; severe infections, 3.1 grams every 4 hours.

2.3 Renal Impairment
For patients with renal insufficiency, an initial loading dose of 3.1 grams should be followed by doses based on creatinine clearance and type of dialysis as indicated in Table 1.

Table 1. Dosage Adjustments for Renal Impairment

Creatinine Clearance (mL/minute)[a]	Dosage[b]
Over 60	3 grams every 4 hours
30 to 60	2 grams every 4 hours
10 to 30	2 grams every 8 hours
Less than 10	2 grams every 12 hours
Less than 10 with hepatic dysfunction	2 grams every 24 hours
Patients on peritoneal dialysis	3 grams every 12 hours
Patients on hemodialysis	2 grams every 12 hours supplemented with 3 grams after each dialysis

[a] To calculate creatinine clearance[1] from a serum creatinine value use the following formula:
$$C_{cr} = (140 - \text{Age}) \text{ (weight in kg)}/72 \times S_{cr} \text{ (mg/100 mL)}$$
This is the calculated creatinine clearance for adult males; for females it is 15% less.
[b] Based on ticarcillin content.

2.4 Administration and Directions for Use
TIMENTIN should be administered by intravenous infusion over a 30-minute period.
Directions for Reconstitution and Further Dilution:
3.1-gram Glass Vials: The 3.1-gram vial should be reconstituted by adding approximately 13 mL of Sterile Water for Injection, USP, or Sodium Chloride Injection, USP, and shaking well. When dissolved, the concentration of ticarcillin will be approximately 200 mg/mL with a corresponding concentration of 6.7 mg/mL for clavulanic acid. The color of reconstituted solutions of TIMENTIN normally ranges from light to dark yellow, depending on concentration, duration, and temperature of storage.
The dissolved drug should be further diluted to desired volume using the recommended solution listed under Stability *[see Dosage and Administration (2.5)]* to a concentration between 10 mg/mL to 100 mg/mL.
Pharmacy Bulk Package: The container closure may be penetrated only one time utilizing a suitable sterile transfer device or dispensing set that allows measured distribution of the contents. A sterile substance that must be reconstituted prior to use may require a separate closure entry. Restrict use of Pharmacy Bulk Packages to an aseptic area such as a laminar flow hood.
Reconstituted contents of the vial should be withdrawn immediately. However, if this is not possible, aliquoting operations must be completed within 4 hours of reconstitution. Discard the reconstituted stock solution 4 hours after initial entry.
Add 76 mL of Sterile Water for Injection, USP, or Sodium Chloride Injection, USP, to the 31–gram Pharmacy Bulk Package and shake well. For ease of reconstitution, the diluent may be added in 2 portions. Each 1 mL of the resulting concentrated stock solution contains approximately 300 mg of ticarcillin and 10 mg of clavulanic acid.
The desired dosage should be withdrawn from the stock solution and further diluted to desired volume using the recommended solution listed under Stability *[see Dosage and Administration (2.5)]* to a concentration between 10 mg/mL to 100 mg/mL.
Directions for Intravenous Infusion: After reconstitution and further dilution and prior to administration, TIMENTIN should be inspected visually for particulate matter. If particulate matter is present, the solution should be discarded.
The solution of reconstituted drug may be administered over a 30-minute period by direct infusion or through a Y–type intravenous infusion set. If this method of administration is used, it is advisable to temporarily discontinue the administration of any other solutions during the infusion of TIMENTIN.
When TIMENTIN is given in combination with another antimicrobial, such as an aminoglycoside, each drug should be given separately in accordance with the recommended dosage and routes of administration for each drug *[see Drug Interactions (7.1)]*.
GALAXY® Container (PL 2040 Plastic): Prior to administration, TIMENTIN should be inspected visually for particulate matter. If particulate matter is present, the solution should be discarded.
Caution: Do not use plastic containers in series connections. Such use could result in an embolism due to residual air being drawn from the primary container before administration of the fluid from the secondary container is completed.
Preparation for Administration: See How Supplied/Storage and Handling (16) for thawing and handling instructions:
- Suspend the container from eyelet support.
- Remove protector from outlet port at bottom of container.
- Attach administration set. Refer to complete directions accompanying set.

2.5 Stability
NOTE: TIMENTIN is incompatible with Sodium Bicarbonate.

3.1-gram Glass Vials: The concentrated stock solution at 200 mg/mL is stable for up to 6 hours at room temperature 21° to 24°C (70° to 75°F) or up to 72 hours under refrigeration 4°C (40°F).
If the concentrated stock solution (200 mg/mL) is held for up to 6 hours at room temperature 21° to 24°C (70° to 75°F) or up to 72 hours under refrigeration 4°C (40°F) and further diluted to a concentration between 10 mg/mL and 100 mg/mL with any of the diluents listed below, then the following stability periods apply.

STABILITY PERIOD

(3.1–gram Vials)

Intravenous Solution (ticarcillin concentrations of 10 mg/mL to 100 mg/mL)	Room Temperature 21° to 24°C (70° to 75°F)	Refrigerated 4°C (40°F)
Dextrose Injection 5%, USP	24 hours	3 days
Sodium Chloride Injection, USP	24 hours	7 days
Lactated Ringer's Injection, USP	24 hours	7 days

If the concentrated stock solution (200 mg/mL) is stored for up to 6 hours at room temperature and then further diluted to a concentration between 10 mg/mL and 100 mg/mL, solutions of Sodium Chloride Injection, USP, and Lactated Ringer's Injection, USP, may be stored frozen –18°C (0°F) for up to 30 days. Solutions prepared with Dextrose Injection 5%, USP, may be stored frozen –18°C (0°F) for up to 7 days. All thawed solutions should be used within 8 hours or discarded. Once thawed, solutions should not be refrozen.

Unused solutions must be discarded after the time periods listed above.

Pharmacy Bulk Package: Aliquots of the reconstituted stock solution at 300 mg/mL are stable for up to 6 hours between 21° and 24°C (70° and 75°F) or up to 72 hours under refrigeration 4°C (40°F). The reconstituted stock solution should be held under refrigeration 4°C (40°F).

If the aliquots of the reconstituted stock solution (300 mg/mL) are held up to 6 hours between 21° and 24°C (70° and 75°F) or up to 72 hours under refrigeration 4°C (40°F) and further diluted to a concentration between 10 mg/mL and 100 mg/mL with any of the diluents listed below, then the following stability periods apply.

STABILITY PERIOD

(31–gram Pharmacy Bulk Package)

Intravenous Solution (ticarcillin concentrations of 10 mg/mL to 100 mg/mL)	Room Temperature 21° to 24°C (70° to 75°F)	Refrigerated 4°C (40°F)
Dextrose Injection 5%, USP	24 hours	3 days
Sodium Chloride Injection 0.9%, USP	24 hours	4 days
Lactated Ringer's Injection, USP	24 hours	4 days
Sterile Water for Injection, USP	24 hours	4 days

If an aliquot of concentrated stock solution (300 mg/mL) is stored for up to 6 hours between 21° and 24°C (70° and 75°F) and then further diluted to a concentration between 10 mg/mL and 100 mg/mL, solutions of Sodium Chloride Injection, USP, Lactated Ringer's Injection, USP, and Sterile Water for Injection, USP, may be stored frozen –18°C (0°F) for up to 30 days. Solutions prepared with Dextrose Injection 5%, USP, may be stored frozen –18°C (0°F) for up to 7 days. All thawed solutions should be used within 8 hours or discarded. Once thawed, solutions should not be refrozen.

Unused solutions must be discarded after the time periods listed above.

GALAXY Container (PL 2040 Plastic): Do not add supplementary medication to the container. The thawed solution is stable for 24 hours at room temperature 22°C (72°F) or for 7 days under refrigeration at 4°C (39°F).

3 DOSAGE FORMS AND STRENGTHS

The 3.1–gram glass vial of TIMENTIN for Injection is a white to pale yellow sterile powder for reconstitution containing ticarcillin disodium equivalent to 3 grams ticarcillin and clavulanate potassium equivalent to 0.1 gram clavulanic acid.

The 31–gram Pharmacy Bulk Package of TIMENTIN for Injection is a white to pale yellow sterile powder for reconstitution containing ticarcillin disodium equivalent to 30 grams ticarcillin and clavulanate potassium equivalent to 1 gram clavulanic acid.

The 100-mL single-dose GALAXY Container (PL 2040 Plastic) of TIMENTIN is a frozen solution containing ticarcillin disodium equivalent to 3.0 grams ticarcillin and clavulanate potassium equivalent to 0.1 gram clavulanic acid.

4 CONTRAINDICATIONS

TIMENTIN is contraindicated in patients who have a history of hypersensitivity reaction (e.g., anaphylaxis or erythema multiforme) to TIMENTIN or to other β–lactam antibacterials (e.g., penicillins and cephalosporins).

5 WARNINGS AND PRECAUTIONS

5.1 Anaphylactic Reactions

Serious and occasionally fatal hypersensitivity (anaphylactic) reactions have been reported in patients receiving beta-lactam antibacterials. These reactions are more likely to occur in individuals with a history of penicillin hypersensitivity and/or a history of sensitivity to multiple allergens. Before initiating therapy with TIMENTIN, inquire about previous hypersensitivity reactions to penicillins, cephalosporins, or other allergens. If an allergic reaction occurs, discontinue TIMENTIN and institute appropriate therapy.

5.2 *Clostridium difficile* Associated Diarrhea

Clostridium difficile associated diarrhea (CDAD) has been reported with use of nearly all antibacterial agents, including TIMENTIN, and may range in severity from mild diarrhea to fatal colitis. Treatment with antibacterial agents alters the normal flora of the colon leading to overgrowth of *C. difficile*.

C. difficile produces toxins A and B, which contribute to the development of CDAD. Hypertoxin-producing strains of *C. difficile* cause increased morbidity and mortality, as these infections can be refractory to antimicrobial therapy and may require colectomy. CDAD must be considered in all patients who present with diarrhea following antibacterial use. Careful medical history is necessary since CDAD has been reported to occur over 2 months after the administration of antibacterial agents.

If CDAD is suspected or confirmed, ongoing antibacterial use not directed against *C. difficile* may need to be discontinued. Appropriate fluid and electrolyte management, protein supplementation, antibacterial treatment of *C. difficile*, and surgical evaluation should be instituted as clinically indicated.

5.3 Convulsions

Patients may experience convulsions when the dose of TIMENTIN exceeds the recommended dose, especially in the presence of impaired renal function [see Adverse Reactions (6.2), Overdosage (10)].

5.4 Risk of Bleeding

Some patients receiving β-lactam antibacterials have experienced bleeding associated with abnormalities in coagulation tests. These adverse reactions are more likely to occur in patients with renal impairment. If bleeding manifestations appear, treatment with TIMENTIN should be discontinued and appropriate therapy instituted.

5.5 Potential for Microbial Overgrowth or Bacterial Resistance

The possibility of superinfections with fungal or bacterial pathogens should be considered during therapy. If superinfections occur, appropriate measures should be taken.

5.6 Development of Drug-Resistant Bacteria

Prescribing TIMENTIN in the absence of a proven or strongly suspected bacterial infection is unlikely to provide benefit to the patient and increases the risk of the development of drug–resistant bacteria.

5.7 Interference with Laboratory Tests

High urine concentrations of ticarcillin may produce false-positive protein reactions (pseudoproteinuria) [see Drug Interactions (7.4)].

Clavulanic acid may cause a nonspecific binding of IgG and albumin by red cell membranes, leading to a false-positive Coombs test [see Drug Interactions (7.4)].

5.8 Electrolyte Imbalance

Hypokalemia has been reported during treatment with TIMENTIN. Serum potassium should be monitored in patients with fluid and electrolyte imbalance and in patients receiving prolonged therapy. The theoretical sodium content is 4.51 mEq (103.6 mg) per gram of TIMENTIN. This should be considered when treating patients requiring restricted salt intake.

6 ADVERSE REACTIONS

The following are discussed in more detail in other sections of the labeling:
- Anaphylactic Reactions [see Warnings and Precautions (5.1)]
- *Clostridium difficile* Associated Diarrhea [see Warnings and Precautions (5.2)]

6.1 Clinical Trials Experience

Because clinical trials are conducted under widely varying conditions, adverse reaction rates observed in the clinical trials of a drug cannot be directly compared to rates in the clinical trials of another drug and may not reflect the rates observed in practice.

Adverse reactions occurring in ≥1% of 867 patients receiving TIMENTIN 3.1 grams in clinical studies included rash, nausea, diarrhea, and phlebitis at the injection site. The most common laboratory abnormalities (≥3%) were elevations in eosinophils, serum aspartate aminotransferase (AST), and serum alanine aminotransferase (ALT).

Available safety data for pediatric patients treated with TIMENTIN demonstrate a similar adverse event profile to that observed in adult patients.

6.2 Postmarketing Experience

In addition to adverse reactions reported from clinical trials, the following adverse reactions have been identified during postmarketing use of TIMENTIN. Because they are reported voluntarily from a population of unknown size, estimates of frequency cannot be made. These adverse reactions have been chosen for inclusion due to a combination of their seriousness, frequency of reporting, or potential causal connection to TIMENTIN.

Hypersensitivity Reactions: Skin rash, pruritus, urticaria, arthralgia, myalgia, drug fever, chills, chest discomfort, anaphylactic reactions, and bullous reactions (including erythema multiforme, toxic epidermal necrolysis, and Stevens–Johnson syndrome).

Central Nervous System: Headache, giddiness, neuromuscular hyperirritability, or convulsive seizures.

Gastrointestinal Disturbances: Disturbances of taste and smell, stomatitis, flatulence, nausea, vomiting and diarrhea, epigastric pain, and pseudomembranous colitis have been reported. Onset of pseudomembranous colitis symptoms may occur during or after antibacterial treatment [see Warnings and Precautions (5.2)].

Hemic and Lymphatic Systems: Thrombocytopenia, leukopenia, neutropenia, eosinophilia, reduction of hemoglobin or hematocrit, and prolongation of prothrombin time and bleeding time.

Abnormalities of Hepatic Function Tests: Elevation of AST, ALT, serum alkaline phosphatase, serum LDH, and serum bilirubin. There have been reports of transient hepatitis and cholestatic jaundice, as with some other penicillins and some cephalosporins.

Renal and Urinary Effects: Hemorrhagic cystitis, elevation of serum creatinine and/or BUN, hypernatremia, reduction in serum potassium, and uric acid.

Local Reactions: Pain, burning, swelling, and induration at the injection site and thrombophlebitis with intravenous administration.

7 DRUG INTERACTIONS

7.1 Aminoglycosides

The mixing of TIMENTIN with an aminoglycoside in solutions for parenteral administration can result in substantial inactivation of the aminoglycoside.

7.2 Probenecid

Probenecid interferes with the renal tubular secretion of ticarcillin, thereby increasing serum concentrations and prolonging serum half–life of ticarcillin. Probenecid does not affect the serum levels of clavulanic acid.

7.3 Oral Contraceptives

Ticarcillin disodium/clavulanate potassium may affect the gut flora, leading to lower estrogen reabsorption and reduced efficacy of combined oral estrogen/progesterone contraceptives.

7.4 Effects on Laboratory Tests

High urine concentrations of ticarcillin may produce false-positive protein reactions (pseudoproteinuria) with certain methods. The bromphenol blue reagent strip test has been reported to be a reliable method for testing protein reactions [see Warnings and Precautions (5.7)].

Clavulanic acid in TIMENTIN may cause a nonspecific binding of IgG and albumin by red cell membranes, leading to a false–positive Coombs test. A positive Coombs test should be interpreted with caution during treatment with TIMENTIN [see Warnings and Precautions (5.7)].

8 USE IN SPECIFIC POPULATIONS

8.1 Pregnancy

Pregnancy Category B.

Reproduction studies have been performed in rats given doses up to 1,050 mg/kg/day (approximately half of the recommended human dose based on body surface area) and have revealed no evidence of harm to the fetus due to TIMENTIN. There are, however, no adequate and well-controlled studies in pregnant women. Because animal reproduction studies are not always predictive of human response, this drug should be used during pregnancy only if clearly needed.

8.3 Nursing Mothers

It is not known whether ticarcillin or clavulanic acid is excreted in human milk. Because many drugs are excreted in human milk, caution should be exercised when TIMENTIN is administered to a nursing woman.

8.4 Pediatric Use

The safety and effectiveness of TIMENTIN have been established in the age group of 3 months to 16 years. Use of TIMENTIN in these age groups is supported by evidence from adequate and well–controlled studies of TIMENTIN in adults with additional efficacy, safety, and pharmacokinetic data from both comparative and non–comparative studies in pediatric patients. There are insufficient data to support the use of TIMENTIN in pediatric patients under 3 months of age.

If meningitis is suspected or documented, an alternative agent with demonstrated clinical efficacy in this setting should be used.

8.5 Geriatric Use

An analysis of clinical studies of TIMENTIN was conducted to determine whether subjects aged 65 and older respond differently from younger subjects. Of the 1,078 subjects treated with at least one dose of TIMENTIN, 67.5% were <65 years old, and 32.5% were ≥65 years old. No overall differences in safety or efficacy were observed between older and younger subjects, and other reported clinical experience have not identified differences in responses between the elderly and younger patients, but a greater sensitivity of some older individuals cannot be ruled out.

This drug is known to be substantially excreted by the kidney, and the risk of toxic reactions to this drug may be greater in patients with impaired renal function. Because elderly patients are more likely to have decreased renal function, care should be taken in dose selection, and it may be useful to monitor renal function [see Dosage and Administration (2.3)].

TIMENTIN contains 103.6 mg (4.51 mEq) of sodium per gram of TIMENTIN. At the usual recommended doses, patients would receive between 1,285 and 1,927 mg/day (56 and 84 mEq) of sodium. The geriatric population may respond with a blunted natriuresis to salt loading. This may be clinically important with regard to such diseases as congestive heart failure.

8.6 Renal Impairment

Ticarcillin is predominantly excreted by the kidney [see Clinical Pharmacology (12.3)]. Dosage adjustments should be made for patients with renal impairment [see Dosage and Administration (2.3)].

10 OVERDOSAGE

In case of overdosage, discontinue TIMENTIN, treat symptomatically, and institute supportive measures as required. Ticarcillin and clavulanic acid may be removed from circulation by hemodialysis.

11 DESCRIPTION

TIMENTIN (ticarcillin disodium and clavulanate potassium) for Injection, 3.1–gram glass vial, 31–gram Pharmacy Bulk Package, and TIMENTIN (ticarcillin disodium and clavulanate potassium) Injection in the GALAXY Container (PL 2040 Plastic) are a combination of ticarcillin disodium and the β–lactamase inhibitor clavulanate potassium (the potassium salt of clavulanic acid) for intravenous administration. Ticarcillin is derived from the basic penicillin nucleus, 6–amino–penicillanic acid. Chemically, ticarcillin disodium is N-(2-Carboxy-3,3-dimethyl-7-oxo-4-thia-1-azabicyclo[3.2.0]hept-6-yl)-3-thiophenemalonamic acid disodium salt and may be represented as:

Clavulanic acid is produced by the fermentation of Streptomyces clavuligerus. It is a β–lactam structurally related to the penicillins and possesses the ability to inactivate a wide variety of β–lactamases by blocking the active sites of these enzymes. Clavulanic acid is particularly active against the clinically important plasmid–mediated β–lactamases frequently responsible for transferred drug resistance to penicillins and cephalosporins.

Chemically, clavulanic potassium is potassium (Z)-(2R,5R)-3-(2-hydroxyethylidene)-7-oxo-4-oxa-1-azabicyclo[3.2.0]heptane-2-carboxylate and may be represented structurally as:

TIMENTIN (ticarcillin disodium and clavulanate potassium) for Injection, the 3.1–gram glass vial or the 31–gram Pharmacy Bulk Package, are white to pale yellow sterile powders to be reconstituted and diluted for intravenous infusion. The reconstituted solution is clear, colorless or pale yellow, with a pH of 5.5 to 7.5. The 3.1–gram glass vial of TIMENTIN for Injection contains ticarcillin disodium equivalent to 3 grams ticarcillin and clavulanate potassium equivalent to 0.1 gram clavulanic acid. The 31–gram TIMENTIN for Injection Pharmacy Bulk Package contains ticarcillin disodium equivalent to 30 grams ticarcillin and clavulanate potassium equivalent to 1 gram clavulanic acid.

TIMENTIN (ticarcillin disodium and clavulanate potassium) Injection in the GALAXY Container (PL 2040 Plastic) is an iso–osmotic, sterile, nonpyrogenic, frozen solution containing 3.0 grams ticarcillin as ticarcillin disodium and 0.1 gram clavulanic acid as clavulanate potassium. Approximately 0.3 gram sodium citrate hydrous, USP, is added as a buffer. Sodium hydroxide is used to adjust pH and convert ticarcillin monosodium to ticarcillin disodium. The pH may have been adjusted with hydrochloric acid. The solution is intended for intravenous use after thawing to room temperature. The pH of thawed solution ranges from 5.5 to 7.5.

The GALAXY container is fabricated from a specially designed multilayer plastic, PL 2040. Solutions are in contact with the polyethylene layer of this container and can leach out certain chemical components of the plastic in very small amounts within the expiration period. The suitability of the plastic has been confirmed in tests in animals according to the USP biological tests for plastic containers, as well as by tissue culture toxicity studies.

For the 3.1-gram dosage of TIMENTIN, the theoretical sodium content is 4.51 mEq (103.6 mg) per gram of TIMENTIN. The theoretical potassium content is 0.15 mEq (6 mg) per gram of TIMENTIN.

For the 3.1-gram dosage of TIMENTIN in the GALAXY Container, the theoretical total sodium content of the 100-mL solution is 18.7 mEq (429 mg), of which 15.6 mEq (359 mg) is contributed by the ticarcillin disodium component of TIMENTIN. The total theoretical potassium content of the 100-mL solution is 0.50 mEq (19.63 mg).

12 CLINICAL PHARMACOLOGY

12.1 Mechanism of Action

TIMENTIN is an antibacterial drug [see Clinical Pharmacology (12.4)].

12.3 Pharmacokinetics

Absorption: After an intravenous infusion (30 minutes) of 3.1 grams of TIMENTIN, peak serum concentrations of both ticarcillin and clavulanic acid were attained immediately after completion of the infusion. Ticarcillin serum levels were similar to those produced by the administration of equivalent amounts of ticarcillin alone with a mean peak serum level of 324 mcg/mL. The corresponding mean peak serum level for clavulanic acid was 8 mcg/mL. (See Table 2.)

Table 2. Mean Peak Serum Levels (mcg/mL) in Adults After a 30-Minute IV Infusion of 3.1 grams of TIMENTIN

Time	Ticarcillin Peak (Range)	Clavulanic Acid Peak (Range)
0	324 (293 – 388)	8.0 (5.3 – 10.3)
15 minutes	223 (184 – 293)	4.6 (3.0 – 7.6)
30 minutes	176 (135 – 235)	2.6 (1.8 – 3.4)
1 hour	131 (102 – 195)	1.8 (1.6 – 2.2)
1.5 hours	90 (65 – 119)	1.2 (0.8 – 1.6)
3.5 hours	27 (19 – 37)	0.3 (0.2 – 0.3)
5.5 hours	6 (5 – 7)	0

The mean area under the serum concentration curve was 485 mcg•hr/mL for ticarcillin and 8.2 mcg•hr/mL for clavulanic acid.

Distribution: Ticarcillin has been found to be approximately 45% bound to human serum protein and clavulanic acid approximately 25% bound. Ticarcillin can be detected in tissues and interstitial fluid following parenteral administration.

Distribution of ticarcillin into bile and pleural fluid has been demonstrated. The results of experiments involving the administration of clavulanic acid to animals suggest that this compound, like ticarcillin, is well distributed in body tissues.

Elimination: Approximately 60% to 70% of ticarcillin and approximately 35% to 45% of clavulanic acid are excreted unchanged in urine during the first 6 hours after administration of a single dose of TIMENTIN to normal volunteers with normal renal function. Two hours after an intravenous injection of 3.1 grams of TIMENTIN, concentrations of ticarcillin in urine generally exceed 1,500 mcg/mL. The corresponding concentrations of clavulanic acid in urine generally exceed 40 mcg/mL. By 4 to 6 hours after injection, the urine concentrations of ticarcillin and clavulanic acid usually decline to approximately 190 mcg/mL and 2 mcg/mL, respectively.

The mean serum half–life of both ticarcillin and clavulanic acid in healthy volunteers was 1.1 hours.

Pediatrics: In pediatric patients receiving approximately 50 mg/kg of TIMENTIN (30:1 ratio ticarcillin to clavulanate), mean ticarcillin serum half–lives were 4.4

hours in neonates (n = 18) and 1.0 hour in infants and children (n = 41). The corresponding clavulanate serum half–lives averaged 1.9 hours in neonates (n = 14) and 0.9 hour in infants and children (n = 40). Area under the serum concentration time curves averaged 339 mcg•hr/mL in infants and children (n = 41), whereas the corresponding mean clavulanate area under the serum concentration time curves was approximately 7 mcg•hr/mL in the same population (n = 40).

Renal Impairment: An inverse relationship exists between the serum half–life of ticarcillin and creatinine clearance. The half–life of ticarcillin in patients with renal failure is approximately 13 hours. The dosage of TIMENTIN need only be adjusted in cases of severe renal impairment [see Dosage and Administration (2.3)].

Ticarcillin may be removed from patients undergoing dialysis; the actual amount removed depends on the duration and type of dialysis.

12.4 Microbiology

Mechanism of Action: Ticarcillin disrupts bacterial cell wall development by inhibiting peptidoglycan synthesis and/or by interacting with penicillin–binding proteins.

Ticarcillin is susceptible to degradation by β–lactamases, so the spectrum of activity does not normally include organisms which produce these enzymes.

Clavulanic acid is a β–lactam, structurally related to the penicillins, which inactivates some β–lactamase enzymes that are commonly found in bacteria resistant to penicillins and cephalosporins. In particular, it had good activity against the clinically important plasmid–mediated β–lactamases frequently responsible for transferred drug resistance.

The formulation of ticarcillin with clavulanic acid in TIMENTIN protects ticarcillin from degradation by β–lactamase enzymes, effectively extending the antibacterial spectrum of ticarcillin to include many bacteria normally resistant to ticarcillin and other β–lactam antibacterials.

Interaction With Other Antimicrobials: In vitro synergism between TIMENTIN and gentamicin, tobramycin, or amikacin against multi-resistant isolates of Pseudomonas aeruginosa has been demonstrated.

Ticarcillin/clavulanic acid has been shown to be active against most isolates of the following bacteria, both in vitro and in clinical infections [see Indications and Usage (1)].

Susceptibility to ticarcillin/clavulanic acid will vary with geography and time; local susceptibility data should be consulted, if available.

Gram-positive bacteria
Staphylococcus aureus (methicillin-susceptible isolates only)
Staphylococcus epidermidis (methicillin-susceptible isolates only)

Gram-negative bacteria
Citrobacter spp.[a]
Enterobacter spp.[a]
E. cloacae[a]
Escherichia coli[a]
Haemophilus influenzae[b]
Klebsiella spp.[a]
K. pneumoniae[a]
Pseudomonas spp.[a]
P. aeruginosa[a]
Serratia marcescens[a]

Anaerobic bacteria
Bacteroides fragilis group
Prevotella melaninogenicus

[a] Some extended spectrum β–lactamase (ESBL)–producing isolates are resistant to ticarcillin/clavulanic acid. Most carbapenemase-producing isolates are resistant to ticarcillin/clavulanic acid.

[b] β–lactamase–negative, ampicillin–resistant (BLNAR) isolates of H. influenzae must be considered resistant to ticarcillin/clavulanic acid.

The following in vitro data are available, but their clinical significance is unknown. At least 90 percent of the following bacteria exhibit an in vitro minimum inhibitory concentration (MIC) less than or equal to the susceptible breakpoint for ticarcillin/clavulanic acid. However, the efficacy of ticarcillin/clavulanic acid in treating clinical infections due to these bacteria have not been established in adequate and well-controlled clinical trials.

Gram-positive bacteria
Staphylococcus saprophyticus (methicillin-susceptible isolates only)
Streptococcus agalactiae (Group B)
Streptococcus bovis
Streptococcus pneumoniae (penicillin-susceptible isolates only)
Streptococcus pyogenes
Streptococcus spp. viridans group (penicillin-susceptible isolates only)

Gram-negative bacteria
Moraxella catarrhalis
Pasteurella multocida

Anaerobic bacteria

Clostridium spp.
C. perfringens
C. difficile
C. sporogenes
C. ramosum
C. bifermentans
Eubacterium spp.
Fusobacterium spp.
F. nucleatum
F. necrophorum
Peptostreptococcus spp.
Veillonella spp.

Susceptibility Testing: When available, the clinical microbiology laboratory should provide the results of in vitro susceptibility test results for antimicrobial drug products used in local hospitals and practice areas to the physician as periodic reports that describe the susceptibility profile of nosocomial and community-acquired pathogens. These reports should aid the physician in selecting an antibacterial drug product for treatment.

Dilution Techniques: Quantitative methods are used to determine antimicrobial minimum inhibitory concentrations (MICs). These MICs provide estimates of the susceptibility of bacteria to antimicrobial compounds. The MICs should be determined using a standardized test method[2,4] (broth and/or agar). The MIC values should be interpreted according to criteria provided in Table 3.

Diffusion Techniques: Quantitative methods that require measurement of zone diameters can also provide reproducible estimates of the susceptibility of bacteria to antimicrobial compounds. The zone size provides an estimate of the susceptibility of bacteria to antimicrobial compounds. The zone size should be determined using a standardized test method.[3,4] These procedures use paper disks impregnated with 85 mcg of ticarcillin/clavulanate potassium (75 mcg ticarcillin plus 10 mcg clavulanate potassium) to test the susceptibility of bacteria to ticarcillin/clavulanic acid. The disc diffusion interpretive criteria are provided in Table 3.

Anaerobic Techniques: For anaerobic bacteria, susceptibility to ticarcillin/clavulanic acid can be determined by standardized test methods.[4,5] The MIC values obtained should be interpreted according to the criteria in Table 3.

[See table 3 above]

Susceptibility of staphylococci to ticarcillin/clavulanate may be deduced by testing penicillin and either oxacillin or cefoxitin.[4]

A report of "Susceptible" indicates the antimicrobial is likely to inhibit growth of the pathogen if the antimicrobial compound reaches the concentrations at the infection site necessary to inhibit growth of the pathogen. A report of "Intermediate" indicates that the result should be considered equivocal, and, if the bacterium is not fully susceptible to alternative, clinically feasible drugs, the test should be repeated. This category implies possible clinical applicability in body sites where the drug product is physiologically concentrated or in situations where a high dosage of the drug product can be used. This category also provides a buffer zone that prevents small uncontrolled technical factors from causing major discrepancies in interpretation. A report of "Resistant" indicates that the antimicrobial is not likely to inhibit growth of the pathogen if the antimicrobial compound reaches the concentrations usually achievable at the infection site; other therapy should be selected.

Quality Control: Standardized susceptibility test procedures require the use of laboratory controls to monitor and ensure the accuracy and precision of supplies and reagents used in the assay, and the techniques of the individual performing the tests.[2,3,4,5] Standard ticarcillin/clavulanic acid powder should provide the following range of MIC values noted in Table 4. For the diffusion technique using the 85 mcg ticarcillin/clavulanate potassium (75 mcg ticarcillin plus 10 mcg clavulanate potassium), the criteria in Table 4 should be achieved.

[See table 4 above]

13 NONCLINICAL TOXICOLOGY

13.1 Carcinogenesis, Mutagenesis, Impairment of Fertility

Long-term studies in animals have not been performed to evaluate carcinogenic potential. Results from in vitro assays in bacteria (Ames tests), yeast, and human lymphocytes, and in vivo in mouse bone marrow (micronucleus test) indicate TIMENTIN is without genotoxic potential.

Reproduction studies have been performed in rats given doses up to 1,050 mg/kg/day (approximately half of the recommended human dose based on body surface area) and have revealed no evidence of impaired fertility due to TIMENTIN.

14 CLINICAL STUDIES

TIMENTIN has been studied in 296 pediatric patients (excluding neonates and infants less than 3 months) in 6 controlled clinical trials. The majority of patients studied had

Table 3. Susceptibility Test Interpretive Criteria for Ticarcillin/Clavulanic Acid

Microorganism	Minimum Inhibitory Concentration (mcg/mL)			Disc Diffusion (Zone Diameter mm)		
	S	I	R	S	I	R
Anaerobes	≤32/2	64/2	≥128/2	-	-	-
Enterobacteriaceae	≤16/2	32/2 – 64/2	≥128/2	≥20	15 - 19	≤14
Pseudomonas aeruginosa	≤16/2	32/2 - 64/2	≥128/2	≥24	16 - 23	≤15

Table 4. Acceptable Quality Control Ranges for Ticarcillin/Clavulanic Acid

QC Strain	Broth MIC (mcg/mL)	Zone Diameter (mm)	Agar Dilution MIC (mcg/mL)
Bacteroides thetaiotaomicron ATCC 29741	0.5/2 - 2/2	-	0.5/2 - 2/2
Clostridium difficile ATCC 700057	-	-	16/2 - 64/2
Enterococcus faecalis ATCC 29212	16/2 - 64/2	-	-
Escherichia coli ATCC 25922	4/2 - 16/2	24 - 30	-
Escherichia coli ATCC 35218	8/2 - 32/2	21 - 25	-
Eubacterium lentum ATCC 43055	8/2 - 32/2	-	16/2 - 64/2
Pseudomonas aeruginosa ATCC 27853	8/2 - 32/2	20 - 28	-
Staphylococcus aureus ATCC 29213	0.5/2- 2/2	-	-
Staphylococcus aureus ATCC 25923	-	29 - 37	-

ATCC = American Type Culture Collection
MIC = Minimum Inhibitory Concentration

intra-abdominal infections, and the primary comparator was clindamycin and gentamicin with or without ampicillin. At the end-of-therapy visit, comparable efficacy was reported in the trial arms using TIMENTIN and an appropriate comparator.

TIMENTIN was also evaluated in an additional 408 pediatric patients (excluding neonates and infants less than 3 months) in 3 uncontrolled US clinical trials. Patients had a broad range of presenting diagnoses including: Infections in bone and joint, skin and skin structure, lower respiratory tract, urinary tract, as well as intra-abdominal and gynecologic infections. Patients received TIMENTIN, either 300 mg/kg/day (based on the ticarcillin component) divided every 4 hours for severe infection or 200 mg/kg/day (based on the ticarcillin component) divided every 6 hours for mild to moderate infections. Efficacy rates were comparable to those obtained in controlled trials.

The adverse event profile in these 704 pediatric patients treated with TIMENTIN was comparable to that seen in adult patients.

15 REFERENCES

1. Cockcroft, DW, et al. Prediction of creatinine clearance from serum creatinine. *Nephron* 16:31-41, 1976.
2. Clinical and Laboratory Standards Institute (CLSI). Methods for Dilution Antimicrobial Susceptibility Tests for Bacteria that Grow Aerobically; Approved Standard – Ninth Edition. 2012. CLSI document M07-A9. Clinical and Laboratory Standards Institute, 950 West Valley Road, Suite 2500, Wayne, Pennsylvania 19087, USA.
3. Clinical and Laboratory Standards Institute (CLSI). Performance Standards for Antimicrobial Disk Diffusion Susceptibility Tests; Approved Standard – Eleventh Edition. 2012. CLSI document M02-A11. Clinical and Laboratory Standards Institute, 950 West Valley Road, Suite 2500, Wayne, Pennsylvania 19087, USA.
4. Clinical and Laboratory Standards Institute (CLSI). Performance Standards for Antimicrobial Susceptibility Testing; Twenty-fourth Informational Supplement. 2014. CLSI document M100-S24. Clinical and Laboratory Standards Institute, 950 West Valley Road, Suite 2500, Wayne, Pennsylvania 19087, USA.
5. Clinical and Laboratory Standards Institute (CLSI). Methods for Antimicrobial Susceptibility Testing of Anaerobic Bacteria; Approved Standard – Eighth Edition. 2012. CLSI document M11-A8. Clinical and Laboratory Standards Institute, 950 West Valley Road, Suite 2500, Wayne, Pennsylvania 19087, USA.

16 HOW SUPPLIED/STORAGE AND HANDLING

Each 3.1-gram vial of TIMENTIN for Injection contains sterile ticarcillin disodium equivalent to 3 grams ticarcillin and sterile clavulanate potassium equivalent to 0.1 gram clavulanic acid.

NDC 0029-6571-26   3.1-gram Vial

Each 31-gram Pharmacy Bulk Package of TIMENTIN for Injection contains sterile ticarcillin disodium equivalent to 30 grams ticarcillin and sterile clavulanate potassium equivalent to 1 gram clavulanic acid.

NDC 0029-6579-21   31-gram Pharmacy Bulk Package

Each 100-mL single-dose GALAXY Container (PL 2040 Plastic) of TIMENTIN Injection contains ticarcillin disodium equivalent to 3.0 grams ticarcillin and clavulanate potassium equivalent to 0.1 gram clavulanic acid.

NDC 0029-6575-31   100 mL GALAXY Container
                          (PL 2040 Plastic)

3.1-gram Vials and 31-gram Pharmacy Bulk Packages of TIMENTIN for Injection should be stored at or below 25°C (77°F).

GALAXY Containers (PL 2040 Plastic) of TIMENTIN Injection should be stored at or below -20°C (-4°F). Avoid unnecessary handling of containers.

Thawing of Plastic Containers: Thaw frozen container at room temperature 22°C (72°F) or in a refrigerator 4°C (39°F). [Do not force thaw by immersion in water baths or by microwave irradiation.] Check for minute leaks by squeezing container firmly. If leaks are detected discard solution as sterility may be impaired. Do not add supplementary medication.

The container should be visually inspected. Thawed solutions should not be used unless clear; solutions will be light to dark yellow in color. Components of the solution may precipitate in the frozen state and will dissolve upon reaching room temperature with little or no agitation. If, after visual inspection, the solution remains cloudy or if an insoluble precipitate is noted or if any seals or outlet ports are not intact, the container should be discarded.

The thawed solution is stable for 24 hours at room temperature 22°C (72°F) or for 7 days under refrigeration 4°C (39°F).

Do not refreeze.

17 PATIENT COUNSELING INFORMATION

Drug Resistance: Inform patients that antibacterial drugs, including TIMENTIN, should only be used to treat bacterial infections. They do not treat viral infections (e.g., the common cold). When TIMENTIN is prescribed to treat a bacterial infection, inform patients that although it is common to feel better early in the course of therapy, the medication should be taken exactly as directed. Skipping doses or not completing the full course of therapy may: (1) decrease the effectiveness of the immediate treatment, and (2) increase the likelihood that bacteria will develop resistance and will not be treatable by TIMENTIN or other antibacterial drugs in the future.

***Clostridium difficile* Associated Diarrhea:** Inform patients that diarrhea is a common problem caused by antibacterials, and it usually ends when the antibacterial is discontinued. Sometimes after starting treatment with antibacterials, patients can develop watery and bloody stools (with or without stomach cramps and fever) even as late as 2 or more months after having taken their last dose of the antibacterial. If this occurs, advise patients to contact their physician as soon as possible.

Allergic Reactions: Inform patients that TIMENTIN contains a penicillin that can cause allergic reactions in some individuals *[see Warnings and Precautions (5.1)]*.

TIMENTIN is a registered trademark of the GSK group of companies.

GALAXY is a registered trademark of Baxter International Inc.

GlaxoSmithKline

Research Triangle Park, NC 27709

©2014, the GSK group of companies. All rights reserved.

TMN:25PI

TWINRIX   ℞

[*twin'rix*]

[Hepatitis A & Hepatitis B (Recombinant) Vaccine]
Suspension for Intramuscular Injection

HIGHLIGHTS OF PRESCRIBING INFORMATION

These highlights do not include all the information needed to use TWINRIX safely and effectively. See full prescribing information for TWINRIX.

TWINRIX [Hepatitis A & Hepatitis B (Recombinant) Vaccine]
Suspension for Intramuscular Injection
Initial U.S. Approval: 2001

─────── INDICATIONS AND USAGE ───────

TWINRIX is a vaccine indicated for active immunization against disease caused by hepatitis A virus and infection by all known subtypes of hepatitis B virus. TWINRIX is approved for use in persons 18 years of age or older. (1)

─────── DOSAGE AND ADMINISTRATION ───────

• TWINRIX is administered by intramuscular injection. (2.2)
• Standard Dosing: A series of 3 doses (1 mL each) given on a 0-, 1-, and 6-month schedule. (2.3)
• Accelerated Dosing: A series of 4 doses (1 mL each) given on days 0, 7, and 21 to 30 followed by a booster dose at month 12. (2.3)

─────── DOSAGE FORMS AND STRENGTHS ───────

Suspension for injection available in 1-mL single-dose vials and prefilled syringes. (3, 11, 16)

─────── CONTRAINDICATIONS ───────

Severe allergic reaction (e.g., anaphylaxis) after a previous dose of any hepatitis A-containing or hepatitis B-containing vaccine, or to any component of TWINRIX, including yeast and neomycin. (4)

─────── WARNINGS AND PRECAUTIONS ───────

• The tip caps of the prefilled syringes may contain natural rubber latex which may cause allergic reactions in latex-sensitive individuals. (5.1)
• Syncope (fainting) can occur in association with administration of injectable vaccines, including TWINRIX. Procedures should be in place to avoid falling injury and to restore cerebral perfusion following syncope. (5.2)

─────── ADVERSE REACTIONS ───────

Following any dose of TWINRIX, the most common (≥10%) solicited injection site reactions were injection site soreness (35% to 41%) and redness (8% to 11%); the most common solicited systemic adverse events were headache (13% to 22%) and fatigue (11% to 14%). (6.1)
To report SUSPECTED ADVERSE REACTIONS, contact GlaxoSmithKline at 1-888-825-5249 or VAERS at 1-800-822-7967 or www.vaers.hhs.gov

─────── DRUG INTERACTIONS ───────

Do not mix TWINRIX with any other vaccine or product in the same syringe or vial. (7)

─────── USE IN SPECIFIC POPULATIONS ───────

• Safety and effectiveness of TWINRIX have not been established in pregnant women, nursing mothers, and pediatric patients. (8.1, 8.3, 8.4)

• Register women who receive TWINRIX while pregnant in the pregnancy registry by calling 1-888-452-9622. (8.1)
See 17 for PATIENT COUNSELING INFORMATION
Revised: 04/2014

FULL PRESCRIBING INFORMATION

1   INDICATIONS AND USAGE

TWINRIX® is indicated for active immunization against disease caused by hepatitis A virus and infection by all known subtypes of hepatitis B virus. TWINRIX is approved for use in persons 18 years of age or older.

2   DOSAGE AND ADMINISTRATION

2.1   Preparation for Administration

Shake well before use. With thorough agitation, TWINRIX is a slightly turbid white suspension. Do not administer if it appears otherwise. Parenteral drug products should be inspected visually for particulate matter and discoloration prior to administration, whenever solution and container permit. If either of these conditions exists, the vaccine should not be administered.

For the prefilled syringes, attach a sterile needle and administer intramuscularly.

For the vials, use a sterile needle and sterile syringe to withdraw the 1-mL dose and administer intramuscularly. Changing needles between drawing vaccine from a vial and injecting it into a recipient is not necessary unless the needle has been damaged or contaminated. Use a separate sterile needle and syringe for each individual.

2.2   Administration

TWINRIX should be administered by intramuscular injection only as a 1-mL dose. Administer in the deltoid region. Do not administer in the gluteal region; such injections may result in a suboptimal response.

Do not administer this product intravenously, intradermally, or subcutaneously.

2.3   Recommended Dose and Schedule

Standard dosing schedule consists of 3 doses (1 mL each), given intramuscularly at 0, 1, and 6 months. Alternatively, an accelerated schedule of 4 doses (1 mL each), given intramuscularly on days 0, 7, and 21 to 30 followed by a booster dose at month 12 may be used.

3   DOSAGE FORMS AND STRENGTHS

Suspension for injection available in 1-mL single-dose vials and prefilled TIP-LOK® syringes *[see Description (11) and How Supplied/Storage and Handling (16)]*.

4   CONTRAINDICATIONS

Severe allergic reaction (e.g., anaphylaxis) after a previous dose of any hepatitis A-containing or hepatitis B-containing vaccine, or to any component of TWINRIX, including yeast and neomycin, is a contraindication to administration of TWINRIX *[see Description (11)]*.

5   WARNINGS AND PRECAUTIONS

5.1   Latex

The tip caps of the prefilled syringes may contain natural rubber latex which may cause allergic reactions in latex-sensitive individuals.

5.2   Syncope

Syncope (fainting) can occur in association with administration of injectable vaccines, including TWINRIX. Syncope can be accompanied by transient neurological signs such as visual disturbance, paresthesia, and tonic-clonic limb movements. Procedures should be in place to avoid falling injury and to restore cerebral perfusion following syncope.

5.3   Preventing and Managing Allergic Vaccine Reactions

Prior to immunization, the healthcare provider should review the immunization history for possible vaccine sensitivity and previous vaccination-related adverse reactions to allow an assessment of benefits and risks. Appropriate medical treatment and supervision must be available to manage possible anaphylactic reactions following administration of the vaccine. *[See Contraindications (4).]*

5.4   Moderate or Severe Acute Illness

To avoid diagnostic confusion between manifestations of an acute illness and possible vaccine adverse effects, vaccination with TWINRIX should be postponed in persons with moderate or severe acute febrile illness unless they are at immediate risk of hepatitis A or hepatitis B infection.

5.5   Altered Immunocompetence

Immunocompromised persons, including individuals receiving immunosuppressive therapy, may have a diminished immune response to TWINRIX.

5.6   Multiple Sclerosis

Results from 2 clinical studies indicate that there is no association between hepatitis B vaccination and the development of multiple sclerosis,[1] and that vaccination with hepatitis B vaccine does not appear to increase the short-term risk of relapse in multiple sclerosis.[2]

5.7   Limitations of Vaccine Effectiveness

Hepatitis A and hepatitis B have relatively long incubation periods. The vaccine may not prevent hepatitis A or hepatitis B infection in individuals who have an unrecognized hepatitis A or hepatitis B infection at the time of vaccination. Additionally, vaccination with TWINRIX may not protect all individuals.

6   ADVERSE REACTIONS

6.1   Clinical Trials Experience

Because clinical trials are conducted under widely varying conditions, adverse reaction rates observed in the clinical trials of a vaccine cannot be directly compared to rates in the clinical trials of another vaccine and may not reflect the rates observed in practice. As with any vaccine, there is the possibility that broad use of TWINRIX could reveal adverse events not observed in clinical trials.

Following any dose of TWINRIX, the most common (≥10%) solicited injection site reactions were injection site soreness (35% to 41%) and redness (8% to 11%); the most common solicited systemic adverse events were headache (13% to 22%) and fatigue (11% to 14%).

The safety of TWINRIX has been evaluated in clinical trials involving the administration of approximately 7,500 doses to more than 2,500 individuals.

In a US study, 773 subjects (18 to 70 years of age) were randomized 1:1 to receive TWINRIX (0-, 1-, and 6-month schedule) or concurrent administration of ENGERIX-B (0-, 1-, and 6-month schedule) and HAVRIX (0- and 6-month schedule). Solicited local adverse reactions and systemic adverse events were recorded by parents/guardians on diary cards for 4 days (days 0 to 3) after vaccination. Unsolicited adverse events were recorded for 31 days after vaccination. Solicited events reported following the administration of TWINRIX or ENGERIX-B and HAVRIX are presented in Table 1.

[See table 1 at top of next page]

Most solicited local adverse reactions and systemic adverse events seen with TWINRIX were considered by the subjects as mild and self-limiting and did not last more than 48 hours.

In a clinical trial in which TWINRIX was given on a 0-, 7-, and 21- to 30-day schedule followed by a booster dose at 12 months, solicited local adverse reactions or systemic adverse events were comparable to those seen in other clinical trials of TWINRIX given on a 0-, 1-, and 6-month schedule.

Among 2,299 subjects in 14 clinical trials, the following adverse events were reported to occur within 30 days following vaccination:

Incidence 1% to 10% of Injections, Seen in Clinical Trials With TWINRIX:

Infections and Infestations: Upper respiratory tract infections.

General Disorders and Administration Site Conditions: Injection site induration.

Incidence <1% of Injections, Seen in Clinical Trials With TWINRIX:

Infections and Infestations: Respiratory tract illnesses.

Metabolism and Nutrition Disorders: Anorexia.

Psychiatric Disorders: Agitation, insomnia.

Nervous System Disorders: Dizziness, migraine, paresthesia, somnolence, syncope.

Ear and Labyrinth Disorders: Vertigo.

Vascular Disorders: Flushing.

Gastrointestinal Disorders: Abdominal pain, vomiting.

Skin and Subcutaneous Tissue Disorders: Erythema, petechiae, rash, sweating, urticaria.

Musculoskeletal and Connective Tissue Disorders: Arthralgia, back pain, myalgia.

General Disorders and Administration Site Conditions: Injection site ecchymosis, injection site pruritus, influenza-like symptoms, irritability, weakness.

Incidence <1% of Injections, Seen in Clinical Trials With HAVRIX and/or ENGERIX-B:

Blood and Lymphatic System Disorders: Lymphadenopathy.[a+b]

Nervous System Disorders: Dysgeusia,[a] hypertonia,[a] tingling.[b]

Eye Disorders: Photophobia.[a]

Vascular Disorders: Hypotension.[b]

Gastrointestinal Disorders: Constipation.[b]

Investigations: Creatine phosphokinase increased.[a]

[a+b] Following either HAVRIX or ENGERIX-B.

[a] Following HAVRIX.

[b] Following ENGERIX-B.

Adverse events within 30 days of vaccination in the US clinical trial of TWINRIX given on a 0-, 7-, and 21- to 30-day schedule followed by a booster dose at 12 months were comparable to those reported in other clinical trials.

6.2 Postmarketing Experience

The following adverse events have been identified during postapproval use of TWINRIX, HAVRIX, or ENGERIX-B. Because these events are reported voluntarily from a population of uncertain size, it is not possible to reliably estimate their frequency or establish a causal relationship to product exposure.

Postmarketing Experience with TWINRIX: The following list includes serious events or events which have suspected causal connection to components of TWINRIX.

Infections and Infestations: Herpes zoster, meningitis.

Blood and Lymphatic System Disorders: Thrombocytopenia, thrombocytopenic purpura.

Immune System Disorders: Allergic reaction, anaphylactoid reaction, anaphylaxis, serum sickness–like syndrome days to weeks after vaccination (including arthralgia/arthritis, usually transient, fever, urticaria, erythema multiforme, ecchymoses, and erythema nodosum).

Nervous System Disorders: Bell's palsy, convulsions, encephalitis, encephalopathy, Guillain-Barré syndrome, hypoesthesia, myelitis, multiple sclerosis, neuritis, neuropathy, optic neuritis, paralysis, paresis, transverse myelitis.

Eye Disorders: Conjunctivitis, visual disturbances.

Ear and Labyrinth Disorders: Earache, tinnitus.

Cardiac Disorders: Palpitations, tachycardia.

Vascular Disorders: Vasculitis.

Respiratory, Thoracic and Mediastinal Disorders: Bronchospasm including asthma-like symptoms, dyspnea.

Gastrointestinal Disorders: Dyspepsia.

Hepatobiliary Disorders: Hepatitis, jaundice.

Skin and Subcutaneous Tissue Disorders: Alopecia, angioedema, eczema, erythema multiforme, erythema nodosum, hyperhydrosis, lichen planus.

Musculoskeletal and Connective Tissue Disorders: Arthritis, muscular weakness.

General Disorders and Administration Site Conditions: Chills, immediate injection site pain, stinging, and burning sensation, injection site reaction, malaise.

Investigations: Abnormal liver function tests.

Postmarketing Experience With HAVRIX and/or ENGERIX-B: The following list includes serious events or events which have suspected causal connection to components of HAVRIX and/or ENGERIX-B, not already reported above for TWINRIX.

Eye Disorders: Keratitis.[b]

Skin and Subcutaneous Tissue Disorders: Stevens-Johnson syndrome.[b]

Congenital, Familial and Genetic Disorders: Congenital abnormality.[a]

[a] Following HAVRIX.

[b] Following ENGERIX-B.

Table 1. Rates of Local Adverse Reactions and Systemic Adverse Events Within 4 Days of Vaccination[a] With TWINRIX[b] or ENGERIX-B and HAVRIX[c]

Local	TWINRIX			ENGERIX-B			HAVRIX	
	Dose 1	Dose 2	Dose 3	Dose 1	Dose 2	Dose 3	Dose 1	Dose 2
	(N = 385) %	(N = 382) %	(N = 374) %	(N = 382) %	(N = 376) %	(N = 369) %	(N = 382) %	(N = 369) %
Soreness	37	35	41	41	25	30	53	47
Redness	8	9	11	6	7	9	7	9
Swelling	4	4	6	3	5	5	5	5

Systemic	TWINRIX			ENGERIX-B and HAVRIX		
	Dose 1	Dose 2	Dose 3	Dose 1[d]	Dose 2[e]	Dose 3[d]
	(N = 385) %	(N = 382) %	(N = 374) %	(N = 382) %	(N = 376) %	(N = 369) %
Headache	22	15	13	19	12	14
Fatigue	14	13	11	14	9	10
Diarrhea	5	4	6	5	3	3
Nausea	4	3	2	7	3	5
Fever	4	3	2	4	2	4
Vomiting	1	1	0	1	1	1

[a] Within 4 days of vaccination defined as day of vaccination and the next 3 days.

[b] 389 subjects received at least 1 dose of TWINRIX.

[c] 384 subjects received at least 1 dose each of ENGERIX-B and HAVRIX.

[d] Doses 1 and 3 included ENGERIX-B and HAVRIX in the control group receiving separate vaccinations.

[e] Dose 2 included only ENGERIX-B in the control group receiving separate vaccinations.

7 DRUG INTERACTIONS

7.1 Concomitant Administration With Vaccines and Immune Globulin

Do not mix TWINRIX with any other vaccine or product in the same syringe or vial.

When concomitant administration of immunoglobulin is required, it should be given with a different syringe and at a different injection site.

There are no data to assess the concomitant use of TWINRIX with other vaccines.

7.2 Immunosuppressive Therapies

Immunosuppressive therapies, including irradiation, antimetabolites, alkylating agents, cytotoxic drugs, and corticosteroids (used in greater than physiologic doses), may reduce the immune response to TWINRIX.

8 USE IN SPECIFIC POPULATIONS

8.1 Pregnancy

Pregnancy Category C

Animal reproduction studies have not been conducted with TWINRIX. It is also not known whether TWINRIX can cause fetal harm when administered to a pregnant woman or can affect reproduction capacity. TWINRIX should be given to a pregnant woman only if clearly needed.

Pregnancy Registry: GlaxoSmithKline maintains a surveillance registry to collect data on pregnancy outcomes and newborn health status outcomes following vaccination with TWINRIX during pregnancy. Women who receive TWINRIX during pregnancy should be encouraged to contact GlaxoSmithKline directly or their healthcare provider should contact GlaxoSmithKline by calling 1-888-452-9622.

8.3 Nursing Mothers

It is not known whether TWINRIX is excreted in human milk. Because many drugs are excreted in human milk, caution should be exercised when TWINRIX is administered to a nursing woman.

8.4 Pediatric Use

Safety and effectiveness in pediatric patients below the age of 18 years have not been established.

8.5 Geriatric Use

Clinical studies of TWINRIX did not include sufficient numbers of subjects aged 65 years and older to determine whether they respond differently from younger subjects [see Clinical Studies (14.1, 14.3)].

11 DESCRIPTION

TWINRIX [Hepatitis A & Hepatitis B (Recombinant) Vaccine] is a bivalent vaccine containing the antigenic components used in producing HAVRIX® (Hepatitis A Vaccine) and ENGERIX-B® [Hepatitis B Vaccine (Recombinant)]. TWINRIX is a sterile suspension for intramuscular administration that contains inactivated hepatitis A virus (strain HM175) and noninfectious hepatitis B virus surface antigen (HBsAg). The hepatitis A virus is propagated in MRC-5 human diploid cells and inactivated with formalin. The purified HBsAg is obtained by culturing genetically engineered *Saccharomyces cerevisiae* yeast cells, which carry the surface antigen gene of the hepatitis B virus. Bulk preparations of each antigen are adsorbed separately onto aluminum salts and then pooled during formulation.

A 1-mL dose of vaccine contains 720 ELISA Units of inactivated hepatitis A virus and 20 mcg of recombinant HBsAg protein. One dose of vaccine also contains 0.45 mg of aluminum in the form of aluminum phosphate and aluminum hydroxide as adjuvants, amino acids, sodium chloride, phosphate buffer, polysorbate 20, and Water for Injection. From the manufacturing process each 1-mL dose of TWINRIX also contains residual formalin (not more than 0.1 mg), MRC-5 cellular proteins (not more than 2.5 mcg), neomycin sulfate (an aminoglycoside antibiotic included in the cell growth media; not more than 20 ng) and yeast protein (no more than 5%).

TWINRIX is available in vials and prefilled syringes. The tip caps of the prefilled syringes may contain natural rubber latex; the plungers are not made with natural rubber latex. The vial stoppers are not made with natural rubber latex. TWINRIX is formulated without preservatives.

12 CLINICAL PHARMACOLOGY

12.1 Mechanism of Action

Hepatitis A: The course of infection with hepatitis A virus (HAV) is extremely variable, ranging from asymptomatic infection to fulminant hepatitis.[3]

The presence of antibodies to HAV (anti-HAV) confers protection against hepatitis A disease. However, the lowest titer needed to confer protection has not been determined. Natural infection provides lifelong immunity even when antibodies to hepatitis A are undetectable. Seroconversion is defined as antibody titers equal to or greater than the assay cut-off (cut-off values vary depending on the assay used) in those previously seronegative.

Hepatitis B: Infection with hepatitis B virus (HBV) can have serious consequences including acute massive hepatic necrosis and chronic active hepatitis. Chronically infected persons are at increased risk for cirrhosis and hepatocellular carcinoma.

Antibody concentrations ≥10 mIU/mL against HBsAg are recognized as conferring protection against hepatitis B virus infection.[4]

13 NONCLINICAL TOXICOLOGY

13.1 Carcinogenesis, Mutagenesis, Impairment of Fertility

TWINRIX has not been evaluated for its carcinogenic or mutagenic potential, or for impairment of fertility.

14 CLINICAL STUDIES

14.1 Immunogenicity: Standard 0-, 1-, and 6-Month Dosing Schedule

In 11 clinical trials, sera from 1,551 healthy adults 17 to 70 years of age, including 555 male subjects and 996 female subjects, were analyzed following administration of 3 doses of TWINRIX on a 0-, 1-, and 6-month schedule. Seroconversion (defined as equal to or greater than assay cut-off depending on assay used) for antibodies against HAV was elicited in 99.9% of vaccinees, and protective antibodies (defined as ≥10 mIU/mL) against HBV surface antigen were detected in 98.5% of vaccinees, 1 month after completion of the 3-dose series (Table 2).

Table 3. Seroconversion and Seroprotection Rates in a US Clinical Trial

Vaccine	N	Timepoint	% Seroconversion for Hepatitis A[a] (95% CI)	% Seroprotection for Hepatitis B[b] (95% CI)
TWINRIX	264	Month 1	91.6	17.9
		Month 2	97.7	61.2
		Month 7	99.6 (97.9, 100.0)	95.1 (91.7, 97.4)
HAVRIX and ENGERIX-B	269	Month 1	98.1	7.5
		Month 2	98.9	50.4
		Month 7	99.3 (97.3, 99.9)	92.2 (88.3, 95.1)

CI = Confidence Interval
[a] Anti-HAV titer ≥assay cut-off: 33 mIU/mL (ENZYMUN-TEST).
[b] Anti-HBsAg titer ≥10 mIU/mL (AUSAB Test).

Table 4. Geometric Mean Titers in a US Clinical Trial

Vaccine	N	Timepoint	GMT to Hepatitis A (95% CI)	GMT to Hepatitis B (95% CI)
TWINRIX	263	Month 1	335	8
	259	Month 2	636	23
	264	Month 7	4756 (4152, 5448)	2099 (1663, 2649)
HAVRIX and ENGERIX-B	268	Month 1	444	6
	269	Month 2	257	18
	269	Month 7	2948 (2638, 3294)	1871 (1428, 2450)

GMT = Geometric mean titer; CI = Confidence Interval

Table 5. Seroconversion and Seroprotection Rates up to One Month After the Last Dose of Vaccines (According To Protocol Cohort)

	Timepoint	TWINRIX[a]	HAVRIX and ENGERIX-B[b]
		(N = 194-204)	(N = 197-207)
% Seroconversion for Hepatitis A[c] (95% CI)	Day 37	98.5 (95.8, 99.7)	98.6 (95.8, 99.7)
	Day 90	100 (98.2, 100)	95.6 (91.9, 98.0)
	Month 12	96.9 (93.4, 98.9)	86.9 (81.4, 91.2)
	Month 13	100 (98.1, 100)	100 (98.1, 100)
% Seroprotection for Hepatitis B[d] (95% CI)	Day 37	63.2 (56.2, 69.9)	43.5 (36.6, 50.5)
	Day 90	83.2 (77.3, 88.1)	76.7 (70.3, 82.3)
	Month 12	82.1 (75.9, 87.2)	77.8 (71.3, 83.4)
	Month 13	96.4 (92.7, 98.5)	93.4 (89.0, 96.4)

CI = Confidence Interval
[a] TWINRIX given on a 0-, 7-, and 21- to 30-day schedule followed by a booster at month 12.
[b] HAVRIX 1440 EL.U./1 mL given on a 0- and 12-month schedule and ENGERIX-B 20 mcg/1 mL given on a 0-, 1-, 2-, and 12-month schedule.
[c] Anti-HAV titer ≥assay cut-off: 15 mIU/mL (anti-HAV Behring Test).
[d] Anti-HBsAg titer ≥10 mIU/mL (AUSAB Test).

Table 2. Seroconversion and Seroprotection Rates in Worldwide Clinical Trials

TWINRIX Dose	N	% Seroconversion for Hepatitis A[a]	% Seroprotection for Hepatitis B[b]
1	1,587	93.8	30.8
2	1,571	98.8	78.2
3	1,551	99.9	98.5

[a] Anti-HAV titer ≥assay cut-off: 20 mIU/mL (HAVAB Test) or 33 mIU/mL (ENZYMUN-TEST®).
[b] Anti-HBsAg titer ≥10 mIU/mL (AUSAB® Test).

One of the 11 trials was a comparative trial conducted in a US population given either TWINRIX (on a 0-, 1-, and 6-month schedule) or HAVRIX (0- and 6-month schedule) and ENGERIX-B (0-, 1-, and 6-month schedule). The monovalent vaccines were given concurrently in opposite arms. Of the 773 adults (18 to 70 years of age) enrolled in this trial, an immunogenicity analysis was performed in 533 subjects who completed the study according to protocol. Of these, 264 subjects received TWINRIX and 269 subjects received HAVRIX and ENGERIX-B. Seroconversion rates against HAV and seroprotection rates against HBV are presented in Table 3; GMTs are presented in Table 4. The absolute difference in anti-HAV seropositivity rates between groups was 0.36% (90% CI: -1.8, 3.1). Non-inferiority in terms of anti-HAV response was demonstrated (lower limit of the 90% CI was higher than the pre-specified non-inferiority criterion of -4.3%). The absolute difference in anti-HBsAg seroprotection rates between groups was 2.8%

(90% CI: -1.3, 7.7). Non-inferiority in terms of anti-HBV response was demonstrated (lower limit of the 90% CI was higher than the pre-specified non-inferiority criterion of -9.4%).
[See table 3 above]
[See table 4 above]
Since the immune responses to hepatitis A and hepatitis B induced by TWINRIX were non-inferior to the monovalent vaccines, efficacy is expected to be similar to the efficacy for each of the monovalent vaccines.
The antibody titers achieved 1 month after the final dose of TWINRIX were higher than titers achieved 1 month after the final dose of HAVRIX in this clinical trial. This may have been due to a difference in the recommended dosage regimens for these 2 vaccines, whereby TWINRIX vaccinees received 3 doses of 720 EL.U. of hepatitis A antigen at 0, 1, and 6 months, whereas HAVRIX vaccinees received 2 doses of 1440 EL.U. of the same antigen (at 0 and 6 months). However, these differences in peak titer have not been shown to be clinically significant.

14.2   Immunogenicity: Accelerated Dosing Schedule (Day 0-, 7-, and 21-30, Month 12)
In 496 healthy adults, the safety and immunogenicity of TWINRIX given on a 0-, 7-, and 21- to 30-day schedule followed by a booster dose at 12 months (N = 250), was compared to separate vaccinations with monovalent hepatitis A vaccine (HAVRIX at 0 and 12 months) and hepatitis B vaccine (ENGERIX-B at 0, 1, and 12 months) as a control group (N = 246).
Following a booster dose at month 12, seroprotection rates for hepatitis B and seroconversion rates for hepatitis A at month 13 following TWINRIX were non-inferior to the control group. The absolute difference in anti-HBs seroprotec-

tion rates between groups (HAVRIX + ENGERIX-B minus TWINRIX) was -2.99 (95% CI: -7.80, 1.49). Non-inferiority was demonstrated as the upper limit of the 95% CI was lower than the pre-defined limit of 7%. The absolute difference in anti-HAV seroprotection rates between groups (HAVRIX + ENGERIX-B minus TWINRIX) was 0 (95% CI: -1.91, 1.94). Non-inferiority was demonstrated as the upper limit of the 95% CI was lower than the pre-defined limit of 7%. The immune responses are presented in Table 5.
[See table 5 above]
14.3   Immunogenicity in Adults Older Than 40 Years of Age
The effect of age on immune response to TWINRIX was studied in 2 trials. The first trial evaluated subjects 41 to 63 years of age (N = 72; mean age = 50). All subjects were seropositive for anti-HAV antibodies following the third dose of TWINRIX. For the hepatitis B response, 94% of subjects were seroprotected after the third dose of TWINRIX.
The second trial included subjects 19 years of age and older with a comparison between those older than 40 years of age (N = 183, 41 to 70 years of age; mean age = 48) with those 40 years of age or younger (N = 191; 19 to 40 years of age; mean age 33). Over 99% of subjects in both age groups achieved a seropositive response for anti-HAV antibodies and GMTs were comparable between the age groups. In the older subjects who received TWINRIX, 92.9% (95% CI: 88.2, 96.2) achieved seroprotection against hepatitis B compared to 96.9% (95% CI: 93.3, 98.8) of the younger subjects. The GMT was 1,890 mIU/mL in the older subjects compared to 2,285 mIU/mL in the younger subjects.
14.4   Duration of Immunity
Two clinical trials involving a total of 129 subjects demonstrated that antibodies to both HAV and HBV surface antigen persisted for at least 4 years after the first vaccine dose in a 3-dose series of TWINRIX, given on a 0-, 1-, and 6-month schedule. For comparison, after the recommended immunization regimens for HAVRIX and ENGERIX-B, respectively, similar studies involving a total of 114 subjects have shown that seropositivity to HAV and HBV also persists for at least 4 years.

15   REFERENCES
1. Ascherio A, Zhang SM, Hernán MA, et al. Hepatitis B vaccination and the risk of multiple sclerosis. *N Engl J Med.* 2001;344(5):327-332.
2. Confavreux C, Suissa S, Saddier P, et al. Vaccination and the risk of relapse in multiple sclerosis. *N Engl J Med.* 2001;344(5):319-326.
3. Lemon SM. Type A viral hepatitis: new developments in an old disease. *N Engl J Med.* 1985;313(17):1059-1067.
4. Frisch-Niggemeyer W, Ambrosch F, Hofmann H. The assessment of immunity against hepatitis B after vaccination. *J Bio Stand.* 1986;14(3):255-258.

16   HOW SUPPLIED/STORAGE AND HANDLING
TWINRIX is available in 1-mL single-dose vials and 1-mL single-dose prefilled disposable TIP-LOK syringes (packaged without needles) (Preservative Free Formulation):
NDC 58160-815-01 Vial in Package of 10: NDC 58160-815-11
NDC 58160-815-05 Syringe in Package of 1: NDC 58160-815-34
NDC 58160-815-43 Syringe in Package of 10: NDC 58160-815-52
Store refrigerated between 2° and 8°C (36° and 46°F). Do not freeze; discard if product has been frozen.

17   PATIENT COUNSELING INFORMATION
• Inform vaccine recipients of the potential benefits and risks of immunization with TWINRIX.
• Emphasize, when educating vaccine recipients regarding potential side effects, that components of TWINRIX cannot cause hepatitis A or hepatitis B infection.
• Instruct vaccine recipients to report any adverse events to their healthcare provider.
• Inform that safety and efficacy have not been established in pregnant women. Register women who receive TWINRIX while pregnant in the pregnancy registry by calling 1-888-452-9622.
• Give vaccine recipients the Vaccine Information Statements, which are required by the National Childhood Vaccine Injury Act of 1986 to be given prior to immunization. These materials are available free of charge at the Centers for Disease Control and Prevention (CDC) website (www.cdc.gov/vaccines).
TWINRIX, HAVRIX, ENGERIX-B, and TIP-LOK are registered trademarks of the GlaxoSmithKline group of companies. ENZYMUN-TEST is a registered trademark of Boehringer Mannheim Immunodiagnostics. AUSAB is a registered trademark of Abbott Laboratories.
Manufactured by **GlaxoSmithKline Biologicals**
Rixensart, Belgium, US License No. 1617
Distributed by **GlaxoSmithKline**
Research Triangle Park, NC 27709
©2013, GlaxoSmithKline group of companies. All rights reserved.
TWR:22PI

TYKERB
[ti'kerb]
(lapatinib)
tablets

℞

HIGHLIGHTS OF PRESCRIBING INFORMATION

These highlights do not include all the information needed to use TYKERB safely and effectively. See full prescribing information for TYKERB.

TYKERB (lapatinib) tablets, for oral use
Initial U.S. Approval: 2007

————RECENT MAJOR CHANGES————

Indication and Usage (1)	10/2013
Dosage and Administration, Dose Modification Guidelines (2.2)	12/2012
Warnings and Precautions, Diarrhea (5.4)	06/2013

WARNING: HEPATOTOXICITY

See full prescribing information for complete boxed warning.

Hepatotoxicity has been observed in clinical trials and postmarketing experience. The hepatotoxicity may be severe and deaths have been reported. Causality of the deaths is uncertain *[see Warnings and Precautions (5.2)]*.

————INDICATIONS AND USAGE————

TYKERB, a kinase inhibitor, is indicated in combination with: (1)
- capecitabine, for the treatment of patients with advanced or metastatic breast cancer whose tumors overexpress HER2 and who have received prior therapy including an anthracycline, a taxane, and trastuzumab.
 Limitation of Use: Patients should have disease progression on trastuzumab prior to initiation of treatment with TYKERB in combination with capecitabine.
- letrozole for the treatment of postmenopausal women with hormone receptor-positive metastatic breast cancer that overexpresses the HER2 receptor for whom hormonal therapy is indicated.

TYKERB in combination with an aromatase inhibitor has not been compared to a trastuzumab-containing chemotherapy regimen for the treatment of metastatic breast cancer.

————DOSAGE AND ADMINISTRATION————

The recommended dosage of TYKERB for advanced or metastatic breast cancer is 1,250 mg (5 tablets) given orally once daily on Days 1-21 continuously in combination with capecitabine 2,000 mg/m^2/day (administered orally in 2 doses approximately 12 hours apart) on Days 1-14 in a repeating 21-day cycle. (2.1)

The recommended dose of TYKERB for hormone receptor-positive, HER2-positive metastatic breast cancer is 1,500 mg (6 tablets) given orally once daily continuously in combination with letrozole. When TYKERB is coadministered with letrozole, the recommended dose of letrozole is 2.5 mg once daily. (2.1)
- TYKERB should be taken at least one hour before or one hour after a meal. However, capecitabine should be taken with food or within 30 minutes after food. (2.1)
- TYKERB should be taken once daily. Do not divide daily doses of TYKERB. (2.1, 12.3)
- Modify dose for cardiac and other toxicities, severe hepatic impairment, diarrhea, and CYP3A4 drug interactions. (2.2)

————DOSAGE FORMS AND STRENGTHS————

250 mg tablets (3)

————CONTRAINDICATIONS————

Known severe hypersensitivity (e.g., anaphylaxis) to this product or any of its components. (4)

————WARNINGS AND PRECAUTIONS————

- Decreases in left ventricular ejection fraction (LVEF) have been reported. Confirm normal LVEF before starting TYKERB and continue evaluations during treatment. (5.1)
- Lapatinib has been associated with hepatotoxicity. Monitor liver function tests before initiation of treatment, every 4 to 6 weeks during treatment, and as clinically indicated. Discontinue and do not restart TYKERB if patients experience severe changes in liver function tests. (5.2)
- Dose reduction in patients with severe hepatic impairment should be considered. (2.2, 5.3, 8.7)
- Diarrhea, including severe diarrhea, has been reported during treatment. Manage with anti-diarrheal agents, and replace fluids and electrolytes if severe. (5.4)
- Lapatinib has been associated with interstitial lung disease and pneumonitis. Discontinue TYKERB if patients experience severe pulmonary symptoms. (5.5)

- Lapatinib may prolong the QT interval in some patients. Consider ECG and electrolyte monitoring. (5.6, 12.4)
- Fetal harm can occur when administered to a pregnant woman. Women should be advised not to become pregnant when taking TYKERB. (5.7)

————ADVERSE REACTIONS————

The most common (>20%) adverse reactions during treatment with TYKERB plus capecitabine were diarrhea, palmar-plantar erythrodysesthesia, nausea, rash, vomiting, and fatigue. The most common (≥20%) adverse reactions during treatment with TYKERB plus letrozole were diarrhea, rash, nausea, and fatigue. (6.1)

To report SUSPECTED ADVERSE REACTIONS, contact GlaxoSmithKline at 1-888-825-5249 or FDA at 1-800-FDA-1088 or www.fda.gov/medwatch

————DRUG INTERACTIONS————

- TYKERB is likely to increase exposure to concomitantly administered drugs which are substrates of CYP3A4, CYP2C8, or P-glycoprotein (ABCB1). (7.1)
- Avoid strong CYP3A4 inhibitors. If unavoidable, consider dose reduction of TYKERB in patients coadministered a strong CYP3A4 inhibitor. (2.2, 7.2)
- Avoid strong CYP3A4 inducers. If unavoidable, consider gradual dose increase of TYKERB in patients coadministered a strong CYP3A4 inducer. (2.2, 7.2)

See 17 for PATIENT COUNSELING INFORMATION and FDA-approved patient labeling

Revised: 10/2013

FULL PRESCRIBING INFORMATION: CONTENTS*
WARNING: HEPATOTOXICITY

FULL PRESCRIBING INFORMATION

WARNING: HEPATOTOXICITY

Hepatotoxicity has been observed in clinical trials and postmarketing experience. The hepatotoxicity may be severe and deaths have been reported. Causality of the deaths is uncertain *[see Warnings and Precautions (5.2)]*.

---

1   INDICATIONS AND USAGE

TYKERB® is indicated in combination with:
- capecitabine for the treatment of patients with advanced or metastatic breast cancer whose tumors overexpress HER2 and who have received prior therapy including an anthracycline, a taxane, and trastuzumab.
 Limitation of Use: Patients should have disease progression on trastuzumab prior to initiation of treatment with TYKERB in combination with capecitabine.
- letrozole for the treatment of postmenopausal women with hormone receptor-positive metastatic breast cancer that overexpresses the HER2 receptor for whom hormonal therapy is indicated.

TYKERB in combination with an aromatase inhibitor has not been compared to a trastuzumab-containing chemotherapy regimen for the treatment of metastatic breast cancer.

2   DOSAGE AND ADMINISTRATION

2.1   Recommended Dosing

Her2-Positive Metastatic Breast Cancer: The recommended dose of TYKERB is 1,250 mg given orally once daily on Days 1-21 continuously in combination with capecitabine 2,000 mg/m^2/day (administered orally in 2 doses approximately 12 hours apart) on Days 1-14 in a repeating 21-day cycle. TYKERB should be taken at least one hour before or one hour after a meal. The dose of TYKERB should be once daily (5 tablets administered all at once); dividing the daily dose is not recommended *[see Clinical Pharmacology (12.3)]*. Capecitabine should be taken with food or within 30 minutes after food. If a day's dose is missed, the patient should not double the dose the next day. Treatment should be continued until disease progression or unacceptable toxicity occurs.

Hormone Receptor-Positive, HER2-Positive Metastatic Breast Cancer: The recommended dose of TYKERB is 1,500 mg given orally once daily continuously in combination with letrozole. When coadministered with TYKERB, the recommended dose of letrozole is 2.5 mg once daily. TYKERB should be taken at least one hour before or one hour after a meal. The dose of TYKERB should be once daily (6 tablets administered all at once); dividing the daily dose is not recommended *[see Clinical Pharmacology (12.3)]*.

2.2   Dose Modification Guidelines

Cardiac Events: TYKERB should be discontinued in patients with a decreased left ventricular ejection fraction (LVEF) that is Grade 2 or greater by National Cancer Institute Common Terminology Criteria for Adverse Events (NCI CTCAE v3) and in patients with an LVEF that drops below the institution's lower limit of normal *[see Warnings and Precautions (5.1) and Adverse Reactions (6.1)]*. TYKERB in combination with capecitabine may be restarted at a reduced dose (1,000 mg/day) and in combination with letrozole may be restarted at a reduced dose of 1,250 mg/day after a minimum of 2 weeks if the LVEF recovers to normal and the patient is asymptomatic.

Hepatic Impairment: Patients with severe hepatic impairment (Child-Pugh Class C) should have their dose of TYKERB reduced. A dose reduction from 1,250 mg/day to 750 mg/day (HER2-positive metastatic breast cancer indication) or from 1,500 mg/day to 1,000 mg/day (hormone receptor-positive, HER2-positive breast cancer indication) in patients with severe hepatic impairment is predicted to adjust the area under the curve (AUC) to the normal range and should be considered. However, there are no clinical data with this dose adjustment in patients with severe hepatic impairment.

Diarrhea: TYKERB should be interrupted in patients with diarrhea which is NCI CTCAE Grade 3 or Grade 1 or 2 with complicating features (moderate to severe abdominal cramping, nausea or vomiting ≥NCI CTCAE Grade 2, decreased performance status, fever, sepsis, neutropenia, frank bleeding, or dehydration). TYKERB may be reintroduced at a lower dose (reduced from 1,250 mg/day to 1,000 mg/day or from 1,500 mg/day to 1,250 mg/day) when diarrhea resolves to Grade 1 or less. TYKERB should be permanently discontinued in patients with diarrhea which is NCI CTCAE Grade 4 *[see Warnings and Precautions (5.4) and Adverse Reactions (6.1)]*.

Concomitant Strong CYP3A4 Inhibitors: The concomitant use of strong CYP3A4 inhibitors should be avoided (e.g., ketoconazole, itraconazole, clarithromycin, atazanavir, indinavir, nefazodone, nelfinavir, ritonavir, saquinavir, telithromycin, voriconazole). Grapefruit may also increase plasma concentrations of lapatinib and should be avoided. If patients must be coadministered a strong CYP3A4 inhibitor, based on pharmacokinetic studies, a dose reduction to 500 mg/day of lapatinib is predicted to adjust the lapatinib AUC to the range observed without inhibitors and should be considered. However, there are no clinical data with this dose adjustment in patients receiving strong CYP3A4 inhibitors. If the strong inhibitor is discontinued, a washout period of approximately 1 week should be allowed before the lapatinib dose is adjusted upward to the indicated dose *[see Drug Interactions (7.2)]*.

Table 1. Adverse Reactions Occurring in ≥10% of Patients

	TYKERB 1,250 mg/day + Capecitabine 2,000 mg/m²/day (N = 198)			Capecitabine 2,500 mg/m²/day (N = 191)		
	All Grades[a]	Grade 3	Grade 4	All Grades[a]	Grade 3	Grade 4
Reactions	%	%	%	%	%	%
Gastrointestinal disorders						
Diarrhea	65	13	1	40	10	0
Nausea	44	2	0	43	2	0
Vomiting	26	2	0	21	2	0
Stomatitis	14	0	0	11	<1	0
Dyspepsia	11	<1	0	3	0	0
Skin and subcutaneous tissue disorders						
Palmar-plantar erythrodysesthesia	53	12	0	51	14	0
Rash[b]	28	2	0	14	1	0
Dry skin	10	0	0	6	0	0
General disorders and administrative site conditions						
Mucosal inflammation	15	0	0	12	2	0
Musculoskeletal and connective tissue disorders						
Pain in extremity	12	1	0	7	<1	0
Back pain	11	1	0	6	<1	0
Respiratory, thoracic, and mediastinal disorders						
Dyspnea	12	3	0	8	2	0
Psychiatric disorders						
Insomnia	10	<1	0	6	0	0

a   National Cancer Institute Common Terminology Criteria for Adverse Events, version 3.
b   Grade 3 dermatitis acneiform was reported in <1% of patients in the group receiving TYKERB plus capecitabine.

Concomitant Strong CYP3A4 Inducers: The concomitant use of strong CYP3A4 inducers should be avoided (e.g., dexamethasone, phenytoin, carbamazepine, rifampin, rifabutin, rifapentin, phenobarbital, St. John's wort). If patients must be coadministered a strong CYP3A4 inducer, based on pharmacokinetic studies, the dose of lapatinib should be titrated gradually from 1,250 mg/day up to 4,500 mg/day (HER2-positive metastatic breast cancer indication) or from 1,500 mg/day up to 5,500 mg/day (hormone receptor-positive, HER2-positive breast cancer indication) based on tolerability. This dose of lapatinib is predicted to adjust the lapatinib AUC to the range observed without inducers and should be considered. However, there are no clinical data with this dose adjustment in patients receiving strong CYP3A4 inducers. If the strong inducer is discontinued the lapatinib dose should be reduced to the indicated dose [see Drug Interactions (7.2)].

Other Toxicities: Discontinuation or interruption of dosing with TYKERB may be considered when patients develop ≥Grade 2 NCI CTCAE toxicity and can be restarted at the standard dose of 1,250 or 1,500 mg/day when the toxicity improves to Grade 1 or less. If the toxicity recurs, then TYKERB in combination with capecitabine should be restarted at a lower dose (1,000 mg/day) and in combination with letrozole should be restarted at a lower dose of 1,250 mg/day.
See manufacturer's prescribing information for the coadministered product dosage adjustment guidelines in the event of toxicity and other relevant safety information or contraindications.

3   DOSAGE FORMS AND STRENGTHS
250 mg tablets — oval, biconvex, orange, film-coated with GS XJG debossed on one side.

4   CONTRAINDICATIONS
TYKERB is contraindicated in patients with known severe hypersensitivity (e.g., anaphylaxis) to this product or any of its components.

5   WARNINGS AND PRECAUTIONS
5.1   Decreased Left Ventricular Ejection Fraction
TYKERB has been reported to decrease LVEF [see Adverse Reactions (6.1)]. In clinical trials, the majority (>57%) of LVEF decreases occurred within the first 12 weeks of treatment; however, data on long-term exposure are limited. Caution should be taken if TYKERB is to be administered to patients with conditions that could impair left ventricular function. LVEF should be evaluated in all patients prior to initiation of treatment with TYKERB to ensure that the patient has a baseline LVEF that is within the institution's normal limits. LVEF should continue to be evaluated during treatment with TYKERB to ensure that LVEF does not decline below the institution's normal limits [see Dosage and Administration (2.2)].

5.2   Hepatotoxicity
Hepatotoxicity (ALT or AST >3 times the upper limit of normal and total bilirubin >2 times the upper limit of normal) has been observed in clinical trials (<1% of patients) and postmarketing experience. The hepatotoxicity may be severe and deaths have been reported. Causality of the deaths is uncertain. The hepatotoxicity may occur days to several months after initiation of treatment. Liver function tests (transaminases, bilirubin, and alkaline phosphatase) should be monitored before initiation of treatment, every 4 to 6 weeks during treatment, and as clinically indicated. If changes in liver function are severe, therapy with TYKERB should be discontinued and patients should not be retreated with TYKERB [see Adverse Reactions (6.1)].

5.3   Patients With Severe Hepatic Impairment
If TYKERB is to be administered to patients with severe pre-existing hepatic impairment, dose reduction should be considered [see Dosage and Administration (2.2) and Use in Specific Populations (8.7)]. In patients who develop severe hepatotoxicity while on therapy, TYKERB should be discontinued and patients should not be retreated with TYKERB [see Warnings and Precautions (5.2)].

5.4   Diarrhea
Diarrhea has been reported during treatment with TYKERB [see Adverse Reactions (6.1)]. The diarrhea may be severe, and deaths have been reported. Diarrhea generally occurs early during treatment with TYKERB, with almost half of those patients with diarrhea first experiencing it within 6 days. This usually lasts 4 to 5 days. Lapatinib-induced diarrhea is usually low-grade, with severe diarrhea of NCI CTCAE Grades 3 and 4 occurring in <10% and <1% of patients, respectively. Early identification and intervention is critical for the optimal management of diarrhea. Patients should be instructed to report any change in bowel patterns immediately. Prompt treatment of diarrhea with anti-diarrheal agents (such as loperamide) after the first unformed stool is recommended. Severe cases of diarrhea may require administration of oral or intravenous electrolytes and fluids, use of antibiotics such as fluoroquinolones (especially if diarrhea is persistent beyond 24 hours, there is fever, or Grade 3 or 4 neutropenia), and interruption or discontinuation of therapy with TYKERB [see Dosage and Administration (2.2)].

5.5   Interstitial Lung Disease/Pneumonitis
Lapatinib has been associated with interstitial lung disease and pneumonitis in monotherapy or in combination with other chemotherapies [see Adverse Reactions (6.1)]. Patients should be monitored for pulmonary symptoms indicative of interstitial lung disease or pneumonitis. TYKERB should be discontinued in patients who experience pulmonary symptoms indicative of interstitial lung disease/pneumonitis which are ≥Grade 3 (NCI CTCAE).

5.6   QT Prolongation
QT prolongation was observed in an uncontrolled, open-label, dose-escalation study of lapatinib in advanced cancer patients [see Clinical Pharmacology (12.4)]. Lapatinib should be administered with caution to patients who have or may develop prolongation of QTc. These conditions include patients with hypokalemia or hypomagnesemia, with congenital long QT syndrome, patients taking anti-arrhythmic medicines or other medicinal products that lead to QT prolongation, and cumulative high-dose anthracycline therapy. Hypokalemia or hypomagnesemia should be corrected prior to lapatinib administration.

5.7   Use in Pregnancy
TYKERB can cause fetal harm when administered to a pregnant woman. Based on findings in animals, TYKERB is expected to result in adverse reproductive effects. Lapatinib administered to rats during organogenesis and through lactation led to death of offspring within the first 4 days after birth [see Use in Specific Populations (8.1)].
There are no adequate and well-controlled studies with TYKERB in pregnant women. Women should be advised not to become pregnant when taking TYKERB. If this drug is used during pregnancy, or if the patient becomes pregnant while taking this drug, the patient should be apprised of the potential hazard to the fetus.

6   ADVERSE REACTIONS
6.1   Clinical Trials Experience
Because clinical trials are conducted under widely varying conditions, adverse reaction rates observed in the clinical trials of a drug cannot be directly compared to rates in the clinical trials of another drug and may not reflect the rates observed in practice.
HER2-Positive Metastatic Breast Cancer: The safety of TYKERB has been evaluated in more than 12,000 patients in clinical trials. The efficacy and safety of TYKERB in combination with capecitabine in breast cancer was evaluated in 198 patients in a randomized, Phase 3 trial [see Clinical Studies (14.1)]. Adverse reactions which occurred in at least 10% of patients in either treatment arm and were higher in the combination arm are shown in Table 1.
The most common adverse reactions (>20%) during therapy with TYKERB plus capecitabine were gastrointestinal (diarrhea, nausea, and vomiting), dermatologic (palmar-plantar erythrodysesthesia and rash), and fatigue. Diarrhea was the most common adverse reaction resulting in discontinuation of study medication.
The most common Grade 3 and 4 adverse reactions (NCI CTCAE v3) were diarrhea and palmar-plantar erythrodysesthesia. Selected laboratory abnormalities are shown in Table 2.
[See table 1 above]
[See table 2 at top of next page]
Hormone Receptor-Positive, Metastatic Breast Cancer: In a randomized clinical trial of patients (N = 1,286) with hormone receptor-positive, metastatic breast cancer, who had not received chemotherapy for their metastatic disease, patients received letrozole with or without TYKERB. In this trial, the safety profile of TYKERB was consistent with previously reported results from trials of TYKERB in the advanced or metastatic breast cancer population. Adverse reactions which occurred in at least 10% of patients in either treatment arm and were higher in the combination arm are shown in Table 3. Selected laboratory abnormalities are shown in Table 4.

[See table 3 above]

[See table 4 at top of next page]

Decreases in Left Ventricular Ejection Fraction: Due to potential cardiac toxicity with HER2 (ErbB2) inhibitors, LVEF was monitored in clinical trials at approximately 8-week intervals. LVEF decreases were defined as signs or symptoms of deterioration in left ventricular cardiac function that are ≥Grade 3 (NCI CTCAE), or a ≥20% decrease in left ventricular cardiac ejection fraction relative to baseline which is below the institution's lower limit of normal. Among 198 patients who received combination treatment with TYKERB/capecitabine, 3 experienced Grade 2 and one had Grade 3 LVEF adverse reactions (NCI CTCAE v3) *[see Warnings and Precautions (5.1)]*. Among 654 patients who received combination treatment with TYKERB/letrozole, 26 patients experienced Grade 1 or 2 and 6 patients had Grade 3 or 4 LVEF adverse reactions.

Hepatotoxicity: TYKERB has been associated with hepatotoxicity *[see Boxed Warning and Warnings and Precautions (5.2)]*.

Interstitial Lung Disease/Pneumonitis: TYKERB has been associated with interstitial lung disease and pneumonitis in monotherapy or in combination with other chemotherapies *[see Warnings and Precautions (5.5)]*.

6.2 Postmarketing Experience

The following adverse reactions have been identified during post-approval use of TYKERB. Because these reactions are reported voluntarily from a population of uncertain size, it is not always possible to reliably estimate their frequency or establish a causal relationship to drug exposure.

Immune System Disorders: Hypersensitivity reactions including anaphylaxis *[see Contraindications (4)]*.

Skin and Subcutaneous Tissue Disorders: Nail disorders including paronychia.

7 DRUG INTERACTIONS

7.1 Effects of Lapatinib on Drug Metabolizing Enzymes and Drug Transport Systems

Lapatinib inhibits CYP3A4, CYP2C8, and P-glycoprotein (P-gp, ABCB1) in vitro at clinically relevant concentrations and is a weak inhibitor of CYP3A4 in vivo. Caution should be exercised and dose reduction of the concomitant substrate drug should be considered when dosing TYKERB concurrently with medications with narrow therapeutic windows that are substrates of CYP3A4, CYP2C8, or P-gp. Lapatinib did not significantly inhibit the following enzymes in human liver microsomes: CYP1A2, CYP2C9, CYP2C19, and CYP2D6 or UGT enzymes in vitro, however, the clinical significance is unknown.

Midazolam: Following coadministration of TYKERB and midazolam (CYP3A4 substrate), 24-hour systemic exposure (AUC) of orally administered midazolam increased 45%, while 24-hour AUC of intravenously administered midazolam increased 22%.

Paclitaxel: In cancer patients receiving TYKERB and paclitaxel (CYP2C8 and P-gp substrate), 24-hour systemic exposure (AUC) of paclitaxel was increased 23%. This increase in paclitaxel exposure may have been underestimated from the in vivo evaluation due to study design limitations.

Digoxin: Following coadministration of TYKERB and digoxin (P-gp substrate), systemic AUC of an oral digoxin dose increased approximately 2.8-fold. Serum digoxin concentrations should be monitored prior to initiation of TYKERB and throughout coadministration. If digoxin serum concentration is >1.2 ng/mL, the digoxin dose should be reduced by half.

7.2 Drugs That Inhibit or Induce Cytochrome P450 3A4 Enzymes

Lapatinib undergoes extensive metabolism by CYP3A4, and concomitant administration of strong inhibitors or inducers of CYP3A4 alter lapatinib concentrations significantly *(see Ketoconazole and Carbamazepine sections, below)*. Dose adjustment of lapatinib should be considered for patients who must receive concomitant strong inhibitors or concomitant strong inducers of CYP3A4 enzymes *[see Dosage and Administration (2.2)]*.

Ketoconazole: In healthy subjects receiving ketoconazole, a CYP3A4 inhibitor, at 200 mg twice daily for 7 days, systemic exposure (AUC) to lapatinib was increased to approximately 3.6-fold of control and half-life increased to 1.7-fold of control.

Carbamazepine: In healthy subjects receiving the CYP3A4 inducer, carbamazepine, at 100 mg twice daily for 3 days and 200 mg twice daily for 17 days, systemic exposure (AUC) to lapatinib was decreased approximately 72%.

7.3 Drugs That Inhibit Drug Transport Systems

Lapatinib is a substrate of the efflux transporter P-glycoprotein (P-gp, ABCB1). If TYKERB is administered with drugs that inhibit P-gp, increased concentrations of lapatinib are likely, and caution should be exercised.

7.4 Acid-Reducing Agents

The aqueous solubility of lapatinib is pH dependent, with higher pH resulting in lower solubility. However, esomeprazole, a proton pump inhibitor, administered at a dose of 40 mg once daily for 7 days, did not result in a clinically meaningful reduction in lapatinib steady-state exposure.

8 USE IN SPECIFIC POPULATIONS

8.1 Pregnancy

Pregnancy Category D *[see Warnings and Precautions (5.7)]*.

Based on findings in animals, TYKERB can cause fetal harm when administered to a pregnant woman. Lapatinib administered to rats during organogenesis and through lactation led to death of offspring within the first 4 days after birth. When administered to pregnant animals during the period of organogenesis, lapatinib caused fetal anomalies (rats) or abortions (rabbits) at maternally toxic doses. There are no adequate and well-controlled studies with TYKERB in pregnant women. Women should be advised not to become pregnant when taking TYKERB. If this drug is used during pregnancy, or if the patient becomes pregnant while taking this drug, the patient should be apprised of the potential hazard to the fetus.

In a study where pregnant rats were dosed with lapatinib during organogenesis and through lactation, at a dose of 120 mg/kg/day (approximately 6.4 times the human clinical exposure based on AUC following 1,250-mg dose of lapatinib plus capecitabine), 91% of the pups had died by the fourth day after birth, while 34% of the 60 mg/kg/day pups were dead. The highest no-effect dose for this study was 20 mg/kg/day (approximately equal to the human clinical exposure based on AUC).

Table 2. Selected Laboratory Abnormalities

Parameters	TYKERB 1,250 mg/day + Capecitabine 2,000 mg/m²/day			Capecitabine 2,500 mg/m²/day		
	All Grades[a]	Grade 3	Grade 4	All Grades[a]	Grade 3	Grade 4
	%	%	%	%	%	%
Hematologic						
Hemoglobin	56	<1	0	53	1	0
Platelets	18	<1	0	17	<1	<1
Neutrophils	22	3	<1	31	2	1
Hepatic						
Total Bilirubin	45	4	0	30	3	0
AST	49	2	<1	43	2	0
ALT	37	2	0	33	1	0

[a] National Cancer Institute Common Terminology Criteria for Adverse Events, version 3.

Table 3. Adverse Reactions Occurring in ≥10% of Patients

Reactions	TYKERB 1,500 mg/day + Letrozole 2.5 mg/day (N = 654)			Letrozole 2.5 mg/day (N = 624)		
	All Grades[a]	Grade 3	Grade 4	All Grades[a]	Grade 3	Grade 4
	%	%	%	%	%	%
Gastrointestinal disorders						
Diarrhea	64	9	<1	20	<1	0
Nausea	31	<1	0	21	<1	0
Vomiting	17	1	<1	11	<1	<1
Anorexia	11	<1	0	9	<1	0
Skin and subcutaneous tissue disorders						
Rash[b]	44	1	0	13	0	0
Dry skin	13	<1	0	4	0	0
Alopecia	13	<1	0	7	0	0
Pruritus	12	<1	0	9	<1	0
Nail Disorder	11	<1	0	<1	0	0
General disorders and administrative site conditions						
Fatigue	20	2	0	17	<1	0
Asthenia	12	<1	0	11	<1	0
Nervous system disorders						
Headache	14	<1	0	13	<1	0
Respiratory, thoracic, and mediastinal disorders						
Epistaxis	11	<1	0	2	<1	0

[a] National Cancer Institute Common Terminology Criteria for Adverse Events, version 3.
[b] In addition to the rash reported under "Skin and subcutaneous tissue disorders", 3 additional subjects in each treatment arm had rash under "Infections and infestations"; none were Grade 3 or 4.

Table 4. Selected Laboratory Abnormalities

Hepatic Parameters	TYKERB 1,500 mg/day + Letrozole 2.5 mg/day			Letrozole 2.5 mg/day		
	All Grades[a]	Grade 3	Grade 4	All Grades[a]	Grade 3	Grade 4
	%	%	%	%	%	%
AST	53	6	0	36	2	<1
ALT	46	5	<1	35	1	0
Total Bilirubin	22	<1	<1	11	1	<1

[a] National Cancer Institute Common Terminology Criteria for Adverse Events, version 3.

Lapatinib was studied for effects on embryo-fetal development in pregnant rats and rabbits given oral doses of 30, 60, and 120 mg/kg/day. There were no teratogenic effects; however, minor anomalies (left-sided umbilical artery, cervical rib, and precocious ossification) occurred in rats at the maternally toxic dose of 120 mg/kg/day (approximately 6.4 times the human clinical exposure based on AUC following 1,250-mg dose of lapatinib plus capecitabine). In rabbits, lapatinib was associated with maternal toxicity at 60 and 120 mg/kg/day (approximately 0.07 and 0.2 times the human clinical exposure, respectively, based on AUC following 1,250-mg dose of lapatinib plus capecitabine) and abortions at 120 mg/kg/day. Maternal toxicity was associated with decreased fetal body weights and minor skeletal variations.

8.3 Nursing Mothers
It is not known whether lapatinib is excreted in human milk. Because many drugs are excreted in human milk and because of the potential for serious adverse reactions in nursing infants from TYKERB, a decision should be made whether to discontinue nursing or to discontinue the drug, taking into account the importance of the drug to the mother.

8.4 Pediatric Use
The safety and effectiveness of TYKERB in pediatric patients have not been established.

8.5 Geriatric Use
Of the total number of metastatic breast cancer patients in clinical studies of TYKERB in combination with capecitabine (N = 198), 17% were 65 years of age and older, and 1% were 75 years of age and older. Of the total number of hormone receptor-positive, HER2-positive metastatic breast cancer patients in clinical studies of TYKERB in combination with letrozole (N = 642), 44% were 65 years of age and older, and 12% were 75 years of age and older. No overall differences in safety or effectiveness were observed between elderly subjects and younger subjects, and other reported clinical experience has not identified differences in responses between the elderly and younger patients, but greater sensitivity of some older individuals cannot be ruled out.

8.6 Renal Impairment
Lapatinib pharmacokinetics have not been specifically studied in patients with renal impairment or in patients undergoing hemodialysis. There is no experience with TYKERB in patients with severe renal impairment. However, renal impairment is unlikely to affect the pharmacokinetics of lapatinib given that less than 2% (lapatinib and metabolites) of an administered dose is eliminated by the kidneys.

8.7 Hepatic Impairment
The pharmacokinetics of lapatinib were examined in subjects with pre-existing moderate (n = 8) or severe (n = 4) hepatic impairment (Child-Pugh Class B/C, respectively) and in 8 healthy control subjects. Systemic exposure (AUC) to lapatinib after a single oral 100-mg dose increased approximately 14% and 63% in subjects with moderate and severe pre-existing hepatic impairment, respectively. Administration of TYKERB in patients with severe hepatic impairment should be undertaken with caution due to increased exposure to the drug. A dose reduction should be considered for patients with severe pre-existing hepatic impairment *[see Dosage and Administration (2.2)]*. In patients who develop severe hepatotoxicity while on therapy, TYKERB should be discontinued and patients should not be retreated with TYKERB *[see Warnings and Precautions (5.2)]*.

10 OVERDOSAGE
There is no known antidote for overdoses of TYKERB. The maximum oral doses of lapatinib that have been administered in clinical trials are 1,800 mg once daily. More frequent ingestion of TYKERB could result in serum concentrations exceeding those observed in clinical trials and could result in increased toxicity. Therefore, missed doses should not be replaced and dosing should resume with the next scheduled daily dose.

Asymptomatic and symptomatic cases of overdose have been reported. The doses ranged from 2,500 to 9,000 mg daily and where reported, the duration varied between 1 and 17 days. Symptoms observed include lapatinib-associated events *[see Adverse Reactions (6.1)]* and in some cases sore scalp, sinus tachycardia (with otherwise normal ECG), and/or mucosal inflammation.
Because lapatinib is not significantly renally excreted and is highly bound to plasma proteins, hemodialysis would not be expected to be an effective method to enhance the elimination of lapatinib.
Treatment of overdose with TYKERB should consist of general supportive measures.

11 DESCRIPTION
Lapatinib is a small molecule and a member of the 4-anilinoquinazoline class of kinase inhibitors. It is present as the monohydrate of the ditosylate salt, with chemical name N-(3-chloro-4-[[(3-fluorophenyl)methyl]oxy]phenyl]-6-[5-([[2-(methylsulfonyl)ethyl]amino]methyl)-2-furanyl]-4-quinazolinamine bis(4-methylbenzenesulfonate) monohydrate. It has the molecular formula $C_{29}H_{26}ClFN_4O_4S$ $(C_7H_8O_3S)_2$ H_2O and a molecular weight of 943.5. Lapatinib ditosylate monohydrate has the following chemical structure:

Lapatinib is a yellow solid, and its solubility in water is 0.007 mg/mL and in 0.1N HCl is 0.001 mg/mL at 25°C.
Each 250 mg tablet of TYKERB contains 405 mg of lapatinib ditosylate monohydrate, equivalent to 398 mg of lapatinib ditosylate or 250 mg lapatinib free base.
The inactive ingredients of TYKERB are: **Tablet Core:** Magnesium stearate, microcrystalline cellulose, povidone, sodium starch glycolate. **Coating:** Orange film-coat: FD&C yellow No. 6/sunset yellow FCF aluminum lake, hypromellose, macrogol/PEG 400, polysorbate 80, titanium dioxide.

12 CLINICAL PHARMACOLOGY
12.1 Mechanism of Action
Lapatinib is a 4-anilinoquinazoline kinase inhibitor of the intracellular tyrosine kinase domains of both Epidermal Growth Factor Receptor (EGFR [ErbB1]) and of Human Epidermal Receptor Type 2 (HER2 [ErbB2]) receptors (estimated K_i^{app} values of 3nM and 13nM, respectively) with a dissociation half-life of ≥300 minutes. Lapatinib inhibits ErbB-driven tumor cell growth in vitro and in various animal models.
An additive effect was demonstrated in an in vitro study when lapatinib and 5-FU (the active metabolite of capecitabine) were used in combination in the 4 tumor cell lines tested. The growth inhibitory effects of lapatinib were evaluated in trastuzumab-conditioned cell lines. Lapatinib retained significant activity against breast cancer cell lines selected for long-term growth in trastuzumab-containing medium in vitro. These in vitro findings suggest non–cross-resistance between these two agents.
Hormone receptor-positive breast cancer cells (with ER [Estrogen Receptor] and/or PgR [Progesterone Receptor]) that coexpress the HER2 tend to be resistant to established endocrine therapies. Similarly, hormone receptor-positive breast cancer cells that initially lack EGFR or HER2 up-regulate these receptor proteins as the tumor becomes resistant to endocrine therapy.

12.3 Pharmacokinetics
Absorption: Absorption following oral administration of TYKERB is incomplete and variable. Serum concentrations appear after a median lag time of 0.25 hours (range 0 to 1.5 hours). Peak plasma concentrations (C_{max}) of lapatinib are achieved approximately 4 hours after administration. Daily dosing of TYKERB results in achievement of steady state within 6 to 7 days, indicating an effective half-life of 24 hours.
At the dose of 1,250 mg daily, steady-state geometric mean (95% confidence interval) values of C_{max} were 2.43 mcg/mL (1.57 to 3.77 mcg/mL) and AUC were 36.2 mcg.h/mL (23.4 to 56 mcg.h/mL).
Divided daily doses of TYKERB resulted in approximately 2-fold higher exposure at steady state (steady-state AUC) compared to the same total dose administered once daily. Systemic exposure to lapatinib is increased when administered with food. Lapatinib AUC values were approximately 3- and 4-fold higher (C_{max} approximately 2.5- and 3-fold higher) when administered with a low-fat (5% fat-500 calories) or with a high-fat (50% fat-1,000 calories) meal, respectively.
Distribution: Lapatinib is highly bound (>99%) to albumin and alpha-1 acid glycoprotein. In vitro studies indicate that lapatinib is a substrate for the transporters breast cancer-resistance protein (BCRP, ABCG2) and P-glycoprotein (P-gp, ABCB1). Lapatinib has also been shown to inhibit P-gp, BCRP, and the hepatic uptake transporter OATP 1B1, in vitro at clinically relevant concentrations.
Metabolism: Lapatinib undergoes extensive metabolism, primarily by CYP3A4 and CYP3A5, with minor contributions from CYP2C19 and CYP2C8 to a variety of oxidated metabolites, none of which accounts for more than 14% of the dose recovered in the feces or 10% of lapatinib concentration in plasma.
Elimination: At clinical doses, the terminal phase half-life following a single dose was 14.2 hours; accumulation with repeated dosing indicates an effective half-life of 24 hours. Elimination of lapatinib is predominantly through metabolism by CYP3A4/5 with negligible (<2%) renal excretion. Recovery of parent lapatinib in feces accounts for a median of 27% (range 3% to 67%) of an oral dose.
Effects of Age, Gender, or Race: Studies of the effects of age, gender, or race on the pharmacokinetics of lapatinib have not been performed.

12.4 QT Prolongation
The QT prolongation potential of lapatinib was assessed as part of an uncontrolled, open-label, dose-escalation study in advanced cancer patients. Eighty-one patients received daily doses of lapatinib ranging from 175 mg/day to 1,800 mg/day. Serial ECGs were collected on Day 1 and Day 14 to evaluate the effect of lapatinib on QT intervals. Analysis of the data suggested a consistent concentration-dependent increase in QTc interval.

12.5 Pharmacogenomics
The HLA alleles DQA1*02:01 and DRB1*07:01 were associated with hepatotoxicity reactions in a genetic substudy of a monotherapy trial with TYKERB (n = 1,194). Severe liver injury (ALT >5 times the upper limit of normal, NCI CT-CAE Grade 3) occurred in 2% of patients overall; the incidence of severe liver injury among DQA1*02:01 or DRB1*07:01 allele carriers was 8% versus 0.5% in non-carriers. These HLA alleles are present in approximately 15% to 25% of Caucasian, Asian, African, and Hispanic populations and 1% in Japanese populations. Liver function should be monitored in all patients receiving therapy with TYKERB regardless of genotype.

13 NONCLINICAL TOXICOLOGY
13.1 Carcinogenesis, Mutagenesis, Impairment of Fertility
Two-year carcinogenicity studies with lapatinib are ongoing.
Lapatinib was not clastogenic or mutagenic in the Chinese hamster ovary chromosome aberration assay, microbial mutagenesis (Ames) assay, human lymphocyte chromosome aberration assay or the in vivo rat bone marrow chromosome aberration assay at single doses up to 2,000 mg/kg. However, an impurity in the drug product (up to 4 ppm or 8 mcg/day) was genotoxic when tested alone in both in vitro and in vivo assays.
There were no effects on male or female rat mating or fertility at doses up to 120 mg/kg/day in females and 180 mg/kg/day in males (approximately 6.4 times and 2.6 times the expected human clinical exposure based on AUC following 1,250-mg dose of lapatinib plus capecitabine, respectively). The effect of lapatinib on human fertility is unknown. However, when female rats were given oral doses of lapatinib during breeding and through the first 6 days of gestation, a significant decrease in the number of live fetuses was seen at 120 mg/kg/day and in the fetal body weights at ≥60 mg/kg/day (approximately 6.4 times and 3.3 times the expected human clinical exposure based on AUC following 1,250-mg dose of lapatinib plus capecitabine, respectively).

14 CLINICAL STUDIES

14.1 HER2-Positive Metastatic Breast Cancer

The efficacy and safety of TYKERB in combination with capecitabine in breast cancer were evaluated in a randomized, Phase 3 trial. Patients eligible for enrollment had HER2 (ErbB2) overexpressing (IHC 3+ or IHC 2+ confirmed by FISH), locally advanced or metastatic breast cancer, progressing after prior treatment that included anthracyclines, taxanes, and trastuzumab.

Patients were randomized to receive either TYKERB 1,250 mg once daily (continuously) plus capecitabine 2,000 mg/m^2/day on Days 1-14 every 21 days, or to receive capecitabine alone at a dose of 2,500 mg/m^2/day on Days 1-14 every 21 days. The endpoint was time to progression (TTP). TTP was defined as time from randomization to tumor progression or death related to breast cancer. Based on the results of a pre-specified interim analysis, further enrollment was discontinued. Three hundred and ninety-nine (399) patients were enrolled in this study. The median age was 53 years and 14% were older than 65 years. Ninety-one percent (91%) were Caucasian. Ninety-seven percent (97%) had stage IV breast cancer, 48% were estrogen receptor+ (ER+) or progesterone receptor+ (PR+), and 95% were ErbB2 IHC 3+ or IHC 2+ with FISH confirmation. Approximately 95% of patients had prior treatment with anthracyclines, taxanes, and trastuzumab.

Efficacy analyses 4 months after the interim analysis are presented in Table 5, Figure 1, and Figure 2.

[See table 5 above]

Table 5. Efficacy Results

	Independent Assessment[a]		Investigator Assessment	
	TYKERB 1,250 mg/day + Capecitabine 2,000 mg/m^2/day	Capecitabine 2,500 mg/m^2/day	TYKERB 1,250 mg/day + Capecitabine 2,000 mg/m^2/day	Capecitabine 2,500 mg/m^2/day
	(N = 198)	(N = 201)	(N = 198)	(N = 201)
Number of TTP events	82	102	121	126
Median TTP, weeks (25th, 75th, Percentile), weeks	27.1 (17.4, 49.4)	18.6 (9.1, 36.9)	23.9 (12.0, 44.0)	18.3 (6.9, 35.7)
Hazard Ratio (HR) (95% CI) P value	0.57 (0.43, 0.77) 0.00013		0.72 (0.56, 0.92) 0.00762	
Response Rate (%) (95% CI)	23.7 (18.0, 30.3)	13.9 (9.5, 19.5)	31.8 (25.4, 38.8)	17.4 (12.4, 23.4)

TTP = Time to progression.

[a] The time from last tumor assessment to the data cut-off date was >100 days in approximately 30% of patients in the independent assessment. The pre-specified assessment interval was 42 or 84 days.

Figure 1. Kaplan-Meier Estimates for Independent Review Panel-evaluated Time to Progression

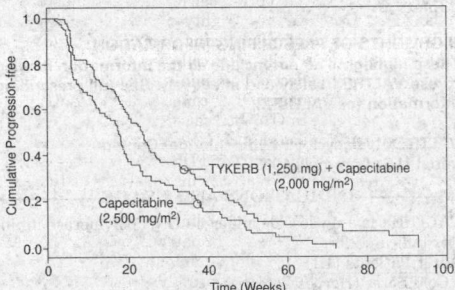

Figure 2. Kaplan-Meier Estimates for Investigator Assessment Time to Progression

At the time of above efficacy analysis, the overall survival data were not mature (32% events). However, based on the TTP results, the study was unblinded and patients receiving capecitabine alone were allowed to cross over to treatment with TYKERB plus capecitabine. The survival data were followed for an additional 2 years to be mature and the analysis is summarized in Table 6.

Table 6: Overall Survival Data

	TYKERB 1,250 mg/day + Capecitabine 2,000 mg/m^2/day (N = 207)	Capecitabine 2,500 mg/m^2/day (N = 201)
Overall Survival		
Died	76%	82%
Median Overall Survival (weeks)	75.0	65.9
Hazard ratio, 95% CI (P value)	0.89 (0.71, 1.10) 0.276	

CI = confidence interval.

Clinical Studies Describing Limitation of Use: In two randomized trials, TYKERB-based chemotherapy regimens have been shown to be less effective than trastuzumab-based chemotherapy regimens. The first randomized, open-label study compared the safety and efficacy of TYKERB in combination with capecitabine relative to trastuzumab in combination with capecitabine in women with HER2-positive metastatic breast cancer (N = 540). The study was stopped early based on the findings of a pre-planned interim analysis showing a low incidence of CNS events (primary endpoint) and superior efficacy of the trastuzumab plus capecitabine. The median progression-free survival was 6.6 months in the group receiving TYKERB in combination with capecitabine compared with 8.0 months in the group receiving the trastuzumab combination [HR = 1.30 (95% CI: 1.04, 1.64)]. Overall survival was analyzed when 26% of deaths occurred in the group receiving TYKERB in combination with capecitabine and 22% in the group receiving the trastuzumab combination [HR = 1.34 (95% CI: 0.95, 1.92)]. The second randomized, open-label study compared the safety and efficacy of taxane-based chemotherapy plus TYKERB to taxane-based chemotherapy plus trastuzumab as first-line therapy in women with HER2-positive, metastatic breast cancer (N = 652). The study was stopped early based on findings from a pre-planned interim analysis. The median progression-free survival was 11.3 months in the trastuzumab combination treatment arm compared to 9.0 months in patients treated with TYKERB in the combination arm for the intent-to-treat population [HR = 1.37 (95% CI: 1.13, 1.65)].

14.2 Hormone Receptor-Positive, HER2-Positive Metastatic Breast Cancer

The efficacy and safety of TYKERB in combination with letrozole were evaluated in a double-blind, placebo-controlled, multi-center study. A total of 1,286 postmenopausal women with hormone receptor-positive (ER-positive and/or PgR-positive) metastatic breast cancer, who had not received prior therapy for metastatic disease, were randomly assigned to receive either TYKERB (1,500 mg once daily) plus letrozole (2.5 mg once daily) (n = 642) or letrozole (2.5 mg once daily) alone (n = 644). Of all patients randomized to treatment, 219 (17%) patients had tumors overexpressing the HER2 receptor, defined as fluorescence in situ hybridization (FISH) (≥2 or 3+ immunohistochemistry (IHC). There were 952 (74%) patients who were HER2-negative and 115 (9%) patients did not have their HER2 receptor status confirmed. The primary objective was to evaluate and compare progression-free survival (PFS) in the HER2-positive population. Progression-free survival was defined as the interval of time between date of randomization and the earlier date of first documented sign of disease progression or death due to any cause.

The baseline demographic and disease characteristics were balanced between the two treatment arms. The median age was 63 years and 45% were 65 years of age or older. Eighty-four percent (84%) of the patients were white. Approximately 50% of the HER2-positive population had prior adjuvant/neo-adjuvant chemotherapy and 56% had prior hormonal therapy. Only 2 patients had prior trastuzumab. In the HER2-positive subgroup (n = 219), the addition of TYKERB to letrozole resulted in an improvement in PFS. In the HER2-negative subgroup, there was no improvement in PFS of the combination of TYKERB plus letrozole compared to the letrozole plus placebo. Overall response rate (ORR)

was also improved with the combination of TYKERB plus letrozole. The overall survival (OS) data were not mature. Efficacy analyses for the hormone receptor-positive, HER2-positive and HER2-negative subgroups are presented in Table 7 and Figure 3.

[See table 7 at top of next page]

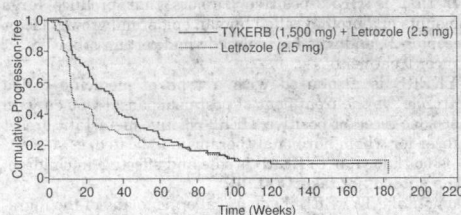

Figure 3. Kaplan-Meier Estimates for Progression-Free Survival for the HER2 Positive Population

16 HOW SUPPLIED/STORAGE AND HANDLING

The 250 mg tablets of TYKERB are oval, biconvex, orange, and film-coated with GS XJG debossed on one side and are available in:

Bottles of 150 tablets: NDC 0173-0752-00

Store at 25°C (77°F); excursions permitted to 15° to 30°C (59° to 86°F) [see USP Controlled Room Temperature].

17 PATIENT COUNSELING INFORMATION

See FDA-approved patient labeling (Patient Information).

17.1 Information for Patients

Patients should be informed of the following:

• TYKERB has been reported to decrease left ventricular ejection fraction which may result in shortness of breath, palpitations, and/or fatigue. Patients should inform their physician if they develop these symptoms while taking TYKERB.

• TYKERB often causes diarrhea which may be severe in some cases. Patients should be told how to manage and/or prevent diarrhea and to inform their physician immediately if there is any change in bowel patterns or severe diarrhea occurs during treatment with TYKERB.

• TYKERB may interact with many drugs; therefore, patients should be advised to report to their healthcare provider the use of any other prescription or nonprescription medication or herbal products.

• TYKERB may interact with grapefruit. Patients should not take TYKERB with grapefruit products.

• TYKERB should be taken at least one hour before or one hour after a meal, in contrast to capecitabine which should be taken with food or within 30 minutes after food.

• The dose of TYKERB should be taken once daily. Dividing the daily dose is not recommended.

TYKERB is a registered trademark of the GlaxoSmithKline group of companies.

GlaxoSmithKline

Research Triangle Park, NC 27709

©2013, GlaxoSmithKline group of companies. All rights reserved.

TKB:13PI

Table 7. Efficacy Results

	HER2-Positive Population		HER2-Negative Population	
	TYKERB 1500 mg/day + Letrozole 2.5 mg/ day	Letrozole 2.5 mg/day	TYKERB 1500 mg/day + Letrozole 2.5 mg/ day	Letrozole 2.5 mg/day
	(N = 111)	(N = 108)	(N = 478)	(N = 474)
Median PFS[a], weeks (95% CI)	35.4 (24.1, 39.4)	13.0 (12.0, 23.7)	59.7 (48.6, 69.7)	58.3 (47.9, 62.0)
Hazard Ratio (95% CI) P value	0.71 (0.53, 0.96) 0.019		0.90 (0.77, 1.05) 0.188	
Response Rate (%) (95% CI)	27.9 (19.8, 37.2)	14.8 (8.7, 22.9)	32.6 (28.4, 37.0)	31.6 (27.5, 36.0)

PFS = progression-free survival; CI = confidence interval.
[a] Kaplan-Meier estimate.

PHARMACIST - DETACH HERE AND GIVE INSTRUCTIONS TO PATIENT

PATIENT INFORMATION
TYKERB® (TIE-curb)
(lapatinib)
tablets
Read this leaflet before you start taking TYKERB and each time you get a refill. There may be new information. This information does not take the place of talking with your doctor about your medical condition or treatment.

What is TYKERB?
TYKERB is used with the medicine capecitabine for the treatment of people with advanced or metastatic breast cancer that is HER2-positive (tumors that produce large amounts of a protein called human epidermal growth factor receptor-2), and who have already had certain other breast cancer treatments.
TYKERB is also used with a type of medicine called letrozole for the treatment of postmenopausal women with hormone receptor-positive, HER2-positive metastatic breast cancer for whom hormonal therapy is indicated.
It is not known if TYKERB is safe and effective in children.
Who should not take TYKERB?
Do not take TYKERB if you are allergic to any of the ingredients in TYKERB. See the end of this leaflet for a complete list of ingredients in TYKERB.
What should I tell my doctor before taking TYKERB?
Before you take TYKERB, tell your doctor if you:
• have heart problems.
• have liver problems. You may need a lower dose of TYKERB.
• have any other medical conditions.
• are pregnant or plan to become pregnant. TYKERB can harm your unborn baby. You should not become pregnant while taking TYKERB. Tell your doctor right away if you become pregnant during treatment with TYKERB.
• are breastfeeding or plan to breastfeed. It is not known if TYKERB passes into your breast milk. You and your doctor should decide if you will take TYKERB or breastfeed. You should not do both.
Tell your doctor about all the medicines you take, including prescription and over-the-counter medicines, vitamins, and herbal supplements. TYKERB may affect the way other medicines work, and other medicines may affect the way TYKERB works.
Especially tell your doctor if you take:
• antibiotics and anti-fungal medicines (used to treat infections)
• HIV medicines
• medicines used to treat seizures
• medicines used to treat heart problems or high blood pressure
• antidepressants
• medicines that reduce stomach acid (antacids)
• St. John's wort
Know the medicines you take. Keep a list of your medicines with you to show your doctor and pharmacist when you get a new medicine. Do not take other medicines during treatment with TYKERB without first talking with your doctor.
How should I take TYKERB?
• Take TYKERB exactly as your doctor tells you to take it. Your doctor may change your dose of TYKERB if needed.
  ○ For people with advanced or metastatic breast cancer, TYKERB and capecitabine are taken in 21-day cycles. The usual dose of TYKERB is 1,250 mg (5 tablets) taken by mouth all at once, **one time a day on days 1 to 21.**
  ○ Your doctor will tell you the dose of capecitabine you should take and when you should take it.
  ○ Take capecitabine with food or within 30 minutes after food.

• For people with hormone receptor-positive, HER2-positive breast cancer, TYKERB and letrozole are taken **every day.** The usual dose of TYKERB is 1,500 mg (6 tablets) taken by mouth all at once, **one time a day.** Your doctor will tell you the dose of letrozole you should take and when you should take it.
• TYKERB should be taken at least 1 hour before, or at least 1 hour after a meal.
• Do not eat or drink grapefruit products during treatment with TYKERB.
• If you miss a dose of TYKERB, take your next dose at your regular time the next day.
• If you take too much TYKERB, call your doctor or go to the nearest hospital emergency room right away.
What are the possible side effects of TYKERB?
TYKERB may cause serious side effects, including:
• **heart problems,** including decreased pumping of blood from the heart and an abnormal heartbeat. Signs and symptoms of an abnormal heartbeat include:
  ○ feeling like your heart is pounding or racing
  ○ dizziness
  ○ tiredness
  ○ feeling lightheaded
  ○ shortness of breath
  Your doctor should check your heart function before you start taking TYKERB and during treatment.
• **liver problems.** Liver problems can be severe and deaths have happened. Signs and symptoms of liver problems include:
  ○ itching
  ○ yellowing of your skin or the white part of your eyes
  ○ dark urine
  ○ pain or discomfort in the right upper stomach area
  Your doctor should do blood tests to check your liver before you start taking TYKERB and during treatment.
• **diarrhea.** Diarrhea is common with TYKERB and may sometimes be severe. Severe diarrhea can cause loss of body fluid (dehydration) and some deaths have happened. Call your doctor right away if you have a change in bowel pattern or if you have severe diarrhea. Follow your doctor's instructions for what to do to help prevent or treat diarrhea.
• **lung problems.** Symptoms of a lung problem with TYKERB include a cough that will not go away or shortness of breath.
Call your doctor right away if you have any of the signs or symptoms of the serious side effects listed above.
Common side effects of TYKERB in combination with capecitabine or letrozole include:
• diarrhea
• red, painful hands and feet
• nausea
• rash
• vomiting
• tiredness or weakness
• mouth sores
• loss of appetite
• indigestion
• unusual hair loss or thinning
• nose bleeds
• headache
• dry skin
• itching
• nail disorders such as nail bed changes, nail pain, infection and swelling of the cuticles.
Tell your doctor if you have any side effect that bothers you or that does not go away.
These are not all the possible side effects of TYKERB. For more information, ask your doctor or pharmacist.
Call your doctor for medical advice about side effects. You may report side effects to FDA at 1-800-FDA-1088.

You may also get side effects from the other medicines taken with TYKERB. Talk to your doctor about possible side effects you may get during treatment.
How should I store TYKERB Tablets?
• Store TYKERB Tablets at room temperature between 68° and 77°F (20° and 25°C).
• Keep the container closed tightly.
• Do not keep medicine that is out of date or that you no longer need.
Keep TYKERB and all medicines out of the reach of children.
General information about TYKERB
Medicines are sometimes prescribed for purposes other than those listed in patient information leaflets. Do not use TYKERB for a condition for which it was not prescribed. Do not give TYKERB to other people, even if they have the same symptoms that you have. It may harm them.
This leaflet summarizes the most important information about TYKERB. If you would like more information, talk with your doctor. You can ask your doctor or pharmacist for information about TYKERB that is written for health professionals.
For more information, call 1-888-825-5249 or go to www.tykerb.com.
What are the ingredients in TYKERB?
Active ingredient: Lapatinib.
Inactive Ingredients: Tablet Core: Magnesium stearate, microcrystalline cellulose, povidone, sodium starch glycolate. **Coating:** Orange film-coat: FD&C yellow No. 6/sunset yellow FCF aluminum lake, hypromellose, macrogol/PEG 400, polysorbate 80, titanium dioxide.
This Patient Information has been approved by the U.S. Food and Drug Administration.
TYKERB is a registered trademark of the GlaxoSmithKline group of companies.
GlaxoSmithKline
Research Triangle Park, NC 27709
©2013, GlaxoSmithKline group of companies. All rights reserved.
Revised: October 2013
TKB:11PIL

VALTREX   ℞
[val'trĕx]
(valacyclovir hydrochloride)
Caplets

HIGHLIGHTS OF PRESCRIBING INFORMATION
These highlights do not include all the information needed to use VALTREX safely and effectively. See full prescribing information for VALTREX.

VALTREX (valacyclovir hydrochloride) Caplets
Initial U.S. Approval: 1995

———————INDICATIONS AND USAGE———————

VALTREX is a nucleoside analogue DNA polymerase inhibitor indicated for:
Adult Patients (1.1)
• Cold Sores (Herpes Labialis)
• Genital Herpes
  • Treatment in immunocompetent patients (initial or recurrent episode)
  • Suppression in immunocompetent or HIV-1-infected patients
  • Reduction of transmission
• Herpes Zoster
Pediatric Patients (1.2)
• Cold Sores (Herpes Labialis)
• Chickenpox
Limitations of Use (1.3)
• The efficacy and safety of VALTREX have not been established in immunocompromised patients other than for the suppression of genital herpes in HIV-1—infected patients.

———————DOSAGE AND ADMINISTRATION———————

Adult Dosage (2.1)	
Cold Sores	2 grams every 12 hours for 1 day
Genital Herpes	
Initial episode	1 gram twice daily for 10 days
Recurrent episodes	500 mg twice daily for 3 days
Suppressive therapy Immunocompetent patients	1 gram once daily

Alternate dose in patients with less than or equal to 9 recurrences/year	500 mg once daily
HIV-1—infected patients	500 mg twice daily
Reduction of transmission	500 mg once daily
Herpes Zoster	1 gram 3 times daily for 7 days

Pediatric Dosage (2.2)

Cold Sores (aged greater than or equal to 12 years)	2 grams every 12 hours for 1 day
Chickenpox (aged 2 to less than 18 years)	20 mg/kg 3 times daily for 5 days; not to exceed 1 gram 3 times daily

Valacyclovir oral suspension (25 mg/mL or 50 mg/mL) can be prepared from the 500 mg VALTREX Caplets. (2.3)

DOSAGE FORMS AND STRENGTHS

Caplets: 500 mg (unscored), 1 gram (partially scored) (3)

CONTRAINDICATIONS

Hypersensitivity to valacyclovir (e.g., anaphylaxis), acyclovir, or any component of the formulation. (4)

WARNINGS AND PRECAUTIONS

- Thrombotic thrombocytopenic purpura/hemolytic uremic syndrome (TTP/HUS): Has occurred in patients with advanced HIV-1 disease and in allogenic bone marrow transplant and renal transplant patients receiving 8 grams per day of VALTREX in clinical trials. Discontinue treatment if clinical symptoms and laboratory findings consistent with TTP/HUS occur. (5.1)
- Acute renal failure: May occur in elderly patients (with or without reduced renal function), patients with underlying renal disease who receive higher than recommended doses of VALTREX for their level of renal function, patients who receive concomitant nephrotoxic drugs, or inadequately hydrated patients. Use with caution in elderly patients and reduce dosage in patients with renal impairment. (2.4, 5.2)
- Central nervous system adverse reactions (e.g., agitation, hallucinations, confusion, and encephalopathy): May occur in both adult and pediatric patients (with or without reduced renal function) and in patients with underlying renal disease who receive higher than recommended doses of VALTREX for their level of renal function. Elderly patients are more likely to have central nervous system adverse reactions. Use with caution in elderly patients and reduce dosage in patients with renal impairment. (2.4,5.3)

ADVERSE REACTIONS

- The most common adverse reactions reported in at least one indication by greater than 10% of adult subjects treated with VALTREX and more commonly than in subjects treated with placebo are headache, nausea, and abdominal pain. (6.1)
- The only adverse reaction occurring in greater than 10% of pediatric subjects less than 18 years of age was headache. (6.2)

To report SUSPECTED ADVERSE REACTIONS, contact GlaxoSmithKline at 1-888-825-5249 or FDA at 1-800-FDA-1088 or www.fda.gov/medwatch.

See 17 for PATIENT COUNSELING INFORMATION and FDA-approved patient labeling

Revised: 12/2013

FULL PRESCRIBING INFORMATION: CONTENTS*

FULL PRESCRIBING INFORMATION

1 INDICATIONS AND USAGE

1.1 Adult Patients

Cold Sores (Herpes Labialis): VALTREX® (valacyclovir hydrochloride) Caplets are indicated for treatment of cold sores (herpes labialis). The efficacy of VALTREX initiated after the development of clinical signs of a cold sore (e.g., papule, vesicle, or ulcer) has not been established.

Genital Herpes: Initial Episode: VALTREX is indicated for treatment of the initial episode of genital herpes in immunocompetent adults. The efficacy of treatment with VALTREX when initiated more than 72 hours after the onset of signs and symptoms has not been established.

Recurrent Episodes: VALTREX is indicated for treatment of recurrent episodes of genital herpes in immunocompetent adults. The efficacy of treatment with VALTREX when initiated more than 24 hours after the onset of signs and symptoms has not been established.

Suppressive Therapy: VALTREX is indicated for chronic suppressive therapy of recurrent episodes of genital herpes in immunocompetent and in HIV-1—infected adults. The efficacy and safety of VALTREX for the suppression of genital herpes beyond 1 year in immunocompetent patients and beyond 6 months in HIV-1—infected patients have not been established.

Reduction of Transmission: VALTREX is indicated for the reduction of transmission of genital herpes in immunocompetent adults. The efficacy of VALTREX for the reduction of transmission of genital herpes beyond 8 months in discordant couples has not been established. The efficacy of VALTREX for the reduction of transmission of genital herpes in individuals with multiple partners and non—heterosexual couples has not been established. Safer sex practices should be used with suppressive therapy (see current Centers for Disease Control and Prevention [CDC] Sexually Transmitted Diseases Treatment Guidelines).

Herpes Zoster: VALTREX is indicated for the treatment of herpes zoster (shingles) in immunocompetent adults. The efficacy of VALTREX when initiated more than 72 hours after the onset of rash and the efficacy and safety of VALTREX for treatment of disseminated herpes zoster have not been established.

1.2 Pediatric Patients

Cold Sores (Herpes Labialis): VALTREX is indicated for the treatment of cold sores (herpes labialis) in pediatric patients aged greater than or equal to 12 years. The efficacy of VALTREX initiated after the development of clinical signs of a cold sore (e.g., papule, vesicle, or ulcer) has not been established.

Chickenpox: VALTREX is indicated for the treatment of chickenpox in immunocompetent pediatric patients aged 2 to less than 18 years. Based on efficacy data from clinical trials with oral acyclovir, treatment with VALTREX should be initiated within 24 hours after the onset of rash [see Clinical Studies (14.4)].

1.3 Limitations of Use

The efficacy and safety of VALTREX have not been established in:
- Immunocompromised patients other than for the suppression of genital herpes in HIV—1—infected patients with a CD4+ cell count greater than or equal to 100 cells/mm³.
- Patients aged less than 12 years with cold sores (herpes labialis).
- Patients aged less than 2 years or greater than or equal to 18 years with chickenpox.
- Patients aged less than 18 years with genital herpes.

- Patients aged less than 18 years with herpes zoster.
- Neonates and infants as suppressive therapy following neonatal herpes simplex virus (HSV) infection.

2 DOSAGE AND ADMINISTRATION

- VALTREX may be given without regard to meals.
- Valacyclovir oral suspension (25 mg/mL or 50 mg/mL) may be prepared extemporaneously from 500-mg VALTREX Caplets for use in pediatric patients for whom a solid dosage form is not appropriate [see Dosage and Administration (2.3)].

2.1 Adult Dosing Recommendations

Cold Sores (Herpes Labialis): The recommended dosage of VALTREX for treatment of cold sores is 2 grams twice daily for 1 day taken 12 hours apart. Therapy should be initiated at the earliest symptom of a cold sore (e.g., tingling, itching, or burning).

Genital Herpes: Initial Episode: The recommended dosage of VALTREX for treatment of initial genital herpes is 1 gram twice daily for 10 days. Therapy was most effective when administered within 48 hours of the onset of signs and symptoms.

Recurrent Episodes: The recommended dosage of VALTREX for treatment of recurrent genital herpes is 500 mg twice daily for 3 days. Initiate treatment at the first sign or symptom of an episode.

Suppressive Therapy: The recommended dosage of VALTREX for chronic suppressive therapy of recurrent genital herpes is 1 gram once daily in patients with normal immune function. In patients with a history of 9 or fewer recurrences per year, an alternative dose is 500 mg once daily. In HIV—1—infected patients with a CD4+ cell count greater than or equal to 100 cells/mm³, the recommended dosage of VALTREX for chronic suppressive therapy of recurrent genital herpes is 500 mg twice daily.

Reduction of Transmission: The recommended dosage of VALTREX for reduction of transmission of genital herpes in patients with a history of 9 or fewer recurrences per year is 500 mg once daily for the source partner.

Herpes Zoster: The recommended dosage of VALTREX for treatment of herpes zoster is 1 gram 3 times daily for 7 days. Therapy should be initiated at the earliest sign or symptom of herpes zoster and is most effective when started within 48 hours of the onset of rash.

2.2 Pediatric Dosing Recommendations

Cold Sores (Herpes Labialis): The recommended dosage of VALTREX for the treatment of cold sores in pediatric patients aged greater than or equal to 12 years is 2 grams twice daily for 1 day taken 12 hours apart. Therapy should be initiated at the earliest symptom of a cold sore (e.g., tingling, itching, or burning).

Chickenpox: The recommended dosage of VALTREX for treatment of chickenpox in immunocompetent pediatric patients aged 2 to less than 18 years is 20 mg/kg administered 3 times daily for 5 days. The total dose should not exceed 1 gram 3 times daily. Therapy should be initiated at the earliest sign or symptom [see Use in Specific Populations (8.4), Clinical Pharmacology (12.3), Clinical Studies (14.4)].

2.3 Extemporaneous Preparation of Oral Suspension

Ingredients and Preparation per USP—NF: VALTREX Caplets 500 mg, cherry flavor, and Suspension Structured Vehicle USP—NF (SSV). Valacyclovir oral suspension (25 mg/mL or 50 mg/mL) should be prepared in lots of 100 mL.

Prepare Suspension at Time of Dispensing as Follows:

- Prepare SSV according to the USP-NF.
- Using a pestle and mortar, grind the required number of VALTREX 500 mg Caplets until a fine powder is produced (5 VALTREX Caplets for 25 mg/mL suspension; 10 VALTREX Caplets for 50 mg/mL suspension).
- Gradually add approximately 5-mL aliquots of SSV to the mortar and triturate the powder until a paste has been produced. Ensure that the powder has been adequately wetted.
- Continue to add approximately 5-mL aliquots of SSV to the mortar, mixing thoroughly between additions, until a concentrated suspension is produced, to a minimum total quantity of 20 mL SSV and a maximum total quantity of 40 mL SSV for both the 25-mg/mL and 50—mg/mL suspensions.
- Transfer the mixture to a suitable 100-mL measuring flask.
- Transfer the cherry flavor* to the mortar and dissolve in approximately 5 mL of SSV. Once dissolved, add to the measuring flask.
- Rinse the mortar at least 3 times with approximately 5-mL aliquots of SSV, transferring the rinsing to the measuring flask between additions.
- Make the suspension to volume (100 mL) with SSV and shake thoroughly to mix.
- Transfer the suspension to an amber glass medicine bottle with a child—resistant closure.
- The prepared suspension should be labeled with the following information "Shake well before using. Store suspension between 2° to 8°C (36° to 46°F) in a refrigerator. Discard after 28 days."

---

*The amount of cherry flavor added is as instructed by the suppliers of the cherry flavor.

Table 1. VALTREX Dosage Recommendations for Adults With Renal Impairment

Indications	Normal Dosage Regimen (Creatinine Clearance ≥50 mL/min)	Creatinine Clearance (mL/min)		
		30-49	10-29	<10
Cold sores (Herpes labialis) Do not exceed 1 day of treatment.	Two 2 gram doses taken 12 hours apart	Two 1 gram doses taken 12 hours apart	Two 500 mg doses taken 12 hours apart	500 mg single dose
Genital herpes: Initial episode	1 gram every 12 hours	no reduction	1 gram every 24 hours	500 mg every 24 hours
Genital herpes: Recurrent episode	500 mg every 12 hours	no reduction	500 mg every 24 hours	500 mg every 24 hours

Genital herpes:
  Suppressive therapy
    Immunocompetent patients
	1 gram every 24 hours	no reduction	500 mg every 24 hours	500 mg every 24 hours

Alternate dose for immunocompetent patients with less than or equal to 9 recurrences/year	500 mg every 24 hours	no reduction	500 mg every 48 hours	500 mg every 48 hours
HIV—1—infected patients	500 mg every 12 hours	no reduction	500 mg every 24 hours	500 mg every 24 hours
Herpes zoster	1 gram every 8 hours	1 gram every 12 hours	1 gram every 24 hours	500 mg every 24 hours

2.4   Patients With Renal Impairment
Dosage recommendations for adult patients with reduced renal function are provided in Table 1 [see Use in Specific Populations (8.5, 8.6), Clinical Pharmacology (12.3)]. Data are not available for the use of VALTREX in pediatric patients with a creatinine clearance less than 50 mL/min/1.73 m².
[See table 1 above]
Hemodialysis: Patients requiring hemodialysis should receive the recommended dose of VALTREX after hemodialysis. During hemodialysis, the half—life of acyclovir after administration of VALTREX is approximately 4 hours. About one-third of acyclovir in the body is removed by dialysis during a 4—hour hemodialysis session.
Peritoneal Dialysis: There is no information specific to administration of VALTREX in patients receiving peritoneal dialysis. The effect of chronic ambulatory peritoneal dialysis (CAPD) and continuous arteriovenous hemofiltration/dialysis (CAVHD) on acyclovir pharmacokinetics has been studied. The removal of acyclovir after CAPD and CAVHD is less pronounced than with hemodialysis, and the pharmacokinetic parameters closely resemble those observed in patients with end—stage renal disease (ESRD) not receiving hemodialysis. Therefore, supplemental doses of VALTREX should not be required following CAPD or CAVHD.

3   DOSAGE FORMS AND STRENGTHS
Caplets:
• 500-mg: blue, film—coated, capsule—shaped tablets printed with "VALTREX 500 mg."
• 1-gram: blue, film—coated, capsule—shaped tablets, with a partial scorebar on both sides, printed with "VALTREX 1 gram."

4   CONTRAINDICATIONS
VALTREX is contraindicated in patients who have had a demonstrated clinically significant hypersensitivity reaction (e.g., anaphylaxis) to valacyclovir, acyclovir, or any component of the formulation [see Adverse Reactions (6.3)].

5   WARNINGS AND PRECAUTIONS
5.1   Thrombotic Thrombocytopenic Purpura/Hemolytic Uremic Syndrome (TTP/HUS)
TTP/HUS, in some cases resulting in death, has occurred in patients with advanced HIV—1 disease and also in allogeneic bone marrow transplant and renal transplant recipients participating in clinical trials of VALTREX at doses of 8 grams per day. Treatment with VALTREX should be stopped immediately if clinical signs, symptoms, and laboratory abnormalities consistent with TTP/HUS occur.
5.2   Acute Renal Failure
Cases of acute renal failure have been reported in:
• Elderly patients with or without reduced renal function. Caution should be exercised when administering VALTREX to geriatric patients, and dosage reduction is recommended for those with impaired renal function [see Dosage and Administration (2.4), Use in Specific Populations (8.5)].
• Patients with underlying renal disease who received higher-than-recommended doses of VALTREX for their level of renal function. Dosage reduction is recommended when administering VALTREX to patients with renal impairment [see Dosage and Administration (2.4), Use in Specific Populations (8.6)].

• Patients receiving other nephrotoxic drugs. Caution should be exercised when administering VALTREX to patients receiving potentially nephrotoxic drugs.
• Patients without adequate hydration. Precipitation of acyclovir in renal tubules may occur when the solubility (2.5 mg/mL) is exceeded in the intratubular fluid. Adequate hydration should be maintained for all patients.
In the event of acute renal failure and anuria, the patient may benefit from hemodialysis until renal function is restored [see Dosage and Administration (2.4), Adverse Reactions (6.3)].
5.3   Central Nervous System Effects
Central nervous system adverse reactions, including agitation, hallucinations, confusion, delirium, seizures, and encephalopathy, have been reported in both adult and pediatric patients with or without reduced renal function and in patients with underlying renal disease who received higher-than-recommended doses of VALTREX for their level of renal function. Elderly patients are more likely to have central nervous system adverse reactions. VALTREX should be discontinued if central nervous system adverse reactions occur [see Adverse Reactions (6.3), Use in Specific Populations (8.5, 8.6)].

6   ADVERSE REACTIONS
The following serious adverse reactions are discussed in greater detail in other sections of the labeling:
• Thrombotic Thrombocytopenic Purpura/Hemolytic Uremic Syndrome [see Warnings and Precautions (5.1)].
• Acute Renal Failure [see Warnings and Precautions (5.2)].
• Central Nervous System Effects [see Warnings and Precautions (5.3)].
The most common adverse reactions reported in at least 1 indication by greater than 10% of adult subjects treated with VALTREX and observed more frequently with VALTREX compared to placebo are headache, nausea, and abdominal pain. The only adverse reaction reported in greater than 10% of pediatric subjects aged less than 18 years was headache.
6.1   Clinical Trials Experience in Adult Subjects
Because clinical trials are conducted under widely varying conditions, adverse reaction rates observed in the clinical trials of a drug cannot be directly compared with rates in the clinical trials of another drug and may not reflect the rates observed in practice.
Cold Sores (Herpes Labialis):   In clinical trials for the treatment of cold sores, the adverse reactions reported by subjects receiving VALTREX 2 grams twice daily (n = 609) or placebo (n = 609) for 1 day, respectively, included headache (14%, 10%) and dizziness (2%, 1%). The frequencies of abnormal ALT (greater than 2 × ULN) were 1.8% for subjects receiving VALTREX compared with 0.8% for placebo. Other laboratory abnormalities (hemoglobin, white blood cells, alkaline phosphatase, and serum creatinine) occurred with similar frequencies in the 2 groups.
Genital Herpes: Initial Episode: In a clinical trial for the treatment of initial episodes of genital herpes, the adverse reactions reported by greater than or equal to 5% of subjects receiving VALTREX 1 gram twice daily for 10 days (n = 318) or oral acyclovir 200 mg 5 times daily for 10 days (n = 318), respectively, included headache (13%, 10%) and nausea (6%, 6%). For the incidence of laboratory abnormalities see Table 2.
Recurrent Episodes: In 3 clinical trials for the episodic treatment of recurrent genital herpes, the adverse reactions

reported by greater than or equal to 5% of subjects receiving VALTREX 500 mg twice daily for 3 days (n = 402), VALTREX 500 mg twice daily for 5 days (n = 1,136) or placebo (n = 259), respectively, included headache (16%, 11%, 14%) and nausea (5%, 4%, 5%). For the incidence of laboratory abnormalities see Table 2.
Suppressive Therapy: Suppression of Recurrent Genital Herpes in Immunocompetent Adults: In a clinical trial for the suppression of recurrent genital herpes infections, the adverse reactions reported by subjects receiving VALTREX 1 gram once daily (n = 269), VALTREX 500 mg once daily (n = 266), or placebo (n = 134), respectively, included headache (35%, 38%, 34%), nausea (11%, 11%, 8%), abdominal pain (11%, 9%, 6%), dysmenorrhea (8%, 5%, 4%), depression (7%, 5%, 5%), arthralgia (6%, 5%, 4%), vomiting (3%, 3%, 2%), and dizziness (4%, 2%, 1%). For the incidence of laboratory abnormalities see Table 2.
Suppression of Recurrent Genital Herpes in HIV—1-Infected Subjects: In HIV—1-infected subjects, frequently reported adverse reactions for VALTREX (500 mg twice daily; n = 194, median days on therapy = 172) and placebo (n = 99, median days on therapy = 59), respectively, included headache (13%, 8%), fatigue (8%, 5%), and rash (8%, 1%). Post-randomization laboratory abnormalities that were reported more frequently in valacyclovir subjects versus placebo included elevated alkaline phosphatase (4%, 2%), elevated ALT (14%, 10%), elevated AST (16%, 11%), decreased neutrophil counts (18%, 10%), and decreased platelet counts (3%, 0%), respectively.
Reduction of Transmission: In a clinical trial for the reduction of transmission of genital herpes, the adverse reactions reported by subjects receiving VALTREX 500 mg once daily (n = 743) or placebo once daily (n = 741), respectively, included headache (29%, 26%), nasopharyngitis (16%, 15%), and upper respiratory tract infection (9%, 10%).
Herpes Zoster: In 2 clinical trials for the treatment of herpes zoster, the adverse reactions reported by subjects receiving VALTREX 1 gram 3 times daily for 7 to 14 days (n = 967) or placebo (n = 195), respectively, included nausea (15%, 8%), headache (14%, 12%), vomiting (6%, 3%), dizziness (3%, 2%), and abdominal pain (3%, 2%). For the incidence of laboratory abnormalities see Table 2.
[See table 2 at top of next page]
6.2   Clinical Trials Experience in Pediatric Subjects
The safety profile of VALTREX has been studied in 177 pediatric subjects aged 1 month to less than 18 years. Sixty-five of these pediatric subjects, aged 12 to less than 18 years, received oral caplets for 1 to 2 days for treatment of cold sores. The remaining 112 pediatric subjects, aged 1 month to less than 12 years, participated in 3 pharmacokinetic and safety trials and received valacyclovir oral suspension. Fifty-one of these 112 pediatric subjects received oral suspension for 3 to 6 days. The frequency, intensity, and nature of clinical adverse reactions and laboratory abnormalities were similar to those seen in adults.
Pediatric Subjects Aged 12 to Less Than 18 Years (Cold Sores):   In clinical trials for the treatment of cold sores, the adverse reactions reported by adolescent subjects receiving VALTREX 2 grams twice daily for 1 day, or VALTREX 2 grams twice daily for 1 day followed by 1 gram twice daily for 1 day (n = 65, across both dosing groups), or placebo (n = 30), respectively, included headache (17%, 3%) and nausea (8%, 0%).
Pediatric Subjects Aged 1 Month to Less Than 12 Years: Adverse events reported in more than 1 subject across the 3 pharmacokinetic and safety trials in children aged 1 month to less than 12 years were diarrhea (5%), pyrexia (4%), dehydration (2%), herpes simplex (2%), and rhinorrhea (2%). No clinically meaningful changes in laboratory values were observed.
6.3   Postmarketing Experience
In addition to adverse events reported from clinical trials, the following events have been identified during postmarketing use of VALTREX. Because they are reported voluntarily from a population of unknown size, estimates of frequency cannot be made. These events have been chosen for inclusion due to a combination of their seriousness, frequency of reporting, or potential causal connection to VALTREX.
General: Facial edema, hypertension, tachycardia.
Allergic: Acute hypersensitivity reactions including anaphylaxis, angioedema, dyspnea, pruritus, rash, and urticaria [see Contraindications (4)].
CNS Symptoms: Aggressive behavior; agitation; ataxia; coma; confusion; decreased consciousness; dysarthria; encephalopathy; mania; and psychosis, including auditory and visual hallucinations, seizures, tremors [see Warnings and Precautions (5.3), Use in Specific Populations (8.5, 8.6)].
Eye: Visual abnormalities.
Gastrointestinal: Diarrhea.
Hepatobiliary Tract and Pancreas: Liver enzyme abnormalities, hepatitis.

Renal: Renal failure, renal pain (may be associated with renal failure) [see Warnings and Precautions (5.2), Use in Specific Populations (8.5, 8.6)].

Hematologic: Thrombocytopenia, aplastic anemia, leukocytoclastic vasculitis, TTP/HUS [see Warnings and Precautions (5.1)].

Skin: Erythema multiforme, rashes including photosensitivity, alopecia.

7 DRUG INTERACTIONS

No clinically significant drug-drug or drug-food interactions with VALTREX are known [see Clinical Pharmacology (12.3)].

8 USE IN SPECIFIC POPULATIONS

8.1 Pregnancy

Pregnancy Category B. There are no adequate and well-controlled trials of VALTREX or acyclovir in pregnant women. Based on prospective pregnancy registry data on 749 pregnancies, the overall rate of birth defects in infants exposed to acyclovir in-utero appears similar to the rate for infants in the general population. VALTREX should be used during pregnancy only if the potential benefit justifies the potential risk to the fetus.

A prospective epidemiologic registry of acyclovir use during pregnancy was established in 1984 and completed in April 1999. There were 749 pregnancies followed in women exposed to systemic acyclovir during the first trimester of pregnancy resulting in 756 outcomes. The occurrence rate of birth defects approximates that found in the general population. However, the small size of the registry is insufficient to evaluate the risk for less common defects or to permit reliable or definitive conclusions regarding the safety of acyclovir in pregnant women and their developing fetuses.

Animal reproduction studies performed at oral doses that provided up to 10 and 7 times the human plasma levels during the period of major organogenesis in rats and rabbits, respectively, revealed no evidence of teratogenicity.

8.3 Nursing Mothers

Following oral administration of a 500—mg dose of VALTREX to 5 nursing mothers, peak acyclovir concentrations (C_{max}) in breast milk ranged from 0.5 to 2.3 times (median 1.4) the corresponding maternal acyclovir serum concentrations. The acyclovir breast milk AUC ranged from 1.4 to 2.6 times (median 2.2) maternal serum AUC. A 500—mg maternal dosage of VALTREX twice daily would provide a nursing infant with an oral acyclovir dosage of approximately 0.6 mg/kg/day. This would result in less than 2% of the exposure obtained after administration of a standard neonatal dose of 30 mg/kg/day of intravenous acyclovir to the nursing infant. Unchanged valacyclovir was not detected in maternal serum, breast milk, or infant urine. Caution should be exercised when VALTREX is administered to a nursing woman.

8.4 Pediatric Use

VALTREX is indicated for treatment of cold sores in pediatric patients aged greater than or equal to 12 years and for treatment of chickenpox in pediatric patients aged 2 to less than 18 years [see Indications and Usage (1.2), Dosage and Administration (2.2)].

The use of VALTREX for treatment of cold sores is based on 2 double-blind, placebo-controlled clinical trials in healthy adults and adolescents (aged greater than or equal to 12 years) with a history of recurrent cold sores [see Clinical Studies (14.1)].

The use of VALTREX for treatment of chickenpox in pediatric patients aged 2 to less than 18 years is based on single—dose pharmacokinetic and multiple—dose safety data from an open—label trial with valacyclovir and supported by efficacy and safety data from 3 randomized, double—blind, placebo—controlled trials evaluating oral acyclovir in pediatric subjects with chickenpox [see Dosage and Administration (2.2), Adverse Reactions (6.2), Clinical Pharmacology (12.3), Clinical Studies (14.4)].

The efficacy and safety of valacyclovir have not been established in pediatric patients:

• aged less than 12 years with cold sores
• aged less than 18 years with genital herpes
• aged less than 18 years with herpes zoster
• aged less than 2 years with chickenpox
• for suppressive therapy following neonatal HSV infection.

The pharmacokinetic profile and safety of valacyclovir oral suspension in children aged less than 12 years were studied in 3 open-label trials. No efficacy evaluations were conducted in any of the 3 trials.

Trial 1 was a single—dose pharmacokinetic, multiple—dose safety trial in 27 pediatric subjects aged 1 to less than 12 years with clinically suspected varicella-zoster virus (VZV) infection [see Dosage and Administration (2.2), Adverse Reactions (6.2), Clinical Pharmacology (12.3), Clinical Studies (14.4)].

Trial 2 was a single—dose pharmacokinetic and safety trial in pediatric subjects aged 1 month to less than 6 years who had an active herpes virus infection or who were at risk for herpes virus infection. Fifty—seven subjects were enrolled and received a single dose of 25 mg/kg valacyclovir oral suspension. In infants and children aged 3 months to less than 6 years, this dose provided comparable systemic acyclovir exposures to that from a 1—gram dose of valacyclovir in adults (historical data). In infants aged 1 month to less than 3 months, mean acyclovir exposures resulting from a 25—mg/kg dose were higher (C_{max}: ↑30%, AUC: ↑60%) than acyclovir exposures following a 1—gram dose of valacyclovir in adults. Acyclovir is not approved for suppressive therapy in infants and children following neonatal HSV infections; therefore valacyclovir is not recommended for this indication because efficacy cannot be extrapolated from acyclovir. Trial 3 was a single—dose pharmacokinetic, multiple—dose safety trial in 28 pediatric subjects aged 1 to less than 12 years with clinically suspected HSV infection. None of the subjects enrolled in this trial had genital herpes. Each subject was dosed with valacyclovir oral suspension, 10 mg/kg twice daily for 3 to 5 days. Acyclovir systemic exposures in pediatric subjects following valacyclovir oral suspension were compared with historical acyclovir systemic exposures in immunocompetent adults receiving the solid oral dosage form of valacyclovir or acyclovir for the treatment of recurrent genital herpes. The mean projected daily acyclovir systemic exposures in pediatric subjects across all age–groups (1 to less than 12 years) were lower (C_{max}: ↓20%, AUC: ↓33%) compared with the acyclovir systemic exposures in adults receiving valacyclovir 500 mg twice daily, but were higher (daily AUC: ↑16%) than systemic exposures in adults receiving acyclovir 200 mg 5 times daily. Insufficient data are available to support valacyclovir for the treatment of recurrent genital herpes in this age–group because clinical information on recurrent genital herpes in young children is limited; therefore, extrapolating efficacy data from adults to this population is not possible. Moreover, valacyclovir has not been studied in children aged 1 to less than 12 years with recurrent genital herpes.

8.5 Geriatric Use

[Of the total number of subjects in clinical trials of VALTREX, 906 were 65 and over, and 352 were 75 and over. In a clinical trial of herpes zoster, the duration of pain after healing (post-herpetic neuralgia) was longer in subjects 65 and older compared with younger adults. Elderly patients are more likely to have reduced renal function and require dose reduction. Elderly patients are also more likely to have renal or CNS adverse events [see Dosage and Administration (2.4), Warnings and Precautions (5.2, 5.3), Clinical Pharmacology (12.3)].

8.6 Renal Impairment

Dosage reduction is recommended when administering VALTREX to patients with renal impairment [see Dosage and Administration (2.4), Warnings and Precautions (5.2, 5.3)].

10 OVERDOSAGE

Caution should be exercised to prevent inadvertent overdose [see Use in Specific Populations (8.5, 8.6)]. Precipitation of acyclovir in renal tubules may occur when the solubility (2.5 mg/mL) is exceeded in the intratubular fluid. In the event of acute renal failure and anuria, the patient may benefit from hemodialysis until renal function is restored [see Dosage and Administration (2.4)].

11 DESCRIPTION

VALTREX (valacyclovir hydrochloride) is the hydrochloride salt of the L—valyl ester of the antiviral drug acyclovir.

VALTREX Caplets are for oral administration. Each caplet contains valacyclovir hydrochloride equivalent to 500 mg or 1 gram valacyclovir and the inactive ingredients carnauba wax, colloidal silicon dioxide, crospovidone, FD&C Blue No. 2 Lake, hypromellose, magnesium stearate, microcrystalline cellulose, polyethylene glycol, polysorbate 80, povidone, and titanium dioxide. The blue, film—coated caplets are printed with edible white ink.

The chemical name of valacyclovir hydrochloride is L-valine, 2-[(2-amino-1,6-dihydro-6-oxo-9H-purin-9-yl)methoxy]ethyl ester, monohydrochloride. It has the following structural formula:

Valacyclovir hydrochloride is a white to off—white powder with the molecular formula $C_{13}H_{20}N_6O_4 \bullet HCl$ and a molecular weight of 360.80. The maximum solubility in water at 25°C is 174 mg/mL. The pk_as for valacyclovir hydrochloride are 1.90, 7.47, and 9.43.

12 CLINICAL PHARMACOLOGY

12.1 Mechanism of Action

Valacyclovir is an antiviral drug [see Clinical Pharmacology (12.4)].

12.3 Pharmacokinetics

The pharmacokinetics of valacyclovir and acyclovir after oral administration of VALTREX have been investigated in 14 volunteer trials involving 283 adults and in 3 trials involving 112 pediatric subjects aged 1 month to less than 12 years.

Pharmacokinetics in Adults: *Absorption and Bioavailability:* After oral administration, valacyclovir hydrochloride is rapidly absorbed from the gastrointestinal tract and nearly completely converted to acyclovir and L—valine by first-pass intestinal and/or hepatic metabolism.

The absolute bioavailability of acyclovir after administration of VALTREX is 54.5% ± 9.1% as determined following a 1-gram oral dose of VALTREX and a 350-mg intravenous acyclovir dose to 12 healthy volunteers. Acyclovir bioavailability from the administration of VALTREX is not altered by administration with food (30 minutes after an 873 Kcal breakfast, which included 51 grams of fat).

Acyclovir pharmacokinetic parameter estimates following administration of VALTREX to healthy adult volunteers are presented in Table 3. There was a less than dose—proportional increase in acyclovir maximum concentration (C_{max}) and area under the acyclovir concentration—time curve (AUC) after single—dose and multiple—dose administration (4 times daily) of VALTREX from doses between 250 mg to 1 gram.

There is no accumulation of acyclovir after the administration of valacyclovir at the recommended dosage regimens in adults with normal renal function.

[See table 3 at top of next page]

Distribution: The binding of valacyclovir to human plasma proteins ranges from 13.5% to 17.9%. The binding of acyclovir to human plasma proteins ranges from 9% to 33%.

Metabolism: Valacyclovir is converted to acyclovir and L—valine by first—pass intestinal and/or hepatic metabolism.

Table 2. Incidence (%) of Laboratory Abnormalities in Herpes Zoster and Genital Herpes Trial Populations

Laboratory Abnormality	Herpes Zoster		Genital Herpes Treatment			Genital Herpes Suppression		
	VALTREX 1 gram 3 Times Daily (n = 967)	Placebo (n = 195)	VALTREX 1 gram Twice Daily (n = 1,194)	VALTREX 500 mg Dwice Daily (n = 1,159)	Placebo (n = 439)	VALTREX 1 gram Once Daily (n = 269)	VALTREX 500 mg Once Daily (n = 266)	Placebo (n = 134)
Hemoglobin (<0.8 × LLN)	0.8%	0%	0.3%	0.2%	0%	0%	0.8%	0.8%
White blood cells (<0.75 × LLN)	1.3%	0.6%	0.7%	0.6%	0.2%	0.7%	0.8%	1.5%
Platelet count (<100,000/mm³)	1.0%	1.2%	0.3%	0.1%	0.7%	0.4%	1.1%	1.5%
AST (SGOT) (>2 × ULN)	1.0%	0%	1.0%	a	0.5%	4.1%	3.8%	3.0%
Serum creatinine (>1.5 × ULN)	0.2%	0%	0.7%	0%	0%	0%	0%	0%

a Data were not collected prospectively.
LLN = Lower limit of normal.
ULN = Upper limit of normal.

Table 3. Mean (±SD) Plasma Acyclovir Pharmacokinetic Parameters Following Administration of VALTREX to Healthy Adult Volunteers

Dose	Single—Dose Administration (N = 8)		Multiple—Dose Administration[a] (N = 24, 8 per treatment arm)	
	C_{max} (±SD) (mcg/mL)	AUC (±SD) (h·mcg/mL)	C_{max} (±SD) (mcg/mL)	AUC (±SD) (h·mcg/mL)
100 mg	0.83 (±0.14)	2.28 (±0.40)	ND	ND
250 mg	2.15 (±0.50)	5.76 (±0.60)	2.11 (±0.33)	5.66 (±1.09)
500 mg	3.28 (±0.83)	11.59 (±1.79)	3.69 (±0.87)	9.88 (±2.01)
750 mg	4.17 (±1.14)	14.11 (±3.54)	ND	ND
1,000 mg	5.65 (±2.37)	19.52 (±6.04)	4.96 (±0.64)	15.70 (±2.27)

[a] Administered 4 times daily for 11 days.
ND = not done.

Table 4. Mean (±SD) Plasma Acyclovir Pharmacokinetic Parameter Estimates Following First-Dose Administration of 20 mg/kg Valacyclovir Oral Suspension to Pediatric Subjects vs. 1-Gram Single Dose of VALTREX to Adults

Parameter	Pediatric Subjects (20 mg/kg Oral Suspension)			Adults 1—gram Solid Dose of VALTREX[a] (N = 15)
	1 -<2 yr (N = 6)	2 -<6 yr (N = 12)	6 -<12 yr (N = 8)	
AUC (mcg·h/mL)	14.4 (±6.26)	10.1 (±3.35)	13.1 (±3.43)	17.2 (±3.10)
C_{max} (mcg/mL)	4.03 (±1.37)	3.75 (±1.14)	4.71 (±1.20)	4.72 (±1.37)

[a] Historical estimates using pediatric pharmacokinetic sampling schedule.

Acyclovir is converted to a small extent to inactive metabolites by aldehyde oxidase and by alcohol and aldehyde dehydrogenase. Neither valacyclovir nor acyclovir is metabolized by cytochrome P450 enzymes. Plasma concentrations of unconverted valacyclovir are low and transient, generally becoming non-quantifiable by 3 hours after administration. Peak plasma valacyclovir concentrations are generally less than 0.5 mcg/mL at all doses. After single—dose administration of 1 gram of VALTREX, average plasma valacyclovir concentrations observed were 0.5, 0.4, and 0.8 mcg/mL in subjects with hepatic dysfunction, renal insufficiency, and in healthy subjects who received concomitant cimetidine and probenecid, respectively.

Elimination: The pharmacokinetic disposition of acyclovir delivered by valacyclovir is consistent with previous experience from intravenous and oral acyclovir. Following the oral administration of a single 1 gram dose of radiolabeled valacyclovir to 4 healthy subjects, 46% and 47% of administered radioactivity was recovered in urine and feces, respectively, over 96 hours. Acyclovir accounted for 89% of the radioactivity excreted in the urine. Renal clearance of acyclovir following the administration of a single 1-gram dose of VALTREX to 12 healthy subjects was approximately 255 ± 86 mL/min which represents 42% of total acyclovir apparent plasma clearance.

The plasma elimination half–life of acyclovir typically averaged 2.5 to 3.3 hours in all trials of VALTREX in subjects with normal renal function.

Specific Populations: *Renal Impairment:* Reduction in dosage is recommended in patients with renal impairment *[see Dosage and Administration (2.4), Use in Specific Populations (8.5, 8.6)].*

Following administration of VALTREX to subjects with ESRD, the average acyclovir half–life is approximately 14 hours. During hemodialysis, the acyclovir half–life is approximately 4 hours. Approximately one–third of acyclovir in the body is removed by dialysis during a 4–hour hemodialysis session. Apparent plasma clearance of acyclovir in subjects on dialysis was 86.3 ± 21.3 mL/min/1.73 m² compared with 679.16 ± 162.76 mL/min/1.73 m² in healthy subjects.

Hepatic Impairment: Administration of VALTREX to subjects with moderate (biopsy—proven cirrhosis) or severe (with and without ascites and biopsy—proven cirrhosis) liver disease indicated that the rate but not the extent of conversion of valacyclovir to acyclovir is reduced, and the acyclovir half–life is not affected. Dosage modification is not recommended for patients with cirrhosis.

HIV-1 Disease: In 9 subjects with HIV-1 disease and CD4+ cell counts less than 150 cells/mm³ who received VALTREX at a dosage of 1 gram 4 times daily for 30 days, the pharmacokinetics of valacyclovir and acyclovir were not different from that observed in healthy subjects.

Geriatrics: After single-dose administration of 1 gram of VALTREX in healthy geriatric subjects, the half–life of acyclovir was 3.11 ± 0.51 hours, compared with 2.91 ± 0.63 hours in healthy younger adult subjects. The pharmacokinetics of acyclovir following single– and multiple–dose oral administration of VALTREX in geriatric subjects varied with renal function. Dose reduction may be required in geriatric patients, depending on the underlying renal status of the patient *[see Dosage and Administration (2.4), Use in Specific Populations (8.5, 8.6)].*

Pediatrics: Acyclovir pharmacokinetics have been evaluated in a total of 98 pediatric subjects (aged 1 month to less than 12 years) following administration of the first dose of an extemporaneous oral suspension of valacyclovir *[see Adverse Reactions (6.2), Use in Specific Populations (8.4)].* Acyclovir pharmacokinetic parameter estimates following a 20—mg/kg dose are provided in Table 4.

[See table 4 above]

Drug Interactions: When VALTREX is coadministered with antacids, cimetidine and/or probenicid, digoxin, or thiazide diuretics in patients with normal renal function, the effects are not considered to be of clinical significance (see below). Therefore, when VALTREX is coadministered with these drugs in patients with normal renal function, no dosage adjustment is recommended.

Antacids: The pharmacokinetics of acyclovir after a single dose of VALTREX (1 gram) were unchanged by coadministration of a single dose of antacids (Al^{3+} or Mg^{++}).

Cimetidine: Acyclovir C_{max} and AUC following a single dose of VALTREX (1 gram) increased by 8% and 32%, respectively, after a single dose of cimetidine (800 mg).

Cimetidine Plus Probenecid: Acyclovir C_{max} and AUC following a single dose of VALTREX (1 gram) increased by 30% and 78%, respectively, after a combination of cimetidine and probenecid, primarily due to a reduction in renal clearance of acyclovir.

Digoxin: The pharmacokinetics of digoxin were not affected by coadministration of VALTREX 1 gram 3 times daily, and the pharmacokinetics of acyclovir after a single dose of VALTREX (1 gram) was unchanged by coadministration of digoxin (2 doses of 0.75 mg).

Probenecid: Acyclovir C_{max} and AUC following a single dose of VALTREX (1 gram) increased by 22% and 49%, respectively, after probenecid (1 gram).

Thiazide Diuretics: The pharmacokinetics of acyclovir after a single dose of VALTREX (1 gram) were unchanged by coadministration of multiple doses of thiazide diuretics.

12.4   Microbiology

Mechanism of Action: Valacyclovir is a nucleoside analogue DNA polymerase inhibitor. Valacyclovir hydrochloride is rapidly converted to acyclovir which has demonstrated antiviral activity against HSV types 1 (HSV—1) and 2 (HSV—2) and VZV both in cell culture and in vivo.

The inhibitory activity of acyclovir is highly selective due to its affinity for the enzyme thymidine kinase (TK) encoded by HSV and VZV. This viral enzyme converts acyclovir into acyclovir monophosphate, a nucleotide analogue. The monophosphate is further converted into diphosphate by cellular guanylate kinase and into triphosphate by a number of cellular enzymes. In biochemical assays, acyclovir triphosphate inhibits replication of herpes viral DNA. This is accomplished in 3 ways: 1) competitive inhibition of viral DNA polymerase, 2) incorporation and termination of the growing viral DNA chain, and 3) inactivation of the viral DNA polymerase. The greater antiviral activity of acyclovir against HSV compared with VZV is due to its more efficient phosphorylation by the viral TK.

Antiviral Activities: The quantitative relationship between the cell culture susceptibility of herpesviruses to antivirals and the clinical response to therapy has not been established in humans, and virus sensitivity testing has not been standardized. Sensitivity testing results, expressed as the concentration of drug required to inhibit by 50% the growth of virus in cell culture (EC_{50}), vary greatly depending upon a number of factors. Using plaque-reduction assays, the EC_{50} values against herpes simplex virus isolates range from 0.09 to 60 µM (0.02 to 13.5 mcg/mL) for HSV—1 and from 0.04 to 44 µM (0.01 to 9.9 mcg/mL) for HSV—2. The EC_{50} values for acyclovir against most laboratory strains and clinical isolates of VZV range from 0.53 to 48 µM (0.12 to 10.8 mcg/mL). Acyclovir also demonstrates activity against the Oka vaccine strain of VZV with a mean EC_{50} of 6 µM (1.35 mcg/mL).

Resistance: Resistance of HSV and VZV to acyclovir can result from qualitative and quantitative changes in the viral TK and/or DNA polymerase. Clinical isolates of VZV with reduced susceptibility to acyclovir have been recovered from patients with AIDS. In these cases, TK-deficient mutants of VZV have been recovered.

Resistance of HSV and VZV to acyclovir occurs by the same mechanisms. While most of the acyclovir—resistant mutants isolated thus far from immunocompromised patients have been found to be TK—deficient mutants, other mutants involving the viral TK gene (TK partial and TK altered) and DNA polymerase have also been isolated. TK—negative mutants may cause severe disease in immunocompromised patients. The possibility of viral resistance to valacyclovir (and therefore, to acyclovir) should be considered in patients who show poor clinical response during therapy.

13   NONCLINICAL TOXICOLOGY
13.1   Carcinogenesis, Mutagenesis, Impairment of Fertility

The data presented below include references to the steady—state acyclovir AUC observed in humans treated with 1 gram VALTREX given orally 3 times a day to treat herpes zoster. Plasma drug concentrations in animal studies are expressed as multiples of human exposure to acyclovir *[see Clinical Pharmacology (12.3)].*

Valacyclovir was noncarcinogenic in lifetime carcinogenicity bioassays at single daily doses (gavage) of valacyclovir giving plasma acyclovir concentrations equivalent to human levels in the mouse bioassay and 1.4 to 2.3 times human levels in the rat bioassay. There was no significant difference in the incidence of tumors between treated and control animals, nor did valacyclovir shorten the latency of tumors. Valacyclovir was tested in 5 genetic toxicity assays. An Ames assay was negative in the absence or presence of metabolic activation. Also negative were an in vitro cytogenetic study with human lymphocytes and a rat cytogenetic study. In the mouse lymphoma assay, valacyclovir was not mutagenic in the absence of metabolic activation. In the presence of metabolic activation (76% to 88% conversion to acyclovir), valacyclovir was mutagenic.

Valacyclovir was mutagenic in a mouse micronucleus assay. Valacyclovir did not impair fertility or reproduction in rats at 6 times human plasma levels.

14   CLINICAL STUDIES
14.1   Cold Sores (Herpes Labialis)

Two double–blind, placebo–controlled clinical trials were conducted in 1,856 healthy adults and adolescents (aged greater than or equal to 12 years) with a history of recurrent cold sores. Subjects self–initiated therapy at the earliest symptoms and prior to any signs of a cold sore. The majority of subjects initiated treatment within 2 hours of onset of symptoms. Subjects were randomized to VALTREX 2 grams twice daily on Day 1 followed by placebo on Day 2, VALTREX 2 grams twice daily on Day 1 followed by 1 gram twice daily on Day 2, or placebo on Days 1 and 2.

The mean duration of cold sore episodes was about 1 day shorter in treated subjects as compared with placebo. The 2—day regimen did not offer additional benefit over the 1—day regimen.

No significant difference was observed between subjects receiving VALTREX or placebo in the prevention of progression of cold sore lesions beyond the papular stage.

14.2 Genital Herpes Infections

Initial Episode: Six hundred forty—three immunocompetent adults with first—episode genital herpes who presented within 72 hours of symptom onset were randomized in a double—blind trial to receive 10 days of VALTREX 1 gram twice daily (n = 323) or oral acyclovir 200 mg 5 times a day (n = 320). For both treatment groups the median time to lesion healing was 9 days, the median time to cessation of pain was 5 days, and the median time to cessation of viral shedding was 3 days.

Recurrent Episodes: Three double—blind trials (2 of them placebo—controlled) in immunocompetent adults with recurrent genital herpes were conducted. Subjects self—initiated therapy within 24 hours of the first sign or symptom of a recurrent genital herpes episode.

In 1 trial, subjects were randomized to receive 5 days of treatment with either VALTREX 500 mg twice daily (n = 360) or placebo (n = 259). The median time to lesion healing was 4 days in the group receiving VALTREX 500 mg versus 6 days in the placebo group, and the median time to cessation of viral shedding in subjects with at least 1 positive culture (42% of the overall trial population) was 2 days in the group receiving VALTREX 500 mg versus 4 days in the placebo group. The median time to cessation of pain was 3 days in the group receiving VALTREX 500 mg versus 4 days in the placebo group. Results supporting efficacy were replicated in a second trial.

In a third trial, subjects were randomized to receive VALTREX 500 mg twice daily for 5 days (n = 398) or VALTREX 500 mg twice daily for 3 days (and matching placebo twice daily for 2 additional days) (n = 402). The median time to lesion healing was about 4½ days in both treatment groups. The median time to cessation of pain was about 3 days in both treatment groups.

Suppressive Therapy: Two clinical trials were conducted, one in immunocompetent adults and one in HIV-1—infected adults.

A double—blind, 12—month, placebo— and active—controlled trial enrolled immunocompetent adults with a history of 6 or more recurrences per year. Outcomes for the overall trial population are shown in Table 5.

[See table 5 above]

Subjects with 9 or fewer recurrences per year showed comparable results with VALTREX 500 mg once daily.

In a second trial, 293 HIV-1-infected adults on stable antiretroviral therapy with a history of 4 or more recurrences of ano—genital herpes per year were randomized to receive either VALTREX 500 mg twice daily (n = 194) or matching placebo (n = 99) for 6 months. The median duration of recurrent genital herpes in enrolled subjects was 8 years, and the median number of recurrences in the year prior to enrollment was 5. Overall, the median pretrial HIV-1 RNA was 2.6 $\log_{10}$ copies/mL. Among subjects who received VALTREX, the pretrial median CD4+ cell count was 336 cells/mm³; 11% had less than 100 cells/mm³, 16% had 100 to 199 cells/mm³, 42% had 200 to 499 cells/mm³, and 31% had greater than or equal to 500 cells/mm³. Outcomes for the overall trial population are shown in Table 6.

Table 6. Recurrence Rates in HIV—1—Infected Adults at 6 Months

Outcome	VALTREX 500 mg Twice Daily (n = 194)	Placebo (n = 99)
Recurrence free	65%	26%
Recurrences	17%	57%
Unknown[a]	18%	17%

[a] Includes lost to follow-up, discontinuations due to adverse events, and consent withdrawn.

Reduction of Transmission of Genital Herpes: A double—blind, placebo—controlled trial to assess transmission of genital herpes was conducted in 1,484 monogamous, heterosexual, immunocompetent adult couples. The couples were discordant for HSV—2 infection. The source partner had a history of 9 or fewer genital herpes episodes per year. Both partners were counseled on safer sex practices and were advised to use condoms throughout the trial period. Source partners were randomized to treatment with either VALTREX 500 mg once daily or placebo once daily for 8 months. The primary efficacy endpoint was symptomatic acquisition of HSV—2 in susceptible partners. Overall HSV—2 acquisition was defined as symptomatic HSV—2 acquisition and/or HSV—2 seroconversion in susceptible partners. The efficacy results are summarized in Table 7.

Table 5. Recurrence Rates in Immunocompetent Adults at 6 and 12 Months

Outcome	6 Months			12 Months		
	VALTREX 1 gram Once Daily (n = 269)	Oral Acyclovir 400 mg Twice Daily (n = 267)	Placebo (n = 134)	VALTREX 1 gram Once Daily (n = 269)	Oral Acyclovir 400 mg Twice Daily (n = 267)	Placebo (n = 134)
Recurrence free	55%	54%	7%	34%	34%	4%
Recurrences	35%	36%	83%	46%	46%	85%
Unknown[a]	10%	10%	10%	19%	19%	10%

[a] Includes lost to follow-up, discontinuations due to adverse events, and consent withdrawn.

Table 7. Percentage of Susceptible Partners Who Acquired HSV-2 Defined by the Primary and Selected Secondary Endpoints

Endpoint	VALTREX[a] (n = 743)	Placebo (n = 741)
Symptomatic HSV—2 acquisition	4 (0.5%)	16 (2.2%)
HSV—2 seroconversion	12 (1.6%)	24 (3.2%)
Overall HSV—2 acquisition	14 (1.9%)	27 (3.6%)

[a] Results show reductions in risk of 75% (symptomatic HSV—2 acquisition), 50% (HSV—2 seroconversion), and 48% (overall HSV—2 acquisition) with VALTREX versus placebo. Individual results may vary based on consistency of safer sex practices.

14.3 Herpes Zoster

Two randomized double–blind clinical trials in immunocompetent adults with localized herpes zoster were conducted. VALTREX was compared with placebo in subjects aged less than 50 years, and with oral acyclovir in subjects aged greater than 50 years. All subjects were treated within 72 hours of appearance of zoster rash. In subjects aged less than 50 years, the median time to cessation of new lesion formation was 2 days for those treated with VALTREX compared with 3 days for those treated with placebo. In subjects aged greater than 50 years, the median time to cessation of new lesions was 3 days in subjects treated with either VALTREX or oral acyclovir. In subjects aged less than 50 years, no difference was found with respect to the duration of pain after healing (post—herpetic neuralgia) between the recipients of VALTREX and placebo. In subjects aged greater than 50 years, among the 83% who reported pain after healing (post—herpetic neuralgia), the median duration of pain after healing [95% confidence interval] in days was: 40 [31, 51], 43 [36, 55], and 59 [41, 77] for 7—day VALTREX, 14—day VALTREX, and 7—day oral acyclovir, respectively.

14.4 Chickenpox

The use of VALTREX for treatment of chickenpox in pediatric subjects aged 2 to less than 18 years is based on single—dose pharmacokinetic and multiple—dose safety data from an open—label trial with valacyclovir and supported by safety and extrapolated efficacy data from 3 randomized, double—blind, placebo—controlled trials evaluating oral acyclovir in pediatric subjects.

The single—dose pharmacokinetic and multiple—dose safety trial enrolled 27 pediatric subjects aged 1 to less than 12 years with clinically suspected VZV infection. Each subject was dosed with valacyclovir oral suspension, 20 mg/kg 3 times daily for 5 days. Acyclovir systemic exposures in pediatric subjects following valacyclovir oral suspension were compared with historical acyclovir systemic exposures in immunocompetent adults receiving the solid oral dosage form of valacyclovir or acyclovir for the treatment of herpes zoster. The mean projected daily acyclovir exposures in pediatric subjects across all age—groups (1 to less than 12 years) were lower (C_{max}: ↓13%, AUC: ↓30%) than the mean daily historical exposures in adults receiving valacyclovir 1 gram 3 times daily, but were higher (daily AUC: ↑50%) than the mean daily historical exposures in adults receiving acyclovir 800 mg 5 times daily. The projected daily exposures in pediatric subjects were greater (daily AUC approximately 100% greater) than the exposures seen in immunocompetent pediatric subjects receiving acyclovir 20 mg/kg 4 times daily for the treatment of chickenpox. Based on the pharmacokinetic and safety data from this trial and the safety and extrapolated efficacy data from the acyclovir trials, oral valacyclovir 20 mg/kg 3 times a day for 5 days (not to exceed 1 gram 3 times daily) is recommended for the treatment of chickenpox in pediatric patients aged 2 to less than 18 years. Because the efficacy and safety of acyclovir for the treatment of chickenpox in children aged less than 2 years have not been established, efficacy data cannot be extrapolated to support valacyclovir treatment in children aged less than 2 years with chickenpox. Valacyclovir is also not recommended for the treatment of herpes zoster in children because safety data up to 7 days' duration are not available [see Use in Specific Populations (8.4)].

16   HOW SUPPLIED/STORAGE AND HANDLING

VALTREX Caplets (blue, film—coated, capsule—shaped tablets) containing valacyclovir hydrochloride equivalent to 500 mg valacyclovir and printed with "VALTREX 500 mg."
Bottle of 30 (NDC 0173-0933-08).
Bottle of 90 (NDC 0173-0933-10).
Unit dose pack of 100 (NDC 0173-0933-56).
VALTREX Caplets (blue, film—coated, capsule—shaped tablets, with a partial scorebar on both sides) containing valacyclovir hydrochloride equivalent to 1 gram valacyclovir and printed with "VALTREX 1 gram."
Bottle of 30 (NDC 0173-0565-04).
Bottle of 90 (NDC 0173-0565-10).

Storage:
Store at 15° to 25°C (59° to 77°F). Dispense in a well-closed container as defined in the USP.

17   PATIENT COUNSELING INFORMATION

Advise the patient to read the FDA–Approved Patient Labeling (Patient Information).

Importance of Adequate Hydration: Patients should be advised to maintain adequate hydration.

Cold Sores (Herpes Labialis): Patients should be advised to initiate treatment at the earliest symptom of a cold sore (e.g., tingling, itching, or burning). There are no data on the effectiveness of treatment initiated after the development of clinical signs of a cold sore (e.g., papule, vesicle, or ulcer). Patients should be instructed that treatment for cold sores should not exceed 1 day (2 doses) and that their doses should be taken about 12 hours apart. Patients should be informed that VALTREX is not a cure for cold sores.

Genital Herpes: Patients should be informed that VALTREX is not a cure for genital herpes. Because genital herpes is a sexually transmitted disease, patients should avoid contact with lesions or intercourse when lesions and/or symptoms are present to avoid infecting partners. Genital herpes is frequently transmitted in the absence of symptoms through asymptomatic viral shedding. Therefore, patients should be counseled to use safer sex practices in combination with suppressive therapy with VALTREX. Sex partners of infected persons should be advised that they might be infected even if they have no symptoms. Type-specific serologic testing of asymptomatic partners of persons with genital herpes can determine whether risk for HSV–2 acquisition exists.

VALTREX has not been shown to reduce transmission of sexually transmitted infections other than HSV–2.

If medical management of a genital herpes recurrence is indicated, patients should be advised to initiate therapy at the first sign or symptom of an episode.

There are no data on the effectiveness of treatment initiated more than 72 hours after the onset of signs and symptoms of a first episode of genital herpes or more than 24 hours after the onset of signs and symptoms of a recurrent episode.

There are no data on the safety or effectiveness of chronic suppressive therapy of more than 1 year's duration in otherwise healthy patients. There are no data on the safety or effectiveness of chronic suppressive therapy of more than 6 months' duration in HIV-1-infected patients.

Herpes Zoster: There are no data on treatment initiated more than 72 hours after onset of the zoster rash. Patients should be advised to initiate treatment as soon as possible after a diagnosis of herpes zoster.

Chickenpox: Patients should be advised to initiate treatment at the earliest sign or symptom of chickenpox.

VALTREX is a registered trademark of the GlaxoSmithKline group of companies.

Distributed by:
GlaxoSmithKline
Research Triangle Park, NC 27709
©2013, GlaxoSmithKline group of companies. All rights reserved.
VTX:6PI

PATIENT INFORMATION
VALTREX® (VAL-trex)
(valacyclovir hydrochloride) Caplets

Read the Patient Information that comes with VALTREX before you start using it and each time you get a refill. There may be new information. This information does not take the place of talking to your healthcare provider about your medical condition or treatment. Ask your healthcare provider or pharmacist if you have questions.

What is VALTREX?

VALTREX is a prescription antiviral medicine. VALTREX lowers the ability of herpes viruses to multiply in your body. VALTREX is used in adults:

- to treat cold sores (also called fever blisters or herpes labialis)
- to treat shingles (also called herpes zoster)
- to treat or control genital herpes outbreaks in adults with normal immune systems
- to control genital herpes outbreaks in adults infected with the human immunodeficiency virus (HIV-1) with CD4+ cell count greater than 100 cells/mm^3
- with safer sex practices to lower the chances of spreading genital herpes to others. Even with safer sex practices, it is still possible to spread genital herpes.

VALTREX used daily with the following safer sex practices can lower the chances of passing genital herpes to your partner.

- **Do not have sexual contact with your partner when you have any symptom or outbreak of genital herpes.**
- **Use a condom** made of latex or polyurethane whenever you have sexual contact.

VALTREX is used in children:

- to treat cold sores (for children aged greater than or equal to 12 years)
- to treat chickenpox (for children aged 2 to less than 18 years).

VALTREX does not cure herpes infections (cold sores, chickenpox, shingles, or genital herpes).

The efficacy of VALTREX has not been studied in children who have not reached puberty.

What are cold sores, chickenpox, shingles, and genital herpes?

Cold sores are caused by a herpes virus that may be spread by kissing or other physical contact with the infected area of the skin. They are small, painful ulcers that you get in or around your mouth. It is not known if VALTREX can stop the spread of cold sores to others.

Chickenpox is caused by a herpes virus. It causes an itchy rash of multiple small, red bumps that look like pimples or insect bites usually appearing first on the abdomen or back and face. It can spread to almost everywhere else on the body and may be accompanied by flu-like symptoms.

Shingles is caused by the same herpes virus that causes chickenpox. It causes small, painful blisters that happen on your skin. Shingles occurs in people who have already had chickenpox. Shingles can be spread to people who have not had chickenpox or the chickenpox vaccine by contact with the infected areas of the skin. It is not known if VALTREX can stop the spread of shingles to others.

Genital herpes is a sexually transmitted disease. It causes small, painful blisters on your genital area. You can spread genital herpes to others, even when you have no symptoms. If you are sexually active, you can still pass herpes to your partner, even if you are taking VALTREX. VALTREX, taken every day as prescribed and used with the following **safer sex practices**, can lower the chances of passing genital herpes to your partner.

- Do not have sexual contact with your partner when you have any symptom or outbreak of genital herpes.
- Use a condom made of latex or polyurethane whenever you have sexual contact.

Ask your healthcare provider for more information about safer sex practices.

Who should not take VALTREX?

Do not take VALTREX if you are allergic to any of its ingredients or to acyclovir. The active ingredient is valacyclovir. See the end of this leaflet for a complete list of ingredients in VALTREX.

Before taking VALTREX, tell your healthcare provider:

About all of your medical conditions, including:

- **if you have had a bone marrow transplant or kidney transplant, or if you have advanced HIV-1 disease or "AIDS".** Patients with these conditions may have a higher chance for getting a blood disorder called thrombotic thrombocytopenic purpura/hemolytic uremic syndrome (TTP/HUS). TTP/HUS can result in death.
- **if you have kidney problems.** Patients with kidney problems may have a higher chance for getting side effects or more kidney problems with VALTREX. Your healthcare provider may give you a lower dose of VALTREX.
- **if you are aged 65 years or older.** Elderly patients have a higher chance of certain side effects. Also, elderly patients are more likely to have kidney problems. Your healthcare provider may give you a lower dose of VALTREX.

- **if you are pregnant or planning to become pregnant.** Talk with your healthcare provider about the risks and benefits of taking prescription drugs (including VALTREX) during pregnancy.
- **if you are breastfeeding.** VALTREX may pass into your milk and it may harm your baby. Talk with your healthcare provider about the best way to feed your baby if you are taking VALTREX.
- **about all the medicines you take,** including prescription and non-prescription medicines, vitamins, and herbal supplements. VALTREX may affect other medicines, and other medicines may affect VALTREX. It is a good idea to keep a complete list of all the medicines you take. Show this list to your healthcare provider and pharmacist any time you get a new medicine.

How should I take VALTREX?

Take VALTREX exactly as prescribed by your healthcare provider. Your dose of VALTREX and length of treatment will depend on the type of herpes infection that you have and any other medical problems that you have.

- Do not stop VALTREX or change your treatment without talking to your healthcare provider.
- VALTREX can be taken with or without food.
- If you are taking VALTREX to treat cold sores, chickenpox, shingles, or genital herpes, you should start treatment as soon as possible after your symptoms start. VALTREX may not help you if you start treatment too late.
- If you miss a dose of VALTREX, take it as soon as you remember and then take your next dose at its regular time. However, if it is almost time for your next dose, do not take the missed dose. Wait and take the next dose at the regular time.
- Do not take more than the prescribed number of VALTREX Caplets each day. Call your healthcare provider right away if you take too much VALTREX.

What are the possible side effects of VALTREX?

Kidney failure and nervous system problems are not common, but can be serious in some patients taking VALTREX. Nervous system problems include aggressive behavior, unsteady movement, shaky movements, confusion, speech problems, hallucinations (seeing or hearing things that are really not there), seizures, and coma. Kidney failure and nervous system problems have happened in patients who already have kidney disease and in elderly patients whose kidneys do not work well due to age. **Always tell your healthcare provider if you have kidney problems before taking VALTREX. Call your doctor right away if you get a nervous system problem while you are taking VALTREX.**

Common side effects of VALTREX in adults include headache, nausea, stomach pain, vomiting, and dizziness. Side effects in HIV-1-infected adults include headache, tiredness, and rash. These side effects usually are mild and do not cause patients to stop taking VALTREX.

Other less common side effects in adults include painful periods in women, joint pain, depression, low blood cell counts, and changes in tests that measure how well the liver and kidneys work.

The most common side effect seen in children aged less than 18 years was headache.

Talk to your healthcare provider if you develop any side effects that concern you.

These are not all the side effects of VALTREX. For more information ask your healthcare provider or pharmacist.

How should I store VALTREX?

- Store VALTREX Caplets at room temperature, 59° to 77°F (15° to 25°C).
- Store VALTREX suspension between 2° to 8°C (36° to 46°F) in a refrigerator. Discard after 28 days.
- Keep VALTREX in a tightly closed container.
- Do not keep medicine that is out of date or that you no longer need.
- Keep VALTREX and all medicines out of the reach of children.

General information about VALTREX

Medicines are sometimes prescribed for conditions that are not mentioned in patient information leaflets. Do not use VALTREX for a condition for which it was not prescribed. Do not give VALTREX to other people, even if they have the same symptoms you have. It may harm them.

This leaflet summarizes the most important information about VALTREX. If you would like more information, talk with your healthcare provider. You can ask your healthcare provider or pharmacist for information about VALTREX that is written for health professionals. More information is available at www.VALTREX.com.

What are the ingredients in VALTREX?

Active Ingredient: valacyclovir hydrochloride

Inactive Ingredients: carnauba wax, colloidal silicon dioxide, crospovidone, FD&C Blue No. 2 Lake, hypromellose, magnesium stearate, microcrystalline cellulose, polyethylene glycol, polysorbate 80, povidone, and titanium dioxide.

VALTREX is a registered trademark of the GlaxoSmithKline group of companies.

Distributed by:
GlaxoSmithKline
Research Triangle Park, NC 27709
©2013, GlaxoSmithKline group of companies. All rights reserved.
November 2013
VTX:5PIL

VENTOLIN HFA   ℞
[vent'ō-lin]
(albuterol sulfate)
Inhalation Aerosol

HIGHLIGHTS OF PRESCRIBING INFORMATION
These highlights do not include all the information needed to use VENTOLIN HFA safely and effectively. See full prescribing information for VENTOLIN HFA.
VENTOLIN HFA (albuterol sulfate) Inhalation Aerosol
Initial U.S. Approval: 1981

——————INDICATIONS AND USAGE——————

VENTOLIN HFA is a beta$_2$-adrenergic agonist indicated for:
- Treatment or prevention of bronchospasm in patients 4 years of age and older with reversible obstructive airway disease. (1.1)
- Prevention of exercise-induced bronchospasm in patients 4 years of age and older. (1.2)

———————DOSAGE AND ADMINISTRATION———————

FOR ORAL INHALATION ONLY.
- Treatment or prevention of bronchospasm in adults and children 4 years of age and older: 2 inhalations every 4 to 6 hours. For some patients, 1 inhalation every 4 hours may be sufficient. (2.1)
- Prevention of exercise-induced bronchospasm in adults and children 4 years of age and older: 2 inhalations 15 to 30 minutes before exercise. (2.2)
- Priming information: Prime VENTOLIN HFA before using for the first time, when the inhaler has not been used for more than 2 weeks, or when the inhaler has been dropped. To prime VENTOLIN HFA, release 4 sprays into the air away from the face, shaking well before each spray. (2.3)
- Cleaning information: At least once a week, wash the actuator with warm water and let it air-dry completely. (2.3)

————DOSAGE FORMS AND STRENGTHS————

Inhalation aerosol: 108 mcg albuterol sulfate (90 mcg albuterol base) from mouthpiece per actuation. Supplied in 18-g canister containing 200 actuations and 8-g canister containing 60 actuations. (3)

———————CONTRAINDICATIONS———————

Hypersensitivity to albuterol sulfate or any of the ingredients of VENTOLIN HFA. (4)

—————WARNINGS AND PRECAUTIONS—————

- Paradoxical bronchospasm may occur and should be treated immediately with alternative therapy. (5.1)
- Need for more doses of VENTOLIN HFA than usual may be a sign of deterioration of asthma and requires re-evaluation of treatment. (5.2)
- Cardiovascular effects may occur with beta-adrenergic agonists use. Consider discontinuation of VENTOLIN HFA if these effects occur. Use with caution in patients with underlying cardiovascular disorders. (5.4)
- Immediate hypersensitivity reactions may occur. Discontinue VENTOLIN HFA if immediate hypersensitivity reactions occur. (5.6)

———————ADVERSE REACTIONS———————

Most common adverse reactions (incidence ≥3%) are throat irritation, viral respiratory infections, upper respiratory inflammation, cough, and musculoskeletal pain. (6)
To report SUSPECTED ADVERSE REACTIONS, contact GlaxoSmithKline at 1-888-825-5249 or FDA at 1-800-FDA-1088 or www.fda.gov/medwatch.

———————DRUG INTERACTIONS———————

- Beta-blockers: May block bronchodilatory effects of beta-agonists and produce severe bronchospasm. Patients with asthma should not normally be treated with beta-blockers. (7.1)
- Diuretics: Electrocardiographic changes and/or hypokalemia associated with diuretics may worsen with concomitant beta-agonists. Consider monitoring potassium levels. (7.2)
- Monoamine oxidase inhibitors (MAOs) or tricyclic antidepressants: May potentiate effect of albuterol on the vascular system. Consider alternative therapy in patients taking MAOs or tricyclic antidepressants. (7.4)

See 17 for PATIENT COUNSELING INFORMATION and FDA-approved patient labeling
Revised: 10/2012

FULL PRESCRIBING INFORMATION

1   INDICATIONS AND USAGE
1.1   Bronchospasm
VENTOLIN® HFA is indicated for the treatment or prevention of bronchospasm in patients 4 years of age and older with reversible obstructive airway disease.
1.2   Exercise-Induced Bronchospasm
VENTOLIN HFA is indicated for the prevention of exercise-induced bronchospasm in patients 4 years of age and older.

2   DOSAGE AND ADMINISTRATION
Administer VENTOLIN HFA by oral inhalation only. Shake VENTOLIN HFA well before each spray.
2.1   Bronchospasm
For treatment of acute episodes of bronchospasm or prevention of symptoms associated with bronchospasm, the usual dosage for adults and children is 2 inhalations repeated every 4 to 6 hours; in some patients, 1 inhalation every 4 hours may be sufficient. More frequent administration or a larger number of inhalations is not recommended.
2.2   Exercise-Induced Bronchospasm
The usual dosage for adults and children 4 years of age and older is 2 inhalations 15 to 30 minutes before exercise.
2.3   Administration Information
Priming: Priming VENTOLIN HFA is essential to ensure appropriate albuterol content in each actuation. Prime VENTOLIN HFA before using for the first time, when the inhaler has not been used for more than 2 weeks, or when the inhaler has been dropped. To prime VENTOLIN HFA, release 4 sprays into the air away from the face, shaking well before each spray.
Cleaning: To ensure proper dosing and to prevent actuator orifice blockage, wash the actuator with warm water and let it air-dry completely at least once a week.
Dose Counter: VENTOLIN HFA has a dose counter attached to the canister that starts at 204 or 64 and counts

down each time a spray is released *[see Dosage Forms and Strengths (3)]*. When the counter reads 020, the patient should contact the pharmacist for a refill of medication or consult the physician to determine whether a prescription refill is needed.
VENTOLIN HFA comes in a moisture-protective foil pouch, which should be removed prior to use. Discard VENTOLIN HFA when the counter reads 000 or 12 months after removal from the moisture-protective foil pouch, whichever comes first *[see Dosage Forms and Strengths (3)]*.
See Patient Information tear-off leaflet for instructions on how to prime and clean the inhaler to ensure proper dosing and to prevent actuator orifice blockage.

3   DOSAGE FORMS AND STRENGTHS
VENTOLIN HFA is an inhalation aerosol. Each actuation contains 108 mcg albuterol sulfate (90 mcg albuterol base) from the mouthpiece. VENTOLIN HFA is supplied as an 18-g pressurized aluminum canister with dose counter fitted with a blue plastic actuator and a blue strapcap; this canister contains 200 actuations. VENTOLIN HFA is also supplied as an 8-g pressurized aluminum canister with dose counter fitted with a blue plastic actuator and a blue strapcap; this canister contains 60 actuations.

4   CONTRAINDICATIONS
VENTOLIN HFA is contraindicated in patients with a history of hypersensitivity to albuterol or any other components of VENTOLIN HFA. Rare cases of hypersensitivity reactions, including urticaria, angioedema, and rash have been reported after the use of albuterol sulfate.

5   WARNINGS AND PRECAUTIONS
5.1   Paradoxical Bronchospasm
Inhaled albuterol sulfate can produce paradoxical bronchospasm, which may be life threatening. If paradoxical bronchospasm occurs, VENTOLIN HFA should be discontinued immediately and alternative therapy instituted. It should be recognized that paradoxical bronchospasm, when associated with inhaled formulations, frequently occurs with the first use of a new canister.
5.2   Deterioration of Asthma
Asthma may deteriorate acutely over a period of hours or chronically over several days or longer. If the patient needs more doses of VENTOLIN HFA than usual, this may be a marker of destabilization of asthma and requires re-evaluation of the patient and treatment regimen, giving special consideration to the possible need for anti-inflammatory treatment, e.g., corticosteroids.
5.3   Use of Anti-inflammatory Agents
The use of beta-adrenergic agonist bronchodilators alone may not be adequate to control asthma in many patients. Early consideration should be given to adding anti-inflammatory agents, e.g., corticosteroids, to the therapeutic regimen.
5.4   Cardiovascular Effects
VENTOLIN HFA, like all other beta$_2$-adrenergic agonists, can produce clinically significant cardiovascular effects in some patients such as changes in pulse rate or blood pressure. If such effects occur, VENTOLIN HFA may need to be discontinued. In addition, beta-agonists have been reported to produce electrocardiogram (ECG) changes, such as flattening of the T wave, prolongation of the QTc interval, and ST segment depression. The clinical relevance of these findings is unknown. Therefore, VENTOLIN HFA, like all other sympathomimetic amines, should be used with caution in patients with underlying cardiovascular disorders, especially coronary insufficiency, cardiac arrhythmias, and hypertension.

5.5   Do Not Exceed Recommended Dose
Fatalities have been reported in association with excessive use of inhaled sympathomimetic drugs in patients with asthma. The exact cause of death is unknown, but cardiac arrest following an unexpected development of a severe acute asthmatic crisis and subsequent hypoxia is suspected.
5.6   Immediate Hypersensitivity Reactions
Immediate hypersensitivity reactions may occur after administration of albuterol sulfate inhalation aerosol, as demonstrated by cases of urticaria, angioedema, rash, bronchospasm, anaphylaxis, and oropharyngeal edema. Discontinue VENTOLIN HFA if immediate hypersensitivity reactions occur.
5.7   Coexisting Conditions
VENTOLIN HFA, like other sympathomimetic amines, should be used with caution in patients with convulsive disorders, hyperthyroidism, or diabetes mellitus and in patients who are unusually responsive to sympathomimetic amines. Large doses of intravenous albuterol have been reported to aggravate preexisting diabetes mellitus and ketoacidosis.
5.8   Hypokalemia
As with other beta-agonists, albuterol may produce significant hypokalemia in some patients, possibly through intracellular shunting, which has the potential to produce adverse cardiovascular effects. The decrease is usually transient, not requiring supplementation.

6   ADVERSE REACTIONS
Use of VENTOLIN HFA may be associated with the following:
• Paradoxical bronchospasm *[see Warnings and Precautions (5.1)]*
• Cardiovascular effects *[see Warnings and Precautions (5.4)]*
• Immediate hypersensitivity reactions *[see Warnings and Precautions (5.6)]*
• Hypokalemia *[see Warnings and Precautions (5.8)]*
6.1   Clinical Trials Experience
The safety data described below reflects exposure to VENTOLIN HFA in 248 patients treated with VENTOLIN HFA in 3 placebo-controlled clinical trials of 2 to 12 weeks' duration. The data from adults and adolescents is based upon 2 clinical trials in which 202 patients with asthma 12 years of age and older were treated with VENTOLIN HFA 2 inhalations 4 times daily for 12 weeks' duration. The adult/adolescent population was 92 female, 110 male and 163 white, 19 black, 18 Hispanic, 2 other. The data from pediatric patients are based upon 1 clinical trial in which 46 patients with asthma 4 to 11 years of age were treated with VENTOLIN HFA 2 inhalations 4 times daily for 2 weeks' duration. The population was 21 female, 25 male and 25 white, 17 black, 3 Hispanic, 1 other.
Because clinical trials are conducted under widely varying conditions, adverse reaction rates observed in the clinical trials of a drug cannot be directly compared to rates in the clinical trials of another drug and may not reflect the rates observed in practice.
Adults and Adolescents 12 Years of Age and Older: The two 12-week, randomized, double-blind studies in 610 adolescent and adult patients with asthma that compared VENTOLIN HFA, a CFC 11/12-propelled albuterol inhaler, and an HFA-134a placebo inhaler. Overall, the incidence and nature of the adverse reactions reported for VENTOLIN HFA and a CFC 11/12-propelled albuterol inhaler were comparable. Table 1 lists the incidence of all adverse reactions (whether considered by the investigator to be related or unrelated to drug) from these studies that

Table 1. Overall Adverse Reactions With ≥3% Incidence in 2 Large 12-Week Clinical Trials in Adolescents and Adults[a]

Adverse Reaction	Percent of Patients		
	VENTOLIN HFA (n = 202) %	CFC 11/12-Propelled Albuterol Inhaler (n = 207) %	Placebo HFA-134a (n = 201) %
Ear, nose, and throat			
Throat irritation	10	6	7
Upper respiratory inflammation	5	5	2
Lower respiratory			
Viral respiratory infections	7	4	4
Cough	5	2	2
Musculoskeletal			
Musculoskeletal pain	5	5	4

[a]This table includes all adverse reactions (whether considered by the investigator to be drug-related or unrelated to drug) that occurred at an incidence rate of at least 3.0% in the group treated with VENTOLIN HFA and more frequently in the group treated with VENTOLIN HFA than in the HFA-134a placebo inhaler group.

Table 2. In Vitro Medication Delivery Through AeroChamber Plus® Valved Holding Chamber With a Facemask

Age	Facemask	Flow Rate (L/min)	Holding Time (seconds)	Mean Medication Delivery Through AeroChamber Plus (mcg/actuation)	Body Weight 50th Percentile (kg)[a]	Medication Delivered per Actuation (mcg/kg)[b]
6 to 12 Months	Small	4.9	0	18.2	7.5-9.9	1.8-2.4
			2	19.8		2.0-2.6
			5	13.8		1.4-1.8
			10	15.4		1.6-2.1
2 to 5 Years	Small	8.0	0	17.8	12.3-18.0	1.0-1.4
			2	16.0		0.9-1.3
			5	16.3		0.9-1.3
			10	18.3		1.0-1.5
2 to 5 Years	Medium	8.0	0	21.1	12.3-18.0	1.2-1.7
			2	15.3		0.8-1.2
			5	18.3		1.0-1.5
			10	18.2		1.0-1.5
>5 Years	Medium	12.0	0	26.8	18.0	1.5
			2	20.9		1.2
			5	19.6		1.1
			10	20.3		1.1

[a]Centers for Disease Control growth charts, developed by the National Center for Health Statistics in collaboration with the National Center for Chronic Disease Prevention and Health Promotion (2000). Ranges correspond to the average of the 50th percentile weight for boys and girls at the ages indicated.
[b]A single inhalation of VENTOLIN HFA in a 70-kg adult without use of a valved holding chamber and facemask delivers approximately 90 mcg, or 1.3 mcg/kg.

occurred at a rate of 3% or greater in the group treated with VENTOLIN HFA and more frequently in the group treated with VENTOLIN HFA than in the HFA-134a placebo inhaler group.
[See table 1 at top of previous page]
Adverse reactions reported by less than 3% of the adolescent and adult patients receiving VENTOLIN HFA and by a greater proportion of patients receiving VENTOLIN HFA than receiving HFA-134a placebo inhaler and that have the potential to be related to VENTOLIN HFA include diarrhea, laryngitis, oropharyngeal edema, cough, lung disorders, tachycardia, and extrasystoles. Palpitation and dizziness have also been observed with VENTOLIN HFA.
Pediatric Patients: Results from the 2-week pediatric clinical study in patients with asthma 4 to 11 years of age showed that this pediatric population had an adverse reaction profile similar to that of the adolescent and adult populations.
Three studies have been conducted to evaluate the safety and efficacy of VENTOLIN HFA in patients between birth and 4 years of age. The results of these studies did not establish the efficacy of VENTOLIN HFA in this age-group [see Pediatric Use (8.4)]. Since the efficacy of VENTOLIN HFA has not been demonstrated in children between birth and 48 months of age, the safety of VENTOLIN HFA in this age-group cannot be established. However, the safety profile observed in the pediatric population under 4 years of age was comparable to that observed in the older pediatric patients and in adolescents and adults. Where adverse reaction incidence rates were greater in patients under 4 years of age compared with older patients, the higher incidence rates were noted in all treatment arms, including placebo. These adverse reactions included upper respiratory tract infection, nasopharyngitis, pyrexia, and tachycardia.

6.2   Postmarketing Experience
In addition to the adverse reactions listed in section 6.1, the following adverse reactions have been identified during postapproval use of VENTOLIN HFA. Because these reactions are reported voluntarily from a population of uncertain size, it is not always possible to reliably estimate their frequency or establish a causal relationship to drug exposure.
Cases of paradoxical bronchospasm, hoarseness, arrhythmias (including atrial fibrillation, supraventricular tachycardia), and hypersensitivity reactions (including urticaria, angioedema, rash) have been reported after the use of VENTOLIN HFA.
In addition, albuterol, like other sympathomimetic agents, can cause adverse reactions such as hypokalemia, hypertension, peripheral vasodilatation, angina, tremor, central nervous system stimulation, hyperactivity, sleeplessness, headache, muscle cramps, drying or irritation of the oropharynx, and metabolic acidosis.

7   DRUG INTERACTIONS
Other short-acting sympathomimetic aerosol bronchodilators should not be used concomitantly with albuterol. If additional adrenergic drugs are to be administered by any route, they should be used with caution to avoid deleterious cardiovascular effects.

7.1   Beta-Blockers
Beta-adrenergic receptor blocking agents not only block the pulmonary effect of beta-agonists, such as VENTOLIN HFA, but may produce severe bronchospasm in patients with asthma. Therefore, patients with asthma should not normally be treated with beta-blockers. However, under certain circumstances, e.g., as prophylaxis after myocardial infarction, there may be no acceptable alternatives to the use of beta-adrenergic blocking agents in patients with asthma. In this setting, cardioselective beta-blockers should be considered, although they should be administered with caution.

7.2   Diuretics
The ECG changes and/or hypokalemia that may result from the administration of nonpotassium-sparing diuretics (such as loop or thiazide diuretics) can be acutely worsened by beta-agonists, especially when the recommended dose of the beta-agonist is exceeded. Although the clinical relevance of these effects is not known, caution is advised in the coadministration of beta-agonists with nonpotassium-sparing diuretics. Consider monitoring potassium levels.

7.3   Digoxin
Mean decreases of 16% to 22% in serum digoxin levels were demonstrated after single-dose intravenous and oral administration of albuterol, respectively, to normal volunteers who had received digoxin for 10 days. The clinical relevance of these findings for patients with obstructive airway disease who are receiving inhaled albuterol and digoxin on a chronic basis is unclear. Nevertheless, it would be prudent to carefully evaluate the serum digoxin levels in patients who are currently receiving digoxin and albuterol.

7.4   Monoamine Oxidase Inhibitors or Tricyclic Antidepressants
VENTOLIN HFA should be administered with extreme caution to patients being treated with monoamine oxidase inhibitors or tricyclic antidepressants, or within 2 weeks of discontinuation of such agents, because the action of albuterol on the vascular system may be potentiated. Consider alternative therapy in patients taking MAOs or tricyclic antidepressants.

8   USE IN SPECIFIC POPULATIONS
8.1   Pregnancy
Teratogenic Effects: Pregnancy Category C.
There are no adequate and well-controlled studies of VENTOLIN HFA or albuterol sulfate in pregnant women. During worldwide marketing experience, various congenital anomalies, including cleft palate and limb defects, have been reported in the offspring of patients being treated with albuterol. Some of the mothers were taking multiple medications during their pregnancies. No consistent pattern of defects can be discerned, and a relationship between albuterol use and congenital anomalies has not been established. Animal reproduction studies in mice and rabbits revealed evidence of teratogenicity. VENTOLIN HFA should be used during pregnancy only if the potential benefit justifies the potential risk to the fetus.
In a mouse reproduction study, subcutaneously administered albuterol sulfate produced cleft palate formation in 5 of 111 (4.5%) fetuses at exposures approximately equal to the maximum recommended human dose (MRHD) for

adults on a mg/m² basis and in 10 of 108 (9.3%) fetuses at approximately 8 times the MRHD. Similar effects were not observed at approximately one eleventh of the MRHD. Cleft palate also occurred in 22 of 72 (30.5%) fetuses from females treated subcutaneously with isoproterenol (positive control). In a rabbit reproduction study, orally administered albuterol sulfate produced cranioschisis in 7 of 19 fetuses (37%) at approximately 680 times the MRHD.
In another rabbit study, an albuterol sulfate/HFA-134a formulation administered by inhalation produced enlargement of the frontal portion of the fetal fontanelles at approximately one third of the MRHD [see Animal Toxicology and/or Pharmacology (13.2)].

8.2   Labor and Delivery
Because of the potential for beta-agonist interference with uterine contractility, use of VENTOLIN HFA for relief of bronchospasm during labor should be restricted to those patients in whom the benefits clearly outweigh the risk.

8.3   Nursing Mothers
Plasma levels of albuterol sulfate and HFA-134a after inhaled therapeutic doses are very low in humans, but it is not known whether the components of VENTOLIN HFA are excreted in human milk. Because of the potential for tumorigenicity shown for albuterol in animal studies and lack of experience with the use of VENTOLIN HFA by nursing mothers, a decision should be made whether to discontinue nursing or to discontinue the drug, taking into account the importance of the drug to the mother. Caution should be exercised when VENTOLIN HFA is administered to a nursing woman.

8.4   Pediatric Use
The safety and effectiveness of VENTOLIN HFA in children 4 years of age and older has been established based upon two 12-week clinical trials in patients 12 years of age and older with asthma and one 2-week clinical trial in patients 4 to 11 years of age with asthma [see Clinical Studies (14.1), Adverse Reactions (6.1)]. The safety and effectiveness of VENTOLIN HFA in children under 4 years of age has not been established. Three studies have been conducted to evaluate the safety and efficacy of VENTOLIN HFA in patients under 4 years of age and the findings are described below.
Two 4-week randomized, double-blind, placebo-controlled studies were conducted in 163 pediatric patients from birth to 48 months of age with symptoms of bronchospasm associated with obstructive airway disease (presenting symptoms included: wheeze, cough, dyspnea, or chest tightness). VENTOLIN HFA or placebo HFA was delivered with either an AeroChamber Plus® Valved Holding Chamber or an Optichamber® Valved Holding Chamber with mask 3 times daily. In one study, VENTOLIN HFA 90 mcg (N = 26), VENTOLIN HFA 180 mcg (N = 25), and placebo HFA (N = 26) were administered to children between 24 and 48 months of age. In the second study, VENTOLIN HFA 90 mcg (N = 29), VENTOLIN HFA 180 mcg (N = 29), and placebo HFA (N = 28) were administered to children between birth and 24 months of age. Over the 4-week treatment period, there were no treatment differences in asthma symptom scores between the groups receiving VENTOLIN HFA 90 mcg, VENTOLIN HFA 180 mcg, and placebo in either study.
In a third study, VENTOLIN HFA was evaluated in 87 pediatric patients younger than 24 months of age for the treatment of acute wheezing. VENTOLIN HFA was delivered with an AeroChamber Plus Valved Holding Chamber in this study. There were no significant differences in asthma symptom scores and mean change from baseline in an asthma symptom score between VENTOLIN HFA 180 mcg and VENTOLIN HFA 360 mcg.
In vitro dose characterization studies were performed to evaluate the delivery of VENTOLIN HFA via holding chambers with facemasks. The studies were conducted with 2 different holding chambers with facemasks (small and medium size). The in vitro study data when simulated to patients suggest that the dose of VENTOLIN HFA presented for inhalation via a valved holding chamber with facemask will be comparable to the dose delivered in adults without a spacer and facemask per kilogram of body weight (Table 2). However, clinical studies in children under 4 years of age described above suggest that either the optimal dose of VENTOLIN HFA has not been defined in this age-group or VENTOLIN HFA is not effective in this age-group. The safety and effectiveness of VENTOLIN HFA administered with or without a spacer device in children under 4 years of age has not been demonstrated.
[See table 2 above]

8.5   Geriatric Use
Clinical studies of VENTOLIN HFA did not include sufficient numbers of subjects aged 65 and over to determine whether they respond differently from younger subjects. Other reported clinical experience has not identified differences in responses between the elderly and younger patients. In general, dose selection for an elderly patient should be cautious, usually starting at the low end of the

dosing range, reflecting the greater frequency of decreased hepatic, renal, or cardiac function, and of concomitant disease or other drug therapy.

10 OVERDOSAGE

The expected symptoms with overdosage are those of excessive beta-adrenergic stimulation and/or occurrence or exaggeration of any of the symptoms listed under ADVERSE REACTIONS, e.g., seizures, angina, hypertension or hypotension, tachycardia with rates up to 200 beats/min, arrhythmias, nervousness, headache, tremor, dry mouth, palpitation, nausea, dizziness, fatigue, malaise, sleeplessness. Hypokalemia and metabolic acidosis may also occur.

As with all sympathomimetic aerosol medications, cardiac arrest and even death may be associated with abuse of VENTOLIN HFA. Treatment consists of discontinuation of VENTOLIN HFA together with appropriate symptomatic therapy. The judicious use of a cardioselective beta-receptor blocker may be considered, bearing in mind that such medication can produce bronchospasm. There is insufficient evidence to determine if dialysis is beneficial for overdosage of VENTOLIN HFA.

The oral median lethal dose of albuterol sulfate in mice is greater than 2,000 mg/kg (approximately 6,800 times the maximum recommended daily inhalation dose for adults on a mg/m² basis and approximately 3,200 times the maximum recommended daily inhalation dose for children on a mg/m² basis). In mature rats, the subcutaneous median lethal dose of albuterol sulfate is approximately 450 mg/kg (approximately 3,000 times the maximum recommended daily inhalation dose for adults on a mg/m² basis and approximately 1,400 times the maximum recommended daily inhalation dose for children on a mg/m² basis). In young rats, the subcutaneous median lethal dose is approximately 2,000 mg/kg (approximately 14,000 times the maximum recommended daily inhalation dose for adults on a mg/m² basis and approximately 6,400 times the maximum recommended daily inhalation dose for children on a mg/m² basis). The inhalation median lethal dose has not been determined in animals.

11 DESCRIPTION

The active component of VENTOLIN HFA is albuterol sulfate, USP, the racemic form of albuterol and a relatively selective beta₂-adrenergic bronchodilator. Albuterol sulfate has the chemical name α¹-[(tert-butylamino)methyl]-4-hydroxy-m-xylene-α, α′-diol sulfate (2:1)(salt) and the following chemical structure:

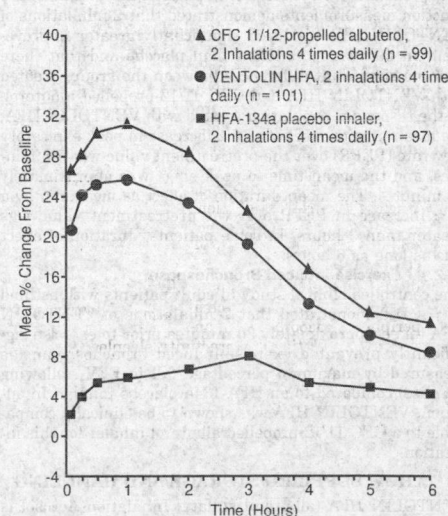

Albuterol sulfate is a white crystalline powder with a molecular weight of 576.7, and the empirical formula is $(C_{13}H_{21}NO_3)_2 \cdot H_2SO_4$. It is soluble in water and slightly soluble in ethanol.

The World Health Organization recommended name for albuterol base is salbutamol.

VENTOLIN HFA is a pressurized metered-dose aerosol unit fitted with a counter. VENTOLIN HFA is intended for oral inhalation only. Each unit contains a microcrystalline suspension of albuterol sulfate in propellant HFA-134a (1,1,1,2-tetrafluoroethane). It contains no other excipients.

Priming VENTOLIN HFA is essential to ensure appropriate albuterol content in each actuation. To prime the inhaler, release 4 sprays into the air away from the face, shaking well before each spray. The inhaler should be primed before using it for the first time, when it has not been used for more than 2 weeks, or when it has been dropped.

After priming, each actuation of the inhaler delivers 120 mcg of albuterol sulfate, USP in 75 mg of suspension from the valve and 108 mcg of albuterol sulfate, USP from the mouthpiece (equivalent to 90 mcg of albuterol base from the mouthpiece).

Each 18-g canister provides 200 inhalations. Each 8-g canister provides 60 inhalations.

This product does not contain chlorofluorocarbons (CFCs) as the propellant.

12 CLINICAL PHARMACOLOGY

12.1 Mechanism of Action

In vitro studies and in vivo pharmacologic studies have demonstrated that albuterol has a preferential effect on beta₂-adrenergic receptors compared with isoproterenol. While it is recognized that beta₂-adrenergic receptors are the predominant receptors in bronchial smooth muscle, data indicate that there is a population of beta₂-receptors in the human heart existing in a concentration between 10% and 50% of cardiac beta-adrenergic receptors. The precise function of these receptors has not been established [see Warnings and Precautions (5.4)].

Activation of beta₂-adrenergic receptors on airway smooth muscle leads to the activation of adenylcyclase and to an increase in the intracellular concentration of cyclic-3′,5′-adenosine monophosphate (cyclic AMP). This increase of cyclic AMP leads to the activation of protein kinase A, which inhibits the phosphorylation of myosin and lowers intracellular ionic calcium concentrations, resulting in relaxation. Albuterol relaxes the smooth muscles of all airways, from the trachea to the terminal bronchioles. Albuterol acts as a functional antagonist to relax the airway irrespective of the spasmogen involved, thus protecting against all bronchoconstrictor challenges. Increased cyclic AMP concentrations are also associated with the inhibition of release of mediators from mast cells in the airway.

Albuterol has been shown in most controlled clinical trials to have more effect on the respiratory tract, in the form of bronchial smooth muscle relaxation, than isoproterenol at comparable doses while producing fewer cardiovascular effects. Controlled clinical studies and other clinical experience have shown that inhaled albuterol, like other beta-adrenergic agonist drugs, can produce a significant cardiovascular effect in some patients, as measured by pulse rate, blood pressure, symptoms, and/or electrocardiographic changes [see Warnings and Precautions (5.4)].

12.2 Pharmacokinetics

The systemic levels of albuterol are low after inhalation of recommended doses. A study conducted in 12 healthy male and female subjects using a higher dose (1,080 mcg of albuterol base) showed that mean peak plasma concentrations of approximately 3 ng/mL occurred at that dosing when albuterol was delivered using propellant HFA-134a. The mean time to peak concentrations (T_{max}) was delayed after administration of VENTOLIN HFA (T_{max} = 0.42 hours) as compared to CFC-propelled albuterol inhaler (T_{max} = 0.17 hours). Apparent terminal plasma half-life of albuterol is approximately 4.6 hours. No further pharmacokinetic studies for VENTOLIN HFA were conducted in neonates, children, or elderly subjects.

13 NONCLINICAL TOXICOLOGY

13.1 Carcinogenesis, Mutagenesis, Impairment of Fertility

In a 2-year study in Sprague-Dawley rats, albuterol sulfate caused a dose-related increase in the incidence of benign leiomyomas of the mesovarium at and above dietary doses of 2.0 mg/kg (approximately 14 times the maximum recommended daily inhalation dose for adults on a mg/m² basis and approximately 6 times the maximum recommended daily inhalation dose for children on a mg/m² basis). In another study this effect was blocked by the coadministration of propranolol, a non-selective beta-adrenergic antagonist. In an 18-month study in CD-1 mice, albuterol sulfate showed no evidence of tumorigenicity at dietary doses of up to 500 mg/kg (approximately 1,700 times the maximum recommended daily inhalation dose for adults on a mg/m² basis and approximately 800 times the maximum recommended daily inhalation dose for children on a mg/m² basis). In a 22-month study in Golden hamsters, albuterol sulfate showed no evidence of tumorigenicity at dietary doses of up to 50 mg/kg (approximately 225 times the maximum recommended daily inhalation dose for adults on a mg/m² basis and approximately 110 times the maximum recommended daily inhalation dose for children on a mg/m² basis).

Albuterol sulfate was not mutagenic in the Ames test or a mutation test in yeast. Albuterol sulfate was not clastogenic in a human peripheral lymphocyte assay or in an AH1 strain mouse micronucleus assay.

Reproduction studies in rats demonstrated no evidence of impaired fertility at oral doses of albuterol sulfate up to 50 mg/kg (approximately 340 times the maximum recommended daily inhalation dose for adults on a mg/m² basis).

13.2 Animal Toxicology and/or Pharmacology

Preclinical: Intravenous studies in rats with albuterol sulfate have demonstrated that albuterol crosses the blood-brain barrier and reaches brain concentrations amounting to approximately 5.0% of the plasma concentrations. In structures outside the blood-brain barrier (pineal and pituitary glands), albuterol concentrations were found to be 100 times those in the whole brain.

Studies in laboratory animals (minipigs, rodents, and dogs) have demonstrated the occurrence of cardiac arrhythmias and sudden death (with histologic evidence of myocardial necrosis) when beta-agonists and methylxanthines are administered concurrently. The clinical relevance of these findings is unknown.

Propellant HFA-134a is devoid of pharmacological activity except at very high doses in animals (380 to 1,300 times the maximum human exposure based on comparisons of AUC values), primarily producing ataxia, tremors, dyspnea, or salivation. These are similar to effects produced by the structurally related CFCs, which have been used extensively in metered-dose inhalers.

In animals and humans, propellant HFA-134a was found to be rapidly absorbed and rapidly eliminated, with an elimination half-life of 3 to 27 minutes in animals and 5 to 7 minutes in humans. Time to maximum plasma concentration (T_{max}) and mean residence time are both extremely short, leading to a transient appearance of HFA-134a in the blood with no evidence of accumulation.

Reproductive Toxicology Studies: A study in CD-1 mice given albuterol sulfate subcutaneously showed cleft palate formation in 5 of 111 (4.5%) fetuses at 0.25 mg/kg (less than the maximum recommended daily inhalation dose for adults on a mg/m² basis) and in 10 of 108 (9.3%) fetuses at 2.5 mg/kg (approximately 8 times the maximum recommended daily inhalation dose for adults on a mg/m² basis). The drug did not induce cleft palate formation at a dose of 0.025 mg/kg (less than the maximum recommended daily inhalation dose for adults on a mg/m² basis). Cleft palate also occurred in 22 of 72 (30.5%) fetuses from females treated subcutaneously with 2.5 mg/kg of isoproterenol (positive control).

A reproduction study in Stride Dutch rabbits revealed cranioschisis in 7 of 19 fetuses (37%) when albuterol sulfate was administered orally at a 50 mg/kg dose (approximately 680 times the maximum recommended daily inhalation dose for adults on a mg/m² basis).

In an inhalation reproduction study in New Zealand white rabbits, albuterol sulfate/HFA-134a formulation exhibited enlargement of the frontal portion of the fetal fontanelles at and above inhalation doses of 0.0193 mg/kg (less than the maximum recommended daily inhalation dose for adults on a mg/m² basis).

A study in which pregnant rats were dosed with radiolabeled albuterol sulfate demonstrated that drug-related material is transferred from the maternal circulation to the fetus.

14 CLINICAL STUDIES

14.1 Bronchospasm Associated With Asthma

Adult and Adolescent Patients 12 Years of Age and Older: The efficacy of VENTOLIN HFA was evaluated in two 12-week, randomized, double-blind, placebo controlled trials in patients 12 years of age and older with mild to moderate asthma. These trials included a total of 610 patients (323 males, 287 females). In each trial, patients received 2 inhalations of VENTOLIN HFA, CFC 11/12-propelled albuterol, or HFA-134a placebo 4 times daily for 12 weeks' duration. Patients taking the HFA-134a placebo inhaler also took VENTOLIN HFA for asthma symptom relief on an as-needed basis. Some patients who participated in these clinical trials were using concomitant inhaled steroid therapy. Efficacy was assessed by serial forced expiratory volume in 1 second (FEV₁). In each of these trials, 2 inhalations of VENTOLIN HFA produced significantly greater improvement in FEV₁ over the pretreatment value than placebo. Results from the 2 clinical trials are described below.

In a 12-week, randomized, double-blind study, VENTOLIN HFA (101 patients) was compared to CFC 11/12-propelled albuterol (99 patients) and an HFA-134a placebo inhaler (97 patients) in adolescent and adult patients 12 to 76 years of age with mild to moderate asthma. Serial FEV₁ measurements [shown below as percent change from test-day baseline at Day 1 (n = 297) and at Week 12 (n = 249)] demonstrated that 2 inhalations of VENTOLIN HFA produced significantly greater improvement in FEV₁ over the pretreatment value than placebo.

FEV₁ as Percent Change From Predose in a Large, 12-Week Clinical Trial

Day 1

Week 12

In the responder population (≥15% increase in FEV_1 within 30 minutes postdose) treated with VENTOLIN HFA, the mean time to onset of a 15% increase in FEV_1 over the pretreatment value was 5.4 minutes, and the mean time to peak effect was 56 minutes. The mean duration of effect as measured by a 15% increase in FEV_1 over the pretreatment value was approximately 4 hours. In some patients, duration of effect was as long as 6 hours.

The second 12-week randomized, double-blind study was conducted to evaluate the efficacy and safety of switching patients from CFC 11/12-propelled albuterol to VENTOLIN HFA. During the 3-week run-in phase of the study, all patients received CFC 11/12-propelled albuterol. During the double-blind treatment phase, VENTOLIN HFA (91 patients) was compared to CFC 11/12-propelled albuterol (100 patients) and an HFA-134a placebo inhaler (95 patients) in adolescent and adult patients with mild to moderate asthma. Serial FEV_1 measurements demonstrated that 2 inhalations of VENTOLIN HFA produced significantly greater improvement in pulmonary function than placebo. The switching from CFC 11/12-propelled albuterol inhaler to VENTOLIN HFA did not reveal any clinically significant changes in the efficacy profile.

In the 2 adult studies, the efficacy results from VENTOLIN HFA were significantly greater than placebo and were clinically comparable to those achieved with CFC 11/12-propelled albuterol, although small numerical differences in mean FEV_1 response and other measures were observed. Physicians should recognize that individual responses to beta-adrenergic agonists administered via different propellants may vary and that equivalent responses in individual patients should not be assumed.

Pediatric Patients 4 Years of Age: The efficacy of VENTOLIN HFA was evaluated in one 2-week, randomized, double-blind, placebo-controlled trial in 135 pediatric patients 4 to 11 years of age with mild to moderate asthma. In this trial, patients received VENTOLIN HFA, CFC 11/12-propelled albuterol, or HFA-134a placebo. Serial pulmonary function measurements demonstrated that 2 inhalations of VENTOLIN HFA produced significantly greater improvement in pulmonary function than placebo and that there were no significant differences between the groups treated with VENTOLIN HFA and CFC 11/12-propelled albuterol. In the responder population treated with VENTOLIN HFA, the mean time to onset of a 15% increase in peak expiratory flow rate (PEFR) over the pretreatment value was 7.8 minutes, and the mean time to peak effect was approximately 90 minutes. The mean duration of effect as measured by a 15% increase in PEFR over the pretreatment value was greater than 3 hours. In some patients, duration of effect was as long as 6 hours.

14.2 Exercise-Induced Bronchospasm
One controlled clinical study in adult patients with asthma (N = 24) demonstrated that 2 inhalations of VENTOLIN HFA taken approximately 30 minutes prior to exercise significantly prevented exercise-induced bronchospasm (as measured by maximum percentage fall in FEV_1 following exercise) compared to an HFA-134a placebo inhaler. In addition, VENTOLIN HFA was shown to be clinically comparable to a CFC 11/12-propelled albuterol inhaler for this indication.

16 HOW SUPPLIED/STORAGE AND HANDLING
VENTOLIN HFA (albuterol sulfate) Inhalation Aerosol is supplied in the following packs as a pressurized aluminum canister fitted with a counter with a blue plastic actuator and a blue strapcap packaged within a moisture-protective foil pouch that also contains a desiccant:
NDC 0173-0682-20 18-g canister containing 200 actuations
NDC 0173-0682-21 8-g canister containing 60 actuations
NDC 0173-0682-24 8-g institutional pack canister containing 60 actuations

Before using, VENTOLIN HFA should be removed from the moisture-protective foil pouch. The pouch and desiccant should be discarded. VENTOLIN HFA should be discarded 12 months after removal from the pouch.

Priming VENTOLIN HFA is essential to ensure appropriate albuterol content in each actuation. To prime the inhaler, release 4 sprays into the air away from the face, shaking well before each spray. The inhaler should be primed before using it for the first time, when the inhaler has not been used for more than 2 weeks, or when it has been dropped.

After priming, each actuation delivers 120 mcg of albuterol sulfate, USP in 75 mg of suspension from the valve and 108 mcg of albuterol sulfate, USP from the mouthpiece (equivalent to 90 mcg of albuterol base from the mouthpiece).

To ensure proper dosing and to prevent actuator orifice blockage, wash the actuator with warm water and let it air-dry completely at least once a week [see the Patient Information tear–off leaflet].

The blue actuator supplied with VENTOLIN HFA should not be used with any other product canisters, and actuators from other products should not be used with a VENTOLIN HFA canister.

VENTOLIN HFA has a counter attached to the canister. The counter starts at 204 or 64 and counts down each time a spray is released. The correct amount of medication in each inhalation cannot be assured after the counter reads 000, even though the canister is not completely empty and will continue to operate. VENTOLIN HFA should be discarded when the counter reads 000 or 12 months after removal from the moisture-protective foil pouch, whichever comes first. Never immerse the canister in water to determine the amount of drug remaining in the canister.

Keep out of reach of children. Avoid spraying in eyes.

Contents Under Pressure: Do not puncture. Do not use or store near heat or open flame. Exposure to temperatures above 120°F may cause bursting. Never throw container into fire or incinerator.

Store between 15° and 25°C (59° and 77°F). Store the inhaler with the mouthpiece down. For best results, the inhaler should be at room temperature before use. SHAKE WELL BEFORE EACH SPRAY.

VENTOLIN HFA does not contain chlorofluorocarbons (CFCs) as the propellant.

17 PATIENT COUNSELING INFORMATION
See FDA-approved patient labeling (Patient Information and Instructions for Use).

17.1 Frequency of Use
The action of VENTOLIN HFA should last up to 4 to 6 hours. VENTOLIN HFA should not be used more frequently than recommended. Do not increase the dose or frequency of doses of VENTOLIN HFA without consulting the physician. If patients find that treatment with VENTOLIN HFA becomes less effective for symptomatic relief, symptoms become worse, and/or they need to use the product more frequently than usual, they should seek medical attention immediately.

17.2 Priming and Cleaning
Priming: Patients should be instructed that priming VENTOLIN HFA is essential to ensure appropriate albuterol content in each actuation. Patients should prime VENTOLIN HFA before using for the first time, when the inhaler has not been used for more than 2 weeks, or when the inhaler has been dropped. To prime VENTOLIN HFA, patients should release 4 sprays into the air away from the face, shaking well before each spray.

Cleaning: To ensure proper dosing and to prevent actuator orifice blockage, patients should be instructed to wash the actuator and dry thoroughly at least once a week. Patients should be informed that detailed cleaning instructions are included in the Patient Information leaflet.

17.3 Dose Counter
Patients should be informed that VENTOLIN HFA has a dose counter that starts at 204 or 64 and counts down each time a spray is released. Patients should be informed to discard VENTOLIN HFA when the counter reads 000 or 12 months after removal from the moisture-protective foil pouch, whichever comes first. When the counter reads 020, the patient should contact the pharmacist for a refill of medication or consult the physician to determine whether a prescription refill is needed. Patients should never try to alter the numbers or remove the counter from the metal canister. Patients should never immerse the canister in water to determine the amount of drug remaining in the canister.

17.4 Paradoxical Bronchospasm
Patients should be informed that VENTOLIN HFA can produce paradoxical bronchospasm. If paradoxical bronchospasm occurs, patients should discontinue VENTOLIN HFA.

17.5 Concomitant Drug Use
While patients are using VENTOLIN HFA, other inhaled drugs and asthma medications should be taken only as directed by the physician.

17.6 Common Adverse Effects
Common adverse effects of treatment with inhaled albuterol include palpitations, chest pain, rapid heart rate, tremor, and nervousness.

17.7 Pregnancy
Patients who are pregnant or nursing should contact their physicians about the use of VENTOLIN HFA.

VENTOLIN is a registered trademark of GlaxoSmithKline.
AeroChamber Plus is a registered trademark of Monaghan Medical Inc.
OptiChamber is a registered trademark of Respironics Inc.
GlaxoSmithKline
Research Triangle Park, NC 27709
©2012, GlaxoSmithKline. All rights reserved.
VNT:8PI
PHARMACIST—DETACH HERE AND GIVE LEAFLET TO PATIENT
Patient Information
VENTOLIN® HFA *(vent' o-lin)*
(albuterol sulfate)
Inhalation Aerosol
Read this Patient Information before you start using VENTOLIN HFA and each time you get a refill. There may be new information. This information does not take the place of talking to your healthcare provider about your medical condition or your treatment.
What is VENTOLIN HFA?
VENTOLIN HFA is a prescription medicine used in people 4 years of age and older to:
• treat or prevent bronchospasm in people who have reversible obstructive airway disease
• prevent exercise-induced bronchospasm
It is not known if VENTOLIN HFA is safe and effective in children under 4 years of age.
Who should not use VENTOLIN HFA?
Do not use VENTOLIN HFA if you are allergic to albuterol sulfate or any of the ingredients in VENTOLIN HFA. See the end of this Patient Information leaflet for a complete list of ingredients in VENTOLIN HFA.
What should I tell my healthcare provider before I use VENTOLIN HFA?
Before you use VENTOLIN HFA, tell your healthcare provider if you:
• have heart problems
• have high blood pressure (hypertension)
• have convulsions (seizures)
• have thyroid problems
• have diabetes
• have low potassium levels in your blood
• are pregnant or plan to become pregnant. It is not known if VENTOLIN HFA will harm your unborn baby. Talk to your healthcare provider if you are pregnant or plan to become pregnant.
• are breastfeeding or plan to breastfeed. It is not known if VENTOLIN HFA passes into your breast milk. Talk to your healthcare provider about the best way to feed your baby if you are using VENTOLIN HFA.
Tell your healthcare provider about all the medicines you take, including prescription and nonprescription medicines, vitamins, and herbal supplements.
VENTOLIN HFA and other medicines may affect each other and cause side effects. VENTOLIN HFA may affect the way other medicines work, and other medicines may affect the way VENTOLIN HFA works.
Especially tell your healthcare provider if you take:
• other inhaled medicines or asthma medicines
• beta-blocker medicines
• diuretics
• digoxin
• monoamine oxidase inhibitors
• tricyclic antidepressants
Ask your healthcare provider or pharmacist for a list of these medicines if you are not sure.
Know the medicines you take. Keep a list of them to show your healthcare provider and pharmacist when you get a new medicine.
How should I use VENTOLIN HFA?
• For detailed instructions, see "**Instructions for Use**" at the end of this Patient Information.
• Use VENTOLIN HFA exactly as your healthcare provider tells you to use it.
• **Do not** increase your dose or take extra doses of VENTOLIN HFA without first talking to your healthcare provider.

- If your child needs to use VENTOLIN HFA, watch your child closely to make sure your child uses the inhaler correctly. Your healthcare provider will show you how your child should use VENTOLIN HFA.
- Each dose of VENTOLIN HFA should last up to 4 hours to 6 hours.
- Get medical help right away if VENTOLIN HFA no longer helps your symptoms.
- Get medical help right away if your symptoms get worse or if you need to use your inhaler more often.
- While you are using VENTOLIN HFA, use other inhaled medicines and asthma medicines only as directed by your healthcare provider.
- Call your healthcare provider if your asthma symptoms like wheezing and trouble breathing become worse over a few hours or days. Your healthcare provider may need to give you another medicine to treat your symptoms.

What are the possible side effects of VENTOLIN HFA?
VENTOLIN HFA may cause serious side effects, including:
- **worsening trouble breathing, coughing, and wheezing (paradoxical bronchospasm).** If this happens, stop using VENTOLIN HFA and call your healthcare provider or get emergency help right away. Paradoxical bronchospasm is more likely to happen with your first use of a new canister of medicine.
- **heart problems, including faster heart rate and higher blood pressure**
- **possible death in people with asthma who use too much VENTOLIN HFA**
- **allergic reactions.** Call your healthcare provider right away if you have any of the following symptoms of an allergic reaction:
  ◦ itchy skin
  ◦ swelling beneath your skin or in your throat
  ◦ rash
  ◦ worsening trouble breathing
- **low potassium levels in your blood**
- **worsening of other medical problems in people who also use VENTOLIN HFA, including increases in blood sugar**

Common side effects of VENTOLIN HFA include:
- your heart feels like it is pounding or racing (palpitations)
- chest pain
- fast heart rate
- shakiness
- nervousness
- headache
- pain
- dizziness
- sore throat
- runny nose

Tell your healthcare provider if you have any side effect that bothers you or that does not go away.

These are not all the possible side effects of VENTOLIN HFA. For more information, ask your healthcare provider or pharmacist.

Call your doctor for medical advice about side effects. You may report side effects to FDA at 1-800-FDA-1088.

How should I store VENTOLIN HFA?
- Store VENTOLIN HFA at room temperature between 59°F and 77°F (15°C and 25°C) with the mouthpiece down.
- Avoid exposure to extreme heat and cold.
- Shake the VENTOLIN HFA canister well before use.
- **Do not** puncture the VENTOLIN HFA canister.
- **Do not** store the VENTOLIN HFA canister near heat or a flame. Temperatures above 120°F may cause the canister to burst.
- **Do not** throw the VENTOLIN HFA canister into a fire or an incinerator.
- Avoid spraying VENTOLIN HFA in your eyes.

Keep VENTOLIN HFA and all medicines out of the reach of children.

General information about the safe and effective use of VENTOLIN HFA
Medicines are sometimes prescribed for purposes other than those listed in a Patient Information leaflet. Do not use VENTOLIN HFA for a condition for which it was not prescribed. Do not give VENTOLIN HFA to other people, even if they have the same symptoms that you have. It may harm them.

This Patient Information leaflet summarizes the most important information about VENTOLIN HFA. If you would like more information, talk with your healthcare provider. You can ask your pharmacist or healthcare provider for information about VENTOLIN HFA that is written for healthcare professionals.

For more information, go to www.ventolin.com or call 1-888-825-5249.

What are the ingredients in VENTOLIN HFA?
Active ingredient: albuterol sulfate
Inactive ingredient: propellant HFA-134a

Instructions for Use
VENTOLIN® HFA *(vent' o-lin)*
(albuterol sulfate)
Inhalation Aerosol
Read this Instructions for Use before you start using VENTOLIN HFA and each time you get a refill. There may

be new information. This information does not take the place of talking to your healthcare provider about your medical condition or your treatment.

The parts of your VENTOLIN HFA inhaler:
There are 2 main parts of your VENTOLIN HFA inhaler:
- the blue plastic actuator that sprays the medicine into your mouth. See Figure A.
- the metal canister that holds the medicine. See Figure A.

Figure A

The actuator has a protective cap that covers the mouthpiece. The strap on the cap will stay attached to the actuator.
Do not use this actuator with a canister of medicine from any other inhaler.
Do not use this canister of medicine with an actuator from any other inhaler.
The canister has a counter that shows you how many sprays of medicine you have left. The number shows through a window in the back of the actuator. The counter starts at either 204 or 64, depending on which size inhaler you have. See Figure B.

Figure B

Priming your VENTOLIN HFA inhaler:
Your VENTOLIN HFA inhaler must be primed before you use it for the first time, when it has not been used for more than 14 days in a row, or if it has been dropped. Do not prime your VENTOLIN HFA every day.
- Remove your VENTOLIN HFA inhaler from its packaging.
- Throw away the pouch and the drying packet that comes inside the pouch.
- Remove the protective cap from the mouthpiece.
- Shake the inhaler well, and spray it into the air away from your face. See Figure C.

Figure C

- Shake and spray the inhaler like this 3 more times to finish priming it. After you prime the actuator for the first time, the dose counter in the window on the back of the actuator should show the number 200 or 60, depending on which size inhaler you have. See Figure D.

Figure D

Each time you use your VENTOLIN HFA inhaler:
- Make sure the canister fits firmly in the plastic actuator.
- Look into the mouthpiece to make sure there are no foreign objects there, especially if the strap is no longer attached to the actuator or the cap has not been used to cover the mouthpiece.

Reading the dose counter on your VENTOLIN HFA actuator:
- The dose counter will count down by 1 number each time you spray the inhaler.

- The dose counter stops counting when it reaches **000**. It will continue to show **000**.
- The dose counter cannot be reset, and it is permanently attached to the metal canister. **Never** try to change the numbers for the dose counter or take the counter off the metal canister.
- **Do not** remove the canister from the plastic actuator except during cleaning to prevent accidently spraying a dose of VENTOLIN HFA into the air.

Using your VENTOLIN HFA inhaler:
Step 1. **Shake the inhaler well** before each spray. Take the cap off the mouthpiece of the actuator.
Step 2. Hold the inhaler with the mouthpiece down. See Figure E.

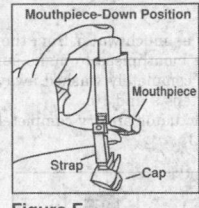

Figure E

Step 3. Breathe out through your mouth and push as much air from your lungs as you can. Put the mouthpiece in your mouth and close your lips around it. See Figure F.

Figure F

Step 4. Push the top of the canister all the way down while you breathe in deeply and slowly through your mouth. See Figure F.
Step 5. Right after the spray comes out, take your finger off the canister. After you have breathed in all the way, take the inhaler out of your mouth and close your mouth.
Step 6. **Hold your breath as long as you can,** up to 10 seconds, then breathe normally.
If your healthcare provider has told you to use more sprays, wait 1 minute and shake the inhaler again. Repeat Steps 2 through Step 6.
Step 7. Put the cap back on the mouthpiece after every time you use the inhaler. Make sure the cap snaps firmly into place.

Cleaning your VENTOLIN HFA actuator:
It is very important to keep the plastic actuator clean so the medicine will not build-up and block the spray. See Figure G.

Figure G

- **Do not try to clean the metal canister or let it get wet.** The inhaler may stop spraying if it is not cleaned correctly.
- **Wash the actuator** at least once a week as follows:
Step 8. Take the canister out of the actuator, and take the cap off the mouthpiece. The strap on the cap will stay attached to the actuator.
Step 9. Hold the actuator under the faucet and run warm water through it for about 30 seconds. See Figure H.

Figure H

Step 10. Turn the actuator upside down and run warm water through the mouthpiece for about 30 seconds. See Figure I.

Figure I

Step 11. Shake off as much water from the actuator as you can. Look into the mouthpiece to make sure any medicine build-up has been completely washed away. If there is any build-up, repeat Steps 9 and 10.

Step 12. Let the actuator air-dry completely, such as overnight. See Figure J.

Figure J

Step 13. When the actuator is dry, put the canister in the actuator and make sure it fits firmly. Shake the inhaler well and spray it once into the air away from your face. (The counter will count down by 1 number.) Put the cap back on the mouthpiece.

If you need to use your inhaler before the actuator is completely dry:

• Shake as much water off the actuator as you can.
• Put the canister in the actuator and make sure it fits firmly.
• Shake the inhaler well and spray it once into the air away from your face.
• Take your VENTOLIN HFA dose as prescribed.
• Follow cleaning Steps 8 through 13 above.

Replacing your VENTOLIN HFA inhaler:

• **When the dose counter on the actuator shows the number 020,** you need to refill your prescription or ask your doctor for another prescription for VENTOLIN HFA.
• **Throw the VENTOLIN HFA inhaler away** as soon as the dose counter shows **000,** after the expiration date on the VENTOLIN HFA packaging, or 12 months after you open the foil pouch, whichever comes first. You should not keep using the inhaler after the dose counter shows **000** even though the canister may not be completely empty. You cannot be sure you will receive the right amount of medicine.

VENTOLIN is a registered trademark of GlaxoSmithKline.
This Patient Information and Instructions for Use has been approved by the U.S. Food and Drug Administration.
GlaxoSmithKline
Research Triangle Park, NC 27709
©2012, GlaxoSmithKline. All rights reserved.
October 2012
VNT:8PIL

VERAMYST   ℞
[ver' ə-mist]
(fluticasone furoate)
Nasal Spray

HIGHLIGHTS OF PRESCRIBING INFORMATION
These highlights do not include all the information needed to use VERAMYST safely and effectively. See full prescribing information for VERAMYST.
VERAMYST (fluticasone furoate) Nasal Spray
Initial U.S. Approval: 2007

————**RECENT MAJOR CHANGES**————

Use in Specific Populations, Pediatric Use (8.4)	August 2012

————**INDICATIONS AND USAGE**————

VERAMYST Nasal Spray is a corticosteroid indicated for treatment of symptoms of seasonal and perennial allergic rhinitis in adults and children ≥2 years. (1.1)

————**DOSAGE AND ADMINISTRATION**————

For intranasal use only. Usual starting dosages:
• Adults and adolescents ≥12 years: 110 mcg (2 sprays per nostril) once daily. (2.1)
• Children 2-11 years: 55 mcg (1 spray per nostril) once daily. (2.2)
• Priming information: Prime VERAMYST Nasal Spray before using for the first time, when not used for more than 30 days, or if the cap has been left off the bottle for 5 days or longer. (2)

————**DOSAGE FORMS AND STRENGTHS**————

Nasal spray: 27.5 mcg of fluticasone furoate in each 50-microliter spray. (3)
Supplied in 10-g bottle containing 120 sprays. (16)

————**CONTRAINDICATIONS**————

Hypersensitivity to ingredients. (4)

————**WARNINGS AND PRECAUTIONS**————

• Epistaxis, nasal ulceration, *Candida albicans* infection, nasal septal perforation, impaired wound healing. Monitor patients periodically for signs of adverse effects on the nasal mucosa. Avoid use in patients with recent nasal ulcers, nasal surgery, or nasal trauma. (5.1)
• Development of glaucoma or posterior subcapsular cataracts. Monitor patients closely with a change in vision or with a history of increased intraocular pressure, glaucoma, and/or cataracts. (5.2)
• Hypersensitivity reactions, including anaphylaxis, angioedema, rash, and urticaria, may occur after administration of VERAMYST Nasal Spray. (5.3)
• Potential worsening of existing tuberculosis; fungal, bacterial, viral, or parasitic infections; or ocular herpes simplex. More serious or even fatal course of chickenpox or measles in susceptible patients. Use caution in patients with the above because of the potential for worsening of these infections. (5.4)
• Hypercorticism and adrenal suppression with very high dosages or at the regular dosage in susceptible individuals. If such changes occur, discontinue VERAMYST Nasal Spray slowly. (5.5)
• Potential reduction in growth velocity in children. Monitor growth routinely in pediatric patients receiving VERAMYST Nasal Spray. (5.7, 8.4)

————**ADVERSE REACTIONS**————

The most common adverse reactions (>1% incidence) included headache, epistaxis, pharyngolaryngeal pain, nasal ulceration, back pain, pyrexia, and cough. (6.1)
To report SUSPECTED ADVERSE REACTIONS, contact GlaxoSmithKline at 1-888-825-5249 or FDA at 1-800-FDA-1088 or www.fda.gov/medwatch.

————**DRUG INTERACTIONS**————

Potent inhibitors of cytochrome P450 3A4 (CYP3A4) may increase exposure to fluticasone furoate.
• Coadministration of ritonavir is not recommended. (5.6, 7)
• Use caution with coadministration of other potent CYP3A4 inhibitors, such as ketoconazole. (5.6, 7)

————**USE IN SPECIFIC POPULATIONS**————

Hepatic impairment may increase exposure to fluticasone furoate. Use with caution in patients with severe hepatic impairment. (8.6)
See 17 for PATIENT COUNSELING INFORMATION and FDA-approved patient labeling

                                            Revised: 08/2012

FULL PRESCRIBING INFORMATION

1   INDICATIONS AND USAGE
1.1   Treatment of Allergic Rhinitis

VERAMYST® (fluticasone furoate) Nasal Spray is indicated for the treatment of the symptoms of seasonal and perennial allergic rhinitis in patients aged 2 years and older.

2   DOSAGE AND ADMINISTRATION

Administer VERAMYST Nasal Spray by the intranasal route only. Prime VERAMYST Nasal Spray before using for the first time by shaking the contents well and releasing 6 sprays into the air away from the face. When VERAMYST Nasal Spray has not been used for more than 30 days or if the cap has been left off the bottle for 5 days or longer, prime the pump again until a fine mist appears. Shake VERAMYST Nasal Spray well before each use.
Titrate an individual patient to the minimum effective dosage to reduce the possibility of side effects.

2.1   Adults and Adolescents Aged 12 Years and Older

The recommended starting dosage is 110 mcg once daily administered as 2 sprays (27.5 mcg/spray) in each nostril. When the maximum benefit has been achieved and symptoms have been controlled, reducing the dosage to 55 mcg (1 spray in each nostril) once daily may be effective in maintaining control of allergic rhinitis symptoms.

2.2   Children Aged 2 to 11 Years

The recommended starting dosage in children is 55 mcg once daily administered as 1 spray (27.5 mcg/spray) in each nostril. Children not adequately responding to 55 mcg may use 110 mcg (2 sprays in each nostril) once daily. Once symptoms have been controlled, dosage reduction to 55 mcg once daily is recommended.

3   DOSAGE FORMS AND STRENGTHS

VERAMYST Nasal Spray is a nasal spray suspension. Each spray (50 microliters) delivers 27.5 mcg of fluticasone furoate.

4   CONTRAINDICATIONS

VERAMYST Nasal Spray is contraindicated in patients with hypersensitivity to any of its ingredients *[see Warnings and Precautions (5.3)]*.

5   WARNINGS AND PRECAUTIONS
5.1   Local Nasal Effects

Epistaxis and Nasal Ulceration: In clinical studies of 2 to 52 weeks' duration, epistaxis and nasal ulcerations were observed more frequently and some epistaxis events were more severe in patients treated with VERAMYST Nasal Spray than those who received placebo *[see Adverse Reactions (6.1)]*.
Candida Infection: Evidence of localized infections of the nose with *Candida albicans* was seen on nasal exams in 7 of 2,745 patients treated with VERAMYST Nasal Spray during clinical trials and was reported as an adverse event in 3 patients. When such an infection develops, it may require treatment with appropriate local therapy and discontinuation of VERAMYST Nasal Spray. Therefore, patients using VERAMYST Nasal Spray over several months or longer should be examined periodically for evidence of *Candida* infection or other signs of adverse effects on the nasal mucosa.
Nasal Septal Perforation: Postmarketing cases of nasal septal perforation have been reported in patients following the intranasal application of VERAMYST Nasal Spray *[see Adverse Reactions (6.2)]*.

Impaired Wound Healing: Because of the inhibitory effect of corticosteroids on wound healing, patients who have experienced recent nasal ulcers, nasal surgery, or nasal trauma should not use VERAMYST Nasal Spray until healing has occurred.

5.2 Glaucoma and Cataracts
Nasal and inhaled corticosteroids may result in the development of glaucoma and/or cataracts. Therefore, close monitoring is warranted in patients with a change in vision or with a history of increased intraocular pressure (IOP), glaucoma, and/or cataracts.

Glaucoma and cataract formation was evaluated with intraocular pressure measurements and slit lamp examinations in 1 controlled 12-month study in 806 adolescent and adult patients aged 12 years and older and in 1 controlled 12-week study in 558 children aged 2 to 11 years. The patients had perennial allergic rhinitis and were treated with either VERAMYST Nasal Spray (110 mcg once daily in adult and adolescent patients and 55 or 110 mcg once daily in pediatric patients) or placebo. Intraocular pressure remained within the normal range (<21 mmHg) in ≥98% of the patients in any treatment group in both studies. However, in the 12-month study in adolescents and adults, 12 patients, all treated with VERAMYST Nasal Spray 110 mcg once daily, had intraocular pressure measurements that increased above normal levels (≥21 mmHg). In the same study, 7 patients (6 treated with VERAMYST Nasal Spray 110 mcg once daily and 1 patient treated with placebo) had cataracts identified during the study that were not present at baseline.

5.3 Hypersensitivity Reactions, Including Anaphylaxis
Hypersensitivity reactions, including anaphylaxis, angioedema, rash, and urticaria, may occur after administration of VERAMYST Nasal Spray. Discontinue VERAMYST Nasal Spray if such reactions occur [see Contraindications (4)].

5.4 Immunosuppression
Persons who are using drugs that suppress the immune system are more susceptible to infections than healthy individuals. Chickenpox and measles, for example, can have a more serious or even fatal course in susceptible children or adults using corticosteroids. In children or adults who have not had these diseases or have not been properly immunized, particular care should be taken to avoid exposure. How the dose, route, and duration of corticosteroid administration affect the risk of developing a disseminated infection is not known. The contribution of the underlying disease and/or prior corticosteroid treatment to the risk is also not known. If a patient is exposed to chickenpox, prophylaxis with varicella zoster immune globulin (VZIG) may be indicated. If a patient is exposed to measles, prophylaxis with pooled intramuscular immunoglobulin (IG) may be indicated. (See the respective package inserts for complete VZIG and IG prescribing information.) If chickenpox or measles develops, treatment with antiviral agents may be considered.

Corticosteroids should be used with caution, if at all, in patients with active or quiescent tuberculous infections of the respiratory tract, untreated local or systemic fungal or bacterial infections, systemic viral or parasitic infections, or ocular herpes simplex because of the potential for worsening of these infections.

5.5 Hypothalamic-Pituitary-Adrenal Axis Effects
Hypercorticism and Adrenal Suppression: When intranasal steroids are used at higher than recommended dosages or in susceptible individuals at recommended dosages, systemic corticosteroid effects such as hypercorticism and adrenal suppression may appear. If such changes occur, the dosage of VERAMYST Nasal Spray should be discontinued slowly, consistent with accepted procedures for discontinuing oral corticosteroid therapy.

The replacement of a systemic corticosteroid with a topical corticosteroid can be accompanied by signs of adrenal insufficiency. In addition, some patients may experience symptoms of corticosteroid withdrawal, e.g., joint and/or muscular pain, lassitude, depression. Patients previously treated for prolonged periods with systemic corticosteroids and transferred to topical corticosteroids should be carefully monitored for acute adrenal insufficiency in response to stress. In those patients who have asthma or other clinical conditions requiring long-term systemic corticosteroid treatment, rapid decreases in systemic corticosteroid dosages may cause a severe exacerbation of their symptoms.

5.6 Use of Cytochrome P450 3A4 Inhibitors
Coadministration with ritonavir is not recommended because of the risk of systemic effects secondary to increased exposure to fluticasone furoate. Use caution with the coadministration of VERAMYST Nasal Spray and other potent cytochrome P450 3A4(CYP3A4) inhibitors, such as ketoconazole [see Drug Interactions (7)].

5.7 Effect on Growth
Corticosteroids may cause a reduction in growth velocity when administered to pediatric patients. Monitor the growth routinely of pediatric patients receiving

Table 1. Adverse Reactions With >1% Incidence in Controlled Clinical Trials of 2 to 6 Weeks' Duration With VERAMYST Nasal Spray in Adult and Adolescent Patients With Seasonal or Perennial Allergic Rhinitis

Adverse Event	Adult and Adolescent Patients Aged 12 Years and Older	
	Vehicle Placebo (n = 774)	VERAMYST Nasal Spray 110 mcg Once Daily (n = 768)
Headache	54 (7%)	72 (9%)
Epistaxis	32 (4%)	45 (6%)
Pharyngolaryngeal pain	8 (1%)	15 (2%)
Nasal ulceration	3 (<1%)	11 (1%)
Back pain	7 (<1%)	9 (1%)

Table 2. Adverse Reactions With >3% Incidence in Controlled Clinical Trials of 2 to 12 Weeks' Duration With VERAMYST Nasal Spray in Pediatric Patients With Seasonal or Perennial Allergic Rhinitis

Adverse Event	Pediatric Patients Aged 2 to <12 Years		
	Vehicle Placebo (n = 429)	VERAMYST Nasal Spray 55 mcg Once Daily (n = 369)	VERAMYST Nasal Spray 110 mcg Once Daily (n = 426)
Headache	31 (7%)	28 (8%)	33 (8%)
Nasopharyngitis	21 (5%)	20 (5%)	21 (5%)
Epistaxis	19 (4%)	17 (5%)	17 (4%)
Pyrexia	7 (2%)	17 (5%)	19 (4%)
Pharyngolaryngeal pain	14 (3%)	16 (4%)	12 (3%)
Cough	12 (3%)	12 (3%)	16 (4%)

VERAMYST Nasal Spray. To minimize the systemic effects of intranasal corticosteroids, including VERAMYST Nasal Spray, titrate each patient's dose to the lowest dosage that effectively controls his/her symptoms [see Use in Specific Populations (8.4)].

6 ADVERSE REACTIONS
Systemic and local corticosteroid use may result in the following:
- Epistaxis, ulcerations, Candida albicans infection, impaired wound healing, and nasal septal perforation [see Warnings and Precautions (5.1)]
- Cataracts and glaucoma [see Warnings and Precautions (5.2)]
- Immunosuppression [see Warnings and Precautions (5.4)]
- Hypothalamic-pituitary-adrenal (HPA) axis effects, including growth reduction [see Warnings and Precautions (5.5), Use in Specific Populations (8.4)]

6.1 Clinical Trials Experience
The safety data described below reflect exposure to VERAMYST Nasal Spray in 1,563 patients with seasonal or perennial allergic rhinitis in 9 controlled clinical trials of 2 to 12 weeks' duration. The data from adults and adolescents are based upon 6 clinical trials in which 768 patients with seasonal or perennial allergic rhinitis (473 females and 295 males aged 12 years and older) were treated with VERAMYST Nasal Spray 110 mcg once daily for 2 to 6 weeks. The racial distribution of adult and adolescent patients receiving VERAMYST Nasal Spray was 82% white, 5% black, and 13% other. The data from pediatric patients are based upon 3 clinical trials in which 795 children with seasonal or perennial rhinitis (352 females and 443 males aged 2 to 11 years) were treated with VERAMYST Nasal Spray 55 or 110 mcg once daily for 2 to 12 weeks. The racial distribution of pediatric patients receiving VERAMYST Nasal Spray was 75% white, 11% black, and 14% other.

Because clinical trials are conducted under widely varying conditions, adverse reaction rates observed in the clinical trials of a drug cannot be directly compared with rates in the clinical trials of another drug and may not reflect the rates observed in practice.

Adults and Adolescents Aged 12 Years and Older: Overall adverse reactions were reported with approximately the same frequency by patients treated with VERAMYST Nasal Spray and those receiving placebo. Less than 3% of patients in clinical trials discontinued treatment because of adverse reactions. The rate of withdrawal among patients receiving VERAMYST Nasal Spray was similar or lower than the rate among patients receiving placebo.

Table 1 displays the common adverse reactions (>1% in any patient group receiving VERAMYST Nasal Spray) that occurred more frequently in patients aged 12 years and older treated with VERAMYST Nasal Spray compared with placebo-treated patients.

[See table 1 above]

There were no differences in the incidence of adverse reactions based on gender or race. Clinical trials did not include sufficient numbers of patients aged 65 years and older to determine whether they respond differently from younger subjects.

Pediatric Patients Aged 2 to 11 Years: In the 3 clinical trials in pediatric patients aged 2 to <12 years, overall adverse reactions were reported with approximately the same frequency by patients treated with VERAMYST Nasal Spray and those receiving placebo. Table 2 displays the common adverse reactions (>3% in any patient group receiving VERAMYST Nasal Spray) that occurred more frequently in patients aged 2 to 11 years treated with VERAMYST Nasal Spray compared with placebo-treated patients.

[See table 2 above]

There were no differences in the incidence of adverse reactions based on gender or race. Pyrexia occurred more frequently in children aged 2 to <6 years compared with children aged 6 to <12 years.

Long-Term (52-Week) Safety Trial: In a 52-week, placebo-controlled, long-term safety trial, 605 patients (307 females and 298 males aged 12 years and older) with perennial allergic rhinitis were treated with VERAMYST Nasal Spray 110 mcg once daily for 12 months and 201 were treated with placebo nasal spray. While most adverse reactions were similar in type and rate between the treatment groups, epistaxis occurred more frequently in patients who received VERAMYST Nasal Spray (123/605, 20%) than in patients who received placebo (17/201, 8%). Epistaxis tended to be more severe in patients treated with VERAMYST Nasal Spray. All 17 reports of epistaxis that occurred in patients who received placebo were of mild intensity, while 83, 39, and 1 of the total 123 epistaxis events in patients treated with VERAMYST Nasal Spray were of mild, moderate, and severe intensity, respectively. No patient experienced a nasal septal perforation during this trial.

6.2 Postmarketing Experience
In addition to adverse reactions reported from clinical trials, the following adverse reactions have been identified during postmarketing use of VERAMYST Nasal Spray. Because these reactions are reported voluntarily from a population of uncertain size, it is not always possible to reliably estimate their frequency or establish a causal relationship to drug exposure. These events have been chosen for inclusion due to either their seriousness, frequency of reporting, or causal connection to fluticasone furoate or a combination of these factors.

Immune System Disorders: Hypersensitivity reactions, including anaphylaxis, angioedema, rash, and urticaria.
Respiratory, Thoracic, and Mediastinal Disorders: Rhinalgia, nasal discomfort (including nasal burning, nasal irritation, and nasal soreness), nasal dryness, and nasal septal perforation.

7 DRUG INTERACTIONS
Fluticasone furoate is cleared by extensive first-pass metabolism mediated by CYP3A4. In a drug interaction study of intranasal fluticasone furoate and the CYP3A4 inhibitor ketoconazole given as a 200-mg once-daily dose for 7 days, 6 of 20 subjects receiving fluticasone furoate had measurable but low levels of fluticasone furoate compared with 1 of 20 receiving fluticasone furoate and placebo. Based on this study and the low systemic exposure, there was a 5% reduction in 24-hour serum cortisol levels with

ketoconazole compared with placebo. The data from this study should be carefully interpreted because the study was conducted with ketoconazole 200 mg once daily rather than 400 mg, which is the maximum recommended dosage. Therefore, caution is required with the coadministration of VERAMYST Nasal Spray and ketoconazole or other potent CYP3A4 inhibitors.

Based on data with another glucocorticoid, fluticasone propionate, metabolized by CYP3A4, coadministration of VERAMYST Nasal Spray with the potent CYP3A4 inhibitor ritonavir is not recommended because of the risk of systemic effects secondary to increased exposure to fluticasone furoate. High exposure to corticosteroids increases the potential for systemic side effects, such as cortisol suppression.

Enzyme induction and inhibition data suggest that fluticasone furoate is unlikely to significantly alter the cytochrome P450-mediated metabolism of other compounds at clinically relevant intranasal dosages.

8 USE IN SPECIFIC POPULATIONS

8.1 Pregnancy

Teratogenic Effects: Pregnancy Category C. Corticosteroids have been shown to be teratogenic in laboratory animals when administered systemically at relatively low dosage levels.

There were no teratogenic effects in rats and rabbits at inhaled fluticasone furoate dosages of up to 91 and 8 mcg/kg/day, respectively (approximately 7 and 1 times, respectively, the maximum recommended daily intranasal dose in adults on a mcg/m^2 basis). There was also no effect on pre- or postnatal development in rats treated with up to 27 mcg/kg/day by inhalation during gestation and lactation (approximately 2 times the maximum recommended daily intranasal dose in adults on a mcg/m^2 basis).

There are no adequate and well-controlled studies in pregnant women. VERAMYST Nasal Spray should be used during pregnancy only if the potential benefit justifies the potential risk to the fetus.

Nonteratogenic Effects: Hypoadrenalism may occur in infants born of mothers receiving corticosteroids during pregnancy. Such infants should be carefully monitored.

8.3 Nursing Mothers

It is not known whether fluticasone furoate is excreted in human breast milk. However, other corticosteroids have been detected in human milk. Since there are no data from controlled trials on the use of intranasal fluticasone furoate by nursing mothers, caution should be exercised when VERAMYST Nasal Spray is administered to a nursing woman.

8.4 Pediatric Use

Controlled clinical trials with VERAMYST Nasal Spray included 1,224 patients aged 2 to 11 years and 344 adolescent patients aged 12 to 17 years [see Clinical Studies (14)]. The safety and effectiveness of VERAMYST Nasal Spray in children younger than 2 years have not been established.

Controlled clinical studies have shown that intranasal corticosteroids may cause a reduction in growth velocity in pediatric patients. This effect has been observed in the absence of laboratory evidence of HPA axis suppression, suggesting that growth velocity is a more sensitive indicator of systemic corticosteroid exposure in pediatric patients than some commonly used tests of HPA axis function. The long-term effects of reduction in growth velocity associated with intranasal corticosteroids, including the impact on final adult height, are unknown. The potential for "catch-up" growth following discontinuation of treatment with intranasal corticosteroids has not been adequately studied. The growth of pediatric patients receiving intranasal corticosteroids, including VERAMYST Nasal Spray, should be monitored routinely (e.g., via stadiometry). The potential growth effects of prolonged treatment should be weighed against the clinical benefits obtained and the risks/benefits of treatment alternatives. To minimize the systemic effects of intranasal corticosteroids, including VERAMYST Nasal Spray, each patient's dose should be titrated to the lowest dosage that effectively controls his/her symptoms.

A randomized, double-blind, parallel-group, multicenter, 1-year placebo-controlled clinical growth study evaluated the effect of 110 mcg of VERAMYST Nasal Spray once daily on growth velocity in 474 prepubescent children (girls aged 5 to 7.5 years and boys aged 5 to 8.5 years) with stadiometry. Mean growth velocity over the 52-week treatment period was lower in the patients receiving VERAMYST Nasal Spray (5.19 cm/year compared with placebo (5.46 cm/year). The mean treatment difference was -0.27 cm/year [95% CI: -0.48 to -0.06] [see Warnings and Precautions (5.7)].

8.5 Geriatric Use

Clinical studies of VERAMYST Nasal Spray did not include sufficient numbers of subjects aged 65 years and older to determine whether they respond differently from younger subjects. Other reported clinical experience has not identified differences in responses between the elderly and younger patients. In general, dose selection for an elderly patient should be cautious, usually starting at the low end of the dosing range, reflecting the greater frequency of decreased hepatic, renal, or cardiac function, and of concomitant disease or other drug therapy.

8.6 Hepatic Impairment

Use VERAMYST Nasal Spray with caution in patients with severe hepatic impairment [see Clinical Pharmacology (12.3)].

8.7 Renal Impairment

No dosage adjustment is required in patients with renal impairment [see Clinical Pharmacology (12.3)].

10 OVERDOSAGE

Chronic overdosage may result in signs/symptoms of hypercorticism [see Warnings and Precautions (5.5)]. There are no data on the effects of acute or chronic overdosage with VERAMYST Nasal Spray. Because of low systemic bioavailability and an absence of acute drug-related systemic findings in clinical studies (with dosages of up to 440 mcg/day for 2 weeks [4 times the maximum recommended daily dose]), overdose is unlikely to require any therapy other than observation.

Intranasal administration of up to 2,640 mcg/day (24 times the recommended adult dose) of fluticasone furoate was administered to healthy human volunteers for 3 days. Single- and repeat-dose studies with orally inhaled fluticasone furoate doses of 50 to 4,000 mcg have shown decreased mean serum cortisol at doses of 500 mcg or higher. The oral median lethal dose in mice and rats was >2,000 mg/kg (approximately 74,000 and 147,000 times, respectively, the maximum recommended daily intranasal dose in adults and 52,000 and 105,000 times, respectively, the maximum recommended daily intranasal dose in children, on a mcg/m^2 basis).

Acute overdosage with the intranasal dosage form is unlikely since 1 bottle of VERAMYST Nasal Spray contains approximately 3 mg of fluticasone furoate, and the bioavailability of fluticasone furoate is <1% for 2.64 mg/day given intranasally and 1% for 2 mg/day given as an oral solution.

11 DESCRIPTION

Fluticasone furoate, the active component of VERAMYST Nasal Spray, is a synthetic fluorinated corticosteroid having the chemical name (6α,11β,16α,17α)-6,9-difluoro-17-{[(fluoro-methyl)thio]carbonyl}-11-hydroxy-16-methyl-3-oxoandrosta-1,4-dien-17-yl 2-furancarboxylate and the following chemical structure:

Fluticasone furoate is a white powder with a molecular weight of 538.6, and the empirical formula is $C_{27}H_{29}F_3O_6S$. It is practically insoluble in water.

VERAMYST Nasal Spray is an aqueous suspension of micronized fluticasone furoate for topical administration to the nasal mucosa by means of a metering (50 microliters), atomizing spray pump. After initial priming [see Dosage and Administration (2)], each actuation delivers 27.5 mcg of fluticasone furoate in a volume of 50 microliters of nasal spray suspension. VERAMYST Nasal Spray also contains 0.015% w/w benzalkonium chloride, dextrose anhydrous, edetate disodium, microcrystalline cellulose and carboxymethylcellulose sodium, polysorbate 80, and purified water. It has a pH of approximately 6.

12 CLINICAL PHARMACOLOGY

12.1 Mechanism of Action

Fluticasone furoate is a synthetic trifluorinated corticosteroid with potent anti-inflammatory activity. The precise mechanism through which fluticasone furoate affects rhinitis symptoms is not known. Corticosteroids have been shown to have a wide range of actions on multiple cell types (e.g., mast cells, eosinophils, neutrophils, macrophages, lymphocytes) and mediators (e.g., histamine, eicosanoids, leukotrienes, cytokines) involved in inflammation. Specific effects of fluticasone furoate demonstrated in in vitro and in vivo models included activation of the glucocorticoid response element, inhibition of pro-inflammatory transcription factors such as NFkB, and inhibition of antigen-induced lung eosinophilia in sensitized rats.

Fluticasone furoate has been shown in vitro to exhibit a binding affinity for the human glucocorticoid receptor that is approximately 29.9 times that of dexamethasone and 1.7 times that of fluticasone propionate. The clinical relevance of these findings is unknown.

12.2 Pharmacodynamics

Adrenal Function: The effects of VERAMYST Nasal Spray on adrenal function have been evaluated in 4 controlled clinical trials in patients with perennial allergic rhinitis. Two 6-week clinical trials were designed specifically to assess the effect of VERAMYST Nasal Spray on the HPA axis with assessments of both 24-hour urinary cortisol excretion and serum cortisol levels in domiciled patients. In addition, one 52-week safety study and one 12-week safety and efficacy study included assessments of 24-hour urinary cortisol excretion. Details of the studies and results are described below. In all 4 studies, since serum fluticasone determinations were generally below the limit of quantification, compliance was assured by efficacy assessments.

Clinical Trials Specifically Designed to Assess Hypothalamic-Pituitary-Adrenal Axis Effect: In a 6-week randomized, double-blind, parallel-group study in adult and adolescent patients aged 12 years and older with perennial allergic rhinitis, VERAMYST Nasal Spray 110 mcg was compared with both placebo nasal spray and prednisone as a positive-control group that received prednisone 10 mg orally once daily for the final 7 days of the treatment period. Adrenal function was assessed by 24-hour urinary cortisol excretion before and after 6 weeks of treatment and by serial serum cortisol levels. Patients were domiciled for collection of 24-hour urinary cortisol. After 6 weeks of treatment, there was a change from baseline in the mean 24-hour urinary cortisol excretion in the group treated with VERAMYST Nasal Spray (n = 43) of -1.16 mcg/day compared with -3.48 mcg/day in the placebo group (n = 42). The difference from placebo in the group treated with VERAMYST Nasal Spray was 2.32 mcg/day (95% CI: -6.76, 11.39). Urinary cortisol data were not available for the positive-control (prednisone) treatment group. For serum cortisol levels, after 6 weeks of treatment there was a change from baseline in the mean (0-24 hours) of -0.38 and 0.08 mcg/dL for the group treated with VERAMYST Nasal Spray (n = 43) and the placebo group (n = 44), respectively, with a difference between the group treated with VERAMYST Nasal Spray and the placebo group of -0.47 mcg/dL (95% CI: -1.31, 0.37). For comparison, in the positive-control (prednisone, n = 12) treatment group, there was a change in mean serum cortisol (0-24 hours) from baseline of -4.49 mcg/dL with a difference between the prednisone and placebo group of -4.57 mcg/dL (95% CI: -5.83, -3.31).

The second 6-week study conducted in children aged 2 to 11 years was of similar design to the adult study, including adrenal function assessments, but did not include a prednisone positive-control arm. Patients were treated once daily with VERAMYST Nasal Spray 110 mcg or placebo nasal spray. After 6 weeks of treatment, there was a change in the mean 24-hour urinary cortisol excretion in the group treated with VERAMYST Nasal Spray (n = 43) of 0.49 mcg/day compared with 1.92 mcg/day in the placebo group (n = 41), with a difference between the group treated with VERAMYST Nasal Spray and the placebo group of -1.43 mcg/day (95% CI: -5.21, 2.35). For serum cortisol levels, after 6 weeks, there was a change from baseline in mean (0-24 hours) of -0.34 and -0.23 mcg/dL for the group treated with VERAMYST Nasal Spray (n = 48) and for the placebo group (n = 47), respectively, with a difference between the group treated with VERAMYST Nasal Spray and the placebo group of -0.11 mcg/dL (95% CI: -0.88, 0.66).

Additional Hypothalamic-Pituitary-Adrenal Axis Assessments: In the 52-week safety trial in adolescents and adults aged 12 years and older with perennial allergic rhinitis, VERAMYST Nasal Spray 110 mcg (n = 605) was compared with placebo nasal spray (n = 201). Adrenal function was assessed by 24-hour urinary cortisol excretion in a subset of patients who received VERAMYST Nasal Spray (n = 370) or placebo (n = 120) before and after 52 weeks of treatment. After 52 weeks of treatment, the mean change from baseline 24-hour urinary cortisol excretion was 5.84 mcg/day in the group treated with VERAMYST Nasal Spray and 3.34 mcg/day in the placebo group. The difference from placebo in mean change from baseline 24-hour urinary cortisol excretion was 2.50 mcg/day (95% CI: -5.49, 10.49). In the 12-week safety and efficacy trial in children aged 2 to 11 years with perennial allergic rhinitis, VERAMYST Nasal Spray 55 mcg (n = 185) and VERAMYST Nasal Spray 110 mcg (n = 185) were compared with placebo nasal spray (n = 188). Adrenal function was assessed by measurement of 24-hour urinary free cortisol in a subset of patients who were aged 6 to 11 years (103 to 109 patients per group) before and after 12 weeks of treatment. After 12 weeks of treatment, there was a decrease in mean 24-hour urinary cortisol excretion from baseline in the group treated with VERAMYST Nasal Spray 55 mcg (n = 109) of -2.93 mcg/day and in the group treated with VERAMYST Nasal Spray 110 mcg (n = 103) of -2.07 mcg/day compared with an increase in the placebo group (n = 107) of 0.08 mcg/day. The difference from placebo in mean change from baseline in 24-hour urinary cortisol excretion for the group treated with VERAMYST Nasal Spray 55 mcg was -3.01 mcg/day (95% CI: -6.16, 0.13) and -2.14 mcg/day (95% CI: -5.33, 1.04) for the group treated with VERAMYST Nasal Spray 110 mcg.

When the results of the HPA axis assessments described above are taken as a whole, an effect of intranasal fluticasone furoate on adrenal function cannot be ruled out, especially in pediatric patients.

Cardiac Effects: A QT/QTc study did not demonstrate an effect of fluticasone furoate administration on the QTc interval. The effect of a single dose of 4,000 mcg of orally inhaled fluticasone furoate on the QTc interval was evaluated over 24 hours in 40 healthy male and female subjects in a placebo and positive (a single dose of 400 mg oral moxifloxacin) controlled cross-over study. The QTcF maximal mean change from baseline following fluticasone furoate was similar to that observed with placebo with a treatment difference of 0.788 msec (90% CI: -1.802, 3.378). In contrast, moxifloxacin given as a 400-mg tablet resulted in prolongation of the QTcF maximal mean change from baseline compared with placebo with a treatment difference of 9.929 msec (90% CI: 7.339, 12.520). While a single dose of fluticasone furoate had no effect on the QTc interval, the effects of fluticasone furoate may not be at steady state following single dose. The effect of fluticasone furoate on the QTc interval following multiple dose administration is unknown.

12.3 Pharmacokinetics

Absorption: Following intranasal administration of fluticasone furoate, most of the dose is eventually swallowed and undergoes incomplete absorption and extensive first-pass metabolism in the liver and gut, resulting in negligible systemic exposure. At the highest recommended intranasal dosage of 110 mcg once daily for up to 12 months in adults and up to 12 weeks in children, plasma concentrations of fluticasone furoate are typically not quantifiable despite the use of a sensitive HPLC-MS/MS assay with a lower limit of quantification (LOQ) of 10 pg/mL. However, in a few isolated cases (<0.3%) fluticasone furoate was detected in high concentrations above 500 pg/mL, and in a single case the concentration was as high as 1,430 pg/mL in the 52-week study. There was no relationship between these concentrations and cortisol levels in these subjects. The reasons for these high concentrations are unknown.

Absolute bioavailability was evaluated in 16 male and female subjects following supratherapeutic dosages of fluticasone furoate (880 mcg given intranasally at 8-hour intervals for 10 doses, or 2,640 mcg/day). The average absolute bioavailability was 0.50% (90% CI: 0.34%, 0.74%).

Due to the low bioavailability by the intranasal route, the majority of the pharmacokinetic data was obtained via other routes of administration. Studies using oral solution and intravenous dosing of radiolabeled drug have demonstrated that at least 30% of fluticasone furoate is absorbed and then rapidly cleared from plasma. Oral bioavailability is on average 1.26%, and the majority of the circulating radioactivity is due to inactive metabolites.

Distribution: Following intravenous administration, the mean volume of distribution at steady state is 608 L.

Binding of fluticasone furoate to human plasma proteins is greater than 99%.

Metabolism: In vivo studies have revealed no evidence of cleavage of the furoate moiety to form fluticasone. Fluticasone furoate is cleared (total plasma clearance of 58.7 L/h) from systemic circulation principally by hepatic metabolism via CYP3A4. The principal route of metabolism is hydrolysis of the S-fluoromethyl carbothioate function to form the inactive 17β-carboxylic acid metabolite.

Elimination: Fluticasone furoate and its metabolites are eliminated primarily in the feces, accounting for approximately 101% and 90% of the orally and intravenously administered dose, respectively. Urinary excretion accounted for approximately 1% and 2% of the orally and intravenously administered dose, respectively. The elimination phase half-life averaged 15.1 hours following intravenous administration.

Population Pharmacokinetics: Fluticasone furoate is typically not quantifiable in plasma following intranasal dosing of 110 mcg once daily with the exception of isolated cases of very high plasma levels (see Absorption). Overall, quantifiable levels (>10 pg/mL) were observed in <31% of patients aged 12 years and older and in <16% of children (aged 2 to 11 years) following intranasal dosing of 110 mcg once daily and in <7% of children following intranasal dosing of 55 mcg once daily. There was no evidence to suggest that the presence or absence of detectable levels of fluticasone furoate was related to gender, age, or race.

Hepatic Impairment: Reduced liver function may affect the elimination of corticosteroids. Since fluticasone furoate undergoes extensive first-pass metabolism by the hepatic CYP3A4, the pharmacokinetics of fluticasone furoate may be altered in patients with hepatic impairment. A study of a single 400-mcg dose of orally inhaled fluticasone furoate in patients with moderate hepatic impairment (Child-Pugh

Class B) resulted in increased C_{max} (42%) and $AUC_{(0-\infty)}$ (172%), resulting in an approximately 20% reduction in serum cortisol level in patients with hepatic impairment compared with healthy subjects. The systemic exposure would be expected to be higher than that observed had the study been conducted after multiple doses and/or in patients with severe hepatic impairment. Therefore, use VERAMYST Nasal Spray with caution in patients with severe hepatic impairment.

Renal Impairment: Fluticasone furoate is not detectable in urine from healthy subjects following intranasal dosing. Less than 1% of dose-related material is excreted in urine. No dosage adjustment is required in patients with renal impairment.

13 NONCLINICAL TOXICOLOGY

13.1 Carcinogenesis, Mutagenesis, Impairment of Fertility

Fluticasone furoate produced no treatment-related increases in the incidence of tumors in 2-year inhalation studies in rats and mice at doses of up to 9 and 19 mcg/kg/day, respectively (less than the maximum recommended daily intranasal dose in adults and children on a mcg/m^2 basis). Fluticasone furoate did not induce gene mutation in bacteria or chromosomal damage in a mammalian cell mutation test in mouse lymphoma L5178Y cells in vitro. There was also no evidence of genotoxicity in the in vivo micronucleus test in rats.

No evidence of impairment of fertility was observed in reproductive studies conducted in male and female rats at inhaled fluticasone furoate doses of up to 24 and 91 mcg/kg/day, respectively (approximately 2 and 7 times, respectively, the maximum recommended daily intranasal dose in adults on a mcg/m^2 basis).

14 CLINICAL STUDIES

14.1 Seasonal and Perennial Allergic Rhinitis

Adult and Adolescent Patients Aged 12 Years and Older: The efficacy and safety of VERAMYST Nasal Spray was evaluated in 5 randomized, double-blind, parallel-group, multicenter, placebo-controlled clinical trials of 2 to 4 weeks' duration in adult and adolescent patients aged 12 years and older with symptoms of seasonal or perennial allergic rhinitis. The 5 clinical trials included one 2-week dose-ranging trial in patients with seasonal allergic rhinitis, three 2-week confirmatory efficacy trials in patients with seasonal allergic rhinitis, and one 4-week efficacy trial in patients with perennial allergic rhinitis. These trials included 1,829 patients (697 males and 1,132 females). About 75% of patients were Caucasian, and the mean age was 36 years. Of these patients, 722 received VERAMYST Nasal Spray 110 mcg once daily administered as 2 sprays in each nostril.

Assessment of efficacy was based on total nasal symptom score (TNSS). TNSS is calculated as the sum of the patients' scoring of the 4 individual nasal symptoms (rhinorrhea, nasal congestion, sneezing, and nasal itching) on a 0 to 3 categorical severity scale (0 = absent, 1 = mild, 2 = moderate, 3 = severe) as reflective(rTNSS) or instantaneous (iTNSS). rTNSS required the patients to record symptom severity over the previous 12 hours; iTNSS required patients to record symptom severity at the time immediately prior to the next dose. Morning and evening rTNSS scores were averaged over the treatment period and the difference from placebo in the change from baseline rTNSS was the primary efficacy endpoint. The morning iTNSS (AM iTNSS) reflects the TNSS at the end of the 24-hour dosing interval and is an indication of whether the effect was maintained over the 24-hour dosing interval.

Additional secondary efficacy variables were assessed, including the total ocular symptom score (TOSS) and the Rhinoconjunctivitis Quality of Life Questionnaire (RQLQ). TOSS is calculated as the sum of the patients' scoring of the 3 individual ocular symptoms (itching/burning, tearing/watering, and redness) on a 0 to 3 categorical severity scale (0 = absent, 1 = mild, 2 = moderate, 3 = severe) as reflective (rTOSS) or instantaneous scores (iTOSS). To assess

Table 3. Mean Change From Baseline in Reflective Total Nasal Symptom Score Over 2 Weeks in Patients With Seasonal Allergic Rhinitis

Treatment	n	Baseline (AM + PM)	Change From Baseline	Difference From Placebo		
				LS Mean	95% CI	P Value
Fluticasone furoate 440 mcg	130	9.6	-4.02	-2.19	-2.75, -1.62	<0.001
Fluticasone furoate 220 mcg	129	9.5	-3.19	-1.36	-1.93, -0.79	<0.001
Fluticasone furoate 110 mcg	127	9.5	-3.84	-2.01	-2.58, -1.44	<0.001
Fluticasone furoate 55 mcg	125	9.6	-3.50	-1.68	-2.25, -1.10	<0.001
Placebo	128	9.6	-1.83			

Table 4. Mean Changes in Efficacy Variables in Adult and Adolescent Patients With Seasonal or Perennial Allergic Rhinitis

Treatment	n	Baseline	Change From Baseline – LS Mean	Difference From Placebo		
				LS Mean	95% CI	P Value
Reflective Total Nasal Symptom Scores						
Seasonal allergic rhinitis trial						
Fluticasone furoate 110 mcg	151	9.6	-3.55	-1.47	-2.01, -0.94	<0.001
Placebo	147	9.9	-2.07			
Perennial allergic rhinitis trial						
Fluticasone furoate 110 mcg	149	8.6	-2.78	-0.71	-1.20, -0.21	0.005
Placebo	153	8.7	-2.08			
Instantaneous Total Nasal Symptom Scores						
Seasonal allergic rhinitis trial						
Fluticasone furoate 110 mcg	151	9.4	-2.90	-1.38	-1.90, -0.85	<0.001
Placebo	147	9.3	-1.53			
Perennial allergic rhinitis trial						
Fluticasone furoate 110 mcg	149	8.2	-2.45	-0.71	-1.20, -0.21	0.006
Placebo	153	8.3	-1.75			
Reflective Total Ocular Symptom Scores						
Seasonal allergic rhinitis trial						
Fluticasone furoate 110 mcg	151	6.6	-2.23	-0.60	-1.01, -0.19	0.004
Placebo	147	6.5	-1.63			
Perennial allergic rhinitis trial						
Fluticasone furoate 110 mcg	149	4.8	-1.39	-0.15	-0.52, 0.22	0.428
Placebo	153	5.0	-1.24			
Rhinoconjunctivitis Quality of Life Questionnaire						
Seasonal allergic rhinitis trial						
Fluticasone furoate 110 mcg	144	3.9	-1.77	-0.60	-0.93, -0.28	<0.001
Placebo	144	3.9	-1.16			
Perennial allergic rhinitis trial						
Fluticasone furoate 110 mcg	143	3.5	-1.41	-0.23	-0.59, 0.13	0.214
Placebo	151	3.4	-1.18			

Table 5. Mean Changes in Efficacy Variables in Pediatric Patients Aged 6 to <12 Years With Seasonal or Perennial Allergic Rhinitis

Treatment	n	Baseline	Change From Baseline – LS Mean	Difference From Placebo		
				LS Mean	95% CI	P Value
Reflective Total Nasal Symptom Scores						
Seasonal allergic rhinitis trial						
Fluticasone furoate 55 mcg	151	8.6	-2.71	-0.16	-0.69, 0.37	0.553
Fluticasone furoate 110 mcg	146	8.5	-3.16	-0.62	-1.15, -0.08	0.025
Placebo	149	8.4	-2.54			
Perennial allergic rhinitis trial						
Fluticasone furoate 55 mcg	144	8.5	-4.16	-0.75	-1.24, -0.27	0.003
Fluticasone furoate 110 mcg	140	8.6	-3.86	-0.45	-0.95, 0.04	0.073
Placebo	147	8.5	-3.41			
Instantaneous Total Nasal Symptom Scores						
Seasonal allergic rhinitis trial						
Fluticasone furoate 55 mcg	151	8.4	-2.37	-0.23	-0.77, 0.30	0.389
Fluticasone furoate 110 mcg	146	8.3	-2.80	-0.67	-1.21, -0.13	0.015
Placebo	149	8.4	-2.13			
Perennial allergic rhinitis trial						
Fluticasone furoate 55 mcg	144	8.3	-3.62	-0.75	-1.24, -0.27	0.002
Fluticasone furoate 110 mcg	140	8.3	-3.52	-0.65	-1.14, -0.16	0.009
Placebo	147	8.3	-2.87			
Reflective Total Ocular Symptom Scores						
Seasonal allergic rhinitis trial						
Fluticasone furoate 55 mcg	151	4.4	-1.26	0.04	-0.33, 0.41	0.826
Fluticasone furoate 110 mcg	146	4.1	-1.45	-0.15	-0.52, 0.22	0.426
Placebo	149	3.8	-1.30			

efficacy, rTOSS and AM iTOSS were evaluated as described above for the TNSS. Patients' perceptions of disease-specific quality of life were evaluated through use of the RQLQ, which assesses the impact of allergic rhinitis treatment through 28 items in 7 domains (activities, sleep, non-nose/eye symptoms, practical problems, nasal symptoms, eye symptoms, and emotional) on a 7-point scale where 0 = no impairment and 6 = maximum impairment. An overall RQLQ score is calculated from the mean of all items in the instrument. An absolute difference of ≥0.5 in mean change from baseline over placebo is considered the minimally important difference (MID) for the RQLQ.

Dose-Ranging Trial: The dose-ranging trial was a 2-week trial that evaluated the efficacy of 4 dosages of fluticasone furoate nasal spray (440, 220, 110, and 55 mcg) in patients with seasonal allergic rhinitis. In this trial, each of the 4 dosages of fluticasone furoate nasal spray demonstrated greater decreases in the rTNSS than placebo, and the difference was statistically significant (Table 3).
[See table 3 at top of previous page]
Each of the 4 dosages of fluticasone furoate nasal spray also demonstrated greater decreases in the AM iTNSS than placebo, and the difference between each of the 4 fluticasone furoate treatment groups and placebo was statistically significant, indicating that the effect was maintained over the 24-hour dosing interval.

Seasonal Allergic Rhinitis Trials: Three clinical trials were designed to evaluate the efficacy of VERAMYST Nasal Spray 110 mcg once daily compared with placebo in patients with seasonal allergic rhinitis over a 2-week treatment period. In all 3 trials, VERAMYST Nasal Spray 110 mcg demonstrated a greater decrease from baseline in the rTNSS and AM iTNSS than placebo, and the difference from placebo was statistically significant. In terms of ocular symptoms, in all 3 seasonal allergic rhinitis trials, VERAMYST Nasal Spray 110 mcg demonstrated a greater decrease from baseline in the rTOSS than placebo and the difference from placebo was statistically significant. For the RQLQ in all 3 seasonal allergic rhinitis trials, VERAMYST Nasal Spray 110 mcg demonstrated greater decrease from baseline in the overall RQLQ than placebo, and the differ-

ence from placebo was statistically significant. The difference in the overall RQLQ score mean change from baseline between the groups treated with VERAMYST Nasal Spray and placebo ranged from -0.60 to -0.70 in the 3 trials, meeting the minimally important difference criterion. Table 4 displays the efficacy results from a representative trial in patients with seasonal allergic rhinitis.
Perennial Allergic Rhinitis Trials: One clinical trial was designed to evaluate the efficacy of VERAMYST Nasal Spray 110 mcg once daily compared with placebo in patients with perennial allergic rhinitis over a 4-week treatment period. VERAMYST Nasal Spray 110 mcg demonstrated a greater decrease from baseline in the rTNSS and AM iTNSS than placebo, and the difference from placebo was statistically significant. Similar to patients with seasonal allergic rhinitis, the improvement of nasal symptoms with VERAMYST Nasal Spray in patients with perennial allergic rhinitis persisted for a full 24 hours, as evaluated by AM iTNSS immediately prior to the next dose. However, unlike the trials in patients with seasonal allergic rhinitis, patients with perennial allergic rhinitis who were treated with VERAMYST Nasal Spray 110 mcg did not demonstrate statistically significant improvement from baseline in rTOSS or in disease-specific quality of life as measured by the RQLQ compared with placebo. In addition, the overall RQLQ score mean change from baseline difference between the group treated with VERAMYST Nasal Spray and the placebo group was -0.23, which did not meet the minimally important difference of ≥0.5. Table 4 displays the efficacy results from the clinical trial in patients with perennial allergic rhinitis.
[See table 4 at top of previous page]
Onset of action was evaluated by frequent instantaneous TNSS assessments after the first dose in the clinical trials in patients with seasonal allergic rhinitis and perennial allergic rhinitis. Onset of action was generally observed within 24 hours in patients with seasonal allergic rhinitis. In patients with perennial rhinitis, onset of action was observed after 4 days of treatment. Continued improvement in symptoms was observed over approximately 1 and 3 weeks in patients with seasonal or perennial allergic rhinitis, respectively.

Pediatric Patients Aged 2 to 11 Years: The efficacy and safety of VERAMYST Nasal Spray were evaluated in 1,112 children (633 boys and 479 girls), mean age of 8 years with seasonal or perennial allergic rhinitis in 2 controlled clinical trials. The pediatric patients were treated with VERAMYST Nasal Spray 55 or 110 mcg once daily for 2 to 12 weeks (n = 369 for each dose). The trials were similar in design to the trials conducted in adolescents and adults; however, the efficacy determination was made from patient- or parent/guardian-reported TNSS for children aged 6 to <12 years. Children treated with VERAMYST Nasal Spray generally exhibited greater decreases in nasal symptoms than placebo-treated patients. In seasonal allergic rhinitis, the difference in rTNSS was statistically significant only for the 110-mcg dose. In perennial allergic rhinitis, the difference in rTNSS was statistically significant only for the 55-mcg dose. Changes in rTOSS in the seasonal allergic rhinitis trial were not statistically significant compared with placebo for either dose. rTOSS was not assessed in the perennial allergic rhinitis trial. Table 5 displays the efficacy results from the clinical trials in patients with perennial allergic rhinitis and seasonal allergic rhinitis in children aged 6 to <12 years. Efficacy in children aged 2 to <6 years was supported by a numerical decrease in the rTNSS.
[See table 5 above]

16   HOW SUPPLIED/STORAGE AND HANDLING

VERAMYST Nasal Spray, 27.5 mcg per spray, is supplied in a brown glass bottle enclosed in a nasal device with a nozzle and a mist-release button to actuate the spray in a box of 1 (NDC 0173-0753-00) with FDA-Approved Patient Labeling (see Patient Instructions for Use for proper actuation of the device). Each bottle contains a net fill weight of 10 g of white, liquid suspension and will provide 120 metered sprays. After priming *[see Dosage and Administration (2)]*, each spray delivers a fine mist containing 27.5 mcg of fluticasone furoate in 50 microliters of formulation through the nozzle. The contents of the bottle can be viewed through an indicator window. Shake the contents well before each use. The correct amount of medication in each spray cannot be assured before the initial priming and after 120 sprays have been used, even though the bottle is not completely empty. The nasal device should be discarded after 120 sprays have been used.
Store the device in the upright position with the cap in place between 15° and 30°C (59° and 86°F). Do not freeze or refrigerate.

17   PATIENT COUNSELING INFORMATION

See FDA-approved patient labeling (Patient Information and Instructions for Use).
17.1   Local Nasal Effects
Patients should be informed that treatment with VERAMYST Nasal Spray may lead to adverse reactions, which include epistaxis and nasal ulceration. *Candida* infection may also occur with treatment with VERAMYST Nasal Spray. In addition, nasal corticosteroids are associated with nasal septal perforation and impaired wound healing. Patients who have experienced recent nasal ulcers, nasal surgery, or nasal trauma should not use VERAMYST Nasal Spray until healing has occurred *[see Warnings and Precautions (5.1)]*.
17.2   Cataracts and Glaucoma
Patients should be informed that glaucoma and cataracts are associated with nasal and inhaled corticosteroid use. Patients should inform his/her health care provider if a change in vision is noted while using VERAMYST Nasal Spray *[see Warnings and Precautions (5.2)]*.
17.3   Hypersensitivity Reactions, Including Anaphylaxis
Patients should be aware that hypersensitivity reactions, including anaphylaxis, angioedema, rash, and urticaria, may occur after administration of VERAMYST Nasal Spray. If such reactions occur, patients should discontinue use of VERAMYST Nasal Spray *[see Warnings and Precautions (5.3)]*.
17.4   Immunosuppression
Patients who are on immunosuppressant doses of corticosteroids should be warned to avoid exposure to chickenpox or measles and, if exposed, to consult their physician without delay. Patients should be informed of potential worsening of existing tuberculosis, fungal, bacterial, viral or parasitic infections, or ocular herpes simplex *[see Warnings and Precautions (5.4)]*.
17.5   Effect on Growth
Parents should be advised that VERAMYST Nasal Spray may slow growth in children. A child taking VERAMYST Nasal Spray should have his/her growth checked regularly *[see Warnings and Precautions (5.7) and Pediatric Use (8.4)]*.
17.6   Use Daily for Best Effect
Patients should use VERAMYST Nasal Spray on a regular once-daily basis for optimal effect. VERAMYST Nasal Spray, like other corticosteroids, does not have an immediate effect on rhinitis symptoms. Although significant improvement is usually achieved within 24 hours in patients

with seasonal allergic rhinitis and 4 days in patients with perennial allergic rhinitis, maximum benefit may not be reached for several days. The patient should not increase the prescribed dosage but should contact the physician if symptoms do not improve or if the condition worsens.

17.7   Keep Spray Out of Eyes
Patients should be informed to avoid spraying VERAMYST Nasal Spray in their eyes.

17.8   Potential Drug Interactions
Patients should be advised that coadministration of VERAMYST Nasal Spray and ritonavir is not recommended and to be cautious if coadministrating with ketoconazole.

GlaxoSmithKline
Research Triangle Park, NC 27709
©2012, GlaxoSmithKline. All rights reserved.
VRM:9PI

Patient Information
VERAMYST® *[VAIR-uh-mist]*
(fluticasone furoate)
Nasal Spray
For Intranasal Use Only

Read the Patient Information that comes with VERAMYST Nasal Spray carefully before you start using it and each time you get a refill. There may be new information. Keep the leaflet for reference because it gives you a summary of important information about VERAMYST Nasal Spray. This leaflet does not take the place of talking to your healthcare provider about your medical condition or your treatment.

What is VERAMYST Nasal Spray?
VERAMYST Nasal Spray is a medicine that treats seasonal and year-round allergy symptoms in adults and children 2 years old and older.

VERAMYST Nasal Spray contains fluticasone furoate, which is a man-made (synthetic) corticosteroid. When you spray VERAMYST Nasal Spray into your nose, it helps reduce the nasal symptoms of allergic rhinitis (inflammation of the lining of the nose), such as stuffy nose, runny nose, nasal itching, and sneezing. VERAMYST Nasal Spray may also help red, itchy, and watery eyes in adults and teenagers with seasonal allergic rhinitis.

Your healthcare provider has prescribed VERAMYST Nasal Spray to treat your symptoms of allergic rhinitis.

It is not known if VERAMYST Nasal Spray is safe and effective in children under 2 years of age.

Who should not use VERAMYST Nasal Spray?
Do not use VERAMYST Nasal Spray if you are allergic to fluticasone furoate or any of the ingredients in VERAMYST Nasal Spray. See the end of this Patient Information leaflet for a complete list of ingredients in VERAMYST Nasal Spray.

What should I tell my healthcare provider before taking VERAMYST Nasal Spray?
Tell your healthcare provider about all of your medical conditions, including if you:
- have had recent nasal sores, nasal surgery, or nasal injury
- have eye or vision problems, such as cataracts or glaucoma (increased pressure in your eye)
- have tuberculosis or any untreated fungal, bacterial, viral infections, or eye infections caused by herpes
- are exposed to chickenpox or measles.
- are feeling unwell or have any symptoms that you do not understand.
- are pregnant or plan to become pregnant. It is not known if VERAMYST Nasal Spray will harm your unborn baby. Talk to your healthcare provider if you are pregnant or plan to become pregnant.
- are breastfeeding or plan to breastfeed. It is not known if VERAMYST Nasal Spray can pass into your breast milk. Talk to your healthcare provider about the best way to feed your baby if you take VERAMYST Nasal Spray.

Tell your healthcare provider about all the medicines you take, including prescription and non-prescription medicines, vitamins, and herbal products. VERAMYST Nasal Spray and other medicines may affect each other, causing side effects. **Be certain to tell your healthcare provider if you are taking a medicine that contains ritonavir (commonly used to treat HIV infection or AIDS).**

How should I use VERAMYST Nasal Spray?
- This medicine is for use in the nose only. Do not spray it in your eyes or mouth.
- An adult should help a young child use this medicine.
- This medicine has been prescribed for you by your healthcare provider. Do not give this medicine to anyone else.
- Use VERAMYST Nasal Spray exactly as your healthcare provider tells you to. Do not take more of your medicine or take it more often than your healthcare provider tells you. The prescription label will usually tell you how many sprays to take and how often. If it does not or if you are not sure, ask your healthcare provider or pharmacist.

- **For people aged 12 years and older,** the usual starting dosage is **2 sprays in each nostril, 1 time a day.** After you begin to feel better, your healthcare provider may tell you that 1 spray in each nostril 1 time a day may be enough for you.
- **For children aged 2 to 11 years,** the usual starting dosage is **1 spray in each nostril, 1 time a day.** Your healthcare provider may tell you to take 2 sprays in each nostril 1 time a day. After you begin to feel better, your healthcare provider may change the dosage to 1 spray in each nostril 1 time a day. An adult should help a young child use this medicine.
- Do not use VERAMYST Nasal Spray after 120 sprays (plus the initial priming sprays) have been used or after the expiration date, whichever comes first. (The sample bottle contains 30 sprays.) The bottle may not be completely empty. The expiration date is printed as "EXP" on the product label and box. Before you throw away VERAMYST Nasal Spray, talk to your healthcare provider to see if you need a refill of your prescription. If your healthcare provider tells you to continue using VERAMYST Nasal Spray, throw away the empty or expired bottle and use a new bottle of VERAMYST Nasal Spray. Follow the **Instructions for Use** below.
- Do not take extra doses or stop taking VERAMYST Nasal Spray without telling your healthcare provider.
- VERAMYST Nasal Spray may begin to work within 24 hours after you take your first dose. It may take several days before it has its greatest effect. If your symptoms do not improve or get worse, call your healthcare provider.
- You will get the best results if you keep using VERAMYST Nasal Spray regularly each day without missing a dose. If you miss a dose by several hours, just take your next dose at the usual time. Do not take an extra dose.

What are the possible side effects of VERAMYST Nasal Spray?
VERAMYST Nasal Spray may cause serious side effects, including:
- **thrush (candidiasis), a fungal infection in your mouth and throat.** Tell your healthcare provider if you have any redness or white colored patches in your mouth or throat.
- **hole in the cartilage in the nose (nasal septal perforation).** Symptoms of nasal septal perforation may include:
  ○ crusting in the nose
  ○ nosebleeds
  ○ runny nose
  ○ whistling sound when you breathe
- **slow wound healing.** You should not use VERAMYST Nasal Spray until your nose has healed if you have a sore in your nose, have had surgery on your nose, or if your nose has been injured.
- **eye problems such as glaucoma and cataracts.** If you have a history of glaucoma or cataracts or have a family history of these eye problems, you should have regular eye exams while you use VERAMYST Nasal Spray.
- **serious allergic reactions.** Serious allergic reactions can happen with VERAMYST Nasal Spray. **Stop using VERAMYST Nasal Spray and call your healthcare provider right away if you have any of the following signs of a serious allergic reaction:**
- shortness of breath or trouble breathing
- skin rash, redness, or swelling
- severe itching
- swelling of the lips, tongue, or face
- **immune system problems that may increase your risk of infections.** You are more likely to get infections if you take medicines that may weaken your body's ability to fight infections. Avoid contact with people who have contagious diseases such as chicken pox or measles while you use VERAMYST Nasal Spray. Symptoms of an infection may include:
  ○ fever
  ○ pain
  ○ aches
  ○ chills
  ○ feeling tired
  ○ nausea
  ○ vomiting
- **adrenal insufficiency.** Adrenal insufficiency is a condition in which the adrenal glands do not make enough steroid hormones. Symptoms of adrenal insufficiency may include:
  ○ tiredness
  ○ weakness
  ○ dizziness
  ○ nausea
  ○ vomiting
- **slowed or delayed growth in children.** A child's growth should be checked regularly while using VERAMYST Nasal Spray.

The most common side effects of VERAMYST Nasal Spray include:
- **adults and adolescents 12 years of age and older**
  ○ headaches

  ○ nose bleeds
  ○ sore throat
  ○ nose sores
  ○ back pain
- **children 2 to 12 years of age**
  ○ headaches
  ○ sore throat
  ○ nose bleeds
  ○ fever
  ○ cough

Tell your healthcare provider if you have any side effect that bothers you or does not go away.

These are not all of the possible side effects of VERAMYST Nasal Spray. For more information, ask your healthcare provider or pharmacist.

Call your doctor for medical advice about side effects. You may report side effects to FDA at 1-800-FDA-1088.

What should I know about allergic rhinitis?
"Rhinitis" means inflammation of the lining of the nose. It is sometimes called "hay fever." Allergic rhinitis can be caused by allergies to pollen, animal dander, house dust mite, and mold spores. If you have allergic rhinitis, your nose becomes stuffy, runny, and itchy. You may also sneeze a lot. You may also have red, itchy, watery eyes; itchy throat; or blocked, itchy ears.

What are the ingredients in VERAMYST Nasal Spray?
Active ingredient: fluticasone furoate
Inactive ingredients: 0.015% w/w benzalkonium chloride, dextrose anhydrous, edetate disodium, microcrystalline cellulose, carboxymethylcellulose sodium, polysorbate 80, and purified water

Instructions for Use
Read this leaflet carefully before you start to use VERAMYST Nasal Spray. If you have any questions, ask your healthcare provider or pharmacist.

The parts of the VERAMYST Nasal Spray
VERAMYST Nasal Spray comes in a brown glass bottle inside a nasal device. It contains 120 sprays (or 30 sprays if it is a sample) plus the first priming sprays. Be careful not to drop it. If you accidentally drop the device, check it for damage. If the device is damaged, return it to your pharmacist.

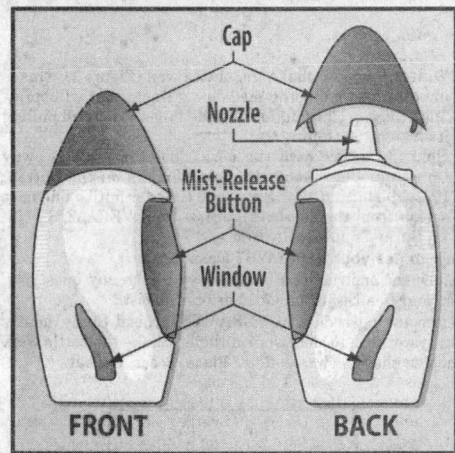

The **Cap** has a tab that keeps the **Mist-Release Button** from being pressed accidentally. It also helps keep the nozzle clean. Do not throw the cap away. Always keep the cap on the device when you are not using it.

The **Nozzle** is small and short, so it will fit inside your nose. The medicine comes out of the nozzle.

Pressing the **Mist-Release Button** sprays a measured amount of medicine from the nozzle as a gentle, fine mist. Because the button is on the side of the device, you can keep the nozzle in the right place in your nose while you press the button.

The **Window** lets you see if there is medicine left in the bottle when you hold it in front of a bright light. (You may not be able to see the medicine in a full bottle because the liquid level is above the window.)

How to prime your VERAMYST Nasal Spray
Priming helps to make sure you always get the same full dose of medicine. You need to prime VERAMYST Nasal Spray:
- before you use a new bottle for the first time.
- if you have not used your VERAMYST Nasal Spray for 30 days or longer.
- if the cap has been left off the bottle for 5 days or longer.
- if the device does not seem to be working right.

To prime VERAMYST Nasal Spray:

Figure 1

Figure 2

Figure 3

1. With the cap on, shake the device well (Figure 1). This is important to make the medicine a liquid that will spray.
2. Take the cap off by **squeezing** the finger grips and pulling it straight off (Figure 2).
3. Hold the device with the nozzle pointing up and away from you. Place your thumb or fingers on the button. Press the button all the way in 6 times or until a fine mist sprays from the nozzle (Figure 3). Your VERAMYST Nasal Spray is now ready to use.

How to use your VERAMYST Nasal Spray

Follow the instructions below. If you have any questions, ask your healthcare provider or pharmacist.

Before taking a dose of VERAMYST Nasal Spray, gently blow your nose to clear your nostrils. Shake the bottle well. Then do these 3 simple steps: **Place, Press, Repeat.**

Figure 4

Figure 5

Figure 6

Figure 7

1. PLACE

Tilt your head forward a little bit. Hold the device upright. **PLACE** the nozzle in one of your nostrils (Figure 4).

Point the end of the nozzle toward the side of your nose, away from the center of your nose (septum). This helps get the medicine to the right part of your nose.

2. PRESS

PRESS the button all the way in 1 time to spray the medicine in your nose while you are breathing in (Figure 5).

Do not get any spray in your eyes. If you do, rinse your eyes well with water.

Take the nozzle out of your nose. Breathe out through your mouth (Figure 6).

3. REPEAT

To deliver the medicine to the other nostril, **REPEAT** Steps 1 and 2 in the other nostril (Figure 7).

If your healthcare provider has told you to take 2 sprays in each nostril, do Steps 1-3 again.

Put the cap back on the device after you have finished taking your dose.

How to clean your VERAMYST Nasal Spray

After each use: wipe the nozzle with a clean, dry tissue (Figure 8). **Never try to clean the nozzle with a pin or anything sharp because this will damage the nozzle.** Do not use water to clean the nozzle.

Figure 8

Once a week: clean the inside of the cap with a clean, dry tissue (Figure 9). This will help keep the nozzle from getting blocked.

Figure 9

How to store your VERAMYST Nasal Spray

• Keep your VERAMYST Nasal Spray and all medicines out of the reach of children.
• Store between 59°F and 86°F (15°C and 30°C). Do not refrigerate or freeze.
• Store with the cap on.
• Store in an upright position.

This Patient Information has been approved by the U.S. Food and Drug Administration.

GlaxoSmithKline
Research Triangle Park, NC 27709
©2012, GlaxoSmithKline. All rights reserved.
August 2012
VRM:9PIL

VOTRIENT ℞
[vo' tre-ent]
(pazopanib)
tablets, for oral use

HIGHLIGHTS OF PRESCRIBING INFORMATION
These highlights do not include all the information needed to use VOTRIENT safely and effectively. See full prescribing information for VOTRIENT.
VOTRIENT (pazopanib) tablets, for oral use
Initial U.S. Approval: 2009

—————RECENT MAJOR CHANGES—————

Dosage and Administration, Dose Modification Guidelines (2.2)	08/2013
Warnings and Precautions, Thrombotic Microangiopathy (5.7)	08/2013

> **WARNING: HEPATOTOXICITY**
> *See full prescribing information for complete boxed warning.*
> Severe and fatal hepatotoxicity has been observed in clinical trials. Monitor hepatic function and interrupt, reduce, or discontinue dosing as recommended *[see Warnings and Precautions (5.1)]*.

—————INDICATIONS AND USAGE—————

VOTRIENT is a kinase inhibitor indicated for the treatment of patients with:
• advanced renal cell carcinoma. (1)
• advanced soft tissue sarcoma who have received prior chemotherapy. (1)

Limitation of Use: The efficacy of VOTRIENT for the treatment of patients with adipocytic soft tissue sarcoma or gastrointestinal stromal tumors has not been demonstrated.

—————DOSAGE AND ADMINISTRATION—————

• 800 mg orally once daily without food (at least 1 hour before or 2 hours after a meal). (2.1)
• Baseline moderate hepatic impairment – 200 mg orally once daily. Not recommended in patients with severe hepatic impairment. (2.2)

—————DOSAGE FORMS AND STRENGTHS—————

200 mg tablets (3)

—————CONTRAINDICATIONS—————

None (4)

—————WARNINGS AND PRECAUTIONS—————

• Increases in serum transaminase levels and bilirubin were observed. Severe and fatal hepatotoxicity has occurred. Measure liver chemistries before the initiation of treatment and regularly during treatment. (5.1)
• Prolonged QT intervals and torsades de pointes have been observed. Use with caution in patients at higher risk of developing QT interval prolongation. Monitoring electrocardiograms and electrolytes should be considered. (5.2)
• Cardiac dysfunction such as congestive heart failure and decreased left ventricular ejection fraction (LVEF) have occurred. Monitor blood pressure and manage hypertension promptly. Baseline and periodic evaluation of LVEF is recommended in patients at risk of cardiac dysfunction. (5.3)
• Fatal hemorrhagic events have been reported. VOTRIENT has not been studied in patients who have a history of hemoptysis, cerebral, or clinically significant gastrointestinal hemorrhage in the past 6 months and should not be used in those patients. (5.4)
• Arterial thromboembolic events have been observed and can be fatal. Use with caution in patients who are at increased risk for these events. (5.5)
• Venous thromboembolic events (VTE) have been observed, including fatal pulmonary emboli (PE). Monitor for signs and symptoms of VTE and PE. (5.6)
• Thrombotic microangiopathy (TMA), including thrombotic thrombocytopenic purpura (TTP) and hemolytic uremic syndrome (HUS) has been observed. Permanently discontinue VOTRIENT if TMA occurs. (5.7)

- Gastrointestinal perforation or fistula has occurred. Fatal perforation events have occurred. Use with caution in patients at risk for gastrointestinal perforation or fistula. (5.8)
- Reversible Posterior Leukoencephalopathy Syndrome (RPLS) has been observed and can be fatal. Permanently discontinue VOTRIENT in patients developing RPLS. (5.9)
- Hypertension including hypertensive crisis has been observed. Blood pressure should be well controlled prior to initiating VOTRIENT. Monitor blood pressure within one week after starting VOTRIENT and frequently thereafter. (5.10)
- Interruption of therapy with VOTRIENT is recommended in patients undergoing surgical procedures. (5.11)
- Hypothyroidism may occur. Monitoring of thyroid function tests is recommended. (5.12)
- Proteinuria: Monitor urine protein. Interrupt treatment for 24-hour urine protein ≥3 grams and discontinue for repeat episodes despite dose reductions. (5.13)
- Infection: Serious infections (with or without neutropenia), some with fatal outcome, have been reported. Monitor for signs and symptoms and treat active infection promptly. Interrupt or discontinue VOTRIENT. (5.14)
- Animal studies have demonstrated VOTRIENT can severely affect organ growth and maturation during early post-natal development. The safety and effectiveness in pediatric patients have not been established. (5.16)
- VOTRIENT can cause fetal harm when administered to a pregnant woman. Women of childbearing potential should be advised of the potential hazard to the fetus and to avoid becoming pregnant while taking VOTRIENT. (5.17, 8.1)

---ADVERSE REACTIONS---

The most common adverse reactions in patients with advanced renal cell carcinoma (≥20%) are diarrhea, hypertension, hair color changes (depigmentation), nausea, anorexia, and vomiting. (6.1)

The most common adverse reactions in patients with advanced soft tissue sarcoma (≥20%) are fatigue, diarrhea, nausea, decreased weight, hypertension, decreased appetite, hair color changes, vomiting, tumor pain, dysgeusia, headache, musculoskeletal pain, myalgia, gastrointestinal pain, and dyspnea. (6.1)

To report SUSPECTED ADVERSE REACTIONS, contact GlaxoSmithKline at 1-888-825-5249 or FDA at 1-800-FDA-1088 or www.fda.gov/medwatch

---DRUG INTERACTIONS---

- CYP3A4 Inhibitors: Avoid use of strong CYP3A4 inhibitors. If coadministration is warranted, reduce the dose of VOTRIENT to 400 mg. (7.1)
- CYP3A4 Inducers: Consider an alternate concomitant medication with no or minimal enzyme induction potential or avoid VOTRIENT. (7.1)
- CYP Substrates: Concomitant use of VOTRIENT with agents with narrow therapeutic windows that are metabolized by CYP3A4, CYP2D6, or CYP2C8 is not recommended. (7.3)
- Concomitant use of VOTRIENT and simvastatin increases the risk of ALT elevations and should be undertaken with caution and close monitoring. (7.4)
- Drugs That Raise Gastric pH: Avoid concomitant use of VOTRIENT with drugs that raise gastric pH. Consider short-acting antacids in place of proton pump inhibitors (PPIs) and H2 receptor antagonists. Separate antacid and pazopanib dosing by several hours. (7.5)

See 17 for PATIENT COUNSELING INFORMATION and Medication Guide

Revised: 06/2014

FULL PRESCRIBING INFORMATION: CONTENTS*

FULL PRESCRIBING INFORMATION

> **WARNING: HEPATOTOXICITY**
>
> Severe and fatal hepatotoxicity has been observed in clinical trials. Monitor hepatic function and interrupt, reduce, or discontinue dosing as recommended *[see Warnings and Precautions (5.1)]*.

1   INDICATIONS AND USAGE

VOTRIENT® is indicated for the treatment of patients with advanced renal cell carcinoma (RCC).

VOTRIENT is indicated for the treatment of patients with advanced soft tissue sarcoma (STS) who have received prior chemotherapy.

Limitation of Use: The efficacy of VOTRIENT for the treatment of patients with adipocytic STS or gastrointestinal stromal tumors has not been demonstrated.

2   DOSAGE AND ADMINISTRATION

2.1   Recommended Dosing

The recommended starting dose of VOTRIENT is 800 mg orally once daily without food (at least 1 hour before or 2 hours after a meal) *[see Clinical Pharmacology (12.3)]*. The dose of VOTRIENT should not exceed 800 mg.

Do not crush tablets due to the potential for increased rate of absorption which may affect systemic exposure *[see Clinical Pharmacology (12.3)]*.

If a dose is missed, it should not be taken if it is less than 12 hours until the next dose.

2.2   Dose Modification Guidelines

In RCC, the initial dose reduction should be 400 mg, and additional dose decrease or increase should be in 200 mg steps based on individual tolerability.

In STS, a decrease or increase should be in 200 mg steps based on individual tolerability.

Hepatic Impairment: No dose adjustment is required in patients with mild hepatic impairment. In patients with moderate hepatic impairment, alternatives to VOTRIENT should be considered. If VOTRIENT is used in patients with moderate hepatic impairment, the dose should be reduced to 200 mg per day. VOTRIENT is not recommended in patients with severe hepatic impairment *[see Use in Specific Populations (8.6) and Clinical Pharmacology (12.3)]*.

Concomitant Strong CYP3A4 Inhibitors: The concomitant use of strong CYP3A4 inhibitors (e.g., ketoconazole, ritonavir, clarithromycin) increases pazopanib concentrations and should be avoided. Consider an alternate concomitant medication with no or minimal potential to inhibit CYP3A4. If coadministration of a strong CYP3A4 inhibitor is warranted, reduce the dose of VOTRIENT to 400 mg. Further dose reductions may be needed if adverse effects occur during therapy *[see Drug Interactions (7.1) and Clinical Pharmacology (12.3)]*.

Concomitant Strong CYP3A4 Inducer: The concomitant use of strong CYP3A4 inducers (e.g., rifampin) may decrease pazopanib concentrations and should be avoided. Consider an alternate concomitant medication with no or minimal enzyme induction potential. VOTRIENT should not be used in patients who cannot avoid chronic use of strong CYP3A4 inducers *[see Drug Interactions (7.1)]*.

3   DOSAGE FORMS AND STRENGTHS

200 mg tablets of VOTRIENT — modified capsule-shaped, gray, film-coated with GS JT debossed on one side. Each tablet contains 216.7 mg of pazopanib hydrochloride equivalent to 200 mg of pazopanib.

4   CONTRAINDICATIONS

None.

5   WARNINGS AND PRECAUTIONS

5.1   Hepatic Toxicity and Hepatic Impairment

In clinical trials with VOTRIENT, hepatotoxicity, manifested as increases in serum transaminases (ALT, AST) and bilirubin, was observed. This hepatotoxicity can be severe and fatal. Transaminase elevations occur early in the course of treatment (92.5% of all transaminase elevations of any grade occurred in the first 18 weeks) *[see Dosage and Administration (2.2)]*.

In the randomized RCC trial, ALT >3 × ULN was reported in 18% and 3% of the VOTRIENT and placebo groups, respectively. ALT >10 × ULN was reported in 4% of patients who received VOTRIENT and in <1% of patients who received placebo. Concurrent elevation in ALT >3 × ULN and bilirubin >2 × ULN in the absence of significant alkaline phosphatase >3 × ULN occurred in 2% (5/290) of patients on VOTRIENT and 1% (2/145) on placebo.

In the randomized STS trial, ALT >3 × ULN was reported in 18% and 5% of the VOTRIENT and placebo groups, respectively. ALT >8 × ULN was reported in 5% and 2% of the VOTRIENT and placebo groups, respectively. Concurrent elevation in ALT >3 × ULN and bilirubin >2 × ULN in the absence of significant alkaline phosphatase >3 × ULN occurred in 2% (4/240) of patients on VOTRIENT and <1% (1/123) on placebo.

Two-tenths percent of the patients (2/977) from trials that supported the RCC indication died with disease progression and hepatic failure and 0.4% of patients (1/240) in the randomized STS trial died of hepatic failure.

- Monitor serum liver tests before initiation of treatment with VOTRIENT and at Weeks 3, 5, 7, and 9. Thereafter, monitor at Month 3 and at Month 4, and as clinically indicated. Periodic monitoring should then continue after Month 4.
- Patients with isolated ALT elevations between 3 × ULN and 8 × ULN may be continued on VOTRIENT with weekly monitoring of liver function until ALT return to Grade 1 or baseline.
- Patients with isolated ALT elevations of >8 × ULN should have VOTRIENT interrupted until they return to Grade 1 or baseline. If the potential benefit for reinitiating treatment with VOTRIENT is considered to outweigh the risk for hepatotoxicity, then reintroduce VOTRIENT at a reduced dose of no more than 400 mg once daily and measure serum liver tests weekly for 8 weeks *[see Dosage and Administration (2.2)]*. Following reintroduction of VOTRIENT, if ALT elevations >3 × ULN recur, then VOTRIENT should be permanently discontinued.
- If ALT elevations >3 × ULN occur concurrently with bilirubin elevations >2 × ULN, VOTRIENT should be permanently discontinued. Patients should be monitored until resolution. VOTRIENT is a UGT1A1 inhibitor. Mild, indirect (unconjugated) hyperbilirubinemia may occur in patients with Gilbert's syndrome *[see Clinical Pharmacology (12.5)]*. Patients with only a mild indirect hyperbilirubinemia, known Gilbert's syndrome, and elevation in ALT >3 × ULN should be managed as per the recommendations outlined for isolated ALT elevations.

Concomitant use of VOTRIENT and simvastatin increases the risk of ALT elevations and should be undertaken with caution and close monitoring *[see Drug Interactions (7.4)]*. Insufficient data are available to assess the risk of concomitant administration of alternative statins and VOTRIENT.

In patients with pre-existing moderate hepatic impairment, the starting dose of VOTRIENT should be reduced or alternatives to VOTRIENT should be considered. Treatment with VOTRIENT is not recommended in patients with pre-existing severe hepatic impairment, defined as total bilirubin >3 × ULN with any level of ALT *[see Dosage and Administration (2.2), Use in Specific Populations (8.6), and Clinical Pharmacology (12.3)]*.

5.2   QT Prolongation and Torsades de Pointes

In the RCC trials of VOTRIENT, QT prolongation (≥500 msec) was identified on routine electrocardiogram monitoring in 2% (11/558) of patients. Torsades de pointes occurred in <1% (2/977) of patients who received VOTRIENT in the monotherapy trials.

In the randomized RCC and STS trials, 1% (3/290) of patients and 0.4% (1/240) of patients, respectively, who received VOTRIENT had post-baseline values between 500 to 549 msec. Post-baseline QT data were only collected in the STS trial if ECG abnormalities were reported as an adverse reaction. None of the 268 patients who received placebo on the two trials had post-baseline QTc values ≥500 msec. VOTRIENT should be used with caution in patients with a history of QT interval prolongation, in patients taking anti-arrhythmics or other medications that may prolong QT interval, and those with relevant pre-existing cardiac disease. When using VOTRIENT, baseline and periodic monitoring of electrocardiograms and maintenance of electrolytes (e.g., calcium, magnesium, potassium) within the normal range should be performed.

5.3 Cardiac Dysfunction
In clinical trials with VOTRIENT, events of cardiac dysfunction such as decreased left ventricular ejection fraction (LVEF) and congestive heart failure have occurred. In the overall safety population with VOTRIENT (N = 586), cardiac dysfunction was observed in 0.6% (4/586) of patients without routine on-study LVEF monitoring. In the randomized STS trial, myocardial dysfunction was defined as symptoms of cardiac dysfunction or ≥15% absolute decline in LVEF compared to baseline or a decline in LVEF of ≥10% compared to baseline that is also below the lower limit of normal. In patients who had baseline and follow up LVEF measurements, myocardial dysfunction occurred in 11% (16/142) of patients on VOTRIENT compared to 5% (2/40) of patients on placebo. One percent (3/240) of patients on VOTRIENT in the STS trial had congestive heart failure which did not resolve in one patient.

Fourteen of the 16 patients with myocardial dysfunction treated with VOTRIENT in the STS trial had concurrent hypertension which may have exacerbated cardiac dysfunction in patients at risk (e.g., those with prior anthracycline therapy) possibly by increasing cardiac afterload. Blood pressure should be monitored and managed promptly using a combination of anti-hypertensive therapy and dose modification of VOTRIENT (interruption and re-initiation at a reduced dose based on clinical judgment) [see Warnings and Precautions (5.10)]. Patients should be carefully monitored for clinical signs or symptoms of congestive heart failure. Baseline and periodic evaluation of LVEF is recommended in patients at risk of cardiac dysfunction including previous anthracycline exposure.

5.4 Hemorrhagic Events
Fatal hemorrhage occurred in 0.9% (5/586) in the RCC trials; there were no reports of fatal hemorrhage in the STS trials. In the randomized RCC trial, 13% (37/290) of patients treated with VOTRIENT and 5% (7/145) of patients on placebo experienced at least 1 hemorrhagic event. The most common hemorrhagic events in the patients treated with VOTRIENT were hematuria (4%), epistaxis (2%), hemoptysis (2%), and rectal hemorrhage (1%). Nine of 37 patients treated with VOTRIENT who had hemorrhagic events experienced serious events including pulmonary, gastrointestinal, and genitourinary hemorrhage. One percent (4/290) of patients treated with VOTRIENT died from hemorrhage compared with no (0/145) patients on placebo. In the overall safety population in RCC (N = 586), cerebral/intracranial hemorrhage was observed in <1% (2/586) of patients treated with VOTRIENT.

In the randomized STS trial, 22% (53/240) of patients treated with VOTRIENT compared to 8% (10/123) treated with placebo experienced at least 1 hemorrhagic event. The most common hemorrhagic events were epistaxis (8%), mouth hemorrhage (3%), and anal hemorrhage (2%). Grade 4 hemorrhagic events in the STS population occurred in 1% (3/240) of patients and included intracranial hemorrhage, subarachnoid hemorrhage, and peritoneal hemorrhage.

VOTRIENT has not been studied in patients who have a history of hemoptysis, cerebral, or clinically significant gastrointestinal hemorrhage in the past 6 months and should not be used in these patients.

5.5 Arterial Thromboembolic Events
Fatal arterial thromboembolic events were observed in 0.3% (2/586) of patients in the RCC trials and in no patients in the STS trials. In the randomized RCC trial, 2% (5/290) of patients receiving VOTRIENT experienced myocardial infarction or ischemia, 0.3% (1/290) had a cerebrovascular accident and 1% (4/290) had an event of transient ischemic attack. In the randomized STS trial, 2% (4/240) of patients receiving VOTRIENT experienced a myocardial infarction or ischemia, 0.4% (1/240) had a cerebrovascular accident and there were no incidents of transient ischemic attack. No arterial thromboembolic events were reported in patients who received placebo in either trial. VOTRIENT should be used with caution in patients who are at increased risk for these events or who have had a history of these events. VOTRIENT has not been studied in patients who have had an arterial thromboembolic event within the previous 6 months and should not be used in those patients.

5.6 Venous Thromboembolic Events
In RCC and STS trials of VOTRIENT, venous thromboembolic events (VTE) including venous thrombosis and fatal pulmonary embolus (PE) have occurred. In the randomized STS trial, venous thromboembolic events were reported in 5% of patients treated with VOTRIENT compared to 2% with placebo. In the randomized RCC trial, the rate was 1% in both arms. Fatal pulmonary embolus occurred in 1% (2/240) of STS patients receiving VOTRIENT and in no patients receiving placebo. There were no fatal pulmonary emboli in the RCC trial. Monitor for signs and symptoms of VTE and PE.

5.7 Thrombotic Microangiopathy
Thrombotic microangiopathy (TMA), including thrombotic thrombocytopenic purpura (TTP) and hemolytic uremic syndrome (HUS) has been reported in clinical trials of VOTRIENT as monotherapy, in combination with bevacizumab, and in combination with topotecan. VOTRIENT is not indicated for use in combination with other agents. Six of the 7 TMA cases occurred within 90 days of the initiation of VOTRIENT. Improvement of TMA was observed after treatment was discontinued. Monitor for signs and symptoms of TMA. Permanently discontinue VOTRIENT in patients developing TMA. Manage as clinically indicated.

5.8 Gastrointestinal Perforation and Fistula
In the RCC and STS trials, gastrointestinal perforation or fistula occurred in 0.9% (5/586) and 1% (4/382) of patients receiving VOTRIENT, respectively. Fatal perforations occurred in 0.3% (2/586) of these patients in the RCC trials and in 0.3% (1/382) of these patients in the STS trials. Monitor for signs and symptoms of gastrointestinal perforation or fistula.

5.9 Reversible Posterior Leukoencephalopathy Syndrome
Reversible Posterior Leukoencephalopathy Syndrome (RPLS) has been reported in patients receiving VOTRIENT and may be fatal.

RPLS is a neurological disorder which can present with headache, seizure, lethargy, confusion, blindness, and other visual and neurologic disturbances. Mild to severe hypertension may be present. The diagnosis of RPLS is optimally confirmed by magnetic resonance imaging. Permanently discontinue VOTRIENT in patients developing RPLS.

5.10 Hypertension
In clinical trials, hypertension (systolic blood pressure ≥150 or diastolic blood pressure ≥100 mm Hg) and hypertensive crisis were observed in patients treated with VOTRIENT. Blood pressure should be well controlled prior to initiating VOTRIENT. Hypertension occurs early in the course of treatment (40% of cases occurred by Day 9 and 90% of cases occurred in the first 18 weeks). Blood pressure should be monitored early after starting treatment (no longer than one week) and frequently thereafter to ensure blood pressure control. Approximately 40% of patients who received VOTRIENT experienced hypertension. Grade 3 hypertension was reported in 4% to 7% of patients receiving VOTRIENT [see Adverse Reactions (6.1)].

Increased blood pressure should be treated promptly with standard anti-hypertensive therapy and dose reduction or interruption of VOTRIENT as clinically warranted. VOTRIENT should be discontinued if there is evidence of hypertensive crisis or if hypertension is severe and persistent despite anti-hypertensive therapy and dose reduction. Approximately 1% of patients required permanent discontinuation of VOTRIENT because of hypertension [see Dosage and Administration (2.2)].

5.11 Wound Healing
No formal trials on the effect of VOTRIENT on wound healing have been conducted. Since vascular endothelial growth factor receptor (VEGFR) inhibitors such as pazopanib may impair wound healing, treatment with VOTRIENT should be stopped at least 7 days prior to scheduled surgery. The decision to resume VOTRIENT after surgery should be based on clinical judgment of adequate wound healing. VOTRIENT should be discontinued in patients with wound dehiscence.

5.12 Hypothyroidism
Hypothyroidism, confirmed based on a simultaneous rise of TSH and decline of T4, was reported in 7% (19/290) of patients treated with VOTRIENT in the randomized RCC trial and in 5% (11/240) of patients treated with VOTRIENT in the randomized STS trial. No patients on the placebo arm of either trial had hypothyroidism. In RCC and STS trials of VOTRIENT, hypothyroidism was reported as an adverse reaction in 4% (26/586) and 5% (20/382) of patients, respectively. Proactive monitoring of thyroid function tests is recommended.

5.13 Proteinuria
In the randomized RCC trial, proteinuria was reported as an adverse reaction in 9% (27/290) of patients receiving VOTRIENT and in no patients receiving placebo. In 2 patients, proteinuria led to discontinuation of treatment with VOTRIENT. In the randomized STS trial, proteinuria was reported as an adverse reaction in 1% (2/240) of patients, and nephrotic syndrome was reported in 1 patient treated with VOTRIENT compared to none in patients receiving placebo. Treatment was withdrawn in the patient with nephrotic syndrome.

Baseline and periodic urinalysis during treatment is recommended with follow up measurement of 24-hour urine protein as clinically indicated. Interrupt VOTRIENT and dose reduce for 24-hour urine protein ≥3 grams; discontinue VOTRIENT for repeat episodes despite dose reductions [see Dosage and Administration (2.2)].

5.14 Infection
Serious infections (with or without neutropenia), including some with fatal outcome, have been reported. Monitor patients for signs and symptoms of infection. Institute appropriate anti-infective therapy promptly and consider interruption or discontinuation of VOTRIENT for serious infections.

5.15 Increased Toxicity With Other Cancer Therapy
VOTRIENT is not indicated for use in combination with other agents. Clinical trials of VOTRIENT in combination with pemetrexed and lapatinib were terminated early due to concerns over increased toxicity and mortality. The fatal toxicities observed included pulmonary hemorrhage, gastrointestinal hemorrhage, and sudden death. A safe and effective combination dose has not been established with these regimens.

5.16 Increased Toxicity in Developing Organs
The safety and effectiveness of VOTRIENT in pediatric patients have not been established. VOTRIENT is not indicated for use in pediatric patients. Based on its mechanism of action, pazopanib may have severe effects on organ growth and maturation during early post-natal development. Administration of pazopanib to juvenile rats less than 21 days old resulted in toxicity to the lungs, liver, heart, and kidney and in death at doses significantly lower than the clinically recommended dose or doses tolerated in older animals. VOTRIENT may potentially cause serious adverse effects on organ development in pediatric patients, particularly in patients younger than 2 years of age [see Use in Specific Populations (8.4)].

5.17 Pregnancy
VOTRIENT can cause fetal harm when administered to a pregnant woman. Based on its mechanism of action, VOTRIENT is expected to result in adverse reproductive effects. In pre-clinical studies in rats and rabbits, pazopanib was teratogenic, embryotoxic, fetotoxic, and abortifacient. There are no adequate and well-controlled studies of VOTRIENT in pregnant women. If this drug is used during pregnancy, or if the patient becomes pregnant while taking this drug, the patient should be apprised of the potential hazard to the fetus. Women of childbearing potential should be advised to avoid becoming pregnant while taking VOTRIENT [see Use in Specific Populations (8.1)].

6 ADVERSE REACTIONS
6.1 Clinical Trials Experience
Because clinical trials are conducted under widely varying conditions, adverse reaction rates observed in the clinical trials of a drug cannot be directly compared to rates in the clinical trials of another drug and may not reflect the rates observed in practice.

Potentially serious adverse reactions with VOTRIENT included:
- Hepatotoxicity [see Warnings and Precautions (5.1)]
- QT prolongation and torsades de pointes [see Warnings and Precautions (5.2)]
- Cardiac dysfunction [see Warnings and Precautions (5.3)]
- Hemorrhagic events [see Warnings and Precautions (5.4)]
- Arterial and venous thromboembolic events [see Warnings and Precautions (5.5 and 5.6)]
- Thrombotic microangiopathy [see Warnings and Precautions (5.7)]
- Gastrointestinal perforation and fistula [see Warnings and Precautions (5.8)]
- Reversible Posterior Leukoencephalopathy Syndrome (RPLS) [see Warnings and Precautions (5.9)]
- Hypertension [see Warnings and Precautions (5.10)]
- Infection [see Warnings and Precautions (5.14)]
- Increased toxicity with other cancer therapies [see Warnings and Precautions (5.15)]

Renal Cell Carcinoma: The safety of VOTRIENT has been evaluated in 977 patients in the monotherapy trials which included 586 patients with RCC at the time of NDA submission. With a median duration of treatment of 7.4 months (range 0.1 to 27.6), the most commonly observed adverse reactions (≥20%) in the 586 patients were diarrhea, hypertension, hair color change, nausea, fatigue, anorexia, and vomiting.

The data described below reflect the safety profile of VOTRIENT in 290 RCC patients who participated in a randomized, double-blind, placebo-controlled trial [see Clinical Studies (14.1)]. The median duration of treatment was 7.4 months (range 0 to 23) for patients who received VOTRIENT and 3.8 months (range 0 to 22) for the placebo arm. Forty-two percent of patients on VOTRIENT required a dose interruption. Thirty-six percent of patients on VOTRIENT were dose reduced. Table 1 presents the most common adverse reactions occurring in ≥10% of patients who received VOTRIENT.

[See table 1 above]
Other adverse reactions observed more commonly in patients treated with VOTRIENT than placebo and that occurred in <10% (any grade) were alopecia (8% versus <1%), chest pain (5% versus 1%), dysgeusia (altered taste) (8% versus <1%), dyspepsia (5% versus <1%), dysphonia (4% versus <1%), facial edema (1% versus 0%), palmar-plantar erythrodysesthesia (hand-foot syndrome) (6% versus <1%), proteinuria (9% versus 0%), rash (8% versus 3%), skin depigmentation (3% versus 0%), and weight decreased (9% versus 3%).

Additional adverse reactions from other clinical trials in RCC patients treated with VOTRIENT are listed below:
Musculoskeletal and Connective Tissue Disorders: Arthralgia, muscle spasms.

Table 2 presents the most common laboratory abnormalities occurring in >10% of patients who received VOTRIENT and more commonly (≥5%) in patients who received VOTRIENT versus placebo.

[See table 2 above]

Soft Tissue Sarcoma: The safety of VOTRIENT has been evaluated in 382 patients with advanced soft tissue sarcoma, with a median duration of treatment of 3.6 months (range 0 to 53). The most commonly observed adverse reactions (≥20%) in the 382 patients were fatigue, diarrhea, nausea, decreased weight, hypertension, decreased appetite, vomiting, tumor pain, hair color changes, musculoskeletal pain, headache, dysgeusia, dyspnea, and skin hypopigmentation.

The data described below reflect the safety profile of VOTRIENT in 240 patients who participated in a randomized, double-blind, placebo-controlled trial *[see Clinical Studies (14.2)]*. The median duration of treatment was 4.5 months (range 0 to 24) for patients who received VOTRIENT and 1.9 months (range 0 to 24) for the placebo arm. Fifty-eight percent of patients on VOTRIENT required a dose interruption. Thirty-eight percent of patients on VOTRIENT had their dose reduced. Seventeen percent of patients who received VOTRIENT discontinued therapy due to adverse reactions. Table 3 presents the most common adverse reactions occurring in ≥10% of patients who received VOTRIENT.

[See table 3 at top of next page]

Other adverse reactions observed more commonly in patients treated with VOTRIENT that occurred in ≥5% of patients and at an incidence of more than 2% difference from placebo included insomnia (9% versus 6%), hypothyroidism (8% versus 0%), dysphonia (8% versus 2%), epistaxis (8% versus 2%), left ventricular dysfunction (8% versus 4%), dyspepsia (7% versus 2%), dry skin (6% versus <1%), chills (5% versus 1%), vision blurred (5% versus 2%), and nail disorder (5% versus 0%).

Table 4 presents the most common laboratory abnormalities occurring in >10% of patients who received VOTRIENT and more commonly (≥5%) in patients who received VOTRIENT versus placebo.

[See table 4 at top of page 1237]

Diarrhea: Diarrhea occurred frequently and was predominantly mild to moderate in severity in both the RCC and STS clinical trials. Patients should be advised how to manage mild diarrhea and to notify their healthcare provider if moderate to severe diarrhea occurs so appropriate management can be implemented to minimize its impact.

Lipase Elevations: In a single-arm RCC trial, increases in lipase values were observed for 27% (48/181) of patients. Elevations in lipase as an adverse reaction were reported for 4% (10/225) of patients and were Grade 3 for 6 patients and Grade 4 for 1 patient. In the RCC trials of VOTRIENT, clinical pancreatitis was observed in <1% (4/586) of patients.

Pneumothorax: Two of 290 patients treated with VOTRIENT and no patient on the placebo arm in the randomized RCC trial developed a pneumothorax. In the randomized trial of VOTRIENT for the treatment of STS, pneumothorax occurred in 3% (8/240) of patients treated with VOTRIENT and in no patients on the placebo arm.

Bradycardia: In the randomized trial of VOTRIENT for the treatment of RCC, bradycardia based on vital signs (<60 beats per minute) was observed in 19% (52/280) of patients treated with VOTRIENT and in 11% (16/144) of patients on the placebo arm. Bradycardia was reported as an adverse reaction in 2% (7/290) of patients treated with VOTRIENT compared to <1% (1/145) of patients treated with placebo. In the randomized trial of VOTRIENT for the treatment of STS, bradycardia based on vital signs (<60 beats per minute) was observed in 19% (45/238) of patients treated with VOTRIENT and in 4% (5/121) of patients on the placebo arm. Bradycardia was reported as an adverse reaction in 2% (4/240) of patients treated with VOTRIENT compared to <1% (1/123) of patients treated with placebo.

6.2 Postmarketing Experience

The following adverse reactions have been identified during post approval use of VOTRIENT. Because these reactions are reported voluntarily from a population of uncertain size it is not always possible to reliably estimate the frequency or establish a causal relationship to drug exposure.
Gastrointestinal Disorders: Pancreatitis

7 DRUG INTERACTIONS

7.1 Drugs That Inhibit or Induce Cytochrome P450 3A4 Enzymes

In vitro studies suggested that the oxidative metabolism of pazopanib in human liver microsomes is mediated primarily by CYP3A4, with minor contributions from CYP1A2 and CYP2C8. Therefore, inhibitors and inducers of CYP3A4 may alter the metabolism of pazopanib.
CYP3A4 Inhibitors: Coadministration of pazopanib with strong inhibitors of CYP3A4 (e.g., ketoconazole, ritonavir, clarithromycin) increases pazopanib concentrations and should be avoided. Consider an alternate concomitant medication with no or minimal potential to inhibit CYP3A4 *[see Clinical Pharmacology (12.3)]*. If coadministration of a strong CYP3A4 inhibitor is warranted, reduce the dose of VOTRIENT to 400 mg *[see Dosage and Administration (2.2)]*. Grapefruit or grapefruit juice should be avoided as it inhibits CYP3A4 activity and may also increase plasma concentrations of pazopanib.
CYP3A4 Inducers: CYP3A4 inducers such as rifampin may decrease plasma pazopanib concentrations. Consider an alternate concomitant medication with no or minimal enzyme induction potential. VOTRIENT should not be used if chronic use of strong CYP3A4 inducers cannot be avoided *[see Dosage and Administration (2.2)]*.

7.2 Drugs That Inhibit Transporters

In vitro studies suggested that pazopanib is a substrate of P-glycoprotein (Pgp) and breast cancer resistance protein (BCRP). Therefore, absorption and subsequent elimination of pazopanib may be influenced by products that affect Pgp and BCRP.
Concomitant treatment with strong inhibitors of Pgp or breast cancer resistance protein (BCRP) should be avoided due to risk of increased exposure to pazopanib. Selection of alternative concomitant medicinal products with no or minimal potential to inhibit Pgp or BCRP should be considered.

Table 1. Adverse Reactions Occurring in ≥10% of Patients With RCC who Received VOTRIENT

	VOTRIENT			Placebo		
	(N = 290)			(N = 145)		
	All Grades[a]	Grade 3	Grade 4	All Grades[a]	Grade 3	Grade 4
Adverse Reactions	%	%	%	%	%	%
Diarrhea	52	3	<1	9	<1	0
Hypertension	40	4	0	10	<1	0
Hair color changes	38	<1	0	3	0	0
Nausea	26	<1	0	9	0	0
Anorexia	22	2	0	10	<1	0
Vomiting	21	2	<1	8	2	0
Fatigue	19	2	0	8	1	1
Asthenia	14	3	0	8	0	0
Abdominal pain	11	2	0	1	0	0
Headache	10	0	0	5	0	0

[a] National Cancer Institute Common Terminology Criteria for Adverse Events, version 3.

Table 2. Selected Laboratory Abnormalities Occurring in >10% of Patients With RCC who Received VOTRIENT and More Commonly (≥5%) in Patients who Received VOTRIENT Versus Placebo

	VOTRIENT			Placebo		
	(N = 290)			(N = 145)		
	All Grades[a]	Grade 3	Grade 4	All Grades[a]	Grade 3	Grade 4
Parameters	%	%	%	%	%	%
Hematologic						
Leukopenia	37	0	0	6	0	0
Neutropenia	34	1	<1	6	0	0
Thrombocytopenia	32	<1	<1	5	0	<1
Lymphocytopenia	31	4	<1	24	1	0
Chemistry						
ALT increased	53	10	2	22	1	0
AST increased	53	7	<1	19	<1	0
Glucose increased	41	<1	0	33	1	0
Total bilirubin increased	36	3	<1	10	1	<1
Phosphorus decreased	34	4	0	11	0	0
Sodium decreased	31	4	1	24	4	0
Magnesium decreased	26	<1	1	14	0	0
Glucose decreased	17	0	<1	3	0	0

[a] National Cancer Institute Common Terminology Criteria for Adverse Events, version 3.

Table 3. Adverse Reactions Occurring in ≥10% of Patients With STS who Received VOTRIENT

Adverse Reactions	VOTRIENT (N = 240)			Placebo (N = 123)		
	All Grades[a]	Grade 3	Grade 4	All Grades[a]	Grade 3	Grade 4
	%	%	%	%	%	%
Fatigue	65	13	1	48	4	1
Diarrhea	59	5	0	15	1	0
Nausea	56	3	0	22	2	0
Weight decreased	48	4	0	15	0	0
Hypertension	42	7	0	6	0	0
Appetite decreased	40	6	0	19	0	0
Hair color changes	39	0	0	2	0	0
Vomiting	33	3	0	11	1	0
Tumor pain	29	8	0	21	7	2
Dysgeusia	28	0	0	3	0	0
Headache	23	1	0	8	0	0
Musculoskeletal pain	23	2	0	20	2	0
Myalgia	23	2	0	9	0	0
Gastrointestinal pain	23	3	0	9	4	0
Dyspnea	20	5	<1	17	5	1
Exfoliative rash	18	<1	0	9	0	0
Cough	17	<1	0	12	<1	0
Peripheral edema	14	2	0	9	2	0
Mucositis	12	2	0	2	0	0
Alopecia	12	0	0	1	0	0
Dizziness	11	1	0	4	0	0
Skin disorder[b]	11	2	0	1	0	0
Skin hypopigmentation	11	0	0	0	0	0
Stomatitis	11	<1	0	3	0	0
Chest pain	10	2	0	6	0	0

[a] National Cancer Institute Common Terminology Criteria for Adverse Events, version 3.
[b] 27 of the 28 cases of skin disorder were palmar-plantar erythrodysesthesia.

7.3 Effects of Pazopanib on CYP Substrates

Results from drug-drug interaction trials conducted in cancer patients suggest that pazopanib is a weak inhibitor of CYP3A4, CYP2C8, and CYP2D6 in vivo, but had no effect on CYP1A2, CYP2C9, or CYP2C19 [see Clinical Pharmacology (12.3)].

Concomitant use of VOTRIENT with agents with narrow therapeutic windows that are metabolized by CYP3A4, CYP2D6, or CYP2C8 is not recommended. Coadministration may result in inhibition of the metabolism of these products and create the potential for serious adverse events [see Clinical Pharmacology (12.3)].

7.4 Effect of Concomitant use of VOTRIENT and Simvastatin

Concomitant use of VOTRIENT and simvastatin increases the incidence of ALT elevations. Across monotherapy studies with VOTRIENT, ALT >3 × ULN was reported in 126/895 (14%) of patients who did not use statins, compared with 11/41 (27%) of patients who had concomitant use of simvastatin. If a patient receiving concomitant simvastatin develops ALT elevations, follow dosing guidelines for VOTRIENT or consider alternatives to VOTRIENT [see Warnings and Precautions (5.1)]. Alternatively, consider discontinuing simvastatin [see Warnings and Precautions (5.1)]. Insufficient data are available to assess the risk of concomitant administration of alternative statins and VOTRIENT.

7.5 Drugs That Raise Gastric pH

In a drug interaction trial in patients with solid tumors, concomitant administration of pazopanib with esomeprazole, a proton pump inhibitor (PPI), decreased the exposure of pazopanib by approximately 40% (AUC and C_{max}). There-fore, concomitant use of VOTRIENT with drugs that raise gastric pH should be avoided. If such drugs are needed, short-acting antacids should be considered in place of PPIs and H2 receptor antagonists. Separate antacid and pazopanib dosing by several hours to avoid a reduction in pazopanib exposure [see Clinical Pharmacology (12.3)].

8 USE IN SPECIFIC POPULATIONS

8.1 Pregnancy

Pregnancy Category D [see Warnings and Precautions (5.17)].

VOTRIENT can cause fetal harm when administered to a pregnant woman. There are no adequate and well-controlled studies of VOTRIENT in pregnant women.

In pre-clinical studies in rats and rabbits, pazopanib was teratogenic, embryotoxic, fetotoxic, and abortifacient. Administration of pazopanib to pregnant rats during organogenesis at a dose level of ≥3 mg/kg/day (approximately 0.1 times the human clinical exposure based on AUC) resulted in teratogenic effects including cardiovascular malformations (retroesophageal subclavian artery, missing innominate artery, changes in the aortic arch) and incomplete or absent ossification. In addition, there was reduced fetal body weight, and pre- and post-implantation embryolethality in rats administered pazopanib at doses ≥3 mg/kg/day. In rabbits, maternal toxicity (reduced food consumption, increased post-implantation loss, and abortion) was observed at doses ≥30 mg/kg/day (approximately 0.007 times the human clinical exposure). In addition, severe maternal body weight loss and 100% litter loss were observed at doses ≥100 mg/kg/day (0.02 times the human clinical exposure), while fetal weight was reduced at doses ≥3 mg/kg/day (AUC not calculated).

If this drug is used during pregnancy, or if the patient becomes pregnant while taking this drug, the patient should be apprised of the potential hazard to the fetus. Women of childbearing potential should be advised to avoid becoming pregnant while taking VOTRIENT.

8.3 Nursing Mothers

It is not known whether this drug is excreted in human milk. Because many drugs are excreted in human milk and because of the potential for serious adverse reactions in nursing infants from VOTRIENT, a decision should be made whether to discontinue nursing or to discontinue the drug, taking into account the importance of the drug to the mother.

8.4 Pediatric Use

The safety and effectiveness of VOTRIENT in pediatric patients have not been established.

In rats, weaning occurs at day 21 postpartum which approximately equates to a human pediatric age of 2 years. In a juvenile animal toxicology study performed in rats, when animals were dosed from day 9 through day 14 postpartum (pre-weaning), pazopanib caused abnormal organ growth/maturation in the kidney, lung, liver, and heart at approximately 0.1 times the clinical exposure, based on AUC in adult patients receiving VOTRIENT. At approximately 0.4 times the clinical exposure (based on the AUC in adult patients), pazopanib administration resulted in mortality.

In repeat-dose toxicology studies in rats including 4-week, 13-week, and 26-week administration, toxicities in bone, teeth, and nail beds were observed at doses ≥3 mg/kg/day (approximately 0.07 times the human clinical exposure based on AUC). Doses of 300 mg/kg/day (approximately 0.8 times the human clinical exposure based on AUC) were not tolerated in 13- and 26-week studies and animals required dose reductions due to body weight loss and morbidity. Hypertrophy of epiphyseal growth plates, nail abnormalities (including broken, overgrown, or absent nails) and tooth abnormalities in growing incisor teeth (including excessively long, brittle, broken and missing teeth, and dentine and enamel degeneration and thinning) were observed in rats at doses ≥30 mg/kg/day (approximately 0.35 times the human clinical exposure based on AUC) at 26 weeks, with the onset of tooth and nail bed alterations noted clinically after 4 to 6 weeks. Similar findings were noted in repeat-dose studies in juvenile rats dosed with pazopanib beginning day 21 postpartum (post-weaning). In the post-weaning animals, the occurrence of changes in teeth and bones occurred earlier and with greater severity than in older animals. There was evidence of tooth degeneration and decreased bone growth at doses ≥30 mg/kg (approximately 0.1 to 0.2 times the AUC in human adults at the clinically recommended dose). Pazopanib exposure in juvenile rats was lower than that seen at the same dose levels in adult animals, based on comparative AUC values. At pazopanib doses approximately 0.5 to 0.7 times the exposure in adult patients at the clinically recommended dose, decreased bone growth in juvenile rats persisted even after the end of the dosing period. Finally, despite lower pazopanib exposures than those reported in adult animals or adult humans, juvenile animals administered 300 mg/kg/dose pazopanib required dose reduction within 4 weeks of dosing initiation due to significant toxicity, although adult animals could tolerate this same dose for at least 3 times as long [see Warnings and Precautions (5.16)].

8.5 Geriatric Use

In clinical trials with VOTRIENT for the treatment of RCC, 33% (196/582) of patients were aged ≥65 years. No overall differences in safety or effectiveness of VOTRIENT were observed between these patients and younger patients. However, patients >60 years of age may be at greater risk for an ALT >3 × ULN. In the STS trials, 24% (93/382) of patients were aged ≥65 years. Patients ≥65 years had increased Grade 3 or 4 fatigue (19% versus 12% for <65), hypertension (10% versus 6%), decreased appetite (11% versus 2%), and ALT (3% versus 2%) or AST elevations (4% versus 1%). Other reported clinical experience has not identified differences in responses between elderly and younger patients, but greater sensitivity of some older individuals cannot be ruled out.

8.6 Hepatic Impairment

In clinical studies for VOTRIENT, patients with total bilirubin ≤1.5 × ULN and AST and ALT ≤2 × ULN were included [see Warnings and Precautions (5.1)].

An analysis of data from a pharmacokinetic study of pazopanib in patients with varying degrees of hepatic dysfunction suggested that no dose adjustment is required in patients with mild hepatic impairment [either total bilirubin within normal limit (WNL) with ALT >ULN or bilirubin >1 × to 1.5 × ULN regardless of the ALT value]. The maximum tolerated dose in patients with moderate hepatic impairment (total bilirubin >1.5 × to 3 × ULN regardless of the ALT value) was 200 mg per day (N = 11). The median steady-state C_{max} and $AUC_{(0-24)}$ achieved at this dose was approximately 40% and 29%, respectively, of that seen in patients with normal hepatic function at the recommended daily dose of 800 mg. The maximum dose explored in patients with severe hepatic impairment (total bilirubin >3 × ULN regardless of the ALT value) was 200 mg per day (N = 14). This dose was not well tolerated. Median exposures achieved at this dose were approximately 18% and 15% of those seen in patients with normal liver function at the recommended daily dose of 800 mg. Therefore, VOTRIENT is not recommended in these patients [see Clinical Pharmacology (12.3)].

8.7 Renal Impairment

Patients with renal cell cancer and mild/moderate renal impairment (creatinine clearance ≥30 mL/min) were included in clinical trials for VOTRIENT.

There are no clinical or pharmacokinetic data in patients with severe renal impairment or in patients undergoing peritoneal dialysis or hemodialysis. However, renal impairment is unlikely to significantly affect the pharmacokinetics of pazopanib since <4% of a radiolabeled oral dose was recovered in the urine. In a population pharmacokinetic analysis using 408 patients with various cancers, creatinine clearance (30-150 mL/min) did not influence clearance of pazopanib. Therefore, renal impairment is not expected to influence pazopanib exposure, and dose adjustment is not necessary.

10 OVERDOSAGE

Pazopanib doses up to 2,000 mg have been evaluated in clinical trials. Dose-limiting toxicity (Grade 3 fatigue) and Grade 3 hypertension were each observed in 1 of 3 patients dosed at 2,000 mg daily and 1,000 mg daily, respectively.

Treatment of overdose with VOTRIENT should consist of general supportive measures. There is no specific antidote for overdosage of VOTRIENT.

Hemodialysis is not expected to enhance the elimination of VOTRIENT because pazopanib is not significantly renally excreted and is highly bound to plasma proteins.

11 DESCRIPTION

VOTRIENT (pazopanib) is a tyrosine kinase inhibitor (TKI). Pazopanib is presented as the hydrochloride salt, with the chemical name 5-[[4-[(2,3-dimethyl-2H-indazol-6-yl)methyl]amino]-2-pyrimidinyl]amino]-2-methylbenzenesulfonamide monohydrochloride. It has the molecular formula $C_{21}H_{23}N_7O_2S \cdot HCl$ and a molecular weight of 473.99. Pazopanib hydrochloride has the following chemical structure:

Pazopanib hydrochloride is a white to slightly yellow solid. It is very slightly soluble at pH 1 and practically insoluble above pH 4 in aqueous media.

Tablets of VOTRIENT are for oral administration. Each 200 mg tablet of VOTRIENT contains 216.7 mg of pazopanib hydrochloride, equivalent to 200 mg of pazopanib free base.

The inactive ingredients of VOTRIENT are: **Tablet Core:** Magnesium stearate, microcrystalline cellulose, povidone, sodium starch glycolate. **Coating:** Gray film-coat: Hypromellose, iron oxide black, macrogol/polyethylene glycol 400 (PEG 400), polysorbate 80, titanium dioxide.

12 CLINICAL PHARMACOLOGY

12.1 Mechanism of Action

Pazopanib is a multi-tyrosine kinase inhibitor of vascular endothelial growth factor receptor (VEGFR)-1, VEGFR-2, VEGFR-3, platelet-derived growth factor receptor (PDGFR)-α and -β, fibroblast growth factor receptor (FGFR)-1 and -3, cytokine receptor (Kit), interleukin-2 receptor inducible T-cell kinase (Itk), leukocyte-specific protein tyrosine kinase (Lck), and transmembrane glycoprotein receptor tyrosine kinase (c-Fms). In vitro, pazopanib inhibited ligand-induced autophosphorylation of VEGFR-2, Kit and PDGFR-β receptors. In vivo, pazopanib inhibited VEGF-induced VEGFR-2 phosphorylation in mouse lungs, angiogenesis in a mouse model, and the growth of some human tumor xenografts in mice.

12.2 Pharmacodynamics

Increases in blood pressure have been observed and are related to steady-state trough plasma pazopanib concentrations.

The QT prolongation potential of pazopanib was assessed in a randomized, blinded, parallel trial (N = 96) using moxifloxacin as a positive control. Pazopanib 800 mg was dosed under fasting conditions on Days 2 to 8 and 1,600 mg was dosed on Day 9 after a meal in order to increase exposure to

Table 4. Selected Laboratory Abnormalities Occurring in >10% of Patients With STS who Received VOTRIENT and More Commonly (≥5%) in Patients who Received VOTRIENT Versus Placebo

	VOTRIENT			Placebo		
	(N = 240)			(N = 123)		
Parameters	All Grades[a]	Grade 3	Grade 4	All Grades[a]	Grade 3	Grade 4
	%	%	%	%	%	%
Hematologic						
Leukopenia	44	1	0	15	0	0
Lymphocytopenia	43	10	0	36	9	2
Thrombocytopenia	36	3	1	6	0	0
Neutropenia	33	4	0	7	0	0
Chemistry						
AST increased	51	5	3	22	2	0
ALT increased	46	8	2	18	2	1
Glucose increased	45	<1	0	35	0	0
Albumin decreased	34	1	0	21	0	0
Alkaline phosphatase increased	32	3	0	23	1	0
Sodium decreased	31	4	0	20	3	0
Total bilirubin increased	29	1	0	7	2	0
Potassium increased	16	1	0	11	0	0

[a] National Cancer Institute Common Terminology Criteria for Adverse Events, version 3.

Table 5. Efficacy Results in RCC Patients by Independent Assessment

Endpoint/Trial Population	VOTRIENT	Placebo	HR (95% CI)
PFS			
Overall ITT	N = 290	N = 145	
Median (months)	9.2	4.2	0.46[a] (0.34, 0.62)
Treatment-naïve subgroup	N = 155 (53%)	N = 78 (54%)	
Median (months)	11.1	2.8	0.40 (0.27, 0.60)
Cytokine pre-treated subgroup	N = 135 (47%)	N = 67 (46%)	
Median (months)	7.4	4.2	0.54 (0.35, 0.84)
Response Rate (CR + PR)	N = 290	N = 145	
% (95% CI)	30 (25.1, 35.6)	3 (0.5, 6.4)	—
Duration of response			
Median (weeks) (95% CI)	58.7 (52.1, 68.1)	_b	

HR = Hazard Ratio; ITT = Intent to Treat; PFS = Progression-free Survival; CR = Complete Response; PR = Partial Response
[a] P value <0.001
[b] There were only 5 objective responses.

pazopanib and its metabolites. No large changes (i.e., >20 msec) in QTc interval following the treatment of pazopanib were detected in this QT trial. The trial was not able to exclude small changes (<10 msec) in QTc interval, because assay sensitivity below this threshold (<10 msec) was not established in this trial [see Warnings and Precautions (5.2)].

12.3 Pharmacokinetics

Absorption: Pazopanib is absorbed orally with median time to achieve peak concentrations of 2 to 4 hours after the dose. Daily dosing at 800 mg results in geometric mean AUC and C_{max} of 1,037 mcg•hr/mL and 58.1 mcg/mL (equivalent to 132 μM), respectively. There was no consistent increase in AUC or C_{max} at pazopanib doses above 800 mg. Administration of a single pazopanib 400 mg crushed tablet increased $AUC_{(0-72)}$ by 46% and C_{max} by approximately 2 fold and decreased t_{max} by approximately 2 hours compared to administration of the whole tablet. These results indicate that the bioavailability and the rate of pazopanib oral absorption are increased after administration of the crushed tablet relative to administration of the whole tablet. Therefore, due to this potential for increased exposure, tablets of VOTRIENT should not be crushed.

Systemic exposure to pazopanib is increased when administered with food. Administration of pazopanib with a high-fat or low-fat meal results in an approximately 2 fold increase in AUC and C_{max}. Therefore, pazopanib should be administered at least 1 hour before or 2 hours after a meal [see Dosage and Administration (2.1)].

Distribution: Binding of pazopanib to human plasma protein in vivo was greater than 99% with no concentration dependence over the range of 10 to 100 mcg/mL. In vitro studies suggest that pazopanib is a substrate for P-glycoprotein (Pgp) and breast cancer resistant protein (BCRP).

Metabolism: In vitro studies demonstrated that pazopanib is metabolized by CYP3A4 with a minor contribution from CYP1A2 and CYP2C8.

Elimination: Pazopanib has a mean half-life of 30.9 hours after administration of the recommended dose of 800 mg. Elimination is primarily via feces with renal elimination accounting for <4% of the administered dose.

Hepatic Impairment: Mild hepatic impairment was defined as either total bilirubin WNL with ALT >ULN or bilirubin >1 × to 1.5 × ULN regardless of the ALT value. The median steady-state pazopanib C_{max} and $AUC_{(0-24)}$ after a once daily dose of 800 mg/day in patients (N = 12) with mild impairment were 34 mcg/mL (range 11 to 104) and 774 mcg•hr/mL (range 215 to 2,034), respectively. These were in a similar range as the median steady-state pazopanib C_{max} and $AUC_{(0-24)}$ in patients (N = 18) with no hepatic impairment (52 mcg/mL, range 17 to 86 and 888 mcg•hr/mL, range 346 to 1,482, respectively) [see Dosage and Administration (2.2)].

Table 6. Efficacy Results in STS Patients by Independent Assessment

Endpoint/Trial Population	VOTRIENT	Placebo	HR (95% CI)
PFS			
Overall ITT	N = 246	N = 123	0.35[a]
Median (months)	4.6	1.6	(0.26, 0.48)
Leiomyosarcoma subgroup	N = 109	N = 49	0.37
Median (months)	4.6	1.9	(0.23, 0.60)
Synovial sarcoma subgroup	N = 25	N = 13	0.43
Median (months)	4.1	0.9	(0.19, 0.98)
'Other soft tissue sarcoma' subgroup	N = 112	N = 61	0.39
Median (months)	4.6	1.0	(0.25, 0.60)
Response Rate (CR + PR)			
% (95% CI)	4 (2.3, 7.9)[b]	0 (0.0, 3.0)	–
Duration of response			
Median (months) (95% CI)	9.0 (3.9, 9.2)		

HR = Hazard Ratio; ITT = Intent to Treat; PFS = Progression-free Survival; CR = Complete Response; PR = Partial Response
[a] P value <0.001
[b] There were 11 partial responses and 0 complete responses.

Moderate hepatic impairment was defined as total bilirubin >1.5 × to 3 × ULN regardless of the ALT value. The maximum tolerated pazopanib dose in patients with moderate impairment was 200 mg once daily. The median (N = 11) steady-state C_{max} with that regimen was 22 mcg/mL (range 4.2 to 33), and the median $AUC_{(0-24)}$ was 257 mcg•hr/mL (range 66 to 488). These values were approximately 43% and 29% of the corresponding median values after administration of 800 mg once daily in patients with normal hepatic function (N = 18) [see Dosage and Administration (2.2)].
Severe hepatic impairment was defined as total bilirubin >3 × ULN regardless of the ALT value. Median exposures in patients with severe hepatic impairment receiving 200 mg once daily (N = 14) were unexpectedly lower than those observed in patients with moderate hepatic impairment receiving 200 mg once daily. The median steady-state C_{max} was 9.4 mcg/mL (range 2.4 to 24), and the median $AUC_{(0-24)}$ was 131 mcg•hr/mL (range 47 to 473). These values were approximately 18% and 15% of the corresponding median values after administration of 800 mg once daily in patients with normal hepatic function. Despite the observed concentrations, the dose of 200 mg was not well tolerated in patients with severe hepatic impairment. Use of VOTRIENT is not recommended in patients with severe hepatic impairment [see Use in Specific Populations (8.6)].
Drug Interactions: Coadministration of multiple doses of oral pazopanib 400 mg with multiple doses of oral ketoconazole 400 mg (strong CYP3A4/P-gp inhibitor) resulted in a 1.7 fold increase in the $AUC_{(0-24)}$ and a 1.5 fold increase in the C_{max} of pazopanib compared to when pazopanib was administered alone. Concurrent administration of a single dose of pazopanib eye drops with ketoconazole in healthy volunteers resulted in a 2 fold and 1.5 fold increase in mean $AUC_{(0-t)}$ and C_{max} values, respectively [see Dosage and Administration (2.2) and Drug Interactions (7.1)].
Administration of 1,500 mg lapatinib, a substrate and weak inhibitor of CYP3A4, Pgp, and BCRP, with 800 mg pazopanib resulted in an approximately 50% to 60% increase in mean pazopanib $AUC_{(0-24)}$ and C_{max} compared to administration of 800 mg pazopanib alone.
In vitro studies with human liver microsomes showed that pazopanib inhibited the activities of CYP enzymes 1A2, 3A4, 2B6, 2C8, 2C9, 2C19, 2D6, and 2E1. Potential induction of human CYP3A4 was demonstrated in an in vitro human PXR assay. Clinical pharmacology studies, using pazopanib 800 mg once daily, have demonstrated that pazopanib does not have a clinically relevant effect on the pharmacokinetics of caffeine (CYP1A2 probe substrate), warfarin (CYP2C9 probe substrate), or omeprazole (CYP2C19 probe substrate) in cancer patients. Pazopanib resulted in an increase of approximately 30% in the mean AUC and C_{max} of midazolam (CYP3A4 probe substrate) and increases of 33% to 64% in the ratio of dextromethorphan to dextrorphan concentrations in the urine after oral administration of dextromethorphan (CYP2D6 probe substrate). Coadministration of pazopanib 800 mg once daily and paclitaxel 80 mg/m^2 (CYP3A4 and CYP2C8 substrate) once weekly resulted in a mean increase of 26% and 31% in paclitaxel AUC and C_{max}, respectively [see Drug Interactions (7.3)].
Pazopanib exhibits pH dependent solubility. In a drug interaction trial in patients with solid tumors, concomitant administration of pazopanib with esomeprazole, a PPI, decreased the exposure of pazopanib by approximately 40% (AUC and C_{max}).
In vitro studies also showed that pazopanib inhibits UGT1A1 and OATP1B1 with IC50s of 1.2 and 0.79 μM, respectively. Pazopanib may increase concentrations of drugs eliminated by UGT1A1 and OATP1B1.

12.5   Pharmacogenomics
Pazopanib can increase serum total bilirubin levels [see Warnings and Precautions (5.1)]. In vitro studies showed that pazopanib inhibits UGT1A1, which glucuronidates bilirubin for elimination. A pooled pharmacogenetic analysis of 236 Caucasian patients evaluated the TA repeat polymorphism of UGT1A1 and its potential association with hyperbilirubinemia during pazopanib treatment. In this analysis, the (TA)7/(TA)7 genotype (UGT1A1*28/*28) (underlying genetic susceptibility to Gilbert's syndrome) was associated with a statistically significant increase in the incidence of hyperbilirubinemia relative to the (TA)6/(TA)6 and (TA)6/(TA)7 genotypes.

13   NONCLINICAL TOXICOLOGY
13.1   Carcinogenesis, Mutagenesis, Impairment of Fertility
Carcinogenicity studies with pazopanib have not been conducted. However, in a 13-week study in mice, proliferative lesions in the liver including eosinophilic foci in 2 females and a single case of adenoma in another female was observed at doses of 1,000 mg/kg/day (approximately 2.5 times the human clinical exposure based on AUC).
Pazopanib did not induce mutations in the microbial mutagenesis (Ames) assay and was not clastogenic in both the in vitro cytogenetic assay using primary human lymphocytes and in the in vivo rat micronucleus assay.
Pazopanib may impair fertility in humans. In female rats, reduced fertility including increased pre-implantation loss and early resorptions were noted at dosages ≥30 mg/kg/day (approximately 0.4 times the human clinical exposure based on AUC). Total litter resorption was seen at 300 mg/kg/day (approximately 0.8 times the human clinical exposure based on AUC). Post-implantation loss, embryolethality, and decreased fetal body weight were noted in females administered doses ≥10 mg/kg/day (approximately 0.3 times the human clinical exposure based on AUC). Decreased corpora lutea and increased cysts were noted in mice given ≥100 mg/kg/day for 13 weeks and ovarian atrophy was noted in rats given ≥300 mg/kg/day for 26 weeks (approximately 1.3 and 0.85 times the human clinical exposure based on AUC, respectively). Decreased corpora lutea was also noted in monkeys given 500 mg/kg/day for up to 34 weeks (approximately 0.4 times the human clinical exposure based on AUC).
Pazopanib did not affect mating or fertility in male rats. However, there were reductions in sperm production rates and testicular sperm concentrations at doses ≥3 mg/kg/day, epididymal sperm concentrations at doses ≥30 mg/kg/day, and sperm motility at ≥100 mg/kg/day following 15 weeks of dosing. Following 15 and 26 weeks of dosing, there were decreased testicular and epididymal weights at doses of ≥30 mg/kg/day (approximately 0.35 times the human clinical exposure based on AUC); atrophy and degeneration of the testes with aspermia, hypospermia and cribiform change in the epididymis was also observed at this dose in the 6-month toxicity studies in male rats.

14   CLINICAL STUDIES
14.1   Renal Cell Carcinoma
The safety and efficacy of VOTRIENT in renal cell carcinoma (RCC) were evaluated in a randomized, double-blind, placebo-controlled, multicenter, Phase 3 trial. Patients (N = 435) with locally advanced and/or metastatic RCC who had received either no prior therapy or one prior cytokine-based systemic therapy were randomized (2:1) to receive VOTRIENT 800 mg once daily or placebo once daily. The primary objective of the trial was to evaluate and compare the 2 treatment arms for progression-free survival (PFS); the secondary endpoints included overall survival (OS), overall response rate (RR), and duration of response.

Of the total of 435 patients enrolled in this trial, 233 patients had no prior systemic therapy (treatment-naïve subgroup) and 202 patients received one prior IL-2 or INFα-based therapy (cytokine-pretreated subgroup). The baseline demographic and disease characteristics were balanced between the VOTRIENT and placebo arms. The majority of patients were male (71%) with a median age of 59 years. Eighty-six percent of patients were Caucasian, 14% were Asian, and less than 1% were other. Forty-two percent were ECOG performance status 0 and 58% were ECOG performance status 1. All patients had clear cell histology (90%) or predominantly clear cell histology (10%). Approximately 50% of all patients had 3 or more organs involved with metastatic disease. The most common metastatic sites at baseline were lung (74%), lymph nodes (56%), bone (27%), and liver (25%).
A similar proportion of patients in each arm were treatment-naïve and cytokine-pretreated (see Table 5). In the cytokine-pretreated subgroup, the majority (75%) had received interferon-based treatment. Similar proportions of patients in each arm had prior nephrectomy (89% and 88% for VOTRIENT and placebo, respectively).
The analysis of the primary endpoint PFS was based on disease assessment by independent radiological review in the entire trial population. Efficacy results are presented in Table 5 and Figure 1.
[See table 5 at top of previous page]

Figure 1. Kaplan-Meier Curve for Progression-Free Survival in RCC by Independent Assessment for the Overall Population (Treatment-Naïve and Cytokine Pre-Treated Populations)

At the protocol-specified final analysis of OS, the median OS was 22.9 months for patients randomized to VOTRIENT and 20.5 months for the placebo arm [HR = 0.91 (95% CI: 0.71, 1.16)]. The median OS for the placebo arm includes 79 patients (54%) who discontinued placebo treatment because of disease progression and crossed over to treatment with VOTRIENT. In the placebo arm, 95 (66%) patients received at least one systemic anti-cancer treatment after progression compared to 88 (30%) patients randomized to VOTRIENT.
14.2   Soft Tissue Sarcoma
The safety and efficacy of VOTRIENT in patients with STS were evaluated in a randomized, double-blind, placebo-controlled, multicenter trial. Patients (N = 369) with metastatic STS who had received prior chemotherapy, including anthracycline treatment, or were unsuited for such therapy, were randomized (2:1) to receive VOTRIENT 800 mg once daily or placebo. Patients with gastrointestinal stromal tumors (GIST) or adipocytic sarcoma were excluded from the trial. Randomization was stratified by the factors of WHO performance status (WHO PS) 0 or 1 at baseline and the number of lines of prior systemic therapy for advanced disease (0 or 1 versus 2+). Progression-free survival (PFS) was assessed by independent radiological review. Other efficacy endpoints included overall survival (OS), overall response rate, and duration of response.
The majority of patients were female (59%) with a median age of 55 years. Seventy-two percent of patients were Caucasian, 22% were Asian, and 6% were other. Forty-three percent of patients had leiomyosarcoma, 10% had synovial sarcoma, and 47% had other soft tissue sarcomas. Fifty-six percent of patients had received 2 or more lines of prior systemic therapy and 44% had received 0 or 1 lines of prior systemic therapy. The median duration of treatment was 4.5 months for patients on the pazopanib arm and 1.9 months for patients on the placebo arm.
Efficacy results are presented in Table 6 and Figure 2.
[See table 6 above]
[See figure 2 at top of next column]
At the protocol-specified final analysis of OS, the median OS was 12.6 months for patients randomized to VOTRIENT and 10.7 months for the placebo arm [HR = 0.87 (95% CI: 0.67, 1.12)].

16   HOW SUPPLIED/STORAGE AND HANDLING
The 200 mg tablets of VOTRIENT are modified capsule-shaped, gray, film-coated with GS JT debossed on one side and are available in:

Figure 2. Kaplan-Meier Curve for Progression-Free Survival in STS by Independent Assessment for the Overall Population

Bottles of 120 tablets: NDC 0173-0804-09
Store at room temperature between 20°C and 25°C (68°F to 77°F); excursions permitted to 15°C to 30°C (59°F to 86°F) [see USP Controlled Room Temperature].

17   PATIENT COUNSELING INFORMATION

The Medication Guide is contained in a separate leaflet that accompanies the product [see FDA-approved patient labeling (Medication Guide)].
However, inform patients of the following:

• Therapy with VOTRIENT may result in hepatobiliary laboratory abnormalities. Monitor serum liver tests (ALT, AST, and bilirubin) prior to initiation of VOTRIENT and at Weeks 3, 5, 7, and 9. Thereafter, monitor at Month 3 and at Month 4, and as clinically indicated. Inform patients that they should report signs and symptoms of liver dysfunction to their healthcare provider right away.

• Prolonged QT intervals and torsades de pointes have been observed. Patients should be advised that ECG monitoring may be performed. Patients should be advised to inform their physicians of concomitant medications.

• Cardiac dysfunction (such as CHF and LVEF decrease) has been observed in patients at risk (e.g., prior anthracycline therapy) particularly in association with development or worsening of hypertension. Patients should be advised to report hypertension or signs and symptoms of congestive heart failure.

• Serious hemorrhagic events have been reported. Patients should be advised to report unusual bleeding.

• Arterial thrombotic events have been reported. Patients should be advised to report signs or symptoms of an arterial thrombosis.

• Reports of pneumothorax and venous thromboembolic events including pulmonary embolus have been reported. Patients should be advised to report if new onset of dyspnea, chest pain, or localized limb edema occurs.

• Advise patients to inform their doctor if they have worsening of neurological function consistent with RPLS (headache, seizure, lethargy, confusion, blindness, and other visual and neurologic disturbances).

• Hypertension and hypertensive crisis have been reported. Patients should be advised to monitor blood pressure early in the course of therapy and frequently thereafter and report increases of blood pressure or symptoms such as blurred vision, confusion, severe headache, or nausea and vomiting.

• GI perforation or fistula has occurred. Advise patients to report signs and symptoms of a GI perforation or fistula.

• VEGFR inhibitors such as VOTRIENT may impair wound healing. Advise patients to stop VOTRIENT at least 7 days prior to a scheduled surgery.

• Hypothyroidism and proteinuria have been reported. Advise patients that thyroid function testing and urinalysis will be performed during treatment.

• Serious infections including some with fatal outcomes have been reported. Advise patients to promptly report any signs or symptoms of infection.

• Women of childbearing potential should be advised of the potential hazard to the fetus and to avoid becoming pregnant.

• Gastrointestinal adverse reactions such as diarrhea, nausea, and vomiting have been reported with VOTRIENT. Patients should be advised how to manage diarrhea and to notify their healthcare provider if moderate to severe diarrhea occurs.

• Patients should be advised to inform their healthcare providers of all concomitant medications, vitamins, or dietary and herbal supplements.

• Patients should be advised that depigmentation of the hair or skin may occur during treatment with VOTRIENT.

• Patients should be advised to take VOTRIENT without food (at least 1 hour before or 2 hours after a meal).

VOTRIENT is a registered trademark of the GSK group of companies.
GlaxoSmithKline
Research Triangle Park, NC 27709
©2014, the GSK group of companies. All rights reserved.
VTR:12PI

MEDICATION GUIDE
VOTRIENT® (VO-tree-ent)
(pazopanib)
tablets

Read the Medication Guide that comes with VOTRIENT before you start taking it and each time you get a refill. There may be new information. This Medication Guide does not take the place of talking with your healthcare provider about your medical condition or treatment.

What is the most important information I should know about VOTRIENT?
• **VOTRIENT can cause serious liver problems including death.** Your healthcare provider will do blood tests to check your liver before you start and while you take VOTRIENT.

Tell your healthcare provider right away if you get any of these signs of liver problems during treatment with VOTRIENT:
• yellowing of your skin or the whites of your eyes (jaundice)
• dark urine
• tiredness
• nausea or vomiting
• loss of appetite
• pain on the right side of your stomach area (abdomen)
• bruise easily

Your healthcare provider may need to prescribe a lower dose of VOTRIENT for you or tell you to stop taking VOTRIENT if you develop liver problems during treatment.

What is VOTRIENT?
VOTRIENT is a prescription medicine used to treat people with:
• advanced renal cell cancer (RCC)
• advanced soft tissue sarcoma (STS) who have received chemotherapy in the past
It is not known if VOTRIENT is effective in treating certain soft tissue sarcomas or certain gastrointestinal tumors.
It is not known if VOTRIENT is safe and effective in children under 18 years of age.

What should I tell my healthcare provider before taking VOTRIENT?

Before you take VOTRIENT, tell your healthcare provider if you:
• have or had liver problems. You may need a lower dose of VOTRIENT or your healthcare provider may prescribe a different medicine to treat your advanced renal cell cancer or advanced soft tissue sarcoma.
• have high blood pressure
• have heart problems or an irregular heartbeat including QT prolongation
• have a history of a stroke
• have headaches, seizures, or vision problems
• have coughed up blood in the last 6 months
• had bleeding of your stomach or intestines in the last 6 months
• have a history of a tear (perforation) in your stomach or intestine, or an abnormal connection between two parts of your gastrointestinal tract (fistula)
• have had blood clots in a vein or in the lung
• have thyroid problems
• had recent surgery (within the last 7 days) or are going to have surgery
• have any other medical conditions
• are pregnant or plan to become pregnant. VOTRIENT can harm your unborn baby. You should not become pregnant while you are taking VOTRIENT.
• are breastfeeding or plan to breastfeed. It is not known if VOTRIENT passes into your breast milk. You and your healthcare provider should decide if you will take VOTRIENT or breastfeed. You should not do both.

Tell your healthcare provider about all the medicines you take including prescription and non-prescription medicines, vitamins, and herbal supplements. VOTRIENT may affect the way other medicines work and other medicines may affect how VOTRIENT works.

Especially, tell your healthcare provider if you:
• take medicines that can affect how your liver enzymes work such as:
  ○ certain antibiotics (used to treat infections)
  ○ certain medicines used to treat HIV
  ○ certain medicines used to treat depression
  ○ medicines used to treat irregular heart beats
• take a medicine that contains simvastatin to treat high cholesterol levels
• take medicines that reduce stomach acid (e.g., esomeprazole)
• drink grapefruit juice
Ask your healthcare provider if you are not sure if your medicine is one that is listed above.
Know the medicines you take. Keep a list of them and show it to your healthcare provider and pharmacist when you get a new medicine.

How should I take VOTRIENT?
• Take VOTRIENT exactly as your healthcare provider tells you. Your healthcare provider will tell you how much VOTRIENT to take.
• Your healthcare provider may change your dose.
• Take VOTRIENT on an empty stomach, at least 1 hour before or 2 hours after food.
• Do not crush VOTRIENT tablets.
• Do not eat grapefruit or drink grapefruit juice during treatment with VOTRIENT. Grapefruit products may increase the amount of VOTRIENT in your body.
• If you miss a dose, take it as soon as you remember. Do not take it if it is close (within 12 hours) to your next dose. Just take the next dose at your regular time. Do not take more than 1 dose of VOTRIENT at a time.
• Your healthcare provider will test your urine, blood, and heart before you start and while you take VOTRIENT.
• Tell your healthcare provider if you plan to have surgery while taking VOTRIENT. You will need to stop taking VOTRIENT at least 7 days before surgery because VOTRIENT may affect healing after surgery.

What are the possible side effects of VOTRIENT?
VOTRIENT may cause serious side effects including:
• See "What is the most important information I should know about VOTRIENT?"
• **irregular or fast heartbeat or fainting**
• **heart failure.** This is a condition where your heart does not pump as well as it should and may cause you to have shortness of breath.
• **heart attack or stroke.** Heart attack and stroke can happen with VOTRIENT and may cause death.
  Symptoms may include: chest pain or pressure, pain in your arms, back, neck or jaw, shortness of breath, numbness or weakness on one side of your body, trouble talking, headache, or dizziness.
• **blood clots.** Blood clots may form in a vein, especially in your legs (deep vein thrombosis or DVT). Pieces of a blood clot may travel to your lungs (pulmonary embolism). This may be life-threatening and cause death.
  Symptoms may include: new chest pain, trouble breathing or shortness of breath that starts suddenly, leg pain, and swelling of the arms and hands, or legs and feet, a cool or pale arm or leg.
• **thrombotic microangiopathy (TMA) including thrombotic thrombocytopenia purpura (TTP) and hemolytic uremic syndrome (HUS):** TMA is a condition involving blood clots that can happen while taking VOTRIENT. TMA is accompanied by a decrease in red blood cells and cells that are involved in clotting. TMA may harm organs such as the brain and kidneys.
• **bleeding problems.** These bleeding problems may be severe and cause death.
  Symptoms may include: unusual bleeding, bruising, or wounds that do not heal.
• **tear in your stomach or intestinal wall (perforation) or an abnormal connection between two parts of your gastro-intestinal tract (fistula).**
  Symptoms may include: pain, swelling in your stomach-area, vomiting blood, and black sticky stools.
• **Reversible Posterior Leukoencephalopathy Syndrome (RPLS).** RPLS is a condition that can happen while taking VOTRIENT that may cause death.
  Symptoms may include: headaches, seizures, lack of energy, confusion, high blood pressure, loss of speech, blindness or changes in vision, and problems thinking.
• **high blood pressure. High blood pressure can happen with VOTRIENT, including a sudden and severe rise in blood pressure which may be life-threatening.** These blood pressure increases usually happen in the first several months of treatment. Your blood pressure should be well controlled before you start taking VOTRIENT. Your healthcare provider should begin checking your blood pressure within 1 week of you starting VOTRIENT and often during treatment to make sure that your blood pressure is well controlled.
Have someone call your healthcare provider or get medical help right away for you, if you get symptoms of a severe increase in blood pressure, including: severe chest pain, severe headache, blurred vision, confusion, nausea and vomiting, severe anxiety, shortness of breath, seizures, or you pass out (become unconscious).
• **thyroid problems.** Your healthcare provider should check you for this during treatment with VOTRIENT.
• **protein in your urine.** Your healthcare provider will check you for this problem. If there is too much protein in your urine, your healthcare provider may tell you to stop taking VOTRIENT.
• **serious infections.** Serious infections can happen with VOTRIENT and can cause death.
  Symptoms of an infection may include: fever, cold symptoms, such as runny nose or sore throat that do not go away, flu symptoms, such as cough, tiredness, and body aches, pain when urinating, cuts, scrapes or wounds that are red, warm, swollen or painful.
• **collapsed lung (pneumothorax).** A collapsed lung can happen with VOTRIENT. Air may get trapped in the space between your lung and chest wall. This may cause you to have shortness of breath.

Call your healthcare provider right away, if you have any of the symptoms listed above.

The most common side effects in people who take VOTRIENT include:

- diarrhea
- change in hair color
- nausea or vomiting
- loss of appetite

Other common side effects in people with advanced soft tissue sarcoma who take VOTRIENT include:

- feeling tired
- decreased weight
- tumor pain
- muscle or bone pain
- headache
- taste changes
- trouble breathing
- change in skin color

Tell your healthcare provider if you have any side effect that bothers you or that does not go away.

These are not all the possible side effects of VOTRIENT. For more information, ask your healthcare provider or pharmacist.

Call your doctor for medical advice about side effects. You may report side effects to FDA at 1-800-FDA-1088.

How should I store VOTRIENT tablets?
Store VOTRIENT at room temperature between 68°F and 77°F (20°C to 25°C).

Keep VOTRIENT and all medicines out of the reach of children.

General information about the safe and effective use of VOTRIENT.

Medicines are sometimes prescribed for purposes other than those listed in a Medication Guide. Do not use VOTRIENT for a condition for which it was not prescribed. Do not give VOTRIENT to other people even if they have the same symptoms that you have. It may harm them.

This Medication Guide summarizes the most important information about VOTRIENT. If you would like more information, talk with your healthcare provider. You can ask your pharmacist or healthcare provider for information about VOTRIENT that is written for healthcare professionals. For more information, go to www.VOTRIENT.com or call 1-888-825-5249.

What are the ingredients in VOTRIENT?
Active ingredient: pazopanib.
Inactive ingredients: Tablet core: Magnesium stearate, microcrystalline cellulose, povidone, sodium starch glycolate. **Coating:** Gray film-coat: Hypromellose, iron oxide black, macrogol/polyethylene glycol 400 (PEG 400), polysorbate 80, titanium dioxide.

This Medication Guide has been approved by the U.S. Food and Drug Administration.

GlaxoSmithKline
Research Triangle Park, NC 27709
Revised: June 2014
VOTRIENT is a registered trademark of the GSK group of companies.
©2014, the GSK group of companies. All rights reserved.
VTR:8MG

WELLBUTRIN   ℞
(bupropion hydrochloride)
Tablets, for oral use

HIGHLIGHTS OF PRESCRIBING INFORMATION
These highlights do not include all the information needed to use WELLBUTRIN safely and effectively. See full prescribing information for WELLBUTRIN.
WELLBUTRIN (bupropion hydrochloride) Tablets, for oral use
Initial U.S. Approval: 1985

——————RECENT MAJOR CHANGES——————

Warnings and Precautions (5.7)   07/2014

WARNING: SUICIDAL THOUGHTS AND BEHAVIORS; AND NEUROPSYCHIATRIC REACTIONS
See full prescribing information for complete boxed warning.
- Increased risk of suicidal thinking and behavior in children, adolescents, and young adults taking antidepressants. (5.1)
- Monitor for worsening and emergence of suicidal thoughts and behaviors. (5.1)
- Serious neuropsychiatric events have been reported in patients taking bupropion for smoking cessation. (5.2)

——————INDICATIONS AND USAGE——————
WELLBUTRIN is an aminoketone antidepressant, indicated for the treatment of major depressive disorder (MDD). (1)

——————DOSAGE AND ADMINISTRATION——————
- Starting dose: 200 mg per day given as 100 mg twice daily (2.1)
- General: Increase dose gradually to reduce seizure risk. (2.1, 5.3)
- After 3 days, may increase the dose to 300 mg per day, given as 100 mg 3 times daily at an interval of at least 6 hours between doses. (2.1)
- Usual target dose: 300 mg per day as 100 mg 3 times daily. (2.1)
- Maximum dose: 450 mg per day given as 150 mg 3 times daily. (2.1)
- Periodically reassess the dose and need for maintenance treatment. (2.1)
- Moderate to severe hepatic impairment: 75 mg once daily. (2.2, 8.7)
- Mild hepatic impairment: Consider reducing the dose and/or frequency of dosing. (2.2, 8.7)
- Renal impairment: Consider reducing the dose and/or frequency. (2.3, 8.6)

——————DOSAGE FORMS AND STRENGTHS——————
Tablets: 75 mg and 100 mg. (3)

——————CONTRAINDICATIONS——————
- Seizure disorder. (4, 5.3)
- Current or prior diagnosis of bulimia or anorexia nervosa. (4, 5.3)
- Abrupt discontinuation of alcohol, benzodiazepines, barbiturates, antiepileptic drugs. (4, 5.3)
- Monoamine Oxidase Inhibitors (MAOIs): Do not use MAOIs intended to treat psychiatric disorders with WELLBUTRIN or within 14 days of stopping treatment with WELLBUTRIN. Do not use WELLBUTRIN within 14 days of stopping an MAOI intended to treat psychiatric disorders. In addition, do not start WELLBUTRIN in a patient who is being treated with linezolid or intravenous methylene blue. (4, 7.6)
- Known hypersensitivity to bupropion or other ingredients of WELLBUTRIN. (4, 5.8)

——————WARNINGS AND PRECAUTIONS——————
- Seizure risk: The risk is dose-related. Can minimize risk by gradually increasing the dose and limiting daily dose to 450 mg. Discontinue if seizure occurs. (4, 5.3, 7.3)
- Hypertension: WELLBUTRIN can increase blood pressure. Monitor blood pressure before initiating treatment and periodically during treatment. (5.4)
- Activation of mania/hypomania: Screen patients for bipolar disorder and monitor for these symptoms. (5.5)
- Psychosis and other neuropsychiatric reactions: Instruct patients to contact a healthcare professional if such reactions occur. (5.6)
- Angle-closure glaucoma: Angle-closure glaucoma has occurred in patients with untreated anatomically narrow angles treated with antidepressants. (5.7)

——————ADVERSE REACTIONS——————
Most common adverse reactions (incidence ≥5% and ≥1% more than placebo rate) are: agitation, dry mouth, constipation, headache/migraine, nausea/vomiting, dizziness, excessive sweating, tremor, insomnia, blurred vision, tachycardia, confusion, rash, hostility, cardiac arrhythmias, and auditory disturbance. (6.1)

To report SUSPECTED ADVERSE REACTIONS, contact GlaxoSmithKline at 1-888-825-5249 or FDA at 1-800-FDA-1088 or www.fda.gov/medwatch

——————DRUG INTERACTIONS——————
- CYP2B6 inducers: Dose increase may be necessary if co-administered with CYP2B6 inducers (e.g., ritonavir, lopinavir, efavirenz, carbamazepine, phenobarbital, and phenytoin) based on clinical response, but should not exceed the maximum recommended dose. (7.1)
- Drugs metabolized by CYP2D6: Bupropion inhibits CYP2D6 and can increase concentrations of: antidepressants (e.g., venlafaxine, nortriptyline, imipramine, desipramine, paroxetine, fluoxetine, sertraline), antipsychotics (e.g., haloperidol, risperidone, thioridazine), beta-blockers (e.g., metoprolol), and Type 1C antiarrhythmics (e.g., propafenone, flecainide). Consider dose reduction when using with bupropion. (7.2)
- Drugs that lower seizure threshold: Dose WELLBUTRIN with caution. (5.3, 7.3)
- Dopaminergic drugs (levodopa and amantadine): CNS toxicity can occur when used concomitantly with WELLBUTRIN. (7.4)
- MAOIs: Increased risk of hypertensive reactions can occur when used concomitantly with WELLBUTRIN. (7.6)

- Drug-laboratory test interactions: WELLBUTRIN can cause false-positive urine test results for amphetamines. (7.7)

——————USE IN SPECIFIC POPULATIONS——————
- Pregnancy: Use only if benefit outweighs potential risk to the fetus. (8.1)

See 17 for PATIENT COUNSELING INFORMATION and Medication Guide

Revised: 07/2014

FULL PRESCRIBING INFORMATION: CONTENTS*
WARNING: SUICIDAL THOUGHTS AND BEHAVIORS; AND NEUROPSYCHIATRIC REACTIONS

FULL PRESCRIBING INFORMATION

WARNING: SUICIDAL THOUGHTS AND BEHAVIORS; AND NEUROPSYCHIATRIC REACTIONS
SUICIDALITY AND ANTIDEPRESSANT DRUGS
Antidepressants increased the risk of suicidal thoughts and behavior in children, adolescents, and young adults in short-term trials. These trials did not show an increase in the risk of suicidal thoughts and behavior with antidepressant use in subjects over age 24; there was a reduction in risk with antidepressant use in subjects aged 65 and older *[see Warnings and Precautions (5.1)]*.
In patients of all ages who are started on antidepressant therapy, monitor closely for worsening, and for

emergence of suicidal thoughts and behaviors. Advise families and caregivers of the need for close observation and communication with the prescriber *[see Warnings and Precautions (5.1)]*.

NEUROPSYCHIATRIC REACTIONS IN PATIENTS TAKING BUPROPION FOR SMOKING CESSATION
Serious neuropsychiatric reactions have occurred in patients taking bupropion for smoking cessation *[see Warnings and Precautions (5.2)]*. The majority of these reactions occurred during bupropion treatment, but some occurred in the context of discontinuing treatment. In many cases, a causal relationship to bupropion treatment is not certain, because depressed mood may be a symptom of nicotine withdrawal. However, some of the cases occurred in patients taking bupropion who continued to smoke. Although WELLBUTRIN® is not approved for smoking cessation, observe all patients for neuropsychiatric reactions. Instruct the patient to contact a healthcare provider if such reactions occur *[see Warnings and Precautions (5.2)]*.

1 INDICATIONS AND USAGE

WELLBUTRIN (bupropion hydrochloride)is indicated for the treatment of major depressive disorder(MDD), as defined by the Diagnostic and Statistical Manual (DSM).
The efficacy of WELLBUTRIN in the treatment of a major depressive episode was established in two 4-week controlled inpatient trials and one 6-week controlled outpatient trial of adult subjects with MDD *[see Clinical Studies (14)]*.

2 DOSAGE AND ADMINISTRATION

2.1 General Instructions for Use

To minimize the risk of seizure, increase the dose gradually *[see Warnings and Precautions (5.3)]*. Increases in dose should not exceed 100 mg per day in a 3–day period. WELLBUTRIN Tablets should be swallowed whole and not crushed, divided, or chewed. WELLBUTRIN may be taken with or without food.
The recommended starting dose is 200 mg per day, given as 100 mg twice daily. After 3 days of dosing, the dose may be increased to 300 mg per day, given as 100 mg 3 times daily, with at least 6 hours between successive doses. Dosing above 300 mg per day may be accomplished using the 75- or 100-mg tablets.
A maximum of 450 mg per day, given in divided doses of not more than 150 mg each, may be considered for patients who show no clinical improvement after several weeks of treatment at 300 mg per day. Administer the 100–mg tablet 4 times daily to not exceed the limit of 150 mg in a single dose.
It is generally agreed that acute episodes of depression require several months or longer of antidepressant drug treatment beyond the response in the acute episode. It is unknown whether the dose of WELLBUTRIN needed for maintenance treatment is identical to the dose that provided an initial response. Periodically reassess the need for maintenance treatment and the appropriate dose for such treatment.

2.2 Dose Adjustment in Patients With Hepatic Impairment

In patients with moderate to severe hepatic impairment (Child-Pugh score: 7 to 15), the maximum dose of WELLBUTRIN is 75 mg per day. In patients with mild hepatic impairment (Child-Pugh score: 5 to 6), consider reducing the dose and/or frequency of dosing *[see Use in Specific Populations (8.7), Clinical Pharmacology (12.3)]*.

2.3 Dose Adjustment in Patients With Renal Impairment

Consider reducing the dose and/or frequency of WELLBUTRIN in patients with renal impairment (Glomerular Filtration Rate <90 mL/min) *[see Use in Specific Populations (8.6), Clinical Pharmacology (12.3)]*.

2.4 Switching a Patient To or From a Monoamine Oxidase Inhibitor (MAOI) Antidepressant

At least 14 days should elapse between discontinuation of an MAOI intended to treat depression and initiation of therapy with WELLBUTRIN. Conversely, at least 14 days should be allowed after stopping WELLBUTRIN before starting an MAOI antidepressant *[see Contraindications (4), Drug Interactions (7.6)]*.

2.5 Use of WELLBUTRIN With Reversible MAOIs Such as Linezolid or Methylene Blue

Do not start WELLBUTRIN in a patient who is being treated with a reversible MAOI such as linezolid or intravenous methylene blue. Drug interactions can increase the risk of hypertensive reactions. In a patient who requires more urgent treatment of a psychiatric condition, non-pharmacological interventions, including hospitalization, should be considered *[see Contraindications (4), Drug Interactions (7.6)]*.
In some cases, a patient already receiving therapy with WELLBUTRIN may require urgent treatment with linezo-

lid or intravenous methylene blue. If acceptable alternatives to linezolid or intravenous methylene blue treatment are not available and the potential benefits of linezolid or intravenous methylene blue treatment are judged to outweigh the risks of hypertensive reactions in a particular patient, WELLBUTRIN should be stopped promptly, and linezolid or intravenous methylene blue can be administered. The patient should be monitored for 2 weeks or until 24 hours after the last dose of linezolid or intravenous methylene blue, whichever comes first. Therapy with WELLBUTRIN may be resumed 24 hours after the last dose of linezolid or intravenous methylene blue.
The risk of administering methylene blue by non-intravenous routes (such as oral tablets or by local injection) or in intravenous doses much lower than 1 mg/kg with WELLBUTRIN is unclear. The clinician should, nevertheless, be aware of the possibility of a drug interaction with such use *[see Contraindications (4), Drug Interactions (7.6)]*.

3 DOSAGE FORMS AND STRENGTHS

- 75 mg – yellow–gold, round, biconvex tablets printed with "WELLBUTRIN 75".
- 100 mg – red, round, biconvex tablets printed with "WELLBUTRIN 100".

4 CONTRAINDICATIONS

- WELLBUTRIN is contraindicated in patients with a seizure disorder.
- WELLBUTRIN is contraindicated in patients with a current or prior diagnosis of bulimia or anorexia nervosa as a higher incidence of seizures was observed in such patients treated with WELLBUTRIN *[see Warnings and Precautions (5.3)]*.
- WELLBUTRIN is contraindicated in patients undergoing abrupt discontinuation of alcohol, benzodiazepines, barbiturates, and antiepileptic drugs *[see Warnings and Precautions (5.3), Drug Interactions (7.3)]*.
- The use of MAOIs (intended to treat psychiatric disorders) concomitantly with WELLBUTRIN or within 14 days of discontinuing treatment with WELLBUTRIN is contraindicated. There is an increased risk of hypertensive reactions when WELLBUTRIN is used concomitantly with MAOIs. The use of WELLBUTRIN within 14 days of discontinuing treatment with an MAOI is also contraindicated. Starting WELLBUTRIN in a patient treated with reversible MAOIs such as linezolid or intravenous methylene blue is contraindicated *[see Dosage and Administration (2.4, 2.5), Warnings and Precautions (5.4), Drug Interactions (7.6)]*.
- WELLBUTRIN is contraindicated in patients with known hypersensitivity to bupropion or other ingredients of WELLBUTRIN. Anaphylactoid/anaphylactic reactions and Stevens-Johnson syndrome have been reported *[see Warnings and Precautions (5.8)]*.

5 WARNINGS AND PRECAUTIONS

5.1 Suicidal Thoughts and Behaviors in Children, Adolescents, and Young Adults

Patients with MDD, both adult and pediatric, may experience worsening of their depression and/or the emergence of suicidal ideation and behavior (suicidality) or unusual changes in behavior, whether or not they are taking antidepressant medications, and this risk may persist until significant remission occurs. Suicide is a known risk of depression and certain other psychiatric disorders, and these disorders themselves are the strongest predictors of suicide. There has been a long-standing concern that antidepressants may have a role in inducing worsening of depression and the emergence of suicidality in certain patients during the early phases of treatment.
Pooled analyses of short–term placebo–controlled trials of antidepressant drugs (selective serotonin reuptake inhibitors [SSRIs] and others) show that these drugs increase the risk of suicidal thinking and behavior (suicidality) in children, adolescents, and young adults (ages 18 to 24) with MDD and other psychiatric disorders. Short-term clinical trials did not show an increase in the risk of suicidality with antidepressants compared with placebo in adults beyond age 24; there was a reduction with antidepressants compared with placebo in adults aged 65 and older.
The pooled analyses of placebo-controlled trials in children and adolescents with MDD, obsessive compulsive disorder (OCD), or other psychiatric disorders included a total of 24 short–term trials of 9 antidepressant drugs in over 4,400 subjects. The pooled analyses of placebo–controlled trials in adults with MDD or other psychiatric disorders included a total of 295 short–term trials (median duration of 2 months) of 11 antidepressant drugs in over 77,000 subjects. There was considerable variation in risk of suicidality among drugs, but a tendency toward an increase in the younger subjects for almost all drugs studied. There were differences in absolute risk of suicidality across the different indications, with the highest incidence in MDD. The risk differences (drug vs. placebo), however, were relatively stable within age strata and across indications. These risk differ-

ences (drug-placebo difference in the number of cases of suicidality per 1,000 subjects treated) are provided in Table 1.

Table 1. Risk Differences in the Number of Suicidality Cases by Age Group in the Pooled Placebo-Controlled Trials of Antidepressants in Pediatric and Adult Subjects

Age Range	Drug-Placebo Difference in Number of Cases of Suicidality per 1,000 Subjects Treated
Increases Compared With Placebo	
<18	14 additional cases
18-24	5 additional cases
Decreases Compared With Placebo	
25-64	1 fewer case
≥65	6 fewer cases

No suicides occurred in any of the pediatric trials. There were suicides in the adult trials, but the number was not sufficient to reach any conclusion about drug effect on suicide.
It is unknown whether the suicidality risk extends to longer-term use, i.e., beyond several months. However, there is substantial evidence from placebo-controlled maintenance trials in adults with depression that the use of antidepressants can delay the recurrence of depression.
All patients being treated with antidepressants for any indication should be monitored appropriately and observed closely for clinical worsening, suicidality, and unusual changes in behavior, especially during the initial few months of a course of drug therapy, or at times of dose changes, either increases or decreases *[see Boxed Warning]*.
The following symptoms, anxiety, agitation, panic attacks, insomnia, irritability, hostility, aggressiveness, impulsivity, akathisia (psychomotor restlessness), hypomania, and mania, have been reported in adult and pediatric patients being treated with antidepressants for major depressive disorder as well as for other indications, both psychiatric and nonpsychiatric. Although a causal link between the emergence of such symptoms and either the worsening of depression and/or the emergence of suicidal impulses has not been established, there is concern that such symptoms may represent precursors to emerging suicidality.
Consideration should be given to changing the therapeutic regimen, including possibly discontinuing the medication, in patients whose depression is persistently worse, or who are experiencing emergent suicidality or symptoms that might be precursors to worsening depression or suicidality, especially if these symptoms are severe, abrupt in onset, or were not part of the patient's presenting symptoms.
Families and caregivers of patients being treated with antidepressants for MDD or other indications, both psychiatric and nonpsychiatric, should be alerted about the need to monitor patients for the emergence of agitation, irritability, unusual changes in behavior, and the other symptoms described above, as well as the emergence of suicidality, and to report such symptoms immediately to healthcare providers. Such monitoring should include daily observation by families and caregivers. Prescriptions for WELLBUTRIN should be written for the smallest quantity of tablets consistent with good patient management, in order to reduce the risk of overdose.

5.2 Neuropsychiatric Symptoms and Suicide Risk in Smoking Cessation Treatment

WELLBUTRIN is not approved for smoking cessation treatment; however, bupropion HCl sustained-release is approved for this use. Serious neuropsychiatric symptoms have been reported in patients taking bupropion for smoking cessation. These have included changes in mood (including depression and mania), psychosis, hallucinations, paranoia, delusions, homicidal ideation, hostility, agitation, aggression, anxiety, and panic, as well as suicidal ideation, suicide attempt, and completed suicide *[see Boxed Warning, Adverse Reactions (6.2)]*. Observe patients for the occurrence of neuropsychiatric reactions. Instruct patients to contact a healthcare professional if such reactions occur.
In many of these cases, a causal relationship to bupropion treatment is not certain, because depressed mood can be a symptom of nicotine withdrawal. However, some of the cases occurred in patients taking bupropion who continued to smoke.

5.3 Seizure

WELLBUTRIN can cause seizure. The risk of seizure is dose-related. The dose should not exceed 450 mg per day. Increase the dose gradually. Discontinue WELLBUTRIN and do not restart treatment if the patient experiences a seizure.
The risk of seizures is also related to patient factors, clinical situations, and concomitant medications that lower the sei-

zure threshold. Consider these risks before initiating treatment with WELLBUTRIN. WELLBUTRIN is contraindicated in patients with a seizure disorder, current or prior diagnosis of anorexia nervosa or bulimia, or undergoing abrupt discontinuation of alcohol, benzodiazepines, barbiturates, and antiepileptic drugs [see Contraindications (4), Drug Interactions (7.3)]. The following conditions can also increase the risk of seizure: severe head injury; arteriovenous malformation; CNS tumor or CNS infection; severe stroke; concomitant use of other medications that lower the seizure threshold (e.g., other bupropion products, antipsychotics, tricyclic antidepressants, theophylline, and systemic corticosteroids); metabolic disorders (e.g., hypoglycemia, hyponatremia, severe hepatic impairment, and hypoxia); use of illicit drugs (e.g., cocaine); or abuse or misuse of prescription drugs such as CNS stimulants. Additional predisposing conditions include diabetes mellitus treated with oral hypoglycemic drugs or insulin; use of anorectic drugs; and excessive use of alcohol, benzodiazepines, sedative/hypnotics, or opiates.

Incidence of Seizure With Bupropion Use: Bupropion is associated with seizures in approximately 0.4% (4/1,000) of patients treated at doses up to 450 mg per day. The estimated seizure incidence for WELLBUTRIN increases almost 10-fold between 450 and 600 mg per day.

The risk of seizure can be reduced if the dose of WELLBUTRIN does not exceed 450 mg per day, given as 150 mg 3 times daily, and the titration rate is gradual.

5.4 Hypertension

Treatment with WELLBUTRIN can result in elevated blood pressure and hypertension. Assess blood pressure before initiating treatment with WELLBUTRIN, and monitor periodically during treatment. The risk of hypertension is increased if WELLBUTRIN is used concomitantly with MAOIs or other drugs that increase dopaminergic or noradrenergic activity [see Contraindications (4)].

Data from a comparative trial of the sustained-release formulation of bupropion HCl, nicotine transdermal system (NTS), the combination of sustained-release bupropion plus NTS, and placebo as an aid to smoking cessation suggest a higher incidence of treatment-emergent hypertension in patients treated with the combination of sustained-release bupropion and NTS. In this trial, 6.1% of subjects treated with the combination of sustained-release bupropion and NTS had treatment–emergent hypertension compared to 2.5%, 1.6%, and 3.1% of subjects treated with sustained-release bupropion, NTS, and placebo, respectively. The majority of these subjects had evidence of pre-existing hypertension. Three subjects (1.2%) treated with the combination of sustained-release bupropion and NTS and 1 subject (0.4%) treated with NTS had study medication discontinued due to hypertension compared with none of the subjects treated with sustained-release bupropion or placebo. Monitoring of blood pressure is recommended in patients who receive the combination of bupropion and nicotine replacement.

In a clinical trial of bupropion immediate-release in MDD subjects with stable congestive heart failure (N = 36), bupropion was associated with an exacerbation of pre-existing hypertension in 2 subjects, leading to discontinuation of bupropion treatment. There are no controlled trials assessing the safety of bupropion in patients with a recent history of myocardial infarction or unstable cardiac disease.

5.5 Activation of Mania/Hypomania

Antidepressant treatment can precipitate a manic, mixed, or hypomanic manic episode. The risk appears to be increased in patients with bipolar disorder or who have risk factors for bipolar disorder. Prior to initiating WELLBUTRIN, screen patients for a history of bipolar disorder and the presence of risk factors for bipolar disorder (e.g., family history of bipolar disorder, suicide, or depression). WELLBUTRIN is not approved for use in treating bipolar depression.

5.6 Psychosis and Other Neuropsychiatric Reactions

Depressed patients treated with WELLBUTRIN have had a variety of neuropsychiatric signs and symptoms, including delusions, hallucinations, psychosis, concentration disturbance, paranoia, and confusion. Some of these patients had a diagnosis of bipolar disorder. In some cases, these symptoms abated upon dose reduction and/or withdrawal of treatment. Instruct patients to contact a healthcare professional if such reactions occur.

5.7 Angle-Closure Glaucoma

The pupillary dilation that occurs following use of many antidepressant drugs including WELLBUTRIN may trigger an angle-closure attack in a patient with anatomically narrow angles who does not have a patent iridectomy.

5.8 Hypersensitivity Reactions

Anaphylactoid/anaphylactic reactions have occurred during clinical trials with bupropion. Reactions have been characterized by pruritus, urticaria, angioedema, and dyspnea requiring medical treatment. In addition, there have been rare, spontaneous postmarketing reports of erythema multiforme, Stevens–Johnson syndrome, and anaphylactic shock associated with bupropion. Instruct patients to discontinue WELLBUTRIN and consult a healthcare provider if they develop an allergic or anaphylactoid/anaphylactic reaction (e.g., skin rash, pruritus, hives, chest pain, edema, and shortness of breath) during treatment.

There are reports of arthralgia, myalgia, fever with rash and other serum sickness-like symptoms suggestive of delayed hypersensitivity.

6 ADVERSE REACTIONS

The following adverse reactions are discussed in greater detail in other sections of the labeling:

- Suicidal thoughts and behaviors in adolescents and young adults [see Boxed Warning, Warnings and Precautions (5.1)]
- Neuropsychiatric symptoms and suicide risk in smoking cessation treatment [see Boxed Warning, Warnings and Precautions (5.2)]
- Seizure [see Warnings and Precautions (5.3)]
- Hypertension [see Warnings and Precautions (5.4)]
- Activation of mania or hypomania [see Warnings and Precautions (5.5)]
- Psychosis and other neuropsychiatric reactions [see Warnings and Precautions (5.6)]
- Angle-closure glaucoma [see Warnings and Precautions (5.7)]
- Hypersensitivity reactions [see Warnings and Precautions (5.8)]

6.1 Clinical Trials Experience

Because clinical trials are conducted under widely varying conditions, adverse reaction rates observed in the clinical trials of a drug cannot be directly compared with rates in the clinical trials of another drug and may not reflect the rates observed in clinical practice.

Adverse Reactions Leading to Discontinuation of Treatment: Adverse reactions were sufficiently troublesome to cause discontinuation of treatment with WELLBUTRIN in approximately 10% of the 2,400 subjects and healthy volunteers who participated in clinical trials during the product's initial development. The more common events causing discontinuation include neuropsychiatric disturbances (3.0%), primarily agitation and abnormalities in mental status; gastrointestinal disturbances (2.1%), primarily nausea and vomiting; neurological disturbances (1.7%), primarily seizures, headaches, and sleep disturbances; and dermatologic problems (1.4%), primarily rashes. It is important to note, however, that many of these events occurred at doses that exceed the recommended daily dose.

Commonly Observed Adverse Reactions: Adverse reactions commonly encountered in subjects treated with WELLBUTRIN are agitation, dry mouth, insomnia, headache/migraine, nausea/vomiting, constipation, tremor, dizziness, excessive sweating, blurred vision, tachycardia, confusion, rash, hostility, cardiac arrhythmia, and auditory disturbance.

Table 2 summarizes the adverse reactions that occurred in placebo-controlled trials at an incidence of at least 1% of subjects receiving WELLBUTRIN and more frequently in these subjects than in the placebo group.

Table 2. Adverse Reactions Reported by at Least 1% of Subjects and at a Greater Frequency Than Placebo in Controlled Clinical Trials

Adverse Reaction	WELLBUTRIN (n = 323) %	Placebo (n = 185) %
Cardiovascular		
Cardiac arrhythmias	5.3	4.3
Dizziness	22.3	16.2
Hypertension	4.3	1.6
Hypotension	2.5	2.2
Palpitations	3.7	2.2
Syncope	1.2	0.5
Tachycardia	10.8	8.6
Dermatologic		
Pruritus	2.2	0.0
Rash	8.0	6.5
Gastrointestinal		
Appetite increase	3.7	2.2
Constipation	26.0	17.3
Dyspepsia	3.1	2.2
Nausea/vomiting	22.9	18.9
Genitourinary		
Impotence	3.4	3.1
Menstrual complaints	4.7	1.1
Urinary frequency	2.5	2.2
Musculoskeletal		
Arthritis	3.1	2.7
Neurological		
Akathisia	1.5	1.1
Cutaneous temperature disturbance	1.9	1.6
Dry mouth	27.6	18.4
Excessive sweating	22.3	14.6
Headache/migraine	25.7	22.2
Impaired sleep quality	4.0	1.6
Insomnia	18.6	15.7
Sedation	19.8	19.5
Sensory disturbance	4.0	3.2
Tremor	21.1	7.6
Neuropsychiatric		
Agitation	31.9	22.2
Anxiety	3.1	1.1
Confusion	8.4	4.9
Decreased libido	3.1	1.6
Delusions	1.2	1.1
Euphoria	1.2	0.5
Hostility	5.6	3.8
Nonspecific		
Fever/chills	1.2	0.5
Special Senses		
Auditory disturbance	5.3	3.2
Blurred vision	14.6	10.3
Gustatory disturbance	3.1	1.1

Other Adverse Reactions Observed During the Clinical Development of WELLBUTRIN: The conditions and duration of exposure to WELLBUTRIN varied greatly, and a substantial proportion of the experience was gained in open and uncontrolled clinical settings. During this experience, numerous adverse events were reported; however, without appropriate controls, it is impossible to determine with certainty which events were or were not caused by WELLBUTRIN. The following enumeration is organized by organ system and describes events in terms of their relative frequency of reporting in the database.

The following definitions of frequency are used: Frequent adverse reactions are defined as those occurring in at least 1/100 subjects. Infrequent adverse reactions are those occurring in 1/100 to 1/1,000 subjects, while rare events are those occurring in less than 1/1,000 subjects.

Cardiovascular: Frequent was edema; infrequent were chest pain, electrocardiogram (ECG) abnormalities (premature beats and nonspecific ST–T changes), and shortness of breath/dyspnea; rare were flushing, and myocardial infarction.

Dermatologic: Infrequent was alopecia.

Endocrine: Infrequent was gynecomastia; rare was glycosuria.

Gastrointestinal: Infrequent were dysphagia, thirst disturbance, and liver damage/jaundice; rare was intestinal perforation.

Genitourinary: Frequent was nocturia; infrequent were vaginal irritation, testicular swelling, urinary tract infection, painful erection, and retarded ejaculation; rare were enuresis, and urinary incontinence.

Neurological: Frequent were ataxia/incoordination, seizure, myoclonus, dyskinesia, and dystonia; infrequent were mydriasis, vertigo, and dysarthria; rare were electroencephalogram (EEG) abnormality, and impaired attention.

Neuropsychiatric: Frequent were mania/hypomania, increased libido, hallucinations, decrease in sexual function, and depression; infrequent were memory impairment, depersonalization, psychosis, dysphoria, mood instability, paranoia, formal thought disorder, and frigidity; rare was suicidal ideation.

Oral Complaints: Frequent was stomatitis; infrequent were toothache, bruxism, gum irritation, and oral edema.

Respiratory: Infrequent were bronchitis and shortness of breath/dyspnea; rare was pulmonary embolism.

Special Senses: Infrequent was visual disturbance; rare was diplopia.

Nonspecific: Frequent were flu–like symptoms; infrequent was nonspecific pain; rare was overdose.

Altered Appetite and Weight: A weight loss of greater than 5 lbs occurred in 28% of subjects receiving WELLBUTRIN. This incidence is approximately double that seen in comparable subjects treated with tricyclics or placebo. Furthermore, while 35% of subjects receiving tricyclic antidepressants gained weight, only 9.4% of subjects treated with WELLBUTRIN did. Consequently, if weight loss is a major presenting sign of a patient's depressive illness, the anorectic and/or weight reducing potential of WELLBUTRIN should be considered.

6.2 Postmarketing Experience

The following adverse reactions have been identified during post-approval use of WELLBUTRIN and are not described elsewhere in the label. Because these reactions are reported voluntarily from a population of uncertain size, it is not always possible to reliably estimate their frequency or establish a causal relationship to drug exposure.

Body (General): Arthralgia, myalgia, and fever with rash and other symptoms suggestive of delayed hypersensitivity. These symptoms may resemble serum sickness [see Warnings and Precautions (5.8)].

Cardiovascular: Hypertension (in some cases severe), orthostatic hypotension, third degree heart block.

Endocrine: Syndrome of inappropriate antidiuretic hormone secretion, hyperglycemia, hypoglycemia.

Gastrointestinal: Esophagitis, hepatitis.

Hemic and Lymphatic: Ecchymosis, leukocytosis, leukopenia, thrombocytopenia. Altered PT and/or INR, infrequently associated with hemorrhagic or thrombotic complications, were observed when bupropion was coadministered with warfarin.

Musculoskeletal: Muscle rigidity/fever/rhabdomyolysis, muscle weakness.

Nervous System: Aggression, coma, completed suicide, delirium, dream abnormalities, paranoid ideation, paresthesia, restlessness, suicide attempt, unmasking of tardive dyskinesia.

Skin and Appendages: Stevens–Johnson syndrome, angioedema, exfoliative dermatitis, urticaria.

Special Senses: Tinnitus, increased intraocular pressure.

7 DRUG INTERACTIONS

7.1 Potential for Other Drugs to Affect WELLBUTRIN

Bupropion is primarily metabolized to hydroxybupropion by CYP2B6. Therefore, the potential exists for drug interactions between WELLBUTRIN and drugs that are inhibitors or inducers of CYP2B6.

Inhibitors of CYP2B6: *Ticlopidine and Clopidogrel:* Concomitant treatment with these drugs can increase bupropion exposure but decrease hydroxybupropion exposure. Based on clinical response, dosage adjustment of WELLBUTRIN may be necessary when coadministered with CYP2B6 inhibitors (e.g., ticlopidine or clopidogrel) [see Clinical Pharmacology (12.3)].

Inducers of CYP2B6: *Ritonavir, Lopinavir, and Efavirenz:* Concomitant treatment with these drugs can decrease bupropion and hydroxybupropion exposure. Dosage increase of WELLBUTRIN may be necessary when coadministered with ritonavir, lopinavir, or efavirenz [see Clinical Pharmacology (12.3)] but should not exceed the maximum recommended dose.

Carbamazepine, Phenobarbital, Phenytoin: While not systematically studied, these drugs may induce the metabolism of bupropion and may decrease bupropion exposure [see Clinical Pharmacology (12.3)]. If bupropion is used concomitantly with a CYP inducer, it may be necessary to increase the dose of bupropion, but the maximum recommended dose should not be exceeded.

7.2 Potential for WELLBUTRIN to Affect Other Drugs

Drugs Metabolized by CYP2D6: Bupropion and its metabolites (erythrohydrobupropion, threohydrobupropion, hydroxybupropion) are CYP2D6 inhibitors. Therefore, coadministration of WELLBUTRIN with drugs that are metabolized by CYP2D6 can increase the exposures of drugs that are substrates of CYP2D6. Such drugs include certain antidepressants (e.g., venlafaxine, nortriptyline, imipramine, desipramine, paroxetine, fluoxetine, and sertraline), antipsychotics (e.g., haloperidol, risperidone, thioridazine), beta-blockers (e.g., metoprolol), and Type 1C antiarrhythmics (e.g., propafenone and flecainide). When used concomitantly with WELLBUTRIN, it may be necessary to decrease the dose of these CYP2D6 substrates, particularly for drugs with a narrow therapeutic index.

Drugs that require metabolic activation by CYP2D6 to be effective (e.g., tamoxifen) theoretically could have reduced efficacy when administered concomitantly with inhibitors of CYP2D6 such as bupropion. Patients treated concomitantly with WELLBUTRIN and such drugs may require increased doses of the drug [see Clinical Pharmacology (12.3)].

7.3 Drugs That Lower Seizure Threshold

Use extreme caution when coadministering WELLBUTRIN with other drugs that lower seizure threshold (e.g., other bupropion products, antipsychotics, antidepressants, theophylline, or systemic corticosteroids). Use low initial doses and increase the dose gradually [see Contraindications (4), Warnings and Precautions (5.3)].

7.4 Dopaminergic Drugs (Levodopa and Amantadine)

Bupropion, levodopa, and amantadine have dopamine agonist effects. CNS toxicity has been reported when bupropion was coadministered with levodopa or amantadine. Adverse reactions have included restlessness, agitation, tremor, ataxia, gait disturbance, vertigo, and dizziness. It is presumed that the toxicity results from cumulative dopamine agonist effects. Use caution when administering WELLBUTRIN concomitantly with these drugs.

7.5 Use With Alcohol

In postmarketing experience, there have been rare reports of adverse neuropsychiatric events or reduced alcohol tolerance in patients who were drinking alcohol during treatment with WELLBUTRIN. The consumption of alcohol during treatment with WELLBUTRIN should be minimized or avoided.

7.6 MAO Inhibitors

Bupropion inhibits the reuptake of dopamine and norepinephrine. Concomitant use of MAOIs and bupropion is contraindicated because there is an increased risk of hypertensive reactions if bupropion is used concomitantly with MAOIs. Studies in animals demonstrate that the acute toxicity of bupropion is enhanced by the MAO inhibitor phenelzine. At least 14 days should elapse between discontinuation of an MAOI intended to treat depression and initiation of treatment with WELLBUTRIN. Conversely, at least 14 days should be allowed after stopping WELLBUTRIN before starting an MAOI antidepressant [see Dosage and Administration (2.4, 2.5), Contraindications (4)].

7.7 Drug-Laboratory Test Interactions

False-positive urine immunoassay screening tests for amphetamines have been reported in patients taking bupropion. This is due to lack of specificity of some screening tests. False-positive test results may result even following discontinuation of bupropion therapy. Confirmatory tests, such as gas chromatography/mass spectrometry, will distinguish bupropion from amphetamines.

8 USE IN SPECIFIC POPULATIONS

8.1 Pregnancy

Pregnancy Category C

Risk Summary: Data from epidemiological studies of pregnant women exposed to bupropion in the first trimester indicate no increased risk of congenital malformations overall. All pregnancies, regardless of drug exposure, have a background rate of 2% to 4% for major malformations, and 15% to 20% for pregnancy loss. No clear evidence of teratogenic activity was found in reproductive developmental studies conducted in rats and rabbits; however, in rabbits, slightly increased incidences of fetal malformations and skeletal variations were observed at doses approximately equal to the maximum recommended human dose (MRHD) and greater and decreased fetal weights were seen at doses twice the MRHD and greater. WELLBUTRIN should be used during pregnancy only if the potential benefit justifies the potential risk to the fetus.

Clinical Considerations: Consider the risks of untreated depression when discontinuing or changing treatment with antidepressant medications during pregnancy and postpartum.

Human Data: Data from the international bupropion Pregnancy Registry (675 first-trimester exposures) and a retrospective cohort study using the United Healthcare database (1,213 first trimester exposures) did not show an increased risk for malformations overall.

No increased risk for cardiovascular malformations overall has been observed after bupropion exposure during the first trimester. The prospectively observed rate of cardiovascular malformations in pregnancies with exposure to bupropion in the first trimester from the international Pregnancy Registry was 1.3% (9 cardiovascular malformations/675 first-trimester maternal bupropion exposures), which is similar to the background rate of cardiovascular malformations (approximately 1%). Data from the United Healthcare database and a case-control study (6,853 infants with cardiovascular malformations and 5,763 with non-cardiovascular malformations) from the National Birth Defects Prevention Study (NBDPS) did not show an increased risk for cardiovascular malformations overall after bupropion exposure during the first trimester.

Study findings on bupropion exposure during the first trimester and risk for left ventricular outflow tract obstruction (LVOTO) are inconsistent and do not allow conclusions regarding a possible association. The United Healthcare database lacked sufficient power to evaluate this association; the NBDPS found increased risk for LVOTO (n = 10; adjusted OR = 2.6; 95% CI: 1.2, 5.7), and the Slone Epidemiology case control study did not find increased risk for LVOTO.

Study findings on bupropion exposure during the first trimester and risk for ventricular septal defect (VSD) are inconsistent and do not allow conclusions regarding a possible association. The Slone Epidemiology Study found an increased risk for VSD following first trimester maternal bupropion exposure (n = 17; adjusted OR = 2.5; 95% CI: 1.3, 5.0) but did not find increased risk for any other cardiovascular malformations studied (including LVOTO as above). The NBDPS and United Healthcare database study did not find an association between first trimester maternal bupropion exposure and VSD.

For the findings of LVOTO and VSD, the studies were limited by the small number of exposed cases, inconsistent findings among studies, and the potential for chance findings from multiple comparisons in case control studies.

Animal Data: In studies conducted in rats and rabbits, bupropion was administered orally during the period of organogenesis at doses of up to 450 and 150 mg/kg/day, respectively (approximately 11 and 7 times the MRHD, respectively, on a mg/m² basis). No clear evidence of teratogenic activity was found in either species; however, in rabbits, slightly increased incidences of fetal malformations and skeletal variations were observed at the lowest dose tested (25 mg/kg/day, approximately equal to the MRHD on a mg/m² basis) and greater. Decreased fetal weights were observed at 50 mg/kg and greater.

When rats were administered bupropion at oral doses of up to 300 mg/kg/day (approximately 7 times the MRHD on a mg/m² basis) prior to mating and throughout pregnancy and lactation, there were no apparent adverse effects on offspring development.

8.3 Nursing Mothers

Bupropion and its metabolites are present in human milk. In a lactation study of 10 women, levels of orally dosed bupropion and its active metabolites were measured in expressed milk. The average daily infant exposure (assuming 150 mL/kg daily consumption) to bupropion and its active metabolites was 2% of the maternal weight-adjusted dose. Exercise caution when WELLBUTRIN is administered to a nursing woman.

8.4 Pediatric Use

Safety and effectiveness in the pediatric population have not been established [see Boxed Warning, Warnings and Precautions (5.1)].

8.5 Geriatric Use

Of the approximately 6,000 subjects who participated in clinical trials with bupropion sustained-release tablets (depression and smoking cessation trials), 275 were aged ≥65 years and 47 were aged ≥75 years. In addition, several hundred subjects aged ≥65 years participated in clinical trials using the immediate-release formulation of bupropion (depression trials). No overall differences in safety or effectiveness were observed between these subjects and younger subjects. Reported clinical experience has not identified differences in responses between the elderly and younger patients, but greater sensitivity of some older individuals cannot be ruled out.

Bupropion is extensively metabolized in the liver to active metabolites, which are further metabolized and excreted by the kidneys. The risk of adverse reactions may be greater in patients with impaired renal function. Because elderly patients are more likely to have decreased renal function, it may be necessary to consider this factor in dose selection; it may be useful to monitor renal function [see Dosage and Administration (2.3), Use in Specific Populations (8.6), Clinical Pharmacology (12.3)].

8.6 Renal Impairment

Consider a reduced dose and/or dosing frequency of WELLBUTRIN in patients with renal impairment (Glomerular Filtration Rate: <90 mL/min). Bupropion and its metabolites are cleared renally and may accumulate in such patients to a greater extent than usual. Monitor closely for adverse reactions that could indicate high bupropion or metabolite exposures [see Dosage and Administration (2.3), Clinical Pharmacology (12.3)].

8.7 Hepatic Impairment

In patients with moderate to severe hepatic impairment (Child-Pugh score: 7 to 15), the maximum dose of WELLBUTRIN is 75 mg daily. In patients with mild hepatic impairment (Child-Pugh score: 5 to 6), consider reducing the dose and/or frequency of dosing [see Dosage and Administration (2.2), Clinical Pharmacology (12.3)].

9 DRUG ABUSE AND DEPENDENCE

9.1 Controlled Substance

Bupropion is not a controlled substance.

9.2 Abuse

Humans: Controlled clinical trials conducted in normal volunteers, in subjects with a history of multiple drug abuse, and in depressed subjects showed some increase in motor activity and agitation/excitement.

In a population of individuals experienced with drugs of abuse, a single dose of 400 mg of bupropion produced mild amphetamine–like activity as compared with placebo on the Morphine–Benzedrine Subscale of the Addiction Research Center Inventories (ARCI) and a score intermediate between placebo and amphetamine on the Liking Scale of the ARCI. These scales measure general feelings of euphoria and drug desirability.

Findings in clinical trials, however, are not known to reliably predict the abuse potential of drugs. Nonetheless, evidence from single–dose trials does suggest that the recommended daily dosage of bupropion when administered in divided doses is not likely to be significantly reinforcing to amphetamine or CNS stimulant abusers. However, higher doses (that could not be tested because of the risk of seizure) might be modestly attractive to those who abuse CNS stimulant drugs.

Animals: Studies in rodents and primates demonstrated that bupropion exhibits some pharmacologic actions common to psychostimulants. In rodents, it has been shown to increase locomotor activity, elicit a mild stereotyped behav-

Table 3. Pharmacokinetics of Bupropion and Metabolites in Patients With Severe Hepatic Cirrhosis: Ratio Relative to Healthy Matched Controls

	C_{max}	AUC	$t_{1/2}$	T_{max}[a]
Bupropion	1.69	3.12	1.43	0.5 h
Hydroxybupropion	0.31	1.28	3.88	19 h
Threo/erythrohydrobupropion amino alcohol	0.69	2.48	1.96	20 h

[a] = Difference

ior response, and increase rates of responding in several schedule–controlled behavior paradigms. In primate models assessing the positive reinforcing effects of psychoactive drugs, bupropion was self-administered intravenously. In rats, bupropion produced amphetamine-like and cocaine-like discriminative stimulus effects in drug discrimination paradigms used to characterize the subjective effects of psychoactive drugs.

10 OVERDOSAGE

10.1 Human Overdose Experience
Overdoses of up to 30 grams or more of bupropion have been reported. Seizure was reported in approximately one-third of all cases. Other serious reactions reported with overdoses of bupropion alone included hallucinations, loss of consciousness, sinus tachycardia, and ECG changes such as conduction disturbances (including QRS prolongation) or arrhythmias. Fever, muscle rigidity, rhabdomyolysis, hypotension, stupor, coma, and respiratory failure have been reported mainly when bupropion was part of multiple drug overdoses.

Although most patients recovered without sequelae, deaths associated with overdoses of bupropion alone have been reported in patients ingesting large doses of the drug. Multiple uncontrolled seizures, bradycardia, cardiac failure, and cardiac arrest prior to death were reported in these patients.

10.2 Overdosage Management
Consult a Certified Poison Control Center for up-to-date guidance and advice. Telephone numbers for certified poison control centers are listed in the Physician's Desk Reference (PDR). Call 1-800-222-1222 or refer to www.poison.org.

There are no known antidotes for bupropion. In case of an overdose, provide supportive care, including close medical supervision and monitoring. Consider the possibility of multiple drug overdose. Ensure an adequate airway, oxygenation, and ventilation. Monitor cardiac rhythm and vital signs. Induction of emesis is not recommended.

11 DESCRIPTION
WELLBUTRIN (bupropion hydrochloride), an antidepressant of the aminoketone class, is chemically unrelated to tricyclic, tetracyclic, selective serotonin re–uptake inhibitor, or other known antidepressant agents. Its structure closely resembles that of diethylpropion; it is related to phenylethylamines. It is designated as (±)-1-(3-chlorophenyl)-2-[(1,1-dimethylethyl)amino]-1-propanone hydrochloride. The molecular weight is 276.2. The molecular formula is $C_{13}H_{18}ClNO \cdot HCl$. Bupropion hydrochloride powder is white, crystalline, and highly soluble in water. It has a bitter taste and produces the sensation of local anesthesia on the oral mucosa. The structural formula is

WELLBUTRIN is supplied for oral administration as 75–mg (yellow–gold) and 100–mg (red) film–coated tablets. Each tablet contains the labeled amount of bupropion hydrochloride and the inactive ingredients: 75–mg tablet – D&C Yellow No. 10 Lake, FD&C Yellow No. 6 Lake, hydroxypropyl cellulose, hypromellose, microcrystalline cellulose, polyethylene glycol, talc, and titanium dioxide; 100–mg tablet – FD&C Red No. 40 Lake, FD&C Yellow No. 6 Lake, hydroxypropyl cellulose, hypromellose, microcrystalline cellulose, polyethylene glycol, talc, and titanium dioxide.

12 CLINICAL PHARMACOLOGY

12.1 Mechanism of Action
The exact mechanism of the antidepressant action of bupropion is not known, but is presumed to be related to noradrenergic and/or dopaminergic mechanisms. Bupropion is a relatively weak inhibitor of the neuronal reuptake of norepinephrine and dopamine, and does not inhibit the reuptake of serotonin. Bupropion does not inhibit monoamine oxidase.

12.3 Pharmacokinetics
Bupropion is a racemic mixture. The pharmacological activity and pharmacokinetics of the individual enantiomers

have not been studied. The mean elimination half-life (±SD) of bupropion after chronic dosing is 21 (±9) hours, and steady-state plasma concentrations of bupropion are reached within 8 days.

Absorption: The absolute bioavailability of WELLBUTRIN in humans has not been determined because an intravenous formulation for human use is not available. However, it appears likely that only a small proportion of any orally administered dose reaches the systemic circulation intact. In rat and dog studies, the bioavailability of bupropion ranged from 5% to 20%.

In humans, following oral administration of WELLBUTRIN, peak plasma bupropion concentrations are usually achieved within 2 hours. Plasma concentrations are dose–proportional following single doses of 100 to 250 mg; however, it is not known if the proportionality between dose and plasma level is maintained in chronic use.

Distribution: In vitro tests show that bupropion is 84% bound to human plasma proteins at concentrations up to 200 mcg/mL. The extent of protein binding of the hydroxybupropion metabolite is similar to that for bupropion, whereas the extent of protein binding of the threohydrobupropion metabolite is about half that seen with bupropion.

Metabolism: Bupropion is extensively metabolized in humans. Three metabolites are active: hydroxybupropion, which is formed via hydroxylation of the *tert*-butyl group of bupropion, and the amino-alcohol isomers threohydrobupropion and erythrohydrobupropion, which are formed via reduction of the carbonyl group. In vitro findings suggest that CYP2B6 is the principal isoenzyme involved in the formation of hydroxybupropion, while cytochrome P450 enzymes are not involved in the formation of threohydrobupropion. Oxidation of the bupropion side chain results in the formation of a glycine conjugate of meta-chlorobenzoic acid, which is then excreted as the major urinary metabolite. The potency and toxicity of the metabolites relative to bupropion have not been fully characterized. However, it has been demonstrated in an antidepressant screening test in mice that hydroxybupropion is one–half as potent as bupropion, while threohydrobupropion and erythrohydrobupropion are 5-fold less potent than bupropion. This may be of clinical importance because the plasma concentrations of the metabolites are as high as or higher than those of bupropion. Following a single dose in humans, peak plasma concentrations of hydroxybupropion occur approximately 3 hours after administration of WELLBUTRIN and are approximately 10 times the peak level of the parent drug at steady state. The elimination half–life of hydroxybupropion is approximately 20 (±5) hours, and its AUC at steady state is about 17 times that of bupropion. The times to peak concentrations for the erythrohydrobupropion and threohydrobupropion metabolites are similar to that of the hydroxybupropion metabolite. However, their elimination half–lives are longer, 33 (±10) and 37 (±13) hours, respectively, and steady–state AUCs are 1.5 and 7 times that of bupropion, respectively.

Bupropion and its metabolites exhibit linear kinetics following chronic administration of 300 to 450 mg per day.

Elimination: Following oral administration of 200 mg of ^{14}C-bupropion in humans, 87% and 10% of the radioactive dose were recovered in the urine and feces, respectively. Only 0.5% of the oral dose was excreted as unchanged bupropion.

Population Subgroups: Factors or conditions altering metabolic capacity (e.g., liver disease, congestive heart failure [CHF], age, concomitant medications, etc.) or elimination may be expected to influence the degree and extent of accumulation of the active metabolites of bupropion. The elimination of the major metabolites of bupropion may be affected by reduced renal or hepatic function because they are moderately polar compounds and are likely to undergo further metabolism or conjugation in the liver prior to urinary excretion.

Renal Impairment: There is limited information on the pharmacokinetics of bupropion in patients with renal impairment. An inter-trial comparison between normal subjects and subjects with end-stage renal failure demonstrated that the parent drug C_{max} and AUC values were comparable in the 2 groups, whereas the hydroxybupropion and threohydrobupropion metabolites had a 2.3- and

2.8-fold increase, respectively, in AUC for subjects with end-stage renal failure. A second trial, comparing normal subjects and subjects with moderate–to–severe renal impairment (GFR 30.9 ± 10.8 mL/min) showed that after a single 150-mg dose of sustained-release bupropion, exposure to bupropion was approximately 2-fold higher in subjects with impaired renal function, while levels of the hydroxybupropion and threo/erythrohydrobupropion (combined) metabolites were similar in the 2 groups. Bupropion is extensively metabolized in the liver to active metabolites, which are further metabolized and subsequently excreted by the kidneys. The elimination of the major metabolites of bupropion may be reduced by impaired renal function. WELLBUTRIN should be used with caution in patients with renal impairment and a reduced frequency and/or dose should be considered *[see Use in Specific Populations (8.6)]*.

Hepatic Impairment: The effect of hepatic impairment on the pharmacokinetics of bupropion was characterized in 2 single-dose trials, one in subjects with alcoholic liver disease and one in subjects with mild-to-severe cirrhosis. The first trial demonstrated that the half–life of hydroxybupropion was significantly longer in 8 subjects with alcoholic liver disease than in 8 healthy volunteers (32 ± 14 hours versus 21 ± 5 hours, respectively). Although not statistically significant, the AUCs for bupropion and hydroxybupropion were more variable and tended to be greater (by 53% to 57%) in volunteers with alcoholic liver disease. The differences in half–life for bupropion and the other metabolites in the 2 groups were minimal.

The second trial demonstrated no statistically significant differences in the pharmacokinetics of bupropion and its active metabolites in 9 subjects with mild-to-moderate hepatic cirrhosis compared with 8 healthy volunteers. However, more variability was observed in some of the pharmacokinetic parameters for bupropion (AUC, C_{max}, and T_{max}) and its active metabolites ($t_{1/2}$) in subjects with mild-to-moderate hepatic cirrhosis. In subjects with severe hepatic cirrhosis, significant alterations in the pharmacokinetics of bupropion and its metabolites were seen (Table 3).

[See table 3 above]

Left Ventricular Dysfunction: During a chronic dosing trial with bupropion in 14 depressed subjects with left ventricular dysfunction (history of CHF or an enlarged heart on x-ray), there was no apparent effect on the pharmacokinetics of bupropion or its metabolites, compared with healthy volunteers.

Age: The effects of age on the pharmacokinetics of bupropion and its metabolites have not been fully characterized, but an exploration of steady–state bupropion concentrations from several depression efficacy trials involving subjects dosed in a range of 300 to 750 mg per day, on a 3 times daily schedule, revealed no relationship between age (18 to 83 years) and plasma concentration of bupropion. A single–dose pharmacokinetic trial demonstrated that the disposition of bupropion and its metabolites in elderly subjects was similar to that of younger subjects. These data suggest there is no prominent effect of age on bupropion concentration; however, another single- and multiple-dose pharmacokinetics trial suggested that the elderly are at increased risk for accumulation of bupropion and its metabolites *[see Use in Specific Populations (8.5)]*.

Gender: Pooled analysis of bupropion pharmacokinetic data from 90 healthy male and 90 healthy female volunteers revealed no sex-related differences in the peak plasma concentrations of bupropion. The mean systemic exposure (AUC) was approximately 13% higher in male volunteers compared with female volunteers. The clinical significance of this finding is unknown.

Smokers: The effects of cigarette smoking on the pharmacokinetics of bupropion were studied in 34 healthy male and female volunteers; 17 were chronic cigarette smokers and 17 were nonsmokers. Following oral administration of a single 150-mg dose of bupropion, there were no statistically significant differences in C_{max}, half-life, T_{max}, AUC, or clearance of bupropion or its active metabolites between smokers and nonsmokers.

Drug Interactions: *Potential for Other Drugs to Affect WELLBUTRIN:* In vitro studies indicate that bupropion is primarily metabolized to hydroxybupropion by CYP2B6. Therefore, the potential exists for drug interactions between WELLBUTRIN and drugs that are inhibitors or inducers of CYP2B6. In addition, in vitro studies suggest that paroxetine, sertraline, norfluoxetine, fluvoxamine, and nelfinavir inhibit the hydroxylation of bupropion.

Inhibitors of CYP2B6: Ticlopidine, Clopidogrel: In a trial in healthy male volunteers, clopidogrel 75 mg once daily or ticlopidine 250 mg twice daily increased exposures (C_{max} and AUC) of bupropion by 40% and 60% for clopidogrel, and by 38% and 85% for ticlopidine, respectively. The exposures (C_{max} and AUC) of hydroxybupropion were decreased 50% and 52%, respectively, by clopidogrel, and 78% and 84%, respectively, by ticlopidine. This effect is thought to be due to the inhibition of the CYP2B6-catalyzed bupropion hydroxylation.

Prasugrel: Prasugrel is a weak inhibitor of CYP2B6. In healthy subjects, prasugrel increased bupropion C_{max} and AUC values by 14% and 18%, respectively, and decreased C_{max} and AUC values of hydroxybupropion, an active metabolite of bupropion, by 32% and 24%, respectively.

Cimetidine: The threohydrobupropion metabolite of bupropion does not appear to be produced by cytochrome P450 enzymes. The effects of concomitant administration of cimetidine on the pharmacokinetics of bupropion and its active metabolites were studied in 24 healthy young male volunteers. Following oral administration of bupropion 300 mg with and without cimetidine 800 mg, the pharmacokinetics of bupropion and hydroxybupropion were unaffected. However, there were 16% and 32% increases in the AUC and C_{max}, respectively of the combined moieties of threohydrobupropion and erythrohydrobupropion.

Citalopram: Citalopram did not affect the pharmacokinetics of bupropion and its three metabolites.

Inducers of CYP2B6: Ritonavir and Lopinavir: In a healthy volunteer trial, ritonavir 100 mg twice daily reduced the AUC and C_{max} of bupropion by 22% and 21%, respectively. The exposure of the hydroxybupropion metabolite was decreased by 23%, the threohydrobupropion decreased by 38%, and the erythrohydrobupropion decreased by 48%.

In a second healthy volunteer trial, ritonavir 600 mg twice daily decreased the AUC and the C_{max} of bupropion by 66% and 62%, respectively. The exposure of the hydroxybupropion metabolite was decreased by 78%, the threohydrobupropion decreased by 50%, and the erythrohydrobupropion decreased by 68%.

In another healthy volunteer trial, lopinavir 400 mg/ritonavir 100 mg twice daily decreased bupropion AUC and C_{max} by 57%. The AUC and C_{max} of hydroxybupropion were decreased by 50% and 31%, respectively.

Efavirenz: In a trial in healthy volunteers, efavirenz 600 mg once daily for 2 weeks reduced the AUC and C_{max} of bupropion by approximately 55% and 34%, respectively. The AUC of hydroxybupropion was unchanged, whereas C_{max} of hydroxybupropion was increased by 50%.

Carbamazepine, Phenobarbital, Phenytoin: While not systematically studied, these drugs may induce the metabolism of bupropion.

Potential for WELLBUTRIN to Affect Other Drugs: Animal data indicated that bupropion may be an inducer of drug-metabolizing enzymes in humans. In one trial, following chronic administration of bupropion 100 mg three times daily to 8 healthy male volunteers for 14 days, there was no evidence of induction of its own metabolism. Nevertheless, there may be potential for clinically important alterations of blood levels of co-administered drugs.

Drugs Metabolized by CYP2D6: In vitro, bupropion and its metabolites (erythrohydrobupropion, threohydrobupropion, hydroxybupropion) are CYP2D6 inhibitors. In a clinical trial of 15 male subjects (ages 19 to 35 years) who were extensive metabolizers of CYP2D6, bupropion 300 mg per day followed by a single dose of 50 mg desipramine increased the C_{max}, AUC, and $t_{1/2}$ of desipramine by an average of approximately 2-, 5-, and 2-fold, respectively. The effect was present for at least 7 days after the last dose of bupropion. Concomitant use of bupropion with other drugs metabolized by CYP2D6 has not been formally studied.

Citalopram: Although citalopram is not primarily metabolized by CYP2D6, in one trial bupropion increased the C_{max} and AUC of citalopram by 30% and 40%, respectively.

Lamotrigine: Multiple oral doses of bupropion had no statistically significant effects on the single-dose pharmacokinetics of lamotrigine in 12 healthy volunteers.

13 NONCLINICAL TOXICOLOGY

13.1 Carcinogenesis, Mutagenesis, Impairment of Fertility

Lifetime carcinogenicity studies were performed in rats and mice at bupropion doses up to 300 and 150 mg/kg/day, respectively. These doses are approximately 7 and 2 times the MRHD, respectively, on a mg/m^2 basis. In the rat study there was an increase in nodular proliferative lesions of the liver at doses of 100 to 300 mg/kg/day (approximately 2 to 7 times the MRHD on a mg/m^2 basis); lower doses were not tested. The question of whether or not such lesions may be precursors of neoplasms of the liver is currently unresolved. Similar liver lesions were not seen in the mouse study, and no increase in malignant tumors of the liver and other organs was seen in either study.

Bupropion produced a positive response (2 to 3 times control mutation rate) in 2 of 5 strains in the Ames bacterial mutagenicity assay. Bupropion produced an increase in chromosomal aberrations in 1 of 3 in vivo rat bone marrow cytogenetic studies.

A fertility study in rats at doses up to 300 mg/kg/day revealed no evidence of impaired fertility.

14 CLINICAL STUDIES

The efficacy of WELLBUTRIN in the treatment of major depressive disorder was established in two 4-week, placebo-

Table 4. Efficacy of WELLBUTRIN for the Treatment of Major Depressive Disorder

Trial Number	Treatment Group	Primary Efficacy Measure: HDRS		
		Mean Baseline Score (SD)	LS Mean Score at Endpoint Visit (SE)	Placebo-subtracted Difference[a] (95% CI)
Trial 1	WELLBUTRIN 300-600 mg/day[b] (n = 48)	28.5 (5.1)	14.9 (1.3)	-4.7 (-8.8, -0.6)
	Placebo (n = 27)	29.3 (7.0)	19.6 (1.6)	--
		Mean Baseline Score (SD)	LS Mean Change from Baseline (SE)	Placebo-subtracted Difference[a] (95% CI)
Trial 2	WELLBUTRIN 300 mg/day (n = 36)	32.4 (5.9)	-15.5 (1.7)	-4.1
	WELLBUTRIN 450 mg/day[b] (n = 34)	34.8 (4.6)	-17.4 (1.7)	-5.9 (-10.5, -1.4)
	Placebo (n=39)	32.9 (5.4)	-11.5 (1.6)	--
Trial 3	WELLBUTRIN 300 mg/day[b] (n = 110)	26.5 (4.3)	-12.0 (NA)	-3.9 (-5.7, -1.0)
	Placebo (n = 106)	27.0 (3.5)	-8.7 (NA)	--

n: sample size; SD: standard deviation; SE: standard error; LS Mean: least-squares mean; CI: unadjusted confidence interval included for doses that were demonstrated to be effective; NA: not available.
[a] Difference (drug minus placebo) in least-squares estimates with respect to the primary efficacy parameter. For Trial 1, it refers to the mean score at the endpoint visit; for Trials 2 and 3, it refers to the mean change from baseline to the endpoint visit.
[b] Doses that are demonstrated to be statistically significantly superior to placebo.

controlled trials in adult inpatients with MDD (Trials 1 and 2 in Table 4) and in one 6-week, placebo-controlled trial in adult outpatients with MDD (Trial 3 in Table 4). In the first trial, the dose range of WELLBUTRIN was 300 mg to 600 mg per day administered in 3 divided doses; 78% of subjects were treated with doses of 300 mg to 450 mg per day. The trial demonstrated the efficacy of WELLBUTRIN as measured by the Hamilton Depression Rating Scale (HDRS) total score, the HDRS depressed mood item (item 1), and the Clinical Global Impressions-severity score (CGI-S). The second trial included 2 doses of WELLBUTRIN (300 and 450 mg per day) and placebo. This trial demonstrated the effectiveness of WELLBUTRIN for only the 450-mg-per-day dose. The efficacy results were statistically significant for the HDRS total score and the CGI-S score, but not for HDRS item 1. In the third trial, outpatients were treated with 300 mg per day of WELLBUTRIN. This trial demonstrated the efficacy of WELLBUTRIN as measured by the HDRS total score, the HDRS item 1, the Montgomery-Asberg Depression Rating Scale (MADRS), the CGI-S score, and the CGI-Improvement Scale (CGI-I) score. Effectiveness of WELLBUTRIN in long-term use, that is, for more than 6 weeks, has not been systematically evaluated in controlled trials.
[See table 4 above]

16 HOW SUPPLIED/STORAGE AND HANDLING

WELLBUTRIN Tablets, 75 mg of bupropion hydrochloride, are yellow-gold, round, biconvex tablets printed with "WELLBUTRIN 75" in bottles of 100 (NDC 0173-0177-55). WELLBUTRIN Tablets, 100 mg of bupropion hydrochloride, are red, round, biconvex tablets printed with "WELLBUTRIN 100" in bottles of 100 (NDC 0173-0178-55). Store at room temperature, 20° to 25°C (68° to 77°F); excursions permitted between 15°C and 30°C (59°F and 86°F) [See USP Controlled Room Temperature]. Protect from light and moisture.

17 PATIENT COUNSELING INFORMATION

Advise the patient to read the FDA-approved patient labeling (Medication Guide).
Inform patients, their families, and their caregivers about the benefits and risks associated with treatment with WELLBUTRIN and counsel them in its appropriate use.
A patient Medication Guide about "Antidepressant Medicines, Depression and Other Serious Mental Illnesses, and Suicidal Thoughts or Actions," "Quitting Smoking, Quit-Smoking Medications, Changes in Thinking and Behavior, Depression, and Suicidal Thoughts or Actions," and "What Other Important Information Should I Know About WELLBUTRIN?" is available for WELLBUTRIN. Instruct patients, their families, and their caregivers to read the Medication Guide and assist them in understanding its contents. Patients should be given the opportunity to discuss the contents of the Medication Guide and to obtain answers to any questions they may have. The complete text of the Medication Guide is reprinted at the end of this document. Advise patients regarding the following issues and to alert their prescriber if these occur while taking WELLBUTRIN.

Suicidal Thoughts and Behaviors: Instruct patients, their families, and/or their caregivers to be alert to the emergence of anxiety, agitation, panic attacks, insomnia, irritability, hostility, aggressiveness, impulsivity, akathisia (psychomotor restlessness), hypomania, mania, other unusual changes in behavior, worsening of depression, and suicidal ideation, especially early during antidepressant treatment and when the dose is adjusted up or down. Advise families and caregivers of patients to observe for the emergence of such symptoms on a day-to-day basis, since changes may be abrupt. Such symptoms should be reported to the patient's prescriber or healthcare professional, especially if they are severe, abrupt in onset, or were not part of the patient's presenting symptoms. Symptoms such as these may be associated with an increased risk for suicidal thinking and behavior and indicate a need for very close monitoring and possibly changes in the medication.

Neuropsychiatric Symptoms and Suicide Risk in Smoking Cessation Treatment: Although WELLBUTRIN is not indicated for smoking cessation treatment, it contains the same active ingredient as ZYBAN® which is approved for this use. Advise patients, families and caregivers that quitting smoking, with or without ZYBAN, may trigger nicotine withdrawal symptoms (e.g., including depression or agitation), or worsen pre-existing psychiatric illness. Some patients have experienced changes in mood (including depression and mania), psychosis, hallucinations, paranoia, delusions, homicidal ideation, aggression, anxiety, and panic, as well as suicidal ideation, suicide attempt, and completed suicide when attempting to quit smoking while taking ZYBAN. If patients develop agitation, hostility, depressed mood, or changes in thinking or behavior that are not typical for them, or if patients develop suicidal ideation or behavior, they should be urged to report these symptoms to their healthcare provider immediately.

Severe Allergic Reactions: Educate patients on the symptoms of hypersensitivity and to discontinue WELLBUTRIN if they have a severe allergic reaction.

Seizure: Instruct patients to discontinue and not restart WELLBUTRIN if they experience a seizure while on treatment. Advise patients that the excessive use or abrupt discontinuation of alcohol, benzodiazepines, antiepileptic drugs, or sedatives/hypnotics can increase the risk of seizure. Advise patients to minimize or avoid use of alcohol.

Angle-Closure Glaucoma: Patients should be advised that taking WELLBUTRIN can cause mild pupillary dilation, which in susceptible individuals, can lead to an episode of angle-closure glaucoma. Pre-existing glaucoma is almost always open-angle glaucoma because angle-closure glaucoma, when diagnosed, can be treated definitively with iridectomy. Open-angle glaucoma is not a risk factor for angle-closure glaucoma. Patients may wish to be examined to determine whether they are susceptible to angle closure, and have a prophylactic procedure (e.g., iridectomy), if they are susceptible [see Warnings and Precautions (5.7)].

Bupropion-Containing Products: Educate patients that WELLBUTRIN contains the same active ingredient (bupropion hydrochloride) found in ZYBAN, which is used

Help Patients Save on Rx Drugs: PDR.net/PharmacyDiscountCard

as an aid to smoking cessation treatment, and that WELLBUTRIN should not be used in combination with ZYBAN or any other medications that contain bupropion (such as WELLBUTRIN SR®, the sustained-release formulation and WELLBUTRIN XL® or FORFIVO XL™, the extended-release formulations, and APLENZIN®, the extended-release formulation of bupropion hydrobromide). In addition, there are a number of generic bupropion HCl products for the immediate-, sustained-, and extended-release formulations.

Potential for Cognitive and Motor Impairment: Advise patients that any CNS–active drug like WELLBUTRIN may impair their ability to perform tasks requiring judgment or motor and cognitive skills. Advise patients that until they are reasonably certain that WELLBUTRIN does not adversely affect their performance, they should refrain from driving an automobile or operating complex, hazardous machinery. WELLBUTRIN may lead to decreased alcohol tolerance.

Concomitant Medications: Counsel patients to notify their healthcare provider if they are taking or plan to take any prescription or over–the–counter drugs because WELLBUTRIN and other drugs may affect each others' metabolisms.

Pregnancy: Advise patients to notify their healthcare provider if they become pregnant or intend to become pregnant during therapy.

Precautions for Nursing Mothers: Advise patients that WELLBUTRIN is present in human milk in small amounts.

Storage Information: Instruct patients to store WELLBUTRIN at room temperature, between 59°F and 86°F (15°C to 30°C) and keep the tablets dry and out of the light.

Administration Information: Instruct patients to take WELLBUTRIN in equally divided doses 3 or 4 times a day, with doses separated by least 6 hours to minimize the risk of seizure. Instruct patients if they miss a dose, not to take an extra tablet to make up for the missed dose and to take the next tablet at the regular time because of the dose-related risk of seizure. Instruct patients that WELLBUTRIN Tablets should be swallowed whole and not crushed, divided, or chewed. WELLBUTRIN can be taken with or without food.

WELLBUTRIN, WELLBUTRIN SR, WELLBUTRIN XL, and ZYBAN are registered trademarks of the GSK group of companies. The other brands listed are trademarks of their respective owners and are not trademarks of the GSK group of companies. The makers of these brands are not affiliated with and do not endorse the GSK group of companies or its products.

Manufactured for:
GlaxoSmithKline
Research Triangle Park, NC 27709
©2014, the GSK group of companies. All rights reserved.
WLT:11PI

Medication Guide
WELLBUTRIN® (WELL byu-trin)
(bupropion hydrochloride) Tablets

Read this Medication Guide carefully before you start taking WELLBUTRIN and each time you get a refill. There may be new information. This information does not take the place of talking with your healthcare provider about your medical condition or your treatment. If you have any questions about WELLBUTRIN, ask your healthcare provider or pharmacist.

IMPORTANT: Be sure to read the three sections of this Medication Guide. The first section is about the risk of suicidal thoughts and actions with antidepressant medicines; the second section is about the risk of changes in thinking and behavior, depression and suicidal thoughts or actions with medicines used to quit smoking; and the third section is entitled "What Other Important Information Should I Know About WELLBUTRIN?"

Antidepressant Medicines, Depression and Other Serious Mental Illnesses, and Suicidal Thoughts or Actions

This section of the Medication Guide is only about the risk of suicidal thoughts and actions with antidepressant medicines. **Talk to your healthcare provider or your family member's healthcare provider about:**
- all risks and benefits of treatment with antidepressant medicines
- all treatment choices for depression or other serious mental illness

What is the most important information I should know about antidepressant medicines, depression and other serious mental illnesses, and suicidal thoughts or actions?
1. **Antidepressant medicines may increase suicidal thoughts or actions in some children, teenagers, or young adults within the first few months of treatment.**
2. **Depression or other serious mental illnesses are the most important causes of suicidal thoughts and actions. Some people may have a particularly high risk of having suicidal thoughts or actions.** These include people who

have (or have a family history of) bipolar illness (also called manic-depressive illness) or suicidal thoughts or actions.
3. **How can I watch for and try to prevent suicidal thoughts and actions in myself or a family member?**
- Pay close attention to any changes, especially sudden changes, in mood, behaviors, thoughts, or feelings. This is very important when an antidepressant medicine is started or when the dose is changed.
- Call your healthcare provider right away to report new or sudden changes in mood, behavior, thoughts, or feelings.
- Keep all follow-up visits with your healthcare provider as scheduled. Call the healthcare provider between visits as needed, especially if you have concerns about symptoms.

Call your healthcare provider right away if you or your family member has any of the following symptoms, especially if they are new, worse, or worry you:

• thoughts about suicide or dying	• trouble sleeping (insomnia)
• attempts to commit suicide	• new or worse irritability
• new or worse depression	• acting aggressive, being angry, or violent
• new or worse anxiety	• acting on dangerous impulses
• feeling very agitated or restless	• an extreme increase in activity and talking (mania)
• panic attacks	• other unusual changes in behavior or mood

What else do I need to know about antidepressant medicines?
- **Never stop an antidepressant medicine without first talking to a healthcare provider.** Stopping an antidepressant medicine suddenly can cause other symptoms.
- **Antidepressants are medicines used to treat depression and other illnesses.** It is important to discuss all the risks of treating depression and also the risks of not treating it. Patients and their families or other caregivers should discuss all treatment choices with the healthcare provider, not just the use of antidepressants.
- **Antidepressant medicines have other side effects.** Talk to the healthcare provider about the side effects of the medicine prescribed for you or your family member.
- **Antidepressant medicines can interact with other medicines.** Know all of the medicines that you or your family member takes. Keep a list of all medicines to show the healthcare provider. Do not start new medicines without first checking with your healthcare provider.

It is not known if WELLBUTRIN is safe and effective in children under the age of 18.

Quitting Smoking, Quit-Smoking Medications, Changes in Thinking and Behavior, Depression, and Suicidal Thoughts or Actions

This section of the Medication Guide is only about the risk of changes in thinking and behavior, depression and suicidal thoughts or actions with drugs used to quit smoking. Although WELLBUTRIN is not a treatment for quitting smoking, it contains the same active ingredient (bupropion hydrochloride) as ZYBAN® which is used to help patients quit smoking.

Some people have had changes in behavior, hostility, agitation, depression, suicidal thoughts or actions while taking bupropion to help them quit smoking. These symptoms can develop during treatment with bupropion or after stopping treatment with bupropion.

If you, your family member, or your caregiver notice agitation, hostility, depression, or changes in thinking or behavior that are not typical for you, or you have any of the following symptoms, stop taking bupropion and call your healthcare provider right away:

• thoughts about suicide or dying	• an extreme increase in activity and talking (mania)
• attempts to commit suicide	• abnormal thoughts or sensations
• new or worse depression	• seeing or hearing things that are not there (hallucinations)
• new or worse anxiety	
• panic attacks	• feeling people are against you (paranoia)
• feeling very agitated or restless	• feeling confused
• acting aggressive, being angry, or violent	• other unusual changes in behavior or mood
• acting on dangerous impulses	

When you try to quit smoking, with or without bupropion, you may have symptoms that may be due to nicotine withdrawal, including urge to smoke, depressed mood, trouble sleeping, irritability, frustration, anger, feeling anxious, dif-

ficulty concentrating, restlessness, decreased heart rate, and increased appetite or weight gain. Some people have even experienced suicidal thoughts when trying to quit smoking without medication. Sometimes quitting smoking can lead to worsening of mental health problems that you already have, such as depression.

Before taking bupropion, tell your healthcare provider if you have ever had depression or other mental illnesses. You should also tell your healthcare provider about any symptoms you had during other times you tried to quit smoking, with or without bupropion.

What Other Important Information Should I Know About WELLBUTRIN?
- **Seizures: There is a chance of having a seizure (convulsion, fit) with WELLBUTRIN, especially in people:**
  - with certain medical problems.
  - who take certain medicines.

The chance of having seizures increases with higher doses of WELLBUTRIN. For more information, see the sections "Who should not take WELLBUTRIN?" and "What should I tell my healthcare provider before taking WELLBUTRIN?" Tell your healthcare provider about all of your medical conditions and all the medicines you take. **Do not take any other medicines while you are taking WELLBUTRIN unless your healthcare provider has said it is okay to take them. If you have a seizure while taking WELLBUTRIN, stop taking the tablets and call your healthcare provider right away.** Do not take WELLBUTRIN again if you have a seizure.

- **High blood pressure (hypertension). Some people get high blood pressure that can be severe, while taking WELLBUTRIN.** The chance of high blood pressure may be higher if you also use nicotine replacement therapy (such as a nicotine patch) to help you stop smoking.
- **Manic episodes. Some people may have periods of mania while taking WELLBUTRIN, including:**
  - Greatly increased energy
  - Severe trouble sleeping
  - Racing thoughts
  - Reckless behavior
  - Unusually grand ideas
  - Excessive happiness or irritability
  - Talking more or faster than usual

If you have any of the above symptoms of mania, call your healthcare provider.

- **Unusual thoughts or behaviors. Some patients have unusual thoughts or behaviors while taking WELLBUTRIN,** including delusions (believe you are someone else), hallucinations (seeing or hearing things that are not there), paranoia (feeling that people are against you), or feeling confused. If this happens to you, call your healthcare provider.

- **Visual problems.**
  - eye pain
  - changes in vision
  - swelling or redness in or around the eye

Only some people are at risk for these problems. You may want to undergo an eye examination to see if you are at risk and receive preventative treatment if you are.

- **Severe allergic reactions. Some people can have severe allergic reactions to WELLBUTRIN. Stop taking WELLBUTRIN and call your healthcare provider right away** if you get a rash, itching, hives, fever, swollen lymph glands, painful sores in the mouth or around the eyes, swelling of the lips or tongue, chest pain, or have trouble breathing. These could be signs of a serious allergic reaction.

What is WELLBUTRIN?
WELLBUTRIN is a prescription medicine used to treat adults with a certain type of depression called major depressive disorder.

Who should not take WELLBUTRIN?
Do not take WELLBUTRIN if you
- have or had a seizure disorder or epilepsy.
- have or had an eating disorder such as anorexia nervosa or bulimia.
- **are taking any other medicines that contain bupropion, including ZYBAN** (used to help people stop smoking) **APLENZIN®, FORFIVO XL™, WELLBUTRIN SR®, or WELLBUTRIN XL®.** Bupropion is the same active ingredient that is in WELLBUTRIN.
- drink a lot of alcohol and abruptly stop drinking, or use medicines called sedatives (these make you sleepy), benzodiazepines, or anti-seizure medicines, and you stop using them all of a sudden.
- take a monoamine oxidase inhibitor (MAOI). Ask your healthcare provider or pharmacist if you are not sure if you take an MAOI, including the antibiotic linezolid.
- do not take an MAOI within 2 weeks of stopping WELLBUTRIN unless directed to do so by your healthcare provider.
- do not start WELLBUTRIN if you stopped taking an MAOI in the last 2 weeks unless directed to do so by your healthcare provider.

Register at PDR.net to Receive Email Drug Alerts

- are allergic to the active ingredient in WELLBUTRIN, bupropion, or to any of the inactive ingredients. See the end of this Medication Guide for a complete list of ingredients in WELLBUTRIN.

What should I tell my healthcare provider before taking WELLBUTRIN?

Tell your healthcare provider if you have ever had depression, suicidal thoughts or actions, or other mental health problems. See "Antidepressant Medicines, Depression and Other Serious Mental Illnesses, and Suicidal Thoughts or Actions."

Tell your healthcare provider about your other medical conditions including if you:

- have liver problems, especially cirrhosis of the liver.
- have kidney problems.
- have, or have had, an eating disorder, such as anorexia nervosa or bulimia.
- have had a head injury.
- have had a seizure (convulsion, fit).
- have a tumor in your nervous system (brain or spine).
- have had a heart attack, heart problems, or high blood pressure.
- are a diabetic taking insulin or other medicines to control your blood sugar.
- drink alcohol.
- abuse prescription medicines or street drugs.
- are pregnant or plan to become pregnant.
- are breastfeeding. WELLBUTRIN passes into your milk in small amounts.

Tell your healthcare provider about all the medicines you take, including prescription, over-the-counter medicines, vitamins, and herbal supplements. Many medicines increase your chances of having seizures or other serious side effects if you take them while you are taking WELLBUTRIN.

How should I take WELLBUTRIN?

- Take WELLBUTRIN exactly as prescribed by your healthcare provider.
- Take WELLBUTRIN at the same time each day.
- Take your doses of WELLBUTRIN at least 6 hours apart.
- **Do not chew, cut, or crush WELLBUTRIN tablets.**
- You may take WELLBUTRIN with or without food.
- If you miss a dose, do not take an extra dose to make up for the dose you missed. Wait and take your next dose at the regular time. **This is very important.** Too much WELLBUTRIN can increase your chance of having a seizure.
- If you take too much WELLBUTRIN, or overdose, call your local emergency room or poison control center right away.
- **Do not take any other medicines while taking WELLBUTRIN unless your healthcare provider has told you it is okay.**
- If you are taking WELLBUTRIN for the treatment of major depressive disorder, it may take several weeks for you to feel that WELLBUTRIN is working. Once you feel better, it is important to keep taking WELLBUTRIN exactly as directed by your healthcare provider. Call your healthcare provider if you do not feel WELLBUTRIN is working for you.
- Do not change your dose or stop taking WELLBUTRIN without talking with your healthcare provider first.

What should I avoid while taking WELLBUTRIN?

- Limit or avoid using alcohol during treatment with WELLBUTRIN. If you usually drink a lot of alcohol, talk with your healthcare provider before suddenly stopping. If you suddenly stop drinking alcohol, you may increase your risk of having seizures.
- Do not drive a car or use heavy machinery until you know how WELLBUTRIN affects you. WELLBUTRIN can affect your ability to do these things safely.

What are possible side effects of WELLBUTRIN?

See "What Other Important Information Should I Know About WELLBUTRIN?"

WELLBUTRIN can cause serious side effects.

The most common side effects of WELLBUTRIN include:

- Nervousness
- Dry mouth
- Constipation
- Headache
- Nausea or vomiting
- Dizziness
- Heavy sweating
- Shakiness (tremor)
- Trouble sleeping
- Blurred vision
- Fast heartbeat

If you have nausea, take your medicine with food. If you have trouble sleeping, do not take your medicine too close to bedtime.

Tell your healthcare provider right away about any side effects that bother you.

These are not all the possible side effects of WELLBUTRIN. For more information, ask your healthcare provider or pharmacist.

Call your healthcare provider for medical advice about side effects. You may report side effects to FDA at 1-800-FDA-1088.

You may also report side effects to GlaxoSmithKline at 1-888-825-5249.

How should I store WELLBUTRIN?

- Store WELLBUTRIN at room temperature between 59°F and 86°F (15°C to 30°C).
- Keep WELLBUTRIN Tablets dry and out of the light.

Keep WELLBUTRIN and all medicines out of the reach of children.

General Information about WELLBUTRIN.

Medicines are sometimes prescribed for purposes other than those listed in a Medication Guide. Do not use WELLBUTRIN for a condition for which it was not prescribed. Do not give WELLBUTRIN to other people, even if they have the same symptoms you have. It may harm them. If you take a urine drug screening test, WELLBUTRIN may make the test result positive for amphetamines. If you tell the person giving you the drug screening test that you are taking WELLBUTRIN, they can do a more specific drug screening test that should not have this problem.

This Medication Guide summarizes important information about WELLBUTRIN. If you would like more information, talk with your healthcare provider. You can ask your healthcare provider or pharmacist for information about WELLBUTRIN that is written for healthcare professionals. For more information about WELLBUTRIN, go to www.wellbutrin.com or call 1-888-825-5249.

What are the ingredients in WELLBUTRIN?

Active ingredient: bupropion hydrochloride.

Inactive ingredients: 75-mg tablet – D&C Yellow No. 10 Lake, FD&C Yellow No. 6 Lake, hydroxypropyl cellulose, hypromellose, microcrystalline cellulose, polyethylene glycol, talc, and titanium dioxide; 100-mg tablet – FD&C Red No. 40 Lake, FD&C Yellow No. 6 Lake, hydroxypropyl cellulose, hypromellose, microcrystalline cellulose, polyethylene glycol, talc, and titanium dioxide.

This Medication Guide has been approved by the U.S. Food and Drug Administration.

WELLBUTRIN, WELLBUTRIN SR, WELLBUTRIN XL, and ZYBAN are registered trademarks of the GSK group of companies.

The other brands listed are trademarks of their respective owners and are not trademarks of the GSK group of companies. The makers of these brands are not affiliated with and do not endorse the GSK group of companies or its products.

Manufactured by:
GlaxoSmithKline
Research Triangle Park, NC 27709
©2014, the GSK group of companies. All rights reserved.
July 2014
WLT:10MG

WELLBUTRIN SR®

[wel′byü-trin]
(bupropion hydrochloride)
Sustained-Release Tablets

℞

HIGHLIGHTS OF PRESCRIBING INFORMATION

These highlights do not include all the information needed to use WELLBUTRIN SR safely and effectively. See full prescribing information for WELLBUTRIN SR.

WELLBUTRIN SR (bupropion hydrochloride) Sustained-Release Tablets, for oral use
Initial U.S. Approval: 1985

WARNING: SUICIDAL THOUGHTS AND BEHAVIORS; AND NEUROPSYCHIATRIC REACTIONS
See full prescribing information for complete boxed warning.

- **Increased the risk of suicidal thinking and behavior in children, adolescents, and young adults taking antidepressants. (5.1)**
- **Monitor worsening and emergence of suicidal thoughts and behavior (5.1)**
- **Serious neuropsychiatric events have been reported in patients taking bupropion for smoking cessation. (5.2)**

———**RECENT MAJOR CHANGES**———

Warnings and Precautions (5.7)   07/2014

———**INDICATIONS AND USAGE**———

- WELLBUTRIN SR is an aminoketone antidepressant, indicated for the treatment of major depressive disorder (MDD). (1)

———**DOSAGE AND ADMINISTRATION**———

- Starting dose: 150 mg per day. (2.1)
- General: Increase dose gradually to reduce seizure risk. (2.1, 5.3)

- After 3 days, may increase the dose to 300 mg per day, given as 150 mg twice daily at an interval of at least 8 hours. (2.1)
- Usual target dose: 300 mg per day as 150 mg twice daily. (2.1)
- Maximum dose: 400 mg per day, given as 200 mg twice daily, for patients not responding to 300 mg per day. (2.1)
- Periodically reassess the dose and need for maintenance treatment. (2.1)
- Moderate to severe hepatic impairment: 100 mg daily or 150 mg every other day. (2.2, 8.7)
- Mild hepatic impairment: Consider reducing the dose and/or frequency of dosing (2.2, 8.7)
- Renal impairment: Consider reducing the dose and/or frequency. (2.3, 8.6)

———**DOSAGE FORMS AND STRENGTHS**———

Tablets: 100 mg, 150 mg, 200 mg. (3)

———**CONTRAINDICATIONS**———

- Seizure disorder. (4, 5.3)
- Current or prior diagnosis of bulimia or anorexia nervosa. (4, 5.3)
- Abrupt discontinuation of alcohol, benzodiazepines, barbiturates, antiepileptic drugs. (4, 5.3)
- Monoamine Oxidase Inhibitors (MAOIs): Do not use MAOIs intended to treat psychiatric disorders with WELLBUTRIN SR or within 14 days of stopping treatment with WELLBUTRIN SR. Do not use WELLBUTRIN SR within 14 days of stopping an MAOI intended to treat psychiatric disorders. In addition, do not start WELLBUTRIN SR in a patient who is being treated with linezolid or intravenous methylene blue. (4, 7.6)
- Known hypersensitivity to bupropion or other ingredients of WELLBUTRIN SR. (4, 5.8)

———**WARNINGS AND PRECAUTIONS**———

- Seizure risk: The risk is dose-related. Can minimize risk by gradually increasing the dose and limiting daily dose to 400 mg. Discontinue if seizure occurs. (4, 5.3, 7.3)
- Hypertension: WELLBUTRIN SR can increase blood pressure. Monitor blood pressure before initiating treatment and periodically during treatment. (5.4)
- Activation of mania/hypomania: Screen patients for bipolar disorder and monitor for these symptoms. (5.5)
- Psychosis and other neuropsychiatric reactions: Instruct patients to contact a healthcare professional if such reactions occur. (5.6)
- Angle-closure glaucoma: Angle-closure glaucoma has occurred in patients with untreated anatomically narrow angles treated with antidepressants. (5.7)

———**ADVERSE REACTIONS**———

Most common adverse reactions (incidence ≥5% and ≥2% more than placebo rate) are: headache, dry mouth, nausea, insomnia, dizziness, pharyngitis, constipation, agitation, anxiety, abdominal pain, tinnitus, tremor, palpitation, myalgia, sweating, rash, and anorexia. (6.1)

To report SUSPECTED ADVERSE REACTIONS, contact GlaxoSmithKline at 1-888-825-5249 or FDA at 1-800-FDA-1088 or www.fda.gov/medwatch.

———**DRUG INTERACTIONS**———

- CYP2B6 inducers: Dose increase may be necessary if coadministered with CYP2B6 inducers (e.g., ritonavir, lopinavir, efavirenz, carbamazepine, phenobarbital, and phenytoin) based on clinical response, but should not exceed the maximum recommended dose. (7.1)
- Drugs metabolized by CYP2D6: Bupropion inhibits CYP2D6 and can increase concentrations of: antidepressants (e.g., venlafaxine, nortriptyline, imipramine, desipramine, paroxetine, fluoxetine, sertraline), antipsychotics (e.g., haloperidol, risperidone, thioridazine), betablockers (e.g., metoprolol), and Type 1C antiarrhythmics (e.g., propafenone, flecainide). Consider dose reduction when using with bupropion. (7.2)
- Drugs that lower seizure threshold: Dose WELLBUTRIN SR with caution. (5.3, 7.3)
- Dopaminergic drugs (levodopa and amantadine): CNS toxicity can occur when used concomitantly with WELLBUTRIN SR. (7.4)
- MAOIs: Increased risk of hypertensive reactions can occur when used concomitantly with WELLBUTRIN SR. (7.6)
- Drug-laboratory test interactions: WELLBUTRIN SR can cause false-positive urine test results for amphetamines. (7.7)

———**USE IN SPECIFIC POPULATIONS**———

- Pregnancy: Use only if benefit outweighs potential risk to the fetus. (8.1)

See 17 for PATIENT COUNSELING INFORMATION and Medication Guide

Revised: 07/2014

FULL PRESCRIBING INFORMATION: CONTENTS*
WARNING: SUICIDAL THOUGHTS AND BEHAV-IORS; AND NEUROPSYCHIATRIC REACTIONS

FULL PRESCRIBING INFORMATION

WARNING: SUICIDAL THOUGHTS AND BE-HAVIORS; AND NEUROPSYCHIATRIC REAC-TIONS
SUICIDALITY AND ANTIDEPRESSANT DRUGS
Antidepressants increased the risk of suicidal thoughts and behavior in children, adolescents, and young adults in short-term trials. These trials did not show an increase in the risk of suicidal thoughts and behavior with antidepressant use in subjects over age 24; there was a reduction in risk with antidepressant use in subjects aged 65 and older [see Warnings and Precautions (5.1)].
In patients of all ages who are started on antidepressant therapy, monitor closely for worsening, and for emergence of suicidal thoughts and behaviors. Advise families and caregivers of the need for close observation and communication with the prescriber [see Warnings and Precautions (5.1)].
NEUROPSYCHIATRIC REACTIONS IN PATIENTS TAK-ING BUPROPION FOR SMOKING CESSATION
Serious neuropsychiatric reactions have occurred in patients taking bupropion for smoking cessation [see Warnings and Precautions (5.2)]. The major-

ity of these reactions occurred during bupropion treatment, but some occurred in the context of discontinuing treatment. In many cases, a causal relationship to bupropion treatment is not certain, because depressed mood may be a symptom of nicotine withdrawal. However, some of the cases occurred in patients taking bupropion who continued to smoke. Although WELLBUTRIN® SR is not approved for smoking cessation, observe all patients for neuropsychiatric reactions. Instruct the patient to contact a healthcare provider if such reactions occur [see Warnings and Precautions (5.2)].

1   INDICATIONS AND USAGE

WELLBUTRIN SR (bupropion hydrochloride) is indicated for the treatment of major depressive disorder (MDD), as defined by the Diagnostic and Statistical Manual (DSM).
The efficacy of bupropion in the treatment of a major depressive episode was established in two 4-week controlled inpatient trials and one 6-week controlled outpatient trial of adult subjects with MDD [see Clinical Studies (14)].
The efficacy of WELLBUTRIN SR in maintaining an antidepressant response for up to 44 weeks following 8 weeks of acute treatment was demonstrated in a placebo-controlled trial [see Clinical Studies (14)].

2   DOSAGE AND ADMINISTRATION

2.1   General Instructions for Use

To minimize the risk of seizure, increase the dose gradually [see Warnings and Precautions (5.3)]. WELLBUTRIN SR Tablets should be swallowed whole and not crushed, divided, or chewed. WELLBUTRIN SR may be taken with or without food.
The usual adult target dose for WELLBUTRIN SR is 300 mg per day, given as 150 mg twice daily. Initiate dosing with 150 mg per day given as a single daily dose in the morning. After 3 days of dosing, the dose may be increased to the 300-mg-per-day target dose, given as 150 mg twice daily. There should be an interval of at least 8 hours between successive doses. A maximum of 400 mg per day, given as 200 mg twice daily, may be considered for patients in whom no clinical improvement is noted after several weeks of treatment at 300 mg per day. To avoid high peak concentrations of bupropion and/or its metabolites, do not exceed 200 mg in any single dose.
It is generally agreed that acute episodes of depression require several months or longer of antidepressant drug treatment beyond the response in the acute episode. It is unknown whether the dose of WELLBUTRIN SR needed for maintenance treatment is identical to the dose that provided an initial response. Periodically reassess the need for maintenance treatment and the appropriate dose for such treatment.

2.2   Dose Adjustment in Patients With Hepatic Impairment

In patients with moderate to severe hepatic impairment (Child-Pugh score: 7 to 15), the maximum dose of WELLBUTRIN SR is 100 mg per day or 150 mg every other day. In patients with mild hepatic impairment (Child-Pugh score: 5 to 6), consider reducing the dose and/or frequency of dosing [see Use in Specific Populations (8.7), Clinical Pharmacology (12.3)].

2.3   Dose Adjustment in Patients With Renal Impairment

Consider reducing the dose and/or frequency of WELLBUTRIN SR in patients with renal impairment (Glomerular Filtration Rate <90 mL/min) [see Use in Specific Populations (8.6), Clinical Pharmacology (12.3)].

2.4   Switching a Patient To or From a Monoamine Oxidase Inhibitor (MAOI) Antidepressant

At least 14 days should elapse between discontinuation of an MAOI intended to treat depression and initiation of therapy with WELLBUTRIN SR. Conversely, at least 14 days should be allowed after stopping WELLBUTRIN SR before starting an MAOI antidepressant [see Contraindications (4), Drug Interactions (7.6)].

2.5   Use of WELLBUTRIN SR With Reversible MAOIs Such as Linezolid or Methylene Blue

Do not start WELLBUTRIN SR in a patient who is being treated with a reversible MAOI such as linezolid or intravenous methylene blue. Drug interactions can increase the risk of hypertensive reactions. In a patient who requires more urgent treatment of a psychiatric condition, nonpharmacological interventions, including hospitalization, should be considered [see Contraindications (4), Drug Interactions (7.6)].
In some cases, a patient already receiving therapy with WELLBUTRIN SR may require urgent treatment with linezolid or intravenous methylene blue. If acceptable alternatives to linezolid or intravenous methylene blue treatment are not available and the potential benefits of linezolid or intravenous methylene blue treatment are judged to out-

weigh the risks of hypertensive reactions in a particular patient, WELLBUTRIN SR should be stopped promptly, and linezolid or intravenous methylene blue can be administered. The patient should be monitored for 2 weeks or until 24 hours after the last dose of linezolid or intravenous methylene blue, whichever comes first. Therapy with WELLBUTRIN SR may be resumed 24 hours after the last dose of linezolid or intravenous methylene blue.
The risk of administering methylene blue by non-intravenous routes (such as oral tablets or by local injection) or in intravenous doses much lower than 1 mg/kg with WELLBUTRIN SR is unclear. The clinician should, nevertheless, be aware of the possibility of a drug interaction with such use [see Contraindications (4), Drug Interactions (7.6)].

3   DOSAGE FORMS AND STRENGTHS

- 100 mg – blue, round, biconvex, film-coated, sustained-release tablets printed with "WELLBUTRIN SR 100".
- 150 mg – purple, round, biconvex, film-coated, sustained-release tablets printed with "WELLBUTRIN SR 150".
- 200 mg – light pink, round, biconvex, film-coated, sustained-release tablets printed with "WELLBUTRIN SR 200".

4   CONTRAINDICATIONS

- WELLBUTRIN SR is contraindicated in patients with a seizure disorder.
- WELLBUTRIN SR is contraindicated in patients with a current or prior diagnosis of bulimia or anorexia nervosa as a higher incidence of seizures was observed in such patients treated with the immediate-release formulation of bupropion [see Warnings and Precautions (5.3)].
- WELLBUTRIN SR is contraindicated in patients undergoing abrupt discontinuation of alcohol, benzodiazepines, barbiturates, and antiepileptic drugs [see Warnings and Precautions (5.3), Drug Interactions (7.3)].
- The use of MAOIs (intended to treat psychiatric disorders) concomitantly with WELLBUTRIN SR or within 14 days of discontinuing treatment with WELLBUTRIN SR is contraindicated. There is an increased risk of hypertensive reactions when WELLBUTRIN SR is used concomitantly with MAOIs. The use of WELLBUTRIN SR within 14 days of discontinuing treatment with an MAOI is also contraindicated. Starting WELLBUTRIN SR in a patient treated with reversible MAOIs such as linezolid or intravenous methylene blue is contraindicated [see Dosage and Administration (2.4, 2.5), Warnings and Precautions (5.4), Drug Interactions (7.6)].
- WELLBUTRIN SR is contraindicated in patients with known hypersensitivity to bupropion or other ingredients of WELLBUTRIN SR. Anaphylactoid/anaphylactic reactions and Stevens-Johnson syndrome have been reported [see Warnings and Precautions (5.8)].

5   WARNINGS AND PRECAUTIONS

5.1   Suicidal Thoughts and Behaviors in Children, Adolescents, and Young Adults

Patients with MDD, both adult and pediatric, may experience worsening of their depression and/or the emergence of suicidal ideation and behavior (suicidality) or unusual changes in behavior, whether or not they are taking antidepressant medications, and this risk may persist until significant remission occurs. Suicide is a known risk of depression and certain other psychiatric disorders, and these disorders themselves are the strongest predictors of suicide. There has been a long-standing concern that antidepressants may have a role in inducing worsening of depression and the emergence of suicidality in certain patients during the early phases of treatment.
Pooled analyses of short-term placebo-controlled trials of antidepressant drugs (selective serotonin reuptake inhibitors [SSRIs] and others) show that these drugs increase the risk of suicidal thinking and behavior (suicidality) in children, adolescents, and young adults (ages 18 to 24) with MDD and other psychiatric disorders. Short-term clinical trials did not show an increase in the risk of suicidality with antidepressants compared with placebo in adults beyond age 24; there was a reduction with antidepressants compared with placebo in adults aged 65 and older.
The pooled analyses of placebo-controlled trials in children and adolescents with MDD, obsessive compulsive disorder (OCD), or other psychiatric disorders included a total of 24 short-term trials of 9 antidepressant drugs in over 4,400 subjects. The pooled analyses of placebo-controlled trials in adults with MDD or other psychiatric disorders included a total of 295 short-term trials (median duration of 2 months) of 11 antidepressant drugs in over 77,000 subjects. There was considerable variation in risk of suicidality among drugs, but a tendency toward an increase in the younger subjects for almost all drugs studied. There were differences in absolute risk of suicidality across the different indications, with the highest incidence in MDD. The risk differences (drug vs. placebo), however, were relatively stable within age strata and across indications. These risk differ-

ences (drug-placebo difference in the number of cases of suicidality per 1,000 subjects treated) are provided in Table 1.

Table 1. Risk Differences in the Number of Suicidality Cases by Age Group in the Pooled Placebo-Controlled Trials of Antidepressants in Pediatric and Adult Subjects

Age Range	Drug-Placebo Difference in Number of Cases of Suicidality per 1,000 Subjects Treated
Increases Compared With Placebo	
<18	14 additional cases
18-24	5 additional cases
Decreases Compared With Placebo	
25-64	1 fewer case
≥65	6 fewer cases

No suicides occurred in any of the pediatric trials. There were suicides in the adult trials, but the number was not sufficient to reach any conclusion about drug effect on suicide.

It is unknown whether the suicidality risk extends to longer-term use, i.e., beyond several months. However, there is substantial evidence from placebo-controlled maintenance trials in adults with depression that the use of antidepressants can delay the recurrence of depression.

All patients being treated with antidepressants for any indication should be monitored appropriately and observed closely for clinical worsening, suicidality, and unusual changes in behavior, especially during the initial few months of a course of drug therapy, or at times of dose changes, either increases or decreases [see Boxed Warning].

The following symptoms, anxiety, agitation, panic attacks, insomnia, irritability, hostility, aggressiveness, impulsivity, akathisia (psychomotor restlessness), hypomania, and mania, have been reported in adult and pediatric patients being treated with antidepressants for major depressive disorder as well as for other indications, both psychiatric and nonpsychiatric. Although a causal link between the emergence of such symptoms and either the worsening of depression and/or the emergence of suicidal impulses has not been established, there is concern that such symptoms may represent precursors to emerging suicidality.

Consideration should be given to changing the therapeutic regimen, including possibly discontinuing the medication, in patients whose depression is persistently worse, or who are experiencing emergent suicidality or symptoms that might be precursors to worsening depression or suicidality, especially if these symptoms are severe, abrupt in onset, or were not part of the patient's presenting symptoms.

Families and caregivers of patients being treated with antidepressants for MDD or other indications, both psychiatric and nonpsychiatric, should be alerted about the need to monitor patients for the emergence of agitation, irritability, unusual changes in behavior, and the other symptoms described above, as well as the emergence of suicidality, and to report such symptoms immediately to healthcare providers. Such monitoring should include daily observation by families and caregivers. Prescriptions for WELLBUTRIN SR should be written for the smallest quantity of tablets consistent with good patient management, in order to reduce the risk of overdose.

5.2   Neuropsychiatric Symptoms and Suicide Risk in Smoking Cessation Treatment
WELLBUTRIN SR is not approved for smoking cessation treatment; however, ZYBAN® is approved for this use. Serious neuropsychiatric symptoms have been reported in patients taking bupropion for smoking cessation. These have included changes in mood (including depression and mania), psychosis, hallucinations, paranoia, delusions, homicidal ideation, hostility, agitation, aggression, anxiety, and panic, as well as suicidal ideation, suicide attempt, and completed suicide [see Boxed Warning, Adverse Reactions (6.2)]. Observe patients for the occurrence of neuropsychiatric reactions. Instruct patients to contact a healthcare professional if such reactions occur.

In many of these cases, a causal relationship to bupropion treatment is not certain, because depressed mood can be a symptom of nicotine withdrawal. However, some of the cases occurred in patients taking bupropion who continued to smoke.

5.3   Seizure
WELLBUTRIN SR can cause seizure. The risk of seizure is dose-related. The dose should not exceed 400 mg per day. Increase the dose gradually. Discontinue WELLBUTRIN SR and do not restart treatment if the patient experiences a seizure.

The risk of seizures is also related to patient factors, clinical situations, and concomitant medications that lower the sei-

zure threshold. Consider these risks before initiating treatment with WELLBUTRIN SR. WELLBUTRIN SR is contraindicated in patients with a seizure disorder, current or prior diagnosis of anorexia nervosa or bulimia, or undergoing abrupt discontinuation of alcohol, benzodiazepines, barbiturates, and antiepileptic drugs [see Contraindications (4), Drug Interactions (7.3)]. The following conditions can also increase the risk of seizure: severe head injury; arteriovenous malformation; CNS tumor or CNS infection; severe stroke; concomitant use of other medications that lower the seizure threshold (e.g., other bupropion products, antipsychotics, tricyclic antidepressants, theophylline, and systemic corticosteroids); metabolic disorders (e.g., hypoglycemia, hyponatremia, severe hepatic impairment, and hypoxia); use of illicit drugs (e.g., cocaine); or abuse or misuse of prescription drugs such as CNS stimulants. Additional predisposing conditions include diabetes mellitus treated with oral hypoglycemic drugs or insulin; use of anorectic drugs; and excessive use of alcohol, benzodiazepines, sedative/hypnotics, or opiates.

Incidence of Seizure With Bupropion Use: When WELLBUTRIN SR is dosed up to 300 mg per day, the incidence of seizure is approximately 0.1% (1/1,000) and increases to approximately 0.4% (4/1,000) at the maximum recommended dose of 400 mg per day.

The risk of seizure can be reduced if the dose of WELLBUTRIN SR does not exceed 400 mg per day, given as 200 mg twice daily, and the titration rate is gradual.

5.4   Hypertension
Treatment with WELLBUTRIN SR can result in elevated blood pressure and hypertension. Assess blood pressure before initiating treatment with WELLBUTRIN SR, and monitor periodically during treatment. The risk of hypertension is increased if WELLBUTRIN SR is used concomitantly with MAOIs or other drugs that increase dopaminergic or noradrenergic activity [see Contraindications (4)].

Data from a comparative trial of the sustained-release formulation of bupropion HCl, nicotine transdermal system (NTS), the combination of sustained-release bupropion plus NTS, and placebo as an aid to smoking cessation suggest a higher incidence of treatment-emergent hypertension in patients treated with the combination of sustained-release bupropion and NTS. In this trial, 6.1% of subjects treated with the combination of sustained-release bupropion and NTS had treatment-emergent hypertension compared with 2.5%, 1.6%, and 3.1% of subjects treated with sustained-release bupropion, NTS, and placebo, respectively. The majority of these subjects had evidence of pre-existing hypertension. Three subjects (1.2%) treated with the combination of sustained-release bupropion and NTS and 1 subject (0.4%) treated with NTS had study medication discontinued due to hypertension compared with none of the subjects treated with sustained-release bupropion or placebo. Monitoring of blood pressure is recommended in patients who receive the combination of bupropion and nicotine replacement.

In a clinical trial of bupropion immediate-release in MDD subjects with stable congestive heart failure (N = 36), bupropion was associated with an exacerbation of pre-existing hypertension in 2 subjects, leading to discontinuation of bupropion treatment. There are no controlled trials assessing the safety of bupropion in patients with a recent history of myocardial infarction or unstable cardiac disease.

5.5   Activation of Mania/Hypomania
Antidepressant treatment can precipitate a manic, mixed, or hypomanic manic episode. The risk appears to be increased in patients with bipolar disorder or who have risk factors for bipolar disorder. Prior to initiating WELLBUTRIN SR, screen patients for a history of bipolar disorder and the presence of risk factors for bipolar disorder (e.g., family history of bipolar disorder, suicide, or depression). WELLBUTRIN SR is not approved for use in treating bipolar depression.

5.6   Psychosis and Other Neuropsychiatric Reactions
Depressed patients treated with WELLBUTRIN SR have had a variety of neuropsychiatric signs and symptoms, including delusions, hallucinations, psychosis, concentration disturbance, paranoia, and confusion. Some of these patients had a diagnosis of bipolar disorder. In some cases, these symptoms abated upon dose reduction and/or withdrawal of treatment. Instruct patients to contact a healthcare professional if such reactions occur.

5.7   Angle-Closure Glaucoma
The pupillary dilation that occurs following use of many antidepressant drugs including WELLBUTRIN SR may trigger an angle-closure attack in a patient with anatomically narrow angles who does not have a patent iridectomy.

5.8   Hypersensitivity Reactions
Anaphylactoid/anaphylactic reactions have occurred during clinical trials with bupropion. Reactions have been characterized by pruritus, urticaria, angioedema, and dyspnea requiring medical treatment. In addition, there have been rare, spontaneous postmarketing reports of erythema multiforme, Stevens–Johnson syndrome, and anaphylactic

shock associated with bupropion. Instruct patients to discontinue WELLBUTRIN SR and consult a healthcare provider if they develop an allergic or anaphylactoid/anaphylactic reaction (e.g., skin rash, pruritus, hives, chest pain, edema, and shortness of breath) during treatment.

There are reports of arthralgia, myalgia, fever with rash and other serum sickness-like symptoms suggestive of delayed hypersensitivity.

6   ADVERSE REACTIONS
The following adverse reactions are discussed in greater detail in other sections of the labeling:
- Suicidal thoughts and behaviors in adolescents and young adults [see Boxed Warning, Warnings and Precautions (5.1)]
- Neuropsychiatric symptoms and suicide risk in smoking cessation treatment [see Boxed Warning, Warnings and Precautions (5.2)]
- Seizure [see Warnings and Precautions (5.3)]
- Hypertension [see Warnings and Precautions (5.4)]
- Activation of mania or hypomania [see Warnings and Precautions (5.5)]
- Psychosis and other neuropsychiatric reactions [see Warnings and Precautions (5.6)]
- Angle-closure glaucoma [see Warnings and Precautions (5.7)]
- Hypersensitivity reactions [see Warnings and Precautions (5.8)]

6.1   Clinical Trials Experience
Because clinical trials are conducted under widely varying conditions, adverse reaction rates observed in the clinical trials of a drug cannot be directly compared with rates in the clinical trials of another drug and may not reflect the rates observed in clinical practice.

Adverse Reactions Leading to Discontinuation of Treatment: In placebo-controlled clinical trials, 4%, 9%, and 11% of the placebo, 300-mg-per-day, and 400-mg-per-day groups, respectively, discontinued treatment due to adverse reactions. The specific adverse reactions leading to discontinuation in at least 1% of the 300-mg-per-day or 400-mg-per-day groups and at a rate at least twice the placebo rate are listed in Table 2.

Table 2. Treatment Discontinuations Due to Adverse Reactions in Placebo-Controlled Trials

Adverse Reaction	Placebo (n = 385)	WELLBUTRIN SR 300 mg/day (n = 376)	WELLBUTRIN SR 400 mg/day (n = 114)
Rash	0.0%	2.4%	0.9%
Nausea	0.3%	0.8%	1.8%
Agitation	0.3%	0.3%	1.8%
Migraine	0.3%	0.0%	1.8%

Commonly Observed Adverse Reactions: Adverse reactions from Table 3 occurring in at least 5% of subjects treated with WELLBUTRIN SR and at a rate at least twice the placebo rate are listed below for the 300- and 400-mg-per-day dose groups.

WELLBUTRIN SR 300 mg per day: Anorexia, dry mouth, rash, sweating, tinnitus, and tremor.

WELLBUTRIN SR 400 mg per day: Abdominal pain, agitation, anxiety, dizziness, dry mouth, insomnia, myalgia, nausea, palpitation, pharyngitis, sweating, tinnitus, and urinary frequency.

Adverse reactions reported in placebo-controlled trials are presented in Table 3. Reported adverse reactions were classified using a COSTART–based Dictionary.

[See table 3 at top of next page]

Other Adverse Reactions Observed During the Clinical Development of Bupropion: In addition to the adverse reactions noted above, the following adverse reactions have been reported in clinical trials with the sustained–release formulation of bupropion in depressed subjects and in nondepressed smokers, as well as in clinical trials with the immediate–release formulation of bupropion.

Adverse reaction frequencies represent the proportion of subjects who experienced a treatment–emergent adverse reaction on at least one occasion in placebo-controlled clinical trials for depression (n = 987) or smoking cessation (n = 1,013), or subjects who experienced an adverse reaction requiring discontinuation of treatment in an open–label surveillance trial with WELLBUTRIN SR (n = 3,100). All treatment–emergent adverse reactions are included except those listed in Table 3, those listed in other safety–related sections of the prescribing information, those subsumed under COSTART terms that are either overly general or excessively specific so as to be uninformative, those not reasonably associated with the use of the drug, and those that were not serious and occurred in fewer than 2 subjects.

Adverse reactions are further categorized by body system and listed in order of decreasing frequency according to the following definitions of frequency: Frequent adverse reactions are defined as those occurring in at least 1/100 subjects. Infrequent adverse reactions are those occurring in 1/100 to 1/1,000 subjects, while rare events are those occurring in less than 1/1,000 subjects.

Body (General): Infrequent were chills, facial edema, and photosensitivity. Rare was malaise.

Cardiovascular: Infrequent were postural hypotension, stroke, tachycardia, and vasodilation. Rare were syncope and myocardial infarction.

Digestive: Infrequent were abnormal liver function, bruxism, gastric reflux, gingivitis, increased salivation, jaundice, mouth ulcers, stomatitis, and thirst. Rare was edema of tongue.

Hemic and Lymphatic: Infrequent was ecchymosis.

Metabolic and Nutritional: Infrequent were edema and peripheral edema.

Musculoskeletal: Infrequent were leg cramps.

Nervous System: Infrequent were abnormal coordination, decreased libido, depersonalization, dysphoria, emotional lability, hostility, hyperkinesia, hypertonia, hypesthesia, suicidal ideation, and vertigo. Rare were amnesia, ataxia, derealization, and hypomania.

Respiratory: Rare was bronchospasm.

Special Senses: Infrequent were accommodation abnormality and dry eye.

Urogenital: Infrequent were impotence, polyuria, and prostate disorder.

Changes in Body Weight: In placebo–controlled trials, subjects experienced weight gain or weight loss as shown in Table 4.

Table 4. Incidence of Weight Gain and Weight Loss (≥5 lbs.) in Placebo-Controlled Trials

Weight Change	WELLBUTRIN SR 300 mg/day (n = 339)	WELLBUTRIN SR 400 mg/day (n = 112)	Placebo (n = 347)
Gained >5 lbs	3%	2%	4%
Lost >5 lbs	14%	19%	6%

In clinical trials conducted with the immediate–release formulation of bupropion, 35% of subjects receiving tricyclic antidepressants gained weight, compared with 9% of subjects treated with the immediate–release formulation of bupropion. If weight loss is a major presenting sign of a patient's depressive illness, the anorectic and/or weight–reducing potential of WELLBUTRIN SR should be considered.

6.2   Postmarketing Experience
The following adverse reactions have been identified during post-approval use of WELLBUTRIN SR and are not described elsewhere in the label. Because these reactions are reported voluntarily from a population of uncertain size, it is not always possible to reliably estimate their frequency or establish a causal relationship to drug exposure.

Body (General): Arthralgia, myalgia, and fever with rash and other symptoms suggestive of delayed hypersensitivity. These symptoms may resemble serum sickness *[see Warnings and Precautions (5.8)]*.

Cardiovascular: Complete atrioventricular block, extrasystoles, hypotension, hypertension (in some cases severe), phlebitis, and pulmonary embolism.

Digestive: Colitis, esophagitis, gastrointestinal hemorrhage, gum hemorrhage, hepatitis, intestinal perforation, pancreatitis, and stomach ulcer.

Endocrine: Hyperglycemia, hypoglycemia, and syndrome of inappropriate antidiuretic hormone.

Hemic and Lymphatic: Anemia, leukocytosis, leukopenia, lymphadenopathy, pancytopenia, and thrombocytopenia. Altered PT and/or INR, infrequently associated with hemorrhagic or thrombotic complications, were observed when bupropion was coadministered with warfarin.

Metabolic and Nutritional: Glycosuria.

Musculoskeletal: Muscle rigidity/fever/rhabdomyolysis and muscle weakness.

Nervous System: Abnormal electroencephalogram (EEG), aggression, akinesia, aphasia, coma, completed suicide, delirium, delusions, dysarthria, dyskinesia, dystonia, euphoria, extrapyramidal syndrome, hallucinations, hypokinesia, increased libido, manic reaction, neuralgia, neuropathy, paranoid ideation, restlessness, suicide attempt, and unmasking tardive dyskinesia.

Respiratory: Pneumonia.

Skin: Alopecia, angioedema, exfoliative dermatitis, hirsutism, and Stevens-Johnson syndrome.

Special Senses: Deafness, increased intraocular pressure, and mydriasis.

Urogenital: Abnormal ejaculation, cystitis, dyspareunia, dysuria, gynecomastia, menopause, painful erection, salpingitis, urinary incontinence, urinary retention, and vaginitis.

Table 3. Adverse Reactions Reported by at Least 1% of Subjects and at a Greater Frequency Than Placebo in Controlled Clinical Trials

Body System/ Adverse Reaction	WELLBUTRIN SR 300 mg/day (n = 376)	WELLBUTRIN SR 400 mg/day (n = 114)	Placebo (n = 385)
Body (General)			
Headache	26%	25%	23%
Infection	8%	9%	6%
Abdominal pain	3%	9%	2%
Asthenia	2%	4%	2%
Chest pain	3%	4%	1%
Pain	2%	3%	2%
Fever	1%	2%	—
Cardiovascular			
Palpitation	2%	6%	2%
Flushing	1%	4%	—
Migraine	1%	4%	1%
Hot flashes	1%	3%	1%
Digestive			
Dry mouth	17%	24%	7%
Nausea	13%	18%	8%
Constipation	10%	5%	7%
Diarrhea	5%	7%	6%
Anorexia	5%	3%	2%
Vomiting	4%	2%	2%
Dysphagia	0%	2%	0%
Musculoskeletal			
Myalgia	2%	6%	3%
Arthralgia	1%	4%	1%
Arthritis	0%	2%	0%
Twitch	1%	2%	—
Nervous system			
Insomnia	11%	16%	6%
Dizziness	7%	11%	5%
Agitation	3%	9%	2%
Anxiety	5%	6%	3%
Tremor	6%	3%	1%
Nervousness	5%	3%	3%
Somnolence	2%	3%	2%
Irritability	3%	2%	2%
Memory decreased	—	3%	1%
Paresthesia	1%	2%	1%
Central nervous system stimulation	2%	1%	1%
Respiratory			
Pharyngitis	3%	11%	2%
Sinusitis	3%	1%	2%
Increased cough	1%	2%	1%
Skin			
Sweating	6%	5%	2%
Rash	5%	4%	1%
Pruritus	2%	4%	2%
Urticaria	2%	1%	0%
Special senses			
Tinnitus	6%	6%	2%
Taste perversion	2%	4%	—
Blurred vision or diplopia	3%	2%	2%
Urogenital			
Urinary frequency	2%	5%	2%
Urinary urgency	—	2%	0%
Vaginal hemorrhage[a]	0%	2%	—
Urinary tract infection	1%	0%	—

[a]Incidence based on the number of female subjects.
— Hyphen denotes adverse events occurring in greater than 0 but less than 0.5% of subjects.

7   DRUG INTERACTIONS
7.1   Potential for Other Drugs to Affect WELLBUTRIN SR
Bupropion is primarily metabolized to hydroxybupropion by CYP2B6. Therefore, the potential exists for drug interactions between WELLBUTRIN SR and drugs that are inhibitors or inducers of CYP2B6.

Inhibitors of CYP2B6: Ticlopidine and Clopidogrel: Concomitant treatment with these drugs can increase bupropion exposure but decrease hydroxybupropion exposure. Based on clinical response, dosage adjustment of WELLBUTRIN SR may be necessary when coadministered with CYP2B6 inhibitors (e.g., ticlopidine or clopidogrel) *[see Clinical Pharmacology (12.3)]*.

Inducers of CYP2B6: Ritonavir, Lopinavir, and Efavirenz: Concomitant treatment with these drugs can decrease bupropion and hydroxybupropion exposure. Dosage increase of WELLBUTRIN SR may be necessary when coadministered with ritonavir, lopinavir, or efavirenz *[see Clinical Pharmacology (12.3)]* but should not exceed the maximum recommended dose.

Carbamazepine, Phenobarbital, Phenytoin: While not systematically studied, these drugs may induce the metabolism of bupropion and may decrease bupropion exposure *[see Clinical Pharmacology (12.3)]*. If bupropion is used concomitantly with a CYP inducer, it may be necessary to increase the dose of bupropion, but the maximum recommended dose should not be exceeded.

7.2   Potential for WELLBUTRIN SR to Affect Other Drugs
Drugs Metabolized by CYP2D6: Bupropion and its metabolites (erythrohydrobupropion, threohydrobupropion, hydroxybupropion) are CYP2D6 inhibitors. Therefore, coadministration of WELLBUTRIN SR with drugs that are metabolized by CYP2D6 can increase the exposures of drugs that are substrates of CYP2D6. Such drugs include certain

antidepressants (e.g., venlafaxine, nortriptyline, imipramine, desipramine, paroxetine, fluoxetine, and sertraline), antipsychotics (e.g., haloperidol, risperidone, thioridazine), beta-blockers (e.g., metoprolol), and Type 1C antiarrhythmics (e.g., propafenone and flecainide). When used concomitantly with WELLBUTRIN SR, it may be necessary to decrease the dose of these CYP2D6 substrates, particularly for drugs with a narrow therapeutic index.

Drugs that require metabolic activation by CYP2D6 to be effective (e.g., tamoxifen) theoretically could have reduced efficacy when administered concomitantly with inhibitors of CYP2D6 such as bupropion. Patients treated concomitantly with WELLBUTRIN SR and such drugs may require increased doses of the drug [see Clinical Pharmacology (12.3)].

7.3 Drugs That Lower Seizure Threshold

Use extreme caution when coadministering WELLBUTRIN SR with other drugs that lower seizure threshold (e.g., other bupropion products, antipsychotics, antidepressants, theophylline, or systemic corticosteroids). Use low initial doses and increase the dose gradually [see Contraindications (4), Warnings and Precautions (5.3)].

7.4 Dopaminergic Drugs (Levodopa and Amantadine)

Bupropion, levodopa, and amantadine have dopamine agonist effects. CNS toxicity has been reported when bupropion was coadministered with levodopa or amantadine. Adverse reactions have included restlessness, agitation, tremor, ataxia, gait disturbance, vertigo, and dizziness. It is presumed that the toxicity results from cumulative dopamine agonist effects. Use caution when administering WELLBUTRIN SR concomitantly with these drugs.

7.5 Use With Alcohol

In postmarketing experience, there have been rare reports of adverse neuropsychiatric events or reduced alcohol tolerance in patients who were drinking alcohol during treatment with WELLBUTRIN SR. The consumption of alcohol during treatment with WELLBUTRIN SR should be minimized or avoided.

7.6 MAO Inhibitors

Bupropion inhibits the reuptake of dopamine and norepinephrine. Concomitant use of MAOIs and bupropion is contraindicated because there is an increased risk of hypertensive reactions if bupropion is used concomitantly with MAOIs. Studies in animals demonstrate that the acute toxicity of bupropion is enhanced by the MAO inhibitor phenelzine. At least 14 days should elapse between discontinuation of an MAOI intended to treat depression and initiation of treatment with WELLBUTRIN SR. Conversely, at least 14 days should be allowed after stopping WELLBUTRIN SR before starting an MAOI antidepressant [see Dosage and Administration (2.4, 2.5), Contraindications (4)].

7.7 Drug-Laboratory Test Interactions

False-positive urine immunoassay screening tests for amphetamines have been reported in patients taking bupropion. This is due to lack of specificity of some screening tests. False-positive test results may result even following discontinuation of bupropion therapy. Confirmatory tests, such as gas chromatography/mass spectrometry, will distinguish bupropion from amphetamines.

8 USE IN SPECIFIC POPULATIONS

8.1 Pregnancy

Pregnancy Category C

Risk Summary: Data from epidemiological studies of pregnant women exposed to bupropion in the first trimester indicate no increased risk of congenital malformations overall. All pregnancies, regardless of drug exposure, have a background rate of 2% to 4% for major malformations, and 15% to 20% for pregnancy loss. No clear evidence of teratogenic activity was found in reproductive developmental studies conducted in rats and rabbits; however, in rabbits, slightly increased incidences of fetal malformations and skeletal variations were observed at doses approximately equal to the maximum recommended human dose (MRHD) and greater and decreased fetal weights were seen at doses twice the MRHD and greater. WELLBUTRIN SR should be used during pregnancy only if the potential benefit justifies the potential risk to the fetus.

Clinical Considerations: Consider the risks of untreated depression when discontinuing or changing treatment with antidepressant medications during pregnancy and postpartum.

Human Data: Data from the international bupropion Pregnancy Registry (675 first trimester exposures) and a retrospective cohort study using the United Healthcare database (1,213 first trimester exposures) did not show an increased risk for malformations overall.

No increased risk for cardiovascular malformations overall has been observed after bupropion exposure during the first trimester. The prospectively observed rate of cardiovascular malformations in pregnancies with exposure to bupropion in the first trimester from the international Pregnancy Registry was 1.3% (9 cardiovascular malformations/675 first-trimester maternal bupropion exposures), which is similar to the background rate of cardiovascular malformations (ap-

proximately 1%). Data from the United Healthcare database and a case-control study (6,853 infants with cardiovascular malformations and 5,763 with non-cardiovascular malformations) from the National Birth Defects Prevention Study (NBDPS) did not show an increased risk for cardiovascular malformations overall after bupropion exposure during the first trimester.

Study findings on bupropion exposure during the first trimester and risk for left ventricular outflow tract obstruction (LVOTO) are inconsistent and do not allow conclusions regarding a possible association. The United Healthcare database lacked sufficient power to evaluate this association; the NBDPS found increased risk for LVOTO (n = 10; adjusted OR = 2.6; 95% CI: 1.2, 5.7), and the Slone Epidemiology case control study did not find increased risk for LVOTO.

Study findings on bupropion exposure during the first trimester and risk for ventricular septal defect (VSD) are inconsistent and do not allow conclusions regarding a possible association. The Slone Epidemiology Study found an increased risk for VSD following first trimester maternal bupropion exposure (n = 17; adjusted OR = 2.5; 95% CI: 1.3, 5.0) but did not find increased risk for any other cardiovascular malformations studied (including LVOTO as above). The NBDPS and United Healthcare database study did not find an association between first trimester maternal bupropion exposure and VSD.

For the findings of LVOTO and VSD, the studies were limited by the small number of exposed cases, inconsistent findings among studies, and the potential for chance findings from multiple comparisons in case control studies.

Animal Data: In studies conducted in rats and rabbits, bupropion was administered orally during the period of organogenesis at doses of up to 450 and 150 mg/kg/day, respectively (approximately 11 and 7 times the MRHD, respectively, on a mg/m² basis). No clear evidence of teratogenic activity was found in either species; however, in rabbits, slightly increased incidences of fetal malformations and skeletal variations were observed at the lowest dose tested (25 mg/kg/day, approximately equal to the MRHD on a mg/m² basis) and greater. Decreased fetal weights were observed at 50 mg/kg and greater.

When rats were administered bupropion at oral doses of up to 300 mg/kg/day (approximately 7 times the MRHD on a mg/m² basis) prior to mating and throughout pregnancy and lactation, there were no apparent adverse effects on offspring development.

8.3 Nursing Mothers

Bupropion and its metabolites are present in human milk. In a lactation study of 10 women, levels of orally dosed bupropion and its active metabolites were measured in expressed milk. The average daily infant exposure (assuming 150 mL/kg daily consumption) to bupropion and its active metabolites was 2% of the maternal weight-adjusted dose. Exercise caution when WELLBUTRIN SR is administered to a nursing woman.

8.4 Pediatric Use

Safety and effectiveness in the pediatric population have not been established [see Boxed Warning, Warnings and Precautions (5.1)].

8.5 Geriatric Use

Of the approximately 6,000 subjects who participated in clinical trials with bupropion sustained-release tablets (depression and smoking cessation trials), 275 were aged ≥65 years and 47 were aged ≥75 years. In addition, several hundred subjects aged ≥65 years participated in clinical trials using the immediate-release formulation of bupropion (depression trials). No overall differences in safety or effectiveness were observed between these subjects and younger subjects. Reported clinical experience has not identified differences in responses between the elderly and younger patients, but greater sensitivity of some older individuals cannot be ruled out.

Bupropion is extensively metabolized in the liver to active metabolites, which are further metabolized and excreted by the kidneys. The risk of adverse reactions may be greater in patients with impaired renal function. Because elderly patients are more likely to have decreased renal function, it may be necessary to consider this factor in dose selection; it may be useful to monitor renal function [see Dosage and Administration (2.3), Use in Specific Populations (8.6), Clinical Pharmacology (12.3)].

8.6 Renal Impairment

Consider a reduced dose and/or dosing frequency of WELLBUTRIN SR in patients with renal impairment (Glomerular Filtration Rate: <90 mL/min). Bupropion and its metabolites are cleared renally and may accumulate in such patients to a greater extent than usual. Monitor closely for adverse reactions that could indicate high bupropion or metabolite exposures [see Dosage and Administration (2.3), Clinical Pharmacology (12.3)].

8.7 Hepatic Impairment

In patients with moderate to severe hepatic impairment (Child-Pugh score: 7 to 15), the maximum dose of WELLBUTRIN SR is 100 mg per day or 150 mg every other

day. In patients with mild hepatic impairment (Child-Pugh score: 5 to 6), consider reducing the dose and/or frequency of dosing [see Dosage and Administration (2.2), Clinical Pharmacology (12.3)].

9 DRUG ABUSE AND DEPENDENCE

9.1 Controlled Substance

Bupropion is not a controlled substance.

9.2 Abuse

Humans: Controlled clinical trials of bupropion (immediate-release formulation) conducted in normal volunteers, in subjects with a history of multiple drug abuse, and in depressed subjects showed some increase in motor activity and agitation/excitement.

In a population of individuals experienced with drugs of abuse, a single dose of 400 mg of bupropion produced mild amphetamine-like activity as compared with placebo on the Morphine-Benzedrine Subscale of the Addiction Research Center Inventories (ARCI) and a score intermediate between placebo and amphetamine on the Liking Scale of the ARCI. These scales measure general feelings of euphoria and drug desirability.

Findings in clinical trials, however, are not known to reliably predict the abuse potential of drugs. Nonetheless, evidence from single-dose trials does suggest that the recommended daily dosage of bupropion when administered in divided doses is not likely to be significantly reinforcing to amphetamine or CNS stimulant abusers. However, higher doses (that could not be tested because of the risk of seizure) might be modestly attractive to those who abuse CNS stimulant drugs.

Animals: Studies in rodents and primates demonstrated that bupropion exhibits some pharmacologic actions common to psychostimulants. In rodents, it has been shown to increase locomotor activity, elicit a mild stereotyped behavior response, and increase rates of responding in several schedule-controlled behavior paradigms. In primate models assessing the positive reinforcing effects of psychoactive drugs, bupropion was self-administered intravenously. In rats, bupropion produced amphetamine-like and cocaine-like discriminative stimulus effects in drug discrimination paradigms used to characterize the subjective effects of psychoactive drugs.

10 OVERDOSAGE

10.1 Human Overdose Experience

Overdoses of up to 30 grams or more of bupropion have been reported. Seizure was reported in approximately one-third of all cases. Other serious reactions reported with overdoses of bupropion alone included hallucinations, loss of consciousness, sinus tachycardia, and ECG changes such as conduction disturbances (including QRS prolongation) or arrhythmias. Fever, muscle rigidity, rhabdomyolysis, hypotension, stupor, coma, and respiratory failure have been reported mainly when bupropion was part of multiple drug overdoses.

Although most patients recovered without sequelae, deaths associated with overdoses of bupropion alone have been reported in patients ingesting large doses of the drug. Multiple uncontrolled seizures, bradycardia, cardiac failure, and cardiac arrest prior to death were reported in these patients.

10.2 Overdosage Management

Consult a Certified Poison Control Center for up-to-date guidance and advice. Telephone numbers for certified poison control centers are listed in the Physician's Desk Reference (PDR). Call 1-800-222-1222 or refer to www.poison.org.

There are no known antidotes for bupropion. In case of an overdose, provide supportive care, including close medical supervision and monitoring. Consider the possibility of multiple drug overdose. Ensure an adequate airway, oxygenation, and ventilation. Monitor cardiac rhythm and vital signs. Induction of emesis is not recommended.

11 DESCRIPTION

WELLBUTRIN SR (bupropion hydrochloride), an antidepressant of the aminoketone class, is chemically unrelated to tricyclic, tetracyclic, selective serotonin re-uptake inhibitor, or other known antidepressant agents. Its structure closely resembles that of diethylpropion; it is related to phenylethylamines. It is designated as (±)-1-(3-chlorophenyl)-2-[(1,1-dimethylethyl)amino]-1-propanone hydrochloride. The molecular weight is 276.2. The molecular formula is $C_{13}H_{18}ClNO \cdot HCl$. Bupropion hydrochloride powder is white, crystalline, and highly soluble in water. It has a bitter taste and produces the sensation of local anesthesia on the oral mucosa. The structural formula is:

WELLBUTRIN SR is supplied for oral administration as 100–mg (blue), 150–mg (purple), and 200–mg (light pink), film–coated, sustained–release tablets. Each tablet contains the labeled amount of bupropion hydrochloride and the inactive ingredients: carnauba wax, cysteine hydrochloride, hypromellose, magnesium stearate, microcrystalline cellulose, polyethylene glycol, polysorbate 80, and titanium dioxide and is printed with edible black ink. In addition, the 100–mg tablet contains FD&C Blue No. 1 Lake, the 150–mg tablet contains FD&C Blue No. 2 Lake and FD&C Red No. 40 Lake, and the 200–mg tablet contains FD&C Red No. 40 Lake.

12 CLINICAL PHARMACOLOGY

12.1 Mechanism of Action

The exact mechanism of the antidepressant action of bupropion is not known, but is presumed to be related to noradrenergic and/or dopaminergic mechanisms. Bupropion is a relatively weak inhibitor of the neuronal reuptake of norepinephrine and dopamine, and does not inhibit the reuptake of serotonin. Bupropion does not inhibit monoamine oxidase.

12.3 Pharmacokinetics

Bupropion is a racemic mixture. The pharmacological activity and pharmacokinetics of the individual enantiomers have not been studied. The mean elimination half–life (±SD) of bupropion after chronic dosing is 21 (±9) hours, and steady-state plasma concentrations of bupropion are reached within 8 days.

Absorption: The absolute bioavailability of WELLBUTRIN SR in humans has not been determined because an intravenous formulation for human use is not available. However, it appears likely that only a small proportion of any orally administered dose reaches the systemic circulation intact. In rat and dog studies, the bioavailability of bupropion ranged from 5% to 20%.

In humans, following oral administration of WELLBUTRIN SR, peak plasma concentration (C_{max}) of bupropion is usually achieved within 3 hours.

In a trial comparing chronic dosing with WELLBUTRIN SR 150 mg twice daily to bupropion immediate–release formulation 100 mg 3 times daily, the steady state C_{max} for bupropion after WELLBUTRIN SR administration was approximately 85% of those achieved after bupropion immediate-release formulation administration. Exposure (AUC) to bupropion was equivalent for both formulations. Bioequivalence was also demonstrated for all three major active metabolites (i.e., hydroxybupropion, threohydrobupropion and erythrohydrobupropion) for both C_{max} and AUC. Thus, at steady state, WELLBUTRIN SR given twice daily, and the immediate–release formulation of bupropion given 3 times daily, are essentially bioequivalent for both bupropion and the 3 quantitatively important metabolites. WELLBUTRIN SR can be taken with or without food. Bupropion C_{max} and AUC was increased by 11% to 35% and 16% to 19%, respectively, when WELLBUTRIN SR was administered with food to healthy volunteers in three trials. The food effect is not considered clinically significant.

Distribution: In vitro tests show that bupropion is 84% bound to human plasma proteins at concentrations up to 200 mcg/mL. The extent of protein binding of the hydroxybupropion metabolite is similar to that for bupropion; whereas, the extent of protein binding of the threohydrobupropion metabolite is about half that seen with bupropion.

Metabolism: Bupropion is extensively metabolized in humans. Three metabolites are active: hydroxybupropion, which is formed via hydroxylation of the tert–butyl group of bupropion, and the amino–alcohol isomers, threohydrobupropion and erythrohydrobupropion, which are formed via reduction of the carbonyl group. In vitro findings suggest that CYP2B6 is the principal isoenzyme involved in the formation of hydroxybupropion, while cytochrome P450 enzymes are not involved in the formation of threohydrobupropion. Oxidation of the bupropion side chain results in the formation of a glycine conjugate of meta–chlorobenzoic acid, which is then excreted as the major urinary metabolite. The potency and toxicity of the metabolites relative to bupropion have not been fully characterized. However, it has been demonstrated in an antidepressant screening test in mice that hydroxybupropion is one-half as potent as bupropion, while threohydrobupropion and erythrohydrobupropion are 5-fold less potent than bupropion. This may be of clinical importance because the plasma concentrations of the metabolites are as high as or higher than those of bupropion. Following a single dose administration of WELLBUTRIN SR in humans, C_{max} of hydroxybupropion occurs approximately 6 hours post–dose and is approximately 10 times the peak level of the parent drug at steady state. The elimination half–life of hydroxybupropion is approximately 20 (±5) hours and its AUC at steady state is about 17 times that of bupropion. The times to peak concentrations for the erythrohydrobupropion and threohydrobupropion metabolites are similar to that of the hydroxybupropion metabolite. However, their elimination half–lives are longer, 33 (±10) and 37 (±13) hours, respectively, and steady–state AUCs are 1.5 and 7 times that of bupropion, respectively.

Bupropion and its metabolites exhibit linear kinetics following chronic administration of 300 to 450 mg per day.

Elimination: Following oral administration of 200 mg of ^{14}C–bupropion in humans, 87% and 10% of the radioactive dose were recovered in the urine and feces, respectively. Only 0.5% of the oral dose was excreted as unchanged bupropion.

Population Subgroups: Factors or conditions altering metabolic capacity (e.g., liver disease, congestive heart failure [CHF], age, concomitant medications, etc.) or elimination may be expected to influence the degree and extent of accumulation of the active metabolites of bupropion. The elimination of the major metabolites of bupropion may be affected by reduced renal or hepatic function because they are moderately polar compounds and are likely to undergo further metabolism or conjugation in the liver prior to urinary excretion.

Renal Impairment: There is limited information on the pharmacokinetics of bupropion in patients with renal impairment. An inter-trial comparison between normal subjects and subjects with end-stage renal failure demonstrated that the parent drug C_{max} and AUC values were comparable in the 2 groups, whereas the hydroxybupropion and threohydrobupropion metabolites had a 2.3- and 2.8-fold increase, respectively, in AUC for subjects with end-stage renal failure. A second trial, comparing normal subjects and subjects with moderate–to–severe renal impairment (GFR 30.9 ± 10.8 mL/min), showed that after a single 150-mg dose of sustained-release bupropion, exposure to bupropion was approximately 2-fold higher in subjects with impaired renal function, while levels of the hydroxybupropion and threo/erythrohydrobupropion (combined) metabolites were similar in the 2 groups. Bupropion is extensively metabolized in the liver to active metabolites, which are further metabolized and subsequently excreted by the kidneys. The elimination of the major metabolites of bupropion may be reduced by impaired renal function. WELLBUTRIN SR should be used with caution in patients with renal impairment and a reduced frequency and/or dose should be considered [see Use in Specific Populations (8.6)].

Hepatic Impairment: The effect of hepatic impairment on the pharmacokinetics of bupropion was characterized in 2 single-dose trials, one in subjects with alcoholic liver disease and one in subjects with mild-to-severe cirrhosis. The first trial demonstrated that the half–life of hydroxybupropion was significantly longer in 8 subjects with alcoholic liver disease than in 8 healthy volunteers (32 ± 14 hours versus 21 ± 5 hours, respectively). Although not statistically significant, the AUCs for bupropion and hydroxybupropion were more variable and tended to be greater (by 53% to 57%) in volunteers with alcoholic liver disease. The differences in half–life for bupropion and the other metabolites in the 2 groups were minimal.

The second trial demonstrated no statistically significant differences in the pharmacokinetics of bupropion and its active metabolites in 9 subjects with mild-to-moderate hepatic cirrhosis compared with 8 healthy volunteers. However, more variability was observed in some of the pharmacokinetic parameters for bupropion (AUC, C_{max}, and T_{max}) and its active metabolites ($t_{1/2}$) in subjects with mild-to-moderate hepatic cirrhosis. In subjects with severe hepatic cirrhosis, significant alterations in the pharmacokinetics of bupropion and its metabolites were seen (Table 5).

Table 5. Pharmacokinetics of Bupropion and Metabolites in Patients With Severe Hepatic Cirrhosis: Ratio Relative to Healthy Matched Controls

	C_{max}	AUC	$t_{1/2}$	T_{max} [a]
Bupropion	1.69	3.12	1.43	0.5 h
Hydroxybupropion	0.31	1.28	3.88	19 h
Threo/ erythrohydrobupropion amino alcohol	0.69	2.48	1.96	20 h

[a] = Difference.

Left Ventricular Dysfunction: During a chronic dosing trial with bupropion in 14 depressed subjects with left ventricular dysfunction (history of CHF or an enlarged heart on x-ray), there was no apparent effect on the pharmacokinetics of bupropion or its metabolites, compared with healthy volunteers.

Age: The effects of age on the pharmacokinetics of bupropion and its metabolites have not been fully characterized, but an exploration of steady–state bupropion concentrations from several depression efficacy trials involving subjects dosed in a range of 300 to 750 mg per day, on a 3 times daily schedule, revealed no relationship between age (18 to 83 years) and plasma concentration of bupropion. A single–dose pharmacokinetic trial demonstrated that the

disposition of bupropion and its metabolites in elderly subjects was similar to that of younger subjects. These data suggest there is no prominent effect of age on bupropion concentration; however, another single- and multiple-dose pharmacokinetics trial suggested that the elderly are at increased risk for accumulation of bupropion and its metabolites [see Use in Specific Populations (8.5)].

Gender: Pooled analysis of bupropion pharmacokinetic data from 90 healthy male and 90 healthy female volunteers revealed no sex–related differences in the peak plasma concentrations of bupropion. The mean systemic exposure (AUC) was approximately 13% higher in male volunteers compared with female volunteers. The clinical significance of this finding is unknown.

Smokers: The effects of cigarette smoking on the pharmacokinetics of bupropion were studied in 34 healthy male and female volunteers; 17 were chronic cigarette smokers and 17 were nonsmokers. Following oral administration of a single 150–mg dose of bupropion, there were no statistically significant differences in C_{max}, half-life, T_{max}, AUC, or clearance of bupropion or its active metabolites between smokers and nonsmokers.

Drug Interactions: Potential for Other Drugs to Affect WELLBUTRIN SR: In vitro studies indicate that bupropion is primarily metabolized to hydroxybupropion by CYP2B6. Therefore, the potential exists for drug interactions between WELLBUTRIN SR and drugs that are inhibitors or inducers of CYP2B6. In addition, in vitro studies suggest that paroxetine, sertraline, norfluoxetine, fluvoxamine, and nelfinavir inhibit the hydroxylation of bupropion.

Inhibitors of CYP2B6: Ticlopidine, Clopidogrel: In a trial in healthy male volunteers, clopidogrel 75 mg once daily or ticlopidine 250 mg twice daily increased exposures (C_{max} and AUC) of bupropion by 40% and 60% for clopidogrel, and by 38% and 85% for ticlopidine, respectively. The exposures (C_{max} and AUC) of hydroxybupropion were decreased 50% and 52%, respectively, by clopidogrel, and 78% and 84%, respectively, by ticlopidine. This effect is thought to be due to the inhibition of the CYP2B6-catalyzed bupropion hydroxylation.

Prasugrel: Prasugrel is a weak inhibitor of CYP2B6. In healthy subjects, prasugrel increased bupropion C_{max} and AUC values by 14% and 18%, respectively, and decreased C_{max} and AUC values of hydroxybupropion, an active metabolite of bupropion, by 32% and 24%, respectively.

Cimetidine: The threohydrobupropion metabolite of bupropion does not appear to be produced by cytochrome P450 enzymes. The effects of concomitant administration of cimetidine on the pharmacokinetics of bupropion and its active metabolites were studied in 24 healthy young male volunteers. Following oral administration of bupropion 300 mg with and without cimetidine 800 mg, the pharmacokinetics of bupropion and hydroxybupropion were unaffected. However, there were 16% and 32% increases in the AUC and C_{max}, respectively, of the combined moieties of threohydrobupropion and erythrohydrobupropion.

Citalopram: Citalopram did not affect the pharmacokinetics of bupropion and its three metabolites.

Inducers of CYP2B6: Ritonavir and Lopinavir: In a healthy volunteer trial, ritonavir 100 mg twice daily reduced the AUC and C_{max} of bupropion by 22% and 21%, respectively. The exposure of the hydroxybupropion metabolite was decreased by 23%, the threohydrobupropion decreased by 38%, and the erythrohydrobupropion decreased by 48%.

In a second healthy volunteer trial, ritonavir 600 mg twice daily decreased the AUC and the C_{max} of bupropion by 66% and 62%, respectively. The exposure of the hydroxybupropion metabolite was decreased by 78%, the threohydrobupropion decreased by 50%, and the erythrohydrobupropion decreased by 68%.

In another healthy volunteer trial, lopinavir 400 mg/ritonavir 100 mg twice daily decreased bupropion AUC and C_{max} by 57%. The AUC and C_{max} of hydroxybupropion were decreased by 50% and 31%, respectively.

Efavirenz: In a trial in healthy volunteers, efavirenz 600 mg once daily for 2 weeks reduced the AUC and Cmax of bupropion by approximately 55% and 34%, respectively. The AUC of hydroxybupropion was unchanged, whereas Cmax of hydroxybupropion was increased by 50%.

Carbamazepine, Phenobarbital, Phenytoin: While not systematically studied, these drugs may induce the metabolism of bupropion.

Potential for WELLBUTRIN SR to Affect Other Drugs: Animal data indicated that bupropion may be an inducer of drug-metabolizing enzymes in humans. In one trial, following chronic administration of bupropion 100 mg three times daily to 8 healthy male volunteers for 14 days, there was no evidence of induction of its own metabolism. Nevertheless, there may be potential for clinically important alterations of blood levels of co-administered drugs.

Drugs Metabolized by CYP2D6: In vitro, bupropion and its metabolites (erythrohydrobupropion, threohydrobupropion, hydroxybupropion) are CYP2D6 inhibitors. In a clinical trial of 15 male subjects (ages 19 to 35 years) who were extensive metabolizers of CYP2D6, bupropion 300 mg per day followed by a single dose of 50 mg desipramine increased the C_{max}, AUC, and t1/2 of desipramine by an average of approximately 2-, 5-, and 2-fold, respectively. The effect was present for at least 7 days after the last dose of bupropion. Concomitant use of bupropion with other drugs metabolized by CYP2D6 has not been formally studied.

Citalopram: Although citalopram is not primarily metabolized by CYP2D6, in one trial bupropion increased the C_{max} and AUC of citalopram by 30% and 40%, respectively.

Lamotrigine: Multiple oral doses of bupropion had no statistically significant effects on the single-dose pharmacokinetics of lamotrigine in 12 healthy volunteers.

13 NONCLINICAL TOXICOLOGY

13.1 Carcinogenesis, Mutagenesis, Impairment of Fertility

Lifetime carcinogenicity studies were performed in rats and mice at bupropion doses up to 300 and 150 mg/kg/day, respectively. These doses are approximately 7 and 2 times the MRHD, respectively, on a mg/m^2 basis. In the rat study there was an increase in nodular proliferative lesions of the liver at doses of 100 to 300 mg/kg/day (approximately 2 to 7 times the MRHD on a mg/m^2 basis); lower doses were not tested. The question of whether or not such lesions may be precursors of neoplasms of the liver is currently unresolved. Similar liver lesions were not seen in the mouse study, and no increase in malignant tumors of the liver and other organs was seen in either study.

Bupropion produced a positive response (2 to 3 times control mutation rate) in 2 of 5 strains in the Ames bacterial mutagenicity assay. Bupropion produced an increase in chromosomal aberrations in 1 of 3 in vivo rat bone marrow cytogenetic studies.

A fertility study in rats at doses up to 300 mg/kg/day revealed no evidence of impaired fertility.

14 CLINICAL STUDIES

The efficacy of the immediate–release formulation of bupropion in the treatment of major depressive disorder was established in two 4–week, placebo–controlled trials in adult inpatients with MDD (Trials 1 and 2 in Table 6) and in one 6–week, placebo–controlled trial in adult outpatients with MDD (Trial 3 in Table 6). In the first trial, the dose range of bupropion was 300 mg to 600 mg per day administered in divided doses; 78% of subjects were treated with doses of 300 mg to 450 mg per day. This trial demonstrated the effectiveness of the immediate–release formulation of bupropion by the Hamilton Depression Rating Scale (HDRS) total score, the HDRS depressed mood item (item 1), and the Clinical Global Impressions severity score (CGI-S). The second trial included 2 doses of the immediate–release formulation of bupropion (300 and 450 mg per day) and placebo. This trial demonstrated the effectiveness of the immediate–release formulation of bupropion, but only at the 450–mg-per-day dose. The efficacy results were significant for the HDRS total score and the CGI-S score, but not for HDRS item 1. In the third trial, outpatients were treated with 300 mg per day of the immediate–release formulation of bupropion. This trial demonstrated the efficacy of the immediate–release formulation of bupropion as measured by the HDRS total score, the HDRS item 1, the Montgomery–Asberg Depression Rating Scale (MADRS), the CGI-S score, and the CGI-Improvement Scale (CGI-I) score.

[See table 6 above]

Although there are not as yet independent trials demonstrating the antidepressant effectiveness of the sustained–release formulation of bupropion, trials have demonstrated the bioequivalence of the immediate–release and sustained–release forms of bupropion under steady–state conditions, i.e., bupropion sustained–release 150 mg twice daily was shown to be bioequivalent to 100 mg 3 times daily of the immediate–release formulation of bupropion, with regard to both rate and extent of absorption, for parent drug and metabolites.

In a longer-term trial, outpatients meeting DSM-IV criteria for major depressive disorder, recurrent type, who had responded during an 8-week open trial on WELLBUTRIN SR (150 mg twice daily) were randomized to continuation of their same dose of WELLBUTRIN SR or placebo for up to 44 weeks of observation for relapse. Response during the open phase was defined as CGI Improvement score of 1 (very much improved) or 2 (much improved) for each of the final 3 weeks. Relapse during the double-blind phase was defined as the investigator's judgment that drug treatment was needed for worsening depressive symptoms. Patients receiving continued treatment with WELLBUTRIN SR experienced significantly lower relapse rates over the subsequent 44 weeks compared with those receiving placebo.

16 HOW SUPPLIED/STORAGE AND HANDLING

WELLBUTRIN SR Sustained–Release Tablets, 100 mg of bupropion hydrochloride, are blue, round, biconvex, film–coated tablets printed with "WELLBUTRIN SR 100" in bottles of 60 (NDC 0173-0947-55) tablets.

Table 6. Efficacy of Immediate-Release Bupropion for the Treatment of Major Depressive Disorder

Trial Number	Treatment Group	Primary Efficacy Measure: HDRS		
		Mean Baseline Score (SD)	LS Mean Score at Endpoint Visit (SE)	Placebo-subtracted Difference[a] (95% CI)
Trial 1	Immediate-Release Bupropion 300-600 mg/day[b] (n = 48)	28.5 (5.1)	14.9 (1.3)	-4.7 (-8.8, -0.6)
	Placebo (n = 27)	29.3 (7.0)	19.6 (1.6)	--
		Mean Baseline Score (SD)	LS Mean Change from Baseline (SE)	Placebo-subtracted Difference[a] (95% CI)
Trial 2	Immediate-Release Bupropion 300 mg/day (n = 36)	32.4 (5.9)	-15.5 (1.7)	-4.1
	Immediate-Release Bupropion 450 mg/day[b] (n = 34)	34.8 (4.6)	-17.4 (1.7)	-5.9 (-10.5, -1.4)
	Placebo (n = 39)	32.9 (5.4)	-11.5 (1.6)	--
Trial 3	Immediate-Release Bupropion 300 mg/day[b] (n = 110)	26.5 (4.3)	-12.0 (NA)	-3.9 (-5.7, -1.0)
	Placebo (n = 106)	27.0 (3.5)	-8.7 (NA)	--

n: sample size; SD: standard deviation; SE: standard error; LS Mean: least-squares mean; CI: unadjusted confidence interval included for doses that were demonstrated to be effective; NA: not available.
[a]Difference (drug minus placebo) in least-squares estimates with respect to the primary efficacy parameter. For Trial 1, it refers to the mean score at the endpoint visit; for Trials 2 and 3, it refers to the mean change from baseline to the endpoint visit.
[b]Doses that are demonstrated to be statistically significantly superior to placebo.

WELLBUTRIN SR Sustained–Release Tablets, 150 mg of bupropion hydrochloride, are purple, round, biconvex, film–coated tablets printed with "WELLBUTRIN SR 150" in bottles of 60 (NDC 0173-0135-55) tablets.

WELLBUTRIN SR Sustained-Release Tablets, 200 mg of bupropion hydrochloride, are light pink, round, biconvex, film-coated tablets printed with "WELLBUTRIN SR 200" in bottles of 60 (NDC 0173-0722-00) tablets.

Store at room temperature, 20° to 25°C (68° to 77°F); excursions permitted between 15°C and 30°C (59°F and 86°F) [see USP Controlled Room Temperature]. Protect from light and moisture.

17 PATIENT COUNSELING INFORMATION

Advise the patient to read the FDA-approved patient labeling (Medication Guide).

Inform patients, their families, and their caregivers about the benefits and risks associated with treatment with WELLBUTRIN SR and counsel them in its appropriate use. A patient Medication Guide about "Antidepressant Medicines, Depression and Other Serious Mental Illnesses, and Suicidal Thoughts or Actions," "Quitting Smoking, Quit-Smoking Medications, Changes in Thinking and Behavior, Depression, and Suicidal Thoughts or Actions," and "What Other Important Information Should I Know About WELLBUTRIN SR?" is available for WELLBUTRIN SR. Instruct patients, their families, and their caregivers to read the Medication Guide and assist them in understanding its contents. Patients should be given the opportunity to discuss the contents of the Medication Guide and to obtain answers to any questions they may have. The complete text of the Medication Guide is reprinted at the end of this document.

Advise patients regarding the following issues and to alert their prescriber if these occur while taking WELLBUTRIN SR.

Suicidal Thoughts and Behaviors: Instruct patients, their families, and/or their caregivers to be alert to the emergence of anxiety, agitation, panic attacks, insomnia, irritability, hostility, aggressiveness, impulsivity, akathisia (psychomotor restlessness), hypomania, mania, other unusual changes in behavior, worsening of depression, and suicidal ideation, especially early during antidepressant treatment and when the dose is adjusted up or down. Advise families and caregivers of patients to observe for the emergence of such symptoms on a day-to-day basis, since changes may be abrupt. Such symptoms should be reported to the patient's prescriber or healthcare professional, especially if they are severe, abrupt in onset, or were not part of the patient's presenting symptoms. Symptoms such as these may be associated with an increased risk for suicidal thinking and behavior and indicate a need for very close monitoring and possibly changes in the medication.

Neuropsychiatric Symptoms and Suicide Risk in Smoking Cessation Treatment: Although WELLBUTRIN SR is not indicated for smoking cessation treatment, it contains the same active ingredient as ZYBAN which is approved for this use. Advise patients, families and caregivers that quitting smoking, with or without ZYBAN, may trigger nicotine withdrawal symptoms (e.g., including depression or agitation), or worsen pre-existing psychiatric illness. Some patients have experienced changes in mood (including depression and mania), psychosis, hallucinations, paranoia, delusions, homicidal ideation, aggression, anxiety, and panic, as well as suicidal ideation, suicide attempt, and completed suicide when attempting to quit smoking while taking ZYBAN. If patients develop agitation, hostility, depressed mood, or changes in thinking or behavior that are not typical for them, or if patients develop suicidal ideation or behavior, they should be urged to report these symptoms to their healthcare provider immediately.

Severe Allergic Reactions: Educate patients on the symptoms of hypersensitivity and to discontinue WELLBUTRIN SR if they have a severe allergic reaction.

Seizure: Instruct patients to discontinue and not restart WELLBUTRIN SR if they experience a seizure while on treatment. Advise patients that the excessive use or abrupt discontinuation of alcohol, benzodiazepines, antiepileptic drugs, or sedatives/hypnotics can increase the risk of seizure. Advise patients to minimize or avoid use of alcohol.

As the dose is increased during initial titration to doses above 150 mg per day, instruct patients to take WELLBUTRIN SR in 2 divided doses, preferably with at least 8 hours between successive doses, to minimize the risk of seizures.

Angle-Closure Glaucoma: Patients should be advised that taking WELLBUTRIN SR can cause mild pupillary dilation, which in susceptible individuals, can lead to an episode of angle-closure glaucoma. Pre-existing glaucoma is almost always open-angle glaucoma because angle-closure glaucoma, when diagnosed, can be treated definitively with iridectomy. Open-angle glaucoma is not a risk factor for angle-closure glaucoma. Patients may wish to be examined to determine whether they are susceptible to angle closure, and have a prophylactic procedure (e.g., iridectomy), if they are susceptible *[see Warnings and Precautions (5.7)]*.

Bupropion-Containing Products: Educate patients that WELLBUTRIN SR contains the same active ingredient (bupropion hydrochloride) found in ZYBAN, which is used as an aid to smoking cessation treatment, and that WELLBUTRIN SR should not be used in combination with ZYBAN or any other medications that contain bupropion (such as WELLBUTRIN®, the immediate-release formulation and WELLBUTRIN XL® or FORFIVO XL™, the extended-release formulations, and APLENZIN®, the extended-release formulation of bupropion hydrobromide). In addition, there are a number of generic bupropion HCl products for the immediate-, sustained-, and extended-release formulations.

Potential for Cognitive and Motor Impairment: Advise patients that any CNS–active drug like WELLBUTRIN SR may impair their ability to perform tasks requiring judgment or motor and cognitive skills. Advise patients that until they are reasonably certain that WELLBUTRIN SR does not adversely affect their performance, they should refrain from driving an automobile or operating complex, hazardous machinery. WELLBUTRIN SR may lead to decreased alcohol tolerance.

Concomitant Medications: Counsel patients to notify their healthcare provider if they are taking or plan to take any prescription or over–the–counter drugs because WELLBUTRIN SR Sustained-Release Tablets and other drugs may affect each others' metabolisms.

Pregnancy: Advise patients to notify their healthcare provider if they become pregnant or intend to become pregnant during therapy.

Precautions for Nursing Mothers: Advise patients that WELLBUTRIN SR is present in human milk in small amounts.

Storage Information: Instruct patients to store WELLBUTRIN SR at room temperature, between 59°F and 86°F (15°C to 30°C) and keep the tablets dry and out of the light.

Administration Information: Instruct patients to swallow WELLBUTRIN SR Tablets whole so that the release rate is not altered. Do not chew, divide, or crush tablets; they are designed to slowly release drug in the body. When patients take more than 150 mg per day, instruct them to take WELLBUTRIN SR in 2 doses at least 8 hours apart, to minimize the risk of seizures. Instruct patients if they miss a dose, not to take an extra tablet to make up for the missed dose and to take the next tablet at the regular time because of the dose-related risk of seizure. Instruct patients that WELLBUTRIN SR Tablets may have an odor. WELLBUTRIN SR can be taken with or without food.

WELLBUTRIN, WELLBUTRIN SR, WELLBUTRIN XL, and ZYBAN are registered trademarks of the GSK group of companies. The other brands listed are trademarks of their respective owners and are not trademarks of the GSK group of companies. The makers of these brands are not affiliated with and do not endorse the GSK group of companies or its products.

GlaxoSmithKline
Research Triangle Park, NC 27709
©2014, the GSK group of companies. All rights reserved.
WLS:12PI

Medication Guide
WELLBUTRIN® SR (WELL byu-trin)
(bupropion hydrochloride) Sustained–Release Tablets
Read this Medication Guide carefully before you start taking WELLBUTRIN SR and each time you get a refill. There may be new information. This information does not take the place of talking with your healthcare provider about your medical condition or your treatment. If you have any questions about WELLBUTRIN SR, ask your healthcare provider or pharmacist.

IMPORTANT: Be sure to read the three sections of this Medication Guide. The first section is about the risk of suicidal thoughts and actions with antidepressant medicines; the second section is about the risk of changes in thinking and behavior, depression and suicidal thoughts or actions with medicines used to quit smoking; and the third section is entitled "What Other Important Information Should I Know About WELLBUTRIN SR?"

Antidepressant Medicines, Depression and Other Serious Mental Illnesses, and Suicidal Thoughts or Actions
This section of the Medication Guide is only about the risk of suicidal thoughts and actions with antidepressant medicines. **Talk to your healthcare provider or your family member's healthcare provider about:**
• all risks and benefits of treatment with antidepressant medicines
• all treatment choices for depression or other serious mental illness

What is the most important information I should know about antidepressant medicines, depression and other serious mental illnesses, and suicidal thoughts or actions?
1. **Antidepressant medicines may increase suicidal thoughts or actions in some children, teenagers, or young adults within the first few months of treatment.**
2. **Depression or other serious mental illnesses are the most important causes of suicidal thoughts and actions. Some people may have a particularly high risk of having suicidal thoughts or actions.** These include people who have (or have a family history of) bipolar illness (also called manic-depressive illness) or suicidal thoughts or actions.
3. **How can I watch for and try to prevent suicidal thoughts and actions in myself and a family member?**
• Pay close attention to any changes, especially sudden changes, in mood, behaviors, thoughts, or feelings. This is very important when an antidepressant medicine is started or when the dose is changed.

• Call your healthcare provider right away to report new or sudden changes in mood, behavior, thoughts, or feelings.
• Keep all follow-up visits with your healthcare provider as scheduled. Call the healthcare provider between visits as needed, especially if you have concerns about symptoms.

Call your healthcare provider right away if you or your family member has any of the following symptoms, especially if they are new, worse, or worry you:

• thoughts about suicide or dying
• attempts to commit suicide
• new or worse depression
• new or worse anxiety
• feeling very agitated or restless
• panic attacks

• trouble sleeping (insomnia)
• new or worse irritability
• acting aggressive, being angry, or violent
• acting on dangerous impulses
• an extreme increase in activity and talking (mania)
• other unusual changes in behavior or mood

What else do I need to know about antidepressant medicines?
• **Never stop an antidepressant medicine without first talking to a healthcare provider.** Stopping an antidepressant medicine suddenly can cause other symptoms.
• **Antidepressants are medicines used to treat depression and other illnesses.** It is important to discuss all the risks of treating depression and also the risks of not treating it. Patients and their families or other caregivers should discuss all treatment choices with the healthcare provider, not just the use of antidepressants.
• **Antidepressant medicines have other side effects.** Talk to the healthcare provider about the side effects of the medicine prescribed for you or your family member.
• **Antidepressant medicines can interact with other medicines.** Know all of the medicines that you or your family member takes. Keep a list of all medicines to show the healthcare provider. Do not start new medicines without first checking with your healthcare provider.

It is not known if WELLBUTRIN SR is safe and effective in children under the age of 18.

Quitting Smoking, Quit-Smoking Medications, Changes in Thinking and Behavior, Depression, and Suicidal Thoughts or Actions
This section of the Medication Guide is only about the risk of changes in thinking and behavior, depression and suicidal thoughts or actions with drugs used to quit smoking. Although WELLBUTRIN SR is not a treatment for quitting smoking, it contains the same active ingredient (bupropion hydrochloride) as ZYBAN® which is used to help patients quit smoking.

Some people have had changes in behavior, hostility, agitation, depression, suicidal thoughts or actions while taking bupropion to help them quit smoking. These symptoms can develop during treatment with bupropion or after stopping treatment with bupropion.

If you, your family member, or your caregiver notice agitation, hostility, depression, or changes in thinking or behavior that are not typical for you, or you have any of the following symptoms, stop taking bupropion and call your healthcare provider right away:

• thoughts about suicide or dying
• attempts to commit suicide
• new or worse depression
• new or worse anxiety
• panic attacks
• feeling very agitated or restless
• acting aggressive, being angry, or violent
• acting on dangerous impulses

• an extreme increase in activity and talking (mania)
• abnormal thoughts or sensations
• seeing or hearing things that are not there (hallucinations)
• feeling people are against you (paranoia)
• feeling confused
• other unusual changes in behavior or mood

When you try to quit smoking, with or without bupropion, you may have symptoms that may be due to nicotine withdrawal, including urge to smoke, depressed mood, trouble sleeping, irritability, frustration, anger, feeling anxious, difficulty concentrating, restlessness, decreased heart rate, and increased appetite or weight gain. Some people have even experienced suicidal thoughts when trying to quit smoking without medication. Sometimes quitting smoking can lead to worsening of mental health problems that you already have, such as depression.

Before taking bupropion, tell your healthcare provider if you have ever had depression or other mental illnesses. You should also tell your healthcare provider about any symptoms you had during other times you tried to quit smoking, with or without bupropion.

What Other Important Information Should I Know About WELLBUTRIN SR?
• **Seizures: There is a chance of having a seizure (convulsion, fit) with WELLBUTRIN SR, especially in people:**
• with certain medical problems.
• who take certain medicines.
The chance of having seizures increases with higher doses of WELLBUTRIN SR. For more information, see the sections "Who should not take WELLBUTRIN SR?" and "What should I tell my healthcare provider before taking WELLBUTRIN SR?" Tell your healthcare provider about all of your medical conditions and all the medicines you take. **Do not take any other medicines while you are taking WELLBUTRIN SR unless your healthcare provider has said it is okay to take them.**
If you have a seizure while taking WELLBUTRIN SR, stop taking the tablets and call your healthcare provider right away. Do not take WELLBUTRIN SR again if you have a seizure.
• **High blood pressure (hypertension). Some people get high blood pressure, that can be severe, while taking WELLBUTRIN SR.** The chance of high blood pressure may be higher if you also use nicotine replacement therapy (such as a nicotine patch) to help you stop smoking.
• **Manic episodes. Some people may have periods of mania while taking WELLBUTRIN SR, including:**
• Greatly increased energy
• Severe trouble sleeping
• Racing thoughts
• Reckless behavior
• Unusually grand ideas
• Excessive happiness or irritability
• Talking more or faster than usual
If you have any of the above symptoms of mania, call your healthcare provider.
• **Unusual thoughts or behaviors. Some patients have unusual thoughts or behaviors while taking WELLBUTRIN, including delusions (believe you are someone else), hallucinations (seeing or hearing things that are not there), paranoia (feeling that people are against you), or feeling confused. If this happens to you, call your healthcare provider.**
• **Visual problems.**
• eye pain
• changes in vision
• swelling or redness in or around the eye
Only some people are at risk for these problems. You may want to undergo an eye examination to see if you are at risk and receive preventative treatment if you are.
• **Severe allergic reactions. Some people can have severe allergic reactions to WELLBUTRIN SR. Stop taking WELLBUTRIN SR and call your healthcare provider right away** if you get a rash, itching, hives, fever, swollen lymph glands, painful sores in the mouth or around the eyes, swelling of the lips or tongue, chest pain, or have trouble breathing. These could be signs of a serious allergic reaction.

What is WELLBUTRIN SR?
WELLBUTRIN SR is a prescription medicine used to treat adults with a certain type of depression called major depressive disorder.

Who should not take WELLBUTRIN SR?
Do not take WELLBUTRIN SR if you
• have or had a seizure disorder or epilepsy.
• have or had an eating disorder such as anorexia nervosa or bulimia.
• **are taking any other medicines that contain bupropion, ZYBAN** (used to help people stop smoking) **APLENZIN®, FORFIVO XL™, WELLBUTRIN®, or WELLBUTRIN XL®.** Bupropion is the same active ingredient that is in WELLBUTRIN SR.
• drink a lot of alcohol and abruptly stop drinking, or use medicines called sedatives (these make you sleepy), benzodiazepines, or anti-seizure medicines, and you stop using them all of a sudden.
• take a monoamine oxidase inhibitor (MAOI). Ask your healthcare provider or pharmacist if you are not sure if you take an MAOI, including the antibiotic linezolid.
  • do not take an MAOI within 2 weeks of stopping WELLBUTRIN SR unless directed to do so by your healthcare provider.
  • do not start WELLBUTRIN SR if you stopped taking an MAOI in the last 2 weeks unless directed to do so by your healthcare provider.
• are allergic to the active ingredient in WELLBUTRIN SR, bupropion, or to any of the inactive ingredients. See the end of this Medication Guide for a complete list of ingredients in WELLBUTRIN SR.

What should I tell my healthcare provider before taking WELLBUTRIN SR?
Tell your healthcare provider if you have ever had depression, suicidal thoughts or actions, or other mental health problems. See "Antidepressant Medicines, Depression and Other Serious Mental Illnesses, and Suicidal Thoughts or Actions."

Tell your healthcare provider about your other medical conditions including if you:
• have liver problems, especially cirrhosis of the liver.
• have kidney problems.
• have, or have had, an eating disorder, such as anorexia nervosa or bulimia.
• have had a head injury.
• have had a seizure (convulsion, fit).
• have a tumor in your nervous system (brain or spine).
• have had a heart attack, heart problems, or high blood pressure.
• are a diabetic taking insulin or other medicines to control your blood sugar.
• drink alcohol.
• abuse prescription medicines or street drugs.
• are pregnant or plan to become pregnant.
• are breastfeeding. WELLBUTRIN passes into your milk in small amounts.

Tell your healthcare provider about all the medicines you take, including prescription, over-the-counter medicines, vitamins, and herbal supplements. Many medicines increase your chances of having seizures or other serious side effects if you take them while you are taking WELLBUTRIN SR.

How should I take WELLBUTRIN SR?
• Take WELLBUTRIN SR exactly as prescribed by your healthcare provider.
• **Swallow WELLBUTRIN SR Tablets whole. Do not chew, cut, or crush WELLBUTRIN SR Tablets.** If you do, the medicine will be released into your body too quickly. If this happens you may be more likely to get side effects including seizures. **Tell your healthcare provider if you cannot swallow tablets.**
• Take WELLBUTRIN SR at the same time each day.
• Take your doses of WELLBUTRIN SR at least 8 hours apart.
• You may take WELLBUTRIN SR with or without food.
• If you miss a dose, do not take an extra dose to make up for the dose you missed. Wait and take your next dose at the regular time. **This is very important.** Too much WELLBUTRIN SR can increase your chance of having a seizure.
• If you take too much WELLBUTRIN SR, or overdose, call your local emergency room or poison control center right away.
• **Do not take any other medicines while taking WELLBUTRIN SR unless your healthcare provider has told you it is okay.**
• If you are taking WELLBUTRIN SR for the treatment of major depressive disorder, it may take several weeks for you to feel that WELLBUTRIN SR is working. Once you feel better, it is important to keep taking WELLBUTRIN SR exactly as directed by your healthcare provider. Call your healthcare provider if you do not feel WELLBUTRIN SR is working for you.
• Do not change your dose or stop taking WELLBUTRIN SR without talking with your healthcare provider first.

What should I avoid while taking WELLBUTRIN SR?
• Limit or avoid using alcohol during treatment with WELLBUTRIN SR. If you usually drink a lot of alcohol, talk with your healthcare provider before suddenly stopping. If you suddenly stop drinking alcohol, you may increase your chance of having seizures.
• Do not drive a car or use heavy machinery until you know how WELLBUTRIN SR affects you. WELLBUTRIN SR can affect your ability to do these things safely.

What are possible side effects of WELLBUTRIN SR?
See "**What Other Important Information Should I Know About WELLBUTRIN SR?**"
WELLBUTRIN SR can cause serious side effects.
The most common side effects of WELLBUTRIN SR include:
• Headache
• Dry mouth
• Nausea
• Trouble sleeping
• Dizziness
• Sore throat
• Constipation
If you have nausea, take your medicine with food. If you have trouble sleeping, do not take your medicine too close to bedtime.
Tell your healthcare provider right away about any side effects that bother you.
These are not all the possible side effects of WELLBUTRIN SR. For more information, ask your healthcare provider or pharmacist.
Call your doctor for medical advice about side effects. You may report side effects to FDA at 1–800-FDA-1088.
You may also report side effects to GlaxoSmithKline at 1-888-825-5249.

How should I store WELLBUTRIN SR?
• Store WELLBUTRIN SR at room temperature between 59°F and 86°F (15°C to 30°C).
• Keep WELLBUTRIN SR dry and out of the light.
• WELLBUTRIN SR Tablets may have an odor.

Keep WELLBUTRIN SR and all medicines out of the reach of children.

General Information about WELLBUTRIN SR.
Medicines are sometimes prescribed for purposes other than those listed in a Medication Guide. Do not use WELLBUTRIN SR for a condition for which it was not prescribed. Do not give WELLBUTRIN SR to other people, even if they have the same symptoms you have. It may harm them.
If you take a urine drug screening test, WELLBUTRIN SR may make the test result positive for amphetamines. If you tell the person giving you the drug screening test that you are taking WELLBUTRIN SR, they can do a more specific drug screening test that should not have this problem.
This Medication Guide summarizes important information about WELLBUTRIN SR. If you would like more information, talk with your healthcare provider. You can ask your healthcare provider or pharmacist for information about WELLBUTRIN SR that is written for healthcare professionals.
For more information about WELLBUTRIN SR, go to www.wellbutrin.com or call 1-888-825-5249.

What are the ingredients in WELLBUTRIN SR?
Active ingredient: bupropion hydrochloride.
Inactive ingredients: carnauba wax, cysteine hydrochloride, hypromellose, magnesium stearate, microcrystalline cellulose, polyethylene glycol, polysorbate 80, and titanium dioxide. In addition, the 100–mg tablet contains FD&C Blue No. 1 Lake, the 150–mg tablet contains FD&C Blue No. 2 Lake and FD&C Red No. 40 Lake, and the 200–mg tablet contains FD&C Red No. 40 Lake. The tablets are printed with edible black ink.
This Medication Guide has been approved by the U.S. Food and Drug Administration.
WELLBUTRIN, WELLBUTRIN SR, WELLBUTRIN XL, and ZYBAN are registered trademarks of the GSK group of companies. The other brands listed are trademarks of their respective owners and are not trademarks of the GSK group of companies. The makers of these brands are not affiliated with and do not endorse the GSK group of companies or its products.
GlaxoSmithKline
Research Triangle Park, NC 27709
©2014, the GSK group of companies. All rights reserved.
July 2014
WLS: 11MG

ZANTAC® 150
(ranitidine hydrochloride)
Tablets, USP   ℞

ZANTAC® 300
(ranitidine hydrochloride)
Tablets, USP   ℞

ZANTAC®
(ranitidine hydrochloride)
Syrup, USP   ℞

DESCRIPTION
The active ingredient in ZANTAC 150 Tablets, ZANTAC 300 Tablets, and ZANTAC Syrup is ranitidine hydrochloride (HCl), USP, a histamine H_2-receptor antagonist. Chemically it is N[2-[[[5-[(dimethylamino)methyl]-2-furanyl]methyl]thio]ethyl]-N′-methyl-2-nitro-1,1-ethenediamine, HCl. It has the following structure:

$(CH_3)_2NCH_2$ — — $CH_2SCH_2CH_2NH$ — $NHCH_3 \bullet HCl$
                O   CHNO_2

The empirical formula is $C_{13}H_{22}N_4O_3S \bullet HCl$, representing a molecular weight of 350.87.
Ranitidine HCl is a white to pale yellow, granular substance that is soluble in water. It has a slightly bitter taste and sulfur-like odor.
Each ZANTAC 150 Tablet for oral administration contains 168 mg of ranitidine HCl equivalent to 150 mg of ranitidine. Each tablet also contains the inactive ingredients FD&C

Yellow No. 6 Aluminum Lake, hypromellose, magnesium stearate, microcrystalline cellulose, titanium dioxide, triacetin, and yellow iron oxide.
Each ZANTAC 300 Tablet for oral administration contains 336 mg of ranitidine HCl equivalent to 300 mg of ranitidine. Each tablet also contains the inactive ingredients croscarmellose sodium, D&C Yellow No. 10 Aluminum Lake, hypromellose, magnesium stearate, microcrystalline cellulose, titanium dioxide, and triacetin.
Each 1 mL of ZANTAC Syrup contains 16.8 mg of ranitidine HCl equivalent to 15 mg of ranitidine. ZANTAC Syrup also contains the inactive ingredients alcohol (7.5%), butylparaben, dibasic sodium phosphate, hypromellose, peppermint flavor, monobasic potassium phosphate, propylparaben, purified water, saccharin sodium, sodium chloride, and sorbitol.

CLINICAL PHARMACOLOGY
ZANTAC is a competitive, reversible inhibitor of the action of histamine at the histamine H_2-receptors, including receptors on the gastric cells. ZANTAC does not lower serum Ca++ in hypercalcemic states. ZANTAC is not an anticholinergic agent.
Pharmacokinetics
Absorption: ZANTAC is 50% absorbed after oral administration, compared to an intravenous (IV) injection with mean peak levels of 440 to 545 ng/mL occurring 2 to 3 hours after a 150-mg dose. The syrup is bioequivalent to the tablets. Absorption is not significantly impaired by the administration of food or antacids. Propantheline slightly delays and increases peak blood levels of ranitidine, probably by delaying gastric emptying and transit time. In one study, simultaneous administration of high-potency antacid (150 mmol) in fasting subjects has been reported to decrease the absorption of ZANTAC.
Distribution: The volume of distribution is about 1.4 L/kg. Serum protein binding averages 15%.
Metabolism: In humans, the N-oxide is the principal metabolite in the urine; however, this amounts to <4% of the dose. Other metabolites are the S-oxide (1%) and the desmethyl ranitidine (1%). The remainder of the administered dose is found in the stool. Studies in patients with hepatic dysfunction (compensated cirrhosis) indicate that there are minor, but clinically insignificant, alterations in ranitidine half-life, distribution, clearance, and bioavailability.
Excretion: The principal route of excretion is the urine, with approximately 30% of the orally administered dose collected in the urine as unchanged drug in 24 hours. Renal clearance is about 410 mL/min, indicating active tubular excretion. The elimination half-life is 2.5 to 3 hours. Four patients with clinically significant renal function impairment (creatinine clearance 25 to 35 mL/min) administered 50 mg of ranitidine intravenously had an average plasma half-life of 4.8 hours, a ranitidine clearance of 29 mL/min, and a volume of distribution of 1.76 L/kg. In general, these parameters appear to be altered in proportion to creatinine clearance (see DOSAGE AND ADMINISTRATION).
Geriatrics: The plasma half-life is prolonged and total clearance is reduced in the elderly population due to a decrease in renal function. The elimination half-life is 3 to 4 hours. Peak levels average 526 ng/mL following a 150-mg twice-daily dose and occur in about 3 hours (see PRECAUTIONS: Geriatric Use and DOSAGE AND ADMINISTRATION: Dosage Adjustment for Patients With Impaired Renal Function).
Pediatrics: There are no significant differences in the pharmacokinetic parameter values for ranitidine in pediatric patients (from 1 month up to 16 years of age) and healthy adults when correction is made for body weight. The average bioavailability of ranitidine given orally to pediatric patients is 48%, which is comparable to the bioavailability of ranitidine in the adult population. All other pharmacokinetic parameter values ($t_{1/2}$, Vd, and CL) are similar to those observed with intravenous ranitidine use in pediatric patients. Estimates of C_{max} and T_{max} are displayed in Table 1.
[See table 1 below]
Plasma clearance measured in 2 neonatal patients (younger than 1 month of age) was considerably lower (3 mL/min/kg)

Table 1. Ranitidine Pharmacokinetics in Pediatric Patients Following Oral Dosing

Population (age)	n	Dosage Form (dose)	C_{max} (ng/mL)	T_{max} (hours)
Gastric or duodenal ulcer (3.5 to 16 years)	12	Tablets (1 to 2 mg/kg)	54 to 492	2.0
Otherwise healthy requiring ZANTAC (0.7 to 14 years, Single dose)	10	Syrup (2 mg/kg)	244	1.61
Otherwise healthy requiring ZANTAC (0.7 to 14 years, Multiple dose)	10	Syrup (2 mg/kg)	320	1.66

Table 2. Effect of Oral ZANTAC on Gastric Acid Secretion

	Time After Dose, hours	% Inhibition of Gastric Acid Output by Dose, mg			
		75-80	100	150	200
Basal	Up to 4		99	95	
Nocturnal	Up to 13	95	96	92	
Betazole	Up to 3		97	99	
Pentagastrin	Up to 5	58	72	72	80
Meal	Up to 3		73	79	95

Table 3. Duodenal Ulcer Patient Healing Rates

	ZANTAC[a]		Placebo[a]	
	Number Entered	Healed/ Evaluable	Number Entered	Healed/ Evaluable
Outpatients Week 2	195	69/182 (38%)[b]	188	31/164 (19%)
Week 4		137/187 (73%)[b]		76/168 (45%)

[a]All patients were permitted antacids as needed for relief of pain.
[b]$P<0.0001$.

Table 5. Duodenal Ulcer Prevalence

Double-Blind, Multicenter, Placebo-Controlled Trials

Multicenter Trial	Drug	Duodenal Ulcer Prevalence			No. of Patients
		0-4 Months	0-8 Months	0-12 Months	
USA	RAN	20%[a]	24%	35%[a]	138
	PLC	44%	54%	59%	139
Foreign	RAN	12%[a]	21%[a]	28%[a]	174
	PLC	56%	64%	68%	165

% = Life table estimate.
[a] = $P<0.05$ (ZANTAC versus comparator).
RAN = ranitidine (ZANTAC).
PLC = placebo.

Table 6. Gastric Ulcer Patient Healing Rates

	ZANTAC[a]		Placebo[a]	
	Number Entered	Healed/ Evaluable	Number Entered	Healed/ Evaluable
Outpatients Week 2	92	16/83 (19%)	94	10/83 (12%)
Week 6		50/73 (68%)[b]		35/69 (51%)

[a]All patients were permitted antacids as needed for relief of pain.
[b]$P= 0.009$.

than children or adults and is likely due to reduced renal function observed in this population (see PRECAUTIONS: Pediatric Use and DOSAGE AND ADMINISTRATION: Pediatric Use).

Pharmacodynamics
Serum concentrations necessary to inhibit 50% of stimulated gastric acid secretion are estimated to be 36 to 94 ng/mL. Following a single oral dose of 150 mg, serum concentrations of ranitidine are in this range up to 12 hours. However, blood levels bear no consistent relationship to dose or degree of acid inhibition.
Antisecretory Activity: 1. Effects on Acid Secretion: ZANTAC inhibits both daytime and nocturnal basal gastric

acid secretions as well as gastric acid secretion stimulated by food, betazole, and pentagastrin, as shown in Table 2.
[See table 2 above]
It appears that basal-, nocturnal-, and betazole-stimulated secretions are most sensitive to inhibition by ZANTAC, responding almost completely to doses of 100 mg or less, while pentagastrin- and food-stimulated secretions are more difficult to suppress.

2. Effects on Other Gastrointestinal Secretions:
Pepsin: Oral ZANTAC does not affect pepsin secretion. Total pepsin output is reduced in proportion to the decrease in volume of gastric juice.

Intrinsic Factor: Oral ZANTAC has no significant effect on pentagastrin-stimulated intrinsic factor secretion.
Serum Gastrin: ZANTAC has little or no effect on fasting or postprandial serum gastrin.
Other Pharmacologic Actions:
1. Gastric bacterial flora—increase in nitrate-reducing organisms, significance not known.
2. Prolactin levels—no effect in recommended oral or IV dosage, but small, transient, dose-related increases in serum prolactin have been reported after IV bolus injections of 100 mg or more.
3. Other pituitary hormones—no effect on serum gonadotropins, TSH, or GH. Possible impairment of vasopressin release.
4. No change in cortisol, aldosterone, androgen, or estrogen levels.
5. No antiandrogenic action.
6. No effect on count, motility, or morphology of sperm.
Pediatrics: Oral doses of 6 to 10 mg/kg/day in 2 or 3 divided doses maintain gastric pH >4 throughout most of the dosing interval.
Clinical Trials
Active Duodenal Ulcer: In a multicenter, double-blind, controlled, US study of endoscopically diagnosed duodenal ulcers, earlier healing was seen in the patients treated with ZANTAC as shown in Table 3.
[See table 3 above]
In these studies, patients treated with ZANTAC reported a reduction in both daytime and nocturnal pain, and they also consumed less antacid than the placebo-treated patients.

Table 4. Mean Daily Doses of Antacid

	Ulcer Healed	Ulcer Not Healed
ZANTAC	0.06	0.71
Placebo	0.71	1.43

Foreign studies have shown that patients heal equally well with 150 mg twice daily and 300 mg at bedtime (85% versus 84%, respectively) during a usual 4-week course of therapy. If patients require extended therapy of 8 weeks, the healing rate may be higher for 150 mg twice daily as compared to 300 mg at bedtime (92% versus 87%, respectively).
Studies have been limited to short-term treatment of acute duodenal ulcer. Patients whose ulcers healed during therapy had recurrences of ulcers at the usual rates.
Maintenance Therapy in Duodenal Ulcer: Ranitidine has been found to be effective as maintenance therapy for patients following healing of acute duodenal ulcers. In 2 independent, double-blind, multicenter, controlled trials, the number of duodenal ulcers observed was significantly less in patients treated with ZANTAC (150 mg at bedtime) than in patients treated with placebo over a 12-month period.
[See table 5 above]
As with other H$_2$-antagonists, the factors responsible for the significant reduction in the prevalence of duodenal ulcers include prevention of recurrence of ulcers, more rapid healing of ulcers that may occur during maintenance therapy, or both.

Gastric Ulcer: In a multicenter, double-blind, controlled, US study of endoscopically diagnosed gastric ulcers, earlier healing was seen in the patients treated with ZANTAC as shown in Table 6.
[See table 6 above]
In this multicenter trial, significantly more patients treated with ZANTAC became pain free during therapy.
Maintenance of Healing of Gastric Ulcers: In 2 multicenter, double-blind, randomized, placebo-controlled, 12-month trials conducted in patients whose gastric ulcers had been previously healed, ZANTAC 150 mg at bedtime was significantly more effective than placebo in maintaining healing of gastric ulcers.
Pathological Hypersecretory Conditions (such as Zollinger-Ellison syndrome): ZANTAC inhibits gastric acid secretion and reduces occurrence of diarrhea, anorexia, and pain in patients with pathological hypersecretion associated with Zollinger-Ellison syndrome, systemic mastocytosis, and other pathological hypersecretory conditions (e.g., postoperative, "short-gut" syndrome, idiopathic). Use of ZANTAC was followed by healing of ulcers in 8 of 19 (42%) patients who were intractable to previous therapy.
Gastroesophageal Reflux Disease (GERD): In 2 multicenter, double-blind, placebo-controlled, 6-week trials performed in the United States and Europe, ZANTAC 150 mg twice daily was more effective than placebo for the relief of heartburn and other symptoms associated with GERD. Ranitidine-treated patients consumed significantly less antacid than did placebo-treated patients.
The US trial indicated that ZANTAC 150 mg twice daily significantly reduced the frequency of heartburn attacks and severity of heartburn pain within 1 to 2 weeks after starting therapy. The improvement was maintained throughout the 6-week trial period. Moreover, patient response rates demonstrated that the effect on heartburn extends through both the day and night time periods.

In 2 additional US multicenter, double-blind, placebo-controlled, 2-week trials, ZANTAC 150 mg twice daily was shown to provide relief of heartburn pain within 24 hours of initiating therapy and a reduction in the frequency of severity of heartburn.

Erosive Esophagitis: In 2 multicenter, double-blind, randomized, placebo-controlled, 12-week trials performed in the United States, ZANTAC 150 mg daily was significantly more effective than placebo in healing endoscopically diagnosed erosive esophagitis and in relieving associated heartburn. The erosive esophagitis healing rates were as follows:

Table 7. Erosive Esophagitis Patient Healing Rates

	Healed/Evaluable	
	Placebo[a] n = 229	ZANTAC 150 mg 4 times daily[a] n = 215
Week 4	43/198 (22%)	96/206 (47%)[b]
Week 8	63/176 (36%)	142/200 (71%)[b]
Week 12	92/159 (58%)	162/192 (84%)[b]

[a]All patients were permitted antacids as needed for relief of pain.
[b]$P<0.001$ versus placebo.

No additional benefit in healing of esophagitis or in relief of heartburn was seen with a ranitidine dose of 300 mg 4 times daily.

Maintenance of Healing of Erosive Esophagitis: In 2 multicenter, double-blind, randomized, placebo-controlled, 48-week trials conducted in patients whose erosive esophagitis had been previously healed, ZANTAC 150 mg twice daily was significantly more effective than placebo in maintaining healing of erosive esophagitis.

INDICATIONS AND USAGE

ZANTAC is indicated in:
1. Short-term treatment of active duodenal ulcer. Most patients heal within 4 weeks. Studies available to date have not assessed the safety of ranitidine in uncomplicated duodenal ulcer for periods of more than 8 weeks.
2. Maintenance therapy for duodenal ulcer patients at reduced dosage after healing of acute ulcers. No placebo-controlled comparative studies have been carried out for periods of longer than 1 year.
3. The treatment of pathological hypersecretory conditions (e.g., Zollinger-Ellison syndrome and systemic mastocytosis).
4. Short-term treatment of active, benign gastric ulcer. Most patients heal within 6 weeks and the usefulness of further treatment has not been demonstrated. Studies available to date have not assessed the safety of ranitidine in uncomplicated, benign gastric ulcer for periods of more than 6 weeks.
5. Maintenance therapy for gastric ulcer patients at reduced dosage after healing of acute ulcers. Placebo-controlled studies have been carried out for 1 year.
6. Treatment of GERD. Symptomatic relief commonly occurs within 24 hours after starting therapy with ZANTAC 150 mg twice daily.
7. Treatment of endoscopically diagnosed erosive esophagitis. Symptomatic relief of heartburn commonly occurs within 24 hours of therapy initiation with ZANTAC 150 mg 4 times daily.
8. Maintenance of healing of erosive esophagitis. Placebo-controlled trials have been carried out for 48 weeks.

Concomitant antacids should be given as needed for pain relief to patients with active duodenal ulcer; active, benign gastric ulcer; hypersecretory states; GERD; and erosive esophagitis.

CONTRAINDICATIONS

ZANTAC is contraindicated for patients known to have hypersensitivity to the drug or any of the ingredients (see PRECAUTIONS).

PRECAUTIONS

General:
1. Symptomatic response to therapy with ZANTAC does not preclude the presence of gastric malignancy.
2. Since ZANTAC is excreted primarily by the kidney, dosage should be adjusted in patients with impaired renal function (see DOSAGE AND ADMINISTRATION). Caution should be observed in patients with hepatic dysfunction since ZANTAC is metabolized in the liver.
3. Rare reports suggest that ZANTAC may precipitate acute porphyric attacks in patients with acute porphyria. ZANTAC should therefore be avoided in patients with a history of acute porphyria.

Laboratory Tests
False-positive tests for urine protein with MULTISTIX® may occur during therapy with ZANTAC, and therefore testing with sulfosalicylic acid is recommended.

Drug Interactions
Ranitidine has been reported to affect the bioavailability of other drugs through several different mechanisms such as competition for renal tubular secretion, alteration of gastric pH, and inhibition of cytochrome P450 enzymes.

Procainamide: Ranitidine, a substrate of the renal organic cation transport system, may affect the clearance of other drugs eliminated by this route. High doses of ranitidine (e.g., such as those used in the treatment of Zollinger-Ellison syndrome) have been shown to reduce the renal excretion of procainamide and N-acetylprocainamide resulting in increased plasma levels of these drugs. Although this interaction is unlikely to be clinically relevant at usual ranitidine doses, it may be prudent to monitor for procainamide toxicity when administered with oral ranitidine at a dose exceeding 300 mg per day.

Warfarin: There have been reports of altered prothrombin time among patients on concomitant warfarin and ranitidine therapy. Due to the narrow therapeutic index, close monitoring of increased or decreased prothrombin time is recommended during concurrent treatment with ranitidine.

Ranitidine may alter the absorption of drugs in which gastric pH is an important determinant of bioavailability. This can result in either an increase in absorption (e.g., triazolam, midazolam, glipizide) or a decrease in absorption (e.g., ketoconazole, atazanavir, delaviridine, gefitinib). Appropriate clinical monitoring is recommended.

Atazanavir: Atazanavir absorption may be impaired based on known interactions with other agents that increase gastric pH. Use with caution. See atazanavir label for specific recommendations.

Delaviridine: Delaviridine absorption may be impaired based on known interactions with other agents that increase gastric pH. Chronic use of H_2-receptor antagonists with delaviridine is not recommended.

Gefitinib: Gefitinib exposure was reduced by 44% with the coadministration of ranitidine and sodium bicarbonate (dosed to maintain gastric pH above 5.0). Use with caution.

Glipizide: In diabetic patients, glipizide exposure was increased by 34% following a single 150-mg dose of oral ranitidine. Use appropriate clinical monitoring when initiating or discontinuing ranitidine.

Ketoconazole: Oral ketoconazole exposure was reduced by up to 95% when oral ranitidine was coadministered in a regimen to maintain a gastric pH of 6 or above. The degree of interaction with usual dose of ranitidine (150 mg twice daily) is unknown.

Midazolam: Oral midazolam exposure in 5 healthy volunteers was increased by up to 65% when administered with oral ranitidine at a dose of 150 mg twice daily. However, in another interaction study in 8 volunteers receiving IV midazolam, a 300 mg oral dose of ranitidine increased midazolam exposure by about 9%. Monitor patients for excessive or prolonged sedation when ranitidine is coadministered with oral midazolam.

Triazolam: Triazolam exposure in healthy volunteers was increased by approximately 30% when administered with oral ranitidine at a dose of 150 mg twice daily. Monitor patients for excessive or prolonged sedation.

Carcinogenesis, Mutagenesis, Impairment of Fertility
There was no indication of tumorigenic or carcinogenic effects in life-span studies in mice and rats at dosages up to 2,000 mg/kg/day.

Ranitidine was not mutagenic in standard bacterial tests (Salmonella, Escherichia coli) for mutagenicity at concentrations up to the maximum recommended for these assays. In a dominant lethal assay, a single oral dose of 1,000 mg/kg to male rats was without effect on the outcome of 2 matings per week for the next 9 weeks.

Pregnancy
Teratogenic Effects: Pregnancy Category B. Reproduction studies have been performed in rats and rabbits at doses up to 160 times the human dose and have revealed no evidence of impaired fertility or harm to the fetus due to ZANTAC. There are, however, no adequate and well-controlled studies in pregnant women. Because animal reproduction studies are not always predictive of human response, this drug should be used during pregnancy only if clearly needed.

Nursing Mothers
Ranitidine is secreted in human milk. Caution should be exercised when ZANTAC is administered to a nursing mother.

Pediatric Use
The safety and effectiveness of ZANTAC have been established in the age-group of 1 month to 16 years for the treatment of duodenal and gastric ulcers, gastroesophageal reflux disease and erosive esophagitis, and the maintenance of healed duodenal and gastric ulcer. Use of ZANTAC in this age-group is supported by adequate and well-controlled studies in adults, as well as additional pharmacokinetic data in pediatric patients and an analysis of the published literature (see CLINICAL PHARMACOLOGY: Pediatrics and DOSAGE AND ADMINISTRATION: Pediatric Use). Safety and effectiveness in pediatric patients for the treatment of pathological hypersecretory conditions or the maintenance of healing of erosive esophagitis have not been established.

Safety and effectiveness in neonates (younger than 1 month of age) have not been established (see CLINICAL PHARMACOLOGY: Pediatrics).

Geriatric Use
Of the total number of subjects enrolled in US and foreign controlled clinical trials of oral formulations of ZANTAC, for which there were subgroup analyses, 4,197 were aged 65 and older, while 899 were aged 75 and older. No overall differences in safety or effectiveness were observed between these subjects and younger subjects, and other reported clinical experience has not identified differences in responses between the elderly and younger patients, but greater sensitivity of some older individuals cannot be ruled out.

This drug is known to be substantially excreted by the kidney and the risk of toxic reactions to this drug may be greater in patients with impaired renal function. Because elderly patients are more likely to have decreased renal function, caution should be exercised in dose selection, and it may be useful to monitor renal function (see CLINICAL PHARMACOLOGY: Pharmacokinetics: Geriatrics and DOSAGE AND ADMINISTRATION: Dosage Adjustment for Patients With Impaired Renal Function).

ADVERSE REACTIONS

The following have been reported as events in clinical trials or in the routine management of patients treated with ZANTAC. The relationship to therapy with ZANTAC has been unclear in many cases. Headache, sometimes severe, seems to be related to administration of ZANTAC.

Central Nervous System
Rarely, malaise, dizziness, somnolence, insomnia, and vertigo. Rare cases of reversible mental confusion, agitation, depression, and hallucinations have been reported, predominantly in severely ill elderly patients. Rare cases of reversible blurred vision suggestive of a change in accommodation have been reported. Rare reports of reversible involuntary motor disturbances have been received.

Cardiovascular
As with other H_2-blockers, rare reports of arrhythmias such as tachycardia, bradycardia, atrioventricular block, and premature ventricular beats.

Gastrointestinal
Constipation, diarrhea, nausea/vomiting, abdominal discomfort/pain, and rare reports of pancreatitis.

Hepatic
There have been occasional reports of hepatocellular, cholestatic, or mixed hepatitis, with or without jaundice. In such circumstances, ranitidine should be immediately discontinued. These events are usually reversible, but in rare circumstances death has occurred. Rare cases of hepatic failure have also been reported. In normal volunteers, SGPT values were increased to at least twice the pretreatment levels in 6 of 12 subjects receiving 100 mg intravenously 4 times daily for 7 days, and in 4 of 24 subjects receiving 50 mg intravenously 4 times daily for 5 days.

Musculoskeletal
Rare reports of arthralgias and myalgias.

Hematologic
Blood count changes (leukopenia, granulocytopenia, and thrombocytopenia) have occurred in a few patients. These were usually reversible. Rare cases of agranulocytosis, pancytopenia, sometimes with marrow hypoplasia, and aplastic anemia and exceedingly rare cases of acquired immune hemolytic anemia have been reported.

Endocrine
Controlled studies in animals and man have shown no stimulation of any pituitary hormone by ZANTAC and no antiandrogenic activity, and cimetidine-induced gynecomastia and impotence in hypersecretory patients have resolved when ZANTAC has been substituted. However, occasional cases of impotence and loss of libido have been reported in male patients receiving ZANTAC, but the incidence did not differ from that in the general population. Rare cases of breast symptoms and conditions, including galactorrhea and gynecomastia, have been reported in both males and females.

Integumentary
Rash, including rare cases of erythema multiforme. Rare cases of alopecia and vasculitis.

Respiratory
A large epidemiological study suggested an increased risk of developing pneumonia in current users of histamine-2-receptor antagonists (H_2RAs) compared to patients who had stopped H_2RA treatment, with an observed adjusted relative risk of 1.63 (95% CI, 1.07–2.48). However, a causal relationship between use of H_2RAs and pneumonia has not been established.

Other
Rare cases of hypersensitivity reactions (e.g., bronchospasm, fever, rash, eosinophilia), anaphylaxis, angioneurotic edema, acute interstitial nephritis, and small increases in serum creatinine.

OVERDOSAGE

There has been limited experience with overdosage. Reported acute ingestions of up to 18 g orally have been associated with transient adverse effects similar to those encountered in normal clinical experience (see ADVERSE REACTIONS). In addition, abnormalities of gait and hypotension have been reported.

When overdosage occurs, the usual measures to remove unabsorbed material from the gastrointestinal tract, clinical monitoring, and supportive therapy should be employed. Studies in dogs receiving dosages of ZANTAC in excess of 225 mg/kg/day have shown muscular tremors, vomiting, and rapid respiration. Single oral doses of 1,000 mg/kg in mice and rats were not lethal. Intravenous LD_{50} values in mice and rats were 77 and 83 mg/kg, respectively.

DOSAGE AND ADMINISTRATION

Active Duodenal Ulcer
The current recommended adult oral dosage of ZANTAC for duodenal ulcer is 150 mg or 10 mL of syrup (2 teaspoonfuls of syrup equivalent to 150 mg of ranitidine) twice daily. An alternative dosage of 300 mg or 20 mL of syrup (4 teaspoonfuls of syrup equivalent to 300 mg of ranitidine) once daily after the evening meal or at bedtime can be used for patients in whom dosing convenience is important. The advantages of one treatment regimen compared to the other in a particular patient population have yet to be demonstrated (see Clinical Trials: Active Duodenal Ulcer). Smaller doses have been shown to be equally effective in inhibiting gastric acid secretion in US studies, and several foreign trials have shown that 100 mg twice daily is as effective as the 150-mg dose.

Antacid should be given as needed for relief of pain (see CLINICAL PHARMACOLOGY: Pharmacokinetics).

Maintenance of Healing of Duodenal Ulcers
The current recommended adult oral dosage is 150 mg or 10 mL of syrup (2 teaspoonfuls of syrup equivalent to 150 mg of ranitidine) at bedtime.

Pathological Hypersecretory Conditions (such as Zollinger-Ellison syndrome)
The current recommended adult oral dosage is 150 mg or 10 mL of syrup (2 teaspoonfuls of syrup equivalent to 150 mg of ranitidine) twice daily. In some patients it may be necessary to administer ZANTAC 150-mg doses more frequently. Dosages should be adjusted to individual patient needs, and should continue as long as clinically indicated. Dosages up to 6 g/day have been employed in patients with severe disease.

Benign Gastric Ulcer
The current recommended adult oral dosage is 150 mg or 10 mL of syrup (2 teaspoonfuls of syrup equivalent to 150 mg of ranitidine) twice daily.

Maintenance of Healing of Gastric Ulcers
The current recommended adult oral dosage is 150 mg or 10 mL of syrup (2 teaspoonfuls of syrup equivalent to 150 mg of ranitidine) at bedtime.

GERD
The current recommended adult oral dosage is 150 mg or 10 mL of syrup (2 teaspoonfuls of syrup equivalent to 150 mg of ranitidine) twice daily.

Erosive Esophagitis
The current recommended adult oral dosage is 150 mg or 10 mL of syrup (2 teaspoonfuls of syrup equivalent to 150 mg of ranitidine) 4 times daily.

Maintenance of Healing of Erosive Esophagitis
The current recommended adult oral dosage is 150 mg or 10 mL of syrup (2 teaspoonfuls of syrup equivalent to 150 mg of ranitidine) twice daily.

Pediatric Use
The safety and effectiveness of ZANTAC have been established in the age-group of 1 month to 16 years. There is insufficient information about the pharmacokinetics of ZANTAC in neonatal patients (younger than 1 month of age) to make dosing recommendations.

The following 3 subsections provide dosing information for each of the pediatric indications.

Treatment of Duodenal and Gastric Ulcers: The recommended oral dose for the treatment of active duodenal and gastric ulcers is 2 to 4 mg/kg twice daily to a maximum of 300 mg/day. This recommendation is derived from adult clinical studies and pharmacokinetic data in pediatric patients.

Maintenance of Healing of Duodenal and Gastric Ulcers: The recommended oral dose for the maintenance of healing of duodenal and gastric ulcers is 2 to 4 mg/kg once daily to a maximum of 150 mg/day. This recommendation is derived from adult clinical studies and pharmacokinetic data in pediatric patients.

Treatment of GERD and Erosive Esophagitis: Although limited data exist for these conditions in pediatric patients, published literature supports a dosage of 5 to 10 mg/kg/day, usually given as 2 divided doses.

Dosage Adjustment for Patients With Impaired Renal Function
On the basis of experience with a group of subjects with severely impaired renal function treated with ZANTAC, the recommended dosage in patients with a creatinine clearance <50 mL/min is 150 mg or 10 mL of syrup (2 teaspoon-

fuls of syrup equivalent to 150 mg of ranitidine) every 24 hours. Should the patient's condition require, the frequency of dosing may be increased to every 12 hours or even further with caution. Hemodialysis reduces the level of circulating ranitidine. Ideally, the dosing schedule should be adjusted so that the timing of a scheduled dose coincides with the end of hemodialysis.

Elderly patients are more likely to have decreased renal function, therefore caution should be exercised in dose selection, and it may be useful to monitor renal function (see CLINICAL PHARMACOLOGY: Pharmacokinetics: Geriatrics and PRECAUTIONS: Geriatric Use).

HOW SUPPLIED
ZANTAC 150 Tablets (ranitidine HCl equivalent to 150 mg of ranitidine) are peach, film-coated, 5-sided tablets embossed with "ZANTAC 150" on one side and "Glaxo" on the other. They are available in bottles of 60 (NDC 0173-0344-42) and 500 (NDC 0173-0344-14) tablets.

ZANTAC 300 Tablets (ranitidine HCl equivalent to 300 mg of ranitidine) are yellow, film-coated, capsule-shaped tablets embossed with "ZANTAC 300" on one side and "Glaxo" on the other. They are available in bottles of 30 (NDC 0173-0393-40) tablets.

Store between 15° and 30°C (59° and 86°F) in a dry place. Protect from light. Replace cap securely after each opening.

ZANTAC Syrup, a clear, pale yellow, peppermint-flavored liquid, contains 16.8 mg of ranitidine HCl equivalent to 15 mg of ranitidine per 1 mL (75 mg/5 mL) in bottles of 16 fluid ounces (1 pint) (NDC 0173-0383-54).

Store between 4° and 25°C (39° and 77°F). Dispense in tight, light-resistant containers as defined in the USP/NF.

GlaxoSmithKline
Research Triangle Park, NC 27709
ZANTAC is a registered trademarks of Warner-Lambert Company, used under license.
MULTISTIX is a registered trademark of Bayer Healthcare LLC.
©2013, GlaxoSmithKline. All rights reserved.
July 2013
ZNT:7PI

ZOFRAN®
[zō' fran]
**(ondansetron hydrochloride)
injection for intravenous use**

HIGHLIGHTS OF PRESCRIBING INFORMATION
These highlights do not include all the information needed to use ZOFRAN safely and effectively. See full prescribing information for ZOFRAN.

ZOFRAN® (ondansetron hydrochloride) injection for intravenous use
Initial U.S. Approval: 1991

INDICATIONS AND USAGE
ZOFRAN Injection is a 5-HT$_3$ receptor antagonist indicated:
• Prevention of nausea and vomiting associated with initial and repeat courses of emetogenic cancer chemotherapy. (1.1)
• Prevention of postoperative nausea and/or vomiting. (1.2)

DOSAGE AND ADMINISTRATION
Prevention of nausea and vomiting associated with initial and repeat courses of emetogenic cancer chemotherapy (2.1):
• Adults and Pediatric patients (6 months to 18 years): Three 0.15 mg/kg doses, up to a maximum of 16 mg per dose, infused intravenously over 15 minutes. The first dose should be administered 30 minutes before the start of chemotherapy. Subsequent doses are administered 4 and 8 hours after the first dose.
Prevention of postoperative nausea and/or vomiting (2.2):

Population	Age	ZOFRAN Injection Dosage	Intravenous Infusion Rate
Adults	> 12 yrs	4 mg × 1	over 2 - 5 min
Pediatrics (> 40 kg)	1 mo. – 12 yrs	4 mg × 1	over 2 - 5 min
Pediatrics (≤ 40 kg)	1 mo. – 12 yrs	0.1 mg/kg × 1	over 2 - 5 min

• In patients with severe hepatic impairment, a total daily dose of 8 mg should not be exceeded. (2.4)

DOSAGE FORMS AND STRENGTHS
ZOFRAN Injection (2 mg/mL): 20 mL multidose vials. (3)

CONTRAINDICATIONS
• Patients known to have hypersensitivity (e.g., anaphylaxis) to this product or any of its components. (4)
• Concomitant use of apomorphine. (4)

WARNINGS AND PRECAUTIONS
• Hypersensitivity reactions including anaphylaxis and bronchospasm, have been reported in patients who have exhibited hypersensitivity to other selective 5-HT$_3$ receptor antagonists. (5.1)
• QT prolongation occurs in a dose-dependent manner. Cases of Torsade de Pointes have been reported. Avoid ZOFRAN in patients with congenital long QT syndrome. (5.2)
• Use in patients following abdominal surgery or in patients with chemotherapy-induced nausea and vomiting may mask a progressive ileus and/or gastric distention. (5.3)(5.4)

ADVERSE REACTIONS
Chemotherapy-Induced Nausea and Vomiting –
• The most common adverse reactions (≥ 7%) in adults are diarrhea, headache, and fever. (6.1)
Postoperative Nausea and Vomiting –
• The most common adverse reaction (≥ 10%) which occurs at a higher frequency compared to placebo in adults is headache. (6.1)
• The most common adverse reaction (≥ 2%) which occurs at a higher frequency compared to placebo in pediatric patients 1 to 24 months of age is diarrhea. (6.1)

To report SUSPECTED ADVERSE REACTIONS, contact GlaxoSmithKline at 1-888-825-5249 or FDA at 1-800-FDA-1088 or www.fda.gov/medwatch

DRUG INTERACTIONS
• Apomorphine – profound hypotension and loss of consciousness. Concomitant use with ondansetron is contraindicated. (7.2)

See 17 for PATIENT COUNSELING INFORMATION

Revised: 12/2013

FULL PRESCRIBING INFORMATION: CONTENTS*

14 CLINICAL STUDIES

14.1 Chemotherapy-Induced Nausea and Vomiting

14.2 Prevention of Postoperative Nausea and/or Vomiting

14.3 Prevention of Further Postoperative Nausea and Vomiting

16 HOW SUPPLIED/STORAGE AND HANDLING
17 PATIENT COUNSELING INFORMATION

* Sections or subsections omitted from the full prescribing information are not listed

---

FULL PRESCRIBING INFORMATION

1 INDICATIONS AND USAGE

1.1 Prevention of Nausea and Vomiting Associated with Initial and Repeat Courses of Emetogenic Cancer Chemotherapy

ZOFRAN Injection is indicated for the prevention of nausea and vomiting associated with initial and repeat courses of emetogenic cancer chemotherapy, including high-dose cisplatin [see Clinical Studies (14.1)].

ZOFRAN is approved for patients aged 6 months and older.

1.2 Prevention of Postoperative Nausea and/or Vomiting

ZOFRAN Injection is indicated for the prevention of postoperative nausea and/or vomiting. As with other antiemetics, routine prophylaxis is not recommended for patients in whom there is little expectation that nausea and/or vomiting will occur postoperatively. In patients in whom nausea and/or vomiting must be avoided postoperatively, ZOFRAN Injection is recommended even when the incidence of postoperative nausea and/or vomiting is low. For patients who do not receive prophylactic ZOFRAN Injection and experience nausea and/or vomiting postoperatively, ZOFRAN Injection may be given to prevent further episodes [see Clinical Studies (14.3)].

ZOFRAN is approved for patients aged 1 month and older.

2 DOSAGE AND ADMINISTRATION

2.1 Prevention of Nausea and Vomiting Associated with Initial and Repeat Courses of Emetogenic Chemotherapy

ZOFRAN Injection should be diluted in 50 mL of 5% Dextrose Injection or 0.9% Sodium Chloride Injection before administration.

Adults

The recommended adult intravenous dosage of ZOFRAN is three 0.15-mg/kg doses up to a maximum of 16 mg per dose [see Clinical Pharmacology (12.2)]. The first dose is infused over 15 minutes beginning 30 minutes before the start of emetogenic chemotherapy. Subsequent doses (0.15 mg/kg up to a maximum of 16 mg per dose) are administered 4 and 8 hours after the first dose of ZOFRAN.

Pediatrics

For pediatric patients 6 months through 18 years of age, the intravenous dosage of ZOFRAN is three 0.15-mg/kg doses up to a maximum of 16 mg per dose [see Clinical Studies (14.1) and Clinical Pharmacology (12.2 and 12.3)]. The first dose is to be administered 30 minutes before the start of moderately to highly emetogenic chemotherapy. Subsequent doses (0.15 mg/kg up to a maximum of 16 mg per dose) are administered 4 and 8 hours after the first dose of ZOFRAN. The drug should be infused intravenously over 15 minutes.

2.2 Prevention of Postoperative Nausea and Vomiting

ZOFRAN Injection should not be mixed with solutions for which physical and chemical compatibility have not been established. In particular, this applies to alkaline solutions as a precipitate may form.

Adults

The recommended adult intravenous dosage of ZOFRAN is 4 mg *undiluted* administered intravenously in not less than 30 seconds, preferably over 2 to 5 minutes, immediately before induction of anesthesia, or postoperatively if the patient did not receive prophylactic antiemetics and experiences nausea and/or vomiting occurring within 2 hours after surgery. Alternatively, 4 mg *undiluted* may be administered intramuscularly as a single injection for adults. While recommended as a fixed dose for patients weighing more than 40 kg or less, or a single 4-mg dose for patients weighing more than 40 kg. The rate of administration should be not less than 30 seconds, preferably over 2 to 5 minutes immediately prior to or following anesthesia induction, or postoperatively if the patient did not receive prophylactic antiemetics and experiences nausea and/or vomiting occurring

shortly after surgery. Prevention of further nausea and vomiting was only studied in patients who had not received prophylactic ZOFRAN.

2.3 Stability and Handling

After dilution, do not use beyond 24 hours. Although ZOFRAN Injection is chemically and physically stable when diluted as recommended, sterile precautions should be observed because diluents generally do not contain preservative.

ZOFRAN Injection is stable at room temperature under normal lighting conditions for 48 hours after dilution with the following intravenous fluids: 0.9% Sodium Chloride Injection, 5% Dextrose Injection, 5% Dextrose and 0.9% Sodium Chloride Injection, 5% Dextrose and 0.45% Sodium Chloride Injection, and 3% Sodium Chloride Injection.

Note: Parenteral drug products should be inspected visually for particulate matter and discoloration before administration whenever solution and container permit.

Precaution: Occasionally, ondansetron precipitates at the stopper/vial interface in vials stored upright. Potency and safety are not affected. If a precipitate is observed, resolubilize by shaking the vial vigorously.

2.4 Dosage Adjustment for Patients with Impaired Hepatic Function

In patients with severe hepatic impairment (Child-Pugh score of 10 or greater), a single maximal daily dose of 8 mg infused over 15 minutes beginning 30 minutes before the start of the emetogenic chemotherapy is recommended. There is no experience beyond first-day administration of ondansetron in these patients [see Clinical Pharmacology (12.3)].

3 DOSAGE FORMS AND STRENGTHS

ZOFRAN Injection, 2 mg/mL is a clear, colorless, nonpyrogenic, sterile solution available as a 20 mL multidose vial.

4 CONTRAINDICATIONS

ZOFRAN Injection is contraindicated for patients known to have hypersensitivity (e.g., anaphylaxis) to this product or any of its components. Anaphylactic reactions have been reported in patients taking ondansetron. [See Adverse Reactions (6.2)].

The concomitant use of apomorphine with ondansetron is contraindicated based on reports of profound hypotension and loss of consciousness when apomorphine was administered with ondansetron.

5 WARNINGS AND PRECAUTIONS

5.1 Hypersensitivity Reactions

Hypersensitivity reactions, including anaphylaxis and bronchospasm, have been reported in patients who have exhibited hypersensitivity to other selective 5-HT$_3$ receptor antagonists.

5.2 QT Prolongation

Ondansetron prolongs the QT interval in a dose-dependent manner [see Clinical Pharmacology (12.2)]. In addition, post-marketing cases of Torsade de Pointes have been reported in patients using ondansetron. Avoid ZOFRAN in patients with congenital long QT syndrome. ECG monitoring is recommended in patients with electrolyte abnormalities (e.g., hypokalemia or hypomagnesemia), congestive heart failure, bradyarrhythmias, or patients taking other medicinal products that lead to QT prolongation.

5.3 Masking of Progressive Ileus and Gastric Distension

The use of ZOFRAN in patients following abdominal surgery or in patients with chemotherapy-induced nausea and vomiting may mask a progressive ileus and gastric distention.

5.4 Effect on Peristalsis

ZOFRAN is not a drug that stimulates gastric or intestinal peristalsis. It should not be used instead of nasogastric suction.

6 ADVERSE REACTIONS

6.1 Clinical Trials Experience

Because clinical trials are conducted under widely varying conditions, adverse reaction rates observed in the clinical trials of a drug cannot be directly compared to rates in the clinical trials of another drug and may not reflect the rates observed in clinical practice.

The following adverse reactions have been reported in clinical trials of adult patients treated with ondansetron, the active ingredient of intravenous ZOFRAN across a range of dosages. A causal relationship to therapy with ZOFRAN (ondansetron) was unclear in many cases.

Chemotherapy-Induced Nausea and Vomiting

Table 1. Adverse Reactions Reported in > 5% of Adult Patients Who Received Ondansetron at a Dosage of Three 0.15-mg/kg Doses

	Number of Adult Patients With Reaction		
Adverse Reaction	ZOFRAN Injection 0.15 mg/kg × 3 n = 419	Metoclopramide n = 156	Placebo n = 34
Diarrhea	16%	44%	18%
Headache	17%	7%	15%
Fever	8%	5%	3%

Cardiovascular

Rare cases of angina (chest pain), electrocardiographic alterations, hypotension, and tachycardia have been reported.

Gastrointestinal

Constipation has been reported in 11% of chemotherapy patients receiving multiday ondansetron.

Hepatic

In comparative trials in cisplatin chemotherapy patients with normal baseline values of aspartate transaminase (AST) and alanine transaminase (ALT), these enzymes have been reported to exceed twice the upper limit of normal in approximately 5% of patients. The increases were transient and did not appear to be related to dose or duration of therapy. On repeat exposure, similar transient elevations in transaminase values occurred in some courses, but symptomatic hepatic disease did not occur.

Integumentary

Rash has occurred in approximately 1% of patients receiving ondansetron.

Neurological

There have been rare reports consistent with, but not diagnostic of, extrapyramidal reactions in patients receiving ZOFRAN Injection, and rare cases of grand mal seizure.

Other

Rare cases of hypokalemia have been reported.

Postoperative Nausea and Vomiting

The adverse reactions in Table 2 have been reported in ≥ 2% of adults receiving ondansetron at a dosage of 4 mg intravenous over 2 to 5 minutes in clinical trials.

Table 2. Adverse Reactions Reported in ≥ 2% (and With Greater Frequency than the Placebo Group) of Adult Patients Receiving Ondansetron at a Dosage of 4 mg Intravenous over 2 to 5 Minutes

Adverse Reaction[a,b]	ZOFRAN Injection 4 mg Intravenous n = 547 patients	Placebo n = 547 patients
Headache	92 (17%)	77 (14%)
Drowsiness/sedation	44 (8%)	37 (7%)
Injection site reaction	21 (4%)	18 (3%)
Fever	10 (2%)	6 (1%)
Cold sensation	9 (2%)	8 (1%)
Pruritus	9 (2%)	3 (< 1%)
Paresthesia	9 (2%)	2 (< 1%)

[a] Adverse Reactions: Rates of these reactions were not significantly different in the ondansetron and placebo groups

[b] Patients were receiving multiple concomitant perioperative and postoperative medications

Pediatric Use

Rates of adverse reactions were similar in both the ondansetron and placebo groups in pediatric patients receiving ondansetron (a single 0.1-mg/kg dose for pediatric patients weighing 40 kg or less, or 4 mg for pediatric patients weighing more than 40 kg) administered intravenously over at least 30 seconds. Diarrhea was seen more frequently in patients taking ZOFRAN (2%) compared to placebo (<1%) in the 1 month to 24 month age group. These patients were receiving multiple concomitant perioperative and postoperative medications.

6.2 Postmarketing Experience

The following adverse reactions have been identified during post-approval use of ondansetron. Because these reactions are reported voluntarily from a population of uncertain size, it is not always possible to reliably estimate their frequency or establish a causal relationship to drug exposure. The reactions have been chosen for inclusion due to a combination of their seriousness, frequency of reporting, or potential causal connection to ondansetron.

Cardiovascular

Arrhythmias (including ventricular and supraventricular tachycardia, premature ventricular contractions, and atrial fibrillation), bradycardia, electrocardiographic alterations (including second-degree heart block, QT/QTc interval prolongation, and ST segment depression), palpitations, and syncope. Rarely and predominantly with intravenous

Table 3. Pharmacokinetics in Normal Adult Volunteers

Age-group (years)	n	Peak Plasma Concentration (ng/mL)	Mean Elimination Half-life (h)	Plasma Clearance (L/h/kg)
19-40	11	102	3.5	0.381
61-74	12	106	4.7	0.319
≥ 75	11	170	5.5	0.262

ondansetron, transient ECG changes including QT/QTc interval prolongation have been reported [see Warnings and Precautions (5.2)].

General
Flushing. Rare cases of hypersensitivity reactions, sometimes severe (e.g., anaphylactic reactions, angioedema, bronchospasm, cardiopulmonary arrest, hypotension, laryngeal edema, laryngospasm, shock, shortness of breath, stridor) have also been reported. A positive lymphocyte transformation test to ondansetron has been reported, which suggests immunologic sensitivity to ondansetron.

Hepatobiliary
Liver enzyme abnormalities have been reported. Liver failure and death have been reported in patients with cancer receiving concurrent medications including potentially hepatotoxic cytotoxic chemotherapy and antibiotics.

Local Reactions
Pain, redness, and burning at site of injection.

Lower Respiratory
Hiccups

Neurological
Oculogyric crisis, appearing alone, as well as with other dystonic reactions. Transient dizziness during or shortly after intravenous infusion.

Skin
Urticaria, Stevens-Johnson syndrome, and toxic epidermal necrolysis.

Eye Disorders
Cases of transient blindness, predominantly during intravenous administration, have been reported. These cases of transient blindness were reported to resolve within a few minutes up to 48 hours. Transient blurred vision, in some cases associated with abnormalities of accommodation, have also been reported.

7 DRUG INTERACTIONS
7.1 Drugs Affecting Cytochrome P-450 Enzymes
Ondansetron does not appear to induce or inhibit the cytochrome P-450 drug-metabolizing enzyme system of the liver. Because ondansetron is metabolized by hepatic cytochrome P-450 drug-metabolizing enzymes (CYP3A4, CYP2D6, CYP1A2), inducers or inhibitors of these enzymes may change the clearance and, hence, the half-life of ondansetron [see Clinical Pharmacology (12.3)]. On the basis of limited available data, no dosage adjustment is recommended for patients on these drugs.

7.2 Apomorphine
Based on reports of profound hypotension and loss of consciousness when apomorphine was administered with ondansetron, the concomitant use of apomorphine with ondansetron is contraindicated [see Contraindications (4)].

7.3 Phenytoin, Carbamazepine, and Rifampin
In patients treated with potent inducers of CYP3A4 (i.e., phenytoin, carbamazepine, and rifampin), the clearance of ondansetron was significantly increased and ondansetron blood concentrations were decreased. However, on the basis of available data, no dosage adjustment for ondansetron is recommended for patients on these drugs [see Clinical Pharmacology (12.3)].

7.4 Tramadol
Although there are no data on pharmacokinetic drug interactions between ondansetron and tramadol, data from two small studies indicate that concomitant use of ondansetron may result in reduced analgesic activity of tramadol. Patients on concomitant ondansetron self administered tramadol more frequently in these studies, leading to an increased cumulative dose in patient controlled administration (PCA) of tramadol.

7.5 Chemotherapy
In humans, carmustine, etoposide, and cisplatin do not affect the pharmacokinetics of ondansetron.
In a crossover study in 76 pediatric patients, intravenous ondansetron did not increase blood levels of high-dose methotrexate.

7.6 Temazepam
The coadministration of ondansetron had no effect on the pharmacokinetics and pharmacodynamics of temazepam.

7.7 Alfentanil and Atracurium
Ondansetron does not alter the respiratory depressant effects produced by alfentanil or the degree of neuromuscular blockade produced by atracurium. Interactions with general or local anesthetics have not been studied.

8 USE IN SPECIFIC POPULATIONS
8.1 Pregnancy
Pregnancy Category B. Reproduction studies have been performed in pregnant rats and rabbits at intravenous doses up to 4 mg/kg per day (approximately 1.4 and 2.9 times the recommended human intravenous dose of 0.15 mg/kg given three times a day, respectively, based on body surface area) and have revealed no evidence of impaired fertility or harm to the fetus due to ondansetron. There are, however, no adequate and well-controlled studies in pregnant women. Because animal reproduction studies are not always predictive of human response, this drug should be used during pregnancy only if clearly needed.

8.3 Nursing Mothers
Ondansetron is excreted in the breast milk of rats. It is not known whether ondansetron is excreted in human milk. Because many drugs are excreted in human milk, caution should be exercised when ondansetron is administered to a nursing woman.

8.4 Pediatric Use
Little information is available about the use of ondansetron in pediatric surgical patients younger than 1 month of age. [See Clinical Studies (14.2)]. Little information is available about the use of ondansetron in pediatric cancer patients younger than 6 months of age. [see Clinical Studies (14.1) and Dosage and Administration (2)].
The clearance of ondansetron in pediatric patients 1 month to 4 months of age is slower and the half-life is ~2.5 fold longer than patients who are > 4 to 24 months of age. As a precaution, it is recommended that patients less than 4 months of age receiving this drug be closely monitored. [See Clinical Pharmacology (12.3)].

8.5 Geriatric Use
Of the total number of subjects enrolled in cancer chemotherapy-induced and postoperative nausea and vomiting in US- and foreign-controlled clinical trials, 862 were 65 years of age and over. No overall differences in safety or effectiveness were observed between these subjects and younger subjects, and other reported clinical experience has not identified differences in responses between the elderly and younger patients, but greater sensitivity of some older individuals cannot be ruled out. Dosage adjustment is not needed in patients over the age of 65 [see Clinical Pharmacology (12.3)].

8.6 Hepatic Impairment
In patients with severe hepatic impairment (Child-Pugh score of 10 or greater), clearance is reduced and apparent volume of distribution is increased with a resultant increase in plasma half-life [see Clinical Pharmacology (12.3)]. In such patients, a total daily dose of 8 mg should not be exceeded [see Dosage and Administration (2.3)].

8.7 Renal Impairment
Although plasma clearance is reduced in patients with severe renal impairment (creatinine clearance < 30 mL/min), no dosage adjustment is recommended [see Clinical Pharmacology (12.3)].

9 DRUG ABUSE AND DEPENDENCE
Animal studies have shown that ondansetron is not discriminated as a benzodiazepine nor does it substitute for benzodiazepines in direct addiction studies.

10 OVERDOSAGE
There is no specific antidote for ondansetron overdose. Patients should be managed with appropriate supportive therapy. Individual intravenous doses as large as 150 mg and total daily intravenous doses as large as 252 mg have been inadvertently administered without significant adverse events. These doses are more than 10 times the recommended daily dose.
In addition to the adverse reactions listed above, the following events have been described in the setting of ondansetron overdose: "Sudden blindness" (amaurosis) of 2 to 3 minutes' duration plus severe constipation occurred in one patient that was administered 72 mg of ondansetron intravenously as a single dose. Hypotension (and faintness) occurred in another patient that took 48 mg of ondansetron hydrochloride tablets. Following infusion of 32 mg over only a 4-minute period, a vasovagal episode with transient second-degree heart block was observed. In all instances, the events resolved completely.

11 DESCRIPTION
The active ingredient of ZOFRAN Injection is ondansetron hydrochloride, a selective blocking agent of the serotonin 5-HT$_3$ receptor type. Its chemical name is (±) 1, 2, 3, 9-tetrahydro-9-methyl-3-[(2-methyl-1H-imidazol-1-yl)methyl]-4H-carbazol-4-one, monohydrochloride, dihydrate. It has the following structural formula:

The empirical formula is $C_{18}H_{19}N_3O \cdot HCl \cdot 2H_2O$, representing a molecular weight of 365.9.
Ondansetron HCl is a white to off-white powder that is soluble in water and normal saline.
Each 1 mL of aqueous solution in the 20 mL multidose vial contains 2 mg of ondansetron as the hydrochloride dihydrate; 8.3 mg of sodium chloride, USP; 0.5 mg of citric acid monohydrate, USP and 0.25 mg of sodium citrate dihydrate, USP as buffers; and 1.2 mg of methylparaben, NF and 0.15 mg of propylparaben, NF as preservatives in Water for Injection, USP.
ZOFRAN Injection is a clear, colorless, nonpyrogenic, sterile solution for intravenous use. The pH of the injection solution is 3.3 to 4.0.

12 CLINICAL PHARMACOLOGY
12.1 Mechanism of Action
Ondansetron is a selective 5-HT$_3$ receptor antagonist. While ondansetron's mechanism of action has not been fully characterized, it is not a dopamine-receptor antagonist.

12.2 Pharmacodynamics
QTc interval prolongation was studied in a double blind, single intravenous dose, placebo- and positive-controlled, crossover study in 58 healthy subjects. The maximum mean (95% upper confidence bound) difference in QTcF from placebo after baseline-correction was 19.5 (21.8) ms and 5.6 (7.4) ms after 15 minute intravenous infusions of 32mg and 8 mg ZOFRAN, respectively. A significant exposure-reponse relationship was identified between ondansetron concentration and ΔΔQTcF. Using the established exposure-response relationship, 24 mg infused intravenously over 15 min had a mean predicted (95% upper prediction interval) ΔΔQTcF of 14.0 (16.3) ms. In contrast, 16 mg infused intravenously over 15 min using the same model had a mean predicted (95% upper prediction interval) ΔΔQTcF of 9.1 (11.2) ms.
In normal volunteers, single intravenous doses of 0.15 mg/kg of ondansetron had no effect on esophageal motility, gastric motility, lower esophageal sphincter pressure, or small intestinal transit time. In another study in six normal male volunteers, a 16-mg dose infused over 5 minutes showed no effect of the drug on cardiac output, heart rate, stroke volume, blood pressure, or electrocardiogram (ECG). Multiday administration of ondansetron has been shown to slow colonic transit in normal volunteers. Ondansetron has no effect on plasma prolactin concentrations. In a gender-balanced pharmacodynamic study (n = 56), ondansetron 4 mg administered intravenously or intramuscularly was dynamically similar in the prevention of nausea and vomiting using the ipecacuanha model of emesis.

12.3 Pharmacokinetics
In normal adult volunteers, the following mean pharmacokinetic data have been determined following a single 0.15-mg/kg intravenous dose.
[See table 3 above]

Absorption
A study was performed in normal volunteers (n = 56) to evaluate the pharmacokinetics of a single 4-mg dose administered as a 5-minute infusion compared to a single intramuscular injection. Systemic exposure as measured by mean AUC were equivalent, with values of 156 [95% CI 136, 180] and 161 [95% CI 137, 190] ng•h/mL for intravenous and intramuscular groups, respectively. Mean peak plasma concentrations were 42.9 [95% CI 33.8, 54.4] ng/mL at 10 minutes after intravenous infusion and 31.9 [95% CI 26.3, 38.6] ng/mL at 41 minutes after intramuscular injection.

Distribution
Plasma protein binding of ondansetron as measured in vitro was 70% to 76%, over the pharmacologic concentration range of 10 to 500 ng/mL. Circulating drug also distributes into erythrocytes.

Metabolism
Ondansetron is extensively metabolized in humans, with approximately 5% of a radiolabeled dose recovered as the

parent compound from the urine. The primary metabolic pathway is hydroxylation on the indole ring followed by subsequent glucuronide or sulfate conjugation.

Although some nonconjugated metabolites have pharmacologic activity, these are not found in plasma at concentrations likely to significantly contribute to the biological activity of ondansetron. The metabolites are observed in the urine.

In vitro metabolism studies have shown that ondansetron is a substrate for multiple human hepatic cytochrome P-450 enzymes, including CYP1A2, CYP2D6, and CYP3A4. In terms of overall ondansetron turnover, CYP3A4 plays a predominant role while formation of the major in vivo metabolites is apparently mediated by CYP1A2. The role of CYP2D6 in ondansetron in vivo metabolism is relatively minor.

The pharmacokinetics of intravenous ondansetron did not differ between subjects who were poor metabolisers of CYP2D6 and those who were extensive metabolisers of CYP2D6, further supporting the limited role of CYP2D6 in ondansetron disposition in vivo.

Elimination

In adult cancer patients, the mean ondansetron elimination half-life was 4.0 hours, and there was no difference in the multidose pharmacokinetics over a 4-day period. In a dose proportionality study, systemic exposure to 32 mg of ondansetron was not proportional to dose as measured by comparing dose-normalized AUC values to an 8-mg dose. This is consistent with a small decrease in systemic clearance with increasing plasma concentrations.

Geriatrics

A reduction in clearance and increase in elimination half-life are seen in patients over 75 years of age. In clinical trials with cancer patients, safety and efficacy were similar in patients over 65 years of age and those under 65 years of age; there was an insufficient number of patients over 75 years of age to permit conclusions in that age-group. No dosage adjustment is recommended in the elderly.

Pediatrics

Pharmacokinetic samples were collected from 74 cancer patients 6 to 48 months of age, who received a dose of 0.15 mg/kg of intravenous ondansetron every 4 hours for 3 doses during a safety and efficacy trial. These data were combined with sequential pharmacokinetics data from 41 surgery patients 1 month to 24 months of age, who received a single dose of 0.1 mg/kg of intravenous ondansetron prior to surgery with general anesthesia, and a population pharmacokinetic analysis was performed on the combined data set. The results of this analysis are included in Table 4 and are compared to the pharmacokinetic results in cancer patients 4 to 18 years of age.

Table 4. Pharmacokinetics in Pediatric Cancer Patients 1 Month to 18 Years of Age

Subjects and Age Group	N	CL (L/h/kg)	Vd$_{ss}$ (L/kg)	T$_{1/2}$ (h)
		Geometric Mean		Mean
Pediatric Cancer Patients 4 to 18 years of age	N = 21	0.599	1.9	2.8
Population PK Patients[a] 1 month to 48 months of age	N = 115	0.582	3.65	4.9

[a] Population PK (Pharmacokinetic) Patients: 64% cancer patients and 36% surgery patients.

Based on the population pharmacokinetic analysis, cancer patients 6 to 48 months of age who receive a dose of 0.15 mg/kg of intravenous ondansetron every 4 hours for 3 doses would be expected to achieve a systemic exposure (AUC) consistent with the exposure achieved in previous pediatric studies in cancer patients (4 to 18 years of age) at similar doses.

In a study of 21 pediatric patients (3 to 12 years of age) who were undergoing surgery requiring anesthesia for a duration of 45 minutes to 2 hours, a single intravenous dose of ondansetron, 2 mg (3 to 7 years) or 4 mg (8 to 12 years), was administered immediately prior to anesthesia induction. Mean weight-normalized clearance and volume of distribution values in these pediatric surgical patients were similar to those previously reported for young adults. Mean terminal half-life was slightly reduced in pediatric patients (range, 2.5 to 3 hours) in comparison with adults (range, 3 to 3.5 hours).

In a study of 51 pediatric patients (1 month to 24 months of age) who were undergoing surgery requiring general anesthesia, a single intravenous dose of ondansetron, 0.1 or 0.2 mg/kg, was administered prior to surgery. As shown in

Table 5, the 41 patients with pharmacokinetic data were divided into 2 groups, patients 1 month to 4 months of age and patients 5 to 24 months of age, and are compared to pediatric patients 3 to 12 years of age.

Table 5. Pharmacokinetics in Pediatric Surgery Patients 1 Month to 12 Years of Age

Subjects and Age Group	N	CL (L/h/kg)	Vd$_{ss}$ (L/kg)	T$_{1/2}$ (h)
		Geometric Mean		Mean
Pediatric Surgery Patients 3 to 12 years of age	N = 21	0.439	1.65	2.9
Pediatric Surgery Patients 5 to 24 months of age	N = 22	0.581	2.3	2.9
Pediatric Surgery Patients 1 month to 4 months of age	N = 19	0.401	3.5	6.7

In general, surgical and cancer pediatric patients younger than 18 years tend to have a higher ondansetron clearance compared to adults leading to a shorter half-life in most pediatric patients. In patients 1 month to 4 months of age, a longer half-life was observed due to the higher volume of distribution in this age group.

In a study of 21 pediatric cancer patients (4 to 18 years of age) who received three intravenous doses of 0.15 mg/kg of

Table 6. Therapeutic Response in Prevention of Chemotherapy-Induced Nausea and Vomiting in Single-Day Cisplatin Therapy[a] in Adults

	Zofran Injection (0.15 mg/kg × 3)	Placebo	P Value[b]
Number of patients	14	14	
Treatment response			
0 Emetic episodes	2 (14%)	0 (0%)	
1-2 Emetic episodes	8 (57%)	0 (0%)	
3-5 Emetic episodes	2 (14%)	1 (7%)	
More than 5 emetic episodes/rescued	2 (14%)	13 (93%)	0.001
Median number of emetic episodes	1.5	Undefined[c]	
Median time to first emetic episode (h)	11.6	2.8	0.001
Median nausea scores (0-100)[d]	3	59	0.034
Global satisfaction with control of nausea and vomiting (0-100)[e]	96	10.5	0.009

[a] Chemotherapy was high dose (100 and 120 mg/m^2; ZOFRAN Injection n = 6, placebo n = 5) or moderate dose (50 and 80 mg/m^2; ZOFRAN Injection n = 8, placebo n = 9). Other chemotherapeutic agents included fluorouracil, doxorubicin, and cyclophosphamide. There was no difference between treatments in the types of chemotherapy that would account for differences in response.
[b] Efficacy based on "all patients treated" analysis.
[c] Median undefined since at least 50% of the patients were rescued or had more than five emetic episodes.
[d] Visual analog scale assessment of nausea: 0 = no nausea, 100 = nausea as bad as it can be.
[e] Visual analog scale assessment of satisfaction: 0 = not at all satisfied, 100 = totally satisfied.

Table 7. Therapeutic Response in Prevention of Vomiting Induced by Cisplatin (≥ 100 mg/m^2) Single-Day Therapy[a] in Adults

	Zofran Injection 0.15 mg/kg × 3	Metoclopramide 2 mg/kg × 6	P Value
Dose Number of patients in efficacy population	136	138	
Treatment response			
0 Emetic episodes	54 (40%)	41 (30%)	
1-2 Emetic episodes	34 (25%)	30 (22%)	
3-5 Emetic episodes	19 (14%)	18 (13%)	
More than 5 emetic episodes/rescued	29 (21%)	49 (36%)	
Comparison of treatments with respect to			
0 Emetic episodes	54/136	41/138	0.083
More than 5 emetic episodes/rescued	29/136	49/138	0.009
Median number of emetic episodes	1	2	0.005
Median time to first emetic episode (h)	20.5	4.3	< 0.001
Global satisfaction with control of nausea and vomiting (0-100)[b]	85	63	0.001
Acute dystonic reactions	0	8	0.005
Akathisia	0	10	0.002

[a] In addition to cisplatin, 68% of patients received other chemotherapeutic agents, including cyclophosphamide, etoposide, and fluorouracil. There was no difference between treatments in the types of chemotherapy that would account for differences in response.
[b] Visual analog scale assessment: 0 = not at all satisfied, 100 = totally satisfied.

ondansetron at 4-hour intervals, patients older than 15 years of age exhibited ondansetron pharmacokinetic parameters similar to those of adults.

Renal Impairment

Due to the very small contribution (5%) of renal clearance to the overall clearance, renal impairment was not expected to significantly influence the total clearance of ondansetron. However, ondansetron mean plasma clearance was reduced by about 41% in patients with severe renal impairment (creatinine clearance < 30 mL/min). This reduction in clearance is variable and was not consistent with an increase in half-life. No reduction in dose or dosing frequency in these patients is warranted.

Hepatic Impairment

In patients with mild-to-moderate hepatic impairment, clearance is reduced 2-fold and mean half-life is increased to 11.6 hours compared to 5.7 hours in those without hepatic impairment. In patients with severe hepatic impairment (Child-Pugh score of 10 or greater), clearance is reduced 2-fold to 3-fold and apparent volume of distribution is increased with a resultant increase in half-life to 20 hours. In patients with severe hepatic impairment, a total daily dose of 8 mg should not be exceeded.

13 NONCLINICAL TOXICOLOGY

13.1 Carcinogenesis, Mutagenesis, Impairment of Fertility

Carcinogenic effects were not seen in 2-year studies in rats and mice with oral ondansetron doses up to 10 and 30 mg/kg per day, respectively (approximately 3.6 and 5.4 times the recommended human intravenous dose of 0.15 mg/kg given three times a day, based on body surface area). Ondansetron was not mutagenic in standard tests for mutagenicity.

Table 8. Therapeutic Response in Prevention of Chemotherapy-Induced Nausea and Vomiting in Single-Day Cyclophosphamide Therapy[a] in Adults

	Zofran Injection (0.15 mg/kg × 3)	Placebo	P Value[b]
Number of patients	10	10	
Treatment response			
0 Emetic episodes	7 (70%)	0 (0%)	0.001
1-2 Emetic episodes	0 (0%)	2 (20%)	
3-5 Emetic episodes	2 (20%)	4 (40%)	
More than 5 emetic episodes/rescued	1 (10%)	4 (40%)	0.131
Median number of emetic episodes	0	4	0.008
Median time to first emetic episode (h)	Undefined[c]	8.79	
Median nausea scores (0-100)[d]	0	60	0.001
Global satisfaction with control of nausea and vomiting (0-100)[e]	100	52	0.008

[a] Chemotherapy consisted of cyclophosphamide in all patients, plus other agents, including fluorouracil, doxorubicin, methotrexate, and vincristine. There was no difference between treatments in the type of chemotherapy that would account for differences in response.
[b] Efficacy based on "all patients treated" analysis.
[c] Median undefined since at least 50% of patients did not have any emetic episodes.
[d] Visual analog scale assessment of nausea: 0 = no nausea, 100 = nausea as bad as it can be.
[e] Visual analog scale assessment of satisfaction: 0 = not at all satisfied, 100 = totally satisfied.

Table 9. Therapeutic Response in Prevention of Postoperative Nausea and Vomiting in Adult Patients

	Ondansetron 4 mg Intravenous	Placebo	P Value
Study 1			
Emetic episodes:			
Number of patients	136	139	
Treatment response over 24-h postoperative period			
0 Emetic episodes	103 (76%)	64 (46%)	< 0.001
1 Emetic episode	13 (10%)	17 (12%)	
More than 1 emetic episode/rescued	20 (15%)	58 (42%)	
Nausea assessments:			
Number of patients	134	136	
No nausea over 24-h postoperative period	56 (42%)	39 (29%)	
Study 2			
Emetic episodes:			
Number of patients	136	143	
Treatment response over 24-h postoperative period			
0 Emetic episodes	85 (63%)	63 (44%)	0.002
1 Emetic episode	16 (12%)	29 (20%)	
More than 1 emetic episode/rescued	35 (26%)	51 (36%)	
Nausea assessments:			
Number of patients	125	133	
No nausea over 24-h postoperative period	48 (38%)	42 (32%)	

Oral administration of ondansetron up to 15 mg/kg per day (approximately 3.8 times the recommended human intravenous dose, based on body surface area) did not affect fertility or general reproductive performance of male and female rats.

14   CLINICAL STUDIES

The clinical efficacy of ondansetron hydrochloride, the active ingredient of ZOFRAN, was assessed in clinical trials as described below.

14.1   Chemotherapy-Induced Nausea and Vomiting

Adults

In a double-blind study of three different dosing regimens of ZOFRAN Injection, 0.015 mg/kg, 0.15 mg/kg, and 0.30 mg/kg, each given three times during the course of cancer chemotherapy, the 0.15-mg/kg dosing regimen was more effective than the 0.015-mg/kg dosing regimen. The 0.30-mg/kg dosing regimen was not shown to be more effective than the 0.15-mg/kg dosing regimen.

Cisplatin-Based Chemotherapy

In a double-blind study in 28 patients, ZOFRAN Injection (three 0.15-mg/kg doses) was significantly more effective than placebo in preventing nausea and vomiting induced by cisplatin-based chemotherapy. Therapeutic response was as shown in Table 6.

[See table 6 at top of previous page]

Ondansetron injection (0.15-mg/kg × 3 doses) was compared with metoclopramide (2 mg/kg × 6 doses) in a single-blind trial in 307 patients receiving cisplatin ≥ 100 mg/m² with or without other chemotherapeutic agents. Patients received

the first dose of ondansetron or metoclopramide 30 minutes before cisplatin. Two additional ondansetron doses were administered 4 and 8 hours later, or five additional metoclopramide doses were administered 2, 4, 7, 10, and 13 hours later. Cisplatin was administered over a period of 3 hours or less. Episodes of vomiting and retching were tabulated over the period of 24 hours after cisplatin. The results of this study are summarized in Table 7.

[See table 7 at top of previous page]

Cyclophosphamide-Based Chemotherapy

In a double-blind, placebo-controlled study of ZOFRAN Injection (three 0.15-mg/kg doses) in 20 patients receiving cyclophosphamide (500 to 600 mg/m²) chemotherapy, ZOFRAN Injection was significantly more effective than placebo in preventing nausea and vomiting. The results are summarized in Table 8.

[See table 8 above]

Re-treatment

In uncontrolled trials, 127 patients receiving cisplatin (median dose, 100 mg/m²) and ondansetron who had two or fewer emetic episodes were re-treated with ondansetron and chemotherapy, mainly cisplatin, for a total of 269 re-treatment courses (median, 2; range, 1 to 10). No emetic episodes occurred in 160 (59%), and two or fewer emetic episodes occurred in 217 (81%) re-treatment courses.

Pediatrics

Four open-label, noncomparative (one US, three foreign) trials have been performed with 209 pediatric cancer patients 4 to 18 years of age given a variety of cisplatin or noncisplatin regimens. In the three foreign trials, the initial ZOFRAN

Injection dose ranged from 0.04 to 0.87 mg/kg for a total dose of 2.16 to 12 mg. This was followed by the oral administration of ondansetron ranging from 4 to 24 mg daily for 3 days. In the US trial, ZOFRAN was administered intravenously (only) in three doses of 0.15 mg/kg each for a total daily dose of 7.2 to 39 mg. In these studies, 58% of the 196 evaluable patients had a complete response (no emetic episodes) on day 1. Thus, prevention of vomiting in these pediatric patients was essentially the same as for patients older than 18 years of age.

An open-label, multicenter, noncomparative trial has been performed in 75 pediatric cancer patients 6 to 48 months of age receiving at least one moderately or highly emetogenic chemotherapeutic agent. Fifty-seven percent (57%) were females; 67% were white, 18% were American Hispanic, and 15% were black patients. ZOFRAN was administered intravenously over 15 minutes in three doses of 0.15 mg/kg. The first dose was administered 30 minutes before the start of chemotherapy, the second and third doses were administered 4 and 8 hours after the first dose, respectively. Eighteen patients (25%) received routine prophylactic dexamethasone (i.e., not given as rescue). Of the 75 evaluable patients, 56% had a complete response (no emetic episodes) on day 1. Thus, prevention of vomiting in these pediatric patients was comparable to the prevention of vomiting in patients 4 years of age and older.

14.2   Prevention of Postoperative Nausea and/or Vomiting

Adults

Adult surgical patients who received ondansetron immediately before the induction of general balanced anesthesia (barbiturate: thiopental, methohexital, or thiamylal; opioid: alfentanil or fentanyl; nitrous oxide; neuromuscular blockade: succinylcholine/curare and/or vecuronium or atracurium; and supplemental isoflurane) were evaluated in two double-blind US studies involving 554 patients. ZOFRAN Injection (4 mg) intravenous given over 2 to 5 minutes was significantly more effective than placebo. The results of these studies are summarized in Table 9.

[See table 9 above]

The study populations in Table 9 consisted mainly of females undergoing laparoscopic procedures.

In a placebo-controlled study conducted in 468 males undergoing outpatient procedures, a single 4-mg intravenous ondansetron dose prevented postoperative vomiting over a 24-hour study period in 79% of males receiving drug compared to 63% of males receiving placebo (P < 0.001).

Two other placebo-controlled studies were conducted in 2,792 patients undergoing major abdominal or gynecological surgeries to evaluate a single 4-mg or 8-mg intravenous ondansetron dose for prevention of postoperative nausea and vomiting over a 24-hour study period. At the 4-mg dosage, 59% of patients receiving ondansetron versus 45% receiving placebo in the first study (P < 0.001) and 41% of patients receiving ondansetron versus 30% receiving placebo in the second study (P = 0.001) experienced no emetic episodes. No additional benefit was observed in patients who received intravenous ondansetron 8 mg compared to patients who received intravenous ondansetron 4 mg.

Pediatrics

Three double-blind, placebo-controlled studies have been performed (one US, two foreign) in 1,049 male and female patients (2 to 12 years of age) undergoing general anesthesia with nitrous oxide. The surgical procedures included tonsillectomy with or without adenoidectomy, strabismus surgery, herniorrhaphy, and orchidopexy. Patients were randomized to either single intravenous doses of ondansetron (0.1 mg/kg for pediatric patients weighing 40 kg or less, 4 mg for pediatric patients weighing more than 40 kg) or placebo. Study drug was administered over at least 30 seconds, immediately prior to or following anesthesia induction. Ondansetron was significantly more effective than placebo in preventing nausea and vomiting. The results of these studies are summarized in Table 10.

Table 10. Therapeutic Response in Prevention of Postoperative Nausea and Vomiting in Pediatric Patients 2 to 12 Years of Age

Treatment Response Over 24 Hours	Ondansetron n (%)	Placebo n (%)	P Value
Study 1			
Number of patients	205	210	
0 Emetic episodes	140 (68%)	82 (39%)	0.001
Failure[a]	65 (32%)	128 (61%)	
Study 2			
Number of patients	112	110	
0 Emetic episodes	68 (61%)	38 (35%)	0.001
Failure[a]	44 (39%)	72 (65%)	
Study 3			
Number of patients	206	206	
0 Emetic episodes	123 (60%)	96 (47%)	0.01
Failure[a]	83 (40%)	110 (53%)	

Table 11. Therapeutic Response in Prevention of Further Postoperative Nausea and Vomiting in Adult Patients

	Ondansetron 4 mg Intravenous	Placebo	P Value
Study 1			
Emetic episodes:			
Number of patients	104	117	
Treatment response 24 h after study drug			
0 Emetic episodes	49 (47%)	19 (16%)	< 0.001
1 Emetic episode	12 (12%)	9 (8%)	
More than 1 emetic episode/rescued	43 (41%)	89 (76%)	
Median time to first emetic episode (min)[a]	55.0	43.0	
Nausea assessments:			
Number of patients	98	102	
Mean nausea score over 24-h postoperative period[b]	1.7	3.1	
Study 2			
Emetic episodes:			
Number of patients	112	108	
Treatment response 24 h after study drug			
0 Emetic episodes	49 (44%)	28 (26%)	0.006
1 Emetic episode	14 (13%)	3 (3%)	
More than 1 emetic episode/rescued	49 (44%)	77 (71%)	
Median time to first emetic episode (min)[a]	60.5	34.0	
Nausea assessments:			
Number of patients	105	85	
Mean nausea score over 24-h postoperative period[b]	1.9	2.9	

[a] After administration of study drug.
[b] Nausea measured on a scale of 0-10 with 0 = no nausea, 10 = nausea as bad as it can be.

Nausea assessments[b]:			
Number of patients	185	191	
None	119 (64%)	99 (52%)	0.01

[a] Failure was one or more emetic episodes, rescued, or withdrawn.
[b] Nausea measured as none, mild, or severe.

A double-blind, multicenter, placebo-controlled study was conducted in 670 pediatric patients 1 month to 24 months of age who were undergoing routine surgery under general anesthesia. Seventy-five percent (75%) were males; 64% were white, 15% were black, 13% were American Hispanic, 2% were Asian, and 6% were "other race" patients. A single 0.1-mg/kg intravenous dose of ondansetron administered within 5 minutes following induction of anesthesia was statistically significantly more effective than placebo in preventing vomiting. In the placebo group, 28% of patients experienced vomiting compared to 11% of subjects who received ondansetron ($P \le 0.01$). Overall, 32 (10%) of placebo patients and 18 (5%) of patients who received ondansetron received antiemetic rescue medication(s) or prematurely withdrew from the study.

14.3   Prevention of Further Postoperative Nausea and Vomiting

Adults

Adult surgical patients receiving general balanced anesthesia (barbiturate: thiopental, methohexital, or thiamylal; opioid: alfentanil or fentanyl; nitrous oxide; neuromuscular blockade: succinylcholine/curare and/or vecuronium or atracurium; and supplemental isoflurane) who received no prophylactic antiemetics and who experienced nausea and/or vomiting within 2 hours postoperatively were evaluated in two double-blind US studies involving 441 patients. Patients who experienced an episode of postoperative nausea and/or vomiting were given ZOFRAN Injection (4 mg) intravenous over 2 to 5 minutes, and this was significantly more effective than placebo. The results of these studies are summarized in Table 11.

[See table 11 above]

The study populations in Table 11 consisted mainly of women undergoing laparoscopic procedures.

Repeat Dosing in Adults

In patients who do not achieve adequate control of postoperative nausea and vomiting following a single, prophylactic, preinduction, intravenous dose of ondansetron 4 mg, administration of a second intravenous dose of ondansetron 4 mg postoperatively does not provide additional control of nausea and vomiting.

Pediatrics

One double-blind, placebo-controlled, US study was performed in 351 male and female outpatients (2 to 12 years of age) who received general anesthesia with nitrous oxide and no prophylactic antiemetics. Surgical procedures were unrestricted. Patients who experienced two or more emetic episodes within 2 hours following discontinuation of nitrous oxide were randomized to either single intravenous doses of ondansetron (0.1 mg/kg for pediatric patients weighing 40 kg or less, 4 mg for pediatric patients weighing more than 40 kg) or placebo administered over at least 30 seconds. Ondansetron was significantly more effective than placebo in preventing further episodes of nausea and vomiting. The results of the study are summarized in Table 12.

Table 12. Therapeutic Response in Prevention of Further Postoperative Nausea and Vomiting in Pediatric Patients 2 to 12 Years of Age

Treatment Response Over 24 Hours	Ondansetron n (%)	Placebo n (%)	P Value
Number of patients	180	171	
0 Emetic episodes	96 (53%)	29 (17%)	0.001
Failure[a]	84 (47%)	142 (83%)	

[a] Failure was one or more emetic episodes, rescued, or withdrawn.

16   HOW SUPPLIED/STORAGE AND HANDLING

ZOFRAN Injection, 2 mg/mL, is supplied as follows:
NDC 0173-0442-00   20-mL multidose vials (Singles)
Storage: Store vials between 2° and 30°C (36° and 86°F). Protect from light.

17   PATIENT COUNSELING INFORMATION

- Patients should be informed that ZOFRAN may cause serious cardiac arrhythmias such as QT prolongation. Patients should be instructed to tell their healthcare provider right away if they perceive a change in their heart rate, if they feel lightheaded, or if they have a syncopal episode.
- Patients should be informed that the chances of developing severe cardiac arrhythmias such as QT prolongation and Torsade de Pointes are higher in the following people:
- Patients with a personal or family history of abnormal heart rhythms, such as congenital long QT syndrome;
- Patients who take medications, such as diuretics, which may cause electrolyte abnormalities
- Patients with hypokalemia or hypomagnesemia
ZOFRAN should be avoided in these patients, since they may be more at risk for cardiac arrhythmias such as QT prolongation and Torsade de Pointes.
- Inform patients that ZOFRAN may cause hypersensitivity reactions, some as severe as anaphylaxis and bronchospasm. The patient should report any signs and symptoms of hypersensitivity reactions, including fever, chills, rash, or breathing problems.
- The patient should report the use of all medications, especially apomorphine, to their healthcare provider. Concomitant use of apomorphine and ZOFRAN may cause a significant drop in blood pressure and loss of consciousness.
- Inform patients that ZOFRAN may cause headache, drowsiness/sedation, constipation, fever and diarrhea.

GlaxoSmithKline
Research Triangle Park, NC 27709
©2013, GlaxoSmithKline. All rights reserved.
ZFJ:8PI

ZOFRAN®
(ondansetron hydrochloride)
Tablets

ZOFRAN ODT®
(ondansetron)
Orally Disintegrating Tablets

ZOFRAN®
(ondansetron hydrochloride)
Oral Solution

℞

DESCRIPTION

The active ingredient in ZOFRAN® Tablets and ZOFRAN® Oral Solution is ondansetron hydrochloride (HCl) as the dihydrate, the racemic form of ondansetron and a selective blocking agent of the serotonin 5-HT$_3$ receptor type. Chemically it is (±) 1, 2, 3, 9-tetrahydro-9-methyl-3-[(2-methyl-1H-imidazol-1-yl)methyl]-4H-carbazol-4-one, monohydrochloride, dihydrate. It has the following structural formula:

The empirical formula is $C_{18}H_{19}N_3O \cdot HCl \cdot 2H_2O$, representing a molecular weight of 365.9.

Ondansetron HCl dihydrate is a white to off-white powder that is soluble in water and normal saline.

The active ingredient in ZOFRAN ODT® Orally Disintegrating Tablets is ondansetron base, the racemic form of ondansetron, and a selective blocking agent of the serotonin 5-HT$_3$ receptor type. Chemically it is (±) 1, 2, 3, 9-tetrahydro-9-methyl-3-[(2-methyl-1H-imidazol-1-yl)methyl]-4H-carbazol-4-one. It has the following structural formula:

The empirical formula is $C_{18}H_{19}N_3O$ representing a molecular weight of 293.4.

Each 4-mg ZOFRAN Tablet for oral administration contains ondansetron HCl dihydrate equivalent to 4 mg of ondansetron. Each 8-mg ZOFRAN Tablet for oral administration contains ondansetron HCl dihydrate equivalent to 8 mg of ondansetron. Each tablet also contains the inactive ingredients lactose, microcrystalline cellulose, pregelatinized starch, hypromellose, magnesium stearate, titanium dioxide, triacetin, and iron oxide yellow (8-mg tablet only). Each 4-mg ZOFRAN ODT Orally Disintegrating Tablet for oral administration contains 4 mg ondansetron base. Each 8-mg ZOFRAN ODT Orally Disintegrating Tablet for oral administration contains 8 mg ondansetron base. Each ZOFRAN ODT Tablet also contains the inactive ingredients aspartame, gelatin, mannitol, methylparaben sodium, propylparaben sodium, and strawberry flavor. ZOFRAN ODT Tablets are a freeze-dried, orally administered formulation of ondansetron which rapidly disintegrates on the tongue and does not require water to aid dissolution or swallowing. Each 5 mL of ZOFRAN Oral Solution contains 5 mg of ondansetron HCl dihydrate equivalent to 4 mg of ondansetron. ZOFRAN Oral Solution contains the inactive ingredients citric acid anhydrous, purified water, sodium benzoate, sodium citrate, sorbitol, and strawberry flavor.

CLINICAL PHARMACOLOGY
Pharmacodynamics

Ondansetron is a selective 5-HT$_3$ receptor antagonist. While its mechanism of action has not been fully characterized, ondansetron is not a dopamine-receptor antagonist. Serotonin receptors of the 5-HT$_3$ type are present both peripherally on vagal nerve terminals and centrally in the chemoreceptor trigger zone of the area postrema. It is not certain whether ondansetron's antiemetic action is mediated centrally, peripherally, or in both sites. However, cytotoxic chemotherapy appears to be associated with release of serotonin from the enterochromaffin cells of the small intestine. In humans, urinary 5-HIAA (5-hydroxyindoleacetic acid) excretion increases after cisplatin administration in parallel with the onset of emesis. The released serotonin may stimulate the vagal afferents through the 5-HT$_3$ receptors and initiate the vomiting reflex.

In animals, the emetic response to cisplatin can be prevented by pretreatment with an inhibitor of serotonin synthesis, bilateral abdominal vagotomy and greater splanchnic nerve section, or pretreatment with a serotonin 5-HT$_3$ receptor antagonist.

Table 1. Pharmacokinetics in Normal Volunteers: Single 8-mg ZOFRAN Tablet Dose

Age-group (years)	Mean Weight (kg)	n	Peak Plasma Concentration (ng/mL)	Time of Peak Plasma Concentration (h)	Mean Elimination Half-life (h)	Systemic Plasma Clearance L/h/kg	Absolute Bioavailability
18-40 M	69.0	6	26.2	2.0	3.1	0.403	0.483
F	62.7	5	42.7	1.7	3.5	0.354	0.663
61-74 M	77.5	6	24.1	2.1	4.1	0.384	0.585
F	60.2	6	52.4	1.9	4.9	0.255	0.643
≥ 75 M	78.0	5	37.0	2.2	4.5	0.277	0.619
F	67.6	6	46.1	2.1	6.2	0.249	0.747

Table 2. Pharmacokinetics in Normal Volunteers: Single 24-mg ZOFRAN Tablet Dose

Age-group (years)	Mean Weight (kg)	n	Peak Plasma Concentration (ng/mL)	Time of Peak Plasma Concentration (h)	Mean Elimination Half-life (h)
18-43 M	84.1	8	125.8	1.9	4.7
F	71.8	8	194.4	1.6	5.8

Table 3. Emetic Episodes: Treatment Response

	Ondansetron 8-mg b.i.d. ZOFRAN Tablets[a]	Placebo	P Value
Number of patients	33	34	
Treatment response			
0 Emetic episodes	20 (61%)	2 (6%)	< 0.001
1-2 Emetic episodes	6 (18%)	8 (24%)	
More than 2 emetic episodes/withdrawn	7 (21%)	24 (71%)	< 0.001
Median number of emetic episodes	0.0	Undefined[b]	
Median time to first emetic episode (h)	Undefined[c]	6.5	

[a] The first dose was administered 30 minutes before the start of emetogenic chemotherapy, with a subsequent dose 8 hours after the first dose. An 8-mg ZOFRAN Tablet was administered twice a day for 2 days after completion of chemotherapy.
[b] Median undefined since at least 50% of the patients were withdrawn or had more than 2 emetic episodes.
[c] Median undefined since at least 50% of patients did not have any emetic episodes.

In normal volunteers, single intravenous doses of 0.15 mg/kg of ondansetron had no effect on esophageal motility, gastric motility, lower esophageal sphincter pressure, or small intestinal transit time. Multiday administration of ondansetron has been shown to slow colonic transit in normal volunteers. Ondansetron has no effect on plasma prolactin concentrations.

Ondansetron does not alter the respiratory depressant effects produced by alfentanil or the degree of neuromuscular blockade produced by atracurium. Interactions with general or local anesthetics have not been studied.

Pharmacokinetics
Ondansetron is well absorbed from the gastrointestinal tract and undergoes some first-pass metabolism. Mean bioavailability in healthy subjects, following administration of a single 8-mg tablet, is approximately 56%.

Ondansetron systemic exposure does not increase proportionately to dose. AUC from a 16-mg tablet was 24% greater than predicted from an 8-mg tablet dose. This may reflect some reduction of first-pass metabolism at higher oral doses. Bioavailability is also slightly enhanced by the presence of food but unaffected by antacids.

Ondansetron is extensively metabolized in humans, with approximately 5% of a radiolabeled dose recovered as the parent compound from the urine. The primary metabolic pathway is hydroxylation on the indole ring followed by subsequent glucuronide or sulfate conjugation. Although some nonconjugated metabolites have pharmacologic activity, these are not found in plasma at concentrations likely to significantly contribute to the biological activity of ondansetron.

In vitro metabolism studies have shown that ondansetron is a substrate for human hepatic cytochrome P-450 enzymes, including CYP1A2, CYP2D6, and CYP3A4. In terms of overall ondansetron turnover, CYP3A4 played the predominant role. Because of the multiplicity of metabolic enzymes capable of metabolizing ondansetron, it is likely that inhibition or loss of one enzyme (e.g., CYP2D6 genetic deficiency) will be compensated by others and may result in little change in overall rates of ondansetron elimination. Ondansetron elimination may be affected by cytochrome P-450 inducers. In a pharmacokinetic study of 16 epileptic patients maintained chronically on CYP3A4 inducers, carbamazepine, or phenytoin, reduction in AUC, C_{max}, and $T_{1/2}$ of ondansetron was observed.[1] This resulted in a significant increase in clearance. However, on the basis of available data, no dosage adjustment for ondansetron is recommended (see PRECAUTIONS: Drug Interactions).

In humans, carmustine, etoposide, and cisplatin do not affect the pharmacokinetics of ondansetron.

Gender differences were shown in the disposition of ondansetron given as a single dose. The extent and rate of ondansetron's absorption is greater in women than men. Slower clearance in women, a smaller apparent volume of distribution (adjusted for weight), and higher absolute bioavailability resulted in higher plasma ondansetron levels. These higher plasma levels may in part be explained by differences in body weight between men and women. It is not known whether these gender-related differences were clinically important. More detailed pharmacokinetic information is contained in Tables 1 and 2 taken from 2 studies.
[See table 1 above]
[See table 2 above]
A reduction in clearance and increase in elimination half-life are seen in patients over 75 years of age. In clinical trials with cancer patients, safety and efficacy were similar in patients over 65 years of age and those under 65 years of age; there was an insufficient number of patients over 75 years of age to permit conclusions in that age-group. No dosage adjustment is recommended in the elderly.

In patients with mild-to-moderate hepatic impairment, clearance is reduced 2-fold and mean half-life is increased to 11.6 hours compared to 5.7 hours in normals. In patients with severe hepatic impairment (Child-Pugh[2] score of 10 or greater), clearance is reduced 2-fold to 3-fold and apparent volume of distribution is increased with a resultant increase in half-life to 20 hours. In patients with severe hepatic impairment, a total daily dose of 8 mg should not be exceeded.

Due to the very small contribution (5%) of renal clearance to the overall clearance, renal impairment was not expected to significantly influence the total clearance of ondansetron. However, ondansetron oral mean plasma clearance was reduced by about 50% in patients with severe renal impairment (creatinine clearance < 30 mL/min). This reduction in clearance is variable and was not consistent with an increase in half-life. No reduction in dose or dosing frequency in these patients is warranted.

Plasma protein binding of ondansetron as measured in vitro was 70% to 76% over the concentration range of 10 to 500 ng/mL. Circulating drug also distributes into erythrocytes.

Four- and 8-mg doses of either ZOFRAN Oral Solution or ZOFRAN ODT Orally Disintegrating Tablets are bioequivalent to corresponding doses of ZOFRAN Tablets and may be used interchangeably. One 24-mg ZOFRAN Tablet is bioequivalent to and interchangeable with three 8-mg ZOFRAN Tablets.

CLINICAL TRIALS
Chemotherapy-Induced Nausea and Vomiting
Highly Emetogenic Chemotherapy
In 2 randomized, double-blind, monotherapy trials, a single 24-mg ZOFRAN Tablet was superior to a relevant historical placebo control in the prevention of nausea and vomiting associated with highly emetogenic cancer chemotherapy, including cisplatin ≥ 50 mg/m². Steroid administration was excluded from these clinical trials. More than 90% of patients receiving a cisplatin dose ≥ 50 mg/m² in the historical placebo comparator experienced vomiting in the absence of antiemetic therapy.

The first trial compared oral doses of ondansetron 24 mg once a day, 8 mg twice a day, and 32 mg once a day in 357 adult cancer patients receiving chemotherapy regimens containing cisplatin ≥ 50 mg/m². A total of 66% of patients in the ondansetron 24-mg once-a-day group, 55% in the ondansetron 8-mg twice-a-day group, and 55% in the ondansetron 32-mg once-a-day group completed the 24-hour study period with 0 emetic episodes and no rescue antiemetic medications, the primary endpoint of efficacy. Each of the 3 treatment groups was shown to be statistically significantly superior to a historical placebo control.

In the same trial, 56% of patients receiving oral ondansetron 24 mg once a day experienced no nausea during the 24-hour study period, compared with 36% of patients in the oral ondansetron 8-mg twice-a-day group (P = 0.001) and 50% in the oral ondansetron 32-mg once-a-day group.

In a second trial, efficacy of the oral ondansetron 24-mg once-a-day regimen in the prevention of nausea and vomiting associated with highly emetogenic cancer chemotherapy, including cisplatin ≥ 50 mg/m², was confirmed.

Moderately Emetogenic Chemotherapy
In 1 double-blind US study in 67 patients, ZOFRAN Tablets 8 mg administered twice a day were significantly more effective than placebo in preventing vomiting induced by cyclophosphamide-based chemotherapy containing doxorubicin. Treatment response was based on the total number of emetic episodes over the 3-day study period. The results of this study are summarized in Table 3:
[See table 3 above]
In 1 double-blind US study in 336 patients, ZOFRAN Tablets 8 mg administered twice a day were as effective as ZOFRAN Tablets 8 mg administered 3 times a day in preventing nausea and vomiting induced by cyclophosphamide-based chemotherapy containing either methotrexate or doxorubicin. Treatment response was based on the total number of emetic episodes over the 3-day study period. The results of this study are summarized in Table 4:
[See table 4 at top of next page]

Re-treatment
In uncontrolled trials, 148 patients receiving cyclophosphamide-based chemotherapy were re-treated with ZOFRAN Tablets 8 mg 3 times daily during subsequent chemotherapy for a total of 396 re-treatment courses. No emetic episodes occurred in 314 (79%) of the re-treatment courses, and only 1 to 2 emetic episodes occurred in 43 (11%) of the re-treatment courses.

Pediatric Studies
Three open-label, uncontrolled, foreign trials have been performed with 182 pediatric patients 4 to 18 years old with cancer who were given a variety of cisplatin or noncisplatin regimens. In these foreign trials, the initial dose of ZOFRAN® (ondansetron HCl) Injection ranged from 0.04 to 0.87 mg/kg for a total dose of 2.16 to 12 mg. This was followed by the administration of ZOFRAN Tablets ranging from 4 to 24 mg daily for 3 days. In these studies, 58% of the 170 evaluable patients had a complete response (no emetic episodes) on day 1. Two studies showed the response rates for patients less than 12 years of age who received ZOFRAN Tablets 4 mg 3 times a day to be similar to those in patients 12 to 18 years of age who received ZOFRAN Tablets 8 mg 3 times daily. Thus, prevention of emesis in these pediatric

patients was essentially the same as for patients older than 18 years of age. Overall, ZOFRAN Tablets were well tolerated in these pediatric patients.

Radiation-Induced Nausea and Vomiting

Total Body Irradiation

In a randomized, double-blind study in 20 patients, ZOFRAN Tablets (8 mg given 1.5 hours before each fraction of radiotherapy for 4 days) were significantly more effective than placebo in preventing vomiting induced by total body irradiation. Total body irradiation consisted of 11 fractions (120 cGy per fraction) over 4 days for a total of 1,320 cGy. Patients received 3 fractions for 3 days, then 2 fractions on day 4.

Single High-Dose Fraction Radiotherapy

Ondansetron was significantly more effective than metoclopramide with respect to complete control of emesis (0 emetic episodes) in a double-blind trial in 105 patients receiving single high-dose radiotherapy (800 to 1,000 cGy) over an anterior or posterior field size of ≥ 80 cm^2 to the abdomen. Patients received the first dose of ZOFRAN Tablets (8 mg) or metoclopramide (10 mg) 1 to 2 hours before radiotherapy. If radiotherapy was given in the morning, 2 additional doses of study treatment were given (1 tablet late afternoon and 1 tablet before bedtime). If radiotherapy was given in the afternoon, patients took only 1 further tablet that day before bedtime. Patients continued the oral medication on a 3 times a day basis for 3 days.

Daily Fractionated Radiotherapy

Ondansetron was significantly more effective than prochlorperazine with respect to complete control of emesis (0 emetic episodes) in a double-blind trial in 135 patients receiving a 1- to 4-week course of fractionated radiotherapy (180 cGy doses) over a field size of ≥ 100 cm^2 to the abdomen. Patients received the first dose of ZOFRAN Tablets (8 mg) or prochlorperazine (10 mg) 1 to 2 hours before the patient received the first daily radiotherapy fraction, with 2 subsequent doses on a 3 times a day basis. Patients continued the oral medication on a 3 times a day basis on each day of radiotherapy.

Postoperative Nausea and Vomiting

Surgical patients who received ondansetron 1 hour before the induction of general balanced anesthesia (barbiturate: thiopental, methohexital, or thiamylal; opioid: alfentanil, sufentanil, morphine, or fentanyl; nitrous oxide; neuromuscular blockade: succinylcholine/curare or gallamine and/or vecuronium, pancuronium, or atracurium; and supplemental isoflurane or enflurane) were evaluated in 2 double-blind studies (1 US study, 1 foreign) involving 865 patients. ZOFRAN Tablets (16 mg) were significantly more effective than placebo in preventing postoperative nausea and vomiting.

The study populations in all trials thus far consisted of women undergoing inpatient surgical procedures. No studies have been performed in males. No controlled clinical study comparing ZOFRAN Tablets to ZOFRAN Injection has been performed.

INDICATIONS AND USAGE

1. Prevention of nausea and vomiting associated with highly emetogenic cancer chemotherapy, including cisplatin ≥ 50 mg/m^2.
2. Prevention of nausea and vomiting associated with initial and repeat courses of moderately emetogenic cancer chemotherapy.
3. Prevention of nausea and vomiting associated with radiotherapy in patients receiving either total body irradiation, single high-dose fraction to the abdomen, or daily fractions to the abdomen.
4. Prevention of postoperative nausea and/or vomiting. As with other antiemetics, routine prophylaxis is not recommended for patients in whom there is little expectation that nausea and/or vomiting will occur postoperatively. In patients where nausea and/or vomiting must be avoided postoperatively, ZOFRAN Tablets, ZOFRAN ODT Orally Disintegrating Tablets, and ZOFRAN Oral Solution are recommended even where the incidence of postoperative nausea and/or vomiting is low.

CONTRAINDICATIONS

The concomitant use of apomorphine with ondansetron is contraindicated based on reports of profound hypotension and loss of consciousness when apomorphine was administered with ondansetron.

ZOFRAN Tablets, ZOFRAN ODT Orally Disintegrating Tablets, and ZOFRAN Oral Solution are contraindicated for patients known to have hypersensitivity to the drug.

WARNINGS

Hypersensitivity reactions have been reported in patients who have exhibited hypersensitivity to other selective 5-HT$_3$ receptor antagonists.

ECG changes including QT interval prolongation has been seen in patients receiving ondansetron. In addition, postmarketing cases of Torsade de Pointes have been reported in patients using ondansetron. Avoid ZOFRAN in patients

Table 4. Emetic Episodes: Treatment Response

	Ondansetron	
	8-mg b.i.d. ZOFRAN Tablets[a]	8-mg t.i.d. ZOFRAN Tablets[b]
Number of patients	165	171
Treatment response		
0 Emetic episodes	101 (61%)	99 (58%)
1-2 Emetic episodes	16 (10%)	17 (10%)
More than 2 emetic episodes/withdrawn	48 (29%)	55 (32%)
Median number of emetic episodes	0.0	0.0
Median time to first emetic episode (h)	Undefined[c]	Undefined[c]
Median nausea scores (0-100)[d]	6	6

[a] The first dose was administered 30 minutes before the start of emetogenic chemotherapy, with a subsequent dose 8 hours after the first dose. An 8-mg ZOFRAN Tablet was administered twice a day for 2 days after completion of chemotherapy.

[b] The first dose was administered 30 minutes before the start of emetogenic chemotherapy, with subsequent doses 4 and 8 hours after the first dose. An 8-mg ZOFRAN Tablet was administered 3 times a day for 2 days after completion of chemotherapy.

[c] Median undefined since at least 50% of patients did not have any emetic episodes.

[d] Visual analog scale assessment: 0 = no nausea, 100 = nausea as bad as it can be.

with congenital long QT syndrome. ECG monitoring is recommended in patients with electrolyte abnormalities (e.g., hypokalemia or hypomagnesemia), congestive heart failure, bradyarrhythmias or patients taking other medicinal products that lead to QT prolongation.

PRECAUTIONS

General

Ondansetron is not a drug that stimulates gastric or intestinal peristalsis. It should not be used instead of nasogastric suction. The use of ondansetron in patients following abdominal surgery or in patients with chemotherapy-induced nausea and vomiting may mask a progressive ileus and/or gastric distension.

Information for Patients

Phenylketonurics

Phenylketonuric patients should be informed that ZOFRAN ODT Orally Disintegrating Tablets contain phenylalanine (a component of aspartame). Each 4-mg and 8-mg orally disintegrating tablet contains < 0.03 mg phenylalanine.

Patients should be instructed not to remove ZOFRAN ODT Tablets from the blister until just prior to dosing. The tablet should not be pushed through the foil. With dry hands, the blister backing should be peeled completely off the blister. The tablet should be gently removed and immediately placed on the tongue to dissolve and be swallowed with the saliva. Peelable illustrated stickers are affixed to the product carton that can be provided with the prescription to ensure proper use and handling of the product.

Drug Interactions

Ondansetron does not itself appear to induce or inhibit the cytochrome P-450 drug-metabolizing enzyme system of the liver (see CLINICAL PHARMACOLOGY, Pharmacokinetics). Because ondansetron is metabolized by hepatic cytochrome P-450 drug-metabolizing enzymes (CYP3A4, CYP2D6, CYP1A2), inducers or inhibitors of these enzymes may change the clearance and, hence, the half-life of ondansetron. On the basis of available data, no dosage adjustment is recommended for patients on these drugs.

Apomorphine

Based on reports of profound hypotension and loss of consciousness when apomorphine was administered with ondansetron, concomitant use of apomorphine with ondansetron is contraindicated (see CONTRAINDICATIONS).

Phenytoin, Carbamazepine, and Rifampicin

In patients treated with potent inducers of CYP3A4 (i.e., phenytoin, carbamazepine, and rifampicin), the clearance of ondansetron was significantly increased and ondansetron blood concentrations were decreased. However, on the basis of available data, no dosage adjustment for ondansetron is recommended for patients on these drugs.[1,3]

Tramadol

Although no pharmacokinetic drug interaction between ondansetron and tramadol has been observed, data from 2 small studies indicate that ondansetron may be associated with an increase in patient controlled administration of tramadol.[4,5]

Chemotherapy

Tumor response to chemotherapy in the P-388 mouse leukemia model is not affected by ondansetron. In humans, carmustine, etoposide, and cisplatin do not affect the pharmacokinetics of ondansetron.

In a crossover study in 76 pediatric patients, I.V. ondansetron did not increase blood levels of high-dose methotrexate.

Use in Surgical Patients

The coadministration of ondansetron had no effect on the pharmacokinetics and pharmacodynamics of temazepam.

Carcinogenesis, Mutagenesis, Impairment of Fertility

Carcinogenic effects were not seen in 2-year studies in rats and mice with oral ondansetron doses up to 10 and 30 mg/kg/day, respectively. Ondansetron was not mutagenic in standard tests for mutagenicity. Oral administration of ondansetron up to 15 mg/kg/day did not affect fertility or general reproductive performance of male and female rats.

Pregnancy

Teratogenic Effects

Pregnancy Category B. Reproduction studies have been performed in pregnant rats and rabbits at daily oral doses up to 15 and 30 mg/kg/day, respectively, and have revealed no evidence of impaired fertility or harm to the fetus due to ondansetron. There are, however, no adequate and well-controlled studies in pregnant women. Because animal reproduction studies are not always predictive of human response, this drug should be used during pregnancy only if clearly needed.

Nursing Mothers

Ondansetron is excreted in the breast milk of rats. It is not known whether ondansetron is excreted in human milk. Because many drugs are excreted in human milk, caution should be exercised when ondansetron is administered to a nursing woman.

Pediatric Use

Little information is available about dosage in pediatric patients 4 years of age or younger (see CLINICAL PHARMACOLOGY and DOSAGE AND ADMINISTRATION sections for use in pediatric patients 4 to 18 years of age).

Geriatric Use

Of the total number of subjects enrolled in cancer chemotherapy-induced and postoperative nausea and vomiting in US- and foreign-controlled clinical trials, for which there were subgroup analyses, 938 were 65 years of age and over. No overall differences in safety or effectiveness were observed between these subjects and younger subjects, and other reported clinical experience has not identified differences in responses between the elderly and younger patients, but greater sensitivity of some older individuals cannot be ruled out. Dosage adjustment is not needed in patients over the age of 65 (see CLINICAL PHARMACOLOGY).

ADVERSE REACTIONS

The following have been reported as adverse events in clinical trials of patients treated with ondansetron, the active ingredient of ZOFRAN. A causal relationship to therapy with ZOFRAN has been unclear in many cases.

Chemotherapy-Induced Nausea and Vomiting

The adverse events in Table 5 have been reported in $\geq 5\%$ of adult patients receiving a single 24-mg ZOFRAN Tablet in 2 trials. These patients were receiving concurrent highly emetogenic cisplatin-based chemotherapy regimens (cisplatin dose ≥ 50 mg/m^2).

Table 5. Principal Adverse Events in US Trials: Single Day Therapy With 24-mg ZOFRAN Tablets (Highly Emetogenic Chemotherapy)

Event	Ondansetron 24 mg q.d. n = 300	Ondansetron 8 mg b.i.d. n = 124	Ondansetron 32 mg q.d. n = 117
Headache	33 (11%)	16 (13%)	17 (15%)
Diarrhea	13 (4%)	9 (7%)	3 (3%)

The adverse events in Table 6 have been reported in ≥ 5% of adults receiving either 8 mg of ZOFRAN Tablets 2 or 3 times a day for 3 days or placebo in 4 trials. These patients were receiving concurrent moderately emetogenic chemotherapy, primarily cyclophosphamide-based regimens.

Table 6. Principal Adverse Events in US Trials: 3 Days of Therapy With 8-mg ZOFRAN Tablets (Moderately Emetogenic Chemotherapy)

Event	Ondansetron 8 mg b.i.d. n = 242	Ondansetron 8 mg t.i.d. n = 415	Placebo n = 262
Headache	58 (24%)	113 (27%)	34 (13%)
Malaise/fatigue	32 (13%)	37 (9%)	6 (2%)
Constipation	22 (9%)	26 (6%)	1 (<1%)
Diarrhea	15 (6%)	16 (4%)	10 (4%)
Dizziness	13 (5%)	18 (4%)	12 (5%)

Central Nervous System
There have been rare reports consistent with, but not diagnostic of, extrapyramidal reactions in patients receiving ondansetron.

Hepatic
In 723 patients receiving cyclophosphamide-based chemotherapy in US clinical trials, AST and/or ALT values have been reported to exceed twice the upper limit of normal in approximately 1% to 2% of patients receiving ZOFRAN Tablets. The increases were transient and did not appear to be related to dose or duration of therapy. On repeat exposure, similar transient elevations in transaminase values occurred in some courses, but symptomatic hepatic disease did not occur. The role of cancer chemotherapy in these biochemical changes cannot be clearly determined.
There have been reports of liver failure and death in patients with cancer receiving concurrent medications including potentially hepatotoxic cytotoxic chemotherapy and antibiotics. The etiology of the liver failure is unclear.

Integumentary
Rash has occurred in approximately 1% of patients receiving ondansetron.

Other
Rare cases of anaphylaxis, bronchospasm, tachycardia, angina (chest pain), hypokalemia, electrocardiographic alterations, vascular occlusive events, and grand mal seizures have been reported. Except for bronchospasm and anaphylaxis, the relationship to ZOFRAN was unclear.

Radiation-Induced Nausea and Vomiting
The adverse events reported in patients receiving ZOFRAN Tablets and concurrent radiotherapy were similar to those reported in patients receiving ZOFRAN Tablets and concurrent chemotherapy. The most frequently reported adverse events were headache, constipation, and diarrhea.

Postoperative Nausea and Vomiting
The adverse events in Table 7 have been reported in ≥ 5% of patients receiving ZOFRAN Tablets at a dosage of 16 mg orally in clinical trials. With the exception of headache, rates of these events were not significantly different in the ondansetron and placebo groups. These patients were receiving multiple concomitant perioperative and postoperative medications.

Table 7. Frequency of Adverse Events From Controlled Studies With ZOFRAN Tablets (Postoperative Nausea and Vomiting)

Adverse Event	Ondansetron 16 mg (n = 550)	Placebo (n = 531)
Wound problem	152 (28%)	162 (31%)
Drowsiness/sedation	112 (20%)	122 (23%)
Headache	49 (9%)	27 (5%)
Hypoxia	49 (9%)	35 (7%)

Pyrexia	45 (8%)	34 (6%)
Dizziness	36 (7%)	34 (6%)
Gynecological disorder	36 (7%)	33 (6%)
Anxiety/agitation	33 (6%)	29 (5%)
Bradycardia	32 (6%)	30 (6%)
Shiver(s)	28 (5%)	30 (6%)
Urinary retention	28 (5%)	18 (3%)
Hypotension	27 (5%)	32 (6%)
Pruritus	27 (5%)	20 (4%)

Preliminary observations in a small number of subjects suggest a higher incidence of headache when ZOFRAN ODT Orally Disintegrating Tablets are taken with water, when compared to without water.

Observed During Clinical Practice
In addition to adverse events reported from clinical trials, the following events have been identified during post-approval use of oral formulations of ZOFRAN. Because they are reported voluntarily from a population of unknown size, estimates of frequency cannot be made. The events have been chosen for inclusion due to a combination of their seriousness, frequency of reporting, or potential causal connection to ZOFRAN.

Cardiovascular
Rarely and predominantly with intravenous ondansetron, transient ECG changes including QT interval prolongation have been reported.

General
Flushing. Rare cases of hypersensitivity reactions, sometimes severe (e.g., anaphylaxis/anaphylactoid reactions, angioedema, bronchospasm, shortness of breath, hypotension, laryngeal edema, stridor) have also been reported. Laryngospasm, shock, and cardiopulmonary arrest have occurred during allergic reactions in patients receiving injectable ondansetron.

Hepatobiliary
Liver enzyme abnormalities

Lower Respiratory
Hiccups

Neurology:
Oculogyric crisis, appearing alone, as well as with other dystonic reactions

Skin
Urticaria, Stevens-Johnson syndrome, and toxic epidermal necrolysis

Special Senses
Eye Disorders
Cases of transient blindness, predominantly during intravenous administration, have been reported. These cases of transient blindness were reported to resolve within a few minutes up to 48 hours.

DRUG ABUSE AND DEPENDENCE
Animal studies have shown that ondansetron is not discriminated as a benzodiazepine nor does it substitute for benzodiazepines in direct addiction studies.

OVERDOSAGE
There is no specific antidote for ondansetron overdose. Patients should be managed with appropriate supportive therapy. Individual intravenous doses as large as 150 mg and total daily intravenous doses as large as 252 mg have been inadvertently administered without significant adverse events. These doses are more than 10 times the recommended daily dose.
In addition to the adverse events listed above, the following events have been described in the setting of ondansetron overdose: "Sudden blindness" (amaurosis) of 2 to 3 minutes' duration plus severe constipation occurred in 1 patient that was administered 72 mg of ondansetron intravenously as a single dose. Hypotension (and faintness) occurred in a patient that took 48 mg of ZOFRAN Tablets. Following infusion of 32 mg over only a 4-minute period, a vasovagal episode with transient second-degree heart block was observed. In all instances, the events resolved completely.

DOSAGE AND ADMINISTRATION
Instructions for Use/Handling ZOFRAN ODT Orally Disintegrating Tablets
Do not attempt to push ZOFRAN ODT Tablets through the foil backing. With dry hands, PEEL BACK the foil backing of 1 blister and GENTLY remove the tablet. IMMEDIATELY place the ZOFRAN ODT Tablet on top of the tongue where it will dissolve in seconds, then swallow with saliva. Administration with liquid is not necessary.

Prevention of Nausea and Vomiting Associated With Highly Emetogenic Cancer Chemotherapy
The recommended adult oral dosage of ZOFRAN is 24 mg given as three 8-mg tablets administered 30 minutes before the start of single-day highly emetogenic chemotherapy, including cisplatin ≥ 50 mg/m². Multiday, single-dose administration of a 24 mg dosage has not been studied.
Pediatric Use
There is no experience with the use of a 24 mg dosage in pediatric patients.
Geriatric Use
The dosage recommendation is the same as for the general population.
Prevention of Nausea and Vomiting Associated With Moderately Emetogenic Cancer Chemotherapy
The recommended adult oral dosage is one 8-mg ZOFRAN Tablet or one 8-mg ZOFRAN ODT Tablet or 10 mL (2 teaspoonfuls equivalent to 8 mg of ondansetron) of ZOFRAN Oral Solution given twice a day. The first dose should be administered 30 minutes before the start of emetogenic chemotherapy, with a subsequent dose 8 hours after the first dose. One 8-mg ZOFRAN Tablet or one 8-mg ZOFRAN ODT Tablet or 10 mL (2 teaspoonfuls equivalent to 8 mg of ondansetron) of ZOFRAN Oral Solution should be administered twice a day (every 12 hours) for 1 to 2 days after completion of chemotherapy.
Pediatric Use
For pediatric patients 12 years of age and older, the dosage is the same as for adults. For pediatric patients 4 through 11 years of age, the dosage is one 4-mg ZOFRAN Tablet or one 4-mg ZOFRAN ODT Tablet or 5 mL (1 teaspoonful equivalent to 4 mg of ondansetron) of ZOFRAN Oral Solution given 3 times a day. The first dose should be administered 30 minutes before the start of emetogenic chemotherapy, with subsequent doses 4 and 8 hours after the first dose. One 4-mg ZOFRAN Tablet or one 4-mg ZOFRAN ODT Tablet or 5 mL (1 teaspoonful equivalent to 4 mg of ondansetron) of ZOFRAN Oral Solution should be administered 3 times a day (every 8 hours) for 1 to 2 days after completion of chemotherapy.
Geriatric Use
The dosage is the same as for the general population.
Prevention of Nausea and Vomiting Associated With Radiotherapy, Either Total Body Irradiation, or Single High-Dose Fraction or Daily Fractions to the Abdomen
The recommended oral dosage is one 8-mg ZOFRAN Tablet or one 8-mg ZOFRAN ODT Tablet or 10 mL (2 teaspoonfuls equivalent to 8 mg of ondansetron) of ZOFRAN Oral Solution given 3 times a day.
For total body irradiation, one 8-mg ZOFRAN Tablet or one 8-mg ZOFRAN ODT Tablet or 10 mL (2 teaspoonfuls equivalent to 8 mg of ondansetron) of ZOFRAN Oral Solution should be administered 1 to 2 hours before each fraction of radiotherapy administered each day.
For single high-dose fraction radiotherapy to the abdomen, one 8-mg ZOFRAN Tablet or one 8-mg ZOFRAN ODT Tablet or 10 mL (2 teaspoonfuls equivalent to 8 mg of ondansetron) of ZOFRAN Oral Solution should be administered 1 to 2 hours before radiotherapy, with subsequent doses every 8 hours after the first dose for 1 to 2 days after completion of radiotherapy.
For daily fractionated radiotherapy to the abdomen, one 8-mg ZOFRAN Tablet or one 8-mg ZOFRAN ODT Tablet or 10 mL (2 teaspoonfuls equivalent to 8 mg of ondansetron) of ZOFRAN Oral Solution should be administered 1 to 2 hours before radiotherapy, with subsequent doses every 8 hours after the first dose for each day radiotherapy is given.
Pediatric Use
There is no experience with the use of ZOFRAN Tablets, ZOFRAN ODT Tablets, or ZOFRAN Oral Solution in the prevention of radiation-induced nausea and vomiting in pediatric patients.
Geriatric Use
The dosage recommendation is the same as for the general population.
Postoperative Nausea and Vomiting
The recommended dosage is 16 mg given as two 8-mg ZOFRAN Tablets or two 8-mg ZOFRAN ODT Tablets or 20 mL (4 teaspoonfuls equivalent to 16 mg of ondansetron) of ZOFRAN Oral Solution 1 hour before induction of anesthesia.
Pediatric Use
There is no experience with the use of ZOFRAN Tablets, ZOFRAN ODT Tablets, or ZOFRAN Oral Solution in the prevention of postoperative nausea and vomiting in pediatric patients.
Geriatric Use
The dosage is the same as for the general population.
Dosage Adjustment for Patients With Impaired Renal Function
The dosage recommendation is the same as for the general population. There is no experience beyond first-day administration of ondansetron.

Dosage Adjustment for Patients With Impaired Hepatic Function

In patients with severe hepatic impairment (Child-Pugh[2] score of 10 or greater), clearance is reduced and apparent volume of distribution is increased with a resultant increase in plasma half-life. In such patients, a total daily dose of 8 mg should not be exceeded.

HOW SUPPLIED

ZOFRAN Tablets, 4 mg (ondansetron HCl dihydrate equivalent to 4 mg of ondansetron) are white, oval, film-coated tablets engraved with "Zofran" on one side and "4" on the other in bottles of 30 tablets (NDC 0173-0446-00).

Store between 2° and 30°C (36° and 86°F). Protect from light. Dispense in tight, light-resistant container as defined in the USP.

ZOFRAN Tablets, 8 mg (ondansetron HCl dihydrate equivalent to 8 mg of ondansetron), are yellow, oval, film-coated tablets engraved with "Zofran" on one side and "8" on the other in daily unit dose packs of 3 tablets (NDC 0173-0447-04), and bottles of 30 tablets (NDC 0173-0447-00).

Bottles: Store between 2° and 30°C (36° and 86°F). Dispense in tight container as defined in the USP.

Unit Dose Packs: Store between 2° and 30°C (36° and 86°F).

ZOFRAN ODT Orally Disintegrating Tablets, 4 mg (as 4 mg ondansetron base) are white, round and plano-convex tablets debossed with a "Z4" on one side in unit dose packs of 30 tablets (NDC 0173-0569-00).

ZOFRAN ODT Orally Disintegrating Tablets, 8 mg (as 8 mg ondansetron base) are white, round and plano-convex tablets debossed with a "Z8" on one side in unit dose packs of 30 tablets (NDC 0173-0570-00).

Store between 2° and 30°C (36° and 86°F).

ZOFRAN Oral Solution, a clear, colorless to light yellow liquid with a characteristic strawberry odor, contains 5 mg of ondansetron HCl dihydrate equivalent to 4 mg of ondansetron per 5 mL in amber glass bottles of 50 mL with child-resistant closures (NDC 0173-0489-00).

Store upright between 15° and 30°C (59° and 86°F). Protect from light. Store bottles upright in cartons.

REFERENCES

1. Britto MR, Hussey EK, Mydlow P, et al. Effect of enzyme inducers on ondansetron (OND) metabolism in humans. *Clin Pharmacol Ther.* 1997;61:228.
2. Pugh RNH, Murray-Lyon IM, Dawson JL, Pietroni MC, Williams R. Transection of the oesophagus for bleeding oesophageal varices. *Brit J Surg.* 1973;60:646-649.
3. Villikka K, Kivisto KT, Neuvonen PJ. The effect of rifampin on the pharmacokinetics of oral and intravenous ondansetron. *Clin Pharmacol Ther.* 1999;65:377-381.
4. De Witte JL, Schoenmaekers B, Sessler DI, et al. *Anesth Analg.* 2001;92:1319-1321.
5. Arcioni R, della Rocca M, Romanò R, et al. *Anesth Analg.* 2002;94:1553-1557.

GlaxoSmithKline
Research Triangle Park, NC 27709
ZOFRAN Tablets and Oral Solution:
GlaxoSmithKline
Research Triangle Park, NC 27709
ZOFRAN ODT Orally Disintegrating Tablets:
Manufactured for GlaxoSmithKline
Research Triangle Park, NC 27709
by Catalent UK Swindon Zydis Ltd.
Blagrove, Swindon, Wiltshire, UK SN5 8RU
©2013, GlaxoSmithKline. All rights reserved.
December 2013
ZFT:6PI

ZYBAN®

[zī'ban]

(bupropion hydrochloride)
Sustained-Release Tablets   ℞

HIGHLIGHTS OF PRESCRIBING INFORMATION

These highlights do not include all the information needed to use ZYBAN safely and effectively. See full prescribing information for ZYBAN.

ZYBAN (bupropion hydrochloride) Sustained-Release Tablets for oral use
Initial U.S. Approval: 1985

RECENT MAJOR CHANGES

Dosage and Administration (2.8)	03/2014
• Contraindications (4)	• 03/2014

WARNING: NEUROPSYCHIATRIC REACTIONS; AND SUICIDAL THOUGHTS AND BEHAVIORS

See full prescribing information for complete boxed warning.

- Serious neuropsychiatric events have been reported in patients taking bupropion for smoking cessation. (5.1)
- Increased risk of suicidal thinking and behavior in children, adolescents, and young adults taking antidepressants. (5.2)
- Monitor for worsening and emergence of suicidal thoughts and behaviors. (5.2)

INDICATIONS AND USAGE

ZYBAN is an aminoketone agent indicated as an aid to smoking cessation treatment. (1)

DOSAGE AND ADMINISTRATION

- Starting dose: 150 mg per day for first 3 days. (2.1)
- General: Increase dose gradually to reduce seizure risk. (2.1, 5.3)
- Begin dosing one week before quit day (2.1)
- After 3 days, increase the dose to 300 mg per day, given as 150 mg twice daily at an interval of at least 8 hours. (2.1)
- May be used with a nicotine transdermal system. (2.5)
- Moderate to severe hepatic impairment: 150 mg every other day. (2.6, 8.7)
- Mild hepatic impairment: Consider reducing the dose and/or frequency of dosing (2.6, 8.7)
- Renal Impairment: Consider reducing the dose and/or frequency. (2.7, 8.6)

DOSAGE FORMS AND STRENGTHS

- Tablets: 150 mg. (3)

CONTRAINDICATIONS

- Seizure disorder. (4, 5.3)
- Current or prior diagnosis of bulimia or anorexia nervosa. (4, 5.3)
- Abrupt discontinuation of alcohol, benzodiazepines, barbiturates, antiepileptic drugs. (4, 5.3)
- Monoamine Oxidase Inhibitors (MAOIs): Do not use MAOIs intended to treat psychiatric disorders with ZYBAN or within 14 days of stopping treatment with ZYBAN. Do not use ZYBAN within 14 days of stopping an MAOI intended to treat psychiatric disorders. In addition, do not start ZYBAN in a patient who is being treated with linezolid or intravenous methylene blue. (4, 7.6)
- Known hypersensitivity to bupropion or other ingredients of ZYBAN. (4, 5.7)

WARNINGS AND PRECAUTIONS

- Seizure risk: The risk is dose-related. Can minimize risk by gradually increasing the dose and limiting daily dose to 300 mg. Discontinue if seizure occurs. (4, 5.3, 7.3)
- Hypertension: ZYBAN can increase blood pressure. Monitor blood pressure before initiating treatment and periodically during treatment, especially if used with nicotine replacement. (5.4)
- Activation of mania/hypomania: Screen patients for bipolar disorder and monitor for these symptoms. (5.5)
- Psychosis and other neuropsychiatric reactions. Instruct patients to contact a healthcare professional if reactions occur. (5.6)

ADVERSE REACTIONS

Most common adverse reactions (incidence ≥5% and ≥1% more than placebo rate) are: insomnia, rhinitis, dry mouth, dizziness, nervous disturbance, anxiety, nausea, constipation, and arthralgia. (6.1)

To report SUSPECTED ADVERSE REACTIONS, contact GlaxoSmithKline at 1-888-825-5249 or FDA at 1-800-FDA-1088 or www.fda.gov/medwatch

DRUG INTERACTIONS

- CYP2B6 inducers: Dose increase may be necessary if co-administered with CYP2B6 inducers (e.g., ritonavir, lopinavir, efavirenz, carbamazepine, phenobarbital and phenytoin) based on clinical response, but should not exceed the maximum recommended dose. (7.1)
- Drugs metabolized by CYP2D6: Bupropion inhibits CYP2D6 and can increase concentrations of: antidepressants (e.g., venlafaxine, nortriptyline, imipramine, desipramine, paroxetine, fluoxetine, sertraline), antipsychotics (e.g., haloperidol, risperidone, thioridazine), beta-blockers (e.g., metoprolol), and Type 1C antiarrhythmics (e.g., propafenone, flecainide). Consider dose reduction when using with bupropion. (7.2)
- Drugs that lower seizure threshold: Dose ZYBAN with caution. (5.3, 7.3)
- Dopaminergic drugs (levodopa and amantadine): CNS toxicity can occur when used concomitantly with ZYBAN. (7.4)

- MAOIs: Increased risk of hypertensive reactions can occur when used concomitantly with ZYBAN. (7.6)
- Drug-laboratory test interactions: ZYBAN can cause false-positive urine test results for amphetamines. (7.8)

USE IN SPECIFIC POPULATIONS

- Pregnancy: Use only if benefit outweighs potential risk to the fetus. (8.1)

See 17 for PATIENT COUNSELING INFORMATION and Medication Guide

Revised: 03/2014

FULL PRESCRIBING INFORMATION: CONTENTS*
WARNING: NEUROPSYCHIATRIC REACTIONS; AND SUICIDAL THOUGHTS AND BEHAVIORS

* Sections or subsections omitted from the full prescribing information are not listed

---

FULL PRESCRIBING INFORMATION

WARNING: NEUROPSYCHIATRIC REACTIONS; AND SUICIDAL THOUGHTS AND BEHAVIORS

NEUROPSYCHIATRIC REACTIONS IN PATIENTS TAKING BUPROPION FOR SMOKING CESSATION

Serious neuropsychiatric reactions have occurred in patients taking ZYBAN® for smoking cessation *[see Warnings and Precautions (5.1)]*. The majority of these reactions occurred during bupropion treatment, but some occurred in the context of discontinuing treatment. In many cases, a causal relationship to bupropion treatment is not certain, because depressed mood may be a symptom of nicotine withdrawal. However, some of these symptoms have occurred in patients taking ZYBAN who continued to smoke.

The risks of ZYBAN should be weighed against the benefits of its use. ZYBAN has been demonstrated to increase the likelihood of abstinence from smoking for as long as 6 months compared with treatment with placebo. The health benefits of quitting smoking are immediate and substantial.

SUICIDALITY AND ANTIDEPRESSANT DRUGS
Although ZYBAN is not indicated for treatment of depression, it contains the same active ingredient as the antidepressant medications WELLBUTRIN®, WELLBUTRIN® SR, and WELLBUTRIN XL®. Antidepressants increased the risk of suicidal thoughts and behavior in children, adolescents, and young adults in short-term trials. These trials did not show an increase in the risk of suicidal thoughts and behavior with antidepressant use in subjects over age 24; there was a reduction in risk with antidepressant use in subjects aged 65 and older *[see Warnings and Precautions (5.2)]*.

In patients of all ages who are started on antidepressant therapy, monitor closely for worsening, and for emergence of suicidal thoughts and behaviors. Advise families and caregivers of the need for close observation and communication with the prescriber *[see Warnings and Precautions (5.2)]*.

1   INDICATIONS AND USAGE
ZYBAN is indicated as an aid to smoking cessation treatment.

2   DOSAGE AND ADMINISTRATION
2.1   Usual Dosage
Treatment with ZYBAN should be initiated **before** the patient's planned quit day, **while the patient is still smoking**, because it takes approximately 1 week of treatment to achieve steady-state blood levels of bupropion. The patient should set a "target quit date" within the first 2 weeks of treatment with ZYBAN.

Dosing: To minimize the risk of seizure:
- Begin dosing with one 150-mg tablet per day for 3 days.
- Increase dose to 300 mg/day given as one 150-mg tablet twice each day with an interval of at least 8 hours between each dose.
- Do not exceed 300 mg/day.

ZYBAN should be swallowed whole and not crushed, divided, or chewed, as this may lead to an increased risk of adverse effects including seizures *[see Warnings and Precautions (5.3)]*.

ZYBAN may be taken with or without food *[see Clinical Pharmacology (12.3)]*.

2.2   Duration of Treatment
Treatment with ZYBAN should be continued for 7 to 12 weeks. If the patient has not quit smoking after 7 to 12 weeks, it is unlikely that he or she will quit during that attempt so treatment with ZYBAN should probably be discontinued and the treatment plan reassessed. The goal of therapy with ZYBAN is complete abstinence.

Discuss discontinuing treatment with ZYBAN after 12 weeks if the patient feels ready but consider whether the patient may benefit from ongoing treatment. Patients who successfully quit after 12 weeks of treatment but do not feel ready to discontinue treatment should be considered for ongoing therapy with ZYBAN; longer treatment should be guided by the relative benefits and risks for individual patients.

It is important that patients continue to receive counseling and support throughout treatment with ZYBAN and for a period of time thereafter.

2.3   Individualization of Therapy
Patients are more likely to quit smoking and remain abstinent if they are seen frequently and receive support from their physicians or other healthcare professionals. It is important to ensure that patients read the instructions provided to them and have their questions answered. Physicians should review the patient's overall smoking cessation program that includes treatment with ZYBAN. Patients should be advised of the importance of participating in the behavioral interventions, counseling, and/or support services to be used in conjunction with ZYBAN *[see Medication Guide]*.

Patients who fail to quit smoking during an attempt may benefit from interventions to improve their chances for success on subsequent attempts. Patients who are unsuccessful should be evaluated to determine why they failed. A new quit attempt should be encouraged when factors that contributed to failure can be eliminated or reduced, and conditions are more favorable.

2.4   Maintenance
Tobacco dependence is a chronic condition. Some patients may need on-going treatment. Whether to continue treatment with ZYBAN for periods longer than 12 weeks for smoking cessation must be determined for individual patients.

2.5   Combination Treatment With ZYBAN and a Nicotine Transdermal System (NTS)
Combination treatment with ZYBAN and NTS may be prescribed for smoking cessation. The prescriber should review the complete prescribing information for both ZYBAN and NTS before using combination treatment *[see Clinical Studies (14)]*. Monitoring for treatment-emergent hypertension in patients treated with the combination of ZYBAN and NTS is recommended.

2.6   Dose Adjustment in Patients With Hepatic Impairment
In patients with moderate to severe hepatic impairment (Child-Pugh score: 7 to 15), the maximum dose should not exceed 150 mg every other day. In patients with mild hepatic impairment (Child-Pugh score: 5 to 6), consider reducing the dose and/or frequency of dosing *[see Use in Specific Populations (8.7) and Clinical Pharmacology (12.3)]*.

2.7   Dose Adjustment in Patients With Renal Impairment
Consider reducing the dose and/or frequency of ZYBAN in patients with renal impairment (Glomerular Filtration Rate <90 mL/min) *[see Use in Specific Populations (8.6) and Clinical Pharmacology (12.3)]*.

2.8   Use of ZYBAN With Reversible MAOIs Such as Linezolid or Methylene Blue
Do not start ZYBAN in a patient who is being treated with a reversible MAOI such as linezolid or intravenous methylene blue. Drug interactions can increase the risk of hypertensive reactions *[see Contraindications (4) and Drug Interactions (7.6)]*.

In some cases, a patient already receiving therapy with ZYBAN may require urgent treatment with linezolid or intravenous methylene blue. If acceptable alternatives to linezolid or intravenous methylene blue treatment are not available and the potential benefits of linezolid or intravenous methylene blue treatment are judged to outweigh the risks of hypertensive reactions in a particular patient, ZYBAN should be stopped promptly, and linezolid or intravenous methylene blue can be administered. The patient should be monitored for 2 weeks or until 24 hours after the last dose of linezolid or intravenous methylene blue, whichever comes first. Therapy with ZYBAN may be resumed 24 hours after the last dose of linezolid or intravenous methylene blue.

The risk of administering methylene blue by non-intravenous routes (such as oral tablets or by local injection) or in intravenous doses much lower than 1 mg/kg with ZYBAN is unclear. The clinician should, nevertheless, be aware of the possibility of a drug interaction with such use *[see Contraindications (4) and Drug Interactions (7.6)]*.

3   DOSAGE FORMS AND STRENGTHS
150 mg – purple, round, biconvex, film-coated, sustained-release tablets printed with "ZYBAN 150".

4   CONTRAINDICATIONS
- ZYBAN is contraindicated in patients with a seizure disorder.
- ZYBAN is contraindicated in patients with a current or prior diagnosis of bulimia or anorexia nervosa as a higher incidence of seizures was observed in such patients treated with the immediate-release formulation of bupropion *[see Warnings and Precautions (5.3)]*.
- ZYBAN is contraindicated in patients undergoing abrupt discontinuation of alcohol, benzodiazepines, barbiturates, and antiepileptic drugs *[see Warnings and Precautions (5.3) and Drug Interactions (7.3)]*.
- The use of MAOIs (intended to treat psychiatric disorders) concomitantly with ZYBAN or within 14 days of discontinuing treatment with ZYBAN is contraindicated. There is an increased risk of hypertensive reactions when ZYBAN is used concomitantly with MAOIs. The use of ZYBAN within 14 days of discontinuing treatment with an MAOI is also contraindicated. Starting ZYBAN in a patient treated with reversible MAOIs such as linezolid or intravenous methylene blue is contraindicated *[see Dosage and Administration (2.8), Warnings and Precautions (5.4), and Drug Interactions (7.6)]*.
- ZYBAN is contraindicated in patients with a known hypersensitivity to bupropion or other ingredients of ZYBAN. Anaphylactoid/anaphylactic reactions and Stevens-Johnson syndrome have been reported *[see Warnings and Precautions (5.7)]*.

5   WARNINGS AND PRECAUTIONS
5.1   Neuropsychiatric Symptoms and Suicide Risk in Smoking Cessation Treatment
Serious neuropsychiatric symptoms have been reported in patients taking ZYBAN for smoking cessation. These have included changes in mood (including depression and mania), psychosis, hallucinations, paranoia, delusions, homicidal ideation, hostility, agitation, aggression, anxiety, and panic, as well as suicidal ideation, suicide attempt, and completed suicide *[see Boxed Warning and Adverse Reactions (6.2)]*. Observe patients for the occurrence of neuropsychiatric reactions. Instruct patients to contact a healthcare professional if such reactions occur.

In many of these cases, a causal relationship to bupropion treatment is not certain, because depressed mood can be a symptom of nicotine withdrawal. However, some of the cases occurred in patients taking ZYBAN who continued to smoke.

The risks of ZYBAN should be weighed against the benefits of its use. ZYBAN has been demonstrated to increase the likelihood of abstinence from smoking for as long as 6 months compared with treatment with placebo. The health benefits of quitting smoking are immediate and substantial.

5.2   Suicidal Thoughts and Behaviors in Children, Adolescents, and Young Adults
Patients with MDD, both adult and pediatric, may experience worsening of their depression and/or the emergence of suicidal ideation and behavior (suicidality) or unusual changes in behavior, whether or not they are taking antidepressant medications, and this risk may persist until significant remission occurs. Suicide is a known risk of depression and certain other psychiatric disorders, and these disorders themselves are the strongest predictors of suicide. There has been a long-standing concern that antidepressants may have a role in inducing worsening of depression and the emergence of suicidality in certain patients during the early phases of treatment.

Pooled analyses of short-term placebo-controlled trials of antidepressant drugs (selective serotonin reuptake inhibitors [SSRIs] and others) show that these drugs increase the risk of suicidal thinking and behavior (suicidality) in children, adolescents, and young adults (ages 18 to 24) with MDD and other psychiatric disorders. Short-term clinical trials did not show an increase in the risk of suicidality with antidepressants compared with placebo in adults beyond age 24; there was a reduction with antidepressants compared with placebo in adults aged 65 and older.

The pooled analyses of placebo-controlled trials in children and adolescents with MDD, obsessive compulsive disorder (OCD), or other psychiatric disorders included a total of 24 short-term trials of 9 antidepressant drugs in over 4,400 subjects. The pooled analyses of placebo-controlled trials in adults with MDD or other psychiatric disorders included a total of 295 short-term trials (median duration of 2 months) of 11 antidepressant drugs in over 77,000 subjects. There was considerable variation in risk of suicidality among drugs, but a tendency toward an increase in the younger subjects for almost all drugs studied. There were differences in absolute risk of suicidality across the different indications, with the highest incidence in MDD. The risk differences (drug vs. placebo), however, were relatively stable within age strata and across indications. These risk differences (drug-placebo difference in the number of cases of suicidality per 1,000 subjects treated) are provided in Table 1.

Table 1. Risk Differences in the Number of Suicidality Cases by Age Group in the Pooled Placebo-Controlled Trials of Antidepressants in Pediatric and Adult Subjects

Age Range	Drug-Placebo Difference in Number of Cases of Suicidality per 1,000 Subjects Treated
Increases Compared With Placebo	
<18	14 additional cases
18-24	5 additional cases
Decreases Compared With Placebo	
25-64	1 fewer case
≥65	6 fewer cases

No suicides occurred in any of the pediatric trials. There were suicides in the adult trials, but the number was not sufficient to reach any conclusion about drug effect on suicide.

It is unknown whether the suicidality risk extends to longer-term use, i.e., beyond several months. However, there is substantial evidence from placebo-controlled maintenance trials in adults with depression that the use of antidepressants can delay the recurrence of depression.

All patients being treated with antidepressants for any indication should be monitored appropriately and observed closely for clinical worsening, suicidality, and unusual changes in behavior, especially during the initial few

months of a course of drug therapy, or at times of dose changes, either increases or decreases [see Boxed Warning]. The following symptoms, anxiety, agitation, panic attacks, insomnia, irritability, hostility, aggressiveness, impulsivity, akathisia (psychomotor restlessness), hypomania, and mania, have been reported in adult and pediatric patients being treated with antidepressants for major depressive disorder as well as for other indications, both psychiatric and nonpsychiatric. Although a causal link between the emergence of such symptoms and either the worsening of depression and/or the emergence of suicidal impulses has not been established, there is concern that such symptoms may represent precursors to emerging suicidality.

Consideration should be given to changing the therapeutic regimen, including possibly discontinuing the medication, in patients whose depression is persistently worse, or who are experiencing emergent suicidality or symptoms that might be precursors to worsening depression or suicidality, especially if these symptoms are severe, abrupt in onset, or were not part of the patient's presenting symptoms.

Families and caregivers of patients being treated with antidepressants for MDD or other indications, both psychiatric and nonpsychiatric, should be alerted about the need to monitor patients for the emergence of agitation, irritability, unusual changes in behavior, and the other symptoms described above, as well as the emergence of suicidality, and to report such symptoms immediately to healthcare providers. Such monitoring should include daily observation by families and caregivers.Prescriptions for ZYBAN should be written for the smallest quantity of tablets consistent with good patient management, in order to reduce the risk of overdose.

5.3 Seizure

ZYBAN can cause seizure. The risk of seizure is dose-related. The dose of ZYBAN should not exceed 300 mg per day [see Dosage and Administration (2.1)]. Discontinue ZYBAN and do not restart treatment if the patient experiences a seizure.

The risk of seizures is also related to patient factors, clinical situations, and concomitant medications that lower the seizure threshold. Consider these risks before initiating treatment with ZYBAN. ZYBAN is contraindicated in patients with a seizure disorder, current or prior diagnosis of anorexia nervosa or bulimia, or undergoing abrupt discontinuation of alcohol, benzodiazepines, barbiturates, and antiepileptic drugs [see Contraindications (4) and Drug Interactions (7.3)]. The following conditions can also increase the risk of seizure: severe head injury; arteriovenous malformation; CNS tumor or CNS infection; severe stroke; concomitant use of other medications that lower the seizure threshold (e.g., other bupropion products, antipsychotics, tricyclic antidepressants, theophylline, and systemic corticosteroids), metabolic disorders (e.g., hypoglycemia, hyponatremia, severe hepatic impairment, and hypoxia), use of illicit drugs (e.g., cocaine), or abuse or misuse of prescription drugs such as CNS stimulants. Additional predisposing conditions include diabetes mellitus treated with oral hypoglycemic drugs or insulin; use of anorectic drugs; and excessive use of alcohol, benzodiazepines, sedative/hypnotics, or opiates.

Incidence of Seizure With Bupropion Use: Doses for smoking cessation should not exceed 300 mg per day. The seizure rate associated with doses of sustained-release bupropion in depressed patients up to 300 mg per day is approximately 0.1% (1/1,000) and increases to approximately 0.4% (4/1000) at doses up to 400 mg per day.

The risk of seizure can be reduced if the dose of ZYBAN for smoking cessation does not exceed 300 mg per day, given as 150 mg twice daily, and titration rate is gradual.

5.4 Hypertension

Treatment with ZYBAN can result in elevated blood pressure and hypertension. Assess blood pressure before initiating treatment with ZYBAN, and monitor periodically during treatment. The risk of hypertension is increased if ZYBAN is used concomitantly with MAOIs or other drugs that increase dopaminergic or noradrenergic activity [see Contraindications (4)].

Data from a comparative trial of ZYBAN, nicotine transdermal system (NTS), the combination of ZYBAN plus NTS, and placebo as an aid to smoking cessation suggest a higher incidence of treatment-emergent hypertension in patients treated with the combination of ZYBAN and NTS. In this trial, 6.1% of subjects treated with the combination of ZYBAN and NTS had treatment-emergent hypertension compared to 2.5%, 1.6%, and 3.1% of subjects treated with ZYBAN, NTS, and placebo, respectively. The majority of these subjects had evidence of pre-existing hypertension. Three subjects (1.2%) treated with the combination of ZYBAN and NTS and 1 subject (0.4%) treated with NTS had study medication discontinued due to hypertension compared with none of the subjects treated with ZYBAN or placebo. Monitoring of blood pressure is recommended in patients who receive the combination of bupropion and nicotine replacement.

In a clinical trial of bupropion immediate-release in MDD subjects with stable congestive heart failure (N = 36), bupropion was associated with an exacerbation of pre-existing hypertension in 2 subjects, leading to discontinuation of bupropion treatment. There are no controlled trials assessing the safety of bupropion in patients with a recent history of myocardial infarction or unstable cardiac disease.

5.5 Activation of Mania/Hypomania

Antidepressant treatment can precipitate a manic, mixed, or hypomanic episode. The risk appears to be increased in patients with bipolar disorder or who have risk factors for bipolar disorder. There were no reports of activation of psychosis or mania in clinical trials with ZYBAN conducted in nondepressed smokers. Bupropion is not approved for use in treating bipolar depression.

5.6 Psychosis and Other Neuropsychiatric Reactions

Depressed patients treated with bupropion in depression trials have had a variety of neuropsychiatric signs and symptoms, including delusions, hallucinations, psychosis, concentration disturbance, paranoia, and confusion. Some of these patients had a diagnosis of bipolar disorder. In some cases, these symptoms abated upon dose reduction and/or withdrawal of treatment. Instruct patients to contact a healthcare professional if such reactions occur.

In clinical trials with ZYBAN conducted in nondepressed smokers, the incidence of neuropsychiatric side effects was generally comparable to placebo. However, in the post-marketing experience, patients taking ZYBAN to quit smoking have reported similar types of neuropsychiatric symptoms to those reported by patients in the clinical trials of bupropion for depression.

5.7 Hypersensitivity Reactions

Anaphylactoid/anaphylactic reactions have occurred during clinical trials with bupropion. Reactions have been characterized by pruritus, urticaria, angioedema, and dyspnea requiring medical treatment. In addition, there have been rare, spontaneous postmarketing reports of erythema multiforme, Stevens-Johnson syndrome, and anaphylactic shock associated with bupropion. Instruct patients to discontinue ZYBAN and consult a healthcare provider if they develop an allergic or anaphylactoid/anaphylactic reaction (e.g., skin rash, pruritus, hives, chest pain, edema, and shortness of breath) during treatment.

There are reports of arthralgia, myalgia, fever with rash and other serum sickness-like symptoms suggestive of delayed hypersensitivity.

6 ADVERSE REACTIONS

The following adverse reactions are discussed in greater detail in other sections of the labeling:

- Neuropsychiatric symptoms and suicide risk in smoking cessation treatment [see Boxed Warning and Warnings and Precautions (5.1)]
- Suicidal thoughts and behaviors in adolescents and young adults [see Boxed Warning and Warnings and Precautions (5.2)]
- Seizure [see Warnings and Precautions (5.3)]
- Hypertension [see Warnings and Precautions (5.4)]
- Activation of mania or hypomania [see Warnings and Precautions (5.5)]
- Psychosis and other neuropsychiatric reactions [see Warnings and Precautions (5.6)]
- Hypersensitivity reactions [see Warnings and Precautions (5.7)]

6.1 Clinical Trials Experience

Because clinical trials are conducted under widely varying conditions, adverse reaction rates observed in the clinical trials of a drug cannot be directly compared with rates in the clinical trials of another drug and may not reflect the rates observed in clinical practice.

Adverse Reactions Leading to Discontinuation of Treatment: Adverse reactions were sufficiently troublesome to cause discontinuation of treatment in 8% of the 706 subjects treated with ZYBAN and 5% of the 313 patients treated with placebo. The more common events leading to discontinuation of treatment with ZYBAN included nervous system disturbances (3.4%), primarily tremors, and skin disorders (2.4%), primarily rashes.

Commonly Observed Adverse Reactions: The most commonly observed adverse reactions consistently associated with the use of ZYBAN were dry mouth and insomnia. The incidence of dry mouth and insomnia may be related to the dose of ZYBAN. The occurrence of these adverse reactions may be minimized by reducing the dose of ZYBAN. In addition, insomnia may be minimized by avoiding bedtime doses.

Adverse reactions reported in the dose-response and comparator trials are presented in Table 2 and Table 3, respectively. Reported adverse reactions were classified using a COSTART-based dictionary.

Table 2. Adverse Reactions Reported by at Least 1% of Subjects and at a Greater Frequency Than Placebo in the Dose-Response Trial

Adverse Reaction	ZYBAN 100 to 300 mg/day (n = 461) %	Placebo (n = 150) %
Body (General)		
Neck pain	2	<1
Allergic reaction	1	0
Cardiovascular		
Hot flashes	1	0
Hypertension	1	<1
Digestive		
Dry mouth	11	5
Increased appetite	2	<1
Anorexia	1	<1
Musculoskeletal		
Arthralgia	4	3
Myalgia	2	1
Nervous system		
Insomnia	31	21
Dizziness	8	7
Tremor	2	1
Somnolence	2	1
Thinking abnormality	1	0
Respiratory		
Bronchitis	2	0
Skin		
Pruritus	3	<1
Rash	3	<1
Dry skin	2	0
Urticaria	1	0
Special senses		
Taste perversion	2	<1

[See table 3 at top of next page]

Adverse reactions in a 1-year maintenance trial and a 12-week COPD trial with ZYBAN were quantitatively and qualitatively similar to those observed in the dose-response and comparator trials.

Other Adverse Reactions Observed During the Clinical Development of Bupropion: In addition to the adverse reactions noted above, the following adverse reactions have been reported in clinical trials with the sustained-release formulation of bupropion in depressed subjects and in nondepressed smokers, as well as in clinical trials with the immediate-release formulation of bupropion.

Adverse reaction frequencies represent the proportion of subjects who experienced a treatment-emergent adverse reaction on at least one occasion in placebo-controlled trials for depression (n = 987) or smoking cessation (n = 1,013), or subjects who experienced an adverse reaction requiring discontinuation of treatment in an open-label surveillance trial with bupropion sustained-release tablets (n = 3,100). All treatment-emergent adverse reactions are included except those listed in Tables 2 and 3, those listed in other safety-related sections of the prescribing information, those subsumed under COSTART terms that are either overly general or excessively specific so as to be uninformative, those not reasonably associated with the use of the drug, and those that were not serious and occurred in fewer than 2 subjects.

Adverse reactions are further categorized by body system and listed in order of decreasing frequency according to the following definitions of frequency: Frequent adverse reactions are defined as those occurring in at least 1/100 subjects. Infrequent adverse reactions are those occurring in 1/100 to 1/1,000 subjects, while rare events are those occurring in less than 1/1,000 subjects.

Body (General): Frequent were asthenia, fever, and headache. Infrequent were chills, inguinal hernia, and photosensitivity. Rare was malaise.

Cardiovascular: Infrequent were flushing, migraine, postural hypotension, stroke, tachycardia, and vasodilation. Rare was syncope.

Digestive: Frequent were dyspepsia and vomiting. Infrequent were abnormal liver function, bruxism, dysphagia, gastric reflux, gingivitis, jaundice, and stomatitis.

Hemic and Lymphatic: Infrequent was ecchymosis.

Table 3. Adverse Reactions Reported by at Least 1% of Subjects on Active Treatment and at a Greater Frequency Than Placebo in the Comparator Trial

Adverse Experience (Costart Term)	ZYBAN 300 mg/day (n = 243) %	Nicotine Transdermal System (NTS) 21 mg/day (n = 243) %	ZYBAN and NTS (n = 244) %	Placebo (n = 159) %
Body				
Abdominal pain	3	4	1	1
Accidental injury	2	2	1	1
Chest pain	<1	1	3	1
Neck pain	2	1	<1	0
Facial edema	<1	0	1	0
Cardiovascular				
Hypertension	1	<1	2	0
Palpitations	2	0	1	0
Digestive				
Nausea	9	7	11	4
Dry mouth	10	4	9	4
Constipation	8	4	9	3
Diarrhea	4	4	3	1
Anorexia	3	1	5	1
Mouth ulcer	2	1	1	1
Thirst	<1	<1	2	0
Musculoskeletal				
Myalgia	4	3	5	3
Arthralgia	5	3	3	2
Nervous system				
Insomnia	40	28	45	18
Dream abnormality	5	18	13	3
Anxiety	8	6	9	6
Disturbed concentration	9	3	9	4
Dizziness	10	2	8	6
Nervousness	4	<1	2	2
Tremor	1	<1	2	0
Dysphoria	<1	1	2	1
Respiratory				
Rhinitis	12	11	9	8
Increased cough	3	5	<1	1
Pharyngitis	3	2	3	0
Sinusitis	2	2	2	1
Dyspnea	1	0	2	1
Epistaxis	2	1	1	0
Skin				
Application site reaction[a]	11	17	15	7
Rash	4	3	3	2
Pruritus	3	1	5	1
Urticaria	2	0	2	0
Special Senses				
Taste perversion	3	1	3	2
Tinnitus	1	0	<1	0

[a] Subjects randomized to ZYBAN or placebo received placebo patches.

Metabolic and Nutritional: Infrequent were edema and peripheral edema.
Musculoskeletal: Infrequent were leg cramps and twitching.
Nervous System: Frequent were agitation, depression, and irritability. Infrequent were abnormal coordination, CNS stimulation, confusion, decreased libido, decreased memory, depersonalization, emotional lability, hostility, hyperkinesia, hypertonia, hypesthesia, paresthesia, suicidal ideation, and vertigo. Rare were amnesia, ataxia, derealization, and hypomania.
Respiratory: Rare was bronchospasm.
Skin: Frequent was sweating.
Special Senses: Frequent was blurred vision or diplopia. Infrequent were accommodation abnormality and dry eye.
Urogenital: Frequent was urinary frequency. Infrequent were impotence, polyuria, and urinary urgency.

6.2 Postmarketing Experience
The following adverse reactions have been identified during post-approval use of ZYBAN and are not described elsewhere in the label. Because these reactions are reported voluntarily from a population of uncertain size, it is not always possible to reliably estimate their frequency or establish a relationship to drug exposure.
Body (General): Arthralgia, myalgia, and fever with rash and other symptoms suggestive of delayed hypersensitivity. These symptoms may resemble serum sickness.
Cardiovascular: Cardiovascular disorder, complete AV block, extrasystoles, hypotension, myocardial infarction, phlebitis, and pulmonary embolism.

Digestive: Colitis, esophagitis, gastrointestinal hemorrhage, gum hemorrhage, hepatitis, increased salivation, intestinal perforation, liver damage, pancreatitis, stomach ulcer, and stool abnormality.
Endocrine: Hyperglycemia, hypoglycemia, and syndrome of inappropriate antidiuretic hormone.
Hemic and Lymphatic: Anemia, leukocytosis, leukopenia, lymphadenopathy, pancytopenia, and thrombocytopenia. Altered PT and/or INR, infrequently associated with hemorrhagic or thrombotic complications, were observed when bupropion was coadministered with warfarin.
Metabolic and Nutritional: Glycosuria.
Musculoskeletal: Arthritis and muscle rigidity/fever/rhabdomyolysis, and muscle weakness.
Nervous System: Abnormal electroencephalogram (EEG), aggression, akinesia, aphasia, coma, completed suicide, delirium, delusions, dysarthria, dyskinesia, dystonia, euphoria, extrapyramidal syndrome, hallucinations, hypokinesia, increased libido, manic reaction, neuralgia, neuropathy, paranoid ideation, restlessness, suicide attempt, and unmasking tardive dyskinesia.
Respiratory: Pneumonia.
Skin: Alopecia, angioedema, exfoliative dermatitis, hirsutism, and Stevens-Johnson syndrome.
Special Senses: Deafness, increased intraocular pressure, and mydriasis.
Urogenital: Abnormal ejaculation, cystitis, dyspareunia, dysuria, gynecomastia, menopause, painful erection, prostate disorder, salpingitis, urinary incontinence, urinary retention, urinary tract disorder, and vaginitis.

7 DRUG INTERACTIONS
7.1 Potential for Other Drugs to Affect ZYBAN
Bupropion is primarily metabolized to hydroxybupropion by CYP2B6. Therefore, the potential exists for drug interactions between ZYBAN and drugs that are inhibitors or inducers of CYP2B6.
Inhibitors of CYP2B6: *Ticlopidine and Clopidogrel:* Concomitant treatment with these drugs can increase bupropion exposure but decrease hydroxybupropion exposure. Based on clinical response, dosage adjustment of ZYBAN may be necessary when coadministered with CYP2B6 inhibitors (e.g., ticlopidine or clopidogrel) *[see Clinical Pharmacology (12.3)].*
Inducers of CYP2B6: *Ritonavir, Lopinavir, and Efavirenz:* Concomitant treatment with these drugs can decrease bupropion and hydroxybupropion exposure. Dosage increase of ZYBAN may be necessary when coadministered with ritonavir, lopinavir, or efavirenz *[see Clinical Pharmacology (12.3)]* but should not exceed the maximum recommended dose.
Carbamazepine, Phenobarbital, Phenytoin: While not systematically studied, these drugs may induce the metabolism of bupropion and may decrease bupropion exposure *[see Clinical Pharmacology (12.3)].* If bupropion is used concomitantly with a CYP inducer, it may be necessary to increase the dose of bupropion, but the maximum recommended dose should not be exceeded.
7.2 Potential for ZYBAN to Affect Other Drugs
Drugs Metabolized by CYP2D6: Bupropion and its metabolites (erythrohydrobupropion, threohydrobupropion, hydroxybupropion) are CYP2D6 inhibitors. Therefore, coadministration of ZYBAN with drugs that are metabolized by CYP2D6 can increase the exposures of drugs that are substrates of CYP2D6. Such drugs include certain antidepressants (e.g., venlafaxine, nortriptyline, imipramine, desipramine, paroxetine, fluoxetine, and sertraline), antipsychotics (e.g., haloperidol, risperidone, thioridazine), beta-blockers (e.g., metoprolol), and Type 1C antiarrhythmics (e.g., propafenone and flecainide). When used concomitantly with ZYBAN, it may be necessary to decrease the dose of these CYP2D6 substrates, particularly for drugs with a narrow therapeutic index.
Drugs that require metabolic activation by CYP2D6 to be effective (e.g., tamoxifen) theoretically could have reduced efficacy when administered concomitantly with inhibitors of CYP2D6 such as bupropion. Patients treated concomitantly with ZYBAN and such drugs may require increased doses of the drug *[see Clinical Pharmacology (12.3)].*
7.3 Drugs That Lower Seizure Threshold
Use extreme caution when coadministering ZYBAN with other drugs that lower seizure threshold (e.g., other bupropion products, antipsychotics, antidepressants, theophylline, or systemic corticosteroids). Use low initial doses and increase the dose gradually *[see Contraindications (4) and Warnings and Precautions (5.3)].*
7.4 Dopaminergic Drugs (Levodopa and Amantadine)
Bupropion, levodopa, and amantadine have dopamine agonist effects. CNS toxicity has been reported when bupropion was coadministered with levodopa or amantadine. Adverse reactions have included restlessness, agitation, tremor, ataxia, gait disturbance, vertigo, and dizziness. It is presumed that the toxicity results from cumulative dopamine agonist effects. Use caution when administering ZYBAN concomitantly with these drugs.
7.5 Use With Alcohol
In postmarketing experience, there have been rare reports of adverse neuropsychiatric events or reduced alcohol tolerance in patients who were drinking alcohol during treatment with ZYBAN. The consumption of alcohol during treatment with ZYBAN should be minimized or avoided.
7.6 MAO Inhibitors
Bupropion inhibits the reuptake of dopamine and norepinephrine. Concomitant use of MAOIs and bupropion is contraindicated because there is an increased risk of hypertensive reactions if bupropion is used concomitantly with MAOIs. Studies in animals demonstrate that the acute toxicity of bupropion is enhanced by the MAO inhibitor phenelzine. At least 14 days should elapse between discontinuation of an MAOI and initiation of treatment with ZYBAN. Conversely, at least 14 days should be allowed after stopping ZYBAN before starting an MAOI intended to treat psychiatric disorders *[see Dosage and Administration (2.8) and Contraindications (4)].*
7.7 Smoking Cessation
Physiological changes resulting from smoking cessation, with or without treatment with ZYBAN, may alter the pharmacokinetics or pharmacodynamics of certain drugs (e.g., theophylline, warfarin, insulin) for which dosage adjustment may be necessary.
7.8 Drug-Laboratory Test Interactions
False-positive urine immunoassay screening tests for amphetamines have been reported in patients taking

bupropion. This is due to lack of specificity of some screening tests. False-positive test results may result even following discontinuation of bupropion therapy. Confirmatory tests, such as gas chromatography/mass spectrometry, will distinguish bupropion from amphetamines.

8 USE IN SPECIFIC POPULATIONS

8.1 Pregnancy
Pregnancy Category C.

Risk Summary: Data from epidemiological studies of pregnant women exposed to bupropion in the first trimester indicate no increased risk of congenital malformations overall. All pregnancies, regardless of drug exposure, have a background rate of 2% to 4% for major malformations, and 15% to 20% for pregnancy loss. No clear evidence of teratogenic activity was found in reproductive developmental studies conducted in rats and rabbits; however, in rabbits, slightly increased incidences of fetal malformations and skeletal variations were observed at doses approximately 2 times the maximum recommended human dose (MRHD) and greater and decreased fetal weights were seen at doses three times the MRHD and greater. ZYBAN should be used during pregnancy only if the potential benefit justifies the potential risk to the fetus.

Clinical Considerations: Pregnant smokers should be encouraged to attempt cessation using educational and behavioral interventions before pharmacological approaches are used.

Human Data: Data from the international bupropion Pregnancy Registry (675 first trimester exposures) and a retrospective cohort study using the United Healthcare database (1,213 first trimester exposures) did not show an increased risk for malformations overall.

No increased risk for cardiovascular malformations overall has been observed after bupropion exposure during the first trimester. The prospectively observed rate of cardiovascular malformations in pregnancies with exposure to bupropion in the first trimester from the international Pregnancy Registry was 1.3% (9 cardiovascular malformations/675 first trimester maternal bupropion exposures), which is similar to the background rate of cardiovascular malformations (approximately 1%). Data from the United Healthcare database and a case-control study (6,853 infants with cardiovascular malformations and 5,763 with non-cardiovascular malformations) from the National Birth Defects Prevention Study (NBDPS) did not show an increased risk for cardiovascular malformations overall after bupropion exposure during the first trimester.

Study findings on bupropion exposure during the first trimester and risk for left ventricular outflow tract obstruction (LVOTO) are inconsistent and do not allow conclusions regarding a possible association. The United Healthcare database lacked sufficient power to evaluate this association; the NBDPS found increased risk for LVOTO (n = 10; adjusted OR = 2.6; 95% CI: 1.2, 5.7), and the Slone Epidemiology case-control study did not find increased risk for LVOTO. Study findings on bupropion exposure during the first trimester and risk for ventricular septal defect (VSD) are inconsistent and do not allow conclusions regarding a possible association. The Slone Epidemiology Study found an increased risk for VSD following first trimester maternal bupropion exposure (n = 17; adjusted OR = 2.5; 95% CI: 1.3, 5.0) but did not find increased risk for any other cardiovascular malformations studied (including LVOTO as above). The NBDPS and United Healthcare database study did not find an association between first trimester maternal bupropion exposure and VSD.

For the findings of LVOTO and VSD, the studies were limited by the small number of exposed cases, inconsistent findings among studies, and the potential for chance findings from multiple comparisons in case control studies.

Animal Data: In studies conducted in rats and rabbits, bupropion was administered orally during the period of organogenesis at doses of up to 450 and 150 mg/kg/day, respectively (approximately 15 and 10 times the MRHD respectively, on a mg/m2 basis). No clear evidence of teratogenic activity was found in either species; however, in rabbits, slightly increased incidences of fetal malformations and skeletal variations were observed at the lowest dose tested (25 mg/kg/day, approximately 2 times the MRHD on a mg/m2 basis) and greater. Decreased fetal weights were observed at 50 mg/kg and greater.

When rats were administered bupropion at oral doses of up to 300 mg/kg/day (approximately 10 times the MRHD on a mg/m2 basis) prior to mating and throughout pregnancy and lactation, there were no apparent adverse effects on offspring development.

8.3 Nursing Mothers
Bupropion and its metabolites are present in human milk. In a lactation study of 10 women, levels of orally dosed bupropion and its active metabolites were measured in expressed milk. The average daily infant exposure (assuming 150 mL/kg daily consumption) to bupropion and its active metabolites was 2% of the maternal weight-adjusted dose. Exercise caution when ZYBAN is administered to a nursing woman.

8.4 Pediatric Use
Safety and effectiveness in the pediatric population have not been established [see Boxed Warning and Warnings and Precautions (5.2)].

8.5 Geriatric Use
Of the approximately 6,000 subjects who participated in clinical trials with bupropion sustained-release tablets (depression and smoking cessation trials), 275 were aged ≥65 years and 47 were aged ≥75 years. In addition, several hundred subjects aged ≥65 years participated in clinical trials using the immediate-release formulation of bupropion (depression trials). No overall differences in safety or effectiveness were observed between these subjects and younger subjects. Reported clinical experience has not identified differences in responses between the elderly and younger patients, but greater sensitivity of some older individuals cannot be ruled out.

Bupropion is extensively metabolized in the liver to active metabolites, which are further metabolized and excreted by the kidneys. The risk of adverse reactions may be greater in patients with impaired renal function. Because elderly patients are more likely to have decreased renal function, it may be necessary to consider this factor in dose selection; it may be useful to monitor renal function [see Dosage and Administration (2.7), Use in Specific Populations (8.6), and Clinical Pharmacology (12.3)].

8.6 Renal Impairment
Consider a reduced dose and/or dosing frequency of ZYBAN in patients with renal impairment (Glomerular Filtration Rate: <90 mL/min). Bupropion and its metabolites are cleared renally and may accumulate in such patients to a greater extent than usual. Monitor closely for adverse reactions that could indicate high bupropion or metabolite exposures [see Dosage and Administration (2.7) and Clinical Pharmacology (12.3)].

8.7 Hepatic Impairment
In patients with moderate to severe hepatic impairment (Child-Pugh score: 7 to 15), the maximum dose of ZYBAN is 150 mg every other day. In patients with mild hepatic impairment (Child-Pugh score: 5 to 6), consider reducing the dose and/or frequency of dosing [see Dosage and Administration (2.6) and Clinical Pharmacology (12.3)].

9 DRUG ABUSE AND DEPENDENCE

9.1 Controlled Substance
Bupropion is not a controlled substance.

9.2 Abuse
Humans: Controlled clinical trials of bupropion (immediate-release formulation) conducted in normal volunteers, in subjects with a history of multiple drug abuse, and in depressed subjects showed some increase in motor activity and agitation/excitement.

In a population of individuals experienced with drugs of abuse, a single dose of 400 mg of bupropion produced mild amphetamine-like activity as compared with placebo on the Morphine-Benzedrine Subscale of the Addiction Research Center Inventories (ARCI) and a score intermediate between placebo and amphetamine on the Liking Scale of the ARCI. These scales measure general feelings of euphoria and drug desirability.

Findings in clinical trials, however, are not known to reliably predict the abuse potential of drugs. Nonetheless, evidence from single-dose trials does suggest that the recommended daily dosage of bupropion when administered in divided doses is not likely to be significantly reinforcing to amphetamine or CNS stimulant abusers. However, higher doses (that could not be tested because of the risk of seizure) might be modestly attractive to those who abuse CNS stimulant drugs.

Animals: Studies in rodents and primates demonstrated that bupropion exhibits some pharmacologic actions common to psychostimulants. In rodents, it has been shown to increase locomotor activity, elicit a mild stereotyped behavior response, and increase rates of responding in several schedule-controlled behavior paradigms. In primate models assessing the positive reinforcing effects of psychoactive drugs, bupropion was self-administered intravenously. In rats, bupropion produced amphetamine-like and cocaine-like discriminative stimulus effects in drug discrimination paradigms used to characterize the subjective effects of psychoactive drugs.

The possibility that bupropion may induce dependence should be kept in mind when evaluating the desirability of including the drug in smoking cessation programs of individual patients.

10 OVERDOSAGE

10.1 Human Overdose Experience
Overdoses of up to 30 grams or more of bupropion have been reported. Seizure was reported in approximately one-third of all cases. Other serious reactions reported with overdoses of bupropion alone included hallucinations, loss of consciousness, sinus tachycardia, and ECG changes such as conduction disturbances (including QRS prolongation) or arrhythmias. Fever, muscle rigidity, rhabdomyolysis, hypotension, stupor, coma, and respiratory failure have been reported mainly when bupropion was part of multiple drug overdoses.

Although most patients recovered without sequelae, deaths associated with overdoses of bupropion alone have been reported in patients ingesting large doses of the drug. Multiple uncontrolled seizures, bradycardia, cardiac failure, and cardiac arrest prior to death were reported in these patients.

10.2 Overdosage Management
Consult a Certified Poison Control Center for up-to-date guidance and advice. Telephone numbers for certified poison control centers are listed in the Physicians' Desk Reference (PDR). Call 1-800-222-1222 or refer to www.poison.org.

There are no known antidotes for bupropion. In case of an overdose, provide supportive care, including close medical supervision and monitoring. Consider the possibility of multiple drug overdose. Ensure an adequate airway, oxygenation, and ventilation. Monitor cardiac rhythm and vital signs. Induction of emesis is not recommended.

11 DESCRIPTION

ZYBAN (bupropion hydrochloride) Sustained-Release Tablets are a non-nicotine aid to smoking cessation. ZYBAN is chemically unrelated to nicotine or other agents currently used in the treatment of nicotine addiction. Initially developed and marketed as an antidepressant (WELLBUTRIN [bupropion hydrochloride] Tablets and WELLBUTRIN SR [bupropion hydrochloride] Sustained-Release Tablets), ZYBAN is also chemically unrelated to tricyclic, tetracyclic, selective serotonin re-uptake inhibitor, or other known antidepressant agents. Its structure closely resembles that of diethylpropion; it is related to phenylethylamines. It is designated as $(\pm)$-1-(3-chlorophenyl)-2-[(1,1-dimethylethyl)-amino]-1-propanone hydrochloride. The molecular weight is 276.2. The molecular formula is $C_{13}H_{18}ClNO \cdot HCl$. Bupropion hydrochloride powder is white, crystalline, and highly soluble in water. It has a bitter taste and produces the sensation of local anesthesia on the oral mucosa. The structural formula is:

ZYBAN is supplied for oral administration as 150-mg (purple), film-coated, sustained-release tablets. Each tablet contains the labeled amount of bupropion hydrochloride and the inactive ingredients carnauba wax, cysteine hydrochloride, hypromellose, magnesium stearate, microcrystalline cellulose, polyethylene glycol, polysorbate 80, and titanium dioxide and is printed with edible black ink. In addition, the 150-mg tablet contains FD&C Blue No. 2 Lake and FD& C Red No. 40 Lake.

12 CLINICAL PHARMACOLOGY

12.1 Mechanism of Action
The exact mechanism by which ZYBAN enhances the ability of patients to abstain from smoking is not known but is presumed to be related to noradrenergic and/or dopaminergic mechanisms. Bupropion is a relatively weak inhibitor of the neuronal reuptake of norepinephrine and dopamine, and does not inhibit the reuptake of serotonin. Bupropion does not inhibit monoamine oxidase.

12.3 Pharmacokinetics
Bupropion is a racemic mixture. The pharmacological activity and pharmacokinetics of the individual enantiomers have not been studied. The mean elimination half-life $(\pm SD)$ of bupropion after chronic dosing is 21 (± 9) hours, and steady-state plasma concentrations of bupropion are reached within 8 days.

Absorption: The absolute bioavailability of ZYBAN in humans has not been determined because an intravenous formulation for human use is not available. However, it appears likely that only a small proportion of any orally administered dose reaches the systemic circulation intact. In rat and dog studies, the bioavailability of bupropion ranged from 5% to 20%.

In humans, following oral administration of ZYBAN, peak plasma concentration (C_{max}) of bupropion is usually achieved within 3 hours.

ZYBAN can be taken with or without food. Bupropion C_{max} and AUC was increased by 11% to 35%, and 16% to 19%, respectively, when ZYBAN was administered with food to

Table 4. Pharmacokinetics of Bupropion and Metabolites in Patients With Severe Hepatic Cirrhosis: Ratio Relative to Healthy Matched Controls

	C_{max}	AUC	$t_{1/2}$	T_{max}[a]
Bupropion	1.69	3.12	1.43	0.5 h
Hydroxybupropion	0.31	1.28	3.88	19 h
Threo/erythrohydrobupropion amino alcohol	0.69	2.48	1.96	20 h

[a] = Difference.

healthy volunteers in three trials. The food effect is not considered clinically significant.

Distribution: In vitro tests show that bupropion is 84% bound to human plasma proteins at concentrations up to 200 mcg/mL. The extent of protein binding of the hydroxybupropion metabolite is similar to that for bupropion; whereas, the extent of protein binding of the threohydrobupropion metabolite is about half that seen with bupropion.

Metabolism: Bupropion is extensively metabolized in humans. Three metabolites are active: hydroxybupropion, which is formed via hydroxylation of the *tert*-butyl group of bupropion, and the amino-alcohol isomers, threohydrobupropion and erythrohydrobupropion, which are formed via reduction of the carbonyl group. In vitro findings suggest that CYP2B6 is the principal isoenzyme involved in the formation of hydroxybupropion, while cytochrome P450 enzymes are not involved in the formation of threohydrobupropion. Oxidation of the bupropion side chain results in the formation of a glycine conjugate of meta-chlorobenzoic acid, which is then excreted as the major urinary metabolite. The potency and toxicity of the metabolites relative to bupropion have not been fully characterized. However, it has been demonstrated in an antidepressant screening test in mice that hydroxybupropion is one-half as potent as bupropion, while threohydrobupropion and erythrohydrobupropion are 5-fold less potent than bupropion. This may be of clinical importance, because the plasma concentrations of the metabolites are as high as or higher than those of bupropion. Following a single dose administration of ZYBAN in humans, C_{max} of hydroxybupropion occurs approximately 6 hours post-dose and is approximately 10 times the peak level of the parent drug at steady state. The elimination half-life of hydroxybupropion is approximately 20 (±5) hours and its AUC at steady state is about 17 times that of bupropion. The times to peak concentrations for the erythrohydrobupropion and threohydrobupropion metabolites are similar to that of the hydroxybupropion metabolite. However, their elimination half-lives are longer, 33 (±10) and 37 (±13) hours, respectively, and steady-state AUCs are 1.5 and 7 times that of bupropion, respectively.

Bupropion and its metabolites exhibit linear kinetics following chronic administration of 300 to 450 mg per day.

Elimination: Following oral administration of 200 mg of ^{14}C-bupropion in humans, 87% and 10% of the radioactive dose were recovered in the urine and feces, respectively. Only 0.5% of the oral dose was excreted as unchanged bupropion.

Population Subgroups: Factors or conditions altering metabolic capacity (e.g., liver disease, congestive heart failure [CHF], age, concomitant medications, etc.) or elimination may be expected to influence the degree and extent of accumulation of the active metabolites of bupropion. The elimination of the major metabolites of bupropion may be affected by reduced renal or hepatic function because they are moderately polar compounds and are likely to undergo further metabolism or conjugation in the liver prior to urinary excretion.

Renal Impairment: There is limited information on the pharmacokinetics of bupropion in patients with renal impairment. An inter-trial comparison between normal subjects and subjects with end-stage renal failure demonstrated that the parent drug C_{max} and AUC values were comparable in the 2 groups, whereas the hydroxybupropion and threohydrobupropion metabolites had a 2.3- and 2.8-fold increase, respectively, in AUC for subjects with end-stage renal failure. A second trial, comparing normal subjects and subjects with moderate-to-severe renal impairment (GFR 30.9 ± 10.8 mL/min), showed that after a single 150-mg dose of sustained-release bupropion, exposure to bupropion was approximately 2-fold higher in subjects with impaired renal function while levels of the hydroxybupropion and threo/erythrohydrobupropion (combined) metabolites were similar in the 2 groups. Bupropion is extensively metabolized in the liver to active metabolites, which are further metabolized and subsequently excreted by the kidneys. The elimination of the major metabolites of bupropion may be reduced by impaired renal function.

ZYBAN should be used with caution in patients with renal impairment and a reduced frequency and/or dose should be considered [see Use in Specific Populations (8.6)].

Hepatic Impairment: The effect of hepatic impairment on the pharmacokinetics of bupropion was characterized in 2 single-dose trials, one in subjects with alcoholic liver disease and one in subjects with mild-to-severe cirrhosis. The first trial demonstrated that the half-life of hydroxybupropion was significantly longer in 8 subjects with alcoholic liver disease than in 8 healthy volunteers (32 ± 14 hours versus 21 ± 5 hours, respectively). Although not statistically significant, the AUCs for bupropion and hydroxybupropion were more variable and tended to be greater (by 53% to 57%) in volunteers with alcoholic liver disease. The differences in half-life for bupropion and the other metabolites in the 2 groups were minimal.

The second trial demonstrated no statistically significant differences in the pharmacokinetics of bupropion and its active metabolites in 9 subjects with mild-to-moderate hepatic cirrhosis compared with 8 healthy volunteers. However, more variability was observed in some of the pharmacokinetic parameters for bupropion (AUC, C_{max}, and T_{max}) and its active metabolites ($t_{1/2}$) in subjects with mild-to-moderate hepatic cirrhosis. In 8 subjects with severe hepatic cirrhosis, significant alterations in the pharmacokinetics of bupropion and its metabolites were seen (Table 4). [See table 4 above]

Smokers: The effects of cigarette smoking on the pharmacokinetics of bupropion were studied in 34 healthy male and female volunteers; 17 were chronic cigarette smokers and 17 were nonsmokers. Following oral administration of a single 150-mg dose of ZYBAN, there were no statistically significant differences in C_{max}, half-life, T_{max}, AUC, or clearance of bupropion or its major metabolites between smokers and nonsmokers.

In a trial comparing the treatment combination of ZYBAN and NTS versus ZYBAN alone, no statistically significant differences were observed between the 2 treatment groups of combination ZYBAN and NTS (n = 197) and ZYBAN alone (n = 193) in the plasma concentrations of bupropion or its active metabolites at Weeks 3 and 6.

Left Ventricular Dysfunction: During a chronic dosing trial with bupropion in 14 depressed subjects with left ventricular dysfunction (history of CHF or an enlarged heart on x-ray), there was no apparent effect on the pharmacokinetics of bupropion or its metabolites, compared with healthy volunteers.

Age: The effects of age on the pharmacokinetics of bupropion and its metabolites have not been fully characterized, but an exploration of steady-state bupropion concentrations from several depression efficacy trials involving subjects dosed in a range of 300 to 750 mg per day, on a 3-times-daily schedule, revealed no relationship between age (18 to 83 years) and plasma concentration of bupropion. A single-dose pharmacokinetic trial demonstrated that the disposition of bupropion and its metabolites in elderly subjects was similar to that of younger subjects. These data suggest there is no prominent effect of age on bupropion concentration; however, another single- and multiple-dose pharmacokinetics trial suggested that the elderly are at increased risk for accumulation of bupropion and its metabolites [see Use in Specific Populations (8.5)].

Gender: Pooled analysis of bupropion pharmacokinetic data from 90 healthy male and 90 healthy female volunteers revealed no sex-related differences in the peak plasma concentrations of bupropion. The mean systemic exposure (AUC) was approximately 13% higher in male volunteers compared with female volunteers. The clinical significance of this finding is unknown.

Drug Interactions: Potential for Other Drugs to Affect ZYBAN: In vitro studies indicate that bupropion is primarily metabolized to hydroxybupropion by CYP2B6. Therefore, the potential exists for drug interactions between ZYBAN and drugs that are inhibitors or inducers of CYP2B6. In addition, in vitro studies suggest that paroxetine, sertraline, norfluoxetine, fluvoxamine, and nelfinavir inhibit the hydroxylation of bupropion.

Inhibitors of CYP2B6: Ticlopidine, Clopidogrel: In a trial in healthy male volunteers, clopidogrel 75 mg once daily or ticlopidine 250 mg twice daily increased exposures (C_{max} and AUC) of bupropion by 40% and 60% for clopidogrel, and by 38% and 85% for ticlopidine, respectively. The exposures (C_{max} and AUC) of hydroxybupropion were decreased 50% and 52%, respectively, by clopidogrel, and 78% and 84%, respectively, by ticlopidine. This effect is thought to be due to the inhibition of the CYP2B6-catalyzed bupropion hydroxylation.

Prasugrel: Prasugrel is a weak inhibitor of CYP2B6. In healthy subjects, prasugrel increased bupropion C_{max} and AUC values by 14% and 18%, respectively, and decreased C_{max} and AUC values of hydroxybupropion, an active metabolite of bupropion, by 32% and 24%, respectively.

Cimetidine: The threohydrobupropion metabolite of bupropion does not appear to be produced by cytochrome P450 enzymes. The effects of concomitant administration of cimetidine on the pharmacokinetics of bupropion and its active metabolites were studied in 24 healthy young male volunteers. Following oral administration of bupropion 300 mg with and without cimetidine 800 mg, the pharmacokinetics of bupropion and hydroxybupropion were unaffected. However, there were 16% and 32% increases in the AUC and C_{max}, respectively, of the combined moieties of threohydrobupropion and erythrohydrobupropion.

Citalopram: Citalopram did not affect the pharmacokinetics of bupropion and its 3 metabolites.

Inducers of CYP2B6: Ritonavir and Lopinavir: In a healthy volunteer trial, ritonavir 100 mg twice daily reduced the AUC and C_{max} of bupropion by 22% and 21%, respectively. The exposure of the hydroxybupropion metabolite was decreased by 23%, the threohydrobupropion decreased by 38%, and the erythrohydrobupropion decreased by 48%.

In a second healthy volunteer trial, ritonavir at a dose of 600 mg twice daily decreased the AUC and the C_{max} of bupropion by 66% and 62%, respectively. The exposure of the hydroxybupropion metabolite was decreased by 78%, the threohydrobupropion decreased by 50%, and the erythrohydrobupropion decreased by 68%.

In another healthy volunteer trial, lopinavir 400 mg/ritonavir 100 mg twice daily decreased bupropion AUC and C_{max} by 57%. The AUC and C_{max} of hydroxybupropion were decreased by 50% and 31%, respectively.

Efavirenz: In a trial in healthy volunteers, efavirenz 600 mg once daily for 2 weeks reduced the AUC and C_{max} of bupropion by approximately 55% and 34%, respectively. The AUC of hydroxybupropion was unchanged, whereas C_{max} of hydroxybupropion was increased by 50%.

Carbamazepine, Phenobarbital, Phenytoin: While not systematically studied, these drugs may induce the metabolism of bupropion.

Potential for ZYBAN to Affect Other Drugs: Animal data indicated that bupropion may be an inducer of drug-metabolizing enzymes in humans. In one trial, following chronic administration of bupropion 100 mg three times daily to 8 healthy male volunteers for 14 days, there was no evidence of induction of its own metabolism. Nevertheless, there may be potential for clinically important alterations of blood levels of co-administered drugs.

Drugs Metabolized by CYP2D6: In vitro, bupropion and its metabolites (erythrohydrobupropion, threohydrobupropion, hydroxybupropion) are CYP2D6 inhibitors. In a clinical trial of 15 male subjects (ages 19 to 35 years) who were extensive metabolizers of CYP2D6, bupropion 300 mg per day followed by a single dose of 50 mg desipramine increased the C_{max}, AUC, and $t_{1/2}$ of desipramine by an average of approximately 2-, 5- and 2-fold, respectively. The effect was present for at least 7 days after the last dose of bupropion. Concomitant use of bupropion with other drugs metabolized by CYP2D6 has not been formally studied.

Citalopram: Although citalopram is not primarily metabolized by CYP2D6, in one trial bupropion increased the C_{max} and AUC of citalopram by 30% and 40%, respectively.

Lamotrigine: Multiple oral doses of bupropion had no statistically significant effects on the single-dose pharmacokinetics of lamotrigine in 12 healthy volunteers.

13 NONCLINICAL TOXICOLOGY

13.1 Carcinogenesis, Mutagenesis, Impairment of Fertility

Lifetime carcinogenicity studies were performed in rats and mice at bupropion doses up to 300 and 150 mg/kg/day, respectively. These doses are approximately 10 and 2 times the MRHD, respectively, on a mg/m^2 basis. In the rat study there was an increase in nodular proliferative lesions of the liver at doses of 100 to 300 mg/kg/day (approximately 3 to 10 times the MRHD on a mg/m^2 basis); lower doses were not tested. The question of whether or not such lesions may be precursors of neoplasms of the liver is currently unresolved.

Similar liver lesions were not seen in the mouse study, and no increase in malignant tumors of the liver and other organs was seen in either study.

Bupropion produced a positive response (2 to 3 times control mutation rate) in 2 of 5 strains in the Ames bacterial mutagenicity assay. Bupropion produced an increase in chromosomal aberrations in 1 of 3 in vivo rat bone marrow cytogenetic studies.

A fertility study in rats at doses up to 300 mg/kg/day revealed no evidence of impaired fertility.

14   CLINICAL STUDIES

The efficacy of ZYBAN as an aid to smoking cessation was demonstrated in 3 placebo-controlled, double-blind trials in nondepressed chronic cigarette smokers (n = 1,940, ≥15 cigarettes per day). In these trials, ZYBAN was used in conjunction with individual smoking cessation counseling.

The first trial was a dose-response trial conducted at 3 clinical centers. Subjects in this trial were treated for 7 weeks with 1 of 3 doses of ZYBAN (100, 150, or 300 mg per day) or placebo; quitting was defined as total abstinence during the last 4 weeks of treatment (Weeks 4 through 7). Abstinence was determined by subject daily diaries and verified by carbon monoxide levels in expired air.

Results of this dose-response trial with ZYBAN demonstrated a dose-dependent increase in the percentage of subjects able to achieve 4-week abstinence (Weeks 4 through 7). Treatment with ZYBAN at both 150 and 300 mg per day was significantly more effective than placebo in this trial.

Table 5 presents quit rates over time in the multicenter trial by treatment group. The quit rates are the proportions of all subjects initially enrolled (i.e., intent-to-treat analysis) who abstained from Week 4 of the trial through the specified week. Treatment with ZYBAN (150 or 300 mg per day) was more effective than placebo in helping subjects achieve 4-week abstinence. In addition, treatment with ZYBAN (7 weeks at 300 mg per day) was more effective than placebo in helping subjects maintain continuous abstinence through Week 26 (6 months) of the trial.

[See Table 5 above]

The second trial was a comparator trial conducted at 4 clinical centers. Four treatments were evaluated: ZYBAN 300 mg per day, nicotine transdermal system (NTS) 21 mg per day, combination of ZYBAN 300 mg per day plus NTS 21 mg per day, and placebo. Subjects were treated for 9 weeks. Treatment with ZYBAN was initiated at 150 mg per day while the subject was still smoking and was increased after 3 days to 300 mg per day given as 150 mg twice daily. NTS 21 mg per day was added to treatment with ZYBAN after approximately 1 week when the subject reached the target quit date. During Weeks 8 and 9 of the trial, NTS was tapered to 14 and 7 mg per day, respectively. Quitting, defined as total abstinence during Weeks 4 through 7, was determined by subject daily diaries and verified by expired air carbon monoxide levels. In this trial, subjects treated with any of the 3 treatments achieved greater 4-week abstinence rates than subjects treated with placebo.

Table 6 presents quit rates over time by treatment group for the comparator trial.

[See table 6 above]

When subjects in this trial were followed out to 1 year, the superiority of ZYBAN and the combination of ZYBAN and NTS over placebo in helping them to achieve abstinence from smoking was maintained. The continuous abstinence rate was 30% (95% CI: 24 to 35) in the subjects treated with ZYBAN and 33% (95% CI: 27 to 39) for subjects treated with the combination at 26 weeks compared with 13% (95% CI: 7 to 18) in the placebo group. At 52 weeks, the continuous abstinence rate was 23% (95% CI: 18 to 28) in the subjects treated with ZYBAN and 28% (95% CI: 23 to 34) for subjects treated with the combination, compared with 8% (95% CI: 3 to 12) in the placebo group. Although the treatment combination of ZYBAN and NTS displayed the highest rates of continuous abstinence throughout the trial, the quit rates for the combination were not significantly higher (P>0.05) than for ZYBAN alone.

The comparisons between ZYBAN, NTS, and combination treatment in this trial have not been replicated, and, therefore should not be interpreted as demonstrating the superiority of any of the active treatment arms over any other.

The third trial was a long-term maintenance trial conducted at 5 clinical centers. Subjects in this trial received open-label ZYBAN 300 mg per day for 7 weeks. Subjects who quit smoking while receiving ZYBAN (n = 432) were then randomized to ZYBAN 300 mg per day or placebo for a total trial duration of 1 year. Abstinence from smoking was determined by subject self-report and verified by expired air carbon monoxide levels. This trial demonstrated that at 6 months, continuous abstinence rates were significantly higher for subjects continuing to receive ZYBAN than for those switched to placebo (P<0.05; 55% versus 44%).

Table 5. Dose-Response Trial: Quit Rates by Treatment Group

Abstinence From Week 4 Through Specified Week	Treatment Groups			
	Placebo (n = 151) % (95% CI)	ZYBAN 100 mg/day (n = 153) % (95% CI)	ZYBAN 150 mg/day (n = 153) % (95% CI)	ZYBAN 300 mg/day (n = 156) % (95% CI)
Week 7 (4-week quit)	17% (11-23)	22% (15-28)	27%[a] (20-35)	36%[a] (28-43)
Week 12	14% (8-19)	20% (13-26)	20% (14-27)	25%[a] (18-32)
Week 26	11% (6-16)	16% (11-22)	18% (12-24)	19%[a] (13-25)

[a]   Significantly different from placebo (P≤0.05).

Table 6. Comparator Trial: Quit Rates by Treatment Group

Abstinence From Week 4 Through Specified Week	Treatment Groups			
	Placebo (n = 160) % (95% CI)	Nicotine Transdermal System (NTS) 21 mg/day (n = 244) % (95% CI)	ZYBAN 300 mg/day (n = 244) % (95% CI)	ZYBAN 300 mg/day and NTS 21 mg/day (n = 245) % (95% CI)
Week 7 (4-week quit)	23% (17-30)	36% (30-42)	49% (43-56)	58% (51-64)
Week 10	20% (14-26)	32% (26-37)	46% (39-52)	51% (45-58)

Quit rates in clinical trials are influenced by the population selected. Quit rates in an unselected population may be lower than the above rates. Quit rates for ZYBAN were similar in subjects with and without prior quit attempts using nicotine replacement therapy.

Treatment with ZYBAN reduced withdrawal symptoms compared with placebo. Reductions on the following withdrawal symptoms were most pronounced: irritability, frustration, or anger; anxiety; difficulty concentrating; restlessness; and depressed mood or negative affect. Depending on the trial and the measure used, treatment with ZYBAN showed evidence of reduction in craving for cigarettes or urge to smoke compared with placebo.

Use In Patients With Chronic Obstructive Pulmonary Disease (COPD): ZYBAN was evaluated in a randomized, double-blind, comparator trial of 404 subjects with mild-to-moderate COPD defined as $FEV_1 \geq 35\%$, $FEV_1/FVC \leq 70\%$, and a diagnosis of chronic bronchitis, emphysema, and/or small airways disease. Subjects aged 36 to 76 years were randomized to ZYBAN 300 mg per day (n = 204) or placebo (n = 200) and treated for 12 weeks. Treatment with ZYBAN was initiated at 150 mg per day for 3 days while the subject was still smoking and increased to 150 mg twice daily for the remaining treatment period. Abstinence from smoking was determined by subject daily diaries and verified by carbon monoxide levels in expired air. Quitters were defined as subjects who were abstinent during the last 4 weeks of treatment. Table 7 shows quit rates in the COPD Trial.

Table 7. COPD Trial: Quit Rates by Treatment Group

4-Week Abstinence Period	Treatment Groups	
	Placebo (n = 200) % (95% CI)	ZYBAN 300 mg/day (n = 204) % (95% CI)
Weeks 9 through 12	12% (8-16)	22%[a] (17-27)

[a]   Significantly different from placebo (P<0.05).

16   HOW SUPPLIED/STORAGE AND HANDLING

ZYBAN Sustained-Release Tablets, 150 mg of bupropion hydrochloride, are purple, round, biconvex, film-coated tablets printed with "ZYBAN 150" in bottles of 60 (NDC 0173-0556-02) tablets and the ZYBAN Advantage Pack® containing 1 bottle of 60 (NDC 0173-0556-01) tablets.

Store at room temperature, 20° to 25°C (68° to 77°F); excursions permitted between 15°C and 30°C (59°F and 86°F) [see USP Controlled Room Temperature]. Protect from light and moisture.

17   PATIENT COUNSELING INFORMATION

Advise the patient to read the FDA-approved patient labeling (Medication Guide).

Although ZYBAN is not indicated for treatment of depression, it contains the same active ingredient as the antidepressant medications WELLBUTRIN, WELLBUTRIN SR, and WELLBUTRIN XL. Inform patients, their families, and their caregivers about the benefits and risks associated with treatment with ZYBAN and counsel them in its appropriate use.

A patient Medication Guide about "Quitting Smoking, Quit-Smoking Medications, Changes in Thinking and Behavior, Depression, and Suicidal Thoughts or Actions," "Antidepressant Medicines, Depression and Other Serious Mental Illnesses, and Suicidal Thoughts or Actions," and "What Other Important Information Should I Know About ZYBAN?" is available for ZYBAN. Instruct patients, their families, and their caregivers to read the Medication Guide and assist them in understanding its contents. Patients should be given the opportunity to discuss the contents of the Medication Guide and to obtain answers to any questions they may have. The complete text of the Medication Guide is reprinted at the end of this document.

Advise patients regarding the following issues and to alert their prescriber if these occur while taking ZYBAN.

Neuropsychiatric Symptoms and Suicide Risk in Smoking Cessation Treatment: Inform patients that quitting smoking, with or without ZYBAN, may be associated with nicotine withdrawal symptoms (including depression or agitation), or exacerbation of pre-existing psychiatric illness. Furthermore, some patients have experienced changes in mood (including depression and mania), psychosis, hallucinations, paranoia, delusions, homicidal ideation, aggression, anxiety, and panic, as well as suicidal ideation, suicide attempt, and completed suicide when attempting to quit smoking while taking ZYBAN. If patients develop agitation, hostility, depressed mood, or changes in thinking or behavior that are not typical for them, or if patients develop suicidal ideation or behavior, they should be urged to report these symptoms to their healthcare provider immediately.

Suicidal Thoughts and Behaviors: Instruct patients, their families, and/or their caregivers to be alert to the emergence of anxiety, agitation, panic attacks, insomnia, irritability, hostility, aggressiveness, impulsivity, akathisia (psychomotor restlessness), hypomania, mania, other unusual changes in behavior, worsening of depression, and suicidal ideation, especially early during antidepressant treatment and when the dose is adjusted up or down. Advise families and caregivers of patients to observe for the emergence of such symptoms on a day-to-day basis, since changes may be abrupt. Such symptoms should be reported to the patient's prescriber or healthcare professional, especially if they are severe, abrupt in onset, or were not part of the patient's presenting symptoms. Symptoms such as these may be associated with an increased risk for suicidal thinking and behavior and indicate a need for very close monitoring and possibly changes in the medication.

Severe Allergic Reactions: Educate patients on the symptoms of hypersensitivity and to discontinue ZYBAN if they have a severe allergic reaction to ZYBAN.

Seizure: Instruct patients to discontinue ZYBAN and not restart it if they experience a seizure while on treatment. Advise patients that the excessive use or abrupt discontinuation of alcohol, benzodiazepines, antiepileptic drugs, or sedatives/hypnotics can increase the risk of seizure. Advise patients to minimize or avoid use of alcohol.

Bupropion-Containing Products: Educate patients that ZYBAN contains the same active ingredient (bupropion hydrochloride) found in WELLBUTRIN, WELLBUTRIN SR, and WELLBUTRIN XL, which are used to treat depression and that ZYBAN should not be used in conjunction with any other medications that contain bupropion (such as WELLBUTRIN, the immediate-release formulation; WELLBUTRIN SR, the sustained-release formulation; WELLBUTRIN XL or FORFIVO XL™, the extended-release formulations; and APLENZIN®, the extended-release formulation of bupropion hydrobromide). In addition, there are a number of generic bupropion HCl products for the immediate-, sustained-, and extended-release formulations.

Potential for Cognitive and Motor Impairment: Advise patients that any CNS-active drug like ZYBAN may impair their ability to perform tasks requiring judgment or motor and cognitive skills. Advise patients that until they are reasonably certain that ZYBAN does not adversely affect their performance, they should refrain from driving an automobile or operating complex, hazardous machinery. ZYBAN may lead to decreased alcohol tolerance.

Concomitant Medications: Counsel patients to notify their healthcare provider if they are taking or plan to take any prescription or over-the-counter drugs because ZYBAN and other drugs may affect each others' metabolism.

Pregnancy: Advise patients to notify their healthcare provider if they become pregnant or intend to become pregnant during therapy.

Precautions for Nursing Mothers: Advise patients that ZYBAN is present in human milk in small amounts.

Storage Information: Instruct patients to store ZYBAN at room temperature, between 59°F and 86°F (15°C to 30°C) and keep the tablets dry and out of the light.

Administration Information: Instruct patients to swallow ZYBAN Tablets whole so that the release rate is not altered. Do not chew, divide, or crush tablets; they are designed to slowly release drug in the body. When patients take more than 150 mg per day, instruct them to take ZYBAN in 2 doses at least 8 hours apart, to minimize the risk of seizures. Instruct patients if they miss a dose, not to take an extra tablet to make up for the missed dose and to take the next tablet at the regular time because of the dose-related risk of seizure. ZYBAN can be taken with or without food. Advise patients that ZYBAN Tablets may have an odor.

ZYBAN, WELLBUTRIN, WELLBUTRIN SR, WELLBUTRIN XL are registered trademarks of the GSK group of companies. The other brands listed are trademarks of their respective owners and are not trademarks of the GSK group of companies. The makers of these brands are not affiliated with and do not endorse the GSK group of companies or its products.

Manufactured for:
GlaxoSmithKline
Research Triangle Park, NC 27709
©2014, the GSK group of companies. All rights reserved.
ZYB:8PI

MEDICATION GUIDE
ZYBAN® (zi ban)
(bupropion hydrochloride) Sustained-Release Tablets

Read this Medication Guide carefully before you start taking ZYBAN and each time you get a refill. There may be new information. This information does not take the place of talking with your healthcare provider about your medical condition or your treatment. If you have any questions about ZYBAN, ask your healthcare provider or pharmacist.

IMPORTANT: Be sure to read the three sections of this Medication Guide. The first section is about the risk of changes in thinking and behavior, depression and suicidal thoughts or actions with medicines used to quit smoking; the second section is about the risk of suicidal thoughts and actions with antidepressant medicines; and the third section is entitled "What Other Important Information Should I Know About ZYBAN?"

Quitting Smoking, Quit-Smoking Medications, Changes in Thinking and Behavior, Depression, and Suicidal Thoughts or Actions

This section of the Medication Guide is only about the risk of changes in thinking and behavior, depression and sui-

cidal thoughts or actions with drugs used to quit smoking. Talk to your healthcare provider or your family member's healthcare provider about:
• all risks and benefits of quit-smoking medicines.
• all treatment choices for quitting smoking.

Some people have had changes in behavior, hostility, agitation, depression, suicidal thoughts or actions while taking ZYBAN to help them quit smoking. These symptoms can develop during treatment with ZYBAN or after stopping treatment with ZYBAN.

If you, your family member, or your caregiver notice agitation, hostility, depression, or changes in thinking or behavior that are not typical for you, or you have any of the following symptoms, stop taking ZYBAN and call your healthcare provider right away:

• thoughts about suicide or dying
• attempts to commit suicide
• new or worse depression
• new or worse anxiety
• panic attacks
• feeling very agitated or restless
• acting aggressive, being angry, or violent
• acting on dangerous impulses
• an extreme increase in activity and talking (mania)
• abnormal thoughts or sensations
• seeing or hearing things that are not there (hallucinations)
• feeling people are against you (paranoia)
• feeling confused
• other unusual changes in behavior or mood

When you try to quit smoking, with or without ZYBAN, you may have symptoms that may be due to nicotine withdrawal, including urge to smoke, depressed mood, trouble sleeping, irritability, frustration, anger, feeling anxious, difficulty concentrating, restlessness, decreased heart rate, and increased appetite or weight gain. Some people have even experienced suicidal thoughts when trying to quit smoking without medication. Sometimes quitting smoking can lead to worsening of mental health problems that you already have, such as depression.

Before taking ZYBAN, tell your healthcare provider if you have ever had depression or other mental illnesses. You should also tell your healthcare provider about any symptoms you had during other times you tried to quit smoking, with or without ZYBAN.

Antidepressant Medicines, Depression and Other Serious Mental Illnesses, and Suicidal Thoughts or Actions

Although ZYBAN is not a treatment for depression, it contains bupropion, the same active ingredient as the antidepressant medications WELLBUTRIN®, WELLBUTRIN® SR, and WELLBUTRIN XL®.

This section of the Medication Guide is only about the risk of suicidal thoughts and actions with antidepressant medicines.

What is the most important information I should know about antidepressant medicines, depression and other serious mental illnesses, and suicidal thoughts or actions?

1. Antidepressant medicines may increase suicidal thoughts or actions in some children, teenagers, or young adults within the first few months of treatment.

2. Depression or other serious mental illnesses are the most important causes of suicidal thoughts and actions. Some people may have a particularly high risk of having suicidal thoughts or actions. These include people who have (or have a family history of) bipolar illness (also called manic-depressive illness) or suicidal thoughts or actions.

3. How can I watch for and try to prevent suicidal thoughts and actions in myself or a family member?
○ Pay close attention to any changes, especially sudden changes, in mood, behaviors, thoughts, or feelings. This is very important when an antidepressant medicine is started or when the dose is changed.
○ Call your healthcare provider right away to report new or sudden changes in mood, behavior, thoughts, or feelings.
○ Keep all follow-up visits with your healthcare provider as scheduled. Call the healthcare provider between visits as needed, especially if you have concerns about symptoms.

Call your healthcare provider right away if you or your family member has any of the following symptoms, especially if they are new, worse, or worry you:

• thoughts about suicide or dying
• attempts to commit suicide
• new or worse depression
• new or worse anxiety
• feeling very agitated or restless
• panic attacks
• trouble sleeping (insomnia)
• new or worse irritability
• acting aggressive, being angry, or violent
• acting on dangerous impulses
• an extreme increase in activity and talking (mania)
• other unusual changes in behavior or mood

What else do I need to know about antidepressant medicines?

• **Never stop an antidepressant medicine without first talking to a healthcare provider.** Stopping an antidepressant medicine suddenly can cause other symptoms.
• **Antidepressants are medicines used to treat depression and other illnesses.** It is important to discuss all the risks of treating depression and also the risks of not treating it. Patients and their families or other caregivers should discuss all treatment choices with the healthcare provider, not just the use of antidepressants.
• **Antidepressant medicines have other side effects.** Talk to the healthcare provider about the side effects of the medicine prescribed for you or your family member.
• **Antidepressant medicines can interact with other medicines.** Know all of the medicines that you or your family member takes. Keep a list of all medicines to show the healthcare provider. Do not start new medicines without first checking with your healthcare provider.

It is not known if ZYBAN is safe and effective in children under the age of 18.

What other important information should I know about ZYBAN?

• **Seizures: There is a chance of having a seizure (convulsion, fit) with ZYBAN, especially in people:**
○ with certain medical problems.
○ who take certain medicines.

The chance of having seizures increases with higher doses of ZYBAN. For more information, see the sections "Who should not take ZYBAN?" and "What should I tell my healthcare provider before taking ZYBAN?" Tell your healthcare provider about all of your medical conditions and all the medicines you take. **Do not take any other medicines while you are taking ZYBAN unless your healthcare provider has said it is okay to take them.**

If you have a seizure while taking ZYBAN, stop taking the tablets and call your healthcare provider right away. Do not take ZYBAN again if you have a seizure.

• **High blood pressure (hypertension).** Some people get high blood pressure that can be severe, while taking ZYBAN. The chance of high blood pressure may be higher if you also use nicotine replacement therapy (such as a nicotine patch) to help you stop smoking (see the section of this Medication Guide called "How should I take ZYBAN?").

• **Manic episodes.** Some people may have periods of mania while taking ZYBAN, including:
○ Greatly increased energy
○ Severe trouble sleeping
○ Racing thoughts
○ Reckless behavior
○ Unusually grand ideas
○ Excessive happiness or irritability
○ Talking more or faster than usual

If you have any of the above symptoms of mania, call your healthcare provider.

• **Unusual thoughts or behaviors.** Some patients have unusual thoughts or behaviors while taking ZYBAN, including delusions (believe you are someone else), hallucinations (seeing or hearing things that are not there), paranoia (feeling that people are against you), or feeling confused. If this happens to you, call your healthcare provider.

• **Severe allergic reactions.** Some people can have severe allergic reactions to ZYBAN. Stop taking ZYBAN and call your healthcare provider right away if you get a rash, itching, hives, fever, swollen lymph glands, painful sores in the mouth or around the eyes, swelling of the lips or tongue, chest pain, or have trouble breathing. These could be signs of a serious allergic reaction.

What is ZYBAN?
ZYBAN is a prescription medicine to help people quit smoking.

ZYBAN should be used with a patient support program. It is important to participate in the behavioral program, counseling, or other support program your healthcare professional recommends.

Quitting smoking can lower your chances of having lung disease, heart disease, or getting certain types of cancer that are related to smoking.

Who should not take ZYBAN?
Do not take ZYBAN if you:
• have or had a seizure disorder or epilepsy.
• have or had an eating disorder such as anorexia nervosa or bulimia.
• **are taking any other medicines that contain bupropion, including WELLBUTRIN, WELLBUTRIN SR, WELLBUTRIN XL, APLENZIN®, or FORFIVO XL™.** Bupropion is the same active ingredient that is in ZYBAN.

- drink a lot of alcohol and abruptly stop drinking, or take medicines called sedatives (these make you sleepy), benzodiazepines, or anti-seizure medicines, and you stop taking them all of a sudden.
- take a monoamine oxidase inhibitor (MAOI). Ask your healthcare provider or pharmacist if you are not sure if you take an MAOI, including the antibiotic linezolid.
  - do not take an MAOI within 2 weeks of stopping ZYBAN unless directed to do so by your healthcare provider.
  - do not start ZYBAN if you stopped taking an MAOI in the last 2 weeks unless directed to do so by your healthcare provider.
- are allergic to the active ingredient in ZYBAN, bupropion, or to any of the inactive ingredients. See the end of this Medication Guide for a complete list of ingredients in ZYBAN.

What should I tell my healthcare provider before taking ZYBAN?
Tell your healthcare provider if you have ever had depression, suicidal thoughts or actions, or other mental health problems. You should also tell your healthcare provider about any symptoms you had during other times you tried to quit smoking, with or without ZYBAN. See "Quitting Smoking, Quit-Smoking Medications, Changes in Thinking and Behavior, Depression, and Suicidal Thoughts or Actions."

- **Tell your healthcare provider about your other medical conditions, including if you:**
  - have liver problems, especially cirrhosis of the liver.
  - have kidney problems.
  - have, or have had, an eating disorder such as anorexia nervosa or bulimia.
  - have had a head injury.
  - have had a seizure (convulsion, fit).
  - have a tumor in your nervous system (brain or spine).
  - have had a heart attack, heart problems, or high blood pressure.
  - are a diabetic taking insulin or other medicines to control your blood sugar.
  - drink alcohol.
  - abuse prescription medicines or street drugs.
  - are pregnant or plan to become pregnant.
  - are breastfeeding. ZYBAN passes into your milk in small amounts.
- **Tell your healthcare provider about all the medicines you take,** including prescription, over-the-counter medicines, vitamins, and herbal supplements. Many medicines increase your chances of having seizures or other serious side effects if you take them while you are taking ZYBAN.

How should I take ZYBAN?
- Start ZYBAN before you stop smoking to give ZYBAN time to build up in your body. It takes about 1 week for ZYBAN to start working.
- Pick a date to stop smoking that is during the second week you are taking ZYBAN.
- Take ZYBAN exactly as prescribed by your healthcare provider. Do not change your dose or stop taking ZYBAN without talking with your healthcare provider first.
- ZYBAN is usually taken for 7 to 12 weeks. Your healthcare provider may decide to prescribe ZYBAN for longer than 12 weeks to help you stop smoking. Follow your healthcare provider's instructions.
- **Swallow ZYBAN Tablets whole. Do not chew, cut, or crush ZYBAN Tablets.** If you do, the medicine will be released into your body too quickly. If this happens you may be more likely to get side effects including seizures. **Tell your healthcare provider if you cannot swallow tablets.**
- ZYBAN Tablets may have an odor. This is normal.
- Take your doses of ZYBAN at least 8 hours apart.
- You may take ZYBAN with or without food.
- It is not dangerous to smoke and take ZYBAN at the same time. But, you will lower your chance of breaking your smoking habit if you smoke after the date you set to stop smoking.
- You may use ZYBAN and nicotine patches (a type of nicotine replacement therapy) at the same time, following the precautions below.
  - You should only use ZYBAN and nicotine patches together under the care of your healthcare provider. Using ZYBAN and nicotine patches together may raise your blood pressure, and sometimes this can be severe.
  - Tell your healthcare provider if you plan to use nicotine patches. Your healthcare provider should check your blood pressure regularly if you use nicotine patches with ZYBAN to help you quit smoking.
- If you miss a dose, do not take an extra dose to make up for the dose you missed. Wait and take your next dose at the regular time. **This is very important.** Too much ZYBAN can increase your chance of having a seizure.
- If you take too much ZYBAN, or overdose, call your local emergency room or poison control center right away.

Do not take any other medicines while taking ZYBAN unless your healthcare provider has told you it is okay.

What should I avoid while taking ZYBAN?
- Limit or avoid using alcohol during treatment with ZYBAN. If you usually drink a lot of alcohol, talk with your healthcare provider before suddenly stopping. If you suddenly stop drinking alcohol, you may increase your chance of having seizures.
- Do not drive a car or use heavy machinery until you know how ZYBAN affects you. ZYBAN can affect your ability to do these things safely.

What are possible side effects of ZYBAN?
ZYBAN can cause serious side effects. See the sections at the beginning of this Medication Guide for information about serious side effects of ZYBAN.
The most common side effects of ZYBAN include:
- trouble sleeping
- stuffy nose
- dry mouth
- dizziness
- feeling anxious
- nausea
- constipation
- joint aches

If you have trouble sleeping, do not take ZYBAN too close to bedtime.
Tell your healthcare provider right away about any side effects that bother you.
These are not all the possible side effects of ZYBAN. For more information, ask your healthcare provider or pharmacist.
Call your doctor for medical advice about side effects. You may report side effects to FDA at 1-800-FDA-1088.
You may also report side effects to GlaxoSmithKline at 1-888-825-5249.

How should I store ZYBAN?
- Store ZYBAN at room temperature between 59°F and 86°F (15°C to 30°C).
- Keep ZYBAN dry and out of the light.

Keep ZYBAN and all medicines out of the reach of children.
General information about ZYBAN.
Medicines are sometimes prescribed for purposes other than those listed in a Medication Guide. Do not use ZYBAN for a condition for which it was not prescribed. Do not give ZYBAN to other people, even if they have the same symptoms you have. It may harm them.
If you take a urine drug screening test, ZYBAN may make the test result positive for amphetamines. If you tell the person giving you the drug screening test that you are taking ZYBAN, they can do a more specific drug screening test that should not have this problem.
This Medication Guide summarizes important information about ZYBAN. If you would like more information, talk with your healthcare provider. You can ask your healthcare provider or pharmacist for information about ZYBAN that is written for health professionals.
For more information about ZYBAN, call 1-888-825-5249.
What are the ingredients in ZYBAN?
Active ingredient: bupropion hydrochloride.
Inactive ingredients: carnauba wax, cysteine hydrochloride, hypromellose, magnesium stearate, microcrystalline cellulose, polyethylene glycol, polysorbate 80 and titanium dioxide. The tablets are printed with edible black ink. In addition, the 150-mg tablet contains FD&C Blue No. 2 Lake and FD&C Red No. 40 Lake.
This Medication Guide has been approved by the U.S. Food and Drug Administration.
ZYBAN, WELLBUTRIN, WELLBUTRIN SR, and WELLBUTRIN XL are registered trademarks of the GSK group of companies.
The other brands listed are trademarks of their respective owners and are not trademarks of the GSK group of companies. The makers of these brands are not affiliated with and do not endorse the GSK group of companies or its products.
Manufactured for:
GlaxoSmithKline
Research Triangle Park, NC 27709
©2014, the GSK group of companies. All rights reserved.
March 2014
ZYB:8MG

Help your patients save on prescription drugs
with the PDR® Pharmacy Discount Card.
For more, visit PDR.net/PharmacyDiscountCard.

Glenwood
**111 CEDAR LANE
ENGLEWOOD, NJ 07631**

Direct Inquiries to:
Professional Services Department
201 569-0050
800 542-0772
For Medical Information Contact:
In Emergencies:
Professional Services Department
201 569-0050
800 542-0772

POTABA®
**Aminobenzoate Potassium, USP
Systemic ANTIFIBROSIS THERAPY**   ℞

FORMULA: POTABA® is chemically pure potassium p-aminobenzoate.

DESCRIPTION
POTABA® (Aminobenzoate Potassium, USP) is available in Capsules. Each Capsule contains the following inactive ingredients: Colloidal Silicon Dioxide, Stearic Acid. Capsule Shell contains: Gelatin and Titanium Dioxide. The imprinting ink contains Titanium Dioxide.

INDICATIONS
Based on a review of this drug by the National Academy of Sciences-National Research Council and/or other information, FDA has classified the indications as follows:
"Possibly" effective: Potassium aminobenzoate is possibly effective in the treatment of scleroderma, dermatomyositis, morphea, linear scleroderma, pemphigus, and Peyronie's disease.
Final classification of the less-than-effective indications requires further investigation.

ADVANTAGES: POTABA® offers a means of treatment of serious and often chronic entities involving fibrosis and nonsuppurative inflammation.

PHARMACOLOGY
p-Aminobenzoate is considered a member of the vitamin B complex. Small amounts are found in cereal, eggs, milk and meats. Detectable amounts are normally present in human blood, spinal fluid, urine, and sweat. PABA is a component of several biologically important systems, and it participates in a number of fundamental biological processes.
It has been suggested that the antifibrosis action of POTABA® is due to its mediation of increased oxygen uptake at the tissue level. Fibrosis is believed to occur from either too much serotonin or too little monoamine oxidase (MAO) activity over a period of time. Monoamine oxidase requires an adequate supply of oxygen to function properly. By increasing oxygen supply at the tissue level POTABA® may enhance MAO activity and prevent or bring about regression of fibrosis.[3]

CLINICAL USES
PEYRONIE'S DISEASE: 21 patients with Peyronie's disease were placed on POTABA® therapy for periods ranging from 3 months to 2 years. Pain disappeared from 16 of 16 cases in which it had been present. There was objective improvement in penile deformity in 10 of 17 patients, and decrease in plaque size in 16 of 21 patients. The authors suggest that this medication offers no hazard of further local injury as may result from other therapy. There were no significant untoward effects encountered on long-term POTABA® therapy.[5,10]
SCLERODERMA: Of 135 patients with diffuse systemic sclerosis treated with POTABA® every patient but one has shown softening of the involved skin if treatment has been continued for 3 months or longer. The responses have been reported in a number of publications.[9] The treatment program consists of systemic antifibrosis therapy with POTABA®, physical therapy, including deep breathing exercises and dynamic traction splints where indicated, and bethanechol chloride for relief of dysphagia as well as small doses of reserpine for amelioration of Raynaud's phenomena.[1,3]
DERMATOMYOSITIS: Five patients with scleroderma and 2 with dermatomyositis were treated with POTABA®. There was striking clinical improvement in each patient. Doses of 15-20 grams per day were well tolerated, and patients were easily able to take these doses.[6]
MORPHEA and LINEAR SCLERODERMA: All 14 patients with localized forms of scleroderma placed on long-term

POTABA® treatment showed softening of the sclerotic component of their disorder. Treatment is particularly indicated in patients where persistent compressive sclerosis may contribute even greater disfigurement or functional embarrassment from secondary pressure atrophy.[8],[9]

DOSAGE & ADMINISTRATION

The average adult daily dose of POTABA® is 12 grams, usually given in four to six divided doses. Capsules 0.5 gram are given at the rate of 4 capsules 6 times daily, or 6 given four times daily, usually with meals, and at bedtime with a snack.

Children are given 1 gram of POTABA® daily in divided doses for each 10 lbs. of body weight.

SIDE EFFECTS: Anorexia, nausea, fever and rash have occurred infrequently and subside with omission of the drug. Desensitization can be accomplished and treatment resumed.

USAGE IN PREGNANCY: Safety for use in pregnancy or during lactation has not been established.

PRECAUTIONS

Should anorexia or nausea occur, therapy is interrupted until the patient is eating normally again. This permits prompt subsidence of symptoms and also avoids the possible development of hypoglycemia. Give cautiously to patients with renal disease. If hypersensitivity reaction should occur, POTABA® should be stopped.

CONTRAINDICATIONS

POTABA® should not be administered to patients taking sulfonamides.

HOW SUPPLIED

POTABA® (Aminobenzoate Potassium, USP) Capsules 0.5 grams are supplied as No. 0 White/White Opaque Hard Gelatin Capsule Printed "POTABA 51" in black ink.
NDC-0516-0051-10 bottle of 1000
Rx only.

REFERENCES

1. From: Inflammation and Diseases of Connective Tissue, Edited by Drs. Lewis C. Mills and John H. Moyer, Published by W. B. Saunders Company, Phila. 1961.
3. Zarafonetis, Chris J. D.: Treatment of Scleroderma, Annals of Int. Med. 50:343-365 (1959).
5. Zarafonetis, C. J. D., and Horrax, T.M.: Treatment of Peyronie's Disease with POTABA, Journ. of Urology 81:770-772 (June 1959).
6. Grace. William J., Kennedy, Richard J., Formato, Anthony: Therapy of Scleroderma and Dermatomyositis, N.Y. State J. of Med. 63:140-144, 1963.
8. Zarafonetis, C. J. D.: Treatment of Localized Forms of Scleroderma, Am. J. Med. Sci. 243:147-158. 1962.
9. Zarafonetis, Chris J. D.: Antifibrotic Therapy With POTABA, Amer. Jrnl. of Med. Sci. 248: No. 5/551-561 (Nov. 1964).
10. Horrax, Trudeau M.: Peyronie's Disease, Scientific Exhibit, Amer. Urological Assn. Annl. Meet., New Orleans, May 1965.

GLENWOOD, LLC
111 Cedar Lane
Englewood, NJ 07631
REV. 11/10

Shown in Product Identification Guide, page 307

Gordon Laboratories
**6801 LUDLOW STREET
UPPER DARBY, PA 19082**

Direct inquiries to:
Customer Service
(610) 734-2011
Fax (610) 734-2049
Website: http://www.gordonlabs.net
E-mail: gordonlabs@att.net
For medical emergencies contact:
David Dercher   (610) 734-2011
                                Fax (610) 734-2049

FORMADON   ℞

INDICATIONS

Used as a drying agent for pre and postsurgical removal of warts; and as an antiperspirant in the treatment of severe conditions of hyperhidrosis and bromidrosis.

ACTIVE INGREDIENT: Formaldehyde (10% of U.S.P. strength).

DESCRIPTION

Formadon provides a preferable vehicle for the topical application of formalin solution (10% U.S.P. strength formaldehyde). It is formulated with an aqueous perfumed base which helps minimize the characteristic pungent odor.

PHARMACOLOGY

Formalin, a solution of formaldehyde, has been extensively used as a drying agent as well as a disinfectant. Direct topical application of formalin solution has been an extremely useful way of dealing with odor-causing bacteria on the surface of the skin. The elimination of hyperhidrosis is of paramount importance in reducing bacteria associated with odor and wetness. Formalin, in drying the skin surface, reduces bacteria flora which can thrive in moisture.

CONTRAINDICATIONS/WARNINGS

Avoid frequent use. Avoid contact with eyes or mucous membranes. Do not apply to open wounds. Should signs of irritation develop, medication should be discontinued. Irritates eyes, nose, and throat. Avoid breathing vapors. Use with adequate ventilation. In the event of eye contact, flush copiously with water and get medical attention. **Keep out of reach of children. For external use only.** Harmful if swallowed. Contact a local Poison Control Center immediately. **Do not induce vomiting.** If conscious, give eight ounces (240 mL) of milk, water or water with activated charcoal. Keep well closed in a cool place. **Federal law prohibits dispensing without a prescription.**

DIRECTIONS

Apply to feet twice weekly or as prescribed by a Physician.

HOW SUPPLIED

2 oz. sponge tip bottle NDC 10481-1050-05
4 oz. plastic bottle NDC 10481-1050-2
Shown in Product Identification Guide, page 307

GORDOCHOM™ Solution   OTC
[gōrdō'kōm]

DESCRIPTION

Gordochom is an antifungal solution for topical use containing 25% Undecylenic Acid and Chloroxylenol as its active ingredients in a penetrating oil base. Undecylenic Acid is chemically 10 hendecenoic acid having the empirical formula $C_{11}H_{20}O_2$ and the chemical bond structure $CH_2=CH$ $(CH_2)8$ CO_2H.

Undecylenic Acid is a colorless to pale yellow liquid. It is insoluble in water and soluble in alcohol, chloroform and ether.

Chloroxylenol is chemically 2-chloro-5-hydroxy-1,3-dimethylbenzene having the empirical formula C_8H_9ClO.

CLINICAL PHARMACOLOGY

Undecylenic Acid is a fungistatic agent employed in the treatment of tinea pedis, ringworm and dermatophytosis. Chloroxylenol is a topical antiseptic, germicide and antifungal agent effective against a wide variety of causative fungi and yeast organisms. Among those affected by Chloroxylenol are candida albicans, aspergillus niger, aspergillus flavus, trichophyton rubrum, trichophyton mentagrophytes, penicillum luteum and epidermophyton floccosum.

The penetrating oil base vehicle serves as a delivery system, enhancing the impregnation of Undecylenic Acid and Chloroxylenol as antimicrobial agents.

INDICATIONS

Cures athlete's foot (tinea pedis), and ringworm (tinea corporis).

CONTRAINDICATIONS

Gordochom is contraindicated in patients who are sensitive to Undecylenic Acid or Chloroxylenol.

WARNINGS

For external use only. Not for opthalmic or optic use. Avoid inhaling and contact with eyes or other mucous membranes. Not to be applied over blistered, raw or oozing areas of skin or over deep puncture wounds.

PRECAUTIONS

If a reaction suggesting sensitivity or chemical irritation should occur with the use of Gordochom, treatment should be discontinued. Use of Gordochom in pregnancy has not been established. **Keep out of reach of children.**

ADVERSE REACTIONS

No significant adverse reactions have been reported. However, attention should be paid to localized hypersensitivity.

DOSAGE AND ADMINISTRATION

Cleanse and dry affected areas. Apply a thin application twice a day (morning and night) to the affected area, or as recommended by your physician. For athlete's foot, pay spe-cial attention to the spaces between the toes; wear well-fitting, ventilated shoes, and change shoes and socks at least once daily. For athlete's foot and ringworm, use daily for 4 weeks. If condition persists longer, consult a physician. This product has not been proven effective on the scalp or nails.

HOW SUPPLIED

Gordochom is available in 1 oz. bottles with special brush applicator. (NDC 10481-8010-2)
Store at controlled room temperatures (59°–86°F).
Shown in Product Identification Guide, page 307

Halozyme Therapeutics, Inc.
**11388 SORRENTO VALLEY ROAD
SAN DIEGO, CA 92121**

Direct Inquires to:
858-794-8889

HYLENEX RECOMBINANT   ℞
(hyaluronidase human injection)

HIGHLIGHTS OF PRESCRIBING INFORMATION
These highlights do not include all the information needed to use HYLENEX recombinant safely and effectively. See full prescribing information for HYLENEX recombinant.
HYLENEX recombinant (hyaluronidase human injection)
Initial U.S. Approval: 2005

───────INDICATIONS AND USAGE───────

HYLENEX recombinant is a tissue permeability modifier indicated as an adjuvant
• in subcutaneous fluid administration for achieving hydration (1.1)
• to increase the dispersion and absorption of other injected drugs (1.2)
• in subcutaneous urography for improving resorption of radiopaque agents (1.3)

────DOSAGE AND ADMINISTRATION────

• Subcutaneous fluid administration:
Inject 150 U HYLENEX recombinant prior to subcutaneous fluid administration. It will facilitate absorption of 1,000 mL or more of solution. The dosage of subcutaneous fluids administered is dependent upon the age, weight, and clinical condition of the patient as well as laboratory determinations. The rate and volume of subcutaneous fluid administration should not exceed those employed for intravenous infusion. (2.1)
• Increasing dispersion and absorption of injected or subcutaneously infused drugs:
Inject 50-300 U (most typically 150 U) HYLENEX recombinant prior to drug administration. Alternatively, add 50-300 U (most typically 150 U) HYLENEX recombinant to the injection solution. (2.2)
• Subcutaneous Urography:
Inject 75 U HYLENEX recombinant subcutaneously over each scapula, followed by injection of the contrast medium at the same sites. (2.3)

───DOSAGE FORMS AND STRENGTHS───

• 150 USP units/mL single dose vials (3)

──────────CONTRAINDICATIONS──────────

• Hypersensitivity (4)

─────WARNINGS AND PRECAUTIONS─────

• Spread of Localized Infection (5.1)
• Ocular Damage (5.2)
• Enzyme Inactivation with Intravenous Administration (5.3)
• Products Containing Plasma-derived Albumin (5.4)

───────────ADVERSE REACTIONS───────────

• Allergic and anaphylactic-like reactions have been reported, rarely. (6)
To report SUSPECTED ADVERSE REACTIONS, contact Halozyme Therapeutics, Inc. at 1-877-877-1679 or FDA at 1-800-FDA-1088 or www.fda.gov/medwatch.

────────DRUG INTERACTIONS────────

• Furosemide, the benzodiazepines and phenytoin are incompatible with hyaluronidase. (7.1)
• Hyaluronidase should not be used to enhance the dispersion and absorption of dopamine and/or alpha agonist drugs. (7.2)
• Local anesthetics: Hyaluronidase hastens onset and shortens duration of effect, increases incidence of systemic reactions. (7.3)

- Large doses of salicylates, cortisone, ACTH, estrogens or antihistamines may require larger amounts of hyaluronidase for equivalent dispersing effect. (7.4)

—————USE IN SPECIFIC POPULATIONS—————

- Pediatric Use: The dosage of subcutaneous fluids administered is dependent upon the age, weight, and clinical condition of the patient. For premature infants or during the neonatal period, the daily dosage should not exceed 25 mL/kg of body weight, and the rate of administration should not be greater than 2 mL per minute. Special care must be taken in pediatric patients to avoid over hydration by controlling the rate and total volume of the infusion. (2.1, 8.4, 14)

See 17 for PATIENT COUNSELING INFORMATION
Revised: 02/2013

FULL PRESCRIBING INFORMATION: CONTENTS*

* Sections or subsections omitted from the full prescribing information are not listed

FULL PRESCRIBING INFORMATION

1   INDICATIONS AND USAGE
1.1   Subcutaneous Fluid Administration
HYLENEX recombinant is indicated as an adjuvant in subcutaneous fluid administration for achieving hydration.
1.2   Dispersion and Absorption of Injected Drugs
HYLENEX recombinant is indicated as an adjuvant to increase the dispersion and absorption of other injected drugs.
1.3   Subcutaneous Urography
HYLENEX recombinant is indicated as an adjunct in subcutaneous urography for improving resorption of radiopaque agents.

2   DOSAGE AND ADMINISTRATION
Parenteral drug products should be inspected visually for particulate matter and discoloration prior to administration whenever solution and container permit.
Always use aseptic precautions. Lightly pinch the skin up into a small mound and insert the needle/catheter into the subcutaneous space. Inject HYLENEX recombinant through the catheter hub or injection port closest to the needle/catheter. Begin administration of solution. Solution should start in readily.
2.1   Subcutaneous Fluid Administration
150 U of HYLENEX recombinant injected prior to start of subcutaneous fluid administration will facilitate absorption

of 1,000 mL or more of solution. As with all parenteral fluid therapy, observe effect closely, with the same precautions for restoring fluid and electrolyte balance as in intravenous injections. The dose, the rate of injection, and the type of solution (saline, glucose, Ringer's, etc.) must be adjusted carefully to the individual patient. When solutions devoid of inorganic electrolytes are administered subcutaneously, hypovolemia may occur. This may be prevented by using solutions containing adequate amounts of inorganic electrolytes and/or controlling the volume and speed of administration. HYLENEX recombinant may be added to small volumes of solution, such as fluid replacement solutions or solutions of drugs for subcutaneous injection. Subcutaneous fluids should be administered as directed by a physician. The dosage of subcutaneous fluids administered is dependent upon the age, weight, and clinical condition of the patient as well as laboratory determinations. The rate and volume of subcutaneous fluid administration should not exceed those employed for intravenous infusion. For premature infants or during the neonatal period, the daily dosage should not exceed 25 mL/kg of body weight, and the rate of administration should not be greater than 2 mL per minute.
2.2   Dispersion and Absorption of Injected Drugs
Dispersion and absorption of other injected or subcutaneously infused drugs may be enhanced by pre-administration of HYLENEX recombinant or by adding 50-300 U, most typically 150 U hyaluronidase, to the injection solution.
2.3   Subcutaneous Urography
The subcutaneous route of administration of urographic contrast media is indicated when intravenous administration cannot be successfully accomplished, particularly in infants and small children. With the patient prone, 75 U of HYLENEX recombinant is injected subcutaneously over each scapula, followed by injection of the contrast medium at the same sites.

3   DOSAGE FORMS AND STRENGTHS
150 USP units/mL single dose vials

4   CONTRAINDICATIONS
HYLENEX recombinant is contraindicated in patients with known hypersensitivity to hyaluronidase or any of the excipients in HYLENEX recombinant. A preliminary skin test for hypersensitivity to HYLENEX recombinant can be performed. The skin test is made by an intradermal injection of approximately 0.02 mL (3 Units) of a 150 Unit/mL solution. A positive reaction consists of a wheal with pseudopods appearing within 5 minutes and persisting for 20 to 30 minutes and accompanied by localized itching. Transient vasodilation at the site of the test, i.e., erythema, is not a positive reaction. Discontinue HYLENEX recombinant if sensitization occurs.

5   WARNINGS AND PRECAUTIONS
5.1   Spread of Localized Infection
Hyaluronidase should not be injected into or around an infected or acutely inflamed area because of the danger of spreading a localized infection.
Hyaluronidase should not be used to reduce the swelling of bites or stings.
5.2   Ocular Damage
Hyaluronidase should not be applied directly to the cornea. It is not for topical use.
5.3   Enzyme Inactivation with Intravenous Administration
HYLENEX recombinant should not be administered intravenously. Its effects relative to dispersion and absorption of other drugs are not produced when it is administered intravenously because the enzyme is rapidly inactivated.
5.4   Products Containing Plasma-derived Albumin
This product contains albumin, a derivative of human blood. Based on effective donor screening and product manufacturing processes, it carries an extremely remote risk for transmission of viral diseases and variant Creutzfeldt-Jakob disease (vCJD). There is a theoretical risk for transmission of Creutzfeldt-Jakob disease (CJD), but if that risk actually exists, the risk of transmission would also be considered extremely remote. No cases of transmission of viral diseases, CJD, or vCJD have ever been identified for licensed albumin or albumin contained in other licensed products.

6   ADVERSE REACTIONS
The following adverse reactions have been identified during post-approval use of hyaluronidase products. Because these reactions are reported voluntarily from a population of uncertain size, it is not always possible to reliably estimate their frequency or establish a causal relationship to drug exposure.
The most frequently reported adverse reactions have been mild local injection site reactions such as erythema and pain. Hyaluronidase has been reported to enhance the adverse reactions associated with co-administered drug products. Edema has been reported most frequently in association with subcutaneous fluid administration. Allergic reactions (urticaria or angioedema) have been reported in

less than 0.1% of patients receiving hyaluronidase. Anaphylactic-like reactions following retrobulbar block or intravenous injections have occurred, rarely.

7   DRUG INTERACTIONS
It is recommended that appropriate references be consulted regarding physical or chemical incompatibilities before adding HYLENEX recombinant to a solution containing another drug.
7.1   Incompatibilities
Furosemide, the benzodiazepines and phenytoin have been found to be incompatible with hyaluronidase.
7.2   Drug-Specific Precautions
Hyaluronidase should not be used to enhance the dispersion and absorption of dopamine and/or alpha agonist drugs.
When considering the administration of any other drug with hyaluronidase, it is recommended that appropriate references first be consulted to determine the usual precautions for the use of the other drug.
7.3   Local Anesthetics
When hyaluronidase is added to a local anesthetic agent, it hastens the onset of analgesia and tends to reduce the swelling caused by local infiltration, but the wider spread of the local anesthetic solution increases its absorption; this shortens its duration of action and tends to increase the incidence of systemic reaction.
7.4   Salicylates, Cortisone, ACTH, Estrogens and Antihistamines
Patients receiving large doses of salicylates, cortisone, ACTH, estrogens or antihistamines may require larger amounts of hyaluronidase for equivalent dispersing effect, since these drugs apparently render tissues partly resistant to the action of hyaluronidase.

8   USE IN SPECIFIC POPULATIONS
8.1   Pregnancy
Pregnancy Category C. In an embryo-fetal study, mice have been dosed daily by subcutaneous injection with recombinant human hyaluronidase at dose levels up to 2,200,000 U/kg. The study found no evidence of teratogenicity. Reduced fetal weight and increased numbers of fetal resorptions were observed, with no effects found at a daily dose of 360,000 U/kg, which represents several orders of magnitude over the suggested human dose range of 50-300 U of HYLENEX recombinant (0.8-5 U/kg in a 60 kg subject).
In a pre- and postnatal development study, mice have been dosed daily by subcutaneous injection with recombinant human hyaluronidase at dose levels up to 1,100,000 U/kg. The study found no adverse effects on sexual maturation, learning and memory of offspring, or their ability to produce another generation of offspring.
It is also not known whether HYLENEX recombinant can cause fetal harm when administered to a pregnant woman. HYLENEX recombinant should be given to a pregnant woman only if clearly needed.
8.2   Labor and Delivery
Administration of hyaluronidase during labor was reported to cause no complications: no increase in blood loss or differences in cervical trauma were observed.
8.3   Nursing Mothers
It is not known whether hyaluronidase is excreted in human milk. Because many drugs are excreted in human milk, caution should be exercised when hyaluronidase is administered to a nursing woman.
8.4   Pediatric Use
Clinical hydration requirements for children can be achieved through administration of subcutaneous fluids facilitated with HYLENEX recombinant.
The dosage of subcutaneous fluids administered is dependent upon the age, weight, and clinical condition of the patient as well as laboratory determinations. The potential for chemical or physical incompatibilities should be kept in mind [see Drug Interactions (7)].
The rate and volume of subcutaneous fluid administration should not exceed those employed for intravenous infusion. For premature infants or during the neonatal period, the daily dosage should not exceed 25 mL/kg of body weight, and the rate of administration should not be greater than 2 mL per minute.
During subcutaneous fluid administration, special care must be taken in pediatric patients to avoid over hydration by controlling the rate and total volume of the infusion [see Dosage and Administration (2.1)].
8.5   Geriatric Use
No overall differences in safety or effectiveness have been observed between elderly and younger adult patients.

11   DESCRIPTION
HYLENEX recombinant is a purified preparation of the enzyme recombinant human hyaluronidase. HYLENEX recombinant is produced by genetically engineered Chinese Hamster Ovary (CHO) cells containing a DNA plasmid encoding for a soluble fragment of human hyaluronidase

(PH20). The purified hyaluronidase glycoprotein contains 447 amino acids with an approximate molecular weight of 61,000 Daltons.

HYLENEX recombinant is supplied as a sterile, clear, colorless, nonpreserved, ready for use solution. Each mL contains 150 USP units of recombinant human hyaluronidase with 8.5 mg sodium chloride, 1.4 mg dibasic sodium phosphate, 1 mg albumin human, 0.9 mg edetate disodium, 0.3 mg calcium chloride, and sodium hydroxide added for pH adjustment.

HYLENEX recombinant has an approximate pH of 7.0 and an osmolality of 290 to 350 mOsm.

12 CLINICAL PHARMACOLOGY
12.1 Mechanism of Action
Hyaluronidase is a dispersion agent, which modifies the permeability of connective tissue through the hydrolysis of hyaluronic acid, a polysaccharide found in the intercellular ground substance of connective tissue, and of certain specialized tissues, such as the umbilical cord and vitreous humor. Hyaluronic acid is also present in the capsules of type A and C hemolytic streptococci. Hyaluronidase hydrolyzes hyaluronic acid by splitting the glucosaminidic bond between C1 of an N-acetylglucosamine moiety and C4 of a glucuronic acid moiety. This temporarily decreases the viscosity of the cellular cement and promotes dispersion of injected fluids or of localized transudates or exudates, thus facilitating their absorption.

Hyaluronidase cleaves glycosidic bonds of hyaluronic acid and, to a variable degree, some other acid mucopolysaccharides of the connective tissue. The activity is measured in vitro by monitoring the decrease in the amount of an insoluble serum albumin-hyaluronic acid complex as the enzyme cleaves the hyaluronic acid component.

12.2 Pharmacodynamics
In the absence of hyaluronidase, material injected subcutaneously disperses very slowly. Hyaluronidase facilitates dispersion, provided local interstitial pressure is adequate to furnish the necessary mechanical impulse. Such an impulse is normally initiated by injected solutions. The rate and extent of dispersion and absorption is proportionate to the amount of hyaluronidase and the volume of solution.

The reconstitution of the dermal barrier removed by intradermal injection of hyaluronidase (20, 2, 0.2, 0.02, and 0.002 U/mL) to adult humans indicated that at 24 hours the restoration of the barrier is incomplete and inversely related to the dosage of hyaluronidase; at 48 hours, the barrier is completely restored in all treated areas.

Results from an experimental study, in humans, on the influence of hyaluronidase in bone repair support the conclusion that hyaluronidase alone, in the usual clinical dosage, does not deter bone healing.

12.3 Pharmacokinetics
Knowledge of the mechanisms involved in the disappearance of injected hyaluronidase is limited. It is known, however, that the components in blood of a number of mammalian species bring about the inactivation of hyaluronidase. Studies have demonstrated that hyaluronidase is antigenic; repeated injections of relatively large amounts of hyaluronidase preparations may result in the formation of neutralizing antibodies.

13 NONCLINICAL TOXICOLOGY
13.1 Carcinogenesis, Mutagenesis, Impairment of Fertility
Hyaluronidase is found in most tissues of the body. Long-term animal studies have not been performed to assess the carcinogenic or mutagenic potential of hyaluronidase.

Human studies on the effect of intravaginal hyaluronidase in sterility due to oligospermia indicated that hyaluronidase may have aided conception. Thus, it appears that hyaluronidase may not adversely affect fertility in females. In addition, when recombinant human hyaluronidase was administered to cynomolgus monkeys for 39 weeks at dose levels up to 220,000 U/kg, no evidence of toxicity to the male or female reproductive system was found through periodic monitoring of in-life parameters, e.g., semen analyses, hormone levels, menstrual cycles, and also from gross pathology, histopathology and organ weight data.

14 CLINICAL STUDIES
HYLENEX recombinant facilitated the administration of subcutaneous fluids in pediatric patients with mild to moderate dehydration in an open-label, multicenter, single arm study in fifty-one (51) patients. A subcutaneous injection of 1 mL (150 U) of HYLENEX recombinant was immediately followed by subcutaneous infusion of isotonic fluids in either the mid-anterior thigh or the inter-scapular area of the upper back.

The safety and flow rate of subcutaneously administered Lactated Ringer's (LR) solution with and without HYLENEX recombinant was evaluated in a prospective, randomized, double-blinded, placebo-controlled, within-subject, single-center study in fifty-four (54) healthy volun-

teers. The mean HYLENEX recombinant facilitated infusion rate was 464 mL/hr versus 118 mL/hr for the saline control (p < 0.001, paired t-test).

16 HOW SUPPLIED/STORAGE AND HANDLING
HYLENEX recombinant is supplied sterile as 150 USP units of nonpreserved recombinant human hyaluronidase per mL in a single-use glass vial.
HYLENEX recombinant is supplied in the following packaging:
1 mL Single Dose Vial (NDC 18657-102-01) available in boxes of 4 (NDC 18657-102-04) or 10 (NDC 18657-102-10)
Store unopened in a refrigerator at 2° to 8°C (36° to 46° F). DO NOT FREEZE.

17 PATIENT COUNSELING INFORMATION
17.1 Important Precautions Regarding HYLENEX recombinant
Instruct patient that HYLENEX recombinant is being used to increase the dispersion and absorption of fluids or other injected drugs, as appropriate to the intended use.
Instruct patient that there may be mild local injection site signs and symptoms, such as redness, swelling, itching, or pain localized to the site of injection.

17.2 What Patients Should Know About Adverse Reactions
Patients should be advised that the most frequently reported adverse reactions have been mild local injection site reactions such as redness, swelling, itching, or pain.
Anaphylactic-like reactions, and allergic reactions, such as hives, have been reported rarely in patients receiving hyaluronidases.

17.3 Patients Should Inform Their Doctors If Taking Other Medications
Instruct patients that they may not receive furosemide, the benzodiazepines, phenytoin, dopamine and/or alpha agonists with HYLENEX recombinant. These medications have been found to be incompatible with hyaluronidase.
Patients should be advised that if they are taking salicylates (e.g., aspirin), steroids (e.g., cortisone or estrogens), or antihistamines, they may need to be prescribed larger amounts of hyaluronidase for equivalent dispersing effect.
Halozyme and Hylenex are registered trademarks of Halozyme, Inc.
U.S. Patent No. 7,767,429
Manufactured for and Marketed by: Halozyme Therapeutics, Inc.
San Diego, CA 92121
For Product Inquiry: 1-855-495-3639
Rev. February 2013
LBL293-05

Shown in Product Identification Guide, page 307

Heel
10421 Research Road SE
Albuquerque, NM 87123

Direct Inquiries to:
Medical Department
(800) 621-7644
Fax: (800) 217-6934
www.heelusa.com
info@heelusa.com

TRAUMEEL®
Injection Solution, Parenteral Use   ℞

HIGHLIGHTS OF PRESCRIBING INFORMATION
Traumeel® Injection Solution, Parenteral Use Rx Only

These highlights do not include all the information needed to use **Traumeel® Injection Solution** safely and effectively. See full prescribing information for Traumeel®.

—————INDICATIONS AND USAGE—————
Traumeel® Injection Solution is a homeopathic drug indicated:
- As a mono-therapy, for the treatment of injuries, inflammatory and degenerative conditions of the musculoskeletal system and for the relief of associated symptoms such as pain. (1.1)
- In combination with Zeel® Injection Solution, for the treatment of inflammatory and degenerative conditions of the musculoskeletal system, such as arthrosis/osteoarthritis and/or rheumatic joint diseases, and for the relief of symptoms including pain, swelling, and joint stiffness. (1.2)

————DOSAGE AND ADMINISTRATION————
- Standard Dosage:
  Adults and children 12 years and older:
  1 ampule 1 to 3 times per 7 days

Children 6 to 11 years:
⅔ of an ampule 1 to 3 times per 7 days
Children 2 to 5 years:
½ ampule 1 to 3 times per 7 days (2)
- Acute Dosage:
  Adults and children 12 years and older:
  1 ampule daily, and then continue with standard dosage.
  Children 6 to 11 years: ⅔ of an ampule daily, and then continue with standard dosage.
  Children 2 to 5 years: ½ ampule daily, and then continue with standard dosage. (2)
- When co-administered with Zeel® Injection Solution, the two products may be mixed 1:1.

———DOSAGE FORMS AND STRENGTHS———
- 1 ampule containing 2.2 ml each containing the active ingredients in the strengths listed under Description. (10)

—————CONTRAINDICATIONS—————
- Traumeel® Injection Solution is contraindicated in patients with known hypersensitivity to Traumeel® or any of its ingredients. (4)

———WARNINGS AND PRECAUTIONS———
- Keep out of reach of children. (5)

—————ADVERSE REACTIONS—————
- Allergic (hypersensitivity) reactions, (e.g. skin allergies, redness/swelling at the injection site, even up to anaphylaxis) may occur in isolated cases. (6)
- To report SUSPECTED ADVERSE REACTIONS, contact Heel Inc. at 1.800.920.9203 or info@heelusa.com or FDA at 1-800-FDA-1088 or www.fda.gov/medwatch.

—————DRUG INTERACTIONS—————
- None known (7)

———USE IN SPECIFIC POPULATIONS———
- No studies have been conducted with Traumeel® Injection Solution on pregnant or lactating women, children, or elderly. (8)

Revised: 01/2014

FULL PRESCRIBING INFORMATION
1 Indications and Usage
1.1 Treatment of injuries and various conditions of the musculoskeletal system.
- Traumeel® Injection Solution is a homeopathic drug product indicated for the treatment of injuries, inflammatory and degenerative conditions of the musculoskeletal system and for the relief of associated symptoms such as pain.

1.2 Co-administration Therapy with Zeel® Injection Solution for the treatment of inflammatory and degenerative conditions of the musculoskeletal system.

- Traumeel® Injection Solution is a homeopathic drug product indicated, in combination with Zeel® Injection Solution, for the treatment of inflammatory and degenerative conditions of the musculoskeletal system, such as arthrosis/osteoarthritis and/or rheumatic joint diseases, and for the relief of symptoms including pain, swelling, and joint stiffness.

2 Dosage and Administration

2.1 General Considerations

- The dosage schedules listed below can be used as a general guide for the administration of Traumeel® Injection Solution.
- If co-administration with a local anesthetic is desired, Traumeel® Injection Solution may be mixed with lidocaine or similar agents at the discretion of the physician.
- Traumeel® Injection solution may be administered s.c., i.d., i.m., i.a. or i.v.
- The interval between injections is left to the discretion of the HCP, but should not exceed 1 ampule in 24 hours.
- Parenteral drug products should be inspected visually for particulate matter and discoloration prior to administration, whenever solution and container permit. Draw up the contents of the ampule into the syringe. Discard half or one third of the contents, depending on the required dosage, before administering.

2.2 Standard Dosage

for the treatment of injuries, inflammatory and degenerative conditions of the musculoskeletal system and for the relief of associated symptoms such as pain.

Adults and children 12 years and older:
1 ampule 1 to 3 times per 7 days
Children 6 to 11 years:
⅔ of an ampule 1 to 3 times per 7 days
Children 2 to 5 years:
½ ampule 1 to 3 times per 7 days

2.3 Acute Dosage

for the treatment of injuries, inflammatory and degenerative conditions of the musculoskeletal system and for the relief of associated symptoms such as pain.

Adults and children 12 years and older:
1 ampule daily, and then continue with standard dosage.
Children 6 to 11 years:
⅔ of an ampule daily, and then continue with standard dosage.
Children 2 to 5 years:
½ ampule daily, and then continue with standard dosage.

2.4 Co-administration therapy with Zeel® Injection Solution

for the treatment of inflammatory and degenerative conditions of the musculoskeletal system, such as arthrosis/osteoarthritis and/or rheumatic joint diseases, and for the relief of symptoms including pain, swelling, and joint stiffness.

- In the treatment of musculoskeletal conditions, if co-administration with another homeopathic medicinal product is desired, Traumeel® Injection Solution may be mixed in a ratio of 1:1 with Zeel® Injection Solution.
- For convenience, the daily dose of Traumeel® Injection Solution may be administered at the same time as a Zeel® Injection Solution, according to the dosing recommendations for each medication.

2.5 Instructions for Opening Glass Ampule

- Cutting open the glass ampule is not necessary. Hold the ampule up at an angle, and tap/shake down the solution contained in the ampule head. Then break off the ampule head by applying pressure away from the color dot. Discard unused solution.

3 Dosage Forms and Strength

One ampule containing 2.2 ml each containing the active ingredients in the strengths listed under Description. (10)

4 Contraindications

- Traumeel® Injection Solution is contraindicated in patients with known hypersensitivity to Traumeel® or any of its ingredients.
- When Traumeel® Injection Solution is co-administered with Zeel® Injection Solution, refer to the *Contraindications* section of the respective Zeel® Injection Solution labeling.

5 Warnings and Precautions

Keep out of reach of children.

Active Ingredients:

Ingredient name	Potency	Quantity	Final dilution
Aconitum napellus	2X	1.32 µl	5.22X
Arnica montana, radix	2X	2.20 µl	5.00X
Bellis perennis	2X	1.10 µl	5.30X
Belladonna	2X	2.20 µl	5.00X
Calendula officinalis	2X	2.20 µl	5.00X
Chamomilla	3X	2.20 µl	6.00X
Echinacea	2X	0.55 µl	5.60X
Echinacea purpurea	2X	0.55 µl	5.60X
Hamamelis virginiana	1X	0.22 µl	5.00X
Hepar sulphuris calcareum	6X	2.20 µl	9.00X
Hypericum perforatum	2X	0.66 µl	5.52X
Mercurius solubilis	6X	1.10 µl	9.30X
Millefolium	3X	2.20 µl	6.00X
Symphytum officinale	6X	2.20 µl	9.00X

6 Adverse Reactions

6.1 Post-marketing Experience

- The following adverse events have been identified during post-marketing use of Traumeel® Injection Solution. Because these events are reported voluntarily from a population of uncertain size, it is not always possible to reliably estimate their frequency or establish a causal relationship to drug exposure.
- Adverse event rates observed in Monotherapy use of Traumeel® Injection Solution: Allergic (hypersensitivity) reactions (e.g. skin allergies, redness/swelling at the injection site, even up to anaphylaxis) may occur in isolated cases.
- Adverse event rates observed in the Monotherapy use of Zeel® Injection Solution: Allergic (hypersensitivity) skin reactions may occur in isolated cases.

7 Drug Interactions

No interactions have been reported, and none are expected due to the homeopathic dilutions.

8 Use in Specific Populations

8.1 Pregnancy

8.1.1 Teratogenic effects

Pregnancy Category C. Some ingredients in Traumeel® Injection Solution have been shown to be teratogenic in various animal species when given in doses several thousand times the human dose. There are no adequate and well-controlled studies in pregnant women. Traumeel® Injection solution should be used during pregnancy only if the potential benefit justifies the potential risk to the fetus. When Traumeel® Injection Solution is administered with Zeel® Injection Solution in a woman of childbearing age, refer to the pregnancy category and product labelling for Zeel® Injection Solution.

8.1.2 Non-teratogenic effects

No known non-teratogenic effects.

8.2 Labor and Delivery

No recognized use in labor or delivery.

8.3 Nursing Mothers:

It is not known whether this drug is excreted in human milk. Because many drugs are excreted in human milk, caution should be exercised when Traumeel® Injection Solution is administered to a nursing woman.

8.4 Pediatric Use

Safety and effectiveness in pediatric patients have not been established. However, traditional homeopathic use of the ingredients in Traumeel® Injection Solution has not identified differences in responses between adults and pediatric patients.

8.5 Geriatric Use

Safety and effectiveness in geriatric patients have not been established. However, traditional homeopathic use of the of the ingredients in Traumeel® Injection Solution has not identified differences in responses between adults and geriatric patients.

9 Overdosage

No negative effects of an overdose have been reported and none are expected due to the homeopathic dilutions.

10 Description

10.1 Ingredients

- Each 2.2 ml ampule contains:
[See table above]
Inactive Ingredients:
Water for injection   2,179.10 µl
Sodium Chloride   19.40 µl

10.2 Pharmaceutical Form

- Injection solution

10.3 Route of Administration

- Parenteral: s.c., i.d., i.m., i.a. or i.v

11 Clinical Pharmacology

11.1 Mechanism of Action

The exact mechanism of Traumeel® Injection Solution is not fully understood.

11.2 Pharmacodynamics

Not applicable for homeopathic medicinal products.

12 References

- Homeopathic Pharmacopeia of the United States Revision Service

13 How Supplied / Storage and handling

13.1 Dosage forms and package sizes

- 1 ampule of 2.2 ml in packs of 10 ampules
- NDC 50114-7004-1

13.2 Storage and handling

- Store at room temperature. Protect from light.
  Shown in Product Identification Guide, page 307

ZEEL®   ℞

Injection Solution, Parenteral Use

HIGHLIGHTS OF PRESCRIBING INFORMATION

Zeel® Injection Solution, Parenteral Use Rx Only

These highlights do not include all the information needed to use **Zeel® Injection Solution** safely and effectively. See full prescribing information for Zeel®.

——INDICATIONS AND USAGE——

Zeel® Injection Solution is a homeopathic drug indicated:
- As a mono-therapy, for the treatment of arthrosis/osteoarthritis, and/or rheumatic joint diseases and for the relief of symptoms such as pain and joint stiffness. (1.1)
- In combination with Traumeel® Injection Solution, for the treatment of inflammatory and degenerative conditions of the musculoskeletal system, such as arthrosis /osteoarthritis and/or rheumatic joint diseases, and for the relief of symptoms including pain, swelling, and joint stiffness. (1.2)

DOSAGE AND ADMINISTRATION

- Standard Dosage:
  Adults and children 12 years and older:
  1 ampule 1 to 3 times per 7 days
  Children 6 to 11 years:
  ⅔ of an ampule 1 to 3 times per 7 days (2)
- Acute Dosage:
  Adults and children 12 years and older:
  1 ampule daily, and then continue with standard dosage.
  Children 6 to 11 years:
  ⅔ of an ampule daily, and then continue with standard dosage. (2)
- When co-administered with Traumeel® Injection Solution, the two products may be mixed 1:1.

DOSAGE FORMS AND STRENGTHS

- 1 ampule containing 2.0 ml each containing the active ingredients in the strengths listed under Description. (10)

CONTRAINDICATIONS

- Zeel® Injection Solution is contraindicated in patients with known hypersensitivity to Zeel® or any of its ingredients. (4)

WARNINGS AND PRECAUTIONS

- Keep out of reach of children. (5)

ADVERSE REACTIONS

- Allergic (hypersensitivity) skin reactions may occur in isolated cases. (6)
- To report SUSPECTED ADVERSE REACTIONS, contact Heel Inc. at 1.800.920.9203 info@heelusa.com or FDA at 1-800-FDA-1088 or www.fda.gov/medwatch.

DRUG INTERACTIONS

- None known (7)

USE IN SPECIFIC POPULATIONS

- No studies have been conducted with Zeel® Injection Solution on pregnant or lactating women, children, or elderly. (8)

Revised: 01/2014

FULL PRESCRIBING INFORMATION: CONTENTS*

FULL PRESCRIBING INFORMATION

1 Indications and Usage

1.1 Treatment of arthrosis/osteoarthritis, and/or rheumatic joint diseases

- Zeel® Injection Solution is a homeopathic drug product indicated for the treatment of arthrosis/osteoarthritis, and/or rheumatic joint diseases and for the relief of symptoms such as pain and joint stiffness.

1.2 Co-administration Therapy with Traumeel® Injection Solution for the treatment of inflammatory and degenerative conditions of the musculoskeletal system.

- Zeel® Injection Solution is a homeopathic drug product indicated, in combination with Traumeel® Injection Solution, for the treatment of inflammatory and degenerative conditions of the musculoskeletal system, such as arthrosis/osteoarthritis and/or rheumatic joint diseases, and for the relief of symptoms including pain, swelling, and joint stiffness.

2 Dosage and Administration

2.1 General Considerations

- The dosage schedules listed below can be used as a general guide for the administration of Zeel® Injection Solution.
- If co-administration with a local anesthetic is desired, Zeel® Injection Solution may be mixed with lidocaine or similar agents at the discretion of the physician.
- Zeel® Injection solution may be administered s.c., i.d., i.m., i.a. or i.v.
- The interval between injections is left to the discretion of the HCP, but should not exceed 1 ampule in 24 hours.
- Parenteral drug products should be inspected visually for particulate matter and discoloration prior to administration, whenever solution and container permit. Draw up the contents of the ampule into the syringe. Discard half or one third of the contents, depending on the required dosage, before administering.

2.2 Standard Dosage

for the treatment of arthrosis/osteoarthritis, and/or rheumatic joint diseases and for the relief of symptoms such as pain and joint stiffness.

Adults and children 12 years and older:
1 ampule 1 to 3 times per 7 days
Children 6 to 11 years:
⅔ of an ampule 1 to 3 times per 7 days

2.3 Acute Dosage

for the treatment of arthrosis/osteoarthritis, and/or rheumatic joint diseases and for the relief of symptoms such as pain and joint stiffness.

Adults and children 12 years and older:
1 ampule daily, and then continue with standard dosage.
Children 6 to 11 years:
⅔ of an ampule daily, and then continue with standard dosage.

2.4 Co-administration therapy with Traumeel® Injection Solution

for the treatment of inflammatory and degenerative conditions of the musculoskeletal system, such as arthrosis/osteoarthritis and/or rheumatic joint diseases, and for the relief of symptoms including pain, swelling, and joint stiffness.

- In the treatment of musculoskeletal conditions, if co-administration with another homeopathic medicinal product is desired, Zeel® Injection Solution may be mixed in a ratio of 1:1 with Traumeel® Injection Solution.
- For convenience, the daily dose of Zeel® Injection Solution may be administered at the same time as a Traumeel® Injection Solution, according to the dosing recommendations for each medication.

2.5 Instructions for Opening Glass Ampule

- Cutting open the glass ampule is not necessary. Hold the ampule up at an angle, and tap/shake down the solution contained in the ampule head. Then break off the ampule head by applying pressure away from the color dot. Discard unused solution.

3 Dosage Forms and Strength

One ampule containing 2.0 ml each containing the active ingredients in the strengths listed under Description. (10)

4 Contraindications

- Zeel® Injection Solution is contraindicated in patients with known hypersensitivity to Zeel® or any of its ingredients.
- When Zeel® Injection Solution is co-administered with Traumeel® Injection Solution, refer to the *Contraindications* section of the respective Traumeel® Injection Solution labeling.

5 Warnings and Precautions

Keep out of reach of children.

6 Adverse Reactions

6.1 Post-marketing Experience

- The following adverse events have been identified during post-marketing use of Zeel® Injection Solution. Because these events are reported voluntarily from a population of uncertain size, it is not always possible to reliably estimate their frequency or establish a causal relationship to drug exposure.
- Adverse event rates observed in Monotherapy use of Zeel® Injection Solution: Allergic (hypersensitivity) skin reactions may occur in isolated cases.
- Adverse event rates observed in Monotherapy use of Traumeel® Injection Solution: Allergic (hypersensitivity) reactions (e.g. skin allergies, redness/swelling at the injection site, even up to anaphylaxis) may occur in isolated cases.

7 Drug Interactions

No interactions have been reported, and none are expected due to the homeopathic dilutions.

8 Use in Specific Populations

8.1 Pregnancy

8.1.1 Teratogenic effects

Pregnancy Category C. Some ingredients in Zeel® Injection Solution have been shown to be teratogenic in various animal species when given in doses several thousand times the human dose. There are no adequate and well-controlled studies in pregnant women. Zeel® Injection solution should be used during pregnancy only if the potential benefit justifies the potential risk to the fetus.

When Zeel® Injection Solution is administered with Traumeel® Injection Solution in a woman of childbearing age, refer to the pregnancy category and product labelling for Traumeel® Injection Solution.

8.1.2 Non-teratogenic effects

No known non-teratogenic effects.

8.2 Labor and delivery

No recognized use in labor or delivery.

8.3 Nursing Mothers:

It is not known whether this drug is excreted in human milk. Because many drugs are excreted in human milk, caution should be exercised when Zeel® Injection Solution is administered to a nursing woman.

8.4 Pediatric use

Safety and effectiveness in pediatric patients have not been established. However, traditional homeopathic use of the ingredients in Zeel® Injection Solution has not identified differences in responses between adults and pediatric patients.

8.5 Geriatric use

Safety and effectiveness in geriatric patients have not been established. However, traditional homeopathic use of the ingredients in Zeel® Injection Solution has not identified differences in responses between adults and geriatric patients.

9 Overdosage

No negative effects of an overdose have been reported and none are expected due to the homeopathic dilutions.

10 Description

10.1 Ingredients

- Each 2.0 ml ampule contains:

Active Ingredients:			
Ingredient name	Potency	Quantity	Final dilution
a-Lipoicum acidum	8X	2.0 µl	10.99X
Arnica montana, radix	4X	200.0 µl	5.00X
Cartilago suis	6X	2.0 µl	9.00X
Coenzyme A	8X	2.0 µl	10.99X
Dulcamara	3X	10.0 µl	5.30X
Embryo totalis suis	6X	2.0 µl	9.00X
Funiculus umbilicalis suis	6X	2.0 µl	9.00X
Nadidum	8X	2.0 µl	10.99X
Natrum oxalaceticum	8X	2.0 µl	10.99X
Placenta suis	6X	2.0 µl	9.00X
Rhus toxicodendron	2X	10.0 µl	4.30X
Sanguinaria canadensis	4X	3.0 µl	6.82X
Sulphur	6X	3.6 µl	8.74X
Symphytum officinale	6X	10.0 µl	8.30X

Inactive Ingredients:

Water for injection	1,747.4 µl
Sodium Chloride	17.6 µl

10.2 Pharmaceutical Form

- Injection solution

10.3 Route of Administration

- Parenteral: s.c., i.d., i.m., i.a. or i.v

11 Clinical Pharmacology

11.1 Mechanism of Action

The exact mechanism of Zeel® Injection Solution is not fully understood.

11.2 Pharmacodynamics

Not applicable for homeopathic medicinal products.

12 References

- Homeopathic Pharmacopeia of the United States Revision Service

13 How Supplied / Storage and handling
13.1 Dosage forms and package sizes
• 1 ampule of 2.0 ml in packs of 10 ampules
• NDC 50114-7030-1
13.2 Storage and handling
• Store at room temperature. Protect from light.
Shown in Product Identification Guide, page 307

High Chemical Company
3901 NEBRASKA AVENUE, SUITE A
LEVITTOWN, PA 19056 - 3333

Phone: 800-447-8792, 215-788-3113
Email: highchemical@sarapin.com

SARAPIN ℞

DESCRIPTION
A sterile aqueous solution of soluble salts of the volatile bases from Sarraceniaceae (Pitcher Plant). Benzyl Alcohol 0.75%.

ACTIONS
The painful syndromes most commonly encountered in general practice which are relieved by SARAPIN® treatment are as follows:
Sciatic Pain
Intercostal Neuralgia
Occipital Neuritis
Brachial Plexus Neuralgia
Meralgia Paresthetica
Lumbar Neuralgia
Trigeminal Neuralgia

ADMINISTRATION
These and allied conditions may be treated with success in a majority of cases by nerve block or local infiltration:
Paravertebral—Careful localization of the zone of tenderness permits a determination of the corresponding trunk levels to be injected.
Perineural—In some instances, as in sciatica, the affected nerve can be injected at a site distant from its origin.
Local Infiltration—Multiple injections throughout an area of tenderness provide for diffusion into all the affected parts.

DOSAGE AND ADMINISTRATION
Paravertebral Injections

Cervical	2–3 ml
Thoracic	5–10 ml
Lumbar	5–10 ml
Sacral	3–5 ml
Sciatic Nerve	10 ml
Local Infiltration	5–10 ml

WARNINGS
Withdraw plunger of syringe to make sure the needle point is not in a blood vessel.

PRECAUTIONS
Procedure should be gentle and unhurried.
SARAPIN® is intended only for professional use. Its successful employment depends upon a thorough knowledge of the anatomy involved.

ADVERSE REACTIONS
Patients should be maintained in a recumbent position for 10 to 15 minutes following injection. A local sensation is to be expected, limited to the distribution of the nerve injected, and usually appearing as a temporary feeling of heaviness, although some cases will feel heat or a transitory aggravation of symptoms.

CONTRAINDICATIONS
SARAPIN® is non-toxic, has no side effects other than above and is contraindicated only in areas of infection.

HOW SUPPLIED
50 ml Multiple Dose Vial.

NDC-10541-0012-2

CAUTION: Federal law prohibits dispensing without prescription.

HIGH CHEMICAL COMPANY
3901 Nebraska Avenue, Suite A
Levittown, PA 19056 - 3333
800-447-8792, 215-788-3113
www.sarapin.com
highchemical@sarapin.com
Shown in Product Identification Guide, page 307

Incyte Corporation
Experimental Station
Route 141 & Henry Clay Road
Building E336
Wilmington, DE 19880

Direct Inquiries:
Tel: 1-855-4-INCYTE (1-855-446-2983)
Tel: 302.498.6700
Medical Information Contact
1-855-4-MEDINFO (1-855-463-3463)
medinfo@incyte.com
Normal business hours: 8am to 8pm ET, Mon-Fri

JAKAFI® ℞
(ruxolitinib)
tablets, for oral use

HIGHLIGHTS OF PRESCRIBING INFORMATION
These highlights do not include all the information needed to use JAKAFI safely and effectively. See full prescribing information for JAKAFI.
JAKAFI® (ruxolitinib) tablets, for oral use
Initial U.S. Approval: 2011

————RECENT MAJOR CHANGES————

Dosage and Administration (2.7)	07/2014
Warnings and Precautions (5.2) (5.3)	07/2014

————INDICATIONS AND USAGE————
Jakafi is a kinase inhibitor indicated for treatment of patients with intermediate or high-risk myelofibrosis, including primary myelofibrosis, post-polycythemia vera myelofibrosis and post-essential thrombocythemia myelofibrosis. (1)

————DOSAGE AND ADMINISTRATION————
• The starting dose of Jakafi is 20 mg given orally twice daily for patients with a platelet count greater than 200×10^9/L, and 15 mg twice daily for patients with a platelet count between 100×10^9/L and 200×10^9/L. (2.1)
• The starting dose of Jakafi is 5 mg twice daily for patients with a platelet count between 50×10^9/L and less than 100×10^9/L. (2.1)
• Monitor complete blood counts every 2 to 4 weeks until doses are stabilized, and then as clinically indicated. Modify or interrupt dosing for thrombocytopenia. (2.1) (2.2)
• Increase dose based on response and as recommended to a maximum of 25 mg twice daily for patients with starting platelet counts 100×10^9/L or greater and to a maximum of 10 mg twice daily for patients with starting platelet count between 50×10^9/L and less than 100×10^9/L. Discontinue after 6 months if no spleen reduction or symptom improvement (2.2) (2.5)

————DOSAGE FORMS AND STRENGTHS————
Tablets: 5 mg, 10 mg, 15 mg, 20 mg and 25 mg. (3)

————CONTRAINDICATIONS————
None. (4)

————WARNINGS AND PRECAUTIONS————
• Thrombocytopenia, Anemia and Neutropenia: Manage by dose reduction, or interruption, or transfusion. (5.1)
• Risk of Infection: Assess patients for signs and symptoms of infection and initiate appropriate treatment promptly. Serious infections should have resolved before starting therapy with Jakafi. (5.2)
• Myelofibrosis Symptom Exacerbation Following Interruption or Discontinuation: Manage with supportive care and consider resuming treatment with Jakafi. (5.3)

————ADVERSE REACTIONS————
The most common hematologic adverse reactions (incidence > 20%) are thrombocytopenia and anemia. The most common non-hematologic adverse reactions (incidence >10%) are bruising, dizziness and headache. (6.1)
To report SUSPECTED ADVERSE REACTIONS, contact Incyte Corporation at 1-855-463-3463 or FDA at 1-800-FDA-1088 or www.fda.gov/medwatch.

————DRUG INTERACTIONS————
• Strong CYP3A4 Inhibitors or Fluconazole: Reduce, interrupt, or discontinue Jakafi doses as recommended. (2.7) (7.1). Avoid use of Jakafi with fluconazole doses greater than 200 mg.

————USE IN SPECIFIC POPULATIONS————
• Renal Impairment: Reduce Jakafi starting dose to 10 mg twice daily for patients with moderate (CrCl 30-59 mL/min) or severe renal impairment (CrCl 15-29 mL/min) and a platelet count between 100×10^9/L and 150×10^9/L.

Avoid in patients with end stage renal disease (CrCl less than 15 mL/min) not requiring dialysis. Avoid in patients with moderate or severe renal impairment and a platelet count less than 100×10^9/L. (2.8) (8.6)
• Hepatic Impairment: Reduce Jakafi starting dose to 10 mg twice daily for patients with any degree of hepatic impairment and a platelet count between 100×10^9/L and 150×10^9/L. Avoid in patients with hepatic impairment with platelet counts less than 100×10^9/L. (2.8) (8.7)
• Nursing Mothers: Discontinue nursing or discontinue the drug taking into account the importance of the drug to the mother. (8.3)
See 17 for PATIENT COUNSELING INFORMATION and FDA-approved patient labeling

Revised: 07/2014

FULL PRESCRIBING INFORMATION

1. INDICATIONS AND USAGE
Jakafi is indicated for treatment of patients with intermediate or high-risk myelofibrosis, including primary myelofibrosis, post-polycythemia vera myelofibrosis and post-essential thrombocythemia myelofibrosis.

2. DOSAGE AND ADMINISTRATION
2.1 Recommended Starting Dose
The recommended starting dose of Jakafi is based on platelet count (*Table 1*). A complete blood count (CBC) and platelet count must be performed before initiating therapy, every 2 to 4 weeks until doses are stabilized, and then as clinically indicated [*see Warnings and Precautions (5.1)*]. Doses may be titrated based on safety and efficacy.

Table 1: Proposed Jakafi Starting Doses

Platelet Count	Starting Dose
Greater than 200×10^9/L	20 mg orally twice daily
100×10^9/L to 200×10^9/L	15 mg orally twice daily
50×10^9/L to less than 100×10^9/L	5 mg orally twice daily

2.2   Dose Modification Guidelines for Hematologic Toxicity for Patients Starting Treatment with a Platelet Count of 100×10^9/L or Greater

Treatment Interruption and Restarting Dosing
Interrupt treatment for platelet counts less than 50×10^9/L or absolute neutrophil count (ANC) less than 0.5×10^9/L. After recovery of platelet counts above 50×10^9/L and ANC above 0.75×10^9/L, dosing may be restarted. Table 2 illustrates the maximum allowable dose that may be used in restarting Jakafi after a previous interruption.

Table 2: Maximum Restarting Doses for Jakafi After Safety Interruption for Thrombocytopenia for Patients Starting Treatment with a Platelet Count of 100×10^9/L or Greater

Current Platelet Count	Maximum Dose When Restarting Jakafi Treatment*
Greater than or equal to 125×10^9/L	20 mg twice daily
100 to less than 125×10^9/L	15 mg twice daily
75 to less than 100×10^9/L	10 mg twice daily for at least 2 weeks; if stable, may increase to 15 mg twice daily
50 to less than 75×10^9/L	5 mg twice daily for at least 2 weeks; if stable, may increase to 10 mg twice daily
Less than 50×10^9/L	Continue hold

*Maximum doses are displayed. When restarting, begin with a dose at least 5 mg twice daily below the dose at interruption.

Following treatment interruption for ANC below 0.5×10^9/L, after ANC recovers to 0.75×10^9/L or greater, restart dosing at the higher of 5 mg once daily or 5 mg twice daily below the largest dose in the week prior to the treatment interruption.

Dose Reductions
Dose reductions should be considered if the platelet counts decrease as outlined in Table 3 with the goal of avoiding dose interruptions for thrombocytopenia.
[See table 3 above]

2.3   Dose Modification Based on Insufficient Response for Patients Starting Treatment with a Platelet Count of 100×10^9/L or Greater
If the response is insufficient and platelet and neutrophil counts are adequate, doses may be increased in 5 mg twice daily increments to a maximum of 25 mg twice daily. Doses should not be increased during the first 4 weeks of therapy and not more frequently than every 2 weeks.
Consider dose increases in patients who meet all of the following conditions:
a. Failure to achieve a reduction from pretreatment baseline in either palpable spleen length of 50% or a 35% reduction in spleen volume as measured by CT or MRI;
b. Platelet count greater than 125×10^9/L at 4 weeks and platelet count never below 100×10^9/L;
c. ANC Levels greater than 0.75×10^9/L.
Based on limited clinical data, long-term maintenance at a 5 mg twice daily dose has not shown responses and continued use at this dose should be limited to patients in whom the benefits outweigh the potential risks. Discontinue Jakafi if there is no spleen size reduction or symptom improvement after 6 months of therapy.

2.4   Dose Modifications for Hematologic Toxicity for Patients Starting Treatment with Platelet Counts of 50×10^9/L to Less Than 100×10^9/L
This section applies only to patients with platelet counts of 50×10^9/L to less than 100×10^9/L prior to any treatment with ruxolitinib. See Section 2.2 for dose modifications for

Table 3: Dosing Recommendations for Thrombocytopenia for Patients Starting Treatment with a Platelet Count of 100×10^9/L or Greater

Platelet Count	Dose at Time of Platelet Decline				
	25 mg twice daily	20 mg twice daily	15 mg twice daily	10 mg twice daily	5 mg twice daily
	New Dose	New Dose	New Dose	New Dose	New Dose
100 to less than 125×10^9/L	20 mg twice daily	15 mg twice daily	No Change	No Change	No Change
75 to less than 100×10^9/L	10 mg twice daily	10 mg twice daily	10 mg twice daily	No Change	No Change
50 to less than 75×10^9/L	5 mg twice daily	5 mg twice daily	5 mg twice daily	5 mg twice daily	No Change
Less than 50×10^9/L	Hold	Hold	Hold	Hold	Hold

hematological toxicity in patients whose platelet counts were 100×10^9/L or more prior to starting treatment with ruxolitinib.

Treatment Interruption and Restarting Dosing
Interrupt treatment for platelet counts less than 25×10^9/L or ANC less than 0.5×10^9/L.
After recovery of platelet counts above 35×10^9/L and ANC above 0.75×10^9/L, dosing may be restarted. Restart dosing at the higher of 5 mg once daily or 5 mg twice daily below the largest dose in the week prior to the decrease in platelet count below 25×10^9/L or ANC below 0.5×10^9/L that led to dose interruption.

Dose Reductions
Reduce the dose of ruxolitinib for platelet counts less than 35×10^9/L as described in Table 4.

Table 4: Dosing Modifications for Thrombocytopenia for Patients with Starting Platelet Count of 50×10^9/L to Less Than 100×10^9/L

Platelet Count	Dosing Recommendations
Less than 25×10^9/L	• Interrupt dosing.
25×10^9/L to less than 35×10^9/L AND the platelet count decline is less than 20% during the prior four weeks	• Decrease dose by 5 mg once daily. • For patients on 5 mg once daily, maintain dose at 5 mg once daily.
25×10^9/L to less than 35×10^9/L AND the platelet count decline is 20% or greater during the prior four weeks	• Decrease dose by 5 mg twice daily. • For patients on 5 mg twice daily, decrease the dose to 5 mg once daily. • For patients on 5 mg once daily, maintain dose at 5 mg once daily.

2.5   Dose Modifications Based on Insufficient Response for Patients with Starting Platelet Count of 50×10^9/L to Less Than 100×10^9/L
Do not increase doses during the first 4 weeks of therapy, and do not increase the dose more frequently than every 2 weeks.
If the response is insufficient as defined in Section 2.3, doses may be increased by increments of 5 mg daily to a maximum of 10 mg twice daily if:
a) the platelet count has remained at least 40×10^9/L, and
b) the platelet count has not fallen by more than 20% in the prior 4 weeks, and
c) the ANC is more than 1×10^9/L, and
d) the dose has not been reduced or interrupted for an adverse event or hematological toxicity in the prior 4 weeks.
Continuation of treatment for more than 6 months should be limited to patients in whom the benefits outweigh the potential risks. Discontinue Jakafi if there is no spleen size reduction or symptom improvement after 6 months of therapy.

2.6   Dose Modification for Bleeding
Interrupt treatment for bleeding requiring intervention regardless of current platelet count. Once the bleeding event has resolved, consider resuming treatment at the prior dose

if the underlying cause of bleeding has been controlled. If the bleeding event has resolved but the underlying cause persists, consider resuming treatment with Jakafi at a lower dose.

2.7   Dose Modification for Drug Interactions
Concomitant Use with Strong CYP3A4 Inhibitors or Fluconazole
Modify the dose of Jakafi when given concomitantly with strong CYP3A4 inhibitors (such as but not limited to boceprevir, clarithromycin, conivaptan, grapefruit juice, indinavir, itraconazole, ketoconazole, lopinavir/ritonavir, mibefradil, nefazodone, nelfinavir, posaconazole, ritonavir, saquinavir, telaprevir, telithromycin, voriconazole) and fluconazole doses less than or equal to 200 mg as follows [see *Drug Interactions* (7.1)]:
• Starting dose, platelet count greater than or equal to 100×10^9/L: 10 mg twice daily
• Starting dose, platelet counts 50 to less than 100×10^9/L: 5 mg once daily
• Patients on stable Jakafi dose of greater than or equal to 10 mg twice daily: Reduce dose by 50% (rounded up to the closest available tablet strength).
• Patients on stable Jakafi dose of 5 mg twice daily: Reduce dose to 5 mg once daily.
• Patients on stable Jakafi dose of 5 mg once daily: Avoid strong CYP3A4 inhibitor or fluconazole treatment or interrupt Jakafi treatment for the duration of strong CYP3A4 inhibitor or fluconazole use.
Avoid the use of fluconazole doses of greater than 200 mg daily concomitantly with Jakafi.
Additional dose modifications should be made with careful monitoring of safety and efficacy.

2.8   Organ Impairment
Renal Impairment
On the basis of pharmacokinetic studies in volunteers with renal impairment, the recommended starting dose is 10 mg twice daily for patients with a platelet count between 100×10^9/L and 150×10^9/L and moderate (CrCl 30-59 mL/min) or severe renal impairment (CrCl 15-29 mL/min). Additional dose modifications should be made with careful monitoring of safety and efficacy.
The recommended starting dose for patients with end stage renal disease on dialysis is 15 mg once after a dialysis session for patients with a platelet count between 100×10^9/L and 200×10^9/L or 20 mg for patients with a platelet count of greater than 200×10^9/L. Subsequent doses should be administered on dialysis days following each dialysis session. Additional dose modifications should be made with frequent monitoring of safety and efficacy.
Avoid use of Jakafi in patients with end stage renal disease (CrCl less than 15 mL/min) not requiring dialysis and in patients with moderate or severe renal impairment with platelet counts less than 100×10^9/L [see *Use in Specific Populations* (8.6)].

Hepatic Impairment
On the basis of pharmacokinetic studies in volunteers with hepatic impairment, the recommended starting dose is 10 mg twice daily for patients with a platelet count between 100×10^9/L and 150×10^9/L. Additional dose modifications should be made with careful monitoring of safety and efficacy.
Avoid use of Jakafi in patients with hepatic impairment with platelet counts less than 100×10^9/L [see *Use in Specific Populations* (8.7)].

2.9   Method of Administration

Jakafi is dosed orally and can be administered with or without food.

If a dose is missed, the patient should not take an additional dose, but should take the next usual prescribed dose.

When discontinuing Jakafi therapy for reasons other than thrombocytopenia, gradual tapering of the dose of Jakafi may be considered, for example by 5 mg twice daily each week.

For patients unable to ingest tablets, Jakafi can be administered through a nasogastric tube (8 French or greater) as follows:

• Suspend one tablet in approximately 40 mL of water with stirring for approximately 10 minutes.
• Within 6 hours after the tablet has dispersed, the suspension can be administered through a nasogastric tube using an appropriate syringe.

The tube should be rinsed with approximately 75 mL of water. The effect of tube feeding preparations on Jakafi exposure during administration through a nasogastric tube has not been evaluated.

3.   DOSAGE FORMS AND STRENGTHS

5 mg tablets - round and white with "INCY" on one side and "5" on the other.

10 mg tablets - round and white with "INCY" on one side and "10" on the other.

15 mg tablets - oval and white with "INCY" on one side and "15" on the other.

20 mg tablets - capsule-shaped and white with "INCY" on one side and "20" on the other.

25 mg tablets - oval and white with "INCY" on one side and "25" on the other.

4.   CONTRAINDICATIONS

None.

5.   WARNINGS AND PRECAUTIONS

5.1   Thrombocytopenia, Anemia and Neutropenia

Treatment with Jakafi can cause thrombocytopenia, anemia and neutropenia. [see Dosage and Administration (2.1)].

Manage thrombocytopenia by reducing the dose or temporarily interrupting Jakafi. Platelet transfusions may be necessary [see Dosage and Administration (2.2), and Adverse Reactions (6.1)].

Patients developing anemia may require blood transfusions and/or dose modifications of Jakafi.

Severe neutropenia (ANC less than 0.5×10^9/L) was generally reversible by withholding Jakafi until recovery [see Adverse Reactions (6.1)].

Perform a pre-treatment complete blood count (CBC) and monitor CBCs every 2 to 4 weeks until doses are stabilized, and then as clinically indicated. [see Dosage and Administration (2.2), and Adverse Reactions (6.1)].

5.2   Risk of Infection

Serious bacterial, mycobacterial, fungal and viral infections have occurred. Delay starting therapy with Jakafi until active serious infections have resolved. Observe patients receiving Jakafi for signs and symptoms of infection and manage promptly.

Tuberculosis

Tuberculosis infection has been reported in patients receiving Jakafi. Observe patients receiving Jakafi for signs and symptoms of active tuberculosis and manage promptly.

Prior to initiating Jakafi, patients should be evaluated for tuberculosis risk factors, and those at higher risk should be tested for latent infection. Risk factors include, but are not limited to, prior residence in or travel to countries with a high prevalence of tuberculosis, close contact with a person with active tuberculosis, and a history of active or latent tuberculosis where an adequate course of treatment cannot be confirmed.

For patients with evidence of active or latent tuberculosis, consult a physician with expertise in the treatment of tuberculosis before starting Jakafi. The decision to continue Jakafi during treatment of active tuberculosis should be based on the overall risk-benefit determination.

PML

Progressive multifocal leukoencephalopathy (PML) has occurred with ruxolitinib treatment for myelofibrosis. If PML is suspected, stop Jakafi and evaluate.

Herpes Zoster

Advise patients about early signs and symptoms of herpes zoster and to seek treatment as early as possible if suspected [see Adverse Reactions (6.1)].

5.3   Myelofibrosis Symptom Exacerbation Following Interruption or Discontinuation of Treatment with Jakafi

Following discontinuation of Jakafi, symptoms of myelofibrosis generally return to pretreatment levels over a period of approximately one week. Some patients have experienced one or more of the following adverse events after discontinuing Jakafi: fever, respiratory distress, hypotension, DIC, or multi-organ failure. If one or more of these occur after discontinuation of, or while tapering the dose of Jakafi, evaluate for and treat any intercurrent illness and consider restarting or increasing the dose of Jakafi. Instruct patients not to interrupt or discontinue Jakafi therapy without consulting their physician. When discontinuing or interrupting therapy with Jakafi for reasons other than thrombocytopenia or neutropenia [see Dosage and Administration (2.9)], consider tapering the dose of Jakafi gradually rather than discontinuing abruptly.

6.   ADVERSE REACTIONS

The following serious adverse reactions are discussed in greater detail in other sections of the labeling:

• Myelosuppression [see Warnings and Precautions (5.1)]
• Risk of Infection [see Warnings and Precautions (5.2)]
• Myelofibrosis Symptom Exacerbation Following Interruption or Discontinuation of Treatment with Jakafi [see Warnings and Precautions (5.3)]

6.1   Clinical Trials Experience

Because clinical trials are conducted under widely varying conditions, adverse reaction rates observed in the clinical trials of a drug cannot be directly compared to rates in the clinical trials of another drug and may not reflect the rates observed in practice.

The safety of Jakafi was assessed in 617 patients in six clinical studies with a median duration of follow-up of 10.9 months, including 301 patients with myelofibrosis in two Phase 3 studies.

In these two Phase 3 studies, patients had a median duration of exposure to Jakafi of 9.5 months (range 0.5 to 17 months), with 88.7% of patients treated for more than 6 months and 24.6% treated for more than 12 months. One hundred and eleven (111) patients started treatment at 15 mg twice daily and 190 patients started at 20 mg twice daily. In patients starting treatment with 15 mg twice daily (pretreatment platelet counts of 100 to 200×10^9/L) and 20 mg twice daily (pretreatment platelet counts greater than 200×10^9/L), 65% and 25% of patients, respectively, required a dose reduction below the starting dose within the first 8 weeks of therapy.

In a double-blind, randomized, placebo-controlled study of Jakafi, among the 155 patients treated with Jakafi, the most frequent adverse drug reactions were thrombocytopenia and anemia [see Table 6]. Thrombocytopenia, anemia and neutropenia are dose related effects. The three most frequent non-hematologic adverse reactions were bruising, dizziness and headache [see Table 5].

Discontinuation for adverse events, regardless of causality, was observed in 11% of patients treated with Jakafi and 10.6% of patients treated with placebo.

Table 5 presents the most common adverse reactions occurring in patients who received Jakafi in the double-blind, placebo-controlled study during randomized treatment. [See table 5 above]

Description of Selected Adverse Drug Reactions

Anemia

In the two Phase 3 clinical studies, median time to onset of first CTCAE Grade 2 or higher anemia was approximately 6 weeks. One patient (0.3%) discontinued treatment because of anemia. In patients receiving Jakafi, mean decreases in hemoglobin reached a nadir of approximately 1.5 to 2.0 g/dL below baseline after 8 to 12 weeks of therapy and then gradually recovered to reach a new steady state that was approximately 1.0 g/dL below baseline. This pattern was observed in patients regardless of whether they had received transfusions during therapy.

In the randomized, placebo-controlled study, 60% of patients treated with Jakafi and 38% of patients receiving placebo received red blood cell transfusions during randomized treatment. Among transfused patients, the median number of units transfused per month was 1.2 in patients treated with Jakafi and 1.7 in placebo treated patients.

Thrombocytopenia

In the two Phase 3 clinical studies, in patients who developed Grade 3 or 4 thrombocytopenia, the median time to onset was approximately 8 weeks. Thrombocytopenia was generally reversible with dose reduction or dose interruption. The median time to recovery of platelet counts above 50×10^9/L was 14 days. Platelet transfusions were administered to 4.7% of patients receiving Jakafi and to 4.0% of patients receiving control regimens. Discontinuation of treatment because of thrombocytopenia occurred in 0.7% of patients receiving Jakafi and 0.9% of patients receiving control regimens. Patients with a platelet count of 100×10^9/L to 200×10^9/L before starting Jakafi had a higher frequency of Grade 3 or 4 thrombocytopenia compared to patients with a platelet count greater than 200×10^9/L (16.5% versus 7.2%).

Neutropenia

In the two Phase 3 clinical studies, 1.0% of patients reduced or stopped Jakafi because of neutropenia.

Table 6 provides the frequency and severity of clinical hematology abnormalities reported for patients receiving treatment with Jakafi or placebo in the placebo-controlled study.

[See table 6 at top of next page]

Additional Data from the Placebo-controlled Study

25.2% of patients treated with Jakafi and 7.3% of patients treated with placebo developed newly occurring or worsening Grade 1 abnormalities in alanine transaminase (ALT). The incidence of greater than or equal to Grade 2 elevations was 1.9% for Jakafi with 1.3% Grade 3 and no Grade 4 ALT elevations.

17.4% of patients treated with Jakafi and 6.0% of patients treated with placebo developed newly occurring or worsening Grade 1 abnormalities in aspartate transaminase (AST). The incidence of Grade 2 AST elevations was 0.6% for Jakafi with no Grade 3 or 4 AST elevations.

16.8% of patients treated with Jakafi and 0.7% of patients treated with placebo developed newly occurring or worsening Grade 1 elevations in cholesterol. The incidence of Grade 2 cholesterol elevations was 0.6% for Jakafi with no Grade 3 or 4 cholesterol elevations.

7.   DRUG INTERACTIONS

7.1   Drugs That Inhibit or Induce Cytochrome P450 Enzymes

Ruxolitinib is metabolized by CYP3A4 and to a lesser extent by CYP2C9.

CYP3A4 inhibitors: The C_{max} and AUC of ruxolitinib increased 33% and 91%, respectively following concomitant administration with the strong CYP3A4 inhibitor ketoconazole in healthy subjects. Concomitant administration with mild or moderate CYP3A4 inhibitors did not result in an exposure change requiring intervention [see Pharmacokinetics (12.3)].

Table 5:   Adverse Reactions Occurring in Patients on Jakafi in the Double-blind, Placebo-controlled Study During Randomized Treatment

Adverse Reactions	Jakafi (N=155)			Placebo (N=151)		
	All Grades[a] (%)	Grade 3 (%)	Grade 4 (%)	All Grades (%)	Grade 3 (%)	Grade 4 (%)
Bruising[b]	23.2	0.6	0	14.6	0	0
Dizziness[c]	18.1	0.6	0	7.3	0	0
Headache	14.8	0	0	5.3	0	0
Urinary Tract Infections[d]	9.0	0	0	5.3	0.7	0.7
Weight Gain[e]	7.1	0.6	0	1.3	0.7	0
Flatulence	5.2	0	0	0.7	0	0
Herpes Zoster[f]	1.9	0	0	0.7	0	0

[a] National Cancer Institute Common Terminology Criteria for Adverse Events (CTCAE), version 3.0
[b] includes contusion, ecchymosis, hematoma, injection site hematoma, periorbital hematoma, vessel puncture site hematoma, increased tendency to bruise, petechiae, purpura
[c] includes dizziness, postural dizziness, vertigo, balance disorder, Meniere's Disease, labyrinthitis
[d] includes urinary tract infection, cystitis, urosepsis, urinary tract infection bacterial, kidney infection, pyuria, bacteria urine, bacteria urine identified, nitrite urine present
[e] includes weight increased, abnormal weight gain
[f] includes herpes zoster and post-herpetic neuralgia

Table 6: Worst Hematology Laboratory Abnormalities in the Placebo-controlled Study[a]

Laboratory Parameter	Jakafi (N=155)			Placebo (N=151)		
	All Grades[b] (%)	Grade 3 (%)	Grade 4 (%)	All Grades (%)	Grade 3 (%)	Grade 4 (%)
Thrombocytopenia	69.7	9.0	3.9	30.5	1.3	0
Anemia	96.1	34.2	11.0	86.8	15.9	3.3
Neutropenia	18.7	5.2	1.9	4.0	0.7	1.3

[a] Presented values are worst Grade values regardless of baseline
[b] National Cancer Institute Common Terminology Criteria for Adverse Events, version 3.0

When administering Jakafi with strong CYP3A4 inhibitors, consider dose reduction [see *Dosage and Administration (2.7)*].

Fluconazole: The AUC of ruxolitinib is predicted to increase by approximately 100% to 300% following concomitant administration with the combined CYP3A4 and CYP2C9 inhibitor fluconazole at doses of 100 mg to 400 mg once daily, respectively [see *Pharmacokinetics (12.3)*]. Avoid the concomitant use of Jakafi with fluconazole doses of greater than 200 mg daily [see *Dosage and Administration (2.7)*].

CYP3A4 inducers: The C_{max} and AUC of ruxolitinib decreased 32% and 61%, respectively, following concomitant administration with the strong CYP3A4 inducer rifampin in healthy subjects. No dose adjustment is recommended; however, monitor patients frequently and adjust the Jakafi dose based on safety and efficacy [see *Pharmacokinetics (12.3)*].

8. USE IN SPECIFIC POPULATIONS
8.1 Pregnancy
Pregnancy Category C
Risk Summary
There are no adequate and well-controlled studies of Jakafi in pregnant women. In embryofetal toxicity studies, treatment with ruxolitinib resulted in an increase in late resorptions and reduced fetal weights at maternally toxic doses. Jakafi should be used during pregnancy only if the potential benefit justifies the potential risk to the fetus.
Animal Data
Ruxolitinib was administered orally to pregnant rats or rabbits during the period of organogenesis, at doses of 15, 30 or 60 mg/kg/day in rats and 10, 30 or 60 mg/kg/day in rabbits. There was no evidence of teratogenicity. However, decreases of approximately 9% in fetal weights were noted in rats at the highest and maternally toxic dose of 60 mg/kg/day. This dose results in an exposure (AUC) that is approximately 2 times the clinical exposure at the maximum recommended dose of 25 mg twice daily. In rabbits, lower fetal weights of approximately 8% and increased late resorptions were noted at the highest and maternally toxic dose of 60 mg/kg/day. This dose is approximately 7% the clinical exposure at the maximum recommended dose.
In a pre- and post-natal development study in rats, pregnant animals were dosed with ruxolitinib from implantation through lactation at doses up to 30 mg/kg/day. There were no drug-related adverse findings in pups for fertility indices or for maternal or embryofetal survival, growth and development parameters at the highest dose evaluated (34% the clinical exposure at the maximum recommended dose of 25 mg twice daily).

8.3 Nursing Mothers
It is not known whether ruxolitinib is excreted in human milk. Ruxolitinib and/or its metabolites were excreted in the milk of lactating rats with a concentration that was 13-fold the maternal plasma. Because many drugs are excreted in human milk and because of the potential for serious adverse reactions in nursing infants from Jakafi, a decision should be made to discontinue nursing or to discontinue the drug, taking into account the importance of the drug to the mother.

8.4 Pediatric Use
The safety and effectiveness of Jakafi in pediatric patients have not been established.

8.5 Geriatric Use
Of the total number of myelofibrosis patients in clinical studies with Jakafi, 51.9% were 65 years of age and older. No overall differences in safety or effectiveness of Jakafi were observed between these patients and younger patients.

8.6 Renal Impairment
The safety and pharmacokinetics of single dose Jakafi (25 mg) were evaluated in a study in healthy subjects [CrCl 72-164 mL/min (N=8)] and in subjects with mild [CrCl 53-83 mL/min (N=8)], moderate [CrCl 38-57 mL/min (N=8)], or severe renal impairment [CrCl 15-51 mL/min (N=8)]. Eight (8) additional subjects with end stage renal disease requiring hemodialysis were also enrolled.

The pharmacokinetics of ruxolitinib was similar in subjects with various degrees of renal impairment and in those with normal renal function. However, plasma AUC values of ruxolitinib metabolites increased with increasing severity of renal impairment. This was most marked in the subjects with end stage renal disease requiring hemodialysis. The change in the pharmacodynamic marker, pSTAT3 inhibition, was consistent with the corresponding increase in metabolite exposure. Ruxolitinib is not removed by dialysis; however, the removal of some active metabolites by dialysis cannot be ruled out.

When administering Jakafi to patients with moderate (CrCl 30-59 mL/min) or severe renal impairment (CrCl 15-29 mL/min) with a platelet count between 100×10^9/L and 150×10^9/L and patients with end stage renal disease on dialysis a dose reduction is recommended [see *Dosage and Administration (2.8)*].

8.7 Hepatic Impairment
The safety and pharmacokinetics of single dose Jakafi (25 mg) were evaluated in a study in healthy subjects (N=8) and in subjects with mild [Child-Pugh A (N=8)], moderate [Child-Pugh B (N=8)], or severe hepatic impairment [Child-Pugh C (N=8)]. The mean AUC for ruxolitinib was increased by 87%, 28% and 65%, respectively, in patients with mild, moderate and severe hepatic impairment compared to patients with normal hepatic function. The terminal elimination half-life was prolonged in patients with hepatic impairment compared to healthy controls (4.1-5.0 hours versus 2.8 hours). The change in the pharmacodynamic marker, pSTAT3 inhibition, was consistent with the corresponding increase in ruxolitinib exposure except in the severe (Child-Pugh C) hepatic impairment cohort where the pharmacodynamic activity was more prolonged in some subjects than expected based on plasma concentrations of ruxolitinib.

When administering Jakafi to patients with any degree of hepatic impairment and with a platelet count between 100×10^9/L and 150×10^9/L, a dose reduction is recommended [see *Dosage and Administration (2,8)*].

10. OVERDOSAGE
There is no known antidote for overdoses with Jakafi. Single doses up to 200 mg have been given with acceptable acute tolerability. Higher than recommended repeat doses are associated with increased myelosuppression including leukopenia, anemia and thrombocytopenia. Appropriate supportive treatment should be given.
Hemodialysis is not expected to enhance the elimination of ruxolitinib.

11. DESCRIPTION
Ruxolitinib phosphate is a kinase inhibitor with the chemical name (R)-3-(4-(7H-pyrrolo[2,3-d]pyrimidin-4-yl)-1H-pyrazol-1-yl)-3-cyclopentylpropanenitrile phosphate and a molecular weight of 404.36. Ruxolitinib phosphate has the following structural formula:

Ruxolitinib phosphate is a white to off-white to light pink powder and is soluble in aqueous buffers across a pH range of 1 to 8.
Jakafi (ruxolitinib) Tablets are for oral administration. Each tablet contains ruxolitinib phosphate equivalent to 5 mg, 10 mg, 15 mg, 20 mg and 25 mg of ruxolitinib free base together with microcrystalline cellulose, lactose monohydrate, magnesium stearate, colloidal silicon dioxide, sodium starch glycolate, povidone and hydroxypropyl cellulose.

12. CLINICAL PHARMACOLOGY
12.1 Mechanism of Action
Ruxolitinib, a kinase inhibitor, inhibits Janus Associated Kinases (JAKs) JAK1 and JAK2 which mediate the signaling of a number of cytokines and growth factors that are important for hematopoiesis and immune function. JAK signaling involves recruitment of STATs (signal transducers and activators of transcription) to cytokine receptors, activation and subsequent localization of STATs to the nucleus leading to modulation of gene expression.
Myelofibrosis (MF) is a myeloproliferative neoplasm (MPN) known to be associated with dysregulated JAK1 and JAK2 signaling. In a mouse model of JAK2V617F-positive MPN, oral administration of ruxolitinib prevented splenomegaly, preferentially decreased JAK2V617F mutant cells in the spleen and decreased circulating inflammatory cytokines (eg, TNF-α, IL-6).

12.2 Pharmacodynamics
Ruxolitinib inhibits cytokine induced STAT3 phosphorylation in whole blood from healthy subjects and MF patients. Jakafi administration resulted in maximal inhibition of STAT3 phosphorylation 2 hours after dosing which returned to near baseline by 10 hours in both healthy subjects and myelofibrosis patients.

12.3 Pharmacokinetics
Absorption
In clinical studies, ruxolitinib is rapidly absorbed after oral Jakafi administration with maximal plasma concentration (C_{max}) achieved within 1 to 2 hours post-dose. Based on a mass balance study in humans, oral absorption of ruxolitinib was estimated to be at least 95%. Mean ruxolitinib C_{max} and total exposure (AUC) increased proportionally over a single dose range of 5 to 200 mg. There were no clinically relevant changes in the pharmacokinetics of ruxolitinib upon administration of Jakafi with a high-fat meal, with the mean C_{max} moderately decreased (24%) and the mean AUC nearly unchanged (4% increase).

Distribution
The apparent volume of distribution of ruxolitinib at steady-state is 53 to 65 L in myelofibrosis patients. Binding to plasma proteins *in vitro* is approximately 97%, mostly to albumin.

Metabolism
In vitro studies suggest that ruxolitinib is metabolized by CYP3A4 and to a lesser extent by CYP2C9.

Elimination
Following a single oral dose of [^{14}C]-labeled ruxolitinib in healthy adult subjects, elimination was predominately through metabolism with 74% of radioactivity excreted in urine and 22% excretion via feces. Unchanged drug accounted for less than 1% of the excreted total radioactivity. The mean elimination half-life of ruxolitinib is approximately 3 hours and the mean half-life of ruxolitinib + metabolites is approximately 5.8 hours.

Effects of Age, Gender, or Race
In healthy subjects, no significant differences in ruxolitinib pharmacokinetics were observed with regard to gender and race. In a population pharmacokinetic evaluation in myelofibrosis patients, no relationship was apparent between oral clearance and patient age or race, and in women, clearance was 17.7 L/h and in men, 22.1 L/h with 39% inter-subject variability.

Drug Interactions
Strong CYP3A4 inhibitors: In a trial of 16 healthy volunteers, a single dose of 10 mg of Jakafi was administered alone on Day 1and a single dose of 10 mg of Jakafi was administered on Day 5 in combination with 200 mg of ketoconazole (a strong CYP3A4 inhibitor, given twice daily on Days 2 to 5). Ketoconazole increased ruxolitinib C_{max} and AUC by 33% and 91%, respectively. Ketoconazole also prolonged ruxolitinib half-life from 3.7 to 6.0 hours [see *Dosage and Administration (2.7) and Drug Interactions (7.1)*].
Fluconazole: Simulations using physiologically-based pharmacokinetic (PBPK) models suggested that fluconazole (a dual CYP3A4 and CYP2C9 inhibitor) increases steady state ruxolitinib AUC by approximately 100% to 300% following concomitant administration of 10 mg of Jakafi twice daily with 100 mg to 400 mg of fluconazole once daily, respectively [see *Dosage and Administration (2.7) and Drug Interactions (7.1)*].
Mild or moderate CYP3A4 inhibitors: In a trial of 15 healthy volunteers, a single dose of 10 mg of Jakafi was administered alone on Day 1 and a single dose of 10 mg of Jakafi was administered on Day 5 in combination with 500 mg of erythromycin (a moderate CYP3A4 inhibitor,

given twice daily on Days 2 to 5). Erythromycin increased ruxolitinib C_{max} and AUC by 8% and 27%, respectively [see Drug Interactions (7.1)].

CYP3A4 inducers: In a trial of 12 healthy volunteers, a single dose of 50 mg of Jakafi was administered alone on Day 1 and a single dose of 50 mg of Jakafi was administered on Day 13 in combination with 600 mg of rifampin (a strong CYP3A4 inducer, given once daily on Days 3 to 13). Rifampin decreased ruxolitinib C_{max} and AUC by 32% and 61%, respectively. In addition, the relative exposure to ruxolitinib's active metabolites increased approximately 100% [see Drug Interactions (7.1)].

In vitro studies: In vitro, ruxolitinib and its M18 metabolite do not inhibit CYP1A2, CYP2B6, CYP2C8, CYP2C9, CYP2C19, CYP2D6 or CYP3A4. Ruxolitinib is not an inducer of CYP1A2, CYP2B6 or CYP3A4 at clinically relevant concentrations.

In vitro, ruxolitinib and its M18 metabolite do not inhibit the P-gp, BCRP, OATP1B1, OATP1B3, OCT1, OCT2, OAT1 or OAT3 transport systems at clinically relevant concentrations. Ruxolitinib is not a substrate for the P-gp transporter.

12.4 Thorough QT Study

The effect of single dose ruxolitinib 25 mg and 200 mg on QTc interval was evaluated in a randomized, placebo-, and active-controlled (moxifloxacin 400 mg) four-period crossover thorough QT study in 47 healthy subjects. In a study with demonstrated ability to detect small effects, the upper bound of the one-sided 95% confidence interval for the largest placebo adjusted, baseline-corrected QTc based on Fridericia correction method (QTcF) was below 10 ms, the threshold for regulatory concern. The dose of 200 mg is adequate to represent the high exposure clinical scenario.

13. NONCLINICAL TOXICOLOGY

13.1 Carcinogenesis, Mutagenesis, Impairment of Fertility

Ruxolitinib was not carcinogenic in the 6-month Tg.rasH2 transgenic mouse model or in a 2-year carcinogenicity study in the rat.

Ruxolitinib was not mutagenic in a bacterial mutagenicity assay (Ames test) or clastogenic in in vitro chromosomal aberration assay (cultured human peripheral blood lymphocytes) or in vivo in a rat bone marrow micronucleus assay. In a fertility study, ruxolitinib was administered to male rats prior to and throughout mating and to female rats prior to mating and up to the implantation day (gestation day 7). Ruxolitinib had no effect on fertility or reproductive function in male or female rats at doses of 10, 30 or 60 mg/kg/day. However, in female rats doses of greater than or equal to 30 mg/kg/day resulted in increased postimplantation loss. The exposure (AUC) at the dose of 30 mg/kg/day is approximately 34% the clinical exposure at the maximum recommended dose of 25 mg twice daily.

14. CLINICAL STUDIES

Two randomized Phase 3 studies (Studies 1 and 2) were conducted in patients with myelofibrosis (either primary myelofibrosis, post-polycythemia vera myelofibrosis or post-essential thrombocythemia-myelofibrosis). In both studies, patients had palpable splenomegaly at least 5 cm below the costal margin and risk category of intermediate 2 (2 prognostic factors) or high risk (3 or more prognostic factors) based on the International Working Group Consensus Criteria (IWG).

The starting dose of Jakafi was based on platelet count. Patients with a platelet count between 100 and $200 \times 10^9/L$ were started on Jakafi 15 mg twice daily and patients with a platelet count greater than $200 \times 10^9/L$ were started on Jakafi 20 mg twice daily. Doses were then individualized based upon tolerability and efficacy with maximum doses of 20 mg twice daily for patients with platelet counts between 100 to less than or equal to $125 \times 10^9/L$, of 10 mg twice daily for patients with platelet counts between 75 to less than or equal to $100 \times 10^9/L$, and of 5 mg twice daily for patients with platelet counts between 50 to less than or equal to $75 \times 10^9/L$.

Study 1

Study 1 was a double-blind, randomized, placebo-controlled study in 309 patients who were refractory to or were not candidates for available therapy. The median age was 68 years (range 40 to 91 years) with 61% of patients older than 65 years and 54% were male. Fifty percent (50%) of patients had primary myelofibrosis, 31% had post-polycythemia vera myelofibrosis and 18% had post-essential thrombocythemia myelofibrosis. Twenty-one percent (21%) of patients had red blood cell transfusions within 8 weeks of enrollment in the study. The median hemoglobin count was 10.5 g/dL and the median platelet count was $251 \times 10^9/L$. Patients had a median palpable spleen length of 16 cm below the costal margin, with 81% having a spleen length 10 cm or greater below the costal margin. Patients had a median spleen volume as measured by magnetic resonance imaging (MRI) or computed tomography (CT) of 2595 cm^3 (range 478 cm^3 to 8881 cm^3). (The upper limit of normal is approximately 300 cm^3).

Patients were dosed with Jakafi or matching placebo. The primary efficacy endpoint was the proportion of patients achieving greater than or equal to a 35% reduction from

baseline in spleen volume at Week 24 as measured by MRI or CT.

Secondary endpoints included duration of a 35% or greater reduction in spleen volume and proportion of patients with a 50% or greater reduction in Total Symptom Score from baseline to Week 24 as measured by the modified Myelofibrosis Symptom Assessment Form (MFSAF) v2.0 diary.

Study 2

Study 2 was an open-label, randomized study in 219 patients. Patients were randomized 2:1 to Jakafi versus best available therapy. Best available therapy was selected by the investigator on a patient-by-patient basis. In the best available therapy arm, the medications received by more than 10% of patients were hydroxyurea (47%) and glucocorticoids (16%). The median age was 66 years (range 35 to 85 years) with 52% of patients older than 65 years and 57% were male. Fifty-three percent (53%) of patients had primary myelofibrosis, 31% had post-polycythemia vera myelofibrosis and 16% had post-essential thrombocythemia myelofibrosis. Twenty-one percent (21%) of patients had red blood cell transfusions within 8 weeks of enrollment in the study. The median hemoglobin count was 10.4 g/dL and the median platelet count was $236 \times 10^9/L$. Patients had a median palpable spleen length of 15 cm below the costal margin, with 70% having a spleen length 10 cm or greater below the costal margin. Patients had a median spleen volume as measured by MRI or CT of 2381 cm^3 (range 451 cm^3 to 7765 cm^3).

The primary efficacy endpoint was the proportion of patients achieving 35% or greater reduction from baseline in spleen volume at Week 48 as measured by MRI or CT.

A secondary endpoint in Study 2 was the proportion of patients achieving a 35% or greater reduction of spleen volume as measured by MRI or CT from baseline to Week 24.

Study 1 and 2 Efficacy Results

Efficacy analyses of the primary endpoint in Studies 1 and 2 are presented in Table 7 below. A significantly larger proportion of patients in the Jakafi group achieved a 35% or greater reduction in spleen volume from baseline in both studies compared to placebo in Study 1 and best available therapy in Study 2. A similar proportion of patients in the Jakafi group achieved a 50% or greater reduction in palpable spleen length.

[See table 7 above]

Figure 1 shows the percent change from baseline in spleen volume for each patient at Week 24 (Jakafi N=139, placebo

N=106) or the last evaluation prior to Week 24 for patients who did not complete 24 weeks of randomized treatment (Jakafi N=16, placebo N=47). One (1) patient (placebo) with a missing baseline spleen volume is not included.

[See figure 1 above]

In Study 1, myelofibrosis symptoms were a secondary endpoint and were measured using the modified Myelofibrosis Symptom Assessment Form (MFSAF) v2.0 diary. The modified MFSAF is a daily diary capturing the core symptoms of myelofibrosis (abdominal discomfort, pain under left ribs, night sweats, itching, bone/muscle pain and early satiety). Symptom scores ranged from 0 to 10 with 0 representing symptoms "absent" and 10 representing "worst imaginable" symptoms. These scores were added to create the daily total score, which has a maximum of 60.

Table 8 presents assessments of Total Symptom Score from baseline to Week 24 in Study 1 including the proportion of patients with at least a 50% reduction (ie, improvement in symptoms). At baseline, the mean Total Symptom Score was 18.0 in the Jakafi group and 16.5 in the placebo group. A higher proportion of patients in the Jakafi group had a 50% or greater reduction in Total Symptom Score than in the placebo group, with a median time to response of less than 4 weeks.

Table 7: Percent of Patients with 35% or Greater Reduction from Baseline in Spleen Volume at Week 24 in Study 1 and at Week 48 in Study 2 (Intent to Treat)

	Study 1		Study 2	
	Jakafi (N=155)	Placebo (N=154)	Jakafi (N=146)	Best Available Therapy (N=73)
Time Points	Week 24		Week 48	
Number (%) of Patients with Spleen Volume Reduction by 35% or More	65 (41.9)	1 (0.7)	41 (28.5)	0
P-value	< 0.0001		< 0.0001	

Figure 1: Percent Change from Baseline in Spleen Volume at Week 24 or Last Observation for Each Patient (Study 1)

Table 8: Improvement in Total Symptom Score

	Jakafi (N=148)	Placebo (N=152)
Number (%) of Patients with 50% or Greater Reduction in Total Symptom Score by Week 24	68 (45.9)	8 (5.3)
P-value	< 0.0001	

Figure 2 shows the percent change from baseline in Total Symptom Score for each patient at Week 24 (Jakafi N=129, placebo N=103) or the last evaluation on randomized therapy prior to Week 24 for patients who did not complete 24 weeks of randomized treatment (Jakafi N=16, placebo N=42). Results are excluded for 5 patients with a baseline Total Symptom Score of zero, 8 patients with missing baseline and 6 patients with insufficient post-baseline data.

Figure 2: Percent Change from Baseline in Total Symptom Score at Week 24 or Last Observation for Each Patient (Study 1)

Worsening of Total Sympton Score is truncated at 150%.

Figure 4: Overall Survival - Kaplan-Meier Curves by Treatment Group in Study 1

	Jakafi (n=155)	Placebo (n=154)
% 1-year Survival	91%	84%
% 2-year Survival	60%	69%
% 3-year Survival	70%	61%

Number at Risk:

Jakafi	155	145	134	122	111	102	29	0
Placebo	154	142	117	101	92	82	32	0

[See figure 2 above]
Figure 3 displays the proportion of patients with at least a 50% improvement in each of the individual symptoms that comprise the Total Symptom Score indicating that all 6 of the symptoms contributed to the higher Total Symptom Score response rate in the group treated with Jakafi.

Figure 3: Proportion of Patients With 50% or Greater Reduction in Individual Symptom Scores at Week 24

Overall survival was a secondary endpoint in both Study 1 and Study 2. Patients in the control groups were eligible for crossover in both studies, and the median times to crossover were 9 months in Study 1 and 17 months in Study 2. Figure 4 and Figure 5 show Kaplan-Meier curves of overall survival at prospectively planned analyses after all patients remaining on study had completed 144 weeks on study.
[See figure 4 above]
[See figure 5 at top of next page]

16. HOW SUPPLIED/STORAGE AND HANDLING
Jakafi (ruxolitinib) Tablets are available as follows:
[See table at top of next page]

17. PATIENT COUNSELING INFORMATION
See FDA-approved patient labeling (Patient Information). Discuss the following with patients prior to treatment with Jakafi:

17.1 Thrombocytopenia, Anemia and Neutropenia
Inform patients that Jakafi is associated with thrombocytopenia, anemia and neutropenia, and of the need to monitor complete blood counts before and during treatment. Advise patients to observe for and report bleeding.

17.2 Infections
Inform patients of the signs and symptoms of infection and to report any such signs and symptoms promptly.
Inform patients regarding the early signs and symptoms of herpes zoster and of progressive multifocal leukoencephalopathy, and advise patients to seek advice of a clinician if such symptoms are observed.

17.3 Drug-drug Interactions
Advise patients to inform their healthcare providers of all medications they are taking, including over-the-counter medications, herbal products and dietary supplements.

17.4 Dialysis
Inform patients on dialysis that their dose should not be taken before dialysis but only following dialysis.

17.5 Compliance
Patients should be advised to continue taking Jakafi every day for as long as their physician tells them and that this is a long-term treatment. Patients should not change dose or stop taking Jakafi without first consulting their physician. Patients should be aware that after discontinuation of treatment, myelofibrosis signs and symptoms are expected to return.

Manufactured for:
Incyte Corporation
Wilmington, DE 19880
Jakafi is a registered trademark of Incyte Corporation. All rights reserved.
U.S. Patent No. 7,598,257; 8,415,362; 8,722,693
© 2011-2014 Incyte Corporation. All rights reserved.

Patient Information
Jakafi® (JAK-ah-fye)
(ruxolitinib) Tablets
Read this Patient Information before you start taking Jakafi and each time you get a refill. There may be new information. This information does not take the place of talking to your healthcare provider about your medical condition or treatment.
What is Jakafi?
Jakafi is a prescription medicine used to treat people with intermediate or high-risk myelofibrosis, including primary myelofibrosis, post-polycythemia vera myelofibrosis and post-essential thrombocythemia myelofibrosis.
It is not known if Jakafi is safe or effective in children.
What should I tell my healthcare provider before taking Jakafi?
Before taking Jakafi, tell your healthcare provider if you:
• have an infection.
• have or have had liver or kidney problems.
• are on dialysis. Jakafi should be taken after your dialysis.
• have any other medical conditions.
• are pregnant, or plan to become pregnant. It is not known if Jakafi will harm your unborn baby.
• are breast-feeding or plan to breast-feed. It is not known if Jakafi passes into your breast milk. You and your healthcare provider should decide if you will take Jakafi or breast-feed. You should not do both.
Tell your healthcare provider about all the medicines you take including prescription and non-prescription medicines, vitamins and herbal supplements. Taking Jakafi with certain other medicines may affect how Jakafi works.
Especially tell your healthcare provider if you take medicine for:
• Fungal infections
• Bacterial infections
• HIV-AIDS
Ask your healthcare provider or pharmacist if you are not sure if your medicine is one listed above.
Know the medicines you take. Keep a list of them to show your healthcare provider and pharmacist when you get a new medicine.
How should I take Jakafi?
• Take Jakafi exactly as your healthcare provider tells you.
• Do not change your dose or stop taking Jakafi without first talking to your healthcare provider.
• You can take Jakafi with or without food.
• Jakafi may also be given through certain nasogastric tubes.
  ◦ Tell your healthcare provider if you cannot take Jakafi by mouth. Your healthcare provider will decide if you can take Jakafi through a nasogastric tube.
  ◦ Ask your healthcare provider to give you specific instruction on how to properly take Jakafi through a nasogastric tube.
• Do not drink grapefruit juice while taking Jakafi. Grapefruit juice can affect the amount of Jakafi in your blood.
• If you take too much Jakafi call your healthcare provider or go to the nearest hospital emergency room department right away. Take the bottle of Jakafi with you.
• If you miss a dose of Jakafi, take your next dose at your regular time. Do not take 2 doses at the same time.
• You will have regular blood tests during your treatment with Jakafi. Your healthcare provider may change your dose of Jakafi or stop your treatment based on the results of your blood tests.
What are the possible side effects of Jakafi?
Jakafi can cause serious side effects including:
Low blood cell counts: Jakafi may cause low platelet counts (thrombocytopenia), low red blood cell counts (anemia), and low white blood cell counts (neutropenia). If you develop bleeding, stop Jakafi and call your doctor. Your healthcare provider will do a blood test to check your blood cell counts before you start Jakafi and regularly during your treatment with Jakafi. Tell your healthcare provider right away if you develop any of these symptoms:
• unusual bleeding
• bruising
• fatigue
• shortness of breath
• fever
Infection: You may be at risk for developing a serious infection while taking Jakafi. Tell your healthcare provider if you have:
• chills
• aches
• fever
• nausea
• vomiting
• weakness
• painful skin rash or blisters

Figure 5: Overall Survival - Kaplan-Meier Curves by Treatment Group in Study 2

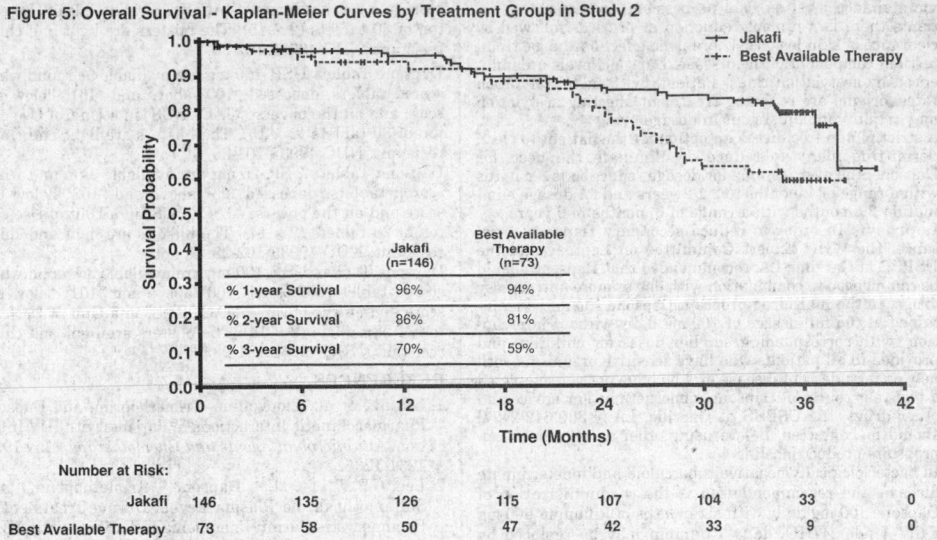

	Jakafi (n=146)	Best Available Therapy (n=73)
% 1-year Survival	96%	94%
% 2-year Survival	86%	81%
% 3-year Survival	70%	59%

Number at Risk:

Jakafi	146	135	126	115	107	104	33	0
Best Available Therapy	73	58	50	47	42	33	9	0

Jakafi Trade Presentations

NDC Number	Strength	Description	Tablets per Bottle
50881-005-60	5 mg	Round tablet with "INCY" on one side and "5" on the other	60
50881-010-60	10 mg	Round tablet with "INCY" on one side and "10" on the other	60
50881-015-60	15 mg	Oval tablet with "INCY" on one side and "15" on the other	60
50881-020-60	20 mg	Capsule shaped tablet with "INCY" on one side and "20" on the other	60
50881-025-60	25 mg	Oval tablet with "INCY" on one side and "25" on the other	60

Store at room temperature 20°C to 25°C (68°F to 77°F); excursions permitted between 15°C and 30°C (59°F and 86°F) [see USP Controlled Room Temperature].

The most common side effects of Jakafi include:
- dizziness
- headache

Tell your healthcare provider about any side effect that bothers you or that does not go away.

These are not all the possible side effects of Jakafi. Ask your healthcare provider or pharmacist for more information.

Call your doctor for medical advice about side effects. You may report side effects to Incyte Corporation at 1-855-463-3463 or FDA at 1-800-FDA-1088 or www.fda.gov/medwatch.

How should I store Jakafi?
- Store Jakafi at room temperature between 68°F and 77°F (20°C and 25°C).

Keep this and all medicines out of the reach of children.
General information about the safe and effective use of Jakafi:

Medicines are sometimes prescribed for purposes other than those listed in Patient Information. Do not use Jakafi for a condition for which it is not prescribed. Do not give Jakafi to other people, even if they have the same symptoms you have. It may harm them.

This Patient Information leaflet summarizes the most important information about Jakafi. If you would like more information, talk with your healthcare provider. You can ask your healthcare provider or pharmacist for information that is written for healthcare professionals.

For more information call 1-855-463-3463 or go to www.jakafi.com.

What are the ingredients in Jakafi?

Active ingredient: ruxolitinib.

Inactive ingredients: microcrystalline cellulose, lactose monohydrate, magnesium stearate, colloidal silicon dioxide, sodium starch glycolate, povidone and hydroxypropyl cellulose.

This Patient Information has been approved by the U.S. Food and Drug Administration.

Jakafi is a registered trademark of Incyte Corporation. All rights reserved.

U.S. Patent No. 7,598,257; 8,415,362; 8,722,693
© 2011-2014 Incyte Corporation. All rights reserved.
Issued: July 2014

Jacobus Pharmaceutical Co., Inc.

37 CLEVELAND LANE
P.O. BOX 5290
PRINCETON, NJ 08540

Direct All Inquiries to:
(609) 921-7447
FAX: (609) 799-1176

DAPSONE ℞
[dap 'sōne]
Tablets, USP
25 mg & 100 mg

DESCRIPTION

Dapsone-USP, 4,4′-diaminodiphenylsulfone (DDS), is a primary treatment for Dermatitis herpetiformis. It is an antibacterial drug for susceptible cases of leprosy. It is a white, odorless crystalline powder, practically insoluble in water and insoluble in fixed and vegetable oils.

Dapsone is issued on prescription in tablets of 25 and 100 mg for oral use.

$$NH_2 \text{—} \bigcirc \text{—} SO_2 \text{—} \bigcirc \text{—} NH_2$$

Inactive Ingredients: Colloidal silicone dioxide, magnesium stearate, microcrystalline cellulose and corn starch.

CLINICAL PHARMACOLOGY

Actions: The mechanism of action in Dermatitis herpetiformis has not been established. By the kinetic method in mice, Dapsone is bactericidal as well as bacteriostatic against *Mycobacterium leprae*.

Absorption and Excretion: Dapsone, when given orally, is rapidly and almost completely absorbed. About 85 percent of the daily intake is recoverable from the urine mainly in the form of water-soluble metabolites. Excretion of the drug is slow and a constant blood level can be maintained with the usual dosage.

Blood Levels: Detected a few minutes after ingestion, the drug reaches peak concentration in 4-8 hours. Daily administration for at least eight days is necessary to achieve a plateau level. With doses of 200 mg daily, this level averaged 2.3 µg/ml with a range of 0.1-7.0 µg/ml. The half-life in the plasma in different individuals varies from ten hours to fifty hours and averages twenty-eight hours. Repeat tests in the same individual are constant. Daily administration (50-100 mg) in leprosy patients will provide blood levels in excess of the usual minimum inhibitory concentration even for patients with a short Dapsone half-life.

INDICATIONS AND USAGE

Dermatitis herpetiformis: (D.H.)
Leprosy: All forms of leprosy except for cases of proven Dapsone resistance.

CONTRAINDICATION

Hypersensitivity to Dapsone and/or its derivatives.

WARNINGS

The patient should be warned to respond to the presence of clinical signs such as sore throat, fever, pallor, purpura or jaundice. Deaths associated with the administration of Dapsone have been reported from agranulocytosis, aplastic anemia and other blood dyscrasias. Complete blood counts should be done frequently in patients receiving Dapsone. The FDA Dermatology Advisory Committee recommended that, when feasible, counts should be done weekly for the first month, monthly for six months and semi-annually thereafter. If a significant reduction in leucocytes, platelets or hemopoiesis is noted, Dapsone should be discontinued and the patient followed intensively. Folic acid antagonists have similar effects and may increase the incidence of hematologic reactions; if co-administered with Dapsone the patient should be monitored more frequently. Patients on weekly pyrimethamine and Dapsone have developed agranulocytosis during the second and third month of therapy. Severe anemia should be treated prior to initiation of therapy and hemoglobin monitored. Hemolysis and methemoglobin may be poorly tolerated by patients with severe cardiopulmonary disease.

Cutaneous reactions, especially bullous, include exfoliative dermatitis and are probably one of the most serious, though rare, complications of sulfone therapy. They are directly due to drug sensitization. Such reactions include toxic erythema, erythema multiforme, toxic epidermal necrolysis, morbilliform and scarlatiniform reactions, urticaria and erythema nodosum. If new or toxic dermatologic reactions occur, sulfone therapy must be promptly discontinued and appropriate therapy instituted. Leprosy reactional states, including cutaneous, are not hypersensitivity reactions to Dapsone and do not require discontinuation. See special section.

PRECAUTIONS

General: Hemolysis and Heinz body formation may be exaggerated in individuals with a glucose-6-phosphate dehydrogenase (G6PD) deficiency, or methemoglobin reductase deficiency, or hemoglobin M. This reaction is frequently dose-related. Dapsone should be given with caution to these patients or if the patient is exposed to other agents or conditions such as infection or diabetic ketosis capable of producing hemolysis. Drugs or chemicals which have produced significant hemolysis in G6PD or methemoglobin reductase deficient patients include Dapsone, sulfanilamide, nitrite, aniline, phenylhydrazine, napthalene, niridazole, nitrofurantoin and 8-amino-antimalarials such as primaquine. Toxic hepatitis and cholestatic jaundice have been reported early in therapy. Hyperbilirubinemia may occur more often in G6PD deficient patients. When feasible, baseline and subsequent monitoring of liver function is recommended; if abnormal, Dapsone should be discontinued until the source of the abnormality is established.

Drug Interactions: Rifampin lowers Dapsone levels 7 to 10-fold by accelerating plasma clearance; in leprosy this reduction has not required a change in dosage. Folic acid antagonists such as pyrimethamine may increase the likelihood of hematologic reactions.

A modest interaction has been reported for patients receiving 100 mg Dapsone daily in combination with trimethoprim 5 mg/kg q6h. On Day 7, the serum Dapsone levels averaged 2.1 ± 1.0 µg/mL in comparison to 1.5 ± 0.5 µg/mL for Dapsone alone. On Day 7, trimethoprim levels averaged 18.4 ± 5.2 µg/mL in comparison to 12.4 ± 4.5 µg/mL for patients not receiving Dapsone. Thus, there is a mutual interaction between Dapsone and trimethoprim in which each raises the level of the other about 1.5 times.

A crossover study[1] designed to assess the potential of a drug interaction between Dapsone, 100 mg/day and trimethoprim, 200 mg every 12 hours, in eight asymptomatic HIV positive volunteers (average CD4 count 524 cells/mm[3]) demonstrated that there was not a significant drug interaction between Dapsone and trimethoprim. However, an earlier report[2] also by Lee et al, in 78 HIV infected patients with acute *Pneumocystis carinii* pneumonia, receiving Dapsone, 100 mg/day and higher trimethoprim dose, 20 mg/kg/day, demonstrated that the serum levels of Dapsone were increased by 40% and trimethoprim levels were increased by 48% when the drugs were administered concurrently.

Carcinogenesis, mutagenesis: Dapsone has been found carcinogenic (sarcomagenic) for male rats and female mice causing mesenchymal tumors in the spleen and peritoneum, and thyroid carcinoma in female rats. Dapsone is not mutagenic with or without microsomal activation in *S. typhimurium* tester strains 1535, 1537, 1538, 98, or 100.

Pregnancy: Teratogenic Effects. Pregnancy Category C: Animal reproduction studies have not been conducted with Dapsone. Extensive, but uncontrolled experience and two published surveys on the use of Dapsone in pregnant women have not shown that Dapsone increases the risk of fetal abnormalities if administered during all trimesters of pregnancy or can affect reproduction capacity. Because of the lack of animal studies or controlled human experience, Dapsone should be given to a pregnant woman only if clearly needed. In general, for leprosy, USPHS at Carville recommends maintenance of Dapsone. Dapsone has been important for the management of some pregnant D.H. patients.

Nursing Mothers: Dapsone is excreted in breast milk in substantial amounts. Hemolytic reactions can occur in neonates. See section on hemolysis. Because of the potential for tumorgenicity shown for Dapsone in animal studies a decision should be made whether to discontinue nursing or discontinue the drug taking into account the importance of drug to the mother.

Pediatric Use: Pediatric patients are treated on the same schedule as adults but with correspondingly smaller doses. Dapsone is generally not considered to have an effect on the later growth, development and functional development of the pediatric patient.

ADVERSE REACTIONS

In addition to the warnings listed above, the following syndromes and serious reactions have been reported in patients on Dapsone.

Hematologic Effects: Dose-related hemolysis is the most common adverse effect and is seen in patients with or without G6PD deficiency. Almost all patients demonstrate the inter-related changes of a loss of 1-2g of hemoglobin, an increase in the reticulocytes (2-12%), a shortened red cell life span and a rise in methemoglobin. G6PD deficient patients have greater responses.

Nervous System Effects: Peripheral neuropathy is a definite but unusual complication of Dapsone therapy in non-leprosy patients. Motor loss is predominant. If muscle weakness appears, Dapsone should be withdrawn. Recovery on withdrawal is usually substantially complete. The mechanism of recovery is reported by axonal regeneration. Some recovered patients have tolerated retreatment at reduced dosage. In leprosy this complication may be difficult to distinguish from a leprosy reactional state.

Body As A Whole: In addition to the warnings and adverse effects reported above, additional adverse reactions include: nausea, vomiting, abdominal pains, pancreatitis, vertigo, blurred vision, tinnitus, insomnia, fever, headache, psychosis, phototoxicity, pulmonary eosinophilia, tachycardia, albuminuria, the nephrotic syndrome, hypoalbuminemia without proteinuria, renal papillary necrosis, male infertility, drug-induced Lupus erythematosus and an infectious mononucleosis-like syndrome. In general, with the exception of the complications of severe anoxia from overdosage (retinal and optic nerve damage, etc.) these adverse reactions have regressed off drug.

OVERDOSAGE

Nausea, vomiting, hyperexcitability can appear a few minutes up to 24 hours after ingestion of an overdosage. Methemoglobin induced depression, convulsions or severe cyanosis requires prompt treatment. In normal and methemoglobin reductase deficient patients, methylene blue, 1-2 mg/kg of body weight, given slowly intravenously, is the treatment of choice. The effect is complete in 30 minutes, but may have to be repeated if methemoglobin reaccumulates. For non-emergencies, if treatment is needed, methylene blue may be given orally in doses of 3-5 mg/kg every 4-6 hours. Methylene blue reduction depends on G6PD and should not be given to fully expressed G6PD deficient patients.

DOSAGE AND ADMINISTRATION

Dermatitis herpetiformis: The dosage should be individually titrated starting in adults with 50 mg daily and correspondingly smaller doses in children. If full control is not achieved within the range of 50-300 mg daily, higher doses may be tried. Dosage should be reduced to a minimum

maintenance level as soon as possible. In responsive patients there is a prompt reduction in pruritus followed by clearance of skin lesions. There is no effect on the gastrointestinal component of the disease. Dapsone levels are influenced by acetylation rates. Patients with high acetylation rates, or who are receiving treatment affecting acetylation may require an adjustment in dosage.

A strict gluten free diet is an option for the patient to elect, permitting many to reduce or eliminate the need for Dapsone; the average time for dosage reduction is 8 months with a range of 4 months to 2 1/2 years and for dosage elimination 29 months with a range of 6 months to 9 years.

Leprosy: In order to reduce secondary Dapsone resistance, the WHO Expert Committee on Leprosy and the USPHS at Carville, LA, recommended that Dapsone should be commenced in combination with one or more anti-leprosy drugs. In the multidrug program Dapsone should be maintained at the full dosage of 100 mg daily without interruption (with corresponding smaller doses for children) and provided to all patients who have sensitive organisms with new or recrudescent disease or who have not yet completed a two year course of Dapsone monotherapy. For advice and other drugs, the USPHS at Carville, LA (1-800-642-2477) should be contacted. Before using other drugs consult appropriate product labeling.

In bacteriologically negative tuberculoid and indeterminate disease, the recommendation is the coadministration of Dapsone 100 mg daily with six months of Rifampin 600 mg daily. Under WHO, daily Rifampin may be replaced by 600 mg Rifampin monthly, if supervised. The Dapsone is continued until all signs of clinical activity are controlled - usually after an additional six months. Then Dapsone should be continued for an additional three years for tuberculoid and indeterminate patients and for five years for borderline tuberculoid patients.

In lepromatous and borderline lepromatous patients, the recommendation is the co-administration of Dapsone 100 mg daily with two years of Rifampin 600 mg daily. Under WHO daily Rifampin may be replaced by 600 mg Rifampin monthly, if supervised. One may elect the concurrent administration of a third anti-leprosy drug, usually either Clofazamine 50-100 mg daily or Ethionamide 250-500 mg daily. Dapsone 100 mg daily is continued 3-10 years until all signs of clinical activity are controlled with skin scrapings and biopsies negative for one year. Dapsone should then be continued for an additional 10 years for borderline patients and for life for lepromatous patients.

Secondary Dapsone resistance should be suspected whenever a lepromatous or borderline lepromatous patient receiving Dapsone treatment relapses clinically and bacteriologically, solid staining bacilli being found in the smears taken from the new active lesions. If such cases show no response to regular and supervised Dapsone therapy within three to six months or good compliance for the past 3-6 months can be assured, Dapsone resistance should be considered confirmed clinically. Determination of drug sensitivity using the mouse footpad method is recommended and, after prior arrangement, is available without charge from the USPHS, Carville, LA. Patients with proven Dapsone resistance should be treated with other drugs.

LEPROSY REACTIONAL STATES

Abrupt changes in clinical activity occur in leprosy with any effective treatment and are known as reactional states. The majority can be classified into two groups. The "Reversal" reaction (Type 1) may occur in borderline or tuberculoid leprosy patients often soon after chemotherapy is started. The mechanism is presumed to result from a reduction in the antigenic load: the patient is able to mount an enhanced delayed hypersensitivity response to residual infection leading to swelling ("Reversal") of existing skin and nerve lesions. If severe, or if neuritis is present, large doses of steroids should always be used. If severe, the patient should be hospitalized. In general anti-leprosy treatment is continued and therapy to suppress the reaction is indicated such as analgesics, steroids, or surgical decompression of swollen nerve trunks. USPHS at Carville, LA should be contacted for advice in management.

Erythema nodosum leprosum (ENL) (lepromatous reaction) (Type 2 reaction) occurs mainly in lepromatous patients and small numbers of borderline patients. Approximately 50% of treated patients show this reaction in the first year. The principal clinical features are fever and tender erythematous skin nodules sometimes associated with malaise, neuritis, orchitis, albuminuria, joint swelling, iritis, epistaxis or depression. Skin lesions can become pustular and/or ulcerate. Histologically there is a vasculitis with an intense polymorphonuclear infiltrate. Elevated circulating immune complexes are considered to be the mechanism of reaction. If severe, patients should be hospitalized. In general, anti-leprosy treatment is continued. Analgesics, steroids, and other agents available from USPHS, Carville, LA, are used to suppress the reaction.

HOW SUPPLIED

Dapsone Tablets USP, 25 mg are available as round white scored tablets, debossed "25" above and "102" below the

score and on the obverse "JACOBUS" in a Unit of Use carton of 30 tablets (2 × 15). The blisters are light and child-resistant. NDC 49938-102-30.

Dapsone Tablets USP, 100 mg are available as round white scored tablets, debossed "100" above and "101" below the score and on the obverse "JACOBUS" in a Unit of Use carton of 30 tablets (2 × 15). The blisters are light and child-resistant. NDC 49938-101-30.

Dapsone Tablets USP, 25 mg are available as round white scored tablets, debossed "25" above and "102" below the score and on the obverse "JACOBUS" in a Unit of Use carton of 28 tablets (2 × 14). The blisters are light and child-resistant. NDC 49938-102-28.

Dapsone Tablets USP, 100 mg are available as round white scored tablets, debossed "100" above and "101" below the score and on the obverse "JACOBUS" in a Unit of Use carton of 28 tablets (2 × 14). The blisters are light and child-resistant. NDC 49938-101-28.

REFERENCES

1. Lee, B., et al., Zidovudine, Trimethoprim, and Dapsone Pharmacokinetic Interactions in Patients with HIV Infection. *Antimicrobial Agents and Chemotherapy*, May 1996; 1231-1236.
2. Lee, B., et al., Dapsone, Trimethoprim, and Sulfamethoxazole Plasma Levels During Treatment of Pneumocystis Carinii Pneumonia in Patients with AIDS, *Annals of Internal Medicine*, 1989; 110:606-611.

Store at 20°-25° C (68°-77°F). [see USP Controlled Room Temperature]. Protect from light.

Rx only. Keep this and all medication out of the reach of children.

JACOBUS PHARMACEUTICAL CO., INC.
P.O. Box 5290
Princeton, NJ 08540
Revised August 2009
0826A09

PASER® GRANULES ℞
[Pa - ser]
(4 grams aminosalicylic acid delayed-release granules)

DESCRIPTION

PASER granules are a delayed release granule preparation of aminosalicylic acid (p-aminosalicylic acid; 4-aminosalicylic acid) for use with other anti-tuberculosis drugs for the treatment of all forms of active tuberculosis due to susceptible strains of tubercle bacilli. The granules are designed for gradual release to avoid high peak levels not useful (and perhaps toxic) with bacteriostatic drugs. Aminosalicylic acid is rapidly degraded in acid media; the protective acid-resistant outer coating is rapidly dissolved in neutral media so a mildly acidic food such as orange, apple or tomato juice, yogurt or apple sauce should be used. Aminosalicylic acid (p-aminosalicylic acid) is 4-Amino-2-hydroxybenzoic acid. PASER granules are the free base of aminosalicylic acid and do NOT contain sodium or a sugar. The molecular formula is $C_7H_7NO_3$ with a molecular weight of 153.14. With heat p-aminosalicylic acid is decarboxylated to produce CO_2 and m-aminophenol. If the airtight packets are swollen, storage has been improper. DO NOT USE if packets are swollen or the granules have lost their tan color and are dark brown or purple.

The structural formula is:

PASER granules are supplied as off-white tan colored granules with an average diameter of 1.5 mm and an average content of 60% aminosalicylic acid by weight. The acid resistant outer coating will be completely removed by a few minutes at a neutral pH. The inert ingredients are:
- colloidal silicon dioxide
- dibutyl sebacate
- hydroxypropyl methyl cellulose
- methacrylic acid copolymer
- microcrystalline cellulose
- talc

The packets contain 4 grams of aminosalicylic acid for oral administration three times a day by sprinkling on apple sauce or yogurt to be eaten without chewing. Suspension in an acidic fruit drink such as orange juice or tomato juice will protect the coating for at least 2 hours. Swirling the juice in the glass will help resuspend the granules if they sink.

CLINICAL PHARMACOLOGY

Mechanism of Action: Aminosalicylic acid is bacteriostatic against Mycobacterium tuberculosis. It inhibits the onset of bacterial resistance to streptomycin and isoniazid. The mechanism of action has been postulated to be inhibition of folic acid synthesis (but without potentiation with antifolic compounds) and/or inhibition of synthesis of the cell wall component, mycobactin, thus reducing iron uptake by M. tuberculosis.

Characteristics: The two major considerations in the clinical pharmacology of aminosalicylic acid are the prompt production of a toxic inactive metabolite under acid conditions and the short serum half life of one hour for the free drug. Both are discussed below.

After two hours in simulated gastric fluid, 10% of unprotected aminosalicylic acid is decarboxylated to form meta-aminophenol, a known hepatotoxin. The acid-resistant coating of the PASER granules protects against degradation in the stomach. The small granules are designed to escape the usual restriction on gastric emptying of large particles. Under neutral conditions such as are found in the small intestine or in neutral foods, the acid-resistant coating is dissolved within one minute. Care must be taken in the administration of these granules to protect the acid-resistant coating by maintaining the granules in an acidic food during dosage administration. Patients who have neutralized gastric acid with antacids will not need to protect the acid resistant coating with an acidic food since no acid is present to spoil the drug. Antacids may influence the absorption of other medications and are not necessary for PASER consumed with an acidic food.

Because PASER granules are protected by an enteric coating absorption does not commence until they leave the stomach; the soft skeletons of the granules remain and may be seen in the stool.

Absorption and excretion: In a single 4 gram pharmacokinetic study with food in normal volunteers the initial time to a $2\mu g/mL$ serum level of aminosalicylic acid was 2 hours with a range of 45 minutes to 24 hours; the median time to peak was 6 hours with a range of 1.5 to 24 hours; the mean peak level was 20 $\mu g/mL$ with a range of 9 to 35 $\mu g/mL$; a level of 2 $\mu g/mL$ was maintained for an average of 7.9 hours with a range of 5 to 9; a level of 1 $\mu g/mL$ was maintained for an average of 8.8 hours with a range of 6 to 11.5 hours. The recommended schedule is 4 grams every 8 hours.

80% of aminosalicylic acid is excreted in the urine, with 50% or more of the dosage excreted in acetylated form. The acetylation process is not genetically determined as is the case for isoniazid. Aminosalicylic acid is excreted by glomerular filtration; although previously reported otherwise, probenecid, a tubular blocking agent, does not enhance plasma concentration. In a 1954 study thyroxine synthesis but not iodide uptake was reported reduced about 40% when the sodium salt (not PASER granules) of aminosalicylic acid was administered one hour before radio-iodine; the sodium salt typically produces a serum level over 120 $\mu g/mL$ at one hour lasting one hour. Occasional goiter development can be prevented by the administration of thyroxine but not iodide. Penetration into the cerebrospinal fluid occurs only if the meninges are inflamed.

Approximately 50-60% of aminosalicylic acid is protein bound; binding is reported to be reduced 50% in kwashiorkor.

Microbiology: The aminosalicylic acid MIC for M. tuberculosis in 7H11 agar was less than 1.0 $\mu g/mL$ for nine strains including three multidrug resistant strains, but 4 and 8 $\mu g/mL$ for two other multidrug resistant strains. The 90% inhibition in 7H12 broth (Bactec) showed little dose response but was interpreted as being less than or equal to 0.12-0.25 $\mu g/mL$ for eight strains of which three were multiresistant, 0.50 $\mu g/mL$ for one resistant strain, questionable for four non-resistant strains and greater than 1$\mu g/mL$ for one non-resistant and three resistant strains. Aminosalicylic acid is not active in vitro against M. avium.

INDICATIONS AND USAGE

PASER is indicated for the treatment of tuberculosis in combination with other active agents. It is most commonly used in patients with Multi-drug Resistant TB (MDR-TB) or in situations when therapy with isoniazid and rifampin is not possible due to a combination of resistance and/or intolerance. When PASER is added to the treatment regimen in patients proven or suspected drug resistance, it should be accompanied by at least one and preferably two other new agents to which the patient's organism is known or expected to be susceptible.

CONTRAINDICATIONS

Hypersensitivity to any component of this medication.
Severe renal disease.

Patients with severe renal disease will accumulate aminosalicylic acid and its acetyl metabolite but will continue to acetylate, thus leading exclusively to the inactive acetylated form; deacetylation, if any, is not significant.

The half life of free aminosalicylic acid in renal disease is 30.8 minutes in comparison to 26.4 minutes in normal volunteers, but the half life of the inactive metabolite is 309 minutes in uremic patients in comparison to 51 minutes in normal volunteers. Although aminosalicylic acid passes di-

alysis membranes, the frequency of dialysis usually is not comparable to the half-life of 50 minutes for the free acid. Patients with end stage renal disease should not receive aminosalicylic acid.

WARNINGS
Liver Function

In one retrospective study of 7492 patients on rapidly absorbed aminosalicylic acid preparations, drug-induced hepatitis occurred in 38 patients (0.5%); in these 38 the first symptom usually appeared within three months of the start of therapy with a rash as the most common event followed by fever and much less frequently by GI disturbances of anorexia, nausea or diarrhea. Only one patient was diagnosed on routine biochemistry.

Premonitory symptoms in 90% of these 38 patients preceded jaundice by a few days to several weeks with the mean time of onset 33 days with a range of 7-90 days. Half of the adverse reactions occurred during the third, fourth or fifth weeks. When aminosalicylic acid-induced hepatitis was diagnosed, hepatomegaly was invariably present with lymphadenopathy in 46%, leucocytosis in 79%, and eosinophilia in 55%. Prompt recognition with discontinuation led to the recovery of all 38 patients. If recognized in the premonitory stage, the reaction is reported to "settle" in 24 hours and no jaundice ensues. From other reported studies failure to recognize the reaction can result in a mortality of up to 21%. The patient must be monitored carefully during the first three months of therapy and treatment must be discontinued immediately at the first sign of a rash, fever or other premonitory signs of intolerance.

PRECAUTIONS
(1) General:

All drugs should be stopped at the first sign suggesting a hypersensitivity reaction. They may be restarted one at a time in very small but gradually increasing doses to determine whether the manifestations are drug-induced and, if so, which drug is responsible.

Desensitization has been accomplished successfully in 15 of 17 patients starting with 10 mg aminosalicylic acid given as a single dose. The dosage is doubled every 2 days until reaching a total of 1 gram after which the dosage is divided to follow the regular schedule of administration. If a mild temperature rise or skin reaction develops, the increment is to be dropped back one level or the progression held for one cycle. Reactions are rare after a total dosage of 1.5 grams. Patients with hepatic disease may not tolerate aminosalicylic acid as well as normal patients, even though the metabolism in patients with hepatic disease has been reported to be comparable to that in normal volunteers.

(2) Information for Patients:

The patient should be advised that the first signs of hypersensitivity include a rash, often followed by fever, and much less frequently, GI disturbances of anorexia, nausea or diarrhea. If such symptoms develop, the patient should immediately cease taking the medication and arrange for a prompt clinical visit.

Patients should be advised that poor compliance in taking anti-TB medication often leads to treatment failure, and, not infrequently, to the development of resistance of the organisms in the individual patient.

Patients should be advised that the skeleton of the granules may be seen in the stool.

The coating to protect the PASER granules dissolves promptly under neutral conditions; the granules therefore should be administered by sprinkling on acidic foods such as apple sauce or yogurt or by suspension in a fruit drink which will protect the coating, but the granules sink and will have to be swirled. The coating will last at least 2 hours in either system. All juices tested to date have been satisfactory; tested are: tomato, orange, grapefruit, grape, cranberry, apple, "fruit punch".

Patients should be advised to store PASER in a refrigerator or freezer. PASER packets may be stored at room temperature for short periods of time.

Patients should be advised NOT to use if the packets are swollen or the granules have lost their tan color and are dark brown or purple. The patient should inform the pharmacist or physician immediately and return the medication.

(3) Laboratory Tests:

Aminosalicylic acid has been reported to interfere technically with the serum determinations of albumin by dye-binding, SGOT by the azoene dye method and with qualitative urine tests for ketones, bilirubin, urobilinogen or porphobilinogen.

(4) Drug Interactions:

Aminosalicylic acid at a dosage of 12 grams in a rapidly available form has been reported to produce a 20 percent reduction in the acetylation of isoniazid, especially in patients who are rapid acetylators; INH serum levels, half lives and excretions in fast acetylators still remain half of the levels seen in slow acetylators with or without p-aminosalicylic acid. The effect is dose related and, while it

has not been studied with the current delayed release preparation, the lower serum levels with this preparation will result in a reduced effect on the acetylation of INH.

Aminosalicylic acid has previously been reported to block the absorption of rifampin. A subsequent report has shown that this blockade was due to an excipient not included in PASER granules. Oral administration of a solution containing both aminosalicylic acid and rifampin showed full absorption of each product.

As a result of competition, Vitamin B_{12} absorption has been reduced 55% by 5 grams of aminosalicylic acid with clinically significant erythrocyte abnormalities developing after depletion; patients on therapy of more than one month should be considered for maintenance B_{12}.

A malabsorption syndrome can develop in patients on aminosalicylic acid but is usually not complete. The complete syndrome includes steatorrhea, an abnormal small bowel pattern on x-ray, villus atrophy, depressed cholesterol, reduced D-xylose and iron absorption. Triglyceride absorption always is normal.

In one literature report 8 hours after the last dosage of aminosalicylic acid at 2 gm qid serum digoxin levels were reduced 40% in two of ten patients but not changed in the remaining eight.

(5) Carcinogenesis, mutagenesis, impairment of fertility:

Sodium aminosalicylate produced an occipital bone defect, probably with a dose response, when administered to ten pregnant Wistar rats at five doses from 3.85 to 385 mg/kg from days 6 to 14. There were no significant changes from controls in any group in corpora lutea, early resorptions, total resorptions, fetal death, litter size, or hematomas. For all except the 77 mg/kg group, fetal weights were significantly greater than controls. Chinchilla rabbits on 5 mg/kg from days 7 to 14 did not show any significant differences as compared to controls for the same parameters studied.

Sodium aminosalicylic acid was not mutagenic in Ames tester strain TA 100. In human lymphocyte cultures in-vitro clastogenic effects of achromatic, chromatid, isochromatic breaks or chromatid translocations were not seen at 153 or 600 $\mu g/mL$. At 1500 and 3000 $\mu g/mL$ there was a dose related increase in chromatid aberrations.

Patients on isoniazid and aminosalicylic acid have been reported to have an increased number of chromosomal aberrations as compared to controls.

(6) Pregnancy: Pregnancy Category C:

Aminosalicylic acid has been reported to produce occipital malformations in rats when given at doses within the human dose range. Although there probably is a dose response, the frequency of abnormalities was comparable to controls at the highest level tested (two times the human dosage). When administered to rabbits at 5 mg/kg, throughout all three trimesters, no teratologic or embryocidal effects were seen. Literature reports on aminosalicylic acid in pregnant women always report coadministration of other medications. Because there are no adequate and well controlled studies of aminosalicylic acid in humans, PASER granules should be given to a pregnant woman only if clearly needed.

(8) Nursing mothers:

After administration of a different preparation of aminosalicylic acid to one patient, the maximum concentration in the milk was 1 $\mu g/mL$ at 3 hours with a half-life of 2.5 hours; the maximum maternal plasma concentration was 70 $\mu g/mL$ at two hours.

ADVERSE EFFECTS

The most common side effect is gastrointestinal intolerance manifested by nausea, vomiting, diarrhea, and abdominal pain.

Hypersensitivity reactions: Fever, skin eruptions of various types, including exfoliative dermatitis, infectious mononucleosis-like, or lymphoma-like syndrome, leucopenia, agranulocytosis, thrombocytopenia, Coombs' positive hemolytic anemia, jaundice, hepatitis, pericarditis, hypoglycemia, optic neuritis, encephalopathy, Leoffler's syndrome, vasculitis and a reduction in prothrombin.

Crystalluria may be prevented by the maintenance of urine at a neutral or an alkaline pH.

OVERDOSAGE

Overdosage has not been reported.

DOSAGE AND ADMINISTRATION

PASER granules should be administered with other drugs to which the organism is known or expected to be susceptible. It is most commonly administered to patients with Multi-drug Resistant TB (MDR-TB) or in other situations in which therapy with isoniazid or rifampin is not possible due to a combination of resistance and/or intolerance. The adult dosage of four grams (one packet) three times per day or correspondingly smaller doses in children should be given by sprinkling on apple sauce or yogurt or by swirling in the glass to suspend the granules in an acidic drink such as tomato or orange juice.

DO NOT USE if packet is swollen or the granules have lost their tan color, turning dark brown or purple.

HOW SUPPLIED

Carton of 30 PASER packets (NDC 49938-107-04).

Each packet contains four grams aminosalicylic acid.

PASER granules are supplied in packets containing 4 grams of aminosalicylic acid for administration three times a day by suspension in an acidic drink or food with a pH less than 5. Examples include apple sauce, yogurt, tomato or orange juice.

Distributors and Pharmacists: Store below 59°F (15°C) (in a refrigerator or freezer).

Patients are urged to store PASER in a refrigerator or freezer. PASER packets may be stored at room temperature for short periods of time.

AVOID EXCESSIVE HEAT. DO NOT USE if packet is swollen or the granules have lost their tan color, turning dark brown or purple.

JACOBUS PHARMACEUTICAL CO. INC.

P.O. Box 5290

Princeton, NJ 08540

2A JULY, 1996

Janssen Pharmaceuticals, Inc.

1000 ROUTE 202 S
RARITAN, NJ 08869-0602
and
1125 TRENTON-HARBOURTON ROAD
TITUSVILLE, NJ 08560-0200
http://www.janssenpharmaceuticalsinc.com

Direct General Inquiries to:
(800) 526-7736
Medical Emergency Contact:
Ph: (800) 457-6399 or 908-218-7325
For Medical Information/Adverse Experience Reporting Contact:
Ph: (800) 457-6399

NUCYNTA®   ℂ ℞

[new-sinn'-tah]
(tapentadol)
immediate-release oral tablets C-II

HIGHLIGHTS OF PRESCRIBING INFORMATION

These highlights do not include all the information needed to use NUCYNTA® safely and effectively. See full prescribing information for NUCYNTA®.

NUCYNTA® (tapentadol) immediate-release oral tablets C-II
Initial U.S. Approval: 2008

RECENT MAJOR CHANGES

Contraindications (4)	07/2013
Warnings and Precautions (5)	07/2013

INDICATIONS AND USAGE

NUCYNTA® is an opioid analgesic indicated for the management of moderate to severe acute pain in adults. (1)

DOSAGE AND ADMINISTRATION

- Individualize dosing according to the severity of pain being treated, the previous experience with similar drugs and the ability to monitor the patient. (2.1)
- Initiate NUCYNTA® with or without food at a dose of 50 mg, 75 mg, or 100 mg every 4 to 6 hours depending upon pain intensity. On the first day of dosing, the second dose may be administered as soon as one hour after the first dose, if adequate pain relief is not attained with the first dose. Subsequent dosing is 50 mg, 75 mg, or 100 mg every 4 to 6 hours and should be adjusted to maintain adequate analgesia with acceptable tolerability. Daily doses greater than 700 mg on the first day of therapy and 600 mg on subsequent days have not been studied and are, therefore, not recommended. (2.2)

DOSAGE FORMS AND STRENGTHS

Tablets: 50 mg, 75 mg, 100 mg (3)

CONTRAINDICATIONS

- Significant respiratory depression (4)
- Acute or severe bronchial asthma, hypercarbia (4)
- Known or suspected paralytic ileus (4)
- Hypersensitivity to tapentadol or to any other ingredients of the product (4)
- Concurrent use of monoamine oxidase (MAO) inhibitors or use within the last 14 days. (4)

WARNINGS AND PRECAUTIONS

- Misuse, Abuse and Diversion: NUCYNTA® is a Schedule II controlled substance with abuse liability similar to other opioids: monitor patients closely for signs of misuse, abuse and addiction. (5.1)
- Elderly, cachectic, and debilitated patients and patients with chronic pulmonary disease: Monitor closely because of increased risk of respiratory depression. (5.5)
- Interaction with CNS depressants including other opioids, sedatives, alcohol, and illicit drugs: Consider dose reduction of one or both drugs because of additive effects. (5.7)
- Hypotensive effect: Monitor for signs of hypotension.(5.8)
- Patients with head injury or increased intracranial pressure: Monitor for sedation and respiratory depression. Avoid use of NUCYNTA® in patients with impaired consciousness or coma susceptible to intracranial effects of CO_2 retention. (5.9)
- Seizures: Use with caution in patients with a history of seizures. (5.10)
- Serotonin Syndrome: Potentially life-threatening condition could result from concomitant serotonergic administration. (5.11)
- Withdrawal: Withdrawal symptoms may occur if NUCYNTA® is discontinued abruptly. (5.13)
- Impaired mental/physical abilities: Caution must be used with potentially hazardous activities. (5.14)

ADVERSE REACTIONS

The most common (≥10%) adverse reactions were nausea, dizziness, vomiting and somnolence. (6)

To report SUSPECTED ADVERSE REACTIONS, contact Janssen Pharmaceuticals, Inc. at 1-800-526-7736 (1-800-JANSSEN) or FDA at 1-800-FDA-1088 or www.fda.gov/medwatch

DRUG INTERACTIONS

- CNS depressants: Increased risk of respiratory depression, hypotension, profound sedation, coma or death. When combined therapy with CNS depressant is contemplated, the dose of one or both agents should be reduced. (7.3)
- Mixed agonist/antagonist opioids (i.e., pentazocine, nalbuphine, and butorphanol): May reduce analgesic effect and/or precipitate withdrawal symptoms. (7.5)
- Monitor for signs of serotonin syndrome when NUCYNTA® is used concurrently with SSRIs, SNRIs, tricyclic antidepressants, or triptans. (7.4)

USE IN SPECIFIC POPULATIONS

- Pregnancy: Based on animal data, may cause fetal harm. (8.1)
- Nursing mothers: Closely monitor infants of nursing women receiving NUCYNTA®. (8.3)
- Renal or hepatic impairment: not recommended in patients with severe renal or hepatic impairment. Reduce dose in patients with moderate hepatic impairment. (8.7, 8.8)

See 17 for PATIENT COUNSELING INFORMATION
Revised: 09/2013

FULL PRESCRIBING INFORMATION: CONTENTS*

FULL PRESCRIBING INFORMATION

1   INDICATIONS AND USAGE

NUCYNTA® (tapentadol) is indicated for the management of moderate to severe acute pain in adults.

2   DOSAGE AND ADMINISTRATION

2.1   Individualization of Dosage

As with any opioid drug product, adjust the dosing regimen for each patient individually, taking into account the patient's prior analgesic treatment experience. In the selection of the initial dose of tapentadol, give attention to the following:

- the total daily dose, potency and specific characteristics of the opioid the patient has been taking previously;
- the reliability of the relative potency estimate used to calculate the equivalent morphine sulfate dose needed;
- the patient's degree of opioid tolerance;
- the general condition and medical status of the patient;
- concurrent medications;
- the type and severity of the patient's pain;
- risk factors for abuse, addiction or diversion, including a prior history of abuse, addiction or diversion.

The following dosing recommendations, therefore, can only be considered suggested approaches to what is actually a series of clinical decisions over time in the management of the pain of each individual patient.

Continual re-evaluation of the patient receiving tapentadol is important, with special attention to the maintenance of pain control and the relative incidence of side effects associated with therapy.

During chronic therapy, especially for non-cancer-related pain, periodically re-assess the continued need for the use of opioid analgesics.

During periods of changing analgesic requirements, including initial titration, frequent contact is recommended between physician, other members of the healthcare team, patient, and the caregiver/family. Monitor the patient for signs of respiratory or central nervous system depression.

2.2   Initiation of Therapy

The dose is 50 mg, 75 mg, or 100 mg every 4 to 6 hours depending upon pain intensity.

On the first day of dosing, the second dose may be administered as soon as one hour after the first dose, if adequate pain relief is not attained with the first dose. Subsequent dosing is 50 mg, 75 mg, or 100 mg every 4 to 6 hours and should be adjusted to maintain adequate analgesia with acceptable tolerability.

Daily doses greater than 700 mg on the first day of therapy and 600 mg on subsequent days have not been studied and are not recommended.

NUCYNTA® may be given with or without food [see Clinical Pharmacology (12.3)].

2.3 Renal Impairment
Use of NUCYNTA® in patients with severe renal impairment is not recommended [see Warnings and Precautions (5.16) and Clinical Pharmacology (12.3)].
No dosage adjustment is recommended in patients with mild or moderate renal impairment.

2.4 Hepatic Impairment
The safety and efficacy of NUCYNTA® has not been studied in patients with severe hepatic impairment (Child-Pugh Score 10–15) and use in this population is not recommended [see Warnings and Precautions (5.15)].
Initiate treatment of patients with moderate hepatic impairment (Child-Pugh Score 7 to 9) with 50 mg no more frequently than once every 8 hours (maximum of three doses in 24 hours). Further treatment should reflect maintenance of analgesia with acceptable tolerability, to be achieved by either shortening or lengthening the dosing interval [see Clinical Pharmacology (12.3)].
No dosage adjustment is recommended in patients with mild hepatic impairment (Child-Pugh Score 5 to 6) [see Clinical Pharmacology (12.3)].

2.5 Elderly Patients
In general, recommended dosing for elderly patients with normal renal and hepatic function is the same as for younger adult patients with normal renal and hepatic function. Because elderly patients are more likely to have decreased renal and hepatic function, consideration should be given to starting elderly patients with the lower range of recommended doses.

2.6 Cessation of Therapy
When the patient no longer requires therapy with tapentadol, gradually taper the dose to prevent signs and symptoms of withdrawal in the physically dependent patient [see Warnings and Precautions (5.13)].

3 DOSAGE FORMS AND STRENGTHS
NUCYNTA® Tablets are round, biconvex and film-coated and are available in the following strengths, colors, and debossings: 50 mg of tapentadol (yellow with "O-M" on one side and "50" on the other side), 75 mg of tapentadol (yellow-orange with "O-M" on one side and "75" on the other side), and 100 mg of tapentadol (orange with "O-M" on one side and "100" on the other side) [see Description (11) and How Supplied/Storage and Handling (16)].

4 CONTRAINDICATIONS
NUCYNTA® is contraindicated in:
- Patients with significant respiratory depression
- Patients with acute or severe bronchial asthma or hypercarbia in an unmonitored setting or in the absence of resuscitative equipment
- Patients with known or suspected paralytic ileus
- Patients with hypersensitivity (e.g. anaphylaxis, angioedema) to tapentadol or to any other ingredients of the product [see Adverse Reactions (6.2)].
- Patients who are receiving monoamine oxidase (MAO) inhibitors or who have taken them within the last 14 days due to potential additive effects on norepinephrine levels which may result in adverse cardiovascular events [see Drug Interactions (7.2)].

5 WARNINGS AND PRECAUTIONS

5.1 Abuse Potential
NUCYNTA® contains tapentadol, an opioid agonist and a Schedule II controlled substance. Tapentadol can be abused in a manner similar to other opioid agonists legal or illicit. Opioid agonists are sought by drug abusers and people with addiction disorders and are subject to criminal diversion. Consider these risks when prescribing or dispensing NUCYNTA® in situations where there is concern about increased risks of misuse, abuse, or diversion. Concerns about abuse, addiction, and diversion should not, however, prevent the proper management of pain.
Assess each patient's risk for opioid abuse or addiction prior to prescribing NUCYNTA®. The risk for opioid abuse is increased in patients with a personal or family history of substance abuse (including drug or alcohol abuse or addiction) or mental illness (e.g., major depression). Patients at increased risk may still be appropriately treated with opioids; however these patients will require intensive monitoring for signs of misuse, abuse, or addiction. Routinely monitor all patients receiving opioids for signs of misuse, abuse, and addiction because these drugs carry a risk for addiction even under appropriate medical use.
Misuse or abuse of NUCYNTA® by crushing, chewing, snorting or injecting will pose a significant risk that could result in overdose and death [see Overdosage (10)].
Contact local state professional licensing board or state controlled substances authority for information on how to prevent and detect abuse or diversion of this product [see Drug Abuse and Dependence (9)].

5.2 Life Threatening Respiratory Depression
Respiratory depression is the chief hazard of opioid agonists, including NUCYNTA®. Respiratory depression, if not immediately recognized and treated, may lead to respiratory arrest and death. Respiratory depression from opioids is manifested by a reduced urge to breathe and a decreased rate of respiration, often associated with a "sighing" pattern of breathing (deep breaths separated by abnormally long pauses). Carbon dioxide (CO_2) retention from opioid-induced respiratory depression can exacerbate the sedating effects of opioids. Management of respiratory depression may include close observation, supportive measures, and use of opioid antagonists, depending on the patient's clinical status [see Overdosage (10)].
Instruct patients against use by individuals other than the patient for whom NUCYNTA® was prescribed and to keep NUCYNTA® out of the reach of children, as such inappropriate use may result in fatal respiratory depression.
Patients with conditions accompanied by hypoxia, hypercarbia or decreased respiratory reserve such as: asthma, chronic obstructive pulmonary disease or cor pulmonale, central nervous system (CNS) depression, or coma may be at increased risk for increased airway resistance and decreased respiratory drive to the point of apnea even with usual therapeutic doses of NUCYNTA®. Consider the use of alternative non-mu-opioid agonist analgesics and use NUCYNTA® only under careful medical supervision at the lowest effective dose in such patients. If respiratory depression occurs, treat the patient for mu-opioid agonist-induced respiratory depression [see Overdosage (10.2)]. To reduce the risk of respiratory depression, proper dosing of NUCYNTA® is essential [see Dosage and Administration (2)].

5.3 Accidental Exposure
Accidental ingestion of NUCYNTA®, especially in children, can result in a fatal overdose of tapentadol.

5.4 Interactions with Alcohol, Other Opioids, and Drugs of Abuse
Due to its mu-opioid agonist activity, NUCYNTA® may be expected to have additive effects when used in conjunction with alcohol, other opioids, or illicit drugs that cause central nervous system depression, respiratory depression, hypotension, and profound sedation, coma or death [see Drug Interactions (7.3)]. Instruct patients not to consume alcoholic beverages or use prescription or non-prescription products containing alcohol, other opioids, or drugs of abuse while on NUCYNTA® therapy [see Drug Interactions (7.1)].

5.5 Elderly, Cachectic, and Debilitated Patients
Respiratory depression is more likely to occur in elderly, cachectic, or debilitated patients as they may have altered pharmacokinetics or altered clearance compared to younger, healthier patients. Therefore, closely monitor such patients, particularly when NUCYNTA® is given concomitantly with other drugs that depress respiration [see Warnings and Precautions (5.2)].

5.6 Use in Patients with Chronic Pulmonary Disease
Monitor for respiratory depression those patients with significant chronic obstructive pulmonary disease or cor pulmonale, and patients having a substantially decreased respiratory reserve, hypoxia, hypercarbia, or pre-existing respiratory depression, as in these patients, even usual therapeutic doses of NUCYNTA® may decrease respiratory drive to the point of apnea [see Warnings and Precautions (5.2)]. Consider the use of alternative non-opioid analgesics in these patients if possible.

5.7 Interactions with CNS Depressants and Illicit Drugs
Hypotension, and profound sedation, coma or respiratory depression may result if NUCYNTA® is used concomitantly with other CNS depressants (e.g., sedatives, anxiolytics, hypnotics, neuroleptics, muscle relaxants, other opioids and illicit drugs). When considering the use of NUCYNTA® in a patient taking a CNS depressant, assess the duration of use of the CNS depressant and the patient's response, including the degree of tolerance that has developed to CNS depression. Additionally, consider the patient's use, if any, of alcohol and/or illicit drugs that can cause CNS depression. If NUCYNTA® therapy is to be initiated in a patient taking a CNS depressant, start with a lower NUCYNTA® dose than usual and monitor patients for signs of sedation and respiratory depression and consider using a lower dose of the concomitant CNS depressant [see Drug Interactions (7.3)].

5.8 Hypotensive Effect
NUCYNTA® may cause severe hypotension. There is an increased risk in patients whose ability to maintain blood pressure has already been compromised by a reduced blood volume or concurrent administration of certain CNS depressant drugs (e.g., phenothiazines or general anesthetics) [see Drug Interactions (7.3)]. Monitor these patients for signs of hypotension after the dose of NUCYNTA®. In patients with circulatory shock, NUCYNTA® may cause vasodilation that can further reduce cardiac output and blood pressure. Avoid the use of NUCYNTA® in patients with circulatory shock.

5.9 Use in Patients with Head Injury or Increased Intracranial Pressure
Monitor patients taking NUCYNTA® who may be susceptible to the intracranial effects of CO_2 retention (e.g., those with evidence of increased intracranial pressure or brain tumors) for signs of sedation and respiratory depression. NUCYNTA® may reduce respiratory drive, and the resultant CO_2 retention can further increase intracranial pressure. Opioids may also obscure the clinical course in a patient with a head injury.
Avoid the use of NUCYNTA® in patients with impaired consciousness or coma.

5.10 Seizures
NUCYNTA® has not been evaluated in patients with a predisposition to a seizure disorder, and such patients were excluded from clinical studies. The active ingredient tapentadol in NUCYNTA® may aggravate convulsions in patients with convulsive disorders, and may induce or aggravate seizures in some clinical settings. Monitor patients with a history of seizure disorders for worsened seizure control during NUCYNTA® therapy.

5.11 Serotonin Syndrome Risk
Cases of life-threatening serotonin syndrome have been reported with the concurrent use of tapentadol and serotonergic drugs. Serotonergic drugs comprise Selective Serotonin Reuptake Inhibitors (SSRIs), Serotonin and Norepinephrine Reuptake Inhibitors (SNRIs), tricyclic antidepressants (TCAs), triptans, drugs that affect the serotonergic neurotransmitter system (e.g. mirtazapine, trazodone, and tramadol), and drugs that impair metabolism of serotonin (including MAOIs). This may occur within the recommended dose. Serotonin syndrome may include mental-status changes (e.g., agitation, hallucinations, coma), autonomic instability (e.g., tachycardia, labile blood pressure, hyperthermia), neuromuscular aberrations (e.g., hyperreflexia, incoordination) and/or gastrointestinal symptoms (e.g., nausea, vomiting, diarrhea) and can be fatal [see Drug Interactions (7.4)].

5.12 Use in Patients with Gastrointestinal Conditions
NUCYNTA® is contraindicated in patients with GI obstruction, including paralytic ileus. The tapentadol in NUCYNTA® may cause spasm of the sphincter of Oddi. Monitor patients with biliary tract disease, including acute pancreatitis, for worsening symptoms.

5.13 Withdrawal
Withdrawal symptoms may occur if NUCYNTA® is discontinued abruptly. These symptoms may include: anxiety, sweating, insomnia, rigors, pain, nausea, tremors, diarrhea, upper respiratory symptoms, piloerection, and rarely, hallucinations. Withdrawal symptoms may be reduced by tapering NUCYNTA® [see Drug Abuse and Dependence (9.3)].

5.14 Driving and Operating Heavy Machinery
NUCYNTA® may impair the mental or physical abilities needed to perform potentially hazardous activities such as driving a car or operating machinery. Warn patients not to drive or operate dangerous machinery unless they are tolerant to the effects of NUCYNTA® and know how they will react to the medication.

5.15 Hepatic Impairment
A study with NUCYNTA® in subjects with hepatic impairment showed higher serum concentrations of tapentadol than in those with normal hepatic function. Avoid use of NUCYNTA® in patients with severe hepatic impairment. Reduce the dose of NUCYNTA® in patients with moderate hepatic impairment [see Dosage and Administration (2.4) and Clinical Pharmacology (12.3)]. Closely monitor patients with moderate hepatic impairment for respiratory and central nervous system depression when receiving NUCYNTA®.

5.16 Renal Impairment
Use of NUCYNTA® in patients with severe renal impairment is not recommended due to accumulation of a metabolite formed by glucuronidation of tapentadol. The clinical relevance of the elevated metabolite is not known [see Clinical Pharmacology (12.3)].

6 ADVERSE REACTIONS
The following adverse reactions are discussed in more detail in other sections of the labeling:
- Respiratory Depression [see Warnings and Precautions (5.2)]
- Interaction with Alcohol [see Warnings and Precautions (5.4)]
- Chronic Pulmonary Disease [see Warnings and Precautions (5.6)]
- Hypotensive Effects [see Warnings and Precautions (5.8)]
- Interactions with Other CNS Depressants [see Warnings and Precautions (5.7)]
- Drug abuse, addiction, and dependence [see Drug Abuse and Dependence (9.2, 9.3)]
- Gastrointestinal Effects [see Warnings and Precautions (5.12)]
- Seizures [see Warnings and Precautions (5.10)]
- Serotonin Syndrome [see Warnings and Precautions (5.11)]

6.1 Clinical Studies Experience
Because clinical trials are conducted under widely varying conditions, adverse reaction rates observed in the clinical trials of a drug cannot be directly compared to rates in the clinical trials of another drug and may not reflect the rates observed in clinical practice.

Based on data from nine Phase 2/3 studies that administered multiple doses (seven placebo- and/or active-controlled, one noncontrolled and one Phase 3 active-controlled safety study) the most common adverse reactions (reported by ≥10% in any NUCYNTA® dose group) were: nausea, dizziness, vomiting and somnolence.

The most common reasons for discontinuation due to adverse reactions in the studies described above (reported by ≥1% in any NUCYNTA® dose group) were dizziness (2.6% vs. 0.5%), nausea (2.3% vs. 0.6%), vomiting (1.4% vs. 0.2%), somnolence (1.3% vs. 0.2%) and headache (0.9% vs. 0.2%) for NUCYNTA®- and placebo-treated patients, respectively. Seventy-six percent of NUCYNTA®-treated patients from the nine studies experienced adverse events.

NUCYNTA® was studied in multiple-dose, active- or placebo-controlled studies, or noncontrolled studies (n = 2178), in single-dose studies (n = 870), in open-label study extension (n = 483) and in Phase 1 studies (n = 597). Of these, 2034 patients were treated with doses of 50 mg to 100 mg of NUCYNTA® dosed every 4 to 6 hours.

The data described below reflect exposure to NUCYNTA® in 3161 patients, including 449 exposed for 45 days. NUCYNTA® was studied primarily in placebo- and active-controlled studies (n = 2266, and n = 2944, respectively). The population was 18 to 85 years old (mean age 46 years), 68% were female, 75% white and 67% were postoperative. Most patients received NUCYNTA® doses of 50 mg, 75 mg, or 100 mg every 4 to 6 hours.

Table 1 Adverse Reactions Reported by ≥1% of NUCYNTA®-Treated Patients In Seven Phase 2/3 Placebo- and/or Oxycodone-Controlled, One Non-controlled, and One Phase 3 Oxycodone-Controlled Safety, Multiple-Dose Clinical Studies

System/Organ Class MedDRA Preferred Term	NUCYNTA® 21 mg – 120 mg (n=2178) %	Placebo (n=619) %
Gastrointestinal disorders		
Nausea	30	13
Vomiting	18	4
Constipation	8	3
Dry mouth	4	<1
Dyspepsia	2	<1
General disorders and administration site conditions		
Fatigue	3	<1
Feeling hot	1	<1
Infections and infestations		
Nasopharyngitis	1	<1
Upper respiratory tract infection	1	<1
Urinary tract infection	1	<1
Metabolism and nutrition disorders		
Decreased appetite	2	0
Nervous system disorders		
Dizziness	24	8
Somnolence	15	3
Tremor	1	<1
Lethargy	1	<1
Psychiatric disorders		
Insomnia	2	<1
Confusional state	1	0
Abnormal dreams	1	<1
Anxiety	1	<1
Skin and subcutaneous tissue disorders		
Pruritus	5	1
Hyperhidrosis	3	<1
Pruritus generalized	3	<1
Rash	1	<1
Vascular disorders		
Hot flush	1	<1

The following adverse drug reactions occurred in less than 1% of NUCYNTA®-treated patients in the pooled safety data from nine Phase 2/3 clinical studies:

Cardiac disorders: heart rate increased, heart rate decreased

Eye disorders: visual disturbance

Gastrointestinal disorders: abdominal discomfort, impaired gastric emptying

General disorders and administration site conditions: irritability, edema, drug withdrawal syndrome, feeling drunk

Immune system disorders: hypersensitivity

Investigations: gamma-glutamyltransferase increased, alanine aminotransferase increased, aspartate aminotransferase increased

Musculoskeletal and connective tissue disorders: involuntary muscle contractions, sensation of heaviness

Nervous system disorders: hypoesthesia, paresthesia, disturbance in attention, sedation, dysarthria, depressed level of consciousness, memory impairment, ataxia, presyncope, syncope, coordination abnormal, seizure

Psychiatric disorders: euphoric mood, disorientation, restlessness, agitation, nervousness, thinking abnormal

Renal and urinary disorders: urinary hesitation, pollakiuria

Respiratory, thoracic and mediastinal disorders: oxygen saturation decreased, cough, dyspnea, respiratory depression

Skin and subcutaneous tissue disorders: urticaria

Vascular disorders: blood pressure decreased

In the pooled safety data, the overall incidence of adverse reactions increased with increased dose of NUCYNTA®, as did the percentage of patients with adverse reactions of nausea, dizziness, vomiting, somnolence, and pruritus.

6.2 Post-marketing Experience

The following additional adverse reactions have been identified during post-approval use of NUCYNTA®. Because these reactions are reported voluntarily from a population of uncertain size, it is not always possible to estimate their frequency reliably.

Gastrointestinal disorders: diarrhea

Nervous system disorders: headache

Psychiatric disorders: hallucination, suicidal ideation

Cardiac disorders: palpitations

Anaphylaxis, angioedema, and anaphylactic shock have been reported very rarely with ingredients contained in NUCYNTA®. Advise patients how to recognize such reactions and when to seek medical attention.

7 DRUG INTERACTIONS

NUCYNTA® is mainly metabolized by glucuronidation. The following substances have been included in a set of interaction studies without any clinically significant finding: acetaminophen, acetylsalicylic acid, naproxen and probenecid [see Clinical Pharmacology (12.3)].

The pharmacokinetics of tapentadol were not affected when gastric pH or gastrointestinal motility were increased by omeprazole and metoclopramide, respectively [see Clinical Pharmacology (12.3)].

7.1 Alcohol, Other Opioids, and Drugs of Abuse

Due to its mu-opioid agonist activity, NUCYNTA® may be expected to have additive effects when used in conjunction with alcohol, other opioids, or illicit drugs that cause central nervous system depression, respiratory depression, hypotension, and profound sedation, coma or death. Instruct patients not to consume alcoholic beverages or use prescription or non-prescription products containing alcohol, other opioids, or drugs of abuse while on NUCYNTA® therapy [see Warnings and Precautions (5.4)].

7.2 Monoamine Oxidase Inhibitors

NUCYNTA® is contraindicated in patients who are receiving monoamine oxidase (MAO) inhibitors or who have taken them within the last 14 days due to potential additive effects on norepinephrine levels which may result in adverse cardiovascular events [see Contraindications (4)].

7.3 CNS Depressants

Concurrent use of NUCYNTA® and other central nervous system (CNS) depressants including sedatives or hypnotics, general anesthetics, phenothiazines, tranquilizers, and alcohol can increase the risk of respiratory depression, hypotension, profound sedation or coma. Monitor patients receiving CNS depressants and NUCYNTA® for signs of respiratory depression and hypotension. When such combined therapy is contemplated, start NUCYNTA® at ⅓ to ½ of the usual dosage and consider using a lower dose of the concomitant CNS depressant [see Warnings and Precautions (5.7)].

7.4 Serotonergic Drugs

There have been post-marketing reports of serotonin syndrome with the concomitant use of tapentadol and serotonergic drugs (e.g., SSRIs and SNRIs). Caution is advised when NUCYNTA® is co-administered with other drugs that may affect serotonergic neurotransmitter systems such as SSRIs, SNRIs, MAOIs, and triptans. If concomitant treatment of NUCYNTA® with a drug affecting the serotonergic neurotransmitter system is clinically warranted, careful observation of the patient is advised [see Warning and Precautions (5.11)].

7.5 Mixed Agonist/Antagonist Opioid Analgesics

The concomitant use of NUCYNTA® with mixed agonist/antagonists (e.g., butorphanol, nalbuphine, and pentazocine) and partial agonists (e.g., buprenorphine) may precipitate withdrawal symptoms. Avoid the use of agonist/antagonists and partial agonists with NUCYNTA®.

7.6 Anticholinergics

The use of NUCYNTA® with anticholinergic products may increase the risk of urinary retention and/or severe constipation, which may lead to paralytic ileus.

8 USE IN SPECIFIC POPULATIONS

8.1 Pregnancy

Pregnancy Category C: There are no adequate and well-controlled studies of NUCYNTA® in pregnant women. NUCYNTA® should be used during pregnancy only if the potential benefit justifies the potential risk to the fetus.

Tapentadol HCl was evaluated for teratogenic effects in pregnant rats and rabbits following intravenous and subcutaneous exposure during the period of embryofetal organogenesis. When tapentadol was administered twice daily by the subcutaneous route in rats at dose levels of 10, 20, or 40 mg/kg/day [producing up to 1 times the plasma exposure at the maximum recommended human dose (MRHD) of 700 mg/day based on an area under the time-curve (AUC) comparison], no teratogenic effects were observed. Evidence of embryofetal toxicity included transient delays in skeletal maturation (i.e. reduced ossification) at the 40 mg/kg/day dose which was associated with significant maternal toxicity. Administration of tapentadol HCl in rabbits at doses of 4, 10, or 24 mg/kg/day by subcutaneous injection [producing 0.2, 0.6, and 1.85 times the plasma exposure at the MRHD based on an AUC comparison] revealed embryofetal toxicity at doses ≥10 mg/kg/day. Findings included reduced fetal viability, skeletal delays and other variations. In addition, there were multiple malformations including gastroschisis/thoracogastroschisis, amelia/phocomelia, and cleft palate at doses ≥10 mg/kg/day and above, and ablepharia, encephalopathy, and spina bifida at the high dose of 24 mg/kg/day. Embryofetal toxicity, including malformations, may be secondary to the significant maternal toxicity observed in the study.

In a study of pre- and postnatal development in rats, oral administration of tapentadol at doses of 20, 50, 150, or 300 mg/kg/day to pregnant and lactating rats during the late gestation and early postnatal period [resulting in up to 1.7 times the plasma exposure at the MRHD on an AUC basis] did not influence physical or reflex development, the outcome of neurobehavioral tests or reproductive parameters. Treatment-related developmental delay was observed, including incomplete ossification, and significant reductions in pup body weights and body weight gains at doses associated with maternal toxicity (150 mg/kg/day and above). At maternal tapentadol doses ≥150 mg/kg/day, a dose-related increase in pup mortality was observed through postnatal Day 4.

8.2 Labor and Delivery

NUCYNTA® is not for use in women during and immediately prior to labor. Occasionally, opioid analgesics may prolong labor by temporarily reducing the strength, duration, and frequency of uterine contractions. However, these effects are not consistent and may be offset by an increased rate of cervical dilatation which tends to shorten labor.

Opioids cross the placenta and may produce respiratory depression and psychophysiologic effects in neonates. Closely observe neonates whose mothers received opioid analgesics during labor for signs of respiratory depression. An opioid antagonist, such as naloxone, should be available for reversal of opioid-induced respiratory depression in the neonate in such situations.

8.3 Nursing Mothers

There is insufficient/limited information on the excretion of tapentadol in human or animal breast milk. Physicochemical and available pharmacodynamic/toxicological data on tapentadol point to excretion in breast milk and risk to the breastfeeding child cannot be excluded.

Because of the potential for adverse reactions in nursing infants from NUCYNTA®, a decision should be made whether to discontinue nursing or discontinue the drug, taking into account the importance of the drug to the mother.

Withdrawal symptoms can occur in breast-feeding infants when maternal administration of NUCYNTA® is stopped.

8.4 Pediatric Use

The safety and effectiveness of NUCYNTA® in pediatric patients less than 18 years of age have not been established.

8.5 Geriatric Use

Of the total number of patients in Phase 2/3 double-blind, multiple-dose clinical studies of NUCYNTA®, 19% were 65 and over, while 5% were 75 and over. No overall differences in effectiveness were observed between these patients and younger patients. The rate of constipation was higher in subjects greater than or equal to 65 years than those less than 65 years (12% vs. 7%).

In general, recommended dosing for elderly patients with normal renal and hepatic function is the same as for younger adult patients with normal renal and hepatic function. Because elderly patients are more likely to have decreased renal and hepatic function, consideration should be given to starting elderly patients with the lower range of recommended doses [see Clinical Pharmacology (12.3)].

8.6 Neonatal Withdrawal Syndrome

Chronic maternal use of NUCYNTA® during pregnancy can affect the neonate with subsequent withdrawal signs. Neonatal withdrawal syndrome presents as irritability, hyperactivity and abnormal sleep pattern, high pitched cry, tremor, vomiting, diarrhea and failure to gain weight. The onset, duration and severity of neonatal withdrawal syndrome vary based on the drug used, duration of use, the dose of last maternal use, and rate of elimination drug by the newborn. Neonatal opioid withdrawal syndrome may be life-threatening and should be treated according to protocols developed by neonatology experts.

8.7 Renal Impairment

The safety and effectiveness of NUCYNTA® has not been established in patients with severe renal impairment (CLCR <30 mL/min). Use of NUCYNTA® in patients with severe renal impairment is not recommended due to accumulation of a metabolite formed by glucuronidation of tapentadol. The clinical relevance of the elevated metabolite is not known [see Clinical Pharmacology (12.3)].

8.8 Hepatic Impairment

Administration of tapentadol resulted in higher exposures and serum levels of tapentadol in subjects with impaired hepatic function compared to subjects with normal hepatic function [see Clinical Pharmacology (12.3)]. The dose of NUCYNTA® should be reduced in patients with moderate hepatic impairment (Child-Pugh Score 7 to 9) [see Dosage and Administration (2.2)].

Use of NUCYNTA® is not recommended in patients with severe hepatic impairment (Child-Pugh Score 10 to 15) [see Warnings and Precautions (5.15)].

9 DRUG ABUSE AND DEPENDENCE

9.1 Controlled Substance

NUCYNTA® contains tapentadol, a Schedule II controlled substance with a high potential for abuse similar to fentanyl, methadone, morphine, oxycodone, and oxymorphone. NUCYNTA® is subject to misuse, abuse, addiction, and criminal diversion [see Warnings and Precautions (5.1)].

9.2 Abuse

All patients treated with opioids require careful monitoring for signs of abuse and addiction, because use of opioid analgesic products carries the risk of addiction even under appropriate medical use.

Drug abuse is the intentional non-therapeutic use of an over-the-counter or prescription drug, even once, for its rewarding psychological or physiological effects. Drug abuse includes, but is not limited to the following examples: the use of a prescription or over-the-counter drug to get "high", or the use of steroids for performance enhancement and muscle build up.

Drug addiction is a cluster of behavioral, cognitive, and physiological phenomena that develop after repeated substance use and include: a strong desire to take the drug, difficulties in controlling its use, persisting in its use despite harmful consequences, a higher priority given to drug use than to other activities and obligations, increased tolerance, and sometimes a physical withdrawal.

"Drug seeking" behavior is very common in addicts, and drug abusers. Drug-seeking tactics include emergency calls or visits near the end of office hours, refusal to undergo appropriate examination, testing or referral, repeated claims of loss of prescriptions, tampering with prescriptions and reluctance to provide prior medical records or contact information for other treating physician(s). "Healthcare professional shopping" (visiting multiple prescribers) to obtain

additional prescriptions is common among drug abusers, people suffering from untreated addiction and criminals seeking drugs to sell.

Abuse and addiction are separate and distinct from physical dependence and tolerance. Physicians should be aware that addiction may not be accompanied by concurrent tolerance and symptoms of physical dependence in all addicts. In addition, abuse of opioids can occur in the absence of true addiction and is characterized by misuse for non-medical purposes, often in combination with other psychoactive substances.

NUCYNTA® can be diverted for non-medical use into illicit channels of distribution. Careful record-keeping of prescribing information, including quantity, frequency, and renewal requests, as required by law, is strongly advised.

Proper assessment of the patient, proper prescribing practices, periodic re-evaluation of therapy, and proper dispensing and storage are appropriate measures that help to limit abuse of opioid drugs.

9.3 Dependence

Both tolerance and physical dependence can develop during chronic opioid therapy. Tolerance is the need for increasing doses of opioids to maintain a defined effect such as analgesia (in the absence of disease progression or other external factors). Tolerance may occur to both the desired and undesired effects of drugs, and may develop at different rates for different effects.

Physical dependence results in withdrawal symptoms after abrupt discontinuation or a significant dose reduction of a drug. Withdrawal also may be precipitated through the administration of drugs with opioid antagonist activity, e.g., naloxone, nalmefene, or mixed agonist/antagonist analgesics (pentazocine, butorphanol, buprenorphine, nalbuphine). Physical dependence may not occur to a clinically significant degree until after several days to weeks of continued opioid usage. Some or all of the following can characterize this syndrome: restlessness, lacrimation, rhinorrhea, yawning, perspiration, chills, piloerection, myalgia, mydriasis, irritability, anxiety, backache, joint pain, weakness, abdominal cramps, insomnia, nausea, anorexia, vomiting, diarrhea, increased blood pressure, respiratory rate, or heart rate. Withdrawal symptoms may be reduced by tapering NUCYNTA®.

Infants born to mothers physically dependent on opioids will also be physically dependent and may exhibit respiratory difficulties and withdrawal symptoms [see Use in Specific Populations (8.1, 8.2)].

10 OVERDOSAGE

10.1 Clinical Presentation

Acute overdosage with opioids can be manifested by respiratory depression, somnolence progressing to stupor or coma, skeletal muscle flaccidity, cold and clammy skin, constricted pupils, and sometimes pulmonary edema, bradycardia, hypotension and death. Marked mydriasis rather than miosis may be seen due to severe hypoxia in overdose situations.

10.2 Management

In case of overdose, priorities are the re-establishment of a patent and protected airway and institution of assisted or controlled ventilation if needed. Employ other supportive measures (including oxygen, vasopressors) in the management of circulatory shock and pulmonary edema as indicated. Cardiac arrest or arrhythmias will require advanced life support techniques.

The opioid antagonists, naloxone or nalmefene, are specific antidotes to respiratory depression resulting from opioid overdose. Opioid antagonists should not be administered in the absence of clinically significant respiratory or circulatory depression secondary to tapentadol overdose. Such agents should be administered cautiously to patients who are known, or suspected to be, physically dependent on NUCYNTA®. In such cases, an abrupt or complete reversal of opioid effects may precipitate an acute withdrawal syndrome.

Because the duration of reversal would be expected to be less than the duration of action of tapentadol in NUCYNTA®, carefully monitor the patient until spontaneous respiration is reliably re-established. If the response to opioid antagonists is suboptimal or not sustained, additional antagonist should be given as directed in the product's prescribing information.

In an individual physically dependent on opioids, administration of an opioid receptor antagonist may precipitate an acute withdrawal. The severity of the withdrawal produced will depend on the degree of physical dependence and the dose of the antagonist administered. If a decision is made to treat serious respiratory depression in the physically dependent patient, administration of the antagonist should be begun with care and by titration with smaller than usual doses of the antagonist.

11 DESCRIPTION

NUCYNTA® (tapentadol) is a mu-opioid receptor agonist, supplied in immediate-release film-coated tablets for oral

administration, containing 58.24, 87.36 and 116.48 mg of tapentadol hydrochloride in each tablet strength, corresponding to 50, 75, and 100 mg of tapentadol free-base, respectively. The chemical name is 3-[(1R,2R)-3-(dimethylamino)-1-ethyl-2-methylpropyl]phenol monohydrochloride. The structural formula is:

The molecular weight of tapentadol HCl is 257.80, and the molecular formula is $C_{14}H_{23}NO \cdot HCl$. The n-octanol:water partition coefficient log P value is 2.87. The pKa values are 9.34 and 10.45.

In addition to the active ingredient tapentadol HCl, NUCYNTA® tablets also contain the following inactive ingredients: croscarmellose sodium, lactose monohydrate, magnesium stearate, microcrystalline cellulose, povidone. The film coatings for all tablet strengths contain polyvinyl alcohol, titanium dioxide, polyethylene glycol, talc, and the colorant FD&C Yellow #6 aluminum lake; the film coatings for the 50 mg and 75 mg tablets also contain the additional colorant D&C Yellow #10 aluminum lake.

12 CLINICAL PHARMACOLOGY

12.1 Mechanism of Action

Tapentadol is a centrally-acting synthetic analgesic. The exact mechanism of action is unknown. Although the clinical relevance is unclear, preclinical studies have shown that tapentadol is a mu-opioid receptor (MOR) agonist and a norepinephrine reuptake inhibitor (NRI). Analgesia in animal models is derived from both of these properties.

12.2 Pharmacodynamics

Tapentadol is 18 times less potent than morphine in binding to the human mu-opioid receptor and is 2–3 times less potent in producing analgesia in animal models. Tapentadol has been shown to inhibit norepinephrine reuptake in the brains of rats resulting in increased norepinephrine concentrations. In preclinical models, the analgesic activity due to the mu-opioid receptor agonist activity of tapentadol can be antagonized by selective mu-opioid antagonists (e.g., naloxone), whereas the norepinephrine reuptake inhibition is sensitive to norepinephrine modulators. Tapentadol exerts its analgesic effects without a pharmacologically active metabolite.

Concentration-Efficacy Relationships

The minimum effective plasma concentration of tapentadol for analgesia varies widely among patients, especially among patients who have been previously treated with agonist opioids.

Concentration-Adverse Experience Relationships

There is a general relationship between increasing opioid plasma concentration and increasing frequency of adverse experiences such as nausea, vomiting, CNS effects, and respiratory depression.

Effects on the Cardiovascular System

There was no effect of therapeutic and supratherapeutic doses of tapentadol on the QT interval. In a randomized, double-blind, placebo- and positive-controlled crossover study, healthy subjects were administered five consecutive doses of NUCYNTA® 100 mg every 6 hours, NUCYNTA® 150 mg every 6 hours, placebo and a single oral dose of moxifloxacin. Similarly, NUCYNTA® had no relevant effect on other ECG parameters (heart rate, PR interval, QRS duration, T-wave or U-wave morphology).

Tapentadol produces peripheral vasodilation which may result in orthostatic hypotension.

Effects on the Central Nervous System (CNS)

The principal therapeutic action of tapentadol is analgesia. Tapentadol causes respiratory depression, in part by a direct effect on the brainstem respiratory centers. The respiratory depression involves a reduction in the responsiveness of the brain stem respiratory centers to both increases in carbon dioxide tension and electrical stimulation. Tapentadol depresses the cough reflex by direct effect on the cough center in the medulla.

Tapentadol causes miosis, even in total darkness. Pinpoint pupils are a sign of opioid overdose but are not pathognomonic (e.g., pontine lesions of hemorrhagic or ischemic origin may produce similar findings). Marked mydriasis rather than miosis may be seen with hypoxia in overdose situations [see Overdosage (10)]. Other effects of tapentadol include anxiolysis, euphoria, and feeling of relaxation, drowsiness and changes in mood.

Effects on the Gastrointestinal Tract and on Other Smooth Muscle

Gastric, biliary and pancreatic secretions are decreased by tapentadol. Tapentadol causes a reduction in motility and is associated with an increase in tone in the antrum of the stomach and duodenum. Digestion of food in the small intestine is delayed and propulsive contractions are decreased. Propulsive peristaltic waves in the colon are decreased, while tone is increased to the point of spasm. The end result is constipation. Tapentadol can cause a marked increase in biliary tract pressure as a result of spasm of the sphincter of Oddi, and transient elevations in serum amylase. Tapentadol may also cause spasm of the sphincter of the urinary bladder.

Effects on the Endocrine System
Opioid agonists have been shown to have a variety of effects on the secretion of hormones. Opioids inhibit the secretion of ACTH, cortisol, and luteinizing hormone (LH) in humans. They also stimulate prolactin, growth hormone (GH) secretion, and pancreatic secretion of insulin and glucagon.

Effects on the Immune System
Opioids have been shown to have a variety of effects on components of the immune system in *in vitro* and animal models. The clinical significance of these findings is unknown.

CNS Depressant/Alcohol Interaction
Additive pharmacodynamic effects may be expected when NUCYNTA® is used in conjunction with alcohol, other opioids, or illicit drugs that cause central nervous system depression.

12.3 Pharmacokinetics
Absorption
The mean absolute bioavailability after single-dose administration (fasting) of NUCYNTA® is approximately 32% due to extensive first-pass metabolism. Maximum serum concentrations of tapentadol are typically observed at around 1.25 hours after dosing.

Dose-proportional increases in the C_{max} and AUC values of tapentadol have been observed over the 50 to 150 mg dose range.

A multiple (every 6 hour) dose study with doses ranging from 75 to 175 mg tapentadol showed a mean accumulation factor of 1.6 for the parent drug and 1.8 for the major metabolite tapentadol-O-glucuronide, which are primarily determined by the dosing interval and apparent half-life of tapentadol and its metabolite.

Food Effect
The AUC and C_{max} increased by 25% and 16%, respectively, when NUCYNTA® was administered after a high-fat, high-calorie breakfast. NUCYNTA® may be given with or without food.

Distribution
Tapentadol is widely distributed throughout the body. Following intravenous administration, the volume of distribution (Vz) for tapentadol is 540 +/- 98 L. The plasma protein binding is low and amounts to approximately 20%.

Metabolism and Elimination
In humans, about 97% of the parent compound is metabolized. Tapentadol is mainly metabolized via Phase 2 pathways, and only a small amount is metabolized by Phase 1 oxidative pathways. The major pathway of tapentadol metabolism is conjugation with glucuronic acid to produce glucuronides. After oral administration approximately 70% (55% O-glucuronide and 15% sulfate of tapentadol) of the dose is excreted in urine in the conjugated form. A total of 3% of drug was excreted in urine as unchanged drug. Tapentadol is additionally metabolized to N-desmethyl tapentadol (13%) by CYP2C9 and CYP2C19 and to hydroxy tapentadol (2%) by CYP2D6, which are further metabolized by conjugation. Therefore, drug metabolism mediated by cytochrome P450 system is of less importance than phase 2 conjugation.

None of the metabolites contribute to the analgesic activity. Tapentadol and its metabolites are excreted almost exclusively (99%) via the kidneys. The terminal half-life is on average 4 hours after oral administration. The total clearance is 1530 +/- 177 mL/min.

Special Populations
Geriatric Patients
The mean exposure (AUC) to tapentadol was similar in elderly subjects compared to young adults, with a 16% lower mean C_{max} observed in the elderly subject group compared to young adult subjects.

Renal Impairment
AUC and C_{max} of tapentadol were comparable in subjects with varying degrees of renal function (from normal to severely impaired). In contrast, increasing exposure (AUC) to tapentadol-O-glucuronide was observed with increasing degree of renal impairment. In subjects with mild (CL_{CR} = 50 to <80 mL/min), moderate (CL_{CR} = 30 to <50 mL/min), and severe (CL_{CR} = <30 mL/min) renal impairment, the AUC of tapentadol-O-glucuronide was 1.5-, 2.5-, and 5.5-fold higher compared with normal renal function, respectively.

Hepatic Impairment
Administration of NUCYNTA® resulted in higher exposures and serum levels to tapentadol in subjects with impaired hepatic function compared to subjects with normal hepatic function. The ratio of tapentadol pharmacokinetic parameters for the mild hepatic impairment group (Child-Pugh Score 5 to 6) and moderate hepatic impairment group (Child-Pugh Score 7 to 9) in comparison to the normal he-

patic function group were 1.7 and 4.2, respectively, for AUC; 1.4 and 2.5, respectively, for C_{max}; and 1.2 and 1.4, respectively, for $t_{1/2}$. The rate of formation of tapentadol-O-glucuronide was lower in subjects with increased liver impairment.

Pharmacokinetic Drug Interactions
Tapentadol is mainly metabolized by Phase 2 glucuronidation, a high capacity/low affinity system; therefore, clinically relevant interactions caused by Phase 2 metabolism are unlikely to occur. Naproxen and probenecid increased the AUC of tapentadol by 17% and 57%, respectively. These changes are not considered clinically relevant and no change in dose is required.

No changes in the pharmacokinetic parameters of tapentadol were observed when acetaminophen and acetylsalicylic acid were given concomitantly.

In vitro studies did not reveal any potential of tapentadol to either inhibit or induce cytochrome P450 enzymes. Furthermore, a minor amount of NUCYNTA® is metabolized via the oxidative pathway. Thus, clinically relevant interactions mediated by the cytochrome P450 system are unlikely to occur.

The pharmacokinetics of tapentadol were not affected when gastric pH or gastrointestinal motility were increased by omeprazole and metoclopramide, respectively.

Plasma protein binding of tapentadol is low (approximately 20%). Therefore, the likelihood of pharmacokinetic drug-drug interactions by displacement from the protein binding site is low.

13 NON-CLINICAL TOXICOLOGY
13.1 Carcinogenesis, Mutagenesis, Impairment of Fertility
Carcinogenesis
Tapentadol was administered to rats (diet) and mice (oral gavage) for two years.

In mice, tapentadol HCl was administered by oral gavage at dosages of 50, 100 and 200 mg/kg/day for 2 years (up to 0.2 times the plasma exposure at the maximum recommended human dose [MRHD] on an area under the time-curve [AUC] basis). No increase in tumor incidence was observed at any dose level.

In rats, tapentadol HCl was administered in diet at dosages of 10, 50, 125 and 250 mg/kg/day for two years (up to 0.2 times in the male rats and 0.6 times in the female rats the MRHD on an AUC basis). No increase in tumor incidence was observed at any dose level.

Mutagenesis
Tapentadol did not induce gene mutations in bacteria, but was clastogenic with metabolic activation in a chromosomal aberration test in V79 cells. The test was repeated and was negative in the presence and absence of metabolic activation. The one positive result for tapentadol was not confirmed *in vivo* in rats, using the two endpoints of chromosomal aberration and unscheduled DNA synthesis, when tested up to the maximum tolerated dose.

Impairment of Fertility
Tapentadol HCl was administered intravenously to male or female rats at dosages of 3, 6, or 12 mg/kg/day (representing exposures of up to approximately 0.4 times the exposure at the MRHD on an AUC basis, based on extrapolation from toxicokinetic analyses in a separate 4-week intravenous study in rats). Tapentadol did not alter fertility at any dose level. Maternal toxicity and adverse effects on embryonic development, including decreased number of implantations, decreased numbers of live conceptuses, and increased pre- and post-implantation losses occurred at dosages ≥6 mg/kg/day.

13.2 Animal Toxicology and/or Pharmacology
In toxicological studies with tapentadol, the most common systemic effects of tapentadol were related to the mu-opioid receptor agonist and norepinephrine reuptake inhibition pharmacodynamic properties of the compound. Transient, dose-dependent and predominantly CNS-related findings were observed, including impaired respiratory function and convulsions, the latter occurring in the dog at plasma levels (C_{max}) which are in the range associated with the maximum recommended human dose (MRHD).

14 CLINICAL STUDIES
The efficacy and safety of NUCYNTA® in the treatment of moderate to severe acute pain has been established in two randomized, double-blind, placebo- and active-controlled studies of moderate to severe pain from first metatarsal bunionectomy and end-stage degenerative joint disease.

14.1 Orthopedic Surgery – Bunionectomy
A randomized, double-blind, parallel-group, active- and placebo-controlled, multiple-dose study demonstrated the efficacy of 50 mg, 75 mg, and 100 mg NUCYNTA® given every 4 to 6 hours for 72 hours in patients aged 18 to 80 years experiencing moderate to severe pain following unilateral, first metatarsal bunionectomy surgery. Patients who qualified for the study with a baseline pain score of ≥4 on an 11-point rating scale ranging from 0 to 10 were randomized to

1 of 5 treatments. Patients were allowed to take a second dose of study medication as soon as 1 hour after the first dose on study Day 1, with subsequent dosing every 4 to 6 hours. If rescue analgesics were required, the patients were discontinued for lack of efficacy. Efficacy was evaluated by comparing the sum of pain intensity difference over the first 48 hours (SPID48) versus placebo. NUCYNTA® at each dose provided a greater reduction in pain compared to placebo based on SPID48 values.

For various degrees of improvement from baseline to the 48-hour endpoint, Figure 1 shows the fraction of patients achieving that level of improvement. The figures are cumulative, such that every patient that achieves a 50% reduction in pain from baseline is included in every level of improvement below 50%. Patients who did not complete the 48-hour observation period in the study were assigned 0% improvement.

Figure 1: Percentage of Patients Achieving Various Levels of Pain Relief as Measured by Pain Severity at 48 Hours Compared to Baseline- Post Operative Bunionectomy

The proportions of patients who showed reduction in pain intensity at 48 hours of 30% or greater, or 50% or greater were significantly higher in patients treated with NUCYNTA® at each dose versus placebo.

14.2 End-Stage Degenerative Joint Disease
A randomized, double-blind, parallel-group, active- and placebo-controlled, multiple-dose study evaluated the efficacy and safety of 50 mg and 75 mg NUCYNTA® given every 4 to 6 hours during waking hours for 10 days in patients aged 18 to 80 years, experiencing moderate to severe pain from end stage degenerative joint disease of the hip or knee, defined as a 3-day mean pain score of ≥5 on an 11-point pain intensity scale, ranging from 0 to 10. Pain scores were assessed twice daily and assessed the pain the patient had experienced over the previous 12 hours. Patients were allowed to continue non-opioid analgesic therapy for which they had been on a stable regimen before screening throughout the study. Eighty-three percent (83%) of patients in the tapentadol treatment groups and the placebo group took such analgesia during the study. The 75 mg treatment group was dosed at 50 mg for the first day of the study, followed by 75 mg for the remaining nine days. Patients requiring rescue analgesics other than study medication were discontinued for lack of efficacy. Efficacy was evaluated by comparing the sum of pain intensity difference (SPID) versus placebo over the first five days of treatment. NUCYNTA® 50 mg and 75 mg provided improvement in pain compared with placebo based on the 5-Day SPID.

For various degrees of improvement from baseline to the Day 5 endpoint, Figure 2 shows the fraction of patients achieving that level of improvement. The figures are cumulative, such that every patient that achieves a 50% reduction in pain from baseline is included in every level of improvement below 50%. Patients who did not complete the 5-day observation period in the study were assigned 0% improvement.

Figure 2: Percentage of Patients Achieving Various Levels of Pain Relief as Measured by Average Pain Severity for the Previous 12 hours, Measured on Study Day 5 Compared to Baseline — End Stage Degenerative Joint Disease

The proportions of patients who showed reduction in pain intensity at 5 days of 30% or greater, or 50% or greater were significantly higher in patients treated with NUCYNTA® at each dose versus placebo.

16 HOW SUPPLIED/STORAGE AND HANDLING

NUCYNTA® Tablets are available in the following strengths and packages. All tablets are round and biconvex-shaped.
50 mg tablets are yellow and debossed with "O-M" on one side and "50" on the other side, and are available in bottles of 100 (NDC 50458-820-04) and hospital unit dose blister packs of 10 (NDC 50458-820-02).
75 mg tablets are yellow-orange and debossed with "O-M" on one side and "75" on the other side, and are available in bottles of 100 (NDC 50458-830-04) and hospital unit dose blister packs of 10 (NDC 50458-830-02).
100 mg tablets are orange and debossed with "O-M" on one side and "100" on the other side, and are available in bottles of 100 (NDC 50458-840-04) and hospital unit dose blister packs of 10 (NDC 50458-840-02).
Storage and Handling
Store up to 25°C (77°F); excursions permitted to 15° – 30°C (59° – 86°F) [see USP Controlled Room Temperature]. Protect from moisture.
Keep NUCYNTA® in a secure place out of reach of children. NUCYNTA® tablets that are no longer needed should be destroyed by flushing down the toilet.

17 PATIENT COUNSELING INFORMATION

Instruct patients to take NUCYNTA® only as prescribed.
Abuse Potential
Inform patients that NUCYNTA® contains tapentadol, a Schedule II controlled substance that is subject to abuse. Instruct patients not to share NUCYNTA® with others and to take steps to protect NUCYNTA® from theft or misuse.
Life-threatening Respiratory Depression
Discuss the risk of respiratory depression with patients, explaining that the risk is greatest when starting NUCYNTA® or when the dose is increased. Advise patients how to recognize respiratory depression and to seek medical attention if they are experiencing breathing difficulties.
Accidental Exposure
Instruct patients to take steps to store NUCYNTA® securely. Accidental exposure, especially in children, may results in serious harm or death. Advise patients to dispose of unused NUCYNTA® by flushing the tablets down the toilet.
Important Administration Instructions
Instruct patients how to properly take NUCYNTA®, including the following:
• Using NUCYNTA® exactly as prescribed to reduce the risk of life-threatening adverse reactions (e.g., respiratory depression).
• Not discontinuing NUCYNTA® without first discussing the need for a tapering regimen with the prescriber.
Risks from Concomitant Use of Alcohol and other CNS Depressants
Inform patients that the concomitant use of alcohol with NUCYNTA® can increase the risk of life-threatening respiratory depression. Instruct patients not to consume alcoholic beverages, as well as prescription and over-the-counter drug products that contain alcohol, during treatment with NUCYNTA®.
Inform patients that potentially serious additive effects may occur if NUCYNTA® is used with other CNS depressants, and not to use such drugs unless supervised by a health care provider.
Concurrent use of MAOI
Inform patients not to take NUCYNTA® while using any drugs that inhibit monoamine oxidase. Patients should not start any new medications while taking NUCYNTA®.
Seizures
Inform patients that NUCYNTA® could cause seizures if they are at risk for seizures or have epilepsy. Patients should be advised to stop taking NUCYNTA® if they have a seizure while taking NUCYNTA® and call their healthcare provider right away.
Serotonin Syndrome
Inform patients that NUCYNTA® could cause a rare but potentially life-threatening condition resulting from concomitant administration of serotonergic drugs (including Serotonin Reuptake Inhibitors, Serotonin and Norepinephrine Reuptake Inhibitors and tricyclic antidepressants). Warn patients of the symptoms of serotonin syndrome and to seek medical attention right away if symptoms develop.
Instruct patients to inform their physicians if they are taking or plan to take additional medications, including CNS Depressants, MAO inhibitors, mixed agonists/antagonist opioid analgesics, anticholinergics, SSRIs, SNRIs, or tricyclic antidepressants.
Hypotension
Inform patients that NUCYNTA® may cause orthostatic hypotension and syncope. Instruct patients how to recognize symptoms of low blood pressure and how to reduce the risk

of serious consequences should hypotension occur (e.g., sit or lie down, carefully rise from a sitting or lying position).
Driving or Operating Heavy Machinery
Inform patients that NUCYNTA® may impair the ability to perform potentially hazardous activities such as driving a car or operating heavy machinery. Advise patients not to perform such tasks until they know how they will react to the medication.
Constipation
Advise patients of the potential for severe constipation, including management instructions and when to seek medical attention.
Anaphylaxis
Inform patients that anaphylaxis has been reported with ingredients contained in NUCYNTA®. Advise patients how to recognize such a reaction and when to seek medical attention.
Pregnancy
Advise female patients that NUCYNTA® can cause fetal harm and to inform the prescriber if they are pregnant or plan to become pregnant.
Manufactured by:
Janssen Ortho, LLC
Gurabo, PR 00778
Manufactured for:
Janssen Pharmaceuticals, Inc.
Titusville, NJ 08560
Revised: September 2013
© Janssen Pharmaceuticals, Inc. 2009
Shown in Product Identification Guide, page 307

NUCYNTA® ER   ℂ ℞
[*new-SINN-tah E-R*]
(tapentadol)
extended-release oral tablets

HIGHLIGHTS OF PRESCRIBING INFORMATION
These highlights do not include all the information needed to use NUCYNTA® ER safely and effectively. See full prescribing information for NUCYNTA® ER.
NUCYNTA®ER (tapentadol) extended-release oral tablets C-II
Initial U.S. Approval: 2008

> **WARNING: ADDICTION, ABUSE, AND MISUSE; LIFE-THREATENING RESPIRATORY DEPRESSION; ACCIDENTAL INGESTION; NEONATAL OPIOID WITHDRAWAL SYNDROME; and INTERACTION WITH ALCOHOL**
> *See full prescribing information for complete boxed warning.*
> • NUCYNTA® ER exposes users to risks of addiction, abuse, and misuse, which can lead to overdose and death. Assess each patient's risk before prescribing, and monitor regularly for development of these behaviors or conditions. (5.1)
> • Serious, life-threatening, or fatal respiratory depression may occur. Monitor closely, especially upon initiation or following a dose increase. Instruct patients to swallow NUCYNTA® ER tablets whole to avoid exposure to a potentially fatal dose of tapentadol. (5.2)
> • Accidental ingestion of NUCYNTA® ER, especially in children, can result in fatal overdose of tapentadol. (5.2)
> • Prolonged use of NUCYNTA® ER during pregnancy can result in neonatal opioid withdrawal syndrome, which may be life-threatening if not recognized and treated. If opioid use is required for a prolonged period in a pregnant woman, advise the patient of the risk of neonatal opioid withdrawal syndrome and ensure that appropriate treatment will be available (5.3).
> • Instruct patients not to consume alcohol or any products containing alcohol while taking NUCYNTA® ER because co-ingestion can result in fatal plasma tapentadol levels. (5.4)

RECENT MAJOR CHANGES

Boxed Warning	04/2014
Indications and Usage (1)	04/2014
Dosage and Administration (2)	04/2014
Warnings and Precautions (5)	04/2014

INDICATIONS AND USAGE

NUCYNTA® ER is an opioid agonist indicated for the management of:
• pain severe enough to require daily, around-the-clock, long-term opioid treatment and for which alternative treatment options are inadequate (1)
• neuropathic pain associated with diabetic peripheral neuropathy (DPN) in adults severe enough to require daily,

around-the-clock, long-term opioid treatment and for which alternative treatment options are inadequate. (1)
Limitations of Use
• Because of the risks of addiction, abuse, and misuse with opioids, even at recommended doses, and because of the greater risks of overdose and death with extended-release opioid formulations, reserve NUCYNTA® ER for use in patients for whom alternative treatment options (e.g., non-opioid analgesics or immediate-release opioids) are ineffective, not tolerated, or would be otherwise inadequate to provide sufficient management of pain.
• NUCYNTA® ER is not indicated as an as-needed (prn) analgesic. (1)

DOSAGE AND ADMINISTRATION

• Individualize dosing based on patient's prior analgesic treatment experience and risk factors for addiction, abuse, and misuse; titrate as needed to provide adequate analgesia and minimize adverse reactions. (2.1, 2.2)
• For use as the first opioid and in opioid non-tolerant patients, initiate with 50 mg tablet orally twice daily (approximately every 12 hours). (2.1)
• To convert to NUCYNTA® ER from another opioid, use available conversion factors to obtain estimated dose. (2.1)
• Titrate patients with dose increases of 50 mg no more than twice daily every three days. (2.2)
• Maximum daily dose is 500 mg per day. (2.1)
• Use a gradual downward titration when NUCYNTA® ER is discontinued in a physically dependent patient. (2.3, 5.12)
• Reduce the dose of NUCYNTA® ER in patients with moderate hepatic impairment. (2.4)
• NUCYNTA® ER use in patients with severe renal impairment is not recommended. (2.5)
• Conservative initial dosing of NUCYNTA® ER in elderly patients is recommended due to possible decreased renal and hepatic function. (2.6)
• Instruct patients to swallow NUCYNTA® ER tablets whole. (2.7)

DOSAGE FORMS AND STRENGTHS

• Extended-release tablets: 50 mg, 100 mg, 150 mg, 200 mg, 250 mg (3)

CONTRAINDICATIONS

• Significant respiratory depression (4)
• Acute or severe bronchial asthma (4)
• Known or suspected paralytic ileus (4)
• Hypersensitivity to tapentadol or to any other ingredients of the product (4)
• Concurrent use of monoamine oxidase inhibitors (MAOI) or use within the last 14 days. (4)

WARNINGS AND PRECAUTIONS

See Boxed WARNINGS
• Interaction with CNS depressants: Concomitant use may cause profound sedation, respiratory depression, and death. If co-administration is required, consider dose reduction of one or both drugs because of additive pharmacological effects. (5.4, 7.3)
• Elderly, cachectic, debilitated patients, and those with chronic pulmonary disease: Monitor closely because of increased risk for life-threatening respiratory depression. (5.5, 5.6)
• Hypotensive effect: Monitor during dose initiation and titration. (5.7)
• Patients with head injury or increased intracranial pressure: Monitor for sedation and respiratory depression. Avoid use of NUCYNTA® ER in patients with impaired consciousness or coma susceptible to intracranial effects of CO_2 retention. (5.8)
• Seizures: Use with caution in patients with a history of seizures. (5.9)
• Serotonin Syndrome: Potentially life-threatening condition could result from concomitant administration of drugs with serotonergic activity. (5.10)

ADVERSE REACTIONS

The most common (≥10%) adverse reactions were nausea, constipation, dizziness, headache, and somnolence. (6)
To report SUSPECTED ADVERSE REACTIONS, contact Janssen Pharmaceuticals, Inc. at 1-800-526-7736 (1-800-JANSSEN) or FDA at 1-800-FDA-1088 or www.fda.gov/medwatch.

DRUG INTERACTIONS

• Monitor for signs of serotonin syndrome when NUCYNTA® ER is used concurrently with SSRIs, SNRIs, tricyclic antidepressants, or triptans. (7.4)
• Mixed agonist/antagonist opioids (i.e., pentazocine, nalbuphine, and butorphanol): May reduce analgesic effect and/or precipitate withdrawal symptoms. (7.6)

USE IN SPECIFIC POPULATIONS

• Pregnancy: Based on animal data, may cause fetal harm. (8.1)

- Nursing mothers: Closely monitor infants of nursing women receiving NUCYNTA® ER. (8.3)
- Renal or hepatic impairment: Not recommended in patients with severe renal or hepatic impairment. Reduce dose in patients with moderate hepatic impairment. (8.6, 8.7)

See 17 for PATIENT COUNSELING INFORMATION and Medication Guide

Revised: 04/2014

FULL PRESCRIBING INFORMATION: CONTENTS*
WARNING: ADDICTION, ABUSE, AND MISUSE;
LIFE-THREATENING RESPIRATORY DEPRESSION;
ACCIDENTAL INGESTION; NEONATAL OPIOID
WITHDRAWAL SYNDROME; and INTERACTION
WITH ALCOHOL

* Sections or subsections omitted from the full prescribing information are not listed

---

FULL PRESCRIBING INFORMATION
**WARNING: ADDICTION, ABUSE, AND MIS-
USE; LIFE-THREATENING RESPIRATORY DE-
PRESSION; ACCIDENTAL INGESTION; NEO-
NATAL OPIOID WITHDRAWAL SYNDROME;
and INTERACTION WITH ALCOHOL**

Addiction, Abuse, and Misuse
NUCYNTA® ER exposes patients and other users to the risks of opioid addiction, abuse, and misuse, which can lead to overdose and death. Assess each patient's risk prior to prescribing NUCYNTA® ER, and monitor all patients regularly for the development of these behaviors or conditions [see Warnings and Precautions (5.1)].

Life-threatening Respiratory Depression
Serious, life-threatening, or fatal respiratory depression may occur with use of NUCYNTA® ER. Monitor for respiratory depression, especially during initiation of NUCYNTA® ER or following a dose increase. Instruct patients to swallow NUCYNTA® ER tablets whole; crushing, chewing, or dissolving NUCYNTA® ER tablets can cause rapid release and absorption of a potentially fatal dose of tapentadol [see Warnings and Precautions (5.2)].

Accidental Ingestion
Accidental ingestion of even one dose of NUCYNTA® ER, especially by children, can result in a fatal overdose of tapentadol [see Warnings and Precautions (5.2)].

Neonatal Opioid Withdrawal Syndrome
Prolonged use of NUCYNTA® ER during pregnancy can result in neonatal opioid withdrawal syndrome, which may be life-threatening if not recognized and treated, and requires management according to protocols developed by neonatology experts. If opioid use is required for a prolonged period in a pregnant woman, advise the patient of the risk of neonatal opioid withdrawal syndrome and ensure that appropriate treatment will be available [see Warnings and Precautions (5.3)].

Interaction with Alcohol
Instruct patients not to consume alcoholic beverages or use prescription or non-prescription products that contain alcohol while taking NUCYNTA® ER. The co-ingestion of alcohol with NUCYNTA® ER may result in increased plasma tapentadol levels and a potentially fatal overdose of tapentadol [see Warnings and Precautions (5.4)].

---

1 INDICATIONS AND USAGE
NUCYNTA® ER (tapentadol) is indicated for the management of:
- pain severe enough to require daily, around-the-clock, long-term opioid treatment and for which alternative treatment options are inadequate
- neuropathic pain associated with diabetic peripheral neuropathy (DPN) in adults severe enough to require daily, around-the-clock, long-term opioid treatment and for which alternative treatment options are inadequate.

Limitations of Usage
- Because of the risks of addiction, abuse, and misuse with opioids, even at recommended doses, and because of the greater risks of overdose and death with extended-release opioid formulations, reserve NUCYNTA® ER for use in patients for whom alternative treatment options (e.g., non-opioid analgesics or immediate-release opioids) are ineffective, not tolerated, or would be otherwise inadequate to provide sufficient management of pain.
- NUCYNTA® ER is not indicated as an as-needed (prn) analgesic.

2 DOSAGE AND ADMINISTRATION
2.1 Initial Dosing
NUCYNTA® ER should be prescribed only by healthcare professionals who are knowledgeable in the use of potent opioids for the management of chronic pain.
Initiate the dosing regimen for each patient individually, taking into account the patient's prior analgesic treatment experience and risk factors for addiction, abuse, and misuse [see Warnings and Precautions (5.1)]. Monitor patients closely for respiratory depression, especially within the first 24–72 hours of initiating therapy with NUCYNTA® ER [see Warnings and Precautions (5.2)].
NUCYNTA® ER tablets must be taken whole. Crushing, chewing, or dissolving NUCYNTA® ER tablets will result in uncontrolled delivery of tapentadol and can lead to overdose or death [see Warnings and Precautions (5.2)].
NUCYNTA® ER is administered at a frequency of twice daily (every 12 hours).
Discontinue all other tapentadol and tramadol products when beginning and while taking NUCYNTA® ER [see

---

Warnings and Precautions (5.10)]. Although the maximum approved total daily dose of NUCYNTA® immediate-release formulation is 600 mg per day, the maximum total daily dose of NUCYNTA® ER is 500 mg. Do not exceed a total daily dose of NUCYNTA® ER of 500 mg.
Use of NUCYNTA® ER as the First Opioid Analgesic
Initiate treatment with NUCYNTA® ER with the 50 mg tablet orally twice daily (approximately every 12 hours).
Use of NUCYNTA® ER in Patients who are not Opioid Tolerant
The starting dose for patients who are not opioid tolerant is NUCYNTA® ER 50 mg orally twice daily (approximately every 12 hours). Use of higher starting doses in patients who are not opioid tolerant may cause fatal respiratory depression. Patients who are opioid tolerant are those receiving, for one week or longer, at least 60 mg oral morphine per day, 25 mcg transdermal fentanyl per hour, 30 mg oral oxycodone per day, 8 mg oral hydromorphone per day, 25 mg oral oxymorphone per day or an equianalgesic dose of another opioid.
Conversion from NUCYNTA® to NUCYNTA® ER
Patients can be converted from NUCYNTA® to NUCYNTA® ER using the equivalent total daily dose of NUCYNTA® and dividing it into two equal doses of NUCYNTA® ER separated by approximately 12-hour intervals. As an example, a patient receiving 50 mg of NUCYNTA® four times per day (200 mg/day) may be converted to 100 mg NUCYNTA® ER twice a day.
Conversion from Other Opioids to NUCYNTA® ER
There are no established conversion ratios for conversion from other opioid to NUCYNTA® ER defined by clinical trials. Discontinue all other around-the-clock opioid drugs when NUCYNTA® ER therapy is initiated.
While there are useful tables of opioid equivalents readily available, there is substantial inter-patient variability in the relative potency of different opioid drugs and products. As such, it is safer to underestimate a patient's 24-hour oral tapentadol requirements and provide rescue medication (e.g., immediate-release opioid) than to overestimate the 24-hour oral tapentadol requirements which could result in adverse reactions.
In general, as with other opioid analgesics, begin with half of the estimated daily tapentadol requirement as the initial dose, managing inadequate analgesia by supplementation with immediate-release rescue medication.
Conversion from Methadone to NUCYNTA® ER
Close monitoring is of particular importance when converting from methadone to other opioid agonists. The ratio between methadone and other opioid agonists may vary widely as a function of previous dose exposure. Methadone has a long half-life and can accumulate in the plasma.
2.2 Titration and Maintenance of Therapy
Individually titrate NUCYNTA® ER to a dose that provides adequate analgesia and minimizes adverse reactions. Continually reevaluate patients receiving NUCYNTA® ER to assess the maintenance of pain control and the relative incidence of adverse reactions, as well as monitoring for the development of addiction, abuse, or misuse. Frequent communication is important among the prescriber, other members of the healthcare team, the patient, and the caregiver/family during periods of changing analgesic requirements, including initial titration. During chronic therapy, periodically reassess the continued need for opioid analgesics.
Titrate patients to adequate analgesia with dose increases of 50 mg no more than twice daily every three days. In clinical studies, efficacy with NUCYNTA® ER was demonstrated relative to placebo in the dosage range of 100 mg to 250 mg twice daily [see Clinical Studies (14)].
Patients who experience breakthrough pain may require a dose increase of NUCYNTA® ER, or may need rescue medication with an appropriate dose of an immediate-release analgesic. If the level of pain increases after dose stabilization, attempt to identify the source of increased pain before increasing the NUCYNTA® ER dose.
If unacceptable opioid-related adverse reactions are observed, the subsequent doses may be reduced. Adjust the dose to obtain an appropriate balance between management of pain and opioid-related adverse reactions.
2.3 Discontinuation of NUCYNTA® ER
When the patient no longer requires therapy with NUCYNTA® ER tablets, use a gradual downward titration of the dose to prevent signs and symptoms of withdrawal in the physically-dependent patient.
2.4 Patients with Hepatic Impairment
The use of NUCYNTA® ER in patients with severe hepatic impairment (Child-Pugh Score 10–15) is not recommended. In patients with moderate hepatic impairment (Child-Pugh Score 7 to 9), initiate treatment using 50 mg NUCYNTA® ER and administer no more frequently than once every 24 hours. The maximum recommended dose for patients with moderate hepatic impairment is 100 mg of NUCYNTA® ER per day [see Clinical Pharmacology (12.3)].

No dosage adjustment is recommended in patients with mild hepatic impairment (Child-Pugh Score 5 to 6) [see Warnings and Precautions (5.14) and Clinical Pharmacology (12.3)].

2.5 Patients with Renal Impairment

No dosage adjustment is recommended in patients with mild or moderate renal impairment. Use of NUCYNTA® ER in patients with severe renal impairment is not recommended [see Warnings and Precautions (5.15) and Clinical Pharmacology (12.3)].

2.6 Elderly Patients

In general, recommended dosing for elderly patients with normal renal and hepatic function is the same as for younger adult patients with normal renal and hepatic function. Because elderly patients are more likely to have decreased renal and hepatic function, consideration should be given to starting elderly patients with the lower range of recommended doses [see Clinical Pharmacology (12.3)].

2.7 Administration of NUCYNTA® ER

Instruct patients to swallow NUCYNTA® ER tablets whole. The tablets are not to be cut, crushed, dissolved, or chewed due to the risk of rapid release and absorption of a potentially fatal dose of tapentadol [see Warnings and Precautions (5.1, 5.2)].

Instruct patients to take NUCYNTA® ER one tablet at a time and with enough water to ensure complete swallowing immediately after placing in the mouth [see Warnings and Precautions (5.2), and Patient Counseling Information (17)].

3 DOSAGE FORMS AND STRENGTHS

NUCYNTA® ER 50 mg, 100 mg, 150 mg, 200 mg and 250 mg extended-release tablets are available in the following colors and prints:
- 50 mg extended-release tablets are white oblong-shaped with a black print "OMJ 50" on one side
- 100 mg extended-release tablets are light-blue oblong-shaped with a black print "OMJ 100" on one side
- 150 mg extended-release tablets are blue-green oblong-shaped with a black print "OMJ 150" on one side
- 200 mg extended-release tablets are blue oblong-shaped with a depression in the middle running lengthwise on each side and a black print "OMJ 200" on one side
- 250 mg extended-release tablets are dark blue oblong-shaped with a depression in the middle running lengthwise on each side and a white print "OMJ 250" on one side.

4 CONTRAINDICATIONS

NUCYNTA® ER is contraindicated in:
- Patients with significant respiratory depression
- Patients with acute or severe bronchial asthma or hypercarbia in an unmonitored setting or in the absence of resuscitative equipment
- Patients with known or suspected paralytic ileus
- Patients with hypersensitivity (e.g. anaphylaxis, angioedema) to tapentadol or to any other ingredients of the product [see Adverse Reactions (6.2)].
- Patients who are receiving monoamine oxidase inhibitors (MAOI) or who have taken them within the last 14 days due to potential additive effects on norepinephrine levels which may result in adverse cardiovascular events [see Drug Interactions (7.2)].

5 WARNINGS AND PRECAUTIONS

5.1 Addiction, Abuse, and Misuse

NUCYNTA® ER contains tapentadol, a Schedule II controlled substance. As an opioid, NUCYNTA® ER exposes users to the risks of addiction, abuse, and misuse [see Drug Abuse and Dependence (9)]. As modified-release products such as NUCYNTA® ER deliver the opioid over an extended period of time, there is a greater risk for overdose and death due to the larger amount of tapentadol present.

Although the risk of addiction in any individual is unknown, it can occur in patients appropriately prescribed NUCYNTA® ER and in those who obtain the drug illicitly. Addiction can occur at recommended doses and if the drug is misused or abused.

Assess each patient's risk for opioid addiction, abuse, or misuse prior to prescribing NUCYNTA® ER, and monitor all patients receiving NUCYNTA® ER for the development of these behaviors or conditions. Risks are increased in patients with a personal or family history of substance abuse (including drug or alcohol addiction or abuse) or mental illness (e.g., major depression). The potential for these risks should not, however, prevent the prescribing of NUCYNTA® ER for the proper management of pain in any given patient. Patients at increased risk may be prescribed modified-release opioid formulations such as NUCYNTA® ER, but use in such patients necessitates intensive counseling about the risks and proper use of NUCYNTA® ER along with intensive monitoring for signs of addiction, abuse, and misuse.

Abuse or misuse of NUCYNTA® ER by crushing, chewing, snorting, or injecting the dissolved product will result in the uncontrolled delivery of tapentadol and can result in overdose and death [see Overdosage (10)].

Opioid agonists such as NUCYNTA® ER are sought by drug abusers and people with addiction disorders and are subject to criminal diversion. Consider these risks when prescribing or dispensing NUCYNTA® ER. Strategies to reduce these risks include prescribing the drug in the smallest appropriate quantity and advising the patient on the proper disposal of unused drug [see Patient Counseling Information (17)]. Contact local state professional licensing board or state controlled substances authority for information on how to prevent and detect abuse or diversion of this product.

5.2 Life-Threatening Respiratory Depression

Serious, life-threatening, or fatal respiratory depression has been reported with the use of modified-release opioids, even when used as recommended. Respiratory depression from opioid use, if not immediately recognized and treated, may lead to respiratory arrest and death. Management of respiratory depression may include close observation, supportive measures, and use of opioid antagonists, depending on the patient's clinical status [see Overdosage (10)]. Carbon dioxide (CO_2) retention from opioid-induced respiratory depression can exacerbate the sedating effects of opioids.

While serious, life-threatening, or fatal respiratory depression can occur at any time during the use of NUCYNTA® ER, the risk is greatest during the initiation of therapy or following a dose increase. Closely monitor patients for respiratory depression when initiating therapy with NUCYNTA® ER and following dose increases.

To reduce the risk of respiratory depression, proper dosing and titration of NUCYNTA® ER are essential [see Dosage and Administration (2)]. Overestimating the NUCYNTA® ER dose when converting patients from another opioid product can result in fatal overdose with the first dose.

Accidental ingestion of even one dose of NUCYNTA® ER, especially by children, can result in respiratory depression and death due to an overdose of tapentadol.

5.3 Neonatal Opioid Withdrawal Syndrome

Prolonged use of NUCYNTA® ER during pregnancy can result in withdrawal signs in the neonate. Neonatal opioid withdrawal syndrome, unlike opioid withdrawal syndrome in adults, may be life-threatening if not recognized and treated, and requires management according to protocols developed by neonatology experts. If opioid use is required for a prolonged period in a pregnant woman, advise the patient of the risk of neonatal opioid withdrawal syndrome and ensure that appropriate treatment will be available.

Neonatal opioid withdrawal syndrome presents as irritability, hyperactivity and abnormal sleep pattern, high pitched cry, tremor, vomiting, diarrhea and failure to gain weight. The onset, duration, and severity of neonatal opioid withdrawal syndrome vary based on the specific opioid used, duration of use, timing and amount of last maternal use, and rate of elimination of the drug by the newborn.

5.4 Interactions with Central Nervous System Depressants

Patients must not consume alcoholic beverages or prescription or non-prescription products containing alcohol while on NUCYNTA® ER therapy. The co-ingestion of alcohol with NUCYNTA® ER may result in increased plasma tapentadol levels and a potentially fatal overdose of tapentadol [see Clinical Pharmacology (12.3)].

Hypotension, profound sedation, coma, respiratory depression, and death may result if NUCYNTA® ER is used concomitantly with alcohol or other central nervous system (CNS) depressants (e.g., sedatives, anxiolytics, hypnotics, neuroleptics, other opioids).

When considering the use of NUCYNTA® ER in a patient taking a CNS depressant, assess the duration of use of the CNS depressant and the patient's response, including the degree of tolerance that has developed to CNS depression. Additionally, evaluate the patient's use of alcohol or illicit drugs that cause CNS depression. If the decision to begin NUCYNTA® ER is made, start with NUCYNTA® ER 50 mg every 12 hours, monitor patients for signs of sedation and respiratory depression, and consider using a lower dose of the concomitant CNS depressant [see Drug Interactions (7.3)].

5.5 Use in Elderly, Cachectic, and Debilitated Patients

Life-threatening respiratory depression is more likely to occur in elderly, cachectic, or debilitated patients as they may have altered pharmacokinetics or altered clearance compared to younger, healthier patients. Therefore, closely monitor such patients, particularly when initiating and titrating NUCYNTA® ER and when NUCYNTA® ER is given concomitantly with other drugs that depress respiration [see Warnings and Precautions (5.2)].

5.6 Use in Patients with Chronic Pulmonary Disease

Monitor for respiratory depression those patients with significant chronic obstructive pulmonary disease or cor pulmonale, and patients having a substantially decreased respiratory reserve, hypoxia, hypercarbia, or pre-existing respiratory depression, particularly when initiating therapy and titrating with NUCYNTA® ER, as in these patients, even usual therapeutic doses of NUCYNTA® ER may de-

crease respiratory drive to the point of apnea [see Warnings and Precautions (5.2)]. Consider the use of alternative non-opioid analgesics in these patients if possible.

5.7 Hypotensive Effect

NUCYNTA® ER may cause severe hypotension. There is an increased risk in patients whose ability to maintain blood pressure has already been compromised by a reduced blood volume or concurrent administration of certain CNS depressant drugs (e.g., phenothiazines or general anesthetics) [see Drug Interactions (7.3)]. Monitor these patients for signs of hypotension after initiating or titrating the dose of NUCYNTA® ER. In patients with circulatory shock, NUCYNTA® ER may cause vasodilation that can further reduce cardiac output and blood pressure. Avoid the use of NUCYNTA® ER in patients with circulatory shock.

5.8 Use in Patients with Head Injury or Increased Intracranial Pressure

Monitor patients taking NUCYNTA® ER who may be susceptible to the intracranial effects of CO_2 retention (e.g., those with evidence of increased intracranial pressure or brain tumors) for signs of sedation and respiratory depression, particularly when initiating therapy with NUCYNTA® ER. NUCYNTA® ER may reduce respiratory drive, and the resultant CO_2 retention can further increase intracranial pressure. Opioids may also obscure the clinical course in a patient with a head injury.

Avoid the use of NUCYNTA® ER in patients with impaired consciousness or coma.

5.9 Seizures

NUCYNTA® ER has not been evaluated in patients with a predisposition to a seizure disorder, and such patients were excluded from clinical studies. The active ingredient tapentadol in NUCYNTA® ER may aggravate convulsions in patients with convulsive disorders, and may induce or aggravate seizures in some clinical settings. Monitor patients with a history of seizure disorders for worsened seizure control during NUCYNTA® ER therapy.

5.10 Serotonin Syndrome

Cases of life-threatening serotonin syndrome have been reported with the concurrent use of tapentadol and serotonergic drugs. Serotonergic drugs comprise Selective Serotonin Reuptake Inhibitors (SSRIs), Serotonin and Norepinephrine Reuptake Inhibitors (SNRIs), tricyclic antidepressants (TCAs), triptans, drugs that affect the serotonergic neurotransmitter system (e.g. mirtazapine, trazodone, and tramadol), and drugs that impair metabolism of serotonin (including MAOIs). This may occur within the recommended dose. Serotonin syndrome may include mental-status changes (e.g., agitation, hallucinations, coma), autonomic instability (e.g., tachycardia, labile blood pressure, hyperthermia), neuromuscular aberrations (e.g., hyperreflexia, incoordination) and/or gastrointestinal symptoms (e.g., nausea, vomiting, diarrhea) and can be fatal [see Drug Interactions (7.4)].

5.11 Use in Patients with Gastrointestinal Conditions

NUCYNTA® ER is contraindicated in patients with GI obstruction, including paralytic ileus. The tapentadol in NUCYNTA® ER may cause spasm of the sphincter of Oddi. Monitor patients with biliary tract disease, including acute pancreatitis, for worsening symptoms.

5.12 Avoidance of Withdrawal

Avoid the use of mixed agonist/antagonist (i.e., pentazocine, nalbuphine, and butorphanol) or partial agonist (buprenorphine) analgesics in patients who have received or are receiving a course of therapy with a full opioid agonist analgesic, including NUCYNTA® ER. In these patients, mixed agonists/antagonists and partial agonist analgesics may reduce the analgesic effect and/or may precipitate withdrawal symptoms.

When discontinuing NUCYNTA® ER, gradually taper the dose [see Dosage and Administration (2.3)].

5.13 Driving and Operating Heavy Machinery

NUCYNTA® ER may impair the mental or physical abilities needed to perform potentially hazardous activities such as driving a car or operating machinery. Warn patients not to drive or operate dangerous machinery unless they are tolerant to the effects of NUCYNTA® ER and know how they will react to the medication.

5.14 Hepatic Impairment

A study with an immediate-release formulation of tapentadol in subjects with hepatic impairment showed higher serum concentrations of tapentadol than in those with normal hepatic function. Avoid use of NUCYNTA® ER in patients with severe hepatic impairment. Reduce the dose of NUCYNTA® ER in patients with moderate hepatic impairment [see Dosage and Administration (2.4) and Clinical Pharmacology (12.3)]. Closely monitor patients with moderate hepatic impairment for respiratory and central nervous system depression when initiating and titrating NUCYNTA® ER.

5.15 Renal Impairment

Use of NUCYNTA® ER in patients with severe renal impairment is not recommended due to accumulation of a metabolite formed by glucuronidation of tapentadol. The clinical relevance of the elevated metabolite is not known [see Clinical Pharmacology (12.3)].

6   ADVERSE REACTIONS

The following serious adverse reactions are discussed elsewhere in the labeling:

- Addiction, Abuse, and Misuse [see Warnings and Precautions (5.1)]
- Life-Threatening Respiratory Depression [see Warnings and Precautions (5.2)]
- Neonatal Opioid Withdrawal Syndrome [see Warnings and Precautions (5.3)]
- Interaction with Other CNS Depressants [see Warnings and Precautions (5.4)]
- Hypotensive Effects [see Warnings and Precautions (5.7)]
- Gastrointestinal Effects [see Warnings and Precautions (5.11)]
- Seizures [see Warnings and Precautions (5.9)]
- Serotonin Syndrome [see Warnings and Precautions (5.10)]

6.1   Clinical Trial Experience

Because clinical trials are conducted under widely varying conditions, adverse reaction rates observed in the clinical trials of a drug cannot be directly compared to rates in the clinical trials of another drug and may not reflect the rates observed in clinical practice.

Commonly-Observed Adverse Reactions in Clinical Studies with NUCYNTA® ER in Patients with Chronic Pain due to Low Back Pain or Osteoarthritis

The safety data described in Table 1 below are based on three pooled, randomized, double-blind, placebo-controlled, parallel group, 15-week studies of NUCYNTA® ER (dosed 100 to 250 mg BID after a 50 mg BID starting dose) in patients with chronic pain due to low back pain (LBP) and osteoarthritis (OA). These trials included 980 NUCYNTA® ER-treated patients and 993 placebo-treated patients. The mean age was 57 years old; 63% were female and 37% were male; 83% were White, 10% were Black, and 5% were Hispanic.

The most common adverse reactions (reported by ≥10% in any NUCYNTA® ER dose group) were: nausea, constipation, dizziness, headache, and somnolence.

The most common reasons for discontinuation due to adverse reactions in eight Phase 2/3 pooled studies reported by ≥1% in any NUCYNTA® ER dose group for NUCYNTA® ER- and placebo-treated patients were nausea (4% vs. 1%), dizziness (3% vs. <1%), vomiting (3% vs. <1%), somnolence (2% vs. <1%), constipation (1% vs. <1%), headache (1% vs. <1%), and fatigue (1% vs. <1%), respectively.

Table 1 Adverse Drug Reactions Reported by ≥ 1% of NUCYNTA® ER-Treated Patients and Greater than Placebo-Treated Patients in Pooled Parallel-Group Trials*

	NUCYNTA® ER 50 to 250 mg BID† (n=980)	Placebo (n=993)
Nausea	21%	7%
Constipation	17%	7%
Dizziness	17%	6%
Headache	15%	13%
Somnolence	12%	4%
Fatigue	9%	4%
Vomiting	8%	3%
Dry mouth	7%	2%
Hyperhidrosis	5%	<1%
Pruritus	5%	2%
Insomnia	4%	2%
Dyspepsia	3%	2%
Lethargy	2%	<1%
Asthenia	2%	<1%
Anxiety	2%	1%
Decreased appetite	2%	<1%
Vertigo	2%	<1%
Hot flush	2%	<1%
Disturbance in attention	1%	<1%
Tremor	1%	<1%
Chills	1%	0%
Abnormal dreams	1%	<1%
Depression	1%	<1%
Vision blurred	1%	<1%
Erectile dysfunction	1%	<1%

* MedDRA preferred terms. The trials included forced titration during the first week of dosing.
† NUCYNTA® ER dosed between 100 and 250 mg BID after a starting dose of 50 mg BID

Commonly-Observed Adverse Reactions in Clinical Studies with NUCYNTA® ER in Patients with Neuropathic Pain Associated with Diabetic Peripheral Neuropathy

The types of adverse reactions seen in the studies of patients with painful diabetic peripheral neuropathy (DPN) were similar to what was seen in the low back pain and osteoarthritis trials. The safety data described in Table 2 below are based on two pooled, randomized withdrawal, double-blind, placebo-controlled, 12-week studies of NUCYNTA® ER (dosed 100 to 250 mg BID) in patients with neuropathic pain associated with diabetic peripheral neuropathy. These trials included 1040 NUCYNTA® ER-treated patients and 343 placebo-treated patients. The mean age was 60 years old; 40% were female and 60% were male; 76% were White, 12% were Black, and 12% were "Other". The most commonly reported ADRs (incidence ≥ 10% in NUCYNTA® ER-treated subjects) were: nausea, constipation, vomiting, dizziness, somnolence, and headache.

Table 2 lists the common adverse reactions reported in 1% or more of NUCYNTA® ER-treated patients and greater than placebo-treated patients with neuropathic pain associated with diabetic peripheral neuropathy in the two pooled studies.

Table 2: Adverse Drug Reactions Reported by ≥ 1% of NUCYNTA® ER-Treated Patients and Greater than Placebo-Treated Patients in Pooled Trials (Studies DPN-1 and DPN-2)*

	NUCYNTA® ER 50 to 250 mg BID† (n=1040)	Placebo‡ (n=343)
Nausea	27%	8%
Dizziness	18%	2%
Somnolence	14%	<1%
Constipation	13%	<1%
Vomiting	12%	3%
Headache	10%	5%
Fatigue	9%	<1%
Pruritus	8%	0%
Dry mouth	7%	<1%
Diarrhea	7%	5%
Decreased appetite	6%	<1%
Anxiety	5%	4%
Insomnia	4%	3%
Hyperhidrosis	3%	2%
Hot flush	3%	2%
Tremor§	3%	3%
Abnormal dreams	2%	0%
Lethargy	2%	0%
Asthenia	2%	<1%
Irritability	2%	1%
Dyspnea	1%	0%
Nervousness	1%	0%
Sedation	1%	0%
Vision blurred	1%	0%
Pruritus generalized	1%	0%
Vertigo	1%	<1%
Abdominal discomfort	1%	<1%
Hypotension	1%	<1%
Dyspepsia	1%	<1%
Hypoesthesia	1%	<1%
Depression	1%	<1%
Rash	1%	<1%
Chills§	1%	1%
Feeling cold§	1%	1%
Drug withdrawal syndrome	1%	<1%

* MedDRA preferred terms.
† NUCYNTA® ER dosed between 100 and 250 mg BID after a starting dose of 50 mg BID. It includes ADR reported in the open-label titration period for all subjects and in the double-blind maintenance period for the subjects who were randomized to NUCYNTA® ER.
‡ It includes ADR reported in the double-blind maintenance period for the subjects who were randomized to placebo after receiving NUCYNTA® ER during the open-label titration period.
§ Tremor was observed in 3.4% of NUCYNTA® ER-treated subjects vs. 3.2% in placebo group, chills- in 1.3% vs.1.2% in placebo, and feeling cold- in 1.3% vs.1.2% in placebo.

Other Adverse Reactions Observed During the Premarketing Evaluation of NUCYNTA® ER

The following additional adverse drug reactions occurred in less than 1% of NUCYNTA® ER-treated patients in ten Phase 2/3 clinical studies:

Nervous system disorders: paresthesia, balance disorder, syncope, memory impairment, mental impairment, depressed level of consciousness, dysarthria, presyncope, coordination abnormal

Gastrointestinal disorders: impaired gastric emptying

General disorders and administration site conditions: feeling abnormal, feeling drunk

Psychiatric disorders: perception disturbances, disorientation, confusional state, agitation, euphoric mood, drug dependence, thinking abnormal, nightmare

Skin and subcutaneous tissue disorders: urticaria

Metabolism and nutrition disorders: weight decreased

Cardiac disorders: heart rate increased, palpitations, heart rate decreased, left bundle branch block

Vascular disorder: blood pressure decreased

Respiratory, thoracic and mediastinal disorders: respiratory depression

Renal and urinary disorders: urinary hesitation, pollakiuria

Reproductive system and breast disorders: sexual dysfunction

Eye disorders: visual disturbance

Immune system disorders: drug hypersensitivity

6.2   Postmarketing Experience

The following adverse reactions, not noted in Section 6.1 above, have been identified during post approval use of tapentadol. Because these reactions are reported voluntarily from a population of uncertain size, it is not always possible to reliably estimate their frequency or establish a causal relationship to drug exposure.

Psychiatric disorders: hallucination, suicidal ideation, panic attack

Anaphylaxis, angioedema, and anaphylactic shock have been reported very rarely with ingredients contained in NUCYNTA® ER. Advise patients how to recognize such reactions and when to seek medical attention.

7   DRUG INTERACTIONS

7.1   Alcohol

Concomitant use of alcohol with NUCYNTA® ER can result in an increase of tapentadol plasma levels and potentially fatal overdose of tapentadol. Instruct patients not to consume alcoholic beverages or use prescription or nonprescription products containing alcohol while on NUCYNTA® ER therapy [see Clinical Pharmacology (12.3)].

7.2   Monoamine Oxidase Inhibitors

NUCYNTA® ER is contraindicated in patients who are receiving monoamine oxidase inhibitors (MAOI) or who have taken them within the last 14 days due to potential additive effects on norepinephrine levels, which may result in adverse cardiovascular events [see Contraindications (4)].

7.3 CNS Depressants
The concomitant use of NUCYNTA® ER with other CNS depressants including sedatives, hypnotics, tranquilizers, general anesthetics, phenothiazines, other opioids, and alcohol can increase the risk of respiratory depression, profound sedation, coma and death. Monitor patients receiving CNS depressants and NUCYNTA® ER for signs of respiratory depression, sedation and hypotension.

When combined therapy with any of the above medications is considered, the dose of one or both agents should be reduced [see Dosage and Administration (2.2) and Warnings and Precautions (5.4)].

7.4 Serotonergic Drugs
There have been post-marketing reports of serotonin syndrome with the concomitant use of tapentadol and serotonergic drugs (e.g., SSRIs and SNRIs). Caution is advised when NUCYNTA® ER is co-administered with other drugs that may affect serotonergic neurotransmitter systems such as SSRIs, SNRIs, MAOIs, and triptans. If concomitant treatment of NUCYNTA® ER with a drug affecting the serotonergic neurotransmitter system is clinically warranted, careful observation of the patient is advised, particularly during treatment initiation and dose increases [see Warning and Precautions (5.10)].

7.5 Muscle Relaxants
Tapentadol may enhance the neuromuscular blocking action of skeletal muscle relaxants and produce an increased degree of respiratory depression. Monitor patients receiving muscle relaxants and NUCYNTA® ER for signs of respiratory depression that may be greater than otherwise expected.

7.6 Mixed Agonist/Antagonist Opioid Analgesics
Mixed agonist/antagonist analgesics (i.e., pentazocine, nalbuphine, and butorphanol) and partial agonists (e.g., buprenorphine) may reduce the analgesic effect of NUCYNTA® ER or precipitate withdrawal symptoms. Avoid the use of mixed agonist/antagonist analgesics in patients receiving NUCYNTA® ER.

7.7 Anticholinergics
The use of NUCYNTA® ER with anticholinergic products may increase the risk of urinary retention and/or severe constipation, which may lead to paralytic ileus.

8 USE IN SPECIFIC POPULATIONS

8.1 Pregnancy
Clinical Considerations
Fetal/neonatal adverse reactions
Prolonged use of opioid analgesics during pregnancy for medical or nonmedical purposes can result in physical dependence in the neonate and neonatal opioid withdrawal syndrome shortly after birth. Observe newborns for symptoms of neonatal opioid withdrawal syndrome, such as poor feeding, diarrhea, irritability, tremor, rigidity, and seizures, and manage accordingly [see Warnings and Precautions (5.3)].

Teratogenic Effects - Pregnancy Category C
There are no adequate and well-controlled studies in pregnant women. NUCYNTA® ER should be used during pregnancy only if the potential benefit justifies the potential risk to the fetus.

Tapentadol HCl was evaluated for teratogenic effects in pregnant rats and rabbits following intravenous and subcutaneous exposure during the period of embryofetal organogenesis. When tapentadol was administered twice daily by the subcutaneous route in rats at dose levels of 10, 20, or 40 mg/kg/day [producing up to 1.36 times the plasma exposure at the maximum recommended human dose (MRHD) of 500 mg/day for NUCYNTA® ER based on an area under the time-curve (AUC) comparison], no teratogenic effects were observed. Evidence of embryofetal toxicity included transient delays in skeletal maturation (i.e., reduced ossification) at the 40 mg/kg/day dose which was associated with significant maternal toxicity. Administration of tapentadol HCl in rabbits at doses of 4, 10, or 24 mg/kg/day by subcutaneous injection [producing 0.3, 0.8, and 2.5 times the plasma exposure at the MRHD based on an AUC comparison, respectively] revealed embryofetal toxicity at doses ≥10 mg/kg/day. Findings included reduced fetal viability, skeletal delays and other variations. In addition, there were multiple malformations including gastroschisis/thoracogastroschisis, amelia/phocomelia, and cleft palate at doses ≥10 mg/kg/day and above, and ablepharia, encephalopathy, and spina bifida at the high dose of 24 mg/kg/day. Embryofetal toxicity, including malformations, may be secondary to the significant maternal toxicity observed in the study.

In a study of pre- and postnatal development in rats, oral administration of tapentadol at doses of 20, 50, 150, or 300 mg/kg/day to pregnant and lactating rats during the late gestation and early postnatal period [resulting in up to 2.28 times the plasma exposure at the MRHD on an AUC basis] did not influence physical or reflex development, the outcome of neurobehavioral tests or reproductive parameters. At maternal tapentadol doses ≥150 mg/kg/day, a dose-related increase in pup mortality was observed to postnatal Day 4. Treatment-related developmental delay was observed in the dead pups, including incomplete ossification. In addition, significant reductions in pup body weights and body weight gains at doses associated with maternal toxicity (150 mg/kg/day and above) were seen throughout lactation.

8.2 Labor and Delivery
Opioids cross the placenta and may produce respiratory depression and psychophysiologic effects in neonates. NUCYNTA® ER is not for use in women during and immediately prior to labor, when shorter acting analgesics or other analgesic techniques are more appropriate. Opioid analgesics can prolong labor through actions that temporarily reduce the strength, duration, and frequency of uterine contractions. However this effect is not consistent and may be offset by an increased rate of cervical dilatation, which tends to shorten labor.

8.3 Nursing Mothers
There is insufficient/limited information on the excretion of tapentadol in human or animal breast milk. Physicochemical and available pharmacodynamic/toxicological data on tapentadol point to excretion in breast milk and risk to the breastfeeding child cannot be excluded.

Because of the potential for adverse reactions in nursing infants from NUCYNTA® ER, a decision should be made whether to discontinue nursing or discontinue the drug, taking into account the importance of the drug to the mother.

Withdrawal symptoms can occur in breast-feeding infants when maternal administration of NUCYNTA® ER is stopped.

8.4 Pediatric Use
The safety and efficacy of NUCYNTA® ER in pediatric patients less than 18 years of age have not been established.

8.5 Geriatric Use
Of the total number of patients in Phase 2/3 double-blind, multiple-dose clinical studies of NUCYNTA® ER, 28% (1023/3613) were 65 years and over, while 7% (245/3613) were 75 years and over. No overall differences in effectiveness or tolerability were observed between these patients and younger patients.

In general, recommended dosing for elderly patients with normal renal and hepatic function is the same as for younger adult patients with normal renal and hepatic function. Because elderly patients are more likely to have decreased renal and hepatic function, consideration should be given to starting elderly patients with the lower range of recommended doses [see Clinical Pharmacology (12.3)].

8.6 Renal Impairment
The safety and effectiveness of NUCYNTA® ER have not been established in patients with severe renal impairment (CL_{CR} <30 mL/min). Use of NUCYNTA® ER in patients with severe renal impairment is not recommended due to accumulation of a metabolite formed by glucuronidation of tapentadol. The clinical relevance of the elevated metabolite is not known [see Clinical Pharmacology (12.3)].

8.7 Hepatic Impairment
Administration of tapentadol resulted in higher exposures and serum levels of tapentadol in subjects with impaired hepatic function compared to subjects with normal hepatic function [see Clinical Pharmacology (12.3)]. The dose of NUCYNTA® ER should be reduced in patients with moderate hepatic impairment (Child-Pugh Score 7 to 9) [see Dosage and Administration (2.4)].

Use of NUCYNTA® ER is not recommended in severe hepatic impairment (Child-Pugh Score 10 to 15) [see Warnings and Precautions (5.14)].

9 DRUG ABUSE AND DEPENDENCE

9.1 Controlled Substance
NUCYNTA® ER contains tapentadol, a Schedule II controlled substance with a high potential for abuse similar to fentanyl, methadone, morphine, oxycodone, and oxymorphone. NUCYNTA® ER can be abused and is subject to misuse, addiction, and criminal diversion [see Warnings and Precautions (5.1)]. The high drug content in the extended release formulation adds to the risk of adverse outcomes from abuse and misuse.

9.2 Abuse
All patients treated with opioids require careful monitoring for signs of abuse and addiction, because use of opioid analgesic products carries the risk of addiction even under appropriate medical use.

Drug abuse is the intentional non-therapeutic use of an over-the-counter or prescription drug, even once, for its rewarding psychological or physiological effects. Drug abuse includes, but is not limited to the following examples: the use of a prescription or over-the-counter drug to get "high", or the use of steroids for performance enhancement and muscle build up.

Drug addiction is a cluster of behavioral, cognitive, and physiological phenomena that develop after repeated substance use and include: a strong desire to take the drug, difficulties in controlling its use, persisting in its use despite harmful consequences, a higher priority given to drug use than to other activities and obligations, increased tolerance, and sometimes a physical withdrawal.

"Drug-seeking" behavior is very common to addicts and drug abusers. Drug-seeking tactics include emergency calls or visits near the end of office hours, refusal to undergo appropriate examination, testing or referral, repeated claims of loss of prescriptions, tampering with prescriptions and reluctance to provide prior medical records or contact information for other treating physician(s). "Doctor shopping" (visiting multiple prescribers) to obtain additional prescriptions is common among drug abusers, and people suffering from untreated addiction. Preoccupation with achieving pain relief can be appropriate behavior in a patient with poor pain control.

Abuse and addiction are separate and distinct from physical dependence and tolerance. Physicians should be aware that addiction may not be accompanied by concurrent tolerance and symptoms of physical dependence in all addicts. In addition, abuse of opioids can occur in the absence of true addiction.

NUCYNTA® ER, like other opioids, can be diverted for non-medical use into illicit channels of distribution. Careful record-keeping of prescribing information, including quantity, frequency, and renewal requests, as required by law, is strongly advised.

Proper assessment of the patient, proper prescribing practices, periodic re-evaluation of therapy, and proper dispensing and storage are appropriate measures that help to limit abuse of opioid drugs.

9.3 Dependence
Both tolerance and physical dependence can develop during chronic opioid therapy. Tolerance is the need for increasing doses of opioids to maintain a defined effect such as analgesia (in the absence of disease progression or other external factors). Tolerance may occur to both the desired and undesired effects of drugs, and may develop at different rates for different effects.

Physical dependence results in withdrawal symptoms after abrupt discontinuation or a significant dose reduction of a drug. Withdrawal also may be precipitated through the administration of drugs with opioid antagonist activity, e.g., naloxone, nalmefene, mixed agonist/antagonist analgesics (pentazocine, butorphanol, nalbuphine), or partial agonists (buprenorphine). Physical dependence may not occur to a clinically significant degree until after several days to weeks of continued opioid usage.

NUCYNTA® ER should not be abruptly discontinued [see Dosage and Administration (2.3)]. If NUCYNTA® ER is abruptly discontinued in a physically-dependent patient, an abstinence syndrome may occur. Some or all of the following can characterize this syndrome: restlessness, lacrimation, rhinorrhea, yawning, perspiration, chills, piloerection, myalgia, mydriasis, irritability, anxiety, backache, joint pain, weakness, abdominal cramps, insomnia, nausea, anorexia, vomiting, diarrhea, increased blood pressure, respiratory rate, or heart rate.

Infants born to mothers physically dependent on opioids will also be physically dependent and may exhibit respiratory difficulties and withdrawal symptoms [see Use in Specific Populations (8.1, 8.2)].

10 OVERDOSAGE

10.1 Clinical Presentation
Acute overdosage with opioids can be manifested by respiratory depression, somnolence progressing to stupor or coma, skeletal muscle flaccidity, cold and clammy skin, constricted pupils, and sometimes pulmonary edema, bradycardia, hypotension and death. Marked mydriasis rather than miosis may be seen due to severe hypoxia in overdose situations.

10.2 Treatment of Overdose
In case of overdose, priorities are the re-establishment of a patent and protected airway and institution of assisted or controlled ventilation if needed. Employ other supportive measures (including oxygen, vasopressors) in the management of circulatory shock and pulmonary edema as indicated. Cardiac arrest or arrhythmias will require advanced life support techniques.

The opioid antagonists, naloxone or nalmefene, are specific antidotes to respiratory depression resulting from opioid overdose. Opioid antagonists should not be administered in the absence of clinically significant respiratory or circulatory depression secondary to tapentadol overdose. Such agents should be administered cautiously to patients who are known, or suspected to be, physically dependent on NUCYNTA® ER. In such cases, an abrupt or complete reversal of opioid effects may precipitate an acute withdrawal syndrome.

Because the duration of reversal would be expected to be less than the duration of action of tapentadol in

NUCYNTA® ER, carefully monitor the patient until spontaneous respiration is reliably re-established. NUCYNTA® ER will continue to release tapentadol adding to the tapentadol load for up to 24 hours after administration necessitating prolonged monitoring. If the response to opioid antagonists is suboptimal or not sustained, additional antagonist should be given as directed in the product's prescribing information.

In an individual physically dependent on opioids, administration of an opioid receptor antagonist may precipitate an acute withdrawal. The severity of the withdrawal produced will depend on the degree of physical dependence and the dose of the antagonist administered. If a decision is made to treat serious respiratory depression in the physically dependent patient, administration of the antagonist should be begun with care and by titration with smaller than usual doses of the antagonist.

11 DESCRIPTION

NUCYNTA® ER (tapentadol) is a mu-opioid receptor agonist, supplied in extended-release film-coated tablets for oral administration, containing 58.24, 116.48, 174.72, 232.96, and 291.20 mg of tapentadol hydrochloride in each tablet strength, corresponding to 50, 100, 150, 200, and 250 mg of tapentadol free-base, respectively. The chemical name is 3-[(1R,2R)-3-(dimethylamino)-1-ethyl-2-methyl-propyl]phenol monohydrochloride. The structural formula is:

. HCl

The molecular weight of tapentadol HCl is 257.80, and the molecular formula is $C_{14}H_{23}NO \cdot HCl$. The n-octanol: water partition coefficient log P value is 2.89. The pKa values are 9.36 and 10.45. In addition to the active ingredient tapentadol HCl, tablets also contain the following inactive ingredients: alpha-tocopherol (vitamin E), hypromellose, polyethylene glycol, and polyethylene oxide. The film coating is comprised of polyvinyl alcohol, polyethylene glycol, talc, titanium dioxide, and the colorant FD&C Blue #2 aluminum lake is used for 100, 150, 200, and 250 mg strengths; and additionally, yellow iron oxide is used in 150 mg tablets. Printing inks contain shellac glaze and propylene glycol for all strengths, and black iron oxide (50, 100, 150 and 200 mg tablets) or titanium dioxide (250 mg tablets).

12 CLINICAL PHARMACOLOGY

12.1 Mechanism of Action

Tapentadol is a centrally-acting synthetic analgesic. The exact mechanism of action is unknown. Although the clinical relevance is unclear, preclinical studies have shown that tapentadol is a mu-opioid receptor (MOR) agonist and a norepinephrine reuptake inhibitor (NRI). Analgesia in animal models is derived from both of these properties.

12.2 Pharmacodynamics

Tapentadol is 18 times less potent than morphine in binding to the human mu-opioid receptor and is 2–3 times less potent in producing analgesia in animal models. Tapentadol has been shown to inhibit norepinephrine reuptake in the brains of rats resulting in increased norepinephrine concentrations. In preclinical models, the analgesic activity due to the mu-opioid receptor agonist activity of tapentadol can be antagonized by selective mu-opioid antagonists (e.g., naloxone), whereas the norepinephrine reuptake inhibition is sensitive to norepinephrine modulators. Tapentadol exerts its analgesic effects without a pharmacologically active metabolite.

Concentration-Efficacy Relationships

The minimum effective plasma concentration of tapentadol for analgesia varies widely among patients, especially among patients who have been previously treated with agonist opioids. As a result, individually titrate patients to achieve a balance between therapeutic and adverse effects. The minimum effective analgesic concentration of tapentadol for any individual patient may increase over time due to an increase in pain, progression of disease, development of a new pain syndrome and/or potential development of analgesic tolerance.

Concentration-Adverse Experience Relationships

There is a general relationship between increasing opioid plasma concentration and increasing frequency of adverse experiences such as nausea, vomiting, CNS effects, and respiratory depression.

Effects on the Cardiovascular System

There was no effect of therapeutic and supratherapeutic doses of tapentadol on the QT interval. In a randomized, double-blind, placebo- and positive-controlled crossover study, healthy subjects were administered five consecutive immediate-release formulation doses of tapentadol 100 mg every 6 hours, tapentadol 150 mg every 6 hours, placebo

and a single oral dose of moxifloxacin. Similarly, the immediate-release formulation tapentadol had no relevant effect on other ECG parameters (heart rate, PR interval, QRS duration, T-wave or U-wave morphology).

Tapentadol produces peripheral vasodilation which may result in orthostatic hypotension.

Effects on the Central Nervous System (CNS)

The principal therapeutic action of tapentadol is analgesia. Tapentadol causes respiratory depression, in part by a direct effect on the brainstem respiratory centers. The respiratory depression involves a reduction in the responsiveness of the brain stem respiratory centers to both increases in carbon dioxide tension and electrical stimulation. Tapentadol depresses the cough reflex by direct effect on the cough center in the medulla.

Tapentadol causes miosis, even in total darkness. Pinpoint pupils are a sign of opioid overdose but are not pathognomonic (e.g., pontine lesions of hemorrhagic or ischemic origin may produce similar findings). Marked mydriasis rather than miosis may be seen with hypoxia in overdose situations [see Overdosage (10)]. Other effects of tapentadol include anxiolysis, euphoria, and feeling of relaxation, drowsiness and changes in mood.

Effects on the Gastrointestinal Tract and on Other Smooth Muscle

Gastric, biliary and pancreatic secretions are decreased by tapentadol. Tapentadol causes a reduction in motility and is associated with an increase in tone in the antrum of the stomach and duodenum. Digestion of food in the small intestine is delayed and propulsive contractions are decreased. Propulsive peristaltic waves in the colon are decreased, while tone is increased to the point of spasm. The end result is constipation. Tapentadol can cause a marked increase in biliary tract pressure as a result of spasm of the sphincter of Oddi, and transient elevations in serum amylase. Tapentadol may also cause spasm of the sphincter of the urinary bladder.

Effects on the Endocrine System

Opioid agonists have been shown to have a variety of effects on the secretion of hormones. Opioids inhibit the secretion of ACTH, cortisol, and luteinizing hormone (LH) in humans. They also stimulate prolactin, growth hormone (GH) secretion, and pancreatic secretion of insulin and glucagon.

Effects on the Immune System

Opioids have been shown to have a variety of effects on components of the immune system in in vitro and animal models. The clinical significance of these findings is unknown.

CNS Depressant/Alcohol Interaction

Additive pharmacodynamic effects may be expected when NUCYNTA® ER is used in conjunction with alcohol, other opioids, or illicit drugs that cause central nervous system depression.

12.3 Pharmacokinetics

Absorption

The mean absolute bioavailability after single-dose administration (fasting) of NUCYNTA® ER is approximately 32% due to extensive first-pass metabolism. Maximum serum concentrations of tapentadol are observed between 3 and 6 hours after administration of NUCYNTA® ER. Dose proportional increases for AUC have been observed after administration of NUCYNTA® ER over the therapeutic dose range. Steady-state exposure of tapentadol is attained after the third dose (i.e., 24 hours after first twice daily multiple dose administration). Following dosing with 250 mg every 12 hours, minimal accumulation was observed.

Food Effect

The AUC and C_{max} increased by 6% and 17%, respectively, when NUCYNTA® ER tablet was administered after a high-fat, high-calorie breakfast. NUCYNTA® ER may be given with or without food.

Distribution

Tapentadol is widely distributed throughout the body. Following intravenous administration, the volume of distribution (Vz) for tapentadol is 540 +/- 98 L. The plasma protein binding is low and amounts to approximately 20%.

Metabolism

In humans, about 97% of the parent compound is metabolized. Tapentadol is mainly metabolized via Phase 2 pathways, and only a small amount is metabolized by Phase 1 oxidative pathways. The major pathway of tapentadol metabolism is conjugation with glucuronic acid to produce glucuronides. After oral administration approximately 70% (55% O-glucuronide and 15% sulfate of tapentadol) of the dose is excreted in urine in the conjugated form. A total of 3% of drug was excreted in urine as unchanged drug. Tapentadol is additionally metabolized to N-desmethyl tapentadol (13%) by CYP2C9 and CYP2C19 and to hydroxy tapentadol (2%) by CYP2D6, which are further metabolized by conjugation. Therefore, drug metabolism mediated by cytochrome P450 system is of less importance than phase 2 conjugation.

None of the metabolites contribute to the analgesic activity.

Excretion

Tapentadol and its metabolites are excreted almost exclusively (99%) via the kidneys. The terminal half-life is on average 5 hours after oral administration. The total clearance of tapentadol is 1603 +/-227 mL/min.

Specific Populations

Geriatric Patients

The mean exposure (AUC) to tapentadol was similar in elderly subjects compared to young adults, with a 16% lower mean C_{max} observed in the elderly subject group compared to young adult subjects.

Renal Impairment

AUC and C_{max} of tapentadol were comparable in subjects with varying degrees of renal function (from normal to severely impaired). In contrast, increasing exposure (AUC) to tapentadol-O-glucuronide was observed with increasing degree of renal impairment. In subjects with mild (CL_{CR}= 50 to <80 mL/min), moderate (CL_{CR}= 30 to <50 mL/min), and severe (CL_{CR}= <30 mL/min) renal impairment, the AUC of tapentadol-O-glucuronide was 1.5-, 2.5-, and 5.5-fold higher compared with normal renal function, respectively.

Hepatic Impairment

Administration of tapentadol resulted in higher exposures and serum levels to tapentadol in subjects with impaired hepatic function compared to subjects with normal hepatic function. The ratio of tapentadol pharmacokinetic parameters for the mild hepatic impairment group (Child-Pugh Score 5 to 6) and moderate hepatic impairment group (Child-Pugh Score 7 to 9) in comparison to the normal hepatic function group were 1.7 and 4.2, respectively, for AUC; 1.4 and 2.5, respectively, for C_{max}; and 1.2 and 1.4, respectively, for $t_{1/2}$. The rate of formation of tapentadol-O-glucuronide was lower in subjects with increased liver impairment.

Pharmacokinetic Drug Interactions

Tapentadol is mainly metabolized by Phase 2 glucuronidation, a high capacity/low affinity system; therefore, clinically relevant interactions caused by Phase 2 metabolism are unlikely to occur. Naproxen and probenecid increased the AUC of tapentadol by 17% and 57%, respectively. These changes are not considered clinically relevant and no change in dose is required.

No changes in the pharmacokinetic parameters of tapentadol were observed when acetaminophen and acetylsalicylic acid were given concomitantly.

In vitro studies did not reveal any potential of tapentadol to either inhibit or induce cytochrome P450 enzymes. Only a minor amount of tapentadol is metabolized via the oxidative pathway. Thus, clinically relevant interactions mediated by the cytochrome P450 system are unlikely to occur.

The pharmacokinetics of tapentadol were not affected when gastric pH or gastrointestinal motility were increased by omeprazole and metoclopramide, respectively.

Plasma protein binding of tapentadol is low (approximately 20%). Therefore, the likelihood of pharmacokinetic drug-drug interactions by displacement from the protein binding site is low.

Drug Interaction/Alcohol Interaction

NUCYNTA® ER may be expected to have additive effects when used in conjunction with alcohol, other opioids, or illicit drugs that cause central nervous system depression, because respiratory depression, hypotension, hypertension, and profound sedation, coma or death may result [see Warnings and Precautions (5.4)].

An in vivo study examined the effect of alcohol (240 mL of 40%) on the bioavailability of a single dose of 100 mg and 250 mg of NUCYNTA® ER tablet in healthy, fasted volunteers. After co-administration of a 100 mg NUCYNTA® ER tablet and alcohol, the mean C_{max} value increased by 48% compared to control with a range of 0.99-fold to 4.38-fold. The mean tapentadol AUC_{last} and AUC_{inf} were increased by 17%; the T_{max} and $t_{1/2}$ were unchanged. After co-administration of a 250 mg NUCYNTA® ER tablet and alcohol, the mean C_{max} value increased by 28% compared to control with a range of 0.90-fold to 2.67-fold. The mean tapentadol AUC_{last} and AUC_{inf} were increased by 16%; the T_{max} and $t_{1/2}$ were unchanged.

13 NONCLINICAL TOXICOLOGY

13.1 Carcinogenesis, Mutagenesis, Impairment of Fertility

Carcinogenesis

Tapentadol was administered to rats (diet) and mice (oral gavage) for two years.

In mice, tapentadol HCl was administered by oral gavage at dosages of 50, 100 and 200 mg/kg/day for 2 years (up to 0.34 times in the male mice and 0.25 times in the female mice the plasma exposure at the maximum recommended human dose [MRHD] for NUCYNTA® ER on an area under the time-curve [AUC] basis). No increase in tumor incidence was observed at any dose level.

In rats, tapentadol HCl was administered in diet at dosages of 10, 50, 125 and 250 mg/kg/day for two years (up to 0.20 times in the male rats and 0.75 times in the female rats the plasma exposure at the MRHD on an AUC basis). No increase in tumor incidence was observed at any dose level.

Mutagenesis

Tapentadol did not induce gene mutations in bacteria, but was clastogenic with metabolic activation in a chromosomal aberration test in V79 cells. The test was repeated and was negative in the presence and absence of metabolic activation. The one positive result for tapentadol was not confirmed *in vivo* in rats, using the two endpoints of chromosomal aberration and unscheduled DNA synthesis, when tested up to the maximum tolerated dose.

Impairment of Fertility

Tapentadol HCl was administered intravenously to male or female rats at dosages of 3, 6, or 12 mg/kg/day (representing exposures of up to approximately 0.56 times in the male rats and 0.50 times in the female rats the exposure at the MRHD on an AUC basis, based on extrapolation from toxicokinetic analyses in a separate 4-week intravenous study in rats). Tapentadol did not alter fertility at any dose level. Maternal toxicity and adverse effects on embryonic development, including decreased number of implantations, decreased numbers of live conceptuses, and increased pre- and post-implantation losses occurred at dosages ≥6 mg/kg/day.

13.2 Animal Toxicology and/or Pharmacology

In toxicological studies with tapentadol, the most common systemic effects of tapentadol were related to the mu-opioid receptor agonist and norepinephrine reuptake inhibition pharmacodynamic properties of the compound. Transient, dose-dependent and predominantly CNS-related findings were observed, including impaired respiratory function and convulsions, the latter occurring in the dog at plasma levels (C_{max}), which are in the range associated with the maximum recommended human dose (MRHD).

14 CLINICAL STUDIES

The efficacy of NUCYNTA® ER was studied in five studies in patients with moderate to severe chronic pain and DPN. Efficacy was demonstrated in one randomized, double-blind, placebo- and active-controlled study in patients with chronic low back pain (LBP), and two randomized, double-blind, placebo-controlled studies in patients with pain related to diabetic peripheral neuropathy (DPN-1 and DPN-2).

14.1 Moderate to Severe Chronic Low Back Pain

In the LBP study, patients 18 years of age or older with chronic low back pain and a baseline pain score of ≥5 on an 11-point numerical rating scale (NRS), ranging from 0 to 10 were enrolled and randomized to 1 of 3 treatments: NUCYNTA® ER, active-control (an extended-release Schedule II opioid analgesic), or placebo.

Patients randomized to NUCYNTA® ER initiated therapy with a dose of 50 mg twice daily for three days. After three days, the dose was increased to 100 mg twice daily. Subsequent titration was allowed over a 3-week titration period to a dose up to 250 mg twice daily, followed by a 12-week maintenance period. There were 981 patients randomized. The mean age of the study population was 50 (range 18 to 89) years; the mean baseline pain intensity score was 8 (SD 1). Approximately half of the patients were opioid-naïve (had not taken opioids during the three months prior to the screening visit).

The number of patients completing the study was 51% in the placebo group, 54% in the NUCYNTA® ER group and 43% in the active-control group. Lack of efficacy was the most common reason for discontinuation among placebo-treated patients (21%), whereas adverse events were the most common reason for discontinuation among the active treatment groups (17% and 32% for NUCYNTA® ER and active-control, respectively).

After 15 weeks of treatment, patients taking NUCYNTA® ER had a significantly greater pain reduction compared to placebo. The proportion of patients with various degrees of improvement is shown in Figure 1. The figure is cumulative, such that patients, whose change from baseline is, for example 50%, are also included at every level of improvement below 50%. Patients who did not complete the study were assigned 0% improvement.

[See figure 1 at top of next column]

14.2 Neuropathic Pain Associated with Diabetic Peripheral Neuropathy

In the two DPN studies, patients 18 years of age or older with pain due to diabetic peripheral neuropathy and a pain score of ≥5 on an 11-point numerical rating scale (NRS) ranging from 0 (no pain) to 10 (worst possible pain) were enrolled. Following an open-label treatment period in which NUCYNTA® ER was administered to all patients for three weeks and titrated to an individually stable dose, patients who had tolerated the drug and demonstrated at least a 1-point improvement in pain intensity on the NRS at the end of the open-label titration period were randomized to either continue the NUCYNTA® ER dose (100 mg to 250 mg twice a day) reached during the open-label titration period, or receive placebo for 12 weeks of maintenance treatment. During the first 4 days of the double-blind maintenance period patients were permitted to take tapentadol ER 25 mg

Figure 1: Percentage of Patients Achieving Various Levels of Improvement in Pain Intensity - Study LBP*

Percent Improvement in Pain from Baseline at Week 15 of the Treatment Period

* The last week of Study LBP was Week 15.

up to two times a day as additional medication. After the first 4 days, patients were allowed to take tapentadol ER 25 mg once daily as needed for pain, in addition to the patient's assigned study drug. Patients recorded their pain in a diary twice daily.

Study DPN-1: A total of 591 patients entered open-label treatment and 389 patients met the criteria for randomization into the double-blind treatment period. The mean age of the randomized population was 60 (range 29 to 87) years; approximately two-thirds of the patients were opioid-naïve (had not taken opioids during the three months prior to the screening visit).

During the titration period, 34% of patients discontinued open-label NUCYNTA® ER. The most common reasons for discontinuation in the double-blind treatment period were lack of efficacy in the placebo group (14%) and adverse events in the NUCYNTA® ER group (15%).

After 12 weeks of treatment, NUCYNTA® ER provided a significantly greater reduction in pain intensity from baseline to the end of the 12-week double-blind period compared to placebo. Figure 2 displays the proportion of randomized patients achieving various degrees of improvement in pain intensity from the start of the open-label titration period to the last week of the randomized withdrawal period. The figure is cumulative, such that patients, whose change from baseline is, for example 50%, are also included at every level of improvement below 50%. Patients who did not complete the study were assigned 0% improvement.

Figure 2: Percentage of Patients Achieving Various Levels of Improvement in Pain Intensity - DPN-1

Percent Improvement in Pain from Baseline at Week 12 of the DB Period

Study DPN-2: A total of 459 patients entered open-label treatment and 320 patients met the criteria for randomization into the double-blind treatment period. The mean age of the randomized population was 59 (range 28 to 83) years; approximately two-thirds of the patients were opioid-naïve (had not taken opioids during the three months prior to the screening visit).

During the titration period, 22% of patients discontinued open-label NUCYNTA® ER and 6% of patients were not subsequently randomized because they failed to have at least 1-point improvement in pain intensity. The most common reason for discontinuation in the double-blind treatment period was adverse events in both the placebo group (9%) and the NUCYNTA® ER group (14%).

After 12 weeks of treatment, NUCYNTA® ER provided a significantly greater reduction in pain intensity from baseline to the end of the 12-week double-blind period compared to placebo. Figure 3 displays the proportion of randomized patients achieving various degrees of improvement in pain intensity from the start of the open-label titration period to the last week of the randomized withdrawal period. The figure is cumulative, such that patients, whose change from baseline is, for example 50%, are also included at every level of improvement below 50%. Patients who did not complete the study were assigned 0% improvement.

[See figure 3 at top of next column]

16 HOW SUPPLIED/STORAGE AND HANDLING

NUCYNTA® ER tablets are available in the following strengths and packages:

Figure 3: Percentage of Patients Achieving Various Levels of Improvement in Pain Intensity-DPN-2

Percent Improvement in Pain from Baseline at Week 12 of the DB Period

50 mg extended-release tablets are white oblong-shaped with a black print "OMJ 50" on one side and are available in bottles of 60 with child-resistant closure (NDC 50458-860-01) and unit dose blister packs of 100 (10 blister strips of 10 tablets each), for hospital use only (NDC 50458-860-02).

100 mg extended-release tablets are light-blue oblong-shaped with a black print "OMJ 100" on one side and are available in bottles of 60 with child-resistant closure (NDC 50458-861-01) and unit dose blister packs of 100 (10 blister strips of 10 tablets each), for hospital use only (NDC 50458-861-02).

150 mg extended-release tablets are blue-green oblong-shaped with a black print "OMJ 150" on one side and are available in bottles of 60 with child-resistant closure (NDC 50458-862-01) and unit dose blister packs of 100 (10 blister strips of 10 tablets each), for hospital use only (NDC 50458-862-02).

200 mg extended-release tablets are blue oblong-shaped with a depression in the middle running lengthwise on each side and with a black print "OMJ 200" on one side, and are available in bottles of 60 with child-resistant closure (NDC 50458-863-01) and unit dose blister packs of 100 (10 blister strips of 10 tablets each), for hospital use only (NDC 50458-863-02).

250 mg extended-release tablets are dark blue oblong-shaped with a depression in the middle running lengthwise on each side and with a white print "OMJ 250" on one side, and are available in bottles of 60 with child-resistant closure (NDC 50458-864-01) and unit dose blister packs of 100 (10 blister strips of 10 tablets each), for hospital use only (NDC 50458-864-02).

Storage and Handling

Store up to 25°C (77°F); excursions permitted to 15° – 30°C (59° – 86°F) [see USP Controlled Room Temperature].

Protect from moisture.

Keep NUCYNTA® ER in a secure place out of reach of children.

NUCYNTA® ER tablets that are no longer needed should be destroyed by flushing down the toilet.

17 PATIENT COUNSELING INFORMATION

Advise the patient to read the FDA-approved patient labeling (Medication Guide).

Addiction, Abuse, and Misuse

Inform patients that the use of NUCYNTA® ER, even when taken as recommended, can result in addiction, abuse, and misuse, which can lead to overdose or death *[see Warnings and Precautions (5.1)]*. Instruct patients not to share NUCYNTA® ER with others and to take steps to protect NUCYNTA® ER from theft or misuse.

Life-threatening Respiratory Depression

Inform patients of the risk of life-threatening respiratory depression, including information that the risk is greatest when starting NUCYNTA® ER or when the dose is increased, and that it can occur even at recommended doses *[see Warnings and Precautions (5.2)]*. Advise patients how to recognize respiratory depression and to seek medical attention if breathing difficulties develop.

Accidental Ingestion

Inform patients that accidental ingestion, especially by children, may result in respiratory depression or death *[see Warnings and Precautions (5.2)]*. Instruct patients to take steps to store NUCYNTA® ER securely and to dispose of unused NUCYNTA® ER by flushing the tablets down the toilet.

Neonatal Opioid Withdrawal Syndrome

Inform female patients of reproductive potential that prolonged use of NUCYNTA® ER during pregnancy can result in neonatal opioid withdrawal syndrome, which may be life-threatening if not recognized and treated *[see Warnings and Precautions (5.3)]*.

Interactions with Alcohol and other CNS Depressants

Instruct patients not to consume alcoholic beverages, as well as prescription and over-the-counter products that contain alcohol, during treatment with NUCYNTA® ER. The co-ingestion of alcohol with NUCYNTA® ER may result in increased plasma tapentadol levels and a potentially fatal overdose of tapentadol [see Warnings and Precautions (5.4)]. Inform patients that potentially serious additive effects may occur if NUCYNTA® ER is used with alcohol or other CNS depressants, and not to use such drugs unless supervised by a health care provider.

Concurrent use of MAOI
Inform patients not to take NUCYNTA® ER while using any drugs that inhibit monoamine oxidase. Patients should not start MAOIs while taking NUCYNTA® ER.

Seizures
Inform patients that NUCYNTA® ER could cause seizures if they are at risk for seizures or have epilepsy. Patients should be advised to stop taking NUCYNTA® ER if they have a seizure while taking NUCYNTA® ER and call their healthcare provider right away.

Serotonin Syndrome
Inform patients that NUCYNTA® ER could cause a rare but potentially life-threatening condition resulting from concomitant administration of serotonergic drugs (including Serotonin Reuptake Inhibitors, Serotonin and Norepinephrine Reuptake Inhibitors and tricyclic antidepressants). Warn patients of the symptoms of serotonin syndrome and to seek medical attention right away if symptoms develop. Instruct patients to inform their physicians if they are taking, or plan to take additional medications including CNS Depressants, MAO inhibitors, mixed agonists/antagonist opioid analgesics, anticholinergics, SSRIs, SNRIs, or tricyclic antidepressants.

Important Administration Instructions
Instruct patients how to properly take NUCYNTA® ER, including the following:
• Swallowing NUCYNTA® ER tablets whole
• Not cutting, crushing, chewing, or dissolving the tablets
• Using NUCYNTA® ER exactly as prescribed to reduce the risk of life-threatening adverse reactions (e.g., respiratory depression)
• Not discontinuing NUCYNTA® ER without first discussing the need for a tapering regimen with the prescriber
• To take each tablet with enough water to ensure complete swallowing immediately after placing in mouth.

Hypotension
Inform patients that NUCYNTA® ER may cause orthostatic hypotension and syncope. Instruct patients how to recognize symptoms of low blood pressure and how to reduce the risk of serious consequences should hypotension occur (e.g., sit or lie down, carefully rise from a sitting or lying position).

Driving or Operating Heavy Machinery
Inform patients that NUCYNTA® ER may impair the ability to perform potentially hazardous activities such as driving a car or operating heavy machinery. Advise patients not to perform such tasks until they know how they will react to the medication.

Constipation
Advise patients of the potential for severe constipation, including management instructions and when to seek medical attention.

Anaphylaxis
Inform patients that anaphylaxis has been reported with ingredients contained in NUCYNTA® ER. Advise patients how to recognize such a reaction and when to seek medical attention.

Pregnancy
Advise female patients that NUCYNTA® ER can cause fetal harm and to inform the prescriber if they are pregnant or plan to become pregnant.

Disposal of Unused NUCYNTA® ER
Advise patients to flush the unused tablets down the toilet when NUCYNTA® ER is no longer needed.

Manufactured by:
Janssen Ortho, LLC
Gurabo, PR 00778
Manufactured for:
Janssen Pharmaceuticals, Inc.
Titusville, NJ 08560
© Janssen Pharmaceuticals, Inc. 2011
Revised: April 2014

Medication Guide
NUCYNTA®ER (new-SINN-tah E-R) (tapentadol)
extended-release oral tablets, CII

NUCYNTA® ER is:
• A strong prescription pain medicine that contains an opioid (narcotic) that is used to manage pain severe enough to require daily around-the-clock, long-term treatment with an opioid, when other pain treatments such as non-opioid pain medicines or immediate-release opioid medicines do not treat your pain well enough or you cannot tolerate them.

• Also used to manage pain from damaged nerves (neuropathic pain) that happens with diabetes and is severe enough to require daily around-the-clock, long-term treatment with an opioid, when other pain treatments such as non-opioid pain medicines do not treat your pain well enough or you cannot tolerate them.
• A long-acting (extended-release) opioid pain medicine that can put you at risk for overdose and death. Even if you take your dose correctly as prescribed you are at risk for opioid addiction, abuse, and misuse that can lead to death.
• Not used to treat pain that is not around-the-clock pain.

Important information about NUCYNTA® ER:
• **Get emergency help right away if you take too much NUCYNTA® ER (overdose).** When you first start taking NUCYNTA® ER, when your dose is changed, or if you take too much (overdose), serious or life threatening breathing problems that can lead to death may occur.
• Never give anyone your NUCYNTA® ER. They could die from taking it. Store NUCYNTA® ER away from children and in a safe place to prevent stealing or abuse. Selling or giving away NUCYNTA® ER is against the law.

Do not take NUCYNTA® ER if you have:
• severe asthma, trouble breathing, or other lung problems.
• a bowel blockage or have narrowing of the stomach or intestines.

Before taking NUCYNTA® ER, tell your healthcare provider if you have a history of:

• head injury, seizures	• liver, kidney, thyroid problems
• problems urinating	• pancreas or gallbladder problems

• abuse of street or prescription drugs, alcohol addiction, or mental health problems.

Tell your healthcare provider if you are:
• **pregnant or planning to become pregnant.** Prolonged use of NUCYNTA® ER during pregnancy can cause withdrawal symptoms in your newborn baby that could be life-threatening if not recognized and treated.
• **breastfeeding.** NUCYNTA® ER passes into breast milk and may harm your baby.
• taking prescription or over-the-counter medicines, vitamins, or herbal supplements. Taking NUCYNTA® ER with certain other medicines can cause serious side effects.

When taking NUCYNTA® ER:
• Do not change your dose. Take NUCYNTA® ER exactly as prescribed by your healthcare provider.
• Take your prescribed dose every 12 hours, at the same time every day. Do not take more than your prescribed dose in 24 hours. If you miss a dose, take your next dose at your usual time.
• Swallow NUCYNTA® ER whole. Do not cut, break, chew, crush, dissolve, snort, or inject NUCYNTA® ER because this may cause you to overdose and die.
• **Call your healthcare provider if the dose you are taking does not control your pain.**
• **Do not stop taking NUCYNTA® ER without talking to your healthcare provider.**
  • After you stop taking NUCYNTA® ER, flush any unused tablets down the toilet.

While taking NUCYNTA® ER DO NOT:
• Drive or operate heavy machinery until you know how NUCYNTA® ER affects you. NUCYNTA® ER can make you sleepy, dizzy, or lightheaded.
• Drink alcohol, or use prescription or over-the-counter medicines containing alcohol. Using products containing alcohol during treatment with NUCYNTA® ER may cause you to overdose and die.

The possible side effects of NUCYNTA® ER are:
• constipation, nausea, sleepiness, vomiting, tiredness, headache, dizziness, abdominal pain. Call your healthcare provider if you have any of these symptoms and they are severe.
Get emergency medical help if you have:
• trouble breathing, shortness of breath, fast heartbeat, chest pain, swelling of your face, tongue or throat, extreme drowsiness, light-headedness when changing positions, or you are feeling faint.
• agitation, hallucinations, coma, feeling overheated, or heavy sweating.
These are not all the possible side effects of NUCYNTA® ER. Call your doctor for medical advice about side effects. You may report side effects to FDA at 1-800-FDA-1088.
For more information go to dailymed.nlm.nih.gov

Manufactured for: Janssen Pharmaceuticals, Inc. Titusville, NJ 08560, www.Nucynta.com or call 1-800-526-7736

This Medication Guide has been approved by the U.S. Food and Drug Administration
Revised: April 2014
Shown in Product Identification Guide, page 307

Jazz Pharmaceuticals, Inc.
3180 PORTER DRIVE
PALO ALTO, CA 94304

Direct Inquiries to:
Phone: (650) 496-3777
Fax: (650) 496-3781
E-mail: customercare@jazzpharma.com
For medical information:
E-mail: jazzpharma@medcomsol.com
For media information:
E-mail: mediainfo@jazzpharma.com

XYREM® ⒸⒾⒾⒾ Ŗ
(sodium oxybate) oral solution
Rx only

HIGHLIGHTS OF PRESCRIBING INFORMATION
These highlights do not include all the information needed to use XYREM safely and effectively. See full prescribing information for XYREM.
Xyrem® (sodium oxybate) oral solution CIII
Initial U.S. Approval: 2002

WARNING: CENTRAL NERVOUS SYSTEM (CNS) DEPRESSION AND MISUSE AND ABUSE.
See full prescribing information for complete boxed warning.
• Respiratory depression can occur with Xyrem use (5.4)
• Xyrem is a Schedule III controlled substance and is the sodium salt of gamma hydroxybutyrate (GHB), a Schedule I controlled substance. Abuse or misuse of illicit GHB is associated with CNS adverse reactions, including seizure, respiratory depression, decreased consciousness, coma and death (5.2, 9.2)
• Because of the risks of CNS depression, abuse, and misuse, Xyrem is available only through a restricted distribution program called the Xyrem Success Program® using a centralized pharmacy. Prescribers and patients must enroll in the program. (5.3)

————**RECENT MAJOR CHANGES**————
Dosage and Administration,
  Dose Adjustment with Co-administration of
  Divalproex Sodium (2.4)   04/2014

————**INDICATIONS AND USAGE**————
Xyrem is a central nervous system depressant indicated for the treatment of:
• Cataplexy in narcolepsy (1.1)
• Excessive daytime sleepiness (EDS) in narcolepsy (1.2)
Xyrem may only be dispensed to patients enrolled in the Xyrem Success Program (1).

————**DOSAGE AND ADMINISTRATION**————
• Initiate dose at 4.5 grams (g) per night administered orally in two equal, divided doses: 2.25 g at bedtime and 2.25 g taken 2.5 to 4 hours later (2.1)
• Titrate to effect in increments of 1.5 g per night at weekly intervals (0.75 g at bedtime and 0.75 g taken 2.5 to 4 hours later) (2.1).
• Recommended dose range: 6 g to 9 g per night orally (2.1).

Total Nightly Dose	Take at Bedtime	Take 2.5 to 4 Hours Later
4.5 g per night	2.25 g	2.25 g
6 g per night	3 g	3 g
7.5 g per night	3.75 g	3.75 g
9 g per night	4.5 g	4.5 g

• Take each dose while in bed and lie down after dosing (2.2).
• Allow 2 hours after eating before dosing (2.2).

- Prepare both doses prior to bedtime; dilute each dose with approximately ¼ cup of water in pharmacy-provided vials (2.2).
- Patients with Hepatic Impairment: starting dose is 2.25 g per night administered orally in two equal, divided doses of approximately 1.13 g at bedtime and approximately 1.13 g taken 2.5 to 4 hours later (2.3).
- Concomitant use with divalproex sodium: an initial reduction in Xyrem dose of at least 20% is recommended (2.4, 7.2).

————————DOSAGE FORMS AND STRENGTHS————————

Oral solution, 0.5 g per mL (3)

————————CONTRAINDICATIONS————————

- Succinic semialdehyde dehydrogenase deficiency (4)
- In combination with sedative hypnotics or alcohol (4)

————————WARNINGS AND PRECAUTIONS————————

- CNS depression: Use caution when considering the concurrent use of Xyrem with other CNS depressants (5.1).
- Caution patients against hazardous activities requiring complete mental alertness or motor coordination within the first 6 hours of dosing or after first initiating treatment until certain that Xyrem does not affect them adversely (5.1).
- Depression and suicidality: Monitor patients for emergent or increased depression and suicidality (5.5).
- Confusion/Anxiety: Monitor for impaired motor/cognitive function (5.6).
- Parasomnias: Evaluate episodes of sleepwalking (5.7).
- High sodium content in Xyrem: Monitor patients with heart failure, hypertension, or impaired renal function (5.8).

————————ADVERSE REACTIONS————————

Most common adverse reactions (≥ 5% and at least twice the incidence with placebo) were nausea, dizziness, vomiting, somnolence, enuresis, and tremor (6.1).
To report SUSPECTED ADVERSE REACTIONS, contact Jazz Pharmaceuticals at 1-800-520-5568, or FDA at 1-800-FDA-1088 or www.fda.gov/Medwatch.

————————USE IN SPECIFIC POPULATIONS————————

- Pregnancy: Based on animal data, may cause fetal harm (8.1).
- Geriatric patients: Monitor for impaired motor and/or cognitive function when taking Xyrem (8.5).

See 17 for PATIENT COUNSELING INFORMATION and Medication Guide

Revised: 04/2014

FULL PRESCRIBING INFORMATION: CONTENTS*
WARNING: CENTRAL NERVOUS SYSTEM (CNS) DEPRESSION and MISUSE AND ABUSE.

FULL PRESCRIBING INFORMATION

> **WARNING: CENTRAL NERVOUS SYSTEM (CNS) DEPRESSION and MISUSE AND ABUSE.**
>
> Xyrem (sodium oxybate) is a CNS depressant. In clinical trials at recommended doses obtundation and clinically significant respiratory depression occurred in Xyrem-treated patients. Almost all of the patients who received Xyrem during clinical trials in narcolepsy were receiving central nervous system stimulants *[see Warnings and Precautions (5.1)]*.
> Xyrem® (sodium oxybate) is the sodium salt of gamma hydroxybutyrate (GHB). Abuse of GHB, either alone or in combination with other CNS depressants, is associated with CNS adverse reactions, including seizure, respiratory depression, decreases in the level of consciousness, coma, and death *[see Warnings and Precautions (5.2)]*.
> Because of the risks of CNS depression, abuse, and misuse, Xyrem is available only through a restricted distribution program called the Xyrem Success Program®, using a centralized pharmacy. Prescribers and patients must enroll in the program. For further information go to www.XYREM.com or call 1-866-XYREM88® (1-866-997-3688) *[see Warnings and Precautions (5.3)]*.

1   INDICATIONS AND USAGE

Limitations of Use
Xyrem may only be dispensed to patients enrolled in the Xyrem Success Program *[see Warnings and Precautions (5.3)]*.

1.1   Cataplexy in Narcolepsy
Xyrem (sodium oxybate) oral solution is indicated for the treatment of cataplexy in narcolepsy.

1.2   Excessive Daytime Sleepiness in Narcolepsy
Xyrem (sodium oxybate) oral solution is indicated for the treatment of excessive daytime sleepiness (EDS) in narcolepsy.

2   DOSAGE AND ADMINISTRATION

Healthcare professionals who prescribe Xyrem must enroll in the Xyrem Success Program and must comply with the requirements to ensure safe use of Xyrem *[see Warnings and Precautions (5.3)]*.

2.1   Dosing Information
The recommended starting dose is 4.5 grams (g) per night administered orally in two equal, divided doses: 2.25 g at bedtime and 2.25 g taken 2.5 to 4 hours later (see Table 1). Increase the dose by 1.5 g per night at weekly intervals (additional 0.75 g at bedtime and 0.75 g taken 2.5 to 4 hours later) to the effective dose range of 6 g to 9 g per night orally. Doses higher than 9 g per night have not been studied and should not ordinarily be administered.

Table 1: Xyrem Dose Regimen (g = grams)

If A Patient's Total Nightly Dose is:	Take at Bedtime:	Take 2.5 to 4 Hours Later:
4.5 g per night	2.25 g	2.25 g
6 g per night	3 g	3 g
7.5 g per night	3.75 g	3.75 g
9 g per night	4.5 g	4.5 g

2.2   Important Administration Instructions
Take the first dose of Xyrem at least 2 hours after eating because food significantly reduces the bioavailability of sodium oxybate.

Prepare both doses of Xyrem prior to bedtime. Prior to ingestion, each dose of Xyrem should be diluted with approximately ¼ cup (approximately 60 mL) of water in the empty pharmacy vials provided. Patients should take both doses of Xyrem while in bed and lie down immediately after dosing as Xyrem may cause them to fall asleep abruptly without first feeling drowsy. Patients will often fall asleep within 5 minutes of taking Xyrem, and will usually fall asleep within 15 minutes, though the time it takes any individual patient to fall asleep may vary from night to night. Patients should remain in bed following ingestion of the first and second doses, and should not take the second dose until 2.5 to 4 hours after the first dose. Patients may need to set an alarm to awaken for the second dose. Rarely, patients may take up to 2 hours to fall asleep.

2.3   Dose Modification in Patients with Hepatic Impairment
The recommended starting dose in patients with hepatic impairment is 2.25 g per night administered orally in two equal, divided doses: approximately 1.13 g at bedtime and approximately 1.13 g taken 2.5 to 4 hours later *[see Use in Specific Populations (8.6); Clinical Pharmacology (12.3)]*.

2.4   Dose Adjustment with Co-administration of Divalproex Sodium
Pharmacokinetic and pharmacodynamics interactions have been observed when Xyrem is co-administered with divalproex sodium. For patients already stabilized on Xyrem, it is recommended that addition of divalproex sodium should be accompanied by an initial reduction in the nightly dose of Xyrem by at least 20%. For patients already taking divalproex sodium, it is recommended that prescribers use a lower starting Xyrem dose with introducing Xyrem. Prescribers should monitor patient response and adjust dose accordingly *[see Drug Interactions (7.2) and Clinical Pharmacology (12.3)]*.

3   DOSAGE FORMS AND STRENGTHS

Xyrem is a clear to slightly opalescent oral solution, in a concentration of 0.5 g per mL.

4   CONTRAINDICATIONS

- Xyrem is contraindicated in patients being treated with sedative hypnotic agents.
- Patients should not drink alcohol when using Xyrem.
- Xyrem is contraindicated in patients with succinic semialdehyde dehydrogenase deficiency. This is a rare disorder of inborn error of metabolism variably characterized by mental retardation, hypotonia, and ataxia.

5   WARNINGS AND PRECAUTIONS

5.1   Central Nervous System Depression
Xyrem is a central nervous system (CNS) depressant. Alcohol and sedative hypnotics are contraindicated in patients who are using Xyrem. The concurrent use of Xyrem with other CNS depressants, including but not limited to opioid analgesics, benzodiazepines, sedating antidepressants or antipsychotics, sedating anti-epileptic drugs, general anesthetics, muscle relaxants, and/or illicit CNS depressants, may increase the risk of respiratory depression, hypotension, profound sedation, syncope, and death. If use of these CNS depressants in combination with Xyrem is required, dose reduction or discontinuation of one or more CNS depressants (including Xyrem) should be considered. In addition, if short-term use of an opioid (e.g. post- or perioperative) is required, interruption of treatment with Xyrem should be considered.

Healthcare providers should caution patients about operating hazardous machinery, including automobiles or airplanes, until they are reasonably certain that Xyrem does not affect them adversely (e.g., impair judgment, thinking, or motor skills). Patients should not engage in hazardous occupations or activities requiring complete mental alertness or motor coordination, such as operating machinery or a motor vehicle or flying an airplane, for at least 6 hours after taking the second nightly dose of Xyrem. Patients should be queried about CNS depression–related events upon initiation of Xyrem therapy and periodically thereafter *[see Warnings and Precautions (5.3)]*.

5.2   Abuse and Misuse
Xyrem is a Schedule III controlled substance. The active ingredient of Xyrem, sodium oxybate or gamma-hydroxybutyrate (GHB), is a Schedule I controlled substance. Abuse of illicit GHB, either alone or in combination with other CNS depressants, is associated with CNS adverse reactions, including seizure, respiratory depression, decreases in the level of consciousness, coma, and death. The rapid onset of sedation, coupled with the amnestic features of Xyrem, particularly when combined with alcohol, has proven to be dangerous for the voluntary and involuntary user (e.g., assault victim). Because illicit use and abuse

of GHB have been reported, physicians should carefully evaluate patients for a history of drug abuse and follow such patients closely, observing them for signs of misuse or abuse of GHB (e.g. increase in size or frequency of dosing, drug-seeking behavior, feigned cataplexy) *[see Warnings and Precautions (5.3) and Drug Abuse and Dependence (9.2)]*.

5.3   Xyrem Success Program

Because of the risks of central nervous system depression and abuse/misuse, Xyrem is available only through a restricted distribution program called the Xyrem Success Program.

Required components of the Xyrem Success Program are:

• Use of a centralized pharmacy
• Healthcare Providers who prescribe Xyrem must complete the enrollment forms and comply with the requirements.
• To receive Xyrem, patients must understand the risks and benefits of Xyrem.

Further information is available at www.XYREM.com or **1-866-XYREM88® (1-866-997-3688).**

5.4   Respiratory Depression and Sleep-Disordered Breathing

Xyrem may impair respiratory drive, especially in patients with compromised respiratory function. In overdoses, life-threatening respiratory depression has been reported *[see Overdosage (10)]*.

In a study assessing the respiratory-depressant effects of Xyrem at doses up to 9 g per night in 21 patients with narcolepsy, no dose-related changes in oxygen saturation were demonstrated in the group as a whole. One of the four patients with preexisting, moderate-to-severe sleep apnea had significant worsening of the apnea/hypopnea index during treatment.

In a study assessing the effects of Xyrem 9 g per night in 50 patients with obstructive sleep apnea, Xyrem did not increase the severity of sleep-disordered breathing and did not adversely affect the average duration and severity of oxygen desaturation overall. However, there was a significant increase in the number of central apneas in patients taking Xyrem, and clinically significant oxygen desaturation (≤55%) was measured in three patients (6%) after Xyrem administration, with one patient withdrawing from the study and two continuing after single brief instances of desaturation. Prescribers should be aware that increased central apneas and clinically relevant desaturation events have been observed with Xyrem administration.

In clinical trials in 128 patients with narcolepsy, two subjects had profound CNS depression, which resolved after supportive respiratory intervention. Two other patients discontinued sodium oxybate because of severe difficulty breathing and an increase in obstructive sleep apnea. In two controlled trials assessing polysomnographic (PSG) measures in patients with narcolepsy, 40 of 477 patients were included with a baseline apnea/hypopnea index of 16 to 67 events per hour, indicative of mild to severe sleep-disordered breathing. None of the 40 patients had a clinically significant worsening of respiratory function as measured by apnea/hypopnea index and pulse oximetry at doses of 4.5 g to 9 g per night.

Prescribers should be aware that sleep-related breathing disorders tend to be more prevalent in obese patients and in postmenopausal women not on hormone replacement therapy as well as among patients with narcolepsy.

5.5   Depression and Suicidality

In clinical trials in patients with narcolepsy (n=781), there were two suicides and two attempted suicides in Xyrem-treated patients, including three patients with a previous history of depressive psychiatric disorder. Of the two suicides, one patient used Xyrem in conjunction with other drugs. Xyrem was not involved in the second suicide. Adverse reactions of depression were reported by 7% of 781 Xyrem-treated patients, with four patients (< 1%) discontinuing because of depression. In most cases, no change in Xyrem treatment was required.

In a controlled trial, with patients randomized to fixed doses of 3 g, 6 g, or 9 g per night Xyrem or placebo, there was a single event of depression at the 3 g per night dose. In another controlled trial, with patients titrated from an initial 4.5 g per night starting dose, the incidences of depression were 1 (1.7%), 1 (1.5%), 2 (3.2%), and 2 (3.6%) for the placebo, 4.5 g, 6 g, and 9 g per night doses, respectively.

The emergence of depression in patients treated with Xyrem requires careful and immediate evaluation. Patients with a previous history of a depressive illness and/or suicide attempt should be monitored carefully for the emergence of depressive symptoms while taking Xyrem.

5.6   Other Behavioral or Psychiatric Adverse Reactions

During clinical trials in narcolepsy, 3% of 781 patients treated with Xyrem experienced confusion, with incidence generally increasing with dose.

Less than 1% of patients discontinued the drug because of confusion. Confusion was reported at all recommended doses from 6 g to 9 g per night. In a controlled trial where patients were randomized to fixed total daily doses of 3 g, 6 g, or 9 g per night or placebo, a dose-response relationship

for confusion was demonstrated, with 17% of patients at 9 g per night experiencing confusion. In all cases in that controlled trial, the confusion resolved soon after termination of treatment. In Trial 3 where sodium oxybate was titrated from an initial 4.5 g per night dose, there was a single event of confusion in one patient at the 9 g per night dose. In the majority of cases in all clinical trials in narcolepsy, confusion resolved either soon after termination of dosing or with continued treatment. However, patients treated with Xyrem who become confused should be evaluated fully, and appropriate intervention considered on an individual basis.

Anxiety occurred in 5.8% of the 874 patients receiving Xyrem in clinical trials in another population. The emergence of or increase in anxiety in patients taking Xyrem should be carefully monitored.

Other neuropsychiatric reactions reported in Xyrem clinical trials included hallucinations, paranoia, psychosis, and agitation. The emergence of thought disorders and/or behavior abnormalities requires careful and immediate evaluation.

5.7   Parasomnias

Sleepwalking, defined as confused behavior occurring at night and at times associated with wandering, was reported in 6% of 781 patients with narcolepsy treated with Xyrem in controlled and long-term open-label studies, with < 1% of patients discontinuing due to sleepwalking. Rates of sleepwalking were similar for patients taking placebo and patients taking Xyrem in controlled trials. It is unclear if some or all of the reported sleepwalking episodes correspond to true somnambulism, which is a parasomnia occurring during non-REM sleep, or to any other specific medical disorder. Five instances of significant injury or potential injury were associated with sleepwalking during a clinical trial of Xyrem in patients with narcolepsy.

Parasomnias including sleepwalking have been reported in postmarketing experience with Xyrem. Therefore, episodes of sleepwalking should be fully evaluated and appropriate interventions considered.

5.8   Use in Patients Sensitive to High Sodium Intake

Xyrem has a high salt content. In patients sensitive to salt intake (e.g., those with heart failure, hypertension, or renal impairment) consider the amount of daily sodium intake in each dose of Xyrem. Table 2 provides the approximate sodium content per Xyrem dose.

Table 2
Approximate Sodium Content per Total Nightly Dose of Xyrem (g = grams)

Xyrem Dose	Sodium Content/Total Nightly Exposure
3 g per night	550 mg
4.5 g per night	820 mg
6 g per night	1100 mg
7.5 g per night	1400 mg
9 g per night	1640 mg

6   ADVERSE REACTIONS

The following adverse reactions appear in other sections of the labeling:

• CNS depression *[see Warnings and Precautions (5.1)]*
• Abuse and Misuse *[see Warnings and Precautions (5.2)]*
• Respiratory Depression and Sleep-disordered Breathing *[see Warnings and Precautions (5.4)]*
• Depression and Suicidality *[see Warnings and Precautions (5.5)]*
• Other Behavioral or Psychiatric Adverse Reactions *[see Warnings and Precautions (5.6)]*
• Parasomnias *[see Warnings and Precautions (5.7)]*
• Use in Patients Sensitive to High Sodium Intake *[see Warnings and Precautions (5.8)]*

6.1   Clinical Trials Experience

Because clinical trials are conducted under widely varying conditions, adverse reaction rates observed in the clinical trials of a drug cannot be directly compared to rates in the clinical trials of another drug and may not reflect the rates observed in clinical practice.

Xyrem was studied in three placebo-controlled clinical trials (Trials N1, N3, and N4, described in Sections 14.1 and 14.2) in 611 patients with narcolepsy (398 subjects treated with Xyrem, and 213 with placebo). A total of 781 patients with narcolepsy were treated with Xyrem in controlled and uncontrolled clinical trials.

Section 6.1 and Table 3 presents adverse reactions from three pooled, controlled trials (N1, N3, N4) in patients with narcolepsy.

Adverse Reactions Leading to Treatment Discontinuation:
Of the 398 Xyrem-treated patients with narcolepsy, 10.3% of patients discontinued because of adverse reactions com-

pared with 2.8% of patients receiving placebo. The most common adverse reaction leading to discontinuation was nausea (2.8%). The majority of adverse reactions leading to discontinuation began during the first few weeks of treatment.

CommonlyObserved Adverse Reactions in Controlled Clinical Trials:
The most common adverse reactions (incidence ≥ 5% and twice the rate seen with placebo) in Xyrem-treated patients were nausea, dizziness, vomiting, somnolence, enuresis, and tremor.

Adverse Reactions Occurring at an Incidence of 2% or greater:
Table 3 lists adverse reactions that occurred at a frequency of 2% or more in any treatment group for three controlled trials and were more frequent in any Xyrem treatment group than with placebo. Adverse reactions are summarized by dose at onset. Almost all patients in these studies initiated treatment at 4.5 g per night. In patients who remained on treatment, adverse reactions tended to occur early and to diminish over time.

[See table 3 at top of next page]

Dose-Response Information
In clinical trials in narcolepsy, a dose-response relationship was observed for nausea, vomiting, paresthesia, disorientation, irritability, disturbance in attention, feeling drunk, sleepwalking, and enuresis. The incidence of all these reactions was notably higher at 9 g per night.

In controlled trials in narcolepsy, discontinuations of treatment due to adverse reactions were greater at higher doses of Xyrem.

6.2   Postmarketing Experience

The following additional adverse reactions that have a likely causal relationship to Xyrem exposure have been identified during postmarketing use of Xyrem. These adverse reactions include: arthralgia, decreased appetite, fall, fluid retention, hangover, headache, hypersensitivity, hypertension, memory impairment, panic attack, vision blurred, and weight decreased. Because these reactions are reported voluntarily, it is not always possible to reliably estimate their frequency.

7   DRUG INTERACTIONS

7.1   Alcohol, Sedative Hypnotics, and CNS Depressants

Xyrem should not be used in combination with alcohol or sedative hypnotics. Use of other CNS depressants may potentiate the CNS-depressant effects of Xyrem.

7.2   Divalproex Sodium

Concomitant use of Xyrem with divalproex sodium resulted in a 25% mean increase in systemic exposure to Xyrem (AUC ratio range of 0.8 to 1.7) and in a greater impairment on some tests of attention and working memory. An initial Xyrem dose reduction of at least 20% is recommended if divalproex sodium is prescribed to patients already taking Xyrem *[see Dosage and Administration (2.4) and Clinical Pharmacology (12.3)]*. Prescribers are advised to monitor patient response closely and adjust dose accordingly if concomitant use of Xyrem and divalproex sodium is warranted.

8   USE IN SPECIFIC POPULATIONS

8.1   Pregnancy

Pregnancy Category C
There are no adequate and well-controlled studies in pregnant women. Xyrem should be used during pregnancy only if the potential benefit justifies the potential risk to the fetus. Oral administration of sodium oxybate to pregnant rats (150, 350, or 1,000 mg/kg/day) or rabbits (300, 600, or 1,200 mg/kg/day) throughout organogenesis produced no clear evidence of developmental toxicity. The highest doses tested in rats and rabbits were approximately 1 and 3 times, respectively, the maximum recommended human dose (MRHD) of 9 g per night on a body surface area (mg/m²) basis.

Oral administration of sodium oxybate (150, 350, or 1,000 mg/kg/day) to rats throughout pregnancy and lactation resulted in increased stillbirths and decreased offspring postnatal viability and body weight gain at the highest dose tested. The no-effect dose for pre- and post-natal developmental toxicity in rats is less than the MRHD on a mg/m² basis.

8.2   Labor and Delivery

Xyrem has not been studied in labor or delivery. In obstetric anesthesia using an injectable formulation of sodium oxybate, newborns had stable cardiovascular and respiratory measures but were very sleepy, causing a slight decrease in Apgar scores. There was a fall in the rate of uterine contractions 20 minutes after injection. Placental transfer is rapid, but umbilical vein levels of sodium oxybate were no more than 25% of the maternal concentration. No sodium oxybate was detected in the infant's blood 30 minutes after delivery. Elimination curves of sodium oxybate between a 2-day-old infant and a 15-year-old patient were similar. Subsequent effects of sodium oxybate on later growth, development, and maturation in humans are unknown.

8.3 Nursing Mothers

It is not known whether sodium oxybate is excreted in human milk. Because many drugs are excreted in human milk, caution should be exercised when Xyrem is administered to a nursing woman.

8.4 Pediatric Use

Safety and effectiveness in pediatric patients have not been established.

8.5 Geriatric Use

Clinical studies of Xyrem in patients with narcolepsy did not include sufficient numbers of subjects age 65 years and older to determine whether they respond differently from younger subjects. In controlled trials in another population, 39 (5%) of 874 patients were 65 years or older. Discontinuations of treatment due to adverse reactions were increased in the elderly compared to younger adults (20.5% v. 18.9%). Frequency of headaches was markedly increased in the elderly (38.5% v. 18.9%). The most common adverse reactions were similar in both age categories. In general, dose selection for an elderly patient should be cautious, usually starting at the low end of the dosing range, reflecting the greater frequency of decreased hepatic, renal, or cardiac function, and of concomitant disease or other drug therapy.

8.6 Hepatic Impairment

The starting dose of Xyrem should be reduced by one-half in patients with liver impairment [see Dosage and Administration (2.3) and Clinical Pharmacology (12.3)].

9 DRUG ABUSE AND DEPENDENCE

9.1 Controlled Substance

Xyrem is a Schedule III controlled substance under the Federal Controlled Substances Act. Non-medical use of Xyrem could lead to penalties assessed under the higher Schedule I controls.

9.2 Abuse

Xyrem (sodium oxybate), the sodium salt of GHB, produces dose-dependent central nervous system effects, including hypnotic and positive subjective reinforcing effects. The onset of effect is rapid, enhancing its potential for abuse or misuse.

The rapid onset of sedation, coupled with the amnestic features of Xyrem, particularly when combined with alcohol, has proven to be dangerous for the voluntary and involuntary user (e.g., assault victim).

Illicit GHB is abused in social settings primarily by young adults. Some of the doses estimated to be abused are in a similar dosage range to that used for treatment of patients with cataplexy. GHB has some commonalities with ethanol over a limited dose range, and some cross tolerance with ethanol has been reported as well. Cases of severe dependence and craving for GHB have been reported when the drug is taken around the clock. Patterns of abuse indicative of dependence include: 1) the use of increasingly large doses, 2) increased frequency of use, and 3) continued use despite adverse consequences.

Because illicit use and abuse of GHB have been reported, physicians should carefully evaluate patients for a history of drug abuse and follow such patients closely, observing them for signs of misuse or abuse of GHB (e.g. increase in size or frequency of dosing, drug-seeking behavior, feigned cataplexy). Dispose of Xyrem according to state and federal regulations. It is safe to dispose of Xyrem down the sanitary sewer.

9.3 Dependence

There have been case reports of withdrawal, ranging from mild to severe, following discontinuation of illicit use of GHB at frequent repeated doses (18 g to 250 g per day) in excess of the therapeutic dose range. Signs and symptoms of GHB withdrawal following abrupt discontinuation included insomnia, restlessness, anxiety, psychosis, lethargy, nausea, tremor, sweating, muscle cramps, tachycardia, headache, dizziness, rebound fatigue and sleepiness, confusion, and, particularly in the case of severe withdrawal, visual hallucinations, agitation, and delirium. These symptoms generally abated in 3 to 14 days. In cases of severe withdrawal, hospitalization may be required. The discontinuation effects of Xyrem have not been systematically evaluated in controlled clinical trials. In the clinical trial experience with Xyrem in narcolepsy/cataplexy patients at therapeutic doses, two patients reported anxiety and one reported insomnia following abrupt discontinuation at the termination of the clinical trial; in the two patients with anxiety, the frequency of cataplexy had increased markedly at the same time.

Tolerance

Tolerance to Xyrem has not been systematically studied in controlled clinical trials. There have been some case reports of symptoms of tolerance developing after illicit use at dosages far in excess of the recommended Xyrem dosage regimen. Clinical studies of sodium oxybate in the treatment of alcohol withdrawal suggest a potential cross-tolerance with alcohol. The safety and effectiveness of Xyrem in the treatment of alcohol withdrawal have not been established.

Table 3
Adverse Reactions Occurring in ≥2% of Patients and More Frequently with Xyrem than Placebo in Three Controlled Trials (N1, N3, N4) by Body System and Dose at Onset

System Organ Class/MedDRA Preferred Term	Placebo (n=213) %	Xyrem 4.5g (n=185) %	Xyrem 6g (n=258) %	Xyrem 9g (n=178) %
ANY ADVERSE REACTION	62	45	55	70
GASTROINTESTINAL DISORDERS				
Nausea	3	8	13	20
Vomiting	1	2	4	11
Diarrhea	2	4	3	4
Abdominal pain upper	2	3	1	2
Dry mouth	2	1	2	1
GENERAL DISORDERS AND ADMINISTRATIVE SITE CONDITIONS				
Pain	1	1	< 1	3
Feeling drunk	1	0	< 1	3
Edema peripheral	1	3	0	0
MUSCULOSKELETAL AND CONNECTIVE TISSUE DISORDERS				
Pain in extremity	1	3	1	1
Cataplexy	1	1	1	2
Muscle spasms	2	2	< 1	2
NERVOUS SYSTEM DISORDERS				
Dizziness	4	9	11	15
Somnolence	4	1	3	8
Tremor	0	0	2	5
Paresthesia	1	2	1	3
Disturbance in attention	0	1	0	4
Sleep paralysis	1	0	1	3
PSYCHIATRIC DISORDERS				
Disorientation	1	1	2	3
Anxiety	1	1	1	2
Irritability	1	0	< 1	3
Sleep walking	0	0	0	3
RENAL AND URINARY DISORDERS				
Enuresis	1	3	3	7
SKIN AND SUBCUTANEOUS TISSUE DISORDERS				
Hyperhidrosis	0	1	1	3

10 OVERDOSAGE

10.1 Human Experience

Information regarding overdose with Xyrem is derived largely from reports in the medical literature that describe symptoms and signs in individuals who have ingested GHB illicitly. In these circumstances the co-ingestion of other drugs and alcohol was common, and may have influenced the presentation and severity of clinical manifestations of overdose.

In clinical trials two cases of overdose with Xyrem were reported. In the first case, an estimated dose of 150 g, more than 15 times the maximum recommended dose, caused a patient to be unresponsive with brief periods of apnea and to be incontinent of urine and feces. This individual recovered without sequelae. In the second case, death was reported following a multiple drug overdose consisting of Xyrem and numerous other drugs.

10.2 Signs and Symptoms

Information about signs and symptoms associated with overdosage with Xyrem derives from reports of its illicit use. Patient presentation following overdose is influenced by the dose ingested, the time since ingestion, the co-ingestion of other drugs and alcohol, and the fed or fasted state. Patients have exhibited varying degrees of depressed consciousness that may fluctuate rapidly between a confusional, agitated combative state with ataxia and coma. Emesis (even when obtunded), diaphoresis, headache, and impaired psychomotor skills have been observed. No typical pupillary changes have been described to assist in diagnosis; pupillary reactivity to light is maintained. Blurred vision has been reported. An increasing depth of coma has been observed at higher doses. Myoclonus and tonic-clonic seizures have been reported. Respiration may be unaffected or compromised in rate and depth. Cheyne-Stokes respiration and apnea have been observed. Bradycardia and hypothermia may accompany unconsciousness, as well as muscular hypotonia, but tendon reflexes remain intact.

10.3 Recommended Treatment of Overdose

General symptomatic and supportive care should be instituted immediately, and gastric decontamination may be considered if co-ingestants are suspected. Because emesis may occur in the presence of obtundation, appropriate posture (left lateral recumbent position) and protection of the airway by intubation may be warranted. Although the gag reflex may be absent in deeply comatose patients, even unconscious patients may become combative to intubation, and rapid-sequence induction (without the use of sedative) should be considered. Vital signs and consciousness should be closely monitored. The bradycardia reported with GHB overdose has been responsive to atropine intravenous administration. No reversal of the central depressant effects of Xyrem can be expected from naloxone or flumazenil administration. The use of hemodialysis and other forms of extra-corporeal drug removal have not been studied in GHB overdose. However, due to the rapid metabolism of sodium oxybate, these measures are not warranted.

10.4 Poison Control Center

As with the management of all cases of drug overdosage, the possibility of multiple drug ingestion should be considered. The healthcare provider is encouraged to collect urine and blood samples for routine toxicologic screening, and to consult with a regional poison control center (1-800-222-1222) for current treatment recommendations.

11 DESCRIPTION

Sodium oxybate, a CNS depressant, is the active ingredient in Xyrem. The chemical name for sodium oxybate is sodium 4-hydroxybutyrate. The molecular formula is C4H7NaO3, and the molecular weight is 126.09 g/mole. The chemical structure is:

$$Na^+ O^- C(=O) - CH_2 - CH_2 - CH_2 - O - H$$

Sodium oxybate is a white to off-white, crystalline powder that is very soluble in aqueous solutions. Each mL of Xyrem contains 0.5 g of sodium oxybate in USP Purified Water, neutralized to pH 7.5 with malic acid.

12 CLINICAL PHARMACOLOGY

12.1 Mechanism of Action

Xyrem is a CNS depressant. The mechanism of action of Xyrem in the treatment of narcolepsy is unknown. Sodium oxybate is the sodium salt of gamma hydroxybutyrate, an endogenous compound and metabolite of the neurotransmitter GABA. It is hypothesized that the therapeutic effects of Xyrem on cataplexy and excessive daytime sleepiness are mediated through $GABA_B$ actions at noradrenergic and dopaminergic neurons, as well as at thalamocortical neurons.

12.3 Pharmacokinetics

Pharmacokinetics of sodium oxybate are nonlinear and are similar following single or repeat dosing.

Absorption

Following oral administration, sodium oxybate is absorbed rapidly across the clinical dose range, with an absolute bioavailability of about 88%. The average peak plasma concentrations (C_{max}) following administration of each of the two 2.25 g doses given under fasting conditions 4 hours apart were similar. The average time to peak plasma concentration (T_{max}) ranged from 0.5 to 1.25 hours. Following oral administration, the plasma levels of sodium oxybate increased more than dose-proportionally, with blood levels increasing 3.7–fold as total daily dose was doubled from 4.5 g to 9 g. Single doses greater than 4.5 g have not been studied. Administration of Xyrem immediately after a high-fat meal resulted in delayed absorption (average T_{max} increased from 0.75 hr to 2 hr) and a reduction in C_{max} by a mean of 59% and of systemic exposure (AUC) by 37%.

Distribution

Sodium oxybate is a hydrophilic compound with an apparent volume of distribution averaging 190 mL/kg to 384 mL/kg. At sodium oxybate concentrations ranging from 3 mcg/mL to 300 mcg/mL, less than 1% is bound to plasma proteins.

Metabolism

Animal studies indicate that metabolism is the major elimination pathway for sodium oxybate, producing carbon dioxide and water via the tricarboxylic acid (Krebs) cycle and secondarily by beta-oxidation. The primary pathway involves a cytosolic NADP+-linked enzyme, GHB dehydrogenase, that catalyzes the conversion of sodium oxybate to succinic semialdehyde, which is then biotransformed to succinic acid by the enzyme succinic semialdehyde dehydrogenase. Succinic acid enters the Krebs cycle where it is metabolized to carbon dioxide and water. A second mitochondrial oxidoreductase enzyme, a transhydrogenase, also catalyzes the conversion to succinic semialdehyde in the presence of α-ketoglutarate. An alternate pathway of biotransformation involves β-oxidation via 3,4–dihydroxybutyrate to carbon dioxide and water. No active metabolites have been identified.

Elimination

The clearance of sodium oxybate is almost entirely by biotransformation to carbon dioxide, which is then eliminated by expiration. On average, less than 5% of unchanged drug appears in human urine within 6 to 8 hours after dosing. Fecal excretion is negligible. Sodium oxybate has an elimination half-life of 0.5 to 1 hour.

Specific Populations

Geriatric

There is limited experience with Xyrem in the elderly. Results from a pharmacokinetic study (n=20) in another studied population indicate that the pharmacokinetic characteristics of sodium oxybate are consistent among younger (age 48 to 64 years) and older (age 65 to 75 years) adults.

Pediatric

Table 4
Median Number of Cataplexy Attacks in Trials N1 and N2

Trial/Dosage Group	Baseline	Median Change from Baseline	Comparison to Placebo (p-value)
Trial N1 (Prospective, Randomized, Parallel Group Trial)			
		(median attacks/week)	
Placebo (n=33)	20.5	-4	–
Xyrem 6 g per night (n=31)	23.0	-10	0.0451
Xyrem 9 g per night (n=33)	23.5	-16	0.0016
Trial N2 (Randomized Withdrawal Trial)			
		(median attacks/2 weeks)	
Placebo (n=29)	4.0	21	–
Xyrem (n=26)	1.9	0	< 0.001

The pharmacokinetics of sodium oxybate in patients younger than 18 years of age have not been studied.

Gender

In a study of 18 female and 18 male healthy adult volunteers, no gender differences were detected in the pharmacokinetics of sodium oxybate oral solution following a single oral dose of 4.5 g.

Race

There are insufficient data to evaluate any pharmacokinetic differences among races.

Renal Impairment

No pharmacokinetic study in patients with renal impairment has been conducted.

Hepatic Impairment

The pharmacokinetics of Xyrem in 16 cirrhotic patients, half without ascites (Child's Class A) and half with ascites (Child's Class C), were compared to the kinetics in 8 subjects with normal hepatic function after a single oral dose of 25 mg/kg. AUC values were double in the cirrhotic patients, with apparent oral clearance reduced from 9.1 mL/min/kg in healthy adults to 4.5 and 4.1 mL/min/kg in Class A and Class C patients, respectively. Elimination half-life was significantly longer in Class C and Class A patients than in control patients (mean $t_{1/2}$ of 59 and 32 minutes, respectively, versus 22 minutes). The starting dose of Xyrem should be reduced by one-half in patients with liver impairment *[see Dosage and Administration (2.3); Use in Specific Populations (8.6)].*

Drug Interactions Studies

Studies *in vitro* with pooled human liver microsomes indicate that sodium oxybate does not significantly inhibit the activities of the human isoenzymes CYP1A2, CYP2C9, CYP2C19, CYP2D6, CYP2E1, or CYP3A up to the concentration of 3 mM (378 mcg/mL), a level considerably higher than levels achieved with therapeutic doses.

Drug interaction studies in healthy adults (age 18 to 50 years) were conducted with Xyrem and divalproex sodium, diclofenac, and ibuprofen.

- Divalproex sodium: Co-administration of Xyrem (6 g per day as two equal doses of 3 grams dosed four hours apart) with divalproex sodium (valproic acid, 1250 mg per day) increased mean systemic exposure to sodium oxybate as shown by AUC by approximately 25%, while C_{max} was comparable. Co-administration did not appear to affect the pharmacokinetics of valproic acid. A greater impairment on some tests of attention and working memory was observed with co-administration of both drugs than with either drug alone *[see Drug Interactions (7.2) and Dosage and Administration (2.4)].*

- Diclofenac: Co-administration of Xyrem (6 g per day as two equal doses of 3 grams dosed four hours apart) with diclofenac (50 mg/dose twice per day) showed no significant differences in systemic exposure to sodium oxybate. Co-administration did not appear to affect the pharmacokinetics of diclofenac.

- Ibuprofen: Co-administration of Xyrem (6 g per day as two equal doses of 3 grams dosed four hours apart) with ibuprofen (800 mg/dose four times per day also dosed four hours apart) resulted in comparable systemic exposure to sodium oxybate as shown by plasma C_{max} and AUC values. Co-administration did not affect the pharmacokinetics of ibuprofen.

Drug interaction studies in healthy adults demonstrated no pharmacokinetic interactions between sodium oxybate and protriptyline hydrochloride, zolpidem tartrate, and modafinil. Also, there were no pharmacokinetic interactions with the alcohol dehydrogenase inhibitor fomepizole. However, pharmacodynamic interactions with these drugs cannot be ruled out. Alteration of gastric pH with omeprazole

produced no significant change in the oxybate kinetics. In addition, drug interaction studies in healthy adults demonstrated no pharmacokinetic or clinically significant pharmacodynamic interactions between sodium oxybate and the SNRI duloxetine HCl.

13 NONCLINICAL TOXICOLOGY

13.1 Carcinogenesis, Mutagenesis, Impairment of Fertility

Carcinogenesis

Administration of sodium oxybate to rats at oral doses of up to 1,000 mg/kg/day for 83 (males) or 104 (females) weeks resulted in no increase in tumors. Plasma exposure (AUC) at the highest dose tested was 2 times that in humans at the maximum recommended human dose (MRHD) of 9 g per night.

The results of 2-year carcinogenicity studies in mouse and rat with gamma-butyrolactone, a compound that is metabolized to sodium oxybate *in vivo*, showed no clear evidence of carcinogenic activity. The plasma AUCs of sodium oxybate achieved at the highest doses tested in these studies were less than that in humans at the MRHD.

Mutagenesis

Sodium oxybate was negative in the *in vitro* bacterial gene mutation assay, an *in vitro* chromosomal aberration assay in mammalian cells, and in an *in vivo* rat micronucleus assay.

Impairment of Fertility

Oral administration of sodium oxybate (150, 350, or 1,000 mg/kg/day) to male and female rats prior to and throughout mating and continuing in females through early gestation resulted in no adverse effects on fertility. The highest dose tested is approximately equal to the MRHD on a mg/m² basis.

14 CLINICAL STUDIES

14.1 Cataplexy in Narcolepsy

The effectiveness of Xyrem in the treatment of cataplexy was established in two randomized, double-blind, placebo-controlled, multicenter, parallel-group trials (Trials N1 and N2) in patients with narcolepsy (see Table 4). In Trials N1 and N2, 85% and 80% of patients, respectively, were also being treated with CNS stimulants. The high percentages of concomitant stimulant use make it impossible to assess the efficacy and safety of Xyrem independent of stimulant use. In each trial, the treatment period was 4 weeks and the total nightly Xyrem doses ranged from 3 g to 9 g, with the total nightly dose administered as two equal doses. The first dose each night was taken at bedtime and the second dose was taken 2.5 to 4 hours later. There were no restrictions on the time between food consumption and dosing.

Trial N1 enrolled 136 narcoleptic patients with moderate to severe cataplexy (median of 21 cataplexy attacks per week) at baseline. Prior to randomization, medications with possible effects on cataplexy were withdrawn, but stimulants were continued at stable doses. Patients were randomized to receive placebo, Xyrem 3 g per night, Xyrem 6 g per night, or Xyrem 9 g per night.

Trial N2 was a randomized withdrawal trial with 55 narcoleptic patients who had been taking open-label Xyrem for 7 to 44 months prior to study entry. To be included, patients were required to have a history of at least 5 cataplexy attacks per week prior to any treatment for cataplexy. Patients were randomized to continued treatment with Xyrem at their stable dose (ranging from 3 g to 9 g per night) or to placebo for 2 weeks. Trial N2 was designed specifically to evaluate the continued efficacy of sodium oxybate after long-term use.

The primary efficacy measure in Trials N1 and N2 was the frequency of cataplexy attacks.

[See table 4 at top of previous page]

In Trial N1, both the 6 g and 9 g per night Xyrem doses resulted in statistically significant reductions in the frequency of cataplexy attacks. The 3 g per night dose had little effect. In Trial N2, patients randomized to placebo after discontinuing long-term open-label Xyrem therapy experienced a significant increase in cataplexy attacks (p < 0.001), providing evidence of long-term efficacy of Xyrem. In Trial N2, the response was numerically similar for patients treated with doses of 6 g to 9 g per night, but there was no effect seen in patients treated with doses less than 6 g per night, suggesting little effect at these doses.

14.2 Excessive Daytime Sleepiness in Narcolepsy

The effectiveness of Xyrem in the treatment of excessive daytime sleepiness in patients with narcolepsy was established in two randomized, double-blind, placebo-controlled trials (Trials N3 and N4) (see Tables 7 to 9). Seventy-eight percent of patients in Trial N3 were also being treated with CNS stimulants.

Trial N3 was a multicenter randomized, double-blind, placebo-controlled, parallel-group trial that evaluated 228 patients with moderate to severe symptoms at entry into the study including a median Epworth Sleepiness Scale (see below) score of 18, and a Maintenance of Wakefulness Test (see below) score of 8.3 minutes. Patients were randomized to one of 4 treatment groups: placebo, Xyrem 4.5 g per night, Xyrem 6 g per night, or Xyrem 9 g per night. The period of double-blind treatment in this trial was 8 weeks. Antidepressants were withdrawn prior to randomization; stimulants were continued at stable doses.

The primary efficacy measures in Trial N3 were the Epworth Sleepiness Scale and the Clinical Global Impression of Change. The Epworth Sleepiness Scale is intended to evaluate the extent of sleepiness in everyday situations by asking the patient a series of questions. In these questions, patients were asked to rate their chances of dozing during each of 8 activities on a scale from 0-3 (0=never; 1=slight; 2=moderate; 3=high). Higher total scores indicate a greater tendency to sleepiness. The Clinical Global Impression of Change is evaluated on a 7-point scale, centered at *No Change*, and ranging from *Very Much Worse* to *Very Much Improved*. In Trial N3, patients were rated by evaluators who based their assessments on the severity of narcolepsy at baseline.

In Trial N3, statistically significant improvements were seen on the Epworth Sleepiness Scale score at Week 8 and on the Clinical Global Impression of Change score at Week 8 with the 6 g and 9 g per night doses of Xyrem compared to the placebo group.

[See table 5 above]

Table 6
Proportion of patients with a very much or much improved Clinical Global Impression of Change in Daytime and Nighttime Symptoms in Trial N3

Treatment Group	Percentages of Responders (Very Much Improved or Much Improved)	Change from Baseline Significance Compared to Placebo (p-value)
Placebo (59)	22%	-
Xyrem 6 g per night (n=58)	52%	< 0.001
Xyrem 9 g per night (n=47)	64%	< 0.001

Trial N4 was a multicenter randomized, double-blind, placebo-controlled, parallel-group trial that evaluated 222 patients with moderate to severe symptoms at entry into the study including a median Epworth Sleepiness Scale score of 15, and a Maintenance of Wakefulness Test (see below) score of 10.3 minutes. At entry, patients had to be taking modafinil at stable doses of 200 mg, 400 mg, or 600 mg daily for at least 1 month prior to randomization. The patients enrolled in the study were randomized to one of 4 treatment groups: placebo, Xyrem, modafinil, or Xyrem plus modafinil. Xyrem was administered in a dose of 6 g per night for 4 weeks, followed by 9 g per night for 4 weeks. Modafinil was continued in the modafinil alone and the Xyrem plus modafinil treatment groups at the patient's prior dose. Trial N4 was not designed to compare the effects of Xyrem to modafinil because patients receiving modafinil were not titrated to a maximal dose. Patients randomized to placebo or to Xyrem treatment were withdrawn from their stable dose of modafinil. Patients taking antidepressants could continue these medications at stable doses.

The primary efficacy measure in Trial N4 was the Maintenance of Wakefulness Test. The Maintenance of Wakefulness Test measures latency to sleep onset (in minutes) av-

eraged over 4 sessions at 2-hour intervals following nocturnal polysomnography. For each test session, the subject was asked to remain awake without using extraordinary measures. Each test session is terminated after 20 minutes if no sleep occurs, or after 10 minutes, if sleep occurs. The overall score is the mean sleep latency for the 4 sessions.

In Trial N4, a statistically significant improvement in the change in the Maintenance of Wakefulness Test score from baseline at Week 8 was seen in the Xyrem and Xyrem plus modafinil groups compared to the placebo group.

This trial was not designed to compare the effects of Xyrem to modafinil, because patients receiving modafinil were not titrated to a maximally effective dose.

[See table 7 above]

16 HOW SUPPLIED/STORAGE AND HANDLING

16.1 How Supplied

Xyrem is a clear to slightly opalescent oral solution. Each prescription includes a carton containing one bottle of Xyrem, a press-in-bottle-adaptor, an oral measuring device (plastic syringe), and a Medication Guide. The pharmacy provides two empty vials with child-resistant caps with each Xyrem shipment.

Each amber bottle contains Xyrem oral solution at a concentration of 0.5 g per mL and has a child-resistant cap.

Carton containing one 180 mL bottle   NDC 68727-100-01

16.2 Storage

Keep out of reach of children.

Xyrem should be stored at 25°C (77°F); excursions permitted to 15° to 30°C (59° to 86°F) (see USP Controlled Room Temperature).

Dispense in tight containers.

Solutions prepared following dilution should be consumed within 24 hours.

16.3 Handling and Disposal

Xyrem is a Schedule III drug under the Controlled Substances Act. Xyrem should be handled according to state and federal regulations. It is safe to dispose of Xyrem down the sanitary sewer.

17 PATIENT COUNSELING INFORMATION

See FDA-approved patient labeling (Medication Guide).

Xyrem Success Program

Inform patients that Xyrem is available only through a restricted distribution program called the Xyrem Success Program.

The contents of the Xyrem Medication Guide and educational materials are reviewed with every patient before initiating treatment with Xyrem.

Patients must read and understand the materials in the Xyrem Success Program prior to initiating treatment. Inform the patient that they should be seen by the prescriber frequently to review dose titration, symptom response, and adverse reactions; a follow-up of every three months is recommended.

Discuss safe and proper use of Xyrem and dosing information with patients prior to the initiation of treatment. Instruct patients to store Xyrem bottles and Xyrem doses in a secure place, out of the reach of children and pets.

Alcohol or Sedative Hypnotics

Advise patients not to drink alcohol or take other sedative hypnotics if they are taking Xyrem.

Sedation

Inform patients that after taking Xyrem they are likely to fall asleep quickly (often within 5 and usually within 15 minutes), but the time it takes to fall asleep can vary from night to night. The sudden onset of sleep, including in a standing position or while rising from bed, has led to falls complicated by injuries, in some cases requiring hospitalization. Instruct patients to remain in bed following ingestion of the first and second doses. Instruct patients not to take the second dose until 2.5 to 4 hours after the first dose.

Food Effects on Xyrem

Inform patients to take the first dose at least 2 hours after eating.

Respiratory Depression

Inform patients that Xyrem can be associated with respiratory depression.

Operating Hazardous Machinery

Inform patients that until they are reasonably certain that Xyrem does not affect them adversely (e.g., impair judgment, thinking, or motor skills) they should not operate hazardous machinery, including automobiles or airplanes.

Suicidality

Instruct patients or families to contact a healthcare provider immediately if the patient develops depressed mood, markedly diminished interest or pleasure in usual activities, significant change in weight and/or appetite, psychomotor agitation or retardation, increased fatigue, feelings of guilt or worthlessness, slowed thinking or impaired concentration, or suicidal ideation.

Sleepwalking

Instruct patients and their families that Xyrem has been associated with sleepwalking and to contact their healthcare provider if this occurs.

Sodium Intake

Instruct patients who are sensitive to salt intake (e.g., those with heart failure, hypertension, or renal impairment) that Xyrem contains a significant amount of sodium and they should limit their sodium intake.

Distributed By:

Jazz Pharmaceuticals, Inc.
Palo Alto, CA 94304

Protected by U.S. Patent Nos. 6,472,431; 6,780,889; 7,262,219; 7,851,506; 8,263,650; 8,324,275; 8,461,203

MEDICATION GUIDE

Xyrem® (ZIE-rem)

(sodium oxybate)

oral solution CIII

Read this Medication Guide carefully before you start taking Xyrem and each time you get a refill. There may be new information. This information does not take the place of talking to your doctor about your medical condition or your treatment.

What is the most important information I should know about Xyrem?

Xyrem can cause serious side effects including slow breathing or changes in your alertness. Do not drink alcohol or take medicines intended to make you fall asleep while you are taking Xyrem because they can make these side effects worse. Call your doctor right away if you have any of these serious side effects.

Table 5
Change from Baseline in Daytime Sleepiness Score (Epworth Sleepiness Scale) at Week 8 in Trial N3 (Range 0-24)

Treatment Group	Baseline	Week 8	Median Change from Baseline at Week 8	p-value
Placebo (n=59)	17.5	17.0	-0.5	-
Xyrem 6 g per night (n=58)	19.0	16.0	-2.0	< 0.001
Xyrem 9 g per night (n=47)	19.0	12.0	-5.0	< 0.001

Table 7
Change in Baseline in the Maintenance of Wakefulness Test Score (in minutes) at Week 8 in Trial N4

Treatment Group	Baseline	Week 8	Mean Change from Baseline at Week 8	p-value
Placebo (modafinil withdrawn) (n=55)	9.7	6.9	-2.7	-
Xyrem (modafinil withdrawn) (n=50)	11.3	12.0	0.6	< 0.001
Xyrem plus modafinil (n=54)	10.4	13.2	2.7	< 0.001

- The active ingredient of Xyrem is a form of gamma-hydroxybutyrate (GHB). GHB is a chemical that has been abused and misused. Abuse and misuse of Xyrem can cause serious medical problems, including:
  - seizures
  - trouble breathing
  - changes in alertness
  - coma
  - death
- Do not drive a car, use heavy machinery, fly an airplane, or do anything that is dangerous or that requires you to be fully awake for at least 6 hours after you take Xyrem. You should not do those activities until you know how Xyrem affects you.
- Xyrem is available only by prescription and filled through the central pharmacy in the Xyrem Success Program. Before you receive Xyrem, your doctor or pharmacist will make sure that you understand how to use Xyrem safely and effectively. If you have any questions about Xyrem, ask your doctor or call the Xyrem Success Program® at 1-866-997-3688.

What is Xyrem?
Xyrem is a prescription medicine used to treat the following symptoms in people who fall asleep frequently during the day, often at unexpected times (narcolepsy):
- suddenly weak or paralyzed muscles when they feel strong emotions (cataplexy)
- excessive daytime sleepiness (EDS) in people who have narcolepsy

It is not known if Xyrem is safe and effective in children.
Xyrem is a controlled substance (CIII) because it contains sodium oxybate that can be a target for people who abuse prescription medicines or street drugs. Keep your Xyrem in a safe place to protect it from theft. Never give your Xyrem to anyone else because it may cause death or harm them. Selling or giving away this medicine is against the law.

Who should not take Xyrem?
Do not take Xyrem if you:
- take other sleep medicines or sedatives (medicines that cause sleepiness)
- drink alcohol
- have a rare problem called succinic semialdehyde dehydrogenase deficiency

Before you take Xyrem, tell your doctor if you:
- have short periods of not breathing while you sleep (sleep apnea)
- snore, have trouble breathing, or have lung problems. You may have a higher chance of having serious breathing problems when you take Xyrem.
- have or had depression or have tried to harm yourself. You should be watched carefully for new symptoms of depression.
- have liver problems
- are on a salt-restricted diet. Xyrem contains a lot of sodium (salt) and may not be right for you.
- have high blood pressure
- have heart failure
- have kidney problems
- are pregnant or plan to become pregnant. It is not known if Xyrem can harm your unborn baby.
- are breastfeeding or plan to breastfeed. It is not known if Xyrem passes into your breast milk. You and your doctor should decide if you will take Xyrem or breastfeed.

Tell your doctor about all the medicines you take, including prescription and non-prescription medicines, vitamins, and herbal supplements.

Especially, tell your doctor if you take other medicines to help you sleep (sedatives). Do not take medicines that make you sleepy with Xyrem.

Know the medicines you take. Keep a list of them to show your doctor and pharmacist when you get a new medicine.

How should I take Xyrem?
- Read the **Instructions for Use** at the end of this Medication Guide for detailed instructions on how to take Xyrem.
- Take Xyrem exactly as your doctor tells you to take it.
- Never change your Xyrem dose without talking to your doctor.
- Xyrem can cause sleep very quickly. You should fall asleep soon. Some patients fall asleep within 5 minutes and most fall asleep within 15 minutes. Some patients take less time to fall asleep and some take more time. The time it takes you to fall asleep might be different from night to night.
- Take your first Xyrem dose at bedtime while you are in bed. Take your second Xyrem dose 2 ½ to 4 hours after you take your first Xyrem dose. You may want to set an alarm clock to make sure you wake up to take your second Xyrem dose. You should remain in bed after taking the first and second doses of Xyrem.
- If you miss your second Xyrem dose, skip that dose and do not take Xyrem again until the next night. Never take 2 Xyrem doses at 1 time.
- Wait at least 2 hours after eating before you take Xyrem.

- You should see your doctor every 3 months for a check-up while taking Xyrem. Your doctor should check to see if Xyrem is helping to lessen your symptoms and if you feel any side effects while you take Xyrem.
- If you take too much Xyrem, call your doctor or go to the nearest hospital emergency room right away.

What are the possible side effects of Xyrem?
Xyrem can cause serious side effects, including:
- See "What is the most important information I should know about Xyrem?"
- **Breathing problems, including:**
  - slower breathing
  - trouble breathing
  - short periods of not breathing while sleeping (sleep apnea). People who already have breathing or lung problems have a higher chance of having breathing problems when they use Xyrem.
- **Mental health problems, including:**
  - confusion
  - seeing or hearing things that are not real (hallucinations)
  - unusual or disturbing thoughts (abnormal thinking)
  - feeling anxious or upset
  - depression
  - thoughts of killing yourself or trying to kill yourself

Call your doctor right away if you have symptoms of mental health problems.
- **Sleepwalking.** Sleepwalking can cause injuries. Call your doctor if you start sleepwalking. Your doctor should check you.

The most common side effects of Xyrem include:
- nausea
- dizziness
- vomiting
- bedwetting
- diarrhea

Your side effects may increase when you take higher doses of Xyrem.

Xyrem can cause physical dependence and craving for the medicine when it is not taken as directed.

These are not all the possible side effects of Xyrem. For more information, ask your doctor or pharmacist.

Call your doctor for medical advice about side effects. You may report side effects to FDA at 1-800-FDA-1088.

How should I store Xyrem?
- Always store Xyrem in the original bottle or in pharmacy containers with child-resistant caps provided by the pharmacy.
- Keep Xyrem in a safe place out of the reach of children and pets.
- Get emergency medical help right away if a child drinks your Xyrem.
- Store Xyrem between 68°F to 77°F (20°C to 24°C). When you have finished using a Xyrem bottle:
  - empty any unused Xyrem down the sink drain
  - cross out the label on the Xyrem bottle with a marker
  - place the empty Xyrem bottle in the trash

General information about the safe and effective use of Xyrem
Medicines are sometimes prescribed for purposes other than those listed in a Medication Guide. Do not use Xyrem for a condition for which it was not prescribed. Do not give Xyrem to other people, even if they have the same symptoms that you have. It may harm them.

This Medication Guide summarizes the most important information about Xyrem. If you would like more information, talk with your doctor. You can ask your pharmacist or doctor for information about Xyrem that is written for health professionals.

For more information, go to www.XYREM.com or call the Xyrem Success Program at 1-866-997-3688.

What are the ingredients in Xyrem?
Active Ingredients: sodium oxybate

Inactive Ingredients: purified water and malic acid

This Medication Guide has been approved by the U.S. Food and Drug Administration.

Distributed By:
Jazz Pharmaceuticals, Inc.
Palo Alto, CA 94304
Revised: April 2014

Instructions for Use
Xyrem® (ZIE-rem)
(sodium oxybate)
oral solution CIII

Read these Instructions for Use carefully before you start taking Xyrem and each time you get a refill. There may be new information. This information does not take the place of talking to your doctor about your medical condition or your treatment.

Note:
- **You will need to split your prescribed Xyrem dose into 2 separate pharmacy containers for mixing.**

- **You will need to mix Xyrem with water before you take your dose.**
- Take your dose within 24 hours after mixing Xyrem with water. If you do not take your dose within this time, you will need to throw the mixture away.

Supplies you will need for mixing and taking Xyrem: See Figure A.
- bottle of your Xyrem medicine
- press-in-bottle-adaptor with straw attached
- syringe for drawing up your Xyrem dose
- a measuring cup containing about ¼ cup of water (not provided with your Xyrem prescription)
- 2 **empty** pharmacy containers with child-resistant caps
- alarm clock by your bedside (alarm clock may be included in your first shipment of Xyrem)

*Please note that the measuring cup and water for dilution are not provided with your Xyrem prescription

Alarm clock not included in every Xyrem shipment

Figure A

Step 1. Take the Xyrem bottle, press-in-bottle-adaptor, and syringe out of the box.
Step 2. Remove the bottle cap from the Xyrem bottle by pushing down while turning the cap counterclockwise (to the left). See Figure B.

Figure B

Step 3.
- The press-in-bottle-adaptor may already be put in place by the pharmacy. If it is not already in place, you will have to do it yourself. After removing the cap from the Xyrem bottle, set the bottle upright on a tabletop.
- While holding the Xyrem bottle in its upright position, insert the press-in-bottle-adaptor into the neck of the Xyrem bottle. See Figure C.

Figure C

- Tilt the straw toward the edge of the bottom of the bottle to be sure you can draw out your dose of the medicine. You only need to do this the first time you open the bottle. See Figure D.

Figure D

- After you draw out your dose of the medicine, leave the adaptor in the bottle for all your future uses. See Figure E.

Figure E

Step 4.
- Take the syringe out of the plastic wrapper. Use only the syringe provided with your Xyrem prescription.
- While holding the Xyrem bottle upright on the tabletop, insert the tip of the syringe into the opening on top of the Xyrem bottle and press down firmly. See Figure F.

Figure F

Step 5.
- Hold the bottle and syringe down with one hand, and draw up one-half (1/2) of your total prescribed nightly dose with the other hand by pulling up on the plunger. For example, if your total nightly dose of Xyrem is 4.5 grams a night, you will need to draw up 2 separate doses of 2.25 grams each, one for each pharmacy container. See Figure G.
Note: The Xyrem medicine will not flow into the syringe unless you keep the bottle upright.

Figure G

Step 6.
- After you draw up each separate Xyrem dose, remove the syringe from the opening of the Xyrem bottle. Put the tip into 1 of the **empty** containers with child-resistant caps provided by the pharmacy.
- **Make sure the pharmacy container is empty and does not contain any medicine from your previous night's dose.**
- Empty each separate Xyrem dose into 1 of the **empty** pharmacy containers by pushing down on the plunger. (See Figure H).
- Using a measuring cup, pour about ¼ cup of water into **each** container. Be careful to add only water to each container and not more Xyrem. All shipped bottles of Xyrem contain the concentrated medicine. Water for mixing the medicine is not provided in the shipment.

Figure H

Step 7.
- Place the child-resistant caps provided on the filled pharmacy containers and turn each cap clockwise (to the right) until it clicks and locks into its child-resistant position. See Figure I.

Figure I

- Put the cap back on the Xyrem bottle and store it in a safe and secure place. Store in a locked place if needed. Keep Xyrem out of the reach of children and pets.
- Rinse the syringe out with water and squirt the liquid into the sink drain.

Step 8.
- At bedtime, and before you take your first Xyrem dose, put your second Xyrem dose in a safe place near your bed.
- You may want to set an alarm clock to make sure you wake up to take the second dose.
- When it is time to take your first Xyrem dose, remove the cap from the container by pressing down on the child-resistant locking tab and turning the cap counterclockwise (to the left).
- Drink all of your first Xyrem dose at bedtime. Put the cap back on the first container before lying down to sleep.
- You should fall asleep soon. Some patients fall asleep within 5 minutes and most fall asleep within 15 minutes. Some patients take less time to fall asleep, and some take more time. The time it takes you to fall asleep might be different from night to night.

Step 9.
- When you wake up 2½ to 4 hours later, take the cap off the second pharmacy container.
- If you wake up before the alarm and it has been at least 2½ hours since your first Xyrem dose, turn off your alarm and take your second Xyrem dose.
- While sitting in bed, drink all of the second Xyrem dose and put the cap back on the second pharmacy container before lying down to continue sleeping.

Distributed By:
Jazz Pharmaceuticals, Inc.
Palo Alto, CA 94304
These Instructions for Use have been approved by the U.S. Food and Drug Administration.
Revised: April 2014

Kowa Pharmaceuticals America, Inc.
530 INDUSTRIAL PARK BOULEVARD
MONTGOMERY, AL 36117

Tel: 334.288.1288
Fax: 334.288.2788
info@KowaPharma.com

LIVALO®   ℞
(pitavastatin)
Tablet, Film Coated for Oral use

HIGHLIGHTS OF PRESCRIBING INFORMATION
These highlights do not include all the information needed to use LIVALO® safely and effectively. See full prescribing information for LIVALO.
LIVALO (pitavastatin) Tablet, Film Coated for Oral use
Initial U.S. Approval: 2009

──────RECENT MAJOR CHANGES──────
None

──────INDICATIONS AND USAGE──────
LIVALO is a HMG-CoA reductase inhibitor indicated for:
- Patients with primary hyperlipidemia or mixed dyslipidemia as an adjunctive therapy to diet to reduce elevated total cholesterol (TC), low-density lipoprotein cholesterol (LDL-C), apolipoprotein B (Apo B), triglycerides (TG), and to increase high-density lipoprotein cholesterol (HDL-C) (1.1)

Limitations of Use (1.2):
- Doses of LIVALO greater than 4 mg once daily were associated with an increased risk for severe myopathy in pre-marketing clinical studies. Do not exceed 4 mg once daily dosing of LIVALO.
- The effect of LIVALO on cardiovascular morbidity and mortality has not been determined.
- LIVALO has not been studied in Fredrickson Type I, III, and V dyslipidemias.

──────DOSAGE AND ADMINISTRATION──────
- LIVALO can be taken with or without food, at any time of day (2.1) Dose Range: 1 mg to 4 mg once daily (2.1)
- **Primary hyperlipidemia and mixed dyslipidemia:** Starting dose 2 mg. When lowering of LDL-C is insufficient, the dosage may be increased to a maximum of 4 mg per day. (2.1)
- **Moderate and severe renal impairment (glomerular filtration rate 30 – 59 and 15 - 29 mL/min/1.73 m², respectively) as well as end-stage renal disease on hemodialysis:** Starting dose of 1 mg once daily and maximum dose of 2 mg once daily (2.2)

──────DOSAGE FORMS AND STRENGTHS──────
- Tablets: 1 mg, 2 mg, and 4 mg (3)

──────CONTRAINDICATIONS──────
- Known hypersensitivity to product components (4)
- Active liver disease, which may include unexplained persistent elevations in hepatic transaminase levels (4)
- Women who are pregnant or may become pregnant (4, 8.1)
- Nursing mothers (4, 8.3)
- Co-administration with cyclosporine (4, 7.1, 12.3)

──────WARNINGS AND PRECAUTIONS──────
- **Skeletal muscle effects (e.g., myopathy and rhabdomyolysis):** Risks increase in a dose-dependent manner, with advanced age (≥65), renal impairment, and inadequately treated hypothyroidism. Advise patients to promptly report unexplained and/or persistent muscle pain, tenderness, or weakness, and discontinue LIVALO (5.1)
- **Liver enzyme abnormalities:** Persistent elevations in hepatic transaminases can occur. Check liver enzyme tests before initiating therapy and as clinically indicated thereafter (5.2)

──────ADVERSE REACTIONS──────
The most frequent adverse reactions (rate ≥2.0% in at least one marketed dose) were myalgia, back pain, diarrhea, constipation and pain in extremity. (6)
To report SUSPECTED ADVERSE REACTIONS, contact Kowa Pharmaceuticals America, Inc. at 1-877-334-3464 or FDA at 1-800-FDA-1088 or www.fda.gov/medwatch.

──────DRUG INTERACTIONS──────
- **Erythromycin:** Combination increases pitavastatin exposure. Limit LIVALO to 1 mg once daily (2.3, 7.2)
- **Rifampin:** Combination increases pitavastatin exposure. Limit LIVALO to 2 mg once daily (2.4, 7.3)
- **Concomitant lipid-lowering therapies:** Use with fibrates or lipid-modifying doses (≥1 g/day) of niacin increases the risk of adverse skeletal muscle effects. Caution should be used when prescribing with LIVALO. (5.1, 7.4, 7.5)

──────USE IN SPECIFIC POPULATIONS──────
- **Pediatric use:** Safety and effectiveness have not been established. (8.4)
- **Renal impairment:** Limitation of a starting dose of LIVALO 1 mg once daily and a maximum dose of LIVALO 2 mg once daily for patients with moderate and severe renal impairment as well as patients receiving hemodialysis (2.2, 8.6)

See 17 for PATIENT COUNSELING INFORMATION
Revised: 10/2013

FULL PRESCRIBING INFORMATION: CONTENTS*

FULL PRESCRIBING INFORMATION

1 INDICATIONS AND USAGE

Drug therapy should be one component of multiple-risk-factor intervention in individuals who require modifications of their lipid profile. Lipid-altering agents should be used in addition to a diet restricted in saturated fat and cholesterol only when the response to diet and other nonpharmacological measures has been inadequate.

1.1 Primary Hyperlipidemia and Mixed Dyslipidemia

LIVALO® is indicated as an adjunctive therapy to diet to reduce elevated total cholesterol (TC), low-density lipoprotein cholesterol (LDL-C), apolipoprotein B (Apo B), triglycerides (TG), and to increase HDL-C in adult patients with primary hyperlipidemia or mixed dyslipidemia.

1.2 Limitations of Use

Doses of LIVALO greater than 4 mg once daily were associated with an increased risk for severe myopathy in premarketing clinical studies. Do not exceed 4 mg once daily dosing of LIVALO.

The effect of LIVALO on cardiovascular morbidity and mortality has not been determined.

LIVALO has not been studied in Fredrickson Type I, III, and V dyslipidemias.

2 DOSAGE AND ADMINISTRATION

2.1 General Dosing Information

The dose range for LIVALO is 1 to 4 mg orally once daily at any time of the day with or without food. The recommended starting dose is 2 mg and the maximum dose is 4 mg. The starting dose and maintenance doses of LIVALO should be individualized according to patient characteristics, such as goal of therapy and response.

After initiation or upon titration of LIVALO, lipid levels should be analyzed after 4 weeks and the dosage adjusted accordingly.

2.2 Dosage in Patients with Renal Impairment

Patients with moderate and severe renal impairment (glomerular filtration rate 30 – 59 mL/min/1.73 m² and 15 – 29 mL/min/1.73 m² not receiving hemodialysis, respectively) as well as end-stage renal disease receiving hemodialysis should receive a starting dose of LIVALO 1 mg once daily and a maximum dose of LIVALO 2 mg once daily.

2.3 Use with Erythromycin

In patients taking erythromycin, a dose of LIVALO 1 mg once daily should not be exceeded [see Drug Interactions (7.2)].

2.4 Use with Rifampin

In patients taking rifampin, a dose of LIVALO 2 mg once daily should not be exceeded [see Drug Interactions (7.3)].

3 DOSAGE FORMS AND STRENGTHS

1 mg: Round white film-coated tablet. Debossed "KC" on one side and "1" on the other side of the tablet.

2 mg: Round white film-coated tablet. Debossed "KC" on one side and "2" on the other side of the tablet.

4 mg: Round white film-coated tablet. Debossed "KC" on one side and "4" on the other side of the tablet.

4 CONTRAINDICATIONS

The use of LIVALO is contraindicated in the following conditions:

- Patients with a known hypersensitivity to any component of this product. Hypersensitivity reactions including rash, pruritus, and urticaria have been reported with LIVALO [see Adverse Reactions (6.1)].
- Patients with active liver disease which may include unexplained persistent elevations of hepatic transaminase levels [see Warnings and Precautions (5.2), Use in Specific Populations (8.7)].
- Women who are pregnant or may become pregnant. Because HMG-CoA reductase inhibitors decrease cholesterol synthesis and possibly the synthesis of other biologically active substances derived from cholesterol, LIVALO may cause fetal harm when administered to pregnant women. Additionally, there is no apparent benefit to therapy during pregnancy, and safety in pregnant women has not been established. If the patient becomes pregnant while taking this drug, the patient should be apprised of the potential hazard to the fetus and the lack of known clinical benefit with continued use during pregnancy [see Use in Specific Populations (8.1) and Nonclinical Toxicology (13.2)].
- Nursing mothers. Animal studies have shown that LIVALO passes into breast milk. Since HMG-CoA reductase inhibitors have the potential to cause serious adverse reactions in nursing infants, LIVALO, like other HMG-CoA reductase inhibitors, is contraindicated in pregnant or nursing mothers [see Use in Specific Populations (8.3) and Nonclinical Toxicology (13.2)].
- Co-administration with cyclosporine [see Drug Interactions (7.1) and Clinical Pharmacology (12.3)].

5 WARNINGS AND PRECAUTIONS

5.1 Skeletal Muscle Effects

Cases of myopathy and rhabdomyolysis with acute renal failure secondary to myoglobinuria have been reported with HMG-CoA reductase inhibitors, including LIVALO. These risks can occur at any dose level, but increase in a dose-dependent manner.

LIVALO should be prescribed with caution in patients with predisposing factors for myopathy. These factors include advanced age (≥65 years), renal impairment, and inadequately treated hypothyroidism. The risk of myopathy may also be increased with concurrent administration of fibrates or lipid-modifying doses of niacin. LIVALO should be administered with caution in patients with impaired renal function, in elderly patients, or when used concomitantly with fibrates or lipid-modifying doses of niacin [see Drug Interactions (7.6), Use in Specific Populations (8.5, 8.6) and Clinical Pharmacology (12.3)].

Cases of myopathy, including rhabdomyolysis, have been reported with HMG-CoA reductase inhibitors coadministered with colchicine, and caution should be exercised when prescribing LIVALO with colchicine [see Drug Interactions (7.7)].

There have been rare reports of immune-mediated necrotizing myopathy (IMNM), an autoimmune myopathy, associated with statin use. IMNM is characterized by: proximal muscle weakness and elevated serum creatine kinase, which persist despite discontinuation of statin treatment; muscle biopsy showing necrotizing myopathy without significant inflammation; improvement with immunosuppressive agents.

LIVALO therapy should be discontinued if markedly elevated creatine kinase (CK) levels occur or myopathy is diagnosed or suspected. LIVALO therapy should also be temporarily withheld in any patient with an acute, serious condition suggestive of myopathy or predisposing to the development of renal failure secondary to rhabdomyolysis (e.g., sepsis, hypotension, dehydration, major surgery, trauma, severe metabolic, endocrine, and electrolyte disorders, or uncontrolled seizures). All patients should be advised to promptly report unexplained muscle pain, tenderness, or weakness, particularly if accompanied by malaise or fever or if muscle signs and symptoms persist after discontinuing LIVALO.

5.2 Liver Enzyme Abnormalities

Increases in serum transaminases (aspartate aminotransferase [AST]/serum glutamic-oxaloacetic transaminase, or alanine aminotransferase [ALT]/serum glutamic-pyruvic transaminase) have been reported with HMG-CoA reductase inhibitors, including LIVALO. In most cases, the elevations were transient and resolved or improved on continued therapy or after a brief interruption in therapy.

In placebo-controlled Phase 2 studies, ALT >3 times the upper limit of normal was not observed in the placebo, LIVALO 1 mg, or LIVALO 2 mg groups. One out of 202 patients (0.5%) administered LIVALO 4 mg had ALT >3 times the upper limit of normal.

It is recommended that liver enzyme tests be performed before the initiation of LIVALO and if signs or symptoms of liver injury occur.

There have been rare postmarketing reports of fatal and non-fatal hepatic failure in patients taking statins, including pitavastatin. If serious liver injury with clinical symptoms and/or hyperbilirubinemia or jaundice occurs during treatment with LIVALO, promptly interrupt therapy. If an alternate etiology is not found do not restart LIVALO.

As with other HMG-CoA reductase inhibitors, LIVALO should be used with caution in patients who consume substantial quantities of alcohol. Active liver disease, which may include unexplained persistent transaminase elevations, is a contraindication to the use of LIVALO [see Contraindications (4)].

5.3 Endocrine Function

Increases in HbA1c and fasting serum glucose levels have been reported with HMG-CoA reductase inhibitors, including LIVALO.

6 ADVERSE REACTIONS

The following serious adverse reactions are discussed in greater detail in other sections of the label:

- Rhabdomyolysis with myoglobinuria and acute renal failure and myopathy (including myositis) [see Warnings and Precautions (5.1)].
- Liver Enzyme Abnormalities [see Warning and Precautions (5.2)].

Of 4,798 patients enrolled in 10 controlled clinical studies and 4 subsequent open-label extension studies, 3,291 patients were administered pitavastatin 1 mg to 4 mg daily. The mean continuous exposure of pitavastatin (1 mg to 4 mg) was 36.7 weeks (median 51.1 weeks). The mean age of the patients was 60.9 years (range; 18 years – 89 years) and the gender distribution was 48% males and 52% females. Approximately 93% of the patients were Caucasian, 7% were Asian/Indian, 0.2% were African American and 0.3% were Hispanic and other.

6.1 Clinical Studies Experience

Because clinical studies on LIVALO are conducted in varying study populations and study designs, the frequency of adverse reactions observed in the clinical studies of LIVALO cannot be directly compared with that in the clinical studies of other HMG-CoA reductase inhibitors and may not reflect the frequency of adverse reactions observed in clinical practice.

Adverse reactions reported in ≥ 2% of patients in controlled clinical studies and at a rate greater than or equal to placebo are shown in Table 1. These studies had treatment duration of up to 12 weeks.

[See table 1 below]

Other adverse reactions reported from clinical studies were arthralgia, headache, influenza, and nasopharyngitis.

The following laboratory abnormalities have also been reported: elevated creatine phosphokinase, transaminases, alkaline phosphatase, bilirubin, and glucose.

In controlled clinical studies and their open-label extensions, 3.9% (1 mg), 3.3% (2 mg), and 3.7% (4 mg) of pitavastatin-treated patients were discontinued due to adverse reactions. The most common adverse reactions that

Table 1. Adverse Reactions* Reported by ≥2.0% of Patients Treated with LIVALO and > Placebo in Short-Term Controlled Studies

Adverse Reactions*	Placebo N= 208	LIVALO 1 mg N=309	LIVALO 2 mg N=951	LIVALO 4 mg N=1540
Back Pain	2.9%	3.9%	1.8%	1.4%
Constipation	1.9%	3.6%	1.5%	2.2%
Diarrhea	1.9%	2.6%	1.5%	1.9%
Myalgia	1.4%	1.9%	2.8%	3.1%
Pain in extremity	1.9%	2.3%	0.6%	0.9%

* Adverse reactions by MedDRA preferred term.

led to treatment discontinuation were: elevated creatine phosphokinase (0.6% on 4 mg) and myalgia (0.5% on 4 mg). Hypersensitivity reactions including rash, pruritus, and urticaria have been reported with LIVALO.

6.2 Postmarketing Experience

The following adverse reactions have been identified during postapproval use of LIVALO. Because these reactions are reported voluntarily from a population of uncertain size, it is not always possible to reliably estimate their frequency or establish a causal relationship to drug exposure.

Adverse reactions associated with LIVALO therapy reported since market introduction, regardless of causality assessment, include the following: abdominal discomfort, abdominal pain, dyspepsia, nausea, asthenia, fatigue, malaise, hepatitis, jaundice, fatal and non-fatal hepatic failure, dizziness, hypoesthesia, insomnia, depression, interstitial lung disease, erectile dysfunction and muscle spasms. There have been rare postmarketing reports of cognitive impairment (e.g., memory loss, forgetfulness, amnesia, memory impairment, confusion) associated with statin use. These cognitive issues have been reported for all statins. The reports are generally nonserious, and reversible upon statin discontinuation, with variable times to symptom onset (1 day to years) and symptom resolution (median of 3 weeks).

There have been rare reports of immune-mediated necrotizing myopathy associated with statin use [see *Warnings and Precautions (5.1)*].

7 DRUG INTERACTIONS

7.1 Cyclosporine

Cyclosporine significantly increased pitavastatin exposure. Co-administration of cyclosporine with LIVALO is contraindicated [see *Contraindications (4) and Clinical Pharmacology (12.3)*].

7.2 Erythromycin

Erythromycin significantly increased pitavastatin exposure. In patients taking erythromycin, a dose of LIVALO 1 mg once daily should not be exceeded [see *Dosage and Administration (2.3) and Clinical Pharmacology (12.3)*].

7.3 Rifampin

Rifampin significantly increased pitavastatin exposure. In patients taking rifampin, a dose of LIVALO 2 mg once daily should not be exceeded [see *Dosage and Administration (2.4) and Clinical Pharmacology (12.3)*].

7.4 Gemfibrozil

Due to an increased risk of myopathy/rhabdomyolysis when HMG-CoA reductase inhibitors are coadministered with gemfibrozil, concomitant administration of LIVALO with gemfibrozil should be avoided.

7.5 Other Fibrates

Because it is known that the risk of myopathy during treatment with HMG-CoA reductase inhibitors is increased with concurrent administration of other fibrates, LIVALO should be administered with caution when used concomitantly with other fibrates [see *Warnings and Precautions (5.1), and Clinical Pharmacology (12.3)*].

7.6 Niacin

The risk of skeletal muscle effects may be enhanced when LIVALO is used in combination with niacin; a reduction in LIVALO dosage should be considered in this setting [see *Warnings and Precautions (5.1)*].

7.7 Colchicine

Cases of myopathy, including rhabdomyolysis, have been reported with HMG-CoA reductase inhibitors coadministered with colchicine, and caution should be exercised when prescribing LIVALO with colchicine.

7.8 Warfarin

LIVALO had no significant pharmacokinetic interaction with R- and S- warfarin. LIVALO had no significant effect on prothrombin time (PT) and international normalized ratio (INR) when administered to patients receiving chronic warfarin treatment [see *Clinical Pharmacology (12.3)*]. However, patients receiving warfarin should have their PT and INR monitored when pitavastatin is added to their therapy.

8 USE IN SPECIFIC POPULATIONS

8.1 Pregnancy

Teratogenic effects: Pregnancy Category X

LIVALO is contraindicated in women who are or may become pregnant. Serum cholesterol and TG increase during normal pregnancy, and cholesterol products are essential for fetal development. Atherosclerosis is a chronic process and discontinuation of lipid-lowering drugs during pregnancy should have little impact on long-term outcomes of primary hyperlipidemia therapy [see *Contraindications (4)*].

There are no adequate and well-controlled studies of LIVALO in pregnant women, although, there have been rare reports of congenital anomalies following intrauterine exposure to HMG-CoA reductase inhibitors. In a review of about 100 prospectively followed pregnancies in women exposed to other HMG-CoA reductase inhibitors, the incidences of congenital anomalies, spontaneous abortions, and fetal deaths/stillbirths did not exceed the rate expected in the general population. However, this study was only able to exclude a three-to-four-fold increased risk of congenital anomalies over background incidence. In 89% of these cases, drug treatment started before pregnancy and stopped during the first trimester when pregnancy was identified.

Reproductive toxicity studies have shown that pitavastatin crosses the placenta in rats and is found in fetal tissues at ≤36% of maternal plasma concentrations following a single dose of 1 mg/kg/day during gestation.

Embryo-fetal developmental studies were conducted in pregnant rats treated with 3, 10, 30 mg/kg/day pitavastatin by oral gavage during organogenesis. No adverse effects were observed at 3 mg/kg/day, systemic exposures 22 times human systemic exposure at 4 mg/day based on AUC.

Embryo-fetal developmental studies were conducted in pregnant rabbits treated with 0.1, 0.3, 1 mg/kg/day pitavastatin by oral gavage during the period of fetal organogenesis. Maternal toxicity consisting of reduced body weight and abortion was observed at all doses tested (4 times human systemic exposure at 4 mg/day based on AUC).

In perinatal/postnatal studies in pregnant rats given oral gavage doses of pitavastatin at 0.1, 0.3, 1, 3, 10, 30 mg/kg/day from organogenesis through weaning, maternal toxicity consisting of mortality at ≥0.3 mg/kg/day and impaired lactation at all doses contributed to the decreased survival of neonates in all dose groups (0.1 mg/kg/day represents approximately 1 time human systemic exposure at 4 mg/day dose based on AUC).

LIVALO may cause fetal harm when administered to a pregnant woman. If the patient becomes pregnant while taking LIVALO, the patient should be apprised of the potential risks to the fetus and the lack of known clinical benefit with continued use during pregnancy.

8.3 Nursing Mothers

It is not known whether pitavastatin is excreted in human milk, however, it has been shown that a small amount of another drug in this class passes into human milk. Rat studies have shown that pitavastatin is excreted into breast milk. Because another drug in this class passes into human milk and HMG-CoA reductase inhibitors have a potential to cause serious adverse reactions in nursing infants, women who require LIVALO treatment should be advised not to nurse their infants or to discontinue LIVALO [see *Contraindications (4)*].

8.4 Pediatric Use

Safety and effectiveness of LIVALO in pediatric patients have not been established.

8.5 Geriatric Use

Of the 2,800 patients randomized to LIVALO 1 mg to 4 mg in controlled clinical studies, 1,209 (43%) were 65 years and older. No significant differences in efficacy or safety were observed between elderly patients and younger patients. However, greater sensitivity of some older individuals cannot be ruled out.

8.6 Renal Impairment

Patients with moderate and severe renal impairment (glomerular filtration rate 30 − 59 mL/min/1.73 m^2 and 15 − 29 mL/min/1.73 m^2 not receiving hemodialysis, respectively) as well as end-stage renal disease receiving hemodialysis should receive a starting dose of LIVALO 1 mg once daily and a maximum dose of LIVALO 2 mg once daily [see *Dosage and Administration (2.2) and Clinical Pharmacology (12.3)*].

8.7 Hepatic Impairment

LIVALO is contraindicated in patients with active liver disease which may include unexplained persistent elevations of hepatic transaminase levels.

10 OVERDOSAGE

There is no known specific treatment in the event of overdose of pitavastatin. In the event of overdose, the patient should be treated symptomatically and supportive measures instituted as required. Hemodialysis is unlikely to be of benefit due to high protein binding ratio of pitavastatin.

11 DESCRIPTION

LIVALO (pitavastatin) is an inhibitor of HMG-CoA reductase. It is a synthetic lipid-lowering agent for oral administration.

The chemical name for pitavastatin is (+)monocalcium *bis*[(3R, 5S, 6E)-7-[2-cyclopropyl-4-(4-fluorophenyl)-3-quinolyl]-3,5-dihydroxy-6-heptenoate]. The structural formula is:

[See chemical structure at top of next column]

The empirical formula for pitavastatin is $C_{50}H_{46}CaF_2N_2O_8$ and the molecular weight is 880.98. Pitavastatin is odorless and occurs as white to pale-yellow powder. It is freely soluble in pyridine, chloroform, dilute hydrochloric acid, and tetrahydrofuran, soluble in ethylene glycol, sparingly soluble in octanol, slightly soluble in methanol, very slightly soluble in water or ethanol, and practically insoluble in acetonitrile or diethyl ether. Pitavastatin is hygroscopic and slightly unstable in light.

Each film-coated tablet of LIVALO contains 1.045 mg, 2.09 mg, or 4.18 mg of pitavastatin calcium, which is equivalent to 1 mg, 2 mg, or 4 mg, respectively of free base and the following inactive ingredients: lactose monohydrate, low substituted hydroxypropylcellulose, hypromellose, magnesium aluminometasilicate, magnesium stearate, and film coating containing the following inactive ingredients: hypromellose, titanium dioxide, triethyl citrate, and colloidal anhydrous silica.

12 CLINICAL PHARMACOLOGY

12.1 Mechanism of Action

Pitavastatin competitively inhibits HMG-CoA reductase, which is a rate-determining enzyme involved with biosynthesis of cholesterol, in a manner of competition with the substrate so that it inhibits cholesterol synthesis in the liver. As a result, the expression of LDL-receptors followed by the uptake of LDL from blood to liver is accelerated and then the plasma TC decreases. Further, the sustained inhibition of cholesterol synthesis in the liver decreases levels of very low density lipoproteins.

12.2 Pharmacodynamics

In a randomized, double-blind, placebo-controlled, 4-way parallel, active-comparator study with moxifloxacin in 174 healthy participants, LIVALO was not associated with clinically meaningful prolongation of the QTc interval or heart rate at daily doses up to 16 mg (4 times the recommended maximum daily dose).

12.3 Pharmacokinetics

Absorption: Pitavastatin peak plasma concentrations are achieved about 1 hour after oral administration. Both C_{max} and AUC_{0-inf} increased in an approximately dose-proportional manner for single LIVALO doses from 1 to 24 mg once daily. The absolute bioavailability of pitavastatin oral solution is 51%. Administration of LIVALO with a high fat meal (50% fat content) decreases pitavastatin C_{max} by 43% but does not significantly reduce pitavastatin AUC. The C_{max} and AUC of pitavastatin did not differ following evening or morning drug administration. In healthy volunteers receiving 4 mg pitavastatin, the percent change from baseline for LDL-C following evening dosing was slightly greater than that following morning dosing. Pitavastatin was absorbed in the small intestine but very little in the colon.

Distribution: Pitavastatin is more than 99% protein bound in human plasma, mainly to albumin and alpha 1-acid glycoprotein, and the mean volume of distribution is approximately 148 L. Association of pitavastatin and/or its metabolites with the blood cells is minimal.

Metabolism: Pitavastatin is marginally metabolized by CYP2C9 and to a lesser extent by CYP2C8. The major metabolite in human plasma is the lactone which is formed via an ester-type pitavastatin glucuronide conjugate by uridine 5'-diphosphate (UDP) glucuronosyltransferase (UGT1A3 and UGT2B7).

Excretion: A mean of 15% of radioactivity of orally administered, single 32 mg ^{14}C-labeled pitavastatin dose was excreted in urine, whereas a mean of 79% of the dose was excreted in feces within 7 days. The mean plasma elimination half-life is approximately 12 hours.

Race: In pharmacokinetic studies pitavastatin C_{max} and AUC were 21 and 5% lower, respectively in Black or African American healthy volunteers compared with those of Caucasian healthy volunteers. In pharmacokinetic comparison between Caucasian volunteers and Japanese volunteers, there were no significant differences in C_{max} and AUC.

Gender: In a pharmacokinetic study which compared healthy male and female volunteers, pitavastatin C_{max} and AUC were 60 and 54% higher, respectively in females. This had no effect on the efficacy or safety of LIVALO in women in clinical studies.

Geriatric: In a pharmacokinetic study which compared healthy young and elderly (≥65 years) volunteers, pitavastatin C_{max} and AUC were 10 and 30% higher, respectively, in the elderly. This had no effect on the efficacy or safety of LIVALO in elderly subjects in clinical studies.

Renal Impairment: In patients with moderate renal impairment (glomerular filtration rate of 30 − 59 mL/min/1.73 m^2) and end stage renal disease receiving hemodialysis, pitavastatin AUC_{0-inf} is 102 and 86% higher than those of healthy volunteers, respectively, while pitavastatin C_{max} is 60 and 40% higher than those of healthy volunteers, re-

Table 2. Effect of Co-Administered Drugs on Pitavastatin Systemic Exposure

Co-administered drug	Dose regimen	Change in AUC*	Change in C_{max}*
Cyclosporine	Pitavastatin 2 mg QD for 6 days + cyclosporine 2 mg/kg on Day 6	↑ 4.6 fold†	↑ 6.6 fold †
Erythromycin	Pitavastatin 4 mg single dose on Day 4 + erythromycin 500 mg 4 times daily for 6 days	↑ 2.8 fold †	↑ 3.6 fold †
Rifampin	Pitavastatin 4 mg QD + rifampin 600 mg QD for 5 days	↑ 29%	↑ 2.0 fold
Atazanavir	Pitavastatin 4 mg QD + atazanavir 300 mg daily for 5 days	↑ 31%	↑ 60%
Darunavir/Ritonavir	Pitavastatin 4mg QD on Days 1-5 and 12-16 + darunavir/ritonavir 800mg/100 mg QD on Days 6-16	↓ 26%	↓ 4%
Lopinavir/Ritonavir	Pitavastatin 4 mg QD on Days 1-5 and 20-24 + lopinavir/ritonavir 400 mg/100 mg BID on Days 9 – 24	↓ 20%	↓4 %
Gemfibrozil	Pitavastatin 4 mg QD + gemfibrozil 600 mg BID for 7 days	↑ 45%	↑ 31%
Fenofibrate	Pitavastatin 4 mg QD + fenofibrate 160 mg QD for 7 days	↑18%	↑ 11%
Ezetimibe	Pitavastatin 2 mg QD + ezetimibe 10 mg for 7 days	↓ 2%	↓0.2%
Enalapril	Pitavastatin 4 mg QD + enalapril 20 mg daily for 5 days	↑ 6%	↓ 7%
Digoxin	Pitavastatin 4 mg QD + digoxin 0.25 mg for 7 days	↑ 4%	↓ 9%
Diltiazem LA	Pitavastatin 4 mg QD on Days 1-5 and 11-15 and diltiazem LA 240 mg on Days 6-15	↑10%	↑15%
Grapefruit Juice	Pitavastatin 2 mg single dose on Day 3 + grapefruit juice for 4 days	↑ 15%	↓ 12%
Itraconazole	Pitavastatin 4 mg single dose on Day 4 + itraconazole 200 mg daily for 5 days	↓ 23%	↓ 22%

*Data presented as x-fold change represent the ratio between co-administration and pitavastatin alone (i.e., 1-fold = no change). Data presented as % change represent % difference relative to pitavastatin alone (i.e., 0% = no change).
† Considered clinically significant [see Dosage and Administration (2) and Drug Interactions (7)]
BID = twice daily; QD = once daily; LA = Long Acting

Table 3. Effect of Pitavastatin Co-Administration on Systemic Exposure to Other Drugs

Co-administered drug	Dose regimen		Change in AUC*	Change in C_{max}*
Atazanavir	Pitavastatin 4 mg QD + atazanavir 300 mg daily for 5 days		↑ 6%	↑ 13%
Darunavir	Pitavastatin 4mg QD on Days 1-5 and 12-16 + darunavir/ritonavir 800mg/100 mg QD on Days 6-16		↑ 3%	↑ 6%
Lopinavir	Pitavastatin 4 mg QD on Days 1-5 and 20-24 + lopinavir/ritonavir 400 mg/100 mg BID on Days 9 – 24		↓ 9%	↓ 7%
Ritonavir	Pitavastatin 4 mg QD on Days 1-5 and 20-24 + lopinavir/ritonavir 400 mg/100 mg BID on Days 9 – 24		↓ 11%	↓ 11%
Ritonavir	Pitavastatin 4mg QD on Days 1-5 and 12-16 + darunavir/ritonavir 800mg/100 mg QD on Days 6-16		↑ 8%	↑ 2%
Enalapril	Pitavastatin 4 mg QD + enalapril 20 mg daily for 5 days	Enalapril	↑ 12%	↑ 12%
		Enalaprilat	↓ 1%	↓ 1%
Warfarin	Individualized maintenance dose of warfarin (2 - 7 mg) for 8 days + pitavastatin 4 mg QD for 9 days	R-warfarin	↑ 7%	↑ 3%
		S-warfarin	↑ 6%	↑ 3%
Ezetimibe	Pitavastatin 2 mg QD + ezetimibe 10 mg for 7 days		↑ 9%	↑ 2%
Digoxin	Pitavastatin 4 mg QD + digoxin 0.25 mg for 7 days		↓ 3%	↓ 4%
Diltiazem LA	Pitavastatin 4 mg QD on Days 1-5 and 11-15 and diltiazem LA 240 mg on Days 6-15		↓ 2%	↓ 7%
Rifampin	Pitavastatin 4 mg QD + rifampin 600 mg QD for 5 days		↓ 15%	↓ 18%

*Data presented as % change represent % difference relative to the investigated drug alone (i.e., 0% = no change).
BID = twice daily; QD = once daily; LA = Long Acting

spectively. Patients received hemodialysis immediately before pitavastatin dosing and did not undergo hemodialysis during the pharmacokinetic study. Hemodialysis patients have 33 and 36% increases in the mean unbound fraction of pitavastatin as compared to healthy volunteers and patients with moderate renal impairment, respectively.

In another pharmacokinetic study, patients with severe renal impairment (glomerular filtration rate 15 – 29 mL/min/1.73 m²) not receiving hemodialysis were administered a single dose of LIVALO 4 mg. The AUC_{0-inf} and the C_{max} were 36 and 18% higher, respectively, compared with those of healthy volunteers. For both patients with severe renal impairment and healthy volunteers, the mean percentage of protein-unbound pitavastatin was approximately 0.6%.

The effect of mild renal impairment on pitavastatin exposure has not been studied.

Hepatic Impairment: The disposition of pitavastatin was compared in healthy volunteers and patients with various degrees of hepatic impairment. The ratio of pitavastatin C_{max} between patients with moderate hepatic impairment (Child-Pugh B disease) and healthy volunteers was 2.7. The ratio of pitavastatin AUC_{inf} between patients with moderate hepatic impairment and healthy volunteers was 3.8. The ratio of pitavastatin C_{max} between patients with mild hepatic impairment (Child-Pugh A disease) and healthy volunteers was 1.3. The ratio of pitavastatin AUC_{inf} between patients with mild hepatic impairment and healthy volunteers was 1.6. Mean pitavastatin $t_½$ for moderate hepatic impairment, mild hepatic impairment, and healthy were 15, 10, and 8 hours, respectively.

Drug-Drug Interactions: The principal route of pitavastatin metabolism is glucuronidation via liver UGTs with subsequent formation of pitavastatin lactone. There is only minimal metabolism by the cytochrome P450 system.

Warfarin: The steady-state pharmacodynamics (international normalized ratio [INR] and prothrombin time [PT]) and pharmacokinetics of warfarin in healthy volunteers were unaffected by the co-administration of LIVALO 4 mg daily. However, patients receiving warfarin should have their PT time or INR monitored when pitavastatin is added to their therapy.

[See table 2 above]
[See table 3 above]

13 NONCLINICAL TOXICOLOGY

13.1 Carcinogenesis, Mutagenesis, Impairment of Fertility

In a 92-week carcinogenicity study in mice given pitavastatin, at the maximum tolerated dose of 75 mg/kg/day with systemic maximum exposures (AUC) 26 times the clinical maximum exposure at 4 mg/day, there was an absence of drug-related tumors.

In a 92-week carcinogenicity study in rats given pitavastatin at 1, 5, 25 mg/kg/day by oral gavage there was a significant increase in the incidence of thyroid follicular cell tumors at 25 mg/kg/day, which represents 295 times human systemic exposures based on AUC at the 4 mg/day maximum human dose.

In a 26-week transgenic mouse (Tg rasH2) carcinogenicity study where animals were given pitavastatin at 30, 75, and 150 mg/kg/day by oral gavage, no clinically significant tumors were observed.

Pitavastatin was not mutagenic in the Ames test with *Salmonella typhimurium* and *Escherichia coli* with and without metabolic activation, the micronucleus test following a single administration in mice and multiple administrations in rats, the unscheduled DNA synthesis test in rats, and a Comet assay in mice. In the chromosomal aberration test, clastogenicity was observed at the highest doses tested which also elicited high levels of cytotoxicity.

Pitavastatin had no adverse effects on male and female rat fertility at oral doses of 10 and 30 mg/kg/day, respectively, at systemic exposures 56- and 354-times clinical exposure at 4 mg/day based on AUC.

Pitavastatin treatment in rabbits resulted in mortality in males and females given 1 mg/kg/day (30-times clinical systemic exposure at 4 mg/day based on AUC) and higher during a fertility study. Although the cause of death was not determined, rabbits had gross signs of renal toxicity (kidneys whitened) indicative of possible ischemia. Lower doses (15-times human systemic exposure) did not show significant toxicity in adult males and females. However, decreased implantations, increased resorptions, and decreased viability of fetuses were observed.

13.2 Animal Toxicology and/or Pharmacology

Central Nervous System Toxicity

CNS vascular lesions, characterized by perivascular hemorrhages, edema, and mononuclear cell infiltration of perivascular spaces, have been observed in dogs treated with several other members of this drug class. A chemically similar drug in this class produced dose-dependent optic nerve degeneration (Wallerian degeneration of retinogeniculate fibers) in dogs, at a dose that produced plasma drug levels about 30 times higher than the mean drug level in humans taking the highest recommended dose. Wallerian degeneration has not been observed with pitavastatin. Cataracts and lens opacities were seen in dogs treated for 52 weeks at a dose level of 1 mg/kg/day (9 times clinical exposure at the maximum human dose of 4 mg/day based on AUC comparisons.

14 CLINICAL STUDIES

14.1 Primary Hyperlipidemia or Mixed Dyslipidemia

Dose-ranging study: A multicenter, randomized, double-blind, placebo-controlled, dose-ranging study was performed to evaluate the efficacy of LIVALO compared with placebo in 251 patients with primary hyperlipidemia (Table 4). LIVALO given as a single daily dose for 12 weeks significantly reduced plasma LDL-C, TC, TG, and Apo-B compared to placebo and was associated with variable increases in HDL-C across the dose range.
[See table 4 above]

Active-controlled study with atorvastatin (NK-104-301): LIVALO was compared with the HMG-CoA reductase inhibitor atorvastatin in a randomized, multicenter, double-blind, double-dummy, active-controlled, non-inferiority Phase 3 study of 817 patients with primary hyperlipidemia or mixed dyslipidemia. Patients entered a 6- to 8-week wash-out/dietary lead-in period and then were randomized to a 12-week treatment with either LIVALO or atorvastatin (Table 5). Non-inferiority of pitavastatin to a given dose of atorvastatin was considered to be demonstrated if the lower bound of the 95% CI for the mean treatment difference was greater than -6% for the mean percent change in LDL-C.

Lipid results are shown in Table 5. For the percent change from baseline to endpoint in LDL-C, LIVALO was non-inferior to atorvastatin for the two pairwise comparisons: LIVALO 2 mg vs. atorvastatin 10 mg and LIVALO 4 mg vs. atorvastatin 20 mg. Mean treatment differences (95% CI) were 0% (-3%, 3%) and 1% (-2%, 4%), respectively.
[See table 5 above]

Active-controlled study with simvastatin (NK-104-302): LIVALO was compared with the HMG-CoA reductase inhibitor simvastatin in a randomized, multicenter, double-blind, double-dummy, active-controlled, non-inferiority Phase 3 study of 843 patients with primary hyperlipidemia or mixed dyslipidemia. Patients entered a 6- to 8-week wash-out/dietary lead-in period and then were randomized to a 12 week treatment with either LIVALO or simvastatin (Table 6). Non-inferiority of pitavastatin to a given dose of simvastatin was considered to be demonstrated if the lower bound of the 95% CI for the mean treatment difference was greater than -6% for the mean percent change in LDL-C.

Lipid results are shown in Table 6. For the percent change from baseline to endpoint in LDL-C, LIVALO was non-inferior to simvastatin for the two pairwise comparisons: LIVALO 2 mg vs. simvastatin 20 mg and LIVALO 4 mg vs. simvastatin 40 mg. Mean treatment differences (95% CI) were 4% (1%, 7%) and 1% (-2%, 4%), respectively.
[See table 6 above]

Active-controlled study with pravastatin in elderly (NK-104-306): LIVALO was compared with the HMG-CoA reductase inhibitor pravastatin in a randomized, multicenter, double-blind, double-dummy, parallel group, active-controlled non-inferiority Phase 3 study of 942 elderly patients (≥65 years) with primary hyperlipidemia or mixed dyslipidemia. Patients entered a 6- to 8-week wash-out/dietary lead-in period, and then were randomized to a once daily dose of LIVALO or pravastatin for 12 weeks (Table 7). Non-inferiority of LIVALO to a given dose of pravastatin was assumed if the lower bound of the 95% CI for the treatment difference was greater than -6% for the mean percent change in LDL-C.

Lipid results are shown in Table 7. LIVALO significantly reduced LDL-C compared to pravastatin as demonstrated by the following pairwise dose comparisons: LIVALO 1 mg vs. pravastatin 10 mg, LIVALO 2 mg vs. pravastatin 20 mg and LIVALO 4 mg vs. pravastatin 40 mg. Mean treatment differences (95% CI) were 9% (6%, 12%), 10% (7%, 13%) and 10% (7%, 13%), respectively.
[See table 7 above]

Active-controlled study with simvastatin in patients with ≥2 risk factors for coronary heart disease (NK-104-304): LIVALO was compared with the HMG-CoA reductase inhibitor simvastatin in a randomized, multicenter, double-blind, double-dummy, active-controlled, non-inferiority Phase 3 study of 351 patients with primary hyperlipidemia or mixed dyslipidemia with ≥2 risk factors for coronary heart disease. After a 6- to 8-week wash-out/dietary lead-in period, patients were randomized to a 12-week treatment with either LIVALO or simvastatin (Table 8). Non-inferiority of LIVALO to simvastatin was considered to be demonstrated if the lower bound of the 95% CI for the mean treatment difference was greater than -6% for the mean percent change in LDL-C.

Lipid results are shown in Table 8. LIVALO 4 mg was non-inferior to simvastatin 40 mg for percent change from baseline to endpoint in LDL-C. The mean treatment difference (95% CI) was 0% (-2%, 3%).
[See table 8 at top of next page]

Active-controlled study with atorvastatin in patients with type II diabetes mellitus (NK-104-305): LIVALO was compared with the HMG-CoA reductase inhibitor atorvastatin

in a randomized, multicenter, double-blind, double-dummy, parallel group, active-controlled, non-inferiority Phase 3 study of 410 subjects with type II diabetes mellitus and combined dyslipidemia. Patients entered a 6- to 8-week washout/dietary lead-in period and were randomized to a once daily dose of LIVALO or atorvastatin for 12 weeks. Non-inferiority of LIVALO was considered to be demonstrated if the lower bound of the 95% CI for the mean treatment difference was greater than -6% for the mean percent change in LDL-C.

Lipid results are shown in Table 9. The treatment difference (95% CI) for LDL-C percent change from baseline was -2% (-6.2%, 1.5%). The two treatment groups were not statistically different on LDL-C. However, the lower limit of the CI was -6.2%, slightly exceeding the -6% non-inferiority limit so that the non-inferiority objective was not achieved.
[See table 9 at top of next page]

The treatment differences in efficacy in LDL-C change from baseline between LIVALO and active controls in the Phase 3 studies are summarized in Figure 1.

[See figure 1 at top of next page]

16 HOW SUPPLIED/STORAGE AND HANDLING

LIVALO tablets for oral administration are provided as white, film-coated tablets that contain 1 mg, 2 mg, or 4 mg of pitavastatin. Each tablet has "KC" debossed on one side and a code number specific to the tablet strength on the other.

Packaging

LIVALO (pitavastatin) Tablets are supplied as;
- NDC 66869-104-90 : 1 mg. Round white film-coated tablet debossed "KC" on one face and "1" on the reverse; HDPE bottles of 90 tablets
- NDC 66869-204-90 : 2 mg. Round white film-coated tablet debossed "KC" on one face and "2" on the reverse; HDPE bottles of 90 tablets
- NDC 66869-404-90 : 4 mg. Round white film-coated tablet debossed "KC" on one face and "4" on the reverse; HDPE bottles of 90 tablets

Storage

Store at room temperature between 15°C and 30°C (59° to 86° F) [see USP]. Protect from light.

Table 4. Dose-Response in Patients with Primary Hypercholesterolemia (Adjusted Mean % Change from Baseline at Week 12)

Treatment	N	LDL-C	Apo-B	TC	TG	HDL-C
Placebo	53	-3	-2	-2	1	0
LIVALO 1mg	52	-32	-25	-23	-15	8
LIVALO 2mg	49	-36	-30	-26	-19	7
LIVALO 4mg	51#	-43	-35	-31	-18	5

The number of subjects for Apo-B was 49

Table 5. Response by Dose of LIVALO and Atorvastatin in Patients with Primary Hyperlipidemia or Mixed Dyslipidemia (Mean % Change from Baseline at Week 12)

Treatment	N	LDL-C	Apo-B	TC	TG	HDL-C	non-HDL-C
LIVALO 2 mg daily	315	-38	-30	-28	-14	4	-35
LIVALO 4 mg daily	298	-45	-35	-32	-19	5	-41
Atorvastatin 10 mg daily	102	-38	-29	-28	-18	3	-35
Atorvastatin 20 mg daily	102	-44	-36	-33	-22	2	-41
Atorvastatin 40 mg daily				----Not Studied----			
Atorvastatin 80 mg daily				----Not Studied----			

Table 6. Response by Dose of LIVALO and Simvastatin in Patients with Primary Hyperlipidemia or Mixed Dyslipidemia (Mean % Change from Baseline at Week 12)

Treatment	N	LDL-C	Apo-B	TC	TG	HDL-C	non-HDL-C
LIVALO 2 mg daily	307	-39	-30	-28	-16	6	-36
LIVALO 4 mg daily	319	-44	-35	-32	-17	6	-41
Simvastatin 20 mg daily	107	-35	-27	-25	-16	6	-32
Simvastatin 40 mg daily	110	-43	-34	-31	-16	7	-39
Simvastatin 80 mg				----Not Studied----			

Table 7. Response by Dose of LIVALO and Pravastatin in Patients with Primary Hyperlipidemia or Mixed Dyslipidemia (Mean % Change from Baseline at Week 12)

Treatment	N	LDL-C	Apo-B	TC	TG	HDL-C	non-HDL-C
LIVALO 1 mg daily	207	-31	-25	-22	-13	1	-29
LIVALO 2 mg daily	224	-39	-31	-27	-15	2	-36
LIVALO 4 mg daily	210	-44	-37	-31	-22	4	-41
Pravastatin 10 mg daily	103	-22	-17	-15	-5	0	-20
Pravastatin 20 mg daily	96	-29	-22	-21	-11	-1	-27
Pravastatin 40 mg daily	102	-34	-28	-24	-15	1	-32
Pravastatin 80 mg daily				----Not Studied----			

Table 8. Response by Dose of LIVALO and Simvastatin in Patients with Primary Hyperlipidemia or Mixed Dyslipidemia with ≥2 Risk Factors for Coronary Heart Disease (Mean % Change from Baseline at Week 12)

Treatment	N	LDL-C	Apo-B	TC	TG	HDL-C	non-HDL-C
LIVALO 4 mg daily	233	-44	-34	-31	-20	7	-40
Simvastatin 40 mg daily	118	-44	-34	-31	-15	5	-39
Simvastatin 80 mg daily			-------------------------Not Studied-------------------------				

Table 9. Response by Dose of LIVALO and Atorvastatin in Patients with Type II Diabetes Mellitus and Combined Dyslipidemia (Mean % Change from Baseline at Week 12)

Treatment	N	LDL-C	Apo-B	TC	TG	HDL-C	non-HDL-C
LIVALO 4 mg daily	274	-41	-32	-28	-20	7	-36
Atorvastatin 20 mg daily	136	-43	-34	-32	-27	8	-40
Atorvastatin 40 mg daily			-------------------Not Studied-------------------				
Atorvastatin 80 mg daily			-------------------Not Studied-------------------				

Figure 1. Treatment Difference in Adjusted Mean Percent Change in LDL-C

NL=non-inferiority limit.

17   PATIENT COUNSELING INFORMATION

The patient should be informed of the following:

17.1   Dosing Time

LIVALO can be taken at any time of the day with or without food.

17.2   Muscle Pain

Patients should be advised to promptly notify their physician of any unexplained muscle pain, tenderness, or weakness particularly if accompanied by malaise or fever, or if these muscle signs or symptoms persist after discontinuing LIVALO. They should discuss all medication, both prescription and over the counter, with their physician.

17.3   Pregnancy

Women of childbearing age should use an effective method of birth control to prevent pregnancy while using LIVALO. Discuss future pregnancy plans with your healthcare professional, and discuss when to stop LIVALO if you are trying to conceive. If you are pregnant, stop taking LIVALO and call your healthcare professional.

17.4   Breastfeeding

Women who are breastfeeding should not use LIVALO. If you have a lipid disorder and are breastfeeding, stop taking LIVALO and consult with your healthcare professional.

17.5   Liver Enzymes

It is recommended that liver enzyme tests be checked before the initiation of LIVALO and if signs or symptoms of liver injury occur. All patients treated with LIVALO should be advised to report promptly any symptoms that may indicate liver injury, including fatigue, anorexia, right upper abdominal discomfort, dark urine or jaundice.

LIVALO is a trademark of the Kowa group of companies.
© Kowa Pharmaceuticals America, Inc. (2009)
Manufactured under license from: Kowa Company, Limited Tokyo 103-8433 Japan
Product of Japan
Manufactured into tablets by: Patheon, Inc. Cincinnati, OH 45237 USA or by Kowa Company, LTD Nagoya, 462-0024 Japan
Marketed by: Kowa Pharmaceuticals America, Inc. Montgomery, AL 36117 USATo request additional information or if you have questions concerning LIVALO please phone Kowa Pharmaceuticals America, Inc. at 877-8-LIVALO (877-854-8256) or fax your inquiry to 800-689-0244

Shown in Product Identification Guide, page 307

MannKind Corporation

1 CASPER STREET
DANBURY, CT 06810

Phone Number:
1-800-633-1610

AFREZZA®   Rx
[uh-FREZZ-uh]
(insulin human)
Inhalation Powder

HIGHLIGHTS OF PRESCRIBING INFORMATION
These highlights do not include all the information needed to use AFREZZA® safely and effectively. See full prescribing information for AFREZZA.
AFREZZA® (insulin human) Inhalation Powder.
Initial U.S. Approval: 06/2014

> **WARNING: RISK OF ACUTE BRONCHOSPASM IN PATIENTS WITH CHRONIC LUNG DISEASE**
> *See full prescribing information for complete boxed warning.*
> - Acute bronchospasm has been observed in patients with asthma and COPD using AFREZZA. (5.1)
> - AFREZZA is contraindicated in patients with chronic lung disease such as asthma or COPD. (4)
> - Before initiating AFREZZA, perform a detailed medical history, physical examination, and spirometry (FEV$_1$) to identify potential lung disease in all patients. (2.5), (5.1)

———INDICATIONS AND USAGE———

- AFREZZA® is a rapid acting inhaled insulin indicated to improve glycemic control in adult patients with diabetes mellitus. (1)

Important limitations of use:
- In patients with type 1 diabetes, must use with a long-acting insulin. (1)
- Not recommended for the treatment of diabetic ketoacidosis. (1)
- Not recommended in patients who smoke (1)

———DOSAGE AND ADMINISTRATION———

- Administer using a single inhalation per cartridge (2.1)
- Administer at the beginning of a meal (2.2)
- Dosing must be individualized (2.2)
- Before initiating, perform a detailed medical history, physical examination, and spirometry (FEV$_1$) in all patients to identify potential lung disease (2.5)

———DOSAGE FORMS AND STRENGTHS———

AFREZZA is available as single-use cartridges of: (3)
- 4 units
- 8 units

———CONTRAINDICATIONS———

- During episodes of hypoglycemia (4)
- Chronic lung disease, such as asthma, or chronic obstructive pulmonary disease (4)
- Hypersensitivity to regular human insulin or any of the AFREZZA excipients (4)

WARNINGS AND PRECAUTIONS

- *Acute Bronchospasm:* Acute bronchospasm has been observed in patients with asthma and COPD. Before initiating, perform spirometry (FEV$_1$) in all patients. Do not use in patients with chronic lung disease (2.5, 4, 5.1)
- *Change in Insulin Regimen:* Carry out under close medical supervision and increase frequency of blood glucose monitoring. (5.2)
- *Hypoglycemia:* May be life-threatening. Increase frequency of glucose monitoring with changes to: insulin dosage, co-administered glucose lowering medications, meal pattern, physical activity; and in patients with renal or hepatic impairment and hypoglycemia unawareness. (5.3, 6, 7, 8.5, 8.6)
- *Decline in Pulmonary Function:* Assess pulmonary function (e.g., spirometry) before initiating, after 6 months of therapy, and annually, even in the absence of pulmonary symptoms. (2.5, 5.4)
- *Lung Cancer:* AFREZZA should not be used in patients with active lung cancer. In patients with a history of lung cancer or at risk for lung cancer, the benefit of AFREZZA use should outweigh this potential risk. (5.5)
- *Diabetic Ketoacidosis:* More patients using AFREZZA experienced diabetic ketoacidosis in clinical trials. In patients at risk for DKA, monitor and change to alternate route of insulin delivery, if indicated. (5.6)
- *Hypersensitivity Reactions:* Severe, life-threatening, generalized allergy, including anaphylaxis, can occur with insulin products, including AFREZZA. Discontinue AFREZZA, monitor and treat if indicated. (5.7)
- *Hypokalemia:* May be life-threatening. Monitor potassium levels in patients at risk of hypokalemia and treat if indicated. (5.8)
- *Fluid Retention and Heart Failure with Concomitant Use of Thiazolidinediones (TZDs):* Observe for signs and symptoms of heart failure; consider dosage reduction or discontinuation if heart failure occurs. (5.9)

ADVERSE REACTIONS

The most common adverse reactions associated with AFREZZA (2% or greater incidence) are hypoglycemia, cough, and throat pain or irritation (6)

To report SUSPECTED ADVERSE REACTIONS, contact Sanofi US 1-800-633-1610 or FDA at (1-800-FDA-1088) or www.fda.gov/medwatch.

DRUG INTERACTIONS

Drugs that Affect Glucose Metabolism: Adjustment of insulin dosage may be needed. (7.1, 7.2, 7.3)
Anti-Adrenergic Drugs (e.g., beta-blockers, clonidine, guanethidine, and reserpine): Signs and symptoms of hypoglycemia may be reduced or absent. (7.3, 7.4)

See 17 for PATIENT COUNSELING INFORMATION and Medication Guide

Revised: 07/2014

FULL PRESCRIBING INFORMATION: CONTENTS*
WARNING: RISK OF ACUTE BRONCHOSPASM IN PATIENTS WITH CHRONIC LUNG DISEASE

FULL PRESCRIBING INFORMATION

WARNING: RISK OF ACUTE BRONCHOSPASM IN PATIENTS WITH CHRONIC LUNG DISEASE

- Acute bronchospasm has been observed in patients with asthma and COPD using AFREZZA. *[see Warnings and Precautions (5.1)]*
- AFREZZA is contraindicated in patients with chronic lung disease such as asthma or COPD. *[see Contraindications (4)]*
- Before initiating AFREZZA, perform a detailed medical history, physical examination, and spirometry (FEV$_1$) to identify potential lung disease in all patients *[see Dosage and Administration (2.5), Warnings and Precautions (5.1)]*

---

1   INDICATIONS AND USAGE

AFREZZA® is a rapid acting inhaled insulin indicated to improve glycemic control in adult patients with diabetes mellitus.

Limitations of Use:

- AFREZZA is not a substitute for long-acting insulin. AFREZZA must be used in combination with long-acting insulin in patients with type 1 diabetes mellitus.
- AFREZZA is not recommended for the treatment of diabetic ketoacidosis *[see Warning and Precautions (5.6)]*.
- The safety and efficacy of AFREZZA in patients who smoke has not been established. The use of AFREZZA is not recommended in patients who smoke or who have recently stopped smoking.

2   DOSAGE AND ADMINISTRATION

2.1   Route of Administration

AFREZZA should only be administered via oral inhalation using the AFREZZA Inhaler. AFREZZA is administered using a single inhalation per cartridge.

2.2   Dosage Information

Administer AFREZZA at the beginning of the meal.
Dosage adjustment may be needed when switching from another insulin to AFREZZA *[see Warnings and Precautions (5.2)]*.

Starting Mealtime Dose:

- *Insulin Naive Individuals:* Start on 4 units of AFREZZA at each meal.
- *Individuals Using Subcutaneous Mealtime (Prandial) Insulin:* Determine the appropriate AFREZZA dose for each meal by converting from the injected dose using Figure 1.
- *Individuals Using Subcutaneous Pre-mixed Insulin:* Estimate the mealtime injected dose by dividing half of the total daily injected pre-mixed insulin dose equally among the three meals of the day. Convert each estimated injected mealtime dose to an appropriate AFREZZA dose using Figure 1. Administer half of the total daily injected pre-mixed dose as an injected basal insulin dose.

[See figure 1 at top of next column]

Mealtime Dose Adjustment

Adjust the dosage of AFREZZA based on the individual's metabolic needs, blood glucose monitoring results and glycemic control goal.

Figure 1. Mealtime AFREZZA Dose Conversion Table

Injected Mealtime Insulin Dose	AFREZZA® Dose	# of 4 unit (blue) cartridges needed	# of 8 unit (green) cartridges needed
up to 4 units	4 units		
5-8 units	8 units		
9-12 units	12 units	✓ +	
13-16 units	16 units		
17-20 units	20 units	✓ +	
21-24 units	24 units		

Dosage adjustments may be needed with changes in physical activity, changes in meal patterns (i.e., macronutrient content or timing of food intake), changes in renal or hepatic function or during acute illness *[see Warnings and Precautions (5.3), and Use in Specific Populations (8.5, 8.6)]*.

Carefully monitor blood glucose control in patients requiring high doses of AFREZZA. If, in these patients, blood glucose control is not achieved with increased AFREZZA doses, consider use of subcutaneous mealtime insulin.

2.3   AFREZZA Administration for Doses Exceeding 8 units

For AFREZZA doses exceeding 8 units, inhalations from multiple cartridges are necessary. To achieve the required total mealtime dose, patients should use a combination of 4 unit and 8 unit cartridges. Examples of cartridge combinations for doses of up to 24 units are shown in Figure 1. For doses above 24 units, combinations of different multiple cartridges can be used.

2.4   Dosage Adjustment due to Drug Interactions

Dosage adjustment may be needed when AFREZZA is coadministered with certain drugs *[see Drug Interactions (7)]*.

2.5   Lung Function Assessment Prior to Administration

AFREZZA is contraindicated in patients with chronic lung disease because of the risk of acute bronchospasm in these patients. Before initiating AFREZZA, perform a medical history, physical examination and spirometry (FEV$_1$) in all patients to identify potential lung disease *[see Contraindications (4) and Warnings and Precautions (5.1)]*.

2.6   Important Administration Instructions

See Patient Instructions for Use for complete administration instructions with illustrations.

Keep the inhaler level and white mouthpiece on top and purple base on the bottom after a cartridge has been inserted into the inhaler. Loss of drug effect can occur if the inhaler is turned upside down, held with the mouthpiece pointing down, shaken (or dropped) after the cartridge has been inserted but before the dose has been administered. If any of the above occur, the cartridge should be replaced before use.

3   DOSAGE FORMS AND STRENGTHS

AFREZZA (insulin human) Inhalation Powder is available as 4 unit and 8 unit single use cartridges to be administered via oral inhalation with the AFREZZA Inhaler only. *[see How Supplied/Storage and Handling (16)]*.

4   CONTRAINDICATIONS

AFREZZA is contraindicated in patients with the following:
- During episodes of hypoglycemia
- Chronic lung disease, such as asthma or chronic obstructive pulmonary disease (COPD), because of the risk of acute bronchospasm *[see Warnings and Precautions (5.1)]*.
- Hypersensitivity to regular human insulin or any of the AFREZZA excipients *[see Warnings and Precautions (5.7)]*.

5   WARNINGS AND PRECAUTIONS

5.1   Acute Bronchospasm in Patients with Chronic Lung Disease

Because of the risk of acute bronchospasm, AFREZZA is contraindicated in patients with chronic lung disease such as asthma or COPD *[see Contraindications (4)]*.

Before initiating therapy with AFREZZA, evaluate all patients with a medical history, physical examination and spirometry (FEV$_1$) to identify potential underlying lung disease.

Acute bronchospasm has been observed following AFREZZA dosing in patients with asthma and patients with COPD. In a study of patients with asthma, bronchoconstriction and wheezing following AFREZZA dosing was reported in 29% (5 out of 17) and 0% (0 out of 13) of patients with and without a diagnosis of asthma, respectively. In this study, a mean decline in FEV$_1$ of 400 mL was observed 15 minutes after a single dose in patients with asthma. In a study of patients with COPD (n=8), a mean decline in FEV$_1$ of 200 mL was observed 18 minutes after a single dose of AFREZZA. The long-term safety and efficacy of AFREZZA in patients with chronic lung disease have not been established.

5.2   Changes in Insulin Regimen

Glucose monitoring is essential for patients receiving insulin therapy. Changes in insulin strength, manufacturer, type, or method of administration may affect glycemic con-

Table 1. Common Adverse Reactions in Patients with Type 2 Diabetes Mellitus (excluding Hypoglycemia) Treated with AFREZZA

	Placebo* (n = 290)	AFREZZA (n = 1991)	Non-placebo comparators (n=1363)
Cough	19.7%	25.6%	5.4%
Throat pain or irritation	3.8%	4.4%	0.9%
Headache	2.8%	3.1%	1.8%
Diarrhea	1.4%	2.7%	2.2%
Productive cough	1.0%	2.2%	0.9%
Fatigue	0.7%	2.0%	0.6%
Nausea	0.3%	2.0%	1.0%

*Carrier particle without insulin was used as placebo [Description (11)].

trol and predispose to hypoglycemia [see Warnings and Precautions (5.3)] or hyperglycemia. These changes should be made under close medical supervision and the frequency of blood glucose monitoring should be increased. Concomitant oral antidiabetic treatment may need to be adjusted.

5.3 Hypoglycemia

Hypoglycemia is the most common adverse reaction associated with insulins, including AFREZZA. Severe hypoglycemia can cause seizures, may be life-threatening, or cause death. Hypoglycemia can impair concentration ability and reaction time; this may place an individual and others at risk in situations where these abilities are important (e.g., driving or operating other machinery).

The timing of hypoglycemia usually reflects the time-action profile of the administered insulin formulation. AFREZZA has a distinct time action profile [see Clinical Pharmacology (12)], which impacts the timing of hypoglycemia. Hypoglycemia can happen suddenly and symptoms may differ across individuals and change over time in the same individual. Symptomatic awareness of hypoglycemia may be less pronounced in patients with longstanding diabetes, in patients with diabetic nerve disease, in patients using certain medications [see Drug Interactions (7)], or in patients who experience recurrent hypoglycemia. Other factors which may increase the risk of hypoglycemia include changes in meal pattern (e.g., macronutrient content or timing of meals), changes in level of physical activity, or changes to co-administered medication [see Drug Interactions (7)]. Patients with renal or hepatic impairment may be at higher risk of hypoglycemia [see Use in Specific Populations (8.5, 8.6)].

Risk Mitigation Strategies for Hypoglycemia

Patients and caregivers must be educated to recognize and manage hypoglycemia. Self-monitoring of blood glucose plays an essential role in the prevention and management of hypoglycemia. In patients at higher risk for hypoglycemia and patients who have reduced symptomatic awareness of hypoglycemia, increased frequency of blood glucose monitoring is recommended.

5.4 Decline in Pulmonary Function

AFREZZA causes a decline in lung function over time as measured by FEV_1. In clinical trials excluding patients with chronic lung disease and lasting up to 2 years, AFREZZA-treated patients experienced a small [40 mL (95% CI: -80, -1)] but greater FEV_1 decline than comparator-treated patients. The FEV_1 decline was noted within the first 3 months, and persisted for the entire duration of therapy (up to 2 years of observation). In this population, the annual rate of FEV_1 decline did not appear to worsen with increased duration of use. The effects of AFREZZA on pulmonary function for treatment duration longer than 2 years has not been established. There are insufficient data in long term studies to draw conclusions regarding reversal of the effect on FEV_1 after discontinuation of AFREZZA. The observed changes in FEV_1 were similar in patients with type 1 and type 2 diabetes.

Assess pulmonary function (e.g., spirometry) at baseline, after the first 6 months of therapy, and annually thereafter, even in the absence of pulmonary symptoms. In patients who have a decline of ≥ 20% in FEV_1 from baseline, consider discontinuing AFREZZA. Consider more frequent monitoring of pulmonary function in patients with pulmonary symptoms such as wheezing, bronchospasm, breathing difficulties, or persistent or recurring cough. If symptoms persist, discontinue AFREZZA. [see Adverse Reactions (6)].

5.5 Lung Cancer

In clinical trials, two cases of lung cancer, one in controlled trials and one in uncontrolled trials (2 cases in 2,750 patient-years of exposure), were observed in participants exposed to AFREZZA while no cases of lung cancer were observed in comparators (0 cases in 2,169 patient-years of exposure). In both cases, a prior history of heavy tobacco use was identified as a risk factor for lung cancer. Two additional cases of lung cancer (squamous cell) occurred in non-smokers exposed to AFREZZA and were reported by investigators after clinical trial completion. These data are insufficient to determine whether AFREZZA has an effect on lung or respiratory tract tumors. In patients with active lung cancer, a prior history of lung cancer, or in patients at risk for lung cancer, consider whether the benefits of AFREZZA use outweigh this potential risk.

5.6 Diabetic Ketoacidosis

In clinical trials enrolling subjects with type 1 diabetes, diabetic ketoacidosis (DKA) was more common in subjects receiving AFREZZA (0.43%; n=13) than in subjects receiving comparators (0.14%; n=3). In patients at risk for DKA, such as those with an acute illness or infection, increase the frequency of glucose monitoring and consider delivery of insulin using an alternate route of administration if indicated [see Limitations of Use (1)].

5.7 Hypersensitivity Reactions

Severe, life-threatening, generalized allergy, including anaphylaxis, can occur with insulin products, including AFREZZA. If hypersensitivity reactions occur, discontinue AFREZZA, treat per standard of care and monitor until symptoms and signs resolve [see Adverse Reactions (6)]. AFREZZA is contraindicated in patients who have had hypersensitivity reactions to AFREZZA or any of its excipients [see Contraindications (4)].

5.8 Hypokalemia

All insulin products, including AFREZZA, cause a shift in potassium from the extracellular to intracellular space, possibly leading to hypokalemia. Untreated hypokalemia may cause respiratory paralysis, ventricular arrhythmia, and death. Monitor potassium levels in patients at risk for hypokalemia (e.g., patients using potassium-lowering medications, patients taking medications sensitive to serum potassium concentrations and patients receiving intravenously administered insulin).

5.9 Fluid Retention and Heart Failure with Concomitant Use of PPAR-gamma Agonists

Thiazolidinediones (TZDs), which are peroxisome proliferator-activated receptor (PPAR)-gamma agonists, can cause dose-related fluid retention, particularly when used in combination with insulin. Fluid retention may lead to or exacerbate heart failure. Patients treated with insulin, including AFREZZA, and a PPAR-gamma agonist should be observed for signs and symptoms of heart failure. If heart failure develops, it should be managed according to current standards of care, and discontinuation or dose reduction of the PPAR-gamma agonist must be considered.

6 ADVERSE REACTIONS

The following serious adverse reactions are described below and elsewhere in the labeling:
- Acute bronchospasm in patients with chronic lung disease [see Warnings and Precautions (5.1)]
- Hypoglycemia [see Warnings and Precautions (5.3)]
- Decline in pulmonary function [see Warnings and Precautions (5.4)]
- Lung cancer [see Warnings and Precautions (5.5)]
- Diabetic ketoacidosis [see Warnings and Precautions (5.6)]
- Hypersensitivity reactions [see Warnings and Precautions (5.7)]

6.1 Clinical Trials Experience

Because clinical trials are conducted under widely varying designs, the incidence of adverse reactions reported in one clinical trial may not be easily compared to the incidence reported in another clinical trial, and may not reflect what is observed in clinical practice.

The data described below reflect exposure of 3017 patients to AFREZZA and include 1026 patients with type 1 diabetes and 1991 patients with type 2 diabetes. The mean exposure duration was 8.17 months for the overall population and 8.16 months and 8.18 months for type 1 and 2 diabetes patients, respectively. In the overall population, 1874 were exposed to AFREZZA for 6 months and 724 for greater than one year. 620 and 1254 patients with type 1 and type 2 diabetes, respectively, were exposed to AFREZZA for up to 6 months. 238 and 486 patients with type 1 and type 2 diabetes, respectively, were exposed to AFREZZA for greater than one year (median exposure = 1.8 years). AFREZZA was studied in placebo and active-controlled trials (n = 3 and n = 10, respectively).

The mean age of the population was 50.2 years and 20 patients were older than 75 years of age. 50.8% of the population were men; 82.6% were White, 1.8% were Asian, 4.9% were Black or African American. 9.7% were Hispanic. At baseline, the type 1 diabetes population had diabetes for an average of 16.6 years and had a mean HbA1c of 8.3%, and the type 2 diabetes population had diabetes for an average of 10.7 years and had a mean HbA1c of 8.8%. At baseline, 33.4% of the population reported peripheral neuropathy, 32.0% reported retinopathy and 19.6% had a history of cardiovascular disease.

Table 1 shows common adverse reactions, excluding hypoglycemia, associated with the use of AFREZZA in the pool of controlled trials in type 2 diabetes patients. These adverse reactions were not present at baseline, occurred more commonly on AFREZZA than on placebo and/or comparator and occurred in at least 2% of patients treated with AFREZZA. [See table 1 above]

Table 2 shows common adverse reactions, excluding hypoglycemia, associated with the use of AFREZZA in the pool of active-controlled trials in type 1 diabetes patients. These adverse reactions were not present at baseline, occurred more commonly on AFREZZA than on comparator, and occurred in at least 2% of patients treated with AFREZZA.

Table 2. Common Adverse Reactions in Patients with Type 1 Diabetes Mellitus (excluding Hypoglycemia) Treated with AFREZZA

	Subcutaneous Insulin (n = 835)	AFREZZA (n = 1026)
Cough	4.9%	29.4%
Throat pain or irritation	1.9%	5.5%
Headache	2.8%	4.7%
Pulmonary function test decreased	1.0%	2.8%
Bronchitis	2.0%	2.5%
Urinary tract infection	1.9%	2.3%

Hypoglycemia

Hypoglycemia is the most commonly observed adverse reaction in patients using insulin, including AFREZZA [see Warnings and Precautions (5.3)]. The incidence of severe and non-severe hypoglycemia of AFREZZA versus placebo in patients with type 2 diabetes is shown in Table 3. A hypoglycemic episode was recorded if a patient reported symptoms of hypoglycemia with or without a blood glucose value consistent with hypoglycemia. Severe hypoglycemia was defined as an event with symptoms consistent with hypoglycemia requiring the assistance of another person and associated with either a blood glucose value consistent with hypoglycemia or prompt recovery after treatment for hypoglycemia.

Table 3. Incidence of Severe and Non-Severe Hypoglycemia in a Placebo-Controlled Study of Patients with Type 2 Diabetes

	Placebo (n = 176)	AFREZZA (n = 177)
Severe Hypoglycemia	1.7%	5.1%
Non-Severe Hypoglycemia	30%	67%

Cough

Approximately 27% of patients treated with AFREZZA reported cough, compared to approximately 5.2% of patients treated with comparator. In clinical trials, cough was the most common reason for discontinuation of AFREZZA therapy (2.8% of AFREZZA-treated patients).

Pulmonary Function Decline

In clinical trials lasting up to 2 years, excluding patients with chronic lung disease, patients treated with AFREZZA had a 40 mL (95% CI: -80, -1) greater decline from baseline in forced expiratory volume in one second (FEV_1) compared to patients treated with comparator anti-diabetes treat-

ments. The decline occurred during the first 3 months of therapy and persisted over 2 years (Figure 2). A decline in FEV_1 of ≥ 15% occurred in 6% of AFREZZA-treated subjects compared to 3% of comparator-treated subjects.
[See figure 2 above]

Weight gain

Weight gain may occur with some insulin therapies, including AFREZZA. Weight gain has been attributed to the anabolic effects of insulin and the decrease in glycosuria. In a clinical trial of patients with type 2 diabetes [see Clinical Studies (14.3)], there was a mean 0.49 kg weight gain among AFREZZA-treated patients compared with a mean 1.13 kg weight loss among placebo-treated patients.

Antibody Production

Increases in anti-insulin antibody concentrations have been observed in patients treated with AFREZZA. Increases in anti-insulin antibodies are observed more frequently with AFREZZA than with subcutaneously injected mealtime insulins. Presence of antibody did not correlate with reduced efficacy, as measured by HbA1c and fasting plasma glucose, or specific adverse reactions.

7   DRUG INTERACTIONS

7.1   Drugs That May Increase the Risk of Hypoglycemia

The risk of hypoglycemia associated with AFREZZA use may be increased with antidiabetic agents, ACE inhibitors, angiotensin II receptor blocking agents, disopyramide, fibrates, fluoxetine, monoamine oxidase inhibitors, pentoxifylline, pramlintide, propoxyphene, salicylates, somatostatin analogs (e.g., octreotide), and sulfonamide antibiotics. Dose adjustment and increased frequency of glucose monitoring may be required when AFREZZA is co-administered with these drugs.

7.2   Drugs That May Decrease the Blood Glucose Lowering Effect of AFREZZA

The glucose lowering effect of AFREZZA may be decreased when co-administered with atypical antipsychotics (e.g., olanzapine and clozapine), corticosteroids, danazol, diuretics, estrogens, glucagon, isoniazid, niacin, oral contraceptives, phenothiazines, progestogens (e.g., in oral contraceptives), protease inhibitors, somatropin, sympathomimetic agents (e.g., albuterol, epinephrine, terbutaline) and thyroid hormones. Dose adjustment and increased frequency of glucose monitoring may be required when AFREZZA is co-administered with these drugs.

7.3   Drugs That May Increase or Decrease the Blood Glucose Lowering Effect of AFREZZA

The glucose lowering effect of AFREZZA may be increased or decreased when co-administered with alcohol, beta-blockers, clonidine, and lithium salts. Pentamidine may cause hypoglycemia, which may sometimes be followed by hyperglycemia. Dose adjustment and increased frequency of glucose monitoring may be required when AFREZZA is co-administered with these drugs.

7.4   Drugs That May Affect Hypoglycemia Signs and Symptoms

The signs and symptoms of hypoglycemia may be blunted when beta-blockers, clonidine, guanethidine, and reserpine are co-administered with AFREZZA.

8   USE IN SPECIFIC POPULATIONS

8.1   Pregnancy Teratogenic Effects: Pregnancy Category C

AFREZZA has not been studied in pregnant women. AFREZZA should not be used during pregnancy unless the potential benefit justifies the potential risk to the fetus.

In pregnant rats given subcutaneous doses of 10, 30, and 100 mg/kg/day of carrier particles (vehicle without insulin) from gestation day 6 through 17 (organogenesis), no major malformations were observed at up to 100 mg/kg/day (a systemic exposure 14-21 times the human systemic exposure, resulting from the maximum recommended daily dose of 99 mg AFREZZA based on AUC).

In pregnant rabbits given subcutaneous doses of 2, 10, and 100 mg/kg/day of carrier particles (vehicle without insulin) from gestation day 7 through 19 (organogenesis), adverse maternal effects were observed at all dose groups (at human systemic exposure following a 99 mg AFREZZA dose, based on AUC).

In pregnant rats given subcutaneous doses of 10, 30, and 100 mg/kg/day of carrier particles (vehicle without insulin) from gestation day 7 through lactation day 20 (weaning), decreased epididymis and testes weights, however, no decrease in fertility was noted, and impaired learning were observed in pups at ≥ 30 mg/kg/day (a systemic exposure 6 times human systemic exposure at the maximum daily AFREZZA dose of 99 mg based on AUC).

8.2   Nursing Mothers

Many drugs are excreted in human milk. A study in rats indicated that the carrier is excreted in milk at approximately 10% of maternal exposure levels. It is therefore highly likely that the insulin and carrier in AFREZZA is excreted in human milk. A decision should be made whether to discontinue nursing or suspend use of the drug since AFREZZA has not been studied in lactating women.

Figure 2. Mean (+/-SE) Change in FEV_1 (Liters) from Baseline for Type 1 and Type 2 Diabetes Patients

Visit						
Baseline	Month3	Month 6	Month 9	Month 12	Month 18	Month 24
(n1=1532)	(n1=1173)	(n1=1058)	(n1=454)	(n1=801)	(n1=507)	(n1=380)
(n2=1542)	(n2=1262)	(n2=1202)	(n2=519)	(n2=957)	(n2=674)	(n2=596)

8.3   Pediatric Use

AFREZZA has not been studied in patients younger than 18 years of age.

8.4   Geriatric Use

In the AFREZZA clinical studies, 381 patients were 65 years of age or older, of which 20 were 75 years of age or older. No overall differences in safety or effectiveness were observed between patients over 65 and younger patients. Pharmacokinetic/pharmacodynamic studies to assess the effect of age have not been conducted.

8.5   Hepatic Impairment

The effect of hepatic impairment on the pharmacokinetics of AFREZZA has not been studied. Frequent glucose monitoring and dose adjustment may be necessary for AFREZZA in patients with hepatic impairment [see Warnings and Precautions (5.3)].

8.6   Renal Impairment

The effect of renal impairment on the pharmacokinetics of AFREZZA has not been studied. Some studies with human insulin have shown increased circulating levels of insulin in patients with renal failure. Frequent glucose monitoring and dose adjustment may be necessary for AFREZZA in patients with renal impairment [see Warnings and Precautions (5.3)].

10   OVERDOSAGE

Excess insulin administration may cause hypoglycemia and hypokalemia [see Warnings and Precautions (5.3), (5.8)].

Mild episodes of hypoglycemia can usually be treated with oral glucose. Adjustments in drug dosage, meal patterns, or exercise, may be needed.

Severe episodes of hypoglycemia with coma, seizure, or neurologic impairment may be treated with intramuscular / subcutaneous glucagon or concentrated intravenous glucose. After apparent clinical recovery from hypoglycemia, continued observation and additional carbohydrate intake may be necessary to avoid recurrence of hypoglycemia. Hypokalemia must be corrected appropriately.

11   DESCRIPTION

11.1   AFREZZA Cartridges

AFREZZA consists of single-use plastic cartridges filled with a white powder containing insulin (human), which is administered via oral inhalation using the AFREZZA Inhaler only.

AFREZZA cartridges contain human insulin produced by recombinant DNA technology utilizing a non-pathogenic laboratory strain of Escherichia coli (K12). Chemically, human insulin has the empirical formula $C_{257}H_{383}N_{65}O_{77}S_6$ and a molecular weight of 5808. Human insulin has the following primary amino acid sequence:

[See chemical structure above]

Insulin is adsorbed onto carrier particles consisting of fumaryl diketopiperazine (FDKP) and polysorbate 80.

AFREZZA Inhalation Powder is a dry powder supplied as 4 unit or 8 unit cartridges. The 4 unit cartridge contains 0.35 mg of insulin. The 8 unit cartridge contains 0.7 mg of insulin.

11.2   AFREZZA Inhaler

The AFREZZA Inhaler is breath-powered by the patient. When the patient inhales through the device, the powder is aerosolized and delivered to the lung. The amount of AFREZZA delivered to the lung will depend on individual patient factors.

12   CLINICAL PHARMACOLOGY

12.1   Mechanism of Action

Insulin lowers blood glucose levels by stimulating peripheral glucose uptake by skeletal muscle and fat, and by inhibiting hepatic glucose production. Insulin inhibits lipolysis in adipocytes, inhibits proteolysis, and enhances protein synthesis.

12.2   Pharmacodynamics

The pharmacodynamic profile for orally inhaled AFREZZA 8 units relative to subcutaneously administered insulin lispro 8 units from a study in 12 patients with type 1 diabetes is shown in Figure 3(A). The median time to maximum effect of AFREZZA (measured by the peak rate of glucose infusion) was approximately 53 minutes (standard deviation of 74 minutes) and the effect then declined to near baseline levels by about 160 minutes.

[See figure 3 at top of next page]

12.3   Pharmacokinetics

The insulin contained in AFREZZA is regular human insulin. Following pulmonary absorption into systemic circulation, the metabolism and elimination are comparable to regular human insulin.

Absorption: The pharmacokinetic profiles for orally inhaled AFREZZA 8 units relative to subcutaneously admin-

Figure 3. Baseline-Corrected Glucose Infusion Rate (A) and Baseline-Corrected Serum Insulin Concentrations (B) after Administration of AFREZZA or Subcutaneous Insulin Lispro in Type 1 Diabetes Patients*

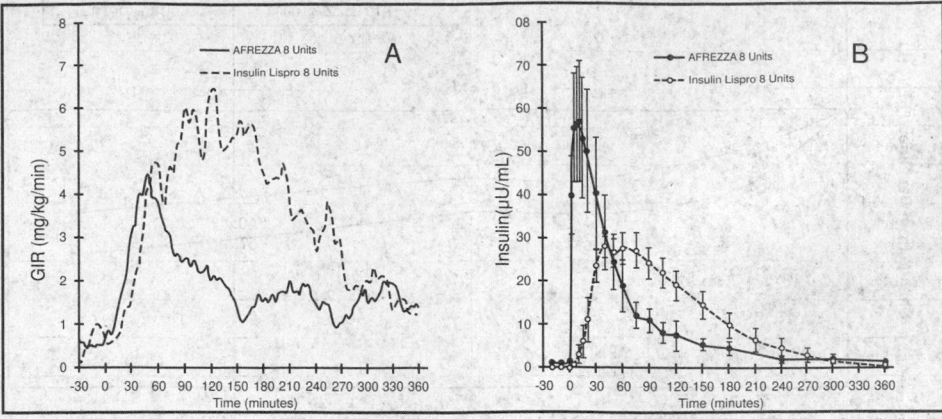

* Despite the faster absorption of insulin (PK) from Afrezza, the onset of activity (PD) was comparable to insulin lispro.

Table 4. Results at Week 24 in an Active-Controlled Study of Mealtime AFREZZA plus Basal Insulin in Adults with Type 1 Diabetes

Efficacy Parameter	AFREZZA + Basal Insulin	Insulin Aspart + Basal Insulin
	(N=174)	(N=170)
HbA$_{1c}$ (%)		
Baseline (adjusted mean[a])	7.94	7.92
Change from baseline (adjusted mean[a,b])	-0.21	-0.40
Difference from insulin aspart (adjusted mean[a,b]) (95% CI)	0.19 (0.02, 0.36)	
Percentage of patients achieving HbA1c ≤ 7%[c]	13.8	27.1
Fasting Plasma Glucose (mg/dL) Mean		
Baseline (adjusted mean[a])	153.9	151.6
Change from baseline (adjusted mean[a])[b]	-25.3	10.2
Difference from insulin aspart (adjusted mean[a,b]) (95% CI)	-35.4 (-56.3, -14.6)	

[a] Adjusted mean was obtained using a Mixed Model Repeated Measures (MMRM) approach with HbA1c or FPG as the dependent variable and treatment, visit, region, basal insulin stratum, and treatment by visit interaction as fixed factors, and corresponding baseline as a covariate. An autoregression (1) [AR(1)] covariance structure was used.

[b] Data at 24 weeks were available from 131 (75 %) and 150 (88%) subjects randomized to the AFREZZA and insulin aspart groups, respectively.

[c] The percentage was calculated based on the number of patients randomized to the trial.

istered insulin lispro 8 units from a study in 12 patients with type 1 diabetes are shown in Figure 3(B). The maximum serum insulin concentration was reached by 12-15 minutes after inhalation of AFREZZA 8 units and serum insulin concentrations declined to baseline by approximately 180 minutes. However, the faster absorption of insulin from Afrezza [see Figure 3(B)] did not result in a faster onset of activity compared to insulin lispro [see Figure 3(A)].

Disposition: Systemic insulin disposition (median terminal half-life) following oral inhalation of AFREZZA 4 and 32 units was 28-39 minutes, and 145 minutes for subcutaneous regular human insulin 15 units.

Carrier Particles
Clinical pharmacology studies showed that carrier particles [see Description (11)] are not metabolized and are eliminated unchanged in the urine following the lung absorption. Following oral inhalation of AFREZZA, a mean of 39% of the inhaled dose of carrier particles was distributed to the lungs and a mean of 7% of the dose was swallowed. The swallowed fraction was not absorbed from the GI tract and was eliminated unchanged in the feces.

Drug Interaction: Bronchodilators and Inhaled Steroids
Albuterol increased the AUC insulin administered by AFREZZA by 25% in patients with asthma. Effect of fluticasone on insulin exposures following AFREZZA administra-tion has not been evaluated in patients with asthma; however, no significant change in insulin exposure was observed in a study in healthy volunteers. Frequent glucose monitoring and dose reduction may be necessary for AFREZZA if it is co-administered with albuterol.

13 NONCLINICAL TOXICOLOGY

In a 104 week carcinogenicity study, rats were given doses up to 46 mg/kg/day of the carrier and up to 1.23 mg/kg/day of insulin, by nose-only inhalation. No increased incidence of tumors was observed at systemic exposures equivalent to the insulin at a maximum daily AFREZZA dose of 99 mg based on a comparison of relative body surface areas across species.

In a 26 week carcinogenicity study, transgenic mice (Tg-ras-H2) given doses up to 75 mg/kg/day of carrier and up to 5 mg/kg/day of AFREZZA. No increased incidence of tumors was observed.

AFREZZA was not genotoxic in Ames bacterial mutagenicity assay and in the chromosome aberration assay, using human peripheral lymphocytes with or without metabolic activation. The carrier alone was not genotoxic in the in vivo mouse micronucleus assay.

In female rats given subcutaneous doses of 10, 30, and 100 mg/kg/day of carrier (vehicle without insulin) beginning 2 weeks prior to mating until gestation day 7, there were no adverse effects on male fertility at doses up to 100 mg/kg/day (a systemic exposure 14-21 times that following the maximum daily AFREZZA dose of 99 mg based on AUC). In female rats there was increased pre- and post-implantation loss at 100 mg/kg/day but not at 30 mg/kg/day (14-21 times higher systemic exposure than the maximum daily AFREZZA dose of 99 mg based on AUC).

14 CLINICAL STUDIES

14.1 Overview of Clinical Studies of AFREZZA for Diabetes Mellitus
AFREZZA has been studied in adults with type 1 diabetes in combination with basal insulin. The efficacy of AFREZZA in type 1 diabetes patients was compared to insulin aspart in combination with basal insulin. AFREZZA has been studied in adults with type 2 diabetes in combination with oral antidiabetic drugs. The efficacy of AFREZZA in type 2 diabetes patients was compared to placebo inhalation.

14.2 Type 1 Diabetes
Patients with inadequately controlled type 1 diabetes participated in a 24-week, open-label, active-controlled study to evaluate the glucose lowering effect of mealtime AFREZZA used in combination with a basal insulin. Following a 4-week basal insulin optimization period, 344 patients were randomized to AFREZZA (n=174) or insulin aspart (n=170)administered at each meal of the day. Mealtime insulin doses were titrated to glycemic goals for the first 12 weeks and kept stable for the last 12 weeks of the study. At Week 24, treatment with basal insulin and mealtime AFREZZA provided a mean reduction in HbA1c that met the pre-specified non-inferiority margin of 0.4%. AFREZZA provided less HbA1c reduction than insulin aspart, and the difference was statistically significant. More subjects in the insulin aspart group achieved the HbA1c target of ≤7% (Table 4).
[See table 4 above]

14.3 Type 2 Diabetes
A total of 479 adult patients with type 2 diabetes inadequately controlled on optimal/maximally tolerated doses of metformin only, or 2 or more oral antidiabetic (OAD) agents participated in a 24-week, double-blind, placebo-controlled study. Following a 6-week run-in period, 353 patients were randomized to AFREZZA (n=177) or an inhaled placebo powder without insulin (n=176). Insulin doses were titrated for the first 12 weeks and kept stable for the last 12 weeks of the study. OADs doses were kept stable. At Week 24, treatment with AFREZZA plus OADs provided a mean reduction in HbA1c that was statistically significantly greater compared to the HbA1c reduction observed in the placebo group (Table 5).
[See table 5 at top of next page]

16 HOW SUPPLIED/STORAGE AND HANDLING

AFREZZA (insulin human) Inhalation Powder is available as 4 unit and 8 unit single-use cartridges. Three cartridges are contained in a single cavity of a blister strip. Each card contains 5 blister strips separated by perforations for a total of 15 cartridges. For convenience, the perforation allows users to remove a single strip containing 3 cartridges. Two cards of the same cartridge strength are packaged in a foil laminate overwrap (30 cartridges per foil package).

The cartridges are color-coded, blue for 4 units and green for 8 units. Each cartridge is marked with "afrezza" and "4 units" or "8 units".

The AFREZZA Inhaler is individually packaged in a translucent overwrap. The inhaler is fully assembled with a removable mouthpiece cover. The AFREZZA Inhaler can be used for up to 15 days from the date of first use. After 15 days of use, the inhaler must be discarded and replaced with a new inhaler.

AFREZZA is available in the following configurations:

• NDC 47918-004-02, AFREZZA (insulin human [rDNA origin]) Inhalation Powder:
  60 – 4 unit cartridges and 2 inhalers
• NDC 47918-004-03, AFREZZA (insulin human [rDNA origin]) Inhalation Powder:
  90 – 4 unit cartridges and 2 inhalers
• NDC 47918-008-03, AFREZZA (insulin human [rDNA origin]) Inhalation Powder:
  90 – 8 unit cartridges and 2 inhalers
• NDC 47918-048-21, AFREZZA (insulin human [rDNA origin]) Inhalation Powder:
  90 cartridges; 60 – 4 unit cartridges and 30 – 8 unit cartridges and 2 inhalers
• NDC 47918-084-21, AFREZZA (insulin human [rDNA origin]) Inhalation Powder:
  90 cartridges; 30 – 4 unit cartridges and 60 – 8 unit cartridges and 2 inhalers
• NDC 47918-840-33, AFREZZA (insulin human [rDNA origin]) Inhalation Powder:
  180 cartridges; 90 – 4 unit cartridges and 90 – 8 unit cartridges and 2 inhalers

Storage

Not in Use: Refrigerated Storage 2-8°C (36-46°F)

Sealed (Unopened) Foil Package	May be stored until the Expiration Date*

* If a foil package is not refrigerated, the contents must be used within 10 days.

In Use: Room Temperature Storage 25°C (77°F), excursions permitted 15-30°C (59-86°F)

Sealed (Unopened) Blister Cards + Strips	Must be used within 10 days
Opened Strips	Must be used within 3 days

Inhaler Storage:

Store at 2-25°C (36-77°F); excursions permitted. Inhaler may be stored refrigerated, but should be at room temperature before use.

Handling:

Before use, cartridges should be at room temperature for 10 minutes.

17 PATIENT COUNSELING INFORMATION

See FDA-approved patient labeling (Medication Guide)

Instructions

Instruct patients to read the Medication Guide before starting AFREZZA therapy and to reread it each time the prescription is renewed, because information may change. Instruct patients to inform their healthcare provider or pharmacist if they develop any unusual symptom, or if any known symptom persists or worsens.

Inform patients of the potential risks and benefits of AFREZZA and of alternative modes of therapy. Inform patients about the importance of adherence to dietary instructions, regular physical activity, periodic blood glucose monitoring and HbA1c testing, recognition and management of hypoglycemia and hyperglycemia, and assessment for diabetes complications. Advise patients to seek medical advice promptly during periods of stress such as fever, trauma, infection, or surgery, as medication requirements may change. Instruct patients to use AFREZZA only with the AFREZZA inhaler.

Inform patients that the most common adverse reactions associated with the use of AFREZZA are hypoglycemia, cough, and throat pain or irritation.

Advise women with diabetes to inform their physician if they are pregnant or are planning to become pregnant while using AFREZZA.

Acute Bronchospasm in Patients with Chronic Lung Disease

Advise patients to inform their physicians if they have a history of lung disease, because AFREZZA should not be used in patients with chronic lung disease (e.g., asthma, COPD, or other chronic lung disease(s)) *[see Contraindications (4) and Warnings and Precautions (5.1)]*.

Advise patients that if they experience any respiratory difficulty after inhalation of AFREZZA, they should report it to their physician immediately for assessment.

Hypoglycemia

Instruct patients on self-management procedures including glucose monitoring, proper inhalation technique, and management of hypoglycemia and hyperglycemia especially at initiation of AFREZZA therapy. Instruct patients on handling of special situations such as intercurrent conditions (illness, stress, or emotional disturbances), an inadequate or skipped insulin dose, inadvertent administration of an increased insulin dose, inadequate food intake, and skipped meals.

Instruct patients on the management of hypoglycemia. Inform patients that their ability to concentrate and react may be impaired as a result of hypoglycemia. Advise patients who have frequent hypoglycemia or reduced or absent warning signs of hypoglycemia to use caution when driving or operating machinery *[see Warnings and Precautions (5.3)]*.

Decline in Pulmonary Function and Monitoring

Inform patients that AFREZZA can cause a decline in lung function and their lung function will be evaluated by spirometry before initiation of AFREZZA treatment *[see Warnings and Precautions (5.4)]*.

Lung Cancer

Inform patients to promptly report any signs or symptoms potentially related to lung cancer *[see Warnings and Precautions (5.5)]*.

Table 5. Results at Week 24 in a Placebo-Controlled Study of AFREZZA in Adults with Type 2 Diabetes Inadequately Controlled on Oral Antidiabetic Agents

Efficacy Parameter	AFREZZA + Oral Anti-Diabetic Agents	Placebo + Oral Anti-Diabetic Agents
	(N=177)	(N=176)
HbA$_{1c}$ (%)		
Baseline (adjusted mean[a])	8.25	8.27
Change from baseline (adjusted mean[a,b])	-0.82	-0.42
Difference from placebo (adjusted mean[a,b]) (95% CI)	-0.40 (-0.57, -0.23)	
Percentage of patients achieving HbA$_{1c}$ ≤ 7%[c]	32.2	15.3
Fasting Plasma Glucose (mg/dL) Mean		
Baseline (adjusted mean[a])	175.9	175.2
Change from baseline (adjusted mean[a])[b]	-11.2	-3.8
Difference from placebo (adjusted mean[a,b]) (95% CI)	-7.4 (-18.0, 3.2)	

[a] Adjusted mean was obtained using a Mixed Model Repeated Measures (MMRM) approach with HbA1c or FPG as the dependent variable and treatment, visit, region, basal insulin stratum, and treatment by visit interaction as fixed factors, and corresponding baseline as a covariate. An autoregression (1) [AR(1)] covariance structure was used.
[b] Data at 24 weeks without rescue therapy were available from 139 (79%) and 129 (73%) subjects randomized to the AFREZZA and placebo groups, respectively.
[c] The percentage was calculated based on the number of patients randomized to the trial.

Diabetic Ketoacidosis

Instruct patients to carefully monitor their blood glucose during illness, infection, and other risk situations for diabetic ketoacidosis and to contact their healthcare provider if their blood glucose control worsens *[see Warnings and Precautions (5.6)]*.

Hypersensitivity Reactions

Advise patients that hypersensitivity reactions can occur with insulin therapy including AFREZZA. Inform patients on the symptoms of hypersensitivity reactions *[see Warnings and Precautions (5.7)]*.

Registered trademark owned by MannKind Corporation
Patented: http://www.mannkindcorp.com/our-technology-patent-notices.htm

Distributed by:
Sanofi-Aventis US LLC
Bridgewater, NJ 08807
A SANOFI COMPANY

Manufactured by:
MannKind Corporation
Danbury, CT 06810
06/2014

17.1 Medication Guide

Medication Guide

AFREZZA® (uh-FREZZ-uh)

(insulin human) inhalation powder

What is the most important information I should know about AFREZZA?

AFREZZA can cause serious side effects, including:

- Sudden lung problems (bronchospasms). Do not use AFREZZA if you have long-term (chronic) lung problems such as asthma or chronic obstructive pulmonary disease (COPD). Before starting AFREZZA, your healthcare provider will give you a breathing test to check how your lungs are working.

What is AFREZZA?

- AFREZZA is a man-made insulin that is breathed-in through your lungs (inhaled) and is used to control high blood sugar in adults with diabetes mellitus.
- AFREZZA is not for use in place of long-acting insulin. AFREZZA must be used with long-acting insulin in people who have type 1 diabetes mellitus.
- AFREZZA is not for use to treat diabetic ketoacidosis.
- It is not known if AFREZZA is safe and effective for use in people who smoke. AFREZZA is not for use in people who smoke or have recently stopped smoking (less than 6 months).

- It is not known if AFREZZA is safe and effective in children under 18 years of age.

Who should not use AFREZZA?

Do not use AFREZZA if you:

- have chronic lung problems such as asthma or COPD.
- are allergic to regular human insulin or any of the ingredients in AFREZZA. See the end of this Medication Guide for a complete list of ingredients in AFREZZA.

What should I tell my healthcare provider before using AFREZZA?

Before using AFREZZA, tell your healthcare provider about all your medical conditions, including if you:

- have lung problems such as asthma or COPD
- have or have had lung cancer
- are using any inhaled medications
- smoke or have recently stopped smoking
- have kidney or liver problems
- are pregnant, planning to become pregnant, or are breastfeeding. AFREZZA may harm your unborn or breastfeeding baby.

Tell your healthcare provider about all the medicines you take, including prescription and over-the-counter medicines, vitamins or herbal supplements.

Before you start using AFREZZA, talk to your healthcare provider about low blood sugar and how to manage it.

How should I use AFREZZA?

- Read the detailed **Instructions for Use** that comes with your AFREZZA.
- Take AFREZZA exactly as your healthcare provider tells you to. Your healthcare provider should tell you how much AFREZZA to use and when to use it.
- Know the strength of AFREZZA you use. **Do not** change the amount of AFREZZA you use unless your healthcare provider tells you to.
- Take AFREZZA at the beginning of your meal.
- **Check your blood sugar levels.** Ask your healthcare provider what your blood sugar should be and when you should check your blood sugar levels.
- **Keep AFREZZA and all medicines out of the reach of children.**

Your dose of AFREZZA may need to change because of:

- Change in level of physical activity or exercise, weight gain or loss, increased stress, illness, change in diet, or because of other medicines you take.

What should I avoid while using AFREZZA?

While using AFREZZA do not:

- drive or operate heavy machinery, until you know how AFREZZA affects you
- drink alcohol or use over-the-counter medicines that contain alcohol
- smoke

What are the possible side effects of AFREZZA?
AFREZZA may cause serious side effects that can lead to death, including:
See "What is the most important information I should know about AFREZZA?"

- **low blood sugar (hypoglycemia).** Signs and symptoms that may indicate low blood sugar include:
  - dizziness or light-headedness, sweating, confusion, headache, blurred vision, slurred speech, shakiness, fast heartbeat, anxiety, irritability or mood change, hunger.
- **decreased lung function.** Your healthcare provider should check how your lungs are working before you start using AFREZZA, 6 months after you start using it and yearly after that.
- **lung cancer.** In studies of AFREZZA in people with diabetes, lung cancer occurred in a few more people who were taking AFREZZA than in people who were taking other diabetes medications. There were too few cases to know if lung cancer was related to AFREZZA. If you have lung cancer, you and your healthcare provider should decide if you should use AFREZZA.
- **diabetic ketoacidosis.** Talk to your healthcare provider if you have an illness. Your AFREZZA dose or how often you check your blood sugar may need to be changed.
- **severe allergic reaction (whole body reaction). Get medical help right away if you have any of these signs or symptoms of a severe allergic reaction:**
  - a rash over your whole body, trouble breathing, a fast heartbeat, or sweating.
- **low potassium in your blood (hypokalemia).**
- **heart failure.** Taking certain diabetes pills called thiazolidinediones or "TZDs" with AFREZZA may cause heart failure in some people. This can happen even if you have never had heart failure or heart problems before. If you already have heart failure it may get worse while you take TZDs with AFREZZA. Your healthcare provider should monitor you closely while you are taking TZDs with AFREZZA. Tell your healthcare provider if you have any new or worse symptoms of heart failure including:
  - shortness of breath, swelling of your ankles or feet, sudden weight gain.

Treatment with TZDs and AFREZZA may need to be changed or stopped by your healthcare provider if you have new or worse heart failure.

Get emergency medical help if you have:
- trouble breathing, shortness of breath, fast heartbeat, swelling of your face, tongue, or throat, sweating, extreme drowsiness, dizziness, confusion.

The most common side effects of AFREZZA include:
- low blood sugar (hypoglycemia), cough, sore throat

These are not all the possible side effects of AFREZZA. Call your doctor for medical advice about side effects. You may report side effects to FDA at 1-800-FDA-1088 (1-800-332-1088).

General information about the safe and effective use of AFREZZA.
Medicines are sometimes prescribed for purposes other than those listed in a Medication Guide. Do not use AFREZZA for a condition for which it was not prescribed. Do not give AFREZZA to other people, even if they have the same symptoms that you have. It may harm them.

This Medication Guide summarizes the most important information about AFREZZA. If you would like more information, talk with your healthcare provider. You can ask your pharmacist or healthcare provider for information about AFREZZA that is written for health professionals. For more information, go to www.AFREZZA.com or call **Sanofi US 1-800-633-1610.**

What are the ingredients in AFREZZA?
Active ingredient: human insulin
Inactive ingredients: fumaryl diketopiperazine, polysorbate 80

Registered trademark owned by MannKind Corporation Patented: http://www.mannkindcorp.com/our-technology-patent-notices.htm

Distributed by:
Sanofi-Aventis US LLC
Bridgewater, NJ 08807
A SANOFI COMPANY

Manufactured by:
MannKind Corporation
Danbury, CT 06810

06/2014

17.2 Instruction for Use
Instructions for Use
AFREZZA® (uh-FREZZ-uh)
(insulin human) inhalation powder
Read this Instructions for Use before you start using AFREZZA and each time you get a new AFREZZA inhaler.

There may be new information. This information does not take the place of talking to your healthcare provider about your medical condition or your treatment.
Your healthcare provider should show you how to use your AFREZZA inhaler the right way before you use it for the first time.
Important information about AFREZZA:

- **AFREZZA comes in 2 strengths** (See Figure A):
  - 4 units (blue cartridge)
  - 8 units (green cartridge)

(Figure A)

- If your prescribed AFREZZA dose is higher than 8 units, you will need to use more than 1 cartridge.
- If you need to use more than 1 cartridge for your dose, throw away the used cartridge before getting a new one. You can tell when a cartridge has been used, because the cup has moved to the center.
- **Do not try to open the AFREZZA cartridges.** The AFREZZA Inhaler opens the cartridge automatically during use.
- **AFREZZA cartridges should only be used with the AFREZZA Inhaler. Do not** try to breathe in the AFREZZA insulin powder in any other way. **Do not** put cartridges in your mouth and **do not** swallow cartridges.
- Use only 1 AFREZZA Inhaler at a time. The same inhaler should be used for the 4 unit or 8 unit cartridges.
- Throw away your AFREZZA Inhaler after 15 days and get a new one.

If you are having problems with your AFREZZA inhaler or if it breaks and you need a new one, call 1-877-323-8505.
Know your AFREZZA® inhaler:

removable purple mouthpiece cover
white mouthpiece
cartridge
white cartridge cup
top of inhaler
purple base
bottom of inhaler

Know your AFREZZA® cartridges:

1 foil package   2 blister cards per package (5 strips per blister card)   3 cartridges per strip

There are two strengths of AFREZZA® cartridges:

One blue cartridge approximates 4 units of injected insulin.

One green cartridge approximates 8 units of injected insulin.

How to take your dose of AFREZZA:
Always be sure you have the right number of AFREZZA cartridges for your dose available before you start. AFREZZA cartridges must only be used with the AFREZZA Inhaler.

Step 1: Select the AFREZZA cartridges for your dose

 If your prescribed AFREZZA® dose is 4 units, use... 1 blue cartridge.

 If your prescribed AFREZZA® dose is 8 units, use... 1 green cartridge.

If your prescribed AFREZZA® dose is more than 8 units you will need to use **more than 1 cartridge** to get your right dose.

Use the dosage chart below to determine the least number of AFREZZA® cartridges you can use for your dose. Other cartridge combinations can be used.

AFREZZA® Dose	# of **4 unit** (blue) cartridges needed	# of **8 unit** (green) cartridges needed
4 units		
8 units		
12 units	+	
16 units		
20 units	+	
24 units		

(Figure B)

Example
If you need to take **12 units** of AFREZZA® you can use...

1 blue (4 unit) cartridge + 1 green (8 unit) cartridge

Select Cartridges
Important: Use the AFREZZA dose chart above (See Figure B) to help you choose the right number of AFREZZA cartridges needed for your dose.

Open Packages
Remove a blister card from the foil package. Tear along perforation to remove one strip.

Push Cartridges to Remove
Remove a cartridge from the strip by pressing on the clear side to push the cartridge out. Remove the right number of cartridges for your dose. Pushing on the cup will not damage the cartridge.
AFREZZA cartridges left over in an opened strip must be used within 3 days.

 Before use, cartridges and inhaler should be at room temperature for 10 minutes. ROOM TEMPERATURE 10 mins.

Before Proceeding:
Check that you have the right AFREZZA cartridge(s) for your dose.
Use only 1 inhaler for multiple cartridges. Throw away your AFREZZA inhaler after 15 days and get a new one.

Step 2: Loading a cartridge

Hold Inhaler
Hold the inhaler level in one (1) hand with the white mouthpiece on the top and purple base on the bottom.

Open Inhaler
Open the inhaler by lifting the white mouthpiece to a vertical position.
Before you put the AFREZZA cartridge in your inhaler, make sure it has been at **room temperature for 10 minutes.**

Place Cartridge
Hold the cartridge with the cup facing down. Line up the cartridge with the opening in the inhaler. The pointed end of the cartridge should line up with the pointed end in the inhaler. Place the cartridge into the inhaler. Be sure that the cartridge lies flat in the inhaler.

KEEP INHALER LEVEL

Keep Level Once Loaded!
Now that the cartridge is loaded, keep the inhaler level from this point forward to avoid loss of drug powder.

DO NOT turn inhaler upside down.

DO NOT point the mouthpiece down.

DO NOT shake or drop the inhaler.

This can result in loss of drug powder.

If any of these occur, throw away the cartridge and load a new cartridge.

Close Inhaler
Lower the mouthpiece to close the inhaler (this will open the drug cartridge).
You should feel a snap when the inhaler is closed.

Step 3: Inhaling AFREZZA

Remove the Mouthpiece Cover
Important: Keep the inhaler level during and after removal of the purple mouthpiece cover.

Check that you are ready to inhale:
- ✓ Purple mouthpiece cover is removed.
- ✓ Inhaler is held level.
- ✓ Fully review the following A-B-C steps prior to beginning the inhale process.

A

Exhale
Hold the inhaler away from your mouth and fully blow out (exhale).

B

Position Inhaler in Mouth
Keeping your head level, place the mouthpiece in your mouth and **tilt the inhaler down towards your chin, as shown.**
Close your lips around the mouthpiece to form a seal.
Tilt the inhaler downward while keeping your head level.

C

Inhale Deeply and Hold Breath
With your mouth closed around the mouthpiece, **inhale deeply through the inhaler.**
Hold your breath for as long as comfortable and at the same time remove the inhaler from your mouth. After holding your breath, exhale and continue to breathe normally.

Step 4: Removing a used cartridge

Replace Mouthpiece Cover
Place the purple mouthpiece cover back onto the inhaler.

Open Inhaler
Open the inhaler by lifting up the white mouthpiece.

Remove Cartridge
Remove the cartridge from the purple base.

TRASH

Throw away the Cartridge
Throw away the used cartridge in your regular household trash.

Multiple cartridge dosing

If you need more than one (1) AFREZZA cartridge for your dose, See the AFREZZA dosage chart above (Figure B).

Repeat steps 2 through 4 for each AFREZZA cartridge you need for your prescribed AFREZZA dose.

⚠ Be careful not to mix NEW cartridges with USED cartridges.

✓ NEW

⊘ USED

The white cup moves to the middle of the cartridge when it has been used.

How should I store AFREZZA?

Not In Use: Refrigerated Storage
Sealed Foil Packages
Store unopened drug in a refrigerator 36 – 46°F (2 – 8°C).

	Refrigerated
Sealed (Unopened)	May be used until the **Expiration Date***

*If a foil package is not refrigerated, the contents must be used within 10 days.

In Use: Room Temperature Storage
Opened Foil Packages
Once a foil package has been opened, see chart below...

		Room Temperature
Blister Cards + Strips	Sealed (Unopened)	Must be used **within 10 Days**
Strips	Opened	Must be used **within 3 Days**

⚠ Before use, cartridges and inhaler should be at room temperature for 10 minutes. ROOM TEMPERATURE 10 mins.

Caring for your AFREZZA inhaler:
Storage Instructions
Once you have taken your full dose, make sure the purple mouthpiece cover has been replaced and the inhaler is closed.

- **Keep the inhaler in a clean, dry place** with the mouthpiece cover on until your next dose.
- May be stored refrigerated, but must be at room temperature before use.
- Never leave or store cartridges in the inhaler.
- Keep out of reach of children.

Care Instructions

CALENDAR
EVERY 15 DAYS

- **Use one inhaler at a time. The same inhaler should be used to take 4 unit or 8 unit cartridges. Rplace the inhaler every 15 days to maintain drug delivery**
Keep track of 15 days from when you start using the inhaler with a calendar, or use the chart on the back of the inhaler box.
- After taking your dose, powder residue in the mouthpiece is normal, this does not affect your dose.
The outside of the inhaler can be wiped with a clean, dry cloth if needed. Never wash the inhaler. Keep it dry.

[See table at top of next page]

Switching between AFREZZA and injected insulin:

Contact your healthcare provide before switching insulins.
AFREZZA® is a mealtime insulin.
Do not switch from AFREZZA to a long acting insulin.
Do not switch from a long acting insulin to AFREZZA®.

This Medication Guide and Instructions for Use has been approved by the U.S. Food and Drug Administration.
Patented: See http://www.mannkindcorp.com/our-technology-patent-notices.htm

Distributed by:
Sanofi-Aventis US LLC
Bridgewater, NJ 08807
A SANOFI COMPANY

Manufactured by:
MannKind Corporation
Danbury, CT 06810

06/2014

Shown in Product Identification Guide, page 307

Merck

ONE MERCK DRIVE
P.O. BOX 100
WHITEHOUSE STATION, NJ 08889-0100 USA

For updates to the product information listed below, please check the Merck Web site, http://www.merck.com.

U.S. Healthcare Professionals
To speak with a Merck health care professional about Merck products or to report an adverse experience with a specific Merck product, please call the Merck National Service Center at (800) 444-2080. The Merck National Service Center is pleased to assist you Monday through Friday from 8 AM to 7 PM ET.

Adverse experiences and product-related emergencies can be reported at any time by dialing (800) 444-2080.

Merck U.S. operating companies include: Merck, Sharp & Dohme Corp.

AMINOHIPPURATE SODIUM "PAH" R_x
[am-ino-hip-pur-ate]
Injection

DESCRIPTION

Aminohippurate sodium[1] is an agent to measure effective renal plasma flow (ERPF). It is the sodium salt of para-aminohippuric acid, commonly abbreviated "PAH". It is water soluble, lipid-insoluble, and has a pKa of 3.83. The empirical formula of the anhydrous salt is $C_9H_9N_2NaO_3$ and its structural formula is:

$$H_2N-\text{—}-CONHCH_2COONa$$

It is provided as a sterile, non-preserved 20 percent aqueous solution for injection, with a pH of 6.7 to 7.6. Each 10 mL contains: Aminohippurate sodium 2 g. Inactive ingredients: Sodium hydroxide to adjust pH, water for injection, q.s.

---

[1] Formerly referred to as Sodium para-Aminohippurate.

CLINICAL PHARMACOLOGY

PAH is filtered by the glomeruli and is actively secreted by the proximal tubules. At low plasma concentrations (1.0 to 2.0 mg/100 mL), an average of 90 percent of PAH is cleared by the kidneys from the renal blood stream in a single circulation. It is ideally suited for measurement of ERPF since it has a high clearance, is essentially nontoxic at the plasma concentrations reached with recommended doses, and its analytical determination is relatively simple and accurate. PAH is also used to measure the functional capacity of the renal tubular secretory mechanism or transport maximum (Tm_{PAH}). This is accomplished by elevating the plasma concentration to levels (40-60 mg/100 mL) sufficient to saturate the maximal capacity of the tubular cells to secrete PAH. Inulin clearance is generally measured during Tm_{PAH} determinations since glomerular filtration rate (GFR) must be known before calculations of secretory Tm measurements can be done (see DOSAGE AND ADMINISTRATION, Calculations).

INDICATIONS AND USAGE

Estimation of effective renal plasma flow.
Measurement of the functional capacity of the renal tubular secretory mechanism.

CONTRAINDICATIONS

Hypersensitivity to this product or to its components.

PRECAUTIONS

General
Intravenous solutions must be given with caution to patients with low cardiac reserve, since a rapid increase in plasma volume can precipitate congestive heart failure.
For measurement of ERPF, small doses of PAH are used. However, in research procedures to measure Tm_{PAH}, high plasma levels are required to saturate the capacity of the tubular cells. During these procedures, the intravenous administration of PAH solutions should be carried out slowly and with caution. The patient should be continuously observed for any adverse reactions.
Use caution when injecting this product into latex-sensitive individuals, since the vial stopper contains dry natural latex rubber that may cause allergic reactions.

Drug Interactions
Renal clearance measurements of PAH cannot be made with any significant accuracy in patients receiving sulfonamides, procaine, or thiazolesulfone. These compounds interfere with chemical color development essential to the analytical procedures.
Probenecid depresses tubular secretion of certain weak acids such as PAH. Therefore, patients receiving probenecid will have erroneously low ERPF and Tm_{PAH} values.

Carcinogenesis, Mutagenesis, Impairment of Fertility
Long-term studies in animals have not been done to evaluate any effects upon fertility or carcinogenic potential of PAH.

Pregnancy
Pregnancy Category C
Animal reproduction studies have not been done with PAH. It is also not known whether PAH can cause fetal harm when given to a pregnant woman or can affect reproduction capacity. PAH should be given to a pregnant woman only if clearly needed.

Nursing Mothers
It is not known whether this drug is excreted in human milk. Because many drugs are excreted in human milk, caution should be exercised when PAH is administered to a nursing woman.

Pediatric Use
Safety and effectiveness in pediatric patients have not been established.

Geriatric Use
Clinical studies of PAH did not include sufficient numbers of subjects aged 65 and over to determine whether they respond differently from younger subjects. Other reported clinical experience has not identified differences in responses between the elderly and younger patients.

ADVERSE REACTIONS

Hypersensitivity reactions including anaphylaxis, angioedema, urticaria, vasomotor disturbances, flushing, tingling, nausea, vomiting, and cramps may occur.
Patients may have a sensation of warmth or the desire to defecate or urinate during or shortly following initiation of infusion.

OVERDOSE

The intravenous LD_{50} in female mice is 7.22 g/kg.

DOSAGE AND ADMINISTRATION

For intravenous use only
Clearance measurements using single injection techniques are generally inaccurate, particularly in the measurement of ERPF. For this reason, intravenous infusions at fixed rates are used to sustain the plasma PAH concentration at the desired level.
To measure ERPF, the concentration of PAH in the plasma should be maintained at 2 mg per 100 mL, which can be achieved with a priming dose of 6 to 10 mg/kg and an infusion dose of 10 to 24 mg/min.
As a research procedure for the measurement of Tm_{PAH}, the plasma level of PAH must be sufficient to saturate the capacity of the tubular secretory cells. Concentrations from 40 to 60 mg per 100 mL are usually necessary.
Technical details of these tests may be found in Smith {1}; Wesson {2}; Bauer {3}; Pitts{4}; and Schnurr {5}.
Parenteral drug products should be inspected visually for particulate matter and discoloration prior to use, whenever solution and container permit. NOTE: The normal color range for this product is a colorless to yellow/brown solution. The efficacy is not affected by color changes within this range.

Calculations
Effective Renal Plasma Flow (ERPF)
The clearance of PAH, which is extracted almost completely from the plasma during its passage through the renal circulation, constitutes a measure of ERPF. Hence:
$ERPF = U_{PAH}V/P_{PAH}$
Where U_{PAH} = concentration of PAH (mg/mL) in the urine
V = rate of urine excretion (mL/min), and
P_{PAH} = plasma concentration of PAH (mg/mL).
Example:
$U_{PAH} = 8.0$ mg/mL
$V = 1.5$ mL/min
$P_{PAH} = 0.02$ mg/mL
$ERPF = 8.0 \times 1.5/0.02 = 600$ mL/min
Based on PAH clearance studies, the normal values for ERPF are:
men 675 ± 150 mL/min
women 595 ± 125 mL/min
Maximum Tubular Secretory
(Tm_{PAH}) Mechanism
The quantity of PAH secreted by the tubules (Tm_{PAH}) is given by the difference between the total rate of excretion ($U_{PAH}V$) and the quantity filtered by the glomeruli (GFR × P_{PAH}). Hence:
$Tm_{PAH} = U_{PAH}V - (GFR \times P_{PAH} \times 0.83)$
The factor, 0.83, corrects for that portion of PAH which is bound to plasma protein and hence is unfilterable.
Example:
$U_{PAH} = 9.55$ mg/mL
$V = 16.68$ mL/min
$GFR = 120$ mL/min
$P_{PAH} = 0.60$ mg/mL
Then $Tm_{PAH} = 9.55 \times 16.68 - (120 \times 0.60 \times 0.83) = 100$ mg/min.
Average normal values of Tm_{PAH} are 80-90 mg/min.
The value of the expression $U_{PAH}V$, used in calculations of ERPF and Tm_{PAH}, may be found by determining the amount of PAH in a measured volume of urine excreted within a specific period of time.
These calculations are based on a body surface area of 1.73 m². Corrections for variations in surface area are made by multiplying the values obtained for ERPF and Tm_{PAH} by 1.73/A, where A is the subject surface area.

HOW SUPPLIED

No. 95 — Aminohippurate Sodium, 20 percent sterile solution for intravenous injection, is supplied as follows:
NDC 0006-3395-11 in 10 mL vials.
Storage
Store at 25°C (77°F); excursions permitted to 15-30°C (59-86°F) [see USP Controlled Room Temperature].

REFERENCES

1. Smith, H.W.: Lectures on the kidney, University Extension Division, University of Kansas, Lawrence, Kansas, 1943.
2. Wesson, L.G., Jr.: "Physiology of the Human Kidney," New York, Grune & Stratton, 1969, pp. 632-655.
3. Bauer, J.D.; Ackermann, P.G.; Toro, G.: "Brays Clinical Laboratory Methods," ed. 7, St. Louis, Mosby, 1968.
4. Pitts, R.F.: "Physiology of the Kidney and Body Fluids," ed. 2, Chicago, Year Book Medical Publishers, 1968.
5. Schnurr, E.; Lahme, W.; Kuppers, H.: Measurement of renal clearance of inulin and PAH in the steady state without urine collection; Clinical Nephrology, *13*(1): (26-29), 1980.

Merck Sharp & Dohme Corp., a subsidiary of
MERCK & CO., INC., Whitehouse Station, NJ 08889, USA
Issued January 2011
Printed in USA
9051026
Copyright © 1983 Merck Sharp & Dohme Corp., a subsidiary of **Merck & Co., Inc.**
All rights reserved

ASMANEX TWISTHALER   ℞

[ăs-măn-ĕcks]
110 mcg, 220 mcg
(mometasone furoate inhalation powder)

HIGHLIGHTS OF PRESCRIBING INFORMATION

These highlights do not include all the information needed to use ASMANEX TWISTHALER safely and effectively. See full prescribing information for ASMANEX TWISTHALER.
ASMANEX TWISTHALER 110 mcg, 220 mcg (mometasone furoate inhalation powder)
Initial U.S. Approval: 1987

——INDICATIONS AND USAGE——

ASMANEX TWISTHALER is a corticosteroid indicated for:
• Maintenance treatment of asthma as prophylactic therapy in patients 4 years of age and older. (1.1)
ASMANEX TWISTHALER is NOT indicated for the relief of acute bronchospasm (1.1, 5.2) or in children less than 4 years of age. (1.1, 8.4).

——DOSAGE AND ADMINISTRATION——

• FOR ORAL INHALATION ONLY. (2)
• Instruct patients to inhale rapidly and deeply and to rinse mouth after inhalation. (2)
[See table above]

——DOSAGE FORMS AND STRENGTHS——

• 220 mcg TWISTHALER: delivers 200 mcg mometasone furoate per actuation. (3)
• 110 mcg TWISTHALER: delivers 100 mcg mometasone furoate per actuation. (3)

——CONTRAINDICATIONS——

• Patients with status asthmaticus or other acute episodes of asthma where intensive measures are required. (4.1)
• Patients with a *known* hypersensitivity to milk proteins or any ingredients of ASMANEX TWISTHALER. (4.2)

——WARNINGS AND PRECAUTIONS——

• *Candida albicans* infection of the mouth and pharynx. Monitor patients periodically for signs of adverse effects in the mouth and pharynx.
  Advise patients to rinse mouth after inhalation. (5.1)
• Deterioration of asthma or acute episodes: ASMANEX TWISTHALER should not be used for relief of acute symptoms. Patients require immediate re-evaluation during rapidly deteriorating asthma. (5.2)
• Hypersensitivity reactions including anaphylaxis, angioedema, pruritus, and rash have been reported with the use of ASMANEX TWISTHALER. Discontinue ASMANEX TWISTHALER if such reactions occur. (5.3)
• Potential worsening of existing tuberculosis; fungal, bacterial, viral, or parasitic infection; or ocular herpes simplex. More serious or even fatal course of chickenpox or measles in susceptible patients. Use caution in patients with the above because of the potential for worsening of these infections. (5.4)
• Risk of impaired adrenal function when transferring from oral steroids to inhaled corticosteroids. Taper patients slowly from systemic corticosteroids if transferring to ASMANEX TWISTHALER. (5.5)

Recommended Dosages for ASMANEX TWISTHALER Treatment

Previous Therapy	Recommended Starting Dose	Highest Recommended Daily Dose
Patients ≥12 years who received bronchodilators alone	220 mcg once daily in the evening*	440 mcg†
Patients ≥12 years who received inhaled corticosteroids	220 mcg once daily in the evening*	440 mcg†
Patients ≥12 years who received oral corticosteroids‡	440 mcg twice daily	880 mcg
Children 4-11 years of age§	110 mcg once daily in the evening*	110 mcg*

*,†,‡,§Please refer to section 2.1 for full dosage recommendations and details.

• Hypercorticism, suppression of hypothalamic-pituitary-adrenal (HPA) function, with very high dosages or at the regular dosage in susceptible individuals. If such changes occur discontinue ASMANEX TWISTHALER slowly. (5.6)
• Reduction in bone mineral density with long-term administration. Monitor patients with major risk factors for decreased bone mineral content. (5.7)
• Suppression of growth in children. Monitor growth routinely in pediatric patients receiving ASMANEX TWISTHALER. (5.8)
• Development of glaucoma, increased intraocular pressure, and posterior subcapsular cataracts. Monitor patients with a change in vision or with a history of increased intraocular pressure, glaucoma, and/or cataracts closely. (5.9)
• Paradoxical bronchospasm may occur with ASMANEX TWISTHALER. Treat bronchospasm immediately with a fast-acting inhaled bronchodilator and discontinue use of ASMANEX TWISTHALER. (5.10)

——ADVERSE REACTIONS——

The most common adverse reactions (incidence ≥5%) are headache, allergic rhinitis, pharyngitis, upper respiratory tract infection, sinusitis, oral candidiasis, dysmenorrhea, musculoskeletal pain, back pain, and dyspepsia. (6.1)
To report SUSPECTED ADVERSE REACTIONS, contact Merck Sharp & Dohme Corp., a subsidiary of Merck & Co., Inc., at 1-877-888-4231 or FDA at 1-800-FDA-1088 or www.fda.gov/medwatch.
See 17 for PATIENT COUNSELING INFORMATION and FDA-approved patient labeling

Revised: 01/2013

FULL PRESCRIBING INFORMATION: CONTENTS*

1   **INDICATIONS AND USAGE**
    1.1   Treatment of Asthma
2   **DOSAGE AND ADMINISTRATION**
    2.1   Recommended Dosages in Patients 4 Years of Age and Older
3   **DOSAGE FORMS AND STRENGTHS**
4   **CONTRAINDICATIONS**
    4.1   Status Asthmaticus
    4.2   Hypersensitivity
5   **WARNINGS AND PRECAUTIONS**
    5.1   Local Effects
    5.2   Acute Asthma Episodes
    5.3   Hypersensitivity Reactions Including Anaphylaxis
    5.4   Immunosuppression
    5.5   Transferring Patients from Systemic Corticosteroid Therapy
    5.6   Hypercorticism and Adrenal Suppression
    5.7   Reduction in Bone Mineral Density
    5.8   Effect on Growth
    5.9   Glaucoma and Cataracts
    5.10   Paradoxical Bronchospasm
6   **ADVERSE REACTIONS**
    6.1   Clinical Studies Experience
    6.2   Postmarketing Experience
7   **DRUG INTERACTIONS**
    7.1   Inhibitors of Cytochrome P450 3A4
8   **USE IN SPECIFIC POPULATIONS**
    8.1   Pregnancy
    8.3   Nursing Mothers
    8.4   Pediatric Use
    8.5   Geriatric Use
    8.6   Hepatic Impairment
10   **OVERDOSAGE**
11   **DESCRIPTION**
12   **CLINICAL PHARMACOLOGY**
    12.1   Mechanism of Action
    12.2   Pharmacodynamics
    12.3   Pharmacokinetics
13   **NONCLINICAL TOXICOLOGY**
    13.1   Carcinogenesis, Mutagenesis, Impairment of Fertility
    13.2   Animal Toxicology and/or Pharmacology
14   **CLINICAL STUDIES**
    14.1   Asthma
16   **HOW SUPPLIED/STORAGE AND HANDLING**
17   **PATIENT COUNSELING INFORMATION**
    17.1   Oral Candidiasis
    17.2   Acute Asthma Episodes
    17.3   Hypersensitivity Reactions Including Anaphylaxis
    17.4   Immunosuppression
    17.5   Hypercorticism and Adrenal Suppression
    17.6   Reduction in Bone Mineral Density
    17.7   Reduced Growth Velocity
    17.8   Use Daily for Best Effect
    17.9   Instructions for Use
* Sections or subsections omitted from the full prescribing information are not listed

---

FULL PRESCRIBING INFORMATION

1   INDICATIONS AND USAGE

1.1   Treatment of Asthma
ASMANEX® TWISTHALER® is indicated for the maintenance treatment of asthma as prophylactic therapy in patients 4 years of age and older.
Important Limitations of Use
ASMANEX TWISTHALER is NOT indicated for the relief of acute bronchospasm.
ASMANEX TWISTHALER is NOT indicated in children less than 4 years of age.

2   DOSAGE AND ADMINISTRATION

Administer ASMANEX TWISTHALER by the orally inhaled route only. Instruct patients to inhale rapidly and deeply. Advise patients to rinse the mouth after inhalation. Individual patients will experience a variable time to onset and degree of symptom relief. Maximum benefit may not be achieved for 1 to 2 weeks or longer after initiation of treatment. After asthma stability has been achieved, it is desirable to titrate to the lowest effective dosage to reduce the possibility of side effects. For patients ≥12 years of age who do not respond adequately to the starting dose after 2 weeks of therapy, higher doses may provide additional asthma control. The safety and efficacy of ASMANEX TWISTHALER when administered in excess of recommended doses have not been established.
2.1   Recommended Dosages in Patients 4 Years of Age and Older
The recommended starting doses and highest recommended daily dose for ASMANEX TWISTHALER treatment based on prior asthma therapy are provided in **Table 1**.
[See table 1 at top of next page]

3   DOSAGE FORMS AND STRENGTHS

ASMANEX TWISTHALER is a dry powder for inhalation that is available in 2 strengths.
ASMANEX TWISTHALER 220 mcg delivers 200 mcg mometasone furoate per actuation from the mouthpiece.
ASMANEX TWISTHALER 110 mcg delivers 100 mcg mometasone furoate per actuation from the mouthpiece.

4   CONTRAINDICATIONS

4.1   Status Asthmaticus
ASMANEX TWISTHALER therapy is contraindicated in the primary treatment of status asthmaticus or other acute episodes of asthma where intensive measures are required.
4.2   Hypersensitivity
ASMANEX TWISTHALER is contraindicated in patients with *known* hypersensitivity to milk proteins or any ingredients of ASMANEX TWISTHALER [see Warnings and Precautions (5.3) and Description (11)].

Table 1: Recommended Dosages for ASMANEX TWISTHALER Treatment

Previous Therapy	Recommended Starting Dose	Highest Recommended Daily Dose
Patients ≥12 years who received bronchodilators alone	220 mcg once daily in the evening*	440 mcg†
Patients ≥12 years who received inhaled corticosteroids	220 mcg once daily in the evening*	440 mcg†
Patients ≥12 years who received oral corticosteroids‡	440 mcg twice daily	880 mcg
Children 4-11 years of age§	110 mcg once daily in the evening*	110 mcg*

* When administered once daily, ASMANEX TWISTHALER should be taken only in the evening.
† The 440 mcg daily dose may be administered in divided doses of 220 mcg twice daily or as 440 mcg once daily.
‡ **For Patients Currently Receiving Chronic Oral Corticosteroid Therapy:** Prednisone should be reduced no faster than 2.5 mg/day on a weekly basis, beginning after at least 1 week of ASMANEX TWISTHALER therapy. Monitor patients carefully for signs of asthma instability, including serial objective measures of airflow, and for signs of adrenal insufficiency during steroid taper and following discontinuation of oral corticosteroid therapy *[see Warnings and Precautions (5.5)]*.
§ Recommended pediatric dosage is 110 mcg once daily in the evening regardless of prior therapy.

5 WARNINGS AND PRECAUTIONS

5.1 Local Effects
In clinical trials, the development of localized infections of the mouth and pharynx with *Candida albicans* occurred in 195 of 3007 patients treated with ASMANEX TWISTHALER. If oropharyngeal candidiasis develops, it should be treated with appropriate local or systemic (i.e., oral) antifungal therapy while remaining on treatment with ASMANEX TWISTHALER therapy, but at times therapy with the ASMANEX TWISTHALER may need to be interrupted. Advise patients to rinse the mouth after inhalation of ASMANEX TWISTHALER.

5.2 Acute Asthma Episodes
ASMANEX TWISTHALER is not a bronchodilator and is not indicated for rapid relief of bronchospasm or other acute episodes of asthma. Instruct patients to contact their physician immediately if episodes of asthma that are not responsive to bronchodilators occur during the course of treatment with ASMANEX TWISTHALER. During such episodes, patients may require therapy with oral corticosteroids.

5.3 Hypersensitivity Reactions Including Anaphylaxis
Hypersensitivity reactions including rash, pruritus, angioedema, and anaphylactic reaction have been reported with use of ASMANEX TWISTHALER. Discontinue ASMANEX TWISTHALER if such reactions occur *[see Contraindications (4.2) and Postmarketing Experience (6.2)]*.
ASMANEX TWISTHALER contains small amounts of lactose, which contains trace levels of milk proteins. In postmarketing experience with ASMANEX TWISTHALER, anaphylactic reactions in patients with milk protein allergy have been reported *[see Contraindications (4.2) and Postmarketing Experience (6.2)]*.

5.4 Immunosuppression
Persons who are using drugs that suppress the immune system are more susceptible to infections than healthy individuals. Chickenpox and measles, for example, can have a more serious or even fatal course in susceptible children or adults using corticosteroids. In such children or adults who have not had these diseases or who are not properly immunized, particular care should be taken to avoid exposure. How the dose, route, and duration of corticosteroid administration affect the risk of developing a disseminated infection is not known. The contribution of the underlying disease and/or prior corticosteroid treatment to the risk is also not known. If exposed to chickenpox, prophylaxis with varicella zoster immune globulin (VZIG) may be indicated. If exposed to measles, prophylaxis with pooled intramuscular immunoglobulin (IG) may be indicated. (See the respective package inserts for complete VZIG and IG prescribing information.) If chickenpox develops, treatment with antiviral agents may be considered.
Inhaled corticosteroids should be used with caution, if at all, in patients with active or quiescent tuberculosis infection of the respiratory tract; untreated systemic fungal, bacterial, viral, or parasitic infections; or ocular herpes simplex.

5.5 Transferring Patients from Systemic Corticosteroid Therapy
Particular care is needed for patients who are transferred from systemically active corticosteroids to ASMANEX TWISTHALER because deaths due to adrenal insufficiency have occurred in asthmatic patients during and after transfer from systemic corticosteroids to less systemically available inhaled corticosteroids. After withdrawal from systemic corticosteroids, a number of months are required for recovery of hypothalamic-pituitary-adrenal (HPA) function. Patients who have been previously maintained on 20 mg or more per day of prednisone (or its equivalent) may be most susceptible, particularly when their systemic corticosteroids

have been almost completely withdrawn. During this period of HPA suppression, patients may exhibit signs and symptoms of adrenal insufficiency when exposed to trauma, surgery, or infection (particularly gastroenteritis) or other conditions associated with severe electrolyte loss. Although ASMANEX TWISTHALER may improve control of asthma symptoms during these episodes, in recommended doses it supplies less than normal physiological amounts of corticosteroid systemically and does NOT provide the mineralocorticoid activity necessary for coping with these emergencies. During periods of stress or severe asthma attack, patients who have been withdrawn from systemic corticosteroids should be instructed to resume oral corticosteroids (in large doses) immediately and to contact their physicians for further instruction. These patients should also be instructed to carry a medical identification card indicating that they may need supplementary systemic corticosteroids during periods of stress or severe asthma attack.
Patients requiring oral corticosteroids should be weaned slowly from systemic corticosteroid use after transferring to ASMANEX TWISTHALER. Prednisone reduction can be accomplished by reducing the daily prednisone dose by 2.5 mg on a weekly basis during treatment with ASMANEX TWISTHALER *[see Dosage and Administration (2.1)]*. Lung function (FEV$_1$ or PEFR), beta-agonist use, and asthma symptoms should be carefully monitored during withdrawal of oral corticosteroids. In addition to monitoring asthma signs and symptoms, patients should be observed for signs and symptoms of adrenal insufficiency such as fatigue, lassitude, weakness, nausea and vomiting, and hypotension.
Transfer of patients from systemic corticosteroid therapy to ASMANEX TWISTHALER may unmask allergic conditions previously suppressed by the systemic corticosteroid therapy, e.g., rhinitis, conjunctivitis, eczema, arthritis, and eosinophilic conditions.
During withdrawal from oral corticosteroids, some patients may experience symptoms of systemically active corticosteroid withdrawal, e.g., joint and/or muscular pain, lassitude, and depression, despite maintenance or even improvement of respiratory function.

5.6 Hypercorticism and Adrenal Suppression
ASMANEX TWISTHALER will often help control asthma symptoms with less suppression of HPA function than therapeutically similar oral doses of prednisone. Since individual sensitivity to effects on cortisol production exists, physicians should consider this information when prescribing ASMANEX TWISTHALER. Particular care should be taken in observing patients postoperatively or during periods of stress for evidence of inadequate adrenal response. It is possible that systemic corticosteroid effects such as hypercorticism and adrenal suppression may appear in a small number of patients, particularly when ASMANEX TWISTHALER is administered at higher than recommended doses over prolonged periods of time. If such effects occur, the dosage of ASMANEX TWISTHALER should be reduced slowly, consistent with accepted procedures for reducing systemic corticosteroids and for management of asthma.

5.7 Reduction in Bone Mineral Density
Decreases in bone mineral density (BMD) have been observed with long-term administration of products containing inhaled corticosteroids, including mometasone furoate. The clinical significance of small changes in BMD with regard to long-term outcomes is unknown. Patients with major risk factors for decreased bone mineral content, such as prolonged immobilization, family history of osteoporosis, or

chronic use of drugs that can reduce bone mass (e.g., anticonvulsants and corticosteroids) should be monitored and treated with established standards of care.
In a 2-year double-blind study in 103 male and female asthma patients 18 to 50 years of age previously maintained on bronchodilator therapy (baseline FEV$_1$ 85%–88% predicted), treatment with ASMANEX TWISTHALER 220 mcg twice daily resulted in significant reductions in lumbar spine (LS) BMD at the end of the treatment period compared to placebo. The mean change from baseline to endpoint in the lumbar spine BMD was -0.015 (-1.43%) for the ASMANEX TWISTHALER group compared to 0.002 (0.25%) for the placebo group. In another 2-year double-blind study in 87 male and female asthma patients 18 to 50 years of age previously maintained on bronchodilator therapy (baseline FEV$_1$ 82%–83% predicted), treatment with ASMANEX TWISTHALER 440 mcg twice daily demonstrated no statistically significant changes in lumbar spine BMD at the end of the treatment period compared to placebo. The mean change from baseline to endpoint in the lumbar spine BMD was -0.018 (-1.57%) for the ASMANEX TWISTHALER group compared to -0.006 (-0.43%) for the placebo group.

5.8 Effect on Growth
Orally inhaled corticosteroids, including ASMANEX TWISTHALER, may cause a reduction in growth velocity when administered to pediatric patients. Monitor the growth of pediatric patients receiving ASMANEX TWISTHALER routinely (e.g., via stadiometry). To minimize the systemic effects of orally inhaled corticosteroids, including ASMANEX TWISTHALER, titrate each patient's dose to the lowest dosage that effectively controls his/her symptoms *[see Use in Specific Populations (8.4)]*.

5.9 Glaucoma and Cataracts
In clinical trials, glaucoma, increased intraocular pressure, and cataracts have been reported in 8 of 3007 patients following the administration of ASMANEX TWISTHALER. Close monitoring is warranted in patients with a change in vision or with a history of increased intraocular pressure, glaucoma, and/or cataracts.

5.10 Paradoxical Bronchospasm
As with other inhaled asthma medications, bronchospasm may occur with an immediate increase in wheezing after dosing. If bronchospasm occurs following dosing with ASMANEX TWISTHALER, it should be treated immediately with a fast-acting inhaled bronchodilator.
Treatment with ASMANEX TWISTHALER should be discontinued and alternative therapy instituted.

6 ADVERSE REACTIONS
Systemic and local corticosteroid use may result in the following:
• *Candida albicans* infection *[see Warnings and Precautions (5.1)]*
• Immunosuppression *[see Warnings and Precautions (5.4)]*
• Hypercorticism and adrenal suppression *[see Warnings and Precautions (5.6)]*
• Growth effects *[see Warnings and Precautions (5.8) and Use in Specific Populations (8.4)]*
• Glaucoma and cataracts *[see Warnings and Precautions (5.9)]*

6.1 Clinical Studies Experience
The safety data described below reflect exposure to ASMANEX TWISTHALER in 2380 patients with asthma exposed for 8 to 12 weeks and 627 patients with asthma exposed for 1 year in a total of 17 clinical trials.
In adult and adolescent patients 12 years of age and older, ASMANEX TWISTHALER was studied in 10 placebo-controlled clinical trials of 8 to 12 weeks duration with a total of 1750 patients receiving ASMANEX TWISTHALER. There were also 3 trials with a total of 475 patients receiving ASMANEX TWISTHALER for 1 year. In the 8- to 12-week clinical trials, the population was 12 to 83 years of age; 38% males and 62% females; and 83% Caucasian, 8% black, 6% Hispanic, and 3% other race/ethnicity. Patients received ASMANEX TWISTHALER 110 mcg twice daily (n=133), 220 mcg once daily in the morning (n=209), 220 mcg once daily in the evening (n=232), 220 mcg twice daily (n=433), 440 mcg once daily in the morning (n=419), 440 mcg once daily in the evening (n=250), or 440 mcg twice daily (n=74). In 3 long-term safety trials (two 9-month extensions of efficacy trials and one 52-week active-controlled safety trial), 475 patients with asthma (12-83 years of age, 44% males, 56% females, 87% Caucasian, 8% black, 4% Hispanic, and 1% other race/ethnicity) received various doses of ASMANEX TWISTHALER for 1 year.
In pediatric patients 4 to 11 years of age, ASMANEX TWISTHALER was studied in 3 placebo-controlled clinical trials of 12 weeks duration with a total of 630 patients receiving ASMANEX TWISTHALER and a 52-week, active-

controlled safety trial with a total of 152 patients receiving ASMANEX TWISTHALER. In the 12-week clinical trials, the population was 4 to 11 years of age; 63% males and 37% females; and 67% Caucasian, 13% black, 17% Hispanic, and 3% other race/ethnicity. Patients received ASMANEX TWISTHALER 110 mcg once daily in the evening (n=98), 110 mcg once daily in the morning (n=181), 110 mcg twice daily (n=179), or 220 mcg once daily in the morning (n=172). In the long-term active-controlled safety trial (n=152), patients with asthma (4 to 11 years of age, 60% males and 40% females, 84% Caucasian, 11% Black, and 5% Hispanic) received ASMANEX TWISTHALER 110 mcg twice daily or 220 mcg once daily in the morning for 52 weeks.

Because clinical trials are conducted under widely varying conditions, adverse reaction rates observed in the clinical trials of a drug cannot be directly compared to rates in the clinical trials of another drug and may not reflect the rates observed in practice.

Adults and Adolescents 12 Years of Age and Older: The safety results of the 10 trials that were 8 to 12 weeks in duration were pooled because patients with asthma in these studies were previously maintained on bronchodilators and/or inhaled corticosteroids. The safety results of the one 12-week clinical trial in patients with asthma previously treated with oral corticosteroids are presented separately. In the pooled 8- to 12-week clinical trials, adverse reactions were reported in 70% of patients treated with ASMANEX TWISTHALER (n=1750) compared to 65% of patients taking placebo (n=720). **Table 2** displays the common adverse reactions (≥3% in any patient group receiving ASMANEX TWISTHALER) that occurred more frequently in patients treated with ASMANEX TWISTHALER compared to patients treated with placebo.

[See table 2 above]

The following other adverse reactions occurred in these clinical trials with an incidence of at least 1% but less than 3% and were more common on ASMANEX TWISTHALER therapy than on placebo:

Body as a Whole: fatigue, flu-like symptoms, pain
Gastrointestinal: gastroenteritis, vomiting, anorexia
Hearing, Vestibular: earache
Resistance Mechanism: infection
Respiratory: dysphonia, epistaxis, nasal irritation, respiratory disorder, throat dry

In the 12-week clinical trial in adult asthmatics who previously required oral corticosteroids, the effects of ASMANEX TWISTHALER therapy administered as two 220-mcg inhalations twice daily (n=46) were compared with those of placebo (n=43). Adverse reactions, whether considered drug-related or not by the investigators, reported in more than 3 patients in the ASMANEX TWISTHALER treatment group, and which occurred more frequently than in placebo were (ASMANEX TWISTHALER % vs. placebo %): musculoskeletal pain (22% vs. 14%), oral candidiasis (22% vs. 9%), sinusitis (22% vs. 19%), allergic rhinitis (20% vs. 5%), upper respiratory infection (15% vs. 14%), arthralgia (13% vs. 7%), fatigue (13% vs. 2%), depression (11% vs. 0%), and sinus congestion (9% vs. 0%). In considering these data, an increased duration of exposure for patients on ASMANEX TWISTHALER treatment (77 days vs. 58 days on placebo) should be taken into account.

Long-Term Clinical Trials Experience - 12 Years of Age and Older: In 3 long-term safety trials, 475 patients with asthma 12 years of age and older were treated with ASMANEX TWISTHALER 220 mcg twice daily (n=60), 220 mcg once daily in the morning (n=41), 220 mcg once daily in the evening (n=40), 440 mcg once daily in the morning (n=44), 440 mcg once daily in the evening (n=41), 440 mcg twice daily (n=62), 880 mcg once daily (n=59), or at variable doses (n=128) for 52 weeks. The safety profile of ASMANEX TWISTHALER in the 52-week trials was similar to the findings in the 8- to 12-week clinical trials. In patients previously on inhaled corticosteroids, cataracts were reported in 3 patients (0.9%) treated with ASMANEX TWISTHALER, compared to 1 patient (1.7%) treated with the active comparator medication. Increased ocular pressure at the end of the study was observed in 2 patients, both on ASMANEX TWISTHALER 880 mcg once daily in the morning. Oral candidiasis, dysphonia, and dysmenorrhea were seen at a higher frequency with long-term administration than in the 8- to 12-week clinical trials.

Pediatric Patients 4 to 11 Years of Age: In the three 12-week clinical trials in pediatric patients 4 to 11 years of age, patients with asthma were previously maintained on bronchodilators and/or inhaled corticosteroids. The safety results from 1 trial are described in **Table 3** for ASMANEX TWISTHALER 110 mcg once daily in the evening. The safety results from the other 2 trials showed similar findings.

Overall adverse reactions were reported with approximately the same frequency by patients treated with ASMANEX TWISTHALER and those receiving placebo. **Table 3** displays the common adverse reactions (≥2% in any patient group receiving ASMANEX TWISTHALER) that occurred

Table 2: Adverse Reactions with ≥3% Incidence in 10 Controlled Clinical Trials with ASMANEX TWISTHALER in Patients 12 Years of Age and Older Previously on Bronchodilators and/or Inhaled Corticosteroids

| | (%) of Patients | | | |
| | ASMANEX TWISTHALER | | | |
Adverse Reaction	220 mcg twice daily (n=433)	440 mcg once daily (n=497)	220 mcg once daily in the evening (n=232)	Placebo (n=720)
Headache	22	17	20	20
Allergic Rhinitis	15	11	14	13
Pharyngitis	11	8	13	7
Upper Respiratory Infection	10	8	15	7
Sinusitis	6	6	5	5
Candidiasis, oral	6	4	4	2
Dysmenorrhea*	9	4	4	4
Musculoskeletal Pain	8	4	4	5
Back Pain	6	3	3	4
Dyspepsia	5	3	3	3
Myalgia	3	2	3	2
Abdominal Pain	3	2	3	2
Nausea	3	1	3	2
Average Duration of Exposure (Days)	81	70	80	62

* Percentages are based on the number of female patients.

more frequently in patients 4 to 11 years of age treated with ASMANEX TWISTHALER compared with placebo-treated patients.

Table 3: Adverse Reactions with ≥2% Incidence in a 12-Week Study with ASMANEX TWISTHALER in Patients 4 to 11 Years of Age Previously on Bronchodilators and/or Inhaled Corticosteroids

| | (%) of Patients | |
| | ASMANEX TWISTHALER | |
Adverse Reaction	110 mcg once daily in the evening (n=98)	Placebo (n=99)
Fever	7	5
Allergic Rhinitis	4	3
Abdominal Pain	6	2
Vomiting	3	2
Urinary Tract Infection	2	1
Bruise	2	0
Average Duration of Exposure (Days)	72	68

Long-Term Clinical Trials Experience in Children 4 to 11 Years of Age: In a 52-week, active-controlled, long-term safety trial, 152 patients with asthma 4 to 11 years of age were treated with ASMANEX TWISTHALER 110 mcg twice daily (n=74) or 220 mcg once daily (n=78). The safety profile for ASMANEX TWISTHALER in the 52-week trial was similar to the findings in the 12-week clinical trials.

6.2 Postmarketing Experience

The following adverse reactions have been reported during post-approval use of ASMANEX TWISTHALER. Because they are reported voluntarily from a population of uncertain size, it is not always possible to reliably estimate their frequency or establish a causal relationship to drug exposure.
Immune System Disorders: Immediate and delayed hypersensitivity reactions including rash, pruritus, angioedema and anaphylactic reaction *[see Warnings and Precautions (5.3) and Contraindications (4.2)]*.
Respiratory, Thoracic and Mediastinal Disorders: Asthma aggravation, which may include cough, dyspnea, wheezing and bronchospasm.

7 DRUG INTERACTIONS

In clinical studies, the concurrent administration of ASMANEX TWISTHALER and other drugs commonly used in the treatment of asthma was not associated with any unusual adverse reactions.

7.1 Inhibitors of Cytochrome P450 3A4

Ketoconazole, a strong inhibitor of cytochrome P450 3A4, may increase plasma levels of mometasone furoate during concomitant dosing *[see Clinical Pharmacology (12.3)]*.

8 USE IN SPECIFIC POPULATIONS

8.1 Pregnancy

Pregnancy Category C:
There are no adequate and well-controlled studies of ASMANEX TWISTHALER use in pregnant women. Animal reproduction studies in mice, rats, and rabbits revealed evidence of teratogenicity. Asthma is a serious and potentially life-threatening condition. Poorly controlled asthma during pregnancy is associated with adverse outcomes for mother and fetus. ASMANEX TWISTHALER should be used during pregnancy only if the potential benefit justifies the potential risk to the fetus.

There is a natural increase in corticosteroid production during pregnancy; therefore, most women require a lower exogenous corticosteroid dose and may not need corticosteroid treatment during pregnancy. Infants born to mothers taking substantial oral corticosteroid doses during pregnancy should be monitored for signs of hypoadrenalism.

When administered to pregnant mice, rats, and rabbits, mometasone furoate increased fetal malformations and decreased fetal growth (measured by lower fetal weights and/or delayed ossification). Dystocia and related complications were also observed when mometasone furoate was administered to rats late in gestation. However, experience with oral corticosteroids suggests that rodents are more prone to teratogenic effects from corticosteroid exposure than humans.

In a mouse reproduction study, subcutaneous mometasone furoate produced cleft palate at approximately one-third of the maximum recommended daily human dose (MRHD) for adults on an mcg/m^2 basis and decreased fetal survival at approximately 1 times the MRHD. No toxicity was observed at approximately one-tenth of the MRHD.

In a rat reproduction study, mometasone furoate produced umbilical hernia at topical dermal doses approximately 6 times the MRHD and delays in ossification at approximately 3 times the MRHD.

In another study, rats received subcutaneous doses of mometasone furoate throughout pregnancy or late in gestation. Treated animals had prolonged and difficult labor, fewer live births, lower birth weight, and reduced early pup survival at a dose that was approximately 6 times the MRHD for adults on an area under the curve (AUC) basis. Similar effects were not observed at approximately 3 times the MRHD.

In rabbits, mometasone furoate caused multiple malformations (e.g., flexed front paws, gallbladder agenesis, umbilical hernia, hydrocephaly) at topical dermal doses approximately 3 times the maximum recommended daily inhalation dose in adults on an mcg/m^2 basis. In an oral study, mometasone furoate increased resorptions and caused cleft palate and/or head malformations (hydrocephaly and domed head) at a dose less than the MRHD for adults based on AUC. At a dose approximately 2 times the MRHD in adults based on AUC, most litters were aborted or resorbed [see Nonclinical Toxicology (13.2)].

8.3   Nursing Mothers

Systemic absorption of a single inhaled 400 mcg mometasone dose was less than 1%. It is not known if mometasone furoate is excreted in human milk. Because other corticosteroids are excreted in human milk, caution should be used when ASMANEX TWISTHALER is administered to nursing women.

8.4   Pediatric Use

The safety and effectiveness of ASMANEX TWISTHALER have been established in children 4 years of age and older. Use of ASMANEX TWISTHALER in children 12 years of age and older is supported by evidence from adequate and well-controlled clinical trials in this patient population [see Clinical Studies (14.1) and Adverse Reactions (6.1)]. Use of ASMANEX TWISTHALER in pediatric patients 4 to 11 years of age is supported by evidence from adequate and well-controlled clinical trials of 12 weeks duration in 630 patients 4 to 11 years of age receiving ASMANEX TWISTHALER and one 52-week safety trial in 152 patients [see Clinical Studies (14.1) and Adverse Reactions (6.1)].

Controlled clinical studies have shown that inhaled corticosteroids may cause a reduction in growth in pediatric patients. In these studies, the mean reduction in growth velocity was approximately 1 cm per year (range: 0.3–1.8 per year) and appears to depend upon dose and duration of exposure. This effect was observed in the absence of laboratory evidence of HPA axis suppression, suggesting that growth velocity is a more sensitive indicator of systemic corticosteroid exposure in pediatric patients than some commonly used tests of HPA axis function. The long-term effects of this reduction in growth velocity associated with orally inhaled corticosteroids, including the impact on final adult height, are unknown. The potential for "catch-up" growth following discontinuation of treatment with orally inhaled corticosteroids has not been adequately studied. The growth of children and adolescents (4 years of age and older) receiving orally inhaled corticosteroids, including ASMANEX TWISTHALER, should be monitored routinely (e.g., via stadiometry).

A 52-week, placebo-controlled, parallel-group study was conducted to assess the potential growth effects of ASMANEX TWISTHALER in 187 prepubescent children (131 males and 56 females) 4 to 9 years of age with asthma who were previously maintained on an inhaled beta-agonist. Treatment groups included ASMANEX TWISTHALER 110 mcg twice daily (n=44), 220 mcg once daily in the morning (n=50), 110 mcg once daily in the morning (n=48), and placebo (n=45). For each patient, an average growth rate was determined using an individual regression approach. The mean growth rates, expressed as least-squares mean in cm per year, for ASMANEX TWISTHALER 110 mcg twice daily, 220 mcg once daily in the morning, 110 mcg once daily in the morning, and placebo were 5.34, 5.93, 6.15, and 6.44, respectively. The differences from placebo and the corresponding 2-sided 95% CI of growth rates for ASMANEX TWISTHALER 110 mcg twice daily, 220 mcg once daily in the morning, and 110 mcg once daily in the morning were -1.11 (95% CI: -2.34, 0.12), -0.51 (95% CI: -1.69, 0.67), and -0.30 (95% CI: -1.48, 0.89), respectively.

The potential growth effects of prolonged treatment with orally inhaled corticosteroids should be weighed against clinical benefits obtained and the availability of safe and effective noncorticosteroid treatment alternatives. To minimize the systemic effects of orally inhaled corticosteroids, including ASMANEX TWISTHALER, each patient should be titrated to his/her lowest effective dose.

8.5   Geriatric Use

A total of 175 patients 65 years of age and over (23 of whom were 75 years of age and older) have been treated with ASMANEX TWISTHALER in controlled clinical trials. No overall differences in safety or effectiveness were observed between these and younger patients, and other reported clinical experience has not identified differences in responses between the elderly and younger patients, but greater sensitivity of some older individuals cannot be ruled out.

8.6   Hepatic Impairment

Concentrations of mometasone furoate appear to increase with severity of hepatic impairment [see Clinical Pharmacology (12.3)].

10   OVERDOSAGE

Chronic overdosage may result in signs/symptoms of hypercorticism [see Warnings and Precautions (5.6)]. Because of low systemic bioavailability and an absence of acute drug-related systemic findings in clinical studies, acute overdose is unlikely to require any treatment other than observation. Single daily doses as high as 1200 mcg per day for 28 days were well tolerated and did not cause a significant reduction in plasma cortisol AUC (94% of placebo AUC). Single oral doses up to 8000 mcg have been studied on human volunteers with no adverse reactions reported.

11   DESCRIPTION

Mometasone furoate, the active component of the ASMANEX TWISTHALER product, is a corticosteroid with the chemical name 9,21-dichloro-11(Beta),17-dihydroxy-16(alpha)-methylpregna-1,4-diene-3,20-dione 17-(2-furoate) and the following chemical structure:

Mometasone furoate is a white powder with an empirical formula of $C_{27}H_{30}Cl_2O_6$, and molecular weight of 521.44 Daltons.

The ASMANEX TWISTHALER 110 mcg and 220 mcg products are cap-activated, inhalation-driven, multidose dry powder inhalers containing mometasone furoate and anhydrous lactose (which contains trace amounts of milk proteins).

Each actuation of the ASMANEX TWISTHALER 110 mcg or 220 mcg inhaler provides a measured dose of approximately 0.75 or 1.5 mg mometasone furoate inhalation powder, containing 110 or 220 mcg of mometasone furoate, respectively. This results in delivery of 100 or 200 mcg mometasone furoate from the mouthpiece, respectively, based on in vitro testing at flow rates of 30 L/min and 60 L/min with constant volume of 2 L. The amount of mometasone furoate emitted from the inhaler in vitro does not differ significantly for flow rates ranging from 28.3 L/min to 70 L/min at a constant volume of 2 L. However, the amount of drug delivered to the lung will depend on patient factors such as inspiratory flow and peak inspiratory flow through the device. In adult and adolescent patients (aged ≥12 years) with varied asthma severity, mean peak inspiratory flow rate through the device was 69 L/min (range: 54–77 L/min). In pediatric patients (aged 5-12 years) diagnosed with asthma, mean peak inspiratory flow rate in the 5- to 8-year-old subgroup was >50 L/min (minimum of 46 L/min) and for the 9- to 12-year-old subgroup was >60 L/min (minimum of 48 L/min).

12   CLINICAL PHARMACOLOGY

12.1   Mechanism of Action

Mometasone furoate is a corticosteroid demonstrating potent anti-inflammatory activity. The precise mechanism of corticosteroid action on asthma is not known. Inflammation is an important component in the pathogenesis of asthma. Corticosteroids have been shown to have a wide range of inhibitory effects on multiple cell types (e.g., mast cells, eosinophils, neutrophils, macrophages, and lymphocytes) and mediators (e.g., histamine, eicosanoids, leukotrienes, and cytokines) involved in inflammation and in the asthmatic response. These anti-inflammatory actions of corticosteroids may contribute to their efficacy in asthma.

Mometasone furoate has been shown in vitro to exhibit a binding affinity for the human glucocorticoid receptor, which is approximately 12 times that of dexamethasone, 7 times that of triamcinolone acetonide, 5 times that of budesonide, and 1.5 times that of fluticasone. The clinical significance of these findings is unknown.

Though effective for the treatment of asthma, corticosteroids do not affect asthma symptoms immediately. Maximum improvement in symptoms following inhaled administration of mometasone furoate may not be achieved for 1 to 2 weeks or longer after starting treatment. When corticosteroids are discontinued, asthma stability may persist for several days or longer.

12.2   Pharmacodynamics

Adrenal Function: The effects of ASMANEX TWISTHALER on adrenal function have been evaluated in 2 clinical studies: 1 in adults 18 years of age and older and 1 in pediatric patients 6 to 11 years of age. Both clinical studies were specifically designed to assess the effect of ASMANEX TWISTHALER on adrenal function.

In a 29-day, randomized, double-blind, placebo-controlled study in 64 adult and adolescent patients 18 years of age and older with asthma, ASMANEX TWISTHALER 440 mcg twice daily and 880 mcg twice daily (twice the highest recommended daily dose) were compared to both placebo and prednisone 10 mg once daily as a positive control. The 30-minute post-Cosyntropin stimulation serum cortisol concentration on Day 29 was 23.2 mcg/dL for the ASMANEX 440 mcg twice daily group (n=16) and 20.8 mcg/dL for the ASMANEX 880 mcg twice daily group (n=16), compared to 14.5 mcg/dL for the oral prednisone 10-mg group (n=16) and 25 mcg/dL for the placebo group (n=16). The difference between ASMANEX 880 mcg twice daily (twice the maximum recommended dose) and placebo was statistically significant.

In a 29-day, randomized, double-blind, placebo-controlled, parallel-group clinical trial in 50 pediatric patients 6 to 11 years of age with asthma, ASMANEX TWISTHALER 110 mcg twice daily, 220 mcg twice daily, and 440 mcg twice daily (2-8 times the highest pediatric daily recommended daily dose) were compared to placebo. HPA-axis function was assessed by 12-hour plasma cortisol AUC and 24-hour urinary-free cortisol concentrations. After 29 days of treatment, the mean changes in plasma cortisol AUC_{0-12h} from baseline were -0.11, -19.5, -21.3, and -3.47 mcg•hr/dL for the treatment groups of ASMANEX TWISTHALER 110 mcg twice daily (n=12), 220 mcg twice daily (n=12), 440 mcg twice daily (n=11), and placebo (n=7), respectively. The mean differences from placebo in the groups treated with ASMANEX TWISTHALER 110 mcg twice daily, 220 mcg twice daily, and 440 mcg twice daily were 3.4 mcg•hr/dL (95% CI: -14.0, 20.7), -16.0 mcg•hr/dL (95% CI: -33.9, 1.9), and -17.9 mcg•hr/dL (95% CI: -35.8, 0.0), respectively. For 24-hour urinary-free cortisol, after 29 days of treatment, the mean changes from baseline were -1.53, -1.33, -6.70, and -4.68 mcg/day for the groups treated with ASMANEX TWISTHALER 110 mcg twice daily (n=12), 220 mcg twice daily (n=12), 440 mcg twice daily (n=12), and placebo (n=10), respectively. The mean differences in urinary-free cortisol changes from baseline compared to placebo were 3.1 mcg/day (95% CI: -3.3, 9.6), 3.3 mcg/day (95% CI: -3.0, 9.7), and -2.0 mcg/day (95% CI: -8.6, 4.6) for the groups treated with 110 mcg twice daily, 220 mcg twice daily, and 440 mcg twice daily, respectively.

12.3   Pharmacokinetics

Absorption: Following a 1000 mcg inhaled dose of tritiated mometasone furoate inhalation powder to 6 healthy human subjects, plasma concentrations of unchanged mometasone furoate were shown to be very low compared to the total radioactivity in plasma. Following an inhaled single 400 mcg dose of ASMANEX TWISTHALER treatment to 24 healthy subjects, plasma concentrations for most subjects were near or below the lower limit of quantitation for the assay (50 pcg/mL). The mean absolute systemic bioavailability of the above single inhaled 400 mcg dose, compared to an intravenous 400 mcg dose of mometasone furoate, was determined to be less than 1%. Following administration of the recommended highest inhaled dose (400 mcg twice daily) to 64 patients for 28 days, concentration-time profiles were discernible, but with large intersubject variability. The coefficient of variation for C_{max} and AUC ranged from approximately 50% to 100%. The mean peak plasma concentrations at steady state ranged from approximately 94 to 114 pcg/mL and the mean time to peak levels ranged from approximately 1.0 to 2.5 hours.

Distribution: Based on the study employing a 1000 mcg inhaled dose of tritiated mometasone furoate inhalation powder in humans, no appreciable accumulation of mometasone furoate in the red blood cells was found. Following an intravenous 400 mcg dose of mometasone furoate, the plasma concentrations showed a biphasic decline, with a mean terminal half-life of about 5 hours and the mean steady-state volume of distribution of 152 L. The in vitro protein binding for mometasone furoate was reported to be 98% to 99% (in a concentration range of 5–500 ng/mL).

Metabolism: Studies have shown that mometasone furoate is primarily and extensively metabolized in the liver of all species investigated and undergoes extensive metabolism to multiple metabolites. In vitro studies have confirmed the primary role of CYP 3A4 in the metabolism of this compound; however, no major metabolites were identified.

Excretion: Following an intravenous dosing, the terminal half-life was reported to be about 5 hours. Following the inhaled dose of tritiated 1000 mcg mometasone furoate, the radioactivity is excreted mainly in the feces (a mean of 74%), and to a small extent in the urine (a mean of 8%) up to 7 days. No radioactivity was associated with unchanged mometasone furoate in the urine.

Special Populations:

Hepatic Impairment: Administration of a single inhaled dose of 400 mcg mometasone furoate to subjects with mild (n=4), moderate (n=4), and severe (n=4) hepatic impairment resulted in only 1 or 2 subjects in each group having detectable peak plasma concentrations of mometasone furoate (ranging from 50–105 pcg/mL). The observed peak plasma concentrations appear to increase with severity of hepatic impairment; however, the numbers of detectable levels were few.

Renal Impairment: The effects of renal impairment on mometasone furoate pharmacokinetics have not been adequately investigated.

Pediatric: Mometasone furoate pharmacokinetics have not been investigated in the pediatric population *[see Use in Specific Populations (8.4)]*.

Gender: The effects of gender on mometasone furoate pharmacokinetics have not been adequately investigated.

Race: The effects of race on mometasone furoate pharmacokinetics have not been adequately investigated.

Drug-Drug Interaction: Inhibitors of Cytochrome P450 3A4: In a drug interaction study, an inhaled dose of mometasone furoate 400 mcg was given to 24 healthy subjects twice daily for 9 days and ketoconazole 200 mg (as well as placebo) were given twice daily concomitantly on Days 4 to 9. Mometasone furoate plasma concentrations were <150 pcg/mL on Day 3 prior to coadministration of ketoconazole or placebo. Following concomitant administration of ketoconazole, 4 out of 12 subjects in the ketoconazole treatment group (n=12) had peak plasma concentrations of mometasone furoate >200 pcg/mL on Day 9 (211–324 pcg/mL).

13 NONCLINICAL TOXICOLOGY

13.1 Carcinogenesis, Mutagenesis, Impairment of Fertility

In a 2-year carcinogenicity study in Sprague Dawley® rats, mometasone furoate demonstrated no statistically significant increase in the incidence of tumors at inhalation doses up to 67 mcg/kg (approximately 8 times the maximum recommended daily inhalation dose in adults on an AUC basis and 2 times the maximum recommended daily inhalation dose in pediatric patients based on an mcg/m² basis). In a 19-month carcinogenicity study in Swiss CD-1 mice, mometasone furoate demonstrated no statistically significant increase in the incidence of tumors at inhalation doses up to 160 mcg/kg (approximately 10 times the maximum recommended daily inhalation dose in adults on an AUC basis and 2 times the maximum recommended daily inhalation dose in pediatric patients based on an mcg/m² basis).

Mometasone furoate increased chromosomal aberrations in an *in vitro* Chinese hamster ovary cell assay, but did not have this effect in an *in vitro* Chinese hamster lung cell assay. Mometasone furoate was not mutagenic in the Ames test or mouse lymphoma assay, and was not clastogenic in an *in vivo* mouse micronucleus assay, a rat bone marrow chromosomal aberration assay, or a mouse male germ-cell chromosomal aberration assay. Mometasone furoate also did not induce unscheduled DNA synthesis *in vivo* in rat hepatocytes.

In reproductive studies in rats, impairment of fertility was not produced by subcutaneous doses up to 15 mcg/kg (approximately 6 times the maximum recommended daily inhalation dose in adults on an AUC basis).

13.2 Animal Toxicology and/or Pharmacology

Reproductive Toxicology Studies: In mice, mometasone furoate caused cleft palate at subcutaneous doses of 60 mcg/kg and above (less than the maximum recommended daily inhalation dose in adults on an mcg/m² basis). Fetal survival was reduced at 180 mcg/kg (approximately equal to the maximum recommended daily inhalation dose in adults on an mcg/m² basis). No toxicity was observed at 20 mcg/kg (less than the maximum recommended daily inhalation dose in adults on an mcg/m² basis).

In rats, mometasone furoate produced umbilical hernia at topical dermal doses of 600 mcg/kg and above (approximately 6 times the maximum recommended daily inhalation dose in adults on an mcg/m² basis). A dose of 300 mcg/kg (approximately 3 times the maximum recommended daily inhalation dose in adults on an mcg/m² basis) produced delays in ossification but no malformations.

When rats received subcutaneous doses of mometasone furoate throughout pregnancy or during the later stages of pregnancy, 15 mcg/kg (approximately 6 times the maximum recommended daily inhalation dose in adults on an AUC basis) caused prolonged and difficult labor and reduced the number of live births, birth weight, and early pup survival. Similar effects were not observed at 7.5 mcg/kg (approximately 3 times the maximum recommended daily inhalation dose in adults on an AUC basis).

In rabbits, mometasone furoate caused multiple malformations (e.g., flexed front paws, gallbladder agenesis, umbilical hernia, hydrocephaly) at topical dermal doses of 150 mcg/kg and above (approximately 3 times the maximum recommended daily inhalation dose in adults on an mcg/m² basis). In an oral study, mometasone furoate increased resorptions and caused cleft palate and/or head malformations (hydrocephaly and domed head) at 700 mcg/kg (less than the maximum recommended daily inhalation dose in adults on an area under the curve [AUC] basis). At 2800 mcg/kg (approximately 2 times the maximum recommended daily inhalation dose in adults on an AUC basis) most litters were aborted or resorbed. No toxicity was observed at 140 mcg/kg (less than the maximum recommended daily inhalation dose in adults on an AUC basis).

14 CLINICAL STUDIES

14.1 Asthma

Adults and Adolescents 12 Years of Age and Older: The efficacy of ASMANEX TWISTHALER in patients with asthma 12 years and older was evaluated in ten 8- to 12-week, randomized, double-blind, placebo-controlled, parallel-group clinical trials. These trials included 1750 patients ranging from 12 to 83 years of age; 38% male and 62% female; and 83% Caucasian, 8% black, 6% Hispanic, and 3% other race/ethnicity. Patients received ASMANEX TWISTHALER 110 mcg twice daily (n=133), 220 mcg once daily in the morning (n=209), 220 mcg once daily in the evening (n=232), 220 mcg twice daily (n=433), 440 mcg once daily in the morning (n=419), 440 mcg once daily in the evening (n=250), or 440 mcg twice daily (n=74). The results of the clinical trials are presented based upon previous asthma therapy.

Patients ≥12 Years of Age Previously Maintained on Bronchodilators Alone: ASMANEX TWISTHALER was studied in three 12-week, double-blind trials in 737 patients with mild to moderate asthma (mean baseline FEV₁≥2.6 L, 72% of predicted normal) who were maintained on short-acting beta₂-agonists alone. The first 2 trials evaluated doses of 440 mcg administered as 2 inhalations once daily in the morning and 1 of these studies also evaluated 220 mcg twice daily. In both trials, AM predose FEV₁ was significantly improved at endpoint (last observation) following treatment with 440 mcg ASMANEX TWISTHALER once daily in the morning as compared to placebo (14% vs. 2.5%, respectively, in 1 trial and 16% vs. 5.5% in the other). There was also a significant improvement in AM predose FEV₁ at endpoint following treatment with ASMANEX TWISTHALER 220 mcg twice daily. Other measures of lung function (AM and PM PEFR) also showed improvement compared to placebo. Patients receiving ASMANEX TWISTHALER treatment had reduced frequency of beta₂-agonist rescue medication use compared to those on placebo (mean reductions at endpoint 2.2 and 0.5 puffs per day, respectively, from a baseline of 4.1 puffs/day). Additionally, fewer patients receiving ASMANEX TWISTHALER 440 mcg once daily experienced asthma worsening than did patients receiving placebo.

In the third trial, 195 asthmatic patients were treated with ASMANEX TWISTHALER 220 mcg once daily in the evening or placebo. The AM FEV₁ at endpoint was significantly improved compared to placebo (mean change at endpoint 0.43 L or 16.8% vs. 0.16 L or 6%, respectively, see **Figure 1**). Evening PEF increased 24.96 L/min (7%) from baseline in the ASMANEX TWISTHALER group compared to 8.67 L/min (4%) in placebo.

FIGURE 1: A 12-Week Trial in Patients Previously Maintained on Inhaled Beta₂-agonists

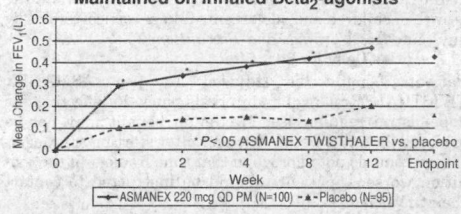

*P<.05 ASMANEX TWISTHALER vs. placebo
—■— ASMANEX 220 mcg QD PM (N=100) --▲-- Placebo (N=95)

Patients ≥12 Years of Age Previously Maintained on Inhaled Corticosteroids: The efficacy and safety of ASMANEX TWISTHALER in doses ranging from 110 mcg twice daily to 440 mcg twice daily was evaluated in 3 trials in 1072 patients previously maintained on inhaled corticosteroids. In the first 2 trials, asthmatic patients (mean baseline FEV₁ ~2.6 L, 76% predicted) were previously on either beclomethasone dipropionate [84–1200 mcg/day], flunisolide [100–2000 mcg/day], fluticasone propionate [110–880 mcg/day], or triamcinolone acetonide [300–2400 mcg/day]. The first trial included 307 patients who were treated in an open-label fashion with ASMANEX TWISTHALER 220 mcg (110 mcg × 2 inhalations) twice daily for 2 weeks followed by 12 weeks of double-blind treatment with ASMANEX TWISTHALER 440 mcg once daily in the morning or placebo. The second trial involved 365 patients who continued on their previous dose of inhaled corticosteroids during a 2-week screening period before being switched to ASMANEX TWISTHALER 440 mcg twice daily, 220 mcg twice daily, 110 mcg twice daily, beclomethasone dipropionate 168 mcg twice daily, or placebo for 12 weeks.

In the first trial, AM predose FEV₁ was effectively maintained (-1.4% change from baseline to endpoint) over the 12 weeks in the patients who were randomized to ASMANEX TWISTHALER 440 mcg once daily in the morning, while decreasing 10% at endpoint in those switched to placebo. In addition, fewer patients treated with ASMANEX TWISTHALER experienced worsening of asthma compared to placebo.

In the second trial, AM predose FEV₁ was significantly increased at endpoint when patients were switched to ASMANEX TWISTHALER 220 mcg twice daily (7% increase) or 440 mcg twice daily (6.2% increase) as compared to a decrease of 7% when switched to placebo. Additionally,

beta₂-agonist rescue medication use was decreased for patients who received ASMANEX TWISTHALER treatment relative to those on placebo (mean reduction from baseline to endpoint 1.1 puffs/day vs. increase of 0.7 puffs/day). Fewer patients receiving ASMANEX TWISTHALER treatment experienced asthma worsening than did patients receiving placebo.

The third trial evaluated the efficacy and safety of ASMANEX TWISTHALER compared to placebo in 400 asthmatic patients (mean FEV₁ 67% predicted at baseline) previously maintained on beclomethasone dipropionate (hydrofluoroalkane [HFA] or chlorofluorocarbon [CFC]) 168–600 mcg/day, budesonide 200–1200 mcg/day, flunisolide 500–2000 mcg/day, fluticasone propionate 88–880 mcg/day, or triamcinolone acetonide 400–1600 mcg/day. Following a 28-day inhaled corticosteroid dose-reduction phase, patients were randomized to ASMANEX TWISTHALER 440 mcg once daily in the evening, 220 mcg once daily in the evening, 220 mcg twice daily, or placebo. At endpoint, patients who received ASMANEX TWISTHALER 220 mcg once daily in the evening, 440 mcg once daily in the evening, or 220 mcg twice daily had a significant improvement in AM FEV₁ [0.41 L (19%), 0.49 L (22%), and 0.51 L (24%) in the 220 mcg once daily in the evening, 440 mcg once daily in the evening, and 220 mcg twice daily treatment group, respectively] compared to placebo [0.16 L (8%)] (see **Figure 2**). Evening PEF increased 15.65 L/min (4.1%) with the 220 mcg once daily in the evening dose, 39.26 L/min (10.7%) with the 440 mcg once daily in the evening dose, and 36.7 L/min (10.8%) with the 220 mcg twice daily dose, respectively, compared to a 1.4 L/min (1%) increase with placebo. Patients receiving all doses of ASMANEX TWISTHALER treatment had reduced frequency of beta₂-agonist rescue medication use compared to those on placebo (mean reductions at endpoint of 1.4–1.8 puffs/day from a baseline of more than 3 puffs/day compared to an increase in use by 0.5 puffs/day for placebo). In addition, fewer patients receiving ASMANEX TWISTHALER experienced asthma worsening than did those on placebo.

FIGURE 2: A 12-Week Trial in Patients Previously Maintained on Inhaled Corticosteroids

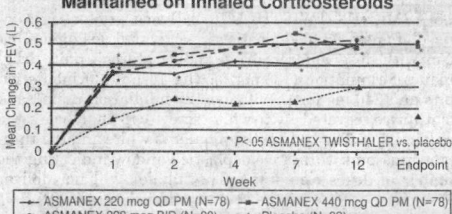

*P<.05 ASMANEX TWISTHALER vs. placebo
—■— ASMANEX 220 mcg QD PM (N=78) --▲-- ASMANEX 440 mcg QD PM (N=78)
—●— ASMANEX 220 mcg BID (N=80) ...◆... Placebo (N=83)

Patients ≥12 Years of Age Previously Maintained on Oral Corticosteroids: The efficacy of ASMANEX TWISTHALER 440 mcg and 880 mcg twice daily was evaluated in one 12-week, double-blind trial in patients previously maintained on oral corticosteroids. A total of 132 patients requiring oral prednisone (baseline mean daily oral prednisone requirement approximately 12 mg; baseline FEV₁ of 1.8 L, 59% of predicted normal), most of whom were also on inhaled corticosteroids (baseline inhaled steroid: beclomethasone dipropionate [168–840 mcg/day], budesonide [800–1600 mcg/day], flunisolide [1000–2000 mcg/day], fluticasone propionate [440–1760 mcg/day], or triamcinolone acetonide [400–2400 mcg/day]) were studied. Patients who received ASMANEX TWISTHALER 440 mcg twice daily had a significant reduction in their oral prednisone (46%) as compared to placebo (164% increase in oral prednisone dose). Additionally, 40% of patients on ASMANEX TWISTHALER 440 mcg twice daily were able to completely discontinue their use of prednisone, whereas 60% of patients on placebo had an increase in daily prednisone use. Patients on ASMANEX TWISTHALER had significant improvement in lung function (14% increase) compared to a 12% decrease in FEV₁ in the placebo group. Additionally, mean rescue beta₂-agonist use was reduced to approximately 3 puffs/day from a baseline of 4–5 puffs/day with ASMANEX TWISTHALER treatment, compared to an increase of 0.3 puffs/day on placebo. Patients who received ASMANEX TWISTHALER 880 mcg twice daily experienced no additional benefit beyond that seen with 440 mcg twice daily.

Pediatric Patients 4 to 11 Years of Age: The efficacy of ASMANEX TWISTHALER in patients with asthma 4 to 11 years of age was evaluated in three 12-week, randomized, double-blind, placebo-controlled, parallel-group clinical trials. These trials included 630 patients receiving ASMANEX TWISTHALER, ranging from 4 to 11 years of age; 63% male and 37% female; and 67% Caucasian, 13% black, 17% Hispanic, and 3% other race/ethnicity. Patients received ASMANEX TWISTHALER 110 mcg once daily in the evening (n=98), 110 mcg once daily in the morning (n=181), 110 mcg twice daily (n=179), or 220 mcg once daily in the morning (n=172). The results for 1 clinical trial are described below. The other 2 clinical trials support the efficacy of ASMANEX TWISTHALER.

A 12-week, placebo-controlled trial of 296 patients 4 to 11 years of age with asthma of at least 6 months duration (mean % predicted FEV_1 at baseline ranging from 77.3%–79.7%) was conducted to demonstrate the efficacy of the ASMANEX TWISTHALER in the treatment of asthma. Patients were treated with ASMANEX TWISTHALER 110 mcg once daily in the evening (n=98) or placebo (n=99) for 12 weeks. Assessment of efficacy was based upon morning predose FEV_1. The primary endpoint was the mean change from baseline to endpoint in percent-predicted FEV_1. For the primary endpoint, improvement in the ASMANEX TWISTHALER 110 mcg once daily in the evening treatment group (4.73) was statistically significant compared to placebo (-1.77). **Figure 3** displays the results for % predicted FEV_1 change from baseline at endpoint.

In this study, secondary endpoints of morning and evening peak expiratory flow and rescue medication use were supportive of efficacy of ASMANEX TWISTHALER.

FIGURE 3: A 12-Week Trial in Children 4 to 11 Years of Age: % Predicted FEV_1 Change from Baseline Over Time and at Endpoint by Treatment Group

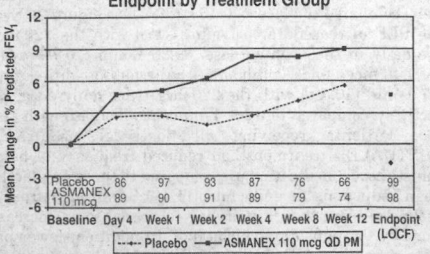

Note: Endpoint=last available data for each subject

16   HOW SUPPLIED/STORAGE AND HANDLING

The ASMANEX TWISTHALER 220 mcg product is comprised of an assembled plastic cap–activated dosing mechanism with dose counter, drug-product storage unit, drug-product formulation (135 mg for the 14 and 30 inhalation units and 240 mg for the 60 and 120 inhalation units), and mouthpiece, covered by a white screw cap that bears the product label. The body of the inhaler is white and the turning grip is pink with a clear plastic window indicating the number of doses remaining. The inhaler will not deliver subsequent doses once the counter reaches zero ("00").

The ASMANEX TWISTHALER 110 mcg product is comprised of an assembled plastic cap–activated dosing mechanism with dose counter, drug-product storage unit, drug-product formulation (135 mg), and mouthpiece, covered by a white screw cap that bears the product label. The body of the inhaler is white and the turning grip is gray with a clear plastic window indicating the number of doses remaining. The inhaler will not deliver subsequent doses once the counter reaches zero ("00").

The ASMANEX TWISTHALER product is available as:

ASMANEX TWISTHALER 220 mcg, which delivers 200 mcg mometasone furoate from the mouthpiece: 14 inhalation units (Institutional Use Only; NDC# 0085-1341-04 and NDC# 0085-1341-06); 30 inhalation units (NDC# 0085-1341-03 and NDC# 0085-1341-07); 60 inhalation units (for more than 1 inhalation daily; NDC# 0085-1341-02); or 120 inhalation units (for more than 2 inhalations daily; NDC# 0085-1341-01).

ASMANEX TWISTHALER 110 mcg, which delivers 100 mcg mometasone furoate from the mouthpiece: 7 inhalation units (Institutional Use Only; NDC# 0085-1461-07); 30 inhalation units (NDC# 0085-1461-02).

Each inhaler is supplied in a protective foil pouch with Patient's Instructions for Use.

Store in a dry place at 25°C (77°F); excursions permitted to 15–30°C (59–86°F) [see USP Controlled Room Temperature].

Discard the inhaler 45 days after opening the foil pouch or when dose counter reads "00", whichever comes first.

17   PATIENT COUNSELING INFORMATION

See FDA-Approved Patient Labeling (Patient Information).

17.1   Oral Candidiasis

Patients should be advised that localized infections with *Candida albicans* occurred in the mouth and pharynx in some patients. If oropharyngeal candidiasis develops, it should be treated with appropriate local or systemic (i.e., oral) antifungal therapy while still continuing with ASMANEX TWISTHALER therapy, but at times therapy with ASMANEX TWISTHALER may need to be temporarily interrupted under close medical supervision. Rinsing the mouth after inhalation is advised *[see Warnings and Precautions (5.1)].*

17.2   Acute Asthma Episodes

Patients should be advised that ASMANEX TWISTHALER is not a bronchodilator and should not be used to treat status asthmaticus or to relieve acute asthma symptoms. Acute asthma symptoms should be treated with an inhaled, short-acting $beta_2$-agonist such as albuterol *[see Warnings and Precautions (5.2)].*

17.3   Hypersensitivity Reactions Including Anaphylaxis

Hypersensitivity reactions including rash, pruritus, angioedema and anaphylactic reaction have been reported with use of ASMANEX TWISTHALER. Discontinue ASMANEX TWISTHALER if such reactions occur *[see Contraindications (4.2), Warnings and Precautions 5.3, and Postmarketing Experience (6.2)].*

ASMANEX TWISTHALER contains small amounts of lactose, which contains trace levels of milk proteins. In postmarketing experience with ASMANEX TWISTHALER, anaphylactic reactions in patients with milk protein allergy have been reported *[see Contraindications (4.2) and Postmarketing Experience (6.2)].*

17.4   Immunosuppression

Patients who are on immunosuppressant doses of corticosteroids should be warned to avoid exposure to chickenpox or measles and, if exposed, to consult their physician without delay. Patients should be informed of potential worsening of existing tuberculosis; fungal, bacterial, viral, or parasitic infections; or ocular herpes simplex *[see Warnings and Precautions (5.4)].*

17.5   Hypercorticism and Adrenal Suppression

Patients should be advised that ASMANEX TWISTHALER may cause systemic corticosteroid effects of hypercorticism and adrenal suppression. Additionally, patients should be instructed that deaths due to adrenal insufficiency have occurred during and after transfer from systemic corticosteroids. Patients should taper slowly from systemic corticosteroids if transferring to ASMANEX TWISTHALER *[see Warnings and Precautions (5.6)].*

17.6   Reduction in Bone Mineral Density

Patients who are at an increased risk for decreased BMD should be advised that the use of corticosteroids may pose an additional risk and should be monitored and, where appropriate, be treated for this condition *[see Warnings and Precautions (5.7)].*

17.7   Reduced Growth Velocity

Patients should be informed that orally inhaled corticosteroids, including mometasone furoate inhalation powder, may cause a reduction in growth velocity when administered to pediatric patients. Physicians should closely follow the growth of children and adolescents taking corticosteroids by any route *[see Warnings and Precautions (5.8)].*

17.8   Use Daily for Best Effect

Patients should be advised to use ASMANEX TWISTHALER at regular intervals, since its effectiveness depends on regular use. Maximum benefit may not be achieved for 1 to 2 weeks or longer after starting treatment. If symptoms do not improve in that time frame or if the condition worsens, patients should be instructed to contact their physician.

17.9   Instructions for Use

Patients should be instructed to record the date of pouch opening on the cap label and discard the inhaler 45 days after opening the foil pouch or when the dose counter reads "00" and the final dose has been inhaled, whichever comes first. The inhaler should be held upright while removing the cap. The medication should be taken as directed, breathing rapidly and deeply, and patients should not breathe out through the inhaler. The mouthpiece should be wiped dry and the cap replaced immediately following each inhalation and rotated fully until the click is heard. Rinsing of mouth after inhalation is advised. Patients should store the unit as instructed. The dose counter displays the doses remaining. When the dose counter indicates zero, the cap will lock and the unit must be discarded. Patients should be advised that if the dose counter is not working correctly, the unit should not be used and it should be brought to their physician or pharmacist.

Manufactured for: Merck Sharp & Dohme Corp., a subsidiary of
MERCK & CO., INC., Whitehouse Station, NJ 08889, USA
Manufactured by:
MSD International GmbH (Singapore Branch)
Singapore 638030, Singapore
Or
Merck Sharp & Dohme Corp., a subsidiary of
Merck & Co., Inc., Whitehouse Station, NJ 08889, USA
U.S. Patent Nos. 5,687,710; 5,829,434; 6,240,918; and 6,503,537.
Copyright © 2008, 2011 Merck Sharp & Dohme Corp., a subsidiary of **Merck & Co., Inc.**
All rights reserved.
Revised: 01/2013
032088-AS-PwIH-USPI.14

Patient Information
ASMANEX® TWISTHALER® 220 mcg (mometasone furoate inhalation powder)
ASMANEX® TWISTHALER® 110 mcg (mometasone furoate inhalation powder)
FOR ORAL INHALATION ONLY
Please read this leaflet carefully before taking ASMANEX® TWISTHALER®.
This leaflet does not contain the complete information about this medication. If you have any questions about ASMANEX TWISTHALER, ask your health care provider or pharmacist.

IMPORTANT POINTS TO REMEMBER ABOUT ASMANEX TWISTHALER

• Your health care provider has prescribed ASMANEX TWISTHALER for you or your child. It contains a medicine called mometasone furoate, which is a man-made corticosteroid. This medicine is used as maintenance treatment that helps prevent and control asthma symptoms.
• ASMANEX TWISTHALER is not a bronchodilator and should not be used for sudden symptoms of shortness of breath. Use an inhaled short-acting bronchodilator such as albuterol to relieve sudden symptoms of shortness of breath.
• Your health care provider may prescribe bronchodilators such as albuterol for emergency relief if an acute asthma attack occurs.
• Use your ASMANEX TWISTHALER regularly and at the same time each day, as prescribed by your health care provider. You or your child may not get the most benefit for 1 to 2 weeks or longer after starting ASMANEX. If you or your child's symptoms do not improve in that time frame or if your condition gets worse, contact your health care provider.
• The cap is needed to use the ASMANEX TWISTHALER. Do not twist the mouthpiece with your hand. When the cap is removed from the TWISTHALER, the dose counter will count down by one, and show the number of doses available after this use.
• The inhaler delivers your medicine as a very fine powder that **you or your child may not taste, smell, or feel.** Do not take or give extra doses unless your health care provider has told you to.
• It is important to replace the cap after each inhalation to protect the inhaler from moisture.
• Do not use the inhaler if you notice that it is not working correctly. Take it to your health care provider or pharmacist.

WHO SHOULD NOT USE ASMANEX TWISTHALER
Do not use ASMANEX TWISTHALER:
• To treat sudden, severe symptoms of asthma.
• If you have an allergy to milk proteins. Ask your health care provider if you are not sure.

HOW TO USE ASMANEX TWISTHALER OR GIVE TO YOUR CHILD
• **Remove the ASMANEX TWISTHALER from its foil pouch** and write the date on the cap label.
• **Throw away the inhaler 45 days after this date or when the dose counter reads "00", indicating the final dose has been inhaled, whichever comes first.**
• **Follow steps 1 and 2 below each time you inhale a dose from your ASMANEX TWISTHALER.**

Inhaler Parts:
See Figures 1 and 2 below to become familiar with the inhaler parts.

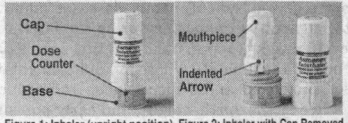

Figure 1: Inhaler (upright position)   Figure 2: Inhaler with Cap Removed

Step 1:   Open inhaler
Hold the inhaler straight up (upright position) with the colored portion (the base) on the bottom *(see Figure 3 below).* It is important that you remove the cap of the TWISTHALER while it is in this upright position to make sure that you get the right amount of medicine with each dose.
Holding the colored base, twist the cap in a counterclockwise direction to remove it *(see Figure 3 below).* As you lift off the cap, the dose counter on the base will count down by one. Removing the cap loads the TWISTHALER with the medicine that you are now ready to inhale.

Figure 3: Cap Removal Loads Dose

IT IS IMPORTANT TO NOTE that the indented arrow (located on the white portion of the TWISTHALER, directly above the colored base) is pointing to the dose counter (see Figure 2).

Step 2: Inhale dose
Breathe out fully. Then bring the TWISTHALER up to your mouth or your child's mouth with the mouthpiece facing toward you or your child. Place the mouthpiece in your mouth or your child's mouth, holding it in a horizontal (on its side) position as shown below (see Figure 4). Firmly close your lips around the mouthpiece and take in a fast, deep breath. Since the medicine is a very fine powder, you may not be able to taste, smell, or feel it after inhalation. Do not cover the ventilation holes while inhaling the dose.

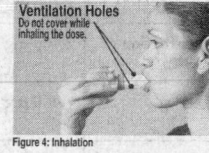

Figure 4: Inhalation

Remove the TWISTHALER from your mouth and hold your breath for about 10 seconds, or as long as you comfortably can.

IMPORTANT: DO NOT BREATHE OUT (EXHALE) INTO THE INHALER.
After you take your medicine, it is important that you wipe the mouthpiece dry, if needed, and then **REPLACE THE CAP**, firmly closing the TWISTHALER right away (see Figures 5 and 6 below).
Be sure that the indented arrow is in line with the dose counter. Put the cap back onto the inhaler and turn it in a clockwise direction, as you gently press down. You'll hear a "click" to let you know that the cap is fully closed. This is the only way to be sure that your next dose is loaded the right way.

Indented Arrow should line up with Dose Counter.

Replace cap and turn clockwise until "click".

Indented Arrow
Dose Counter

Figure 5: Closing the Inhaler

You'll hear a "click" to let you know that the cap is fully closed.

This is the only way to be sure that your next dose is properly loaded.

Figure 6: Closed Inhaler

IT IS IMPORTANT TO REPEAT STEPS 1 AND 2 EACH TIME YOU INHALE.
Rinse your mouth after using.
STORING YOUR INHALER
• Keep your inhaler clean and dry at all times. If the mouthpiece needs cleaning, gently wipe the mouthpiece with a dry cloth or tissue as needed. Do not wash the inhaler. Avoid contact with any liquids.
• **Store in a dry place at 25°C (77°F) [may range between 15–30°C (59–86°F)].**
• Keep your inhaler out of the reach of children.
HOW TO KNOW WHEN YOUR INHALER IS EMPTY
The inhaler has a dose counter on the colored base, which shows the number of doses left to use. As you lift off the cap to take your dose, the dose counter on the base will count down by one (if you began with the dose counter reading "30" this will cause the dose counter to now read "29"). Read the numbers from top to bottom.
When the unit reads "01" this indicates the last remaining dose. After dose "01" the counter will read "00". When you replace the cap, the unit will lock and then must be thrown away. Start using a new ASMANEX TWISTHALER as instructed by your health care provider.
POSSIBLE SIDE EFFECTS WITH ASMANEX TWISTHALER
Serious Side Effects may include:
• **Fungal infections in the mouth and throat.** Patients who use inhaled steroid medicines for asthma may develop a fungal infection of the mouth. Rinse your mouth after using ASMANEX TWISTHALER.
• Worsening asthma or sudden asthma attacks.
• **Serious allergic reactions.** Call your health care provider or get emergency medical care if you get any symptoms of a serious allergic reaction, including:

• Rash
• Swelling of the face, mouth and tongue
• Breathing problems
• **Possible increased risk of infection due to a weakened immune system with using steroid medicines.** Tell your health care provider if you or your child have or had TB, are exposed to anyone with chickenpox or measles, or about any other infections you or your child had before or while using ASMANEX TWISTHALER.
• **Adrenal insufficiency (your adrenal gland cannot produce enough steroids since you were on oral steroid medicine).** If you or your child took steroids by mouth and are having them decreased (tapered) or you are being switched to ASMANEX TWISTHALER, you should be followed closely by your health care professional.
Death can occur. Tell your health care professional right away about any symptoms such as feeling tired or exhausted, weakness, nausea, vomiting, or symptoms of low blood pressure (such as dizziness or faintness). If you or your child is under stress, such as with surgery, after surgery or trauma, you may need steroids by mouth again.
• **Decreased bone mass (bone mineral density).** Patients who use inhaled steroid medicines for a long time may have an increased risk of decreased bone mass, which can affect bone strength. Talk with your health care provider about any questions about bone health.
The most common side effects with ASMANEX TWISTHALER include: headache, nasal allergy symptoms, sore throat, upper respiratory tract infection, sinus infection, fungal infections in the mouth, painful menstrual periods, muscle and bone pain, back pain, and upset stomach. Tell your health care professional about any side effects that bother you or do not go away. These are not all of the possible side effects with ASMANEX TWISTHALER. For more information, ask your health care professional.
Manufactured for: Merck Sharp & Dohme Corp., a subsidiary of
MERCK & CO., INC., Whitehouse Station, NJ 08889, USA
Manufactured by:
MSD International GmbH (Singapore Branch)
Singapore 638030, Singapore
Or
Merck Sharp & Dohme Corp., a subsidiary of
Merck & Co., Inc., Whitehouse Station, NJ 08889, USA
U.S. Patent Nos. 5,687,710; 5,829,434; 6,240,918; and 6,503,537.
Copyright © 2008, 2011 Merck Sharp & Dohme Corp., a subsidiary of **Merck & Co., Inc.**
All rights reserved.
Revised: 01/2013
032088-AS-PwIH-PPI.9

AVELOX
[ă'vĕ-lŏks]
(moxifloxacin hydrochloride)
Tablet, film-coated
AVELOX
(moxifloxacin hydrochloride)
Injection, solution for IV use

Rx

HIGHLIGHTS OF PRESCRIBING INFORMATION
These highlights do not include all the information needed to use AVELOX safely and effectively. See full prescribing information for AVELOX.
AVELOX (moxifloxacin) hydrochloride Tablet, film-coated
AVELOX (moxifloxacin) hydrochloride Injection, solution for IV use
Initial U.S. Approval: 1999

WARNING:
Fluoroquinolones, including AVELOX®, are associated with an increased risk of tendinitis and tendon rupture in all ages. This risk is further increased in older patients usually over 60 years of age, in patients taking corticosteroid drugs, and in patients with kidney, heart or lung transplants *[see Warnings and Precautions (5.1)]*.
Fluoroquinolones, including AVELOX, may exacerbate muscle weakness in persons with myasthenia gravis. Avoid AVELOX in patients with known history of myasthenia gravis *[see Warnings and Precautions (5.2).]*

To reduce the development of drug-resistant bacteria and maintain the effectiveness of AVELOX and other antibacterial drugs, AVELOX should be used only to treat or prevent infections that are proven or strongly suspected to be caused by susceptible bacteria. (1)

——————RECENT MAJOR CHANGES——————
Warnings and Precautions, Peripheral Neuropathy (5.8)
8/13

——————INDICATIONS AND USAGE——————
AVELOX is a fluoroquinolone antibacterial indicated for treating infections in adults ≥ 18 years of age caused by designated, susceptible bacteria. (1, 12.4)
• Acute Bacterial Sinusitis (1.1)
• Acute Bacterial Exacerbation of Chronic Bronchitis (1.2)
• Community Acquired Pneumonia (1.3)
• Skin and Skin Structure Infections: Uncomplicated (1.4) and Complicated (1.5)
• Complicated Intra-Abdominal Infections (1.6)

——————DOSAGE AND ADMINISTRATION——————

Type of Infection	Dose Every 24 hours	Duration (days)
Acute Bacterial Sinusitis (1.1)	400 mg	10
Acute Bacterial Exacerbation of Chronic Bronchitis (1.2)	400 mg	5
Community Acquired Pneumonia (1.3)	400 mg	7-14
Uncomplicated Skin and Skin Structure Infections (SSSI) (1.4)	400 mg	7
Complicated SSSI (1.5)	400 mg	7-21
Complicated Intra-Abdominal Infections (1.6)	400 mg	5-14

• No dosage adjustment in patients with renal or hepatic impairment. (8.6, 8.7)
• AVELOX Tablets: Administer 4 hours before or 8 hours after antacids, sucralfate, multivitamins and other products with multivalent cations. (2.2)
• AVELOX IV: Slow IV infusion over 60 minutes. Avoid rapid or bolus IV. (2.3)
• Do not mix with other medications in IV bag or in IV line (2.3)

——————DOSAGE FORMS AND STRENGTHS——————
• AVELOX Tablets 400 mg moxifloxacin hydrochloride
• AVELOX IV 250 mL flexibag containing 400 mg moxifloxacin hydrochloride in sodium chloride injection (3.2)

——————CONTRAINDICATIONS——————
Known hypersensitivity to AVELOX or other quinolones (4, 5.4)

——————WARNINGS AND PRECAUTIONS——————
• Increased risk of tendinitis and tendon rupture. This risk is further increased in older patients usually over 60 years of age, in patients taking corticosteroids, and in patients with kidney, heart or lung transplants. Discontinue if pain or inflammation in a tendon occurs. (5.1, 8.5)
• Prolongation of the QT interval and isolated cases of torsade de pointes has been reported. Avoid use in patients with known prolongation, hypokalemia, and with drugs that prolong the QT interval. (5.3, 7.4, 8.5). Use caution in patients with proarrhythmic conditions such as clinically significant bradycardia or acute myocardial ischemia. (5.3)
• Serious and sometimes fatal hypersensitivity reactions, including anaphylactic reactions, may occur after first or subsequent doses. Discontinue drug use at first sign of skin rash, jaundice or any other sign of hypersensitivity. (5.4, 5.5)
• Central nervous system (CNS) events including dizziness, confusion, hallucination, depression, and rarely suicidal thoughts or acts may occur after first dose. Use caution in patients with known or suspected CNS disorders that may predispose to seizures or lower the seizure threshold. (5.6)
• Clostridium difficile-associated diarrhea: Evaluate if diarrhea occurs. (5.7)
• Peripheral neuropathy: Discontinue if symptoms occur. (5.8)

——————ADVERSE REACTIONS——————
Most common reactions (≥3%) were nausea, diarrhea, headache, and dizziness (6.2)
To report SUSPECTED ADVERSE REACTIONS, contact Bayer HealthCare Pharmaceuticals Inc. at 1-888-842-2937 or FDA at 1-800-FDA-1088 or www.fda.gov/medwatch

——————DRUG INTERACTIONS——————

Interacting Drug	Interaction
Antacids, sucralfate, multivitamins, and other products containing multivalent cations	Moxifloxacin absorption is decreased. Administer AVELOX Tablet at least 4 hours before or 8 hours after these products. (2.2, 7.1, 12.3, 17.2)
Warfarin	Anticoagulant effect of warfarin may be enhanced. Monitor prothrombin time/INR, watch for bleeding. (6.4, 7.2, 12.3)

| Class IA and Class III antiarrhythmics: | Proarrhythmic effect may be enhanced. Avoid concomitant use. (5.3, 7.4) |

USE IN SPECIFIC POPULATIONS

- **Pregnancy:** Based on animal data may cause fetal harm (8.1)
- **Geriatrics:** Increased risk for severe tendon disorders further increased by concomitant corticosteroid therapy and increased risk of prolongation of the QT interval. (5.1, 5.3, 8.5)

See 17 for PATIENT COUNSELING INFORMATION and FDA-approved patient labeling

Revised: 08/2013

FULL PRESCRIBING INFORMATION

> **WARNING:**
> Fluoroquinolones, including AVELOX®, are associated with an increased risk of tendinitis and tendon rupture in all ages. This risk is further increased in older patients usually over 60 years of age, in patients taking corticosteroid drugs, and in patients with kidney, heart or lung transplants. *[see Warnings and Precautions (5.1)].*
> Fluoroquinolones, including AVELOX, may exacerbate muscle weakness in persons with myasthenia gravis. Avoid AVELOX in patients with known history of myasthenia gravis *[see Warnings and Precautions (5.2)].*

1 INDICATIONS AND USAGE

To reduce the development of drug-resistant bacteria and maintain the effectiveness of AVELOX® and other antibacterial drugs, AVELOX should be used only to treat or prevent infections that are proven or strongly suspected to be caused by susceptible bacteria. When culture and susceptibility information are available, they should be considered in selecting or modifying antibacterial therapy. In the absence of such data, local epidemiology and susceptibility patterns may contribute to the empiric selection of therapy. AVELOX® Tablets and IV are indicated for the treatment of adults (≥ 18 years of age) with infections caused by susceptible isolates of the designated microorganisms in the conditions listed below *[see Dosage and Administration (2) and Use In Specific Populations (8.5)].*

Culture and Susceptibility Testing
Appropriate culture and susceptibility tests should be performed before treatment in order to isolate and identify organisms causing infection and to determine their susceptibility to moxifloxacin *[see Clinical Pharmacology (12.4)].* Therapy with AVELOX may be initiated before results of these tests are known; once results become available, appropriate therapy should be continued.

1.1 Acute Bacterial Sinusitis
AVELOX is indicated for the treatment of Acute Bacterial Sinusitis caused by *Streptococcus pneumoniae, Haemophilus influenzae,* or *Moraxella catarrhalis [see Clinical Studies (14.4)].*

1.2 Acute Bacterial Exacerbation of Chronic Bronchitis
AVELOX is indicated for the treatment of Acute Bacterial Exacerbation of Chronic Bronchitis caused by *Streptococcus pneumoniae, Haemophilus influenzae, Haemophilus parainfluenzae, Klebsiella pneumoniae,* methicillin-susceptible *Staphylococcus aureus,* or *Moraxella catarrhalis [see Clinical Studies (14.1)].*

1.3 Community Acquired Pneumonia
AVELOX is indicated for the treatment of Community Acquired Pneumonia caused by *Streptococcus pneumoniae* (including multi-drug resistant isolates*), *Haemophilus influenzae, Moraxella catarrhalis,* methicillin-susceptible *Staphylococcus aureus, Klebsiella pneumoniae, Mycoplasma pneumoniae,* or *Chlamydophila pneumoniae.*

* MDRSP, Multi-drug resistant *Streptococcus pneumoniae* includes isolates previously known as PRSP (Penicillin-resistant *S. pneumoniae*), and are isolates resistant to two or more of the following antibiotics: penicillin (minimum inhibitory concentrations [MIC] ≥ 2 mcg/mL), 2nd generation cephalosporins (for example, cefuroxime), macrolides, tetracyclines, and trimethoprim/sulfamethoxazole *[see Clinical Studies (14.2)].*

1.4 Uncomplicated Skin and Skin Structure Infections
AVELOX is indicated for the treatment of Uncomplicated Skin and Skin Structure Infections caused by methicillin-susceptible *Staphylococcus aureus* or *Streptococcus pyogenes [see Clinical Studies (14.5)].*

1.5 Complicated Skin and Skin Structure Infections
AVELOX is indicated for the treatment of Complicated Skin and Skin Structure Infections caused by methicillin-susceptible *Staphylococcus aureus, Escherichia coli, Klebsiella pneumoniae,* or *Enterobacter cloacae [see Clinical Studies (14.6)].*

1.6 Complicated Intra-Abdominal Infections
AVELOX is indicated for the treatment of Complicated Intra-Abdominal Infections including polymicrobial infections such as abscess caused by *Escherichia coli, Bacteroides fragilis, Streptococcus anginosus, Streptococcus constel-* *latus, Enterococcus faecalis, Proteus mirabilis, Clostridium perfringens, Bacteroides thetaiotaomicron,* or *Peptostreptococcusspecies [see Clinical Studies (14.7)].*

2 DOSAGE AND ADMINISTRATION

2.1 Dosage in Adult Patients
The dose of AVELOX is 400 mg (orally or as an intravenous infusion) once every 24 hours. The duration of therapy depends on the type of infection as described in **Table 1.**

Table 1 Dosage and Duration of Therapy in Adult Patients

Type of Infection*	Dose Every 24 hours	Duration (days)
Acute Bacterial Sinusitis (1.1)	400 mg	10
Acute Bacterial Exacerbation of Chronic Bronchitis (1.2)	400 mg	5
Community Acquired Pneumonia (1.3)	400 mg	7–14
Uncomplicated Skin and Skin Structure Infections (SSSI) (1.4)	400 mg	7
Complicated SSSI (1.5)	400 mg	7–21
Complicated Intra-Abdominal Infections (1.6)	400 mg	5–14

* Due to the designated pathogens *[see Indications and Usage (1), for IV use, see Use in Specific Populations (8.5)].*

Intravenous formulation is indicated when it offers a route of administration advantageous to the patient (for example, patient cannot tolerate an oral dosage form). When switching from intravenous to oral formulation, no dosage adjustment is necessary. Patients whose therapy is started with AVELOX IV may be switched to AVELOX Tablets when clinically indicated at the discretion of the physician.

2.2 Drug Interactions with Multivalent Cations
Oral doses of AVELOX should be administered at least 4 hours before or 8 hours after products containing magnesium, aluminum, iron or zinc, including antacids, sucralfate, multivitamins and VIDEX® (didanosine) chewable/buffered tablets or the pediatric powder for oral solution *[see Drug Interactions (7.1) and Clinical Pharmacology (12.3)].*

2.3 Administration Instructions
AVELOX Film-Coated Tablets
AVELOX Tablets can be taken with or without food, drink fluids liberally.

AVELOX IV Solution for Infusion
Parenteral drug products should be inspected visually for particulate matter and discoloration prior to administration, whenever solution and container permit.

AVELOX IV should be administered by INTRAVENOUS infusion only. It is not intended for intra-arterial, intramuscular, intrathecal, intraperitoneal, or subcutaneous administration.

AVELOX IV should be administered by intravenous infusion over a period of 60 minutes by direct infusion or through a Y-type intravenous infusion set which may already be in place. Caution: rapid or bolus intravenous infusion must be avoided.

Because only limited data are available on the compatibility of AVELOX intravenous injection with other intravenous substances, additives or other medications should not be added to AVELOX IV or infused simultaneously through the same intravenous line. If the same intravenous line or a Y-type line is used for sequential infusion of other drugs, or if the "piggyback" method of administration is used, the line should be flushed before and after infusion of AVELOX IV with an infusion solution compatible with AVELOX IV as well as with other drug(s) administered via this common line.

AVELOX IV is compatible with the following intravenous solutions at ratios from 1:10 to 10:1

0.9% Sodium Chloride Injection, USP	Sterile Water for Injection, USP
1M Sodium Chloride Injection	10% Dextrose for Injection, USP
5% Dextrose Injection, USP	Lactated Ringer's for Injection

2.4 Preparation for Administration of AVELOX IV
To prepare AVELOX IV injection premix in flexible containers:
1. Close flow control clamp of administration set.
2. Remove cover from port at bottom of container.

3. Insert piercing pin from an appropriate transfer set (for example, one that does not require excessive force, such as ISO compatible administration set) into port with a gentle twisting motion until pin is firmly seated.
NOTE: Refer to complete directions that have been provided with the administration set.

3 DOSAGE FORMS AND STRENGTHS

3.1 AVELOX Tablets
- Containing moxifloxacin hydrochloride (equivalent to 400 mg moxifloxacin)
- Oblong, dull red film-coated tablets
- Imprinted with BAYER on one side and M400 on the other

3.2 AVELOX IV
- Containing 400 mg moxifloxacin in 0.8% saline (moxifloxacin hydrochloride in sodium chloride injection) with pH ranging from 4.1 to 4.6.
- Ready-to-use 250 mL latex-free flexibags. No further dilution is necessary
- Sterile, preservative free, 0.8% sodium chloride aqueous solution of moxifloxacin hydrochloride

4 CONTRAINDICATIONS
AVELOX is contraindicated in persons with a history of hypersensitivity to moxifloxacin or any member of the quinolone class of antimicrobial agents.

5 WARNINGS AND PRECAUTIONS

5.1 Tendinopathy and Tendon Rupture
Fluoroquinolones, including AVELOX, are associated with an increased risk of tendinitis and tendon rupture in all ages. This adverse reaction most frequently involves the Achilles tendon, and rupture of the Achilles tendon may require surgical repair. Tendinitis and tendon rupture in the rotator cuff (the shoulder), the hand, the biceps, the thumb, and other tendon sites have also been reported. The risk of developing fluoroquinolone-associated tendinitis and tendon rupture is further increased in older patients usually over 60 years of age, in patients taking corticosteroid drugs, and in patients with kidney, heart or lung transplants. Factors, in addition to age and corticosteroid use, that may independently increase the risk of tendon rupture include strenuous physical activity, renal failure, and previous tendon disorders such as rheumatoid arthritis. Tendinitis and tendon rupture have also occurred in patients taking fluoroquinolones who do not have the above risk factors. Tendon rupture can occur during or after completion of therapy; cases occurring up to several months after completion of therapy have been reported. AVELOX should be discontinued if the patient experiences pain, swelling, inflammation or rupture of a tendon. Patients should be advised to rest at the first sign of tendinitis or tendon rupture, and to contact their healthcare provider regarding changing to a non-quinolone antimicrobial drug. [see Adverse Reactions (6.4) and Patient Counseling Information (17.3).]

5.2 Exacerbation of Myasthenia Gravis
Fluoroquinolones, including AVELOX, have neuromuscular blocking activity and may exacerbate muscle weakness in persons with myasthenia gravis. Postmarketing serious adverse events, including deaths and requirement for ventilatory support, have been associated with fluoroquinolone use in persons with myasthenia gravis. Avoid AVELOX in patients with known history of myasthenia gravis [see Patient Counseling Information (17.3)].

5.3 QT Prolongation
AVELOX has been shown to prolong the QT interval of the electrocardiogram in some patients. Following oral dosing with 400 mg of AVELOX the mean (± SD) change in QTc from the pre-dose value at the time of maximum drug concentration was 6 msec (± 26) (n = 787). Following a course of daily intravenous dosing (400 mg; 1 hour infusion each day) the mean change in QTc from the Day 1 pre-dose value was 10 msec (±22) on Day 1 (n=667) and 7 msec (± 24) on Day 3 (n = 667).

The drug should be avoided in patients with known prolongation of the QT interval, patients with uncorrected hypokalemia and patients receiving Class IA (for example, quinidine, procainamide) or Class III (for example, amiodarone, sotalol) antiarrhythmic agents, due to the lack of clinical experience with the drug in these patient populations. Pharmacokinetic studies between AVELOX and other drugs that prolong the QT interval such as cisapride, erythromycin, antipsychotics, and tricyclic antidepressants have not been performed. An additive effect of AVELOX and these drugs cannot be excluded; therefore caution should be exercised when AVELOX is given concurrently with these drugs. In premarketing clinical trials, the rate of cardiovascular adverse events was similar in 798 AVELOX and 702 comparator treated patients who received concomitant therapy with drugs known to prolong the QTc interval.

AVELOX should be used with caution in patients with ongoing proarrhythmic conditions, such as clinically significant bradycardia, acute myocardial ischemia. The magnitude of QT prolongation may increase with increasing concentrations of the drug or increasing rates of infusion of the intravenous formulation. Therefore the recommended dose or infusion rate should not be exceeded. QT prolongation may lead to an increased risk for ventricular arrhythmias including torsade de pointes. No excess in cardiovascular morbidity or mortality attributable to QTc prolongation occurred with AVELOX treatment in over 15,500 patients in controlled clinical studies, including 759 patients who were hypokalemic at the start of treatment, and there was no increase in mortality in over 18,000 AVELOX tablet treated patients in a postmarketing observational study in which ECGs were not performed. Elderly patients using IV AVELOX may be more susceptible to drug-associated QT prolongation. [see Use In Specific Populations, (8.5).] In addition, AVELOX should be used with caution in patients with mild, moderate, or severe liver cirrhosis. [See Clinical Pharmacology (12.3) and Patient Counseling Information (17.3).]

5.4 Hypersensitivity Reactions
Serious anaphylactic reactions, some following the first dose, have been reported in patients receiving quinolone therapy, including AVELOX. Some reactions were accompanied by cardiovascular collapse, loss of consciousness, tingling, pharyngeal or facial edema, dyspnea, urticaria, and itching. Serious anaphylactic reactions require immediate emergency treatment with epinephrine. AVELOX should be discontinued at the first appearance of a skin rash or any other sign of hypersensitivity. Oxygen, intravenous steroids, and airway management, including intubation, may be administered as indicated. [see Adverse Reactions (6) and Patient Counseling Information (17.3).]

5.5 Other Serious and Sometimes Fatal Reactions
Other serious and sometimes fatal events, some due to hypersensitivity, and some due to uncertain etiology, have been reported rarely in patients receiving therapy with quinolones, including AVELOX. These events may be severe and generally occur following the administration of multiple doses. Clinical manifestations may include one or more of the following:
- Fever, rash, or severe dermatologic reactions (for example, toxic epidermal necrolysis, Stevens-Johnson syndrome)
- Vasculitis; arthralgia; myalgia; serum sickness
- Allergic pneumonitis
- Interstitial nephritis; acute renal insufficiency or failure
- Hepatitis; jaundice; acute hepatic necrosis or failure
- Anemia, including hemolytic and aplastic; thrombocytopenia, including thrombotic thrombocytopenic purpura; leukopenia; agranulocytosis; pancytopenia; and/or other hematologic abnormalities

The drug should be discontinued immediately at the first appearance of a skin rash, jaundice, or any other sign of hypersensitivity and supportive measures instituted [see Patient Counseling Information (17.3) and Adverse Reactions (6.4).

5.6 Central Nervous System Effects
Fluoroquinolones, including AVELOX, may cause central nervous system (CNS) events, including: nervousness, agitation, insomnia, anxiety, nightmares or paranoia [see Adverse Reactions (6.2, 6.4)].

Convulsions and increased intracranial pressure (including pseudotumor cerebri) have been reported in patients receiving fluoroquinolones. Fluoroquinolones may also cause central nervous system (CNS) events including: dizziness, confusion, tremors, hallucinations, depression, and, rarely, suicidal thoughts or acts. These reactions may occur following the first dose. If these reactions occur in patients receiving AVELOX, the drug should be discontinued and appropriate measures instituted. As with all fluoroquinolones, AVELOX should be used with caution in patients with known or suspected CNS disorders (for example, severe cerebral arteriosclerosis, epilepsy) or in the presence of other risk factors that may predispose to seizures or lower the seizure threshold. [See Drug Interactions (7.4) Adverse Reactions (6.2, 6.4) and Patient Counseling Information (17.3).]

5.7 Clostridium Difficile-Associated Diarrhea
Clostridium difficile-associated diarrhea (CDAD) has been reported with use of nearly all antibacterial agents, including AVELOX, and may range in severity from mild diarrhea to fatal colitis. Treatment with antibacterial agents alters the normal flora of the colon leading to overgrowth of C. difficile.
C. difficile produces toxins A and B which contribute to the development of CDAD. Hypertoxin producing strains of C. difficile cause increased morbidity and mortality, as these infections can be refractory to antimicrobial therapy and may require colectomy. CDAD must be considered in all patients who present with diarrhea following antibiotic use. Careful medical history is necessary since CDAD has been reported to occur over two months after the administration of antibacterial agents.

If CDAD is suspected or confirmed, ongoing antibiotic use not directed against C. difficile may need to be discontinued. Appropriate fluid and electrolyte management, protein supplementation, antibiotic treatment of C. difficile, and surgical evaluation should be instituted as clinically indicated [see Adverse Reactions (6.2) and Patient Counseling Information (17.3)].

5.8 Peripheral Neuropathy
Cases of sensory or sensorimotor axonal polyneuropathy affecting small and/or large axons resulting in paresthesias, hypoesthesias, dysesthesias and weakness have been reported in patients receiving fluoroquinolones including AVELOX. Symptoms may occur soon after initiation of AVELOX and may be irreversible. AVELOX should be discontinued immediately if the patient experiences symptoms of peripheral neuropathy including pain, burning, tingling, numbness, and/or weakness or other alterations of sensation including light touch, pain, temperature, position sense, and vibratory sensation [see Adverse Reactions (6.2, 6.4) and Patient Counseling Information (17.3)].

5.9 Arthropathic Effects in Animals
The oral administration of AVELOX caused lameness in immature dogs. Histopathological examination of the weight-bearing joints of these dogs revealed permanent lesions of the cartilage. Related quinolone-class drugs also produce erosions of cartilage of weight-bearing joints and other signs of arthropathy in immature animals of various species. [See Animal Toxicology and/or Pharmacology (13.2).]

5.10 Photosensitivity/Phototoxicity
Moderate to severe photosensitivity/phototoxicity reactions, the latter of which may manifest as exaggerated sunburn reactions (for example, burning, erythema, exudation, vesicles, blistering, edema) involving areas exposed to light (typically the face, "V" area of the neck, extensor surfaces of the forearms, dorsa of the hands), can be associated with the use of quinolone antibiotics after sun or UV light exposure. Therefore, excessive exposure to these sources of light should be avoided. Drug therapy should be discontinued if phototoxicity occurs. [see Adverse Reactions (6.4) and Pharmacokinetics (12.3).]

5.11 Development of Drug Resistant Bacteria
Prescribing AVELOX in the absence of a proven or strongly suspected bacterial infection or a prophylactic indication is unlikely to provide benefit to the patient and increases the risk of the development of drug-resistant bacteria [see Patient Counseling Information (17.1)].

6 ADVERSE REACTIONS

6.1 Serious and Otherwise Important Adverse Reactions
The following serious and otherwise important adverse reactions are discussed in greater detail in the warnings and precautions section of the label:
- Tendinopathy and Tendon Rupture [see Warnings and Precautions (5.1)]
- QT Prolongation [see Warnings and Precautions (5.3)]
- Hypersensitivity Reactions [see Warnings and Precautions (5.4)]
- Other Serious and Sometimes Fatal Reactions [see Warnings and Precautions (5.5)]
- Central Nervous System Effects [see Warnings and Precautions (5.6)]
- Clostridium difficile-Associated Diarrhea [see Warnings and Precautions (5.7)]
- Peripheral Neuropathy that may be irreversible [see Warnings and Precautions (5.8)]
- Photosensitivity/Phototoxicity [see Warnings and Precautions (5.10)]
- Development of Drug Resistant Bacteria [see Warnings and Precautions (5.11)]

6.2 Clinical Trial Experience
Because clinical trials are conducted under widely varying conditions, adverse reaction rates observed in the clinical trials of a drug cannot be directly compared to rates in the clinical trials of another drug and may not reflect the rates observed in practice.
The data described below reflect exposure to AVELOX in 14981 patients in 71 active controlled Phase II- IV clinical trials in different indications [see Indications and Usage (1).] The population studied had a mean age of 50 years (approximately 73% of the population was <65 years of age), 50% were male, 63% were Caucasian, 12% were Asian and 9% were Black. Patients received AVELOX 400 mg once daily PO, IV, or sequentially (IV followed by PO). Treatment duration was usually 6-10 days, and the mean number of days on therapy was 9 days.
Discontinuation of AVELOX due to adverse events occurred in 5.0% of patients overall, 4.1% of patients treated with 400 mg PO, 3.9% with 400 mg IV and 8.2% with sequential therapy 400 mg PO/IV. The most common adverse events leading to discontinuation with the 400 mg PO doses were nausea (0.8%), diarrhea (0.5%), dizziness (0.5%), and vomiting (0.4%). The most common adverse event leading to dis-

continuation with the 400 mg IV dose was rash (0.5%). The most common adverse events leading to discontinuation with the 400 mg IV/PO sequential dose were diarrhea (0.5%), pyrexia (0.4%).

Adverse reactions occurring in ≥1% of AVELOX-treated patients and less common adverse reactions, occurring in 0.1 to <1% of AVELOX-treated patients, are shown in **Tables 2** and **Table 3**, respectively. The most common adverse drug reactions (≥3%) are nausea, diarrhea, headache, and dizziness.

Table 2 Common (≥ 1.0%) Adverse Reactions Reported in Active-Controlled Clinical Trials with AVELOX

System Organ Class	Adverse Reactions*	% (N=14,981)
Blood and Lymphatic System Disorders	Anemia	1.1
Gastrointestinal Disorders	Nausea	6.9
	Diarrhea	6.0
	Vomiting	2.4
	Constipation	1.9
	Abdominal pain	1.5
	Abdominal pain upper	1.1
	Dyspepsia	1.0
General Disorders and Administration Site Conditions	Pyrexia	1.1
Investigations	Alanine aminotransferase increased	1.1
Metabolism and Nutritional Disorder	Hypokalemia	1
Nervous System Disorders	Headache	4.2
	Dizziness	3.0
Psychiatric Disorders	Insomnia	1.9

* MedDRA Version 12.0

Table 3 Less Common (0.1 to <1.0%) Adverse Reactions Reported in Active-Controlled Clinical Trials with AVELOX (N=14,981)

System Organ Class	Adverse Reactions[a]
Blood and Lymphatic System Disorders	Thrombocythemia Eosinophilia Neutropenia Thrombocytopenia Leukopenia Leukocytosis
Cardiac Disorders	Atrial fibrillation Palpitations Tachycardia Cardiac failure congestive Angina pectoris Cardiac failure Cardiac arrest Bradycardia
Ear and Labyrinth Disorders	Vertigo Tinnitus
Eye Disorders	Vision blurred
Gastrointestinal Disorders	Dry mouth Abdominal discomfort Flatulence Abdominal distention Gastritis Gastroesophageal reflux disease
General Disorders and Administration Site Conditions	Fatigue Chest pain Asthenia Edema peripheral Pain Malaise Infusion site extravasation Edema Chills Chest discomfort Facial pain
Hepatobiliary disorders	Hepatic function abnormal
Infections and Infestations	Vulvovaginal candidiasis Oral candidiasis Vulvovaginal mycotic infection Candidiasis Vaginal infection Oral fungal infection Fungal infection Gastroenteritis
Investigations	Aspartate aminotransferase increased Gamma-glutamyltransferase increased Blood alkaline phosphatase increased Hepatic enzyme increased Electrocardiogram QT prolonged Blood lactate dehydrogenase increased Platelet count increased Blood amylase increased Blood glucose increased Lipase increased Hemoglobin decreased Blood creatinine increased Transaminases increased White blood cell count increased Blood urea increased Liver function test abnormal Hematocrit decreased Prothrombin time prolonged Eosinophil count increased Activated partial thromboplastin time prolonged Blood bilirubin increased Blood triglycerides increased Blood uric acid increased Blood pressure increased
Metabolism and Nutrition Disorders	Hyperglycemia Anorexia Hypoglycemia Hyperlipidemia Decreased appetite Dehydration
Musculoskeletal and Connective Tissue Disorders	Back pain Pain in extremity Arthralgia Myalgia Muscle spasms Musculoskeletal chest pain Musculoskeletal pain
Nervous System Disorders	Dysgeusia Somnolence Tremor Lethargy Paresthesia Tension headache Hypoesthesia Syncope
Psychiatric Disorders	Anxiety Confusional state Agitation Depression Nervousness Restlessness Hallucination Disorientation
Renal and Urinary Disorders	Renal failure Dysuria Renal failure acute
Reproductive System and Breast Disorders	Vulvovaginal pruritus
Respiratory, Thoracic, and Mediastinal Disorders	Dyspnea Asthma Wheezing Bronchospasm
Skin and Subcutaneous Tissue Disorders	Rash Pruritus Hyperhidrosis Erythema Urticaria Dermatitis allergic Night sweats
Vascular Disorders	Hypertension Hypotension Phlebitis

[a]MedDRA Version 12.0

6.3 Laboratory Changes

Changes in laboratory parameters, without regard to drug relationship, which are not listed above and which occurred in ≥ 2% of patients and at an incidence greater than in controls included: increases in MCH, neutrophils, WBCs, PT ratio, ionized calcium, chloride, albumin, globulin, bilirubin; decreases in hemoglobin, RBCs, neutrophils, eosinophils, basophils, PT ratio, glucose, pO$_2$, bilirubin, and amylase. It cannot be determined if any of the above laboratory abnormalities were caused by the drug or the underlying condition being treated.

6.4 Postmarketing Experience

Table 4 lists adverse reactions that have been identified during post-approval use of AVELOX. Because these events are reported voluntarily from a population of uncertain size, it is not always possible to reliably estimate their frequency or establish a causal relationship to drug exposure.

Table 4 Postmarketing Reports of Adverse Drug Reactions

System/Organ Class	Adverse Reaction
Blood and Lymphatic System Disorders	Agranulocytosis Pancytopenia [see Warnings and Precautions (5.5)]
Cardiac Disorders	Ventricular tachyarrhythmias (including in very rare cases cardiac arrest and torsade de pointes, and usually in patients with concurrent severe underlying proarrhythmic conditions)
Ear and Labyrinth Disorders	Hearing impairment, including deafness (reversible in majority of cases)
Eye Disorders	Vision loss (especially in the course of CNS reactions, transient in majority of cases)
Hepatobiliary Disorders	Hepatitis (predominantly cholestatic) Hepatic failure (including fatal cases) Jaundice Acute hepatic necrosis [see Warnings and Precautions (5.5)]

Immune System Disorders	Anaphylactic reaction Anaphylactic shock Angioedema (including laryngeal edema) *[see Warnings and Precautions (5.4, 5.5)]*
Musculoskeletal and Connective Tissue Disorders	Tendon rupture *[see Warnings and Precautions (5.1)]*
Nervous System Disorders	Altered coordination Abnormal gait *[see Warnings and Precautions (5.8)]* Myasthenia gravis (exacerbation of) *[see Warnings and Precautions (5.2)]* Muscle weakness Peripheral neuropathy, (that may be irreversible), polyneuropathy *[see Warnings and Precautions (5.8)]*
Psychiatric Disorders	Psychotic reaction (very rarely culminating in self-injurious behavior, such as suicidal ideation/ thoughts or suicide attempts *[see Warnings and Precautions (5.6)]*
Renal and Urinary Disorders	Renal dysfunction Interstitial nephritis *[see Warnings and Precautions (5.5)]*
Respiratory, Thoracic and Mediastinal Disorders	Allergic pneumonitis *[see Warnings and Precautions (5.5)]*
Skin and Subcutaneous Tissue Disorders	Photosensitivity/ phototoxicity reaction *[see Warnings and Precautions (5.10)]* Stevens-Johnson syndrome Toxic epidermal necrolysis *[see Warnings and Precautions (5.5)]*

7 DRUG INTERACTIONS

7.1 Antacids, Sucralfate, Multivitamins and other products containing Multivalent Cations

Quinolones form chelates with alkaline earth and transition metal cations. Oral administration of quinolones with antacids containing aluminum or magnesium, with sucralfate, with metal cations such as iron, or with multivitamins containing iron or zinc, or with formulations containing divalent and trivalent cations such as VIDEX® (didanosine) chewable/buffered tablets or the pediatric powder for oral solution, may substantially interfere with the absorption of quinolones, resulting in systemic concentrations considerably lower than desired. Therefore, AVELOX should be taken at least 4 hours before or 8 hours after these agents. *[see Dosage and Administration (2.2), Pharmacokinetics (12.3), and Patient Counseling Information (17.2).]*

7.2 Warfarin

Quinolones, including AVELOX, have been reported to enhance the anticoagulant effects of warfarin or its derivatives in the patient population. In addition, infectious disease and its accompanying inflammatory process, age, and general status of the patient are risk factors for increased anticoagulant activity. Therefore the prothrombin time, International Normalized Ratio (INR), or other suitable anticoagulation tests should be closely monitored if a quinolone is administered concomitantly with warfarin or its derivatives. *[see Adverse Reactions (6.2, 6.3), Pharmacokinetics (12.3), and Patient Counseling Information (17.3).]*

7.3 Nonsteroidal Anti-Inflammatory Drugs (NSAIDs)

Although not observed with AVELOX in preclinical and clinical trials, the concomitant administration of a nonsteroidal anti-inflammatory drug with a quinolone may increase the risks of CNS stimulation and convulsions *[see Warnings and Precautions (5.6), and Patient Counseling Information (17.3)].*

7.4 Drugs that Prolong QT

There is limited information available on the potential for a pharmacodynamic interaction in humans between AVELOX and other drugs that prolong the QTc interval of the electrocardiogram. Sotalol, a Class III antiarrhythmic, has been shown to further increase the QTc interval when combined with high doses of intravenous (IV) AVELOX in dogs. Therefore, AVELOX should be avoided with Class IA and Class III antiarrhythmics. *[see Warnings and Precautions, (5.3), Nonclinical Toxicology (13.2), and Patient Counseling Information (17.3).]*

8 USE IN SPECIFIC POPULATIONS

8.1 Pregnancy

Pregnancy Category C.

Because no adequate or well-controlled studies have been conducted in pregnant women, AVELOX should be used during pregnancy only if the potential benefit justifies the potential risk to the fetus.

Moxifloxacin was not teratogenic when administered to pregnant rats during organogenesis at oral doses as high as 500 mg/kg/day or 0.24 times the maximum recommended human dose based on systemic exposure (AUC), but decreased fetal body weights and slightly delayed fetal skeletal development (indicative of fetotoxicity) were observed. Intravenous administration of 80 mg/kg/day (approximately 2 times the maximum recommended human dose based on body surface area (mg/m²) to pregnant rats resulted in maternal toxicity and a marginal effect on fetal and placental weights and the appearance of the placenta. There was no evidence of teratogenicity at intravenous doses as high as 80 mg/kg/day. Intravenous administration of 20 mg/kg/day (approximately equal to the maximum recommended human oral dose based upon systemic exposure) to pregnant rabbits during organogenesis resulted in decreased fetal body weights and delayed fetal skeletal ossification. When rib and vertebral malformations were combined, there was an increased fetal and litter incidence of these effects. Signs of maternal toxicity in rabbits at this dose included mortality, abortions, marked reduction of food consumption, decreased water intake, body weight loss and hypoactivity. There was no evidence of teratogenicity when pregnant cynomolgus monkeys were given oral doses as high as 100 mg/kg/day (2.5 times the maximum recommended human dose based upon systemic exposure). An increased incidence of smaller fetuses was observed at 100 mg/kg/day. In an oral pre- and postnatal development study conducted in rats, effects observed at 500 mg/kg/day included slight increases in duration of pregnancy and prenatal loss, reduced pup birth weight and decreased neonatal survival. Treatment-related maternal mortality occurred during gestation at 500 mg/kg/day in this study.

8.3 Nursing Mothers

Moxifloxacin is excreted in the breast milk of rats. Moxifloxacin may also be excreted in human milk. Because of the potential for serious adverse reactions in infants who are nursing from mothers taking AVELOX, a decision should be made whether to discontinue nursing or to discontinue the drug, taking into account the importance of the drug to the mother.

8.4 Pediatric Use

Safety and effectiveness in pediatric patients and adolescents less than 18 years of age have not been established. AVELOX causes arthropathy in juvenile animals *[see Boxed Warning, Warnings and Precautions (5.9), and Clinical Pharmacology (12.3)].*

8.5 Geriatric Use

Geriatric patients are at increased risk for developing severe tendon disorders including tendon rupture when being treated with a fluoroquinolone such as AVELOX. This risk is further increased in patients receiving concomitant corticosteroid therapy. Tendinitis or tendon rupture can involve the Achilles, hand, shoulder, or other tendon sites and can occur during or after completion of therapy; cases occurring up to several months after fluoroquinolone treatment have been reported. Caution should be used when prescribing AVELOX to elderly patients especially those on corticosteroids. Patients should be informed of this potential side effect and advised to discontinue AVELOX and contact their healthcare provider if any symptoms of tendinitis or tendon rupture occur. *[see Boxed Warning, Warnings and Precautions (5.1), and Adverse Reactions (6.2).]*

In controlled multiple-dose clinical trials, 23% of patients receiving oral AVELOX were greater than or equal to 65 years of age and 9% were greater than or equal to 75 years of age. The clinical trial data demonstrate that there is no difference in the safety and efficacy of oral AVELOX in patients aged 65 or older compared to younger adults.

In trials of intravenous use, 42% of AVELOX patients were greater than or equal to 65 years of age, and 23% were greater than or equal to 75 years of age. The clinical trial data demonstrate that the safety of intravenous AVELOX in patients aged 65 or older was similar to that of comparator-treated patients. In general, elderly patients may be more susceptible to drug-associated effects of the QT interval. Therefore, AVELOX should be avoided in patients taking drugs that can result in prolongation of the QT interval (for example, class IA or class III antiarrhythmics) or in patients with risk factors for torsade de pointes (for example, known QT prolongation, uncorrected hypokalemia). *[see Warnings and Precautions (5.3), Drug Interactions (7.4), and Clinical Pharmacology (12.3).]*

8.6 Renal Impairment

The pharmacokinetic parameters of moxifloxacin are not significantly altered in mild, moderate, severe, or end-stage renal disease. No dosage adjustment is necessary in patients with renal impairment, including those patients requiring hemodialysis (HD) or continuous ambulatory peritoneal dialysis (CAPD) *[see Dosage and Administration (2), and Clinical Pharmacology (12.3).]*

8.7 Hepatic Impairment

No dosage adjustment is recommended for mild, moderate, or severe hepatic insufficiency (Child-Pugh Classes A, B, or C). However, due to metabolic disturbances associated with hepatic insufficiency, which may lead to QT prolongation, AVELOX should be used with caution in these patients *[see Warnings and Precaution (5.3), and Clinical Pharmacology, (12.3)].*

10 OVERDOSAGE

Single oral overdoses up to 2.8 g were not associated with any serious adverse events. In the event of acute overdose, the stomach should be emptied and adequate hydration maintained. ECG monitoring is recommended due to the possibility of QT interval prolongation. The patient should be carefully observed and given supportive treatment. The administration of activated charcoal as soon as possible after oral overdose may prevent excessive increase of systemic moxifloxacin exposure. About 3% and 9% of the dose of moxifloxacin, as well as about 2% and 4.5% of its glucuronide metabolite are removed by continuous ambulatory peritoneal dialysis and hemodialysis, respectively.

Single oral AVELOX doses of 2000, 500, and 1500 mg/kg were lethal to rats, mice, and cynomolgus monkeys, respectively. The minimum lethal intravenous dose in mice and rats was 100 mg/kg. Adverse clinical signs included CNS and gastrointestinal effects such as decreased activity, somnolence, tremor, convulsions, vomiting and diarrhea.

11 DESCRIPTION

AVELOX (moxifloxacin) hydrochloride is a synthetic broad spectrum antibacterial agent for oral and intravenous administration. Moxifloxacin, a fluoroquinolone, is available as the monohydrochloride salt of 1-cyclopropyl-7-[(S,S)-2,8-diazabicyclo[4.3.0]non-8-yl]-6-fluoro-8-methoxy-1,4-dihydro-4-oxo-3 quinoline carboxylic acid. It is a slightly yellow to yellow crystalline substance with a molecular weight of 437.9. Its empirical formula is $C_{21}H_{24}FN_3O_4 \cdot HCl$ and its chemical structure is as follows:

11.1 AVELOX Tablets

- AVELOX Tablets are available as film-coated tablets containing moxifloxacin hydrochloride (equivalent to 400 mg moxifloxacin).
- The inactive ingredients are microcrystalline cellulose, lactose monohydrate, croscarmellose sodium, magnesium stearate, hypromellose, titanium dioxide, polyethylene glycol and ferric oxide.

11.2 AVELOX IV

- AVELOX IV is available in ready-to-use 250 mL latex-free flexibags as a sterile, preservative free, 0.8% sodium chloride aqueous solution of moxifloxacin hydrochloride (containing 400 mg moxifloxacin) with pH ranging from 4.1 to 4.6.
- The appearance of the intravenous solution is yellow. The color does not affect, nor is it indicative of, product stability.
- The inactive ingredients are sodium chloride, USP, Water for Injection, USP, and may include hydrochloric acid and/or sodium hydroxide for pH adjustment.
- AVELOX IV contains approximately 34.2 mEq (787 mg) of sodium in 250 mL.

12 CLINICAL PHARMACOLOGY

12.1 Mechanism of Action

AVELOX is a member of the fluoroquinolone class of antibacterial agents *[see Microbiology (12.4)].*

12.3 Pharmacokinetics

Absorption

Moxifloxacin, given as an oral tablet, is well absorbed from the gastrointestinal tract. The absolute bioavailability of moxifloxacin is approximately 90 percent. Co-administration with a high fat meal (that is, 500 calories from fat) does not affect the absorption of moxifloxacin.

Consumption of 1 cup of yogurt with moxifloxacin does not significantly affect the extent or rate of systemic absorption (AUC).

Table 5 Mean (± SD) C_{max} and AUC values following single and multiple doses of 400 mg moxifloxacin given orally

	C_{max} (mg/L)	AUC (mg·h/L)	Half-life (hr)
Single Dose Oral Healthy (n = 372)	3.1 ± 1	36.1 ± 9.1	11.5–15.6*
Multiple Dose Oral			
Healthy young male/female (n = 15)	4.5 ± 0.5	48 ± 2.7	12.7 ± 1.9
Healthy elderly male (n = 8)	3.8 ± 0.3	51.8 ± 6.7	
Healthy elderly female (n = 8)	4.6 ± 0.6	54.6 ± 6.7	
Healthy young male (n = 8)	3.6 ± 0.5	48.2 ± 9	
Healthy young female (n = 9)	4.2 ± 0.5	49.3 ± 9.5	

* Range of means from different studies

Table 6 Mean (± SD) C_{max} and AUC values following single and multiple doses of 400 mg moxifloxacin given by 1 hour IV infusion

	C_{max} (mg/L)	AUC (mg·h/L)	Half-life (hr)
Single Dose IV			
Healthy young male/female (n = 56)	3.9 ± 0.9	39.3 ± 8.6	8.2 - 15.4*
Patients (n = 118)			
Male (n = 64)	4.4 ± 3.7		
Female (n = 54)	4.5 ± 2		
< 65 years (n = 58)	4.6 ± 4.2		
≥ 65 years (n = 60)	4.3 ± 1.3		
Multiple Dose IV			
Healthy young male (n = 8)	4.2 ± 0.8	38 ± 4.7	14.8 ± 2.2
Healthy elderly (n =12; 8 male, 4 female)	6.1 ± 1.3	48.2 ± 0.9	10.1 ± 1.6
Patients† (n = 107)			
Male (n = 58)	4.2 ± 2.6		
Female (n = 49)	4.6 ± 1.5		
<65 years (n = 52)	4.1 ± 1.4		
≥65 years (n = 55)	4.7 ± 2.7		

* Range of means from different studies
† Expected C_{max} (concentration obtained around the time of the end of the infusion)

Plasma concentrations increase proportionally with dose up to the highest dose tested (1200 mg single oral dose). The mean (± SD) elimination half-life from plasma is 12 ± 1.3 hours; steady-state is achieved after at least three days with a 400 mg once daily regimen.

Figure 1 Mean Steady-State Plasma Concentrations of Moxifloxacin Obtained With Once Daily Dosing of 400 mg Either Orally (n=10) or by IV Infusion (n=12)

Distribution
Moxifloxacin is approximately 30-50% bound to serum proteins, independent of drug concentration. The volume of dis-

Table 7 Moxifloxacin Concentrations (mean ± SD) in Tissues and the Corresponding Plasma Concentrations After a Single 400 mg Oral or Intravenous Dose

Tissue or Fluid	N	Plasma Concentration (mcg/mL)	Tissue or Fluid Concentration (mcg/mL or mcg/g)	Tissue Plasma Ratio
Respiratory				
Alveolar Macrophages	5	3.3 ± 0.7	61.8 ± 27.3	21.2 ± 10
Bronchial Mucosa	8	3.3 ± 0.7	5.5 ± 1.3	1.7 ± 0.3
Epithelial Lining Fluid	5	3.3 ± 0.7	24.4 ± 14.7	8.7 ± 6.1
Sinus				
Maxillary Sinus Mucosa	4	3.7 ± 1.1*	7.6 ± 1.7	2 ± 0.3
Anterior Ethmoid Mucosa	3	3.7 ± 1.1*	8.8 ± 4.3	2.2 ± 0.6
Nasal Polyps	4	3.7 ± 1.1*	9.8 ± 4.5	2.6 ± 0.6
Skin, Musculoskeletal				
Blister Fluid	5	3 ± 0.5†	2.6 ± 0.9	0.9 ± 0.2
Subcutaneous Tissue	6	2.3 ± 0.4‡	0.9 ± 0.3§	0.4 ± 0.6
Skeletal Muscle	6	2.3 ± 0.4‡	0.9 ± 0.2§	0.4 ± 0.1
Intra-Abdominal				
Abdominal tissue	8	2.9 ± 0.5	7.6 ± 2	2.7 ± 0.8
Abdominal exudate	10	2.3 ± 0.5	3.5 ±1.2	1.6 ± 0.7
Abscess fluid	6	2.7 ± 0.7	2.3 ±1.5	0.8 ± 0.4

All moxifloxacin concentrations were measured 3 hours after a single 400 mg dose, except the abdominal tissue and exudate concentrations which were measured at 2 hours post-dose and the sinus concentrations which were measured 3 hours post-dose after 5 days of dosing.

* N = 5
† N = 7
‡ N = 12
§ Reflects only non-protein bound concentrations of drug.

tribution of moxifloxacin ranges from 1.7 to 2.7 L/kg. Moxifloxacin is widely distributed throughout the body, with tissue concentrations often exceeding plasma concentrations. Moxifloxacin has been detected in the saliva, nasal and bronchial secretions, mucosa of the sinuses, skin blister fluid, subcutaneous tissue, skeletal muscle, and abdominal tissues and fluids following oral or intravenous administration of 400 mg. Moxifloxacin concentrations measured post-dose in various tissues and fluids following a 400 mg oral or IV dose are summarized in **Table 7**. The rates of elimination of moxifloxacin from tissues generally parallel the elimination from plasma.
[See table 7 above]

Metabolism
Approximately 52% of an oral or intravenous dose of moxifloxacin is metabolized via glucuronide and sulfate conjugation. The cytochrome P450 system is not involved in moxifloxacin metabolism, and is not affected by moxifloxacin. The sulfate conjugate (M1) accounts for approximately 38% of the dose, and is eliminated primarily in the feces. Approximately 14% of an oral or intravenous dose is converted to a glucuronide conjugate (M2), which is excreted exclusively in the urine. Peak plasma concentrations of M2 are approximately 40% those of the parent drug, while plasma concentrations of M1 are generally less than 10% those of moxifloxacin.
In vitro studies with cytochrome (CYP) P450 enzymes indicate that moxifloxacin does not inhibit CYP3A4, CYP2D6, CYP2C9, CYP2C19, or CYP1A2, suggesting that moxifloxacin is unlikely to alter the pharmacokinetics of drugs metabolized by these enzymes.

Excretion
Approximately 45% of an oral or intravenous dose of moxifloxacin is excreted as unchanged drug (~20% in urine and ~25% in feces). A total of 96% ± 4% of an oral dose is excreted as either unchanged drug or known metabolites. The mean (± SD) apparent total body clearance and renal clearance are 12 ± 2 L/hr and 2.6 ± 0.5 L/hr, respectively.

Pharmacokinetics in Specific Populations
Geriatric
Following oral administration of 400 mg moxifloxacin for 10 days in 16 elderly (8 male; 8 female) and 17 young (8 male; 9 female) healthy volunteers, there were no age-related changes in moxifloxacin pharmacokinetics. In 16 healthy male volunteers (8 young; 8 elderly) given a single 200 mg dose of oral moxifloxacin, the extent of systemic exposure (AUC and C_{max}) was not statistically different between young and elderly males and elimination half-life was unchanged. No dosage adjustment is necessary based on age. In large phase III studies, the concentrations around the time of the end of the infusion in elderly patients following intravenous infusion of 400 mg were similar to those observed in young patients. *[see Use In Specific Populations (8.5).]*

Pediatric
The pharmacokinetics of moxifloxacin in pediatric subjects has not been studied *[see Use In Specific Populations (8.4)].*
Gender
Following oral administration of 400 mg moxifloxacin daily for 10 days to 23 healthy males (19-75 years) and 24 healthy females (19-70 years), the mean AUC and C_{max} were 8% and 16% higher, respectively, in females compared to males. There are no significant differences in moxifloxacin pharmacokinetics between male and female subjects when differences in body weight are taken into consideration.
A 400 mg single dose study was conducted in 18 young males and females. The comparison of moxifloxacin pharmacokinetics in this study (9 young females and 9 young males) showed no differences in AUC or C_{max} due to gender. Dosage adjustments based on gender are not necessary.
Race
Steady-state moxifloxacin pharmacokinetics in male Japanese subjects were similar to those determined in Caucasians, with a mean C_{max} of 4.1 mcg/mL, an AUC_{24} of 47 mcg•h/mL, and an elimination half-life of 14 hours, following 400 mg p.o. daily.
Renal Insufficiency
The pharmacokinetic parameters of moxifloxacin are not significantly altered in mild, moderate, severe, or end-stage renal disease. No dosage adjustment is necessary in patients with renal impairment, including those patients requiring hemodialysis (HD) or continuous ambulatory peritoneal dialysis (CAPD).
In a single oral dose study of 24 patients with varying degrees of renal function from normal to severely impaired, the mean peak concentrations (C_{max}) of moxifloxacin were reduced by 21% and 28% in the patients with moderate ($CL_{CR} \geq 30$ and ≤ 60 mL/min) and severe ($CL_{CR} < 30$ mL/min) renal impairment, respectively. The mean systemic exposure (AUC) in these patients was increased by 13%. In the moderate and severe renally impaired patients, the mean AUC for the sulfate conjugate (M1) increased by 1.7-fold (ranging up to 2.8-fold) and mean AUC and C_{max} for the glucuronide conjugate (M2) increased by 2.8-fold (ranging up to 4.8-fold) and 1.4-fold (ranging up to 2.5-fold), respectively. *[see Use in Specific Populations (8.6).]*
The pharmacokinetics of single dose and multiple dose moxifloxacin were studied in patients with $CL_{CR} < 20$ mL/min on either hemodialysis or continuous ambulatory peritoneal dialysis (8 HD, 8 CAPD). Following a single 400 mg oral dose, the AUC of moxifloxacin in these HD and CAPD patients did not vary significantly from the AUC generally found in healthy volunteers. C_{max} values of moxifloxacin were reduced by about 45% and 33% in HD and CAPD patients, respectively, compared to healthy, historical controls. The exposure (AUC) to the sulfate conjugate (M1) increased by 1.4- to 1.5-fold in these patients. The mean AUC of the glucuronide conjugate (M2) increased by a factor of 7.5,

whereas the mean C_{max} values of the glucuronide conjugate (M2) increased by a factor of 2.5 to 3, compared to healthy subjects. The sulfate and the glucuronide conjugates of moxifloxacin are not microbiologically active, and the clinical implication of increased exposure to these metabolites in patients with renal disease including those undergoing HD and CAPD has not been studied.

Oral administration of 400 mg QD AVELOX for 7 days to patients on HD or CAPD produced mean systemic exposure (AUC_{ss}) to moxifloxacin similar to that generally seen in healthy volunteers. Steady-state C_{max} values were about 22% lower in HD patients but were comparable between CAPD patients and healthy volunteers. Both HD and CAPD removed only small amounts of moxifloxacin from the body (approximately 9% by HD, and 3% by CAPD). HD and CAPD also removed about 4% and 2% of the glucuronide metabolite (M2), respectively.

Hepatic Insufficiency

No dosage adjustment is recommended for mild, moderate, or severe hepatic insufficiency (Child-Pugh Classes A, B, or C). However, due to metabolic disturbances associated with hepatic insufficiency, which may lead to QT prolongation, AVELOX should be used with caution in these patients *[see Warnings and Precautions (5.3), Use in Specific Populations (8.7)]*.

In 400 mg single oral dose studies in 6 patients with mild (Child-Pugh Class A) and 10 patients with moderate (Child-Pugh Class B) hepatic insufficiency, moxifloxacin mean systemic exposure (AUC) was 78% and 102%, respectively, of 18 healthy controls and mean peak concentration (C_{max}) was 79% and 84% of controls.

The mean AUC of the sulfate conjugate of moxifloxacin (M1) increased by 3.9-fold (ranging up to 5.9-fold) and 5.7-fold (ranging up to 8-fold) in the mild and moderate groups, respectively. The mean C_{max} of M1 increased by approximately 3-fold in both groups (ranging up to 4.7- and 3.9-fold). The mean AUC of the glucuronide conjugate of moxifloxacin (M2) increased by 1.5-fold (ranging up to 2.5-fold) in both groups. The mean C_{max} of M2 increased by 1.6- and 1.3-fold (ranging up to 2.7- and 2.1-fold), respectively. The clinical significance of increased exposure to the sulfate and glucuronide conjugates has not been studied. In a subset of patients participating in a clinical trial, the plasma concentrations of moxifloxacin and metabolites determined approximately at the moxifloxacin T_{max} following the first intravenous or oral AVELOX dose in the Child-Pugh Class C patients (n=10) were similar to those in the Child-Pugh Class A/B patients (n=5), and also similar to those observed in healthy volunteer studies.

Photosensitivity Potential

A study of the skin response to ultraviolet (UVA and UVB) and visible radiation conducted in 32 healthy volunteers (8 per group) demonstrated that AVELOX does not show phototoxicity in comparison to placebo. The minimum erythematous dose (MED) was measured before and after treatment with AVELOX (200 mg or 400 mg once daily), lomefloxacin (400 mg once daily), or placebo. In this study, the MED measured for both doses of AVELOX were not significantly different from placebo, while lomefloxacin significantly lowered the MED.

It is difficult to ascribe relative photosensitivity/phototoxicity among various fluoroquinolones during actual patient use because other factors play a role in determining a subject's susceptibility to this adverse event such as: a patient's skin pigmentation, frequency and duration of sun and artificial ultraviolet light (UV) exposure, wearing of sunscreen and protective clothing, the use of other concomitant drugs and the dosage and duration of fluoroquinolone therapy *[see Warnings and Precautions (5.10), Adverse Reactions (6.3), and Patient Counseling Information (17.3)]*.

Drug-Drug Interactions

The following drug interactions were studied in healthy volunteers or patients.

Antacids and iron significantly reduced bioavailability of moxifloxacin, as observed with other quinolones *[see Drug Interactions (7.1)]*.

Calcium, digoxin, itraconazole, morphine, probenecid, ranitidine, theophylline, and warfarin did not significantly affect the pharmacokinetics of moxifloxacin. These results and the data from *in vitro* studies suggest that moxifloxacin is unlikely to significantly alter the metabolic clearance of drugs metabolized by CYP3A4, CYP2D6, CYP2C9, CYP2C19, or CYP1A2 enzymes.

Moxifloxacin had no clinically significant effect on the pharmacokinetics of atenolol, digoxin, glyburide, itraconazole, oral contraceptives, theophylline, and warfarin *[see Drug Interactions (7.2)]*.

Antacids

When moxifloxacin (single 400 mg tablet dose) was administered two hours before, concomitantly, or 4 hours after an aluminum/magnesium-containing antacid (900 mg aluminum hydroxide and 600 mg magnesium hydroxide as a single oral dose) to 12 healthy volunteers there was a 26%, 60% and 23% reduction in the mean AUC of moxifloxacin, respectively. Moxifloxacin should be taken at least 4 hours before or 8 hours after antacids containing magnesium or aluminum, as well as sucralfate, metal cations such as iron, and multivitamin preparations with zinc, or VIDEX® (didanosine) chewable/ buffered tablets or the pediatric powder for oral solution. *[see Dosage and Administration (2.2), Drug Interactions (7.1)]*.

Atenolol

In a crossover study involving 24 healthy volunteers (12 male; 12 female), the mean atenolol AUC following a single oral dose of 50 mg atenolol with placebo was similar to that observed when atenolol was given concomitantly with a single 400 mg oral dose of moxifloxacin. The mean C_{max} of single dose atenolol decreased by about 10% following co-administration with a single dose of moxifloxacin.

Calcium

Twelve healthy volunteers were administered concomitant moxifloxacin (single 400 mg dose) and calcium (single dose of 500 mg Ca^{++} dietary supplement) followed by an additional two doses of calcium 12 and 24 hours after moxifloxacin administration. Calcium had no significant effect on the mean AUC of moxifloxacin. The mean C_{max} was slightly reduced and the time to maximum plasma concentration was prolonged when moxifloxacin was given with calcium compared to when moxifloxacin was given alone (2.5 hours versus 0.9 hours). These differences are not considered to be clinically significant.

Digoxin

No significant effect of moxifloxacin (400 mg once daily for two days) on digoxin (0.6 mg as a single dose) AUC was detected in a study involving 12 healthy volunteers. The mean digoxin C_{max} increased by about 50% during the distribution phase of digoxin. This transient increase in digoxin C_{max} is not viewed to be clinically significant. Moxifloxacin pharmacokinetics were similar in the presence or absence of digoxin. No dosage adjustment for moxifloxacin or digoxin is required when these drugs are administered concomitantly.

Glyburide

In diabetics, glyburide (2.5 mg once daily for two weeks pretreatment and for five days concurrently) mean AUC and C_{max} were 12% and 21% lower, respectively, when taken with moxifloxacin (400 mg once daily for five days) in comparison to placebo. Nonetheless, blood glucose levels were decreased slightly in patients taking glyburide and moxifloxacin in comparison to those taking glyburide alone, suggesting no interference by moxifloxacin on the activity of glyburide. These interaction results are not viewed as clinically significant.

Iron

When moxifloxacin tablets were administered concomitantly with iron (ferrous sulfate 100 mg once daily for two days), the mean AUC and C_{max} of moxifloxacin was reduced by 39% and 59%, respectively. Moxifloxacin should only be taken more than 4 hours before or 8 hours after iron products. *[see Dosage and Administration (2.2), Drug Interactions (7.1)]*.

Itraconazole

In a study involving 11 healthy volunteers, there was no significant effect of itraconazole (200 mg once daily for 9 days), a potent inhibitor of cytochrome P4503A4, on the pharmacokinetics of moxifloxacin (a single 400 mg dose given on the 7th day of itraconazole dosing). In addition, moxifloxacin was shown not to affect the pharmacokinetics of itraconazole.

Morphine

No significant effect of morphine sulfate (a single 10 mg intramuscular dose) on the mean AUC and C_{max} of moxifloxacin (400 mg single dose) was observed in a study of 20 healthy male and female volunteers.

Oral Contraceptives

A placebo-controlled study in 29 healthy female subjects showed that moxifloxacin 400 mg daily for 7 days did not interfere with the hormonal suppression of oral contraception with 0.15 mg levonorgestrel/0.03 mg ethinylestradiol (as measured by serum progesterone, FSH, estradiol, and LH), or with the pharmacokinetics of the administered contraceptive agents.

Probenecid

Probenecid (500 mg twice daily for two days) did not alter the renal clearance and total amount of moxifloxacin (400 mg single dose) excreted renally in a study of 12 healthy volunteers.

Ranitidine

No significant effect of ranitidine (150 mg twice daily for three days as pretreatment) on the pharmacokinetics of moxifloxacin (400 mg single dose) was detected in a study involving 10 healthy volunteers.

Theophylline

No significant effect of moxifloxacin (200 mg every twelve hours for 3 days) on the pharmacokinetics of theophylline (400 mg every twelve hours for 3 days) was detected in a study involving 12 healthy volunteers. In addition, theophylline was not shown to affect the pharmacokinetics of moxifloxacin. The effect of co-administration of a 400 mg dose of moxifloxacin with theophylline has not been studied, but it is not expected to be clinically significant based on *in vitro* metabolic data showing that moxifloxacin does not inhibit the CYP1A2 isoenzyme.

Warfarin

No significant effect of moxifloxacin (400 mg once daily for eight days) on the pharmacokinetics of R- and S-warfarin (25 mg single dose of warfarin sodium on the fifth day) was detected in a study involving 24 healthy volunteers. No significant change in prothrombin time was observed. *[see Adverse Reactions (6.2), Drug Interactions (7.2)]*.

12.4   Microbiology

Mechanism of Action

The bactericidal action of moxifloxacin results from inhibition of the topoisomerase II (DNA gyrase) and topoisomerase IV required for bacterial DNA replication, transcription, repair, and recombination. It appears that the C8-methoxy moiety contributes to enhanced activity and lower selection of resistant mutants of Gram-positive bacteria compared to the C8-H moiety. The presence of the bulky bicycloamine substituent at the C-7 position prevents active efflux, associated with the *NorA* or *pmrA* genes seen in certain Gram-positive bacteria.

Mechanism of Resistance

The mechanism of action for fluoroquinolones, including moxifloxacin, is different from that of macrolides, beta-lactams, aminoglycosides, or tetracyclines; therefore, microorganisms resistant to these classes of drugs may be susceptible to moxifloxacin. Resistance to fluoroquinolones occurs primarily by a mutation in topoisomerase II (DNA gyrase) or topoisomerase IV genes, decreased outer membrane permeability or drug efflux. *In vitro* resistance to moxifloxacin develops slowly via multiple-step mutations. Resistance to

Table 8 Susceptibility Test Interpretive Criteria for Moxifloxacin

Species	MIC (mcg/mL)			Zone Diameter (mm)		
	S	I	R	S	I	R
Enterobacteriacae	≤2	4	≥8	≥19	16–18	≤15
Enterococcus faecalis	≤1	2	≥4	≥18	15–17	≤14
Staphylococcus aureus	≤2	4	≥8	≥19	16–18	≤15
Haemophilus influenzae	≤1	-*	-*	≥18	-*	-*
Haemophilus parainfluenzae	≤1	-*	-*	≥18	-*	-*
Streptococcus pneumoniae	≤1	2	≥4	≥18	15–17	≤14[†]
Streptococcus species	≤1	2	≥4	≥18	15–17	≤14[†]
Anaerobic bacteria	≤2	4	≥8			

S=susceptible, I=Intermediate, and R=resistant.

* The current absence of data on moxifloxacin-resistant isolates precludes defining any results other than "Susceptible".
† Isolates yielding test results (MIC or zone diameter) other than susceptible, should be submitted to a reference laboratory for additional testing.

moxifloxacin occurs *in vitro* at a general frequency of between 1.8×10^{-9} to $< 1 \times 10^{-11}$ for Gram-positive bacteria.

Cross Resistance

Cross-resistance has been observed between moxifloxacin and other fluoroquinolones against Gram-negative bacteria. Gram-positive bacteria resistant to other fluoroquinolones may, however, still be susceptible to moxifloxacin. There is no known cross-resistance between moxifloxacin and other classes of antimicrobials.

Moxifloxacin has been shown to be active against most isolates of the following bacteria, both *in vitro* and in clinical infections. *[see Indications and Usage (1)].*

Gram-positive bacteria
• *Enterococcus faecalis*
• *Staphylococcus aureus*
• *Streptococcus anginosus*
• *Streptococcus constellatus*
• *Streptococcus pneumoniae* (including multi-drug resistant isolates [MDRSP]**)
• *Streptococcus pyogenes*

**MDRSP, Multi-drug resistant *Streptococcus pneumoniae* includes isolates previously known as PRSP (Penicillin-resistant *S. pneumoniae*), and are isolates resistant to two or more of the following antibiotics: penicillin (MIC) ≥2 mcg/mL), 2nd generation cephalosporins (for example, cefuroxime), macrolides, tetracyclines, and trimethoprim/sulfamethoxazole.

Gram-negative bacteria
• *Enterobacter cloacae*
• *Escherichia coli*
• *Haemophilus influenzae*
• *Haemophilus parainfluenzae*
• *Klebsiella pneumoniae*
• *Moraxella catarrhalis*
• *Proteus mirabilis*

Anaerobic bacteria
• *Bacteroides fragilis*
• *Bacteroides thetaiotaomicron*
• *Clostridium perfringens*
• *Peptostreptococcus species*

Other microorganisms
• *Chlamydophila pneumoniae*
• *Mycoplasma pneumoniae*

The following *in vitro* data are available, **but their clinical significance is unknown.** At least 90 percent of the following bacteria exhibit an *in vitro* minimum inhibitory concentration (MIC) less than or equal to the susceptible breakpoint for moxifloxacin. However, the efficacy of AVELOX in treating clinical infections due to these bacteria **has not been** established in adequate and well controlled clinical trials.

Gram-positive bacteria
• *Staphylococcus epidermidis*
• *Streptococcus agalactiae*
• *Streptococcus viridans group*

Gram-negative bacteria
• *Citrobacter freundii*
• *Klebsiellao xytoca*
• *Legionella pneumophila*

Anaerobic bacteria
• *Fusobacterium species*
• *Prevotella species*

Susceptibility Tests Methods

When available, the clinical microbiology laboratory should provide the results of *in vitro* susceptibility test results for antimicrobial drug products used in resident hospitals to the physician as periodic reports that describe the susceptibility profile of nosocomial and community acquired pathogens. These reports should aid the physician in selecting an antibacterial drug product for treatment.

• **Dilution Techniques**

Quantitative methods are used to determine antimicrobial minimum inhibitory concentrations (MICs). These MICs provide estimates of the susceptibility of bacteria to antimicrobial compounds. The MICs should be determined using a standardized procedure. Standardized procedures are based on a dilution method (broth and/or agar).[1] The MIC values should be interpreted according to the criteria in Table 8.

• **Diffusion Techniques**

Quantitative methods that require measurement of zone diameters can also provide reproducible estimates of the susceptibility of bacteria to antimicrobial compounds. The zone size provides an estimate of the susceptibility of bacteria to antimicrobial compounds. The zone size prove should be determined using a standardized test method.[2,3] This procedure uses paper disks impregnated with 5 mcg moxifloxacin to test the susceptibility of bacteria to moxifloxacin. The disc diffusion interpretive criteria are provided in Table 8.

• **Anaerobic Techniques**

For anaerobic bacteria, the susceptibility to moxifloxacin can be determined by a standardized test method.[4] The MIC values obtained should be interpreted according to the criteria provided in Table 8.

[See table 8 at top of previous page]

A report of "Susceptible" indicates that the antimicrobial is likely to inhibit growth of the pathogen if the antimicrobial compound reaches the concentrations at the infection site necessary to inhibit growth of the pathogen. A report of "Intermediate" indicates that the result should be considered equivocal, and, if the microorganism is not fully susceptible to alternative, clinically feasible drugs, the test should be repeated. This category implies possible clinical applicability in body sites where the drug is physiologically concentrated or in situations where a high dosage of the drug product can be used. This category also provides a buffer zone that prevents small uncontrolled technical factors from causing major discrepancies in interpretation. A report of "Resistant" indicates that the antimicrobial is not likely to inhibit growth of the pathogen if the antimicrobial compound reaches the concentrations usually achievable at the infection site; other therapy should be selected.

• **Quality Control**

Standardized susceptibility test procedures require the use of laboratory controls to monitor and ensure the accuracy and precision of supplies and reagents used in the assay and the techniques of the individuals performing the test.[1,2,3,4] Standard moxifloxacin powder should provide the following range of MIC values noted in Table 9. For the diffusion technique using the 5 mcg moxifloxacin disk, the criteria in Table 9 should be achieved.

Table 9 Acceptable Quality Control Ranges for Moxifloxacin

Strains	MIC range (mcg/mL)	Zone Diameter (mm)
Enterococcus faecalis ATCC 29212	0.06–0.5	-
Escherichia coli ATCC 25922	0.008–0.06	28–35
Haemophilus influenzae ATCC 49247	0.008–0.03	31–39
Staphylococcus aureus ATCC29213	0.015–0.06	-
Staphylococcus aureus ATCC25923		28–35
Streptococcus pneumoniae ATCC 49619	0.06–0.25	25–31
Bacteroides fragilis ATCC 25285	0.125–0.5	
Bacteroides thetaiotaomicron ATCC 29741	1–4	
Eubacterium lentum ATCC 43055	0.125–0.5	

13 NONCLINICAL TOXICOLOGY

13.1 Carcinogenesis, Mutagenesis, Impairment of Fertility

Long term studies in animals to determine the carcinogenic potential of moxifloxacin have not been performed.

Moxifloxacin was not mutagenic in 4 bacterial strains (TA 98, TA 100, TA 1535, TA 1537) used in the Ames *Salmonella* reversion assay. As with other quinolones, the positive response observed with moxifloxacin in strain TA 102 using the same assay may be due to the inhibition of DNA gyrase. Moxifloxacin was not mutagenic in the CHO/HGPRT mammalian cell gene mutation assay. An equivocal result was obtained in the same assay when v79 cells were used. Moxifloxacin was clastogenic in the v79 chromosome aberration assay, but it did not induce unscheduled DNA synthesis in cultured rat hepatocytes. There was no evidence of genotoxicity *in vivo* in a micronucleus test or a dominant lethal test in mice.

Moxifloxacin had no effect on fertility in male and female rats at oral doses as high as 500 mg/kg/day, approximately 12 times the maximum recommended human dose based on body surface area (mg/m²), or at intravenous doses as high as 45 mg/kg/day, approximately equal to the maximum recommended human dose based on body surface area (mg/m²). At 500 mg/kg orally there were slight effects on sperm morphology (head-tail separation) in male rats and on the estrous cycle in female rats.

13.2 Animal Toxicology and/or Pharmacology

Quinolones have been shown to cause arthropathy in immature animals. In studies in juvenile dogs oral doses of moxifloxacin ≥ 30 mg/kg/day (approximately 1.5 times the maximum recommended human dose based upon systemic exposure) for 28 days resulted in arthropathy. There was no evidence of arthropathy in mature monkeys and rats at oral doses up to 135 and 500 mg/kg/day, respectively.

Moxifloxacin at an oral dose of 300 mg/kg did not show an increase in acute toxicity or potential for CNS toxicity (for example, seizures) in mice when used in combination with NSAIDs such as diclofenac, ibuprofen, or fenbufen. Some quinolones have been reported to have proconvulsant activity that is exacerbated with concomitant use of nonsteroidal anti-inflammatory drugs (NSAIDs).

A QT-prolonging effect of moxifloxacin was found in dog studies, at plasma concentrations about five times the human therapeutic level. The combined infusion of sotalol, a Class III antiarrhythmic agent, with moxifloxacin induced a higher degree of QTc prolongation in dogs than that induced by the same dose (30 mg/kg) of moxifloxacin alone. Electrophysiological *in vitro* studies suggested an inhibition of the rapid activating component of the delayed rectifier potassium current (I_{Kr}) as an underlying mechanism.

No signs of local intolerability were observed in dogs when moxifloxacin was administered intravenously. After intra-arterial injection, inflammatory changes involving the peri-arterial soft tissue were observed suggesting that intra-arterial administration of AVELOX should be avoided.

14 CLINICAL STUDIES

14.1 Acute Bacterial Exacerbation of Chronic Bronchitis

AVELOX Tablets (400 mg once daily for five days) were evaluated for the treatment of acute bacterial exacerbation of chronic bronchitis in a randomized, double-blind, controlled clinical trial conducted in the US. This study compared AVELOX with clarithromycin (500 mg twice daily for 10 days) and enrolled 629 patients. Clinical success was assessed at 7-17 days post-therapy. The clinical success for AVELOX was 89% (222/250) compared to 89% (224/251) for clarithromycin.

Table 10 Clinical Success Rates at Follow-Up Visit for Clinically Evaluable Patients by Pathogen (Acute Bacterial Exacerbation of Chronic Bronchitis)

PATHOGEN	AVELOX	Clarithromycin
Streptococcus pneumoniae	16/16 (100%)	20/23 (87%)
Haemophilus influenzae	33/37 (89%)	36/41 (88%)
Haemophilus parainfluenzae	16/16 (100%)	14/14 (100%)
Moraxella catarrhalis	29/34 (85%)	24/24 (100%)
Staphylococcus aureus	15/16 (94%)	6/8 (75%)
Klebsiella pneumoniae	18/20 (90%)	10/11 (91%)

The microbiological eradication rates (eradication plus presumed eradication) in AVELOX treated patients were *Streptococcus pneumoniae* 100%, *Haemophilus influenzae* 89%, *Haemophilus parainfluenzae* 100%, *Moraxella catarrhalis* 85%, *Staphylococcus aureus* 94%, and *Klebsiella pneumonia* 85%.

14.2 Community Acquired Pneumonia

A randomized, double-blind, controlled clinical trial was conducted in the US to compare the efficacy of AVELOX Tablets (400 mg once daily) to that of high-dose clarithromycin (500 mg twice daily) in the treatment of patients with clinically and radiologically documented community acquired pneumonia. This study enrolled 474 patients (382 of whom were valid for the efficacy analysis conducted at the 14 - 35 day follow-up visit). Clinical success for clinically evaluable patients was 95% (184/194) for AVELOX and 95% (178/188) for high dose clarithromycin.

A randomized, double-blind, controlled trial was conducted in the US and Canada to compare the efficacy of sequential IV/PO AVELOX 400 mg QD for 7-14 days to an IV/PO fluoroquinolone control (trovafloxacin or levofloxacin) in the treatment of patients with clinically and radiologically documented community acquired pneumonia. This study enrolled 516 patients, 362 of whom were valid for the efficacy analysis conducted at the 7-30 day post-therapy visit. The clinical success rate was 86% (157/182) for AVELOX therapy and 89% (161/180) for the fluoroquinolone comparators. An open-label ex-US study that enrolled 628 patients compared AVELOX to sequential IV/PO amoxicillin/clavulanate (1.2 g IV q8h/625 mg PO q8h) with or without high-dose IV/PO clarithromycin (500 mg BID). The intravenous formulations of the comparators are not FDA approved. The clinical success rate at Day 5-7 for AVELOX therapy was 93% (241/258) and demonstrated superiority to amoxicillin/clavulanate ± clarithromycin (85%, 239/280) [95% C.I. of difference in success rates between moxifloxacin and comparator (2.9%, 13.2%)]. The clinical success rate at the 21-28 days post-therapy visit for AVELOX was 84% (216/258), which also demonstrated superiority to the comparators (74%, 208/280) [95% C.I. of difference in success rates between moxifloxacin and comparator (2.6%, 16.3%)]. The clinical success rates by pathogen across four CAP studies are presented in **Table 11**.

Table 11 Clinical Success Rates By Pathogen (Pooled CAP Studies)

PATHOGEN	AVELOX	
Streptococcus pneumoniae	80/85	(94%)
Staphylococcus aureus	17/20	(85%)
Klebsiella pneumoniae	11/12	(92%)
Haemophilus influenzae	56/61	(92%)
Chlamydophila pneumoniae	119/128	(93%)
Mycoplasma pneumoniae	73/76	(96%)
Moraxella catarrhalis	11/12	(92%)

14.3 Community Acquired Pneumonia caused by Multi-Drug Resistant *Streptococcus pneumoniae* (MDRSP)*

AVELOX was effective in the treatment of community acquired pneumonia (CAP) caused by multi-drug resistant *Streptococcus pneumoniae* MDRSP* isolates. Of 37 microbiologically evaluable patients with MDRSP isolates, 35 patients (95%) achieved clinical and bacteriological success post-therapy. The clinical and bacteriological success rates based on the number of patients treated are shown in **Table 12**.

* MDRSP, Multi-drug resistant *Streptococcus pneumoniae* includes isolates previously known as PRSP (Penicillin-resistant *S. pneumoniae*), and are isolates resistant to two or more of the following antibiotics: penicillin (MIC ≥ 2 mcg/mL), 2nd generation cephalosporins (for example, cefuroxime), macrolides, tetracyclines, and trimethoprim/sulfamethoxazole.

[See table 12 above]

Not all isolates were resistant to all antimicrobial classes tested. Success and eradication rates are summarized in Table 13.

Table 13 Clinical Success Rates and Microbiological Eradication Rates for Resistant Streptococcus pneumoniae (Community Acquired Pneumonia)

S. pneumoniae with MDRSP	Clinical Success	Bacteriological Eradication Rate
Resistant to 2 antimicrobials	12/13 (92.3 %)	12/13 (92.3 %)
Resistant to 3 antimicrobials	10/11 (90.9 %)*	10/11 (90.9 %)*
Resistant to 4 antimicrobials	6/6 (100%)	6/6 (100%)
Resistant to 5 antimicrobials	7/7 (100%)*	7/7 (100%)*
Bacteremia with MDRSP	9/9 (100%)	9/9 (100%)

* One patient had a respiratory isolate resistant to 5 antimicrobials and a blood isolate resistant to 3 antimicrobials. The patient was included in the category resistant to 5 antimicrobials.

14.4 Acute Bacterial Sinusitis

In a controlled double-blind study conducted in the US, AVELOX Tablets (400 mg once daily for ten days) were compared with cefuroxime axetil (250 mg twice daily for ten days) for the treatment of acute bacterial sinusitis. The trial included 457 patients valid for the efficacy analysis. Clinical success (cure plus improvement) at the 7 to 21 day post-therapy test of cure visit was 90% for AVELOX and 89% for cefuroxime.

An additional non-comparative study was conducted to gather bacteriological data and to evaluate microbiological eradication in adult patients treated with AVELOX 400 mg once daily for seven days. All patients (n = 336) underwent antral puncture in this study. Clinical success rates and eradication/presumed eradication rates at the 21 to 37 day follow-up visit were 97% (29 out of 30) for *Streptococcus pneumoniae*, 83% (15 out of 18) for *Moraxella catarrhalis*, and 80% (24 out of 30) for *Haemophilus influenzae*.

14.5 Uncomplicated Skin and Skin Structure Infections

A randomized, double-blind, controlled clinical trial conducted in the US compared the efficacy of AVELOX 400 mg

once daily for seven days with cephalexin HCl 500 mg three times daily for seven days. The percentage of patients treated for uncomplicated abscesses was 30%, furuncles 8%, cellulitis 16%, impetigo 20%, and other skin infections 26%. Adjunctive procedures (incision and drainage or debridement) were performed on 17% of the AVELOX treated patients and 14% of the comparator treated patients. Clinical success rates in evaluable patients were 89% (108/122) for AVELOX and 91% (110/121) for cephalexin HCl.

14.6 Complicated Skin and Skin Structure Infections

Two randomized, active controlled trials of cSSSI were performed. A double-blind trial was conducted primarily in North America to compare the efficacy of sequential IV/PO AVELOX 400 mg QD for 7-14 days to an IV/PO beta-lactam/beta-lactamase inhibitor control in the treatment of patients with cSSSI. This study enrolled 617 patients, 335 of which were valid for the efficacy analysis. A second open-label International study compared AVELOX 400 mg QD for 7-21 days to sequential IV/PO beta-lactam/beta-lactamase inhibitor control in the treatment of patients with cSSSI. This study enrolled 804 patients, 632 of which were valid for the efficacy analysis. Surgical incision and drainage or debridement was performed on 55% of the AVELOX treated and 53% of the comparator treated patients in these studies and formed an integral part of therapy for this indication. Success rates varied with the type of diagnosis ranging from 61% in patients with infected ulcers to 90% in patients with complicated erysipelas. These rates were similar to those seen with comparator drugs. The overall success rates in the evaluable patients and the clinical success by pathogen are shown in **Tables 14 and 15**.

Table 14 Overall Clinical Success Rates in Patients with Complicated Skin and Skin Structure Infections

Study	AVELOX n/ N (%)	Comparator n/N (%)	95% Confidence Interval*
North America	125/162 (77.2%)	141/173 (81.5%)	(-14.4%, 2%)
International	254/315 (80.6%)	268/317 (84.5%)	(-9.4%, 2.2%)

* of difference in success rates between Moxifloxacin and comparator (Moxifloxacin – comparator)

Table 15 Clinical Success Rates by Pathogen in Patients with Complicated Skin and Skin Structure Infections

Pathogen	AVELOX n/ N (%)	Comparator n/N (%)
Staphylococcus aureus (methicillin-susceptible isolates)*	106/129 (82.2%)	120/137 (87.6%)
Escherichia coli	31/38 (81.6%)	28/33 (84.8%)
Klebsiella pneumoniae	11/12 (91.7 %)	7/10 (70%)
Enterobacter cloacae	9/11 (81.8%)	4/7 (57.1%)

* methicillin susceptibility was only determined in the North American Study

14.7 Complicated Intra-Abdominal Infections

Two randomized, active controlled trials of cIAI were performed. A double-blind trial was conducted primarily in

Table 12 Clinical and Bacteriological Success Rates for AVELOX-Treated MDRSP CAP Patients (Population: Valid for Efficacy)

Screening Susceptibility	Clinical Success		Bacteriological Success	
	n/N*	%	n/N†	%
Penicillin-resistant	21/21	100%‡	21/21	100%‡
2nd generation cephalosporin-resistant	25/26	96%‡	25/26	96%‡
Macrolide-resistant§	22/23	96%	22/23	96%
Trimethoprim/sulfamethoxazole-resistant	28/30	93%	28/30	93%
Tetracycline-resistant	17/18	94%	17/18	94%

* n = number of patients successfully treated; N = number of patients with MDRSP (from a total of 37 patients)
† n = number of patients successfully treated (presumed eradication or eradication); N = number of patients with MDRSP (from a total of 37 patients)
‡ One patient had a respiratory isolate that was resistant to penicillin and cefuroxime but a blood isolate that was intermediate to penicillin and cefuroxime. The patient is included in the database based on the respiratory isolate.
§ Azithromycin, clarithromycin, and erythromycin were the macrolide antimicrobials tested.

North America to compare the efficacy of sequential IV/PO AVELOX 400 mg QD for 5-14 days to IV/ piperacillin/tazobactam followed by PO amoxicillin/clavulanic acid in the treatment of patients with cIAI, including peritonitis, abscesses, appendicitis with perforation, and bowel perforation. This study enrolled 681 patients, 379 of which were considered clinically evaluable. A second open-label international study compared AVELOX 400 mg QD for 5-14 days to IV ceftriaxone plus IV metronidazole followed by PO amoxicillin/clavulanic acid in the treatment of patients with cIAI. This study enrolled 595 patients, 511 of which were considered clinically evaluable. The clinically evaluable population consisted of subjects with a surgically confirmed complicated infection, at least 5 days of treatment and a 25-50 day follow-up assessment for patients at the Test of Cure visit. The overall clinical success rates in the clinically evaluable patients are shown in **Table 16**.

Table 16 Clinical Success Rates in Patients with Complicated Intra-Abdominal Infections

Study	AVELOX n/ N (%)	Comparator n/N (%)	95% Confidence Interval*
North America (overall)	146/183 (79.8 %)	153/196 (78.1 %)	(-7.4%, 9.3%)
Abscess	40/57 (70.2 %)	49/63 (77.8 %)†	NA‡
Non-abscess	106/126 (84.1 %)	104/133 (78.2 %)	NA‡
International (overall)	199/246 (80.9 %)	218/265 (82.3 %)	(-8.9 %, 4.2%)
Abscess	73/93 (78.5 %)	86/99 (86.9 %)	NA
Non-abscess	126/153 (82.4 %)	132/166 (79.5 %)	NA

* of difference in success rates between AVELOX and comparator (AVELOX – comparator)
† Excludes 2 patients who required additional surgery within the first 48 hours.
‡ NA - not applicable

15 REFERENCES

1. Clinical and Laboratory Standards Institute (CLSI), Methods for Dilution Antimicrobial Susceptibility Tests for Bacteria That Grow Aerobically 9th edition. Approved Standard CLSI Document M7-A9, CLSI, 950 West Valley Rd., Suite 2500, Wayne, PA 19087, 2012.
2. CLSI , Performance Standards for Antimicrobial Susceptibility Testing 22 Informational Supplement. CLSI Document M100-S22, 2012.
3. CLSI , Performance Standards for Antimicrobial Disk Susceptibility Tests 11th edition. Approved Standard CLSI Document M2-A11, 2012.
4. CLSI , Methods for Antimicrobial Susceptibility Testing of Anaerobic Bacteria 8th edition; Approved Standard CLSI Document M11-A8, 2012

16 HOW SUPPLIED/STORAGE AND HANDLING
16.1 AVELOX Tablets

AVELOX (moxifloxacin) hydrochloride tablets are available as oblong, dull red film-coated tablets containing 400 mg moxifloxacin.

The tablet is coded with the word "BAYER" on one side and "M400" on the reverse side.

Package	NDC Code
Bottles of 30:	0085-1733-01
Unit Dose Pack of 50:	0085-1733-02
ABC Pack of 5:	0085-1733-03

Store at 25°C (77°F); excursions permitted to 15–30°C (59–86°F) [see USP Controlled Room Temperature]. Avoid high humidity.

16.2   AVELOX Intravenous Solution – Premix Bags
AVELOX IV (moxifloxacin) hydrochloride in sodium chloride injection) is available in ready-to-use 250 mL latex-free flexible bags containing 400 mg of moxifloxacin in 0.8% saline. NO FURTHER DILUTION OF THIS PREPARATION IS NECESSARY.

Package	NDC Code
250 mL flexible container	0085-1737-01

Parenteral drug products should be inspected visually for particulate matter prior to administration. Samples containing visible particulates should not be used.
Because the premix flexible containers are for single-use only, any unused portion should be discarded.
Store at 25°C (77°F); excursions permitted to 15–30°C (59–86°F) [see USP Controlled Room Temperature].
DO NOT REFRIGERATE – PRODUCT PRECIPITATES UPON REFRIGERATION.

17   PATIENT COUNSELING INFORMATION
See FDA-Approved Medication Guide
17.1   Antibacterial Resistance
Antibacterial drugs including AVELOX should only be used to treat bacterial infections. They do not treat viral infections (for example, the common cold). When AVELOX is prescribed to treat a bacterial infection, patients should be told that although it is common to feel better early in the course of therapy, the medication should be taken exactly as directed. Skipping doses or not completing the full course of therapy may (1) decrease the effectiveness of the immediate treatment and (2) increase the likelihood that bacteria will develop resistance and will not be treatable by AVELOX or other antibacterial drugs in the future.

17.2   Administration With Food, Fluids, and Drug Products Containing Multivalent Cations
Patients should be informed that AVELOX tablets may be taken with or without food. Patients should be advised to drink fluids liberally.
AVELOX tablets should be taken at least 4 hours before or 8 hours after multivitamins (containing iron or zinc), antacids (containing magnesium or aluminum), sucralfate, or VIDEX® (didanosine) chewable/buffered tablets or the pediatric powder for oral solution.

17.3   Serious and Potentially Serious Adverse Reactions
To assure safe and effective use of AVELOX, patients should be informed of the following serious adverse reactions that have been associated with AVELOX and other fluoroquinolone use:

- **Tendon Disorders:** Patients should contact their healthcare provider if they experience pain, swelling, or inflammation of a tendon, or weakness or inability to use one of their joints; rest and refrain from exercise; and discontinue AVELOX treatment. The risk of severe tendon disorder with fluoroquinolones is higher in older patients usually over 60 years of age, in patients taking corticosteroid drugs, and in patients with kidney, heart or lung transplants.
- **Exacerbation of Myasthenia Gravis:** fluoroquinolones like AVELOX may cause worsening of myasthenia gravis symptoms, including muscle weakness and breathing problems. Patients should call their healthcare provider right away if they have any worsening muscle weakness or breathing problems.
- **Prolongation of the QT interval:** AVELOX may produce changes in the electrocardiogram (QTc interval prolongation). AVELOX should be avoided in patients receiving Class IA (for example quinidine, procainamide) or Class III (for example amiodarone, sotalol) antiarrhythmic agents. AVELOX may add to the QTc prolonging effects of other drugs such as cisapride, erythromycin, antipsychotics, and tricyclic antidepressants. The patients should inform their physician of any personal or family history of QTc prolongation or proarrhythmic conditions such as recent hypokalemia, significant bradycardia, and acute myocardial ischemia. Patients should contact their physician if they experience palpitations or fainting spells while taking AVELOX.
- **Hypersensitivity Reactions:** Patients should be advised that AVELOX may be associated with hypersensitivity reactions, including anaphylactic reactions, even following a single dose. Patients should discontinue AVELOX at the first sign of a skin rash or other signs of an allergic reaction.
- **Convulsions:** Convulsions have been reported in patients receiving quinolones, and they should notify their physician before taking AVELOX if there is a history of this condition. Patients should also inform their physician if they are taking NSAIDs concurrently with AVELOX.
- **Neurologic Adverse Effects (for example, dizziness, lightheadedness):** AVELOX may cause dizziness, lightheadedness and vision disorders; therefore, patients should know how they react to this drug before they operate an automobile or machinery or engage in activities requiring mental alertness or coordination.
- **Psychotic Reaction:** Psychotic reactions sometimes resulting in self-injurious behavior have been reported in patients receiving quinolones. Patients should notify their physician if they have a history of psychiatric illness before taking AVELOX.
- **Peripheral Neuropathies:** Patients should be informed that peripheral neuropathy has been associated with AVELOX use. Symptoms may occur soon after initiation of therapy and may be irreversible. If symptoms of peripheral neuropathy including pain, burning, tingling, numbness, and/or weakness develop, patients should immediately discontinue AVELOX and contact their physician.
- **Photosensitivity/Phototoxicity:** Patients should be informed that photosensitivity/phototoxicity has been reported in patients receiving quinolones. Patients should minimize or avoid exposure to natural or artificial sunlight (tanning beds or UVA/B treatment) while taking quinolones. If patients need to be outdoors while using quinolones, they should wear loose-fitting clothes that protect skin from sun exposure and discuss other sun protection measures with their physician. If a sunburn-like reaction or skin eruption occurs, patients should contact their physician.
- **Diarrhea:** Diarrhea is a common problem caused by antibiotics which usually ends when the antibiotic is discontinued. Sometimes after starting treatment with antibiotics, patients can develop watery and bloody stools (with or without stomach cramps and fever) even as late as two or more months after having taken the last dose of the antibiotic. If this occurs, patients should contact their physician as soon as possible.

FDA-Approved Medication Guide
MEDICATION GUIDE
AVELOX® (AV-eh-locks)
(moxifloxacin hydrochloride)
Tablets
AVELOX® IV (AV-eh-locks)
(moxifloxacin hydrochloride)
Injection Solution for IV use
Read the Medication Guide that comes with AVELOX® before you start taking it and each time you get a refill. There may be new information. This Medication Guide does not take the place of talking to your healthcare provider about your medical condition or your treatment.
What is the most important information I should know about AVELOX?
AVELOX belongs to a class of antibiotics called fluoroquinolones. AVELOX can cause side effects that may be serious or even cause death. If you get any of the following serious side effects, get medical help right away. Talk with your healthcare provider about whether you should continue to take AVELOX.
1. Tendon rupture or swelling of the tendon (tendinitis).
- **Tendon problems can happen in people of all ages who take AVELOX.** Tendons are tough cords of tissue that connect muscles to bones. Symptoms of tendon problems may include:
  - Pain, swelling, tears and inflammation of tendons including the back of the ankle (Achilles), shoulder, hand, or other tendon sites.
- **The risk of getting tendon problems while you take AVELOX is higher if you:**
  - Are over 60 years of age
  - Are taking steroids (corticosteroids)
  - Have a kidney, heart or lung transplant
- Tendon problems can happen in people who do not have the above risk factors when they take AVELOX.
- **Other reasons that can increase your risk of tendon problems can include:**
  - Physical activity or exercise
  - Kidney failure
  - Tendon problems in the past, such as in people with rheumatoid arthritis (RA)
- **Call your healthcare provider right away at the first sign of tendon pain, swelling or inflammation.** Stop taking AVELOX until tendinitis or tendon rupture has been ruled out by your healthcare provider. Avoid exercise and using the affected area. The most common area of pain and swelling is in the Achilles tendon at the back of your ankle. This can also happen with other tendons.

- **Talk to your healthcare provider about the risk of tendon rupture with continued use of AVELOX.** You may need a different antibiotic that is not a fluoroquinolone to treat your infection.
- **Tendon rupture can happen while you are taking or after you have finished taking AVELOX.** Tendon ruptures have happened up to several months after patients have finished taking their fluoroquinolone.
- **Get medical help right away if you get any of the following signs or symptoms of a tendon rupture:**
  - Hear or feel a snap or pop in a tendon area
  - Bruising right after an injury in a tendon area
  - Unable to move the affected area or bear weight
2. Worsening of myasthenia gravis (a disease which causes muscle weakness). Fluoroquinolones like AVELOX may cause worsening of myasthenia gravis symptoms, including muscle weakness and breathing problems. Call your healthcare provider right away if you have any worsening muscle weakness or breathing problems.
See the section "**What are the possible side effects of AVELOX?**" for more information about side effects.
What is AVELOX?
AVELOX is a fluoroquinolone antibiotic medicine used to treat certain types of infections caused by certain germs called bacteria in adults 18 years or older. It is not known if AVELOX is safe and works in people under 18 years of age. Children have a higher chance of getting bone, joint, and tendon (musculoskeletal) problems while taking fluoroquinolone antibiotic medicines.
Sometimes infections are caused by viruses rather than by bacteria. Examples include viral infections in the sinuses and lungs, such as the common cold or flu. Antibiotics, including AVELOX, do not kill viruses.
Call your healthcare provider if you think your condition is not getting better while you are taking AVELOX.
Who should not take AVELOX?
Do not take AVELOX if you have ever had a severe allergic reaction to an antibiotic known as a fluoroquinolone, or if you are allergic to any of the ingredients in AVELOX. Ask your healthcare provider if you are not sure. See the list of ingredients in AVELOX at the end of this Medication Guide.
What should I tell my healthcare provider before taking AVELOX?
See "**What is the most important information I should know about AVELOX?**"
Tell your healthcare provider about all your medical conditions, including if you:
- Have tendon problems
- Have a disease that causes muscle weakness (myasthenia gravis)
- Have central nervous system problems (such as epilepsy)
- Have nerve problems
- Have or anyone in your family has an irregular heartbeat, especially a condition called "QT prolongation"
- Have low blood potassium (hypokalemia)
- Have a slow heartbeat (bradycardia)
- Have a history of seizures
- Have kidney problems
- Have rheumatoid arthritis (RA) or other history of joint problems
- Are pregnant or planning to become pregnant. It is not known if AVELOX will harm your unborn child.
- Are breast-feeding or planning to breast-feed. It is not known if AVELOX passes into breast milk. You and your healthcare provider should decide whether you will take AVELOX or breast-feed.
Tell your healthcare provider about all the medicines you take, including prescription and non-prescription medicines, vitamins and herbal and dietary supplements. AVELOX and other medicines can affect each other causing side effects. Especially tell your healthcare provider if you take:
- An NSAID (Non-Steroidal Anti-Inflammatory Drug). Many common medicines for pain relief are NSAIDs. Taking an NSAID while you take AVELOX or other fluoroquinolones may increase your risk of central nervous system effects and seizures. See "**What are the possible side effects of AVELOX?**"
- A blood thinner (warfarin, Coumadin, Jantoven).
- A medicine to control your heart rate or rhythm (antiarrhythmic) See "**What are the possible side effects of AVELOX?**"
- An anti-psychotic medicine.
- A tricyclic antidepressant.
- Erythromycin.
- A water pill (diuretic).
- A steroid medicine. Corticosteroids taken by mouth or by injection may increase the chance of tendon injury. See "**What is the most important information I should know about AVELOX?**"
- Certain medicines may keep AVELOX from working correctly. Take AVELOX either 4 hours before or 8 hours after taking these products:

- An antacid, multivitamin, or other product that has magnesium, aluminum, iron, or zinc
- Sucralfate (Carafate)
- Didanosine (Videx®, Videx EC®)

Ask your healthcare provider if you are not sure if any of your medicines are listed above.
Know the medicines you take. Keep a list of your medicines and show it to your healthcare provider and pharmacist when you get a new medicine.

How should I take AVELOX?
- Take AVELOX once a day exactly as prescribed by your healthcare provider.
- Take AVELOX at about the same time each day.
- AVELOX Tablets should be swallowed.
- AVELOX can be taken with or without food.
- Drink plenty of fluids while taking AVELOX.
- AVELOX IV is given to you by intravenous (IV) infusion into your vein slowly, over 60 minutes, as prescribed by your healthcare provider.
- Do not skip any doses, or stop taking AVELOX even if you begin to feel better, until you finish your prescribed treatment, unless:
  - You have tendon effects (see **"What is the most important information I should know about AVELOX?"**).
  - You have a serious allergic reaction (see **"What are the possible side effects of AVELOX?"**), or your healthcare provider tells you to stop.
- This will help make sure that all of the bacteria are killed and lower the chance that the bacteria will become resistant to AVELOX. If this happens, AVELOX and other antibiotic medicines may not work in the future.
- If you miss a dose of AVELOX, take it as soon as you remember. Do not take more than 1 dose of AVELOX in one day.
- If you take too much, call your healthcare provider or get medical help immediately.

What should I avoid while taking AVELOX?
- AVELOX can make you feel dizzy and lightheaded. Do not drive, operate machinery, or do other activities that require mental alertness or coordination until you know how AVELOX affects you.
- Avoid sunlamps, tanning beds, and try to limit your time in the sun. AVELOX can make your skin sensitive to the sun (photosensitivity) and the light from sunlamps and tanning beds. You could get severe sunburn, blisters or swelling of your skin. If you get any of these symptoms while taking AVELOX, call your healthcare provider right away. You should use a sunscreen and wear a hat and clothes that cover your skin if you have to be in sunlight.

What are the possible side effects of AVELOX?
AVELOX can cause side effects that may be serious or even cause death. See **"What is the most important information I should know about AVELOX?"**
Other serious side effects of AVELOX include:
- **Central Nervous System effects**
Seizures have been reported in people who take fluoroquinolone antibiotics including AVELOX. Tell your healthcare provider if you have a history of seizures. Ask your healthcare provider whether taking AVELOX will change your risk of having a seizure.
Central Nervous System (CNS) side effects may happen as soon as after taking the first dose of AVELOX. Talk to your healthcare provider right away if you have any of these side effects, or other changes in mood or behavior:
- Feeling dizzy
- Seizures
- Hear voices, see things, or sense things that are not there (hallucinations)
- Feel restless
- Tremors
- Feel anxious or nervous
- Confusion
- Depression
- Trouble sleeping
- Feel more suspicious (paranoia)
- Suicidal thoughts or acts
- Nightmares
- Vision Loss
- **Serious allergic reactions**
Allergic reactions can happen in people taking fluoroquinolones, including AVELOX, even after only one dose. Stop taking AVELOX and get emergency medical help right away if you get any of the following symptoms of a severe allergic reaction:
- Hives
- Trouble breathing or swallowing
- Swelling of the lips, tongue, face
- Throat tightness, hoarseness
- Rapid heartbeat
- Faint
- Yellowing of the skin or eyes. Stop taking AVELOX and tell your healthcare provider right away if you get yellowing of your skin or white part of your eyes, or if you have dark urine. These can be signs of a serious reaction to AVELOX (a liver problem).

- **Skin rash**
Skin rash may happen in people taking AVELOX even after only one dose. Stop taking AVELOX at the first sign of a skin rash and call your healthcare provider. Skin rash may be a sign of a more serious reaction to AVELOX.
- **Serious heart rhythm changes** (QT prolongation and torsade de pointes)
Tell your healthcare provider right away if you have a change in your heart beat (a fast or irregular heartbeat), or if you faint. AVELOX may cause a rare heart problem known as prolongation of the QT interval. This condition can cause an abnormal heartbeat and can be very dangerous. The chances of this event are higher in people:
- Who are elderly
- With a family history of prolonged QT interval
- With low blood potassium (hypokalemia)
- Who take certain medicines to control heart rhythm (antiarrhythmics)
- **Intestine infection** (Pseudomembranous colitis)
Pseudomembranous colitis can happen with most antibiotics, including AVELOX. Call your healthcare provider right away if you get watery diarrhea, diarrhea that does not go away, or bloody stools. You may have stomach cramps and a fever. Pseudomembranous colitis can happen 2 or more months after you have finished your antibiotic.
- **Changes in sensation and nerve damage (Peripheral Neuropathy)**
Damage to the nerves in arms, hands, legs, or feet can happen in people taking fluoroquinolones, including AVELOX. Stop AVELOX and talk with your healthcare provider right away if you get any of the following symptoms of peripheral neuropathy in your arms, hands, legs, or feet:
- Pain
- Burning
- Tingling
- Numbness
- Weakness
The nerve damage may be permanent.
- **Sensitivity to sunlight** (photosensitivity)
See **"What should I avoid while taking AVELOX?"**
The most common side effects of AVELOX include nausea and diarrhea.
These are not all the possible side effects of AVELOX. Tell your healthcare provider about any side effect that bothers you or that does not go away.
Call your doctor for medical advice about side effects. You may report side effects to FDA at 1-800-FDA-1088.

How should I store AVELOX?
AVELOX Tablets
- Store AVELOX 59–86°F (15–30°C)
- Keep AVELOX away from moisture (humidity)
Keep AVELOX and all medicines out of the reach of children.

General Information about AVELOX
Medicines are sometimes prescribed for purposes other than those listed in a Medication Guide. Do not use AVELOX for a condition for which it is not prescribed. Do not give AVELOX to other people, even if they have the same symptoms that you have. It may harm them.
This Medication Guide summarizes the most important information about AVELOX. If you would like more information about AVELOX, talk with your healthcare provider. You can ask your healthcare provider or pharmacist for information about AVELOX that is written for healthcare professionals. For more information go to www.AVELOX.com or call 1-800-526-4099.

What are the ingredients in AVELOX?
- **AVELOX Tablets:**
  - Active ingredient: moxifloxacin hydrochloride
  - Inactive ingredients: microcrystalline cellulose, lactose monohydrate, croscarmellose sodium, magnesium stearate, hypromellose, titanium dioxide, polyethylene glycol, and ferric oxide
- **AVELOX IV:**
  - Active ingredient: moxifloxacin hydrochloride
  - Inactive ingredients: sodium chloride, USP, water for injection, USP, and may include hydrochloric acid and/or sodium hydroxide for pH adjustment
Revised August 2013
This Medication Guide has been approved by the U.S. Food and Drug Administration.
Manufactured for:
Bayer HealthCare Pharmaceuticals Inc.
Wayne, NJ 07470
AVELOX Tablets manufactured in Germany
AVELOX IV manufactured in Germany
or
AVELOX IV manufactured in Norway by
Fresenius Kabi Norge AS
NO-1753 Halden, Norway
Distributed by:
Merck Sharp & Dohme Corp., a subsidiary of
Merck & Co., Inc.
Whitehouse Station, NJ 08889, USA

AVELOX® is a registered trademark of Bayer Aktiengesellschaft and is used under license by Merck Sharp & Dohme Corp., a subsidiary of **Merck & Co.**, Inc.
Rx Only
©2012 Bayer HealthCare Pharmaceuticals Inc.
83680831, R.4
Shown in Product Identification Guide, page 308

CANCIDAS® ℞
[*kan-si-das*]
(caspofungin acetate)
for injection, for intravenous use

HIGHLIGHTS OF PRESCRIBING INFORMATION
These highlights do not include all the information needed to use CANCIDAS safely and effectively. See full prescribing information for CANCIDAS.
CANCIDAS® (caspofungin acetate) for injection, for intravenous use
Initial U.S. Approval: 2001

----RECENT MAJOR CHANGES----
Warnings and Precautions, Hypersensitivity
(5.1)   01/2013

----INDICATIONS AND USAGE----
CANCIDAS is an echinocandin antifungal drug indicated in adults and pediatric patients (3 months and older) for:
- Empirical therapy for presumed fungal infections in febrile, neutropenic patients. (1)
- Treatment of candidemia and the following *Candida* infections: intra-abdominal abscesses, peritonitis and pleural space infections. (1)
- Treatment of esophageal candidiasis. (1)
- Treatment of invasive aspergillosis in patients who are refractory to or intolerant of other therapies (e.g., amphotericin B, lipid formulations of amphotericin B, itraconazole). (1)

----DOSAGE AND ADMINISTRATION----
For All Patients (2.1):
- Administer by slow intravenous (IV) infusion over approximately 1 hour. Not for IV bolus administration.
- Do not mix or co-infuse CANCIDAS with other medications. Do not use diluents containing dextrose (α-D-glucose).
Adults [≥18 years of age] (2.2):
- Administer a single 70-mg loading dose on Day 1, followed by 50 mg once daily for all indications except esophageal candidiasis.
- For esophageal candidiasis, use 50 mg once daily with no loading dose.
Pediatric Patients [3 months to 17 years of age] (2.3):
- Dosing should be based on the patient's body surface area.
- For all indications, administer a single 70-mg/m² loading dose on Day 1, followed by 50 mg/m² once daily thereafter.
- **Maximum loading dose and daily maintenance dose should not exceed 70 mg, regardless of the patient's calculated dose.**
Dosing With Rifampin and Other Inducers of Drug Clearance (2.5):
- Use 70-mg once daily dose for adult patients on rifampin.
- Consider dose increase to 70 mg once daily for adult patients on nevirapine, efavirenz, carbamazepine, dexamethasone, or phenytoin.
- Pediatric patients receiving these same concomitant medications may also require an increase in dose to 70 mg/m² once daily (maximum daily dose not to exceed 70 mg).

----DOSAGE FORMS AND STRENGTHS----
- Vials: 50 or 70 mg lyophilized powder (plus allowance for overfill). (3)

----CONTRAINDICATIONS----
- CANCIDAS is contraindicated in patients with hypersensitivity to any component of this product. (4)

----WARNINGS AND PRECAUTIONS----
- Hypersensitivity:
Anaphylaxis has been reported. If this occurs, CANCIDAS should be discontinued and appropriate treatment administered. Possible histamine-mediated adverse reactions, including rash, facial swelling, angioedema, pruritus, sensation of warmth or bronchospasm have been reported and may require discontinuation and/or administration of appropriate treatment. (5.1)
- Use with cyclosporine: Limit use to patients for whom potential benefit outweighs potential risk. Monitor patients who develop abnormal liver function tests (LFTs) during concomitant therapy and evaluate risk/benefit of continuing CANCIDAS. (5.2)
- Hepatic effects: Can cause abnormalities in LFTs and isolated cases of clinically significant hepatic dysfunction, hepatitis, or hepatic failure. Monitor patients who develop

abnormal LFTs for evidence of worsening hepatic function, and evaluate risk/benefit of continuing CANCIDAS. (5.3)

---------------ADVERSE REACTIONS---------------

- *Adults:* Most common adverse reactions (incidence ≥10%) are diarrhea, pyrexia, ALT/AST increased, blood alkaline phosphatase increased, and blood potassium decreased. (6.1)
- *Pediatric patients:* Most common adverse reactions (incidence ≥10%) are pyrexia, diarrhea, rash, ALT/AST increased, blood potassium decreased, hypotension, and chills. (6.2)

To report SUSPECTED ADVERSE REACTIONS, contact Merck Sharp & Dohme Corp., a subsidiary of Merck & Co., Inc., at 1-877-888-4231 or FDA at 1-800-FDA-1088 or www.fda.gov/medwatch.

---------------USE IN SPECIFIC POPULATIONS---------------

- Pregnancy: Based on animal data, may cause fetal harm. (8.1)
- Pediatric use: Safety and efficacy in neonates and infants less than 3 months old have not been established. (8.4)
- Hepatic impairment: Reduce dose for adult patients with moderate hepatic impairment (35 mg once daily, with a 70-mg loading dose on Day 1 where appropriate). No data are available in adults with severe impairment or in pediatric patients with any degree of impairment. (8.6, 12.3)

See 17 for PATIENT COUNSELING INFORMATION
Revised: 08/2013

FULL PRESCRIBING INFORMATION: CONTENTS*

* Sections or subsections omitted from the full prescribing information are not listed

FULL PRESCRIBING INFORMATION

1 INDICATIONS AND USAGE

CANCIDAS® is indicated in adults and pediatric patients (3 months and older) for:

- Empirical therapy for presumed fungal infections in febrile, neutropenic patients
- Treatment of candidemia and the following *Candida* infections: intra-abdominal abscesses, peritonitis and pleural space infections. CANCIDAS has not been studied in endocarditis, osteomyelitis, and meningitis due to *Candida*.
- Treatment of esophageal candidiasis [see Clinical Studies (14.3)]
- Treatment of invasive aspergillosis in patients who are refractory to or intolerant of other therapies (e.g., amphotericin B, lipid formulations of amphotericin B, itraconazole). CANCIDAS has not been studied as initial therapy for invasive aspergillosis.

2 DOSAGE AND ADMINISTRATION

2.1 Instructions for Use in All Patients

CANCIDAS should be administered by slow intravenous (IV) infusion over approximately 1 hour. CANCIDAS should not be administered by IV bolus administration.

Do not mix or co-infuse CANCIDAS with other medications, as there are no data available on the compatibility of CANCIDAS with other intravenous substances, additives, or medications. DO NOT USE DILUENTS CONTAINING DEXTROSE (α-D-GLUCOSE), as CANCIDAS is not stable in diluents containing dextrose.

2.2 Recommended Dosing in Adult Patients [≥18 years of age]

The usual dose is 50 mg once daily (following a 70-mg loading dose for most indications). The safety and efficacy of a dose of 150 mg daily (range: 1 to 51 days; median: 14 days) have been studied in 100 adult patients with candidemia and other *Candida* infections. The efficacy of CANCIDAS at this higher dose was not significantly better than the efficacy of the 50-mg daily dose of CANCIDAS. The efficacy of doses higher than 50 mg daily in the other adult patients for whom CANCIDAS is indicated is not known [see Clinical Studies (14.2)].

Empirical Therapy

A single 70-mg loading dose should be administered on Day 1, followed by 50 mg once daily thereafter. Duration of treatment should be based on the patient's clinical response. Empirical therapy should be continued until resolution of neutropenia. Patients found to have a fungal infection should be treated for a minimum of 14 days; treatment should continue for at least 7 days after both neutropenia and clinical symptoms are resolved. If the 50-mg dose is well tolerated but does not provide an adequate clinical response, the daily dose can be increased to 70 mg.

Candidemia and Other Candida Infections [see Clinical Studies (14.2)]

A single 70-mg loading dose should be administered on Day 1, followed by 50 mg once daily thereafter. Duration of treatment should be dictated by the patient's clinical and microbiological response. In general, antifungal therapy should continue for at least 14 days after the last positive culture. Patients who remain persistently neutropenic may warrant a longer course of therapy pending resolution of the neutropenia.

Esophageal Candidiasis

The dose is 50 mg once daily for 7 to 14 days after symptom resolution. A 70-mg loading dose has not been studied for this indication. Because of the risk of relapse of oropharyngeal candidiasis in patients with HIV infections, suppressive oral therapy could be considered [see Clinical Studies (14.3)].

Invasive Aspergillosis

A single 70-mg loading dose should be administered on Day 1, followed by 50 mg once daily thereafter. Duration of treatment should be based upon the severity of the patient's underlying disease, recovery from immunosuppression, and clinical response.

2.3 Recommended Dosing in Pediatric Patients [3 months to 17 years of age]

For all indications, a single 70-mg/m² loading dose should be administered on Day 1, followed by 50 mg/m² once daily thereafter. **The maximum loading dose and the daily maintenance dose should not exceed 70 mg, regardless of the patient's calculated dose.** Dosing in pediatric patients (3 months to 17 years of age) should be based on the patient's body surface area (BSA) as calculated by the Mosteller Formula [see References (15)]:

$$BSA\ (m^2) = \sqrt{\frac{Height\ (cm)\ \times\ Weight\ (kg)}{3600}}$$

Following calculation of the patient's BSA, the loading dose in milligrams should be calculated as BSA (m²) × 70 mg/m². The maintenance dose in milligrams should be calculated as BSA (m²) × 50 mg/m².

Duration of treatment should be individualized to the indication, as described for each indication in adults [see Dosage and Administration (2.2)]. If the 50-mg/m² daily dose is well tolerated but does not provide an adequate clinical response, the daily dose can be increased to 70 mg/m² daily (not to exceed 70 mg).

2.4 Patients with Hepatic Impairment

Adult patients with mild hepatic impairment (Child-Pugh score 5 to 6) do not need a dosage adjustment. For adult patients with moderate hepatic impairment (Child-Pugh score 7 to 9), CANCIDAS 35 mg once daily is recommended based upon pharmacokinetic data [see Clinical Pharmacology (12.3)]. However, where recommended, a 70-mg loading dose should still be administered on Day 1. There is no clinical experience in adult patients with severe hepatic impairment (Child-Pugh score >9) and in pediatric patients with any degree of hepatic impairment.

2.5 Patients Receiving Concomitant Inducers of Drug Clearance

Adult patients on rifampin should receive 70 mg of CANCIDAS once daily. Adult patients on nevirapine, efavirenz, carbamazepine, dexamethasone, or phenytoin may require an increase in dose to 70 mg of CANCIDAS once daily [see Drug Interactions (7)].

When CANCIDAS is co-administered to pediatric patients with inducers of drug clearance, such as rifampin, efavirenz, nevirapine, phenytoin, dexamethasone, or carbamazepine, a CANCIDAS dose of 70 mg/m² once daily (not to exceed 70 mg) should be considered [see Drug Interactions (7)].

2.6 Preparation and Reconstitution for Administration

Do not mix or co-infuse CANCIDAS with other medications, as there are no data available on the compatibility of CANCIDAS with other intravenous substances, additives, or medications. DO NOT USE DILUENTS CONTAINING DEXTROSE (α-D-GLUCOSE), as CANCIDAS is not stable in diluents containing dextrose.

Preparation of CANCIDAS for Infusion

A. Equilibrate the refrigerated vial of CANCIDAS to room temperature.

B. Aseptically add 10.8 mL of 0.9% Sodium Chloride Injection, Sterile Water for Injection, Bacteriostatic Water for Injection with methylparaben and propylparaben, or Bacteriostatic Water for Injection with 0.9% benzyl alcohol to the vial.

Each vial of CANCIDAS contains an intentional overfill of CANCIDAS. Thus, the drug concentration of the resulting solution is listed in Table 1 below.

Table 1: Information for Preparation of CANCIDAS

CANCIDAS vial	Total Drug Content (including overfill)	Reconstitution Volume to be added	Resulting Concentration following Reconstitution
50 mg	54.6 mg	10.8 mL	5 mg/mL
70 mg	75.6 mg	10.8 mL	7 mg/mL

The white to off-white cake will dissolve completely. Mix gently until a clear solution is obtained. Visually inspect the reconstituted solution for particulate matter or discoloration during reconstitution and prior to infusion. Do not use if the solution is cloudy or has precipitated.

The reconstituted solution may be stored for up to one hour at ≤25°C (≤77°F).

CANCIDAS vials are for single use only; the remaining solution should be discarded.

C. Aseptically transfer the appropriate volume (mL) of reconstituted CANCIDAS to an IV bag (or bottle) containing 250 mL of 0.9%, 0.45%, or 0.225% Sodium Chloride Injection or Lactated Ringers Injection. Alternatively, the volume (mL) of reconstituted CANCIDAS can be added to a reduced volume of 0.9%, 0.45%, or 0.225% Sodium Chloride Injection or Lactated Ringers Injection, not to exceed a final concentration of 0.5 mg/mL.

This infusion solution must be used within 24 hours if stored at ≤25°C (≤77°F) or within 48 hours if stored refrigerated at 2 to 8°C (36 to 46°F).

Special Considerations for Pediatric Patients >3 Months of Age

Follow the reconstitution procedures described above using either the 70-mg or 50-mg vial to create the reconstituted solution [see Dosage and Administration (2.3)]. From the reconstituted solution in the vial, remove the volume of drug equal to the calculated loading dose or calculated maintenance dose based on a concentration of 7 mg/mL (if reconstituted from the 70-mg vial) or a concentration of 5 mg/mL (if reconstituted from the 50-mg vial).

The choice of vial should be based on total milligram dose of drug to be administered to the pediatric patient. To help ensure accurate dosing, it is recommended for pediatric doses less than 50 mg that 50-mg vials (with a concentration of 5 mg/mL) be used if available. The 70-mg vial should be reserved for pediatric patients requiring doses greater than 50 mg.

The maximum loading dose and the daily maintenance dose should not exceed 70 mg, regardless of the patient's calculated dose.

3 DOSAGE FORMS AND STRENGTHS

CANCIDAS 50 mg is a white to off-white powder/cake for infusion in a vial with a red aluminum band and a plastic cap. CANCIDAS 50-mg vial contains 54.6 mg of caspofungin.

CANCIDAS 70 mg is a white to off-white powder/cake for infusion in a vial with a yellow/orange aluminum band and a plastic cap. CANCIDAS 70-mg vial contains 75.6 mg of caspofungin.

4 CONTRAINDICATIONS

CANCIDAS is contraindicated in patients with hypersensitivity (e.g., anaphylaxis) to any component of this product [see Adverse Reactions (6)].

5 WARNINGS AND PRECAUTIONS

5.1 Hypersensitivity

Anaphylaxis has been reported during administration of CANCIDAS. If this occurs, CANCIDAS should be discontinued and appropriate treatment administered.

Possible histamine-mediated adverse reactions, including rash, facial swelling, angioedema, pruritus, sensation of warmth or bronchospasm have been reported and may require discontinuation and/or administration of appropriate treatment.

5.2 Concomitant Use with Cyclosporine

Concomitant use of CANCIDAS with cyclosporine should be limited to patients for whom the potential benefit outweighs the potential risk. In one clinical study, 3 of 4 healthy adult subjects who received CANCIDAS 70 mg on Days 1 through 10, and also received two 3 mg/kg doses of cyclosporine 12 hours apart on Day 10, developed transient elevations of alanine transaminase (ALT) on Day 11 that were 2 to 3 times the upper limit of normal (ULN). In a separate panel of adult subjects in the same study, 2 of 8 who received CANCIDAS 35 mg daily for 3 days and cyclosporine (two 3 mg/kg doses administered 12 hours apart) on Day 1 had small increases in ALT (slightly above the ULN) on Day 2. In both groups, elevations in aspartate transaminase (AST) paralleled ALT elevations, but were of lesser magnitude. In another clinical study, 2 of 8 healthy men developed transient ALT elevations of less than 2× ULN. In this study, cyclosporine (4 mg/kg) was administered on Days 1 and 12, and CANCIDAS was administered (70 mg) daily on Days 3 through 13. In one subject, the ALT elevation occurred on Days 7 and 9 and, in the other subject, the ALT elevation occurred on Day 19. These elevations returned to normal by Day 27. In all groups, elevations in AST paralleled ALT elevations but were of lesser magnitude. In these clinical studies, cyclosporine (one 4 mg/kg dose or two 3 mg/kg doses) increased the AUC of caspofungin by approximately 35%.

In a retrospective postmarketing study, 40 immunocompromised patients, including 37 transplant recipients, were treated with CANCIDAS and cyclosporine for 1 to 290 days (median 17.5 days). Fourteen patients (35%) developed transaminase elevations >5× upper limit of normal or >3× baseline during concomitant therapy or the 14-day follow-up period; five were considered possibly related to concomitant therapy. One patient had elevated bilirubin considered possibly related to concomitant therapy. No patient developed clinical evidence of hepatotoxicity or serious hepatic events. Discontinuations due to laboratory abnormalities in hepatic enzymes from any cause occurred in four patients. Of these, 2 were considered possibly related to therapy with CANCIDAS and/or cyclosporine as well as to other possible causes.

In the prospective invasive aspergillosis and compassionate use studies, there were 4 adult patients treated with CANCIDAS (50 mg/day) and cyclosporine for 2 to 56 days. None of these patients experienced increases in hepatic enzymes.

Given the limitations of these data, CANCIDAS and cyclosporine should only be used concomitantly in those patients for whom the potential benefit outweighs the potential risk. Patients who develop abnormal liver function tests during concomitant therapy should be monitored and the risk/benefit of continuing therapy should be evaluated.

5.3 Hepatic Effects

Laboratory abnormalities in liver function tests have been seen in healthy volunteers and in adult and pediatric patients treated with CANCIDAS. In some adult and pediatric patients with serious underlying conditions who were receiving multiple concomitant medications with CANCIDAS, isolated cases of clinically significant hepatic dysfunction, hepatitis, and hepatic failure have been reported; a causal relationship to CANCIDAS has not been established. Patients who develop abnormal liver function tests during CANCIDAS therapy should be monitored for evidence of worsening hepatic function and evaluated for risk/benefit of continuing CANCIDAS therapy.

6 ADVERSE REACTIONS

The following serious adverse reactions are discussed in detail in another section of the labeling:

Table 2: Adverse Reactions Among Patients with Persistent Fever and Neutropenia* Incidence ≥7.5% for at Least One Treatment Group by System Organ Class or Preferred Term

Adverse Reaction (MedDRA v10.1 System Organ Class and Preferred Term)	CANCIDAS[†] N=564 (percent)	AmBisome[‡] N=547 (percent)
All Systems, Any Adverse Reaction	95	97
Investigations	58	63
Alanine Aminotransferase Increased	18	20
Blood Alkaline Phosphatase Increased	15	23
Blood Potassium Decreased	15	23
Aspartate Aminotransferase Increased	14	17
Blood Bilirubin Increased	10	14
Blood Albumin Decreased	7	8
Blood Magnesium Decreased	7	9
Blood Glucose Increased	6	9
Bilirubin Conjugated Increased	5	9
Blood Urea Increased	4	8
Blood Creatinine Increased	3	11
General Disorders and Administration Site Conditions	57	63
Pyrexia	27	29
Chills	23	31
Edema Peripheral	11	12
Mucosal Inflammation	6	8
Gastrointestinal Disorders	50	55
Diarrhea	20	16
Nausea	11	20
Abdominal Pain	9	11
Vomiting	9	17
Respiratory, Thoracic and Mediastinal Disorders	47	49
Cough	11	10
Dyspnea	9	10
Rales	7	8
Infections and Infestations	45	42
Pneumonia	11	10
Skin and Subcutaneous Tissue Disorders	42	37
Rash	16	14
Nervous System Disorders	25	27
Headache	11	12
Metabolism and Nutrition Disorders	21	24
Hypokalemia	6	8
Vascular Disorders	20	23
Hypotension	6	10
Cardiac Disorders	16	19
Tachycardia	7	9

Within any system organ class, individuals may experience more than 1 adverse reaction.
* Regardless of causality
† 70 mg on Day 1, then 50 mg once daily for the remainder of treatment; daily dose was increased to 70 mg for 73 patients.
‡ 3 mg/kg/day; daily dose was increased to 5 mg/kg for 74 patients.

• Hepatic effects [see Warnings and Precautions (5.3)]
• Hypersensitivity [see Warnings and Precautions (5.1)]

Because clinical trials are conducted under widely varying conditions, adverse reaction rates observed in clinical trials of CANCIDAS cannot be directly compared to rates in clinical trials of another drug and may not reflect the rates observed in practice. The adverse reaction information from clinical trials does provide a basis for identifying adverse reactions that appear to be related to drug use and for approximating rates.

6.1 Clinical Trials Experience in Adults

The overall safety of CANCIDAS was assessed in 1865 adult individuals who received single or multiple doses of CANCIDAS: 564 febrile, neutropenic patients (empirical therapy study); 382 patients with candidemia and/or intra-abdominal abscesses, peritonitis, or pleural space infections (including 4 patients with chronic disseminated candidiasis); 297 patients with esophageal and/or oropharyngeal candidiasis; 228 patients with invasive aspergillosis; and 394 individuals in phase I studies. In the empirical therapy study patients had undergone hematopoietic stem-cell transplantation or chemotherapy. In the studies involving patients with documented Candida infections, the majority of the patients had serious underlying medical conditions (e.g., hematologic or other malignancy, recent major surgery, HIV) requiring multiple concomitant medications. Patients in the noncomparative Aspergillus studies often had serious predisposing medical conditions (e.g., bone marrow or peripheral stem cell transplants, hematologic malignancy, solid tumors or organ transplants) requiring multiple concomitant medications.

Empirical Therapy

In the randomized, double-blinded empirical therapy study, patients received either CANCIDAS 50 mg/day (following a 70-mg loading dose) or AmBisome® (amphotericin B liposome for injection, 3 mg/kg/day). In this study clinical or laboratory hepatic adverse reactions were reported in 39% and 45% of patients in the CANCIDAS and AmBisome groups, respectively. Also reported was an isolated, serious adverse reaction of hyperbilirubinemia considered possibly related to CANCIDAS. Adverse reactions occurring in ≥7.5% of the patients in either treatment group are presented in Table 2.

[See table 2 above]

Table 3: Adverse Reactions Among Patients with Candidemia or other Candida Infections*, † Incidence ≥10% for at Least One Treatment Group by System Organ Class or Preferred Term

Adverse Reaction (MedDRA v10.1 System Organ Class and Preferred Term)	CANCIDAS 50 mg‡ N=114 (percent)	Amphotericin B N=125 (percent)
All Systems, Any Adverse Reaction	96	99
Investigations	67	82
Blood Potassium Decreased	23	32
Blood Alkaline Phosphatase Increased	21	32
Hemoglobin Decreased	18	23
Alanine Aminotransferase Increased	16	15
Aspartate Aminotransferase Increased	16	14
Blood Bilirubin Increased	13	17
Hematocrit Decreased	13	18
Blood Creatinine Increased	11	28
Red Blood Cells Urine Positive	10	10
Blood Urea Increased	9	23
Bilirubin Conjugated Increased	8	14
Gastrointestinal Disorders	49	53
Vomiting	17	16
Diarrhea	14	10
Nausea	9	17
Infections and Infestations	48	54
Septic Shock	11	9
Pneumonia	4	10
General Disorders and Administration Site Conditions	47	63
Pyrexia	13	33
Edema Peripheral	11	12
Chills	9	30
Respiratory, Thoracic and Mediastinal Disorders	40	54
Respiratory Failure	11	12
Pleural Effusion	9	14
Tachypnea	1	11
Cardiac Disorders	26	34
Tachycardia	8	12
Skin and Subcutaneous Tissue Disorders	25	28
Rash	4	10
Vascular Disorders	25	38
Hypotension	10	16
Blood and Lymphatic System Disorders	15	13
Anemia	11	9

Within any system organ class, individuals may experience more than 1 adverse reaction.
*   Intra-abdominal abscesses, peritonitis and pleural space infections.
†   Regardless of causality
‡   Patients received CANCIDAS 70 mg on Day 1, then 50 mg once daily for the remainder of their treatment.

The proportion of patients who experienced an infusion-related adverse reaction (defined as a systemic event, such as pyrexia, chills, flushing, hypotension, hypertension, tachycardia, dyspnea, tachypnea, rash, or anaphylaxis, that developed during the study therapy infusion and one hour following infusion) was significantly lower in the group treated with CANCIDAS (35%) than in the group treated with AmBisome (52%).

To evaluate the effect of CANCIDAS and AmBisome on renal function, nephrotoxicity was defined as doubling of serum creatinine relative to baseline or an increase of ≥1 mg/dL in serum creatinine if baseline serum creatinine was above the upper limit of the normal range. Among patients whose baseline creatinine clearance was >30 mL/min, the incidence of nephrotoxicity was significantly lower in the group treated with CANCIDAS (3%) than in the group treated with AmBisome (12%). Clinical renal events, regardless of causality, were similar between CANCIDAS (75/564, 13%) and AmBisome (85/547, 16%).

Candidemia and Other Candida Infections
In the randomized, double-blinded invasive candidiasis study, patients received either CANCIDAS 50 mg/day (following a 70-mg loading dose) or amphotericin B 0.6 to 1 mg/kg/day. Adverse reactions occurring in ≥10% of the patients in either treatment group are presented in Table 3.
[See table 3 above]

The proportion of patients who experienced an infusion-related adverse reaction (defined as a systemic event, such as pyrexia, chills, flushing, hypotension, hypertension, tachycardia, dyspnea, tachypnea, rash, or anaphylaxis, that developed during the study therapy infusion and one hour following infusion) was significantly lower in the group treated with CANCIDAS (20%) than in the group treated with amphotericin B (49%).

To evaluate the effect of CANCIDAS and amphotericin B on renal function, nephrotoxicity was defined as doubling of serum creatinine relative to baseline or an increase of ≥1 mg/dL in serum creatinine if baseline serum creatinine was above the upper limit of the normal range. In a subgroup of patients whose baseline creatinine clearance was >30 mL/min, the incidence of nephrotoxicity was significantly lower in the group treated with CANCIDAS than in the group treated with amphotericin B.

In a second randomized, double-blinded invasive candidiasis study, patients received either CANCIDAS 50 mg/day (following a 70-mg loading dose) or CANCIDAS 150 mg/day. The proportion of patients who experienced any adverse reaction was similar in the 2 treatment groups; however, this study was not large enough to detect differences in rare or unexpected adverse events. Adverse reactions occurring in ≥5% of the patients in either treatment group are presented in Table 4.

[See table 4 at top of next page]
Esophageal Candidiasis and Oropharyngeal Candidiasis
Adverse reactions occurring in ≥10% of patients with esophageal and/or oropharyngeal candidiasis are presented in Table 5.
[See table 5 at bottom of next page]
Invasive Aspergillosis
In an open-label, noncomparative aspergillosis study, in which 69 patients received CANCIDAS (70-mg loading dose on Day 1 followed by 50 mg daily), the following treatment-emergent adverse reactions were observed with an incidence of ≥12.5%: blood alkaline phosphatase increased (22%), hypotension (20%), respiratory failure (20%), pyrexia (17%), diarrhea (15%), nausea (15%), headache (15%), rash (13%), aspergillosis (13%), alanine aminotransferase increased (13%), aspartate aminotransferase increased (13%), blood bilirubin increased (13%), and blood potassium decreased (13%). Also reported infrequently in this patient population were pulmonary edema, ARDS (adult respiratory distress syndrome), and radiographic infiltrates.

6.2   Clinical Trials Experience in Pediatric Patients (3 months to 17 years of age)
The overall safety of CANCIDAS was assessed in 171 pediatric patients who received single or multiple doses of CANCIDAS. The distribution among the 153 pediatric patients who were over the age of 3 months was as follows: 104 febrile, neutropenic patients; 38 patients with candidemia and/or intra-abdominal abscesses, peritonitis, or pleural space infections; 1 patient with esophageal candidiasis; and 10 patients with invasive aspergillosis. The overall safety profile of CANCIDAS in pediatric patients is comparable to that in adult patients. Table 6 shows the incidence of adverse reactions reported in ≥7.5% of pediatric patients in clinical studies.
One patient (0.6%) receiving CANCIDAS, and three patients (12%) receiving AmBisome developed a serious drug-related adverse reaction. Two patients (1%) were discontinued from CANCIDAS and three patients (12%) were discontinued from AmBisome due to a drug-related adverse reaction. The proportion of patients who experienced an infusion-related adverse reaction (defined as a systemic event, such as pyrexia, chills, flushing, hypotension, hypertension, tachycardia, dyspnea, tachypnea, rash, or anaphylaxis, that developed during the study therapy infusion and one hour following infusion) was 22% in the group treated with CANCIDAS and 35% in the group treated with AmBisome.
[See table 6 at top of page 1344]
6.3   Overall Safety Experience of CANCIDAS in Clinical Trials
The overall safety of CANCIDAS was assessed in 2036 individuals (including 1642 adult or pediatric patients and 394 volunteers) from 34 clinical studies. These individuals received single or multiple (once daily) doses of CANCIDAS, ranging from 5 mg to 210 mg. Full safety data is available from 1951 individuals, as the safety data from 85 patients enrolled in 2 compassionate use studies was limited solely to serious adverse reactions. Treatment emergent adverse reactions, regardless of causality, which occurred in ≥5% of all individuals who received CANCIDAS in these trials, are shown in Table 7.
Overall, 1665 of the 1951 (85%) patients/volunteers who received CANCIDAS experienced an adverse reaction.

Table 7: Treatment-Emergent* Adverse Reactions in Patients Who Received CANCIDAS in Clinical Trials† Incidence ≥5% for at Least One Treatment Group by System Organ Class or Preferred Term

Adverse Reaction‡ (MedDRA v10 System Organ Class and Preferred Term)	CANCIDAS (N = 1951) n	(%)
All Systems, Any Adverse Reaction	1665	(85)
Investigations	901	(46)
Alanine Aminotransferase Increased	258	(13)
Aspartate Aminotransferase Increased	233	(12)
Blood Alkaline Phosphatase Increased	232	(12)
Blood Potassium Decreased	220	(11)
Blood Bilirubin Increased	117	(6)
General Disorders and Administration Site Conditions	843	(43)
Pyrexia	381	(20)
Chills	192	(10)
Edema Peripheral	110	(6)

Gastrointestinal Disorders	754	(39)
Diarrhea	273	(14)
Nausea	166	(9)
Vomiting	146	(8)
Abdominal Pain	112	(6)
Infections and Infestations	730	(37)
Pneumonia	115	(6)
Respiratory, Thoracic, and Mediastinal Disorders	613	(31)
Cough	111	(6)
Skin and Subcutaneous Tissue Disorders	520	(27)
Rash	159	(8)
Erythema	98	(5)
Nervous System Disorders	412	(21)
Headache	193	(10)
Vascular Disorders	344	(18)
Hypotension	118	(6)

* Defined as an adverse reaction, regardless of causality, while on CANCIDAS or during the 14-day post-CANCIDAS follow-up period.

† Incidence for each preferred term is ≥5% among individuals who received at least 1 dose of CANCIDAS.

‡ Within any system organ class, individuals may experience more than 1 adverse event.

Clinically significant adverse reactions, regardless of causality or incidence which occurred in less than 5% of patients are listed below.

- *Blood and lymphatic system disorders:* anemia, coagulopathy, febrile neutropenia, neutropenia, thrombocytopenia
- *Cardiac disorders:* arrhythmia, atrial fibrillation, bradycardia, cardiac arrest, myocardial infarction, tachycardia
- *Gastrointestinal disorders:* abdominal distension, abdominal pain upper, constipation, dyspepsia
- *General disorders and administration site conditions:* asthenia, fatigue, infusion site pain/pruritus/swelling, mucosal inflammation, edema
- *Hepatobiliary disorders:* hepatic failure, hepatomegaly, hepatotoxicity, hyperbilirubinemia, jaundice
- *Infections and infestations:* bacteremia, sepsis, urinary tract infection
- *Metabolic and nutrition disorders:* anorexia, decreased appetite, fluid overload, hypomagnesemia, hypercalcemia, hyperglycemia, hypokalemia
- *Musculoskeletal, connective tissue, and bone disorders:* arthralgia, back pain, pain in extremity
- *Nervous system disorders:* convulsion, dizziness, somnolence, tremor
- *Psychiatric disorders:* anxiety, confusional state, depression, insomnia
- *Renal and urinary disorders:* hematuria, renal failure
- *Respiratory, thoracic, and mediastinal disorders:* dyspnea, epistaxis, hypoxia, tachypnea
- *Skin and subcutaneous tissue disorders:* erythema, petechiae, skin lesion, urticaria
- *Vascular disorders:* flushing, hypertension, phlebitis

6.4 Postmarketing Experience

The following additional adverse reactions have been identified during the post-approval use of CANCIDAS. Because these reactions are reported voluntarily from a population of uncertain size, it is not always possible to reliably estimate their frequency or establish a causal relationship to drug exposure.

- *Gastrointestinal disorders:* pancreatitis
- *Hepatobiliary disorders:* hepatic necrosis
- *Skin and subcutaneous tissue disorders:* erythema multiforme, Stevens-Johnson, skin exfoliation
- *Renal and urinary disorders:* clinically significant renal dysfunction
- *General disorders and administration site conditions:* swelling and peripheral edema

7 DRUG INTERACTIONS

[See Clinical Pharmacology (12.3).]

In clinical studies, caspofungin did not induce the CYP3A4 metabolism of other drugs. Caspofungin is not a substrate for P-glycoprotein and is a poor substrate for cytochrome P450 enzymes.

Clinical studies in adult healthy volunteers show that the pharmacokinetics of CANCIDAS are not altered by itraconazole, amphotericin B, mycophenolate, nelfinavir, or

Table 4: Adverse Reactions Among Patients with Candidemia or other Candida Infections*, † Incidence ≥5% for at Least One Treatment Group by System Organ Class or Preferred Term

Adverse Reaction (MedDRA v11.0 System Organ Class and Preferred Term)	CANCIDAS 50 mg‡ N=104 (percent)	CANCIDAS 150 mg N=100 (percent)
All Systems, Any Adverse Reaction	83	83
Infections and Infestations	44	43
Septic Shock	13	14
Pneumonia	5	7
Sepsis	5	7
General Disorders and Administration Site Conditions	33	27
Pyrexia	6	6
Gastrointestinal Disorders	30	33
Vomiting	11	6
Diarrhea	6	7
Nausea	5	7
Investigations	28	35
Alkaline Phosphatase Increased	12	9
Aspartate Aminotransferase Increased	6	9
Blood potassium decreased	6	8
Alanine Aminotransferase Increased	4	7
Respiratory, Thoracic and Mediastinal Disorders	23	26
Respiratory Failure	6	2
Vascular Disorders	19	18
Hypotension	7	3
Hypertension	5	6
Skin and Subcutaneous Tissue Disorders	15	15
Decubitus Ulcer	3	5

Within any system organ class, individuals may experience more than 1 adverse event

* Intra-abdominal abscesses, peritonitis and pleural space infections.

† Regardless of causality

‡ Patients received CANCIDAS 70 mg on Day 1, then 50 mg once daily for the remainder of their treatment.

Table 5: Adverse Reactions Among Patients with Esophageal and/or Oropharyngeal Candidiasis* Incidence ≥10% for at Least One Treatment Group by System Organ Class or Preferred Term

Adverse Reaction (MedDRA v10.1 System Organ Class and Preferred Term)	CANCIDAS 50 mg† N=83 (percent)	Fluconazole IV 200 mg† N=94 (percent)
All Systems, Any Adverse Reaction	90	93
Gastrointestinal Disorders	58	50
Diarrhea	27	18
Nausea	15	15
Investigations	53	61
Hemoglobin Decreased	21	16
Hematocrit Decreased	18	16
Aspartate Aminotransferase Increased	13	19
Blood Alkaline Phosphatase Increased	13	17
Alanine Aminotransferase Increased	12	17
White Blood Cell Count Decreased	12	19
General Disorders and Administration Site Conditions	31	36
Pyrexia	21	21
Vascular Disorders	19	15
Phlebitis	18	11
Nervous System Disorders	18	17
Headache	15	9

Within any system organ class, individuals may experience more than 1 adverse reaction.

* Regardless of causality

† Derived from a comparator-controlled clinical study.

tacrolimus. CANCIDAS has no effect on the pharmacokinetics of itraconazole, amphotericin B, or the active metabolite of mycophenolate.

Cyclosporine: In two adult clinical studies, cyclosporine (one 4 mg/kg dose or two 3 mg/kg doses) increased the AUC of caspofungin by approximately 35%. CANCIDAS did not

Table 6: Adverse Reactions Among Pediatric Patients (0 months to 17 years of age)* Incidence ≥7.5% for at Least One Treatment Group by System Organ Class or Preferred Term

Adverse Reaction (MedDRA v10.0 System Organ Class and Preferred Term)	Noncomparative Clinical Studies CANCIDAS Any Dose N=115 (percent)	Comparator-Controlled Clinical Study of Empirical Therapy	
		CANCIDAS 50 mg/m²† N=56 (percent)	AmBisome 3 mg/kg N=26 (percent)
All Systems, Any Adverse Reaction	95	96	89
Investigations	55	41	50
Blood Potassium Decreased	18	9	27
Aspartate Aminotransferase Increased	17	2	12
Alanine Aminotransferase Increased	14	5	12
Blood Potassium Increased	3	0	8
Protein Total Decreased	0	0	8
General Disorders and Administration Site Conditions	47	59	42
Pyrexia	29	30	23
Chills	10	13	8
Mucosal Inflammation	10	4	4
Edema	3	4	8
Respiratory, Thoracic and Mediastinal Disorders	43	32	27
Respiratory Distress	8	0	4
Cough	6	9	8
Gastrointestinal Disorders	42	41	35
Diarrhea	17	7	15
Vomiting	8	11	12
Abdominal Pain	7	4	12
Nausea	4	4	8
Infections and Infestations	40	30	35
Central Line Infection	1	9	0
Skin and Subcutaneous Tissue Disorders	33	41	39
Pruritus	7	6	8
Rash	6	23	8
Erythema	4	9	0
Vascular Disorders	24	21	19
Hypotension	12	9	8
Hypertension	10	9	4
Metabolism and Nutrition Disorders	22	11	23
Hypokalemia	8	5	4
Cardiac Disorders	17	13	19
Tachycardia	4	11	19
Nervous System Disorders	13	16	8
Headache	5	9	4
Musculoskeletal and Connective Tissue Disorders	11	14	12
Back Pain	4	0	8
Blood and Lymphatic System Disorders	10	2	15
Anemia	2	0	8
Immune System Disorders	7	7	12
Graft Versus Host Disease	1	4	8

Within any system organ class, individuals may experience more than 1 adverse reaction.

* Regardless of causality

† 70 mg/m² on Day 1, then 50 mg/m² once daily for the remainder of the treatment.

increase the plasma levels of cyclosporine. There were transient increases in liver ALT and AST when CANCIDAS and cyclosporine were co-administered [see Warnings and Precautions (5.2)].

Tacrolimus: For patients receiving CANCIDAS and tacrolimus, standard monitoring of tacrolimus blood concentrations and appropriate tacrolimus dosage adjustments are recommended.

Rifampin: Adult patients on rifampin should receive 70 mg of CANCIDAS daily.

Other inducers of drug clearance:

Adults: When CANCIDAS is co-administered to adult patients with inducers of drug clearance, such as efavirenz, nevirapine, phenytoin, dexamethasone, or carbamazepine, use of a daily dose of 70 mg of CANCIDAS should be considered.

Pediatric Patients: When CANCIDAS is co-administered to pediatric patients with inducers of drug clearance, such as rifampin, efavirenz, nevirapine, phenytoin, dexamethasone, or carbamazepine, a CANCIDAS dose of 70 mg/m²

daily (not to exceed an actual daily dose of 70 mg) should be considered.

8 USE IN SPECIFIC POPULATIONS

8.1 Pregnancy

Pregnancy Category C

There are no adequate and well-controlled studies with the use of CANCIDAS in pregnant women. In animal studies, caspofungin caused embryofetal toxicity, including increased resorptions, increased peri-implantation loss, and incomplete ossification at multiple fetal sites. CANCIDAS should be used during pregnancy only if the potential benefit justifies the potential risk to the fetus.

In offspring born to pregnant rats treated with caspofungin at doses comparable to the human dose based on body surface area comparisons, there was incomplete ossification of the skull and torso and increased incidences of cervical rib. There was also an increase in resorptions and peri-implantation losses. In pregnant rabbits treated with caspofungin at doses comparable to 2 times the human dose based on body surface area comparisons, there was an increased incidence of incomplete ossification of the talus/calcaneus in offspring and increases in fetal resorptions. Caspofungin crossed the placenta in rats and rabbits and was detectable in fetal plasma.

8.3 Nursing Mothers

It is not known whether caspofungin is present in human milk. Caspofungin was found in the milk of lactating, drug-treated rats. Because many drugs are excreted in human milk, caution should be exercised when caspofungin is administered to a nursing woman.

8.4 Pediatric Use

The safety and effectiveness of CANCIDAS in pediatric patients 3 months to 17 years of age are supported by evidence from adequate and well-controlled studies in adults, pharmacokinetic data in pediatric patients, and additional data from prospective studies in pediatric patients 3 months to 17 years of age for the following indications [see Indications and Usage (1)]:

• Empirical therapy for presumed fungal infections in febrile, neutropenic patients.

• Treatment of candidemia and the following *Candida* infections: intra-abdominal abscesses, peritonitis, and pleural space infections.

• Treatment of esophageal candidiasis.

• Treatment of invasive aspergillosis in patients who are refractory to or intolerant of other therapies (e.g., amphotericin B, lipid formulations of amphotericin B, itraconazole).

The efficacy and safety of CANCIDAS has not been adequately studied in prospective clinical trials involving neonates and infants under 3 months of age. Although limited pharmacokinetic data were collected in neonates and infants below 3 months of age, these data are insufficient to establish a safe and effective dose of caspofungin in the treatment of neonatal candidiasis. Invasive candidiasis in neonates has a higher rate of CNS and multi-organ involvement than in older patients; the ability of CANCIDAS to penetrate the blood-brain barrier and to treat patients with meningitis and endocarditis is unknown.

CANCIDAS has not been studied in pediatric patients with endocarditis, osteomyelitis, and meningitis due to *Candida*. CANCIDAS has also not been studied as initial therapy for invasive aspergillosis in pediatric patients.

In clinical trials, 171 pediatric patients (0 months to 17 years of age), including 18 patients who were less than 3 months of age, were given intravenous CANCIDAS. Pharmacokinetic studies enrolled a total of 66 pediatric patients, and an additional 105 pediatric patients received CANCIDAS in safety and efficacy studies [see Clinical Pharmacology (12.3) and Clinical Studies (14.5)]. The majority of the pediatric patients received CANCIDAS at a once-daily maintenance dose of 50 mg/m² for a mean duration of 12 days (median 9, range 1-87 days). In all studies, safety was assessed by the investigator throughout study therapy and for 14 days following cessation of study therapy. The most common adverse reactions in pediatric patients treated with CANCIDAS were pyrexia (29%), blood potassium decreased (15%), diarrhea (14%), increased aspartate aminotransferase (12%), rash (12%), increased alanine aminotransferase (11%), hypotension (11%), and chills (11%) [see Adverse Reactions (6.2)].

Postmarketing hepatobiliary adverse reactions have been reported in pediatric patients with serious underlying medical conditions [see Warnings and Precautions (5.3)].

8.5 Geriatric Use

Clinical studies of CANCIDAS did not include sufficient numbers of patients aged 65 and over to determine whether they respond differently from younger patients. Although the number of elderly patients was not large enough for a statistical analysis, no overall differences in safety or efficacy were observed between these and younger patients. Plasma concentrations of caspofungin in healthy older men and women (≥65 years of age) were increased slightly (approximately 28% in AUC) compared to young healthy men. A similar effect of age on pharmacokinetics was seen in patients with candidemia or other *Candida* infections (intra-abdominal abscesses, peritonitis, or pleural space infections). No dose adjustment is recommended for the elderly; however, greater sensitivity of some older individuals cannot be ruled out.

8.6 Patients with Hepatic Impairment

Adult patients with mild hepatic impairment (Child-Pugh score 5 to 6) do not need a dosage adjustment. For adult patients with moderate hepatic impairment (Child-Pugh score 7 to 9), CANCIDAS 35 mg once daily is recommended based upon pharmacokinetic data *[see Clinical Pharmacology (12.3)]*. However, where recommended, a 70-mg loading dose should still be administered on Day 1 *[see Dosage and Administration (2.4) and Clinical Pharmacology (12.3)]*. There is no clinical experience in adult patients with severe hepatic impairment (Child-Pugh score >9) and in pediatric patients 3 months to 17 years of age with any degree of hepatic impairment.

8.7 Patients with Renal Impairment

No dosage adjustment is necessary for patients with renal impairment. Caspofungin is not dialyzable; thus, supplementary dosing is not required following hemodialysis *[see Clinical Pharmacology (12.3)]*.

10 OVERDOSAGE

In 6 healthy subjects who received a single 210-mg dose, no significant adverse reactions were reported. Multiple doses above 150 mg daily have not been studied. Caspofungin is not dialyzable. The minimum lethal dose of caspofungin in rats was 50 mg/kg, a dose which is equivalent to 10 times the recommended daily dose based on relative body surface area comparison.

In clinical trials, one pediatric patient (16 years of age) unintentionally received a single dose of caspofungin of 113 mg (on Day 1), followed by 80 mg daily for an additional 7 days. No clinically significant adverse reactions were reported.

11 DESCRIPTION

CANCIDAS is a sterile, lyophilized product for intravenous (IV) infusion that contains a semisynthetic lipopeptide (echinocandin) compound synthesized from a fermentation product of *Glarea lozoyensis*. CANCIDAS is an echinocandin that inhibits the synthesis of β (1,3)-D-glucan, an integral component of the fungal cell wall.

CANCIDAS (caspofungin acetate) is 1-[(4R,5S)-5-[(2-aminoethyl)amino]-N^2-(10,12-dimethyl-1-oxotetradecyl)-4-hydroxy-L-ornithine]-5-[(3R)-3-hydroxy-L-ornithine] pneumocandin B$_0$ diacetate (salt). CANCIDAS 50 mg also contains: 39 mg sucrose, 26 mg mannitol, glacial acetic acid, and sodium hydroxide. CANCIDAS 70 mg also contains 54 mg sucrose, 36 mg mannitol, glacial acetic acid, and sodium hydroxide. Caspofungin acetate is a hygroscopic, white to off-white powder. It is freely soluble in water and methanol, and slightly soluble in ethanol. The pH of a saturated aqueous solution of caspofungin acetate is approximately 6.6. The empirical formula is $C_{52}H_{88}N_{10}O_{15} \cdot 2C_2H_4O_2$ and the formula weight is 1213.42. The structural formula is:

12 CLINICAL PHARMACOLOGY

12.1 Mechanism of Action

Caspofungin is an antifungal drug *[see Clinical Pharmacology (12.4)]*.

12.3 Pharmacokinetics

Adult and pediatric pharmacokinetic parameters are presented in Table 8.

Distribution

Plasma concentrations of caspofungin decline in a polyphasic manner following single 1-hour IV infusions. A short α-phase occurs immediately postinfusion, followed by a β-phase (half-life of 9 to 11 hours) that characterizes much of the profile and exhibits clear log-linear behavior from 6 to 48 hours postdose during which the plasma concentration decreases 10-fold. An additional, longer half-life phase, γ-phase, (half-life of 40-50 hours), also occurs. Distribution, rather than excretion or biotransformation, is the dominant

Table 8: Pharmacokinetic Parameters Following Multiple Doses of CANCIDAS in Pediatric (3 months to 17 years) and Adult Patients

Population	N	Daily Dose	Pharmacokinetic Parameters (Mean ± Standard Deviation)				
			AUC$_{0-24hr}$ (µg·hr/mL)	C$_{1hr}$ (µg/mL)	C$_{24hr}$ (µg/mL)	t$_{1/2}$ (hr)*	Cl (mL/min)
PEDIATRIC PATIENTS							
Adolescents, Aged 12-17 years	8	50 mg/m²	124.9 ± 50.4	14.0 ± 6.9	2.4 ± 1.0	11.2 ± 1.7	12.6 ± 5.5
Children, Aged 2-11 years	9	50 mg/m²	120.0 ± 33.4	16.1 ± 4.2	1.7 ± 0.8	8.2 ± 2.4	6.4 ± 2.6
Young Children, Aged 3-23 months	8	50 mg/m²	131.2 ± 17.7	17.6 ± 3.9	1.7 ± 0.7	8.8 ± 2.1	3.2 ± 0.4
ADULT PATIENTS							
Adults with Esophageal Candidiasis	6†	50 mg	87.3 ± 30.0	8.7 ± 2.1	1.7 ± 0.7	13.0 ± 1.9	10.6 ± 3.8
Adults receiving Empirical Therapy	119‡	50 mg§	--	8.0 ± 3.4	1.6 ± 0.7	--	--

* Harmonic Mean ± jackknife standard deviation
† N=5 for C$_{1hr}$ and AUC$_{0-24hr}$; N=6 for C$_{24hr}$
‡ N=117 for C$_{24hr}$; N=119 for C$_{1hr}$
§ Following an initial 70-mg loading dose on day 1

mechanism influencing plasma clearance. Caspofungin is extensively bound to albumin (~97%), and distribution into red blood cells is minimal. Mass balance results showed that approximately 92% of the administered radioactivity was distributed to tissues by 36 to 48 hours after a single 70-mg dose of [³H] caspofungin acetate. There is little excretion or biotransformation of caspofungin during the first 30 hours after administration.

Metabolism

Caspofungin is slowly metabolized by hydrolysis and N-acetylation. Caspofungin also undergoes spontaneous chemical degradation to an open-ring peptide compound, L-747969. At later time points (≥5 days postdose), there is a low level (≤7 picomoles/mg protein, or ≤1.3% of administered dose) of covalent binding of radiolabel in plasma following single-dose administration of [³H] caspofungin acetate, which may be due to two reactive intermediates formed during the chemical degradation of caspofungin to L-747969. Additional metabolism involves hydrolysis into constitutive amino acids and their degradates, including dihydroxyhomotyrosine and N-acetyl-dihydroxyhomotyrosine. These two tyrosine derivatives are found only in urine, suggesting rapid clearance of these derivatives by the kidneys.

Excretion

Two single-dose radiolabeled pharmacokinetic studies were conducted. In one study, plasma, urine, and feces were collected over 27 days, and in the second study plasma was collected over 6 months. Plasma concentrations of radioactivity and of caspofungin were similar during the first 24 to 48 hours postdose; thereafter drug levels fell more rapidly. In plasma, caspofungin concentrations fell below the limit of quantitation after 6 to 8 days postdose, while radiolabel fell below the limit of quantitation at 22.3 weeks postdose. After single intravenous administration of [³H] caspofungin acetate, excretion of caspofungin and its metabolites in humans was 35% of dose in feces and 41% of dose in urine. A small amount of caspofungin is excreted unchanged in urine (~1.4% of dose). Renal clearance of parent drug is low (~0.15 mL/min) and total clearance of caspofungin is 12 mL/min.

Special Populations

Renal Impairment

In a clinical study of single 70-mg doses, caspofungin pharmacokinetics were similar in healthy adult volunteers with mild renal impairment (creatinine clearance 50 to 80 mL/min) and control subjects. Moderate (creatinine clearance 31 to 49 mL/min), severe (creatinine clearance 5 to 30 mL/min), and end-stage (creatinine clearance <10 mL/min and dialysis dependent) renal impairment moderately increased caspofungin plasma concentrations after single-dose administration (range: 30 to 49% for AUC). However, in adult patients with invasive aspergillosis, candidemia, or other *Candida* infections (intra-abdominal abscesses, peritonitis, or pleural space infections) who received multiple daily doses of CANCIDAS 50 mg, there was no significant effect of mild to end-stage renal impairment on caspofungin concentrations. No dosage adjustment is necessary for patients with renal impairment. Caspofungin is not dialyzable, thus supplementary dosing is not required following hemodialysis.

Hepatic Impairment

Plasma concentrations of caspofungin after a single 70-mg dose in adult patients with mild hepatic impairment (Child-Pugh score 5 to 6) were increased by approximately 55% in AUC compared to healthy control subjects. In a 14-day multiple-dose study (70 mg on Day 1 followed by 50 mg daily thereafter), plasma concentrations in adult patients with mild hepatic impairment were increased modestly (19 to 25% in AUC) on Days 7 and 14 relative to healthy control subjects. No dosage adjustment is recommended for patients with mild hepatic impairment.

Adult patients with moderate hepatic impairment (Child-Pugh score 7 to 9) who received a single 70-mg dose of CANCIDAS had an average plasma caspofungin increase of 76% in AUC compared to control subjects. A dosage reduction is recommended for adult patients with moderate hepatic impairment based upon these pharmacokinetic data *[see Dosage and Administration (2.4)]*.

There is no clinical experience in adult patients with severe hepatic impairment (Child-Pugh score >9) or in pediatric patients with any degree of hepatic impairment.

Gender

Plasma concentrations of caspofungin in healthy adult men and women were similar following a single 70-mg dose. After 13 daily 50-mg doses, caspofungin plasma concentrations in women were elevated slightly (approximately 22% in area under the curve [AUC]) relative to men. No dosage adjustment is necessary based on gender.

Race

Regression analyses of patient pharmacokinetic data indicated that no clinically significant differences in the pharmacokinetics of caspofungin were seen among Caucasians, Blacks, and Hispanics. No dosage adjustment is necessary on the basis of race.

Geriatric Patients

Plasma concentrations of caspofungin in healthy older men and women (≥65 years of age) were increased slightly (approximately 28% AUC) compared to young healthy men after a single 70-mg dose of caspofungin. In patients who were treated empirically or who had candidemia or other *Candida* infections (intra-abdominal abscesses, peritonitis, or pleural space infections), a similar modest effect of age was seen in older patients relative to younger patients. No dosage adjustment is necessary for the elderly *[see Use in Specific Populations (8.5)]*.

Pediatric Patients

CANCIDAS has been studied in five prospective studies involving pediatric patients under 18 years of age, including three pediatric pharmacokinetic studies [initial study in adolescents (12-17 years of age) and children (2-11 years of age) followed by a study in younger patients (3-23 months of age) and then followed by a study in neonates and infants (<3 months)] *[see Use in Specific Populations (8.4)]*.

Pharmacokinetic parameters following multiple doses of CANCIDAS in pediatric and adult patients are presented in Table 8.

[See table 8 above]

Drug Interactions *[see Drug Interactions (7)]*

Studies *in vitro* show that caspofungin acetate is not an inhibitor of any enzyme in the cytochrome P450 (CYP) system. In clinical studies, caspofungin did not induce the CYP3A4 metabolism of other drugs. Caspofungin is not a substrate for P-glycoprotein and is a poor substrate for cytochrome P450 enzymes.

Clinical studies in adult healthy volunteers show that the pharmacokinetics of CANCIDAS are not altered by itraconazole, amphotericin B, mycophenolate, nelfinavir, or tacrolimus. CANCIDAS has no effect on the pharmacokinetics of itraconazole, amphotericin B, or the active metabolite of mycophenolate.

Cyclosporine: In two adult clinical studies, cyclosporine (one 4 mg/kg dose or two 3 mg/kg doses) increased the AUC of caspofungin by approximately 35%. CANCIDAS did not increase the plasma levels of cyclosporine. There were transient increases in liver ALT and AST when CANCIDAS and cyclosporine were co-administered *[see Warnings and Precautions (5.2)]*.

Tacrolimus: CANCIDAS reduced the blood AUC_{0-12} of tacrolimus (FK-506, Prograf®) by approximately 20%, peak blood concentration (C_{max}) by 16%, and 12-hour blood concentration (C_{12hr}) by 26% in healthy adult subjects when tacrolimus (2 doses of 0.1 mg/kg 12 hours apart) was administered on the 10th day of CANCIDAS 70 mg daily, as compared to results from a control period in which tacrolimus was administered alone. For patients receiving both therapies, standard monitoring of tacrolimus blood concentrations and appropriate tacrolimus dosage adjustments are recommended.

Rifampin: A drug-drug interaction study with rifampin in adult healthy volunteers has shown a 30% decrease in caspofungin trough concentrations. Adult patients on rifampin should receive 70 mg of CANCIDAS daily.

Other inducers of drug clearance

Adults: In addition, results from regression analyses of adult patient pharmacokinetic data suggest that coadministration of other inducers of drug clearance (efavirenz, nevirapine, phenytoin, dexamethasone, or carbamazepine) with CANCIDAS may result in clinically meaningful reductions in caspofungin concentrations. It is not known which drug clearance mechanism involved in caspofungin disposition may be inducible. When CANCIDAS is co-administered to adult patients with inducers of drug clearance, such as efavirenz, nevirapine, phenytoin, dexamethasone, or carbamazepine, use of a daily dose of 70 mg of CANCIDAS should be considered.

Pediatric patients: In pediatric patients, results from regression analyses of pharmacokinetic data suggest that coadministration of dexamethasone with CANCIDAS may result in clinically meaningful reductions in caspofungin trough concentrations. This finding may indicate that pediatric patients will have similar reductions with inducers as seen in adults. When CANCIDAS is co-administered to pediatric patients with inducers of drug clearance, such as rifampin, efavirenz, nevirapine, phenytoin, dexamethasone, or carbamazepine, a CANCIDAS dose of 70 mg/m² daily (not to exceed an actual daily dose of 70 mg) should be considered.

12.4 Microbiology

Mechanism of Action

Caspofungin, an echinocandin, inhibits the synthesis of beta (1,3)-D-glucan, an essential component of the cell wall of susceptible *Aspergillus* species and *Candida* species. Beta (1,3)-D-glucan is not present in mammalian cells. Caspofungin has shown activity against *Candida* species and in regions of active cell growth of the hyphae of *Aspergillus fumigatus*.

Drug Resistance

There have been reports of clinical failures in patients receiving caspofungin therapy due to the development of drug resistance. Some of these reports have identified specific mutations in the Fks subunits of the glucan synthase enzyme. These mutations are associated with higher MICs and breakthrough infection. *Candida* species that exhibit reduced susceptibility to caspofungin as a result of an in-

crease in the chitin content of the fungal cell wall have also been identified, although the significance of this phenomenon in vivo is not well known.

Drug Interactions

Studies *in vitro* and *in vivo* of caspofungin, in combination with amphotericin B, suggest no antagonism of antifungal activity against either *A. fumigatus* or *C. albicans*. The clinical significance of these results is unknown.

Activity in Vitro and in Clinical Infections

Caspofungin has been shown to be active **both in vitro and in clinical infections** against most strains of the following microorganisms:

Aspergillus fumigatus
Aspergillus flavus
Aspergillus terreus
Candida albicans
Candida glabrata
Candida guilliermondii
Candida krusei
Candida parapsilosis
Candida tropicalis

Susceptibility Testing Methods

The interpretive standards for caspofungin against *Candida* species are applicable only to tests performed using Clinical Laboratory and Standards Institute (CLSI) microbroth dilution reference methods[2,3] for MIC (partial inhibition endpoint) read at 24 hours. No interpretive criteria have been established for *Aspergillus* species and other filamentous fungi.

When available, the clinical microbiology laboratory should provide the results of *in vitro* susceptibility test results for antimicrobial drug products used in resident hospitals to the physician as periodic reports that describe the susceptibility profile of pathogens. These reports should aid the physician in selecting an antifungal drug product for treatment. The techniques for Broth Microdilution are described below.

Broth Microdilution Techniques

Quantitative methods are used to determine antifungal minimum inhibitory concentrations (MICs). These MICs provide estimates of the susceptibility of *Candida* spp. to antifungal agents. MICs should be determined using a standardized procedure at 24 hours[2,3]. Standardized procedures are based on a microdilution method (broth) with standardized inoculum concentrations and standardized concentrations of caspofungin powder. The MIC values should be interpreted according to the criteria provided in Table 9.

Table 9: Susceptibility Interpretive Criteria for Caspofungin

Pathogen	Broth Microdilution MIC* (mcg/mL) at 24 hours	
	Susceptible (S)	Non-Susceptible (NS)
Candida species	≤2	≥2

* A report of "Susceptible" indicates that the pathogen is likely to be inhibited if the antimicrobial compound in the blood reaches the concentrations usually achievable.

Quality Control

Standardized susceptibility test procedures require the use of quality control organisms to control the technical aspects of the test procedures. Standard caspofungin powder should provide the following range of values noted in Table 10[3]. Quality control microorganisms are specific strains of organisms with intrinsic biological properties relating to resistance mechanisms and their genetic expression within fungi; the specific strains used for microbiological control are not clinically significant.

Table 10: Acceptable Quality Control Ranges for caspofungin to be used in Validation of Susceptibility Test Results

QC Strain	Broth Microdilution (MIC in mcg/mL) at 24 hours*
Candida parapsilosis ATCC 22019	0.25 – 1.0
Candida krusei ATCC 6258	0.12 – 1.0

* The MIC for caspofungin is the lowest concentration at which a score of 2 (prominent decrease in turbidity [> 50% inhibition of growth as compared to the growth control]; see CLSI document M27-A3[2], Section 7.6.3) is observed after 24 hours of incubation.

13 NONCLINICAL TOXICOLOGY

13.1 Carcinogenesis, Mutagenesis, Impairment of Fertility

No long-term studies in animals have been performed to evaluate the carcinogenic potential of caspofungin.

Caspofungin did not show evidence of mutagenic or genotoxic potential when evaluated in the following *in vitro* assays: bacterial (Ames) and mammalian cell (V79 Chinese hamster lung fibroblasts) mutagenesis assays, the alkaline elution/rat hepatocyte DNA strand break test, and the chromosome aberration assay in Chinese hamster ovary cells. Caspofungin was not genotoxic when assessed in the mouse bone marrow chromosomal test at doses up to 12.5 mg/kg (equivalent to a human dose of 1 mg/kg based on body surface area comparisons), administered intravenously.

Fertility and reproductive performance were not affected by the intravenous administration of caspofungin to rats at doses up to 5 mg/kg. At 5 mg/kg exposures were similar to those seen in patients treated with the 70-mg dose.

13.2 Animal Toxicology and/or Pharmacology

In one 5-week study in monkeys at doses which produced exposures approximately 4 to 6 times those seen in adult patients treated with a 70-mg dose, scattered small foci of subcapsular necrosis were observed microscopically in the livers of some animals (2/8 monkeys at 5 mg/kg and 4/8 monkeys at 8 mg/kg); however, this histopathological finding was not seen in another study of 27 weeks duration at similar doses.

No treatment-related findings were seen in a 5-week study in infant monkeys at doses which produced exposures approximately 3 times those achieved in pediatric patients receiving a maintenance dose of 50 mg/m² daily.

14 CLINICAL STUDIES

The results of the adult clinical studies are presented by indications in Section 14.1 to 14.4. Results of pediatric clinical trials are in Section 14.5.

14.1 Empirical Therapy in Febrile, Neutropenic Patients

A double-blind study enrolled 1111 febrile, neutropenic (<500 cells/mm³) patients who were randomized to treatment with daily doses of CANCIDAS (50 mg/day following a 70-mg loading dose on Day 1) or AmBisome (3 mg/kg/day). Patients were stratified based on risk category (high-risk patients had undergone allogeneic stem cell transplantation or had relapsed acute leukemia) and on receipt of prior antifungal prophylaxis. Twenty-four percent of patients were high risk and 56% had received prior antifungal prophylaxis. Patients who remained febrile or clinically deteriorated following 5 days of therapy could receive 70 mg/day of CANCIDAS or 5 mg/kg/day of AmBisome. Treatment was continued to resolution of neutropenia (but not beyond 28 days unless a fungal infection was documented).

An overall favorable response required meeting each of the following criteria: no documented breakthrough fungal infections up to 7 days after completion of treatment, survival for 7 days after completion of study therapy, no discontinuation of the study drug because of drug-related toxicity or lack of efficacy, resolution of fever during the period of neutropenia, and successful treatment of any documented baseline fungal infection.

Based on the composite response rates, CANCIDAS was as effective as AmBisome in empirical therapy of persistent febrile neutropenia (see Table 11).

[See table 11 below]

The rate of successful treatment of documented baseline infections, a component of the primary endpoint, was not statistically different between treatment groups.

The response rates did not differ between treatment groups based on either of the stratification variables: risk category or prior antifungal prophylaxis.

14.2 Candidemia and the Following other *Candida* Infections: Intra-Abdominal Abscesses, Peritonitis and Pleural Space Infections

In a randomized, double-blind study, patients with a proven diagnosis of invasive candidiasis received daily doses of

Table 11: Favorable Response of Patients with Persistent Fever and Neutropenia

	CANCIDAS*	AmBisome*	% Difference (Confidence Interval)[†]
Number of Patients[‡]	556	539	
Overall Favorable Response	190 (33.9%)	181 (33.7%)	0.2 (-5.6, 6.0)
No documented breakthrough fungal infection	527 (94.8%)	515 (95.5%)	-0.8
Survival 7 days after end of treatment	515 (92.6%)	481 (89.2%)	3.4
No discontinuation due to toxicity or lack of efficacy	499 (89.7%)	461 (85.5%)	4.2
Resolution of fever during neutropenia	229 (41.2%)	223 (41.4%)	-0.2

* CANCIDAS: 70 mg on Day 1, then 50 mg once daily for the remainder of treatment (daily dose increased to 70 mg for 73 patients); AmBisome: 3 mg/kg/day (daily dose increased to 5 mg/kg for 74 patients).

[†] Overall Response: estimated % difference adjusted for strata and expressed as CANCIDAS – AmBisome (95.2% CI); Individual criteria presented above are not mutually exclusive. The percent difference calculated as CANCIDAS – AmBisome.

[‡] Analysis population excluded subjects who did not have fever or neutropenia at study entry.

CANCIDAS (50 mg/day following a 70-mg loading dose on Day 1) or amphotericin B deoxycholate (0.6 to 0.7 mg/kg/day for non-neutropenic patients and 0.7 to 1 mg/kg/day for neutropenic patients). Patients were stratified by both neutropenic status and APACHE II score. Patients with *Candida* endocarditis, meningitis, or osteomyelitis were excluded from this study.

Patients who met the entry criteria and received one or more doses of IV study therapy were included in the modified intention-to-treat [MITT] analysis of response at the end of IV study therapy. A favorable response at this time point required both symptom/sign resolution/improvement and microbiological clearance of the *Candida* infection.

Two hundred thirty-nine patients were enrolled. Patient disposition is shown in Table 12.

[See table 12 above]

Of the 239 patients enrolled, 224 met the criteria for inclusion in the MITT population (109 treated with CANCIDAS and 115 treated with amphotericin B). Of these 224 patients, 186 patients had candidemia (92 treated with CANCIDAS and 94 treated with amphotericin B). The majority of the patients with candidemia were non-neutropenic (87%) and had an APACHE II score less than or equal to 20 (77%) in both arms. Most candidemia infections were caused by *C. albicans* (39%), followed by *C. parapsilosis* (20%), *C. tropicalis* (17%), *C. glabrata* (8%), and *C. krusei* (3%).

At the end of IV study therapy, CANCIDAS was comparable to amphotericin B in the treatment of candidemia in the MITT population. For the other efficacy time points (Day 10 of IV study therapy, end of all antifungal therapy, 2-week post-therapy follow-up, and 6- to 8-week post-therapy follow-up), CANCIDAS was as effective as amphotericin B. Outcome, relapse and mortality data are shown in Table 13.

[See table 13 above]

In this study, the efficacy of CANCIDAS in patients with intra-abdominal abscesses, peritonitis and pleural space *Candida* infections was evaluated in 19 non-neutropenic patients. Two of these patients had concurrent candidemia. *Candida* was part of a polymicrobial infection that required adjunctive surgical drainage in 11 of these 19 patients. A favorable response was seen in 9 of 9 patients with peritonitis, 3 of 4 with abscesses (liver, parasplenic, and urinary bladder abscesses), 2 of 2 with pleural space infections, 1 of 2 with mixed peritoneal and pleural infection, 1 of 1 with mixed abdominal abscess and peritonitis, and 0 of 1 with *Candida* pneumonia.

Overall, across all sites of infection included in the study, the efficacy of CANCIDAS was comparable to that of amphotericin B for the primary endpoint.

In this study, the efficacy data for CANCIDAS in neutropenic patients with candidemia were limited. In a separate compassionate use study, 4 patients with hepatosplenic candidiasis received prolonged therapy with CANCIDAS following other long-term antifungal therapy; three of these patients had a favorable response.

In a second randomized, double-blind study, 197 patients with proven invasive candidiasis received CANCIDAS 50 mg/day (following a 70-mg loading dose on Day 1) or CANCIDAS 150 mg/day. The diagnostic criteria, evaluation time points, and efficacy endpoints were similar to those employed in the prior study. Patients with *Candida* endocarditis, meningitis, or osteomyelitis were excluded. Although this study was designed to compare the safety of the two doses, it was not large enough to detect differences in rare or unexpected adverse events [see Adverse Reactions (6.1)]. A significant improvement in efficacy with the 150-mg daily dose was not seen when compared to the 50-mg dose.

14.3 Esophageal Candidiasis (and information on oropharyngeal candidiasis)

The safety and efficacy of CANCIDAS in the treatment of esophageal candidiasis was evaluated in one large, controlled, noninferiority, clinical trial and two smaller dose-response studies.

In all 3 studies, patients were required to have symptoms and microbiological documentation of esophageal candidiasis; most patients had advanced AIDS (with CD4 counts <50/mm³).

Of the 166 patients in the large study who had culture-confirmed esophageal candidiasis at baseline, 120 had *Candida albicans* and 2 had *Candida tropicalis* as the sole baseline pathogen whereas 44 had mixed baseline cultures containing *C. albicans* and one or more additional *Candida* species.

In the large, randomized, double-blind study comparing CANCIDAS 50 mg/day versus intravenous fluconazole 200 mg/day for the treatment of esophageal candidiasis, patients were treated for an average of 9 days (range 7-21 days). Favorable overall response at 5 to 7 days following discontinuation of study therapy required both complete resolution of symptoms and significant endoscopic improvement. The definition of endoscopic response was based on severity of disease at baseline using a 4-grade scale and re-

quired at least a two-grade reduction from baseline endoscopic score or reduction to grade 0 for patients with a baseline score of 2 or less.

The proportion of patients with a favorable overall response was comparable for CANCIDAS and fluconazole as shown in Table 14.

[See table 14 at top of next page]

The proportion of patients with a favorable symptom response was also comparable (90.1% and 89.4% for CANCIDAS and fluconazole, respectively). In addition, the proportion of patients with a favorable endoscopic response was comparable (85.2% and 86.2% for CANCIDAS and fluconazole, respectively).

As shown in Table 15, the esophageal candidiasis relapse rates at the Day 14 post-treatment visit were similar for the two groups. At the Day 28 post-treatment visit, the group treated with CANCIDAS had a numerically higher incidence of relapse; however, the difference was not statistically significant.

[See table 15 at top of next page]

In this trial, which was designed to establish noninferiority of CANCIDAS to fluconazole for the treatment of esophageal candidiasis, 122 (70%) patients also had oropharyngeal candidiasis. A favorable response was defined as complete resolution of all symptoms of oropharyngeal disease and all

visible oropharyngeal lesions. The proportion of patients with a favorable oropharyngeal response at the 5- to 7-day post-treatment visit was numerically lower for CANCIDAS; however, the difference was not statistically significant. Oropharyngeal candidiasis relapse rates at Day 14 and Day 28 post-treatment visits were statistically significantly higher for CANCIDAS than for fluconazole. The results are shown in Table 16.

[See table 16 at top of next page]

The results from the two smaller dose-ranging studies corroborate the efficacy of CANCIDAS for esophageal candidiasis that was demonstrated in the larger study.

CANCIDAS was associated with favorable outcomes in 7 of 10 esophageal *C. albicans* infections refractory to at least 200 mg of fluconazole given for 7 days, although the *in vitro* susceptibility of the infecting isolates to fluconazole was not known.

14.4 Invasive Aspergillosis

Sixty-nine patients between the ages of 18 and 80 with invasive aspergillosis were enrolled in an open-label, noncomparative study to evaluate the safety, tolerability, and efficacy of CANCIDAS. Enrolled patients had previously been refractory to or intolerant of other antifungal therapy(ies). Refractory patients were classified as those who had disease progression or failed to improve despite therapy for at least

---

Table 12: Disposition in Candidemia and Other Candida Infections (Intra-abdominal abscesses, peritonitis, and pleural space infections)

	CANCIDAS*	Amphotericin B
Randomized patients	114	125
Patients completing study†	63 (55.3%)	69 (55.2%)
DISCONTINUATIONS OF STUDY†		
All Study Discontinuations	51 (44.7%)	56 (44.8%)
Study Discontinuations due to clinical adverse events	39 (34.2%)	43 (34.4%)
Study Discontinuations due to laboratory adverse events	0 (0%)	1 (0.8%)
DISCONTINUATIONS OF STUDY THERAPY		
All Study Therapy Discontinuations	48 (42.1%)	58 (46.4%)
Study Therapy Discontinuations due to clinical adverse events	30 (26.3%)	37 (29.6%)
Study Therapy Discontinuations due to laboratory adverse events	1 (0.9%)	7 (5.6%)
Study Therapy Discontinuations due to all drug-related‡ adverse events	3 (2.6%)	29 (23.2%)

* Patients received CANCIDAS 70 mg on Day 1, then 50 mg once daily for the remainder of their treatment.
† Study defined as study treatment period and 6-8 week follow-up period.
‡ Determined by the investigator to be possibly, probably, or definitely drug-related.

Table 13: Outcomes, Relapse, & Mortality in Candidemia and Other Candida Infections (Intra-abdominal abscesses, peritonitis, and pleural space infections)

	CANCIDAS*	Amphotericin B	% Difference† after adjusting for strata (Confidence Interval)‡
Number of MITT§ patients	109	115	
FAVORABLE OUTCOMES (MITT) AT THE END OF IV STUDY THERAPY			
All MITT patients	81/109 (74.3%)	78/115 (67.8%)	7.5 (-5.4, 20.3)
Candidemia	67/92 (72.8%)	63/94 (67.0%)	7.0 (-7.0, 21.1)
Neutropenic	6/14 (43%)	5/10 (50%)	
Non-neutropenic	61/78 (78%)	58/84 (69%)	
Endophthalmitis	0/1	2/3	
Multiple Sites	4/5	4/4	
Blood / Pleural	1/1	1/1	
Blood / Peritoneal	1/1	1/1	
Blood / Urine	-	1/1	
Peritoneal / Pleural	1/2	-	
Abdominal / Peritoneal	-	1/1	
Subphrenic / Peritoneal	1/1	-	
DISSEMINATED INFECTIONS, RELAPSES AND MORTALITY			
Disseminated Infections in neutropenic patients	4/14 (28.6%)	3/10 (30.0%)	
All relapses¶	7/81 (8.6%)	8/78 (10.3%)	
Culture-confirmed relapse	5/81 (6%)	2/78 (3%)	
Overall study# mortality in MITT	36/109 (33.0%)	35/115 (30.4%)	
Mortality during study therapy	18/109 (17%)	13/115 (11%)	
Mortality attributed to *Candida*	4/109 (4%)	7/115 (6%)	

* Patients received CANCIDAS 70 mg on Day 1, then 50 mg once daily for the remainder of their treatment.
† Calculated as CANCIDAS – amphotericin B
‡ 95% CI for candidemia, 95.6% for all patients
§ Modified intention-to-treat
¶ Includes all patients who either developed a culture-confirmed recurrence of *Candida* infection or required antifungal therapy for the treatment of a proven or suspected *Candida* infection in the follow-up period.
# Study defined as study treatment period and 6-8 week follow-up period.

Table 14: Favorable Response Rates for Patients with Esophageal Candidiasis*

	CANCIDAS	Fluconazole	% Difference[†] (95% CI)
Day 5-7 post-treatment	66/81 (81.5%)	80/94 (85.1%)	-3.6 (-14.7, 7.5)

* Analysis excluded patients without documented esophageal candidiasis or patients not receiving at least 1 day of study therapy.
† Calculated as CANCIDAS – fluconazole

Table 15: Relapse Rates at 14 and 28 Days Post-Therapy in Patients with Esophageal Candidiasis at Baseline

	CANCIDAS	Fluconazole	% Difference* (95% CI)
Day 14 post-treatment	7/66 (10.6%)	6/76 (7.9%)	2.7 (-6.9, 12.3)
Day 28 post-treatment	18/64 (28.1%)	12/72 (16.7%)	11.5 (-2.5, 25.4)

* Calculated as CANCIDAS – fluconazole

Table 16: Oropharyngeal Candidiasis Response Rates at 5 to 7 Days Post-Therapy and Relapse Rates at 14 and 28 Days Post-Therapy in Patients with Oropharyngeal and Esophageal Candidiasis at Baseline

	CANCIDAS	Fluconazole	% Difference* (95% CI)
Response Rate Day 5-7 post-treatment	40/56 (71.4%)	55/66 (83.3%)	-11.9 (-26.8, 3.0)
Relapse Rate Day 14 post-treatment	17/40 (42.5%)	7/53 (13.2%)	29.3 (11.5, 47.1)
Relapse Rate Day 28 post-treatment	23/39 (59.0%)	18/51 (35.3%)	23.7 (3.4, 43.9)

* Calculated as CANCIDAS – fluconazole

7 days with amphotericin B, lipid formulations of amphotericin B, itraconazole, or an investigational azole with reported activity against *Aspergillus*. Intolerance to previous therapy was defined as a doubling of creatinine (or creatinine ≥2.5 mg/dL while on therapy), other acute reactions, or infusion-related toxicity. To be included in the study, patients with pulmonary disease must have had definite (positive tissue histopathology or positive culture from tissue obtained by an invasive procedure) or probable (positive radiographic or computed tomography evidence with supporting culture from bronchoalveolar lavage or sputum, galactomannan enzyme-linked immunosorbent assay, and/or polymerase chain reaction) invasive aspergillosis. Patients with extrapulmonary disease had to have definite invasive aspergillosis. The definitions were modeled after the Mycoses Study Group Criteria *[see References (15)]*. Patients were administered a single 70-mg loading dose of CANCIDAS and subsequently dosed with 50 mg daily. The mean duration of therapy was 33.7 days, with a range of 1 to 162 days.

An independent expert panel evaluated patient data, including diagnosis of invasive aspergillosis, response and tolerability to previous antifungal therapy, treatment course on CANCIDAS, and clinical outcome.

A favorable response was defined as either complete resolution (complete response) or clinically meaningful improvement (partial response) of all signs and symptoms and attributable radiographic findings. Stable, nonprogressive disease was considered to be an unfavorable response.

Among the 69 patients enrolled in the study, 63 met entry diagnostic criteria and had outcome data; and of these, 52 patients received treatment for >7 days. Fifty-three (84%) were refractory to previous antifungal therapy and 10 (16%) were intolerant. Forty-five patients had pulmonary disease and 18 had extrapulmonary disease. Underlying conditions were hematologic malignancy (N=24), allogeneic bone marrow transplant or stem cell transplant (N=18), organ transplant (N=8), solid tumor (N=3), or other conditions (N=10). All patients in the study received concomitant therapies for their other underlying conditions. Eighteen patients received tacrolimus and CANCIDAS concomitantly, of whom 8 also received mycophenolate mofetil.

Overall, the expert panel determined that 41% (26/63) of patients receiving at least one dose of CANCIDAS had a favorable response. For those patients who received >7 days of therapy with CANCIDAS, 50% (26/52) had a favorable response. The favorable response rates for patients who were either refractory to or intolerant of previous therapies were 36% (19/53) and 70% (7/10), respectively. The response rates among patients with pulmonary disease and extrapulmonary disease were 47% (21/45) and 28% (5/18), respectively. Among patients with extrapulmonary disease, 2 of 8 patients who also had definite, probable, or possible CNS involvement had a favorable response. Two of these 8 patients had progression of disease and manifested CNS involvement while on therapy.

CANCIDAS is effective for the treatment of invasive aspergillosis in patients who are refractory to or intolerant of itraconazole, amphotericin B, and/or lipid formulations of amphotericin B. However, the efficacy of CANCIDAS for initial treatment of invasive aspergillosis has not been evaluated in comparator-controlled clinical studies.

14.5 Pediatric Patients

The safety and efficacy of CANCIDAS were evaluated in pediatric patients 3 months to 17 years of age in two prospective, multicenter clinical trials.

The first study, which enrolled 82 patients between 2 to 17 years of age, was a randomized, double-blind study comparing CANCIDAS (50 mg/m² IV once daily following a 70-mg/m² loading dose on Day 1 [not to exceed 70 mg daily]) to AmBisome (3 mg/kg IV daily) in a 2:1 treatment fashion (56 on caspofungin, 26 on AmBisome) as empirical therapy in pediatric patients with persistent fever and neutropenia. The study design and criteria for efficacy assessment were similar to the study in adult patients *[see Clinical Studies (14.1)]*. Patients were stratified based on risk category (high-risk patients had undergone allogeneic stem cell transplantation or had relapsed acute leukemia). Twenty-seven percent of patients in both treatment groups were high risk. Favorable overall response rates of pediatric patients with persistent fever and neutropenia are presented in Table 17.

Table 17: Favorable Overall Response Rates of Pediatric Patients with Persistent Fever and Neutropenia

	CANCIDAS	AmBisome*
Number of Patients	56	25
Overall Favorable Response	26/56 (46.4%)	8/25 (32.0%)
High risk	9/15 (60.0%)	0/7 (0.0%)
Low risk	17/41 (41.5%)	8/18 (44.4%)

* One patient excluded from analysis due to no fever at study entry.

The second study was a prospective, open-label, noncomparative study estimating the safety and efficacy of caspofungin in pediatric patients (ages 3 months to 17 years) with candidemia and other *Candida* infections, esophageal candidiasis, and invasive aspergillosis (as salvage therapy). The study employed diagnostic criteria which were based on established EORTC/MSG criteria of proven or probable infection; these criteria were similar to those criteria employed in the adult studies for these various indications. Similarly, the efficacy time points and endpoints used in this study were similar to those employed in the corresponding adult studies *[see Clinical Studies (14.2,14.3, and 14.4)]*. All patients received CANCIDAS at 50 mg/m² IV once daily following a 70-mg/m² loading dose on Day 1 (not to exceed 70 mg daily). Among the 49 enrolled

patients who received CANCIDAS, 48 were included in the efficacy analysis (one patient excluded due to not having a baseline *Aspergillus* or *Candida* infection). Of these 48 patients, 37 had candidemia or other *Candida* infections, 10 had invasive aspergillosis, and 1 patient had esophageal candidiasis. Most candidemia and other *Candida* infections were caused by *C. albicans* (35%), followed by *C. parapsilosis* (22%), *C. tropicalis* (14%), and *C. glabrata* (11%). The favorable response rate, by indication, at the end of caspofungin therapy was as follows: 30/37 (81%) in candidemia or other *Candida* infections, 5/10 (50%) in invasive aspergillosis, and 1/1 in esophageal candidiasis.

15 REFERENCES

1. Mosteller RD: Simplified Calculation of Body Surface Area. N Engl J Med 1987 Oct 22;317(17): 1098 (letter).
2. Clinical and Laboratory Standards Institute (CLSI). *Reference Method for Broth Dilution Antifungal Susceptibility Testing of Yeasts; Approved Standard-Third Edition.* CLSI document M27-A3. Clinical and Laboratory Standards Institute, 940 West Valley Road, Suite 1400, Wayne, Pennsylvania 19087, USA, 2008.
3. Clinical and Laboratory Standards Institute (CLSI). *Reference Method for Broth Dilution Antifungal Susceptibility Testing of Yeasts; Third Informational Supplement.* CLSI document M27-S3. Clinical and Laboratory Standards Institute, 940 West Valley Road, Suite 1400, Wayne, Pennsylvania 19087, USA, 2008.
4. Denning DW, Lee JY, Hostetler JS, et al. NIAID Mycoses Study Group multicenter trial of oral itraconazole therapy for invasive aspergillosis. Am J Med 1994; 97:135-144.

16 HOW SUPPLIED/STORAGE AND HANDLING

How Supplied

CANCIDAS 50 mg is a white to off-white powder/cake for infusion in a vial with a red aluminum band and a plastic cap.

NDC 0006-3822-10 supplied as one single-use vial.

CANCIDAS 70 mg is a white to off-white powder/cake for infusion in a vial with a yellow/orange aluminum band and a plastic cap.

NDC 0006-3823-10 supplied as one single-use vial.

Storage and Handling

Vials

The lyophilized vials should be stored refrigerated at 2° to 8°C (36° to 46°F).

Reconstituted Concentrate

Reconstituted CANCIDAS in the vial may be stored at ≤25°C (≤77°F) for one hour prior to the preparation of the patient infusion solution.

Diluted Product

The final patient infusion solution in the IV bag or bottle can be stored at ≤25°C (≤77°F) for 24 hours or at 2 to 8°C (36 to 46°F) for 48 hours.

17 PATIENT COUNSELING INFORMATION

17.1 Hypersensitivity

Inform patients that anaphylactic reactions have been reported during administration of CANCIDAS. CANCIDAS can cause hypersensitivity reactions, including rash, facial swelling, angioedema, pruritus, sensation of warmth, or bronchospasm. Inform patients to report these signs or symptoms to their healthcare providers.

17.2 Hepatic Effects

Inform patients that there have been isolated reports of serious hepatic effects from CANCIDAS therapy. Physicians will assess the risk/benefit of continuing CANCIDAS therapy if abnormal liver function tests occur during treatment.

Distributed by: Merck Sharp & Dohme Corp., a subsidiary of **MERCK & CO., INC.**, Whitehouse Station, NJ 08889, USA

The trademarks depicted herein are owned by their respective companies.

Copyright © 2001, 2009 Merck Sharp & Dohme Corp., a subsidiary of **Merck & Co., Inc.**

All rights reserved.

Revised: 08/2013

uspi-mk0991-i-1308r003

Shown in Product Identification Guide, page 308

CELESTONE® SOLUSPAN®[1] ℞

brand of betamethasone sodium phosphate and betamethasone acetate

Injectable Suspension USP

6 mg per mL

DESCRIPTION

CELESTONE® SOLUSPAN®[1] Injectable Suspension is a sterile aqueous suspension containing 3 mg per milliliter betamethasone, as betamethasone sodium phosphate, and 3 mg per milliliter betamethasone acetate. Inactive ingredients per mL: 7.1 mg dibasic sodium phosphate; 3.4 mg monobasic sodium phosphate; 0.1 mg edetate disodium; and 0.2 mg benzalkonium chloride as preservative. The pH is adjusted to between 6.8 and 7.2.

The formula for betamethasone sodium phosphate is $C_{22}H_{28}FNa_2O_8P$ and it has a molecular weight of 516.40. Chemically, it is 9-Fluoro-11β,17,21-trihydroxy-16β-methylpregna-1,4-diene-3,20-dione 21-(disodium phosphate).

The formula for betamethasone acetate is $C_{24}H_{31}FO_6$ and it has a molecular weight of 434.50. Chemically, it is 9-Fluoro-11β,17,21-trihydroxy-16β-methylpregna-1,4-diene-3,20-dione 21-acetate.

The chemical structures for betamethasone sodium phosphate and betamethasone acetate are as follows:

betamethasone sodium phosphate

betamethasone acetate

Betamethasone sodium phosphate is a white to practically white, odorless powder, and is hygroscopic. It is freely soluble in water and in methanol, but is practically insoluble in acetone and in chloroform.

Betamethasone acetate is a white to creamy white, odorless powder that sinters and resolidifies at about 165°C, and remelts at about 200°C-220°C with decomposition. It is practically insoluble in water, but freely soluble in acetone, and is soluble in alcohol and in chloroform.

[1] brand of rapid and repository injectable

CLINICAL PHARMACOLOGY

Glucocorticoids, naturally occurring and synthetic, are adrenocortical steroids that are readily absorbed from the gastrointestinal tract.

Naturally occurring glucocorticoids (hydrocortisone and cortisone), which also have salt-retaining properties, are used as replacement therapy in adrenocortical deficiency states. Their synthetic analogs are primarily used for their anti-inflammatory effects in disorders of many organ systems. A derivative of prednisolone, betamethasone has a 16β-methyl group that enhances the anti-inflammatory action of the molecule and reduces the sodium- and water-retaining properties of the fluorine atom bound at carbon 9.

Betamethasone sodium phosphate, a soluble ester, provides prompt activity, while betamethasone acetate is only slightly soluble and affords sustained activity.

INDICATIONS AND USAGE

When oral therapy is not feasible, the **intramuscular use** of CELESTONE® SOLUSPAN®[1] Injectable Suspension is indicated as follows:

Allergic States
Control of severe or incapacitating allergic conditions intractable to adequate trials of conventional treatment in asthma, atopic dermatitis, contact dermatitis, drug hypersensitivity reactions, perennial or seasonal allergic rhinitis, serum sickness, transfusion reactions.

Dermatologic Diseases
Bullous dermatitis herpetiformis, exfoliative erythroderma, mycosis fungoides, pemphigus, severe erythema multiforme (Stevens-Johnson syndrome).

Endocrine Disorders
Congenital adrenal hyperplasia, hypercalcemia associated with cancer, nonsuppurative thyroiditis.
Hydrocortisone or cortisone is the drug of choice in primary or secondary adrenocortical insufficiency. Synthetic analogs may be used in conjunction with mineralocorticoids where applicable; in infancy mineralocorticoid supplementation is of particular importance.

Gastrointestinal Diseases
To tide the patient over a critical period of the disease in regional enteritis and ulcerative colitis.

Hematologic Disorders
Acquired (autoimmune) hemolytic anemia, Diamond-Blackfan anemia, pure red cell aplasia, selected cases of secondary thrombocytopenia.

Miscellaneous
Trichinosis with neurologic or myocardial involvement, tuberculous meningitis with subarachnoid block or impending block when used with appropriate antituberculous chemotherapy.

Neoplastic Diseases
For palliative management of leukemias and lymphomas.

Nervous System
Acute exacerbations of multiple sclerosis; cerebral edema associated with primary or metastatic brain tumor or craniotomy.

Ophthalmic Diseases
Sympathetic ophthalmia, temporal arteritis, uveitis and ocular inflammatory conditions unresponsive to topical corticosteroids.

Renal Diseases
To induce diuresis or remission of proteinuria in idiopathic nephrotic syndrome or that due to lupus erythematosus.

Respiratory Diseases
Berylliosis, fulminating or disseminated pulmonary tuberculosis when used concurrently with appropriate antituberculous chemotherapy, idiopathic eosinophilic pneumonias, symptomatic sarcoidosis.

Rheumatic Disorders As adjunctive therapy for short-term administration (to tide the patient over an acute episode or exacerbation) in acute gouty arthritis; acute rheumatic carditis; ankylosing spondylitis; psoriatic arthritis; rheumatoid arthritis, including juvenile rheumatoid arthritis (selected cases may require low-dose maintenance therapy). For the treatment of dermatomyositis, polymyositis, and systemic lupus erythematosus.

The **intra-articular or soft tissue administration** of CELESTONE SOLUSPAN Injectable Suspension is indicated as adjunctive therapy for short-term administration (to tide the patient over an acute episode or exacerbation) in acute gouty arthritis, acute and subacute bursitis, acute nonspecific tenosynovitis, epicondylitis, rheumatoid arthritis, synovitis of osteoarthritis.

The **intralesional administration** of CELESTONE SOLUSPAN Injectable Suspension is indicated for alopecia areata; discoid lupus erythematosus; keloids; localized hypertrophic, infiltrated, inflammatory lesions of granuloma annulare, lichen planus, lichen simplex chronicus (neurodermatitis), and psoriatic plaques; necrobiosis lipoidica diabeticorum.

CELESTONE SOLUSPAN Injectable Suspension may also be useful in cystic tumors of an aponeurosis or tendon (ganglia).

CONTRAINDICATIONS

CELESTONE® SOLUSPAN®[1] Injectable Suspension is contraindicated in patients who are hypersensitive to any components of this product.
Intramuscular corticosteroid preparations are contraindicated for idiopathic thrombocytopenic purpura.

WARNINGS

CELESTONE® SOLUSPAN®[1] Injectable Suspension should not be administered intravenously.

Serious Neurologic Adverse Reactions with Epidural Administration
Serious neurologic events, some resulting in death, have been reported with epidural injection of corticosteroids. Specific events reported include, but are not limited to, spinal cord infarction, paraplegia, quadriplegia, cortical blindness, and stroke. These serious neurologic events have been reported with and without use of fluoroscopy. The safety and effectiveness of epidural administration of corticosteroids have not been established, and corticosteroids are not approved for this use.

General
Rare instances of anaphylactoid reactions have occurred in patients receiving corticosteroid therapy (see **ADVERSE REACTIONS**).
In patients on corticosteroid therapy subjected to any unusual stress, hydrocortisone or cortisone is the drug of choice as a supplement during and after the event.

Cardio-renal
Average and large doses of corticosteroids can cause elevation of blood pressure, salt and water retention, and increased excretion of potassium. These effects are less likely to occur with the synthetic derivatives except when used in large doses. Dietary salt restriction and potassium supplementation may be necessary. All corticosteroids increase calcium excretion.
Literature reports suggest an apparent association between use of corticosteroids and left ventricular free wall rupture after a recent myocardial infarction; therefore, therapy with corticosteroids should be used with great caution in these patients.

Endocrine
Corticosteroids can produce reversible hypothalamic pituitary adrenal (HPA) axis suppression with the potential for glucocorticosteroid insufficiency after withdrawal of treatment.

Metabolic clearance of corticosteroids is decreased in hypothyroid patients and increased in hyperthyroid patients. Changes in thyroid status of the patient may necessitate adjustment in dosage.

Infections
General
Patients who are on corticosteroids are more susceptible to infections than are healthy individuals. There may be decreased resistance and inability to localize infection when corticosteroids are used. Infection with any pathogen (viral, bacterial, fungal, protozoan, or helminthic) in any location of the body may be associated with the use of corticosteroids alone or in combination with other immunosuppressive agents. These infections may be mild to severe. With increasing doses of corticosteroids, the rate of occurrence of infectious complications increases. Corticosteroids may also mask some signs of current infection.

Fungal Infections
Corticosteroids may exacerbate systemic fungal infections and therefore should not be used in the presence of such infections unless they are needed to control drug reactions. There have been cases reported in which concomitant use of amphotericin B and hydrocortisone was followed by cardiac enlargement and congestive heart failure (see **PRECAUTIONS, Drug Interactions, Amphotericin B Injection and Potassium-Depleting Agents** section).

Special Pathogens
Latent disease may be activated or there may be an exacerbation of intercurrent infections due to pathogens, including those caused by *Amoeba, Candida, Cryptococcus, Mycobacterium, Nocardia, Pneumocystis,* and *Toxoplasma.*
It is recommended that latent amebiasis or active amebiasis be ruled out before initiating corticosteroid therapy in any patient who has spent time in the tropics or in any patient with unexplained diarrhea.
Similarly, corticosteroids should be used with great care in patients with known or suspected Strongyloides (threadworm) infestation. In such patients, corticosteroid-induced immunosuppression may lead to Strongyloides hyperinfection and dissemination with widespread larval migration, often accompanied by severe enterocolitis and potentially fatal gram-negative septicemia.
Corticosteroids should not be used in cerebral malaria.

Tuberculosis
The use of corticosteroids in active tuberculosis should be restricted to those cases of fulminating or disseminated tuberculosis in which the corticosteroid is used for the management of the disease in conjunction with an appropriate antituberculous regimen.
If corticosteroids are indicated in patients with latent tuberculosis or tuberculin reactivity, close observation is necessary as reactivation of the disease may occur. During prolonged corticosteroid therapy, these patients should receive chemoprophylaxis.

Vaccination
Administration of live or live, attenuated vaccines is contraindicated in patients receiving immunosuppressive doses of corticosteroids. Killed or inactivated vaccines may be administered. However, the response to such vaccines cannot be predicted. Immunization procedures may be undertaken in patients who are receiving corticosteroids as replacement therapy, eg, for Addison's disease.

Viral Infections
Chickenpox and measles can have a more serious or even fatal course in pediatric and adult patients on corticosteroids. In pediatric and adult patients who have not had these diseases, particular care should be taken to avoid exposure. The contribution of the underlying disease and/or prior corticosteroid treatment to the risk is also not known. If exposed to chickenpox, prophylaxis with varicella zoster immune globulin (VZIG) may be indicated. If exposed to measles, prophylaxis with immunoglobulin (IG) may be indicated. (See the respective package inserts for complete VZIG and IG prescribing information.) If chickenpox develops, treatment with antiviral agents should be considered.

Neurologic
Reports of severe medical events have been associated with the intrathecal route of administration (see **ADVERSE REACTIONS, Gastrointestinal** and **Neurologic/Psychiatric** sections).
Results from one multicenter, randomized, placebo-controlled study with methylprednisolone hemisuccinate, an IV corticosteroid, showed an increase in early mortality (at 2 weeks) and late mortality (at 6 months) in patients with cranial trauma who were determined not to have other clear indications for corticosteroid treatment. High doses of corticosteroids, including CELESTONE SOLUSPAN, should not be used for the treatment of traumatic brain injury.

Ophthalmic
Use of corticosteroids may produce posterior subcapsular cataracts, glaucoma with possible damage to the optic nerves, and may enhance the establishment of secondary ocular infections due to bacteria, fungi, or viruses. The use

of oral corticosteroids is not recommended in the treatment of optic neuritis and may lead to an increase in the risk of new episodes. Corticosteroids should not be used in active ocular herpes simplex.

PRECAUTIONS
General
This product, like many other steroid formulations, is sensitive to heat. Therefore, it should not be autoclaved when it is desirable to sterilize the exterior of the vial.
The lowest possible dose of corticosteroid should be used to control the condition under treatment. When reduction in dosage is possible, the reduction should be gradual.
Since complications of treatment with glucocorticoids are dependent on the size of the dose and the duration of treatment, a risk/benefit decision must be made in each individual case as to dose and duration of treatment and as to whether daily or intermittent therapy should be used.
Kaposi's sarcoma has been reported to occur in patients receiving corticosteroid therapy, most often for chronic conditions. Discontinuation of corticosteroids may result in clinical improvement.

Cardio-renal
As sodium retention with resultant edema and potassium loss may occur in patients receiving corticosteroids, these agents should be used with caution in patients with congestive heart failure, hypertension, or renal insufficiency.

Endocrine
Drug-induced secondary adrenocortical insufficiency may be minimized by gradual reduction of dosage. This type of relative insufficiency may persist for months after discontinuation of therapy. Therefore, in any situation of stress occurring during that period, naturally occurring glucocorticoids (hydrocortisone cortisone), which also have salt-retaining properties, rather than betamethasone, are the appropriate choices as replacement therapy in adrenocortical deficiency states.

Gastrointestinal
Steroids should be used with caution in active or latent peptic ulcers, diverticulitis, fresh intestinal anastomoses, and nonspecific ulcerative colitis, since they may increase the risk of a perforation.
Signs of peritoneal irritation following gastrointestinal perforation in patients receiving corticosteroids may be minimal or absent.
There is an enhanced effect of corticosteroids in patients with cirrhosis.

Intra-Articular and Soft Tissue Administration
Intra-articular injected corticosteroids may be systemically absorbed.
Appropriate examination of any joint fluid present is necessary to exclude a septic process.
A marked increase in pain accompanied by local swelling, further restriction of joint motion, fever, and malaise are suggestive of septic arthritis. If this complication occurs and the diagnosis of sepsis is confirmed, appropriate antimicrobial therapy should be instituted.
Injection of a steroid into an infected site is to be avoided.
Local injection of a steroid into a previously injected joint is not usually recommended.
Corticosteroid injection into unstable joints is generally not recommended.
Intra-articular injection may result in damage to joint tissues (see ADVERSE REACTIONS, Musculoskeletal section).

Musculoskeletal
Corticosteroids decrease bone formation and increase bone resorption both through their effect on calcium regulation (ie, decreasing absorption and increasing excretion) and inhibition of osteoblast function. This, together with a decrease in the protein matrix of the bone secondary to an increase in protein catabolism, and reduced sex hormone production, may lead to inhibition of bone growth in pediatric patients and the development of osteoporosis at any age. Special consideration should be given to patients at increased risk of osteoporosis (ie, postmenopausal women) before initiating corticosteroid therapy.

Neuro-psychiatric
Although controlled clinical trials have shown corticosteroids to be effective in speeding the resolution of acute exacerbations of multiple sclerosis, they do not show that they affect the ultimate outcome or natural history of the disease. The studies do show that relatively high doses of corticosteroids are necessary to demonstrate a significant effect (see DOSAGE AND ADMINISTRATION).
An acute myopathy has been observed with the use of high doses of corticosteroids, most often occurring in patients with disorders of neuromuscular transmission (eg, myasthenia gravis), or in patients receiving concomitant therapy with neuromuscular blocking drugs (eg, pancuronium). This acute myopathy is generalized, may involve ocular and respiratory muscles, and may result in quadriparesis. Elevation of creatinine kinase may occur. Clinical improvement or recovery after stopping corticosteroids may require weeks to years.

Psychic derangements may appear when corticosteroids are used, ranging from euphoria, insomnia, mood swings, personality changes, and severe depression to frank psychotic manifestations. Also, existing emotional instability or psychotic tendencies may be aggravated by corticosteroids.

Ophthalmic
Intraocular pressure may become elevated in some individuals. If steroid therapy is continued for more than 6 weeks, intraocular pressure should be monitored.

Information for Patients
Patients should be warned not to discontinue the use of corticosteroids abruptly or without medical supervision, to advise any medical attendants that they are taking corticosteroids and to seek medical advice at once should they develop fever or other signs of infection.
Persons who are on corticosteroids should be warned to avoid exposure to chickenpox or measles. Patients should also be advised that if they are exposed, medical advice should be sought without delay.

Drug Interactions
Aminoglutethimide
Aminoglutethimide may lead to a loss of corticosteroid-induced adrenal suppression.
Amphotericin B Injection and Potassium-Depleting Agents
When corticosteroids are administered concomitantly with potassium-depleting agents (ie, amphotericin B, diuretics), patients should be observed closely for development of hypokalemia. There have been cases reported in which concomitant use of amphotericin B and hydrocortisone was followed by cardiac enlargement and congestive heart failure.
Antibiotics
Macrolide antibiotics have been reported to cause a significant decrease in corticosteroid clearance.
Anticholinesterases
Concomitant use of anticholinesterase agents and corticosteroids may produce severe weakness in patients with myasthenia gravis. If possible, anticholinesterase agents should be withdrawn at least 24 hours before initiating corticosteroid therapy.
Anticoagulants, Oral
Coadministration of corticosteroids and warfarin usually results in inhibition of response to warfarin, although there have been some conflicting reports. Therefore, coagulation indices should be monitored frequently to maintain the desired anticoagulant effect.
Antidiabetics
Because corticosteroids may increase blood glucose concentrations, dosage adjustments of antidiabetic agents may be required.
Antitubercular Drugs
Serum concentrations of isoniazid may be decreased.
Cholestyramine
Cholestyramine may increase the clearance of corticosteroids.
Cyclosporine
Increased activity of both cyclosporine and corticosteroids may occur when the two are used concurrently. Convulsions have been reported with this concurrent use.
Digitalis Glycosides
Patients on digitalis glycosides may be at increased risk of arrhythmias due to hypokalemia.
Estrogens, Including Oral Contraceptives
Estrogens may decrease the hepatic metabolism of certain corticosteroids, thereby increasing their effect.
Hepatic Enzyme Inducers (eg, barbiturates, phenytoin, carbamazepine, rifampin)
Drugs which induce hepatic microsomal drug-metabolizing enzyme activity may enhance the metabolism of corticosteroids and require that the dosage of the corticosteroid be increased.
Ketoconazole
Ketoconazole has been reported to decrease the metabolism of certain corticosteroids by up to 60%, leading to an increased risk of corticosteroid side effects.
Nonsteroidal Anti-inflammatory Agents (NSAIDS)
Concomitant use of aspirin (or other nonsteroidal anti-inflammatory agents) and corticosteroids increases the risk of gastrointestinal side effects. Aspirin should be used cautiously in conjunction with corticosteroids in hypoprothrombinemia. The clearance of salicylates may be increased with concurrent use of corticosteroids.

Skin Tests
Corticosteroids may suppress reactions to skin tests.

Vaccines
Patients on prolonged corticosteroid therapy may exhibit a diminished response to toxoids and live or inactivated vaccines due to inhibition of antibody response. Corticosteroids may also potentiate the replication of some organisms contained in live attenuated vaccines. Route administration of vaccines or toxoids should be deferred until corticosteroid therapy is discontinued if possible (see WARNINGS, Infections, Vaccination section).

Carcinogenesis, Mutagenesis, Impairment of Fertility
No adequate studies have been conducted in animals to determine whether corticosteroids have a potential for carcinogenesis or mutagenesis.
Steroids may increase or decrease motility and number of spermatozoa in some patients.

Pregnancy
Teratogenic Effects
Pregnancy Category C
Corticosteroids have been shown to be teratogenic in many species when given in doses equivalent to the human dose. Animal studies in which corticosteroids have been given to pregnant mice, rats, and rabbits have yielded an increased incidence of cleft palate in the offspring. There are no adequate and well-controlled studies in pregnant women. Corticosteroids should be used during pregnancy only if the potential benefit justifies the potential risk to the fetus. Infants born to mothers who have received corticosteroids during pregnancy should be carefully observed for signs of hypoadrenalism.

Nursing Mothers
Systemically administered corticosteroids appear in human milk and could suppress growth, interfere with endogenous corticosteroid production, or cause other untoward effects. Caution should be exercised when corticosteroids are administered to a nursing woman.

Pediatric Use
The efficacy and safety of corticosteroids in the pediatric population are based on the well-established course of effect of corticosteroids, which is similar in pediatric and adult populations. Published studies provide evidence of efficacy and safety in pediatric patients for the treatment of nephrotic syndrome (>2 years of age), and aggressive lymphomas and leukemias (>1 month of age). Other indications for pediatric use of corticosteroids, eg, severe asthma and wheezing, are based on adequate and well-controlled trials conducted in adults, on the premises that the course of the diseases and their pathophysiology are considered to be substantially similar in both populations.
The adverse effects of corticosteroids in pediatric patients are similar to those in adults (see ADVERSE REACTIONS). Like adults, pediatric patients should be carefully observed with frequent measurements of blood pressure, weight, height, intraocular pressure, and clinical evaluation for the presence of infection, psychosocial disturbances, thromboembolism, peptic ulcers, cataracts, and osteoporosis. Pediatric patients who are treated with corticosteroids by any route, including systemically administered corticosteroids, may experience a decrease in their growth velocity. This negative impact of corticosteroids on growth has been observed at low systemic doses and in the absence of laboratory evidence of HPA axis suppression (ie, cosyntropin stimulation and basal cortisol plasma levels). Growth velocity may therefore be a more sensitive indicator of systemic corticosteroid exposure in pediatric patients than some commonly used tests of HPA axis function. The linear growth of pediatric patients treated with corticosteroids should be monitored, and the potential growth effects of prolonged treatment should be weighed against clinical benefits obtained and the availability of treatment alternatives. In order to minimize the potential growth effects of corticosteroids, pediatric patients should be titrated to the lowest effective dose.

Geriatric Use
No overall differences in safety or effectiveness were observed between elderly subjects and younger subjects, and other reported clinical experience has not identified differences in responses between the elderly and young patients, but greater sensitivity of some older individuals cannot be ruled out.

ADVERSE REACTIONS (listed alphabetically, under each subsection)
Allergic Reactions
Anaphylactoid reaction, anaphylaxis, angioedema.
Cardiovascular
Bradycardia, cardiac arrest, cardiac arrhythmias, cardiac enlargement, circulatory collapse, congestive heart failure, fat embolism, hypertension, hypertrophic cardiomyopathy in premature infants, myocardial rupture following recent myocardial infarction (see WARNINGS), pulmonary edema, syncope, tachycardia, thromboembolism, thrombophlebitis, vasculitis.
Dermatologic
Acne, allergic dermatitis, cutaneous and subcutaneous atrophy, dry scaly skin, ecchymoses and petechiae, edema, erythema, hyperpigmentation, hypopigmentation, impaired wound healing, increased sweating, rash, sterile abscess, striae, suppressed reactions to skin tests, thin fragile skin, thinning scalp hair, urticaria.

Endocrine

Decreased carbohydrate and glucose tolerance, development of cushingoid state, glucosuria, hirsutism, hypertrichosis, increased requirements for insulin or oral hypoglycemic adrenocortical and pituitary unresponsiveness (particularly in times of stress, as in trauma, surgery, or illness), suppression of growth in pediatric patients.

Fluid and Electrolyte Disturbances

Congestive heart failure in susceptible patients, fluid retention, hypokalemic alkalosis, potassium loss, sodium retention.

Gastrointestinal

Abdominal distention, bowel/bladder dysfunction (after intrathecal administration), elevation in serum liver enzyme levels (usually reversible upon discontinuation), hepatomegaly, increased appetite, nausea, pancreatitis, peptic ulcer with possible perforation and hemorrhage, perforation of the small and large intestine (particularly in patients with inflammatory bowel disease), ulcerative esophagitis.

Metabolic

Negative nitrogen balance due to protein catabolism.

Musculoskeletal

Aseptic necrosis of femoral and humeral heads, calcinosis (following intra-articular or intralesional use), Charcot-like arthropathy, loss of muscle mass, muscle weakness, osteoporosis, pathologic fracture of long bones, postinjection flare (following intra-articular use), steroid myopathy, tendon rupture, vertebral compression fractures.

Neurologic/Psychiatric

Convulsions, depression, emotional instability, euphoria, headache, increased intracranial pressure with papilledema (pseudotumor cerebri) usually following discontinuation of treatment, insomnia, mood swings, neuritis, neuropathy, paresthesia, personality changes, psychic disorders, vertigo. Arachnoiditis, meningitis, paraparesis/paraplegia, and sensory disturbances have occurred after intrathecal administration (see **WARNINGS, Neurologic** section).

Ophthalmic

Exophthalmos, glaucoma, increased intraocular pressure, posterior subcapsular cataracts, rare instances of blindness associated with periocular injections.

Other

Abnormal fat deposits, decreased resistance to infection, hiccups, increased or decreased motility and number of spermatozoa, malaise, moon face, weight gain.

OVERDOSAGE

Treatment of acute overdose is by supportive and symptomatic therapy. For chronic overdosage in the face of severe disease requiring continuous steroid therapy, the dosage of the corticosteroid may be reduced only temporarily, or alternate day treatment may be introduced.

DOSAGE AND ADMINISTRATION

Benzyl alcohol as a preservative has been associated with a fatal "Gasping Syndrome" in premature infants and infants of low birth weight. Solutions used for further dilution of this product should be preservative-free when used in the neonate, especially the premature infant. The initial dosage of parenterally administered CELESTONE® SOLUSPAN®[1] Injectable Suspension may vary from 0.25 to 9.0 mg per day depending on the specific disease entity being treated. However, in certain overwhelming, acute, life-threatening situations, administrations in dosages exceeding the usual dosages may be justified and may be in multiples of the oral dosages.

It Should Be Emphasized That Dosage Requirements Are Variable and Must Be Individualized on the Basis of the Disease Under Treatment and the Response of the Patient. After a favorable response is noted, the proper maintenance dosage should be determined by decreasing the initial drug dosage in small decrements at appropriate time intervals until the lowest dosage which will maintain an adequate clinical response is reached. Situations which may make dosage adjustments necessary are changes in clinical status secondary to remissions or exacerbations in the disease process, the patient's individual drug responsiveness, and the effect of patient exposure to stressful situations not directly related to the disease entity under treatment. In this latter situation it may be necessary to increase the dosage of the corticosteroid for a period of time consistent with the patient's condition. If after long-term therapy the drug is to be stopped, it is recommended that it be withdrawn gradually rather than abruptly.

In the treatment of acute exacerbations of multiple sclerosis, daily doses of 30 mg of betamethasone for a week followed by 12 mg every other day for 1 month are recommended (see **PRECAUTIONS, Neuro-psychiatric** section). In pediatric patients, the initial dose of betamethasone may vary depending on the specific disease entity being treated. The range of initial doses is 0.02 to 0.3 mg/kg/day in three or four divided doses (0.6 to 9 mg/m² bsa/day).

For the purpose of comparison, the following is the equivalent milligram dosage of the various glucocorticoids:

Cortisone, 25	Triamcinolone, 4
Hydrocortisone, 20	Paramethasone, 2
Prednisolone, 5	Betamethasone, 0.75
Prednisone, 5	Dexamethasone, 0.75
Methylprednisolone, 4	

These dose relationships apply only to oral or intravenous administration of these compounds. When these substances or their derivatives are injected intramuscularly or into joint spaces, their relative properties may be greatly altered.

If coadministration of a local anesthetic is desired, CELESTONE SOLUSPAN Injectable Suspension may be mixed with 1% or 2% lidocaine hydrochloride, using the formulations which do not contain parabens. Similar local anesthetics may also be used. Diluents containing methylparaben, propylparaben, phenol, etc., should be avoided, since these compounds may cause flocculation of the steroid. The required dose of CELESTONE SOLUSPAN Injectable Suspension is first withdrawn from the vial into the syringe. The local anesthetic is then drawn in, and the syringe shaken briefly. **Do not inject local anesthetics into the vial of CELESTONE SOLUSPAN Injectable Suspension.**

Bursitis, Tenosynovitis, Peritendinitis

In acute subdeltoid, subacromial, olecranon, and prepatellar bursitis, one intrabursal injection of 1.0 mL CELESTONE SOLUSPAN Injectable Suspension can relieve pain and restore full range of movement. Several intrabursal injections of corticosteroids are usually required in recurrent acute bursitis and in acute exacerbations of chronic bursitis. Partial relief of pain and some increase in mobility can be expected in both conditions after one or two injections. Chronic bursitis may be treated with reduced dosage once the acute condition is controlled. In tenosynovitis and tendinitis, three or four local injections at intervals of 1 to 2 weeks between injections are given in most cases. Injections should be made into the affected tendon sheaths rather than into the tendons themselves. In ganglions of joint capsules and tendon sheaths, injection of 0.5 mL directly into the ganglion cysts has produced marked reduction in the size of the lesions.

Rheumatoid Arthritis and Osteoarthritis

Following intra-articular administration of 0.5 to 2.0 mL of CELESTONE SOLUSPAN Injectable Suspension, relief of pain, soreness, and stiffness may be experienced. Duration of relief varies widely in both diseases. Intra-articular Injection of CELESTONE SOLUSPAN Injectable Suspension is well tolerated in joints and periarticular tissues. There is virtually no pain on injection, and the "secondary flare" that sometimes occurs a few hours after intra-articular injection of corticosteroids has not been reported with CELESTONE SOLUSPAN Injectable Suspension. Using sterile technique, a 20- to 24-gauge needle on an empty syringe is inserted into the synovial cavity and a few drops of synovial fluid are withdrawn to confirm that the needle is in the joint. The aspirating syringe is replaced by a syringe containing CELESTONE SOLUSPAN Injectable Suspension and injection is then made into the joint.

Recommended Doses for Intra-articular Injection

Size of joint	Location	Dose (mL)
Very large	Hip	1.0-2.0
Large	Knee, ankle, shoulder	1.0
Medium	Elbow, wrist	0.5-1.0
Small (metacarpophalangeal, interphalangeal) (sternoclavicular)	Hand, chest	0.25-0.5

A portion of the administered dose of CELESTONE SOLUSPAN Injectable Suspension is absorbed systemically following intra-articular injection. In patients being treated concomitantly with oral or parenteral corticosteroids, especially those receiving large doses, the systemic absorption of the drug should be considered in determining intra-articular dosage.

Dermatologic Conditions

In intralesional treatment, 0.2 mL/cm² of CELESTONE SOLUSPAN Injectable Suspension is injected intradermally (not subcutaneously) using a tuberculin syringe with a 25-gauge, ½-inch needle. Care should be taken to deposit a uniform depot of medication intradermally. A total of no more than 1.0 mL at weekly intervals is recommended.

Disorders of the Foot

A tuberculin syringe with a 25-gauge, ¾-inch needle is suitable for most injections into the foot. The following doses are recommended at intervals of 3 days to a week.

Diagnosis	CELESTONE SOLUSPAN Injectable Suspension Dose (mL)
Bursitis under heloma durum or heloma molle	0.25-0.5
under calcaneal spur	0.5
over hallux rigidus or digiti quinti varus	0.5
Tenosynovitis, periostitis of cuboid	0.5
Acute gouty arthritis	0.5-1.0

HOW SUPPLIED

CELESTONE® SOLUSPAN®[1] Injectable Suspension, 5-mL multiple-dose vial; box of one (NDC 0085-0566-05). **SHAKE WELL BEFORE USING.**
Store at 25°C (77°F); excursions permitted to 15°-30°C (59°-86°F) [see USP Controlled Room Temperature].
Protect from light.
Rx only
Manufactured for: Merck Sharp & Dohme Corp., a subsidiary of **MERCK & CO., INC.**, Whitehouse Station, NJ 08889, USA
Manufactured by: Patheon UK Limited, Covingham, Swindon, Wiltshire, SN3 5BZ, United Kingdom
For patent information: www.merck.com/product/patent/home.html
Copyright © 1969, 2012 Merck Sharp & Dohme Corp., a subsidiary of **Merck & Co., Inc.**
All rights reserved.
Revised: 05/2014
uspi-mk5166a-soi-1405r006

CLARINEX®

[klă-rĭ-nĕcks]
(desloratadine)
Tablets, RediTabs®, and Oral Solution for oral use

℞

HIGHLIGHTS OF PRESCRIBING INFORMATION

These highlights do not include all the information needed to use CLARINEX safely and effectively. See full prescribing information for CLARINEX.
CLARINEX® (desloratadine) Tablets, RediTabs®, and Oral Solution for oral use
Initial U.S. Approval: 2001

——INDICATIONS AND USAGE——

CLARINEX is an H₁-receptor antagonist indicated for:
- **Seasonal Allergic Rhinitis:** relief of nasal and non-nasal symptoms in patients 2 years of age and older. (1.1)
- **Perennial Allergic Rhinitis:** relief of nasal and non-nasal symptoms in patients 6 months of age and older. (1.2)
- **Chronic Idiopathic Urticaria:** symptomatic relief of pruritus, reduction in the number of hives, and size of hives in patients 6 months of age and older. (1.3)

——DOSAGE AND ADMINISTRATION——

Dosage (by age):
Adults and Adolescents 12 Years of Age and Over:
- CLARINEX Tablets - one 5 mg tablet once daily **or**
- CLARINEX RediTabs Tablets - one 5 mg tablet once daily **or**
- CLARINEX Oral Solution - 2 teaspoonfuls (5 mg in 10 mL) once daily (2)

Children 6 to 11 Years of Age:
- CLARINEX Oral Solution - 1 teaspoonful (2.5 mg in 5 mL) once daily **or**
- CLARINEX RediTabs Tablets - one 2.5 mg tablet once daily (2)

Children 12 Months to 5 Years of Age:
- CLARINEX Oral Solution - 1/2 teaspoonful (1.25 mg in 2.5 mL) once daily (2)

Children 6 to 11 Months of Age:
- CLARINEX Oral Solution - 2 mL (1 mg) once daily (2)

DOSAGE FORMS AND STRENGTHS

- CLARINEX Tablets - 5 mg (3)
- CLARINEX Oral Solution - 0.5 mg/1 mL (3)

CONTRAINDICATIONS

- Hypersensitivity (4, 6.2)

WARNINGS AND PRECAUTIONS

- Hypersensitivity reactions including rash, pruritus, urticaria, edema, dyspnea, and anaphylaxis have been reported. In such cases, stop CLARINEX at once and consider alternative treatments. (5.1)

ADVERSE REACTIONS

- The most common adverse reactions (reported in ≥2% of adult and adolescent patients with allergic rhinitis and greater than placebo) were pharyngitis, dry mouth, myalgia, fatigue, somnolence, dysmenorrhea. (6.1)

To report SUSPECTED ADVERSE REACTIONS, contact Merck Sharp & Dohme Corp., a subsidiary of Merck & Co., Inc., at 1-877-888-4231 or FDA at 1-800-FDA-1088 or www.fda.gov/medwatch.

USE IN SPECIFIC POPULATIONS

- Renal impairment: dosage adjustment is recommended (2.5, 8.6, 12.3)
- Hepatic impairment: dosage adjustment is recommended (2.5, 8.7, 12.3)

See 17 for PATIENT COUNSELING INFORMATION and FDA-approved patient labeling

Revised: 04/2014

FULL PRESCRIBING INFORMATION: CONTENTS*

FULL PRESCRIBING INFORMATION

1 INDICATIONS AND USAGE

1.1 Seasonal Allergic Rhinitis

CLARINEX® is indicated for the relief of the nasal and non-nasal symptoms of seasonal allergic rhinitis in patients 2 years of age and older.

1.2 Perennial Allergic Rhinitis

CLARINEX is indicated for the relief of the nasal and non-nasal symptoms of perennial allergic rhinitis in patients 6 months of age and older.

1.3 Chronic Idiopathic Urticaria

CLARINEX is indicated for the symptomatic relief of pruritus, reduction in the number of hives, and size of hives, in patients with chronic idiopathic urticaria 6 months of age and older.

2 DOSAGE AND ADMINISTRATION

Although an orally disintegrating tablet formulation of desloratadine may be available in the marketplace, CLARINEX® RediTabs® Tablets are no longer marketed. CLARINEX Tablets, Oral Solution, or RediTabs Tablets may be taken without regard to meals. Place CLARINEX (desloratadine) RediTabs Tablets on the tongue and allow to disintegrate before swallowing. Tablet disintegration occurs rapidly. Administer with or without water. Take tablet immediately after opening the blister.

The age-appropriate dose of CLARINEX Oral Solution should be administered with a commercially available measuring dropper or syringe that is calibrated to deliver 2 mL and 2.5 mL (½ teaspoon).

2.1 Adults and Adolescents 12 Years of Age and Over

The recommended dose of CLARINEX Tablets or CLARINEX RediTabs Tablets is one 5-mg tablet once daily. The recommended dose of CLARINEX Oral Solution is 2 teaspoonfuls (5 mg in 10 mL) once daily.

2.2 Children 6 to 11 Years of Age

The recommended dose of CLARINEX Oral Solution is 1 teaspoonful (2.5 mg in 5 mL) once daily. The recommended dose of CLARINEX RediTabs Tablets is one 2.5-mg tablet once daily.

2.3 Children 12 Months to 5 Years of Age

The recommended dose of CLARINEX Oral Solution is ½ teaspoonful (1.25 mg in 2.5 mL) once daily.

2.4 Children 6 to 11 Months of Age

The recommended dose of CLARINEX Oral Solution is 2 mL (1 mg) once daily.

2.5 Adults with Hepatic or Renal Impairment

In adult patients with liver or renal impairment, a starting dose of one 5-mg tablet every other day is recommended based on pharmacokinetic data. Dosing recommendation for children with liver or renal impairment cannot be made due to lack of data [see Clinical Pharmacology (12.3)].

3 DOSAGE FORMS AND STRENGTHS

CLARINEX Tablets are light blue, film-coated tablets embossed with "C5" containing 5 mg desloratadine.

CLARINEX Oral Solution is a clear orange-colored liquid containing 0.5 mg desloratadine/1 mL.

4 CONTRAINDICATIONS

CLARINEX Tablets, RediTabs, and Oral Solution are contraindicated in patients who are hypersensitive to this medication or to any of its ingredients or to loratadine [see Warnings and Precautions (5.1) and Adverse Reactions (6.2)].

5 WARNINGS AND PRECAUTIONS

5.1 Hypersensitivity Reactions

Hypersensitivity reactions including rash, pruritus, urticaria, edema, dyspnea, and anaphylaxis have been reported after administration of desloratadine. If such a reaction occurs, therapy with CLARINEX should be stopped and alternative treatment should be considered. [See Adverse Reactions (6.2).]

6 ADVERSE REACTIONS

The following adverse reactions are discussed in greater detail in other sections of the label:

- Hypersensitivity reactions. [See Warnings and Precautions (5.1).]

6.1 Clinical Trials Experience

Because clinical trials are conducted under widely varying conditions, adverse reaction rates observed in the clinical trials of a drug cannot be directly compared to rates in the clinical trials of another drug and may not reflect the rates observed in clinical practice.

Adults and Adolescents

Allergic Rhinitis: In multiple-dose placebo-controlled trials, 2834 patients ages 12 years or older received CLARINEX Tablets at doses of 2.5 mg to 20 mg daily, of whom 1655 patients received the recommended daily dose of 5 mg. In patients receiving 5 mg daily, the rate of adverse events was similar between CLARINEX and placebo-treated patients. The percent of patients who withdrew prematurely due to adverse events was 2.4% in the CLARINEX group and 2.6% in the placebo group. There were no serious adverse events in these trials in patients receiving desloratadine. All adverse events that were reported by greater than or equal to 2% of patients who received the recommended daily dose of CLARINEX Tablets (5 mg once daily), and that were more common with CLARINEX Tablets than placebo, are listed in Table 1.

Table 1: Incidence of Adverse Events Reported by ≥2% of Adult and Adolescent Allergic Rhinitis Patients Receiving CLARINEX Tablets

Adverse Event	CLARINEX Tablets 5 mg (n=1655)	Placebo (n=1652)
Infections and Infestations		
Pharyngitis	4.1%	2.0%
Nervous System Disorders		
Somnolence	2.1%	1.8%
Gastrointestinal Disorders		
Dry Mouth	3.0%	1.9%
Musculoskeletal and Connective Tissue Disorders		
Myalgia	2.1%	1.8%
Reproductive System and Breast Disorders		
Dysmenorrhea	2.1%	1.6%
General Disorders and Administration Site Conditions		
Fatigue	2.1%	1.2%

The frequency and magnitude of laboratory and electrocardiographic abnormalities were similar in CLARINEX and placebo-treated patients.

There were no differences in adverse events for subgroups of patients as defined by gender, age, or race.

Chronic Idiopathic Urticaria: In multiple-dose, placebo-controlled trials of chronic idiopathic urticaria, 211 patients ages 12 years or older received CLARINEX Tablets and 205 received placebo. Adverse events that were reported by greater than or equal to 2% of patients who received CLARINEX Tablets and that were more common with CLARINEX than placebo were (rates for CLARINEX and placebo, respectively): headache (14%, 13%), nausea (5%, 2%), fatigue (5%, 1%), dizziness (4%, 3%), pharyngitis (3%, 2%), dyspepsia (3%, 1%), and myalgia (3%, 1%).

Pediatrics

Two hundred and forty-six pediatric subjects 6 months to 11 years of age received CLARINEX Oral Solution for 15 days in three placebo-controlled clinical trials. Pediatric subjects aged 6 to 11 years received 2.5 mg once a day, subjects aged 1 to 5 years received 1.25 mg once a day, and subjects 6 to 11 months of age received 1.0 mg once a day.

In subjects 6 to 11 years of age, no individual adverse event was reported by 2 percent or more of the subjects.

In subjects 2 to 5 years of age, adverse events reported for CLARINEX and placebo in at least 2 percent of subjects receiving CLARINEX Oral Solution and at a frequency greater than placebo were fever (5.5%, 5.4%), urinary tract infection (3.6%, 0%) and varicella (3.6%, 0%).

In subjects 12 months to 23 months of age, adverse events reported for the CLARINEX product and placebo in at least 2 percent of subjects receiving CLARINEX Oral Solution and at a frequency greater than placebo were fever (16.9%, 12.9%), diarrhea (15.4%, 11.3%), upper respiratory tract infections (10.8%, 9.7%), coughing (10.8%, 6.5%), appetite increased (3.1%, 1.6%), emotional lability (3.1%, 0%), epistaxis (3.1%, 0%), parasitic infection (3.1%, 0%), pharyngitis (3.1%, 0%), rash maculopapular (3.1%, 0%).

In subjects 6 months to 11 months of age, adverse events reported for CLARINEX and placebo in at least 2 percent of subjects receiving CLARINEX Oral Solution and at a frequency greater than placebo were upper respiratory tract infections (21.2%, 12.9%), diarrhea (19.7%, 8.1%), fever (12.1%, 1.6%), irritability (12.1%, 11.3%), coughing (10.6%, 9.7%), somnolence (9.1%, 8.1%), bronchitis (6.1%, 0%), otitis media (6.1%, 1.6%), vomiting (6.1%, 3.2%), anorexia (4.5%, 1.6%), pharyngitis (4.5%, 1.6%), insomnia (4.5%, 0%), rhinorrhea (4.5%, 3.2%), erythema (3.0%, 1.6%), and nausea (3.0%, 0%).

There were no clinically meaningful changes in any electrocardiographic parameter, including the QTc interval. Only one of the 246 pediatric subjects receiving CLARINEX Oral Solution in the clinical trials discontinued treatment because of an adverse event.

6.2 Post-Marketing Experience

Because adverse events are reported voluntarily from a population of uncertain size, it is not always possible to reliably estimate their frequency or establish a causal relationship to drug exposure. The following spontaneous adverse events have been reported during the marketing of desloratadine: tachycardia, palpitations, rare cases of hypersensitivity reactions (such as rash, pruritus, urticaria, edema, dyspnea, and anaphylaxis), psychomotor hyperactivity, movement disorders (including dystonia, tics, and extrapyramidal symptoms), seizures, and elevated liver enzymes including bilirubin, and very rarely, hepatitis.

7 DRUG INTERACTIONS

7.1 Inhibitors of Cytochrome P450 3A4

In controlled clinical studies co-administration of desloratadine with ketoconazole, erythromycin, or azithromycin resulted in increased plasma concentrations of desloratadine and 3 hydroxydesloratadine, but there were no clinically relevant changes in the safety profile of desloratadine. [See Clinical Pharmacology (12.3).]

7.2 Fluoxetine
In controlled clinical studies co-administration of desloratadine with fluoxetine, a selective serotonin reuptake inhibitor (SSRI), resulted in increased plasma concentrations of desloratadine and 3 hydroxydesloratadine, but there were no clinically relevant changes in the safety profile of desloratadine. [See Clinical Pharmacology (12.3).]

7.3 Cimetidine
In controlled clinical studies co-administration of desloratadine with cimetidine, a histamine H2-receptor antagonist, resulted in increased plasma concentrations of desloratadine and 3 hydroxydesloratadine, but there were no clinically relevant changes in the safety profile of desloratadine. [See Clinical Pharmacology (12.3).]

8 USE IN SPECIFIC POPULATIONS
8.1 Pregnancy
Pregnancy Category C: There are no adequate and well-controlled studies in pregnant women. Because animal reproduction studies are not always predictive of human response, desloratadine should be used during pregnancy only if clearly needed.

Desloratadine was not teratogenic in rats or rabbits at approximately 210 and 230 times, respectively, the area under the concentration-time curve (AUC) in humans at the recommended daily oral dose. An increase in pre-implantation loss and a decreased number of implantations and fetuses were noted, however, in a separate study in female rats at approximately 120 times the AUC in humans at the recommended daily oral dose. Reduced body weight and slow righting reflex were reported in pups at approximately 50 times or greater than the AUC in humans at the recommended daily oral dose. Desloratadine had no effect on pup development at approximately 7 times the AUC in humans at the recommended daily oral dose. The AUCs in comparison referred to the desloratadine exposure in rabbits and the sum of desloratadine and its metabolites exposures in rats, respectively. [See Nonclinical Toxicology (13.2).]

8.3 Nursing Mothers
Desloratadine passes into breast milk; therefore, a decision should be made whether to discontinue nursing or to discontinue desloratadine, taking into account the benefit of the drug to the nursing mother and the possible risk to the child.

8.4 Pediatric Use
The recommended dose of CLARINEX Oral Solution in the pediatric population is based on cross-study comparison of the plasma concentration of CLARINEX in adults and pediatric subjects. The safety of CLARINEX Oral Solution has been established in 246 pediatric subjects aged 6 months to 11 years in three placebo-controlled clinical studies. Since the course of seasonal and perennial allergic rhinitis and chronic idiopathic urticaria and the effects of CLARINEX are sufficiently similar in the pediatric and adult populations, it allows extrapolation from the adult efficacy data to pediatric patients. The effectiveness of CLARINEX Oral Solution in these age groups is supported by evidence from adequate and well-controlled studies of CLARINEX Tablets in adults. The safety and effectiveness of CLARINEX Tablets or CLARINEX Oral Solution have not been demonstrated in pediatric patients less than 6 months of age. [See Clinical Pharmacology (12.3).]

The CLARINEX RediTabs 2.5-mg tablet has not been evaluated in pediatric patients. Bioequivalence of the CLARINEX RediTabs Tablet and the previously marketed RediTabs Tablet was established in adults. In conjunction with the dose-finding studies in pediatrics described, the pharmacokinetic data for CLARINEX RediTabs supports the use of the 2.5-mg dose strength in pediatric patients 6 to 11 years of age.

8.5 Geriatric Use
Clinical studies of desloratadine did not include sufficient numbers of subjects aged 65 and over to determine whether they respond differently from younger subjects. Other reported clinical experience has not identified differences between the elderly and younger patients. In general, dose selection for an elderly patient should be cautious, reflecting the greater frequency of decreased hepatic, renal, or cardiac function, and of concomitant disease or other drug therapy. [See Clinical Pharmacology (12.3).]

8.6 Renal Impairment
Dosage adjustment for patients with renal impairment is recommended [see Dosage and Administration (2.5) and Clinical Pharmacology (12.3)].

8.7 Hepatic Impairment
Dosage adjustment for patients with hepatic impairment is recommended [see Dosage and Administration (2.5) and Clinical Pharmacology (12.3)].

9 DRUG ABUSE AND DEPENDENCE
There is no information to indicate that abuse or dependency occurs with CLARINEX Tablets.

10 OVERDOSAGE
In the event of overdose, consider standard measures to remove any unabsorbed drug. Symptomatic and supportive treatment is recommended. Desloratadine and 3-hydroxydesloratadine are not eliminated by hemodialysis. Information regarding acute overdosage is limited to experience from post-marketing adverse event reports and from clinical trials conducted during the development of the CLARINEX product. In a dose-ranging trial, at doses of 10 mg and 20 mg/day somnolence was reported.

In another study, no clinically relevant adverse events were reported in normal male and female volunteers who were given single daily doses of CLARINEX 45 mg for 10 days [see Clinical Pharmacology (12.2)].

Lethality occurred in rats at oral doses of 250 mg/kg or greater (estimated desloratadine and desloratadine metabolite exposures were approximately 120 times the AUC in humans at the recommended daily oral dose). The oral median lethal dose in mice was 353 mg/kg (estimated desloratadine exposures were approximately 290 times the human daily oral dose on a mg/m² basis). No deaths occurred at oral doses up to 250 mg/kg in monkeys (estimated desloratadine exposures were approximately 810 times the human daily oral dose on a mg/m² basis).

11 DESCRIPTION
CLARINEX (desloratadine) Tablets are light blue, round, film-coated tablets containing 5 mg desloratadine, an antihistamine, to be administered orally. CLARINEX Tablets also contain the following excipients: dibasic calcium phosphate dihydrate USP, microcrystalline cellulose NF, corn starch NF, talc USP, carnauba wax NF, white wax NF, coating material consisting of lactose monohydrate, hypromellose, titanium dioxide, polyethylene glycol, and FD&C Blue #2 Aluminum Lake.

CLARINEX Oral Solution is a clear orange-colored liquid containing 0.5 mg/1 mL desloratadine. The Oral Solution contains the following inactive ingredients: propylene glycol USP, sorbitol solution USP, citric acid (anhydrous) USP, sodium citrate dihydrate USP, sodium benzoate NF, disodium edetate USP, purified water USP. It also contains granulated sugar, natural and artificial flavor for bubble gum, and FDC Yellow #6 dye.

Desloratadine is a white to off-white powder that is slightly soluble in water, but very soluble in ethanol and propylene glycol. It has an empirical formula: $C_{19}H_{19}ClN_2$ and a molecular weight of 310.8. The chemical name is 8-chloro-6,11-dihydro-11-(4-piperdinylidene)-5H-benzo[5,6]cyclohepta-[1,2-b]pyridine and has the following structure:

12 CLINICAL PHARMACOLOGY
12.1 Mechanism of Action
Desloratadine is a long-acting tricyclic histamine antagonist with selective H_1-receptor histamine antagonist activity. Receptor binding data indicates that at a concentration of 2–3 ng/mL (7 nanomolar), desloratadine shows significant interaction with the human histamine H_1-receptor. Desloratadine inhibited histamine release from human mast cells in vitro. Results of a radiolabeled tissue distribution study in rats and a radioligand H_1-receptor binding study in guinea pigs showed that desloratadine did not readily cross the blood brain barrier. The clinical significance of this finding is unknown.

12.2 Pharmacodynamics
Wheal and Flare: Human histamine skin wheal studies following single and repeated 5-mg doses of desloratadine have shown that the drug exhibits an antihistaminic effect by 1 hour; this activity may persist for as long as 24 hours. There was no evidence of histamine-induced skin wheal tachyphylaxis within the desloratadine 5-mg group over the 28-day treatment period. The clinical relevance of histamine wheal skin testing is unknown.

Effects on QT_c: Single daily doses of 45 mg were given to normal male and female volunteers for 10 days. All ECGs obtained in this study were manually read in a blinded fashion by a cardiologist. In CLARINEX-treated subjects, there was an increase in mean heart rate of 9.2 bpm relative to placebo. The QT interval was corrected for heart rate (QT_c) by both the Bazett and Fridericia methods. Using the QT_c (Bazett) there was a mean increase of 8.1 msec in CLARINEX-treated subjects relative to placebo. Using QT_c (Fridericia) there was a mean increase of 0.4 msec in CLARINEX-treated subjects relative to placebo. No clinically relevant adverse events were reported.

12.3 Pharmacokinetics
Absorption
Following oral administration of a desloratadine 5-mg tablet once daily for 10 days to normal healthy volunteers, the mean time to maximum plasma concentrations (T_{max}) occurred at approximately 3 hours post dose and mean steady state peak plasma concentrations (C_{max}) and AUC of 4 ng/mL and 56.9 ng·hr/mL were observed, respectively. Neither food nor grapefruit juice had an effect on the bioavailability (C_{max} and AUC) of desloratadine.

The pharmacokinetic profile of CLARINEX Oral Solution was evaluated in a three-way crossover study in 30 adult volunteers. A single dose of 10 mL of CLARINEX Oral Solution containing 5 mg of desloratadine was bioequivalent to a single dose of 5-mg CLARINEX Tablet. Food had no effect on the bioavailability (AUC and C_{max}) of CLARINEX Oral Solution.

The pharmacokinetic profile of CLARINEX RediTabs Tablets was evaluated in a three-way crossover study in 24 adult volunteers. A single CLARINEX RediTabs Tablet containing 5 mg of desloratadine was bioequivalent to a single 5-mg CLARINEX RediTabs Tablet (original formulation) for both desloratadine and 3-hydroxydesloratadine. Food and water had no effect on the bioavailability (AUC and C_{max}) of CLARINEX RediTabs Tablets.

Distribution
Desloratadine and 3-hydroxydesloratadine are approximately 82% to 87% and 85% to 89% bound to plasma proteins, respectively. Protein binding of desloratadine and 3-hydroxydesloratadine was unaltered in subjects with impaired renal function.

Metabolism
Desloratadine (a major metabolite of loratadine) is extensively metabolized to 3-hydroxydesloratadine, an active metabolite, which is subsequently glucuronidated. The enzyme(s) responsible for the formation of 3-hydroxydesloratadine have not been identified. Data from clinical trials indicate that a subset of the general population has a decreased ability to form 3-hydroxydesloratadine, and are poor metabolizers of desloratadine. In pharmacokinetic studies (n=3748), approximately 6% of subjects were poor metabolizers of desloratadine (defined as a subject with an AUC ratio of 3-hydroxydesloratadine to desloratadine less than 0.1, or a subject with a desloratadine half-life exceeding 50 hours). These pharmacokinetic studies included subjects between the ages of 2 and 70 years, including 977 subjects aged 2 to 5 years, 1575 subjects aged 6 to 11 years, and 1196 subjects aged 12 to 70 years. There was no difference in the prevalence of poor metabolizers across age groups. The frequency of poor metabolizers was higher in Blacks (17%, n=988) as compared to Caucasians (2%, n=1,462) and Hispanics (2%, n=1,063). The median exposure (AUC) to desloratadine in the poor metabolizers was approximately 6-fold greater than in the subjects who are not poor metabolizers. Subjects who are poor metabolizers of desloratadine cannot be prospectively identified and will be exposed to higher levels of desloratadine following dosing with the recommended dose of desloratadine. In multidose clinical safety studies, where metabolizer status was identified, a total of 94 poor metabolizers and 123 normal metabolizers were enrolled and treated with CLARINEX Oral Solution for 15–35 days. In these studies, no overall differences in safety were observed between poor metabolizers and normal metabolizers. Although not seen in these studies, an increased risk of exposure-related adverse events in patients who are poor metabolizers cannot be ruled out.

Elimination
The mean plasma elimination half-life of desloratadine was approximately 27 hours. C_{max} and AUC values increased in a dose proportional manner following single oral doses between 5 and 20 mg. The degree of accumulation after 14 days of dosing was consistent with the half-life and dosing frequency. A human mass balance study documented a recovery of approximately 87% of the ^{14}C-desloratadine dose, which was equally distributed in urine and feces as metabolic products. Analysis of plasma 3-hydroxydesloratadine showed similar T_{max} and half-life values compared to desloratadine.

Special Populations
Geriatric Subjects: In older subjects (≥65 years old; n=17) following multiple-dose administration of CLARINEX Tablets, the mean C_{max} and AUC values for desloratadine were 20% greater than in younger subjects (<65 years old). The oral total body clearance (CL/F) when normalized for body weight was similar between the two age groups. The mean plasma elimination half-life of desloratadine was 33.7 hr in subjects ≥65 years old. The pharmacokinetics for 3-hydroxydesloratadine appeared unchanged in older versus younger subjects. These age-related differences are unlikely to be clinically relevant and no dosage adjustment is recommended in elderly subjects.

Pediatric Subjects: In subjects 6 to 11 years old, a single dose of 5 mL of CLARINEX Oral Solution containing 2.5 mg

Table 2: Changes in Desloratadine and 3-Hydroxydesloratadine Pharmacokinetics in Healthy Male and Female Volunteers

	Desloratadine		3-Hydroxydesloratadine	
	C_{max}	$AUC_{0-24\ hrs}$	C_{max}	$AUC_{0-24\ hrs}$
Erythromycin (500 mg Q8h)	+ 24%	+ 14%	+ 43%	+ 40%
Ketoconazole (200 mg Q12h)	+ 45%	+ 39%	+ 43%	+ 72%
Azithromycin (500 mg day 1, 250 mg QD × 4 days)	+ 15%	+ 5%	+ 15%	+ 4%
Fluoxetine (20 mg QD)	+ 15%	+ 0%	+ 17%	+ 13%
Cimetidine (600 mg Q12h)	+ 12%	+ 19%	- 11%	- 3%

of desloratadine, resulted in desloratadine plasma concentrations similar to those achieved in adults administered a single 5-mg CLARINEX Tablet. In subjects 2 to 5 years old, a single dose of 2.5 mL of CLARINEX Oral Solution containing 1.25 mg of desloratadine, resulted in desloratadine plasma concentrations similar to those achieved in adults administered a single 5-mg CLARINEX Tablet. However, the C_{max} and AUC of the metabolite (3-hydroxydesloratadine) were 1.27 and 1.61 times higher for the 5-mg dose of Oral Solution administered in adults compared to the C_{max} and AUC obtained in children 2 to 11 years of age receiving 1.25–2.5 mg of CLARINEX Oral Solution.

A single dose of either 2.5 mL or 1.25 mL of CLARINEX Oral Solution containing 1.25 mg or 0.625 mg, respectively, of desloratadine was administered to subjects 6 to 11 months of age and 12 to 23 months of age. The results of a population pharmacokinetic analysis indicated that a dose of 1 mg for subjects aged 6 to 11 months and 1.25 mg for subjects 12 to 23 months of age is required to obtain desloratadine plasma concentrations similar to those achieved in adults administered a single 5-mg dose of CLARINEX Oral Solution.

The CLARINEX RediTabs 2.5-mg tablet has not been evaluated in pediatric patients. Bioequivalence of the CLARINEX RediTabs Tablet and the original CLARINEX RediTabs Tablets was established in adults. In conjunction with the dose-finding studies in pediatrics described, the pharmacokinetic data for CLARINEX RediTabs Tablets supports the use of the 2.5-mg dose strength in pediatric patients 6 to 11 years of age.

Renally Impaired: Desloratadine pharmacokinetics following a single dose of 7.5 mg were characterized in patients with mild (n=7; creatinine clearance 51–69 mL/min/1.73 m²), moderate (n=6; creatinine clearance 34–43 mL/min/1.73 m²), and severe (n=6; creatinine clearance 5–29 mL/min/1.73 m²) renal impairment or hemodialysis dependent (n=6) patients. In patients with mild and moderate renal impairment, median C_{max} and AUC values increased by approximately 1.2- and 1.9-fold, respectively, relative to subjects with normal renal function. In patients with severe renal impairment or who were hemodialysis dependent, C_{max} and AUC values increased by approximately 1.7- and 2.5-fold, respectively. Minimal changes in 3-hydroxydesloratadine concentrations were observed. Desloratadine and 3-hydroxydesloratadine were poorly removed by hemodialysis. Plasma protein binding of desloratadine and 3-hydroxydesloratadine was unaltered by renal impairment. No dosage adjustment for patients with renal impairment is recommended [see Dosage and Administration (2.5)].

Hepatically Impaired: Desloratadine pharmacokinetics were characterized following a single oral dose in patients with mild (n=4), moderate (n=4), and severe (n=4) hepatic impairment as defined by the Child-Pugh classification of hepatic function and 8 subjects with normal hepatic function. Patients with hepatic impairment, regardless of severity, had approximately a 2.4-fold increase in AUC as compared with normal subjects. The apparent oral clearance of desloratadine in patients with mild, moderate, and severe hepatic impairment was 37%, 36%, and 28% of that in normal subjects, respectively. An increase in the mean elimination half-life of desloratadine in patients with hepatic impairment was observed. For 3-hydroxydesloratadine, the mean C_{max} and AUC values for patients with hepatic impairment were not statistically significantly different from subjects with normal hepatic function. Dosage adjustment for patients with hepatic impairment is recommended [see Dosage and Administration (2.5)].

Gender: Female subjects treated for 14 days with CLARINEX Tablets had 10% and 3% higher desloratadine C_{max} and AUC values, respectively, compared with male subjects. The 3-hydroxydesloratadine C_{max} and AUC values were also increased by 45% and 48%, respectively, in fe-

males compared with males. However, these apparent differences are not likely to be clinically relevant and therefore no dosage adjustment is recommended.

Race: Following 14 days of treatment with CLARINEX Tablets, the C_{max} and AUC values for desloratadine were 18% and 32% higher, respectively, in Blacks compared with Caucasians. For 3-hydroxydesloratadine there was a corresponding 10% reduction in C_{max} and AUC values in Blacks compared to Caucasians. These differences are not likely to be clinically relevant and therefore no dose adjustment is recommended.

Drug Interactions: In two controlled crossover clinical pharmacology studies in healthy male (n=12 in each study) and female (n=12 in each study) volunteers, desloratadine 7.5 mg (1.5 times the daily dose) once daily was coadministered with erythromycin 500 mg every 8 hours or ketoconazole 200 mg every 12 hours for 10 days. In three separate controlled, parallel group clinical pharmacology studies, desloratadine at the clinical dose of 5 mg has been coadministered with azithromycin 500 mg followed by 250 mg once daily for 4 days (n=18) or with fluoxetine 20 mg once daily for 7 days after a 23-day pretreatment period with fluoxetine (n=18) or with cimetidine 600 mg every 12 hours for 14 days (n=18) under steady-state conditions to normal healthy male and female volunteers. Although increased plasma concentrations (C_{max} and $AUC_{0-24\ hrs}$) of desloratadine and 3-hydroxydesloratadine were observed (see Table 2), there were no clinically relevant changes in the safety profile of desloratadine, as assessed by electrocardiographic parameters (including the corrected QT interval), clinical laboratory tests, vital signs, and adverse events.

[See table 2 above]

13   NONCLINICAL TOXICOLOGY
13.1   Carcinogenesis, Mutagenesis, Impairment of Fertility
Carcinogenicity Studies

The carcinogenic potential of desloratadine was assessed using a loratadine study in rats and a desloratadine study in mice. In a 2-year study in rats, loratadine was administered in the diet at doses up to 25 mg/kg/day (estimated desloratadine and desloratadine metabolite exposures were approximately 30 times the AUC in humans at the recommended daily oral dose). A significantly higher incidence of hepatocellular tumors (combined adenomas and carcinomas) was observed in males given 10 mg/kg/day of loratadine and in males and females given 25 mg/kg/day of loratadine. The estimated desloratadine and desloratadine metabolite exposures in rats given 10 mg/kg of loratadine were approximately 7 times the AUC in humans at the recommended daily oral dose. The clinical significance of these findings during long-term use of desloratadine is not known.

In a 2-year dietary study in mice, males and females given up to 16 mg/kg/day and 32 mg/kg/day desloratadine, respectively, did not show significant increases in the incidence of any tumors. The estimated desloratadine and desloratadine metabolite exposures in mice at these doses were 12 and 27 times, respectively, the AUC in humans at the recommended daily oral dose.

Genotoxicity Studies

In genotoxicity studies with desloratadine, there was no evidence of genotoxic potential in a reverse mutation assay (Salmonella / E. coli mammalian microsome bacterial mutagenicity assay) or in 2 assays for chromosomal aberrations (human peripheral blood lymphocyte clastogenicity assay and mouse bone marrow micronucleus assay).

Impairment of Fertility

There was no effect on female fertility in rats at desloratadine doses up to 24 mg/kg/day (estimated desloratadine and desloratadine metabolite exposures were approximately 130 times the AUC in humans at the recommended daily oral dose). A male specific decrease in fertility,

demonstrated by reduced female conception rates, decreased sperm numbers and motility, and histopathologic testicular changes, occurred at an oral desloratadine dose of 12 mg/kg in rats (estimated desloratadine and desloratadine metabolite exposures were approximately 45 times the AUC in humans at the recommended daily oral dose). Desloratadine had no effect on fertility in rats at an oral dose of 3 mg/kg/day (estimated desloratadine and desloratadine metabolite exposures were approximately 8 times the AUC in humans at the recommended daily oral dose).

13.2   Animal Toxicology and/or Pharmacology
Reproductive Toxicology Studies

Desloratadine was not teratogenic in rats at doses up to 48 mg/kg/day (estimated desloratadine and desloratadine metabolite exposures were approximately 210 times the AUC in humans at the recommended daily oral dose) or in rabbits at doses up to 60 mg/kg/day (estimated desloratadine exposures were approximately 230 times the AUC in humans at the recommended daily oral dose). In a separate study, an increase in pre-implantation loss and a decreased number of implantations and fetuses were noted in female rats at 24 mg/kg (estimated desloratadine and desloratadine metabolite exposures were approximately 120 times the AUC in humans at the recommended daily oral dose). Reduced body weight and slow righting reflex were reported in pups at doses of 9 mg/kg/day or greater (estimated desloratadine and desloratadine metabolite exposures were approximately 50 times or greater than the AUC in humans at the recommended daily oral dose). Desloratadine had no effect on pup development at an oral dose of 3 mg/kg/day (estimated desloratadine and desloratadine metabolite exposures were approximately 7 times the AUC in humans at the recommended daily oral dose).

14   CLINICAL STUDIES
14.1   Seasonal Allergic Rhinitis

The clinical efficacy and safety of CLARINEX Tablets were evaluated in over 2300 patients 12 to 75 years of age with seasonal allergic rhinitis. A total of 1838 patients received 2.5 to 20 mg of CLARINEX in 4 double-blind, randomized, placebo-controlled clinical trials of 2 to 4 weeks' duration conducted in the United States. The results of these studies demonstrated the efficacy and safety of CLARINEX 5 mg in the treatment of adult and adolescent patients with seasonal allergic rhinitis. In a dose-ranging trial, CLARINEX 2.5 to 20 mg/day was studied. Doses of 5, 7.5, 10, and 20 mg/day were superior to placebo, and no additional benefit was seen at doses above 5.0 mg. In the same study, an increase in the incidence of somnolence was observed at doses of 10 mg/day and 20 mg/day (5.2% and 7.6%, respectively), compared to placebo (2.3%).

In two 4-week studies of 924 patients (aged 15 to 75 years) with seasonal allergic rhinitis and concomitant asthma, CLARINEX Tablets 5 mg once daily improved rhinitis symptoms, with no decrease in pulmonary function. This supports the safety of administering CLARINEX Tablets to adult patients with seasonal allergic rhinitis with mild to moderate asthma.

CLARINEX Tablets 5 mg once daily significantly reduced the Total Symptom Score (the sum of individual scores of nasal and non-nasal symptoms) in patients with seasonal allergic rhinitis. See Table 3.

Table 3: TOTAL SYMPTOM SCORE (TSS) Changes in a 2-Week Clinical Trial in Patients with Seasonal Allergic Rhinitis

Treatment Group (n)	Mean Baseline* (SEM)	Change from Baseline† (SEM)	Placebo Comparison (P-value)
CLARINEX 5.0 mg (171)	14.2 (0.3)	-4.3 (0.3)	P<0.01
Placebo (173)	13.7 (0.3)	-2.5 (0.3)	

SEM=Standard Error of the Mean
*At baseline, a total nasal symptom score (sum of 4 individual symptoms) of at least 6 and a total non-nasal symptom score (sum of 4 individual symptoms) of at least 5 (each symptom scored 0 to 3 where 0=no symptom and 3=severe symptoms) was required for trial eligibility. TSS ranges from 0=no symptoms to 24=maximal symptoms.
†Mean reduction in TSS averaged over the 2-week treatment period.

There were no significant differences in the effectiveness of CLARINEX Tablets 5 mg across subgroups of patients defined by gender, age, or race.

14.2   Perennial Allergic Rhinitis

The clinical efficacy and safety of CLARINEX Tablets 5 mg were evaluated in over 1300 patients 12 to 80 years of age with perennial allergic rhinitis. A total of 685 patients received 5 mg/day of CLARINEX in two double-blind, randomized, placebo-controlled clinical trials of 4 weeks' duration conducted in the United States and internationally. In one of these studies CLARINEX Tablets 5 mg once daily was shown to significantly reduce the Total Symptom Score in patients with perennial allergic rhinitis (Table 4).

Table 4: TOTAL SYMPTOM SCORE (TSS) Changes in a 4-Week Clinical Trial in Patients with Perennial Allergic Rhinitis

Treatment Group (n)	Mean Baseline* (SEM)	Change from Baseline[†] (SEM)	Placebo Comparison (P-value)
CLARINEX 5.0 mg (337)	12.37 (0.18)	-4.06 (0.21)	$P=0.01$
Placebo (337)	12.30 (0.18)	-3.27 (0.21)	

SEM=Standard Error of the Mean
*At baseline, average of total symptom score (sum of 5 individual nasal symptoms and 3 non-nasal symptoms, each symptom scored 0 to 3 where 0=no symptom and 3=severe symptoms) of at least 10 was required for trial eligibility. TSS ranges from 0=no symptoms to 24=maximal symptoms.
[†]Mean reduction in TSS averaged over the 4-week treatment period.

14.3   Chronic Idiopathic Urticaria
The efficacy and safety of CLARINEX Tablets 5 mg once daily was studied in 416 chronic idiopathic urticaria patients 12 to 84 years of age, of whom 211 received CLARINEX. In two double-blind, placebo-controlled, randomized clinical trials of six weeks duration, at the pre-specified one-week primary time point evaluation, CLARINEX Tablets significantly reduced the severity of pruritus when compared to placebo (Table 5). Secondary endpoints were also evaluated, and during the first week of therapy CLARINEX Tablets 5 mg reduced the secondary endpoints, "Number of Hives" and the "Size of the Largest Hive," when compared to placebo.

Table 5: PRURITUS SYMPTOM SCORE Changes in the First Week of a Clinical Trial in Patients with Chronic Idiopathic Urticaria

Treatment Group (n)	Mean Baseline (SEM)	Change from Baseline* (SEM)	Placebo Comparison (P-value)
CLARINEX 5.0 mg (115)	2.19 (0.04)	-1.05 (0.07)	$P<0.01$
Placebo (110)	2.21 (0.04)	-0.52 (0.07)	

Pruritus scored 0 to 3 where 0=no symptom to 3=maximal symptom
SEM=Standard Error of the Mean
*Mean reduction in pruritus averaged over the first week of treatment.

The clinical safety of CLARINEX Oral Solution was documented in three, 15-day, double-blind, placebo-controlled safety studies in pediatric subjects with a documented history of allergic rhinitis, chronic idiopathic urticaria, or subjects who were candidates for antihistamine therapy. In the first study, 2.5 mg of CLARINEX Oral Solution was administered to 60 pediatric subjects 6 to 11 years of age. The second study evaluated 1.25 mg of CLARINEX Oral Solution administered to 55 pediatric subjects 2 to 5 years of age. In the third study, 1.25 mg of CLARINEX Oral Solution was administered to 65 pediatric subjects 12 to 23 months of age and 1.0 mg of CLARINEX Oral Solution was administered to 66 pediatric subjects 6 to 11 months of age. The results of these studies demonstrated the safety of CLARINEX Oral Solution in pediatric subjects 6 months to 11 years of age.

16   HOW SUPPLIED/STORAGE AND HANDLING
CLARINEX Tablets: Embossed "C5", light blue, film-coated tablets that are packaged in high-density polyethylene plastic bottles of 100 (NDC 0085-1264-01) and 500 (NDC 0085-1264-02).
CLARINEX Oral Solution: Clear orange-colored liquid containing 0.5 mg/1 mL desloratadine in a 16-ounce Amber glass bottle (NDC 0085-1334-01) and a 4-ounce Amber glass bottle (NDC 0085-1334-02).
Storage
• **CLARINEX Tablets:** Protect Unit-of-Use packaging and Unit-Dose Hospital Pack from excessive moisture. Store at 25°C (77°F); excursions permitted to 15–30°C (59–86°F) [see USP Controlled Room Temperature]. Heat Sensitive. Avoid exposure at or above 30°C (86°F).

• **CLARINEX Oral Solution:** Store at 25°C (77°F); excursions permitted to 15–30°C (59–86°F) [see USP Controlled Room Temperature]. Protect from light.

17   PATIENT COUNSELING INFORMATION
See FDA-Approved Patient Labeling (Patient Information).
17.1   Information for Patients
• Patients should be instructed to use CLARINEX as directed.
• As there are no food effects on bioavailability, patients can be instructed that CLARINEX Tablets, Oral Solution, or RediTabs Tablets may be taken without regard to meals.
• Patients should be advised not to increase the dose or dosing frequency as studies have not demonstrated increased effectiveness at higher doses and somnolence may occur.
• Phenylketonurics: CLARINEX RediTabs Tablets contain phenylalanine.
CLARINEX Tablets and Oral Solution are
Manufactured for: Merck Sharp & Dohme Corp., a subsidiary of
MERCK & CO., INC.,Whitehouse Station, NJ 08889, USA
CLARINEX Tablets are
Manufactured by: Merck Sharp & Dohme Corp., a subsidiary of
Merck & Co., Inc.,Whitehouse Station, NJ 08889, USA
CLARINEX Oral Solution is
Manufactured by: Schering-Plough Canada, Inc., Pointe Claire, Quebec, Canada
For patent information:
www.merck.com/product/patent/home.html
Copyright © 2004, 2005, 2010 Merck Sharp & Dohme Corp., a subsidiary of **Merck & Co., Inc.**
All rights reserved.
uspi-mk4117-mtl-1404r007
PATIENT INFORMATION
CLARINEX®   (CLA-RI-NEX)   (desloratadine)   Tablets, RediTabs®, and Oral Solution
Read the Patient Information that comes with CLARINEX® before you start taking it and each time you get a refill. There may be new information. This leaflet is a summary of the information for patients. Your doctor or pharmacist can give you additional information. This leaflet does not take the place of talking to your doctor about your medical condition or treatment.
What is CLARINEX?
CLARINEX is a prescription medicine that contains the medicine desloratadine (an antihistamine).
CLARINEX is used to help control the symptoms of:
■ seasonal allergic rhinitis (sneezing, stuffy nose, runny nose and itching of the nose) in people 2 years of age and older.
■ perennial allergic rhinitis (sneezing, stuffy nose, runny nose and itching of the nose) in people 6 months of age and older.
■ chronic idiopathic urticaria (long-term itching) and to reduce the number and size of hives in people 6 months of age and older.
CLARINEX is not for children younger than 6 months of age.
Who should not take CLARINEX?
Do not take CLARINEX if you:
■ are allergic to desloratadine or any of the ingredients in CLARINEX Tablets, CLARINEX RediTabs® or CLARINEX Oral Solution. See the end of this leaflet for a complete list of ingredients.
■ are allergic to loratadine (Alavert, Claritin).
Talk to your doctor before taking this medicine if you have any questions about whether or not to take this medicine.
What should I tell my doctor before taking CLARINEX?
Before you take CLARINEX, tell your doctor if you:
■ have liver or kidney problems.
■ have any other medical conditions.
■ are pregnant or plan to become pregnant. It is not known if CLARINEX will harm your unborn baby. Talk to your doctor if you are pregnant or plan to become pregnant.
■ are breast-feeding or plan to breast-feed. CLARINEX **can pass into your breast milk.** Talk to your doctor about the best way to feed your baby if you take CLARINEX.
Tell your doctor about all the medicines you take, including prescription and non-prescription medicines, vitamins and herbal supplements. CLARINEX may affect the way other medicines work, and other medicines may affect how CLARINEX works. Especially tell your doctor if you take:
■ ketoconazole (Nizoral)
■ erythromycin (Ery-tab, Eryc, PCE)
■ azithromycin (Zithromax, Zmax)
■ antihistamines
■ fluoxetine (Prozac)
■ cimetidine (Tagamet)
Know the medicines you take. Keep a list of your medicines and show it to your doctor and pharmacist when you get a new medicine.

How should I take CLARINEX?
■ Take CLARINEX exactly as your doctor tells you to take it.
■ Do not change your dose of CLARINEX or take more often than prescribed.
■ CLARINEX can be taken with or without food.
■ Place CLARINEX RediTabs Tablet on your tongue and allow it to dissolve before swallowing. CLARINEX RediTabs can be taken with or without water. Take your CLARINEX RediTabs Tablet right away after opening the blister.
■ Take CLARINEX Oral Solution with a measuring dropper or oral syringe that can measure 2 mL or 2.5 mL. Ask your pharmacist for a dropper or syringe if you do not have one.
■ If you take too much CLARINEX, call your doctor or get medical attention right away.
What are the possible side effects of CLARINEX Tablets?
CLARINEX may cause serious side effects, including:
■ Allergic reactions. Stop taking CLARINEX and call your doctor right away or get emergency help if you have any of these symptoms:
  ◦ rash
  ◦ itching
  ◦ hives
  ◦ swelling of your lips, tongue, face, and throat
  ◦ shortness of breath or trouble breathing
The most common side effects of CLARINEX in adults and children 12 years of age and older with allergic rhinitis include:
■ sore throat
■ dry mouth
■ muscle pain
■ tiredness
■ sleepiness
■ menstrual pain
Increased sleepiness or tiredness can happen if you take more CLARINEX than your doctor prescribed to you.
Tell your doctor if you have any side effect that bothers you or that does not go away.
These are not all of the possible side effects of CLARINEX. For more information, ask your doctor or pharmacist.
Call your doctor for medical advice about side effects. You may report side effects to FDA at 1-800-FDA-1088.
How should I store CLARINEX?
■ Store CLARINEX Tablets between 59°F to 86°F (15°C to 30°C).
■ CLARINEX Tablets are sensitive to heat. Do not store above 86°F (30°C).
■ Protect CLARINEX Tablets from moisture.
■ Store CLARINEX Oral Solution between 59°F to 86°F (15°C to 30°C). Protect CLARINEX Oral Solution from light.
Keep CLARINEX Tablets, RediTabs Tablets, and **Oral Solution** and all medicines out of the reach of children.
General information about CLARINEX
Medicines are sometimes prescribed for purposes other than those listed in a patient information leaflet. Do not use CLARINEX for a condition for which it was not prescribed. Do not give CLARINEX to other people, even if they have the same condition you have. It may harm them.
This Patient Information leaflet summarizes the most important information about CLARINEX. If you would like more information, talk with your doctor. You can ask your pharmacist or doctor for information about CLARINEX that is written for health professionals.
For more information, go to www.CLARINEX.com
What are the ingredients in CLARINEX?
Active ingredient: desloratadine
Patients with Phenylketonuria: CLARINEX RediTabs Tablets contain phenylalanine.
Inactive ingredients in CLARINEX Tablets: dibasic calcium phosphate dihydrate USP, microcrystalline cellulose NF, corn starch NF, talc USP, carnauba wax NF, white wax NF, coating material consisting of lactose monohydrate, hypromellose, titanium dioxide, polyethylene glycol, and FD&C Blue #2 Aluminum Lake.
Inactive ingredients in CLARINEX Oral Solution: propylene glycol USP, sorbitol solution USP, citric acid (anhydrous) USP, sodium citrate dihydrate USP, sodium benzoate NF, disodium edetate USP, purified water USP. It also contains granulated sugar, natural and artificial flavor for bubble gum and FDC Yellow #6 dye.
CLARINEX Tablets and Oral Solution are
Manufactured for: Merck Sharp & Dohme Corp., a subsidiary of
MERCK & CO., INC.,Whitehouse Station, NJ 08889, USA
CLARINEX Tablets are
Manufactured by: Merck Sharp & Dohme Corp., a subsidiary of
Merck & Co., Inc.,Whitehouse Station, NJ 08889, USA
CLARINEX Oral Solution is
Manufactured by: Schering-Plough Canada, Inc., Pointe Claire, Quebec, Canada
For patent information:
www.merck.com/product/patent/home.html

Help Patients Save on Rx Drugs: PDR.net/PharmacyDiscountCard

The trademarks depicted herein are owned by their respective companies.
Copyright © 2010 Merck Sharp & Dohme Corp., a subsidiary of **Merck & Co., Inc.**
All rights reserved.
Revised: 04/2014
usppi-mk4117-mtl-1404r006
Shown in Product Identification Guide, page 308

CLARINEX-D® 12 HOUR   ℞

[klă-rĭ-něks D]
Extended Release Tablets
(desloratadine/pseudoephedrine sulfate)
for oral use

HIGHLIGHTS OF PRESCRIBING INFORMATION
These highlights do not include all the information needed to use CLARINEX-D 12 HOUR Extended Release Tablets safely and effectively. See full prescribing information for CLARINEX-D 12 HOUR Extended Release Tablets.
CLARINEX-D®12 HOUR Extended Release Tablets
(desloratadine/pseudoephedrine sulfate) for oral use
Initial U.S. Approval: 2005

―――――――INDICATIONS AND USAGE―――――――

CLARINEX-D 12 HOUR is a combination product containing an H₁-receptor antagonist and a sympathomimetic amine indicated for:
• Relief of nasal and non-nasal symptoms of seasonal allergic rhinitis, including nasal congestion, in adults and adolescents 12 years of age and older. (1.1)

―――――――DOSAGE AND ADMINISTRATION―――――――

For oral use only (2)
Adults and adolescents 12 years of age and over: The recommended dose of CLARINEX-D 12 HOUR Extended Release Tablets is one tablet twice a day. (2.1)

―――――――DOSAGE FORMS AND STRENGTHS―――――――

Desloratadine 2.5 mg/Pseudoephedrine sulfate 120 mg tablets. (3)

―――――――CONTRAINDICATIONS―――――――

• Hypersensitivity (4)
• Narrow-Angle Glaucoma (4)
• Urinary Retention (4)
• Patients Receiving MAO Inhibitors or within 14 days of stopping such treatment (4)
• Severe hypertension or severe coronary artery disease. (4)

―――――――WARNINGS AND PRECAUTIONS―――――――

• Cardiovascular and central nervous system effects: Use with caution in patients with cardiovascular disorders. (5.1)
• Coexisting conditions: Use with caution in patients with increased intraocular pressure, prostatic hypertrophy, diabetes mellitus, or hyperthyroidism. (5.2)

―――――――ADVERSE REACTIONS―――――――

• The most common adverse reactions (reported in ≥2% of patients) were insomnia, headache, mouth dry, fatigue, somnolence, pharyngitis, dizziness, nausea, and anorexia. (6.1)

To report SUSPECTED ADVERSE REACTIONS, contact Merck Sharp & Dohme Corp., a subsidiary of Merck & Co., Inc., at 1-877-888-4231 or FDA at 1-800-FDA-1088 or www.fda.gov/medwatch

―――――――DRUG INTERACTIONS―――――――

Monoamine Oxidase (MAO) Inhibitors: Do not use. May potentiate the effect of pseudoephedrine on vascular system. (7.1)

―――――――USE IN SPECIFIC POPULATIONS―――――――

• Renal impairment: Avoid in patients with renal impairment. (8.6)
• Hepatic impairment: Avoid in patients with hepatic impairment. (8.7)
See 17 for PATIENT COUNSELING INFORMATION and FDA-approved patient labeling

Revised: 03/2014

FULL PRESCRIBING INFORMATION: CONTENTS*
* Sections or subsections omitted from the full prescribing information are not listed

―――――――――――――――――――――――

FULL PRESCRIBING INFORMATION
1   INDICATIONS AND USAGE
1.1   Seasonal Allergic Rhinitis
CLARINEX-D® 12 HOUR Extended Release Tablets is indicated for the relief of the nasal and non-nasal symptoms of seasonal allergic rhinitis, including nasal congestion, in adults and adolescents 12 years of age and older. CLARINEX-D 12 HOUR Extended Release Tablets should be administered when the antihistaminic properties of desloratadine and the nasal decongestant properties of pseudoephedrine are desired *[see Clinical Pharmacology (12)].*

2   DOSAGE AND ADMINISTRATION
Administer CLARINEX-D 12 HOUR Extended Release Tablet by the oral route only. Do not break, chew, or crush the tablet. Swallow the tablet whole.
2.1   Adults and Adolescents 12 years of Age and Over
The recommended dose of CLARINEX-D 12 HOUR Extended Release Tablets is 1 tablet twice a day, administered approximately 12 hours apart and with or without a meal. Higher doses or increased dosing frequency of CLARINEX-D 12 HOUR Extended Release Tablets have not demonstrated increased effectiveness. Do not exceed the recommended dose as desloratadine and pseudoephedrine, the active components of CLARINEX-D 12 HOUR Extended Release Tablets have been associated with adverse effects at higher doses *[see Overdosage (10.1) and (10.2)].*

3   DOSAGE FORMS AND STRENGTHS
CLARINEX-D 12 HOUR Extended Release Tablets are oval shaped, blue and white bilayer tablets with "D12" embossed in the blue layer. Each tablet contains 2.5 mg desloratadine in the blue immediate-release layer and 120 mg of pseudoephedrine sulfate USP in the white extended-release layer.

4   CONTRAINDICATIONS
CLARINEX-D 12 HOUR Extended Release Tablets are contraindicated in:
• Patients with hypersensitivity to any of its ingredients, or to loratadine *[see Warnings and Precautions (5.4) and Adverse Reactions (6.2)]*
• Patients with narrow-angle glaucoma
• Patients with urinary retention
• Patients receiving monoamine oxidase (MAO) inhibitor therapy or within fourteen (14) days of stopping such treatment *[see Drug Interactions (7.1)]*
• Patients with severe hypertension or severe coronary artery disease

5   WARNINGS AND PRECAUTIONS
5.1   Cardiovascular and Central Nervous System Effects
The pseudoephedrine sulfate contained in CLARINEX-D 12 HOUR Extended Release Tablets, like other sympathomimetic amines, can produce cardiovascular and central nervous system (CNS) effects in some patients such as insomnia, dizziness, weakness, tremor, or arrhythmias. In addition, central nervous system stimulation with convulsions or cardiovascular collapse with accompanying hypotension has been reported. Therefore, CLARINEX-D 12 HOUR Extended Release Tablets should be used with caution in patients with cardiovascular disorders, and should not be used in patients with severe hypertension or severe coronary artery disease.
5.2   Coexisting Conditions
CLARINEX-D 12 HOUR Extended Release Tablets contain pseudoephedrine sulfate, a sympathomimetic amine, and therefore should be used with caution in patients with diabetes and hyperthyroidism. Also use with caution in patients with prostatic hypertrophy or increased intraocular pressure, as urinary retention and narrow-angle glaucoma may occur *[see Contraindications (4)].*
5.3   Co-Administration with Monoamine Oxidase (MAO) Inhibitors
CLARINEX-D 12 HOUR Extended Release Tablets should not be used in patients receiving monoamine oxidase (MAO) inhibitor therapy or within fourteen (14) days of stopping such treatment as an increase in blood pressure or hypertensive crisis, may occur *[see Contraindications (4) and Drug Interactions (7.1)].*
5.4   Hypersensitivity Reactions
Hypersensitivity reactions including rash, pruritus, urticaria, edema, dyspnea, and anaphylaxis have been reported after administration of desloratadine a component of CLARINEX-D 12 HOUR Extended Release Tablets. If such a reaction occurs, therapy with CLARINEX-D 12 HOUR Extended Release Tablets should be stopped and alternative treatment should be considered *[see Adverse Reactions (6.2)].*
5.5   Renal Impairment
CLARINEX-D 12 HOUR Extended Release Tablets should generally be avoided in patients with renal impairment *[see Clinical Pharmacology (12)].*
5.6   Hepatic Impairment
CLARINEX-D 12 HOUR Extended Release Tablets should generally be avoided in patients with hepatic impairment *[see Clinical Pharmacology (12)].*

6   ADVERSE REACTIONS
The following adverse reactions are discussed in greater detail in other sections of the label:
• Cardiovascular and Central Nervous System effects *[see Warnings and Precautions (5.1)]*
• Increased intraocular pressure *[see Warnings and Precautions (5.2)]*
• Urinary retention in patients with prostatic hypertrophy *[see Warnings and Precautions (5.2)]*
• Hypersensitivity reactions *[see Warnings and Precautions (5.4)]*

6.1   Clinical Trials Experience
Because clinical trials are conducted under widely varying conditions, adverse reaction rates observed in the clinical trials of a drug cannot be directly compared to rates in the clinical trials of another drug and may not reflect the rates observed in clinical practice.
The safety data described below are from 2 clinical trials with CLARINEX-D 12 HOUR Extended Release Tablets that included 1248 patients with seasonal allergic rhinitis, of which 414 patients received CLARINEX-D 12 HOUR Extended Release Tablets twice daily for up to 2 weeks. The majority of patients were between 18 and <65 years of age with a mean age of 35.8 years and were predominantly women (64%). Patient ethnicity was 82% Caucasian, 9% Black, 6% Hispanic and 3% Asian/other ethnicity. The percentage of subjects receiving CLARINEX-D 12 HOUR Extended Release Tablets and who discontinued from the clinical trials because of an adverse event was 3.6%. Adverse reactions that were reported by ≥2% of subjects receiving CLARINEX-D 12 HOUR Extended Release Tablets are shown in **Table 1.**
[See table 1 at top of next page]
There were no relevant differences in adverse reactions for subgroups of patients as defined by gender, age, or race.
6.2   Post-Marketing Experience
In addition to the adverse reactions reported during clinical trials and listed above, adverse events have been identified

during post approval use of CLARINEX-D 12 HOUR Extended Release Tablets. Because these events are reported voluntarily from a population of uncertain size, it is not always possible to reliably estimate their frequency or establish a causal relationship to drug exposure. Adverse events identified from post-marketing surveillance on the use of CLARINEX-D 12 HOUR Extended Release Tablets include tachycardia, palpitations, dyspnea, rash and pruritus.

In addition to these events, the following spontaneous adverse events have been reported during the marketing of desloratadine as a single ingredient product: headache, somnolence, dizziness and rarely hypersensitivity reactions (such as urticaria, edema and anaphylaxis), psychomotor hyperactivity, movement disorders (including dystonia, tics, and extrapyramidal symptoms), seizures, and elevated liver enzymes including bilirubin and, very rarely, hepatitis.

7 DRUG INTERACTIONS

No specific interaction studies have been conducted with CLARINEX-D 12 HOUR Extended Release Tablets.

7.1 Monoamine Oxidase Inhibitors

CLARINEX-D 12 HOUR Extended Release Tablets should not be used in patients receiving monoamine oxidase (MAO) inhibitor therapy or within fourteen (14) days of stopping such treatment because the action of pseudoephedrine a component of CLARINEX-D 12 HOUR Extended Release tablets on the vascular system may be potentiated by these agents [see Contraindications (4) and Warnings and Precautions (5.3)].

7.2 Beta-Adrenergic Blocking Agents

The antihypertensive effects of beta-adrenergic blocking agents, methyldopa, and reserpine, may be reduced by sympathomimetics such as pseudoephedrine. Exercise caution when using CLARINEX-D 12 HOUR Extended Release Tablets with these agents.

7.3 Digitalis

Increased ectopic pacemaker activity can occur when pseudoephedrine is used concomitantly with digitalis. Exercise caution when using CLARINEX-D 12 HOUR Extended Release Tablets with these agents.

7.4 Inhibitors of Cytochrome P450 3A4

In controlled clinical studies co-administration of desloratadine with ketoconazole, erythromycin, or azithromycin resulted in increased plasma concentrations of desloratadine and 3-hydroxydesloratadine but there were no clinically relevant changes in the safety profile of desloratadine [see Clinical Pharmacology (12.3)].

7.5 Fluoxetine

In controlled clinical studies co-administration of desloratadine with fluoxetine, a selective serotonin reuptake inhibitor (SSRI), resulted in increased plasma concentrations of desloratadine and 3-hydroxydesloratadine but there were no clinically relevant changes in the safety profile of desloratadine [see Clinical Pharmacology (12.3)].

7.6 Cimetidine

In controlled clinical studies co-administration of desloratadine with cimetidine a histamine H_2-receptor antagonist resulted in increased plasma concentrations of desloratadine and 3-hydroxydesloratadine but there were no clinically relevant changes in the safety profile of desloratadine [see Clinical Pharmacology (12.3)].

8 USE IN SPECIFIC POPULATIONS

8.1 Pregnancy

Pregnancy Category C: There are no adequate and well-controlled studies of desloratadine and pseudoephedrine in combination in pregnant women. Neither are there animal reproduction studies conducted with the combination of desloratadine and pseudoephedrine. Desloratadine was not teratogenic in rats or rabbits but affected implantation in rats. Because animal reproduction studies are not always predictive of human response, CLARINEX-D 12 HOUR Extended Release Tablets should be used during pregnancy only if clearly needed.

Desloratadine was not teratogenic in rats or rabbits at approximately 210 and 230 times, respectively, the AUC in humans at the recommended daily oral dose. An increase in pre-implantation loss and a decreased number of implantations and fetuses were noted, however, in a separate study in female rats at approximately 120 times the AUC in humans at the recommended daily oral dose. Reduced body weight and slow righting reflex were reported in pups at approximately 50 times or greater than the AUC in humans at the recommended daily oral dose. Desloratadine had no effect on pup development at approximately 7 times the AUC in humans at the recommended daily oral dose. The AUCs in comparison referred to the desloratadine exposure in rabbits and the sum of desloratadine and its metabolites exposures in rats, respectively [see Nonclinical Toxicology (13.2)].

8.3 Nursing Mothers

Desloratadine and pseudoephedrine both pass into breast milk; therefore, a decision should be made whether to discontinue nursing or to discontinue CLARINEX-D 12 HOUR Extended Release Tablets, taking into account the benefit of the drug to the nursing mother and the possible risk to the child.

8.4 Pediatric Use

CLARINEX-D 12 HOUR Extended Release Tablets are not indicated for use in pediatric patients under 12 years of age.

8.5 Geriatric Use

The number of subjects (n=10) ≥65 years old treated with CLARINEX-D 12 HOUR Extended Release Tablets was too limited to make any formal statistical comparison regarding the efficacy or safety of this drug product in this age group, or to determine whether they respond differently from younger subjects. Other reported clinical experience has not identified differences between the elderly and younger patients, although the elderly are more likely to have adverse reactions to sympathomimetic amines. In general, dose selection for an elderly patient should be cautious, reflecting the greater frequency of decreased hepatic, renal, or cardiac function, and of concomitant disease or other drug therapy [see Clinical Pharmacology (12.3)].

Pseudoephedrine, desloratadine, and their metabolites are known to be substantially excreted by the kidney, and the risk of adverse reactions may be greater in patients with renal impairment. Because elderly patients are more likely to have decreased renal function, care should be taken in dose selection, and it may be useful to monitor the patient for adverse events [see Clinical Pharmacology (12.3)].

8.6 Renal Impairment

No studies with CLARINEX-D 12 HOUR Extended Release Tablets were conducted in subjects with renal impairment. CLARINEX-D 12 HOUR Extended Release Tablets should generally be avoided in patients with renal impairment [see Warnings and Precautions (5.5) and Clinical Pharmacology (12.3)].

8.7 Hepatic Impairment

No studies with CLARINEX-D 12 HOUR Extended Release Tablets or pseudoephedrine were conducted in subjects with hepatic impairment. CLARINEX-D 12 HOUR Extended Release Tablets should generally be avoided in patients with hepatic impairment [see Warnings and Precautions (5.6) and Clinical Pharmacology (12.3)].

8.8 Gender

No clinically significant gender-related differences were observed in the pharmacokinetic parameters of desloratadine, 3-hydroxydesloratadine or pseudoephedrine following administration of CLARINEX-D 12 HOUR Extended Release Tablets.

8.9 Race

No studies have been conducted to evaluate the effect of race on the pharmacokinetics of CLARINEX-D 12 HOUR Extended Release Tablets.

9 DRUG ABUSE AND DEPENDENCE

There is no information to indicate that abuse or dependency occurs with CLARINEX or CLARINEX-D 12 HOUR Extended Release Tablets.

10 OVERDOSAGE

In the event of overdose, consider standard measures to remove any unabsorbed drug. Symptomatic and supportive treatment is recommended. Desloratadine and 3-hydroxydesloratadine are not eliminated by hemodialysis.

10.1 Desloratadine

Information regarding acute overdosage with desloratadine is limited to experience from post-marketing adverse event reports and from clinical trials conducted during the development of the CLARINEX product. In the reported cases of overdose, there were no significant adverse events that were attributed to desloratadine. In a dose-ranging trial, at doses of 10 mg and 20 mg/day, somnolence was reported.

In another study, no clinically relevant adverse events were reported in normal male and female volunteers who were given single daily doses of CLARINEX 45 mg for 10 days [see Clinical Pharmacology (12.2)].

Lethality occurred in rats at oral doses of 250 mg/kg or greater (estimated desloratadine and desloratadine metabolite exposures were approximately 120 times the AUC in humans at the recommended daily oral dose). The oral median lethal dose in mice was 353 mg/kg (estimated desloratadine exposure was approximately 290 times the human daily oral dose on an mg/m^2 basis). No deaths occurred at oral doses up to 250 mg/kg in monkeys (estimated desloratadine exposure was approximately 810 times the human daily oral dose on an mg/m^2 basis).

10.2 Sympathomimetics

In large doses, sympathomimetics such as pseudoephedrine may give rise to giddiness, headache, nausea, vomiting, sweating, thirst, tachycardia, precordial pain, palpitations, difficulty in micturition, muscle weakness and tenseness, anxiety, restlessness, and insomnia. Many patients can present a toxic psychosis with delusions and hallucinations. Some may develop cardiac arrhythmias, circulatory collapse, convulsions, coma, and respiratory failure.

11 DESCRIPTION

CLARINEX-D 12 HOUR Extended Release Tablets are oval-shaped blue and white bilayer tablets containing 2.5 mg desloratadine in the blue immediate-release layer and 120 mg of pseudoephedrine sulfate USP in the white extended-release layer which is released slowly, allowing for twice-daily administration.

The inactive ingredients contained in CLARINEX-D 12 HOUR Extended Release Tablets are hypromellose USP, microcrystalline cellulose NF, povidone USP, silicon dioxide NF, magnesium stearate NF, corn starch NF, edetate disodium USP, citric acid anhydrous USP, stearic acid NF, and FD&C Blue No. 2 aluminum lake dye.

Desloratadine, 1 of the 2 active ingredients of CLARINEX-D 12 HOUR Extended Release Tablets, is a white to off-white powder that is slightly soluble in water, but very soluble in ethanol and propylene glycol. It has an empirical formula: $C_{19}H_{19}ClN_2$ and a molecular weight of 310.8. The chemical name is 8-chloro-6,11-dihydro-11-(4-piperidinylidene)-5*H*-benzo[5,6] cyclohepta [1,2-*b*]pyridine and has the following structure:

Table 1: Incidence of Adverse Reactions Reported by ≥2% of Subjects Receiving CLARINEX-D 12 HOUR Extended Release Tablets

Adverse Reaction	CLARINEX-D 12 HOUR BID (N=414)	Desloratadine 5 mg QD (N=412)	Pseudoephedrine 120 mg BID (N=422)
Gastrointestinal Disorders			
Mouth Dry	8%	2%	8%
Nausea	2%	1%	3%
General Disorders and Administration Site Conditions			
Fatigue	4%	2%	2%
Metabolism and Nutrition Disorders			
Anorexia	2%	0%	2%
Nervous System Disorders			
Headache	8%	8%	9%
Somnolence	3%	4%	2%
Dizziness	3%	2%	2%
Psychiatric Disorders			
Insomnia	10%	3%	13%
Respiratory, Thoracic, and Mediastinal Disorders			
Pharyngitis	3%	3%	3%

Pseudoephedrine sulfate, the other active ingredient of CLARINEX-D 12 HOUR Extended Release Tablets, is the synthetic salt of one of the naturally occurring dextrorotatory diastereomers of ephedrine and is classified as an indirect sympathomimetic amine. Pseudoephedrine sulfate is a colorless hygroscopic crystal or white, hygroscopic crystalline powder, practically odorless, with a bitter taste. It is very soluble in water, freely soluble in alcohol, and sparingly soluble in ether. The empirical formula for pseudoephedrine sulfate is $(C_{10}H_{15}NO)_2 \cdot H_2SO_4$; the chemical name is benzenemethanol, α-[1-(methylamino) ethyl]-, [S-(R^*,R^*)]-, sulfate (2:1)(salt); and the chemical structure is:

$$\left[\begin{array}{c} \text{NHCH}_3 \\ \text{H} \quad | \\ | \quad | \\ \text{C} - \text{C} - \text{CH}_3 \\ | \quad | \\ \text{OH} \quad \text{H} \end{array} \right]_2 \cdot H_2SO_4$$

12 CLINICAL PHARMACOLOGY

12.1 Mechanism of Action

Desloratadine is a long acting tricyclic histamine antagonist with selective H_1-receptor histamine antagonist activity. Receptor binding data indicate that at a concentration of 2 to 3 ng/mL (7 nanomolar), desloratadine shows significant interaction with the human histamine H_1 receptor. Desloratadine inhibited histamine release from human mast cells *in vitro*. Results of a radiolabeled tissue distribution study in rats and a radioligand H_1-receptor-binding study in guinea pigs showed that desloratadine does not readily cross the blood brain barrier. The clinical significance of this finding is unknown.

Pseudoephedrine sulfate is an orally active sympathomimetic amine and exerts a decongestant action on the nasal mucosa. Pseudoephedrine sulfate is recognized as an effective agent for the relief of nasal congestion due to allergic rhinitis. Pseudoephedrine produces peripheral effects similar to those of ephedrine and central effects similar to, but less intense than, amphetamines. It has the potential for excitatory side effects.

12.2 Pharmacodynamics

Wheal and Flare: Human histamine skin wheal studies following single and repeated 5 mg doses of desloratadine have shown that the drug exhibits an antihistaminic effect by 1 hour; this activity may persist for as long as 24 hours. There was no evidence of histamine-induced skin wheal tachyphylaxis within the desloratadine 5 mg group over the 28-day treatment period. The clinical relevance of histamine wheal skin testing is unknown.

Effects on QT$_c$: In clinical trials for CLARINEX-D 12 HOUR Extended Release Tablets, ECGs were recorded at baseline and endpoint within 1 to 3 hours after the last dose. The majority of ECGs were normal at both baseline and endpoint. No clinically meaningful changes were observed following treatment with CLARINEX-D 12 HOUR Extended Release Tablets for any ECG parameter, including the QT$_c$ interval. An increase in the ventricular rate of 7.1 and 6.4 bpm was observed in the CLARINEX-D 12 HOUR Extended Release Tablets and pseudoephedrine groups, respectively, compared to an increase of 3.2 bpm in subjects receiving desloratadine alone. Single daily doses of CLARINEX 45 mg were given to normal male and female volunteers for 10 days.

All ECGs obtained in this study were manually read in a blinded fashion by a cardiologist. In the CLARINEX-treated subjects, there was a mean increase in the maximum heart rate of 9.2 bpm relative to placebo. The QT interval was corrected for heart rate (QT$_c$) by both Bazett's and Fridericia methods. Using the QT$_c$ (Bazett), there was a mean increase of 8.1 msec in the CLARINEX-treated subjects relative to placebo. Using QT$_c$ (Fridericia) there was a mean increase of 0.4 msec in CLARINEX-treated subjects relative to placebo. No clinically relevant adverse events were reported.

12.3 Pharmacokinetics

Absorption: In a single dose pharmacokinetic study, the mean time to maximum plasma concentrations (T$_{max}$) for desloratadine occurred at approximately 4 to 5 hours post dose and mean peak plasma concentrations (C$_{max}$) and area under the concentration-time curve (AUC) of approximately 1.09 ng/mL and 31.6 ng·hr/mL, respectively, were observed. In another pharmacokinetic study, food and grapefruit juice had no effect on the bioavailability (C$_{max}$ and AUC) of desloratadine.

For pseudoephedrine, the mean T$_{max}$ occurred at 6 to 7 hours post dose and mean peak plasma concentrations (C$_{max}$) and area under the concentration-time curve (AUC) of approximately 263 ng/mL and 4588 ng·hr/mL, respectively, were observed. Food had no effect on the bioavailability (C$_{max}$ and AUC) of pseudoephedrine.

Following oral administration of CLARINEX-D 12 HOUR Extended Release Tablets twice daily for 14 days in healthy volunteers, steady-state conditions were reached on Day 10 for desloratadine, 3-hydroxydesloratadine and pseudoephedrine. For desloratadine, mean steady-state peak plasma concentrations (C$_{max}$) and area under the concentration-time curve AUC $_{0-12\,hrs}$ of approximately 1.7 ng/mL and 16 ng·hr/mL were observed, respectively. For pseudoephedrine, mean steady-state peak plasma concentrations (C$_{max}$) and AUC $_{0-12\,hrs}$ of 459 ng/mL and 4658 ng·hr/mL were observed.

Distribution: Desloratadine and 3-hydroxydesloratadine are approximately 82% to 87% and 85% to 89%, bound to plasma proteins, respectively. Protein binding of desloratadine and 3-hydroxydesloratadine was unaltered in subjects with impaired renal function.

Metabolism: Desloratadine (a major metabolite of loratadine) is extensively metabolized to 3-hydroxydesloratadine, an active metabolite, which is subsequently glucuronidated. The enzyme(s) responsible for the formation of 3-hydroxydesloratadine have not been identified. Data from clinical trials with desloratadine indicate that a subset of the general population has a decreased ability to form 3-hydroxydesloratadine, and are poor metabolizers of desloratadine. In pharmacokinetic studies (n=3748), approximately 6% of subjects were poor metabolizers of desloratadine (defined as a subject with an AUC ratio of 3-hydroxydesloratadine to desloratadine less than 0.1, or a subject with a desloratadine half-life exceeding 50 hours). These pharmacokinetic studies included subjects between the ages of 2 and 70 years, including 977 subjects aged 2 to 5 years, 1575 subjects aged 6 to 11 years, and 1196 subjects aged 12 to 70 years. There was no difference in the prevalence of poor metabolizers across age groups. The frequency of poor metabolizers was higher in Blacks (17%, n=988) as compared to Caucasians (2%, n=1462) and Hispanics (2%, n=1063). The median exposure (AUC) to desloratadine in the poor metabolizers was approximately 6-fold greater than in the subjects who are not poor metabolizers. Subjects who are poor metabolizers of desloratadine cannot be prospectively identified and will be exposed to higher levels of desloratadine following dosing with the recommended dose of desloratadine. In multidose clinical safety studies, where metabolizer status was prospectively identified, a total of 94 poor metabolizers and 123 normal metabolizers were enrolled and treated with CLARINEX Syrup for 15 to 35 days. In these studies, no overall differences in safety were observed between poor metabolizers and normal metabolizers. Although not seen in these studies, an increased risk of exposure-related adverse events in patients who are poor metabolizers cannot be ruled out.

Pseudoephedrine alone is incompletely metabolized (less than 1%) in the liver by N-demethylation to an inactive metabolite. The drug and its metabolite are excreted in the urine. About 55% to 96% of an administered dose of pseudoephedrine hydrochloride is excreted unchanged in the urine.

Elimination: Following single dose administration of CLARINEX-D 12 HOUR Extended Release Tablets, the mean plasma elimination half-life of desloratadine was approximately 27 hours. In another study, following administration of single oral doses of desloratadine 5 mg, C$_{max}$ and AUC values increased in a dose proportional manner following single oral doses between 5 and 20 mg. The degree of accumulation after 14 days of dosing was consistent with the half-life and dosing frequency. A human mass balance study documented a recovery of approximately 87% of the ^{14}C-desloratadine dose, which was equally distributed in urine and feces as metabolic products. Analysis of plasma 3-hydroxydesloratadine showed similar T$_{max}$ and half-life values compared to desloratadine.

The mean elimination half-life of pseudoephedrine is dependent on urinary pH. The elimination half-life is approximately 3 to 6 or 9 to 16 hours when the urinary pH is 5 or 8, respectively.

Geriatric Subjects: Following multiple-dose administration of CLARINEX Tablets, the mean C$_{max}$ and AUC values for desloratadine were 20% greater than in younger subjects (< 65 years old). The oral total body clearance (CL/F) when normalized for body weight was similar between the 2 age groups. The mean plasma elimination half-life of desloratadine was 33.7 hr in subjects ≥65 years old. The pharmacokinetics for 3-hydroxydesloratadine appeared unchanged in older vs. younger subjects. These age-related differences are unlikely to be clinically relevant and no dosage adjustment is recommended in elderly patients.

Pediatric Subjects: CLARINEX-D 12 HOUR Extended Release Tablets are not an appropriate dosage form for use in pediatric patients below 12 years of age.

Renally Impaired: Following a single dose of desloratadine 7.5 mg, pharmacokinetics were characterized in subjects with mild (n=7; creatinine clearance 51–69 mL/min/1.73 m²), moderate (n=6; creatinine clearance 34–43 mL/min/1.73 m²) and severe (n=6; creatinine clearance 5–29 mL/min/1.73 m²) renal impairment or hemodialysis dependent (n=6) subjects. In subjects with mild and moderate renal impairment, median C$_{max}$ and AUC values increased by approximately 1.2- and 1.9-fold, respectively, relative to subjects with normal renal function. In subjects with severe renal impairment or who were hemodialysis dependent, C$_{max}$ and AUC values increased by approximately 1.7- and 2.5-fold, respectively. Minimal changes in 3-hydroxydesloratadine concentrations were observed. Desloratadine and 3-hydroxydesloratadine were poorly removed by hemodialysis. Plasma protein binding of desloratadine and 3-hydroxydesloratadine was unaltered by renal impairment.

Pseudoephedrine is primarily excreted unchanged in the urine as unchanged drug with the remainder apparently being metabolized in the liver. Therefore, pseudoephedrine may accumulate in patients with renal impairment.

Hepatically Impaired: Following a single oral dose of desloratadine, pharmacokinetics were characterized in subjects with mild (n=4), moderate (n=4) and severe (n=4) hepatic impairment as defined by the Child-Pugh classification of hepatic impairment and 8 subjects with normal hepatic function. Subjects with hepatic impairment, regardless of severity, had approximately a 2.4-fold increase in AUC as compared with normal subjects. The apparent oral clearance of desloratadine in subjects with mild, moderate, and severe hepatic impairment was 37%, 36%, and 28% of that in normal subjects, respectively. An increase in the mean elimination half-life of desloratadine in subjects with hepatic impairment was observed. For 3-hydroxydesloratadine, the mean C$_{max}$ and AUC values for subjects with hepatic impairment combined were not statistically significantly different from subjects with normal hepatic function.

Gender: Female subjects treated for 14 days with CLARINEX Tablets had 10% and 3% higher desloratadine C$_{max}$ and AUC values, respectively, compared with male subjects. The 3-hydroxydesloratadine C$_{max}$ and AUC values were also increased by 45% and 48%, respectively, in females compared with males. However, these apparent differences are not considered to be clinically relevant.

Race: Following 14 days of treatment with CLARINEX Tablets, the C$_{max}$ and AUC values for desloratadine were 18% and 32% higher, respectively in Blacks compared with Caucasians. For 3-hydroxydesloratadine there was a corresponding 10% reduction in C$_{max}$ and AUC values in Blacks compared to Caucasians. These differences are not considered to be clinically relevant.

Drug Interaction: In 2 controlled crossover clinical pharmacology studies in healthy male (n=12 in each study) and female (n=12 in each study) subjects, desloratadine 7.5 mg (1.5 times the daily dose) once daily was co-administered with erythromycin 500 mg every 8 hours or ketoconazole 200 mg every 12 hours for 10 days. In 3 separate controlled, parallel group clinical pharmacology studies, desloratadine at the clinical dose of 5 mg has been co-administered with azithromycin 500 mg followed by 250 mg once daily for 4 days (n=18) or with fluoxetine 20 mg once daily for 7 days after a 23-day pretreatment period with fluoxetine (n=18) or with cimetidine 600 mg every 12 hours for 14 days (n=18) under steady state conditions to healthy male and female subjects. Although increased plasma concentrations (C$_{max}$ and AUC $_{0-24\,hrs}$) of desloratadine and 3-hydroxydesloratadine were observed (see **Table 2**), there were no clinically relevant changes in the safety profile of desloratadine, as assessed by electrocardiographic parameters (including the corrected QT interval), clinical laboratory tests, vital signs and adverse events.
[See table 2 at top of next page]

13 NONCLINICAL TOXICOLOGY

13.1 Carcinogenesis, Mutagenesis, Impairment of Fertility

There are no animal or laboratory studies on the combination product of desloratadine and pseudoephedrine sulfate to evaluate carcinogenesis, mutagenesis, or impairment of fertility.

Carcinogenicity Studies: The carcinogenic potential of desloratadine was assessed using a loratadine study in rats and a desloratadine study in mice. In a 2-year study in rats, loratadine was administered in the diet at doses up to 25 mg/kg/day (estimated desloratadine and desloratadine metabolite exposures were approximately 30 times the AUC in humans at the recommended daily oral dose). A significantly higher incidence of hepatocellular tumors (combined adenomas and carcinomas) was observed in males given 10 mg/kg/day of loratadine and in males and females given 25 mg/kg/day of loratadine. The estimated desloratadine and desloratadine metabolite exposures in rats given

10 mg/kg of loratadine were approximately 7 times the AUC in humans at the recommended daily oral dose. The clinical significance of these findings during long-term use of desloratadine is not known.

In a 2-year dietary study in mice, males and females given up to 16 mg/kg/day and 32 mg/kg/day desloratadine, respectively, did not show significant increases in the incidence of any tumors. The estimated desloratadine and desloratadine metabolite exposures in mice at these doses were 12 and 27 times, respectively, the AUC in humans at the recommended daily oral dose.

Genotoxicity Studies: In genotoxicity studies with desloratadine, there was no evidence of genotoxic potential in a reverse mutation assay (*Salmonella/E. coli* mammalian microsome bacterial mutagenicity assay) or in 2 assays for chromosomal aberrations (human peripheral blood lymphocyte clastogenicity assay and mouse bone marrow micronucleus assay).

Impairment of Fertility: There was no effect on female fertility in rats at desloratadine doses up to 24 mg/kg/day (estimated desloratadine and desloratadine metabolite exposures were approximately 130 times the AUC in humans at the recommended daily oral dose). A male-specific decrease in fertility, demonstrated by reduced female conception rates, decreased sperm numbers and motility, and histopathologic testicular changes, occurred at an oral desloratadine dose of 12 mg/kg (estimated desloratadine and desloratadine metabolite exposures were approximately 45 times the AUC in humans at the recommended daily oral dose). Desloratadine had no effect on fertility in rats at an oral dose of 3 mg/kg/day (estimated desloratadine and desloratadine metabolite exposures were approximately 8 times the AUC in humans at the recommended daily oral dose).

13.2 Animal Toxicology and/or Pharmacology

Reproductive Toxicology Studies: Desloratadine was not teratogenic in rats at doses up to 48 mg/kg/day (estimated desloratadine and desloratadine metabolite exposures were approximately 210 times the AUC in humans at the recommended daily oral dose) or in rabbits at doses up to 60 mg/kg/day (estimated desloratadine exposures were approximately 230 times the AUC in humans at the recommended daily oral dose). In a separate study, an increase in pre-implantation loss and a decreased number of implantations and fetuses were noted in female rats at 24 mg/kg (estimated desloratadine and desloratadine metabolite exposures were approximately 120 times the AUC in humans at the recommended daily oral dose). Reduced body weight and slow righting reflex were reported in pups at doses of 9 mg/kg/day or greater (estimated desloratadine and desloratadine metabolite exposures were approximately 50 times or greater than the AUC in humans at the recommended daily oral dose). Desloratadine had no effect on pup development at an oral dose of 3 mg/kg/day (estimated desloratadine and desloratadine metabolite exposures were approximately 7 times the AUC in humans at the recommended daily oral dose).

14 CLINICAL STUDIES

14.1 Seasonal Allergic Rhinitis

The clinical efficacy and safety of CLARINEX-D 12 HOUR Extended Release Tablets was evaluated in two 2-week multicenter, randomized parallel group clinical trials involving 1248 subjects 12 to 78 years of age with seasonal allergic rhinitis, 414 of whom received CLARINEX-D 12 HOUR Extended Release Tablets. In the 2 trials, subjects were randomized to receive CLARINEX-D 12 HOUR Extended Release Tablets twice daily, CLARINEX Tablets 5 mg once daily, or sustained-release pseudoephedrine tablet 120 mg twice daily for 2 weeks. The majority of patients were between 18 and <65 years of age with a mean age of 35.8 years and were predominantly women (64%). Patient ethnicity was 82% Caucasian, 9% Black, 6% Hispanic and 3% Asian/other ethnicity. Primary efficacy variable was twice-daily reflective patient scoring of 4 nasal symptoms (rhinorrhea, nasal stuffiness/congestion, nasal itching, and sneezing) and four non-nasal symptoms (itching/burning eyes, tearing/watering eyes, redness of eyes, and itching of ears/palate) on a 4 point scale (0=none, 1=mild, 2=moderate, and 3=severe). In both trials, the antihistaminic efficacy of CLARINEX-D 12 HOUR Extended Release Tablets, as measured by total symptom score excluding nasal congestion, was significantly greater than pseudoephedrine alone over the 2-week treatment period; and the decongestant efficacy of CLARINEX-D 12 HOUR Extended Release Tablets, as measured by nasal stuffiness/congestion, was significantly greater than CLARINEX (desloratadine alone) over the 2-week treatment period. Primary efficacy variable results from 1 of 2 trials are shown in **Table 3**.
[See table 3 above]

There were no significant differences in the efficacy of CLARINEX-D 12 HOUR Extended Release Tablets across subgroups of subjects defined by gender, age, or race.

16 HOW SUPPLIED/STORAGE AND HANDLING

CLARINEX-D 12 HOUR Extended Release Tablets are oval-shaped, blue and white bilayer tablets with "D12" embossed in the blue layer, containing 2.5 mg desloratadine in the blue immediate-release layer and 120 mg of pseudoephedrine sulfate USP in the white extended-release layer. CLARINEX-D 12 HOUR Extended Release Tablets are supplied in high-density polyethylene bottles of 100 (NDC 0085-1322-01).

Storage: Store at 25°C (77°F); excursions permitted to 15°–30°C (59°–86°F) [see USP Controlled Room Temperature]. Avoid exposure at or above 30°C (86°F). Protect from excessive moisture. Protect from light.

17 PATIENT COUNSELING INFORMATION

See FDA-approved patient labeling (Patient Information).

17.1 Cardiovascular and Central Nervous System Effects

Patients should be informed that pseudoephedrine, one of the active ingredients in CLARINEX-D 12 HOUR Extended Release Tablets may cause cardiovascular or central nervous system effects such as insomnia, dizziness, tremor, or arrhythmia.

17.2 Dosing

Patients should be advised not to increase the dose or dosing frequency of CLARINEX-D 12 HOUR Extended Release Tablets.

17.3 Additional Antihistamines and/or Decongestants

Patients should be advised against the concurrent use of CLARINEX-D 12 HOUR Extended Release Tablets with other antihistamines and/or decongestants.

17.4 Monoamine Oxidase (MAO) Inhibitors

Patients should be informed that due to its pseudoephedrine component, they should not use CLARINEX-D 12 HOUR with a monoamine oxidase (MAO) inhibitor or within 14 days of stopping use of an MAO inhibitor.

17.5 Coexisting Conditions

Patients with severe hypertension or severe coronary artery disease, narrow-angle glaucoma, or urinary retention should be advised not to use CLARINEX-D 12 HOUR Extended Release Tablets.

17.6 Instructions for Use

Patients should be instructed not to break, crush, or chew the tablet; the tablet should be swallowed whole, and can be taken without regard to meals.

Manufactured for: Merck Sharp & Dohme Corp., a subsidiary of
MERCK & CO., INC., Whitehouse Station, NJ 08889, USA
Manufactured by:
Patheon Inc., Whitby, Ontario
L1N 5Z5, Canada
For patent information:
www.merck.com/product/patent/home.html
Copyright © 2006, 2009 Merck Sharp & Dohme Corp., a subsidiary of **Merck & Co., Inc.**
All rights reserved.
uspi-mk4117a-t-d12-1403r005
PATIENT INFORMATION
CLARINEX-D® (CLA-RI-NEX) 12 Hour Extended Release Tablets
(desloratadine and pseudoephedrine sulfate)
Read the Patient Information that comes with CLARINEX-D 12 Hour Extended Release Tablets before you start taking it and each time you get a refill. There may be new information. This leaflet is a summary of the information for patients. Your doctor or pharmacist can give you additional information. This leaflet does not take the place of talking to your doctor about your medical condition or treatment.

Table 2: Changes in Desloratadine and 3-hydroxydesloratadine Pharmacokinetics in Healthy Male and Female Subjects

	Desloratadine		3-hydroxydesloratadine	
	C_{max}	$AUC_{0-24hrs}$	C_{max}	$AUC_{0-24hrs}$
Erythromycin (500 mg Q8h)	+24%	+14%	+43%	+40%
Ketoconazole (200 mg Q12h)	+45%	+39%	+43%	+72%
Azithromycin (500 mg Day 1, 250 mg QD × 4 days)	+15%	+5%	+15%	+4%
Fluoxetine (20 mg QD)	+15%	+0%	+17%	+13%
Cimetidine (600 mg Q12h)	+12%	+19%	-11%	-3%

Table 3: Changes in Symptoms in a 2-Week Clinical Trial in Subjects With Seasonal Allergic Rhinitis

Treatment Group (n)	Mean Baseline* (SEM)	Change (% Change) from Baseline† (SEM)	CLARINEX-D 12 HOUR Comparison to Components‡ (P-value)
Total Symptom Score (Excluding Nasal Congestion)			
CLARINEX-D 12 HOUR Extended Release Tablets BID (199)	14.18 (0.21)	-6.54 (-46.0) (0.30)	-
Pseudoephedrine tablet 120 mg BID (197)	14.06 (0.21)	-5.07 (-35.9) (0.30)	**P<0.001**
CLARINEX 5 mg Tablets QD (197)	14.82 (0.21)	-5.09 (-33.5) (0.30)	P<0.001
Nasal Stuffiness/Congestion			
CLARINEX-D 12 HOUR Extended Release Tablets BID (199)	2.47 (0.027)	-0.93 (-37.4) (0.046)	-
Pseudoephedrine tablet 120 mg BID (197)	2.46 (0.027)	-0.75 (-31.2) (0.046)	P=0.006
CLARINEX 5 mg Tablets QD (197)	2.50 (0.027)	-0.66 (-26.7) (0.046)	**P<0.001**

SEM=Standard Error of the Mean
* To qualify at Baseline, the sum of the twice-daily diary reflective scores for the 3 days prior to Baseline and the morning of the Baseline visit were to total ≥42 for total nasal symptom score (sum of 4 nasal symptoms of rhinorrhea, nasal stuffiness/congestion, nasal itching, and sneezing) and a total of ≥35 for total non-nasal symptoms score (sum of 4 non-nasal symptoms of itching/burning eyes, tearing/watering eyes, redness of eyes, and itching of ears/palate), and a score of ≥14 for each of the individual symptoms of nasal stuffiness/congestion and rhinorrhea. Each symptom was scored on a 4-point severity scale (0=none, 1=mild, 2=moderate, 3=severe).
† Mean reduction in score averaged over the 2-week treatment period.
‡ The comparison of interest is shown bolded.

What is CLARINEX-D® 12 Hour Extended Release Tablets?

CLARINEX-D 12 Hour Extended Release Tablets is a prescription medicine that contains the medicines desloratadine (an antihistamine) and pseudoephedrine (a nasal decongestant). CLARINEX-D 12 Hour Extended Release Tablets is used to help control the symptoms of seasonal allergic rhinitis (sneezing, stuffy nose, runny nose and itching of the nose) in adults and children 12 years and older.

CLARINEX-D 12 Hour Extended Release Tablets is not for children under 12 years of age.

Who should not take CLARINEX-D® 12 Hour Extended Release Tablets?

Do not take CLARINEX-D 12 Hour Extended Release Tablets if you:

- are allergic to desloratadine or pseudoephedrine sulfate or any of the ingredients in CLARINEX-D 12 Hour Extended Release Tablets. See the end of this leaflet for a complete list of ingredients in CLARINEX-D 12 Hour Extended Release Tablets.
- are allergic to loratadine (Alavert, Claritin)
- have narrow-angle glaucoma
- have problems with urination (urinary retention)
- take a Monoamine Oxidase Inhibitor (MAOI) medicine to treat depression, or if you stopped taking an MAOI medicine within the last 2 weeks. Ask your doctor or pharmacist if you are not sure if you take an MAOI medicine.
- have severe high blood pressure
- have severe heart disease

Talk to your doctor before taking this medicine if you have any of these conditions.

What should I tell my doctor before taking CLARINEX-D® 12 Hour Extended Release Tablets?

Before you take CLARINEX-D 12 Hour Extended Release Tablets, tell your doctor if you:

- have any of the conditions listed in the section "Who should not take CLARINEX-D 12 Hour Extended Release Tablets?"
- diabetes
- hyperthyroidism
- have prostate problems
- have liver or kidney problems
- have any other medical conditions
- are pregnant or plan to become pregnant. It is not known if CLARINEX-D 12 Hour Extended Release Tablets will harm your unborn baby. Talk to your doctor if you are pregnant or plan to become pregnant.
- are breastfeeding or plan to breastfeed. CLARINEX-D 12 Hour Extended Release Tablets **can pass into your breast milk.** Talk to your doctor about the best way to feed your baby if you take CLARINEX-D 12 Hour Extended Release Tablets.

Tell your doctor about all the medicines you take, including prescription and nonprescription medicines, vitamins and herbal supplements. CLARINEX-D® 12 Hour Extended Release Tablets may affect the way other medicines work, and other medicines may affect how CLARINEX-D 12 Hour Extended Release Tablets works. Especially tell your doctor if you take:

- Monoamine Oxidase Inhibitors (MAOIs). You should not use CLARINEX-D 12 Hour Extended Release Tablets if you take an MAOI or within 2 weeks of stopping an MAOI.
- methyldopa
- reserpine (Serpalan)
- digitalis (Digoxin, Lanoxicaps, Lanoxin) ketoconazole (Nizoral)
- erythromycin (Ery-tab, Eryc, PCE)
- azithromycin (Zithromax, Zmax)
- antihistamines
- other decongestant medicines

Know the medicines you take. Keep a list of your medicines and show it to your doctor and pharmacist when you get a new medicine.

How should I take CLARINEX-D® 12 Hour Extended Release Tablets?

Take CLARINEX-D 12 Hour Extended Release Tablets exactly as your doctor tells you to take it.

- CLARINEX-D 12 Hour Extended Release Tablets can be taken with or without food.
- Swallow CLARINEX-D 12 Hour Extended Release Tablets whole. **Do not break, crush, or chew** CLARINEX-D 12 Hour Extended Release Tablets before swallowing. If you cannot swallow CLARINEX-D 12 Hour Extended Release Tablets whole, tell your doctor. You may need a different medicine.
- Take **1** CLARINEX-D 12 Hour Extended Release Tablet 2 times a day (every 12 hours).

What are the possible side effects of CLARINEX-D® 12 Hour Extended Release Tablets?

CLARINEX-D 12 Hour Extended Release Tablets may cause serious side effects, including:

- Cardiovascular and central nervous system effects, such as

  - unable to sleep (insomnia)
  - dizziness
  - weakness
  - tremor
  - irregular heart beat
  - seizure
  - low blood pressure

- Increased sleepiness or tiredness can happen if you take more CLARINEX-D 12 Hour Extended Release Tablets than your doctor prescribed to you.
- Allergic reactions. Stop taking CLARINEX-D 12 Hour Extended Release Tablets and call your doctor right away or get emergency help if you have any of these symptoms:
  - rash
  - itching
  - hives
  - swelling of your lips, tongue, face, and throat
  - shortness of breath or trouble breathing

The most common side effects of CLARINEX-D 12 HOUR Extended Release Tablets include:

- unable to sleep (insomnia)
- sore throat
- headache
- dizziness
- dry mouth
- nausea
- tiredness
- loss of appetite
- sleepiness

Tell your doctor if you have any side effect that bothers you or that does not go away.

These are not all of the possible side effects of CLARINEX-D 12 Hour Extended Release Tablets. For more information, ask your doctor or pharmacist.

Call your doctor for medical advice about side effects. You may report side effects to FDA at 1-800-FDA-1088.

How should I store CLARINEX-D® 12 Hour Extended Release Tablets?

- Store CLARINEX-D 12 Hour Extended Release Tablets at 59°F to 86°F (15°C to 30°C)
- Keep CLARINEX-D 12 Hour Extended Release Tablets dry and out of the light.

Keep CLARINEX-D 12 Hour Extended Release Tablets and all medicines out of the reach of children.

General information about CLARINEX-D® 12 Hour Extended Release Tablets

Medicines are sometimes prescribed for purposes other than those listed in a patient information leaflet. Do not use CLARINEX-D 12 Hour Extended Release Tablets for a condition for which it was not prescribed. Do not give CLARINEX-D 12 Hour Extended Release Tablets to other people, even if they have the same condition you have. It may harm them.

This patient information leaflet summarizes the most important information about CLARINEX-D 12 Hour Extended Release Tablets. If you would like more information, talk with your doctor. You can ask your pharmacist or doctor for information about CLARINEX-D 12 Hour Extended Release Tablets that is written for health professionals.

For more information, go to **www.CLARINEX.com**

What are the ingredients in CLARINEX-D® 12 Hour Extended Release Tablets?

Active ingredients: desloratadine and pseudoephedrine sulfate

Inactive ingredients: hypromellose USP, microcrystalline cellulose NF, povidone USP, silicon dioxide NF, magnesium stearate NF, corn starch NF, edetate disodium USP, citric acid anhydrous USP, stearic acid NF, and FD&C Blue No. 2 aluminum lake dye.

Manufactured for: Merck Sharp & Dohme Corp., a subsidiary of

MERCK & CO., INC.,Whitehouse Station, NJ 08889, USA

Manufactured by:

Patheon Inc., Whitby, Ontario

L1N 5Z5, Canada

For patent information:

www.merck.com/product/patent/home.html

Copyright © 2006, 2009 Merck Sharp & Dohme Corp., a subsidiary of Merck & Co., Inc.

All rights reserved.

Revised: 03/2014

usppi-mk4117a-t-d12-1403r004

Shown in Product Identification Guide, page 308

COMVAX®   ℞

[com-vax]

[Haemophilus b Conjugate (Meningococcal Protein Conjugate) and Hepatitis B (Recombinant) Vaccine]

DESCRIPTION

COMVAX® [Haemophilus b Conjugate (Meningococcal Protein Conjugate) and Hepatitis B (Recombinant) Vaccine]

is a sterile bivalent vaccine made of the antigenic components used in producing PedvaxHIB® [Haemophilus b Conjugate Vaccine (Meningococcal Protein Conjugate)] and RECOMBIVAX HB® [Hepatitis B Vaccine (Recombinant)]. These components are the *Haemophilus influenzae* type b capsular polysaccharide [polyribosylribitol phosphate (PRP)] that is covalently bound to an outer membrane protein complex (OMPC) of *Neisseria meningitidis* and hepatitis B surface antigen (HBsAg) from recombinant yeast cultures.

Haemophilus influenzae type b and *Neisseria meningitidis* serogroup B are grown in complex fermentation media. The primary ingredients of the phenol-inactivated fermentation medium for *Haemophilus influenzae* include an extract of yeast, nicotinamide adenine dinucleotide, hemin chloride, soy peptone, dextrose, and mineral salts and for *Neisseria meningitidis* include an extract of yeast, amino acids and mineral salts. The PRP is purified from the culture broth by purification procedures which include ethanol fractionation, enzyme digestion, phenol extraction and diafiltration. The OMPC from *Neisseria meningitidis* is purified by detergent extraction, ultracentrifugation, diafiltration and sterile filtration.

The PRP-OMPC conjugate is prepared by the chemical coupling of the highly purified PRP (polyribosylribitol phosphate) of *Haemophilus influenzae* type b (Haemophilus b, Ross strain) to an OMPC of the B11 strain of *Neisseria meningitidis* serogroup B. The coupling of the PRP to the OMPC is necessary for enhanced immunogenicity of the PRP. This coupling is confirmed by analysis of the components of the conjugate following chemical treatment which yields a unique amino acid. After conjugation, the aqueous bulk is then adsorbed onto an amorphous aluminum hydroxyphosphate sulfate adjuvant (previously referred to as aluminum hydroxide).

HBsAg is produced in recombinant yeast cells. A portion of the hepatitis B virus gene, coding for HBsAg, is cloned into yeast, and the vaccine for hepatitis B is produced from cultures of this recombinant yeast strain according to methods developed in the Merck Research Laboratories. The antigen is harvested and purified from fermentation cultures of a recombinant strain of the yeast *Saccharomyces cerevisiae* containing the gene for the *adw* subtype of HBsAg. The fermentation process involves growth of *Saccharomyces cerevisiae* on a complex fermentation medium which consists of an extract of yeast, soy peptone, dextrose, amino acids and mineral salts.

The HBsAg protein is released from the yeast cells by mechanical cell disruption and detergent extraction, and purified by a series of physical and chemical methods, which includes ion and hydrophobic chromatography, and diafiltration. The purified protein is treated in phosphate buffer with formaldehyde and then coprecipitated with alum (potassium aluminum sulfate) to form bulk vaccine adjuvanted with amorphous aluminum hydroxyphosphate sulfate. The vaccine contains no detectable yeast DNA, and 1% or less of the protein is of yeast origin.

The individual PRP-OMPC and HBsAg adjuvanted bulks are combined to produce COMVAX. Each 0.5 mL dose of COMVAX is formulated to contain 7.5 mcg PRP conjugated to approximately 125 mcg OMPC, 5 mcg HBsAg, approximately 225 mcg aluminum as amorphous aluminum hydroxyphosphate sulfate, and 35 mcg sodium borate (decahydrate) as a pH stabilizer, in 0.9% sodium chloride. The vaccine contains not more than 0.0004% (w/v) residual formaldehyde.

The potency of the PRP-OMPC component is measured by quantitating the polysaccharide concentration by an HPLC method. The potency of the HBsAg component is measured relative to a standard by an *in vitro* immunoassay.

The product contains no preservative.

COMVAX is a sterile suspension for intramuscular injection.

CLINICAL PHARMACOLOGY

Haemophilus influenzae type b Disease

Prior to the introduction of *Haemophilus b* conjugate vaccines, *Haemophilus influenzae* type b (Hib) was the most frequent cause of bacterial meningitis and a leading cause of serious, systemic bacterial disease in young children worldwide.[1-4]

Hib disease occurred primarily in children under 5 years of age, and in the United States prior to the initiation of a vaccine program was estimated to account for nearly 20,000 cases of invasive infections annually, approximately 12,000 of which were meningitis. The mortality rate from Hib meningitis is about 5%. In addition, up to 35% of survivors develop neurologic sequelae including seizures, deafness, and mental retardation.[5,6] Other invasive diseases caused by this bacterium include cellulitis, epiglottitis, sepsis, pneumonia, septic arthritis, osteomyelitis, and pericarditis.

Prior to the introduction of the vaccine, it was estimated that 17% of all cases of Hib disease occurred in infants less than 6 months of age. The peak incidence of Hib meningitis occurred between 6 to 11 months of age. Forty-seven percent of all cases occurred by one year of age with the remaining 53% of cases occurring over the next four years.[2,20] Among children under 5 years of age, the risk of invasive Hib disease is increased in certain populations including the following:

- Daycare attendees[7,8,9]
- Lower socio-economic groups[10]
- Blacks[11] (especially those who lack the Km(1) immuno-globulin allotype)[12]
- Caucasians who lack the G2m(23) immunoglobulin allo-type[13]
- Native Americans[14-16]
- Household contacts of cases[17]
- Individuals with asplenia, sickle cell disease, or antibody deficiency syndromes.[18,19]

Prevention of Hib Disease with Vaccine

An important virulence factor of the Hib bacterium is its polysaccharide capsule (PRP). Antibody to PRP (anti-PRP) has been shown to correlate with protection against Hib disease.[3,21] While the anti-PRP level associated with protection using conjugated vaccines has not yet been determined, the level of anti-PRP associated with protection in studies using bacterial polysaccharide immune globulin or nonconjugated PRP vaccines ranged from ≥0.15 to ≥1.0 mcg/mL.[22-23]

Nonconjugated PRP vaccines are capable of stimulating B-lymphocytes to produce antibody without the help of T-lymphocytes (T-independent). The responses to many other antigens are augmented by helper T-lymphocytes (T-dependent). PedvaxHIB is a PRP-conjugate vaccine in which the PRP is covalently bound to the OMPC carrier[29] producing an antigen which is postulated to convert the T-independent antigen (PRP alone) into a T-dependent antigen resulting in both an enhanced antibody response and immunologic memory.

Clinical Trials with PedvaxHIB

The protective efficacy of the PRP-OMPC component of COMVAX was demonstrated in a randomized, double-blind, placebo-controlled study involving 3486 Native American (Navajo) infants (The Protective Efficacy Study) who completed the primary two-dose regimen for lyophilized PedvaxHIB. This population has a much higher incidence of Hib disease than the United States population as a whole and also has a lower antibody response to Haemophilus b conjugate vaccines, including PedvaxHIB.[14-16,30,31]

Each infant in this study received two doses of either placebo or lyophilized PedvaxHIB (15 mcg Haemophilus b PRP) with the first dose administered at a mean of 8 weeks of age and the second administered approximately two months later; DTP (Diphtheria and Tetanus Toxoids and whole cell Pertussis Vaccine, Adsorbed) and OPV (Poliovirus Vaccine Live Oral Trivalent) were administered concomitantly. In a subset of 416 subjects, lyophilized PedvaxHIB (15 mcg Haemophilus b PRP) induced anti-PRP levels >0.15 mcg/mL in 88% and >1.0 mcg/mL in 52% with a geometric mean titer (GMT) of 0.95 mcg/mL one to three months after the first dose; the corresponding anti-PRP levels one to three months following the second dose were 91% and 60%, respectively, with a GMT of 1.43 mcg/mL. These antibody responses were associated with a high level of protection.

Most subjects were initially followed until 15 to 18 months of age. During this time, 22 cases of invasive Hib disease occurred in the placebo group (8 cases after the first dose and 14 cases after the second dose) and only 1 case in the vaccine group (none after the first dose and 1 after the second dose). Following the primary two-dose regimen, the protective efficacy of lyophilized PedvaxHIB was calculated to be 93% with a 95% confidence interval (C.I.) of 57-98%. In the two months between the first and second doses, the difference in number of cases of disease between placebo and vaccine recipients (8 vs 0 cases, respectively) was statistically significant (p=0.008). At termination of the study, placebo recipients were then offered vaccine. All original participants were then followed two years and nine months from termination of the study. During this extended follow-up, invasive Hib disease occurred in an additional 7 of the original placebo recipients prior to receiving vaccine and in 1 of the original vaccine recipients (who had received only 1 dose of vaccine). No cases of invasive Hib disease were observed in placebo recipients after they received at least one dose of vaccine. Efficacy for this follow-up period, estimated from person-days at risk, was 96.6% (95 C.I., 72.2-99.9%) in children under 18 months of age and 100% (95 C.I., 23.5-100%) in children over 18 months of age.[31] Thus, in this study, a protective efficacy of 93% was achieved with an anti-PRP level of >1.0 mcg/mL in 60% of vaccinees and a GMT of 1.43 mcg/mL one to three months after the second dose.

Hepatitis B Disease

Hepatitis B virus is an important cause of viral hepatitis. According to the Centers for Disease Control (CDC), there are an estimated 200,000-300,000 new cases of Hepatitis B infection annually in the United States.[32] There is no spe-

cific treatment for this disease. The incubation period for hepatitis B is relatively long; six weeks to six months may elapse between exposure and the onset of clinical symptoms. The prognosis following infection with hepatitis B virus is variable and dependent on at least three factors: (1) Age — infants and younger children usually experience milder initial disease than older persons but are much more likely to remain persistently infected and become at risk of developing serious chronic liver disease; (2) Dose of virus — the higher the dose, the more likely acute icteric hepatitis B will result; and, (3) Severity of associated underlying disease — underlying malignancy or pre-existing hepatic disease predisposes to increased mortality and morbidity.[34] Consequently, carriers of HBsAg frequently give no history of having had recognized acute hepatitis. It has been estimated that more than 285 million people in the world today are persistently infected with hepatitis B virus.[35] The CDC estimates that there are approximately 1 million-1.25 million chronic carriers of hepatitis B virus in the USA.[32] Chronic carriers represent the largest human reservoir of hepatitis B virus.

A serious complication of acute hepatitis B virus infection is massive hepatic necrosis while sequelae of chronic hepatitis B include cirrhosis of the liver, chronic active hepatitis, and hepatocellular carcinoma. Chronic carriers of HBsAg appear to be at increased risk of developing hepatocellular carcinoma. Although a number of etiologic factors are associated with development of hepatocellular carcinoma, the single most important etiologic factor appears to be chronic infection with hepatitis B virus.[36] According to the CDC, hepatitis B vaccine is recognized as the first anti-cancer vaccine because it can prevent primary liver cancer.[67]

The vehicles for transmission of the virus are most often blood and blood products but the viral antigen has also been found in tears, saliva, breast milk, urine, semen, and vaginal secretions. Hepatitis B virus is capable of surviving for days on environmental surfaces exposed to body fluids containing hepatitis B virus. Infection may occur when hepatitis B virus, transmitted by infected body fluids, is implanted via mucous surfaces or percutaneously introduced through accidental or deliberate breaks in the skin. Transmission of hepatitis B virus infection is often associated with close interpersonal contact with an infected individual and with crowded living conditions.[37]

Prevention of Hepatitis B Disease with Vaccine

Hepatitis B infection and disease can be prevented through immunization with vaccines that contain viral surface antigen (HBsAg) and induce formation of protective antibody (anti-HBs).[38-39]

Multiple clinical studies have defined a protective level of anti-HBs as 1) 10 or more sample ratio units (SRU or S/N) as determined by radioimmunoassay or 2) a positive result as determined by enzyme immunoassay.[40-46] Note: 10 SRU is comparable to 10 mIU/mL of antibody.[36] The ACIP and an international group of hepatitis B experts consider an anti-HBs titer ≥10 mIU/mL an adequate response to a complete course of hepatitis B vaccine and protective against clinically significant infection (antigenemia with or without clinical disease).[36,46]

Clinical Trials with RECOMBIVAX HB

In clinical studies, 100% of 92 infants under 1 year of age born of non-carrier mothers developed a protective level of antibody (anti-HBs ≥10 mIU/mL) after receiving three 5-mcg doses of RECOMBIVAX HB at intervals of 0, 1, and 6 months.[31]

In one clinical study of RECOMBIVAX HB (2.5 mcg), which examined a different regimen of RECOMBIVAX HB, protective levels of antibody were achieved in 98% of 52 healthy infants vaccinated at 2, 4, and 12 months of age. Protective anti-HBs levels were achieved in 100% of 50 infants vaccinated at 2, 4, and 15 months of age.[47]

The protective efficacy of three 5-mcg doses of RECOMBIVAX HB, given at birth (with Hepatitis B Immune Globulin), 1, and 6 months of age, has been demonstrated in neonates born of mothers positive for both HBsAg and HBeAg (a core-associated antigenic complex which correlates with high infectivity). In this trial, after nine months of follow-up, chronic infection had not occurred in 96% of 130 infants.[48] The estimated efficacy in prevention of chronic hepatitis B infection was 95% as compared to the infection rate in untreated historical controls.[49]

Immunogenicity of COMVAX

The immunogenicity of COMVAX (7.5 mcg Haemophilus b PRP, 5 mcg HBsAg) was assessed in 1602 infants and children 6 weeks to 15 months of age in 5 clinical studies. In 2 controlled clinical trials (n=684), the immune response of COMVAX was compared with that obtained using the monovalent vaccines, PedvaxHIB (7.5 mcg Haemophilus b PRP) and RECOMBIVAX HB (5 mcg HBsAg) given at separate sites, either concurrently or one month apart. The immunogenicity of COMVAX was further assessed in 2 uncontrolled studies (n=852). In the first, a complete three-dose series of COMVAX was administered concurrently with other routine pediatric vaccines. In the second, COMVAX was administered as the third dose of Haemophilus b PRP and HBsAg concurrently with routine pediatric vaccines. COMVAX was also administered as the control arm in the evaluation of an investigational vaccine (n=66).

These studies demonstrate COMVAX to be highly immunogenic. The antibody responses are summarized below.

Antibody Responses to COMVAX in Infants Not Previously Vaccinated with Hib or Hepatitis B Vaccine

In the pivotal, controlled, multicenter, randomized, open-label study, 882 infants approximately 2 months of age, who had not previously received any Hib or hepatitis B vaccine, were assigned to receive a three-dose regimen of either COMVAX or PedvaxHIB plus RECOMBIVAX HB at approximately 2, 4, and 12-15 months of age. The proportions of evaluable vaccinees developing clinically important levels of anti-PRP (percent with >1.0 mcg/mL after the second dose, n=762) and anti-HBs (percent with ≥10 mIU/mL after the third dose, n=750) were similar in children given COMVAX or concurrent PedvaxHIB and RECOMBIVAX HB (Table 1).

The anti-PRP response after the second dose among infants given COMVAX in this study was 72.4% (C.I. 68.7, 76.0) >1.0 mcg/mL with a GMT=2.5 mcg/mL (C.I. 2.2, 2.8) and was comparable to that of infants given the PedvaxHIB and RECOMBIVAX HB controls which was 76.3% (C.I. 70.2, 82.5) with a GMT=2.8 mcg/mL (C.I. 2.2, 3.5). These responses exceed the response of Native American (Navajo) infants in a previous study of lyophilized PedvaxHIB (60% >1.0 mcg/mL; GMT=1.43 mcg/mL) that was associated with

Table 1: Antibody Responses to COMVAX, PedvaxHIB, and RECOMBIVAX HB in Infants Not Previously Vaccinated with Hib or Hepatitis B Vaccine

Vaccine	Age (months)	Time	n	Anti-PRP % Subjects with >0.15 mcg/mL	Anti-PRP % Subjects with >1.0 mcg/mL	Anti-PRP GMT (mcg/mL)	n	Anti-HBs % Subjects ≥10 mIU/mL	Anti-HBs GMT (mIU/mL)
COMVAX (7.5 mcg PRP, 5 mcg HBsAg) [N=661]		Prevaccination	633	34.4	4.7	0.1	603	10.6	0.6
	2	Dose 1*	620	88.9	51.5	1.0	595	34.3	4.2
	4	Dose 2*	576	94.8	72.4†	2.5†	571	92.1	113.9
	12/15	Dose 3‡	570	99.3	92.6	9.5	571	98.4	4467.5†
PedvaxHIB (7.5 mcg PRP) + RECOMBIVAX HB (5 mcg HBsAg) [N=221]		Prevaccination	208	33.7	5.8	0.1	196	7.1	0.5
	2	Dose 1*	202	90.1	53.5	1.1	198	41.9	5.3
	4	Dose 2*	186	95.2	76.3†	2.8†	185	98.4†	255.7
	12/15	Dose 3‡	181	98.9	92.3	10.2	179	100.0†	6943.9†

* Postvaccination responses were determined approximately two months after doses 1 and 2.
† C.I.'s of comparisons:
  Dose 2 Anti-PRP: 95% C.I. on difference in % >1.0 mcg/mL (-11.2, 3.1); 95% C.I. on ratio of GMT (0.69, 1.17)
  Dose 3 Anti-HBs: 95% C.I. on difference in % ≥10 mIU/mL (-2.9, -0.6); 95% C.I. on ratio of GMT (0.49, 0.91)
‡ Postvaccination responses were determined approximately one month after administration of dose 3.
More than three-quarters of the infants in the study received DTP and OPV concomitantly with the first two doses of COMVAX or PedvaxHIB plus RECOMBIVAX HB, and approximately one-third received M-M-R® II (Measles, Mumps, and Rubella Virus Vaccine Live) with the third dose of these vaccines at 12 or 15 months of age.

Table 2: Antibody Responses to COMVAX in Infants Previously Vaccinated with Hepatitis B Vaccine at Birth

Study	Age (months) at Vaccination	Time	n	Anti-PRP % Subjects with >0.15 mcg/mL	Anti-PRP % Subjects with >1.0 mcg/mL	Anti-PRP GMT (mcg/mL)	n	Anti-HBs % Subjects ≥10 mIU/mL	Anti-HBs GMT (mIU/mL)
		Prevaccination	119	24.4	5.9	0.1	71	25.4	2.9
Study 1	2	Dose 1			--------------Not Measured--------------				
[N=126]	4	Dose 2*	111	94.6	81.1	3.3	111	98.2	417.2
	14/15	Dose 3*	88	100	93.2	11.0	87	98.9	3500.7
		Prevaccination	17	58.8	0	0.2	15	6.7	0.7
Study 2	2	Dose 1†	17	88.2	47.1	0.9	16	81.3	35.2
[N=19]	4	Dose 2†	17	100	76.5	2.8	16	100	281.8
	15	Dose 3†	15	100	100	8.5	16	100	3913.4

* Postvaccination responses were determined approximately 2 months after dose 2 and 1 month after dose 3.
† Postvaccination responses were determined approximately 2 months after doses 1, 2, and 3.
Infants in these studies received DTP and OPV or eIPV (enhanced inactivated poliovirus vaccine) concomitantly with the first two doses of COMVAX, while the third dose of COMVAX was given concomitantly with DTaP (diphtheria and tetanus and acellular pertussis), OPV, and M-M-R® II at 14-15 months of age (Study 1) or with just M-M-R® II at 15 months of age (Study 2).

a 93% reduction in the incidence of invasive Hib disease. The efficacy of COMVAX in the prevention of invasive Hib disease is expected to be similar to that obtained with monovalent lyophilized PedvaxHIB in the Protective Efficacy Trial (see CLINICAL PHARMACOLOGY, Clinical Trials with PedvaxHIB).

The anti-HBs response after the third dose among infants given COMVAX in this study was 98.4% ≥10 mIU/mL (C.I. 97.0, 99.3) with a GMT of 4467.5 (C.I. 3786.3, 5271.3) compared to 100.0% (C.I. 97.9, 100.0) with a GMT of 6943.9 (C.I. 5555.9, 8678.7) among infants given COMVAX or concurrent PedvaxHIB and RECOMBIVAX HB.

Although the difference in anti-HBs GMT is statistically significant (p=0.011), both values are much greater than the level of 10 mIU/mL previously established as marking a protective response to hepatitis B.[42,44-46,51,52] These GMTs are higher than those observed in young infants who received the currently licensed regimen of RECOMBIVAX HB consisting of 5-mcg doses administered on the standard 0, 1, and 6-month schedule (GMT ~ 1359.9 mIU/mL).[53-55] In addition, two studies have shown that infants given 2.5-mcg doses of RECOMBIVAX HB according to the schedule used for COMVAX (2, 4, and 12-15 months of age) developed GMTs of 1245-3424 mIU/mL.[47,64] While a difference in GMT may result in differential retention of ≥10 mIU/mL of anti-HBs after a number of years, this is of no apparent clinical significance because of immunologic memory.[56,57] Because the HBsAg component of COMVAX induces a comparable anti-HBs response to that obtained with RECOMBIVAX HB, the efficacy of COMVAX is expected to be similar (Table 1).
[See table 1 at top of previous page]

Antibody Responses to COMVAX in Infants Previously Vaccinated with Hepatitis B Vaccine at Birth
Two clinical studies assessed antibody responses to a three-dose series of COMVAX in 128 evaluable infants who were previously given a birth dose of hepatitis B vaccine. Table 2 summarizes the anti-PRP and anti-HBs responses of these infants. The antibody responses were clinically comparable to those observed in the pivotal trial of COMVAX (Table 1).
[See table 2 above]

Interchangeability of COMVAX and Licensed Haemophilus b Conjugate Vaccines or Recombinant Hepatitis B Vaccines
Among 58 children previously given a primary course of PedvaxHIB, 90% (95% C.I. 78.8%, 96.1%) developed an anti-PRP response >1 mcg/mL with a GMT of 9.6 mcg/mL (95% C.I. 6.6, 14.1) in response to a dose of COMVAX at 12-15 months of age. Among 683 children previously given a primary course of another HIB or HIB-containing vaccine, 99% (95% C.I. 97.9%, 99.6%) developed an anti-PRP response >1 mcg/mL with a GMT of 14.9 mcg/mL (95% C.I. 13.7, 16.3) in response to a dose of COMVAX at 12-15 months of age.
In another study, COMVAX was administered either concomitantly or six weeks after vaccination with M-M-R® II and VARIVAX® (Varicella Virus Vaccine Live, Oka/Merck). Among 149 children who previously received 2 doses of monovalent Hepatitis B vaccine, 100% (95% C.I. 97.6%, 100.0%) developed an anti-HBs response ≥10 mIU/mL with a GMT of 2194.6 mIU/mL (95% C.I. 1667.8, 2887.8) in response to a dose of COMVAX at 12-15 months of age.

Antibody Responses to COMVAX and Concurrently Administered Vaccines
Immunogenicity results from open-labeled studies indicate that COMVAX can be administered concomitantly with DTP, DTaP, OPV, IPV (inactivated poliomyelitis vaccine), M-M-R II, and VARIVAX using separate sites and syringes for injectable vaccines.

DTP and DTaP
After a primary series of DTP (2, 4, 6 months of age) given concomitantly with COMVAX (2 and 4 months of age), 98.2% of 57 infants developed a 4-fold rise in antibody to diphtheria, 100% of 57 infants developed a 4-fold rise in antibody to tetanus, and 89.5% to 96.5% of 57 infants developed a 4-fold rise in antibody to pertussis antigens, depending on the assay used and adjusted for maternal antibody. In this trial, after 2 doses of COMVAX, 79.0% of 62 infants developed anti-PRP >1.0 mcg/mL and after 3 doses (2, 4, and 15 months of age), 100% of 59 infants developed ≥10 mIU/mL of anti-HBs.
After a primary series of DTaP and COMVAX given concomitantly at 2, 4, and 6 months of age, 100% of 18 infants had ≥0.01 antitoxin units/mL to diphtheria and tetanus and 94.4% to 100% of 18 infants developed a ≥4-fold rise in antibody to pertussis antigens, depending on the assay used and adjusted for maternal antibody. In this trial, after 2 doses of COMVAX, 85.7% of 63 infants developed anti-PRP >1.0 mcg/mL and after 3 doses administered on the compressed schedule of 2, 4, and 6 months of age, 92.9% of 56 infants developed ≥10 mIU/mL of anti-HBs.

OPV and IPV
After a primary series of OPV (2, 4, 6 months of age) given concomitantly with COMVAX (2 and 4 months of age), 98.3% of 60 infants had neutralizing antibody ≥1:4 to poliovirus type 1, 100% of 57 infants had neutralizing antibody ≥1:4 to poliovirus type 2 and 98.1% of 53 infants had neutralizing antibody ≥1:4 to poliovirus type 3. In this trial, after 2 doses of COMVAX, 79.0% of 62 infants developed anti-PRP >1.0 mcg/mL and after 3 doses, 100% of 59 infants developed ≥10 mIU/mL of anti-HBs.
After a primary series of IPV and COMVAX given concomitantly at 2, 4, and 6 months of age, 100% of 38 infants had neutralizing antibody ≥1:4 to poliovirus types 1, 2, and 3. In this trial, after 2 doses of COMVAX, 85.7% of 63 infants developed anti-PRP >1.0 mcg/mL and after 3 doses administered on the compressed schedule of 2, 4, and 6 months of age, 92.9% of 56 infants developed ≥10 mIU/mL of anti-HBs.

M-M-R II and VARIVAX
After concomitant vaccination of M-M-R II and VARIVAX with COMVAX (12 to 15 months of age), 99.4% of 313 children developed antibody to measles, 99.2% of 354 children developed antibody to mumps, 100% of 358 children developed antibody to rubella and 100% of 276 children developed antibody to varicella. In this trial, infants received the primary series of Hib vaccine and the first two doses of Hepatitis B vaccine in the first year of life. After the dose of COMVAX, 97.8% of 368 infants developed >1.0 mcg/mL of anti-PRP and 99.2% developed ≥10 mIU/mL of anti-HBs.

INDICATIONS AND USAGE
COMVAX is indicated for vaccination against invasive disease caused by Haemophilus influenzae type b and against infection caused by all known subtypes of hepatitis B virus in infants 6 weeks to 15 months of age born of HBsAg negative mothers.
Infants born to HBsAg positive mothers should receive Hepatitis B Immune Globulin and Hepatitis B Vaccine (Recombinant) at birth and should complete the hepatitis B vaccination series given according to a particular schedule (see manufacturer's circular for Hepatitis B Vaccine [Recombinant]).
Infants born to mothers of unknown HBsAg status should receive Hepatitis B Vaccine (Recombinant) at birth and should complete the hepatitis B vaccination series given according to a particular schedule (see manufacturer's circular for Hepatitis B Vaccine [Recombinant]).

Vaccination with COMVAX should ideally begin at approximately 2 months of age or as soon thereafter as possible. In order to complete the three-dose regimen of COMVAX, vaccination should be initiated no later than 10 months of age. Infants in whom vaccination with a PRP-OMPC-containing product (i.e., PedvaxHIB, COMVAX) is not initiated until 11 months of age do not require three doses of PRP-OMPC; however, three doses of an HBsAg-containing product are required for complete vaccination against hepatitis B, regardless of age. For infants and children not vaccinated according to the recommended schedule see DOSAGE AND ADMINISTRATION.
COMVAX will not protect against invasive disease caused by Haemophilus influenzae other than type b or against invasive disease (such as meningitis or sepsis) caused by other microorganisms. COMVAX will not prevent hepatitis caused by other viruses known to infect the liver. Because of the long incubation period for hepatitis B, it is possible for unrecognized infection to be present at the time the vaccine is given. The vaccine may not prevent hepatitis B in such patients.
As with other vaccines, COMVAX may not induce protective antibody levels immediately following vaccination and may not result in a protective antibody response in all individuals given the vaccine.

Use With Other Vaccines
Immunogenicity results from open-labeled studies indicate that COMVAX can be administered concomitantly with DTP, DTaP, OPV, IPV, M-M-R II, and VARIVAX using separate sites and syringes for injectable vaccines (see CLINICAL PHARMACOLOGY).

CONTRAINDICATIONS
Hypersensitivity to yeast or any component of the vaccine. The decision to administer or delay vaccination because of current or recent febrile illness depends on the severity of symptoms and on the etiology of the disease. The ACIP has recommended that immunization should be delayed during the course of an acute febrile illness.[63] All vaccines can be administered to persons with minor illnesses such as diarrhea, mild upper-respiratory infection with or without low-grade fever, or other low-grade febrile illness. Persons with moderate or severe febrile illness should be vaccinated as soon as they have recovered from the acute phase of the illness.

WARNINGS
Patients who develop symptoms suggestive of hypersensitivity after an injection should not receive further injections of the vaccine (see CONTRAINDICATIONS).

PRECAUTIONS
General
General care is to be taken by the health-care provider for the safe and effective use of this product.
As for any vaccine, adequate treatment provisions, including epinephrine, should be available for immediate use should an anaphylactic or anaphylactoid reaction occur.
Use caution when vaccinating latex-sensitive individuals since the vial stopper contains dry natural latex rubber that may cause allergic reactions.
As reported with Haemophilus b Polysaccharide Vaccine and another Haemophilus b Conjugate Vaccine, cases of Haemophilus b disease may occur in the week after vaccination, prior to the onset of the protective effects of the vaccines.
The packaging stopper of this product contains natural rubber latex which may cause allergic reactions.
Instructions to Health-care Provider
The health-care provider should determine the current health status and previous vaccination history of the vaccinee.
The health-care provider should question the patient, parent or guardian about reactions to a previous dose of COMVAX, PedvaxHIB or other Haemophilus b conjugate vaccines or RECOMBIVAX HB or other hepatitis B vaccines.
Injection of a blood vessel should be avoided.
COMVAX should be given with caution in infants with bleeding disorders such as hemophilia or thrombocytopenia, with steps taken to avoid the risk of hematoma following the injection.
If COMVAX is used in persons with malignancies or those receiving immunosuppressive therapy or who are otherwise immunocompromised, the expected immune response may not be obtained.
COMVAX is not contraindicated in the presence of HIV infection.[68]
Information for Vaccine Recipients and Parents/Guardians
The health-care provider should provide the vaccine information required to be given with each vaccination to the patient, parent or guardian.
The health-care provider should inform the patient, parent or guardian of the benefits and risks associated with vaccination. For risks associated with vaccination, see WARNINGS, PRECAUTIONS, and ADVERSE REACTIONS.
Laboratory Test Interactions
Sensitive tests (e.g., Latex Agglutination Kits) may detect PRP derived from the vaccine in the urine of some vaccinees for at least 30 days following vaccination with lyophilized PedvaxHIB[58]; in clinical studies with lyophilized Pedvax-

HIB, such children demonstrated a normal immune response to the vaccine. It is not known whether antigenuria will occur after vaccination with COMVAX.

Drug Interaction
Deferral of immunization may be considered in individuals receiving immunosuppressive therapy.

Carcinogenesis, Mutagenesis, Impairment of Fertility
COMVAX has not been evaluated for its carcinogenic or mutagenic potential, or its potential to impair fertility.

Pregnancy
Pregnancy Category C:
Animal reproduction studies have not been conducted with COMVAX. It is also not known whether COMVAX can cause fetal harm when administered to a pregnant woman or can affect reproduction capacity. COMVAX is not recommended for use in women of childbearing age.

Pediatric Use
Safety and effectiveness of COMVAX in infants below the age of 6 weeks and above the age of 15 months have not been established. However, studies have demonstrated that PedvaxHIB is safe and immunogenic when administered to infants and children up to the age of 71 months and RECOMBIVAX HB is safe and immunogenic in persons of all ages.

COMVAX should not be used in infants younger than 6 weeks of age because this will lead to a reduced anti-PRP response and may lead to immune tolerance (impaired ability to respond to subsequent exposure to the PRP antigen).{59-61}

Infants born to HBsAg-positive mothers should not receive COMVAX but instead should receive Hepatitis B Immune Globulin and Hepatitis B Vaccine (Recombinant) at birth and should complete the hepatitis B vaccination series given according to a particular schedule (see manufacturer's circular for Hepatitis B Vaccine [Recombinant]). (See DOSAGE AND ADMINISTRATION.)

Geriatric Use
This vaccine is NOT recommended for use in adult populations.

ADVERSE REACTIONS

In clinical trials involving the administration of 7918 doses of COMVAX to 3561 healthy infants 6 weeks to 15 months of age, COMVAX was generally well tolerated. In these studies, infants received COMVAX with licensed pediatric vaccines (n=1745) or investigational vaccines (n=1816). Serious adverse experience data were available for all 3561 infants and non-serious adverse experience data were available for a subset of 1678 infants.

Pivotal Immunogenicity and Safety Study
In the pivotal, randomized, multicenter study, 882 infants were assigned in a 3:1 ratio to receive either COMVAX or PedvaxHIB plus RECOMBIVAX HB at separate injection sites at 2, 4, and 12-15 months of age. Children may have also received routine pediatric immunizations. The children were monitored daily for five days after each injection for injection-site and systemic adverse experiences. During this time, adverse experiences in infants who received COMVAX were generally similar in type and frequency to those observed in infants who received PedvaxHIB plus RECOMBIVAX HB.

The most frequently cited events were mild, transient signs and symptoms of inflammation at the injection site (i.e., pain/soreness, erythema, and swelling/induration), somnolence, and irritability, all of which were prompted for on report cards filled out by parents of vaccinated children. Table 3 summarizes the frequencies of injection-site and systemic adverse experiences within five days of vaccination that were reported among ≥1.0% of children in this pivotal trial.
[See table 3 above]

Infants Previously Vaccinated with Hepatitis B Vaccine
In a group of infants (N=126) given a three-dose course of COMVAX after previously receiving a dose of Hepatitis B Vaccine (Recombinant) at or shortly after birth, the type, frequency, and severity of adverse experiences did not appear to be greater than those observed in infants in the pivotal study who did not receive hepatitis B vaccine at birth.

Infants 6 Weeks to 15 Months of Age
In clinical trials, 3285 doses of COMVAX were administered to 1678 infants who were monitored for injection-site and systemic adverse experiences from Days 0 to 5 after each injection of vaccine. Of these, 855 infants had safety data following vaccination at approximately 2 months of age, 836 infants at approximately 4 months of age and 1573 infants at 12 to 15 months of age. The most frequently reported adverse experiences (≥1% of subjects for at least one injection), without regard to causality are listed in decreasing order of frequency within each body system:

Injection Site Reactions: Pain/tenderness/soreness, swelling/induration, erythema; *Body as a Whole:* Fever; *Digestive System:* Anorexia, diarrhea, vomiting; *Nervous System/Psychiatric:* Irritability, somnolence, crying; *Respiratory System:* Upper respiratory infection, rhinorrhea, cough, rhinitis; *Skin:* Rash; *Special Senses:* Otitis media.

Table 3: Local Reactions and Systemic Complaints Within 5 Days After Injection Reported to Occur in ≥1.0%* of Children Given a 3-Dose Course of COMVAX Compared to These Events in Children Given Concomitant Injections of PedvaxHIB and RECOMBIVAX HB

Event	Injection 1[†]		Injection 2[†]		Injection 3	
	COMVAX (N=660) %	PedvaxHIB and RECOMBIVAX HB[‡] (N=221) %	COMVAX (N=645) %	PedvaxHIB and RECOMBIVAX HB[‡] (N=213) %	COMVAX (N=593) %	PedvaxHIB and RECOMBIVAX HB[‡] (N=193) %
Injection Site Reactions						
Pain/Soreness[§]	34.5	37.6	24.3	25.8	23.9	21.2
Erythema (>1 in.)[§]	22.4 (2.7)	25.8 (2.7)	25.7 (1.4)	23.5 (3.3)	27.2 (3.0)	24.4 (1.6)
Swelling/Induration (>1 in.)[§]	27.6 (3.0)	33.5 (4.1)	30.4 (2.9)	31.0 (3.8)	27.2 (3.2)	29.5 (4.1)
Systemic Complaints						
Irritability[§]	57.0	46.6	50.7	44.1	32.2	29.0
Somnolence[§]	49.5	47.1	37.4	31.9	21.1	22.3
Crying—						
unusual, high pitched[§]	10.6	8.6	6.7	2.3	2.9	3.6
not otherwise specified	2.3	2.3	1.4	2.3	0.7	1.6
prolonged (>4 hrs.)[§]	2.4	2.3	0.8	1.4	0.2	0
Anorexia	3.9	2.3	2.0	0.9	0.8	0.5
Vomiting	2.1	1.8	2.5	0.9	1.0	1.6
Otitis media	0.5	0	2.0	1.4	2.7	1.6
Fever (°F, rectal equiv.)[¶]						
101.0-102.9	14.2	11.9	13.8	12.2	10.5	6.4
≥103.0	0.8	0	1.6	1.4	2.7	4.3
Diarrhea	1.7	1.8	0.8	0.9	2.2	0.5
Upper respiratory infection	0.5	0.5	1.1	0.9	1.3	0.5
Rash	0.8	0	0.9	0.9	0.8	0.5
Rhinorrhea	0.2	0	1.1	0.9	1.3	2.1
Respiratory congestion	0.6	0.5	1.2	0.9	0.3	0.5
Cough	0.2	0	0.9	0.5	0.2	1.0
Candidiasis, oral	0.3	0.5	0.8	0	0.2	0
Rash, diaper	0.5	0.5	0.5	0.9	0.2	0

* Overall frequency of each event listed above is ≥1% even though the frequency after a given dose may be <1%.
† Most children received DTP and OPV concomitantly with the first two doses of COMVAX or PedvaxHIB and RECOMBIVAX HB.
‡ Injection site reactions for PedvaxHIB and RECOMBIVAX HB based on occurrence with either of the monovalent components.
§ Events prompted for on Vaccination Report Card given to parents/guardians of vaccinees.
¶ N for injections 1, 2, and 3 equals 655, 639, and 588, respectively, for COMVAX; N for injections 1, 2, and 3 equals 218, 213, and 187, respectively, for PedvaxHIB and RECOMBIVAX HB.

Post-Marketing Experience
As with any vaccine, there is the possibility that broad use of COMVAX could reveal adverse experiences not observed in clinical trials. The following additional adverse reactions have been reported with the use of the marketed vaccine.
Hypersensitivity
Anaphylaxis, angioedema, urticaria, erythema multiforme
Hematologic
Thrombocytopenia
Nervous System
Seizure, febrile seizures

Potential Adverse Effects
In addition, a variety of adverse effects have been reported with marketed use of either PedvaxHIB or RECOMBIVAX HB in infants and children through 71 months of age. These adverse effects are listed below.
PedvaxHIB
Hematologic/Lymphatic
Lymphadenopathy
Skin
Sterile injection-site abscess; pain at the injection site
RECOMBIVAX HB
Hypersensitivity
Symptoms of hypersensitivity including reports of rash, pruritus, edema, arthralgia, dyspnea, hypotension, and ecchymoses
Cardiovascular System
Tachycardia; syncope
Digestive System
Elevation of liver enzymes
Hematologic
Increased erythrocyte sedimentation rate
Musculoskeletal System
Arthritis
Nervous System
Bell's Palsy; Guillain-Barré Syndrome
Psychiatric/Behavioral
Agitation; somnolence; irritability
Skin
Stevens-Johnson Syndrome; alopecia
Special Senses
Conjunctivitis; visual disturbances

Adverse Event Reporting
Patients, parents and guardians should be instructed to report any serious adverse reactions to their health-care provider who in turn should report such events to the U.S. Department of Health and Human Services through the Vaccine Adverse Event Reporting System (VAERS), 1-800-822-7967. The health-care provider should inform the parent or guardian of the National Vaccine Injury Compensation Program (NVICP), 1-800-338-2382.

DOSAGE AND ADMINISTRATION
FOR INTRAMUSCULAR ADMINISTRATION
Do not inject intravenously, intradermally, or subcutaneously.

Recommended Schedule
Infants born to HBsAg negative mothers should be vaccinated with three 0.5 mL doses of COMVAX, ideally at 2, 4, and 12-15 months of age. If the recommended schedule cannot be followed, the interval between the first two doses should be at least six weeks and the interval between the second and third dose should be as close as possible to eight to eleven months.

Infants born to HBsAg-positive mothers should receive Hepatitis B Immune Globulin and Hepatitis B Vaccine (Recombinant) at birth and should complete the hepatitis B vaccination series given according to a particular schedule (see manufacturer's circular for Hepatitis B Vaccine [Recombinant]).

Infants born to mothers of unknown HBsAg status should receive Hepatitis B Vaccine (Recombinant) at birth and should complete the hepatitis B vaccination series given according to a particular schedule (see manufacturer's circular for Hepatitis B Vaccine [Recombinant]).

The subsequent administration of COMVAX for completion of the hepatitis B vaccination series in infants who were born to HBsAg positive mothers and received HBIG or infants born to mothers of unknown status has not been studied.

COMVAX should not be administered to any infant before the age of 6 weeks.

Modified Schedules
Children previously vaccinated with one or more doses of either hepatitis B vaccine or Haemophilus b conjugate vaccine

Children who receive one dose of hepatitis B vaccine at or shortly after birth may be administered COMVAX on the schedule of 2, 4, and 12-15 months of age. There are no data to support the use of a three-dose series of COMVAX in infants who have previously received more than one dose of hepatitis B vaccine. However, COMVAX may be administered to children otherwise scheduled to receive concurrent RECOMBIVAX HB and PedvaxHIB.

Children not vaccinated according to recommended schedule for COMVAX

Vaccination schedules for children not vaccinated according to the recommended schedule should be considered on an individual basis. The number of doses of a PRP-OMPC-containing product (i.e., COMVAX, PedvaxHIB) depends on the age that vaccination is begun. An infant 2 to 10 months of age should receive three doses of a product containing PRP-OMPC. An infant 11 to 14 months of age should receive two doses of a product containing PRP-OMPC. A child 15 to 71 months of age should receive one dose of a product containing PRP-OMPC. Infants and children, regardless of age, should receive three doses of an HBsAg-containing product. COMVAX is for intramuscular injection. The *anterolateral thigh* is the recommended site for intramuscular injection in infants. Data suggests that injections given in the buttocks frequently are given into fatty tissue instead of into muscle. Such injections have resulted in a lower seroconversion rate (for hepatitis B vaccine) than was expected.

Injection must be accomplished with a needle long enough to ensure intramuscular deposition of the vaccine. The ACIP has recommended that for intramuscular injections, the needle should be of sufficient length to reach the muscle mass itself. In a clinical trial with COMVAX (see CLINICAL PHARMACOLOGY, Antibody Responses to COMVAX in Infants Not Previously Vaccinated with Hib or Hepatitis B Vaccine, Table 1) vaccination was accomplished with a needle length of 5/8 inches in accordance with ACIP recommendations in effect at that time.[62] ACIP currently recommends that needles of longer length (7/8 to 1 inch) be used.[63]

The vaccine should be used as supplied; no reconstitution is necessary.

Shake well before withdrawal and use. Thorough agitation is necessary to maintain suspension of the vaccine.

Parenteral drug products should be inspected visually for extraneous particulate matter and discoloration prior to administration whenever solution and container permit. After thorough agitation, COMVAX is a slightly opaque, white suspension.

It is important to use a separate sterile syringe and needle for each patient to prevent transmission of infectious agents from one person to another.

Interchangeability of COMVAX and Licensed Haemophilus b Conjugate Vaccines or Recombinant Hepatitis B Vaccines

Since 1990, the Advisory Committee on Immunization Practices (ACIP) and the Committee on Infectious Diseases of the American Academy of Pediatrics (AAP) have recommended routine immunization of infants starting at 2 months of age with a polysaccharide-protein conjugate vaccine to prevent invasive Hib disease.[32,33]

Three Hib vaccines are licensed for infant vaccination: 1) oligosaccharide conjugate Hib vaccine (HbOC) (HibTITER[®1]), 2) polyribosylribitol phosphate-tetanus toxoid conjugate (PRP-T) (ActHIB[®1] and OmniHIB[®1]), and 3) Haemophilus b conjugate vaccine (meningococcal protein conjugate) (PRP-OMPC) (PedvaxHIB). According to the ACIP, these products are now considered interchangeable for primary as well as booster vaccination.[66]

Because vaccination recommendations limited to high-risk individuals have failed to substantially lower the overall incidence of hepatitis B infection, both the Advisory Committee on Immunization Practices (ACIP) and the Committee on Infectious Diseases of the American Academy of Pediatrics (AAP) have endorsed universal infant immunization as part of a comprehensive strategy for the control of hepatitis B infection.[32,50]

---

[1] HibTITER is a registered trademark of Lederle Laboratories, ActHIB is a registered trademark of Aventis Pasteur Inc. and OmniHIB is a registered trademark of GlaxoSmithKline.

HOW SUPPLIED

No. 4898 — COMVAX is supplied as 7.5 mcg PRP polysaccharide conjugated to approximately 125 mcg OMPC and 5 mcg HBsAg in a box of 10 single dose vials.

NDC 0006-4898-00.

Storage

Store vaccine at 2-8°C (36-46°F). Storage above or below the recommended temperature may reduce potency.

DO NOT FREEZE since freezing destroys potency.

REFERENCES

1. Cochi, S.L., et al. JAMA 253: 521-529, 1985.
2. Schlech, W.F., III, et al. JAMA 253: 1749-1754, 1985.
3. Peltola, H., et al. N Engl J Med 310: 1561-1566, 1984.
4. Cardoz, M., et al. Bull WHO 59: 575-584, 1981.
5. Sell, S.H., et al. Pediatr 49: 206-217, 1972.
6. Taylor, H.G., et al. Pediatr 74: 198-205, 1984.
7. Hay, J.W., et al. Pediatr 80(3): 319-329, 1987.
8. Redmond, S.R., et al. JAMA 252: 2581-2584, 1984.
9. Istre, G.R., et al. J Pediatr 106: 190-195, 1985.
10. Fraser, D.W., et al. J Infect Dis 127: 271-277, 1973.
11. Tarr, P.I., et al. J Pediatr 92: 884-888, 1978.
12. Granoff, D.M., et al. J Clin Invest 74: 1708-1714, 1984.
13. Ambrosino, D.M., et al. J Clin Invest 75: 1935-1942, 1985.
14. Coulehan, J.L., et al. Pub Health Rep 99: 404-409, 1984.
15. Losonsky, G.A., et al. Pediatr Infect Dis J 3: 539-547, 1985.
16. Ward, J.I., et al. Lancet 1: 1281-1285, 1981.
17. Ward, J.I., et al. N Engl J Med 301: 122-126, 1979.
18. Ward, J.I., et al. J Pediatr 88: 261-263, 1983.
19. Bartlett, A.V., et al. J Pediatr 102: 55-58, 1983.
20. Centers for Disease Control. MMWR 34(15): 201-205, 1985.
21. Santosham, M., et al. N Engl J Med 317: 923-929, 1987.
22. Siber, G.R., et al. Infect Immun 45: 248-254, 1984.
23. Smith, D.H., et al. Pediatr 52: 637-644, 1973.
24. Robbins, J.B., et al. Pediatr Res 7: 103-110, 1973.
25. Kaythy, H., et al. J Infect Dis 147: 1100, 1983.
26. Peltola, H., et al. Pediatr 60: 730-737, 1977.
27. Ward, J.I., et al. Pediatr 81: 886-893, 1988.
28. Daum, R.S., et al. Pediatr 81: 893-897, 1988.
29. Marburg, S., et al. J Am Chem Soc 108: 5282-5287, 1986.
30. Letson, G.W., et al. Pediatr Infect Dis J 7(111): 747-752, 1988.
31. Data on file at Merck Research Laboratories.
32. Centers for Disease Control. MMWR 40(RR-1):1-25, 1991.
33. Committee on Infectious Disease. Update Pediatrics 88(1): 169-172, 1991.
34. Robinson, W.S. "Principles and Practice of Infectious Diseases," G.L. Mandell; R.G. Douglas; J.E. Bennett (eds), vol. 2, New York, John Wiley & Sons, 1985, pp. 1002-1029.
35. Maynard, J. E., et al. "Viral Hepatitis and Liver Disease", A.J. Zuckerman (ed.), Alan R. Liss, Inc., 1988, pp. 967-969.
36. Centers for Disease Control. MMWR 39(RR-2): 5-26, 1990.
37. Wands, J.R., et al. "Principles of Internal Medicine," G.W. Thorn, R.D. Adams, E. Braunwald, K.J. Isselbacher, R.G. Petersdorf (eds), vol. 2, McGraw-Hill, 1977, pp. 1590-1598.
38. Sitrin, R.D., Wampler, D.E., Ellis, R.W. Survey of licensed hepatitis B vaccines and their production processes. In: Ellis RW, ed. Hepatitis B vaccines in clinical practice. New York: Marcel Dekker, Inc., 1993, pp. 83-101.
39. West, D.J. Scope and design of hepatitis B vaccine clinical trials. In Ellis RW, ed. Hepatitis B vaccines in clinical practice. New York: Marcel Dekker, Inc., 1993, pp. 159-177.
40. Hadler, S.C., et al. NEJM 315(4): 209-214, 1986.
41. Szmuness, W., et al. NEJM 303: 833-841, 1980.
42. Francis, D.P., et al. Ann Int Med 97: 362-366, 1982.
43. Szmuness, W., et al. NEJM 307: 1481-1486, 1982.
44. Szmuness, W., et al. Hepatology 1: 377-385, 1981.
45. Coutinho, R.A., et al. BMJ 286: 1305-1308, 1983.
46. International Group: Immunisation against hepatitis B, Lancet 1(8590): 875-876, 1988.
47. Keyserling, H.L., et al. J Pediatr 125(1): 67-69, 1994.
48. Stevens, C.E.; Taylor, P.E.; Tong, M.J., et al. "Viral Hepatitis and Liver Diseases." A.J. Zuckerman (ed.), Alan R. Liss, Inc., 1988, pp. 982-983.
49. Stevens, C.E., et al. Pediatr 90(1, Part 2): 170-173, 1992.
50. Universal Hepatitis B Immunization, Committee on Infectious Diseases. Pediatr 89(4): 795-800, 1992.
51. Centers for Disease Control. MMWR 34: 313-24, 329-35, 1985.
52. Centers for Disease Control. MMWR 36: 353-60, 366, 1987.
53. West, D.J., et al. Pediatr Clin North Am 37: 585-601, 1990.
54. Seto, D., et al. Pediatr Res 31(4 Pt 2): 179A, 1992.
55. Froehlich, H. Pediatr Res 31(4 Pt 2): 92A, 1992.
56. Jilg, W., et al. Infection 17: 70-6, 1989.
57. West, D.J., et al. Vaccine 14: 1019-27, 1996.
58. Goep, J.G., et al. Pediatr Infect Dis J 1(1): 2-5, 1992.
59. Keyserling, H.L., et al. Program and Abstracts of the 30th ICAAC, 1990. (Abst. 63).
60. Ward, J.I., et al. Program and Abstracts of the 32nd ICAAC, 1992. (Abst. 984).
61. Lieberman, J.M., et al. Infect Dis, 199 (Abst.1028).
62. Centers for Disease Control. MMWR 38(13): 205-228, 1989.
63. Centers for Disease Control. MMWR 43(RR-1): 1994.
64. Reisenger, K.S., et al. Pediatr Res (4 pt. 2): 179A, 1993.
65. Centers for Disease Control. MMWR 46(54): 74, 1998.
66. Centers for Disease Control. MMWR 47(1): 9, 1998.
67. Centers for Disease Control. Federal Register, 64(35):9044-9045, February 23, 1999.
68. Centers for Disease Control. MMWR 42(RR-4): 1-18, April 9, 1993.

Manuf. and Dist. by: Merck Sharp & Dohme Corp., a subsidiary of MERCK & CO., INC., Whitehouse Station, NJ 08889, USA

Issued December 2010

Printed in USA

Copyright © 2001 Merck Sharp & Dohme Corp., a subsidiary of Merck & Co., Inc.

All rights reserved

9882603

COSOPT® PF
(dorzolamide hydrochloride - timolol maleate ophthalmic solution)
2%/0.5%

Rx

HIGHLIGHTS OF PRESCRIBING INFORMATION

These highlights do not include all the information needed to use COSOPT PF safely and effectively. See full prescribing information for COSOPT PF.

COSOPT® PF (dorzolamide hydrochloride-timolol maleate ophthalmic solution) 2%/0.5%

Initial U.S. Approval: 1998

---INDICATIONS AND USAGE---

• COSOPT PF is a carbonic anhydrase inhibitor with a beta-adrenergic receptor blocking agent indicated for the reduction of elevated intraocular pressure (IOP) in patients with open-angle glaucoma or ocular hypertension who are insufficiently responsive to beta-blockers.

• The IOP-lowering of COSOPT twice daily was slightly less than that seen with the concomitant administration of 0.5% timolol twice daily, and 2% dorzolamide three times daily. (1)

---DOSAGE AND ADMINISTRATION---

The dose is one drop of COSOPT PF in the affected eye(s) two times daily. (2)

---DOSAGE FORMS AND STRENGTHS---

Solution containing 20 mg/mL dorzolamide and 5 mg/mL timolol. (3)

---CONTRAINDICATIONS---

COSOPT PF is contraindicated in patients with:

• Bronchial asthma or a history of bronchial asthma, severe chronic obstructive pulmonary disease. (4.1)

• Sinus bradycardia, second or third degree atrioventricular block, overt cardiac failure, cardiogenic shock. (4.2)

• Hypersensitivity to any component of this product. (4.3, 5.3)

---WARNINGS AND PRECAUTIONS---

• Potentiation of Respiratory Reactions Including Asthma (5.1)

• Cardiac Failure (5.2)

• Sulfonamide Hypersensitivity (5.3)

• Obstructive Pulmonary Disease (5.4)

• Increased Reactivity to Allergens (5.5)

• Potentiation of Muscle Weakness (5.6)

• Masking of Hypoglycemic Symptoms in Patients with Diabetes Mellitus (5.7)

• Masking of Thyrotoxicosis (5.8)

• Renal and Hepatic Impairment (5.9)

• Impairment of Beta-Adrenergically Mediated Reflexes During Surgery (5.10)

---ADVERSE REACTIONS---

The most frequently reported adverse reactions were taste perversion (bitter, sour, or unusual taste) or ocular burning and/or stinging in up to 30% of patients. Conjunctival hyperemia, blurred vision, superficial punctate keratitis or eye itching were reported between 5-15% of patients. (6)

To report SUSPECTED ADVERSE REACTIONS, contact Merck Sharp & Dohme Corp., a subsidiary of Merck & Co., Inc., at 1-877-888-4231 or FDA at 1-800-FDA-1088 or www.fda.gov/medwatch

---DRUG INTERACTIONS---

• Potential additive effect of oral carbonic anhydrase inhibitor with COSOPT PF. (7.1)

• Potential acid-base and electrolyte disturbances. (7.2)

• Concomitant use with systemic beta-blockers may potentiate systemic beta-blockade. (7.3)

- Oral or intravenous calcium antagonists may cause atrioventricular conduction disturbances, left ventricular failure, and hypotension. (7.4)
- Catecholamine-depleting drugs may have additive effects and produce hypotension and/or marked bradycardia. (7.5)
- Digitalis and calcium antagonists may have additive effects in prolonging atrioventricular conduction time. (7.6)
- CYP2D6 inhibitors may potentiate systemic beta-blockade. (7.7)

See 17 for PATIENT COUNSELING INFORMATION and FDA-approved patient labeling

Revised: 05/2012

FULL PRESCRIBING INFORMATION

1   INDICATIONS AND USAGE

COSOPT® PF is indicated for the reduction of elevated intraocular pressure (IOP) in patients with open-angle glaucoma or ocular hypertension who are insufficiently responsive to beta-blockers (failed to achieve target IOP determined after multiple measurements over time). The IOP-lowering of COSOPT® administered twice a day was slightly less than that seen with the concomitant administration of 0.5% timolol administered twice a day and 2% dorzolamide administered three times a day [see Clinical Studies (14.1)].

2   DOSAGE AND ADMINISTRATION

The dose is one drop of COSOPT PF in the affected eye(s) two times daily.

If more than one topical ophthalmic drug is being used, the drugs should be administered at least five minutes apart [see Drug Interactions (7.3)].

The solution from one individual unit is to be used immediately after opening for administration to one or both eyes. Since sterility cannot be maintained after the individual unit is opened, the remaining contents should be discarded immediately after administration.

3   DOSAGE FORMS AND STRENGTHS

Solution containing 20 mg/mL dorzolamide (22.26 mg of dorzolamide hydrochloride) and 5 mg/mL timolol (6.83 mg timolol maleate).

4   CONTRAINDICATIONS

4.1   Asthma, COPD

COSOPT PF is contraindicated in patients with bronchial asthma, a history of bronchial asthma, or severe chronic obstructive pulmonary disease [see Warnings and Precautions (5.1)].

4.2   Sinus Bradycardia, AV Block, Cardiac Failure, Cardiogenic Shock

COSOPT PF is contraindicated in patients with sinus bradycardia, second or third degree atrioventricular block, overt cardiac failure, and cardiogenic shock [see Warnings and Precautions (5.2)].

4.3   Hypersensitivity

COSOPT PF is contraindicated in patients who are hypersensitive to any component of this product [see Warnings and Precautions (5.3)].

5   WARNINGS AND PRECAUTIONS

5.1   Potentiation of Respiratory Reactions Including Asthma

COSOPT PF contains timolol maleate, a beta-adrenergic blocking agent; and although administered topically, is absorbed systemically. Therefore, the same types of adverse reactions that are attributable to systemic administration of beta-adrenergic blocking agents may occur with topical administration. For example, severe respiratory reactions, including death due to bronchospasm in patients with asthma, and rarely death in association with cardiac failure, have been reported following systemic or ophthalmic administration of timolol maleate [see Contraindications (4.1) and Patient Counseling Information (17.1)].

5.2   Cardiac Failure

Sympathetic stimulation may be essential for support of the circulation in individuals with diminished myocardial contractility, and its inhibition by beta-adrenergic receptor blockade may precipitate more severe failure.

In patients without a history of cardiac failure continued depression of the myocardium with beta-blocking agents over a period of time can, in some cases, lead to cardiac failure. At the first sign or symptom of cardiac failure, COSOPT PF should be discontinued [see Contraindications (4.2) and Patient Counseling Information (17.2)].

5.3   Sulfonamide Hypersensitivity

COSOPT PF contains dorzolamide, a sulfonamide; and although administered topically, it is absorbed systemically. Therefore, the same types of adverse reactions that are attributable to sulfonamides may occur with topical administration of COSOPT PF. Fatalities have occurred, although rarely, due to severe reactions to sulfonamides including Stevens-Johnson syndrome, toxic epidermal necrolysis, fulminant hepatic necrosis, agranulocytosis, aplastic anemia, and other blood dyscrasias. Sensitization may recur when a sulfonamide is readministered irrespective of the route of administration. If signs of serious reactions or hypersensitivity occur, discontinue the use of this preparation [see Contraindications (4.3) and Patient Counseling Information (17.3)].

5.4   Obstructive Pulmonary Disease

Patients with chronic obstructive pulmonary disease (e.g., chronic bronchitis, emphysema) of mild or moderate severity, bronchospastic disease, or a history of bronchospastic disease (other than bronchial asthma or a history of bronchial asthma, in which COSOPT PF is contraindicated) should, in general, not receive beta-blocking agents, including COSOPT PF [see Contraindications (4.1) and Patient Counseling Information (17.1)].

5.5   Increased Reactivity to Allergens

While taking beta-blockers, patients with a history of atopy or a history of severe anaphylactic reactions to a variety of allergens may be more reactive to repeated accidental, diagnostic, or therapeutic challenge with such allergens. Such patients may be unresponsive to the usual doses of epinephrine used to treat anaphylactic reactions.

5.6   Potentiation of Muscle Weakness

Beta-adrenergic blockade has been reported to potentiate muscle weakness consistent with certain myasthenic symptoms (e.g., diplopia, ptosis, and generalized weakness). Timolol has been reported rarely to increase muscle weakness in some patients with myasthenia gravis or myasthenic symptoms.

5.7   Masking of Hypoglycemic Symptoms in Patients with Diabetes Mellitus

Beta-adrenergic blocking agents should be administered with caution in patients subject to spontaneous hypoglycemia or to diabetic patients (especially those with labile diabetes) who are receiving insulin or oral hypoglycemic agents. Beta-adrenergic receptor blocking agents may mask the signs and symptoms of acute hypoglycemia.

5.8   Masking of Thyrotoxicosis

Beta-adrenergic blocking agents may mask certain clinical signs (e.g., tachycardia) of hyperthyroidism. Patients suspected of developing thyrotoxicosis should be managed carefully to avoid abrupt withdrawal of beta-adrenergic blocking agents that might precipitate a thyroid storm.

5.9   Renal and Hepatic Impairment

Dorzolamide has not been studied in patients with severe renal impairment (CrCl <30 mL/min). Because dorzolamide and its metabolite are excreted predominantly by the kidney, COSOPT PF is not recommended in such patients. Dorzolamide has not been studied in patients with hepatic impairment and should therefore be used with caution in such patients.

5.10   Impairment of Beta-Adrenergically Mediated Reflexes During Surgery

The necessity or desirability of withdrawal of beta-adrenergic blocking agents prior to major surgery is controversial. Beta-adrenergic receptor blockade impairs the ability of the heart to respond to beta-adrenergically mediated reflex stimuli. This may augment the risk of general anesthesia in surgical procedures. Some patients receiving beta-adrenergic receptor blocking agents have experienced protracted severe hypotension during anesthesia. Difficulty in restarting and maintaining the heartbeat has also been reported. For these reasons, in patients undergoing elective surgery, some authorities recommend gradual withdrawal of beta-adrenergic receptor blocking agents.

If necessary during surgery, the effects of beta-adrenergic blocking agents may be reversed by sufficient doses of adrenergic agonists.

5.11   Corneal Endothelium

Carbonic anhydrase activity has been observed in both the cytoplasm and around the plasma membranes of the corneal endothelium. There is an increased potential for developing corneal edema in patients with low endothelial cell counts. Caution should be used when prescribing COSOPT PF to this group of patients.

6   ADVERSE REACTIONS

6.1   Clinical Studies Experience

Because clinical trials are conducted under widely varying conditions, adverse reaction rates observed in the clinical trials of a drug cannot be directly compared to rates in the clinical trials of another drug and may not reflect the rates observed in practice.

COSOPT and COSOPT PF

COSOPT and COSOPT PF were evaluated in patients with elevated intraocular pressure treated for open-angle glaucoma or ocular hypertension for up to 15 months. Approximately 5% of all patients discontinued therapy because of adverse reactions.

The most frequently reported adverse reactions occurring in up to 30% of patients were taste perversion (bitter, sour, or unusual taste) or ocular burning and/or stinging. The following adverse reactions were reported in 5-15% of patients: conjunctival hyperemia, blurred vision, superficial punctate keratitis or eye itching.

The following adverse reactions were reported in 1-5% of patients: abdominal pain, back pain, blepharitis, bronchitis, cloudy vision, conjunctival discharge, conjunctival edema, conjunctival follicles, conjunctival injection, conjunctivitis, corneal erosion, corneal staining, cortical lens opacity, cough, dizziness, dryness of eyes, dyspepsia, eye debris, eye discharge, eye pain, eye tearing, eyelid edema, eyelid erythema, eyelid exudate/scales, eyelid pain or discomfort, foreign body sensation, glaucomatous cupping, headache, hypertension, influenza, lens nucleus coloration, lens opacity, nausea, nuclear lens opacity, pharyngitis, post-subcapsular cataract, sinusitis, upper respiratory infection, urinary tract infection, visual field defect, vitreous detachment.

Other adverse reactions that have been reported with the individual components are listed below:

Dorzolamide 2%

Angioedema, asthenia/fatigue, bronchospasm, contact dermatitis, epistaxis, eyelid crusting, ocular discomfort, photophobia, signs and symptoms of ocular allergic reaction, transient myopia.

Timolol (ocular administration)

Body as a Whole: Asthenia/fatigue; *Cardiovascular:* Arrhythmia, syncope, cerebral ischemia, worsening of angina pectoris, palpitation, cardiac arrest, pulmonary edema, edema, claudication, Raynaud's phenomenon, and cold hands and feet; *Digestive:* Anorexia; *Immunologic:* Systemic lupus erythematosus; *Nervous System/Psychiatric:* Increase in signs and symptoms of myasthenia gravis, somnolence, insomnia, nightmares, behavioral changes and psychic disturbances including confusion, hallucinations, anxiety, disorientation, nervousness, and memory loss; *Skin:* Alopecia, psoriasiform rash or exacerbation of psoriasis; *Hypersensitivity:* Signs and symptoms of systemic allergic reactions, including anaphylaxis, angioedema, urticaria, and localized and generalized rash; *Respiratory:* Bronchospasm (predominantly in patients with pre-existing bronchospastic disease); *Endocrine:* Masked symptoms of hypoglycemia in diabetic patients; *Special Senses:* Ptosis, decreased corneal sensitivity, cystoid macular edema, visual disturbances including refractive changes and diplopia, pseudopemphigoid, and tinnitus; *Urogenital:* Retroperitoneal fibrosis, decreased libido, impotence, and Peyronie's disease.

6.2 Post-Marketing Experience
The following adverse reactions have been identified during post-approval use of COSOPT or COSOPT PF. Because these reactions are reported voluntarily from a population of uncertain size, it is not always possible to reliably estimate their frequency or establish a causal relationship to drug exposure: bradycardia, cardiac failure, cerebral vascular accident, chest pain, choroidal detachment following filtration surgery, depression, diarrhea, dry mouth, dyspnea, heart block, hypotension, iridocyclitis, myocardial infarction, nasal congestion, Stevens-Johnson syndrome, toxic epidermal necrolysis, paresthesia, photophobia, respiratory failure, skin rashes, urolithiasis, and vomiting.

Timolol (oral administration)
The following additional adverse reactions have been reported in clinical experience with ORAL timolol maleate or other ORAL beta-blocking agents and may be considered potential effects of ophthalmic timolol maleate: *Allergic:* Erythematous rash, fever combined with aching and sore throat, laryngospasm with respiratory distress; *Body as a Whole:* Extremity pain, decreased exercise tolerance, weight loss; *Cardiovascular:* Worsening of arterial insufficiency, vasodilatation; *Digestive:* Gastrointestinal pain, hepatomegaly, mesenteric arterial thrombosis, ischemic colitis; *Hematologic:* Nonthrombocytopenic purpura; thrombocytopenic purpura, agranulocytosis; *Endocrine:* Hyperglycemia, hypoglycemia; *Skin:* Pruritus, skin irritation, increased pigmentation, sweating; *Musculoskeletal:* Arthralgia; *Nervous System/Psychiatric:* Vertigo, local weakness, diminished concentration, reversible mental depression progressing to catatonia, an acute reversible syndrome characterized by disorientation for time and place, emotional lability, slightly clouded sensorium, and decreased performance on neuropsychometrics; *Respiratory:* Rales, bronchial obstruction; *Urogenital:* Urination difficulties.

7 DRUG INTERACTIONS
7.1 Oral Carbonic Anhydrase Inhibitors
There is a potential for an additive effect on the known systemic effects of carbonic anhydrase inhibition in patients receiving an oral carbonic anhydrase inhibitor and COSOPT PF. The concomitant administration of COSOPT PF and oral carbonic anhydrase inhibitors is not recommended.

7.2 High-Dose Salicylate Therapy
Although acid-base and electrolyte disturbances were not reported in the clinical trials with dorzolamide hydrochloride ophthalmic solution, these disturbances have been reported with oral carbonic anhydrase inhibitors and have, in some instances, resulted in drug interactions (e.g., toxicity associated with high-dose salicylate therapy). Therefore, the potential for such drug interactions should be considered in patients receiving COSOPT PF.

7.3 Beta-Adrenergic Blocking Agents
Patients who are receiving a beta-adrenergic blocking agent orally and COSOPT PF should be observed for potential additive effects of beta-blockade, both systemic and on intraocular pressure. The concomitant use of two topical beta-adrenergic blocking agents is not recommended.

7.4 Calcium Antagonists
Caution should be used in the coadministration of beta-adrenergic blocking agents, such as COSOPT PF, and oral or intravenous calcium antagonists because of possible atrioventricular conduction disturbances, left ventricular failure, and hypotension. In patients with impaired cardiac function, coadministration should be avoided.

7.5 Catecholamine-Depleting Drugs
Close observation of the patient is recommended when a beta-blocker is administered to patients receiving catecholamine-depleting drugs such as reserpine, because of possible additive effects and the production of hypotension and/or marked bradycardia, which may result in vertigo, syncope, or postural hypotension.

7.6 Digitalis and Calcium Antagonists
The concomitant use of beta-adrenergic blocking agents with digitalis and calcium antagonists may have additive effects in prolonging atrioventricular conduction time.

7.7 CYP2D6 Inhibitors
Potentiated systemic beta-blockade (e.g., decreased heart rate, depression) has been reported during combined treatment with CYP2D6 inhibitors (e.g., quinidine, SSRIs) and timolol.

7.8 Clonidine
Oral beta-adrenergic blocking agents may exacerbate the rebound hypertension which can follow the withdrawal of clonidine. There have been no reports of exacerbation of rebound hypertension with ophthalmic timolol maleate.

8 USE IN SPECIFIC POPULATIONS
8.1 Pregnancy
Teratogenic Effects. Pregnancy Category C. Developmental toxicity studies with dorzolamide hydrochloride in rabbits at oral doses of ≥2.5 mg/kg/day (31 times the recommended human ophthalmic dose) revealed malformations of the vertebral bodies. These malformations occurred at doses that caused metabolic acidosis with decreased body weight gain in dams and decreased fetal weights. No treatment-related malformations were seen at 1 mg/kg/day (13 times the recommended human ophthalmic dose).
Teratogenicity studies with timolol in mice, rats, and rabbits at oral doses up to 50 mg/kg/day (7,000 times the systemic exposure following the maximum recommended human ophthalmic dose) demonstrated no evidence of fetal malformations. Although delayed fetal ossification was observed at this dose in rats, there were no adverse effects on postnatal development of offspring. Doses of 1000 mg/kg/day (142,000 times the systemic exposure following the maximum recommended human ophthalmic dose) were maternotoxic in mice and resulted in an increased number of fetal resorptions. Increased fetal resorptions were also seen in rabbits at doses of 14,000 times the systemic exposure following the maximum recommended human ophthalmic dose, in this case without apparent maternotoxicity.
There are no adequate and well-controlled studies in pregnant women. COSOPT PF should be used during pregnancy only if the potential benefit justifies the potential risk to the fetus.

8.3 Nursing Mothers
It is not known whether dorzolamide is excreted in human milk. Timolol maleate has been detected in human milk following oral and ophthalmic drug administration. Because of the potential for serious adverse reactions from COSOPT PF in nursing infants, a decision should be made whether to discontinue nursing or to discontinue the drug, taking into account the importance of the drug to the mother.

8.4 Pediatric Use
The safety and effectiveness of dorzolamide hydrochloride ophthalmic solution and timolol maleate ophthalmic solution have been established when administered individually in pediatric patients aged 2 years and older. Use of these drug products in these children is supported by evidence from adequate and well-controlled studies in children and adults. Safety and efficacy in pediatric patients below the age of 2 years have not been established.

8.5 Geriatric Use
No overall differences in safety or effectiveness have been observed between elderly and younger patients.

10 OVERDOSAGE
Symptoms consistent with systemic administration of beta-blockers or carbonic anhydrase inhibitors may occur, including electrolyte imbalance, development of an acidotic state, dizziness, headache, shortness of breath, bradycardia, bronchospasm, cardiac arrest and possible central nervous system effects. Serum electrolyte levels (particularly potassium) and blood pH levels should be monitored. *[See Adverse Reactions (6).]*
A study of patients with renal failure showed that timolol did not dialyze readily.

11 DESCRIPTION
COSOPT PF (dorzolamide hydrochloride-timolol maleate ophthalmic solution) is the combination of a topical carbonic anhydrase inhibitor and a topical beta-adrenergic receptor blocking agent.
Dorzolamide hydrochloride is described chemically as: (4*S-trans*)-4-(ethylamino)-5,6-dihydro-6-methyl-4*H*-thieno[2,3-*b*]thiopyran-2-sulfonamide 7,7-dioxide monohydrochloride. Dorzolamide hydrochloride is optically active. The specific rotation is:

$$[\alpha] \quad 25°C \quad (C=1, \text{water}) = \sim -17°.$$
$$405 \text{ nm}$$

Its empirical formula is $C_{10}H_{16}N_2O_4S_3 \cdot HCl$ and its structural formula is:

Dorzolamide hydrochloride has a molecular weight of 360.91. It is a white to off-white, crystalline powder, which is soluble in water and slightly soluble in methanol and ethanol.
Timolol maleate is described chemically as: (-)-1-(*tert*-butylamino)-3-[(4-morpholino-1,2,5-thiadiazol-3-yl)oxy]-2-propanol maleate (1:1) (salt). Timolol maleate possesses an asymmetric carbon atom in its structure and is provided as the levo-isomer. The optical rotation of timolol maleate is:

$$[\alpha] \quad 25°C \quad \text{in 1N HCl } (C = 5) = -12.2°$$
$$405 \text{ nm} \quad (-11.7° \text{ to } -12.5°).$$

Its molecular formula is $C_{13}H_{24}N_4O_3S \cdot C_4H_4O_4$ and its structural formula is:

Timolol maleate has a molecular weight of 432.50. It is a white, odorless, crystalline powder which is soluble in water, methanol, and alcohol. Timolol maleate is stable at room temperature.
COSOPT PF is supplied as a sterile, clear, colorless to nearly colorless, isotonic, buffered, slightly viscous, aqueous solution. The pH of the solution is approximately 5.65, and the osmolarity is 242-323 mOsM. Each mL of COSOPT PF contains 20 mg dorzolamide (22.26 mg of dorzolamide hydrochloride) and 5 mg timolol (6.83 mg timolol maleate). Inactive ingredients are sodium citrate, hydroxyethyl cellulose, sodium hydroxide, mannitol, and water for injection. COSOPT PF does not contain a preservative.

12 CLINICAL PHARMACOLOGY
12.1 Mechanism of Action
COSOPT PF is comprised of two components: dorzolamide hydrochloride and timolol maleate. Each of these two components decreases elevated intraocular pressure, whether or not associated with glaucoma, by reducing aqueous humor secretion. Elevated intraocular pressure is a major risk factor in the pathogenesis of optic nerve damage and glaucomatous visual field loss. The higher the level of intraocular pressure, the greater the likelihood of glaucomatous field loss and optic nerve damage.
Dorzolamide hydrochloride is an inhibitor of human carbonic anhydrase II. Inhibition of carbonic anhydrase in the ciliary processes of the eye decreases aqueous humor secretion, presumably by slowing the formation of bicarbonate ions with subsequent reduction in sodium and fluid transport. Timolol maleate is a beta$_1$ and beta$_2$ (non-selective) adrenergic receptor blocking agent that does not have significant intrinsic sympathomimetic, direct myocardial depressant, or local anesthetic (membrane-stabilizing) activity. The combined effect of these two agents administered as COSOPT PF administered twice daily results in additional intraocular pressure reduction compared to either component administered alone, but the reduction is not as much as when dorzolamide administered three times daily and timolol twice daily are administered concomitantly. *[See Clinical Studies (14).]*

12.3 Pharmacokinetics
Dorzolamide Hydrochloride
When topically applied, dorzolamide reaches the systemic circulation. To assess the potential for systemic carbonic anhydrase inhibition following topical administration, drug and metabolite concentrations in RBCs and plasma and carbonic anhydrase inhibition in RBCs were measured. Dorzolamide accumulates in RBCs during chronic dosing as a result of binding to CA-II. The parent drug forms a single N-desethyl metabolite, which inhibits CA-II less potently than the parent drug but also inhibits CA-I. The metabolite also accumulates in RBCs where it binds primarily to CA-I. Plasma concentrations of dorzolamide and metabolite are generally below the assay limit of quantitation (15nM). Dorzolamide binds moderately to plasma proteins (approximately 33%).
Dorzolamide is primarily excreted unchanged in the urine; the metabolite also is excreted in urine. After dosing is stopped, dorzolamide washes out of RBCs nonlinearly, resulting in a rapid decline of drug concentration initially, followed by a slower elimination phase with a half-life of about four months.
To simulate the systemic exposure after long-term topical ocular administration, dorzolamide was given orally to eight healthy subjects for up to 20 weeks. The oral dose of 2 mg twice daily closely approximates the amount of drug delivered by topical ocular administration of dorzolamide 2% three times daily. Steady state was reached within 8 weeks. The inhibition of CA-II and total carbonic anhydrase

activities was below the degree of inhibition anticipated to be necessary for a pharmacological effect on renal function and respiration in healthy individuals.

Timolol Maleate

In a study of plasma drug concentrations in six subjects, the systemic exposure to timolol was determined following twice daily topical administration of timolol maleate ophthalmic solution 0.5%. The mean peak plasma concentration following morning dosing was 0.46 ng/mL.

13 NONCLINICAL TOXICOLOGY

13.1 Carcinogenesis, Mutagenesis, Impairment of Fertility

In a two-year study of dorzolamide hydrochloride administered orally to male and female Sprague-Dawley rats, urinary bladder papillomas were seen in male rats in the highest dosage group of 20 mg/kg/day (250 times the recommended human ophthalmic dose). Papillomas were not seen in rats given oral doses equivalent to approximately 12 times the recommended human ophthalmic dose. No treatment-related tumors were seen in a 21-month study in female and male mice given oral doses up to 75 mg/kg/day (~900 times the recommended human ophthalmic dose).

The increased incidence of urinary bladder papillomas seen in the high-dose male rats is a class-effect of carbonic anhydrase inhibitors in rats. Rats are particularly prone to developing papillomas in response to foreign bodies, compounds causing crystalluria, and diverse sodium salts. No changes in bladder urothelium were seen in dogs given oral dorzolamide hydrochloride for one year at 2 mg/kg/day (25 times the recommended human ophthalmic dose) or monkeys dosed topically to the eye at 0.4 mg/kg/day (~5 times the recommended human ophthalmic dose) for one year.

In a two-year study of timolol maleate administered orally to rats, there was a statistically significant increase in the incidence of adrenal pheochromocytomas in male rats administered 300 mg/kg/day (approximately 42,000 times the systemic exposure following the maximum recommended human ophthalmic dose). Similar differences were not observed in rats administered oral doses equivalent to approximately 14,000 times the maximum recommended human ophthalmic dose.

In a lifetime oral study of timolol maleate in mice, there were statistically significant increases in the incidence of benign and malignant pulmonary tumors, benign uterine polyps and mammary adenocarcinomas in female mice at 500 mg/kg/day, (approximately 71,000 times the systemic exposure following the maximum recommended human ophthalmic dose), but not at 5 or 50 mg/kg/day (approximately 700 or 7,000, respectively, times the systemic exposure following the maximum recommended human ophthalmic dose). In a subsequent study in female mice, in which post-mortem examinations were limited to the uterus and the lungs, a statistically significant increase in the incidence of pulmonary tumors was again observed at 500 mg/kg/day.

The increased occurrence of mammary adenocarcinomas was associated with elevations in serum prolactin which occurred in female mice administered oral timolol at 500 mg/kg/day, but not at doses of 5 or 50 mg/kg/day. An increased incidence of mammary adenocarcinomas in rodents has been associated with administration of several other therapeutic agents that elevate serum prolactin, but no correlation between serum prolactin levels and mammary tumors has been established in humans. Furthermore, in adult human female subjects who received oral dosages of up to 60 mg of timolol maleate (the maximum recommended human oral dosage), there were no clinically meaningful changes in serum prolactin.

The following tests for mutagenic potential were negative for dorzolamide: (1) *in vivo* (mouse) cytogenetic assay; (2) *in vitro* chromosomal aberration assay; (3) alkaline elution assay; (4) V-79 assay; and (5) Ames test.

Timolol maleate was devoid of mutagenic potential when tested *in vivo* (mouse) in the micronucleus test and cytogenetic assay (doses up to 800 mg/kg) and *in vitro* in a neoplastic cell transformation assay (up to 100 μg/mL). In Ames tests the highest concentrations of timolol employed, 5,000 or 10,000 μg/plate, were associated with statistically significant elevations of revertants observed with tester strain TA100 (in seven replicate assays), but not in the remaining three strains. In the assays with tester strain TA100, no consistent dose response relationship was observed, and the ratio of test to control revertants did not reach 2. A ratio of 2 is usually considered the criterion for a positive Ames test.

Reproduction and fertility studies in rats with either timolol maleate or dorzolamide hydrochloride demonstrated no adverse effect on male or female fertility at doses up to approximately 100 times the systemic exposure following the maximum recommended human ophthalmic dose.

14 CLINICAL STUDIES

14.1 COSOPT Efficacy

Clinical studies of 3 to 15 months duration were conducted to compare the IOP-lowering effect over the course of the day of COSOPT twice daily (dosed morning and bedtime) to individually- and concomitantly-administered 0.5% timolol twice daily and 2.0% dorzolamide twice and three times daily. The IOP-lowering effect of COSOPT twice daily was greater (1-3 mmHg) than that of monotherapy with either 2.0% dorzolamide three times daily or 0.5% timolol twice daily. The IOP-lowering effect of COSOPT twice daily was approximately 1 mmHg less than that of concomitant therapy with 2.0% dorzolamide three times daily and 0.5% timolol twice daily.

Open-label extensions of two studies were conducted for up to 12 months. During this period, the IOP-lowering effect of COSOPT twice daily was consistent during the 12 month follow-up period.

14.2 COSOPT PF Equivalence Study

In an active-treatment controlled, parallel, double-masked study in 261 patients with elevated intraocular pressure ≥22 mmHg in one or both eyes, COSOPT PF had an IOP-lowering effect equivalent to that of COSOPT.

16 HOW SUPPLIED/STORAGE AND HANDLING

COSOPT PF is supplied in a foil pouch containing 15 low density polyethylene 0.2 mL single-use containers.

NDC 0006-3629-60, package of 60 single-use vials.

NDC 0006-3629-62, package of 180 single-use vials.

Store COSOPT PF at 20-25°C (68-77°F). Do not freeze. Store in the original pouch. After the pouch is opened, store the remaining single-use containers in the foil pouch to protect from light. Write down the date you open the foil pouch in the space provided on the pouch. Discard any unused containers 15 days after first opening the pouch.

17 PATIENT COUNSELING INFORMATION

See FDA-Approved Patient Labeling (Patient Information).

17.1 Potential for Exacerbation of Asthma and COPD

COSOPT PF may cause severe worsening of asthma and COPD symptoms including death due to bronchospasm. Patients with bronchial asthma, a history of bronchial asthma, severe chronic obstructive pulmonary disease should be advised not to take this product. *[See Contraindications (4.1).]*

17.2 Potential of Cardiovascular Effects

COSOPT PF may cause worsening of cardiac symptoms. Patients with sinus bradycardia, second or third degree atrioventricular block, or cardiac failure should be advised not to take this product. *[See Contraindications (4.2).]*

17.3 Sulfonamide Reactions

COSOPT PF contains dorzolamide (which is a sulfonamide) and, although administered topically, is absorbed systemically. Therefore the same types of adverse reactions that are attributable to sulfonamides may occur with topical administration, including severe skin reactions. Patients should be advised that if serious or unusual reactions or signs of hypersensitivity occur, they should discontinue the use of the product and seek their physician's advice. *[See Warnings and Precautions (5.3).]*

17.4 Handling the Single-Use Container

COSOPT PF is a sterile solution that does not contain a preservative. The solution from one individual unit is to be used immediately after opening for administration to one or both eyes. Since sterility cannot be maintained after the individual unit is opened, the remaining contents should be discarded immediately after administration.

17.5 Intercurrent Ocular Conditions

Patients also should be advised that if they have ocular surgery or develop an intercurrent ocular condition (e.g., trauma or infection), they should immediately seek their physician's advice concerning the continued use of this product.

17.6 Concomitant Topical Ocular Therapy

If more than one topical ophthalmic drug is being used, the drugs should be administered at least five minutes apart.

Manuf. for: Merck Sharp & Dohme Corp., a subsidiary of **MERCK & CO., INC.,** Whitehouse Station, NJ 08889, USA

By: Catalent Pharma Solutions, LLC Woodstock, IL 60098, USA

Copyright © 2012 Merck Sharp & Dohme Corp., a subsidiary of **Merck & Co., Inc.**

All rights reserved.

Revised: 05/2012

6081301

Patient Information

COSOPT® PF (CO-sopt PEA EHF)

(dorzolamide hydrochloride-timolol maleate ophthalmic solution) 2%/0.5%

Read this information before you start using COSOPT PF and each time you get a refill. There may be new information. This information does not take the place of talking to your doctor about your medical condition or your treatment.

What is COSOPT PF?

COSOPT PF is a prescription sterile eye drop solution that contains 2 medicines, dorzolamide hydrochloride (a sulfonamide carbonic anhydrase inhibitor) and timolol maleate (a beta-adrenergic blocker). COSOPT PF is used to lower the pressure in the eye (intraocular pressure) in people with open-angle glaucoma or ocular hypertension, when their eye pressure is too high and beta-adrenergic blocker medicines alone have not adequately lowered the pressure.

It is not known if COSOPT PF is safe and effective in children under 2 years of age.

Who should not use COSOPT PF?

Do not use COSOPT PF if you:

• have or have had asthma
• have or have had severe lung problems (chronic obstructive pulmonary disease)
• have heart problems, including slow or irregular heartbeat or heart failure
• are allergic to dorzolamide hydrochloride, timolol maleate, or any of the ingredients in COSOPT PF. See the end of this leaflet for a complete list of ingredients in COSOPT PF.

Talk to your healthcare provider before taking this medicine if you have any of these conditions.

What should I tell my doctor before using COSOPT PF?

Before you use COSOPT PF, tell your doctor if you:

• have problems with muscle weakness (myasthenia gravis)
• have diabetes or problems with low blood sugar (hypoglycemia)
• have thyroid, kidney, or liver problems
• are planning to have surgery
• are allergic to sulfa drugs
• have or have had eye problems, including any surgery on your eye or eyes, or are using any other eye medicines
• have any other medical problems
• are pregnant or plan to become pregnant. It is not known if COSOPT PF will harm your unborn baby. If you become pregnant while using COSOPT PF talk to your doctor right away.
• are breastfeeding or plan to breastfeed. It is not known whether dorzolamide passes into your breast milk however, timolol has been detected in breast milk. Talk to your doctor about the best way to feed your baby if you use COSOPT PF.

Tell your doctor about all the medicines you take, including prescription and non-prescription medicines, vitamins, and herbal supplements.

COSOPT PF and other medicines may affect each other causing side effects. COSOPT PF may affect the way other medicines work, and other medicines may affect how COSOPT PF works.

Know the medicines you take. Keep a list of them to show your doctor and pharmacist when you get a new medicine.

How should I use COSOPT PF?

Read the Instructions for Use at the end of this Patient Information leaflet for additional instructions about the right way to use COSOPT PF.

• Use COSOPT PF exactly as your doctor tells you.
• **Use 1 drop of COSOPT PF in your eye (or eyes) in the morning and 1 drop in the evening.**
• If you use other medicines in your eye, wait at least 5 minutes between using COSOPT PF and your other eye medicines.
• Use your COSOPT PF right away after opening. Each COSOPT PF single-use container is sterile and is to be used 1 time then thrown away.
• Do not save any COSOPT PF that may be left over after you use a single-use container. Using COSOPT PF that is not sterile may cause other eye problems.

What are the possible side effects of COSOPT PF?

COSOPT PF may cause serious side effects including:

• **severe breathing problems.** These breathing problems can happen in people who have asthma, chronic obstructive pulmonary disease, or heart failure and can cause death. Tell your doctor right away if you have breathing problems while taking COSOPT PF.
• **heart failure.** This can happen in people who already have heart failure and in people who have never had heart failure before. Tell your doctor right away if you get any of these symptoms of heart failure while taking COSOPT PF:
  ○ shortness of breath
  ○ irregular heartbeat (palpitations)
  ○ swelling of your ankles or feet
  ○ sudden weight gain
• **severe allergic reactions.** These allergic reactions can happen the first time you use COSOPT PF or after you have been using COSOPT PF for a while and may cause death. **Stop taking COSOPT PF and call your doctor right away or get emergency help if you get any of these symptoms of an allergic reaction:**
  ○ swelling of your face, lips, mouth, or tongue
  ○ trouble breathing
  ○ wheezing
  ○ severe itching
  ○ skin rash, redness, or swelling
  ○ dizziness or fainting
  ○ fast heartbeat or pounding in your chest (tachycardia)
  ○ sweating

- **worsening muscle weakness.** COSOPT PF can cause muscle weakness to get worse in people who already have problems with muscle weakness (myasthenia gravis).
- **kidney problems.** Your doctor may do tests to check your kidney function while you use COSOPT PF.
- **swelling of your eye (cornea)**

The most common side effects of COSOPT PF include:
- a bitter, sour, or unusual taste in your mouth after using COSOPT PF
- burning, stinging, redness, or itching of the eye
- blurred vision
- painful, red, watery eyes with increased sensitivity (superficial punctate keratitis)

Tell your doctor if you have any new eye problems while using COSOPT PF including:
- an eye injury
- an eye infection
- a sudden loss of vision
- eye surgery
- swelling and redness of and around your eye (conjunctivitis)
- problems with your eyelids

Tell your doctor if you have any other side effects that bother you.

These are not all the possible side effects of COSOPT PF. For more information, ask your doctor or pharmacist.

Call your doctor about medical advice about side effects. You may report side effects to FDA at 1-800-FDA-1088.

What should I do in case of an overdose?

If you swallow the contents of the container, contact your doctor immediately. Among other effects, you may feel lightheaded, have difficulty breathing, or feel your heart rate has slowed.

How should I store COSOPT PF?
- Store COSOPT PF at room temperature between 68°F to 77°F (20°C to 25°C). Do not freeze.
- Keep the COSOPT PF single-use containers in their original foil pouch to protect from light.
- Write down the date you open the foil pouch in the space provided on the pouch.
- Throw away all unused COSOPT PF single-use containers 15 days after first opening the pouch.

Keep COSOPT PF and all medicines out of the reach of children.

General information about the safe and effective use of COSOPT PF.

Medicines are sometimes prescribed for purposes other than those listed in a Patient Information leaflet. Do not use COSOPT PF for a condition for which it was not prescribed. Do not give COSOPT PF to other people, even if they have the same symptoms you have. It may harm them. This Patient Information leaflet summarizes the most important information about COSOPT PF. If you would like more information, talk with your doctor. You can ask your pharmacist or doctor for information about COSOPT PF that is written for health professionals.

What are the ingredients in COSOPT PF?

Active ingredients: dorzolamide hydrochloride and timolol maleate

Inactive ingredients: sodium citrate, hydroxyethyl cellulose, sodium hydroxide, mannitol, and water for injection.

Instructions for Use

Read these instructions before using your COSOPT PF and each time you get a refill. There may be new information. This leaflet does not take the place of talking with your doctor about your medical condition or your treatment.

Important:
- **COSOPT PF is for the eye only. Do not swallow COSOPT PF.**
- COSOPT PF single-use containers are packaged in a foil pouch.
- Write down the date you open the foil pouch in the space provided on the pouch.

Every time you use COSOPT PF:

Step 1. Wash your hands.
Step 2. Take the strip of single-use containers from the pouch.
Step 3. Pull off 1 single-use container from the strip.
Step 4. Put the remaining strip of single-use containers back in the pouch and fold the edge to close the pouch.

Step 5. Hold the single-use container upright. Make sure that the solution is in the bottom part of the single-use container **(See Figure A).**

(Figure A)

Step 6. Open the single-use container by twisting off the tab **(See Figure B).**

(Figure B)

Step 7. Tilt your head backwards. If you are unable to tilt your head, lie down.
Step 8. Place the tip of the single-use container close to your eye. Be careful not to touch your eye with the tip of the single-use container **(See Figure C).**

(Figure C)

Step 9. Pull the lower eyelid downwards and look up.
Step 10. Gently squeeze the container and let 1 drop of COSOPT PF fall into the space between your lower eyelid and your eye. If a drop misses your eye, try again **(See Figure D).**

(Figure D)

Step 11. Blot any excess solution from the skin around the eye with a tissue.

- If your doctor has told you to use drops in both eyes, repeat steps 7 to 11 for your other eye.
- There is enough COSOPT PF in 1 single-use container for 1 or both of your eyes.
- Throw away the opened single-use container with any remaining COSOPT PF right away.

This Patient Information and Instructions for Use have been approved by the U.S. Food and Drug Administration.

Manuf. for: Merck Sharp & Dohme Corp., a subsidiary of **MERCK & CO., INC.,** Whitehouse Station, NJ 08889, USA
By: Catalent Pharma Solutions, LLC
Woodstock, IL 60098, USA
Copyright © 2012 Merck Sharp & Dohme Corp., a subsidiary of **Merck & Co., Inc.**
All rights reserved.
Issued: May 2012
6081301

Shown in Product Identification Guide, page 308

CRIXIVAN®
(INDINAVIR SULFATE)
CAPSULES

℞

DESCRIPTION

CRIXIVAN® (indinavir sulfate) is an inhibitor of the human immunodeficiency virus (HIV) protease. CRIXIVAN Capsules are formulated as a sulfate salt and are available for oral administration in strengths of 200 and 400 mg of indinavir (corresponding to 250 and 500 mg indinavir sulfate, respectively). Each capsule also contains the inactive ingredients anhydrous lactose and magnesium stearate. The capsule shell has the following inactive ingredients and dyes: gelatin and titanium dioxide.

The chemical name for indinavir sulfate is [1(1S,2R),5(S)]-2,3,5-trideoxy-N-(2,3-dihydro-2-hydroxy-1H-inden-1-yl)-5-[2-[[(1,1-dimethylethyl)amino]carbonyl]-4-(3-pyridinyl-methyl)-1-piperazinyl]-2-(phenylmethyl)-D-*erythro*-pentonamide sulfate (1:1) salt. Indinavir sulfate has the following structural formula:

Indinavir sulfate is a white to off-white, hygroscopic, crystalline powder with the molecular formula $C_{36}H_{47}N_5O_4 \cdot H_2SO_4$ and a molecular weight of 711.88. It is very soluble in water and in methanol.

MICROBIOLOGY

Mechanism of Action:

HIV-1 protease is an enzyme required for the proteolytic cleavage of the viral polyprotein precursors into the individual functional proteins found in infectious HIV-1. Indinavir binds to the protease active site and inhibits the activity of the enzyme. This inhibition prevents cleavage of the viral polyproteins resulting in the formation of immature noninfectious viral particles.

Antiretroviral Activity *In Vitro*:

The *in vitro* activity of indinavir was assessed in cell lines of lymphoblastic and monocytic origin and in peripheral blood lymphocytes. HIV-1 variants used to infect the different cell types include laboratory-adapted variants, primary clinical isolates and clinical isolates resistant to nucleoside analogue and nonnucleoside inhibitors of the HIV-1 reverse transcriptase. The IC_{95} (95% inhibitory concentration) of indinavir in these test systems was in the range of 25 to 100 nM. In drug combination studies with the nucleoside analogues zidovudine and didanosine, indinavir showed synergistic activity in cell culture. The relationship between *in vitro* susceptibility of HIV-1 to indinavir and inhibition of HIV-1 replication in humans has not been established.

Drug Resistance:

Isolates of HIV-1 with reduced susceptibility to the drug have been recovered from some patients treated with indinavir. Viral resistance was correlated with the accumulation of mutations that resulted in the expression of amino acid substitutions in the viral protease. Eleven amino acid residue positions, (L10I/V/R, K20I/M/R, L24I, M46I/L, I54A/V, L63P, I64V, A71T/V, V82A/F/T, I84V, and L90M), at which substitutions are associated with resistance, have been identified. Resistance was mediated by the co-expression of multiple and variable substitutions at these positions. No single substitution was either necessary or sufficient for measurable resistance (≥4-fold increase in IC_{95}). In general, higher levels of resistance were associated with the co-expression of greater numbers of substitutions, although their individual effects varied and were not additive. At least 3 amino acid substitutions must be present for phenotypic resistance to indinavir to reach measurable levels. In addition, mutations in the p7/ p1 and p1/ p6 gag cleavage sites were observed in some indinavir resistant HIV-1 isolates.

In vitro phenotypic susceptibilities to indinavir were determined for 38 viral isolates from 13 patients who experienced virologic rebounds during indinavir monotherapy. Pretreatment isolates from five patients exhibited indinavir IC_{95} values of 50-100 nM. At or following viral RNA rebound (after 12-76 weeks of therapy), IC_{95} values ranged from 25 to >3000 nM, and the viruses carried 2 to 10 mutations in the protease gene relative to baseline.

Cross-Resistance to Other Antiviral Agents:

Varying degrees of HIV-1 cross-resistance have been observed between indinavir and other HIV-1 protease inhibitors. In studies with ritonavir, saquinavir, and amprenavir, the extent and spectrum of cross-resistance varied with the specific mutational patterns observed. In general, the degree of cross-resistance increased with the accumulation of resistance-associated amino acid substitutions. Within a panel of 29 viral isolates from indinavir-treated patients that exhibited measurable (≥4-fold) phenotypic resistance to indinavir, all were resistant to ritonavir. Of the indinavir resistant HIV-1 isolates, 63% showed resistance to saquinavir and 81% to amprenavir.

CLINICAL PHARMACOLOGY

Pharmacokinetics

Absorption:

Indinavir was rapidly absorbed in the fasted state with a time to peak plasma concentration (T_{max}) of 0.8 ± 0.3 hours (mean ± S.D.) (n=11). A greater than dose-proportional increase in indinavir plasma concentrations was observed over the 200-1000 mg dose range. At a dosing regimen of 800 mg every 8 hours, steady-state area under the plasma concentration time curve (AUC) was 30,691 ± 11,407 nM•hour (n=16), peak plasma concentration (C_{max})

was 12,617 ± 4037 nM (n=16), and plasma concentration eight hours post dose (trough) was 251 ± 178 nM (n=16).

Effect of Food on Oral Absorption:

Administration of indinavir with a meal high in calories, fat, and protein (784 kcal, 48.6 g fat, 31.3 g protein) resulted in a 77% ± 8% reduction in AUC and an 84% ± 7% reduction in C_{max} (n=10). Administration with lighter meals (e.g., a meal of dry toast with jelly, apple juice, and coffee with skim milk and sugar or a meal of corn flakes, skim milk and sugar) resulted in little or no change in AUC, C_{max} or trough concentration.

Distribution:

Indinavir was approximately 60% bound to human plasma proteins over a concentration range of 81 nM to 16,300 nM.

Metabolism:

Following a 400-mg dose of ^{14}C-indinavir, 83 ± 1% (n=4) and 19 ± 3% (n=6) of the total radioactivity was recovered in feces and urine, respectively; radioactivity due to parent drug in feces and urine was 19.1% and 9.4%, respectively. Seven metabolites have been identified, one glucuronide conjugate and six oxidative metabolites. *In vitro* studies indicate that cytochrome P-450 3A4 (CYP3A4) is the major enzyme responsible for formation of the oxidative metabolites.

Elimination:

Less than 20% of indinavir is excreted unchanged in the urine. Mean urinary excretion of unchanged drug was 10.4 ± 4.9% (n=10) and 12.0 ± 4.9% (n=10) following a single 700-mg and 1000-mg dose, respectively. Indinavir was rapidly eliminated with a half-life of 1.8 ± 0.4 hours (n=10). Significant accumulation was not observed after multiple dosing at 800 mg every 8 hours.

Special Populations

Hepatic Insufficiency:

Patients with mild to moderate hepatic insufficiency and clinical evidence of cirrhosis had evidence of decreased metabolism of indinavir resulting in approximately 60% higher mean AUC following a single 400-mg dose (n=12). The half-life of indinavir increased to 2.8 ± 0.5 hours. Indinavir pharmacokinetics have not been studied in patients with severe hepatic insufficiency (see DOSAGE AND ADMINISTRATION, Hepatic Insufficiency).

Renal Insufficiency:

The pharmacokinetics of indinavir have not been studied in patients with renal insufficiency.

Gender:

The effect of gender on the pharmacokinetics of indinavir was evaluated in 10 HIV seropositive women who received CRIXIVAN 800 mg every 8 hours with zidovudine 200 mg every 8 hours and lamivudine 150 mg twice a day for one week. Indinavir pharmacokinetic parameters in these women were compared to those in HIV seropositive men (pooled historical control data). Differences in indinavir exposure, peak concentrations, and trough concentrations between males and females are shown in Table 1 below:

[See table 1 above]

The clinical significance of these gender differences in the pharmacokinetics of indinavir is not known.

Race:

Pharmacokinetics of indinavir appear to be comparable in Caucasians and Blacks based on pharmacokinetic studies including 42 Caucasians (26 HIV-positive) and 16 Blacks (4 HIV-positive).

Pediatric:

The optimal dosing regimen for use of indinavir in pediatric patients has not been established. In HIV-infected pediatric patients (age 4-15 years), a dosage regimen of indinavir capsules, 500 mg/m^2 every 8 hours, produced AUC_{0-8hr} of 38,742 ± 24,098 nM•hour (n=34), C_{max} of 17,181 ± 9809 nM (n=34), and trough concentrations of 134 ± 91 nM (n=28). The pharmacokinetic profiles of indinavir in pediatric patients were not comparable to profiles previously observed in HIV-infected adults receiving the recommended dose of 800 mg every 8 hours. The AUC and C_{max} values were slightly higher and the trough concentrations were considerably lower in pediatric patients. Approximately 50% of the pediatric patients had trough values below 100 nM; whereas, approximately 10% of adult patients had trough levels below 100 nM. The relationship between specific trough values and inhibition of HIV replication has not been established.

Pregnant Patients:

The optimal dosing regimen for use of indinavir in pregnant patients has not been established. A CRIXIVAN dose of 800 mg every 8 hours (with zidovudine 200 mg every 8 hours and lamivudine 150 mg twice a day) has been studied in 16 HIV-infected pregnant patients at 14 to 28 weeks of gestation at enrollment (study PACTG 358). The mean indinavir plasma AUC_{0-8hr} at weeks 30-32 of gestation (n=11) was 9231 nM•hr, which is 74% (95% CI: 50%, 86%) lower than that observed 6 weeks postpartum. Six of these 11 (55%) patients had mean indinavir plasma concentrations 8 hours post-dose (C_{min}) below assay threshold of reliable quantification. The pharmacokinetics of indinavir in these 11 patients at 6 weeks postpartum were generally similar to those observed in non-pregnant patients in another study (see PRECAUTIONS, Pregnancy).

Table 1

PK Parameter	% change in PK parameter for females relative to males	90% Confidence Interval
AUC_{0-8h} (nM•hr)	↓13%	(↓32%, ↑12%)
C_{max} (nM)	↓13%	(↓32%, ↑10%)
C_{8h} (nM)	↓22%	(↓47%, ↑15%)

↓Indicates a decrease in the PK parameter; ↑indicates an increase in the PK parameter.

Table 2: Drug Interactions: Pharmacokinetic Parameters for Indinavir in the Presence of the Coadministered Drug (See PRECAUTIONS, Table 9 for Recommended Alterations in Dose or Regimen)

Coadministered drug	Dose of Coadministered drug (mg)	Dose of CRIXIVAN (mg)	n	C_{max}	AUC	C_{min}
Cimetidine	600 twice daily, 6 days	400 single dose	12	1.07 (0.77, 1.49)	0.98 (0.81, 1.19)	0.82 (0.69, 0.99)
Clarithromycin	500 q12h, 7 days	800 three times daily, 7 days	10	1.08 (0.85, 1.38)	1.19 (1.00, 1.42)	1.57 (1.16, 2.12)
Delavirdine	400 three times daily	400 three times daily, 7 days	28	0.64* (0.48, 0.86)	No significant change*	2.18* (1.16, 4.12)
Delavirdine	400 three times daily	600 three times daily, 7 days	28	No significant change	1.53* (1.07, 2.20)	3.98* (2.04, 7.78)
Efavirenz[†]	600 once daily, 10 days	1000 three times daily, 10 days After morning dose After afternoon dose After evening dose	20	No significant change* No significant change* 0.71* (0.57, 0.89)	0.67* (0.61, 0.74) 0.63* (0.54, 0.74) 0.54* (0.46, 0.63)	0.61* (0.49, 0.76) 0.48* (0.43, 0.53) 0.43* (0.37, 0.50)
Fluconazole[†]	400 once daily, 8 days	1000 three times daily, 7 days	11	0.87 (0.72, 1.05)	0.76 (0.59, 0.98)	0.90 (0.72, 1.12)
Grapefruit Juice	8 oz.	400 single dose	10	0.65 (0.53, 0.79)	0.73 (0.60, 0.87)	0.90 (0.71, 1.15)
Isoniazid	300 once daily in the morning, 8 days	800 three times daily, 7 days	11	0.95 (0.88, 1.03)	0.99 (0.87, 1.13)	0.89 (0.75, 1.06)
Itraconazole	200 twice daily, 7 days	600 three times daily, 7 days	12	0.78* (0.69, 0.88)	0.99* (0.91, 1.06)	1.49* (1.28, 1.74)
Ketoconazole	400 once daily, 7 days 400 once daily, 7 days	600 three times daily, 7 days 400 three times daily, 7 days	12 12	0.69* (0.61, 0.78) 0.42* (0.37, 0.47)	0.80* (0.74, 0.87) 0.44* (0.41, 0.48)	1.29* (1.11, 1.51) 0.73* (0.62, 0.85)
Methadone	20-60 once daily in the morning, 8 days	800 three times daily, 8 days	10	See text below for discussion of interaction.		
Quinidine	200 single dose	400 single dose	10	0.96 (0.79, 1.18)	1.07 (0.89, 1.28)	0.93 (0.73, 1.19)
Rifabutin	150 once daily in the morning, 10 days	800 three times daily, 10 days	14	0.80 (0.72, 0.89)	0.68 (0.60, 0.76)	0.60 (0.51, 0.72)
Rifabutin	300 once daily in the morning, 10 days	800 three times daily, 10 days	10	0.75 (0.61, 0.91)	0.66 (0.56, 0.77)	0.61 (0.50, 0.75)
Rifampin	600 once daily in the morning, 8 days	800 three times daily, 7 days	12	0.13 (0.08, 0.22)	0.08 (0.06, 0.11)	Not Done
Ritonavir	100 twice daily, 14 days	800 twice daily, 14 days	10, 16[‡]	See text below for discussion of interaction.		
Ritonavir	200 twice daily, 14 days	800 twice daily, 14 days	9, 16[‡]	See text below for discussion of interaction.		
Sildenafil	25 single dose	800 three times daily	6	See text below for discussion of interaction.		

(Table continued on next page)

Drug Interactions:
(also see CONTRAINDICATIONS, WARNINGS, PRECAUTIONS, Drug Interactions)

Table 2 (cont.): Drug Interactions: Pharmacokinetic Parameters for Indinavir in the Presence of the Coadministered Drug (See PRECAUTIONS, Table 9 for Recommended Alterations in Dose or Regimen)

Coadministered drug	Dose of Coadministered drug (mg)	Dose of CRIXIVAN (mg)	n	Ratio (with/without coadministered drug) of Indinavir Pharmacokinetic Parameters (90% CI); No Effect = 1.00		
				C_{max}	AUC	C_{min}
St. John's wort (*Hypericum perforatum*, standardized to 0.3 % hypericin)	300 three times daily with meals, 14 days	800 three times daily	8	Not Available	0.46 (0.34, 0.58)§	0.19 (0.06, 0.33)§
Stavudine (d4T)[†]	40 twice daily, 7 days	800 three times daily, 7 days	11	0.95 (0.80, 1.11)	0.95 (0.80, 1.12)	1.13 (0.83, 1.53)
Trimethoprim/ Sulfamethoxazole	800 Trimethoprim/ 160 Sulfamethoxazole q12h, 7 days	400 four times daily, 7 days	12	1.12 (0.87, 1.46)	0.98 (0.81, 1.18)	0.83 (0.72, 0.95)
Zidovudine[‡]	200 three times daily, 7 days	1000 three times daily, 7 days	12	1.06 (0.91, 1.25)	1.05 (0.86, 1.28)	1.02 (0.77, 1.35)
Zidovudine/ Lamivudine (3TC)[†]	200/150 three times daily, 7 days	800 three times daily, 7 days	6, 9¶	1.05 (0.83, 1.33)	1.04 (0.67, 1.61)	0.98 (0.56, 1.73)

All interaction studies conducted in healthy, HIV-negative adult subjects, unless otherwise indicated.
* Relative to indinavir 800 mg three times daily alone.
† Study conducted in HIV-positive subjects.
‡ Comparison to historical data on 16 subjects receiving indinavir alone.
§ 95% CI.
¶ Parallel group design; n for indinavir + coadministered drug, n for indinavir alone.

Table 3: Drug Interactions: Pharmacokinetic Parameters for Coadministered Drug in the Presence of Indinavir (See PRECAUTIONS, Table 9 for Recommended Alterations in Dose or Regimen)

Coadministered drug	Dose of Coadministered drug (mg)	Dose of CRIXIVAN (mg)	n	Ratio (with/without CRIXIVAN) of Coadministered Drug Pharmacokinetic Parameters (90% CI); No Effect = 1.00		
				C_{max}	AUC	C_{min}
Clarithromycin	500 twice daily, 7 days	800 three times daily, 7 days	12	1.19 (1.02, 1.39)	1.47 (1.30, 1.65)	1.97 (1.58, 2.46) n=11
Efavirenz	200 once daily, 14 days	800 three times daily, 14 days	20	No significant change	No significant change	--
Ethinyl Estradiol (ORTHO-NOVUM 1/35)*	35 mcg, 8 days	800 three times daily, 8 days	18	1.02 (0.96, 1.09)	1.22 (1.15, 1.30)	1.37 (1.24, 1.51)
Isoniazid	300 once daily in the morning, 8 days	800 three times daily, 8 days	11	1.34 (1.12, 1.60)	1.12 (1.03, 1.22)	1.00 (0.92, 1.08)
Methadone[†]	20-60 once daily in the morning, 8 days	800 three times daily, 8 days	12	0.93 (0.84, 1.03)	0.96 (0.86, 1.06)	1.06 (0.94, 1.19)
Norethindrone (ORTHO-NOVUM 1/35)*	1 mcg, 8 days	800 three times daily, 8 days	18	1.05 (0.95, 1.16)	1.26 (1.20, 1.31)	1.44 (1.32, 1.57)
Rifabutin 150 mg once daily in the morning, 11 days + indinavir compared to 300 mg once daily in the morning, 11 days alone	150 once daily in the morning, 10 days	800 three times daily, 10 days	14	1.29 (1.05, 1.59)	1.54 (1.33, 1.79)	1.99 (1.71, 2.31) n=13
	300 once daily in the morning, 10 days	800 three times daily, 10 days	10	2.34 (1.64, 3.35)	2.73 (1.99, 3.77)	3.44 (2.65, 4.46) n=9

(Table continued on next page)

Indinavir is an inhibitor of the cytochrome P450 isoform CYP3A4. Coadministration of CRIXIVAN and drugs primarily metabolized by CYP3A4 may result in increased plasma concentrations of the other drug, which could increase or prolong its therapeutic and adverse effects (see CONTRAINDICATIONS and WARNINGS). Based on *in vitro* data in human liver microsomes, indinavir does not inhibit CYP1A2, CYP2C9, CYP2E1 and CYP2B6. However, indinavir may be a weak inhibitor of CYP2D6.

Indinavir is metabolized by CYP3A4. Drugs that induce CYP3A4 activity would be expected to increase the clearance of indinavir, resulting in lowered plasma concentrations of indinavir. Coadministration of CRIXIVAN and other drugs that inhibit CYP3A4 may decrease the clearance of indinavir and may result in increased plasma concentrations of indinavir.

Drug interaction studies were performed with CRIXIVAN and other drugs likely to be coadministered and some drugs commonly used as probes for pharmacokinetic interactions. The effects of coadministration of CRIXIVAN on the AUC, C_{max} and C_{min} are summarized in Table 2 (effect of other drugs on indinavir) and Table 3 (effect of indinavir on other drugs). For information regarding clinical recommendations, see Table 9 in PRECAUTIONS.
[See table 2 on previous page and above]
[See table 3 below and on next page]

Delavirdine: Delavirdine inhibits the metabolism of indinavir such that coadministration of 400-mg or 600-mg indinavir three times daily with 400-mg delavirdine three times daily alters indinavir AUC, C_{max} and C_{min} (see Table 2). Indinavir had no effect on delavirdine pharmacokinetics (see DOSAGE AND ADMINISTRATION, Concomitant Therapy, Delavirdine), based on a comparison to historical delavirdine pharmacokinetic data.

Methadone: Administration of indinavir (800 mg every 8 hours) with methadone (20 mg to 60 mg daily) for one week in subjects on methadone maintenance resulted in no change in methadone AUC. Based on a comparison to historical data, there was little or no change in indinavir AUC.

Ritonavir: Compared to historical data in patients who received indinavir 800 mg every 8 hours alone, twice-daily coadministration to volunteers of indinavir 800 mg and ritonavir with food for two weeks resulted in a 2.7-fold increase of indinavir AUC_{24h}, a 1.6-fold increase in indinavir C_{max}, and an 11-fold increase in indinavir C_{min} for a 100-mg ritonavir dose and a 3.6-fold increase of indinavir AUC_{24h}, a 1.8-fold increase in indinavir C_{max}, and a 24-fold increase in indinavir C_{min} for a 200-mg ritonavir dose. In the same study, twice-daily coadministration of indinavir (800 mg) and ritonavir (100 or 200 mg) resulted in ritonavir AUC_{24h} increases versus the same doses of ritonavir alone (see Table 3).

Sildenafil: The results of one published study in HIV-infected men (n=6) indicated that coadministration of indinavir (800 mg every 8 hours chronically) with a single 25-mg dose of sildenafil resulted in an 11% increase in average AUC_{0-8hr} of indinavir and a 48% increase in average indinavir peak concentration (C_{max}) compared to 800 mg every 8 hours alone. Average sildenafil AUC was increased by 340% following coadministration of sildenafil and indinavir compared to historical data following administration of sildenafil alone (see CONTRAINDICATIONS, WARNINGS, Drug Interactions and PRECAUTIONS, Drug Interactions).

Vardenafil: Indinavir (800 mg every 8 hours) coadministered with a single 10-mg dose of vardenafil resulted in a 16-fold increase in vardenafil AUC, a 7-fold increase in vardenafil C_{max}, and a 2-fold increase in vardenafil half-life (see WARNINGS, Drug Interactions and PRECAUTIONS, Drug Interactions).

INDICATIONS AND USAGE

CRIXIVAN in combination with antiretroviral agents is indicated for the treatment of HIV infection.
This indication is based on two clinical trials of approximately 1 year duration that demonstrated: 1) a reduction in the risk of AIDS-defining illnesses or death; 2) a prolonged suppression of HIV RNA.

Description of Studies

In all clinical studies, with the exception of ACTG 320, the AMPLICOR HIV MONITOR assay was used to determine the level of circulating HIV RNA in serum. This is an experimental use of the assay. HIV RNA results should not be directly compared to results from other trials using different HIV RNA assays or using other sample sources.

Study ACTG 320 was a multicenter, randomized, double-blind clinical endpoint trial to compare the effect of CRIXIVAN in combination with zidovudine and lamivudine with that of zidovudine plus lamivudine on the progression to an AIDS-defining illness (ADI) or death. Patients were protease inhibitor and lamivudine naive and zidovudine experienced, with CD4 cell counts of ≤200 cells/mm³. The study enrolled 1156 HIV-infected patients (17% female, 28% Black, 18% Hispanic, mean age 39 years). The mean baseline CD4 cell count was 87 cells/mm³. The mean baseline HIV RNA was 4.95 $\log_{10}$ copies/mL (89,035 copies/mL). The study was terminated after a planned interim analysis, resulting in a median follow-up of 38 weeks and a maximum follow-up of 52 weeks. Results are shown in Table 4 and Figures 1 & 2.

Table 4: ACTG 320

Endpoint	Number (%) of Patients with AIDS-defining Illness or Death	
	IDV+ZDV+L (n=577)	ZDV+L (n=579)
HIV Progression or Death	35 (6.1)	63 (10.9)
Death*	10 (1.7)	19 (3.3)

IDV = Indinavir, ZDV = Zidovudine, L = Lamivudine
* The number of deaths is inadequate to assess the impact of Indinavir on survival.

Study ACTG 320: Figure 1 - Indinavir Protocol ACTG 320 Zidovudine Experienced Plasma Viral RNA - Proportions Below 400 copies/mL

Study ACTG 320: Figure 2 - ACTG 320 Zidovudine Experienced CD4 Cell Counts - Mean Change from Baseline

Study 028, a double-blind, multicenter, randomized, clinical endpoint trial conducted in Brazil, compared the effects of CRIXIVAN plus zidovudine with those of CRIXIVAN alone or zidovudine alone on the progression to an ADI or death, and on surrogate marker responses. All patients were antiretroviral naive with CD4 cell counts of 50 to 250 cells/mm^3. The study enrolled 996 HIV-1 seropositive patients [28% female, 11% Black, 1% Asian/Other, median age 33 years, mean baseline CD4 cell count of 152 cells/mm^3, mean serum viral RNA of 4.44 log$_{10}$ copies/mL (27,824 copies/mL)]. Treatment regimens containing zidovudine were modified in a blinded manner with the optional addition of lamivudine (median time: week 40). The median length of follow-up was 56 weeks with a maximum of 97 weeks. The study was terminated after a planned interim analysis, resulting in a median follow-up of 56 weeks and a maximum follow-up of 97 weeks. Results are shown in Table 5 and Figures 3 and 4.

Table 5: Protocol 028

Endpoint	Number (%) of Patients with AIDS-defining Illness or Death		
	IDV+ZDV (n=332)	IDV (n=332)	ZDV (n=332)
HIV Progression or Death	21 (6.3)	27 (8.1)	62 (18.7)
Death*	8 (2.4)	5 (1.5)	11 (3.3)

* The number of deaths is inadequate to assess the impact of Indinavir on survival.

Study 028: Figure 3 - Indinavir Protocol 028 Zidovudine Naive Viral RNA - Proportions Below 500 Copies/mL in Serum

[See figure at top of next column]
Study 035 was a multicenter, randomized trial in 97 HIV-1 seropositive patients who were zidovudine-experienced (median exposure 30 months), protease-inhibitor- and lamivudine-naive, with mean baseline CD4 count 175 cells/mm^3 and mean baseline serum viral RNA 4.62 log$_{10}$ copies/mL (41,230 copies/mL). Comparisons included CRIXIVAN plus zidovudine plus lamivudine vs. CRIXIVAN alone vs. zidovudine plus lamivudine. After at least 24 weeks of randomized, double-blind therapy, patients were switched to open-label CRIXIVAN plus lamivudine plus zidovudine. Mean changes in log$_{10}$ viral RNA in serum, the proportions of patients with viral RNA below 500 copies/mL in serum, and mean changes in CD4 cell counts, during 24

Table 3 *(cont.):* **Drug Interactions: Pharmacokinetic Parameters for Coadministered Drug in the Presence of Indinavir (See PRECAUTIONS, Table 9 for Recommended Alterations in Dose or Regimen)**

Coadministered drug	Dose of Coadministered drug (mg)	Dose of CRIXIVAN (mg)	n	Ratio (with/without CRIXIVAN) of Coadministered Drug Pharmacokinetic Parameters (90% CI); No Effect = 1.00		
				C$_{max}$	AUC	C$_{min}$
Ritonavir	100 twice daily, 14 days	800 twice daily, 14 days	10, 4‡	1.61 (1.13, 2.29)	1.72 (1.20, 2.48)	1.62 (0.93, 2.85)
	200 twice daily, 14 days	800 twice daily, 14 days	9, 5‡	1.19 (0.85, 1.66)	1.96 (1.39, 2.76)	4.71 (2.66, 8.33) n=9, 4
Saquinavir						
Hard gel formulation	600 single dose	800 three times daily, 2 days	6	4.7 (2.7, 8.1)	6.0 (4.0, 9.1)	2.9 (1.7, 4.7)§
Soft gel formulation	800 single dose	800 three times daily, 2 days	6	6.5 (4.7, 9.1)	7.2 (4.3, 11.9)	5.5 (2.2, 14.1)§
Soft gel formulation	1200 single dose	800 three times daily, 2 days	6	4.0 (2.7, 5.9)	4.6 (3.2, 6.7)	5.5 (3.7, 8.3)§
Sildenafil	25 single dose	800 three times daily	6	See text below for discussion of interaction.		
Stavudine¶	40 twice daily, 7 days	800 three times daily, 7 days	13	0.86 (0.73, 1.03)	1.21 (1.09, 1.33)	Not Done
Theophylline	250 single dose (on Days 1 and 7)	800 three times daily, 6 days (Days 2 to 7)	12, 4‡	0.88 (0.76, 1.03)	1.14 (1.04, 1.24)	1.13 (0.86, 1.49) n=7, 3
Trimethoprim/ Sulfamethoxazole Trimethoprim	800 Trimethoprim/ 160 Sulfamethoxazole q12h, 7 days	400 q6h, 7 days	12	1.18 (1.05, 1.32)	1.18 (1.05, 1.33)	1.18 (1.00, 1.39)
Trimethoprim/ Sulfamethoxazole Sulfamethoxazole	800 Trimethoprim/ 160 Sulfamethoxazole q12h, 7 days	400 q6h, 7 days	12	1.01 (0.95, 1.08)	1.05 (1.01, 1.09)	1.05 (0.97, 1.14)
Vardenafil	10 single dose	800 three times daily	18	See text below for discussion of interaction.		
Zidovudine¶	200 three times daily, 7 days	1000 three times daily, 7 days	12	0.89 (0.73, 1.09)	1.17 (1.07, 1.29)	1.51 (0.71, 3.20) n=4
Zidovudine/ Lamivudine¶ Zidovudine	200/150 three times daily, 7 days	800 three times daily, 7 days	6, 7‡	1.23 (0.74, 2.03)	1.39 (1.02, 1.89)	1.08 (0.77, 1.50) n=5, 5
Zidovudine/ Lamivudine¶ Lamivudine	200/150 three times daily, 7 days	800 three times daily, 7 days	6, 7‡	0.73 (0.52, 1.02)	0.91 (0.66, 1.26)	0.88 (0.59, 1.33)

All interaction studies conducted in healthy, HIV-negative adult subjects, unless otherwise indicated.
* Registered trademark of Ortho Pharmaceutical Corporation.
† Study conducted in subjects on methadone maintenance.
‡ Parallel group design; n for coadministered drug + indinavir, n for coadministered drug alone.
§ C$_{6hr}$
¶ Study conducted in HIV-positive subjects.

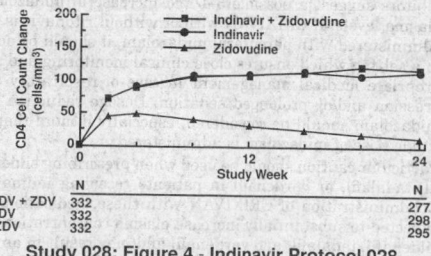

Study 028: Figure 4 - Indinavir Protocol 028 Zidovudine Naive CD4 Cell Counts - Mean Change from Baseline

weeks of randomized, double-blinded therapy are summarized in Figures 5, 6, and 7, respectively. A limited number of patients remained on randomized, double-blind treatment for longer periods; based on this extended treatment experience, it appears that a greater number of subjects randomized to CRIXIVAN plus zidovudine plus lamivudine demonstrated HIV RNA levels below 500 copies/mL during one year of therapy as compared to those in other treatment groups.

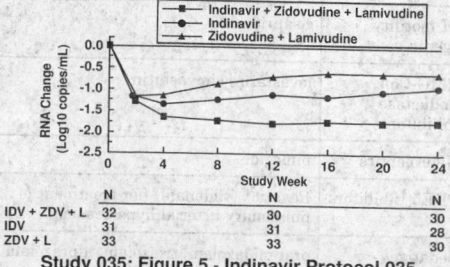

Study 035: Figure 5 - Indinavir Protocol 035 Zidovudine Experienced Viral RNA - Mean Log10 Change from Baseline in Serum

Study 035: Figure 6 - Indinavir Protocol 035 Zidovudine Experienced Viral RNA - Proportions Below 500 Copies/mL in Serum

Study 035: Figure 7 - Indinavir Protocol 035 Zidovudine Experienced CD4 Cell Counts - Mean Change from Baseline

Genotypic Resistance in Clinical Studies

Study 006 (10/15/93-10/12/94) was a dose-ranging study in which patients were initially treated with CRIXIVAN at a dose of <2.4 g/day followed by 2.4 g/day. Study 019 (6/23/94-4/10/95) was a randomized comparison of CRIXIVAN 600 mg every 6 hours, CRIXIVAN plus zidovudine, and zidovudine alone. Table 6 shows the incidence of genotypic resistance at 24 weeks in these studies.

Table 6: Genotypic Resistance at 24 Weeks

Treatment Group	Resistance to IDV n/N*	Resistance to ZDV n/N*
IDV	—	—
<2.4 g/day	31/37 (84%)	—
2.4 g/day	9/21 (43%)	1/17 (6%)
IDV/ZDV	4/22 (18%)	1/22 (5%)
ZDV	1/18 (6%)	11/17 (65%)

* N - includes patients with non-amplifiable virus at 24 weeks who had amplifiable virus at week 0.

CONTRAINDICATIONS

CRIXIVAN is contraindicated in patients with clinically significant hypersensitivity to any of its components.

Inhibition of CYP3A4 by CRIXIVAN can result in elevated plasma concentrations of the following drugs, potentially causing serious or life-threatening reactions:

Table 7: Drug Interactions With Crixivan: Contraindicated Drugs

Drug Class	Drugs Within Class That Are Contraindicated With CRIXIVAN
Alpha 1-adrenoreceptor antagonist	alfuzosin
Antiarrhythmics	amiodarone
Ergot derivatives	dihydroergotamine, ergonovine, ergotamine, methylergonovine
GI motility agents	cisapride
HMG-CoA Reductase Inhibitors	lovastatin, simvastatin
Neuroleptics	pimozide
PDE5 Inhibitors	Revatio* (sildenafil) [for treatment of pulmonary arterial hypertension]
Sedative/ hypnotics	oral midazolam, triazolam, alprazolam

* Registered trademark of Pfizer, Inc.

WARNINGS

ALERT: Find out about medicines that should NOT be taken with CRIXIVAN. This statement is included on the product's bottle label.

Nephrolithiasis/Urolithiasis

Nephrolithiasis/urolithiasis has occurred with CRIXIVAN therapy. The cumulative frequency of nephrolithiasis is substantially higher in pediatric patients (29%) than in adult patients (12.4%; range across individual trials: 4.7% to 34.4%). The cumulative frequency of nephrolithiasis events increases with increasing exposure to CRIXIVAN; however, the risk over time remains relatively constant. In some cases, nephrolithiasis/urolithiasis has been associated with renal insufficiency or acute renal failure, pyelonephritis with or without bacteremia. If signs or symptoms of nephrolithiasis/urolithiasis occur, (including flank pain, with or without hematuria or microscopic hematuria), temporary interruption (e.g., 1-3 days) or discontinuation of therapy may be considered. **Adequate hydration is recommended in all patients treated with CRIXIVAN. (See ADVERSE REACTIONS and DOSAGE AND ADMINISTRATION, Nephrolithiasis/Urolithiasis.)**

Hemolytic Anemia

Acute hemolytic anemia, including cases resulting in death, has been reported in patients treated with CRIXIVAN. Once a diagnosis is apparent, appropriate measures for the treatment of hemolytic anemia should be instituted, including discontinuation of CRIXIVAN.

Hepatitis

Hepatitis including cases resulting in hepatic failure and death has been reported in patients treated with CRIXIVAN. Because the majority of these patients had confounding medical conditions and/or were receiving concomitant therapy(ies), a causal relationship between CRIXIVAN and these events has not been established.

Hyperglycemia

New onset diabetes mellitus, exacerbation of pre-existing diabetes mellitus and hyperglycemia have been reported during post-marketing surveillance in HIV-infected patients receiving protease inhibitor therapy. Some patients required either initiation or dose adjustments of insulin or oral hypoglycemic agents for treatment of these events. In some cases, diabetic ketoacidosis has occurred. In those patients who discontinued protease inhibitor therapy, hyperglycemia persisted in some cases. Because these events have been reported voluntarily during clinical practice, estimates of frequency cannot be made and a causal relationship between protease inhibitor therapy and these events has not been established.

Drug Interactions

Concomitant use of CRIXIVAN with lovastatin or simvastatin is contraindicated due to an increased risk of myopathy including rhabdomyolysis. Caution should be exercised if CRIXIVAN is used concurrently with atorvastatin or rosuvastatin. Titrate the atorvastatin and rosuvastatin doses carefully and use the lowest necessary dose with CRIXIVAN. (See PRECAUTIONS, Drug Interactions.)

Midazolam is extensively metabolized by CYP3A4. Coadministration with CRIXIVAN with or without ritonavir may cause a large increase in the concentration of this benzodiazepine. No drug interaction study has been performed for the co-administration of CRIXIVAN with benzodiazepines. Based on data from other CYP3A4 inhibitors, plasma concentrations of midazolam are expected to be significantly higher when midazolam is given orally. Therefore CRIXIVAN should not be co-administered with orally administered midazolam (see CONTRAINDICATIONS), whereas caution should be used with co-administration of CRIXIVAN and parenteral midazolam. Data from concomitant use of parenteral midazolam with other protease inhibitors suggest a possible 3-4 fold increase in midazolam plasma levels. If CRIXIVAN with or without ritonavir is co-administered with parenteral midazolam, it should be done in a setting which ensures close clinical monitoring and appropriate medical management in case of respiratory depression and/or prolonged sedation. Dosage reduction for midazolam should be considered, especially if more than a single dose of midazolam is administered.

Particular caution should be used when prescribing sildenafil, tadalafil, or vardenafil in patients receiving indinavir. Coadministration of CRIXIVAN with these medications is expected to substantially increase plasma concentrations of sildenafil, tadalafil, and vardenafil and may result in an increase in adverse events, including hypotension, visual changes, and priapism, which have been associated with sildenafil, tadalafil, and vardenafil (see CONTRAINDICATIONS and PRECAUTIONS, Drug Interactions and Information for Patients, and the manufacturer's complete prescribing information for sildenafil, tadalafil, or vardenafil). Concomitant use of CRIXIVAN and St. John's wort (*Hypericum perforatum*) or products containing St. John's wort is not recommended. Coadministration of CRIXIVAN and St. John's wort has been shown to substantially decrease indinavir concentrations (see CLINICAL PHARMACOLOGY, Drug Interactions) and may lead to loss of virologic response and possible resistance to CRIXIVAN or to the class of protease inhibitors.

PRECAUTIONS

General

Indirect hyperbilirubinemia has occurred frequently during treatment with CRIXIVAN and has infrequently been associated with increases in serum transaminases (see also ADVERSE REACTIONS, Clinical Trials and Post-Marketing Experience). It is not known whether CRIXIVAN will exacerbate the physiologic hyperbilirubinemia seen in neonates. (See Pregnancy.)

Tubulointerstitial Nephritis

Reports of tubulointerstitial nephritis with medullary calcification and cortical atrophy have been observed in patients with asymptomatic severe leukocyturia (>100 cells/ high power field). Patients with asymptomatic severe leukocyturia should be followed closely and monitored frequently with urinalyses. Further diagnostic evaluation may be warranted, and discontinuation of CRIXIVAN should be considered in all patients with severe leukocyturia.

Immune reconstitution syndrome has been reported in patients treated with combination antiretroviral therapy, including CRIXIVAN. During the initial phase of combination antiretroviral treatment, patients whose immune system responds may develop an inflammatory response to indolent or residual opportunistic infections (such as *Mycobacterium avium* infection, cytomegalovirus, *Pneumocystis jirovecii* pneumonia [PCP], or tuberculosis), which may necessitate further evaluation and treatment.

Autoimmune disorders (such as Graves' disease, polymyositis, and Guillain-Barré syndrome) have also been reported to occur in the setting of immune reconstitution; however, the time to onset is more variable, and can occur many months after initiation of treatment.

Coexisting Conditions

Patients with hemophilia: There have been reports of spontaneous bleeding in patients with hemophilia A and B treated with protease inhibitors. In some patients, additional factor VIII was required. In many of the reported cases, treatment with protease inhibitors was continued or restarted. A causal relationship between protease inhibitor therapy and these episodes has not been established. (See ADVERSE REACTIONS, Post-Marketing Experience.)

Patients with hepatic insufficiency due to cirrhosis: In these patients, the dosage of CRIXIVAN should be lowered because of decreased metabolism of CRIXIVAN (see DOSAGE AND ADMINISTRATION).

Patients with renal insufficiency: Patients with renal insufficiency have not been studied.

Fat Redistribution

Redistribution/accumulation of body fat including central obesity, dorsocervical fat enlargement (buffalo hump), peripheral wasting, facial wasting, breast enlargement, and "cushingoid appearance" have been observed in patients receiving antiretroviral therapy. The mechanism and long-term consequences of these events are currently unknown. A causal relationship has not been established.

Information for Patients

A statement to patients and health care providers is included on the product's bottle label. **ALERT: Find out about medicines that should NOT be taken with CRIXIVAN.** A Patient Package Insert (PPI) for CRIXIVAN is available for patient information.

CRIXIVAN is not a cure for HIV-1 infection and patients may continue to experience illnesses associated with HIV-1 infection, including opportunistic infections. Patients should remain under the care of a physician when using CRIXIVAN.

Patients should be advised to avoid doing things that can spread HIV-1 infection to others.

- **Do not share needles or other injection equipment.**
- **Do not share personal items that can have blood or body fluids on them, like toothbrushes and razor blades**.
- **Do not have any kind of sex without protection.** Always practice safe sex by using a latex or polyurethane condom to lower the chance of sexual contact with semen, vaginal secretions, or blood.
- **Do not breastfeed.** We do not know if CRIXIVAN can be passed to your baby in your breast milk and whether it could harm your baby. Also, mothers with HIV-1 should not breastfeed because HIV-1 can be passed to the baby in the breast milk.

Patients should be advised to remain under the care of a physician when using CRIXIVAN and should not modify or discontinue treatment without first consulting the physician. Therefore, if a dose is missed, patients should take the next dose at the regularly scheduled time and should not double this dose. Therapy with CRIXIVAN should be initiated and maintained at the recommended dosage.

CRIXIVAN may interact with some drugs; therefore, patients should be advised to report to their doctor the use of any other prescription, non-prescription medication or herbal products, particularly St. John's wort.

For optimal absorption, CRIXIVAN should be administered without food but with water 1 hour before or 2 hours after a meal. Alternatively, CRIXIVAN may be administered with other liquids such as skim milk, juice, coffee, or tea, or with a light meal, e.g., dry toast with jelly, juice, and coffee with skim milk and sugar; or corn flakes, skim milk and sugar (see CLINICAL PHARMACOLOGY, Effect of Food on Oral Absorption and DOSAGE AND ADMINISTRATION). Ingestion of CRIXIVAN with a meal high in calories, fat, and protein reduces the absorption of indinavir.

Patients receiving a phosphodiesterase type 5 (PDE5) inhibitor (sildenafil, tadalafil, or vardenafil) should be advised that they may be at an increased risk of PDE5 inhibitor-associated adverse events including hypotension, visual changes, and priapism, and should promptly report any symptoms to their doctors (see CONTRAINDICATIONS and WARNINGS, Drug Interactions).

Patients should be informed that redistribution or accumulation of body fat may occur in patients receiving antiretroviral therapy and that the cause and long-term health effects of these conditions are not known at this time.

CRIXIVAN Capsules are sensitive to moisture. Patients should be informed that CRIXIVAN should be stored and used in the original container and the desiccant should remain in the bottle.

Drug Interactions

Indinavir is an inhibitor of the cytochrome P450 isoform CYP3A4. Coadministration of CRIXIVAN and drugs primarily metabolized by CYP3A4 may result in increased plasma concentrations of the other drug, which could increase or prolong its therapeutic and adverse effects (see CONTRAINDICATIONS and WARNINGS).

Indinavir is metabolized by CYP3A4. Drugs that induce CYP3A4 activity would be expected to increase the clearance of indinavir, resulting in lowered plasma concentrations of indinavir. Coadministration of CRIXIVAN and other drugs that inhibit CYP3A4 may decrease the clearance of indinavir and may result in increased plasma concentrations of indinavir.

Table 8: Drugs That Should Not Be Coadministered with CRIXIVAN

Drug Class: Drug Name	Clinical Comment
Alpha 1-adrenoreceptor antagonist: alfuzosin	Potentially increased alfuzosin concentrations can result in hypotension.
Antiarrhythmics: amiodarone	CONTRAINDICATED due to potential for serious and/or life-threatening reactions such as cardiac arrhythmias.
Antimycobacterial: rifampin	May lead to loss of virologic response and possible resistance to CRIXIVAN or to the class of protease inhibitors or other coadministered antiretroviral agents.
Ergot derivatives: dihydroergotamine, ergonovine, ergotamine, methylergonovine	CONTRAINDICATED due to potential for serious and/or life-threatening reactions such as acute ergot toxicity characterized by peripheral vasospasm and ischemia of the extremities and other tissues.
GI motility agents: cisapride	CONTRAINDICATED due to potential for serious and/or life-threatening reactions such as cardiac arrhythmias.
Herbal products: St. John's wort (Hypericum perforatum)	May lead to loss of virologic response and possible resistance to CRIXIVAN or to the class of protease inhibitors.
HMG-CoA Reductase inhibitors: lovastatin, simvastatin	CONTRAINDICATED due to an increased risk for serious reactions such as myopathy including rhabdomyolysis.
Neuroleptic: pimozide	CONTRAINDICATED due to potential for serious and/or life-threatening reactions such as cardiac arrhythmias.

PDE5 inhibitor: Revatio* (sildenafil) [for treatment of pulmonary arterial hypertension]	A safe and effective dose has not been established when used with CRIXIVAN. There is increased potential for sildenafil-associated adverse events (which include visual disturbances, hypotension, prolonged erection, and syncope).
Protease inhibitor: atazanavir	Both CRIXIVAN and atazanavir are associated with indirect (unconjugated) hyperbilirubinemia. Combinations of these drugs have not been studied and coadministration of CRIXIVAN and atazanavir is not recommended.
Sedative/hypnotics: Oral midazolam, triazolam, alprazolam	CONTRAINDICATED due to potential for serious and/or life-threatening reactions such as prolonged or increased sedation or respiratory depression.

* Registered trademark of Pfizer, Inc.

[See table 9 on pages 1374 and 1375]

Carcinogenesis, Mutagenesis, Impairment of Fertility

Carcinogenicity studies were conducted in mice and rats. In mice, no increased incidence of any tumor type was observed. The highest dose tested in rats was 640 mg/kg/day; at this dose a statistically significant increased incidence of thyroid adenomas was seen only in male rats. At that dose, daily systemic exposure in rats was approximately 1.3 times higher than daily systemic exposure in humans. No evidence of mutagenicity or genotoxicity was observed in in vitro microbial mutagenesis (Ames) tests, in vitro alkaline elution assays for DNA breakage, in vitro and in vivo chromosomal aberration studies, and in vitro mammalian cell mutagenesis assays. No treatment-related effects on mating, fertility, or embryo survival were seen in female rats and no treatment-related effects on mating performance were seen in male rats at doses providing systemic exposure comparable to or slightly higher than that with the clinical dose. In addition, no treatment-related effects were observed in fecundity or fertility of untreated females mated to treated males.

Pregnancy

Pregnancy Category C:

Developmental toxicity studies were performed in rabbits (at doses up to 240 mg/kg/day), dogs (at doses up to 80 mg/kg/day), and rats (at doses up to 640 mg/kg/day). The highest doses in these studies produced systemic exposures in these species comparable to or slightly greater than human exposure. No treatment-related external, visceral, or skeletal changes were observed in rabbits or dogs. No treatment-related external or visceral changes were observed in rats. Treatment-related increases over controls in the incidence of supernumerary ribs (at exposures at or below those in humans) and of cervical ribs (at exposures comparable to or slightly greater than those in humans) were seen in rats. In all three species, no treatment-related effects on embryonic/fetal survival or fetal weights were observed.

In rabbits, at a maternal dose of 240 mg/kg/day, no drug was detected in fetal plasma 1 hour after dosing. Fetal plasma drug levels 2 hours after dosing were approximately 3% of maternal plasma drug levels. In dogs, at a maternal dose of 80 mg/kg/day, fetal plasma drug levels were approximately 50% of maternal plasma drug levels both 1 and 2 hours after dosing. In rats, at maternal doses of 40 and 640 mg/kg/day, fetal plasma drug levels were approximately 10 to 15% and 10 to 20% of maternal plasma drug levels 1 and 2 hours after dosing, respectively.

Indinavir was administered to Rhesus monkeys during the third trimester of pregnancy (at doses up to 160 mg/kg twice daily) and to neonatal Rhesus monkeys (at doses up to 160 mg/kg twice daily). When administered to neonates, indinavir caused an exacerbation of the transient physiologic hyperbilirubinemia seen in this species after birth; serum bilirubin values were approximately fourfold above controls at 160 mg/kg twice daily. A similar exacerbation did not occur in neonates after in utero exposure to indinavir during the third trimester of pregnancy. In Rhesus monkeys, fetal plasma drug levels were approximately 1 to 2% of maternal plasma drug levels approximately 1 hour after maternal dosing at 40, 80, or 160 mg/kg twice daily.

Hyperbilirubinemia has occurred during treatment with CRIXIVAN (see PRECAUTIONS and ADVERSE REACTIONS). It is unknown whether CRIXIVAN administered to the mother in the perinatal period will exacerbate physiologic hyperbilirubinemia in neonates.

There are no adequate and well-controlled studies in pregnant patients. CRIXIVAN should be used during pregnancy only if the potential benefit justifies the potential risk to the fetus.

A CRIXIVAN dose of 800 mg every 8 hours (with zidovudine 200 mg every 8 hours and lamivudine 150 mg twice a day) has been studied in 16 HIV-infected pregnant patients at 14 to 28 weeks of gestation at enrollment (study PACTG 358). Given the substantially lower antepartum exposures observed and the limited data in this patient population, indinavir use is not recommended in HIV-infected pregnant patients (see CLINICAL PHARMACOLOGY, Pregnant Patients).

Antiretroviral Pregnancy Registry

To monitor maternal-fetal outcomes of pregnant patients exposed to CRIXIVAN, an Antiretroviral Pregnancy Registry has been established. Physicians are encouraged to register patients by calling 1-800-258-4263.

Nursing Mothers

Studies in lactating rats have demonstrated that indinavir is excreted in milk. Although it is not known whether CRIXIVAN is excreted in human milk, there exists the potential for adverse effects from indinavir in nursing infants. Mothers should be instructed to discontinue nursing if they are receiving CRIXIVAN. This is consistent with the recommendation by the U.S. Public Health Service Centers for Disease Control and Prevention that HIV-infected mothers not breast-feed their infants to avoid risking postnatal transmission of HIV.

Pediatric Use

The optimal dosing regimen for use of indinavir in pediatric patients has not been established. A dose of 500 mg/m² every eight hours has been studied in uncontrolled studies of 70 children, 3 to 18 years of age. The pharmacokinetic profiles of indinavir at this dose were not comparable to profiles previously observed in adults receiving the recommended dose (see CLINICAL PHARMACOLOGY, Pediatric). Although viral suppression was observed in some of the 32 children who were followed on this regimen through 24 weeks, a substantially higher rate of nephrolithiasis was reported when compared to adult historical data (see WARNINGS, Nephrolithiasis/Urolithiasis). Physicians considering the use of indinavir in pediatric patients without other protease inhibitor options should be aware of the limited data available in this population and the increased risk of nephrolithiasis.

Geriatric Use

Clinical studies of CRIXIVAN did not include sufficient numbers of subjects aged 65 and over to determine whether they respond differently from younger subjects. In general, dose selection for an elderly patient should be cautious, reflecting the greater frequency of decreased hepatic, renal or cardiac function and of concomitant disease or other drug therapy.

ADVERSE REACTIONS

Clinical Trials in Adults

Nephrolithiasis/urolithiasis, including flank pain with or without hematuria (including microscopic hematuria), has been reported in approximately 12.4% (301/2429; range across individual trials: 4.7% to 34.4%) of patients receiving CRIXIVAN at the recommended dose in clinical trials with a median follow-up of 47 weeks (range: 1 day to 242 weeks; 2238 patient-years follow-up). The cumulative frequency of nephrolithiasis events increases with duration of exposure to CRIXIVAN; however, the risk over time remains relatively constant. Of the patients treated with CRIXIVAN who developed nephrolithiasis/urolithiasis in clinical trials during the double-blind phase, 2.8% (7/246) were reported to develop hydronephrosis and 4.5% (11/246) underwent stent placement. Following the acute episode, 4.9% (12/246) of patients discontinued therapy. (See WARNINGS and DOSAGE AND ADMINISTRATION, Nephrolithiasis/Urolithiasis.)

Asymptomatic hyperbilirubinemia (total bilirubin ≥2.5 mg/dL), reported predominantly as elevated indirect bilirubin, has occurred in approximately 14% of patients treated with CRIXIVAN. In <1% this was associated with elevations in ALT or AST.

Hyperbilirubinemia and nephrolithiasis/urolithiasis occurred more frequently at doses exceeding 2.4 g/day compared to doses ≤2.4 g/day.

Clinical adverse experiences reported in ≥2% of patients treated with CRIXIVAN alone, CRIXIVAN in combination with zidovudine or zidovudine plus lamivudine, zidovudine alone, or zidovudine plus lamivudine are presented in Table 10.

[See table 10 at top of page 1376]

In Phase I and II controlled trials, the following adverse events were reported significantly more frequently by those randomized to the arms containing CRIXIVAN than by those randomized to nucleoside analogues: rash, upper respiratory infection, dry skin, pharyngitis, taste perversion.

Selected laboratory abnormalities of severe or life-threatening intensity reported in patients treated with CRIXIVAN alone, CRIXIVAN in combination with zidovudine or zidovudine plus lamivudine, zidovudine alone, or zidovudine plus lamivudine are presented in Table 11.

[See table 11 on page 1376]

Post-Marketing Experience

Body As A Whole: redistribution/accumulation of body fat (see PRECAUTIONS, Fat Redistribution).

Cardiovascular System: cardiovascular disorders including myocardial infarction and angina pectoris; cerebrovascular disorder.

Digestive System: liver function abnormalities; hepatitis including reports of hepatic failure (see WARNINGS); pancreatitis; jaundice; abdominal distention; dyspepsia.

Hematologic: increased spontaneous bleeding in patients with hemophilia (see PRECAUTIONS); acute hemolytic anemia (see WARNINGS).

Endocrine/Metabolic: new onset diabetes mellitus, exacerbation of pre-existing diabetes mellitus, hyperglycemia (see WARNINGS).

Hypersensitivity: anaphylactoid reactions; urticaria; vasculitis.

Musculoskeletal System: arthralgia, periarthritis.

Nervous System/Psychiatric: oral paresthesia; depression.

Skin and Skin Appendage: rash including erythema multiforme and Stevens-Johnson syndrome; hyperpigmentation; alopecia; ingrown toenails and/or paronychia; pruritus.

Urogenital System: nephrolithiasis/urolithiasis, in some cases resulting in renal insufficiency or acute renal failure, pyelonephritis with or without bacteremia (see WARNINGS); interstitial nephritis sometimes with indinavir crystal deposits; in some patients, the interstitial nephritis did not resolve following discontinuation of CRIXIVAN; renal insufficiency; renal failure; leukocyturia (see PRECAUTIONS); crystalluria; dysuria.

Laboratory Abnormalities

Increased serum triglycerides; increased serum cholesterol.

OVERDOSAGE

There have been more than 60 reports of acute or chronic human overdosage (up to 23 times the recommended total daily dose of 2400 mg) with CRIXIVAN. The most commonly reported symptoms were renal (e.g., nephrolithiasis/urolithiasis, flank pain, hematuria) and gastrointestinal (e.g., nausea, vomiting, diarrhea).

It is not known whether CRIXIVAN is dialyzable by peritoneal or hemodialysis.

DOSAGE AND ADMINISTRATION

The recommended dosage of CRIXIVAN is 800 mg (usually **two** 400-mg capsules) orally every 8 hours.

CRIXIVAN must be taken at intervals of 8 hours. For optimal absorption, CRIXIVAN should be administered without food but with water 1 hour before or 2 hours after a meal. Alternatively, CRIXIVAN may be administered with other liquids such as skim milk, juice, coffee, or tea, or with a light meal, e.g., dry toast with jelly, juice, and coffee with skim milk and sugar; or corn flakes, skim milk and sugar. (See CLINICAL PHARMACOLOGY, Effect of Food on Oral Absorption.)

To ensure adequate hydration, it is recommended that adults drink at least 1.5 liters (approximately 48 ounces) of liquids during the course of 24 hours.

Concomitant Therapy

(See CLINICAL PHARMACOLOGY, Drug Interactions, and/or PRECAUTIONS, Drug Interactions.)

Delavirdine

Dose reduction of CRIXIVAN to 600 mg every 8 hours should be considered when administering delavirdine 400 mg three times a day.

Didanosine

If indinavir and didanosine are administered concomitantly, they should be administered at least one hour apart on an empty stomach (consult the manufacturer's product circular for didanosine).

Itraconazole

Dose reduction of CRIXIVAN to 600 mg every 8 hours is recommended when administering itraconazole 200 mg twice daily concurrently.

Ketoconazole

Dose reduction of CRIXIVAN to 600 mg every 8 hours is recommended when administering ketoconazole concurrently.

Rifabutin

Dose reduction of rifabutin to half the standard dose (consult the manufacturer's product circular for rifabutin) and a dose increase of CRIXIVAN to 1000 mg every 8 hours are recommended when rifabutin and CRIXIVAN are coadministered.

Hepatic Insufficiency

The dosage of CRIXIVAN should be reduced to 600 mg every 8 hours in patients with mild-to-moderate hepatic insufficiency due to cirrhosis.

Nephrolithiasis/Urolithiasis

In addition to adequate hydration, medical management in patients who experience nephrolithiasis/urolithiasis may include temporary interruption (e.g., 1 to 3 days) or discontinuation of therapy.

Table 9: Established and Other Potentially Significant Drug Interactions: Alteration in Dose or Regimen May Be Recommended Based on Drug Interaction Studies or Predicted Interaction (See also CLINICAL PHARMACOLOGY for magnitude of interaction, WARNINGS and DOSAGE AND ADMINISTRATION.)

Drug Name	Effect	Clinical Comment
HIV Antiviral Agents		
Delavirdine	↑ indinavir concentration	Dose reduction of CRIXIVAN to 600 mg every 8 hours should be considered when taking delavirdine 400 mg three times a day.
Didanosine		Indinavir and didanosine formulations containing buffer should be administered at least one hour apart on an empty stomach.
Efavirenz	↓ indinavir concentration	The optimal dose of indinavir, when given in combination with efavirenz, is not known. Increasing the indinavir dose to 1000 mg every 8 hours does not compensate for the increased indinavir metabolism due to efavirenz.
Nelfinavir	↑ indinavir concentration	The appropriate doses for this combination, with respect to efficacy and safety, have not been established.
Nevirapine	↓ indinavir concentration	Indinavir concentrations may be decreased in the presence of nevirapine. The appropriate doses for this combination, with respect to efficacy and safety, have not been established.
Ritonavir	↑ indinavir concentration ↑ ritonavir concentration	The appropriate doses for this combination, with respect to efficacy and safety, have not been established. Preliminary clinical data suggest that the incidence of nephrolithiasis is higher in patients receiving indinavir in combination with ritonavir than those receiving CRIXIVAN 800 mg q8h.
Saquinavir	↑ saquinavir concentration	The appropriate doses for this combination, with respect to efficacy and safety, have not been established.
Other Agents		
Antiarrhythmics: bepridil, lidocaine(systemic) and quinidine	↑ antiarrhythmic agents concentration	Caution is warranted and therapeutic concentration monitoring is recommended for antiarrhythmics when coadministered with CRIXIVAN.
Anticonvulsants: carbamazepine, phenobarbital, phenytoin	↓ indinavir concentration	Use with caution. CRIXIVAN may not be effective due to decreased indinavir concentrations in patients taking these agents concomitantly.
Antidepressant: Trazodone	↑ trazodone concentration	Concomitant use of trazodone and CRIXIVAN may increase plasma concentrations of trazodone. Adverse events of nausea, dizziness, hypotension and syncope have been observed following coadministration of trazodone and ritonavir. If trazodone is used with a CYP3A4 inhibitor such as CRIXIVAN, the combination should be used with caution and a lower dose of trazodone should be considered.
Anti-gout: Colchicine	↑ colchicine concentration	Patients with renal or hepatic impairment should not be given colchicine with CRIXIVAN. *Treatment of gout flares:* Co-administration of colchicine in patients on CRIXIVAN: 0.6 mg (1 tablet) × 1 dose, followed by 0.3 mg (half tablet) 1 hour later. Dose to be repeated no earlier than 3 days. *Prophylaxis of gout flares:* Co-administration of colchicine in patients on CRIXIVAN: If the original colchicine regimen was 0.6 mg twice a day, the regimen should be adjusted to 0.3 mg once a day. If the original colchicine regimen was 0.6 mg once a day, the regimen should be adjusted to 0.3 mg once every other day. *Treatment of familial Mediterranean fever (FMF):* Co-administration of colchicine in patients on CRIXIVAN: Maximum daily dose of 0.6 mg (may be given as 0.3 mg twice a day).
Calcium Channel Blockers, Dihydropyridine: e.g., felodipine, nifedipine, nicardipine	↑ dihydropyridine calcium channel blockers concentration	Caution is warranted and clinical monitoring of patients is recommended.
Clarithromycin	↑ clarithromycin concentration ↑ indinavir concentration	The appropriate doses for this combination, with respect to efficacy and safety, have not been established.
Endothelin receptor antagonist: Bosentan	↑ bosentan concentration	Co-administration of bosentan in patients on CRIXIVAN or co-administration of CRIXIVAN in patients on bosentan: Start at or adjust bosentan to 62.5 mg once daily or every other day based upon individual tolerability.
HMG-CoA Reductase Inhibitors: atorvastatin, rosuvastatin	↑ atorvastatin concentration ↑ rosuvastatin concentration	The atorvastatin and rosuvastatin doses should be carefully titrated; use the lowest dose necessary with careful monitoring during treatment with CRIXIVAN.

(Table continued on next page)

HOW SUPPLIED

CRIXIVAN Capsules are supplied as follows:

No. 3756 — 200 mg capsules: semi-translucent white capsules coded "CRIXIVAN™ 200 mg" in blue. Available as: **NDC** 0006-0571-43 unit-of-use bottles of 360 (with desiccant).

No. 3758 — 400 mg capsules: semi-translucent white capsules coded "CRIXIVAN™ 400 mg" in green. Available as: **NDC** 0006-0573-62 unit-of-use bottles of 180 (with desiccant)

Storage

Bottles: Store in a tightly-closed container at room temperature, 15-30°C (59-86°F). Protect from moisture. CRIXIVAN Capsules are sensitive to moisture. CRIXIVAN should be dispensed and stored in the original container. The desiccant should remain in the original bottle.

Dist. by: Merck Sharp & Dohme Corp., a subsidiary of **MERCK & CO., INC.**, Whitehouse Station, NJ 08889, USA

For patent information:
www.merck.com/product/patent/home.html

Copyright © 1996, 1997, 1998, 1999, 2004 Merck Sharp & Dohme Corp., a subsidiary of **Merck & Co., Inc.**
All rights reserved.
Revised 12/2013
uspi-mk0639-c-1312r016

CRIXIVAN® (indinavir sulfate) Capsules
Patient Information about
CRIXIVAN (KRIK-sih-van)
for HIV (Human Immunodeficiency Virus) Infection
Generic name: indinavir (in-DIH-nuh-veer) sulfate
ALERT: Find out about medicines that should NOT be taken with CRIXIVAN®. Please also read the section "MEDICINES YOU SHOULD NOT TAKE WITH CRIXIVAN".

Please read this information before you start taking CRIXIVAN. Also, read the leaflet each time you renew your prescription, just in case anything has changed. Remember, this leaflet does not take the place of careful discussions with your doctor. You and your doctor should discuss CRIXIVAN when you start taking your medication and at regular checkups. You should remain under a doctor's care when using CRIXIVAN and should not change or stop treatment without first talking with your doctor.

What is CRIXIVAN?

CRIXIVAN is an oral capsule used for the treatment of HIV (Human Immunodeficiency Virus). HIV is the virus that causes AIDS (acquired immune deficiency syndrome). CRIXIVAN is a type of HIV drug called a protease (PRO-tee-ase) inhibitor.

How does CRIXIVAN work?

CRIXIVAN is a protease inhibitor that fights HIV. CRIXIVAN can help reduce your chances of getting illnesses associated with HIV. CRIXIVAN can also help lower the amount of HIV in your body (called "viral load") and raise your CD4 (T) cell count. CRIXIVAN may not have these effects in all patients.

CRIXIVAN is usually prescribed with other anti-HIV drugs such as ZDV (also called AZT), 3TC, ddI, ddC, or d4T. CRIXIVAN works differently from these other anti-HIV drugs. Talk with your doctor about how you should take CRIXIVAN.

How should I take CRIXIVAN?

There are six important things you must do to help you benefit from CRIXIVAN:

1. **Take CRIXIVAN capsules every day as prescribed by your doctor.** Continue taking CRIXIVAN unless your doctor tells you to stop. Take the exact amount of CRIXIVAN that your doctor tells you to take, right from the very start. To help make sure you will benefit from CRIXIVAN, you must not skip doses or take "drug holidays". If you don't take CRIXIVAN as prescribed, the activity of CRIXIVAN may be reduced (due to resistance).

2. **Take CRIXIVAN capsules every 8 hours around the clock, every day.** It may be easier to remember to take CRIXIVAN if you take it at the same time every day. If you have questions about when to take CRIXIVAN, your doctor or health care provider can help you decide what schedule works for you.

3. **If you miss a dose by more than 2 hours, wait and then take the next dose at the regularly scheduled time.** However, if you miss a dose by less than 2 hours, take your missed dose immediately. Then take your next dose at the regularly scheduled time. Do not take more or less than your prescribed dose of CRIXIVAN at any one time.

4. **Take CRIXIVAN with water.** You can also take CRIXIVAN with other beverages such as skim or non-fat milk, juice, coffee, or tea.

5. **Ideally, take each dose of CRIXIVAN without food but with water at least one hour before or two hours after a meal.** Or you can take CRIXIVAN with a light meal. Examples of light meals include:
dry toast with jelly, juice, and coffee (with skim or non-fat milk and sugar if you want)
cornflakes with skim or non-fat milk and sugar
Do not take CRIXIVAN at the same time as any meals that are high in calories, fat, and protein (for example — a bacon and egg breakfast). When taken at the same time

as CRIXIVAN, these foods can interfere with CRIXIVAN being absorbed into your bloodstream and may lessen its effect.

6. **It is critical to drink plenty of fluids while taking CRIXIVAN.** Adults should drink at least six 8-ounce glasses of liquids (preferably water) throughout the day,

Table 9: Established and Other Potentially Significant Drug Interactions: Alteration in Dose or Regimen May Be Recommended Based on Drug Interaction Studies or Predicted Interaction (See also CLINICAL PHARMACOLOGY for magnitude of interaction, WARNINGS and DOSAGE AND ADMINISTRATION.)

Drug Name	Effect	Clinical Comment
Other Agents *(cont.)*		
Immunosuppressants: cyclosporine, tacrolimus, sirolimus	↑ immunosuppressant agents concentration	Plasma concentrations may be increased by CRIXIVAN.
Inhaled beta agonist: Salmeterol	↑ salmeterol	Concurrent administration of salmeterol with CRIXIVAN is not recommended. The combination may result in increased risk of cardiovascular adverse events associated with salmeterol, including QT prolongation, palpitations and sinus tachycardia.
Inhaled/nasal steroid: Fluticasone	↑ fluticasone concentration	Concomitant use of fluticasone propionate and CRIXIVAN may increase plasma concentrations of fluticasone propionate. Use with caution. Consider alternatives to fluticasone propionate, particularly for long-term use. Fluticasone use is not recommended in situations where CRIXIVAN is coadministered with a potent CYP3A4 inhibitor such as ritonavir unless the potential benefit to the patient outweighs the risk of systemic corticosteroid side effects.
Itraconazole	↑ indinavir concentration	Dose reduction of CRIXIVAN to 600 mg every 8 hours is recommended when administering itraconazole concurrently.
Ketoconazole	↑ indinavir concentration	Dose reduction of CRIXIVAN to 600 mg every 8 hours should be considered.
Midazolam (parenteral administration)	↑ midazolam concentration	Concomitant use of parenteral midazolam with CRIXIVAN may increase plasma concentrations of midazolam. Coadministration should be done in a setting which ensures close clinical monitoring and appropriate medical management in case of respiratory depression and/or prolonged sedation. Dosage reduction for midazolam should be considered, especially if more than a single dose of midazolam is administered. Coadministration of oral midazolam with CRIXIVAN is CONTRAINDICATED (see Table 8).
Rifabutin	↓ indinavir concentration ↑ rifabutin concentration	Dose reduction of rifabutin to half the standard dose and a dose increase of CRIXIVAN to 1000 mg every 8 hours are recommended when rifabutin and CRIXIVAN are coadministered.
Sildenafil	↑ sildenafil concentration (only the use of sildenafil at doses used for treatment of erectile dysfunction has been studied with CRIXIVAN)	May result in an increase in PDE5 inhibitor-associated adverse events, including hypotension, syncope, visual disturbances, and priapism. *Use of sildenafil for pulmonary arterial hypertension (PAH):* Use of Revatio* (sildenafil) is contraindicated when used for the treatment of pulmonary arterial hypertension (PAH) [see CONTRAINDICATIONS]. *Use of sildenafil for erectile dysfunction:* Sildenafil dose should not exceed a maximum of 25 mg in a 48-hour period in patients receiving concomitant CRIXIVAN therapy. Use with increased monitoring for adverse events.
Tadalafil	↑ tadalafil concentration	May result in an increase in PDE5 inhibitor-associated adverse events, including hypotension, visual disturbances, and priapism. *Use of tadalafil for pulmonary arterial hypertension (PAH):* The following dose adjustments are recommended for use of Adcirca† (tadalafil) with CRIXIVAN: Co-administration of Adcirca in patients on CRIXIVAN or co-administration of CRIXIVAN in patients on Adcirca: Start at or adjust Adcirca to 20 mg once daily. Increase to 40 mg once daily based upon individual tolerability. *Use of tadalafil for erectile dysfunction:* Tadalafil dose should not exceed a maximum of 10 mg in a 72-hour period in patients receiving concomitant CRIXIVAN therapy. Use with increased monitoring for adverse events.
Vardenafil	↑ vardenafil concentration	Vardenafil dose should not exceed a maximum of 2.5 mg in a 24-hour period in patients receiving concomitant indinavir therapy.
Venlafaxine	↓ indinavir concentration	In a study of 9 healthy volunteers, venlafaxine administered under steady-state conditions at 150 mg/day resulted in a 28% decrease in the AUC of a single 800 mg oral dose of indinavir and a 36% decrease in indinavir C_{max}. Indinavir did not affect the pharmacokinetics of venlafaxine and ODV. The clinical significance of this finding is unknown.

Note: ↑ = increase; ↓ = decrease
* Registered trademark of Pfizer, Inc.
† Registered trademark of Eli Lilly and Company.

Table 10: Clinical Adverse Experiences Reported in ≥2% of Patients

	Study 028 Considered Drug-Related and of Moderate or Severe Intensity			Study ACTG 320 of Unknown Drug Relationship and of Severe or Life-threatening Intensity	
Adverse Experience	CRIXIVAN Percent (n=332)	CRIXIVAN plus Zidovudine Percent (n=332)	Zidovudine Percent (n=332)	CRIXIVAN plus Zidovudine plus Lamivudine Percent (n=571)	Zidovudine plus Lamivudine Percent (n=575)
Body as a Whole					
Abdominal pain	16.6	16.0	12.0	1.9	0.7
Asthenia/fatigue	2.1	4.2	3.6	2.4	4.5
Fever	1.5	1.5	2.1	3.8	3.0
Malaise	2.1	2.7	1.8	0	0
Digestive System					
Nausea	11.7	31.9	19.6	2.8	1.4
Diarrhea	3.3	3.0	2.4	0.9	1.2
Vomiting	8.4	17.8	9.0	1.4	1.4
Acid regurgitation	2.7	5.4	1.8	0.4	0
Anorexia	2.7	5.4	3.0	0.5	0.2
Appetite increase	2.1	1.5	1.2	0	0
Dyspepsia	1.5	2.7	0.9	0	0
Jaundice	1.5	2.1	0.3	0	0
Hemic and Lymphatic System					
Anemia	0.6	1.2	2.1	2.4	3.5
Musculoskeletal System					
Back pain	8.4	4.5	1.5	0.9	0.7
Nervous System / Psychiatric					
Headache	5.4	9.6	6.0	2.4	2.8
Dizziness	3.0	3.9	0.9	0.5	0.7
Somnolence	2.4	3.3	3.3	0	0
Skin and Skin Appendage					
Pruritus	4.2	2.4	1.8	0.5	0
Rash	1.2	0.6	2.4	1.1	0.5
Respiratory System					
Cough	1.5	0.3	0.6	1.6	1.0
Difficulty breathing/ dyspnea/ shortness of breath	0	0.6	0.3	1.8	1.0
Urogenital System					
Nephrolithiasis/urolithiasis*	8.7	7.8	2.1	2.6	0.3
Dysuria	1.5	2.4	0.3	0.4	0.2
Special Senses					
Taste perversion	2.7	8.4	1.2	0.2	0

* Including renal colic, and flank pain with and without hematuria

Table 11: Selected Laboratory Abnormalities of Severe or Life-threatening Intensity Reported in Studies 028 and ACTG 320

	Study 028			Study ACTG 320	
	CRIXIVAN Percent (n=329)	CRIXIVAN plus Zidovudine Percent (n=320)	Zidovudine Percent (n=330)	CRIXIVAN plus Zidovudine plus Lamivudine Percent (n=571)	Zidovudine plus Lamivudine Percent (n=575)
Hematology					
Decreased hemoglobin <7.0 g/dL	0.6	0.9	3.3	2.4	3.5
Decreased platelet count <50 THS/mm³	0.9	0.9	1.8	0.2	0.9
Decreased neutrophils <0.75 THS/mm³	2.4	2.2	6.7	5.1	14.6
Blood chemistry					
Increased ALT >500% ULN*	4.9	4.1	3.0	2.6	2.6
Increased AST >500% ULN	3.7	2.8	2.7	3.3	2.8
Total serum bilirubin >250% ULN	11.9	9.7	0.6	6.1	1.4
Increased serum amylase >200% ULN	2.1	1.9	1.8	0.9	0.3
Increased glucose >250 mg/dL	0.9	0.9	0.6	1.6	1.9
Increased creatinine >300% ULN	0	0	0.6	0.2	0

* Upper limit of the normal range.

every day. Your health care provider will give you further instructions on the amount of fluid that you should drink. **CRIXIVAN can cause kidney stones.** Having enough fluids in your body should help reduce the chances of forming a kidney stone. Call your doctor or other health care provider if you develop kidney pains (middle to lower stomach or back pain) or blood in the urine.

Does CRIXIVAN cure HIV or AIDS?

CRIXIVAN does not cure HIV infection or AIDS and you may continue to experience illnesses associated with HIV-1 infection, including opportunistic infections. You should remain under the care of a doctor when using CRIXIVAN.

Avoid doing things that can spread HIV-1 infection.
• Do not share needles or other injection equipment.
• Do not share personal items that can have blood or body fluids on them, like toothbrushes and razor blades.
• Do not have any kind of sex without protection. Always practice safe sex by using a latex or polyurethane condom to lower the chance of sexual contact with semen, vaginal secretions, or blood.

Who should not take CRIXIVAN?

Do not take CRIXIVAN if you have had a serious allergic reaction to CRIXIVAN or any of its components.

What other medical problems or conditions should I discuss with my doctor?

Talk to your doctor if:
• You are pregnant or if you become pregnant while you are taking CRIXIVAN. We do not yet know how CRIXIVAN affects pregnant women or their developing babies.
• You are breastfeeding. **Do not breastfeed.** We do not know if CRIXIVAN can be passed to your baby in your breast milk and whether it could harm your baby. Also, mothers with HIV-1 should not breastfeed because HIV-1 can be passed to the baby in the breast milk.

Also talk to your doctor if you have:
• Problems with your liver, especially if you have mild or moderate liver disease caused by cirrhosis
• Problems with your kidneys
• Diabetes
• Hemophilia
• High cholesterol and you are taking cholesterol-lowering medicines called "statins"

Tell your doctor about any medicines you are taking or plan to take, including non-prescription medicines, herbal products including St. John's wort (*Hypericum perforatum*), or dietary supplements.

Can CRIXIVAN be taken with other medications?

MEDICINES YOU SHOULD NOT TAKE WITH CRIXIVAN

Oral VERSED® (midazolam)	HALCION® (triazolam)
ORAP® (pimozide)	XANAX® (alprazolam)
PROPULSID® (cisapride)	REVATIO® (sildenafil for the treatment of pulmonary arterial hypertension)
CORDARONE® (amiodarone)	UROXATRAL® (alfuzosin)
HISMANAL® (astemizole)	Ergot medications (e.g., Wigraine®, Cafergot®, D.H.E. 45®, Migranal®, Ergotrate®, and Methergine®)
	ZOCOR® (simvastatin)
	MEVACOR® (lovastatin)

Taking CRIXIVAN with the above medications could result in serious or life-threatening problems (such as irregular heartbeat or excessive sleepiness).

In addition, you should not take CRIXIVAN with the following:
Rifampin, known as RIFADIN®, RIFAMATE®, RIFATER®, or RIMACTANE®.

There is also an increased risk of drug interactions between CRIXIVAN and LIPITOR® (atorvastatin) and CRESTOR® (rosuvastatin); talk to your doctor before you take any of these cholesterol-reducing drugs with CRIXIVAN.

Taking CRIXIVAN with REYATAZ® (atazanavir) is not recommended because they can both sometimes cause increased levels of bilirubin in the blood.

Taking CRIXIVAN with St. John's wort (*Hypericum perforatum*), an herbal product sold as a dietary supplement, or products containing St. John's wort is not recommended. Taking St. John's wort has been shown to decrease CRIXIVAN levels and may lead to increased viral load and possible resistance to CRIXIVAN or cross resistance to other antiretroviral drugs.

Before you take VIAGRA® (sildenafil), CIALIS® (tadalafil), or LEVITRA® (vardenafil) with CRIXIVAN, talk to your doctor about possible drug interactions and side effects. If you take any of these medicines together with CRIXIVAN, you may be at increased risk of side effects such as low blood pressure, visual changes, and penile erection lasting more than 4 hours, which have been associated with sildenafil, tadalafil, and vardenafil. If an erection lasts longer than 4 hours, you should seek immediate medical assistance to avoid permanent damage to your penis. Your doctor can explain these symptoms to you.

MEDICINES YOU CAN TAKE WITH CRIXIVAN

RETROVIR® (zidovudine, ZDV also called AZT)	EPIVIR™ (lamivudine, 3TC)
ZERIT® (stavudine, d4T)	isoniazid (INH)
BACTRIM®/SEPTRA® (trimethoprim/ sulfamethoxazole)	DIFLUCAN® (fluconazole)
BIAXIN® (clarithromycin)	ORTHO-NOVUM 1/35® (oral contraceptive)
TAGAMET® (cimetidine)	Methadone
VIDEX® (didanosine, ddI) — If you take CRIXIVAN with VIDEX, take them at least one hour apart.	

MYCOBUTIN® (rifabutin) — If you take CRIXIVAN with MYCOBUTIN, your doctor may adjust both the dose of MYCOBUTIN and the dose of CRIXIVAN.

NIZORAL® (ketoconazole) — If you take CRIXIVAN with NIZORAL, your doctor may adjust the dose of CRIXIVAN.

RESCRIPTOR® (delavirdine) — If you take CRIXIVAN with RESCRIPTOR, your doctor may adjust the dose of CRIXIVAN.

SPORANOX® (itraconazole) — If you take CRIXIVAN with SPORANOX, your doctor may adjust the dose of CRIXIVAN.

SUSTIVA™ (efavirenz) — If you take CRIXIVAN with SUSTIVA, check with your doctor.

Intravenous VERSED® (midazolam) — If you take CRIXIVAN with Intravenous VERSED®, your doctor may adjust the dose of VERSED®.

Talk to your doctor about any medications you are taking.
Calcium Channel Blockers: Tell your doctor if you are taking calcium channel blockers (e.g., amlodipine, felodipine).
Antiarrhythmics: Tell your doctor if you are taking antiarrhythmics (e.g., quinidine).
Anticonvulsants: Tell your doctor if you are taking anticonvulsants (e.g., phenobarbital, phenytoin, or carbamazepine).
Steroids: Tell your doctor if you are taking steroids (e.g., dexamethasone).

What are the possible side effects of CRIXIVAN?
Like all prescription drugs, CRIXIVAN can cause side effects. The following is **not** a complete list of side effects reported with CRIXIVAN when taken either alone or with other anti-HIV drugs. Do not rely on this leaflet alone for information about side effects. Your doctor can discuss with you a more complete list of side effects.

Some patients treated with CRIXIVAN developed kidney stones. In some of these patients this led to more severe kidney problems, including kidney failure or inflammation of the kidneys or kidney infection which sometimes spread to the blood. Drinking at least six 8-ounce glasses of liquids (preferably water) each day should help reduce the chances of forming a kidney stone (see How should I take CRIXIVAN?). Call your doctor or other health care provider if you develop kidney pains (middle to lower stomach or back pain) or blood in the urine.

Some patients treated with CRIXIVAN have had rapid breakdown of red blood cells (hemolytic anemia) which in some cases was severe or resulted in death.

Some patients treated with CRIXIVAN have had liver problems including liver failure and death. Some patients had other illnesses or were taking other drugs. It is uncertain if CRIXIVAN caused these liver problems.

Diabetes and high blood sugar (hyperglycemia) have occurred in patients taking protease inhibitors. In some of these patients, this led to ketoacidosis, a serious condition caused by poorly controlled blood sugar. Some patients had diabetes before starting protease inhibitors, others did not. Some patients required adjustments to their diabetes medication. Others needed new diabetes medication.

In some patients with hemophilia, increased bleeding has been reported.

Severe muscle pain and weakness have occurred in patients taking protease inhibitors, including CRIXIVAN, together with some of the cholesterol-lowering medicines called "statins". Call your doctor if you develop severe muscle pain or weakness.

Changes in body fat have been seen in some patients taking antiretroviral therapy. These changes may include increased amount of fat in the upper back and neck ("buffalo hump"), breast, and around the trunk. Loss of fat from the legs, arms and face may also happen. The cause and long term health effects of these conditions are not known at this time.

In some patients with advanced HIV infection (AIDS), signs and symptoms of inflammation from opportunistic infections may occur when combination antiretroviral treatment is started.

Clinical Studies

Increases in bilirubin (one laboratory test of liver function) have been reported in approximately 14% of patients. Usually, this finding has not been associated with liver problems. However, on rare occasions, a person may develop yellowing of the skin and/or eyes.

Side effects occurring in 2% or more of patients included: abdominal pain, fatigue or weakness, low red blood cell count, flank pain, painful urination, feeling unwell, nausea, upset stomach, diarrhea, vomiting, acid regurgitation, increased or decreased appetite, back pain, headache, dizziness, taste changes, rash, itchy skin, yellowing of the skin and/or eyes, upper respiratory infection, dry skin, and sore throat.

Swollen kidneys due to blocked urine flow occurred rarely.

Marketing Experience
Other side effects reported since CRIXIVAN has been marketed include: allergic reactions; severe skin reactions; yellowing of the skin and/or eyes; heart problems including heart attack; stroke; abdominal swelling; indigestion; inflammation of the kidneys; decreased kidney function; inflammation of the pancreas; joint pain; depression; itching; hives; change in skin color; hair loss; ingrown toenails with or without infection; crystals in the urine; painful urination; numbness of the mouth; increased cholesterol; pain and difficulty moving shoulder.

Tell your doctor promptly about these or any other unusual symptoms. If the condition persists or worsens, seek medical attention.

How should I store CRIXIVAN capsules?
• Keep CRIXIVAN capsules in the bottle they came in and at room temperature (59°-86°F).
• Keep CRIXIVAN capsules dry by leaving the small desiccant in the bottle. Keep the bottle closed.

This medication was prescribed for your particular condition. Do not use it for any other condition or give it to anybody else. Keep CRIXIVAN and all medicines out of the reach of children. If you suspect that more than the prescribed dose of this medicine has been taken, contact your local poison control center or emergency room immediately.

This leaflet provides a summary of information about CRIXIVAN. If you have any questions or concerns about either CRIXIVAN or HIV, talk to your doctor.

Distributed by:
Merck Sharp & Dohme Corp., a subsidiary of Merck & Co., Inc.
Whitehouse Station, NJ 08889, USA
For patent information:
www.merck.com/product/patent/home.html
The trademarks depicted herein are owned by their respective companies.

Copyright © 1996, 1999 Merck Sharp & Dohme Corp., a subsidiary of Merck & Co., Inc.
All rights reserved.
Revised 12/2013
usppi-mk0639-c-1312r016

Shown in Product Identification Guide, page 308

DIPROLENE® AF ℞
[dĭp-rō-lēn]
**brand of augmented betamethasone dipropionate[1]
Cream 0.05%**
(potency expressed as betamethasone)
[1]Vehicle augments the penetration of the steroid.

For Dermatologic Use Only - Not for Ophthalmic Use

DESCRIPTION
DIPROLENE® AF Cream 0.05% contains betamethasone dipropionate USP, a synthetic adrenocorticosteroid, for dermatologic use in an emollient base. Betamethasone, an analog of prednisolone, has a high degree of corticosteroid activity and a slight degree of mineralocorticoid¹ activity. Betamethasone dipropionate is the 17,21-dipropionate ester of betamethasone.

Chemically, betamethasone dipropionate is 9-fluoro-11β,17,21-trihydroxy-16β-methylpregna-1,4-diene-3,20-dione 17,21-dipropionate, with the empirical formula $C_{28}H_{37}FO_7$, a molecular weight of 504.6, and the following structural formula:

Betamethasone dipropionate is a white to creamy white, odorless crystalline powder, insoluble in water.

Each gram of DIPROLENE AF Cream 0.05% contains: 0.643 mg betamethasone dipropionate USP (equivalent to 0.5 mg betamethasone) in an emollient cream base of purified water; chlorocresol; propylene glycol; white petrolatum; white wax; cyclomethicone; sorbitol solution; glyceryl oleate/propylene glycol; ceteareth-30; carbomer 940; and sodium hydroxide.

CLINICAL PHARMACOLOGY
The corticosteroids are a class of compounds comprising steroid hormones secreted by the adrenal cortex and their synthetic analogs. In pharmacologic doses, corticosteroids are used primarily for their anti-inflammatory and/or immunosuppressive effects.

Topical corticosteroids, such as betamethasone dipropionate, are effective in the treatment of corticosteroid-

responsive dermatoses primarily because of their anti-inflammatory, antipruritic, and vasoconstrictive actions. However, while the physiologic, pharmacologic, and clinical effects of the corticosteroids are well known, the exact mechanisms of their actions in each disease are uncertain. Betamethasone dipropionate, a corticosteroid, has been shown to have topical (dermatologic) and systemic pharmacologic and metabolic effects characteristic of this class of drugs.

Pharmacokinetics
The extent of percutaneous absorption of topical corticosteroids is determined by many factors including the vehicle, the integrity of the epidermal barrier, and the use of occlusive dressings (see **DOSAGE AND ADMINISTRATION**). Topical corticosteroids can be absorbed through normal intact skin. Inflammation and/or other disease processes in the skin may increase percutaneous absorption. Occlusive dressings substantially increase the percutaneous absorption of topical corticosteroids (see **DOSAGE AND ADMINISTRATION**).

Once absorbed through the skin, topical corticosteroids enter pharmacokinetic pathways similar to systemically administered corticosteroids. Corticosteroids are bound to plasma proteins in varying degrees, are metabolized primarily in the liver, and excreted by the kidneys. Some of the topical corticosteroids and their metabolites are also excreted into the bile.

DIPROLENE® AF Cream 0.05% was applied once daily at 7 grams per day for 1 week to diseased skin, in adult patients with psoriasis or atopic dermatitis, to study its effects on the hypothalamic-pituitary-adrenal (HPA) axis. The results suggested that the drug caused a slight lowering of adrenal corticosteroid secretion, although in no case did plasma cortisol levels go below the lower limit of the normal range.

Sixty-seven pediatric patients ages 1 to 12 years, with atopic dermatitis, were enrolled in an open-label, hypothalamic-pituitary-adrenal (HPA) axis safety study. DIPROLENE AF Cream 0.05% was applied twice daily for 2 to 3 weeks over a mean body surface area of 58% (range 35% to 95%). In 19 of 60 (32%) evaluable patients, adrenal suppression was indicated by either a ≤5 mcg/dL pre-stimulation cortisol, or a cosyntropin post-stimulation cortisol ≤18 mcg/dL and/or an increase of <7 mcg/dL from the baseline cortisol. Studies performed with DIPROLENE AF Cream 0.05% indicate that it is in the high range of potency as compared with other topical corticosteroids.

INDICATIONS AND USAGE
DIPROLENE® AF Cream 0.05% is a high-potency corticosteroid indicated for relief of the inflammatory and pruritic manifestations of corticosteroid-responsive dermatoses in patients 13 years and older.

CONTRAINDICATIONS
DIPROLENE® AF Cream 0.05% is contraindicated in patients who are hypersensitive to betamethasone dipropionate, to other corticosteroids, or to any ingredient in this preparation.

PRECAUTIONS
General
Systemic absorption of topical corticosteroids has produced reversible HPA axis suppression, manifestations of Cushing's syndrome, hyperglycemia, and glucosuria in some patients.

Conditions which augment systemic absorption include the application of the more potent corticosteroids, use over large surface areas, prolonged use, and the addition of occlusive dressings. Use of more than one corticosteroid-containing product at the same time may increase total systemic glucocorticoid exposure (see **DOSAGE AND ADMINISTRATION**).

Therefore, patients receiving a large dose of a potent topical steroid applied to a large surface area should be evaluated periodically for evidence of HPA axis suppression by using the urinary-free cortisol and ACTH stimulation tests. If HPA axis suppression is noted, an attempt should be made to withdraw the drug, to reduce the frequency of application, or to substitute a less potent steroid.

Recovery of HPA axis function is generally prompt and complete upon discontinuation of the drug. In an open-label pediatric study of 60 evaluable patients, of the 19 who showed evidence of suppression, 4 patients were tested 2 weeks after discontinuation of DIPROLENE® AF Cream 0.05%, and 3 of the 4 (75%) had complete recovery of HPA axis function. Infrequently, signs and symptoms of steroid withdrawal may occur, requiring supplemental systemic corticosteroids. Children may absorb proportionally larger amounts of topical corticosteroids and thus be more susceptible to systemic toxicity (see **PRECAUTIONS, Pediatric Use** section).

If irritation develops, topical corticosteroids should be discontinued and appropriate therapy instituted.

In the presence of dermatological infections, the use of an appropriate antifungal or antibacterial agent should be instituted. If a favorable response does not occur promptly, the corticosteroid should be discontinued until the infection has been adequately controlled.

Information for Patients

Patients using topical corticosteroids should receive the following information and instructions. This information is intended to aid in the safe and effective use of this medication. It is not a disclosure of all possible adverse or intended effects.

1. This medication is to be used as directed by the physician and should not be used longer than the prescribed time period. It is for external use only. Avoid contact with the eyes.
2. Patients should be advised not to use this medication for any disorder other than that for which it was prescribed.
3. The treated skin area should not be bandaged or otherwise covered or wrapped as to be occlusive (see **DOSAGE AND ADMINISTRATION**).
4. Patients should report any signs of local adverse reactions.
5. Other corticosteroid-containing products should not be used with DIPROLENE AF Cream 0.05% without first talking to your physician.

Laboratory Tests

The following tests may be helpful in evaluating HPA axis suppression:

Urinary-free cortisol test

ACTH stimulation test

Carcinogenesis, Mutagenesis, and Impairment of Fertility

Long-term animal studies have not been performed to evaluate the carcinogenic potential of betamethasone dipropionate.

Betamethasone was negative in the bacterial mutagenicity assay (*Salmonella typhimurium* and *Escherichia coli*), and in the mammalian cell mutagenicity assay (CHO/HGPRT). It was positive in the *in vitro* human lymphocyte chromosome aberration assay, and equivocal in the *in vivo* mouse bone marrow micronucleus assay. This pattern of response is similar to that of dexamethasone and hydrocortisone.

Reproductive studies with betamethasone dipropionate carried out in rabbits at doses of 1.0 mg/kg by the intramuscular route and in mice up to 33 mg/kg by the intramuscular route indicated no impairment of fertility except for dose-related increases in fetal resorption rates in both species. These doses are approximately 5- and 38-fold the human dose based on a mg/m^2 comparison, respectively.

Pregnancy

Teratogenic Effects

Pregnancy Category C

Corticosteroids are generally teratogenic in laboratory animals when administered systemically at relatively low dosage levels.

Betamethasone dipropionate has been shown to be teratogenic in rabbits when given by the intramuscular route at doses of 0.05 mg/kg. This dose is approximately 0.2-fold the maximum human dose based on a mg/m^2 comparison. The abnormalities observed included umbilical hernias, cephalocele, and cleft palates.

Some corticosteroids have been shown to be teratogenic after dermal application in laboratory animals. There are no adequate and well-controlled studies in pregnant women on teratogenic effects from topically applied corticosteroids. Therefore, topical corticosteroids should be used during pregnancy only if the potential benefit justifies the potential risk to the fetus. Drugs of this class should not be used extensively on pregnant patients, in large amounts, or for prolonged periods of time.

Nursing Mothers

It is not known whether topical administration of corticosteroids can result in sufficient systemic absorption to produce detectable quantities in breast milk. Systemically administered corticosteroids are secreted into breast milk in quantities not likely to have a deleterious effect on the infant. Nevertheless, a decision should be made whether to discontinue nursing or to discontinue the drug, taking into account the importance of the drug to the mother.

Pediatric Use

Use of DIPROLENE AF Cream 0.05% in pediatric patients 12 years of age and younger is not recommended (see **CLINICAL PHARMACOLOGY** and **ADVERSE REACTIONS**). In an open-label study, 19 of 60 (32%) evaluable pediatric patients (aged 3 months-12 years old) using DIPROLENE AF Cream 0.05% for treatment of atopic dermatitis demonstrated HPA axis suppression. The proportion of patients with adrenal suppression in this study was progressively greater, the younger the age group (see **CLINICAL PHARMACOLOGY, Pharmacokinetics** section).

Pediatric patients may demonstrate greater susceptibility to topical corticosteroid-induced HPA axis suppression and Cushing's syndrome than mature patients because of a larger skin surface area to body weight ratio. The study described above supports this premise, as adrenal suppression in 9-12 year olds, 6-8 year olds, 2-5 year olds, and 3 months-1 year old was 17%, 32%, 38%, and 50%, respectively.

Hypothalamic-pituitary-adrenal (HPA) axis suppression, Cushing's syndrome, and intracranial hypertension have been reported in children receiving topical corticosteroids. Manifestations of adrenal suppression in children include linear growth retardation, delayed weight gain, low plasma cortisol levels, and absence of response to ACTH stimulation. Manifestations of intracranial hypertension include bulging fontanelles, headaches, and bilateral papilledema. Chronic corticosteroid therapy may interfere with the growth and development of children.

Geriatric Use

Clinical studies of DIPROLENE AF Cream 0.05% included 104 subjects who were 65 years of age and over and 8 subjects who were 75 years of age and over. No overall differences in safety or effectiveness were observed between these subjects and younger subjects, and other reported clinical experience has not identified differences in responses between the elderly and younger patients. However, greater sensitivity of some older individuals cannot be ruled out.

ADVERSE REACTIONS

The only local adverse reaction reported to be possibly or probably related to treatment with DIPROLENE® AF Cream 0.05% during adult-controlled clinical studies was stinging. It occurred in 1 patient, 0.4%, of the 242 patients or subjects involved in the studies.

Adverse reactions reported to be possibly or probably related to treatment with DIPROLENE AF Cream 0.05% during a pediatric clinical study include signs of skin atrophy (telangiectasia, bruising, shininess). Skin atrophy occurred in 7 of 67 (10%) patients, involving all age groups from 3 months – 12 years of age.

The following local adverse reactions are reported infrequently when topical corticosteroids are used as recommended. These reactions are listed in an approximate decreasing order of occurrence: burning, itching, irritation, dryness, folliculitis, hypertrichosis, acneiform eruptions, hypopigmentation, perioral dermatitis, allergic contact dermatitis, maceration of the skin, secondary infection, skin atrophy, striae, miliaria.

Systemic absorption of topical corticosteroids has produced reversible hypothalamic-pituitary-adrenal (HPA) axis suppression, manifestations of Cushing's syndrome, hyperglycemia, and glucosuria in some patients.

OVERDOSAGE

Topically applied corticosteroids can be absorbed in sufficient amounts to produce systemic effects (see **PRECAUTIONS**).

DOSAGE AND ADMINISTRATION

Apply a thin film of DIPROLENE® AF Cream 0.05% to the affected skin areas once or twice daily. Treatment with DIPROLENE AF Cream 0.05% should be limited to 50 g per week.

DIPROLENE AF Cream 0.05% is not to be used with occlusive dressings.

HOW SUPPLIED

DIPROLENE® AF Cream 0.05% is supplied in 15-g (NDC 0085-0517-01) and 50-g (NDC 0085-0517-04) tubes; boxes of one.

Store at 25°C (77°F); excursions permitted to 15-30°C (59-86°F) [see USP Controlled Room Temperature].

Manufactured for: Merck Sharp & Dohme Corp., a subsidiary of

MERCK & CO., INC., Whitehouse Station, NJ 08889, USA

Manufactured by: Schering Plough Canada, Inc.

Pointe Claire, Quebec, Canada

Copyright © 1987, 2001 Merck Sharp & Dohme Corp., a subsidiary of **Merck & Co., Inc.**

All rights reserved.

Rev. 05/12

011460-DPL-CR-USPI.2

DIPROLENE® LOTION 0.05%   ℞

[dĭp-rō-lēn]

brand of augmented betamethasone dipropionate[1]

Lotion 0.05% (potency expressed as betamethasone)

[1]Vehicle augments the penetration of the steroid.

For Dermatologic Use Only

Not for Ophthalmic Use

DESCRIPTION

DIPROLENE® (augmented betamethasone dipropionate) Lotion contains betamethasone dipropionate USP, a synthetic adrenocorticosteroid, for dermatologic use. Betamethasone, an analog of prednisolone, has a high degree of corticosteroid activity and a slight degree of mineralocorticoid activity. Betamethasone dipropionate is the 17, 21-dipropionate ester of betamethasone.

Chemically, betamethasone dipropionate is 9-fluoro-11β,17,21-trihydroxy-16β-methylpregna-1,4-diene-

3,20-dione 17,21-dipropionate, with the empirical formula $C_{28}H_{37}FO_7$, a molecular weight of 504.6, and the following structural formula:

It is a white to creamy-white, odorless powder insoluble in water; freely soluble in acetone and in chloroform; sparingly soluble in alcohol.

Each gram of DIPROLENE Lotion 0.05% contains 0.643 mg betamethasone dipropionate USP (equivalent to 0.5 mg betamethasone), in an augmented lotion base of purified water; isopropyl alcohol (30%); hydroxypropyl cellulose; propylene glycol; sodium phosphate monobasic monohydrate; and phosphoric acid used to adjust the pH.

CLINICAL PHARMACOLOGY

The corticosteroids are a class of compounds comprising steroid hormones secreted by the adrenal cortex and their synthetic analogs. In pharmacologic doses, corticosteroids are used primarily for their anti-inflammatory and/or immunosuppressive effects.

Topical corticosteroids, such as betamethasone dipropionate, are effective in the treatment of corticosteroid-responsive dermatoses primarily because of their anti-inflammatory, antipruritic, and vasoconstrictive actions. However, while the physiologic, pharmacologic, and clinical effects of the corticosteroids are well known, the exact mechanisms of their actions in each disease are uncertain. Betamethasone dipropionate, a corticosteroid, has been shown to have topical (dermatologic) and systemic pharmacologic and metabolic effects characteristic of this class of drugs.

Pharmacokinetics

The extent of percutaneous absorption of topical corticosteroids is determined by many factors including the vehicle, the integrity of the epidermal barrier, and the use of occlusive dressings (see **DOSAGE AND ADMINISTRATION**). Topical corticosteroids can be absorbed through normal intact skin. Inflammation and/or other disease processes in the skin may increase percutaneous absorption. Occlusive dressings substantially increase the percutaneous absorption of topical corticosteroids (see **DOSAGE AND ADMINISTRATION**).

Once absorbed through the skin, topical corticosteroids enter pharmacokinetic pathways similar to systemically administered corticosteroids. Corticosteroids are bound to plasma proteins in varying degrees, are metabolized primarily in the liver, and excreted by the kidneys. Some of the topical corticosteroids and their metabolites are also excreted into the bile.

Studies performed with DIPROLENE® Lotion indicate that it is in the super-high range of potency as compared with other topical corticosteroids.

INDICATIONS AND USAGE

DIPROLENE® Lotion is a super-high potency corticosteroid indicated for the relief of the inflammatory and pruritic manifestations of corticosteroid-responsive dermatoses in patients 13 years of age and older. The total dose should not exceed 50 mL per week because of the potential for the drug to suppress the hypothalamic-pituitary-adrenal (HPA) axis.

CONTRAINDICATIONS

DIPROLENE® Lotion is contraindicated in patients who are hypersensitive to betamethasone dipropionate, to other corticosteroids, or to any ingredient in this preparation.

PRECAUTIONS

General

Systemic absorption of topical corticosteroids has produced reversible HPA axis suppression, manifestations of Cushing's syndrome, hyperglycemia, and glucosuria in some patients.

Conditions which augment systemic absorption include the application of the more potent corticosteroids, use over large surface areas, prolonged use, and the addition of occlusive dressings. Use of more than one corticosteroid-containing product at the same time may increase total systemic glucocorticoid exposure (see **DOSAGE AND ADMINISTRATION**).

Therefore, patients receiving a large dose of a potent topical steroid applied to a large surface area should be evaluated periodically for evidence of HPA axis suppression by using the urinary-free cortisol and ACTH stimulation tests. If HPA axis suppression is noted, an attempt should be made to withdraw the drug, to reduce the frequency of application, or to substitute a less potent steroid.

Recovery of HPA axis function is generally prompt and complete upon discontinuation of the drug. Patients should not be treated with amounts of DIPROLENE® Lotion greater than 50 mL per week because of the potential for the drug to suppress HPA axis. Patients receiving super-potent corticosteroids should not be treated for more than 2 weeks at a time and only small areas should be treated at any one time due to the increased risk of HPA axis suppression.

DIPROLENE Lotion was applied once daily at 7 mL per day for 21 days to diseased scalp and body skin in patients with scalp psoriasis to study its effects on the HPA axis. In 2 out of 11 patients, the drug lowered plasma cortisol levels below normal limits. HPA axis suppression in these patients was transient and returned to normal within a week. In one of these patients, plasma cortisol levels returned to normal while treatment continued.

Infrequently, signs and symptoms of steroid withdrawal may occur, requiring supplemental systemic corticosteroids. Pediatric patients may absorb proportionally larger amounts of topical corticosteroids and thus be more susceptible to systemic toxicity (see **PRECAUTIONS, Pediatric Use** section).

If irritation develops, topical corticosteroids should be discontinued and appropriate therapy instituted.

In the presence of dermatological infections, the use of an appropriate antifungal or antibacterial agent should be instituted. If a favorable response does not occur promptly, the corticosteroid should be discontinued until the infection has been adequately controlled.

DIPROLENE Lotion should not be used in the treatment of rosacea or perioral dermatitis, and it should not be used on the face, groin, or in the axillae.

Information for Patients

Patients using topical corticosteroids should receive the following information and instructions. This information is intended to aid in the safe and effective use of this medication. It is not a disclosure of all possible adverse or intended effects.

1. This medication is to be used as directed by the physician and should not be used longer than the prescribed time period. It is for external use only. Avoid contact with the eyes.
2. This medication should not be used for any disorder other than that for which it was prescribed.
3. The treated skin area should not be bandaged, or otherwise covered or wrapped, so as to be occlusive (see **DOSAGE AND ADMINISTRATION**).
4. Patients should report to their physician any signs of local adverse reactions.
5. Patients should be advised not to use DIPROLENE® Lotion in the treatment of diaper dermatitis. DIPROLENE Lotion should not be applied in the diaper areas as diapers or plastic pants may constitute occlusive dressing (see **DOSAGE AND ADMINISTRATION**).
6. This medication should not be used on the face, underarms, or groin areas unless directed by the physician.
7. As with other corticosteroids, therapy should be discontinued when control is achieved. If no improvement is seen within 2 weeks, contact the physician.
8. Other corticosteroid-containing products should not be used with DIPROLENE Lotion.

Laboratory Tests

The following tests may be helpful in evaluating patients for HPA axis suppression:

ACTH stimulation test
Urinary-free cortisol test

Carcinogenesis, Mutagenesis, and Impairment of Fertility

Long-term animal studies have not been performed to evaluate the carcinogenic potential of betamethasone dipropionate. Betamethasone was negative in the bacterial mutagenicity assay (*Salmonella typhimurium* and *Escherichia coli*), and in the mammalian cell mutagenicity assay (CHO/HGPRT). It was positive in the *in vitro* human lymphocyte chromosome aberration assay, and equivocal in the *in vivo* mouse bone marrow micronucleus assay. This pattern of response is similar to that of dexamethasone and hydrocortisone. Studies in rabbits, mice, and rats using intramuscular doses up to 1, 33, and 2 mg/kg, respectively, resulted in dose-related increases in fetal resorptions in rabbits and mice.

Pregnancy

Teratogenic Effects
Pregnancy Category C
Corticosteroids have been shown to be teratogenic in laboratory animals when administered systemically at relatively low dosage levels. Some corticosteroids have been shown to be teratogenic after dermal application in laboratory animals. Betamethasone dipropionate has been shown to be teratogenic in rabbits when given by the intramuscular route at doses of 0.05 mg/kg. This dose is approximately 0.2 times the human topical dose of DIPROLENE Lotion in mg/m^2 of body surface area, assuming 100% absorption and the use in a 60 kg person of 7 g per day. The abnormalities observed included umbilical hernias, cephalocele, and cleft palate. There are no adequate and well-controlled studies in pregnant women on teratogenic effects from topically applied corticosteroids. DIPROLENE Lotion should be used during pregnancy only if the potential benefit justifies the potential risk to the fetus.

Nursing Mothers

Systemically administered corticosteroids appear in human milk and could suppress growth, interfere with endogenous corticosteroid production, or cause other untoward effects. It is not known whether topical administration of corticosteroids could result in sufficient systemic absorption to produce detectable quantities in human milk. Because many drugs are excreted in human milk, caution should be exercised when DIPROLENE Lotion is administered to a nursing woman.

Pediatric Use

Use of DIPROLENE Lotion, 0.05%, in pediatric patients 12 years of age and younger is not recommended (see **CLINICAL PHARMACOLOGY** and **ADVERSE REACTIONS**). Pediatric patients may demonstrate greater susceptibility to topical corticosteroid-induced HPA axis suppression and Cushing's syndrome than mature patients because of a larger skin surface to body weight ratio.

Hypothalamic-pituitary-adrenal (HPA) axis suppression, Cushing's syndrome, and intracranial hypertension have been reported in children receiving topical corticosteroids. Manifestations of adrenal suppression in children include linear growth retardation, delayed weight gain, low plasma cortisol levels, and absence of response to ACTH stimulation. Manifestations of intracranial hypertension include bulging fontanelles, headaches, and bilateral papilledema. Chronic corticosteroid therapy may interfere with the growth and development of children.

Geriatric Use

Seven clinical studies of DIPROLENE Lotion evaluated 407 subjects of which 56 subjects were 65 years of age and over and 9 subjects were 75 years of age and over. No overall differences in safety or effectiveness were observed in these clinical studies between geriatric subjects and younger subjects. There was a numerical difference for application site reactions (most frequently reported events were burning and stinging) which occurred in 15% (10/65) of geriatric subjects and 11% (38/342) of subjects less than 65 years of age. Other reported clinical experience has not identified differences in responses between the elderly and younger patients. However, greater sensitivity of some older individuals cannot be ruled out.

ADVERSE REACTIONS

The local adverse reactions which were reported with DIPROLENE® Lotion during controlled clinical trials were as follows: erythema, folliculitis, pruritus, and vesiculation each occurring in less than 1% of patients.

The following additional local adverse reactions have been reported with topical corticosteroids, and they may occur more frequently with the use of occlusive dressings and higher potency corticosteroids. These reactions are listed in an approximately decreasing order of occurrence: burning, itching, irritation, dryness, folliculitis, hypertrichosis, acneiform eruptions, hypopigmentation, perioral dermatitis, allergic contact dermatitis, secondary infection, skin atrophy, striae, and miliaria.

Systemic absorption of topical corticosteroids has produced reversible hypothalamic-pituitary-adrenal (HPA) axis suppression, manifestations of Cushing's syndrome, hyperglycemia, and glucosuria in some patients.

OVERDOSAGE

Topically applied DIPROLENE® Lotion can be absorbed in sufficient amounts to produce systemic effects (see **PRECAUTIONS**).

DOSAGE AND ADMINISTRATION

Apply a few drops of DIPROLENE® Lotion to the affected skin once or twice daily and massage lightly until the lotion disappears.

DIPROLENE Lotion is a super-high potency topical corticosteroid. **Treatment with DIPROLENE Lotion should be limited to two weeks, and amounts greater than 50 mL per week should not be used.**

As with other highly active corticosteroids, therapy should be discontinued when control is achieved. If no improvement is seen within 2 weeks, reassessment of diagnosis may be necessary.

DIPROLENE Lotion should not be used with occlusive dressings. DIPROLENE Lotion should not be applied to the diaper area if the patient requires diapers or plastic pants as these garments may constitute occlusive dressing.

HOW SUPPLIED

DIPROLENE® Lotion 0.05% is supplied in 30-mL (29 g) (NDC 0085-0962-01) and 60-mL (58 g) (NDC 0085-0962-02) plastic squeeze bottles; boxes of one.

Store at 25°C (77°F); excursions permitted to 15–30°C (59–86°F) [see USP Controlled Room Temperature].

Manufactured for: Merck Sharp & Dohme Corp., a subsidiary of
MERCK & CO., INC., Whitehouse Station, NJ 08889, USA
Manufactured by: Schering Plough Canada, Inc.,
Pointe Claire, Quebec H9R 1B4, Canada
Copyright © 1988, 2004 Merck Sharp & Dohme Corp., a subsidiary of Merck & Co., Inc.
All rights reserved.
Revised: 10/2012
011460-DPL-LT-USPI.2

DIPROLENE®

℞

[dĭp-rō-lēn]
brand of augmented betamethasone dipropionate[1]
Ointment 0.05%
(potency expressed as betamethasone)

[1]Vehicle augments the penetration of the steroid.
For Dermatologic Use Only - Not for Ophthalmic Use

DESCRIPTION

DIPROLENE® (augmented betamethasone dipropionate) Ointment contains betamethasone dipropionate USP, a synthetic adrenocorticosteroid, for dermatologic use. Betamethasone, an analog of prednisolone, has a high degree of corticosteroid activity and a slight degree of mineralocorticoid activity. Betamethasone dipropionate is the 17, 21-dipropionate ester of betamethasone.

Chemically, betamethasone dipropionate is 9-fluoro-11β, 17,21-trihydroxy-16β-methylpregna-1,4-diene-3,20-dione 17,21-dipropionate, with the empirical formula $C_{28}H_{37}FO_7$, a molecular weight of 504.6 and the following structural formula:

It is a white to creamy-white, odorless powder insoluble in water; freely soluble in acetone and in chloroform; sparingly soluble in alcohol.

Each gram of DIPROLENE Ointment 0.05% contains 0.643 mg betamethasone dipropionate USP (equivalent to 0.5 mg betamethasone), in a vehicle of propylene glycol; propylene glycol stearate; white wax; and white petrolatum.

CLINICAL PHARMACOLOGY

The corticosteroids are a class of compounds comprising steroid hormones secreted by the adrenal cortex and their synthetic analogs. In pharmacologic doses, corticosteroids are used primarily for their anti-inflammatory and/or immunosuppressive effects. Topical corticosteroids, such as betamethasone dipropionate, are effective in the treatment of corticosteroid-responsive dermatoses primarily because of their anti-inflammatory, antipruritic, and vasoconstrictive actions. However, while the physiologic, pharmacologic, and clinical effects of the corticosteroids are well known, the exact mechanisms of their actions in each disease are uncertain. Betamethasone dipropionate, a corticosteroid, has been shown to have topical (dermatologic) and systemic pharmacologic and metabolic effects characteristic of this class of drugs.

Pharmacokinetics

The extent of percutaneous absorption of topical corticosteroids is determined by many factors including the vehicle, the integrity of the epidermal barrier, and the use of occlusive dressings (see **DOSAGE AND ADMINISTRATION**). Topical corticosteroids can be absorbed through normal intact skin. Inflammation and/or other disease processes in the skin may increase percutaneous absorption. Occlusive dressings substantially increase the percutaneous absorption of topical corticosteroids (see **DOSAGE AND ADMINISTRATION**).

Once absorbed through the skin, topical corticosteroids enter pharmacokinetic pathways similar to systemically administered corticosteroids. Corticosteroids are bound to plasma proteins in varying degrees, are metabolized primarily in the liver, and excreted by the kidneys. Some of the topical corticosteroids and their metabolites are also excreted into the bile.

Studies performed with DIPROLENE® Ointment indicate that it is in the super-high range of potency as compared with other topical corticosteroids.

INDICATIONS AND USAGE

DIPROLENE® Ointment is a super-high potency corticosteroid indicated for the relief of the inflammatory and pruritic manifestations of corticosteroid-responsive dermatoses in patients 13 years of age and older. The total dose should not exceed 50 g per week because of the potential for the drug to suppress the hypothalamic-pituitary-adrenal (HPA) axis.

CONTRAINDICATIONS

DIPROLENE® Ointment is contraindicated in patients who are hypersensitive to betamethasone dipropionate, to other corticosteroids, or to any ingredient in this preparation.

PRECAUTIONS
General

Systemic absorption of topical corticosteroids has produced reversible HPA axis suppression, manifestations of Cushing's syndrome, hyperglycemia, and glucosuria in some patients. Conditions which augment systemic absorption include the application of the more potent corticosteroids, use over large surface areas, prolonged use, and the addition of occlusive dressings. Use of more than one corticosteroid-containing product at the same time may increase total systemic glucocorticoid exposure (see **DOSAGE AND ADMINISTRATION**).

Therefore, patients receiving a large dose of a potent topical steroid applied to a large surface area should be evaluated periodically for evidence of HPA axis suppression by using the urinary-free cortisol and ACTH stimulation tests. If HPA axis suppression is noted, an attempt should be made to withdraw the drug, to reduce the frequency of application, or to substitute a less potent steroid.

Recovery of HPA axis function is generally prompt and complete upon discontinuation of the drug. Patients should not be treated with amounts of DIPROLENE® Ointment greater than 50 g per week because of the potential for the drug to suppress HPA axis. Patients receiving super-potent corticosteroids should not be treated for more than 2 weeks at a time and only small areas should be treated at any one time due to the increased risk of HPA suppression.

At 14 g per day DIPROLENE Ointment was shown to depress the plasma levels of adrenal cortical hormones following repeated application to diseased skin in patients with psoriasis. These effects were reversible upon discontinuation of treatment. At 7 g per day DIPROLENE Ointment was shown to cause minimal inhibition of the HPA axis when applied 2 times daily for 2 to 3 weeks in healthy patients and in patients with psoriasis and eczematous disorders.

With 6 to 7 g of DIPROLENE Ointment applied once daily for 3 weeks, no significant inhibition of the HPA axis was observed in patients with psoriasis and atopic dermatitis, as measured by plasma cortisol and 24-hour urinary 17-hydroxy-corticosteroid levels. Infrequently, signs and symptoms of steroid withdrawal may occur, requiring supplemental systemic corticosteroids.

Pediatric patients may absorb proportionally larger amounts of topical corticosteroids and thus be more susceptible to systemic toxicity (see **PRECAUTIONS, Pediatric Use** section).

If irritation develops, topical corticosteroids should be discontinued and appropriate therapy instituted.

In the presence of dermatological infections, the use of an appropriate antifungal or antibacterial agent should be instituted. If a favorable response does not occur promptly, the corticosteroid should be discontinued until the infection has been adequately controlled. DIPROLENE Ointment should not be used in the treatment of rosacea or perioral dermatitis, and it should not be used on the face, groin, or in the axillae.

Information for Patients

Patients using topical corticosteroids should receive the following information and instructions. This information is intended to aid in the safe and effective use of this medication. It is not a disclosure of all possible adverse or intended effects.

1. This medication is to be used as directed by the physician and should not be used longer than the prescribed time period. It is for external use only. Avoid contact with the eyes.
2. This medication should not be used for any disorder other than that for which it was prescribed.
3. The treated skin area should not be bandaged, otherwise covered or wrapped, so as to be occlusive (see **DOSAGE AND ADMINISTRATION**).
4. Patients should report to their physician any signs of local adverse reactions.
5. Patients should be advised not to use DIPROLENE Ointment in the treatment of diaper dermatitis. DIPROLENE Ointment should not be applied in the diaper areas as diapers or plastic pants may constitute occlusive dressing (see **DOSAGE AND ADMINISTRATION**).
6. This medication should not be used on the face, underarms, or groin areas unless directed by the physician.
7. As with other corticosteroids, therapy should be discontinued when control is achieved. If no improvement is seen within 2 weeks, contact the physician.
8. Other corticosteroid-containing products should not be used with DIPROLENE Ointment.

Laboratory Tests

The following tests may be helpful in evaluating patients for HPA axis suppression:
ACTH stimulation test
Urinary-free cortisol test

Carcinogenesis, Mutagenesis, and Impairment of Fertility

Long-term animal studies have not been performed to evaluate the carcinogenic potential of betamethasone dipropionate. Betamethasone was negative in the bacterial mutagenicity assay (*Salmonella typhimurium* and *Escherichia coli*), and in the mammalian cell mutagenicity assay (CHO/HGPRT). It was positive in the *in vitro* human lymphocyte chromosome aberration assay, and equivocal in the *in vivo* mouse bone marrow micronucleus assay. This pattern of response is similar to that of dexamethasone and hydrocortisone. Studies in rabbits, mice, and rats using intramuscular doses up to 1, 33, and 2 mg/kg, respectively, resulted in dose-related increases in fetal resorptions in rabbits and mice.

Pregnancy
Teratogenic Effects
Pregnancy Category C

Corticosteroids have been shown to be teratogenic in laboratory animals when administered systemically at relatively low dosage levels. Some corticosteroids have been shown to be teratogenic after dermal application in laboratory animals. Betamethasone dipropionate has been shown to be teratogenic in rabbits when given by the intramuscular route at doses of 0.05 mg/kg. This dose is approximately 0.2 times the human topical dose of DIPROLENE Ointment in mg/m² of body surface area, assuming 100% absorption and the use in a 60 kg person of 7 g per day. The abnormalities observed included umbilical hernias, cephalocele, and cleft palate. There are no adequate and well-controlled studies in pregnant women on teratogenic effects from topically applied corticosteroids. DIPROLENE Ointment should be used during pregnancy only if the potential benefit justifies the potential risk to the fetus.

Nursing Mothers

Systemically administered corticosteroids appear in human milk and could suppress growth, interfere with endogenous corticosteroid production, or cause other untoward effects. It is not known whether topical administration of corticosteroids could result in sufficient systemic absorption to produce detectable quantities in human milk. Because many drugs are excreted in human milk, caution should be exercised when DIPROLENE Ointment is administered to a nursing woman.

Pediatric Use

Use of DIPROLENE Ointment, 0.05%, in pediatric patients 12 years of age and younger is not recommended (see **CLINICAL PHARMACOLOGY** and **ADVERSE REACTIONS**).

Pediatric patients may demonstrate greater susceptibility to topical corticosteroid-induced HPA axis suppression and Cushing's syndrome than mature patients because of a larger skin surface area to body weight ratio.

Hypothalamic-pituitary-adrenal (HPA) axis suppression, Cushing's syndrome, and intracranial hypertension have been reported in children receiving topical corticosteroids. Manifestations of adrenal suppression in children include linear growth retardation, delayed weight gain, low plasma cortisol levels, and an absence of response to ACTH stimulation. Manifestations of intracranial hypertension include bulging fontanelles, headaches, and bilateral papilledema. Chronic corticosteroid therapy may interfere with the growth and development of children.

Geriatric Use

Clinical studies of DIPROLENE Ointment included 225 subjects who were 65 years of age and over and 46 subjects who were 75 years of age and over. No overall differences in safety or effectiveness were observed between these subjects and younger subjects, and other reported clinical experience has not identified differences in responses between the elderly and younger patients. However, greater sensitivity of some older individuals cannot be ruled out.

ADVERSE REACTIONS

The local adverse reactions which were reported with DIPROLENE® Ointment during controlled clinical trials were as follows: erythema, folliculitis, pruritus, and vesiculation each occurring in less than 1% of patients.

The following additional local adverse reactions have been reported with topical corticosteroids, and they may occur more frequently with the use of occlusive dressings and higher potency corticosteroids. These reactions are listed in an approximately decreasing order of occurrence: burning, itching, irritation, dryness, folliculitis, hypertrichosis, acneiform eruptions, hypopigmentation, perioral dermatitis, allergic contact dermatitis, secondary infection, skin atrophy, striae, and miliaria.

Systemic absorption of topical corticosteroids has produced reversible hypothalamic-pituitary-adrenal (HPA) axis suppression, manifestations of Cushing's syndrome, hyperglycemia, and glucosuria in some patients.

OVERDOSAGE

Topically applied DIPROLENE® Ointment can be absorbed in sufficient amounts to produce systemic effects (see **PRECAUTIONS**).

DOSAGE AND ADMINISTRATION

Apply a thin film of DIPROLENE® Ointment to the affected skin once or twice daily. DIPROLENE Ointment is a super-high potency topical corticosteroid. **Treatment with DIPROLENE Ointment should be limited to 50 g per week.** As with other corticosteroids, therapy should be discontinued when control is achieved. If no improvement is seen within 2 weeks, reassessment of diagnosis may be necessary.

DIPROLENE Ointment should not be used with occlusive dressings. DIPROLENE Ointment should not be applied to the diaper area if the patient requires diapers or plastic pants as these garments may constitute occlusive dressing.

HOW SUPPLIED

DIPROLENE® Ointment 0.05% is supplied in 15-g (NDC 0085-0575-02) and 50-g (NDC 0085-0575-05) tubes; boxes of one.

Store at 25°C (77°F); excursions permitted to 15-30°C (59-86°F) [see USP Controlled Room Temperature].

Manufactured for: Merck Sharp & Dohme Corp., a subsidiary of **MERCK & CO., INC.**, Whitehouse Station, NJ 08889, USA
Manufactured by: Schering Plough Canada, Inc.
Pointe Claire, Quebec, Canada
Copyright © 1983, 2004 Merck Sharp & Dohme Corp., a subsidiary of **Merck & Co., Inc.**
All rights reserved.
Rev. 05/12
011460-DPL-OT-USPI.2

DULERA® 100 mcg/5 mcg ℞
[*dew-LAIR-ah*]
(mometasone furoate 100 mcg and formoterol fumarate dihydrate 5 mcg)
Inhalation Aerosol

DULERA® 200 mcg/5 mcg
(mometasone furoate 200 mcg and formoterol fumarate dihydrate 5 mcg)
Inhalation Aerosol
FOR ORAL INHALATION

HIGHLIGHTS OF PRESCRIBING INFORMATION

These highlights do not include all the information needed to use DULERA safely and effectively. See full prescribing information for DULERA.

DULERA® 100 mcg/5 mcg (mometasone furoate 100 mcg and formoterol fumarate dihydrate 5 mcg) Inhalation Aerosol

DULERA® 200 mcg/5 mcg (mometasone furoate 200 mcg and formoterol fumarate dihydrate 5 mcg) Inhalation Aerosol

FOR ORAL INHALATION
Initial U.S. Approval: 2010

> **WARNING: ASTHMA-RELATED DEATH**
> *See full prescribing information for complete boxed warning.*
> - Long-acting beta₂-adrenergic agonists (LABA), such as formoterol, one of the active ingredients in DULERA, increase the risk of asthma-related death. Data from a large placebo-controlled U.S. study that compared the safety of another LABA (salmeterol) or placebo added to usual asthma therapy showed an increase in asthma-related deaths in patients receiving salmeterol. This finding of an increased risk of asthma-related death is considered a class effect of the LABA, including formoterol. Currently available data are inadequate to determine whether concurrent use of inhaled corticosteroids or other long-term asthma control drugs mitigates the increased risk of asthma-related death from LABA. Available data from controlled clinical trials suggest that LABA increase the risk of asthma-related hospitalization in pediatric and adolescent patients.
> - When treating patients with asthma, prescribe DULERA only for patients with asthma not adequately controlled on a long-term asthma control medication, such as an inhaled corticosteroid or whose disease severity clearly warrants initiation of treatment with both an inhaled corticosteroid and LABA. Once asthma control is achieved and maintained, assess the patient at regular intervals and step down therapy (e.g., discontinue DULERA) if possible without loss of asthma control, and maintain the patient on a long-term asthma control medication, such as an inhaled corticosteroid. Do not

use DULERA for patients whose asthma is adequately controlled on low or medium dose inhaled corticosteroids. (1.1, 5.1)

---RECENT MAJOR CHANGES---

Warnings and Precautions, Coexisting   07/2013
Conditions (5.15)

---INDICATIONS AND USAGE---

DULERA is a combination product containing a corticosteroid and a long-acting beta₂-adrenergic agonist indicated for:
• Treatment of asthma in patients 12 years of age and older. (1.1)
Important limitations:
• Not indicated for the relief of acute bronchospasm. (1.1)

---DOSAGE AND ADMINISTRATION---

For oral inhalation only. (2.1)
Treatment of asthma in patients ≥12 years: 2 inhalations twice daily of DULERA 100 mcg/5 mcg or 200 mcg/5 mcg. Starting dosage is based on prior asthma therapy. (2.2)

---DOSAGE FORMS AND STRENGTHS---

Inhalation aerosol containing a combination of mometasone furoate (100 or 200 mcg) and formoterol fumarate dihydrate (5 mcg) per actuation. (3)

---CONTRAINDICATIONS---

• Primary treatment of status asthmaticus or acute episodes of asthma requiring intensive measures. (4.1)
• Hypersensitivity to any of the ingredients of DULERA. (4.2)

---WARNINGS AND PRECAUTIONS---

• Asthma-related death: Long-acting beta₂-adrenergic agonists increase the risk. Prescribe only for recommended patient populations. (5.1)
• Deterioration of disease and acute episodes: Do not initiate in acutely deteriorating asthma or to treat acute symptoms. (5.2)
• Use with additional long-acting beta₂-agonist: Do not use in combination because of risk of overdose. (5.3)
• Localized infections: Candida albicans infection of the mouth and throat may occur. Monitor patients periodically for signs of adverse effects on the oral cavity. Advise patients to rinse the mouth following inhalation. (5.4)
• Immunosuppression: Potential worsening of existing tuberculosis, fungal, bacterial, viral, or parasitic infection; or ocular herpes simplex infections. More serious or even fatal course of chickenpox or measles can occur in susceptible patients. Use with caution in patients with these infections because of the potential for worsening of these infections. (5.5)
• Transferring patients from systemic corticosteroids: Risk of impaired adrenal function when transferring from oral steroids. Taper patients slowly from systemic corticosteroids if transferring to DULERA. (5.6)
• Hypercorticism and adrenal suppression: May occur with very high dosages or at the regular dosage in susceptible individuals. If such changes occur, discontinue DULERA slowly. (5.7)
• Strong cytochrome P450 3A4 inhibitors (e.g., ritonavir): Risk of increased systemic corticosteroid effects. Exercise caution when used with DULERA. (5.8)
• Paradoxical bronchospasm: Discontinue DULERA and institute alternative therapy if paradoxical bronchospasm occurs. (5.9)
• Patients with cardiovascular disorders: Use with caution because of beta-adrenergic stimulation. (5.11)
• Decreases in bone mineral density: Monitor patients with major risk factors for decreased bone mineral content. (5.12)
• Effects on growth: Monitor growth of pediatric patients. (5.13)
• Glaucoma and cataracts: Monitor patients with change in vision or with a history of increased intraocular pressure, glaucoma, and/or cataracts closely. (5.14)
• Coexisting conditions: Use with caution in patients with aneurysm, pheochromocytoma, convulsive disorders, thyrotoxicosis, diabetes mellitus, and ketoacidosis. (5.15)
• Hypokalemia and hyperglycemia: Be alert to hypokalemia and hyperglycemia. (5.16)

---ADVERSE REACTIONS---

Most common adverse reactions (reported in ≥3% of patients) included:
• Nasopharyngitis, sinusitis and headache. (6.1)
To report SUSPECTED ADVERSE REACTIONS, contact Merck Sharp & Dohme Corp., a subsidiary of Merck & Co., Inc., at 1-877-888-4231 or FDA at 1-800-FDA-1088 or www.fda.gov/medwatch.

---DRUG INTERACTIONS---

• Strong cytochrome P450 3A4 inhibitors (e.g., ritonavir): Use with caution. May cause increased systemic corticosteroid effects. (7.1)

• Adrenergic agents: Use with caution. Additional adrenergic drugs may potentiate sympathetic effects. (7.2)
• Xanthine derivatives and diuretics: Use with caution. May potentiate ECG changes and/or hypokalemia. (7.3, 7.4)
• MAO inhibitors, tricyclic antidepressants, macrolides, and drugs that prolong QTc interval: Use with extreme caution. May potentiate effect on the cardiovascular system. (7.5)
• Beta-blockers: Use with caution and only when medically necessary. May decrease effectiveness and produce severe bronchospasm. (7.6)
• Halogenated hydrocarbons: There is an elevated risk of arrhythmias in patients receiving concomitant anesthesia with halogenated hydrocarbons. (7.7)

---USE IN SPECIFIC POPULATIONS---

• Hepatic impairment: Monitor patients for signs of increased drug exposure. (8.6)
See 17 for PATIENT COUNSELING INFORMATION and Medication Guide

Revised: 04/2014

FULL PRESCRIBING INFORMATION

WARNING: ASTHMA-RELATED DEATH

Long-acting beta₂-adrenergic agonists (LABA), such as formoterol, one of the active ingredients in DULERA, increase the risk of asthma-related death. Data from a large placebo-controlled U.S. study that compared the safety of another long-acting beta₂-adrenergic agonist (salmeterol) or placebo added to usual asthma therapy showed an increase in asthma-related deaths in patients receiving salmeterol. This finding with salmeterol is considered a class effect of the LABA, including formoterol. Currently available data are inadequate to determine whether concurrent use of inhaled corticosteroids or other long-term asthma control drugs mitigates the increased risk of asthma-related death from LABA. Available data from controlled clinical trials suggest that LABA increase the risk of asthma-related hospitalization in pediatric and adolescent patients. Therefore, when treating patients with asthma, DULERA should only be used for patients not adequately controlled on a long-term asthma control medication, such as an inhaled corticosteroid or whose disease severity clearly warrants initiation of treatment with both an inhaled corticosteroid and LABA. Once asthma control is achieved and maintained, assess the patient at regular intervals and step down therapy (e.g., discontinue DULERA) if possible without loss of asthma control, and maintain the patient on a long-term asthma control medication, such as an inhaled corticosteroid. Do not use DULERA for patients whose asthma is adequately controlled on low or medium dose inhaled corticosteroids. [See Warnings and Precautions (5.1).]

1   INDICATIONS AND USAGE
1.1   Treatment of Asthma
DULERA is indicated for the treatment of asthma in patients 12 years of age and older.
Long-acting beta₂-adrenergic agonists, such as formoterol, one of the active ingredients in DULERA, increase the risk of asthma-related death. Available data from controlled clinical trials suggest that LABA increase the risk of asthma-related hospitalization in pediatric and adolescent patients [see Warnings and Precautions (5.1)]. Therefore, when treating patients with asthma, DULERA should only be used for patients not adequately controlled on a long-term asthma control medication, such as an inhaled corticosteroid or whose disease severity clearly warrants initiation of treatment with both an inhaled corticosteroid and LABA. Once asthma control is achieved and maintained, assess the patient at regular intervals and step down therapy (e.g., discontinue DULERA) if possible without loss of asthma control, and maintain the patient on a long-term asthma control medication, such as an inhaled corticosteroid. Do not use DULERA for patients whose asthma is adequately controlled on low or medium dose inhaled corticosteroids.
Important Limitation of Use
• DULERA is NOT indicated for the relief of acute bronchospasm.

2   DOSAGE AND ADMINISTRATION
2.1   General
DULERA should be administered only by the orally inhaled route (see Patient Instructions for Use in the Medication Guide). After each dose, the patient should be advised to rinse his/her mouth with water without swallowing.
The cap from the mouthpiece of the actuator should be removed before using DULERA.
DULERA should be primed before using for the first time by releasing 4 test sprays into the air, away from the face, shaking well before each spray. In cases where the inhaler has not been used for more than 5 days, prime the inhaler again by releasing 4 test sprays into the air, away from the face, shaking well before each spray.
The DULERA canister should only be used with the DULERA actuator. The DULERA actuator should not be used with any other inhalation drug product. Actuators from other products should not be used with the DULERA canister.
2.2   Dosing
DULERA should be administered as two inhalations twice daily every day (morning and evening) by the orally inhaled route.

Table 1: Recommended Dosages for DULERA

Previous Therapy	Recommended Dose	Maximum Recommended Daily Dose
Inhaled medium dose corticosteroids	DULERA 100 mcg/5 mcg, 2 inhalations twice daily	400 mcg/20 mcg
Inhaled high dose corticosteroids	DULERA 200 mcg/5 mcg, 2 inhalations twice daily	800 mcg/20 mcg

Shake well prior to each inhalation.

The recommended starting dosages for DULERA treatment are based on prior asthma therapy.

[See table 1 above]

The maximum daily recommended dose is two inhalations of DULERA 200 mcg/5 mcg twice daily. Do not use more than two inhalations twice daily of the prescribed strength of DULERA as some patients are more likely to experience adverse effects with higher doses of formoterol. If symptoms arise between doses, an inhaled short-acting beta$_2$-agonist should be taken for immediate relief.

If a previously effective dosage regimen of DULERA fails to provide adequate control of asthma, the therapeutic regimen should be re-evaluated and additional therapeutic options, e.g., replacing the current strength of DULERA with a higher strength, adding additional inhaled corticosteroid, or initiating oral corticosteroids, should be considered.

The maximum benefit may not be achieved for 1 week or longer after beginning treatment. Individual patients may experience a variable time to onset and degree of symptom relief. For patients ≥12 years of age who do not respond adequately after 2 weeks of therapy, higher strength may provide additional asthma control.

3   DOSAGE FORMS AND STRENGTHS

DULERA is a pressurized metered dose inhaler that is available in 2 strengths.

DULERA 100 mcg/5 mcg delivers 100 mcg of mometasone furoate and 5 mcg of formoterol fumarate dihydrate per actuation.

DULERA 200 mcg/5 mcg delivers 200 mcg of mometasone furoate and 5 mcg of formoterol fumarate dihydrate per actuation.

4   CONTRAINDICATIONS

4.1   Status Asthmaticus

DULERA is contraindicated in the primary treatment of status asthmaticus or other acute episodes of asthma where intensive measures are required.

4.2   Hypersensitivity

DULERA is contraindicated in patients with known hypersensitivity to mometasone furoate, formoterol fumarate, or any of the ingredients in DULERA [see Warnings and Precautions (5.10)].

5   WARNINGS AND PRECAUTIONS

5.1   Asthma-Related Death

Long-acting beta$_2$-adrenergic agonists, such as formoterol, one of the active ingredients in DULERA, increase the risk of asthma-related death. Currently available data are inadequate to determine whether concurrent use of inhaled corticosteroids or other long-term asthma control drugs mitigates the increased risk of asthma-related death from LABA. Available data from controlled clinical trials suggest that LABA increase the risk of asthma-related hospitalization in pediatric and adolescent patients. Therefore, when treating patients with asthma, physicians should only prescribe DULERA for patients with asthma not adequately controlled on a long-term asthma control medication, such as an inhaled corticosteroid or whose disease severity clearly warrants initiation of treatment with both an inhaled corticosteroid and LABA. Once asthma control is achieved and maintained, assess the patient at regular intervals and step down therapy (e.g., discontinue DULERA) if possible without loss of asthma control, and maintain the patient on a long-term asthma control medication, such as an inhaled corticosteroid. Do not use DULERA for patients whose asthma is adequately controlled on low or medium dose inhaled corticosteroids.

A 28-week, placebo-controlled US study comparing the safety of salmeterol with placebo, each added to usual asthma therapy, showed an increase in asthma-related deaths in patients receiving salmeterol (13/13,176 in patients treated with salmeterol vs. 3/13,179 in patients treated with placebo; RR 4.37, 95% CI 1.25, 15.34). This finding with salmeterol is considered a class effect of the LABAs, including formoterol, one of the active ingredients in DULERA. No study adequate to determine whether the rate of asthma-related death is increased with DULERA has been conducted.

Clinical studies with formoterol suggested a higher incidence of serious asthma exacerbations in patients who received formoterol fumarate than in those who received placebo. The sizes of these studies were not adequate to precisely quantify the differences in serious asthma exacerbation rates between treatment groups.

5.2   Deterioration of Disease and Acute Episodes

DULERA should not be initiated in patients during rapidly deteriorating or potentially life-threatening episodes of asthma. DULERA has not been studied in patients with acutely deteriorating asthma. The initiation of DULERA in this setting is not appropriate.

Increasing use of inhaled, short-acting beta$_2$-agonists is a marker of deteriorating asthma. In this situation, the patient requires immediate re-evaluation with reassessment of the treatment regimen, giving special consideration to the possible need for replacing the current strength of DULERA with a higher strength, adding additional inhaled corticosteroid, or initiating systemic corticosteroids. Patients should not use more than 2 inhalations twice daily (morning and evening) of DULERA.

DULERA is not indicated for the relief of acute symptoms, i.e., as rescue therapy for the treatment of acute episodes of bronchospasm. An inhaled, short-acting beta$_2$-agonist, not DULERA, should be used to relieve acute symptoms such as shortness of breath. When prescribing DULERA, the physician must also provide the patient with an inhaled, short-acting beta$_2$-agonist (e.g., albuterol) for treatment of acute symptoms, despite regular twice-daily (morning and evening) use of DULERA.

When beginning treatment with DULERA, patients who have been taking oral or inhaled, short-acting beta$_2$-agonists on a regular basis (e.g., 4 times a day) should be instructed to discontinue the regular use of these drugs.

5.3   Excessive Use of DULERA and Use with Other Long-Acting Beta$_2$-Agonists

As with other inhaled drugs containing beta$_2$-adrenergic agents, DULERA should not be used more often than recommended, at higher doses than recommended, or in conjunction with other medications containing long-acting beta$_2$-agonists, as an overdose may result. Clinically significant cardiovascular effects and fatalities have been reported in association with excessive use of inhaled sympathomimetic drugs. Patients using DULERA should not use an additional long-acting beta$_2$-agonist (e.g., salmeterol, formoterol fumarate, arformoterol tartrate) for any reason, including prevention of exercise-induced bronchospasm (EIB) or the treatment of asthma.

5.4   Local Effects

In clinical trials, the development of localized infections of the mouth and pharynx with *Candida albicans* has occurred in patients treated with DULERA. If oropharyngeal candidiasis develops, it should be treated with appropriate local or systemic (i.e., oral) antifungal therapy while remaining on treatment with DULERA therapy, but at times therapy with DULERA may need to be interrupted. Advise patients to rinse the mouth after inhalation of DULERA.

5.5   Immunosuppression

Persons who are using drugs that suppress the immune system are more susceptible to infections than healthy individuals.

Chickenpox and measles, for example, can have a more serious or even fatal course in susceptible children or adults using corticosteroids. In such children or adults who have not had these diseases or who are not properly immunized, particular care should be taken to avoid exposure. How the dose, route, and duration of corticosteroid administration affect the risk of developing a disseminated infection is not known. The contribution of the underlying disease and/or prior corticosteroid treatment to the risk is also not known. If exposed to chickenpox, prophylaxis with varicella zoster immune globulin (VZIG) or pooled intravenous immunoglobulin (IVIG) may be indicated. If exposed to measles, prophylaxis with pooled intramuscular immunoglobulin (IG) may be indicated. (See the respective package inserts for complete VZIG and IG prescribing information.) If chickenpox develops, treatment with antiviral agents may be considered.

DULERA should be used with caution, if at all, in patients with active or quiescent tuberculosis infection of the respiratory tract, untreated systemic fungal, bacterial, viral, or parasitic infections; or ocular herpes simplex.

5.6   Transferring Patients from Systemic Corticosteroid Therapy

Particular care is needed for patients who are transferred from systemically active corticosteroids to DULERA because deaths due to adrenal insufficiency have occurred in asthmatic patients during and after transfer from systemic corticosteroids to less systemically available inhaled corticosteroids. After withdrawal from systemic corticosteroids, a number of months are required for recovery of hypothalamic-pituitary-adrenal (HPA) function.

Patients who have been previously maintained on 20 mg or more per day of prednisone (or its equivalent) may be most susceptible, particularly when their systemic corticosteroids have been almost completely withdrawn. During this period of HPA suppression, patients may exhibit signs and symptoms of adrenal insufficiency when exposed to trauma, surgery, or infection (particularly gastroenteritis) or other conditions associated with severe electrolyte loss. Although DULERA may improve control of asthma symptoms during these episodes, in recommended doses it supplies less than normal physiological amounts of corticosteroid systemically and does NOT provide the mineralocorticoid activity necessary for coping with these emergencies.

During periods of stress or severe asthma attack, patients who have been withdrawn from systemic corticosteroids should be instructed to resume oral corticosteroids (in large doses) immediately and to contact their physicians for further instruction. These patients should also be instructed to carry a medical identification card indicating that they may need supplementary systemic corticosteroids during periods of stress or severe asthma attack.

Patients requiring systemic corticosteroids should be weaned slowly from systemic corticosteroid use after transferring to DULERA. Lung function (FEV$_1$ or PEF), beta-agonist use, and asthma symptoms should be carefully monitored during withdrawal of systemic corticosteroids. In addition to monitoring asthma signs and symptoms, patients should be observed for signs and symptoms of adrenal insufficiency such as fatigue, lassitude, weakness, nausea and vomiting, and hypotension.

Transfer of patients from systemic corticosteroid therapy to DULERA may unmask allergic conditions previously suppressed by the systemic corticosteroid therapy, e.g., rhinitis, conjunctivitis, eczema, arthritis, and eosinophilic conditions.

During withdrawal from oral corticosteroids, some patients may experience symptoms of systemically active corticosteroid withdrawal, e.g., joint and/or muscular pain, lassitude, and depression, despite maintenance or even improvement of respiratory function.

5.7   Hypercorticism and Adrenal Suppression

Mometasone furoate, a component of DULERA, will often help control asthma symptoms with less suppression of HPA function than therapeutically equivalent oral doses of prednisone. Since mometasone furoate is absorbed into the circulation and can be systemically active at higher doses, the beneficial effects of DULERA in minimizing HPA dysfunction may be expected only when recommended dosages are not exceeded and individual patients are titrated to the lowest effective dose.

Because of the possibility of systemic absorption of inhaled corticosteroids, patients treated with DULERA should be observed carefully for any evidence of systemic corticosteroid effects. Particular care should be taken in observing patients postoperatively or during periods of stress for evidence of inadequate adrenal response.

It is possible that systemic corticosteroid effects such as hypercorticism and adrenal suppression (including adrenal crisis) may appear in a small number of patients, particularly when mometasone furoate is administered at higher than recommended doses over prolonged periods of time. If such effects occur, the dosage of DULERA should be reduced slowly, consistent with accepted procedures for reducing systemic corticosteroids and for management of asthma symptoms.

5.8   Drug Interactions with Strong Cytochrome P450 3A4 Inhibitors

Caution should be exercised when considering the coadministration of DULERA with ketoconazole, and other known strong CYP3A4 inhibitors (e.g., ritonavir, atazanavir, clarithromycin, indinavir, itraconazole, nefazodone, nelfinavir, saquinavir, telithromycin) because adverse effects related to increased systemic exposure to mometasone furoate may occur [see Drug Interactions (7.1) and Clinical Pharmacology (12.3)].

5.9   Paradoxical Bronchospasm and Upper Airway Symptoms

DULERA may produce inhalation induced bronchospasm with an immediate increase in wheezing after dosing that may be life-threatening. If inhalation induced bronchospasm occurs, it should be treated immediately with an inhaled, short-acting bronchodilator. DULERA should be discontinued immediately and alternative therapy instituted.

5.10   Immediate Hypersensitivity Reactions

Immediate hypersensitivity reactions may occur after administration of DULERA, as demonstrated by cases of urticaria, flushing, allergic dermatitis, and bronchospasm.

5.11 Cardiovascular and Central Nervous System Effects

Excessive beta-adrenergic stimulation has been associated with seizures, angina, hypertension or hypotension, tachycardia with rates up to 200 beats/min, arrhythmias, nervousness, headache, tremor, palpitation, nausea, dizziness, fatigue, malaise, and insomnia. Therefore, DULERA should be used with caution in patients with cardiovascular disorders, especially coronary insufficiency, cardiac arrhythmias, and hypertension.

Formoterol fumarate, a component of DULERA, can produce a clinically significant cardiovascular effect in some patients as measured by pulse rate, blood pressure, and/or symptoms. Although such effects are uncommon after administration of DULERA at recommended doses, if they occur, the drug may need to be discontinued. In addition, beta-agonists have been reported to produce ECG changes, such as flattening of the T wave, prolongation of the QTc interval, and ST segment depression. The clinical significance of these findings is unknown. Fatalities have been reported in association with excessive use of inhaled sympathomimetic drugs.

5.12 Reduction in Bone Mineral Density

Decreases in bone mineral density (BMD) have been observed with long-term administration of products containing inhaled corticosteroids, including mometasone furoate, one of the components of DULERA. The clinical significance of small changes in BMD with regard to long-term outcomes, such as fracture, is unknown. Patients with major risk factors for decreased bone mineral content, such as prolonged immobilization, family history of osteoporosis, or chronic use of drugs that can reduce bone mass (e.g., anticonvulsants and corticosteroids) should be monitored and treated with established standards of care.

In a 2-year double-blind study in 103 male and female asthma patients 18 to 50 years of age previously maintained on bronchodilator therapy (Baseline FEV_1 85%–88% predicted), treatment with mometasone furoate dry powder inhaler 200 mcg twice daily resulted in significant reductions in lumbar spine (LS) BMD at the end of the treatment period compared to placebo. The mean change from Baseline to Endpoint in the lumbar spine BMD was -0.015 (-1.43%) for the mometasone furoate group compared to 0.002 (0.25%) for the placebo group. In another 2-year double-blind study in 87 male and female asthma patients 18 to 50 years of age previously maintained on bronchodilator therapy (Baseline FEV_1 82%–83% predicted), treatment with mometasone furoate 400 mcg twice daily demonstrated no statistically significant changes in lumbar spine BMD at the end of the treatment period compared to placebo. The mean change from Baseline to Endpoint in the lumbar spine BMD was -0.018 (-1.57%) for the mometasone furoate group compared to -0.006 (-0.43%) for the placebo group.

5.13 Effect on Growth

Orally inhaled corticosteroids, including DULERA, may cause a reduction in growth velocity when administered to pediatric patients. Monitor the growth of pediatric patients receiving DULERA routinely (e.g., via stadiometry). To minimize the systemic effects of orally inhaled corticosteroids, including DULERA, titrate each patient's dose to the lowest dosage that effectively controls his/her symptoms *[see Use in Specific Populations (8.4)]*.

5.14 Glaucoma and Cataracts

Glaucoma, increased intraocular pressure, and cataracts have been reported following the use of long-term administration of inhaled corticosteroids, including mometasone furoate, a component of DULERA. Therefore, close monitoring is warranted in patients with a change in vision or with a history of increased intraocular pressure, glaucoma, and/or cataracts *[see Adverse Reactions (6)]*.

5.15 Coexisting Conditions

DULERA, like other medications containing sympathomimetic amines, should be used with caution in patients with aneurysm, pheochromocytoma, convulsive disorders, or thyrotoxicosis; and in patients who are unusually responsive to sympathomimetic amines. Doses of the related beta-agonist albuterol, when administered intravenously, have been reported to aggravate preexisting diabetes mellitus and ketoacidosis.

5.16 Hypokalemia and Hyperglycemia

Beta-agonist medications may produce significant hypokalemia in some patients, possibly through intracellular shunting, which has the potential to produce adverse cardiovascular effects. The decrease in serum potassium is usually transient, not requiring supplementation. Clinically significant changes in blood glucose and/or serum potassium were seen infrequently during clinical studies with DULERA at recommended doses.

6 ADVERSE REACTIONS

Long-acting beta-adrenergic agonists, such as formoterol, one of the active ingredients in DULERA, increase the risk of asthma-related death. Currently available data are inadequate to determine whether concurrent use of inhaled cor-

---

Table 2: Treatment-Emergent Adverse Reactions in DULERA Groups Occurring at an Incidence of ≥3% and More Commonly than Placebo

Adverse Reactions	DULERA*		Mometasone Furoate*		Formoterol*	Placebo*
	100 mcg/5 mcg n=424 n (%)	200 mcg/5 mcg n=255 n (%)	100 mcg n=192 n (%)	200 mcg n=240 n (%)	5 mcg n=202 n (%)	n=196 n (%)
Nasopharyngitis	20 (4.7)	12 (4.7)	15 (7.8)	13 (5.4)	13 (6.4)	7 (3.6)
Sinusitis	14 (3.3)	5 (2.0)	6 (3.1)	4 (1.7)	7 (3.5)	2 (1.0)
Headache	19 (4.5)	5 (2.0)	10 (5.2)	8 (3.3)	6 (3.0)	7 (3.6)
Average Duration of Exposure (days)	116	81	165	79	131	138

*All treatments were administered as two inhalations twice daily.

---

ticosteroids or other long-term asthma control drugs mitigates the increased risk of asthma-related death from LABA. Available data from controlled clinical trials suggest that LABA increase the risk of asthma-related hospitalization in pediatric and adolescent patients. Data from a large placebo-controlled US trial that compared the safety of another long-acting beta-adrenergic agonist (salmeterol) or placebo added to usual asthma therapy showed an increase in asthma-related deaths in patients receiving salmeterol *[see Warnings and Precautions (5.1)]*.

Systemic and local corticosteroid use may result in the following:

- *Candida albicans* infection *[see Warnings and Precautions (5.4)]*
- Immunosuppression *[see Warnings and Precautions (5.5)]*
- Hypercorticism and adrenal suppression *[see Warnings and Precautions (5.7)]*
- Growth effects in pediatrics *[see Warnings and Precautions (5.13)]*
- Glaucoma and cataracts *[see Warnings and Precautions (5.14)]*

Because clinical trials are conducted under widely varying conditions, adverse reaction rates observed in the clinical trials of a drug cannot be directly compared to rates in the clinical trials of another drug and may not reflect the rates observed in practice.

6.1 Clinical Trials Experience

The safety data described below is based on 3 clinical trials which randomized 1913 patients 12 years of age and older with asthma, including 679 patients exposed to DULERA for 12 to 26 weeks and 271 patients exposed for 1 year. DULERA was studied in two placebo- and active-controlled trials (n=781 and n=728, respectively) and in a long-term 52-week safety trial (n=404). In the 12 to 26-week clinical trials, the population was 12 to 84 years of age, 41% male and 59% female, 73% Caucasians, 27% non-Caucasians. Patients received two inhalations twice daily of DULERA (100 mcg/5 mcg or 200 mcg/5 mcg), mometasone furoate MDI (100 mcg or 200 mcg), formoterol MDI (5 mcg) or placebo. In the long-term 52-week active-comparator safety trial, the population was 12 years to 75 years of age with asthma, 37% male and 63% female, 47% Caucasians, 53% non-Caucasians and received two inhalations twice daily of DULERA 100 mcg/5 mcg or 200 mcg/5 mcg, or an active comparator.

The incidence of treatment emergent adverse reactions associated with DULERA in Table 2 below is based upon pooled data from 2 clinical trials 12 to 26 weeks in duration in patients 12 years and older treated with two inhalations twice daily of DULERA (100 mcg/5 mcg or 200 mcg/5 mcg), mometasone furoate MDI (100 mcg or 200 mcg), formoterol MDI (5mcg) or placebo.

[See table 2 above]

Oral candidiasis has been reported in clinical trials at an incidence of 0.7% in patients using DULERA 100 mcg/5 mcg, 0.8% in patients using DULERA 200 mcg/5 mcg and 0.5% in the placebo group.

Long-Term Clinical Trial Experience

In a long-term safety trial in patients 12 years and older treated for 52 weeks with DULERA 100 mcg/5 mcg (n=141), DULERA 200 mcg/5 mcg (n=130) or an active comparator (n=133), safety outcomes in general were similar to those observed in the shorter 12 to 26 week controlled trials. No asthma-related deaths were observed. Dysphonia was observed at a higher frequency in the longer term treatment trial at a reported incidence of 7/141 (5%) patients receiving DULERA 100 mcg/5 mcg and 5/130 (3.8%) patients receiving DULERA 200 mcg/5 mcg. No clinically significant changes in blood chemistry, hematology, or ECG were observed.

6.2 Postmarketing Experience

The following adverse reactions have been reported during post-approval use of DULERA or post-approval use with inhaled mometasone furoate or inhaled formoterol fumarate. Because these reactions are reported voluntarily from a population of uncertain size, it is not always possible to reliably estimate their frequency or establish a causal relationship to drug exposure.

Cardiac disorders: angina pectoris, cardiac arrhythmias, e.g., atrial fibrillation, ventricular extrasystoles, tachyarrhythmia

Immune system disorders: immediate and delayed hypersensitivity reactions including anaphylactic reaction, angioedema, severe hypotension, rash, pruritus

Investigations: electrocardiogram QT prolonged, blood pressure increased (including hypertension)

Metabolism and nutrition disorders: hypokalemia, hyperglycemia

Respiratory, thoracic and mediastinal disorders: asthma aggravation, which may include cough, dyspnea, wheezing and bronchospasm

7 DRUG INTERACTIONS

In clinical trials, concurrent administration of DULERA and other drugs, such as short-acting beta-agonist and intranasal corticosteroids have not resulted in an increased frequency of adverse drug reactions. No formal drug interaction studies have been performed with DULERA. The drug interactions of the combination are expected to reflect those of the individual components.

7.1 Inhibitors of Cytochrome P450 3A4

The main route of metabolism of corticosteroids, including mometasone furoate, a component of DULERA, is via cytochrome P450 (CYP) isoenzyme 3A4 (CYP3A4). After oral administration of ketoconazole, a strong inhibitor of CYP3A4, the mean plasma concentration of orally inhaled mometasone furoate increased. Concomitant administration of CYP3A4 inhibitors may inhibit the metabolism of, and increase the systemic exposure to, mometasone furoate. Caution should be exercised when considering the coadministration of DULERA with long-term ketoconazole and other known strong CYP3A4 inhibitors (e.g., ritonavir, atazanavir, clarithromycin, indinavir, itraconazole, nefazodone, nelfinavir, saquinavir, telithromycin) *[see Warnings and Precautions (5.8) and Clinical Pharmacology (12.3)]*.

7.2 Adrenergic Agents

If additional adrenergic drugs are to be administered by any route, they should be used with caution because the pharmacologically predictable sympathetic effects of formoterol, a component of DULERA, may be potentiated.

7.3 Xanthine Derivatives

Concomitant treatment with xanthine derivatives may potentiate any hypokalemic effect of formoterol, a component of DULERA.

7.4 Diuretics

Concomitant treatment with diuretics may potentiate the possible hypokalemic effect of adrenergic agonists. The ECG changes and/or hypokalemia that may result from the administration of non-potassium-sparing diuretics (such as loop or thiazide diuretics) can be acutely worsened by beta-agonists, especially when the recommended dose of the beta-agonist is exceeded. Although the clinical significance of these effects is not known, caution is advised in the coadministration of DULERA with non-potassium-sparing diuretics.

7.5 Monoamine Oxidase Inhibitors, Tricyclic Antidepressants, and Drugs Known to Prolong the QTc Interval

DULERA should be administered with caution to patients being treated with monoamine oxidase inhibitors, tricyclic antidepressants, macrolides, or drugs known to prolong the

QTc interval or within 2 weeks of discontinuation of such agents, because the action of formoterol, a component of DULERA, on the cardiovascular system may be potentiated by these agents. Drugs that are known to prolong the QTc interval have an increased risk of ventricular arrhythmias.

7.6 Beta-Adrenergic Receptor Antagonists

Beta-adrenergic receptor antagonists (beta-blockers) and formoterol may inhibit the effect of each other when administered concurrently. Beta-blockers not only block the therapeutic effects of beta$_2$-agonists, such as formoterol, a component of DULERA, but may produce severe bronchospasm in patients with asthma. Therefore, patients with asthma should not normally be treated with beta-blockers. However, under certain circumstances, e.g., as prophylaxis after myocardial infarction, there may be no acceptable alternatives to the use of beta-blockers in patients with asthma. In this setting, cardioselective beta-blockers could be considered, although they should be administered with caution.

7.7 Halogenated Hydrocarbons

There is an elevated risk of arrhythmias in patients receiving concomitant anesthesia with halogenated hydrocarbons.

8 USE IN SPECIFIC POPULATIONS

8.1 Pregnancy

DULERA: Teratogenic Effects: Pregnancy Category C
There are no adequate and well-controlled studies of DULERA, mometasone furoate only or formoterol fumarate only in pregnant women. Animal reproduction studies of mometasone furoate and formoterol in mice, rats, and/or rabbits revealed evidence of teratogenicity as well as other developmental toxic effects. Because animal reproduction studies are not always predictive of human response, DULERA should be used during pregnancy only if the potential benefit justifies the potential risk to the fetus.

Mometasone Furoate: Teratogenic Effects
When administered to pregnant mice, rats, and rabbits, mometasone furoate increased fetal malformations and decreased fetal growth (measured by lower fetal weights and/or delayed ossification). Dystocia and related complications were also observed when mometasone furoate was administered to rats late in gestation. However, experience with oral corticosteroids suggests that rodents are more prone to teratogenic effects from corticosteroid exposure than humans.

In a mouse reproduction study, subcutaneous mometasone furoate produced cleft palate at approximately one-third of the maximum recommended daily human dose (MRHD) on a mcg/m^2 basis and decreased fetal survival at approximately 1 time the MRHD. No toxicity was observed at approximately one-tenth of the MRHD on a mcg/m^2 basis.

In a rat reproduction study, mometasone furoate produced umbilical hernia at topical dermal doses approximately 6 times the MRHD on a mcg/m^2 basis and delays in ossification at approximately 3 times the MRHD on a mcg/m^2 basis. In another study, rats received subcutaneous doses of mometasone furoate throughout pregnancy or late in gestation. Treated animals had prolonged and difficult labor, fewer live births, lower birth weight, and reduced early pup survival at a dose that was approximately 8 times the MRHD on an area under the curve (AUC) basis. Similar effects were not observed at approximately 4 times MRHD on an AUC basis.

In rabbits, mometasone furoate caused multiple malformations (e.g., flexed front paws, gallbladder agenesis, umbilical hernia, hydrocephaly) at topical dermal doses approximately 3 times the MRHD on a mcg/m^2 basis. In an oral study, mometasone furoate increased resorptions and caused cleft palate and/or head malformations (hydrocephaly and domed head) at a dose less than the MRHD based on AUC. At a dose approximately 2 times the MRHD based on AUC, most litters were aborted or resorbed [see Nonclinical Toxicology (13.2)].

Nonteratogenic Effects:
Hypoadrenalism may occur in infants born to women receiving corticosteroids during pregnancy. Infants born to mothers taking substantial corticosteroid doses during pregnancy should be monitored for signs of hypoadrenalism.

Formoterol Fumarate: Teratogenic Effects
Formoterol fumarate administered throughout organogenesis did not cause malformations in rats or rabbits following oral administration. When given to rats throughout organogenesis, oral doses of approximately 80 times the MRHD on a mcg/m^2 basis and above delayed ossification of the fetus, and doses of approximately 2400 times the MRHD on a mcg/m^2 basis and above decreased fetal weight. Formoterol fumarate has been shown to cause stillbirth and neonatal mortality at oral doses of approximately 2400 times the MRHD on a mcg/m^2 basis and above in rats receiving the drug during the late stage of pregnancy. These effects, however, were not produced at a dose of approximately 80 times the MRHD on a mcg/m^2 basis.

In another testing laboratory, formoterol was shown to be teratogenic in rats and rabbits. Umbilical hernia, a malformation, was observed in rat fetuses at oral doses approxi-

mately 1200 times and greater than the MRHD on a mcg/m^2 basis. Brachygnathia, a skeletal malformation, was observed in rat fetuses at an oral dose approximately 6100 times the MRHD on a mcg/m^2 basis. In another study in rats, no teratogenic effects were seen at inhalation doses up to approximately 500 times the MRHD on a mcg/m^2 basis. Subcapsular cysts on the liver were observed in rabbit fetuses at an oral dose approximately 49,000 times the MRHD on a mcg/m^2 basis. No teratogenic effects were observed at oral doses up to approximately 3000 times the MRHD on a mcg/m^2 basis [see Nonclinical Toxicology (13.2)].

8.2 Labor and Delivery

There are no adequate and well-controlled human studies that have studied the effects of DULERA during labor and delivery.

Because beta-agonists may potentially interfere with uterine contractility, DULERA should be used during labor only if the potential benefit justifies the potential risk [see Nonclinical Toxicology (13.2)].

8.3 Nursing Mothers

DULERA: It is not known whether DULERA is excreted in human milk. Because many drugs are excreted in human milk, caution should be exercised when DULERA is administered to a nursing woman.

Since there are no data from well-controlled human studies on the use of DULERA on nursing mothers, based on data for the individual components, a decision should be made whether to discontinue nursing or to discontinue DULERA, taking into account the importance of DULERA to the mother.

Mometasone Furoate: It is not known if mometasone furoate is excreted in human milk. However, other corticosteroids are excreted in human milk.

Formoterol Fumarate: In reproductive studies in rats, formoterol was excreted in the milk. It is not known whether formoterol is excreted in human milk.

8.4 Pediatric Use

The safety and effectiveness of DULERA have been established in patients 12 years of age and older in 3 clinical trials up to 52 weeks in duration. In the 3 clinical trials, 101 patients 12 to 17 years of age were treated with DULERA. Patients in this age-group demonstrated efficacy results similar to those observed in patients 18 years of age and older. There were no obvious differences in the type or frequency of adverse drug reactions reported in this age group compared to patients 18 years of age and older. Similar efficacy and safety results were observed in an additional 22 patients 12 to 17 years of age who were treated with DULERA in another clinical trial. The safety and efficacy of DULERA have not been established in children less than 12 years of age.

Controlled clinical studies have shown that inhaled corticosteroids may cause a reduction in growth velocity in pediatric patients. In these studies, the mean reduction in growth velocity was approximately 1 cm per year (range 0.3 to 1.8 per year) and appears to depend upon dose and duration of exposure. This effect was observed in the absence of laboratory evidence of hypothalamic-pituitary-adrenal (HPA) axis suppression, suggesting that growth velocity is a more sensitive indicator of systemic corticosteroid exposure in pediatric patients than some commonly used tests of HPA axis function. The long-term effects of this reduction in growth velocity associated with orally inhaled corticosteroids, including the impact on final adult height, are unknown. The potential for "catch up" growth following discontinuation of treatment with orally inhaled corticosteroids has not been adequately studied.

The growth of children and adolescents receiving orally inhaled corticosteroids, including DULERA, should be monitored routinely (e.g., via stadiometry). If a child or adolescent on any corticosteroid appears to have growth suppression, the possibility that he/she is particularly sensitive to this effect should be considered. The potential growth effects of prolonged treatment should be weighed against clinical benefits obtained and the risks associated with alternative therapies. To minimize the systemic effects of orally inhaled corticosteroids, including DULERA, each patient should be titrated to his/her lowest effective dose [see Dosage and Administration (2.2)].

8.5 Geriatric Use

A total of 77 patients 65 years of age and older (11 of whom were 75 years and older) have been treated with DULERA in 3 clinical trials up to 52 weeks in duration. Similar efficacy and safety results were observed in an additional 28 patients 65 years of age and older who were treated with DULERA in another clinical trial. No overall differences in safety or effectiveness were observed between these patients and younger patients, but greater sensitivity of some older individuals cannot be ruled out. As with other products containing beta$_2$-agonists, special caution should be observed when using DULERA in geriatric patients who have concomitant cardiovascular disease that could be adversely

affected by beta$_2$-agonists. Based on available data for DULERA or its active components, no adjustment of dosage of DULERA in geriatric patients is warranted.

8.6 Hepatic Impairment

Concentrations of mometasone furoate appear to increase with severity of hepatic impairment [see Clinical Pharmacology (12.3)].

10 OVERDOSAGE

10.1 Signs and Symptoms

DULERA: DULERA contains both mometasone furoate and formoterol fumarate; therefore, the risks associated with overdosage for the individual components described below apply to DULERA.

Mometasone Furoate: Chronic overdosage may result in signs/symptoms of hypercorticism [see Warnings and Precautions (5.7)]. Single oral doses up to 8000 mcg of mometasone furoate have been studied on human volunteers with no adverse reactions reported.

Formoterol Fumarate: The expected signs and symptoms with overdosage of formoterol are those of excessive beta-adrenergic stimulation and/or occurrence or exaggeration of any of the following signs and symptoms: angina, hypertension or hypotension, tachycardia, with rates up to 200 beats/min., arrhythmias, nervousness, headache, tremor, seizures, muscle cramps, dry mouth, palpitation, nausea, dizziness, fatigue, malaise, hypokalemia, hyperglycemia, and insomnia. Metabolic acidosis may also occur. Cardiac arrest and even death may be associated with an overdose of formoterol.

The minimum acute lethal inhalation dose of formoterol fumarate in rats is 156 mg/kg (approximately 63,000 times the MRHD on a mcg/m^2 basis). The median lethal oral doses in Chinese hamsters, rats, and mice provide even higher multiples of the MRHD.

10.2 Treatment

DULERA: Treatment of overdosage consists of discontinuation of DULERA together with institution of appropriate symptomatic and/or supportive therapy. The judicious use of a cardioselective beta-receptor blocker may be considered, bearing in mind that such medication can produce bronchospasm. There is insufficient evidence to determine if dialysis is beneficial for overdosage of DULERA. Cardiac monitoring is recommended in cases of overdosage.

11 DESCRIPTION

DULERA 100 mcg/5 mcg and DULERA 200 mcg/5 mcg are combinations of mometasone furoate and formoterol fumarate dihydrate for oral inhalation only.

One active component of DULERA is mometasone furoate, a corticosteroid having the chemical name 9,21-dichloro-11(Beta),17-dihydroxy-16 (alpha)-methylpregna-1,4-diene-3,20-dione 17-(2-furoate) with the following chemical structure:

Mometasone furoate is a white powder with an empirical formula of C$_{27}$H$_{30}$Cl$_2$O$_6$, and molecular weight 521.44. It is practically insoluble in water; slightly soluble in methanol, ethanol, and isopropanol; soluble in acetone.

One active component of DULERA is formoterol fumarate dihydrate, a racemate. Formoterol fumarate dihydrate is a selective beta$_2$-adrenergic bronchodilator having the chemical name of (±)-2-hydroxy-5-[(1RS)-1-hydroxy-2-[[(1RS)-2-(4-methoxyphenyl)-1-methylethyl]-amino]ethyl]formanilide fumarate dihydrate with the following chemical structure:

Formoterol fumarate dihydrate has a molecular weight of 840.9, and its empirical formula is (C$_{19}$H$_{24}$N$_2$O$_4$)$_2$•C$_4$H$_4$O$_4$•2H$_2$O. Formoterol fumarate dihydrate is a white to yellowish powder, which is freely soluble in glacial acetic acid, soluble in methanol, sparingly soluble in ethanol and isopropanol, slightly soluble in water, and practically insoluble in acetone, ethyl acetate, and diethyl ether.

Each DULERA 100 mcg/5 mcg and 200 mcg/5 mcg is a hydrofluoroalkane (HFA-227) propelled pressurized metered dose inhaler containing sufficient amount of drug for 60 or 120 inhalations [see How Supplied/Storage and Handling (16)]. After priming, each actuation of the inhaler delivers

115 or 225 mcg of mometasone furoate and 5.5 mcg of formoterol fumarate dihydrate in 69.6 mg of suspension from the valve and delivers 100 or 200 mcg of mometasone furoate and 5 mcg of formoterol fumarate dihydrate from the actuator. The actual amount of drug delivered to the lung may depend on patient factors, such as the coordination between actuation of the device and inspiration through the delivery system. DULERA also contains anhydrous alcohol as a cosolvent and oleic acid as a surfactant. DULERA should be primed before using for the first time by releasing 4 test sprays into the air, away from the face, shaking well before each spray. In cases where the inhaler has not been used for more than 5 days, prime the inhaler again by releasing 4 test sprays into the air, away from the face, shaking well before each spray.

12   CLINICAL PHARMACOLOGY
12.1   Mechanism of Action
DULERA: DULERA contains both mometasone furoate and formoterol fumarate; therefore, the mechanisms of actions described below for the individual components apply to DULERA. These drugs represent two different classes of medications (a synthetic corticosteroid and a selective long-acting beta$_2$-adrenergic receptor agonist) that have different effects on clinical, physiological, and inflammatory indices of asthma.

Mometasone furoate: Mometasone furoate is a corticosteroid demonstrating potent anti-inflammatory activity. The precise mechanism of corticosteroid action on asthma is not known. Inflammation is an important component in the pathogenesis of asthma. Corticosteroids have been shown to have a wide range of inhibitory effects on multiple cell types (e.g., mast cells, eosinophils, neutrophils, macrophages, and lymphocytes) and mediators (e.g., histamine, eicosanoids, leukotrienes, and cytokines) involved in inflammation and in the asthmatic response. These anti-inflammatory actions of corticosteroids may contribute to their efficacy in asthma. Mometasone furoate has been shown in vitro to exhibit a binding affinity for the human glucocorticoid receptor, which is approximately 12 times that of dexamethasone, 7 times that of triamcinolone acetonide, 5 times that of budesonide, and 1.5 times that of fluticasone. The clinical significance of these findings is unknown.

Formoterol fumarate: Formoterol fumarate is a long-acting selective beta$_2$-adrenergic receptor agonist (beta$_2$-agonist). Inhaled formoterol fumarate acts locally in the lung as a bronchodilator. In vitro studies have shown that formoterol has more than 200-fold greater agonist activity at beta$_2$-receptors than at beta$_1$-receptors. Although beta$_2$-receptors are the predominant adrenergic receptors in bronchial smooth muscle and beta$_1$-receptors are the predominant receptors in the heart, there are also beta$_2$-receptors in the human heart comprising 10% to 50% of the total beta-adrenergic receptors. The precise function of these receptors has not been established, but they raise the possibility that even highly selective beta$_2$-agonists may have cardiac effects.

The pharmacologic effects of beta$_2$-adrenoceptor agonist drugs, including formoterol, are at least in part attributable to stimulation of intracellular adenyl cyclase, the enzyme that catalyzes the conversion of adenosine triphosphate (ATP) to cyclic-3', 5'-adenosine monophosphate (cyclic AMP). Increased cyclic AMP levels cause relaxation of bronchial smooth muscle and inhibition of release of mediators of immediate hypersensitivity from cells, especially from mast cells.

In vitro tests show that formoterol is an inhibitor of the release of mast cell mediators, such as histamine and leukotrienes, from the human lung. Formoterol also inhibits histamine-induced plasma albumin extravasation in anesthetized guinea pigs and inhibits allergen-induced eosinophil influx in dogs with airway hyper-responsiveness. The relevance of these in vitro and animal findings to humans is unknown.

12.2   Pharmacodynamics
Cardiovascular Effects:
DULERA:
In a single-dose, double-blind placebo-controlled crossover trial in 25 patients with asthma, single-dose treatment of 10 mcg formoterol fumarate in combination with 400 mcg of mometasone furoate delivered via DULERA 200 mcg/5 mcg were compared to formoterol fumarate 10 mcg MDI, formoterol fumarate 12 mcg dry powder inhaler (DPI; nominal dose of formoterol fumarate delivered 10 mcg), or placebo. The degree of bronchodilation at 12 hours after dosing with DULERA was similar to formoterol fumarate delivered alone via MDI or DPI.

ECGs and blood samples for glucose and potassium were obtained prior to dosing and post dose. No downward trend in serum potassium was observed and values were within the normal range and appeared to be similar across all treatments over the 12 hour period. Mean blood glucose appeared similar across all groups for each time point. There was no evidence of significant hypokalemia or hyperglycemia in response to formoterol treatment.

No relevant changes in heart rate or changes in ECG data were observed with DULERA in the trial. No patients had a QTcB (QTc corrected by Bazett's formula) ≥500 msec during treatment.

In a single-dose crossover trial involving 24 healthy subjects, single dose of formoterol fumarate 10, 20, or 40 mcg in combination with 400 mcg of mometasone furoate delivered via DULERA were evaluated for safety (ECG, blood potassium and glucose changes). ECGs and blood samples for glucose and potassium were obtained at baseline and post dose. Decrease in mean serum potassium was similar across all three treatment groups (approximately 0.3 mmol/L) and values were within the normal range. No clinically significant increases in mean blood glucose values or heart rate were observed. No subjects had a QTcB >500 msec during treatment.

Three active- and placebo-controlled trials (study duration ranging from 12, 26, and 52 weeks) evaluated 1913 patients 12 years of age and older with asthma. No clinically meaningful changes were observed in potassium and glucose values, vital signs, or ECG parameters in patients receiving DULERA.

HPA Axis Effects:
The effects of inhaled mometasone furoate administered via DULERA on adrenal function were evaluated in two clinical trials in patients with asthma. HPA-axis function was assessed by 24-hour plasma cortisol AUC. Although both these trials have open-label design and contain small number of subjects per treatment arm, results from these trials taken together demonstrated suppression of 24-hour plasma cortisol AUC for DULERA 200 mcg/5 mcg compared to placebo consistent with the known systemic effects of inhaled corticosteroid.

In a 42-day, open-label, placebo and active-controlled study 60 patients with asthma 18 years of age and older were randomized to receive two inhalations twice daily of 1 of the following treatments: DULERA 100 mcg/5 mcg, DULERA 200 mcg/5 mcg, fluticasone propionate/salmeterol xinafoate 230 mcg/21 mcg, or placebo. At Day 42, the mean change from baseline plasma cortisol AUC$_{(0-24\ hr)}$ was 8%, 22% and 34% lower compared to placebo for the DULERA 100 mcg/5 mcg (n=13), DULERA 200 mcg/5 mcg (n=15) and fluticasone propionate/salmeterol xinafoate 230 mcg/21 mcg (n=16) treatment groups, respectively.

In a 52-week, open-label safety study, primary analysis of the plasma cortisol 24-hour AUC was performed on 57 patients with asthma who received 2 inhalations twice daily of DULERA 100 mcg/5 mcg, DULERA 200 mcg/5 mcg, fluticasone propionate/salmeterol xinafoate 125/25 mcg, or fluticasone propionate/salmeterol xinafoate 250/25 mcg. At Week 52, the mean plasma cortisol AUC$_{(0-24\ hr)}$ was 2.2%, 29.6%, 16.7%, and 32.2% lower from baseline for the DULERA 100 mcg/5 mcg (n=18), DULERA 200 mcg/5 mcg (n=20), fluticasone propionate/salmeterol xinafoate 125/25 mcg (n=8), and fluticasone propionate/salmeterol xinafoate 250/25 mcg (n=11) treatment groups, respectively.

Other Mometasone Products
HPA Axis Effects:
The potential effect of mometasone furoate via a dry powder inhaler (DPI) on the HPA axis was assessed in a 29-day study. A total of 64 adult patients with mild to moderate asthma were randomized to one of 4 treatment groups: mometasone furoate DPI 440 mcg twice daily, mometasone furoate DPI 880 mcg twice daily, oral prednisone 10 mg once daily, or placebo. The 30-minute post-Cosyntropin stimulation serum cortisol concentration on Day 29 was 23.2 mcg/dl for the mometasone furoate DPI 440 mcg twice daily group and 20.8 mcg/dl for the mometasone furoate DPI 880 mcg twice daily group, compared to 14.5 mcg/dl for the oral prednisone 10 mg group and 25 mcg/dl for the placebo group. The difference between mometasone furoate DPI 880 mcg twice daily (twice the maximum recommended dose) and placebo was statistically significant.

12.3   Pharmacokinetics
Absorption
Mometasone furoate:
Healthy Subjects: The systemic exposures to mometasone furoate from DULERA versus mometasone furoate delivered via DPI were compared. Following oral inhalation of single and multiple doses of the DULERA, mometasone furoate was absorbed in healthy subjects with median T$_{max}$ values ranging from 0.50 to 4 hours. Following single-dose administration of higher than recommended dose of DULERA (4 inhalations of DULERA 200 mcg/5 mcg) in healthy subjects, the arithmetic mean (CV%) C$_{max}$ and AUC$_{(0-12\ hr)}$ values for MF were 67.8 (49) pg/mL and 650 (51) pg·hr/mL, respectively while the corresponding estimates following 5 days of BID dosing of DULERA 800 mcg/20 mcg were 241 (36) pg/mL and 2200 (35) pg·hr/mL. Exposure to mometasone furoate increased with increasing inhaled dose of DULERA 100 mcg/5 mcg to 200 mcg/5 mcg. Studies using oral dosing of labeled and unlabeled drug have demonstrated that the oral systemic bioavailability of mometasone furoate is negligible (<1%).

The above study demonstrated that the systemic exposure to mometasone furoate (based on AUC) was approximately 52% and 25% lower on Day 1 and Day 5, respectively, following DULERA administration compared to mometasone furoate via a DPI.

Asthma Patients: Following oral inhalation of single and multiple doses of the DULERA, mometasone furoate was absorbed in asthma patients with median T$_{max}$ values ranging from 1 to 2 hours. Following single-dose administration of DULERA 400 mcg/10 mcg, the arithmetic mean (CV%) C$_{max}$ and AUC$_{(0-12\ hr)}$ values for MF were 20 (88) pg/mL and 170 (94) pg·hr/mL, respectively while the corresponding estimates following BID dosing of DULERA 400 mcg/10 mcg at steady-state were 60 (36) pg/mL and 577 (40) pg·hr/mL.

Formoterol fumarate:
Healthy Subjects: When DULERA was administered to healthy subjects, formoterol was absorbed with median T$_{max}$ values ranging from 0.167 to 0.5 hour. In a single-dose study with DULERA 400 mcg/10 mcg in healthy subjects, arithmetic mean (CV%) C$_{max}$ and AUC for formoterol were 15 (50) pmol/L and 81 (51) pmol*h/L, respectively. Over the dose range of 10 to 40 mcg for formoterol from DULERA, the exposure to formoterol was dose proportional.

Asthma Patients: When DULERA was administered to patients with asthma, formoterol was absorbed with median T$_{max}$ values ranging from 0.58 to 1.97 hours. In a single-dose study with DULERA 400 mcg/10 mcg in patients with asthma, arithmetic mean (CV%) C$_{max}$ and AUC$_{(0-12\ hr)}$ for formoterol were 22 (29) pmol/L and 125 (42) pmol*h/L, respectively. Following multiple-dose administration of DULERA 400 mcg/10 mcg, the steady-state arithmetic mean (CV%) C$_{max}$ and AUC$_{(0-12\ hr)}$ for formoterol were 41 (59) pmol/L and 226 (54) pmol*hr/L.

Distribution
Mometasone furoate: Based on the study employing a 1000 mcg inhaled dose of tritiated mometasone furoate inhalation powder in humans, no appreciable accumulation of mometasone furoate in the red blood cells was found. Following an intravenous 400 mcg dose of mometasone furoate, the plasma concentrations showed a biphasic decline, with a mean steady-state volume of distribution of 152 liters. The in vitro protein binding for mometasone furoate was reported to be 98% to 99% (in a concentration range of 5 to 500 ng/mL).

Formoterol fumarate: The binding of formoterol to human plasma proteins in vitro was 61% to 64% at concentrations from 0.1 to 100 ng/mL. Binding to human serum albumin in vitro was 31% to 38% over a range of 5 to 500 ng/mL. The concentrations of formoterol used to assess the plasma protein binding were higher than those achieved in plasma following inhalation of a single 120 mcg dose.

Metabolism
Mometasone furoate: Studies have shown that mometasone furoate is primarily and extensively metabolized in the liver of all species investigated and undergoes extensive metabolism to multiple metabolites. In-vitro studies have confirmed the primary role of human liver cytochrome P-450 3A4 (CYP3A4) in the metabolism of this compound, however, no major metabolites were identified. Human liver CYP3A4 metabolizes mometasone furoate to 6-beta hydroxy mometasone furoate.

Formoterol fumarate: Formoterol is metabolized primarily by direct glucuronidation at either the phenolic or aliphatic hydroxyl group or O-demethylation followed by glucuronide conjugation at either phenolic hydroxyl groups. Minor pathways involve sulfate conjugation of formoterol and deformylation followed by sulfate conjugation. The most prominent pathway involves direct conjugation at the phenolic hydroxyl group. The second major pathway involves O-demethylation followed by conjugation at the phenolic 2'-hydroxyl group. Four cytochrome P450 isozymes (CYP2D6, CYP2C19, CYP2C9 and CYP2A6) are involved in the O-demethylation of formoterol. Formoterol did not inhibit CYP450 enzymes at therapeutically relevant concentrations. Some patients may be deficient in CYP2D6 or 2C19 or both. Whether a deficiency in one or both of these isozymes results in elevated systemic exposure to formoterol or systemic adverse effects has not been adequately explored.

Excretion
Mometasone furoate: Following an intravenous dosing, the terminal half-life was reported to be about 5 hours. Following the inhaled dose of tritiated 1000 mcg mometasone furoate, the radioactivity is excreted mainly in the feces (a mean of 74%), and to a small extent in the urine (a mean of 8%) up to 7 days. No radioactivity was associated with unchanged mometasone furoate in the urine. Absorbed mometasone furoate is cleared from plasma at a rate of approximately 12.5 mL/min/kg, independent of dose. The effective t½ for mometasone furoate following inhalation with DULERA was 25 hours in healthy subjects and in patients with asthma.

Formoterol fumarate: Following oral administration of 80 mcg of radiolabeled formoterol fumarate to 2 healthy subjects, 59% to 62% of the radioactivity was eliminated in the urine and 32% to 34% in the feces over a period of 104 hours. In an oral inhalation study with DULERA, renal clearance of formoterol from the blood was 217 mL/min. In single-dose studies, the mean t½ values for formoterol in plasma were 9.1 hours and 10.8 hours from the urinary excretion data. The accumulation of formoterol in plasma after multiple dose administration was consistent with the increase expected with a drug having a terminal t½ of 9 to 11 hour.

Following single inhaled doses ranging from 10 to 40 mcg to healthy subjects from the MFF MDI, 6.2% to 6.8% of the formoterol dose was excreted in urine unchanged. The (R,R) and (S,S)-enantiomers accounted, respectively, for 37% and 63% of the formoterol recovered in urine. From urinary excretion rates measured in healthy subjects, the mean terminal elimination half-lives for the (R,R)- and (S,S)-enantiomers were determined to be 13 and 9.5 hours, respectively. The relative proportion of the two enantiomers remained constant over the dose range studied.

Special Populations
Hepatic/Renal Impairment: There are no data regarding the specific use of DULERA in patients with hepatic or renal impairment.

A study evaluating the administration of a single inhaled dose of 400 mcg mometasone furoate by a dry powder inhaler to subjects with mild (n=4), moderate (n=4), and severe (n=4) hepatic impairment resulted in only 1 or 2 subjects in each group having detectable peak plasma concentrations of mometasone furoate (ranging from 50–105 pcg/mL). The observed peak plasma concentrations appear to increase with severity of hepatic impairment; however, the numbers of detectable levels were few.

Gender and Race: Specific studies to examine the effects of gender and race on the pharmacokinetics of DULERA have not been specifically studied.

Geriatrics: The pharmacokinetics of DULERA have not been specifically studied in the elderly population.

Drug-Drug Interactions
A single-dose crossover study was conducted to compare the pharmacokinetics of 4 inhalations of the following: mometasone furoate MDI, formoterol MDI, DULERA (mometasone furoate/formoterol fumarate MDI), and mometasone furoate MDI plus formoterol fumarate MDI administered concurrently. The results of the study indicated that there was no evidence of a pharmacokinetic interaction between the two components of DULERA.

Inhibitors of Cytochrome P450 Enzymes: *Ketoconazole:* In a drug interaction study, an inhaled dose of mometasone furoate 400 mcg delivered by a dry powder inhaler was given to 24 healthy subjects twice daily for 9 days and ketoconazole 200 mg (as well as placebo) were given twice daily concomitantly on Days 4 to 9. Mometasone furoate plasma concentrations were <150 pcg/mL on Day 3 prior to coadministration of ketoconazole or placebo. Following concomitant administration of ketoconazole, 4 out of 12 subjects in the ketoconazole treatment group (n=12) had peak plasma concentrations of mometasone furoate >200 pcg/mL on Day 9 (211–324 pcg/mL). Mometasone furoate plasma levels appeared to increase and plasma cortisol levels appeared to decrease upon concomitant administration of ketoconazole.

Specific drug-drug interaction studies with formoterol have not been performed.

13 NONCLINICAL TOXICOLOGY
13.1 Carcinogenesis, Mutagenesis, Impairment of Fertility
Mometasone furoate: In a 2-year carcinogenicity study in Sprague Dawley® rats, mometasone furoate demonstrated no statistically significant increase in the incidence of tumors at inhalation doses up to 67 mcg/kg (approximately 14 times the MRHD on an AUC basis). In a 19-month carcinogenicity study in Swiss CD-1 mice, mometasone furoate demonstrated no statistically significant increase in the incidence of tumors at inhalation doses up to 160 mcg/kg (approximately 9 times the MRHD on an AUC basis).

Mometasone furoate increased chromosomal aberrations in an *in vitro* Chinese hamster ovary cell assay, but did not have this effect in an *in vitro* Chinese hamster lung cell assay. Mometasone furoate was not mutagenic in the Ames test or mouse lymphoma assay, and was not clastogenic in an *in vivo* mouse micronucleus assay, a rat bone marrow chromosomal aberration assay, or a mouse male germ-cell chromosomal aberration assay. Mometasone furoate also did not induce unscheduled DNA synthesis *in vivo* in rat hepatocytes.

In reproductive studies in rats, impairment of fertility was not produced by subcutaneous doses up to 15 mcg/kg (approximately 8 times the MRHD on an AUC basis).

Formoterol fumarate: The carcinogenic potential of formoterol fumarate has been evaluated in 2-year drinking water and dietary studies in both rats and mice. In rats, the incidence of ovarian leiomyomas was increased at doses of 15 mg/kg and above in the drinking water study and at

20 mg/kg in the dietary study, but not at dietary doses up to 5 mg/kg (AUC exposure approximately 265 times human exposure at the MRHD). In the dietary study, the incidence of benign ovarian theca-cell tumors was increased at doses of 0.5 mg/kg and above (AUC exposure at the low dose of 0.5 mg/kg was approximately 27 times human exposure at the MRHD). This finding was not observed in the drinking water study, nor was it seen in mice (see below).

In mice, the incidence of adrenal subcapsular adenomas and carcinomas was increased in males at doses of 69 mg/kg and above in the drinking water study, but not at doses up to 50 mg/kg (AUC exposure approximately 350 times human exposure at the MRHD) in the dietary study. The incidence of hepatocarcinomas was increased in the dietary study at doses of 20 and 50 mg/kg in females and 50 mg/kg in males, but not at doses up to 5 mg/kg in either males or females (AUC exposure approximately 35 times human exposure at the MRHD). Also in the dietary study, the incidence of uterine leiomyomas and leiomyosarcomas was increased at doses of 2 mg/kg and above (AUC exposure at the low dose of 2 mg/kg was approximately 14 times human exposure at the MRHD). Increases in leiomyomas of the rodent female genital tract have been similarly demonstrated with other beta-agonist drugs.

Formoterol fumarate was not mutagenic or clastogenic in the following tests: mutagenicity tests in bacterial and mammalian cells, chromosomal analyses in mammalian cells, unscheduled DNA synthesis repair tests in rat hepatocytes and human fibroblasts, transformation assay in mammalian fibroblasts and micronucleus tests in mice and rats. Reproduction studies in rats revealed no impairment of fertility at oral doses up to 3 mg/kg (approximately 1200 times the MRHD on a mcg/m² basis).

13.2 Animal Toxicology and/or Pharmacology
Animal Pharmacology
Formoterol fumarate: Studies in laboratory animals (minipigs, rodents, and dogs) have demonstrated the occurrence of cardiac arrhythmias and sudden death (with histologic evidence of myocardial necrosis) when beta-agonists and methylxanthines are administered concurrently. The clinical significance of these findings is unknown.

Reproductive Toxicology Studies
Mometasone furoate: In mice, mometasone furoate caused cleft palate at subcutaneous doses of 60 mcg/kg and above (approximately 1/3 of the maximum recommended human dose MRHD on a mcg/m² basis). Fetal survival was reduced at 180 mcg/kg (approximately equal to the MRHD on a mcg/m² basis). No toxicity was observed at 20 mcg/kg (approximately one-tenth of the MRHD on a mcg/m² basis). In rats, mometasone furoate produced umbilical hernia at topical dermal doses of 600 mcg/kg and above (approximately 6 times the MRHD on a mcg/m² basis). A dose of 300 mcg/kg (approximately 3 times the MRHD on a mcg/m² basis) produced delays in ossification, but no malformations.

When rats received subcutaneous doses of mometasone furoate throughout pregnancy or during the later stages of pregnancy, 15 mcg/kg (approximately 8 times the MRHD on an AUC basis) caused prolonged and difficult labor and reduced the number of live births, birth weight, and early pup survival. Similar effects were not observed at 7.5 mcg/kg (approximately 4 times the MRHD on an AUC basis).

In rabbits, mometasone furoate caused multiple malformations (e.g., flexed front paws, gallbladder agenesis, umbilical hernia, hydrocephaly) at topical dermal doses of 150 mcg/kg and above (approximately 3 times the MRHD on a mcg/m² basis). In an oral study, mometasone furoate increased resorptions and caused cleft palate and/or head malformations (hydrocephaly and domed head) at 700 mcg/kg (less than the MRHD on an area under the curve [AUC] basis). At 2800 mcg/kg (approximately 2 times the MRHD on an AUC basis) most litters were aborted or resorbed. No toxicity was observed at 140 mcg/kg (less than the MRHD on an AUC basis).

Formoterol fumarate: Formoterol fumarate administered throughout organogenesis did not cause malformations in rats or rabbits following oral administration. When given to rats throughout organogenesis, oral doses of 0.2 mg/kg (approximately 80 times the MRHD on a mcg/m² basis) and above delayed ossification of the fetus, and doses of 6 mg/kg (approximately 2400 times the MRHD on a mcg/m² basis) and above decreased fetal weight. Formoterol fumarate has been shown to cause stillbirth and neonatal mortality at oral doses of 6 mg/kg (approximately 2400 times the MRHD on a mcg/m² basis) and above in rats receiving the drug during the late stage of pregnancy. These effects, however, were not produced at a dose of 0.2 mg/kg (approximately 80 times the MRHD on a mcg/m² basis).

In another testing laboratory, formoterol fumarate was shown to be teratogenic in rats and rabbits. Umbilical hernia, a malformation, was observed in rat fetuses at oral doses of 3 mg/kg/day and above (approximately 1200 times greater than the MRHD on a mcg/m² basis). Brachygnathia, a skeletal malformation, was observed for rat fetuses at an

oral dose of 15 mg/kg/day (approximately 6100 times the MRHD on a mcg/m² basis). In another study in rats, no teratogenic effects were seen at inhalation doses up to 1.2 mg/kg/day (approximately 500 times the MRHD on a mcg/m² basis). Subcapsular cysts on the liver were observed for rabbit fetuses at an oral dose of 60 mg/kg (approximately 49,000 times the MRHD on a mcg/m² basis). No teratogenic effects were observed at oral doses up to 3.5 mg/kg (approximately 3000 times the MRHD on a mcg/m² basis).

14 CLINICAL STUDIES
14.1 Asthma
The safety and efficacy of DULERA were demonstrated in two randomized, double-blind, parallel group, multicenter clinical trials of 12 to 26 weeks in duration involving 1509 patients 12 years of age and older with persistent asthma uncontrolled on medium or high dose inhaled corticosteroids (baseline FEV₁ means of 66% to 73% of predicted normal). These studies included a 2 to 3-week run-in period with mometasone furoate to establish a certain level of asthma control. One clinical trial compared DULERA to placebo and the individual components, mometasone furoate and formoterol (Trial 1) and one clinical trial compared two different strengths of DULERA to mometasone furoate alone (Trial 2).

Trial 1: Clinical Trial with DULERA 100 mcg/5 mcg
This 26-week, placebo-controlled trial evaluated 781 patients 12 years of age and older comparing DULERA 100 mcg/5 mcg (n=191 patients), mometasone furoate 100 mcg (n=192 patients), formoterol fumarate 5 mcg (n=202 patients) and placebo (n=196 patients); each administered as 2 inhalations twice daily by metered dose inhalation aerosols. All other maintenance therapies were discontinued. This study included a 2 to 3-week run-in period with mometasone furoate 100 mcg, 2 inhalations twice daily. This trial included patients ranging from 12 to 76 years of age, 41% male and 59% female, and 72% Caucasian and 28% non-Caucasian. Patients had persistent asthma and were not well controlled on medium dose of inhaled corticosteroids prior to randomization. All treatment groups were balanced with regard to baseline characteristics. Mean FEV₁ and mean percent predicted FEV₁ were similar among all treatment groups (2.33 L, 73%). Eight (4%) patients receiving DULERA 100 mcg/5 mcg, 13 (7%) patients receiving mometasone furoate 100 mcg, 47 (23%) patients receiving formoterol fumarate 5 mcg and 46 (23%) patients receiving placebo discontinued the study early due to treatment failure.

FEV₁ AUC$_{(0-12 hr)}$ was assessed as a co-primary efficacy endpoint to evaluate the contribution of the formoterol component to DULERA. Patients receiving DULERA 100 mcg/5 mcg had significantly higher increases from baseline at Week 12 in mean FEV₁ AUC$_{(0-12 hr)}$ compared to mometasone furoate 100 mcg (the primary treatment comparison) and vs. placebo (both p<0.001) (Figure 1). These differences were maintained through Week 26. Figure 1 shows the change from baseline post-dose serial FEV₁ evaluations in Trial 1.

Figure 1

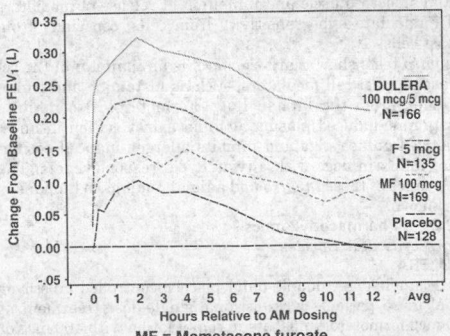

Trial 1 - DULERA 100 mcg/5 mcg - FEV₁ Serial Evaluations for Observed Cases at Week 12 Change from Baseline by Treatment

MF = Mometasone furoate
F = Formoterol fumarate
Mean FEV₁ over 12 hours at Week 12 (shown as AVG)

Clinically judged deteriorations in asthma or reductions in lung function were assessed as another primary endpoint to evaluate the contribution of mometasone furoate 100 mcg to DULERA 100 mcg/5 mcg (primary treatment comparison DULERA vs. formoterol). Deteriorations in asthma were defined as any of the following: a 20% decrease in FEV₁; a 30% decrease in PEF on two or more consecutive days; emergency treatment, hospitalization, or treatment with systemic corticosteroids or other asthma medications not allowed per protocol. Fewer patients who received DULERA 100 mcg/5 mcg reported an event compared to patients who received formoterol 5 mcg (p<0.001).

[See table 3 above]

The change in mean trough FEV$_1$ from baseline to Week 12 was assessed as another endpoint to evaluate the contribution of mometasone furoate 100 mcg to DULERA 100 mcg/5 mcg. A significantly greater increase in mean trough FEV$_1$ was observed for DULERA 100 mcg/5 mcg compared to formoterol 5 mcg (the primary treatment comparison) as well as to placebo (Table 4).

[See table 4 above]

The effect of DULERA 100 mcg/5 mcg, two inhalations twice daily on selected secondary efficacy endpoints, including proportion of nights with nocturnal awakenings (-60% vs. -15%), change in total rescue medication use (-0.6 vs. +1.1 puffs/day), change in morning peak flow (+18.1 vs. -28.4 L/min) and evening peak flow (+10.8 vs. -32.1 L/min) further supports the efficacy of DULERA 100 mcg/5 mcg compared to placebo.

The subjective impact of asthma on patients' health-related quality of life was evaluated by the Asthma Quality of Life Questionnaire (AQLQ(S)) (based on a 7-point scale where 1 = maximum impairment and 7 = no impairment). A change from baseline ≥0.5 points is considered a clinically meaningful improvement. The mean difference in AQLQ between patients receiving DULERA 100 mcg/5 mcg and placebo was 0.5 [95% CI 0.32, 0.68].

Trial 2: Clinical Trial With DULERA 200 mcg/5 mcg

This 12-week double-blind trial evaluated 728 patients 12 years of age and older comparing DULERA 200 mcg/5 mcg (n=255 patients) with DULERA 100 mcg/5 mcg (n=233 patients) and mometasone furoate 200 mcg (n=240 patients), each administered as 2 inhalations twice daily by metered dose inhalation aerosols. All other maintenance therapies were discontinued. This trial included a 2 to 3-week run-in period with mometasone furoate 200 mcg, 2 inhalations twice daily. Patients had persistent asthma and were uncontrolled on high dose inhaled corticosteroids prior to study entry. All treatment groups were balanced with regard to baseline characteristics. This trial included patients ranging from 12 to 84 years of age, 44% male and 56% female, and 89% Caucasian and 11% non-Caucasian. Mean FEV$_1$ and mean percent predicted FEV$_1$ values were similar among all treatment groups (2.05 L, 66%). Eleven (5%) patients receiving DULERA 100 mcg/5 mcg, 8 (3%) patients receiving DULERA 200 mcg/5 mcg and 13 (5%) patients receiving mometasone furoate 200 mcg discontinued the trial early due to treatment failure.

The primary efficacy endpoint was the mean change in FEV$_1$ AUC$_{(0-12 \text{ hr})}$ from baseline to Week 12. Patients receiving DULERA 100 mcg/5 mcg and DULERA 200 mcg/5 mcg had significantly greater increases from baseline at Day 1 in mean FEV$_1$ AUC$_{(0-12 \text{ hr})}$ compared to mometasone furoate 200 mcg. The difference was maintained over 12 weeks of therapy.

Mean change in trough FEV$_1$ from baseline to Week 12 was also assessed to evaluate the relative contribution of mometasone furoate to DULERA 100 mcg/5 mcg and DULERA 200 mcg/5 mcg (Table 5). A greater numerical increase in the mean trough FEV$_1$ was observed for DULERA 200 mcg/5 mcg compared to DULERA 100 mcg/5 mcg and mometasone furoate 200 mcg.

Table 5: Trial 2 – Change in Trough FEV$_1$ from Baseline to Week 12

Treatment Arm	N	Baseline (L)	Change from Baseline at Week 12 (L)
DULERA 100 mcg/5 mcg	232	2.10	0.14
DULERA 200 mcg/5 mcg	255	2.05	0.19
Mometasone furoate 200 mcg	239	2.07	0.10

Clinically judged deterioration in asthma or reduction in lung function was assessed as an additional endpoint. Fewer patients who received DULERA 200 mcg/5 mcg or DULERA 100/5 mcg compared to mometasone furoate 200 mcg alone reported an event, defined as in Trial 1 by any of the following: a 20% decrease in FEV$_1$; a 30% decrease in PEF on two or more consecutive days; emergency treatment, hospitalization, or treatment with systemic corticosteroids or other asthma medications not allowed per protocol.

[See table 6 at top of next page]

Other Studies

In addition to Trial 1 and Trial 2, the safety and efficacy of the individual components, mometasone furoate MDI 100 mcg and 200 mcg, in comparison to placebo were demonstrated in three other, 12-week, placebo controlled trials which evaluated the mean change in FEV$_1$ from baseline as

Table 3: Trial 1 - Clinically Judged Deterioration in Asthma or Reduction in Lung Function*

	DULERA 100 mcg/ 5 mcg[†] (n=191)	Mometasone Furoate 100 mcg[†] (n=192)	Formoterol 5 mcg[†] (n=202)	Placebo[†] (n=196)
Clinically judged deterioration in asthma or reduction in lung function*	58 (30%)	65 (34%)	109 (54%)	109 (56%)
Decrease in FEV$_1$[‡]	18 (9%)	19 (10%)	31 (15%)	41 (21%)
Decrease in PEF[§]	37 (19%)	41 (21%)	62 (31%)	61 (31%)
Emergency treatment	0	1 (<1%)	4 (2%)	1 (<1%)
Hospitalization	1 (<1%)	0	0	0
Treatment with excluded asthma medication[¶]	2 (1%)	4 (2%)	17 (8%)	8 (4%)

* Includes only the first event day for each patient. Patients could have experienced more than one event criterion.
† Two inhalations, twice daily.
‡ Decrease in absolute FEV$_1$ below the treatment period stability limit (defined as 80% of the average of the two predose FEV$_1$ measurements taken 30 minutes and immediately prior to the first dose of randomized trial medication).
§ Decrease in AM or PM peak expiratory flow (PEF) on 2 or more consecutive days below the treatment period stability limit (defined as 70% of the AM or PM PEF obtained over the last 7 days of the run-in period).
¶ Thirty patients received glucocorticosteroids; 1 patient received formoterol via dry powder inhaler in the Formoterol 5 mcg group.

Table 4: Trial 1 – Change in Trough FEV$_1$ from Baseline to Week 12

Treatment Arm	N	Baseline (L)	Change From Baseline at Week 12 (L)	Treatment Difference from Placebo (L)	P-Value vs. Placebo	P-Value vs. Formoterol
DULERA 100 mcg/5 mcg	167	2.33	0.13	0.18	<0.001	<0.001
Mometasone furoate 100 mcg	175	2.36	0.07	0.12	<0.001	0.058
Formoterol fumarate 5 mcg	141	2.29	0.00	0.05	0.170	
Placebo	145	2.30	-0.05			

LS means and p-values are from Week 12 estimates of a longitudinal analysis model.

a primary endpoint. The safety and efficacy of formoterol MDI 5 mcg alone in comparison to placebo was replicated in another 26-week trial that evaluated a lower dose of mometasone furoate MDI in combination with formoterol.

16 HOW SUPPLIED/STORAGE AND HANDLING

16.1 How Supplied

DULERA is available in two strengths and supplied in the following package sizes (Table 7):

Table 7

Package	NDC
DULERA 100 mcg/5 mcg 120 inhalations	0085-7206-01
DULERA 100 mcg/5 mcg 60 inhalations (institutional pack)	0085-7206-07
DULERA 200 mcg/5 mcg 120 inhalations	0085-4610-01
DULERA 200 mcg/5 mcg 60 inhalations (institutional pack)	0085-4610-05

Each strength is supplied as a pressurized aluminum canister that has a blue plastic actuator integrated with a dose counter and a green dust cap. Each 120-inhalation canister has a net fill weight of 13 grams and each 60-inhalation canister has a net fill weight of 8.8 grams. Each canister is placed into a carton. Each carton contains 1 canister and a Medication Guide.

Initially the dose counter will display "64" or "124" actuations. After the initial priming with 4 actuations, the dose counter will read "60" or "120" and the inhaler is now ready for use.

16.2 Storage and Handling

The DULERA canister should only be used with the DULERA actuator. The DULERA actuator should not be used with any other inhalation drug product. Actuators from other products should not be used with the DULERA canister.

The canister should not be removed from the actuator because the correct amount of medication may not be discharged; the dose counter may not function properly; reinsertion may cause the dose counter to count down by 1 and discharge a puff.

The correct amount of medication in each inhalation cannot be ensured after the labeled number of actuations from the canister has been used, even though the inhaler may not feel completely empty and may continue to operate. The inhaler should be discarded when the labeled number of actuations has been used (the dose counter will read "0").

Store at controlled room temperature 20–25°C (68–77°F); excursions permitted to 15–30°C (59–86°F) [see USP Controlled Room Temperature].

The 120-inhalation inhaler does not require specific storage orientation. For the 60-inhalation inhaler, after priming, store the inhaler with the mouthpiece down or in a horizontal position.

For best results, the canister should be at room temperature before use. Shake well and remove the cap from the mouthpiece of the actuator before using. Keep out of reach of children. Avoid spraying in eyes.

Contents Under Pressure: Do not puncture. Do not use or store near heat or open flame. Exposure to temperatures above 120°F may cause bursting. Never throw container into fire or incinerator.

17 PATIENT COUNSELING INFORMATION

See FDA-Approved Patient Labeling (Medication Guide).

17.1 Asthma-Related Death

Patients should be informed that formoterol, one of the active ingredients in DULERA, increases the risk of asthma-related death. In pediatric and adolescent patients, formoterol may increase the risk of asthma-related hospitalization. They should also be informed that data are not adequate to determine whether the concurrent use of inhaled

Help Patients Save on Rx Drugs: PDR.net/PharmacyDiscountCard

Table 6: Trial 2 - Clinically Judged Deterioration in Asthma or Reduction in Lung Function*

	DULERA 100 mcg/ 5 mcg[†] (n=233)	DULERA 200 mcg/ 5 mcg[†] (n=255)	Mometasone Furoate 200 mcg[†] (n=240)
Clinically judged deterioration in asthma or reduction in lung function*	29 (12%)	31 (12%)	44 (18%)
Decrease in FEV_1[‡]	23 (10%)	17 (7%)	33 (14%)
Decrease in PEF on two consecutive days[§]	2 (1%)	4 (2%)	3 (1%)
Emergency treatment	2 (1%)	1 (<1%)	1 (<1%)
Hospitalization	0	1 (<1%)	0
Treatment with excluded asthma medication[¶]	5 (2%)	8 (3%)	12 (5%)

* Includes only the first event day for each patient. Patients could have experienced more than one event criterion.
† Two inhalations, twice daily.
‡ Decrease in absolute FEV_1 below the treatment period stability limit (defined as 80% of the average of the two predose FEV_1 measurements taken 30 minutes and immediately prior to the first dose of randomized trial medication).
§ Decrease in AM or PM peak expiratory flow (PEF) below the treatment period stability limit (defined as 70% of the AM or PM PEF obtained over the last 7 days of the run-in period).
¶ Twenty four patients received glucocorticosteroids; 1 patient received albuterol in the DULERA 200 mcg / 5 mcg group.

corticosteroids, the other component of DULERA, or other long-term asthma-control therapy mitigates or eliminates this risk [see Warnings and Precautions (5.1)].

17.2   Not for Acute Symptoms
DULERA is not indicated to relieve acute asthma symptoms and extra doses should not be used for that purpose. Acute symptoms should be treated with an inhaled, short-acting, beta₂-agonist (the health care provider should prescribe the patient with such medication and instruct the patient in how it should be used).
Patients should be instructed to seek medical attention immediately if they experience any of the following:
• If their symptoms worsen
• Significant decrease in lung function as outlined by the physician
• If they need more inhalations of a short-acting beta₂-agonist than usual
Patients should be advised not to increase the dose or frequency of DULERA. The daily dosage of DULERA should not exceed two inhalations twice daily. If they miss a dose, they should be instructed to take their next dose at the same time they normally do. DULERA provides bronchodilation for up to 12 hours.
Patients should not stop or reduce DULERA therapy without physician/provider guidance since symptoms may recur after discontinuation [see Warnings and Precautions (5.2)].

17.3   Do Not Use Additional Long-Acting Beta₂-Agonists
When patients are prescribed DULERA, other long-acting beta₂-agonists should not be used [see Warnings and Precautions (5.3)].

17.4   Risks Associated With Corticosteroid Therapy
Local Effects: Patients should be advised that localized infections with Candida albicans occurred in the mouth and pharynx in some patients. If oropharyngeal candidiasis develops, it should be treated with appropriate local or systemic (i.e., oral) antifungal therapy while still continuing with DULERA therapy, but at times therapy with DULERA may need to be temporarily interrupted under close medical supervision. Rinsing the mouth after inhalation is advised [see Warnings and Precautions (5.4)].
Immunosuppression: Patients who are on immunosuppressant doses of corticosteroids should be warned to avoid exposure to chickenpox or measles and, if exposed, to consult their physician without delay. Patients should be informed of potential worsening of existing tuberculosis, fungal, bacterial, viral, or parasitic infections, or ocular herpes simplex [see Warnings and Precautions (5.5)].
Hypercorticism and Adrenal Suppression: Patients should be advised that DULERA may cause systemic corticosteroid effects of hypercorticism and adrenal suppression. Additionally, patients should be instructed that deaths due to adrenal insufficiency have occurred during and after transfer from systemic corticosteroids. Patients should taper slowly from systemic corticosteroids if transferring to DULERA [see Warnings and Precautions (5.7)].
Reduction in Bone Mineral Density: Patients who are at an increased risk for decreased BMD should be advised that

the use of corticosteroids may pose an additional risk and should be monitored and, where appropriate, be treated for this condition [see Warnings and Precautions (5.12)].
Reduced Growth Velocity: Patients should be informed that orally inhaled corticosteroids, a component of DULERA, may cause a reduction in growth velocity when administered to pediatric patients. Physicians should closely follow the growth of pediatric patients taking corticosteroids by any route [see Warnings and Precautions (5.13)].
Glaucoma and Cataracts: Long-term use of inhaled corticosteroids may increase the risk of some eye problems (glaucoma or cataracts); regular eye examinations should be considered [see Warnings and Precautions (5.14)].

17.5   Risks Associated With Beta-Agonist Therapy
Patients should be informed that treatment with beta₂-agonists may lead to adverse events which include palpitations, chest pain, rapid heart rate, tremor or nervousness [see Warnings and Precautions (5.11)].

17.6   Instructions for Use
Patients should be instructed regarding the following:
• Read the Medication Guide before use and follow the Instructions for Use carefully.
• Patients should be reminded to:
  ∘ Remove the cap from the mouthpiece of the actuator before use.
  ∘ Not remove the canister from the actuator.
  ∘ Not wash inhaler in water. The mouthpiece should be cleaned using a dry wipe after every 7 days of use.
Manufactured for: Merck Sharp & Dohme Corp., a subsidiary of
MERCK & CO., INC., Whitehouse Station, NJ 08889, USA
Manufactured by: 3M Health Care Ltd., Loughborough, United Kingdom.
For patent information: www.merck.com/product/patent/home.html
The trademarks depicted herein are owned by their respective companies.
Copyright © 2010 Merck Sharp & Dohme Corp., a subsidiary of **Merck & Co., Inc.**
All rights reserved.
uspi-mk0887a-ao-1404r022

Medication Guide
DULERA® [dew-LAIR-ah] 100 mcg/5 mcg
(mometasone furoate 100 mcg and formoterol fumarate dihydrate 5 mcg) Inhalation Aerosol
DULERA® 200 mcg/5 mcg
(mometasone furoate 200 mcg and formoterol fumarate dihydrate 5 mcg) Inhalation Aerosol
Read the Medication Guide that comes with DULERA® before you start using it and each time you get a refill. There may be new information. This Medication Guide does not take the place of talking to your healthcare provider about your medical condition or treatment.

What is the most important information I should know about DULERA?
DULERA can cause serious side effects, including:
1. People with asthma who take long-acting beta₂-adrenergic agonist (LABA) medicines such as formoterol (one of the medicines in DULERA), have an increased risk of death from asthma problems. It is not known whether mometasone furoate, the other medicine in DULERA, reduces the risk of death from asthma problems seen with formoterol.
   • Call your healthcare provider if breathing problems worsen over time while using DULERA. You may need different treatment.
   • Get emergency medical care if:
     • breathing problems worsen quickly, and
     • you use your rescue inhaler medicine, but it does not relieve your breathing problems.
2. DULERA should be used only if your healthcare provider decides that your asthma is not well controlled with a long-term asthma control medicine, such as an inhaled corticosteroid.
3. When your asthma is well controlled, your healthcare provider may tell you to stop taking DULERA. Your healthcare provider will decide if you can stop DULERA without loss of asthma control. Your healthcare provider may prescribe a different long-term asthma-control medicine for you, such as an inhaled corticosteroid.
4. Children and adolescents who take LABA medicines may have an increased risk of being hospitalized for asthma problems.

What is DULERA?
DULERA combines an inhaled corticosteroid medicine, mometasone furoate (the same medicine found in ASMANEX TWISTHALER), and a long-acting beta₂-agonist medicine (LABA), formoterol (the same medicine found in FORADIL® AEROLIZER®).
• Inhaled corticosteroids help to decrease inflammation in the lungs. Inflammation in the lungs can lead to asthma symptoms.
• LABA medicines are used in people with asthma. LABA medicines help the muscles around the airways in your lungs stay relaxed to prevent asthma symptoms, such as wheezing and shortness of breath. These symptoms can happen when the muscles around the airways tighten. This makes it hard to breathe. In severe cases, wheezing can stop your breathing and may lead to death if not treated right away.
DULERA is used to control symptoms of asthma and prevent symptoms such as wheezing in people 12 years of age and older.
DULERA should not be used as a rescue inhaler.
DULERA contains formoterol (the same medicine found in FORADIL AEROLIZER). LABA medicines such as formoterol increase the risk of death from asthma problems.
DULERA is not for children and adults with asthma who:
• are well controlled with an asthma-control medicine, such as a low to medium dose of an inhaled corticosteroid medicine
• only need a rescue inhaler once in awhile
It is not known if DULERA is safe and effective in children less than 12 years of age.

Who should not use DULERA?
Do not use DULERA:
• to treat sudden severe symptoms of asthma
• if you are allergic to any of the ingredients in DULERA. See the end of the Medication Guide for a list of ingredients in DULERA.

What should I tell my healthcare provider before using DULERA?
Tell your healthcare provider about all of your health conditions, including if you:
• have heart problems
• have high blood pressure
• have seizures
• have thyroid problems
• have diabetes
• have liver problems
• have osteoporosis
• have an immune system problem
• have eye problems such as increased pressure in the eye, glaucoma, or cataracts
• are allergic to any medicines
• are exposed to chickenpox or measles
• have an aneurysm (swelling of an artery)
• have a pheochromocytoma (a tumor of the adrenal gland that can affect your blood pressure)
• are scheduled to have surgery
• have any other medical problems
• are pregnant or planning to become pregnant. It is not known if DULERA may harm your unborn baby.
• are breastfeeding. It is not known if DULERA passes into your milk and if it can harm your baby. You and your healthcare provider should decide if you will take DULERA while breastfeeding.

Tell your healthcare provider about all the medicines you take including prescription and non-prescription medicines, vitamins, and herbal supplements. DULERA and certain other medicines may interact with each other. This may cause serious side effects.

Especially, tell your healthcare provider if you take antifungal medicines, such as ketoconazole, or anti-HIV medicines, such as ritonavir. The anti-HIV medicines NORVIR® (ritonavir capsules) Soft Gelatin, NORVIR® (ritonavir oral solution), and KALETRA® (lopinavir/ritonavir) Tablets contain ritonavir.

Know the medicines you take. Keep a list and show it to your healthcare provider and pharmacist each time you get a new medicine.

How should I use DULERA?
See the step-by-step instructions for using DULERA at the end of this Medication Guide. Do not use DULERA unless your healthcare provider has taught you and you understand everything. Ask your healthcare provider or pharmacist if you have any questions.

- Use DULERA exactly as prescribed. **Do not use DULERA more often than prescribed.** DULERA comes in 2 strengths. Your healthcare provider has prescribed the strength that is best for you. Note the differences between DULERA and your other inhaled medications, including the differences in prescribed use and physical appearance.
- DULERA should be taken every day as 2 puffs in the morning and 2 puffs in the evening.
- If you miss a dose of DULERA, skip your missed dose and take your next dose at your regular time. Do not take DULERA more often or use more puffs than you have been prescribed.
- **While you are using DULERA 2 times each day, do not use other medicines that contain a long-acting beta₂-agonist (LABA) for any reason.** Ask your healthcare provider or pharmacist if any of your other medicines are LABA medicines.
- If you take more DULERA than your healthcare provider has prescribed, get medical help right away if you have any unusual symptoms, such as problems breathing, palpitations, chest pain, increased heart rate, nervousness or shakiness.
- Do not change or stop using DULERA or other asthma medicines used to control or treat your breathing problems unless told to do so by your healthcare provider. Your healthcare provider will change your medicines as needed.
- DULERA does not relieve sudden asthma symptoms. Always have a rescue inhaler with you to treat sudden symptoms. Use your rescue inhaler if you have breathing problems between doses of DULERA. If you do not have a rescue inhaler, call your healthcare provider to have one prescribed for you.
- **Remove the cap from the mouthpiece of the actuator before using DULERA.**
- DO NOT remove the canister from the actuator because:
  ○ You may not receive the correct amount of medication.
  ○ The dose counter may not function properly.
  ○ Reinsertion may cause the dose counter to count down by 1 and may discharge a puff.
- Rinse your mouth with water after each dose (2 puffs) of DULERA. This will help to lessen the chance of getting a yeast infection (thrush) in the mouth and throat.
- Do not spray DULERA in your eyes. If you accidentally get DULERA in your eyes, rinse your eyes with water and if redness or irritation continues, call your healthcare provider.
- **Call your healthcare provider or get medical care right away if:**
  - your breathing problems worsen with DULERA
  - you need to use your rescue inhaler more often than usual
  - your rescue inhaler does not work as well for you at relieving symptoms
  - you need to use 4 or more inhalations of your rescue inhaler for 2 or more days in a row
  - you use 1 whole canister of your rescue inhaler in 8 weeks' time
  - your peak flow meter results decrease. Your healthcare provider will tell you the numbers that are right for you.
  - you have asthma and your symptoms do not improve after using DULERA regularly for 1 to 2 weeks

What are the possible side effects of DULERA?
DULERA can cause serious side effects, including:
- **See "What is the most important information I should know about DULERA?"**
- **Thrush in the mouth and throat.** You may develop a yeast infection (Candida albicans) in your mouth or throat. Rinse your mouth with water after using DULERA to help prevent an infection in your mouth or throat.
- **Immune system effects and a higher chance for infections.**
- Tell your healthcare provider about any signs of infection such as:
  - fever
  - feeling tired

- pain
- nausea
- body aches
- vomiting
- chills
- **Adrenal insufficiency.** Adrenal insufficiency is a condition in which the adrenal glands do not make enough steroid hormones. This can happen when you stop taking oral corticosteroid medicines and start inhaled corticosteroid medicines.
- **Increased wheezing right after taking DULERA.** Always have a rescue inhaler with you to treat sudden wheezing.
- **Serious allergic reactions.** Call your healthcare provider or get emergency medical care if you get any of the following symptoms of a serious allergic reaction:
  - rash
  - hives
  - swelling, including swelling of the face, mouth, and tongue
  - breathing problems
- Using too much of a LABA medicine may cause:
  - **chest pain**
  - **increased or decreased blood pressure**
  - **a fast and irregular heartbeat**
  - **headache**
  - **tremor**
  - **nervousness**
  - **dizziness**
  - **weakness**
  - **seizures**
  - **electrocardiogram (ECG) changes**
- **Lower bone mineral density.** This may be a problem for people who already have a higher chance for low bone density (osteoporosis).
- **Slowed growth in children.** A child's growth should be checked often.
- **Eye problems including glaucoma and cataracts.** You should have regular eye exams while using DULERA.
- **Decreases in blood potassium levels (hypokalemia)**
- **Increases in blood sugar levels (hyperglycemia)**

The most common side effects of DULERA include:
- inflammation of the nose and throat (nasopharyngitis)
- inflammation of the sinuses (sinusitis)
- headache

Other side effects:
- Worsening asthma or sudden asthma attacks have been reported with the use of inhaled mometasone furoate (one of the medicines in DULERA).

Tell your healthcare provider about any side effect that bothers you or that does not go away.

These are not all the side effects with DULERA. Ask your healthcare provider or pharmacist for more information.

Call your doctor for medical advice about side effects. You may report side effects to FDA at 1-800-FDA-1088.

You may also report side effects to Merck Sharp & Dohme Corp., a subsidiary of Merck & Co., Inc., at 1-877-888-4231.

How do I store DULERA?
- Store DULERA at room temperature between 59°F to 86°F (15°C to 30°C).
- The 120-actuation inhaler can be stored in any position. For the 60-actuation inhaler, after priming, store the inhaler with the mouthpiece down or sideways.
- The contents of your DULERA are under pressure. Do not puncture. Do not use or store near heat or open flame. Storage above 120°F may cause the canister to burst.
- Do not throw container into fire or incinerator.
- **Keep DULERA and all medicines out of the reach of children.**

General Information about DULERA
Medicines are sometimes prescribed for purposes other than those listed in a Medication Guide. Do not use DULERA for a condition for which it was not prescribed. Do not give your DULERA to other people, even if they have the same condition. It may harm them.

This Medication Guide summarizes the most important information about DULERA. If you would like more information, talk with your healthcare provider. You can ask your healthcare provider or pharmacist for information about DULERA that was written for healthcare professionals. For more information about DULERA, go to www.DULERA.com or call 1-800-622-4477.

What are the ingredients in DULERA?
Active ingredients: mometasone furoate and formoterol fumarate dihydrate

Inactive ingredients: hydrofluoroalkane (HFA-227), anhydrous alcohol and oleic acid

Patient Instructions for Use
DULERA®
DULERA® 100 mcg/5 mcg
(mometasone furoate 100 mcg and formoterol fumarate dihydrate 5 mcg) Inhalation Aerosol

DULERA® 200 mcg/5 mcg
(mometasone furoate 200 mcg and formoterol fumarate dihydrate 5 mcg) Inhalation Aerosol

How to use your DULERA
Before using your DULERA, read the complete instructions and use only as directed.

The parts of your DULERA:
There are 2 main parts to your DULERA inhaler – the metal canister that holds the medicine and the blue plastic actuator that sprays the medicine from the canister. The inhaler also has a green cap that covers the mouthpiece of the actuator (see **Figure 1**). The cap from the mouthpiece must be removed before use. The inhaler contains 60 or 120 actuations (puffs).

Figure 1

The inhaler comes with dose counter located on the plastic actuator. See **Figure 1**. The counter display will show the number of actuations (puffs) of medicine remaining. The dose counter will initially display "64" or "124" actuations remaining. Each time you press the canister, a puff of medicine is released and the counter will count down by 1. The counter will stop counting at 0.

- **YOU SHOULD NOT REMOVE THE CANISTER FROM THE ACTUATOR** because:
  ○ You may not receive the correct amount of medication.
  ○ The dose counter may not function properly.
  ○ Reinsertion may cause the counter to count down by 1 and may discharge a puff.
- Use the DULERA canister only with the actuator supplied with the product. Do not use parts of the DULERA inhaler with parts from any other inhalation medicine.

Before using your DULERA:
REMOVE THE CAP FROM THE MOUTHPIECE OF THE ACTUATOR (see **Figure 2**). Check the mouthpiece for objects before use. Make sure the canister is fully inserted into the actuator.

Figure 2

Priming your DULERA Inhaler:
Before you use DULERA for the first time, you must prime the inhaler.
1. To prime the inhaler, hold it in the upright position and release 4 actuations (puffs) into the air, away from your face.
2. Shake the inhaler well before each of the priming actuations. After priming 4 times, the dose counter should read either "60" or "120".
3. **If you do not use your DULERA for more than 5 days, you will need to prime it again before use.**

Using your DULERA
4. **REMOVE THE CAP FROM THE MOUTHPIECE OF THE ACTUATOR** (see **Figure 3**). Check the mouthpiece for objects before use. Make sure the canister is fully inserted into the actuator.
5. Shake the inhaler well before each use.
6. Breathe out as fully as you comfortably can through your mouth. Push out as much air from your lungs as possible. Hold the inhaler in the upright position and place the mouthpiece into your mouth (see **Figure 4**). Close your lips around the mouthpiece.

FOR ORAL INHALATION ONLY

Figure 3　　　　　**Figure 4**

7. Take a deep breath (inhale) in slowly through your mouth. While doing this, press down firmly and fully on the top of the canister until it stops moving in the actuator. Take your finger off the canister.

8. When you have finished breathing in, hold your breath as long as you comfortably can, up to 10 seconds. Then remove the inhaler from your mouth and breathe out through your nose, while keeping your lips closed.

9. Wait at least **30 seconds** to take your second puff of DULERA.

10. Shake the inhaler well again and repeat steps 6 through 8 to take your second puff of DULERA.

After using your DULERA inhaler:

11. Replace the cap over the mouthpiece right away after use (see **Figure 5**).

Figure 5

12. After you finish taking DULERA (2 puffs), rinse your mouth with water.

Reading the counter

• The dose counter identifies the number of inhalations (puffs) left in your inhaler.

• The counter will count down each time you release a puff of medicine (either when preparing your DULERA inhaler for use or when taking the medicine).

When to replace your DULERA:

• It is important that you pay attention to the number of inhalations (puffs) left in your DULERA inhaler by reading the counter.

• When the counter reads 20, you should refill your prescription or ask your healthcare provider if you need a new prescription for DULERA.

• Throw away DULERA after the counter reaches 0, indicating that you have used the number of actuations on the product label and box. Your inhaler may not feel empty and it may continue to operate, but you will not get the right amount of medicine if you keep using it.

• Never try to change the numbers on the counter or remove the counter from the actuator.

• Do not use the inhaler after the expiration date.

How do I store DULERA?

• Store DULERA at room temperature between 59°F to 86°F (15°C to 30°C).

• The 120-actuation inhaler can be stored in any position. For the 60-actuation inhaler, after priming, store the inhaler with the mouthpiece down or sideways.

• The contents of your DULERA canister are under pressure. Do not puncture or throw the canister into a fire or incinerator. Do not use or store it near heat or open flame. Storage above 120°F (50°C) may cause the canister to burst.

• Keep DULERA and all medicines out of the reach of children.

How to clean your DULERA:

The mouthpiece should be cleaned using a dry wipe after every 7 days of use.

Routine cleaning instructions:

• Remove the cap off the mouthpiece. Wipe the inside and outside surfaces of the actuator mouthpiece with a clean, dry, lint-free tissue or cloth. **Do not wash or put any parts of your inhaler in water.** Put the cap back on the mouthpiece after cleaning.

• Do not remove the canister from the actuator.

• Do not attempt to unblock the actuator with a sharp object, such as a pin.

Manufactured for:　Merck Sharp & Dohme Corp., a subsidiary of

MERCK & CO., INC., Whitehouse Station, NJ 08889, USA

Manufactured by:　3M Health Care Ltd., Loughborough, United Kingdom.

This Medication Guide has been approved by the U.S. Food and Drug Administration.

For patent information:　www.merck.com/product/patent/home.html

The trademarks depicted herein are owned by their respective companies.

Copyright © 2010 Merck Sharp & Dohme Corp., a subsidiary of **Merck & Co., Inc.**

All rights reserved.

Revised:　4/2014

usmg-mk0887a-ao-1404r017

Shown in Product Identification Guide, page 308

───────────────

ELOCON®　　　　　　　　　　　　　　　　　℞

[ĕl′ō-cŏn]

(mometasone furoate)

Cream, 0.1% for topical use

HIGHLIGHTS OF PRESCRIBING INFORMATION

These highlights do not include all the information needed to use ELOCON Cream safely and effectively. See full prescribing information for ELOCON Cream.

ELOCON®(mometasone furoate) Cream, 0.1% for topical use

Initial U.S. Approval: 1987

─────────INDICATIONS AND USAGE─────────

ELOCON Cream is a corticosteroid indicated for the relief of the inflammatory and pruritic manifestations of corticosteroid-responsive dermatoses in patients ≥2 years of age. (1)

────────DOSAGE AND ADMINISTRATION────────

• Apply a thin film to the affected skin areas once daily. (2)
• Discontinue therapy when control is achieved. (2)
• If no improvement is seen within 2 weeks, reassess diagnosis. (2)
• The safety and efficacy of ELOCON Cream, 0.1% in pediatric patients for more than 3 weeks of use have not been established. (2)
• Do not use with occlusive dressings unless directed by a physician. (2)

───────DOSAGE FORMS AND STRENGTHS───────

• Cream, 0.1%. (3)

─────────────CONTRAINDICATIONS─────────────

• None. (4)

────────WARNINGS AND PRECAUTIONS────────

• Reversible HPA axis suppression with the potential for glucocorticosteroid insufficiency after withdrawal of treatment, Cushing's syndrome, and hyperglycemia may occur due to systemic absorption. Patients applying a topical steroid to a large surface area or to areas under occlusion should be evaluated periodically for evidence of HPA axis suppression. Modify use should HPA axis suppression develop. Pediatric patients may be more susceptible to systemic toxicity. (5.1, 8.4)

─────────────ADVERSE REACTIONS─────────────

Most common adverse reactions are:　burning, pruritus, and skin atrophy. (6)

To report SUSPECTED ADVERSE REACTIONS, contact Merck Sharp & Dohme Corp., a subsidiary of Merck & Co., Inc., at 1-877-888-4231 or FDA at 1-800-FDA-1088 or www.fda.gov/medwatch.

See 17 for PATIENT COUNSELING INFORMATION

Revised: 04/2013

FULL PRESCRIBING INFORMATION: CONTENTS*

FULL PRESCRIBING INFORMATION

1　INDICATIONS AND USAGE

ELOCON® Cream is a corticosteroid indicated for the relief of the inflammatory and pruritic manifestations of corticosteroid-responsive dermatoses in patients 2 years of age or older.

2　DOSAGE AND ADMINISTRATION

Apply a thin film of ELOCON Cream to the affected skin areas once daily. ELOCON Cream may be used in pediatric patients 2 years of age or older. Since safety and efficacy of ELOCON Cream have not been established in pediatric patients below 2 years of age; use in this age group is not recommended *[see Warnings and Precautions (5.1) and Use in Specific Populations (8.4)].*

Therapy should be discontinued when control is achieved. If no improvement is seen within 2 weeks, reassessment of diagnosis may be necessary. Safety and efficacy of ELOCON Cream in pediatric patients for more than 3 weeks of use have not been established.

ELOCON Cream should not be used with occlusive dressings unless directed by a physician. ELOCON Cream should not be applied in the diaper area if the child still requires diapers or plastic pants, as these garments may constitute occlusive dressing.

ELOCON Cream is for topical use only. It is not for oral, ophthalmic, or intravaginal use.

Avoid use on the face, groin, or axillae.

3　DOSAGE FORMS AND STRENGTHS

Cream, 0.1%. Each gram of ELOCON Cream contains 1 mg of mometasone furoate in a white to off-white smooth and homogenous cream base.

4　CONTRAINDICATIONS

None.

5　WARNINGS AND PRECAUTIONS

5.1　Effects on Endocrine System

Systemic absorption of topical corticosteroids can produce reversible hypothalamic-pituitary-adrenal (HPA) axis suppression with the potential for glucocorticosteroid insufficiency. This may occur during treatment or after withdrawal of treatment. Manifestations of Cushing's syndrome, hyperglycemia, and glucosuria can also be produced in some patients by systemic absorption of topical corticosteroids while on treatment. Factors that predispose a patient using a topical corticosteroid to HPA axis suppression include the use of high-potency steroids, large treatment surface areas, prolonged use, use of occlusive dressings, altered skin barrier, liver failure and young age.

Because of the potential for systemic absorption, use of topical corticosteroids may require that patients be periodically evaluated for HPA axis suppression. This may be done by using the adrenocorticotropic hormone (ACTH) stimulation test.

In a study evaluating the effects of mometasone furoate cream on the HPA axis, 15 grams were applied twice daily for 7 days to six adult subjects with psoriasis or atopic dermatitis. The results show that the drug caused a slight lowering of adrenal corticosteroid secretion.

If HPA axis suppression is noted, an attempt should be made to gradually withdraw the drug, to reduce the frequency of application, or to substitute a less potent corticosteroid. Recovery of HPA axis function is generally prompt upon discontinuation of topical corticosteroids. Infrequently, signs and symptoms of glucocorticosteroid insufficiency may occur, requiring supplemental systemic corticosteroids. Pediatric patients may be more susceptible to systemic toxicity from equivalent doses due to their larger skin surface to body mass ratios *[see Use in Specific Populations (8.4)]*.

5.2 Allergic Contact Dermatitis

If irritation develops, ELOCON Cream should be discontinued and appropriate therapy instituted. Allergic contact dermatitis with corticosteroids is usually diagnosed by observing a failure to heal rather than noting a clinical exacerbation as with most topical products not containing corticosteroids. Such an observation should be corroborated with appropriate diagnostic patch testing.

5.3 Concomitant Skin Infections

If concomitant skin infections are present or develop, an appropriate antifungal or antibacterial agent should be used. If a favorable response does not occur promptly, use of ELOCON Cream should be discontinued until the infection has been adequately controlled.

6 ADVERSE REACTIONS

Because clinical trials are conducted under widely varying conditions, adverse reaction rates observed in the clinical trials of a drug cannot be directly compared to rates in the clinical trials of another drug and may not reflect the rates observed in clinical practice.

In controlled clinical trials involving 319 subjects, the incidence of adverse reactions associated with the use of ELOCON Cream was 1.6%. Reported reactions included burning, pruritus, and skin atrophy. Reports of rosacea associated with the use of ELOCON Cream have also been received. In controlled clinical trials (n=74) involving pediatric subjects 2 to 12 years of age, the incidence of adverse experiences associated with the use of ELOCON Cream was approximately 7%. Reported reactions included stinging, pruritus, and furunculosis.

The following adverse reactions were reported to be possibly or probably related to treatment with ELOCON Cream during clinical trials in 4% of 182 pediatric subjects 6 months to 2 years of age: decreased glucocorticoid levels, 2; paresthesia, 2; folliculitis, 1; moniliasis, 1; bacterial infection, 1; skin depigmentation, 1. The following signs of skin atrophy were also observed among 97 subjects treated with ELOCON Cream in a clinical trial: shininess, 4; telangiectasia, 1; loss of elasticity, 4; loss of normal skin markings, 4; thinness, 1; and bruising, 1.

The following additional local adverse reactions have been reported with topical corticosteroids, but may occur more frequently with the use of occlusive dressings. These reactions are: irritation, dryness, folliculitis, hypertrichosis, acneiform eruptions, hypopigmentation, perioral dermatitis, allergic contact dermatitis, secondary infection, striae, and miliaria.

7 DRUG INTERACTIONS

No drug-drug interaction studies have been conducted with ELOCON Cream.

8 USE IN SPECIFIC POPULATIONS

8.1 Pregnancy

Teratogenic Effects Pregnancy Category C:

There are no adequate and well-controlled studies in pregnant women. Therefore, ELOCON Cream should be used during pregnancy only if the potential benefit justifies the potential risk to the fetus.

Corticosteroids have been shown to be teratogenic in laboratory animals when administered systemically at relatively low dosage levels. Some corticosteroids have been shown to be teratogenic after dermal application in laboratory animals.

When administered to pregnant rats, rabbits, and mice, mometasone furoate increased fetal malformations. The doses that produced malformations also decreased fetal growth, as measured by lower fetal weights and/or delayed ossification. Mometasone furoate also caused dystocia and related complications when administered to rats during the end of pregnancy.

In mice, mometasone furoate caused cleft palate at subcutaneous doses of 60 mcg/kg and above. Fetal survival was reduced at 180 mcg/kg. No toxicity was observed at 20 mcg/kg. (Doses of 20, 60, and 180 mcg/kg in the mouse are approximately 0.01, 0.02, and 0.05 times the estimated maximum clinical topical dose from ELOCON Cream on a mcg/m² basis.)

In rats, mometasone furoate produced umbilical hernias at topical doses of 600 mcg/kg and above. A dose of 300 mcg/kg produced delays in ossification, but no malformations. (Doses of 300 and 600 mcg/kg in the rat are approximately 0.2 and 0.4 times the estimated maximum clinical topical dose from ELOCON Cream on a mcg/m² basis.)

In rabbits, mometasone furoate caused multiple malformations (e.g., flexed front paws, gallbladder agenesis, umbilical

hernia, hydrocephaly) at topical doses of 150 mcg/kg and above (approximately 0.2 times the estimated maximum clinical topical dose from ELOCON Cream on a mcg/m² basis). In an oral study, mometasone furoate increased resorptions and caused cleft palate and/or head malformations (hydrocephaly and domed head) at 700 mcg/kg. At 2800 mcg/kg most litters were aborted or resorbed. No toxicity was observed at 140 mcg/kg. (Doses at 140, 700, and 2800 mcg/kg in the rabbit are approximately 0.2, 0.9, and 3.6 times the estimated maximum clinical topical dose from ELOCON Cream on a mcg/m² basis.)

When rats received subcutaneous doses of mometasone furoate throughout pregnancy or during the later stages of pregnancy, 15 mcg/kg caused prolonged and difficult labor and reduced the number of live births, birth weight, and early pup survival. Similar effects were not observed at 7.5 mcg/kg. (Doses of 7.5 and 15 mcg/kg in the rat are approximately 0.005 and 0.01 times the estimated maximum clinical topical dose from ELOCON Cream on a mcg/m² basis.)

8.3 Nursing Mothers

Systemically administered corticosteroids appear in human milk and could suppress growth, interfere with endogenous corticosteroid production, or cause other untoward effects. It is not known whether topical administration of corticosteroids could result in sufficient systemic absorption to produce detectable quantities in human milk. Because many drugs are excreted in human milk, caution should be exercised when ELOCON Cream is administered to a nursing woman.

8.4 Pediatric Use

ELOCON Cream may be used with caution in pediatric patients 2 years of age or older, although the safety and efficacy of drug use for longer than 3 weeks have not been established. Since safety and efficacy of ELOCON Cream have not been established in pediatric patients below 2 years of age, its use in this age group is not recommended.

In a pediatric trial, 24 atopic dermatitis subjects, of whom 19 subjects were age 2 to 12 years, were treated with ELOCON Cream once daily. The majority of subjects cleared within 3 weeks.

ELOCON Cream caused HPA axis suppression in approximately 16% of pediatric subjects ages 6 to 23 months, who showed normal adrenal function by Cortrosyn test before starting treatment, and were treated for approximately 3 weeks over a mean body surface area of 41% (range 15%-94%). The criteria for suppression were: basal cortisol level of ≤5 mcg/dL, 30-minute post-stimulation level of ≤18 mcg/dL, or an increase of <7 mcg/dL. Follow-up testing 2 to 4 weeks after trial completion, available for 5 of the subjects, demonstrated suppressed HPA axis function in 1 subject, using these same criteria. Long-term use of topical corticosteroids has not been studied in this population *[see Clinical Pharmacology (12.2)]*.

Because of a higher ratio of skin surface area to body mass, pediatric patients are at a greater risk than adults of HPA axis suppression and Cushing's syndrome when they are treated with topical corticosteroids. They are, therefore, also at greater risk of adrenal insufficiency during and/or after withdrawal of treatment. Pediatric patients may be more susceptible than adults to skin atrophy, including striae, when they are treated with topical corticosteroids. Pediatric patients applying topical corticosteroids to greater than 20% of body surface are at higher risk of HPA axis suppression.

HPA axis suppression, Cushing's syndrome, linear growth retardation, delayed weight gain, and intracranial hypertension have been reported in pediatric patients receiving topical corticosteroids. Manifestations of adrenal suppression in children include low plasma cortisol levels and an absence of response to ACTH stimulation. Manifestations of intracranial hypertension include bulging fontanelles, headaches, and bilateral papilledema.

ELOCON Cream should not be used in the treatment of diaper dermatitis.

8.5 Geriatric Use

Clinical studies of ELOCON Cream included 190 subjects who were 65 years of age and over and 39 subjects who were 75 years of age and over. No overall differences in safety or effectiveness were observed between these subjects and younger subjects, and other reported clinical experience has not identified differences in responses between the elderly and younger patients. However, greater sensitivity of some older individuals cannot be ruled out.

10 OVERDOSAGE

Topically applied ELOCON Cream can be absorbed in sufficient amounts to produce systemic effects *[see Warnings and Precautions (5.1)]*.

11 DESCRIPTION

ELOCON (mometasone furoate) Cream, 0.1% contains mometasone furoate for topical use. Mometasone furoate is a synthetic corticosteroid with anti-inflammatory activity. Chemically, mometasone furoate is 9α,21-dichloro-11β,17-dihydroxy-16α-methylpregna-1,4-diene-3,20-dione 17-(2-

furoate), with the empirical formula $C_{27}H_{30}Cl_2O_6$, a molecular weight of 521.4 and the following structural formula:

Mometasone furoate is a white to off-white powder practically insoluble in water, slightly soluble in octanol, and moderately soluble in ethyl alcohol.

Each gram of ELOCON Cream, 0.1% contains 1 mg mometasone furoate in a white to off-white cream base of aluminum starch octenylsuccinate (Gamma Irradiated), hexylene glycol, hydrogenated soybean lecithin, phosphoric acid, purified water, titanium dioxide, white soft paraffin, and white wax.

12 CLINICAL PHARMACOLOGY

12.1 Mechanism of Action

Like other topical corticosteroids, mometasone furoate has anti-inflammatory, antipruritic, and vasoconstrictive properties. The mechanism of the anti-inflammatory activity of the topical steroids, in general, is unclear. However, corticosteroids are thought to act by the induction of phospholipase A₂ inhibitory proteins, collectively called lipocortins. It is postulated that these proteins control the biosynthesis of potent mediators of inflammation such as prostaglandins and leukotrienes by inhibiting the release of their common precursor arachidonic acid. Arachidonic acid is released from membrane phospholipids by phospholipase A₂.

12.2 Pharmacodynamics

Studies performed with ELOCON Cream indicate that it is in the medium range of potency as compared with other topical corticosteroids.

In a study evaluating the effects of mometasone furoate cream on the HPA axis, 15 grams were applied twice daily for 7 days to six adult subjects with psoriasis or atopic dermatitis. The cream was applied without occlusion to at least 30% of the body surface. The results showed that the drug caused a slight lowering of adrenal corticosteroid secretion *[see Warnings and Precautions (5.1)]*.

Ninety-seven pediatric subjects ages 6 to 23 months with atopic dermatitis were enrolled in an open-label HPA axis safety study. ELOCON Cream was applied once daily for approximately 3 weeks over a mean body surface area of 41% (range 15%-94%). In approximately 16% of subjects who showed normal adrenal function by Cortrosyn test before starting treatment, adrenal suppression was observed at the end of treatment with ELOCON Cream. The criteria for suppression were: basal cortisol level of ≤5 mcg/dL, 30-minute post-stimulation level of ≤18 mcg/dL, or an increase of <7 mcg/dL. Follow-up testing 2 to 4 weeks after stopping treatment, available for 5 of the subjects, demonstrated suppressed HPA axis function in one subject, using these same criteria *[see Use in Specific Populations (8.4)]*.

12.3 Pharmacokinetics

The extent of percutaneous absorption of topical corticosteroids is determined by many factors including the vehicle and the integrity of the epidermal barrier. Studies in humans indicate that approximately 0.4% of the applied dose of ELOCON Cream enters the circulation after 8 hours of contact on normal skin without occlusion. Inflammation and/or other disease processes in the skin may increase percutaneous absorption.

13 NONCLINICAL TOXICOLOGY

13.1 Carcinogenesis, Mutagenesis, Impairment of Fertility

Long-term animal studies have not been performed to evaluate the carcinogenic potential of ELOCON Cream. Long-term carcinogenicity studies of mometasone furoate were conducted by the inhalation route in rats and mice. In a 2-year carcinogenicity study in Sprague Dawley rats, mometasone furoate demonstrated no statistically significant increase of tumors at inhalation doses up to 67 mcg/kg (approximately 0.04 times the estimated maximum clinical topical dose from ELOCON Cream on a mcg/m² basis). In a 19-month carcinogenicity study in Swiss CD-1 mice, mometasone furoate demonstrated no statistically significant increase in the incidence of tumors at inhalation doses up to 160 mcg/kg (approximately 0.05 times the estimated maximum clinical topical dose from ELOCON Cream on a mcg/m² basis).

Mometasone furoate increased chromosomal aberrations in an *in vitro* Chinese hamster ovary cell assay, but did not increase chromosomal aberrations in an *in vitro* Chinese hamster lung cell assay. Mometasone furoate was not mutagenic in the Ames test or mouse lymphoma assay, and was not clastogenic in an *in vivo* mouse micronucleus assay, a rat bone marrow chromosomal aberration assay, or a mouse male germ-cell chromosomal aberration assay. Mometasone furoate also did not induce unscheduled DNA synthesis *in vivo* in rat hepatocytes.

In reproductive studies in rats, impairment of fertility was not produced in male or female rats by subcutaneous doses up to 15 mcg/kg (approximately 0.01 times the estimated maximum clinical topical dose from ELOCON Cream on a mcg/m² basis).

14 CLINICAL STUDIES

The safety and efficacy of the ELOCON Cream for the treatment of corticosteroid-responsive dermatoses were evaluated in two randomized, double-blind, vehicle-controlled clinical trials, one in psoriasis and one in atopic dermatitis. A total 366 subjects (12-81 years of age), of whom 177 received ELOCON Cream and 181 subjects received vehicle cream, were evaluated in these trials. ELOCON Cream or the vehicle cream were applied once daily for 21 days.
The two trials showed ELOCON Cream is effective in the treatment of psoriasis and atopic dermatitis.

16 HOW SUPPLIED/STORAGE AND HANDLING

ELOCON Cream is white to off-white in color and supplied in 15-gram (NDC 0085-3149-01) and 50-gram (NDC 0085-3149-03) tubes.
Store at 25°C (77°F); excursions permitted to 15-30°C (59-86°F) [see USP Controlled Room Temperature]. Avoid excessive heat.

17 PATIENT COUNSELING INFORMATION

Inform patients of the following:
• Use ELOCON Cream as directed by the physician. It is for external use only.
• Avoid contact with the eyes.
• Do not use ELOCON Cream on the face, underarms, or groin areas unless directed by the physician.
• Do not use ELOCON Cream for any disorder other than that for which it was prescribed.
• The treated skin area should not be bandaged or otherwise covered or wrapped so as to be occlusive, unless directed by the physician.
• Report any signs of local adverse reactions to the physician.
• Advise patients not to use ELOCON Cream in the treatment of diaper dermatitis. Do not apply ELOCON Cream in the diaper area, as diapers or plastic pants may constitute occlusive dressing.
• Discontinue therapy when control is achieved. If no improvement is seen within 2 weeks, contact the physician.
• Do not use other corticosteroid-containing products with ELOCON Cream without first consulting with the physician.

Manufactured for: Merck Sharp & Dohme Corp., a subsidiary of
MERCK & CO., INC., Whitehouse Station, NJ 08889, USA
Manufactured by:
Schering-Plough Labo NV
Heist-op-den-Berg, Belgium
Copyright © 1987, 2008, 2012 Merck Sharp & Dohme Corp., a subsidiary of **Merck & Co., Inc.**
All rights reserved.
032088-EL-CR-USPI.7

ELOCON® LOTION   ℞
[ĕl'ō-cŏn]
mometasone furoate
Lotion, 0.1% for topical use

HIGHLIGHTS OF PRESCRIBING INFORMATION
These highlights do not include all the information needed to use ELOCON Lotion safely and effectively. See full prescribing information for ELOCON Lotion.
ELOCON® (mometasone furoate) Lotion, 0.1% for topical use
Initial U.S. Approval: 1987

————INDICATIONS AND USAGE————
ELOCON Lotion is a corticosteroid indicated for the relief of the inflammatory and pruritic manifestations of corticosteroid-responsive dermatoses in patients ≥12 years of age. (1)

————DOSAGE AND ADMINISTRATION————
• Apply a few drops to the affected skin areas once daily and massage lightly until it disappears. (2)
• Discontinue therapy when control is achieved. (2)
• If no improvement is seen within 2 weeks, reassess diagnosis. (2)
• Do not use with occlusive dressings unless directed by a physician. (2)

————DOSAGE FORMS AND STRENGTHS————
• Lotion, 0.1%. (3)

————CONTRAINDICATIONS————
• None. (4)

————WARNINGS AND PRECAUTIONS————
• Reversible HPA axis suppression with the potential for glucocorticosteroid insufficiency after withdrawal of treatment, Cushing's syndrome, and hyperglycemia may occur due to systemic absorption. Patients applying a topical steroid to a large surface area or to areas under occlusion should be evaluated periodically for evidence of HPA axis suppression. Modify use should HPA axis suppression develop. Pediatric patients may be more susceptible to systemic toxicity. (5.1, 8.4)

————ADVERSE REACTIONS————
Most common adverse reactions included are acneiform reaction, burning, itching and folliculitis. (6)
To report SUSPECTED ADVERSE REACTIONS, contact Merck Sharp & Dohme Corp., a subsidiary of Merck & Co., Inc., at 1-877-888-4231 or FDA at 1-800-FDA-1088 or www.fda.gov/medwatch
See 17 for PATIENT COUNSELING INFORMATION
Revised: 03/2013

FULL PRESCRIBING INFORMATION: CONTENTS*

FULL PRESCRIBING INFORMATION

1 INDICATIONS AND USAGE

ELOCON® Lotion is a corticosteroid indicated for the relief of the inflammatory and pruritic manifestations of corticosteroid-responsive dermatoses in patients 12 years of age or older.

2 DOSAGE AND ADMINISTRATION

Apply a few drops of ELOCON Lotion to the affected skin areas once daily and massage lightly until it disappears. Therapy should be discontinued when control is achieved. If no improvement is seen within 2 weeks, reassessment of diagnosis may be necessary [see Warnings and Precautions (5.1) and Use in Specific Populations (8.4)].
ELOCON Lotion should not be used with occlusive dressings unless directed by a physician. ELOCON Lotion should not be applied in the diaper area if the patient still requires diapers or plastic pants, as these garments may constitute occlusive dressing.
ELOCON Lotion is for topical use only. It is not for oral, ophthalmic, or intravaginal use.
Avoid use on the face, groin, or axillae.

3 DOSAGE FORMS AND STRENGTHS

Lotion, 0.1%. Each gram of ELOCON Lotion contains 1 mg of mometasone furoate in a colorless, clear to translucent lotion base.

4 CONTRAINDICATIONS

None.

5 WARNINGS AND PRECAUTIONS
5.1 Effects on Endocrine System

Systemic absorption of topical corticosteroids can produce reversible hypothalamic-pituitary-adrenal (HPA) axis suppression with the potential for glucocorticosteroid insufficiency. This may occur during treatment or after withdrawal of treatment. Manifestations of Cushing's syndrome, hyperglycemia, and glucosuria can also be produced in some patients by systemic absorption of topical corticosteroids while on treatment. Factors that predispose a patient using a topical corticosteroid to HPA axis suppression include the use of high potency steroids, large treatment surface areas, prolonged use, use of occlusive dressing, altered skin barrier, liver failure and young age.
Because of the potential for systemic absorption, use of topical corticosteroids may require that patients be periodically evaluated for HPA axis suppression. This may be done by using the adrenocorticotropic hormone (ACTH) stimulation test.
In a study evaluating the effects of mometasone furoate lotion on the HPA axis, 15 mL were applied without occlusion twice daily (30 mL per day) for 7 days to 4 adult subjects with scalp and body psoriasis. At the end of treatment, the plasma cortisol levels for each of the 4 subjects remained within the normal range and changed little from baseline.
If HPA axis suppression is documented, an attempt should be made to gradually withdraw the drug, to reduce the frequency of application, or to substitute a less potent corticosteroid. Recovery of HPA axis function is generally prompt upon discontinuation of topical corticosteroids. Infrequently, signs and symptoms of glucocorticosteroid insufficiency may occur, requiring supplemental systemic corticosteroids.
Pediatric patients may be more susceptible to systemic toxicity from equivalent doses due to their larger skin surface to body mass ratios [see Use in Specific Populations (8.4)].

5.2 Allergic Contact Dermatitis

If irritation develops, ELOCON Lotion should be discontinued and appropriate therapy instituted. Allergic contact dermatitis with corticosteroids is usually diagnosed by observing failure to heal rather than noting a clinical exacerbation. Such an observation should be corroborated with appropriate diagnostic patch testing.

5.3 Concomitant Skin Infections

If concomitant skin infections are present or develop, an appropriate antifungal or antibacterial agent should be used. If a favorable response does not occur promptly, use of ELOCON Lotion should be discontinued until the infection has been adequately controlled.

6 ADVERSE REACTIONS

Because clinical trials are conducted under widely varying conditions, adverse reaction rates observed in the clinical trials of a drug cannot be directly compared to rates in the clinical trials of another drug and may not reflect the rates observed in clinical practice.
In clinical trials involving 209 subjects, the incidence of adverse reactions associated with the use of ELOCON Lotion was 3%. Reported reactions included acneiform reaction, 2; burning, 4; and itching, 1. In an irritation/sensitization study involving 156 normal subjects, the incidence of folliculitis was 3% (4 subjects).
The following adverse reactions were reported to be possibly or probably related to treatment with ELOCON Lotion during a clinical trial in 14% of 65 pediatric subjects 6 months to 2 years of age: decreased glucocorticoid levels, 4; paresthesia, 2; dry mouth,1; an unspecified endocrine disorder, 1; pruritus, 1; and an unspecified skin disorder, 1. The following signs of skin atrophy were also observed among 65 subjects treated with ELOCON Lotion in a clinical trial: shininess, 4; telangiectasia, 2; loss of elasticity, 2; and loss of normal skin markings, 3.
The following additional local adverse reactions have been reported with topical corticosteroids, but may occur more frequently with the use of occlusive dressings. These reactions are: irritation, dryness, hypertrichosis, hypopigmentation, perioral dermatitis, allergic contact dermatitis, secondary infection, skin atrophy, striae, and miliaria.

7 DRUG INTERACTIONS

No drug-drug interaction studies have been conducted with ELOCON Lotion.

8 USE IN SPECIFIC POPULATIONS
8.1 Pregnancy

Teratogenic Effects Pregnancy Category C:
There are no adequate and well-controlled studies in pregnant women. Therefore, ELOCON Lotion should be used during pregnancy only if the potential benefit justifies the potential risk to the fetus.
Corticosteroids have been shown to be teratogenic in laboratory animals when administered systemically at relatively low dosage levels. Some corticosteroids have been shown to be teratogenic after dermal application in laboratory animals.
When administered to pregnant rats, rabbits, and mice, mometasone furoate increased fetal malformations. The doses that produced malformations also decreased fetal growth, as measured by lower fetal weights and/or delayed ossification. Mometasone furoate also caused dystocia and related complications when administered to rats during the end of pregnancy.

In mice, mometasone furoate caused cleft palate at subcutaneous doses of 60 mcg/kg and above. Fetal survival was reduced at 180 mcg/kg. No toxicity was observed at 20 mcg/kg. (Doses of 20, 60, and 180 mcg/kg in the mouse are approximately 0.01, 0.02, and 0.05 times the estimated maximum clinical topical dose from ELOCON Lotion on a mcg/m^2 basis.)

In rats, mometasone furoate produced umbilical hernias at topical doses of 600 mcg/kg and above. A dose of 300 mcg/kg produced delays in ossification, but no malformations. (Doses of 300 and 600 mcg/kg in the rat are approximately 0.2 and 0.4 times the estimated maximum clinical topical dose from ELOCON Lotion on a mcg/m^2 basis.)

In rabbits, mometasone furoate caused multiple malformations (e.g., flexed front paws, gallbladder agenesis, umbilical hernia, hydrocephaly) at topical doses of 150 mcg/kg and above (approximately 0.2 times the estimated maximum clinical topical dose from ELOCON Lotion on a mcg/m^2 basis). In an oral study, mometasone furoate increased resorptions and caused cleft palate and/or head malformations (hydrocephaly and domed head) at 700 mcg/kg. At 2800 mcg/kg most litters were aborted or resorbed. No toxicity was observed at 140 mcg/kg. (Doses at 140, 700, and 2800 mcg/kg in the rabbit are approximately 0.2, 0.9, and 3.6 times the estimated maximum clinical topical dose from ELOCON Lotion on a mcg/m^2 basis.)

When rats received subcutaneous doses of mometasone furoate throughout pregnancy or during the later stages of pregnancy, 15 mcg/kg caused prolonged and difficult labor and reduced the number of live births, birth weight, and early pup survival. Similar effects were not observed at 7.5 mcg/kg. (Doses of 7.5 and 15 mcg/kg in the rat are approximately 0.005 and 0.01 times the estimated maximum clinical topical dose from ELOCON Lotion on a mcg/m^2 basis.)

8.3 Nursing Mothers

Systemically administered corticosteroids appear in human milk and could suppress growth, interfere with endogenous corticosteroid production, or cause other untoward effects. It is not known whether topical administration of corticosteroids could result in sufficient systemic absorption to produce detectable quantities in human milk. Because many drugs are excreted in human milk, caution should be exercised when ELOCON Lotion is administered to a nursing woman.

8.4 Pediatric Use

Since safety and efficacy of ELOCON Lotion have not been established in pediatric patients below 12 years of age, its use in this age group is not recommended.

ELOCON Lotion caused HPA axis suppression in approximately 29% of pediatric subjects ages 6 to 23 months, who showed normal adrenal function by Cortrosyn test before starting treatment, and were treated for approximately 3 weeks over a mean body surface area of 40% (range 16%-90%). The criteria for suppression were: basal cortisol level of ≤5 mcg/dL, 30-minute post-stimulation level of ≤18 mcg/dL, or an increase of <7 mcg/dL. Follow-up testing 2 to 4 weeks after stopping treatment, available for 8 of the subjects, demonstrated suppressed HPA axis function in 1 subject, using these same criteria. Long-term use of topical corticosteroids has not been studied in this population [see Clinical Pharmacology (12.2)].

Because of a higher ratio of skin surface area to body mass, pediatric patients are at a greater risk than adults of HPA axis suppression and Cushing's syndrome when they are treated with topical corticosteroids. They are, therefore, also at greater risk of adrenal insufficiency during and/or after withdrawal of treatment. Pediatric patients may be more susceptible than adults to skin atrophy, including striae, when they are treated with topical corticosteroids. Pediatric patients applying topical corticosteroids to greater than 20% of body surface are at higher risk of HPA axis suppression.

HPA axis suppression, Cushing's syndrome, linear growth retardation, delayed weight gain, and intracranial hypertension have been reported in pediatric patients receiving topical corticosteroids. Manifestations of adrenal suppression in children include low plasma cortisol levels and absence of response to ACTH stimulation. Manifestations of intracranial hypertension include bulging fontanelles, headaches, and bilateral papilledema.

ELOCON Lotion should not be used in the treatment of diaper dermatitis.

8.5 Geriatric Use

Clinical trials of ELOCON Lotion did not include sufficient numbers of subjects aged 65 and over to determine whether they respond differently from younger subjects. Other reported clinical experience has not identified differences in responses between the elderly and younger patients. In general, dose selection for an elderly patient should be cautious, usually starting at the low end of the dosing range.

10 OVERDOSAGE

Topically applied ELOCON Lotion can be absorbed in sufficient amounts to produce systemic effects [see Warnings and Precautions (5.1)].

11 DESCRIPTION

ELOCON (mometasone furoate) Lotion, 0.1% contains mometasone furoate for topical use. Mometasone furoate is a synthetic corticosteroid with anti-inflammatory activity. Chemically, mometasone furoate is 9α, 21-dichloro-11β,17-dihydroxy-16α-methylpregna-1,4-diene-3,20-dione 17-(2-furoate), with the empirical formula $C_{27}H_{30}Cl_2O_6$, a molecular weight of 521.4 and the following structural formula:

Mometasone furoate is a white to off-white powder practically insoluble in water, slightly soluble in octanol, and moderately soluble in ethyl alcohol.

Each gram of ELOCON Lotion, 0.1% contains 1 mg mometasone furoate in a colorless, clear to translucent lotion base of hydroxypropyl cellulose, isopropyl alcohol (40%), propylene glycol, purified water and sodium phosphate monobasic monohydrate. May also contain phosphoric acid used to adjust the pH to approximately 4.5.

12 CLINICAL PHARMACOLOGY

12.1 Mechanism of Action

Like other topical corticosteroids, mometasone furoate has anti-inflammatory, antipruritic, and vasoconstrictive properties. The mechanism of the anti-inflammatory activity of the topical steroids, in general, is unclear. However, corticosteroids are thought to act by the induction of phospholipase A_2 inhibitory proteins, collectively called lipocortins. It is postulated that these proteins control the biosynthesis of potent mediators of inflammation such as prostaglandins and leukotrienes by inhibiting the release of their common precursor arachidonic acid. Arachidonic acid is released from membrane phospholipids by phospholipase A_2.

12.2 Pharmacodynamics

Studies performed with ELOCON Lotion indicate that it is in the medium range of potency as compared with other topical corticosteroids.

In a study evaluating the effects of mometasone furoate lotion on the HPA axis, 15 mL were applied without occlusion twice daily (30 mL per day) for 7 days to 4 adult subjects with scalp and body psoriasis. At the end of treatment, the plasma cortisol levels for each of the 4 subjects remained within the normal range and changed little from baseline [see Warnings and Precautions (5.1)].

Sixty-five pediatric subjects ages 6 to 23 months, with atopic dermatitis, were enrolled in an open-label, HPA axis safety trial. ELOCON Lotion was applied once daily for approximately 3 weeks over a mean body surface area of 40% (range 16%-90%). In approximately 29% of subjects who showed normal adrenal function by Cortrosyn test before starting treatment, adrenal suppression was observed at the end of treatment with ELOCON Lotion. The criteria for suppression were: basal cortisol level of ≤5 mcg/dL, 30-minute post-stimulation level of ≤18 mcg/dL, or an increase of <7 mcg/dL. Follow-up testing 2 to 4 weeks after stopping treatment, available for 8 of the subjects, demonstrated suppressed HPA axis function in 1 subject, using these same criteria [see Use in Specific Populations (8.4)].

12.3 Pharmacokinetics

The extent of percutaneous absorption of topical corticosteroids is determined by many factors including the vehicle and the integrity of the epidermal barrier. Studies in humans indicate that approximately 0.7% of the applied dose of ELOCON Lotion enters the circulation after 8 hours of contact on normal skin without occlusion. A similar minimal degree of absorption of the corticosteroid from the lotion formulation would be anticipated. Inflammation and/or other disease processes in the skin may increase percutaneous absorption.

13 NONCLINICAL TOXICOLOGY

13.1 Carcinogenesis, Mutagenesis, Impairment of Fertility

Long-term animal studies have not been performed to evaluate the carcinogenic potential of ELOCON Lotion. Long-term carcinogenicity studies of mometasone furoate were conducted by the inhalation route in rats and mice. In a 2-year carcinogenicity study in Sprague Dawley rats, mometasone furoate demonstrated no statistically significant increase of tumors at inhalation doses up to 67 mcg/kg (approximately 0.04 times the estimated maximum clinical topical dose from ELOCON Lotion on a mcg/m^2 basis). In a 19-month carcinogenicity study in Swiss CD-1 mice, mometasone furoate demonstrated no statistically significant increase in the incidence of tumors at inhalation doses up to 160 mcg/kg (approximately 0.05 times the estimated maximum clinical topical dose from ELOCON Lotion on a mcg/m^2 basis).

Mometasone furoate increased chromosomal aberrations in an *in vitro* Chinese hamster ovary cell assay, but did not increase chromosomal aberrations in an *in vitro* Chinese hamster lung cell assay. Mometasone furoate was not mutagenic in the Ames test or mouse lymphoma assay, and was not clastogenic in an *in vivo* mouse micronucleus assay, a rat bone marrow chromosomal aberration assay, or a mouse male germ-cell chromosomal aberration assay. Mometasone furoate also did not induce unscheduled DNA synthesis *in vivo* in rat hepatocytes.

In reproductive studies in rats, impairment of fertility was not produced in male or female rats by subcutaneous doses up to 15 mcg/kg (approximately 0.01 times the estimated maximum clinical topical dose from ELOCON Lotion on a mcg/m^2 basis).

14 CLINICAL STUDIES

The safety and efficacy of ELOCON Lotion, 0.1% for the treatment of corticosteroid-responsive dermatoses was demonstrated in two vehicle-controlled trials, one in scalp psoriasis and one in seborrheic dermatitis. A total of 405 subjects (age range: 12-95 years) received ELOCON Lotion (205 subjects) or the vehicle lotion applied once daily for 21 days.

16 HOW SUPPLIED/STORAGE AND HANDLING

ELOCON Lotion is colorless, clear to translucent and supplied in 30-mL (27.5 gram) (NDC 0085-0854-01) and 60-mL (55 gram) (NDC 0085-0854-02) bottles; boxes of one.

Store ELOCON Lotion, 0.1% at 25°C (77°F); excursions permitted to 15-30°C (59-86°F) [see USP Controlled Room Temperature].

17 PATIENT COUNSELING INFORMATION

Inform patients of the following:

• Use ELOCON Lotion as directed by the physician. It is for external use only.
• Avoid contact with the eyes.
• Do not use ELOCON Lotion on the face, underarms, or groin areas.
• Do not use ELOCON Lotion for any disorder other than that for which it was prescribed.
• The treated skin area should not be bandaged or otherwise covered or wrapped so as to be occlusive, unless directed by the physician.
• Report any signs of local adverse reactions to the physician.
• Advise patients not to use ELOCON Lotion in the treatment of diaper dermatitis. Do not apply ELOCON Lotion in the diaper area, as diapers or plastic pants may constitute occlusive dressing.
• Discontinue therapy when control is achieved. If no improvement is seen within 2 weeks, contact the physician.
• Do not use other corticosteroid-containing products with ELOCON Lotion without first consulting with the physician.

Manufactured for: Merck Sharp & Dohme Corp., a subsidiary of **MERCK & CO., INC.**, Whitehouse Station, NJ 08889, USA
Manufactured by: Schering Plough Canada, Inc.
Pointe Claire, Quebec, Canada.
Copyright © 1989, 2008, 2012 Merck Sharp & Dohme Corp., a subsidiary of Merck & Co., Inc.
All rights reserved.
032088-EL-LT-USPI.6

ELOCON®

℞

[el'ō-cŏn]

(mometasone furoate)
Ointment, 0.1% for topical use

HIGHLIGHTS OF PRESCRIBING INFORMATION

These highlights do not include all the information needed to use ELOCON Ointment safely and effectively. See full prescribing information for ELOCON Ointment.
ELOCON® (mometasone furoate) Ointment, 0.1% for topical use
Initial U.S. Approval: 1987

INDICATIONS AND USAGE

ELOCON Ointment is a corticosteroid indicated for the relief of the inflammatory and pruritic manifestations of corticosteroid-responsive dermatoses in patients ≥2 years of age (1)

DOSAGE AND ADMINISTRATION

• Apply a thin film to the affected skin areas once daily. (2)
• Discontinue therapy when control is achieved. (2)
• If no improvement is seen within 2 weeks, reassess diagnosis. (2)
• The safety and efficacy of ELOCON Ointment in pediatric patients for more than 3 weeks of use have not been established. (2)
• Do not use with occlusive dressings unless directed by a physician. (2)

——————DOSAGE FORMS AND STRENGTHS——————

• Ointment, 0.1%. (3)

——————CONTRAINDICATIONS——————

• None. (4)

——————WARNINGS AND PRECAUTIONS——————

• Reversible HPA axis suppression with the potential for glucocorticosteroid insufficiency after withdrawal of treatment, Cushing's syndrome, and hyperglycemia may occur due to systemic absorption. Patients applying a topical steroid to a large surface area or to areas under occlusion should be evaluated periodically for evidence of HPA axis suppression. Modify use should HPA axis suppression develop. Pediatric patients may be more susceptible to systemic toxicity. (5.1, 8.4)

——————ADVERSE REACTIONS——————

Most common adverse reactions are burning, pruritus, skin atrophy, tingling/stinging and furunculosis. (6)

To report SUSPECTED ADVERSE REACTIONS, contact Merck Sharp & Dohme Corp., a subsidiary of Merck & Co., Inc., at 1-877-888-4231 or FDA at 1-800-FDA-1088 or www.fda.gov/medwatch.

See 17 for PATIENT COUNSELING INFORMATION
Revised: 03/2013

FULL PRESCRIBING INFORMATION: CONTENTS*

FULL PRESCRIBING INFORMATION

1   INDICATIONS AND USAGE

ELOCON® Ointment is a corticosteroid indicated for the relief of the inflammatory and pruritic manifestations of corticosteroid-responsive dermatoses in patients 2 years of age or older.

2   DOSAGE AND ADMINISTRATION

Apply a thin film of ELOCON Ointment to the affected skin areas once daily.

Therapy should be discontinued when control is achieved. If no improvement is seen within 2 weeks, reassessment of diagnosis may be necessary.

Safety and efficacy of ELOCON Ointment in pediatric patients for more than 3 weeks of use have not been established [see Warnings and Precautions (5.1) and Use in Specific Populations (8.4)].

ELOCON Ointment should not be used with occlusive dressings unless directed by a physician. ELOCON Ointment should not be applied in the diaper area if the child still requires diapers or plastic pants, as these garments may constitute occlusive dressing.

ELOCON Ointment is for topical use only. It is not for oral, ophthalmic, or intravaginal use.

Avoid use on the face, groin, or axillae.

3   DOSAGE FORMS AND STRENGTHS

Ointment, 0.1%. Each gram of ELOCON Ointment contains 1 mg of mometasone furoate in a white to off-white uniform ointment base.

4   CONTRAINDICATIONS

None.

5   WARNINGS AND PRECAUTIONS
5.1   Effects on Endocrine System

Systemic absorption of topical corticosteroids can produce reversible hypothalamic-pituitary-adrenal (HPA) axis suppression with the potential for glucocorticosteroid insufficiency. This may occur during treatment or after withdrawal of treatment. Manifestations of Cushing's syndrome, hyperglycemia, and glucosuria can also be produced in some patients by systemic absorption of topical corticosteroids while on treatment. Factors that predispose a patient using a topical corticosteroid to HPA axis suppression include the use of high-potency steroids, large treatment surface areas, prolonged use, use of occlusive dressings, altered skin barrier, liver failure, and young age.

Because of the potential for systemic absorption, use of topical corticosteroids may require that patients be periodically evaluated for HPA axis suppression. This may be done by using the adrenocorticotropic hormone (ACTH) stimulation test.

In a study evaluating the effects of mometasone furoate ointment on the HPA axis, 15 grams were applied twice daily for 7 days to 6 adult subjects with psoriasis or atopic dermatitis. The results show that the drug caused a slight lowering of adrenal corticosteroid secretion.

If HPA axis suppression is documented, an attempt should be made to gradually withdraw the drug, to reduce the frequency of application, or to substitute a less potent corticosteroid. Recovery of HPA axis function is generally prompt upon discontinuation of topical corticosteroids. Infrequently, signs and symptoms of glucocorticosteroid insufficiency may occur, requiring supplemental systemic corticosteroids.

Pediatric patients may be more susceptible to systemic toxicity from equivalent doses due to their larger skin surface to body mass ratios [see Use in Specific Populations (8.4)].

5.2   Allergic Contact Dermatitis

If irritation develops, ELOCON Ointment should be discontinued and appropriate therapy instituted. Allergic contact dermatitis with corticosteroids is usually diagnosed by observing failure to heal rather than noting a clinical exacerbation. Such an observation should be corroborated with appropriate diagnostic patch testing.

5.3   Concomitant Skin Infections

If concomitant skin infections are present or develop, an appropriate antifungal or antibacterial agent should be used. If a favorable response does not occur promptly, use of ELOCON Ointment should be discontinued until the infection has been adequately controlled.

6   ADVERSE REACTIONS

Because clinical trials are conducted under widely varying conditions, adverse reaction rates observed in the clinical trials of a drug cannot be directly compared to rates in the clinical trials of another drug and may not reflect the rates observed in clinical practice.

In controlled clinical trials involving 812 subjects, the incidence of adverse reactions associated with the use of ELOCON Ointment was 4.8%. Reported reactions included burning, pruritus, skin atrophy, tingling/stinging, and furunculosis. Cases of rosacea associated with the use of ELOCON Ointment have been reported.

The following adverse reactions were reported to be possibly or probably related to treatment with ELOCON Ointment during a clinical study in 5% of 63 pediatric subjects 6 months to 2 years of age: decreased glucocorticoid levels, 1; an unspecified skin disorder, 1; and a bacterial skin infection, 1. The following signs of skin atrophy were also observed among 63 subjects treated with ELOCON Ointment in a clinical trial: shininess, 4; telangiectasia, 1; loss of elasticity, 4; loss of normal skin markings, 4; and thinness, 1. The following additional local adverse reactions have been reported with topical corticosteroids, but may occur more frequently with the use of occlusive dressings. These reactions are: irritation, dryness, folliculitis, hypertrichosis, acneiform eruptions, hypopigmentation, perioral dermatitis, allergic contact dermatitis, secondary infection, skin atrophy, striae, and miliaria.

7   DRUG INTERACTIONS

No drug-drug interaction studies have been conducted with ELOCON Ointment.

8   USE IN SPECIFIC POPULATIONS
8.1   Pregnancy

Teratogenic Effects Pregnancy Category C:

There are no adequate and well-controlled studies in pregnant women. Therefore, ELOCON Ointment should be used during pregnancy only if the potential benefit justifies the potential risk to the fetus.

Corticosteroids have been shown to be teratogenic in laboratory animals when administered systemically at relatively low dosage levels. Some corticosteroids have been shown to be teratogenic after dermal application in laboratory animals.

When administered to pregnant rats, rabbits, and mice, mometasone furoate increased fetal malformations. The

doses that produced malformations also decreased fetal growth, as measured by lower fetal weights and/or delayed ossification. Mometasone furoate also caused dystocia and related complications when administered to rats during the end of pregnancy.

In mice, mometasone furoate caused cleft palate at subcutaneous doses of 60 mcg/kg and above. Fetal survival was reduced at 180 mcg/kg. No toxicity was observed at 20 mcg/kg. (Doses of 20, 60, and 180 mcg/kg in the mouse are approximately 0.01, 0.02, and 0.05 times the estimated maximum clinical topical dose from ELOCON Ointment on a mcg/m² basis.)

In rats, mometasone furoate produced umbilical hernias at topical doses of 600 mcg/kg and above. A dose of 300 mcg/kg produced delays in ossification, but no malformations. (Doses of 300 and 600 mcg/kg in the rat are approximately 0.2 and 0.4 times the estimated maximum clinical topical dose from ELOCON Ointment on a mcg/m² basis.)

In rabbits, mometasone furoate caused multiple malformations (e.g., flexed front paws, gallbladder agenesis, umbilical hernia, hydrocephaly) at topical doses of 150 mcg/kg and above (approximately 0.2 times the estimated maximum clinical topical dose from ELOCON Ointment on a mcg/m² basis). In an oral study, mometasone furoate increased resorptions and caused cleft palate and/or head malformations (hydrocephaly and domed head) at 700 mcg/kg. At 2800 mcg/kg most litters were aborted or resorbed. No toxicity was observed at 140 mcg/kg. (Doses of 140, 700, and 2800 mcg/kg in the rabbit are approximately 0.2, 0.9, and 3.6 times the estimated maximum clinical topical dose from ELOCON Ointment on a mcg/m² basis.)

When rats received subcutaneous doses of mometasone furoate throughout pregnancy or during the later stages of pregnancy, 15 mcg/kg caused prolonged and difficult labor and reduced the number of live births, birth weight, and early pup survival. Similar effects were not observed at 7.5 mcg/kg. (Doses of 7.5 and 15 mcg/kg in the rat are approximately 0.005 and 0.01 times the estimated maximum clinical topical dose from ELOCON Ointment on a mcg/m² basis.)

8.3   Nursing Mothers

Systemically administered corticosteroids appear in human milk and could suppress growth, interfere with endogenous corticosteroid production, or cause other untoward effects. It is not known whether topical administration of corticosteroids could result in sufficient systemic absorption to produce detectable quantities in human milk. Because many drugs are excreted in human milk, caution should be exercised when ELOCON Ointment is administered to a nursing woman.

8.4   Pediatric Use

ELOCON Ointment may be used with caution in pediatric patients 2 years of age or older, although the safety and efficacy of drug use for longer than 3 weeks have not been established. Since safety and efficacy of ELOCON Ointment have not been established in pediatric patients below 2 years of age, its use in this age group is not recommended. ELOCON Ointment caused HPA axis suppression in approximately 27% of pediatric subjects ages 6 to 23 months, who showed normal adrenal function by Cortrosyn test before starting treatment, and were treated for approximately 3 weeks over a mean body surface area of 39% (range 15%-99%). The criteria for suppression were: basal cortisol level of ≤5 mcg/dL, 30-minute post-stimulation level of ≤18 mcg/dL, or an increase of <7 mcg/dL. Follow-up testing 2 to 4 weeks after stopping treatment, available for 8 of the subjects, demonstrated suppressed HPA axis function in 3 subjects, using these same criteria. Long-term use of topical corticosteroids has not been studied in this population [see Clinical Pharmacology (12.2)].

Because of a higher ratio of skin surface area to body mass, pediatric patients are at a greater risk than adults of HPA axis suppression and Cushing's syndrome when they are treated with topical corticosteroids. They are, therefore, also at greater risk of glucocorticosteroid insufficiency during and/or after withdrawal of treatment. Pediatric patients may be more susceptible than adults to skin atrophy, including striae, when they are treated with topical corticosteroids. Pediatric patients applying topical corticosteroids to greater than 20% of body surface are at higher risk of HPA axis suppression.

HPA axis suppression, Cushing's syndrome, linear growth retardation, delayed weight gain, and intracranial hypertension have been reported in children receiving topical corticosteroids. Manifestations of adrenal suppression in children include low plasma cortisol levels and absence of response to ACTH stimulation. Manifestations of intracranial hypertension include bulging fontanelles, headaches, and bilateral papilledema.

ELOCON Ointment should not be used in the treatment of diaper dermatitis.

8.5   Geriatric Use

Clinical trials of ELOCON Ointment included 310 subjects who were 65 years of age and over and 57 subjects who were

75 years of age and over. No overall differences in safety or effectiveness were observed between these subjects and younger subjects, and other reported clinical experience has not identified differences in responses between the elderly and younger subjects. However, greater sensitivity of some older individuals cannot be ruled out.

10 OVERDOSAGE

Topically applied ELOCON Ointment can be absorbed in sufficient amounts to produce systemic effects [see Warnings and Precautions (5.1)].

11 DESCRIPTION

ELOCON (mometasone furoate) Ointment, 0.1% contains mometasone furoate for topical use. Mometasone furoate is a synthetic corticosteroid with anti-inflammatory activity. Chemically, mometasone furoate is $9\alpha,21$-dichloro-$11\beta,17$-dihydroxy-16α-methylpregna-1,4-diene-3,20-dione 17-(2-furoate), with the empirical formula $C_{27}H_{30}Cl_2O_6$, a molecular weight of 521.4 and the following structural formula:

Mometasone furoate is a white to off-white powder practically insoluble in water, slightly soluble in octanol, and moderately soluble in ethyl alcohol.

Each gram of ELOCON Ointment, 0.1% contains 1 mg mometasone furoate in a white to off-white uniform ointment base of hexylene glycol, phosphoric acid, propylene glycol stearate (55% monoester), purified water, white wax, and white petrolatum.

12 CLINICAL PHARMACOLOGY

12.1 Mechanism of Action

Like other topical corticosteroids, mometasone furoate has anti-inflammatory, antipruritic, and vasoconstrictive properties. The mechanism of the anti-inflammatory activity of the topical steroids, in general, is unclear. However, corticosteroids are thought to act by the induction of phospholipase A_2 inhibitory proteins, collectively called lipocortins. It is postulated that these proteins control the biosynthesis of potent mediators of inflammation such as prostaglandins and leukotrienes by inhibiting the release of their common precursor arachidonic acid. Arachidonic acid is released from membrane phospholipids by phospholipase A_2

12.2 Pharmacodynamics

Studies performed with ELOCON Ointment indicate that it is in the medium range of potency as compared with other topical corticosteroids.

In a study evaluating the effects of mometasone furoate ointment on the HPA axis, 15 grams were applied twice daily for 7 days to 6 adult subjects with psoriasis or atopic dermatitis. The ointment was applied without occlusion to at least 30% of the body surface. The results showed that the drug caused a slight lowering of adrenal corticosteroid secretion [see Warnings and Precautions (5.1)].

Sixty-three pediatric subjects ages 6 to 23 months, with atopic dermatitis, were enrolled in an open-label HPA axis safety study. ELOCON Ointment was applied once daily for approximately 3 weeks over a mean body surface area of 39% (range 15%-99%). In approximately 27% of subjects who showed normal adrenal function by Cortrosyn test before starting treatment, adrenal suppression was observed at the end of treatment with ELOCON Ointment. The criteria for suppression were: basal cortisol level of ≤5 mcg/dL, 30-minute post-stimulation level of ≤18 mcg/dL, or an increase of <7 mcg/dL. Follow-up testing 2 to 4 weeks after stopping treatment, available for 8 of the subjects, demonstrated suppressed HPA axis function in 3 subjects, using these same criteria [see Use in Specific Populations (8.4)].

12.3 Pharmacokinetics

The extent of percutaneous absorption of topical corticosteroids is determined by many factors including the vehicle and the integrity of the epidermal barrier. Studies in humans indicate that approximately 0.7% of the applied dose of ELOCON Ointment enters the circulation after 8 hours of contact with normal skin without occlusion. Inflammation and/or other disease processes in the skin may increase percutaneous absorption.

13 NONCLINICAL TOXICOLOGY

13.1 Carcinogenesis, Mutagenesis, Impairment of Fertility

Long-term animal studies have not been performed to evaluate the carcinogenic potential of ELOCON Ointment. Long-term carcinogenicity studies of mometasone furoate were conducted by the inhalation route in rats and mice. In a 2-year carcinogenicity study in Sprague Dawley rats, mometasone furoate demonstrated no statistically signifi-

cant increase of tumors at inhalation doses up to 67 mcg/kg (approximately 0.04 times the estimated maximum clinical topical dose from ELOCON Ointment on a mcg/m² basis). In a 19-month carcinogenicity study in Swiss CD-1 mice, mometasone furoate demonstrated no statistically significant increase in the incidence of tumors at inhalation doses up to 160 mcg/kg (approximately 0.05 times the estimated maximum clinical topical dose from ELOCON Ointment on a mcg/m² basis).

Mometasone furoate increased chromosomal aberrations in an in vitro Chinese hamster ovary cell assay, but did not increase chromosomal aberrations in an in vitro Chinese hamster lung cell assay. Mometasone furoate was not mutagenic in the Ames test or mouse lymphoma assay, and was not clastogenic in an in vivo mouse micronucleus assay, a rat bone marrow chromosomal aberration assay, or a mouse male germ-cell chromosomal aberration assay. Mometasone furoate also did not induce unscheduled DNA synthesis in vivo in rat hepatocytes.

In reproductive studies in rats, impairment of fertility was not produced in male or female rats by subcutaneous doses up to 15 mcg/kg (approximately 0.01 times the estimated maximum clinical topical dose from ELOCON Ointment on a mcg/m² basis).

14 CLINICAL STUDIES

The safety and efficacy of ELOCON Ointment, 0.1% for the treatment of corticosteroid-responsive dermatoses was demonstrated in two vehicle-controlled trials, one in psoriasis and one in atopic dermatitis. A total of 218 subjects received ELOCON Ointment (109 subjects) or the vehicle ointment applied once daily for 21 days.

16 HOW SUPPLIED/STORAGE AND HANDLING

ELOCON Ointment is a white to off-white uniform ointment and supplied in 15-gram (NDC 0085-0370-01) and 45-gram (NDC 0085-0370-02) tubes; boxes of one.
Store at 25°C (77°F); excursions permitted to 15-30°C (59-86°F) [see USP Controlled Room Temperature].

17 PATIENT COUNSELING INFORMATION

Inform patients of the following:
- Use ELOCON Ointment as directed by the physician. It is for external use only.
- Avoid contact with the eyes.
- Do not use ELOCON Ointment on the face, underarms, or groin areas.
- Do not use ELOCON Ointment for any disorder other than that for which it was prescribed.
- The treated skin area should not be bandaged or otherwise covered or wrapped so as to be occlusive, unless directed by the physician.
- Report any signs of local adverse reactions to the physician.
- Advise patients not to use ELOCON Ointment in the treatment of diaper dermatitis. Do not apply ELOCON Ointment in the diaper area, as diapers or plastic pants may constitute occlusive dressing.
- Discontinue therapy when control is achieved. If no improvement is seen within 2 weeks, contact the physician.
- Do not use other corticosteroid-containing products with ELOCON Ointment without first consulting with the physician.

Manufactured for: Merck Sharp & Dohme Corp., a subsidiary of
MERCK & CO., INC., Whitehouse Station, NJ 08889, USA
Manufactured by: Schering Plough Canada, Inc.
Pointe Claire, Quebec H9R 1B4, Canada
Copyright © 1987, 2008, 2012 Merck Sharp & Dohme Corp., a subsidiary of Merck & Co., Inc.
All rights reserved.
032088-EL-OT-USPI.6

EMEND®
[ē' mĕnd]
(aprepitant)
capsules, for oral use   Rx

HIGHLIGHTS OF PRESCRIBING INFORMATION

These highlights do not include all the information needed to use EMEND safely and effectively. See full prescribing information for EMEND.
EMEND (aprepitant) capsules, for oral use
Initial U.S. Approval: 2003

——INDICATIONS AND USAGE——

EMEND® is a substance P/neurokinin 1 (NK₁) receptor antagonist, indicated:
- in combination with other antiemetic agents for the:
  ◦ prevention of acute and delayed nausea and vomiting associated with initial and repeat courses of highly emetogenic cancer chemotherapy (HEC) including high-dose cisplatin (1.1)

  ◦ prevention of nausea and vomiting associated with initial and repeat courses of moderately emetogenic cancer chemotherapy (MEC) (1.1)
- for the prevention of postoperative nausea and vomiting (PONV) (1.2)
Limitations of Use (1.3)
- Not studied for the treatment of established nausea and vomiting.
- Chronic continuous administration is not recommended.

——DOSAGE AND ADMINISTRATION——

Prevention of Chemotherapy Induced Nausea and Vomiting (2.1)
- EMEND is given for 3 days as part of the chemotherapy induced nausea and vomiting (CINV) regimen that includes a corticosteroid and a 5-HT₃ antagonist. (2.1)
  ◦ The recommended dose of EMEND is 125 mg orally 1 hour prior to chemotherapy treatment (Day 1) and 80 mg orally once daily in the morning on Days 2 and 3. (2.1)
  ◦ EMEND (fosaprepitant dimeglumine) for Injection may be substituted for oral EMEND (125 mg) on Day 1 only as part of the CINV regimen. (2.1)
Prevention of Postoperative Nausea and Vomiting (2.2)
- The recommended oral dosage of EMEND for the postoperative nausea and vomiting (PONV) indication is 40 mg within 3 hours prior to induction of anesthesia. (2.2)

——DOSAGE FORMS AND STRENGTHS——

Capsules: 40 mg; 80 mg; 125 mg (3)

——CONTRAINDICATIONS——

- Hypersensitivity to any component of this medication. (4, 6.2)
- EMEND should not be used concurrently with pimozide, terfenadine, astemizole, or cisapride, since inhibition of CYP3A4 by aprepitant could result in elevated plasma concentrations of these drugs, potentially causing serious or life-threatening reactions. (4)

——WARNINGS AND PRECAUTIONS——

- Coadministration of aprepitant with warfarin (a CYP2C9 substrate) may result in a clinically significant decrease in International Normalized Ratio (INR) of prothrombin time. (5.2)
- The efficacy of hormonal contraceptives during and for 28 days following the last dose of EMEND may be reduced. Alternative or back-up methods of contraception should be used. (5.3, 7.1)
- EMEND is a dose-dependent inhibitor of CYP3A4, and should be used with caution in patients receiving concomitant medications that are primarily metabolized through CYP3A4. (5.1)
- Caution should be exercised when administered in patients with severe hepatic impairment. (2.5, 5.4, 12.3)

——ADVERSE REACTIONS——

- Clinical adverse experiences for the CINV regimen in conjunction with highly and moderately emetogenic chemotherapy (incidence >10%) are: alopecia, anorexia, asthenia/fatigue, constipation, diarrhea, headache, hiccups, nausea. (6.1)
- Clinical adverse experiences for the PONV regimen (incidence >5%) are: constipation, hypotension, nausea, pruritus, pyrexia. (6.1)

To report SUSPECTED ADVERSE REACTIONS, contact Merck Sharp & Dohme Corp., a subsidiary of Merck & Co., Inc., at 1-877-888-4231 or FDA at 1-800-FDA-1088 or www.fda.gov/medwatch.

——DRUG INTERACTIONS——

- Aprepitant is a substrate for CYP3A4; therefore, coadministration of EMEND with drugs that inhibit or induce CYP3A4 activity may result in increased or reduced plasma concentrations of aprepitant, respectively. (5.1, 7.1, 7.2).
- Aprepitant is an inducer of CYP2C9; therefore, coadministration of EMEND with drugs that are metabolized by CYP2C9 (e.g., warfarin, tolbutamide), may result in lower plasma concentrations of these drugs. (5.2, 7.1)

See 17 for PATIENT COUNSELING INFORMATION and FDA-approved patient labeling

Revised: 08/2014

FULL PRESCRIBING INFORMATION: CONTENTS*

	Day 1	Day 2	Day 3	Day 4
EMEND*	125 mg orally	80 mg orally	80 mg orally	none
Dexamethasone†	12 mg orally	8 mg orally	8 mg orally	8 mg orally
5-HT₃ antagonist	See the package insert for the selected 5-HT₃ antagonist for appropriate dosing information.	none	none	none

* EMEND is administered orally 1 hour prior to chemotherapy treatment on Day 1 and in the morning on Days 2 and 3.
† Dexamethasone is administered 30 minutes prior to chemotherapy treatment on Day 1 and in the morning on Days 2 through 4. The dose of dexamethasone accounts for drug interactions.

	Day 1	Day 2	Day 3
EMEND*	125 mg orally	80 mg orally	80 mg orally
Dexamethasone†	12 mg orally	none	none
5-HT₃ antagonist	See the package insert for the selected 5-HT₃ antagonist for appropriate dosing information.	none	none

* EMEND is administered orally 1 hour prior to chemotherapy treatment on Day 1 and in the morning on Days 2 and 3.
† Dexamethasone is administered 30 minutes prior to chemotherapy treatment on Day 1. The dose of dexamethasone accounts for drug interactions.

FULL PRESCRIBING INFORMATION

1   INDICATIONS AND USAGE
1.1   Prevention of Chemotherapy Induced Nausea and Vomiting (CINV)
EMEND®, in combination with other antiemetic agents, is indicated for the:
• prevention of acute and delayed nausea and vomiting associated with initial and repeat courses of highly emetogenic cancer chemotherapy (HEC) including high-dose cisplatin

• prevention of nausea and vomiting associated with initial and repeat courses of moderately emetogenic cancer chemotherapy (MEC) [see Dosage and Administration (2.1)].

1.2   Prevention of Postoperative Nausea and Vomiting (PONV)
EMEND is indicated for the prevention of postoperative nausea and vomiting [see Dosage and Administration (2.2)].

1.3   Limitations of Use
EMEND has not been studied for the treatment of established nausea and vomiting.
Chronic continuous administration is not recommended [see Warnings and Precautions (5.5)].

2   DOSAGE AND ADMINISTRATION
2.1   Prevention of Chemotherapy Induced Nausea and Vomiting (CINV)
Capsules of EMEND (aprepitant) are given for 3 days as part of a regimen that includes a corticosteroid and a 5-HT₃ antagonist. The recommended dose of EMEND is 125 mg orally 1 hour prior to chemotherapy treatment (Day 1) and 80 mg orally once daily in the morning on Days 2 and 3.
The package insert for the co-administered 5-HT₃ antagonist must be consulted prior to initiation of treatment with EMEND.
EMEND may be taken with or without food.
EMEND (fosaprepitant dimeglumine) for Injection (115 mg) is a prodrug of aprepitant and may be substituted for oral EMEND (125 mg), 30 minutes prior to chemotherapy, on Day 1 only of the CINV regimen as an intravenous infusion administered over 15 minutes.
The following regimen should be used for the prevention of nausea and vomiting associated with highly emetogenic cancer chemotherapy:
[See first table above]
The following regimen should be used for the prevention of nausea and vomiting associated with moderately emetogenic cancer chemotherapy:
[See second table above]
2.2   Prevention of Postoperative Nausea and Vomiting (PONV)
The recommended oral dosage of EMEND is 40 mg within 3 hours prior to induction of anesthesia.
EMEND may be taken with or without food.
2.3   Geriatric Patients
No dosage adjustment is necessary for the elderly.
2.4   Patients with Renal Impairment
No dosage adjustment is necessary for patients with renal impairment or for patients with end stage renal disease (ESRD) undergoing hemodialysis.
2.5   Patients with Hepatic Impairment
No dosage adjustment is necessary for patients with mild to moderate hepatic impairment (Child-Pugh score 5 to 9). There are no clinical data in patients with severe hepatic impairment (Child-Pugh score >9).

2.6   Coadministration with Other Drugs
For additional information on dose adjustment for corticosteroids when coadministered with EMEND, see Drug Interactions (7.1).
Refer to the full prescribing information for coadministered antiemetic agents.

3   DOSAGE FORMS AND STRENGTHS
• Capsules EMEND 40 mg are opaque, hard, gelatin capsules, with white body and mustard yellow cap with "464" and "40 mg" printed radially in black ink on the body.
• Capsules EMEND 80 mg are white, opaque, hard, gelatin capsules, with "461" and "80 mg" printed radially in black ink on the body.
• Capsules EMEND 125 mg are opaque, hard, gelatin capsules, with white body and pink cap with "462" and "125 mg" printed radially in black ink on the body.

4   CONTRAINDICATIONS
EMEND is contraindicated in patients who are hypersensitive to any component of the product.
EMEND is a dose-dependent inhibitor of cytochrome P450 isoenzyme 3A4 (CYP3A4). EMEND should not be used concurrently with pimozide, terfenadine, astemizole, or cisapride. Inhibition of CYP3A4 by aprepitant could result in elevated plasma concentrations of these drugs, potentially causing serious or life-threatening reactions [see Drug Interactions (7.1)].

5   WARNINGS AND PRECAUTIONS
5.1   CYP3A4 Interactions
EMEND (aprepitant), a dose-dependent inhibitor of CYP3A4, should be used with caution in patients receiving concomitant medications that are primarily metabolized through CYP3A4.
Moderate inhibition of CYP3A4 by aprepitant, 125-mg/80-mg regimen, could result in elevated plasma concentrations of these concomitant medications.
Weak inhibition of CYP3A4 by a single 40-mg dose of aprepitant is not expected to alter the plasma concentrations of concomitant medications that are primarily metabolized through CYP3A4 to a clinically significant degree.
When aprepitant is used concomitantly with another CYP3A4 inhibitor, aprepitant plasma concentrations could be elevated. When EMEND is used concomitantly with medications that induce CYP3A4 activity, aprepitant plasma concentrations could be reduced and this may result in decreased efficacy of EMEND [see Drug Interactions (7.1)].
Chemotherapy agents that are known to be metabolized by CYP3A4 include docetaxel, paclitaxel, etoposide, irinotecan, ifosfamide, imatinib, vinorelbine, vinblastine and vincristine. In clinical studies, EMEND (125-mg/80-mg regimen) was administered commonly with etoposide, vinorelbine, or paclitaxel. The doses of these agents were not adjusted to account for potential drug interactions.
In separate pharmacokinetic studies, no clinically significant change in docetaxel or vinorelbine pharmacokinetics was observed when EMEND (125-mg/80-mg regimen) was co-administered.
Due to the small number of patients in clinical studies who received the CYP3A4 substrates vinblastine, vincristine, or ifosfamide, particular caution and careful monitoring are advised in patients receiving these agents or other chemotherapy agents metabolized primarily by CYP3A4 that were not studied [see Drug Interactions (7.1)].
5.2   Coadministration with Warfarin (a CYP2C9 substrate)
Coadministration of EMEND with warfarin may result in a clinically significant decrease in International Normalized Ratio (INR) of prothrombin time. In patients on chronic warfarin therapy, the INR should be closely monitored in the 2-week period, particularly at 7 to 10 days, following initiation of the 3-day regimen of EMEND with each chemotherapy cycle, or following administration of a single 40-mg dose of EMEND for the prevention of postoperative nausea and vomiting [see Drug Interactions (7.1)].
5.3   Coadministration with Hormonal Contraceptives
Upon coadministration with EMEND, the efficacy of hormonal contraceptives during and for 28 days following the last dose of EMEND may be reduced. Alternative or back-up methods of contraception should be used during treatment with EMEND and for 1 month following the last dose of EMEND [see Drug Interactions (7.1)].
5.4   Patients with Severe Hepatic Impairment
There are no clinical or pharmacokinetic data in patients with severe hepatic impairment (Child-Pugh score >9). Therefore, caution should be exercised when EMEND is administered in these patients [see Clinical Pharmacology (12.3) and Dosage and Administration (2.5)].
5.5   Chronic Continuous Use
Chronic continuous use of EMEND for prevention of nausea and vomiting is not recommended because it has not been

studied; and because the drug interaction profile may change during chronic continuous use.

6   ADVERSE REACTIONS

The overall safety of aprepitant was evaluated in approximately 5300 individuals.

Because clinical trials are conducted under widely varying conditions, adverse reaction rates observed in the clinical trials of a drug cannot be directly compared to rates in the clinical trials of another drug and may not reflect the rates observed in clinical practice.

6.1   Clinical Trials Experience

Chemotherapy Induced Nausea and Vomiting
Highly Emetogenic Chemotherapy
In 2 well-controlled clinical trials in patients receiving highly emetogenic cancer chemotherapy, 544 patients were treated with aprepitant during Cycle 1 of chemotherapy and 413 of these patients continued into the Multiple-Cycle extension for up to 6 cycles of chemotherapy. EMEND was given in combination with ondansetron and dexamethasone.

In Cycle 1, clinical adverse experiences were reported in approximately 69% of patients treated with the aprepitant regimen compared with approximately 68% of patients treated with standard therapy. Table 1 shows the percent of patients with clinical adverse experiences reported at an incidence ≥3%.

Table 1: Percent of Patients Receiving Highly Emetogenic Chemotherapy with Clinical Adverse Experiences (Incidence ≥3%) — Cycle 1

	Aprepitant Regimen (N = 544)	Standard Therapy (N = 550)
Body as a Whole/Site Unspecified		
Asthenia/Fatigue	17.8	11.8
Dizziness	6.6	4.4
Dehydration	5.9	5.1
Abdominal Pain	4.6	3.3
Fever	2.9	3.5
Mucous Membrane Disorder	2.6	3.1
Digestive System		
Nausea	12.7	11.8
Constipation	10.3	12.2
Diarrhea	10.3	7.5
Vomiting	7.5	7.6
Heartburn	5.3	4.9
Gastritis	4.2	3.1
Epigastric Discomfort	4.0	3.1
Eyes, Ears, Nose, and Throat		
Tinnitus	3.7	3.8
Hemic and Lymphatic System		
Neutropenia	3.1	2.9
Metabolism and Nutrition		
Anorexia	10.1	9.5
Nervous System		
Headache	8.5	8.7
Insomnia	2.9	3.1
Respiratory System		
Hiccups	10.8	5.6

In addition, isolated cases of serious adverse experiences, regardless of causality, of bradycardia, disorientation, and perforating duodenal ulcer were reported in highly emetogenic CINV clinical studies.

Moderately Emetogenic Chemotherapy
During Cycle 1 of 2 moderately emetogenic chemotherapy studies, 868 patients were treated with the aprepitant regimen and 686 of these patients continued into extensions for up to 4 cycles of chemotherapy. In the combined analysis of Cycle 1 data for these 2 studies, adverse experiences were reported in approximately 69% of patients treated with the aprepitant regimen compared with approximately 72% of patients treated with standard therapy.

In the combined analysis of Cycle 1 data for these 2 studies, the adverse experience profile in both moderately emetogenic chemotherapy studies was generally comparable to the highly emetogenic chemotherapy studies. Table 2 shows the percent of patients with clinical adverse experiences reported at an incidence ≥3%.

Table 2: Percent of Patients Receiving Moderately Emetogenic Chemotherapy with Clinical Adverse Experiences (Incidence ≥3%) — Cycle 1

	Aprepitant Regimen (N = 868)	Standard Therapy (N = 846)
Blood and Lymphatic System Disorders		
Neutropenia	5.8	5.6
Metabolism and Nutrition Disorders		
Anorexia	6.2	7.2
Psychiatric Disorders		
Insomnia	2.6	3.7
Nervous System Disorders		
Headache	13.2	14.3
Dizziness	2.8	3.4
Gastrointestinal Disorders		
Constipation	10.3	15.5
Diarrhea	7.6	8.7
Dyspepsia	5.8	3.8
Nausea	5.8	5.1
Stomatitis	3.1	2.7
Skin and Subcutaneous Tissue Disorders		
Alopecia	12.4	11.9
General Disorders and General Administration Site Conditions		
Fatigue	15.4	15.6
Asthenia	4.7	4.6

In a combined analysis of these two studies, isolated cases of serious adverse experiences were similar in the two treatment groups.

Highly and Moderately Emetogenic Chemotherapy
The following additional clinical adverse experiences (incidence >0.5% and greater than standard therapy), regardless of causality, were reported in patients treated with aprepitant regimen in either HEC or MEC studies:

Infections and infestations: candidiasis, herpes simplex, lower respiratory infection, oral candidiasis, pharyngitis, septic shock, upper respiratory infection, urinary tract infection.

Neoplasms benign, malignant and unspecified (including cysts and polyps): malignant neoplasm, non-small cell lung carcinoma.

Blood and lymphatic system disorders: anemia, febrile neutropenia, thrombocytopenia.

Metabolism and nutrition disorders: appetite decreased, diabetes mellitus, hypokalemia.

Psychiatric disorders: anxiety disorder, confusion, depression.

Nervous system: peripheral neuropathy, sensory neuropathy, taste disturbance, tremor.

Eye disorders: conjunctivitis.

Cardiac disorders: myocardial infarction, palpitations, tachycardia.

Vascular disorders: deep venous thrombosis, flushing, hot flush, hypertension, hypotension.

Respiratory, thoracic and mediastinal disorders: cough, dyspnea, nasal secretion, pharyngolaryngeal pain, pneumonitis, pulmonary embolism, respiratory insufficiency, vocal disturbance.

Gastrointestinal disorders: abdominal pain upper, acid reflux, deglutition disorder, dry mouth, dysgeusia, dysphagia, eructation, flatulence, obstipation, salivation increased.

Skin and subcutaneous tissue disorders: acne, diaphoresis, pruritus, rash.

Musculoskeletal and connective tissue disorders: arthralgia, back pain, muscular weakness, musculoskeletal pain, myalgia.

Renal and urinary disorders: dysuria, renal insufficiency.

Reproductive system and breast disorders: pelvic pain.

General disorders and administrative site conditions: edema, malaise, pain, rigors.

Investigations: weight loss.

Stevens-Johnson syndrome was reported as a serious adverse experience in a patient receiving aprepitant with cancer chemotherapy in another CINV study.

Laboratory Adverse Experiences
Table 3 shows the percent of patients with laboratory adverse experiences reported at an incidence ≥3% in patients receiving highly emetogenic chemotherapy.

Table 3: Percent of Patients Receiving Highly Emetogenic Chemotherapy with Laboratory Adverse Experiences (Incidence ≥3%) — Cycle 1

	Aprepitant Regimen (N = 544)	Standard Therapy (N = 550)
Proteinuria	6.8	5.3
ALT Increased	6.0	4.3
Blood Urea Nitrogen Increased	4.7	3.5
Serum Creatinine Increased	3.7	4.3
AST Increased	3.0	1.3

The following additional laboratory adverse experiences (incidence >0.5% and greater than standard therapy), regardless of causality, were reported in patients treated with aprepitant regimen: alkaline phosphatase increased, hyperglycemia, hyponatremia, leukocytes increased, erythrocyturia, leukocyturia.

The adverse experience profiles in the Multiple-Cycle extensions of HEC and MEC studies for up to 6 cycles of chemotherapy were generally similar to that observed in Cycle 1.

Postoperative Nausea and Vomiting
In well-controlled clinical studies in patients receiving general anesthesia, 564 patients were administered 40-mg aprepitant orally and 538 patients were administered 4-mg ondansetron IV.

Clinical adverse experiences were reported in approximately 60% of patients treated with 40-mg aprepitant compared with approximately 64% of patients treated with 4-mg ondansetron IV. Table 4 shows the percent of patients with clinical adverse experiences reported at an incidence ≥3% of the combined studies.

Table 4: Percent of Patients Receiving General Anesthesia with Clinical Adverse Experiences (Incidence ≥3%)

	Aprepitant 40 mg (N = 564)	Ondansetron (N = 538)
Infections and Infestations		
Urinary Tract Infection	2.3	3.2
Blood and Lymphatic System Disorders		
Anemia	3.0	4.3
Psychiatric Disorders		
Insomnia	2.1	3.3
Nervous System Disorders		
Headache	5.0	6.5
Cardiac Disorders		
Bradycardia	4.4	3.9
Vascular Disorders		
Hypotension	5.7	4.6
Hypertension	2.1	3.2
Gastrointestinal Disorders		
Nausea	8.5	8.6
Constipation	8.5	7.6
Flatulence	4.1	5.8
Vomiting	2.5	3.9
Skin and Subcutaneous Tissue Disorders		
Pruritus	7.6	8.4
General Disorders and General Administration Site Conditions		
Pyrexia	5.9	10.6

The following additional clinical adverse experiences (incidence >0.5% and greater than ondansetron), regardless of causality, were reported in patients treated with aprepitant:

Infections and infestations: postoperative infection

Metabolism and nutrition disorders: hypokalemia, hypovolemia.

Nervous system disorders: dizziness, hypoesthesia, syncope.

Vascular disorders: hematoma

Respiratory, thoracic and mediastinal disorders: dyspnea, hypoxia, respiratory depression.

Gastrointestinal disorders: abdominal pain, abdominal pain upper, dry mouth, dyspepsia.

Skin and subcutaneous tissue disorders: urticaria

General disorders and administrative site conditions: hypothermia, pain.

Investigations: blood pressure decreased

Injury, poisoning and procedural complications: operative hemorrhage, wound dehiscence.

Other adverse experiences (incidence ≤0.5%) reported in patients treated with aprepitant 40 mg for postoperative nausea and vomiting included:

Nervous system disorders: dysarthria, sensory disturbance.

Eye disorders: miosis, visual acuity reduced.

Respiratory, thoracic and mediastinal disorders: wheezing

Gastrointestinal disorders: bowel sounds abnormal, stomach discomfort.

There were no serious adverse drug-related experiences reported in the postoperative nausea and vomiting clinical studies in patients taking 40-mg aprepitant.

Laboratory Adverse Experiences

One laboratory adverse experience, hemoglobin decreased (40-mg aprepitant 3.8%, ondansetron 4.2%), was reported at an incidence ≥3% in a patient receiving general anesthesia. The following additional laboratory adverse experiences (incidence >0.5% and greater than ondansetron), regardless of causality, were reported in patients treated with aprepitant 40 mg: blood albumin decreased, blood bilirubin increased, blood glucose increased, blood potassium decreased, glucose urine present.

The adverse experience of ALT increased occurred with similar incidence in patients treated with aprepitant 40 mg (1.1%) as in patients treated with ondansetron 4 mg (1.0%).

Other Studies

In addition, two serious adverse experiences were reported in postoperative nausea and vomiting (PONV) clinical studies in patients taking a higher dose of aprepitant: one case of constipation, and one case of sub-ileus.

Angioedema and urticaria were reported as serious adverse experiences in a patient receiving aprepitant in a non-CINV/non-PONV study.

6.2 Postmarketing Experience

The following adverse reactions have been identified during postmarketing use of aprepitant. Because these reactions are reported voluntarily from a population of uncertain size, it is generally not possible to reliably estimate their frequency or establish a causal relationship to drug exposure.

Skin and subcutaneous tissue disorders: pruritus, rash, urticaria, rarely Stevens-Johnson syndrome/toxic epidermal necrolysis.

Immune system disorders: hypersensitivity reactions including anaphylactic reactions.

Nervous system disorders: Events of ifosfamide-induced neurotoxicity have been reported after aprepitant and ifosfamide coadministration.

7 DRUG INTERACTIONS

Aprepitant is a substrate, a weak-to-moderate (dose-dependent) inhibitor, and an inducer of CYP3A4. Aprepitant is also an inducer of CYP2C9.

7.1 Effect of Aprepitant on the Pharmacokinetics of Other Agents

CYP3A4 substrates:

Weak inhibition of CYP3A4 by a single 40-mg dose of aprepitant is not expected to alter the plasma concentrations of concomitant medications that are primarily metabolized through CYP3A4 to a clinically significant degree. However, higher aprepitant doses or repeated dosing at any aprepitant dose may have a clinically significant effect.

As a moderate inhibitor of CYP3A4 at a dose of 125 mg/80 mg, aprepitant can increase plasma concentrations of concomitantly administered oral medications that are metabolized through CYP3A4 *[see Contraindications (4)]*. The use of fosaprepitant may increase CYP3A4 substrate plasma concentrations to a lesser degree than the use of oral aprepitant (125 mg).

5-HT₃ antagonists: In clinical drug interaction studies, aprepitant did not have clinically important effects on the pharmacokinetics of ondansetron, granisetron, or hydrodolasetron (the active metabolite of dolasetron).

Corticosteroids:

Dexamethasone: EMEND, when given as a regimen of 125 mg with dexamethasone coadministered orally as 20 mg on Day 1, and EMEND when given as 80 mg/day with dexamethasone coadministered orally as 8 mg on Days 2 through 5, increased the AUC of dexamethasone, a CYP3A4 substrate, by 2.2-fold on Days 1 and 5. The oral dexamethasone doses should be reduced by approximately 50% when coadministered with EMEND (125-mg/80-mg regimen), to achieve exposures of dexamethasone similar to those obtained when it is given without EMEND. The daily

dose of dexamethasone administered in clinical chemotherapy induced nausea and vomiting studies with EMEND reflects an approximate 50% reduction of the dose of dexamethasone *[see Dosage and Administration (2.1)]*. A single dose of EMEND (40 mg) when coadministered with a single oral dose of dexamethasone 20 mg, increased the AUC of dexamethasone by 1.45-fold. Therefore, no dose adjustment is recommended.

Methylprednisolone: EMEND, when given as a regimen of 125 mg on Day 1 and 80 mg/day on Days 2 and 3, increased the AUC of methylprednisolone, a CYP3A4 substrate, by 1.34-fold on Day 1 and by 2.5-fold on Day 3, when methylprednisolone was coadministered intravenously as 125 mg on Day 1 and orally as 40 mg on Days 2 and 3. The IV methylprednisolone dose should be reduced by approximately 25%, and the oral methylprednisolone dose should be reduced by approximately 50% when coadministered with EMEND (125-mg/80-mg regimen) to achieve exposures of methylprednisolone similar to those obtained when it is given without EMEND. Although the concomitant administration of methylprednisolone with the single 40-mg dose of aprepitant has not been studied, a single 40-mg dose of EMEND produces a weak inhibition of CYP3A4 (based on midazolam interaction study) and it is not expected to alter the plasma concentrations of methylprednisolone to a clinically significant degree. Therefore, no dose adjustment is recommended.

Chemotherapeutic agents:

Docetaxel: In a pharmacokinetic study, EMEND (125-mg/80-mg regimen) did not influence the pharmacokinetics of docetaxel.

Vinorelbine: In a pharmacokinetic study, EMEND (125-mg/80-mg regimen) did not influence the pharmacokinetics of vinorelbine to a clinically significant degree.

Other Chemotherapeutic Agents: EMEND should be used with caution in patients receiving other chemotherapeutic agents that are primarily metabolized through CYP3A4 *[see Warnings and Precautions (5.1) and Adverse Reactions (6.2)]*.

CYP2C9 substrates (Warfarin, Tolbutamide):

Aprepitant has been shown to induce the metabolism of S(-) warfarin and tolbutamide, which are metabolized through CYP2C9. Coadministration of EMEND with these drugs or other drugs that are known to be metabolized by CYP2C9, such as phenytoin, may result in lower plasma concentrations of these drugs.

Warfarin: A single 125-mg dose of EMEND was administered on Day 1 and 80 mg/day on Days 2 and 3 to healthy subjects who were stabilized on chronic warfarin therapy. Although there was no effect of EMEND on the plasma AUC of R(+) or S(-) warfarin determined on Day 3, there was a 34% decrease in S(-) warfarin (a CYP2C9 substrate) trough concentration accompanied by a 14% decrease in the prothrombin time (reported as International Normalized Ratio or INR) 5 days after completion of dosing with EMEND. In patients on chronic warfarin therapy, the prothrombin time (INR) should be closely monitored in the 2-week period, particularly at 7 to 10 days, following initiation of the 3-day regimen of EMEND with each chemotherapy cycle, or following administration of a single 40-mg dose of EMEND for the prevention of postoperative nausea and vomiting.

Tolbutamide: EMEND, when given as 125 mg on Day 1 and 80 mg/day on Days 2 and 3, decreased the AUC of tolbutamide (a CYP2C9 substrate) by 23% on Day 4, 28% on Day 8, and 15% on Day 15, when a single dose of tolbutamide 500 mg was administered orally prior to the administration of the 3-day regimen of EMEND and on Days 4, 8, and 15.

EMEND, when given as a 40-mg single oral dose on Day 1, decreased the AUC of tolbutamide (a CYP2C9 substrate) by 8% on Day 2, 16% on Day 4, 15% on Day 8, and 10% on Day 15, when a single dose of tolbutamide 500 mg was administered orally prior to the administration of EMEND 40 mg and on Days 2, 4, 8, and 15. This effect was not considered clinically important.

Oral contraceptives: Aprepitant, when given once daily for 14 days as a 100-mg capsule with an oral contraceptive containing 35 mcg of ethinyl estradiol and 1 mg of norethindrone, decreased the AUC of ethinyl estradiol by 43%, and decreased the AUC of norethindrone by 8%.

In another study, a daily dose of an oral contraceptive containing ethinyl estradiol and norethindrone was administered on Days 1 through 21, and EMEND was given as a 3-day regimen of 125 mg on Day 8 and 80 mg/day on Days 9 and 10 with ondansetron 32 mg IV on Day 8 and oral dexamethasone given as 12 mg on Day 8 and 8 mg/day on Days 9, 10, and 11. In the study, the AUC of ethinyl estradiol decreased by 19% on Day 10 and there was as much as a 64% decrease in ethinyl estradiol trough concentrations during Days 9 through 21. While there was no effect of EMEND on the AUC of norethindrone on Day 10, there was as much as a 60% decrease in norethindrone trough concentrations during Days 9 through 21.

In another study, a daily dose of an oral contraceptive containing ethinyl estradiol and norgestimate (which is converted to norelgestromin) was administered on Days 1 through 21, and EMEND 40 mg was given on Day 8. In the study, the AUC of ethinyl estradiol decreased by 4% and 29% on Day 8 and Day 12, respectively, while the AUC of norelgestromin increased by 18% on Day 8 and decreased by 10% on Day 12. In addition, the trough concentrations of ethinyl estradiol and norelgestromin on Days 8 through 21 were generally lower following coadministration of the oral contraceptive with EMEND 40 mg on Day 8 compared to the trough levels following administration of the oral contraceptive alone.

The coadministration of EMEND may reduce the efficacy of hormonal contraceptives (these can include birth control pills, skin patches, implants, and certain IUDs) during and for 28 days after administration of the last dose of EMEND. Alternative or back-up methods of contraception should be used during treatment with EMEND and for 1 month following the last dose of EMEND.

Midazolam: EMEND increased the AUC of midazolam, a sensitive CYP3A4 substrate, by 2.3-fold on Day 1 and 3.3-fold on Day 5, when a single oral dose of midazolam 2 mg was coadministered on Day 1 and Day 5 of a regimen of EMEND 125 mg on Day 1 and 80 mg/day on Days 2 through 5. The potential effects of increased plasma concentrations of midazolam or other benzodiazepines metabolized via CYP3A4 (alprazolam, triazolam) should be considered when coadministering these agents with EMEND (125 mg/80 mg). A single dose of EMEND (40 mg) increased the AUC of midazolam by 1.2-fold on Day 1, when a single oral dose of midazolam 2 mg was coadministered on Day 1 with EMEND 40 mg; this effect was not considered clinically important.

In another study with intravenous administration of midazolam, EMEND was given as 125 mg on Day 1 and 80 mg/day on Days 2 and 3, and midazolam 2 mg IV was given prior to the administration of the 3-day regimen of EMEND and on Days 4, 8, and 15. EMEND increased the AUC of midazolam by 25% on Day 4 and decreased the AUC of midazolam by 19% on Day 8 relative to the dosing of EMEND on Days 1 through 3. These effects were not considered clinically important. The AUC of midazolam on Day 15 was similar to that observed at baseline.

An additional study was completed with intravenous administration of midazolam and EMEND. Intravenous midazolam 2 mg was given 1 hour after oral administration of a single dose of EMEND 125 mg. The plasma AUC of midazolam was increased by 1.5-fold. Depending on clinical situations (e.g., elderly patients) and degree of monitoring available, dosage adjustment for intravenous midazolam may be necessary when it is coadministered with EMEND for the chemotherapy induced nausea and vomiting indication (125 mg on Day 1 followed by 80 mg on Days 2 and 3).

7.2 Effect of Other Agents on the Pharmacokinetics of Aprepitant

Aprepitant is a substrate for CYP3A4; therefore, coadministration of EMEND with drugs that inhibit CYP3A4 activity may result in increased plasma concentrations of aprepitant. Consequently, concomitant administration of EMEND with strong CYP3A4 inhibitors (e.g., ketoconazole, itraconazole, nefazodone, troleandomycin, clarithromycin, ritonavir, nelfinavir) should be approached with caution. Because moderate CYP3A4 inhibitors (e.g., diltiazem) result in a 2-fold increase in plasma concentrations of aprepitant, concomitant administration should also be approached with caution.

Aprepitant is a substrate for CYP3A4; therefore, coadministration of EMEND with drugs that strongly induce CYP3A4 activity (e.g., rifampin, carbamazepine, phenytoin) may result in reduced plasma concentrations of aprepitant that may result in decreased efficacy of EMEND.

Ketoconazole: When a single 125-mg dose of EMEND was administered on Day 5 of a 10-day regimen of 400 mg/day of ketoconazole, a strong CYP3A4 inhibitor, the AUC of aprepitant increased approximately 5-fold and the mean terminal half-life of aprepitant increased approximately 3-fold. Concomitant administration of EMEND with strong CYP3A4 inhibitors should be approached cautiously.

Rifampin: When a single 375-mg dose of EMEND was administered on Day 9 of a 14-day regimen of 600 mg/day of rifampin, a strong CYP3A4 inducer, the AUC of aprepitant decreased approximately 11-fold and the mean terminal half-life decreased approximately 3-fold.

Coadministration of EMEND with drugs that induce CYP3A4 activity may result in reduced plasma concentrations and decreased efficacy of EMEND.

7.3 Additional Interactions

EMEND is unlikely to interact with drugs that are substrates for the P-glycoprotein transporter, as demonstrated by the lack of interaction of EMEND with digoxin in a clinical drug interaction study.

Diltiazem: In patients with mild to moderate hypertension, administration of aprepitant once daily, as a tablet formulation comparable to 230 mg of the capsule formulation, with diltiazem 120 mg 3 times daily for 5 days, resulted in a 2-fold increase of aprepitant AUC and a simultaneous 1.7-fold increase of diltiazem AUC. These pharmacokinetic effects did not result in clinically meaningful changes in ECG, heart rate or blood pressure beyond those changes induced by diltiazem alone.

Paroxetine: Coadministration of once daily doses of aprepitant, as a tablet formulation comparable to 85 mg or 170 mg of the capsule formulation, with paroxetine 20 mg once daily, resulted in a decrease in AUC by approximately 25% and C_{max} by approximately 20% of both aprepitant and paroxetine.

8 USE IN SPECIFIC POPULATIONS

8.1 Pregnancy
Teratogenic effects
Pregnancy Category B: Reproduction studies have been performed in rats at oral doses up to 1000 mg/kg twice daily (plasma AUC_{0-24hr} of 31.3 mcg•hr/mL, about 1.6 times the human exposure at the recommended dose) and in rabbits at oral doses up to 25 mg/kg/day (plasma AUC_{0-24hr} of 26.9 mcg•hr/mL, about 1.4 times the human exposure at the recommended dose) and have revealed no evidence of impaired fertility or harm to the fetus due to aprepitant. There are, however, no adequate and well-controlled studies in pregnant women. Because animal reproduction studies are not always predictive of human response, this drug should be used during pregnancy only if clearly needed.

8.3 Nursing Mothers
Aprepitant is excreted in the milk of rats. It is not known whether this drug is excreted in human milk. Because many drugs are excreted in human milk and because of the potential for possible serious adverse reactions in nursing infants from aprepitant and because of the potential for tumorigenicity shown for aprepitant in rodent carcinogenicity studies, a decision should be made whether to discontinue nursing or to discontinue the drug, taking into account the importance of the drug to the mother.

8.4 Pediatric Use
Safety and effectiveness of EMEND in pediatric patients have not been established.

8.5 Geriatric Use
In 2 well-controlled chemotherapy-induced nausea and vomiting clinical studies, of the total number of patients (N=544) treated with EMEND, 31% were 65 and over, while 5% were 75 and over. In well-controlled postoperative nausea and vomiting clinical studies, of the total number of patients (N=1120) treated with EMEND, 7% were 65 and over, while 2% were 75 and over. No overall differences in safety or effectiveness were observed between these subjects and younger subjects. Greater sensitivity of some older individuals cannot be ruled out. Dosage adjustment in the elderly is not necessary.

10 OVERDOSAGE
No specific information is available on the treatment of overdosage.

Drowsiness and headache were reported in one patient who ingested 1440 mg of aprepitant.

In the event of overdose, EMEND should be discontinued and general supportive treatment and monitoring should be provided. Because of the antiemetic activity of aprepitant, drug-induced emesis may not be effective.

Aprepitant cannot be removed by hemodialysis.

11 DESCRIPTION
EMEND (aprepitant) is a substance P/neurokinin 1 (NK_1) receptor antagonist, chemically described as 5-[[(2*R*, 3*S*)-2-[(1*R*)-1-[3,5-bis(trifluoromethyl)phenyl]ethoxy]-3-(4-fluorophenyl)-4-morpholinyl]methyl]-1,2-dihydro-3*H*-1,2,4-triazol-3-one.

Its empirical formula is $C_{23}H_{21}F_7N_4O_3$, and its structural formula is:

Aprepitant is a white to off-white crystalline solid, with a molecular weight of 534.43. It is practically insoluble in water. Aprepitant is sparingly soluble in ethanol and isopropyl acetate and slightly soluble in acetonitrile.

Each capsule of EMEND for oral administration contains either 40 mg, 80 mg, or 125 mg of aprepitant and the following inactive ingredients: sucrose, microcrystalline cellulose, hydroxypropyl cellulose and sodium lauryl sulfate. The capsule shell excipients are gelatin, titanium dioxide, and may contain sodium lauryl sulfate and silicon dioxide. The 40-mg

capsule shell also contains yellow ferric oxide, and the 125-mg capsule also contains red ferric oxide and yellow ferric oxide.

12 CLINICAL PHARMACOLOGY

12.1 Mechanism of Action
Aprepitant is a selective high-affinity antagonist of human substance P/neurokinin 1 (NK_1) receptors. Aprepitant has little or no affinity for serotonin (5-HT_3), dopamine, and corticosteroid receptors, the targets of existing therapies for chemotherapy-induced nausea and vomiting (CINV) and postoperative nausea and vomiting (PONV).

Aprepitant has been shown in animal models to inhibit emesis induced by cytotoxic chemotherapeutic agents, such as cisplatin, via central actions. Animal and human Positron Emission Tomography (PET) studies with aprepitant have shown that it crosses the blood brain barrier and occupies brain NK_1 receptors. Animal and human studies show that aprepitant augments the antiemetic activity of the 5-HT_3-receptor antagonist ondansetron and the corticosteroid dexamethasone and inhibits both the acute and delayed phases of cisplatin-induced emesis.

12.2 Pharmacodynamics
NK_1 Receptor Occupancy
In two single-blind, multiple-dose, randomized, and placebo-controlled studies, healthy young men received oral aprepitant doses of 10 mg (N=2), 30 mg (N=3), 100 mg (N=3) or 300 mg (N=5) once daily for 14 days with 2 or 3 subjects on placebo. Both plasma aprepitant concentration and NK_1 receptor occupancy in the corpus striatum by positron emission tomography were evaluated, at predose and 24 hours after the last dose. At aprepitant plasma concentrations of ~10 ng/mL and ~100 ng/mL, the NK_1 receptor occupancies were ~50% and ~90%, respectively. The oral aprepitant regimen for CINV produces mean trough plasma aprepitant concentrations >500 ng/mL, which would be expected to, based on the fitted curve with the Hill equation, result in >95% brain NK_1 receptor occupancy. However, the receptor occupancy for either CINV or PONV dosing regimen has not been determined. In addition, the relationship between NK_1 receptor occupancy and the clinical efficacy of aprepitant has not been established.

Cardiac Electrophysiology
In a randomized, double-blind, positive-controlled, thorough QTc study, a single 200-mg dose of fosaprepitant had no effect on the QTc interval. QT prolongation with the oral dosing regimens for CINV and PONV are not expected.

12.3 Pharmacokinetics
Absorption
Following oral administration of a single 40-mg dose of EMEND in the fasted state, mean area under the plasma concentration-time curve ($AUC_{0-\infty}$) was 7.8 mcg•hr/mL and mean peak plasma concentration (C_{max}) was 0.7 mcg/mL, occurring at approximately 3 hours postdose (T_{max}). The absolute bioavailability at the 40-mg dose has not been determined.

Following oral administration of a single 125-mg dose of EMEND on Day 1 and 80 mg once daily on Days 2 and 3, the AUC_{0-24hr} was approximately 19.6 mcg•hr/mL and 21.2 mcg•hr/mL on Day 1 and Day 3, respectively. The C_{max} of 1.6 mcg/mL and 1.4 mcg/mL were reached in approximately 4 hours (T_{max}) on Day 1 and Day 3, respectively. At the dose range of 80-125 mg, the mean absolute oral bioavailability of aprepitant is approximately 60 to 65%. Oral administration of the capsule with a standard high-fat breakfast had no clinically meaningful effect on the bioavailability of aprepitant.

The pharmacokinetics of aprepitant are non-linear across the clinical dose range. In healthy young adults, the increase in $AUC_{0-\infty}$ was 26% greater than dose proportional between 80-mg and 125-mg single doses administered in the fed state.

Distribution
Aprepitant is greater than 95% bound to plasma proteins. The mean apparent volume of distribution at steady state (Vd_{ss}) is approximately 70 L in humans.

Aprepitant crosses the placenta in rats and rabbits and crosses the blood brain barrier in humans [see Clinical Pharmacology (12.1)].

Metabolism
Aprepitant undergoes extensive metabolism. *In vitro* studies using human liver microsomes indicate that aprepitant is metabolized primarily by CYP3A4 with minor metabolism by CYP1A2 and CYP2C19. Metabolism is largely via oxidation at the morpholine ring and its side chains. No metabolism by CYP2D6, CYP2C9, or CYP2E1 was detected. In healthy young adults, aprepitant accounts for approximately 24% of the radioactivity in plasma over 72 hours following a single oral 300-mg dose of [^{14}C]-aprepitant, indicating a substantial presence of metabolites in the plasma. Seven metabolites of aprepitant, which are only weakly active, have been identified in human plasma.

Excretion
Following administration of a single IV 100-mg dose of [^{14}C]-aprepitant prodrug to healthy subjects, 57% of the radioactivity was recovered in urine and 45% in feces. A study was not conducted with radiolabeled capsule formulation. The results after oral administration may differ.

Aprepitant is eliminated primarily by metabolism; aprepitant is not renally excreted. The apparent plasma clearance of aprepitant ranged from approximately 62 to 90 mL/min. The apparent terminal half-life ranged from approximately 9 to 13 hours.

Specific Populations
Gender
Following oral administration of a single dose of EMEND, the AUC_{0-24hr} and C_{max} are 14% and 22% higher in females as compared with males. The half-life of aprepitant is 25% lower in females as compared with males and T_{max} occurs at approximately the same time. These differences are not considered clinically meaningful. No dosage adjustment is necessary based on gender.

Geriatric
Following oral administration of a single 125-mg dose of EMEND on Day 1 and 80 mg once daily on Days 2 through 5, the AUC_{0-24hr} of aprepitant was 21% higher on Day 1 and 36% higher on Day 5 in elderly (≥65 years) relative to younger adults. The C_{max} was 10% higher on Day 1 and 24% higher on Day 5 in elderly relative to younger adults. These differences are not considered clinically meaningful. No dosage adjustment is necessary in elderly patients.

Race
Following oral administration of a single dose of EMEND, the AUC_{0-24hr} and C_{max} are approximately 42% and 29% higher in Hispanics as compared with Caucasians. The AUC_{0-24hr} and C_{max} are 62% and 41% higher in Asians as compared to Caucasians. There was no difference in AUC_{0-24hr} or C_{max} between Caucasians and Blacks. These differences are not considered clinically meaningful. No dosage adjustment is necessary based on race.

Body Mass Index (BMI)
For every 5 kg/m² increase in BMI, AUC_{0-24hr} and C_{max} of aprepitant decrease by 10%. BMI of subjects in the analysis ranged from 18 kg/m² to 36 kg/m². This change is not considered clinically meaningful. No dosage adjustment is necessary based on BMI.

Hepatic Insufficiency
Following administration of a single 125-mg dose of EMEND on Day 1 and 80 mg once daily on Days 2 and 3 to patients with mild hepatic impairment (Child-Pugh score 5 to 6), the AUC_{0-24hr} of aprepitant was 11% lower on Day 1 and 36% lower on Day 3, as compared with healthy subjects given the same regimen. In patients with moderate hepatic impairment (Child-Pugh score 7 to 9), the AUC_{0-24hr} of aprepitant was 10% higher on Day 1 and 18% higher on Day 3, as compared with healthy subjects given the same regimen. These differences in AUC_{0-24hr} are not considered clinically meaningful; therefore, no dosage adjustment is necessary in patients with mild to moderate hepatic impairment. There are no clinical or pharmacokinetic data in patients with severe hepatic impairment (Child-Pugh score >9) [see Warnings and Precautions (5.4)].

Renal Insufficiency
A single 240-mg dose of EMEND was administered to patients with severe renal impairment (creatinine clearance <30 mL/min/1.73 m² as measured by 24-hour urinary creatinine clearance) and to patients with end stage renal disease (ESRD) requiring hemodialysis.

In patients with severe renal impairment, the $AUC_{0-\infty}$ of total aprepitant (unbound and protein bound) decreased by 21% and C_{max} decreased by 32%, relative to healthy subjects (creatinine clearance >80 mL/min estimated by Cockcroft-Gault method). In patients with ESRD undergoing hemodialysis, the $AUC_{0-\infty}$ of total aprepitant decreased by 42% and C_{max} decreased by 32%. Due to modest decreases in protein binding of aprepitant in patients with renal disease, the AUC of pharmacologically active unbound drug was not significantly affected in patients with renal impairment compared with healthy subjects. Hemodialysis conducted 4 or 48 hours after dosing had no significant effect on the pharmacokinetics of aprepitant; less than 0.2% of the dose was recovered in the dialysate.

No dosage adjustment is necessary for patients with renal impairment or for patients with ESRD undergoing hemodialysis.

13 NONCLINICAL TOXICOLOGY

13.1 Carcinogenesis, Mutagenesis, Impairment of Fertility
Carcinogenicity studies were conducted in Sprague-Dawley rats and in CD-1 mice for 2 years. In the rat carcinogenicity studies, animals were treated with oral doses ranging from 0.05 to 1000 mg/kg twice daily. The highest dose produced a systemic exposure to aprepitant (plasma AUC_{0-24hr}) of 0.7 to

Table 5: Treatment Regimens in Highly Emetogenic Chemotherapy Trials*

Treatment Regimen	Day 1	Days 2 to 4
Aprepitant	Aprepitant 125 mg PO Dexamethasone 12 mg PO 5-HT$_3$ antagonist†	Aprepitant 80 mg PO Daily (Days 2 and 3 only) Dexamethasone 8 mg PO Daily (morning)
Standard Therapy	Dexamethasone 20 mg PO 5-HT$_3$ antagonist†	Dexamethasone 8 mg PO Daily (morning) Dexamethasone 8 mg PO Daily (evening)

* Aprepitant placebo and dexamethasone placebo were used to maintain blinding.
† Ondansetron 32 mg I.V. was used in the clinical trials of EMEND. Although this dose was used in clinical trials, this is no longer the currently recommended dose. Refer to the ondansetron package insert for the current dosing.

1.6 times the human exposure (AUC$_{0-24hr}$ = 19.6 mcg•hr/mL) at the recommended dose of 125 mg/day. Treatment with aprepitant at doses of 5 to 1000 mg/kg twice daily caused an increase in the incidences of thyroid follicular cell adenomas and carcinomas in male rats. In female rats, it produced hepatocellular adenomas at 5 to 1000 mg/kg twice daily and hepatocellular carcinomas and thyroid follicular cell adenomas at 125 to 1000 mg/kg twice daily. In the mouse carcinogenicity studies, the animals were treated with oral doses ranging from 2.5 to 2000 mg/kg/day. The highest dose produced a systemic exposure of about 2.8 to 3.6 times the human exposure at the recommended dose. Treatment with aprepitant produced skin fibrosarcomas at 125 and 500 mg/kg/day doses in male mice.
Aprepitant was not genotoxic in the Ames test, the human lymphoblastoid cell (TK6) mutagenesis test, the rat hepatocyte DNA strand break test, the Chinese hamster ovary (CHO) cell chromosome aberration test and the mouse micronucleus test.
Aprepitant did not affect the fertility or general reproductive performance of male or female rats at doses up to the maximum feasible dose of 1000 mg/kg twice daily (providing exposure in male rats lower than the exposure at the recommended human dose and exposure in female rats at about 1.6 times the human exposure.

14 CLINICAL STUDIES
14.1 Prevention of Chemotherapy Induced Nausea and Vomiting (CINV)
Oral administration of EMEND in combination with ondansetron and dexamethasone (aprepitant regimen) has been shown to prevent acute and delayed nausea and vomiting associated with highly emetogenic chemotherapy including high-dose cisplatin, and nausea and vomiting associated with moderately emetogenic chemotherapy.
Highly Emetogenic Chemotherapy (HEC)
In 2 multicenter, randomized, parallel, double-blind, controlled clinical studies, the aprepitant regimen (see Table 6) was compared with standard therapy in patients receiving a chemotherapy regimen that included cisplatin >50 mg/m^2 (mean cisplatin dose = 80.2 mg/m^2). Of the 550 patients who were randomized to receive the aprepitant regimen, 42% were women, 58% men, 59% White, 3% Asian, 5% Black, 12% Hispanic American, and 21% Multi-Racial. The aprepitant-treated patients in these clinical studies ranged from 14 to 84 years of age, with a mean age of 56 years. 170 patients were 65 years or older, with 29 patients being 75 years or older.
Patients (N = 1105) were randomized to either the aprepitant regimen (N = 550) or standard therapy (N = 555). The treatment regimens are defined in Table 5. [See table 5 above]
During these studies, 95% of the patients in the aprepitant group received a concomitant chemotherapeutic agent in addition to protocol-mandated cisplatin. The most common chemotherapeutic agents and the number of aprepitant patients exposed follows: etoposide (106), fluorouracil (100), gemcitabine (89), vinorelbine (82), paclitaxel (52), cyclophosphamide (50), doxorubicin (38), docetaxel (11).
The antiemetic activity of EMEND was evaluated during the acute phase (0 to 24 hours post-cisplatin treatment), the delayed phase (25 to 120 hours post-cisplatin treatment) and overall (0 to 120 hours post-cisplatin treatment) in Cycle 1. Efficacy was based on evaluation of the following endpoints:
Primary endpoint:
• complete response (defined as no emetic episodes and no use of rescue therapy)
Other prespecified endpoints:
• complete protection (defined as no emetic episodes, no use of rescue therapy, and a maximum nausea visual analogue scale [VAS] score <25 mm on a 0 to 100 mm scale)
• no emesis (defined as no emetic episodes regardless of use of rescue therapy)
• no nausea (maximum VAS <5 mm on a 0 to 100 mm scale)
• no significant nausea (maximum VAS <25 mm on a 0 to 100 mm scale)
A summary of the key study results from each individual study analysis is shown in Table 6 and in Table 7.

Table 6: Percent of Patients Receiving Highly Emetogenic Chemotherapy Responding by Treatment Group and Phase for Study 1 — Cycle 1

ENDPOINTS	Aprepitant Regimen (N = 260)* %	Standard Therapy (N = 261)* %	p-Value
PRIMARY ENDPOINT			
Complete Response			
Overall†	73	52	<0.001
OTHER PRESPECIFIED ENDPOINTS			
Complete Response			
Acute phase‡	89	78	<0.001
Delayed phase§	75	56	<0.001
Complete Protection			
Overall	63	49	0.001
Acute phase	85	75	NS¶
Delayed phase	66	52	<0.001
No Emesis			
Overall	78	55	<0.001
Acute phase	90	79	0.001
Delayed phase	81	59	<0.001
No Nausea			
Overall	48	44	NS#
Delayed phase	51	48	NS#
No Significant Nausea			
Overall	73	66	NS#
Delayed phase	75	69	NS#

Visual analogue scale (VAS) score range: 0 mm = no nausea; 100 mm = nausea as bad as it could be.
* N: Number of patients (older than 18 years of age) who received cisplatin, study drug, and had at least one post-treatment efficacy evaluation.
† Overall: 0 to 120 hours post-cisplatin treatment.
‡ Acute phase: 0 to 24 hours post-cisplatin treatment.
§ Delayed phase: 25 to 120 hours post-cisplatin treatment.
¶ Not statistically significant when adjusted for multiple comparisons.
\# Not statistically significant.

Table 7: Percent of Patients Receiving Highly Emetogenic Chemotherapy Responding by Treatment Group and Phase for Study 2 — Cycle 1

ENDPOINTS	Aprepitant Regimen (N = 261)* %	Standard Therapy (N = 263)* %	p-Value
PRIMARY ENDPOINT			
Complete Response			
Overall†	63	43	<0.001
OTHER PRESPECIFIED ENDPOINTS			
Complete Response			
Acute phase‡	83	68	<0.001
Delayed phase§	68	47	<0.001

(continued top right)

Table (Study 2 continued)

	Aprepitant Regimen	Standard Therapy	p-Value
Complete Protection			
Overall	56	41	<0.001
Acute phase	80	65	<0.001
Delayed phase	61	44	<0.001
No Emesis			
Overall	66	44	<0.001
Acute phase	84	69	<0.001
Delayed phase	72	48	<0.001
No Nausea			
Overall	49	39	NS¶
Delayed phase	53	40	NS¶
No Significant Nausea			
Overall	71	64	NS#
Delayed phase	73	65	NS#

Visual analogue scale (VAS) score range: 0 mm = no nausea; 100 mm = nausea as bad as it could be.
* N: Number of patients (older than 18 years of age) who received cisplatin, study drug, and had at least one post-treatment efficacy evaluation.
† Overall: 0 to 120 hours post-cisplatin treatment.
‡ Acute phase: 0 to 24 hours post-cisplatin treatment.
§ Delayed phase: 25 to 120 hours post-cisplatin treatment.
¶ Not statistically significant when adjusted for multiple comparisons.
\# Not statistically significant.

In both studies, a statistically significantly higher proportion of patients receiving the aprepitant regimen in Cycle 1 had a complete response in the overall phase (primary endpoint), compared with patients receiving standard therapy. A statistically significant difference in complete response in favor of the aprepitant regimen was also observed when the acute phase and the delayed phase were analyzed separately.
In both studies, the estimated time to first emesis after initiation of cisplatin treatment was longer with the aprepitant regimen, and the incidence of first emesis was reduced in the aprepitant regimen group compared with standard therapy group as depicted in the Kaplan-Meier curves in Figure 1.

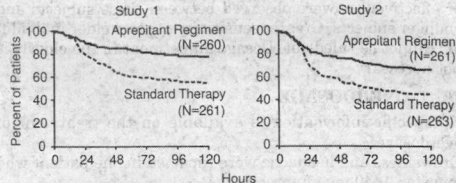

p-Value <0.001 based on a log rank test for Study 1 and Study 2; nominal p-values not adjusted for multiplicity.

Figure 1: Percent of Patients Receiving Highly Emetogenic Chemotherapy Who Remain Emesis Free Over Time — Cycle 1

Patient-Reported Outcomes: The impact of nausea and vomiting on patients' daily lives was assessed in Cycle 1 of both Phase III studies using the Functional Living Index–Emesis (FLIE), a validated nausea- and vomiting-specific patient-reported outcome measure. Minimal or no impact of nausea and vomiting on patients' daily lives is defined as a FLIE total score >108. In each of the 2 studies, a higher proportion of patients receiving the aprepitant regimen reported minimal or no impact of nausea and vomiting on daily life (Study 1: 74% versus 64%; Study 2: 75% versus 64%).
Multiple-Cycle Extension: In the same 2 clinical studies, patients continued into the Multiple-Cycle extension for up to 5 additional cycles of chemotherapy. The proportion of patients with no emesis and no significant nausea by treatment group at each cycle is depicted in Figure 2. Antiemetic effectiveness for the patients receiving the aprepitant regimen is maintained throughout repeat cycles for those patients continuing in each of the multiple cycles.
[See figure 2 at top of next column]
Moderately Emetogenic Chemotherapy (MEC)
In a multicenter, randomized, double-blind, parallel-group, clinical study in breast cancer patients, the aprepitant regimen (see Table 9) was compared with a standard of care therapy in patients receiving a moderately emetogenic chemotherapy regimen that included cyclophosphamide 750-1500 mg/m^2; or cyclophosphamide 500-1500 mg/m^2 and doxorubicin (≤60 mg/m^2) or epirubicin (≤100 mg/m^2).

Figure 2: Proportion of Patients Receiving Highly Emetogenic Chemotherapy with No Emesis and No Significant Nausea by Treatment Group and Cycle

	2	3	4	5	6
Aprepitant (N)	158	122	81	54	40
Standard (N)	177	111	68	37	29
Aprepitant (N)	191	148	103	63	43
Standard (N)	216	167	112	74	43

In this study, the most common combinations were cyclophosphamide + doxorubicin (60.6%); and cyclophosphamide + epirubicin + fluorouracil (21.6%).

Of the 438 patients who were randomized to receive the aprepitant regimen, 99.5% were women. Of these, approximately 80% were White, 8% Black, 8% Asian, 4% Hispanic, and <1% Other. The aprepitant-treated patients in this clinical study ranged from 25 to 78 years of age, with a mean age of 53 years; 70 patients were 65 years or older, with 12 patients being over 74 years.

Patients (N = 866) were randomized to either the aprepitant regimen (N = 438) or standard therapy (N = 428). The treatment regimens are defined in Table 8.

[See table 8 above]

The antiemetic activity of EMEND was evaluated based on the following endpoints:

Primary endpoint:
• complete response (defined as no emetic episodes and no use of rescue therapy) in the overall phase (0 to 120 hours post-chemotherapy)

Other prespecified endpoints:
• no emesis (defined as no emetic episodes regardless of use of rescue therapy)
• no nausea (maximum VAS <5 mm on a 0 to 100 mm scale)
• no significant nausea (maximum VAS <25 mm on a 0 to 100 mm scale)
• complete protection (defined as no emetic episodes, no use of rescue therapy, and a maximum nausea visual analogue scale [VAS] score <25 mm on a 0 to 100 mm scale)
• complete response during the acute and delayed phases
A summary of the key results from this study is shown in Table 9.

Table 9: Percent of Patients Receiving Moderately Emetogenic Chemotherapy Responding by Treatment Group and Phase — Cycle 1

ENDPOINTS	Aprepitant Regimen (N = 433)* %	Standard Therapy (N = 424)* %	p-Value
PRIMARY ENDPOINT†			
Complete Response	51	42	0.015
OTHER PRESPECIFIED ENDPOINTS†			
No Emesis	76	59	NS‡
No Nausea	33	33	NS
No Significant Nausea	61	56	NS
No Rescue Therapy	59	56	NS
Complete Protection	43	37	NS

* N: Number of patients included in the primary analysis of complete response.
† Overall: 0 to 120 hours post-chemotherapy treatment.
‡ NS when adjusted for prespecified multiple comparisons rule; unadjusted p-value <0.001.

In this study, a statistically significantly (p=0.015) higher proportion of patients receiving the aprepitant regimen (51%) in Cycle 1 had a complete response (primary endpoint) during the overall phase compared with patients receiving standard therapy (42%). The difference between treatment groups was primarily driven by the "No Emesis Endpoint", a principal component of this composite primary endpoint. In addition, a higher proportion of patients receiving the aprepitant regimen in Cycle 1 had a complete response during the acute (0-24 hours) and delayed (25-120 hours) phases compared with patients receiving standard therapy; however, the treatment group differences failed to reach statistical significance, after multiplicity adjustments.

Table 8: Treatment Regimens in Moderately Emetogenic Chemotherapy Trials

Treatment Regimen	Day 1	Days 2 to 3
Aprepitant	Aprepitant 125 mg PO* Dexamethasone 12 mg PO† Ondansetron 8 mg PO × 2 doses‡	Aprepitant 80 mg PO Daily
Standard Therapy	Dexamethasone 20 mg PO Ondansetron 8 mg PO × 2 doses	Ondansetron 8 mg PO Daily (every 12 hours)

Aprepitant placebo and dexamethasone placebo were used to maintain blinding.
* 1 hour prior to chemotherapy.
† 30 minutes prior to chemotherapy.
‡ 30 to 60 minutes prior to chemotherapy and 8 hours after first ondansetron dose.

Patient-Reported Outcomes: In a phase III study in patients receiving moderately emetogenic chemotherapy, the impact of nausea and vomiting on patients' daily lives was assessed in Cycle 1 using the FLIE. A higher proportion of patients receiving the aprepitant regimen reported minimal or no impact on daily life (64% versus 56%). This difference between treatment groups was primarily driven by the "No Vomiting Domain" of this composite endpoint.

Multiple-Cycle Extension: Patients receiving moderately emetogenic chemotherapy were permitted to continue into the Multiple-Cycle extension of the study for up to 3 additional cycles of chemotherapy. Antiemetic effect for patients receiving the aprepitant regimen is maintained during all cycles.

Postmarketing Trial: In a postmarketing, multicenter, randomized, double-blind, parallel-group, clinical study in 848 cancer patients, the aprepitant regimen (N=430) was compared with a standard of care therapy (N=418) in patients receiving a moderately emetogenic chemotherapy regimen that included any IV dose of oxaliplatin, carboplatin, epirubicin, idarubicin, ifosfamide, irinotecan, daunorubicin, doxorubicin; cyclophosphamide IV (<1500 mg/m²); or cytarabine IV (>1 g/m²).

Of the 430 patients who were randomized to receive the aprepitant regimen, 76% were women and 24% were men. The distribution by race was 67% White, 6% Black or African American, 11% Asian, and 12% multiracial. Classified by ethnicity, 36% were Hispanic and 64% were non-Hispanic. The aprepitant-treated patients in this clinical study ranged from 22 to 85 years of age, with a mean age of 57 years; approximately 59% of the patients were 55 years or older with 32 patients being over 74 years. Patients receiving the aprepitant regimen were receiving chemotherapy for a variety of tumor types including 50% with breast cancer, 21% with gastrointestinal cancers including colorectal cancer, 13% with lung cancer and 6% with gynecological cancers.

The antiemetic activity of EMEND was evaluated based on no vomiting (with or without rescue therapy) in the overall period (0 to 120 hours post-chemotherapy) and complete response (defined as no vomiting and no use of rescue therapy) in the overall period.
A summary of the key results from this study is shown in Table 10.

Table 10: Percent of Patients Receiving Moderately Emetogenic Chemotherapy Responding by Treatment Group for Study 2 — Cycle 1

ENDPOINTS	Aprepitant Regimen (N = 430)* %	Standard Therapy (N = 418)* %	p-Value
No Vomiting Overall	76	62	<0.0001
Complete Response Overall	69	56	0.0003

* N = Number of patients who received chemotherapy treatment, study drug, and had at least one post-treatment efficacy evaluation.

In this study, a statistically significantly higher proportion of patients receiving the aprepitant regimen (76%) in Cycle 1 had no vomiting during the overall phase compared with patients receiving standard therapy (62%). In addition, a higher proportion of patients receiving the aprepitant regimen (69%) in Cycle 1 had a complete response in the overall phase (0-120 hours) compared with patients receiving standard therapy (56%). In the acute phase (0 to 24 hours following initiation of chemotherapy), a higher proportion of patients receiving aprepitant compared to patients receiving standard therapy were observed to have no vomiting (92% and 84%, respectively) and complete response (89% and 80%, respectively). In the delayed phase (25 to 120 hours following initiation of chemotherapy), a higher proportion of patients receiving aprepitant compared to pa-

tients receiving standard therapy were observed to have no vomiting (78% and 67%, respectively) and complete response (71% and 61%, respectively).
In a subgroup analysis by tumor type, a numerically higher proportion of patients receiving aprepitant were observed to have no vomiting and complete response compared to patients receiving standard therapy. For gender, the difference in complete response rates between the aprepitant and standard regimen groups was similar in females (64.5% and 50.3%, respectively) and 4% in males (82.2% and 78.2%, respectively) during the overall phase. A similar difference for gender was observed for the no vomiting endpoint.

14.2 Prevention of Postoperative Nausea and Vomiting (PONV)

In two multicenter, randomized, double-blind, active comparator-controlled, parallel-group clinical studies (PONV Studies 1 and 2), aprepitant was compared with ondansetron for the prevention of postoperative nausea and vomiting in 1658 patients undergoing open abdominal surgery. Patients were randomized to receive 40-mg aprepitant, 125-mg aprepitant, or 4-mg ondansetron. Aprepitant was given orally with 50 mL of water 1 to 3 hours before anesthesia. Ondansetron was given intravenously immediately before induction of anesthesia. A comparison between the 125-mg dose and the 40-mg dose did not demonstrate any additional clinical benefit. The remainder of this section will focus on the results in the 40-mg aprepitant dose recommended for PONV.

Of the 564 patients who received 40-mg aprepitant, 92% were women and 8% were men; of these, 58% were White, 13% Hispanic American, 7% Multi-Racial, 14% Black, 6% Asian, and 2% Other. The age of patients treated with 40-mg aprepitant ranged from 19 to 84 years, with a mean age of 46.1 years. 46 patients were 65 years or older, with 13 patients being 75 years or older.

The antiemetic activity of EMEND was evaluated during the 0 to 48 hour period following the end of surgery. The two pivotal studies were of similar design; however, they differed in terms of study hypothesis, efficacy analyses and geographic location. PONV Study 1 was a multinational study including the U.S., whereas, PONV Study 2 was conducted entirely in the U.S.

Efficacy measures in PONV Study 1 included:
• no emesis (defined as no emetic episodes regardless of use of rescue therapy) in the 0 to 24 hours following the end of surgery (primary)
• complete response (defined as no emetic episodes and no use of rescue therapy) in the 0 to 24 hours following the end of surgery (primary)
• no emesis (defined as no emetic episodes regardless of use of rescue therapy) in the 0 to 48 hours following the end of surgery (secondary)
• time to first use of rescue medication in the 0 to 24 hours following the end of surgery (exploratory)
• time to first emesis in the 0 to 48 hours following the end of surgery (exploratory).
A closed testing procedure was applied to control the type I error for the primary endpoints.
The results of the primary and secondary endpoints for 40-mg aprepitant and 4-mg ondansetron are described in Table 11:
[See table 11 at top of next page]
The use of aprepitant did not affect the time to first use of rescue medication when compared to ondansetron. However, compared to the ondansetron group, use of aprepitant delayed the time to first vomiting, as depicted in Figure 3.
[See figure 3 at top of next column]
Efficacy measures in PONV Study 2 included:
• complete response (defined as no emetic episodes and no use of rescue therapy) in the 0 to 24 hours following the end of surgery (primary)
• no emesis (defined as no emetic episodes regardless of use of rescue therapy) in the 0 to 24 hours following the end of surgery (secondary)
• no use of rescue therapy in the 0 to 24 hours following the end of surgery (secondary)
• no emesis (defined as no emetic episodes regardless of use of rescue therapy) in the 0 to 48 hours following the end of surgery (secondary).

Figure 3: Percent of Patients Who Remain Emesis Free During the 48 Hours Following End of Surgery

PONV Study 2 failed to satisfy its primary hypothesis that aprepitant is superior to ondansetron in the prevention of PONV as measured by the proportion of patients with complete response in the 24 hours following end of surgery. The study demonstrated that both dose levels of aprepitant had a clinically meaningful effect with respect to the secondary endpoint "no vomiting" during the first 24 hours after surgery and showed that the use of 40-mg aprepitant was associated with a 16% improvement over ondansetron for the no vomiting endpoint.
[See table 12 above]

16   HOW SUPPLIED/STORAGE AND HANDLING

No. 3854 — 80-mg capsules: White, opaque, hard gelatin capsule with "461" and "80 mg" printed radially in black ink on the body. They are supplied as follows:
NDC 0006-0461-02 unit-of-use BiPack of 2
NDC 0006-0461-06 unit-dose package of 6.
No. 3855 — 125-mg capsules: Opaque, hard gelatin capsule with white body and pink cap with "462" and "125 mg" printed radially in black ink on the body. They are supplied as follows:
NDC 0006-0462-06 unit-dose package of 6.
No. 3862 — Unit-of-use TriPack containing one 125-mg capsule and two 80-mg capsules.
NDC 0006-3862-03.
No. 6741 — 40-mg capsules: Opaque, hard gelatin capsule with white body and mustard yellow cap with "464" and "40 mg" printed radially in black ink on the body. They are supplied as follows:
NDC 0006-0464-10 unit-of-use package of 1
NDC 0006-0464-05 unit-dose package of 5.
Storage
Store at 20-25°C (68-77°F) [see USP Controlled Room Temperature].

17   PATIENT COUNSELING INFORMATION

"See FDA-Approved Patient Labeling (Patient Information)"
Physicians should instruct their patients to read the patient package insert before starting therapy with EMEND and to reread it each time the prescription is renewed.
Patients should be instructed to take EMEND only as prescribed. For the prevention of chemotherapy induced nausea and vomiting (CINV), patients should be advised to take their first dose (125 mg) of EMEND 1 hour prior to chemotherapy treatment. For the prevention of postoperative nausea and vomiting (PONV), patients should receive their medication (40-mg capsule of EMEND) within 3 hours prior to induction of anesthesia.
Allergic reactions, which may be serious, and may include hives, rash and itching and cause difficulty in breathing or swallowing, have been reported in general use with EMEND. Physicians should instruct their patients to stop taking EMEND and call their doctor right away if they experience an allergic reaction. In addition, severe skin reactions may occur rarely.
EMEND may interact with some drugs including chemotherapy; therefore, patients should be advised to report to their doctor the use of any other prescription, nonprescription medication or herbal products.
Patients on chronic warfarin therapy should be instructed to have their clotting status closely monitored in the 2-week period, particularly at 7 to 10 days, following initiation of the 3-day regimen of EMEND 125 mg/80 mg with each chemotherapy cycle, or following administration of a single 40-mg dose of EMEND for the prevention of postoperative nausea and vomiting.
Administration of EMEND may reduce the efficacy of hormonal contraceptives. Patients should be advised to use alternative or back-up methods of contraception during treatment with EMEND and for 1 month following the last dose of EMEND.
Distributed by:
Merck Sharp & Dohme Corp., a subsidiary of **MERCK & CO., INC.,** Whitehouse Station, NJ 08889, USA
U.S. Patent Nos.: 5,719,147; 6,096,742

Table 11: PONV Study 1 – Response Rates for Select Efficacy Endpoints (Modified-Intention-to-Treat Population)

Treatment	n/m (%)	Aprepitant vs Ondansetron		
		Δ	Odds ratio*	Analysis
Primary Endpoints				
No Vomiting 0 to 24 hours (Superiority) (no emetic episodes)				
Aprepitant 40 mg	246/293 (84.0)	12.6%	2.1	P<0.001†
Ondansetron	200/280 (71.4)			
Complete Response (Non-inferiority: If LB‡ >0.65) (no emesis and no rescue therapy, 0 to 24 hours)				
Aprepitant 40 mg	187/293 (63.8)	8.8%	1.4	LB=1.02
Ondansetron	154/280 (55.0)			
Complete Response (Superiority: If LB >1.0) (no emesis and no rescue therapy, 0 to 24 hours)				
Aprepitant 40 mg	187/293 (63.8)	8.8%	1.4	LB=1.02§
Ondansetron	154/280 (55.0)			
Secondary Endpoint				
No Vomiting 0 to 48 hours (Superiority) (no emetic episodes)				
Aprepitant 40 mg	238/292 (81.5)	15.2%	2.3	P<0.001†
Ondansetron	185/279 (66.3)			

n/m = Number of responders/number of patients in analysis.
Δ Difference (%): Aprepitant 40 mg minus Ondansetron.
* Estimated odds ratio for Aprepitant versus Ondansetron. A value of >1 favors Aprepitant over Ondansetron.
† P-value of two-sided test <0.05.
‡ LB= lower bound of 1-sided 97.5% confidence interval for the odds ratio.
§ Based on the prespecified fixed sequence multiplicity strategy, Aprepitant 40 mg was not superior to Ondansetron.

Table 12: PONV Study 2 (Modified-Intention-to-Treat Population)

Treatment	n/m(%)	Aprepitant vs Ondansetron		
		Δ	Odds ratio*	p-Value
Primary Endpoint				
Complete Response (no emesis and no rescue therapy, 0 to 24 hours)				
Aprepitant 40 mg	111/248 (44.8)	2.5%	1.1	0.61
Ondansetron	104/246 (42.3)			
Secondary Endpoints				
No Vomiting (no emetic episodes, 0 to 24 hours)				
Aprepitant 40 mg	223/248 (89.9)	16.3%	3.2	<0.001†
Ondansetron	181/246 (73.6)			
No Use of Rescue Medication (for established emesis or nausea, 0 to 24 hours)				
Aprepitant 40 mg	112/248 (45.2)	-0.7%	1.0	0.83
Ondansetron	113/246 (45.9)			
No Vomiting 0 to 48 hours (Superiority) (no emetic episodes, 0 to 48 hours)				
Aprepitant 40 mg	209/247 (84.6)	17.7%	2.7	<0.001†
Ondansetron	164/245 (66.9)			

n/m = Number of responders/number of patients in analysis.
Δ Difference (%): Aprepitant 40 mg minus Ondansetron.
* Estimated odds ratio: Aprepitant 40 mg versus Ondansetron.
† Not statistically significant after pre-specified multiplicity adjustment.

Copyright © 2003, 2005, 2006 Merck Sharp & Dohme Corp., a subsidiary of **Merck & Co., Inc.**

All rights reserved.
uspi-mk0869-c-1408r007

Patient Information
EMEND® (EE mend)
(aprepitant)
Capsules

Read the Patient Information that comes with EMEND before you start taking it and each time you refill your prescription. There may be new information. This leaflet does not take the place of talking with your doctor about your medical condition or treatment.

What is EMEND?

EMEND is a prescription medicine used in adults to prevent nausea and vomiting:
• caused by certain anti-cancer (chemotherapy) medicines. When used for this purpose, EMEND is always used with other medicines.
• after surgery.

EMEND is not used to treat nausea and vomiting that you already have.

EMEND should not be used continuously for a long time (chronic use).

It is not known if EMEND is safe and effective in children.

Who should not take EMEND?

Do not take EMEND if you:
• are taking any of the following medicines:
  ◦ ORAP® (pimozide)
  ◦ SELDANE® (terfenadine)
  ◦ HISMANAL® (astemizole)
  ◦ PROPULSID® (cisapride)

Taking EMEND with any of these medicines could cause serious or life-threatening problems.
• are allergic to any of the ingredients in EMEND. See the end of this leaflet for a list of all the ingredients in EMEND.

What should I tell my doctor before and during treatment with EMEND?

Before you take EMEND, tell your doctor if you:
• have liver problems
• are pregnant or plan to become pregnant. It is not known if EMEND can harm your unborn baby.
Women who use birth control medicines containing hormones to prevent pregnancy (birth control pills, skin patches, implants, and certain IUDs) should also use a back-up method of birth control during treatment with EMEND and for up to 1 month after using EMEND to prevent pregnancy.
• are breast-feeding. It is not known if EMEND passes into your milk and if it can harm your baby.

Tell your doctor about all the medicines you are taking or plan to take, including prescription and non-prescription medicines, vitamins, and herbal supplements.

EMEND may cause serious life-threatening reactions if used with certain medicines. See the section "Who should not take EMEND?"

EMEND may affect how other medicines work, and other medicines may affect how EMEND works. Ask your doctor or pharmacist before you take any new medicine. They can tell you if it is safe to take the medicine with EMEND.

Know the medicines you take. Keep a list of them to show your doctor or pharmacist when you get a new medicine.

How should I take EMEND?
• Take EMEND exactly as prescribed.
• If you take too much EMEND, call your doctor, local emergency department or poison control center right away.
• If you are receiving cancer chemotherapy, EMEND is taken as 3 doses over 3 days - starting on the day you have chemotherapy, and the two days after chemotherapy. There are two ways that your doctor may prescribe EMEND for you:
1. Capsules of EMEND by mouth for all 3 doses:
  ◦ You should get a package that has three capsules of EMEND.
  ◦ Day 1 (Day of chemotherapy): Take one 125-mg capsule of EMEND (white and pink) by mouth 1 hour before you start your chemotherapy treatment.
  ◦ Day 2 and Day 3 (the two days after chemotherapy): Take one 80-mg capsule of EMEND (white) by mouth, each morning for the 2 days after your chemotherapy treatment.
  Or
2. Intravenous (IV) injection into a vein the first day, then capsules by mouth on the two days after chemotherapy:
  ◦ Day 1 (Day of chemotherapy):   EMEND will be given to you by intravenous (IV) injection in your vein 30 minutes before you start your chemotherapy treatment.
  ◦ You should get a package that has two capsules of EMEND.
  ◦ Day 2 and Day 3 (the two days after chemotherapy): Take one 80-mg capsule of EMEND (white) by mouth, each morning for the 2 days after your chemotherapy treatment.
• If you are receiving chemotherapy, EMEND may be taken with or without food.
• If you are having surgery:

◦ Your doctor will prescribe a 40-mg capsule of EMEND for you before surgery. You take EMEND within three hours before surgery.
◦ Follow your doctor's instructions about restrictions on eating and drinking before surgery.
• If you take the blood thinner medicine warfarin sodium (COUMADIN®, JANTOVEN®), your doctor may do blood tests after you take EMEND to check your blood clotting.

What are the possible side effects of EMEND?

EMEND may cause serious side effects, including:
• **Serious allergic reactions.** Allergic reactions can happen with EMEND and may be serious. Stop taking EMEND and call your doctor right away if you have any of these signs or symptoms of an allergic reaction:
  ◦ hives
  ◦ rash
  ◦ itching
  ◦ trouble breathing or swallowing.
• Severe skin reactions may occur rarely.

In people taking EMEND to prevent nausea and vomiting caused by chemotherapy, the most common side effects of EMEND include:
• tiredness
• nausea
• hiccups
• constipation
• diarrhea
• loss of appetite
• headache
• hair loss

In people taking EMEND to prevent nausea and vomiting after surgery, the most common side effects are:
• constipation
• nausea
• itch
• fever
• low blood pressure
• headache

Tell your doctor if you have any side effect that bothers you or that does not go away. These are not all of the possible side effects of EMEND. For more information ask your doctor or pharmacist.

Call your doctor for medical advice about side effects. You may report side effects to FDA at 1-800-FDA-1088.

How should I store EMEND?
• Store EMEND at room temperature, between 68°F and 77°F (20°C and 25°C).
• **Keep EMEND and all medicines out of the reach of children.**

General information about EMEND

Medicines are sometimes prescribed for conditions that are not mentioned in patient information leaflets. Do not use EMEND for a condition for which it was not prescribed. Do not give EMEND to other people, even if they have the same symptoms you have. It may harm them.

This Patient Information leaflet summarizes the most important information about EMEND. If you would like to know more information, talk with your doctor. You can ask your doctor or pharmacist for information about EMEND that is written for health professionals. For more information about EMEND call 1-800-622-4477 or go to www.emend.com.

What are the ingredients in EMEND?

Active ingredient: aprepitant

Inactive ingredients: sucrose, microcrystalline cellulose, hydroxypropyl cellulose and sodium lauryl sulfate. The capsule shell excipients are gelatin, titanium dioxide, and may contain sodium lauryl sulfate and silicon dioxide. The 125-mg capsule shell also contains red ferric oxide and yellow ferric oxide. The 40-mg capsule shell also contains yellow ferric oxide.

Distributed by:

Merck Sharp & Dohme Corp., a subsidiary of **MERCK & CO., INC.**, Whitehouse Station, NJ 08889, USA

U.S. Patent Nos.: 5,719,147; 6,096,742

The brands listed in the above sections "Who should not take EMEND?" and "How should I take EMEND?" are the registered trademarks of their respective owners and are not trademarks of Merck Sharp & Dohme Corp., a subsidiary of Merck & Co., Inc.

Copyright © 2003, 2005, 2006 Merck Sharp & Dohme Corp., a subsidiary of **Merck & Co., Inc.**

All rights reserved.

Revised: 07/2012

USPPI-C-08691207R004

Shown in Product Identification Guide, page 308

EMEND   ℞
[ĕ′mĕnd]
(fosaprepitant dimeglumine)
for Injection, for intravenous use

HIGHLIGHTS OF PRESCRIBING INFORMATION

These highlights do not include all the information needed to use EMEND safely and effectively. See full prescribing information for EMEND.

EMEND (fosaprepitant dimeglumine) for Injection,
for intravenous use
Initial U.S. Approval: 2008

———INDICATIONS AND USAGE———

EMEND® for Injection is a substance P/neurokinin-1 (NK₁) receptor antagonist, in combination with other antiemetic agents, is indicated in adults for the (1):
• prevention of acute and delayed nausea and vomiting associated with initial and repeat courses of highly emetogenic cancer chemotherapy (HEC) including high-dose cisplatin
• prevention of nausea and vomiting associated with initial and repeat courses of moderately emetogenic cancer chemotherapy (MEC)
Limitations of Use (1)
• Chronic continuous administration is not recommended.

———DOSAGE AND ADMINISTRATION———

• *HEC (Single Dose Regimen):* EMEND for Injection (150 mg) is administered on Day 1 only as an infusion **over 20-30 minutes** initiated approximately 30 minutes prior to chemotherapy. No capsules of EMEND are administered on Days 2 and 3. EMEND for Injection is part of a regimen to prevent nausea and vomiting induced by HEC that includes a corticosteroid and a 5-HT₃ antagonist. (2.1)
• *HEC and MEC (3-Day Dosing Regimen):* EMEND for Injection (115 mg) is administered on Day 1 as an infusion **over 15 minutes** initiated approximately 30 minutes prior to chemotherapy. EMEND capsules (80 mg) are given orally on Days 2 and 3. EMEND for Injection and EMEND capsules are part of a regimen to prevent nausea and vomiting induced by HEC or MEC that includes a corticosteroid and a 5-HT₃ antagonist. (2.1, 2.2)

———DOSAGE FORMS AND STRENGTHS———

One single dose glass vial supplied as sterile lyophilized powder for intravenous use only after reconstitution and dilution: 150 mg and 115 mg (3)

———CONTRAINDICATIONS———

• Known hypersensitivity to any component of this drug. (4)
• Do not use concurrently with pimozide or cisapride, since inhibition of CYP3A4 by aprepitant may result in elevated plasma concentrations of these drugs, potentially causing serious or life-threatening reactions. (4)

———WARNINGS AND PRECAUTIONS———

• Fosaprepitant should be used with caution in patients receiving concomitant medications that are primarily metabolized through CYP3A4. (5.1)
• Immediate hypersensitivity reactions may occur during infusion. Patients have generally responded to discontinuation. It is not recommended to reinitiate the infusion. (5.2)
• Coadministration of fosaprepitant or aprepitant with warfarin (a CYP2C9 substrate) may result in a clinically significant decrease in International Normalized Ratio (INR) of prothrombin time. (5.3)
• The efficacy of hormonal contraceptives during and for 28 days following the last dose of fosaprepitant or aprepitant may be reduced. Alternative or back-up methods of contraception should be used. (5.4)

———ADVERSE REACTIONS———

• Adverse reactions for the CINV oral aprepitant regimen in conjunction with highly and moderately emetogenic chemotherapy (incidence ≥1% and greater than standard therapy) are: hiccups, asthenia/fatigue, AST/ALT increased, headache, constipation, anorexia, dyspepsia, diarrhea, eructation. (6.1)
• Adverse reactions reported for EMEND for Injection were generally similar to that seen in prior HEC studies with oral aprepitant. In addition, infusion site reactions (3%) occurred with EMEND for Injection. (6.1)

To report SUSPECTED ADVERSE REACTIONS, contact Merck Sharp & Dohme Corp., a subsidiary of Merck & Co., Inc., at 1-877-888-4231 or FDA at 1-800-FDA-1088 or www.fda.gov/medwatch.

———DRUG INTERACTIONS———

• Coadministration of fosaprepitant or aprepitant with drugs that inhibit or induce CYP3A4 activity may result in increased or reduced plasma concentrations of aprepitant, respectively. (7.1, 7.2)
• Coadministration of EMEND for Injection with drugs that are metabolized by CYP2C9 (e.g., warfarin, tolbutamide), may result in lower plasma concentrations of these drugs. (7.1)

See 17 for PATIENT COUNSELING INFORMATION and FDA-approved patient labeling

Revised: 08/2014

FULL PRESCRIBING INFORMATION: CONTENTS*
1   INDICATIONS AND USAGE
2   DOSAGE AND ADMINISTRATION
        2.1   Prevention of Nausea and Vomiting Associated with Highly Emetogenic Chemotherapy (HEC)

Table 1: Recommended dosing (Single Dose Regimen of EMEND) for the prevention of nausea and vomiting associated with highly emetogenic cancer chemotherapy

	Day 1	Day 2	Day 3	Day 4
EMEND	150 mg intravenous	none	none	none
Dexamethasone*	12 mg orally	8 mg orally	8 mg orally twice daily	8 mg orally twice daily
5-HT₃ antagonist	See the package insert for the selected 5-HT₃ antagonist for appropriate dosing information.	none	none	none

* Dexamethasone should be administered 30 minutes prior to chemotherapy treatment on Day 1 and in the morning on Days 2 through 4. The dose of dexamethasone accounts for drug interactions.

Table 2: Recommended dosing (3-Day Dosing Regimen of EMEND) for the prevention of nausea and vomiting associated with highly emetogenic cancer chemotherapy

	Day 1	Day 2	Day 3	Day 4
EMEND	115 mg intravenous	80 mg orally	80 mg orally	none
Dexamethasone*	12 mg orally	8 mg orally	8 mg orally once daily	8 mg orally once daily
5-HT₃ antagonist	See the package insert for the selected 5-HT₃ antagonist for appropriate dosing information.	none	none	none

* Dexamethasone should be administered 30 minutes prior to chemotherapy treatment on Day 1 and in the morning on Days 2 through 4. The dose of dexamethasone accounts for drug interactions.

FULL PRESCRIBING INFORMATION

1 INDICATIONS AND USAGE

EMEND® for Injection is a substance P/neurokinin-1 (NK₁) receptor antagonist indicated in adults for use in combination with other antiemetic agents for the:

- prevention of acute and delayed nausea and vomiting associated with initial and repeat courses of highly emetogenic cancer chemotherapy (HEC) including high-dose cisplatin *[see Dosage and Administration (2.1)]*
- prevention of nausea and vomiting associated with initial and repeat courses of moderately emetogenic cancer chemotherapy (MEC) *[see Dosage and Administration (2.2)]*.

Limitations of Use

EMEND for Injection has not been studied for the treatment of established nausea and vomiting.

Chronic continuous administration is not recommended *[see Warnings and Precautions (5.5)]*.

2 DOSAGE AND ADMINISTRATION

2.1 Prevention of Nausea and Vomiting Associated with Highly Emetogenic Chemotherapy (HEC)

EMEND for Injection 150 mg (Single Dose Regimen of EMEND):

EMEND for Injection 150 mg is administered intravenously on Day 1 only as an infusion **over 20-30 minutes** initiated approximately 30 minutes prior to chemotherapy. No capsules of EMEND are administered on Days 2 and 3. EMEND for Injection should be administered in conjunction with a corticosteroid and a 5-HT₃ antagonist as specified in Table 1. The recommended dosage of dexamethasone with EMEND for Injection 150 mg differs from the recommended dosage of dexamethasone with EMEND for Injection 115 mg on Days 3 and 4. The package insert for the co-administered 5-HT₃ antagonist must be consulted prior to initiation of treatment with EMEND for Injection.

[See table 1 above]

EMEND for Injection 115 mg (3-Day Dosing Regimen of EMEND):

EMEND for Injection 115 mg is administered on Day 1 only as an infusion **over 15 minutes** initiated 30 minutes prior to chemotherapy. Capsules of EMEND 80 mg should be administered on Days 2 and 3. EMEND for Injection 115 mg should be administered in conjunction with a corticosteroid and a 5-HT₃ antagonist as specified in Table 2. The recommended dosage of dexamethasone with EMEND for Injection 115 mg differs from the recommended dosage of dexamethasone with EMEND for Injection 150 mg on Days 3 and 4. The package insert for the co-administered 5-HT₃ antagonist must be consulted prior to initiation of treatment with EMEND for Injection.

Capsules of EMEND 125 mg may be substituted for EMEND for Injection 115 mg on Day 1.

[See table 2 above]

2.2 Prevention of Nausea and Vomiting Associated with Moderately Emetogenic Chemotherapy (MEC)

EMEND for Injection 115 mg (3-Day Dosing Regimen of EMEND):

EMEND for Injection 115 mg is administered on Day 1 only as an infusion **over 15 minutes** initiated 30 minutes prior to

chemotherapy. Capsules of EMEND 80 mg should be administered on Days 2 and 3. EMEND for Injection 115 mg should be administered in conjunction with a corticosteroid and a 5-HT₃ antagonist as specified in Table 3. The recommended dosage of dexamethasone with EMEND for Injection 115 mg differs from the recommended dosage of dexamethasone with EMEND for Injection 150 mg on Days 3 and 4. The package insert for the co-administered 5-HT₃ antagonist must be consulted prior to initiation of treatment with EMEND for Injection.

Capsules of EMEND 125 mg may be substituted for EMEND for Injection 115 mg on Day 1.

Table 3: Recommended dosing (3-Day Dosing Regimen of EMEND) for the prevention of nausea and vomiting associated with moderately emetogenic cancer chemotherapy

	Day 1	Day 2	Day 3
EMEND	115 mg intravenous	80 mg orally	80 mg orally
Dexamethasone*	12 mg orally	none	none
5-HT₃ antagonist	See the package insert for the selected 5-HT₃ antagonist for appropriate dosing information.	none	none

* Dexamethasone should be administered 30 minutes prior to chemotherapy treatment on Day 1. The dose of dexamethasone accounts for drug interactions.

2.3 Preparation of EMEND for Injection

Table 4: Preparation Instructions for EMEND for Injection (115 mg and 150 mg)

	115 mg	150 mg
Step 1	Aseptically inject 5 mL 0.9% Sodium Chloride for Injection (normal saline) into the vial. Assure that normal saline is added to the vial along the vial wall in order to prevent foaming. Swirl the vial gently. Avoid shaking and jetting saline into the vial.	Aseptically inject 5 mL 0.9% Sodium Chloride for Injection (normal saline) into the vial. Assure that normal saline is added to the vial along the vial wall in order to prevent foaming. Swirl the vial gently. Avoid shaking and jetting saline into the vial.
Step 2	Aseptically prepare an infusion bag filled with **110 mL** of normal saline.	Aseptically prepare an infusion bag filled with **145 mL** of normal saline.
Step 3	Aseptically withdraw the entire volume from the vial and transfer it into the infusion bag containing **110 mL** of normal saline to yield a total volume of **115 mL** and a final concentration of 1 mg/1 mL.	Aseptically withdraw the entire volume from the vial and transfer it into the infusion bag containing **145 mL** of normal saline to yield a total volume of **150 mL** and a final concentration of 1 mg/1 mL.
Step 4	Gently invert the bag 2-3 times.	Gently invert the bag 2-3 times.

Note: *The differences in preparation for each dose are displayed as bolded text.*

The reconstituted final drug solution is stable for 24 hours at ambient room temperature (at or below 25°C).

Parenteral drug products should be inspected visually for particulate matter and discoloration before administration whenever solution and container permit.

Caution: EMEND for Injection should not be mixed or reconstituted with solutions for which physical and chemical compatibility have not been established. EMEND for Injection is incompatible with any solutions containing divalent cations (e.g., Ca²⁺, Mg²⁺), including Lactated Ringer's Solution and Hartmann's Solution.

3 DOSAGE FORMS AND STRENGTHS

One 150-mg single dose glass vial: White to off-white lyophilized solid (Sterile lyophilized powder for intravenous use only after reconstitution and dilution).

One 115-mg single dose glass vial: White to off-white lyophilized solid (Sterile lyophilized powder for intravenous use only after reconstitution and dilution).

4 CONTRAINDICATIONS
4.1 Hypersensitivity
EMEND for Injection is contraindicated in patients who are hypersensitive to EMEND for Injection, aprepitant, polysorbate 80 or any other components of the product. Known hypersensitivity reactions include: flushing, erythema, dyspnea, and anaphylactic reactions [see Adverse Reactions (6.2)].

4.2 Concomitant Use with Pimozide or Cisapride
Aprepitant, when administered orally, is a moderate cytochrome P450 isoenzyme 3A4 (CYP3A4) inhibitor following the 3-day antiemetic dosing regimen for CINV. Since fosaprepitant is rapidly converted to aprepitant, do not use fosaprepitant concurrently with pimozide or cisapride. Inhibition of CYP3A4 by aprepitant could result in elevated plasma concentrations of these drugs, potentially causing serious or life-threatening reactions [see Drug Interactions (7.1)].

5 WARNINGS AND PRECAUTIONS
5.1 CYP3A4 Interactions
Fosaprepitant is rapidly converted to aprepitant, which is a moderate inhibitor of CYP3A4 when administered as a 3-day antiemetic dosing regimen for CINV. Fosaprepitant should be used with caution in patients receiving concomitant medications that are primarily metabolized through CYP3A4. Inhibition of CYP3A4 by aprepitant or fosaprepitant could result in elevated plasma concentrations of these concomitant medications. When fosaprepitant is used concomitantly with another CYP3A4 inhibitor, aprepitant plasma concentrations could be elevated. When aprepitant is used concomitantly with medications that induce CYP3A4 activity, aprepitant plasma concentrations could be reduced, and this may result in decreased efficacy of aprepitant [see Drug Interactions (7.1)].

Chemotherapy agents that are known to be metabolized by CYP3A4 include docetaxel, paclitaxel, etoposide, irinotecan, ifosfamide, imatinib, vinorelbine, vinblastine and vincristine. In clinical studies, the oral aprepitant regimen was administered commonly with etoposide, vinorelbine, or paclitaxel. The doses of these agents were not adjusted to account for potential drug interactions.

In separate pharmacokinetic studies, no clinically significant change in docetaxel or vinorelbine pharmacokinetics was observed when the oral aprepitant regimen was coadministered.

Due to the small number of patients in clinical studies who received the CYP3A4 substrates vinblastine, vincristine, or ifosfamide, particular caution and careful monitoring are advised in patients receiving these agents or other chemotherapy agents metabolized primarily by CYP3A4 that were not studied [see Drug Interactions (7.1)].

5.2 Hypersensitivity Reactions
Isolated reports of immediate hypersensitivity reactions including flushing, erythema, dyspnea, and anaphylaxis have occurred during infusion of fosaprepitant. These hypersensitivity reactions have generally responded to discontinuation of the infusion and administration of appropriate therapy. Reinitiation of the infusion is not recommended in patients who experience these symptoms during first-time use.

5.3 Coadministration with Warfarin (a CYP2C9 substrate)
Coadministration of fosaprepitant or aprepitant with warfarin may result in a clinically significant decrease in International Normalized Ratio (INR) of prothrombin time. In patients on chronic warfarin therapy, the INR should be closely monitored in the 2-week period, particularly at 7 to 10 days, following initiation of fosaprepitant with each chemotherapy cycle [see Drug Interactions (7.1)].

5.4 Coadministration with Hormonal Contraceptives
Upon coadministration with fosaprepitant or aprepitant, the efficacy of hormonal contraceptives may be reduced during and for 28 days following the last dose of either fosaprepitant or aprepitant. Alternative or back-up methods of contraception should be used during treatment with and for 1 month following the last dose of fosaprepitant or aprepitant [see Drug Interactions (7.1)].

5.5 Chronic Continuous Use
Chronic continuous use of EMEND for Injection for prevention of nausea and vomiting is not recommended because it has not been studied; and because the drug interaction profile may change during chronic continuous use.

6 ADVERSE REACTIONS
6.1 Clinical Trials Experience
Because clinical trials are conducted under widely varying conditions, adverse reaction rates observed in the clinical trials of a drug cannot be directly compared to rates in the clinical trials of another drug and may not reflect the rates observed in clinical practice.

Since EMEND for Injection is converted to aprepitant, those adverse reactions associated with aprepitant might also be expected to occur with EMEND for Injection.

The overall safety of fosaprepitant was evaluated in approximately 1100 individuals and the overall safety of aprepitant was evaluated in approximately 6500 individuals.

Oral Aprepitant
Highly Emetogenic Chemotherapy (HEC)
In 2 well-controlled clinical trials in patients receiving highly emetogenic cancer chemotherapy, 544 patients were treated with aprepitant during Cycle 1 of chemotherapy and 413 of these patients continued into the Multiple-Cycle extension for up to 6 cycles of chemotherapy. Oral aprepitant was given in combination with ondansetron and dexamethasone.

In Cycle 1, adverse reactions were reported in approximately 17% of patients treated with the aprepitant regimen compared with approximately 13% of patients treated with standard therapy. Treatment was discontinued due to adverse reactions in 0.6% of patients treated with the aprepitant regimen compared with 0.4% of patients treated with standard therapy.

The most common adverse reactions reported in patients treated with the aprepitant regimen with an incidence ≥1% and greater than standard therapy are listed in Table 5.

Table 5: Adverse Reactions (incidence ≥1%) in patients receiving HEC with a greater incidence in the Aprepitant Regimen relative to Standard Therapy

	Aprepitant Regimen (N=544)	Standard Therapy (N=550)
Respiratory System		
hiccups	4.6	2.9
Body as a Whole/ Site Unspecified		
asthenia/fatigue	2.9	1.6
Investigations		
ALT increased	2.8	1.5
AST increased	1.1	0.9
Digestive System		
constipation	2.2	2.0
dyspepsia	1.5	0.7
diarrhea	1.1	0.9
Nervous System		
headache	2.2	1.8
Metabolism and Nutrition		
anorexia	2.0	0.5

A listing of adverse reactions in the aprepitant regimen (incidence <1%) that occurred at a greater incidence than standard therapy are presented in the *Less Common Adverse Reactions* subsection below.

In an additional active-controlled clinical study in 1169 patients receiving aprepitant and highly emetogenic chemotherapy, the adverse experience profile was generally similar to that seen in the other HEC studies with aprepitant.
Moderately Emetogenic Chemotherapy (MEC)
In 2 well-controlled clinical trials in patients receiving moderately emetogenic cancer chemotherapy, 868 patients were treated with the aprepitant regimen during Cycle 1 of chemotherapy and 686 of these patients continued into extensions for up to 4 cycles of chemotherapy. In both studies, oral aprepitant was given in combination with ondansetron and dexamethasone (aprepitant regimen).
In the combined analysis of Cycle 1 data for these 2 studies, adverse reactions were reported in approximately 14% of patients treated with the aprepitant regimen compared with approximately 15% of patients treated with standard therapy. Treatment was discontinued due to adverse reactions in 0.7% of patients treated with the aprepitant regimen compared with 0.2% of patients treated with standard therapy.
The most common adverse reactions reported in patients treated with the aprepitant regimen with an incidence ≥1% and greater than standard therapy are listed in Table 6.

Table 6: Adverse Reactions (incidence ≥1%) in patients receiving MEC with a greater incidence in the Aprepitant Regimen relative to Standard Therapy

	Aprepitant Regimen (N=868)	Standard Therapy (N=846)
Gastrointestinal disorders		
eructation	1.0	0.1
General disorders and administration site conditions		
fatigue	1.4	0.9

A listing of adverse reactions in the aprepitant regimen (incidence <1%) that occurred at a greater incidence than standard therapy are presented in the *Less Common Adverse Reactions* subsection below.
Less Common Adverse Reactions
Adverse reactions reported in either HEC or MEC studies in patients treated with the aprepitant regimen with an incidence <1% and greater than standard therapy are listed in Table 7.

Table 7: Adverse Reactions (incidence <1%) in patients observed in either HEC or MEC Studies with a greater incidence in the Aprepitant Regimen relative to Standard Therapy

Infection and infestations	candidiasis, staphylococcal infection
Blood and the lymphatic system disorders	anemia, febrile neutropenia
Metabolism and nutrition disorders	weight gain, polydipsia
Psychiatric disorders	disorientation, euphoria, anxiety
Nervous system disorders	dizziness, dream abnormality, cognitive disorder, lethargy, somnolence
Eye disorders	conjunctivitis
Ear and labyrinth disorders	tinnitus
Cardiac disorders	bradycardia, cardiovascular disorder, palpitations
Vascular disorders	hot flush, flushing
Respiratory, thoracic and mediastinal disorders	pharyngitis, sneezing, cough, postnasal drip, throat irritation
Gastrointestinal disorders	nausea, acid reflux, dysgeusia, epigastric discomfort, obstipation, gastroesophageal reflux disease, perforating duodenal ulcer, vomiting, abdominal pain, dry mouth, abdominal distension, faeces hard, neutropenic colitis, flatulence, stomatitis
Skin and subcutaneous tissue disorders	rash, acne, photosensitivity, hyperhidrosis, oily skin, pruritus, skin lesion
Musculoskeletal and connective tissue disorders	muscle cramp, myalgia, muscular weakness
Renal and urinary disorders	polyuria, dysuria, pollakiuria
General disorders and administration site condition	edema, chest discomfort, malaise, thirst, chills, gait disturbance
Investigations	alkaline phosphatase increased, hyperglycemia, microscopic hematuria, hyponatremia, weight decreased, neutrophil count decreased

In another chemotherapy induced nausea and vomiting (CINV) study, Stevens-Johnson syndrome was reported as a serious adverse reaction in a patient receiving aprepitant with cancer chemotherapy.

The adverse experience profiles in the Multiple-Cycle extensions of HEC and MEC studies for up to 6 cycles of chemotherapy were similar to that observed in Cycle 1.

Fosaprepitant
In an active-controlled clinical study in patients receiving highly emetogenic chemotherapy, safety was evaluated for 1143 patients receiving the 1-day regimen of EMEND for Injection 150 mg compared to 1169 patients receiving the 3-day regimen of EMEND (aprepitant). The safety profile was generally similar to that seen in prior HEC studies with aprepitant. However, infusion-site reactions occurred at a higher incidence in patients in the fosaprepitant group (3.0%) compared to those in the aprepitant group (0.5%). The reported infusion-site reactions included infusion-site erythema, infusion-site pruritus, infusion-site pain, infusion-site induration, and infusion-site thrombophlebitis.

The following additional adverse reactions occurred with fosaprepitant 150 mg and were not reported in the corresponding section above.

Table 8: Adverse Reactions (incidence >0.1%) in patients receiving Fosaprepitant 150 mg and not reported above for the Oral Aprepitant Regimen

General disorders and administration site conditions	infusion site erythema, infusion site pruritus, infusion site induration, infusion site pain
Investigations	blood pressure increased
Skin and subcutaneous tissue disorders	erythema
Vascular disorders	thrombophlebitis (predominantly, infusion-site thrombophlebitis)

Other Studies with Postoperative Nausea and Vomiting
In well-controlled clinical studies in patients receiving general balanced anesthesia, 564 patients were administered 40-mg aprepitant orally and 538 patients were administered 4-mg ondansetron intravenously.

Adverse reactions were reported in approximately 4% of patients treated with 40-mg aprepitant compared with approximately 6% of patients treated with 4-mg ondansetron intravenously.

In patients treated with aprepitant, increased ALT (1.1%) was seen at a greater incidence than with ondansetron (1.0%). The following additional adverse reactions were observed in patients treated with aprepitant at an incidence <1% and greater than with ondansetron.

Table 9: Adverse Reactions (incidence <1%) in patients receiving Aprepitant 40 mg with a greater incidence in the Aprepitant group relative to ondansetron

Psychiatric disorders	insomnia
Nervous system disorders	dysarthria, hypoesthesia, sensory disturbance
Eye disorders	miosis, visual acuity reduced
Cardiac disorders	bradycardia
Respiratory, thoracic and mediastinal disorders	dyspnea, wheezing
Gastrointestinal disorders	abdominal pain upper, bowel sounds abnormal, dry mouth, nausea, stomach discomfort

In addition, two serious adverse reactions were reported in postoperative nausea and vomiting (PONV) clinical studies in patients taking a higher dose of aprepitant: one case of constipation, and one case of subileus.

Other Studies
Angioedema and urticaria were reported as serious adverse reactions in a patient receiving aprepitant in a non-CINV/non-PONV study.

6.2 Postmarketing Experience
The following adverse reactions have been identified during post approval use of fosaprepitant and aprepitant. Because these reactions are reported voluntarily from a population of uncertain size, it is not always possible to reliably estimate their frequency or establish a causal relationship to drug exposure.

Skin and subcutaneous tissue disorders: pruritus, rash, urticaria, rarely Stevens-Johnson syndrome/toxic epidermal necrolysis.
Immune system disorders: hypersensitivity reactions including anaphylactic reactions.
Nervous system disorders: Events of ifosfamide-induced neurotoxicity have been reported after aprepitant and ifosfamide coadministration.

7 DRUG INTERACTIONS
Drug interactions following administration of fosaprepitant are likely to occur with drugs that interact with oral aprepitant.

Aprepitant is a substrate, a moderate inhibitor, and an inducer of CYP3A4 when administered as a 3-day antiemetic dosing regimen for CINV. Aprepitant is also an inducer of CYP2C9.

Fosaprepitant 150 mg, given as a single dose, is a weak inhibitor of CYP3A4, and does not induce CYP3A4. Fosaprepitant or aprepitant is unlikely to interact with drugs that are substrates for the P-glycoprotein transporter. The following information was derived from data with oral aprepitant, two studies conducted with fosaprepitant and oral midazolam, and one study conducted with fosaprepitant and dexamethasone.

7.1 Effect of Fosaprepitant/Aprepitant on the Pharmacokinetics of Other Agents
CYP3A4 substrates:
Aprepitant, as a moderate inhibitor of CYP3A4, and fosaprepitant 150 mg, as a weak inhibitor of CYP3A4, can increase plasma concentrations of concomitantly coadministered oral medications that are metabolized through CYP3A4 *[see Contraindications (4)]*.
5-HT$_3$ antagonists:
In clinical drug interaction studies, aprepitant did not have clinically important effects on the pharmacokinetics of ondansetron, granisetron, or hydrodolasetron (the active metabolite of dolasetron).
Corticosteroids:
Dexamethasone: Fosaprepitant 150 mg administered as a single intravenous dose on Day 1 increased the AUC$_{0-24hr}$ of dexamethasone, administered as a single 8-mg oral dose on Days 1, 2, and 3, by approximately 2-fold on Days 1 and 2. The oral dexamethasone dose on Days 1 and 2 should be reduced by approximately 50% when coadministered with fosaprepitant 150-mg intravenous on Day 1.
An oral aprepitant regimen of 125 mg on Day 1, and 80 mg/day on Days 2 through 5, coadministered with 20-mg oral dexamethasone on Day 1 and 8-mg oral dexamethasone on Days 2 through 5, increased the AUC of dexamethasone by 2.2-fold on Days 1 and 5. The oral dexamethasone doses should be reduced by approximately 50% when coadministered with a regimen of fosaprepitant 115 mg followed by aprepitant.
Methylprednisolone: An oral aprepitant regimen of 125 mg on Day 1 and 80 mg/day on Days 2 and 3 increased the AUC of methylprednisolone by 1.34-fold on Day 1 and by 2.5-fold on Day 3, when methylprednisolone was coadministered intravenously as 125 mg on Day 1 and orally as 40 mg on Days 2 and 3. The intravenous methylprednisolone dose should be reduced by approximately 25%, and the oral methylprednisolone dose should be reduced by approximately 50% when coadministered with a regimen of fosaprepitant 115 mg followed by aprepitant.
Chemotherapeutic agents:
Docetaxel: In a pharmacokinetic study, oral aprepitant (CINV regimen) did not influence the pharmacokinetics of docetaxel.
Vinorelbine: In a pharmacokinetic study, oral aprepitant (CINV regimen) did not influence the pharmacokinetics of vinorelbine to a clinically significant degree.
Other Chemotherapeutic Agents: EMEND for Injection should be used with caution in patients receiving other chemotherapeutic agents that are primarily metabolized through CYP3A4 *[see Warnings and Precautions (5.1) and Adverse Reactions (6.2)]*.
Oral contraceptives: When oral aprepitant, ondansetron, and dexamethasone were coadministered with an oral contraceptive containing ethinyl estradiol and norethindrone, the trough concentrations of both ethinyl estradiol and norethindrone were reduced by as much as 64% for 3 weeks post-treatment.
The coadministration of fosaprepitant or aprepitant may reduce the efficacy of hormonal contraceptives (these can include birth control pills, skin patches, implants, and certain IUDs) during and for 28 days after administration of the last dose of fosaprepitant or aprepitant. Alternative or back-up methods of contraception should be used during treatment with and for 1 month following the last dose of fosaprepitant or aprepitant.
Midazolam:
Interactions between aprepitant or fosaprepitant and coadministered midazolam are listed in the table below (increase is indicated as "↑", decrease as "↓", no change as "↔").

Table 10: Pharmacokinetic Interaction Data for Fosaprepitant/Aprepitant and Coadministered Midazolam

Dose of fosaprepitant/ aprepitant	Dose of Midazolam	Observed Drug Interactions
fosaprepitant 150 mg on Day 1	oral 2 mg on Days 1 and 4	AUC ↑ 1.8-fold on Day 1 and AUC ↔ on Day 4
fosaprepitant 100 mg on Day 1	oral 2 mg	oral midazolam AUC ↑ 1.6-fold
oral aprepitant 125 mg on Day 1 and 80 mg on Days 2 to 5	oral 2 mg SD on Days 1 and 5	oral midazolam AUC ↑ 2.3-fold on Day 1 and ↑ 3.3-fold on Day 5
oral aprepitant 125 mg on Day 1 and 80 mg on Days 2 and 3	intravenous 2 mg prior to 3-day regimen of aprepitant and on Days 4, 8 and 15	intravenous midazolam AUC ↑ 25% on Day 4, AUC ↓ 19% on Day 8 and AUC ↓ 4% on Day 15
oral aprepitant 125 mg	intravenous 2 mg given 1 hour after aprepitant	intravenous midazolam AUC ↑ 1.5-fold

A difference of less than 2-fold increase of midazolam AUC was not considered clinically important.
The potential effects of increased plasma concentrations of midazolam or other benzodiazepines metabolized via CYP3A4 (alprazolam, triazolam) should be considered when coadministering these agents with fosaprepitant or aprepitant.
CYP2C9 substrates (Warfarin, Tolbutamide):
Warfarin: A single 125-mg dose of oral aprepitant was administered on Day 1 and 80 mg/day on Days 2 and 3 to healthy subjects who were stabilized on chronic warfarin therapy. Although there was no effect of oral aprepitant on the plasma AUC of R(+) or S(-) warfarin determined on Day 3, there was a 34% decrease in S(-) warfarin trough concentration accompanied by a 14% decrease in the prothrombin time (reported as International Normalized Ratio or INR) 5 days after completion of dosing with oral aprepitant. In patients on chronic warfarin therapy, the prothrombin time (INR) should be closely monitored in the 2-week period, particularly at 7 to 10 days, following initiation of fosaprepitant with each chemotherapy cycle.
Tolbutamide: Oral aprepitant, when given as 125 mg on Day 1 and 80 mg/day on Days 2 and 3, decreased the AUC of tolbutamide by 23% on Day 4, 28% on Day 8, and 15% on Day 15, when a single dose of tolbutamide 500 mg was administered orally prior to the administration of the 3-day regimen of oral aprepitant and on Days 4, 8, and 15.
7.2 Effect of Other Agents on the Pharmacokinetics of Aprepitant
Aprepitant is a substrate for CYP3A4; therefore, coadministration of fosaprepitant or aprepitant with drugs that inhibit CYP3A4 activity may result in increased plasma concentrations of aprepitant. Consequently, concomitant administration of fosaprepitant or aprepitant with strong CYP3A4 inhibitors (e.g., ketoconazole, itraconazole, nefazodone, troleandomycin, clarithromycin, ritonavir, nelfinavir) should be approached with caution. Because moderate CYP3A4 inhibitors (e.g., diltiazem) result in a 2-fold increase in plasma concentrations of aprepitant, concomitant administration should also be approached with caution.
Aprepitant is a substrate for CYP3A4; therefore, coadministration of fosaprepitant or aprepitant with drugs that strongly induce CYP3A4 activity (e.g., rifampin, carbamazepine, phenytoin) may result in reduced plasma concentrations and decreased efficacy.
Ketoconazole: When a single 125-mg dose of oral aprepitant was administered on Day 5 of a 10-day regimen of 400 mg/day of ketoconazole, a strong CYP3A4 inhibitor, the AUC of aprepitant increased approximately 5-fold and the mean terminal half-life of aprepitant increased approximately 3-fold. Concomitant administration of fosaprepitant or aprepitant with strong CYP3A4 inhibitors should be approached cautiously.
Rifampin: When a single 375-mg dose of oral aprepitant was administered on Day 9 of a 14-day regimen of 600 mg/day of rifampin, a strong CYP3A4 inducer, the AUC of aprepitant decreased approximately 11-fold and the mean terminal half-life decreased approximately 3-fold.
Coadministration of fosaprepitant or aprepitant with drugs that induce CYP3A4 activity may result in reduced plasma concentrations and decreased efficacy.
7.3 Additional Interactions
Diltiazem: In a study in 10 patients with mild to moderate hypertension, intravenous infusion of 100 mg of

fosaprepitant with diltiazem 120 mg 3 times daily, resulted in a 1.5-fold increase of aprepitant AUC and a 1.4-fold increase in diltiazem AUC. It also resulted in a small but clinically meaningful further maximum decrease in diastolic blood pressure [mean (SD) of 24.3 (± 10.2) mm Hg with fosaprepitant versus 15.6 (± 4.1) mm Hg without fosaprepitant] and resulted in a small further maximum decrease in systolic blood pressure [mean (SD) of 29.5 (± 7.9) mm Hg with fosaprepitant versus 23.8 (± 4.8) mm Hg without fosaprepitant], which may be clinically meaningful, but did not result in a clinically meaningful further change in heart rate or PR interval, beyond those changes induced by diltiazem alone.

In the same study, administration of aprepitant once daily, as a tablet formulation comparable to 230 mg of the capsule formulation, with diltiazem 120 mg 3 times daily for 5 days, resulted in a 2-fold increase of aprepitant AUC and a simultaneous 1.7-fold increase of diltiazem AUC. These pharmacokinetic effects did not result in clinically meaningful changes in ECG, heart rate or blood pressure beyond those changes induced by diltiazem alone.

Paroxetine: Coadministration of once daily doses of aprepitant, as a tablet formulation comparable to 85 mg or 170 mg of the capsule formulation, with paroxetine 20 mg once daily, resulted in a decrease in AUC by approximately 25% and C_{max} by approximately 20% of both aprepitant and paroxetine.

8 USE IN SPECIFIC POPULATIONS

8.1 Pregnancy

Teratogenic effects

Pregnancy Category B: In the reproduction studies conducted with fosaprepitant and aprepitant, the highest systemic exposures to aprepitant were obtained following oral administration of aprepitant. Reproduction studies performed in rats at oral doses of aprepitant up to 1000 mg/kg twice daily (plasma AUC_{0-24hr} of 31.3 mcg•hr/mL, about 1.6 times the human exposure at the recommended dose) and in rabbits at oral doses up to 25 mg/kg/day (plasma AUC_{0-24hr} of 26.9 mcg•hr/mL, about 1.4 times the human exposure at the recommended dose) revealed no evidence of impaired fertility or harm to the fetus due to aprepitant. There are, however, no adequate and well-controlled studies in pregnant women. Because animal reproduction studies are not always predictive of human response, this drug should be used during pregnancy only if clearly needed.

8.3 Nursing Mothers

Aprepitant is excreted in the milk of rats. It is not known whether this drug is excreted in human milk. Because many drugs are excreted in human milk and because of the potential for possible serious adverse reactions in nursing infants from aprepitant and because of the potential for tumorigenicity shown for aprepitant in rodent carcinogenicity studies, a decision should be made whether to discontinue nursing or to discontinue the drug, taking into account the importance of the drug to the mother.

8.4 Pediatric Use

Safety and effectiveness of EMEND for Injection in pediatric patients have not been established.

8.5 Geriatric Use

In 2 well-controlled chemotherapy-induced nausea and vomiting clinical studies, of the total number of patients (N=544) treated with oral aprepitant, 31% were 65 and over, while 5% were 75 and over. No overall differences in safety or effectiveness were observed between these subjects and younger subjects. Greater sensitivity of some older individuals cannot be ruled out. Dosage adjustment in the elderly is not necessary *[see Clinical Pharmacology (12.3)].*

8.6 Patients with Severe Hepatic Impairment

There are no clinical or pharmacokinetic data in patients with severe hepatic impairment (Child-Pugh score >9). Therefore, caution should be exercised when fosaprepitant or aprepitant is administered in these patients *[see Clinical Pharmacology (12.3)].*

10 OVERDOSAGE

There is no specific information on the treatment of overdosage with fosaprepitant or aprepitant.

In the event of overdose, fosaprepitant and/or oral aprepitant should be discontinued and general supportive treatment and monitoring should be provided. Because of the antiemetic activity of aprepitant, drug-induced emesis may not be effective.

Aprepitant cannot be removed by hemodialysis.

Thirteen patients in the randomized controlled trial of EMEND for Injection received both fosaprepitant 150 mg and at least one dose of oral aprepitant, 125 mg or 80 mg. Three patients reported adverse reactions that were similar to those experienced by the total study population.

11 DESCRIPTION

EMEND (fosaprepitant dimeglumine) for Injection is a sterile, lyophilized prodrug of aprepitant, a substance P/neurokinin-1 (NK_1) receptor antagonist, and is chemically described as 1-Deoxy-1-(methylamino)-D-glucitol[3-[[(2R,

3S)-2-[(1R)-1-[3,5-bis(trifluoromethyl)phenyl]ethoxy]-3-(4-fluorophenyl)-4-morpholinyl]methyl]-2,5-dihydro-5-oxo-1*H*-1,2,4-triazol-1-yl]phosphonate (2:1) (salt).

Its empirical formula is $C_{23}H_{22}F_7N_4O_6P$ • $2(C_7H_{17}NO_5)$ and its structural formula is:

Fosaprepitant dimeglumine is a white to off-white amorphous powder with a molecular weight of 1004.83. It is freely soluble in water.

EMEND for Injection is a lyophilized prodrug of aprepitant containing polysorbate 80 (PS80), to be administered intravenously as an infusion.

Each vial of EMEND for Injection 115 mg for intravenous administration contains 188 mg of fosaprepitant dimeglumine equivalent to 115 mg of fosaprepitant free acid and the following inactive ingredients: edetate disodium (14.4 mg), polysorbate 80 (57.5 mg), lactose anhydrous (287.5 mg), sodium hydroxide and/or hydrochloric acid (for pH adjustment). Each vial of EMEND for Injection 150 mg for intravenous administration contains 245.3 mg of fosaprepitant dimeglumine equivalent to 150 mg of fosaprepitant free acid and the following inactive ingredients: edetate disodium (18.8 mg), polysorbate 80 (75 mg), lactose anhydrous (375 mg), sodium hydroxide and/or hydrochloric acid (for pH adjustment). Fosaprepitant dimeglumine hereafter will be referred to as fosaprepitant.

12 CLINICAL PHARMACOLOGY

Fosaprepitant, a prodrug of aprepitant, when administered intravenously is rapidly converted to aprepitant, a substance P/neurokinin 1 (NK_1) receptor antagonist. Plasma concentrations of fosaprepitant are below the limits of quantification (10 ng/mL) within 30 minutes of the completion of infusion *[see Clinical Pharmacology (12.3)].* Upon conversion of 188 mg of fosaprepitant dimeglumine (equivalent to 115-mg fosaprepitant free acid) to aprepitant, 18.3 mg of phosphoric acid and 73 mg of meglumine are liberated. Upon conversion of 245.3 mg of fosaprepitant dimeglumine (equivalent to 150-mg fosaprepitant free acid) to aprepitant, 23.9 mg of phosphoric acid and 95.3 mg of meglumine are liberated.

12.1 Mechanism of Action

Fosaprepitant is a prodrug of aprepitant and accordingly, its antiemetic effects are attributable to aprepitant.

Aprepitant is a selective high-affinity antagonist of human substance P/neurokinin 1 (NK_1) receptors. Aprepitant has little or no affinity for serotonin (5-HT_3), dopamine, and corticosteroid receptors, the targets of existing therapies for chemotherapy-induced nausea and vomiting (CINV). Aprepitant has been shown in animal models to inhibit emesis induced by cytotoxic chemotherapeutic agents, such as cisplatin, via central actions. Animal and human Positron Emission Tomography (PET) studies with aprepitant have shown that it crosses the blood brain barrier and occupies brain NK_1 receptors. Animal and human studies show that aprepitant augments the antiemetic activity of the 5-HT_3-receptor antagonist ondansetron and the corticosteroid dexamethasone and inhibits both the acute and delayed phases of cisplatin-induced emesis.

12.2 Pharmacodynamics

NK₁ Receptor Occupancy

In two single-blind, multiple-dose, randomized, and placebo control studies, healthy young men received oral aprepitant doses of 10 mg (N=2), 30 mg (N=3), 100 mg (N=3) or 300 mg (N=5) once daily for 14 days with 2 or 3 subjects on placebo. Both plasma aprepitant concentration and NK_1 receptor occupancy in the corpus striatum by positron emission tomography were evaluated, at predose and 24 hours after the last dose. At aprepitant plasma concentrations of ~10 ng/mL and ~100 ng/mL, the NK_1 receptor occupancies were ~50% and ~90%, respectively. The oral aprepitant regimen for CINV produces mean trough plasma aprepitant concentrations >500 ng/mL, which would be expected to, based on the fitted curve with the Hill equation, result in >95% brain NK_1 receptor occupancy. However, the receptor occupancy for either CINV or PONV dosing regimen has not been determined. In addition, the relationship between NK_1 receptor occupancy and the clinical efficacy of aprepitant has not been established.

Cardiac Electrophysiology

In a randomized, double-blind, positive-controlled, thorough QTc study, a single 200-mg dose of fosaprepitant had no effect on the QTc interval.

12.3 Pharmacokinetics

Aprepitant after Fosaprepitant Administration

Following a single intravenous 115-mg dose of fosaprepitant administered as a 15-minute infusion to healthy volunteers

the mean $AUC_{0-\infty}$ of aprepitant was 31.7 (± 14.3) mcg•hr/mL and the mean maximal aprepitant concentration (C_{max}) was 3.27 (± 1.16) mcg/mL. The mean aprepitant plasma concentration at 24 hours postdose was similar between the 125-mg oral aprepitant dose and the 115-mg intravenous fosaprepitant dose. (See Figure 1.)

Figure 1: Mean Plasma Concentration of Aprepitant Following 125-mg Oral Aprepitant and 115-mg Intravenous Fosaprepitant

Following a single, intravenous 150-mg dose of fosaprepitant administered as a 20-minute infusion to healthy volunteers, the mean $AUC_{0-\infty}$ of aprepitant was 37.38 (± 14.75) mcg•hr/mL and the mean maximal aprepitant concentration (C_{max}) was 4.15 (± 1.15) mcg/mL.

Distribution

Fosaprepitant is rapidly converted to aprepitant. Aprepitant is greater than 95% bound to plasma proteins. The mean apparent volume of distribution at steady state (Vd_{ss}) is approximately 70 L in humans.

Aprepitant crosses the placenta in rats and rabbits and crosses the blood brain barrier in humans *[see Clinical Pharmacology (12.1)].*

Metabolism

Fosaprepitant was rapidly converted to aprepitant in *in vitro* incubations with liver preparations from nonclinical species (rat and dog) and humans. Furthermore, fosaprepitant underwent rapid and nearly complete conversion to aprepitant in S9 preparations from multiple other human tissues including kidney, lung and ileum. Thus, it appears that the conversion of fosaprepitant to aprepitant can occur in multiple extrahepatic tissues in addition to the liver. In humans, fosaprepitant administered intravenously was rapidly converted to aprepitant within 30 minutes following the end of infusion.

Aprepitant undergoes extensive metabolism. *In vitro* studies using human liver microsomes indicate that aprepitant is metabolized primarily by CYP3A4 with minor metabolism by CYP1A2 and CYP2C19. Metabolism is largely via oxidation at the morpholine ring and its side chains. No metabolism by CYP2D6, CYP2C9, or CYP2E1 was detected. In healthy young adults, aprepitant accounts for approximately 24% of the radioactivity in plasma over 72 hours following a single oral 300-mg dose of [^{14}C]-aprepitant, indicating a substantial presence of metabolites in the plasma. Seven metabolites of aprepitant, which are only weakly active, have been identified in human plasma.

Excretion

Following administration of a single intravenous 100-mg dose of [^{14}C]-fosaprepitant to healthy subjects, 57% of the radioactivity was recovered in urine and 45% in feces.

Aprepitant is eliminated primarily by metabolism; aprepitant is not renally excreted. The apparent terminal half-life ranged from approximately 9 to 13 hours.

Specific Populations

Gender

Following oral administration of a single dose of aprepitant, the AUC_{0-24hr} and C_{max} are 14% and 22% higher in females as compared with males. The half-life of aprepitant is 25% lower in females as compared with males and T_{max} occurs at approximately the same time. These differences are not considered clinically meaningful. No dosage adjustment is necessary based on gender.

Geriatric

Following oral administration of a single 125-mg dose of aprepitant on Day 1 and 80 mg once daily on Days 2 through 5, the AUC_{0-24hr} of aprepitant was 21% higher on Day 1 and 36% higher on Day 5 in elderly (≥65 years) relative to younger adults. The C_{max} was 10% higher on Day 1 and 24% higher on Day 5 in elderly relative to younger adults. These differences are not considered clinically meaningful. No dosage adjustment is necessary in elderly patients.

Race

Following oral administration of a single dose of aprepitant, the AUC_{0-24hr} and C_{max} are approximately 42% and 29% higher in Hispanics as compared with Caucasians. The AUC_{0-24hr} and C_{max} are 62% and 41% higher in Asians as

Table 11: Treatment Regimens — Highly Emetogenic Chemotherapy Trials*

	Day 1	Day 2	Day 3	Day 4
CINV Aprepitant Regimen				
Aprepitant	125 mg orally	80 mg orally	80 mg orally	none
Dexamethasone	12 mg orally	8 mg orally	8 mg orally	8 mg orally
5-HT$_3$ antagonist[†]	See package insert	none	none	none
CINV Standard Therapy				
Dexamethasone	20 mg orally	8 mg orally twice daily	8 mg orally twice daily	8 mg orally twice daily
5-HT$_3$ antagonist[†]	See package insert	none	none	none

* Aprepitant placebo and dexamethasone placebo were used to maintain blinding.
† Ondansetron 32 mg I.V. was used in the clinical trials of aprepitant. Although this dose was used in clinical trials, this is no longer the currently recommended dose. Refer to the ondansetron package insert for the current dosing.

compared to Caucasians. There was no difference in AUC_{0-24hr} or C_{max} between Caucasians and Blacks. These differences are not considered clinically meaningful. No dosage adjustment is necessary based on race.

Body Mass Index (BMI)
For every 5 kg/m^2 increase in BMI, AUC_{0-24hr} and C_{max} of aprepitant decrease by 11%. BMI of subjects in the analysis ranged from 18 kg/m^2 to 36 kg/m^2. This change is not considered clinically meaningful. No dosage adjustment is necessary based on BMI.

Hepatic Insufficiency
Fosaprepitant is metabolized in various extrahepatic tissues; therefore hepatic impairment is not expected to alter the conversion of fosaprepitant to aprepitant.
Following administration of a single 125-mg dose of oral aprepitant on Day 1 and 80 mg once daily on Days 2 and 3 to patients with mild hepatic impairment (Child-Pugh score 5 to 6), the AUC_{0-24hr} of aprepitant was 11% lower on Day 1 and 36% lower on Day 3, as compared with healthy subjects given the same regimen. In patients with moderate hepatic impairment (Child-Pugh score 7 to 9), the AUC_{0-24hr} of aprepitant was 10% higher on Day 1 and 18% higher on Day 3, as compared with healthy subjects given the same regimen. These differences in AUC_{0-24hr} are not considered clinically meaningful; therefore, no dosage adjustment is necessary in patients with mild to moderate hepatic impairment.
There are no clinical or pharmacokinetic data in patients with severe hepatic impairment (Child-Pugh score >9) [see *Use in Specific Populations (8.6)*].

Renal Insufficiency
A single 240-mg dose of oral aprepitant was administered to patients with severe renal impairment (creatinine clearance <30 mL/min/1.73 m^2 as measured by 24-hour urinary creatinine clearance) and to patients with end stage renal disease (ESRD) requiring hemodialysis.
In patients with severe renal impairment, the $AUC_{0-\infty}$ of total aprepitant (unbound and protein bound) decreased by 21% and C_{max} decreased by 32%, relative to healthy subjects (creatinine clearance >80 mL/min estimated by Cockcroft-Gault method). In patients with ESRD undergoing hemodialysis, the $AUC_{0-\infty}$ of total aprepitant decreased by 42% and C_{max} decreased by 32%. Due to modest decreases in protein binding of aprepitant in patients with renal disease, the AUC of pharmacologically active unbound drug was not significantly affected in patients with renal impairment compared with healthy subjects. Hemodialysis conducted 4 or 48 hours after dosing had no significant effect on the pharmacokinetics of aprepitant; less than 0.2% of the dose was recovered in the dialysate.
No dosage adjustment is necessary for patients with renal impairment or for patients with ESRD undergoing hemodialysis.

13 NONCLINICAL TOXICOLOGY

13.1 Carcinogenesis, Mutagenesis, Impairment of Fertility

Carcinogenicity studies were conducted in Sprague-Dawley rats and in CD-1 mice for 2 years. In the rat carcinogenicity studies, animals were treated with oral doses ranging from 0.05 to 1000 mg/kg twice daily. The highest dose produced a systemic exposure to aprepitant (plasma AUC_{0-24hr} of 0.7 to 1.6 times the human exposure (AUC_{0-24hr} = 19.6 mcg•hr/mL) at the recommended dose of 125 mg/day. Treatment with aprepitant at doses of 5 to 1000 mg/kg twice daily caused an increase in the incidences of thyroid follicular cell adenomas and carcinomas in male rats. In female rats, it produced hepatocellular adenomas at 5 to 1000 mg/kg twice daily and hepatocellular carcinomas and thyroid follicular cell adenomas at 125 to 1000 mg/kg twice daily. In the mouse carcinogenicity studies, the animals were treated with oral doses ranging from 2.5 to

2000 mg/kg/day. The highest dose produced a systemic exposure of about 2.8 to 3.6 times the human exposure at the recommended dose. Treatment with aprepitant produced skin fibrosarcomas at 125 and 500 mg/kg/day doses in male mice. Carcinogenicity studies were not conducted with fosaprepitant.
Aprepitant and fosaprepitant were not genotoxic in the Ames test, the human lymphoblastoid cell (TK6) mutagenesis test, the rat hepatocyte DNA strand break test, the Chinese hamster ovary (CHO) cell chromosome aberration test and the mouse micronucleus test.
Fosaprepitant, when administered intravenously, is rapidly converted to aprepitant. In the fertility studies conducted with fosaprepitant and aprepitant, the highest systemic exposures to aprepitant were obtained following oral administration of aprepitant. Oral aprepitant did not affect the fertility or general reproductive performance of male or female rats at doses up to the maximum feasible dose of 1000 mg/kg twice daily (providing exposure in male rats lower than the exposure at the recommended human dose and exposure in female rats at about 1.6 times the human exposure).

14 CLINICAL STUDIES

Fosaprepitant, a prodrug of aprepitant, when administered intravenously is rapidly converted to aprepitant.
Oral administration of aprepitant in combination with ondansetron and dexamethasone (aprepitant regimen) has been shown to prevent acute and delayed nausea and vomiting associated with highly emetogenic chemotherapy including high-dose cisplatin, and nausea and vomiting associated with moderately emetogenic chemotherapy.

14.1 Highly Emetogenic Chemotherapy (HEC)

EMEND for Injection 115 mg (3-Day Dosing Regimen of EMEND)
Fosaprepitant 115 mg intravenous infused over 15 minutes can be substituted for 125 mg oral aprepitant on Day 1 of a 3-day regimen. Efficacy studies with the 3-day regimen were conducted with oral aprepitant.
In 2 multicenter, randomized, parallel, double-blind, controlled clinical studies, the aprepitant regimen (see Table 11) was compared with standard therapy in patients receiving a chemotherapy regimen that included cisplatin >50 mg/m^2 (mean cisplatin dose = 80.2 mg/m^2). Of the 550 patients who were randomized to receive the aprepitant regimen, 42% were women, 58% men, 59% White, 3% Asian, 5% Black, 12% Hispanic American, and 21% Multi-Racial. The aprepitant-treated patients in these clinical studies ranged from 14 to 84 years of age, with a mean age of 56 years. 170 patients were 65 years or older, with 29 patients being 75 years or older.
Patients (N = 1105) were randomized to either the aprepitant regimen (N = 550) or standard therapy (N = 555). The treatment regimens are defined in Table 11.
[See table 11 above]
During these studies, 95% of the patients in the aprepitant group received a concomitant chemotherapeutic agent in addition to protocol-mandated cisplatin. The most common chemotherapeutic agents and the number of aprepitant patients exposed follow: etoposide (106), fluorouracil (100), gemcitabine (89), vinorelbine (82), paclitaxel (52), cyclophosphamide (50), doxorubicin (38), docetaxel (11).
The antiemetic activity of oral aprepitant was evaluated during the acute phase (0 to 24 hours post-cisplatin treatment), the delayed phase (25 to 120 hours post-cisplatin treatment) and overall (0 to 120 hours post-cisplatin treatment) in Cycle 1. Efficacy was based on evaluation of the following endpoints in which emetic episodes included vomiting, retching, or dry heaves:
Primary endpoint:
● complete response (defined as no emetic episodes and no use of rescue therapy as recorded in patient diaries)

Other prespecified endpoints:
● complete protection (defined as no emetic episodes, no use of rescue therapy, and a maximum nausea visual analogue scale [VAS] score <25 mm on a 0 to 100 mm scale)
● no emesis (defined as no emetic episodes regardless of use of rescue therapy)
● no nausea (maximum VAS <5 mm on a 0 to 100 mm scale)
● no significant nausea (maximum VAS <25 mm on a 0 to 100 mm scale)
A summary of the key study results from each individual study analysis is shown in Table 12 and in Table 13.

Table 12: Percent of Patients Receiving Highly Emetogenic Chemotherapy Responding by Treatment Group and Phase for Study 1 — Cycle 1

ENDPOINTS	Aprepitant Regimen (N = 260)* %	Standard Therapy (N = 261)* %	p-Value
PRIMARY ENDPOINT			
Complete Response			
Overall[†]	73	52	<0.001
OTHER PRESPECIFIED ENDPOINTS			
Complete Response			
Acute phase[‡]	89	78	<0.001
Delayed phase[§]	75	56	<0.001
Complete Protection			
Overall	63	49	0.001
Acute phase	85	75	NS[¶]
Delayed phase	66	52	<0.001
No Emesis			
Overall	78	55	<0.001
Acute phase	90	79	0.001
Delayed phase	81	59	<0.001
No Nausea			
Overall	48	44	NS[#]
Delayed phase	51	48	NS[#]
No Significant Nausea			
Overall	73	66	NS[#]
Delayed phase	75	69	NS[#]

Visual analogue scale (VAS) score range: 0 mm = no nausea; 100 mm = nausea as bad as it could be.
* N: Number of patients (older than 18 years of age) who received cisplatin, study drug, and had at least one post-treatment efficacy evaluation.
† Overall: 0 to 120 hours post-cisplatin treatment.
‡ Acute phase: 0 to 24 hours post-cisplatin treatment.
§ Delayed phase: 25 to 120 hours post-cisplatin treatment.
¶ Not statistically significant when adjusted for multiple comparisons.
# Not statistically significant.

Table 13: Percent of Patients Receiving Highly Emetogenic Chemotherapy Responding by Treatment Group and Phase for Study 2 — Cycle 1

ENDPOINTS	Aprepitant Regimen (N = 261)* %	Standard Therapy (N = 263)* %	p-Value
PRIMARY ENDPOINT			
Complete Response			
Overall[†]	63	43	<0.001
OTHER PRESPECIFIED ENDPOINTS			
Complete Response			
Acute phase[‡]	83	68	<0.001
Delayed phase[§]	68	47	<0.001
Complete Protection			
Overall	56	41	<0.001
Acute phase	80	65	<0.001
Delayed phase	61	44	<0.001

No Emesis

Overall	66	44	<0.001
Acute phase	84	69	<0.001
Delayed phase	72	48	<0.001

No Nausea

Overall	49	39	NS¶
Delayed phase	53	40	NS¶

No Significant Nausea

Overall	71	64	NS#
Delayed phase	73	65	NS#

Visual analogue scale (VAS) score range: 0 mm = no nausea; 100 mm = nausea as bad as it could be.
* N: Number of patients (older than 18 years of age) who received cisplatin, study drug, and had at least one post-treatment efficacy evaluation.
† Overall: 0 to 120 hours post-cisplatin treatment.
‡ Acute phase: 0 to 24 hours post-cisplatin treatment.
§ Delayed phase: 25 to 120 hours post-cisplatin treatment.
¶ Not statistically significant when adjusted for multiple comparisons.
# Not statistically significant.

In both studies, a statistically significantly higher proportion of patients (both p<0.001) receiving the aprepitant regimen in Cycle 1 had a complete response in the overall phase (primary endpoint), compared with patients receiving standard therapy. A statistically significant difference in complete response in favor of the aprepitant regimen was also observed when the acute phase and the delayed phase were analyzed separately.

In both studies, the estimated time to first emesis after initiation of cisplatin treatment was longer with the aprepitant regimen, and the incidence of first emesis was reduced in the aprepitant regimen group compared with standard therapy group as depicted in the Kaplan-Meier curves in Figure 2.

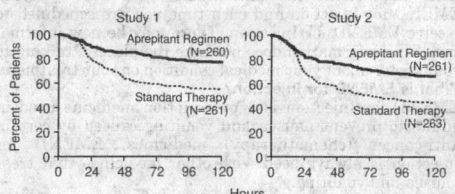

p-Value <0.001 based on a log rank test for Study 1 and Study 2; nominal p-values not adjusted for multiplicity.

Figure 2: Percent of Patients Receiving Highly Emetogenic Chemotherapy Who Remain Emesis Free Over Time — Cycle 1

Additional Patient-Reported Outcomes: The impact of nausea and vomiting on patients' daily lives was assessed in Cycle 1 of both phase 3 studies using the Functional Living Index–Emesis (FLIE), a validated nausea- and vomiting-specific patient-reported outcome measure. Minimal or no impact of nausea and vomiting on patients' daily lives is defined as a FLIE total score >108. In each of the 2 studies, a higher proportion of patients receiving the aprepitant regimen reported minimal or no impact of nausea and vomiting on daily life (Study 1: 74% versus 64%; Study 2: 75% versus 64%).

Multiple-Cycle Extension: In the same 2 clinical studies, patients continued into the Multiple-Cycle extension for up to 5 additional cycles of chemotherapy. The proportion of patients with no emesis and no significant nausea by treatment group at each cycle is depicted in Figure 3.

Aprepitant (N)	158	122	81	54	40
Standard (N)	177	111	68	37	29
	191	148	103	63	43
	216	167	112	74	43

Figure 3: Proportion of Patients Receiving Highly Emetogenic Chemotherapy with No Emesis and No Significant Nausea by Treatment Group and Cycle

Table 14: Treatment Regimens — Highly Emetogenic Chemotherapy Trial*

	Day 1	Day 2	Day 3	Day 4
CINV Fosaprepitant Regimen				
Fosaprepitant	150 mg intravenously	none	none	none
Dexamethasone	12 mg orally	8 mg orally	8 mg orally twice daily	8 mg orally twice daily
5-HT₃ antagonist†	See package insert	none	none	none
CINV Aprepitant Regimen				
Aprepitant	125 mg orally	80 mg orally	80 mg orally	none
Dexamethasone	12 mg orally	8 mg orally	8 mg orally	8 mg orally
5-HT₃ antagonist†	See package insert	none	none	none

* Fosaprepitant placebo, aprepitant placebo and dexamethasone placebo (in the evenings on Days 3 and 4) were used to maintain blinding.
† Ondansetron 32 mg I.V. was used in the clinical trial of EMEND for Injection. Although this dose was used in the clinical trial, this is no longer the currently recommended dose. Refer to the ondansetron package insert for the current dosing.

Table 15: Percent of Patients Receiving Highly Emetogenic Chemotherapy Responding by Treatment Group and Phase — Cycle 1

ENDPOINTS	Fosaprepitant Regimen (N = 1106)* %	Aprepitant Regimen (N = 1134)* %	Difference† (95% CI)
PRIMARY ENDPOINT			
Complete Response‡			
Overall§	71.9	72.3	-0.4 (-4.1, 3.3)
SECONDARY ENDPOINTS			
Complete Response‡			
Delayed phase¶	74.3	74.2	0.1 (-3.5, 3.7)
No Vomiting			
Overall§	72.9	74.6	-1.7 (-5.3, 2.0)

* N: Number of patients included in the primary analysis of complete response.
† Difference and Confidence interval (CI) were calculated using the method proposed by Miettinen and Nurminen and adjusted for Gender.
‡ Complete Response = no vomiting and no use of rescue therapy.
§ Overall = 0 to 120 hours post-initiation of cisplatin chemotherapy.
¶ Delayed phase = 25 to 120 hours post-initiation of cisplatin chemotherapy.

EMEND for Injection 150 mg (Single Dose Regimen of EMEND)
EMEND for Injection 150 mg infused over 20-30 minutes is administered on Day 1 only and can be substituted for the 3-day dosing regimen of EMEND for the prevention of nausea and vomiting induced by HEC.

In a randomized, parallel, double-blind, active-controlled study, EMEND for Injection 150 mg (N=1147) was compared with a 3-day oral aprepitant regimen (N=1175) (see Table 14 below) in patients receiving a highly emetogenic chemotherapy regimen that included cisplatin (≥70 mg/m²). Patient demographics were similar between the two treatment groups. Of the total 2322 patients receiving EMEND for Injection or oral aprepitant, 63% were men, 56% White, 26% Asian, 3% American Indian/Alaska Native, 2% Black, 13% Multi-Racial, and 33% Hispanic/Latino ethnicity. Patient ages ranged from 19 to 86 years of age, with a mean age of 56 years. Other concomitant chemotherapy agents were administered similar to those in prior HEC studies described above.

[See table 14 above]

The efficacy of fosaprepitant 150 mg was evaluated based on the primary and secondary endpoints listed in Table 15 below and was shown to be non-inferior to that of the 3-day oral aprepitant regimen with regard to complete response in each of the evaluated phases. The pre-specified non-inferiority margin for complete response in the overall phase was 7%. The pre-specified non-inferiority margin for complete response in the delayed phase was 7.3%. The pre-specified non-inferiority margin for no vomiting in the overall phase was 8.2%.

[See table 15 above]

14.2 Moderately Emetogenic Chemotherapy (MEC)
In a multicenter, randomized, double-blind, parallel-group, clinical study in breast cancer patients, the aprepitant regimen (see Table 16) was compared with a standard of care therapy in patients receiving a moderately emetogenic chemotherapy regimen that included cyclophosphamide 750-1500 mg/m²; or cyclophosphamide 500-1500 mg/m² and doxorubicin (≤60 mg/m²) or epirubicin (≤100 mg/m²).

In this study, the most common combinations were cyclophosphamide + doxorubicin (60.6%); and cyclophosphamide + epirubicin + fluorouracil (21.6%).

Of the 438 patients who were randomized to receive the aprepitant regimen, 99.5% were women. Of these, approximately 80% were White, 8% Black, 8% Asian, 4% Hispanic, and <1% Other. The aprepitant-treated patients in this clinical study ranged from 25 to 78 years of age, with a mean age of 53 years; 70 patients were 65 years or older, with 12 patients being over 74 years.

Patients (N = 866) were randomized to either the aprepitant regimen (N = 438) or standard therapy (N = 428). The treatment regimens are defined in Table 16.

Table 16: Treatment Regimens — Moderately Emetogenic Chemotherapy Trial*

	Day 1	Day 2	Day 3
CINV Aprepitant Regimen			
Aprepitant	125 mg orally†	80 mg orally	80 mg orally
Dexamethasone	12 mg orally‡	none	none
Ondansetron	8 mg orally × 2 doses§	none	none

CINV Standard Therapy			
Dexamethasone	20 mg orally	none	none
Ondansetron	8 mg orally × 2 doses	8 mg orally twice daily	8 mg orally twice daily

* Aprepitant placebo and dexamethasone placebo were used to maintain blinding.
† 1 hour prior to chemotherapy.
‡ Dexamethasone was administered 30 minutes prior to chemotherapy treatment on Day 1.
§ Ondansetron was administered 30 to 60 minutes prior to chemotherapy treatment on Day 1 and 8 hours after first ondansetron dose.

The antiemetic activity of oral aprepitant was evaluated based on the following endpoints in which emetic episodes included vomiting, retching, or dry heaves:
Primary endpoint:
• complete response (defined as no emetic episodes and no use of rescue therapy as recorded in patient diaries) in the overall phase (0 to 120 hours post-chemotherapy)
Other prespecified endpoints:
• no emesis (defined as no emetic episodes regardless of use of rescue therapy)
• no nausea (maximum VAS <5 mm on a 0 to 100 mm scale)
• no significant nausea (maximum VAS <25 mm on a 0 to 100 mm scale)
• complete protection (defined as no emetic episodes, no use of rescue therapy, and a maximum nausea visual analogue scale [VAS] score <25 mm on a 0 to 100 mm scale)
• complete response during the acute and delayed phases.
A summary of the key results from this study is shown in Table 17.

Table 17: Percent of Patients Receiving Moderately Emetogenic Chemotherapy Responding by Treatment Group and Phase — Cycle 1

ENDPOINTS	Aprepitant Regimen (N = 433)* %	Standard Therapy (N = 424)* %	p-Value
PRIMARY ENDPOINT†			
Complete Response	51	42	0.015
OTHER PRESPECIFIED ENDPOINTS†			
No Emesis	76	59	NS‡
No Nausea	33	33	NS
No Significant Nausea	61	56	NS
No Rescue Therapy	59	56	NS
Complete Protection	43	37	NS

* N: Number of patients included in the primary analysis of complete response.
† Overall: 0 to 120 hours post-chemotherapy treatment.
‡ NS when adjusted for prespecified multiple comparisons rule; unadjusted p-value <0.001.

In this study, a statistically significantly (p=0.015) higher proportion of patients receiving the aprepitant regimen in Cycle 1 had a complete response (primary endpoint) during the overall phase compared with patients receiving standard therapy. The difference between treatment groups was primarily driven by the "No Emesis Endpoint", a principal component of this composite primary endpoint. In addition, a higher proportion of patients receiving the aprepitant regimen in Cycle 1 had a complete response during the acute (0-24 hours) and delayed (25-120 hours) phases compared with patients receiving standard therapy; however, the treatment group differences failed to reach statistical significance, after multiplicity adjustments.
Additional Patient-Reported Outcomes: In a phase 3 study in patients receiving moderately emetogenic chemotherapy, the impact of nausea and vomiting on patients' daily lives was assessed in Cycle 1 using the FLIE. A higher proportion of patients receiving the aprepitant regimen reported minimal or no impact on daily life (64% versus 56%). This difference between treatment groups was primarily driven by the "No Vomiting Domain" of this composite endpoint.
Multiple-Cycle Extension: Patients receiving moderately emetogenic chemotherapy were permitted to continue into the Multiple-Cycle extension of the study for up to 3 additional cycles of chemotherapy. Antiemetic effect for patients receiving the aprepitant regimen is maintained during all cycles.

Postmarketing Trial: In a postmarketing, multicenter, randomized, double-blind, parallel-group, clinical study in 848 cancer patients, the aprepitant regimen (N=430) was compared with a standard of care therapy (N=418) in patients receiving a moderately emetogenic chemotherapy regimen that included any IV dose of oxaliplatin, carboplatin, epirubicin, idarubicin, ifosfamide, irinotecan, daunorubicin, doxorubicin; cyclophosphamide IV (<1500 mg/m²); or cytarabine IV (>1 g/m²).
Of the 430 patients who were randomized to receive the aprepitant regimen, 76% were women and 24% were men. The distribution by race was 67% White, 6% Black or African American, 11% Asian, and 12% multiracial. Classified by ethnicity, 36% were Hispanic and 64% were non-Hispanic. The aprepitant-treated patients in this clinical study ranged from 22 to 85 years of age, with a mean age of 57 years; approximately 59% of the patients were 55 years or older with 32 patients being over 74 years. Patients receiving the aprepitant regimen were receiving chemotherapy for a variety of tumor types including 50% with breast cancer, 21% with gastrointestinal cancers including colorectal cancer, 13% with lung cancer and 6% with gynecological cancers.
The antiemetic activity of EMEND was evaluated based on no vomiting (with or without rescue therapy) in the overall period (0 to 120 hours post-chemotherapy) and complete response (defined as no vomiting and no use of rescue therapy) in the overall period.
A summary of the key results from this study is shown in Table 18.

Table 18: Percent of Patients Receiving Moderately Emetogenic Chemotherapy Responding by Treatment Group for Study 2 — Cycle 1

ENDPOINTS	Aprepitant Regimen (N = 430)* %	Standard Therapy (N = 418)* %	p-Value
No Vomiting Overall	76	62	<0.0001
Complete Response Overall	69	56	0.0003

* N = Number of patients who received chemotherapy treatment, study drug, and had at least one post-treatment efficacy evaluation.

In this study, a statistically significantly higher proportion of patients receiving the aprepitant regimen (76%) in Cycle 1 had no vomiting during the overall phase compared with patients receiving standard therapy (62%). In addition, a higher proportion of patients receiving the aprepitant regimen (69%) in Cycle 1 had a complete response in the overall phase (0-120 hours) compared with patients receiving standard therapy (56%). In the acute phase (0 to 24 hours following initiation of chemotherapy), a higher proportion of patients receiving aprepitant compared to patients receiving standard therapy were observed to have no vomiting (92% and 84%, respectively) and complete response (89% and 80%, respectively). In the delayed phase (25 to 120 hours following initiation of chemotherapy), a higher proportion of patients receiving aprepitant compared to patients receiving standard therapy were observed to have no vomiting (78% and 67%, respectively) and complete response (71% and 61%, respectively).
In a subgroup analysis by tumor type, a numerically higher proportion of patients receiving aprepitant were observed to have no vomiting and complete response compared to patients receiving standard therapy. For gender, the difference in complete response rates between the aprepitant and standard regimen groups was 14% in females (64.5% and 50.3%, respectively) and 4% in males (82.2% and 78.2%, respectively) during the overall phase. A similar difference for gender was observed for the no vomiting endpoint.

16   HOW SUPPLIED/STORAGE AND HANDLING

No. 3884 — One 115-mg single dose glass vial: White to off-white lyophilized solid. Supplied as follows:
NDC 0006-3884-32 1 vial per carton.
No. 3941 — One 150-mg single dose glass vial: White to off-white lyophilized solid. Supplied as follows:
NDC 0006-3941-32 1 vial per carton.
Storage
Vials: Store at 2-8°C (36-46°F).
Sterile lyophilized powder for intravenous use only after reconstitution and dilution.

17   PATIENT COUNSELING INFORMATION

"See FDA-Approved Patient Labeling (Patient Information)"

Physicians should instruct their patients to read the patient package insert before starting therapy with EMEND for Injection and to reread it each time the prescription is renewed.
Patients should follow the physician's instructions for the EMEND for Injection regimen.
Allergic reactions, which may be sudden and/or serious, and may include hives, rash, itching, redness of the face/skin and may cause difficulty in breathing or swallowing, have been reported. Physicians should instruct their patients to stop using EMEND and call their doctor right away if they experience an allergic reaction. In addition, severe skin reactions may occur rarely.
Patients who develop an infusion site reaction such as erythema, edema, pain, or thrombophlebitis should be instructed on how to care for the local reaction and when to seek further evaluation.
EMEND for Injection may interact with some drugs including chemotherapy; therefore, patients should be advised to report to their doctor the use of any other prescription, nonprescription medication or herbal products.
Patients on chronic warfarin therapy should be instructed to have their clotting status closely monitored in the 2-week period, particularly at 7 to 10 days, following initiation of fosaprepitant with each chemotherapy cycle.
Administration of EMEND for Injection may reduce the efficacy of hormonal contraceptives. Patients should be advised to use alternative or back-up methods of contraception during treatment with and for 1 month following the last dose of fosaprepitant or aprepitant.
Manufactured for:
Merck Sharp & Dohme Corp., a subsidiary of **MERCK & CO., INC.,** Whitehouse Station, NJ 08889, USA
Manufactured by:
DSM Pharmaceuticals, Inc., 5900 Martin Luther King Jr. Highway, Greenville, NC 27834, USA
U.S. Patent Nos.: 5,512,570; 5,691,336
Copyright © 2008, 2009 Merck Sharp & Dohme Corp., a subsidiary of **Merck & Co., Inc.**
All rights reserved.
uspi-mk0517-iv-1408r011
Patient Information
EMEND® (EE mend)
(fosaprepitant dimeglumine)
for Injection
Read this Patient Information before you start receiving EMEND for Injection and each time you are scheduled to receive EMEND for Injection. There may be new information. This information does not take the place of talking to your doctor about your medical condition or your treatment.
What is EMEND for Injection?
EMEND for Injection is a prescription medicine used in adults to prevent nausea and vomiting caused by certain anti-cancer (chemotherapy) medicines. EMEND for Injection is always used with other medicines that treat nausea and vomiting.
EMEND for Injection is not used to treat nausea and vomiting that you already have.
EMEND for Injection should not be used continuously for a long time (chronic use).
It is not known if EMEND for Injection is safe and effective in children.
Who should not take EMEND for Injection?
Do not take EMEND for Injection if you:
• are taking any of the following medicines:
  ○ pimozide (ORAP®)
  ○ cisapride (PROPULSID®)
Taking EMEND for Injection with any of these medicines could cause serious or life-threatening problems.
• are allergic to any of the ingredients in EMEND for Injection. See the end of this leaflet for a list of all the ingredients in EMEND for Injection.
What should I tell my doctor before receiving EMEND for Injection?
Before you receive EMEND for Injection, tell your doctor if you:
• have liver problems.
• are pregnant or plan to become pregnant. It is not known if EMEND for Injection can harm your unborn baby.
  Women who use birth control medicines containing hormones to prevent pregnancy (birth control pills, skin patches, implants, and certain IUDs) should also use a backup method of birth control during treatment with EMEND for Injection and for up to 1 month after using EMEND for Injection to prevent pregnancy.
• are breastfeeding or plan to breastfeed. It is not known if EMEND for Injection passes into your milk and if it can harm your baby. You and your doctor should decide if you will take EMEND for Injection or breastfeed. You should not do both.
Tell your doctor about all the medicines you take, including prescription and non-prescription medicines, vitamins, and herbal supplements.
EMEND for Injection may cause serious life-threatening reactions if used with certain medicines. See the section "Who should not take EMEND for Injection?".
EMEND for Injection may affect how other medicines work, and other medicines may affect how EMEND for Injection

works. Ask your doctor or pharmacist before you take any new medicine. They can tell you if it is safe to take the medicine with EMEND for Injection.

Know the medicines you take. Keep a list of them to show your doctor or pharmacist when you get a new medicine.

How will I receive EMEND for Injection?

You will receive EMEND for Injection in one of two ways:

1. EMEND for Injection 150 mg given on Day 1 only.
- Day 1 (Day of chemotherapy): EMEND for Injection 150 mg will be given to you by infusion in your vein (intravenous) about 30 minutes before you start your chemotherapy treatment.

Or

2. EMEND for Injection 115 mg given along with capsules of EMEND.
- Day 1 (Day of chemotherapy): EMEND for Injection 115 mg will be given to you by infusion in your vein (intravenous) about 30 minutes before you start your chemotherapy treatment.
- You will get a prescription for two capsules of EMEND.
- Day 2 and Day 3 (the two days after chemotherapy): Take one 80-mg capsule of EMEND (white) by mouth, each morning for the 2 days after your chemotherapy treatment.
- If you take the blood thinner medicine warfarin sodium (COUMADIN®, JANTOVEN®), your doctor may do blood tests after you take EMEND to check your blood clotting.

What are the possible side effects of EMEND for Injection?
EMEND for Injection may cause serious side effects, including:
- **Serious allergic reactions.** Allergic reactions can happen suddenly with EMEND for Injection and may be serious. Tell your doctor or nurse right away if you have flushing or redness of your face or skin, or trouble breathing during or soon after you receive EMEND for Injection.
- Severe skin reactions may occur rarely.

EMEND capsules can also cause allergic reactions. If you receive EMEND for Injection on Day 1, and then take EMEND capsules on Days 2 and 3, stop taking the EMEND capsules and call your doctor right away if you have any of these signs or symptoms of an allergic reaction:
  ◦ hives
  ◦ rash
  ◦ itching
  ◦ redness of the face or skin
  ◦ trouble breathing or swallowing.

The most common side effects of EMEND for Injection include:
- hiccups
- weakness or tiredness
- changes in liver function blood test results. Your doctor will check you for this.
- headache
- constipation
- loss of appetite
- indigestion
- diarrhea
- belching

Infusion-site side effects with EMEND for Injection may include pain, hardening, redness or itching at the site of infusion. Swelling (inflammation) of a vein caused by a blood clot can also happen at the infusion site. Tell your doctor if you get any infusion-site side effects.

Tell your doctor if you have any side effect that bothers you or that does not go away. These are not all of the possible side effects of EMEND for Injection. For more information ask your doctor or pharmacist.

Call your doctor for medical advice about side effects. You may report side effects to FDA at 1-800-FDA-1088.

General information about EMEND for Injection

This Patient Information leaflet summarizes the most important information about EMEND for Injection. If you would like to know more information, talk with your doctor. You can ask your doctor or pharmacist for information about EMEND for Injection that is written for health professionals. For more information about EMEND for Injection call 1-800-622-4477 or go to www.emend.com.

What are the ingredients in EMEND for Injection?
Active ingredient: fosaprepitant dimeglumine
Inactive ingredients: edetate disodium, polysorbate 80, lactose anhydrous, sodium hydroxide and/or hydrochloric acid (for pH adjustment).
Manufactured for:
Merck Sharp & Dohme Corp., a subsidiary of
MERCK & CO., INC., Whitehouse Station, NJ 08889, USA
Manufactured by:
DSM Pharmaceuticals, Inc., 5900 Martin Luther King Jr. Highway, Greenville, NC 27834, USA
U.S. Patent Nos.: 5,512,570; 5,691,336
The brands listed in the above sections "Who should not take EMEND for Injection?" and "How will I receive EMEND for Injection?" are the registered trademarks of

their respective owners and are not trademarks of Merck Sharp & Dohme Corp., a subsidiary of Merck & Co., Inc. Copyright © 2008, 2009 Merck Sharp & Dohme Corp., a subsidiary of **Merck & Co., Inc.**
All rights reserved.
Revised: 07/2012
USPPI-IV-05171207R008

FOLLISTIM® AQ CARTRIDGE   ℞
[Fol-lis-tim]
(follitropin beta injection)
for subcutaneous use

HIGHLIGHTS OF PRESCRIBING INFORMATION
These highlights do not include all the information needed to use FOLLISTIM® AQ Cartridge safely and effectively. See full prescribing information for FOLLISTIM® AQ Cartridge. FOLLISTIM® AQ Cartridge (follitropin beta injection) for subcutaneous use
Initial U.S. Approval:1997

———————**INDICATIONS AND USAGE**———————
Follistim AQ Cartridge is a gonadotropin indicated:
In Women for:
- Induction of Ovulation and Pregnancy in Anovulatory Infertile Women in Whom the Cause of Infertility is Functional and Not Due to Primary Ovarian Failure (1.1)
- Pregnancy in Normal Ovulatory Women Undergoing Controlled Ovarian Stimulation as Part of an In Vitro Fertilization (IVF) or Intracytoplasmic Sperm Injection (ICSI) Cycle (1.2)
In Men for:
- Induction of Spermatogenesis in Men with Primary and Secondary Hypogonadotropic Hypogonadism (HH) in Whom the Cause of Infertility is Not Due to Primary Testicular Failure (1.3)

———————**DOSAGE AND ADMINISTRATION**———————
See Dose Conversion Table 1 for Follistim AQ Cartridge with Pen Injector (2.1)
In Anovulatory Women Undergoing Ovulation Induction (2.2):
- Starting daily dose of 50 international units of Follistim AQ Cartridge is administered subcutaneously for at least the first 7 days. The dose is increased by 25 or 50 international units at weekly intervals until follicular growth and/or serum estradiol levels indicate an adequate response.
  ▪ When an acceptable pre-ovulatory state is achieved, final oocyte maturation is achieved with 5,000 to 10,000 international units of human chorionic gonadotropin (hCG).
  ▪ The woman and her partner should have intercourse daily, beginning on the day prior to the administration of hCG and until ovulation becomes apparent.
In Normal Ovulatory Women Undergoing Controlled Ovarian Stimulation as Part of an In Vitro Fertilization or Intracytoplasmic Sperm Injection Cycle (2.3):
- Starting dose of 200 international units (actual cartridge doses) of Follistim AQ Cartridge is administered subcutaneously for at least the first 7 days of treatment. Subsequent doses can be adjusted down or up based upon ovarian response as determined by ultrasound evaluation of follicular growth and serum estradiol levels. Dosage reduction in high responders can be considered from the 6th day of treatment onward according to individual response.
  ▪ Final oocyte maturation is induced with a dose of 5,000-10,000 international units of hCG.
  ▪ Oocyte (egg) retrieval is performed 34 to 36 hours later.
Induction of Spermatogenesis in Men (2.4):
- Pretreatment with hCG alone (1,500 international units twice weekly) is required. If serum testosterone levels have not normalized after 8 weeks of hCG treatment, the dose may be increased to 3,000 international units twice a week.
- After normalization of serum testosterone levels, administer 450 international units per week (225 international units twice weekly or 150 international units three times weekly) of Follistim AQ Cartridge subcutaneously with the same pre-treatment hCG dose used to normalize testosterone levels.

———————**DOSAGE FORMS AND STRENGTHS**———————
Injection: Follistim AQ Cartridge 175 IU per 0.210 mL (3)
Injection: Follistim AQ Cartridge 350 IU per 0.420 mL (3)
Injection: Follistim AQ Cartridge 650 IU per 0.780 mL (3)
Injection: Follistim AQ Cartridge 975 IU per 1.170 mL (3)

———————**CONTRAINDICATIONS**———————
Women and men who exhibit:
- Prior hypersensitivity to recombinant hFSH products (4)
- High levels of FSH indicating primary gonadal failure (4)
- Presence of uncontrolled non-gonadal endocrinopathies (4)

- Hypersensitivity reactions related to streptomycin or neomycin (4)
- Tumors of the ovary, breast, uterus, testis, hypothalamus or pituitary gland (4)
Women who exhibit:
- Pregnancy (4, 8.1)
- Heavy or irregular vaginal bleeding of undetermined origin (4)
- Ovarian cysts or enlargement not due to polycystic ovary syndrome (PCOS) (4)

———————**WARNINGS AND PRECAUTIONS**———————
Treatment with Follistim AQ may result in:
- Abnormal Ovarian Enlargement (5.1)
- Ovarian Hyperstimulation Syndrome (OHSS) (5.2)
- Pulmonary and Vascular Complications (5.3)
- Ovarian Torsion (5.4)
- Multi-fetal Gestation and Birth (5.5)
- Congenital Anomalies (5.6)
- Ectopic Pregnancy (5.7)
- Spontaneous Abortion (5.8)
- Ovarian Neoplasms (5.9)

———————**ADVERSE REACTIONS**———————
The most common adverse reactions (≥2%) in women undergoing ovulation induction are ovarian hyperstimulation syndrome, ovarian cyst, abdominal discomfort, abdominal pain and lower abdominal pain. (6.1)
The most common adverse reactions (≥2%) in women undergoing controlled ovarian stimulation as part of an IVF or ICSI cycle are pelvic discomfort, headache, ovarian hyperstimulation syndrome, pelvic pain, nausea and fatigue. (6.1)
The most common (≥2%) adverse reactions in men undergoing induction of spermatogenesis are headache, acne, injection site reaction, injection site pain, gynecomastia, rash and dermoid cyst. (6.1)
To report SUSPECTED ADVERSE REACTIONS, contact Merck Sharp & Dohme Corp., a subsidiary of Merck & Co., Inc., at 1-877-888-4231 or FDA at 1-800-FDA-1088 or www.fda.gov/medwatch.

———————**USE IN SPECIFIC POPULATIONS**———————
Nursing Mothers: It is not known whether this drug is excreted in human milk. (8.3)
See 17 for PATIENT COUNSELING INFORMATION and FDA-approved patient labeling
                                                     Revised: 10/2013

FULL PRESCRIBING INFORMATION: CONTENTS*
1 INDICATIONS AND USAGE
  1.1 Induction of Ovulation and Pregnancy in Anovulatory Infertile Women in Whom the Cause of Infertility is Functional and Not Due to Primary Ovarian Failure
  1.2 Pregnancy in Normal Ovulatory Women Undergoing Controlled Ovarian Stimulation as Part of an In Vitro Fertilization (IVF) or Intracytoplasmic Sperm Injection (ICSI) Cycle
  1.3 Induction of Spermatogenesis in Men with Primary and Secondary Hypogonadotropic Hypogonadism (HH) in Whom the Cause of Infertility is Not Due to Primary Testicular Failure
2 DOSAGE AND ADMINISTRATION
  2.1 General Dosing Information
  2.2 Recommended Dosing in Anovulatory Women Undergoing Ovulation Induction
  2.3 Recommended Dosing in Normal Ovulatory Women Undergoing Controlled Ovarian Stimulation as Part of an In Vitro Fertilization (IVF) or Intracytoplasmic Sperm Injection (ICSI) Cycle
  2.4 Recommended Dosing for Induction of Spermatogenesis in Men
3 DOSAGE FORMS AND STRENGTHS
4 CONTRAINDICATIONS
5 WARNINGS AND PRECAUTIONS
  5.1 Abnormal Ovarian Enlargement
  5.2 Ovarian Hyperstimulation Syndrome (OHSS)
  5.3 Pulmonary and Vascular Complications
  5.4 Ovarian Torsion
  5.5 Multi-fetal Gestation and Birth
  5.6 Congenital Anomalies
  5.7 Ectopic Pregnancy
  5.8 Spontaneous Abortion
  5.9 Ovarian Neoplasms
  5.10 Laboratory Tests
  5.11 Follistim Pen
6 ADVERSE REACTIONS
  6.1 Clinical Study Experience
  6.2 Postmarketing Experience

FULL PRESCRIBING INFORMATION

1   INDICATIONS AND USAGE

Follistim® AQ (follitropin beta injection) Cartridge is indicated:

In Women for:

1.1   Induction of Ovulation and Pregnancy in Anovulatory Infertile Women in Whom the Cause of Infertility is Functional and Not Due to Primary Ovarian Failure

Prior to initiation of treatment with Follistim AQ Cartridge:
- Women should have a complete gynecologic and endocrinologic evaluation.
- Primary ovarian failure should be excluded.
- The possibility of pregnancy should be excluded.
- Tubal patency should be demonstrated.
- The fertility status of the male partner should be evaluated.

1.2   Pregnancy in Normal Ovulatory Women Undergoing Controlled Ovarian Stimulation as Part of an In Vitro Fertilization (IVF) or Intracytoplasmic Sperm Injection (ICSI) Cycle

Prior to initiation of treatment with Follistim AQ Cartridge:
- Women should have a complete gynecologic and endocrinologic evaluation and diagnosis of cause of infertility.
- The possibility of pregnancy should be excluded.
- The fertility status of the male partner should be evaluated.

In Men for:

1.3   Induction of Spermatogenesis in Men with Primary and Secondary Hypogonadotropic Hypogonadism (HH) in Whom the Cause of Infertility is Not Due to Primary Testicular Failure

Prior to initiation of treatment with Follistim AQ Cartridge:
- Men should have a complete medical and endocrinologic evaluation.
- Hypogonadotropic hypogonadism should be confirmed and primary testicular failure should be excluded.
- Serum testosterone levels should be normalized with human chorionic gonadotropin (hCG) treatment.
- The fertility status of the female partner should be evaluated.

2   DOSAGE AND ADMINISTRATION

2.1   General Dosing Information

- Parenteral drug products should be inspected visually for particulate matter and discoloration prior to administration, whenever solution and container permit. If the solution is not clear and colorless or has particles in it, the solution should not be used.
- Do not add any other medicines into the Follistim AQ Cartridge.
- Follistim AQ Cartridge with the pen injector device delivers on average an 18% higher amount of follitropin beta when compared to reconstituted Follistim delivered with a conventional syringe and needle. When administering Follistim AQ Cartridge, a lower starting dose and lower dose adjustments (as compared to reconstituted Follistim) should be considered. For that purpose the following Dose Conversion Table is provided:

Table 1: Follistim AQ Cartridge Administered Subcutaneously With the Follistim Pen Dose Conversion Table*

Lyophilized recombinant FSH dosing with ampules or vials, using conventional syringe	Follistim AQ Cartridge dosing with the Follistim Pen
75 IU	50 IU
150 IU	125 IU
225 IU	175 IU
300 IU	250 IU
375 IU	300 IU
450 IU	375 IU

* Each value represents an 18% difference rounded to the nearest 25 IU increment.

2.2   Recommended Dosing in Anovulatory Women Undergoing Ovulation Induction

The dosing scheme is stepwise and is individualized for each woman [see Clinical Studies (14.1)].
- A starting daily dose of 50 international units of Follistim AQ Cartridge is administered [see Dosage and Administration (2.1)] subcutaneously daily for at least the first 7 days.
- Subsequent dosage adjustments are made at weekly intervals based upon ovarian response. If an increase in dose is indicated by the ovarian response, the increase should be made by 25 or 50 international units of Follistim AQ Cartridge at weekly intervals until follicular growth and/or serum estradiol levels indicate an adequate ovarian response.
The following should be considered when planning the woman's individualized dose:
    ■ Appropriate Follistim AQ Cartridge dose adjustment(s) should be used to prevent multiple follicular growth and cycle cancellation.
    ■ The maximum, individualized, daily dose of Follistim AQ Cartridge is 250 international units.
- Treatment should continue until ultrasonic visualizations and/or serum estradiol determinations approximate the pre-ovulatory conditions seen in normal individuals.
- When pre-ovulatory conditions are reached, 5,000 to 10,000 international units of hCG are used to induce final oocyte maturation and ovulation.
The administration of hCG must be withheld in cases where the ovarian monitoring suggests an increased risk of OHSS on the last day of Follistim AQ Cartridge therapy [see Warnings and Precautions (5.1, 5.2, 5.10)].
- The woman and her partner should be encouraged to have intercourse daily, beginning on the day prior to the administration of hCG and until ovulation becomes apparent [see Warnings and Precautions (5.10)].
- During treatment with Follistim AQ Cartridge and during a two-week post-treatment period, the woman should be assessed at least every other day for signs of excessive ovarian stimulation.
It is recommended that Follistim AQ Cartridge administration be stopped if the ovarian monitoring suggests an increased risk of OHSS or abdominal pain occurs. Most OHSS occurs after treatment has been discontinued and reaches its maximum at about seven to ten days post-ovulation.

2.3   Recommended Dosing in Normal Ovulatory Women Undergoing Controlled Ovarian Stimulation as Part of an In Vitro Fertilization (IVF) or Intracytoplasmic Sperm Injection (ICSI) Cycle

The dosing scheme follows a stepwise approach and is individualized for each woman.
- A starting dose of 200 international units (actual cartridge doses) of Follistim AQ Cartridge is administered [see Dosage and Administration (2.1)] subcutaneously daily for at least the first 7 days of treatment.
- Subsequent to the first 7 days of treatment, the dose can be adjusted down or up based upon the woman's ovarian response as determined by ultrasound evaluation of follicular growth and serum estradiol levels. Dosage reduction in high responders can be considered from the 6th day of treatment onward according to individual response.
The following should be considered when planning the woman's individualized dose:
    ■ For most normal responding women, the daily starting dose can be continued until pre-ovulatory conditions are achieved (seven to twelve days).
    ■ For low or poor responding women, the daily dose should be increased according to the ovarian response. The maximum, individualized, daily dose of Follistim AQ Cartridge is 500 international units.

    ■ For high responding women [those at particular risk of abnormal ovarian enlargement and/or ovarian hyperstimulation syndrome (OHSS)], decrease or temporarily stop the daily dose, or discontinue the cycle according to individual response [see Warnings and Precautions (5.1, 5.2, 5.10)].
- When a sufficient number of follicles of adequate size are present, dosing of Follistim AQ Cartridge is stopped and final maturation of the oocytes is induced by administering hCG at a dose of 5,000 to 10,000 international units. The administration of hCG should be withheld in cases where the ovarian monitoring suggests an increased risk of OHSS on the last day of Follistim AQ Cartridge therapy [see Warnings and Precautions (5.1, 5.2, 5.10)].
- Oocyte (egg) retrieval should be performed 34 to 36 hours following the administration of hCG.

2.4   Recommended Dosing for Induction of Spermatogenesis in Men

- Pretreatment with hCG is required prior to concomitant therapy with Follistim AQ Cartridge and hCG. An initial dosage of 1,500 international units of hCG should be administered at twice weekly intervals to normalize serum testosterone levels. If serum testosterone levels have not normalized after 8 weeks of hCG treatment, the hCG dose can be increased to 3,000 international units twice weekly [see Clinical Studies (14.3)].
- After normal serum testosterone levels have been reached, Follistim AQ Cartridge should be administered by subcutaneous injection concomitantly with hCG treatment. Follistim is given at a dosage of 450 international units per week, as either 225 international units twice weekly or 150 international units three times per week, in combination with the same hCG dose used to normalize testosterone levels. Based on delivery of a higher dose of follitropin beta with the Follistim AQ Cartridge and pen injector [see Dosage and Administration (2.1)], a lower dose of Follistim AQ Cartridge may be considered. The concomitant therapy should be continued for at least 3 to 4 months before any improvement in spermatogenesis can be expected. If a man has not responded after this period, the combination therapy may be continued. Treatment response has been noted at up to 12 months.

3   DOSAGE FORMS AND STRENGTHS

Injection: Follistim AQ Cartridge 175 international units per 0.210 mL
Injection: Follistim AQ Cartridge 350 international units per 0.420 mL
Injection: Follistim AQ Cartridge 650 international units per 0.780 mL
Injection: Follistim AQ Cartridge 975 international units per 1.170 mL

4   CONTRAINDICATIONS

Follistim AQ Cartridge is contraindicated in women and men who exhibit:
- Prior hypersensitivity to recombinant hFSH products
- High levels of FSH indicating primary gonadal failure
- Presence of uncontrolled non-gonadal endocrinopathies (e.g., thyroid, adrenal, or pituitary disorders) [see Indications and Usage (1.1, 1.2, 1.3)]
- Hypersensitivity reactions to streptomycin or neomycin. Follistim AQ may contain traces of these antibiotics
- Tumors of the ovary, breast, uterus, testis, hypothalamus or pituitary gland

Follistim AQ Cartridge is also contraindicated in women who exhibit:
- Pregnancy [see Use in Specific Populations (8.1)]
- Heavy or irregular vaginal bleeding of undetermined origin
- Ovarian cysts or enlargement not due to polycystic ovary syndrome (PCOS)

5   WARNINGS AND PRECAUTIONS

Follistim AQ Cartridge should be used only by physicians who are experienced in infertility treatment. Follistim AQ Cartridge contains a potent gonadotropic substance capable of causing Ovarian Hyperstimulation Syndrome (OHSS) [see Warnings and Precautions (5.2)] with or without pulmonary or vascular complications [see Warnings and Precautions (5.3)] and multiple births [see Warnings and Precautions (5.5)]. Gonadotropin therapy requires the availability of appropriate monitoring facilities [see Warnings and Precautions (5.10)].
Careful attention should be given to the diagnosis of infertility and in the selection of candidates for Follistim AQ Cartridge therapy [see Indications and Usage (1.1, 1.2, 1.3) and Dosage and Administration (2.2, 2.3, 2.4)].
Switching to Follistim AQ Cartridge from other brands (manufacturer), types (recombinant, urinary), and/or methods of administration (Follistim Pen, conventional syringe) may necessitate an adjustment of the dose [see Dosage and Administration (2)].

5.1   Abnormal Ovarian Enlargement

In order to minimize the hazards associated with abnormal ovarian enlargement that may occur with Follistim AQ therapy, treatment should be individualized and the lowest effective dose should be used [see Dosage and Administration (2.2, 2.3)]. Use of ultrasound monitoring of ovarian response and/or measurement of serum estradiol levels is important to minimize the risk of overstimulation [see Warnings and Precautions (5.8)].

If the ovaries are abnormally enlarged on the last day of Follistim AQ therapy, hCG should not be administered in order to reduce the chances of developing Ovarian Hyperstimulation Syndrome (OHSS). Intercourse should be prohibited in patients with significant ovarian enlargement after ovulation because of the danger of hemoperitoneum resulting from ruptured ovarian cysts [see Warnings and Precautions (5.3)].

5.2 Ovarian Hyperstimulation Syndrome (OHSS)

OHSS is a medical entity distinct from uncomplicated ovarian enlargement and may progress rapidly to become a serious medical condition. OHSS is characterized by a dramatic increase in vascular permeability, which can result in a rapid accumulation of fluid in the peritoneal cavity, thorax, and potentially, the pericardium. The early warning signs of OHSS developing are severe pelvic pain, nausea, vomiting, and weight gain. Abdominal pain, abdominal distension, gastrointestinal symptoms including nausea, vomiting and diarrhea, severe ovarian enlargement, weight gain, dyspnea, and oliguria have been reported with OHSS. Clinical evaluation may reveal hypovolemia, hemoconcentration, electrolyte imbalances, ascites, hemoperitoneum, pleural effusions, hydrothorax, acute pulmonary distress, and thromboembolic reactions [see Warnings and Precautions (5.3)]. Transient liver function test abnormalities suggestive of hepatic dysfunction with or without morphologic changes on liver biopsy have also been reported in association with OHSS.

OHSS occurs after gonadotropin treatment has been discontinued, and it can develop rapidly, reaching its maximum about seven to ten days following treatment. Usually, OHSS resolves spontaneously with the onset of menses. If there is a risk for OHSS evident prior to hCG administration [see Warnings and Precautions (5.1)], the hCG must be withheld. Cases of OHSS are more common, more severe, and more protracted if pregnancy occurs; therefore, women should be assessed for the development of OHSS for at least two weeks after hCG administration.

If serious OHSS occurs, gonadotropins, including hCG, should be stopped and consideration should be given as to whether the patient needs to be hospitalized. Treatment is primarily symptomatic and overall should consist of bed rest, fluid and electrolyte management, and analgesics (if needed). Because the use of diuretics can accentuate the diminished intravascular volume, diuretics should be avoided except in the late phase of resolution as described below. The management of OHSS may be divided into three phases as follows:

■ Acute Phase:

Management should be directed at preventing hemoconcentration due to loss of intravascular volume to the third space and minimizing the risk of thromboembolic phenomena and kidney damage. Fluid intake and output, weight, hematocrit, serum and urinary electrolytes, urine specific gravity, BUN and creatinine, total proteins with albumin: globulin ratio, coagulation studies, electrocardiogram to monitor for hyperkalemia, and abdominal girth should be thoroughly assessed daily or more often based on the clinical need. Treatment, consisting of limited intravenous fluids, electrolytes, and human serum albumin is intended to normalize electrolytes while maintaining an acceptable but somewhat reduced intravascular volume. Full correction of the intravascular volume deficit may lead to an unacceptable increase in the amount of third space fluid accumulation.

■ Chronic Phase:

After the acute phase is successfully managed as above, excessive fluid accumulation in the third space should be limited by instituting severe potassium, sodium, and fluid restriction.

■ Resolution Phase:

As third space fluid returns to the intravascular compartment, a fall in hematocrit and increasing urinary output are observed in the absence of any increase in intake. Peripheral and/or pulmonary edema may result if the kidneys are unable to excrete third space fluid as rapidly as it is mobilized. Diuretics may be indicated during the resolution phase, if necessary, to combat pulmonary edema.

OHSS increases the risk of injury to the ovary. The ascitic, pleural, and pericardial fluid should not be removed unless there is the necessity to relieve symptoms such as pulmonary distress or cardiac tamponade. Pelvic examination may cause rupture of an ovarian cyst, which may result in hemoperitoneum, and should therefore be avoided. If bleeding occurs and requires surgical intervention, the clinical objective should be to control the bleeding and retain as much ovarian tissue as possible.

During clinical trials with Follistim or Follistim AQ Cartridge therapy, OHSS occurred in 7.6% of 105 women (OI) and 6.4% of 751 women (IVF or ICSI) treated with Follistim and Follistim AQ Cartridge, respectively.

5.3 Pulmonary and Vascular Complications

Serious pulmonary conditions (e.g., atelectasis, acute respiratory distress syndrome) have been reported in women treated with gonadotropins. In addition, thromboembolic reactions both in association with, and separate from OHSS have been reported following gonadotropin therapy. Intravascular thrombosis, which may originate in venous or arterial vessels, can result in reduced blood flow to vital organs or the extremities. Women with generally recognized risk factors for thrombosis, such as a personal or family history, severe obesity, or thrombophilia, may have an increased risk of venous or arterial thromboembolic events, during or following treatment with gonadotropins. Sequelae of such reactions have included venous thrombophlebitis, pulmonary embolism, pulmonary infarction, cerebral vascular occlusion (stroke), and arterial occlusion resulting in loss of limb and rarely in myocardial infarction. In rare cases, pulmonary complications and/or thromboembolic reactions have resulted in death. In women with recognized risk factors, the benefits of ovulation induction, in vitro fertilization (IVF) or intracytoplasmic sperm injection (ICSI) treatment need to be weighed against the risks. It should be noted, that pregnancy itself also carries an increased risk of thrombosis.

5.4 Ovarian Torsion

Ovarian torsion has been reported after treatment with Follistim AQ Cartridge and after intervention with other gonadotropins. This may be related to OHSS, pregnancy, previous abdominal surgery, past history of ovarian torsion, previous or current ovarian cyst and polycystic ovaries. Damage to the ovary due to reduced blood supply can be limited by early diagnosis and immediate detorsion.

5.5 Multi-fetal Gestation and Birth

Multi-fetal gestation and births have been reported with all gonadotropin treatments including Follistim AQ Cartridge treatment. The woman and her partner should be advised of the potential risk of multi-fetal gestation and births before starting treatment.

5.6 Congenital Anomalies

The incidence of congenital malformations after IVF or ICSI may be slightly higher than after spontaneous conception. This slightly higher incidence is thought to be related to differences in parental characteristics (e.g., maternal age, sperm characteristics) and to the higher incidence of multifetal gestations after IVF or ICSI. There are no indications that the use of gonadotropins during IVF or ICSI is associated with an increased risk of congenital malformations.

5.7 Ectopic Pregnancy

Since infertile women undergoing IVF or ICSI often have tubal abnormalities, the incidence of ectopic pregnancies might be increased. Early confirmation of an intrauterine pregnancy should be determined by β-hCG testing and transvaginal ultrasound.

5.8 Spontaneous Abortion

The risk of spontaneous abortions (miscarriage) is increased with gonadotropin products. However, causality has not been established. The increased risk may be a factor of the underlying infertility.

5.9 Ovarian Neoplasms

There have been infrequent reports of ovarian neoplasms, both benign and malignant, in women who have undergone multiple drug regimens for controlled ovarian stimulation; however, a causal relationship has not been established.

5.10 Laboratory Tests

For Women:

In most instances, treatment with Follistim AQ Cartridge will result only in follicular growth and maturation. In order to complete the final phase of follicular maturation and to induce ovulation, hCG must be given following the administration of Follistim AQ Cartridge or when clinical assessment indicates that sufficient follicular maturation has occurred. The degree of follicular maturation and the timing of hCG administration can both be determined with the use of sonographic visualization of the ovaries and endometrial lining in conjunction with measurement of serum estradiol levels. The combination of transvaginal ultrasonography and measurement of serum estradiol levels is also useful for minimizing the risk of OHSS and multi-fetal gestations. The clinical confirmation of ovulation is obtained by the following direct or indirect indices of progesterone production as well as sonographic evidence of ovulation.

Direct or indirect indices of progesterone production are:
■ Urinary or serum luteinizing hormone (LH) rise
■ A rise in basal body temperature
■ Increase in serum progesterone
■ Menstruation following the shift in basal body temperature

The following provide sonographic evidence of ovulation:
■ Collapsed follicle
■ Fluid in the cul-de-sac

■ Features consistent with corpus luteum formation
Sonographic evaluation of the early pregnancy is also important to rule out ectopic pregnancy.

For Men:

Clinical monitoring for spermatogenesis utilizes the following indirect or direct measures:
■ Serum testosterone level
■ Semen analysis

5.11 Follistim Pen

The Follistim Pen is intended only for use with Follistim AQ Cartridge. The Follistim Pen is not recommended for the blind or visually impaired without the assistance of an individual with good vision who is trained in the proper use of the injection device.

6 ADVERSE REACTIONS

The following serious adverse reactions are discussed elsewhere in the labeling:

• Ovarian Hyperstimulation Syndrome [see Warnings and Precautions (5.2)]
• Atelectasis [see Warnings and Precautions (5.3)]
• Thromboembolism [see Warnings and Precautions (5.3)]
• Ovarian Torsion [see Warnings and Precautions (5.4)]
• Multi-fetal Gestation and Birth [see Warnings and Precautions (5.5)]
• Congenital Anomalies [see Warnings and Precautions (5.6)]
• Ectopic Pregnancy [see Warnings and Precautions (5.7)]
• Spontaneous Abortion [see Warnings and Precautions (5.8)]

6.1 Clinical Study Experience

Because clinical trials are conducted under widely varying conditions, adverse reactions rates observed in the clinical trials of a drug cannot be directly compared to rates in the clinical trial of another drug and may not reflect the rates observed in practice.

Ovulation Induction

In a single cycle, multi-center, assessor-blind, parallel group, comparative study, a total of 172 chronic anovulatory women who had failed to ovulate and/or conceive with clomiphene citrate therapy, were randomized and treated with Follistim (105) or a urofollitropin comparator. Adverse reactions with an incidence of greater than 2% in either treatment group are listed in Table 2.

Table 2: Common Adverse Reactions Reported at a Frequency of ≥2% in an Assessor-Blind, Comparative Study of Anovulatory Women Receiving Ovulation Induction

System Organ Class/Adverse Reactions	Treatment Number (%) of Women	
	Follistim N=105 n (%)	Comparator N=67 n (%)
Gastrointestinal disorders		
Abdominal discomfort	3 (2.9)	1 (1.5)
Abdominal pain	3 (2.9)	2 (3.0)
Abdominal pain lower	3 (2.9)	1 (1.5)
Reproductive system and breast disorders		
Ovarian cyst	3 (2.9)	2 (3.0)
Ovarian hyperstimulation syndrome	8 (7.6)	3 (4.5)
General disorders and administration site conditions		
Pyrexia	0 (0.0)	2 (3.0)

Adverse reactions reported commonly (greater than or equal to 2% of women treated with Follistim) in other ovulation induction clinical trials were headache, abdominal distension, constipation, diarrhea, nausea, pelvic pain, uterine enlargement, vaginal hemorrhage and injection site reaction.

In Vitro Fertilization/Intracytoplasmic Sperm Injection

In a single cycle, multi-center, double-blind, parallel group, comparative study, a total of 1509 women were randomized to receive controlled ovarian stimulation with either Follistim AQ Cartridge (751 women were treated with Follistim AQ Cartridge) or a comparator and pituitary suppression with a gonadotropin releasing hormone (GnRH) antagonist as part of an in vitro fertilization (IVF) or intracytoplasmic sperm injection (ICSI) cycle. Table 3 lists adverse reactions with an incidence of greater than 2% in the group of women treated with Follistim AQ Cartridge.

Table 3: Common Adverse Reactions Reported At a Frequency of ≥2% in a Randomized, Double-blind, Active-controlled, Comparative Study of Normal Ovulatory Women Undergoing Controlled Ovarian Stimulation as Part of an In Vitro Fertilization or Intracytoplasmic Sperm Injection Cycle

System Organ Class/Adverse Reactions	Follistim AQ Cartridge Treatment N = 751 n* (%)
Nervous System disorders	
Headache	55 (7.3%)
Gastrointestinal disorders	
Nausea	29 (3.9%)
Reproductive system and breast disorders	
Ovarian Hyperstimulation Syndrome	48 (6.4%)
Pelvic discomfort	62 (8.3%)
Pelvic Pain	41 (5.5%)
General disorders and Administration site conditions	
Fatigue	17 (2.3%)

* n = number of women with the adverse reaction

Induction of Spermatogenesis
In an open-label, non-comparative clinical trial, 49 men with hypogonadotropic hypogonadism were enrolled to receive pretreatment with hCG, followed by combination therapy with hCG and Follistim for induction of spermatogenesis. Of the 49 men, 30 received weekly Follistim doses of 450 international units; 24 of these 30 men received a total of 48 weeks of treatment with Follistim. Adverse reactions occurring with an incidence of greater than 2% in the 30 men treated with Follistim are listed in Table 4.

Table 4: Common Adverse Reactions Reported At a Frequency of ≥2% in an Open-Label Clinical Trial in Men with Hypogonadotropic Hypogonadism

System Organ Class/Adverse Reactions	Follistim Treatment N=30 n (%)
Nervous system disorders	
Headache	2 (6.7)
General disorders and administration site disorders	
Injection site reaction	2 (6.7)
Injection site pain	2 (6.7)
Skin and cutaneous tissue disorders	
Acne	2 (6.7)
Rash	1 (3.3)
Reproductive system and breast disorders	
Gynecomastia	1 (3.3)
Neoplasms benign, malignant and unspecified	
Dermoid cyst	1 (3.3)

6.2   Postmarketing Experience
The following adverse reactions have been identified during post approval use of Follistim and/or Follistim AQ Cartridge. Because these reactions are reported voluntarily from a population of uncertain size, it is not always possible to reliably estimate their frequency or establish a causal relationship to drug exposure.

Gastrointestinal disorders
Abdominal distension, abdominal pain, constipation, diarrhea
General disorders and administration site conditions
Injection site reaction
Reproductive system and breast disorders
Breast tenderness, metrorrhagia, ovarian enlargement, vaginal hemorrhage
Skin and subcutaneous tissue disorders
Rash
Vascular disorders
Thromboembolism [see Warnings and Precautions (5.3)]

7   DRUG INTERACTIONS
No drug-drug interaction studies have been performed.

8   USE IN SPECIFIC POPULATIONS
8.1   Pregnancy
Pregnancy Category X: Follistim AQ Cartridge should not be used during pregnancy [see Contraindications (4)].
8.3   Nursing Mothers
It is not known whether this drug is excreted in human milk. Because many drugs are excreted in human milk and because of the potential for serious adverse reactions in the nursing infant from Follistim AQ Cartridge, a decision should be made whether to discontinue nursing or to discontinue the drug, taking into account the importance of the drug to the mother.
8.4   Pediatric Use
Safety and effectiveness in pediatric patients have not been established.
8.5   Geriatric Use
Clinical studies of Follistim did not include subjects aged 65 and over.

10   OVERDOSAGE
Aside from the possibility of Ovarian Hyperstimulation Syndrome [see Warnings and Precautions (5.2, 5.3)] and multiple gestations [see Warnings and Precautions (5.5)], there is no additional information concerning the consequences of acute overdosage with Follistim AQ Cartridge.

11   DESCRIPTION
Follistim AQ Cartridge contains human follicle-stimulating hormone (hFSH), a glycoprotein hormone which is manufactured by recombinant DNA (rDNA) technology. The active drug substance, follitropin beta, has a dimeric structure containing two glycoprotein subunits (alpha and beta). Both the 92 amino acid alpha-chain and the 111 amino acid beta-chain have complex heterogeneous structures arising from two N-linked oligosaccharide chains. Follitropin beta is synthesized in a Chinese hamster ovary (CHO) cell line that has been transfected with a plasmid containing the two subunit DNA sequences encoding for hFSH. The purification process results in a highly purified preparation with a consistent hFSH isoform profile and high specific activity [as determined by the Ph. Eur. test for FSH *in vivo* bioactivity and on the basis of the molar extinction coefficient at 277 nm ($\epsilon_s \cdot mg^{-1} cm^{-1}$) = 1.066].
The biological activity is determined by measuring the increase in ovary weight in female rats. The intrinsic luteinizing hormone (LH) activity in follitropin beta is less than 1 international unit per 40,000 international units FSH. The compound is considered to contain no LH activity.
The amino acid sequence and tertiary structure of the product are indistinguishable from that of hFSH of urinary source. Also, based on available data derived from physicochemical tests and bioassay, follitropin beta and follitropin alfa, another recombinant follicle-stimulating hormone product, are indistinguishable.
Follistim AQ Cartridge is a ready for use, prefilled with solution, disposable cartridge containing either 175 IU of follitropin beta in 0.210 mL (833 IU/mL), 350 IU in 0.420 mL (833 IU/mL), 650 IU in 0.780 mL (833 IU/mL) or 975 IU in 1.170 mL (833 IU/mL) of aqueous solution for multiple dose use, with a maximal deliverable dose of either 150 IU, 300 IU, 600 IU or 900 IU, respectively. Inactive ingredients in the cartridges include: benzyl alcohol NF 10 mg/mL; L-methionine USP 0.5 mg/mL; polysorbate 20

NF 0.2 mg/mL; sodium citrate (dihydrate) USP 14.7 mg/mL; sucrose NF 50 mg/mL; and water for injection USP. Hydrochloric acid NF and/or sodium hydroxide NF are used to adjust the pH to 7.
Follistim AQ Cartridge is for use only with the Follistim Pen, which features an adjustable dosing system for administering the drug in a microvolume of solution. The Follistim Pen with Follistim AQ Cartridge is intended for SUBCUTANEOUS USE ONLY. The recombinant protein in Follistim AQ Cartridge has been standardized for FSH *in vivo* bioactivity in terms of the WHO International Standard for Follicle Stimulating Hormone (FSH) Recombinant, Human for Bioassay (code 92/642), issued by the World Health Organization Expert Committee on Biological Standardization (1995). Under current storage conditions, Follistim AQ may contain up to 11% of oxidized follitropin beta.
In clinical trials with Follistim, serum antibodies to FSH or anti-CHO cell derived proteins were not detected in any of the treated patients after exposure to Follistim for up to three cycles.

12   CLINICAL PHARMACOLOGY
12.1   Mechanism of Action
Women:
Follicle-stimulating hormone (FSH), the active component in Follistim AQ Cartridge, is required for normal follicular growth, maturation, and gonadal steroid production.
In women, the level of FSH is critical for the onset and duration of follicular development, and consequently for the timing and number of follicles reaching maturity. Follistim AQ Cartridge stimulates ovarian follicular growth in women who do not have primary ovarian failure. In order to effect the final phase of follicle maturation, resumption of meiosis and rupture of the follicle in the absence of an endogenous LH surge, human chorionic gonadotropin (hCG) must be given following treatment with Follistim AQ Cartridge when patient monitoring indicates appropriate follicular development parameters have been reached.
Men:
Follistim when administered with hCG stimulates spermatogenesis in men with hypogonadotropic hypogonadism. FSH, the active component of Follistim, is the pituitary hormone responsible for spermatogenesis.
12.3   Pharmacokinetics
Pharmacokinetic parameters for Follistim AQ Cartridge were evaluated in an open-label, single-center, randomized study in 20 healthy women. Serum FSH values from a single subcutaneous injection of reconstituted Follistim lyophilized powder administered by conventional syringe were compared to those values following a single subcutaneous injection of Follistim AQ Cartridge administered with the Follistim Pen injector. Administration of follitropin beta with the Follistim Pen resulted an 18% increase in $AUC_{0-\infty}$ and C_{max}. The 18% difference in serum FSH concentrations resulting from administration of the two formulations was due to differences between the anticipated and actual volume delivered with the conventional syringe. The pharmacokinetic parameters for Follistim AQ Cartridge are as follows:
[See table 5 below]
Absorption:
Women:
The bioavailability of Follistim following subcutaneous and intramuscular administration was investigated in healthy, pituitary-suppressed women given a single 300 international units dose. In these women, the area under the curve (AUC), expressed as the mean ± SD, was equivalent between the subcutaneous (455.6 ± 141.4 IU*h/L) and intramuscular (445.7 ± 135.7 IU*h/L) routes of administration. However, equivalence could not be established with respect to the peak serum FSH levels (C_{max}). The C_{max} achieved after subcutaneous administration and intramuscular administration was 5.41 ± 0.72 international units/L and 6.86 ± 2.90 international units/L, respectively. After subcutaneous or intramuscular injection the apparent dose absorbed was 77.8% and 76.4%, respectively.
The pharmacokinetics and pharmacodynamics of a single, intramuscular dose (300 international units) of Follistim were also investigated in a group (n=8) of gonadotropin-deficient, but otherwise healthy women. In these women, FSH (mean ± SD) AUC was 339 ± 105 international units*h/L, C_{max} was 4.3 ± 1.7 international units/L. C_{max} occurred at approximately 27 ± 5.4 hours after intramuscular administration.
A multiple dose, dose proportionality, pharmacokinetic study of Follistim was completed in healthy, pituitary-suppressed, female subjects given subcutaneous doses of 75, 150, or 225 international units for 7 days. Steady-state blood concentrations of FSH were reached with all doses after 5 days of treatment based on the trough concentrations of FSH just prior to dosing (C_{trough}). Peak blood concentrations with the 75, 150, and 225 international units dose were 4.30 ± 0.60 international units/L, 8.51 ± 1.16 international units/L and 13.92 ± 1.81 international units/L, respectively.

Table 5: Mean (SD) Pharmacokinetic Parameters of a Single Subcutaneous Injection of 150 IU of Follistim AQ Cartridge (n=20)

	$AUC_{0-\infty}$ (IU/L*h)	C_{max} (IU/L)	t_{max} (h)	$t_{1/2}$ (h)	CL_{app} (L/h/kg)
Follistim AQ Cartridge	215.1 (45.8)	3.4 (0.7)	12.9 (6.2)	33.4 (4.2)	0.01 (0.003)

$AUC_{0-\infty}$ Area under the curve
C_{max} Maximum concentration
t_{max} Time to maximum concentration
$t_{1/2}$ Elimination half-life
CL_{app} Clearance

Men:
No PK studies were conducted using Follistim AQ Cartridge in men. Exposures of follitropin beta from Follistim AQ Cartridge and Follistim are expected to be equivalent after adjusting for the 18% difference in dose *[see Dosage and Administration (2)].*

Serum levels of FSH were measured in a clinical study that compared the effects of two different dosing schedules of Follistim (150 international units three times a week or 225 international units twice a week) administered by subcutaneous injection concurrently with chorionic gonadotropin for induction of spermatogenesis in hypogonadotropic hypogonadal men. Administration of Follistim was started at Week 17. Mean serum trough concentrations of FSH remained fairly constant over the treatment period. At the end of treatment (Week 64), the mean serum trough concentrations of FSH were 2.09 international units/L in the 150 international units group and 3.22 international units/L in the 225 international units group. Serum trough concentrations of FSH measured prior to the first Follistim injection on the Mondays of active treatment period (Weeks 17 to 64) and one week after the end of treatment period are presented in Figure 1.

Figure 1: Mean (SD) Serum Trough Concentrations of FSH in Men Following Subcutaneous Administration of Follistim Using Two Different Dosing Schedules (150 International Units Three Times a Week or 225 International Units Twice a Week)

Distribution:
The volume of distribution of Follistim in healthy, pituitary-suppressed, women following intravenous administration of a 300 international units dose was approximately 8 L.

Metabolism:
The recombinant FSH in Follistim AQ Cartridge is biochemically very similar to urinary FSH and it is therefore anticipated that it is metabolized in the same manner.

Elimination:
The elimination half-life ($t_{1/2}$) following a single subcutaneous injection of 150 IU of Follistim AQ Cartridge in women was 33.4 (4.2) hours. The clearance was 0.01 (0.003) L/h/kg.

Use in Specific Populations:
Body weight: The effect of body weight on the pharmacokinetics of Follistim was evaluated in a group of European and Japanese women who were significantly different in terms of body weight. The European women had a body weight of (mean ± SD) 67.4 ± 13.5 kg and the Japanese subjects were 46.8 ± 11.6 kg. Following a single intramuscular dose of 300 international units of Follistim, the AUC was significantly smaller in European women (339 ± 105 international units*h/L) than in Japanese women (544 ± 201 international units*h/L). However, clearance per kg of body weight was essentially the same for the respective groups (0.014 and 0.013 L/hr/kg).

Geriatric Use: The pharmacokinetics of Follistim has not been studied in geriatric subjects.

Pediatric Use: The pharmacokinetics of Follistim has not been studied in pediatric subjects.

Renal Impairment: The effect of renal impairment on the pharmacokinetics of Follistim has not been studied.

Hepatic Impairment: The effect of hepatic impairment on the pharmacokinetics of Follistim has not been studied.

13 NONCLINICAL TOXICOLOGY

13.1 Carcinogenesis, Mutagenesis, Impairment of Fertility

Long-term toxicity studies in animals have not been performed with Follistim to evaluate the carcinogenic potential of the drug. Follistim was not mutagenic in the Ames test using *S. typhimurium* and *E. coli* tester strains and did not produce chromosomal aberrations in an in vitro assay using human lymphocytes.

14 CLINICAL STUDIES

14.1 Ovulation Induction

The efficacy of Follistim for ovulation induction was evaluated in a randomized, assessor-blind, parallel-group comparative, multicenter safety and efficacy study of 172 chronic anovulatory women (105 subjects on Follistim) who

Table 9: Number of Men Receiving Follistim Who Achieved a Mean Sperm Density of ≥10^6/mL on Their Last Two Treatment Assessments

	Follistim 150 international units three times a week (n=15)		Follistim 225 international units twice a week (n=15)		Overall (n=30)	
Sperm Density of ≥10^6/mL	n	%	n	%	n	%
Yes	6	40	7	47	13	43
No	9	60	8	53	17	57

had previously failed to ovulate and/or conceive during clomiphene citrate treatment. The study results for ovulation rates are summarized in Table 6 and those for pregnancy rates are summarized in Table 7.

Table 6: Cumulative Ovulation Rates

Cycle	Follistim (n=105)
First treatment cycle	72%
Second treatment cycle	82%
Third treatment cycle	85%

Table 7: Cumulative Ongoing*,† Pregnancy Rates

Cycle	Follistim (n=105)
First treatment cycle	14%
Second treatment cycle	19%
Third treatment cycle	23%

* All ongoing pregnancies were confirmed after at least 12 weeks after the hCG injection.
† Study was not powered to demonstrate this outcome.

14.2 Controlled Ovarian Stimulation as Part of an In Vitro Fertilization (IVF) or Intracytoplasmic Sperm Injection (ICSI) Cycle

The efficacy of Follistim AQ Cartridge was evaluated in a randomized, double-blind, active-controlled study of 1,509 healthy normal ovulatory women (mean age, body weight, and body mass index of 32 years, 68 kg and 25 kg/m², respectively) treated for one cycle with controlled ovarian stimulation and pituitary suppression with a GnRH antagonist as part of an in vitro fertilization or intracytoplasmic sperm injection cycle. This 2008 study was conducted in Europe and North America (United States and Canada). Approximately 54% of the subjects were from North America. The overall results, as well as the results from North America only, for clinical pregnancy are summarized in Table 8.

Table 8: Pregnancy Results from Treatment With Follistim AQ Cartridge and a GnRH Antagonist in Normal Ovulatory Women Undergoing Controlled Ovarian Stimulation as Part of an In Vitro Fertilization or Intracytoplasmic Sperm Injection Cycle.* Intent-to-Treat Population (ITT)

Parameter	Follistim AQ Cartridge Overall data (n=750)	Follistim AQ Cartridge North American data (n=403)
Clinical pregnancy rate/ cycle initiation†	41.1%	48.9%

* single treatment cycle results
† Clinical pregnancy was assessed ≥6 weeks after transfer of one or two embryos.

14.3 Induction of Spermatogenesis

The safety and efficacy of Follistim administered by subcutaneous injection concomitantly with chorionic gonadotropin for injection (hCG) has been examined in a multicenter, open-label, non-comparator clinical study for induction of spermatogenesis in hypogonadotropic hypogonadal men. The study compared the effects of two different Follistim dosing schedules on semen parameters and serum levels of follicle stimulating hormone (FSH). The multicenter study involved a 16-week pretreatment phase with hCG at a dosage of 1,500 international units twice a week to normalize serum testosterone levels. If serum testosterone levels did not normalize after 8 weeks of hCG treatment, the hCG

dose could have been increased to 3,000 international units twice a week. This phase was followed by a 48-week treatment phase. Men who were still azoospermic after the pretreatment phase were randomized to receive either 225 international units Follistim together with 1,500 international units hCG twice a week or 150 international units Follistim three times a week together with 1,500 international units hCG twice weekly. Men who required 3,000 international units of hCG twice a week in the pretreatment phase were continued on that dosage during the treatment phase. The mean age of patients in both treatment groups was approximately 30 years (range 18 to 47 years). At baseline, mean left and right testis volumes were 4.61 ± 2.94 mL and 4.57 ± 3.00 mL, respectively, in the group receiving three weekly injections of Follistim. For the group receiving two weekly injections of Follistim, the mean left and right testis volumes were 6.54 ± 2.45 mL and 7.21 ± 2.94 mL, respectively, at baseline. The primary efficacy endpoint was the percentage of patients with a mean sperm density of ≥1 × 10^6/mL on their last two treatment assessments. The outcomes of treatment in the 30 men enrolled in the treatment phase are summarized in Table 9.
[See table 9 above]

Overall, the median time to reach a sperm concentration of 10^6 per mL was 165 days (range 25 to 327 days) in patients who demonstrated a sperm concentration of at least 10^6 per mL. The median time to reach a sperm concentration of at least 10^6 per mL was 186 days (range 25 to 327 days) for the 150 international units group and 141 days (range 43 to 204 days) for the 225 international units group. No pregnancy data were collected during the trial.

The local tolerance data were comparable between the two treatment groups. The mean percentage of days without pain calculated for all subjects in the treatment period was 91.3% for patients in the 150 international units (three times a week) and 76.0% for patients in the 225 international units (two times a week) Follistim treatment groups. In the 225 international units (twice per week) group, local symptoms judged as severe by the investigator were: itching in 1 patient (7%), pain in 2 patients (13%), bruising in 2 patients (13%), swelling in 2 patients (13%), and redness in 1 patient (7%). In the 150 international units (three times per week) group, 1 event in 1 patient (bruising, 7%) was judged as severe. No patient discontinued treatment due to injection site reaction or injection site pain.

16 HOW SUPPLIED/STORAGE AND HANDLING

Follistim AQ Cartridge is supplied in a box containing disposable, 29 gauge, ultra-fine, ½-inch, sterile BD Micro-Fine™ Pen Needles (for use with Follistim Pen available separately) and one disposable, blister packed, prefilled 1.5 mL colorless glass cartridge, with grey rubber piston and an aluminum crimp-cap with black rubber inlay and in the following presentations:

NDC 0052-0303-01 Follistim AQ Cartridge 175 international units per 0.210 mL (delivering 150 international units) with orange crimp-caps and 3 BD Micro-Fine Pen Needles

NDC 0052-0313-01 Follistim AQ Cartridge 350 international units per 0.420 mL (delivering 300 international units) with silver crimp-caps and 5 BD Micro-Fine Pen Needles

NDC 0052-0316-01 Follistim AQ Cartridge 650 international units per 0.780 mL (delivering 600 international units) with gold crimp-caps and 7 BD Micro-Fine Pen Needles

NDC 0052-0326-01 Follistim AQ Cartridge 975 international units per 1.170 mL (delivering 900 international units) with blue crimp-caps and 10 BD Micro-Fine Pen Needles

Store refrigerated 2-8°C (36-46°F) until dispensed. Upon dispensing, the product may be stored by the patient at 2-8°C (36-46°F) until the expiration date, or at 25°C (77°F) for 3 months or until expiration date, whichever occurs first. Once the rubber inlay of the Follistim AQ Cartridge has been pierced by a needle, the product can only be stored for a maximum of 28 days at 2-25°C (36-77°F). Protect from light. Do not freeze.

17 PATIENT COUNSELING INFORMATION

"See FDA-Approved Patient Labeling (Patient Information)"

17.1 Dosing and Use of Follistim AQ Cartridge with Pen

Instruct women and men on the correct usage and dosing of Follistim AQ Cartridge in conjunction with the Follistim Pen. Make sure that individuals who have used other gonadotropin products delivered by a syringe are aware of differences arising from use of the pen. Women and men should read and follow all instructions in the Follistim Pen "Instructions for Use" Manual prior to administration of Follistim AQ Cartridge.

Advise women and men of the number of doses which can be extracted from the full unused Follistim AQ Cartridge that you have prescribed.

17.2 Therapy Duration and Necessary Monitoring in Women and Men Undergoing Treatment

Prior to beginning therapy with Follistim AQ Cartridge, inform women and men about the time commitment and monitoring procedures necessary to undergo treatment *[see Dosage and Administration (2), Warnings and Precautions (5.10)]*.

17.3 Instructions on a Missed Dose

Inform women and men that if they miss or forget to take a dose of Follistim AQ Cartridge, the next dose should not be doubled and they should call the healthcare provider for further dosing instructions.

17.4 Ovarian Hyperstimulation Syndrome

Inform women regarding the risks with use of Follistim AQ Cartridge of Ovarian Hyperstimulation Syndrome *[see Warnings and Precautions (5.2)]* and associated symptoms including lung and blood vessel problems *[see Warnings and Precautions (5.3)]* and ovarian torsion *[see Warnings and Precautions (5.4)]*.

17.5 Multi-fetal Gestation and Birth

Inform women regarding the risk of multi-fetal gestations with the use of Follistim AQ Cartridge *[see Warnings and Precautions (5.5)]*.

Manufactured for: Merck Sharp & Dohme Corp., a subsidiary of
MERCK & CO., INC., Whitehouse Station, NJ 08889, USA
Manufactured by: Vetter Pharma-Fertigung GmbH & Co. KG, Ravensburg, Germany
BD, BD Logo and BD Micro-Fine are trademarks of Becton, Dickinson and Company
For patent information: www.merck.com/product/patent/home.html
Copyright © 2004, 2010, 2011 Merck Sharp & Dohme B.V., a subsidiary of Merck & Co., Inc.
All rights reserved.
Revised: 10/2013
uspi-mk8328-SOi-1310R011

PATIENT INFORMATION

**Follistim® (Fol'-lis-tim) AQ Cartridge
(follitropin beta injection)**

Read the Patient Information that comes with Follistim® AQ Cartridge before you start using it and each time you get a refill. There may be new information. This information does not take the place of talking with your healthcare provider about your medical condition or treatment.

What is Follistim AQ Cartridge?

Follistim AQ is a prescription medicine that contains follicle-stimulating hormone (FSH). The medicine is taken with the Follistim Pen®.

Follistim AQ Cartridge is used:

In women:
• to help healthy ovaries to develop (mature) and release eggs
• as part of treatment programs that use special techniques (skills) to help women get pregnant by causing their ovaries to produce more mature eggs

In men:
• to help bring about the production and development of sperm

Who should not take Follistim AQ Cartridge?

Do not take Follistim AQ Cartridge if you are a Woman or Man who:
• is allergic to recombinant human FSH products
• has a high level of FSH in your blood indicating that your ovaries (women only) or testes (men only) may be permanently damaged and do not work at all
• has uncontrolled thyroid, pituitary, or adrenal gland problems
• is allergic to streptomycin or neomycin (types of antibiotics)
• has a tumor of the hypothalamus, pituitary gland, breast, uterus (women only), ovary (women only), or testis (men only)

Do not take Follistim AQ Cartridge if you are a Woman who:
• is pregnant or think you may be pregnant
• has heavy or irregular vaginal bleeding and the cause is not known
• has ovarian cysts or enlarged ovaries, not due to polycystic ovary syndrome (PCOS)

Talk to your healthcare provider before taking this medicine if you have any of the conditions listed above.

What should I tell my healthcare provider before taking Follistim AQ Cartridge?

Before you take Follistim AQ, tell your healthcare provider if you:
• have an increased risk of blood clots (thrombosis)
• have ever had a blood clot (thrombosis), or anyone in your immediate family has ever had a blood clot (thrombosis)
• had stomach (abdominal) surgery
• had twisting of your ovary (ovarian torsion)
• had or have a cyst in your ovary
• have polycystic ovary disease
• have any other medical conditions
• are breastfeeding or plan to breastfeed. It is not known if the medicine in Follistim AQ Cartridge passes into your breast milk. You and your healthcare provider should decide if you will take Follistim AQ Cartridge or breastfeed. You should not do both.

Tell your healthcare provider about all the medicines you take, including prescription and non-prescription medicines, vitamins, and herbal supplements.

Know the medicines you take. Keep a list of them and show your healthcare provider and pharmacist when you get a new medicine.

How should I use Follistim AQ Cartridge?

• Be sure that you read, understand, and follow the "Patient Instructions for Use" that come with Follistim AQ Cartridge.
• Use Follistim AQ Cartridge exactly as your healthcare provider tells you to.
• Your healthcare provider will tell you how much Follistim AQ Cartridge to use, how to inject it, and how often it should be injected.
• Do not inject Follistim AQ Cartridge at home until your healthcare provider has taught you the right way to put the cartridge and pen device together and to inject yourself.
• Do not mix any other medicines into the cartridge.
• Do not change your dose of Follistim AQ Cartridge unless your healthcare provider tells you to.
• Call your healthcare provider immediately if you use too much Follistim AQ Cartridge.
• If you miss or forget to take a dose, do not double your next dose. Ask your healthcare provider for instructions.
• Use Follistim AQ Cartridge only with the Follistim Pen.
• Do not use the Follistim Pen if you are blind or visually impaired unless you have assistance from an individual with good vision who is trained in the right way to use the pen.
• Do not re-use the BD Micro-Fine™ Pen Needle.
• Your healthcare provider will do blood and urine hormone tests while you are taking Follistim AQ Cartridge. Make sure you follow-up with your healthcare provider to have your blood and urine tested when told to do so.

Women:
• Your healthcare provider may do ultrasound scans of your ovaries. Make sure you follow-up with your healthcare provider to have your ultrasound scans.

Men:
• Your healthcare provider may test your semen while you are taking Follistim AQ Cartridge. Make sure you follow-up with your healthcare provider to give a semen sample for testing.

What are the possible side effects of Follistim AQ Cartridge?

Follistim AQ Cartridge may cause serious side effects.
Serious side effects in women include:
• Ovarian enlargement
• Ovarian hyperstimulation syndrome (OHSS). OHSS is a serious medical problem that can happen when the ovaries are over stimulated. In rare cases it has caused death. OHSS causes fluid to build up suddenly in your stomach and chest areas and can cause blood clots to form. Call your healthcare provider right away if you have:
  • pain in your lower stomach area
  • nausea
  • vomiting
  • weight gain
  • diarrhea
  • decreased urine output
  • trouble breathing
• Lung problems. Follistim AQ Cartridge can cause you to have fluid in your lungs (atelectasis) and trouble breathing (acute respiratory distress syndrome).
• Blood clots. Follistim AQ Cartridge may increase your chance of having blood clots in your blood vessels. Blood clots can cause:
  • blood vessel problems (thrombophlebitis)
  • stroke
  • loss of your arm or leg
  • blood clot in your lungs (pulmonary embolus)
  • heart attack
• Ovarian torsion. Follistim AQ Cartridge may increase the chance of twisting of the ovaries in women with certain conditions such as OHSS, pregnancy and previous abdominal surgery. Twisting of the ovary could cause the blood flow to the ovary to be cut off.
• Pregnancy and birth of multiple babies. Having a pregnancy with more than one baby at a time increases the health risk for you and your babies. Discuss your chances of multiple births with your healthcare provider.

• Birth defects. A woman's age, certain sperm problems, genetic background of both parents and a pregnancy with multiple babies can increase the chance that your baby might have birth defects.
• Ectopic pregnancy (pregnancy outside of the womb). The chance of a pregnancy outside of the womb is increased in women with damaged fallopian tubes.
• Miscarriage. The chance of loss of an early pregnancy may be increased in women who have difficulty with becoming pregnant at all.

The most common side effects of Follistim AQ Cartridge include:

In women:
• headache
• nausea
• stomach pain
• discomfort or pain in the lower stomach area
• cyst (closed sac) in the ovary
• feeling tired

In men:
• headache
• pain at the injection site
• bruising, swelling or redness at the injection site
• breast enlargement
• acne

These are not all the possible side effects of Follistim AQ Cartridge. For more information, ask your healthcare provider or pharmacist.

Call your healthcare provider immediately if you get worsening or strong pain in the lower stomach area (abdomen). Also, call your healthcare provider immediately if this happens some days after the last injection has been given.

Tell your healthcare provider if you have any side effect that bothers you or that does not go away.

Call your doctor for medical advice about side effects. You may report side effects to FDA at 1-800-FDA-1088.

How should I store Follistim AQ Cartridge?

• Store Follistim AQ Cartridge in the refrigerator between 2-8°C (36-46°F) until the expiration date.
• Follistim AQ can be stored at or below 25°C (77°F) for 3 months or until the expiration date, whichever comes first. Once the rubber inlay of the Follistim AQ Cartridge has been pierced by a needle, the product may be stored only for a maximum of 28 days at 2-25°C (36-77°F).
• Keep Follistim AQ Cartridge away from light.
• Do not freeze.

Keep Follistim AQ Cartridge and all medicines out of the reach of children.

General information about Follistim AQ Cartridge

Medicines are sometimes prescribed for purposes other than those listed in the Patient Information leaflet. Do not use Follistim AQ for a condition for which it was not prescribed. Do not give Follistim AQ Cartridge to other people, even if they have the same condition that you have. It may harm them.

This Patient Information leaflet summarizes the most important information about Follistim AQ Cartridge. If you would like more information, talk with your healthcare provider. You can ask your pharmacist or healthcare provider for more information about Follistim AQ Cartridge that is written for healthcare professionals.

For more information, go to **www.follistim.com** or call 1-866-836-5633.

What are the ingredients in Follistim AQ Cartridge?

Active ingredient: follitropin beta
Inactive ingredients: sucrose, sodium citrate, benzyl alcohol NF-10 mg/mL, L-methionine, polysorbate 20, water for injection, hydrochloric acid, and/or sodium hydroxide.
Manufactured for: Merck Sharp & Dohme Corp., a subsidiary of
MERCK & CO., INC., Whitehouse Station, NJ 08889, USA
Manufactured by: Vetter Pharma-Fertigung GmbH & Co. KG, Ravensburg, Germany
BD, BD Logo and BD Micro-Fine are trademarks of Becton, Dickinson and Company.
For patent information: www.merck.com/product/patent/home.html
Copyright © 2004, 2010, 2011 Merck Sharp & Dohme B.V., a subsidiary of Merck & Co., Inc.
All rights reserved.
Revised: 10/2013
usppi-mk8328-SOi-1310R012

PATIENT INSTRUCTIONS FOR USE

**Follistim® (Fol'-lis-tim) AQ Cartridge
(follitropin beta injection)**

Read the Patient Instructions for Use that comes with Follistim® AQ Cartridge before you start using it and each time you get a refill. There may be new information. This information does not take the place of talking with your healthcare provider about your medical condition or treatment.

A. Getting Ready

• Follistim Pen is not recommended for the blind or visually impaired user without the assistance of an individual with good vision, trained in the proper use of the injection device.

- Learn about all of the parts of the Follistim Pen (See Figure 1), Follistim AQ Cartridge (Figure 2) and the BD Micro-Fine™ Pen Needle (Figure 3). You will need to recognize these parts to follow the directions.

Figure 1. Follistim Pen and its Parts

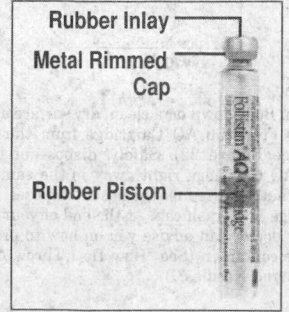

Figure 2. Parts of Follistim AQ Cartridge

Figure 3. Parts of BD Micro-Fine Pen Needle Unit

- Remove the Cartridge out of the refrigerator.
- Injecting cold drug is likely to cause discomfort. Therefore, it is recommended you allow the drug to reach room temperature before taking the injection.
- Check the liquid in the cartridge. It should appear clear and colorless. If the solution is not clear and colorless or has particles in it, **do not use it.**
- **Gather the supplies you will need for your injection. You will need:**
  - a clean dry surface
  - alcohol
  - cotton balls or alcohol pads
  - sterile gauze
  - a puncture-proof container to throw away the used syringe and needle
- Wash your hands with soap and water and dry them before you use Follistim Pen or when you replace the cartridge.

B. Loading the Follistim Pen with the Follistim AQ Cartridge

- Holding the Pen Body firmly with one hand, pull off the Protective Cap with your other hand (See Figure 4). Put the cap aside on a clean, dry surface.

Figure 4

- Unscrew the entire Pen Body from the Cartridge Holder (See Figure 5). Place the Cartridge Holder and the Pen Body aside on a clean, dry surface.

Figure 5

- Take the Follistim AQ Cartridge out of its package. Clean the rubber inlay on the cartridge with an alcohol pad. Pick up the Cartridge Holder. Put the Cartridge into the Cartridge Holder (See Figure 6). The metal rimmed cap goes in first.

Figure 6

- Pick up the Pen Body and lower it into the Cartridge Holder. The black rod must press against the Rubber Piston on the cartridge. Screw the Pen Body fully onto the Cartridge Holder (See Figure 7). Make sure there is no gap between the Pen Body and the Cartridge Holder. The arrow (▲) on the Cartridge Holder should point to the middle of the yellow alignment mark (■■) on the blue Pen Body.

Figure 7

- Clean the open end of the Cartridge Holder with an alcohol pad (See Figure 8).

Figure 8

- Pick up a new BD Micro-Fine Pen Needle that is in its Outer Needle Shield. Peel off the protective paper seal (See Figure 9). Do **not** touch the needle. Do not place the open needle on any surface. **Use Only the BD Micro-Fine 0.33 mm × 12.7 mm (29G) Pen Needles as supplied with the Follistim AQ Cartridge.**
- You must use a new BD Micro-Fine Pen Needle with each injection. Never reuse a needle. Attach a new BD Micro-Fine Pen Needle after you make sure there is a Follistim AQ Cartridge in the Cartridge.

Figure 9

- Hold the Outer Needle Shield firmly in one hand while holding the Cartridge Holder firmly in the other hand. Push the end of the Cartridge Holder into the Outer Needle Shield. Screw them tightly together (See Figure 10).

Place your Follistim Pen with the loaded cartridge and attached needle, flat on a clean, dry surface.

Figure 10

C. Preparing the Injection Site

- Follistim AQ Cartridge can be injected directly into a layer of fat under your skin (subcutaneously).
- When giving a subcutaneous injection, follow your healthcare provider's instructions about changing the site for each injection. This will help lower your chances of having a skin reaction.
- **Do not** inject Follistim AQ Cartridge into an area that is tender, red, bruised, or hard.
- The recommended site for injecting Follistim AQ Cartridge subcutaneously is:
  - just below your belly button (navel) (See Figure 11)

Figure 11

  - the upper outer area of your thigh (See Figure 12)

Figure 12

- Clean the skin with an alcohol wipe where the injection is to be made. Clean about two inches around the injection site where the needle will be inserted. Do not touch the cleaned area of skin.

D. Dialing the Dose Before You Give the Injection

- Your healthcare provider will decide on the dose of Follistim AQ Cartridge to be given. This dose may be increased or decreased as your treatment progresses depending on your individual type of treatment.
- Follistim AQ Cartridge using Follistim Pen can be administered subcutaneously (beneath the skin) in prescribed doses from 50 International Units (IU) up to 450 IU, in marked 25 IU increments. The Dosage Scale on the Pen has numbers and audible clicks to help you set the correct dose.
- Pull off the outer needle shield. Leave the Inner Needle Shield in place over the needle attached to the Pen (See Figure 13). Do not throw the Outer Needle Shield away, you will need it later when you throw the needle away.

Figure 13

- Carefully remove the Inner Needle Shield and discard it (See Figure 14). Do not touch the needle or let it touch any surface while uncapped.

Figure 14

- Hold the Follistim Pen with the needle pointing upwards. Tap the Cartridge Holder gently with your finger to help air bubbles rise to the top of the needle. The small amount of air bubble will not affect the amount of medicine you receive.
- With a loaded new, unused cartridge:
  1. Dial the Dosage Knob until you hear one click. With the needle pointing upwards, push in the Injection Button.
  2. Look for a droplet at the tip of the needle (See Figure 15). If you see the droplet, then you can dial in your dose.
  3. If you do **not** see a droplet, repeat Step 1 (as above) until you see droplet.

  You must **make sure you see a droplet** of medicine (**check the flow of medicine**) or you may **not** inject the correct amount of medicine.

Figure 15

- With a partially used cartridge, to give yourself another dose of medicine you will need to attach a new BD Micro-Fine Pen Needle and look for a droplet forming at the tip of the needle (See Figure 15 above). If you see a droplet, then you can dial in your dose.
  If **no** droplet:
  1. Dial the Dosage Knob until you hear one click. With the needle pointing upwards, push in the Injection Button.
  2. Look for a droplet at the tip of the needle. If you see the droplet, then you can dial in your dose.
- Your Follistim AQ Cartridge should be one of the following:
  - Orange Metal Cap – 150 international units
  - Silver Metal Cap – 300 international units
  - Gold Metal Cap – 600 international units
  - Blue Metal Cap – 900 international units

If you did **not** understand that you should have one of the cartridges above, please contact your healthcare provider.

- For doses of 50 IU up to 450 IU, turn the Dosage Knob until the correct dosage aligns with the dosage markers on each side of the Dosage Window (see Figure 16).

Figure 16

- If by mistake you dial past the correct number, do not try to turn the Dosage Knob backward to fix the mistake. Continue to turn the Dosage Knob in the same direction past the 450 IU mark, as far as it will turn. The Dosage Scale must move freely. Push the Injection Button in all the way. See Figure 17. Start to dial again starting from "0" upwards. By following these directions, you will not lose any medicine from the Follistim AQ Cartridge (See "Checking the Medicine Level Remaining").

Figure 17

- If you turn the Dosage Knob backward to correct the mistake, it will not damage the Pen, but you will lose some medication from the Follistim AQ Cartridge.
- Never dial your dose or try to correct a dialing mistake when the needle is still in your skin as this may result in your receiving an incorrect dose.
- If your prescribed dose exceeds the deliverable dose of Follistim Pen or exceeds the amount remaining in the cartridge, you will need to give yourself more than one injection.

E. Giving Yourself an Injection

- Pinch a fold of skin at the cleaned injection site. **Do not** touch the cleaned area of skin.
- With the other hand hold the entire Pen with Cartridge loaded and Needle on like you would a pencil. Use a quick "dart-like" motion to insert the needle straight up and down (90-degree angle).
- Press the injection button all the way in to make sure you give yourself a full injection. (See Figure 18). Wait for five seconds before pulling the needle out of the skin. The middle of the Dosage Window should display a dot next to the "0".

Figure 18

If the injection button does **not** push in all the way, and the number in the Dosage Window does not read "0", it means there is not enough medication left in the cartridge to complete your prescribed dose. The number in the Dosage Window will give you the amount of medicine needed to complete your dose. Write this number down. This will be the number you dial for the completion of your dose. **Start over** with a new Follistim AQ Cartridge and a new needle and follow all the instructions up to this step. Make sure you choose a different injection site to complete your dose of Follistim AQ Cartridge.

- Pull out the BD Micro-Fine Needle and firmly press down on the injection site with an alcohol swab. Use the BD Micro-Fine Pen Needle for one injection only.
- Place the Outer Needle Shield on a flat table surface with the opening pointing up. The opening of the Outer Needle Shield is the wider end with the rim. Without holding on to the Outer Needle Shield, carefully insert the needle (attached to the Follistim Pen) into the opening of the Outer Needle Shield and push down firmly. The Outer Needle Shield should now be attached to the Cartridge Holder and covering the needle (See Figure 19).

Figure 19

- Grip the Outer Needle Shield and use it to unscrew the needle from the Cartridge Holder (See Figure 20). If there is Follistim AQ Cartridge medicine left for more injections, put the Pen Cap back on the Pen Body and store your Follistim Pen in a safe place in the refrigerator (not in the freezer) or at room temperature. Never store the Follistim Pen with a needle attached to it. If you are giving an injection to another person, be very careful when removing the needle from the skin. Accidental needle sticks can transmit potentially serious or grave infectious diseases. [See figure 20 at top of next column]
- Throw away the Outer Needle Shield with the used needle right away. Do not throw away in a trash can. Place it in a "special" container. (See " How Do I Throw Away Used Cartridges and Needles?")
- If there is Follistim AQ Cartridge medicine left for more injections, put the Pen Cap back on the Pen Body and store your Follistim Pen in a safe place in the refrigerator (not in the freezer) or at room temperature. Never store the Follistim Pen with a needle attached to it. If you are

Figure 20

giving an injection to another person, be very careful when removing the needle from the skin. Accidental needle sticks can lead to serious infections.

- Unscrew the Pen Body from the Cartridge Holder with the **empty** Follistim AQ Cartridge (See Figure 21).

Figure 21

- Put the Pen Body down on a clean, dry surface and remove the empty Follistim AQ Cartridge from the Cartridge Holder (See Figure 22). Safely, dispose of the empty Follistim AQ Cartridge right away in the same "special" container that you used for the needle disposal. Do not put the cartridge in a trash can. At the end of your treatment cycle, your doctor can advise you on how to properly dispose of the container. (See "How Do I Throw Away Used Cartridges and Needles?")

Figure 22

F. Checking the Medicine Level Remaining
For women and men:
Your healthcare provider should advise you of the number of prescribed doses which can be extracted from the full unused Follistim AQ Cartridge.

- **Do not** use the cartridge beyond the advised number of doses. Otherwise, you will run the risk that there will not be enough volume of drug for your prescribed dose.

For women only:
- Keep a Follistim Pen Treatment Diary as follows:
  1. Record the Follistim AQ Cartridge content on Day 1. This will either be 150, 300, 600 or 900 international units depending on what your healthcare provider has prescribed for you.
  2. Record the dose you have been prescribed for your injection.
  3. Subtract your Day 1 dose from the Follistim AQ Cartridge content (150, 300, 600 or 900 international units). (See example – Figure 23.) This will give you the **remaining** Follistim AQ Cartridge content after the Day 1 dose is taken.
  4. Place the number determined as the content after Day 1 (see number 3) in the box as the Follistim AQ Cartridge content **available** for Day 2. (See example – Figure 23.)
  5. Subtract your Day 2 dose from the Follistim AQ Cartridge content you recorded in Step 4. This will give you the **remaining** Follistim AQ Cartridge content after Day 2. Record this number of units. (See example – Figure 23.)
  6. Repeat the steps to determine the Follistim AQ Cartridge content **available** and Follistim AQ Cartridge **remaining** for each day of use.

Day	Date	Dose Prescribed	Follistim AQ Cartridge Content Available	Follistim AQ Cartridge Content Remaining
1	month/day/year	150	600	450
2	month/day/year	150	450	300
3	month/day/year	150	300	150
4	month/day/year	150	150	0

Figure 23. Example of Treatment Diary Starting with a 600 International Unit Cartridge

If you do not know if there is not enough medicine left in the Follistim AQ Cartridge for your next prescribed dose, see section "If There is Not Enough Follistim AQ in the Cartridge".

G. If There is Not Enough Follistim AQ in the Cartridge

1. If you realize **before** you inject that you do not have enough medicine remaining in your Follistim AQ Cartridge for your complete dose, follow either Option 1 or Option 2, but **not** both.
   - Option 1:
     - Dial your dose and inject the remaining content in the Follistim AQ Cartridge. The Dosage Knob Injection Button will not push in all the way (do not try to force down the button) and the Dosage Window number will not read "0" but will read the number of units you will need to complete your prescribed dose.
     - Write down the number of units needed to complete your dose.
     - Remove the needle and dispose of it properly (see "How Do I Throw Away Used Cartridges and Needles?").
     - Using the Dosage Knob, reset the Dial Window to "0" by turning the Dosage Knob past the 450 IU mark as far as it will turn and push the Injection Button in all the way.
     - Before attempting to replace a Follistim AQ Cartridge, be sure that a BD Micro-Fine Pen Needle is not attached to the Follistim Pen.
     - Insert a new cartridge into the Follistim Pen and attach a new BD Micro-Fine needle.
     - Dial to the number of units you have written down to complete your prescribed dose.
     - Prepare a different injection site and inject the remaining drug to complete your dose (See "Giving Yourself an Injection").
   - Option 2
     - Remove the Follistim AQ Cartridge.
     - **Start over** with a new Follistim AQ Cartridge and Insert into the Follistim Pen.
     - Follow the instructions for "Dialing the Dose" and "Giving Yourself an Injection."

2. If you realize **after** you have inserted the needle at the injection site that you do not have enough medicine remaining in your Follistim AQ Cartridge for your complete dose:
   - Inject the remaining content in the Follistim AQ Cartridge. The Injection Button will not push in all the way and the number in the Dosage Window will not read "0" but will read the number of units you will need to complete your dose.
   - Wait 5 seconds before withdrawing the needle from your skin and gently apply pressure to the injection site with an alcohol pad.
   - Dispose of the used needle (See "How Do I Throw Away Used Cartridges and Needles?").
   - Write down the number of units needed to complete your dose.
   - Using the Dosage Knob, reset the Dial Window to "0" by turning the Dosage Knob past the 450 IU mark as it will turn and push the Injection Button in all the way.
   - Insert a new cartridge into the Follistim Pen and attach a new BD Micro-Fine needle.
   - Dial to the number you have recorded to complete your prescribed dose.
   - Prepare a different injection site and inject the remaining drug to complete your dose (See "Giving Yourself an Injection").

H. How to Solve Problems with Follistim AQ Cartridge and Follistim Pen

If you have problems with using the Follistim AQ Cartridge and the Follistim Pen, see the following chart. If you still have problems after following the chart or if your problem is not on the chart, contact your healthcare provider.
[See table above]
Important: If you have a question, always mention the Lot number of your Follistim Pen as printed on the Pen Body. If you have a complaint, please do not discard any product or packaging.
For questions on information contained in this leaflet, call 1-866-836-5633.
www.follistim.com

How Do I Throw Away Used Cartridges and Needles?

Check with your healthcare provider or pharmacist for instructions about the right way to throw away used cartridges and needles. There may be special local or state laws about how to throw away used syringes and needles.
- **Do not** throw away used cartridges and needles in the household trash and do not recycle them.
- Put used and empty cartridges and needles in a closeable, puncture-resistant container. You may use a sharps container (such as a red bio-hazard container), a hard plastic container with a screw-on cap (such as an empty detergent bottle) or in a metal container with a plastic lid, (such as a coffee can).
- When the container is full, tape around the cap or lid to make sure the cap or lid does not come off.
- When your injection is given by another person, this person must also be careful when removing the cartridge and needle and disposing of the cartridge and needle to

PROBLEM	POSSIBLE CAUSES	WHAT TO DO
The Pen Body will not screw tightly into the Cartridge Holder.	Is something in the way?	Take out the Follistim Cartridge and check the Cartridge Holder to see if anything is in the way. Follow the instructions in this pamphlet to Screw the Pen Body fully onto the Cartridge Holder.
No drug is coming out while checking the flow.	The Cartridge Holder and the Pen Body are not properly screwed together.	Remove the current needle; tighten the Pen Body to the Cartridge Holder ensuring the arrow on the Cartridge Holder is pointing to the middle of the yellow alignment mark on the blue Pen Body. Attach a new needle to the Pen. Recheck the flow as follows: a. Dial the Dosage Knob until you hear one click. With needle pointing upwards, push in the Injection Button. b. Look for a droplet at the tip of the needle.
	Is the Follistim Cartridge empty?	Change to a new cartridge.
	Has the needle been properly attached to the Follistim Pen?	Remove needle and replace with a new one, ensuring that the needle is screwed on tightly to the Pen. Recheck the flow as follows: a. Dial the Dosage Knob until you hear one click. With needle pointing upwards, push in the Injection Button. b. Look for a droplet at the tip of the needle.
You are concerned that you can turn the Dosage Knob to the next number without clicking and the injection button spins freely.	This is not a problem.	The system is in the reset mode. The Injection Button and Dosage Knob must be pushed all the way down to '0' to re-engage the mechanism and the correct dose can now be set. A click will be heard for each setting in the viewing window.
The Dosage Knob does not go back to '0' while you are injecting.	Is the Follistim Cartridge empty?	Change to a new cartridge.
	Is the needle blocked?	a. Remove the needle from the skin and dispose of safely. b. Check the Dosage Window and note how much remaining drug to inject. c. Attach a new needle. Recheck the flow as follows: a. Dial the Dosage Knob until you hear one click. With needle pointing upwards, push in the Injection Button. b. Look for a droplet at the tip of the needle. c. Dial remaining dose.
Some of the drug is dripping out of the needle when you withdraw it from your skin.	Did you take the needle out of your skin before waiting 5 seconds as directed in Step 15?	If this happens you should inform your doctor. To avoid this problem again, you should always wait 5 seconds after you push the Injection Button before you withdraw the needle from your skin.
The needle is left on the Follistim Pen.	Have you missed any of the instructions?	Dispose of the needle in a properly secured container as instructed by your doctor. Change to a new Follistim Cartridge and a new needle.
After your last injection, a remaining volume may be left in the cartridge in addition to the normal quantity of drug dispensed.	The cartridge contains extra volume for checking the drug flow.	This is not a problem.
You cannot get the cartridge out of the Follistim Pen.	Is the needle attached?	Remove the needle from the Follistim Pen and dispose of properly. (Unscrew the Cartridge Holder from the Pen Body and take out the cartridge.)
You are not sure how much drug is left in the cartridge and you do not want to start an injection and then find out that there is not enough drug.	Have you kept good records of your doses?	In case of any doubt, you should load a new, unused Follistim Cartridge into the Follistim Pen. See **"If There is Not Enough Follistim AQ in the Cartridge."** To avoid this problem again, you should record your injections. (Women should use a treatment diary.)

prevent accidental needle stick injury and passing infection.

How Do I Care for the Follistim Pen?
1. Clean all exposed surfaces of the Follistim Pen with a clean, damp cloth such as a paper towel. Never wash it in water, detergent or strong medical cleaners.
2. Handle the Follistim Pen carefully to avoid causing damage. You could damage the Follistim Pen by dropping it or handling it roughly.
3. Keep the Follistim Pen away from dust and dirt.
4. Never store the Follistim Pen with a needle attached to it. If you store the Follistim Pen with the needle attached, the drug could leak out and there is risk of contamination.
5. If the Follistim Pen breaks or is damaged, do not try to fix it yourself. Contact your healthcare provider.
6. Do not share your Follistim Pen with another person.

How should I store Follistim AQ Cartridge?
- Store Follistim AQ Cartridge in the refrigerator between 2-8°C (36-46°F) until the expiration date.

- Follistim AQ can be stored at or below 25°C (77°F) for 3 months or until the expiration date, whichever comes first. Once the rubber inlay of the Follistim AQ Cartridge has been pierced by a needle, the product may be stored only for a maximum of 28 days at 2-25°C (36-77°F).
- Keep Follistim AQ Cartridge away from light.
- Do not freeze.

Keep Follistim AQ Cartridge, needles, and the disposal container, out of the reach of children.
Manufactured for: Merck Sharp & Dohme Corp., a subsidiary of
MERCK & CO., INC., Whitehouse Station, NJ 08889, USA
Manufactured by: Vetter Pharma-Fertigung GmbH & Co. KG, Ravensburg, Germany
BD, BD Logo and BD Micro-Fine are trademarks of Becton, Dickinson and Company.
For patent information: www.merck.com/product/patent/home.html
Copyright © 2004, 2010, 2011 Merck Sharp & Dohme B.V., a subsidiary of **Merck & Co., Inc.**
All rights reserved.
Revised: 10/2013
usppi-mk8328-SOi-1310R012

FOLLISTIM AQ   ℞
(follitropin beta injection)
for subcutaneous or intramuscular use

HIGHLIGHTS OF PRESCRIBING INFORMATION
These highlights do not include all the information needed to use Follistim® AQ safely and effectively. See full prescribing information for Follistim AQ.
Follistim AQ (follitropin beta injection) for subcutaneous or intramuscular use
Initial U.S. Approval: 1997

———————**INDICATIONS AND USAGE**———————
Follistim AQ is a gonadotropin indicated:
In Women for:
- Induction of ovulation and pregnancy in anovulatory infertile women in whom the cause of infertility is functional and not due to primary ovarian failure (1.1)
- Development of multiple follicles in ovulatory women participating in an Assisted Reproductive Technology (ART) program (1.2)

In Men for:
- Induction of spermatogenesis in men with primary and secondary hypogonadotropic hypogonadism (HH) in whom the cause of infertility is not due to primary testicular failure (1.3)

———————**DOSAGE AND ADMINISTRATION**———————
Ovulation Induction in Women (2.2)
- Starting daily dose of 75 international units of Follistim AQ is administered subcutaneously or intramuscularly for at least the first 7 days. The dose is increased by 25 or 50 international units at weekly intervals until follicular growth and/or serum estradiol levels indicate an adequate response.
  - When an acceptable pre-ovulatory state is achieved, final oocyte maturation is achieved with 5000 to 10,000 international units of human chorionic gonadotropin (hCG).
  - The woman and her partner should have intercourse daily, beginning on the day prior to the administration of hCG and until ovulation becomes apparent.

Assisted Reproductive Technology (ART) in Women (2.3)
- Starting dose of 150 to 225 international units of Follistim AQ is administered subcutaneously or intramuscularly for at least the first 4 days of treatment. Subsequent doses are adjusted based upon ovarian response as determined by ultrasound evaluation of follicular growth and serum estradiol levels.
  - Final oocyte maturation is induced with a dose of 5000-10,000 international units of hCG.
  - Oocyte (egg) retrieval is performed 34 to 36 hours later.

Induction of Spermatogenesis in Men (2.4)
- Pretreatment with hCG alone (1500 international units twice weekly) is required. If serum testosterone levels have not normalized after 8 weeks of hCG treatment, the dose may be increased to 3000 international units twice a week.
- After normalization of serum testosterone levels, administer 450 international units per week (225 international units twice weekly or 150 international units three times weekly) of Follistim AQ subcutaneously (only) with the same pre-treatment hCG dose used to normalize testosterone levels.

———————**DOSAGE FORMS AND STRENGTHS**———————
Single-Use Vial 75 international units per 0.5 mL (3)
Single-Use Vial 150 international units per 0.5 mL (3)

———————**CONTRAINDICATIONS**———————
Women and men who exhibit:
- Prior hypersensitivity to recombinant hFSH products (4)
- High levels of FSH indicating primary gonadal failure (4)

- Presence of uncontrolled non-gonadal endocrinopathies (4)
- Hypersensitivity reactions related to streptomycin or neomycin (4)
- Tumor of the ovary, breast, uterus, testis, hypothalamus or pituitary gland (4)

Women who exhibit:
- Pregnancy (4, 8.1)
- Heavy or irregular vaginal bleeding of undetermined origin (4)
- Ovarian cysts or enlargement not due to polycystic ovary syndrome (PCOS) (4)

———————**WARNINGS AND PRECAUTIONS**———————
Treatment with Follistim AQ may result in:
- Abnormal Ovarian Enlargement (5.1)
- Ovarian Hyperstimulation Syndrome (OHSS) (5.2)
- Pulmonary and Vascular Complications (5.3)
- Ovarian Torsion (5.4)
- Multi-fetal Gestation and Birth (5.5)
- Congenital Anomalies (5.6)
- Ectopic Pregnancy (5.7)
- Spontaneous Abortion (5.8)
- Ovarian Neoplasms (5.9)

———————**ADVERSE REACTIONS**———————
The most common adverse reactions (≥2%) in women undergoing ovulation induction are: ovarian hyperstimulation syndrome, ovarian cyst, abdominal discomfort, abdominal pain and lower abdominal pain. (6.1)
The most common adverse reactions (≥2%) in women receiving ART are ovarian hyperstimulation syndrome and abdominal pain. (6.1)
The most common (≥2%) adverse reactions in men undergoing induction of spermatogenesis are headache, acne, injection site reaction, injection site pain, gynecomastia, rash and dermoid cyst. (6.1)
To report SUSPECTED ADVERSE REACTIONS, contact Merck Sharp & Dohme Corp., a subsidiary of Merck & Co., Inc., at 1-877-888-4231 or FDA at 1-800-FDA-1088 or www.fda.gov/medwatch.

———————**USE IN SPECIFIC POPULATIONS**———————
Nursing Mothers: It is not known whether this drug is excreted in human milk. (8.3)
See 17 for PATIENT COUNSELING INFORMATION and FDA-approved patient labeling

Revised: 12/2013

FULL PRESCRIBING INFORMATION: CONTENTS*

FULL PRESCRIBING INFORMATION

1   INDICATIONS AND USAGE
Follistim® AQ (follitropin beta injection) is indicated:
In Women for:
1.1   Induction of ovulation and pregnancy in anovulatory infertile women in whom the cause of infertility is functional and not due to primary ovarian failure
Prior to initiation of treatment with Follistim AQ:
- Women should have a complete gynecologic and endocrinologic evaluation.
- Primary ovarian failure should be excluded.
- The possibility of pregnancy should be excluded.
- Tubal patency should be demonstrated.
- The fertility status of the male partner should be evaluated.

1.2   Development of multiple follicles in ovulatory women participating in an Assisted Reproductive Technology (ART) program
Prior to initiation of treatment with Follistim AQ:
- Women should have a complete gynecologic and endocrinologic evaluation and diagnosis of cause of infertility.
- The possibility of pregnancy should be excluded.
- The fertility status of the male partner should be evaluated.

In Men for:
1.3   Induction of spermatogenesis in men with primary and secondary hypogonadotropic hypogonadism (HH) in whom the cause of infertility is not due to primary testicular failure
Prior to initiation of treatment with Follistim AQ:
- Men should have a complete medical and endocrinologic evaluation.
- Hypogonadotropic hypogonadism should be confirmed and primary testicular failure should be excluded.
- Serum testosterone levels should be normalized with human chorionic gonadotropin (hCG) treatment.
- The fertility status of the female partner should be evaluated.

2   DOSAGE AND ADMINISTRATION
2.1   General Dosing
- Parenteral drug products should be inspected visually for particulate matter and discoloration prior to administration, whenever solution and container permit. If the solution is not clear and colorless or has particles in it, the solution should not be used.
- Do not mix Follistim AQ with any other medicines in the same vial or in the same syringe.

2.2   Recommended Dosing for Ovulation Induction
The dosing scheme is stepwise and is individualized for each woman [see Clinical Studies (14.1)].
- A starting daily dose of 75 international units of Follistim AQ is administered for at least the first 7 days.
- Subsequent dosage adjustments are made at weekly intervals based upon ovarian response. If an increase in dose is indicated by the ovarian response, the increase should be made by 25 or 50 international units of Follistim AQ at weekly intervals until follicular growth and/or serum estradiol levels indicate an adequate ovarian response.
The following should be considered when planning the woman's individualized dose:
  - Appropriate Follistim AQ dose adjustment(s) should be used to prevent multiple follicular growth and cycle cancellation.
  - The maximum, individualized, daily dose of Follistim AQ is 300 international units.
- Treatment should continue until ultrasonic visualizations and/or serum estradiol determinations approximate the pre-ovulatory conditions seen in normal individuals.
- When pre-ovulatory conditions are reached, 5000 to 10,000 international units of hCG are used to induce final oocyte maturation and ovulation.
The administration of hCG must be withheld in cases where the ovarian monitoring suggests an increased risk of OHSS on the last day of Follistim AQ therapy [see Warnings and Precautions (5.1, 5.2, 5.10)].
- The woman and her partner should be encouraged to have intercourse daily, beginning on the day prior to the administration of hCG and until ovulation becomes apparent [see Warnings and Precautions (5.10)].

• During treatment with Follistim AQ and during a two-week post-treatment period, the woman should be assessed at least every other day for signs of excessive ovarian stimulation.

It is recommended that Follistim AQ administration be stopped if the ovarian monitoring suggests an increased risk of OHSS or abdominal pain occurs. Most OHSS occurs after treatment has been discontinued and reaches its maximum at about seven to ten days post-ovulation.

2.3 Recommended Dosing for ART

The dosing scheme follows a stepwise approach and is individualized for each woman.

• A starting dose of 150 to 225 international units of Follistim AQ is administered subcutaneously or intramuscularly daily for at least the first 4 days of treatment.

• Subsequent dosing beyond the first 4 days of treatment is adjusted based upon the woman's ovarian response as determined by ultrasound evaluation of follicular growth and serum estradiol levels.

The following should be considered when planning the woman's individualized dose:

■ For most normal responding women, the daily starting dose can be continued until pre-ovulatory conditions are achieved (six to twelve days).

■ For low or poor responding women, the daily dose should be increased according to the ovarian response. The maximum, individualized, daily dose of Follistim AQ is 600 international units.

■ For high responding women [those at particular risk of abnormal ovarian enlargement and/or ovarian hyperstimulation syndrome (OHSS)], decrease or temporarily stop the daily dose, or discontinue the cycle according to individual response [see Warnings and Precautions (5.1, 5.2, 5.10)].

• When a sufficient number of follicles of adequate size are present, dosing of Follistim AQ is stopped and final maturation of the oocytes is induced by administering hCG at a dose of 5000 to 10,000 international units. The administration of hCG should be withheld in cases where the ovarian monitoring suggests an increased risk of OHSS on the last day of Follistim AQ therapy [see Warnings and Precautions (5.1, 5.2, 5.10)].

• Oocyte (egg) retrieval should be performed 34 to 36 hours following the administration of hCG.

2.4 Recommended Dosing for Induction of Spermatogenesis in Men

• Pretreatment with hCG is required prior to concomitant therapy with Follistim AQ and hCG. An initial dosage of 1500 international units of hCG should be administered at twice weekly intervals to normalize serum testosterone levels. If serum testosterone levels have not normalized after 8 weeks of hCG treatment, the hCG dose can be increased to 3000 international units twice weekly [see Clinical Studies (14.3)].

• After normal serum testosterone levels have been reached, Follistim AQ should be administered by subcutaneous injection concomitantly with hCG treatment. Follistim AQ should be given at a dosage of 450 international units per week, as either 225 international units twice weekly or 150 international units three times per week, in combination with the same hCG dose used to normalize testosterone levels.

The concomitant therapy should be continued for at least 3 to 4 months before any improvement in spermatogenesis can be expected. If a man has not responded after this period, the combination therapy may be continued. Treatment response has been noted at up to 12 months.

3 DOSAGE FORMS AND STRENGTHS

Follistim AQ Single-Use Vial 75 international units per 0.5 mL
Follistim AQ Single-Use Vial 150 international units per 0.5 mL

4 CONTRAINDICATIONS

Follistim AQ is contraindicated in women and men who exhibit:

• Prior hypersensitivity to recombinant hFSH products
• High levels of FSH indicating primary gonadal failure
• Presence of uncontrolled non-gonadal endocrinopathies (e.g., thyroid, adrenal, or pituitary disorders) [see Indications and Usage (1.1, 1.2, 1.3)]
• Hypersensitivity reactions to streptomycin or neomycin. Follistim AQ may contain traces of these antibiotics.
• Tumor of the ovary, breast, uterus, testis, hypothalamus or pituitary gland

Follistim AQ is also contraindicated in women who exhibit:

• Pregnancy [see Use in Specific Populations (8.1)]
• Heavy or irregular vaginal bleeding of undetermined origin
• Ovarian cysts or enlargement not due to polycystic ovary syndrome (PCOS)

5 WARNINGS AND PRECAUTIONS

Follistim AQ should be used only by physicians who are experienced in infertility treatment. Follistim AQ is a potent gonadotropic substance capable of causing Ovarian Hyperstimulation Syndrome (OHSS) [see Warnings and Precautions (5.2)] with or without pulmonary or vascular complications [see Warnings and Precautions (5.3)] and multiple births [see Warnings and Precautions (5.5)]. Gonadotropin therapy requires the availability of appropriate monitoring facilities [see Warnings and Precautions (5.10)].

Careful attention should be given to the diagnosis of infertility and in the selection of candidates for Follistim AQ therapy [see Indications and Usage (1.1, 1.2, 1.3) and Dosage and Administration (2.2, 2.3, 2.4)].

5.1 Abnormal Ovarian Enlargement

In order to minimize the hazards associated with abnormal ovarian enlargement that may occur with Follistim AQ therapy, treatment should be individualized and the lowest effective dose should be used [see Dosage and Administration (2.2, 2.3)]. Use of ultrasound monitoring of ovarian response and/or measurement of serum estradiol levels is important to minimize the risk of overstimulation [see Warnings and Precautions (5.8)].

If the ovaries are abnormally enlarged on the last day of Follistim AQ therapy, hCG should not be administered in order to reduce the chances of developing Ovarian Hyperstimulation Syndrome (OHSS). Intercourse should be prohibited in patients with significant ovarian enlargement after ovulation because of the danger of hemoperitoneum resulting from ruptured ovarian cysts [see Warnings and Precautions (5.3)].

5.2 Ovarian Hyperstimulation Syndrome (OHSS)

OHSS is a medical entity distinct from uncomplicated ovarian enlargement and may progress rapidly to become a serious medical condition. OHSS is characterized by a dramatic increase in vascular permeability, which can result in a rapid accumulation of fluid in the peritoneal cavity, thorax, and potentially, the pericardium. The early warning signs of OHSS developing are severe pelvic pain, nausea, vomiting, and weight gain. Abdominal pain, abdominal distension, gastrointestinal symptoms including nausea, vomiting and diarrhea, severe ovarian enlargement, weight gain, dyspnea, and oliguria have been reported with OHSS. Clinical evaluation may reveal hypovolemia, hemoconcentration, electrolyte imbalances, ascites, hemoperitoneum, pleural effusions, hydrothorax, acute pulmonary distress, and thromboembolic reactions [see Warnings and Precautions (5.3)]. Transient liver function test abnormalities suggestive of hepatic dysfunction with or without morphologic changes on liver biopsy have also been reported in association with OHSS.

OHSS occurs after gonadotropin treatment has been discontinued and it can develop rapidly, reaching its maximum about seven to ten days following treatment. Usually, OHSS resolves spontaneously with the onset of menses. If there is evidence that OHSS may be developing prior to hCG administration [see Warnings and Precautions (5.1)], the hCG must be withheld. Cases of OHSS are more common, more severe, and more protracted if pregnancy occurs; therefore, women should be assessed for the development of OHSS for at least two weeks after hCG administration.

If serious OHSS occurs, treatment should be stopped and the patient should be hospitalized. Treatment is primarily symptomatic and overall should consist of bed rest, fluid and electrolyte management, and analgesics (if needed). Because the use of diuretics can accentuate the diminished intravascular volume, diuretics should be avoided except in the late phase of resolution as described below. The management of OHSS may be divided into three phases as follows:

■ Acute Phase:

Management should be directed at preventing hemoconcentration due to loss of intravascular volume to the third space and minimizing the risk of thromboembolic phenomena and kidney damage. Fluid intake and output, weight, hematocrit, serum and urinary electrolytes, urine specific gravity, BUN and creatinine, total proteins with albumin: globulin ratio, coagulation studies, electrocardiogram to monitor for hyperkalemia, and abdominal girth should be thoroughly assessed daily or more often based on the clinical need. Treatment, consisting of limited intravenous fluids, electrolytes, human serum albumin, is intended to normalize electrolytes while maintaining an acceptable but somewhat reduced intravascular volume. Full correction of the intravascular volume deficit may lead to an unacceptable increase in the amount of third space fluid accumulation

■ Chronic Phase:

After the acute phase is successfully managed as above, excessive fluid accumulation in the third space should be limited by instituting severe potassium, sodium, and fluid restriction

■ Resolution Phase:

As third space fluid returns to the intravascular compartment, a fall in hematocrit and increasing urinary output are observed in the absence of any increase in intake. Peripheral and/or pulmonary edema may result if the kidneys are unable to excrete third space fluid as rapidly as it is mobilized. Diuretics may be indicated during the resolution phase, if necessary, to combat pulmonary edema

OHSS increases the risk of injury to the ovary. The ascitic, pleural, and pericardial fluid should not be removed unless there is the necessity to relieve symptoms such as pulmonary distress or cardiac tamponade. Pelvic examination may cause rupture of an ovarian cyst, which may result in hemoperitoneum, and should therefore be avoided. If bleeding occurs and requires surgical intervention, the clinical objective should be to control the bleeding and retain as much ovarian tissue as possible.

During clinical trials with Follistim therapy, OHSS occurred in 7.6% of 105 women (OI) and 5.2% of 591 women (ART) treated with Follistim.

5.3 Pulmonary and Vascular Complications

Serious pulmonary conditions (e.g., atelectasis, acute respiratory distress syndrome) have been reported in women treated with gonadotropins. In addition, thromboembolic reactions both in association with, and separate from, OHSS have been reported following gonadotropin therapy. Intravascular thrombosis, which may originate in venous or arterial vessels, can result in reduced blood flow to vital organs or the extremities. Women with generally recognized risk factors for thrombosis, such as a personal or family history, severe obesity, or thrombophilia, may have an increased risk of venous or arterial thromboembolic events, during or following treatment with gonadotropins. Sequelae of such reactions have included venous thrombophlebitis, pulmonary embolism, pulmonary infarction, cerebral vascular occlusion (stroke), and arterial occlusion resulting in loss of limb and rarely in myocardial infarction. In rare cases, pulmonary complications and/or thromboembolic reactions have resulted in death. In women with recognized risk factors, the benefits of ovulation induction or in vitro fertilization (IVF) treatment need to be weighed against the risks. It should be noted that pregnancy itself also carries an increased risk of thrombosis.

5.4 Ovarian Torsion

Ovarian torsion has been reported after treatment with Follistim AQ and after intervention with other gonadotropins. This may be related to OHSS, pregnancy, previous abdominal surgery, past history of ovarian torsion, previous or current ovarian cyst and polycystic ovaries. Damage to the ovary due to reduced blood supply can be limited by early diagnosis and immediate detorsion.

5.5 Multi-fetal Gestation and Birth

Multi-fetal gestation and births have been reported with all gonadotropin treatments including Follistim AQ treatment. The woman and her partner should be advised of the potential risk of multi-fetal gestation and births before starting treatment.

5.6 Congenital Anomalies

The incidence of congenital malformations after ART may be slightly higher than after spontaneous conception. This slightly higher incidence is thought to be related to differences in parental characteristics (e.g., maternal age, sperm characteristics) and to the higher incidence of multi-fetal gestations after ART. There are no indications that the use of gonadotropins during ART is associated with an increased risk of congenital malformations.

5.7 Ectopic Pregnancy

Since infertile women undergoing ART, and particularly IVF, often have tubal abnormalities the incidence of ectopic pregnancies might be increased. Early confirmation of an intrauterine pregnancy should be determined by hCG testing and transvaginal ultrasound.

5.8 Spontaneous Abortion

The risk of spontaneous abortions (miscarriage) is increased with gonadotropin products. However, causality has not been established. The increased risk may be a factor of the underlying infertility.

5.9 Ovarian Neoplasms

There have been infrequent reports of ovarian neoplasms, both benign and malignant, in women who have undergone multiple drug regimens for ovulation induction; however, a causal relationship has not been established.

5.10 Laboratory Tests

For Women:

In most instances, treatment with Follistim AQ will result only in follicular growth and maturation. In order to complete the final phase of follicular maturation and to induce ovulation, hCG must be given following the administration of Follistim AQ or when clinical assessment indicates that sufficient follicular maturation has occurred. The degree of follicular maturation and the timing of hCG administration can both be determined with the use of sonographic visualization of the ovaries and endometrial lining in conjunction with measurement of serum estradiol levels. The combination of transvaginal ultrasonography and measurement of serum estradiol levels is also useful for minimizing the risk of OHSS and multi-fetal gestations.

The clinical confirmation of ovulation is obtained by the following direct or indirect indices of progesterone production as well as sonographic evidence of ovulation.

Direct or indirect indices of progesterone production are:
- Urinary or serum luteinizing hormone (LH) rise
- A rise in basal body temperature
- Increase in serum progesterone
- Menstruation following the shift in basal body temperature

The following provide sonographic evidence of ovulation:
- Collapsed follicle
- Fluid in the cul-de-sac
- Features consistent with corpus luteum formation

Sonographic evaluation of the early pregnancy is also important to rule out ectopic pregnancy.

For Men:
Clinical monitoring for spermatogenesis utilizes the following indirect or direct measures:
- Serum testosterone level
- Semen analysis

6 ADVERSE REACTIONS

The following serious adverse reactions are discussed elsewhere in the labeling:
- Ovarian Hyperstimulation Syndrome [see Warnings and Precautions (5.2)]
- Atelectasis [see Warnings and Precautions (5.3)]
- Thromboembolism [see Warnings and Precautions (5.3)]
- Ovarian Torsion [see Warnings and Precautions (5.4)]
- Multi-fetal Gestation and Birth [see Warnings and Precautions (5.5)]
- Congenital Anomalies [see Warnings and Precautions (5.6)]
- Ectopic Pregnancy [see Warnings and Precautions (5.7)]
- Spontaneous Abortion [see Warnings and Precautions (5.8)]

6.1 Clinical Study Experience
Because clinical trials are conducted under widely varying conditions, adverse reaction rates observed in the clinical trials of a drug cannot be directly compared to rates in the clinical trials of another drug and may not reflect the rates observed in clinical practice.

Ovulation Induction
In a single cycle, multi-center, assessor-blind, parallel group, comparative study, a total of 172 chronic anovulatory women who had failed to ovulate and/or conceive with clomiphene citrate therapy, were randomized and treated with Follistim (105) or a urofollitropin comparator. Adverse reactions with an incidence of greater than 2% in either treatment group are listed in Table 1.

TABLE 1: Common Adverse Reactions Reported at a Frequency of ≥2% in an Assessor-Blind, Comparative Study of Women Receiving Ovulation Induction

System Organ Class/Adverse Reactions	Treatment Number (%) of Women	
	Follistim N=105 n (%)	Comparator N=67 n (%)
Gastrointestinal disorders		
Abdominal discomfort	3 (2.9)	1 (1.5)
Abdominal pain	3 (2.9)	2 (3.0)
Abdominal pain lower	3 (2.9)	1 (1.5)
Reproductive system and breast disorders		
Ovarian cyst	3 (2.9)	2 (3.0)
Ovarian hyperstimulation syndrome	8 (7.6)	3 (4.5)
General disorders and administration site conditions		
Pyrexia	0 (0.0)	2 (3.0)

Adverse reactions reported commonly (greater than or equal to 2% of women treated with Follistim) in other ovulation induction clinical trials were headache, abdominal distension, constipation, diarrhea, nausea, pelvic pain, uterine enlargement, vaginal hemorrhage and injection site reaction. The following medical events have been reported subsequent to pregnancies resulting from Follistim AQ therapy:
- Ectopic pregnancy [see Warnings and Precautions (5.7)]
- Spontaneous abortion [see Warnings and Precautions (5.8)]

ART
In a multiple cycle, multi-center, assessor-blind, parallel group, comparative study, after pituitary suppression with a gonadotropin release hormone (GnRH) agonist, a total of 989 women were randomized and treated with Follistim (N=591) or a urofollitropin comparator as part of *in vitro*

fertilization therapy (IVF). Adverse reactions with an incidence of greater than 2% in either treatment group are listed in Table 2.

TABLE 2: Common Adverse Reactions Reported at a Frequency of ≥2% in an Assessor-Blind, Comparative Study of Women Receiving In Vitro Fertilization (IVF)

System Organ Class/Adverse Reactions	Treatment Number (%) of Women	
	Follistim N=591 n (%)	Comparator N=398 n (%)
Gastrointestinal disorders		
Abdominal pain	13 (2.2)	4 (1.0)
Reproductive system and breast disorders		
Ovarian hyperstimulation syndrome	31 (5.2)	17 (4.3)

Adverse reactions reported commonly (greater than or equal to 2% of women treated with Follistim) in other IVF clinical trials were headache, abdominal distension, constipation, diarrhea, nausea, pelvic pain, breast tenderness, metrorrhagia, ovarian enlargement, vaginal hemorrhage, injection site reaction and rash.

The following medical events have been reported subsequent to pregnancies resulting from Follistim AQ therapy:
- Ectopic pregnancy [see Warnings and Precautions (5.7)]
- Spontaneous abortion [see Warnings and Precautions (5.8)]

Induction of Spermatogenesis
In an open-label, non-comparative clinical trial, 49 men with hypogonadotropic hypogonadism were enrolled to received pretreatment with hCG, followed by combination therapy with hCG and Follistim for induction of spermatogenesis. Of the 49 men, 30 received weekly Follistim doses of 450 international units; 24 of these 30 men received a total of 48 weeks of treatment with Follistim. Adverse reactions occurring with an incidence of greater than 2% in the 30 men treated with Follistim are listed in Table 3.

TABLE 3: Common Adverse Reactions Reported at a Frequency of ≥2% in an Open-Label Clinical Trial in Men with Hypogonadotropic Hypogonadism

System Organ Class/Adverse Reactions	Follistim Treatment N=30 n (%)
Nervous system disorders	
Headache	2 (6.7)
General disorders and administration site disorders	
Injection site reaction	2 (6.7)
Injection site pain	2 (6.7)
Skin and subcutaneous tissue disorders	
Acne	2 (6.7)
Rash	1 (3.3)
Reproductive system and breast disorders	
Gynecomastia	1 (3.3)
Neoplasms benign, malignant and unspecified	
Dermoid cyst	1 (3.3)

6.2 Postmarketing Experience
The following adverse reactions have been identified during post approval use of Follistim and/or Follistim AQ. Because these reactions are reported voluntarily from a population of uncertain size, it is not always possible to reliably estimate their frequency or establish a causal relationship to drug exposure.

Vascular disorders:
Thromboembolism [see Warnings and Precautions (5.3)]

7 DRUG INTERACTIONS
No drug-drug interaction studies have been performed.

8 USE IN SPECIFIC POPULATIONS
8.1 Pregnancy
Pregnancy Category X: Follistim AQ should not be used during pregnancy [see Contraindications (4)].
8.3 Nursing Mothers
It is not known whether this drug is excreted in human milk. Because many drugs are excreted in human milk and

because of the potential for serious adverse reactions in the nursing infant from Follistim AQ, a decision should be made whether to discontinue nursing or to discontinue the drug, taking into account the importance of the drug to the mother.
8.4 Pediatric Use
Safety and effectiveness in pediatric patients have not been established.
8.5 Geriatric Use
Clinical studies of Follistim did not include subjects aged 65 and over.

10 OVERDOSAGE
Aside from the possibility of Ovarian Hyperstimulation Syndrome [see Warnings and Precautions (5.2, 5.3)] and multiple gestations [see Warnings and Precautions (5.5)], there is no additional information concerning the consequences of acute overdosage with Follistim AQ.

11 DESCRIPTION
Follistim AQ contains human follicle-stimulating hormone (hFSH), a glycoprotein hormone which is manufactured by recombinant DNA (rDNA) technology. The active drug substance, follitropin beta, has a dimeric structure containing two glycoprotein subunits (alpha and beta). Both the 92 amino acid alpha-chain and the 111 amino acid beta-chain have complex heterogeneous structures arising from two N-linked oligosaccharide chains. Follitropin beta is synthesized in a Chinese hamster ovary (CHO) cell line that has been transfected with a plasmid containing the two subunit DNA sequences encoding for hFSH. The purification process results in a highly purified preparation with a consistent hFSH isoform profile and high specific activity [as determined by the Ph. Eur. test for FSH *in vivo* bioactivity and on the basis of the molar extinction coefficient at 277 nm ($\epsilon_s:mg^{-1}cm^{-1}$)=1.066].
The biological activity is determined by measuring the increase in ovary weight in female rats. The intrinsic luteinizing hormone (LH) activity in follitropin beta is less than 1 international unit per 40,000 international units FSH. The compound is considered to contain no LH activity.
The amino acid sequence and tertiary structure of the product are indistinguishable from that of hFSH of urinary source. Also, based on available data derived from physicochemical tests and bioassay, follitropin beta and follitropin alfa, another recombinant follicle-stimulating hormone product, are indistinguishable.
Follistim AQ is presented as a sterile aqueous solution intended for subcutaneous (in men and women) or intramuscular (women only) administration. Each single-use vial of Follistim AQ contains the following per 0.5 mL: 75 international units or 150 international units of FSH activity; 25 mg sucrose NF; 7.35 mg sodium citrate (dihydrate) USP; 0.25 mg L-methionine USP; 0.1 mg polysorbate 20 NF; and water for injection USP. Hydrochloric acid NF and/or sodium hydroxide NF are used to adjust the pH to 7.
The recombinant protein in Follistim AQ has been standardized for FSH *in vivo* bioactivity in terms of the WHO International Standard for Follicle Stimulating Hormone (FSH) Recombinant, Human for Bioassay (code 92/642), issued by the World Health Organization Expert Committee on Biological Standardization (1995). Under current storage conditions, Follistim AQ may contain up to 11% of oxidized follitropin beta.
In clinical trials with Follistim, serum antibodies to FSH or anti-CHO cell derived proteins were not detected in any of the treated patients after exposure to Follistim for up to three cycles.
Therapeutic Class: Infertility.

12 CLINICAL PHARMACOLOGY
12.1 Mechanism of Action
Women:
Follicle-stimulating hormone (FSH), the active component in Follistim AQ, is required for normal follicular growth, maturation, and gonadal steroid production.
In women, the level of FSH is critical for the onset and duration of follicular development, and consequently for the timing and number of follicles reaching maturity. Follistim AQ stimulates ovarian follicular growth in women who do not have primary ovarian failure. In order to effect the final phase of follicle maturation, resumption of meiosis and rupture of the follicle in the absence of an endogenous LH surge, human chorionic gonadotropin (hCG) must be given following treatment with Follistim AQ when patient monitoring indicates appropriate follicular development parameters have been reached.
Men:
Follistim when administered with hCG stimulates spermatogenesis in men with hypogonadotropic hypogonadism. FSH, the active component of Follistim, is the pituitary hormone responsible for spermatogenesis.
12.3 Pharmacokinetics
Exposures of follitropin beta from Follistim AQ and Follistim are expected to be equivalent. The following information is based on studies conducted with Follistim.
Absorption:
Women:
The bioavailability of Follistim following subcutaneous and intramuscular administration was investigated in healthy,

pituitary-suppressed, women given a single 300 international units dose. In these women, the area under the curve (AUC), expressed as the mean ± SD, was equivalent between the subcutaneous (455.6 ± 141.4 IU*h/L) and intramuscular (445.7 ± 135.7 IU*h/L) routes of administration. However, equivalence could not be established with respect to the peak serum FSH levels (C_{max}). The C_{max} achieved after subcutaneous administration and intramuscular administration was 5.41 ± 0.72 international units/L and 6.86 ± 2.90 international units/L, respectively. After subcutaneous or intramuscular injection the apparent dose absorbed was 77.8% and 76.4%, respectively.

The pharmacokinetics and pharmacodynamics of a single, intramuscular dose (300 international units) of Follistim were also investigated in a group (n=8) of gonadotropin-deficient, but otherwise healthy women. In these women, FSH (mean ± SD) AUC was 339 ± 105 international units*h/L, C_{max} was 4.3 ± 1.7 international units/L. C_{max} occurred at approximately 27 ± 5.4 hours after intramuscular administration.

A multiple dose, dose proportionality, pharmacokinetic study of Follistim was completed in healthy, pituitary-suppressed, women given subcutaneous doses of 75, 150, or 225 international units for 7 days. Steady-state blood concentrations of FSH were reached with all doses after 5 days of treatment based on the trough concentrations of FSH just prior to dosing (C_{trough}). Peak blood concentrations with the 75, 150, and 225 international units dose were 4.30 ± 0.60 international units/L, 8.51 ± 1.16 international units/L and 13.92 ± 1.81 international units/L, respectively.

A multiple dose, dose proportionality, pharmacokinetic study of Follistim was completed in healthy, pituitary-suppressed, women given intramuscular doses of 75, 150, or 225 international units for 7 days. Steady-state blood concentrations of FSH were reached with all doses after 4 days of treatment based on the minimum concentrations of FSH just prior to dosing (C_{min}). Peak blood concentrations with the 75, 150, and 225 international units dose were 4.65 ± 1.49 international units/L, 9.46 ± 2.57 international units/L and 11.30 ± 1.77 international units/L, respectively.

Men:
Serum levels of FSH were measured in a clinical study that compared the effects of two different dosing schedules of Follistim (150 international units three times a week or 225 international units twice a week) administered by subcutaneous injection concurrently with chorionic gonadotropin for injection for induction of spermatogenesis in hypogonadotropic hypogonadal men. Administration of Follistim was started at Week 17. Mean serum trough concentrations of FSH remained fairly constant over the treatment period. At the end of treatment (Week 64), the mean serum trough concentrations of FSH were 2.09 international units/L in the 150 international units group and 3.22 international units/L in the 225 international units group. Serum trough concentrations of FSH measured prior to the first Follistim injection on the Mondays of active treatment period (Weeks 17 to 64) and one week after the end of treatment period are presented in **Figure 1**.

FIGURE 1: Mean (SD) Serum Trough Concentrations of FSH in Men Following Subcutaneous Administration of Follistim Using Two Different Dosing Schedules (150 International Units Three Times a Week or 225 International Units Twice a Week)

Distribution:
The volume of distribution of Follistim in healthy, pituitary-suppressed, women following intravenous administration of a 300 international units dose was approximately 8 L.
Metabolism:
The recombinant FSH in Follistim AQ is biochemically very similar to urinary FSH and it is therefore anticipated that it is metabolized in the same manner.
Elimination:
The elimination half-life ($t_{1/2}$) following a single intramuscular dose (300 international units) of Follistim in women was 43.9 ± 14.1 hours (mean ± SD). The elimination half-life

following a 7-day intramuscular treatment of women with 75, 150, or 225 international units was 26.9 ± 7.8 hours (mean ± SD), 30.1 ± 6.2 and 28.9 ± 6.5, respectively.
Use in Specific Populations:
Body weight: The effect of body weight on the pharmacokinetics of Follistim was evaluated in a group of European and Japanese women who were significantly different in terms of body weight. The European women had a body weight of (mean ± SD) 67.4 ± 13.5 kg and the Japanese subjects were 46.8 ± 11.6 kg. Following a single intramuscular dose of 300 international units of Follistim, the AUC was significantly smaller in European women (339 ± 105 international units*h/L) than in Japanese women (544 ± 201 international units*h/L). However, clearance per kg of body weight was essentially the same for the respective groups (0.014 and 0.013 L/hr/kg).
Geriatric Use: The pharmacokinetics of Follistim has not been studied in geriatric subjects.
Pediatric Use: The pharmacokinetics of Follistim has not been studied in pediatric subjects.
Renal Impairment: The effect of renal impairment on the pharmacokinetics of Follistim has not been studied.
Hepatic Impairment: The effect of hepatic impairment on the pharmacokinetics of Follistim has not been studied.

13 NONCLINICAL TOXICOLOGY
13.1 Carcinogenesis, Mutagenesis, Impairment of Fertility
Long-term toxicity studies in animals have not been performed with Follistim to evaluate the carcinogenic potential of the drug. Follistim was not mutagenic in the Ames test using *S. typhimurium* and *E. coli* tester strains and did not produce chromosomal aberrations in an *in vitro* assay using human lymphocytes.

14 CLINICAL STUDIES
14.1 Ovulation Induction
The efficacy of Follistim for Ovulation Induction was evaluated in a randomized, assessor-blind, parallel-group comparative, multicenter safety and efficacy study of 172 chronic anovulatory women (105 subjects on Follistim) who had previously failed to ovulate and/or conceive during clomiphene citrate treatment. The study results for ovulation rates are summarized in **Table 4** and those for pregnancy rates are summarized in **Table 5**.

TABLE 4: Cumulative Ovulation Rates

Cycle	Follistim (n=105)
First treatment cycle	72%
Second treatment cycle	82%
Third treatment cycle	85%

TABLE 5: Cumulative Ongoing*,† Pregnancy Rates

Cycle	Follistim (n=105)
First treatment cycle	14%
Second treatment cycle	19%
Third treatment cycle	23%

* All ongoing pregnancies were confirmed after at least 12 weeks after the hCG injection.
† Study was not powered to demonstrate this outcome.

14.2 Assisted Reproductive Technology (ART)
The efficacy of Follistim as part of an Assisted Reproductive Technology (ART) program was established in three studies, two of which are described below.
Follistim was evaluated in a randomized, assessor-blind, parallel-group, comparative, multicenter safety and efficacy study of 981 healthy normal ovulatory infertile women (mean age 32) treated for multiple cycles with *in vitro* fertilization and controlled ovarian stimulation with Follistim (n=585) or urofollitropin (n=396) after pituitary suppression with a GnRH agonist. The first cycle results with Follistim are summarized in **Table 6**.

TABLE 6: Results of First Cycle Treatment of Infertile Women With Follistim and In Vitro Fertilization After Pituitary Suppression With a GnRH Agonist*

Parameter	Follistim (n=585)
Total number of oocytes recovered	10.9
Ongoing† pregnancy rate/attempt‡	22.2%

Ongoing† pregnancy rate/transfer‡, §	26.0%

* All values are means.
† A single vital or multiple vital pregnancy was termed ongoing when a pregnancy, at least 12 weeks after embryo transfer (ET), was confirmed by the investigator.
‡ Study was not powered to demonstrate these secondary endpoints.
§ Transfers were limited to a maximum of three embryos.

Follistim was also evaluated in a randomized, assessor-blind, parallel-group, comparative, single center safety and efficacy study in 89 infertile healthy normal ovulatory women (mean age 32) treated for one cycle with *in vitro* fertilization and controlled ovarian stimulation with Follistim (n=54) or menotropins (n=35) without pituitary suppression with a GnRH agonist. The results with Follistim are summarized in **Table 7**.

TABLE 7: Results of Single Cycle Treatment of Infertile Women Treated With In Vitro Fertilization and Follistim Without Pituitary Suppression*

Parameter	Follistim (n=54)
Total number of oocytes recovered	9.9
Ongoing† pregnancy rate/attempt‡	22.2%
Ongoing† pregnancy rate/transfer‡,§	30.8%

* All values are means.
† A single vital or multiple vital pregnancy was termed ongoing when a pregnancy, at least 12 weeks after embryo transfer (ET), was confirmed by the investigator.
‡ Study was not powered to demonstrate these secondary endpoints.
§ Transfers were limited to a maximum of three embryos.

14.3 Induction of Spermatogenesis
The safety and efficacy of Follistim administered by subcutaneous injection concomitantly with chorionic gonadotropin for injection (hCG) has been examined in a multicenter, open-label, non-comparator clinical study for induction of spermatogenesis in hypogonadotropic hypogonadal men. The study compared the effects of two different Follistim dosing schedules on semen parameters and serum levels of follicle stimulating hormone (FSH). The multicenter study involved a 16-week pretreatment phase with hCG at a dosage of 1500 international units twice a week to normalize serum testosterone levels. If serum testosterone levels did not normalize after 8 weeks of hCG treatment, the hCG dose could have been increased to 3000 international units twice a week. This phase was followed by a 48-week treatment phase. Men who were still azoospermic after the pretreatment phase were randomized to receive either 225 international units Follistim together with 1500 international units hCG twice a week or 150 international units Follistim three times a week together with 1500 international units hCG twice weekly. Men who required 3000 international units of hCG twice a week in the pretreatment phase were continued on that dosage during the treatment phase. The mean age of patients in both treatment groups was approximately 30 years (range 18 to 47 years). At baseline, mean left and right testis volumes were 4.61 ± 2.94 mL and 4.57 ± 3.00 mL, respectively, in the group receiving three weekly injections of Follistim. For the group receiving two weekly injections of Follistim, the mean left and right testis volumes were 6.54 ± 2.45 mL and 7.21 ± 2.94 mL, respectively, at baseline. The primary efficacy endpoint was the percentage of patients with a mean sperm density of ≥1 × 10^6/mL on their last two treatment assessments. The outcomes of treatment in the 30 men enrolled in the treatment phase are summarized in **Table 8**.
[See table 8 at top of next page]
Overall, the median time to reach a sperm concentration of 10^6 per mL was 165 days (range 25 to 327 days) in patients who demonstrated a sperm concentration of at least 10^6 per mL. The median time to reach a sperm concentration of at least 10^6 per mL was 186 days (range 25 to 327 days) for the 150 international units group and 141 days (range 43 to 204 days) for the 225 international units group. No pregnancy data were collected during the trial.
The local tolerance data were comparable between the two treatment groups. The mean percentage of days without pain calculated for all subjects in the treatment period was 91.3% for patients in the 150 international units (three times a week) and 76.0% for patients in the 225 international units (two times a week) Follistim treatment groups. In the 225 international units (twice per week) group, local symptoms judged as severe by the investigator were: itching in 1 patient (7%), pain in 2 patients (13%), bruising in 2

TABLE 8: Number of Men Receiving Follistim Who Achieved a Mean Sperm Density of ≥10^6/mL on Their Last Two Treatment Assessments

	Follistim 150 international units three times a week (n=15)		Follistim 225 international units twice a week (n=15)		Overall (n=30)	
Sperm Density of ≥10^6/mL	n	%	n	%	n	%
Yes	6	40	7	47	13	43
No	9	60	8	53	17	57

patients (13%), swelling in 2 patients (13%), and redness in 1 patient (7%). In the 150 international units (three times per week) group, 1 event in 1 patient (bruising, 7%) was judged as severe. No patient discontinued treatment due to injection site reaction or injection site pain.

16 HOW SUPPLIED/STORAGE AND HANDLING

Follistim AQ (follitropin beta injection) is supplied as a sterile aqueous solution in a 2-mL vial to deliver 0.5 mL of the drug in the following concentrations and packaging:
Follistim AQ Single-Use Vial 75 international units per 0.5 mL

    Box of 1   NDC 0052-0308-02

Follistim AQ Single-Use Vial 150 international units per 0.5 mL

    Box of 1   NDC 0052-0309-02

Store refrigerated, 2° - 8°C (36° - 46°F) until dispensed. Upon dispensing, the product may be stored by the patient at 2° - 8°C (36° - 46°F) until the expiration date, or at or below 25°C (77°F) for 3 months or until expiration date, whichever occurs first. Protect from light, keep container in carton. Do not freeze.

17 PATIENT COUNSELING INFORMATION

See FDA-Approved Patient Labeling

17.1 Therapy Duration and Necessary Monitoring in Women and Men Undergoing Treatment

Prior to beginning therapy with Follistim AQ, inform women and men about the time commitment and monitoring procedures necessary to undergo treatment *[see Dosage and Administration (2), Warnings and Precautions (5.10)]*.

17.2 Instructions on a Missed Dose

Inform women and men that if they miss or forget to take a dose of Follistim AQ, the next dose should not be doubled and they should call the healthcare provider for further dosing instructions.

17.3 Ovarian Hyperstimulation Syndrome

Inform women regarding the risks with use of Follistim AQ of Ovarian Hyperstimulation Syndrome *[see Warnings and Precautions (5.2)]* and associated symptoms including lung and blood vessel problems *[see Warnings and Precautions (5.3)]* and ovarian torsion *[see Warnings and Precautions (5.4)]*.

17.4 Multi-fetal Gestation and Birth

Inform women regarding the risk of multi-fetal gestations with the use of Follistim AQ *[see Warnings and Precautions (5.5)]*.

Manufactured for: Merck Sharp & Dohme Corp., a subsidiary of
MERCK & CO., INC., Whitehouse Station, NJ 08889, USA
Manufactured by: N.V. Organon, Oss, The Netherlands, a subsidiary of
Merck & Co., Inc., Whitehouse Station, NJ 08889, USA
For patent information: www.merck.com/product/patent/home.html
Copyright © 2005, 2010 Merck Sharp & Dohme B.V., a subsidiary of **Merck & Co., Inc.** All rights reserved.
Revised: 12/2013
uspi-mk8328-SOi-1312R006

PATIENT INFORMATION LEAFLET
Follistim® (Fol'-lis-tim) AQ
(follitropin beta injection)
Single-Use Vial

Read the Patient Information that comes with Follistim® AQ before you start using it and each time you get a refill. There may be new information. This information does not take the place of talking with your healthcare provider about your medical condition or treatment.

What is Follistim AQ?
Follistim AQ is a prescription medicine that contains follicle-stimulating hormone (FSH).

Follistim AQ is used:
In women:
• to help healthy ovaries to develop (mature) and release eggs
• as part of an Assisted Reproductive Technology (ART) program to help the ovaries produce more mature eggs

In men:
• to help bring about the production and development of sperm

Who should not take Follistim AQ?
Do not take Follistim AQ if you are a Woman or Man who:
• is allergic to recombinant human FSH products
• has a high level of FSH in your blood indicating that your ovaries (women only) or testes (men only) may be permanently damaged and do not work at all
• has uncontrolled thyroid, pituitary, or adrenal gland problems
• is allergic to streptomycin or neomycin (types of antibiotics)
• has a tumor of the hypothalamus, pituitary gland, breast, uterus (women only), ovary (women only), or testis (men only)

Do not take Follistim AQ if you are a Woman who:
• is pregnant or think you may be pregnant
• has heavy or irregular vaginal bleeding and the cause is not known
• has ovarian cysts or enlarged ovaries, not due to polycystic ovary syndrome (PCOS)

Talk to your healthcare provider before taking this medicine if you have any of the conditions listed above.

What should I tell my healthcare provider before taking Follistim AQ?
Before you take Follistim AQ, tell your healthcare provider if you:
• have an increased risk of blood clots (thrombosis)
• have ever had a blood clot (thrombosis), or anyone in your immediate family has ever had a blood clot (thrombosis)
• had stomach (abdominal) surgery
• had twisting of your ovary (ovarian torsion)
• had or have a cyst in your ovary
• have polycystic ovary disease
• have any other medical conditions
• are breastfeeding or plan to breastfeed. It is not known if Follistim AQ passes into your breast milk. You and your healthcare provider should decide if you will take Follistim AQ or breastfeed. You should not do both.

Tell your healthcare provider about all the medicines you take, including prescription and non-prescription medicines, vitamins, and herbal supplements.
Know the medicines you take. Keep a list of them and show your healthcare provider and pharmacist when you get a new medicine.

How should I use Follistim AQ?
• Be sure that you read, understand, and follow the "Patient Instructions for Use" that come with Follistim AQ.
• Use Follistim AQ exactly as your healthcare provider tells you to.
• Your healthcare provider will tell you how much Follistim AQ to use, how to inject it, and how often it should be injected.
• Do not inject Follistim AQ at home until your healthcare provider has taught you the right way.
• Do not mix Follistim AQ with any other medicines in the same vial or in the same syringe.
• Do not change your dose of Follistim AQ unless your healthcare provider tells you to.
• **Call your healthcare provider immediately** if you use too much Follistim AQ.
• If you miss or forget to take a dose, do not double your next dose. Ask your healthcare provider for instructions.
• Your healthcare provider will do blood and urine hormone tests while you are taking Follistim AQ. Make sure you follow-up with your healthcare provider to have your blood and urine tested when told to do so.

Women:
• Your healthcare provider may do ultrasound scans of your ovaries. Make sure you follow-up with your healthcare provider to have your ultrasound scans.

Men:
• Your healthcare provider may test your semen while you are taking Follistim AQ. Make sure you follow-up with your healthcare provider to give a semen sample for testing.

What are the possible side effects of Follistim AQ?
Follistim AQ may cause serious side effects.
Serious side effects in women include:
• **Ovarian enlargement**
• **Ovarian hyperstimulation syndrome (OHSS).** OHSS is a serious medical problem that can happen when the ovaries are over stimulated. In rare cases it has caused death. OHSS causes fluid to build up suddenly in your stomach and chest areas and can cause blood clots to form. Call your healthcare provider right away if you have:
  • pain in your lower stomach area
  • nausea
  • vomiting
  • weight gain
  • diarrhea
  • decreased urine output
  • trouble breathing
• **Lung problems.** Follistim AQ can cause you to have fluid in your lungs (atelectasis) and trouble breathing (acute respiratory distress syndrome).
• **Blood clots.** Follistim AQ may increase your chance of having blood clots in your blood vessels. Blood clots can cause:
  • blood vessel problems (thrombophlebitis)
  • stroke
  • loss of your arm or leg
  • blood clot in your lungs (pulmonary embolus)
  • heart attack
• **Ovarian torsion.** Follistim AQ may increase the chance of twisting of the ovaries in women with certain conditions such as OHSS, pregnancy and previous abdominal surgery. Twisting of the ovary could cause the blood flow to the ovary to be cut off.
• **Pregnancy and birth of multiple babies.** Having a pregnancy with more than one baby at a time increases the health risk for you and your babies. Discuss your chances of multiple births with your healthcare provider.
• **Birth defects.** A woman's age, certain sperm problems, genetic background of both parents and a pregnancy with multiple babies can increase the chance that your baby might have birth defects.
• **Ectopic pregnancy (pregnancy outside of the womb).** The chance of a pregnancy outside of the womb is increased in women with damaged fallopian tubes.
• **Miscarriage.** The chance of loss of an early pregnancy may be increased in women who have difficulty with becoming pregnant at all.

The most common side effects of Follistim AQ include:
In women:
• cyst in the ovary
• stomach pain
In men:
• headache
• pain at the injection site
• bruising, swelling or redness at the injection site
• breast enlargement
• acne

These are not all the possible side effects of Follistim AQ. For more information, ask your healthcare provider or pharmacist.

Call your healthcare provider immediately if you get worsening or strong abdominal pain. Also, call your healthcare provider immediately if this happens some days after the last injection has been given. Tell your healthcare provider if you have any side effect that bothers you or that does not go away.

Call your doctor for medical advice about side effects. You may report side effects to FDA at 1-800-FDA-1088.

How should I store Follistim AQ?
• Store Follistim AQ in the refrigerator between 2° - 8°C (36° - 46°F) until the expiration date.
• Follistim AQ can be stored at or below 25°C (77°F) for 3 months or until the expiration date, whichever comes first.
• Keep Follistim AQ away from light.
• Do not freeze.

Keep Follistim AQ and all medicines out of the reach of children.

General information about Follistim AQ
Medicines are sometimes prescribed for purposes other than those listed in the Patient Information leaflet. Do not use Follistim AQ for a condition for which it was not prescribed. Do not give Follistim AQ to other people, even if they have the same condition that you have. It may harm them.
This Patient Information leaflet summarizes the most important information about Follistim AQ. If you would like more information, talk with your healthcare provider. You can ask your pharmacist or healthcare provider for more information about Follistim AQ that is written for healthcare professionals.
For more information, go to **www.follistim.com** or call 1-866-836-5633.

What are the ingredients in Follistim AQ?

Active ingredient: follitropin beta

Inactive ingredients: sucrose, sodium citrate, L-methionine, polysorbate 20, water for injection, hydrochloric acid, and/or sodium hydroxide.

Manufactured for: Merck Sharp & Dohme Corp., a subsidiary of **MERCK & CO., INC.,** Whitehouse Station, NJ 08889, USA

Manufactured by: N.V. Organon, Oss, The Netherlands, a subsidiary of **Merck & Co., Inc.,** Whitehouse Station, NJ 08889, USA

For patent information: www.merck.com/product/patent/home.html

Copyright © 2005, 2010 Merck Sharp & Dohme B.V., a subsidiary of **Merck & Co., Inc.** All rights reserved.

Revised: 12/2013

usppi-mk8328-SOi-1312R006

PATIENT INSTRUCTIONS FOR USE

Follistim® (Fol´-lis-tim) AQ

(follitropin beta injection)

Single-Use Vial

Read the Patient Instructions for Use that comes with Follistim® AQ before you start using it and each time you get a refill. There may be new information. This information does not take the place of talking with your healthcare provider about your medical condition or treatment.

A. Getting Ready

• Remove the vial from the refrigerator.

• Check the liquid in the vial. It should appear clear and colorless. If the solution is not clear and colorless or has particles in it, **do not use it.**

• **Gather the supplies you will need for your injection. You will need:**

  ◦ a clean dry surface
  ◦ alcohol
  ◦ cotton balls or alcohol pads
  ◦ sterile gauze
  ◦ a puncture-proof container to throw away the used syringe and needle

• Wash your hands and dry them.

B. Preparing your Follistim AQ Injection

• Flip off the protective cap on the top of the vial. **Do not** remove the rubber stopper. Wipe the top of the rubber stopper with an alcohol wipe.

• Use a syringe and needle that has been recommended by your healthcare provider, attach a needle to the syringe.

C. Draw up your Dose

• Carefully remove the needle cover (cap) from the needle (See Figure 1).

Figure 1

• Pull back on the plunger to draw the amount of air into the syringe equal to the dose needed.

• With the vial on a flat work surface, insert the needle straight down through the rubber stopper of the Follistim AQ vial.

• Push the plunger of the syringe down to inject the air from the syringe into the vial of Follistim AQ. The air injected into the vial will allow Follistim AQ to be easily withdrawn into the syringe.

• Keep the needle inside the vial. Turn the vial and syringe upside down. Be sure that the tip of the Follistim AQ needle is in the liquid. Slowly pull back on the plunger to fill the syringe with Follistim AQ liquid to the number (mL or cc) that matches the dose your healthcare provider prescribed (See Figure 2).

Figure 2

D. Remove the Air

• Hold the syringe with the needle pointed up. Check for air bubbles in the syringe. A small amount of air will not hurt you. If you see large air bubbles, gently tap the side of the syringe with your finger until the air bubbles rise to the top of the syringe.

• Slowly push the plunger to force the air bubbles out of the syringe. You will see a drop of liquid on the tip of the needle (See Figure 3).

Figure 3

• Double-check that you have the right dose in the syringe. Lay the syringe down on its side until you have selected and prepared your injection site.

E. Selecting and Preparing the Injection Site

• Follistim AQ can be injected into your body using two different ways (routes) as described below. Follow your healthcare provider's instructions about how you should inject Follistim AQ.

1. Subcutaneous Route:

For women and men:

• Follistim AQ can be injected directly into a layer of fat under your skin (subcutaneously).

• When giving a subcutaneous injection, follow your healthcare provider's instructions about changing the site for each injection. This will help lower your chances of having a skin reaction.

• **Do not** inject Follistim AQ into an area that is tender, red, bruised, or hard.

• Recommended sites for injecting Follistim AQ subcutaneously are:

  ◦ Just below your belly button (navel) (See Figure 4)
  ◦ The upper outer area of your thigh (See Figure 4)

Belly Button (navel)   Upper Outer area of the thigh

Figure 4

• Clean the skin with an alcohol wipe where the injection is to be made. Be careful not to touch the skin that has been wiped clean.

• Pick up the prepared syringe and needle and hold it in the hand that you will use to inject the medicine.

• Use the other hand to pinch a fold of skin at the cleaned injection site. **Do not** touch the cleaned area of skin.

• Hold the syringe like you would a pencil. Use a quick "dart-like" motion to insert the needle either straight up and down (90-degree angle) or at a slight angle (45-degree angle) (See Figure 5).

Figure 5

• Let go of the syringe and slowly pull back on the plunger. If blood comes into the syringe, **Do not** inject Follistim AQ because the needle might have entered a blood vessel.

• If no blood is seen and the needle is properly placed, push the plunger slowly and steadily to inject the Follistim AQ solution.

• Once you have injected the entire content of the syringe, pull the needle out of your skin and press a cotton ball or gauze over the injection site and hold it there for several seconds (See Figure 6).

• Gently massage the site while still maintaining pressure. This will help disperse the Follistim AQ solution and may relieve any discomfort.

• **Do not** put the needle cover (cap) back on the needle.

[See figure 6 at top of next column]

• Throw away the used needle and syringe in your puncture-proof container. (See "How Do I Throw Away Used Syringes and Needles?")

• For each injection, prepare a new syringe of Follistim AQ using the instructions above. Clean a new area of skin. In this new area of clean skin, again insert a new needle (as

Figure 6

you did before), and again pull the plunger back slightly. If blood does not enter the syringe, inject the Follistim AQ by slowly pushing the plunger all the way down.

• Pull the needle out of your skin and press a cotton ball or gauze over the injection site and hold it there for several seconds. Do not put the needle cover (cap) back on the needle.

• Throw away the used needle and syringe in your puncture-proof container. (See "How Do I Throw Away Used Syringes and Needles?")

2. Intramuscular Route:

For women only:

◦ You will need to ask another person to give you your Follistim AQ injection intramuscularly (IM).

• Follistim AQ can be injected directly into your muscle (intramuscularly).

• When giving an intramuscular injection, follow your healthcare provider's instructions about changing the site for each injection. This will help lower your chances of having a skin reaction.

• **Do not** inject Follistim AQ into an area that is tender, red, bruised, or hard.

• Recommended site for injecting Follistim AQ intramuscularly is:

  ◦ The upper outer area of the buttock (See Figure 7).

Figure 7

• Relax the muscle first by shifting your weight to the leg opposite of the side that the medicine will be injected into.

• Clean the skin with an alcohol wipe where the injection is to be made. Be careful not to touch the skin that has been wiped clean.

Instructions for giving an IM injection to the patient:

• Pick up the prepared syringe and needle and hold it in the hand that you will use to inject the medicine.

• Use the other hand to stretch a fold of skin at the cleaned injection site. Stretching the skin helps the needle to go in more easily and pushes the tissue beneath the skin out of the way. **Do not** touch the cleaned area of skin (See Figure 8).

• Hold the syringe like you would a pencil. Use a quick "dart-like" motion to insert the needle straight up and down (90-degree angle) (See Figure 8).

Figure 8

• Let go of the syringe and slowly pull back on the plunger. If blood comes into the syringe, **Do not** inject Follistim AQ because the needle might have entered a blood vessel.

• Pull the needle out of your skin and press a cotton ball or gauze over the injection site and hold it there for several seconds (See Figure 6).

• Gently massage the site while still maintaining pressure. This will help disperse the Follistim AQ solution and may relieve any discomfort.

• **Do not** put the needle cover (cap) back on the needle.

• Throw away the used needle and syringe in your puncture-proof container. (See "How Do I Throw Away Used Syringes and Needles?")

• For each injection, prepare a new syringe of Follistim AQ using the instructions above. Clean a new area of skin. In this new area of clean skin, again insert a new needle (as

you did before), and again pull the plunger back slightly. If blood does not enter the syringe, inject the Follistim AQ by slowly pushing the plunger all the way down.
- Pull the needle out of your skin and press a cotton ball or gauze over the injection site and hold it there for several seconds.
- **Do not** put the needle cover (cap) back on the needle.
- Throw away the used needle and syringe in your puncture-proof container. (See "How Do I Throw Away Used Syringes and Needles?")

How Do I Throw Away Used Syringes and Needles?
Check with your healthcare provider or pharmacist for instructions about the right way to throw away used syringes and needles. There may be special local or state laws about how to throw away used syringes and needles.
- **Do not** throw away used syringes and needles in the household trash and do not recycle them.
- Put used and empty Follistim AQ syringes, needles, and vials in a closeable, puncture-resistant container. You may use a sharps container (such as a red bio-hazard container), a hard plastic container with a screw-on cap (such as an empty detergent bottle) or in a metal container with a plastic lid, (such as a coffee can).
- When the container is full, tape around the cap or lid to make sure the cap or lid does not come off.
- When your injection is given by another person, this person must also be careful when removing the syringe and needle and disposing of the syringe and needle to prevent accidental needle stick injury and passing infection.

How should I store Follistim AQ?
- Store Follistim AQ in the refrigerator at 2° - 8°C (36° - 46°F) until the expiration date.
- Follistim AQ can be stored at or below 25°C (77°F) for 3 months or until the expiration date, whichever comes first.
- Keep Follistim AQ away from light.
- Do not freeze.
Keep Follistim AQ, syringes, needles, and the disposal container out of the reach of children.
Manufactured for: Merck Sharp & Dohme Corp., a subsidiary of
MERCK & CO., INC., Whitehouse Station, NJ 08889, USA
Manufactured by: N.V. Organon, Oss, The Netherlands, a subsidiary of
Merck & Co., Inc., Whitehouse Station, NJ 08889, USA
For patent information: www.merck.com/product/patent/home.html
Copyright © 2005, 2010 Merck Sharp & Dohme B.V., a subsidiary of **Merck & Co., Inc.** All rights reserved.
Revised: 12/2013
usppi-mk8328-SOi-1312R006

FORADIL® AEROLIZER®   ℞
[fōr-ă-dĭl]
(formoterol fumarate inhalation powder)
FOR ORAL INHALATION ONLY

HIGHLIGHTS OF PRESCRIBING INFORMATION
These highlights do not include all the information needed to use FORADIL® AEROLIZER® safely and effectively. See full prescribing information for FORADIL AEROLIZER.
FORADIL AEROLIZER (formoterol fumarate inhalation powder)
FOR ORAL INHALATION ONLY
Initial U.S. Approval: 2001

> **WARNING: ASTHMA-RELATED DEATH**
> *See full prescribing information for complete boxed warning*
> - Long-acting beta₂-adrenergic agonists (LABA), such as formoterol the active ingredient in FORADIL, increase the risk of asthma-related death. A large placebo-controlled study with another LABA (salmeterol) showed an increase in asthma-related deaths in patients receiving salmeterol. This finding with salmeterol is considered a class effect of LABA, including formoterol. (5.1)
> - Prescribe FORADIL AEROLIZER only as additional therapy for patients with asthma who are currently taking but are inadequately controlled on a long-term asthma control medication, such as an inhaled corticosteroid. Once asthma control is achieved and maintained, assess the patient at regular intervals and step down therapy (e.g., discontinue FORADIL AEROLIZER) if possible without loss of asthma control and maintain the patient on a long-term asthma control medication, such as an inhaled corticosteroid. Do not use FORADIL AEROLIZER for patients whose asthma is adequately controlled on low- or medium-dose inhaled corticosteroids. (1.1, 5.1).

- Available data from controlled clinical trials suggest that LABA increase the risk of asthma-related hospitalization in pediatric and adolescent patients. (5.1)

---RECENT MAJOR CHANGES---
Warnings and Precautions,
 Coexisting Conditions (5.8) 09/2012

---INDICATIONS AND USAGE---
FORADIL AEROLIZER is a LABA indicated for:
- Treatment of asthma in patients ≥5 years as an add-on to a long-term asthma control medication such as an inhaled corticosteroid. (1.1)
- Prevention of exercise-induced bronchospasm (EIB) in patients ≥5 years. (1.2)
- Maintenance treatment of bronchoconstriction in patients with chronic obstructive pulmonary disease (COPD). (1.3)
Important limitations of use:
- NOT indicated for the relief of acute bronchospasm. (1.1, 1.3)

---DOSAGE AND ADMINISTRATION---
For oral inhalation only. **DO NOT** swallow Foradil capsule. Foradil capsule should be **always** used with Aerolizer inhaler **ONLY**.
- Treatment of asthma in patients ≥5 years: Inhalation of one capsule every 12 hours in addition to concomitant treatment with a long-term control medication such as an inhaled corticosteroid. (2.1)
- EIB: Inhalation of one capsule at least 15 minutes before exercise Additional doses should not be used for 12 hours. (2.2)
- Maintenance treatment of bronchoconstriction in patients with COPD: Inhalation of one capsule every 12 hours. (2.3)

---DOSAGE FORMS AND STRENGTHS---
Foradil capsules for oral inhalation: 12 mcg formoterol fumarate powder, for use with Aerolizer inhaler. (3)

---CONTRAINDICATIONS---
- Asthma: Without concomitant use of a long-term asthma control medication such as an inhaled corticosteroid. (4)
- Hypersensitivity to formoterol fumarate or any components of this product. (4)

---WARNINGS AND PRECAUTIONS---
- Asthma-related deaths and asthma-related hospitalizations: LABA increase the risk. Prescribe for asthma only as concomitant therapy with a long-term control medication such as an inhaled corticosteroid. (5.1)
- Deterioration of asthma and acute episodes: Do not initiate during acutely deteriorating asthma. Do not use to treat acute symptoms. (5.2)
- Corticosteroids: Not a substitute for corticosteroids. Corticosteroids should not be stopped or reduced when FORADIL AEROLIZER is initiated. (5.3)
- Use with additional long-acting beta₂-agonist: Do not use in combination because of risk of overdose. (5.4)
- Paradoxical bronchospasm: Discontinue FORADIL AEROLIZER and institute alternative therapy if paradoxical bronchospasm occurs. (5.5)
- Patients with cardiovascular or central nervous system disorders: Use with caution because of beta-adrenergic stimulation. (5.6)
- Coexisting conditions: Use with caution in patients with convulsive disorders, thyrotoxicosis, diabetes mellitus, ketoacidosis, aneurysm, and pheochromocytoma. (5.8)
- Metabolic effects: Be alert to hypokalemia and hyperglycemia. (5.9)

---ADVERSE REACTIONS---
Most common adverse reactions (incidence ≥1% and more common than placebo) are:
- Asthma: viral infection, bronchitis, chest infection, dyspnea, chest pain, tremor, dizziness, insomnia, tonsillitis, rash, dysphonia, and serious asthma exacerbation. (6.1, 6.3)
- COPD: Upper respiratory tract infection, back pain, pharyngitis, chest pain, sinusitis, fever, leg cramps, muscle cramps, anxiety, pruritus, increased sputum, and dry mouth. (6.2)
To report SUSPECTED ADVERSE REACTIONS, contact Merck Sharp & Dohme Corporation, a subsidiary of Merck & Co., Inc. at 1-877-888-4231 or FDA at 1-800-FDA-1088 or www.fda.gov/medwatch.

---DRUG INTERACTIONS---
- Adrenergic agents: Use with caution. Additional adrenergic drugs may potentiate sympathetic effects. (7.1)
- Xanthine derivatives, systemic corticosteroids, and non-potassium sparing diuretics: Use with caution. May potentiate hypokalemia or ECG changes. (7.2, 7.3)

- MAO inhibitors, tricyclic antidepressants, macrolides, and drugs that prolong QTc interval: Use with extreme caution. May potentiate effect on cardiovascular system. (7.4)
- Beta-blockers: Use with caution and only when medically necessary. May decrease effectiveness and produce severe bronchospasm. (7.5)
- Halogenated hydrocarbons: There is an elevated risk of arrhythmias in patients receiving concomitant anesthesia with halogenated hydrocarbons. (7.6)

See 17 for PATIENT COUNSELING INFORMATION and Medication Guide

Revised: 11/2012

FULL PRESCRIBING INFORMATION: CONTENTS*
WARNING: ASTHMA-RELATED DEATH

FULL PRESCRIBING INFORMATION

> **WARNING: ASTHMA-RELATED DEATH**
> Long-acting beta₂-adrenergic agonists (LABA), such as formoterol the active ingredient in FORADIL

AEROLIZER, increase the risk of asthma-related death. Data from a large placebo controlled US study that compared the safety of another LABA (salmeterol) or placebo added to usual asthma therapy showed an increase in asthma-related deaths in patients receiving salmeterol. This finding with salmeterol is considered a class effect of LABA, including formoterol [see *Warnings and Precautions (5.1)*]. Currently available data are inadequate to determine whether concurrent use of inhaled corticosteroids or other long-term asthma control drugs mitigates the increased risk of asthma-related death from LABA.

Because of this risk, use of FORADIL AEROLIZER for the treatment of asthma without a concomitant long-term asthma control medication, such as an inhaled corticosteroid, is contraindicated. Use FORADIL AEROLIZER only as additional therapy for patients with asthma who are currently taking but are inadequately controlled on the long-term asthma control medication, such as an inhaled corticosteroid. Once asthma control is achieved and maintained, assess the patient at regular intervals and step down therapy (e.g., discontinue FORADIL AEROLIZER) if possible without loss of asthma control, and maintain the patient on a long-term asthma control medication, such as an inhaled corticosteroid. Do not use FORADIL AEROLIZER for patients whose asthma is adequately controlled on low or medium dose inhaled corticosteroids.

Pediatric and Adolescent Patients

Available data from controlled clinical trials suggest that LABA increase the risk of asthma-related hospitalization in pediatric and adolescent patients. For pediatric and adolescent patients with asthma who require addition of a LABA to an inhaled corticosteroid, a fixed-dose combination product containing both an inhaled corticosteroid and LABA should ordinarily be considered to ensure adherence with both drugs. In cases where use of a separate long-term asthma control medication (e.g., inhaled corticosteroid) and LABA is clinically indicated, appropriate steps must be taken to ensure adherence with both treatment components. If adherence cannot be assured, a fixed-dose combination product containing both an inhaled corticosteroid and LABA is recommended.

1 INDICATIONS AND USAGE
1.1 Treatment of Asthma
FORADIL AEROLIZER is indicated for the treatment of asthma and in the prevention of bronchospasm only as concomitant therapy with a long-term asthma control medication, such as an inhaled corticosteroid, in adults and children 5 years of age and older with reversible obstructive airways disease, including patients with symptoms of nocturnal asthma.

Long acting beta$_2$-adrenergic agonists (LABA), such as formoterol, the active ingredient in FORADIL AEROLIZER, increase the risk of asthma-related death. Use of FORADIL AEROLIZER for the treatment of asthma without concomitant use of a long-term asthma control medication, such as an inhaled corticosteroid, is contraindicated. Use FORADIL AEROLIZER only as additional therapy for patients with asthma who are currently taking but are inadequately controlled on a long-term asthma control medication, such as an inhaled corticosteroid. Once asthma control is achieved and maintained, assess the patient at regular intervals and step down therapy (e.g., discontinue FORADIL AEROLIZER) if possible without loss of asthma control, and maintain the patient on a long-term asthma control medication, such as an inhaled corticosteroid. Do not use FORADIL AEROLIZER for patients whose asthma is adequately controlled on low or medium dose inhaled corticosteroids [see *Contraindications (4) and Warnings and Precautions (5.1)*].

Pediatric and Adolescent Patients

Available data from controlled clinical trials suggest that LABA increase the risk of asthma-related hospitalization in pediatric and adolescent patients. For pediatric and adolescent patients with asthma who require addition of a LABA to an inhaled corticosteroid, a fixed-dose combination product containing both an inhaled corticosteroid and LABA should ordinarily be used to ensure adherence with both drugs. In cases where use of a separate long-term asthma control medication (e.g., inhaled corticosteroid) and LABA is clinically indicated, appropriate steps must be taken to ensure adherence with both treatment components. If adherence cannot be assured, a fixed-dose combination product containing both an inhaled corticosteroid and LABA is recommended [see *Warnings and Precautions (5.1)*].

Important Limitation of Use

FORADIL AEROLIZER is NOT indicated for the relief of acute bronchospasm.

1.2 Prevention of Exercise-Induced Bronchospasm
FORADIL AEROLIZER is also indicated for the acute prevention of exercise-induced bronchospasm in adults and children 5 years of age and older, when administered on an occasional, as-needed basis. Use of FORADIL AEROLIZER as a single agent for the prevention of exercise-induced bronchospasm may be clinically indicated in patients who do not have persistent asthma. In patients with persistent asthma, use of FORADIL AEROLIZER for the prevention of exercise-induced bronchospasm may be clinically indicated, but the treatment of asthma should include a long-term asthma control medication, such as an inhaled corticosteroid.

1.3 Maintenance Treatment of Chronic Obstructive Pulmonary Disease
FORADIL AEROLIZER is indicated for the long-term, twice daily (morning and evening) administration in the maintenance treatment of bronchoconstriction in patients with Chronic Obstructive Pulmonary Disease including chronic bronchitis and emphysema.

Important Limitation of Use

FORADIL AEROLIZER is NOT indicated for the relief of acute bronchospasm.

2 DOSAGE AND ADMINISTRATION
FORADIL capsules should be administered only by the oral inhalation route and only using the AEROLIZER Inhaler (see the accompanying Medication Guide). **FORADIL capsules should not be swallowed.** FORADIL capsules should always be stored in the blister, and only removed IMMEDIATELY BEFORE USE.

2.1 Asthma
Long-acting beta$_2$-adrenergic agonists (LABA), such as formoterol, the active ingredient in FORADIL AEROLIZER, increase the risk of asthma-related death [see *Warnings and Precautions (5.1)*]. Because of this risk, use of FORADIL AEROLIZER for the treatment of asthma without concomitant use of a long-term asthma control medication, such as an inhaled corticosteroid, is contraindicated. Use FORADIL AEROLIZER only as additional therapy for patients with asthma who are currently taking but are inadequately controlled on a long-term asthma control medication, such as an inhaled corticosteroid. Once asthma control is achieved and maintained, assess the patient at regular intervals and step down therapy (e.g., discontinue FORADIL AEROLIZER) if possible without loss of asthma control, and maintain the patient on a long-term asthma control medication, such as an inhaled corticosteroid. Do not use FORADIL AEROLIZER for patients whose asthma is adequately controlled on low or medium dose inhaled corticosteroids.

Pediatric and Adolescent Patients

For adults and children 5 years of age and older, the usual dosage is the inhalation of the contents of one 12-mcg FORADIL capsule every 12 hours using the AEROLIZER Inhaler. The patient must not exhale into the device. The total daily dose of FORADIL should not exceed one capsule twice daily (24 mcg total daily dose). More frequent administration or administration of a larger number of inhalations is not recommended. If symptoms arise between doses, an inhaled short-acting beta2-agonist should be taken for immediate relief.

Available data from controlled clinical trials suggest that LABA increase the risk of asthma-related hospitalization in pediatric and adolescent patients. For patients with asthma less than 18 years of age who require addition of a LABA to an inhaled corticosteroid, a fixed-dose combination product containing both an inhaled corticosteroid and LABA should ordinarily be used to ensure adherence with both drugs. In cases where use of a separate long-term asthma control medication (e.g., inhaled corticosteroid) and LABA is clinically indicated, appropriate steps must be taken to ensure adherence with both treatment components. If adherence cannot be assured, a fixed-dose combination product containing both an inhaled corticosteroid and LABA is recommended.

2.2 Exercise-Induced Bronchospasm (EIB)
Use of FORADIL AEROLIZER as a single agent for the prevention of exercise induced bronchospasm may be clinically indicated in patients who do not have persistent asthma. In patients with persistent asthma, use of FORADIL AEROLIZER for the prevention of exercise induced bronchospasm may be clinically indicated, but the treatment of asthma should include a long-term asthma control medication, such as an inhaled corticosteroid. For adults and children 5 years of age or older, the usual dosage is the inhalation of the contents of one 12-mcg FORADIL capsule at least 15 minutes before exercise administered on an occasional as needed basis. When used intermittently as needed for prevention, protection may last up to 12 hours. Additional doses of FORADIL AEROLIZER should not be used for 12 hours after the administration of this drug. Regular, twice-daily dosing has not been studied in preventing EIB. Patients who are receiving FORADIL AEROLIZER

twice daily for treatment of their asthma should not use additional doses for prevention of EIB and may require a short-acting bronchodilator.

2.3 Chronic Obstructive Pulmonary Disease (COPD)
For maintenance treatment of bronchoconstriction in patients with COPD (including chronic bronchitis and emphysema) the usual dosage is the inhalation of the contents of one 12 mcg FORADIL capsule every 12 hours using the AEROLIZER inhaler.

A total daily dose of greater than 24 mcg is not recommended.

3 DOSAGE FORMS AND STRENGTHS
FORADIL AEROLIZER consists of FORADIL capsules and an AEROLIZER inhaler. FORADIL capsules contain 12 mcg dry powder formulation of formoterol fumarate in a clear, hard gelatin capsule for inhalation use with the AEROLIZER inhaler only.

4 CONTRAINDICATIONS
- Because of the risk of asthma-related death and hospitalization, use of FORADIL AEROLIZER for the treatment of asthma without concomitant use of a long-term asthma control medication, such as an inhaled corticosteroid, is contraindicated [see *Warnings and Precautions (5.1)*].
- FORADIL AEROLIZER is contraindicated as primary treatment of status asthmaticus or other acute episodes of asthma or COPD where intensive measures are required [see *Warnings and Precautions (5.2)*].
- FORADIL (formoterol fumarate) is contraindicated in patients with a history of hypersensitivity to formoterol fumarate or to any components of this product [see *Warnings and Precautions (5.7)*].

5 WARNINGS AND PRECAUTIONS
5.1 Asthma-Related Death
Long-acting beta$_2$-adrenergic agonists, such as formoterol, the active ingredient in FORADIL AEROLIZER, increase the risk of asthma-related death. Currently available data are inadequate to determine whether concurrent use of inhaled corticosteroids or other long-term asthma control drugs mitigates the increased risk of asthma-related death from LABA.

Because of this risk, use of FORADIL AEROLIZER for the treatment of asthma without concomitant use of a long-term asthma control medication, such as an inhaled corticosteroid, is contraindicated. Once asthma control is achieved and maintained, assess the patient at regular intervals and step down therapy (e.g., discontinue FORADIL AEROLIZER) if possible without loss of asthma control, and maintain the patient on a long-term asthma control medication, such as an inhaled corticosteroid. Do not use FORADIL AEROLIZER for patients whose asthma is adequately controlled on low or medium dose inhaled corticosteroids.

Pediatric and Adolescent Patients

Available data from controlled clinical trials suggest that LABA increase the risk of asthma-related hospitalization in pediatric and adolescent patients. For pediatric and adolescent patients with asthma who require addition of a LABA to an inhaled corticosteroid, a fixed-dose combination product containing both an inhaled corticosteroid and LABA should ordinarily be considered to ensure adherence with both drugs. In cases where use of a separate long-term asthma control medication (e.g., inhaled corticosteroid) and LABA is clinically indicated, appropriate steps must be taken to ensure adherence with both treatment components. If adherence cannot be assured, a fixed-dose combination product containing both an inhaled corticosteroid and LABA is recommended.

A 28-week, placebo-controlled US study comparing the safety of salmeterol with placebo, each added to usual asthma therapy, showed an increase in asthma-related deaths in patients receiving salmeterol (13/13,176 in patients treated with salmeterol vs. 3/13,179 in patients treated with placebo; RR 4.37, 95% CI 1.25, 15.34). The increased risk of asthma-related death is considered a class effect of the long-acting beta2-adrenergic agonists, including formoterol. No study adequate to determine whether the rate of asthma-related death is increased with FORADIL AEROLIZER has been conducted.

Clinical studies with FORADIL AEROLIZER suggested a higher incidence of serious asthma exacerbations in patients who received FORADIL AEROLIZER than in those who received placebo [see *Adverse Reactions (6.2, 6.3)*]. The sizes of these studies were not adequate to precisely quantify the differences in serious asthma exacerbation rates between treatment groups.

The studies described above enrolled patients with asthma. No studies have been conducted that were adequate to determine whether the rate of death in patients with COPD is increased by long-acting beta$_2$-adrenergic agonists.

5.2 Deterioration of Disease and Acute Episodes
FORADIL AEROLIZER should not be initiated in patients with significantly worsening, acutely deteriorating, or po-

Number and Frequency of Serious Asthma Exacerbations in Patients 12 Years of Age and Older from Two 12-Week Controlled Clinical Trials

	Foradil 12 mcg twice daily	Foradil 24 mcg twice daily	Albuterol 180 mcg four times daily	Placebo
Trial #1 Serious asthma exacerbations	0/136 (0)	4/135 (3.0%)[1]	2/134 (1.5%)	0/136 (0)
Trial #2 Serious asthma exacerbations	1/139 (0.7%)	5/136 (3.7%)[2]	0/138 (0)	2/141 (1.4%)

[1] patient required intubation
[2] patients had respiratory arrest; 1 of the patients died

tentially life-threatening episodes of asthma or COPD. The use of FORADIL AEROLIZER in this setting is not appropriate [see Indications and Usage (1.1, 1.3)].
Asthma may deteriorate acutely over a period of hours or chronically over several days or longer. It is important to watch for signs of worsening asthma, such as increasing use of inhaled, short-acting beta₂-adrenergic agonists or a significant decrease in peak expiratory flow (PEF) or lung function. Such findings require immediate evaluation. Patients should be advised to seek immediate attention should their condition deteriorate. Increasing the daily dosage of FORADIL AEROLIZER beyond the recommended dose in this situation is not appropriate. FORADIL AEROLIZER should not be used more frequently than twice daily (morning and evening) at the recommended dose.
FORADIL AEROLIZER should not be used to treat acute symptoms. FORADIL AEROLIZER has not been studied in the relief of acute symptoms and extra doses should not be used for that purpose. When prescribing FORADIL AEROLIZER, the physician should also provide the patient with an inhaled, short-acting beta₂-agonist for treatment of symptoms that occur acutely, despite regular twice-daily (morning and evening) use of FORADIL AEROLIZER. Patients should also be cautioned that increasing inhaled beta₂-agonist use is a signal of deteriorating asthma [see Information for Patients (17) and the accompanying Medication Guide.]
When beginning treatment with FORADIL AEROLIZER, patients who have been taking inhaled, short-acting beta₂-agonists on a regular basis (e.g., four times a day) should be instructed to discontinue the regular use of these drugs and use them only for symptomatic relief of acute symptoms.

5.3 FORADIL AEROLIZER is not a substitute for corticosteroids
There are no data demonstrating that FORADIL has any clinical anti-inflammatory effect and therefore it cannot be expected to take the place of corticosteroids. Corticosteroids should not be stopped or reduced at the time FORADIL AEROLIZER is initiated. Patients who already require oral or inhaled corticosteroids for treatment of asthma should be continued on this type of treatment even if they feel better as a result of initiating FORADIL AEROLIZER. Any change in corticosteroid dosage, in particular a reduction, should be made ONLY after clinical evaluation [see Patient Counseling Information (17.2)].

5.4 Excessive Use and Use with Other Long-Acting Beta₂-Agonists
FORADIL AEROLIZER should not be used more often or at doses higher than recommended, or in conjunction with other medications containing LABA, as an overdose may result. Patients using FORADIL AEROLIZER should not use an additional LABA (e.g., salmeterol xinafoate, arformoterol tartrate) for any reason. Fatalities have been reported in association with excessive use of inhaled sympathomimetic drugs in patients with asthma. The exact cause of death is unknown, but cardiac arrest following an unexpected development of a severe acute asthmatic crisis and subsequent hypoxia is suspected. In addition, data from clinical trials with FORADIL AEROLIZER suggest that the use of doses higher than recommended is associated with an increased risk of serious asthma exacerbations [see Adverse Reactions (6.2, 6.3)].

5.5 Paradoxical Bronchospasm
As with other inhaled beta₂-agonists, formoterol can produce paradoxical bronchospasm that may be life-threatening. If paradoxical bronchospasm occurs, FORADIL AEROLIZER should be discontinued immediately and alternative therapy instituted.

5.6 Cardiovascular and Central Nervous System Effects
Excessive beta-adrenergic stimulation has been associated with seizures, angina, hypertension or hypotension, tachycardia with rates up to 200 beats/min, arrhythmias, nervousness, headache, tremor, palpitation, nausea, dizziness, fatigue, malaise, and insomnia. Fatalities have been reported in association with excessive use of inhaled sympathomimetic drugs [see Overdosage (10)].

Formoterol fumarate, like other beta₂-agonists, can produce a clinically significant cardiovascular effect in some patients as measured by increases in pulse rate, blood pressure, and/or symptoms. Although such effects are uncommon after administration of FORADIL AEROLIZER at recommended doses, if they occur, the drug may need to be discontinued. In addition, beta-agonists have been reported to produce ECG changes, such as flattening of the T wave, prolongation of the QTc interval, and ST segment depression. The clinical significance of these findings is unknown. Therefore, formoterol fumarate, like other sympathomimetic amines, should be used with caution in patients with cardiovascular disorders, especially coronary insufficiency, cardiac arrhythmias, and hypertension.

5.7 Immediate Hypersensitivity Reactions
Immediate hypersensitivity reactions may occur after administration of FORADIL AEROLIZER, as demonstrated by cases of anaphylactic reactions, urticaria, angioedema, rash, and bronchospasm.
FORADIL AEROLIZER contains lactose, which contains trace levels of milk proteins. Allergic reactions to products containing milk proteins may occur in patients with severe milk protein allergy.

5.8 Coexisting Conditions
Formoterol fumarate, like other sympathomimetic amines, should be used with caution in patients with cardiovascular disorders, especially coronary insufficiency, cardiac arrhythmias, hypertension, aneurysm, and pheochromocytoma; in patients with convulsive disorders or thyrotoxicosis; and in patients who are unusually responsive to sympathomimetic amines. Doses of the related beta2-agonist albuterol, when administered intravenously, have been reported to aggravate preexisting diabetes mellitus and ketoacidosis.

5.9 Hypokalemia and Hyperglycemia
Beta-agonist medications may produce significant hypokalemia in some patients, possibly through intracellular shunting, which has the potential to produce adverse cardiovascular effects. The decrease in serum potassium is usually transient, not requiring supplementation.
Clinically significant changes in blood glucose and/or serum potassium were infrequent during clinical studies with long-term administration of FORADIL AEROLIZER at the recommended dose.

5.10 Inappropriate Route of Administration
FORADIL capsules should ONLY be used with the AEROLIZER Inhaler and SHOULD NOT be swallowed. FORADIL capsules should always be stored in the blister, and only removed IMMEDIATELY before use.

6 ADVERSE REACTIONS
Long-acting beta₂-adrenergic agonists (LABA), including formoterol, the active ingredient in FORADIL AEROLIZER, increase the risk of asthma-related death and may increase the risk of asthma-related hospitalizations in pediatric and adolescent patients. Clinical trials with FORADIL AEROLIZER suggested a higher incidence of serious asthma exacerbations in patients who received FORADIL AEROLIZER than in those who received placebo [see Warnings and Precautions (5.1)].
Adverse reactions common to LABA drugs include: angina, hypertension or hypotension, tachycardia, arrhythmias, nervousness, headache, tremor, dry mouth, palpitation, muscle cramps, nausea, dizziness, fatigue, malaise, hypokalemia, hyperglycemia, metabolic acidosis, and insomnia.
Because clinical trials are conducted under widely varying conditions, adverse reaction rates observed in the clinical trials of a drug cannot be directly compared to rates in the clinical trials of another drug and may not reflect the rates observed in clinical trials.

6.1 Asthma
Of the 5824 patients in multiple-dose controlled clinical trials, 1985 were treated with FORADIL AEROLIZER at the recommended dose of 12 mcg twice daily. The following table shows treatment-emergent adverse reactions where the frequency was greater than or equal to 1% in the FORADIL

twice daily group and where the rates in the FORADIL group exceeded placebo. Three treatment-emergent adverse reactions showed dose ordering among tested doses of 6, 12, and 24 mcg administered twice daily; tremor, dizziness and dysphonia.

Number and Frequency of Treatment-Emergent Adverse Reactions in Patients 5 Years of Age and Older from Multiple-Dose Controlled Clinical Trials

Treatment-Emergent Adverse Reaction	Foradil Aerolizer 12 mcg twice daily		Placebo	
	n	(%)	n	(%)
Total Patients	1985	(100)	969	(100)
Infection viral	341	(17.2)	166	(17.1)
Bronchitis	92	(4.6)	42	(4.3)
Chest infection	54	(2.7)	4	(0.4)
Dyspnea	42	(2.1)	16	(1.7)
Chest pain	37	(1.9)	13	(1.3)
Tremor	37	(1.9)	4	(0.4)
Dizziness	31	(1.6)	15	(1.5)
Insomnia	29	(1.5)	8	(0.8)
Tonsilitis	23	(1.2)	7	(0.7)
Rash	22	(1.1)	7	(0.7)
Dysphonia	19	(1.0)	9	(0.9)

In patients 5-12 years of age, the numbers and percent of patients who reported treatment-emergent adverse reactions were comparable in the 12 mcg twice daily and placebo groups. In general, the pattern of the treatment-emergent adverse reactions observed in children differed from the usual pattern seen in adults. Treatment-emergent adverse reactions that were more frequent in the formoterol group than in the placebo group reflected infection/inflammation (viral infection, rhinitis, tonsillitis, gastroenteritis) or abdominal complaints (abdominal pain, nausea, dyspepsia).

Serious Asthma Exacerbations in Adolescents and Adults 12 Years of Age and Older
In two 12-week controlled trials with combined enrollment of 1095 patients 12 years of age and older, FORADIL AEROLIZER 12 mcg twice daily was compared to FORADIL AEROLIZER 24 mcg twice daily, albuterol 180 mcg four times daily, and placebo. Serious asthma exacerbations (acute worsening of asthma resulting in hospitalization) occurred more commonly with FORADIL AEROLIZER 24 mcg twice daily than with the recommended dose of FORADIL AEROLIZER 12 mcg twice daily, albuterol, or placebo. The results are shown in the following table.
[See table above]
In a 16-week, randomized, multi-center, double-blind, parallel-group trial, patients who received either 24 mcg twice daily or 12 mcg twice daily doses of FORADIL AEROLIZER experienced more serious asthma exacerbations than patients who received placebo [see Clinical Trials (14.1)]. The results are shown in the following table.

Number and Frequency of Serious Asthma Exacerbations in Patients 12 Years of Age and Older from a 16-Week Trial

	Foradil 12 mcg twice daily	Foradil 24 mcg twice daily	Placebo
Serious asthma exacerbations	3/527 (0.6%)	2/527 (0.4%)	1/514 (0.2%)

Serious Asthma Exacerbations in Children 5-11 Years of Age
The safety of FORADIL AEROLIZER 12 mcg twice daily compared to FORADIL AEROLIZER 24 mcg twice daily and placebo was investigated in one large, multicenter, randomized, double-blind, 52-week clinical trial in 518 children with asthma (ages 5-12 years) in need of daily bronchodilators and anti-inflammatory treatment. More children who received FORADIL AEROLIZER 24 mcg twice daily than children who received FORADIL AEROLIZER 12 mcg twice daily or placebo experienced serious asthma exacerbations, as shown in the next table.

Number and Frequency of Serious Asthma Exacerbations in Patients 5-12 Years of Age from a 52-Week Trial

	Foradil 12 mcg twice daily	Foradil 24 mcg twice daily	Placebo
Serious asthma exacerbations	8/171 (4.7%)	11/171 (6.4%)	0/176 (0)

6.2 COPD
Of the 1634 patients in two pivotal multiple-dose Chronic Obstructive Pulmonary Disease (COPD) controlled trials, 405 were treated with FORADIL AEROLIZER 12 mcg twice

daily. Treatment-emergent adverse reactions reported were similar to those seen in asthmatic patients, but with a higher incidence of COPD-related events in both placebo and formoterol treated patients.

The following table shows treatment-emergent adverse reactions where the frequency was greater than or equal to 1% in the FORADIL AEROLIZER group and where the rates in the FORADIL AEROLIZER group exceeded placebo. The two clinical trials included doses of 12 mcg and 24 mcg, administered twice daily. Seven treatment-emergent adverse reactions showed dose ordering among tested doses of 12 and 24 mcg administered twice daily; pharyngitis, fever, muscle cramps, increased sputum, dysphonia, myalgia, and tremor.

Number and Frequency of Treatment-Emergent Adverse Reactions in Adult COPD Patients Treated in Multiple-Dose Controlled Clinical Trials

Treatment-Emergent Adverse Reaction	Foradil Aerolizer 12 mcg twice daily		Placebo	
Total Patients	n	(%)	n	(%)
	405	(100)	420	(100)
Upper respiratory tract infection	30	(7.4)	24	(5.7)
Pain back	17	(4.2)	17	(4.0)
Pharyngitis	14	(3.5)	10	(2.4)
Pain chest	13	(3.2)	9	(2.1)
Sinusitis	11	(2.7)	7	(1.7)
Fever	9	(2.2)	6	(1.4)
Cramps leg	7	(1.7)	2	(0.5)
Cramps muscle	7	(1.7)	0	
Anxiety	6	(1.5)	5	(1.2)
Pruritis	6	(1.5)	4	(1.0)
Sputum increased	6	(1.5)	5	(1.2)
Mouth dry	5	(1.2)	4	(1.0)

Overall, the frequency of all cardiovascular treatment-emergent adverse reactions in the two pivotal studies was 6.4% for FORADIL AEROLIZER 12 mcg twice daily, and 6.0% for placebo. There were no frequently-occurring specific cardiovascular treatment-emergent adverse reactions for FORADIL AEROLIZER (frequency greater than or equal to 1% and greater than placebo).

6.3   Postmarketing Experience
The following adverse reactions have been identified during post approval use of FORADIL. Because these reactions are reported voluntarily from a population of uncertain size, it is not always possible to reliably estimate their frequency or establish a causal relationship to drug exposure.

In extensive worldwide marketing experience with FORADIL, serious exacerbations of asthma, including some that have been fatal, have been reported. While most of these cases have been in patients with severe or acutely deteriorating asthma [see Warnings and Precautions (5.1, 5.2)], a few have occurred in patients with less severe asthma. It is not possible to determine from these individual case reports whether FORADIL AEROLIZER contributed to the events.

Immune system disorders: rare reports of anaphylactic reactions, including severe hypotension and angioedema
Metabolism and nutrition disorders: Hypokalemia, hyperglycemia
Respiratory, thoracic and mediastinal disorders: Cough
Skin and subcutaneous tissue disorders: Rash
Cardiac disorders: Angina pectoris, cardiac arrhythmias, e.g., atrial fibrillation, ventricular extrasystoles, tachyarrhythmia
Investigations: Electrocardiogram QT prolonged, blood pressure increased (including hypertension)

7   DRUG INTERACTIONS
7.1   Adrenergic Drugs
If additional adrenergic drugs are to be administered by any route, they should be used with caution because the pharmacologically predictable sympathetic effects of formoterol may be potentiated.

7.2   Xanthine Derivatives or Systemic Corticosteroids
Concomitant treatment with xanthine derivatives or systemic corticosteroids may potentiate any hypokalemic effect of adrenergic agonists.

7.3   Diuretics
The ECG changes or hypokalemia that may result from the administration of non-potassium sparing diuretics (such as loop or thiazide diuretics) can be acutely worsened by beta-agonists, especially when the recommended dose of the beta-agonist is exceeded. Although the clinical significance of these effects is not known, caution is advised in the coadministration of beta-agonist with non-potassium sparing diuretics.

7.4   Monoamine Oxidase Inhibitors and Tricyclic Antidepressants, QTc Prolonging Drugs
Formoterol, as with other beta₂-agonists, should be administered with extreme caution to patients being treated with monoamine oxidase inhibitors, tricyclic antidepressants, macrolides or drugs known to prolong the QTc interval because the action of adrenergic agonists on the cardiovascular system may be potentiated by these agents. Drugs that are known to prolong the QTc interval have an increased risk of ventricular arrhythmias.

7.5   Beta-blockers
Beta-adrenergic receptor antagonists (beta-blockers) and formoterol may inhibit the effect of each other when administered concurrently. Beta-blockers not only block the therapeutic effects of beta₂-agonists, such as formoterol, but may produce severe bronchospasm in asthmatic patients. Therefore, patients with asthma should not normally be treated with beta-blockers. However, under certain circumstances, e.g., as prophylaxis after myocardial infarction, there may be no acceptable alternatives to the use of beta-blockers in patients with asthma. In this setting, cardioselective beta-blockers could be considered, although they should be administered with caution.

7.6   Halogenated Hydrocarbons
There is an elevated risk of arrhythmias in patients receiving concomitant anesthesia with halogenated hydrocarbons.

8   USE IN SPECIFIC POPULATIONS
8.1   Pregnancy
Pregnancy Category C.
Teratogenic Effects: There are no adequate and well-controlled studies of FORADIL AEROLIZER in pregnant women. Animal reproduction studies of formoterol fumarate in rats and rabbits revealed evidence of teratogenicity as well as other developmental toxic effects. Because there are no adequate and well-controlled studies in pregnant women, FORADIL AEROLIZER should be used during pregnancy only if the potential benefit justifies the potential risk to the fetus.

Formoterol fumarate administered throughout organogenesis did not cause malformations in rats or rabbits following oral administration. When given to rats throughout organogenesis, oral doses equal to or greater than 80 times the maximum recommended human dose (MRHD) for adults (on a mcg/m² basis for maternal doses of 0.2 mg/kg and above) delayed ossification of the fetus and doses equal to or greater than 2400 times the MRHD for adults (on a mcg/m² basis for maternal doses of 6 mg/kg and above) decreased fetal weight. Formoterol fumarate has been shown to cause stillbirth and neonatal mortality at oral doses equal to or greater than 2400 times the MRHD for adults (on a mcg/m² basis for maternal doses of 6 mg/kg and above) in rats receiving the drug during the late stage of pregnancy. These effects, however, were not produced at a dose equal to 80 times the MRHD for adults (on a mcg/m² basis for a maternal dose of 0.2 mg/kg).

In another testing laboratory, formoterol fumarate was shown to be teratogenic in rats and rabbits. Umbilical hernia, a malformation, was observed in rat fetuses at oral doses equal to or greater than 1200 times the MRHD for adults (on a mcg/m² basis for maternal doses of 3 mg/kg/day and above). Brachygnathia, a skeletal malformation, was observed for rat fetuses at an oral dose equal to 6100 times the MRHD for adults (on a mcg/m² basis for a maternal dose of 15 mg/kg/day). In another study in rats, no teratogenic effects were seen at inhalation doses up to 500 times the MRHD for adults (on a mcg/m² basis for maternal doses up to 1.2 mg/kg/day). Subcapsular cysts on the liver were observed for rabbit fetuses at an oral dose equal to 49000 times the MRHD for adults (on a mcg/m² basis for a maternal dose of 60 mg/kg). No teratogenic effects were observed at oral doses up to 3000 times the MRHD for adults (on a mcg/m² basis for maternal doses up to 3.5 mg/kg).

8.2   Labor and Delivery
There are no adequate and well-controlled human studies that have investigated the effects of FORADIL AEROLIZER during labor and delivery.

Because beta-agonists may potentially interfere with uterine contractility, FORADIL AEROLIZER should be used during labor only if the potential benefit justifies the potential risk.

Formoterol fumarate has been shown to cause stillbirth and neonatal mortality at oral doses equal to or greater than 2400 times the MRHD for adults (on a mcg/m² basis for maternal doses of 6 mg/kg and above) in rats receiving the drug for several days at the end of pregnancy. These effects were not produced at a dose 80 times the MRHD for adults (on a mcg/m² basis for a maternal dose of 0.2 mg/kg).

8.3   Nursing Mothers
In reproductive studies in rats, formoterol was excreted in the milk. It is not known whether formoterol is excreted in human milk, but because many drugs are excreted in human milk, caution should be exercised if FORADIL AEROLIZER is administered to nursing women. There are no well-controlled human studies of the use of FORADIL AEROLIZER in nursing mothers.

8.4   Pediatric Use
Asthma
Available data from controlled clinical trials suggest that LABA increase the risk of asthma-related hospitalization in pediatric and adolescent patients. For pediatric and adolescent patients with asthma who require addition of a LABA to an inhaled corticosteroid, a fixed-dose combination product containing both an inhaled corticosteroid and LABA should ordinarily be used to ensure adherence with both drugs [see Indications and Usage (1.1) and Warnings and Precautions (5.1)].

A total of 776 children 5 years of age and older with asthma were studied in three multiple-dose controlled clinical trials. Of the 512 children who received formoterol, 508 were 5-12 years of age, and approximately one third were 5-8 years of age [see Adverse Reactions (6.2, 6.3)].
Exercise-Induced Bronchospasm
A total of 25 pediatric patients, 4-11 years of age, were studied in two well-controlled single-dose clinical trials.
The safety and effectiveness of FORADIL AEROLIZER in pediatric patients below 5 years of age has not been established [see Clinical Trials (14.3), and Adverse Reaction (6.2)].

8.5   Geriatric Use
Of the total number of patients who received FORADIL AEROLIZER in adolescent and adult chronic dosing asthma clinical trials, 318 were 65 years of age or older and 39 were 75 years of age and older. Of the 811 patients who received FORADIL AEROLIZER in two pivotal multiple-dose controlled clinical studies in patients with COPD, 395 (48.7%) were 65 years of age or older while 62 (7.6%) were 75 years of age or older. No overall differences in safety or effectiveness were observed between these subjects and younger subjects. A slightly higher frequency of chest infection was reported in the 39 asthma patients 75 years of age and older, although a causal relationship with FORADIL has not been established. Other reported clinical experience has not identified differences in responses between the elderly and younger adult patients, but greater sensitivity of some older individuals cannot be ruled out.

10   OVERDOSAGE
The expected signs and symptoms with overdosage of FORADIL AEROLIZER are those of excessive beta-adrenergic stimulation and/or occurrence or exaggeration of any of the signs and symptoms listed under ADVERSE REACTIONS, e.g., angina, hypertension or hypotension, tachycardia, with rates up to 200 beats/min., arrhythmias, nervousness, headache, tremor, seizures, muscle cramps, dry mouth, palpitation, nausea, dizziness, fatigue, malaise, hypokalemia, hyperglycemia, and insomnia. Metabolic acidosis may also occur. Cardiac arrest and even death may be associated with an overdose of FORADIL AEROLIZER.

Treatment of overdosage consists of discontinuation of FORADIL AEROLIZER together with institution of appropriate symptomatic and/or supportive therapy. The judicious use of a cardioselective beta-receptor blocker may be considered, bearing in mind that such medication can produce bronchospasm. There is insufficient evidence to determine if dialysis is beneficial for overdosage of FORADIL AEROLIZER. Cardiac monitoring is recommended in cases of overdosage.

11   DESCRIPTION
FORADIL AEROLIZER consists of a dry powder formulation of formoterol fumarate intended for oral inhalation only with the AEROLIZER Inhaler. The inhalation powder is packaged in clear hard gelatin capsules.

Each capsule contains a dry powder blend of 12 mcg of formoterol fumarate and 25 mg of lactose (which contains trace levels of milk proteins) as a carrier.

The active component of FORADIL is formoterol fumarate, a racemate. Formoterol fumarate is a selective beta₂-adrenergic agonist. Its chemical name is (±)-2-hydroxy-5-[(1RS)-1-hydroxy-2-[[(1RS)-2-(4-methoxyphenyl)-1-methylethyl]-amino]ethyl]formanilide fumarate dihydrate; its structural formula is:

Formoterol fumarate has a molecular weight of 840.9, and its empirical formula is $(C_{19}H_{24}N_2O_4)_2 \cdot C_4H_4O_4 \cdot 2H_2O$. Formoterol fumarate is a white to yellowish crystalline powder, which is freely soluble in glacial acetic acid, soluble in methanol, sparingly soluble in ethanol and isopropanol, slightly soluble in water, and practically insoluble in acetone, ethyl acetate, and diethyl ether.

The AEROLIZER Inhaler is a plastic device used for inhaling FORADIL. The amount of drug delivered to the lung will depend on patient factors, such as inspiratory flow rate and inspiratory time. Under standardized *in vitro* testing at a fixed flow rate of 60 L/min for 2 seconds, the AEROLIZER Inhaler delivered 10 mcg of formoterol fumarate from the mouthpiece. Peak inspiratory flow rates (PIFR) achievable through the AEROLIZER Inhaler were evaluated in 33 adult and adolescent patients and 32 pediatric patients with mild-to-moderate asthma. Mean PIFR was 117.82 L/min (range 34-188 L/min) for adult and adolescent patients, and 99.66 L/min (range 43-187 L/min) for pediatric patients. Approximately ninety percent of each population studied generated a PIFR through the device exceeding 60 L/min.

To use the delivery system, a FORADIL capsule is placed in the well of the AEROLIZER Inhaler, and the capsule is pierced by pressing and releasing the buttons on the side of the device. The formoterol fumarate formulation is dispersed into the air stream when the patient inhales rapidly and deeply through the mouthpiece.

12 CLINICAL PHARMACOLOGY

12.1 Mechanism of Action

Formoterol fumarate is a long-acting beta$_2$-adrenergic receptor agonist (beta$_2$-agonist). Inhaled formoterol fumarate acts locally in the lung as a bronchodilator. *In vitro* studies have shown that formoterol has more than 200-fold greater agonist activity at beta$_2$-receptors than at beta$_1$-receptors. Although beta^2-receptors are the predominant adrenergic receptors in bronchial smooth muscle and beta$_1$-receptors are the predominant receptors in the heart, there are also beta$_2$-receptors in the human heart comprising 10%-50% of the total beta-adrenergic receptors. The precise function of these receptors has not been established, but they raise the possibility that even highly selective beta$_2$-agonists may have cardiac effects.

The pharmacologic effects of beta$_2$-adrenoceptor agonist drugs, including formoterol, are at least in part attributable to stimulation of intracellular adenyl cyclase, the enzyme that catalyzes the conversion of adenosine triphosphate (ATP) to cyclic-3', 5'-adenosine monophosphate (cyclic AMP). Increased cyclic AMP levels cause relaxation of bronchial smooth muscle and inhibition of release of mediators of immediate hypersensitivity from cells, especially from mast cells.

In vitro tests show that formoterol is an inhibitor of the release of mast cell mediators, such as histamine and leukotrienes, from the human lung. Formoterol also inhibits histamine-induced plasma albumin extravasation in anesthetized guinea pigs and inhibits allergen-induced eosinophil influx in dogs with airway hyper-responsiveness. The relevance of these *in vitro* and animal findings to humans is unknown.

12.2 Pharmacodynamics

Systemic Safety and Pharmacokinetic/Pharmacodynamic Relationships

The major adverse effects of inhaled beta$_2$-agonists occur as a result of excessive activation of the systemic beta-adrenergic receptors. The most common adverse effects in adults and adolescents include skeletal muscle tremor and cramps, insomnia, tachycardia, decreases in plasma potassium, and increases in plasma glucose.

Pharmacokinetic/pharmacodynamic (PK/PD) relationships between heart rate, ECG parameters, and serum potassium levels and the urinary excretion of formoterol were evaluated in 10 healthy male volunteers (25 to 45 years of age) following inhalation of single doses containing 12, 24, 48, or 96 mcg of formoterol fumarate. There was a linear relationship between urinary formoterol excretion and decreases in serum potassium, increases in plasma glucose, and increases in heart rate.

In a second study, PK/PD relationships between plasma formoterol levels and pulse rate, ECG parameters, and plasma potassium levels were evaluated in 12 healthy volunteers following inhalation of a single 120 mcg dose of formoterol fumarate (10 times the recommended clinical dose). Reductions of plasma potassium concentration were observed in all subjects. Maximum reductions from baseline ranged from 0.55 to 1.52 mmol/L with a median maximum reduction of 1.01 mmol/L. The formoterol plasma concentration was highly correlated with the reduction in plasma potassium concentration. Generally, the maximum effect on plasma potassium was noted 1 to 3 hours after peak formoterol plasma concentrations were achieved. A mean maximum increase of pulse rate of 26 bpm was observed 6 hours post dose. The maximum increase of mean corrected QT interval (QTc) was 25 msec when calculated using Bazett's correction and was 8 msec when calculated using Fridericia's correction. The QTc returned to baseline within 12-24 hours post-dose. Formoterol plasma concentrations were weakly correlated with pulse rate and increase of QTc duration. The effects on plasma potassium, pulse rate, and QTc interval are known pharmacological effects of this class of study drug and were not unexpected at the very high formoterol dose (120 mcg single dose, 10 times the recommended single dose) tested in this study. These effects were well-tolerated by the healthy volunteers.

The electrocardiographic and cardiovascular effects of FORADIL AEROLIZER were compared with those of albuterol and placebo in two pivotal 12-week double-blind studies of patients with asthma. A subset of patients underwent continuous electrocardiographic monitoring during three 24-hour periods. No important differences in ventricular or supraventricular ectopy between treatment groups were observed. In these two studies, the total number of patients with asthma exposed to any dose of FORADIL AEROLIZER who had continuous electrocardiographic monitoring was about 200.

Continuous electrocardiographic monitoring was performed in an 8-week, randomized, double-blind, and placebo controlled trial in 204 COPD patients treated with FORADIL AEROLIZER 12 mcg twice daily or placebo. Holter monitoring was used to evaluate predefined proarrhythmic events. Non-sustained ventricular tachycardia occurred in 2 (2.2%) of FORADIL AEROLIZER treated patients compared to none in the placebo group. An increase in ventricular premature beats (VPB) occurred in 3 (3.3 %) of FORADIL AEROLIZER treated patients compared to 2 (1.9%) in the placebo group. There were no events of sustained ventricular tachycardia, ventricular flutter or fibrillation, or symptomatic runs of VPB. One patient in the FORADIL AEROLIZER group had a serious adverse event of atrial flutter.

The electrocardiographic effects of FORADIL AEROLIZER were evaluated versus placebo in a 12-month pivotal double-blind study of patients with COPD. An analysis of ECG intervals was performed for patients who participated at study sites in the United States, including 46 patients treated with FORADIL AEROLIZER 12 mcg twice daily, and 50 patients treated with FORADIL AEROLIZER 24 mcg twice daily. ECGs were performed predose, and at 5-15 minutes and 2 hours post-dose at study baseline and after 3, 6, and 12 months of treatment. The results showed that there was no clinically meaningful acute or chronic effect on ECG intervals, including QTc, resulting from treatment with FORADIL AEROLIZER.

Tachyphylaxis/Tolerance

In a clinical study in 19 adult patients with mild asthma, the bronchoprotective effect of formoterol, as assessed by methacholine challenge, was studied following an initial dose of 24 mcg (twice the recommended dose) and after 2 weeks of 24 mcg twice daily. Tolerance to the bronchoprotective effects of formoterol was observed as evidenced by a diminished bronchoprotective effect on FEV$_1$ after 2 weeks of dosing, with loss of protection at the end of the 12 hour dosing period.

Rebound bronchial hyper-responsiveness after cessation of chronic formoterol therapy has not been observed.

In three large clinical trials in patients with asthma, while efficacy of formoterol versus placebo was maintained, a slightly reduced bronchodilatory response (as measured by 12-hour FEV$_1$ AUC) was observed within the formoterol arms over time, particularly with the 24 mcg twice daily dose (twice the daily recommended dose). A similarly reduced FEV$_1$ AUC over time was also noted in the albuterol treatment arms (180 mcg four times daily by metered-dose inhaler).

12.3 Pharmacokinetics

Information on the pharmacokinetics of formoterol in plasma has been obtained in healthy subjects by oral inhalation of doses higher than the recommended range and in Chronic Obstructive Pulmonary Disease (COPD) patients after oral inhalation of doses at and above the therapeutic dose. Urinary excretion of unchanged formoterol was used as an indirect measure of systemic exposure. Plasma drug disposition data parallel urinary excretion, and the elimination half-lives calculated for urine and plasma are similar.

Absorption

Following inhalation of a single 120 mcg dose of formoterol fumarate by 12 healthy subjects, formoterol was rapidly absorbed into plasma, reaching a maximum drug concentration of 92 pg/mL within 5 minutes of dosing. In COPD patients treated for 12 weeks with formoterol fumarate 12 or 24 mcg twice daily, the mean plasma concentrations of formoterol obtained at 10 min, 2 h, and 6 h post inhalation ranged between 4.0 and 8.8 pg/mL and 8.0 and 17.3 pg/mL, respectively.

Following inhalation of 12 to 96 mcg of formoterol fumarate by 10 healthy males, urinary excretion of both (R,R)- and (S,S)-enantiomers of formoterol increased proportionally to the dose. Thus, absorption of formoterol following inhalation appeared linear over the dose range studied.

In a study in patients with asthma, when formoterol 12 or 24 mcg twice daily was given by oral inhalation for 4 weeks or 12 weeks, the accumulation index, based on the urinary excretion of unchanged formoterol ranged from 1.63 to 2.08 in comparison with the first dose. For COPD patients, when formoterol 12 or 24 mcg twice daily was given by oral inhalation for 12 weeks, the accumulation index, based on the urinary excretion of unchanged formoterol was 1.19 - 1.38. This suggests some accumulation of formoterol in

plasma with multiple dosing. The excreted amounts of formoterol at steady-state were close to those predicted based on single-dose kinetics. As with many drug products for oral inhalation, it is likely that the majority of the inhaled formoterol fumarate delivered is swallowed and then absorbed from the gastrointestinal tract.

Distribution

The binding of formoterol to human plasma proteins *in vitro* was 61%-64% at concentrations from 0.1 to 100 ng/mL. Binding to human serum albumin *in vitro* was 31%-38% over a range of 5 to 500 ng/mL. The concentrations of formoterol used to assess the plasma protein binding were higher than those achieved in plasma following inhalation of a single 120 mcg dose.

Metabolism

Formoterol is metabolized primarily by direct glucuronidation at either the phenolic or aliphatic hydroxyl group and O-demethylation followed by glucuronide conjugation at either phenolic hydroxyl groups. Minor pathways involve sulfate conjugation of formoterol and deformylation followed by sulfate conjugation. The most prominent pathway involves direct conjugation at the phenolic hydroxyl group. The second major pathway involves O-demethylation followed by conjugation at the phenolic 2'-hydroxyl group. Four cytochrome P450 isozymes (CYP2D6, CYP2C19, CYP2C9, and CYP2A6) are involved in the O-demethylation of formoterol. Formoterol did not inhibit CYP450 enzymes at therapeutically relevant concentrations. Some patients may be deficient in CYP2D6 or 2C19 or both. Whether a deficiency in one or both of these isozymes results in elevated systemic exposure to formoterol or systemic adverse effects has not been adequately explored.

Excretion

Following oral administration of 80 mcg of radiolabeled formoterol fumarate to 2 healthy subjects, 59%-62% of the radioactivity was eliminated in the urine and 32%-34% in the feces over a period of 104 hours. Renal clearance of formoterol from blood in these subjects was about 150 mL/min. Following inhalation of a 12 mcg or 24 mcg dose by 16 patients with asthma, about 10% and 15%-18% of the total dose was excreted in the urine as unchanged formoterol and direct conjugates of formoterol, respectively. Following inhalation of 12 mcg or 24 mcg dose by 18 patients with COPD the corresponding values were 7% and 6-9% of the dose, respectively.

Based on plasma concentrations measured following inhalation of a single 120 mcg dose by 12 healthy subjects, the mean terminal elimination half-life was determined to be 10 hours. From urinary excretion rates measured in these subjects, the mean terminal elimination half-lives for the (R,R)- and (S,S)-enantiomers were determined to be 13.9 and 12.3 hours, respectively. The (R,R)- and (S,S)-enantiomers represented about 40% and 60% of unchanged drug excreted in the urine, respectively, following single inhaled doses between 12 and 120 mcg in healthy volunteers and single and repeated doses of 12 and 24 mcg in patients with asthma. Thus, the relative proportion of the two enantiomers remained constant over the dose range studied and there was no evidence of relative accumulation of one enantiomer over the other after repeated dosing.

Special Populations

Gender: After correction for body weight, formoterol pharmacokinetics did not differ significantly between males and females.

Geriatric and Pediatric: The pharmacokinetics of formoterol have not been studied in the elderly population, and limited data are available in pediatric patients.

In a study of children with asthma who were 5 to 12 years of age, when formoterol fumarate 12 or 24 mcg was given twice daily by oral inhalation for 12 weeks, the accumulation index ranged from 1.18 to 1.84 based on urinary excretion of unchanged formoterol. Hence, the accumulation in children did not exceed that in adults, where the accumulation index ranged from 1.63 to 2.08 (see above). Approximately 6% and 6.5% to 9% of the dose was recovered in the urine of the children as unchanged and conjugated formoterol, respectively.

Hepatic/Renal Impairment

The pharmacokinetics of formoterol have not been studied in subjects with hepatic or renal impairment.

13 NONCLINICAL TOXICOLOGY

13.1 Carcinogenesis, Mutagenesis, Impairment of Fertility

The carcinogenic potential of formoterol fumarate has been evaluated in 2-year drinking water and dietary studies in both rats and mice. In rats, the incidence of ovarian leiomyomas was increased at doses of 15 mg/kg and above in the drinking water study and at 20 mg/kg in the dietary study, but not at dietary doses up to 5 mg/kg (AUC exposure approximately 450 times human exposure at the maximum recommended human dose [MRHD]). In the dietary study, the incidence of benign ovarian theca-cell tumors was increased at doses of 0.5 mg/kg and above (AUC exposure at the low dose of 0.5 mg/kg was approximately 45 times human exposure at the MRHD). This finding was not observed in the drinking water study, nor was it seen in mice (see below).

In mice, the incidence of adrenal subcapsular adenomas and carcinomas was increased in males at doses of 69 mg/kg and above in the drinking water study, but not at doses up to 50 mg/kg (AUC exposure approximately 590 times human exposure at the MRHD) in the dietary study. The incidence of hepatocarcinomas was increased in the dietary study at doses of 20 and 50 mg/kg in females and 50 mg/kg in males, but not at doses up to 5 mg/kg in either males or females (AUC exposure approximately 60 times human exposure at the MRHD). Also in the dietary study, the incidence of uterine leiomyomas and leiomyosarcomas was increased at doses of 2 mg/kg and above (AUC exposure at the low dose of 2 mg/kg was approximately 25 times human exposure at the MRHD). Increases in leiomyomas of the rodent female genital tract have been similarly demonstrated with other beta-agonist drugs.

Formoterol fumarate was not mutagenic or clastogenic in the following tests: mutagenicity tests in bacterial and mammalian cells, chromosomal analyses in mammalian cells, unscheduled DNA synthesis repair tests in rat hepatocytes and human fibroblasts, transformation assay in mammalian fibroblasts and micronucleus tests in mice and rats. Reproduction studies in rats revealed no impairment of fertility at oral doses up to 3 mg/kg (approximately 1200 times the MRHD on a mcg/m^2 basis).

13.2 Animal Toxicology and/or Pharmacology

Studies in laboratory animals (minipigs, rodents, and dogs) have demonstrated the occurrence of cardiac arrhythmias and sudden death (with histologic evidence of myocardial necrosis) when beta-agonists and methylxanthines are administered concurrently. The clinical significance of these findings is unknown.

14 CLINICAL STUDIES

14.1 Asthma

Adults and Adolescents 12 Years of Age and Older

In a placebo-controlled, single-dose clinical trial, the onset of bronchodilation (defined as a 15% or greater increase from baseline in FEV$_1$) was similar for FORADIL AEROLIZER and albuterol 180 mcg by metered-dose inhaler.

In single-dose and multiple-dose clinical trials, the maximum improvement in FEV$_1$ for FORADIL AEROLIZER 12 mcg generally occurred within 1 to 3 hours, and an increase in FEV$_1$ above baseline was observed for 12 hours in most patients.

FORADIL AEROLIZER 12 mcg twice daily was compared to FORADIL AEROLIZER 24 mcg twice daily, albuterol 180 mcg four times daily by metered-dose inhaler, and placebo in a total of 1095 adult and adolescent patients 12 years of age and above with mild-to-moderate asthma (defined as FEV$_1$ 40%-80% of the patient's predicted normal value) who participated in two pivotal, 12-week, multicenter, randomized, double-blind, parallel group trials.

The results of both clinical trials showed that FORADIL AEROLIZER 12 mcg twice daily resulted in significantly greater post-dose bronchodilation (as measured by serial FEV$_1$ for 12 hours post-dose) throughout the 12-week treatment period. There was no significant difference in post-dose bronchodilation between FORADIL AEROLIZER 12 mcg twice daily and FORADIL AEROLIZER 24 mcg twice daily, but serious asthma exacerbations occurred more commonly in the higher dose group [*see Warnings and Precautions (5.1) and Adverse Reactions (6.2)*]. Mean FEV$_1$ measurements from both studies are shown below for the first and last treatment days (see Figures 1 and 2).

[See figures 1a and 1b at top of next column]
[See figures 2a and 2b at top of next column]

Compared with placebo and albuterol, patients treated with FORADIL AEROLIZER 12 mcg demonstrated improvement in many secondary efficacy endpoints, including improved combined and nocturnal asthma symptom scores, fewer nighttime awakenings, fewer nights in which patients used rescue medication, and higher morning and evening peak flow rates. FORADIL AEROLIZER 24 mcg twice daily did not provide any additional improvements in these secondary endpoints compared to FORADIL AEROLIZER 12 mcg twice daily.

A 16-week, randomized, multi-center, double-blind, parallel-group trial enrolled 1568 patients 12 years of age and older with mild-to-moderate asthma (defined as FEV$_1$ ≥40% of the patient's predicted normal value) in three treatment groups: FORADIL AEROLIZER 12 mcg twice daily, FORADIL AEROLIZER 24 mcg twice daily, and placebo. The trial's primary endpoint was the incidence of serious asthma-related adverse events. Serious asthma exacerbations occurred in 3 (0.6%) patients who received FORADIL AEROLIZER 12 mcg twice daily, 2 (0.4%) patients who received FORADIL AEROLIZER 24 mcg twice daily, and 1 (0.2%) patient who received placebo. The size of this trial

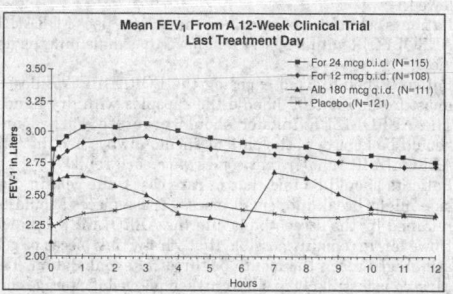

Figures 1a and 1b: Mean FEV$_1$ from Clinical Trial A

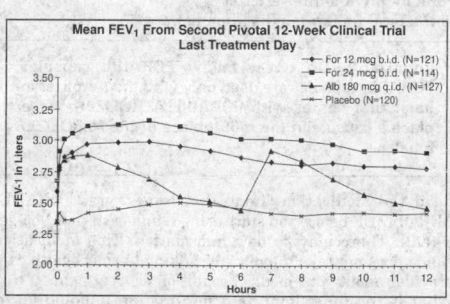

Figures 2a and 2b: Mean FEV$_1$ from Clinical Trial B

was not adequate to precisely quantify the differences in serious asthma exacerbation rates between treatment groups. All serious asthma exacerbations resulted in hospitalizations. While there were no deaths in the trial, the duration and size of this trial were not adequate to quantify the rate of asthma-related death. See [*Warnings and Precautions (5.1)*] for information about a trial that compared another long-acting beta$_2$-adrenergic agonist to placebo.

Children 5-11 Years of Age

A 12-month, multi-center, randomized, double-blind, parallel-group, trial compared FORADIL AEROLIZER 12 mcg twice daily and FORADIL AEROLIZER 24 mcg twice daily to placebo in a total of 518 children with asthma (ages 5-12 years) who required daily bronchodilators and anti-inflammatory treatment. Efficacy was evaluated on the first day of treatment, at Week 12, and at the end of treatment.

FORADIL AEROLIZER 12 mcg twice daily demonstrated a greater 12-hour FEV$_1$ AUC compared to placebo on the first day of treatment, after twelve weeks of treatment, and after one year of treatment. FORADIL AEROLIZER 24 mcg twice daily did not result in any additional improvement in 12-hour FEV$_1$ AUC compared to FORADIL AEROLIZER 12 mcg twice daily.

14.2 Exercise-Induced Bronchospasm

The effect of FORADIL AEROLIZER on exercise-induced bronchospasm (defined as >20% fall in FEV$_1$) was examined in four randomized, single-dose, double-blind, crossover trials in a total of 77 patients 4 to 41 years of age with exercise-induced bronchospasm. Exercise challenge testing was conducted 15 minutes, and 4, 8, and 12 hours following

administration of a single dose of study drug (FORADIL AEROLIZER 12 mcg, albuterol 180 mcg by metered-dose inhaler, or placebo) on separate test days. FORADIL AEROLIZER 12 mcg and albuterol 180 mcg were each superior to placebo for FEV$_1$ measurements obtained 15 minutes after study drug administration. FORADIL AEROLIZER 12 mcg maintained superiority over placebo at 4, 8, and 12 hours after administration. Most subjects were protected from exercise-induced bronchospasm for up to 12 hours following administration of FORADIL AEROLIZER, however, some were not. The efficacy of FORADIL AEROLIZER in the prevention of exercise-induced bronchospasm when dosed on a regular twice daily regimen has not been studied.

14.3 COPD

In multiple-dose clinical trials in patients with COPD, FORADIL AEROLIZER 12 mcg was shown to provide onset of significant bronchodilation (defined as 15% or greater increase from baseline in FEV$_1$) within 5 minutes of oral inhalation after the first dose. Bronchodilation was maintained for at least 12 hours.

FORADIL AEROLIZER was studied in two pivotal, double-blind, placebo-controlled, randomized, multi-center, parallel-group trials in a total of 1634 adult patients (age range: 34-88 years; mean age: 63 years) with COPD who had a mean FEV$_1$ that was 46% of predicted. The diagnosis of COPD was based upon a prior clinical diagnosis of COPD, a smoking history (greater than 10 pack-years), age (at least 40 years), spirometry results (prebronchodilator baseline FEV$_1$ less than 70% of the predicted value, and at least 0.75 liters, with the FEV$_1$/VC being less than 88% for men and less than 89% for women), and symptom score (greater than zero on at least four of the seven days prior to randomization). These studies included approximately equal numbers of patients with and without baseline bronchodilator reversibility, defined as a 15% or greater increase FEV$_1$ after inhalation of 200 mcg of albuterol sulfate. A total of 405 patients received FORADIL AEROLIZER 12 mcg, administered twice daily. Each trial compared FORADIL AEROLIZER 12 mcg twice daily and FORADIL AEROLIZER 24 mcg twice daily with placebo and an active control drug. The active control drug was ipratropium bromide in COPD Trial A, and slow-release theophylline in COPD Trial B (the theophylline arm in this study was open-label). The treatment period was 12 weeks in COPD Trial A, and 12 months in COPD Trial B.

The results showed that FORADIL AEROLIZER 12 mcg twice daily resulted in significantly greater post-dose bronchodilation (as measured by serial FEV$_1$ for 12 hours post-dose; the primary efficacy analysis) compared to placebo when evaluated after 12 weeks of treatment in both trials, and after 12 months of treatment in the 12-month trial (COPD Trial B). Compared to FORADIL AEROLIZER 12 mcg twice daily, FORADIL AEROLIZER 24 mcg twice daily did not provide any additional benefit on a variety of endpoints including FEV$_1$.

Mean FEV$_1$ measurements after 12 weeks of treatment for one of the two major efficacy trials are shown in the figure below.

Figure 3 Mean FEV$_1$ After 12 Weeks of Treatment from COPD Trial A

FORADIL AEROLIZER 12 mcg twice daily was statistically superior to placebo at all post-dose timepoints tested (from 5 minutes to 12 hours post-dose) throughout the 12-week (COPD Trial A) and 12-month (COPD Trial B) treatment periods.

In both pivotal trials compared with placebo, patients treated with FORADIL AEROLIZER 12 mcg demonstrated improved morning premedication peak expiratory flow rates and took fewer puffs of rescue albuterol.

16 HOW SUPPLIED/STORAGE AND HANDLING

16.1 How Supplied

FORADIL AEROLIZER contains: aluminum blister-packaged 12-mcg FORADIL (formoterol fumarate) clear gelatin capsules with "CG" printed on one end and "FXF" printed on the opposite end; one AEROLIZER Inhaler; and Medication Guide.

Unit Dose (blister pack)
Box of 12 (strips of 6)   NDC 0085-1402-01
Unit Dose (blister pack)
Box of 60 (strips of 6)   NDC 0085-1401-01

16.2 Storage and Handling

Prior to dispensing: Store in a refrigerator, 2°C to 8°C (36°F to 46°F)

After dispensing to patient: Store at 20°C to 25°C (68°F to 77°F) [*see USP Controlled Room Temperature*]. Protect from heat and moisture. **Capsules should always be stored in the blister and only removed from the blister immediately before use.**

FORADIL capsules should be used with the AEROLIZER Inhaler only. The AEROLIZER Inhaler should not be used with any other capsules.

Always discard the FORADIL capsules and AEROLIZER Inhaler by the "Use by" date and always use the new AEROLIZER Inhaler provided with each new prescription. Keep out of the reach of children.

17 PATIENT COUNSELING INFORMATION

See FDA-approved **patient labeling** (Medication Guide and Instructions for Use)

Patients should be instructed to read the accompanying Medication Guide with each new prescription and refill. The complete text of the Medication Guide is reprinted at the end of this document. Patients should be given the following information:

17.1 Asthma-Related Death

Patients should be informed that long-acting beta$_2$-adrenergic agonists (LABA), including formoterol, the active ingredient in FORADIL AEROLIZER, increase the risk of asthma-related death and may increase the risk of asthma-related hospitalizations in pediatric and adolescent patients. Currently available data are inadequate to determine whether concurrent use of inhaled corticosteroids or other long-term asthma control drugs mitigates the increased risk of asthma- related death from LABA.

Patients should be informed that FORADIL AEROLIZER should not be the only therapy for the treatment of asthma and must only be used as additional therapy when a long-term asthma control medication (e.g., inhaled corticosteroids) do not adequately control asthma symptoms. Patients should be informed that when FORADIL AEROLIZER is added to their treatment regimen they must continue to use their long-term asthma control medication.

17.2 Not for Acute Symptoms

FORADIL AEROLIZER is not indicated to relieve acute asthma symptoms or exacerbations of COPD and extra doses should not be used for that purpose. Acute symptoms should be treated with an inhaled, short-acting, beta$_2$-agonist (the health-care provider should prescribe the patient with such medication and instruct the patient in how it should be used). Patients should be instructed to seek medical attention if their symptoms worsen, if FORADIL AEROLIZER treatment becomes less effective, or if they need more inhalations of a short-acting beta$_2$-agonist than usual. Patients should not inhale more than the contents of one capsule at any one time. The daily dosage of FORADIL AEROLIZER should not exceed one capsule twice daily (24 mcg total daily dose).

17.3 Required Concomitant Therapy

Patients with asthma should be advised that FORADIL AEROLIZER must always be used with a long-term asthma control medication such as an inhaled corticosteroid. FORADIL AEROLIZER should not be used as a substitute for oral or inhaled corticosteroids. The dosage of these medications should not be changed and they should not be stopped without consulting the physician, even if the patient feels better after initiating treatment with FORADIL AEROLIZER.

17.4 Common Adverse Reactions

Patients should be informed that treatment with beta$_2$-agonists may lead to adverse events which include palpitations, chest pain, rapid heart rate, tremor or nervousness.

17.5 Appropriate Dosing

The active ingredient of FORADIL (formoterol fumarate) is a long-acting, bronchodilator used for the treatment of asthma, including nocturnal asthma, for the prevention of exercise-induced bronchospasm, and for the maintenance treatment of bronchoconstriction in patients with Chronic Obstructive Pulmonary Disease including chronic bronchitis and emphysema. FORADIL AEROLIZER provides bronchodilation for up to 12 hours. Patients should be advised not to increase the dose or frequency of FORADIL AEROLIZER without consulting the prescribing physician. Patients should be warned not to stop or reduce concomitant asthma therapy without medical advice.

For asthma and COPD, the usual dose is one FORADIL capsule inhaled through the AEROLIZER inhaler 2 times each day (morning and evening). The 2 doses should be about 12 hours apart. Patients should be advised not to use other LABA when using FORADIL AEROLIZER.

When FORADIL AEROLIZER is used for the prevention of EIB, the contents of one capsule should be taken at least 15 minutes prior to exercise. Additional doses of FORADIL AEROLIZER should not be used for 12 hours. Prevention of EIB has not been studied in patients who are receiving

chronic FORADIL AEROLIZER administration twice daily and these patients should not use additional FORADIL AEROLIZER for prevention of EIB.

17.6 Instructions for Administration

It is important for patients to understand how to correctly administer FORADIL capsules using the AEROLIZER Inhaler and how FORADIL should be used in relation to other asthma medications they are taking (see the accompanying Medication Guide).

Patients should be instructed that FORADIL capsules should only be administered via the AEROLIZER device and the AEROLIZER device should not be used for administering other medications. The contents of FORADIL capsules are for oral inhalation only and must not be swallowed.

Patients should be informed never to use FORADIL AEROLIZER with a spacer and never to exhale into the device.

Patients should avoid exposing the FORADIL capsules to moisture and should handle the capsules with dry hands. The AEROLIZER Inhaler should never be washed and should be kept dry. The patient should always use the new AEROLIZER Inhaler that comes with each refill.

Patients should be told that in rare cases, the gelatin capsule might break into small pieces. These pieces should be retained by the screen built into the AEROLIZER Inhaler. However, it remains possible that rarely, tiny pieces of gelatin might reach the mouth or throat after inhalation. The capsule is less likely to shatter when pierced if: storage conditions are strictly followed, capsules are removed from the blister immediately before use, and the capsules are only pierced once.

Women should be advised to contact their physician if they become pregnant or if they are nursing.

Manufactured for: Merck Sharp & Dohme Corp., a subsidiary of

MERCK & CO., INC., Whitehouse Station, NJ 08889, USA

Manufactured by:

Novartis Pharma AG, Basle, Switzerland

Copyright © 2010 Merck Sharp & Dohme Corporation, a subsidiary of **Merck & Co., Inc.**

All rights reserved.

T2012-217

November 2012

MEDICATION GUIDE

Foradil® [FOR-a-dil] Aerolizer®
(formoterol fumarate inhalation powder)

Important: Do not swallow FORADIL capsules. FORADIL capsules are used only with the Aerolizer inhaler that comes with FORADIL AEROLIZER. Never place a capsule in the mouthpiece of the AEROLIZER Inhaler.

Read the Medication Guide that comes with FORADIL AEROLIZER before you start using it and each time you get a refill. There may be new information. This Medication Guide does not take the place of talking to your health care provider about your medical condition or treatment.

What is the most important information I should know about FORADIL AEROLIZER?

FORADIL AEROLIZER can cause serious side effects, including:

1. People with asthma who take long-acting beta$_2$-adrenergic agonist (LABA) medicines, such as formoterol fumarate inhalation powder (FORADIL AEROLIZER), have an increased risk of death from asthma problems.

- Call your healthcare provider if breathing problems worsen over time while using FORADIL AEROLIZER. You may need a different treatment.
- Get emergency medical care if:
  - breathing problems worsen quickly, and
  - you use your rescue inhaler medicine, but it does not relieve your breathing problems.

2. Do not use FORADIL AEROLIZER as your only asthma medicine. FORADIL AEROLIZER must only be used with a long-term asthma control medicine, such as an inhaled corticosteroid.

3. When your asthma is well controlled, your healthcare provider may tell you to stop taking FORADIL AEROLIZER. Your healthcare provider will decide if you can stop FORADIL AEROLIZER without loss of asthma control. You will continue taking your long-term asthma control medicine, such as an inhaled corticosteroid.

4. Children and adolescents who take LABA medicines may have an increased risk of being hospitalized for asthma problems.

What is FORADIL AEROLIZER?

FORADIL AEROLIZER is a long-acting beta$_2$-agonist (LABA). LABA medicines help the muscles around the airways in your lungs stay relaxed to prevent asthma symptoms, such as wheezing and shortness of breath. These symptoms can happen when the muscles around the air-

ways tighten. This makes it hard to breathe. In severe cases, wheezing can stop your breathing and cause death if not treated right away.

FORADIL AEROLIZER is used for asthma, exercise-induced bronchospasm (EIB) and chronic obstructive pulmonary disease (COPD) as follows:

Asthma

FORADIL AEROLIZER is used with a long-term asthma control medicine, such as an inhaled corticosteroid, in adults and children ages 5 and older:

- to control symptoms of asthma, and
- to prevent symptoms such as wheezing

LABA medicines, such as FORADIL AEROLIZER, increase the risk of death from asthma problems. FORADIL AEROLIZER is not for adults and children with asthma who are well controlled with long-term asthma control medicine, such as low to medium dose of an inhaled corticosteroid medicine.

Exercise-Induced Bronchospasm (EIB)

FORADIL AEROLIZER is used to prevent wheezing caused by exercise in adults and children 5 years of age and older.

- If you have EIB only, your healthcare provider may prescribe only FORADIL AEROLIZER for your condition
- If you have EIB and asthma, your healthcare provider should also prescribe a long-term asthma control medicine, such as an inhaled corticosteroid

Chronic Obstructive Pulmonary Disease (COPD)

FORADIL AEROLIZER is used long-term, 2 times each day (morning and evening), to control symptoms of COPD and prevent wheezing in adults with COPD.

It is not known if FORADIL AEROLIZER is safe and effective in children under 5 years of age.

Who should not use FORADIL AEROLIZER?

Do not take FORADIL AEROLIZER:

- to treat your asthma without a long-term asthma control medicine, such as an inhaled corticosteroid
- to treat sudden symptoms of asthma or COPD
- if you are allergic to formoterol fumarate or any of the ingredients in FORADIL AEROLIZER. Ask your healthcare provider if you are not sure. See the end of this Medication Guide for a complete list of ingredients in FORADIL AEROLIZER.

What should I tell my healthcare provider before using FORADIL AEROLIZER?

Tell your healthcare provider about all of your health conditions, including if you:

- have heart problems
- have high blood pressure
- have seizures
- have thyroid problems
- have diabetes
- have an aneurysm (swelling of an artery)
- have a pheochromocytoma (a tumor of the adrenal gland that can affect your blood pressure)
- are scheduled to have surgery
- are pregnant or planning to become pregnant. It is not known if FORADIL AEROLIZER may harm your unborn baby.
- are breastfeeding. It is not known if FORADIL AEROLIZER passes into your milk and if it can harm your baby.
- are allergic to FORADIL AEROLIZER, any other medicines, or food products.

FORADIL AEROLIZER contains lactose (milk sugar) and a small amount of milk proteins. It is possible that allergic reactions may happen in patients who have a severe milk protein allergy.

Tell your healthcare provider about all the medicines you take including prescription and non-prescription medicines, vitamins, and herbal supplements. FORADIL AEROLIZER and certain other medicines may interact with each other. This may cause serious side effects.

Know the medicines you take. Keep a list and show it to your healthcare provider and pharmacist each time you get a new medicine.

How do I use FORADIL capsules with the Aerolizer inhaler?

See the step-by-step instructions for using FORADIL Capsules with the Aerolizer inhaler at the end of this Medication Guide.

- Do not use FORADIL unless your healthcare provider has taught you and you understand everything. Ask your healthcare provider or pharmacist if you have any questions.
- Children should use FORADIL AEROLIZER with an adult's help, as instructed by the child's healthcare provider.
- Use FORADIL AEROLIZER exactly as prescribed. **Do not use FORADIL AEROLIZER more often than prescribed.**
- For asthma and COPD, the usual dose is 1 FORADIL capsule inhaled through the AEROLIZER inhaler 2 times each day (morning and evening). The 2 doses should be about 12 hours apart.

- For preventing exercise-induced bronchospasm, the usual dose is 1 FORADIL capsule inhaled through the AEROLIZER inhaler at least 15 minutes before exercise, as needed. Do not use FORADIL AEROLIZER more often than every 12 hours. Do not use extra FORADIL AEROLIZER before exercise if you already use it 2 times each day.
- If you miss a dose of FORADIL AEROLIZER, just skip that dose. Take your next dose at your usual time. Never take 2 doses at one time.
- Do not use a spacer device with FORADIL AEROLIZER.
- Do not breathe into FORADIL AEROLIZER.
- While you are using FORADIL AEROLIZER 2 times each day, do not use other medicines that contain a long-acting beta₂-agonist (LABA) for any reason. Ask your healthcare provider or pharmacist for a list of these medicines.
- Do not stop using FORADIL AEROLIZER or any of your asthma medicines unless told to do so by your healthcare provider because your symptoms might get worse. Your healthcare provider will change your medicines as needed.
- FORADIL AEROLIZER does not relieve sudden symptoms. Always have a rescue inhaler medicine with you to treat sudden symptoms. If you do not have an inhaled, short-acting bronchodilator, contact your healthcare provider to have one prescribed for you.

Call your healthcare provider or get medical care right away if:

- your breathing problems worsen with FORADIL AEROLIZER
- you need to use your rescue inhaler medicine more often than usual
- your rescue inhaler medicine does not work as well for you at relieving symptoms
- you need to use 4 or more inhalations of your rescue inhaler medicine for 2 or more days in a row
- you use 1 whole canister of your rescue inhaler medicine in 8 weeks time
- your peak flow meter results decrease. Your healthcare provider will tell you the numbers that are right for you.
- you have asthma and your symptoms do not improve after using FORADIL AEROLIZER regularly for 1 week.

What are the possible side effects with FORADIL AEROLIZER?

FORADIL AEROLIZER may cause serious side effects, including:

See "What is the most important information I should know about FORADIL AEROLIZER?"

- **Sudden breathing problems immediately after inhaling your medicine** (wheezing or coughing and difficulty breathing)
- **Fast or irregular heart beat** (palpitations)
- **Serious allergic reactions including rash, hives, swelling of the face, mouth, and tongue, and breathing problems.** Call your healthcare provider or get emergency medical care if you get any symptoms of a serious allergic reaction.
- **Low blood potassium** (which may cause symptoms of muscle spasm, muscle weakness or abnormal heart rhythm)
- **Increases in blood sugar levels** (hyperglycemia)
- Using too much of a LABA medicine may cause:
  ○ chest pain
  ○ increased blood pressure
  ○ a fast or irregular heart beat
  ○ headache
  ○ tremor
  ○ nervousness
  ○ dizziness
  ○ weakness
  ○ trouble sleeping
  ○ electrocardiogram (ECG) changes
  ○ seizures

Common side effects with FORADIL AEROLIZER include:

Asthma in Adults and Adolescents:

- headache
- tremor
- chest infection
- chest pain
- trouble sleeping

Asthma in Children 5-12 Years of Age:

- viral infections
- runny nose
- tonsillitis
- gastroenteritis
- abdominal pain
- nausea
- dyspepsia

COPD:

- respiratory infection
- throat infection
- chest pain
- sinus infection
- fever
- leg cramps
- muscle cramps

Tell your healthcare provider about any side effect that bothers you or that does not go away.

These are not all the side effects with FORADIL AEROLIZER. Ask your healthcare provider or pharmacist for more information.

Call your doctor for medical advice about side effects. You may report side effects to FDA at 1-800-FDA-1088.

How do I store FORADIL AEROLIZER?

- Store FORADIL AEROLIZER at room temperature between 68°F and 77°F (20°C to 25°C).
- Protect FORADIL AEROLIZER from heat and moisture.
- Do not remove FORADIL capsules from their foil blister package until just before use.
- Always discard the old AEROLIZER inhaler by the "Use by" date and use the new one provided with each new prescription.
- Safely discard FORADIL capsules and the Aerolizer inhaler if no longer needed or is out-of-date.

Keep FORADIL AEROLIZER and all medicines out of the reach of children.

General Information about FORADIL AEROLIZER

Medicines are sometimes prescribed for purposes other than those listed in a Medication Guide. Do not use FORADIL AEROLIZER for a condition for which it was not prescribed. Do not give FORADIL AEROLIZER to other people, even if they have the same condition. It may harm them.

This Medication Guide summarizes the most important information about FORADIL AEROLIZER. If you would like more information, talk with your healthcare provider. You can ask your healthcare provider or pharmacist for information about FORADIL AEROLIZER that was written for healthcare professionals. If you have any questions about the use of FORADIL AEROLIZER, call (toll-free) 1-800-622-4477 or go to www.foradil.us.

What are the ingredients in FORADIL AEROLIZER?

Active ingredient: formoterol fumarate

Inactive ingredients: lactose (contains milk proteins), gelatin (capsule shell)

T2012-118

November 2012

INSTRUCTIONS FOR USE

Do not swallow FORADIL capsules.

Follow the instructions below for using your FORADIL AEROLIZER. **You will breathe-in (inhale) the medicine in the FORADIL capsules from the FORADIL AEROLIZER.** If you have any questions, ask your healthcare provider or pharmacist.

FORADIL AEROLIZER

- **FORADIL AEROLIZER consists of FORADIL capsules and a AEROLIZER Inhaler.**
- **FORADIL capsules come on blister cards.**
- **Keep your FORADIL and AEROLIZER Inhaler dry. Handle with DRY hands.**

Foil blister card

The Aerolizer consists of the following parts:
1. A cap to protect the mouthpiece of the base
2. A base that allows the proper release of medicine from the capsule. The base consists of:
3. A mouth piece
4. A capsule chamber
5. A button with "winglets" (projecting side pieces) and pins on each side
6. An air inlet channel.

With each new prescription of FORADIL AEROLIZER or refill, your pharmacist should have written the "Use by" date on the sticker on the outside of the FORADIL AEROLIZER box. Remove the "Use by" sticker on the box and place it on the AEROLIZER Inhaler cover that comes with FORADIL. If the sticker is blank, count 4 months from the date you got your FORADIL AEROLIZER from the pharmacy and write this date on the sticker. Also, check the expiration date stamped on the box. If this date is less than 4 months from your purchase date, write this date on the sticker.

Do not use FORADIL capsules with any other capsule inhaler, and do not use the AEROLIZER inhaler to take any other capsule medicine.

Taking a dose of FORADIL AEROLIZER requires the following steps:

1. Do not remove a FORADIL capsule from the blister card until you are ready for a dose.
2. Pull off the AEROLIZER Inhaler cover. (Figure A)

Figure A

3. Hold the base of the AEROLIZER Inhaler firmly and twist the mouthpiece in the direction of the arrow to open. (Figure B) Push the buttons in on each side to make sure that you can see 4 pins in the capsule well of the AEROLIZER Inhaler.

Figure B

4. Separate one FORADIL capsule blister by tearing at the precut lines. (Figure C)

Figure C

5. Peel the paper backing that covers one FORADIL capsule on the blister card. Push the FORADIL capsule through the foil. (Figure D)

Figure D

PEEL BACK

6. Place the FORADIL capsule in the capsule-chamber in the base of the AEROLIZER Inhaler. **Never place a capsule directly into the mouthpiece.** (Figure E)

Figure E

7. Twist the mouthpiece back to the closed position. (Figure F)
[See figure F at top of next column]

8. Hold the mouthpiece of the AEROLIZER Inhaler upright and press both buttons at the same time. Only press the buttons **ONCE.** You should hear a click as the FORADIL capsule is being pierced. (Figure G)
[See figure G at top of next column]

9. Release the buttons. If the buttons stay stuck, grasp the wings on the buttons and pull them out of the stuck position before the next step. Do not push the buttons a second time. This may cause the FORADIL capsule to break into small pieces. There is a screen built into the AEROLIZER Inhaler to hold these small pieces. It is possible that tiny pieces of a FORADIL capsule might reach your mouth or throat when

Figure F

Figure G

you inhale the medicine. This will not harm you, but to avoid this, only pierce the capsule once. The FORADIL capsules are also less likely to break into small pieces if you store them the right way (See "How do I store FORADIL AEROLIZER?").

10. Breathe out (exhale) fully. **Do not exhale into the AEROLIZER mouthpiece.** (Figure H)

Figure H

EXHALE

11. Tilt your head back slightly. Keep the AEROLIZER Inhaler level, with the blue buttons to the left and right (**not up and down**). Place the mouthpiece in your mouth and close your lips around the mouthpiece. (Figures I and J)

CORRECT   INCORRECT
Figure I   **Figure J**

12. Breathe in quickly and deeply (Figure K). This will cause the FORADIL capsule to spin around in the chamber and deliver your dose of medicine. You should hear a whirring noise and experience a sweet taste in your mouth. If you do not hear the whirring noise, the capsule may be stuck. If this occurs, open the AEROLIZER Inhaler and loosen the capsule allowing it to spin freely. **Do not try to loosen the capsule by pressing the buttons again.** (You will have to repeat steps 10 to 12 again to get your dose.)

Figure K

13. Remove the AEROLIZER Inhaler from your mouth. Continue to hold your breath as long as you can and then exhale.

14. Open the AEROLIZER Inhaler to see if any powder is still in the capsule. If any powder remains in the capsule repeat steps 10 to 13. Most people are able to empty the capsule in one or two inhalations.

---

15. After use, open the AEROLIZER Inhaler, remove and discard the empty capsule. Do not leave a used capsule in the chamber.

16. Close the mouthpiece and replace the cover.

Remember:
- Never breathe into the AEROLIZER Inhaler.
- Never take the AEROLIZER Inhaler apart.
- Never place a FORADIL capsule directly into the mouthpiece of the AEROLIZER Inhaler.
- Never leave a used FORADIL capsule in the AEROLIZER Inhaler chamber.
- Always use the AEROLIZER Inhaler in a level position.
- Never wash the AEROLIZER Inhaler. **Keep it dry.**
- Always keep the AEROLIZER Inhaler and FORADIL capsules in a dry place.
- Always use the new AEROLIZER Inhaler that comes with your refill.

This Medication Guide and Instructions for Use has been approved by the U.S. Food and Drug Administration.

FORADIL® is a registered trademark of Astellas Pharma Inc.

AEROLIZER® is a registered trademark of Novartis AG.

Manufactured for: Merck Sharp & Dohme Corp., a subsidiary of

MERCK & CO., INC., Whitehouse Station, NJ 08889, USA

Manufactured by:

Novartis Pharma AG, Basle, Switzerland

Copyright © 2010 Merck Sharp & Dohme Corporation, a subsidiary of **Merck & Co., Inc.**

All rights reserved.

T2012-219

November 2012

Shown in Product Identification Guide, page 308

FOSAMAX® ℞
[*FOSS-ah-max*]
(alendronate sodium)
tablets, for oral use

FOSAMAX® ℞
(alendronate sodium)
oral solution

HIGHLIGHTS OF PRESCRIBING INFORMATION

These highlights do not include all the information needed to use FOSAMAX safely and effectively. See full prescribing information for FOSAMAX.

FOSAMAX® (alendronate sodium) tablets, for oral use
FOSAMAX® (alendronate sodium) oral solution
Initial U.S. Approval: 1995

———RECENT MAJOR CHANGES———

Dosage and Administration (2)   12/2013

———INDICATIONS AND USAGE———

FOSAMAX is a bisphosphonate indicated for:
- Treatment and prevention of osteoporosis in postmenopausal women (1.1, 1.2)
- Treatment to increase bone mass in men with osteoporosis (1.3)
- Treatment of glucocorticoid-induced osteoporosis (1.4)
- Treatment of Paget's disease of bone (1.5)

Limitations of use:
Optimal duration of use has not been determined. For patients at low-risk for fracture, consider drug discontinuation after 3 to 5 years of use. (1.6)

———DOSAGE AND ADMINISTRATION———

- Treatment of osteoporosis in postmenopausal women and in men: 10 mg daily or 70 mg (tablet or oral solution) once weekly. (2.1, 2.3)
- Prevention of osteoporosis in postmenopausal women: 5 mg daily or 35 mg once weekly. (2.2)
- Glucocorticoid-induced osteoporosis: 5 mg daily; or 10 mg daily in postmenopausal women not receiving estrogen. (2.4)
- Paget's disease: 40 mg daily for six months. (2.5)
- Instruct patients to: (2.6)
  ◦ Swallow tablets whole with 6-8 ounces plain water at least 30 minutes before the first food, drink, or medication of the day.
  ◦ Swallow oral solution followed by at least 2 ounces of water.
  ◦ Not lie down for at least 30 minutes after taking FOSAMAX and until after food.

———DOSAGE FORMS AND STRENGTHS———

Tablets: 70 mg (3)

———CONTRAINDICATIONS———

- Abnormalities of the esophagus which delay emptying such as stricture or achalasia (4, 5.1)
- Inability to stand/sit upright for at least 30 minutes (2.6, 4, 5.1)

- Do not administer FOSAMAX oral solution to patients at increased risk of aspiration. (4)
- Hypocalcemia (4, 5.2)
- Hypersensitivity to any component of this product (4, 6.2)

———WARNINGS AND PRECAUTIONS———

- *Upper Gastrointestinal Adverse Reactions* can occur. Instruct patients to follow dosing instructions. Discontinue if new or worsening symptoms occur. (5.1)
- *Hypocalcemia* can worsen and must be corrected prior to use. (5.2)
- *Severe Bone, Joint, Muscle Pain* may occur. Discontinue use if severe symptoms develop. (5.3)
- *Osteonecrosis of the Jaw* has been reported. (5.4)
- *Atypical Femur Fractures* have been reported. Patients with new thigh or groin pain should be evaluated to rule out an incomplete femoral fracture. (5.5)

———ADVERSE REACTIONS———

Most common adverse reactions (greater than or equal to 3%) are abdominal pain, acid regurgitation, constipation, diarrhea, dyspepsia, musculoskeletal pain, nausea. (6.1)

To report SUSPECTED ADVERSE REACTIONS, contact Merck Sharp & Dohme Corp., a subsidiary of Merck & Co., Inc., at 1-877-888-4231 or FDA at 1-800-FDA-1088 or www.fda.gov/medwatch.

———DRUG INTERACTIONS———

- Calcium supplements, antacids, or oral medications containing multivalent cations interfere with absorption of alendronate. (2.6, 7.1)
- Use caution when co-prescribing aspirin/nonsteroidal anti-inflammatory drugs that may worsen gastrointestinal irritation. (7.2, 7.3)

———USE IN SPECIFIC POPULATIONS———

- FOSAMAX is not indicated for use in pediatric patients. (8.4)
- FOSAMAX is not recommended in patients with renal impairment (creatinine clearance less than 35 mL/min). (5.6, 8.6)

See 17 for PATIENT COUNSELING INFORMATION and Medication Guide

Revised: 05/2014

FULL PRESCRIBING INFORMATION: CONTENTS*

FULL PRESCRIBING INFORMATION

1   INDICATIONS AND USAGE

1.1   Treatment of Osteoporosis in Postmenopausal Women

FOSAMAX® is indicated for the treatment of osteoporosis in postmenopausal women. In postmenopausal women, FOSAMAX increases bone mass and reduces the incidence of fractures, including those of the hip and spine (vertebral compression fractures). [See Clinical Studies (14.1).]

1.2   Prevention of Osteoporosis in Postmenopausal Women

FOSAMAX is indicated for the prevention of postmenopausal osteoporosis [see Clinical Studies (14.2)].

1.3   Treatment to Increase Bone Mass in Men with Osteoporosis

FOSAMAX is indicated for treatment to increase bone mass in men with osteoporosis [see Clinical Studies (14.3)].

1.4   Treatment of Glucocorticoid-Induced Osteoporosis

FOSAMAX is indicated for the treatment of glucocorticoid-induced osteoporosis in men and women receiving glucocorticoids in a daily dosage equivalent to 7.5 mg or greater of prednisone and who have low bone mineral density [see Clinical Studies (14.4)].

1.5   Treatment of Paget's Disease of Bone

FOSAMAX is indicated for the treatment of Paget's disease of bone in men and women. Treatment is indicated in patients with Paget's disease of bone who have alkaline phosphatase at least two times the upper limit of normal, or those who are symptomatic, or those at risk for future complications from their disease. [See Clinical Studies (14.5).]

1.6   Important Limitations of Use

The optimal duration of use has not been determined. The safety and effectiveness of FOSAMAX for the treatment of osteoporosis are based on clinical data of four years duration. All patients on bisphosphonate therapy should have the need for continued therapy re-evaluated on a periodic basis. Patients at low-risk for fracture should be considered for drug discontinuation after 3 to 5 years of use. Patients who discontinue therapy should have their risk for fracture re-evaluated periodically.

2   DOSAGE AND ADMINISTRATION

Although alendronate tablets 5 mg, 10 mg, 35 mg, and 40 mg are available in the marketplace, FOSAMAX is no longer marketed in the 5 mg, 10 mg, 35 mg, and 40 mg strengths.

Although an oral solution of alendronate may be available in the marketplace, FOSAMAX oral solution is no longer marketed.

2.1   Treatment of Osteoporosis in Postmenopausal Women

The recommended dosage is:
• one 70 mg tablet once weekly
    or
• one bottle of 70 mg oral solution once weekly
    or
• one 10 mg tablet once daily

2.2   Prevention of Osteoporosis in Postmenopausal Women

The recommended dosage is:
• one 35 mg tablet once weekly
    or
• one 5 mg tablet once daily

2.3   Treatment to Increase Bone Mass in Men with Osteoporosis

The recommended dosage is:
• one 70 mg tablet once weekly
    or
• one bottle of 70 mg oral solution once weekly
    or
• one 10 mg tablet once daily

2.4   Treatment of Glucocorticoid-Induced Osteoporosis

The recommended dosage is one 5 mg tablet once daily, except for postmenopausal women not receiving estrogen, for whom the recommended dosage is one 10 mg tablet once daily.

2.5   Treatment of Paget's Disease of Bone

The recommended treatment regimen is 40 mg once a day for six months.

Re-treatment of Paget's Disease

Re-treatment with FOSAMAX may be considered, following a six-month post-treatment evaluation period in patients who have relapsed, based on increases in serum alkaline phosphatase, which should be measured periodically. Re-treatment may also be considered in those who failed to normalize their serum alkaline phosphatase.

2.6   Important Administration Instructions

Instruct patients to do the following:
• Take FOSAMAX *at least* one-half hour before the first food, beverage, or medication of the day with plain water only [see Patient Counseling Information (17.2)]. Other beverages (including mineral water), food, and some medications are likely to reduce the absorption of FOSAMAX [see Drug Interactions (7.1)]. Waiting less than 30 minutes, or taking FOSAMAX with food, beverages (other than plain water) or other medications will lessen the effect of FOSAMAX by decreasing its absorption into the body.
• Take FOSAMAX upon arising for the day. To facilitate delivery to the stomach and thus reduce the potential for esophageal irritation, a FOSAMAX tablet should be swallowed with a full glass of water (6-8 ounces). To facilitate gastric emptying FOSAMAX oral solution should be followed by at least 2 ounces (a quarter of a cup) of water. Patients should not lie down for at least 30 minutes and until after their first food of the day. FOSAMAX should not be taken at bedtime or before arising for the day. Failure to follow these instructions may increase the risk of esophageal adverse experiences [see Warnings and Precautions (5.1) and Patient Counseling Information (17.2)].

2.7   Recommendations for Calcium and Vitamin D Supplementation

Instruct patients to take supplemental calcium if dietary intake is inadequate [see Warnings and Precautions (5.2)]. Patients at increased risk for vitamin D insufficiency (e.g., over the age of 70 years, nursing home-bound, or chronically ill) may need vitamin D supplementation. Patients with gastrointestinal malabsorption syndromes may require higher doses of vitamin D supplementation and measurement of 25-hydroxyvitamin D should be considered.

Patients treated with glucocorticoids should receive adequate amounts of calcium and vitamin D.

2.8   Administration Instructions for Missed Doses

If a once-weekly dose of FOSAMAX is missed, instruct patients to take one dose on the morning after they remember. They should not take two doses on the same day but should return to taking one dose once a week, as originally scheduled on their chosen day.

3   DOSAGE FORMS AND STRENGTHS

• 70 mg tablets are white, oval, uncoated tablets with code 31 on one side and an outline of a bone image on the other.

4   CONTRAINDICATIONS

FOSAMAX is contraindicated in patients with the following conditions:
• Abnormalities of the esophagus which delay esophageal emptying such as stricture or achalasia [see Warnings and Precautions (5.1)]
• Inability to stand or sit upright for at least 30 minutes [see Dosage and Administration (2.6); Warnings and Precautions (5.1)]
• Do not administer FOSAMAX oral solution to patients at increased risk of aspiration.
• Hypocalcemia [see Warnings and Precautions (5.2)]
• Hypersensitivity to any component of this product. Hypersensitivity reactions including urticaria and angioedema have been reported [see Adverse Reactions (6.2)].

5   WARNINGS AND PRECAUTIONS

5.1   Upper Gastrointestinal Adverse Reactions

FOSAMAX, like other bisphosphonates administered orally, may cause local irritation of the upper gastrointestinal mucosa. Because of these possible irritant effects and a potential for worsening of the underlying disease, caution should be used when FOSAMAX is given to patients with active upper gastrointestinal problems (such as known Barrett's esophagus, dysphagia, other esophageal diseases, gastritis, duodenitis, or ulcers).

Esophageal adverse experiences, such as esophagitis, esophageal ulcers and esophageal erosions, occasionally with bleeding and rarely followed by esophageal stricture or perforation, have been reported in patients receiving treatment with oral bisphosphonates including FOSAMAX. In some cases these have been severe and required hospitalization. Physicians should therefore be alert to any signs or symptoms signaling a possible esophageal reaction and patients should be instructed to discontinue FOSAMAX and seek medical attention if they develop dysphagia, odynophagia, retrosternal pain or new or worsening heartburn.

The risk of severe esophageal adverse experiences appears to be greater in patients who lie down after taking oral bisphosphonates including FOSAMAX and/or who fail to swallow oral bisphosphonates including FOSAMAX with the recommended full glass (6-8 ounces) of water, and/or who continue to take oral bisphosphonates including FOSAMAX after developing symptoms suggestive of esophageal irritation. Therefore, it is very important that the full dosing instructions are provided to, and understood by, the patient [see Dosage and Administration (2.6)]. In patients who cannot comply with dosing instructions due to mental disability, therapy with FOSAMAX should be used under appropriate supervision.

There have been post-marketing reports of gastric and duodenal ulcers with oral bisphosphonate use, some severe and with complications, although no increased risk was observed in controlled clinical trials [see Adverse Reactions (6.2)].

5.2   Mineral Metabolism

Hypocalcemia must be corrected before initiating therapy with FOSAMAX [see Contraindications (4)]. Other disorders affecting mineral metabolism (such as vitamin D deficiency) should also be effectively treated. In patients with these conditions, serum calcium and symptoms of hypocalcemia should be monitored during therapy with FOSAMAX.

Presumably due to the effects of FOSAMAX on increasing bone mineral, small, asymptomatic decreases in serum calcium and phosphate may occur, especially in patients with Paget's disease, in whom the pretreatment rate of bone turnover may be greatly elevated, and in patients receiving glucocorticoids, in whom calcium absorption may be decreased.

Ensuring adequate calcium and vitamin D intake is especially important in patients with Paget's disease of bone and in patients receiving glucocorticoids.

5.3   Musculoskeletal Pain

In post-marketing experience, severe and occasionally incapacitating bone, joint, and/or muscle pain has been reported in patients taking bisphosphonates that are approved for the prevention and treatment of osteoporosis [see Adverse Reactions (6.2)]. This category of drugs includes FOSAMAX (alendronate). Most of the patients were postmenopausal women. The time to onset of symptoms varied from one day to several months after starting the drug. Discontinue use if severe symptoms develop. Most patients had relief of symptoms after stopping. A subset had recurrence of symptoms when rechallenged with the same drug or another bisphosphonate.

In placebo-controlled clinical studies of FOSAMAX, the percentages of patients with these symptoms were similar in the FOSAMAX and placebo groups.

5.4   Osteonecrosis of the Jaw

Osteonecrosis of the jaw (ONJ), which can occur spontaneously, is generally associated with tooth extraction and/or local infection with delayed healing, and has been reported in patients taking bisphosphonates, including FOSAMAX. Known risk factors for osteonecrosis of the jaw include invasive dental procedures (e.g., tooth extraction, dental implants, boney surgery), diagnosis of cancer, concomitant therapies (e.g., chemotherapy, corticosteroids), poor oral hygiene, and co-morbid disorders (e.g., periodontal and/or other pre-existing dental disease, anemia, coagulopathy, infection, ill-fitting dentures). The risk of ONJ may increase with duration of exposure to bisphosphonates.

For patients requiring invasive dental procedures, discontinuation of bisphosphonate treatment may reduce the risk for ONJ. Clinical judgment of the treating physician and/or oral surgeon should guide the management plan of each patient based on individual benefit/risk assessment.

Patients who develop osteonecrosis of the jaw while on bisphosphonate therapy should receive care by an oral surgeon. In these patients, extensive dental surgery to treat ONJ may exacerbate the condition. Discontinuation of bisphosphonate therapy should be considered based on individual benefit/risk assessment.

5.5   Atypical Subtrochanteric and Diaphyseal Femoral Fractures

Atypical, low-energy, or low trauma fractures of the femoral shaft have been reported in bisphosphonate-treated patients. These fractures can occur anywhere in the femoral shaft from just below the lesser trochanter to above the supracondylar flare and are transverse or short oblique in orientation without evidence of comminution. Causality has not been established as these fractures also occur in osteoporotic patients who have not been treated with bisphosphonates.

Atypical femur fractures most commonly occur with minimal or no trauma to the affected area. They may be bilateral

Table 1: Osteoporosis Treatment Studies in Postmenopausal Women Adverse Reactions Considered Possibly, Probably, or Definitely Drug Related by the Investigators and Reported in Greater Than or Equal to 1% of Patients

	United States/Multinational Studies		Fracture Intervention Trial	
	FOSAMAX* % (n=196)	Placebo % (n=397)	FOSAMAX† % (n=3236)	Placebo % (n=3223)
Gastrointestinal				
abdominal pain	6.6	4.8	1.5	1.5
nausea	3.6	4.0	1.1	1.5
dyspepsia	3.6	3.5	1.1	1.2
constipation	3.1	1.8	0.0	0.2
diarrhea	3.1	1.8	0.6	0.3
flatulence	2.6	0.5	0.2	0.3
acid regurgitation	2.0	4.3	1.1	0.9
esophageal ulcer	1.5	0.0	0.1	0.1
vomiting	1.0	1.5	0.2	0.3
dysphagia	1.0	0.0	0.1	0.1
abdominal distention	1.0	0.8	0.0	0.0
gastritis	0.5	1.3	0.6	0.7
Musculoskeletal				
musculoskeletal (bone, muscle or joint) pain	4.1	2.5	0.4	0.3
muscle cramp	0.0	1.0	0.2	0.1
Nervous System / Psychiatric				
headache	2.6	1.5	0.2	0.2
dizziness	0.0	1.0	0.0	0.1
Special Senses				
taste perversion	0.5	1.0	0.1	0.0

* 10 mg/day for three years
† 5 mg/day for 2 years and 10 mg/day for either 1 or 2 additional years

Table 3: Osteoporosis Prevention Studies in Postmenopausal Women Adverse Reactions Considered Possibly, Probably, or Definitely Drug Related by the Investigators and Reported in Greater Than or Equal to 1% of Patients

	Two/Three-Year Studies		One-Year Study	
	FOSAMAX 5 mg/day % (n=642)	Placebo % (n=648)	FOSAMAX 5 mg/day % (n=361)	Once Weekly FOSAMAX 35 mg % (n=362)
Gastrointestinal				
dyspepsia	1.9	1.4	2.2	1.7
abdominal pain	1.7	3.4	4.2	2.2
acid regurgitation	1.4	2.5	4.2	4.7
nausea	1.4	1.4	2.5	1.4
diarrhea	1.1	1.7	1.1	0.6
constipation	0.9	0.5	1.7	0.3
abdominal distention	0.2	0.3	1.4	1.1
Musculoskeletal				
musculoskeletal (bone, muscle or joint) pain	0.8	0.9	1.9	2.2

and many patients report prodromal pain in the affected area, usually presenting as dull, aching thigh pain, weeks to months before a complete fracture occurs. A number of reports note that patients were also receiving treatment with glucocorticoids (e.g. prednisone) at the time of fracture.

Any patient with a history of bisphosphonate exposure who presents with thigh or groin pain should be suspected of having an atypical fracture and should be evaluated to rule out an incomplete femur fracture. Patients presenting with an atypical fracture should also be assessed for symptoms and signs of fracture in the contralateral limb. Interruption of bisphosphonate therapy should be considered, pending a risk/benefit assessment, on an individual basis.

5.6   Renal Impairment
FOSAMAX is not recommended for patients with creatinine clearance less than 35 mL/min.

5.7   Glucocorticoid-Induced Osteoporosis
The risk versus benefit of FOSAMAX for treatment at daily dosages of glucocorticoids less than 7.5 mg of prednisone or equivalent has not been established [see Indications and Usage (1.4)]. Before initiating treatment, the gonadal hormonal status of both men and women should be ascertained and appropriate replacement considered.

A bone mineral density measurement should be made at the initiation of therapy and repeated after 6 to 12 months of combined FOSAMAX and glucocorticoid treatment.

6   ADVERSE REACTIONS
6.1   Clinical Trials Experience
Because clinical trials are conducted under widely varying conditions, adverse reaction rates observed in the clinical trials of a drug cannot be directly compared to rates in the clinical trials of another drug and may not reflect the rates observed in clinical practice.

Treatment of Osteoporosis in Postmenopausal Women
Daily Dosing
The safety of FOSAMAX in the treatment of postmenopausal osteoporosis was assessed in four clinical trials that enrolled 7453 women aged 44-84 years. Study 1 and Study 2 were identically designed, three-year, placebo-controlled, double-blind, multicenter studies (United States and Multinational n=994); Study 3 was the three-year vertebral fracture cohort of the Fracture Intervention Trial [FIT] (n=2027) and Study 4 was the four-year clinical fracture cohort of FIT (n=4432). Overall, 3620 patients were exposed to placebo and 3432 patients exposed to FOSAMAX. Patients with pre-existing gastrointestinal disease and concomitant use of non-steroidal anti-inflammatory drugs were included in these clinical trials. In Study 1 and Study 2 all women received 500 mg elemental calcium as carbonate. In Study 3 and Study 4 all women with dietary calcium intake less than 1000 mg per day received 500 mg calcium and 250 international units Vitamin D per day.

Among patients treated with alendronate 10 mg or placebo in Study 1 and Study 2, and all patients in Study 3 and Study 4, the incidence of all-cause mortality was 1.8% in the placebo group and 1.8% in the FOSAMAX group. The incidence of serious adverse event was 30.7% in the placebo group and 30.9% in the FOSAMAX group. The percentage of patients who discontinued the study due to any clinical adverse event was 9.5% in the placebo group and 8.9% in the FOSAMAX group. Adverse reactions from these studies considered by the investigators as possibly, probably, or definitely drug related in greater than or equal to 1% of patients treated with either FOSAMAX or placebo are presented in Table 1.
[See table 1 above]

Rash and erythema have occurred.
Gastrointestinal Adverse Reactions: One patient treated with FOSAMAX (10 mg/day), who had a history of peptic ulcer disease and gastrectomy and who was taking concomitant aspirin, developed an anastomotic ulcer with mild hemorrhage, which was considered drug related. Aspirin and FOSAMAX were discontinued and the patient recovered. In the Study 1 and Study 2 populations, 49-54% had a history of gastrointestinal disorders at baseline and 54-89% used nonsteroidal anti-inflammatory drugs or aspirin at some time during the studies. [See Warnings and Precautions (5.1).]

Laboratory Test Findings: In double-blind, multicenter, controlled studies, asymptomatic, mild, and transient decreases in serum calcium and phosphate were observed in approximately 18% and 10%, respectively, of patients taking FOSAMAX versus approximately 12% and 3% of those taking placebo. However, the incidences of decreases in serum calcium to less than 8.0 mg/dL (2.0 mM) and serum phosphate to less than or equal to 2.0 mg/dL (0.65 mM) were similar in both treatment groups.

Weekly Dosing
The safety of FOSAMAX 70 mg once weekly for the treatment of postmenopausal osteoporosis was assessed in a one-year, double-blind, multicenter study comparing FOSAMAX 70 mg once weekly and FOSAMAX 10 mg daily. The overall safety and tolerability profiles of once weekly FOSAMAX 70 mg and FOSAMAX 10 mg daily were similar. The adverse reactions considered by the investigators as possibly, probably, or definitely drug related in greater than or equal to 1% of patients in either treatment group are presented in Table 2.

Table 2: Osteoporosis Treatment Studies in Postmenopausal Women Adverse Reactions Considered Possibly, Probably, or Definitely Drug Related by the Investigators and Reported in Greater Than or Equal to 1% of Patients

	Once Weekly FOSAMAX 70 mg % (n=519)	FOSAMAX 10 mg/day % (n=370)
Gastrointestinal		
abdominal pain	3.7	3.0
dyspepsia	2.7	2.2
acid regurgitation	1.9	2.4
nausea	1.9	2.4
abdominal distention	1.0	1.4
constipation	0.8	1.6
flatulence	0.4	1.6
gastritis	0.2	1.1
gastric ulcer	0.0	1.1
Musculoskeletal		
musculoskeletal (bone, muscle, joint) pain	2.9	3.2
muscle cramp	0.2	1.1

Prevention of Osteoporosis in Postmenopausal Women
Daily Dosing
The safety of FOSAMAX 5 mg/day in postmenopausal women 40-60 years of age has been evaluated in three double-blind, placebo-controlled studies involving over 1,400 patients randomized to receive FOSAMAX for either two or three years. In these studies the overall safety profiles of FOSAMAX 5 mg/day and placebo were similar. Discontinuation of therapy due to any clinical adverse event occurred in 7.5% of 642 patients treated with FOSAMAX 5 mg/day and 5.7% of 648 patients treated with placebo.
Weekly Dosing
The safety of FOSAMAX 35 mg once weekly compared to FOSAMAX 5 mg daily was evaluated in a one-year, double-blind, multicenter study of 723 patients. The overall safety and tolerability profiles of once weekly FOSAMAX 35 mg and FOSAMAX 5 mg daily were similar.

The adverse reactions from these studies considered by the investigators as possibly, probably, or definitely drug related in greater than or equal to 1% of patients treated with either once weekly FOSAMAX 35 mg, FOSAMAX 5 mg/day or placebo are presented in Table 3.
[See table 3 above]

Concomitant Use with Estrogen / Hormone Replacement Therapy
In two studies (of one and two years' duration) of postmenopausal osteoporotic women (total: n=853), the safety and tolerability profile of combined treatment with FOSAMAX 10 mg once daily and estrogen ± progestin (n=354) was consistent with those of the individual treatments.

Osteoporosis in Men
In two placebo-controlled, double-blind, multicenter studies in men (a two-year study of FOSAMAX 10 mg/day and a one-year study of once weekly FOSAMAX 70 mg) the rates

of discontinuation of therapy due to any clinical adverse event were 2.7% for FOSAMAX 10 mg/day vs. 10.5% for placebo, and 6.4% for once weekly FOSAMAX 70 mg vs. 8.6% for placebo. The adverse reactions considered by the investigators as possibly, probably, or definitely drug related in greater than or equal to 2% of patients treated with either FOSAMAX or placebo are presented in Table 4.
[See table 4 above]

Glucocorticoid-Induced Osteoporosis
In two, one-year, placebo-controlled, double-blind, multicenter studies in patients receiving glucocorticoid treatment, the overall safety and tolerability profiles of FOSAMAX 5 and 10 mg/day were generally similar to that of placebo. The adverse reactions considered by the investigators as possibly, probably, or definitely drug related in greater than or equal to 1% of patients treated with either FOSAMAX 5 or 10 mg/day or placebo are presented in Table 5.

Table 5: One-Year Studies in Glucocorticoid-Treated Patients Adverse Reactions Considered Possibly, Probably, or Definitely Drug Related by the Investigators and Reported in Greater Than or Equal to 1% of Patients

	FOSAMAX 10 mg/day % (n=157)	FOSAMAX 5 mg/day % (n=161)	Placebo % (n=159)
Gastrointestinal			
abdominal pain	3.2	1.9	0.0
acid regurgitation	2.5	1.9	1.3
constipation	1.3	0.6	0.0
melena	1.3	0.0	0.0
nausea	0.6	1.2	0.6
diarrhea	0.0	0.6	1.3
Nervous System/ Psychiatric			
headache	0.6	0.0	1.3

The overall safety and tolerability profile in the glucocorticoid-induced osteoporosis population that continued therapy for the second year of the studies (FOSAMAX: n=147) was consistent with that observed in the first year.

Paget's Disease of Bone
In clinical studies (osteoporosis and Paget's disease), adverse events reported in 175 patients taking FOSAMAX 40 mg/day for 3-12 months were similar to those in postmenopausal women treated with FOSAMAX 10 mg/day. However, there was an apparent increased incidence of upper gastrointestinal adverse reactions in patients taking FOSAMAX 40 mg/day (17.7% FOSAMAX vs. 10.2% placebo). One case of esophagitis and two cases of gastritis resulted in discontinuation of treatment.
Additionally, musculoskeletal (bone, muscle or joint) pain, which has been described in patients with Paget's disease treated with other bisphosphonates, was considered by the investigators as possibly, probably, or definitely drug related in approximately 6% of patients treated with FOSAMAX 40 mg/day versus approximately 1% of patients treated with placebo, but rarely resulted in discontinuation of therapy. Discontinuation of therapy due to any clinical adverse events occurred in 6.4% of patients with Paget's disease treated with FOSAMAX 40 mg/day and 2.4% of patients treated with placebo.

6.2 Post-Marketing Experience
The following adverse reactions have been identified during post-approval use of FOSAMAX. Because these reactions are reported voluntarily from a population of uncertain size, it is not always possible to reliably estimate their frequency or establish a causal relationship to drug exposure.
Body as a Whole: hypersensitivity reactions including urticaria and angioedema. Transient symptoms of myalgia, malaise, asthenia and fever have been reported with FOSAMAX, typically in association with initiation of treatment. Symptomatic hypocalcemia has occurred, generally in association with predisposing conditions. Peripheral edema.
Gastrointestinal: esophagitis, esophageal erosions, esophageal ulcers, esophageal stricture or perforation, and oropharyngeal ulceration. Gastric or duodenal ulcers, some severe and with complications, have also been reported *[see Dosage and Administration (2.6); Warnings and Precautions (5.1)].*
Localized osteonecrosis of the jaw, generally associated with tooth extraction and/or local infection with delayed healing, has been reported *[see Warnings and Precautions (5.4)].*
Musculoskeletal: bone, joint, and/or muscle pain, occasionally severe, and incapacitating *[see Warnings and Precautions (5.3)];* joint swelling; low-energy femoral shaft and subtrochanteric fractures *[see Warnings and Precautions (5.5)].*
Nervous System: dizziness and vertigo.
Pulmonary: acute asthma exacerbations.

Table 4: Osteoporosis Studies in Men Adverse Reactions Considered Possibly, Probably, or Definitely Drug Related by the Investigators and Reported in Greater Than or Equal to 2% of Patients

	Two-year Study		One-year Study	
	FOSAMAX 10 mg/day % (n=146)	Placebo % (n=95)	Once Weekly FOSAMAX 70 mg % (n=109)	Placebo % (n=58)
Gastrointestinal				
acid regurgitation	4.1	3.2	0.0	0.0
flatulence	4.1	1.1	0.0	0.0
gastroesophageal reflux disease	0.7	3.2	2.8	0.0
dyspepsia	3.4	0.0	2.8	1.7
diarrhea	1.4	1.1	2.8	0.0
abdominal pain	2.1	1.1	0.9	3.4
nausea	2.1	0.0	0.0	0.0

Skin: rash (occasionally with photosensitivity), pruritus, alopecia, severe skin reactions, including Stevens-Johnson syndrome and toxic epidermal necrolysis.
Special Senses: uveitis, scleritis or episcleritis.

7 DRUG INTERACTIONS
7.1 Calcium Supplements/Antacids
Co-administration of FOSAMAX and calcium, antacids, or oral medications containing multivalent cations will interfere with absorption of FOSAMAX. Therefore, instruct patients to wait at least one-half hour after taking FOSAMAX before taking any other oral medications.
7.2 Aspirin
In clinical studies, the incidence of upper gastrointestinal adverse events was increased in patients receiving concomitant therapy with daily doses of FOSAMAX greater than 10 mg and aspirin-containing products.
7.3 Nonsteroidal Anti-Inflammatory Drugs
FOSAMAX may be administered to patients taking nonsteroidal anti-inflammatory drugs (NSAIDs). In a 3-year, controlled, clinical study (n=2027) during which a majority of patients received concomitant NSAIDs, the incidence of upper gastrointestinal adverse events was similar in patients taking FOSAMAX 5 or 10 mg/day compared to those taking placebo. However, since NSAID use is associated with gastrointestinal irritation, caution should be used during concomitant use with FOSAMAX.

8 USE IN SPECIFIC POPULATIONS
8.1 Pregnancy
Pregnancy Category C:
There are no studies in pregnant women. FOSAMAX should be used during pregnancy only if the potential benefit justifies the potential risk to the mother and fetus.
Bisphosphonates are incorporated into the bone matrix, from which they are gradually released over a period of years. The amount of bisphosphonate incorporated into adult bone, and hence, the amount available for release back into the systemic circulation, is directly related to the dose and duration of bisphosphonate use. There are no data on fetal risk in humans. However, there is a theoretical risk of fetal harm, predominantly skeletal, if a woman becomes pregnant after completing a course of bisphosphonate therapy. The impact of variables such as time between cessation of bisphosphonate therapy to conception, the particular bisphosphonate used, and the route of administration (intravenous versus oral) on the risk has not been studied.
Reproduction studies in rats showed decreased postimplantation survival and decreased body weight gain in normal pups at doses less than half of the recommended clinical dose. Sites of incomplete fetal ossification were statistically significantly increased in rats beginning at approximately 3 times the clinical dose in vertebral (cervical, thoracic, and lumbar), skull, and sternebral bones. No similar fetal effects were seen when pregnant rabbits were treated with doses approximately 10 times the clinical dose.
Both total and ionized calcium decreased in pregnant rats at approximately 4 times the clinical dose resulting in delays and failures of delivery. Protracted parturition due to maternal hypocalcemia occurred in rats at doses as low as one tenth the clinical dose when rats were treated from before mating through gestation. Maternotoxicity (late pregnancy deaths) also occurred in the female rats treated at approximately 4 times the clinical dose for varying periods of time ranging from treatment only during pre-mating to treatment only during early, middle, or late gestation; these deaths were lessened but not eliminated by cessation of treatment. Calcium supplementation either in the drinking water or by minipump could not ameliorate the hypocalcemia or prevent maternal and neonatal deaths due to delays in delivery; intravenous calcium supplementation prevented maternal, but not fetal deaths.

Exposure multiples based on surface area, mg/m^2, were calculated using a 40-mg human daily dose. Animal dose ranged between 1 and 15 mg/kg/day in rats and up to 40 mg/kg/day in rabbits.
8.3 Nursing Mothers
It is not known whether alendronate is excreted in human milk. Because many drugs are excreted in human milk, caution should be exercised when FOSAMAX is administered to nursing women.
8.4 Pediatric Use
FOSAMAX is not indicated for use in pediatric patients.
The safety and efficacy of FOSAMAX were examined in a randomized, double-blind, placebo-controlled two-year study of 139 pediatric patients, aged 4-18 years, with severe osteogenesis imperfecta (OI). One-hundred-and-nine patients were randomized to 5 mg FOSAMAX daily (weight less than 40 kg) or 10 mg FOSAMAX daily (weight greater than or equal to 40 kg) and 30 patients to placebo. The mean baseline lumbar spine BMD Z-score of the patients was -4.5. The mean change in lumbar spine BMD Z-score from baseline to Month 24 was 1.3 in the FOSAMAX-treated patients and 0.1 in the placebo-treated patients. Treatment with FOSAMAX did not reduce the risk of fracture. Sixteen percent of the FOSAMAX patients who sustained a radiologically-confirmed fracture by Month 12 of the study had delayed fracture healing (callus remodeling) or fracture non-union when assessed radiographically at Month 24 compared with 9% of the placebo-treated patients. In FOSAMAX-treated patients, bone histomorphometry data obtained at Month 24 demonstrated decreased bone turnover and delayed mineralization time; however, there were no mineralization defects. There were no statistically significant differences between the FOSAMAX and placebo groups in reduction of bone pain. The oral bioavailability in children was similar to that observed in adults.
The overall safety profile of FOSAMAX in osteogenesis imperfecta patients treated for up to 24 months was generally similar to that of adults with osteoporosis treated with FOSAMAX. However, there was an increased occurrence of vomiting in osteogenesis imperfecta patients treated with FOSAMAX compared to placebo. During the 24-month treatment period, vomiting was observed in 32 of 109 (29.4%) patients treated with FOSAMAX and 3 of 30 (10%) patients treated with placebo.
In a pharmacokinetic study, 6 of 24 pediatric osteogenesis imperfecta patients who received a single oral dose of FOSAMAX 35 or 70 mg developed fever, flu-like symptoms, and/or mild lymphocytopenia within 24 to 48 hours after administration. These events, lasting no more than 2 to 3 days and responding to acetaminophen, are consistent with an acute-phase response that has been reported in patients receiving bisphosphonates, including FOSAMAX. *[See Adverse Reactions (6.2).]*
8.5 Geriatric Use
Of the patients receiving FOSAMAX in the Fracture Intervention Trial (FIT), 71% (n=2302) were greater than or equal to 65 years of age and 17% (n=550) were greater than or equal to 75 years of age. Of the patients receiving FOSAMAX in the United States and Multinational osteoporosis treatment studies in women, osteoporosis studies in men, glucocorticoid-induced osteoporosis studies, and Paget's disease studies *[see Clinical Studies (14.1), (14.3), (14.4), (14.5)],* 45%, 54%, 37%, and 70%, respectively, were 65 years of age or over. No overall differences in efficacy or safety were observed between these patients and younger patients, but greater sensitivity of some older individuals cannot be ruled out.
8.6 Renal Impairment
FOSAMAX is not recommended for patients with creatinine clearance less than 35 mL/min. No dosage adjustment is necessary in patients with creatinine clearance values between 35-60 mL/min *[see Clinical Pharmacology (12.3)].*

8.7 Hepatic Impairment

As there is evidence that alendronate is not metabolized or excreted in the bile, no studies were conducted in patients with hepatic impairment. No dosage adjustment is necessary [see Clinical Pharmacology (12.3)].

10 OVERDOSAGE

Significant lethality after single oral doses was seen in female rats and mice at 552 mg/kg (3256 mg/m^2) and 966 mg/kg (2898 mg/m^2), respectively. In males, these values were slightly higher, 626 and 1280 mg/kg, respectively. There was no lethality in dogs at oral doses up to 200 mg/kg (4000 mg/m^2).

No specific information is available on the treatment of overdosage with FOSAMAX. Hypocalcemia, hypophosphatemia, and upper gastrointestinal adverse events, such as upset stomach, heartburn, esophagitis, gastritis, or ulcer, may result from oral overdosage. Milk or antacids should be given to bind alendronate. Due to the risk of esophageal irritation, vomiting should not be induced and the patient should remain fully upright.

Dialysis would not be beneficial.

11 DESCRIPTION

FOSAMAX (alendronate sodium) is a bisphosphonate that acts as a specific inhibitor of osteoclast-mediated bone resorption. Bisphosphonates are synthetic analogs of pyrophosphate that bind to the hydroxyapatite found in bone. Alendronate sodium is chemically described as (4-amino-1-hydroxybutylidene) bisphosphonic acid monosodium salt trihydrate.

The empirical formula of alendronate sodium is C$_4$H$_{12}$NNaO$_7$P$_2$•3H$_2$O and its formula weight is 325.12. The structural formula is:

$$\begin{array}{c} NH_2 \\ | \\ CH_2 \\ | \\ CH_2 \\ | \\ CH_2 \\ | \\ O \quad CH_2 \quad O \\ || \quad | \quad || \\ HO-P-C-P-ONa \cdot 3H_2O \\ | \quad | \quad | \\ OH \quad OH \quad OH \end{array}$$

Alendronate sodium is a white, crystalline, nonhygroscopic powder. It is soluble in water, very slightly soluble in alcohol, and practically insoluble in chloroform.

FOSAMAX tablets for oral administration contain 91.37 mg of alendronate monosodium salt trihydrate, which is the molar equivalent of 70 mg of free acid, and the following inactive ingredients: microcrystalline cellulose, anhydrous lactose, croscarmellose sodium, and magnesium stearate.

12 CLINICAL PHARMACOLOGY

12.1 Mechanism of Action

Animal studies have indicated the following mode of action. At the cellular level, alendronate shows preferential localization to sites of bone resorption, specifically under osteoclasts. The osteoclasts adhere normally to the bone surface but lack the ruffled border that is indicative of active resorption. Alendronate does not interfere with osteoclast recruitment or attachment, but it does inhibit osteoclast activity. Studies in mice on the localization of radioactive [^{3}H]alendronate in bone showed about 10-fold higher uptake on osteoclast surfaces than on osteoblast surfaces. Bones examined 6 and 49 days after [^{3}H]alendronate administration in rats and mice, respectively, showed that normal bone was formed on top of the alendronate, which was incorporated inside the matrix. While incorporated in bone matrix, alendronate is not pharmacologically active. Thus, alendronate must be continuously administered to suppress osteoclasts on newly formed resorption surfaces. Histomorphometry in baboons and rats showed that alendronate treatment reduces bone turnover (i.e., the number of sites at which bone is remodeled). In addition, bone formation exceeds bone resorption at these remodeling sites, leading to progressive gains in bone mass.

12.2 Pharmacodynamics

Alendronate is a bisphosphonate that binds to bone hydroxyapatite and specifically inhibits the activity of osteoclasts, the bone-resorbing cells. Alendronate reduces bone resorption with no direct effect on bone formation, although the latter process is ultimately reduced because bone resorption and formation are coupled during bone turnover.

Osteoporosis in Postmenopausal Women

Osteoporosis is characterized by low bone mass that leads to an increased risk of fracture. The diagnosis can be confirmed by the finding of low bone mass, evidence of fracture on x-ray, a history of osteoporotic fracture, or height loss or kyphosis, indicative of vertebral (spinal) fracture. Osteoporosis occurs in both males and females but is most common among women following the menopause, when bone turnover increases and the rate of bone resorption exceeds that of bone formation. These changes result in progressive bone loss and lead to osteoporosis in a significant proportion of women over age 50. Fractures, usually of the spine, hip, and

wrist, are the common consequences. From age 50 to age 90, the risk of hip fracture in white women increases 50-fold and the risk of vertebral fracture 15- to 30-fold. It is estimated that approximately 40% of 50-year-old women will sustain one or more osteoporosis-related fractures of the spine, hip, or wrist during their remaining lifetimes. Hip fractures, in particular, are associated with substantial morbidity, disability, and mortality.

Daily oral doses of alendronate (5, 20, and 40 mg for six weeks) in postmenopausal women produced biochemical changes indicative of dose-dependent inhibition of bone resorption, including decreases in urinary calcium and urinary markers of bone collagen degradation (such as deoxypyridinoline and cross-linked N-telopeptides of type I collagen). These biochemical changes tended to return toward baseline values as early as 3 weeks following the discontinuation of therapy with alendronate and did not differ from placebo at 7 months.

Long-term treatment of osteoporosis with FOSAMAX 10 mg/day (for up to five years) reduced urinary excretion of markers of bone resorption, deoxypyridinoline and cross-linked N-telopeptides of type I collagen, by approximately 50% and 70%, respectively, to reach levels similar to those seen in healthy premenopausal women. Similar decreases were seen in patients in osteoporosis prevention studies who received FOSAMAX 5 mg/day. The decrease in the rate of bone resorption indicated by these markers was evident as early as one month and at three to six months reached a plateau that was maintained for the entire duration of treatment with FOSAMAX. In osteoporosis treatment studies FOSAMAX 10 mg/day decreased the markers of bone formation, osteocalcin and bone specific alkaline phosphatase by approximately 50%, and total serum alkaline phosphatase by approximately 25 to 30% to reach a plateau after 6 to 12 months. In osteoporosis prevention studies FOSAMAX 5 mg/day decreased osteocalcin and total serum alkaline phosphatase by approximately 40% and 15%, respectively. Similar reductions in the rate of bone turnover were observed in postmenopausal women during one-year studies with once weekly FOSAMAX 70 mg for the treatment of osteoporosis and once weekly FOSAMAX 35 mg for the prevention of osteoporosis. These data indicate that the rate of bone turnover reached a new steady-state, despite the progressive increase in the total amount of alendronate deposited within bone.

As a result of inhibition of bone resorption, asymptomatic reductions in serum calcium and phosphate concentrations were also observed following treatment with FOSAMAX. In the long-term studies, reductions from baseline in serum calcium (approximately 2%) and phosphate (approximately 4 to 6%) were evident the first month after the initiation of FOSAMAX 10 mg. No further decreases in serum calcium were observed for the five-year duration of treatment; however, serum phosphate returned toward prestudy levels during years three through five. Similar reductions were observed with FOSAMAX 5 mg/day. In one-year studies with once weekly FOSAMAX 35 and 70 mg, similar reductions were observed at 6 and 12 months. The reduction in serum phosphate may reflect not only the positive bone mineral balance due to FOSAMAX but also a decrease in renal phosphate reabsorption.

Osteoporosis in Men

Treatment of men with osteoporosis with FOSAMAX 10 mg/day for two years reduced urinary excretion of cross-linked N-telopeptides of type I collagen by approximately 60% and bone-specific alkaline phosphatase by approximately 40%. Similar reductions were observed in a one-year study in men with osteoporosis receiving once weekly FOSAMAX 70 mg.

Glucocorticoid-Induced Osteoporosis

Sustained use of glucocorticoids is commonly associated with development of osteoporosis and resulting fractures (especially vertebral, hip, and rib). It occurs both in males and females of all ages. Osteoporosis occurs as a result of inhibited bone formation and increased bone resorption resulting in net bone loss. Alendronate decreases bone resorption without directly inhibiting bone formation.

In clinical studies of up to two years' duration, FOSAMAX 5 and 10 mg/day reduced cross-linked N-telopeptides of type I collagen (a marker of bone resorption) by approximately 60% and reduced bone-specific alkaline phosphatase and total serum alkaline phosphatase (markers of bone formation) by approximately 15 to 30% and 8 to 18%, respectively. As a result of inhibition of bone resorption, FOSAMAX 5 and 10 mg/day induced asymptomatic decreases in serum calcium (approximately 1 to 2%) and serum phosphate (approximately 1 to 8%).

Paget's Disease of Bone

Paget's disease of bone is a chronic, focal skeletal disorder characterized by greatly increased and disorderly bone remodeling. Excessive osteoclastic bone resorption is followed by osteoblastic new bone formation, leading to the replacement of the normal bone architecture by disorganized, enlarged, and weakened bone structure.

Clinical manifestations of Paget's disease range from no symptoms to severe morbidity due to bone pain, bone deformity, pathological fractures, and neurological and other complications. Serum alkaline phosphatase, the most frequently used biochemical index of disease activity, provides an objective measure of disease severity and response to therapy.

FOSAMAX decreases the rate of bone resorption directly, which leads to an indirect decrease in bone formation. In clinical trials, FOSAMAX 40 mg once daily for six months produced significant decreases in serum alkaline phosphatase as well as in urinary markers of bone collagen degradation. As a result of the inhibition of bone resorption, FOSAMAX induced generally mild, transient, and asymptomatic decreases in serum calcium and phosphate.

12.3 Pharmacokinetics

Absorption

Relative to an intravenous reference dose, the mean oral bioavailability of alendronate in women was 0.64% for doses ranging from 5 to 70 mg when administered after an overnight fast and two hours before a standardized breakfast. Oral bioavailability of the 10 mg tablet in men (0.59%) was similar to that in women when administered after an overnight fast and 2 hours before breakfast.

FOSAMAX 70 mg oral solution and FOSAMAX 70 mg tablet are equally bioavailable.

A study examining the effect of timing of a meal on the bioavailability of alendronate was performed in 49 postmenopausal women. Bioavailability was decreased (by approximately 40%) when 10 mg alendronate was administered either 0.5 or 1 hour before a standardized breakfast, when compared to dosing 2 hours before eating. In studies of treatment and prevention of osteoporosis, alendronate was effective when administered at least 30 minutes before breakfast.

Bioavailability was negligible whether alendronate was administered with or up to two hours after a standardized breakfast. Concomitant administration of alendronate with coffee or orange juice reduced bioavailability by approximately 60%.

Distribution

Preclinical studies (in male rats) show that alendronate transiently distributes to soft tissues following 1 mg/kg intravenous administration but is then rapidly redistributed to bone or excreted in the urine. The mean steady-state volume of distribution, exclusive of bone, is at least 28 L in humans. Concentrations of drug in plasma following therapeutic oral doses are too low (less than 5 ng/mL) for analytical detection. Protein binding in human plasma is approximately 78%.

Metabolism

There is no evidence that alendronate is metabolized in animals or humans.

Excretion

Following a single intravenous dose of [^{14}C]alendronate, approximately 50% of the radioactivity was excreted in the urine within 72 hours and little or no radioactivity was recovered in the feces. Following a single 10 mg intravenous dose, the renal clearance of alendronate was 71 mL/min (64, 78; 90% confidence interval [CI]), and systemic clearance did not exceed 200 mL/min. Plasma concentrations fell by more than 95% within 6 hours following intravenous administration. The terminal half-life in humans is estimated to exceed 10 years, probably reflecting release of alendronate from the skeleton. Based on the above, it is estimated that after 10 years of oral treatment with FOSAMAX (10 mg daily) the amount of alendronate released daily from the skeleton is approximately 25% of that absorbed from the gastrointestinal tract.

Specific Populations

Gender: Bioavailability and the fraction of an intravenous dose excreted in urine were similar in men and women.

Geriatric: Bioavailability and disposition (urinary excretion) were similar in elderly and younger patients. No dosage adjustment is necessary in elderly patients.

Race: Pharmacokinetic differences due to race have not been studied.

Renal Impairment: Preclinical studies show that, in rats with kidney failure, increasing amounts of drug are present in plasma, kidney, spleen, and tibia. In healthy controls, drug that is not deposited in bone is rapidly excreted in the urine. No evidence of saturation of bone uptake was found after 3 weeks dosing with cumulative intravenous doses of 35 mg/kg in young male rats. Although no formal renal impairment pharmacokinetic study has been conducted in patients, it is likely that, as in animals, elimination of alendronate via the kidney will be reduced in patients with impaired renal function. Therefore, somewhat greater accumulation of alendronate in bone might be expected in patients with impaired renal function.

No dosage adjustment is necessary for patients with creatinine clearance 35 to 60 mL/min. FOSAMAX is not recommended for patients with creatinine clearance less than 35 mL/min due to lack of experience with alendronate in renal failure.

Hepatic Impairment: As there is evidence that alendronate is not metabolized or excreted in the bile, no studies were conducted in patients with hepatic impairment. No dosage adjustment is necessary.

Drug Interactions

Intravenous ranitidine was shown to double the bioavailability of oral alendronate. The clinical significance of this increased bioavailability and whether similar increases will occur in patients given oral H_2-antagonists is unknown.

In healthy subjects, oral prednisone (20 mg three times daily for five days) did not produce a clinically meaningful change in the oral bioavailability of alendronate (a mean increase ranging from 20 to 44%).

Products containing calcium and other multivalent cations are likely to interfere with absorption of alendronate.

13 NONCLINICAL TOXICOLOGY

13.1 Carcinogenesis, Mutagenesis, Impairment of Fertility

Harderian gland (a retro-orbital gland not present in humans) adenomas were increased in high-dose female mice (p=0.003) in a 92-week oral carcinogenicity study at doses of alendronate of 1, 3, and 10 mg/kg/day (males) or 1, 2, and 5 mg/kg/day (females). These doses are equivalent to approximately 0.1 to 1 times a maximum recommended daily dose of 40 mg (Paget's disease) based on surface area, mg/m^2. The relevance of this finding to humans is unknown. Parafollicular cell (thyroid) adenomas were increased in high-dose male rats (p=0.003) in a 2-year oral carcinogenicity study at doses of 1 and 3.75 mg/kg body weight. These doses are equivalent to approximately 0.3 and 1 times a 40 mg human daily dose based on surface area, mg/m^2. The relevance of this finding to humans is unknown.

Alendronate was not genotoxic in the *in vitro* microbial mutagenesis assay with and without metabolic activation, in an *in vitro* mammalian cell mutagenesis assay, in an *in vitro* alkaline elution assay in rat hepatocytes, and in an *in vivo* chromosomal aberration assay in mice. In an *in vitro* chromosomal aberration assay in Chinese hamster ovary cells, however, alendronate gave equivocal results.

Alendronate had no effect on fertility (male or female) in rats at oral doses up to 5 mg/kg/day (approximately 1 times a 40 mg human daily dose based on surface area, mg/m^2).

13.2 Animal Toxicology and/or Pharmacology

The relative inhibitory activities on bone resorption and mineralization of alendronate and etidronate were compared in the Schenk assay, which is based on histological examination of the epiphyses of growing rats. In this assay, the lowest dose of alendronate that interfered with bone mineralization (leading to osteomalacia) was 6000-fold the antiresorptive dose. The corresponding ratio for etidronate was one to one. These data suggest that alendronate administered in therapeutic doses is highly unlikely to induce osteomalacia.

14 CLINICAL STUDIES

14.1 Treatment of Osteoporosis in Postmenopausal Women

Daily Dosing

The efficacy of FOSAMAX 10 mg daily was assessed in four clinical trials. Study 1, a three-year, multicenter, double-blind, placebo-controlled, US clinical study enrolled 478 patients with a BMD T-score at or below minus 2.5 with or without a prior vertebral fracture; Study 2, a three-year, multicenter, double-blind, placebo-controlled Multinational clinical study enrolled 516 patients with a BMD T-score at or below minus 2.5 with or without a prior vertebral fracture; Study 3, the Three-Year Study of the Fracture Intervention Trial (FIT) a study which enrolled 2027 postmenopausal patients with at least one baseline vertebral fracture; and Study 4, the Four-Year Study of FIT: a study which enrolled 4432 postmenopausal patients with low bone mass but without a baseline vertebral fracture.

Effect on Fracture Incidence

To assess the effects of FOSAMAX on the incidence of vertebral fractures (detected by digitized radiography; approximately one third of these were clinically symptomatic), the U.S. and Multinational studies were combined in an analysis that compared placebo to the pooled dosage groups of FOSAMAX (5 or 10 mg for three years or 20 mg for two years followed by 5 mg for one year). There was a statistically significant reduction in the proportion of patients treated with FOSAMAX experiencing one or more new vertebral fractures relative to those treated with placebo (3.2% vs. 6.2%; a 48% relative risk reduction). A reduction in the total number of new vertebral fractures (4.2 vs. 11.3 per 100 patients) was also observed. In the pooled analysis, patients who received FOSAMAX had a loss in stature that was statistically significantly less than was observed in those who received placebo (-3.0 mm vs. -4.6 mm).

The Fracture Intervention Trial (FIT) consisted of two studies in postmenopausal women: the Three-Year Study of pa-

tients who had at least one baseline radiographic vertebral fracture and the Four-Year Study of patients with low bone mass but without a baseline vertebral fracture. In both studies of FIT, 96% of randomized patients completed the studies (i.e., had a closeout visit at the scheduled end of the study); approximately 80% of patients were still taking study medication upon completion.

Fracture Intervention Trial: Three-Year Study (patients with at least one baseline radiographic vertebral fracture)

This randomized, double-blind, placebo-controlled, 2027-patient study (FOSAMAX, n=1022; placebo, n=1005) demonstrated that treatment with FOSAMAX resulted in statistically significant reductions in fracture incidence at three years as shown in Table 6.

[See table 6 above]

Furthermore, in this population of patients with baseline vertebral fracture, treatment with FOSAMAX significantly reduced the incidence of hospitalizations (25.0% vs. 30.7%). In the Three-Year Study of FIT, fractures of the hip occurred in 22 (2.2%) of 1005 patients on placebo and 11 (1.1%) of 1022 patients on FOSAMAX, p=0.047. Figure 1 displays the cumulative incidence of hip fractures in this study.

[See figure 1 at top of next column]

Fracture Intervention Trial: Four-Year Study (patients with low bone mass but without a baseline radiographic vertebral fracture)

This randomized, double-blind, placebo-controlled, 4432-patient study (FOSAMAX, n=2214; placebo, n=2218) further investigated the reduction in fracture incidence due to FOSAMAX. The intent of the study was to recruit women with osteoporosis, defined as a baseline femoral neck BMD at least two standard deviations below the mean for young adult women. However, due to subsequent revisions to the normative values for femoral neck BMD, 31% of patients were found not to meet this entry criterion and thus this study included both osteoporotic and non-osteoporotic women. The results are shown in Table 7 for the patients with osteoporosis.

[See table 7 above]

Fracture Results Across Studies

In the Three-Year Study of FIT, FOSAMAX reduced the percentage of women experiencing at least one new radiographic vertebral fracture from 15.0% to 7.9% (47% relative

risk reduction, p<0.001); in the Four-Year Study of FIT, the percentage was reduced from 3.8% to 2.1% (44% relative risk reduction, p=0.001); and in the combined U.S./Multinational studies, from 6.2% to 3.2% (48% relative risk reduction, p=0.034).

FOSAMAX reduced the percentage of women experiencing multiple (two or more) new vertebral fractures from 4.2% to 0.6% (87% relative risk reduction, p<0.001) in the combined U.S./Multinational studies and from 4.9% to 0.5% (90% relative risk reduction, p<0.001) in the Three-Year Study of FIT. In the Four-Year Study of FIT, FOSAMAX reduced the percentage of osteoporotic women experiencing multiple vertebral fractures from 0.6% to 0.1% (78% relative risk reduction, p=0.035).

Thus, FOSAMAX reduced the incidence of radiographic vertebral fractures in osteoporotic women whether or not they had a previous radiographic vertebral fracture.

Effect on Bone Mineral Density

The bone mineral density efficacy of FOSAMAX 10 mg once daily in postmenopausal women, 44 to 84 years of age, with

Table 6: Effect of FOSAMAX on Fracture Incidence in the Three-Year Study of FIT (patients with vertebral fracture at baseline)

| | Percent of Patients | | | |
	FOSAMAX (n=1022)	Placebo (n=1005)	Absolute Reduction in Fracture Incidence	Relative Reduction in Fracture Risk %
Patients with:				
Vertebral fractures (diagnosed by X-ray)*				
≥1 new vertebral fracture	7.9	15.0	7.1	47[†]
≥2 new vertebral fractures	0.5	4.9	4.4	90[†]
Clinical (symptomatic) fractures				
Any clinical (symptomatic) fracture	13.8	18.1	4.3	26[‡]
≥1 clinical (symptomatic) vertebral fracture	2.3	5.0	2.7	54[§]
Hip fracture	1.1	2.2	1.1	51[¶]
Wrist (forearm) fracture	2.2	4.1	1.9	48[¶]

* Number evaluable for vertebral fractures: FOSAMAX, n=984; placebo, n=966
† p<0.001,
‡ p=0.007,
§ p<0.01,
¶ p<0.05

Table 7: Effect of FOSAMAX on Fracture Incidence in Osteoporotic* Patients in the Four-Year Study of FIT (patients without vertebral fracture at baseline)

| | Percent of Patients | | | |
	FOSAMAX (n=1545)	Placebo (n=1521)	Absolute Reduction in Fracture Incidence	Relative Reduction in Fracture Risk (%)
Patients with:				
Vertebral fractures (diagnosed by X-ray)[†]				
≥1 new vertebral fracture	2.5	4.8	2.3	48[‡]
≥2 new vertebral fractures	0.1	0.6	0.5	78[§]
Clinical (symptomatic) fractures				
Any clinical (symptomatic) fracture	12.9	16.2	3.3	22[¶]
≥1 clinical (symptomatic) vertebral fracture	1.0	1.6	0.6	41 (NS)[#]
Hip fracture	1.0	1.4	0.4	29 (NS)[#]
Wrist (forearm) fracture	3.9	3.8	-0.1	NS[#]

* Baseline femoral neck BMD at least 2 SD below the mean for young adult women
† Number evaluable for vertebral fractures: FOSAMAX, n=1426; placebo, n=1428
‡ p<0.001,
§ p=0.035,
¶ p=0.01
# Not significant. This study was not powered to detect differences at these sites.

Figure 1:

Cumulative Incidence of Hip Fractures in the Three-Year Study of FIT (patients with radiographic vertebral fracture at baseline)

osteoporosis (lumbar spine bone mineral density [BMD] of at least 2 standard deviations below the premenopausal mean) was demonstrated in four double-blind, placebo-controlled clinical studies of two or three years' duration. Figure 2 shows the mean increases in BMD of the lumbar spine, femoral neck, and trochanter in patients receiving FOSAMAX 10 mg/day relative to placebo-treated patients at three years for each of these studies.

Figure 2:

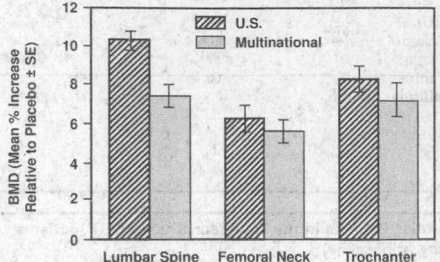

Osteoporosis Treatment Studies in Postmenopausal Women

Increase in BMD
FOSAMAX 10 mg/day at Three Years

At three years significant increases in BMD, relative both to baseline and placebo, were seen at each measurement site in each study in patients who received FOSAMAX 10 mg/day. Total body BMD also increased significantly in each study, suggesting that the increases in bone mass of the spine and hip did not occur at the expense of other skeletal sites. Increases in BMD were evident as early as three months and continued throughout the three years of treatment. (See Figure 3 for lumbar spine results.) In the two-year extension of these studies, treatment of 147 patients with FOSAMAX 10 mg/day resulted in continued increases in BMD at the lumbar spine and trochanter (absolute additional increases between years 3 and 5: lumbar spine, 0.94%; trochanter, 0.88%). BMD at the femoral neck, forearm and total body were maintained. FOSAMAX was similarly effective regardless of age, race, baseline rate of bone turnover, and baseline BMD in the range studied (at least 2 standard deviations below the premenopausal mean).

Figure 3:

Osteoporosis Treatment Studies in Postmenopausal Women

Time Course of Effect of FOSAMAX 10 mg/day Versus Placebo:
Lumbar Spine BMD Percent Change From Baseline

In patients with postmenopausal osteoporosis treated with FOSAMAX 10 mg/day for one or two years, the effects of treatment withdrawal were assessed. Following discontinuation, there were no further increases in bone mass and the rates of bone loss were similar to those of the placebo groups.

Bone Histology
Bone histology in 270 postmenopausal patients with osteoporosis treated with FOSAMAX at doses ranging from 1 to 20 mg/day for one, two, or three years revealed normal mineralization and structure, as well as the expected decrease in bone turnover relative to placebo. These data, together with the normal bone histology and increased bone strength observed in rats and baboons exposed to long-term alendronate treatment, support the conclusion that bone formed during therapy with FOSAMAX is of normal quality.
Effect on Height
FOSAMAX, over a three- or four-year period, was associated with statistically significant reductions in loss of height vs. placebo in patients with and without baseline radiographic vertebral fractures. At the end of the FIT studies, the between-treatment group differences were 3.2 mm in the Three-Year Study and 1.3 mm in the Four-Year Study.
Weekly Dosing
The therapeutic equivalence of once-weekly FOSAMAX 70 mg (n=519) and FOSAMAX 10 mg daily (n=370) was demonstrated in a one-year, double-blind, multicenter study of postmenopausal women with osteoporosis. In the primary analysis of completers, the mean increases from baseline in lumbar spine BMD at one year were 5.1% (4.8, 5.4%; 95%

CI) in the 70-mg once-weekly group (n=440) and 5.4% (5.0, 5.8%; 95% CI) in the 10-mg daily group (n=330). The two treatment groups were also similar with regard to BMD increases at other skeletal sites. The results of the intention-to-treat analysis were consistent with the primary analysis of completers.
Concomitant Use with Estrogen/Hormone Replacement Therapy (HRT)
The effects on BMD of treatment with FOSAMAX 10 mg once daily and conjugated estrogen (0.625 mg/day) either alone or in combination were assessed in a two-year, double-blind, placebo-controlled study of hysterectomized postmenopausal osteoporotic women (n=425). At two years, the increases in lumbar spine BMD from baseline were significantly greater with the combination (8.3%) than with either estrogen or FOSAMAX alone (both 6.0%).
The effects on BMD when FOSAMAX was added to stable doses (for at least one year) of HRT (estrogen ± progestin) were assessed in a one-year, double-blind, placebo-controlled study in postmenopausal osteoporotic women (n=428). The addition of FOSAMAX 10 mg once daily to HRT produced, at one year, significantly greater increases in lumbar spine BMD (3.7%) vs. HRT alone (1.1%).
In these studies, significant increases or favorable trends in BMD for combined therapy compared with HRT alone were seen at the total hip, femoral neck, and trochanter. No significant effect was seen for total body BMD.
Histomorphometric studies of transiliac biopsies in 92 subjects showed normal bone architecture. Compared to placebo there was a 98% suppression of bone turnover (as assessed by mineralizing surface) after 18 months of combined treatment with FOSAMAX and HRT, 94% on FOSAMAX alone, and 78% on HRT alone. The long-term effects of combined FOSAMAX and HRT on fracture occurrence and fracture healing have not been studied.

14.2   Prevention of Osteoporosis in Postmenopausal Women
Daily Dosing
Prevention of bone loss was demonstrated in two double-blind, placebo-controlled studies of postmenopausal women 40-60 years of age. One thousand six hundred nine patients (FOSAMAX 5 mg/day; n=498) who were at least six months postmenopausal were entered into a two-year study without regard to their baseline BMD. In the other study, 447 patients (FOSAMAX 5 mg/day; n=88), who were between six months and three years postmenopause, were treated for up to three years. In the placebo-treated patients BMD losses of approximately 1% per year were seen at the spine, hip (femoral neck and trochanter) and total body. In contrast, FOSAMAX 5 mg/day prevented bone loss in the majority of patients and induced significant increases in mean bone mass at each of these sites (see Figure 4). In addition, FOSAMAX 5 mg/day reduced the rate of bone loss at the forearm by approximately half relative to placebo. FOSAMAX 5 mg/day was similarly effective in this population regardless of age, time since menopause, race and baseline rate of bone turnover.

Figure 4:

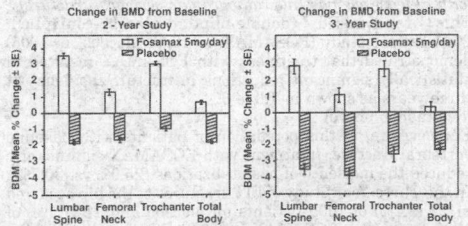

Osteoporosis Prevention Studies in Postmenopausal Women

Bone Histology
Bone histology was normal in the 28 patients biopsied at the end of three years who received FOSAMAX at doses of up to 10 mg/day.
Weekly Dosing
The therapeutic equivalence of once weekly FOSAMAX 35 mg (n=362) and FOSAMAX 5 mg daily (n=361) was demonstrated in a one-year, double-blind, multicenter study of postmenopausal women without osteoporosis. In the primary analysis of completers, the mean increases from baseline in lumbar spine BMD at one year were 2.9% (2.6, 3.2%; 95% CI) in the 35-mg once-weekly group (n=307) and 3.2% (2.9, 3.5%; 95% CI) in the 5-mg daily group (n=298). The two treatment groups were also similar with regard to BMD increases at other skeletal sites. The results of the intention-to-treat analysis were consistent with the primary analysis of completers.

14.3   Treatment to Increase Bone Mass in Men with Osteoporosis
The efficacy of FOSAMAX in men with hypogonadal or idiopathic osteoporosis was demonstrated in two clinical studies.

Daily Dosing
A two-year, double-blind, placebo-controlled, multicenter study of FOSAMAX 10 mg once daily enrolled a total of 241 men between the ages of 31 and 87 (mean, 63). All patients in the trial had either a BMD T-score less than or equal to -2 at the femoral neck and less than or equal to -1 at the lumbar spine, or a baseline osteoporotic fracture and a BMD T-score less than or equal to -1 at the femoral neck. At two years, the mean increases relative to placebo in BMD in men receiving FOSAMAX 10 mg/day were significant at the following sites: lumbar spine, 5.3%; femoral neck, 2.6%; trochanter, 3.1%; and total body, 1.6%. Treatment with FOSAMAX also reduced height loss (FOSAMAX, -0.6 mm vs. placebo, -2.4 mm).
Weekly Dosing
A one-year, double-blind, placebo-controlled, multicenter study of once weekly FOSAMAX 70 mg enrolled a total of 167 men between the ages of 38 and 91 (mean, 66). Patients in the study had either a BMD T-score less than or equal to -2 at the femoral neck and less than or equal to -1 at the lumbar spine, or a BMD T-score less than or equal to -2 at the lumbar spine and less than or equal to -1 at the femoral neck, or a baseline osteoporotic fracture and a BMD T-score less than or equal to -1 at the femoral neck. At one year, the mean increases relative to placebo in BMD in men receiving FOSAMAX 70 mg once weekly were significant at the following sites: lumbar spine, 2.8%; femoral neck, 1.9%; trochanter, 2.0%; and total body, 1.2%. These increases in BMD were similar to those seen at one year in the 10 mg once-daily study.
In both studies, BMD responses were similar regardless of age (greater than or equal to 65 years vs. less than 65 years), gonadal function (baseline testosterone less than 9 ng/dL vs. greater than or equal to 9 ng/dL), or baseline BMD (femoral neck and lumbar spine T-score less than or equal to -2.5 vs. greater than -2.5).

14.4   Treatment of Glucocorticoid-Induced Osteoporosis
The efficacy of FOSAMAX 5 and 10 mg once daily in men and women receiving glucocorticoids (at least 7.5 mg/day of prednisone or equivalent) was demonstrated in two, one-year, double-blind, randomized, placebo-controlled, multicenter studies of virtually identical design, one performed in the United States and the other in 15 different countries (Multinational [which also included FOSAMAX 2.5 mg/day]). These studies enrolled 232 and 328 patients, respectively, between the ages of 17 and 83 with a variety of glucocorticoid-requiring diseases. Patients received supplemental calcium and vitamin D. Figure 5 shows the mean increases relative to placebo in BMD of the lumbar spine, femoral neck, and trochanter in patients receiving FOSAMAX 5 mg/day for each study.

Figure 5:

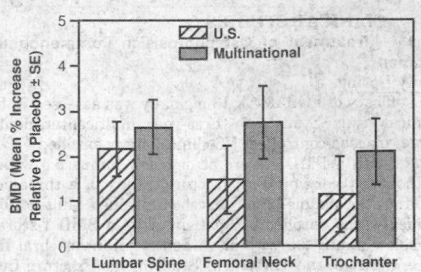

Studies in Glucocorticoid - Treated Patients
Increase in BMD
FOSAMAX 5 mg/day at One Year

After one year, significant increases relative to placebo in BMD were seen in the combined studies at each of these sites in patients who received FOSAMAX 5 mg/day. In the placebo-treated patients, a significant decrease in BMD occurred at the femoral neck (-1.2%), and smaller decreases were seen at the lumbar spine and trochanter. Total body BMD was maintained with FOSAMAX 5 mg/day. The increases in BMD with FOSAMAX 10 mg/day were similar to those with FOSAMAX 5 mg/day in all patients except for postmenopausal women not receiving estrogen therapy. In these women, the increases (relative to placebo) with FOSAMAX 10 mg/day were greater than those with FOSAMAX 5 mg/day at the lumbar spine (4.1% vs. 1.6%) and trochanter (2.8% vs. 1.7%), but not at other sites. FOSAMAX was effective regardless of dose or duration of glucocorticoid use. In addition, FOSAMAX was similarly effective regardless of age (less than 65 vs. greater than or equal to 65 years), race (Caucasian vs. other races), gender, underlying disease, baseline BMD, baseline bone turnover, and use with a variety of common medications.
Bone histology was normal in the 49 patients biopsied at the end of one year who received FOSAMAX at doses of up to 10 mg/day.

Of the original 560 patients in these studies, 208 patients who remained on at least 7.5 mg/day of prednisone or equivalent continued into a one-year double-blind extension. After two years of treatment, spine BMD increased by 3.7% and 5.0% relative to placebo with FOSAMAX 5 and 10 mg/day, respectively. Significant increases in BMD (relative to placebo) were also observed at the femoral neck, trochanter, and total body.

After one year, 2.3% of patients treated with FOSAMAX 5 or 10 mg/day (pooled) vs. 3.7% of those treated with placebo experienced a new vertebral fracture (not significant). However, in the population studied for two years, treatment with FOSAMAX (pooled dosage groups: 5 or 10 mg for two years or 2.5 mg for one year followed by 10 mg for one year) significantly reduced the incidence of patients with a new vertebral fracture (FOSAMAX 0.7% vs. placebo 6.8%).

14.5 Treatment of Paget's Disease of Bone

The efficacy of FOSAMAX 40 mg once daily for six months was demonstrated in two double-blind clinical studies of male and female patients with moderate to severe Paget's disease (alkaline phosphatase at least twice the upper limit of normal): a placebo-controlled, multinational study and a U.S. comparative study with etidronate disodium 400 mg/day. Figure 6 shows the mean percent changes from baseline in serum alkaline phosphatase for up to six months of randomized treatment.

Figure 6:

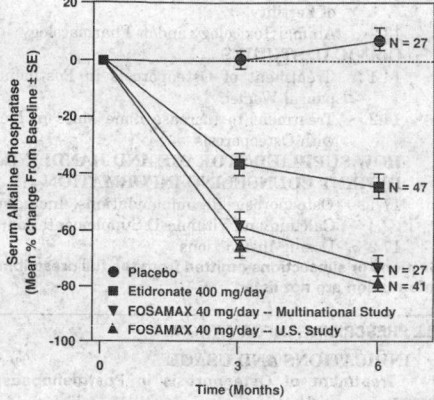

Studies in Paget's Disease of Bone

Effect on Serum Alkaline Phosphatase of FOSAMAX 40 mg/day
Versus Placebo or Etidronate 400 mg/day

At six months the suppression in alkaline phosphatase in patients treated with FOSAMAX was significantly greater than that achieved with etidronate and contrasted with the complete lack of response in placebo-treated patients. Response (defined as either normalization of serum alkaline phosphatase or decrease from baseline greater than or equal to 60%) occurred in approximately 85% of patients treated with FOSAMAX in the combined studies vs. 30% in the etidronate group and 0% in the placebo group. FOSAMAX was similarly effective regardless of age, gender, race, prior use of other bisphosphonates, or baseline alkaline phosphatase within the range studied (at least twice the upper limit of normal).

Bone histology was evaluated in 33 patients with Paget's disease treated with FOSAMAX 40 mg/day for 6 months. As in patients treated for osteoporosis *[see Clinical Studies (14.1)]*, FOSAMAX did not impair mineralization, and the expected decrease in the rate of bone turnover was observed. Normal lamellar bone was produced during treatment with FOSAMAX, even where preexisting bone was woven and disorganized. Overall, bone histology data support the conclusion that bone formed during treatment with FOSAMAX is of normal quality.

16 HOW SUPPLIED/STORAGE AND HANDLING

How Supplied
No. 3814 — FOSAMAX Tablets, 70 mg, are white, oval, uncoated tablets with code 31 on one side and an outline of a bone image on the other.
• **NDC** 0006-0031-44 unit-of-use blister package of 4.
Storage
FOSAMAX Tablets:
Store in a well-closed container at room temperature, 15-30°C (59-86°F).

17 PATIENT COUNSELING INFORMATION

See FDA-approved patient labeling (Medication Guide).
Instruct patients to read the Medication Guide before starting therapy with FOSAMAX and to reread it each time the prescription is renewed.

17.1 Osteoporosis Recommendations, Including Calcium and Vitamin D Supplementation

Instruct patients to take supplemental calcium and vitamin D, if daily dietary intake is inadequate. Weight-bearing exercise should be considered along with the modification of certain behavioral factors, such as cigarette smoking and/or excessive alcohol consumption, if these factors exist.

17.2 Dosing Instructions

Instruct patients that the expected benefits of FOSAMAX may only be obtained when it is taken with plain water the first thing upon arising for the day at least 30 minutes before the first food, beverage, or medication of the day. Even dosing with orange juice or coffee has been shown to markedly reduce the absorption of FOSAMAX *[see Clinical Pharmacology (12.3)]*.

Instruct patients not to chew or suck on the tablet because of a potential for oropharyngeal ulceration.

Instruct patients to swallow each tablet of FOSAMAX with a full glass of water (6-8 ounces) to facilitate delivery to the stomach and thus reduce the potential for esophageal irritation. Instruct patients to drink at least 2 ounces (a quarter of a cup) of water after taking FOSAMAX oral solution, to facilitate gastric emptying.

Instruct patients not to lie down for at least 30 minutes and until after their first food of the day.

Instruct patients not to take FOSAMAX at bedtime or before arising for the day. Patients should be informed that failure to follow these instructions may increase their risk of esophageal problems.

Instruct patients that if they develop symptoms of esophageal disease (such as difficulty or pain upon swallowing, retrosternal pain or new or worsening heartburn) they should stop taking FOSAMAX and consult their physician. If patients miss a dose of once weekly FOSAMAX, instruct patients to take one dose on the morning after they remember. They should not take two doses on the same day but should return to taking one dose once a week, as originally scheduled on their chosen day.

Distributed by:
Merck Sharp & Dohme Corp., a subsidiary of
MERCK & CO., INC., Whitehouse Station, NJ 08889, USA
Manufactured by:
Merck Sharp & Dohme Corp., a subsidiary of **Merck & Co., Inc.**
Whitehouse Station, NJ 08889, USA
FOSAMAX Tablets, 70 mg, are also manufactured by:
Merck Sharp & Dohme (Italia) S.p.A.
Via Emilia, 21, 27100 - Pavia, Italy
For patent information:
www.merck.com/product/patent/home.html
Copyright © 1995, 1997, 2000, 2010, 2012 Merck Sharp & Dohme Corp., a subsidiary of **Merck & Co., Inc.**
All rights reserved.
uspi-mk0217-mf-1405r019

MEDICATION GUIDE

FOSAMAX® (FOSS-ah-max)
(alendronate sodium)
Tablets
Read the Medication Guide that comes with FOSAMAX® before you start taking it and each time you get a refill. There may be new information. This Medication Guide does not take the place of talking with your doctor about your medical condition or treatment. Talk to your doctor if you have any questions about FOSAMAX.

What is the most important information I should know about FOSAMAX?
FOSAMAX can cause serious side effects including:
1. Esophagus problems
2. Low calcium levels in your blood (hypocalcemia)
3. Bone, joint, or muscle pain
4. Severe jaw bone problems (osteonecrosis)
5. Unusual thigh bone fractures

1. Esophagus problems.
   Some people who take FOSAMAX may develop problems in the esophagus (the tube that connects the mouth and the stomach). These problems include irritation, inflammation, or ulcers of the esophagus which may sometimes bleed.
   • It is important that you take FOSAMAX exactly as prescribed to help lower your chance of getting esophagus problems. (See the section "How should I take FOSAMAX?")
   • Stop taking FOSAMAX and call your doctor right away if you get chest pain, new or worsening heartburn, or have trouble or pain when you swallow.

2. Low calcium levels in your blood (hypocalcemia).
   FOSAMAX may lower the calcium levels in your blood. If you have low blood calcium before you start taking FOSAMAX, it may get worse during treatment. Your low blood calcium must be treated before you take FOSAMAX. Most people with low blood calcium levels do not have symptoms, but some people may have symptoms. Call your doctor right away if you have symptoms of low blood calcium such as:

• Spasms, twitches, or cramps in your muscles
• Numbness or tingling in your fingers, toes, or around your mouth
Your doctor may prescribe calcium and vitamin D to help prevent low calcium levels in your blood, while you take FOSAMAX. Take calcium and vitamin D as your doctor tells you to.

3. Bone, joint, or muscle pain.
Some people who take FOSAMAX develop severe bone, joint, or muscle pain.

4. Severe jaw bone problems (osteonecrosis).
Severe jaw bone problems may happen when you take FOSAMAX. Your doctor should examine your mouth before you start FOSAMAX. Your doctor may tell you to see your dentist before you start FOSAMAX. It is important for you to practice good mouth care during treatment with FOSAMAX.

5. Unusual thigh bone fractures.
Some people have developed unusual fractures in their thigh bone. Symptoms of a fracture may include new or unusual pain in your hip, groin, or thigh.

Call your doctor right away if you have any of these side effects.

What is FOSAMAX?
FOSAMAX is a prescription medicine used to:
• Treat or prevent osteoporosis in women after menopause. It helps reduce the chance of having a hip or spinal fracture (break).
• Increase bone mass in men with osteoporosis.
• Treat osteoporosis in either men or women who are taking corticosteroid medicines.
• Treat certain men and women who have Paget's disease of the bone.
It is not known how long FOSAMAX works for the treatment and prevention of osteoporosis. You should see your doctor regularly to determine if FOSAMAX is still right for you.
FOSAMAX is not for use in children.

Who should not take FOSAMAX?
Do not take FOSAMAX if you:
• Have certain problems with your esophagus, the tube that connects your mouth with your stomach
• Cannot stand or sit upright for at least 30 minutes
• Have low levels of calcium in your blood
• Are allergic to FOSAMAX or any of its ingredients. A list of ingredients is at the end of this leaflet.

What should I tell my doctor before taking FOSAMAX?
Before you start FOSAMAX, be sure to talk to your doctor if you:
• Have problems with swallowing
• Have stomach or digestive problems
• Have low blood calcium
• Plan to have dental surgery or teeth removed
• Have kidney problems
• Have been told you have trouble absorbing minerals in your stomach or intestines (malabsorption syndrome)
• Are pregnant, or plan to become pregnant. It is not known if FOSAMAX can harm your unborn baby.
• Are breast-feeding or plan to breast-feed. It is not known if FOSAMAX passes into your milk and may harm your baby.
Especially tell your doctor if you take:
• antacids
• aspirin
• Nonsteroidal Anti-Inflammatory (NSAID) medicines
Tell your doctor about all the medicines you take, including prescription and non-prescription medicines, vitamins, and herbal supplements. Certain medicines may affect how FOSAMAX works.
Know the medicines you take. Keep a list of them and show it to your doctor and pharmacist each time you get a new medicine.

How should I take FOSAMAX?
• Take FOSAMAX exactly as your doctor tells you.
• **FOSAMAX works only if taken on an empty stomach.**
• Take FOSAMAX, **after** you get up for the day and **before** taking your first food, drink, or other medicine.
• Take FOSAMAX while you are sitting or standing.
• **Do not chew or suck on a tablet of FOSAMAX.**
• Swallow FOSAMAX tablet with a full glass (6-8 oz) of plain water only.
• **Do not** take FOSAMAX with mineral water, coffee, tea, soda, or juice.
  • If you take **Alendronate Daily:**
    • Take 1 alendronate tablet one time a day, every day **after** you get up for the day and **before** taking your first food, drink, or other medicine.
  • If you take **Once Weekly FOSAMAX:**
    • Choose the day of the week that best fits your schedule.
    • Take 1 dose of FOSAMAX every week on your chosen day **after** you get up for the day and **before** taking your first food, drink, or other medicine.
After swallowing FOSAMAX tablet, wait at least 30 minutes:
• Before you lie down. You may sit, stand or walk, and do normal activities like reading.

- Before you take your first food or drink except for plain water.
- Before you take other medicines, including antacids, calcium, and other supplements and vitamins.

Do not lie down for at least 30 minutes after you take FOSAMAX and after you eat your first food of the day.
If you miss a dose of FOSAMAX, do not take it later in the day. Take your missed dose on the next morning after you remember and then return to your normal schedule. Do not take 2 doses on the same day.
If you take too much FOSAMAX, call your doctor. Do not try to vomit. Do not lie down.

What are the possible side effects of FOSAMAX?
FOSAMAX may cause serious side effects.
- See "What is the most important information I should know about FOSAMAX?"

The most common side effects of FOSAMAX are:
- Stomach area (abdominal) pain
- Heartburn
- Constipation
- Diarrhea
- Upset stomach
- Pain in your bones, joints, or muscles
- Nausea

You may get allergic reactions, such as hives or swelling of your face, lips, tongue, or throat.
Worsening of asthma has been reported.
Tell your doctor if you have any side effect that bothers you or that does not go away.
These are not all the possible side effects of FOSAMAX. For more information, ask your doctor or pharmacist.
Call your doctor for medical advice about side effects. You may report side effects to FDA at 1-800-FDA-1088.

How do I store FOSAMAX?
- Store FOSAMAX at room temperature, 59°F to 86°F (15°C to 30°C).
- Keep FOSAMAX in a tightly closed container.

Keep FOSAMAX and all medicines out of the reach of children.

General information about the safe and effective use of FOSAMAX.
Medicines are sometimes prescribed for purposes other than those listed in a Medication Guide. Do not use FOSAMAX for a condition for which it was not prescribed. Do not give FOSAMAX to other people, even if they have the same symptoms you have. It may harm them.
This Medication Guide summarizes the most important information about FOSAMAX. If you would like more information, talk with your doctor. You can ask your doctor or pharmacist for information about FOSAMAX that is written for health professionals. For more information, go to: www.FOSAMAX.com or call 1-800-622-4477 (toll-free).

What are the ingredients in FOSAMAX?
Tablets:
Active ingredient: alendronate sodium
Inactive ingredients: microcrystalline cellulose, anhydrous lactose, croscarmellose sodium, magnesium stearate.
Distributed by:
Merck Sharp & Dohme Corp., a subsidiary of
MERCK & CO., INC., Whitehouse Station, NJ 08889, USA
Manufactured by: Merck Sharp & Dohme Corp., a subsidiary of **Merck & Co., Inc.**
Whitehouse Station, NJ 08889, USA
FOSAMAX Tablets, 70 mg, are also manufactured by:
Merck Sharp & Dohme (Italia) S.p.A.
Via Emilia, 21, 27100 - Pavia, Italy
For patent information:
www.merck.com/product/patent/home.html
Copyright © 2010, 2012 Merck Sharp & Dohme Corp., a subsidiary of **Merck & Co., Inc.**
All rights reserved.
Revised: 12/2013
usmg-mk0217-mf-1312r017
This Medication Guide has been approved by the U.S. Food and Drug Administration.
Shown in Product Identification Guide, page 308

FOSAMAX® PLUS D   ℞
[FOSS-ah-max PLUS D]
(alendronate sodium/cholecalciferol) tablets

HIGHLIGHTS OF PRESCRIBING INFORMATION
These highlights do not include all the information needed to use FOSAMAX PLUS D safely and effectively. See full prescribing information for FOSAMAX PLUS D.
FOSAMAX® PLUS D
(alendronate sodium/cholecalciferol) tablets
Initial U.S. Approval: 2005

————INDICATIONS AND USAGE————
FOSAMAX PLUS D is a combination of a bisphosphonate and vitamin D indicated for:
- Treatment of osteoporosis in postmenopausal women (1.1)

- Treatment to increase bone mass in men with osteoporosis (1.2)
Limitations of use:
- FOSAMAX PLUS D alone should not be used to treat vitamin D deficiency. (1.3)
- Optimal duration of use has not been determined. For patients at low-risk for fracture, consider drug discontinuation after 3 to 5 years of use. (1.3)

————DOSAGE AND ADMINISTRATION————
- 70 mg alendronate/2800 international units vitamin D$_3$ or 70 mg alendronate/5600 international units vitamin D$_3$ tablet once weekly. (2.1, 2.2)
- Instruct patients to: (2.3)
  ○ Swallow tablets whole with 6-8 ounces plain water at least 30 minutes before the first food, drink, or medication of the day.
  ○ Not lie down for at least 30 minutes after taking FOSAMAX PLUS D and until after food.

————DOSAGE FORMS AND STRENGTHS————
Tablets: 70 mg/2800 international units and 70 mg/5600 international units (3)

————CONTRAINDICATIONS————
- Abnormalities of the esophagus which delay emptying such as stricture or achalasia (4, 5.1)
- Inability to stand/sit upright for at least 30 minutes (4, 5.1)
- Hypocalcemia (4, 5.2)
- Hypersensitivity to any component of this product (4, 6.2)

————WARNINGS AND PRECAUTIONS————
- *Upper Gastrointestinal Adverse Reactions* can occur. Instruct patients to follow dosing instructions. Discontinue if new or worsening symptoms occur. (5.1)
- *Hypocalcemia* can worsen and must be corrected prior to use. (5.2)
- *Severe Bone, Joint, Muscle Pain* may occur. Discontinue use if severe symptoms develop. (5.3)
- *Osteonecrosis of the Jaw* has been reported. (5.4)
- *Atypical Femur Fractures* have been reported. Patients with new thigh or groin pain should be evaluated to rule out an incomplete femoral fracture. (5.5)

————ADVERSE REACTIONS————
Most common adverse reactions (greater than or equal to 3%) for alendronate are: abdominal pain, acid regurgitation, constipation, diarrhea, dyspepsia, musculoskeletal pain, nausea. (6.1)
To report SUSPECTED ADVERSE REACTIONS, contact Merck Sharp & Dohme Corp., a subsidiary of Merck & Co., Inc., at 1-877-888-4231 or FDA at 1-800-FDA-1088 or www.fda.gov/medwatch.

————DRUG INTERACTIONS————
- Calcium supplements/antacids or oral medications containing multivalent cations interfere with absorption of alendronate. (2.3, 7.1)
- Use caution when co-prescribing aspirin/nonsteroidal anti-inflammatory drugs that may worsen gastrointestinal irritation. (7.2, 7.3)
- Some drugs may impair the absorption or increase the catabolism of cholecalciferol (vitamin D$_3$). Additional vitamin D supplementation should be considered. (7.4, 7.5, 12.3)

————USE IN SPECIFIC POPULATIONS————
- FOSAMAX PLUS D is not indicated for use in pediatric patients. (8.4)
- FOSAMAX PLUS D is not recommended in patients with severe renal impairment (creatinine clearance less than 35 mL/min). (5.6, 8.6)
See 17 for PATIENT COUNSELING INFORMATION and Medication Guide

Revised: 05/2014

FULL PRESCRIBING INFORMATION: CONTENTS*

FULL PRESCRIBING INFORMATION

1   INDICATIONS AND USAGE
1.1   Treatment of Osteoporosis in Postmenopausal Women
FOSAMAX® PLUS D is indicated for the treatment of osteoporosis in postmenopausal women. In postmenopausal women, FOSAMAX PLUS D increases bone mass and reduces the incidence of fractures, including those of the hip and spine (vertebral compression fractures). *[See Clinical Studies (14.1).]*
1.2   Treatment to Increase Bone Mass in Men with Osteoporosis
FOSAMAX PLUS D is indicated for treatment to increase bone mass in men with osteoporosis *[see Clinical Studies (14.2)].*
1.3   Important Limitations of Use
FOSAMAX PLUS D alone should not be used to treat vitamin D deficiency.
The optimal duration of use has not been determined. The safety and effectiveness of FOSAMAX PLUS D for the treatment of osteoporosis are based on clinical data of four years duration. All patients on bisphosphonate therapy should have the need for continued therapy re-evaluated on a periodic basis. Patients at low-risk for fracture should be considered for drug discontinuation after 3 to 5 years of use. Patients who discontinue therapy should have their risk for fracture re-evaluated periodically.

2   DOSAGE AND ADMINISTRATION
2.1   Treatment of Osteoporosis in Postmenopausal Women
The recommended dosage is one 70 mg alendronate/2800 international units vitamin D$_3$ or one 70 mg alendronate/5600 international units vitamin D$_3$ tablet once weekly. For most osteoporotic women, the appropriate dose is FOSAMAX PLUS D (70 mg alendronate/5600 international units vitamin D$_3$) once weekly.
2.2   Treatment to Increase Bone Mass in Men with Osteoporosis
The recommended dosage is one 70 mg alendronate/2800 international units vitamin D$_3$ or one 70 mg alendronate/5600 international units vitamin D$_3$ tablet once weekly. For most osteoporotic men, the appropriate dose is FOSAMAX PLUS D (70 mg alendronate/5600 international units vitamin D$_3$) once weekly.

2.3 Important Administration Instructions

Instruct patients to do the following:

• Take FOSAMAX PLUS D *at least* one-half hour before the first food, beverage, or medication of the day with plain water only *[see Patient Counseling Information (17.2)]*. Other beverages (including mineral water), food, and some medications are likely to reduce the absorption of alendronate *[see Drug Interactions (7.1)]*. Waiting less than 30 minutes, or taking FOSAMAX PLUS D with food, beverages (other than plain water) or other medications will lessen the effect of alendronate by decreasing its absorption into the body.

• Take FOSAMAX PLUS D upon arising for the day. To facilitate delivery to the stomach and thus reduce the potential for esophageal irritation, a FOSAMAX PLUS D tablet should be swallowed with a full glass of water (6-8 ounces). Patients should not lie down for at least 30 minutes and until after their first food of the day. FOSAMAX PLUS D should not be taken at bedtime or before arising for the day. Failure to follow these instructions may increase the risk of esophageal adverse experiences *[see Warnings and Precautions (5.1) and Patient Counseling Information (17.2)]*.

2.4 Recommendations for Calcium and Vitamin D Supplementation

Instruct patients to take supplemental calcium if dietary intake is inadequate *[see Warnings and Precautions (5.2)]*. Patients at increased risk for vitamin D insufficiency (e.g., over the age of 70 years, nursing home bound, or chronically ill) may need additional vitamin D supplementation. Patients with gastrointestinal malabsorption syndromes may require higher doses of vitamin D supplementation and measurement of 25-hydroxyvitamin D should be considered. The recommended intake of vitamin D is 400-800 international units daily. FOSAMAX PLUS D 70 mg/2800 international units and 70 mg/5600 international units are intended to provide seven days' worth of 400 or 800 international units daily vitamin D in a single, once-weekly dose, respectively.

2.5 Administration Instructions for Missed Doses

If a once-weekly dose of FOSAMAX PLUS D is missed, instruct patients to take one tablet on the morning after they remember. They should not take two tablets on the same day but should return to taking one tablet once a week, as originally scheduled on their chosen day.

3 DOSAGE FORMS AND STRENGTHS

• 70 mg/2800 international units tablets are white to off-white, modified capsule-shaped tablets with code 710 on one side and an outline of a bone image on the other.
• 70 mg/5600 international units tablets are white to off-white, modified rectangle-shaped tablets with code 270 on one side and an outline of a bone image on the other.

4 CONTRAINDICATIONS

FOSAMAX PLUS D is contraindicated in patients with the following conditions:

• Abnormalities of the esophagus which delay esophageal emptying such as stricture or achalasia *[see Warnings and Precautions (5.1)]*
• Inability to stand or sit upright for at least 30 minutes *[see Dosage and Administration (2.3), Warnings and Precautions (5.1)]*
• Hypocalcemia *[see Warnings and Precautions (5.2)]*
• Hypersensitivity to any component of this product. Hypersensitivity reactions including urticaria and angioedema have been reported *[see Adverse Reactions (6.2)]*.

5 WARNINGS AND PRECAUTIONS

5.1 Upper Gastrointestinal Adverse Reactions

FOSAMAX PLUS D, like other bisphosphonates administered orally, may cause local irritation of the upper gastrointestinal mucosa. Because of these possible irritant effects and a potential for worsening of the underlying disease, caution should be used when FOSAMAX PLUS D is given to patients with active upper gastrointestinal problems (such as known Barrett's esophagus, dysphagia, other esophageal diseases, gastritis, duodenitis, or ulcers).

Esophageal adverse experiences, such as esophagitis, esophageal ulcers and esophageal erosions, occasionally with bleeding and rarely followed by esophageal stricture or perforation, have been reported in patients receiving treatment with oral bisphosphonates including FOSAMAX PLUS D. In some cases these have been severe and required hospitalization. Physicians should therefore be alert to any signs or symptoms signaling a possible esophageal reaction and patients should be instructed to discontinue FOSAMAX PLUS D and seek medical attention if they develop dysphagia, odynophagia, retrosternal pain or new or worsening heartburn.

The risk of severe esophageal adverse experiences appears to be greater in patients who lie down after taking oral bisphosphonates including FOSAMAX PLUS D and/or who fail to swallow oral bisphosphonates including FOSAMAX PLUS D with the recommended full glass (6-8 ounces) of

water, and/or who continue to take oral bisphosphonates including FOSAMAX PLUS D after developing symptoms suggestive of esophageal irritation. Therefore, it is very important that the full dosing instructions are provided to, and understood by, the patient *[see Dosage and Administration (2.3)]*. In patients who cannot comply with dosing instructions due to mental disability, therapy with FOSAMAX PLUS D should be used under appropriate supervision.

There have been post-marketing reports of gastric and duodenal ulcers with oral bisphosphonate use, some severe and with complications, although no increased risk was observed in controlled clinical trials *[see Adverse Reactions (6.2)]*.

5.2 Mineral Metabolism

Alendronate Sodium

Hypocalcemia must be corrected before initiating therapy with FOSAMAX PLUS D *[see Contraindications (4)]*. Other disorders affecting mineral metabolism (such as vitamin D deficiency) should also be effectively treated. In patients with these conditions, serum calcium and symptoms of hypocalcemia should be monitored during therapy with FOSAMAX PLUS D.

Presumably due to the effects of alendronate on increasing bone mineral, small, asymptomatic decreases in serum calcium and phosphate may occur.

Cholecalciferol

FOSAMAX PLUS D alone should not be used to treat vitamin D deficiency (commonly defined as 25-hydroxyvitamin D level below 9 ng/mL). Patients at increased risk for vitamin D insufficiency may require higher doses of vitamin D supplementation *[see Dosage and Administration (2.4)]*. Patients with gastrointestinal malabsorption syndromes may require higher doses of vitamin D supplementation and measurement of 25-hydroxyvitamin D should be considered.

Vitamin D_3 supplementation may worsen hypercalcemia and/or hypercalciuria when administered to patients with diseases associated with unregulated overproduction of 1,25 dihydroxyvitamin D (e.g., leukemia, lymphoma, sarcoidosis). Urine and serum calcium should be monitored in these patients.

5.3 Musculoskeletal Pain

In post-marketing experience, severe and occasionally incapacitating bone, joint, and/or muscle pain has been reported in patients taking bisphosphonates that are approved for the prevention and treatment of osteoporosis *[see Adverse Reactions (6.2)]*. This category of drugs includes alendronate. Most of the patients were postmenopausal women. The time to onset of symptoms varied from one day to several months after starting the drug. Discontinue use if severe symptoms develop. Most patients had relief of symptoms after stopping. A subset had recurrence of symptoms when rechallenged with the same drug or another bisphosphonate.

In placebo-controlled clinical studies of FOSAMAX, the percentages of patients with these symptoms were similar in the FOSAMAX and placebo groups.

5.4 Osteonecrosis of the Jaw

Osteonecrosis of the jaw (ONJ), which can occur spontaneously, is generally associated with tooth extraction and/or local infection with delayed healing, and has been reported in patients taking bisphosphonates, including FOSAMAX PLUS D. Known risk factors for osteonecrosis of the jaw include invasive dental procedures (e.g., tooth extraction, dental implants, boney surgery), diagnosis of cancer, concomitant therapies (e.g., chemotherapy, corticosteroids), poor oral hygiene, and co-morbid disorders (e.g., periodontal and/or other pre-existing dental disease, anemia, coagulopathy, infection, ill-fitting dentures). The risk of ONJ may increase with duration of exposure to bisphosphonates.

For patients requiring invasive dental procedures, discontinuation of bisphosphonate treatment may reduce the risk for ONJ. Clinical judgment of the treating physician and/or oral surgeon should guide the management plan of each patient based on individual benefit/risk assessment.

Patients who develop osteonecrosis of the jaw while on bisphosphonate therapy should receive care by an oral surgeon. In these patients, extensive dental surgery to treat ONJ may exacerbate the condition. Discontinuation of bisphosphonate therapy should be considered based on individual benefit/risk assessment.

5.5 Atypical Subtrochanteric and Diaphyseal Femoral Fractures

Atypical, low-energy, or low trauma fractures of the femoral shaft have been reported in bisphosphonate-treated patients. These fractures can occur anywhere in the femoral shaft from just below the lesser trochanter to above the supracondylar flare and are transverse or short oblique in orientation without evidence of comminution. Causality has not been established as these fractures also occur in osteoporotic patients who have not been treated with bisphosphonates.

Atypical femur fractures most commonly occur with minimal or no trauma to the affected area. They may be bilateral and many patients report prodromal pain in the affected area, usually presenting as dull, aching thigh pain, weeks to months before a complete fracture occurs. A number of reports note that patients were also receiving treatment with glucocorticoids (e.g. prednisone) at the time of fracture.

Any patient with a history of bisphosphonate exposure who presents with thigh or groin pain should be suspected of having an atypical fracture and should be evaluated to rule out an incomplete femur fracture. Patients presenting with an atypical fracture should also be assessed for symptoms and signs of fracture in the contralateral limb. Interruption of bisphosphonate therapy should be considered, pending a risk/benefit assessment, on an individual basis.

5.6 Renal Impairment

FOSAMAX PLUS D is not recommended for patients with creatinine clearance less than 35 mL/min.

6 ADVERSE REACTIONS

6.1 Clinical Trials Experience

Because clinical trials are conducted under widely varying conditions, adverse reaction rates observed in the clinical

Table 1: Osteoporosis Treatment Studies in Postmenopausal Women Adverse Reactions Considered Possibly, Probably, or Definitely Drug Related by the Investigators and Reported in Greater Than or Equal to 1% of Patients

| | United States/Multinational Studies | | Fracture Intervention Trial | |
	FOSAMAX* % (n=196)	Placebo % (n=397)	FOSAMAX[†] % (n=3236)	Placebo % (n=3223)
Gastrointestinal				
abdominal pain	6.6	4.8	1.5	1.5
nausea	3.6	4.0	1.1	1.5
dyspepsia	3.6	3.5	1.1	1.2
constipation	3.1	1.8	0.0	0.2
diarrhea	3.1	1.8	0.6	0.3
flatulence	2.6	0.5	0.2	0.3
acid regurgitation	2.0	4.3	1.1	0.9
esophageal ulcer	1.5	0.0	0.1	0.1
vomiting	1.0	1.5	0.2	0.3
dysphagia	1.0	0.0	0.1	0.1
abdominal distention	1.0	0.8	0.0	0.0
gastritis	0.5	1.3	0.6	0.7
Musculoskeletal				
musculoskeletal (bone, muscle or joint) pain	4.1	2.5	0.4	0.3
muscle cramp	0.0	1.0	0.2	0.1
Nervous System/Psychiatric				
headache	2.6	1.5	0.2	0.2
dizziness	0.0	1.0	0.0	0.1
Special Senses				
taste perversion	0.5	1.0	0.1	0.0

* 10 mg/day for three years
† 5 mg/day for 2 years and 10 mg/day for either 1 or 2 additional years

trials of a drug cannot be directly compared to rates in the clinical trials of another drug and may not reflect the rates observed in clinical practice.

FOSAMAX
Treatment of Osteoporosis in Postmenopausal Women
FOSAMAX Daily
The safety of FOSAMAX in the treatment of postmenopausal osteoporosis was assessed in four clinical trials that enrolled 7453 women aged 44-84 years. Study 1 and Study 2 were identically designed, three-year, placebo-controlled, double-blind, multicenter studies (United States and Multinational; n=994); Study 3 was the three-year vertebral fracture cohort of the Fracture Intervention Trial [FIT] (n=2027); and Study 4 was the four-year clinical fracture cohort of FIT (n=4432). Overall, 3620 patients were exposed to placebo and 3432 patients exposed to FOSAMAX. Patients with pre-existing gastrointestinal disease and concomitant use of non-steroidal anti-inflammatory drugs were included in these clinical trials. In Study 1 and Study 2 all women received 500 mg elemental calcium as carbonate. In Study 3 and Study 4 all women with dietary calcium intake less than 1000 mg per day received 500 mg calcium and 250 international units Vitamin D per day.

Among patients treated with alendronate 10 mg or placebo in Study 1 and Study 2, and all patients in Study 3 and Study 4, the incidence of all-cause mortality was 1.8% in the placebo group and 1.8% in the FOSAMAX group. The incidence of serious adverse event was 30.7% in the placebo group and 30.9% in the FOSAMAX group. The percentage of patients who discontinued the study due to any clinical adverse event was 9.5% in the placebo group and 8.9% in the FOSAMAX group. Adverse reactions from these studies considered by the investigators as possibly, probably, or definitely drug related in greater than or equal to 1% of patients treated with either FOSAMAX or placebo are presented in Table 1.

[See table 1 at top of previous page]

Rash and erythema have occurred.

Gastrointestinal Adverse Reactions: One patient treated with FOSAMAX (10 mg/day), who had a history of peptic ulcer disease and gastrectomy and who was taking concomitant aspirin, developed an anastomotic ulcer with mild hemorrhage, which was considered drug related. Aspirin and FOSAMAX were discontinued and the patient recovered. In the Study 1 and Study 2 populations, 49-54% had a history of gastrointestinal disorders at baseline, and 54-89% used nonsteroidal anti-inflammatory drugs or aspirin at some time during the studies. *[See Warnings and Precautions (5.1).]*

Laboratory Test Findings: In double-blind, multicenter, controlled studies, asymptomatic, mild, and transient decreases in serum calcium and phosphate were observed in approximately 18% and 10%, respectively, of patients taking FOSAMAX versus approximately 12% and 3% of those taking placebo. However, the incidences of decreases in serum calcium to less than 8.0 mg/dL (2.0 mM) and serum phosphate to less than or equal to 2.0 mg/dL (0.65 mM) were similar in both treatment groups.

FOSAMAX Once-Weekly
The safety of FOSAMAX 70 mg once weekly for the treatment of postmenopausal osteoporosis was assessed in a one-year, double-blind, multicenter study comparing FOSAMAX 70 mg once weekly and FOSAMAX 10 mg daily. The overall safety and tolerability profiles of once weekly FOSAMAX 70 mg and FOSAMAX 10 mg daily were similar. The adverse reactions considered by the investigators as possibly, probably, or definitely drug related in greater than or equal to 1% of patients in either treatment group are presented in Table 2.

Table 2: Osteoporosis Treatment Studies in Postmenopausal Women Adverse Reactions Considered Possibly, Probably, or Definitely Drug Related by the Investigators and Reported in Greater Than or Equal to 1% of Patients

	Once Weekly FOSAMAX 70 mg % (n=519)	FOSAMAX 10 mg/day % (n=370)
Gastrointestinal		
abdominal pain	3.7	3.0
dyspepsia	2.7	2.2
acid regurgitation	1.9	2.4
nausea	1.9	2.4
abdominal distention	1.0	1.4
constipation	0.8	1.6
flatulence	0.4	1.6
gastritis	0.2	1.1
gastric ulcer	0.0	1.1

Table 3: Osteoporosis Studies in Men Adverse Reactions Considered Possibly, Probably, or Definitely Drug Related by the Investigators and Reported in Greater Than or Equal to 2% of Patients

	Two-year Study		One-year Study	
	FOSAMAX 10 mg/day % (n=146)	Placebo % (n=95)	Once Weekly FOSAMAX 70 mg % (n=109)	Placebo % (n=58)
Gastrointestinal				
acid regurgitation	4.1	3.2	0.0	0.0
flatulence	4.1	1.1	0.0	0.0
gastroesophageal reflux disease	0.7	3.2	2.8	0.0
dyspepsia	3.4	0.0	2.8	1.7
diarrhea	1.4	1.1	2.8	0.0
abdominal pain	2.1	1.1	0.9	3.4
nausea	2.1	0.0	0.0	0.0
Musculoskeletal				
musculoskeletal (bone, muscle, joint) pain	2.9	3.2		
muscle cramp	0.2	1.1		

Concomitant Use With Estrogen/Hormone Replacement Therapy
In two studies (of one and two years' duration) of postmenopausal osteoporotic women (total: n=853), the safety and tolerability profile of combined treatment with FOSAMAX 10 mg once daily and estrogen ± progestin (n=354) was consistent with those of the individual treatments.

Osteoporosis in Men
In two placebo-controlled, double-blind, multicenter studies in men (a two-year study of FOSAMAX 10 mg/day and a one-year study of once weekly FOSAMAX 70 mg) the rates of discontinuation of therapy due to any clinical adverse event were 2.7% for FOSAMAX 10 mg/day vs. 10.5% for placebo, and 6.4% for once weekly FOSAMAX 70 mg vs. 8.6% for placebo. The adverse reactions considered by the investigators as possibly, probably, or definitely drug related in greater than or equal to 2% of patients treated with either FOSAMAX or placebo are presented in Table 3.
[See table 3 above]

FOSAMAX PLUS D
In a fifteen-week double-blind, multinational study in osteoporotic postmenopausal women (n=682) and men (n=35), the safety profile of FOSAMAX PLUS D (70 mg/2800 international units) was similar to that of FOSAMAX once weekly 70 mg. In the 24-week double-blind extension study in women (n=619) and men (n=33), the safety profile of FOSAMAX PLUS D (70 mg/2800 international units) administered with an additional 2800 international units vitamin D_3 was similar to that of FOSAMAX PLUS D (70 mg/2800 international units).

6.2 Post-Marketing Experience
The following adverse reactions have been identified during post-approval use of FOSAMAX and FOSAMAX PLUS D. Because these reactions are reported voluntarily from a population of uncertain size, it is not always possible to reliably estimate their frequency or establish a causal relationship to drug exposure.
Body as a Whole: hypersensitivity reactions including urticaria and angioedema. Transient symptoms of myalgia, malaise, asthenia and rarely, fever have been reported with alendronate, typically in association with initiation of treatment. Symptomatic hypocalcemia has occurred, generally in association with predisposing conditions. Peripheral edema.
Gastrointestinal: esophagitis, esophageal erosions, esophageal ulcers, esophageal stricture or perforation, and oropharyngeal ulceration. Gastric or duodenal ulcers, some severe and with complications have also been reported *[see Dosage and Administration (2.3) and Warnings and Precautions (5.1)].*
Localized osteonecrosis of the jaw, generally associated with tooth extraction and/or local infection with delayed healing, has been reported *[see Warnings and Precautions (5.4)].*
Musculoskeletal: bone, joint, and/or muscle pain, occasionally severe, and incapacitating *[see Warnings and Precautions (5.3)];* joint swelling; low-energy femoral shaft and subtrochanteric fractures *[see Warnings and Precautions (5.5)].*
Nervous System: dizziness and vertigo.
Pulmonary: acute asthma exacerbations.
Skin: rash (occasionally with photosensitivity), pruritus, alopecia, severe skin reactions, including Stevens-Johnson syndrome and toxic epidermal necrolysis.
Special Senses: uveitis, scleritis or episcleritis.

7 DRUG INTERACTIONS
7.1 Calcium Supplements/Antacids
Co-administration of FOSAMAX PLUS D and calcium, antacids, or oral medications containing multivalent cations will interfere with absorption of alendronate. Therefore, instruct patients to wait at least one-half hour after taking FOSAMAX PLUS D before taking any other oral medications.
7.2 Aspirin
In clinical studies, the incidence of upper gastrointestinal adverse events was increased in patients receiving concomitant therapy with daily doses of FOSAMAX greater than 10 mg and aspirin-containing products.
7.3 Nonsteroidal Anti-Inflammatory Drugs
FOSAMAX PLUS D may be administered to patients taking nonsteroidal anti-inflammatory drugs (NSAIDs). In a 3-year, controlled, clinical study (n=2027) during which a majority of patients received concomitant NSAIDs, the incidence of upper gastrointestinal adverse events was similar in patients taking FOSAMAX 5 or 10 mg/day compared to those taking placebo. However, since NSAID use is associated with gastrointestinal irritation, caution should be used during concomitant use with FOSAMAX PLUS D.
7.4 Drugs that May Impair the Absorption of Cholecalciferol
Olestra, mineral oils, orlistat, and bile acid sequestrants (e.g., cholestyramine, colestipol) may impair the absorption of vitamin D. Additional vitamin D supplementation should be considered *[see Clinical Pharmacology (12.3)].*
7.5 Drugs that May Increase the Catabolism of Cholecalciferol
Anticonvulsants, cimetidine, and thiazides may increase the catabolism of vitamin D. Additional vitamin D supplementation should be considered *[see Clinical Pharmacology (12.3)].*

8 USE IN SPECIFIC POPULATIONS
8.1 Pregnancy
Pregnancy Category C:
There are no studies in pregnant women. FOSAMAX PLUS D should be used during pregnancy only if the potential benefit justifies the potential risk to the mother and fetus.
Alendronate Sodium
Bisphosphonates are incorporated into the bone matrix, from which they are gradually released over a period of years. The amount of bisphosphonate incorporated into adult bone, and hence, the amount available for release back into the systemic circulation, is directly related to the dose and duration of bisphosphonate use. There are no data on fetal risk in humans. However, there is a theoretical risk of fetal harm, predominantly skeletal, if a woman becomes pregnant after completing a course of bisphosphonate therapy. The impact of variables such as time between cessation of bisphosphonate therapy to conception, the particular bisphosphonate used, and the route of administration (intravenous versus oral) on the risk has not been studied.
Reproduction studies in rats showed decreased postimplantation survival and decreased body weight gain in normal pups at doses less than half of the recommended clinical dose. Sites of incomplete fetal ossification were statistically significantly increased in rats beginning at approximately 3 times the clinical dose in vertebral (cervical, thoracic, and lumbar), skull, and sternebral bones. No similar fetal effects were seen when pregnant rabbits were treated with doses approximately 10 times the clinical dose.
Both total and ionized calcium decreased in pregnant rats at approximately 4 times the clinical dose resulting in delays and failures of delivery. Protracted parturition due to maternal hypocalcemia occurred in rats at doses as low as one tenth the clinical dose when rats were treated from before mating through gestation. Maternotoxicity (late pregnancy deaths) also occurred in the female rats treated at approximately 4 times the clinical dose for varying periods of time ranging from treatment only during pre-mating to treatment only during early, middle, or late gestation; these deaths were lessened but not eliminated by cessation of treatment. Calcium supplementation either in the drinking water or by minipump could not ameliorate the hypocalcemia or prevent maternal and neonatal deaths due to delays in delivery; intravenous calcium supplementation prevented maternal, but not fetal deaths.

Cholecalciferol
No data are available for cholecalciferol (vitamin D_3). Administration of high doses (greater than or equal to 10,000 international units/every other day) of ergocalciferol (vitamin D_2) to pregnant rabbits resulted in abortions and an increased incidence of fetal aortic stenosis. Administration of vitamin D_2 (40,000 international units/day) to pregnant rats resulted in neonatal death, decreased fetal weight, and impaired osteogenesis of long bones postnatally.

8.3   Nursing Mothers
Cholecalciferol and some of its active metabolites pass into breast milk. It is not known whether alendronate is excreted in human milk. Because many drugs are excreted in human milk, caution should be exercised when FOSAMAX PLUS D is administered to nursing women.

8.4   Pediatric Use
FOSAMAX PLUS D is not indicated for use in pediatric patients.
The safety and efficacy of alendronate were examined in a randomized, double-blind, placebo-controlled two-year study of 139 pediatric patients, aged 4-18 years, with severe osteogenesis imperfecta (OI). One-hundred-and-nine patients were randomized to 5 mg alendronate daily (weight less than 40 kg) or 10 mg alendronate daily (weight greater than or equal to 40 kg) and 30 patients to placebo. The mean baseline lumbar spine BMD Z-score of the patients was -4.5. The mean change in lumbar spine BMD Z-score from baseline to Month 24 was 1.3 in the alendronate-treated patients and 0.1 in the placebo-treated patients. Treatment with alendronate did not reduce the risk of fracture. Sixteen percent of the alendronate patients who sustained a radiologically-confirmed fracture by Month 12 of the study had delayed fracture healing (callus remodeling) or fracture non-union when assessed radiographically at Month 24 compared with 9% of the placebo-treated patients. In alendronate-treated patients, bone histomorphometry data obtained at Month 24 demonstrated decreased bone turnover and delayed mineralization time; however, there were no mineralization defects. There were no statistically significant differences between the alendronate and placebo groups in reduction of bone pain. The oral bioavailability of alendronate in children was similar to that observed in adults.

8.5   Geriatric Use
Of the patients receiving FOSAMAX in the Fracture Intervention Trial (FIT), 71% (n=2302) were greater than or equal to 65 years of age and 17% (n=550) were greater than or equal to 75 years of age. Of the patients receiving FOSAMAX in the United States and Multinational osteoporosis treatment studies in women, and osteoporosis studies in men *[see Clinical Studies (14.1, 14.2)]*, 45% and 54%, respectively, were 65 years of age or over. No overall differences in efficacy or safety were observed between these patients and younger patients, but greater sensitivity of some older individuals cannot be ruled out. Dietary requirements of vitamin D_3 are increased in the elderly.

8.6   Renal Impairment
FOSAMAX PLUS D is not recommended for patients with creatinine clearance less than 35 mL/min. No dosage adjustment is necessary in patients with creatinine clearance values between 35-60 mL/min *[see Clinical Pharmacology (12.3)]*.

8.7   Hepatic Impairment
Alendronate Sodium
As there is evidence that alendronate is not metabolized or excreted in the bile, no studies were conducted in patients with hepatic impairment. No dosage adjustment is necessary *[see Clinical Pharmacology (12.3)]*.
Cholecalciferol
Vitamin D_3 may not be adequately absorbed in patients who have malabsorption due to inadequate bile production.

10   OVERDOSAGE
Alendronate Sodium
Significant lethality after single oral doses with alendronate was seen in female rats and mice at 552 mg/kg (3256 mg/m²) and 966 mg/kg (2898 mg/m²), respectively. In males, these values were slightly higher, 626 and 1280 mg/kg, respectively. There was no lethality in dogs at oral doses up to 200 mg/kg (4000 mg/m²).
No specific information is available on the treatment of overdosage with alendronate. Hypocalcemia, hypophosphatemia, and upper gastrointestinal adverse events, such as upset stomach, heartburn, esophagitis, gastritis, or ulcer, may result from oral overdosage. Milk or antacids should be given to bind alendronate. Due to the risk of esophageal irritation, vomiting should not be induced and the patient should remain fully upright.
Dialysis would not be beneficial.
Cholecalciferol
Significant lethality occurred in mice treated with a single high oral dose of calcitriol (4 mg/kg), the hormonal metabolite of cholecalciferol.

There is limited information regarding doses of cholecalciferol associated with acute toxicity, although intermittent (yearly or twice yearly) single doses of ergocalciferol (vitamin D_2) as high as 600,000 international units have been given without reports of toxicity. Signs and symptoms of vitamin D toxicity include hypercalcemia, hypercalciuria, anorexia, nausea, vomiting, polyuria, polydipsia, weakness, and lethargy. Serum and urine calcium levels should be monitored in patients with suspected vitamin D toxicity. Standard therapy includes restriction of dietary calcium, hydration, and systemic glucocorticoids in patients with severe hypercalcemia.
Dialysis to remove vitamin D would not be beneficial.

11   DESCRIPTION
FOSAMAX PLUS D contains alendronate sodium, a bisphosphonate, and cholecalciferol (vitamin D_3).
Alendronate sodium is a bisphosphonate that acts as a specific inhibitor of osteoclast-mediated bone resorption. Bisphosphonates are synthetic analogs of pyrophosphate that bind to the hydroxyapatite found in bone.
Alendronate sodium is chemically described as (4-amino-1-hydroxybutylidene) bisphosphonic acid monosodium salt trihydrate.
The empirical formula of alendronate sodium is $C_4H_{12}NNaO_7P_2 \cdot 3H_2O$ and its formula weight is 325.12. The structural formula is:

$$\begin{array}{c} NH_2 \\ | \\ CH_2 \\ | \\ CH_2 \\ | \\ O \quad CH_2 \quad O \\ \| \quad | \quad \| \\ HO-P-C-P-ONa \cdot 3H_2O \\ | \quad | \quad | \\ OH \quad OH \quad OH \end{array}$$

Alendronate sodium is a white, crystalline, nonhygroscopic powder. It is soluble in water, very slightly soluble in alcohol, and practically insoluble in chloroform.
Cholecalciferol (vitamin D_3) is a secosterol that is the natural precursor of the calcium-regulating hormone calcitriol (1,25 dihydroxyvitamin D_3).
The chemical name of cholecalciferol is $(3\beta,5Z,7E)$-9,10-secocholesta-5,7,10(19)-trien-3-ol. The empirical formula of cholecalciferol is $C_{27}H_{44}O$ and its molecular weight is 384.6. The structural formula is:

Cholecalciferol is a white, crystalline, odorless powder. Cholecalciferol is practically insoluble in water, freely soluble in usual organic solvents, and slightly soluble in vegetable oils.
FOSAMAX PLUS D for oral administration contains 91.37 mg of alendronate monosodium salt trihydrate, the molar equivalent of 70 mg of free acid, and 70 or 140 mcg of cholecalciferol, equivalent to 2800 or 5600 international units vitamin D, respectively. Each tablet contains the following inactive ingredients: microcrystalline cellulose, lactose anhydrous, medium chain triglycerides, gelatin, croscarmellose sodium, sucrose, colloidal silicon dioxide, magnesium stearate, butylated hydroxytoluene, modified food starch, and sodium aluminum silicate.

12   CLINICAL PHARMACOLOGY
12.1   Mechanism of Action
Alendronate Sodium
Animal studies have indicated the following mode of action. At the cellular level, alendronate shows preferential localization to sites of bone resorption, specifically under osteoclasts. The osteoclasts adhere normally to the bone surface but lack the ruffled border that is indicative of active resorption. Alendronate does not interfere with osteoclast recruitment or attachment, but it does inhibit osteoclast activity. Studies in mice on the localization of radioactive [³H]alendronate in bone showed about 10-fold higher uptake on osteoclast surfaces than on osteoblast surfaces. Bones examined 6 and 49 days after [³H]alendronate administration in rats and mice, respectively, showed that normal bone was formed on top of the alendronate, which was incorporated inside the matrix. While incorporated in bone matrix, alendronate is not pharmacologically active. Thus, alendronate must be continuously administered to suppress osteoclasts on newly formed resorption surfaces. Histomor-

phometry in baboons and rats showed that alendronate treatment reduces bone turnover (i.e., the number of sites at which bone is remodeled). In addition, bone formation exceeds bone resorption at these remodeling sites, leading to progressive gains in bone mass.
Cholecalciferol
Vitamin D_3 is produced in the skin by photochemical conversion of 7-dehydrocholesterol to previtamin D_3 by ultraviolet light. This is followed by non-enzymatic isomerization to vitamin D_3. In the absence of adequate sunlight exposure, vitamin D_3 is an essential dietary nutrient. Vitamin D_3 in skin and dietary vitamin D_3 (absorbed into chylomicrons) is converted to 25-hydroxyvitamin D_3 in the liver. Conversion to the active calcium-mobilizing hormone 1,25-dihydroxyvitamin D_3 (calcitriol) in the kidney is stimulated by both parathyroid hormone and hypophosphatemia. The principal action of 1,25-dihydroxyvitamin D_3 is to increase intestinal absorption of both calcium and phosphate as well as regulate serum calcium, renal calcium and phosphate excretion, bone formation and bone resorption.
Vitamin D is required for normal bone formation. Vitamin D insufficiency develops when both sunlight exposure and dietary intake are inadequate. Insufficiency is associated with negative calcium balance, increased parathyroid hormone levels, bone loss, and increased risk of skeletal fracture. In severe cases, deficiency results in more severe hyperparathyroidism, hypophosphatemia, proximal muscle weakness, bone pain and osteomalacia.

12.2   Pharmacodynamics
Alendronate Sodium
Alendronate is a bisphosphonate that binds to bone hydroxyapatite and specifically inhibits the activity of osteoclasts, the bone-resorbing cells. Alendronate reduces bone resorption with no direct effect on bone formation, although the latter process is ultimately reduced because bone resorption and formation are coupled during bone turnover.
Daily oral doses of alendronate (5, 20, and 40 mg for six weeks) in postmenopausal women produced biochemical changes indicative of dose-dependent inhibition of bone resorption, including decreases in urinary calcium and urinary markers of bone collagen degradation (such as deoxypyridinoline and cross-linked N-telopeptides of type I collagen). These biochemical changes tended to return toward baseline values as early as 3 weeks following the discontinuation of therapy with alendronate and did not differ from placebo after 7 months.
Long-term treatment of osteoporosis with FOSAMAX 10 mg/day (for up to five years) reduced urinary excretion of markers of bone resorption, deoxypyridinoline and cross-linked N-telopeptides of type I collagen, by approximately 50% and 70%, respectively, to reach levels similar to those seen in healthy premenopausal women. The decrease in the rate of bone resorption indicated by these markers was evident as early as one month and at three to six months reached a plateau that was maintained for the entire duration of treatment with FOSAMAX. In osteoporosis treatment studies FOSAMAX 10 mg/day decreased the markers of bone formation, osteocalcin and bone specific alkaline phosphatase by approximately 50%, and total serum alkaline phosphatase by approximately 25 to 30% to reach a plateau after 6 to 12 months. Similar reductions in the rate of bone turnover were observed in postmenopausal women during one-year studies with once weekly FOSAMAX 70 mg for the treatment of osteoporosis. These data indicate that the rate of bone turnover reached a new steady-state, despite the progressive increase in the total amount of alendronate deposited within bone.
As a result of inhibition of bone resorption, asymptomatic reductions in serum calcium and phosphate concentrations were also observed following treatment with FOSAMAX. In the long-term studies, reductions from baseline in serum calcium (approximately 2%) and phosphate (approximately 4 to 6%) were evident the first month after the initiation of FOSAMAX 10 mg. No further decreases in serum calcium were observed for the five-year duration of treatment; however, serum phosphate returned toward prestudy levels during years three through five. In one-year studies with once weekly FOSAMAX 70 mg, similar reductions were observed at 6 and 12 months. The reduction in serum phosphate may reflect not only the positive bone mineral balance due to FOSAMAX but also a decrease in renal phosphate reabsorption.
Osteoporosis in Men
Treatment of men with osteoporosis with FOSAMAX 10 mg/day for two years reduced urinary excretion of cross-linked N-telopeptides of type I collagen by approximately 60% and bone-specific alkaline phosphatase by approximately 40%. Similar reductions were observed in a one-year study in men with osteoporosis receiving once weekly FOSAMAX 70 mg.
Cholecalciferol
Vitamin D is required for normal bone formation. Vitamin D insufficiency is associated with negative calcium balance, leading to increased parathyroid hormone levels and worsening of bone loss associated with osteoporosis. When taken without vitamin D, alendronate is also associated with a re-

Table 4: 25-hydroxyvitamin D Levels after Treatment with FOSAMAX PLUS D (70 mg/2800 international units) or FOSAMAX 70 mg at Week 15*

25-hydroxyvitamin D Ranges (ng/mL)	<9	9-14	15-19	20-24	25-29	30-62
			Number (%) of Patients			
FOSAMAX PLUS D (70 mg/2800 international units) (N=357)	4 (1.1)	37 (10.4)	87 (24.4)	84 (23.5)	82 (23.0)	63 (17.7)
FOSAMAX 70 mg (N=351)	46 (13.1)	66 (18.8)	108 (30.8)	58 (16.5)	37 (10.5)	36 (10.3)

* Patients who were vitamin D deficient (25-hydroxyvitamin D less than 9 ng/mL) at baseline were excluded.

Table 5: 25-hydroxyvitamin D Levels after Treatment with FOSAMAX PLUS D at Week 39

25-hydroxyvitamin D Ranges (ng/mL)	<9	9-14	15-19	20-24	25-29	30-59
			Number (%) of Patients			
FOSAMAX PLUS D (Vitamin D_3 5600 international units group)* (N=321)	0	10 (3.1)	29 (9.0)	79 (24.6)	87 (27.1)	116 (36.1)
FOSAMAX PLUS D (Vitamin D_3 2800 international units group)† (N=320)	1 (0.3)	17 (5.3)	56 (17.5)	80 (25.0)	74 (23.1)	92 (28.8)

* Patients received FOSAMAX 70 mg or FOSAMAX PLUS D (70 mg/2800 international units) for the 15-week base study followed by FOSAMAX PLUS D (70 mg/2800 international units) and 2800 international units additional vitamin D_3 for the 24-week extension study.

† Patients received FOSAMAX 70 mg or FOSAMAX PLUS D (70 mg/2800 international units) for 15-week base study followed by FOSAMAX PLUS D (70 mg/2800 international units) and placebo for the additional vitamin D_3 for 24-week extension study.

duction in serum calcium concentrations and increased parathyroid hormone levels. In a 15-week trial, 717 postmenopausal women and men, mean age 67 years, with osteoporosis (lumbar spine bone mineral density [BMD] of at least 2.5 standard deviations below the premenopausal mean) were randomized to receive either weekly FOSAMAX PLUS D 70 mg/2800 international units vitamin D or weekly FOSAMAX 70 mg alone with no vitamin D supplementation. Patients who were vitamin D deficient (25-hydroxyvitamin D less than 9 ng/mL) at baseline were excluded. Treatment with FOSAMAX PLUS D 70 mg/2800 international units resulted in a smaller reduction in serum calcium levels (-0.9%) when compared to FOSAMAX 70 mg alone (-1.4%). As well, treatment with FOSAMAX PLUS D 70 mg/2800 international units resulted in a significantly smaller increase in parathyroid hormone levels when compared to FOSAMAX 70 mg alone (14% and 24%, respectively).

The sufficiency of patients' vitamin D status is best assessed by measuring 25-hydroxyvitamin D levels. In the 15-week trial mentioned above, baseline 25-hydroxyvitamin D levels were 22.2 ng/mL in the FOSAMAX PLUS D group and 22.1 ng/mL in the FOSAMAX only group. After 15 weeks of treatment, the mean levels were 23.1 ng/mL and 18.4 ng/mL in the FOSAMAX PLUS D and FOSAMAX only groups, respectively. The final levels of 25-hydroxyvitamin D at Week 15 are summarized in Table 4.
[See table 4 above]

Patients (n=652) who completed the above 15-week trial continued in a 24-week extension in which all received FOSAMAX PLUS D (70 mg/2800 international units) and were randomly assigned to receive either additional once weekly vitamin D_3 2800 international units (Vitamin D_3 5600 international units group) or matching placebo (Vitamin D_3 2800 international units group). After 24 weeks of extended treatment (Week 39 from original baseline), the mean levels of 25-hydroxyvitamin D were 27.9 ng/mL and 25.6 ng/mL in the vitamin D_3 5600 international units group and vitamin D_3 2800 international units group, respectively. The percentage of patients with hypercalciuria at Week 39 was not statistically different between treatment groups.

The distribution of the final levels of 25-hydroxyvitamin D at Week 39 is summarized in Table 5.
[See table 5 above]

12.3 Pharmacokinetics

Absorption
Alendronate Sodium
Relative to an intravenous reference dose, the mean oral bioavailability of alendronate in women was 0.64% for doses ranging from 5 to 70 mg when administered after an overnight fast and two hours before a standardized breakfast. Oral bioavailability of the 10-mg tablet in men (0.59%) was similar to that in women when administered after an overnight fast and 2 hours before breakfast.

In a study, the alendronate in the FOSAMAX PLUS D (70 mg/2800 international units) tablet and the FOSAMAX (alendronate sodium) 70-mg tablet were found to be equally bioavailable. In a separate study, the alendronate in the FOSAMAX PLUS D (70 mg/5600 international units) tablet was found to be equally bioavailable to the alendronate in the FOSAMAX (alendronate sodium) 70-mg tablet.

A study examining the effect of timing of a meal on the bioavailability of alendronate was performed in 49 postmenopausal women. Bioavailability was decreased (by approximately 40%) when 10 mg alendronate was administered either 0.5 or 1 hour before a standardized breakfast, when compared to dosing 2 hours before eating. In studies of treatment and prevention of osteoporosis, alendronate was effective when administered at least 30 minutes before breakfast.

Bioavailability was negligible whether alendronate was administered with or up to two hours after a standardized breakfast. Concomitant administration of alendronate with coffee or orange juice reduced bioavailability by approximately 60%.

Cholecalciferol
Following administration of FOSAMAX PLUS D (70 mg/2800 international units) after an overnight fast and two hours before a standard meal, the baseline adjusted mean area under the serum-concentration-time curve ($AUC_{0-120 hrs}$) for vitamin D_3 was 120.7 ng-hr/mL. The baseline adjusted mean maximal serum concentration (C_{max}) of vitamin D_3 was 4.0 ng/mL, and the baseline adjusted mean time to maximal serum concentration (T_{max}) was 10.6 hrs. The bioavailability of the 2800 international units vitamin D_3 in FOSAMAX PLUS D is similar to 2800 international units vitamin D_3 administered alone.

In a separate study, the baseline adjusted mean $AUC_{0-80 hrs}$ and baseline adjusted mean C_{max} for vitamin D_3 were 355.6 ng-hr/mL and 10.8 ng/mL, respectively. The baseline adjusted mean T_{max} was 9.2 hrs. The bioavailability of the 5600 international units vitamin D_3 in the FOSAMAX PLUS D is similar to 5600 international units vitamin D_3 administered as two 2800 international units vitamin D_3 tablets.

Distribution
Alendronate Sodium
Preclinical studies (in male rats) show that alendronate transiently distributes to soft tissues following 1 mg/kg intravenous administration but is then rapidly redistributed to bone or excreted in the urine. The mean steady-state volume of distribution, exclusive of bone, is at least 28 L in humans. Concentrations of drug in plasma following therapeutic oral doses are too low (less than 5 ng/mL) for analytical detection. Protein binding in human plasma is approximately 78%.

Cholecalciferol
Following absorption, vitamin D_3 enters the blood as part of chylomicrons. Vitamin D_3 is rapidly distributed mostly to the liver where it undergoes metabolism to 25-hydroxyvitamin D_3, the major storage form. Lesser amounts are distributed to adipose tissue and stored as vitamin D_3 at these sites for later release into the circulation. Circulating vitamin D_3 is bound to vitamin D-binding protein.

Metabolism
Alendronate Sodium
There is no evidence that alendronate is metabolized in animals or humans.

Cholecalciferol
Vitamin D_3 is rapidly metabolized by hydroxylation in the liver to 25-hydroxyvitamin D_3, and subsequently metabolized in the kidney to 1,25-dihydroxyvitamin D_3, which represents the biologically active form. Further hydroxylation occurs prior to elimination. A small percentage of vitamin D_3 undergoes glucuronidation prior to elimination.

Excretion
Alendronate Sodium
Following a single intravenous dose of [^{14}C]alendronate, approximately 50% of the radioactivity was excreted in the urine within 72 hours and little or no radioactivity was recovered in the feces. Following a single 10-mg intravenous dose, the renal clearance of alendronate was 71 mL/min (64, 78; 90% confidence interval [CI]), and systemic clearance did not exceed 200 mL/min. Plasma concentrations fell by more than 95% within 6 hours following intravenous administration. The terminal half-life in humans is estimated to exceed 10 years, probably reflecting release of alendronate from the skeleton. Based on the above, it is estimated that after 10 years of oral treatment with FOSAMAX (10 mg daily) the amount of alendronate released daily from the skeleton is approximately 25% of that absorbed from the gastrointestinal tract.

Cholecalciferol
When radioactive vitamin D_3 was intravenously administered to healthy subjects, the mean urinary excretion of radioactivity after 48 hours was 2.4% of the administered dose, and the mean fecal excretion of radioactivity after 48 hours was 4.9% of the administered dose. In both cases, the excreted radioactivity was almost exclusively as metabolites of the parent. The mean half-life of baseline adjusted vitamin D_3 in the serum following an oral dose of FOSAMAX PLUS D is approximately 14 hours.

Specific Populations
Gender: Bioavailability and the fraction of an intravenous dose of alendronate excreted in urine were similar in men and women.

Geriatric:
Alendronate Sodium
Bioavailability and disposition of alendronate (urinary excretion) were similar in elderly and younger patients. No dosage adjustment of alendronate is necessary.

Cholecalciferol
Dietary requirements of vitamin D_3 are increased in the elderly.

Race: Pharmacokinetic differences due to race have not been studied.

Renal Impairment:
Alendronate Sodium
Preclinical studies show that, in rats with kidney failure, increasing amounts of drug are present in plasma, kidney, spleen, and tibia. In healthy controls, drug that is not deposited in bone is rapidly excreted in the urine. No evidence of saturation of bone uptake was found after 3 weeks dosing with cumulative intravenous doses of 35 mg/kg in young male rats. Although no formal renal impairment pharmacokinetic study has been conducted in patients, it is likely that, as in animals, elimination of alendronate via the kidney will be reduced in patients with impaired renal function. Therefore, somewhat greater accumulation of alendronate in bone might be expected in patients with impaired renal function.

No dosage adjustment is necessary for patients with creatinine clearance 35 to 60 mL/min. FOSAMAX PLUS D is not recommended for patients with creatinine clearance less than 35 mL/min due to lack of experience with alendronate in renal failure.

Cholecalciferol
Patients with renal insufficiency will have decreased ability to form the active 1,25-dihydroxyvitamin D_3 metabolite.

Hepatic Impairment:
Alendronate Sodium
As there is evidence that alendronate is not metabolized or excreted in the bile, no studies were conducted in patients with hepatic impairment. No dosage adjustment is necessary.

Cholecalciferol
Vitamin D_3 may not be adequately absorbed in patients who have malabsorption due to inadequate bile production.

Drug Interactions
Alendronate Sodium
Intravenous ranitidine was shown to double the bioavailability of oral alendronate. The clinical significance of this

increased bioavailability and whether similar increases will occur in patients given oral H_2-antagonists is unknown.

In healthy subjects, oral prednisone (20 mg three times daily for five days) did not produce a clinically meaningful change in the oral bioavailability of alendronate (a mean increase ranging from 20 to 44%).

Products containing calcium and other multivalent cations are likely to interfere with absorption of alendronate.

Cholecalciferol

Olestra, mineral oils, orlistat, and bile acid sequestrants (e.g., cholestyramine, colestipol) may impair the absorption of vitamin D. Anticonvulsants, cimetidine, and thiazides may increase the catabolism of vitamin D.

13 NONCLINICAL TOXICOLOGY

13.1 Carcinogenesis, Mutagenesis, Impairment of Fertility

The following data are based on findings for the individual components of FOSAMAX PLUS D.

Alendronate Sodium

Harderian gland (a retro-orbital gland not present in humans) adenomas were increased in high-dose female mice (p=0.003) in a 92-week oral carcinogenicity study at doses of alendronate of 1, 3, and 10 mg/kg/day (males) or 1, 2, and 5 mg/kg/day (females). These doses are equivalent to 0.5 to 4 times a maximum recommended daily dose of 10 mg based on surface area, mg/m². The relevance of this finding to humans is unknown.

Parafollicular cell (thyroid) adenomas were increased in high-dose male rats (p=0.003) in a 2-year oral carcinogenicity study at doses of 1 and 3.75 mg/kg body weight. These doses are equivalent to 1 and 4 times a 10-mg human daily dose based on surface area, mg/m². The relevance of this finding to humans is unknown.

Alendronate was not genotoxic in the *in vitro* microbial mutagenesis assay with and without metabolic activation, in an *in vitro* mammalian cell mutagenesis assay, in an *in vitro* alkaline elution assay in rat hepatocytes, and in an *in vivo* chromosomal aberration assay in mice. In an *in vitro* chromosomal aberration assay in Chinese hamster ovary cells, however, alendronate gave equivocal results.

Alendronate had no effect on fertility (male or female) in rats at oral doses up to 5 mg/kg/day (4 times a 10-mg human daily dose based on surface area, mg/m²).

Cholecalciferol

The carcinogenic potential of cholecalciferol (vitamin D_3) has not been studied in rodents. Calcitriol, the hormonal metabolite of cholecalciferol, was not genotoxic in the Ames microbial mutagenesis assay with or without metabolic activation, and in an *in vivo* micronucleus assay in mice.

Ergocalciferol (vitamin D_2) at high doses (150,000 to 200,000 international units/kg/day) administered prior to mating resulted in altered estrous cycle and inhibition of pregnancy in rats. The potential effect of cholecalciferol on male fertility is unknown in rats.

13.2 Animal Toxicology and/or Pharmacology

The relative inhibitory activities on bone resorption and mineralization of alendronate and etidronate were compared in the Schenk assay, which is based on histological examination of the epiphyses of growing rats. In this assay, the lowest dose of alendronate that interfered with bone mineralization (leading to osteomalacia) was 6000-fold the antiresorptive dose. The corresponding ratio for etidronate was one to one. These data suggest that alendronate administered in therapeutic doses is highly unlikely to induce osteomalacia.

14 CLINICAL STUDIES

14.1 Treatment of Osteoporosis in Postmenopausal Women

FOSAMAX Daily

The efficacy of FOSAMAX 10 mg daily was assessed in four clinical trials. Study 1, a three-year, multicenter, double-blind, placebo-controlled, US clinical study enrolled 478 patients with a BMD T-score at or below minus 2.5 with or without a prior vertebral fracture; Study 2, a three-year, multicenter, double-blind, placebo-controlled, Multinational clinical study enrolled 516 patients with a BMD T-score at or below minus 2.5 with or without a prior vertebral fracture; Study 3, the Three-Year Study of the Fracture Intervention Trial (FIT), a study which enrolled 2027 postmenopausal patients with at least one baseline vertebral fracture; and Study 4, the Four-Year Study of FIT, a study which enrolled 4432 postmenopausal patients with low bone mass but without a baseline vertebral fracture.

Effect on Fracture Incidence

To assess the effects of FOSAMAX on the incidence of vertebral fractures (detected by digitized radiography; approximately one third of these were clinically symptomatic), the U.S. and Multinational studies were combined in an analysis that compared placebo to the pooled dosage groups of FOSAMAX (5 or 10 mg for three years or 20 mg for two years followed by 5 mg for one year). There was a statistically significant reduction in the proportion of patients treated with FOSAMAX experiencing one or more new ver-

Table 6: Effect of FOSAMAX on Fracture Incidence in the Three-Year Study of FIT (patients with vertebral fracture at baseline)

	Percent of Patients		Absolute Reduction in Fracture Incidence	Relative Reduction in Fracture Risk %
	FOSAMAX (n=1022)	Placebo (n=1005)		
Patients with:				
Vertebral fractures (diagnosed by X-ray)*				
≥1 new vertebral fracture	7.9	15.0	7.1	47[†]
≥2 new vertebral fractures	0.5	4.9	4.4	90[†]
Clinical (symptomatic) fractures				
Any clinical (symptomatic) fracture	13.8	18.1	4.3	26[‡]
≥1 clinical (symptomatic) vertebral fracture	2.3	5.0	2.7	54[§]
Hip fracture	1.1	2.2	1.1	51[¶]
Wrist (forearm) fracture	2.2	4.1	1.9	48[¶]

* Number evaluable for vertebral fractures: FOSAMAX, n=984; placebo, n=966
[†] p<0.001
[‡] p=0.007
[§] p<0.01
[¶] p<0.05

Table 7: Effect of FOSAMAX on Fracture Incidence in Osteoporotic* Patients in the Four-Year Study of FIT (patients without vertebral fracture at baseline)

	Percent of Patients		Absolute Reduction in Fracture Incidence	Relative Reduction in Fracture Risk (%)
	FOSAMAX (n=1545)	Placebo (n=1521)		
Patients with:				
Vertebral fractures (diagnosed by X-ray)[†]				
≥1 new vertebral fracture	2.5	4.8	2.3	48[‡]
≥2 new vertebral fractures	0.1	0.6	0.5	78[§]
Clinical (symptomatic) fractures				
Any clinical (symptomatic) fracture	12.9	16.2	3.3	22[¶]
≥1 clinical (symptomatic) vertebral fracture	1.0	1.6	0.6	41 (NS)[#]
Hip fracture	1.0	1.4	0.4	29 (NS)[#]
Wrist (forearm) fracture	3.9	3.8	-0.1	NS[#]

* Baseline femoral neck BMD at least 2 SD below the mean for young adult women
[†] Number evaluable for vertebral fractures: FOSAMAX, n=1426; placebo, n=1428
[‡] p<0.001
[§] p=0.035
[¶] p=0.01
[#] Not significant. This study was not powered to detect differences at these sites.

tebral fractures relative to those treated with placebo (3.2% vs. 6.2%; a 48% relative risk reduction). A reduction in the total number of new vertebral fractures (4.2 vs. 11.3 per 100 patients) was also observed. In the pooled analysis, patients who received FOSAMAX had a loss in stature that was statistically significantly less than was observed in those who received placebo (-3.0 mm vs. -4.6 mm).

The Fracture Intervention Trial (FIT) consisted of two studies in postmenopausal women: the Three-Year Study of patients who had at least one baseline radiographic vertebral fracture and the Four-Year Study of patients with low bone mass but without a baseline vertebral fracture. In both studies of FIT, 96% of randomized patients completed the studies (i.e., had a closeout visit at the scheduled end of the study); approximately 80% of patients were still taking study medication upon completion.

Fracture Intervention Trial: Three-Year Study (patients with at least one baseline radiographic vertebral fracture)

This randomized, double-blind, placebo-controlled, 2027-patient study (FOSAMAX, n=1022; placebo, n=1005) demonstrated that treatment with FOSAMAX resulted in statistically significant reductions in fracture incidence at three years as shown in Table 6.

[See table 6 above]

Furthermore, in this population of patients with baseline vertebral fracture, treatment with FOSAMAX significantly reduced the incidence of hospitalizations (25.0% vs. 30.7%). In the Three-Year Study of FIT, fractures of the hip occurred in 22 (2.2%) of 1005 patients on placebo and 11 (1.1%) of 1022 patients on FOSAMAX, p=0.047. Figure 1 displays the cumulative incidence of hip fractures in this study.

[See figure 1 at top of next column]

Fracture Intervention Trial: Four-Year Study (patients with low bone mass but without a baseline radiographic vertebral fracture)

This randomized, double-blind, placebo-controlled, 4432-patient study (FOSAMAX, n=2214; placebo, n=2218) further investigated the reduction in fracture incidence due to FOSAMAX. The intent of the study was to recruit women with osteoporosis, defined as a baseline femoral neck BMD at least two standard deviations below the mean for young adult women. However, due to subsequent revisions to the

Figure 1: **Cumulative Incidence of Hip Fractures in the Three-Year Study of FIT (patients with radiographic vertebral fracture at baseline)**

normative values for femoral neck BMD, 31% of patients were found not to meet this entry criterion and thus this study included both osteoporotic and non-osteoporotic women. The results are shown in Table 7 below for the patients with osteoporosis.

[See table 7 above]

Fracture Results Across Studies

In the Three-Year Study of FIT, FOSAMAX reduced the percentage of women experiencing at least one new radiographic vertebral fracture from 15.0% to 7.9% (47% relative risk reduction, p<0.001); in the Four-Year Study of FIT, the percentage was reduced from 3.8% to 2.1% (44% relative risk reduction, p=0.001); and in the combined U.S./Multinational studies, from 6.2% to 3.2% (48% relative risk reduction, p=0.034).

FOSAMAX reduced the percentage of women experiencing multiple (two or more) new vertebral fractures from 4.2% to 0.6% (87% relative risk reduction, p<0.001) in the combined U.S./Multinational studies and from 4.9% to 0.5% (90% relative risk reduction, p<0.001) in the Three-Year Study of FIT. In the Four-Year Study of FIT, FOSAMAX reduced the percentage of osteoporotic women experiencing multiple vertebral fractures from 0.6% to 0.1% (78% relative risk reduction, p=0.035).

Thus, FOSAMAX reduced the incidence of radiographic vertebral fractures in osteoporotic women whether or not they had a previous radiographic vertebral fracture.

Effect on Bone Mineral Density

The bone mineral density efficacy of FOSAMAX 10 mg once daily in postmenopausal women, 44 to 84 years of age, with osteoporosis (lumbar spine bone mineral density [BMD] of at least 2 standard deviations below the premenopausal mean) was demonstrated in four double-blind, placebo-controlled clinical studies of two or three years' duration. Figure 2 shows the mean increases in BMD of the lumbar spine, femoral neck, and trochanter in patients receiving FOSAMAX 10 mg/day relative to placebo-treated patients at three years for each of these studies.

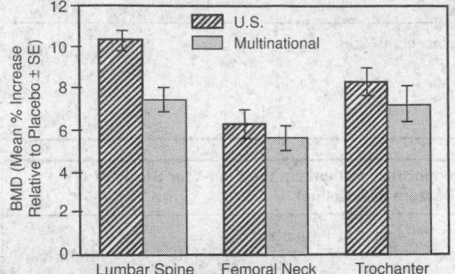

Figure 2: Osteoporosis Treatment Studies in Postmenopausal Women: Increase in BMD: FOSAMAX 10 mg/day at Three Years

At three years significant increases in BMD, relative both to baseline and placebo, were seen at each measurement site in each study in patients who received FOSAMAX 10 mg/day. Total body BMD also increased significantly in each study, suggesting that the increases in bone mass of the spine and hip did not occur at the expense of other skeletal sites. Increases in BMD were evident as early as three months and continued throughout the three years of treatment. (See figure 3 for lumbar spine results.) In the two-year extension of these studies, treatment of 147 patients with FOSAMAX 10 mg/day resulted in continued increases in BMD at the lumbar spine and trochanter (absolute additional increases between years 3 and 5: lumbar spine, 0.94%; trochanter, 0.88%). BMD at the femoral neck, forearm and total body were maintained. FOSAMAX was similarly effective regardless of age, race, baseline rate of bone turnover, and baseline BMD in the range studied (at least 2 standard deviations below the premenopausal mean).

Figure 3: Osteoporosis Treatment Studies in Postmenopausal Women: Time Course of Effect of FOSAMAX 10 mg/day Versus Placebo: Lumbar Spine BMD Percent Change From Baseline

In patients with postmenopausal osteoporosis treated with FOSAMAX 10 mg/day for one or two years, the effects of treatment withdrawal were assessed. Following discontinuation, there were no further increases in bone mass and the rates of bone loss were similar to those of the placebo groups.

Bone Histology

Bone histology in 270 postmenopausal patients with osteoporosis treated with FOSAMAX at doses ranging from 1 to 20 mg/day for one, two, or three years revealed normal mineralization and structure, as well as the expected decrease in bone turnover relative to placebo. These data, together with the normal bone histology and increased bone strength observed in rats and baboons exposed to long-term alendronate treatment, support the conclusion that bone formed during therapy with FOSAMAX is of normal quality.

Effect on Height

FOSAMAX, over a three- or four-year period, was associated with statistically significant reductions in loss of height vs. placebo in patients with and without radiographic vertebral fractures. At the end of the FIT studies, the between-treatment group differences were 3.2 mm in the Three-Year Study and 1.3 mm in the Four-Year Study.

FOSAMAX Once-Weekly

The therapeutic equivalence of once-weekly FOSAMAX 70 mg (n=519) and FOSAMAX 10 mg daily (n=370) was demonstrated in a one-year, double-blind, multicenter study of postmenopausal women with osteoporosis. In the primary analysis of completers, the mean increases from baseline in lumbar spine BMD at one year were 5.1% (4.8, 5.4%; 95% CI) in the 70-mg once-weekly group (n=440) and 5.4% (5.0, 5.8%; 95% CI) in the 10-mg daily group (n=330). The two treatment groups were also similar with regard to BMD increases at other skeletal sites. The results of the intention-to-treat analysis were consistent with the primary analysis of completers.

Concomitant Use with Estrogen Hormone Replacement Therapy

The effects on BMD of treatment with FOSAMAX 10 mg once daily and conjugated estrogen (0.625 mg/day) either alone or in combination were assessed in a two-year, double-blind, placebo-controlled study of hysterectomized postmenopausal osteoporotic women (n=425). At two years, the increases in lumbar spine BMD from baseline were significantly greater with the combination (8.3%) than with either estrogen or FOSAMAX alone (both 6.0%).

The effects on BMD when FOSAMAX was added to stable doses (for at least one year) of HRT (estrogen ± progestin) were assessed in a one-year, double-blind, placebo-controlled study in postmenopausal osteoporotic women (n=428). The addition of FOSAMAX 10 mg once daily to HRT produced, at one year, significantly greater increases in lumbar spine BMD (3.7%) than HRT alone (1.1%).

In these studies, significant increases or favorable trends in BMD for combined therapy compared with HRT alone were seen at the total hip, femoral neck, and trochanter. No significant effect was seen for total body BMD.

Histomorphometric studies of transiliac biopsies in 92 subjects showed normal bone architecture. Compared to placebo there was a 98% suppression of bone turnover (as assessed by mineralizing surface) after 18 months of combined treatment with FOSAMAX and HRT, 94% on FOSAMAX alone, and 78% on HRT alone. The long-term effects of combined FOSAMAX and HRT on fracture occurrence and fracture healing have not been studied.

14.2 Treatment to Increase Bone Mass in Men with Osteoporosis

The efficacy of FOSAMAX in men with hypogonadal or idiopathic osteoporosis was demonstrated in two clinical studies.

FOSAMAX Daily

A two-year, double-blind, placebo-controlled, multicenter study of FOSAMAX 10 mg once daily enrolled a total of 241 men between the ages of 31 and 87 (mean, 63). All patients in the trial had either a BMD T-score less than or equal to -2 at the femoral neck and less than or equal to -1 at the lumbar spine, or a baseline osteoporotic fracture and a BMD T-score less than or equal to -1 at the femoral neck. At two years, the mean increases relative to placebo in BMD in men receiving FOSAMAX 10 mg/day were significant at the following sites: lumbar spine, 5.3%; femoral neck, 2.6%; trochanter, 3.1%; and total body, 1.6%. Treatment with FOSAMAX also reduced height loss (FOSAMAX, -0.6 mm vs. placebo, -2.4 mm).

FOSAMAX Once-Weekly

A one-year, double-blind, placebo-controlled, multicenter study of once weekly FOSAMAX 70 mg enrolled a total of 167 men between the ages of 38 and 91 (mean, 66). Patients in the study had either a BMD T-score less than or equal to -2 at the femoral neck and less than or equal to -1 at the lumbar spine, or a BMD T-score less than or equal to -2 at the lumbar spine and less than or equal to -1 at the femoral neck, or a baseline osteoporotic fracture and a BMD T-score less than or equal to -1 at the femoral neck. At one year, the mean increases relative to placebo in BMD in men receiving FOSAMAX 70 mg once weekly were significant at the following sites: lumbar spine, 2.8%; femoral neck, 1.9%; trochanter, 2.0%; and total body, 1.2%. These increases in BMD were similar to those seen at one year in the 10 mg once-daily study.

In both studies, BMD responses were similar regardless of age (greater than or equal to 65 years vs. less than 65 years), gonadal function (baseline testosterone less than 9 ng/dL vs. greater than or equal to 9 ng/dL), or baseline BMD (femoral neck and lumbar spine T-score less than or equal to -2.5 vs. greater than -2.5).

16 HOW SUPPLIED/STORAGE AND HANDLING

No. 3870 — Tablets FOSAMAX PLUS D 70 mg/2800 international units are white to off-white, modified capsule-shaped tablets with code 710 on one side and an outline of a bone image on the other. They are supplied as follows:
NDC 0006-0710-44 unit of use blister packages of 4.

No. 6746 — Tablets FOSAMAX PLUS D 70 mg/5600 international units are white to off-white, modified rectangle-shaped tablets with code 270 on one side and an outline of a bone image on the other. They are supplied as follows:

NDC 0006-0270-44 unit of use blister packages of 4
NDC 0006-0270-21 unit dose packages of 20.

Storage

Store at 20-25°C (68-77°F), excursions between 15-30°C (59-86°F) are allowed. [See USP Controlled Room Temperature.] Protect from moisture and light. Store tablets in the original blister package until use.

17 PATIENT COUNSELING INFORMATION

See FDA-approved patient labeling (Medication Guide). Instruct patients to read the Medication Guide before starting therapy with FOSAMAX PLUS D and to reread it each time the prescription is renewed.

17.1 Osteoporosis Recommendations, Including Calcium and Vitamin D Supplementation

Instruct patients to take supplemental calcium if intake is inadequate. Patients at increased risk for vitamin D insufficiency (e.g., over the age of 70 years, nursing home bound, or chronically ill) should take additional vitamin D if needed *[see Dosage and Administration (2.4)]*. Patients with gastrointestinal malabsorption syndromes may require additional vitamin D supplementation. Weight-bearing exercise should be considered along with the modification of certain behavioral factors, such as cigarette smoking and/or excessive alcohol consumption, if these factors exist.

17.2 Dosing Instructions

Instruct patients that the expected benefits of FOSAMAX PLUS D may only be obtained when it is taken with plain water the first thing upon arising for the day at least 30 minutes before the first food, beverage, or medication of the day. Even dosing with orange juice or coffee has been shown to markedly reduce the absorption of alendronate *[see Clinical Pharmacology (12.3)]*.

Instruct patients not to chew or suck on the tablet because of a potential for oropharyngeal ulceration.

Instruct patients to swallow each tablet of FOSAMAX PLUS D with a full glass of water (6-8 ounces) and not to lie down for at least 30 minutes and until after their first food of the day to facilitate delivery to the stomach and thus reduce the potential for esophageal irritation.

Instruct patients not to take FOSAMAX PLUS D at bedtime or before arising for the day. Patients should be informed that failure to follow these instructions may increase their risk of esophageal problems.

Instruct patients that if they develop symptoms of esophageal disease (such as difficulty or pain upon swallowing, retrosternal pain or new or worsening heartburn) they should stop taking FOSAMAX PLUS D and consult their physician.

If patients miss a dose of FOSAMAX PLUS D, instruct patients to take one tablet on the morning after they remember. They should not take two tablets on the same day but should return to taking one tablet once a week, as originally scheduled on their chosen day.

Manuf. for: Merck Sharp & Dohme Corp., a subsidiary of **MERCK & CO., INC.**, Whitehouse Station, NJ 08889, USA
By:
FROSST IBERICA, S.A.
28805 Alcalá de Henares
Madrid, Spain
For patent information:
www.merck.com/product/patent/home.html
Copyright © 2005, 2007, 2010, 2012 Merck Sharp & Dohme Corp., a subsidiary of **Merck & Co., Inc.**
All rights reserved.
uspi-mk0217a-t-1405r016

MEDICATION GUIDE
FOSAMAX® PLUS D (FOSS-ah-max PLUS D)
(alendronate sodium/cholecalciferol)
Tablets

Read the Medication Guide that comes with FOSAMAX® PLUS D before you start taking it and each time you get a refill. There may be new information. This Medication Guide does not take the place of talking with your doctor about your medical condition or treatment. Talk to your doctor if you have any questions about FOSAMAX PLUS D.

What is the most important information I should know about FOSAMAX PLUS D?
FOSAMAX PLUS D can cause serious side effects including:
1. Esophagus problems
2. Low calcium levels in your blood (hypocalcemia)
3. Bone, joint, or muscle pain
4. Severe jaw bone problems (osteonecrosis)
5. Unusual thigh bone fractures
1. **Esophagus problems.**
   Some people who take FOSAMAX PLUS D may develop problems in the esophagus (the tube that connects the mouth and the stomach). These problems include irritation, inflammation, or ulcers of the esophagus which may sometimes bleed.
   • It is important that you take FOSAMAX PLUS D exactly as prescribed to help lower your chance of getting esophagus problems. (See the section "How should I take FOSAMAX PLUS D tablet?")

○ Stop taking FOSAMAX PLUS D and call your doctor right away if you get chest pain, new or worsening heartburn, or have trouble or pain when you swallow.

2. **Low calcium levels in your blood (hypocalcemia).**
FOSAMAX PLUS D may lower the calcium levels in your blood. If you have low blood calcium before you start taking FOSAMAX PLUS D, it may get worse during treatment. Your low blood calcium must be treated before you take FOSAMAX PLUS D. Most people with low blood calcium levels do not have symptoms, but some people may have symptoms. Call your doctor right away if you have symptoms of low blood calcium such as:
   ○ Spasms, twitches, or cramps in your muscles
   ○ Numbness or tingling in your fingers, toes, or around your mouth
   Your doctor may prescribe calcium and vitamin D to help prevent low calcium levels in your blood, while you take FOSAMAX PLUS D. Take calcium and vitamin D as your doctor tells you to.

3. **Bone, joint, or muscle pain.**
Some people who take FOSAMAX PLUS D develop severe bone, joint, or muscle pain.

4. **Severe jaw bone problems (osteonecrosis).**
Severe jaw bone problems may happen when you take FOSAMAX PLUS D. Your doctor should examine your mouth before you start FOSAMAX PLUS D. Your doctor may tell you to see your dentist before you start FOSAMAX PLUS D. It is important for you to practice good mouth care during treatment with FOSAMAX PLUS D.

5. **Unusual thigh bone fractures.**
Some people have developed unusual fractures in their thigh bone. Symptoms of a fracture may include new or unusual pain in your hip, groin, or thigh.

Call your doctor right away if you have any of these side effects.

What is FOSAMAX PLUS D?
FOSAMAX PLUS D is a prescription medicine used to:
• Treat osteoporosis in women after menopause. FOSAMAX PLUS D helps increase bone mass and reduces the chance of having a hip or spinal fracture (break).
• Increase bone mass in men with osteoporosis.
FOSAMAX PLUS D should not be used to treat vitamin D deficiency.
It is not known how long FOSAMAX PLUS D works for the treatment of osteoporosis. You should see your doctor regularly to determine if FOSAMAX PLUS D is still right for you.
FOSAMAX PLUS D is not for use in children.

Who should not take FOSAMAX PLUS D?
Do not take FOSAMAX PLUS D if you:
• Have certain problems with your esophagus, the tube that connects your mouth with your stomach
• Cannot stand or sit upright for at least 30 minutes
• Have low levels of calcium in your blood
• Are allergic to FOSAMAX PLUS D or any of its ingredients. A list of ingredients is at the end of this leaflet.

What should I tell my doctor before taking FOSAMAX PLUS D?
Before you start FOSAMAX PLUS D, be sure to talk to your doctor if you:
• Have problems with swallowing
• Have stomach or digestive problems
• Have low blood calcium
• Plan to have dental surgery or teeth removed
• Have kidney problems
• Have sarcoidosis, leukemia, lymphoma. These conditions may cause changes in vitamin D.
• Have been told you have trouble absorbing minerals in your stomach or intestines (malabsorption syndrome)
• Are pregnant or plan to become pregnant. It is not known if FOSAMAX PLUS D can harm your unborn baby.
• Are breast-feeding or plan to breast-feed. It is not known if FOSAMAX PLUS D passes into your milk and may harm your baby.
Especially tell your doctor if you take:
• antacids
• aspirin
• Nonsteroidal Anti-Inflammatory (NSAID) medicines
Tell your doctor about all the medicines you take, including prescription and non-prescription medicines, vitamins, and herbal supplements. Certain medicines may affect how FOSAMAX PLUS D works.
Know the medicines you take. Keep a list of them and show it to your doctor and pharmacist each time you get a new medicine.

How should I take FOSAMAX PLUS D tablet?
• Take FOSAMAX PLUS D exactly as your doctor tells you.
• **FOSAMAX PLUS D works only if taken on an empty stomach.**
• Take 1 dose of FOSAMAX PLUS D 1 time a week, **after** you get up for the day and **before** taking your first food, drink, or other medicine.

• Take FOSAMAX PLUS D while you are sitting or standing.
• Take your FOSAMAX PLUS D tablet with a full glass (6-8 oz) of plain water.
• **Do not chew or suck on a tablet of FOSAMAX PLUS D.**
• **Do not** take FOSAMAX PLUS D with mineral water, coffee, tea, soda, or juice.
• Do not take FOSAMAX PLUS D at bedtime.
After swallowing FOSAMAX PLUS D, wait at least 30 minutes:
• Before you lie down. You may sit, stand or walk, and do normal activities like reading.
• Before you take your first food or drink except for plain water.
• Before you take other medicines, including antacids, calcium, and other supplements and vitamins.
Do not lie down for at least 30 minutes after you take FOSAMAX PLUS D and after you eat your first food of the day.
If you miss a dose of FOSAMAX PLUS D, do not take it later in the day. Take your missed dose on the next morning after you remember and then return to your normal schedule. Do not take 2 doses on the same day.
If you take too much FOSAMAX PLUS D, call your doctor. Do not try to vomit. Do not lie down.

What are the possible side effects of FOSAMAX PLUS D?
FOSAMAX PLUS D may cause serious side effects.
• See "What is the most important information I should know about FOSAMAX PLUS D?"
The most common side effects of FOSAMAX PLUS D are:
• Stomach area (abdominal) pain
• Heartburn
• Constipation
• Diarrhea
• Upset stomach
• Pain in your bones, joints, or muscles
• Nausea
You may get allergic reactions, such as hives or swelling of your face, lips, tongue, or throat.
Worsening of asthma has been reported.
Tell your doctor if you have any side effect that bothers you or that does not go away.
These are not all the possible side effects of FOSAMAX PLUS D. For more information, ask your doctor or pharmacist.
Call your doctor for medical advice about side effects. You may report side effects to FDA at 1-800-FDA-1088.

How do I store FOSAMAX PLUS D?
• Store FOSAMAX PLUS D at room temperature, 68°F to 77°F (20°C to 25°C).
• Keep FOSAMAX PLUS D away from light.
• Keep FOSAMAX PLUS D package and tablets dry.
• Store FOSAMAX PLUS D in the original package.
Keep FOSAMAX PLUS D and all medicines out of the reach of children.

General information about the safe and effective use of FOSAMAX PLUS D.
Medicines are sometimes prescribed for purposes other than those listed in a Medication Guide. Do not use FOSAMAX PLUS D for a condition for which it was not prescribed. Do not give FOSAMAX PLUS D to other people, even if they have the same symptoms you have. It may harm them.
This Medication Guide summarizes the most important information about FOSAMAX PLUS D. If you would like more information, talk with your doctor. You can ask your doctor or pharmacist for information about FOSAMAX PLUS D that is written for health professionals. For more information, go to: www.fosamaxplusd.com or call 1-800-622-4477 (toll-free).

What are the ingredients in FOSAMAX PLUS D?
Active ingredients: alendronate sodium and cholecalciferol (vitamin D_3).
Inactive ingredients: cellulose, lactose, medium chain triglycerides, gelatin, croscarmellose sodium, sucrose, colloidal silicon dioxide, magnesium stearate, butylated hydroxytoluene, modified food starch, and sodium aluminum silicate.
Manuf. for: Merck Sharp & Dohme Corp., a subsidiary of **MERCK & CO., INC.,** Whitehouse Station, NJ 08889, USA
By:
FROSST IBERICA, S.A.
28805 Alcalá de Henares
Madrid, Spain
For patent information:
www.merck.com/product/patent/home.html
Copyright © 2010 Merck Sharp & Dohme Corp., a subsidiary of Merck & Co., Inc.
All rights reserved.
Revised: 11/2013
usmg-mk0217a-t-1311r015
This Medication Guide has been approved by the U.S. Food and Drug Administration.

Shown in Product Identification Guide, page 308

GANIRELIX ACETATE INJECTION

℞

FOR SUBCUTANEOUS USE ONLY

DESCRIPTION

Ganirelix Acetate Injection is a synthetic decapeptide with high antagonistic activity against naturally occurring gonadotropin-releasing hormone (GnRH). Ganirelix Acetate is derived from native GnRH with substitutions of amino acids at positions 1, 2, 3, 6, 8, and 10 to form the following molecular formula of the peptide: N-acetyl-3-(2-naphthyl)-D-alanyl-4-chloro-D-phenylalanyl-3-(3-pyridyl)-D-alanyl-L-seryl-L-tyrosyl-N^9,N^{10}-diethyl-D-homoarginyl-L-leucyl-N^9,N^{10}-diethyl-L-homoarginyl-L-prolyl-D-alanylamide acetate. The molecular weight for Ganirelix Acetate is 1570.4 as an anhydrous free base. The structural formula is as follows:

Ganirelix Acetate Injection is supplied as a colorless, sterile, ready-to-use, aqueous solution intended for SUBCUTANEOUS administration only. Each sterile, prefilled syringe contains 250 mcg/0.5 mL of Ganirelix Acetate, 0.1 mg glacial acetic acid, 23.5 mg mannitol, and water for injection adjusted to pH 5.0 with acetic acid, NF and/or sodium hydroxide, NF.

CLINICAL PHARMACOLOGY

The pulsatile release of GnRH stimulates the synthesis and secretion of luteinizing hormone (LH) and follicle-stimulating hormone (FSH). The frequency of LH pulses in the mid and late follicular phase is approximately 1 pulse per hour. These pulses can be detected as transient rises in serum LH. At midcycle, a large increase in GnRH release results in an LH surge. The midcycle LH surge initiates several physiologic actions including: ovulation, resumption of meiosis in the oocyte, and luteinization. Luteinization results in a rise in serum progesterone with an accompanying decrease in estradiol levels.
Ganirelix Acetate acts by competitively blocking the GnRH receptors on the pituitary gonadotroph and subsequent transduction pathway. It induces a rapid, reversible suppression of gonadotropin secretion. The suppression of pituitary LH secretion by Ganirelix Acetate is more pronounced than that of FSH. An initial release of endogenous gonadotropins has not been detected with Ganirelix Acetate, which is consistent with an antagonist effect. Upon discontinuation of Ganirelix Acetate, pituitary LH and FSH levels are fully recovered within 48 hours.

Pharmacokinetics
The pharmacokinetic parameters of single and multiple injections of Ganirelix Acetate Injection in healthy adult females are summarized in Table I. Steady-state serum concentrations are reached after 3 days of treatment. The pharmacokinetics of Ganirelix Acetate are dose-proportional in the dose range of 125 to 500 mcg.
[See table I at top of next page]
Absorption
Ganirelix Acetate is rapidly absorbed following subcutaneous injection with maximum serum concentrations reached approximately one hour after dosing. The mean absolute bioavailability of Ganirelix Acetate following a single 250 mcg subcutaneous injection to healthy female volunteers is 91.1%.
Distribution
The mean (SD) volume of distribution of Ganirelix Acetate in healthy females following intravenous administration of a single 250-mcg dose is 43.7 (11.4) liters (L). *In vitro* protein binding to human plasma is 81.9%.
Metabolism
Following single-dose intravenous administration of radiolabeled Ganirelix Acetate to healthy female volunteers, Ganirelix Acetate is the major compound present in the plasma (50–70% of total radioactivity in the plasma) up to 4 hours and urine (17.1–18.4% of administered dose) up to 24 hours. Ganirelix Acetate is not found in the feces. The 1–4 peptide and 1–6 peptide of Ganirelix Acetate are the primary metabolites observed in the feces.
Excretion
On average, 97.2% of the total radiolabeled Ganirelix Acetate dose is recovered in the feces and urine (75.1% and 22.1%, respectively) over 288 h following intravenous single dose administration of 1 mg [^{14}C]-Ganirelix Acetate. Urinary excretion is virtually complete in 24 h, whereas fecal excretion starts to plateau 192 h after dosing.

TABLE I: Mean (SD) pharmacokinetic parameters of 250 mcg of Ganirelix Acetate following a single subcutaneous (SC) injection (n=15) and daily SC injections (n=15) for seven days.

	t_{max} h	$t_{1/2}$ h	C_{max} ng/mL	AUC ng·h/mL	CL/F L/h	V_d/F L
Ganirelix Acetate single dose	1.1 (0.3)	12.8 (4.3)	14.8 (3.2)	96 (12)	2.4 (0.2)*	43.7 (11.4)*
Ganirelix Acetate multiple dose	1.1 (0.2)	16.2 (1.6)	11.2 (2.4)	77.1 (9.8)	3.3 (0.4)	76.5 (10.3)

t_{max} Time to maximum concentration
$t_{1/2}$ Elimination half-life
C_{max} Maximum serum concentration
AUC Area under the curve; Single dose: $AUC_{0-\infty}$; multiple dose: AUC_{0-24}
V_d Volume of distribution
CL Clearance = Dose/$AUC_{0-\infty}$
F Absolute bioavailability
* Based on intravenous administration

TABLE II: Results from the multicenter, double-blind, randomized, dose-finding study to assess the efficacy of Ganirelix Acetate Injection to prevent premature LH surges in women undergoing COH with recombinant FSH.

	Daily dose (mcg) of Ganirelix Acetate Injection					
	62.5 mcg	125 mcg	250 mcg	500 mcg	1000 mcg	2000 mcg
No. subjects receiving Ganirelix Acetate	31	66	70	69	66	30
No. subjects with ET*	27	61	62	54	61	27
No. of subjects with LH rise ≥ 10 mIU/mL[†]	4	6	1	0	0	0
Serum LH (mIU/mL) on day of hCG[‡] 5th–95th percentiles	3.6 0.6–19.9	2.5 0.6–11.4	1.7 < 0.25–6.4	1.0 0.4–4.7	0.6 < 0.25–2.2	0.3 < 0.25–0.8
Serum E_2 (pg/mL) on day of hCG[‡] 5th–95th percentiles	1475 645–3720	1110 424–3780	1160 384–3910	823 279–2720	703 284–2360	441 166–1940
Vital pregnancy rate[§]						
per attempt, n (%)	7 (22.6)	17 (25.8)	25 (35.7)	8 (11.6)	9 (13.6)	2 (6.7)
per transfer, n (%)	7 (25.9)	17 (27.9)	25 (40.3)	8 (14.8)	9 (14.8)	2 (7.4)
Implantation rate (%)[¶]	14.2 (26.8)	16.3 (30.5)	21.9 (30.6)	9.0 (23.7)	8.5 (21.7)	4.9 (20.1)

(Protocol 38602)
* ET: Embryo Transfer
† Following initiation of Ganirelix Acetate therapy. Includes subjects who have complied with daily injections
‡ Median values
§ As evidenced by ultrasound at 5–6 weeks following ET
¶ Mean (standard deviation)

TABLE III: Results from the multicenter, open-label, randomized study to assess the efficacy and safety of Ganirelix Acetate Injection in women undergoing COH.

	Ganirelix Acetate 250 mcg
No. subjects treated	463
Duration of GnRH analog (days)*[†]	5.4 (2.0)
Duration of recombinant FSH (days)*[†]	9.6 (2.0)
Serum E_2 (pg/mL) on day of hCG[‡] 5th–95th percentiles	1190 373–3105
Serum LH (mIU/mL) on day of hCG[‡] 5th–95th percentiles	1.6 0.6–6.9
No. of subjects with LH rise ≥ 10 mIU/mL[§]	13
No. of follicles > 11 mm*[†]	10.7 (5.3)
No. of subjects with oocyte retrieval	440
No. of oocytes[†]	8.7 (5.6)
Fertilization rate	62.1%
No. subjects with ET[¶]	399
No. of embryos transferred[†]	2.2 (0.6)
No. of embryos[†]	6.0 (4.5)
Ongoing pregnancy rate[#]*[ ]	
per attempt, n (%)[Þ]	94 (20.3)
per transfer, n (%)	93 (23.3)
Implantation rate (%)[†]	15.7 (29)

(Protocol 38607)
Some centers were limited to the transfer of ≤ 2 embryos based on local practice standards
* Restricted to subjects with hCG injection
† Mean (standard deviation)
‡ Median values
§ Following initiation of Ganirelix Acetate therapy
¶ ET: Embryo Transfer
# As evidenced by ultrasound at 12–16 weeks following ET
Þ Includes one patient who achieved pregnancy with intrauterine induction

The mean number of days of Ganirelix Acetate treatment was 5.4 (2–14).

LH Surges
The midcycle LH surge initiates several physiologic actions including: ovulation, resumption of meiosis in the oocyte, and luteinization. In 463 subjects administered Ganirelix Acetate Injection 250 mcg, a premature LH surge prior to hCG administration, (LH rise ≥ 10 mIU/mL with a significant rise in serum progesterone > 2 ng/mL, or a significant decline in serum estradiol) occurred in less than 1% of subjects.

INDICATIONS AND USAGE

Ganirelix Acetate Injection is indicated for the inhibition of premature LH surges in women undergoing controlled ovarian hyperstimulation.

CONTRAINDICATIONS

Ganirelix Acetate Injection is contraindicated under the following conditions:
• Known hypersensitivity to Ganirelix Acetate or to any of its components.
• Known hypersensitivity to GnRH or any other GnRH analog.
• Known or suspected pregnancy (see PRECAUTIONS).

WARNINGS

Ganirelix Acetate Injection should be prescribed by physicians who are experienced in infertility treatment. Before

Special Populations
The pharmacokinetics of Ganirelix Acetate Injection have not been determined in special populations such as geriatric, pediatric, renally impaired and hepatically impaired patients (see PRECAUTIONS).
Drug-Drug Interactions
Formal *in vivo* or *in vitro* drug-drug interaction studies have not been conducted (see PRECAUTIONS). Since Ganirelix Acetate can suppress the secretion of pituitary gonadotropins, dose adjustments of exogenous gonadotropins may be necessary when used during controlled ovarian hyperstimulation (COH).

Clinical Studies
The efficacy of Ganirelix Acetate Injection was established in two adequate and well-controlled clinical studies which included women with normal endocrine and pelvic ultrasound parameters. The studies intended to exclude subjects with polycystic ovary syndrome (PCOS) and subjects with low or no ovarian reserve. One cycle of study medication was administered to each randomized subject. For both studies, the administration of exogenous recombinant FSH [Follistim® (follitropin beta for injection)] 150 IU daily was initiated on the morning of Day 2 or 3 of a natural menstrual cycle. Ganirelix Acetate Injection was administered on the morning of Day 7 or 8 (Day 6 of recombinant FSH administration). The dose of recombinant FSH administered was adjusted according to individual responses starting on the day of initiation of Ganirelix Acetate. Both recombinant FSH and Ganirelix Acetate were continued daily until at least three follicles were 17 mm or greater in diameter at which time hCG [Pregnyl® (chorionic gonadotropin for injection, USP)] was administered. Following hCG administration, Ganirelix Acetate and recombinant FSH administration were discontinued. Oocyte retrieval, followed by *in vitro* fertilization (IVF) or intracytoplasmic sperm injection (ICSI), was subsequently performed.
In a multicenter, double-blind, randomized, dose-finding study, the safety and efficacy of Ganirelix Acetate Injection were evaluated for the prevention of LH surges in women undergoing COH with recombinant FSH. Ganirelix Acetate Injection doses ranging from 62.5 mcg to 2000 mcg and recombinant FSH were administered to 332 patients undergoing COH for IVF (see TABLE II). Median serum LH on the day of hCG administration decreased with increasing doses of Ganirelix Acetate. Median serum E_2 (17β-estradiol) on the day of hCG administration was 1475, 1110, and 1160 pg/mL for the 62.5-, 125-, and 250-mcg doses, respectively. Lower peak serum E_2 levels of 823, 703, and 441 pg/mL were seen at higher doses of Ganirelix Acetate 500, 1000, and 2000 mcg, respectively. The highest pregnancy and implantation rates were achieved with the 250-mcg dose of Ganirelix Acetate Injection as summarized in Table II.
[See table II above]
Transient LH rises alone were not deleterious to achieving pregnancy with Ganirelix Acetate at doses of 125 mcg (3/6 subjects) and 250 mcg (1/1 subjects). In addition, none of the subjects with LH rises ≥ 10 mIU/mL had premature luteinization indicated by a serum progesterone above 2 ng/mL.
A multicenter, open-label, randomized study was conducted to assess the efficacy and safety of Ganirelix Acetate Injection in women undergoing COH. Follicular phase treatment with Ganirelix Acetate 250 mcg was studied using a luteal phase GnRH agonist as a reference treatment. A total of 463 subjects were treated with Ganirelix Acetate by subcutaneous injection once daily starting on Day 6 of recombinant FSH treatment. Recombinant FSH was maintained at 150 IU for the first 5 days of ovarian stimulation and was then adjusted by the investigator on the sixth day of gonadotropin use according to individual responses. The results for the Ganirelix Acetate arm are summarized in Table III.

starting treatment with Ganirelix Acetate, pregnancy must be excluded. Safe use of Ganirelix Acetate during pregnancy has not been established (see CONTRAINDICATIONS and PRECAUTIONS).

PRECAUTIONS

General

Special care should be taken in women with signs and symptoms of active allergic conditions. Cases of hypersensitivity reactions, including anaphylactoid reactions, have been reported, as early as with the first dose, during post-marketing surveillance (see ADVERSE REACTIONS). In the absence of clinical experience, Ganirelix Acetate treatment is not advised in women with severe allergic conditions.

The packaging of this product contains natural rubber latex which may cause allergic reactions (see HOW SUPPLIED).

Information for Patients

Prior to therapy with Ganirelix Acetate Injection, patients should be informed of the duration of treatment and monitoring procedures that will be required. The risk of possible adverse reactions should be discussed (see ADVERSE REACTIONS).

Ganirelix Acetate should not be prescribed if the patient is pregnant.

Laboratory Tests

A neutrophil count $\geq 8.3 (\times 10^9/L)$ was noted in 11.9% (up to $16.8 \times 10^9/L$) of all subjects treated within the adequate and well-controlled clinical trials. In addition, downward shifts within the Ganirelix Acetate Injection group were observed for hematocrit and total bilirubin. The clinical significance of these findings was not determined.

Drug Interactions

No formal drug-drug interaction studies have been performed.

Carcinogenesis and Mutagenesis, Impairment of Fertility

Long-term toxicity studies in animals have not been performed with Ganirelix Acetate Injection to evaluate the carcinogenic potential of the drug. Ganirelix Acetate did not induce a mutagenic response in the Ames test (*S. typhimurium* and *E. coli*) or produce chromosomal aberrations in *in vitro* assay using Chinese Hamster Ovary cells.

Pregnancy

Pregnancy Category X

Ganirelix Acetate Injection is contraindicated in pregnant women. When administered from Day 7 to near term to pregnant rats and rabbits at doses up to 10 and 30 mcg/day (approximately 0.4 to 3.2 times the human dose based on body surface area), Ganirelix Acetate increased the incidence of litter resorption. There was no increase in fetal abnormalities. No treatment-related changes in fertility, physical, or behavioral characteristics were observed in the offspring of female rats treated with Ganirelix Acetate during pregnancy and lactation.

The effects on fetal resorption are logical consequences of the alteration in hormonal levels brought about by the antigonadotropic properties of this drug and could result in fetal loss in humans. Therefore, this drug should not be used in pregnant women (see CONTRAINDICATIONS).

Nursing Mothers

Ganirelix Acetate Injection should not be used by lactating women. It is not known whether this drug is excreted in human milk.

Geriatric Use

Clinical studies with Ganirelix Acetate Injection did not include a sufficient number of subjects aged 65 and over.

ADVERSE REACTIONS

The safety of Ganirelix Acetate Injection was evaluated in two randomized, parallel-group, multicenter controlled clinical studies. Treatment duration for Ganirelix Acetate ranged from 1 to 14 days. Table IV represents adverse events (AEs) from first day of Ganirelix Acetate administration until confirmation of pregnancy by ultrasound at an incidence of $\geq 1\%$ in Ganirelix Acetate-treated subjects without regard to causality.

TABLE IV: Incidence of common adverse events (Incidence ≥ 1% in Ganirelix Acetate-treated subjects). Completed controlled clinical studies (All-subjects-treated group).

Adverse Events Occurring in ≥ 1%	Ganirelix Acetate N=794 % (n)
Abdominal Pain (gynecological)	4.8 (38)
Death Fetal	3.7 (29)
Headache	3.0 (24)
Ovarian Hyperstimulation Syndrome	2.4 (19)
Vaginal Bleeding	1.8 (14)
Injection Site Reaction	1.1 (9)
Nausea	1.1 (9)
Abdominal Pain (gastrointestinal)	1.0 (8)

During post-marketing surveillance, rare cases of hypersensitivity reactions, including anaphylactoid reactions, have been reported, as early as with the first dose (see PRECAUTIONS).

Congenital Anomalies

Ongoing clinical follow-up studies of 283 newborns of women administered Ganirelix Acetate Injection were reviewed. There were three neonates with major congenital anomalies and 18 neonates with minor congenital anomalies. The major congenital anomalies were: hydrocephalus/meningocele, omphalocele, and Beckwith-Wiedemann Syndrome. The minor congenital anomalies were: nevus, skin tags, sacral sinus, hemangioma, torticollis/asymmetric skull, talipes, supernumerary digit finger, hip subluxation, torticollis/high palate, occiput/abnormal hand crease, hernia umbilicalis, hernia inguinalis, hydrocele, undescended testis, and hydronephrosis. The causal relationship between these congenital anomalies and Ganirelix Acetate is unknown. Multiple factors, genetic and others (including, but not limited to ICSI, IVF, gonadotropins, progesterone) may confound ART (Assisted Reproductive Technology) procedures.

OVERDOSAGE

There have been no reports of overdosage with Ganirelix Acetate Injection in humans.

DOSAGE AND ADMINISTRATION

After initiating FSH therapy on Day 2 or 3 of the cycle, Ganirelix Acetate Injection 250 mcg may be administered subcutaneously once daily during the mid to late portion of the follicular phase. By taking advantage of endogenous pituitary FSH secretion, the requirement for exogenously administered FSH may be reduced. Treatment with Ganirelix Acetate should be continued daily until the day of hCG administration. When a sufficient number of follicles of adequate size are present, as assessed by ultrasound, final maturation of follicles is induced by administering hCG. The administration of hCG should be withheld in cases where the ovaries are abnormally enlarged on the last day of FSH therapy to reduce the chance of developing OHSS (Ovarian Hyperstimulation Syndrome).

Directions for Using Ganirelix Acetate Injection

1. Ganirelix Acetate Injection is supplied in a sterile, prefilled syringe and is intended for SUBCUTANEOUS administration only.
2. Wash hands thoroughly with soap and water.
3. The most convenient sites for SUBCUTANEOUS injection are in the abdomen around the navel or upper thigh.
4. The injection site should be swabbed with a disinfectant to remove any surface bacteria. Clean about two inches around the point where the needle will be inserted and let the disinfectant dry for at least one minute before proceeding.
5. With syringe held upward, remove needle cover.
6. Pinch up a large area of skin between the finger and thumb. Vary the injection site a little with each injection.
7. The needle should be inserted at the base of the pinched-up skin at an angle of 45–90° to the skin surface.
8. When the needle is correctly positioned, it will be difficult to draw back on the plunger. If any blood is drawn into the syringe, the needle tip has penetrated a vein or artery. If this happens, withdraw the needle slightly and reposition the needle without removing it from the skin. Alternatively, remove the needle and use a new, sterile, prefilled syringe. Cover the injection site with a swab containing disinfectant and apply pressure; the site should stop bleeding within one or two minutes.
9. Once the needle is correctly placed, depress the plunger slowly and steadily, so the solution is correctly injected and the skin is not damaged.
10. Pull the syringe out quickly and apply pressure to the site with a swab containing disinfectant.
11. Use the sterile, prefilled syringe only once and dispose of it properly.

HOW SUPPLIED

Ganirelix Acetate Injection is supplied in:
Disposable, sterile, ready for use, prefilled 1 mL glass syringes containing 250 mcg/0.5 mL aqueous solution of Ganirelix Acetate closed with a rubber piston that does not contain latex. Each Ganirelix Acetate sterile, prefilled syringe is affixed with a 27 gauge × ½-inch needle **closed by a needle shield of natural rubber latex** and is blister-packed. (See PRECAUTIONS, General.)

Single syringe   NDC 0052-0301-51

Storage

Store at 25°C (77°F); excursions permitted to 15–30°C (59–86°F) [see USP Controlled Room Temperature]. Protect from light.

Manufactured for: Merck Sharp & Dohme Corp., a subsidiary of **MERCK & CO., INC.,** Whitehouse Station, NJ 08889, USA

Manufactured by: Vetter Pharma-Fertigung GmbH & Co. KG, Ravensburg, Germany

For patent information: www.merck.com/product/patent/home.html

Copyright © 1999, 2008 Merck Sharp & Dohme B.V., a subsidiary of **Merck & Co., Inc.**

All rights reserved.

Revised: 12/2013

uspi-mk8761-soi-1312r003

Rx only

GARDASIL

[*GARD-ah-sill*]

[Human Papillomavirus Quadrivalent (Types 6, 11, 16, and 18) Vaccine, Recombinant]

Suspension for Intramuscular Injection

HIGHLIGHTS OF PRESCRIBING INFORMATION

These highlights do not include all the information needed to use GARDASIL safely and effectively. See full prescribing information for GARDASIL.

GARDASIL®

[Human Papillomavirus Quadrivalent (Types 6, 11, 16, and 18) Vaccine, Recombinant]

Suspension for intramuscular injection

Initial U.S. Approval: 2006

——INDICATIONS AND USAGE——

GARDASIL is a vaccine indicated in girls and women 9 through 26 years of age for the prevention of the following diseases caused by Human Papillomavirus (HPV) types included in the vaccine:

- Cervical, vulvar, vaginal, and anal cancer caused by HPV types 16 and 18 (1.1)
- Genital warts (condyloma acuminata) caused by HPV types 6 and 11 (1.1)

And the following precancerous or dysplastic lesions caused by HPV types 6, 11, 16, and 18:

- Cervical intraepithelial neoplasia (CIN) grade 2/3 and Cervical adenocarcinoma *in situ* (AIS) (1.1)
- Cervical intraepithelial neoplasia (CIN) grade 1 (1.1)
- Vulvar intraepithelial neoplasia (VIN) grade 2 and grade 3 (1.1)
- Vaginal intraepithelial neoplasia (VaIN) grade 2 and grade 3 (1.1)
- Anal intraepithelial neoplasia (AIN) grades 1, 2, and 3 (1.1)

GARDASIL is indicated in boys and men 9 through 26 years of age for the prevention of the following diseases caused by HPV types included in the vaccine:

- Anal cancer caused by HPV types 16 and 18 (1.2)
- Genital warts (condyloma acuminata) caused by HPV types 6 and 11 (1.2)

And the following precancerous or dysplastic lesions caused by HPV types 6, 11, 16, and 18:

- Anal intraepithelial neoplasia (AIN) grades 1, 2, and 3. (1.2)

Limitations of GARDASIL Use and Effectiveness:

- GARDASIL does not eliminate the necessity for women to continue to undergo recommended cervical cancer screening. (1.3, 17)
- Recipients of GARDASIL should not discontinue anal cancer screening if it has been recommended by a health care provider. (1.3, 17)
- GARDASIL has not been demonstrated to provide protection against disease from vaccine and non-vaccine HPV types to which a person has previously been exposed through sexual activity. (1.3, 14.4, 14.5)
- GARDASIL is not intended to be used for treatment of active external genital lesions; cervical, vulvar, vaginal, and anal cancers; CIN; VIN; VaIN; or AIN. (1.3)
- GARDASIL has not been demonstrated to protect against diseases due to HPV types not contained in the vaccine. (1.3, 14.4, 14.5)
- Not all vulvar, vaginal, and anal cancers are caused by HPV, and GARDASIL protects only against those vulvar, vaginal, and anal cancers caused by HPV 16 and 18. (1.3)
- GARDASIL does not protect against genital diseases not caused by HPV. (1.3)
- Vaccination with GARDASIL may not result in protection in all vaccine recipients. (1.3)
- GARDASIL has not been demonstrated to prevent HPV-related CIN 2/3 or worse in women older than 26 years of age. (14.7)

Table 3: Postdose Evaluation of Injection-Site Adverse Reactions in Girls and Women 9 Through 26 Years of Age (1 to 5 Days Postvaccination)

Adverse Reaction	GARDASIL (% occurrence)			AAHS Control* (% occurrence)			Saline Placebo (% occurrence)		
	Post-dose 1 N† = 5011	Post-dose 2 N = 4924	Post-dose 3 N = 4818	Post-dose 1 N = 3410	Post-dose 2 N = 3351	Post-dose 3 N = 3295	Post-dose 1 N = 315	Post-dose 2 N = 301	Post-dose 3 N = 300
Pain	63.4	60.7	62.7	57.0	47.8	49.6	33.7	20.3	27.3
Mild/Moderate	62.5	59.7	61.2	56.6	47.3	48.9	33.3	20.3	27.0
Severe	0.9	1.0	1.5	0.4	0.5	0.6	0.3	0.0	0.3
Swelling‡	10.2	12.8	15.1	8.2	7.5	7.6	4.4	3.0	3.3
Mild/Moderate	9.6	11.9	14.2	8.1	7.2	7.3	4.4	3.0	3.3
Severe	0.6	0.8	0.9	0.2	0.2	0.2	0.0	0.0	0.0
Erythema‡	9.2	12.1	14.7	9.8	8.4	8.9	7.3	5.3	5.7
Mild/Moderate	9.0	11.7	14.3	9.5	8.4	8.8	7.3	5.3	5.7
Severe	0.2	0.3	0.4	0.3	0.1	0.1	0.0	0.0	0.0

* AAHS Control = Amorphous Aluminum Hydroxyphosphate Sulfate
† N = Number of individuals with follow-up
‡ Intensity of swelling and erythema was measured by size (inches): Mild = 0 to ≤1; Moderate = >1 to ≤2; Severe = >2.

Table 4: Postdose Evaluation of Injection-Site Adverse Reactions in Boys and Men 9 Through 26 Years of Age (1 to 5 Days Postvaccination)

Adverse Reaction	GARDASIL (% occurrence)			AAHS Control* (% occurrence)			Saline Placebo (% occurrence)		
	Post-dose 1 N† = 3003	Post-dose 2 N = 2898	Post-dose 3 N = 2826	Post-dose 1 N = 1950	Post-dose 2 N = 1854	Post-dose 3 N = 1799	Post-dose 1 N = 269	Post-dose 2 N = 263	Post-dose 3 N = 259
Pain	44.7	36.9	34.4	38.4	28.2	25.8	27.5	20.5	16.2
Mild/Moderate	44.5	36.4	34.1	37.9	28.2	25.5	27.5	20.2	16.2
Severe	0.2	0.5	0.3	0.4	0.1	0.3	0.0	0.4	0.0
Swelling‡	5.6	6.6	7.7	5.6	4.5	4.1	4.8	1.5	3.5
Mild/Moderate	5.3	6.2	7.1	5.4	4.5	4.0	4.8	1.5	3.1
Severe	0.2	0.3	0.5	0.2	0.0	0.1	0.0	0.0	0.4
Erythema‡	7.2	8.0	8.7	8.3	6.3	5.7	7.1	5.7	5.0
Mild/Moderate	6.8	7.7	8.3	8.0	6.2	5.6	7.1	5.7	5.0
Severe	0.3	0.2	0.3	0.2	0.1	0.1	0.0	0.0	0.0

* AAHS Control = Amorphous Aluminum Hydroxyphosphate Sulfate
† N = Number of individuals with follow-up
‡ Intensity of swelling and erythema was measured by size (inches): Mild = 0 to ≤1; Moderate = >1 to ≤2; Severe = >2.

DOSAGE AND ADMINISTRATION

0.5-mL suspension for intramuscular injection at the following schedule: 0, 2 months, 6 months. (2.1)

DOSAGE FORMS AND STRENGTHS

• 0.5-mL suspension for injection as a single-dose vial and prefilled syringe. (3, 11)

CONTRAINDICATIONS

• Hypersensitivity, including severe allergic reactions to yeast (a vaccine component), or after a previous dose of GARDASIL. (4, 11)

WARNINGS AND PRECAUTIONS

• Because vaccinees may develop syncope, sometimes resulting in falling with injury, observation for 15 minutes after administration is recommended. Syncope, sometimes associated with tonic-clonic movements and other seizure-like activity, has been reported following vaccination with GARDASIL. When syncope is associated with tonic-clonic movements, the activity is usually transient and typically responds to restoring cerebral perfusion by maintaining a supine or Trendelenburg position. (5.1)

ADVERSE REACTIONS

The most common adverse reaction was headache. Common adverse reactions (frequency of at least 1.0% and greater than AAHS control or saline placebo) are fever, nausea, dizziness; and injection-site pain, swelling, erythema, pruritus, and bruising. (6.1)

To report SUSPECTED ADVERSE REACTIONS, contact Merck Sharp & Dohme Corp., a subsidiary of Merck & Co., Inc., at 1-877-888-4231 or VAERS at 1-800-822-7967 or www.vaers.hhs.gov.

DRUG INTERACTIONS

GARDASIL may be administered concomitantly with RECOMBIVAX HB® (7.1) or with Menactra and Adacel. (7.2)

USE IN SPECIFIC POPULATIONS

Safety and effectiveness of GARDASIL have not been established in the following populations:

• Pregnant women. Women who receive GARDASIL during pregnancy are encouraged to contact Merck Sharp & Dohme Corp., a subsidiary of Merck & Co., Inc., at 1-877-888-4231. (8.1)
• Children below the age of 9 years. (8.4)
• Immunocompromised individuals. Response to GARDASIL may be diminished. (8.6)

See 17 for PATIENT COUNSELING INFORMATION and FDA-approved patient labeling

Revised: 06/2014

FULL PRESCRIBING INFORMATION: CONTENTS*

1   **INDICATIONS AND USAGE**
   1.1   Girls and Women
   1.2   Boys and Men
   1.3   Limitations of GARDASIL Use and Effectiveness
2   **DOSAGE AND ADMINISTRATION**
   2.1   Dosage
   2.2   Method of Administration
3   **DOSAGE FORMS AND STRENGTHS**
4   **CONTRAINDICATIONS**
5   **WARNINGS AND PRECAUTIONS**
   5.1   Syncope
   5.2   Managing Allergic Reactions
6   **ADVERSE REACTIONS**
   6.1   Clinical Trials Experience
   6.2   Postmarketing Experience
7   **DRUG INTERACTIONS**
   7.1   Use with RECOMBIVAX HB
   7.2   Use with Menactra and Adacel
   7.3   Use with Hormonal Contraceptives
   7.4   Use with Systemic Immunosuppressive Medications
8   **USE IN SPECIFIC POPULATIONS**
   8.1   Pregnancy
   8.3   Nursing Mothers
   8.4   Pediatric Use
   8.5   Geriatric Use
   8.6   Immunocompromised Individuals
10   **OVERDOSAGE**
11   **DESCRIPTION**
12   **CLINICAL PHARMACOLOGY**
   12.1   Mechanism of Action

13   **NONCLINICAL TOXICOLOGY**
   13.1   Carcinogenesis, Mutagenesis, Impairment of Fertility
14   **CLINICAL STUDIES**
   14.1   Prophylactic Efficacy – HPV Types 6, 11, 16, and 18 in Girls and Women 16 Through 26 Years of Age
   14.2   Prophylactic Efficacy – HPV Types 6, 11, 16, and 18 in Boys and Men 16 Through 26 Years of Age
   14.3   Prophylactic Efficacy – Anal Disease Caused by HPV Types 6, 11, 16, and 18 in Boys and Men 16 Through 26 Years of Age in the MSM Sub-study
   14.4   Population Impact in Girls and Women 16 Through 26 Years of Age
   14.5   Population Impact in Boys and Men 16 Through 26 Years of Age
   14.6   Overall Population Impact
   14.7   Studies in Women 27 Through 45 Years of Age
   14.8   Immunogenicity
   14.9   Studies with RECOMBIVAX HB [hepatitis B vaccine (recombinant)]
   14.10   Studies with Menactra [Meningococcal (Groups A, C, Y and W-135) Polysaccharide Diphtheria Toxoid Conjugate Vaccine] and Adacel [Tetanus Toxoid, Reduced Diphtheria Toxoid and Acellular Pertussis Vaccine Adsorbed (Tdap)]
16   **HOW SUPPLIED/STORAGE AND HANDLING**
17   **PATIENT COUNSELING INFORMATION**

* Sections or subsections omitted from the full prescribing information are not listed

FULL PRESCRIBING INFORMATION

1   **INDICATIONS AND USAGE**

1.1   Girls and Women

GARDASIL® is a vaccine indicated in girls and women 9 through 26 years of age for the prevention of the following diseases caused by Human Papillomavirus (HPV) types included in the vaccine:

• Cervical, vulvar, vaginal, and anal cancer caused by HPV types 16 and 18

Table 7: Postdose Evaluation of Fever in Girls and Women 9 Through 26 Years of Age (1 to 5 Days Postvaccination)

Temperature (°F)	GARDASIL (% occurrence)			AAHS Control* or Saline Placebo (% occurrence)		
	Postdose 1 N[†] = 4945	Postdose 2 N = 4804	Postdose 3 N = 4671	Postdose 1 N = 3681	Postdose 2 N = 3564	Postdose 3 N = 3467
≥100 to <102	3.7	4.1	4.4	3.1	3.8	3.6
≥102	0.3	0.5	0.5	0.2	0.4	0.5

* AAHS Control = Amorphous Aluminum Hydroxyphosphate Sulfate
† N = Number of individuals with follow-up

Table 8: Postdose Evaluation of Fever in Boys and Men 9 Through 26 Years of Age (1 to 5 Days Postvaccination)

Temperature (°F)	GARDASIL (% occurrence)			AAHS Control* or Saline Placebo (% occurrence)		
	Postdose 1 N[†] = 2972	Postdose 2 N = 2849	Postdose 3 N = 2792	Postdose 1 N = 2194	Postdose 2 N = 2079	Postdose 3 N = 2046
≥100 to <102	2.4	2.5	2.3	2.1	2.2	1.6
≥102	0.6	0.5	0.5	0.5	0.3	0.3

* AAHS Control = Amorphous Aluminum Hydroxyphosphate Sulfate
† N = Number of individuals with follow-up

- Genital warts (condyloma acuminata) caused by HPV types 6 and 11

And the following precancerous or dysplastic lesions caused by HPV types 6, 11, 16, and 18:

- Cervical intraepithelial neoplasia (CIN) grade 2/3 and Cervical adenocarcinoma in situ (AIS)
- Cervical intraepithelial neoplasia (CIN) grade 1
- Vulvar intraepithelial neoplasia (VIN) grade 2 and grade 3
- Vaginal intraepithelial neoplasia (VaIN) grade 2 and grade 3
- Anal intraepithelial neoplasia (AIN) grades 1, 2, and 3

1.2 Boys and Men
GARDASIL is indicated in boys and men 9 through 26 years of age for the prevention of the following diseases caused by HPV types included in the vaccine:

- Anal cancer caused by HPV types 16 and 18
- Genital warts (condyloma acuminata) caused by HPV types 6 and 11

And the following precancerous or dysplastic lesions caused by HPV types 6, 11, 16, and 18:

- Anal intraepithelial neoplasia (AIN) grades 1, 2, and 3

1.3 Limitations of GARDASIL Use and Effectiveness
The health care provider should inform the patient, parent, or guardian that vaccination does not eliminate the necessity for women to continue to undergo recommended cervical cancer screening. Women who receive GARDASIL should continue to undergo cervical cancer screening per standard of care. [See Patient Counseling Information (17).]
Recipients of GARDASIL should not discontinue anal cancer screening if it has been recommended by a health care provider. [See Patient Counseling Information (17).]
GARDASIL has not been demonstrated to provide protection against disease from vaccine and non-vaccine HPV types to which a person has previously been exposed through sexual activity. [See Clinical Studies (14.4, 14.5).]
GARDASIL is not intended to be used for treatment of active external genital lesions; cervical, vulvar, vaginal, and anal cancers; CIN; VIN; VaIN; or AIN.
GARDASIL has not been demonstrated to protect against diseases due to HPV types not contained in the vaccine. [See Clinical Studies (14.4, 14.5).]
Not all vulvar, vaginal, and anal cancers are caused by HPV, and GARDASIL protects only against those vulvar, vaginal, and anal cancers caused by HPV 16 and 18.
GARDASIL does not protect against genital diseases not caused by HPV.
Vaccination with GARDASIL may not result in protection in all vaccine recipients.
GARDASIL has not been demonstrated to prevent HPV-related CIN 2/3 or worse in women older than 26 years of age. [See Clinical Studies (14.7).]

2 DOSAGE AND ADMINISTRATION
2.1 Dosage
GARDASIL should be administered intramuscularly as a 0.5-mL dose at the following schedule: 0, 2 months, 6 months. [See Clinical Studies (14.8).]
2.2 Method of Administration
For intramuscular use only.
Shake well before use. Thorough agitation immediately before administration is necessary to maintain suspension of the vaccine. GARDASIL should not be diluted or mixed with other vaccines. After thorough agitation, GARDASIL is a white, cloudy liquid. Parenteral drug products should be inspected visually for particulate matter and discoloration prior to administration. Do not use the product if particulates are present or if it appears discolored.
GARDASIL should be administered intramuscularly in the deltoid region of the upper arm or in the higher anterolateral area of the thigh.
Syncope has been reported following vaccination with GARDASIL and may result in falling with injury; observation for 15 minutes after administration is recommended. [See Warnings and Precautions (5.1).]
Single-Dose Vial Use
Withdraw the 0.5-mL dose of vaccine from the single-dose vial using a sterile needle and syringe and use promptly.
Prefilled Syringe Use
This package does not contain a needle. Shake well before use. Attach the needle by twisting in a clockwise direction until the needle fits securely on the syringe. Administer the entire dose as per standard protocol.

3 DOSAGE FORMS AND STRENGTHS
GARDASIL is a suspension for intramuscular administration available in 0.5-mL single dose vials and prefilled syringes. See *Description (11)* for the complete listing of ingredients.

4 CONTRAINDICATIONS
Hypersensitivity, including severe allergic reactions to yeast (a vaccine component), or after a previous dose of GARDASIL. [See Description (11).]

5 WARNINGS AND PRECAUTIONS
5.1 Syncope
Because vaccinees may develop syncope, sometimes resulting in falling with injury, observation for 15 minutes after administration is recommended. Syncope, sometimes associated with tonic-clonic movements and other seizure-like activity, has been reported following vaccination with GARDASIL. When syncope is associated with tonic-clonic movements, the activity is usually transient and typically responds to restoring cerebral perfusion by maintaining a supine or Trendelenburg position.
5.2 Managing Allergic Reactions
Appropriate medical treatment and supervision must be readily available in case of anaphylactic reactions following the administration of GARDASIL.

6 ADVERSE REACTIONS
Overall Summary of Adverse Reactions
Headache, fever, nausea, and dizziness; and local injection site reactions (pain, swelling, erythema, pruritus, and bruising) occurred after administration with GARDASIL. Syncope, sometimes associated with tonic-clonic movements and other seizure-like activity, has been reported following vaccination with GARDASIL and may result in falling with injury; observation for 15 minutes after administration is recommended. [See Warnings and Precautions (5.1).]
Anaphylaxis has been reported following vaccination with GARDASIL.
6.1 Clinical Trials Experience
Because clinical trials are conducted under widely varying conditions, adverse reaction rates observed in the clinical trials of a vaccine cannot be directly compared to rates in the clinical trials of another vaccine and may not reflect the rates observed in practice.
Studies in Girls and Women (9 Through 45 Years of Age) and Boys and Men (9 Through 26 Years of Age)
In 7 clinical trials (5 Amorphous Aluminum Hydroxyphosphate Sulfate [AAHS]-controlled, 1 saline placebo-controlled, and 1 uncontrolled), 18,083 individuals were administered GARDASIL or AAHS control or saline placebo on the day of enrollment, and approximately 2 and 6 months thereafter, and safety was evaluated using vaccination report cards (VRC)-aided surveillance for 14 days after each injection of GARDASIL or AAHS control or saline placebo in these individuals. The individuals who were monitored using VRC-aided surveillance included 10,088 individuals 9 through 45 years of age at enrollment who received GARDASIL and 7,995 individuals who received AAHS control or saline placebo. Few individuals (0.2%) discontinued due to adverse reactions. The race distribution of the 9- through 26-year-old girls and women in the safety population was as follows: 62.3% White; 17.6% Hispanic (Black and White); 6.8% Asian; 6.7% Other; 6.4% Black; and 0.3% American Indian. The race distribution of the 24- through 45-year-old women in the safety population of Study 6 was as follows: 20.6% White; 43.2% Hispanic (Black and White); 0.2% Other; 4.8% Black; 31.2% Asian; and 0.1% American Indian. The race distribution of the 9- through 26-year-old boys and men in the safety population was as follows: 42.0% White; 19.7% Hispanic (Black and White); 11.0% Asian; 11.2% Other; 15.9% Black; and 0.1% American Indian.
Common Injection-Site Adverse Reactions in Girls and Women 9 Through 26 Years of Age
The injection site adverse reactions that were observed among recipients of GARDASIL at a frequency of at least 1.0% and also at a greater frequency than that observed among AAHS control or saline placebo recipients were shown in Table 1.

Table 1: Injection-Site Adverse Reactions in Girls and Women 9 Through 26 Years of Age*

Adverse Reaction (1 to 5 Days Postvaccination)	GARDASIL (N = 5088) %	AAHS Control[†] (N = 3470) %	Saline Placebo (N = 320) %
Injection Site			
Pain	83.9	75.4	48.6
Swelling	25.4	15.8	7.3
Erythema	24.7	18.4	12.1
Pruritus	3.2	2.8	0.6
Bruising	2.8	3.2	1.6

* The injection-site adverse reactions that were observed among recipients of GARDASIL were at a frequency of at least 1.0% and also at a greater frequency than that observed among AAHS control or saline placebo recipients.
† AAHS Control = Amorphous Aluminum Hydroxyphosphate Sulfate

Common Injection-Site Adverse Reactions in Boys and Men 9 Through 26 Years of Age
The injection site adverse reactions that were observed among recipients of GARDASIL at a frequency of at least 1.0% and also at a greater frequency than that observed among AAHS control or saline placebo recipients are shown in Table 2.

Table 2: Injection-Site Adverse Reactions in Boys and Men 9 Through 26 Years of Age*

Adverse Reaction (1 to 5 Days Postvaccination)	GARDASIL (N = 3093) %	AAHS Control[†] (N = 2029) %	Saline Placebo (N = 274) %
Injection Site			
Pain	61.4	50.8	41.6
Erythema	16.7	14.1	14.5
Swelling	13.9	9.6	8.2
Hematoma	1.0	0.3	3.3

* The injection-site adverse reactions that were observed among recipients of GARDASIL were at a frequency of at least 1.0% and also at a greater frequency than that observed among AAHS control or saline placebo recipients.
† AAHS Control = Amorphous Aluminum Hydroxyphosphate Sulfate

Evaluation of Injection-Site Adverse Reactions by Dose in Girls and Women 9 Through 26 Years of Age
An analysis of injection-site adverse reactions in girls and women by dose is shown in Table 3. Of those girls and

Table 11: Analysis of Efficacy of GARDASIL in the PPE* Population† of 16- Through 26-Year-Old Girls and Women for Vaccine HPV Types

Population	GARDASIL		AAHS Control		% Efficacy (95% CI)
	N	Number of cases	N	Number of cases	
HPV 16- or 18-related CIN 2/3 or AIS					
Study 1‡	755	0	750	12	100.0 (65.1, 100.0)
Study 2	231	0	230	1	100.0 (-3744.9, 100.0)
Study 3	2201	0	2222	36	100.0 (89.2, 100.0)
Study 4	5306	2	5262	63	96.9 (88.2, 99.6)
Combined Protocols§	8493	2	8464	112	98.2 (93.5, 99.8)
HPV 16-related CIN 2/3 or AIS					
Combined Protocols§	7402	2	7205	93	97.9 (92.3, 99.8)
HPV 18-related CIN 2/3 or AIS					
Combined Protocols§	7382	0	7316	29	100.0 (86.6, 100.0)
HPV 16- or 18-related VIN 2/3					
Study 2	231	0	230	0	Not calculated
Study 3	2219	0	2239	6	100.0 (14.4, 100.0)
Study 4	5322	0	5275	4	100.0 (-50.3, 100.0)
Combined Protocols§	7772	0	7744	10	100.0 (55.5, 100.0)
HPV 16- or 18-related VaIN 2/3					
Study 2	231	0	230	0	Not calculated
Study 3	2219	0	2239	5	100.0 (-10.1, 100.0)
Study 4	5322	0	5275	4	100.0 (-50.3, 100.0)
Combined Protocols§	7772	0	7744	9	100.0 (49.5, 100.0)
HPV 6-, 11-, 16-, or 18-related CIN (CIN 1, CIN 2/3) or AIS					
Study 2	235	0	233	3	100.0 (-138.4, 100.0)
Study 3	2241	0	2258	77	100.0 (95.1, 100.0)
Study 4	5388	9	5374	145	93.8 (88.0, 97.2)
Combined Protocols§	7864	9	7865	225	96.0 (92.3, 98.2)
HPV 6-, 11-, 16-, or 18-related Genital Warts					
Study 2	235	0	233	3	100.0 (-139.5, 100.0)
Study 3	2261	0	2279	58	100.0 (93.5, 100.0)
Study 4	5404	2	5390	132	98.5 (94.5, 99.8)
Combined Protocols§	7900	2	7902	193	99.0 (96.2, 99.9)
HPV 6- and 11-related Genital Warts					
Combined Protocols§	6932	2	6856	189	99.0 (96.2, 99.9)

N = Number of individuals with at least 1 follow-up visit after Month 7
CI = Confidence Interval
Note 1: Point estimates and confidence intervals are adjusted for person-time of follow-up.
Note 2: The first analysis in the table (i.e., HPV 16- or 18-related CIN 2/3, AIS or worse) was the primary endpoint of the vaccine development plan.
Note 3: Table 11 does not include cases due to non-vaccine HPV types.
AAHS Control = Amorphous Aluminum Hydroxyphosphate Sulfate
* The PPE population consisted of individuals who received all 3 vaccinations within 1 year of enrollment, did not have major deviations from the study protocol, and were naïve (PCR negative and seronegative) to the relevant HPV type(s) (Types 6, 11, 16, and 18) prior to dose 1 and through 1 month postdose 3 (Month 7).
† See Table 14 for analysis of vaccine impact in the general population.
‡ Evaluated only the HPV 16 L1 VLP vaccine component of GARDASIL
§ Analyses of the combined trials were prospectively planned and included the use of similar study entry criteria.

women who reported an injection-site reaction, 94.3% judged their injection-site adverse reaction to be mild or moderate in intensity.
[See table 3 at top of page 1452]
Evaluation of Injection-Site Adverse Reactions by Dose in Boys and Men 9 Through 26 Years of Age
An analysis of injection-site adverse reactions in boys and men by dose is shown in Table 4. Of those boys and men who

reported an injection-site reaction, 96.4% judged their injection-site adverse reaction to be mild or moderate in intensity.
[See table 4 at top of page 1452]
Common Systemic Adverse Reactions in Girls and Women 9 Through 26 Years of Age
Headache was the most commonly reported systemic adverse reaction in both treatment groups (GARDASIL =

28.2% and AAHS control or saline placebo = 28.4%). Fever was the next most commonly reported systemic adverse reaction in both treatment groups (GARDASIL = 13.0% and AAHS control or saline placebo = 11.2%).
Adverse reactions that were observed among recipients of GARDASIL, at a frequency of greater than or equal to 1.0% where the incidence in the GARDASIL group was greater than or equal to the incidence in the AAHS control or saline placebo group, are shown in Table 5.

Table 5: Common Systemic Adverse Reactions in Girls and Women 9 Through 26 Years of Age (GARDASIL ≥Control)*

Adverse Reactions (1 to 15 Days Postvaccination)	GARDASIL (N = 5088) %	AAHS Control† or Saline Placebo (N = 3790) %
Pyrexia	13.0	11.2
Nausea	6.7	6.5
Dizziness	4.0	3.7
Diarrhea	3.6	3.5
Vomiting	2.4	1.9
Cough	2.0	1.5
Toothache	1.5	1.4
Upper respiratory tract infection	1.5	1.5
Malaise	1.4	1.2
Arthralgia	1.2	0.9
Insomnia	1.2	0.9
Nasal congestion	1.1	0.9

* The adverse reactions in this table are those that were observed among recipients of GARDASIL at a frequency of at least 1.0% and greater than or equal to those observed among AAHS control or saline placebo recipients.
† AAHS Control = Amorphous Aluminum Hydroxyphosphate Sulfate

Common Systemic Adverse Reactions in Boys and Men 9 Through 26 Years of Age
Headache was the most commonly reported systemic adverse reaction in both treatment groups (GARDASIL = 12.3% and AAHS control or saline placebo = 11.2%). Fever was the next most commonly reported systemic adverse reaction in both treatment groups (GARDASIL = 8.3% and AAHS control or saline placebo = 6.5%).
Adverse reactions that were observed among recipients of GARDASIL, at a frequency of greater than or equal to 1.0% where the incidence in the group that received GARDASIL was greater than or equal to the incidence in the AAHS control or saline placebo group, are shown in Table 6.

Table 6: Common Systemic Adverse Reactions in Boys and Men 9 Through 26 Years of Age (GARDASIL ≥Control)*

Adverse Reactions (1 to 15 Days Postvaccination)	GARDASIL (N = 3093) %	AAHS Control† or Saline Placebo (N = 2303) %
Headache	12.3	11.2
Pyrexia	8.3	6.5
Oropharyngeal pain	2.8	2.1
Diarrhea	2.7	2.2
Nasopharyngitis	2.6	2.6
Nausea	2.0	1.0
Upper respiratory tract infection	1.5	1.0
Abdominal pain upper	1.4	1.4
Myalgia	1.3	0.7
Dizziness	1.2	0.9
Vomiting	1.0	0.8

* The adverse reactions in this table are those that were observed among recipients of GARDASIL at a frequency of at least 1.0% and greater than or equal to those observed among AAHS control or saline placebo recipients.
† AAHS Control = Amorphous Aluminum Hydroxyphosphate Sulfate

Evaluation of Fever by Dose in Girls and Women 9 Through 26 Years of Age
An analysis of fever in girls and women by dose is shown in Table 7.
[See table 7 at top of previous page]

Table 12: Analysis of Efficacy of GARDASIL in the PPE* Population of 16- Through 26-Year-Old Boys and Men for Vaccine HPV Types

Endpoint	GARDASIL		AAHS Control		% Efficacy (95% CI)
	N[†]	Number of cases	N	Number of cases	
External Genital Lesions HPV 6-, 11-, 16-, or 18- related					
External Genital Lesions	1394	3	1404	32	90.6 (70.1, 98.2)
Condyloma	1394	3	1404	28	89.3 (65.3, 97.9)
PIN 1/2/3	1394	0	1404	4	100.0 (-52.1, 100.0)

CI = Confidence Interval
AAHS Control = Amorphous Aluminum Hydroxyphosphate Sulfate
* The PPE population consisted of individuals who received all 3 vaccinations within 1 year of enrollment, did not have major deviations from the study protocol, and were naïve (PCR negative and seronegative) to the relevant HPV type(s) (Types 6, 11, 16, and 18) prior to dose 1 and through 1 month postdose 3 (Month 7).
† N = Number of individuals with at least 1 follow-up visit after Month 7

Table 13: Analysis of Efficacy of GARDASIL for Anal Disease in the PPE* Population of 16- Through 26-Year-Old Boys and Men in the MSM Sub-study for Vaccine HPV Types

HPV 6-, 11-, 16-, or 18- related Endpoint	GARDASIL		AAHS Control		% Efficacy (95% CI)
	N[†]	Number of cases	N	Number of cases	
AIN 1/2/3	194	5	208	24	77.5 (39.6, 93.3)
AIN 2/3	194	3	208	13	74.9 (8.8, 95.4)
AIN 1	194	4	208	16	73.0 (16.3, 93.4)
Condyloma Acuminatum	194	0	208	6	100.0 (8.2, 100.0)
Non-acuminate	194	4	208	11	60.4 (-33.5, 90.8)

CI = Confidence Interval
AAHS Control = Amorphous Aluminum Hydroxyphosphate Sulfate
* The PPE population consisted of individuals who received all 3 vaccinations within 1 year of enrollment, did not have major deviations from the study protocol, and were naïve (PCR negative and seronegative) to the relevant HPV type(s) (Types 6, 11, 16, and 18) prior to dose 1 and through 1 month postdose 3 (month 7).
† N = Number of individuals with at least 1 follow-up visit after Month 7

Table 14: Effectiveness of GARDASIL in Prevention of HPV 6, 11, 16, or 18-Related Genital Disease in Girls and Women 16 Through 26 Years of Age, Regardless of Current or Prior Exposure to Vaccine HPV Types

Endpoint	Analysis	GARDASIL or HPV 16 L1 VLP Vaccine		AAHS Control		% Reduction (95% CI)
		N	Cases	N	Cases	
HPV 16- or 18-related CIN 2/3 or AIS	Prophylactic Efficacy*	9346	4	9407	155	97.4 (93.3, 99.3)
	HPV 16 and/or HPV 18 Positive at Day 1[†]	2870	142	2898	148[‡]	--[§]
	Girls and Women Regardless of Current or Prior Exposure to HPV 16 or 18[¶]	9836	146	9904	303	51.8 (41.1, 60.7)
HPV 16- or 18-related VIN 2/3 or VaIN 2/3	Prophylactic Efficacy*	8642	1	8673	34	97.0 (82.4, 99.9)
	HPV 16 and/or HPV 18 Positive at Day 1[†]	1880	8	1876	4	--[§]
	Girls and Women Regardless of Current or Prior Exposure to HPV 16 or 18[¶]	8955	9	8968	38	76.3 (50.0, 89.9)
HPV 6-, 11-, 16-, 18-related CIN (CIN 1, CIN 2/3) or AIS	Prophylactic Efficacy*	8630	16	8680	309	94.8 (91.5, 97.1)
	HPV 6, HPV 11, HPV 16, and/or HPV 18 Positive at Day 1[†]	2466	186[#]	2437	213[#]	--[§]
	Girls and Women Regardless of Current or Prior Exposure to Vaccine HPV Types[¶]	8819	202	8854	522	61.5 (54.6, 67.4)

(Table continued on next page)

Evaluation of Fever by Dose in Boys and Men 9 Through 26 Years of Age
An analysis of fever in boys and men by dose is shown in Table 8.
[See table 8 at top of page 1453]
Serious Adverse Reactions in the Entire Study Population
Across the clinical studies, 258 individuals (GARDASIL N = 128 or 0.8%; placebo N = 130 or 1.0%) out of 29,323 (GARDASIL N = 15,706; AAHS control N = 13,023; or saline placebo N = 594) individuals (9- through 45-year-old girls and women; and 9- through 26-year-old boys and men) reported a serious systemic adverse reaction.
Of the entire study population (29,323 individuals), 0.04% of the reported serious systemic adverse reactions were judged to be vaccine related by the study investigator. The most frequently (frequency of 4 cases or greater with either

GARDASIL, AAHS control, saline placebo, or the total of all three) reported serious systemic adverse reactions, regardless of causality, were:
Headache [0.02% GARDASIL (3 cases) vs. 0.02% AAHS control (2 cases)],
Gastroenteritis [0.02% GARDASIL (3 cases) vs. 0.02% AAHS control (2 cases)],
Appendicitis [0.03% GARDASIL (5 cases) vs. 0.01% AAHS control (1 case)],
Pelvic inflammatory disease [0.02% GARDASIL (3 cases) vs. 0.03% AAHS control (4 cases)],
Urinary tract infection [0.01% GARDASIL (2 cases) vs. 0.02% AAHS control (2 cases)],
Pneumonia [0.01% GARDASIL (2 cases) vs. 0.02% AAHS control (2 cases)],
Pyelonephritis [0.01% GARDASIL (2 cases) vs. 0.02% AAHS control (3 cases)],
Pulmonary embolism [0.01% GARDASIL (2 cases) vs. 0.02% AAHS control (2 cases)].
One case (0.006% GARDASIL; 0.0% AAHS control or saline placebo) of bronchospasm; and 2 cases (0.01% GARDASIL; 0.0% AAHS control or saline placebo) of asthma were reported as serious systemic adverse reactions that occurred following any vaccination visit.
In addition, there was 1 individual in the clinical trials, in the group that received GARDASIL, who reported two injection-site serious adverse reactions (injection-site pain and injection-site joint movement impairment).
Deaths in the Entire Study Population
Across the clinical studies, 40 deaths (GARDASIL N = 21 or 0.1%; placebo N = 19 or 0.1%) were reported in 29,323 (GARDASIL N = 15,706; AAHS control N = 13,023, saline placebo N = 594) individuals (9- through 45-year-old girls and women; and 9- through 26-year-old boys and men). The events reported were consistent with events expected in healthy adolescent and adult populations. The most common cause of death was motor vehicle accident (5 individuals who received GARDASIL and 4 individuals who received AAHS control), followed by drug overdose/suicide (2 individuals who received GARDASIL and 6 individuals who received AAHS control), gunshot wound (1 individual who received GARDASIL and 3 individuals who received AAHS control), and pulmonary embolus/deep vein thrombosis (1 individual who received GARDASIL and 1 individual who received AAHS control). In addition, there were 2 cases of sepsis, 1 case of pancreatic cancer, 1 case of arrhythmia, 1 case of pulmonary tuberculosis, 1 case of hyperthyroidism, 1 case of post-operative pulmonary embolism and acute renal failure, 1 case of traumatic brain injury/cardiac arrest, 1 case of systemic lupus erythematosus, 1 case of cerebrovascular accident, 1 case of breast cancer, and 1 case of nasopharyngeal cancer in the group that received GARDASIL; 1 case of asphyxia, 1 case of acute lymphocytic leukemia, 1 case of chemical poisoning, and 1 case of myocardial ischemia in the AAHS control group; and 1 case of medulloblastoma in the saline placebo group.
Systemic Autoimmune Disorders in Girls and Women 9 Through 26 Years of Age
In the clinical studies, 9- through 26-year-old girls and women were evaluated for new medical conditions that occurred over the course of follow-up. New medical conditions potentially indicative of a systemic autoimmune disorder seen in the group that received GARDASIL, AAHS control or saline placebo are shown in Table 9. This population includes all girls and women who received at least one dose of GARDASIL or AAHS control or saline placebo, and had safety data available.

Table 9: Summary of Girls and Women 9 Through 26 Years of Age Who Reported an Incident Condition Potentially Indicative of a Systemic Autoimmune Disorder After Enrollment in Clinical Trials of GARDASIL, Regardless of Causality

Conditions	GARDASIL (N = 10,706)	AAHS Control* or Saline Placebo (N = 9412)
	n (%)	n (%)
Arthralgia/Arthritis/Arthropathy[†]	120 (1.1)	98 (1.0)
Autoimmune Thyroiditis	4 (0.0)	1 (0.0)
Celiac Disease	10 (0.1)	6 (0.1)
Diabetes Mellitus Insulin-dependent	2 (0.0)	2 (0.0)
Erythema Nodosum	2 (0.0)	4 (0.0)
Hyperthyroidism[‡]	27 (0.3)	21 (0.2)
Hypothyroidism[§]	35 (0.3)	38 (0.4)
Inflammatory Bowel Disease[¶]	7 (0.1)	10 (0.1)
Multiple Sclerosis	2 (0.0)	4 (0.0)
Nephritis[#]	2 (0.0)	5 (0.1)
Optic Neuritis	2 (0.0)	0 (0.0)
Pigmentation Disorder[b]	4 (0.0)	3 (0.0)

Psoriasis[ß]	13 (0.1)	15 (0.2)
Raynaud's Phenomenon	3 (0.0)	4 (0.0)
Rheumatoid Arthritis[à]	6 (0.1)	2 (0.0)
Scleroderma/Morphea	2 (0.0)	1 (0.0)
Stevens-Johnson Syndrome	1 (0.0)	0 (0.0)
Systemic Lupus Erythematosus	1 (0.0)	3 (0.0)
Uveitis	3 (0.0)	1 (0.0)
All Conditions	**245 (2.3)**	**218 (2.3)**

N = Number of individuals enrolled
n = Number of individuals with specific new Medical Conditions
NOTE: Although an individual may have had two or more new Medical Conditions, the individual is counted only once within a category. The same individual may appear in different categories.
* AAHS Control = Amorphous Aluminum Hydroxyphosphate Sulfate
† Arthralgia/Arthritis/Arthropathy includes the following terms: Arthralgia, Arthritis, Arthritis reactive, and Arthropathy
‡ Hyperthyroidism includes the following terms: Basedow's disease, Goiter, Toxic nodular goiter, and Hyperthyroidism
§ Hypothyroidism includes the following terms: Hypothyroidism and thyroiditis
¶ Inflammatory bowel disease includes the following terms: Colitis ulcerative, Crohn's disease, and Inflammatory bowel disease
# Nephritis includes the following terms: Nephritis, Glomerulonephritis minimal lesion, Glomerulonephritis proliferative
Þ Pigmentation disorder includes the following terms: Pigmentation disorder, Skin depigmentation, and Vitiligo
ß Psoriasis includes the following terms: Psoriasis, Pustular psoriasis, and Psoriatic arthropathy
à Rheumatoid arthritis includes juvenile rheumatoid arthritis. One woman counted in the rheumatoid arthritis group reported rheumatoid arthritis as an adverse experience at Day 130.

Systemic Autoimmune Disorders in Boys and Men 9 Through 26 Years of Age
In the clinical studies, 9- through 26-year-old boys and men were evaluated for new medical conditions that occurred over the course of follow-up. New medical conditions potentially indicative of a systemic autoimmune disorder seen in the group that received GARDASIL or AAHS control or saline placebo are shown in Table 10. This population includes all boys and men who received at least one dose of GARDASIL or AAHS control or saline placebo, and had safety data available.

Table 10: Summary of Boys and Men 9 Through 26 Years of Age Who Reported an Incident Condition Potentially Indicative of a Systemic Autoimmune Disorder After Enrollment in Clinical Trials of GARDASIL, Regardless of Causality

Conditions	GARDASIL (N = 3093)	AAHS Control* or Saline Placebo (N = 2303)
	n (%)	n (%)
Alopecia Areata	2 (0.1)	0 (0.0)
Ankylosing Spondylitis	1 (0.0)	2 (0.1)
Arthralgia/Arthritis/ Reactive Arthritis	30 (1.0)	17 (0.7)
Autoimmune Thrombocytopenia	1 (0.0)	0 (0.0)
Diabetes Mellitus Type 1	3 (0.1)	2 (0.1)
Hyperthyroidism	0 (0.0)	1 (0.0)
Hypothyroidism[†]	3 (0.1)	0 (0.0)
Inflammatory Bowel Disease[‡]	1 (0.0)	2 (0.1)
Myocarditis	1 (0.0)	1 (0.0)
Proteinuria	1 (0.0)	0 (0.0)
Psoriasis	0 (0.0)	4 (0.2)
Skin Depigmentation	1 (0.0)	0 (0.0)
Vitiligo	2 (0.1)	5 (0.2)
All Conditions	**46 (1.5)**	**34 (1.5)**

N = Number of individuals who received at least one dose of either vaccine or placebo

Table 14 *(cont.)*: Effectiveness of GARDASIL in Prevention of HPV 6, 11, 16, or 18-Related Genital Disease in Girls and Women 16 Through 26 Years of Age, Regardless of Current or Prior Exposure to Vaccine HPV Types

Endpoint	Analysis	GARDASIL or HPV 16 L1 VLP Vaccine		AAHS Control		% Reduction (95% CI)
		N	Cases	N	Cases	
HPV 6-, 11-, 16-, or 18-related Genital Warts	Prophylactic Efficacy*	8761	10	8792	252	96.0 (92.6, 98.1)
	HPV 6, HPV 11, HPV 16, and/or HPV 18 Positive at Day 1[†]	2501	51[Þ]	2475	55[Þ]	--[§]
	Girls and Women Regardless of Current or Prior Exposure to Vaccine HPV Types[¶]	8955	61	8968	307	80.3 (73.9, 85.3)
HPV 6- or 11-related Genital Warts	Prophylactic Efficacy*	7769	9	7792	246	96.4 (93.0, 98.4)
	HPV 6 and/or HPV 11 Positive at Day 1[†]	1186	51	1176	54	--[§]
	Girls and Women Regardless of Current or Prior Exposure to Vaccine HPV Types[¶]	8955	60	8968	300	80.1 (73.7, 85.2)

CI = Confidence Interval
N = Number of individuals who have at least one follow-up visit after Day 1
Note 1: The 16- and 18-related CIN 2/3 or AIS composite endpoint included data from studies 1, 2, 3, and 4. All other endpoints only included data from studies 2, 3, and 4.
Note 2: Positive status at Day 1 denotes PCR positive and/or seropositive for the respective type at Day 1.
Note 3: Table 14 does not include disease due to non-vaccine HPV types.
AAHS Control = Amorphous Aluminum Hydroxyphosphate Sulfate
* Includes all individuals who received at least 1 vaccination and who were HPV-naïve (i.e., seronegative and PCR negative) at Day 1 to the vaccine HPV type being analyzed. Case counting started at 1 month postdose 1.
† Includes all individuals who received at least 1 vaccination and who were HPV positive or had unknown HPV status at Day 1, to at least one vaccine HPV type. Case counting started at Day 1.
‡ Out of the 148 AAHS control cases of 16/18 CIN 2/3, 2 women were missing serology or PCR results for Day 1.
§ There is no expected efficacy since GARDASIL has not been demonstrated to provide protection against disease from vaccine HPV types to which a person has previously been exposed through sexual activity.
¶ Includes all individuals who received at least 1 vaccination (regardless of baseline HPV status at Day 1). Case counting started at 1 month postdose 1.
# Includes 2 AAHS control women with missing serology/PCR data at Day 1.
Þ Includes 1 woman with missing serology/PCR data at Day 1.

n = Number of individuals with specific new Medical Conditions
NOTE: Although an individual may have had two or more new Medical Conditions, the individual is counted only once within a category. The same individual may appear in different categories.
* AAHS Control = Amorphous Aluminum Hydroxyphosphate Sulfate
† Hypothyroidism includes the following terms: Hypothyroidism and Autoimmune thyroiditis
‡ Inflammatory bowel disease includes the following terms: Colitis ulcerative and Crohn's disease

Safety in Concomitant Use with RECOMBIVAX HB® [hepatitis B vaccine (recombinant)] in Girls and Women 16 Through 23 Years of Age
The safety of GARDASIL when administered concomitantly with RECOMBIVAX HB® [hepatitis B vaccine (recombinant)] was evaluated in an AAHS-controlled study of 1871 girls and women with a mean age of 20.4 years *[see Clinical Studies (14.9)]*. The race distribution of the study individuals was as follows: 61.6% White; 23.8% Other; 11.9% Black; 1.6% Hispanic (Black and White); 0.8% Asian; and 0.3% American Indian. The rates of systemic and injection-site adverse reactions were similar among girls and women who received concomitant vaccination as compared with those who received GARDASIL or RECOMBIVAX HB [hepatitis B vaccine (recombinant)].
Safety in Concomitant Use with Menactra [Meningococcal (Groups A, C, Y and W-135) Polysaccharide Diphtheria Toxoid Conjugate Vaccine] and Adacel [Tetanus Toxoid, Reduced Diphtheria Toxoid and Acellular Pertussis Vaccine Adsorbed (Tdap)]
The safety of GARDASIL when administered concomitantly with Menactra [Meningococcal (Groups A, C, Y and W-135) Polysaccharide Diphtheria Toxoid Conjugate Vaccine] and Adacel [Tetanus Toxoid, Reduced Diphtheria Toxoid and Acellular Pertussis Vaccine Adsorbed (Tdap)] was evaluated in a randomized study of 1040 boys and girls with a mean age of 12.6 years *[see Clinical Studies (14.10)]*. The race distribution of the study subjects was as follows: 77.7% White; 1.4% Multi-racial; 12.3% Black; 6.8% Hispanic (Black and White); 1.2% Asian; 0.4% American Indian, and 0.2% Indian.
There was an increase in injection-site swelling reported at the injection site for GARDASIL (concomitant = 10.9%, non-concomitant = 6.9%) when GARDASIL was administered concomitantly with Menactra and Adacel as compared to

non-concomitant (separated by 1 month) vaccination. The majority of injection-site swelling adverse experiences were reported as being mild to moderate in intensity.
Safety in Women 27 Through 45 Years of Age
The adverse reaction profile in women 27 through 45 years of age was comparable to the profile seen in girls and women 9 through 26 years of age.

6.2   Postmarketing Experience
The following adverse events have been spontaneously reported during post-approval use of GARDASIL. Because these events were reported voluntarily from a population of uncertain size, it is not possible to reliably estimate their frequency or to establish a causal relationship to vaccine exposure.
Blood and lymphatic system disorders: Autoimmune hemolytic anemia, idiopathic thrombocytopenic purpura, lymphadenopathy.
Respiratory, thoracic and mediastinal disorders: Pulmonary embolus.
Gastrointestinal disorders: Nausea, pancreatitis, vomiting.
General disorders and administration site conditions: Asthenia, chills, death, fatigue, malaise.
Immune system disorders: Autoimmune diseases, hypersensitivity reactions including anaphylactic/anaphylactoid reactions, bronchospasm, and urticaria.
Musculoskeletal and connective tissue disorders: Arthralgia, myalgia.
Nervous system disorders: Acute disseminated encephalomyelitis, dizziness, Guillain-Barré syndrome, headache, motor neuron disease, paralysis, seizures, syncope (including syncope associated with tonic-clonic movements and other seizure-like activity) sometimes resulting in falling with injury, transverse myelitis.
Infections and infestations: cellulitis.
Vascular disorders: Deep venous thrombosis.

7   DRUG INTERACTIONS
7.1   Use with RECOMBIVAX HB
Results from clinical studies indicate that GARDASIL may be administered concomitantly (at a separate injection site) with RECOMBIVAX HB [hepatitis B vaccine (recombinant)] *[see Clinical Studies (14.9)]*.
7.2   Use with Menactra and Adacel
Results from clinical studies indicate that GARDASIL may be administered concomitantly (at a separate injection site)

with Menactra [Meningococcal (Groups A, C, Y and W-135) Polysaccharide Diphtheria Toxoid Conjugate Vaccine] and Adacel [Tetanus Toxoid, Reduced Diphtheria Toxoid and Acellular Pertussis Vaccine Adsorbed (Tdap)] [see Clinical Studies (14.10)].

7.3 Use with Hormonal Contraceptives

In clinical studies of 16- through 26-year-old women, 13,912 (GARDASIL N = 6952; AAHS control or saline placebo N = 6960) who had post-Month 7 follow-up used hormonal contraceptives for a total of 33,859 person-years (65.8% of the total follow-up time in the studies).

In one clinical study of 24- through 45-year-old women, 1357 (GARDASIL N = 690; AAHS control N = 667) who had post-Month 7 follow-up used hormonal contraceptives for a total of 3400 person-years (31.5% of the total follow-up time in the study). Use of hormonal contraceptives or lack of use of hormonal contraceptives among study participants did not impair the immune response in the per protocol immunogenicity (PPI) population.

7.4 Use with Systemic Immunosuppressive Medications

Immunosuppressive therapies, including irradiation, antimetabolites, alkylating agents, cytotoxic drugs, and corticosteroids (used in greater than physiologic doses), may reduce the immune responses to vaccines [see Use in Specific Populations (8.6)].

8 USE IN SPECIFIC POPULATIONS

8.1 Pregnancy

Pregnancy Category B:

Reproduction studies have been performed in female rats at doses equivalent to the recommended human dose and have revealed no evidence of impaired female fertility or harm to the fetus due to GARDASIL. There are, however, no adequate and well-controlled studies in pregnant women. Because animal reproduction studies are not always predictive of human responses, GARDASIL should be used during pregnancy only if clearly needed.

An evaluation of the effect of GARDASIL on embryo-fetal, pre- and postweaning development was conducted using rats. One group of rats was administered GARDASIL twice prior to gestation, during the period of organogenesis (gestation Day 6) and on lactation Day 7. A second group of pregnant rats was administered GARDASIL during the period of organogenesis (gestation Day 6) and on lactation Day 7 only. GARDASIL was administered at 0.5 mL/rat/occasion (120 mcg total protein which is equivalent to the recommended human dose) by intramuscular injection. No adverse effects on mating, fertility, pregnancy, parturition, lactation, embryo-fetal or pre- and postweaning development were observed. There were no vaccine-related fetal malformations or other evidence of teratogenesis noted in this study. In addition, there were no treatment-related effects on developmental signs, behavior, reproductive performance, or fertility of the offspring.

Clinical Studies in Humans

In clinical studies, women underwent urine pregnancy testing prior to administration of each dose of GARDASIL. Women who were found to be pregnant before completion of a 3-dose regimen of GARDASIL were instructed to defer completion of their vaccination regimen until resolution of the pregnancy.

GARDASIL is not indicated for women 27 years of age or older. However, safety data in women 16 through 45 years of age was collected, and 3819 women (GARDASIL N = 1894 vs. AAHS control or saline placebo N = 1925) reported at least 1 pregnancy each.

The overall proportions of pregnancies that resulted in an adverse outcome, defined as the combined numbers of spontaneous abortion, late fetal death, and congenital anomaly cases out of the total number of pregnancy outcomes for which an outcome was known (and excluding elective terminations), were 22.6% (446/1973) in women who received GARDASIL and 23.1% (460/1994) in women who received AAHS control or saline placebo.

Overall, 55 and 65 women in the group that received GARDASIL or AAHS control or saline placebo, respectively (2.9% and 3.4% of all women who reported a pregnancy in the respective vaccination groups), experienced a serious adverse reaction during pregnancy. The most common events reported were conditions that can result in Caesarean section (e.g., failure of labor, malpresentation, cephalopelvic disproportion), premature onset of labor (e.g., threatened abortions, premature rupture of membranes), and pregnancy-related medical problems (e.g., pre-eclampsia, hyperemesis). The proportions of pregnant women who experienced such events were comparable between the groups receiving GARDASIL and AAHS control or saline placebo. There were 45 cases of congenital anomaly in pregnancies that occurred in women who received GARDASIL and 34 cases of congenital anomaly in pregnancies that occurred in women who received AAHS control or saline placebo. Further sub-analyses were conducted to evaluate pregnancies with estimated onset within 30 days or more than 30

days from administration of a dose of GARDASIL or AAHS control or saline placebo. For pregnancies with estimated onset within 30 days of vaccination, 5 cases of congenital anomaly were observed in the group that received GARDASIL compared to 1 case of congenital anomaly in the group that received AAHS control or saline placebo. The congenital anomalies seen in pregnancies with estimated onset within 30 days of vaccination included pyloric stenosis, congenital megacolon, congenital hydronephrosis, hip dysplasia, and club foot. Conversely, in pregnancies with onset more than 30 days following vaccination, 40 cases of congenital anomaly were observed in the group that received GARDASIL compared with 33 cases of congenital anomaly in the group that received AAHS control or saline placebo.

Women who receive GARDASIL during pregnancy are encouraged to contact Merck Sharp & Dohme Corp., a subsidiary of Merck & Co., Inc., at 1-877-888-4231 or VAERS at 1-800-822-7967 or www.vaers.hhs.gov.

8.3 Nursing Mothers

Women 16 Through 45 Years of Age

It is not known whether GARDASIL is excreted in human milk. Because many drugs are excreted in human milk, caution should be exercised when GARDASIL is administered to a nursing woman.

GARDASIL or AAHS control were given to a total of 1133 women (vaccine N = 582, AAHS control N = 551) during the relevant Phase III clinical studies.

Table 15: Effectiveness of GARDASIL in Prevention of Any HPV Type Related Genital Disease in Girls and Women 16 Through 26 Years of Age, Regardless of Current or Prior Infection with Vaccine or Non-Vaccine HPV Types

Endpoints Caused by Vaccine or Non-vaccine HPV Types	Analysis	GARDASIL		AAHS Control		% Reduction (95% CI)
		N	Cases	N	Cases	
CIN 2/3 or AIS	Prophylactic Efficacy*	4616	77	4680	136	42.7 (23.7, 57.3)
	Girls and Women Regardless of Current or Prior Exposure to Vaccine or Non-Vaccine HPV Types†	8559	421	8592	516	18.4 (7.0, 28.4)
VIN 2/3 and VaIN 2/3	Prophylactic Efficacy*	4688	7	4735	31	77.1 (47.1, 91.5)
	Girls and Women Regardless of Current or Prior Exposure to Vaccine or Non-Vaccine HPV Types†	8688	30	8701	61	50.7 (22.5, 69.3)
CIN (Any Grade) or AIS	Prophylactic Efficacy*	4616	272	4680	390	29.7 (17.7, 40.0)
	Girls and Women Regardless of Current or Prior Exposure to Vaccine or Non-Vaccine HPV Types†	8559	967	8592	1189	19.1 (11.9, 25.8)
Genital Warts	Prophylactic Efficacy*	4688	29	4735	169	82.8 (74.3, 88.8)
	Girls and Women Regardless of Current or Prior Exposure to Vaccine or Non-Vaccine HPV Types†	8688	132	8701	350	62.5 (54.0, 69.5)

CI = Confidence Interval

AAHS Control = Amorphous Aluminum Hydroxyphosphate Sulfate

* Includes all individuals who received at least 1 vaccination and who had a Pap test that was negative for SIL [Squamous Intraepithelial Lesion] at Day 1 and were naïve to 14 common HPV types at Day 1. Case counting started at 1 month postdose 1.

† Includes all individuals who received at least 1 vaccination (regardless of baseline HPV status or Pap test result at Day 1). Case counting started at 1 month postdose 1.

Table 16: Effectiveness of GARDASIL in Prevention of HPV Types 6-, 11-, 16-, or 18-Related Anogenital Disease in Boys and Men 16 Through 26 Years of Age, Regardless of Current or Prior Exposure to Vaccine HPV Types

Endpoint	Analysis	GARDASIL		AAHS Control		% Reduction (95% CI)
		N	Cases	N	Cases	
External Genital Lesions	Prophylactic Efficacy*	1775	13	1770	54	76.3 (56.0, 88.1)
	HPV 6, HPV 11, HPV 16, and/or HPV 18 Positive at Day 1†	460	14	453	26	--‡
	Boys and Men Regardless of Current or Prior Exposure to Vaccine or Non-Vaccine HPV Types§	1943	27	1937	80	66.7 (48.0, 79.3)
Condyloma	Prophylactic Efficacy*	1775	10	1770	49	80.0 (59.9, 90.9)
	HPV 6, HPV 11, HPV 16, and/or HPV 18 Positive at Day 1†	460	14	453	25	--†
	Boys and Men Regardless of Current or Prior Exposure to Vaccine or Non-Vaccine HPV Types§	1943	24	1937	74	68.1 (48.8, 80.7)

(Table continued on next page)

Table 16 (cont.): Effectiveness of GARDASIL in Prevention of HPV Types 6-, 11-, 16-, or 18-Related Anogenital Disease in Boys and Men 16 Through 26 Years of Age, Regardless of Current or Prior Exposure to Vaccine HPV Types

Endpoint	Analysis	GARDASIL		AAHS Control		% Reduction (95% CI)
		N	Cases	N	Cases	
PIN 1/2/3	Prophylactic Efficacy*	1775	4	1770	5	20.7 (-268.4, 84.3)
	HPV 6, HPV 11, HPV 16, and/or HPV 18 Positive at Day 1†	460	2	453	1	--‡
	Boys and Men Regardless of Current or Prior Exposure to Vaccine or Non-Vaccine HPV Types§	1943	6	1937	6	0.3 (-272.8, 73.4)
AIN 1/2/3	Prophylactic Efficacy*	259	9	261	39	76.9 (51.4, 90.1)
	HPV 6, HPV 11, HPV 16, and/or HPV 18 Positive at Day 1†	103	29	116	38	--‡
	Boys and Men Regardless of Current or Prior Exposure to Vaccine or Non-Vaccine HPV Types§	275	38	276	77	50.3 (25.7, 67.2)
AIN 2/3	Prophylactic Efficacy*	259	7	261	19	62.5 (6.9, 86.7)
	HPV 6, HPV 11, HPV 16, and/or HPV 18 Positive at Day 1†	103	11	116	20	--‡
	Boys and Men Regardless of Current or Prior Exposure to Vaccine or Non-Vaccine HPV Types§	275	18	276	39	54.2 (18.0, 75.3)

CI = Confidence Interval
AAHS Control = Amorphous Aluminum Hydroxyphosphate Sulfate
* Includes all individuals who received at least 1 vaccination and who were HPV-naïve (i.e., seronegative and PCR negative) at Day 1 to the vaccine HPV type being analyzed. Case counting started at Day 1.
† Includes all individuals who received at least 1 vaccination and who were HPV positive or had unknown HPV status at Day 1, to at least one vaccine HPV type. Case counting started at Day 1.
‡ There is no expected efficacy since GARDASIL has not been demonstrated to provide protection against disease from vaccine HPV types to which a person has previously been exposed through sexual activity.
§ Includes all individuals who received at least 1 vaccination. Case counting started at Day 1.

Table 17: Effectiveness of GARDASIL in Prevention of Any HPV Type Related Anogenital Disease in Boys and Men 16 Through 26 Years of Age, Regardless of Current or Prior Infection with Vaccine or Non-Vaccine HPV Types

Endpoint	Analysis	GARDASIL		AAHS Control		% Reduction (95% CI)
		N	Cases	N	Cases	
External Genital Lesions	Prophylactic Efficacy*	1275	7	1270	37	81.5 (58.0, 93.0)
	Boys and Men Regardless of Current or Prior Exposure to Vaccine or Non-Vaccine HPV Types†	1943	38	1937	92	59.3 (40.0, 72.9)
Condyloma	Prophylactic Efficacy*	1275	5	1270	33	85.2 (61.8, 95.5)
	Boys and Men Regardless of Current or Prior Exposure to Vaccine or Non-Vaccine HPV Types†	1943	33	1937	85	61.8 (42.3, 75.3)
PIN 1/2/3	Prophylactic Efficacy*	1275	2	1270	4	50.7 (-244.3, 95.5)
	Boys and Men Regardless of Current or Prior Exposure to Vaccine or Non-Vaccine HPV Types†	1943	8	1937	7	-13.9 (-269.0, 63.9)
AIN 1/2/3	Prophylactic Efficacy*	129	12	126	28	54.9 (8.4, 79.1)
	Boys and Men Regardless of Current or Prior Exposure to Vaccine or Non-Vaccine HPV Types†	275	74	276	103	25.7 (-1.1, 45.6)
AIN 2/3	Prophylactic Efficacy*	129	8	126	18	52.5 (-14.8, 82.1)
	Boys and Men Regardless of Current or Prior Exposure to Vaccine or Non-Vaccine HPV Types†	275	44	276	59	24.3 (-13.8, 50.0)

CI = Confidence Interval
AAHS Control = Amorphous Aluminum Hydroxyphosphate Sulfate
* Includes all individuals who received at least 1 vaccination and who were seronegative and PCR negative at enrollment to HPV 6, 11, 16 and 18, and PCR negative at enrollment to HPV 31, 33, 35, 39, 45, 51, 52, 56, 58 and 59. Case counting started at Day 1.
† Includes all individuals who received at least 1 vaccination. Case counting started at Day 1.

Overall, 27 and 13 infants of women who received GARDASIL or AAHS control, respectively (representing 4.6% and 2.4% of the total number of women who were breast-feeding during the period in which they received GARDASIL or AAHS control, respectively), experienced a serious adverse reaction.

In a post-hoc analysis of clinical studies, a higher number of breast-feeding infants (n = 7) whose mothers received GARDASIL had acute respiratory illnesses within 30 days post vaccination of the mother as compared to infants (n = 2) whose mothers received AAHS control.

8.4 Pediatric Use
Safety and effectiveness have not been established in pediatric patients below 9 years of age.

8.5 Geriatric Use
The safety and effectiveness of GARDASIL have not been evaluated in a geriatric population, defined as individuals aged 65 years and over.

8.6 Immunocompromised Individuals
The immunologic response to GARDASIL may be diminished in immunocompromised individuals [see Drug Interactions (7.4)].

10 OVERDOSAGE
There have been reports of administration of higher than recommended doses of GARDASIL.
In general, the adverse event profile reported with overdose was comparable to recommended single doses of GARDASIL.

11 DESCRIPTION
GARDASIL, Human Papillomavirus Quadrivalent (Types 6, 11, 16, and 18) Vaccine, Recombinant, is a non-infectious recombinant quadrivalent vaccine prepared from the purified virus-like particles (VLPs) of the major capsid (L1) protein of HPV Types 6, 11, 16, and 18. The L1 proteins are produced by separate fermentations in recombinant Saccharomyces cerevisiae and self-assembled into VLPs. The fermentation process involves growth of S. cerevisiae on chemically-defined fermentation media which include vitamins, amino acids, mineral salts, and carbohydrates. The VLPs are released from the yeast cells by cell disruption and purified by a series of chemical and physical methods. The purified VLPs are adsorbed on preformed aluminum-containing adjuvant (Amorphous Aluminum Hydroxyphosphate Sulfate). The quadrivalent HPV VLP vaccine is a sterile liquid suspension that is prepared by combining the adsorbed VLPs of each HPV type and additional amounts of the aluminum-containing adjuvant and the final purification buffer.

GARDASIL is a sterile suspension for intramuscular administration. Each 0.5-mL dose contains approximately 20 mcg of HPV 6 L1 protein, 40 mcg of HPV 11 L1 protein, 40 mcg of HPV 16 L1 protein, and 20 mcg of HPV 18 L1 protein.

Each 0.5-mL dose of the vaccine contains approximately 225 mcg of aluminum (as Amorphous Aluminum Hydroxyphosphate Sulfate adjuvant), 9.56 mg of sodium chloride, 0.78 mg of L-histidine, 50 mcg of polysorbate 80, 35 mcg of sodium borate, <7 mcg yeast protein/dose, and water for injection. The product does not contain a preservative or antibiotics.

After thorough agitation, GARDASIL is a white, cloudy liquid.

12 CLINICAL PHARMACOLOGY
12.1 Mechanism of Action
HPV only infects human beings. Animal studies with analogous animal papillomaviruses suggest that the efficacy of L1 VLP vaccines may involve the development of humoral immune responses. Human beings develop a humoral immune response to the vaccine, although the exact mechanism of protection is unknown.

13 NONCLINICAL TOXICOLOGY
13.1 Carcinogenesis, Mutagenesis, Impairment of Fertility
GARDASIL has not been evaluated for the potential to cause carcinogenicity or genotoxicity.

GARDASIL administered to female rats at a dose of 120 mcg total protein, which is equivalent to the recommended human dose, had no effects on mating performance, fertility, or embryonic/fetal survival.

The effect of GARDASIL on male fertility has been studied in male rats at an intramuscular dose of 0.5 mL/rat/occasion (120 mcg total protein which is equivalent to the recommended human dose). One group of male rats was administered GARDASIL once, 3 days prior to cohabitation, and a second group of male rats was administered GARDASIL three times, at 6 weeks, 3 weeks, and 3 days prior to cohabitation. There were no treatment-related effects on reproductive performance including fertility, sperm count, and sperm motility. There were no treatment-related gross or histomorphologic and weight changes on the testes.

14 CLINICAL STUDIES
CIN 2/3 and AIS are the immediate and necessary precursors of squamous cell carcinoma and adenocarcinoma of the

cervix, respectively. Their detection and removal has been shown to prevent cancer; thus, they serve as surrogate markers for prevention of cervical cancer. In the clinical studies in girls and women aged 16 through 26 years, cases of CIN 2/3 and AIS were the efficacy endpoints to assess prevention of cervical cancer. In addition, cases of VIN 2/3 and VaIN 2/3 were the efficacy endpoints to assess prevention of HPV-related vulvar and vaginal cancers, and observations of external genital lesions were the efficacy endpoints for the prevention of genital warts.

In clinical studies in boys and men aged 16 through 26 years, efficacy was evaluated using the following endpoints: external genital warts and penile/perineal/perianal intraepithelial neoplasia (PIN) grades 1/2/3 or penile/perineal/perianal cancer. In addition, cases of AIN grades 1/2/3 and anal cancer made up the composite efficacy endpoint used to assess prevention of HPV-related anal cancer.

Anal HPV infection, AIN, and anal cancer were not endpoints in the studies conducted in women. The similarity of HPV-related anal disease in men and women supports bridging the indication of prevention of AIN and anal cancer to women.

Efficacy was assessed in 6 AAHS-controlled, double-blind, randomized Phase II and III clinical studies. The first Phase II study evaluated the HPV 16 component of GARDASIL (Study 1, N = 2391 16- through 26-year-old girls and women) and the second evaluated all components of GARDASIL (Study 2, N = 551 16- through 26-year-old girls and women). Two Phase III studies evaluated GARDASIL in 5442 (Study 3) and 12,157 (Study 4) 16- through 26-year-old girls and women. A third Phase III study, Study 5, evaluated GARDASIL in 4055 16- through 26-year-old boys and men, including a subset of 598 (GARDASIL = 299; placebo = 299) men who self-identified as having sex with men (MSM population). A fourth Phase III study, Study 6, evaluated GARDASIL in 3817 24- through 45-year-old women. Together, these six studies evaluated 28,413 individuals (20,541 girls and women 16 through 26 years of age at enrollment with a mean age of 20.0 years, 4055 boys and men 16 through 26 years of age at enrollment with a mean age of 20.5 years, and 3817 women 24 through 45 years of age at enrollment with a mean age of 34.3 years). The race distribution of the 16- through 26-year-old girls and women in the clinical trials was as follows: 70.4% White; 12.2% Hispanic (Black and White); 8.8% Other; 4.6% Black; 3.8% Asian; and 0.2% American Indian. The race distribution of the 16-through 26-year-old boys and men in the clinical trials was as follows: 35.2% White; 20.5% Hispanic (Black and White); 14.4% Other; 19.8% Black; 10.0% Asian; and 0.1% American Indian. The race distribution of the 24- through 45-year-old women in the clinical trials was as follows: 20.6% White; 43.2% Hispanic (Black and White); 0.2% Other; 4.8% Black; 31.2% Asian; and 0.1% American Indian.

The median duration of follow-up was 4.0, 3.0, 3.0, 3.0, 2.3, and 4.0 years for Study 1, Study 2, Study 3, Study 4, Study 5, and Study 6, respectively. Individuals received vaccine or AAHS control on the day of enrollment and 2 and 6 months thereafter. Efficacy was analyzed for each study individually and for all studies in girls and women combined according to a prospective clinical plan.

Overall, 73% of 16- through 26-year-old girls and women, 67% of 24- through 45-year-old women, and 83% of 16-through 26-year-old boys and men were naïve (i.e., PCR [Polymerase Chain Reaction] negative and seronegative for all 4 vaccine HPV types) to all 4 vaccine HPV types at enrollment.

A total of 27% of 16- through 26-year-old girls and women, 33% of 24- through 45-year-old women, and 17% of 16-through 26-year-old boys and men had evidence of prior exposure to or ongoing infection with at least 1 of the 4 vaccine HPV types. Among these individuals, 74% of 16- through 26-year-old girls and women, 71% of 24- through 45-year-old women, and 78% of 16- through 26-year-old boys and men had evidence of prior exposure to or ongoing infection with only 1 of the 4 vaccine HPV types and were naïve (PCR negative and seronegative) to the remaining 3 types.

In 24- through 45-year-old individuals, 0.4% had been exposed to all 4 vaccine HPV types.

In individuals who were naïve (PCR negative and seronegative) to all 4 vaccine HPV types, CIN, genital warts, VIN, VaIN, PIN, and persistent infection caused by any of the 4 vaccine HPV types were counted as endpoints.

Among individuals who were positive (PCR positive and/or seropositive) for a vaccine HPV type at Day 1, endpoints related to that type were not included in the analyses of prophylactic efficacy. Endpoints related to the remaining types for which the individual was naïve (PCR negative and seronegative) were counted.

For example, in individuals who were HPV 18 positive (PCR positive and/or seropositive) at Day 1, lesions caused by HPV 18 were not counted in the prophylactic efficacy evaluations. Lesions caused by HPV 6, 11, and 16 were included in the prophylactic efficacy evaluations. The same approach was used for the other types.

Table 18: Summary of Month 7 Anti-HPV cLIA Geometric Mean Titers in the PPI* Population of Girls and Women

Population	N†	n‡	% Seropositive (95% CI)	GMT (95% CI) mMU§/mL
Anti-HPV 6				
9- through 15-year-old girls	1122	917	99.9 (99.4, 100.0)	929.2 (874.6, 987.3)
16- through 26-year-old girls and women	9859	3329	99.8 (99.6, 99.9)	545.0 (530.1, 560.4)
27- through 34-year-old women	667	439	98.4 (96.7, 99.4)	435.6 (393.4, 482.4)
35- through 45-year-old women	957	644	98.1 (96.8, 99.0)	397.3 (365.2, 432.2)
Anti-HPV 11				
9- through 15-year-old girls	1122	917	99.9 (99.4, 100.0)	1304.6 (1224.7, 1389.7)
16- through 26-year-old girls and women	9859	3353	99.8 (99.5, 99.9)	748.9 (726.0, 772.6)
27- through 34-year-old women	667	439	98.2 (96.4, 99.2)	577.9 (523.8, 637.5)
35- through 45-year-old women	957	644	97.7 (96.2, 98.7)	512.8 (472.9, 556.1)
Anti-HPV 16				
9- through 15-year-old girls	1122	915	99.9 (99.4, 100.0)	4918.5 (4556.6, 5309.1)
16- through 26-year-old girls and women	9859	3249	99.8 (99.6, 100.0)	2409.2 (2309.0, 2513.8)
27- through 34-year-old women	667	435	99.3 (98.0, 99.9)	2342.5 (2119.1, 2589.6)
35- through 45-year-old women	957	657	98.2 (96.8, 99.1)	2129.5 (1962.7, 2310.5)
Anti-HPV 18				
9- through 15-year-old girls	1122	922	99.8 (99.2, 100.0)	1042.6 (967.6, 1123.3)
16- through 26-year-old girls and women	9859	3566	99.4 (99.1, 99.7)	475.2 (458.8, 492.1)
27- through 34-year-old women	667	501	98.0 (96.4, 99.0)	385.8 (347.6, 428.1)
35- through 45-year-old women	957	722	96.4 (94.8, 97.6)	324.6 (297.6, 354.0)

cLIA = Competitive Luminex Immunoassay
CI = Confidence Interval
GMT = Geometric Mean Titers
* The PPI population consisted of individuals who received all 3 vaccinations within pre-defined day ranges, did not have major deviations from the study protocol, met predefined criteria for the interval between the Month 6 and Month 7 visit, and were naïve (PCR negative and seronegative) to the relevant HPV type(s) (types 6, 11, 16, and 18) prior to dose 1 and through 1 month Postdose 3 (Month 7).
† Number of individuals randomized to the respective vaccination group who received at least 1 injection.
‡ Number of individuals contributing to the analysis.
§ mMU = milli-Merck Units

14.1 Prophylactic Efficacy – HPV Types 6, 11, 16, and 18 in Girls and Women 16 Through 26 Years of Age

GARDASIL was administered without prescreening for presence of HPV infection and the efficacy trials allowed enrollment of girls and women regardless of baseline HPV status (i.e., PCR status or serostatus). Girls and women with current or prior HPV infection with an HPV type contained in the vaccine were not eligible for prophylactic efficacy evaluations for that type.

The primary analyses of efficacy with respect to HPV types 6, 11, 16, and 18 were conducted in the per-protocol efficacy (PPE) population, consisting of girls and women who received all 3 vaccinations within 1 year of enrollment, did not have major deviations from the study protocol, and were naïve (PCR negative in cervicovaginal specimens and seronegative) to the relevant HPV type(s) (Types 6, 11, 16, and 18) prior to dose 1 and through 1 month Postdose 3 (Month 7). Efficacy was measured starting after the Month 7 visit.

GARDASIL was efficacious in reducing the incidence of CIN (any grade including CIN 2/3); AIS; genital warts; VIN (any grade); and VaIN (any grade) related to vaccine HPV types 6, 11, 16, or 18 in those who were PCR negative and seronegative at baseline (Table 11).

In addition, girls and women who were already infected with 1 or more vaccine-related HPV types prior to vaccination were protected from precancerous cervical lesions and external genital lesions caused by the other vaccine HPV types.

[See table 11 at top of page 1454]

Prophylactic efficacy against overall cervical and genital disease related to HPV 6, 11, 16, and 18 in an extension phase of Study 2, that included data through Month 60, was noted to be 100% (95% CI: 12.3%, 100.0%) among girls and women in the per protocol population naïve to the relevant HPV types.

GARDASIL was efficacious against HPV disease caused by HPV types 6, 11, 16, and 18 in girls and women who were naïve for those specific HPV types at baseline.

14.2 Prophylactic Efficacy – HPV Types 6, 11, 16, and 18 in Boys and Men 16 Through 26 Years of Age

The primary analyses of efficacy were conducted in the per-protocol efficacy (PPE) population. This population consisted of boys and men who received all 3 vaccinations within 1 year of enrollment, did not have major deviations from the study protocol, and were naïve (PCR negative and seronegative) to the relevant HPV type(s) (Types 6, 11, 16, and 18) prior to dose 1 and through 1 month postdose 3 (Month 7). Efficacy was measured starting after the Month 7 visit.

GARDASIL was efficacious in reducing the incidence of genital warts related to vaccine HPV types 6 and 11 in those boys and men who were PCR negative and seronegative at baseline (Table 12). Efficacy against penile/perineal/perianal intraepithelial neoplasia (PIN) grades 1/2/3 or penile/perineal/perianal cancer was not demonstrated as the number of cases was too limited to reach statistical significance. [See table 12 at top of page 1455]

14.3 Prophylactic Efficacy – Anal Disease Caused by HPV Types 6, 11, 16, and 18 in Boys and Men 16 Through 26 Years of Age in the MSM Sub-study

A sub-study of Study 5 evaluated the efficacy of GARDASIL against anal disease (anal intraepithelial neoplasia and anal cancer) in a population of 598 MSM. The primary analyses of efficacy were conducted in the per-protocol efficacy (PPE) population of Study 5.

Table 19: Summary of Month 7 Anti-HPV cLIA Geometric Mean Titers in the PPI* Population of Boys and Men

Population	N†	n‡	% Seropositive (95% CI)	GMT (95% CI) mMU§/mL
Anti-HPV 6				
9- through 15-year-old boys	1072	884	99.9 (99.4, 100.0)	1037.5 (963.5, 1117.3)
16- through 26-year-old boys and men	2026	1093	98.9 (98.1, 99.4)	447.8 (418.9, 478.6)
Anti-HPV 11				
9- through 15-year-old boys	1072	885	99.9 (99.4, 100.0)	1386.8 (1298.5, 1481.0)
16- through 26-year-old boys and men	2026	1093	99.2 (98.4, 99.6)	624.3 (588.4, 662.3)
Anti-HPV 16				
9- through 15-year-old boys	1072	882	99.8 (99.2, 100.0)	6056.5 (5601.3, 6548.7)
16- through 26-year-old boys and men	2026	1136	98.8 (97.9, 99.3)	2403.3 (2243.4, 2574.6)
Anti-HPV 18				
9- through 15-year-old boys	1072	887	99.8 (99.2, 100)	1357.4 (1249.4, 1474.7)
16- through 26-year-old boys and men	2026	1175	97.4 (96.3, 98.2)	402.6 (374.6, 432.7)

cLIA = Competitive Luminex Immunoassay
CI = Confidence Interval
GMT = Geometric Mean Titers
* The PPI population consisted of individuals who received all 3 vaccinations within pre-defined day ranges, did not have major deviations from the study protocol, met predefined criteria for the interval between the Month 6 and Month 7 visit, and were naïve (PCR negative and seronegative) to the relevant HPV type(s) (types 6, 11, 16, and 18) prior to dose 1 and through 1 month Postdose 3 (Month 7).
† Number of individuals randomized to the respective vaccination group who received at least 1 injection.
‡ Number of individuals contributing to the analysis.
§ mMU = milli-Merck Units

GARDASIL was efficacious in reducing the incidence of anal intraepithelial neoplasia (AIN) grades 1 (both condyloma and non-acuminate), 2, and 3 related to vaccine HPV types 6, 11, 16, and 18 in those boys and men who were PCR negative and seronegative at baseline (Table 13).
[See table 13 at top of page 1455]

14.4   Population Impact in Girls and Women 16 Through 26 Years of Age
Effectiveness of GARDASIL in Prevention of HPV Types 6-, 11-, 16-, or 18-Related Genital Disease in Girls and Women 16 Through 26 Years of Age, Regardless of Current or Prior Exposure to Vaccine HPV Types
The clinical trials included girls and women regardless of current or prior exposure to vaccine HPV types, and additional analyses were conducted to evaluate the impact of GARDASIL with respect to HPV 6-, 11-, 16-, and 18-related cervical and genital disease in these girls and women. Here, analyses included events arising among girls and women regardless of baseline PCR status and serostatus, including HPV infections that were present at the start of vaccination as well as events that arose from infections that were acquired after the start of vaccination.
The impact of GARDASIL in girls and women regardless of current or prior exposure to a vaccine HPV type is shown in Table 14. Impact was measured starting 1 month Postdose 1. Prophylactic efficacy denotes the vaccine's efficacy in girls and women who are naïve (PCR negative and seronegative) to the relevant HPV types at Day 1. Vaccine impact in girls and women who were positive for vaccine HPV infection, as well as vaccine impact among girls and women regardless of baseline vaccine HPV PCR status and serostatus are also presented. The majority of CIN and genital warts, VIN, and VaIN related to a vaccine HPV type detected in the group that received GARDASIL occurred as a consequence of HPV infection with the relevant HPV type that was already present at Day 1.
There was no clear evidence of protection from disease caused by HPV types for which girls and women were PCR positive regardless of serostatus at baseline.
[See table 14 on pages 1455 and 1456]
Effectiveness of GARDASIL in Prevention of Any HPV Type Related Genital Disease in Girls and Women 16 Through 26 Years of Age, Regardless of Current or Prior Infection with Vaccine or Non-Vaccine HPV Types
The impact of GARDASIL against the overall burden of dysplastic or papillomatous cervical, vulvar, and vaginal disease regardless of HPV detection, results from a combination of prophylactic efficacy against vaccine HPV types, disease contribution from vaccine HPV types present at time of vaccination, the disease contribution from HPV types not contained in the vaccine, and disease in which HPV was not detected.
Additional efficacy analyses were conducted in 2 populations: (1) a generally HPV-naïve population (negative to 14 common HPV types and had a Pap test that was negative for SIL [Squamous Intraepithelial Lesion] at Day 1), approximating a population of sexually-naïve girls and women and (2) the general study population of girls and women regardless of baseline HPV status, some of whom had HPV-related disease at Day 1.
Among generally HPV-naïve girls and women and among all girls and women in the study population (including girls and women with HPV infection at Day 1), GARDASIL reduced the overall incidence of CIN 2/3 or AIS; of VIN 2/3 or VaIN 2/3; of CIN (any grade) or AIS; and of Genital Warts (Table 15). These reductions were primarily due to reductions in lesions caused by HPV types 6, 11, 16, and 18 in girls and women naïve (seronegative and PCR negative) for the specific relevant vaccine HPV type. Infected girls and women may already have CIN 2/3 or AIS at Day 1 and some will develop CIN 2/3 or AIS during follow-up, either related to a vaccine or non-vaccine HPV type present at the time of vaccination or related to a non-vaccine HPV type not present at the time of vaccination.
[See table 15 at top of page 1457]

14.5   Population Impact in Boys and Men 16 Through 26 Years of Age
Effectiveness of GARDASIL in Prevention of HPV Types 6-, 11-, 16-, or 18-Related Anogenital Disease in Boys and Men 16 Through 26 Years of Age, Regardless of Current or Prior Exposure to Vaccine HPV Types
Study 5 included boys and men regardless of current or prior exposure to vaccine HPV types, and additional analyses were conducted to evaluate the impact of GARDASIL with respect to HPV 6-, 11-, 16-, and 18-related anogenital disease in these boys and men. Here, analyses included events arising among boys and men regardless of baseline PCR status and serostatus, including HPV infections that were present at the start of vaccination as well as events that arose from infections that were acquired after the start of vaccination.
The impact of GARDASIL in boys and men regardless of current or prior exposure to a vaccine HPV type is shown in Table 16. Impact was measured starting at Day 1. Prophylactic efficacy denotes the vaccine's efficacy in boys and men who are naïve (PCR negative and seronegative) to the relevant HPV types at Day 1. Vaccine impact in boys and men who were positive for vaccine HPV infection, as well as vaccine impact among boys and men regardless of baseline vaccine HPV PCR status and serostatus are also presented. The majority of anogenital disease related to a vaccine HPV type detected in the group that received GARDASIL occurred as a consequence of HPV infection with the relevant HPV type that was already present at Day 1.
There was no clear evidence of protection from disease caused by HPV types for which boys and men were PCR positive regardless of serostatus at baseline.
[See table 16 on pages 1457 and 1458]

Effectiveness of GARDASIL in Prevention of Any HPV Type Related Anogenital Disease in Boys and Men 16 Through 26 Years of Age, Regardless of Current or Prior Infection with Vaccine or Non-Vaccine HPV Types
The impact of GARDASIL against the overall burden of dysplastic or papillomatous anogenital disease regardless of HPV detection, results from a combination of prophylactic efficacy against vaccine HPV types, disease contribution from vaccine HPV types present at time of vaccination, the disease contribution from HPV types not contained in the vaccine, and disease in which HPV was not detected.
Additional efficacy analyses from Study 5 were conducted in 2 populations: (1) a generally HPV-naïve population that consisted of boys and men who are seronegative and PCR negative to HPV 6, 11, 16, and 18 and PCR negative to HPV 31, 33, 35, 39, 45, 51, 52, 56, 58 and 59 at Day 1, approximating a population of sexually-naïve boys and men and (2) the general study population of boys and men regardless of baseline HPV status, some of whom had HPV-related disease at Day 1.
Among generally HPV-naïve boys and men and among all boys and men in Study 5 (including boys and men with HPV infection at Day 1), GARDASIL reduced the overall incidence of anogenital disease (Table 17). These reductions were primarily due to reductions in lesions caused by HPV types 6, 11, 16, and 18 in boys and men naïve (seronegative and PCR negative) for the specific relevant vaccine HPV type. Infected boys and men may already have anogenital disease at Day 1 and some will develop anogenital disease during follow-up, either related to a vaccine or non-vaccine HPV type present at the time of vaccination or related to a non-vaccine HPV type not present at the time of vaccination.
[See table 17 at top of page 1458]

14.6   Overall Population Impact
The subject characteristics (e.g. lifetime sex partners, geographic distribution of the subjects) influence the HPV prevalence of the population and therefore the population benefit can vary widely.
The overall efficacy of GARDASIL will vary with the baseline prevalence of HPV infection and disease, the incidence of infections against which GARDASIL has shown protection, and those infections against which GARDASIL has not been shown to protect.
The efficacy of GARDASIL for HPV types not included in the vaccine (i.e., cross-protective efficacy) is a component of the overall impact of the vaccine on rates of disease caused by HPV. Cross-protective efficacy was not demonstrated against disease caused by non-vaccine HPV types in the combined database of the Study 3 and Study 4 trials.
GARDASIL does not protect against genital disease not related to HPV. One woman who received GARDASIL in Study 3 developed an external genital well-differentiated squamous cell carcinoma at Month 24. No HPV DNA was detected in the lesion or in any other samples taken throughout the study.
In 18,150 girls and women enrolled in Study 2, Study 3, and Study 4, GARDASIL reduced definitive cervical therapy procedures by 23.9% (95% CI: 15.2%, 31.7%).

14.7   Studies in Women 27 Through 45 Years of Age
Study 6 evaluated efficacy in 3253 women 27 through 45 years of age based on a combined endpoint of HPV 6-, 11-, 16- or 18-related persistent infection, genital warts, vulvar and vaginal dysplastic lesions of any grade, CIN of any grade, AIS, and cervical cancer. These women were randomized 1:1 to receive either GARDASIL or AAHS control. The efficacy for the combined endpoint was driven primarily by prevention of persistent infection. There was no statistically significant efficacy demonstrated for CIN 2/3, AIS, or cervical cancer. In post hoc analyses conducted to assess the impact of GARDASIL on the individual components of the combined endpoint, the results in the population of women naïve to the relevant HPV type at baseline were as follows: prevention of HPV 6-, 11-, 16- or 18-related persistent infection (80.5% [95% CI: 68.3, 88.6]), prevention of HPV 6-, 11-, 16- or 18-related CIN (any grade) (85.8% [95% CI: 52.4, 97.3]), and prevention of HPV 6-, 11-, 16- or 18-related genital warts (87.6% [95% CI: 7.3, 99.7]).
Efficacy for disease endpoints was diminished in a population impact assessment of women who were vaccinated regardless of baseline HPV status (full analysis set). In the full analysis set (FAS), efficacy was not demonstrated for the following endpoints: prevention of HPV 16- and 18-related CIN 2/3, AIS, or cervical cancer and prevention of HPV 6- and 11-related condyloma. No efficacy was demonstrated against CIN 2/3, AIS, or cervical cancer in the general population irrespective of HPV type (FAS any type analysis).

14.8   Immunogenicity
Assays to Measure Immune Response
The minimum anti-HPV titer that confers protective efficacy has not been determined.
Because there were few disease cases in individuals naïve (PCR negative and seronegative) to vaccine HPV types at

baseline in the group that received GARDASIL, it has not been possible to establish minimum anti-HPV 6, anti-HPV 11, anti-HPV 16, and anti-HPV 18 antibody levels that protect against clinical disease caused by HPV 6, 11, 16, and/or 18.

The immunogenicity of GARDASIL was assessed in 23,951 9- through 45-year-old girls and women (GARDASIL N = 12,634; AAHS control or saline placebo N = 11,317) and 5417 9- through 26-year-old boys and men (GARDASIL N = 3109; AAHS control or saline placebo N = 2308).

Type-specific immunoassays with type-specific standards were used to assess immunogenicity to each vaccine HPV type. These assays measured antibodies against neutralizing epitopes for each HPV type. The scales for these assays are unique to each HPV type; thus, comparisons across types and to other assays are not appropriate.

Immune Response to GARDASIL

The primary immunogenicity analyses were conducted in a per-protocol immunogenicity (PPI) population. This population consisted of individuals who were seronegative and PCR negative to the relevant HPV type(s) at enrollment, remained HPV PCR negative to the relevant HPV type(s) through 1 month postdose 3 (Month 7), received all 3 vaccinations, and did not deviate from the study protocol in ways that could interfere with the effects of the vaccine.

Immunogenicity was measured by (1) the percentage of individuals who were seropositive for antibodies against the relevant vaccine HPV type, and (2) the Geometric Mean Titer (GMT).

In clinical studies in 16- through 26-year-old girls and women, 99.8%, 99.8%, 99.8%, and 99.4% who received GARDASIL became anti-HPV 6, anti-HPV 11, anti-HPV 16, and anti-HPV 18 seropositive, respectively, by 1 month postdose 3 across all age groups tested.

In clinical studies in 27- through 45-year-old women, 98.2%, 97.9%, 98.6%, and 97.1% who received GARDASIL became anti-HPV 6, anti-HPV 11, anti-HPV 16, and anti-HPV 18 seropositive, respectively, by 1 month postdose 3 across all age groups tested.

In clinical studies in 16- through 26-year-old boys and men, 98.9%, 99.2%, 98.8%, and 97.4% who received GARDASIL became anti-HPV 6, anti-HPV 11, anti-HPV 16, and anti-HPV 18 seropositive, respectively, by 1 month postdose 3 across all age groups tested.

Across all populations, anti-HPV 6, anti-HPV 11, anti-HPV 16, and anti-HPV 18 GMTs peaked at Month 7 (Table 18 and Table 19). GMTs declined through Month 24 and then stabilized through Month 36 at levels above baseline. Tables 20 and 21 display the persistence of anti-HPV cLIA geometric mean titers by gender and age group. The duration of immunity following a complete schedule of immunization with GARDASIL has not been established.

[See table 18 at top of page 1459]
[See table 19 at top of previous page]
[See table 20 above]
[See table 21 at top of next page]

Tables 18 and 19 display the Month 7 immunogenicity data for girls and women and boys and men. Anti-HPV responses 1 month postdose 3 among 9- through 15-year-old adolescent girls were non-inferior to anti-HPV responses in 16- through 26-year-old girls and women in the combined database of immunogenicity studies for GARDASIL. Anti-HPV responses 1 month postdose 3 among 9- through 15-year-old adolescent boys were non-inferior to anti-HPV responses in 16- through 26-year-old boys and men in Study 5.

On the basis of this immunogenicity bridging, the efficacy of GARDASIL in 9- through 15-year-old adolescent girls and boys is inferred.

GMT Response to Variation in Dosing Regimen in 18- Through 26-Year-Old Women

Girls and women evaluated in the PPE population of clinical studies received all 3 vaccinations within 1 year of enrollment. An analysis of immune response data suggests that flexibility of ±1 month for Dose 2 (i.e., Month 1 to Month 3 in the vaccination regimen) and flexibility of ±2 months for Dose 3 (i.e., Month 4 to Month 8 in the vaccination regimen) do not impact the immune responses to GARDASIL.

Duration of the Immune Response to GARDASIL

The duration of immunity following a complete schedule of immunization with GARDASIL has not been established. The peak anti-HPV GMTs for HPV types 6, 11, 16, and 18 occurred at Month 7. Anti-HPV GMTs for HPV types 6, 11, 16, and 18 were similar between measurements at Month 24 and Month 60 in Study 2.

14.9   Studies with RECOMBIVAX HB [hepatitis B vaccine (recombinant)]

The safety and immunogenicity of co-administration of GARDASIL with RECOMBIVAX HB [hepatitis B vaccine (recombinant)] (same visit, injections at separate sites) were evaluated in a randomized, double-blind, study of 1871 women aged 16 through 24 years at enrollment. The race distribution of the girls and women in the clinical trial was

as follows: 61.6% White; 1.6% Hispanic (Black and White); 23.8% Other; 11.9% Black; 0.8% Asian; and 0.3% American Indian.

Subjects either received GARDASIL and RECOMBIVAX HB (n = 466), GARDASIL and RECOMBIVAX HB-matched placebo (n = 468), RECOMBIVAX HB and GARDASIL-matched placebo (n = 467) or RECOMBIVAX-matched placebo and GARDASIL-matched placebo (n = 470) at Day 1, Month 2 and Month 6. Immunogenicity was assessed for all vaccines 1 month post completion of the vaccination series. Concomitant administration of GARDASIL with RECOMBIVAX HB [hepatitis B vaccine (recombinant)] did not interfere with the antibody response to any of the vaccine antigens when GARDASIL was given concomitantly with RECOMBIVAX HB or separately.

14.10   Studies with Menactra [Meningococcal (Groups A, C, Y and W-135) Polysaccharide Diphtheria Toxoid Conjugate Vaccine] and Adacel [Tetanus Toxoid, Reduced Diphtheria Toxoid and Acellular Pertussis Vaccine Adsorbed (Tdap)]

The safety and immunogenicity of co-administration of GARDASIL with Menactra [Meningococcal (Groups A, C, Y and W-135) Polysaccharide Diphtheria Toxoid Conjugate Vaccine] and Adacel [Tetanus Toxoid, Reduced Diphtheria Toxoid and Acellular Pertussis Vaccine Adsorbed (Tdap)] (same visit, injections at separate sites) were evaluated in an open-labeled, randomized, controlled study of 1040 boys and girls 11 through 17 years of age at enrollment. The race distribution of the subjects in the clinical trial was as fol-

Table 20: Persistence of Anti-HPV cLIA Geometric Mean Titers in 9- Through 45-Year-Old Girls and Women

Assay (cLIA)/ Time Point	9- to 15-Year-Old Girls (N* = 1122)		16- to 26-Year-Old Girls and Women (N* = 9859)		27- to 34-Year-Old Women (N* = 667)		35- to 45-Year-Old Women (N* = 957)	
	n[†]	GMT (95% CI) mMU[‡]/mL	n[†]	GMT (95% CI) mMU[‡]/mL	n[†]	GMT (95% CI) mMU[‡]/mL	n[†]	GMT (95% CI) mMU[‡]/mL
Anti-HPV 6								
Month 07	917	929.2 (874.6, 987.3)	3329	545.0 (530.1, 560.4)	439	435.6 (393.4, 482.4)	644	397.3 (365.2, 432.2)
Month 24	214	156.1 (135.6, 179.6)	2788	109.1 (105.2, 113.1)	421	70.7 (63.8, 78.5)	628	69.3 (63.7, 75.4)
Month 36[§]	356	129.4 (115.6, 144.8)	-	-	399	79.5 (72.0, 87.7)	618	81.1 (75.0, 87.8)
Month 48[¶]	-	-	2514	73.8 (70.9, 76.8)	391	58.8 (52.9, 65.3)	616	62.0 (57.0, 67.5)
Anti-HPV 11								
Month 07	917	1304.6 (1224.7, 1389.7)	3353	748.9 (726.0, 772.6)	439	577.9 (523.8, 637.5)	644	512.8 (472.9, 556.1)
Month 24	214	218.0 (188.3, 252.4)	2817	137.1 (132.1, 142.3)	421	79.3 (71.5, 87.8)	628	73.4 (67.4, 79.8)
Month 36[§]	356	148.0 (131.1, 167.1)	-	-	399	81.8 (74.3, 90.1)	618	77.4 (71.6, 83.6)
Month 48[¶]	-	-	2538	89.4 (85.9, 93.1)	391	67.4 (60.9, 74.7)	616	62.7 (57.8, 68.0)
Anti-HPV 16								
Month 07	915	4918.5 (4556.6, 5309.1)	3249	2409.2 (2309.0, 2513.8)	435	2342.5 (2119.1, 2589.6)	657	2129.5 (1962.7, 2310.5)
Month 24	211	944.2 (804.4, 1108.3)	2721	442.6 (425.0, 460.9)	416	285.9 (254.4, 321.2)	642	271.4 (247.1, 298.1)
Month 36[§]	353	642.2 (562.8, 732.8)	-	-	399	291.5 (262.5, 323.8)	631	276.7 (254.5, 300.8)
Month 48[¶]	-	-	2474	326.2 (311.8, 341.3)	394	211.8 (189.5, 236.8)	628	192.8 (176.5, 210.6)
Anti-HPV 18								
Month 07	922	1042.6 (967.6, 1123.3)	3566	475.2 (458.8, 492.1)	501	385.8 (347.6, 428.1)	722	324.6 (297.6, 354.0)
Month 24	214	137.7 (114.8, 165.1)	3002	50.8 (48.2, 53.5)	478	31.8 (28.1, 36.0)	705	26.0 (23.5, 28.8)
Month 36[§]	357	87.0 (74.8, 101.2)	-	-	453	32.1 (28.5, 36.3)	689	27.0 (24.5, 29.8)
Month 48[¶]	-	-	2710	33.2 (31.5, 35.0)	444	25.2 (22.3, 28.5)	688	21.2 (19.2, 23.4)

cLIA = Competitive Luminex Immunoassay
CI = Confidence Interval
GMT = Geometric Mean Titers
* N = Number of individuals randomized in the respective group who received at least 1 injection.
† n = Number of individuals in the indicated immunogenicity population.
‡ mMU = milli-Merck Units
§ Month 37 for 9- to 15-year-old girls. No serology samples were collected at this time point for 16- to 26-year-old girls and women.
¶ Month 48/End-of-study visits for 16- to 26-year-old girls and women were generally scheduled earlier than Month 48. Mean visit timing was Month 44. The studies in 9- to 15-year-old girls were planned to end prior to 48 months and therefore no serology samples were collected.

Table 21: Persistence of Anti-HPV cLIA Geometric Mean Titers in 9- Through 26-Year-Old Boys and Men

Assay (cLIA)/ Time Point	9- to 15-Year-Old Boys (N* = 1072)		16- to 26-Year-Old Boys and Men (N* = 2026)	
	n[†]	GMT (95% CI) mMU[‡]/mL	n[†]	GMT (95% CI) mMU[‡]/mL
Anti-HPV 6				
Month 07	884	1037.5 (963.5, 1117.3)	1094	447.2 (418.4, 477.9)
Month 24	323	134.1 (119.5, 150.5)	907	80.3 (74.9, 86.0)
Month 36[§]	342	126.6 (111.9, 143.2)	654	72.4 (68.0, 77.2)
Month 48[¶]	-	-	-	-
Anti-HPV 11				
Month 07	885	1386.8 (1298.5, 1481.0)	1094	624.5 (588.6, 662.5)
Month 24	324	188.5 (168.4, 211.1)	907	94.6 (88.4, 101.2)
Month 36[§]	342	148.8 (131.1, 169.0)	654	80.3 (75.7, 85.2)
Month 48[¶]	-	-	-	-
Anti-HPV 16				
Month 07	882	6056.5 (5601.4, 6548.6)	1137	2401.5 (2241.8, 2572.6)
Month 24	322	938.2 (825.0, 1067.0)	938	347.7 (322.5, 374.9)
Month 36[§]	341	708.8 (613.9, 818.3)	672	306.7 (287.5, 327.1)
Month 48[¶]	-	-	-	-
Anti-HPV 18				
Month 07	887	1357.4 (1249.4, 1474.7)	1176	402.6 (374.6, 432.6)
Month 24	324	131.9 (112.1, 155.3)	967	38.7 (35.2, 42.5)
Month 36[§]	343	113.0 (94.7, 135.0)	690	33.4 (30.9, 36.1)
Month 48[¶]	-	-	-	-

cLIA = Competitive Luminex Immunoassay
CI = Confidence Interval
GMT = Geometric Mean Titers
* N = Number of individuals randomized in the respective group who received at least 1 injection.
† n = Number of individuals in the indicated immunogenicity population.
‡ mMU = milli-Merck Units
§ Month 36 time point for 16- to 26-year-old boys and men; Month 37 for 9- to 15-year-old boys.
¶ The studies in 9- to 15-year-old boys and girls and 16- to 26-year-old boys and men were planned to end prior to 48 months and therefore no serology samples were collected.

lows: 77.7% White; 6.8% Hispanic (Black and White); 1.4% Multi-racial; 12.3% Black; 1.2% Asian; 0.2% Indian; and 0.4% American Indian.

One group received GARDASIL in one limb and both Menactra and Adacel, as separate injections, in the opposite limb concomitantly on Day 1 (n = 517). The second group received the first dose of GARDASIL on Day 1 in one limb then Menactra and Adacel, as separate injections, at Month 1 in the opposite limb (n = 523). Subjects in both vaccination groups received the second dose of GARDASIL at Month 2 and the third dose at Month 6. Immunogenicity was assessed for all vaccines 1 month post completion of the vaccination series (1 dose for Menactra and Adacel and 3 doses for GARDASIL).

Concomitant administration of GARDASIL with Menactra [Meningococcal (Groups A, C, Y and W-135) Polysaccharide Diphtheria Toxoid Conjugate Vaccine] and Adacel [Tetanus Toxoid, Reduced Diphtheria Toxoid and Acellular Pertussis Vaccine Adsorbed (Tdap)] did not interfere with the antibody response to any of the vaccine antigens when GARDASIL was given concomitantly with Menactra and Adacel or separately.

16 HOW SUPPLIED/STORAGE AND HANDLING

All presentations for GARDASIL contain a suspension of 120 mcg L1 protein from HPV types 6, 11, 16, and 18 in a 0.5-mL dose. GARDASIL is supplied in vials and syringes.
Carton of one 0.5-mL single-dose vial. **NDC** 0006-4045-00.
Carton of ten 0.5-mL single-dose vials. **NDC** 0006-4045-41.
Carton of six 0.5-mL single-dose prefilled Luer-Lok® syringes with tip caps. **NDC** 0006-4109-09.
Carton of ten 0.5-mL single-dose prefilled Luer-Lok® syringes with tip caps. **NDC** 0006-4109-02.
Store refrigerated at 2 to 8°C (36 to 46°F). Do not freeze. Protect from light.
GARDASIL should be administered as soon as possible after being removed from refrigeration.
GARDASIL can be out of refrigeration (at temperatures at or below 25°C/77°F), for a total time of not more than 72 hours.

17 PATIENT COUNSELING INFORMATION

Advise the patient to read the FDA-approved patient labeling (Patient Information).
Inform the patient, parent, or guardian:
• Vaccination does not eliminate the necessity for women to continue to undergo recommended cervical cancer screen-ing. Women who receive GARDASIL should continue to undergo cervical cancer screening per standard of care.
• Recipients of GARDASIL should not discontinue anal cancer screening if it has been recommended by a health care provider.
• GARDASIL has not been demonstrated to provide protection against disease from vaccine and non-vaccine HPV types to which a person has previously been exposed through sexual activity.
• Since syncope has been reported following vaccination sometimes resulting in falling with injury, observation for 15 minutes after administration is recommended.
• Vaccine information is required to be given with each vaccination to the patient, parent, or guardian.
• Information regarding benefits and risks associated with vaccination.
• GARDASIL is not recommended for use in pregnant women.
• Importance of completing the immunization series unless contraindicated.
• Report any adverse reactions to their health care provider.

Manuf. and Dist. by: Merck Sharp & Dohme Corp., a subsidiary of **MERCK & CO., INC.,** Whitehouse Station, NJ 08889, USA

For patent information:
www.merck.com/product/patent/home.html

The trademarks depicted herein are owned by their respective companies.
Copyright © 2006, 2009, 2010, 2011 Merck Sharp & Dohme Corp., a subsidiary of **Merck & Co., Inc.**
All rights reserved.
uspi-v501-i-1406r020
Printed in USA

USPPI
Patient Information about
GARDASIL® (pronounced "gard-Ah-sill")
Generic name: [Human Papillomavirus Quadrivalent (Types 6, 11, 16, and 18) Vaccine, Recombinant]
Read this information with care before getting GARDASIL[1]. You (the person getting GARDASIL) will need 3 doses of the vaccine. It is important to read this leaflet when you get each dose. This leaflet does not take the place of talking with your health care provider about GARDASIL.

What is GARDASIL?
GARDASIL is a vaccine (injection/shot) that is used for girls and women 9 through 26 years of age to help protect against the following diseases caused by Human Papillomavirus (HPV):
• Cervical cancer
• Vulvar and vaginal cancers
• Anal cancer
• Genital warts
• Precancerous cervical, vaginal, vulvar, and anal lesions
GARDASIL is used for boys and men 9 through 26 years of age to help protect against the following diseases caused by HPV:
• Anal cancer
• Genital warts
• Precancerous anal lesions
  • The diseases listed above have many causes, and GARDASIL only protects against diseases caused by certain kinds of HPV (called Type 6, Type 11, Type 16, and Type 18). Most of the time, these 4 types of HPV are responsible for the diseases listed above.
  • GARDASIL cannot protect you from a disease that is caused by other types of HPV, other viruses, or bacteria.
  • GARDASIL does not treat HPV infection.
  • You cannot get HPV or any of the above diseases from GARDASIL.

What important information about GARDASIL should I know?
• You should continue to get routine cervical cancer screening.
• GARDASIL may not fully protect everyone who gets the vaccine.
• GARDASIL will not protect against HPV types that you already have.

Who should not get GARDASIL?
You should not get GARDASIL if you have, or have had:
• an allergic reaction after getting a dose of GARDASIL.
• a severe allergic reaction to yeast, amorphous aluminum hydroxyphosphate sulfate, polysorbate 80.

What should I tell my health care provider before getting GARDASIL?
Tell your health care provider if you:
• are pregnant or planning to get pregnant. GARDASIL is not recommended for use in pregnant women.
• have immune problems, like HIV infection, cancer, or you take medicines that affect your immune system.
• have a fever over 100°F (37.8°C).
• had an allergic reaction to another dose of GARDASIL.
• take any medicines, even those you can buy over the counter.
Your health care provider will help decide if you should get the vaccine.

How is GARDASIL given?

GARDASIL is a shot that is usually given in the arm muscle. You will need 3 shots given on the following schedule:
- Dose 1: at a date you and your health care provider choose.
- Dose 2: 2 months after Dose 1.
- Dose 3: 6 months after Dose 1.

Fainting can happen after getting GARDASIL. Sometimes people who faint can fall and hurt themselves. For this reason, your health care provider may ask you to sit or lie down for 15 minutes after you get GARDASIL. Some people who faint might shake or become stiff. This may require evaluation or treatment by your health care provider.

Make sure that you get all 3 doses on time so that you get the best protection. If you miss a dose, talk to your health care provider.

Can other vaccines and medications be given at the same time as GARDASIL?

GARDASIL can be given at the same time as RECOMBIVAX HB®1 [hepatitis B vaccine (recombinant)] or Menactra [Meningococcal (Groups A, C, Y and W-135) Polysaccharide Diphtheria Toxoid Conjugate Vaccine] and Adacel [Tetanus Toxoid, Reduced Diphtheria Toxoid and Acellular Pertussis Vaccine Adsorbed (Tdap)].

What are the possible side effects of GARDASIL?

The most common side effects with GARDASIL are:
- pain, swelling, itching, bruising, and redness at the injection site
- headache
- fever
- nausea
- dizziness
- vomiting
- fainting

There was no increase in side effects when GARDASIL was given at the same time as RECOMBIVAX HB [hepatitis B vaccine (recombinant)].

There was more injection-site swelling at the injection site for GARDASIL when GARDASIL was given at the same time as Menactra [Meningococcal (Groups A, C, Y and W-135) Polysaccharide Diphtheria Toxoid Conjugate Vaccine] and Adacel [Tetanus Toxoid, Reduced Diphtheria Toxoid and Acellular Pertussis Vaccine Adsorbed (Tdap)].

Tell your health care provider if you have any of the following problems because these may be signs of an allergic reaction:
- difficulty breathing
- wheezing (bronchospasm)
- hives
- rash

Tell your health care provider if you have:
- swollen glands (neck, armpit, or groin)
- joint pain
- unusual tiredness, weakness, or confusion
- chills
- generally feeling unwell
- leg pain
- shortness of breath
- chest pain
- aching muscles
- muscle weakness
- seizure
- bad stomach ache
- bleeding or bruising more easily than normal
- skin infection

Contact your health care provider right away if you get any symptoms that concern you, even several months after getting the vaccine.

For a more complete list of side effects, ask your health care provider.

What are the ingredients in GARDASIL?

The ingredients are proteins of HPV Types 6, 11, 16, and 18, amorphous aluminum hydroxyphosphate sulfate, yeast protein, sodium chloride, L-histidine, polysorbate 80, sodium borate, and water for injection.

This leaflet is a summary of information about GARDASIL. If you would like more information, please talk to your health care provider or visit www.gardasil.com.

Manufactured and Distributed by: Merck Sharp & Dohme Corp., a subsidiary of Merck & Co., Inc.

Whitehouse Station, NJ 08889, USA

Issued April 2011

9883616

1Registered trademark of Merck Sharp & Dohme Corp., a subsidiary of **Merck & Co., Inc.**

Copyright © 2006, 2009 Merck Sharp & Dohme Corp., a subsidiary of **Merck & Co., Inc.**

All rights reserved

GRASTEK®

Rx

(Timothy Grass Pollen Allergen Extract)
Tablet for Sublingual Use

HIGHLIGHTS OF PRESCRIBING INFORMATION

These highlights do not include all the information needed to use GRASTEK safely and effectively. See full prescribing information for GRASTEK.

GRASTEK® (Timothy Grass Pollen Allergen Extract)
Tablet for Sublingual Use
Initial U.S. Approval: 2014

WARNING: SEVERE ALLERGIC REACTIONS
See full prescribing information for complete boxed warning.
- **GRASTEK can cause life-threatening allergic reactions such as anaphylaxis and severe laryngopharyngeal restriction. (5.1)**
- **Do not administer GRASTEK to patients with severe, unstable or uncontrolled asthma. (4)**
- **Observe patients in the office for at least 30 minutes following the initial dose. (5.1)**
- **Prescribe auto-injectable epinephrine, instruct and train patients on its appropriate use, and instruct patients to seek immediate medical care upon its use. (5.2)**
- **GRASTEK may not be suitable for patients with certain underlying medical conditions that may reduce their ability to survive a serious allergic reaction. (5.2)**
- **GRASTEK may not be suitable for patients who may be unresponsive to epinephrine or inhaled bronchodilators, such as those taking beta-blockers. (5.2)**

——INDICATIONS AND USAGE——

GRASTEK is an allergen extract indicated as immunotherapy for the treatment of grass pollen-induced allergic rhinitis with or without conjunctivitis confirmed by positive skin test or *in vitro* testing for pollen-specific IgE antibodies for Timothy grass or cross-reactive grass pollens. GRASTEK is approved for use in persons 5 through 65 years of age. (1)

——DOSAGE AND ADMINISTRATION——

For sublingual use only. (2)
- One tablet daily. (2.1)
- Initiate treatment at least 12 weeks before the expected onset of each grass pollen season and continue treatment throughout the season. For sustained effectiveness for one grass pollen season after cessation of treatment, GRASTEK may be taken daily for three consecutive years. (2.2)
- Place the tablet immediately under the tongue. Allow it to remain there until completely dissolved. Do not swallow for at least 1 minute. (2.2)
- Administer the first dose of GRASTEK under the supervision of a physician with experience in the diagnosis and treatment of allergic diseases. Observe patients in the office for at least 30 minutes following the initial dose. (2.2)

——DOSAGE FORMS AND STRENGTHS——

- Tablet, 2800 Bioequivalent Allergy Units (BAUs) (3)

——CONTRAINDICATIONS——

- Severe, unstable or uncontrolled asthma. (4)
- History of any severe systemic allergic reaction or any severe local reaction to sublingual allergen immunotherapy. (4)
- A history of eosinophilic esophagitis. (4)
- Hypersensitivity to any of the inactive ingredients contained in this product. (4)

——WARNINGS AND PRECAUTIONS——

- Inform patients of the signs and symptoms of serious allergic reactions and instruct them to seek immediate medical care and discontinue therapy should any of these occur. (5.1)
- In case of oral inflammation or wounds, stop treatment with GRASTEK to allow complete healing of the oral cavity. (5.7)

——ADVERSE REACTIONS——

- Adverse reactions reported in ≥5% of patients were: ear pruritus, oral pruritus, tongue pruritus, mouth edema, throat irritation. (6)

To report SUSPECTED ADVERSE REACTIONS, contact Merck Sharp & Dohme Corp., a subsidiary of Merck & Co., Inc., at 1-877-888-4231 or FDA at 1-800-FDA-1088 or www.fda.gov/medwatch.

See 17 for PATIENT COUNSELING INFORMATION

Revised: 06/2014

FULL PRESCRIBING INFORMATION: CONTENTS*

FULL PRESCRIBING INFORMATION

WARNING: SEVERE ALLERGIC REACTIONS
- **GRASTEK can cause life-threatening allergic reactions such as anaphylaxis and severe laryngopharyngeal restriction. (5.1)**
- **Do not administer GRASTEK to patients with severe, unstable or uncontrolled asthma. (4)**
- **Observe patients in the office for at least 30 minutes following the initial dose. (5.1)**
- **Prescribe auto-injectable epinephrine, instruct and train patients on its appropriate use, and instruct patients to seek immediate medical care upon its use. (5.2)**
- **GRASTEK may not be suitable for patients with certain underlying medical conditions that may reduce their ability to survive a serious allergic reaction. (5.2)**
- **GRASTEK may not be suitable for patients who may be unresponsive to epinephrine or inhaled bronchodilators, such as those taking beta-blockers. (5.2)**

1   INDICATIONS AND USAGE

GRASTEK® is an allergen extract indicated as immunotherapy for the treatment of grass pollen-induced allergic rhinitis with or without conjunctivitis confirmed by positive skin test or *in vitro* testing for pollen-specific IgE antibodies for Timothy grass or cross-reactive grass pollens. GRASTEK is approved for use in persons 5 through 65 years of age. GRASTEK is not indicated for the immediate relief of allergic symptoms.

2   DOSAGE AND ADMINISTRATION

For sublingual use only.

2.1   Dose

One GRASTEK tablet daily.

2.2   Administration

Administer the first dose of GRASTEK in a healthcare setting under the supervision of a physician with experience in the diagnosis and treatment of allergic diseases. After receiving the first dose of GRASTEK, observe the patient for at least 30 minutes to monitor for signs or symptoms of a severe systemic or a severe local allergic reaction. If the patient tolerates the first dose, the patient may take subsequent doses at home.

Administer GRASTEK to children under adult supervision.

Take the tablet from the blister unit after carefully removing the foil with dry hands.

Place the tablet immediately under the tongue. Allow it to remain there until completely dissolved. Do not swallow for at least 1 minute.

Wash hands after handling the tablet.

Do not take the tablet with food or beverage. Food or beverage should not be taken for the following 5 minutes after taking the tablet.

Initiate treatment at least 12 weeks before the expected onset of each grass pollen season and continue treatment throughout the season. For sustained effectiveness for one grass pollen season after cessation of treatment, GRASTEK may be taken daily for three consecutive years (including the intervals between the grass pollen seasons). The safety and efficacy of initiating treatment in season have not been established.

Data regarding the safety of restarting treatment after missing a dose of GRASTEK are limited. In the clinical trials, treatment interruptions for up to seven days were allowed.

Prescribe auto-injectable epinephrine to patients prescribed GRASTEK and instruct them in the proper use of emergency self-injection of epinephrine *[See Warnings and Precautions (5.2)].*

3 DOSAGE FORMS AND STRENGTHS

GRASTEK is available as 2800 Bioequivalent Allergy Unit (BAU) tablets that are white to off-white, circular with a debossed round detail on one side.

4 CONTRAINDICATIONS

GRASTEK is contraindicated in patients with:
- Severe, unstable or uncontrolled asthma
- A history of any severe systemic allergic reaction
- A history of any severe local reaction after taking any sublingual allergen immunotherapy
- A history of eosinophilic esophagitis
- Hypersensitivity to any of the inactive ingredients [gelatin, mannitol and sodium hydroxide] contained in this product *[See Description (11)].*

5 WARNINGS AND PRECAUTIONS

5.1 Severe Allergic Reactions

GRASTEK can cause systemic allergic reactions including anaphylaxis which may be life-threatening. In addition, GRASTEK can cause severe local reactions, including laryngopharyngeal swelling, which can compromise breathing and be life-threatening. Educate patients to recognize the signs and symptoms of these allergic reactions and instruct them to seek immediate medical care and discontinue therapy should any of these occur. Allergic reactions may require treatment with epinephrine. *[See Warnings and Precautions (5.2)]*

Administer the initial dose of GRASTEK in a healthcare setting under the supervision of a physician with experience in the diagnosis and treatment of allergic diseases and prepared to manage a life-threatening systemic or local allergic reaction. Observe patients in the office for at least 30 minutes following the initial dose of GRASTEK.

5.2 Epinephrine

Prescribe auto-injectable epinephrine to patients receiving GRASTEK. Instruct patients to recognize the signs and symptoms of a severe allergic reaction and in the proper use of emergency auto-injectable epinephrine. Instruct patients to seek immediate medical care upon use of auto-injectable epinephrine and to stop treatment with GRASTEK. *[See Patient Counseling Information (17).]*

See the epinephrine package insert for complete information.

GRASTEK may not be suitable for patients with certain medical conditions that may reduce the ability to survive a serious allergic reaction or increase the risk of adverse reactions after epinephrine administration. Examples of these medical conditions include but are not limited to: markedly compromised lung function (either chronic or acute), unstable angina, recent myocardial infarction, significant arrhythmia, and uncontrolled hypertension.

GRASTEK may not be suitable for patients who are taking medications that can potentiate or inhibit the effect of epinephrine. These medications include:

Beta-adrenergic blockers: Patients taking beta-adrenergic blockers may be unresponsive to the usual doses of epinephrine used to treat serious systemic reactions, including anaphylaxis. Specifically, beta-adrenergic blockers antagonize the cardiostimulating and bronchodilating effects of epinephrine.

Alpha-adrenergic blockers, ergot alkaloids: Patients taking alpha-adrenergic blockers may be unresponsive to the usual doses of epinephrine used to treat serious systemic reactions, including anaphylaxis. Specifically, alpha-adrenergic blockers antagonize the vasoconstricting and hypertensive effects of epinephrine. Similarly, ergot alkaloids may reverse the pressor effects of epinephrine.

Tricyclic antidepressants, levothyroxine sodium, monoamine oxidase inhibitors and certain antihistamines: The adverse effects of epinephrine may be potentiated in patients taking tricyclic antidepressants, levothyroxine sodium, monoamine oxidase inhibitors, and the antihistamines chlorpheniramine, and diphenhydramine.

Cardiac glycosides, diuretics: Patients who receive epinephrine while taking cardiac glycosides or diuretics should be observed carefully for the development of cardiac arrhythmias.

5.3 Upper Airway Compromise

GRASTEK can cause local reactions in the mouth or throat that could compromise the upper airway *[See Adverse Reactions (6.1 and 6.2)].* Consider discontinuation of GRASTEK in patients who experience persistent and escalating adverse reactions in the mouth or throat.

5.4 Eosinophilic Esophagitis

Eosinophilic esophagitis has been reported in association with sublingual tablet immunotherapy *[See Contraindica-*

tions (4) and Adverse Reactions (6.2)]. Discontinue GRASTEK and consider a diagnosis of eosinophilic esophagitis in patients who experience severe or persistent gastroesophageal symptoms including dysphagia or chest pain.

5.5 Asthma

GRASTEK has not been studied in subjects with moderate or severe asthma or any subjects who required daily medication to treat asthma.

Withhold immunotherapy with GRASTEK if the patient is experiencing an acute asthma exacerbation. Reevaluate patients who have recurrent asthma exacerbations and consider discontinuation of GRASTEK.

5.6 Concomitant Allergen Immunotherapy

GRASTEK has not been studied in subjects who are receiving concomitant allergen immunotherapy. Concomitant dosing with other allergen immunotherapy may increase the likelihood of local or systemic adverse reactions to either subcutaneous or sublingual allergen immunotherapy.

5.7 Oral Inflammation

Stop treatment with GRASTEK to allow complete healing of the oral cavity in patients with oral inflammation (e.g., oral lichen planus, mouth ulcers or thrush) or oral wounds, such as those following oral surgery or dental extraction.

6 ADVERSE REACTIONS

Adverse reactions reported in ≥5% of patients were: ear pruritus, oral pruritus, tongue pruritus, mouth edema, and throat irritation.

6.1 Clinical Trials Experience

Because clinical trials are conducted under widely varying conditions, adverse reaction rates observed in the clinical trials of a drug cannot be directly compared to rates in the clinical trials of another drug and may not reflect the rates observed in clinical practice.

Adults

The safety data described below are based on 6 clinical trials which randomized 3589 subjects 18 through 65 years of age with Timothy grass pollen induced rhinitis with or without conjunctivitis, including 1669 subjects who were exposed to at least one dose of GRASTEK. Of the subjects treated with GRASTEK, 25% had mild asthma and 80% were sensitized to other allergens in addition to grass. The subject population was 88% White, 7% African American, and 3% Asian. Subjects were 52% male, and 88% of subjects were between 18 and 50 years of age. Subject demographics in placebo-treated subjects were similar to the active group.

The most common adverse reactions reported in subjects treated with GRASTEK were oral pruritus (26.7% vs 3.5% placebo), throat irritation (22.6% vs 2.8%), ear pruritus (12.5% vs 1.1%) and mouth edema (11.1% vs 0.8%). The percentage of subjects who discontinued from the clinical trials because of an adverse reaction while exposed to GRASTEK or placebo was 4.9% and 0.9%, respectively. The most common adverse reactions that led to study discontinuation in subjects who were exposed to GRASTEK were pharyngeal edema and oral pruritus.

Seven adult subjects (7/1669; 0.4%) who received GRASTEK experienced treatment-related systemic allergic reactions that led to discontinuation of GRASTEK in four out of the seven subjects.

- Five of the seven subjects had reactions on Day 1 of treatment with GRASTEK. Symptoms included swelling of lips/mouth; oral/pharyngeal itching; ear itching, sneezing, rhinorrhea, throat irritation, dysphonia, dysphagia, chest discomfort, and rash. Three of the five subjects received treatment with epinephrine and antihistamines, and one of the three also received oral corticosteroids. One of the five subjects who had a reaction on Day 1 of treatment with GRASTEK also had a reaction on Day 2 of treatment with GRASTEK. Symptoms on Day 2 included oral burning sensation; rhinorrhea; and throat irritation.
- One of the seven subjects had a reaction on Day 2 after tolerating treatment with GRASTEK on Day 1. Symptoms included edema of the lower lip, epigastric discomfort and dizziness.
- One of the seven subjects developed chest tightness and shortness of breath on Day 42 of treatment with GRASTEK.

Adverse reactions reported in ≥1% of subjects treated with GRASTEK are shown in Table 1.

Table 1: Adverse Reactions Reported in ≥1% of Adults Treated with GRASTEK

Adverse Reaction	GRASTEK (N=1669)	PLACEBO (N=1645)
Nervous System Disorders		
Headache	2.1%	1.3%
Ear and Labyrinth Disorders		
Ear pruritus	12.5%	1.1%

	GRASTEK	PLACEBO
Respiratory, Thoracic and Mediastinal Disorders		
Throat irritation	22.6%	2.8%
Pharyngeal edema	3.4%	0.1%
Dry throat	1.7%	0.4%
Oropharyngeal pain	1.6%	1.0%
Nasal discomfort	1.6%	1.0%
Throat tightness	1.4%	0.2%
Dyspnea	1.1%	0.4%
Gastrointestinal Disorders		
Oral pruritus	26.7%	3.5%
Mouth edema	11.1%	0.8%
Paraesthesia oral	9.8%	2.0%
Tongue pruritus	5.7%	0.5%
Lip swelling	4.0%	0.2%
Swollen tongue	2.8%	0.1%
Dyspepsia	2.3%	0.1%
Hypoesthesia oral	2.3%	1.0%
Nausea	1.9%	0.6%
Oral discomfort	1.6%	0.3%
Oral mucosal erythema	1.5%	0.6%
Lip edema	1.3%	0.1%
Glossitis	1.3%	0.1%
Stomatitis	1.1%	0.3%
Tongue disorder	1.1%	0.2%
Tongue edema	1.1%	0.4%
Glossodynia	1.0%	0.3%
Dysphagia	1.0%	0.2%
Palatal edema	1.0%	0.1%
Skin and Subcutaneous Tissue Disorders		
Pruritus	2.4%	1.0%
Urticaria	1.7%	0.9%
General Disorders and Administration Site Conditions		
Chest discomfort	1.6%	0.5%
Fatigue	1.4%	0.4%

Adverse reactions of interest that occurred in ≤1% of GRASTEK recipients include abdominal pain and gastroesophageal reflux.

Pediatrics

Safety data are based on 3 clinical trials which randomized 881 subjects between 5 and 17 years of age with grass pollen induced rhinitis with or without conjunctivitis. Overall, 445 subjects received at least one dose of GRASTEK. Of the subjects treated with GRASTEK, 31% had mild asthma and 86% were sensitized to other allergens in addition to grass. The subject population was 86% White, 7% African American and 3% multi-racial. The majority (66%) of subjects were male. The mean age of subjects was 11.7 years. Subject demographics in placebo-treated subjects were similar to the active group.

The most common adverse reactions in pediatric subjects treated with GRASTEK were oral pruritus (24.4% vs 2.1% placebo), throat irritation (21.3% vs 2.5%) and mouth edema (9.8% vs 0.2%). The percentage of subjects who discontinued from the clinical trials because of an adverse reaction while exposed to GRASTEK or placebo was 6.3% and 0.7%, respectively.

One pediatric subject (1/447; 0.2%) who received GRASTEK experienced a treatment-related systemic allergic reaction consisting of lip angioedema, slight dysphagia due to the sensation of a lump in the throat, and intermittent cough which was of moderate intensity on Day 1. The subject was treated with epinephrine, recovered, and was discontinued from the trial.

Adverse reactions reported in ≥1% of subjects treated with GRASTEK are shown in Table 2.

Table 2: Adverse Reactions Reported in ≥1% of Pediatric Subjects Treated with GRASTEK

Adverse Reaction	GRASTEK (N=447)	PLACEBO (N=434)
Nervous System Disorders		
Headache	3.4%	1.8%
Ear and Labyrinth Disorders		
Ear pruritus	7.2%	0.5%
Eye Disorders		
Eye pruritus	3.4%	2.1%
Respiratory, Thoracic and Mediastinal Disorders		
Throat irritation	21.3%	2.5%
Oropharyngeal pain	4.0%	1.4%
Pharyngeal erythema	3.6%	0.7%

Pharyngeal edema	2.9%	0%
Cough	2.7%	1.2%
Dyspnea	2.0%	0.5%
Nasal discomfort	1.6%	0.9%
Nasal congestion	1.6%	0.5%
Sneezing	1.6%	0.7%
Gastrointestinal Disorders		
Oral pruritus	24.4%	2.1%
Mouth edema	9.8%	0.2%
Tongue pruritus	9.2%	0.9%
Lip swelling	7.2%	0.5%
Paraesthesia oral	5.4%	1.2%
Oral mucosal erythema	4.9%	0.9%
Lip pruritus	2.9%	0.2%
Swollen tongue	2.5%	0%
Dysphagia	2.0%	0%
Nausea	1.6%	0.5%
Oral discomfort	1.6%	0.2%
Stomatitis	1.3%	0%
Hypoesthesia oral	1.1%	0.2%
Glossodynia	1.1%	0.2%
Skin and Subcutaneous Tissue Disorders		
Urticaria	1.8%	0.2%
General Disorders and Administration Site Conditions		
Chest discomfort	2.0%	0.5%

Table 3: Total Combined Scores (TCS), Rhinoconjunctivitis Daily Symptom Scores (DSS), and Daily Medication Scores (DMS) During the Grass Pollen Season

Endpoint*	GRASTEK (N)[†] Score[‡]	Placebo (N)[†] Score[‡]	Treatment Difference (GRASTEK − Placebo)	Difference Relative to Placebo[§] Estimate (95% CI)
TCS Entire Season	(629) 3.24	(672) 4.22	-0.98	-23% (-36.0, -13.0)
TCS Peak Season	(620) 3.33	(663) 4.67	-1.33	-29% (-39.0, -15.0)
DSS Entire Season	(629) 2.49	(672) 3.13	-0.64	-20% (-32.0, -10.0)
DMS Entire Season	(629) 0.88	(672) 1.36	-0.48	-35% (-49.3, -20.8)

TCS=Total Combined Score (DSS + DMS); DSS=Daily Symptom Score; DMS=Daily Medication Score.
* Non-parametric analysis for TCS and DSS endpoints: Parametric analysis using zero-inflated log-normal model for DMS.
† Number of subjects in analyses.
‡ For TCS and DSS endpoints the group medians are reported, treatment difference and that relative to placebo is based on group medians. For DMS, the group means are reported and difference relative to placebo is based on estimated group means.
§ Difference relative to placebo computed as: (GRASTEK - placebo)/placebo × 100.

6.2 Postmarketing Experience
Postmarketing Safety Studies
In European post-approval studies which included 1,666 patients treated with GRASTEK (marketed under the name GRAZAX), reported serious adverse reactions assessed as related to GRASTEK use included anaphylactic reaction, asthma exacerbation, hoarseness, laryngitis, oral ulceration, and ulcerative colitis exacerbation.
Spontaneous Postmarketing Reports
The following adverse reactions have been identified during post-approval use of GRASTEK (marketed under the name GRAZAX in Europe). Because these reactions are reported voluntarily from a population of uncertain size, it is not always possible to reliably estimate their frequency or establish a causal relationship to drug exposure. These include: altered state of consciousness, anaphylactic shock, angioedema, asthma exercise induced, chest pressure, diarrhea, difficulty speaking, dizziness, drowsiness, eosinophilic esophagitis, erythema facial, face edema, forced expiratory volume decreased, heart rate increased, heart rate irregular, hyperventilation, hypotension, laryngeal discomfort, oral pain, oxygen saturation decreased, peak expiratory flow rate decreased, pneumonia, rash, respiratory distress, sensation of foreign body, status asthmaticus, swelling of neck, throat pruritus, tremor, vital capacity decreased, vomiting, and wheezing. Included in these reports was an adult male with asthma who experienced anaphylactic shock within two minutes of administration of GRASTEK. The patient experienced depressed level of consciousness, hypotension, increased heart rate, wheezing, urticaria, and face edema.
Eosinophilic esophagitis has been reported following treatment with GRASTEK (marketed under the name GRAZAX). The clinical details of some postmarketing reports are consistent with a drug-induced effect, including at least one case with resolution of symptoms upon discontinuation of GRASTEK, relapse after resuming GRASTEK and resolution again after discontinuation of GRASTEK.

8 USE IN SPECIFIC POPULATIONS
8.1 Pregnancy
Pregnancy Category B: Reproductive and developmental toxicity studies performed in female mice have revealed no evidence of harm to the fetus due to GRASTEK. In these studies, the effect of Timothy grass (*Phleum pratense*) pollen allergen extract, the active component of GRASTEK, on embryo-fetal development was evaluated. Mice were administered approximately 460,000 BAU/kg/day of Timothy grass pollen allergen extract by oral gavage on days 0 to 15 of gestation. A dose of 460,000 BAU/kg/day of Timothy grass pollen allergen extract corresponds to approximately 8,200-fold a human dose on a BAU/kg/day basis. No adverse effects on embryo-fetal development were observed. There are, however, no adequate and well-controlled studies in pregnant women. Because animal reproduction studies are not always predictive of human response, GRASTEK should be used during pregnancy only if clearly needed.
Because systemic and local adverse reactions with immunotherapy may be poorly tolerated during pregnancy, GRASTEK should be used during pregnancy only if clearly needed.

8.3 Nursing Mothers
It is not known if GRASTEK is excreted in human milk. Because many drugs are excreted in human milk, caution should be exercised when GRASTEK is administered to a nursing woman.

8.4 Pediatric Use
Efficacy and safety of GRASTEK have been established in children and adolescents 5 through 17 years of age. The safety and efficacy in pediatric patients below 5 years of age have not been established.
8.5 Geriatric Use
There is no clinical trial experience with GRASTEK in patients over 65 years of age.

11 DESCRIPTION
GRASTEK tablets contain pollen allergen extract from Timothy grass (*Phleum pratense*). GRASTEK is a sublingual tablet.
GRASTEK is available as a tablet of 2800 BAU of Timothy grass pollen allergen extract.
Inactive ingredients: gelatin NF (fish source), mannitol USP and sodium hydroxide NF.

12 CLINICAL PHARMACOLOGY
12.1 Mechanism of Action
The precise mechanisms of action of allergen immunotherapy are not known.

13 NONCLINICAL TOXICOLOGY
13.1 Carcinogenesis, Mutagenesis, Impairment of Fertility
No studies have been performed in animals to evaluate the carcinogenic potential of GRASTEK.
There were no positive findings in the *in vitro* mouse lymphoma and the bacterial reverse mutation assays for mutagenicity using Timothy grass (*Phleum pratense*) pollen allergen extract.
A fertility study in mice revealed no evidence of impaired fertility due to Timothy grass pollen allergen extract.

14 CLINICAL STUDIES
The efficacy of GRASTEK in the treatment of allergic rhinitis with or without conjunctivitis in Timothy grass pollen allergic subjects 5 years of age and older, with or without mild asthma, was evaluated during the first grass pollen season in two trials of approximately 24 weeks treatment duration. The sustained effect of GRASTEK was evaluated in one trial conducted over 5 grass pollen seasons. All three trials were randomized, double-blind, parallel group, multicenter clinical trials. Subjects had a history of grass pollen induced rhinitis with or without conjunctivitis and sensitivity to Timothy grass pollen as determined by specific testing (IgE). In these three studies, subjects initiated GRASTEK or placebo approximately 12 weeks prior to the pollen season. In the long-term study, subjects received GRASTEK or placebo daily for 3 consecutive years and were followed for 2 years without treatment.
Efficacy was established by self-reporting of rhinoconjunctivitis daily symptom scores (DSS) and daily medication scores (DMS). Daily rhinoconjunctivitis symptoms included four nasal symptoms (runny nose, stuffy nose, sneezing, and itchy nose), and two ocular symptoms (gritty/itchy eyes and watery eyes). The rhinoconjunctivitis symptoms were measured on a scale of 0 (none) to 3 (severe). Subjects in clinical trials were allowed to take symptom-relieving medications (including systemic and topical antihistamines and topical and oral corticosteroids) as needed. The daily medication score measured the use of standard open-label allergy medications. Predefined values were assigned to each class of medication. Generally, systemic and topical antihistamines were given the lowest score, topical steroids an intermedi-

ate score, and oral corticosteroids the highest score. The sums of the DSS and DMS were combined into the Total Combined Score (TCS) which was averaged over the entire grass pollen season.

14.1 First Season Efficacy
Adults and Children
This placebo-controlled trial evaluated 1501 subjects 5 through 65 years of age (approximately 80% were 18 years and older) comparing GRASTEK (N=752) and placebo (N=749) administered as a sublingual tablet daily for approximately 24 weeks. The subject population was 84% White, 9% African American and 4% Asian. The majority of subjects were male (52%). In this study, approximately 25% of subjects had mild, intermittent asthma and 85% of all subjects were sensitized to other allergens in addition to grass pollen. Subjects with a clinical history of symptomatic allergies to non-grass pollen allergens that required treatment during the grass pollen season were excluded from the studies. All treatment groups were balanced with regard to baseline characteristics.
Subjects treated with GRASTEK had a decrease in the TCS throughout the grass pollen season compared to placebo-treated subjects. Similarly, the DSS and DMS were decreased in subjects treated with GRASTEK compared to placebo throughout the grass pollen season, and the TCS was decreased compared to placebo during the peak grass pollen season (see Table 3).
[See table 3 above]
Children
This double-blind clinical trial of approximately 24 weeks duration evaluated 344 pediatric subjects 5 to 17 years of age who were treated with either GRASTEK or placebo once daily. The subject population was 88% White, 7% African American, and 2% Asian. The majority (65%) of subjects were male. The mean age of subjects was 12.3 years. In this study, 26% of subjects had mild intermittent asthma and most subjects (89%) were sensitized to other allergens in addition to grass pollen. Subjects with a clinical history of symptomatic allergies to non-grass pollen allergens that required treatment during the grass pollen season were excluded from the studies. All treatment groups were balanced with regard to baseline characteristics.
Pediatric subjects treated with GRASTEK had a decrease in TCS throughout the grass pollen season compared to placebo treated subjects (see Table 4). Similarly, the DSS and DMS were decreased in GRASTEK compared to placebo throughout the grass pollen season.
[See table 4 at top of next page]
14.2 Sustained Effect
Adult Subjects 18 Years and Older
The sustained effect of GRASTEK was measured in a 5-year double-blind study. The study included 634 randomized subjects between 18 and 65 years of age. The subject population was 96% White, 2% Asian and 1% African American. The majority (59%) of subjects were male. The mean age of subjects was 34 years. Subjects received either GRASTEK or placebo daily for 3 consecutive years and were then observed for 2 subsequent years during which they did not receive study drug. Subjects treated with GRASTEK had a decrease in TCS throughout the grass pollen season during the three years of active treatment. This effect was sustained during the grass pollen season in the first year after discontinuation of GRASTEK (see Table 5), but not in the second year.

Table 4: Total Combined Scores (TCS), Rhinoconjunctivitis Daily Symptom Scores (DSS) and Daily Medication Scores (DMS) During the Entire Grass Pollen Season

Endpoint*	GRASTEK (N=149)[†] Score[‡]	Placebo (N=158)[†] Score[‡]	Treatment Difference (GRASTEK – Placebo)	Difference Relative to Placebo[§] Estimate (95% CI)
TCS	4.62	6.25	-1.63	-26% (-38.2, -10.1)
DSS	3.71	4.91	-1.20	-24% (-36.4, -9.1)
DMS	0.91	1.33	-0.42	-32% (-57.7, 4.0)

TCS=Total combined score (DSS + DMS); DSS=Daily Symptom Score; DMS=Daily Medication Score.
* Parametric analysis using analysis of variance model for all endpoints.
† Number of subjects in analyses.
‡ The estimated group means are reported and difference relative to placebo is based on estimated group means.
§ Difference relative to placebo computed as: (GRASTEK - placebo)/placebo × 100.

Table 5: Rhinoconjunctivitis Total Combined Score (TCS), Daily Symptom Score (DSS), and Daily Medication Score (DMS) During the Entire Grass Pollen Season from the 5-Year Study

Endpoint	Difference Relative to Placebo* (95% CI)			
	Treatment Year 1 N=568[†]	Treatment Year 2[‡] N=316[†]	Treatment Year 3 N=287[†]	Post Treatment Year 1 N=257[†]
TCS	-34.2% (-42.0%, -26.3%)	-40.9% (-51.8%, -29.5%)	-34.0% (-45.5%, -21.4%)	-27.2% (-39.9%, -12.4%)
DSS	-31.2% (-38.8%, -23.4%)	-36.2% (-46.5%, -26.2%)	-29.0% (-40.3%, -16.3%)	-26.2% (-37.6%, -12.2%)
DMS	-38.4% (-49.8%, -26.5%)	-45.5% (-60.4%, -28.2%)	-40.1% (-55.4%, -21.2%)	-28.6% (-46.3%, -6.0%)

TCS=Total Combined Score (DSS + DMS); DSS=Daily Symptom Score; DMS=Daily Medication Score.
* Difference relative to placebo computed as: (GRASTEK - placebo)/placebo × 100.
† Number of subjects in analyses.
‡ Study extended from 1 to 5 years (site closures, subject unwillingness to participate beyond 1 year).

[See table 5 above]

16 HOW SUPPLIED/STORAGE AND HANDLING

GRASTEK 2800 BAU tablets are white to off-white, circular sublingual tablets with a debossed round detail on one side. GRASTEK is supplied as follows:
3 blister packages of 10 tablets (30 tablets total). NDC 0006-4229-30
Store at controlled room temperature 20°C-25°C (68°F-77°F); excursions permitted between 15°C-30°C (59°F-86°F). Store in the original package until use to protect from moisture.

17 PATIENT COUNSELING INFORMATION

Advise patients to read the FDA-approved patient labeling (Medication Guide) and to keep GRASTEK and all medicines out of the reach of children.
Severe Allergic Reactions
Advise patients that GRASTEK may cause life-threatening systemic or local allergic reactions, including anaphylaxis. Educate patients about the signs and symptoms of these allergic reactions *[See Warnings and Precautions (5.1).]*. The signs and symptoms of a severe allergic reaction may include: syncope, dizziness, hypotension, tachycardia, dyspnea, wheezing, bronchospasm, chest discomfort, cough, abdominal pain, vomiting, diarrhea, rash, pruritus, flushing, and urticaria.
Ensure that patients have auto-injectable epinephrine and instruct patients in its proper use. Instruct patients who experience a severe allergic reaction to seek immediate medical care, discontinue GRASTEK, and resume treatment only when advised by a physician to do so. *[See Warnings and Precautions (5.2).]*
Advise patients to read the patient information for epinephrine.
Inform patients that the first dose of GRASTEK must be administered in a healthcare setting under the supervision of a physician and that they will be monitored for at least 30 minutes to watch for signs and symptoms of a life-threatening systemic or local allergic reaction *[See Warnings and Precautions (5.1).]*
Because of the risk of upper airway compromise, instruct patients with persistent and escalating adverse reactions in the mouth or throat to discontinue GRASTEK and to contact their healthcare professional. *[See Warnings and Precautions (5.3).]*

Because of the risk of eosinophilic esophagitis, instruct patients with severe or persistent symptoms of esophagitis to discontinue GRASTEK and to contact their healthcare professional. *[See Warnings and Precautions (5.4)].*
Inform parents/guardians that GRASTEK should only be administered to children under adult supervision *[See Dosage and Administration (2.2)].*
Asthma
Instruct patients with asthma that if they have difficulty breathing or if their asthma becomes difficult to control, they should stop taking GRASTEK and contact their healthcare professional immediately *[See Warnings and Precautions (5.5)].*
Administration Instructions
Instruct patients to carefully remove the foil from the blister unit with dry hands and then take the sublingual tablet immediately by placing it under the tongue where it will dissolve. Also instruct patients to wash their hands after handling the tablet, and to avoid food or beverages for 5 minutes after taking the tablet. *[See Dosage and Administration (2.2).]*
Manufactured for: Merck Sharp & Dohme Corp., a subsidiary of **MERCK & CO., INC.,** Whitehouse Station, NJ 08889, USA
Manufactured by:
Catalent Pharma Solutions Limited, Blagrove, Swindon, Wiltshire, SN5 8RU UK
For patent information:
www.merck.com/product/patent/home.html
Copyright © 2014 Merck Sharp & Dohme Corp., a subsidiary of **Merck & Co., Inc.**
All rights reserved.
uspi-mk7243-sb-1406r001
MEDICATION GUIDE
GRASTEK® (GRAS-tek)
(Timothy Grass Pollen Allergen Extract)
Carefully read this Medication Guide before you or your child start taking GRASTEK and each time you get a refill. This Medication Guide does not take the place of talking to your doctor about your medical condition or treatment. Talk with your doctor or pharmacist if there is something you do not understand or you want to learn more about GRASTEK.

What is the Most Important Information I Should Know about GRASTEK?
GRASTEK can cause severe allergic reactions that may be life-threatening. Stop taking GRASTEK and get medical treatment right away if you or your child has any of the following symptoms after taking GRASTEK:
• Trouble breathing
• Throat tightness or swelling
• Trouble swallowing or speaking
• Dizziness or fainting
• Rapid or weak heartbeat
• Severe stomach cramps or pain, vomiting, or diarrhea
• Severe flushing or itching of the skin
For home administration of GRASTEK, your doctor will prescribe auto-injectable epinephrine, a medicine you can inject if you or your child has a severe allergic reaction after taking GRASTEK. Your doctor will train and instruct you on the proper use of auto-injectable epinephrine.
Talk to your doctor or read the epinephrine patient information if you have any questions about the use of auto-injectable epinephrine.
What is GRASTEK?
GRASTEK is a prescription medicine used for sublingual (under the tongue) immunotherapy to treat Timothy and related grass pollen allergies that can cause sneezing, runny or itchy nose, stuffy or congested nose, or itchy and watery eyes. GRASTEK may be prescribed for persons 5 through 65 years of age who are allergic to grass pollen.
GRASTEK is taken for about 12 weeks before grass pollen season and throughout grass pollen season. GRASTEK may also be taken daily for 3 years to provide a sustained effect for a fourth year in which you do not have to take GRASTEK.
GRASTEK is NOT a medication that gives immediate relief for symptoms of grass allergy.
Who Should Not Take GRASTEK?
You or your child should not take GRASTEK if:
• You or your child has severe, unstable or uncontrolled asthma
• You or your child had a severe allergic reaction in the past that included any of these symptoms:
  ○ Trouble breathing
  ○ Dizziness or fainting
  ○ Rapid or weak heartbeat
• You or your child has ever had difficulty with breathing due to swelling of the throat or upper airway after using any sublingual immunotherapy before.
• You or your child has ever been diagnosed with eosinophilic esophagitis.
• You or your child is allergic to any of the inactive ingredients contained in GRASTEK. The inactive ingredients contained in GRASTEK are: gelatin, mannitol and sodium hydroxide.
What Should I Tell My Doctor Before Taking GRASTEK?
Your doctor may decide that GRASTEK is not the best treatment if:
• You or your child has asthma, depending on how severe it is.
• You or your child suffers from lung disease such as chronic obstructive pulmonary disease (COPD)
• You or your child suffers from heart disease such as coronary artery disease, an irregular heart rhythm, or you have hypertension that is not well controlled.
• You or your daughter is pregnant, plans to become pregnant during the time you will be taking GRASTEK, or is breast-feeding.
• You or your child is unable or unwilling to administer auto-injectable epinephrine to treat a severe allergic reaction to GRASTEK.
• You or your child is taking certain medicines that enhance the likelihood of a severe reaction, or interfere with the treatment of a severe reaction. These medicines include:
  ○ beta blockers and alpha-blockers (prescribed for high blood pressure)
  ○ cardiac glycosides (prescribed for heart failure or problems with heart rhythm)
  ○ diuretics (prescribed for heart conditions and high blood pressure)
  ○ ergot alkaloids (prescribed for migraine headache)
  ○ monoamine oxidase inhibitors or tricyclic antidepressants (prescribed for depression)
  ○ thyroid hormone (prescribed for low thyroid activity).
You should tell your doctor if you or your child is taking or has recently taken any other medicines, including medicines obtained without a prescription and herbal supplements. Keep a list of them and show it to your doctor and pharmacist each time you get a new supply of GRASTEK. Ask your doctor or pharmacist for advice before taking GRASTEK.
Are there any reasons to stop taking GRASTEK?
Stop GRASTEK and contact your doctor if you or your child has any of the following after taking GRASTEK:
• Any type of a serious allergic reaction

- Throat tightness that worsens or swelling of the tongue or throat that causes trouble speaking, breathing or swallowing
- Asthma or any other breathing condition that gets worse
- Dizziness or fainting
- Rapid or weak heartbeat
- Severe stomach cramps or pain, vomiting, or diarrhea
- Severe flushing or itching of the skin
- Heartburn, difficulty swallowing, pain with swallowing, or chest pain that does not go away or worsens

Also, stop taking GRASTEK following: mouth surgery procedures (such as tooth removal), or if you develop any mouth infections, ulcers or cuts in the mouth or throat.

How should I take GRASTEK?

Take GRASTEK exactly as your doctor tells you. GRASTEK is a prescription medicine that is placed under the tongue.

- Take the tablet from the blister package after carefully removing the foil with dry hands.
- Place the tablet immediately under the tongue. Allow it to remain there until completely dissolved. Do not swallow for at least 1 minute.
- Do not take GRASTEK with food or beverage. Food and beverage should not be taken for the following 5 minutes.
- Wash hands after taking the tablet.

Take the first tablet of GRASTEK in your doctor's office. After taking the first tablet, you or your child will be watched for at least 30 minutes for symptoms of a serious allergic reaction.

If you tolerate the first dose of GRASTEK, you or your child will continue GRASTEK therapy at home by taking one tablet every day. Children should be given each tablet of GRASTEK by an adult who will watch for any symptoms of a serious allergic reaction.

Take GRASTEK as prescribed by your doctor until the end of the treatment course. If you forget to take GRASTEK, do not take a double dose. Take the next dose at your normal scheduled time the next day. If you miss more than one dose of GRASTEK, contact your healthcare provider before restarting.

What are the possible side effects of GRASTEK?

In children and adults, the most commonly reported side effects were itching of the mouth, lips, or tongue, swelling under the tongue, or throat irritation. These side effects, by themselves, were not dangerous or life-threatening.

GRASTEK can cause severe allergic reactions that may be life-threatening. Symptoms of allergic reactions to GRASTEK include:

- Trouble breathing
- Throat tightness or swelling
- Trouble swallowing or speaking
- Dizziness or fainting
- Rapid or weak heartbeat
- Severe stomach cramps or pain, vomiting, or diarrhea
- Severe flushing or itching of the skin

For additional information on the possible side effects of GRASTEK, talk with your doctor or pharmacist. You may report side effects to the U.S. Food and Drug Administration (FDA) at 1-800-FDA-1088 or www.fda.gov/medwatch.

How should I store GRASTEK?

Keep GRASTEK out of the reach of children.

Throw away any unused GRASTEK after the expiration date which is stated on the carton and blister pack after "EXP."

Store GRASTEK in a dry place at room temperature, 15°C to 30°C (59°F to 86°F), in the original package.

General information about GRASTEK

Medicines are sometimes prescribed for purposes other than those listed in a Medication Guide. Do not use GRASTEK for a condition for which it was not prescribed. Do not give GRASTEK to other people, even if they have the same symptoms. It may harm them.

This Medication Guide summarizes the most important information about GRASTEK. If you would like more information, talk with your doctor. You can ask your doctor or pharmacist for information about GRASTEK that was written for healthcare professionals. For more information go to www.grastek.com or call toll-free at 1-800-622-4477.

This Medication Guide has been approved by the U.S. Food and Drug Administration.

Manufactured for: Merck Sharp & Dohme Corp., a subsidiary of **MERCK & CO., INC.,** Whitehouse Station, NJ 08889, USA
Manufactured by:
Catalent Pharma Solutions Limited, Blagrove, Swindon, Wiltshire, SN5 8RU UK
For patent information:
www.merck.com/product/patent/home.html
Copyright © 2014 Merck Sharp & Dohme Corp., a subsidiary of Merck & Co., Inc.
All rights reserved.
Revised: 04/2014
usmg-mk7243-sb-1404r000

Shown in Product Identification Guide, page 308

IMPLANON®
(etonogestrel implant)
for subdermal use

℞

HIGHLIGHTS OF PRESCRIBING INFORMATION
These highlights do not include all the information needed to use IMPLANON safely and effectively. See full prescribing information for IMPLANON.
IMPLANON® (etonogestrel implant), for subdermal use
Initial U.S. Approval: 2001

———INDICATIONS AND USAGE———

IMPLANON is a progestin indicated for use by women to prevent pregnancy. (1)

———DOSAGE AND ADMINISTRATION———

Insert one IMPLANON subdermally just under the skin at the inner side of the non-dominant upper arm. IMPLANON must be removed no later than by the end of the third year. (2)

———DOSAGE FORMS AND STRENGTHS———

IMPLANON consists of a single, rod-shaped implant, containing 68 mg etonogestrel, pre-loaded in the needle of a disposable applicator. (3)

———CONTRAINDICATIONS———

- Known or suspected pregnancy (4)
- Current or past history of thrombosis or thromboembolic disorders (4, 5.4)
- Liver tumors, benign or malignant, or active liver disease (4, 5.7)
- Undiagnosed abnormal genital bleeding (4, 5.2)
- Known or suspected breast cancer, personal history of breast cancer, or other progestin-sensitive cancer, now or in the past (4, 5.6)
- Allergic reaction to any of the components of IMPLANON (4, 6)

———WARNINGS AND PRECAUTIONS———

- Insertion and removal complications: Pain, paresthesias, bleeding, hematoma, scarring or infection may occur. (5.1)
- Menstrual bleeding pattern: Counsel women regarding changes in bleeding frequency, intensity, or duration. (5.2)
- Ectopic pregnancies: Be alert to the possibility of an ectopic pregnancy in women using IMPLANON who become pregnant or complain of lower abdominal pain. (5.3)
- Thrombotic and other vascular events: The IMPLANON implant should be removed in the event of a thrombosis. (5.4)
- Liver disease: Remove the IMPLANON implant if jaundice occurs. (5.7)
- Elevated blood pressure: The IMPLANON implant should be removed if blood pressure rises significantly and becomes uncontrolled. (5.9)
- Carbohydrate and lipid metabolic effects: Monitor prediabetic and diabetic women using IMPLANON. (5.11)

———ADVERSE REACTIONS———

Most common (≥10%) adverse reactions reported in clinical trials were change in menstrual bleeding pattern, headache, vaginitis, weight increase, acne, breast pain, abdominal pain, and pharyngitis. (6.1)

To report SUSPECTED ADVERSE REACTIONS, contact Merck Sharp & Dohme Corp., a subsidiary of Merck & Co., Inc., at 1-877-888-4231 or FDA at 1-800-FDA-1088 or *www.fda.gov/medwatch*.

———DRUG INTERACTIONS———

Drugs or herbal products that induce certain enzymes, such as CYP3A4, may decrease the effectiveness of progestin hormonal contraceptives or increase breakthrough bleeding. (7.1)

———USE IN SPECIFIC POPULATIONS———

- Pregnant women: IMPLANON should be removed if maintaining a pregnancy. (8.1)
- Overweight women: IMPLANON may become less effective in overweight women over time, especially in the presence of other factors that decrease etonogestrel concentrations, such as concomitant use of hepatic enzyme inducers. (8.8)

See 17 for PATIENT COUNSELING INFORMATION and FDA-approved patient labeling

Revised: 07/2014

FULL PRESCRIBING INFORMATION

1   INDICATIONS AND USAGE

IMPLANON® is indicated for use by women to prevent pregnancy.

2   DOSAGE AND ADMINISTRATION

The efficacy of IMPLANON does not depend on daily, weekly or monthly administration.

All healthcare providers should receive instruction and training prior to performing insertion and/or removal of IMPLANON.

A single IMPLANON implant is inserted subdermally in the upper arm. To reduce the risk of neural or vascular injury, the implant should be inserted at the inner side of the non-dominant upper arm about 8-10 cm (3-4 inches) above the medial epicondyle of the humerus. The implant should be inserted subdermally just under the skin to avoid the large blood vessels and nerves that lie deeper in the subcutaneous tissues in the sulcus between the triceps and biceps muscles. IMPLANON must be inserted by the expiration date stated on the packaging. IMPLANON is a long-acting (up to 3 years), reversible, hormonal contraceptive method. The implant must be removed by the end of the third year and may be replaced by a new implant at the time of removal, if continued contraceptive protection is desired.

2.1   Initiating Contraception with IMPLANON
IMPORTANT: Rule out pregnancy before inserting the implant.

Timing of insertion depends on the woman's recent contraceptive history, as follows:

- No preceding hormonal contraceptive use in the past month

    IMPLANON should be inserted between Day 1 (first day of menstrual bleeding) and Day 5 of the menstrual cycle, even if the woman is still bleeding.

If inserted as recommended, back-up contraception is not necessary. If deviating from the recommended timing of insertion, the woman should be advised to use a barrier method until 7 days after insertion. If intercourse has already occurred, pregnancy should be excluded.

• Switching contraceptive method to IMPLANON

Combination hormonal contraceptives:

IMPLANON should preferably be inserted on the day after the last active tablet of the previous combined oral contraceptive or on the day of the removal of the vaginal ring or transdermal patch. At the latest, IMPLANON should be inserted on the day following the usual tablet-free, ring-free, patch-free or placebo tablet interval of the previous combined hormonal contraceptive.

If inserted as recommended, back-up contraception is not necessary. If deviating from the recommended timing of insertion, the woman should be advised to use a barrier method until 7 days after insertion. If intercourse has already occurred, pregnancy should be excluded.

Progestin-only contraceptives:

There are several types of progestin-only methods. IMPLANON should be inserted as follows:

• Injectable Contraceptives: Insert IMPLANON on the day the next injection is due.

• Minipill: A woman may switch to IMPLANON on any day of the month. IMPLANON should be inserted within 24 hours after taking the last tablet.

• Contraceptive implant or intrauterine system (IUS): Insert IMPLANON on the same day as the previous contraceptive implant or IUS is removed.

If inserted as recommended, back-up contraception is not necessary. If deviating from the recommended timing of insertion, the woman should be advised to use a barrier method until 7 days after insertion. If intercourse has already occurred, pregnancy should be excluded.

• Following abortion or miscarriage

• First Trimester: IMPLANON should be inserted within 5 days following a first trimester abortion or miscarriage.

• Second Trimester: Insert IMPLANON between 21 to 28 days following second trimester abortion or miscarriage.

If inserted as recommended, back-up contraception is not necessary. If deviating from the recommended timing of insertion, the woman should be advised to use a barrier method until 7 days after insertion. If intercourse has already occurred, pregnancy should be excluded.

• Postpartum

• Not Breastfeeding: IMPLANON should be inserted between 21 to 28 days postpartum. If inserted as recommended, back-up contraception is not necessary. If deviating from the recommended timing of insertion, the woman should be advised to use a barrier method until 7 days after insertion. If intercourse has already occurred, pregnancy should be excluded.

• Breastfeeding: IMPLANON should be inserted after the fourth postpartum week [see Use in Specific Populations (8.3)]. The woman should be advised to use a barrier method until 7 days after insertion. If intercourse has already occurred, pregnancy should be excluded.

2.2   Insertion of IMPLANON

The basis for successful use and subsequent removal of IMPLANON is a correct and carefully performed subdermal insertion of the single, rod-shaped implant in accordance with the instructions. Both the healthcare provider and the woman should be able to feel the implant under the skin after placement.

All healthcare providers performing insertions and/or removals of IMPLANON should receive instructions and training prior to inserting or removing the implant. Information concerning the insertion and removal of IMPLANON will be sent upon request free of charge [1-877-IMPLANON (1-877-467-5266)].

Preparation

Prior to inserting IMPLANON carefully read the instructions for insertion as well as the full prescribing information.

Before insertion of IMPLANON, the healthcare provider should confirm that:

• The woman is not pregnant nor has any other contraindication for the use of IMPLANON [see Contraindications (4)].

• The woman has had a medical history and physical examination, including a gynecologic examination, performed.

• The woman understands the benefits and risks of IMPLANON.

• The woman has received a copy of the Patient Labeling included in packaging.

• The woman has reviewed and completed a consent form to be maintained with the woman's chart.

• The woman does not have allergies to the antiseptic and anesthetic to be used during insertion.

Insert IMPLANON under aseptic conditions.

The following equipment is needed for the implant insertion:

• An examination table for the woman to lie on

• Sterile surgical drapes, sterile gloves, antiseptic solution, sterile marker (optional)

• Local anesthetic, needles, and syringe

• Sterile gauze, adhesive bandage, pressure bandage

An applicator and its parts are shown below (Figures 1a and 1b).

Figure 1a (Not to scale)

applicator seal — applicator
Grooved tip — obturator support — obturator
needle — cannula
location of IMPLANON
IMPLANON
4 cm
needle shield

Figure 1b

Grooved tip

Grooved tip of obturator (enlarged)

The procedure used for IMPLANON insertion is opposite from that of an injection. The obturator keeps IMPLANON in place while the cannula is retracted. The obturator must remain fixed in place while the cannula with needle is retracted from the arm. Do not push the obturator.

Insertion Procedure

Step 1. Have the woman lie on her back on the examination table with her non-dominant arm flexed at the elbow and externally rotated so that her wrist is parallel to her ear or her hand is positioned next to her head (Figure 2).

Figure 2

Step 2. Identify the insertion site, which is at the inner side of the non-dominant upper arm about 8-10 cm (3-4 inches) above the medial epicondyle of the humerus (Figure 3). **The implant should be inserted subdermally just under the skin to avoid the large blood vessels and nerves that lie deeper in the subcutaneous tissue in the sulcus between the triceps and biceps muscles** [see Warnings and Precautions (5.1)].

Step 3. Make two marks with a sterile marker: first, mark the spot where the etonogestrel implant will be inserted, and second, mark a spot a few centimeters proximal to the first mark (Figure 3). This second mark will later serve as a direction guide during insertion.

Guiding Mark

8–10 cm

Medial Epicondyle

Insertion Site

Figure 3

Step 4. Clean the insertion site with an antiseptic solution.

Step 5. Anesthetize the insertion area (for example, with anesthetic spray or by injecting 2 mL of 1% lidocaine just under the skin along the planned insertion tunnel).

Step 6. Remove the sterile pre-loaded disposable IMPLANON applicator carrying the implant from its blister. Keep the IMPLANON needle and rod sterile. The applicator should not be used if sterility is in question. If contamination occurs, use a new package of IMPLANON with a new sterile applicator.

Step 7. Keep the shield on the needle and look for the IMPLANON rod, seen as a white cylinder inside the needle tip.

Step 8. If you don't see the IMPLANON rod, tap the top of the needle shield against a firm surface to bring the implant into the needle tip.

Step 9. Following visual confirmation, lower the IMPLANON rod back into the needle by tapping it back into the needle tip. Then remove the needle shield, while holding the applicator upright.

Step 10. **Note that IMPLANON can fall out of the needle.** Therefore, after you remove the needle shield, keep the applicator in the upright position until the moment of insertion

Step 11. With your free hand, stretch the skin around the insertion site with thumb and index finger (Figure 4).

Figure 4

Step 12. At a slight angle (not greater than 20°), insert **only** the tip of the needle with the beveled side up into the insertion site (Figure 5).

20°

Figure 5

Step 13. Lower the applicator to a horizontal position. Lift the skin up with the tip of the needle, but **keep the needle in the subdermal connective tissue** (Figure 6).

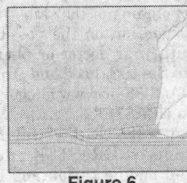

Figure 6

Step 14. While "tenting" (lifting) the skin, gently insert the needle to its full length. Keep the needle parallel to the surface of the skin during insertion (Figure 7).

Figure 7

Step 15. **If IMPLANON is placed too deeply, the removal process can be difficult or impossible. If the needle is not inserted to its full length, the implant may protrude from the insertion site and fall out.**

Step 16. Break the seal of the applicator by pressing the obturator support (Figure 8).

[See figure 8 at top of next column]

Step 17. Turn the obturator 90° in either direction with respect to the needle (Figure 9).

[See figure 9 at top of next column]

Step 18. While holding the obturator fixed in place on the arm, fully retract the cannula (Figure 10). **Note: This procedure is opposite from an injection. Do not push the obturator. By holding the obturator fixed in place on the arm and fully retracting the cannula, the implant will be left in its correct subdermal position. Do not simulta-**

Figure 8

Figure 9

neously retract the obturator and cannula from the patient's arm.

Figure 10

In this figure, the right hand is holding the obturator in place while the left hand is retracting the cannula.

Step 19. Confirm that the implant has been inserted by checking the tip of the needle for the absence of the implant. After insertion of the implant, the grooved tip of the obturator will be visible inside the needle (Figure 11).

Grooved tip

Figure 11

Step 20. **Always verify the presence of the implant in the woman's arm immediately after insertion by palpation.** By palpating both ends of the implant, you should be able to confirm the presence of the 4-cm rod (Figure 12).

Figure 12

If you cannot feel the implant or are in doubt of its presence,
• Check the tip of the needle for the absence of the implant. After insertion of the implant, the grooved tip of the obturator will be visible inside the needle.
• Use other methods to confirm the presence of the implant. Suitable methods to locate are: ultrasound (US) with a high-frequency linear array transducer (10 MHz or greater) or magnetic resonance imaging (MRI). Please note that the IMPLANON rod is not radiopaque and cannot be seen by X-ray or CT scan. If ultrasound and MRI fail, call 1-877-IMPLANON (1-877-467-5266) for information on the procedure for measuring etonogestrel blood levels.

Until the presence of the implant has been verified, the woman should be advised to use a non-hormonal contraceptive method, such as condoms.

Step 21. Place a small adhesive bandage over the insertion site. Request that the woman palpate the implant.

Step 22. Apply a pressure bandage with sterile gauze to minimize bruising. The woman may remove the pressure bandage in 24 hours and the small bandage over the insertion site in 3 to 5 days.

Step 23. Complete the USER CARD and give it to the woman to keep. Also, complete the PATIENT CHART LABEL and affix it to the woman's medical record.

Step 24. The applicator is for single use only and should be disposed in accordance with the Center for Disease Control and Prevention guidelines for handling of hazardous waste.

2.3 Removal of IMPLANON
Preparation

Before initiating the removal procedure, the healthcare provider should carefully read the instructions for removal and consult the USER CARD and/or the PATIENT CHART LABEL for the location of the implant. The exact location of the implant in the arm should be verified by palpation. If the implant is not palpable, ultrasound with a high-frequency linear array transducer (10 MHz or greater) or magnetic resonance imaging can be performed to verify its presence. A non-palpable implant should always be first located prior to removal. Suitable methods for localization include ultrasound with a high-frequency linear array transducer (10 MHz or greater) or magnetic resonance imaging. If these imaging methods fail to locate the implant, etonogestrel blood level determination can be used for verification of the presence of the implant. For details on etonogestrel blood level determination, call 1-877-IMPLANON (1-877-467-5266) for further instructions.

After localization of a non-palpable implant, consider conducting removal with ultrasound guidance.

There have been occasional reports of migration of the implant; usually this involves minor movement relative to the original position. This may complicate localization of the implant by palpation, ultrasound or magnetic resonance imaging, and removal may require a larger incision and more time.

Exploratory surgery without knowledge of the exact location of the implant is strongly discouraged. Removal of deeply inserted implants should be conducted with caution in order to prevent injury to deeper neural or vascular structures in the arm and be performed by healthcare providers familiar with the anatomy of the arm.

Before removal of the implant, the healthcare provider should confirm that:
• The woman does not have allergies to the antiseptic or anesthetic to be used.

Remove the implant under aseptic conditions.

The following equipment is needed for removal of the implant:
• An examination table for the woman to lie on
• Sterile surgical drapes, sterile gloves, antiseptic solution, sterile marker (optional)
• Local anesthetic, needles, and syringe
• Sterile scalpel, forceps (straight and curved mosquito)
• Skin closure, sterile gauze, adhesive bandage and pressure bandages

Removal Procedure

Step 1. Clean the site where the incision will be made and apply an antiseptic. Locate the implant by palpation and mark the distal end (end closest to the elbow), for example, with a sterile marker (Figure 13).

Figure 13

Step 2. Anesthetize the arm, for example, with 0.5 to 1 mL 1% lidocaine at the marked site where the incision will be made (Figure 14). Be sure to inject the local anesthetic **under** the implant to keep it close to the skin surface.

Figure 14

Step 3. Push down the proximal end of the implant (Figure 15) to stabilize it; a bulge may appear indicating the distal end of the implant. Starting at the distal tip of the implant, make a longitudinal incision of 2 mm towards the elbow.

Figure 15

Step 4. Gently push the implant towards the incision until the tip is visible. Grasp the implant with forceps (preferably curved mosquito forceps) and gently remove the implant (Figure 16).

Figure 16

Step 5. If the implant is encapsulated, make an incision into the tissue sheath and then remove the implant with the forceps (Figures 17 and 18).

Figure 17   **Figure 18**

Step 6. If the tip of the implant does not become visible in the incision, gently insert a forceps into the incision (Figure 19). Flip the forceps over into your other hand (Figure 20).

Figure 19   **Figure 20**

Step 7. With a second pair of forceps carefully dissect the tissue around the implant and grasp the implant (Figure 21). The implant can then be removed.

Figure 21

Step 8. Confirm that the entire implant, which is 4 cm long, has been removed by measuring its length. If a partial implant (less than 4 cm) is removed, the remaining piece should be removed by following the instructions in section 2.3. *[See Dosage and Administration (2.3).]* If the woman would like to continue using IMPLANON, a new implant may be inserted immediately after the old implant is removed using the same incision *[see Dosage and Administration (2.4)]*.

Step 9. After removing the implant, close the incision with a steri-strip and apply an adhesive bandage.

Step 10. Apply a pressure bandage with sterile gauze to minimize bruising. The woman may remove the pressure bandage in 24 hours and the small bandage in 3 to 5 days.

2.4 Replacing IMPLANON

Immediate replacement can be done after removal of the previous implant and is similar to the insertion procedure described in section 2.2 Insertion of IMPLANON.

The new implant may be inserted in the same arm, and through the same incision from which the previous implant was removed. If the same incision is being used to insert a new implant, anesthetize the insertion site [for example, 2 mL lidocaine (1%)] applying it just under the skin along the 'insertion canal.'

Follow the subsequent steps in the insertion instructions [see Dosage and Administration (2.2)].

3 DOSAGE FORMS AND STRENGTHS

Single, off-white, soft, flexible, ethylene vinylacetate (EVA) implant, 4 cm in length and 2 mm in diameter containing 68 mg etonogestrel.

4 CONTRAINDICATIONS

IMPLANON should not be used in women who have
• Known or suspected pregnancy
• Current or past history of thrombosis or thromboembolic disorders
• Liver tumors, benign or malignant, or active liver disease
• Undiagnosed abnormal genital bleeding
• Known or suspected breast cancer, personal history of breast cancer, or other progestin-sensitive cancer, now or in the past
• Allergic reaction to any of the components of IMPLANON [see Adverse Reactions (6)]

5 WARNINGS AND PRECAUTIONS

The following information is based on experience with either IMPLANON, other progestin-only contraceptives, or experience with combination (estrogen plus progestin) oral contraceptives.

5.1 Complications of Insertion and Removal

IMPLANON should be inserted subdermally so that it will be palpable after insertion, and this should be confirmed by palpation immediately after insertion. Failure to insert IMPLANON properly may go unnoticed unless it is palpated immediately after insertion. Undetected failure to insert the implant may lead to an unintended pregnancy. Complications related to insertion and removal procedures, such as pain, paresthesias, bleeding, hematoma, scarring or infection, may occur. Occasionally in post-marketing use, implant insertions have failed because the implant fell out of the needle or remained in the needle during insertion.

If IMPLANON is inserted too deeply (intramuscular or in the fascia), neural or vascular injury may occur. To reduce the risk of neural or vascular injury, IMPLANON should be inserted at the inner side of the non-dominant upper arm about 8-10 cm (3-4 inches) above the medial epicondyle of the humerus. IMPLANON should be inserted subdermally just under the skin to avoid the large blood vessels and nerves that lie deeper in the subcutaneous tissues in the sulcus between the triceps and biceps muscles. Deep insertions of IMPLANON have been associated with paraesthesia (due to neural injury) and migration of the implant (due to intramuscular or fascial insertion), and in a very few cases with intravascular insertion. If infection develops at the insertion site, start suitable treatment. If the infection persists, the implant should be removed. Incomplete insertions or infections may lead to expulsion. In postmarketing use there have been cases of failure to localize and remove the implant, probably due to deep insertion. There has been 1 case of an intravascular insertion reported post-marketing which led to inability to remove the implant.

Implant removal may be difficult or impossible if the implant is not inserted correctly, is inserted too deeply, not palpable, encased in fibrous tissue, or has migrated. Deep insertions may lead to difficult localization of the implant and may also result in the need for a surgical procedure in an operating room in order to remove the implant. Exploratory surgery without knowledge of the exact location of the implant is strongly discouraged. Removal of deeply inserted implants should be conducted with caution in order to prevent injury to deeper neural or vascular structures in the arm and be performed by healthcare providers familiar with the anatomy of the arm. Failure to remove the implant may result in continued effects of etonogestrel, such as compromised fertility, ectopic pregnancy, or persistence or occurrence of a drug-related adverse event.

5.2 Changes in Menstrual Bleeding Patterns

After starting IMPLANON, women are likely to have a change from their normal menstrual bleeding pattern. These may include changes in bleeding frequency (absent, less, more frequent or continuous), intensity (reduced or increased) or duration. In clinical trials, bleeding patterns ranged from amenorrhea (1 in 5 women) to frequent and/or prolonged bleeding (1 in 5 women). The bleeding pattern experienced during the first three months of IMPLANON use is broadly predictive of the future bleeding pattern for many women. Women should be counseled regarding the bleeding pattern changes they may experience so that they know what to expect. Abnormal bleeding should be evaluated as needed to exclude pathologic conditions or pregnancy.

In clinical studies of IMPLANON, reports of changes in bleeding pattern were the most common reason for stopping treatment (11.1%). Irregular bleeding (10.8%) was the single most common reason women stopped treatment, while amenorrhea (0.3%) was cited less frequently. In these stud-

ies, women had an average of 17.7 days of bleeding or spotting every 90 days (based on 3,315 intervals of 90 days recorded by 780 patients). The percentages of patients having 0, 1-7, 8-21, or >21 days of spotting or bleeding over a 90-day interval while using the IMPLANON implant are shown in Table 1.

Table 1: Percentages of Patients with 0, 1 - 7, 8 - 21, or >21 Days of Spotting or Bleeding Over a 90-Day Interval While Using IMPLANON

Total Days of Spotting or Bleeding	Percentage of Patients		
	Treatment Days 91-180 (N = 745)	Treatment Days 271-360 (N = 657)	Treatment Days 631-720 (N = 547)
0 Days	19%	24%	17%
1-7 Days	15%	13%	12%
8-21 Days	30%	30%	37%
>21 Days	35%	33%	35%

Bleeding patterns observed with use of IMPLANON for up to 2 years, and the proportion of 90-day intervals with these bleeding patterns, are summarized in Table 2.

Table 2: Bleeding Patterns Using IMPLANON during the First 2 Years of Use*

BLEEDING PATTERNS	DEFINITIONS	%[†]
Infrequent	Less than three bleeding and/or spotting episodes in 90 days (excluding amenorrhea)	33.6
Amenorrhea	No bleeding and/or spotting in 90 days	22.2
Prolonged	Any bleeding and/or spotting episode lasting more than 14 days in 90 days	17.7
Frequent	More than 5 bleeding and/or spotting episodes in 90 days	6.7

* Based on 3,315 recording periods of 90 day's duration in 780 women, excluding the first 90 days after implant insertion
† % = Percentage of 90-day intervals with this pattern

In case of undiagnosed, persistent, or recurrent abnormal vaginal bleeding, appropriate measures should be conducted to rule out malignancy.

5.3 Ectopic Pregnancies

As with all progestin-only contraceptive products, be alert to the possibility of an ectopic pregnancy among women using IMPLANON who become pregnant or complain of lower abdominal pain. Although ectopic pregnancies are uncommon among women using IMPLANON, a pregnancy that occurs in a woman using IMPLANON may be more likely to be ectopic than a pregnancy occurring in a woman using no contraception.

5.4 Thrombotic and Other Vascular Events

The use of combination hormonal contraceptives (progestin plus estrogen) increases the risk of vascular events, including arterial events (strokes and myocardial infarctions) or deep venous thrombotic events (venous thromboembolism, deep venous thrombosis, retinal vein thrombosis, and pulmonary embolism). IMPLANON is a progestin-only contraceptive. It is unknown whether this increased risk is applicable to etonogestrel alone. It is recommended, however, that women with risk factors known to increase the risk of venous and arterial thromboembolism be carefully assessed.

There have been postmarketing reports of serious arterial and venous thromboembolic events, including cases of pulmonary emboli (some fatal), deep vein thrombosis, myocardial infarction, and strokes, in women using IMPLANON. IMPLANON should be removed in the event of a thrombosis.

Due to the risk of thromboembolism associated with pregnancy and immediately following delivery, IMPLANON should not be used prior to 21 days postpartum. Women with a history of thromboembolic disorders should be made aware of the possibility of a recurrence.

Evaluate for retinal vein thrombosis immediately if there is unexplained loss of vision, proptosis, diplopia, papilledema, or retinal vascular lesions.

Consider removal of the IMPLANON implant in case of long-term immobilization due to surgery or illness.

5.5 Ovarian Cysts

If follicular development occurs, atresia of the follicle is sometimes delayed, and the follicle may continue to grow beyond the size it would attain in a normal cycle. Generally, these enlarged follicles disappear spontaneously. On rare occasion, surgery may be required.

5.6 Carcinoma of the Breast and Reproductive Organs

Women who currently have or have had breast cancer should not use hormonal contraception because breast cancer may be hormonally sensitive [see Contraindications (4)]. Some studies suggest that the use of combination hormonal contraceptives might increase the incidence of breast cancer; however, other studies have not confirmed such findings.

Some studies suggest that the use of combination hormonal contraceptives is associated with an increase in the risk of cervical cancer or intraepithelial neoplasia. However, there is controversy about the extent to which such findings are due to differences in sexual behavior and other factors.

Women with a family history of breast cancer or who develop breast nodules should be carefully monitored.

5.7 Liver Disease

Disturbances of liver function may necessitate the discontinuation of hormonal contraceptive use until markers of liver function return to normal. Remove IMPLANON if jaundice develops.

Hepatic adenomas are associated with combination hormonal contraceptives use. An estimate of the attributable risk is 3.3 cases per 100,000 for combination hormonal contraceptives users. It is not known whether a similar risk exists with progestin-only methods like IMPLANON.

The progestin in IMPLANON may be poorly metabolized in women with liver impairment. Use of IMPLANON in women with active liver disease or liver cancer is contraindicated [see Contraindications (4)].

5.8 Weight Gain

In clinical studies, mean weight gain in US IMPLANON users was 2.8 pounds after 1 year and 3.7 pounds after 2 years. How much of the weight gain was related to the implant is unknown. In studies, 2.3% of the users reported weight gain as the reason for having the implant removed.

5.9 Elevated Blood Pressure

Women with a history of hypertension-related diseases or renal disease should be discouraged from using hormonal contraception. For women with well-controlled hypertension, use of IMPLANON can be considered. Women with hypertension using IMPLANON should be closely monitored. If sustained hypertension develops during the use of IMPLANON, or if a significant increase in blood pressure does not respond adequately to antihypertensive therapy, IMPLANON should be removed.

5.10 Gallbladder Disease

Studies suggest a small increased relative risk of developing gallbladder disease among combination hormonal contraceptive users. It is not known whether a similar risk exists with progestin-only methods like IMPLANON.

5.11 Carbohydrate and Lipid Metabolic Effects

Use of IMPLANON may induce mild insulin resistance and small changes in glucose concentrations of unknown clinical significance. Carefully monitor prediabetic and diabetic women using IMPLANON.

Women who are being treated for hyperlipidemia should be followed closely if they elect to use IMPLANON. Some progestins may elevate LDL levels and may render the control of hyperlipidemia more difficult.

5.12 Depressed Mood

Women with a history of depressed mood should be carefully observed. Consideration should be given to removing IMPLANON in patients who become significantly depressed.

5.13 Return to Ovulation

In clinical trials with IMPLANON, the etonogestrel levels in blood decreased below sensitivity of the assay by one week after removal of the implant. In addition, pregnancies were observed to occur as early as 7 to 14 days after removal. Therefore, a woman should re-start contraception immediately after removal of the implant if continued contraceptive protection is desired.

5.14 Fluid Retention

Hormonal contraceptives may cause some degree of fluid retention. They should be prescribed with caution, and only with careful monitoring, in patients with conditions which might be aggravated by fluid retention. It is unknown if IMPLANON causes fluid retention.

5.15 Contact Lenses

Contact lens wearers who develop visual changes or changes in lens tolerance should be assessed by an ophthalmologist.

5.16 Monitoring

A woman who is using IMPLANON should have a yearly visit with her healthcare provider for a blood pressure check and for other indicated health care.

5.17 Drug-Laboratory Test Interactions

Sex hormone-binding globulin concentrations may be decreased for the first 6 months after IMPLANON insertion followed by a gradual recovery. Thyroxine concentrations may initially be slightly decreased followed by gradual recovery to baseline.

6 ADVERSE REACTIONS

The following adverse reactions reported with the use of hormonal contraception are discussed elsewhere in the labeling:

- Changes in Menstrual Bleeding Patterns [see *Warnings and Precautions (5.2)*]
- Ectopic Pregnancies [see *Warnings and Precautions (5.3)*]
- Thrombotic and Other Vascular Events [see *Warnings and Precautions (5.4)*]
- Liver Disease [see *Warnings and Precautions (5.7)*]

6.1 Clinical Trials Experience

Because clinical trials are conducted under widely varying conditions, adverse reaction rates observed in the clinical trials of a drug cannot be directly compared to rates in the clinical trials of another drug and may not reflect the rates observed in practice.

In clinical trials including 942 women who were evaluated for safety, change in menstrual bleeding patterns (irregular menses) was the most common adverse reaction causing discontinuation of use of IMPLANON (11.1% of women). Adverse reactions that resulted in a rate of discontinuation of ≥1% are shown in Table 3.

Table 3: Adverse Reactions Leading to Discontinuation of Treatment in 1% or More of Subjects in Clinical Trials of IMPLANON

Adverse Reactions	All Studies N = 942
Bleeding Irregularities*	11.1%
Emotional Lability†	2.3%
Weight Increase	2.3%
Headache	1.6%
Acne	1.3%
Depression‡	1.0%

* Includes "frequent", "heavy", "prolonged", "spotting", and other patterns of bleeding irregularity.
† Among US subjects (N=330), 6.1% experienced emotional lability that led to discontinuation.
‡ Among US subjects (N=330), 2.4% experienced depression that led to discontinuation.

Other adverse reactions that were reported by at least 5% of subjects in clinical trials of IMPLANON are listed in Table 4.

Table 4: Common Adverse Reactions Reported by ≥5% of Subjects in Clinical Trials with IMPLANON

Adverse Reaction	All Studies N=942
Headache	24.9%
Vaginitis	14.5%
Weight increase	13.7%
Acne	13.5%
Breast pain	12.8%
Abdominal pain	10.9%
Pharyngitis	10.5%
Leukorrhea	9.6%
Influenza-like symptoms	7.6%
Dizziness	7.2%
Dysmenorrhea	7.2%
Back pain	6.8%
Emotional lability	6.5%
Nausea	6.4%
Pain	5.6%
Nervousness	5.6%
Depression	5.5%
Hypersensitivity	5.4%
Insertion site pain	5.2%

Implant site complications were reported by 3.6% of subjects during any of the assessments in clinical trials. Pain was the most frequent implant site complication, reported during and/or after insertion, occurring in 2.9% of subjects. Additionally, hematoma, redness, and swelling were reported by 0.1%, 0.3%, and 0.3% of patients, respectively [see *Warnings and Precautions (5.1)*].

6.2 Postmarketing Experience

The following additional adverse reactions have been identified during post-approval use of IMPLANON. Because these reactions are reported voluntarily from a population of uncertain size, it is not possible to reliably estimate their frequency or establish a causal relationship to drug exposure.

Gastrointestinal disorders: constipation, diarrhea, flatulence, vomiting.

General disorders and administration site conditions: edema, fatigue, implant site reaction, pyrexia.

Immune system disorders: anaphylactic reactions

Infections and infestations: rhinitis, urinary tract infection.

Investigations: clinically relevant rise in blood pressure, weight decreased.

Metabolism and nutrition disorders: increased appetite.

Musculoskeletal and connective tissue disorders: arthralgia, musculoskeletal pain, myalgia.

Nervous system disorders: convulsions, migraine, somnolence.

Pregnancy, puerperium and perinatal conditions: ectopic pregnancy.

Psychiatric disorders: anxiety, insomnia, libido decreased.

Renal and urinary disorders: dysuria.

Reproductive system and breast disorders: breast discharge, breast enlargement, ovarian cyst, pruritus genital, vulvovaginal discomfort.

Skin and subcutaneous tissue disorders: angioedema, aggravation of angioedema and/or aggravation of hereditary angioedema, alopecia, chloasma, hypertrichosis, pruritus, rash, seborrhea, urticaria.

Vascular disorders: hot flush.

Complications related to insertion or removal of the implant reported include: bruising, slight local irritation, pain or itching, fibrosis at the implant site, paresthesia or paresthesia-like events, scarring and abscess.

7 DRUG INTERACTIONS

7.1 Changes in Contraceptive Effectiveness Associated with Coadministration of Other Products

Drugs or herbal products that induce enzymes, including CYP3A4, that metabolize progestins may decrease the plasma concentrations of progestins, and may decrease the effectiveness of IMPLANON. In women on long-term treatment with hepatic enzyme inducing drugs, it is recommended to remove the implant and to advise a contraceptive method that is unaffected by the interacting drug.

Some of these drugs or herbal products that induce enzymes, including CYP3A4, include:

- barbiturates
- bosentan
- carbamazepine
- felbamate
- griseofulvin
- oxcarbazepine
- phenytoin
- rifampin
- St. John's wort
- Topiramate

HIV Antiretrovirals

Significant changes (increase or decrease) in the plasma levels of progestin have been noted in some cases of coadministration with HIV protease inhibitors or with nonnucleoside reverse transcriptase inhibitors. Consult the labeling of all concurrently-used drugs to obtain further information about interactions with hormonal contraceptives or the potential for enzyme alterations.

7.2 Increase in Plasma Concentrations of Etonogestrel Associated with Coadministered Drugs

CYP3A4 inhibitors such as itraconazole or ketoconazole may increase plasma concentrations of etonogestrel.

7.3 Changes in Plasma Concentrations of Coadministered Drugs

Hormonal contraceptives may affect the metabolism of other drugs. Consequently, plasma concentrations may either increase (for example, cyclosporin) or decrease (for example, lamotrigine). Consult the labeling of all concurrently-used drugs to obtain further information about interactions with hormonal contraceptives or the potential for enzyme alterations.

8 USE IN SPECIFIC POPULATIONS

8.1 Pregnancy

IMPLANON is not indicated for use during pregnancy [see *Contraindications (4)*].

Teratology studies have been performed in rats and rabbits using oral administration up to 390 and 790 times the human IMPLANON dose (based upon body surface) and revealed no evidence of fetal harm due to etonogestrel exposure.

Studies have revealed no increased risk of birth defects in women who have used combination oral contraceptives before pregnancy or during early pregnancy. There is no evidence that the risk associated with IMPLANON is different from that of combination oral contraceptives.

IMPLANON should be removed if maintaining a pregnancy.

8.3 Nursing Mothers

Based on limited clinical data, IMPLANON may be used during breastfeeding after the fourth postpartum week. Use of IMPLANON before the fourth postpartum week has not been studied. Small amounts of etonogestrel are excreted in breast milk. During the first months after insertion of IMPLANON, when maternal blood levels of etonogestrel are highest, about 100 ng of etonogestrel may be ingested by the child per day based on an average daily milk ingestion of 658 mL. Based on daily milk ingestion of 150 mL/kg, the mean daily infant etonogestrel dose one month after insertion of IMPLANON is about 2.2% of the weight-adjusted maternal daily dose, or about 0.2% of the estimated absolute maternal daily dose. The health of breast-fed infants whose mothers began using IMPLANON during the fourth to eighth week postpartum (n=38) was evaluated in a comparative study with infants of mothers using a non-hormonal IUD (n=33). They were breast-fed for a mean duration of 14 months and followed up to 36 months of age. No significant effects and no differences between the groups were observed on the physical and psychomotor development of these infants. No differences between groups in the production or quality of breast milk were detected.

Healthcare providers should discuss both hormonal and non-hormonal contraceptive options, as steroids may not be the initial choice for these patients.

8.4 Pediatric Use

Safety and efficacy of IMPLANON have been established in women of reproductive age. Safety and efficacy of IMPLANON are expected to be the same for postpubertal adolescents. However, no clinical studies have been conducted in women less than 18 years of age. Use of this product before menarche is not indicated.

8.5 Geriatric Use

This product has not been studied in women over 65 years of age and is not indicated in this population.

8.6 Hepatic Impairment

No studies were conducted to evaluate the effect of hepatic disease on the disposition of IMPLANON. The use of IMPLANON in women with active liver disease is contraindicated [see *Contraindications (4)*].

8.7 Renal Impairment

No studies were conducted to evaluate the effect of renal disease on the disposition of IMPLANON.

8.8 Overweight Women

The effectiveness of IMPLANON in women who weighed more than 130% of their ideal body weight has not been defined because such women were not studied in clinical trials. Serum concentrations of etonogestrel are inversely related to body weight and decrease with time after implant insertion. It is therefore possible that IMPLANON may be less effective in overweight women, especially in the presence of other factors that decrease serum etonogestrel concentrations such as concomitant use of hepatic enzyme inducers.

10 OVERDOSAGE

Overdosage may result if more than 1 implant is inserted. In case of suspected overdose, the implant should be removed.

11 DESCRIPTION

IMPLANON (etonogestrel implant) is a progestin-only, soft, flexible implant preloaded in a sterile, disposable applicator for subdermal use. The implant is off-white, non-biodegradable and 4 cm in length with a diameter of 2 mm (see Figure 22). Each implant consists of an ethylene vinylacetate (EVA) copolymer core, containing 68 mg of the synthetic progestin etonogestrel, surrounded by an EVA copolymer skin. Once inserted subdermally, the release rate is 60 to 70 mcg/day in Week 5 to 6 and decreases to approximately 35 to 45 mcg/day at the end of the first year, to approximately 30 to 40 mcg/day at the end of the second year, and then to approximately 25 to 30 mcg/day at the end of the third year. IMPLANON is a progestin-only contraceptive and does not contain estrogen. IMPLANON does not contain latex and is not radio-opaque.

2 mm

4 cm

Figure 22 (Not to scale)

Etonogestrel [13-Ethyl-17-hydroxy-11-methylene-18,19-dinor-17α-pregn-4-en-20-yn-3-one], structurally derived from 19-nortestosterone, is the synthetic biologically active metabolite of the synthetic progestin desogestrel. It has a molecular weight of 324.46 and the following structural formula (Figure 23).

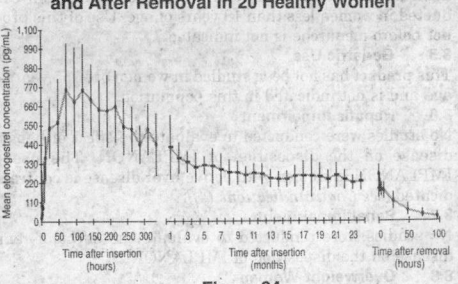

$C_{22}H_{28}O_2$

Figure 23

12 CLINICAL PHARMACOLOGY

12.1 Mechanism of Action
The contraceptive effect of IMPLANON is achieved by suppression of ovulation, increased viscosity of the cervical mucus, and alterations in the endometrium.

12.2 Pharmacodynamics
Exposure-response relationships of IMPLANON are unknown.

12.3 Pharmacokinetics
Absorption
After subdermal insertion of the etonogestrel implant, etonogestrel is released into the circulation and is approximately 100% bioavailable.

The mean peak serum concentrations in 3 pharmacokinetic studies ranged between 781 and 894 pg/mL and were reached within the first few weeks after insertion. The mean serum etonogestrel concentration decreases gradually over time declining to 192 to 261 pg/mL at 12 months (n=41), 154 to 194 pg/mL at 24 months (n=35), and 156 to 177 pg/mL at 36 months (n=17).

The pharmacokinetic profile of IMPLANON from 1 of 3 pharmacokinetic studies is shown in Figure 24.

Figure 24 Mean Serum Concentration-time Profile of Etonogestrel During 2 Years of IMPLANON Use and After Removal in 20 Healthy Women

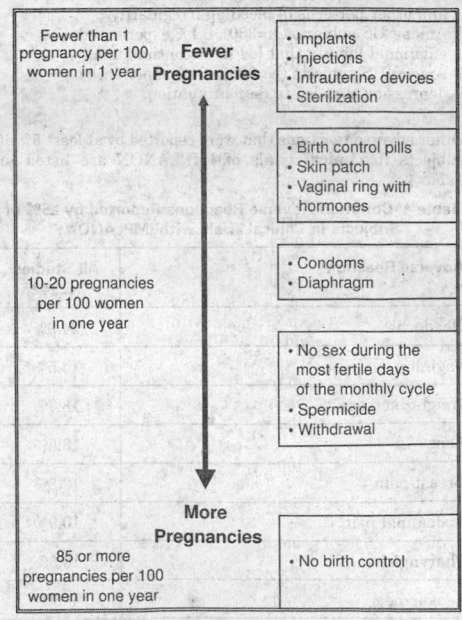

Time after insertion (hours)

Time after insertion (months)

Time after removal (hours)

Figure 24

Distribution
The apparent volume of distribution averages about 201 L. Etonogestrel is approximately 32% bound to sex hormone binding globulin (SHBG) and 66% bound to albumin in blood.

Metabolism
In vitro data shows that etonogestrel is metabolized in liver microsomes by the cytochrome P450 3A4 isoenzyme. The biological activity of etonogestrel metabolites is unknown.

Excretion
The elimination half-life of etonogestrel is approximately 25 hours. Excretion of etonogestrel and its metabolites, either as free steroid or as conjugates, is mainly in urine and to a lesser extent in feces. After removal of the implant, etonogestrel concentrations decreased below sensitivity of the assay by 1 week.

13 NONCLINICAL TOXICOLOGY

13.1 Carcinogenesis, Mutagenesis, Impairment of Fertility
In a 24-month carcinogenicity study in rats with subdermal implants releasing 10 and 20 mcg etonogestrel per day (equal to approximately 1.8-3.6 times the systemic steady state exposure in women using IMPLANON), no drug-related carcinogenic potential was observed. Etonogestrel was not genotoxic in the *in vitro* Ames/Salmonella reverse mutation assay, the chromosomal aberration assay in Chinese hamster ovary cells or in the *in vivo* mouse micronucleus test. Fertility returned after withdrawal from treatment.

14 CLINICAL STUDIES

14.1 Pregnancy
In clinical trials of up to 3 years duration that involved 923 subjects, 18 - 40 years of age at entry, and 1,756 women-years of IMPLANON use, the total exposures expressed as 28-day cycle equivalents by study year were:

Year 1: 10,866 cycles
Year 2: 8,581 cycles
Year 3: 3,442 cycles

The clinical trials excluded women who:
• Weighed more than 130% of their ideal body weight
• Were chronically taking medications that induce liver enzymes

In the subgroup of women 18 to 35 years of age at entry, 6 pregnancies during 20,648 cycles of use were reported. Two pregnancies occurred in each of Years 1, 2 and 3. Each conception was likely to have occurred shortly before or within 2 weeks after IMPLANON removal. With these 6 pregnancies, the cumulative Pearl Index was 0.38 pregnancies per 100 women-years of use.

14.2 Return to Ovulation
In clinical trials with IMPLANON, the etonogestrel levels in blood decreased below sensitivity of the assay by one week after removal of the implant. In addition, pregnancies were observed to occur as early as 7 to 14 days after removal. Therefore, a woman should re-start contraception immediately after removal of the implant if continued contraceptive protection is desired.

16 HOW SUPPLIED/STORAGE AND HANDLING

16.1 How Supplied
One IMPLANON package consists of a single implant containing 68 mg etonogestrel that is 4 cm in length and 2 mm in diameter, which is pre-loaded in the needle of a disposable applicator. The sterile applicator containing the implant is packed in a blister pack.
NDC 0052-0272-01

16.2 Storage and Handling
Store IMPLANON (etonogestrel implant) at 25°C (77°F); excursions permitted to 15°-30°C (59°-86°F) [see USP Controlled Room Temperature]. Protect from light. Avoid storing IMPLANON in direct sunlight or at temperatures above 30°C (86°F).

17 PATIENT COUNSELING INFORMATION

"See FDA-Approved Patient Labeling (Patient Information)"

• Counsel women about the insertion and removal procedure of the IMPLANON implant. Provide the woman with a copy of the Patient Labeling and ensure that she understands the information in the Patient Labeling before insertion and removal. A USER CARD and consent form are included in the packaging. Have the woman complete a consent form and retain it in your records. The USER CARD should be filled out and given to the patient after insertion of the IMPLANON implant so that she will have a record of the location of the implant in the upper arm and when it should be removed.
• Counsel women that IMPLANON does not protect against HIV infection (AIDS) or other sexually transmitted diseases.
• Counsel women that the use of IMPLANON may be associated with changes in their normal menstrual bleeding patterns so that they know what to expect.

FDA-Approved Patient Labeling
See the full patient product information for IMPLANON.
Manufactured for: Merck Sharp & Dohme Corp., a subsidiary of **MERCK & CO., INC.**, Whitehouse Station, NJ 08889, USA
Manufactured by: N.V. Organon, Oss, The Netherlands, a subsidiary of **Merck & Co., Inc.**, Whitehouse Station, NJ 08889, USA
For patent information:
www.merck.com/product/patent/home.html
Copyright © 2006, 2009, 2012 Merck Sharp & Dohme B.V., a subsidiary of **Merck & Co., Inc.**
All rights reserved.
Revised: 07/2014
uspi-mk8415-ipt-1407r009

FDA-Approved Patient Labeling
IMPLANON® (etonogestrel implant)
Subdermal Use

IMPLANON® does not protect against HIV infection (the virus that causes AIDS) or other sexually transmitted diseases. Read this Patient Information leaflet carefully before you decide if IMPLANON is right for you. This information does not take the place of talking with your healthcare provider. If you have any questions about IMPLANON, ask your healthcare provider.

What is IMPLANON?
IMPLANON is a hormone-releasing birth control implant for use by women to prevent pregnancy for up to 3 years. The implant is a flexible plastic rod about the size of a matchstick that contains a progestin hormone called

etonogestrel. Your healthcare provider will insert the implant just under the skin of the inner side of your upper arm. You can use a single IMPLANON implant for up to 3 years. IMPLANON does not contain estrogen.

What if I need birth control for more than 3 years?
The IMPLANON implant must be removed after 3 years. Your healthcare provider can insert a new implant under your skin after taking out the old one if you choose to continue using IMPLANON for birth control.

What if I change my mind about birth control and want to stop using IMPLANON before 3 years?
Your healthcare provider can remove the implant at any time. You may become pregnant as early as the first week after removal of the implant. If you do not want to get pregnant after your healthcare provider removes the IMPLANON implant, you should start another birth control method right away.

How does IMPLANON work?
IMPLANON prevents pregnancy in several ways. The most important way is by stopping the release of an egg from your ovary. IMPLANON also thickens the mucus in your cervix and this change may keep sperm from reaching the egg. IMPLANON also changes the lining of your uterus.

How well does IMPLANON work?
When the IMPLANON implant is placed correctly, your chance of getting pregnant is very low (less than 1 pregnancy per 100 women who use IMPLANON for 1 year). It is not known if IMPLANON is as effective in very overweight women because studies did not include many overweight women.

The following chart shows the chance of getting pregnant for women who use different methods of birth control. Each box on the chart contains a list of birth control methods that are similar in effectiveness. The most effective methods are at the top of the chart. The box on the bottom of the chart shows the chance of getting pregnant for women who do not use birth control and are trying to get pregnant.

Fewer than 1 pregnancy per 100 women in 1 year **Fewer Pregnancies**	• Implants • Injections • Intrauterine devices • Sterilization
	• Birth control pills • Skin patch • Vaginal ring with hormones
10-20 pregnancies per 100 women in one year	• Condoms • Diaphragm
	• No sex during the most fertile days of the monthly cycle • Spermicide • Withdrawal
More Pregnancies 85 or more pregnancies per 100 women in one year	• No birth control

Who should not use IMPLANON?
Do not use IMPLANON if you
• Are pregnant or think you may be pregnant
• Have, or have had serious blood clots, such as blood clots in your legs (deep venous thrombosis), lungs (pulmonary embolism), eyes (total or partial blindness), heart (heart attack), or brain (stroke)
• Have liver disease or a liver tumor
• Have unexplained vaginal bleeding
• Have breast cancer or any other cancer that is sensitive to progestin (a female hormone), now or in the past
• Are allergic to anything in IMPLANON
Tell your healthcare provider if you have or have had any of the conditions listed above. Your healthcare provider can suggest a different method of birth control.

In addition, talk to your healthcare provider about using IMPLANON if you:
- Have diabetes
- Have high cholesterol or triglycerides
- Have headaches
- Have gallbladder or kidney problems
- Have a history of depressed mood
- Have high blood pressure
- Have an allergy to numbing medicines (anesthetics) or medicines used to clean your skin (antiseptics). These medicines will be used when the implant is placed into or removed from your arm.

Interaction with Other Medicines

Tell your healthcare provider about all the medicines you take, including prescription and non-prescription medicines, vitamins and herbal supplements. Certain medicines may make IMPLANON less effective, including:
- barbiturates
- bosentan
- carbamazepine
- felbamate
- griseofulvin
- oxcarbazepine
- phenytoin
- rifampin
- St. John's wort
- topiramate
- HIV medicines

Ask your healthcare provider if you are not sure if your medicine is one listed above.

If there are medicines that you have been taking for a long time, that make IMPLANON less effective, tell your healthcare provider. Your healthcare provider may remove the IMPLANON implant and recommend a birth control method that can be used effectively with these medicines. When you are using IMPLANON, tell all of your healthcare providers that you have IMPLANON in place in your arm.

How is the IMPLANON implant placed and removed?

Your healthcare provider will place and remove the IMPLANON implant in a minor surgical procedure in his or her office. The implant is placed just under the skin on the inner side of your upper arm.

The timing of insertion is important. Your healthcare provider may:
- Perform a pregnancy test before inserting IMPLANON
- Schedule the insertion at a specific time of your menstrual cycle (for example, within the first days of your regular menstrual bleeding)

Immediately after the IMPLANON implant has been placed, you and your healthcare provider should check that the implant is in your arm by feeling for it.

If you and your healthcare provider cannot feel the IMPLANON implant, use a non-hormonal birth control method (such as condoms) until your healthcare provider confirms that the implant is in place. You may need special tests to check that the implant is in place or to help find the implant when it is time to take it out.

Your healthcare provider will cover the site where IMPLANON was placed with 2 bandages. Leave the top bandage on for 24 hours. Keep the smaller bandage clean, dry, and in place for 3 to 5 days.

You will be asked to review and sign a consent form prior to inserting the IMPLANON implant. You will also get a USER CARD to keep at home with your health records. Your healthcare provider will fill out the USER CARD with the date the implant was inserted and the date the implant is to be removed. Keep track of the date the implant is to be removed. Schedule an appointment with your healthcare provider to remove the implant on or before the removal date.

Be sure to have checkups as advised by your healthcare provider.

What are the most common side effects I can expect while using IMPLANON?

- **Changes in Menstrual Bleeding Patterns (menstrual periods)**

  The most common side effect of IMPLANON is a change in your normal menstrual bleeding pattern. In studies, about one out of ten women stopped using the implant because of an unfavorable change in their bleeding pattern. You may experience longer or shorter bleeding during your periods or have no bleeding at all. The time between periods may vary, and in between periods you may also have spotting. Talk with your healthcare provider right away if:
- You think you may be pregnant
- Your menstrual bleeding is heavy and prolonged

Besides changes in menstrual bleeding patterns, other frequent side effects that caused women to stop using the implant include:
- Mood swings
- Weight gain
- Headache
- Acne
- Depressed mood

Other common side effects include:
- Headache
- Vaginitis (inflammation of the vagina)
- Weight gain
- Acne
- Breast pain
- Viral infections such as sore throats or flu-like symptoms
- Stomach pain
- Painful periods
- Mood swings, nervousness, or depressed mood
- Back pain
- Nausea
- Dizziness
- Pain
- Pain at the site of insertion

This is not a complete list of possible side effects. For more information, ask your healthcare provider for advice about any side effects that concern you. You may report side effects to the FDA at 1-800-FDA-1088.

What are the possible risks of using IMPLANON?

- **Problems with Insertion and Removal**

  The implant may not be placed in your arm at all due to a failed insertion or if the implant has fallen out of the needle. If this happens, you may become pregnant. Immediately after insertion, and with help from your healthcare provider, you should be able to feel the implant under your skin. If you can't feel the implant, tell your healthcare provider.

  Removal of the implant may be very difficult or impossible because the implant is not where it should be. Special procedures, including surgery in the hospital, may be needed to remove the implant. If the implant is not removed, then the effects of IMPLANON will continue for a longer period of time.

  Other problems related to insertion and removal are:
  - Pain, irritation, swelling, or bruising at the insertion site
  - Scarring, including a thick scar called a keloid around the insertion site
  - Infection
  - Scar tissue may form around the implant making it difficult to remove
  - The implant may come out by itself. You may become pregnant if the implant comes out by itself. Use a back up birth control method and call your healthcare provider right away if the implant comes out.
  - The need for surgery in the hospital to remove the implant
  - Injury to nerves or blood vessels in your arm
  - The implant breaks making removal difficult

- **Ectopic Pregnancy**

  If you become pregnant while using IMPLANON, you have a slightly higher chance that the pregnancy will be ectopic (occurring outside the womb) than do women who do not use birth control. Unusual vaginal bleeding or lower stomach (abdominal) pain may be a sign of ectopic pregnancy. Ectopic pregnancy is a medical emergency that often requires surgery. Ectopic pregnancies can cause serious internal bleeding, infertility, and even death. Call your healthcare provider right away if you think you are pregnant or have unexplained lower stomach (abdominal) pain.

- **Ovarian Cysts**

  Cysts may develop on the ovaries and usually go away without treatment but sometimes surgery is needed to remove them.

- **Breast Cancer**

  It is not known whether IMPLANON use changes a woman's risk for breast cancer. If you have breast cancer now, or have had it in the past, do not use IMPLANON because some breast cancers are sensitive to hormones.

- **Serious Blood Clots**

  IMPLANON may increase your chance of serious blood clots, especially if you have other risk factors such as smoking. It is possible to die from a problem caused by a blood clot, such as a heart attack or a stroke.

  Some examples of serious blood clots are blood clots in the:
  - Legs (deep vein thrombosis)
  - Lung (pulmonary embolism)
  - Brain (stroke)
  - Heart (heart attack)
  - Eyes (total or partial blindness)

  The risk of serious blood clots is increased in women who smoke. If you smoke and want to use IMPLANON, you should quit. Your healthcare provider may be able to help. Tell your healthcare provider at least 4 weeks before if you are going to have surgery or will need to be on bed rest. You have an increased chance of getting blood clots during surgery or bed rest.

- **Other Risks**

  A few women who use birth control that contains hormones may get:
  - High blood pressure
  - Gallbladder problems
  - Rare cancerous or noncancerous liver tumors

When should I call my healthcare provider?

Call your healthcare provider right away if you have:
- Pain in your lower leg that does not go away
- Severe chest pain or heaviness in the chest
- Sudden shortness of breath, sharp chest pain, or coughing blood
- Symptoms of a severe allergic reaction, such as swollen face, tongue or throat; trouble breathing or swallowing
- Sudden severe headache unlike your usual headaches
- Weakness or numbness in your arm, leg, or trouble speaking
- Sudden partial or complete blindness
- Yellowing of your skin or whites of your eyes, especially with fever, tiredness, loss of appetite, dark colored urine, or light colored bowel movements
- Severe pain, swelling, or tenderness in the lower stomach (abdomen)
- Lump in your breast
- Problems sleeping, lack of energy, tiredness, or you feel very sad
- Heavy menstrual bleeding

What if I become pregnant while using IMPLANON?

You should see your healthcare provider right away if you think that you may be pregnant. It is important to remove the implant and make sure that the pregnancy is not ectopic (occurring outside the womb). Based on experience with other hormonal contraceptives, IMPLANON is not likely to cause birth defects.

Can I use IMPLANON when I am breastfeeding?

If you are breastfeeding your child, you may use IMPLANON if 4 weeks have passed since you had your baby. A small amount of the hormone contained in IMPLANON passes into your breast milk. The health of breast-fed children whose mothers were using the implant has been studied up to 3 years of age in a small number of children. No effects on the growth and development of the children were seen. If you are breastfeeding and want to use IMPLANON, talk with your healthcare provider for more information.

Additional Information

This Patient Information leaflet contains important information about IMPLANON. If you would like more information, talk with your healthcare provider. You can ask your healthcare provider for information about IMPLANON that is written for healthcare professionals. You may also call 1-877-IMPLANON (1-877-467-5266) or visit www.IMPLANON-USA.com

Manufactured for: Merck Sharp & Dohme Corp., a subsidiary of **MERCK & CO., INC.**, Whitehouse Station, NJ 08889, USA

Manufactured by: N.V. Organon, Oss, The Netherlands, a subsidiary of **Merck & Co., Inc.**, Whitehouse Station, NJ 08889, USA

For patent information:
www.merck.com/product/patent/home.html

Copyright © 2012 Merck Sharp & Dohme B.V., a subsidiary of Merck & Co., Inc.
All rights reserved.

Revised: 07/2014
usppi-mk8415-ipt-1407r009

IMPLANON®
(etonogestrel implant)
68 mg For Subdermal Use Only
PATIENT CONSENT FORM

I understand the Patient Labeling for IMPLANON®. I have discussed IMPLANON with my healthcare provider who answered all my questions. I understand that there are benefits as well as risks from using IMPLANON. I understand that there are other birth control methods and that each has its own benefits and risks.

I also understand that this Patient Consent Form is important. I understand that I need to sign this form to show that I am making an informed and careful decision to use IMPLANON, and that I have read and understand the following points.
- IMPLANON helps to keep me from getting pregnant.
- No contraceptive method is 100% effective, including IMPLANON.
- IMPLANON is made of a hormone mixed in a plastic rod.
- It is important to have IMPLANON inserted at the right time of my menstrual cycle.
- **After IMPLANON is inserted, I should check that it is in place by gently pressing my fingertips over the skin in my arm where IMPLANON was inserted. I should be able to feel the small rod.**
- IMPLANON must be removed at the end of 3 years. IMPLANON can be removed sooner if I want.
- If I have trouble finding a healthcare provider to remove IMPLANON, I can call (877) 467-5266 for help.
- IMPLANON is placed under the skin of my arm during a procedure done in my healthcare provider's office. There is a slight risk of getting a scar or an infection from this procedure.

- Removal is usually a small office procedure. However, removal may be difficult. Rarely, IMPLANON cannot be found when it is time to remove it. Special procedures, including surgery in the hospital, may be needed. Difficult removals may cause pain and scarring and may result in damage to nerves and blood vessels. If IMPLANON cannot be found, its effects may continue.
- **Most women have changes in their menstrual bleeding while using IMPLANON. I also will likely have changes in my menstrual bleeding while using IMPLANON. My bleeding may be irregular, lighter or heavier, or my bleeding may completely stop. If I think I am pregnant, I should see my healthcare provider as soon as possible.**
- I understand the warning signs for problems with IMPLANON. I should seek medical attention if any warning signs appear.
- I should tell all my healthcare providers that I am using IMPLANON.
- I need to have a medical checkup regularly and at any time I am having problems.
- IMPLANON does not protect me from HIV infection (AIDS) or any other sexually transmitted disease.

After learning about IMPLANON, I choose to use IMPLANON.

_____
(Name of Healthcare Provider)

_____   _____
(Patient Signature)   (Date)

WITNESSED BY:
The patient above has signed this consent in my presence after I counseled her and answered her questions.

_____   _____
(Healthcare Provider Signature)   (Date)

I have provided an accurate translation of this information to the patient whose signature appears above. She has stated that she understands the information and has had an opportunity to have her questions answered.

_____   _____
(Signature of Translator)   (Date)

Manufactured for: Merck Sharp & Dohme Corp., a subsidiary of **MERCK & CO., INC.,** Whitehouse Station, NJ 08889, USA
Manufactured by: N.V. Organon, Oss, The Netherlands, a subsidiary of **Merck & Co., Inc.,** Whitehouse Station, NJ 08889, USA
For patent information:
www.merck.com/product/patent/home.html
Copyright © 2006, 2009 Merck Sharp & Dohme B.V., a subsidiary of **Merck & Co., Inc.**
All rights reserved.
Revised: 03/2014
pcf-mk8415-ipt-1403r003
Shown in Product Identification Guide, page 308

INTEGRILIN®   ℞
[ĭn-tĕg-rĭl-in]
(eptifibatide)
injection, for intravenous use

HIGHLIGHTS OF PRESCRIBING INFORMATION
These highlights do not include all the information needed to use INTEGRILIN safely and effectively. See full prescribing information for INTEGRILIN.
INTEGRILIN® (eptifibatide) injection, for intravenous use
Initial U.S. Approval: 1998

————INDICATIONS AND USAGE————
INTEGRILIN is a platelet aggregation inhibitor indicated for:
- Treatment of acute coronary syndrome (ACS) managed medically or with percutaneous coronary intervention (PCI) (1.1)
- Treatment of patients undergoing PCI (including intracoronary stenting) (1.2)

————DOSAGE AND ADMINISTRATION————
ACS or PCI: 180 mcg/kg IV bolus as soon as possible after diagnosis followed by infusion at 2 mcg/kg/min. (2.1, 2.2)
PCI: Add a second 180 mcg/kg bolus at 10 minutes. (2.2)
In patients with creatinine clearance less than 50 mL/min, reduce the infusion to 1 mcg/kg/min. (2.1, 2.2, 2.3)

————DOSAGE FORMS AND STRENGTHS————
- 20 mg/10 mL (2 mg/mL) in a single-use vial for bolus injection (3)

- 75 mg/100 mL (0.75 mg/mL) in a single-use vial for infusion (3)
- 200 mg/100 mL (2 mg/mL) in a single-use vial for infusion (3)

————CONTRAINDICATIONS————
- Bleeding diathesis or bleeding within the previous 30 days (4)
- Severe uncontrolled hypertension (4)
- Major surgery within the preceding 6 weeks (4)
- Stroke within 30 days or any history of hemorrhagic stroke (4)
- Coadministration of another parenteral GP IIb/IIIa inhibitor (4)
- Dependency on renal dialysis (4)
- Known hypersensitivity to any component of the product (4)

————WARNINGS AND PRECAUTIONS————
- INTEGRILIN can cause serious bleeding. If bleeding cannot be controlled, discontinue INTEGRILIN immediately. Minimize vascular and other traumas. If heparin is given concomitantly, monitor aPTT or ACT. (5.1)
- Thrombocytopenia: Discontinue INTEGRILIN and heparin. Monitor and treat condition appropriately. (5.2)

————ADVERSE REACTIONS————
Bleeding and hypotension are the most commonly reported adverse reactions. (6.1)
To report SUSPECTED ADVERSE REACTIONS, contact Merck Sharp & Dohme Corp., a subsidiary of Merck & Co., Inc., at 1-877-888-4231 or FDA at 1-800-FDA-1088 or www.fda.gov/medwatch.

————DRUG INTERACTIONS————
- Coadministration of antiplatelet agents, thrombolytics, heparin, aspirin, and chronic NSAID use increases the risk of bleeding. Avoid concomitant use with other glycoprotein (GP) IIb/IIIa inhibitors. (7.1)

————USE IN SPECIFIC POPULATIONS————
- _Geriatric Use:_   Risk of bleeding increases with age. (8.5)
See 17 for PATIENT COUNSELING INFORMATION
Revised: 04/2014

FULL PRESCRIBING INFORMATION: CONTENTS*

FULL PRESCRIBING INFORMATION

1   INDICATIONS AND USAGE
1.1   Acute Coronary Syndrome (ACS)
INTEGRILIN® is indicated to decrease the rate of a combined endpoint of death or new myocardial infarction (MI)

in patients with ACS (unstable angina [UA]/non-ST-elevation myocardial infarction [NSTEMI]), including patients who are to be managed medically and those undergoing percutaneous coronary intervention (PCI).
1.2   Percutaneous Coronary Intervention (PCI)
INTEGRILIN is indicated to decrease the rate of a combined endpoint of death, new MI, or need for urgent intervention in patients undergoing PCI, including those undergoing intracoronary stenting [see Clinical Studies (14.1, 14.2)].

2   DOSAGE AND ADMINISTRATION
Before infusion of INTEGRILIN, the following laboratory tests should be performed to identify pre-existing hemostatic abnormalities: hematocrit or hemoglobin, platelet count, serum creatinine, and PT/aPTT. In patients undergoing PCI, the activated clotting time (ACT) should also be measured.
The activated partial thromboplastin time (aPTT) should be maintained between 50 and 70 seconds unless PCI is to be performed. In patients treated with heparin, bleeding can be minimized by close monitoring of the aPTT and ACT.
2.1   Dosage in Acute Coronary Syndrome (ACS)

Indication	Normal Renal Function	Creatinine Clearance less than 50 mL/min
Patients with ACS	180 mcg/kg intravenous (IV) bolus as soon as possible after diagnosis, followed by continuous infusion of 2 mcg/kg/min	180 mcg/kg IV bolus as soon as possible after diagnosis, followed by continuous infusion of 1 mcg/kg/min

- Infusion should continue until hospital discharge or initiation of coronary artery bypass graft surgery (CABG), up to 72 hours
- If a patient is to undergo PCI, the infusion should be continued until hospital discharge or for up to 18 to 24 hours after the procedure, whichever comes first, allowing for up to 96 hours of therapy
- Aspirin, 160 to 325 mg, should be given daily

INTEGRILIN should be given concomitantly with heparin dosed to achieve the following parameters:
   During Medical Management: Target aPTT 50 to 70 seconds
- If weight greater than or equal to 70 kg, 5000-unit bolus followed by infusion of 1000 units/h.
- If weight less than 70 kg, 60-units/kg bolus followed by infusion of 12 units/kg/h.
   During PCI: Target ACT 200 to 300 seconds
- If heparin is initiated prior to PCI, additional boluses during PCI to maintain an ACT target of 200 to 300 seconds.
- Heparin infusion after the PCI is discouraged.

2.2   Dosage in Percutaneous Coronary Intervention (PCI)

Indication	Normal Renal Function	Creatinine Clearance less than 50 mL/min
Patients with PCI	180 mcg/kg IV bolus immediately before PCI followed by continuous infusion of 2 mcg/kg/min and a second bolus of 180 mcg/kg (given 10 minutes after the first bolus)	180 mcg/kg IV bolus immediately before PCI followed by continuous infusion of 1 mcg/kg/min and a second bolus of 180 mcg/kg (given 10 minutes after the first bolus)

- Infusion should be continued until hospital discharge, or for up to 18 to 24 hours, whichever comes first. A minimum of 12 hours of infusion is recommended.
- In patients who undergo CABG surgery, INTEGRILIN infusion should be discontinued prior to surgery.
- Aspirin, 160 to 325 mg, should be given 1 to 24 hours prior to PCI and daily thereafter

- INTEGRILIN should be given concomitantly with heparin to achieve a target ACT of 200 to 300 seconds. Administer 60-units/kg bolus initially in patients not treated with heparin within 6 hours prior to PCI.
- Additional boluses during PCI to maintain ACT within target.
- Heparin infusion after the PCI is strongly discouraged.

Table 1: INTEGRILIN Dosing Charts by Weight

Patient Weight		180-mcg/kg Bolus Volume	2-mcg/kg/min Infusion Volume (CrCl greater than or equal to 50 mL/min)		1-mcg/kg/min Infusion Volume (CrCl less than 50 mL/min)	
(kg)	(lb)	(from 2-mg/mL vial)	(from 2-mg/mL 100-mL vial)	(from 0.75-mg/mL 100-mL vial)	(from 2-mg/mL 100-mL vial)	(from 0.75-mg/mL 100-mL vial)
37-41	81-91	3.4 mL	2 mL/h	6 mL/h	1 mL/h	3 mL/h
42-46	92-102	4 mL	2.5 mL/h	7 mL/h	1.3 mL/h	3.5 mL/h
47-53	103-117	4.5 mL	3 mL/h	8 mL/h	1.5 mL/h	4 mL/h
54-59	118-130	5 mL	3.5 mL/h	9 mL/h	1.8 mL/h	4.5 mL/h
60-65	131-143	5.6 mL	3.8 mL/h	10 mL/h	1.9 mL/h	5 mL/h
66-71	144-157	6.2 mL	4 mL/h	11 mL/h	2 mL/h	5.5 mL/h
72-78	158-172	6.8 mL	4.5 mL/h	12 mL/h	2.3 mL/h	6 mL/h
79-84	173-185	7.3 mL	5 mL/h	13 mL/h	2.5 mL/h	6.5 mL/h
85-90	186-198	7.9 mL	5.3 mL/h	14 mL/h	2.7 mL/h	7 mL/h
91-96	199-212	8.5 mL	5.6 mL/h	15 mL/h	2.8 mL/h	7.5 mL/h
97-103	213-227	9 mL	6 mL/h	16 mL/h	3.0 mL/h	8 mL/h
104-109	228-240	9.5 mL	6.4 mL/h	17 mL/h	3.2 mL/h	8.5 mL/h
110-115	241-253	10.2 mL	6.8 mL/h	18 mL/h	3.4 mL/h	9 mL/h
116-121	254-267	10.7 mL	7 mL/h	19 mL/h	3.5 mL/h	9.5 mL/h
>121	>267	11.3 mL	7.5 mL/h	20 mL/h	3.7 mL/h	10 mL/h

Patients requiring thrombolytic therapy should discontinue INTEGRILIN.

2.3 Important Administration Instructions

1. Inspect INTEGRILIN for particulate matter and discoloration prior to administration, whenever solution and container permit.
2. May administer INTEGRILIN in the same intravenous line as alteplase, atropine, dobutamine, heparin, lidocaine, meperidine, metoprolol, midazolam, morphine, nitroglycerin, or verapamil. Do not administer INTEGRILIN through the same intravenous line as furosemide.
3. May administer INTEGRILIN in the same IV line with 0.9% NaCl or 0.9% NaCl/5% dextrose. With either vehicle, the infusion may also contain up to 60 mEq/L of potassium chloride.
4. Withdraw the bolus dose(s) of INTEGRILIN from the 10-mL vial into a syringe. Administer the bolus dose(s) by IV push.
5. Immediately following the bolus dose administration, initiate a continuous infusion of INTEGRILIN. When using an intravenous infusion pump, administer INTEGRILIN undiluted directly from the 100-mL vial. Spike the 100-mL vial with a vented infusion set. Center the spike within the circle on the stopper top.
6. Discard any unused portion left in the vial.

Administer INTEGRILIN by volume according to patient weight (see Table 1).
[See table 1 above]

3 DOSAGE FORMS AND STRENGTHS

- Injection: 20 mg of INTEGRILIN in 10 mL (2 mg/mL), for intravenous bolus
- Injection: 75 mg of INTEGRILIN in 100 mL (0.75 mg/mL), for intravenous infusion
- Injection: 200 mg of INTEGRILIN in 100 mL (2 mg/mL), for intravenous infusion

4 CONTRAINDICATIONS

Treatment with INTEGRILIN is contraindicated in patients with:
- A history of bleeding diathesis, or evidence of active abnormal bleeding within the previous 30 days
- Severe hypertension (systolic blood pressure >200 mm Hg or diastolic blood pressure >110 mm Hg) not adequately controlled on antihypertensive therapy
- Major surgery within the preceding 6 weeks
- History of stroke within 30 days or any history of hemorrhagic stroke
- Current or planned administration of another parenteral GP IIb/IIIa inhibitor
- Dependency on renal dialysis
- Hypersensitivity to INTEGRILIN or any component of the product (hypersensitivity reactions that occurred included anaphylaxis and urticaria)

5 WARNINGS AND PRECAUTIONS

5.1 Bleeding

Bleeding is the most common complication encountered during INTEGRILIN therapy. Administration of INTEGRILIN is associated with an increase in major and minor bleeding, as classified by the criteria of the Thrombolysis in Myocardial Infarction Study group (TIMI) *[see Adverse Reactions (6.1)]*. Most major bleeding associated with INTEGRILIN has been at the arterial access site for cardiac catheterization or from the gastrointestinal or genitourinary tract. Minimize the use of arterial and venous punctures, intramuscular injections, and the use of urinary catheters, the

nasotracheal intubation, and nasogastric tubes. When obtaining intravenous access, avoid non-compressible sites (e.g., subclavian or jugular veins).

Use of Thrombolytics, Anticoagulants, and Other Antiplatelet Agents

Risk factors for bleeding include older age, a history of bleeding disorders, and concomitant use of drugs that increase the risk of bleeding (thrombolytics, oral anticoagulants, nonsteroidal anti-inflammatory drugs, and $P2Y_{12}$ inhibitors). Concomitant treatment with other inhibitors of platelet receptor glycoprotein (GP) IIb/IIIa should be avoided. In patients treated with heparin, bleeding can be minimized by close monitoring of the aPTT and ACT *[see Dosage and Administration (2)]*.

Care of the Femoral Artery Access Site in Patients Undergoing Percutaneous Coronary Intervention (PCI)

In patients undergoing PCI, treatment with INTEGRILIN is associated with an increase in major and minor bleeding at the site of arterial sheath placement. After PCI, INTEGRILIN infusion should be continued until hospital discharge or up to 18 to 24 hours, whichever comes first. Heparin use is discouraged after the PCI procedure. Early sheath removal is encouraged while INTEGRILIN is being infused. Prior to removing the sheath, it is recommended that heparin be discontinued for 3 to 4 hours and an aPTT of <45 seconds or ACT <150 seconds be achieved. In any case, both heparin and INTEGRILIN should be discontinued and sheath hemostasis should be achieved at least 2 to 4 hours before hospital discharge. If bleeding at access site cannot be controlled with pressure, infusion of INTEGRILIN and heparin should be discontinued immediately.

5.2 Thrombocytopenia

There have been reports of acute, profound thrombocytopenia (immune-mediated and non-immune mediated) with INTEGRILIN. In the event of acute profound thrombocytopenia or a confirmed platelet decrease to <100,000/mm³, discontinue INTEGRILIN and heparin (unfractionated or low-molecular weight). Monitor serial platelet counts, assess the presence of drug-dependent antibodies, and treat as appropriate *[see Adverse Reactions (6.1)]*.

There has been no clinical experience with INTEGRILIN initiated in patients with a baseline platelet count <100,000/mm³. If a patient with low platelet counts is receiving INTEGRILIN, their platelet count should be monitored closely.

6 ADVERSE REACTIONS

The following serious adverse reaction is also discussed elsewhere in the labeling:
- Bleeding *[see Contraindications (4) and Warnings and Precautions (5.1)]*

6.1 Clinical Trials Experience

Because clinical studies are conducted under widely varying conditions, adverse reaction rates observed in the clinical studies of a drug cannot be directly compared to rates in the clinical trials of another drug and may not reflect the rates observed in clinical practice.

A total of 16,782 patients were treated in the Phase III clinical trials (PURSUIT, ESPRIT, and IMPACT II) *[see Clinical Trials (14)]*. These 16,782 patients had a mean age of 62 years (range: 20-94 years). Eighty-nine percent of the patients were Caucasian, with the remainder being predominantly Black (5%) and Hispanic (5%). Sixty-eight percent were men. Because of the different regimens used in PURSUIT, IMPACT II, and ESPRIT, data from the 3 studies were not pooled.

Bleeding and hypotension were the most commonly reported adverse reactions (incidence ≥5% and greater than placebo) in the INTEGRILIN controlled clinical trial database.

Bleeding

The incidence of bleeding and transfusions in the PURSUIT and ESPRIT studies are shown in Table 2. Bleeding was classified as major or minor by the criteria of the TIMI study group. Major bleeding consisted of intracranial hemorrhage and other bleeding that led to decreases in hemoglobin greater than 5 g/dL. Minor bleeding included spontaneous gross hematuria, spontaneous hematemesis, other observed blood loss with a hemoglobin decrease of more than 3 g/dL, and other hemoglobin decreases that were greater than 4 g/dL but less than 5 g/dL. In patients who received transfusions, the corresponding loss in hemoglobin was estimated through an adaptation of the method of Landefeld et al.

Table 2: Bleeding and Transfusions in the PURSUIT and ESPRIT Studies

	Placebo n (%)	INTEGRILIN 180/2 n (%)
PURSUIT (ACS)		
Patients	4696	4679
Major bleeding*	425 (9.3%)	498 (10.8%)
Minor bleeding*	347 (7.6%)	604 (13.1%)
Requiring transfusions†	490 (10.4%)	601 (12.8%)

	Placebo n (%)	INTEGRILIN 180/2/180 n (%)
ESPRIT (PCI)		
Patients	1024	1040
Major bleeding*	4 (0.4%)	13 (1.3%)
Minor bleeding*	18 (2%)	29 (3%)
Requiring transfusions†	11 (1.1%)	16 (1.5%)

Note: Denominator is based on patients for whom data are available.

* For major and minor bleeding, patients are counted only once according to the most severe classification.

† Includes transfusions of whole blood, packed red blood cells, fresh frozen plasma, cryoprecipitate, platelets, and autotransfusion during the initial hospitalization.

The majority of major bleeding reactions in the ESPRIT study occurred at the vascular access site (1 and 8 patients, or 0.1% and 0.8% in the placebo and INTEGRILIN groups, respectively). Bleeding at "other" locations occurred in 0.2% and 0.4% of patients, respectively.

In the PURSUIT study, the greatest increase in major bleeding in INTEGRILIN-treated patients compared to placebo-treated patients was also associated with bleeding at the femoral artery access site (2.8% versus 1.3%). Oropharyngeal (primarily gingival), genitourinary, gastrointestinal, and retroperitoneal bleeding were also seen more commonly in INTEGRILIN-treated patients compared to placebo-treated patients.

Among patients experiencing a major bleed in the IMPACT II study, an increase in bleeding on INTEGRILIN versus placebo was observed only for the femoral artery access site (3.2% versus 2.8%).

Table 3 displays the incidence of TIMI major bleeding according to the cardiac procedures carried out in the PURSUIT study. The most common bleeding complications were related to cardiac revascularization (CABG-related or femoral artery access site bleeding). A corresponding table for ESPRIT is not presented, as every patient underwent PCI in the ESPRIT study and only 11 patients underwent CABG.

Table 3: Major Bleeding by Procedures in the PURSUIT Study

	Placebo n (%)	INTEGRILIN 180/2 n (%)
Patients	4577	4604
Overall incidence of major bleeding	425 (9.3%)	498 (10.8%)
Breakdown by procedure:		
CABG	375 (8.2%)	377 (8.2%)
Angioplasty without CABG	27 (0.6%)	64 (1.4%)
Angiography without angioplasty or CABG	11 (0.2%)	29 (0.6%)
Medical therapy only	12 (0.3%)	28 (0.6%)

Note: Denominators are based on the total number of patients whose TIMI classification was resolved.

In the PURSUIT and ESPRIT studies, the risk of major bleeding with INTEGRILIN increased as patient weight decreased. This relationship was most apparent for patients weighing less than 70 kg.

Bleeding resulting in discontinuation of the study drug was more frequent among patients receiving INTEGRILIN than placebo (4.6% versus 0.9% in ESPRIT, 8% versus 1% in PURSUIT, 3.5% versus 1.9% in IMPACT II).

Intracranial Hemorrhage and Stroke
Intracranial hemorrhage was rare in the PURSUIT, IMPACT II, and ESPRIT clinical studies. In the PURSUIT study, 3 patients in the placebo group, 1 patient in the group treated with INTEGRILIN 180/1.3, and 5 patients in the group treated with INTEGRILIN 180/2 experienced a hemorrhagic stroke. The overall incidence of stroke was 0.5% in patients receiving INTEGRILIN 180/1.3, 0.7% in patients receiving INTEGRILIN 180/2, and 0.8% in placebo patients. In the IMPACT II study, intracranial hemorrhage was experienced by 1 patient treated with INTEGRILIN 135/0.5, 2 patients treated with INTEGRILIN 135/0.75, and 2 patients in the placebo group. The overall incidence of stroke was 0.5% in patients receiving 135/0.5 INTEGRILIN, 0.7% in patients receiving INTEGRILIN 135/0.75, and 0.7% in the placebo group.

In the ESPRIT study, there were 3 hemorrhagic strokes, 1 in the placebo group and 2 in the INTEGRILIN group. In addition there was 1 case of cerebral infarction in the INTEGRILIN group.

Immunogenicity/Thrombocytopenia
The potential for development of antibodies to eptifibatide has been studied in 433 subjects. INTEGRILIN was nonantigenic in 412 patients receiving a single administration of INTEGRILIN (135-mcg/kg bolus followed by a continuous infusion of either 0.5 mcg/kg/min or 0.75 mcg/kg/min), and in 21 subjects to whom INTEGRILIN (135-mcg/kg bolus followed by a continuous infusion of 0.75 mcg/kg/min) was administered twice, 28 days apart. In both cases, plasma for antibody detection was collected approximately 30 days after each dose. The development of antibodies to eptifibatide at higher doses has not been evaluated.

In patients with suspected INTEGRILIN-related immune-mediated thrombocytopenia, IgG antibodies that react with the GP IIb/IIIa complex were identified in the presence of eptifibatide and in INTEGRILIN-naïve patients. These findings suggest acute thrombocytopenia after the administration of INTEGRILIN can develop as a result of naturally occurring drug-dependent antibodies or those induced by prior exposure to INTEGRILIN. Similar antibodies were identified with other GP IIb/IIIa ligand-mimetic agents. Immune-mediated thrombocytopenia with INTEGRILIN may be associated with hypotension and/or other signs of hypersensitivity.

In the PURSUIT and IMPACT II studies, the incidence of thrombocytopenia (<100,000/mm^3 or ≥50% reduction from baseline) and the incidence of platelet transfusions were similar between patients treated with INTEGRILIN and placebo. In the ESPRIT study, the incidence was 0.6% in the placebo group and 1.2% in the INTEGRILIN group.

Other Adverse Reactions
In the PURSUIT and ESPRIT studies, the incidence of serious nonbleeding adverse reactions was similar in patients receiving placebo or INTEGRILIN (19% and 19%, respectively, in PURSUIT; 6% and 7%, respectively, in ESPRIT). In PURSUIT, the only serious nonbleeding adverse reaction that occurred at a rate of at least 1% and was more common with INTEGRILIN than placebo (7% versus 6%) was hypotension. Most of the serious nonbleeding adverse reactions consisted of cardiovascular reactions typical of a UA population. In the IMPACT II study, serious nonbleeding adverse reactions that occurred in greater than 1% of patients were uncommon and similar in incidence between placebo- and INTEGRILIN-treated patients.

Discontinuation of study drug due to adverse reactions other than bleeding was uncommon in the PURSUIT, IMPACT II, and ESPRIT studies, with no single reaction occurring in >0.5% of the study population (except for "other" in the ESPRIT study).

6.2 Postmarketing Experience
Because the reactions below are reported voluntarily from a population of uncertain size, it is generally not possible to reliably estimate their frequency or establish a causal relationship to drug exposure.

The following adverse reactions have been reported in postmarketing experience, primarily with INTEGRILIN in combination with heparin and aspirin: cerebral, GI, and pulmonary hemorrhage. Fatal bleeding reactions have been reported. Acute profound thrombocytopenia, as well as immune-mediated thrombocytopenia, has been reported *[see Adverse Reactions (6.1)].*

7 DRUG INTERACTIONS
7.1 Use of Thrombolytics, Anticoagulants, and Other Antiplatelet Agents
Coadministration of antiplatelet agents, thrombolytics, heparin, aspirin, and chronic NSAID use increases the risk of bleeding. Concomitant treatment with other inhibitors of platelet receptor GP IIb/IIIa should be avoided.

8 USE IN SPECIFIC POPULATIONS
8.1 Pregnancy
Pregnancy Category B
Teratology studies have been performed by continuous intravenous infusion of eptifibatide in pregnant rats at total daily doses of up to 72 mg/kg/day (about 4 times the recommended maximum daily human dose on a body surface area basis) and in pregnant rabbits at total daily doses of up to 36 mg/kg/day (also about 4 times the recommended maximum daily human dose on a body surface area basis). These studies revealed no evidence of harm to the fetus due to eptifibatide. There are, however, no adequate and well-controlled studies in pregnant women with INTEGRILIN. Because animal reproduction studies are not always predictive of human response, INTEGRILIN should be used during pregnancy only if clearly needed.

8.3 Nursing Mothers
It is not known whether eptifibatide is excreted in human milk. Because many drugs are excreted in human milk, caution should be exercised when INTEGRILIN is administered to a nursing mother.

8.4 Pediatric Use
Safety and effectiveness of INTEGRILIN in pediatric patients have not been studied.

8.5 Geriatric Use
The PURSUIT and IMPACT II clinical studies enrolled patients up to the age of 94 years (45% were age 65 and over; 12% were age 75 and older). There was no apparent difference in efficacy between older and younger patients treated with INTEGRILIN. The incidence of bleeding complications was higher in the elderly in both placebo and INTEGRILIN groups, and the incremental risk of INTEGRILIN-associated bleeding was greater in the older patients. No dose adjustment was made for elderly patients, but patients over 75 years of age had to weigh at least 50 kg to be enrolled in the PURSUIT study; no such limitation was stipulated in the ESPRIT study *[see Adverse Reactions (6.1)].*

8.6 Renal Impairment
Approximately 50% of eptifibatide is cleared by the kidney in patients with normal renal function. Total drug clearance is decreased by approximately 50% and steady-state plasma INTEGRILIN concentrations are doubled in patients with an estimated CrCl <50 mL/min (using the Cockcroft-Gault equation). Therefore, the infusion dose should be reduced to 1 mcg/kg/min in such patients *[see Dosage and Administration (2)].* The safety and efficacy of INTEGRILIN in patients dependent on dialysis has not been established.

10 OVERDOSAGE
There has been only limited experience with overdosage of INTEGRILIN. There were 8 patients in the IMPACT II study, 9 patients in the PURSUIT study, and no patients in the ESPRIT study who received bolus doses and/or infusion doses more than double those called for in the protocols. None of these patients experienced an intracranial bleed or other major bleeding.

Eptifibatide was not lethal to rats, rabbits, or monkeys when administered by continuous intravenous infusion for 90 minutes at a total dose of 45 mg/kg (about 2 to 5 times the recommended maximum daily human dose on a body surface area basis). Symptoms of acute toxicity were loss of righting reflex, dyspnea, ptosis, and decreased muscle tone in rabbits and petechial hemorrhages in the femoral and abdominal areas of monkeys.

From *in vitro* studies, eptifibatide is not extensively bound to plasma proteins and thus may be cleared from plasma by dialysis.

11 DESCRIPTION
Eptifibatide is a cyclic heptapeptide containing 6 amino acids and 1 mercaptopropionyl (des-amino cysteinyl) residue. An interchain disulfide bridge is formed between the cysteine amide and the mercaptopropionyl moieties. Chemically it is N^6-(aminoiminomethyl)-N^2-(3-mercapto-1-oxopropyl)-L-lysylglycyl-L-α-aspartyl-L-tryptophyl-L-prolyl-L-cysteinamide, cyclic (1→6)-disulfide. Eptifibatide binds to the platelet receptor glycoprotein (GP) IIb/IIIa of human platelets and inhibits platelet aggregation.

The eptifibatide peptide is produced by solution-phase peptide synthesis, and is purified by preparative reverse-phase liquid chromatography and lyophilized. The structural formula is:
[See chemical structure at top of next column]
INTEGRILIN Injection is a clear, colorless, sterile, non-pyrogenic solution for intravenous (IV) use with an empirical formula of $C_{35}H_{49}N_{11}O_9S_2$ and a molecular weight of 831.96. Each 10-mL vial contains 2 mg/mL of INTEGRILIN and each 100-mL vial contains either 0.75 mg/mL of INTEGRILIN or 2 mg/mL of INTEGRILIN. Each vial of either size also contains 5.25 mg/mL citric acid and sodium hydroxide to adjust the pH to 5.35.

12 CLINICAL PHARMACOLOGY
12.1 Mechanism of Action
Eptifibatide reversibly inhibits platelet aggregation by preventing the binding of fibrinogen, von Willebrand factor, and other adhesive ligands to GP IIb/IIIa. When administered intravenously, eptifibatide inhibits *ex vivo* platelet aggregation in a dose- and concentration-dependent manner. Platelet aggregation inhibition is reversible following cessation of the eptifibatide infusion; this is thought to result from dissociation of eptifibatide from the platelet.

12.2 Pharmacodynamics
Infusion of eptifibatide into baboons caused a dose-dependent inhibition of *ex vivo* platelet aggregation, with complete inhibition of aggregation achieved at infusion rates greater than 5 mcg/kg/min. In a baboon model that is refractory to aspirin and heparin, doses of eptifibatide that inhibit aggregation prevented acute thrombosis with only a modest prolongation (2- to 3-fold) of the bleeding time. Platelet aggregation in dogs was also inhibited by infusions of eptifibatide, with complete inhibition at 2 mcg/kg/min. This infusion dose completely inhibited canine coronary thrombosis induced by coronary artery injury (Folts model). Human pharmacodynamic data were obtained in healthy subjects and in patients presenting with UA or NSTEMI and/or undergoing percutaneous coronary intervention. Studies in healthy subjects enrolled only males; patient studies enrolled approximately one-third women. In these studies, INTEGRILIN inhibited *ex vivo* platelet aggregation induced by adenosine diphosphate (ADP) and other agonists in a dose- and concentration-dependent manner. The effect of INTEGRILIN was observed immediately after administration of a 180-mcg/kg intravenous bolus. Table 4 shows the effects of dosing regimens of INTEGRILIN used in the IMPACT II and PURSUIT studies on *ex vivo* platelet aggregation induced by 20 µM ADP in PPACK-anticoagulated platelet-rich plasma and on bleeding time. The effects of the dosing regimen used in ESPRIT on platelet aggregation have not been studied.

Table 4: Platelet Inhibition and Bleeding Time

	PURSUIT 180/2*
Inhibition of platelet aggregation 15 min after bolus	84%
Inhibition of platelet aggregation at steady state	>90%
Bleeding-time prolongation at steady state	<5×
Inhibition of platelet aggregation 4h after infusion discontinuation	<50%
Bleeding-time prolongation 6h after infusion discontinuation	1.4×

* 180-mcg/kg bolus followed by a continuous infusion of 2 mcg/kg/min.

The INTEGRILIN dosing regimen used in the ESPRIT study included two 180-mcg/kg bolus doses given 10 minutes apart combined with a continuous 2-mcg/kg/min infusion.

When administered alone, INTEGRILIN has no measurable effect on PT or aPTT.

There were no important differences between men and women or between age groups in the pharmacodynamic properties of eptifibatide. Differences among ethnic groups have not been assessed.

12.3 Pharmacokinetics
The pharmacokinetics of eptifibatide are linear and dose-proportional for bolus doses ranging from 90 to 250 mcg/kg and infusion rates from 0.5 to 3 mcg/kg/min. Plasma elimination half-life is approximately 2.5 hours. Administration of a single 180-mcg/kg bolus combined with an infusion pro-

duces an early peak level, followed by a small decline prior to attaining steady state (within 4-6 hours). This decline can be prevented by administering a second 180-mcg/kg bolus 10 minutes after the first. The extent of eptifibatide binding to human plasma protein is about 25%. Clearance in patients with coronary artery disease is about 55 mL/kg/h. In healthy subjects, renal clearance accounts for approximately 50% of total body clearance, with the majority of the drug excreted in the urine as eptifibatide, deaminated eptifibatide, and other, more polar metabolites. No major metabolites have been detected in human plasma.

Special Populations

Geriatric

Patients in clinical studies were older (range: 20-94 years) than those in the clinical pharmacology studies. Elderly patients with coronary artery disease demonstrated higher plasma levels and lower total body clearance of eptifibatide when given the same dose as younger patients. Limited data are available on lighter weight (<50 kg) patients over 75 years of age.

Renal Impairment

In patients with moderate to severe renal insufficiency (CrCl <50 mL/min using the Cockcroft-Gault equation), the clearance of eptifibatide is reduced by approximately 50% and steady-state plasma levels approximately doubled [see Use in Specific Populations (8.6) and Dosage and Administration (2)].

Hepatic Impairment

No studies have been conducted in patients with hepatic impairment.

Gender

Males and females have not demonstrated any clinically significant differences in the pharmacokinetics of eptifibatide.

13   NONCLINICAL TOXICOLOGY

13.1   Carcinogenesis, Mutagenesis, Impairment of Fertility

No long-term studies in animals have been performed to evaluate the carcinogenic potential of eptifibatide. Eptifibatide was not genotoxic in the Ames test, the mouse lymphoma cell (L 5178Y, TK+/-) forward mutation test, the human lymphocyte chromosome aberration test, or the mouse micronucleus test. Administered by continuous intravenous infusion at total daily doses up to 72 mg/kg/day (about 4 times the recommended maximum daily human dose on a body surface area basis), eptifibatide had no effect on fertility and reproductive performance of male and female rats.

14   CLINICAL STUDIES

INTEGRILIN was studied in 3 placebo-controlled, randomized studies. PURSUIT evaluated patients with acute coronary syndromes: UA or NSTEMI. Two other studies, ESPRIT and IMPACT II, evaluated patients about to undergo a PCI. Patients underwent primarily balloon angioplasty in IMPACT II and intracoronary stent placement, with or without angioplasty, in ESPRIT.

14.1   Non-ST-Segment Elevation Acute Coronary Syndrome

Non-ST-segment elevation acute coronary syndrome is defined as prolonged (≥10 minutes) symptoms of cardiac ischemia within the previous 24 hours associated with either ST-segment changes (elevations between 0.6 mm and 1 mm or depression >0.5 mm), T-wave inversion (>1 mm), or positive CK-MB. This definition includes "unstable angina" and "NSTEMI" but excludes MI that is associated with Q waves or greater degrees of ST-segment elevation.

PURSUIT (Platelet Glycoprotein IIb/IIIa in Unstable Angina: Receptor Suppression Using INTEGRILIN Therapy)

PURSUIT was a 726-center, 27-country, double-blind, randomized, placebo-controlled study in 10,948 patients presenting with UA or NSTEMI. Patients could be enrolled only if they had experienced cardiac ischemia at rest (≥10 minutes) within the previous 24 hours and had either ST-segment changes (elevations between 0.6 mm and 1 mm or depression >0.5 mm), T-wave inversion (>1 mm), or increased CK-MB. Important exclusion criteria included a history of bleeding diathesis, evidence of abnormal bleeding within the previous 30 days, uncontrolled hypertension, major surgery within the previous 6 weeks, stroke within the previous 30 days, any history of hemorrhagic stroke, serum creatinine >2 mg/dL, dependency on renal dialysis, or platelet count <100,000/mm³.

Patients were randomized to placebo, to INTEGRILIN 180-mcg/kg bolus followed by a 2-mcg/kg/min infusion (180/2), or to INTEGRILIN 180-mcg/kg bolus followed by a 1.3-mcg/kg/min infusion (180/1.3). The infusion was continued for 72 hours, until hospital discharge, or until the time of CABG, whichever occurred first, except that if PCI was performed, the INTEGRILIN infusion was continued for 24 hours after the procedure, allowing for a duration of infusion up to 96 hours.

Table 5: Clinical Events in the PURSUIT Study

Death or MI	Placebo (n=4739) n (%)	INTEGRILIN (180 mcg/kg bolus then 2 mcg/kg/min infusion) (n=4722) n (%)	p-value
3 days	359 (7.6%)	279 (5.9%)	0.001
7 days	552 (11.6%)	477 (10.1%)	0.016
30 days			
Death or MI (primary endpoint)	745 (15.7%)	672 (14.2%)	0.042
Death	177 (3.7%)	165 (3.5%)	
Nonfatal MI	568 (12%)	507 (10.7%)	

Table 6: Clinical Events (Death or MI) in the PURSUIT Study Within 72 Hours of Randomization

	Placebo	INTEGRILIN (180 mcg/kg bolus then 2 mcg/kg/min infusion)
Overall patient population	n=4739	n=4722
– At 72 hours	7.6%	5.9%
Patients undergoing early PCI	n=631	n=619
– Pre-procedure (nonfatal MI only)	5.5%	1.8%
– At 72 hours	14.4%	9%
Patients not undergoing early PCI	n=4108	n=4103
– At 72 hours	6.5%	5.4%

The lower-infusion-rate arm was stopped after the first interim analysis when the 2 active-treatment arms appeared to have the same incidence of bleeding.

Patient age ranged from 20 to 94 (mean 63) years, and 65% were male. The patients were 89% Caucasian, 6% Hispanic, and 5% Black, recruited in the United States and Canada (40%), Western Europe (39%), Eastern Europe (16%), and Latin America (5%).

This was a "real world" study; each patient was managed according to the usual standards of the investigational site; frequencies of angiography, PCI, and CABG therefore differed widely from site to site and from country to country. Of the patients in PURSUIT, 13% were managed with PCI during drug infusion, of whom 50% received intracoronary stents; 87% were managed medically (without PCI during drug infusion).

The majority of patients received aspirin (75-325 mg once daily). Heparin was administered intravenously or subcutaneously, at the physician's discretion, most commonly as an intravenous bolus of 5000 units followed by a continuous infusion of 1000 units/h. For patients weighing less than 70 kg, the recommended heparin bolus dose was 60 units/kg followed by a continuous infusion of 12 units/kg/h. A target aPTT of 50 to 70 seconds was recommended. A total of 1250 patients underwent PCI within 72 hours after randomization, in which case they received intravenous heparin to maintain an ACT of 300 to 350 seconds.

The primary endpoint of the study was the occurrence of death from any cause or new MI (evaluated by a blinded Clinical Endpoints Committee) within 30 days of randomization.

Compared to placebo, INTEGRILIN administered as a 180-mcg/kg bolus followed by a 2-mcg/kg/min infusion significantly (p=0.042) reduced the incidence of endpoint events (see Table 6). The reduction in the incidence of endpoint events in patients receiving INTEGRILIN was evident early during treatment, and this reduction was maintained through at least 30 days (see Figure 1). Table 5 also shows the incidence of the components of the primary endpoint, death (whether or not preceded by an MI) and new MI in surviving patients at 30 days.

[See table 5 above]

Figure 1: Kaplan-Meier Plot of Time to Death or Myocardial Infarction Within 30 Days of Randomization in the PURSUIT Study

Treatment: —— INTEGRILIN ---- Placebo

Treatment with INTEGRILIN prior to determination of patient management strategy reduced clinical events regard-

less of whether patients ultimately underwent diagnostic catheterization, revascularization (i.e., PCI or CABG surgery) or continued to receive medical management alone. Table 6 shows the incidence of death or MI within 72 hours. [See table 6 above]

All of the effect of INTEGRILIN was established within 72 hours (during the period of drug infusion), regardless of management strategy. Moreover, for patients undergoing early PCI, a reduction in events was evident prior to the procedure.

An analysis of the results by sex suggests that women who would not routinely be expected to undergo PCI receive less benefit from INTEGRILIN (95% confidence limits for relative risk of 0.94 - 1.28) than do men (0.72 - 0.9). This difference may be a true treatment difference, the effect of other differences in these subgroups, or a statistical anomaly. No differential outcomes were seen between male and female patients undergoing PCI (see results for ESPRIT).

Follow-up data were available through 165 days for 10,611 patients enrolled in the PURSUIT trial (96.9% of the initial enrollment). This follow-up included 4566 patients who received INTEGRILIN at the 180/2 dose. As reported by the investigators, the occurrence of death from any cause or new MI for patients followed for at least 165 days was reduced from 13.6% with placebo to 12.1% with INTEGRILIN 180/2.

14.2   Percutaneous Coronary Intervention (PCI)

IMPACT II (INTEGRILIN to Minimize Platelet Aggregation and Prevent Coronary Thrombosis II)

IMPACT II was a multicenter, double-blind, randomized, placebo-controlled study conducted in the United States in 4010 patients undergoing PCI. Major exclusion criteria included a history of bleeding diathesis, major surgery within 6 weeks of treatment, gastrointestinal bleeding within 30 days, any stroke or structural CNS abnormality, uncontrolled hypertension, PT >1.2 times control, hematocrit <30%, platelet count <100,000/mm³, and pregnancy.

Patient age ranged from 24 to 89 (mean 60) years, and 75% were male. The patients were 92% Caucasian, 5% Black, and 3% Hispanic. Forty-one percent of the patients underwent PCI for ongoing ACS. Patients were randomly assigned to 1 of 3 treatment regimens, each incorporating a bolus dose initiated immediately prior to PCI followed by a continuous infusion lasting 20 to 24 hours:

1) 135-mcg/kg bolus followed by a continuous infusion of 0.5 mcg/kg/min of INTEGRILIN (135/0.5);
2) 135-mcg/kg bolus followed by a continuous infusion of 0.75 mcg/kg/min of INTEGRILIN (135/0.75); or
3) a matching placebo bolus followed by a matching placebo continuous infusion.

Each patient received aspirin and an intravenous heparin bolus of 100 units/kg, with additional bolus infusions of up to 2000 additional units of heparin every 15 minutes to maintain an ACT of 300 to 350 seconds.

The primary endpoint was the composite of death, MI, or urgent revascularization, analyzed at 30 days after randomization in all patients who received at least 1 dose of study drug.

As shown in Table 7, each INTEGRILIN regimen reduced the rate of death, MI, or urgent intervention, although at 30 days, this finding was statistically significant only in the lower-dose INTEGRILIN group. As in the PURSUIT study, the effects of INTEGRILIN were seen early and persisted throughout the 30-day period.

Table 7: Clinical Events in the IMPACT II Study

	Placebo n (%)	INTEGRILIN (135 mcg/kg bolus then 0.5 mcg/kg/min infusion) n (%)	INTEGRILIN (135 mcg/kg bolus then 0.75 mcg/kg/min infusion) n (%)
Patients	1285	1300	1286
Abrupt Closure	65 (5.1%)	36 (2.8%)	43 (3.3%)
p-value versus placebo		0.003	0.03
Death, MI, or Urgent Intervention			
24 hours	123 (9.6%)	86 (6.6%)	89 (6.9%)
p-value versus placebo		0.006	0.014
48 hours	131 (10.2%)	99 (7.6%)	102 (7.9%)
p-value versus placebo		0.021	0.045
30 days (primary endpoint)	149 (11.6%)	118 (9.1%)	128 (10%)
p-value versus placebo		0.035	0.179
Death or MI			
30 days	110 (8.6%)	89 (6.8%)	95 (7.4%)
p-value versus placebo		0.102	0.272
6 months	151 (11.9%)*	136 (10.6%)*	130 (10.3%)*
p-value versus placebo		0.297	0.182

* Kaplan-Meier estimate of event rate.

Table 8: Clinical Events in the ESPRIT Study

	Placebo (n=1024)	INTEGRILIN* (n=1040)	Relative Risk (95% CI)	p-value
Death, MI, UTVR, or Thrombotic "Bailout"				
48 hours (primary endpoint)	108 (10.5%)	69 (6.6%)	0.629 (0.471, 0.84)	0.0015
30 days	120 (11.7%)	78 (7.5%)	0.64 (0.488, 0.84)	0.0011
Death, MI, or UTVR				
48 hours	95 (9.3%)	62 (6%)	0.643 (0.472, 0.875)	0.0045
30 days (key secondary endpoint)	107 (10.4%)	71 (6.8%)	0.653 (0.49, 0.871)	0.0034
Death or MI				
48 hours	94 (9.2%)	57 (5.5%)	0.597 (0.435, 0.82)	0.0013
30 days	104 (10.2%)	66 (6.3%)	0.625 (0.465, 0.84)	0.0016

* INTEGRILIN was administered as 180 mcg/kg boluses at times 0 and 10 minutes and an infusion at 2 mcg/kg/min.

Table 9: Clinical Events at 6 Months and 1 Year in the ESPRIT Study

	Placebo (n=1024)	INTEGRILIN (n=1040)	Hazard Ratio (95% CI)
Death, MI, or Target Vessel Revascularization			
6 months	187 (18.5%)	146 (14.3%)	0.744 (0.599, 0.924)
1 year	222 (22.1%)	178 (17.5%)	0.762 (0.626, 0.929)
Death, MI			
6 months	117 (11.5%)	77 (7.4%)	0.631 (0.473, 0.841)
1 year	126 (12.4%)	83 (8%)	0.63 (0.478, 0.832)

Percentages are Kaplan-Meier event rates.

[See table 7 above]

ESPRIT (Enhanced Suppression of the Platelet IIb/IIIa Receptor with INTEGRILIN Therapy)
The ESPRIT study was a multicenter, double-blind, randomized, placebo-controlled study conducted in the United States and Canada that enrolled 2064 patients undergoing elective or urgent PCI with intended intracoronary stent placement. Exclusion criteria included MI within the previous 24 hours, ongoing chest pain, administration of any oral antiplatelet or oral anticoagulant other than aspirin within 30 days of PCI (although loading doses of thienopyridine on the day of PCI were encouraged), planned PCI of a saphenous vein graft or subsequent "staged" PCI, prior stent placement in the target lesion, PCI within the previous 90 days, a history of bleeding diathesis, major surgery within 6 weeks of treatment, gastrointestinal bleeding within 30 days, any stroke or structural CNS abnormality, uncontrolled hypertension, PT >1.2 times control, hematocrit <30%, platelet count <100,000/mm^3, and pregnancy. Patient age ranged from 24 to 93 (mean 62) years, and 73% of patients were male. The study enrolled 90% Caucasian, 5% African American, 2% Hispanic, and 1% Asian patients. Patients received a wide variety of stents. Patients were randomized either to placebo or INTEGRILIN administered as an intravenous bolus of 180 mcg/kg followed immediately by a continuous infusion of 2 mcg/kg/min, and a second bolus of 180 mcg/kg administered 10 minutes later (180/2/180). INTEGRILIN infusion was continued for 18 to 24 hours after PCI or until hospital discharge, whichever came first. Each patient received at least 1 dose of aspirin (162-325 mg) and 60 units/kg of heparin as a bolus (not to exceed 6000 units) if not already receiving a heparin infusion. Additional boluses of heparin (10-40 units/kg) could be administered in order to reach a target ACT between 200 and 300 seconds.
The primary endpoint of the ESPRIT study was the composite of death, MI, urgent target vessel revascularization (UTVR), and "bailout" to open-label INTEGRILIN due to a thrombotic complication of PCI (TBO) (e.g., visible thrombus, "no reflow," or abrupt closure) at 48 hours. MI, UTVR, and TBO were evaluated by a blinded Clinical Events Committee.
As shown in Table 8, the incidence of the primary endpoint and selected secondary endpoints was significantly reduced in patients who received INTEGRILIN. A treatment benefit in patients who received INTEGRILIN was seen by 48 hours and at the end of the 30-day observation period.
[See table 8 above]
The need for thrombotic "bailout" was significantly reduced with INTEGRILIN at 48 hours (2.1% for placebo, 1% for INTEGRILIN; p=0.029). Consistent with previous studies of GP IIb/IIIa inhibitors, most of the benefit achieved acutely with INTEGRILIN was in the reduction of MI. INTEGRILIN reduced the occurrence of MI at 48 hours from 9% for placebo to 5.4% (p=0.0015) and maintained that effect with significance at 30 days.
There was no treatment difference with respect to sex in ESPRIT. INTEGRILIN reduced the incidence of the primary endpoint in both men (95% confidence limits for relative risk: 0.54, 1.07) and women (0.24, 0.72) at 48 hours.
Follow-up (12-month) mortality data were available for 2024 patients (1017 on INTEGRILIN) enrolled in the ESPRIT trial (98.1% of the initial enrollment). Twelve-month clinical event data were available for 1964 patients (988 on

INTEGRILIN), representing 95.2% of the initial enrollment. As shown in Table 9, the treatment effect of INTEGRILIN seen at 48 hours and 30 days appeared preserved at 6 months and 1 year. Most of the benefit was in reduction of MI.
[See table 9 above]

16 HOW SUPPLIED/STORAGE AND HANDLING
16.1 How Supplied
INTEGRILIN (eptifibatide) injection is supplied as a sterile solution in 10-mL vials containing 20 mg of INTEGRILIN (NDC 0085-1177-01) and 100-mL vials containing either 75 mg of INTEGRILIN (NDC 0085-1136-01) or 200 mg of INTEGRILIN (NDC 0085-1177-02).
16.2 Storage
Vials should be stored refrigerated at 2-8°C (36-46°F). Vials may be transferred to room temperature storage[1] for a period not to exceed 2 months. Upon transfer, vial cartons must be marked by the dispensing pharmacist with a "DISCARD BY" date (2 months from the transfer date or the labeled expiration date, whichever comes first).
Protect from light until administration.

---
[1] Store at 25°C (77°F); excursions permitted to 15-30°C (59-86°F) [see USP Controlled Room Temperature].

17 PATIENT COUNSELING INFORMATION
Instruct patients to inform the doctor or healthcare provider about any medical conditions, medications, and allergies.
Manufactured for: Merck Sharp & Dohme Corp., a subsidiary of
MERCK & CO., INC., Whitehouse Station, NJ 08889, USA
Manufactured by:
Patheon Italia S.p.A, Ferentino, 03013, Italy
For patent information: www.merck.com/product/patent/home.html
INTEGRILIN is a registered trademark of Millennium Pharmaceuticals, Inc.
uspi-mk6936-iv-1404r012
Shown in Product Identification Guide, page 308

INTRON® A   ℞
Interferon alfa-2b, recombinant
For Injection

> **WARNING**
> Alpha interferons, including INTRON®A, cause or aggravate fatal or life-threatening neuropsychiatric, autoimmune, ischemic, and infectious disorders. Patients should be monitored closely with periodic clinical and laboratory evaluations. Patients with persistently severe or worsening signs or symptoms of these conditions should be withdrawn from therapy. In many but not all cases these disorders resolve after stopping INTRON A therapy. See **WARNINGS** and **ADVERSE REACTIONS.**

DESCRIPTION
INTRON® A (Interferon alfa-2b) for intramuscular, subcutaneous, intralesional, or intravenous Injection is a purified sterile recombinant interferon product.
INTRON A recombinant for Injection has been classified as an alpha interferon and is a water-soluble protein with a molecular weight of 19,271 daltons produced by recombinant DNA techniques. It is obtained from the bacterial fermentation of a strain of *Escherichia coli* bearing a genetically engineered plasmid containing an interferon alfa-2b gene from human leukocytes. The fermentation is carried out in a defined nutrient medium containing the antibiotic tetracycline hydrochloride at a concentration of 5 to 10 mg/L; the presence of this antibiotic is not detectable in the final product. The specific activity of interferon alfa-2b, recombinant is approximately 2.6×10^8 IU/mg protein as measured by the HPLC assay.
[See first table at top of next page]
Prior to administration, the INTRON A Powder for Injection is to be reconstituted with the provided Diluent for INTRON A (Sterile Water for Injection USP) (see **DOSAGE AND ADMINISTRATION**). INTRON A Powder for Injection is a white to cream-colored powder.
[See second table at top of next page]
These packages do not require reconstitution prior to administration (see **DOSAGE AND ADMINISTRATION**). INTRON A Solution for Injection is a clear, colorless solution.

CLINICAL PHARMACOLOGY
General
The interferons are a family of naturally occurring small proteins and glycoproteins with molecular weights of approximately 15,000 to 27,600 daltons produced and secreted by cells in response to viral infections and to synthetic or biological inducers.

Preclinical Pharmacology

Interferons exert their cellular activities by binding to specific membrane receptors on the cell surface. Once bound to the cell membrane, interferons initiate a complex sequence of intracellular events. *In vitro* studies demonstrated that these include the induction of certain enzymes, suppression of cell proliferation, immunomodulating activities such as enhancement of the phagocytic cytotoxicity of macrophages and augmentation of the specific cytotoxicity of lymphocytes for target cells, and inhibition of virus replication in virus-infected cells.

In a study using human hepatoblastoma cell line HB 611, the *in vitro* antiviral activity of alpha interferon was demonstrated by its inhibition of hepatitis B virus (HBV) replication.

The correlation between these *in vitro* data and the clinical results is unknown. Any of these activities might contribute to interferon's therapeutic effects.

Pharmacokinetics

The pharmacokinetics of INTRON® A were studied in 12 healthy male volunteers following single doses of 5 million IU/m^2 administered intramuscularly, subcutaneously, and as a 30-minute intravenous infusion in a crossover design.

The mean serum INTRON A concentrations following intramuscular and subcutaneous injections were comparable. The maximum serum concentrations obtained via these routes were approximately 18 to 116 IU/mL and occurred 3 to 12 hours after administration. The elimination half-life of INTRON A following both intramuscular and subcutaneous injections was approximately 2 to 3 hours. Serum concentrations were undetectable by 16 hours after the injections. After intravenous administration, serum INTRON A concentrations peaked (135–273 IU/mL) by the end of the 30-minute infusion, then declined at a slightly more rapid rate than after intramuscular or subcutaneous drug administration, becoming undetectable 4 hours after the infusion. The elimination half-life was approximately 2 hours.

Urine INTRON A concentrations following a single dose (5 million IU/m^2) were not detectable after any of the parenteral routes of administration. This result was expected since preliminary studies with isolated and perfused rabbit kidneys have shown that the kidney may be the main site of interferon catabolism.

There are no pharmacokinetic data available for the intralesional route of administration.

Serum Neutralizing Antibodies

In INTRON A-treated patients tested for antibody activity in clinical trials, serum anti-interferon neutralizing antibodies were detected in 0% (0/90) of patients with hairy cell leukemia, 0.8% (2/260) of patients treated intralesionally for condylomata acuminata, and 4% (1/24) of patients with AIDS-Related Kaposi's Sarcoma. Serum neutralizing antibodies have been detected in less than 3% of patients treated with higher INTRON A doses in malignancies other than hairy cell leukemia or AIDS-Related Kaposi's Sarcoma. The clinical significance of the appearance of serum anti-interferon neutralizing activity in these indications is not known.

Serum anti-interferon neutralizing antibodies were detected in 7% (12/168) of patients either during treatment or after completing 12 to 48 weeks of treatment with 3 million IU TIW of INTRON A therapy for chronic hepatitis C and in 13% (6/48) of patients who received INTRON A therapy for chronic hepatitis B at 5 million IU QD for 4 months, and in 3% (1/33) of patients treated at 10 million IU TIW. Serum anti-interferon neutralizing antibodies were detected in 9% (5/53) of pediatric patients who received INTRON A therapy for chronic hepatitis B at 6 million IU/m^2 TIW. Among all chronic hepatitis B or C patients, pediatrics and adults with detectable serum neutralizing antibodies, the titers detected were low (22/24 with titers less than or equal to 1:40 and 2/24 with titers less than or equal to 1:160). The appearance of serum anti-interferon neutralizing activity did not appear to affect safety or efficacy.

Hairy Cell Leukemia

In clinical trials in patients with hairy cell leukemia, there was depression of hematopoiesis during the first 1 to 2 months of INTRON A treatment, resulting in reduced numbers of circulating red and white blood cells, and platelets. Subsequently, both splenectomized and nonsplenectomized patients achieved substantial and sustained improvements in granulocytes, platelets, and hemoglobin levels in 75% of treated patients and at least some improvement (minor responses) occurred in 90%. INTRON A treatment resulted in a decrease in bone marrow hypercellularity and hairy cell infiltrates. The hairy cell index (HCI), which represents the percent of bone marrow cellularity times the percent of hairy cell infiltrate, was greater than or equal to 50% at the beginning of the study in 87% of patients. The percentage of patients with such an HCI decreased to 25% after 6 months and to 14% after 1 year. These results indicate that even though hematologic improvement had occurred earlier, prolonged INTRON A treatment may be required to obtain maximal reduction in tumor cell infiltrates in the bone marrow.

The percentage of patients with hairy cell leukemia who required red blood cell or platelet transfusions decreased significantly during treatment and the percentage of patients with confirmed and serious infections declined as granulocyte counts improved. Reversal of splenomegaly and of clinically significant hypersplenism was demonstrated in some patients.

A study was conducted to assess the effects of extended INTRON A treatment on duration of response for patients who responded to initial therapy. In this study, 126 responding patients were randomized to receive additional INTRON A treatment for 6 months or observation for a comparable period, after 12 months of initial INTRON A therapy. During this 6-month period, 3% (2/66) of INTRON A-treated patients relapsed compared with 18% (11/60) who were not treated. This represents a significant difference in time to relapse in favor of continued INTRON A treatment (P=0.006/0.01, Log Rank/Wilcoxon). Since a small proportion of the total population had relapsed, median time to relapse could not be estimated in either group. A similar pattern in relapses was seen when all randomized treatment, including that beyond 6 months, and available follow-up data were assessed. The 15% (10/66) relapses among INTRON A patients occurred over a significantly longer period of time than the 40% (24/60) with observation (P=0.0002/0.0001, Log Rank/Wilcoxon). Median time to relapse was estimated, using the Kaplan-Meier method, to be 6.8 months in the observation group but could not be estimated in the INTRON A group.

Subsequent follow-up with a median time of approximately 40 months demonstrated an overall survival of 87.8%. In a comparable historical control group followed for 24 months, overall median survival was approximately 40%.

Malignant Melanoma

The safety and efficacy of INTRON A was evaluated as adjuvant to surgical treatment in patients with melanoma who were free of disease (post surgery) but at high risk for systemic recurrence. These included patients with lesions of Breslow thickness greater than 4 mm, or patients with lesions of any Breslow thickness with primary or recurrent nodal involvement. In a randomized, controlled trial in 280 patients, 143 patients received INTRON A therapy at 20 million IU/m^2 intravenously five times per week for 4 weeks (induction phase) followed by 10 million IU/m^2 subcutaneously three times per week for 48 weeks (maintenance phase). In the clinical trial, the median daily INTRON A dose administered to patients was 19.1 million IU/m^2 during the induction phase and 9.1 million IU/m^2 during the maintenance phase. INTRON A therapy was begun less than or equal to 56 days after surgical resection. The remaining 137 patients were observed.

INTRON A therapy produced a significant increase in relapse-free and overall survival. Median time to relapse for the INTRON A-treated patients versus observation patients was 1.72 years versus 0.98 years (P<0.01, stratified Log Rank). The estimated 5-year relapse-free survival rate, using the Kaplan-Meier method, was 37% for INTRON A-treated patients versus 26% for observation patients. Median overall survival time for INTRON A-treated patients versus observation patients was 3.82 years versus 2.78 years (P=0.047, stratified Log Rank). The estimated 5-year overall survival rate, using the Kaplan-Meier method, was 46% for INTRON A-treated patients versus 37% for observation patients.

In a second study of 642 resected high-risk melanoma patients, subjects were randomized equally to one of three groups: high-dose INTRON A therapy for 1 year (same schedule as above), low-dose INTRON A therapy for 2 years (3 MU/d TIW SC), and observation. Consistent with the earlier trial, high-dose INTRON A therapy demonstrated an improvement in relapse-free survival (3-year estimated RFS 48% versus 41%; median RFS 2.4 versus 1.6 years, P=not significant). Relapse-free survival in the low-dose INTRON A arm was similar to that seen in the observation arm. Neither high-dose nor low-dose INTRON A therapy showed a benefit in overall survival as compared to observation in this study.

Follicular Lymphoma

The safety and efficacy of INTRON A in conjunction with CHVP, a combination chemotherapy regimen, was evaluated as initial treatment in patients with clinically aggressive, large tumor burden, Stage III/IV follicular Non-Hodgkin's Lymphoma. Large tumor burden was defined by the presence of any one of the following: a nodal or extranodal tumor mass with a diameter of greater than 7 cm; involvement of at least three nodal sites (each with a diameter of greater than 3 cm); systemic symptoms; splenomegaly; serous effusion, orbital or epidural involvement; ureteral compression; or leukemia.

In a randomized, controlled trial, 130 patients received CHVP therapy and 135 patients received CHVP therapy plus INTRON A therapy at 5 million IU subcutaneously three times weekly for the duration of 18 months. CHVP chemotherapy consisted of cyclophosphamide 600 mg/m^2, doxorubicin 25 mg/m^2, and teniposide (VM-26) 60 mg/m^2, administered intravenously on Day 1 and prednisone at a daily dose of 40 mg/m^2 given orally on Days 1 to 5. Treatment consisted of six CHVP cycles administered monthly, followed by an additional six cycles administered every 2 months for 1 year. Patients in both treatment groups received a total of 12 CHVP cycles over 18 months.

The group receiving the combination of INTRON A therapy plus CHVP had a significantly longer progression-free survival (2.9 years versus 1.5 years, P=0.0001, Log Rank test). After a median follow-up of 6.1 years, the median survival for patients treated with CHVP alone was 5.5 years while median survival for patients treated with CHVP plus INTRON A therapy had not been reached (P=0.004, Log Rank test). In three additional published, randomized, controlled studies of the addition of interferon alpha to anthracycline-containing combination chemotherapy regi-

Powder for Injection

Vial Strength Million IU	mL Diluent	Final Concentration after Reconstitution million IU/mL*	mg INTRON A[†] per vial	Route of Administration
10	1	10	0.038	IM, SC, IV, IL
18	1	18	0.069	IM, SC, IV
50	1	50	0.192	IM, SC, IV

* Each mL also contains 20 mg glycine, 2.3 mg sodium phosphate dibasic, 0.55 mg sodium phosphate monobasic, and 1.0 mg human albumin.
† Based on the specific activity of approximately 2.6×10^8 IU/mg protein, as measured by HPLC assay.

Solution Vials for Injection

Vial Strength	Concentration*	mg INTRON A[†] per vial	Route of Administration
18[‡] MIU multidose	3 million IU/0.5 mL	0.088	IM, SC
25[§] MIU multidose	5 million IU/0.5 mL	0.123	IM, SC, IL

* Each mL contains 7.5 mg sodium chloride, 1.8 mg sodium phosphate dibasic, 1.3 mg sodium phosphate monobasic, 0.1 mg edetate disodium, 0.1 mg polysorbate 80, and 1.5 mg m-cresol as a preservative.
† Based on the specific activity of approximately 2.6×10^8 IU/mg protein as measured by HPLC assay.
‡ This is a multidose vial which contains a total of 22.8 million IU of interferon alfa-2b, recombinant per 3.8 mL in order to provide the delivery of six 0.5-mL doses, each containing 3 million IU of INTRON A (for a label strength of 18 million IU).
§ This is a multidose vial which contains a total of 32.0 million IU of interferon alfa-2b, recombinant per 3.2 mL in order to provide the delivery of five 0.5-mL doses, each containing 5 million IU of INTRON A (for a label strength of 25 million IU).

mens,[1–3] the addition of interferon alpha was associated with significantly prolonged progression-free survival. Differences in overall survival were not consistently observed.

Condylomata Acuminata

Condylomata acuminata (venereal or genital warts) are associated with infections of the human papilloma virus (HPV). The safety and efficacy of INTRON A in the treatment of condylomata acuminata were evaluated in three controlled double-blind clinical trials. In these studies, INTRON A doses of 1 million IU per lesion were administered intralesionally three times a week (TIW), in less than or equal to 5 lesions per patient for 3 weeks. The patients were observed for up to 16 weeks after completion of the full treatment course.

INTRON A treatment of condylomata was significantly more effective than placebo, as measured by disappearance of lesions, decreases in lesion size, and by an overall change in disease status. Of 192 INTRON A-treated patients and 206 placebo-treated patients who were evaluable for efficacy at the time of best response during the course of the study, 42% of INTRON A patients versus 17% of placebo patients experienced clearing of all treated lesions. Likewise, 24% of INTRON A patients versus 8% of placebo patients experienced marked (75% to less than 100%) reduction in lesion size, 18% versus 9% experienced moderate (50% to 75%) reduction in lesion size, 10% versus 42% had a slight (less than 50%) reduction in lesion size, 5% versus 24% had no change in lesion size, and 0% versus 1% experienced exacerbation (P<0.001).

In one of these studies, 43% (54/125) of patients in whom multiple (less than or equal to 3) lesions were treated experienced complete clearing of all treated lesions during the course of the study. Of these patients, 81% remained cleared 16 weeks after treatment was initiated.

Patients who did not achieve total clearing of all their treated lesions had these same lesions treated with a second course of therapy. During this second course of treatment, 38% to 67% of patients had clearing of all treated lesions. The overall percentage of patients who had cleared all their treated lesions after two courses of treatment ranged from 57% to 85%.

INTRON A-treated lesions showed improvement within 2 to 4 weeks after the start of treatment in the above study; maximal response to INTRON A therapy was noted 4 to 8 weeks after initiation of treatment.

The response to INTRON A therapy was better in patients who had condylomata for shorter durations than in patients with lesions for a longer duration.

Another study involved 97 patients in whom three lesions were treated with either an intralesional injection of 1.5 million IU of INTRON A per lesion followed by a topical application of 25% podophyllin, or a topical application of 25% podophyllin alone. Treatment was given once a week for 3 weeks. The combined treatment of INTRON A and podophyllin was shown to be significantly more effective than podophyllin alone, as determined by the number of patients whose lesions cleared. This significant difference in response was evident after the second treatment (Week 3) and continued through 8 weeks post-treatment. At the time of the patient's best response, 67% (33/49) of the INTRON A- and podophyllin-treated patients had all three treated lesions clear while 42% (20/48) of the podophyllin-treated patients had all three clear (P=0.003).

AIDS-Related Kaposi's Sarcoma

The safety and efficacy of INTRON A in the treatment of Kaposi's Sarcoma (KS), a common manifestation of the Acquired Immune Deficiency Syndrome (AIDS), were evaluated in clinical trials in 144 patients.

In one study, INTRON A doses of 30 million IU/m[2] were administered subcutaneously three times per week (TIW) to patients with AIDS-Related KS. Doses were adjusted for patient tolerance. The average weekly dose delivered in the first 4 weeks was 150 million IU; at the end of 12 weeks this averaged 110 million IU/week; and by 24 weeks averaged 75 million IU/week.

Forty-four percent of asymptomatic patients responded versus 7% of symptomatic patients. The median time to response was approximately 2 months and 1 month, respectively, for asymptomatic and symptomatic patients. The median duration of response was approximately 3 months and 1 month, respectively, for the asymptomatic and symptomatic patients. Baseline T4/T8 ratios were 0.46 for responders versus 0.33 for nonresponders.

In another study, INTRON A doses of 35 million IU were administered subcutaneously, daily (QD), for 12 weeks. Maintenance treatment, with every other day dosing (QOD), was continued for up to 1 year in patients achieving antitumor and antiviral responses. The median time to response was 2 months and the median duration of response was 5 months in the asymptomatic patients.

In all studies, the likelihood of response was greatest in patients with relatively intact immune systems as assessed by baseline CD4 counts (interchangeable with T4 counts). Results at doses of 30 million IU/m[2] TIW and 35 million IU/QD

were subcutaneously similar and are provided together in TABLE 1. This table demonstrates the relationship of response to baseline CD4 count in both asymptomatic and symptomatic patients in the 30 million IU/m[2] TIW and the 35 million IU/QD treatment groups.

In the 30 million IU study group, 7% (5/72) of patients were complete responders and 22% (16/72) of the patients were partial responders. The 35 million IU study had 13% (3/23 patients) complete responders and 17% (4/23) partial responders.

For patients who received 30 million IU TIW, the median survival time was longer in patients with CD4 greater than 200 (30.7 months) than in patients with CD4 less than or equal to 200 (8.9 months). Among responders, the median survival time was 22.6 months versus 9.7 months in nonresponders.

Chronic Hepatitis C

The safety and efficacy of INTRON A in the treatment of chronic hepatitis C was evaluated in 5 randomized clinical studies in which an INTRON A dose of 3 million IU three times a week (TIW) was assessed. The initial three studies were placebo-controlled trials that evaluated a 6-month (24-week) course of therapy. In each of the three studies, INTRON A therapy resulted in a reduction in serum alanine aminotransferase (ALT) in a greater proportion of patients versus control patients at the end of 6 months of dosing. During the 6 months of follow-up, approximately 50% of the patients who responded maintained their ALT response. A combined analysis comparing pretreatment and post-treatment liver biopsies revealed histological improvement in a statistically significantly greater proportion of INTRON A-treated patients compared to controls.

Two additional studies have investigated longer treatment durations (up to 24 months).[5,6] Patients in the two studies to evaluate longer duration of treatment had hepatitis with or without cirrhosis in the absence of decompensated liver disease. Complete response to treatment was defined as normalization of the final two serum ALT levels during the treatment period. A sustained response was defined as a complete response at the end of the treatment period, with sustained normal ALT values lasting at least 6 months following discontinuation of therapy.

In Study 1, all patients were initially treated with INTRON A 3 million IU TIW subcutaneously for 24 weeks (run-in period). Patients who completed the initial 24-week treatment period were then randomly assigned to receive no further treatment, or to receive 3 million IU TIW for an additional 48 weeks. In Study 2, patients who met the entry criteria were randomly assigned to receive INTRON A 3 million IU TIW subcutaneously for 24 weeks or to receive INTRON A 3 million IU TIW subcutaneously for 96 weeks. In both studies, patient follow-up was variable and some data collection was retrospective.

Results show that longer durations of INTRON A therapy improved the sustained response rate (see TABLE 2). In patients with complete responses (CR) to INTRON A therapy after 6 months of treatment (149/352 [42%]), responses were less often sustained if drug was discontinued (21/70 [30%]) than if it was continued for 18 to 24 months (44/79 [56%]). Of all patients randomized, the sustained response rate in the patients receiving 18 or 24 months of therapy was 22% and 26%, respectively, in the two trials. In patients who did not have a CR by 6 months, additional therapy did not result in significantly more responses, since almost all patients who responded to therapy did so within the first 16 weeks of treatment.

A subset (less than 50%) of patients from the combined extended dosing studies had liver biopsies performed both before and after INTRON A treatment. Improvement in necroinflammatory activity as assessed retrospectively by the Knodell (Study 1) and Scheuer (Study 2) Histology Activity Indices was observed in both studies. A higher number of patients (58%, 45/78) improved with extended therapy than with shorter (6 months) therapy (38%, 34/89) in this subset. Combination treatment with INTRON A and REBETOL® (ribavirin USP) provided a significant reduction in virologic load and improved histologic response in adult patients with compensated liver disease who were treatment-naïve or had relapsed following therapy with alpha interferon alone; pediatric patients previously untreated with alpha interferon experienced a sustained virologic response. See REBETOL prescribing information for additional information.

Chronic Hepatitis B

Adults

The safety and efficacy of INTRON A in the treatment of chronic hepatitis B were evaluated in three clinical trials in which INTRON A doses of 30 to 35 million IU per week were administered subcutaneously (SC), as either 5 million IU daily (QD), or 10 million IU three times a week (TIW) for 16 weeks versus no treatment. All patients were 18 years of age or older with compensated liver disease, and had chronic hepatitis B virus (HBV) infection (serum HBsAg positive for at least 6 months) and HBV replication (serum

HBeAg positive). Patients were also serum HBV-DNA positive, an additional indicator of HBV replication, as measured by a research assay.[7,8] All patients had elevated serum alanine aminotransferase (ALT) and liver biopsy findings compatible with the diagnosis of chronic hepatitis. Patients with the presence of antibody to human immunodeficiency virus (anti-HIV) or antibody to hepatitis delta virus (anti-HDV) in the serum were excluded from the studies.

Virologic response to treatment was defined in these studies as a loss of serum markers of HBV replication (HBeAg and HBV DNA). Secondary parameters of response included loss of serum HBsAg, decreases in serum ALT, and improvement in liver histology.

In each of two randomized controlled studies, a significantly greater proportion of INTRON A-treated patients exhibited a virologic response compared with untreated control patients (see TABLE 3). In a third study without a concurrent control group, a similar response rate to INTRON A therapy was observed. Pretreatment with prednisone, evaluated in two of the studies, did not improve the response rate and provided no additional benefit.

The response to INTRON A therapy was durable. No patient responding to INTRON A therapy at a dose of 5 million IU QD or 10 million IU TIW relapsed during the follow-up period, which ranged from 2 to 6 months after treatment ended. The loss of serum HBeAg and HBV DNA was maintained in 100% of 19 responding patients followed for 3.5 to 36 months after the end of therapy.

In a proportion of responding patients, loss of HBeAg was followed by the loss of HBsAg. HBsAg was lost in 27% (4/15) of patients who responded to INTRON A therapy at a dose of 5 million IU QD, and 35% (8/23) of patients who responded to 10 million IU TIW. No untreated control patient lost HBsAg in these studies.

In an ongoing study to assess the long-term durability of virologic response, 64 patients responding to INTRON A therapy have been followed for 1.1 to 6.6 years after treatment; 95% (61/64) remain serum HBeAg negative, and 49% (30/61) lost serum HBsAg.

INTRON A therapy resulted in normalization of serum ALT in a significantly greater proportion of treated patients compared to untreated patients in each of two controlled studies (see TABLE 4). In a third study without a concurrent control group, normalization of serum ALT was observed in 50% (12/24) of patients receiving INTRON A therapy.

Virologic response was associated with a reduction in serum ALT to normal or near normal (less than or equal to 1.5 × the upper limit of normal) in 87% (13/15) of patients responding to INTRON A therapy at 5 million IU QD, and 100% (23/23) of patients responding to 10 million IU TIW. Improvement in liver histology was evaluated in Studies 1 and 3 by comparison of pretreatment and 6-month post-treatment liver biopsies using the semiquantitative Knodell Histology Activity Index.[9] No statistically significant difference in liver histology was observed in treated patients compared to control patients in Study 1. Although statistically significant histological improvement from baseline was observed in treated patients in Study 3 (P≤0.01), there was no control group for comparison. Of those patients exhibiting a virologic response following treatment with 5 million IU QD or 10 million IU TIW, histological improvement was observed in 85% (17/20) compared to 36% (9/25) of patients who were not virologic responders. The histological improvement was due primarily to decreases in severity of necrosis, degeneration, and inflammation in the periportal, lobular, and portal regions of the liver (Knodell Categories I + II + III). Continued histological improvement was observed in four responding patients who lost serum HBsAg and were followed 2 to 4 years after the end of INTRON A therapy.[10]

Pediatrics

The safety and efficacy of INTRON A in the treatment of chronic hepatitis B was evaluated in one randomized controlled trial of 149 patients ranging from 1 year to 17 years of age. Seventy-two patients were treated with 3 million IU/m[2] of INTRON A therapy administered subcutaneously three times a week (TIW) for 1 week; the dose was then escalated to 6 million IU/m[2] TIW for a minimum of 16 weeks up to 24 weeks. The maximum weekly dosage was 10 million IU TIW. Seventy-seven patients were untreated controls. Study entry and response criteria were identical to those described in the adult patient population.

Patients treated with INTRON A therapy had a better response (loss of HBV DNA and HBeAg at 24 weeks of follow-up) compared to the untreated controls (24% [17/72] versus 10% [8/77] P=0.05). Sixteen of the 17 responders treated with INTRON A therapy remained HBV DNA and HBeAg negative and had a normal serum ALT 12 to 24 months after completion of treatment. Serum HBsAg became negative in 7 out of 17 patients who responded to INTRON A therapy. None of the control patients who had an HBV DNA and HBeAg response became HBsAg negative. At 24 weeks of follow-up, normalization of serum ALT was similar in patients treated with INTRON A therapy (17%, 12/72) and in untreated control patients (16%, 12/77). Patients with a baseline HBV DNA less than 100 pg/mL were more likely to respond to INTRON A therapy than were patients with a baseline HBV DNA greater than 100 pg/mL (35% versus 9%, respectively). Patients who contracted hepatitis B through maternal vertical transmission had lower response rates than those who contracted the disease by other means (5% versus 31%, respectively). There was no evidence that the effects on HBV DNA and HBeAg were limited to specific subpopulations based on age, gender, or race.

[See table 1 above]
[See table 2 above]
[See table 3 above]
[See table 4 above]

INDICATIONS AND USAGE

Hairy Cell Leukemia

INTRON® A is indicated for the treatment of patients 18 years of age or older with hairy cell leukemia.

Malignant Melanoma

INTRON A is indicated as adjuvant to surgical treatment in patients 18 years of age or older with malignant melanoma who are free of disease but at high risk for systemic recurrence, within 56 days of surgery.

Follicular Lymphoma

INTRON A is indicated for the initial treatment of clinically aggressive (see **Clinical Pharmacology**) follicular Non-Hodgkin's Lymphoma in conjunction with anthracycline-containing combination chemotherapy in patients 18 years of age or older. Efficacy of INTRON A therapy in patients with low-grade, low-tumor burden follicular Non-Hodgkin's Lymphoma has not been demonstrated.

Condylomata Acuminata

INTRON A is indicated for intralesional treatment of selected patients 18 years of age or older with condylomata acuminata involving external surfaces of the genital and perianal areas (see **DOSAGE AND ADMINISTRATION**). The use of this product in adolescents has not been studied.

AIDS-Related Kaposi's Sarcoma

INTRON A is indicated for the treatment of selected patients 18 years of age or older with AIDS-Related Kaposi's Sarcoma. The likelihood of response to INTRON A therapy is greater in patients who are without systemic symptoms, who have limited lymphadenopathy and who have a relatively intact immune system as indicated by total CD4 count.

Chronic Hepatitis C

INTRON A is indicated for the treatment of chronic hepatitis C in patients 18 years of age or older with compensated liver disease who have a history of blood or blood-product exposure and/or are HCV antibody positive. Studies in these patients demonstrated that INTRON A therapy can produce clinically meaningful effects on this disease, manifested by normalization of serum alanine aminotransferase (ALT) and reduction in liver necrosis and degeneration.

A liver biopsy should be performed to establish the diagnosis of chronic hepatitis. Patients should be tested for the presence of antibody to HCV. Patients with other causes of chronic hepatitis, including autoimmune hepatitis, should be excluded. Prior to initiation of INTRON A therapy, the physician should establish that the patient has compensated liver disease. The following patient entrance criteria for compensated liver disease were used in the clinical studies and should be considered before INTRON A treatment of patients with chronic hepatitis C:

- No history of hepatic encephalopathy, variceal bleeding, ascites, or other clinical signs of decompensation
- Bilirubin — Less than or equal to 2 mg/dL
- Albumin — Stable and within normal limits
- Prothrombin Time — Less than 3 seconds prolonged
- WBC — Greater than or equal to 3000/mm³
- Platelets — Greater than or equal to 70,000/mm³

Serum creatinine should be normal or near normal.

Prior to initiation of INTRON A therapy, CBC and platelet counts should be evaluated in order to establish baselines for monitoring potential toxicity. These tests should be repeated at Weeks 1 and 2 following initiation of INTRON A therapy, and monthly thereafter. Serum ALT should be evaluated at approximately 3-month intervals to assess response to treatment (see **DOSAGE AND ADMINISTRATION**).

Patients with preexisting thyroid abnormalities may be treated if thyroid-stimulating hormone (TSH) levels can be maintained in the normal range by medication. TSH levels must be within normal limits upon initiation of INTRON A treatment and TSH testing should be repeated at 3 and 6 months (see **PRECAUTIONS, Laboratory Tests**).

INTRON A in combination with REBETOL® is indicated for the treatment of chronic hepatitis C in patients 3 years of age and older with compensated liver disease previously untreated with alpha interferon therapy and in patients 18 years of age and older who have relapsed following alpha interferon therapy. See REBETOL prescribing information for additional information.

Chronic Hepatitis B

INTRON A is indicated for the treatment of chronic hepatitis B in patients 1 year of age or older with compensated liver disease. Patients who have been serum HBsAg positive for at least 6 months and have evidence of HBV replication (serum HBeAg positive) with elevated serum ALT are candidates for treatment. Studies in these patients demonstrated that INTRON A therapy can produce virologic remission of this disease (loss of serum HBeAg) and normalization of serum aminotransferases. INTRON A therapy resulted in the loss of serum HBsAg in some responding patients.

Prior to initiation of INTRON A therapy, it is recommended that a liver biopsy be performed to establish the presence of chronic hepatitis and the extent of liver damage. The physician should establish that the patient has compensated liver disease. The following patient entrance criteria for compensated liver disease were used in the clinical studies and should be considered before INTRON A treatment of patients with chronic hepatitis B:

- No history of hepatic encephalopathy, variceal bleeding, ascites, or other signs of clinical decompensation
- Bilirubin — Normal
- Albumin — Stable and within normal limits
- Prothrombin Time — *Adults* less than 3 seconds prolonged

TABLE 1 RESPONSE BY BASELINE CD4 COUNT* IN AIDS-RELATED KS PATIENTS

	30 million IU/m² TIW, SC and 35 million IU QD, SC			
	Asymptomatic		Symptomatic	
CD4<200	4/14	(29%)	0/19	(0%)
200≤CD4≤400	6/12	(50%)	0/5	(0%)
		} 58%		
CD4>400	5/7	(71%)	0/0	(0%)

* Data for CD4, and asymptomatic and symptomatic classification were not available for all patients.

TABLE 2 SUSTAINED ALT RESPONSE RATE VERSUS DURATION OF THERAPY IN CHRONIC HEPATITIS C PATIENTS INTRON A 3 Million IU TIW

	Treatment Group*- Number of Patients (%)		
Study Number	INTRON A 3 million IU 24 weeks of treatment	INTRON A 3 million IU 72 or 96 weeks of treatment†	Difference (Extended - 24 weeks) (95% CI)‡
	ALT response at the end of follow-up		
1	12/101 (12%)	23/104 (22%)	10% (-3, 24)
2	9/67 (13%)	21/80 (26%)	13% (-4, 30)
Combined Studies	21/168 (12.5%)	44/184 (24%)	11.4% (2, 21)
	ALT response at the end of treatment		
1	40/101 (40%)	51/104 (49%)	--
2	32/67 (48%)	35/80 (44%)	--

* Intent-to-treat groups.
† Study 1: 72 weeks of treatment; Study 2: 96 weeks of treatment.
‡ Confidence intervals adjusted for multiple comparisons due to 3 treatment arms in the study.

TABLE 3 VIROLOGIC RESPONSE* IN CHRONIC HEPATITIS B PATIENTS

	Treatment Group† - Number of Patients (%)						
Study Number	INTRON A 5 million IU QD		INTRON A 10 million IU TIW		Untreated Controls		P‡ Value
1[7]	15/38	(39%)	--	--	3/42	(7%)	0.0009
2	--	--	10/24	(42%)	1/22	(5%)	0.005
3[8]	--	--	13/24§	(54%)	2/27	(7%)§	NA§
All Studies	15/38	(39%)	23/48	(48%)	6/91	(7%)	--

* Loss of HBeAg and HBV DNA by 6 months post-therapy.
† Patients pretreated with prednisone not shown.
‡ INTRON A treatment group versus untreated control.
§ Untreated control patients evaluated after 24-week observation period. A subgroup subsequently received INTRON A therapy. A direct comparison is not applicable (NA).

TABLE 4 ALT RESPONSES* IN CHRONIC HEPATITIS B PATIENTS

	Treatment Group - Number of Patients (%)						
Study Number	INTRON A 5 million IU QD		INTRON A 10 million IU TIW		Untreated Controls		P† Value
1	16/38	(42%)	--	--	8/42	(19%)	0.03
2	--	--	10/24	(42%)	1/22	(5%)	0.0034
3	--	--	12/24‡	(50%)	2/27	(7%)‡	NA‡
All Studies	16/38	(42%)	22/48	(46%)	11/91	(12%)	--

* Reduction in serum ALT to normal by 6 months post-therapy.
† INTRON A treatment group versus untreated control.
‡ Untreated control patients evaluated after 24-week observation period. A subgroup subsequently received INTRON A therapy. A direct comparison is not applicable (NA).

- • WBC
- • Platelets

Pediatrics less than or equal to 2 seconds prolonged

Greater than or equal to 4000/mm^3
Adults greater than or equal to 100,000/mm^3
Pediatrics greater than or equal to 150,000/mm^3

Patients with causes of chronic hepatitis other than chronic hepatitis B or chronic hepatitis C should not be treated with INTRON A. CBC and platelet counts should be evaluated prior to initiation of INTRON A therapy in order to establish baselines for monitoring potential toxicity. These tests should be repeated at treatment Weeks 1, 2, 4, 8, 12, and 16. Liver function tests, including serum ALT, albumin, and bilirubin, should be evaluated at treatment Weeks 1, 2, 4, 8, 12, and 16. HBeAg, HBsAg, and ALT should be evaluated at the end of therapy, as well as 3- and 6-months post-therapy, since patients may become virologic responders during the 6-month period following the end of treatment. In clinical studies in adults, 39% (15/38) of responding patients lost HBeAg 1 to 6 months following the end of INTRON A therapy. Of responding patients who lost HBsAg, 58% (7/12) did so 1 to 6 months post-treatment.

A transient increase in ALT greater than or equal to 2 times baseline value (flare) can occur during INTRON A therapy for chronic hepatitis B. In clinical trials in adults and pediatrics, this flare generally occurred 8 to 12 weeks after initiation of therapy and was more frequent in responders (*adults* 63%, 24/38; *pediatrics* 59%, 10/17) than in nonresponders (*adults* 27%, 13/48; *pediatrics* 35%, 19/55). However, in adults and pediatrics, elevations in bilirubin greater than or equal to 3 mg/dL (greater than or equal to 2 times ULN) occurred infrequently (*adults* 2%, 2/86; *pediatrics* 3%, 2/72) during therapy. When ALT flare occurs, in general, INTRON A therapy should be continued unless signs and symptoms of liver failure are observed. During ALT flare, clinical symptomatology and liver function tests including ALT, prothrombin time, alkaline phosphatase, albumin, and bilirubin, should be monitored at approximately 2-week intervals (see **WARNINGS**).

CONTRAINDICATIONS

INTRON® A is contraindicated in patients with:
- • Hypersensitivity to interferon alpha or any component of the product
- • Autoimmune hepatitis
- • Decompensated liver disease

INTRON A and REBETOL® combination therapy is additionally contraindicated in:
- • Patients with hypersensitivity to ribavirin or any other component of the product
- • Women who are pregnant
- • Men whose female partners are pregnant
- • Patients with hemoglobinopathies (e.g., thalassemia major, sickle cell anemia)
- • Patients with creatinine clearance less than 50 mL/min.

See REBETOL prescribing information for additional information.

WARNINGS

General

Moderate to severe adverse experiences may require modification of the patient's dosage regimen, or in some cases termination of INTRON® A therapy. Because of the fever and other "flu-like" symptoms associated with INTRON A administration, it should be used cautiously in patients with debilitating medical conditions, such as those with a history of pulmonary disease (e.g., chronic obstructive pulmonary disease) or diabetes mellitus prone to ketoacidosis. Caution should also be observed in patients with coagulation disorders (e.g., thrombophlebitis, pulmonary embolism) or severe myelosuppression.

Cardiovascular Disorders

INTRON A therapy should be used cautiously in patients with a history of cardiovascular disease. Those patients with a history of myocardial infarction and/or previous or current arrhythmic disorder who require INTRON A therapy should be closely monitored (see **PRECAUTIONS, Laboratory Tests**). Cardiovascular adverse experiences, which include hypotension, arrhythmia, or tachycardia of 150 beats per minute or greater, and rarely, cardiomyopathy and myocardial infarction have been observed in some INTRON A-treated patients. Some patients with these adverse events had no history of cardiovascular disease. Transient cardiomyopathy was reported in approximately 2% of the AIDS-Related Kaposi's Sarcoma patients treated with INTRON A. Hypotension may occur during INTRON A administration, or up to 2 days post-therapy, and may require supportive therapy including fluid replacement to maintain intravascular volume.

Supraventricular arrhythmias occurred rarely and appeared to be correlated with preexisting conditions and prior therapy with cardiotoxic agents. These adverse experiences were controlled by modifying the dose or discontinuing treatment, but may require specific additional therapy.

Cerebrovascular Disorders

Ischemic and hemorrhagic cerebrovascular events have been observed in patients treated with interferon alpha-based therapies, including INTRON A. Events occurred in patients with few or no reported risk factors for stroke, including patients less than 45 years of age. Because these are spontaneous reports, estimates of frequency cannot be made and a causal relationship between interferon alpha-based therapies and these events is difficult to establish.

Neuropsychiatric Disorders

DEPRESSION AND SUICIDAL BEHAVIOR INCLUDING SUICIDAL IDEATION, SUICIDAL ATTEMPTS, AND COMPLETED SUICIDES, HOMICIDAL IDEATION, AND AGGRESSIVE BEHAVIOR SOMETIMES DIRECTED TOWARDS OTHERS, HAVE BEEN REPORTED IN ASSOCIATION WITH TREATMENT WITH ALPHA INTERFERONS, INCLUDING INTRON A THERAPY. If patients develop psychiatric problems, including clinical depression, it is recommended that the patients be carefully monitored during treatment and in the 6-month follow-up period. INTRON A should be used with caution in patients with a history of psychiatric disorders. INTRON A therapy should be discontinued for any patient developing severe psychiatric disorder during treatment. Obtundation and coma have also been observed in some patients, usually elderly, treated at higher doses. While these effects are usually rapidly reversible upon discontinuation of therapy, full resolution of symptoms has taken up to 3 weeks in a few severe episodes. If psychiatric symptoms persist or worsen, or suicidal ideation or aggressive behavior towards others is identified, it is recommended that treatment with INTRON A be discontinued and the patient followed, with psychiatric intervention as appropriate. Narcotics, hypnotics, or sedatives may be used concurrently with caution and patients should be closely monitored until the adverse effects have resolved. Suicidal ideation or attempts occurred more frequently among pediatric patients, primarily adolescents, compared to adult patients (2.4% versus 1%) during treatment and off-therapy follow-up. Cases of encephalopathy have also been observed in some patients, usually elderly, treated with higher doses of INTRON A.

Treatment with interferons may be associated with exacerbated symptoms of psychiatric disorders in patients with co-occurring psychiatric and substance use disorders. If treatment with interferons is initiated in patients with prior history or existence of psychiatric condition or with a history of substance use disorders, treatment considerations should include the need for drug screening and periodic health evaluation, including psychiatric symptom monitoring. Early intervention for re-emergence or development of neuropsychiatric symptoms and substance use is recommended.

Bone Marrow Toxicity

INTRON A therapy suppresses bone marrow function and may result in severe cytopenias including aplastic anemia. It is advised that complete blood counts (CBC) be obtained pretreatment and monitored routinely during therapy (see **PRECAUTIONS, Laboratory Tests**). INTRON A therapy should be discontinued in patients who develop severe decreases in neutrophil (less than 0.5×10^9/L) or platelet counts (less than 25×10^9/L) (see **DOSAGE AND ADMINISTRATION, Guidelines for Dose Modification**).

Ophthalmologic Disorders

Decrease or loss of vision, retinopathy including macular edema, retinal artery or vein thrombosis, retinal hemorrhages and cotton wool spots; optic neuritis, papilledema, and serous retinal detachment may be induced or aggravated by treatment with interferon alfa-2b or other alpha interferons. All patients should receive an eye examination at baseline. Patients with preexisting ophthalmologic disorders (e.g., diabetic or hypertensive retinopathy) should receive periodic ophthalmologic exams during interferon alpha treatment. Any patient who develops ocular symptoms should receive a prompt and complete eye examination. Interferon alfa-2b treatment should be discontinued in patients who develop new or worsening ophthalmologic disorders.

Endocrine Disorders

Infrequently, patients receiving INTRON A therapy developed thyroid abnormalities, either hypothyroid or hyperthyroid. The mechanism by which INTRON A may alter thyroid status is unknown. Patients with preexisting thyroid abnormalities whose thyroid function cannot be maintained in the normal range by medication should not be treated with INTRON A. Prior to initiation of INTRON A therapy, serum TSH should be evaluated. Patients developing symptoms consistent with possible thyroid dysfunction during the course of INTRON A therapy should have their thyroid function evaluated and appropriate treatment instituted. Therapy should be discontinued for patients developing thyroid abnormalities during treatment whose thyroid function cannot be normalized by medication. Discontinuation of INTRON A therapy has not always reversed thyroid dysfunction occurring during treatment. Diabetes mellitus has been observed in patients treated with alpha interferons. Patients with these conditions who cannot be effectively treated by medication should not begin INTRON A therapy. Patients who develop these conditions during treatment and cannot be controlled with medication should not continue INTRON A therapy.

Gastrointestinal Disorders

Hepatotoxicity, including fatality, has been observed in interferon alpha-treated patients, including those treated with INTRON A. Any patient developing liver function abnormalities during treatment should be monitored closely and if appropriate, treatment should be discontinued.

Pulmonary Disorders

Dyspnea, pulmonary infiltrates, pneumonia, bronchiolitis obliterans, interstitial pneumonitis, pulmonary hypertension, and sarcoidosis, some resulting in respiratory failure and/or patient deaths, may be induced or aggravated by INTRON A or other alpha interferons. Recurrence of respiratory failure has been observed with interferon rechallenge. The etiologic explanation for these pulmonary findings has yet to be established. Any patient developing fever, cough, dyspnea, or other respiratory symptoms should have a chest X-ray taken. If the chest X-ray shows pulmonary infiltrates or there is evidence of pulmonary function impairment, the patient should be closely monitored, and, if appropriate, interferon alpha treatment should be discontinued. While this has been reported more often in patients with chronic hepatitis C treated with interferon alpha, it has also been reported in patients with oncologic diseases treated with interferon alpha.

Autoimmune Disorders

Rare cases of autoimmune diseases including thrombocytopenia, vasculitis, Raynaud's phenomenon, rheumatoid arthritis, lupus erythematosus, and rhabdomyolysis have been observed in patients treated with alpha interferons, including patients treated with INTRON A. In very rare cases the event resulted in fatality. The mechanism by which these events developed and their relationship to interferon alpha therapy is not clear. Any patient developing an autoimmune disorder during treatment should be closely monitored and, if appropriate, treatment should be discontinued.

Human Albumin

The powder formulations of this product contain albumin, a derivative of human blood. Based on effective donor screening and product manufacturing processes, it carries an extremely remote risk for transmission of viral diseases. A theoretical risk for transmission of Creutzfeldt-Jakob disease (CJD) also is considered extremely remote. No cases of transmission of viral diseases or CJD have ever been identified for albumin.

AIDS-Related Kaposi's Sarcoma

INTRON A therapy should not be used for patients with rapidly progressive visceral disease (see **CLINICAL PHARMACOLOGY**). Also of note, there may be synergistic adverse effects between INTRON A and zidovudine. Patients receiving concomitant zidovudine have had a higher incidence of neutropenia than that expected with zidovudine alone. Careful monitoring of the WBC count is indicated in all patients who are myelosuppressed and in all patients receiving other myelosuppressive medications. The effects of INTRON A when combined with other drugs used in the treatment of AIDS-related disease are unknown.

Chronic Hepatitis C and Chronic Hepatitis B

Patients with decompensated liver disease, autoimmune hepatitis or a history of autoimmune disease, and patients who are immunosuppressed transplant recipients should not be treated with INTRON A. There are reports of worsening liver disease, including jaundice, hepatic encephalopathy, hepatic failure, and death following INTRON A therapy in such patients. Therapy should be discontinued for any patient developing signs and symptoms of liver failure. Chronic hepatitis B patients with evidence of decreasing hepatic synthetic functions, such as decreasing albumin levels or prolongation of prothrombin time, who nevertheless meet the entry criteria to start therapy, may be at increased risk of clinical decompensation if a flare of aminotransferases occurs during INTRON A treatment. In such patients, if increases in ALT occur during INTRON A therapy for chronic hepatitis B, they should be followed carefully, including close monitoring of clinical symptomatology and liver function tests including ALT, prothrombin time, alkaline phosphatase, albumin, and bilirubin. In considering these patients for INTRON A therapy, the potential risks must be evaluated against the potential benefits of treatment.

Peripheral Neuropathy

Peripheral neuropathy has been reported when alpha interferons were given in combination with telbivudine. In one clinical trial, an increased risk and severity of peripheral neuropathy was observed with the combination use of telbivudine and pegylated interferon alfa-2a as compared to telbivudine alone. The safety and efficacy of telbivudine in combination with interferons for the treatment of chronic hepatitis B has not been demonstrated.

Use with Ribavirin
(See also REBETOL® prescribing information) REBETOL may cause birth defects and/or death of the unborn child. REBETOL therapy should not be started until a report of a negative pregnancy test has been obtained immediately prior to planned initiation of therapy. Patients should use at least two forms of contraception and have monthly pregnancy tests (see **CONTRAINDICATIONS** and **PRECAUTIONS, Information for Patients**).

Combination treatment with INTRON A and REBETOL was associated with hemolytic anemia. Hemoglobin less than 10 g/dL was observed in approximately 10% of adult and pediatric patients in clinical trials. Anemia occurred within 1 to 2 weeks of initiation of ribavirin therapy. Combination treatment with INTRON A and REBETOL should **not** be used in patients with creatinine clearance less than 50 mL/min. See REBETOL prescribing information for additional information.

PRECAUTIONS
General
Acute serious hypersensitivity reactions (e.g., urticaria, angioedema, bronchoconstriction, anaphylaxis) have been observed rarely in INTRON® A-treated patients; if such an acute reaction develops, the drug should be discontinued immediately and appropriate medical therapy instituted. Transient rashes have occurred in some patients following injection, but have not necessitated treatment interruption. While fever may be related to the flu-like syndrome reported commonly in patients treated with interferon, other causes of persistent fever should be ruled out.

There have been reports of interferon, including INTRON A, exacerbating preexisting psoriasis and sarcoidosis as well as development of new sarcoidosis. Therefore, INTRON A therapy should be used in these patients only if the potential benefit justifies the potential risk.

Variations in dosage, routes of administration, and adverse reactions exist among different brands of interferon. Therefore, do not use different brands of interferon in any single treatment regimen.

Triglycerides
Elevated triglyceride levels have been observed in patients treated with interferons, including INTRON A therapy. Elevated triglyceride levels should be managed as clinically appropriate. Hypertriglyceridemia may result in pancreatitis. Discontinuation of INTRON A therapy should be considered for patients with persistently elevated triglycerides (e.g., triglycerides greater than 1000 mg/dL) associated with symptoms of potential pancreatitis, such as abdominal pain, nausea, or vomiting.

Drug Interactions
Interactions between INTRON A and other drugs have not been fully evaluated. Caution should be exercised when administering INTRON A therapy in combination with other potentially myelosuppressive agents such as zidovudine. Concomitant use of alpha interferon and theophylline decreases theophylline clearance, resulting in a 100% increase in serum theophylline levels.

Information for Patients
Patients receiving INTRON A alone or in combination with REBETOL® should be informed of the risks and benefits associated with treatment and should be instructed on proper use of the product. To supplement your discussion with a patient, you may wish to provide patients with a copy of the **MEDICATION GUIDE**.

Patients should be informed of, and advised to seek medical attention for, symptoms indicative of serious adverse reactions associated with this product. Such adverse reactions may include depression (suicidal ideation), cardiovascular (chest pain), ophthalmologic toxicity (decrease in/or loss of vision), pancreatitis or colitis (severe abdominal pain), and cytopenias (high persistent fevers, bruising, dyspnea). Patients should be advised that some side effects such as fatigue and decreased concentration might interfere with the ability to perform certain tasks. Patients who are taking INTRON A in combination with REBETOL must be thoroughly informed of the risks to a fetus. Female patients and female partners of male patients must be told to use two forms of birth control during treatment and for six months after therapy is discontinued (see **MEDICATION GUIDE**).

Patients should be advised to remain well hydrated during the initial stages of treatment and that use of an antipyretic may ameliorate some of the flu-like symptoms.

If a decision is made to allow a patient to self-administer INTRON A, they should be instructed, based on their treatment, if they should inject a dose of INTRON® A subcutaneously or intramuscularly. If it is too difficult for them to inject themselves, they should be instructed to ask someone who has been trained to give the injection to them. Patients should be instructed on the importance of site selection for self-administering the injection, as well as the importance on rotating the injection sites. A puncture resistant container for the disposal of needles and syringes should be supplied. Patients self-administering INTRON A should be instructed on the proper disposal of needles and syringes and cautioned against reuse.

Dental and Periodontal Disorders
Dental and periodontal disorders have been reported in patients receiving ribavirin and interferon combination therapy. In addition, dry mouth could have a damaging effect on teeth and mucous membranes of the mouth during long-term treatment with the combination of REBETOL and interferon alfa-2b. Patients should brush their teeth thoroughly twice daily and have regular dental examinations. In addition, some patients may experience vomiting. If this reaction occurs, they should be advised to rinse out their mouth thoroughly afterwards.

Laboratory Tests
In addition to those tests normally required for monitoring patients, the following laboratory tests are recommended for all patients on INTRON A therapy, prior to beginning treatment and then periodically thereafter.

• Standard hematologic tests - including hemoglobin, complete and differential white blood cell counts, and platelet count.

• Blood chemistries - electrolytes, liver function tests, and TSH.

Those patients who have preexisting cardiac abnormalities and/or are in advanced stages of cancer should have electrocardiograms taken prior to and during the course of treatment.

Mild-to-moderate leukopenia and elevated serum liver enzyme (SGOT) levels have been reported with intralesional administration of INTRON A (see **ADVERSE REACTIONS**); therefore, the monitoring of these laboratory parameters should be considered.

Baseline chest X-rays are suggested and should be repeated if clinically indicated.

For malignant melanoma patients, differential WBC count and liver function tests should be monitored weekly during the induction phase of therapy and monthly during the maintenance phase of therapy.

For specific recommendations in chronic hepatitis C and chronic hepatitis B, see **INDICATIONS AND USAGE**.

Carcinogenesis, Mutagenesis, Impairment of Fertility
Studies with INTRON A have not been performed to determine carcinogenicity.

Interferon may impair fertility. In studies of interferon administration in nonhuman primates, menstrual cycle abnormalities have been observed. Decreases in serum estradiol and progesterone concentrations have been reported in women treated with human leukocyte interferon.[12] Therefore, fertile women should not receive INTRON A therapy unless they are using effective contraception during the therapy period. INTRON A therapy should be used with caution in fertile men.

Mutagenicity studies have demonstrated that INTRON A is not mutagenic.

Studies in mice (0.1, 1.0 million IU/day), rats (4, 20, 100 million IU/kg/day), and cynomolgus monkeys (1.1 million IU/kg/day; 0.25, 0.75, 2.5 million IU/kg/day) injected with INTRON A for up to 9 days, 3 months, and 1 month, respectively, have revealed no evidence of toxicity. However, in cynomolgus monkeys (4, 20, 100 million IU/kg/day) injected daily for 3 months with INTRON A, toxicity was observed at the mid and high doses and mortality was observed at the high dose.

However, due to the known species-specificity of interferon, the effects in animals are unlikely to be predictive of those in man.

INTRON A in combination with REBETOL should be used with caution in fertile men. See the REBETOL prescribing information for additional information.

Pregnancy Category C
INTRON A has been shown to have abortifacient effects in *Macaca mulatta* (rhesus monkeys) at 15 and 30 million IU/kg (estimated human equivalent of 5 and 10 million IU/kg, based on body surface area adjustment for a 60-kg adult). There are no adequate and well-controlled studies in pregnant women. INTRON A therapy should be used during pregnancy only if the potential benefit justifies the potential risk to the fetus.

Pregnancy Category X applies to combination treatment with INTRON A and REBETOL (see **CONTRAINDICATIONS**). See REBETOL prescribing information for additional information. Significant teratogenic and/or embryocidal effects have been demonstrated in all animal species exposed to ribavirin. REBETOL therapy is contraindicated in women who are pregnant and in the male partners of women who are pregnant. See **CONTRAINDICATIONS** and the REBETOL prescribing information.

Ribavirin Pregnancy Registry: A Ribavirin Pregnancy Registry has been established to monitor maternal-fetal outcomes of pregnancies in female patients and female partners of male patients exposed to ribavirin during treatment and for 6 months following cessation of treatment. Physicians and patients are encouraged to report such cases by calling 1-800-593-2214.

Nursing Mothers
It is not known whether this drug is excreted in human milk. However, studies in mice have shown that mouse interferons are excreted into the milk. Because of the potential for serious adverse reactions from the drug in nursing infants, a decision should be made whether to discontinue nursing or to discontinue INTRON A therapy, taking into account the importance of the drug to the mother.

Pediatric Use
General
Safety and effectiveness in pediatric patients have not been established for indications other than chronic hepatitis B and chronic hepatitis C.

Chronic Hepatitis B
Safety and effectiveness in pediatric patients ranging in age from 1 to 17 years have been established based upon one controlled clinical trial (see **CLINICAL PHARMACOLOGY, INDICATIONS AND USAGE,** and **DOSAGE AND ADMINISTRATION, Chronic Hepatitis B Pediatrics**).

Chronic Hepatitis C
Safety and effectiveness in pediatric patients ranging in age from 3 to 16 years have been established based upon clinical studies in 118 patients. See REBETOL prescribing information for additional information. Suicidal ideation or attempts occurred more frequently among pediatric patients compared to adult patients (2.4% versus 1%) during treatment and off-therapy follow-up (see **WARNINGS, Neuropsychiatric Disorders**). During a 48-week course of therapy there was a decrease in the rate of linear growth (mean percentile assignment decrease of 7%) and a decrease in the rate of weight gain (mean percentile assignment decrease of 9%). A general reversal of these trends was noted during the 24-week post-treatment period.

Long-term data in a limited number of patients suggests that combination therapy may induce a growth inhibition that results in reduced final adult height in some patients (see **ADVERSE REACTIONS, Chronic Hepatitis C Pediatrics**).

Geriatric Use
In all clinical studies of INTRON A, including studies as monotherapy and in combination with REBETOL (ribavirin USP) Capsules, only a small percentage of the subjects were aged 65 and over. These numbers were too few to determine if they respond differently from younger subjects except for the clinical trials of INTRON A in combination with REBETOL, where elderly subjects had a higher frequency of anemia (67%) than did younger patients (28%).

In a database consisting of clinical study and postmarketing reports for various indications, cardiovascular adverse events and confusion were reported more frequently in elderly patients receiving INTRON A therapy compared to younger patients.

In general, INTRON A therapy should be administered to elderly patients cautiously, reflecting the greater frequency of decreased hepatic, renal, bone marrow, and/or cardiac function and concomitant disease or other drug therapy. INTRON A is known to be substantially excreted by the kidney, and the risk of adverse reactions to INTRON A may be greater in patients with impaired renal function. Because elderly patients often have decreased renal function, patients should be carefully monitored during treatment, and dose adjustments made based on symptoms and/or laboratory abnormalities (see **CLINICAL PHARMACOLOGY** and **DOSAGE AND ADMINISTRATION**).

ADVERSE REACTIONS
General
The adverse experiences listed below were reported to be possibly or probably related to INTRON® A therapy during clinical trials. Most of these adverse reactions were mild to moderate in severity and were manageable. Some were transient and most diminished with continued therapy.

The most frequently reported adverse reactions were "flu-like" symptoms, particularly fever, headache, chills, myalgia, and fatigue. More severe toxicities are observed generally at higher doses and may be difficult for patients to tolerate.

[See table on pages 1484 and 1485]

Hairy Cell Leukemia
The adverse reactions most frequently reported during clinical trials in 145 patients with hairy cell leukemia were the "flu-like" symptoms of fever (68%), fatigue (61%), and chills (46%).

Malignant Melanoma
The INTRON A dose was modified because of adverse events in 65% (n=93) of the patients. INTRON A therapy was discontinued because of adverse events in 8% of the patients during induction and 18% of the patients during maintenance. The most frequently reported adverse reaction was fatigue, which was observed in 96% of patients. Other adverse reactions that were recorded in greater than 20% of

TREATMENT-RELATED ADVERSE EXPERIENCES BY INDICATION

Dosing Regimens
Percentage (%) of Patients*

ADVERSE EXPERIENCE	MALIGNANT MELANOMA 20 MIU/m² Induction (IV) 10 MIU/m² Maintenance (SC) N=143	FOLLICULAR LYMPHOMA 5 MIU TIW/SC N=135	HAIRY CELL LEUKEMIA 2 MIU/m² TIW/SC N=145	CONDYLOMATA ACUMINATA 1 MIU/lesion N=352	AIDS-RELATED KAPOSI'S SARCOMA 30 MIU/m² TIW/SC N=74	35 MIU QD/SC N=29	CHRONIC HEPATITIS C† 3 MIU TIW N=183	CHRONIC HEPATITIS B Adults 5 MIU QD N=101	10 MIU TIW N=78	Pediatrics 6 MIU/m²TIW N=116
Application-Site Disorders				20						
injection site inflammation	--	1	--	--	--	--	5	3	--	--
other (≤5%)	burning, injection site bleeding, injection site pain, injection site reaction (5% in chronic hepatitis B pediatrics), itching									
Blood Disorders (<5%)	anemia, anemia hypochromic, granulocytopenia, hemolytic anemia, leukopenia, lymphocytosis, neutropenia (9% in chronic hepatitis C, 14% in chronic hepatitis B pediatrics), thrombocytopenia (10% in chronic hepatitis C) (bleeding 8% in malignant melanoma), thrombocytopenia purpura									
Body as a Whole										
facial edema	--	1	--	<1	--	10	<1	3	1	<1
weight decrease	3	13	<1	1	5	3	10	2	5	3
other (≤5%)	allergic reaction, cachexia, dehydration, earache, hernia, edema, hypercalcemia, hyperglycemia, hypothermia, inflammation nonspecific, lymphadenitis, lymphadenopathy, mastitis, periorbital edema, poor peripheral circulation, peripheral edema (6% in follicular lymphoma), phlebitis superficial, scrotal/penile edema, thirst, weakness, weight increase									
Cardiovascular System Disorders (<5%)	angina, arrhythmia, atrial fibrillation, bradycardia, cardiac failure, cardiomegaly, cardiomyopathy, coronary artery disorder, extrasystoles, heart valve disorder, hematoma, hypertension (9% in chronic hepatitis C), hypotension, palpitations, phlebitis, postural hypotension, pulmonary embolism, Raynaud's disease, tachycardia, thrombosis, varicose vein									
Endocrine System Disorders (<5%)	aggravation of diabetes mellitus, goiter, gynecomastia, hyperglycemia, hyperthyroidism, hypertriglyceridemia, hypothyroidism, virilism									
Flu-like Symptoms										
fever	81	56	68	56	47	55	34	66	86	94
headache	62	21	39	47	36	21	43	61	44	57
chills	54	--	46	45	--	--	34	--	--	--
myalgia	75	16	39	44	34	28	43	59	40	27
fatigue	96	8	61	18	84	48	23	75	69	71
increased sweating	6	13	7	2	4	21	4	1	1	3
asthenia	--	63	7	--	11	--	40	5	15	5
rigors	2	7	--	--	30	14	16	38	42	30
arthralgia	6	8	8	9	--	3	16	19	8	15
dizziness	23	--	12	9	7	24	9	13	10	8
influenza-like symptoms	10	18	37	--	45	79	26	5	--	<1
back pain	--	15	19	6	1	3	--	5	5	--
dry mouth	1	2	19	--	22	28	5	6	5	--
chest pain	2	8	<1	<1	1	28	4	4	--	--
malaise	6	--	--	14	5	--	13	9	6	3
pain (unspecified)	15	9	18	3	3	3	--	--	--	--
other (<5%)	chest pain substernal, hyperthermia, rhinitis, rhinorrhea									
Gastrointestinal System Disorders										
diarrhea	35	19	18	2	18	45	13	19	8	12
anorexia	69	21	19	1	38	41	14	43	53	43
nausea	66	24	21	17	28	21	19	50	33	18
taste alteration	24	2	13	<1	5	7	2	10	--	--
abdominal pain	2	20	<5	1	5	21	16	5	4	23
loose stools	--	1	--	<1	--	10	2	2	--	2
vomiting	‡	32	6	2	11	14	8	7	10	27
constipation	1	14	<1	--	1	10	4	5	--	2
gingivitis	2§	7§	--	--	--	14	--	1	--	--
dyspepsia	--	2	--	2	4	--	7	3	8	3
other (<5%)	abdominal ascites, abdominal distension, colitis, dysphagia, eructation, esophagitis, flatulence, gallstones, gastric ulcer, gastritis, gastroenteritis, gastrointestinal disorder (7% in follicular lymphoma), gastrointestinal hemorrhage, gastrointestinal mucosal discoloration, gingival bleeding, gum hyperplasia, halitosis, hemorrhoids, increased appetite, increased saliva, intestinal disorder, melena, mouth ulceration, mucositis, oral hemorrhage, oral leukoplakia, rectal bleeding after stool, rectal hemorrhage, stomatitis, stomatitis ulcerative, taste loss, tongue disorder, tooth disorder									
Liver and Biliary System Disorders (<5%)	abnormal hepatic function tests, biliary pain, bilirubinemia, hepatitis, increased lactate dehydrogenase, increased transaminases (SGOT/SGPT) (elevated SGOT 63% in malignant melanoma and 24% in follicular lymphoma), jaundice, right upper quadrant pain (15% in chronic hepatitis C), and very rarely, hepatic encephalopathy, hepatic failure, and death									
Musculoskeletal System Disorders										
musculoskeletal pain	--	18	--	--	--	--	21	9	1	10
other (<5%)	arteritis, arthritis, arthritis aggravated, arthrosis, bone disorder, bone pain, carpal tunnel syndrome, hyporeflexia, leg cramps, muscle atrophy, muscle weakness, polyarteritis nodosa, tendinitis, rheumatoid arthritis, spondylitis									

(Table continued on next page)

INTRON A-treated patients included neutropenia (92%), fever (81%), myalgia (75%), anorexia (69%), vomiting/nausea (66%), increased SGOT (63%), headache (62%), chills (54%), depression (40%), diarrhea (35%), alopecia (29%), altered taste sensation (24%), dizziness/vertigo (23%), and anemia (22%).

Adverse reactions classified as severe or life threatening (ECOG Toxicity Criteria grade 3 or 4) were recorded in 66% and 14% of INTRON A-treated patients, respectively. Severe adverse reactions recorded in greater than 10% of INTRON A-treated patients included neutropenia/leukopenia (26%), fatigue (23%), fever (18%), myalgia (17%), headache (17%), chills (16%), and increased SGOT (14%). Grade 4 fatigue was recorded in 4% and grade 4 depression was recorded in 2% of INTRON A-treated patients. No other grade 4 AE was reported in more than 2 INTRON A-treated patients. Lethal hepatotoxicity occurred in 2 INTRON A-treated patients early in the clinical trial. No subsequent

TREATMENT-RELATED ADVERSE EXPERIENCES BY INDICATION (cont.)

Dosing Regimens
Percentage (%) of Patients*

ADVERSE EXPERIENCE	MALIGNANT MELANOMA 20 MIU/m² Induction (IV) 10 MIU/m² Maintenance (SC)	FOLLICULAR LYMPHOMA 5 MIU TIW/SC	HAIRY CELL LEUKEMIA 2 MIU/m² TIW/SC	CONDYLOMATA ACUMINATA 1 MIU/lesion	AIDS-RELATED KAPOSI'S SARCOMA 30 MIU/m² TIW/SC	AIDS-RELATED KAPOSI'S SARCOMA 35 MIU QD/SC	CHRONIC HEPATITIS C† 3 MIU TIW	CHRONIC HEPATITIS B Adults 5 MIU QD	CHRONIC HEPATITIS B Adults 10 MIU TIW	CHRONIC HEPATITIS B Pediatrics 6 MIU/m²TIW
	N=143	N=135	N=145	N=352	N=74	N=29	N=183	N=101	N=78	N=116
Nervous System and Psychiatric Disorders										
depression	40	9	6	3	9	28	19	17	6	4
paresthesia	13	13	6	1	3	21	5	6	3	<1
impaired concentration	--	1	--	<1	3	14	3	8	5	3
amnesia	¶	1	<5	--	--	14	--	--	--	--
confusion	8	2	<5	4	12	10	1	--	--	2
hypoesthesia	--	1	<5	1	--	10	--	--	--	--
irritability	1	1	--	--	--	--	13	16	12	22
somnolence	1	2	<5	3	3	--	33#	14	9	5
anxiety	1	9	5	<1	1	3	5	2	--	3
insomnia	5	4	--	<1	3	3	12	11	6	8
nervousness	1	1	--	1	--	3	2	3	--	3
decreased libido	1	1	<5	--	--	--	1	5	1	--

other (<5%): abnormal coordination, abnormal dreaming, abnormal gait, abnormal thinking, aggravated depression, aggressive reaction, agitation (7% in chronic hepatitis B pediatrics), alcohol intolerance, apathy, aphasia, ataxia, Bell's palsy, CNS dysfunction, coma, convulsions, delirium, dysphonia, emotional lability, extrapyramidal disorder, feeling of ebriety, flushing, hearing disorder, hearing impairment, hot flashes, hyperesthesia, hyperkinesia, hypertonia, hypokinesia, impaired consciousness, labyrinthine disorder, loss of consciousness, manic depression, manic reaction, migraine, neuralgia, neuritis, neuropathy, neurosis, paresis, paroniria, parosmia, personality disorder, polyneuropathy, psychosis, speech disorder, stroke, suicidal ideation, suicide attempt, syncope, tinnitus, tremor, twitching, vertigo (8% in follicular lymphoma)

Reproduction System Disorders (<5%)
amenorrhea (12% in follicular lymphoma), dysmenorrhea, impotence, leukorrhea, menorrhagia, menstrual irregularity, pelvic pain, penis disorder, sexual dysfunction, uterine bleeding, vaginal dryness

Resistance Mechanism Disorders

moniliasis	--	1	--	<1	--	17	--	--	--	--
herpes simplex	1	2	--	1	--	3	1	5	--	--

other (<5%): abscess, conjunctivitis, fungal infection, hemophilus, herpes zoster, infection, infection bacterial, infection nonspecific (7% in follicular lymphoma), infection parasitic, otitis media, sepsis, stye, trichomonas, upper respiratory tract infection, viral infection (7% in chronic hepatitis C)

Respiratory System Disorders

dyspnea	15	14	<1	--	1	34	3	5	--	--
coughing	6	13	<1	--	--	31	1	4	--	5
pharyngitis	2	8	<5	1	1	31	3	7	1	7
sinusitis	1	4	--	--	--	21	2	--	--	--
nonproductive coughing	2	7	--	--	--	14	0	1	--	--
nasal congestion	1	7	--	--	--	10	<1	4	--	--

other (≤5%): asthma, bronchitis (10% in follicular lymphoma), bronchospasm, cyanosis, epistaxis (7% in chronic hepatitis B pediatrics), hemoptysis, hypoventilation, laryngitis, lung fibrosis, pleural effusion, orthopnea, pleural pain, pneumonia, pneumonitis, pneumothorax, rales, respiratory disorder, respiratory insufficiency, sneezing, tonsillitis, tracheitis, wheezing

Skin and Appendages Disorders

dermatitis	1	--	8	--	--	--	2	1	--	--
alopecia	29	23	8	--	12	31	28	26	38	17
pruritus	--	10	11	1	7	--	9	6	4	3
rash	19	13	25	--	9	10	5	8	1	5
dry skin	1	3	9	--	9	10	4	3	--	<1

other (<5%): abnormal hair texture, acne, cellulitis, cyanosis of the hand, cold and clammy skin, dermatitis lichenoides, eczema, epidermal necrolysis, erythema, erythema nodosum, folliculitis, furunculosis, increased hair growth, lacrimal gland disorder, lacrimation, lipoma, maculopapular rash, melanosis, nail disorders, nonherpetic cold sores, pallor, peripheral ischemia, photosensitivity, pruritus genital, psoriasis, psoriasis aggravated, purpura (5% in chronic hepatitis C), rash erythematous, sebaceous cyst, skin depigmentation, skin discoloration, skin nodule, urticaria, vitiligo

Urinary System Disorders (<5%)
albumin/protein in urine, cystitis, dysuria, hematuria, incontinence, increased BUN, micturition disorder, micturition frequency, nocturia, polyuria (10% in follicular lymphoma), renal insufficiency, urinary tract infection (5% in chronic hepatitis C)

Vision Disorders (<5%)
abnormal vision, blurred vision, diplopia, dry eyes, eye pain, nystagmus, photophobia

* Dash (--) indicates not reported
† Percentages based upon a summary of all adverse events during 18 to 24 months of treatment
‡ Vomiting was reported with nausea as a single term
§ Includes stomatitis/mucositis
¶ Amnesia was reported with confusion as a single term
# Predominantly lethargy

lethal hepatotoxicities were observed with adequate monitoring of liver function tests (see **PRECAUTIONS, Laboratory Tests**).
Follicular Lymphoma
Ninety-six percent of patients treated with CHVP plus INTRON A therapy and 91% of patients treated with CHVP alone reported an adverse event of any severity. Asthenia, fever, neutropenia, increased hepatic enzymes, alopecia, headache, anorexia, "flu-like" symptoms, myalgia, dyspnea, thrombocytopenia, paresthesia, and polyuria occurred more frequently in the CHVP plus INTRON A-treated patients than in patients treated with CHVP alone. Adverse reactions classified as severe or life threatening (World Health Organization grade 3 or 4) recorded in greater than 5% of CHVP plus INTRON A-treated patients included neutropenia (34%), asthenia (10%), and vomiting (10%). The incidence of neutropenic infection was 6% in CHVP plus INTRON A versus 2% in CHVP alone. One patient in each treatment group required hospitalization.
Twenty-eight percent of CHVP plus INTRON A-treated patients had a temporary modification/interruption of their INTRON A therapy, but only 13 patients (10%) permanently stopped INTRON A therapy because of toxicity. There were four deaths on study; two patients committed suicide in the CHVP plus INTRON A arm and two patients in the CHVP arm had unwitnessed sudden death. Three patients with hepatitis B (one of whom also had alcoholic cirrhosis) developed hepatotoxicity leading to discontinuation of INTRON A. Other reasons for discontinuation included intolerable asthenia (5/135), severe flu symptoms (2/135), and one patient each with exacerbation of ankylosing spondylitis, psychosis, and decreased ejection fraction.

ABNORMAL LABORATORY TEST VALUES BY INDICATION

Dosing Regimens
Percentage (%) of Patients

Laboratory Tests	MALIGNANT MELANOMA 20 MIU/m² Induction (IV) 10 MIU/m² Maintenance (SC) N=143	FOLLICULAR LYMPHOMA 5 MIU TIW/SC N=135	HAIRY CELL LEUKEMIA 2 MIU/m² TIW/SC N=145	CONDYLOMATA ACUMINATA 1 MIU/lesion N=352	AIDS-RELATED KAPOSI'S SARCOMA 30 MIU/m² TIW/SC N=69–73	35 MIU QD/SC N=26–28	CHRONIC HEPATITIS C 3 MIU TIW N=140–171	CHRONIC HEPATITIS B Adults 5 MIU QD N=96–101	10 MIU TIW N=75–103	Pediatrics 6 MIU/m²TIW N=113–115
Hemoglobin	22	8	NA	--	1	15	26*	32†	23†	17‡
White Blood Cell Count	§	--	NA	17	10	22	26¶	68¶	34¶	9¶
Platelet Count	15	13	NA	--	0	8	15#	12#	5#	1#
Serum Creatinine	3	2	0	--	--	--	6	3	0	3
Alkaline Phosphatase	13	--	4	--	--	--	--	8	4	0
Lactate Dehydrogenase	1	--	0	--	--	--	--	--	--	--
Serum Urea Nitrogen	12	4	0	--	--	--	--	2	0	2
SGOT	63	24	4	12	11	41	--	--	--	--
SGPT	2	--	13	--	10	15	--	--	--	--
Granulocyte Count										
• Total	92	36	NA	--	31	39	45ᵖ	75ᵖ	61ᵖ	70ᵖ
• 1000–<1500/mm³	66	--	--	--	--	--	32	30	32	43
• 750–<1000/mm³	--	21	--	--	--	--	10	24	18	18
• 500–<750/mm³	25	--	--	--	--	--	1	17	9	7
• <500/mm³	1	13	--	--	--	--	2	4	2	2

NA - Not Applicable- Patients' initial hematologic laboratory test values were abnormal due to their condition.

* Decrease of ≥2 g/dL; 20% 2–<3 g/dL; 6% ≥3 g/dL
† Decrease of ≥2 g/dL
‡ Decrease of ≥2 g/dL; 14% 2–<3 g/dL; 3% ≥3 g/dL
§ White Blood Cell Count was reported as neutropenia
¶ Decrease to <3000/mm³
# Decrease to <70,000/mm³
Þ Neutrophils plus bands

Condylomata Acuminata

Eighty-eight percent (311/352) of patients treated with INTRON A for condylomata acuminata who were evaluable for safety reported an adverse reaction during treatment. The incidence of the adverse reactions reported increased when the number of treated lesions increased from one to five. All 40 patients who had five warts treated reported some type of adverse reaction during treatment.

Adverse reactions and abnormal laboratory test values reported by patients who were re-treated were qualitatively and quantitatively similar to those reported during the initial INTRON A treatment period.

AIDS-Related Kaposi's Sarcoma

In patients with AIDS-Related Kaposi's Sarcoma, some type of adverse reaction occurred in 100% of the 74 patients treated with 30 million IU/m² three times a week and in 97% of the 29 patients treated with 35 million IU per day. Of these adverse reactions, those classified as severe (World Health Organization grade 3 or 4) were reported in 27% to 55% of patients. Severe adverse reactions in the 30 million IU/m² TIW study included: fatigue (20%), influenza-like symptoms (15%), anorexia (12%), dry mouth (4%), headache (4%), confusion (3%), fever (3%), myalgia (3%), and nausea and vomiting (1% each). Severe adverse reactions for patients who received the 35 million IU QD included: fever (24%), fatigue (17%), influenza-like symptoms (14%), dyspnea (14%), headache (10%), pharyngitis (7%), and ataxia, confusion, dysphagia, GI hemorrhage, abnormal hepatic function, increased SGOT, myalgia, cardiomyopathy, face edema, depression, emotional lability, suicide attempt, chest pain, and coughing (1 patient each). Overall, the incidence of severe toxicity was higher among patients who received the 35 million IU per day dose.

Chronic Hepatitis C

Adults

Two studies of extended treatment (18–24 months) with INTRON A show that approximately 95% of all patients treated experience some type of adverse event and that patients treated for extended duration continue to experience adverse events throughout treatment. Most adverse events reported are mild to moderate in severity. However, 29/152 (19%) of patients treated for 18 to 24 months experienced a serious adverse event compared to 11/163 (7%) of those treated for 6 months. Adverse events which occur or persist during extended treatment are similar in type and severity to those occurring during short-course therapy.

Of the patients achieving a complete response after 6 months of therapy, 12/79 (15%) subsequently discontinued INTRON A treatment during extended therapy because of adverse events, and 23/79 (29%) experienced severe adverse events (WHO grade 3 or 4) during extended therapy.

In patients using combination treatment with INTRON A and REBETOL, the primary toxicity observed was hemolytic anemia. Reductions in hemoglobin levels occurred within the first 1 to 2 weeks of therapy. Cardiac and pulmonary events associated with anemia occurred in approximately 10% of patients treated with INTRON A/REBETOL therapy. See REBETOL prescribing information for additional information.

Chronic Hepatitis C
Pediatrics

In pediatric patients with chronic hepatitis C treated with INTRON A 3 MIU/m² three times weekly and REBETOL 15 mg/kg per day, all subjects (n=118) had at least one adverse event during 24-48 weeks of treatment, of which 80% were considered to be mild or moderate in severity. Six percent discontinued therapy due to adverse reactions and dose modifications were required in 30% of subjects, most commonly for anemia and neutropenia. Adverse events occurring in more than 50% of subjects included headache, fever, fatigue and anorexia. Adverse events occurring in 20-50% of subjects included influenza-like symptoms, abdominal pain, vomiting, nausea, myalgia, pharyngitis, diarrhea, viral infection, rigors, weight decrease, musculoskeletal pain, alopecia and dizziness. The most common laboratory test abnormalities were neutropenia (34%) and anemia (27%). Depression was reported in 13% (n=15) of children. Three of these subjects had suicidal ideation, and one attempted suicide. Weight loss and slowed growth are common in pediatric patients during combination therapy with INTRON A and REBETOL. Following treatment, rebound growth and weight gain occurred in most subjects. Long-term follow-up data in pediatric subjects, however, indicates that INTRON A in combination with REBETOL may induce a growth inhibition that results in reduced adult height in some patients (see **PRECAUTIONS, Pediatric Use**).

Chronic Hepatitis B
Adults

In patients with chronic hepatitis B, some type of adverse reaction occurred in 98% of the 101 patients treated at 5 million IU QD and 90% of the 78 patients treated at 10 million IU TIW. Most of these adverse reactions were mild to moderate in severity, were manageable, and were reversible following the end of therapy.

Adverse reactions classified as severe (causing a significant interference with normal daily activities or clinical state) were reported in 21% to 44% of patients. The severe adverse reactions reported most frequently were the "flu-like" symptoms of fever (28%), fatigue (15%), headache (5%), myalgia (4%), rigors (4%), and other severe "flu-like" symptoms, which occurred in 1% to 3% of patients. Other severe adverse reactions occurring in more than one patient were alopecia (8%), anorexia (6%), depression (3%), nausea (3%), and vomiting (2%).

To manage side effects, the dose was reduced, or INTRON A therapy was interrupted in 25% to 38% of patients. Five percent of patients discontinued treatment due to adverse experiences.

Chronic Hepatitis B
Pediatrics

In pediatric patients with chronic hepatitis B (n=72) during 16-24 weeks of treatment, the most frequently reported adverse events were those commonly associated with interferon treatment: flu-like symptoms (100%), gastrointestinal system disorders (46%), and nausea and vomiting (40%). Neutropenia (13%) and thrombocytopenia (3%) were also reported. None of the adverse events was life threatening and most were moderate to severe and resolved upon dose reduction or drug discontinuation.

[See table above]

Postmarketing Experience

The following adverse reactions have been identified during postapproval use of INTRON A alone or in combination with REBETOL. Because these reactions are reported voluntarily from a population of uncertain size, it is not always possible to reliably estimate their frequency or establish a causal relationship to drug exposure.

Blood and Lymphatic System Disorders
pancytopenia (concurrent anemia, leukopenia, thrombocytopenia), aplastic anemia, pure red cell aplasia, thrombotic thrombocytopenic purpura, idiopathic thrombocytopenic purpura

Ear and Labyrinth Disorders
hearing loss

Endocrine Disorders
hypopituitarism

Eye Disorders
Vogt-Koyanagi-Harada syndrome, serous retinal detachment

Gastrointestinal Disorders
pancreatitis

General Disorders and Administration Site Conditions
asthenic conditions (including asthenia, malaise, fatigue)

Immune System Disorders
cases of acute hypersensitivity reactions, including anaphylaxis and angioedema, systemic lupus erythematosus, sarcoidosis or exacerbation of sarcoidosis
Musculoskeletal and Connective Tissue Disorders
myositis
Nervous System Disorders
peripheral neuropathy
Psychiatric Disorders
homicidal ideation, psychosis including hallucinations
Renal and Urinary Disorders
renal failure, renal insufficiency, nephrotic syndrome
Respiratory, Thoracic, and Mediastinal Disorders
pulmonary hypertension
Skin and Subcutaneous Tissue Disorders
injection site necrosis, Stevens-Johnson syndrome, toxic epidermal necrolysis, erythema multiforme, urticaria

OVERDOSAGE
There is limited experience with overdosage. Postmarketing surveillance includes reports of patients receiving a single dose as great as 10 times the recommended dose. In general, the primary effects of an overdose are consistent with the effects seen with therapeutic doses of interferon alfa-2b. Hepatic enzyme abnormalities, renal failure, hemorrhage, and myocardial infarction have been reported with single administration overdoses and/or with longer durations of treatment than prescribed (see **ADVERSE REACTIONS**). Toxic effects after ingestion of interferon alfa-2b are not expected because interferons are poorly absorbed orally. Consultation with a poison center is recommended.

Treatment
There is no specific antidote for interferon alfa-2b. Hemodialysis and peritoneal dialysis are not considered effective for treatment of overdose.

DOSAGE AND ADMINISTRATION
General
IMPORTANT: INTRON® A is supplied as 1) Powder for Injection/Reconstitution; 2) Solution for Injection in Vials. **Not all dosage forms and strengths are appropriate for some indications.** It is important that you carefully read the instructions below for the indication you are treating to ensure you are using an appropriate dosage form and strength.
To enhance the tolerability of INTRON A, injections should be administered in the evening when possible.
To reduce the incidence of certain adverse reactions, acetaminophen may be administered at the time of injection.
The solution should be allowed to come to room temperature before using.

Hairy Cell Leukemia
(see DOSAGE AND ADMINISTRATION, General)
Dose
The recommended dose for the treatment of hairy cell leukemia is 2 million IU/m² administered intramuscularly or subcutaneously 3 times a week for up to 6 months. Patients with platelet counts of less than 50,000/mm³ should not be administered INTRON A intramuscularly, but instead by subcutaneous administration. Patients who are responding to therapy may benefit from continued treatment.
[See table above]
NOTE: INTRON A Powder for Injection does not contain a preservative. The vial must be discarded after reconstitution and withdrawal of a single dose.
Dose Adjustment
• If severe adverse reactions develop, the dosage should be modified (50% reduction) or therapy should be temporarily withheld until the adverse reactions abate and then resume at 50% (1 MIU/m² TIW).
• If severe adverse reactions persist or recur following dosage adjustment, INTRON A should be permanently discontinued.
• INTRON A should be discontinued for progressive disease or failure to respond after six months of treatment.

Malignant Melanoma
(see DOSAGE AND ADMINISTRATION, General)
INTRON A adjuvant treatment of malignant melanoma is given in two phases, induction and maintenance.
Induction Recommended Dose
The recommended daily dose of INTRON A in induction is 20 million IU/m² as an intravenous infusion, over 20 minutes, 5 consecutive days per week, for 4 weeks (see Dose Adjustment below).

Dosage Forms for This Indication

Dosage Form	Concentration	Route
Powder 10 MIU	10 MIU/mL	IV
Powder 18 MIU	18 MIU/mL	IV
Powder 50 MIU	50 MIU/mL	IV

Dosage Forms for This Indication

Dosage Form	Concentration	Route	Fixed Doses
Powder 10 MIU (single dose)	10 MIU/mL	IM, SC	N/A
Solution 18 MIU multidose	6 MIU/mL	IM, SC	N/A
Solution 25 MIU multidose	10 MIU/mL	IM, SC	N/A

Dosage Forms for This Indication

Dosage Form	Concentration	Route	Fixed Doses
Powder 10 MIU (single dose)*	10 MIU/mL	SC	N/A
Powder 18 MIU (single dose)†	18 MIU/mL	SC	N/A
Solution 18 MIU multidose	6 MIU/mL	SC	N/A
Solution 25 MIU multidose	10 MIU/mL	SC	N/A

* Patients receiving 50% dose reduction only
† Patients receiving full dose only

NOTE: INTRON A Solution for Injection in vials is NOT recommended for intravenous administration and should not be used for the induction phase of malignant melanoma.
NOTE: INTRON A Powder for Injection does not contain a preservative. The vial must be discarded after reconstitution and withdrawal of a single dose.
Dose Adjustment
NOTE: Regular laboratory testing should be performed to monitor laboratory abnormalities for the purpose of dose modifications (see **PRECAUTIONS, Laboratory Tests**).
• INTRON A should be withheld for severe adverse reactions, including granulocyte counts greater than 250/mm³ but less than 500/mm³ or SGPT/SGOT greater than 5–10× upper limit of normal, until adverse reactions abate. INTRON A treatment should be restarted at 50% of the previous dose.
• INTRON A should be permanently discontinued for:
  ◦ Toxicity that does not abate after withholding INTRON A
  ◦ Severe adverse reactions which recur in patients receiving reduced doses of INTRON A
  ◦ Granulocyte count less than 250/mm³ or SGPT/SGOT of greater than 10× upper limit of normal
Maintenance Recommended Dose
The recommended dose of INTRON A for maintenance is 10 million IU/m² as a subcutaneous injection three times per week for 48 weeks (see Dose Adjustment below).
[See table above]
NOTE: INTRON A Powder for Injection does not contain a preservative. The vial must be discarded after reconstitution and withdrawal of a single dose.
Dose Adjustment
NOTE: Regular laboratory testing should be performed to monitor laboratory abnormalities for the purpose of dose modifications (see **PRECAUTIONS, Laboratory Tests** section).
• INTRON A should be withheld for severe adverse reactions, including granulocyte counts greater than 250/mm³ but less than 500/mm³ or SGPT/SGOT greater than 5–10× upper limit of normal, until adverse reactions abate. INTRON A treatment should be restarted at 50% of the previous dose.
• INTRON A should be permanently discontinued for:
  ◦ Toxicity that does not abate after withholding INTRON A
  ◦ Severe adverse reactions which recur in patients receiving reduced doses of INTRON A
  ◦ Granulocyte count less than 250/mm³ or SGPT/SGOT of greater than 10× upper limit of normal

Follicular Lymphoma
(see DOSAGE and ADMINISTRATION, General)
Dose
The recommended dose of INTRON A for the treatment of follicular lymphoma is 5 million IU subcutaneously three times per week for up to 18 months in conjunction with anthracycline-containing chemotherapy regimen and following completion of the chemotherapy regimen.

Dosage Forms for This Indication

Dosage Form	Concentration	Route	Fixed Doses
Powder 10 MIU (single dose)	10 MIU/mL	SC	N/A
Solution 18 MIU multidose	6 MIU/mL	SC	N/A
Solution 25 MIU multidose	10 MIU/mL	SC	N/A

NOTE: INTRON A Powder for Injection does not contain a preservative. The vial must be discarded after reconstitution and withdrawal of a single dose.
Dose Adjustment
• Doses of myelosuppressive drugs were reduced by 25% from a full-dose CHOP regimen, and cycle length increased by 33% (e.g., from 21 to 28 days) when alpha interferon was added to the regimen.
• Delay chemotherapy cycle if neutrophil count was less than 1500/mm³ or platelet count was less than 75,000/mm³.
• INTRON A should be permanently discontinued if SGOT exceeds greater than 5× the upper limit of normal or serum creatinine greater than 2.0 mg/dL (see **WARNINGS**).
• Administration of INTRON A therapy should be withheld for a neutrophil count less than 1000/mm³, or a platelet count less than 50,000/mm³.
• INTRON A dose should be reduced by 50% (2.5 MIU TIW) for a neutrophil count greater than 1000/mm³, but less than 1500/mm³. The INTRON A dose may be re-escalated to the starting dose (5 million IU TIW) after resolution of hematologic toxicity (ANC greater than 1500/mm³).

Condylomata Acuminata
(see DOSAGE and ADMINISTRATION, General)
Dose
The recommended dose is 1.0 million IU per lesion in a maximum of 5 lesions in a single course. The lesions should be injected three times weekly on alternate days for 3 weeks. An additional course may be administered at 12 to 16 weeks.

Dosage Forms for This Indication

Dosage Form	Concentration	Route
Powder 10 MIU (single dose)	10 MIU/mL	IL
Solution 25 MIU multidose	10 MIU/mL	IL

NOTE: INTRON A Powder for Injection does not contain a preservative. The vial must be discarded after reconstitution and withdrawal of a single dose.
NOTE: Do not use the following formulations for this indication:
• the 18 million or 50 million IU Powder for Injection
• the 18 million IU multidose INTRON A Solution for Injection
Dose Adjustment
None
Technique for Injection
The injection should be administered intralesionally using a Tuberculin or similar syringe and a 25-to 30-gauge needle. The needle should be directed at the center of the base of the wart and at an angle almost parallel to the plane of the skin (approximately that in the commonly used PPD test). This will deliver the interferon to the dermal core of the lesion, infiltrating the lesion and causing a small wheal. Care should be taken not to go beneath the lesion too deeply; subcutaneous injection should be avoided, since this area is below the base of the lesion. Do not inject too superficially since this will result in possible leakage, infiltrating only the keratinized layer and not the dermal core.

AIDS-Related Kaposi's Sarcoma
(see DOSAGE and ADMINISTRATION, General)
Dose
The recommended dose of INTRON A for Kaposi's Sarcoma is 30 million IU/m²/dose administered subcutaneously or intramuscularly three times a week until disease progression or maximal response has been achieved after 16 weeks of treatment. Dose reduction is frequently required (see **Dose Adjustment** below).

INTRON A Dose	White Blood Cell Count	Granulocyte Count	Platelet Count
Reduce 50%	$<1.5 \times 10^9$ /L	$<0.75 \times 10^9$ /L	$<50 \times 10^9$ /L
Permanently Discontinue	$<1.0 \times 10^9$ /L	$<0.5 \times 10^9$ /L	$<25 \times 10^9$ /L

Dosage Forms for This Indication

Dosage Form	Concentration	Route
Powder 50 MIU	50 MIU/mL	IM, SC

NOTE: INTRON A Solution for Injection in vials should NOT be used for AIDS-Related Kaposi's Sarcoma.
NOTE: INTRON A Powder for Injection does not contain a preservative. The vial must be discarded after reconstitution and withdrawal of a single dose.
Dose Adjustment
• INTRON A dose should be reduced by 50% or withheld for severe adverse reactions.
• INTRON A may be resumed at a reduced dose if severe adverse reactions abate with interruption of dosing.
• INTRON A should be permanently discontinued if severe adverse reactions persist or if they recur in patients receiving a reduced dose.

Chronic Hepatitis C
(see **DOSAGE and ADMINISTRATION, General**)
Dose
The recommended dose of INTRON A for the treatment of chronic hepatitis C is 3 million IU three times a week (TIW) administered subcutaneously or intramuscularly. In patients tolerating therapy with normalization of ALT at 16 weeks of treatment, INTRON A therapy should be extended to 18 to 24 months (72 to 96 weeks) at 3 million IU TIW to improve the sustained response rate (see **CLINICAL PHARMACOLOGY, Chronic Hepatitis C**). Patients who do not normalize their ALTs or have persistently high levels of HCV RNA after 16 weeks of therapy rarely achieve a sustained response with extension of treatment. Consideration should be given to discontinuing these patients from therapy.
When INTRON A is administered in combination with REBETOL®, patients with impaired renal function and/or those over the age of 50 should be carefully monitored with respect to the development of anemia. See REBETOL prescribing information for dosing when used in combination with REBETOL for adults and pediatric patients.

Dosage Forms for This Indication

Dosage Form	Concentration	Route	Fixed Doses
Solution 18 MIU multidose	6 MIU/mL	IM, SC	N/A

Dose Adjustment
If severe adverse reactions develop during INTRON A treatment, the dose should be modified (50% reduction) or therapy should be temporarily discontinued until the adverse reactions abate. If intolerance persists after dose adjustment, INTRON A therapy should be discontinued.

Chronic Hepatitis B Adults
(see **DOSAGE and ADMINISTRATION, General**)
Dose
The recommended dose of INTRON A for the treatment of chronic hepatitis B is 30 to 35 million IU per week, administered subcutaneously or intramuscularly, either as 5 million IU daily (QD) or as 10 million IU three times a week (TIW) for 16 weeks.

Dosage Forms for This Indication

Dosage Form	Concentration	Route	Fixed Doses
Powder 10 MIU (single dose)	10 MIU/mL	IM, SC	N/A
Solution 25 MIU multidose	10 MIU/mL	IM, SC	N/A

NOTE: INTRON A Powder for Injection does not contain a preservative. The vial must be discarded after reconstitution and withdrawal of a single dose.

Chronic Hepatitis B Pediatrics
(see **DOSAGE and ADMINISTRATION, General**)
Dose
The recommended dose of INTRON A for the treatment of chronic hepatitis B is 3 million IU/m^2 three times a week (TIW) for the first week of therapy followed by dose escalation to 6 million IU/m^2 TIW (maximum of 10 million IU TIW) administered subcutaneously for a total duration of 16 to 24 weeks.

Dosage Forms for This Indication

Dosage Form	Concentration	Route	Fixed Doses
Powder 10 MIU (single dose)	10 MIU/mL	SC	N/A
Solution 25 MIU multidose	10 MIU/mL	SC	N/A

NOTE: INTRON A Powder for Injection does not contain a preservative. The vial must be discarded after reconstitution and withdrawal of a single dose.
Dose Adjustment
If severe adverse reactions or laboratory abnormalities develop during INTRON A therapy, the dose should be modified (50% reduction) or discontinued if appropriate, until the adverse reactions abate. If intolerance persists after dose adjustment, INTRON A therapy should be discontinued.
For patients with decreases in white blood cell, granulocyte or platelet counts, the following guidelines for dose modification should be followed:
[See table above]
INTRON A therapy was resumed at up to 100% of the initial dose when white blood cell, granulocyte, and/or platelet counts returned to normal or baseline values.

PREPARATION AND ADMINISTRATION
Reconstitution of INTRON® A Powder for Injection
The reconstituted solution is clear and colorless to light yellow. The INTRON A powder reconstituted with Sterile Water for Injection USP is a single-use vial and does not contain a preservative. **DO NOT RE-ENTER VIAL AFTER WITHDRAWING THE DOSE. DISCARD UNUSED PORTION** (see **DOSAGE and ADMINISTRATION**). Once the dose from the single-dose vial has been withdrawn, the sterility of any remaining product can no longer be guaranteed. Pooling of unused portions of some medications has been linked to bacterial contamination and morbidity.

• **Intramuscular, Subcutaneous, or Intralesional Administration**
Inject 1 mL Diluent (Sterile Water for Injection USP) for INTRON A into the INTRON A vial. Swirl gently to hasten complete dissolution of the powder. The appropriate INTRON A dose should then be withdrawn and injected intramuscularly, subcutaneously, or intralesionally (see **MEDICATION GUIDE** for detailed instructions).
Please refer to the **MEDICATION GUIDE** for detailed, step-by-step instructions on how to inject the INTRON A dose. After preparation and administration of the INTRON A injection, it is essential to follow the procedure for proper disposal of syringes and needles (see **MEDICATION GUIDE** for detailed instructions).
Parenteral drug products should be inspected visually for particulate matter and discoloration prior to administration.

• **Intravenous Infusion**
The infusion solution should be prepared immediately prior to use. Based on the desired dose, the appropriate vial strength(s) of INTRON A should be reconstituted with the diluent provided. Inject 1 mL Diluent (Sterile Water for Injection USP) for INTRON A into the INTRON A vial. Swirl gently to hasten complete dissolution of the powder. The appropriate INTRON A dose should then be withdrawn and injected into a 100-mL bag of 0.9% Sodium Chloride Injection USP. The final concentration of INTRON A should not be less than 10 million IU/100 mL.
Please refer to the **MEDICATION GUIDE** for detailed, step-by-step instructions on how to inject the INTRON A dose. After preparation and administration of INTRON A, it is essential to follow the procedure for proper disposal of syringes and needles.

INTRON A Solution for Injection in Vials
INTRON A Solution for Injection is supplied in two multidose vials. The solutions for injection do not require reconstitution prior to administration; the solution is clear and colorless.
The appropriate dose should be withdrawn from the vial and injected intramuscularly, subcutaneously, or intralesionally.

INTRON A Solution for Injection is not recommended for intravenous administration.
Please refer to the **MEDICATION GUIDE** for detailed, step-by-step instructions on how to inject the INTRON A dose. After preparation and administration of INTRON A, it is essential to follow the procedure for proper disposal of syringes and needles.

HOW SUPPLIED
INTRON® A Powder for Injection
INTRON A Powder for Injection, 10 million IU per vial and Diluent for INTRON A (Sterile Water for Injection USP) 1.25 mL per vial; boxes containing 1 INTRON A vial and 1 vial of INTRON A Diluent (NDC 0085-0571-02).
INTRON A Powder for Injection, 18 million IU per vial and Diluent for INTRON A (Sterile Water for Injection USP) 1.25 mL per vial; boxes containing 1 INTRON A vial and 1 vial of INTRON A Diluent (NDC 0085-1110-01).
INTRON A Powder for Injection, 50 million IU per vial and Diluent for INTRON A (Sterile Water for Injection USP) 1.25 mL per vial; boxes containing 1 INTRON A vial and 1 vial of INTRON A Diluent (NDC 0085-0539-01).

INTRON A Solution for Injection in Vials
INTRON A Solution for Injection, 18 million IU multidose vial (22.8 million IU per 3.8 mL per vial); boxes containing 1 vial of INTRON A Solution for Injection (NDC 0085-1168-01).
INTRON A Solution for Injection, 25 million IU multidose vial (32 million IU per 3.2 mL per vial); boxes containing 1 vial of INTRON A Solution for Injection (NDC 0085-1133-01).

Storage
• **INTRON A Powder for Injection/Reconstitution**
INTRON A Powder for Injection should be stored in the refrigerator at 2° to 8°C (36°– 46°F). After reconstitution, the solution should be used immediately, but may be stored up to 24 hours at 2° to 8°C (36°– 46°F). Throw away any medicine left in the vial after you withdraw 1 dose.
• **INTRON A Solution for Injection in Vials**
INTRON A Solution for Injection in vials should be stored in the refrigerator at 2° to 8°C (36°– 46°F).
INTRON A Solution for Injection should not be frozen and should be kept away from heat. Throw away any unused INTRON A Solution for Injection remaining in the vial after one month.

References
1. Smalley R, et al. *N Engl J Med.* 1992;327:1336–1341.
2. Aviles A, et al. *Leukemia and Lymphoma.* 1996;20:495–499.
3. Unterhalt M, et al. *Blood.* 1996;88(10 Suppl 1):1744A.
4. Schiller J, et al. *J Biol Response Mod.* 1989;8:252–261.
5. Poynard T, et al. *N Engl J Med.* 1995;332(22)1457–1462.
6. Lin R, et al. *J Hepatol.* 1995;23:487–496.
7. Perrillo R, et al. *N Engl J Med.* 1990;323:295–301.
8. Perez V, et al. *J Hepatol.* 1990;11:S113–S117.
9. Knodell R, et al. *Hepatology.* 1981;1:431–435.
10. Perrillo R, et al. *Ann Intern Med.* 1991;115:113–115.
11. Kauppila A, et al. *Int J Cancer.* 1982;29:291–294.

Manufactured by: Schering Corporation, a subsidiary of **MERCK & CO., INC.**
Whitehouse Station, NJ 08889, USA
U.S. Patent Nos. 5,935,566 and 6,610,830.
Copyright © 1986, 2011 Schering Corporation, a subsidiary of **Merck & Co., Inc.** All rights reserved.
Rev. 04/2014
uspi-mk2958-mtl-1404r025

MEDICATION GUIDE
INTRON® A (In-tron-aye)
(Interferon alfa-2b, recombinant)
Read this Medication Guide before you start taking INTRON A, and each time you get a refill. There may be new information. This information does not take the place of talking with your healthcare provider about your medical condition or your treatment.
If you are taking INTRON A with REBETOL, also read the Medication Guide for REBETOL® (ribavirin) Capsules and Oral Solution.
INTRON A alone is a treatment for certain types of cancers and hepatitis B virus. INTRON A by itself or with REBETOL is a treatment for some people infected with hepatitis C virus.
What is the most important information I should know about INTRON A?
INTRON A can cause serious side effects that:
• **may cause death, or**
• **may worsen certain serious diseases that you may already have.**
Tell your healthcare provider right away if you have any of the symptoms listed below while taking INTRON A. If symptoms get worse, or become severe and continue, your healthcare provider may tell you to stop taking INTRON A permanently. In many, but not all people, these symptoms go away after they stop taking INTRON A.
1. **Heart problems.** Some people who take INTRON A may develop heart problems, including:
• low blood pressure
• fast heart rate or abnormal heart beats
• trouble breathing or chest pain
• heart attacks or heart muscle problems (cardiomyopathy)

2. **Stroke or symptoms of a stroke. Symptoms may include weakness, loss of coordination, and numbness.** Stroke or symptoms of a stroke may happen in people who have some risk factors **or** no known risk factors for a stroke.

3. **Mental health problems and suicide.** INTRON A may cause you to develop mood or behavior problems that may get worse during treatment with INTRON A or after your last dose, including:
   - irritability (getting upset easily)
   - depression (feeling low, feeling bad about yourself, or feeling hopeless)
   - aggressive behavior
   - thoughts of hurting yourself or others, or suicide
   - former drug addicts may fall back into drug addiction or overdose

   If you have these symptoms, your healthcare provider should carefully monitor you during treatment with INTRON A and for 6 months after your last dose.

4. **New or worsening autoimmune disease.** Some people taking INTRON A develop autoimmune diseases (a condition where the body's immune cells attack other cells or organs in the body), including rheumatoid arthritis, systemic lupus erythematosus, sarcoidosis, and psoriasis. In some people who already have an autoimmune disease, the disease may get worse while on INTRON A.

5. **Infections.** Some people who take INTRON A may get an infection. Symptoms may include:
   - fever
   - chills
   - bloody diarrhea
   - burning or pain with urination
   - urinating often
   - coughing up mucus (phlegm) that is discolored (for example yellow or pink)

While taking INTRON A, you should see a healthcare provider regularly for check-ups and blood tests to make sure that your treatment is working and to check for side effects.

What is INTRON A?

INTRON A is a prescription medicine that is used:
- to treat adults with a blood cancer called hairy cell leukemia
- to treat certain adults with a type of skin cancer called malignant melanoma
- to treat adults with some types of Follicular Non-Hodgkin's Lymphoma along with certain chemotherapy medicines
- to treat certain adults with genital warts (condylomata acuminate), by injecting the medicine directly into the warts
- to treat certain adults with a type of cancer caused by AIDS, called AIDS-related Kaposi's Sarcoma
- alone to treat adults with chronic (lasting a long time) hepatitis C infection with stable liver problems
- with REBETOL to treat chronic (lasting a long time) hepatitis C infection in people 3 years and older with stable liver problems
- to treat chronic (lasting a long time) hepatitis B infection in people 1 year and older with stable liver problems

Who should not take INTRON A?

Do not take INTRON A if you:
- had a serious allergic reaction to another alpha interferon product or are allergic to any of the ingredients in INTRON A. See the end of this Medication Guide for a complete list of ingredients. Ask your healthcare provider if you are not sure.
- have certain types of hepatitis (autoimmune hepatitis)
- have certain other liver problems

Talk to your healthcare provider before taking INTRON A if you have any of these conditions.

What should I tell my healthcare provider before taking INTRON A?

Before you take INTRON A, tell your healthcare provider if you:
- **See "What is the most important information I should know about INTRON A?"**
- have or ever had any problems with your heart, including heart attack or have high blood pressure
- have or ever had bleeding problems or blood clots
- are being treated for a mental illness or had treatment in the past for any mental illness, including depression and suicidal behavior
- have any kind of autoimmune disease (where the body's immune system attacks the body's own cells), such as psoriasis, systemic lupus erythematosus, rheumatoid arthritis
- have or ever had low blood cell counts
- have ever been addicted to drugs or alcohol
- have liver problems (other than hepatitis B or C)
- have or had lung problems, such as chronic obstructive pulmonary disease (COPD)
- have diabetes
- have colitis (inflammation of your intestine)
- have a condition that suppresses your immune system, such as cancer

- have hepatitis B or C infection
- have HIV infection (the virus that causes AIDS)
- have kidney problems
- have high blood triglyceride levels (fat in your blood)
- have an organ transplant and are taking medicine that keeps your body from rejecting your transplant (suppresses your immune system)
- have any other medical conditions
- are pregnant or plan to become pregnant. It is not known if INTRON A will harm your unborn baby. You should use effective birth control during treatment with INTRON A. Talk to your healthcare provider about birth control choices for you during treatment with INTRON A. Tell your healthcare provider if you become pregnant during treatment with INTRON A.
- are breast-feeding or plan to breast-feed. It is not known if INTRON A passes into your breast milk. You and your healthcare provider should decide if you will use INTRON A or breast-feed. You should not do both.

Tell your healthcare provider about all the medicines you take, including prescription and non-prescription medicines, vitamins, and herbal supplements. INTRON A and certain other medicines may affect each other and cause side effects.

Especially tell your healthcare provider if you take:
- the anti-hepatitis B medicine telbivudine (Tyzeka)
- the anti-HIV medicine zidovudine (Retrovir)
- theophylline (Theo-24, Elixophyllin, Uniphyl, Theolair). Your healthcare provider may need to monitor the amount of theophylline in your body and make changes to your theophylline dose.

Know the medicines you take. Keep a list of them and show it to your healthcare provider and pharmacist when you get a new medicine.

How should I take INTRON A?

- INTRON A is given as an injection under the skin (subcutaneous) or into a muscle (intramuscular), into genital lesions, or as an injection into a vein (intravenous), depending on the condition that is being treated.
- Your healthcare provider will decide your dose of INTRON A and how often you will take it.
- If your healthcare provider decides that you can inject INTRON A for your condition, inject it exactly as prescribed, under your skin (subcutaneous injection) or into your muscle (intramuscular injection). Do not change your dose or how you inject INTRON A unless your healthcare provider tells you to.
- Do not take more than your prescribed dose.
- Your healthcare provider should show you how to prepare and measure your dose of INTRON A and how to inject yourself before you use INTRON A for the first time.
- You should not inject INTRON A until your healthcare provider has shown you how to use INTRON A the right way.
- INTRON A comes as:
  - a powder for injection in a vial that is used only 1 time (single-use vial). The powder must be mixed with water for injection (a diluent) before you inject it.
  - a solution for injection in a multi-dose vial
- See the attached Instructions for Use for detailed instructions for preparing and injecting a dose of INTRON A.
- If you miss a dose of INTRON A, take the missed dose as soon as possible during the same day or the next day, then continue on your regular dosing schedule. If several days go by after you miss a dose, check with your healthcare provider to see what to do.
- Do not inject more than 1 dose or take more than your prescribed dose without talking to your healthcare provider.
- If you take too much INTRON A, call your healthcare provider right away. Your healthcare provider may examine you more closely, and do blood tests.
- Your healthcare provider should do regular blood tests before you start INTRON A, and during your treatment to see how well the treatment is working and to check for side effects.

What are the possible side effects of INTRON A?

INTRON A may cause serious side effects including:
- **See "What is the most important information I should know about INTRON A?"**
- **Blood problems.** INTRON A can affect your bone marrow and cause low white blood cell and platelet counts. In some people, these blood counts may fall to dangerously low levels. If your blood cell counts become very low, you can get infections or have bleeding problems.
- **Serious eye problems.** INTRON A may cause eye problems that may lead to vision loss or blindness. You should have an eye exam before you start taking INTRON A. If you have eye problems or have had them in the past, you may need eye exams while taking INTRON A. Tell your healthcare provider or eye doctor right away if you have any vision changes while taking INTRON A.
- **Thyroid problems.** Some people develop changes in the function of their thyroid. Symptoms of thyroid problems include:

  - problems concentrating
  - feeling cold or hot all the time
  - changes in your weight
  - skin changes
- **Blood sugar problems.** Some people may develop high blood sugar or diabetes. If you have high blood sugar or diabetes before starting INTRON A, talk to your healthcare provider before you take INTRON A. If you develop high blood sugar or diabetes while taking INTRON A, your healthcare provider may tell you to stop INTRON A and prescribe a different medicine for you. Symptoms of high blood sugar or diabetes may include:
  - increased thirst
  - tiredness
  - urinating more often than normal
  - increased appetite
  - weight loss
  - your breath smells like fruit
- **Lung problems including:**
  - trouble breathing
  - pneumonia
  - inflammation of lung tissue
  - new or worse high blood pressure of the lungs (pulmonary hypertension). This can be severe and may lead to death.

  You may need to have a chest X-ray or other tests if you develop fever, cough, shortness of breath, or other symptoms of a lung problem during treatment with INTRON A.
- **Severe liver problems, or worsening of liver problems including liver failure and death.** Symptoms may include:
  - nausea
  - loss of appetite
  - tiredness
  - diarrhea
  - yellowing of your skin or the white part of your eyes
  - bleeding more easily than normal
  - swelling of your stomach area (abdomen)
  - confusion
  - sleepiness
  - you cannot be awakened (coma)
- **Serious allergic reactions and skin reactions. Symptoms may include:**

◦ itching	◦ chest pain
◦ swelling of your face,	◦ feeling faint
eyes, lips, tongue, or throat	◦ skin rash, hives, sores in
◦ trouble breathing	your mouth, or your skin
◦ anxiousness	blisters and peels

- **Swelling of your pancreas (pancreatitis) and intestines (colitis).** Symptoms may include:
  - severe stomach area (abdomen) pain
  - severe back pain
  - nausea
  - vomiting
  - fever
- **New or worsening autoimmune disease.** Some patients taking INTRON A develop autoimmune diseases (a condition where the body's immune cells attack other cells or organs in the body), including rheumatoid arthritis, systemic lupus erythematosus, sarcoidosis, and psoriasis. In some patients who already have an autoimmune disease, the disease may worsen while on INTRON A.
- **Nerve problems.** People who take INTRON A or other alpha interferon products with telbivudine (Tyzeka) can develop nerve problems such as continuing numbness, tingling, or burning sensation in the arms or legs (peripheral neuropathy). Call your healthcare provider if you have any of these symptoms.
- **Growth problems in children.** Weight loss and slowed growth are common in children during combination treatment with INTRON A and REBETOL. Most children will go through a growth spurt and gain weight after treatment stops. Some children may not reach the height that they were expected to have before treatment. Talk to your healthcare provider if you are concerned about your child's growth during treatment with INTRON A and REBETOL.
- **Dental and gum problems.**

Tell your healthcare provider right away if you have any of the symptoms listed above.

The most common side effects of INTRON A include:
- **Flu-like symptoms.** Symptoms may include: headache, muscle aches, tiredness, and fever. Some of these symptoms may be decreased by injecting your INTRON A dose in the evening. Talk to your healthcare provider about which over-the-counter medicines you can take to help prevent or decrease some of the symptoms.
- **Tiredness.** Many people become very tired during treatment with INTRON A.
- **Appetite problems.** Nausea, loss of appetite, and weight loss can happen with INTRON A.
- **Skin reactions.** Redness, swelling, and itching are common at the injection site.
- **Hair thinning.**

Tell your healthcare provider if you have any side effect that bothers you or that does not go away.

These are not all the side effects of INTRON A. For more information, ask your healthcare provider or pharmacist. Call your doctor for medical advice about side effects. You may report side effects to the FDA at 1-800-FDA-1088.

How should I store INTRON A?
INTRON A Solution for Injection:
◦ Store in the refrigerator between 36°F to 46°F (2°C to 8°C).
◦ INTRON A Solution for Injection in Multidose vials for injection may be used to give more than 1 injection of medicine.
◦ Do not freeze.
◦ Throw away any unused INTRON A Solution for Injection remaining in the vial after one month.

INTRON A Powder for Injection:
Before mixing, store in the refrigerator between 36°F to 46°F (2°C to 8°C).
◦ After mixing the INTRON A Powder for Injection, use the solution right away or store the solution in the refrigerator for up to 24 hours between 36°F to 46°F (2°C to 8°C).
◦ Throw away any medicine left in the vial after you withdraw 1 dose.
◦ Do not freeze.

Keep INTRON A and all medicines out of the reach of children.

General Information about INTRON A
Medicines are sometimes prescribed for purposes other than those listed in a Medication Guide. Do not use INTRON A for a condition for which it was not prescribed. Do not give INTRON A to other people, even if they have the same symptoms that you have. It may harm them.

This Medication Guide summarizes the most important information about INTRON A. If you would like more information, ask your healthcare provider. You can ask your healthcare provider or pharmacist for information about INTRON A that was written for health care professionals.
◦ For more information, go to www.IntronA.com or call 1-800-622-4477.

What are the ingredients in INTRON A?
Active ingredient: interferon alfa-2b
Inactive ingredients:
◦ **Powder for injection contains:** glycine, sodium phosphate dibasic, sodium phosphate monobasic, human albumin. Sterile water for injection is provided as a diluent.
◦ **Solution Multidose vials for injection contain:** sodium chloride, sodium phosphate dibasic, sodium phosphate monobasic, edetate disodium, polysorbate 80, and m-cresol as a preservative.

The Medication Guide has been approved by the U.S. Food and Drug Administration.
Manufactured by: Schering Corporation, a subsidiary of **Merck & Co., Inc.,** Whitehouse Station, NJ 08889 USA
Copyright © 1996, 2011 Schering Corporation, a subsidiary of Merck & Co., Inc.
All rights reserved.
Revised: 04/2014
usmg-mk2958-mtl-1404r010

Instructions for Use

INTRON® A (In-tron-aye)
(Interferon alfa-2b, recombinant)
Solution for Injection
Be sure that you read, understand and follow these instructions before injecting INTRON A. Your healthcare provider should show you how to prepare, measure and inject INTRON A properly before you use it for the first time. Ask your healthcare provider if you have any questions.

Before starting, collect all of the supplies that you will need to use for preparing and injecting INTRON A. You will need the following supplies:
◦ 1 vial of INTRON A solution
◦ 1 single-use disposable syringe and needle
◦ 1 cotton ball or gauze
◦ 2 alcohol swabs
You will also need a puncture-proof disposable container to throw away used syringes, needles and vials.

Important:
• **Never re-use disposable syringes and needles.**
• Make sure you have the right syringe and needle to use with INTRON A. Your healthcare provider should tell you what syringes and needles to use to inject INTRON A.

How should I prepare a dose of INTRON® A?
1. Find a well lit, clean, flat working surface.
2. Before removing INTRON A from the carton, look at the expiration date printed on the carton. Make sure that the expiration date has not passed. Do not use if the expiration date has passed.
3. Wash your hands well with soap and warm water (See Figure 1). Keep your work area, your hands and injection site clean to decrease the risk of infection.

Figure 1

4. Remove 1 vial of INTRON A solution from the carton (See Figure 2).

Figure 2

5. Look at the vial of INTRON A. The solution should be clear and colorless, without particles. Do not use the vial of INTRON A if the medicine is cloudy, has particles or is not clear and colorless.
6. Remove the protective plastic cap from the top of the INTRON A vial. Clean the rubber stopper on the top of the INTRON A vial with an alcohol swab (See Figure 3).

Figure 3

7. Gently warm the INTRON A solution by slowly rolling the vial in the palms of your hands for about one minute (See Figure 4). Do not shake the vial.

Figure 4

8. Open the package of the syringe you are using (See Figure 5) and if it does not have a needle attached, then attach a new needle to the syringe.

Figure 5

9. Remove the protective cap from the needle of the syringe. Fill the syringe with air by pulling back on the plunger to the mark on the syringe that matches the dose prescribed by your healthcare provider (See Figure 6).

Figure 6

10. Hold the vial of INTRON A Solution for Injection on your flat working surface (See Figure 7). Do not touch the cleaned rubber stopper.

Figure 7

11. Push the needle straight down through the middle of the rubber stopper of the vial containing the INTRON A solution (See Figure 8). Slowly inject all the air from the syringe into the air space above the solution.

Figure 8

12. Keep the needle in the vial. Turn the vial upside down (See Figure 9).
◦ Make sure the tip of the needle is in the INTRON A solution.
◦ Slowly pull the plunger back to fill the syringe with INTRON A solution to the dose (mL or cc) prescribed by your healthcare provider.

Figure 9

13. With the needle still in the vial, check the syringe for air bubbles (See Figure 10).
◦ If there are any air bubbles, gently tap the syringe with your finger until the air bubbles rise to the top of the syringe.
◦ Slowly push the plunger up to remove the air bubbles.
◦ If you push solution back into the vial, slowly pull back on the plunger to draw the dose prescribed by your healthcare provider.

Figure 10

14. Do not remove the needle from the vial. Lay the vial and syringe on its side on your flat work surface until you are ready to inject the INTRON A solution.

How should I choose a site for injection?
Based on your treatment, your healthcare provider will tell you if you should inject a dose of INTRON® A under the skin (subcutaneous injection) or into the muscle (intramuscular injection). If it is too difficult for you to inject, ask someone who has been trained to give injections to help you.

FOR SUBCUTANEOUS INJECTION
The best sites for injection are areas on your body with a layer of fat between skin and muscle such as (See Figure 11):
• the front of your middle thighs
• the outer area of your upper arms
• the abdomen, except around the navel
[See figure 11 at top of next column]
FOR INTRAMUSCULAR INJECTION
The best sites for injection into your muscle are (See Figure 12):

Figure 11

• the front of the middle thighs
• the upper arms
• the upper outer areas of the buttocks

Figure 12

You should use a different site each time you inject INTRON® A to avoid soreness at any one site. Do not inject INTRON A into an area where the skin is irritated, red, bruised, infected or has scars, stretch marks or lumps.

How should I inject a dose of INTRON® A?

15. Clean the injection site with a new alcohol swab. Wait for the area to dry.
16. Pick up the vial and syringe from your flat work surface. Remove the syringe and needle from the vial.
    ∘ Hold the syringe in the hand that you will use to inject INTRON A.
    ∘ Do not touch the needle or allow it to touch the work surface.
17. With your other hand, pinch a fold of the skin at the cleaned injection site.

For subcutaneous injection (under the skin):
∘ Hold the syringe (like a pencil) at a **45-degree angle** to the skin. With a quick "dart-like" motion, push the needle into the skin (See Figure 13).

Figure 13

For intramuscular injection (into the muscle):
∘ Hold the syringe (like a pencil) at a **90-degree angle** to the skin. With a quick "dart-like" motion, push the needle into the muscle (See Figure 14).

Figure 14

18. After the needle is inserted, remove the hand used to pinch the skin. Use it to hold the syringe barrel.
    ∘ Pull the plunger back slightly.
    ∘ **If no blood is present in the syringe,** inject the medicine by gently pressing the plunger all the way down the syringe barrel, until the syringe is empty.
    ∘ **If blood comes into the syringe,** the needle has entered a blood vessel. Do not inject INTRON® A.
    ∘ Withdraw the needle and throw away the syringe and needle in the puncture-proof container. See "How should I dispose of used syringes, needles and vials?"
    ∘ Then, repeat steps 1 through 18 with a new dose of INTRON A and inject the medicine at a new injection site.
19. When the syringe is empty, pull the needle out of the skin.
    ∘ Place a cotton ball or gauze over the injection site and press for several seconds. Do not massage the injection site.
    ∘ If there is bleeding, cover the injection site with a bandage.
20. Throw away the used syringe, needle and vial. See "How should I dispose of used syringes, needles and vials?"

How should I dispose of used syringes, needles and vials?
Throw away used syringes, needles and vials in a puncture-proof container, sharps container or a hard container, like a metal can with a lid. Always place needles facing down. Do not use glass or clear plastic containers for disposal of needles and syringes. **Always keep the puncture-proof container out of the reach of children.**
• Check with your healthcare provider for instructions about the right way to throw away used needles and syringes. There may be local or state laws about how to throw away used needles and syringes. Always follow the instructions of your healthcare provider.
Do not throw away used needles, syringes or the puncture-proof container in household trash and do not recycle them.

How should I store INTRON® A?
INTRON A Solution for Injection:
• Store in the refrigerator at 36°F to 46°F (2°C to 8°C).
• Do not freeze Intron A.
• Allow the INTRON A Solution for Injection to come to room temperature before using. INTRON A Solution in Multidose vials for Injection may be used to give more than 1 injection of medicine.
• Throw away any unused INTRON A Solution for Injection remaining in the vial after 1 month
• Keep away from heat.
• **Keep INTRON A and all medicines out of the reach of children.**

Schering Corporation, a subsidiary of **Merck & Co., Inc.,** Whitehouse Station, NJ 08889 USA
Copyright © 1996, 2001, 2004, Schering Corporation, a subsidiary of **Merck & Co., Inc.**
All rights reserved.
U.S. Patent No. 5,935,566 and 6,610,830.
Rev. 02/2011
B-350339708T

Instructions for Use
INTRON® A (In-tron-aye)
(Interferon alfa-2b, recombinant)
Powder for Solution
Be sure that you read, understand, and follow these instructions before injecting INTRON A. Your healthcare provider should show you how to prepare, measure, and inject INTRON A properly before you use it for the first time. Ask your healthcare provider if you have any questions.
Before starting, collect all of the supplies that you will need to use for preparing and injecting INTRON A. For each injection you will need the following supplies:
∘ 1 vial of INTRON A powder for solution
∘ 1 vial of sterile water for injection (diluent)
∘ 1 single-use disposable syringe and needle
∘ 1 cotton ball or gauze
∘ 2 alcohol swabs
You will also need a puncture-proof disposable container to throw away used syringes, needles and vials.
Important:
∘ **Never re-use disposable syringes and needles.**
∘ The vial of mixed INTRON A should be used right away. Do not mix more than 1 vial of INTRON A at a time. If you do not use the vial of prepared solution right away, store it in a refrigerator and use within 24 hours. See the end of these Instructions for Use for information about "How should I store INTRON A?"
∘ After mixing, throw away (discard) the vial of INTRON A after you withdraw one dose of medicine.
∘ Make sure you have the right syringe and needle to use with INTRON A. Your healthcare provider should tell you what syringes and needles to use to inject INTRON A.

How should I prepare a dose of INTRON A?
Before you inject INTRON A, the powder must be mixed with 1 mL (cc) of the sterile water for injection (diluent) from the INTRON A vial package.
1. Find a clean, well-lit, flat work surface.
2. Get one of your INTRON A vial packages. Check the date printed on the carton. Make sure that the expiration date has not passed.
3. Wash your hands well with soap and water. Keep your work area, your hands, and injection site clean to decrease the risk of infection (See Figure 1).

Figure 1

4. Gently warm the vial of diluent by slowly rolling the vial in the palms of your hands for one minute (See Figure 2).

Figure 2

5. Remove the protective plastic cap from the tops of both vials (INTRON A powder and the diluent). Clean the rubber stopper on the top of both vials with an alcohol swab (See Figure 3).

Figure 3

6. Open the package for the syringe (See Figure 4) you are using and if it does not have a needle attached, then attach a new needle to the syringe.

Figure 4

7. Remove the needle cover from the syringe. Fill the syringe with air by pulling the plunger back to 1 mL (See Figure 5).

Figure 5

8. Hold the diluent vial on your flat work surface. Do not touch the cleaned rubber stopper (See Figure 6).

Figure 6

9. Push the needle straight down through the middle of the rubber stopper of the diluent vial and slowly inject all the air from the syringe into the air space above the diluent (See Figure 7).

Figure 7

10. Keep the needle in the vial. Turn the vial upside down and make sure the tip of the needle is in the diluent.
    ∘ Slowly pull the plunger back to fill the syringe with diluent to the 1 mL mark on the side of the syringe (See Figure 8).
[See figure 8 at top of next column]
11. With the needle still inserted in the vial, check the syringe for air bubbles (See Figure 9).
    ∘ If there are any air bubbles, gently tap the syringe with your finger until the air bubbles rise to the top of the syringe.
    ∘ Slowly push the plunger up to remove the air bubbles.

Figure 8

If you push diluent back into the vial, slowly pull back on the plunger to again draw 1 mL of diluent back into the syringe.

Figure 9

12. Remove the needle from the vial. Do not let the syringe touch anything.
13. Insert the needle through the center of the rubber stopper of the INTRON A powder vial. Do not touch the cleaned rubber stopper.
    ◦ Place the needle tip, at an angle, against the side of the INTRON A powder vial (See Figure 10).

Figure 10

◦ Slowly push the plunger down to inject the diluent into the vial. The stream of liquid should run down the sides of the glass vial.
◦ To prevent bubbles from forming, do not aim the stream of diluent directly on the medicine in the bottom of the vial.
◦ Do not remove the needle from the vial.
14. Gently swirl the INTRON A vial in a circular motion until the powder is completely dissolved (See Figure 11).

Figure 11

◦ Do not shake the vial. If any powder remains undissolved in the vial, gently turn the vial upside down until all of the powder is dissolved.
◦ The solution may look cloudy or bubbly for a few minutes. If air bubbles do form, wait until the solution settles and all bubbles rise to the top. Then withdraw your dose from the vial.
15. After the INTRON A completely dissolves, the solution should be clear and colorless to light yellow, without particles. Do not use the mixed solution if you see particles in it, or it is not clear and colorless to light yellow.
16. With the needle in the vial, turn the vial upside down (See Figure 12).
[See figure 12 at top of next column]
    ◦ Hold the vial with one hand. Be sure the tip of the needle is in the INTRON A solution. Slowly pull the plunger back to fill the syringe with the exact amount of INTRON A into the syringe that your healthcare provider told you to use.
17. With the needle still inserted in the vial, check the syringe for air bubbles. If you see any air bubbles, gently tap the syringe with your finger until the air bubbles rise to the top of the syringe (See Figure 13).
[See figure 13 at top of next column]
18. Slowly push the plunger up to remove the air bubbles. If you push solution back into the vial, slowly pull back on the plunger again to draw the correct amount of INTRON A solution back into the syringe.

Figure 12

Figure 13

19. Do not remove the needle from the vial. Lay the vial and syringe on its side on your flat work surface until you are ready to inject the INTRON A solution.

How should I choose a site for injection?
Based on your treatment, your healthcare provider will tell you if you should inject a dose of INTRON® A under the skin (subcutaneous injection) or into the muscle (intramuscular injection). If it is too difficult for you to inject, ask someone who has been trained to give injections to help you.

FOR SUBCUTANEOUS INJECTION
The best sites for injection are areas on your body with a layer of fat between skin and muscle, such as (See Figure 14):
• the front of your middle thighs
• the outer area of your upper arms
• the abdomen, except around the navel

Figure 14

FOR INTRAMUSCULAR INJECTION
The best sites for injection into your muscle are (See Figure 15):
• the front of the middle thighs
• the upper arms
• the upper outer areas of the buttocks

Figure 15

You should use a different site each time you inject INTRON® A to avoid soreness at any one site. Do not inject INTRON A into an area where the skin is irritated, red, bruised, infected or has scars, stretch marks, or lumps.

How should I inject a dose of INTRON® A?
20. Clean the injection site with a new alcohol swab. Wait for the skin to dry.
21. Pick up the vial and syringe from your flat work surface. Remove the syringe and needle from the vial.
    ◦ Hold the syringe in the hand that you will use to inject INTRON A.
    ◦ Do not touch the needle or allow it to touch the work surface.
22. With one hand, pinch a fold of the skin at the cleaned injection site.
23. **For subcutaneous injection (under the skin):**
    ◦ With the other hand, hold the syringe (like a pencil) at a **45-degree angle** to the skin. With a quick "dart-like" motion, push the needle into the skin (See Figure 16).
[See figure 16 at top of next column]
24. **For intramuscular injection (into the muscle):**
    ◦ Hold the syringe (like a pencil) at a **90-degree angle** to the skin.

Figure 16

◦ With a quick "dart-like" motion, push the needle into the muscle (See Figure 17).

Figure 17

25. After the needle is inserted, remove the hand used to pinch the skin and use it to hold the syringe barrel.
    ◦ Pull the plunger back slightly.
    ◦ **If no blood is present in the syringe**, inject the medicine by gently pushing the plunger all the way down the syringe barrel, until the syringe is empty.
    ◦ **If blood comes into the syringe**, the needle has entered a blood vessel. Do not inject INTRON® A.
      ◦ Withdraw the needle and throw away the syringe and needle in the puncture-proof container. See "How should I dispose of used syringes, needles and vials?".
      ◦ Then, repeat steps 1 through 25 with a new dose of INTRON A and inject the medicine at a new injection site.
26. When the syringe is empty, pull the needle out of the skin.
    ◦ Place a cotton ball or gauze over the injection site and press for several seconds. Do not massage the injection site.
    ◦ If there is bleeding, cover the injection site with a bandage.
27. Throw away the used syringe, needle, and vial. See "How should I dispose of used syringes, needles and vials?".

How should I dispose of used syringes, needles, and vials?
• Throw away used syringes, needles, and vials in a puncture-proof container, such as sharps container, or a hard container like a metal can with a lid. Always place needles facing down. Do not use glass or clear plastic containers for disposal of needles and syringes. **Always keep the puncture-proof container out of the reach of children.**
• Do not throw away used needles, syringes, or the puncture-proof container in household trash and do not recycle them.
• Check with your healthcare provider for instructions about the right way to throw away used needles and syringes. There may be special state and local laws for disposal of used needles and syringes. Always follow the instructions of your healthcare provider.

How should I store INTRON® A?
INTRON A Powder for Injection:
◦ Before mixing, store in the refrigerator between 36°F to 46°F (2°C to 8°C).
◦ After mixing the INTRON A Powder for Injection, use the solution right away or store the solution in the refrigerator for up to 24 hours between 36°F to 46°F (2°C to 8°C). Allow the solution to come to room temperature before using.
◦ Do not freeze Intron A.
◦ Keep away from heat.
◦ Throw away any medicine left in the vial after you withdraw 1 dose.

Keep INTRON A and all medicines out of the reach of children.

Schering Corporation, a subsidiary of **Merck & Co., Inc.**, Whitehouse Station, NJ 08889 USA
Copyright © 1996, 2001, 2004, Schering Corporation, a subsidiary of **Merck & Co., Inc.**
All rights reserved.
Rev. 02/2011
U.S. Patent Nos. 5,935,566 and 6,610,830.
35038302T

Instructions for Use

INTRON® A (In-tron-aye)
(Interferon alfa-2b, recombinant)
Solution for Injection Multidose Pen
Be sure that you read, understand, and follow these instructions about the right way to use your Multidose Pen before injecting INTRON A. Your healthcare provider should show you how to prepare, measure, and inject your INTRON A from the Multidose Pen properly before you use it for the first time. Ask your healthcare provider if you have any questions.

Before starting, collect all of the supplies that you will need to use for preparing and injecting INTRON A from your

Multidose Pen. Make sure you have the right strength of INTRON A Multidose Pen that your healthcare provider prescribed for you. You will need the following supplies:
• the INTRON A Multidose Pen
• 1 Novofine® needle
• 2 alcohol swabs
• 1 cotton ball or gauze

You will also need a puncture-proof disposable container to throw away your used INTRON A Multidose Pen and the Novofine needle.

Important:
◦ **Never re-use needles.**
◦ Make sure that you have the correct INTRON A Multidose Pen prescribed by your healthcare provider. The INTRON A Multidose Pen should only be used with **Novofine** needles. These are the needles that come packaged with the pen. If you use other needles, the pen may not work the right way. You could get the wrong dose of INTRON A.
◦ INTRON A Multidose Pen may be used to give more than 1 injection of medicine.

To prevent spread of infection, do not allow anyone else to use your multidose pen and needles. Figures 1 and 2 below show the different parts of the INTRON A Multidose Pen and the Novofine needle. The parts of the pen you need to know are:

INTRON A Pen   Novofine Needle Assembly

Figure 1   **Figure 2**

• The **color-coded push button** and **push button scale**. These are located at the bottom of the pen when it is held with the cap side up. This tells you the dose that has been set.
• The **color-coding** band. This is located on the INTRON A reservoir. The band lets you know the dose that you are using.
  ◦ **The 3 MIU INTRON A Multidose Pen**: has a brown push button, a brown color-coding band, and color-coded label.
  ◦ **The 5 MIU INTRON A Multidose Pen**: has a light blue push button, a light blue color-coding band, and color-coded label.
  ◦ **The 10 MIU INTRON A Multidose Pen**: has a pink push button, a pink color-coding band, and color-coded label.
• The **cap**. The cap is used for setting the dose and storing the pen. You will not be able to set the dose or completely close the pen unless you line up the **triangle** on the **cap scale** with the **dosage indicator** on the barrel.

How should I prepare a dose of INTRON® A using a Multidose Pen?
1. Find a clean, well-lit, flat work surface.
2. Get one of your INTRON A Multidose Pen packages. Look at the date printed on the carton to make sure that the expiration date has not passed. Do not use if the expiration date has passed.
3. Wash your hands well with soap and warm water (See Figure 3). It is important to keep your work area, your hands, and injection site clean to decrease the risk of infection.

Figure 3

4. Remove the INTRON A Multidose Pen from the carton. Pull the cap off the pen and put the cap on the clean, flat work surface so that the inside of the cap remains clean (you will need to use this cap to recap the INTRON A Multidose pen in step 32 below). Wipe the rubber membrane with one alcohol swab (See Figure 4).

Figure 4

5. Look at the solution inside the pen. The solution should be clear and colorless, without particles. Do not use the INTRON A if the medicine is cloudy, has particles, or is not clear and colorless.
6. Remove the paper backing from the Novofine® needle by pulling the paper tab (See Figure 5). You will see the back of the needle once the paper tab is removed.

Figure 5

7. Keep the needle in its outer, clear needle cap. Gently push the Novofine needle straight into the pen's rubber membrane that you just cleaned. Screw the needle onto the INTRON A Multidose Pen by turning it in the direction of the arrow in the figure below (clockwise) (See Figure 6).

Figure 6

8. With the needle facing up, pull off the outer, clear needle cap (See Figure 7). Set the outer needle cap down on your clean flat work surface for later use and make sure that the inside of the cap remains clean. Next, carefully pull off the white inner needle cap (See Figure 8). The needle can be seen now.

Figure 7

Figure 8

9. Keep the needle facing up and remove any air bubbles that may be in the reservoir by tapping the reservoir with your finger (See Figure 9). If you have any air bubbles, they will rise to the top of the reservoir.

Figure 9

10. Hold the pen by the barrel. Turn the INTRON A reservoir in the direction of the arrow in the figure below (clockwise), until you feel it click into place (See Figure 10).

Figure 10

11. Keep the needle facing up and press the push button all the way up. A drop of INTRON A solution should come out of the tip of the needle (See Figure 11).

Figure 11

12. Put the outer cap you removed in Step 8 above back on the INTRON A Multidose Pen. Make sure you line up the black triangle on the pen cap with the dosage indicator on the pen barrel (See Figure 12). The pen is now ready to set the dose.

Figure 12

How should I set the dose prescribed by my healthcare provider?
13. Hold the pen from side-to-side (horizontally) in the middle of the pen barrel so the push button can move freely with one of your hands. With the other hand, hold the Multidose Pen cap (See Figure 13).

Figure 13

14. Set the dose prescribed by your healthcare provider by turning the cap in the direction of the arrow (clockwise). With each clockwise turn, the push button will start to rise and you will see the push button scale. Do not use force to turn the pen cap or you may damage the pen.
• To set a 3 MIU dose using the 3 MIU Multidose Pen, turn the cap 2 full turns (10 clicks) = 3 MIU (See Figure 14).

Figure 14

• To set a 5 MIU dose using the 5 MIU Multidose Pen, turn the cap 2 full turns (10 clicks) = 5 MIU (See Figure 15).

Figure 15

• To set a 10 MIU dose using the 10 MIU Multidose Pen, turn the cap 2 full turns (10 clicks) = 10 MIU (See Figure 16).

Figure 16

15. After each complete turn, make sure the triangle on the cap is lined up with the dosage indicator on the pen barrel.

If your healthcare provider has prescribed a dose other than 3.0, 5.0, or 10.0 MIU, the dose can be set by turning the cap as many times as shown below:

A dose prescribed other than 3 MIU from the 3 MIU multidose pen
1 full turn (5 clicks) = 1.5 MIU
3 full turns (15 clicks) = 4.5 MIU
4 full turns (20 clicks) = 6 MIU

A dose prescribed other than 5 MIU from the 5 MIU multidose pen
1 full turn (5 clicks) = 2.5 MIU
3 full turns (15 clicks) = 7.5 MIU
4 full turns (20 clicks) = 10 MIU

A dose prescribed other than 10 MIU from the 10 MIU multidose pen
1 full turn (5 clicks) = 5 MIU
3 full turns (15 clicks) = 15 MIU
4 full turns (20 clicks) = 20 MIU

16. Check the push button scale to make sure you have set the correct dose.
17. If you set a wrong dose:
   • Turn the cap back (counterclockwise) as far as you can until the push button is all the way in, and the push button scale is completely covered.
   • Then begin at step 13 again.
18. Gently warm the INTRON® A Multidose Pen by slowly rolling the capped Multidose Pen in the palms of your hands for about one minute (See Figure 17). **Do not shake.**

Figure 17

19. Place the Multidose Pen on your flat work surface until you are ready to inject INTRON A.

How should I choose a site for injection?
INTRON® A is given from the Multidose Pen as an injection under the skin (subcutaneous injection). If it is too difficult for you to inject, ask someone who has been trained to give injections to help you.
The best sites for injection are areas on your body with a layer of fat between skin and muscle (See Figure 18), such as:
• the front of the middle thighs
• the outer area of the upper arms
• the abdomen, except around the navel

Figure 18

You should use a different site each time you inject INTRON A to avoid soreness at any one site. Do not inject INTRON A into an area where the skin is irritated, red, bruised, infected or has scars, stretch marks, or lumps.

How should I inject a dose of INTRON® A?
20. Clean the injection site with a new alcohol swab.
21. Pick up the Multidose Pen from your flat work surface and remove the cap from the needle.
22. With one hand, pinch a fold of the skin at the cleaned injection site.
23. Hold the Multidose Pen (like a pencil) at a **45-degree angle** to the skin. With a quick "dart-like" motion, push the needle into the skin (See Figure 19).

Figure 19

24. After the needle is inserted, remove the hand used to pinch the skin and use it to hold the pen barrel.
   ◦ Pull the plunger back slightly.
   ◦ **If no blood is present in the pen reservoir,** inject the medicine by gently pressing the push button all the way down.

   • **If blood comes into the pen reservoir,** the needle has entered a blood vessel. Do not inject INTRON A.
     ◦ Withdraw the needle and throw away the used INTRON A Multidose Pen and needle in the puncture-proof container. See "How should I dispose of the used INTRON A Multidose Pens and needles?".
     ◦ Then, repeat steps 1 through 24 with a new dose of INTRON A and inject the medicine at a new injection site.
25. Leave the needle in place for a few seconds while holding down the push button.
26. Slowly release the push button and pull the needle out of the skin.
27. Place a cotton ball or gauze over the injection site and press for several seconds.
   ◦ Do not massage the injection site.
   ◦ If there is bleeding, cover the injection site with a bandage.
28. If there is enough solution left in the INTRON A Multidose Pen for another dose of INTRON A, refrigerate the INTRON A Multidose Pen after use.

How should I remove the needle from the Multidose Pen?
29. To remove the needle, you have to recap the needle. Do not hold the cap in your hand, you may hurt yourself. Instead, using a scooping motion, carefully replace the outer, clear needle cap (like capping a pen) (See Figure 20).

Figure 20

30. After you recap the needle, remove the needle by holding the clear outer needle cap with one hand and holding the pen barrel with the other hand. Turn in the direction of the arrow (counterclockwise), as in Figure 21 below.

Figure 21

31. Carefully lift the needle off the pen and throw away the capped needle (See Figure 22). See "How should I dispose of the used INTRON A Multidose Pens and needles?"

Figure 22

32. Replace the pen cap you removed in Step 4 above over the pen reservoir so that the black triangle is lined up with the dosage indicator (See Figure 23).

Figure 23

How should I dispose of the used INTRON A Multidose Pens and needles?
• Throw away all used needles and Multidose Pens in a puncture-proof container, sharps container, or a hard container like a metal can with a lid. Always place needles facing down. Do not use glass or clear plastic containers for disposal of needles and syringes. **Always keep the puncture-proof container out of the reach of children.**
• Check with your healthcare provider for instructions about the right way to throw away used needles and used Multidose Pens. There may be local or state laws about how to throw away used needles and Multidose Pens. Always follow the instructions of your healthcare provider.
• Do not throw away used needles and Multidose Pens in household trash and do not recycle them.

How should I store the INTRON® A Multidose Pen?
INTRON A in Multidose Pens:
Store in the refrigerator at 36°F to 46°F (2°C to 8°C).
◦ INTRON A Solution for Injection in the Multidose Pens may be used to give more than 1 injection of medicine.
Do not throw away used needles, syringes or the puncture-proof container in household trash and do not recycle them.

Keep INTRON A and all medicines out of the reach of children.
Schering Corporation, a subsidiary of **Merck & Co., Inc.,** Whitehouse Station, NJ 08889, USA
Copyright © 1996, 2001, 2006, Schering Corporation, a subsidiary of **Merck & Co., Inc.**
All rights reserved.
U.S. Patent Nos. 5,935,566 and 6,610,830
Novofine® is a registered trademark of Novo Nordisk A/S.
B-35038400T
Rev. 02/2011
Shown in Product Identification Guide, page 308

INVANZ®   ℞
(ertapenem for injection)
for intravenous (IV) or intramuscular (IM) use

HIGHLIGHTS OF PRESCRIBING INFORMATION
These highlights do not include all the information needed to use INVANZ safely and effectively. See full prescribing information for INVANZ.
INVANZ® (ertapenem for injection) for intravenous (IV) or intramuscular (IM) use
Initial U.S. Approval: 2001

To reduce the development of drug-resistant bacteria and maintain the effectiveness of INVANZ and other antibacterial drugs, INVANZ should be used only to treat or prevent infections that are proven or strongly suspected to be caused by susceptible bacteria. (1)

————INDICATIONS AND USAGE————
INVANZ is a penem antibacterial indicated in adult patients and pediatric patients (3 months of age and older) for the treatment of the following moderate to severe infections caused by susceptible bacteria:
• Complicated intra-abdominal infections. (1.1)
• Complicated skin and skin structure infections, including diabetic foot infections without osteomyelitis. (1.2)
• Community-acquired pneumonia. (1.3)
• Complicated urinary tract infections including pyelonephritis. (1.4)
• Acute pelvic infections including postpartum endomyometritis, septic abortion and post surgical gynecologic infections. (1.5)
INVANZ is indicated in adults for the prophylaxis of surgical site infection following elective colorectal surgery. (1.6)

————DOSAGE AND ADMINISTRATION————
Do not mix or co-infuse INVANZ with other medications. Do not use diluents containing dextrose (α–D–glucose). (2.1)
INVANZ should be infused over 30 minutes in both the Treatment and Prophylactic regimens. (2.1)
Dosing considerations should be made in adults with advanced or end-stage renal impairment and those on hemodialysis. (2.4, 2.5)
Treatment regimen:
• Adults and pediatric patients 13 years of age and older. The dosage should be 1 gram once a day intravenously or intramuscularly. (2.2)
• Patients 3 months to 12 years of age should be administered 15 mg/kg twice daily (not to exceed 1 g/day intravenously or intramuscularly.) (2.2)
• Intravenous infusion may be administered in adults and pediatrics for up to 14 days or intramuscular injection for up to 7 days. (2.1)
Prophylaxis regimen for adults:
• 1 gram single dose given 1 hour prior to elective colorectal surgery. (2.3)

————DOSAGE FORMS AND STRENGTHS————
• Vial 1 gram. (3)
• ADD-Vantage® vial: 1 gram. (3)

————CONTRAINDICATIONS————
• Known hypersensitivity to product components or anaphylactic reactions to β-lactams. (4)
• Due to the use of lidocaine HCl as a diluent, INVANZ administered intramuscularly is contraindicated in patients with a known hypersensitivity to local anesthetics of the amide type. (4)

————WARNINGS AND PRECAUTIONS————
• Serious hypersensitivity (anaphylactic) reactions have been reported in patients receiving β-lactams. (5.1)
• Seizures and other central nervous system adverse experiences have been reported during treatment. (5.2)
• Co-administration of INVANZ with valproic acid or divalproex sodium reduces the serum concentration of valproic acid potentially increasing the risk of breakthrough seizures. (5.3)
• *Clostridium difficile*-associated diarrhea (ranging from mild diarrhea to fatal colitis): Evaluate if diarrhea occurs. (5.4)

• Caution should be taken when administering INVANZ intramuscularly to avoid inadvertent injection into a blood vessel. (5.5)

---ADVERSE REACTIONS---

Adults:
The most common adverse reactions (≥5%) in patients treated with INVANZ, including those who were switched to therapy with an oral antimicrobial, were diarrhea, nausea, headache and infused vein complication. (6.1)
In the prophylaxis indication the overall adverse experience profile was generally comparable to that observed for ertapenem in other clinical trials. (6.1)
Pediatrics:
Adverse reactions in this population were comparable to adults. The most common adverse reactions (≥5%) in pediatric patients treated with INVANZ, including those who were switched to therapy with an oral antimicrobial, were diarrhea, vomiting and infusion site pain. (6.1)
To report SUSPECTED ADVERSE REACTIONS, contact Merck Sharp & Dohme Corp., a subsidiary of Merck & Co., Inc., at 1-877-888-4231 or FDA at 1-800-FDA-1088 or www.fda.gov/medwatch.

---DRUG INTERACTIONS---

• Co-administration with probenecid inhibits the renal excretion of ertapenem and is therefore not recommended. (7.1)
• The concomitant use of ertapenem and valproic acid/divalproex sodium is generally not recommended. Antibacterials other than carbapenems should be considered to treat infections in patients whose seizures are well controlled on valproic acid or divalproex sodium. (5.2, 7.2)

---USE IN SPECIFIC POPULATIONS---

• Renal Impairment: Dose adjustment is necessary, if creatinine clearance is ≤30 mL/min/1.73 m^2. (2.4, 8.6, 12.3)
See 17 for PATIENT COUNSELING INFORMATION
Revised: 08/2014

FULL PRESCRIBING INFORMATION: CONTENTS*

* Sections or subsections omitted from the full prescribing information are not listed

Table 1: Treatment Guidelines for Adults and Pediatric Patients With Normal Renal Function* and Body Weight

Infection[†]	Daily Dose (IV or IM) Adults and Pediatric Patients 13 years of age and older	Daily Dose (IV or IM) Pediatric Patients 3 months to 12 years of age	Recommended Duration of Total Antimicrobial Treatment
Complicated intra-abdominal infections	1 g	15 mg/kg twice daily[‡]	5 to 14 days
Complicated skin and skin structure infections, including diabetic foot infections[§]	1 g	15 mg/kg twice daily[‡]	7 to 14 days[¶]
Community acquired pneumonia	1 g	15 mg/kg twice daily[‡]	10 to 14 days[#]
Complicated urinary tract infections, including pyelonephritis	1 g	15 mg/kg twice daily[‡]	10 to 14 days[#]
Acute pelvic infections including postpartum endomyometritis, septic abortion and post surgical gynecologic infections	1 g	15 mg/kg twice daily[‡]	3 to 10 days

* defined as creatinine clearance >90 mL/min/1.73 m^2
† due to the designated pathogens [see Indications and Usage (1)]
‡ not to exceed 1 g/day
§ INVANZ has not been studied in diabetic foot infections with concomitant osteomyelitis [see Clinical Studies (14.1)].
¶ adult patients with diabetic foot infections received up to 28 days of treatment (parenteral or parenteral plus oral switch therapy)
# duration includes a possible switch to an appropriate oral therapy, after at least 3 days of parenteral therapy, once clinical improvement has been demonstrated.

FULL PRESCRIBING INFORMATION

1   INDICATIONS AND USAGE

To reduce the development of drug-resistant bacteria and maintain the effectiveness of INVANZ® and other antibacterial drugs, INVANZ should be used only to treat or prevent infections that are proven or strongly suspected to be caused by susceptible bacteria. When culture and susceptibility information are available, they should be considered in selecting or modifying antibacterial therapy. In the absence of such data, local epidemiology and susceptibility patterns may contribute to the empiric selection of therapy.
Treatment
INVANZ is indicated for the treatment of adult patients and pediatric patients (3 months of age and older) with the following moderate to severe infections caused by susceptible isolates of the designated microorganisms [see Dosage and Administration (2)].

1.1   Complicated Intra-Abdominal Infections
INVANZ is indicated for the treatment of complicated intra-abdominal infections due to *Escherichia coli, Clostridium clostridioforme, Eubacterium lentum, Peptostreptococcus* species, *Bacteroides fragilis, Bacteroides distasonis, Bacteroides ovatus, Bacteroides thetaiotaomicron,* or *Bacteroides uniformis.*

1.2   Complicated Skin and Skin Structure Infections, Including Diabetic Foot Infections without Osteomyelitis
INVANZ is indicated for the treatment of complicated skin and skin structure infections, including diabetic foot infections without osteomyelitis due to *Staphylococcus aureus* (methicillin susceptible isolates only), *Streptococcus agalactiae, Streptococcus pyogenes, Escherichia coli, Klebsiella pneumoniae, Proteus mirabilis, Bacteroides fragilis, Peptostreptococcus* species, *Porphyromonas asaccharolytica,* or *Prevotella bivia.* INVANZ has not been studied in diabetic foot infections with concomitant osteomyelitis [see Clinical Studies (14)].

1.3   Community Acquired Pneumonia
INVANZ is indicated for the treatment of community acquired pneumonia due to *Streptococcus pneumoniae* (penicillin susceptible isolates only) including cases with concurrent bacteremia, *Haemophilus influenzae* (beta-lactamase negative isolates only), or *Moraxella catarrhalis.*

1.4   Complicated Urinary Tract Infections Including Pyelonephritis
INVANZ is indicated for the treatment of complicated urinary tract infections including pyelonephritis due to *Escherichia coli,* including cases with concurrent bacteremia, or *Klebsiella pneumoniae.*

1.5   Acute Pelvic Infections Including Postpartum Endomyometritis, Septic Abortion and Post Surgical Gynecologic Infections
INVANZ is indicated for the treatment of acute pelvic infections including postpartum endomyometritis, septic abortion and post surgical gynecological infections due to *Streptococcus agalactiae, Escherichia coli, Bacteroides fragilis, Porphyromonas asaccharolytica, Peptostreptococcus* species, or *Prevotella bivia.*
Prevention
INVANZ is indicated in adults for:
1.6   Prophylaxis of Surgical Site Infection Following Elective Colorectal Surgery
INVANZ is indicated for the prevention of surgical site infection following elective colorectal surgery.

2   DOSAGE AND ADMINISTRATION
2.1   Instructions for Use in All Patients
For Intravenous or Intramuscular Use
DO NOT MIX OR CO-INFUSE INVANZ WITH OTHER MEDICATIONS. DO NOT USE DILUENTS CONTAINING DEXTROSE (α-D-GLUCOSE).
INVANZ may be administered by intravenous infusion for up to 14 days or intramuscular injection for up to 7 days. When administered intravenously, INVANZ should be infused over a period of 30 minutes. Intramuscular administration of INVANZ may be used as an alternative to intravenous administration in the treatment of those infections for which intramuscular therapy is appropriate.

2.2   Treatment Regimen
13 years of age and older
The dose of INVANZ in patients 13 years of age and older is 1 gram (g) given once a day [see Clinical Pharmacology (12.3)].
3 months to 12 years of age
The dose of INVANZ in patients 3 months to 12 years of age is 15 mg/kg twice daily (not to exceed 1 g/day).
Table 1 presents treatment guidelines for INVANZ.
[See table 1 above]
2.3   Prophylactic Regimen in Adults
Table 2 presents prophylaxis guidelines for INVANZ.

Table 2: Prophylaxis Guidelines for Adults

Indication	Daily Dose (IV) Adults	Recommended Duration of Total Antimicrobial Treatment
Prophylaxis of surgical site infection following elective colorectal surgery	1 g	Single intravenous dose given 1 hour prior to surgical incision

2.4 Patients with Renal Impairment

INVANZ may be used for the treatment of infections in adult patients with renal impairment. In patients whose creatinine clearance is >30 mL/min/1.73 m^2, no dosage adjustment is necessary. Adult patients with severe renal impairment (creatinine clearance ≤30 mL/min/1.73 m^2) and end-stage renal disease (creatinine clearance ≤10 mL/min/1.73 m^2) should receive 500 mg daily. A supplementary dose of 150 mg is recommended if ertapenem is administered within 6 hours prior to hemodialysis. There are no data in pediatric patients with renal impairment.

2.5 Patients on Hemodialysis

When adult patients on hemodialysis are given the recommended daily dose of 500 mg of INVANZ within 6 hours prior to hemodialysis, a supplementary dose of 150 mg is recommended following the hemodialysis session. If INVANZ is given at least 6 hours prior to hemodialysis, no supplementary dose is needed. There are no data in patients undergoing peritoneal dialysis or hemofiltration. There are no data in pediatric patients on hemodialysis. When only the serum creatinine is available, the following formula[1] may be used to estimate creatinine clearance. The serum creatinine should represent a steady state of renal function.

Males: $\dfrac{(\text{weight in kg}) \times (140\text{-age in years})}{(72) \times \text{serum creatinine (mg/100 mL)}}$

Females: (0.85) × (value calculated for males)

[1]Cockcroft and Gault equation: Cockcroft DW, Gault MH. Prediction of creatinine clearance from serum creatinine. Nephron. 1976

2.6 Patients with Hepatic Impairment

No dose adjustment recommendations can be made in patients with hepatic impairment *[see Use in Specific Populations (8.7) and Clinical Pharmacology (12.3)]*.

2.7 Preparation and Reconstitution for Administration

Vials

Adults and pediatric patients 13 years of age and older
Preparation for intravenous administration:

DO NOT MIX OR CO-INFUSE INVANZ WITH OTHER MEDICATIONS. DO NOT USE DILUENTS CONTAINING DEXTROSE (α-D-GLUCOSE).

INVANZ MUST BE RECONSTITUTED AND THEN DILUTED PRIOR TO ADMINISTRATION.

1. Reconstitute the contents of a 1 g vial of INVANZ with 10 mL of one of the following: Water for Injection, 0.9% Sodium Chloride Injection or Bacteriostatic Water for Injection.
2. Shake well to dissolve and immediately transfer contents of the reconstituted vial to 50 mL of 0.9% Sodium Chloride Injection.
3. Complete the infusion within 6 hours of reconstitution.

Preparation for intramuscular administration:

INVANZ MUST BE RECONSTITUTED PRIOR TO ADMINISTRATION.

1. Reconstitute the contents of a 1 g vial of INVANZ with 3.2 mL of 1.0% lidocaine HCl injection[2] (**without epinephrine**). Shake vial thoroughly to form solution.
2. Immediately withdraw the contents of the vial and administer by deep intramuscular injection into a large muscle mass (such as the gluteal muscles or lateral part of the thigh).
3. The reconstituted IM solution should be used within 1 hour after preparation. **NOTE: THE RECONSTITUTED SOLUTION SHOULD NOT BE ADMINISTERED INTRAVENOUSLY.**

Pediatric patients 3 months to 12 years of age
Preparation for intravenous administration:

DO NOT MIX OR CO-INFUSE INVANZ WITH OTHER MEDICATIONS. DO NOT USE DILUENTS CONTAINING DEXTROSE (α-D-GLUCOSE).

INVANZ MUST BE RECONSTITUTED AND THEN DILUTED PRIOR TO ADMINISTRATION.

1. Reconstitute the contents of a 1 g vial of INVANZ with 10 mL of one of the following: Water for Injection, 0.9% Sodium Chloride Injection or Bacteriostatic Water for Injection.
2. Shake well to dissolve and immediately withdraw a volume equal to 15 mg/kg of body weight (not to exceed 1 g/day) and dilute in 0.9% Sodium Chloride Injection to a final concentration of 20 mg/mL or less.
3. Complete the infusion within 6 hours of reconstitution.

Preparation for intramuscular administration:

INVANZ MUST BE RECONSTITUTED PRIOR TO ADMINISTRATION.

1. Reconstitute the contents of a 1 g vial of INVANZ with 3.2 mL of 1.0% lidocaine HCl injection[2] (**without epinephrine**). Shake vial thoroughly to form solution.
2. Immediately withdraw a volume equal to 15 mg/kg of body weight (not to exceed 1 g/day) and administer by deep intramuscular injection into a large muscle mass (such as the gluteal muscles or lateral part of the thigh).

3. The reconstituted IM solution should be used within 1 hour after preparation. **NOTE: THE RECONSTITUTED SOLUTION SHOULD NOT BE ADMINISTERED INTRAVENOUSLY.**

ADD-Vantage®[3] Vials

INVANZ in ADD-Vantage® vials should be reconstituted with ADD-Vantage® diluent containers containing 50 mL or 100 mL of 0.9% Sodium Chloride Injection.

[2]Refer to the prescribing information for lidocaine HCl.
[3]Registered trademark of Hospira Laboratories, Inc.

INSTRUCTIONS FOR USE OF
INVANZ®
(Ertapenem for Injection)
IN ADD-Vantage VIALS
For I.V. Use Only.
To Open Diluent Container:
Peel overwrap from the corner and remove container. Some opacity of the plastic due to moisture absorption during the sterilization process may be observed. This is normal and does not affect the solution quality or safety. The opacity will diminish gradually.
To Assemble Vial and Flexible Diluent Container:
(Use Aseptic Technique)
Remove the protective covers from the top of the vial and the vial port on the diluent container as follows:
To remove the breakaway vial cap, swing the pull ring over the top of the vial and pull down far enough to start the opening. (SEE FIGURE 1.) Pull the ring approximately half way around the cap and then pull straight up to remove the cap. (SEE FIGURE 2.) NOTE: DO NOT ACCESS VIAL WITH SYRINGE.

Fig. 1   Fig. 2

To remove the vial port cover, grasp the tab on the pull ring, pull up to break the three tie strings, then pull back to remove the cover. (SEE FIGURE 3.)
Screw the vial into the vial port until it will go no further. THE VIAL MUST BE SCREWED IN TIGHTLY TO ASSURE A SEAL. This occurs approximately ½ turn (180°) after the first audible click. (SEE FIGURE 4.) The clicking sound does not assure a seal; the vial must be turned as far as it will go. NOTE: Once vial is seated, do not attempt to remove. (SEE FIGURE 4.)
Recheck the vial to assure that it is tight by trying to turn it further in the direction of assembly.
Label appropriately.

Fig. 3   Fig. 4

To Prepare Admixture:
Squeeze the bottom of the diluent container gently to inflate the portion of the container surrounding the end of the drug vial.
With the other hand, push the drug vial down into the container telescoping the walls of the container. Grasp the inner cap of the vial through the walls of the container. (SEE FIGURE 5.)
Pull the inner cap from the drug vial. (SEE FIGURE 6.) Verify that the rubber stopper has been pulled out, allowing the drug and diluent to mix.
Mix container contents thoroughly and use within the specified time.

Fig. 5   Fig. 6

Preparation for Administration:
(Use Aseptic Technique)
Confirm the activation and admixture of vial contents.
Check for leaks by squeezing container firmly. If leaks are found, discard unit as sterility may be impaired.
Close flow control clamp of administration set.
Remove cover from outlet port at bottom of container.
Insert piercing pin of administration set into port with a twisting motion until the pin is firmly seated. NOTE: See full directions on administration set carton.
Lift the free end of the hanger loop on the bottom of the vial, breaking the two tie strings. Bend the loop outward to lock it in the upright position, then suspend container from hanger.
Squeeze and release drip chamber to establish proper fluid level in chamber.
Open flow control clamp and clear air from set. Close clamp. Attach set to venipuncture device. If device is not indwelling, prime and make venipuncture.
Regulate rate of administration with flow control clamp.
WARNING: Do not use flexible container in series connections.
Storage
INVANZ (Ertapenem for Injection) 1 g single dose ADD-Vantage® vials should be prepared with ADD-Vantage® diluent containers containing 50 mL or 100 mL of 0.9% Sodium Chloride Injection. When prepared with this diluent, INVANZ (Ertapenem for Injection) maintains satisfactory potency **for 6 hours at room temperature (25°C) or for 24 hours under refrigeration (5°C) and used within 4 hours after removal from refrigeration. Solutions of INVANZ should not be frozen.**
Before administering, see accompanying package circular for INVANZ (Ertapenem for Injection).
Parenteral drug products should be inspected visually for particulate matter and discoloration prior to use, whenever solution and container permit. Solutions of INVANZ range from colorless to pale yellow. Variations of color within this range do not affect the potency of the product.

3 DOSAGE FORMS AND STRENGTHS

Vials
INVANZ is a sterile lyophilized powder in a vial containing 1.046 g ertapenem sodium equivalent to 1 g ertapenem for intravenous infusion or for intramuscular injection.
ADD-Vantage® Vials
INVANZ is a lyophilized powder in an ADD-Vantage® vial containing 1.046 g ertapenem sodium equivalent to 1 g ertapenem for intravenous infusion.

4 CONTRAINDICATIONS

- INVANZ is contraindicated in patients with known hypersensitivity to any component of this product or to other drugs in the same class or in patients who have demonstrated anaphylactic reactions to beta-lactams.
- Due to the use of lidocaine HCl as a diluent, INVANZ administered intramuscularly is contraindicated in patients with a known hypersensitivity to local anesthetics of the amide type.

5 WARNINGS AND PRECAUTIONS

5.1 Hypersensitivity Reactions

Serious and occasionally fatal hypersensitivity (anaphylactic) reactions have been reported in patients receiving therapy with beta-lactams. These reactions are more likely to occur in individuals with a history of sensitivity to multiple allergens. There have been reports of individuals with a history of penicillin hypersensitivity who have experienced severe hypersensitivity reactions when treated with another beta-lactam. Before initiating therapy with INVANZ, careful inquiry should be made concerning previous hypersensitivity reactions to penicillins, cephalosporins, other beta-lactams and other allergens. If an allergic reaction to INVANZ occurs, discontinue the drug immediately. Serious anaphylactic reactions require immediate emergency treatment as clinically indicated.

5.2 Seizure Potential

Seizures and other central nervous system (CNS) adverse experiences have been reported during treatment with INVANZ *[see Adverse Reactions (6.1)]*. During clinical investigations in adult patients treated with INVANZ (1 g once a day), seizures, irrespective of drug relationship, occurred in 0.5% of patients during study therapy plus 14-day follow-up period *[see Adverse Reactions (6.1)]*. These experiences have occurred most commonly in patients with CNS disorders (e.g., brain lesions or history of seizures) and/or compromised renal function. Close adherence to the recommended dosage regimen is urged, especially in patients with known factors that predispose to convulsive activity. Anticonvulsant therapy should be continued in patients with known seizure disorders. If focal tremors, myoclonus, or seizures occur, patients should be evaluated neurologically, placed on anticonvulsant therapy if not already instituted, and the dosage of INVANZ re-examined to determine whether it should be decreased or discontinued.

5.3 Interaction with Valproic Acid

Case reports in the literature have shown that co-administration of carbapenems, including ertapenem, to patients receiving valproic acid or divalproex sodium results in a reduction in valproic acid concentrations. The valproic acid concentrations may drop below the therapeutic range as a result of this interaction, therefore increasing the risk of breakthrough seizures. Increasing the dose of valproic acid or divalproex sodium may not be sufficient to overcome this interaction. The concomitant use of ertapenem and valproic acid/divalproex sodium is generally not recommended. Anti-bacterials other than carbapenems should be considered to treat infections in patients whose seizures are well controlled on valproic acid or divalproex sodium. If administration of INVANZ is necessary, supplemental anticonvulsant therapy should be considered [see Drug Interactions (7.2)].

5.4 Clostridium difficile-Associated Diarrhea (CDAD)

CDAD has been reported with use of nearly all antibacterial agents, including ertapenem, and may range in severity from mild diarrhea to fatal colitis. Treatment with antibacterial agents alters the normal flora of the colon leading to overgrowth of Clostridium difficile.

Clostridium difficile produces toxins A and B which contribute to the development of CDAD. Hypertoxin producing strains of Clostridium difficile cause increased morbidity and mortality, as these infections can be refractory to antimicrobial therapy and may require colectomy. CDAD must be considered in all patients who present with diarrhea following antibiotic use. Careful medical history is necessary since CDAD has been reported to occur over two months after the administration of antibacterial agents.

If CDAD is suspected or confirmed, ongoing antibiotic use not directed against Clostridium difficile may need to be discontinued. Appropriate fluid and electrolyte management, protein supplementation, antibiotic treatment of Clostridium difficile, and surgical evaluation should be instituted as clinically indicated.

5.5 Caution with Intramuscular Administration

Caution should be taken when administering INVANZ intramuscularly to avoid inadvertent injection into a blood vessel [see Dosage and Administration (2.7)].

5.6 Development of Drug-Resistant Bacteria

As with other antibiotics, prolonged use of INVANZ may result in overgrowth of non-susceptible organisms. Repeated evaluation of the patient's condition is essential. If superinfection occurs during therapy, appropriate measures should be taken.

Prescribing INVANZ in the absence of a proven or strongly suspected bacterial infection or a prophylactic indication is unlikely to provide benefit to the patient and increases the risk of the development of drug-resistant bacteria.

5.7 Laboratory Tests

While INVANZ possesses toxicity similar to the beta-lactam group of antibiotics, periodic assessment of organ system function, including renal, hepatic, and hematopoietic, is advisable during prolonged therapy.

6 ADVERSE REACTIONS

The following are described in greater detail in the Warnings and Precautions section.

• Hypersensitivity Reactions [see Warnings and Precautions (5.1)]
• Seizure Potential [see Warnings and Precautions (5.2)]
• Interaction with Valproic Acid [see Warnings and Precautions (5.3)]
• Clostridium difficile-Associated Diarrhea (CDAD) [see Warnings and Precautions (5.4)]
• Caution with Intramuscular Administration [see Warnings and Precautions (5.5)]
• Development of Drug-Resistant Bacteria [see Warnings and Precautions (5.6)]
• Laboratory Tests [see Warnings and Precautions (5.7)]

6.1 Clinical Trials Experience

Because clinical trials are conducted under widely varying conditions, adverse reaction rates observed in the clinical trials of a drug cannot be directly compared to rates in the clinical trials of another drug and may not reflect the rates observed in practice.

Adults Receiving INVANZ as a Treatment Regimen

Clinical trials enrolled 1954 patients treated with INVANZ; in some of the clinical trials, parenteral therapy was followed by a switch to an appropriate oral antimicrobial [see

Table 3: Incidence (%) of Adverse Experiences Reported During Study Therapy Plus 14-Day Follow-Up in ≥2.0% of Adult Patients Treated With INVANZ in Clinical Trials

Adverse Events	INVANZ* 1 g daily (N=802)	Piperacillin/ Tazobactam* 3.375 g q6h (N=774)	INVANZ† 1 g daily (N=1152)	Ceftriaxone† 1 or 2 g daily (N=942)
Local:				
Infused vein complication	7.1	7.9	5.4	6.7
Systemic:				
Death	2.5	1.6	1.3	1.6
Edema/swelling	3.4	2.5	2.9	3.3
Fever	5.0	6.6	2.3	3.4
Abdominal pain	3.6	4.8	4.3	3.9
Hypotension	2.0	1.4	1.0	1.2
Constipation	4.0	5.4	3.3	3.1
Diarrhea	10.3	12.1	9.2	9.8
Nausea	8.5	8.7	6.4	7.4
Vomiting	3.7	5.3	4.0	4.0
Altered mental status‡	5.1	3.4	3.3	2.5
Dizziness	2.1	3.0	1.5	2.1
Headache	5.6	5.4	6.8	6.9
Insomnia	3.2	5.2	3.0	4.1
Dyspnea	2.6	1.8	1.0	2.4
Pruritus	2.0	2.6	1.0	1.9
Rash	2.5	3.1	2.3	1.5
Vaginitis	1.4	1.0	3.3	3.7

* Includes Phase IIb/III Complicated intra-abdominal infections, Complicated skin and skin structure infections and Acute pelvic infections trials
† Includes Phase IIb/III Community acquired pneumonia and Complicated urinary tract infections, and Phase IIa trials
‡ Includes agitation, confusion, disorientation, decreased mental acuity, changed mental status, somnolence, stupor

Clinical Studies (14)]. Most adverse experiences reported in these clinical trials were described as mild to moderate in severity. INVANZ was discontinued due to adverse experiences in 4.7% of patients. Table 3 shows the incidence of adverse experiences reported in ≥2.0% of patients in these trials. The most common drug-related adverse experiences in patients treated with INVANZ, including those who were switched to therapy with an oral antimicrobial, were diarrhea (5.5%), infused vein complication (3.7%), nausea (3.1%), headache (2.2%), and vaginitis in females (2.1%). [See table 3 above]

In patients treated for complicated intra-abdominal infections, death occurred in 4.7% (15/316) of patients receiving INVANZ and 2.6% (8/307) of patients receiving comparator drug. These deaths occurred in patients with significant comorbidity and/or severe baseline infections. Deaths were considered unrelated to study drugs by investigators.

In clinical trials, seizure was reported during study therapy plus 14-day follow-up period in 0.5% of patients treated with INVANZ, 0.3% of patients treated with piperacillin/tazobactam and 0% of patients treated with ceftriaxone [see Warnings and Precautions (5.2)].

Additional adverse experiences that were reported with INVANZ with an incidence >0.1% within each body system are listed below

Body as a Whole: abdominal distention, pain, chills, septicemia, septic shock, dehydration, gout, malaise, asthenia/fatigue, necrosis, candidiasis, weight loss, facial edema, injection site induration, injection site pain, extravasation, phlebitis/thrombophlebitis, flank pain, syncope

Cardiovascular System: heart failure, hematoma, chest pain, hypertension, tachycardia, cardiac arrest, bradycardia, arrhythmia, atrial fibrillation, heart murmur, ventricular tachycardia, asystole, subdural hemorrhage

Digestive System: acid regurgitation, oral candidiasis, dyspepsia, gastrointestinal hemorrhage, anorexia, flatulence, C. difficile-associated diarrhea, stomatitis, dysphagia, hemorrhoids, ileus, cholelithiasis, duodenitis, esophagitis, gastritis, jaundice, mouth ulcer, pancreatitis, pyloric stenosis

Musculoskeletal System: leg pain

Nervous System & Psychiatric: anxiety, nervousness, seizure [see Warnings and Precautions (5.2)], tremor, depression, hypesthesia, spasm, paresthesia, aggressive behavior, vertigo

Respiratory System: cough, pharyngitis, rales/rhonchi, respiratory distress, pleural effusion, hypoxemia, bronchoconstriction, pharyngeal discomfort, epistaxis, pleuritic pain, asthma, hemoptysis, hiccups, voice disturbance

Skin & Skin Appendage: erythema, sweating, dermatitis, desquamation, flushing, urticaria

Special Senses: taste perversion

Urogenital System: renal impairment, oliguria/anuria, vaginal pruritus, hematuria, urinary retention, bladder dysfunction, vaginal candidiasis, vulvovaginitis.

In a clinical trial for the treatment of diabetic foot infections in which 289 adult diabetic patients were treated with INVANZ, the adverse experience profile was generally similar to that seen in previous clinical trials.

Prophylaxis of Surgical Site Infection following Elective Colorectal Surgery

In a clinical trial in adults for the prophylaxis of surgical site infection following elective colorectal surgery in which 476 patients received a 1 g dose of INVANZ 1 hour prior to surgery and were then followed for safety 14 days post surgery, the overall adverse experience profile was generally comparable to that observed for INVANZ in previous clinical trials. Table 4 shows the incidence of adverse experiences other than those previously described above for INVANZ that were reported regardless of causality in ≥2.0% of patients in this trial.

Table 4: Incidence (%) of Adverse Experiences Reported During Study Therapy Plus 14-Day Follow-Up in ≥2.0% of Adult Patients Treated With INVANZ for Prophylaxis of Surgical Site Infections Following Elective Colorectal Surgery

Adverse Events	INVANZ 1 g (N = 476)	Cefotetan 2 g (N = 476)
Anemia	5.7	6.9
Small intestinal obstruction	2.1	1.9
Pneumonia	2.1	4.0
Postoperative infection	2.3	4.0
Urinary tract infection	3.8	5.5
Wound infection	6.5	12.4
Wound complication	2.9	2.3
Atelectasis	3.4	1.9

Additional adverse experiences that were reported in this prophylaxis trial with INVANZ, regardless of causality, with an incidence >0.5% within each body system are listed below:

Gastrointestinal Disorders: C. difficile infection or colitis, dry mouth, hematochezia

General Disorders and Administration Site Condition: crepitations

Infections and Infestations: cellulitis, abdominal abscess, fungal rash, pelvic abscess

Injury, Poisoning and Procedural Complications: incision site complication, incision site hemorrhage, intestinal stoma complication, anastomotic leak, seroma, wound dehiscence, wound secretion

Musculoskeletal and Connective Tissue Disorders: muscle spasms

Nervous System Disorders: cerebrovascular accident

Renal and Urinary Disorders: dysuria, pollakiuria

Respiratory, Thoracic and Mediastinal Disorders: crackles lung, lung infiltration, pulmonary congestion, pulmonary embolism, wheezing

Pediatric Patients Receiving INVANZ as a Treatment Regimen

Clinical trials enrolled 384 patients treated with INVANZ; in some of the clinical trials, parenteral therapy was followed by a switch to an appropriate oral antimicrobial [see Clinical Studies (14)]. The overall adverse experience profile

Table 5: Incidence (%) of Adverse Experiences Reported During Study Therapy Plus 14-Day Follow-Up in ≥2.0% of Pediatric Patients Treated With INVANZ in Clinical Trials

Adverse Events	INVANZ[*][†] (N=384)	Ceftriaxone* (N=100)	Ticarcillin/Clavulanate[†] (N=24)
Local:			
Infusion Site Erythema	3.9	3.0	8.3
Infusion Site Pain	7.0	4.0	20.8
Systemic:			
Abdominal Pain	4.7	3.0	4.2
Constipation	2.3	0.0	0.0
Diarrhea	11.7	17.0	4.2
Loose Stools	2.1	0.0	0.0
Vomiting	10.2	11.0	8.3
Pyrexia	4.9	6.0	8.3
Upper Respiratory Tract Infection	2.3	3.0	0.0
Headache	4.4	4.0	0.0
Cough	4.4	3.0	0.0
Diaper Dermatitis	4.7	4.0	0.0
Rash	2.9	2.0	8.3

* Includes Phase IIb Complicated skin and skin structure infections, Community acquired pneumonia and Complicated urinary tract infections trials in which patients 3 months to 12 years of age received INVANZ 15 mg/kg IV twice daily up to a maximum of 1 g or ceftriaxone 50 mg/kg/day IV in two divided doses up to a maximum of 2 g, and patients 13 to 17 years of age received INVANZ 1 g IV daily or ceftriaxone 50 mg/kg/day IV in a single daily dose.
† Includes Phase IIb Acute pelvic infections and Complicated intra-abdominal infections trials in which patients 3 months to 12 years of age received INVANZ 15 mg/kg IV twice daily up to a maximum of 1 g and patients 13 to 17 years of age received INVANZ 1 g IV daily or ticarcillin/clavulanate 50 mg/kg for patients <60 kg or ticarcillin/clavulanate 3.0 g for patients >60 kg, 4 or 6 times a day.

Table 6: Incidence* (%) of Laboratory Adverse Experiences Reported During Study Therapy Plus 14-Day Follow-Up in ≥2.0% of Adult Patients Treated With INVANZ in Clinical Trials

Adverse laboratory experiences	INVANZ[†] 1 g daily (n[§]=766)	Piperacillin/ Tazobactam[†] 3.375 g q6h (n[§]=755)	INVANZ[‡] 1 g daily (n[§]=1122)	Ceftriaxone[‡] 1 or 2 g daily (n[§]=920)
ALT increased	8.8	7.3	8.3	6.9
AST increased	8.4	8.3	7.1	6.5
Serum alkaline phosphatase increased	6.6	7.2	4.3	2.8
Eosinophils increased	1.1	1.1	2.1	1.8
Hematocrit decreased	3.0	2.9	3.4	2.4
Hemoglobin decreased	4.9	4.7	4.5	3.5
Platelet count increased	6.5	6.3	4.3	3.5
Urine RBCs increased	2.5	2.9	1.1	1.0
Urine WBCs increased	2.5	3.2	1.6	1.1

* Number of patients with laboratory adverse experiences/Number of patients with the laboratory test
† Includes Phase IIb/III Complicated intra-abdominal infections, Complicated skin and skin structure infections and Acute pelvic infections trials
‡ Includes Phase IIb/III Community acquired pneumonia and Complicated urinary tract infections, and Phase IIa trials
§ Number of patients with one or more laboratory tests

in pediatric patients is comparable to that in adult patients. Table 5 shows the incidence of adverse experiences reported in ≥2.0% of pediatric patients in clinical trials. The most common drug-related adverse experiences in pediatric patients treated with INVANZ, including those who were switched to therapy with an oral antimicrobial, were diarrhea (6.5%), infusion site pain (5.5%), infusion site erythema (2.6%), vomiting (2.1%).

[See table 5 above]

Additional adverse experiences that were reported with INVANZ with an incidence >0.5% within each body system are listed below:

Gastrointestinal Disorders: nausea
General Disorders and Administration Site Condition: hypothermia, chest pain, upper abdominal pain; infusion site pruritus, induration, phlebitis, swelling, and warmth
Infections and Infestations: candidiasis, oral candidiasis, viral pharyngitis, herpes simplex, ear infection, abdominal abscess
Metabolism and Nutrition Disorders: decreased appetite
Musculoskeletal and Connective Tissue Disorders: arthralgia
Nervous System Disorders: dizziness, somnolence
Psychiatric Disorders: insomnia
Reproductive System and Breast Disorders: genital rash
Respiratory, Thoracic and Mediastinal Disorders: wheezing, nasopharyngitis, pleural effusion, rhinitis, rhinorrhea
Skin and Subcutaneous Tissue Disorders: dermatitis, pruritus, rash erythematous, skin lesion
Vascular Disorders: phlebitis

6.2 Post-Marketing Experience
The following additional adverse reactions have been identified during the post-approval use of INVANZ. Because these reactions are reported voluntarily from a population of uncertain size, it is not always possible to reliably estimate their frequency or establish a causal relationship to drug exposure.

Gastrointestinal Disorders: teeth staining
Immune System Disorders: anaphylaxis including anaphylactoid reactions
Musculoskeletal and Connective Tissue Disorders: muscular weakness
Nervous System Disorders: coordination abnormal, depressed level of consciousness, dyskinesia, gait disturbance, myoclonus, tremor
Psychiatric Disorders: altered mental status (including aggression, delirium), hallucinations
Skin and Subcutaneous Tissue Disorders: Drug Rash with Eosinophilia and Systemic Symptoms (DRESS syndrome)

6.3 Adverse Laboratory Changes in Clinical Trials
Adults Receiving INVANZ as Treatment Regimen
Laboratory adverse experiences that were reported during therapy in ≥2.0% of adult patients treated with INVANZ in clinical trials are presented in Table 6. Drug-related laboratory adverse experiences that were reported during therapy in ≥2.0% of adult patients treated with INVANZ, including those who were switched to therapy with an oral antimicrobial, in clinical trials were ALT increased (6.0%), AST increased (5.2%), serum alkaline phosphatase increased (3.4%), and platelet count increased (2.8%). INVANZ was discontinued due to laboratory adverse experiences in 0.3% of patients.

[See table 6 above]

Additional laboratory adverse experiences that were reported during therapy in >0.1% of patients treated with INVANZ in clinical trials include: increases in serum creatinine, serum glucose, BUN, total, direct and indirect serum bilirubin, serum sodium and potassium, PT and PTT; decreases in serum potassium, serum albumin, WBC, platelet count, and segmented neutrophils.

In a clinical trial for the treatment of diabetic foot infections in which 289 adult diabetic patients were treated with INVANZ, the laboratory adverse experience profile was generally similar to that seen in previous clinical trials.

Prophylaxis of Surgical Site Infection following Elective Colorectal Surgery
In a clinical trial in adults for the prophylaxis of surgical site infection elective colorectal surgery in which 476 patients received a 1 g dose of INVANZ 1 hour prior to surgery and were then followed for safety 14 days post surgery, the overall laboratory adverse experience profile was generally comparable to that observed for INVANZ in previous clinical trials.

Pediatric Patients Receiving INVANZ as a Treatment Regimen
Laboratory adverse experiences that were reported during therapy in ≥2.0% of pediatric patients treated with INVANZ in clinical trials are presented in Table 7. Drug-related laboratory adverse experiences that were reported during therapy in ≥2.0% of pediatric patients treated with INVANZ, including those who were switched to therapy with an oral antimicrobial, in clinical trials were neutrophil count decreased (3.0%), ALT increased (2.2%), and AST increased (2.1%).

Table 7: Incidence* (%) of Specific Laboratory Adverse Experiences Reported During Study Therapy Plus 14-Day Follow-Up in ≥2.0% of Pediatric Patients Treated With INVANZ in Clinical Trials

Adverse laboratory experiences	INVANZ (n[†]=379)	Ceftriaxone (n[†]=97)	Ticarcillin/ Clavulanate (n[†]=24)
ALT Increased	3.8	1.1	4.3
AST Increased	3.8	1.1	4.3
Neutrophil Count Decreased	5.8	3.1	0.0

* Number of patients with laboratory adverse experiences/Number of patients with the laboratory test; where at least 300 patients had the test
† Number of patients with one or more laboratory tests

Additional laboratory adverse experiences that were reported during therapy in >0.5% of patients treated with INVANZ in clinical trials include: alkaline phosphatase increased, eosinophil count increased, platelet count increased, white blood cell count decreased and urine protein present.

7 DRUG INTERACTIONS
7.1 Probenecid
Probenecid interferes with the active tubular secretion of ertapenem, resulting in increased plasma concentrations of ertapenem [see Clinical Pharmacology (12.3)]. Co-administration of probenecid with ertapenem is not recommended.

7.2 Valproic Acid
Case reports in the literature have shown that co-administration of carbapenems, including ertapenem, to patients receiving valproic acid or divalproex sodium results in a reduction of valproic acid concentrations. The valproic acid concentrations may drop below the therapeutic range as a result of this interaction, therefore increasing the risk of breakthrough seizures. Although the mechanism of this interaction is unknown, data from in vitro and animal studies suggest that carbapenems may inhibit the hydrolysis of valproic acid's glucuronide metabolite (VPA-g) back to valproic acid, thus decreasing the serum concentrations of valproic acid [see Warnings and Precautions (5.3)].

8 USE IN SPECIFIC POPULATIONS
8.1 Pregnancy
Pregnancy Category B
In mice and rats given intravenous doses of up to 700 mg/kg/day (for mice, approximately 3 times the recommended human dose of 1 g based on body surface area and for rats, approximately 1.2 times the human exposure at the recommended dose of 1 g based on plasma AUCs), there was no evidence of developmental toxicity as assessed by external, visceral, and skeletal examination of the fetuses. However, in mice given 700 mg/kg/day, slight decreases in average fetal weights and an associated decrease in the average number of ossified sacrocaudal vertebrae were observed. Ertapenem crosses the placental barrier in rats.
There are, however, no adequate and well-controlled trials in pregnant women. Because animal reproduction studies are not always predictive of human response, this drug should be used during pregnancy only if clearly needed.

8.2 Labor and Delivery
INVANZ has not been studied for use during labor and delivery.

8.3 Nursing Mothers
Ertapenem is excreted in human breast milk [see Clinical Pharmacology (12.3)]. Caution should be exercised when INVANZ is administered to a nursing woman. INVANZ should be administered to nursing mothers only when the expected benefit outweighs the risk.

8.4 Pediatric Use

Safety and effectiveness of INVANZ in pediatric patients 3 months to 17 years of age are supported by evidence from adequate and well-controlled trials in adults, pharmacokinetic data in pediatric patients, and additional data from comparator-controlled trials in pediatric patients 3 months to 17 years of age [see Indications and Usage (1.1), (1.2), (1.3), (1.4) and (1.5) and Clinical Studies (14.2)].

INVANZ is not recommended in infants under 3 months of age as no data are available.

INVANZ is not recommended in the treatment of meningitis in the pediatric population due to lack of sufficient CSF penetration.

8.5 Geriatric Use

Of the 1,835 patients in Phase 2b/3 trials treated with INVANZ, approximately 26 percent were 65 and over, while approximately 12 percent were 75 and over. No overall differences in safety or effectiveness were observed between these patients and younger patients. Other reported clinical experience has not identified differences in responses between the elderly and younger patients, but greater sensitivity of some older individuals cannot be ruled out.

This drug is known to be substantially excreted by the kidney, and the risk of toxic reactions to this drug may be greater in patients with impaired renal function. Because elderly patients are more likely to have decreased renal function, care should be taken in dose selection, and it may be useful to monitor renal function [see Dosage and Administration (2.2)].

8.6 Patients with Renal Impairment

Dosage adjustment is necessary in patients with creatinine clearance 30 mL/min or less [see Dosage and Administration (2.4) and Clinical Pharmacology (12.3)].

8.7 Patients with Hepatic Impairment

The pharmacokinetics of ertapenem in patients with hepatic impairment have not been established. Of the total number of patients in clinical trials, 37 patients receiving ertapenem 1 g daily and 36 patients receiving comparator drugs were considered to have Child-Pugh Class A, B, or C liver impairment. The incidence of adverse experiences in patients with hepatic impairment was similar between the ertapenem group and the comparator groups.

10 OVERDOSAGE

No specific information is available on the treatment of overdosage with INVANZ. Intentional overdosing of INVANZ is unlikely. Intravenous administration of INVANZ at a dose of 2 g over 30 min or 3 g over 1-2h in healthy adult volunteers resulted in an increased incidence of nausea. In clinical trials in adults, inadvertent administration of three 1 g doses of INVANZ in a 24 hour period resulted in diarrhea and transient dizziness in one patient. In pediatric clinical trials, a single intravenous dose of 40 mg/kg up to a maximum of 2 g did not result in toxicity.

In the event of an overdose, INVANZ should be discontinued and general supportive treatment given until renal elimination takes place.

INVANZ can be removed by hemodialysis; the plasma clearance of the total fraction of ertapenem was increased 30% in subjects with end-stage renal disease when hemodialysis (4 hour session) was performed immediately following administration. However, no information is available on the use of hemodialysis to treat overdosage.

11 DESCRIPTION

INVANZ (Ertapenem for Injection) is a sterile, synthetic, parenteral, 1-β methyl-carbapenem that is structurally related to beta-lactam antibiotics.

Chemically, INVANZ is described as [4R-[3(3S*, 5S*),4α,5β,6β(R*)]]-3-[[5-[[(3-carboxyphenyl)amino]carbonyl]-3-pyrrolidinyl]thio]-6-(1-hydroxyethyl)-4-methyl-7-oxo-1-azabicyclo[3.2.0]hept-2-ene-2-carboxylic acid monosodium salt. Its molecular weight is 497.50. The empirical formula is $C_{22}H_{24}N_3O_7SNa$, and its structural formula is:

Ertapenem sodium is a white to off-white hygroscopic, weakly crystalline powder. It is soluble in water and 0.9% sodium chloride solution, practically insoluble in ethanol, and insoluble in isopropyl acetate and tetrahydrofuran.

INVANZ is supplied as sterile lyophilized powder for intravenous infusion after reconstitution with appropriate diluent [see Dosage and Administration (2.7)] and transfer to 50 mL 0.9% Sodium Chloride Injection or for intramuscular injection following reconstitution with 1% lidocaine hydrochloride. Each vial contains 1.046 grams ertapenem sodium, equivalent to 1 gram ertapenem. The sodium content is approximately 137 mg (approximately 6.0 mEq).

Table 8: Plasma Concentrations of Ertapenem in Adults After Single Dose Administration

Dose/Route	Average Plasma Concentrations (mcg/mL)								
	0.5 hr	1 hr	2 hr	4 hr	6 hr	8 hr	12 hr	18 hr	24 hr
1 g IV*	155	115	83	48	31	20	9	3	1
1 g IM	33	53	67	57	40	27	13	4	2

* Infused at a constant rate over 30 minutes

Table 9: Plasma Concentrations of Ertapenem in Pediatric Patients After Single IV* Dose Administration

Age Group	Dose	Average Plasma Concentrations (mcg/mL)							
		0.5 hr	1 hr	2 hr	4 hr	6 hr	8 hr	12 hr	24 hr
3 to 23 months	15 mg/kg†	103.8	57.3	43.6	23.7	13.5	8.2	2.5	-
	20 mg/kg†	126.8	87.6	58.7	28.4	-	12.0	3.4	0.4
	40 mg/kg‡	199.1	144.1	95.7	58.0	-	20.2	7.7	0.6
2 to 12 years	15 mg/kg†	113.2	63.9	42.1	21.9	12.8	7.6	3.0	-
	20 mg/kg†	147.6	97.6	63.2	34.5	-	12.3	4.9	0.5
	40 mg/kg‡	241.7	152.7	96.3	55.6	-	18.8	7.2	0.6
13 to 17 years	20 mg/kg†	170.4	98.3	67.8	40.4	-	16.0	7.0	1.1
	1 g§	155.9	110.9	74.8	-	24.0	-	6.2	-
	40 mg/kg‡	255.0	188.7	127.9	76.2	-	31.0	15.3	2.1

* Infused at a constant rate over 30 minutes
† up to a maximum dose of 1 g/day
‡ up to a maximum dose of 2 g/day
§ Based on three patients receiving 1 g ertapenem who volunteered for pharmacokinetic assessment in one of the two safety and efficacy trials

Each vial of INVANZ contains the following inactive ingredients: 175 mg sodium bicarbonate and sodium hydroxide to adjust pH to 7.5.

12 CLINICAL PHARMACOLOGY

12.1 Mechanism of Action

Ertapenem sodium is a carbapenem antibiotic [see Clinical Pharmacology (12.4)].

12.3 Pharmacokinetics

Average plasma concentrations (mcg/mL) of ertapenem following a single 30-minute infusion of a 1 g intravenous (IV) dose and administration of a single 1 g intramuscular (IM) dose in healthy young adults are presented in Table 8.
[See table 8 above]

The area under the plasma concentration-time curve (AUC) of ertapenem in adults increased less-than dose-proportional based on total ertapenem concentrations over the 0.5 to 2 g dose range, whereas the AUC increased greater-than dose-proportional based on unbound ertapenem concentrations. Ertapenem exhibits non-linear pharmacokinetics due to concentration-dependent plasma protein binding at the proposed therapeutic dose [see Clinical Pharmacology (12.3)]. There is no accumulation of ertapenem following multiple IV or IM 1 g daily doses in healthy adults.

Average plasma concentrations (mcg/mL) of ertapenem in pediatric patients are presented in Table 9.
[See table 9 above]

Absorption

Ertapenem, reconstituted with 1% lidocaine HCl injection, USP (in saline without epinephrine), is almost completely absorbed following intramuscular (IM) administration at the recommended dose of 1 g. The mean bioavailability is approximately 90%. Following 1 g daily IM administration, mean peak plasma concentrations (C_{max}) are achieved in approximately 2.3 hours (T_{max}).

Distribution

Ertapenem is highly bound to human plasma proteins, primarily albumin. In healthy young adults, the protein binding of ertapenem decreases as plasma concentrations increase, from approximately 95% bound at an approximate plasma concentration of <100 micrograms (mcg)/mL to approximately 85% bound at an approximate plasma concentration of 300 mcg/mL.

The apparent volume of distribution at steady state (V_{ss}) of ertapenem in adults is approximately 0.12 liter/kg, approximately 0.2 liter/kg in pediatric patients 3 months to 12 years of age and approximately 0.16 liter/kg in pediatric patients 13 to 17 years of age.

The concentrations of ertapenem achieved in suction-induced skin blister fluid at each sampling point on the third day of 1 g once daily IV doses are presented in Table 10. The ratio of AUC_{0-24} in skin blister fluid/AUC_{0-24} in plasma is 0.61.

Table 10: Concentrations (mcg/mL) of Ertapenem in Adult Skin Blister Fluid at each Sampling Point on the Third Day of 1-g Once Daily IV Doses

0.5 hr	1 hr	2 hr	4 hr	8 hr	12 hr	24 hr
7	12	17	24	24	21	8

The concentration of ertapenem in breast milk from 5 lactating women with pelvic infections (5 to 14 days postpartum) was measured at random time points daily for 5 consecutive days following the last 1 g dose of intravenous therapy (3-10 days of therapy). The concentration of ertapenem in breast milk within 24 hours of the last dose of therapy in all 5 women ranged from <0.13 (lower limit of quantitation) to 0.38 mcg/mL; peak concentrations were not assessed. By day 5 after discontinuation of therapy, the level of ertapenem was undetectable in the breast milk of 4 women and below the lower limit of quantitation (<0.13 mcg/mL) in 1 woman.

Metabolism

In healthy young adults, after infusion of 1 g IV radiolabeled ertapenem, the plasma radioactivity consists predominantly (94%) of ertapenem. The major metabolite of ertapenem is the inactive ring-opened derivative formed by hydrolysis of the beta-lactam ring.

Elimination

Ertapenem is eliminated primarily by the kidneys. The mean plasma half-life in healthy young adults is approximately 4 hours and the plasma clearance is approximately 1.8 L/hour. The mean plasma half-life in pediatric patients 13 to 17 years of age is approximately 4 hours and approximately 2.5 hours in pediatric patients 3 months to 12 years of age.

Following the administration of 1 g IV radiolabeled ertapenem to healthy young adults, approximately 80% is recovered in urine and 10% in feces. Of the 80% recovered in urine, approximately 38% is excreted as unchanged drug and approximately 37% as the ring-opened metabolite.

In healthy young adults given a 1 g IV dose, the mean percentage of the administered dose excreted in urine was 17.4% during 0-2 hours postdose, 5.4% during 4-6 hours postdose, and 2.4% during 12-24 hours postdose.

Special Populations

Renal Impairment

Total and unbound fractions of ertapenem pharmacokinetics were investigated in 26 adult subjects (31 to 80 years of age) with varying degrees of renal impairment. Following a single 1 g IV dose of ertapenem, the unbound AUC increased 1.5-fold and 2.3-fold in subjects with mild renal impairment (CL_{CR} 60-90 mL/min/1.73 m²) and moderate renal

Table 11: Susceptibility Interpretive Criteria for Ertapenem

Pathogen	Minimum Inhibitory Concentrations* MIC (μg/mL)			Disk Diffusion Zone Diameter (mm)		
	S	I	R	S	I	R
Enterobacteriaceae	≤0.5	1	≥2	≥22	19-21	≤18
Staphylococcus aureus†	≤2.0	4.0	≥8.0	≥19	16-18	≤15
Haemophilus spp.*	≤0.5	-	-	≥19	-	-
Streptococcus pneumoniae‡	≤1.0	2	≥4	-	-	-
Streptococcus spp. Beta Hemolytic Group*,‡,§	≤1.0	-	-	-	-	-
Streptococcus spp. Viridans Group*	≤1.0	-	-	-	-	-
Anaerobes	≤4.0	8.0	≥16.0	-	-	-

* For some organism/antimicrobial combinations, the absence or rare occurrence of resistant strains precludes defining any results categories other than "susceptible". For strains yielding results suggestive of a "non-susceptible" category, organism identification and antimicrobial susceptibility test results should be confirmed.

† For oxacillin-susceptible S. aureus results for carbapenems, including ertapenem, if tested, should be reported according to the results generated using routine interpretive criteria. For oxacillin-resistant S. aureus and coagulase negative staphylococci, other beta lactam agents, including carbapenems, may appear active in vitro but are not effective clinically. Results for beta lactam agents other than cephalosporins with anti-MRSA activity should be reported as resistant or should not be reported.

‡ S. pneumoniae penicillin MICs ≤2 mcg/mL indicate susceptibility to ertapenem.

§ A beta hemolytic Streptococcus spp. (Groups A, B, C, G) isolate susceptible to penicillin (MIC ≤0.12 μg/mL) can be considered susceptible to ertapenem and need not be tested against ertapenem.

impairment (CL_{CR} 31-59 mL/min/1.73 m²), respectively, compared with healthy young subjects (25 to 45 years of age). No dosage adjustment is necessary in patients with CL_{CR} ≥31 mL/min/1.73 m². The unbound AUC increased 4.4-fold and 7.6-fold in subjects with advanced renal impairment (CL_{CR} 5-30 mL/min/1.73 m²) and end-stage renal disease (CL_{CR} <10 mL/min/1.73 m²), respectively, compared with healthy young subjects. The effects of renal impairment on AUC of total drug were of smaller magnitude. The recommended dose of ertapenem in adult patients with CL_{CR} ≤30 mL/min/1.73 m² is 0.5 grams every 24 hours. Following a single 1 g IV dose given immediately prior to a 4 hour hemodialysis session in 5 adult patients with end-stage renal disease, approximately 30% of the dose was recovered in the dialysate. Dose adjustments are recommended for patients with severe renal impairment and end-stage renal disease [see Dosage and Administration (2.4)]. There are no data in pediatric patients with renal impairment.

Hepatic Impairment
The pharmacokinetics of ertapenem in patients with hepatic impairment have not been established. However, ertapenem does not appear to undergo hepatic metabolism based on in vitro studies and approximately 10% of an administered dose is recovered in the feces [see Clinical Pharmacology (12.3) and Dosage and Administration (2.6)].

Gender
The effect of gender on the pharmacokinetics of ertapenem was evaluated in healthy male (n=8) and healthy female (n=8) subjects. The differences observed could be attributed to body size when body weight was taken into consideration. No dose adjustment is recommended based on gender.

Geriatric Patients
The impact of age on the pharmacokinetics of ertapenem was evaluated in healthy male (n=7) and healthy female (n=7) subjects ≥65 years of age. The total and unbound AUC increased 37% and 67%, respectively, in elderly adults relative to young adults. These changes were attributed to age-related changes in creatinine clearance. No dosage adjustment is necessary for elderly patients with normal (for their age) renal function.

Pediatric Patients
Plasma concentrations of ertapenem are comparable in pediatric patients 13 to 17 years of age and adults following a 1 g once daily IV dose.

Following the 20 mg/kg dose (up to a maximum dose of 1 g), the pharmacokinetic parameter values in patients 13 to 17 years of age (N=6) were generally comparable to those in healthy young adults.

Plasma concentrations at the midpoint of the dosing interval following a single 15 mg/kg IV dose of ertapenem in patients 3 months to 12 years of age are comparable to plasma concentrations at the midpoint of the dosing interval following a 1 g once daily IV dose in adults [see Clinical Pharmacology (12.3)]. The plasma clearance (mL/min/kg) of ertapenem in patients 3 months to 12 years of age is approximately 2-fold higher as compared to in adults. At the 15 mg/kg dose, the AUC value (doubled to model a twice daily dosing regimen, i.e., 30 mg/kg/day exposure) in patients 3 months to 12 years of age was comparable to the

AUC value in young healthy adults receiving a 1 g IV dose of ertapenem.

Drug Interactions
When ertapenem is co-administered with probenecid (500 mg p.o. every 6 hours), probenecid competes for active tubular secretion and reduces the renal clearance of ertapenem. Based on total ertapenem concentrations, probenecid increased the AUC of ertapenem by 25%, and reduced the plasma and renal clearance of ertapenem by 20% and 35%, respectively. The half-life of ertapenem was increased from 4.0 to 4.8 hours.

In vitro studies in human liver microsomes indicate that ertapenem does not inhibit metabolism mediated by any of the following cytochrome p450 (CYP) isoforms: 1A2, 2C9, 2C19, 2D6, 2E1 and 3A4.

In vitro studies indicate that ertapenem does not inhibit P-glycoprotein-mediated transport of digoxin or vinblastine and that ertapenem is not a substrate for P-glycoprotein-mediated transport.

12.4   Microbiology
Mechanism of Action
Ertapenem has in vitro activity against Gram-positive and Gram-negative aerobic and anaerobic bacteria. The bactericidal activity of ertapenem results from the inhibition of cell wall synthesis and is mediated through ertapenem binding to penicillin binding proteins (PBPs). In Escherichia coli, it has strong affinity toward PBPs 1a, 1b, 2, 3, 4 and 5 with preference for PBPs 2 and 3.

Mechanism of Resistance
Ertapenem is stable against hydrolysis by a variety of beta-lactamases, including penicillinases, and cephalosporinases and extended spectrum beta-lactamases. Ertapenem is hydrolyzed by metallo-beta-lactamases.

Ertapenem has been shown to be active against most isolates of the following microorganisms both in vitro and in clinical infections as described in the INDICATIONS AND USAGE section:

Gram-positive bacteria:
Staphylococcus aureus (methicillin susceptible isolates only)
Streptococcus agalactiae
Streptococcus pneumoniae (penicillin susceptible isolates only)
Streptococcus pyogenes

Gram-negative bacteria:
Escherichia coli
Haemophilus influenzae (beta-lactamase negative isolates only)
Klebsiella pneumoniae
Moraxella catarrhalis
Proteus mirabilis

Anaerobic bacteria:
Bacteroides fragilis
Bacteroides distasonis
Bacteroides ovatus
Bacteroides thetaiotaomicron
Bacteroides uniformis
Clostridium clostridioforme
Eubacterium lentum

Peptostreptococcus species
Porphyromonas asaccharolytica
Prevotella bivia

The following in vitro data are available, **but their clinical significance is unknown**. At least 90% of the following bacteria exhibit an in vitro minimum inhibitory concentration (MIC) less than or equal to the susceptible breakpoint for ertapenem. However, the efficacy of ertapenem in treating clinical infections due to these bacteria **has not been** established in adequate and well-controlled clinical trials:

Gram-positive bacteria:
Staphylococcus epidermidis (methicillin susceptible isolates only)
Streptococcus pneumoniae (penicillin-intermediate isolates)

Gram-negative bacteria:
Citrobacter freundii
Citrobacter koseri
Enterobacter aerogenes
Enterobacter cloacae
Haemophilus influenzae (beta-lactamase positive isolates only)
Haemophilus parainfluenzae
Klebsiella oxytoca (excluding ESBL producing isolates)
Morganella morganii
Proteus vulgaris
Providencia rettgeri
Providencia stuartii
Serratia marcescens

Anaerobic bacteria:
Bacteroides vulgatus
Clostridium perfringens
Fusobacterium spp.

Susceptibility Test Methods:
When available, the clinical microbiology laboratory should provide the results of in vitro susceptibility tests for antimicrobial drug products used in resident hospitals to the physician as periodic reports which describe the susceptibility profile of nosocomial and community-acquired pathogens. These reports should aid the physician in selecting the most effective antimicrobial.

Dilution Techniques:
Quantitative methods are used to determine antimicrobial minimum inhibitory concentrations (MICs). These MICs provide estimates of the susceptibility of bacteria to antimicrobial compounds. The MICs should be determined using a standardized procedure. Standardized procedures are based on a broth dilution method {1} or equivalent with standardized inoculum concentrations and standardized concentrations of ertapenem powder. The MIC values should be interpreted according to criteria provided in Table 11 and {4}.

Diffusion Techniques:
Quantitative methods that require measurement of zone diameters also provide reproducible estimates of the susceptibility of bacteria to antimicrobial compounds. One such standardized procedure {2} requires the use of standardized inoculum concentrations. This procedure uses paper disks impregnated with 10-μg ertapenem to test the susceptibility of microorganisms to ertapenem. The disk diffusion interpretive criteria should be interpreted according to criteria provided in Table 11 and {4}.

Anaerobic Techniques:
For anaerobic bacteria, the susceptibility to ertapenem as MICs can be determined by standardized test methods {3}. The MIC values obtained should be interpreted according to criteria provided in Table 11 and {4}.

[See table 11 above]

A report of "Susceptible" indicates that the pathogen is likely to be inhibited if the antimicrobial compound at the infection site reaches the concentrations usually achievable. A report of "Intermediate" indicates that the result should be considered equivocal, and, if the microorganism is not fully susceptible to alternative, clinically feasible drugs, the test should be repeated. This category implies possible clinical applicability in body sites where the drug is physiologically concentrated or in situations where high dosage of drug can be used. This category also provides a buffer zone which prevents small uncontrolled technical factors from causing major discrepancies in interpretation. A report of "Resistant" indicates that the pathogen is not likely to be inhibited if the antimicrobial compound at the infection site reaches the concentrations usually achievable; other therapy should be selected.

Quality Control
Standardized susceptibility test procedures require the use of laboratory control microorganisms to ensure the accuracy and precision of supplies and reagents used in the assay, and the techniques of the individuals performing the test. Quality control microorganisms are specific strains of organisms with intrinsic biological properties. QC strains are very stable strains which will give a standard and repeatable susceptibility pattern. The specific strains used for microbiological quality control are not clinically significant. Standard ertapenem powder should provide the following range of values noted in Table 12 and {4,5}.

Table 12: Acceptable Quality Control Ranges for Ertapenem

Microorganism	Minimum Inhibitory Concentrations MIC Range (μg/mL)	Disk Diffusion Zone Diameter (mm)
Escherichia coli ATCC 25922	0.004-0.016	29-36
Haemophilus influenzae ATCC 49766	0.015-0.06	27-33
Staphylococcus aureus ATCC 29213	0.06-0.25	-
Staphylococcus aureus ATCC 25923	-	24-31
Streptococcus pneumoniae ATCC 49619	0.03-0.25	28-35
Bacteroides fragilis ATCC 25285	0.06-0.5 * 0.06-0.25[†]	
Bacteroides thetaiotaomicron ATCC 29741	0.5-2.0 * 0.25-1.0 [†]	
Eubacterium lentum ATCC 43055	0.5-4.0 * 0.5-2.0 [†]	

* Quality control ranges for broth microdilution testing
† Quality control ranges for agar dilution testing

13 NONCLINICAL TOXICOLOGY

13.1 Carcinogenesis, Mutagenesis, Impairment of Fertility

No long-term studies in animals have been performed to evaluate the carcinogenic potential of ertapenem.

Ertapenem was neither mutagenic nor genotoxic in the following in vitro assays: alkaline elution/rat hepatocyte assay, chromosomal aberration assay in Chinese hamster ovary cells, and TK6 human lymphoblastoid cell mutagenesis assay; and in the in vivo mouse micronucleus assay.

In mice and rats, IV doses of up to 700 mg/kg/day (for mice, approximately 3 times the recommended human dose of 1 g based on body surface area and for rats, approximately 1.2 times the human exposure at the recommended dose of 1 g based on plasma AUCs) resulted in no effects on mating performance, fecundity, fertility, or embryonic survival.

13.2 Animal Toxicology and/or Pharmacology

In repeat-dose studies in rats, treatment-related neutropenia occurred at every dose-level tested, including the lowest dose of 2 mg/kg (approximately 2% of the human dose on a body surface area basis).

Studies in rabbits and Rhesus monkeys were inconclusive with regard to the effect on neutrophil counts.

14 CLINICAL STUDIES

14.1 Adults

Complicated Intra-Abdominal Infections

Ertapenem was evaluated in adults for the treatment of complicated intra-abdominal infections in a randomized, double-blind, non-inferiority clinical trial. This trial compared ertapenem (1 g intravenously once a day) with piperacillin/tazobactam (3.375 g intravenously every 6 hours) for 5 to 14 days and enrolled 665 patients with localized complicated appendicitis, and any other complicated intra-abdominal infection including colonic, small intestinal, and biliary infections and generalized peritonitis. The combined clinical and microbiologic success rates in the microbiologically evaluable population at 4 to 6 weeks posttherapy (test-of-cure) were 83.6% (163/195) for ertapenem and 80.4% (152/189) for piperacillin/tazobactam.

Complicated Skin and Skin Structure Infections

Ertapenem was evaluated in adults for the treatment of complicated skin and skin structure infections in a randomized, double-blind, non-inferiority clinical trial. This trial compared ertapenem (1 g intravenously once a day) with piperacillin/tazobactam (3.375 g intravenously every 6 hours) for 7 to 14 days and enrolled 540 patients including patients with deep soft tissue abscess, posttraumatic wound infection and cellulitis with purulent drainage. The clinical success rates at 10 to 21 days posttherapy (test-of-cure) were 83.9% (141/168) for ertapenem and 85.3% (145/170) for piperacillin/tazobactam.

Diabetic Foot Infections

Ertapenem was evaluated in adults for the treatment of diabetic foot infections without concomitant osteomyelitis in a multicenter, randomized, double-blind, non-inferiority clinical trial. This trial compared ertapenem (1 g intravenously once a day) with piperacillin/tazobactam (3.375 g intravenously every 6 hours). Test-of-cure was defined as clinical response between treatment groups in the clinically evaluable population at the 10-day posttherapy follow-up visit. The population at the 10-day posttherapy randomized to ertapenem included 295 patients randomized to ertapenem. Both regimens allowed patients to piperacillin/tazobactam. Both regimens allowed the option to switch to oral amoxicillin/clavulanate for a total of 5 to 28 days of treatment (parenteral and oral). All patients were eligible to receive appropriate adjunctive treatments, such as debridement, as is typically required in the treatment of diabetic foot infections, and most patients received these treatments. Patients with suspected osteomyelitis could be enrolled if all the infected bone was removed within 2 days of initiation of study therapy, and proved within 2 days of initiation of study therapy. Investigators had the option to add open-label vancomycin if enterococci or methicillin-resistant Staphylococcus aureus (MRSA) were among the pathogens isolated or if patients had a history of MRSA infection and additional therapy was indicated in the opinion of the investigator. Two hundred and four (204) patients randomized to ertapenem and 202 patients randomized to piperacillin/tazobactam were clinically evaluable. The clinical success rates at 10 days posttherapy were 75% (153/204) for ertapenem and 70.8% (143/202) for piperacillin/tazobactam.

Community Acquired Pneumonia

Ertapenem was evaluated in adults for the treatment of community acquired pneumonia in two randomized, double-blind, non-inferiority clinical trials. Both trials compared ertapenem (1 g parenterally once a day) with ceftriaxone (1 g parenterally once a day) and enrolled a total of 866 patients. Both regimens allowed the option to switch to oral amoxicillin/clavulanate for a total of 10 to 14 days of treatment (parenteral and oral). In the first trial the primary efficacy parameter was the clinical success rate in the clinically evaluable population and success rates were 92.3% (168/182) for ertapenem and 91.0% (183/201) for ceftriaxone at 7 to 14 days posttherapy (test-of-cure). In the second trial the primary efficacy parameter was the clinical success rate in the microbiologically evaluable population and success rates were 91% (91/100) for ertapenem and 91.8% (45/49) for ceftriaxone at 7 to 14 days posttherapy (test-of-cure).

Complicated Urinary Tract Infections Including Pyelonephritis

Ertapenem was evaluated in adults for the treatment of complicated urinary tract infections including pyelonephritis in two randomized, double-blind, non-inferiority clinical trials. Both trials compared ertapenem (1 g parenterally once a day) with ceftriaxone (1 g parenterally once a day) and enrolled a total of 850 patients. Both regimens allowed the option to switch to oral ciprofloxacin (500 mg twice daily) for a total of 10 to 14 days of treatment (parenteral and oral). The microbiological success rates (combined trials) at 5 to 9 days posttherapy (test-of-cure) were 89.5% (229/256) for ertapenem and 91.1% (204/224) for ceftriaxone.

Acute Pelvic Infections Including Endomyometritis, Septic Abortion and Post-Surgical Gynecological Infections

Ertapenem was evaluated in adults for the treatment of acute pelvic infections in a randomized, double-blind, non-inferiority clinical trial. This trial compared ertapenem (1 g intravenously once a day) with piperacillin/tazobactam (3.375 g intravenously every 6 hours) for 3 to 10 days and enrolled 412 patients including 350 patients with obstetric/postpartum infections and 45 patients with septic abortion. The clinical success rates in the clinically evaluable population at 2 to 4 weeks posttherapy (test-of-cure) were 93.9% (153/163) for ertapenem and 91.5% (140/153) for piperacillin/tazobactam.

Prophylaxis of Surgical Site Infections Following Elective Colorectal Surgery

Ertapenem was evaluated in adults for prophylaxis of surgical site infection following elective colorectal surgery in a multicenter, randomized, double-blind, non-inferiority clinical trial. This trial compared a single intravenous dose of ertapenem (1 g) versus cefotetan (2 g) administered over 30 minutes, 1 hour before elective colorectal surgery. Test-of-prophylaxis was defined as no evidence of surgical site infection, post-operative anastomotic leak, or unexplained antibiotic use in the clinically evaluable population up to and including at the 4-week posttreatment follow-up visit. The trial included 500 patients randomized to ertapenem and 502 patients randomized to cefotetan. The modified intent-to-treat (MITT) population consisted of 451 ertapenem patients and 450 cefotetan patients and included all patients who were randomized, treated, and underwent elective colorectal surgery with adequate bowel preparation. The clinically evaluable population was a subset of the MITT population and consisted of patients who received a complete dose of study therapy no more than two hours prior to surgical incision and no more than six hours before surgical closure. Clinically evaluable patients had sufficient information to determine outcome at the 4-week follow-up assessment and had no confounding factors that interfered with the assessment of that outcome. Examples of confounding factors included prior or concomitant antibiotic violations, the need for a second surgical procedure during the study period, and identification of a distant site infection with concomitant antibiotic administration and no evidence of subsequent wound infection. Three-hundred forty-six (346) patients randomized to ertapenem and 339 patients randomized to cefotetan were clinically evaluable. The prophylactic success rates at 4 weeks posttreatment in the clinically evaluable population were 70.5% (244/346) for ertapenem and 57.2% (194/339) for cefotetan (difference 13.3%, [95% C.I.: 6.1, 20.4], p<0.001). Prophylaxis failure due to surgical site infections occurred in 18.2% (63/346) ertapenem patients and 31.0% (105/339) cefotetan patients. Post-operative anastomotic leak occurred in 2.9% (10/346) ertapenem patients and 4.1% (14/339) cefotetan patients. Unexplained antibiotic use occurred in 8.4% (29/346) ertapenem patients and 7.7% (26/339) cefotetan patients. Though patient numbers were small in some subgroups, in general, clinical response rates by age, gender, and race were consistent with the results found in the clinically evaluable population. In the MITT analysis, the prophylactic success rates at 4 weeks posttreatment were 58.3% (263/451) for ertapenem and 48.9% (220/450) for cefotetan (difference 9.4%, [95% C.I.: 2.9, 15.9], p=0.002). A statistically significant difference favoring ertapenem over cefotetan with respect to the primary endpoint has been observed at a significance level of 5% in this trial. A second adequate and well-controlled trial to confirm these findings has not been conducted; therefore, the clinical superiority of ertapenem over cefotetan has not been demonstrated.

14.2 Pediatric Patients

Ertapenem was evaluated in pediatric patients 3 months to 17 years of age in two randomized, multicenter clinical trials.

The first trial enrolled 404 patients and compared ertapenem (15 mg/kg intravenous (IV) every 12 hours in patients 3 months to 12 years of age, and 1 g IV once a day in patients 13 to 17 years of age) to ceftriaxone (50 mg/kg/day IV in two divided doses in patients 3 months to 12 years of age and 50 mg/kg/day IV as a single daily dose in patients 13 to 17 years of age) for the treatment of complicated urinary tract infection (UTI), skin and soft tissue infection (SSTI), or community-acquired pneumonia (CAP). Both regimens allowed the option to switch to oral amoxicillin/clavulanate for a total of up to 14 days of treatment (parenteral and oral). The microbiological success rates in the evaluable per protocol (EPP) analysis in patients treated for UTI were 87.0% (40/46) for ertapenem and 90.0% (18/20) for ceftriaxone. The clinical success rates in the EPP analysis in patients treated for SSTI were 95.5% (64/67) for ertapenem and 100% (26/26) for ceftriaxone, and in patients treated for CAP were 96.1% (74/77) for ertapenem and 96.4% (27/28) for ceftriaxone.

The second trial enrolled 112 patients and compared ertapenem (15 mg/kg IV every 12 hours in patients 3 months to 12 years of age, and 1 g IV once a day in patients 13 to 17 years of age) to ticarcillin/clavulanate (50 mg/kg for patients <60 kg or 3.0 g for patients >60 kg, 4 or 6 times a day) up to 14 days for the treatment of complicated intra-abdominal infections (IAI) and acute pelvic infections (API). In patients treated for IAI (primarily patients with perforated or complicated appendicitis), the clinical success rates were 83.7% (36/43) for ertapenem and 63.6% (7/11) for ticarcillin/clavulanate in the EPP analysis. In patients treated for API (post-operative or spontaneous obstetrical endomyometritis, or septic abortion), the clinical success rates were 100% (23/23) for ertapenem and 100% (4/4) for ticarcillin/clavulanate in the EPP analysis.

15 REFERENCES

1. Clinical and Laboratory Standards Institute (CLSI). Methods for Dilution Antimicrobial Susceptibility Tests for Bacteria that Grow Aerobically. 9th Edition; CLSI Document M7-A9. CLSI, Wayne, PA, 2012.
2. Clinical and Laboratory Standards Institute (CLSI). Performance Standards for Antimicrobial Disk Susceptibility Tests. 11th Edition; CLSI Document M2-A11. CLSI, Wayne, PA, 2012.
3. Clinical and Laboratory Standards Institute (CLSI). Methods for Antimicrobial Susceptibility Testing of Anaerobic Bacteria – 7th Edition; CLSI Document M11-A7. CLSI, Wayne, PA, 2007.
4. Clinical and Laboratory Standards Institute (CLSI). Performance Standards for Antimicrobial Susceptibility Testing – 22nd Informational Supplement. CLSI Document M100-S22. CLSI, Wayne, PA, 2012.
5. Clinical and Laboratory Standards Institute (CLSI, formerly NCCLS). Performance Standards for Antimicrobial Susceptibility of Anaerobic Bacteria; Informational Supplement. CLSI Document M11-S1. CLSI, Wayne, PA, 2010.

16 HOW SUPPLIED/STORAGE AND HANDLING

16.1 How Supplied

INVANZ is supplied as a sterile lyophilized powder in single dose vials containing ertapenem for intravenous infusion or for intramuscular injection as follows:

No. 3843—1 g ertapenem equivalent
NDC 0006-3843-71 in trays of 10 vials.

INVANZ is supplied as a sterile lyophilized powder in single dose ADD-Vantage® vials containing ertapenem for intravenous infusion as follows:
No. 3845—1 g ertapenem equivalent
NDC 0006-3845-71 in trays of 10 ADD-Vantage® vials.

16.2 Storage and Handling
Before reconstitution
Do not store lyophilized powder above 25°C (77°F).
Reconstituted and infusion solutions
The reconstituted solution, immediately diluted in 0.9% Sodium Chloride Injection [see Dosage and Administration (2.7)], may be stored at room temperature (25°C) and used within 6 hours or stored for 24 hours under refrigeration (5°C) and used within 4 hours after removal from refrigeration. Solutions of INVANZ should not be frozen.

17 PATIENT COUNSELING INFORMATION
17.1 Instructions for Patients
Patients should be advised that allergic reactions, including serious allergic reactions could occur and that serious reactions may require immediate treatment. Advise patients to report any previous hypersensitivity reactions to INVANZ, other beta-lactams or other allergens.
Patients should be counseled to inform their physician if they are taking valproic acid or divalproex sodium. Valproic acid concentrations in the blood may drop below the therapeutic range upon co-administration with INVANZ. If treatment with INVANZ is necessary and continued, alternative or supplemental anti-convulsant medication to prevent and/or treat seizures may be needed.
Patients should be counseled that antibacterial drugs including INVANZ should only be used to treat bacterial infections. They do not treat viral infections (e.g., the common cold). When INVANZ is prescribed to treat a bacterial infection, patients should be told that although it is common to feel better early in the course of therapy, the medication should be taken exactly as directed. Skipping doses or not completing the full course of therapy may (1) decrease the effectiveness of the immediate treatment and (2) increase the likelihood that bacteria will develop resistance and will not be treatable by INVANZ or other antibacterial drugs in the future.
Diarrhea is a common problem caused by antibiotics which usually ends when the antibiotic is discontinued. Sometimes after starting treatment with antibiotics, patients can develop watery and bloody stools (with or without stomach cramps and fever) even as late as two or more months after having taken the last dose of the antibiotic. If this occurs, patients should contact their physician as soon as possible.
Manuf. for: Merck Sharp & Dohme Corp., a subsidiary of **MERCK & CO., INC.**, Whitehouse Station, NJ 08889, USA
By: Laboratoires Merck Sharp & Dohme-Chibret
Clermont Ferrand Cedex 9, 63963, France
Copyright © 2001, 2007, 2011 Merck Sharp & Dohme Corp., a subsidiary of **Merck & Co., Inc.**
All rights reserved
For patent information:
www.merck.com/product/patent/home.html
uspi-mk0826-i-1408r019

ISENTRESS®
(raltegravir)
Film-Coated Tablets, for oral use
ISENTRESS®
(raltegravir)
Chewable Tablets, for oral use
ISENTRESS®
(raltegravir)
for oral suspension

℞

HIGHLIGHTS OF PRESCRIBING INFORMATION
These highlights do not include all the information needed to use ISENTRESS safely and effectively. See full prescribing information for ISENTRESS.
ISENTRESS® (raltegravir) film-coated tablets, for oral use
ISENTRESS® (raltegravir) chewable tablets, for oral use
ISENTRESS® (raltegravir) for oral suspension
Initial U.S. Approval: 2007

---RECENT MAJOR CHANGES---

Indications and Usage (1)	12/2013
Dosage and Administration	
General Dosing Recommendations (2.1)	12/2013
Pediatrics (2.3)	12/2013
Method of Administration (2.4)	12/2013

---INDICATIONS AND USAGE---

ISENTRESS is a human immunodeficiency virus integrase strand transfer inhibitor (HIV-1 INSTI) indicated:
• In combination with other antiretroviral agents for the treatment of HIV-1 infection in patients 4 weeks of age and older (1).
The use of other active agents with ISENTRESS is associated with a greater likelihood of treatment response (14).

---DOSAGE AND ADMINISTRATION---

ISENTRESS can be administered with or without food (2.1).
Do not substitute ISENTRESS chewable tablets or ISENTRESS for oral suspension for the ISENTRESS 400 mg film-coated tablet.
See specific dosing guidance for chewable tablets and the formulation for oral suspension (2.1).
Adults
• 400 mg film-coated tablet orally, twice daily (2.2).
• During coadministration with rifampin in adults, 800 mg twice daily (2.1).
Children and Adolescents
• at least 25 kg: One 400 mg film-coated tablet orally, twice daily. If unable to swallow a tablet, consider the chewable tablet, as specified in Table 1 (2.3).
• at least 3 kg to less than 25 kg: Weight based dosing, as specified in Table 2. For patients weighing between 11 and 20 kg, either the chewable tablet or the formulation for oral suspension can be used, as specified in Table 2 (2.3).

---DOSAGE FORMS AND STRENGTHS---

• Film-Coated Tablets: 400 mg (3).
• Chewable Tablets: 100 mg scored and 25 mg (3).
• For Oral Suspension: Single-use packet of 100 mg (3).

---CONTRAINDICATIONS---

None (4).

---WARNINGS AND PRECAUTIONS---

• Severe, potentially life-threatening and fatal skin reactions have been reported. This includes cases of Stevens-Johnson syndrome, hypersensitivity reaction and toxic epidermal necrolysis. Immediately discontinue treatment with ISENTRESS and other suspect agents if severe hypersensitivity, severe rash, or rash with systemic symptoms or liver aminotransferase elevations develops and monitor clinical status, including liver aminotransferases closely (5.1).
• Monitor for Immune Reconstitution Syndrome (5.2).
• Inform patients with phenylketonuria that the 100 mg and 25 mg chewable tablets contain phenylalanine (5.3).

---ADVERSE REACTIONS---

• The most common adverse reactions of moderate to severe intensity (≥2%) are insomnia, headache, dizziness, nausea and fatigue (6.1).
• Creatine kinase elevations were observed in subjects who received ISENTRESS. Myopathy and rhabdomyolysis have been reported. Use with caution in patients at increased risk of myopathy or rhabdomyolysis, such as patients receiving concomitant medications known to cause these conditions and patients with a history of rhabdomyolysis, myopathy or increased serum creatine kinase (6.2).
To report SUSPECTED ADVERSE REACTIONS, contact Merck Sharp & Dohme Corp., a subsidiary of Merck & Co., Inc., at 1-877-888-4231 or FDA at 1-800-FDA-1088 or www.fda.gov/medwatch.

---DRUG INTERACTIONS---

• Coadministration of ISENTRESS and other drugs may alter the plasma concentration of raltegravir. The potential for drug-drug interactions must be considered prior to and during therapy (7).
• Coadministration of ISENTRESS with drugs that are strong inducers of UGT1A1, such as rifampin, may result in reduced plasma concentrations of raltegravir (2.1, 7.2).

---USE IN SPECIFIC POPULATIONS---

Pregnancy:
• ISENTRESS should be used during pregnancy only if the potential benefit justifies the potential risk to the fetus (8.1).
Nursing Mothers:
• Breastfeeding is not recommended while taking ISENTRESS (8.3).
See 17 for PATIENT COUNSELING INFORMATION and FDA-approved patient labeling

Revised: 08/2014

FULL PRESCRIBING INFORMATION

1 INDICATIONS AND USAGE
ISENTRESS® is indicated in combination with other antiretroviral agents for the treatment of human immunodeficiency virus (HIV-1) infection in patients 4 weeks of age and older.
• The use of other active agents with ISENTRESS is associated with a greater likelihood of treatment response [see Clinical Studies (14)].

2 DOSAGE AND ADMINISTRATION
2.1 General Dosing Recommendations
• ISENTRESS Film-Coated Tablets, Chewable Tablets and For Oral Suspension can be administered with or without food [see Clinical Pharmacology (12.3)].
• Because the formulations are not bioequivalent, do not substitute ISENTRESS chewable tablets or ISENTRESS for oral suspension for the ISENTRESS 400 mg film-coated tablet. See specific dosing guidance for chewable tablets and the formulation for oral suspension.
• During coadministration of ISENTRESS 400 mg film-coated tablets with rifampin, the recommended dosage of ISENTRESS is 800 mg twice daily in adults. There are no data to guide co-administration of ISENTRESS with rifampin in patients below 18 years of age [see Drug Interactions (7.2)].
• Maximum dose of chewable tablets is 300 mg twice daily.
• Maximum dose of oral suspension is 100 mg twice daily.
• Each single-use packet for oral suspension contains 100 mg of raltegravir which is suspended in 5 mL of water giving a final concentration of 20 mg/mL.

2.2 Adults
For the treatment of adult patients with HIV-1 infection, the dosage of ISENTRESS is one 400 mg film-coated tablet administered orally, twice daily.

2.3 Pediatrics
• If at least 25 kg: One 400 mg film-coated tablet orally, twice daily.
• If unable to swallow a tablet, consider the chewable tablet, as specified in Table 1.

Table 1: Alternative Dose* with ISENTRESS Chewable Tablets for Pediatric Patients Weighing at Least 25 kg

Body Weight (kg)	Dose	Number of Chewable Tablets
25 to less than 28	150 mg twice daily	1.5 × 100 mg† twice daily
28 to less than 40	200 mg twice daily	2 × 100 mg twice daily
At least 40	300 mg twice daily	3 × 100 mg twice daily

* The weight-based dosing recommendation for the chewable tablet is based on approximately 6 mg/kg/dose twice daily [see Clinical Pharmacology (12.3)].
† The 100 mg chewable tablet can be divided into equal halves.

Main page (right column)

Psychiatric Disorders

Insomnia	4%	4%

n = total number of subjects per treatment group
* Includes adverse experiences considered by investigators to be at least possibly, probably, or definitely related to the drug.
† Intensities are defined as follows: Moderate (discomfort enough to cause interference with usual activity); Severe (incapacitating with inability to work or do usual activity).

Laboratory Abnormalities

The percentages of adult subjects treated with ISENTRESS 400 mg twice daily or efavirenz in Protocol 021 with selected Grades 2 to 4 laboratory abnormalities that represent a worsening Grade from baseline are presented in Table 4.
[See table 4 at top of next page]

Lipids, Change from Baseline
Changes from baseline in fasting lipids are shown in Table 5.
[See table 5 at top of next page]

Treatment-Experienced Adults
The safety assessment of ISENTRESS in treatment-experienced subjects is based on the pooled safety data from the randomized, double-blind, placebo-controlled trials, BENCHMRK 1 and BENCHMRK 2 (Protocols 018 and 019) in antiretroviral treatment-experienced HIV-1 infected adult subjects. A total of 462 subjects received the recommended dose of ISENTRESS 400 mg twice daily in combination with optimized background therapy (OBT) compared to 237 subjects taking placebo in combination with OBT. The median duration of therapy in these trials was 96 weeks for subjects receiving ISENTRESS and 38 weeks for subjects receiving placebo. The total exposure to ISENTRESS was 708 patient-years versus 244 patient-years on placebo. The rates of discontinuation due to adverse events were 4% in subjects receiving ISENTRESS and 5% in subjects receiving placebo.

Clinical ADRs were considered by investigators to be causally related to ISENTRESS + OBT or placebo + OBT. Clinical ADRs of moderate to severe intensity occurring in ≥2% of subjects treated with ISENTRESS and occurring at a higher rate compared to placebo are presented in Table 6.

Table 6: Adverse Drug Reactions* of Moderate to Severe Intensity† Occurring in ≥2% of Treatment-Experienced Adult Subjects Receiving ISENTRESS and at a Higher Rate Compared to Placebo (96 Week Analysis)

System Organ Class, Adverse Reactions	Randomized Studies Protocol 018 and 019	
	ISENTRESS 400 mg Twice Daily + OBT (n = 462)	Placebo + OBT (n = 237)
Nervous System Disorders		
Headache	2%	<1%

n=total number of subjects per treatment group.
* Includes adverse reactions at least possibly, probably, or definitely related to the drug.
† Intensities are defined as follows: Moderate (discomfort enough to cause interference with usual activity); Severe (incapacitating with inability to work or do usual activity).

Laboratory Abnormalities
The percentages of adult subjects treated with ISENTRESS 400 mg twice daily or placebo in Protocols 018 and 019 with selected Grade 2 to 4 laboratory abnormalities representing a worsening Grade from baseline are presented in Table 7.
[See table 7 at top of page 1505]

Less Common Adverse Reactions Observed in Treatment-Naïve and Treatment-Experienced Studies
The following ADRs occurred in <2% of treatment-naïve or treatment-experienced subjects receiving ISENTRESS in a combination regimen. These events have been included because of their seriousness, increased frequency on ISENTRESS compared with efavirenz or placebo, or investigator's assessment of potential causal relationship.
Gastrointestinal Disorders: abdominal pain, gastritis, dyspepsia, vomiting
General Disorders and Administration Site Conditions: asthenia
Hepatobiliary Disorders: hepatitis
Immune System Disorders: hypersensitivity
Infections and Infestations: genital herpes, herpes zoster

Main page (middle column)

function, including hepatic failure. Discontinue ISENTRESS and other suspect agents immediately if signs symptoms of severe skin reactions or hypersensitivity re-develop (including, but not limited to, severe rash or ...nied by fever, general malaise, fatigue, muscle ...blisters, oral lesions, conjunctivitis, facial ...inophilia, angioedema). Clinical status ...notransferases should be monitored and ...rapy initiated. Delay in stopping ...eatment or other suspect agents after the on-...rash may result in a life-threatening reaction.

Immune Reconstitution Syndrome
...reconstitution syndrome has been reported in pa-...reated with combination antiretroviral therapy, in-...g ISENTRESS. During the initial phase of combina-...antiretroviral treatment, patients whose immune ...stems respond may develop an inflammatory response to ...ndolent or residual opportunistic infections (such as *Mycobacterium avium* infection, cytomegalovirus, *Pneumocystis jiroveci* pneumonia, tuberculosis), which may necessitate further evaluation and treatment.

Autoimmune disorders (such as Graves' disease, polymyositis, and Guillain-Barré syndrome) have also been reported to occur in the setting of immune reconstitution; however, the time to onset is more variable, and can occur many months after initiation of treatment.

5.3 Phenylketonurics
ISENTRESS Chewable Tablets contain phenylalanine, a component of aspartame. Each 25 mg ISENTRESS Chewable Tablet contains approximately 0.05 mg phenylalanine. Each 100 mg ISENTRESS Chewable Tablet contains approximately 0.10 mg phenylalanine. Phenylalanine can be harmful to patients with phenylketonuria.

6 ADVERSE REACTIONS
Because clinical trials are conducted under widely varying conditions, adverse reaction rates observed in the clinical trials of a drug cannot be directly compared to rates in the clinical trials of another drug and ... reflect the rates observed in ... Trials Experience

6 ... Treatment-Naïve Adults
The following safety assessment of ISENTRESS in treatment-naïve subjects is based on the randomized double-blind active controlled study of treatment-naïve subjects, STARTMRK (Protocol 021) with ISENTRESS 400 mg twice daily in combination with a fixed dose of emtricitabine 200 mg (+) tenofovir 300 mg, (N=281) versus efavirenz (EFV) 600 mg at bedtime in combination with emtricitabine (+) tenofovir, (N... During double-blind treatment, the total follow-up ... receiving ISENTRESS 400 mg twice daily ... nofovir was 1104 patient-years a... age, ... subjects receiving efa-...bine (+) tenofovir.
...on of therapy due to ...ng ISENTRESS + ...bjects receiving

gs: PDR.net/PharmacyDiscountCard

...myolysis have been reported. Use ...s at increased risk of myopathy or ...s patients receiving concomitant ...use these conditions and patients ...myolysis, myopathy or increased

...only in treatment-experienced ...ontaining ISENTRESS ...ubjects receiving ISENTRESS + daru-...r darunavir/ritonavir without ...that was considered drug re-...for all three groups. These ...n severity and did not limit ...ions due to rash.
...ns - Adults

...acebo-controlled trials, ... 114/699 or 16%) and ...3 or 6%) with chronic ...d/or hepatitis C virus ...rovided that baseli-...es the upper li...ofile of ISE...patitis C of ...ithout... ...noush ow ...r for a...erienc...

	3 × 25 mg twice daily
...L (100 mg) twice daily	1 × 100 mg twice daily
	1.5 × 100 mg† twice daily

...based dosing recommendation for the ...tablet and oral sus... is based on ...roximately 6 mg/kg/dose twice daily [see *Clinical Pharmacology (12.3)*].
For ... between 11 and ... ...can be used ...
...and 50 mg tablet ... can be divided into equal
‡ The ...00 mg chewable tab... can be divided into equal halves.

...ethod of Administration
2. ...NTRESS Film-Coated Tablets
• Film-Coated Tablets must be swallowed whole
ISENTRESS Chewable Tablets
• Chewable Tablets may be chewed or swallowed whole
ISENTRESS For Oral Suspension
Each single-use ISENTRESS packet for oral suspension contains 100 mg of raltegravir which is to be suspended in 5 mL of water giving a final concentration of 20 m...
• Pour packet contents of ISENTRESS ... into 5 mL of water and mix
• Once mixed, measure the ... suspension with a s... the volume (d...

Lower center torn fragment

...than 2 Years of Age...
...s also been studied in 2... years
...lers 4 weeks to less than 2 years in IMPAAC...
...with other antiretroviral agents in IMPAAC... [see in *Specific Populations (8.4)* and *Clinical* ...]

...infants and toddlers, the frequency, type and ...drug-related adverse reactions through Week 48 ...parable to those observed in adults.
...sh experienced a Grade 3 serious drug-related al-... that resulted in treatment discontinuation.

Postmarketing Experience
...llowing adverse reactions have been identified during ...pproval use of ISENTRESS. Because these reactions ...reported voluntarily from a population of uncertain size, ... not always possible to reliably estimate their frequency ...establish a causal relationship to drug exposure.

Blood and Lymphatic System Disorders: thrombocytope-
Gastrointestinal Disorders: diarrhea
Hepatobiliary Disorders: hepatic failure (with and with-...out associated hypersensitivity) in patients with underlying liver disease and/or concomitant medications
Musculoskeletal and Connective Tissue Disorders: rhabdo-myolysis
Nervous System Disorders: cerebellar ataxia
Psychiatric Disorders: anxiety, paranoia

7 DRUG INTERACTIONS
7.1 Effect of Raltegravir on the Pharmacokinetics of Other Agents
Raltegravir does not inhibit (IC$_{50}$>100 μM) CYP1A2, CYP2B6, CYP2C8, CYP2C9, CYP2C19, CYP2D6 or CYP3A

	5%
	6%

Table 4: Selected Grade 2 to 4 Laboratory Abnormalities Reported in Treatment-Naïve Subjects (240 Week Analysis)

Laboratory Parameter Preferred Term (Unit)	Limit	Randomized Study Protocol 021	
		ISENTRESS 400 mg Twice Daily + Emtricitabine (+) Tenofovir (N = 281)	Efavirenz 600 mg At Bedtime + Emtricitabine (+) Tenofovir (N = 282)
Hematology			
Absolute neutrophil count (10³/μL)			
Grade 2	0.75 - 0.999	3%	5%
Grade 3	0.50 - 0.749	3%	1%
Grade 4	<0.50	1%	1%
Hemoglobin (gm/dL)			
Grade 2	7.5 - 8.4	1%	1%
Grade 3	6.5 - 7.4	1%	1%
Grade 4	<6.5	<1%	0%
Platelet count (10³/μL)			
Grade 2	50 - 99.999	1%	0%
Grade 3	25 - 49.999	<1%	<1%
Grade 4	<25	0%	0%
Blood chemistry			
Fasting (non-random) serum glucose test (mg/dL)			
Grade 2	126 - 250	7%	6%
Grade 3	251 - 500	2%	1%
Grade 4	>500	0%	0%
Total serum bilirubin			
Grade 2	1.6 - 2.5 × ULN	5%	<1%
Grade 3	2.6 - 5.0 × ULN	1%	0%
Grade 4	>5.0 × ULN	<1%	0%
Serum aspartate aminotransferase			
Grade 2	2.6 - 5.0 × ULN	8%	10%
Grade 3	5.1 - 10.0 × ULN	5%	3%
Grade 4	>10.0 × ULN		<1%
Serum alanine aminotransferase			
Grade 2	2.6 - 5.0 × ULN	11%	12%
Grade 3	5.1 - 10.0 × ULN	2%	2%
Grade 4	>10.0 × ULN	2%	1%
Serum alkaline phosphatase			
Grade 2	2.6 - 5.0 × ULN	1%	3%
Grade 3	5.1 - 10.0 × ULN	0%	1%
Grade 4	>10.0 × ULN	<1%	<1%

ULN = Upper limit of normal range

Table 5: Lipid Values, Mean Change from Baseline, Protocol 021

Laboratory Parameter Preferred Term	ISENTRESS 400 mg Twice Daily + Emtricitabine (+) Tenofovir N = 207			Efavirenz 600 mg At Bedtime + Emtricitabine (+) Tenofovir N = 187		
			Change from Baseline at Week 240			Change from Baseline at Week 240
	Baseline Mean (mg/dL)	Week 240 Mean (mg/dL)	Mean Change (mg/dL)	Baseline Mean (mg/dL)	Week 240 Mean (mg/dL)	Mean Change (mg/dL)
LDL-Cholesterol*	96	106	10	93	118	25
HDL-Cholesterol*	38	44	6	38	51	13
Total Cholesterol*	159	175	16	157	201	44
Triglyceride*	128	130	2	141	178	37

Notes:
N = total number of subjects per treatment group with at least one lipid test result available. The analysis is based on all available data.
If subjects initiated or increased serum lipid-reducing agents, the last available lipid values prior to the change in therapy were used in the analysis. If the missing data was due to other reasons, subjects were censored thereafter for the analysis. At baseline, serum lipid-reducing agents were used in 5% of subjects in the group receiving ISENTRESS and 3% in the efavirenz group. Through Week 240, serum lipid-reducing agents were used in 9% of subjects in the group receiving ISENTRESS and 15% in the efavirenz group.
* Fasting (non-random) laboratory tests at Week 240.

Psychiatric Disorders: depression (particularly in subjects with a pre-existing history of psychiatric illness), including suicidal ideation and behaviors
Renal and Urinary Disorders: nephrolithiasis, renal failure
Selected Adverse Events - Adults
Cancers were reported in treatment-experienced subjects who initiated ISENTRESS or placebo, both with OBT, and in treatment-naïve subjects who initiated ISENTRESS or

efavirenz, both with emtricitabine (+) tenofovir; several were recurrent. The types and rates of specific cancers were those expected in a highly immunodeficient population (many had CD4+ counts below 50 cells/mm³ and most had prior AIDS diagnoses). The risk of developing cancer in these studies was similar in the group receiving ISENTRESS and the group receiving the comparator.
Grade 2-4 creatine kinase laboratory abnormalities were observed in subjects treated with ISENTRESS (see Ta

Myopathy and rhabd
with caution in patien
rhabdomyolysis, such
medications known to ca
with a history of rhabd
serum creatine kinase.
Rash occurred more com
subjects receiving regimens
navir/ritonavir compared to
without darunavir/ritonavir
ISENTRESS. However, rash
lated occurred at similar rate
rashes were mild to moderate
therapy; there were no discontin
Patients with Co-existing Condit
Patients Co-infected with Hepat
Virus
In the randomized, double-blind,
treatment-experienced subjects (N
treatment-naïve subjects (N = 34/56
(but not acute) active hepatitis B an
co-infection were permitted to enroll p
liver function tests did not exceed 5 tim
normal (ULN). In general the safety pr
in subjects with hepatitis B and/or he
infection was similar to that in subjects
and/or hepatitis C virus co-infection, alt
AST and ALT abnormalities were highe
with hepatitis B and/or hepatitis C virus
treatment groups. At 96 weeks, in trea
subjects, Grade 2 or higher laboratory
represent a worsening Grade from basel
total bilirubin occurred in 29%, 34% and
of co-infected subjects treated with ISENTR
pared to 11%, 10% and 9% of all other su
ISENTRESS. At 240 weeks, in trea
Grade 2 or higher laboratory abn
worsening Grade from baseline of AST, ALT or to
bin occurred in 22%, respectic co-
infected subjects treated with ISENTRESS as co to
13%, 13% of all other subjects tr with
ISENTRESS

2 to 18 Years of Age
treatment, has been HIV-1 infected
cents 2 to 18 years of age, children an adoles
retroviral agents in IMPAAC combination with other anti-
Populations (8.4) and Clinical Studies [see Use in Specific
patients, 96 received the recommend of
ISENTRESS.
In these 96 children and adolescents, frequency, type and severity of drug related adverse reactions through Week 24 were comparable to those observed in adults.
One patient experienced drug related clinical adverse reactions of Grade 3 psychomotor hyperactivity, abnormal behavior and insomnia; one patient experienced a Grade 2 serious drug related allergic rash.
One patient experienced drug related laboratory abnormalities, Grade 4 AST Grade 3 ALT, which were considered serious.
4 Weeks to less
ISENTRESS h HIV-1 infected in
fants and todd
combination
P1066 [see U
Studies (14.
In these 2
severity of
were com
One pati
lergic ra
6.2
The fo
posta
are
it is
or
B

in vitro. Moreover, *in vitro*, raltegravir did not induce CYP1A2, CYP2B6 or CYP3A4. A midazolam drug interaction study confirmed the low propensity of raltegravir to alter the pharmacokinetics of agents metabolized by CYP3A4 *in vivo* by demonstrating a lack of effect of raltegravir on the pharmacokinetics of midazolam, a sensitive CYP3A4 substrate. Similarly, raltegravir is not an inhibitor (IC_{50}>50 µM) of the UDP-glucuronosyltransferases (UGT) tested (UGT1A1, UGT2B7), and raltegravir does not inhibit P-glycoprotein-mediated transport. Based on these data, ISENTRESS is not expected to affect the pharmacokinetics of drugs that are substrates of these enzymes or P-glycoprotein (e.g., protease inhibitors, NNRTIs, opioid analgesics, statins, azole antifungals, proton pump inhibitors and anti-erectile dysfunction agents).

In drug interaction studies, raltegravir did not have a clinically meaningful effect on the pharmacokinetics of the following: hormonal contraceptives, methadone, lamivudine, tenofovir, etravirine, darunavir/ritonavir, telaprevir, boceprevir.

7.2 Effect of Other Agents on the Pharmacokinetics of Raltegravir

Raltegravir is not a substrate of cytochrome P450 (CYP) enzymes. Based on *in vivo* and *in vitro* studies, raltegravir is eliminated mainly by metabolism via a UGT1A1-mediated glucuronidation pathway.

Rifampin, a strong inducer of UGT1A1, reduces plasma concentrations of ISENTRESS. Therefore, in adults the dose of ISENTRESS should be increased during coadministration with rifampin. There are no data to guide co-administration of ISENTRESS with rifampin in patients below 18 years of age [see Dosage and Administration (2.1)]. The impact of other inducers of drug metabolizing enzymes, such as phenytoin and phenobarbital, on UGT1A1 is unknown.

Coadministration of ISENTRESS with drugs that inhibit UGT1A1 may increase plasma levels of raltegravir.

Coadministration of ISENTRESS with antacids containing divalent metal cations may reduce raltegravir absorption by chelation, resulting in a decrease of raltegravir plasma levels. Taking an aluminum and magnesium antacid within 6 hours of ISENTRESS administration significantly decreased raltegravir plasma levels. Therefore, coadministration of ISENTRESS with aluminum and/or magnesium-containing antacids is not recommended. Coadministration of ISENTRESS with a calcium carbonate antacid decreased raltegravir plasma levels; however, this interaction is not considered clinically meaningful. Therefore, when ISENTRESS is coadministered with calcium carbonate-containing antacids, no dose adjustment is recommended. All interaction studies were performed in adults.

Selected drug interactions are presented in Table 8 [see Clinical Pharmacology (12.3)].

[See table 8 at top of next page]

8 USE IN SPECIFIC POPULATIONS

8.1 Pregnancy

Pregnancy Category C

ISENTRESS should be used during pregnancy only if the potential benefit justifies the potential risk to the fetus. There are no adequate and well-controlled studies in pregnant women. In addition, there have been no pharmacokinetic studies conducted in pregnant patients.

Developmental toxicity studies were performed in rabbits (at oral doses up to 1000 mg/kg/day) and rats (at oral doses up to 600 mg/kg/day). The reproductive toxicity study in rats was performed with pre-, peri-, and postnatal evaluation. The highest doses in these studies produced systemic exposures in these species approximately 3- to 4-fold the exposure at the recommended human dose. In both rabbits and rats, no treatment-related effects on embryonic/fetal survival or fetal weights were observed. In addition, no treatment-related external, visceral, or skeletal changes were observed in rabbits. However, treatment-related increases over controls in the incidence of supernumerary ribs were seen in rats at 600 mg/kg/day (exposures 3-fold the exposure at the recommended human dose).

Placenta transfer of drug was demonstrated in both rats and rabbits. At a maternal dose of 600 mg/kg/day in rats, mean drug concentrations in fetal plasma were approximately 1.5- to 2.5-fold greater than in maternal plasma at 1 hour and 24 hours postdose, respectively. Mean drug concentrations in fetal plasma were approximately 2% of the mean maternal concentration at both 1 and 24 hours postdose at a maternal dose of 1000 mg/kg/day in rabbits.

Antiretroviral Pregnancy Registry

To monitor maternal-fetal outcomes of pregnant patients exposed to ISENTRESS, an Antiretroviral Pregnancy Registry has been established. Physicians are encouraged to register patients by calling 1-800-258-4263.

8.3 Nursing Mothers

Breastfeeding is not recommended while taking ISENTRESS. In addition, it is recommended that HIV-1-infected mothers not breastfeed their infants to avoid risking postnatal transmission of HIV-1.

Table 7: Selected Grade 2 to 4 Laboratory Abnormalities Reported in Treatment-Experienced Subjects (96 Week Analysis)

Laboratory Parameter Preferred Term (Unit)	Limit	Randomized Studies Protocol 018 and 019	
		ISENTRESS 400 mg Twice Daily + OBT (N = 462)	Placebo + OBT (N = 237)
Hematology			
Absolute neutrophil count (10^3/µL)			
Grade 2	0.75 - 0.999	4%	5%
Grade 3	0.50 - 0.749	3%	3%
Grade 4	<0.50	1%	<1%
Hemoglobin (gm/dL)			
Grade 2	7.5 - 8.4	1%	3%
Grade 3	6.5 - 7.4	1%	1%
Grade 4	<6.5	<1%	0%
Platelet count (10^3/µL)			
Grade 2	50 - 99.999	3%	5%
Grade 3	25 - 49.999	1%	<1%
Grade 4	<25	1%	<1%
Blood chemistry			
Fasting (non-random) serum glucose test (mg/dL)			
Grade 2	126 - 250	10%	7%
Grade 3	251 - 500	3%	1%
Grade 4	>500	0%	0%
Total serum bilirubin			
Grade 2	1.6 - 2.5 × ULN	6%	3%
Grade 3	2.6 - 5.0 × ULN	3%.	3%
Grade 4	>5.0 × ULN	1%	0%
Serum aspartate aminotransferase			
Grade 2	2.6 - 5.0 × ULN	9%	7%
Grade 3	5.1 - 10.0 × ULN	4%	3%
Grade 4	>10.0 × ULN	1%	1%
Serum alanine aminotransferase			
Grade 2	2.6 - 5.0 × ULN	9%	9%
Grade 3	5.1 - 10.0 × ULN	4%	2%
Grade 4	>10.0 × ULN	1%	2%
Serum alkaline phosphatase			
Grade 2	2.6 - 5.0 × ULN	2%	<1%
Grade 3	5.1 - 10.0 × ULN	<1%	1%
Grade 4	>10.0 × ULN	1%	<1%
Serum pancreatic amylase test			
Grade 2	1.6 - 2.0 × ULN	2%	1%
Grade 3	2.1 - 5.0 × ULN	4%	3%
Grade 4	>5.0 × ULN	<1%	<1%
Serum lipase test			
Grade 2	1.6 - 3.0 × ULN	5%	4%
Grade 3	3.1 - 5.0 × ULN	2%	1%
Grade 4	>5.0 × ULN	0%	0%
Serum creatine kinase			
Grade 2	6.0 - 9.9 × ULN	2%	2%
Grade 3	10.0 - 19.9 × ULN	4%	3%
Grade 4	≥20.0 × ULN	3%	1%

ULN = Upper limit of normal range

It is not known whether raltegravir is secreted in human milk. However, raltegravir is secreted in the milk of lactating rats. Mean drug concentrations in milk were approximately 3-fold greater than those in maternal plasma at a maternal dose of 600 mg/kg/day in rats. There were no effects in rat offspring attributable to exposure of ISENTRESS through the milk.

8.4 Pediatric Use

The safety, tolerability, pharmacokinetic profile, and efficacy of ISENTRESS were evaluated in HIV-1 infected infants, children and adolescents 4 weeks to 18 years of age in an open-label, multicenter clinical trial, IMPAACT P1066 [see Clinical Pharmacology (12.3) and Clinical Studies (14.3)]. The safety profile was comparable to that observed in adults [see Adverse Reactions (6.1)]. See Dosage and Administration (2.3) for dosing recommendations for children 4 weeks of age and older. The safety and dosing information for ISENTRESS have not been established in infants less than 4 weeks of age.

8.5 Geriatric Use

Clinical studies of ISENTRESS did not include sufficient numbers of subjects aged 65 and over to determine whether they respond differently from younger subjects. Other reported clinical experience has not identified differences in responses between the elderly and younger subjects. In general, dose selection for an elderly patient should be cautious, reflecting the greater frequency of decreased hepatic, renal, or cardiac function, and of concomitant disease or other drug therapy.

8.6 Use in Patients with Hepatic Impairment

No clinically important pharmacokinetic differences between subjects with moderate hepatic impairment and healthy subjects were observed. No dosage adjustment is necessary for patients with mild to moderate hepatic impairment. The effect of severe hepatic impairment on the pharmacokinetics of raltegravir has not been studied [see Clinical Pharmacology (12.3)].

8.7 Use in Patients with Renal Impairment

No clinically important pharmacokinetic differences between subjects with severe renal impairment and healthy subjects were observed. No dosage adjustment is necessary [see Clinical Pharmacology (12.3)].

10 OVERDOSAGE

No specific information is available on the treatment of overdosage with ISENTRESS. Doses as high as 1600-mg single dose and 800-mg twice-daily multiple doses were studied in healthy volunteers without evidence of toxicity. Occasional doses of up to 1800 mg per day were taken in the clinical studies of HIV-1 infected subjects without evidence of toxicity.

Table 8:   Selected Drug Interactions in Adults

Concomitant Drug Class: Drug Name	Effect on Concentration of Raltegravir	Clinical Comment
HIV-1-Antiviral Agents		
atazanavir	↑	Atazanavir, a strong inhibitor of UGT1A1, increases plasma concentrations of raltegravir. However, since concomitant use of ISENTRESS with atazanavir/ritonavir did not result in a unique safety signal in Phase 3 studies, no dose adjustment is recommended.
atazanavir/ritonavir	↑	Atazanavir/ritonavir increases plasma concentrations of raltegravir. However, since concomitant use of ISENTRESS with atazanavir/ritonavir did not result in a unique safety signal in Phase 3 studies, no dose adjustment is recommended.
efavirenz	↓	Efavirenz reduces plasma concentrations of raltegravir. The clinical significance of this interaction has not been directly assessed.
etravirine	↓	Etravirine reduces plasma concentrations of raltegravir. The clinical significance of this interaction has not been directly assessed.
tipranavir/ritonavir	↓	Tipranavir/ritonavir reduces plasma concentrations of raltegravir. However, since comparable efficacy was observed for this combination relative to other ISENTRESS-containing regimens in Phase 3 studies 018 and 019, no dose adjustment is recommended.
Metal-Containing Antacids		
aluminum and/or magnesium-containing antacids	↓	Coadministration or staggered administration of aluminum and/or magnesium hydroxide-containing antacids and ISENTRESS is not recommended.
calcium carbonate antacids	↓	No dose adjustment is recommended when ISENTRESS is coadministered with calcium carbonate-containing antacids.
H2 Blockers and Proton Pump Inhibitors		
omeprazole	↑	Coadministration of medicinal products that increase gastric pH (e.g., omeprazole) may increase raltegravir levels based on increased raltegravir solubility at higher pH. However, since concomitant use of ISENTRESS with proton pump inhibitors and H2 blockers did not result in a unique safety signal in Phase 3 studies, no dose adjustment is recommended.
HCV-Antiviral Agents		
boceprevir	↔	No dose adjustment required for ISENTRESS or boceprevir.
telaprevir	↑	No dose adjustment required for ISENTRESS or telaprevir.
Other Agents		
rifampin	↓	Rifampin, a strong inducer of UGT1A1, reduces plasma concentrations of raltegravir. The recommended dosage of ISENTRESS is 800 mg twice daily during coadministration with rifampin.

In the event of an overdose, it is reasonable to employ the standard supportive measures, e.g., remove unabsorbed material from the gastrointestinal tract, employ clinical monitoring (including obtaining an electrocardiogram), and institute supportive therapy if required. The extent to which ISENTRESS may be dialyzable is unknown.

11   DESCRIPTION

ISENTRESS contains raltegravir potassium, a human immunodeficiency virus integrase strand transfer inhibitor. The chemical name for raltegravir potassium is N-[(4-Fluorophenyl) methyl]-1,6-dihydro-5-hydroxy-1-methyl-2-[1-methyl-1-[[(5-methyl-1,3,4-oxadiazol-2-yl)carbonyl]amino]ethyl]-6-oxo-4-pyrimidinecarboxamide monopotassium salt.

The empirical formula is $C_{20}H_{20}FKN_6O_5$ and the molecular weight is 482.51. The structural formula is:

Raltegravir potassium is a white to off-white powder. It is soluble in water, slightly soluble in methanol, very slightly soluble in ethanol and acetonitrile and insoluble in isopropanol.

Each 400 mg film-coated tablet of ISENTRESS for oral administration contains 434.4 mg of raltegravir (as potassium salt), equivalent to 400 mg of raltegravir free phenol and the following inactive ingredients: calcium phosphate dibasic anhydrous, hypromellose 2208, lactose monohydrate, magnesium stearate, microcrystalline cellulose, poloxamer 407 (contains 0.01% butylated hydroxytoluene as antioxidant), sodium stearyl fumarate. In addition, the film coating contains the following inactive ingredients: black iron oxide, polyethylene glycol 3350, polyvinyl alcohol, red iron oxide, talc and titanium dioxide.

Each 100 mg chewable tablet of ISENTRESS for oral administration contains 108.6 mg of raltegravir (as potassium salt), equivalent to 100 mg of raltegravir free phenol and the following inactive ingredients: ammonium hydroxide, crospovidone, ethylcellulose 20 cP, fructose, hydroxypropyl cellulose, hypromellose 2910/6cP, magnesium stearate, mannitol, medium chain triglycerides, monoammonium glycyrrhizinate, natural and artificial flavors (orange, banana, and masking that contains aspartame), oleic acid, PEG 400, red iron oxide, saccharin sodium, sodium citrate dihydrate, sodium stearyl fumarate, sorbitol, sucralose and yellow iron oxide.

Each 25 mg chewable tablet of ISENTRESS for oral administration contains 27.16 mg of raltegravir (as potassium salt), equivalent to 25 mg of raltegravir free phenol and the following inactive ingredients: ammonium hydroxide, crospovidone, ethylcellulose 20 cP, fructose, hydroxypropyl cellulose, hypromellose 2910/6cP, magnesium stearate, mannitol, medium chain triglycerides, monoammonium glycyrrhizinate, natural and artificial flavors (orange, banana, and masking that contains aspartame), oleic acid, PEG 400, saccharin sodium, sodium citrate dihydrate, sodium stearyl fumarate, sorbitol, sucralose and yellow iron oxide.

Each packet of ISENTRESS for oral suspension 100 mg, contains 108.6 mg of raltegravir (as potassium salt), equivalent to 100 mg of raltegravir free phenol and the following inactive ingredients: ammonium hydroxide, banana with other natural flavors, carboxymethylcellulose sodium, crospovidone, ethylcellulose 20 cP, fructose, hydroxypropyl cellulose, hypromellose 2910/6cP, macrogol/PEG 400, magnesium stearate, maltodextrin, mannitol, medium chain triglycerides, microcrystalline cellulose, monoammonium glycyrrhizinate, oleic acid, sorbitol, sucralose and sucrose.

12   CLINICAL PHARMACOLOGY

12.1   Mechanism of Action

Raltegravir is an HIV-1 antiviral drug [see Microbiology (12.4)].

12.2   Pharmacodynamics

In a monotherapy study raltegravir (400 mg twice daily) demonstrated rapid antiviral activity with mean viral load reduction of 1.66 $\log_{10}$ copies/mL by Day 10.

In the randomized, double-blind, placebo-controlled, dose-ranging trial, Protocol 005, and Protocols 018 and 019, antiviral responses were similar among subjects regardless of dose.

Effects on Electrocardiogram

In a randomized, placebo-controlled, crossover study, 31 healthy subjects were administered a single oral supratherapeutic dose of raltegravir 1600 mg and placebo. Peak raltegravir plasma concentrations were approximately 4-fold higher than the peak concentrations following a 400 mg dose. ISENTRESS did not appear to prolong the QTc interval for 12 hours postdose. After baseline and placebo adjustment, the maximum mean QTc change was -0.4 msec (1-sided 95% upper CI: 3.1 msec).

12.3   Pharmacokinetics

Adults

Absorption

Raltegravir (film-coated tablet) is absorbed with a T_{max} of approximately 3 hours postdose in the fasted state. Raltegravir AUC and C_{max} increase dose proportionally over the dose range 100 mg to 1600 mg. Raltegravir C_{12hr} increases dose proportionally over the dose range of 100 to 800 mg and increases slightly less than dose proportionally over the dose range 100 mg to 1600 mg. With twice-daily dosing, pharmacokinetic steady state is achieved within approximately the first 2 days of dosing. There is little to no accumulation in AUC and C_{max}. The average accumulation ratio for C_{12hr} ranged from approximately 1.2 to 1.6.

The absolute bioavailability of raltegravir has not been established. Based on a formulation comparison study in healthy adult volunteers, the chewable tablet and oral suspension have higher oral bioavailability compared to the 400 mg film-coated tablet.

In subjects who received 400 mg twice daily alone, raltegravir drug exposures were characterized by a geometric mean AUC_{0-12hr} of 14.3 µM·hr and C_{12hr} of 142 nM.

Considerable variability was observed in the pharmacokinetics of raltegravir. For observed C_{12hr} in Protocols 018 and 019, the coefficient of variation (CV) for inter-subject variability = 212% and the CV for intra-subject variability = 122%.

Effect of Food on Oral Absorption

ISENTRESS may be administered with or without food. Raltegravir was administered without regard to food in the pivotal safety and efficacy studies in HIV-1-infected patients. The effect of consumption of low-, moderate- and high-fat meals on steady-state raltegravir pharmacokinetics was assessed in healthy volunteers administered the 400 mg film-coated tablet. Administration of multiple doses of raltegravir following a moderate-fat meal (600 Kcal, 21 g fat) did not affect raltegravir AUC to a clinically meaningful degree with an increase of 13% relative to fasting. Raltegravir C_{12hr} was 66% higher and C_{max} was 5% higher following a moderate-fat meal compared to fasting. Administration of raltegravir following a high-fat meal (825 Kcal, 52 g fat) increased AUC and C_{max} by approximately 2-fold and increased C_{12hr} by 4.1-fold. Administration of raltegravir following a low-fat meal (300 Kcal, 2.5 g fat) decreased AUC and C_{max} by 46% and 52%, respectively; C_{12hr} was essentially unchanged. Food appears to increase pharmacokinetic variability relative to fasting.

Administration of the chewable tablet with a high fat meal led to an average 6% decrease in AUC, 62% decrease in C_{max}, and 188% increase in C_{12hr} compared to administration in the fasted state. Administration of the chewable tablet with a high fat meal does not affect raltegravir pharmacokinetics to a clinically meaningful degree and the chewable tablet can be administered without regard to food. The effect of food on the formulation for oral suspension was not studied.

Distribution

Raltegravir is approximately 83% bound to human plasma protein over the concentration range of 2 to 10 μM.

In one study of HIV-1 infected subjects who received raltegravir 400 mg twice daily, raltegravir was measured in the cerebrospinal fluid. In the study (n=18), the median cerebrospinal fluid concentration was 5.8% (range 1 to 53.5%) of the corresponding plasma concentration. This median proportion was approximately 3-fold lower than the free fraction of raltegravir in plasma. The clinical relevance of this finding is unknown.

Metabolism and Excretion

The apparent terminal half-life of raltegravir is approximately 9 hours, with a shorter α-phase half-life (~1 hour) accounting for much of the AUC. Following administration of an oral dose of radiolabeled raltegravir, approximately 51 and 32% of the dose was excreted in feces and urine, respectively. In feces, only raltegravir was present, most of which is likely derived from hydrolysis of raltegravir-glucuronide secreted in bile as observed in preclinical species. Two components, namely raltegravir and raltegravir-glucuronide, were detected in urine and accounted for approximately 9 and 23% of the dose, respectively. The major circulating entity was raltegravir and represented approximately 70% of the total radioactivity; the remaining radioactivity in plasma was accounted for by raltegravir-glucuronide. Studies using isoform-selective chemical inhibitors and cDNA-expressed UDP-glucuronosyltransferases (UGT) show that UGT1A1 is the main enzyme responsible for the formation of raltegravir-glucuronide. Thus, the data indicate that the major mechanism of clearance of raltegravir in humans is UGT1A1-mediated glucuronidation.

Special Populations

Pediatric

Two pediatric formulations were evaluated in healthy adult volunteers, where the chewable tablet and oral suspension were compared to the 400 mg tablet. The chewable tablet and oral suspension demonstrated higher oral bioavailability, thus higher AUC, compared to the 400 mg tablet. In the same study, the oral suspension resulted in higher oral bioavailability compared to the chewable tablet. These observations resulted in proposed pediatric doses targeting 6 mg/kg/dose for the chewable tablets and oral suspension. As displayed in Table 9, the doses recommended for HIV-infected infants, children and adolescents 4 weeks to 18 years of age [see Dosage and Administration (2.3)] resulted in a pharmacokinetic profile of raltegravir similar to that observed in adults receiving 400 mg twice daily.

Overall, dosing in pediatric patients achieved exposures (C_{trough}) above 45 nM in the majority of subjects, but some differences in exposures between formulations were observed. Pediatric patients above 25 kg administered the chewable tablets had lower trough concentrations (113 nM) compared to pediatric patients above 25 kg administered the 400 mg tablet formulation (233 nM) [see Clinical Studies (14.3)]. As a result, the 400 mg film-coated tablet is the recommended dose in patients weighing at least 25 kg; however, the chewable tablet offers an alternative regimen in patients weighing at least 25 kg who are unable to swallow the film-coated tablet [see Dosage and Administration (2.3)]. In addition, pediatric patients weighing 11 to 25 kg who were administered the chewable tablets had the lowest trough concentrations (82 nM) compared to all other pediatric subgroups.

[See table 9 above]

The pharmacokinetics of raltegravir in infants under 4 weeks of age has not been established.

Age

The effect of age (18 years and older) on the pharmacokinetics of raltegravir was evaluated in the composite analysis. No dosage adjustment is necessary.

Race

The effect of race on the pharmacokinetics of raltegravir in adults was evaluated in the composite analysis. No dosage adjustment is necessary.

Gender

A study of the pharmacokinetics of raltegravir was performed in healthy adult males and females. Additionally, the effect of gender was evaluated in a composite analysis of pharmacokinetic data from 103 healthy subjects and 28 HIV-1 infected subjects receiving raltegravir monotherapy with fasted administration. No dosage adjustment is necessary.

Table 9: Raltegravir Steady State Pharmacokinetic Parameters in Pediatric Patients Following Administration of Recommended Doses

Body Weight	Formulation	Dose	N*	Geometric Mean (%CV†) AUC$_{0-12hr}$ (μM·hr)	Geometric Mean (%CV†) C$_{12hr}$ (nM)
≥25 kg	Film-coated tablet	400 mg twice daily	18	14.1 (121%)	233 (157%)
≥25 kg	Chewable tablet	Weight based dosing, see Table 1	9	22.1 (36%)	113 (80%)
11 to less than 25 kg	Chewable tablet	Weight based dosing, see Table 2	13	18.6 (68%)	82 (123%)
3 to less than 20 kg	Oral suspension	Weight based dosing, see Table 2	19	24.5 (43%)	113 (69%)

* Number of patients with intensive pharmacokinetic (PK) results at the final recommended dose.
† Geometric coefficient of variation.

Hepatic Impairment

Raltegravir is eliminated primarily by glucuronidation in the liver. A study of the pharmacokinetics of raltegravir was performed in adult subjects with moderate hepatic impairment. Additionally, hepatic impairment was evaluated in the composite pharmacokinetic analysis. There were no clinically important pharmacokinetic differences between subjects with moderate hepatic impairment and healthy subjects. No dosage adjustment is necessary for patients with mild to moderate hepatic impairment. The effect of severe hepatic impairment on the pharmacokinetics of raltegravir has not been studied.

Renal Impairment

Renal clearance of unchanged drug is a minor pathway of elimination. A study of the pharmacokinetics of raltegravir was performed in adult subjects with severe renal impairment. Additionally, renal impairment was evaluated in the composite pharmacokinetic analysis. There were no clinically important pharmacokinetic differences between subjects with severe renal impairment and healthy subjects. No dosage adjustment is necessary. Because the extent to which ISENTRESS may be dialyzable is unknown, dosing before a dialysis session should be avoided.

UGT1A1 Polymorphism

There is no evidence that common UGT1A1 polymorphisms alter raltegravir pharmacokinetics to a clinically meaningful extent. In a comparison of 30 adult subjects with *28/*28 genotype (associated with reduced activity of UGT1A1) to 27 adult subjects with wild-type genotype, the geometric mean ratio (90% CI) of AUC was 1.41 (0.96, 2.09).

Drug Interactions [see Drug Interactions (7)]

[See table 10 at top of next page]

12.4   Microbiology

Mechanism of Action

Raltegravir inhibits the catalytic activity of HIV-1 integrase, an HIV-1 encoded enzyme that is required for viral replication. Inhibition of integrase prevents the covalent insertion, or integration, of unintegrated linear HIV-1 DNA into the host cell genome preventing the formation of the HIV-1 provirus. The provirus is required to direct the production of progeny virus, so inhibiting integration prevents propagation of the viral infection. Raltegravir did not significantly inhibit human phosphoryltransferases including DNA polymerases α, β, and γ.

Antiviral Activity in Cell Culture

Raltegravir at concentrations of 31 ± 20 nM resulted in 95% inhibition (EC$_{95}$) of viral spread (relative to an untreated virus-infected culture) in human T-lymphoid cell cultures infected with the cell-line adapted HIV-1 variant H9IIIB. In addition, 5 clinical isolates of HIV-1 subtype B had EC$_{95}$ values ranging from 9 to 19 nM in cultures of mitogen-activated human peripheral blood mononuclear cells. In a single-cycle infection assay, raltegravir inhibited infection of 23 HIV-1 isolates representing 5 non-B subtypes (A, C, D, F, and G) and 5 circulating recombinant forms (AE, AG, BF, BG, and cpx) with EC$_{50}$ values ranging from 5 to 12 nM. Raltegravir also inhibited replication of a HIV-2 isolate when tested in CEMx174 cells (EC$_{95}$ value = 6 nM). Additive to synergistic antiretroviral activity was observed when human T-lymphoid cells infected with the H9IIIB variant of HIV-1 were incubated with raltegravir in combination with non-nucleoside reverse transcriptase inhibitors (delavirdine, efavirenz, or nevirapine); nucleoside analog reverse transcriptase inhibitors (abacavir, didanosine, lamivudine, stavudine, tenofovir, zalcitabine, or zidovudine); protease inhibitors (amprenavir, atazanavir, indinavir, lopinavir, nelfinavir, ritonavir, or saquinavir); or the entry inhibitor enfuvirtide.

Resistance

The mutations observed in the HIV-1 integrase coding sequence that contributed to raltegravir resistance (evolved either in cell culture or in subjects treated with raltegravir) generally included an amino acid substitution at either Y143 (changed to C, H, or R) or Q148 (changed to H, K, or R) or N155 (changed to H) plus one or more additional substitutions (i.e., L74M, E92Q, Q95K/R, T97A, E138A/K, G140A/S, V151I, G163R, H183P, Y226C/D/F/H, S230R, and D232N). E92Q and F121C are occasionally seen in the absence of substitutions at Y143, Q148, or N155 in raltegravir-treatment failure subjects.

Treatment-Naïve Adult Subjects: By Week 96 in the STARTMRK trial, the primary raltegravir resistance-associated substitutions were observed in 4 (2 with Y143H/R and 2 with Q148H/R) of the 10 virologic failure subjects with evaluable genotypic data from paired baseline and raltegravir treatment-failure isolates.

Treatment-Experienced Adult Subjects: By Week 96 in the BENCHMRK trials, at least one of the primary raltegravir resistance-associated substitutions, Y143C/H/R, Q148H/K/R, and N155H, was observed in 76 of the 112 virologic failure subjects with evaluable genotypic data from paired baseline and raltegravir treatment-failure isolates. The emergence of the primary raltegravir resistance-associated substitutions was observed cumulatively in 70 subjects by Week 48 and 78 subjects by Week 96, 15.2% and 17% of the raltegravir recipients, respectively. Some (n=58) of those HIV-1 isolates harboring one or more of the primary raltegravir resistance-associated substitutions were evaluated for raltegravir susceptibility yielding a median decrease of 26.3-fold (mean 48.9 ± 44.8-fold decrease, ranging from 0.8- to 159-fold) compared to the wild-type reference.

13   NONCLINICAL TOXICOLOGY

13.1   Carcinogenesis, Mutagenesis, Impairment of Fertility

Carcinogenicity studies of raltegravir in mice did not show any carcinogenic potential. At the highest dose levels, 400 mg/kg/day in females and 250 mg/kg/day in males, systemic exposure was 1.8-fold (females) or 1.2-fold (males) greater than the AUC (54 μM·hr) at the 400-mg twice daily human dose. Treatment-related squamous cell carcinoma of nose/nasopharynx was observed in female rats dosed with 600 mg/kg/day raltegravir for 104 weeks. These tumors were possibly the result of local irritation and inflammation due to local deposition and/or aspiration of drug in the mucosa of the nose/nasopharynx during dosing. No tumors of the nose/nasopharynx were observed in rats dosed with 150 mg/kg/day (males) and 50 mg/kg/day (females) and the systemic exposure in rats was 1.7-fold (males) to 1.4-fold (females) greater than the AUC (54 μM·hr) at the 400-mg twice daily human dose.

No evidence of mutagenicity or genotoxicity was observed in in vitro microbial mutagenesis (Ames) tests, in vitro alkaline elution assays for DNA breakage, and in vitro and in vivo chromosomal aberration studies.

No effect on fertility was seen in male and female rats at doses up to 600 mg/kg/day which resulted in a 3-fold exposure above the exposure at the recommended human dose.

14   CLINICAL STUDIES

Description of Clinical Studies

The evidence of durable efficacy of ISENTRESS is based on the analyses of 240-week data from a randomized, double-blind, active-control trial, STARTMRK (Protocol 021) in antiretroviral treatment-naïve HIV-1 infected adult subjects and 96-week data from 2 randomized, double-blind, placebo-controlled studies, BENCHMRK 1 and BENCHMRK 2 (Protocols 018 and 019), in antiretroviral treatment-experienced HIV-1 infected adult subjects.

14.1   Treatment-Naïve Adult Subjects

STARTMRK (Protocol 021) is a Phase 3 study to evaluate the safety and antiretroviral activity of ISENTRESS

Table 10: Effect of Other Agents on the Pharmacokinetics of Raltegravir in Adults

Coadministered Drug	Coadministered Drug Dose/ Schedule	Raltegravir Dose/Schedule	Ratio (90% Confidence Interval) of Raltegravir Pharmacokinetic Parameters with/without Coadministered Drug; No Effect = 1.00			
			n	C_{max}	AUC	C_{min}
aluminum and magnesium hydroxide antacid	20 mL single dose given with raltegravir	400 mg twice daily	25	0.56 (0.42, 0.73)	0.51 (0.40, 0.65)	0.37 (0.29, 0.48)
	20 mL single dose given 2 hours before raltegravir		23	0.49 (0.33, 0.71)	0.49 (0.35, 0.67)	0.44 (0.34, 0.55)
	20 mL single dose given 2 hours after raltegravir		23	0.78 (0.53, 1.13)	0.70 (0.50, 0.96)	0.43 (0.34, 0.55)
atazanavir	400 mg daily	100 mg single dose	10	1.53 (1.11, 2.12)	1.72 (1.47, 2.02)	1.95 (1.30, 2.92)
atazanavir/ ritonavir	300 mg/100 mg daily	400 mg twice daily	10	1.24 (0.87, 1.77)	1.41 (1.12, 1.78)	1.77 (1.39, 2.25)
boceprevir	800 mg three times daily	400 mg single dose	22	1.11 (0.91-1.36)	1.04 (0.88-1.22)	0.75 (0.45-1.23)
calcium carbonate antacid	3000 mg single dose given with raltegravir	400 mg twice daily	24	0.48 (0.36, 0.63)	0.45 (0.35, 0.57)	0.68 (0.53, 0.87)
efavirenz	600 mg daily	400 mg single dose	9	0.64 (0.41, 0.98)	0.64 (0.52, 0.80)	0.79 (0.49, 1.28)
etravirine	200 mg twice daily	400 mg twice daily	19	0.89 (0.68, 1.15)	0.90 (0.68, 1.18)	0.66 (0.34, 1.26)
omeprazole	20 mg daily	400 mg single dose	14 (10 for AUC)	4.15 (2.82, 6.10)	3.12 (2.13, 4.56)	1.46 (1.10, 1.93)
rifampin	600 mg daily	400 mg single dose	9	0.62 (0.37, 1.04)	0.60 (0.39, 0.91)	0.39 (0.30, 0.51)
rifampin	600 mg daily	400 mg twice daily when administered alone; 800 mg twice daily when administered with rifampin	14	1.62 (1.12, 2.33)	1.27 (0.94, 1.71)	0.47 (0.36, 0.61)
ritonavir	100 mg twice daily	400 mg single dose	10	0.76 (0.55, 1.04)	0.84 (0.70, 1.01)	0.99 (0.70, 1.40)
telaprevir	750 mg every 8 hours	400 mg twice daily	20	1.26 (0.97, 1.62)	1.31 (1.03, 1.67)	1.78 (1.26, 2.53)
tenofovir	300 mg daily	400 mg twice daily	9	1.64 (1.16, 2.32)	1.49 (1.15, 1.94)	1.03 (0.73, 1.45)
tipranavir/ ritonavir	500 mg/200 mg twice daily	400 mg twice daily	15 (14 for C_{min})	0.82 (0.46, 1.46)	0.76 (0.49, 1.19)	0.45 (0.31, 0.66)

400 mg twice daily + emtricitabine (+) tenofovir versus efavirenz 600 mg at bedtime plus emtricitabine (+) tenofovir in treatment-naïve HIV-1-infected subjects with HIV-1 RNA >5000 copies/mL. Randomization was stratified by screening HIV-1 RNA level (≤50,000 copies/mL; and >50,000 copies/mL) and by hepatitis status.

Table 11 shows the demographic characteristics of subjects in the group receiving ISENTRESS 400 mg twice daily and subjects in the comparator group.

Table 11: Baseline Characteristics

Randomized Study Protocol 021	ISENTRESS 400 mg Twice Daily (N = 281)	Efavirenz 600 mg At Bedtime (N = 282)
Gender		
Male	81%	82%
Female	19%	18%

Race		
White	41%	44%
Black	12%	8%
Asian	13%	11%
Hispanic	21%	24%
Native American	<1%	<1%
Multiracial	12%	13%
Region		
Latin America	35%	34%
Southeast Asia	12%	10%
North America	29%	32%
EU/Australia	23%	23%
Age (years)		
18-64	99%	99%
≥65	1%	1%
Mean (SD)	38 (9)	37 (10)
Median (min, max)	37 (19 to 67)	*36 (19 to 71)
CD4+ Cell Count (cells/microL)		
Mean (SD)	219 (124)	217 (134)
Median (min, max)	212 (1 to 620)	204 (4 to 807)
Plasma HIV-1 RNA (log_{10} copies/mL)		
Mean (SD)	5 (1)	5 (1)
Median (min, max)	5 (3 to 6)	5 (4 to 6)
Plasma HIV-1 RNA (copies/mL)		
Geometric Mean	103205	106215
Median (min, max)	114000 (400 to 750000)	104000 (4410 to 750000)
History of AIDS*		
Yes	19%	21%
Viral Subtype		
Clade B	78%	82%
Non-Clade B[†]	21%	17%
Baseline Plasma HIV-1 RNA		
≤100,000 copies/mL	45%	49%
>100,000 copies/mL	55%	51%
Baseline CD4+ Cell Counts		
≤50 cells/mm³	10%	11%
>50 cells/mm³ and ≤200 cells/mm³	37%	37%
>200 cells/mm³	53%	51%
Hepatitis Status		
Hepatitis B or C Positive[‡]	6%	6%

Notes:
ISENTRESS and Efavirenz were administered with emtricitabine (+) tenofovir
N = Number of subjects in each group.
* Includes additional subjects identified as having a history of AIDS.
† Non-Clade B Subtypes (# of subjects): Clade A (4), A/C (1), A/G (2), A1 (1), AE (29), AG (12), BF (6), C (37), D (2), F (2), F1 (5), G (2), Complex (3).
‡ Evidence of hepatitis B surface antigen or evidence of HCV RNA by polymerase chain reaction (PCR) quantitative test for hepatitis C Virus.

Week 240 outcomes from Protocol 021 are shown in Table 12.
[See table 12 at top of next page]
The mean changes in CD4 count from baseline were 295 cells/mm³ in the group receiving ISENTRESS 400 mg twice daily and 236 cells/mm³ in the group receiving Efavirenz 600 mg at bedtime.

14.2 Treatment-Experienced Adult Subjects
BENCHMRK 1 and BENCHMRK 2 are Phase 3 studies to evaluate the safety and antiretroviral activity of ISENTRESS 400 mg twice daily in combination with an optimized background therapy (OBT), versus OBT alone, in HIV-1-infected subjects, 16 years or older, with documented resistance to at least 1 drug in each of 3 classes (NNRTIs, NRTIs, PIs) of antiretroviral therapies. Randomization was stratified by degree of resistance to PI (1PI vs. >1PI) and the use of enfuvirtide in the OBT. Prior to randomization, OBT was selected by the investigator based on genotypic/ phenotypic resistance testing and prior ART history.
Table 13 shows the demographic characteristics of subjects in the group receiving ISENTRESS 400 mg twice daily and subjects in the placebo group.

Table 13: Baseline Characteristics

Randomized Studies Protocol 018 and 019	ISENTRESS 400 mg Twice Daily + OBT (N = 462)	Placebo + OBT (N = 237)
Gender		
Male	88%	89%
Female	12%	11%

Race

White	65%	73%
Black	14%	11%
Asian	3%	3%
Hispanic	11%	8%
Others	6%	5%

Age (years)

Median (min, max)	45 (16 to 74)	45 (17 to 70)

CD4+ Cell Count

Median (min, max), cells/mm^3	119 (1 to 792)	123 (0 to 759)
≤50 cells/mm^3	32%	33%
>50 and ≤200 cells/mm^3	37%	36%

Plasma HIV-1 RNA

Median (min, max), log$_{10}$ copies/mL	4.8 (2 to 6)	4.7 (2 to 6)
>100,000 copies/mL	36%	33%

History of AIDS

Yes	92%	91%

Prior Use of ART, Median (1st Quartile, 3rd Quartile)

Years of ART Use	10 (7 to 12)	10 (8 to 12)
Number of ART	12 (9 to 15)	12 (9 to 14)

Hepatitis Co-infection*

No Hepatitis B or C virus	83%	84%
Hepatitis B virus only	8%	3%
Hepatitis C virus only	8%	12%
Co-infection of Hepatitis B and C virus	1%	1%

Stratum

Enfuvirtide in OBT	38%	38%
Resistant to ≥2 PI	97%	95%

* Hepatitis B virus surface antigen positive or hepatitis C virus antibody positive.

Table 14 compares the characteristics of optimized background therapy at baseline in the group receiving ISENTRESS 400 mg twice daily and subjects in the control group.

Table 14: Characteristics of Optimized Background Therapy at Baseline

Randomized Studies Protocol 018 and 019	ISENTRESS 400 mg Twice Daily + OBT (N = 462)	Placebo + OBT (N = 237)
Number of ARTs in OBT		
Median (min, max)	4 (1 to 7)	4 (2 to 7)
Number of Active PI in OBT by Phenotypic Resistance Test*		
0	36%	41%
1 or more	60%	58%
Phenotypic Sensitivity Score (PSS)†		
0	15%	18%
1	31%	30%
2	31%	28%
3 or more	18%	20%

Genotypic Sensitivity Score (GSS)†		
0	25%	27%
1	38%	40%
2	24%	21%
3 or more	11%	10%

* Darunavir use in OBT in darunavir-naïve subjects was counted as one active PI.
† The Phenotypic Sensitivity Score (PSS) and the Genotypic Sensitivity Score (GSS) were defined as the total oral ARTs in OBT to which a subject's viral isolate showed phenotypic sensitivity and genotypic sensitivity, respectively, based upon phenotypic and genotypic resistance tests. Enfuvirtide use in OBT in enfuvirtide-naïve subjects was counted as one active drug in OBT in the GSS and PSS. Similarly, darunavir use in OBT in darunavir-naïve subjects was counted as one active drug in OBT.

Week 96 outcomes for the 699 subjects randomized and treated with the recommended dose of ISENTRESS 400 mg twice daily or placebo in the pooled BENCHMRK 1 and 2 studies are shown in Table 15.
[See table 15 above]
The mean changes in CD4 count from baseline were 118 cells/mm^3 in the group receiving ISENTRESS 400 mg twice daily and 47 cells/mm^3 for the control group.
Treatment-emergent CDC Category C events occurred in 4% of the group receiving ISENTRESS 400 mg twice daily and 5% of the control group.
Virologic responses at Week 96 by baseline genotypic and phenotypic sensitivity score are shown in Table 16.
[See table 16 at top of next page]
Switch of Suppressed Subjects from Lopinavir (+) Ritonavir to Raltegravir
The SWITCHMRK 1 & 2 Phase 3 studies evaluated HIV-1 infected subjects receiving suppressive therapy (HIV-1 RNA <50 copies/mL on a stable regimen of lopinavir 200 mg (+) ritonavir 50 mg 2 tablets twice daily plus at least 2 nucleoside reverse transcriptase inhibitors for >3 months) and randomized them 1:1 to either continue lopinavir (+) ritonavir (n=174 and n=178, SWITCHMRK 1 & 2, respectively) or replace lopinavir (+) ritonavir with ISENTRESS 400 mg twice daily (n=174 and n=176, respectively). The primary virology endpoint was the proportion of subjects with HIV-1 RNA less than 50 copies/mL at Week 24 with a prespecified non-inferiority margin of -12% for each study; and the frequency of adverse events up to 24 weeks.
Subjects with a prior history of virological failure were not excluded and the number of previous antiretroviral therapies was not limited.
These studies were terminated after the primary efficacy analysis at Week 24 because they each failed to demonstrate non-inferiority of switching to ISENTRESS versus continuing on lopinavir (+) ritonavir. In the combined analysis of these studies at Week 24, suppression of HIV-1 RNA to less than 50 copies/mL was maintained in 82.3% of the ISENTRESS group versus 90.3% of the lopinavir (+) ritonavir group. Clinical and laboratory adverse events occurred at similar frequencies in the treatment groups.
14.3 Pediatric Subjects
2 to 18 Years of Age
IMPAACT P1066 is a Phase I/II open label multicenter trial to evaluate the pharmacokinetic profile, safety, tolerability, and efficacy of raltegravir in HIV infected children. This study enrolled 126 treatment experienced children and adolescents 2 to 18 years of age. Subjects were stratified by age, enrolling adolescents first and then successively younger children. Subjects were enrolled into cohorts according to age and received the following formulations: Cohort I (12 to less than 18 years old), 400 mg film-coated tablet; Cohort IIa (6 to less than 12 years old), 400 mg film-coated tablet; Cohort IIb (6 to less than 12 years old), chewable tablet; Cohort III (2 to less than 6 years), chewable tablet. Raltegravir was administered with an optimized background regimen.
The initial dose finding stage included intensive pharmacokinetic evaluation. Dose selection was based upon achieving similar raltegravir plasma exposure and trough concentration as seen in adults, and acceptable short term safety. After dose selection, additional subjects were enrolled for evaluation of long term safety, tolerability and efficacy. Of the 126 subjects, 96 received the recommended dose of ISENTRESS [see Dosage and Administration (2.3)].

Table 12: Virologic Outcomes of Randomized Treatment of Protocol 021 at 240 Weeks

	ISENTRESS 400 mg Twice Daily (N = 281)	Efavirenz 600 mg At Bedtime (N = 282)	Difference (ISENTRESS – Efavirenz) (CI)
Subjects with HIV-1 RNA less than 50 copies/mL	66%	60%	6.6% (-1.4%, 14.5%)
Virologic Failure*	8%	15%	
No virologic data at Week 240 Window Reasons			
Discontinued study due to AE or death†	5%	10%	
Discontinued study for other reasons‡	15%	14%	
Missing data during window but on study	6%	2%	

* Includes subjects who discontinued prior to Week 240 for lack of efficacy or subjects who are ≥50 copies/mL in the 240-week window (+/-6-weeks).
† Includes subjects who discontinued due to AE or Death at any time point from Day 1 through the Week 240 window if this resulted in no virologic data on treatment during Week 240 visit window.
‡ Other includes: withdrew consent, loss to follow-up, moved etc., if the viral load at the time of discontinuation was <50 copies/mL.

Table 15: Virologic Outcomes of Randomized Treatment of Protocols 018 and 019 at 96 Weeks (Pooled Analysis)

	ISENTRESS 400 mg Twice Daily + OBT (N = 462)	Placebo + OBT (N = 237)
Subjects with HIV-1 RNA less than 50 copies/mL	55%	27%
Virologic Failure*	35%	66%
No virologic data at Week 96 Window Reasons		
Discontinued study due to AE or death†	3%	3%
Discontinued study for other reasons‡	4%	4%
Missing data during window but on study	4%	<1%

* Includes subjects who switched to open-label raltegravir after Week 16 due to the protocol-defined virologic failure, subjects who discontinued prior to Week 96 for lack of efficacy, subjects changed OBT due to lack of efficacy prior to Week 96, or subjects who were ≥50 copies in the 96 week window.
† Includes subjects who discontinued due to AE or Death at any time point from Day 1 through the Week 96 window if this resulted in no virologic data on treatment during the Week 96 window.
‡ Other includes: withdrew consent, loss to follow-up, moved etc., if the viral load at the time of discontinuation was <50 copies/mL.

Table 16: Virologic Response at 96 Week Window by Baseline Genotypic/Phenotypic Sensitivity Score

| | Percent with HIV-1 RNA <50 copies/mL At Week 96 | | | |
| | ISENTRESS 400 mg Twice Daily + OBT (N = 462) | | Placebo + OBT (N = 237) | |
		n		n
Phenotypic Sensitivity Score (PSS)*				
0	67	43	43	5
1	144	58	71	23
2	142	61	66	32
3 or more	85	48	48	42
Genotypic Sensitivity Score (GSS)*				
0	116	39	65	5
1	177	62	95	26
2	111	61	49	53
3 or more	51	49	23	35

* The Phenotypic Sensitivity Score (PSS) and the Genotypic Sensitivity Score (GSS) were defined as the total oral ARTs in OBT to which a subject's viral isolate showed phenotypic sensitivity and genotypic sensitivity, respectively, based upon phenotypic and genotypic resistance tests. Enfuvirtide use in OBT in enfuvirtide-naïve subjects was counted as one active drug in OBT in the GSS and PSS. Similarly, darunavir use in OBT in darunavir-naïve subjects was counted as one active drug in OBT.

These 96 subjects had a median age of 13 (range 2 to 18) years, were 51% Female, 34% Caucasian, and 59% Black. At baseline, mean plasma HIV-1 RNA was 4.3 $\log_{10}$ copies/mL, median CD4 cell count was 481 cells/mm^3 (range: 0 – 2361) and median CD4% was 23.3% (range: 0 – 44). Overall, 8% had baseline plasma HIV-1 RNA >100,000 copies/mL and 59% had a CDC HIV clinical classification of category B or C. Most subjects had previously used at least one NNRTI (78%) or one PI (83%).

Ninety-three (97%) subjects 2 to 18 years of age completed 24 weeks of treatment (3 discontinued due to non-compliance). At Week 24, 54% achieved HIV RNA <50 copies/mL; 66% achieved HIV RNA <400 copies/mL. The mean CD4 count (percent) increase from baseline to Week 24 was 119 cells/mm^3 (3.8%).

4 Weeks to Less Than 2 Years of Age
IMPAACT P1066 also enrolled HIV-infected, infants and toddlers 4 weeks to less than 2 years of age (Cohorts IV and V) who had received prior antiretroviral therapy either as prophylaxis for prevention of mother-to-child transmission (PMTCT) and/or as combination antiretroviral therapy for treatment of HIV infection. Raltegravir was administered as an oral suspension without regard to food in combination with an optimized background regimen.

The 26 subjects had a median age of 28 weeks (range: 4 -100), were 35% female, 85% Black and 8% Caucasian. At baseline, mean plasma HIV-1 RNA was 5.7 $\log_{10}$ copies/mL (range: 3.1 – 7), median CD4 cell count was 1400 cells/mm^3 (range: 131 – 3648) and median CD4% was 18.6% (range: 3.3 – 39.3). Overall, 69% had baseline plasma HIV-1 RNA exceeding 100,000 copies/mL and 23% had a CDC clinical classification of category B or C. None of the 26 patients were completely treatment naïve. All infants under 6 months of age had received nevirapine or zidovudine for prevention of mother-to-infant transmission, and 43% of patients greater than 6 months of age had received two or more antiretrovirals.

Of the 26 treated subjects, 23 subjects were included in the Week 24 and 48 efficacy analyses, respectively. All 26 treated subjects were included for safety analyses.

At Week 24, 39% achieved HIV RNA <50 copies/mL and 61% achieved HIV RNA <400 copies/mL. The mean CD4 count (percent) increase from baseline to Week 24 was 500 cells/mm^3 (7.5%).

At Week 48, 44% achieved HIV RNA <50 copies/mL and 61% achieved HIV RNA <400 copies/mL. The mean CD4 count (percent) increase from baseline to Week 48 was 492 cells/mm^3 (7.8%).

16   HOW SUPPLIED/STORAGE AND HANDLING

ISENTRESS tablets 400 mg are pink, oval-shaped, film-coated tablets with "227" on one side. They are supplied as follows:

NDC 0006-0227-61 unit-of-use bottles of 60.
No. 3894
ISENTRESS tablets 100 mg are pale orange, oval-shaped, orange-banana flavored, chewable tablets scored on both sides and imprinted on one face with the Merck logo and "477" on opposite sides of the score. They are supplied as follows:

NDC 0006-0477-61 unit-of-use bottles of 60.
No. 3972

ISENTRESS tablets 25 mg are pale yellow, round, orange-banana flavored, chewable tablets with the Merck logo on one side and "473" on the other side. They are supplied as follows:

NDC 0006-0473-61 unit-of-use bottles of 60.
No. 3965
ISENTRESS for oral suspension 100 mg is a white to off-white granular powder that may contain yellow or beige to tan particles, in child resistant single-use foil packets, packaged as a kit with two 5 mL dosing syringes and two mixing cups. It is supplied as follows:

NDC 0006-3603-60 unit of use carton with 60 packets.
NDC 0006-3603-01 individual packet.
No. 3603
Storage and Handling
400 mg Film-coated Tablets, Chewable Tablets and For Oral Suspension
Store at 20-25°C (68-77°F); excursions permitted to 15-30°C (59-86°F). See USP Controlled Room Temperature.
Chewable Tablets
Store in the original package with the bottle tightly closed. Keep the desiccant in the bottle to protect from moisture.
For Oral Suspension
Store in the original container. Do not open foil packet until ready for use.

17   PATIENT COUNSELING INFORMATION

Advise patients to read the FDA-approved patient labeling (Patient Information and Instructions for Use).
General Information
Instruct patients to reread patient labeling each time the prescription is renewed.
Patients should remain under the care of a physician when using ISENTRESS. Instruct patients to inform their physician or pharmacist if they develop any unusual symptom, or if any known symptom persists or worsens.
ISENTRESS is not a cure for HIV-1 infection and patients may continue to experience illnesses associated with HIV-1 infection such as opportunistic infections. Tell patients that sustained decreases in plasma HIV RNA have been associated with a reduced risk of progression to AIDS and death. Patients should remain on continuous HIV therapy to control HIV infection and decrease HIV-related illnesses.
Advise patients to avoid doing things that can spread HIV-1 infection to others.
• Do not share needles or other injection equipment.
• Do not share personal items that can have blood or body fluids on them, like toothbrushes and razor blades.
• Do not have any kind of sex without protection. Always practice safe sex by using a latex or polyurethane condom to lower the chance of sexual contact with semen, vaginal secretions, or blood.
• Do not breastfeed. Mothers with HIV-1 should not breastfeed because HIV-1 can be passed to the baby in the breast milk. Also, it is unknown if ISENTRESS can be passed to the baby through breast milk and whether it could harm the baby.
General Dosing Instructions
Instruct patients that if they miss a dose of ISENTRESS, they should take it as soon as they remember. If they do not remember until it is time for the next dose, instruct them to

skip the missed dose and go back to the regular schedule. Instruct patients not to double their next dose or take more than the prescribed dose.
Film-Coated Tablets and Chewable Tablets
Inform patients that the chewable tablet forms can be chewed or swallowed whole, but the film-coated tablets must be swallowed whole.
For Oral Suspension
Instruct parents and/or caregivers to read the Instructions for Use before preparing and administering ISENTRESS for oral suspension to pediatric patients. Instruct parents and/or caregivers that ISENTRESS for oral suspension should be administered within 30 minutes of mixing.
Severe and Potentially Life-threatening Rash
Inform patients that severe and potentially life-threatening rash has been reported. Advise patients to immediately contact their healthcare provider if they develop rash. Instruct patients to immediately stop taking ISENTRESS and other suspect agents, and seek medical attention if they develop a rash associated with any of the following symptoms as it may be a sign of a more serious reaction such as Stevens-Johnson syndrome, toxic epidermal necrolysis or severe hypersensitivity: fever, generally ill feeling, extreme tiredness, muscle or joint aches, blisters, oral lesions, eye inflammation, facial swelling, swelling of the eyes, lips, mouth, breathing difficulty, and/or signs and symptoms of liver problems (e.g., yellowing of the skin or whites of the eyes, dark or tea colored urine, pale colored stools/bowel movements, nausea, vomiting, loss of appetite, or pain, aching or sensitivity on the right side below the ribs). Inform patients that if severe rash occurs, their physician will closely monitor them, order laboratory tests and initiate appropriate therapy.
Rhabdomyolysis
Before patients begin ISENTRESS, ask them if they have a history of rhabdomyolysis, myopathy or increased creatine kinase or if they are taking medications known to cause these conditions such as statins, fenofibrate, gemfibrozil or zidovudine.
Instruct patients to immediately report to their healthcare provider any unexplained muscle pain, tenderness, or weakness while taking ISENTRESS.
Phenylketonuria
Alert patients with phenylketonuria that ISENTRESS Chewable Tablets contain phenylalanine [see Warnings and Precautions (5.3)].
Drug Interactions
Instruct patients to avoid taking aluminum and/or magnesium containing antacids during treatment with ISENTRESS [see Drug Interactions (7.2)].
Distributed by:
Merck Sharp & Dohme Corp., a subsidiary of **Merck & Co., Inc.**
Whitehouse Station, NJ 08889, USA
For patent information:
www.merck.com/product/patent/home.html
Copyright © 2014 Merck Sharp & Dohme Corp., a subsidiary of **Merck & Co., Inc.**
All rights reserved.
uspi-mk0518-mf-1408r028
Patient Information
ISENTRESS® (eye **sen** tris)
(raltegravir)
film-coated tablets
ISENTRESS® (eye **sen** tris)
(raltegravir)
chewable tablets
ISENTRESS® (eye **sen** tris)
(raltegravir)
for oral suspension
Read this Patient Information before you start taking ISENTRESS and each time you get a refill. There may be new information. This information does not take the place of talking with your doctor about your medical condition or your treatment.
What is ISENTRESS?
ISENTRESS is a prescription HIV medicine used with other antiretroviral medicines to treat Human Immunodeficiency Virus-1 (HIV-1) infection in people 4 weeks of age and older. HIV is the virus that causes AIDS (Acquired Immune Deficiency Syndrome).
It is not known if ISENTRESS is safe and effective in babies under 4 weeks of age.
When used with other HIV medicines to treat HIV-1 infection, ISENTRESS may help:
• reduce the amount of HIV in your blood. This is called "viral load".
• increase the number of white blood cells called CD4+ (T) cells in your blood, which help fight off other infections.

- reduce the amount of HIV-1 and increase the CD4+ (T) cells in your blood, which may help improve your immune system. This may reduce your risk of death or getting infections that can happen when your immune system is weak (opportunistic infections).

ISENTRESS does not cure HIV-1 infection or AIDS.
You must stay on continuous HIV therapy to control HIV-1 infection and decrease HIV-related illnesses.

Avoid doing things that can spread HIV-1 infection to others:
- Do not share or re-use needles or other injection equipment.
- Do not share personal items that can have blood or body fluids on them, like toothbrushes and razor blades.
- Do not have any kind of sex without protection. Always practice safe sex by using a latex or polyurethane condom to lower the chance of sexual contact with any body fluids such as semen, vaginal secretions, or blood.

Ask your doctor if you have any questions on how to prevent passing HIV to other people.

What should I tell my doctor before taking ISENTRESS?
Before you take ISENTRESS, tell your doctor if you:
- have liver problems
- have a history of a muscle disorder called rhabdomyolysis or myopathy
- have increased levels of creatine kinase in your blood
- have phenylketonuria (PKU). ISENTRESS chewable tablets contain phenylalanine as part of the artificial sweetener, aspartame. The artificial sweetener may be harmful to people with PKU.
- have any other medical conditions
- are pregnant or plan to become pregnant. It is not known if ISENTRESS can harm your unborn baby.
  Pregnancy Registry: There is a pregnancy registry for women who take antiviral medicines during pregnancy. The purpose of this registry is to collect information about the health of you and your baby. Talk to your doctor about how you can take part in this registry.
- are breastfeeding or plan to breastfeed. **Do not breastfeed if you take ISENTRESS.**
  ∘ You should not breastfeed if you have HIV-1 because of the risk of passing HIV-1 to your baby.
  ∘ It is not known if ISENTRESS passes into your breast milk.
  ∘ Talk with your doctor about the best way to feed your baby.

Tell your doctor about all the medicines you take, including, prescription and over-the-counter medicines, vitamins, and herbal supplements. ISENTRESS and certain other medicines may affect each other causing serious side effects. ISENTRESS may affect the way other medicines work and other medicines may affect how ISENTRESS works.

Especially tell your doctor if you take any of these medicines:
- rifampin (Rifadin, Rifamate, Rifater, Rimactane)
- an antacid medicine that contains aluminum or magnesium
- a cholesterol lowering medicine (statin)
- a medicine that contains fenofibrate (Antara, Lipofen, Tricor, Trilipix)
- gemfibrozil (Lopid)
- a medicine that contains zidovudine (Combivir, Retrovir, Trizivir)

Ask your doctor or pharmacist if you are not sure if your medicine is one that is listed above.

Know the medicines you take. Keep a list of them to show your doctor and pharmacist when you get a new medicine. Do not start any new medicines while you are taking ISENTRESS without first talking with your doctor.

How should I take ISENTRESS?
- Take ISENTRESS exactly as prescribed by your doctor.
- **Do not** change your dose of ISENTRESS or stop your treatment without talking with your doctor first.
- Stay under the care of your doctor while taking ISENTRESS.
- ISENTRESS film-coated tablets must be swallowed whole.
- ISENTRESS chewable tablets may be chewed or swallowed whole.
- ISENTRESS for oral suspension should be given to your child within 30 minutes of mixing. **See the detailed Instructions for Use that comes with ISENTRESS for oral suspension,** for information about the correct way to mix and give a dose of ISENTRESS for oral suspension. If you have questions about how to mix or give ISENTRESS for oral suspension, talk to your doctor or pharmacist.
- **Do not switch between the film-coated tablet, the chewable tablet, or the oral suspension without talking with your doctor first.**
- **Do not** run out of ISENTRESS. Get a refill of your ISENTRESS from your doctor or pharmacy before you run out.
- If you miss a dose, take it as soon as you remember. If you do not remember until it is time for your next dose, skip

the missed dose and go back to your regular schedule. Do not double your next dose or take more ISENTRESS than prescribed.
- If you take too much ISENTRESS, call your doctor or go to the nearest hospital emergency room right away.

What are the possible side effects of ISENTRESS?
ISENTRESS can cause serious side effects including:
- **Serious skin reactions and allergic reactions.** Some people who take ISENTRESS develop serious skin reactions and allergic reactions that can be severe, and may be life-threatening or lead to death. If you develop a rash with any of the following symptoms, stop using ISENTRESS and call your doctor right away:
  ∘ fever
  ∘ generally ill feeling
  ∘ extreme tiredness
  ∘ muscle or joint aches
  ∘ blisters or sores in mouth
  ∘ blisters or peeling of the skin
  ∘ redness or swelling of the eyes
  ∘ swelling of the mouth or face
  ∘ problems breathing

Sometimes allergic reactions can affect body organs, such as your liver. Call your doctor right away if you have any of the following signs or symptoms of liver problems:
  ∘ yellowing of your skin or whites of your eyes
  ∘ dark or tea colored urine
  ∘ pale colored stools (bowel movements)
  ∘ nausea or vomiting
  ∘ loss of appetite
  ∘ pain, aching, or tenderness on the right side of your stomach area
- **Changes in your immune system (Immune Reconstitution Syndrome)** can happen when you start taking HIV-1 medicines. Your immune system may get stronger and begin to fight infections that have been hidden in your body for a long time. Tell your doctor right away if you start having new symptoms after starting your HIV-1 medicine.

The most common side effects of ISENTRESS include:
- trouble sleeping
- headache
- dizziness
- nausea
- tiredness

Less common side effects of ISENTRESS include:
- depression
- hepatitis
- genital herpes
- herpes zoster including shingles
- kidney failure
- kidney stones
- indigestion or stomach area pain
- vomiting
- suicidal thoughts and actions
- weakness

Tell your doctor right away if you get unexplained muscle pain, tenderness, or weakness while taking ISENTRESS. These may be signs of a rare serious muscle problem that can lead to kidney problems.

Tell your doctor if you have any side effect that bothers you or that does not go away.

These are not all the possible side effects of ISENTRESS. For more information, ask your doctor or pharmacist.

Call your doctor for medical advice about side effects. You may report side effects to FDA at 1-800-FDA-1088.

How should I store ISENTRESS?
Film-Coated Tablets:
- Store ISENTRESS film-coated tablets at room temperature between 68°F to 77°F (20°C to 25°C).

Chewable Tablets:
- Store ISENTRESS chewable tablets at room temperature between 68°F to 77°F (20°C to 25°C).
- Store ISENTRESS chewable tablets in the original package with the bottle tightly closed.
- Keep the drying agent (desiccant) in the bottle to protect from moisture.

For Oral Suspension:
- Store ISENTRESS for oral suspension at room temperature between 68°F to 77°F (20°C to 25°C).
- Store in the original container. Do not open the foil packet until ready for use.

Keep ISENTRESS and all medicines out of the reach of children.

General information about ISENTRESS
Medicines are sometimes prescribed for purposes other than those listed in a Patient Information Leaflet. Do not use ISENTRESS for a condition for which it was not prescribed. Do not give ISENTRESS to other people, even if they have the same symptoms you have. It may harm them.

You can ask your doctor or pharmacist for information about ISENTRESS that is written for health professionals.

For more information go to www.ISENTRESS.com or call 1-800-622-4477.

What are the ingredients in ISENTRESS?
ISENTRESS film-coated tablets:
Active ingredient: raltegravir
Inactive ingredients: calcium phosphate dibasic anhydrous, hypromellose 2208, lactose monohydrate, magnesium stearate, microcrystalline cellulose, poloxamer 407 (contains 0.01% butylated hydroxytoluene as antioxidant), sodium stearyl fumarate.
The film coating contains: black iron oxide, polyethylene glycol 3350, polyvinyl alcohol, red iron oxide, talc and titanium dioxide.
ISENTRESS chewable tablets:
Active ingredient: raltegravir
Inactive ingredients: ammonium hydroxide, crospovidone, ethylcellulose 20 cP, fructose, hydroxypropyl cellulose, hypromellose 2910/6cP, magnesium stearate, mannitol, medium chain triglycerides, monoammonium glycyrrhizinate, natural and artificial flavors (orange, banana, and masking that contains aspartame), oleic acid, PEG 400, saccharin sodium, sodium citrate dihydrate, sodium stearyl fumarate, sorbitol, sucralose and yellow iron oxide. The 100 mg chewable tablet also contains red iron oxide.
ISENTRESS for oral suspension:
Active ingredient: raltegravir
Inactive ingredients: ammonium hydroxide, banana with other natural flavors, carboxymethylcellulose sodium, crospovidone, ethylcellulose 20 cP, fructose, hydroxypropyl cellulose, hypromellose 2910/6cP, macrogol/PEG 400, magnesium stearate, maltodextrin, mannitol, medium chain triglycerides, microcrystalline cellulose, monoammonium glycyrrhizinate, oleic acid, sorbitol, sucralose and sucrose.

This Patient Information has been approved by the U.S. Food and Drug Administration.

Distributed by:

Merck Sharp & Dohme Corp., a subsidiary of **Merck & Co., Inc.**

Whitehouse Station, NJ 08889, USA

Revised December 2013

For patent information:

www.merck.com/product_patent/home.html

Copyright © 2007, 2013 Merck Sharp & Dohme Corp., a subsidiary of **Merck & Co., Inc.**

All rights reserved.

usppi-mk0518-mf-1312r025

Instructions for Use
ISENTRESS® (eye **sen** tris)
(raltegravir)
for oral suspension

Read this Instructions for Use before you mix and give a dose of ISENTRESS for oral suspension to your child for the first time, and each time you get a refill. There may be new information. These instructions will help you to correctly mix and give a dose of ISENTRESS for oral suspension to your child.

See the Patient Information leaflet that comes with ISENTRESS for oral suspension for more information about ISENTRESS.

Your doctor will decide the right dose based on your child's weight.

Ask your doctor or pharmacist if you have any questions about how to mix or give ISENTRESS for oral suspension to your child.

Each ISENTRESS for oral suspension kit contains the following supplies (see Figure A):
- 2 reusable mixing cups with attached lids
- 2 reusable 5 mL dosing syringes
- 60 foil packets containing ISENTRESS for oral suspension

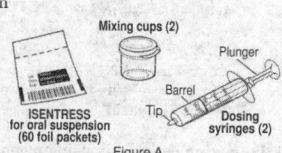

Figure A

For each dose of ISENTRESS for oral suspension you will need the following:
- 1 mixing cup with attached lid
- 1 dosing syringe (5mL)
- 1 foil packet containing the medicine
- Drinking water (not included in kit)

How do I prepare a dose of ISENTRESS for oral suspension?
Step 1. Fill mixing cup about half-way with drinking water (see Figure B).

Figure B

Step 2. Fill the dosing syringe. Start with the plunger pushed all the way inside the barrel of the syringe. Insert the tip of the syringe into the water and pull back on the plunger to the 5 mL marking on the barrel of the syringe (see Figure C).

Figure C

Step 3. Pour out remaining water from mixing cup (see Figure D).

Figure D

Step 4. Add the 5 mL of water from the dosing syringe back into the mixing cup by pressing down on the plunger (see Figure E).

Figure E

Step 5. Open 1 foil packet. There is a notch that you can use to tear open the foil packet, or you may use scissors to cut along the dotted line. Pour entire contents into mixing cup (see Figure F).

Figure F

Step 6. Close the attached lid to seal the mixing cup (see Figure G). It will snap shut.

Figure G

Step 7. Swirl the mixing cup to mix using a gentle circular motion for 30-60 seconds (see Figure H). **Do not** turn the mixing cup upside down. The liquid will be cloudy.

Figure H

Step 8. Open the mixing cup. Put the tip of the syringe into the liquid and **pull back the plunger to the mL marking that matches your child's prescribed dose** (see Figure I). Your child's dose may be different from the one shown in the figure.

Figure I

How should I give a dose of ISENTRESS for oral suspension?
Step 9. Place the tip of the dosing syringe in your child's mouth and turn it toward either cheek. Gently push down on the plunger to give the medicine (see Figure J). Give the dose of ISENTRESS oral suspension to your child within 30 minutes of mixing. If you are not able to give your child's dose within 30 minutes of mixing, pour the unused medicine into the trash. You will need to mix a new dose.

Figure J

How should I dispose of leftover ISENTRESS for oral suspension?
Step 10. Pour any leftover medicine from the mixing cup into the trash (see Figure K).

Figure K

Step 11. Remove plunger from the barrel of the dosing syringe. Hand wash the dosing syringe and mixing cup with warm water and dish soap. Rinse with water and air dry (see Figure L).

Figure L

How should I store ISENTRESS for oral suspension?
• Store ISENTRESS for oral suspension at room temperature between 68°F to 77°F (20°C to 25°C).
• Store in the original container. Do not open the foil packets until ready for use.
Keep ISENTRESS for oral suspension and all medicines out of the reach of children.
For more information go to www.ISENTRESS.com or call 1-800-622-4477.
This Instructions for Use has been approved by the U.S. Food and Drug Administration.
Distributed by:
Merck Sharp & Dohme Corp., a subsidiary of **Merck & Co., Inc.**
Whitehouse Station, NJ 08889, USA
Issued December 2013
For patent information:
www.merck.com/product/patent/home.html
Copyright © 2013 Merck Sharp & Dohme Corp., a subsidiary of **Merck & Co., Inc.**
All rights reserved.
ifu-mk0518-mf-1312r000
Shown in Product Identification Guide, page 308

JANUMET®   ℞
[*JAN-you-met*]
(sitagliptin/metformin HCl)
tablets

HIGHLIGHTS OF PRESCRIBING INFORMATION
These highlights do not include all the information needed to use JANUMET safely and effectively. See full prescribing information for JANUMET.
JANUMET® (sitagliptin and metformin HCl) tablets
Initial U.S. Approval: 2007

WARNING: LACTIC ACIDOSIS
See full prescribing information for complete boxed warning.
• Lactic acidosis can occur due to metformin accumulation. The risk increases with conditions such as sepsis, dehydration, excess alcohol intake, hepatic insufficiency, renal impairment, and acute congestive heart failure. (5.1)
• Symptoms include malaise, myalgias, respiratory distress, increasing somnolence, and nonspecific abdominal distress. Laboratory abnormalities include low pH, increased anion gap and elevated blood lactate. (5.1)
• If acidosis is suspected, discontinue JANUMET and hospitalize the patient immediately. (5.1)

——————RECENT MAJOR CHANGES——————

Contraindications (4)	09/2013
Warnings and Precautions	
Lactic Acidosis (5.1)	09/2013
Assessment of Renal Function (5.4)	09/2013

——————INDICATIONS AND USAGE——————

JANUMET is a dipeptidyl peptidase-4 (DPP-4) inhibitor and biguanide combination product indicated as an adjunct to diet and exercise to improve glycemic control in adults with type 2 diabetes mellitus when treatment with both sitagliptin and metformin is appropriate. (1, 14)
Important Limitations of Use:
• JANUMET should not be used in patients with type 1 diabetes or for the treatment of diabetic ketoacidosis. (1)
• JANUMET has not been studied in patients with a history of pancreatitis. (1, 5.2)

——————DOSAGE AND ADMINISTRATION——————

• Individualize the starting dose of JANUMET based on the patient's current regimen. (2.1)
• May adjust the dosing based on effectiveness and tolerability while not exceeding the maximum recommended daily dose of 100 mg sitagliptin and 2000 mg metformin. (2.1)
• JANUMET should be given twice daily with meals, with gradual dose escalation, to reduce the gastrointestinal (GI) side effects due to metformin. (2.1)

——————DOSAGE FORMS AND STRENGTHS——————

Tablets: 50 mg sitagliptin/500 mg metformin HCl and 50 mg sitagliptin/1000 mg metformin HCl (3)

——————CONTRAINDICATIONS——————

• Renal dysfunction, e.g., serum creatinine ≥1.5 mg/dL [males], ≥1.4 mg/dL [females] or abnormal creatinine clearance. (4, 5.1, 5.4)
• Metabolic acidosis, including diabetic ketoacidosis. (4, 5.1)
• History of a serious hypersensitivity reaction to JANUMET or sitagliptin (one of the components of JANUMET), such as anaphylaxis or angioedema. (5.14, 6.2)

——————WARNINGS AND PRECAUTIONS——————

• Lactic acidosis: Warn against excessive alcohol intake. JANUMET is not recommended in hepatic impairment and is contraindicated in renal impairment. Ensure normal renal function before initiating and at least annually thereafter. (5.1, 5.3, 5.6)
• Temporarily discontinue JANUMET in patients undergoing radiologic studies with intravascular administration of iodinated contrast materials or any surgical procedures necessitating restricted intake of food or fluids. (5.1, 5.3, 5.4, 5.7)
• There have been postmarketing reports of acute pancreatitis, including fatal and non-fatal hemorrhagic or necrotizing pancreatitis. If pancreatitis is suspected, promptly discontinue JANUMET. (5.2)
• There have been postmarketing reports of acute renal failure, sometimes requiring dialysis. Before initiating JANUMET and at least annually thereafter, assess renal function and verify as normal. (4, 5.1, 5.4, 5.10, 6.2)

- Vitamin B_{12} deficiency: Metformin may lower Vitamin B_{12} levels. Measure hematologic parameters annually. (5.5, 6.1)
- When used with an insulin secretagogue (e.g., sulfonylurea) or with insulin, a lower dose of the insulin secretagogue or insulin may be required to reduce the risk of hypoglycemia. (2.1, 5.9)
- There have been postmarketing reports of serious allergic and hypersensitivity reactions in patients treated with sitagliptin (one of the components of JANUMET), such as anaphylaxis, angioedema, and exfoliative skin conditions including Stevens-Johnson syndrome. In such cases, promptly stop JANUMET, assess for other potential causes, institute appropriate monitoring and treatment, and initiate alternative treatment for diabetes. (5.14, 6.2)
- There have been no clinical studies establishing conclusive evidence of macrovascular risk reduction with JANUMET or any other anti-diabetic drug. (5.15)

---ADVERSE REACTIONS---

- The most common adverse reactions reported in ≥5% of patients simultaneously started on sitagliptin and metformin and more commonly than in patients treated with placebo were diarrhea, upper respiratory tract infection, and headache. (6.1)
- Adverse reactions reported in ≥5% of patients treated with sitagliptin in combination with sulfonylurea and metformin and more commonly than in patients treated with placebo in combination with sulfonylurea and metformin were hypoglycemia and headache. (6.1)
- Hypoglycemia was the only adverse reaction reported in ≥5% of patients treated with sitagliptin in combination with insulin and metformin and more commonly than in patients treated with placebo in combination with insulin and metformin. (6.1)

To report SUSPECTED ADVERSE REACTIONS, contact Merck Sharp & Dohme Corp., a subsidiary of Merck & Co., Inc., at 1-877-888-4231 or FDA at 1-800-FDA-1088 or www.fda.gov/medwatch.

---DRUG INTERACTIONS---

- Cationic drugs eliminated by renal tubular secretion: Use with caution. (5.10, 7.2)

---USE IN SPECIFIC POPULATIONS---

- Safety and effectiveness of JANUMET in children under 18 years have not been established. (8.4)
- There are no adequate and well-controlled studies in pregnant women. To report drug exposure during pregnancy call 1-800-986-8999. (8.1)

See 17 for PATIENT COUNSELING INFORMATION and Medication Guide

Revised: 02/2014

FULL PRESCRIBING INFORMATION: CONTENTS*

FULL PRESCRIBING INFORMATION

> **WARNING: LACTIC ACIDOSIS**
>
> **Lactic acidosis is a rare, but serious complication that can occur due to metformin accumulation. The risk increases with conditions such as sepsis, dehydration, excess alcohol intake, hepatic impairment, renal impairment, and acute congestive heart failure.**
>
> **The onset is often subtle, accompanied only by nonspecific symptoms such as malaise, myalgias, respiratory distress, increasing somnolence, and nonspecific abdominal distress.**
>
> **Laboratory abnormalities include low pH, increased anion gap and elevated blood lactate.**
>
> **If acidosis is suspected, JANUMET should be discontinued and the patient hospitalized immediately. [See Warnings and Precautions (5.1).]**

1   INDICATIONS AND USAGE

JANUMET is indicated as an adjunct to diet and exercise to improve glycemic control in adults with type 2 diabetes mellitus when treatment with both sitagliptin and metformin is appropriate. [See Clinical Studies (14).]

Important Limitations of Use

JANUMET should not be used in patients with type 1 diabetes or for the treatment of diabetic ketoacidosis.

JANUMET has not been studied in patients with a history of pancreatitis. It is unknown whether patients with a history of pancreatitis are at increased risk for the development of pancreatitis while using JANUMET. [See Warnings and Precautions (5.2).]

2   DOSAGE AND ADMINISTRATION
2.1   Recommended Dosing

The dosage of JANUMET should be individualized on the basis of the patient's current regimen, effectiveness, and tolerability while not exceeding the maximum recommended daily dose of 100 mg sitagliptin and 2000 mg metformin. Initial combination therapy or maintenance of combination therapy should be individualized and left to the discretion of the health care provider.

JANUMET should generally be given twice daily with meals, with gradual dose escalation, to reduce the gastrointestinal (GI) side effects due to metformin. JANUMET must not be split or divided before swallowing.

The starting dose of JANUMET should be based on the patient's current regimen. JANUMET should be given twice daily with meals. The following doses are available:

50 mg sitagliptin/500 mg metformin hydrochloride
50 mg sitagliptin/1000 mg metformin hydrochloride

The recommended starting dose in patients not currently treated with metformin is 50 mg sitagliptin/500 mg metformin hydrochloride twice daily, with gradual dose escalation recommended to reduce gastrointestinal side effects associated with metformin.

The starting dose in patients already treated with metformin should provide sitagliptin dosed as 50 mg twice daily (100 mg total daily dose) and the dose of metformin already being taken. For patients taking metformin 850 mg twice daily, the recommended starting dose of JANUMET is 50 mg sitagliptin/1000 mg metformin hydrochloride twice daily.

Patients treated with an insulin secretagogue or insulin

Coadministration of JANUMET with an insulin secretagogue (e.g., sulfonylurea) or insulin may require lower doses of the insulin secretagogue or insulin to reduce the risk of hypoglycemia [see Warnings and Precautions (5.9)].

No studies have been performed specifically examining the safety and efficacy of JANUMET in patients previously treated with other oral antihyperglycemic agents and switched to JANUMET. Any change in therapy of type 2 diabetes should be undertaken with care and appropriate monitoring as changes in glycemic control can occur.

3   DOSAGE FORMS AND STRENGTHS

- 50 mg/500 mg tablets are light pink, capsule-shaped, film-coated tablets with "575" debossed on one side.
- 50 mg/1000 mg tablets are red, capsule-shaped, film-coated tablets with "577" debossed on one side.

4   CONTRAINDICATIONS

JANUMET (sitagliptin and metformin HCl) is contraindicated in patients with:

- Renal impairment (e.g., serum creatinine levels greater than or equal to 1.5 mg/dL for men, greater than or equal to 1.4 mg/dL for women or abnormal creatinine clearance), which may also result from conditions such as cardiovascular collapse (shock), acute myocardial infarction, and septicemia [see Warnings and Precautions (5.1)].
- Hypersensitivity to metformin hydrochloride.
- Acute or chronic metabolic acidosis, including diabetic ketoacidosis. Diabetic ketoacidosis should be treated with insulin.
- History of a serious hypersensitivity reaction to JANUMET or sitagliptin (one of the components of JANUMET), such as anaphylaxis or angioedema. [See Warnings and Precautions (5.14); Adverse Reactions (6.2).]

5   WARNINGS AND PRECAUTIONS
5.1   Lactic Acidosis
Metformin hydrochloride

Lactic acidosis is a rare, but serious, metabolic complication that can occur due to metformin accumulation during treatment with JANUMET; when it occurs, it is fatal in approximately 50% of cases. Lactic acidosis may also occur in association with a number of pathophysiologic conditions, including diabetes mellitus, and whenever there is significant tissue hypoperfusion and hypoxemia. Lactic acidosis is characterized by elevated blood lactate levels (>5 mmol/L), decreased blood pH, electrolyte disturbances with an increased anion gap, and an increased lactate/pyruvate ratio. When metformin is implicated as the cause of lactic acidosis, metformin plasma levels >5 µg/mL are generally found. The reported incidence of lactic acidosis in patients receiving metformin hydrochloride is very low (approximately 0.03 cases/1000 patient-years, with approximately 0.015 fatal cases/1000 patient-years). In more than 20,000 patient-years exposure to metformin in clinical trials, there were no reports of lactic acidosis. Reported cases have occurred primarily in diabetic patients with significant renal impairment, including both intrinsic renal disease and renal hypoperfusion, often in the setting of multiple concomitant medical/surgical problems and multiple concomitant medications. Patients with congestive heart failure requiring pharmacologic management, in particular those with unstable or acute congestive heart failure who are at risk of hypoperfusion and hypoxemia, are at increased risk of lactic acidosis. The risk of lactic acidosis increases with the degree of renal dysfunction and the patient's age. The risk of lactic acidosis may, therefore, be significantly decreased by regular monitoring of renal function in patients taking metformin and by use of the minimum effective dose of metformin. In particular, treatment of the elderly should be accompanied by careful monitoring of renal function. In addition, metformin should be promptly withheld in the presence of any condition associated with hypoxemia, dehydration, or sepsis. Because impaired hepatic function may significantly limit the ability to clear lactate, metformin should generally be avoided in patients with clinical or laboratory evidence of hepatic disease. Patients should be cautioned against excessive alcohol intake, either acute or chronic, when taking metformin, since alcohol potentiates the effects of metformin hydrochloride on lactate metabolism. In addition, metformin should be temporarily discontinued prior to any intravascular radiocontrast study and for any surgical procedure [see Warnings and Precautions (5.4, 5.6, 5.7, 5.11)].

The onset of lactic acidosis often is subtle, and accompanied only by nonspecific symptoms such as malaise, myalgias, respiratory distress, increasing somnolence, and nonspecific abdominal distress. There may be associated hypothermia, hypotension, and resistant bradyarrhythmias with more marked acidosis. The patient and the patient's physician must be aware of the possible importance of such symptoms and the patient should be instructed to notify the physician immediately if they occur [see Warnings and Precautions (5.12)]. Metformin should be withdrawn until the situation is clarified. Serum electrolytes, ketones, blood glucose, and if indicated, blood pH, lactate levels, and even blood metformin levels may be useful. Once a patient is stabilized on any dose level of metformin, gastrointestinal symptoms, which are common during initiation of therapy, are unlikely to be drug related. Later occurrence of gastrointestinal symptoms could be due to lactic acidosis or other serious disease.

Levels of fasting venous plasma lactate above the upper limit of normal but less than 5 mmol/L in patients taking metformin do not necessarily indicate impending lactic acidosis and may be explainable by other mechanisms, such as poorly controlled diabetes or obesity, vigorous physical activity, or technical problems in sample handling [see Warnings and Precautions (5.8, 5.13)].

Lactic acidosis should be suspected in any diabetic patient with metabolic acidosis lacking evidence of ketoacidosis (ketonuria and ketonemia).

Table 1: Sitagliptin and Metformin Coadministered to Patients with Type 2 Diabetes Inadequately Controlled on Diet and Exercise: Adverse Reactions Reported (Regardless of Investigator Assessment of Causality) in ≥5% of Patients Receiving Combination Therapy (and Greater than in Patients Receiving Placebo)*

	Number of Patients (%)			
	Placebo	Sitagliptin 100 mg once daily	Metformin 500 mg/ Metformin 1000 mg twice daily[†]	Sitagliptin 50 mg twice daily + Metformin 500 mg/ Metformin 1000 mg twice daily[†]
	N = 176	N = 179	N = 364[†]	N = 372[†]
Diarrhea	7 (4.0)	5 (2.8)	28 (7.7)	28 (7.5)
Upper Respiratory Tract Infection	9 (5.1)	8 (4.5)	19 (5.2)	23 (6.2)
Headache	5 (2.8)	2 (1.1)	14 (3.8)	22 (5.9)

* Intent-to-treat population.
† Data pooled for the patients given the lower and higher doses of metformin.

Lactic acidosis is a medical emergency that must be treated in a hospital setting. In a patient with lactic acidosis who is taking metformin, the drug should be discontinued immediately and general supportive measures promptly instituted. Because metformin hydrochloride is dialyzable (with a clearance of up to 170 mL/min under good hemodynamic conditions), prompt hemodialysis is recommended to correct the acidosis and remove the accumulated metformin. Such management often results in prompt reversal of symptoms and recovery *[see Contraindications (4); Warnings and Precautions (5.6, 5.7, 5.10, 5.11, 5.12)].*

5.2 Pancreatitis
There have been postmarketing reports of acute pancreatitis, including fatal and non-fatal hemorrhagic or necrotizing pancreatitis, in patients taking JANUMET. After initiation of JANUMET, patients should be observed carefully for signs and symptoms of pancreatitis. If pancreatitis is suspected, JANUMET should promptly be discontinued and appropriate management should be initiated. It is unknown whether patients with a history of pancreatitis are at increased risk for the development of pancreatitis while using JANUMET.

5.3 Impaired Hepatic Function
Since impaired hepatic function has been associated with some cases of lactic acidosis, JANUMET should generally be avoided in patients with clinical or laboratory evidence of hepatic disease.

5.4 Assessment of Renal Function
Metformin and sitagliptin are known to be substantially excreted by the kidney.
Metformin hydrochloride
The risk of metformin accumulation and lactic acidosis increases with the degree of impairment of renal function. Therefore, JANUMET is contraindicated in patients with renal impairment.
Before initiation of JANUMET and at least annually thereafter, renal function should be assessed and verified as normal. In patients in whom development of renal dysfunction is anticipated (e.g., elderly), renal function should be assessed more frequently and JANUMET discontinued if evidence of renal impairment is present.
Sitagliptin
There have been postmarketing reports of worsening renal function, including acute renal failure, sometimes requiring dialysis. Before initiation of therapy with JANUMET and at least annually thereafter, renal function should be assessed and verified as normal. In patients in whom development of renal dysfunction is anticipated, particularly in elderly patients, renal function should be assessed more frequently and JANUMET discontinued if evidence of renal impairment is present.

5.5 Vitamin B₁₂ Levels
In controlled clinical trials of metformin of 29 weeks duration, a decrease to subnormal levels of previously normal serum Vitamin B_{12} levels, without clinical manifestations, was observed in approximately 7% of patients. Such decrease, possibly due to interference with B_{12} absorption from the B_{12}-intrinsic factor complex, is, however, very rarely associated with anemia and appears to be rapidly reversible with discontinuation of metformin or Vitamin B_{12} supplementation. Measurement of hematologic parameters on an annual basis is advised in patients on JANUMET and any apparent abnormalities should be appropriately investigated and managed. *[See Adverse Reactions (6.1).]*
Certain individuals (those with inadequate Vitamin B_{12} or calcium intake or absorption) appear to be predisposed to developing subnormal Vitamin B_{12} levels. In these patients, routine serum Vitamin B_{12} measurements at two- to three-year intervals may be useful.

5.6 Alcohol Intake
Alcohol is known to potentiate the effect of metformin on lactate metabolism. Patients, therefore, should be warned against excessive alcohol intake, acute or chronic, while receiving JANUMET.

5.7 Surgical Procedures
Use of JANUMET should be temporarily suspended for any surgical procedure (except minor procedures not associated with restricted intake of food and fluids) and should not be restarted until the patient's oral intake has resumed and renal function has been evaluated as normal.

5.8 Change in Clinical Status of Patients with Previously Controlled Type 2 Diabetes
A patient with type 2 diabetes previously well controlled on JANUMET who develops laboratory abnormalities or clinical illness (especially vague and poorly defined illness) should be evaluated promptly for evidence of ketoacidosis or lactic acidosis. Evaluation should include serum electrolytes and ketones, blood glucose and, if indicated, blood pH, lactate, pyruvate, and metformin levels. If acidosis of either form occurs, JANUMET must be stopped immediately and other appropriate corrective measures initiated.

5.9 Use with Medications Known to Cause Hypoglycemia
Sitagliptin
When sitagliptin was used in combination with a sulfonylurea or with insulin, medications known to cause hypoglycemia, the incidence of hypoglycemia was increased over that of placebo used in combination with a sulfonylurea or with insulin *[see Adverse Reactions (6)].* Therefore, patients also receiving an insulin secretagogue (e.g., sulfonylurea) or insulin may require a lower dose of the insulin secretagogue or insulin to reduce the risk of hypoglycemia *[see Dosage and Administration (2.1)].*
Metformin hydrochloride
Hypoglycemia does not occur in patients receiving metformin alone under usual circumstances of use, but could occur when caloric intake is deficient, when strenuous exercise is not compensated by caloric supplementation, or during concomitant use with other glucose-lowering agents (such as sulfonylureas and insulin) or ethanol. Elderly, debilitated, or malnourished patients, and those with adrenal or pituitary insufficiency or alcohol intoxication are particularly susceptible to hypoglycemic effects. Hypoglycemia may be difficult to recognize in the elderly, and in people who are taking β-adrenergic blocking drugs.

5.10 Concomitant Medications Affecting Renal Function or Metformin Disposition
Concomitant medication(s) that may affect renal function or result in significant hemodynamic change or may interfere with the disposition of metformin, such as cationic drugs that are eliminated by renal tubular secretion *[see Drug Interactions (7.2)],* should be used with caution.

5.11 Radiologic Studies with Intravascular Iodinated Contrast Materials
Intravascular contrast studies with iodinated materials (for example, intravenous urogram, intravenous cholangiography, angiography, and computed tomography (CT) scans with intravascular contrast materials) can lead to acute alteration of renal function and have been associated with lactic acidosis in patients receiving metformin *[see Contraindications (4)].* Therefore, in patients in whom any such study is planned, JANUMET should be temporarily discontinued at the time of or prior to the procedure, and withheld for 48 hours subsequent to the procedure and reinstituted only after renal function has been re-evaluated and found to be normal.

5.12 Hypoxic States
Cardiovascular collapse (shock) from whatever cause, acute congestive heart failure, acute myocardial infarction and other conditions characterized by hypoxemia have been associated with lactic acidosis and may also cause prerenal azotemia. When such events occur in patients on JANUMET therapy, the drug should be promptly discontinued.

5.13 Loss of Control of Blood Glucose
When a patient stabilized on any diabetic regimen is exposed to stress such as fever, trauma, infection, or surgery, a temporary loss of glycemic control may occur. At such times, it may be necessary to withhold JANUMET and temporarily administer insulin. JANUMET may be reinstituted after the acute episode is resolved.

5.14 Hypersensitivity Reactions
There have been postmarketing reports of serious hypersensitivity reactions in patients treated with sitagliptin, one of the components of JANUMET. These reactions include anaphylaxis, angioedema, and exfoliative skin conditions including Stevens-Johnson syndrome. Onset of these reactions occurred within the first 3 months after initiation of treatment with sitagliptin, with some reports occurring after the first dose. If a hypersensitivity reaction is suspected, discontinue JANUMET, assess for other potential causes for the event, and institute alternative treatment for diabetes. *[See Adverse Reactions (6.2).]*
Angioedema has also been reported with other dipeptidyl peptidase-4 (DPP-4) inhibitors. Use caution in a patient with a history of angioedema with another DPP-4 inhibitor because it is unknown whether such patients will be predisposed to angioedema with JANUMET.

5.15 Macrovascular Outcomes
There have been no clinical studies establishing conclusive evidence of macrovascular risk reduction with JANUMET or any other anti-diabetic drug.

6 ADVERSE REACTIONS
6.1 Clinical Trials Experience
Because clinical trials are conducted under widely varying conditions, adverse reaction rates observed in the clinical trials of a drug cannot be directly compared to rates in the clinical trials of another drug and may not reflect the rates observed in practice.
Sitagliptin and Metformin Coadministration in Patients with Type 2 Diabetes Inadequately Controlled on Diet and Exercise
Table 1 summarizes the most common (≥5% of patients) adverse reactions reported (regardless of investigator assessment of causality) in a 24-week placebo-controlled factorial study in which sitagliptin and metformin were coadministered to patients with type 2 diabetes inadequately controlled on diet and exercise.
[See table 1 above]
Sitagliptin Add-on Therapy in Patients with Type 2 Diabetes Inadequately Controlled on Metformin Alone
In a 24-week placebo-controlled trial of sitagliptin 100 mg administered once daily added to a twice daily metformin regimen, there were no adverse reactions reported regardless of investigator assessment of causality in ≥5% of patients and more commonly than in patients given placebo. Discontinuation due to clinical adverse reactions was similar to the placebo treatment group (sitagliptin and metformin, 1.9%; placebo and metformin, 2.5%).
Gastrointestinal Adverse Reactions
The incidences of pre-selected gastrointestinal adverse experiences in patients treated with sitagliptin and metformin were similar to those reported for patients treated with metformin alone. See Table 2.
[See table 2 at top of next page]
Sitagliptin in Combination with Metformin and Glimepiride
In a 24-week placebo-controlled study of sitagliptin 100 mg as add-on therapy in patients with type 2 diabetes inadequately controlled on metformin and glimepiride (sitagliptin, N=116; placebo, N=113), the adverse reactions reported regardless of investigator assessment of causality in ≥5% of patients treated with sitagliptin and more commonly than in patients treated with placebo were: hypoglycemia (Table 3) and headache (6.9%, 2.7%).
Sitagliptin in Combination with Metformin and Rosiglitazone
In a placebo-controlled study of sitagliptin 100 mg as add-on therapy in patients with type 2 diabetes inadequately controlled on metformin and rosiglitazone (sitagliptin, N=181; placebo, N=97), the adverse reactions reported regardless of investigator assessment of causality through Week 18 in ≥5% of patients treated with sitagliptin and more commonly than in patients treated with placebo were: upper respiratory tract infection (sitagliptin, 5.5%; placebo, 5.2%) and nasopharyngitis (6.1%, 4.1%). Through Week 54, the adverse reactions reported regardless of investigator assessment of causality in ≥5% of patients treated with sitagliptin and more commonly than in patients treated with placebo were: upper respiratory tract infection (sitagliptin, 15.5%; placebo, 6.2%), nasopharyngitis (11.0%, 9.3%), peripheral edema (8.3%, 5.2%), and headache (5.5%, 4.1%).

Sitagliptin in Combination with Metformin and Insulin
In a 24-week placebo-controlled study of sitagliptin 100 mg as add-on therapy in patients with type 2 diabetes inadequately controlled on metformin and insulin (sitagliptin, N=229; placebo, N=233), the only adverse reaction reported regardless of investigator assessment of causality in ≥5% of patients treated with sitagliptin and more commonly than in patients treated with placebo was hypoglycemia (Table 3).
Hypoglycemia
In all (N=5) studies, adverse reactions of hypoglycemia were based on all reports of symptomatic hypoglycemia; a concurrent glucose measurement was not required although most (77%) reports of hypoglycemia were accompanied by a blood glucose measurement ≤70 mg/dL. When the combination of sitagliptin and metformin was coadministered with a sulfonylurea or with insulin, the percentage of patients reporting at least one adverse reaction of hypoglycemia was higher than that observed with placebo and metformin coadministered with a sulfonylurea or with insulin (Table 3).
[See table 3 above]
The overall incidence of reported adverse reactions of hypoglycemia in patients with type 2 diabetes inadequately controlled on diet and exercise was 0.6% in patients given placebo, 0.6% in patients given sitagliptin alone, 0.8% in patients given metformin alone, and 1.6% in patients given sitagliptin in combination with metformin. In patients with type 2 diabetes inadequately controlled on metformin alone, the overall incidence of adverse reactions of hypoglycemia was 1.3% in patients given add-on sitagliptin and 2.1% in patients given add-on placebo.
In the study of sitagliptin and add-on combination therapy with metformin and rosiglitazone, the overall incidence of hypoglycemia was 2.2% in patients given add-on sitagliptin and 0.0% in patients given add-on placebo through Week 18. Through Week 54, the overall incidence of hypoglycemia was 3.9% in patients given add-on sitagliptin and 1.0% in patients given add-on placebo.
Vital Signs and Electrocardiograms
With the combination of sitagliptin and metformin, no clinically meaningful changes in vital signs or in ECG (including in QTc interval) were observed.
Pancreatitis
In a pooled analysis of 19 double-blind clinical trials that included data from 10,246 patients randomized to receive sitagliptin 100 mg/day (N=5429) or corresponding (active or placebo) control (N=4817), the incidence of acute pancreatitis was 0.1 per 100 patient-years in each group (4 patients with an event in 4708 patient-years for sitagliptin and 4 patients with an event in 3942 patient-years for control) [See Warnings and Precautions (5.2).]
Sitagliptin
The most common adverse experience in sitagliptin monotherapy reported regardless of investigator assessment of causality in ≥5% of patients and more commonly than in patients given placebo was nasopharyngitis.
Metformin hydrochloride
The most common (>5%) established adverse reactions due to initiation of metformin therapy are diarrhea, nausea/vomiting, flatulence, abdominal discomfort, indigestion, asthenia, and headache.
Laboratory Tests
Sitagliptin
The incidence of laboratory adverse reactions was similar in patients treated with sitagliptin and metformin (7.6%) compared to patients treated with placebo and metformin (8.7%). In most but not all studies, a small increase in white blood cell count (approximately 200 cells/microL difference in WBC vs placebo; mean baseline WBC approximately 6600 cells/microL) was observed due to a small increase in neutrophils. This change in laboratory parameters is not considered to be clinically relevant.
Metformin hydrochloride
In controlled clinical trials of metformin of 29 weeks duration, a decrease to subnormal levels of previously normal serum Vitamin B_{12} levels, without clinical manifestations, was observed in approximately 7% of patients. Such decrease, possibly due to interference with B_{12} absorption from the B_{12}-intrinsic factor complex, is, however, very rarely associated with anemia and appears to be rapidly reversible with discontinuation of metformin or Vitamin B_{12} supplementation. [See Warnings and Precautions (5.5).]
6.2   Postmarketing Experience
Additional adverse reactions have been identified during postapproval use of JANUMET or sitagliptin, one of the components of JANUMET. These reactions have been reported when JANUMET or sitagliptin have been used alone and/or in combination with other antihyperglycemic agents. Because these reactions are reported voluntarily from a population of uncertain size, it is generally not possible to reliably estimate their frequency or establish a causal relationship to drug exposure.
Hypersensitivity reactions including anaphylaxis, angioedema, rash, urticaria, cutaneous vasculitis, and exfoliative skin conditions including Stevens-Johnson syndrome [see Warnings and Precautions (5.14)]; upper respiratory tract infection; hepatic enzyme elevations; acute pancreatitis, including fatal and non-fatal hemorrhagic and necrotizing pancreatitis [see Indications and Usage (1); Warnings and Precautions (5.2)]; worsening renal function, including acute renal failure (sometimes requiring dialysis) [see Warnings and Precautions (5.4)]; constipation; vomiting; headache; arthralgia; myalgia; pain in extremity; back pain.

7   DRUG INTERACTIONS
7.1   Carbonic Anhydrase Inhibitors
Topiramate or other carbonic anhydrase inhibitors (e.g., zonisamide, acetazolamide or dichlorphenamide) frequently decrease serum bicarbonate and induce non-anion gap, hyperchloremic metabolic acidosis. Concomitant use of these drugs may induce metabolic acidosis. Use these drugs with caution in patients treated with JANUMET, as the risk of lactic acidosis may increase.
7.2   Cationic Drugs
Cationic drugs (e.g., amiloride, digoxin, morphine, procainamide, quinidine, quinine, ranitidine, triamterene, trimethoprim, or vancomycin) that are eliminated by renal tubular secretion theoretically have the potential for interaction with metformin by competing for common renal tubular transport systems. Although such interactions remain theoretical (except for cimetidine), careful patient monitoring and dose adjustment of JANUMET and/or the interfering drug is recommended in patients who are taking cationic medications that are excreted via the proximal renal tubular secretory system.
7.3   The Use of Metformin with Other Drugs
Certain drugs tend to produce hyperglycemia and may lead to loss of glycemic control. These drugs include the thiazides and other diuretics, corticosteroids, phenothiazines, thyroid products, estrogens, oral contraceptives, phenytoin, nicotinic acid, sympathomimetics, calcium channel blocking drugs, and isoniazid. When such drugs are administered to a patient receiving JANUMET the patient should be closely observed to maintain adequate glycemic control.

8   USE IN SPECIFIC POPULATIONS
8.1   Pregnancy
Pregnancy Category B:
JANUMET
There are no adequate and well-controlled studies in pregnant women with JANUMET or its individual components; therefore, the safety of JANUMET in pregnant women is not known. JANUMET should be used during pregnancy only if clearly needed.
Merck Sharp & Dohme Corp., a subsidiary of Merck & Co., Inc., maintains a registry to monitor the pregnancy outcomes of women exposed to JANUMET while pregnant. Health care providers are encouraged to report any prenatal exposure to JANUMET by calling the Pregnancy Registry at 1-800-986-8999.
No animal studies have been conducted with the combined products in JANUMET to evaluate effects on reproduction. The following data are based on findings in studies performed with sitagliptin or metformin individually.
Sitagliptin
Reproduction studies have been performed in rats and rabbits. Doses of sitagliptin up to 125 mg/kg (approximately 12 times the human exposure at the maximum recommended human dose) did not impair fertility or harm the fetus. There are, however, no adequate and well-controlled studies with sitagliptin in pregnant women.
Sitagliptin administered to pregnant female rats and rabbits from gestation day 6 to 20 (organogenesis) was not teratogenic at oral doses up to 250 mg/kg (rats) and 125 mg/kg (rabbits), or approximately 30 and 20 times human exposure at the maximum recommended human dose (MRHD) of 100 mg/day based on AUC comparisons. Higher doses in-

Table 2: Pre-selected Gastrointestinal Adverse Reactions (Regardless of Investigator Assessment of Causality) Reported in Patients with Type 2 Diabetes Receiving Sitagliptin and Metformin

Number of Patients (%)

	Study of Sitagliptin and Metformin in Patients Inadequately Controlled on Diet and Exercise				Study of Sitagliptin Add-on in Patients Inadequately Controlled on Metformin Alone	
	Placebo	Sitagliptin 100 mg once daily	Metformin 500 mg/ Metformin 1000 mg twice daily*	Sitagliptin 50 mg twice daily + Metformin 500 mg/ Metformin 1000 mg twice daily*	Placebo and Metformin ≥1500 mg daily	Sitagliptin 100 mg once daily and Metformin ≥1500 mg daily
	N = 176	N = 179	N = 364	N = 372	N = 237	N = 464
Diarrhea	7 (4.0)	5 (2.8)	28 (7.7)	28 (7.5)	6 (2.5)	11 (2.4)
Nausea	2 (1.1)	2 (1.1)	20 (5.5)	18 (4.8)	2 (0.8)	6 (1.3)
Vomiting	1 (0.6)	0 (0.0)	2 (0.5)	8 (2.2)	2 (0.8)	5 (1.1)
Abdominal Pain†	4 (2.3)	6 (3.4)	14 (3.8)	11 (3.0)	9 (3.8)	10 (2.2)

* Data pooled for the patients given the lower and higher doses of metformin.
† Abdominal discomfort was included in the analysis of abdominal pain in the study of initial therapy.

Table 3: Incidence and Rate of Hypoglycemia* (Regardless of Investigator Assessment of Causality) in Placebo-Controlled Clinical Studies of Sitagliptin in Combination with Metformin Coadministered with Glimepiride or Insulin

Add-On to Glimepiride + Metformin (24 weeks)	Sitagliptin 100 mg + Metformin + Glimepiride	Placebo + Metformin + Glimepiride
	N = 116	N = 113
Overall (%)	19 (16.4)	1 (0.9)
Rate (episodes/patient-year)†	0.82	0.02
Severe (%)‡	0 (0.0)	0 (0.0)
Add-On to Insulin + Metformin (24 weeks)	Sitagliptin 100 mg + Metformin + Insulin	Placebo + Metformin + Insulin
	N = 229	N = 233
Overall (%)	35 (15.3)	19 (8.2)
Rate (episodes/patient-year)†	0.98	0.61
Severe (%)‡	1 (0.4)	1 (0.4)

* Adverse reactions of hypoglycemia were based on all reports of symptomatic hypoglycemia; a concurrent glucose measurement was not required: Intent-to-treat population.
† Based on total number of events (i.e., a single patient may have had multiple events).
‡ Severe events of hypoglycemia were defined as those events requiring medical assistance or exhibiting depressed level/loss of consciousness or seizure.

creased the incidence of rib malformations in offspring at 1000 mg/kg, or approximately 100 times human exposure at the MRHD.

Sitagliptin administered to female rats from gestation day 6 to lactation day 21 decreased body weight in male and female offspring at 1000 mg/kg. No functional or behavioral toxicity was observed in offspring of rats.

Placental transfer of sitagliptin administered to pregnant rats was approximately 45% at 2 hours and 80% at 24 hours postdose. Placental transfer of sitagliptin administered to pregnant rabbits was approximately 66% at 2 hours and 30% at 24 hours.

Metformin hydrochloride
Metformin was not teratogenic in rats and rabbits at doses up to 600 mg/kg/day. This represents an exposure of about 2 and 6 times the maximum recommended human daily dose of 2,000 mg based on body surface area comparisons for rats and rabbits, respectively. Determination of fetal concentrations demonstrated a partial placental barrier to metformin.

8.3 Nursing Mothers
No studies in lactating animals have been conducted with the combined components of JANUMET. In studies performed with the individual components, both sitagliptin and metformin are secreted in the milk of lactating rats. It is not known whether sitagliptin is excreted in human milk. Because many drugs are excreted in human milk, caution should be exercised when JANUMET is administered to a nursing woman.

8.4 Pediatric Use
Safety and effectiveness of JANUMET in pediatric patients under 18 years have not been established.

8.5 Geriatric Use
JANUMET
Because sitagliptin and metformin are substantially excreted by the kidney, and because aging can be associated with reduced renal function, JANUMET should be used with caution as age increases. Care should be taken in dose selection and should be based on careful and regular monitoring of renal function. *[See Warnings and Precautions (5.1, 5.4); Clinical Pharmacology (12.3).]*

Sitagliptin
Of the total number of subjects (N=3884) in Phase II and III clinical studies of sitagliptin, 725 patients were 65 years and over, while 61 patients were 75 years and over. No overall differences in safety or effectiveness were observed between subjects 65 years and over and younger subjects. While this and other reported clinical experience have not identified differences in responses between the elderly and younger patients, greater sensitivity of some older individuals cannot be ruled out.

Metformin hydrochloride
Controlled clinical studies of metformin did not include sufficient numbers of elderly patients to determine whether they respond differently from younger patients, although other reported clinical experience has not identified differences in responses between the elderly and young patients. Metformin should only be used in patients with normal renal function. The initial and maintenance dosing of metformin should be conservative in patients with advanced age, due to the potential for decreased renal function in this population. Any dose adjustment should be based on a careful assessment of renal function. *[See Contraindications (4); Warnings and Precautions (5.4); Clinical Pharmacology (12.3).]*

10 OVERDOSAGE
Sitagliptin
During controlled clinical trials in healthy subjects, single doses of up to 800 mg sitagliptin were administered. Maximal mean increases in QTc of 8.0 msec were observed in one study at a dose of 800 mg sitagliptin, a mean effect that is not considered clinically important *[see Clinical Pharmacology (12.2)].* There is no experience with doses above 800 mg in clinical studies. In Phase I multiple-dose studies, there were no dose-related clinical adverse reactions observed with sitagliptin with doses of up to 400 mg per day for periods of up to 28 days.

In the event of an overdose, it is reasonable to employ the usual supportive measures, e.g., remove unabsorbed material from the gastrointestinal tract, employ clinical monitoring (including obtaining an electrocardiogram), and institute supportive therapy as indicated by the patient's clinical status.

Sitagliptin is modestly dialyzable. In clinical studies, approximately 13.5% of the dose was removed over a 3- to 4-hour hemodialysis session. Prolonged hemodialysis may be considered if clinically appropriate. It is not known if sitagliptin is dialyzable by peritoneal dialysis.

Metformin hydrochloride
Overdose of metformin hydrochloride has occurred, including ingestion of amounts greater than 50 grams. Hypoglycemia was reported in approximately 10% of cases, but no causal association with metformin hydrochloride has been

established. Lactic acidosis has been reported in approximately 32% of metformin overdose cases *[see Warnings and Precautions (5.1)].* Metformin is dialyzable with a clearance of up to 170 mL/min under good hemodynamic conditions. Therefore, hemodialysis may be useful for removal of accumulated drug from patients in whom metformin overdosage is suspected.

11 DESCRIPTION
JANUMET (sitagliptin and metformin HCl) tablets contain two oral antihyperglycemic drugs used in the management of type 2 diabetes: sitagliptin and metformin hydrochloride.

Sitagliptin
Sitagliptin is an orally-active inhibitor of the dipeptidyl peptidase-4 (DPP-4) enzyme. Sitagliptin is present in JANUMET tablets in the form of sitagliptin phosphate monohydrate. Sitagliptin phosphate monohydrate is described chemically as 7-[(3R)-3-amino-1-oxo-4-(2,4,5-trifluorophenyl)butyl]-5,6,7,8-tetrahydro-3-(trifluoromethyl)-1,2,4-triazolo[4,3-a]pyrazine phosphate (1:1) monohydrate with an empirical formula of $C_{16}H_{15}F_6N_5O \cdot H_3PO_4 \cdot H_2O$ and a molecular weight of 523.32. The structural formula is:

Sitagliptin phosphate monohydrate is a white to off-white, crystalline, non-hygroscopic powder. It is soluble in water and N,N-dimethyl formamide; slightly soluble in methanol; very slightly soluble in ethanol, acetone, and acetonitrile; and insoluble in isopropanol and isopropyl acetate.

Metformin hydrochloride
Metformin hydrochloride (N,N-dimethylimidodicarbonimidic diamide hydrochloride) is not chemically or pharmacologically related to any other classes of oral antihyperglycemic agents. Metformin hydrochloride is a white to off-white crystalline compound with a molecular formula of $C_4H_{11}N_5 \cdot HCl$ and a molecular weight of 165.63. Metformin hydrochloride is freely soluble in water and is practically insoluble in acetone, ether, and chloroform. The pK_a of metformin is 12.4. The pH of a 1% aqueous solution of metformin hydrochloride is 6.68. The structural formula is as shown:

JANUMET
JANUMET is available for oral administration as tablets containing 64.25 mg sitagliptin phosphate monohydrate and metformin hydrochloride equivalent to: 50 mg sitagliptin as free base and 500 mg metformin hydrochloride (JANUMET 50 mg/500 mg) or 1000 mg metformin hydrochloride (JANUMET 50 mg/1000 mg). Each film-coated tablet of JANUMET contains the following inactive ingredients: microcrystalline cellulose, polyvinylpyrrolidone, sodium lauryl sulfate, and sodium stearyl fumarate. In addition, the film coating contains the following inactive ingredients: polyvinyl alcohol, polyethylene glycol, talc, titanium dioxide, red iron oxide, and black iron oxide.

12 CLINICAL PHARMACOLOGY
12.1 Mechanism of Action
JANUMET
JANUMET combines two antidiabetic medications with complementary mechanisms of action to improve glycemic control in patients with type 2 diabetes: sitagliptin, a dipeptidyl peptidase-4 (DPP-4) inhibitor, and metformin hydrochloride, a member of the biguanide class.

Sitagliptin
Sitagliptin is a DPP-4 inhibitor, which is believed to exert its actions in patients with type 2 diabetes by slowing the inactivation of incretin hormones. Concentrations of the active intact hormones are increased by sitagliptin, thereby increasing and prolonging the action of these hormones. Incretin hormones, including glucagon-like peptide-1 (GLP-1) and glucose-dependent insulinotropic polypeptide (GIP), are released by the intestine throughout the day, and levels are increased in response to a meal. These hormones are rapidly inactivated by the enzyme DPP-4. The incretins are part of an endogenous system involved in the physiologic regulation of glucose homeostasis. When blood glucose concentrations are normal or elevated, GLP-1 and GIP increase insulin synthesis and release from pancreatic beta cells by intracellular signaling pathways involving cyclic AMP. GLP-1 also lowers glucagon secretion from pancreatic alpha cells, leading to reduced hepatic glucose production. By in-

creasing and prolonging active incretin levels, sitagliptin increases insulin release and decreases glucagon levels in the circulation in a glucose-dependent manner. Sitagliptin demonstrates selectivity for DPP-4 and does not inhibit DPP-8 or DPP-9 activity *in vitro* at concentrations approximating those from therapeutic doses.

Metformin hydrochloride
Metformin is an antihyperglycemic agent which improves glucose tolerance in patients with type 2 diabetes, lowering both basal and postprandial plasma glucose. Its pharmacologic mechanisms of action are different from other classes of oral antihyperglycemic agents. Metformin decreases hepatic glucose production, decreases intestinal absorption of glucose, and improves insulin sensitivity by increasing peripheral glucose uptake and utilization. Unlike sulfonylureas, metformin does not produce hypoglycemia in either patients with type 2 diabetes or normal subjects (except in special circumstances *[see Warnings and Precautions (5.9)]*) and does not cause hyperinsulinemia. With metformin therapy, insulin secretion remains unchanged while fasting insulin levels and day-long plasma insulin response may actually decrease.

12.2 Pharmacodynamics
Sitagliptin
General
In patients with type 2 diabetes, administration of sitagliptin led to inhibition of DPP-4 enzyme activity for a 24-hour period. After an oral glucose load or a meal, this DPP-4 inhibition resulted in a 2- to 3-fold increase in circulating levels of active GLP-1 and GIP, decreased glucagon concentrations, and increased responsiveness of insulin release to glucose, resulting in higher C-peptide and insulin concentrations. The rise in insulin with the decrease in glucagon was associated with lower fasting glucose concentrations and reduced glucose excursion following an oral glucose load or a meal.

Sitagliptin and Metformin hydrochloride Coadministration
In a two-day study in healthy subjects, sitagliptin alone increased active GLP-1 concentrations, whereas metformin alone increased active and total GLP-1 concentrations to similar extents. Coadministration of sitagliptin and metformin had an additive effect on active GLP-1 concentrations. Sitagliptin, but not metformin, increased active GIP concentrations. It is unclear what these findings mean for changes in glycemic control in patients with type 2 diabetes.

In studies with healthy subjects, sitagliptin did not lower blood glucose or cause hypoglycemia.

Cardiac Electrophysiology
In a randomized, placebo-controlled crossover study, 79 healthy subjects were administered a single oral dose of sitagliptin 100 mg, sitagliptin 800 mg (8 times the recommended dose), and placebo. At the recommended dose of 100 mg, there was no effect on the QTc interval obtained at the peak plasma concentration, or at any other time during the study. Following the 800-mg dose, the maximum increase in the placebo-corrected mean change in QTc from baseline at 3 hours postdose was 8.0 msec. This increase is not considered to be clinically significant. At the 800-mg dose, peak sitagliptin plasma concentrations were approximately 11 times higher than the peak concentrations following a 100-mg dose.

In patients with type 2 diabetes administered sitagliptin 100 mg (N=81) or sitagliptin 200 mg (N=63) daily, there were no meaningful changes in QTc interval based on ECG data obtained at the time of expected peak plasma concentration.

12.3 Pharmacokinetics
JANUMET
The results of a bioequivalence study in healthy subjects demonstrated that the JANUMET (sitagliptin and metformin HCl) 50 mg/500 mg and 50 mg/1000 mg combination tablets are bioequivalent to coadministration of corresponding doses of sitagliptin (JANUVIA®) and metformin hydrochloride as individual tablets.

Absorption
Sitagliptin
The absolute bioavailability of sitagliptin is approximately 87%. Coadministration of a high-fat meal with sitagliptin had no effect on the pharmacokinetics of sitagliptin.

Metformin hydrochloride
The absolute bioavailability of a metformin hydrochloride 500-mg tablet given under fasting conditions is approximately 50-60%. Studies using single oral doses of metformin hydrochloride tablets 500 mg to 1500 mg, and 850 mg to 2550 mg, indicate that there is a lack of dose proportionality with increasing doses, which is due to decreased absorption rather than an alteration in elimination. Food decreases the extent of and slightly delays the absorption of metformin, as shown by approximately a 40% lower mean peak plasma concentration (C_{max}), a 25% lower area under the plasma concentration versus time curve (AUC), and a 35-minute prolongation of time to peak plasma concentration (T_{max}) following administration of a single 850-mg tablet of

metformin with food, compared to the same tablet strength administered fasting. The clinical relevance of these decreases is unknown.

Distribution
Sitagliptin
The mean volume of distribution at steady state following a single 100-mg intravenous dose of sitagliptin to healthy subjects is approximately 198 liters. The fraction of sitagliptin reversibly bound to plasma proteins is low (38%).

Metformin hydrochloride
The apparent volume of distribution (V/F) of metformin following single oral doses of metformin hydrochloride tablets 850 mg averaged 654 ± 358 L. Metformin is negligibly bound to plasma proteins, in contrast to sulfonylureas, which are more than 90% protein bound. Metformin partitions into erythrocytes, most likely as a function of time. At usual clinical doses and dosing schedules of metformin hydrochloride tablets, steady-state plasma concentrations of metformin are reached within 24-48 hours and are generally <1 mcg/mL. During controlled clinical trials of metformin, maximum metformin plasma levels did not exceed 5 mcg/mL, even at maximum doses.

Metabolism
Sitagliptin
Approximately 79% of sitagliptin is excreted unchanged in the urine with metabolism being a minor pathway of elimination.
Following a [^{14}C]sitagliptin oral dose, approximately 16% of the radioactivity was excreted as metabolites of sitagliptin. Six metabolites were detected at trace levels and are not expected to contribute to the plasma DPP-4 inhibitory activity of sitagliptin. *In vitro* studies indicated that the primary enzyme responsible for the limited metabolism of sitagliptin was CYP3A4, with contribution from CYP2C8.

Metformin hydrochloride
Intravenous single-dose studies in normal subjects demonstrate that metformin is excreted unchanged in the urine and does not undergo hepatic metabolism (no metabolites have been identified in humans) nor biliary excretion.

Excretion
Sitagliptin
Following administration of an oral [^{14}C]sitagliptin dose to healthy subjects, approximately 100% of the administered radioactivity was eliminated in feces (13%) or urine (87%) within one week of dosing. The apparent terminal $t_{1/2}$ following a 100-mg oral dose of sitagliptin was approximately 12.4 hours and renal clearance was approximately 350 mL/min.
Elimination of sitagliptin occurs primarily via renal excretion and involves active tubular secretion. Sitagliptin is a substrate for human organic anion transporter-3 (hOAT-3), which may be involved in the renal elimination of sitagliptin. The clinical relevance of hOAT-3 in sitagliptin transport has not been established. Sitagliptin is also a substrate of p-glycoprotein, which may also be involved in mediating the renal elimination of sitagliptin. However, cyclosporine, a p-glycoprotein inhibitor, did not reduce the renal clearance of sitagliptin.

Metformin hydrochloride
Renal clearance is approximately 3.5 times greater than creatinine clearance, which indicates that tubular secretion is the major route of metformin elimination. Following oral administration, approximately 90% of the absorbed drug is eliminated via the renal route within the first 24 hours, with a plasma elimination half-life of approximately 6.2 hours. In blood, the elimination half-life is approximately 17.6 hours, suggesting that the erythrocyte mass may be a compartment of distribution.

Specific Populations
Renal Impairment
JANUMET
JANUMET should not be used in patients with renal impairment *[see Contraindications (4); Warnings and Precautions (5.4)]*.
Sitagliptin
An approximately 2-fold increase in the plasma AUC of sitagliptin was observed in patients with moderate renal impairment, and an approximately 4-fold increase was observed in patients with severe renal impairment including patients with ESRD on hemodialysis, as compared to normal healthy control subjects.
Metformin hydrochloride
In patients with decreased renal function (based on measured creatinine clearance), the plasma and blood half-life of metformin is prolonged and the renal clearance is decreased in proportion to the decrease in creatinine clearance.

Hepatic Impairment
Sitagliptin
In patients with moderate hepatic impairment (Child-Pugh score 7 to 9), mean AUC and C_{max} of sitagliptin increased approximately 21% and 13%, respectively, compared to

Table 4: Effect of Sitagliptin on Systemic Exposure of Coadministered Drugs

Coadministered Drug	Dose of Coadministered Drug*	Dose of Sitagliptin*	Geometric Mean Ratio (ratio with/without sitagliptin) No Effect = 1.00		
				AUC[†]	C_{max}
No dosing adjustments required for the following:					
Digoxin	0.25 mg[‡] once daily for 10 days	100 mg[‡] once daily for 10 days	Digoxin	1.11[§]	1.18
Glyburide	1.25 mg	200 mg[‡] once daily for 6 days	Glyburide	1.09	1.01
Simvastatin	20 mg	200 mg[‡] once daily for 5 days	Simvastatin	0.85[¶]	0.80
			Simvastatin Acid	1.12[¶]	1.06
Rosiglitazone	4 mg	200 mg[‡] once daily for 5 days	Rosiglitazone	0.98	0.99
Warfarin	30 mg single dose on day 5	200 mg[‡] once daily for 11 days	S(-) Warfarin	0.95	0.89
			R(+) Warfarin	0.99	0.89
Ethinyl estradiol and norethindrone	21 days once daily of 35 µg ethinyl estradiol with norethindrone 0.5 mg × 7 days, 0.75 mg × 7 days, 1.0 mg × 7 days	200 mg[‡] once daily for 21 days	Ethinyl estradiol	0.99	0.97
			Norethindrone	1.03	0.98
Metformin	1000 mg[‡] twice daily for 14 days	50 mg[‡] twice daily for 7 days	Metformin	1.02[#]	0.97

* All doses administered as single dose unless otherwise specified.
† AUC is reported as $AUC_{0-\infty}$ unless otherwise specified.
‡ Multiple dose.
§ AUC_{0-24hr}.
¶ AUC_{0-last}.
# AUC_{0-12hr}.

healthy matched controls following administration of a single 100-mg dose of sitagliptin. These differences are not considered to be clinically meaningful.
There is no clinical experience in patients with severe hepatic impairment (Child-Pugh score >9).
Metformin hydrochloride
No pharmacokinetic studies of metformin have been conducted in patients with hepatic impairment.
Gender
Sitagliptin
Gender had no clinically meaningful effect on the pharmacokinetics of sitagliptin based on a composite analysis of Phase I pharmacokinetic data and on a population pharmacokinetic analysis of Phase I and Phase II data.
Metformin hydrochloride
Metformin pharmacokinetic parameters did not differ significantly between normal subjects and patients with type 2 diabetes when analyzed according to gender. Similarly, in controlled clinical studies in patients with type 2 diabetes, the antihyperglycemic effect of metformin was comparable in males and females.
Geriatric
Sitagliptin
When the effects of age on renal function are taken into account, age alone did not have a clinically meaningful impact on the pharmacokinetics of sitagliptin based on a population pharmacokinetic analysis. Elderly subjects (65 to 80 years) had approximately 19% higher plasma concentrations of sitagliptin compared to younger subjects.
Metformin hydrochloride
Limited data from controlled pharmacokinetic studies of metformin in healthy elderly subjects suggest that total plasma clearance of metformin is decreased, the half life is prolonged, and C_{max} is increased, compared to healthy young subjects. From these data, it appears that the change in metformin pharmacokinetics with aging is primarily accounted for by a change in renal function.
As is true for all patients, JANUMET treatment should not be initiated in geriatric patients unless measurement of creatinine clearance demonstrates that renal function is normal *[see Warnings and Precautions (5.1, 5.4)]*.
Pediatric
No studies with JANUMET have been performed in pediatric patients.
Race
Sitagliptin
Race had no clinically meaningful effect on the pharmacokinetics of sitagliptin based on a composite analysis of available pharmacokinetic data, including subjects of white, Hispanic, black, Asian, and other racial groups.

Metformin hydrochloride
No studies of metformin pharmacokinetic parameters according to race have been performed. In controlled clinical studies of metformin in patients with type 2 diabetes, the antihyperglycemic effect was comparable in whites (n=249), blacks (n=51), and Hispanics (n=24).
Body Mass Index (BMI)
Sitagliptin
Body mass index had no clinically meaningful effect on the pharmacokinetics of sitagliptin based on a composite analysis of Phase I pharmacokinetic data and on a population pharmacokinetic analysis of Phase I and Phase II data.
Drug Interactions
Sitagliptin and Metformin hydrochloride
Coadministration of multiple doses of sitagliptin (50 mg) and metformin (1000 mg) given twice daily did not meaningfully alter the pharmacokinetics of either sitagliptin or metformin in patients with type 2 diabetes.
Pharmacokinetic drug interaction studies with JANUMET have not been performed; however, such studies have been conducted with the individual components of JANUMET (sitagliptin and metformin hydrochloride).
Sitagliptin
In Vitro Assessment of Drug Interactions
Sitagliptin is not an inhibitor of CYP isozymes CYP3A4, 2C8, 2C9, 2D6, 1A2, 2C19 or 2B6, and is not an inducer of CYP3A4. Sitagliptin is a p-glycoprotein substrate, but does not inhibit p-glycoprotein mediated transport of digoxin. Based on these results, sitagliptin is considered unlikely to cause interactions with other drugs that utilize these pathways.
Sitagliptin is not extensively bound to plasma proteins. Therefore, the propensity of sitagliptin to be involved in clinically meaningful drug-drug interactions mediated by plasma protein binding displacement is very low.
In Vivo Assessment of Drug Interactions
[See table 4 above]
[See table 5 at top of next page]
[See table 6 at top of next page]
[See table 7 at top of next page]

13 NONCLINICAL TOXICOLOGY
13.1 Carcinogenesis, Mutagenesis, Impairment of Fertility
JANUMET
No animal studies have been conducted with the combined products in JANUMET to evaluate carcinogenesis, mutagenesis or impairment of fertility. The following data are based on the findings in studies with sitagliptin and metformin individually.

Table 5: Effect of Coadministered Drugs on Systemic Exposure of Sitagliptin

Coadministered Drug	Dose of Coadministered Drug*	Dose of Sitagliptin*	Geometric Mean Ratio (ratio with/without coadministered drug) No Effect = 1.00		
				AUC†	C_{max}
No dosing adjustments required for the following:					
Cyclosporine	600 mg once daily	100 mg once daily	Sitagliptin	1.29	1.68
Metformin	1000 mg‡ twice daily for 14 days	50 mg‡ twice daily for 7 days	Sitagliptin	1.02§	1.05

* All doses administered as single dose unless otherwise specified.
† AUC is reported as $AUC_{0-\infty}$ unless otherwise specified.
‡ Multiple dose.
§ AUC_{0-12hr}.

Table 6: Effect of Metformin on Systemic Exposure of Coadministered Drugs

Coadministered Drug	Dose of Coadministered Drug*	Dose of Metformin*	Geometric Mean Ratio (ratio with/without metformin) No Effect = 1.00		
				AUC†	C_{max}
No dosing adjustments required for the following:					
Cimetidine	400 mg	850 mg	Cimetidine	0.95‡	1.01
Glyburide	5 mg	500 mg§	Glyburide	0.78¶	0.63¶
Furosemide	40 mg	850 mg	Furosemide	0.87¶	0.69¶
Nifedipine	10 mg	850 mg	Nifedipine	1.10‡	1.08
Propranolol	40 mg	850 mg	Propranolol	1.01‡	0.94
Ibuprofen	400 mg	850 mg	Ibuprofen	0.97#	1.01#

* All doses administered as single dose unless otherwise specified.
† AUC is reported as $AUC_{0-\infty}$ unless otherwise specified.
‡ AUC_{0-24hr}.
§ GLUMETZA (metformin hydrochloride extended-release tablets) 500 mg.
¶ Ratio of arithmetic means, p value of difference <0.05.
# Ratio of arithmetic means.

Table 7: Effect of Coadministered Drugs on Systemic Exposure of Metformin

Coadministered Drug	Dose of Coadministered Drug*	Dose of Metformin*	Geometric Mean Ratio (ratio with/without coadministered drug) No Effect = 1.00		
				AUC†	C_{max}
No dosing adjustments required for the following:					
Glyburide	5 mg	500 mg‡	Metformin‡	0.98§	0.99§
Furosemide	40 mg	850 mg	Metformin	1.09§	1.22§
Nifedipine	10 mg	850 mg	Metformin	1.16	1.21
Propranolol	40 mg	850 mg	Metformin	0.90	0.94
Ibuprofen	400 mg	850 mg	Metformin	1.05§	1.07§
Cationic drugs eliminated by renal tubular secretion may reduce metformin elimination: use with caution. [See Warnings and Precautions (5.10) and Drug Interactions (7.2).]					
Cimetidine	400 mg	850 mg	Metformin	1.40	1.61
Carbonic anhydrase inhibitors may cause metabolic acidosis: use with caution. [See Warnings and Precautions (5.1) and Drug Interactions (7.1).]					
Topiramate	100 mg¶	500 mg¶	Metformin	1.25¶	1.17

* All doses administered as single dose unless otherwise specified.
† AUC is reported as $AUC_{0-\infty}$ unless otherwise specified.
‡ GLUMETZA (metformin hydrochloride extended-release tablets) 500 mg.
§ Ratio of arithmetic means.
¶ Steady state 100 mg Topiramate every 12 hr + metformin 500 mg every 12 hr AUC = AUC_{0-12hr}.

Sitagliptin
A two-year carcinogenicity study was conducted in male and female rats given oral doses of sitagliptin of 50, 150, and 500 mg/kg. There was an increased incidence of combined liver adenoma/carcinoma in males and females and of liver carcinoma in females at 500 mg/kg. This dose results in exposures approximately 60 times the human exposure at the maximum recommended daily adult human dose (MRHD) of 100 mg/day based on AUC comparisons. Liver tumors were not observed at 150 mg/kg, approximately 20 times the human exposure at the MRHD. A two-year carcinogenicity study was conducted in male and female mice given oral doses of sitagliptin of 50, 125, 250, and 500 mg/kg/day. There was no increase in the incidence of tu-

mors in any organ up to 500 mg/kg, approximately 70 times human exposure at the MRHD. Sitagliptin was not mutagenic or clastogenic with or without metabolic activation in the Ames bacterial mutagenicity assay, a Chinese hamster ovary (CHO) chromosome aberration assay, an in vitro cytogenetics assay in CHO, an in vitro rat hepatocyte DNA alkaline elution assay, and an in vivo micronucleus assay.
In rat fertility studies with oral gavage doses of 125, 250, and 1000 mg/kg, males were treated for 4 weeks prior to mating, during mating, up to scheduled termination (approximately 8 weeks total), and females were treated 2 weeks prior to mating through gestation day 7. No adverse effect on fertility was observed at 125 mg/kg (approximately 12 times human exposure at the MRHD of 100 mg/day based on AUC comparisons). At higher doses, nondose-related increased resorptions in females were observed (approximately 25 and 100 times human exposure at the MRHD based on AUC comparison).

Metformin hydrochloride
Long-term carcinogenicity studies have been performed in rats (dosing duration of 104 weeks) and mice (dosing duration of 91 weeks) at doses up to and including 900 mg/kg/day and 1500 mg/kg/day, respectively. These doses are both approximately four times the maximum recommended human daily dose of 2000 mg based on body surface area comparisons. No evidence of carcinogenicity with metformin was found in either male or female mice. Similarly, there was no tumorigenic potential observed with metformin in male rats. There was, however, an increased incidence of benign stromal uterine polyps in female rats treated with 900 mg/kg/day.
There was no evidence of a mutagenic potential of metformin in the following in vitro tests: Ames test (S. typhimurium), gene mutation test (mouse lymphoma cells), or chromosomal aberrations test (human lymphocytes). Results in the in vivo mouse micronucleus test were also negative. Fertility of male or female rats was unaffected by metformin when administered at doses as high as 600 mg/kg/day, which is approximately three times the maximum recommended human daily dose based on body surface area comparisons.

14 CLINICAL STUDIES
The coadministration of sitagliptin and metformin has been studied in patients with type 2 diabetes inadequately controlled on diet and exercise and in combination with other antihyperglycemic agents.
None of the clinical efficacy studies described below was conducted with JANUMET; however, bioequivalence of JANUMET with coadministered sitagliptin and metformin hydrochloride tablets was demonstrated.

Sitagliptin and Metformin Coadministration in Patients with Type 2 Diabetes Inadequately Controlled on Diet and Exercise
A total of 1091 patients with type 2 diabetes and inadequate glycemic control on diet and exercise participated in a 24-week, randomized, double-blind, placebo-controlled factorial study designed to assess the efficacy of sitagliptin and metformin coadministration. Patients on an antihyperglycemic agent (N=541) underwent a diet, exercise, and drug washout period of up to 12 weeks duration. After the washout period, patients with inadequate glycemic control (A1C 7.5% to 11%) were randomized after completing a 2-week single-blind placebo run-in period. Patients not on antihyperglycemic agents at study entry (N=550) with inadequate glycemic control (A1C 7.5% to 11%) immediately entered the 2-week single-blind placebo run-in period and then were randomized. Approximately equal numbers of patients were randomized to receive placebo, 100 mg of sitagliptin once daily, 500 mg or 1000 mg of metformin twice daily, or 50 mg of sitagliptin twice daily in combination with 500 mg or 1000 mg of metformin twice daily. Patients who failed to meet specific glycemic goals during the study were treated with glyburide (glibenclamide) rescue.
Sitagliptin and metformin coadministration provided significant improvements in A1C, FPG, and 2-hour PPG compared to placebo, to metformin alone, and to sitagliptin alone (Table 8, Figure 1). Mean reductions from baseline in A1C were generally greater for patients with higher baseline A1C values. For patients not on an antihyperglycemic agent at study entry, mean reductions from baseline in A1C were: sitagliptin 100 mg once daily, -1.1%; metformin 500 mg bid, -1.1%; metformin 1000 mg bid, -1.2%; sitagliptin 50 mg bid with metformin 500 mg bid, -1.6%; sitagliptin 50 mg bid with metformin 1000 mg bid, -1.9%; and for patients receiving placebo, -0.2%. Lipid effects were generally neutral. The decrease in body weight in the groups given sitagliptin in combination with metformin was similar to that in the groups given metformin alone or placebo.
[See table 8 at top of next page]
[See figure 1 at top of next column]
Initial combination therapy or maintenance of combination therapy should be individualized and are left to the discretion of the health care provider.

Figure 1: Mean Change from Baseline for A1C (%) over 24 Weeks with Sitagliptin and Metformin, Alone and in Combination in Patients with Type 2 Diabetes Inadequately Controlled with Diet and Exercise*

o Placebo
□ Metformin 1000 mg b.i.d.
● Sitagliptin 100 mg q.d.
♦ Sitagliptin 50 mg b.i.d. + Metformin 500 mg b.i.d.
◇ Metformin 500 mg b.i.d.
■ Sitagliptin 50 mg b.i.d. + Metformin 1000 mg b.i.d.

*All Patients Treated Population: least squares means adjusted for prior antihyperglycemic therapy and baseline value.

Sitagliptin Add-on Therapy in Patients with Type 2 Diabetes Inadequately Controlled on Metformin Alone

A total of 701 patients with type 2 diabetes participated in a 24-week, randomized, double-blind, placebo-controlled study designed to assess the efficacy of sitagliptin in combination with metformin. Patients already on metformin (N=431) at a dose of at least 1500 mg per day were randomized after completing a 2-week, single-blind placebo run-in period. Patients on metformin and another antihyperglycemic agent (N=229) and patients not on any antihyperglycemic agents (off therapy for at least 8 weeks, N=41) were randomized after a run-in period of approximately 10 weeks on metformin (at a dose of at least 1500 mg per day) in monotherapy. Patients were randomized to the addition of either 100 mg of sitagliptin or placebo, administered once daily. Patients who failed to meet specific glycemic goals during the studies were treated with pioglitazone rescue.

In combination with metformin, sitagliptin provided significant improvements in A1C, FPG, and 2-hour PPG compared to placebo with metformin (Table 9). Rescue glycemic therapy was used in 5% of patients treated with sitagliptin 100 mg and 14% of patients treated with placebo. A similar decrease in body weight was observed for both treatment groups.

Table 9: Glycemic Parameters at Final Visit (24-Week Study) of Sitagliptin as Add-on Combination Therapy with Metformin*

	Sitagliptin 100 mg once daily + Metformin	Placebo + Metformin
A1C (%)	**N = 453**	**N = 224**
Baseline (mean)	8.0	8.0
Change from baseline (adjusted mean†)	-0.7	-0.0
Difference from placebo + metformin (adjusted mean†) (95% CI)	-0.7‡ (-0.8, -0.5)	
Patients (%) achieving A1C <7%	213 (47%)	41 (18%)
FPG (mg/dL)	**N = 454**	**N = 226**
Baseline (mean)	170	174
Change from baseline (adjusted mean†)	-17	9
Difference from placebo + metformin (adjusted mean†) (95% CI)	-25‡ (-31, -20)	
2-hour PPG (mg/dL)	**N = 387**	**N = 182**
Baseline (mean)	275	272
Change from baseline (adjusted mean†)	-62	-11
Difference from placebo + metformin (adjusted mean†) (95% CI)	-51‡ (-61, -41)	

* Intent-to-treat population using last observation on study prior to pioglitazone rescue therapy.
† Least squares means adjusted for prior antihyperglycemic therapy and baseline value.
‡ p<0.001 compared to placebo + metformin.

Table 8: Glycemic Parameters at Final Visit (24-Week Study) for Sitagliptin and Metformin, Alone and in Combination in Patients with Type 2 Diabetes Inadequately Controlled on Diet and Exercise*

	Placebo	Sitagliptin 100 mg once daily	Metformin 500 mg twice daily	Metformin 1000 mg twice daily	Sitagliptin 50 mg twice daily + Metformin 500 mg twice daily	Sitagliptin 50 mg twice daily + Metformin 1000 mg twice daily
A1C (%)	**N = 165**	**N = 175**	**N = 178**	**N = 177**	**N = 183**	**N = 178**
Baseline (mean)	8.7	8.9	8.9	8.7	8.8	8.8
Change from baseline (adjusted mean†)	0.2	-0.7	-0.8	-1.1	-1.4	-1.9
Difference from placebo (adjusted mean†) (95% CI)		-0.8‡ (-1.1, -0.6)	-1.0‡ (-1.2, -0.8)	-1.3‡ (-1.5, -1.1)	-1.6‡ (-1.8, -1.3)	-2.1‡ (-2.3, -1.8)
Patients (%) achieving A1C <7%	15 (9%)	35 (20%)	41 (23%)	68 (38%)	79 (43%)	118 (66%)
% Patients receiving rescue medication	32	21	17	12	8	2
FPG (mg/dL)	**N = 169**	**N = 178**	**N = 179**	**N = 179**	**N = 183**	**N = 180**
Baseline (mean)	196	201	205	197	204	197
Change from baseline (adjusted mean†)	6	-17	-27	-29	-47	-64
Difference from placebo (adjusted mean†) (95% CI)		-23‡ (-33, -14)	-33‡ (-43, -24)	-35‡ (-45, -26)	-53‡ (-62, -43)	-70‡ (-79, -60)
2-hour PPG (mg/dL)	**N = 129**	**N = 136**	**N = 141**	**N = 138**	**N = 147**	**N = 152**
Baseline (mean)	277	285	293	283	292	287
Change from baseline (adjusted mean†)	0	-52	-53	-78	-93	-117
Difference from placebo (adjusted mean†) (95% CI)		-52‡ (-67, -37)	-54‡ (-69, -39)	-78‡ (-93, -63)	-93‡ (-107, -78)	-117‡ (-131, -102)

* Intent-to-treat population using last observation on study prior to glyburide (glibenclamide) rescue therapy.
† Least squares means adjusted for prior antihyperglycemic therapy status and baseline value.
‡ p<0.001 compared to placebo.

Sitagliptin Add-on Therapy in Patients with Type 2 Diabetes Inadequately Controlled on the Combination of Metformin and Glimepiride

A total of 441 patients with type 2 diabetes participated in a 24-week, randomized, double-blind, placebo-controlled study designed to assess the efficacy of sitagliptin in combination with glimepiride, with or without metformin. Patients entered a run-in treatment period on glimepiride (≥4 mg per day) alone or glimepiride in combination with metformin (≥1500 mg per day). After a dose-titration and dose-stable run-in period of up to 16 weeks and a 2-week placebo run-in period, patients with inadequate glycemic control (A1C 7.5% to 10.5%) were randomized to the addition of either 100 mg of sitagliptin or placebo, administered once daily. Patients who failed to meet specific glycemic goals during the studies were treated with pioglitazone rescue.

Patients receiving sitagliptin with metformin and glimepiride had significant improvements in A1C and FPG compared to patients receiving placebo with metformin and glimepiride (Table 10), with mean reductions from baseline relative to placebo in A1C of -0.9% and in FPG of -21 mg/dL. Rescue therapy was used in 8% of patients treated with add-on sitagliptin 100 mg and 29% of patients treated with add-on placebo. The patients treated with add-on sitagliptin had a mean increase in body weight of 1.1 kg vs. add-on placebo (+0.4 kg vs. -0.7 kg). In addition, add-on sitagliptin resulted in an increased rate of hypoglycemia compared to add-on placebo. [See Warnings and Precautions (5.9); Adverse Reactions (6.1).]

Table 10: Glycemic Parameters at Final Visit (24-Week Study) for Sitagliptin in Combination with Metformin and Glimepiride*

	Sitagliptin 100 mg + Metformin and Glimepiride	Placebo + Metformin and Glimepiride
A1C (%)	**N = 115**	**N = 105**
Baseline (mean)	8.3	8.3
Change from baseline (adjusted mean†)	-0.6	0.3
Difference from placebo (adjusted mean†) (95% CI)	-0.9‡ (-1.1, -0.7)	
Patients (%) achieving A1C <7%	26 (23%)	1 (1%)
FPG (mg/dL)	**N = 115**	**N = 109**
Baseline (mean)	179	179
Change from baseline (adjusted mean†)	-8	13
Difference from placebo (adjusted mean†) (95% CI)	-21‡ (-32, -10)	

* Intent-to-treat population using last observation on study prior to pioglitazone rescue therapy.
† Least squares means adjusted for prior antihyperglycemic therapy status and baseline value.
‡ p<0.001 compared to placebo.

Sitagliptin Add-on Therapy in Patients with Type 2 Diabetes Inadequately Controlled on the Combination of Metformin and Rosiglitazone

A total of 278 patients with type 2 diabetes participated in a 54-week, randomized, double-blind, placebo-controlled study designed to assess the efficacy of sitagliptin in combination with metformin and rosiglitazone. Patients on dual therapy with metformin ≥1500 mg/day and rosiglitazone ≥4 mg/day or with metformin ≥1500 mg/day and pioglitazone ≥30 mg/day (switched to rosiglitazone ≥4 mg/day) entered a dose-stable run-in period of 6 weeks. Patients on other dual therapy were switched to metformin ≥1500 mg/day and rosiglitazone ≥4 mg/day in a dose titration/stabilization run-in period of up to 20 weeks in duration. After the run-in period, patients with inadequate glycemic control (A1C 7.5% to 11%) were randomized 2:1 to the addition of either 100 mg of sitagliptin or placebo, administered once daily. Patients who failed to meet specific glycemic goals during the studies were treated with glipizide (or other sulfonylurea) rescue. The primary time point for evaluation of glycemic parameters was Week 18.

In combination with metformin and rosiglitazone, sitagliptin provided significant improvements in A1C, FPG, and 2-hour PPG compared to placebo with metformin and rosiglitazone (Table 11) at Week 18. At Week 54, mean reduction in A1C was -1.0% for patients treated with sitagliptin and -0.3% for patients treated with placebo in an analysis based on the intent-to-treat population. Rescue therapy was used in 18% of patients treated with sitagliptin 100 mg and 40% of patients treated with placebo. There was no significant difference between sitagliptin and placebo in body weight change.

Table 11: Glycemic Parameters at Week 18 for Sitagliptin in Add-on Combination Therapy with Metformin and Rosiglitazone*

	Week 18	
	Sitagliptin 100 mg + Metformin + Rosiglitazone	Placebo + Metformin + Rosiglitazone
A1C (%)	N = 176	N = 93
Baseline (mean)	8.8	8.7
Change from baseline (adjusted mean[†])	-1.0	-0.4
Difference from placebo + rosiglitazone + metformin (adjusted mean[†]) (95% CI)	-0.7[‡] (-0.9, -0.4)	
Patients (%) achieving A1C <7%	39 (22%)	9 (10%)
FPG (mg/dL)	N = 179	N = 94
Baseline (mean)	181	182
Change from baseline (adjusted mean[†])	-30	-11
Difference from placebo + rosiglitazone + metformin (adjusted mean[†]) (95% CI)	-18[‡] (-26, -10)	
2-hour PPG (mg/dL)	N = 152	N = 80
Baseline (mean)	256	248
Change from baseline (adjusted mean[†])	-59	-21
Difference from placebo + rosiglitazone + metformin (adjusted mean[†]) (95% CI)	-39[‡] (-51, -26)	

* Intent-to-treat population using last observation on study prior to glipizide (or other sulfonylurea) rescue therapy.

† Least squares means adjusted for prior antihyperglycemic therapy status and baseline value.

‡ p<0.001 compared to placebo + metformin + rosiglitazone.

Sitagliptin Add-on Therapy in Patients with Type 2 Diabetes Inadequately Controlled on the Combination of Metformin and Insulin

A total of 641 patients with type 2 diabetes participated in a 24-week, randomized, double-blind, placebo-controlled study designed to assess the efficacy of sitagliptin as add-on to insulin therapy. Approximately 75% of patients were also taking metformin. Patients entered a 2-week, single-blind run-in treatment period on pre-mixed, long-acting, or intermediate-acting insulin, with or without metformin (≥1500 mg per day). Patients using short-acting insulins were excluded unless the short-acting insulin was administered as part of a pre-mixed insulin. After the run-in period, patients with inadequate glycemic control (A1C 7.5% to 11%) were randomized to the addition of either 100 mg of sitagliptin (N=229) or placebo (N=233), administered once daily. Patients were on a stable dose of insulin prior to enrollment with no changes in insulin dose permitted during the run-in period. Patients who failed to meet specific glycemic goals during the double-blind treatment period were to have uptitration of the background insulin dose as rescue therapy.

Among patients also receiving metformin, the median daily insulin (pre-mixed, intermediate or long acting) dose at baseline was 40 units in the sitagliptin-treated patients and 42 units in the placebo-treated patients. The median change from baseline in daily dose of insulin was zero for both groups at the end of the study. Patients receiving sitagliptin with metformin and insulin had significant improvements in A1C, FPG and 2-hour PPG compared to patients receiving placebo with metformin and insulin (Table 12). The adjusted mean change from baseline in body weight was -0.3 kg in patients receiving sitagliptin with metformin and insulin and -0.2 kg in patients receiving placebo with metformin and insulin. There was an increased rate of hypoglycemia in patients treated with sitagliptin. [See Warnings and Precautions (5.9); Adverse Reactions (6.1).]

Table 12: Glycemic Parameters at Final Visit (24-Week Study) for Sitagliptin as Add-on Combination Therapy with Metformin and Insulin*

	Sitagliptin 100 mg + Metformin + Insulin	Placebo + Metformin + Insulin
A1C (%)	N = 223	N = 229
Baseline (mean)	8.7	8.6
Change from baseline (adjusted mean[†,‡])	-0.7	-0.1
Difference from placebo (adjusted mean[†]) (95% CI)	-0.5[§] (-0.7, -0.4)	
Patients (%) achieving A1C <7%	32 (14%)	12 (5%)
FPG (mg/dL)	N = 225	N = 229
Baseline (mean)	173	176
Change from baseline (adjusted mean[†])	-22	-4
Difference from placebo (adjusted mean[†]) (95% CI)	-18[§] (-28, -8.4)	
2-hour PPG (mg/dL)	N = 182	N = 189
Baseline (mean)	281	281
Change from baseline (adjusted mean[†])	-39	1
Difference from placebo (adjusted mean[†]) (95% CI)	-40[§] (-53, -28)	

* Intent-to-treat population using last observation on study prior to rescue therapy.

† Least squares means adjusted for insulin use at the screening visit, type of insulin used at the screening visit (pre-mixed vs. non pre-mixed [intermediate- or long-acting]), and baseline value.

‡ Treatment by insulin stratum interaction was not significant (p >0.10).

§ p<0.001 compared to placebo.

Sitagliptin Add-on Therapy vs. Glipizide Add-on Therapy in Patients with Type 2 Diabetes Inadequately Controlled on Metformin

The efficacy of sitagliptin was evaluated in a 52-week, double-blind, glipizide-controlled noninferiority trial in patients with type 2 diabetes. Patients not on treatment or on other antihyperglycemic agents entered a run-in treatment period of up to 12 weeks duration with metformin monotherapy (dose of ≥1500 mg per day) which included washout of medications other than metformin, if applicable. After the run-in period, those with inadequate glycemic control (A1C 6.5% to 10%) were randomized 1:1 to the addition of sitagliptin 100 mg once daily or glipizide for 52 weeks. Patients receiving glipizide were given an initial dosage of 5 mg/day and then electively titrated over the next 18 weeks to a maximum dosage of 20 mg/day as needed to optimize glycemic control. Thereafter, the glipizide dose was to be kept constant, except for down-titration to prevent hypoglycemia. The mean dose of glipizide after the titration period was 10 mg.

After 52 weeks, sitagliptin and glipizide had similar mean reductions from baseline in A1C in the intent-to-treat analysis (Table 13). These results were consistent with the per protocol analysis (Figure 2). A conclusion in favor of the noninferiority of sitagliptin to glipizide may be limited to patients with baseline A1C comparable to those included in the study (over 70% of patients had baseline A1C <8% and over 90% had A1C <9%).

Table 13: Glycemic Parameters in a 52-Week Study Comparing Sitagliptin to Glipizide as Add-On Therapy in Patients Inadequately Controlled on Metformin (Intent-to-Treat Population)*

	Sitagliptin 100 mg + Metformin	Glipizide + Metformin
A1C (%)	N = 576	N = 559
Baseline (mean)	7.7	7.6
Change from baseline (adjusted mean[†])	-0.5	-0.6
FPG (mg/dL)	N = 583	N = 568
Baseline (mean)	166	164
Change from baseline (adjusted mean[†])	-8	-8

* The intent-to-treat analysis used the patients' last observation in the study prior to discontinuation.

† Least squares means adjusted for prior antihyperglycemic therapy status and baseline A1C value.

Figure 2: Mean Change from Baseline for A1C (%) Over 52 Weeks in a Study Comparing Sitagliptin to Glipizide as Add-On Therapy in Patients Inadequately Controlled on Metformin (Per Protocol Population)*

♦ Sitagliptin 100 mg   ○ Glipizide

* The per protocol population (mean baseline A1C of 7.5%) included patients without major protocol violations who had observations at baseline and at Week 52.

The incidence of hypoglycemia in the sitagliptin group (4.9%) was significantly (p<0.001) lower than that in the glipizide group (32.0%). Patients treated with sitagliptin exhibited a significant mean decrease from baseline in body weight compared to a significant weight gain in patients administered glipizide (-1.5 kg vs. +1.1 kg).

16   HOW SUPPLIED/STORAGE AND HANDLING
No. 6747 — Tablets JANUMET, 50 mg/500 mg, are light pink, capsule-shaped, film-coated tablets with "575" debossed on one side. They are supplied as follows:
NDC 0006-0575-61 unit-of-use bottles of 60
NDC 0006-0575-62 unit-of-use bottles of 180
NDC 0006-0575-52 unit dose blister packages of 50
NDC 0006-0575-82 bulk bottles of 1000.
No. 6749 — Tablets JANUMET, 50 mg/1000 mg, are red, capsule-shaped, film-coated tablets with "577" debossed on one side. They are supplied as follows:
NDC 0006-0577-61 unit-of-use bottles of 60
NDC 0006-0577-62 unit-of-use bottles of 180
NDC 0006-0577-52 unit dose blister packages of 50
NDC 0006-0577-82 bulk bottles of 1000.
Store at 20-25°C (68-77°F), excursions permitted to 15-30°C (59-86°F). [See USP Controlled Room Temperature.]

17   PATIENT COUNSELING INFORMATION

See FDA-Approved Patient Labeling (Medication Guide).
17.1   Instructions
Patients should be informed of the potential risks and benefits of JANUMET and of alternative modes of therapy. They should also be informed about the importance of adherence to dietary instructions, regular physical activity, periodic blood glucose monitoring and A1C testing, recognition and management of hypoglycemia and hyperglycemia, and assessment for diabetes complications. During periods of stress such as fever, trauma, infection, or surgery, medication requirements may change and patients should be advised to seek medical advice promptly.
The risks of lactic acidosis due to the metformin component, its symptoms, and conditions that predispose to its development, as noted in Warnings and Precautions (5.1), should be explained to patients. Patients should be advised to discontinue JANUMET immediately and to promptly notify their health practitioner if unexplained hyperventilation, myalgia, malaise, unusual somnolence, dizziness, slow or irregular heart beat, sensation of feeling cold (especially in the extremities) or other nonspecific symptoms occur. Gastrointestinal symptoms are common during initiation of metformin treatment and may occur during initiation of JANUMET therapy; however, patients should consult their physician if they develop unexplained symptoms. Although gastrointestinal symptoms that occur after stabilization are unlikely to be drug related, such an occurrence of symptoms should be evaluated to determine if it may be due to lactic acidosis or other serious disease.
Patients should be counseled against excessive alcohol intake, either acute or chronic, while receiving JANUMET.

Patients should be informed about the importance of regular testing of renal function and hematological parameters when receiving treatment with JANUMET.

Patients should be informed that acute pancreatitis has been reported during postmarketing use of JANUMET. Patients should be informed that persistent severe abdominal pain, sometimes radiating to the back, which may or may not be accompanied by vomiting, is the hallmark symptom of acute pancreatitis. Patients should be instructed to promptly discontinue JANUMET and contact their physician if persistent severe abdominal pain occurs [see Warnings and Precautions (5.2)].

Patients should be informed that the incidence of hypoglycemia is increased when JANUMET is added to an insulin secretagogue (e.g., sulfonylurea) or insulin therapy and that a lower dose of the insulin secretagogue or insulin may be required to reduce the risk of hypoglycemia.

Patients should be informed that allergic reactions have been reported during postmarketing use of sitagliptin, one of the components of JANUMET. If symptoms of allergic reactions (including rash, hives, and swelling of the face, lips, tongue, and throat that may cause difficulty in breathing or swallowing) occur, patients must stop taking JANUMET and seek medical advice promptly.

Patients should be informed that the tablets must never be split or divided before swallowing.

Physicians should instruct their patients to read the Medication Guide before starting JANUMET therapy and to re-read each time the prescription is renewed. Patients should be instructed to inform their doctor if they develop any bothersome or unusual symptom, or if any symptom persists or worsens.

17.2   Laboratory Tests

Response to all diabetic therapies should be monitored by periodic measurements of blood glucose and A1C levels, with a goal of decreasing these levels towards the normal range. A1C is especially useful for evaluating long-term glycemic control.

Initial and periodic monitoring of hematologic parameters (e.g., hemoglobin/hematocrit and red blood cell indices) and renal function (serum creatinine) should be performed, at least on an annual basis. While megaloblastic anemia has rarely been seen with metformin therapy, if this is suspected, Vitamin B_{12} deficiency should be excluded.

Dist. by: Merck Sharp & Dohme Corp., a subsidiary of **MERCK & CO., INC.,** Whitehouse Station, NJ 08889, USA

For patent information: www.merck.com/product/patent/home.html

The trademarks depicted herein are owned by their respective companies.

Copyright © 2007, 2008, 2009, 2010 Merck Sharp & Dohme Corp., a subsidiary of **Merck & Co., Inc.**

All rights reserved.

uspi-mk0431a-t-1402r009

Medication Guide

JANUMET® (JAN-you-met)

(sitagliptin and metformin hydrochloride)

Tablets

Read this Medication Guide carefully before you start taking JANUMET and each time you get a refill. There may be new information. This information does not take the place of talking with your doctor about your medical condition or your treatment. If you have any questions about JANUMET, ask your doctor or pharmacist.

What is the most important information I should know about JANUMET?

Serious side effects can happen in people taking JANUMET, including:

1. Lactic Acidosis. Metformin, one of the medicines in JANUMET, can cause a rare but serious condition called lactic acidosis (a build-up of lactic acid in the blood) that can cause death. Lactic acidosis is a medical emergency and must be treated in the hospital.

Stop taking JANUMET and call your doctor right away if you get any of the following symptoms, which could be signs of lactic acidosis.

You:
• feel very weak or tired.
• have unusual (not normal) muscle pain.
• have trouble breathing.
• have unusual sleepiness or sleep longer than usual.
• have sudden stomach or intestinal problems with nausea and vomiting or diarrhea.
• feel cold, especially in your arms and legs.
• feel dizzy or lightheaded.
• have a slow or irregular heartbeat.

You have a higher chance of getting lactic acidosis if you:
• have kidney problems. People whose kidneys are not working properly should not take JANUMET.
• have liver problems.
• have congestive heart failure that requires treatment with medicines.
• drink alcohol very often, or drink a lot of alcohol in short-term "binge" drinking.

• get dehydrated (lose a large amount of body fluids). This can happen if you are sick with a fever, vomiting, or diarrhea. Dehydration can also happen when you sweat a lot with activity or exercise and do not drink enough fluids.
• have certain x-ray tests with dyes or contrast agents that are injected into your body.
• have surgery.
• have a heart attack, severe infection, or stroke.

2. Pancreatitis (inflammation of the pancreas) which may be severe and lead to death.

Certain medical problems make you more likely to get pancreatitis.

Before you start taking JANUMET:

Tell your doctor if you have ever had
• pancreatitis
• stones in your gallbladder (gallstones)
• a history of alcoholism
• high blood triglyceride levels

Stop taking JANUMET and call your doctor right away if you have pain in your stomach area (abdomen) that is severe and will not go away. The pain may be felt going from your abdomen through to your back. The pain may happen with or without vomiting. These may be symptoms of pancreatitis.

What is JANUMET?

• JANUMET is a prescription medicine that contains two prescription diabetes medicines, sitagliptin (JANUVIA®) and metformin. JANUMET can be used along with diet and exercise to lower blood sugar in adults with type 2 diabetes.
• JANUMET is not for people with type 1 diabetes.
• JANUMET is not for people with diabetic ketoacidosis (increased ketones in your blood or urine).
• If you have had pancreatitis (inflammation of the pancreas) in the past, it is not known if you have a higher chance of getting pancreatitis while you take JANUMET.
• It is not known if JANUMET is safe and effective when used in children under 18 years of age.

Who should not take JANUMET?

Do not take JANUMET if:
• your kidneys are not working properly.
• you are allergic to any of the ingredients in JANUMET. See the end of this Medication Guide for a complete list of ingredients in JANUMET.

Symptoms of a serious allergic reaction to JANUMET may include:
  ◦ rash
  ◦ raised red patches on your skin (hives)
  ◦ swelling of the face, lips, tongue, and throat that may cause difficulty in breathing or swallowing
• you have diabetic ketoacidosis. See "What is JANUMET?"

What should I tell my doctor before taking JANUMET?

Before you take JANUMET, tell your doctor if you:
• have or have had inflammation of your pancreas (pancreatitis).
• have kidney problems.
• have liver problems.
• have heart problems, including congestive heart failure.
• drink alcohol very often, or drink a lot of alcohol in short-term "binge" drinking.
• are going to get an injection of dye or contrast agents for an x-ray procedure; JANUMET will need to be stopped for a short time. Talk to your doctor about when you should stop JANUMET and when you should start JANUMET again. See "What is the most important information I should know about JANUMET?".
• have any other medical conditions.
• are pregnant or plan to become pregnant. It is not known if JANUMET will harm your unborn baby. If you are pregnant, talk with your doctor about the best way to control your blood sugar while you are pregnant.

Pregnancy Registry: If you take JANUMET at any time during your pregnancy, talk with your doctor about how you can join the JANUMET pregnancy registry. The purpose of this registry is to collect information about the health of you and your baby. You can enroll in this registry by calling 1-800-986-8999.
• are breast-feeding or plan to breast-feed. It is not known if JANUMET will pass into your breast milk. Talk with your doctor about the best way to feed your baby if you are taking JANUMET.

Tell your doctor about all the medicines you take, including prescription and non-prescription medicines, vitamins, and herbal supplements. JANUMET may affect how well other drugs work and some drugs can affect how well JANUMET works.

Know the medicines you take. Keep a list of your medicines and show it to your doctor and pharmacist when you get a new medicine.

How should I take JANUMET?
• Take JANUMET exactly as your doctor tells you.
• Your doctor may change your dose of JANUMET if needed.
• Your doctor may tell you to take JANUMET along with certain other diabetes medicines. Low blood sugar can

happen more often when JANUMET is taken with certain other diabetes medicines. See "**What are the possible side effects of JANUMET?**".
• Take JANUMET with meals to lower your chance of having an upset stomach.
• Do not break or cut JANUMET tablets before swallowing. If you cannot swallow JANUMET tablets whole, tell your doctor.
• Continue to take JANUMET as long as your doctor tells you.
• If you take too much JANUMET, call your doctor or local Poison Control Center right away.
• If you miss a dose, take it with food as soon as you remember. If you do not remember until it is time for your next dose, skip the missed dose and go back to your regular schedule. Do not take two doses of JANUMET at the same time.
• You may need to stop taking JANUMET for a short time. Call your doctor for instructions if you:
  ◦ are dehydrated (have lost too much body fluid). Dehydration can occur if you are sick with severe vomiting, diarrhea or fever, or if you drink a lot less fluid than normal.
  ◦ plan to have surgery.
  ◦ are going to get an injection of dye or contrast agent for an x-ray procedure. See "**What is the most important information I should know about JANUMET?**" and "**What should I tell my doctor before taking JANUMET?**"
• When your body is under some types of stress, such as fever, trauma (such as a car accident), infection or surgery, the amount of diabetes medicine that you need may change. Tell your doctor right away if you have any of these problems and follow your doctor's instructions.
• Check your blood sugar as your doctor tells you to.
• Stay on your prescribed diet and exercise program while taking JANUMET.
• Talk to your doctor about how to prevent, recognize and manage low blood sugar (hypoglycemia), high blood sugar (hyperglycemia), and problems you have because of your diabetes.
• Your doctor will check your diabetes with regular blood tests, including your blood sugar levels and your hemoglobin A1C.
• Your doctor will do blood tests to check how well your kidneys are working before and during your treatment with JANUMET.

What are the possible side effects of JANUMET?

Serious side effects have happened in people taking JANUMET.
• See "**What is the most important information I should know about JANUMET?**".
• **Low blood sugar (hypoglycemia).** If you take JANUMET with another medicine that can cause low blood sugar, such as a sulfonylurea or insulin, your risk of getting low blood sugar is higher. The dose of your sulfonylurea medicine or insulin may need to be lowered while you use JANUMET. Signs and symptoms of low blood sugar may include:

• headache	• irritability
• drowsiness	• hunger
• weakness	• fast heart beat
• dizziness	• sweating
• confusion	• feeling jittery

• **Serious allergic reactions.** If you have any symptoms of a serious allergic reaction, stop taking JANUMET and call your doctor right away. See "**Who should not take JANUMET?**". Your doctor may give you a medicine for your allergic reaction and prescribe a different medicine for your diabetes.
• **Kidney problems**, sometimes requiring dialysis.

The most common side effects of JANUMET include:
• stuffy or runny nose and sore throat
• upper respiratory infection
• diarrhea
• nausea and vomiting
• gas, upset stomach, indigestion
• weakness
• headache
• low blood sugar (hypoglycemia) when used in combination with certain medications, such as a sulfonylurea or insulin.

Taking JANUMET with meals can help lessen the common stomach side effects of metformin that usually happen at the beginning of treatment. If you have unusual or sudden stomach problems, talk with your doctor. Stomach problems that start later during treatment may be a sign of something more serious.

JANUMET may have other side effects, including:
• swelling of the hands or legs. Swelling of the hands and legs can happen if you take JANUMET in combination with rosiglitazone (Avandia®). Rosiglitazone is another type of diabetes medicine.

These are not all the possible side effects of JANUMET. For more information, ask your doctor or pharmacist.

Tell your doctor if you have any side effect that bothers you, is unusual, or does not go away.

Call your doctor for medical advice about side effects. You may report side effects to FDA at 1-800-FDA-1088.

How should I store JANUMET?
Store JANUMET at 68°F to 77°F (20°C to 25°C).

Keep JANUMET and all medicines out of the reach of children.

General information about the use of JANUMET
Medicines are sometimes prescribed for purposes other than those listed in Medication Guides. Do not use JANUMET for a condition for which it was not prescribed. Do not give JANUMET to other people, even if they have the same symptoms you have. It may harm them.

This Medication Guide summarizes the most important information about JANUMET. If you would like to know more information, talk with your doctor. You can ask your doctor or pharmacist for additional information about JANUMET that is written for health care professionals. For more information go to www.JANUMET.com or call 1-800-622-4477.

What are the ingredients in JANUMET?
Active ingredients: sitagliptin and metformin hydrochloride

Inactive ingredients: microcrystalline cellulose, polyvinylpyrrolidone, sodium lauryl sulfate, and sodium stearyl fumarate. The tablet film coating contains the following inactive ingredients: polyvinyl alcohol, polyethylene glycol, talc, titanium dioxide, red iron oxide, and black iron oxide.

What is type 2 diabetes?
Type 2 diabetes is a condition in which your body does not make enough insulin, and the insulin that your body produces does not work as well as it should. Your body can also make too much sugar. When this happens, sugar (glucose) builds up in the blood. This can lead to serious medical problems.

High blood sugar can be lowered by diet and exercise, and by certain medicines when necessary.

This Medication Guide has been approved by the U.S. Food and Drug Administration.

Dist. by: Merck Sharp & Dohme Corp., a subsidiary of **MERCK & CO., INC.**, Whitehouse Station, NJ 08889, USA

For patent information: www.merck.com/product/patent/home.html

The trademarks depicted herein are owned by their respective companies.

Copyright © 2010 Merck Sharp & Dohme Corp., a subsidiary of **Merck & Co., Inc.**

All rights reserved.

Revised: 02/2014

usmg-mk0431a-t-1402r009

Shown in Product Identification Guide, page 308

JANUMET® XR ℞
[JAN-you-met]
(sitagliptin and metformin HCl extended-release) tablets

HIGHLIGHTS OF PRESCRIBING INFORMATION
These highlights do not include all the information needed to use JANUMET XR safely and effectively. See full prescribing information for JANUMET XR.

JANUMET® XR (sitagliptin and metformin HCl extended-release) tablets
Initial U.S. Approval: 2012

WARNING: LACTIC ACIDOSIS

See full prescribing information for complete boxed warning.

- **Lactic acidosis can occur due to metformin accumulation. The risk increases with conditions such as sepsis, dehydration, excess alcohol intake, hepatic insufficiency, renal impairment, and acute congestive heart failure. (5.1)**
- **Symptoms include malaise, myalgias, respiratory distress, increasing somnolence, and nonspecific abdominal distress. Laboratory abnormalities include low pH, increased anion gap and elevated blood lactate. (5.1)**
- **If acidosis is suspected, discontinue JANUMET XR and hospitalize the patient immediately. (5.1)**

——RECENT MAJOR CHANGES——

Dosage and Administration
Recommended Dosing (2.1)   02/2014

——INDICATIONS AND USAGE——

JANUMET XR is a dipeptidyl peptidase-4 (DPP-4) inhibitor and biguanide combination product indicated as an adjunct to diet and exercise to improve glycemic control in adults with type 2 diabetes mellitus when treatment with both sitagliptin and metformin extended-release is appropriate. (1, 14)

Important Limitations of Use:
- Not for the treatment of type 1 diabetes or diabetic ketoacidosis. (1)
- Has not been studied in patients with a history of pancreatitis. (1, 5.2)

——DOSAGE AND ADMINISTRATION——

- Individualize the starting dose of JANUMET XR based on the patient's current regimen. (2.1)
- May adjust the dosing based on effectiveness and tolerability while not exceeding the maximum recommended daily dose of 100 mg sitagliptin and 2000 mg metformin extended-release. (2.1)
- Administer once daily with a meal preferably in the evening. Gradually escalate the dose to reduce the gastrointestinal side effects due to metformin. (2.1)
- Maintain the same total daily dose of sitagliptin and metformin when changing between JANUMET and JANUMET XR, without exceeding the maximum recommended daily dose of 2000 mg metformin extended-release. (2.1)

——DOSAGE FORMS AND STRENGTHS——

JANUMET XR Tablets: 100 mg sitagliptin/1000 mg metformin HCl extended-release, 50 mg sitagliptin/500 mg metformin HCl extended-release, and 50 mg sitagliptin/1000 mg metformin HCl extended-release. (3)

——CONTRAINDICATIONS——

- Renal dysfunction, e.g., serum creatinine ≥1.5 mg/dL [males], ≥1.4 mg/dL [females] or abnormal creatinine clearance. (4, 5.1, 5.4)
- Metabolic acidosis, including diabetic ketoacidosis. (4, 5.1)
- History of a serious hypersensitivity reaction (e.g., anaphylaxis or angioedema) to JANUMET XR or to one of its components. (5.14, 6.2)

——WARNINGS AND PRECAUTIONS——

- Lactic acidosis: Warn against excessive alcohol intake. JANUMET XR is not recommended in hepatic impairment and is contraindicated in renal impairment. Ensure normal renal function before initiating and at least annually thereafter.
- Temporarily discontinue JANUMET XR in patients undergoing radiologic studies with intravascular administration of iodinated contrast materials or any surgical procedures necessitating restricted intake of food or fluids. (5.1, 5.3, 5.4, 5.7)
- There have been postmarketing reports of acute pancreatitis, including fatal and non-fatal hemorrhagic or necrotizing pancreatitis in patients treated with sitagliptin (one of the components of JANUMET XR) with or without metformin. If pancreatitis is suspected, promptly discontinue JANUMET XR. (5.2)
- There have been postmarketing reports of acute renal failure in patients treated with sitagliptin with or without metformin, sometimes requiring dialysis. Before initiating JANUMET XR and at least annually thereafter, assess renal function and verify as normal. (4, 5.1, 5.4, 5.10, 6.2)
- Vitamin B$_{12}$ deficiency: Metformin may lower Vitamin B$_{12}$ levels. Measure hematologic parameters annually. (5.5, 6.1)
- When used with an insulin secretagogue (e.g., sulfonylurea) or with insulin, a lower dose of the insulin secretagogue or insulin may be required to minimize the risk of hypoglycemia. (2.1, 5.9)
- There have been postmarketing reports of serious allergic and hypersensitivity reactions in patients treated with sitagliptin, such as anaphylaxis, angioedema, and exfoliative skin conditions including Stevens-Johnson syndrome. In such cases, promptly stop JANUMET XR, assess for other potential causes, institute appropriate monitoring and treatment, and initiate alternative treatment for diabetes. (5.14, 6.2)
- There have been no clinical studies establishing conclusive evidence of macrovascular risk reduction with JANUMET XR or any other anti-diabetic drug. (5.15)

——ADVERSE REACTIONS——

- The most common adverse reactions reported in ≥5% of patients simultaneously started on sitagliptin and metformin and more commonly than in patients treated with placebo were diarrhea, upper respiratory tract infection, and headache. (6.1)
- Adverse reactions reported in ≥5% of patients treated with sitagliptin in combination with sulfonylurea and metformin and more commonly than in patients treated with placebo in combination with sulfonylurea and metformin were hypoglycemia and headache. (6.1)
- Hypoglycemia was the only adverse reaction reported in ≥5% of patients treated with sitagliptin in combination with insulin and metformin and more commonly than in patients treated with placebo in combination with insulin and metformin. (6.1)

To report SUSPECTED ADVERSE REACTIONS, contact Merck Sharp & Dohme Corp., a subsidiary of Merck & Co., Inc., at 1-877-888-4231 or FDA at 1-800-FDA-1088 or www.fda.gov/medwatch.

——DRUG INTERACTIONS——

- Cationic drugs eliminated by renal tubular secretion: Use with caution. (5.10, 7.2)

——USE IN SPECIFIC POPULATIONS——

- Safety and effectiveness of JANUMET XR in children under 18 years have not been established. (8.4)
- There are no adequate and well-controlled studies in pregnant women. To report drug exposure during pregnancy call 1-800-986-8999. (8.1)

See 17 for PATIENT COUNSELING INFORMATION and Medication Guide

Revised: 02/2014

FULL PRESCRIBING INFORMATION

WARNING: LACTIC ACIDOSIS

Lactic acidosis is a rare, but serious complication that can occur due to metformin accumulation. The risk increases with conditions such as sepsis, dehydration, excess alcohol intake, hepatic impairment, renal impairment, and acute congestive heart failure.

The onset of lactic acidosis is often subtle, accompanied only by nonspecific symptoms such as malaise, myalgias, respiratory distress, increasing somnolence, and nonspecific abdominal distress.

Laboratory abnormalities include low pH, increased anion gap and elevated blood lactate.

If acidosis is suspected, JANUMET XR (sitagliptin and metformin HCl extended-release) tablets should be discontinued and the patient hospitalized immediately. *[See Warnings and Precautions (5.1).]*

1 INDICATIONS AND USAGE

JANUMET® XR is indicated as an adjunct to diet and exercise to improve glycemic control in adults with type 2 diabetes mellitus when treatment with both sitagliptin and metformin extended-release is appropriate. *[See Clinical Studies (14).]*

Important Limitations of Use

JANUMET XR should not be used in patients with type 1 diabetes mellitus or for the treatment of diabetic ketoacidosis.

JANUMET XR has not been studied in patients with a history of pancreatitis. It is unknown whether patients with a history of pancreatitis are at increased risk for the development of pancreatitis while using JANUMET XR. *[See Warnings and Precautions (5.2).]*

2 DOSAGE AND ADMINISTRATION

2.1 Recommended Dosing

The dose of JANUMET XR should be individualized on the basis of the patient's current regimen, effectiveness, and tolerability while not exceeding the maximum recommended daily dose of 100 mg sitagliptin and 2000 mg metformin. Initial combination therapy or maintenance of combination therapy should be individualized and left to the discretion of the healthcare provider.

- In patients not currently treated with metformin, the recommended total daily starting dose of JANUMET XR is 100 mg sitagliptin and 1000 mg metformin hydrochloride (HCl) extended-release. Patients with inadequate glycemic control on this dose of metformin can be titrated gradually, to reduce gastrointestinal side effects associated with metformin, up to the maximum recommended daily dose.
- In patients already treated with metformin, the recommended total daily starting dose of JANUMET XR is 100 mg sitagliptin and the previously prescribed dose of metformin.
- For patients taking metformin immediate-release 850 mg twice daily or 1000 mg twice daily, the recommended starting dose of JANUMET XR is two 50 mg sitagliptin/ 1000 mg metformin hydrochloride extended-release tablets taken together once daily.
- Maintain the same total daily dose of sitagliptin and metformin when changing between JANUMET (sitagliptin and metformin HCl immediate-release) and JANUMET XR. Patients with inadequate glycemic control on this dose of metformin can be titrated gradually, to reduce gastrointestinal side effects associated with metformin, up to the maximum recommended daily dose.

JANUMET XR should be administered with food to reduce the gastrointestinal side effects associated with the metformin component. JANUMET XR should be given once daily with a meal preferably in the evening. JANUMET XR should be swallowed whole. The tablets must not be split, crushed, or chewed before swallowing. There have been reports of incompletely dissolved JANUMET XR tablets being eliminated in the feces. It is not known whether this material seen in feces contains active drug. If a patient reports repeatedly seeing tablets in feces, the healthcare provider should assess adequacy of glycemic control *[see Patient Counseling Information (17.1)].*

The 100 mg sitagliptin/1000 mg metformin hydrochloride extended-release tablet should be taken as a single tablet once daily. Patients using two JANUMET XR tablets (such as two 50 mg sitagliptin/500 mg metformin hydrochloride extended-release tablets or two 50 mg sitagliptin/1000 mg metformin hydrochloride extended-release tablets) should take the two tablets together once daily.

Patients treated with an insulin secretagogue or insulin

Coadministration of JANUMET XR with an insulin secretagogue (e.g., sulfonylurea) or insulin may require lower doses of the insulin secretagogue or insulin to reduce the risk of hypoglycemia *[see Warnings and Precautions (5.9)].* No studies have been performed specifically examining the safety and efficacy of JANUMET XR in patients previously treated with other oral antihyperglycemic agents and switched to JANUMET XR. Any change in therapy of type 2 diabetes should be undertaken with care and appropriate monitoring as changes in glycemic control can occur.

3 DOSAGE FORMS AND STRENGTHS

- 100 mg/1000 mg tablets are blue, bi-convex oval, film-coated tablets with "81" debossed on one side.
- 50 mg/500 mg tablets are light blue, bi-convex oval, film-coated tablets with "78" debossed on one side.
- 50 mg/1000 mg tablets are light green, bi-convex oval, film-coated tablets with "80" debossed on one side.

4 CONTRAINDICATIONS

JANUMET XR is contraindicated in patients with:

- Renal impairment (e.g., serum creatinine levels greater than or equal to 1.5 mg/dL for men, greater than or equal to 1.4 mg/dL for women or abnormal creatinine clearance), which may also result from conditions such as cardiovascular collapse (shock), acute myocardial infarction, and septicemia *[see Warnings and Precautions (5.1)].*

- Hypersensitivity to metformin hydrochloride.
- Acute or chronic metabolic acidosis, including diabetic ketoacidosis. Diabetic ketoacidosis should be treated with insulin.
- History of a serious hypersensitivity reaction to JANUMET XR or sitagliptin, such as anaphylaxis or angioedema. *[See Warnings and Precautions (5.14); Adverse Reactions (6.2).]*

5 WARNINGS AND PRECAUTIONS

5.1 Lactic Acidosis

Metformin hydrochloride

Lactic acidosis is a serious, metabolic complication that can occur due to metformin accumulation during treatment with JANUMET XR and is fatal in approximately 50% of cases. Lactic acidosis may also occur in association with a number of pathophysiologic conditions, including diabetes mellitus, and whenever there is significant tissue hypoperfusion and hypoxemia. Lactic acidosis is characterized by elevated blood lactate concentrations (>5 mmol/L), decreased blood pH, electrolyte disturbances with an increased anion gap, and an increased lactate/pyruvate ratio. When metformin is implicated as the cause of lactic acidosis, metformin plasma levels >5 µg/mL are generally found. The reported incidence of lactic acidosis in patients receiving metformin hydrochloride is approximately 0.03 cases/1000 patient-years, with approximately 0.015 fatal cases/1000 patient-years. In more than 20,000 patient-years exposure to metformin in clinical trials, there were no reports of lactic acidosis. Reported cases have occurred primarily in diabetic patients with significant renal impairment, including both intrinsic renal disease and renal hypoperfusion, often in the setting of multiple concomitant medical/surgical problems and multiple concomitant medications. Patients with congestive heart failure requiring pharmacologic management, in particular those with unstable or acute congestive heart failure who are at risk of hypoperfusion and hypoxemia, are at increased risk of lactic acidosis. The risk of lactic acidosis increases with the degree of renal dysfunction and the patient's age. The risk of lactic acidosis may, therefore, be significantly decreased by regular monitoring of renal function in patients taking JANUMET XR. In particular, treatment of the elderly should be accompanied by careful monitoring of renal function. JANUMET XR treatment should not be initiated in any patient unless measurement of creatinine clearance demonstrates that renal function is not reduced. In addition, JANUMET XR should be promptly withheld in the presence of any condition associated with hypoxemia, dehydration, or sepsis. Because impaired hepatic function may significantly limit the ability to clear lactate, JANUMET XR should generally be avoided in patients with clinical or laboratory evidence of hepatic impairment. Patients should be cautioned against excessive alcohol intake when taking JANUMET XR, because alcohol potentiates the effects of metformin on lactate metabolism. In addition, JANUMET XR should be temporarily discontinued prior to any intravascular radiocontrast study and for any surgical procedure necessitating restricted intake of food or fluids. Use of topiramate, a carbonic anhydrase inhibitor, in epilepsy and migraine prophylaxis may frequently cause dose-dependent metabolic acidosis (in controlled trials, 32% and 67% for adjunctive treatment in adults and pediatric patients, respectively, and 15 to 25% for monotherapy of epilepsy, with decrease in serum bicarbonate to less than 20 mEq/L; 3% and 11% for adjunctive treatment in adults and pediatric patients, respectively, and 1 to 7% for monotherapy of epilepsy, with decrease in serum bicarbonate to less than 17 mEq/L) and may exacerbate the risk of metformin-induced lactic acidosis. *[See Drug Interactions (7.1); Clinical Pharmacology (12).]* The onset of lactic acidosis often is subtle, and accompanied only by nonspecific symptoms such as malaise, myalgias, respiratory distress, increasing somnolence, and nonspecific abdominal distress. There may be associated hypothermia, hypotension, and resistant bradyarrhythmias with more marked acidosis. Patients should be educated to promptly report these symptoms to their physician should they occur. If present, JANUMET XR should be withdrawn until lactic acidosis is ruled out. Serum electrolytes, ketones, blood glucose, blood pH, lactate levels, and blood metformin levels may be useful. Once a patient is stabilized on any dose level of JANUMET XR, gastrointestinal symptoms, which are common during initiation of therapy, are unlikely to recur. Later occurrence of gastrointestinal symptoms could be due to lactic acidosis or other serious disease. Levels of fasting venous plasma lactate above the upper limit of normal but less than 5 mmol/L in patients taking JANUMET XR do not necessarily indicate impending lactic acidosis and may be explainable by other mechanisms, such as poorly-controlled diabetes or obesity, vigorous physical activity, or technical problems in sample handling. Lactic acidosis should be suspected in any diabetic patient with metabolic acidosis lacking evidence of ketoacidosis (ketonuria and ketonemia). Lactic acidosis is a medical emergency that must be treated in a hospital setting. In a patient with lactic acidosis who is taking JANUMET XR, the drug should be discontinued immediately and general supportive measures promptly instituted. Because metformin hydrochloride is dialyzable (with a clearance of up to 170 mL/min under good hemodynamic conditions), prompt hemodialysis is recommended to correct the acidosis and remove the accumulated metformin. Such management often results in prompt reversal of symptoms and recovery. *[See Contraindications (4).]*

5.2 Pancreatitis

There have been postmarketing reports of acute pancreatitis, including fatal and non-fatal hemorrhagic or necrotizing pancreatitis, in patients taking sitagliptin with or without metformin. After initiation of JANUMET XR, patients should be observed carefully for signs and symptoms of pancreatitis. If pancreatitis is suspected, JANUMET XR should be promptly discontinued and appropriate management should be initiated. It is unknown whether patients with a history of pancreatitis are at increased risk for the development of pancreatitis while using JANUMET XR.

5.3 Impaired Hepatic Function

Since impaired hepatic function has been associated with some cases of lactic acidosis, JANUMET XR should generally be avoided in patients with clinical or laboratory evidence of hepatic disease.

5.4 Assessment of Renal Function

Metformin and sitagliptin are substantially excreted by the kidney.

Metformin hydrochloride

The risk of metformin accumulation and lactic acidosis increases with the degree of impairment of renal function. Therefore, JANUMET XR is contraindicated in patients with renal impairment.

Before initiation of JANUMET XR and at least annually thereafter, renal function should be assessed and verified as normal. In patients in whom development of renal dysfunction is anticipated (e.g., elderly), renal function should be assessed more frequently and JANUMET XR discontinued if evidence of renal impairment is present.

Sitagliptin

There have been postmarketing reports of worsening renal function in patients taking sitagliptin with or without metformin, including acute renal failure, sometimes requiring dialysis. Before initiation of therapy with JANUMET XR and at least annually thereafter, renal function should be assessed and verified as normal. In patients in whom development of renal dysfunction is anticipated, particularly in elderly patients, renal function should be assessed more frequently and JANUMET XR discontinued if evidence of renal impairment is present.

5.5 Vitamin B$_{12}$ Levels

In controlled clinical trials of metformin of 29 weeks duration, a decrease to subnormal levels of previously normal serum Vitamin B$_{12}$ levels, without clinical manifestations, was observed in approximately 7% of patients. Such decrease, possibly due to interference with B$_{12}$ absorption from the B$_{12}$-intrinsic factor complex, is, however, very rarely associated with anemia and appears to be rapidly reversible with discontinuation of metformin or Vitamin B$_{12}$ supplementation. Measurement of hematologic parameters on an annual basis is advised in patients on JANUMET XR and any apparent abnormalities should be appropriately investigated and managed. *[See Adverse Reactions (6.1).]* Certain individuals (those with inadequate Vitamin B$_{12}$ or calcium intake or absorption) appear to be predisposed to developing subnormal Vitamin B$_{12}$ levels. In these patients, routine serum Vitamin B$_{12}$ measurements at two- to three-year intervals may be useful.

5.6 Alcohol Intake

Alcohol potentiates the effect of metformin on lactate metabolism. Patients should be warned against excessive alcohol intake while receiving JANUMET XR.

5.7 Surgical Procedures

Use of JANUMET XR should be temporarily suspended for any surgical procedure (except minor procedures not associated with restricted intake of food and fluids) and should not be restarted until the patient's oral intake has resumed and renal function has been evaluated as normal.

5.8 Change in Clinical Status of Patients with Previously Controlled Type 2 Diabetes

A patient with type 2 diabetes previously well controlled on JANUMET XR who develops laboratory abnormalities or clinical illness (especially vague and poorly defined illness) should be evaluated promptly for evidence of ketoacidosis or lactic acidosis. Evaluation should include serum electrolytes and ketones, blood glucose and, if indicated, blood pH, lactate, pyruvate, and metformin levels. If acidosis of either form occurs, JANUMET XR must be stopped immediately and other appropriate corrective measures initiated.

5.9 Use with Medications Known to Cause Hypoglycemia

Sitagliptin

When sitagliptin was used in combination with a sulfonylurea or with insulin, medications known to cause hypoglycemia, the incidence of hypoglycemia was increased over

Table 1: Sitagliptin and Metformin Immediate-Release Coadministered to Patients with Type 2 Diabetes Inadequately Controlled on Diet and Exercise: Adverse Reactions Reported (Regardless of Investigator Assessment of Causality) in ≥5% of Patients Receiving Combination Therapy (and Greater than in Patients Receiving Placebo) *

	Number of Patients (%)			
	Placebo	Sitagliptin 100 mg once daily	Metformin Immediate-Release 500 mg or 1000 mg twice daily [†]	Sitagliptin 50 mg twice daily + Metformin Immediate-Release 500 mg or 1000 mg twice daily [†]
	N = 176	N = 179	N = 364[†]	N = 372[†]
Diarrhea	7 (4.0)	5 (2.8)	28 (7.7)	28 (7.5)
Upper Respiratory Tract Infection	9 (5.1)	8 (4.5)	19 (5.2)	23 (6.2)
Headache	5 (2.8)	2 (1.1)	14 (3.8)	22 (5.9)

* Intent-to-treat population.
† Data pooled for the patients given the lower and higher doses of metformin.

Table 2: Pre-selected Gastrointestinal Adverse Reactions (Regardless of Investigator Assessment of Causality) Reported in Patients with Type 2 Diabetes Receiving Sitagliptin and Metformin Immediate-Release

	Number of Patients (%)					
	Study of Sitagliptin and Metformin Immediate-Release in Patients Inadequately Controlled on Diet and Exercise				Study of Sitagliptin Add-on in Patients Inadequately Controlled on Metformin Immediate-Release Alone	
	Placebo	Sitagliptin 100 mg once daily	Metformin Immediate-Release 500 mg or 1000 mg twice daily *	Sitagliptin 50 mg bid + Metformin Immediate-Release 500 mg or 1000 mg twice daily *	Placebo and Metformin Immediate-Release ≥1500 mg daily	Sitagliptin 100 mg once daily and Metformin Immediate-Release ≥1500 mg daily
	N = 176	N = 179	N = 364	N = 372	N = 237	N = 464
Diarrhea	7 (4.0)	5 (2.8)	28 (7.7)	28 (7.5)	6 (2.5)	11 (2.4)
Nausea	2 (1.1)	2 (1.1)	20 (5.5)	18 (4.8)	2 (0.8)	6 (1.3)
Vomiting	1 (0.6)	0 (0.0)	2 (0.5)	8 (2.2)	2 (0.8)	5 (1.1)
Abdominal Pain[†]	4 (2.3)	6 (3.4)	14 (3.8)	11 (3.0)	9 (3.8)	10 (2.2)

* Data pooled for the patients given the lower and higher doses of metformin.
† Abdominal discomfort was included in the analysis of abdominal pain in the study of initial therapy.

that of placebo used in combination with a sulfonylurea or with insulin [see Adverse Reactions (6)]. Therefore, patients also receiving an insulin secretagogue (e.g., sulfonylurea) or insulin may require a lower dose of the insulin secretagogue or insulin to reduce the risk of hypoglycemia [see Dosage and Administration (2.1)].

Metformin hydrochloride
Hypoglycemia does not occur in patients receiving metformin alone under usual circumstances of use, but could occur when caloric intake is deficient, when strenuous exercise is not compensated by caloric supplementation, or during concomitant use with other glucose-lowering agents (such as sulfonylureas and insulin) or ethanol. Elderly, debilitated, or malnourished patients, and those with adrenal or pituitary insufficiency or alcohol intoxication are particularly susceptible to hypoglycemic effects. Hypoglycemia may be difficult to recognize in the elderly, and in people who are taking β-adrenergic blocking drugs.

5.10 Concomitant Medications Affecting Renal Function or Metformin Disposition
Concomitant medication(s) that may affect renal function or result in significant hemodynamic change or may interfere with the disposition of metformin, such as cationic drugs that are eliminated by renal tubular secretion [see Drug Interactions (7.2)], should be used with caution.

5.11 Radiologic Studies with Intravascular Iodinated Contrast Materials
Intravascular contrast studies with iodinated materials (for example, intravenous urogram, intravenous cholangiography, angiography, and computed tomography (CT) scans with intravascular contrast materials) can lead to acute alteration of renal function and have been associated with lactic acidosis in patients receiving metformin [see Contraindications (4)]. Therefore, in patients in whom any such study is planned, JANUMET XR should be temporarily discontinued at the time of or prior to the procedure, and withheld for

48 hours subsequent to the procedure and reinstituted only after renal function has been re-evaluated and found to be normal.

5.12 Hypoxic States
Cardiovascular collapse (shock) from whatever cause, acute congestive heart failure, acute myocardial infarction and other conditions characterized by hypoxemia have been associated with lactic acidosis and may also cause prerenal azotemia. When such events occur in patients on JANUMET XR therapy, the drug should be promptly discontinued.

5.13 Loss of Control of Blood Glucose
When a patient stabilized on any diabetic regimen is exposed to stress such as fever, trauma, infection, or surgery, a temporary loss of glycemic control may occur. At such times, it may be necessary to withhold JANUMET XR and temporarily administer insulin. JANUMET XR may be reinstituted after the acute episode is resolved.

5.14 Hypersensitivity Reactions
There have been postmarketing reports of serious hypersensitivity reactions in patients treated with sitagliptin, one of the components of JANUMET XR. These reactions include anaphylaxis, angioedema, and exfoliative skin conditions including Stevens-Johnson syndrome. Onset of these reactions occurred within the first 3 months after initiation of treatment with sitagliptin, with some reports occurring after the first dose. If a hypersensitivity reaction is suspected, discontinue JANUMET XR, assess for other potential causes for the event, and institute alternative treatment for diabetes. [See Adverse Reactions (6.2).]
Use caution in a patient with a history of angioedema to another dipeptidyl peptidase-4 (DPP4) inhibitor because it is unknown whether such patients will be predisposed to angioedema with JANUMET XR.

5.15 Macrovascular Outcomes
There have been no clinical studies establishing conclusive evidence of macrovascular risk reduction with JANUMET XR or any other anti-diabetic drug.

6 ADVERSE REACTIONS
6.1 Clinical Trials Experience
Because clinical trials are conducted under widely varying conditions, adverse reaction rates observed in the clinical trials of a drug cannot be directly compared to rates in the clinical trials of another drug and may not reflect the rates observed in practice.
Sitagliptin and Metformin Immediate-Release Coadministration in Patients with Type 2 Diabetes Inadequately Controlled on Diet and Exercise
Table 1 summarizes the most common (≥5% of patients) adverse reactions reported (regardless of investigator assessment of causality) in a 24-week placebo-controlled factorial study in which sitagliptin and metformin immediate-release were coadministered to patients with type 2 diabetes inadequately controlled on diet and exercise.
[See table 1 above]
Sitagliptin Add-on Therapy in Patients with Type 2 Diabetes Inadequately Controlled on Metformin Immediate-Release Alone
In a 24-week placebo-controlled trial of sitagliptin 100 mg administered once daily added to a twice daily metformin immediate-release regimen, there were no adverse reactions reported regardless of investigator assessment of causality in ≥5% of patients and more commonly than in patients given placebo. Discontinuation of therapy due to clinical adverse reactions was similar to the placebo treatment group (sitagliptin and metformin immediate-release, 1.9%; placebo and metformin immediate-release, 2.5%).
Gastrointestinal Adverse Reactions
The incidences of pre-selected gastrointestinal adverse experiences in patients treated with sitagliptin and metformin immediate-release were similar to those reported for patients treated with metformin immediate-release alone. See Table 2.
[See table 2 above]
Sitagliptin in Combination with Metformin Immediate-Release and Glimepiride
In a 24-week placebo-controlled study of sitagliptin 100 mg as add-on therapy in patients with type 2 diabetes inadequately controlled on metformin immediate-release and glimepiride (sitagliptin, N=116; placebo, N=113), the adverse reactions reported regardless of investigator assessment of causality in ≥5% of patients treated with sitagliptin and more commonly than in patients treated with placebo were: hypoglycemia (Table 3) and headache (6.9%, 2.7%).
Sitagliptin in Combination with Metformin Immediate-Release and Rosiglitazone
In a placebo-controlled study of sitagliptin 100 mg as add-on therapy in patients with type 2 diabetes inadequately controlled on metformin immediate-release and rosiglitazone (sitagliptin, N=181; placebo, N=97), the adverse reactions reported regardless of investigator assessment of causality through Week 18 in ≥5% of patients treated with sitagliptin and more commonly than in patients treated with placebo were: upper respiratory tract infection (sitagliptin, 5.5%; placebo, 5.2%) and nasopharyngitis (6.1%, 4.1%). Through Week 54, the adverse reactions reported regardless of investigator assessment of causality in ≥5% of patients treated with sitagliptin and more commonly than in patients treated with placebo were: upper respiratory tract infection (sitagliptin, 15.5%; placebo, 6.2%), nasopharyngitis (11.0%, 9.3%), peripheral edema (8.3%, 5.2%), and headache (5.5%, 4.1%).
Sitagliptin in Combination with Metformin Immediate-Release and Insulin
In a 24-week placebo-controlled study of sitagliptin 100 mg as add-on therapy in patients with type 2 diabetes inadequately controlled on metformin immediate-release and insulin (sitagliptin, N=229; placebo, N=233), the only adverse reaction reported regardless of investigator assessment of causality in ≥5% of patients treated with sitagliptin and more commonly than in patients treated with placebo was hypoglycemia (Table 3).
Hypoglycemia
In all (N=5) studies, adverse reactions of hypoglycemia were based on all reports of symptomatic hypoglycemia; a concurrent glucose measurement was not required although most (77%) reports of hypoglycemia were accompanied by a blood glucose measurement ≤70 mg/dL. When the combination of sitagliptin and metformin immediate-release was coadministered with a sulfonylurea or with insulin, the percentage of patients reporting at least one adverse reaction of hypoglycemia was higher than that observed with placebo and metformin immediate-release coadministered with a sulfonylurea or with insulin (Table 3).
[See table 3 at top of next page]
The overall incidence of reported adverse reactions of hypoglycemia in patients with type 2 diabetes inadequately controlled on diet and exercise was 0.6% in patients given placebo, 0.6% in patients given sitagliptin alone, 0.8% in patients given metformin immediate-release alone, and 1.6% in patients given sitagliptin in combination with metformin immediate-release. In patients with type 2 diabetes inadequately controlled on metformin immediate-release alone, the overall incidence of adverse reactions of hypoglycemia was 1.3% in patients given add-on sitagliptin and 2.1% in patients given add-on placebo.

In the study of sitagliptin and add-on combination therapy with metformin immediate-release and rosiglitazone, the overall incidence of hypoglycemia was 2.2% in patients given add-on sitagliptin and 0.0% in patients given add-on placebo through Week 18. Through Week 54, the overall incidence of hypoglycemia was 3.9% in patients given add-on sitagliptin and 1.0% in patients given add-on placebo.

Vital Signs and Electrocardiograms

With the combination of sitagliptin and metformin immediate-release, no clinically meaningful changes in vital signs or in electrocardiogram parameters (including the QTc interval) were observed.

Pancreatitis

In a pooled analysis of 19 double-blind clinical trials that included data from 10,246 patients randomized to receive sitagliptin 100 mg/day (N=5429) or corresponding (active or placebo) control (N=4817), the incidence of acute pancreatitis was 0.1 per 100 patient-years in each group (4 patients with an event in 4708 patient-years for sitagliptin and 4 patients with an event in 3942 patient-years for control). *[See Warnings and Precautions (5.2).]*

Sitagliptin

The most common adverse experience in sitagliptin monotherapy reported regardless of investigator assessment of causality in ≥5% of patients and more commonly than in patients given placebo was nasopharyngitis.

Metformin Extended-Release

In a 24-week clinical trial in which extended-release metformin or placebo was added to glyburide therapy, the most common (>5% and greater than placebo) adverse reactions in the combined treatment group were hypoglycemia (13.7% vs. 4.9%), diarrhea (12.5% vs. 5.6%), and nausea (6.7% vs. 4.2%).

Laboratory Tests

Sitagliptin

The incidence of laboratory adverse reactions was similar in patients treated with sitagliptin and metformin immediate-release (7.6%) compared to patients treated with placebo and metformin (8.7%). In most but not all studies, a small increase in white blood cell count (approximately 200 cells/microL difference in WBC vs. placebo; mean baseline WBC approximately 6600 cells/microL) was observed due to a small increase in neutrophils. This change in laboratory parameters is not considered to be clinically relevant.

Metformin hydrochloride

In controlled clinical trials of metformin of 29 weeks duration, a decrease to subnormal levels of previously normal serum Vitamin B_{12} levels, without clinical manifestations, was observed in approximately 7% of patients. Such decrease, possibly due to interference with B_{12} absorption from the B_{12}-intrinsic factor complex, is, however, very rarely associated with anemia and appears to be rapidly reversible with discontinuation of metformin or Vitamin B_{12} supplementation. *[See Warnings and Precautions (5.5).]*

6.2 Postmarketing Experience

Additional adverse reactions have been identified during postapproval use of sitagliptin with or without metformin, and/or in combination with other antidiabetic medications. Because these reactions are reported voluntarily from a population of uncertain size, it is generally not possible to reliably estimate their frequency or establish a causal relationship to drug exposure.

Hypersensitivity reactions including anaphylaxis, angioedema, rash, urticaria, cutaneous vasculitis, and exfoliative skin conditions including Stevens-Johnson syndrome *[see Warnings and Precautions (5.14)]*; upper respiratory tract infection; hepatic enzyme elevations; acute pancreatitis, including fatal and non-fatal hemorrhagic and necrotizing pancreatitis *[see Indications and Usage (1); Warnings and Precautions (5.2)]*; worsening renal function, including acute renal failure (sometimes requiring dialysis)*[see Warnings and Precautions (5.4)]*; constipation; vomiting; headache; arthralgia; myalgia; pain in extremity; back pain.

7 DRUG INTERACTIONS

7.1 Carbonic Anhydrase Inhibitors

Topiramate or other carbonic anhydrase inhibitors (e.g., zonisamide, acetazolamide or dichlorphenamide) frequently decrease serum bicarbonate and induce non-anion gap, hyperchloremic metabolic acidosis. Concomitant use of these drugs may induce metabolic acidosis. Use these drugs with caution in patients treated with JANUMET XR, as the risk of lactic acidosis may increase.

7.2 Cationic Drugs

Cationic drugs (e.g., amiloride, digoxin, morphine, procainamide, quinidine, quinine, ranitidine, triamterene, trimethoprim, or vancomycin) that are eliminated by renal tubular secretion theoretically have the potential for interaction with metformin by competing for common renal tubular transport systems. Although such interactions remain theoretical (except for cimetidine), careful patient monitoring and dose adjustment of JANUMET XR and/or the interfering drug is recommended in patients who are taking cationic medications that are excreted via the proximal renal tubular secretory system.

Table 3: Incidence and Rate of Hypoglycemia* (Regardless of Investigator Assessment of Causality) in Placebo-Controlled Clinical Studies of Sitagliptin in Combination with Metformin Immediate-Release Coadministered with Glimepiride or Insulin

Add-On to Glimepiride + Metformin Immediate-Release (24 weeks)	Sitagliptin 100 mg + Metformin Immediate-Release + Glimepiride	Placebo + Metformin Immediate-Release + Glimepiride
	N = 116	N = 113
Overall (%)	19 (16.4)	1 (0.9)
Rate (episodes/patient-year) [†]	0.82	0.02
Severe (%)[‡]	0 (0.0)	0 (0.0)
Add-On to Insulin + Metformin Immediate-Release (24 weeks)	**Sitagliptin 100 mg + Metformin Immediate-Release + Insulin**	**Placebo + Metformin Immediate-Release + Insulin**
	N = 229	N = 233
Overall (%)	35 (15.3)	19 (8.2)
Rate (episodes/patient-year) [†]	0.98	0.61
Severe (%)[‡]	1 (0.4)	1 (0.4)

* Adverse reactions of hypoglycemia were based on all reports of symptomatic hypoglycemia; a concurrent glucose measurement was not required: Intent-to-treat population.
[†] Based on total number of events (i.e., a single patient may have had multiple events).
[‡] Severe events of hypoglycemia were defined as those events requiring medical assistance or exhibiting depressed level/loss of consciousness or seizure.

7.3 The Use of Metformin with Other Drugs

Certain drugs tend to produce hyperglycemia and may lead to loss of glycemic control. These drugs include the thiazides and other diuretics, corticosteroids, phenothiazines, thyroid products, estrogens, oral contraceptives, phenytoin, nicotinic acid, sympathomimetics, calcium channel blocking drugs, and isoniazid. When such drugs are administered to a patient receiving JANUMET XR the patient should be closely observed to maintain adequate glycemic control.

8 USE IN SPECIFIC POPULATIONS

8.1 Pregnancy

Pregnancy Category B:

JANUMET XR

There are no adequate and well-controlled studies in pregnant women with JANUMET XR or its individual components; therefore, the safety of JANUMET XR in pregnant women is not known. JANUMET XR should be used during pregnancy only if clearly needed.

Merck Sharp & Dohme Corp., a subsidiary of Merck & Co., Inc., maintains a registry to monitor the pregnancy outcomes of women exposed to JANUMET XR while pregnant. Healthcare providers are encouraged to report any prenatal exposure to JANUMET XR by calling the Pregnancy Registry at 1-800-986-8999.

No animal studies have been conducted with the combined products in JANUMET XR to evaluate effects on reproduction. The following data are based on findings in studies performed with sitagliptin or metformin individually.

Sitagliptin

Reproduction studies have been performed in rats and rabbits. Doses of sitagliptin up to 125 mg/kg (approximately 12 times the human exposure at the maximum recommended human dose) did not impair fertility or harm the fetus. There are, however, no adequate and well-controlled studies with sitagliptin in pregnant women.

Sitagliptin administered to pregnant female rats and rabbits from gestation day 6 to 20 (organogenesis) was not teratogenic at oral doses up to 250 mg/kg (rats) and 125 mg/kg (rabbits), or approximately 30 and 20 times human exposure at the maximum recommended human dose (MRHD) of 100 mg/day based on AUC comparisons. Higher doses increased the incidence of rib malformations in offspring at 1000 mg/kg, or approximately 100 times human exposure at the MRHD.

Sitagliptin administered to female rats from gestation day 6 to lactation day 21 decreased body weight in male and female offspring at 1000 mg/kg. No functional or behavioral toxicity was observed in offspring of rats.

Placental transfer of sitagliptin administered to pregnant rats was approximately 45% at 2 hours and 80% at 24 hours postdose. Placental transfer of sitagliptin administered to pregnant rabbits was approximately 66% at 2 hours and 30% at 24 hours.

Metformin hydrochloride

Metformin was not teratogenic in rats and rabbits at doses up to 600 mg/kg/day, which represent 3 and 6 times the maximum recommended human daily dose of 2000 mg based on body surface area comparison for rats and rabbits, respectively. However, because animal reproduction studies are not always predictive of human response, metformin hydrochloride should not be used during pregnancy unless clearly needed.

8.3 Nursing Mothers

No studies in lactating animals have been conducted with the combined components of JANUMET XR. In studies performed with the individual components, both sitagliptin and metformin are secreted in the milk of lactating rats. It is not known whether sitagliptin or metformin are excreted in human milk. Because many drugs are excreted in human milk, caution should be exercised when JANUMET XR is administered to a nursing woman.

8.4 Pediatric Use

Safety and effectiveness of JANUMET XR in pediatric patients under 18 years have not been established.

8.5 Geriatric Use

JANUMET XR

Because sitagliptin and metformin are substantially excreted by the kidney, and because aging can be associated with reduced renal function, JANUMET XR should be used with caution as age increases. Care should be taken in dose selection and should be based on careful and regular monitoring of renal function. *[See Warnings and Precautions (5.1, 5.4); Clinical Pharmacology (12.3).]*

Sitagliptin

Of the total number of subjects (N=3884) in premarketing Phase II and III clinical studies of sitagliptin, 725 patients were 65 years and over, while 61 patients were 75 years and over. No overall differences in safety or effectiveness were observed between subjects 65 years and over and younger subjects. While this and other reported clinical experience have not identified differences in responses between the elderly and younger patients, greater sensitivity of some older individuals cannot be ruled out.

Metformin hydrochloride

Controlled clinical studies of metformin did not include sufficient numbers of elderly patients to determine whether they respond differently from younger patients, although other reported clinical experience has not identified differences in responses between the elderly and young patients. Metformin should only be used in patients with normal renal function. The initial and maintenance dosing of metformin should be conservative in patients with advanced age, due to the potential for decreased renal function in this population. Any dose adjustment should be based on a careful assessment of renal function. *[See Contraindications (4); Warnings and Precautions (5.4); Clinical Pharmacology (12.3).]*

10 OVERDOSAGE

Sitagliptin

During controlled clinical trials in healthy subjects, single doses of up to 800 mg sitagliptin were administered. Maximal mean increases in QTc of 8.0 msec were observed in one study at a dose of 800 mg sitagliptin, a mean effect that is not considered clinically important *[see Clinical Pharmacology (12.2)]*. There is no experience with doses above 800 mg in clinical studies. In Phase I multiple-dose studies, there were no dose-related clinical adverse reactions observed with sitagliptin with doses of up to 400 mg per day for periods of up to 28 days.

In the event of an overdose, it is reasonable to employ the usual supportive measures, e.g., remove unabsorbed material from the gastrointestinal tract, employ clinical monitoring (including obtaining an electrocardiogram), and institute supportive therapy as indicated by the patient's clinical status.

Sitagliptin is modestly dialyzable. In clinical studies, approximately 13.5% of the dose was removed over a 3- to 4-hour hemodialysis session. Prolonged hemodialysis may be considered if clinically appropriate. It is not known if sitagliptin is dialyzable by peritoneal dialysis.

Metformin hydrochloride

Overdose of metformin hydrochloride has occurred, including ingestion of amounts greater than 50 grams. Hypoglycemia was reported in approximately 10% of cases, but no causal association with metformin hydrochloride has been established. Lactic acidosis has been reported in approximately 32% of metformin overdose cases [see *Warnings and Precautions (5.1)*]. Metformin is dialyzable with a clearance of up to 170 mL/min under good hemodynamic conditions. Therefore, hemodialysis may be useful for removal of accumulated drug from patients in whom metformin overdosage is suspected.

11   DESCRIPTION

JANUMET XR tablets contain two oral antidiabetic medications used in the management of type 2 diabetes: sitagliptin and metformin hydrochloride extended-release.

Sitagliptin

Sitagliptin is an orally-active inhibitor of the dipeptidyl peptidase-4 (DPP-4) enzyme. Sitagliptin phosphate monohydrate drug substance is used to manufacture JANUMET XR. Sitagliptin phosphate monohydrate is described chemically as 7-[(3R)-3-amino-1-oxo-4-(2,4,5-trifluorophenyl)butyl]-5,6,7,8-tetrahydro-3-(trifluoromethyl)-1,2,4-triazolo[4,3-α]pyrazine phosphate (1:1) monohydrate with an empirical formula of $C_{16}H_{15}F_6N_5O•H_3PO_4•H_2O$ and a molecular weight of 523.32. The structural formula is:

Sitagliptin phosphate monohydrate is a white to off-white, crystalline, non-hygroscopic powder. It is soluble in water and N,N-dimethyl formamide; slightly soluble in methanol; very slightly soluble in ethanol, acetone, and acetonitrile; and insoluble in isopropanol and isopropyl acetate.

Metformin hydrochloride

Metformin hydrochloride (N,N-dimethylimidodicarbonimidic diamide hydrochloride) is a white to off-white crystalline compound with a molecular formula of $C_4H_{11}N_5•HCl$ and a molecular weight of 165.63. Metformin hydrochloride is freely soluble in water and is practically insoluble in acetone, ether, and chloroform. The pK_a of metformin is 12.4. The pH of a 1% aqueous solution of metformin hydrochloride is 6.68. The structural formula is as shown:

JANUMET XR

JANUMET XR consists of an extended-release metformin core tablet coated with an immediate-release layer of sitagliptin. The sitagliptin layer is coated with a soluble polymeric film. JANUMET XR is available for oral administration as tablets containing 64.25 mg sitagliptin phosphate monohydrate (equivalent to 50 mg sitagliptin as free base) and either 500 mg metformin hydrochloride extended-release (50 mg/500 mg) or 1000 mg metformin hydrochloride extended-release (50 mg/1000 mg). Additionally, JANUMET XR is available for oral administration as tablets containing 128.5 mg sitagliptin phosphate monohydrate (equivalent to 100 mg sitagliptin as free base) and 1000 mg metformin hydrochloride extended-release (100 mg/1000 mg).

All doses of JANUMET XR contain the following inactive ingredients: povidone, hypromellose, colloidal silicon dioxide, sodium stearyl fumarate, propyl gallate, polyethylene glycol, and kaolin. The JANUMET XR 50 mg/500 mg tablet contains the additional inactive ingredient microcrystalline cellulose. In addition, the film coating for all doses contains the following inactive ingredients: hypromellose, hydroxypropyl cellulose, titanium dioxide, FD&C #2/Indigo Carmine Aluminum Lake and carnauba wax. The JANUMET XR 50 mg/1000 mg tablet film coating also contains the inactive ingredient yellow iron oxide.

Table 4: Effect of Sitagliptin on Systemic Exposure of Coadministered Drugs

Coadministered Drug	Dose of Coadministered Drug*	Dose of Sitagliptin *		Geometric Mean Ratio (ratio with/without sitagliptin) No Effect = 1.00	
				AUC[†]	C_{max}
No dosing adjustments required for the following:					
Digoxin	0.25 mg‡ once daily for 10 days	100 mg‡ once daily for 10 days	Digoxin	1.11[§]	1.18
Glyburide	1.25 mg	200 mg‡ once daily for 6 days	Glyburide	1.09	1.01
Simvastatin	20 mg	200 mg‡ once daily for 5 days	Simvastatin	0.85[¶]	0.80
			Simvastatin Acid	1.12[¶]	1.06
Rosiglitazone	4 mg	200 mg‡ once daily for 5 days	Rosiglitazone	0.98	0.99
Warfarin	30 mg single dose on day 5	200 mg‡ once daily for 11 days	S(-) Warfarin	0.95	0.89
			R(+) Warfarin	0.99	0.89
Ethinyl estradiol and norethindrone	21 days once daily of 35 μg ethinyl estradiol with norethindrone 0.5 mg × 7 days, 0.75 mg × 7 days, 1.0 mg × 7 days	200 mg‡ once daily for 21 days	Ethinyl estradiol	0.99	0.97
			Norethindrone	1.03	0.98
Metformin	1000 mg‡ twice daily for 14 days	50 mg‡ twice daily for 7 days	Metformin	1.02[#]	0.97

*   All doses administered as single dose unless otherwise specified
†   AUC is reported as $AUC_{0-\infty}$ unless otherwise specified
‡   Multiple dose
§ AUC_{0-24hr}
¶ AUC_{0-last}
# AUC_{0-12hr}

12   CLINICAL PHARMACOLOGY

12.1   Mechanism of Action

JANUMET XR

JANUMET XR tablets combine two antidiabetic medications with complementary mechanisms of action to improve glycemic control in adults with type 2 diabetes: sitagliptin, a dipeptidyl peptidase-4 (DPP-4) inhibitor, and metformin hydrochloride extended-release, a member of the biguanide class.

Sitagliptin

Sitagliptin is a DPP-4 inhibitor, which exerts its actions in patients with type 2 diabetes by slowing the inactivation of incretin hormones. Concentrations of the active intact hormones are increased by sitagliptin, thereby increasing and prolonging the action of these hormones. Incretin hormones, including glucagon-like peptide-1 (GLP-1) and glucose-dependent insulinotropic polypeptide (GIP), are released by the intestine throughout the day, and levels are increased in response to a meal. These hormones are rapidly inactivated by the enzyme DPP-4. The incretins are part of an endogenous system involved in the physiologic regulation of glucose homeostasis. When blood glucose concentrations are normal or elevated, GLP-1 and GIP increase insulin synthesis and release from pancreatic beta cells by intracellular signaling pathways involving cyclic AMP. GLP-1 also lowers glucagon secretion from pancreatic alpha cells, leading to reduced hepatic glucose production. By increasing and prolonging active incretin levels, sitagliptin increases insulin release and decreases glucagon levels in the circulation in a glucose-dependent manner. Sitagliptin demonstrates selectivity for DPP-4 and does not inhibit DPP-8 or DPP-9 activity *in vitro* at concentrations approximating those from therapeutic doses.

Metformin hydrochloride

Metformin is a biguanide that improves glycemic control in patients with type 2 diabetes, lowering both basal and postprandial plasma glucose. Metformin decreases hepatic glucose production, decreases intestinal absorption of glucose, and improves insulin sensitivity by increasing peripheral glucose uptake and utilization. Metformin does not produce hypoglycemia in either patients with type 2 diabetes or healthy subjects except in certain circumstances [see *Warnings and Precautions (5.9)*] and does not cause hyperinsulinemia. With metformin therapy, insulin secretion remains unchanged while fasting insulin levels and day-long plasma insulin response may actually decrease.

12.2   Pharmacodynamics

Sitagliptin

In patients with type 2 diabetes, administration of sitagliptin led to inhibition of DPP-4 enzyme activity for a 24-hour period. After an oral glucose load or a meal, this DPP-4 inhibition resulted in a 2- to 3-fold increase in circulating levels of active GLP-1 and GIP, decreased glucagon concentrations, and increased responsiveness of insulin release to glucose, resulting in higher C-peptide and insulin concentrations. The rise in insulin with the decrease in glucagon was associated with lower fasting glucose concentrations and reduced glucose excursion following an oral glucose load or a meal.

Sitagliptin and Metformin hydrochloride Coadministration

In a two-day study in healthy subjects, sitagliptin alone increased active GLP-1 concentrations, whereas metformin alone increased active and total GLP-1 concentrations to similar extents. Coadministration of sitagliptin and metformin had an additive effect on active GLP-1 concentrations. Sitagliptin, but not metformin, increased active GIP concentrations. It is unclear what these findings mean for changes in glycemic control in patients with type 2 diabetes.

In studies with healthy subjects, sitagliptin did not lower blood glucose or cause hypoglycemia.

Cardiac Electrophysiology

In a randomized, placebo-controlled crossover study, 79 healthy subjects were administered a single oral dose of sitagliptin 100 mg, sitagliptin 800 mg (8 times the recommended dose), and placebo. At the recommended dose of 100 mg, there was no effect on the QTc interval obtained at the peak plasma concentration, or at any other time during the study. Following the 800-mg dose, the maximum increase in the placebo-corrected mean change in QTc from baseline at 3 hours postdose was 8.0 msec. This increase is not considered to be clinically significant. At the 800-mg dose, peak sitagliptin plasma concentrations were approximately 11 times higher than the peak concentrations following a 100-mg dose.

In patients with type 2 diabetes administered sitagliptin 100 mg (N=81) or sitagliptin 200 mg (N=63) daily, there were no meaningful changes in QTc interval based on ECG data obtained at the time of expected peak plasma concentration.

12.3   Pharmacokinetics

JANUMET XR

The results of a study in healthy subjects demonstrated that the JANUMET XR (sitagliptin and metformin HCl extended-release) 50 mg/500 mg and 100 mg/1000 mg tablets are bioequivalent to coadministration of corresponding doses of sitagliptin and metformin hydrochloride extended-release.

Bioequivalence between two JANUMET XR 50 mg/500 mg tablets and one JANUMET XR 100 mg/1000 mg tablet was also demonstrated.

After administration of two JANUMET XR 50 mg/1000 mg tablets once daily with the evening meal for 7 days in healthy adult subjects, steady-state for sitagliptin and metformin is reached by Day 4 and 5, respectively. The median T_{max} value for sitagliptin and metformin at steady state is approximately 3 and 8 hours postdose, respectively. The median T_{max} value for sitagliptin and metformin after administration of a single tablet of JANUMET is 3 and 3.5 hours postdose, respectively.

Absorption
JANUMET XR
After administration of JANUMET XR tablets with a high-fat breakfast, the AUC for sitagliptin was not altered. The mean C_{max} was decreased by 17%, although the median T_{max} was unchanged relative to the fasted state. After administration of JANUMET XR with a high-fat breakfast, the AUC for metformin increased 62%, the C_{max} for metformin decreased by 9%, and the median T_{max} for metformin occurred 2 hours later relative to the fasted state.

Sitagliptin
The absolute bioavailability of sitagliptin is approximately 87%. Coadministration of a high-fat meal with sitagliptin had no effect on the pharmacokinetics of sitagliptin.

Distribution
Sitagliptin
The mean volume of distribution at steady state following a single 100-mg intravenous dose of sitagliptin to healthy subjects is approximately 198 liters. The fraction of sitagliptin reversibly bound to plasma proteins is low (38%).

Metformin hydrochloride
Distribution studies with extended-release metformin have not been conducted; however, the apparent volume of distribution (V/F) of metformin following single oral doses of immediate-release metformin hydrochloride tablets 850 mg averaged 654 ± 358 L. Metformin is negligibly bound to plasma proteins. Metformin partitions into erythrocytes, most likely as a function of time. At usual clinical doses and dosing schedules of metformin hydrochloride tablets, steady-state plasma concentrations of metformin are reached within 24-48 hours and are generally <1 mcg/mL. During controlled clinical trials of metformin, maximum metformin plasma levels did not exceed 5 mcg/mL, even at maximum doses.

Metabolism
Sitagliptin
Approximately 79% of sitagliptin is excreted unchanged in the urine with metabolism being a minor pathway of elimination.

Following a [^{14}C]sitagliptin oral dose, approximately 16% of the radioactivity was excreted as metabolites of sitagliptin. Six metabolites were detected at trace levels and are not expected to contribute to the plasma DPP-4 inhibitory activity of sitagliptin. *In vitro* studies indicated that the primary enzyme responsible for the limited metabolism of sitagliptin was CYP3A4, with contribution from CYP2C8.

Metformin hydrochloride
Intravenous single-dose studies in normal subjects demonstrate that metformin is excreted unchanged in the urine and does not undergo hepatic metabolism (no metabolites have been identified in humans) or biliary excretion. Metabolism studies with extended-release metformin tablets have not been conducted.

Excretion
Sitagliptin
Following administration of an oral [^{14}C]sitagliptin dose to healthy subjects, approximately 100% of the administered radioactivity was eliminated in feces (13%) or urine (87%) within one week of dosing. The apparent terminal $t_{1/2}$ following a 100-mg oral dose of sitagliptin was approximately 12.4 hours and renal clearance was approximately 350 mL/min.

Elimination of sitagliptin occurs primarily via renal excretion and involves active tubular secretion. Sitagliptin is a substrate for human organic anion transporter-3 (hOAT-3), which may be involved in the renal elimination of sitagliptin. The clinical relevance of hOAT-3 in sitagliptin transport has not been established. Sitagliptin is also a substrate of p-glycoprotein, which may also be involved in mediating the renal elimination of sitagliptin. However, cyclosporine, a p-glycoprotein inhibitor, did not reduce the renal clearance of sitagliptin.

Metformin hydrochloride
Renal clearance is approximately 3.5 times greater than creatinine clearance, which indicates that tubular secretion

is the major route of metformin elimination. Following oral administration, approximately 90% of the absorbed drug is eliminated via the renal route within the first 24 hours, with a plasma elimination half-life of approximately 6.2 hours. In blood, the elimination half-life is approximately 17.6 hours, suggesting that the erythrocyte mass may be a compartment of distribution.

Specific Populations
Renal Impairment
JANUMET XR
JANUMET XR should not be used in patients with renal impairment [see Contraindications (4); Warnings and Precautions (5.4)].
Sitagliptin
An approximately 2-fold increase in the plasma AUC of sitagliptin was observed in patients with moderate renal impairment, and an approximately 4-fold increase was observed in patients with severe renal impairment including patients with end-stage renal disease (ESRD) on hemodialysis, as compared to normal healthy control subjects.
Metformin hydrochloride
In patients with decreased renal function (based on measured creatinine clearance), the plasma and blood half-life of metformin is prolonged and the renal clearance is decreased in proportion to the decrease in creatinine clearance.

Hepatic Impairment
Sitagliptin
In patients with moderate hepatic impairment (Child-Pugh score 7 to 9), mean AUC and C_{max} of sitagliptin increased approximately 21% and 13%, respectively, compared to healthy matched controls following administration of a single 100-mg dose of sitagliptin. These differences are not considered to be clinically meaningful.
There is no clinical experience in patients with severe hepatic impairment (Child-Pugh score >9).
Metformin hydrochloride
No pharmacokinetic studies of metformin have been conducted in patients with hepatic impairment.

Gender
Sitagliptin
Gender had no clinically meaningful effect on the pharmacokinetics of sitagliptin based on a composite analysis of Phase I pharmacokinetic data and on a population pharmacokinetic analysis of Phase I and Phase II data.
Metformin hydrochloride
Metformin pharmacokinetic parameters did not differ significantly between normal subjects and patients with type 2 diabetes when analyzed according to gender. Similarly, in controlled clinical studies in patients with type 2 diabetes, the antihyperglycemic effect of metformin was comparable in males and females.
Geriatric
Sitagliptin
When the effects of age on renal function are taken into account, age alone did not have a clinically meaningful impact on the pharmacokinetics of sitagliptin based on a population pharmacokinetic analysis. Elderly subjects (65 to 80 years) had approximately 19% higher plasma concentrations of sitagliptin compared to younger subjects.
Metformin hydrochloride
Limited data from controlled pharmacokinetic studies of metformin in healthy elderly subjects suggest that total plasma clearance of metformin is decreased, the half life is prolonged, and C_{max} is increased, compared to healthy young subjects. From these data, it appears that the change in metformin pharmacokinetics with aging is primarily accounted for by a change in renal function.
As is true for all patients, JANUMET XR treatment should not be initiated in geriatric patients unless measurement of creatinine clearance demonstrates that renal function is normal [see Warnings and Precautions (5.1, 5.4)].
Pediatric
No studies with JANUMET XR have been performed in pediatric patients.
Race
Sitagliptin
Race had no clinically meaningful effect on the pharmacokinetics of sitagliptin based on a composite analysis of available pharmacokinetic data, including subjects of white, Hispanic, black, Asian, and other racial groups.

Table 5: Effect of Coadministered Drugs on Systemic Exposure of Sitagliptin

Coadministered Drug	Dose of Coadministered Drug*	Dose of Sitagliptin*	Geometric Mean Ratio (ratio with/without coadministered drug) No Effect = 1.00		
				AUC[†]	C_{max}
No dosing adjustments required for the following:					
Cyclosporine	600 mg once daily	100 mg once daily	Sitagliptin	1.29	1.68
Metformin	1000 mg[‡] twice daily for 14 days	50 mg[‡] twice daily for 7 days	Sitagliptin	1.02[§]	1.05

* All doses administered as single dose unless otherwise specified
† AUC is reported as $AUC_{0-\infty}$ unless otherwise specified
‡ Multiple dose
§ AUC_{0-12hr}

Table 6: Effect of Metformin on Systemic Exposure of Coadministered Drugs

Coadministered Drug	Dose of Coadministered Drug*	Dose of Metformin*	Geometric Mean Ratio (ratio with/without metformin) No Effect = 1.00		
				AUC[†]	C_{max}
No dosing adjustments required for the following:					
Cimetidine	400 mg	850 mg	Cimetidine	0.95[‡]	1.01
Glyburide	5 mg	500 mg[§]	Glyburide	0.78[¶]	0.63[¶]
Furosemide	40 mg	850 mg	Furosemide	0.87[¶]	0.69[¶]
Nifedipine	10 mg	850 mg	Nifedipine	1.10[‡]	1.08
Propranolol	40 mg	850 mg	Propranolol	1.01[‡]	0.94
Ibuprofen	400 mg	850 mg	Ibuprofen	0.97[#]	1.01[#]

* All doses administered as single dose unless otherwise specified
† AUC is reported as $AUC_{0-\infty}$ unless otherwise specified
‡ AUC_{0-24hr}
§ GLUMETZA (metformin hydrochloride extended-release tablets) 500 mg
¶ Ratio of arithmetic means, p value of difference < 0.05
# Ratio of arithmetic means

Table 7: Effect of Coadministered Drugs on Systemic Exposure of Metformin

Coadministered Drug	Dose of Coadministered Drug*	Dose of Metformin*	Geometric Mean Ratio (ratio with/without coadministered drug) No Effect = 1.00		
				AUC[†]	C$_{max}$
No dosing adjustments required for the following:					
Glyburide	5 mg	500 mg[‡]	Metformin[‡]	0.98[§]	0.99[§]
Furosemide	40 mg	850 mg	Metformin	1.09[§]	1.22[§]
Nifedipine	10 mg	850 mg	Metformin	1.16	1.21
Propranolol	40 mg	850 mg	Metformin	0.90	0.94
Ibuprofen	400 mg	850 mg	Metformin	1.05[§]	1.07[§]
Cationic drugs eliminated by renal tubular secretion may reduce metformin elimination: use with caution. [See Warnings and Precautions (5.10) and Drug Interactions (7.2).]					
Cimetidine	400 mg	850 mg	Metformin	1.40	1.61
Carbonic anhydrase inhibitors may cause metabolic acidosis: use with caution. [See Warnings and Precautions (5.1) and Drug Interactions (7.1).]					
Topiramate	100 mg[¶]	500 mg[¶]	Metformin	1.25[¶]	1.17

* All doses administered as single dose unless otherwise specified
† AUC is reported as AUC$_{0-∞}$ unless otherwise specified
‡ GLUMETZA (metformin hydrochloride extended-release tablets) 500 mg
§ Ratio of arithmetic means
¶ Steady state 100 mg Topiramate every 12 hr + metformin 500 mg every 12 hr. AUC = AUC$_{0-12hr}$

Metformin hydrochloride
No studies of metformin pharmacokinetic parameters according to race have been performed. In controlled clinical studies of metformin in patients with type 2 diabetes, the antihyperglycemic effect was comparable in whites (n=249), blacks (n=51), and Hispanics (n=24).

Body Mass Index (BMI)
Sitagliptin
Body mass index had no clinically meaningful effect on the pharmacokinetics of sitagliptin based on a composite analysis of Phase I pharmacokinetic data and on a population pharmacokinetic analysis of Phase I and Phase II data.

Drug Interactions
Sitagliptin and Metformin hydrochloride
Coadministration of multiple doses of sitagliptin (50 mg) and metformin (1000 mg) given twice daily did not meaningfully alter the pharmacokinetics of either sitagliptin or metformin in patients with type 2 diabetes.
Pharmacokinetic drug interaction studies with JANUMET XR have not been performed; however, such studies have been conducted with the individual components of JANUMET XR (sitagliptin and metformin hydrochloride extended-release).

Sitagliptin
In Vitro Assessment of Drug Interactions
Sitagliptin is not an inhibitor of CYP isozymes CYP3A4, 2C8, 2C9, 2D6, 1A2, 2C19 or 2B6, and is not an inducer of CYP3A4. Sitagliptin is a p-glycoprotein substrate, but does not inhibit p-glycoprotein mediated transport of digoxin. Based on these results, sitagliptin is considered unlikely to cause interactions with other drugs that utilize these pathways.
Sitagliptin is not extensively bound to plasma proteins. Therefore, the propensity of sitagliptin to be involved in clinically meaningful drug-drug interactions mediated by plasma protein binding displacement is very low.
In Vivo Assessment of Drug Interactions
[See table 4 at top of page 1526]
[See table 5 at top of previous page]
[See table 6 at top of previous page]
[See table 7 above]

13 NONCLINICAL TOXICOLOGY
13.1 Carcinogenesis, Mutagenesis, Impairment of Fertility
JANUMET XR
No animal studies have been conducted with the combined products in JANUMET XR to evaluate carcinogenesis, mutagenesis or impairment of fertility. The following data are based on the findings in studies with sitagliptin and metformin individually.
Sitagliptin
A two-year carcinogenicity study was conducted in male and female rats given oral doses of sitagliptin of 50, 150, and 500 mg/kg/day. There was an increased incidence of combined liver adenoma/carcinoma in males and females and of liver carcinoma in females at 500 mg/kg. This dose results in exposures approximately 60 times the human exposure at the maximum recommended daily adult human dose (MRHD) of 100 mg/day based on AUC comparisons. Liver tumors were not observed at 150 mg/kg, approximately 20 times the human exposure at the MRHD. A two-year carcinogenicity study was conducted in male and female mice given oral doses of sitagliptin of 50, 125, 250, and 500 mg/kg/day. There was no increase in the incidence of tumors in any organ up to 500 mg/kg, approximately 70 times human exposure at the MRHD. Sitagliptin was not mutagenic or clastogenic with or without metabolic activation in the Ames bacterial mutagenicity assay, a Chinese hamster ovary (CHO) chromosome aberration assay, an *in vitro* cytogenetics assay in CHO, an *in vitro* rat hepatocyte DNA alkaline elution assay, and an *in vivo* micronucleus assay.
In rat fertility studies with oral gavage doses of 125, 250, and 1000 mg/kg, males were treated for 4 weeks prior to mating, during mating, up to scheduled termination (approximately 8 weeks total), and females were treated 2 weeks prior to mating through gestation day 7. No adverse effect on fertility was observed at 125 mg/kg (approximately 12 times human exposure at the MRHD of 100 mg/day based on AUC comparisons). At higher doses, nondose-related increased resorptions in females were observed (approximately 25 and 100 times human exposure at the MRHD based on AUC comparison).
Metformin hydrochloride
Long-term carcinogenicity studies have been performed in Sprague Dawley rats at doses of 150, 300, and 450 mg/kg/day in males and 150, 450, 900, and 1200 mg/kg/day in females. These doses are approximately 2, 4, and 8 times in males, and 3, 7, 12, and 16 times in females of the maximum recommended human daily dose of 2000 mg based on body surface area comparisons. No evidence of carcinogenicity with metformin was found in either male or female rats. A carcinogenicity study was also performed in Tg.AC transgenic mice at doses up to 2000 mg applied dermally. No evidence of carcinogenicity was observed in male or female mice.
Genotoxicity assessments in the Ames test, gene mutation test (mouse lymphoma cells), chromosomal aberrations test (human lymphocytes) and *in vivo* mouse micronucleus tests were negative. Fertility of male or female rats was not affected by metformin when administered at doses up to 600 mg/kg/day, which is approximately 3 times the maximum recommended human daily dose based on body surface area comparisons.

14 CLINICAL STUDIES
The coadministration of sitagliptin and metformin immediate-release has been studied in patients with type 2 diabetes inadequately controlled on diet and exercise and in combination with other antidiabetic medications.
There have been no clinical efficacy or safety studies conducted with JANUMET XR to characterize its effect on hemoglobin A1c (A1C) reduction. Bioequivalence of JANUMET XR tablets with coadministered sitagliptin and extended-release metformin tablets has been demonstrated for all tablet strengths *[see Clinical Pharmacology (12.3)]*.

Metformin Extended-Release Compared to Metformin Immediate-Release in Patients with Type 2 Diabetes
In a multicenter, randomized, double-blind, active-controlled, dose-ranging, parallel group trial extended-release metformin 1500 mg once daily, extended-release metformin 1500 mg per day in divided doses (500 mg in the morning and 1000 mg in the evening), and extended-release metformin 2000 mg once daily were compared to immediate-release metformin 1500 mg per day in divided doses (500 mg in the morning and 1000 mg in the evening). This trial enrolled patients (n = 338) who were newly diagnosed with diabetes, patients treated only with diet and exercise, patients treated with a single anti-diabetic medication (sulfonylureas, alpha-glucosidase inhibitors, thiazolidinediones, or meglitinides), and patients (n = 368) receiving metformin up to 1500 mg/day plus a sulfonylurea at a dose equal to or less than one-half the maximum dose. Patients who were enrolled on monotherapy or combination antidiabetic therapy underwent a 6-week washout. Patients randomized to extended-release metformin began titration from 1000 mg/day up to their assigned treatment dose over 3 weeks. Patients randomized to immediate-release metformin initiated 500 mg twice daily for 1 week followed by 500 mg with breakfast and 1000 mg with dinner for the second week. The 3-week treatment period was followed by an additional 21-week period at the randomized dose. For HbA1c and fasting plasma glucose, each of the extended-release metformin regimens was at least as effective as immediate-release metformin. Additionally, once daily dosing of extended-release metformin was as effective as twice daily dosing of the immediate-release metformin formulation.

Sitagliptin and Metformin Immediate-Release Coadministration in Patients with Type 2 Diabetes Inadequately Controlled on Diet and Exercise
A total of 1091 patients with type 2 diabetes and inadequate glycemic control on diet and exercise participated in a 24-week, randomized, double-blind, placebo-controlled factorial study designed to assess the efficacy of sitagliptin and metformin immediate-release coadministration. Patients on an antihyperglycemic agent (N=541) underwent a diet, exercise, and drug washout period of up to 12 weeks duration. After the washout period, patients with inadequate glycemic control (A1C 7.5% to 11%) were randomized after completing a 2-week single-blind placebo run-in period. Patients not on antihyperglycemic agents at study entry (N=550) with inadequate glycemic control (A1C 7.5% to 11%) immediately entered the 2-week single-blind placebo run-in period and then were randomized. Approximately equal numbers of patients were randomized to receive placebo, 100 mg of sitagliptin once daily, 500 mg or 1000 mg of metformin immediate-release twice daily, or 50 mg of sitagliptin twice daily in combination with 500 mg or 1000 mg of metformin immediate-release twice daily. Patients who failed to meet specific glycemic goals during the study were treated with glyburide (glibenclamide) rescue. Sitagliptin and metformin immediate-release coadministration provided significant improvements in A1C, FPG, and 2-hour PPG compared to placebo, to metformin immediate-release alone, and to sitagliptin alone (Table 8, Figure 1). For patients not on an antihyperglycemic agent at study entry, mean reductions from baseline in A1C were: sitagliptin 100 mg once daily, -1.1%; metformin immediate-release 500 mg bid, -1.1%; metformin immediate-release 1000 mg bid, -1.2%; sitagliptin 50 mg bid with metformin immediate-release 500 mg bid, -1.6%; sitagliptin 50 mg bid with metformin immediate-release 1000 mg bid, -1.9%; and for patients receiving placebo, -0.2%. Lipid effects were generally neutral. The decrease in body weight in the groups given sitagliptin in combination with metformin immediate-release was similar to that in the groups given metformin alone or placebo.
[See table 8 at top of next page]
[See figure 1 at top of next column]
Initial combination therapy or maintenance of combination therapy should be individualized and are left to the discretion of the healthcare provider.

Sitagliptin Add-on Therapy in Patients with Type 2 Diabetes Inadequately Controlled on Metformin Immediate-Release Alone
A total of 701 patients with type 2 diabetes participated in a 24-week, randomized, double-blind, placebo-controlled study designed to assess the efficacy of sitagliptin in combination with metformin immediate-release. Patients already on metformin immediate-release (N=431) at a dose of at least 1500 mg per day were randomized after completing a 2-week, single-blind placebo run-in period. Patients on metformin immediate-release and another antihyperglycemic agent (N=229) and patients not on any antihyperglycemic agents (off therapy for at least 8 weeks, N=41) were randomized after a run-in period of approximately 10 weeks on metformin immediate-release (at a dose of at least 1500 mg per day) in monotherapy. Patients were randomized to the addition of either 100 mg of sitagliptin or placebo, adminis-

Table 8: Glycemic Parameters at Final Visit (24-Week Study) for Sitagliptin and Metformin Immediate-Release, Alone and in Combination in Patients with Type 2 Diabetes Inadequately Controlled on Diet and Exercise*

	Placebo	Sitagliptin 100 mg once daily	Metformin Immediate-Release 500 mg twice daily	Metformin Immediate-Release 1000 mg twice daily	Sitagliptin 50 mg bid + Metformin Immediate-Release 500 mg twice daily	Sitagliptin 50 mg bid + Metformin Immediate-Release 1000 mg twice daily
A1C (%)	N = 165	N = 175	N = 178	N = 177	N = 183	N = 178
Baseline (mean)	8.7	8.9	8.9	8.7	8.8	8.8
Change from baseline (adjusted mean[†])	0.2	-0.7	-0.8	-1.1	-1.4	-1.9
Difference from placebo (adjusted mean[†]) (95% CI)		-0.8[‡] (-1.1, -0.6)	-1.0[‡] (-1.2, -0.8)	-1.3[‡] (-1.5, -1.1)	-1.6[‡] (-1.8, -1.3)	-2.1[‡] (-2.3, -1.8)
Patients (%) achieving A1C <7%	15 (9%)	35 (20%)	41 (23%)	68 (38%)	79 (43%)	118 (66%)
% Patients receiving rescue medication	32	21	17	12	8	2
FPG (mg/dL)	N = 169	N = 178	N = 179	N = 179	N = 183	N = 180
Baseline (mean)	196	201	205	197	204	197
Change from baseline (adjusted mean[†])	6	-17	-27	-29	-47	-64
Difference from placebo (adjusted mean[†]) (95% CI)		-23[‡] (-33, -14)	-33[‡] (-43, -24)	-35[‡] (-45, -26)	-53[‡] (-62, -43)	-70[‡] (-79, -60)
2-hour PPG (mg/dL)	N = 129	N = 136	N = 141	N = 138	N = 147	N = 152
Baseline (mean)	277	285	293	283	292	287
Change from baseline (adjusted mean[†])	0	-52	-53	-78	-93	-117
Difference from placebo (adjusted mean[†]) (95% CI)		-52[‡] (-67, -37)	-54[‡] (-69, -39)	-78[‡] (-93, -63)	-93[‡] (-107, -78)	-117[‡] (-131, -102)

* Intent-to-treat population using last observation on study prior to glyburide (glibenclamide) rescue therapy.
† Least squares means adjusted for prior antihyperglycemic therapy status and baseline value.
‡ p<0.001 compared to placebo.

Figure 1: Mean Change from Baseline for A1C (%) over 24 Weeks with Sitagliptin and Metformin Immediate-Release, Alone and in Combination in Patients with Type 2 Diabetes Inadequately Controlled with Diet and Exercise*

○ Placebo (N=89)
● Sitagliptin 100 mg once daily (N=113)
◆ Metformin Immediate-Release 500 mg twice daily (N=128)
□ Metformin Immediate-Release 1000 mg twice daily (N=139)
✦ Sitagliptin 50 mg twice daily + Metformin Immediate-Release 500 mg twice daily (N=150)
■ Sitagliptin 50 mg twice daily + Metformin Immediate-Release 1000 mg twice daily (N=156)

* The Completers Population: least squares means adjusted for prior antihyperglycemic therapy and baseline value.

tered once daily. Patients who failed to meet specific glycemic goals during the studies were treated with pioglitazone rescue.

In combination with metformin immediate-release, sitagliptin provided significant improvements in A1C, FPG, and 2-hour PPG compared to placebo with metformin immediate-release (Table 9). Rescue glycemic therapy was used in 5% of patients treated with sitagliptin 100 mg and 14% of patients treated with placebo. A similar decrease in body weight was observed for both treatment groups.
[See table 9 at top of next page]

Sitagliptin Add-on Therapy in Patients with Type 2 Diabetes Inadequately Controlled on the Combination of Metformin Immediate-Release and Glimepiride

A total of 441 patients with type 2 diabetes participated in a 24-week, randomized, double-blind, placebo-controlled study designed to assess the efficacy of sitagliptin in combination with glimepiride, with or without metformin immediate-release. Patients entered a run-in treatment period on glimepiride (≥4 mg per day) alone or glimepiride in combination with metformin immediate-release (≥1500 mg per day). After a dose-titration and dose-stable run-in period of up to 16 weeks and a 2-week placebo run-in period, patients with inadequate glycemic control (A1C 7.5% to 10.5%) were randomized to the addition of either 100 mg of sitagliptin or placebo, administered once daily. Patients who failed to meet specific glycemic goals during the studies were treated with pioglitazone rescue.

Patients receiving sitagliptin with metformin immediate-release and glimepiride had significant improvements in A1C and FPG compared to patients receiving placebo with metformin immediate-release and glimepiride (Table 10), with mean reductions from baseline relative to placebo in A1C of -0.9% and in FPG of -21 mg/dL. Rescue therapy was used in 8% of patients treated with add-on sitagliptin 100 mg and 29% of patients treated with add-on placebo. The patients treated with add-on sitagliptin had a mean increase in body weight of 1.1 kg vs. add-on placebo (+0.4 kg vs. -0.7 kg). In addition, add-on sitagliptin resulted in an increased rate of hypoglycemia compared to add-on placebo.
[See Warnings and Precautions (5.9); Adverse Reactions (6.1).]
[See table 10 at top of next page]

Sitagliptin Add-on Therapy in Patients with Type 2 Diabetes Inadequately Controlled on the Combination of Metformin Immediate-Release and Rosiglitazone

A total of 278 patients with type 2 diabetes participated in a 54-week, randomized, double-blind, placebo-controlled study designed to assess the efficacy of sitagliptin in combination with metformin immediate-release and rosiglitazone. Patients on dual therapy with metformin immediate-

release ≥1500 mg/day and rosiglitazone ≥4 mg/day or with metformin immediate-release ≥1500 mg/day and pioglitazone ≥30 mg/day (switched to rosiglitazone ≥4 mg/day) entered a dose-stable run-in period of 6 weeks. Patients on other dual therapy were switched to metformin immediate-release ≥1500 mg/day and rosiglitazone ≥4 mg/day in a dose titration/stabilization run-in period of up to 20 weeks in duration. After the run-in period, patients with inadequate glycemic control (A1C 7.5% to 11%) were randomized 2:1 to the addition of either 100 mg of sitagliptin or placebo, administered once daily. Patients who failed to meet specific glycemic goals during the studies were treated with glipizide (or other sulfonylurea) rescue. The primary time point for evaluation of glycemic parameters was Week 18.

In combination with metformin immediate-release and rosiglitazone, sitagliptin provided significant improvements in A1C, FPG, and 2-hour PPG compared to placebo with metformin immediate-release and rosiglitazone (Table 11) at Week 18. At Week 54, mean reduction in A1C was -1.0% for patients treated with sitagliptin and -0.3% for patients treated with placebo in an analysis based on the intent-to-treat population. Rescue therapy was used in 18% of patients treated with sitagliptin 100 mg and 40% of patients treated with placebo. There was no significant difference between sitagliptin and placebo in body weight change.
[See table 11 at top of page 1531]

Sitagliptin Add-on Therapy in Patients with Type 2 Diabetes Inadequately Controlled on the Combination of Metformin Immediate-Release and Insulin

A total of 641 patients with type 2 diabetes participated in a 24-week, randomized, double-blind, placebo-controlled study designed to assess the efficacy of sitagliptin as add-on to insulin therapy. Approximately 75% of patients were also taking metformin immediate-release. Patients entered a 2-week, single-blind run-in treatment period on pre-mixed, long-acting, or intermediate-acting insulin, with or without metformin immediate-release (≥1500 mg per day). Patients using short-acting insulins were excluded unless the short-acting insulin was administered as part of a pre-mixed insulin. After the run-in period, patients with inadequate gly-

Help Patients Save on Rx Drugs: PDR.net/PharmacyDiscountCard

Table 9: Glycemic Parameters at Final Visit (24-Week Study) of Sitagliptin as Add-on Combination Therapy with Metformin Immediate-Release*

	Sitagliptin 100 mg once daily + Metformin Immediate-Release	Placebo + Metformin Immediate-Release
A1C (%)	N = 453	N = 224
Baseline (mean)	8.0	8.0
Change from baseline (adjusted mean†)	-0.7	-0.0
Difference from placebo + metformin immediate-release (adjusted mean†) (95% CI)	-0.7‡ (-0.8, -0.5)	
Patients (%) achieving A1C <7%	213 (47%)	41 (18%)
FPG (mg/dL)	N = 454	N = 226
Baseline (mean)	170	174
Change from baseline (adjusted mean†)	-17	9
Difference from placebo + metformin immediate-release (adjusted mean†) (95% CI)	-25‡ (-31, -20)	
2-hour PPG (mg/dL)	N = 387	N = 182
Baseline (mean)	275	272
Change from baseline (adjusted mean†)	-62	-11
Difference from placebo + metformin immediate-release (adjusted mean†) (95% CI)	-51‡ (-61, -41)	

* Intent-to-treat population using last observation on study prior to pioglitazone rescue therapy.
† Least squares means adjusted for prior antihyperglycemic therapy and baseline value.
‡ p<0.001 compared to placebo + metformin.

Table 10: Glycemic Parameters at Final Visit (24-Week Study) for Sitagliptin in Combination with Metformin Immediate-Release and Glimepiride*

	Sitagliptin 100 mg + Metformin Immediate-Release and Glimepiride	Placebo + Metformin Immediate-Release and Glimepiride
A1C (%)	N = 115	N = 105
Baseline (mean)	8.3	8.3
Change from baseline (adjusted mean†)	-0.6	0.3
Difference from placebo (adjusted mean†) (95% CI)	-0.9‡ (-1.1, -0.7)	
Patients (%) achieving A1C <7%	26 (23%)	1 (1%)
FPG (mg/dL)	N = 115	N = 109
Baseline (mean)	179	179
Change from baseline (adjusted mean†)	-8	13
Difference from placebo (adjusted mean†) (95% CI)	-21‡ (-32, -10)	

* Intent-to-treat population using last observation on study prior to pioglitazone rescue therapy.
† Least squares means adjusted for prior antihyperglycemic therapy status and baseline value.
‡ p<0.001 compared to placebo.

cemic control (A1C 7.5% to 11%) were randomized to the addition of either 100 mg of sitagliptin (N=229) or placebo (N=233), administered once daily. Patients were on a stable dose of insulin prior to enrollment with no changes in insulin dose permitted during the run-in period. Patients who failed to meet specific glycemic goals during the double-blind treatment period were to have uptitration of the background insulin dose as rescue therapy.

Among patients also receiving metformin immediate-release, the median daily insulin (pre-mixed, intermediate or long acting) dose at baseline was 40 units in the sitagliptin-treated patients and 42 units in the placebo-treated patients. The median change from baseline in daily dose of insulin was zero for both groups at the end of the study. Patients receiving sitagliptin with metformin immediate-release and insulin had significant improvements in A1C, FPG and 2-hour PPG compared to patients receiving placebo with metformin immediate-release and in-

sulin (Table 12). The adjusted mean change from baseline in body weight was -0.3 kg in patients receiving sitagliptin with metformin immediate-release and insulin and -0.2 kg in patients receiving placebo with metformin immediate-release and insulin. There was an increased rate of hypoglycemia in patients treated with sitagliptin. *[See Warnings and Precautions (5.9); Adverse Reactions (6.1).]*
[See table 12 at top of next page]

Sitagliptin Add-on Therapy vs. Glipizide Add-on Therapy in Patients with Type 2 Diabetes Inadequately Controlled on Metformin Immediate-Release
The efficacy of sitagliptin was evaluated in a 52-week, double-blind, glipizide-controlled noninferiority trial in patients with type 2 diabetes. Patients not on treatment or on other antihyperglycemic agents entered a run-in treatment period of up to 12 weeks duration with metformin immediate-release monotherapy (dose of ≥1500 mg per day) which included washout of medications other than

metformin immediate-release, if applicable. After the run-in period, those with inadequate glycemic control (A1C 6.5% to 10%) were randomized 1:1 to the addition of sitagliptin 100 mg once daily or glipizide for 52 weeks. Patients receiving glipizide were given an initial dosage of 5 mg/day and then electively titrated over the next 18 weeks to a maximum dosage of 20 mg/day as needed to optimize glycemic control. Thereafter, the glipizide dose was to be kept constant, except for down-titration to prevent hypoglycemia. The mean dose of glipizide after the titration period was 10 mg.

After 52 weeks, sitagliptin and glipizide had similar mean reductions from baseline in A1C in the intent-to-treat analysis (Table 13). These results were consistent with the per protocol analysis (Figure 2). A conclusion in favor of the non-inferiority of sitagliptin to glipizide may be limited to patients with baseline A1C comparable to those included in the study (over 70% of patients had baseline A1C <8% and over 90% had A1C <9%).
[See table 13 at top of page 1532]

Figure 2: Mean Change from Baseline for A1C (%) Over 52 Weeks in a Study Comparing Sitagliptin to Glipizide as Add-On Therapy in Patients Inadequately Controlled on Metformin Immediate-Release (Per Protocol Population)*

* The per protocol population (mean baseline A1C of 7.5%) included patients without major protocol violations who had observations at baseline and at Week 52.

The incidence of hypoglycemia in the sitagliptin group (4.9%) was significantly (p<0.001) lower than that in the glipizide group (32.0%). Patients treated with sitagliptin exhibited a significant mean decrease from baseline in body weight compared to a significant weight gain in patients administered glipizide (-1.5 kg vs. +1.1 kg).

16 HOW SUPPLIED/STORAGE AND HANDLING
No. 3961 — Tablets JANUMET XR, 50 mg/500 mg, are light blue, bi-convex oval, film-coated tablets with "78" debossed on one side. They are supplied as follows:
NDC 0006-0078-61 unit-of-use bottles of 60
NDC 0006-0078-62 unit-of-use bottles of 180
NDC 0006-0078-82 bulk bottles of 1000.
No. 3962 — Tablets JANUMET XR, 50 mg/1000 mg, are light green, bi-convex oval, film-coated tablets with "80" debossed on one side. They are supplied as follows:
NDC 0006-0080-61 unit-of-use bottles of 60
NDC 0006-0080-62 unit-of-use bottles of 180
NDC 0006-0080-82 bulk bottles of 1000.
No. 3963 — Tablets JANUMET XR, 100 mg/1000 mg, are blue, bi-convex oval, film-coated tablets with "81" debossed on one side. They are supplied as follows:
NDC 0006-0081-31 unit-of-use bottles of 30
NDC 0006-0081-54 unit-of-use bottles of 90
NDC 0006-0081-82 bulk bottles of 1000.
Store at 20-25°C (68-77°F), excursions permitted to 15-30°C (59-86°F). [See USP Controlled Room Temperature.] Store in a dry place with cap tightly closed. When container is subdivided, dispense into a USP tightly closed, moisture-resistant container.

17 PATIENT COUNSELING INFORMATION
See FDA-Approved Patient Labeling (Medication Guide).
17.1 Instructions
Patients should be informed of the potential risks and benefits of JANUMET XR and of alternative modes of therapy. They should also be informed about the importance of adherence to dietary instructions, regular physical activity, periodic blood glucose monitoring and A1C testing, recognition and management of hypoglycemia and hyperglycemia, and assessment for diabetes complications. During periods of stress such as fever, trauma, infection, or surgery, medication requirements may change and patients should be advised to seek medical advice promptly.

Table 11: Glycemic Parameters at Week 18 for Sitagliptin in Add-on Combination Therapy with Metformin Immediate-Release and Rosiglitazone*

	Week 18	
	Sitagliptin 100 mg + Metformin Immediate-Release + Rosiglitazone	Placebo + Metformin Immediate-Release + Rosiglitazone
A1C (%)	N = 176	N = 93
Baseline (mean)	8.8	8.7
Change from baseline (adjusted mean[†])	-1.0	-0.4
Difference from placebo + rosiglitazone + metformin immediate-release (adjusted mean[†]) (95% CI)	-0.7[‡] (-0.9, -0.4)	
Patients (%) achieving A1C <7%	39 (22%)	9 (10%)
FPG (mg/dL)	N = 179	N = 94
Baseline (mean)	181	182
Change from baseline (adjusted mean[†])	-30	-11
Difference from placebo + rosiglitazone + metformin immediate-release (adjusted mean[†]) (95% CI)	-18[‡] (-26, -10)	
2-hour PPG (mg/dL)	N = 152	N = 80
Baseline (mean)	256	248
Change from baseline (adjusted mean[†])	-59	-21
Difference from placebo + rosiglitazone + metformin immediate-release (adjusted mean[†]) (95% CI)	-39[‡] (-51, -26)	

* Intent-to-treat population using last observation on study prior to glipizide (or other sulfonylurea) rescue therapy.
† Least squares means adjusted for prior antihyperglycemic therapy status and baseline value.
‡ p<0.001 compared to placebo + metformin + rosiglitazone.

Table 12: Glycemic Parameters at Final Visit (24-Week Study) for Sitagliptin as Add-on Combination Therapy with Metformin Immediate-Release and Insulin*

	Sitagliptin 100 mg + Metformin Immediate-Release + Insulin	Placebo + Metformin Immediate-Release + Insulin
A1C (%)	N = 223	N = 229
Baseline (mean)	8.7	8.6
Change from baseline (adjusted mean[†, ‡])	-0.7	-0.1
Difference from placebo (adjusted mean[†]) (95% CI)	-0.5[§] (-0.7, -0.4)	
Patients (%) achieving A1C (%) <7%	32 (14%)	12 (5%)
FPG (mg/dL)	N = 225	N = 229
Baseline (mean)	173	176
Change from baseline (adjusted mean[†])	-22	-4
Difference from placebo (adjusted mean[†]) (95% CI)	-18[§] (-28, -8.4)	
2-hour PPG (mg/dL)	N = 182	N = 189
Baseline (mean)	281	281
Change from baseline (adjusted mean[†])	-39	1
Difference from placebo (adjusted mean[†]) (95% CI)	-40[§] (-53, -28)	

* Intent-to-treat population using last observation on study prior to rescue therapy.
† Least squares mean adjusted for insulin use at the screening visit, type of insulin used at the screening visit (pre-mixed vs. non pre-mixed [intermediate- or long-acting]), and baseline value.
‡ Treatment by insulin stratum interaction was not significant (p>0.10).
§ p<0.001 compared to placebo.

The risks of lactic acidosis due to the metformin component, its symptoms, and conditions that predispose to its development, as noted in *Warnings and Precautions (5.1)*, should be explained to patients. Patients should be advised to discontinue JANUMET XR immediately and to promptly notify their health practitioner if unexplained hyperventilation, myalgia, malaise, unusual somnolence, dizziness, slow or irregular heart beat, sensation of feeling cold (especially in the extremities) or other nonspecific symptoms occur. Gastrointestinal symptoms are common during initiation of metformin treatment and may occur during initiation of JANUMET XR therapy; however, patients should consult their physician if they develop unexplained symptoms. Although gastrointestinal symptoms that occur after stabilization are unlikely to be drug related, such an occurrence of symptoms should be evaluated to determine if it may be due to lactic acidosis or other serious disease.

Patients should be advised to notify their health practitioner or call the Poison Control Center immediately in case of JANUMET XR overdose.

Patients should be counseled against excessive alcohol intake, either acute or chronic, while receiving JANUMET XR.

Patients should be informed about the importance of regular testing of renal function and hematological parameters when receiving treatment with JANUMET XR.

Patients should be informed that acute pancreatitis has been reported during postmarketing use of JANUMET. Patients should be informed that persistent severe abdominal pain, sometimes radiating to the back, which may or may not be accompanied by vomiting, is the hallmark symptom of acute pancreatitis. Patients should be instructed to promptly discontinue JANUMET XR and contact their physician if persistent severe abdominal pain occurs [see Warnings and Precautions (5.2)].

Patients should be informed that the incidence of hypoglycemia is increased when sitagliptin with or without metformin is added to an insulin secretagogue (e.g., sulfonylurea) or insulin therapy and that a lower dose of the insulin secretagogue or insulin may be required to reduce the risk of hypoglycemia.

Patients should be informed that allergic reactions have been reported during postmarketing use of sitagliptin, one of the components of JANUMET XR. If symptoms of allergic reactions (including rash, hives, and swelling of the face, lips, tongue, and throat that may cause difficulty in breathing or swallowing) occur, patients must stop taking JANUMET XR and seek medical advice promptly.

Patients should be informed that the tablets must be swallowed whole and never split, crushed or chewed.

Patients should be informed that incompletely dissolved JANUMET XR tablets may be eliminated in the feces. Tell patients that, if they repeatedly see tablets in feces, they should report this finding to their healthcare provider. If a patient reports repeatedly observing tablets in feces, the healthcare provider should assess adequacy of glycemic control.

Physicians should instruct their patients to read the Medication Guide before starting JANUMET XR therapy and to reread each time the prescription is renewed. Patients should be instructed to inform their doctor if they develop any bothersome or unusual symptom, or if any symptom persists or worsens.

17.2   Laboratory Tests
Response to all diabetic therapies should be monitored by periodic measurements of blood glucose and A1C levels, with a goal of decreasing these levels towards the normal range. A1C is especially useful for evaluating long-term glycemic control.

Initial and periodic monitoring of hematologic parameters (e.g., hemoglobin/hematocrit and red blood cell indices) and renal function (serum creatinine) should be performed, at least on an annual basis. While megaloblastic anemia has rarely been seen with metformin therapy, if this is suspected, Vitamin B_{12} deficiency should be excluded.

Manufactured for: Merck Sharp & Dohme Corp., a subsidiary of
MERCK & CO., INC., Whitehouse Station, NJ 08889, USA
Manufactured by:
Merck Sharp & Dohme Corp., a subsidiary of
Merck & Co., Inc., Whitehouse Station, NJ 08889, USA
OR
Patheon Inc., Whitby, Ontario, Canada L1N 5Z5
For patent information: www.merck.com/product/patent/home.html
Copyright © 2012 Merck Sharp & Dohme Corp., a subsidiary of **Merck & Co., Inc.**
All rights reserved.
uspi-mk0431a-xrt-1402r004
Medication Guide
JANUMET® XR (JAN-you-met XR)
(sitagliptin and metformin hydrochloride extended-release) Tablets
Read this Medication Guide carefully before you start taking JANUMET XR and each time you get a refill. There may be new information. This information does not take the place of talking with your doctor about your medical condition or your treatment. If you have any questions about JANUMET XR, ask your doctor or pharmacist.

Table 13: Glycemic Parameters in a 52-Week Study Comparing Sitagliptin to Glipizide as Add-On Therapy in Patients Inadequately Controlled on Metformin Immediate-Release (Intent-to-Treat Population) *

	Sitagliptin 100 mg + Metformin Immediate-Release	Glipizide + Metformin Immediate-Release
A1C (%)	N = 576	N = 559
Baseline (mean)	7.7	7.6
Change from baseline (adjusted mean†)	-0.5	-0.6
FPG (mg/dL)	N = 583	N = 568
Baseline (mean)	166	164
Change from baseline (adjusted mean†)	-8	-8

* The intent-to-treat analysis used the patients' last observation in the study prior to discontinuation.
† Least squares means adjusted for prior antihyperglycemic therapy status and baseline A1C value.

What is the most important information I should know about JANUMET XR?

Serious side effects can happen in people taking JANUMET XR, including:

1. **Lactic Acidosis.** Metformin, one of the medicines in JANUMET XR, can cause a rare but serious condition called lactic acidosis (a build-up of lactic acid in the blood) that can cause death. Lactic acidosis is a medical emergency and must be treated in the hospital.

Stop taking JANUMET XR and call your doctor right away if you get any of the following symptoms, which could be signs of lactic acidosis.
You:
• feel very weak or tired.
• have unusual (not normal) muscle pain.
• have trouble breathing.
• have unusual sleepiness or sleep longer than usual.
• have sudden stomach or intestinal problems with nausea and vomiting or diarrhea.
• feel cold, especially in your arms and legs.
• feel dizzy or lightheaded.
• have a slow or irregular heartbeat
You have a higher chance of getting lactic acidosis if you:
• have kidney problems. People whose kidneys are not working properly should not take JANUMET XR.
• have liver problems.
• have congestive heart failure that requires treatment with medicines.
• drink alcohol very often, or drink a lot of alcohol in short-term "binge" drinking.
• get dehydrated (lose a large amount of body fluids). This can happen if you are sick with a fever, vomiting, or diarrhea. Dehydration can also happen when you sweat a lot with activity or exercise and do not drink enough fluids.
• have certain x-ray tests with dyes or contrast agents that are injected into your body.
• have surgery.
• have a heart attack, severe infection, or stroke.

2. **Pancreatitis** (inflammation of the pancreas) which may be severe and lead to death. Certain medical problems make you more likely to get pancreatitis.

Before you start taking JANUMET XR:

Tell your doctor if you have ever had
• pancreatitis
• stones in your gallbladder (gallstones)
• a history of alcoholism
• high blood triglyceride levels

Stop taking JANUMET XR and call your doctor right away if you have pain in your stomach area (abdomen) that is severe and will not go away. The pain may be felt going from your abdomen through to your back. The pain may happen with or without vomiting. These may be symptoms of pancreatitis.

What is JANUMET XR?

• JANUMET XR is a prescription medicine that contains 2 prescription diabetes medicines, sitagliptin (JANUVIA®) and extended-release metformin hydrochloride. JANUMET XR can be used along with diet and exercise to lower blood sugar in adults with type 2 diabetes.
• JANUMET XR is not for people with type 1 diabetes.
• JANUMET XR is not for people with diabetic ketoacidosis (increased ketones in your blood or urine).
• If you have had pancreatitis (inflammation of the pancreas) in the past, it is not known if you have a higher chance of getting pancreatitis while you take JANUMET XR.
• It is not known if JANUMET XR is safe and effective when used in children under 18 years of age.

Who should not take JANUMET XR?
Do not take JANUMET XR if:
• your kidneys are not working properly.
• you are allergic to any of the ingredients in JANUMET XR. See the end of this Medication Guide for a complete list of ingredients in JANUMET XR.
Symptoms of a serious allergic reaction to JANUMET XR may include:
• rash
• raised red patches on your skin (hives)
• swelling of the face, lips, tongue, and throat that may cause difficulty in breathing or swallowing
• you have diabetic ketoacidosis. See "What is JANUMET XR?".

What should I tell my doctor before taking JANUMET XR?
Before you take JANUMET XR, tell your doctor if you:
• have or have had inflammation of your pancreas (pancreatitis).
• have kidney problems.
• have liver problems.
• have heart problems, including congestive heart failure.
• drink alcohol very often, or drink a lot of alcohol in short-term "binge" drinking.
• are going to get an injection of dye or contrast agents for an x-ray procedure; JANUMET XR will need to be stopped for a short time. Talk to your doctor about when you should stop JANUMET XR and when you should start JANUMET XR again. See "What is the most important information I should know about JANUMET XR?".
• have any other medical conditions.
• are pregnant or plan to become pregnant. It is not known if JANUMET XR will harm your unborn baby. If you are pregnant, talk with your doctor about the best way to control your blood sugar while you are pregnant.
Pregnancy Registry: If you take JANUMET XR at any time during your pregnancy, talk with your doctor about how you can join the JANUMET XR pregnancy registry. The purpose of this registry is to collect information about the health of you and your baby. You can enroll in this registry by calling 1-800-986-8999.
• are breast-feeding or plan to breast-feed. It is not known if JANUMET XR will pass into your breast milk. Talk with your doctor about the best way to feed your baby if you are taking JANUMET XR.

Tell your doctor about all the medicines you take, including prescription and non-prescription medicines, vitamins, and herbal supplements. JANUMET XR may affect how well other drugs work and some drugs can affect how well JANUMET XR works.

Know the medicines you take. Keep a list of your medicines and show it to your doctor and pharmacist when you get a new medicine.

How should I take JANUMET XR?
• Take JANUMET XR exactly as your doctor tells you. Your doctor will tell you how many JANUMET XR tablets to take and when you should take them.
• Your doctor may change your dose of JANUMET XR if needed.
• Your doctor may tell you to take JANUMET XR along with certain other diabetes medicines. Low blood sugar (hypoglycemia) can happen more often when JANUMET XR is taken with certain other diabetes medicines. See "What are the possible side effects of JANUMET XR?".
• Take JANUMET XR 1 time each day with a meal to help to lower your chance of having an upset stomach. It is better to take JANUMET XR with your evening meal.
• Take JANUMET XR tablets whole. Do not break, cut, crush, dissolve, or chew JANUMET XR tablets before swallowing. If you cannot swallow JANUMET XR tablets whole, tell your doctor.

• You may see something that looks like the JANUMET XR tablet in your stool (bowel movement). If you see tablets in your stool several times, talk to your doctor. Do not stop taking JANUMET XR without talking to your doctor.
• Continue to take JANUMET XR as long as your doctor tells you.
• If you take too much JANUMET XR, call your doctor or local Poison Control Center right away.
• If you miss a dose, take it with food as soon as you remember. If you do not remember until it is time for your next dose, skip the missed dose and go back to your regular schedule. Do not take 2 doses of JANUMET XR at the same time.
• You may need to stop taking JANUMET XR for a short time. Call your doctor for instructions if you:
  • are dehydrated (have lost too much body fluid). Dehydration can occur if you are sick with severe vomiting, diarrhea or fever, or if you drink a lot less fluid than normal.
  • plan to have surgery.
  • are going to get an injection of dye or contrast agent for an x-ray procedure. See "What is the most important information I should know about JANUMET XR?" and "What should I tell my doctor before taking JANUMET XR?".
• When your body is under some types of stress, such as fever, trauma (such as a car accident), infection or surgery, the amount of diabetes medicine that you need may change. Tell your doctor right away if you have any of these problems and follow your doctor's instructions.
• Check your blood sugar as your doctor tells you to.
• Stay on your prescribed diet and exercise program while taking JANUMET XR.
• Talk to your doctor about how to prevent, recognize and manage low blood sugar (hypoglycemia), high blood sugar (hyperglycemia), and problems you have because of your diabetes.
• Your doctor will check your diabetes with regular blood tests, including your blood sugar levels and your hemoglobin A1C.
• Your doctor will do blood tests to check how well your kidneys are working before and during your treatment with JANUMET XR.

What are the possible side effects of JANUMET XR?
Serious side effects have happened in people taking JANUMET XR or the individual medicines in JANUMET XR.
• See "What is the most important information I should know about JANUMET XR?".
• **Low blood sugar (hypoglycemia).** If you take JANUMET XR with another medicine that can cause low blood sugar, such as a sulfonylurea or insulin, your risk of getting low blood sugar is higher. The dose of your sulfonylurea medicine or insulin may need to be lowered while you use JANUMET XR. Signs and symptoms of low blood sugar may include:

• headache	• irritability
• drowsiness	• hunger
• weakness	• fast heart beat
• dizziness	• sweating
• confusion	• feeling jittery

• **Serious allergic reactions.** If you have any symptoms of a serious allergic reaction, stop taking JANUMET XR and call your doctor right away. See "Who should not take JANUMET XR?". Your doctor may give you a medicine for your allergic reaction and prescribe a different medicine for your diabetes.
• **Kidney problems,** sometimes requiring dialysis.
The most common side effects of JANUMET XR include:
• stuffy or runny nose and sore throat
• upper respiratory infection
• diarrhea
• nausea and vomiting
• gas, upset stomach, indigestion
• weakness
• headache
• low blood sugar (hypoglycemia) when used in combination with certain medications, such as a sulfonylurea or insulin.

Taking JANUMET XR with meals can help lessen the common stomach side effects of metformin that usually happen at the beginning of treatment. If you have unusual or sudden stomach problems, talk with your doctor. Stomach problems that start later during treatment may be a sign of something more serious.

JANUMET XR may have other side effects, including:
• swelling of the hands or legs. Swelling of the hands and legs can happen if you take JANUMET XR in combination with rosiglitazone (Avandia®). Rosiglitazone is another type of diabetes medicine.

These are not all the possible side effects of JANUMET XR. For more information, ask your doctor or pharmacist.

Tell your doctor if you have any side effect that bothers you, is unusual, or does not go away.

Call your doctor for medical advice about side effects. You may report side effects to FDA at 1-800-FDA-1088.

How should I store JANUMET XR?
Store JANUMET XR at 68°F to 77°F (20°C to 25°C). Store in a dry place and keep cap tightly closed.

Keep JANUMET XR and all medicines out of the reach of children.

General information about the use of JANUMET XR.
Medicines are sometimes prescribed for purposes other than those listed in Medication Guides. Do not use JANUMET XR for a condition for which it was not prescribed. Do not give JANUMET XR to other people, even if they have the same symptoms you have. It may harm them.

This Medication Guide summarizes the most important information about JANUMET XR. If you would like to know more information, talk with your doctor. You can ask your doctor or pharmacist for additional information about JANUMET XR that is written for health care professionals. For more information go to www.janumetxr.com or call 1-800-622-4477.

What are the ingredients in JANUMET XR?
Active ingredients: sitagliptin and metformin hydrochloride extended-release
Inactive ingredients:
• **All doses of JANUMET XR Tablets contain:** povidone, hypromellose, colloidal silicon dioxide, sodium stearyl fumarate, propyl gallate, polyethylene glycol, and kaolin. Film coating contains hypromellose, hydroxypropyl cellulose, titanium dioxide, FD&C #2/Indigo Carmine Aluminum Lake and carnauba wax.
• **In addition the JANUMET XR 50 mg/500 mg Tablets also contain:** microcrystalline cellulose.
• **In addition the JANUMET XR 50 mg/1000 mg Tablets also contain:** yellow iron oxide.

What is type 2 diabetes?
Type 2 diabetes is a condition in which your body does not make enough insulin, and the insulin that your body produces does not work as well as it should. Your body can also make too much sugar. When this happens, sugar (glucose) builds up in the blood. This can lead to serious medical problems.

High blood sugar can be lowered by diet and exercise, and by certain medicines when necessary.

This Medication Guide has been approved by the U.S. Food and Drug Administration.

Manufactured for: Merck Sharp & Dohme Corp., a subsidiary of
MERCK & CO., INC., Whitehouse Station, NJ 08889, USA
Manufactured by:
Merck Sharp & Dohme Corp., a subsidiary of
Merck & Co., Inc., Whitehouse Station, NJ 08889, USA
OR
Patheon Inc., Whitby, Ontario, Canada L1N 5Z5
For patent information: www.merck.com/product/patent/home.html
The trademarks depicted herein are owned by their respective companies.

Copyright © 2012 Merck Sharp & Dohme Corp., a subsidiary of **Merck & Co., Inc.**
All rights reserved.
Revised: 02/2014
usmg-mk0431a-xrt-1402r004
Shown in Product Identification Guide, page 308

JANUVIA®
[ja-new'-vee-a]
(sitagliptin)
Tablets   ℞

HIGHLIGHTS OF PRESCRIBING INFORMATION
These highlights do not include all the information needed to use JANUVIA safely and effectively. See full prescribing information for JANUVIA.
JANUVIA® (sitagliptin) Tablets
Initial U.S. Approval: 2006

————————INDICATIONS AND USAGE————————
JANUVIA is a dipeptidyl peptidase-4 (DPP-4) inhibitor indicated as an adjunct to diet and exercise to improve glycemic control in adults with type 2 diabetes mellitus. (1.1)
Important Limitations of Use:
• JANUVIA should not be used in patients with type 1 diabetes or for the treatment of diabetic ketoacidosis. (1.2)
• JANUVIA has not been studied in patients with a history of pancreatitis. (1.2, 5.1)

————————DOSAGE AND ADMINISTRATION————————
The recommended dose of JANUVIA is 100 mg once daily. JANUVIA can be taken with or without food. (2.1)
Dosage adjustment is recommended for patients with moderate or severe renal insufficiency or end-stage renal disease. (2.2)

Dosage Adjustment in Patients With Moderate, Severe and End Stage Renal Disease (ESRD) (2.2)

50 mg once daily	25 mg once daily
Moderate	Severe and ESRD
CrCl ≥30 to <50 mL/min	CrCl <30 mL/min
~Serum Cr levels [mg/dL]	~Serum Cr levels [mg/dL]
Men: >1.7– ≤3.0;	Men: >3.0;
Women: >1.5– ≤2.5	Women: >2.5; or on dialysis

————DOSAGE FORMS AND STRENGTHS————
Tablets: 100 mg, 50 mg, and 25 mg (3)

————————CONTRAINDICATIONS————————
History of a serious hypersensitivity reaction to sitagliptin, such as anaphylaxis or angioedema (5.4, 6.2)

————————WARNINGS AND PRECAUTIONS————————
• There have been postmarketing reports of acute pancreatitis, including fatal and non-fatal hemorrhagic or necrotizing pancreatitis. If pancreatitis is suspected, promptly discontinue JANUVIA. (5.1)
• There have been postmarketing reports of acute renal failure, sometimes requiring dialysis. Dosage adjustment is recommended in patients with moderate or severe renal insufficiency and in patients with ESRD. Assessment of renal function is recommended prior to initiating JANUVIA and periodically thereafter. (2.2, 5.2, 6.2)
• There is an increased risk of hypoglycemia when JANUVIA is added to an insulin secretagogue (e.g., sulfonylurea) or insulin therapy. Consider lowering the dose of the sulfonylurea or insulin to reduce the risk of hypoglycemia. (2.3, 5.3)
• There have been postmarketing reports of serious allergic and hypersensitivity reactions in patients treated with JANUVIA such as anaphylaxis, angioedema, and exfoliative skin conditions including Stevens-Johnson syndrome. In such cases, promptly stop JANUVIA, assess for other potential causes, institute appropriate monitoring and treatment, and initiate alternative treatment for diabetes. (5.4, 6.2)
• There have been no clinical studies establishing conclusive evidence of macrovascular risk reduction with JANUVIA or any other anti-diabetic drug. (5.5)

————————ADVERSE REACTIONS————————
Adverse reactions reported in ≥5% of patients treated with JANUVIA and more commonly than in patients treated with placebo are: upper respiratory tract infection, nasopharyngitis and headache. In the add-on to sulfonylurea and add-on to insulin studies, hypoglycemia was also more commonly reported in patients treated with JANUVIA compared to placebo. (6.1)

To report SUSPECTED ADVERSE REACTIONS, contact Merck Sharp & Dohme Corp., a subsidiary of Merck & Co., Inc., at 1-877-888-4231 or FDA at 1-800-FDA-1088 or www.fda.gov/medwatch.

————————USE IN SPECIFIC POPULATIONS————————
• Safety and effectiveness of JANUVIA in children under 18 years have not been established. (8.4)
• There are no adequate and well-controlled studies in pregnant women. To report drug exposure during pregnancy call 1-800-986-8999. (8.1)

See 17 for PATIENT COUNSELING INFORMATION and Medication Guide

Revised: 02/2014

FULL PRESCRIBING INFORMATION

1 INDICATIONS AND USAGE
1.1 Monotherapy and Combination Therapy
JANUVIA® is indicated as an adjunct to diet and exercise to improve glycemic control in adults with type 2 diabetes mellitus. *[See Clinical Studies (14).]*
1.2 Important Limitations of Use
JANUVIA should not be used in patients with type 1 diabetes or for the treatment of diabetic ketoacidosis, as it would not be effective in these settings.
JANUVIA has not been studied in patients with a history of pancreatitis. It is unknown whether patients with a history of pancreatitis are at increased risk for the development of pancreatitis while using JANUVIA. *[See Warnings and Precautions (5.1).]*

2 DOSAGE AND ADMINISTRATION
2.1 Recommended Dosing
The recommended dose of JANUVIA is 100 mg once daily. JANUVIA can be taken with or without food.
2.2 Patients with Renal Insufficiency
For patients with mild renal insufficiency (creatinine clearance [CrCl] greater than or equal to 50 mL/min, approximately corresponding to serum creatinine levels of less than or equal to 1.7 mg/dL in men and less than or equal to 1.5 mg/dL in women), no dosage adjustment for JANUVIA is required.
For patients with moderate renal insufficiency (CrCl greater than or equal to 30 to less than 50 mL/min, approximately corresponding to serum creatinine levels of greater than 1.7 to less than or equal to 3.0 mg/dL in men and greater than 1.5 to less than or equal to 2.5 mg/dL in women), the dose of JANUVIA is 50 mg once daily.
For patients with severe renal insufficiency (CrCl less than 30 mL/min, approximately corresponding to serum creatinine levels of greater than 3.0 mg/dL in men and greater than 2.5 mg/dL in women) or with end-stage renal disease (ESRD) requiring hemodialysis or peritoneal dialysis, the dose of JANUVIA is 25 mg once daily. JANUVIA may be administered without regard to the timing of dialysis.
Because there is a need for dosage adjustment based upon renal function, assessment of renal function is recommended prior to initiation of JANUVIA and periodically thereafter. Creatinine clearance can be estimated from serum creatinine using the Cockcroft-Gault formula. *[See Clinical Pharmacology (12.3).]* There have been postmarketing reports of worsening renal function in patients with renal insufficiency, some of whom were prescribed inappropriate doses of sitagliptin.
2.3 Concomitant Use with an Insulin Secretagogue (e.g., Sulfonylurea) or with Insulin
When JANUVIA is used in combination with an insulin secretagogue (e.g., sulfonylurea) or with insulin, a lower dose of the insulin secretagogue or insulin may be required to reduce the risk of hypoglycemia. *[See Warnings and Precautions (5.3).]*

3 DOSAGE FORMS AND STRENGTHS
• 100 mg tablets are beige, round, film-coated tablets with "277" on one side.
• 50 mg tablets are light beige, round, film-coated tablets with "112" on one side.
• 25 mg tablets are pink, round, film-coated tablets with "221" on one side.

4 CONTRAINDICATIONS
History of a serious hypersensitivity reaction to sitagliptin, such as anaphylaxis or angioedema. *[See Warnings and Precautions (5.4); Adverse Reactions (6.2).]*

5 WARNINGS AND PRECAUTIONS

5.1 Pancreatitis

There have been postmarketing reports of acute pancreatitis, including fatal and non-fatal hemorrhagic or necrotizing pancreatitis, in patients taking JANUVIA. After initiation of JANUVIA, patients should be observed carefully for signs and symptoms of pancreatitis. If pancreatitis is suspected, JANUVIA should promptly be discontinued and appropriate management should be initiated. It is unknown whether patients with a history of pancreatitis are at increased risk for the development of pancreatitis while using JANUVIA.

5.2 Renal Impairment

Assessment of renal function is recommended prior to initiating JANUVIA and periodically thereafter. A dosage adjustment is recommended in patients with moderate or severe renal insufficiency and in patients with ESRD requiring hemodialysis or peritoneal dialysis. [See Dosage and Administration (2.2); Clinical Pharmacology (12.3).] Caution should be used to ensure that the correct dose of JANUVIA is prescribed for patients with moderate (creatinine clearance ≥30 to <50 mL/min) or severe (creatinine clearance <30 mL/min) renal impairment.

There have been postmarketing reports of worsening renal function, including acute renal failure, sometimes requiring dialysis. A subset of these reports involved patients with renal insufficiency, some of whom were prescribed inappropriate doses of sitagliptin. A return to baseline levels of renal insufficiency has been observed with supportive treatment and discontinuation of potentially causative agents. Consideration can be given to cautiously reinitiating JANUVIA if another etiology is deemed likely to have precipitated the acute worsening of renal function.

JANUVIA has not been found to be nephrotoxic in preclinical studies at clinically relevant doses, or in clinical trials.

5.3 Use with Medications Known to Cause Hypoglycemia

When JANUVIA was used in combination with a sulfonylurea or with insulin, medications known to cause hypoglycemia, the incidence of hypoglycemia was increased over that of placebo used in combination with a sulfonylurea or with insulin. [See Adverse Reactions (6.1).] Therefore, a lower dose of sulfonylurea or insulin may be required to reduce the risk of hypoglycemia. [See Dosage and Administration (2.3).]

5.4 Hypersensitivity Reactions

There have been postmarketing reports of serious hypersensitivity reactions in patients treated with JANUVIA. These reactions include anaphylaxis, angioedema, and exfoliative skin conditions including Stevens-Johnson syndrome. Onset of these reactions occurred within the first 3 months after initiation of treatment with JANUVIA, with some reports occurring after the first dose. If a hypersensitivity reaction is suspected, discontinue JANUVIA, assess for other potential causes for the event, and institute alternative treatment for diabetes. [See Adverse Reactions (6.2).]

Angioedema has also been reported with other dipeptidyl peptidase-4 (DPP-4) inhibitors. Use caution in a patient with a history of angioedema with another DPP-4 inhibitor because it is unknown whether such patients will be predisposed to angioedema with JANUVIA.

5.5 Macrovascular Outcomes

There have been no clinical studies establishing conclusive evidence of macrovascular risk reduction with JANUVIA or any other anti-diabetic drug.

6 ADVERSE REACTIONS

6.1 Clinical Trials Experience

Because clinical trials are conducted under widely varying conditions, adverse reaction rates observed in the clinical trials of a drug cannot be directly compared to rates in the clinical trials of another drug and may not reflect the rates observed in practice.

In controlled clinical studies as both monotherapy and combination therapy with metformin, pioglitazone, or rosiglitazone and metformin, the overall incidence of adverse reactions, hypoglycemia, and discontinuation of therapy due to

clinical adverse reactions with JANUVIA were similar to placebo. In combination with glimepiride, with or without metformin, the overall incidence of clinical adverse reactions with JANUVIA was higher than with placebo, in part related to a higher incidence of hypoglycemia (see Table 3); the incidence of discontinuation due to clinical adverse reactions was similar to placebo.

Two placebo-controlled monotherapy studies, one of 18- and one of 24-week duration, included patients treated with JANUVIA 100 mg daily, JANUVIA 200 mg daily, and placebo. Five placebo-controlled add-on combination therapy studies were also conducted: one with metformin; one with pioglitazone; one with metformin and rosiglitazone; one with glimepiride (with or without metformin); and one with insulin (with or without metformin). In these trials, patients with inadequate glycemic control on a stable dose of the background therapy were randomized to add-on therapy with JANUVIA 100 mg daily or placebo. The adverse reactions, excluding hypoglycemia, reported regardless of investigator assessment of causality in ≥5% of patients treated with JANUVIA 100 mg daily and more commonly than in patients treated with placebo, are shown in Table 1 for the clinical trials of at least 18 weeks duration. Incidences of hypoglycemia are shown in Table 3.

Table 1: Placebo-Controlled Clinical Studies of JANUVIA Monotherapy or Add-on Combination Therapy with Pioglitazone, Metformin + Rosiglitazone, or Glimepiride +/- Metformin: Adverse Reactions (Excluding Hypoglycemia) Reported in ≥5% of Patients and More Commonly than in Patients Given Placebo, Regardless of Investigator Assessment of Causality*

	Number of Patients (%)	
Monotherapy (18 or 24 weeks)	**JANUVIA 100 mg**	**Placebo**
	N = 443	N = 363
Nasopharyngitis	23 (5.2)	12 (3.3)
Combination with Pioglitazone (24 weeks)	**JANUVIA 100 mg + Pioglitazone**	**Placebo + Pioglitazone**
	N = 175	N = 178
Upper Respiratory Tract Infection	11 (6.3)	6 (3.4)
Headache	9 (5.1)	7 (3.9)
Combination with Metformin + Rosiglitazone (18 weeks)	**JANUVIA 100 mg + Metformin + Rosiglitazone**	**Placebo + Metformin + Rosiglitazone**
	N = 181	N = 97
Upper Respiratory Tract Infection	10 (5.5)	5 (5.2)
Nasopharyngitis	11 (6.1)	4 (4.1)
Combination with Glimepiride (+/- Metformin) (24 weeks)	**JANUVIA 100 mg + Glimepiride (+/- Metformin)**	**Placebo + Glimepiride (+/- Metformin)**
	N = 222	N = 219
Nasopharyngitis	14 (6.3)	10 (4.6)
Headache	13 (5.9)	5 (2.3)

* Intent-to-treat population

In the 24-week study of patients receiving JANUVIA as add-on combination therapy with metformin, there were no adverse reactions reported regardless of investigator assessment of causality in ≥5% of patients and more commonly than in patients given placebo.

In the 24-week study of patients receiving JANUVIA as add-on therapy to insulin (with or without metformin),

there were no adverse reactions reported regardless of investigator assessment of causality in ≥5% of patients and more commonly than in patients given placebo, except for hypoglycemia (see Table 3).

In the study of JANUVIA as add-on combination therapy with metformin and rosiglitazone (Table 1), through Week 54 the adverse reactions reported regardless of investigator assessment of causality in ≥5% of patients treated with JANUVIA and more commonly than in patients treated with placebo were: upper respiratory tract infection (JANUVIA, 15.5%; placebo, 6.2%), nasopharyngitis (11.0%, 9.3%), peripheral edema (8.3%, 5.2%), and headache (5.5%, 4.1%).

In a pooled analysis of the two monotherapy studies, the add-on to metformin study, and the add-on to pioglitazone study, the incidence of selected gastrointestinal adverse reactions in patients treated with JANUVIA was as follows: abdominal pain (JANUVIA 100 mg, 2.3%; placebo, 2.1%), nausea (1.4%, 0.6%), and diarrhea (3.0%, 2.3%).

In an additional, 24-week, placebo-controlled factorial study of initial therapy with sitagliptin in combination with metformin, the adverse reactions reported (regardless of investigator assessment of causality) in ≥5% of patients are shown in Table 2.

[See table 2 below]

In a 24-week study of initial therapy with JANUVIA in combination with pioglitazone, there were no adverse reactions reported (regardless of investigator assessment of causality) in ≥5% of patients and more commonly than in patients given pioglitazone alone.

No clinically meaningful changes in vital signs or in ECG (including in QTc interval) were observed in patients treated with JANUVIA.

In a pooled analysis of 19 double-blind clinical trials that included data from 10,246 patients randomized to receive sitagliptin 100 mg/day (N=5429) or corresponding (active or placebo) control (N=4817), the incidence of acute pancreatitis was 0.1 per 100 patient-years in each group (4 patients with an event in 4708 patient-years for sitagliptin and 4 patients with an event in 3942 patient-years for control). [See Warnings and Precautions (5.1).]

Hypoglycemia

In all (N=9) studies, adverse reactions of hypoglycemia were based on all reports of symptomatic hypoglycemia. A concurrent blood glucose measurement was not required although most (74%) reports of hypoglycemia were accompanied by a blood glucose measurement ≤70 mg/dL. When JANUVIA was co-administered with a sulfonylurea or with insulin, the percentage of patients with at least one adverse reaction of hypoglycemia was higher than in the corresponding placebo group (Table 3).

Table 3: Incidence and Rate of Hypoglycemia* in Placebo-Controlled Clinical Studies when JANUVIA was used as Add-On Therapy to Glimepiride (with or without Metformin) or Insulin (with or without Metformin), Regardless of Investigator Assessment of Causality

Add-On to Glimepiride (+/- Metformin) (24 weeks)	JANUVIA 100 mg + Glimepiride (+/- Metformin)	Placebo + Glimepiride (+/- Metformin)
	N = 222	N = 219
Overall (%)	27 (12.2)	4 (1.8)
Rate (episodes/ patient-year)[†]	0.59	0.24
Severe (%)[‡]	0 (0.0)	0 (0.0)
Add-On to Insulin (+/- Metformin) (24 weeks)	**JANUVIA 100 mg + Insulin (+/- Metformin)**	**Placebo + Insulin (+/- Metformin)**
	N = 322	N = 319
Overall (%)	50 (15.5)	25 (7.8)
Rate (episodes/ patient-year)[†]	1.06	0.51
Severe (%)[‡]	2 (0.6)	1 (0.3)

* Adverse reactions of hypoglycemia were based on all reports of symptomatic hypoglycemia; a concurrent glucose measurement was not required; intent-to-treat population.
† Based on total number of events (i.e., a single patient may have had multiple events).
‡ Severe events of hypoglycemia were defined as those events requiring medical assistance or exhibiting depressed level/loss of consciousness or seizure.

In a pooled analysis of the two monotherapy studies, the add-on to metformin study, and the add-on to pioglitazone

Table 2: Initial Therapy with Combination of Sitagliptin and Metformin: Adverse Reactions Reported (Regardless of Investigator Assessment of Causality) in ≥5% of Patients Receiving Combination Therapy (and Greater than in Patients Receiving Metformin alone, Sitagliptin alone, and Placebo)*

	Number of Patients (%)			
	Placebo	Sitagliptin (JANUVIA) 100 mg QD	Metformin 500 or 1000 mg bid[†]	Sitagliptin 50 mg bid + Metformin 500 or 1000 mg bid[†]
	N = 176	N = 179	N = 364[†]	N = 372[†]
Upper Respiratory Infection	9 (5.1)	8 (4.5)	19 (5.2)	23 (6.2)
Headache	5 (2.8)	2 (1.1)	14 (3.8)	22 (5.9)

* Intent-to-treat population.
† Data pooled for the patients given the lower and higher doses of metformin.

study, the overall incidence of adverse reactions of hypoglycemia was 1.2% in patients treated with JANUVIA 100 mg and 0.9% in patients treated with placebo.

In the study of JANUVIA as add-on combination therapy with metformin and rosiglitazone, the overall incidence of hypoglycemia was 2.2% in patients given add-on JANUVIA and 0.0% in patients given add-on placebo through Week 18. Through Week 54, the overall incidence of hypoglycemia was 3.9% in patients given add-on JANUVIA and 1.0% in patients given add-on placebo.

In the 24-week, placebo-controlled factorial study of initial therapy with JANUVIA in combination with metformin, the incidence of hypoglycemia was 0.6% in patients given placebo, 0.6% in patients given JANUVIA alone, 0.8% in patients given metformin alone, and 1.6% in patients given JANUVIA in combination with metformin.

In the study of JANUVIA as initial therapy with pioglitazone, one patient taking JANUVIA experienced a severe episode of hypoglycemia. There were no severe hypoglycemia episodes reported in other studies except in the study involving co-administration with insulin.

Laboratory Tests

Across clinical studies, the incidence of laboratory adverse reactions was similar in patients treated with JANUVIA 100 mg compared to patients treated with placebo. A small increase in white blood cell count (WBC) was observed due to an increase in neutrophils. This increase in WBC (of approximately 200 cells/microL vs placebo, in four pooled placebo-controlled clinical studies, with a mean baseline WBC count of approximately 6600 cells/microL) is not considered to be clinically relevant. In a 12-week study of 91 patients with chronic renal insufficiency, 37 patients with moderate renal insufficiency were randomized to JANUVIA 50 mg daily, while 14 patients with the same magnitude of renal impairment were randomized to placebo. Mean (SE) increases in serum creatinine were observed in patients treated with JANUVIA [0.12 mg/dL (0.04)] and in patients treated with placebo [0.07 mg/dL (0.07)]. The clinical significance of this added increase in serum creatinine relative to placebo is not known.

6.2 Postmarketing Experience

Additional adverse reactions have been identified during postapproval use of JANUVIA as monotherapy and/or in combination with other antihyperglycemic agents. Because these reactions are reported voluntarily from a population of uncertain size, it is generally not possible to reliably estimate their frequency or establish a causal relationship to drug exposure.

Hypersensitivity reactions including anaphylaxis, angioedema, rash, urticaria, cutaneous vasculitis, and exfoliative skin conditions including Stevens-Johnson syndrome *[see Warnings and Precautions (5.4)]*; hepatic enzyme elevations; acute pancreatitis, including fatal and non-fatal hemorrhagic and necrotizing pancreatitis *[see Indications and Usage (1.2); Warnings and Precautions (5.1)]*; worsening renal function, including acute renal failure (sometimes requiring dialysis) *[see Warnings and Precautions (5.2)]*; constipation; vomiting; headache; arthralgia; myalgia; pain in extremity; back pain.

7 DRUG INTERACTIONS

7.1 Digoxin

There was a slight increase in the area under the curve (AUC, 11%) and mean peak drug concentration (C_{max}, 18%) of digoxin with the co-administration of 100 mg sitagliptin for 10 days. Patients receiving digoxin should be monitored appropriately. No dosage adjustment of digoxin or JANUVIA is recommended.

8 USE IN SPECIFIC POPULATIONS

8.1 Pregnancy

Pregnancy Category B:

Reproduction studies have been performed in rats and rabbits. Doses of sitagliptin up to 125 mg/kg (approximately 12 times the human exposure at the maximum recommended human dose) did not impair fertility or harm the fetus. There are, however, no adequate and well-controlled studies in pregnant women. Because animal reproduction studies are not always predictive of human response, this drug should be used during pregnancy only if clearly needed. Merck Sharp & Dohme Corp., a subsidiary of Merck & Co., Inc., maintains a registry to monitor the pregnancy outcomes of women exposed to JANUVIA while pregnant. Health care providers are encouraged to report any prenatal exposure to JANUVIA by calling the Pregnancy Registry at 1-800-986-8999.

Sitagliptin administered to pregnant female rats and rabbits from gestation day 6 to 20 (organogenesis) was not teratogenic at oral doses up to 250 mg/kg (rats) and 125 mg/kg (rabbits), or approximately 30- and 20-times human exposure at the maximum recommended human dose (MRHD) of 100 mg/day based on AUC comparisons. Higher doses increased the incidence of rib malformations in offspring at 1000 mg/kg, or approximately 100 times human exposure at the MRHD.

Sitagliptin administered to female rats from gestation day 6 to lactation day 21 decreased body weight in male and female offspring at 1000 mg/kg. No functional or behavioral toxicity was observed in offspring of rats.

Placental transfer of sitagliptin administered to pregnant rats was approximately 45% at 2 hours and 80% at 24 hours postdose. Placental transfer of sitagliptin administered to pregnant rabbits was approximately 66% at 2 hours and 30% at 24 hours.

8.3 Nursing Mothers

Sitagliptin is secreted in the milk of lactating rats at a milk to plasma ratio of 4:1. It is not known whether sitagliptin is excreted in human milk. Because many drugs are excreted in human milk, caution should be exercised when JANUVIA is administered to a nursing woman.

8.4 Pediatric Use

Safety and effectiveness of JANUVIA in pediatric patients under 18 years of age have not been established.

8.5 Geriatric Use

Of the total number of subjects (N=3884) in pre-approval clinical safety and efficacy studies of JANUVIA, 725 patients were 65 years and over, while 61 patients were 75 years and over. No overall differences in safety or effectiveness were observed between subjects 65 years and over and younger subjects. While this and other reported clinical experience have not identified differences in responses between the elderly and younger patients, greater sensitivity of some older individuals cannot be ruled out.

This drug is known to be substantially excreted by the kidney. Because elderly patients are more likely to have decreased renal function, care should be taken in dose selection in the elderly, and it may be useful to assess renal function in these patients prior to initiating dosing and periodically thereafter *[see Dosage and Administration (2.2); Clinical Pharmacology (12.3)]*.

10 OVERDOSAGE

During controlled clinical trials in healthy subjects, single doses of up to 800 mg JANUVIA were administered. Maximal mean increases in QTc of 8.0 msec were observed in one study at a dose of 800 mg JANUVIA, a mean effect that is not considered clinically important *[see Clinical Pharmacology (12.2)]*. There is no experience with doses above 800 mg in clinical studies. In Phase I multiple-dose studies, there were no dose-related clinical adverse reactions observed with JANUVIA with doses of up to 600 mg per day for periods of up to 10 days and 400 mg per day for up to 28 days. In the event of an overdose, it is reasonable to employ the usual supportive measures, e.g., remove unabsorbed material from the gastrointestinal tract, employ clinical monitoring (including obtaining an electrocardiogram), and institute supportive therapy as dictated by the patient's clinical status.

Sitagliptin is modestly dialyzable. In clinical studies, approximately 13.5% of the dose was removed over a 3- to 4-hour hemodialysis session. Prolonged hemodialysis may be considered if clinically appropriate. It is not known if sitagliptin is dialyzable by peritoneal dialysis.

11 DESCRIPTION

JANUVIA Tablets contain sitagliptin phosphate, an orally-active inhibitor of the dipeptidyl peptidase-4 (DPP-4) enzyme.

Sitagliptin phosphate monohydrate is described chemically as 7-[(3R)-3-amino-1-oxo-4-(2,4,5-trifluorophenyl)butyl]-5,6,7,8-tetrahydro-3-(trifluoromethyl)-1,2,4-triazolo[4,3-a]pyrazine phosphate (1:1) monohydrate.

The empirical formula is $C_{16}H_{15}F_6N_5O \cdot H_3PO_4 \cdot H_2O$ and the molecular weight is 523.32. The structural formula is:

Sitagliptin phosphate monohydrate is a white to off-white, crystalline, non-hygroscopic powder. It is soluble in water and N,N-dimethyl formamide; slightly soluble in methanol; very slightly soluble in ethanol, acetone, and acetonitrile; and insoluble in isopropanol and isopropyl acetate.

Each film-coated tablet of JANUVIA contains 32.13, 64.25, or 128.5 mg of sitagliptin phosphate monohydrate, which is equivalent to 25, 50, or 100 mg, respectively, of free base and the following inactive ingredients: microcrystalline cellulose, anhydrous dibasic calcium phosphate, croscarmellose sodium, magnesium stearate, and sodium stearyl fumarate. In addition, the film coating contains the following inactive ingredients: polyvinyl alcohol, polyethylene glycol, talc, titanium dioxide, red iron oxide, and yellow iron oxide.

12 CLINICAL PHARMACOLOGY

12.1 Mechanism of Action

Sitagliptin is a DPP-4 inhibitor, which is believed to exert its actions in patients with type 2 diabetes by slowing the inactivation of incretin hormones. Concentrations of the active intact hormones are increased by JANUVIA, thereby increasing and prolonging the action of these hormones. Incretin hormones, including glucagon-like peptide-1 (GLP-1) and glucose-dependent insulinotropic polypeptide (GIP), are released by the intestine throughout the day, and levels are increased in response to a meal. These hormones are rapidly inactivated by the enzyme, DPP-4. The incretins are part of an endogenous system involved in the physiologic regulation of glucose homeostasis. When blood glucose concentrations are normal or elevated, GLP-1 and GIP increase insulin synthesis and release from pancreatic beta cells by intracellular signaling pathways involving cyclic AMP. GLP-1 also lowers glucagon secretion from pancreatic alpha cells, leading to reduced hepatic glucose production. By increasing and prolonging active incretin levels, JANUVIA increases insulin release and decreases glucagon levels in the circulation in a glucose-dependent manner. Sitagliptin demonstrates selectivity for DPP-4 and does not inhibit DPP-8 or DPP-9 activity *in vitro* at concentrations approximating those from therapeutic doses.

12.2 Pharmacodynamics

General

In patients with type 2 diabetes, administration of JANUVIA led to inhibition of DPP-4 enzyme activity for a 24-hour period. After an oral glucose load or a meal, this DPP-4 inhibition resulted in a 2- to 3-fold increase in circulating levels of active GLP-1 and GIP, decreased glucagon concentrations, and increased responsiveness of insulin release to glucose, resulting in higher C-peptide and insulin concentrations. The rise in insulin with the decrease in glucagon was associated with lower fasting glucose concentrations and reduced glucose excursion following an oral glucose load or a meal.

In a two-day study in healthy subjects, sitagliptin alone increased active GLP-1 concentrations, whereas metformin alone increased active and total GLP-1 concentrations to similar extents. Co-administration of sitagliptin and metformin had an additive effect on active GLP-1 concentrations. Sitagliptin, but not metformin, increased active GIP concentrations. It is unclear how these findings relate to changes in glycemic control in patients with type 2 diabetes. In studies with healthy subjects, JANUVIA did not lower blood glucose or cause hypoglycemia.

Cardiac Electrophysiology

In a randomized, placebo-controlled crossover study, 79 healthy subjects were administered a single oral dose of JANUVIA 100 mg, JANUVIA 800 mg (8 times the recommended dose), and placebo. At the recommended dose of 100 mg, there was no effect on the QTc interval obtained at the peak plasma concentration, or at any other time during the study. Following the 800 mg dose, the maximum increase in the placebo-corrected mean change in QTc from baseline was observed at 3 hours postdose and was 8.0 msec. This increase is not considered to be clinically significant. At the 800 mg dose, peak sitagliptin plasma concentrations were approximately 11 times higher than the peak concentrations following a 100 mg dose.

In patients with type 2 diabetes administered JANUVIA 100 mg (N=81) or JANUVIA 200 mg (N=63) daily, there were no meaningful changes in QTc interval based on ECG data obtained at the time of expected peak plasma concentration.

12.3 Pharmacokinetics

The pharmacokinetics of sitagliptin has been extensively characterized in healthy subjects and patients with type 2 diabetes. After oral administration of a 100 mg dose to healthy subjects, sitagliptin was rapidly absorbed, with peak plasma concentrations (median T_{max}) occurring 1 to 4 hours postdose. Plasma AUC of sitagliptin increased in a dose-proportional manner. Following a single oral 100 mg dose to healthy subjects, mean plasma AUC of sitagliptin was 8.52 μM•hr, C_{max} was 950 nM, and apparent terminal half-life ($t_{1/2}$) was 12.4 hours. Plasma AUC of sitagliptin increased approximately 14% following 100 mg doses at steady-state compared to the first dose. The intra-subject and inter-subject coefficients of variation for sitagliptin AUC were small (5.8% and 15.1%). The pharmacokinetics of sitagliptin was generally similar in healthy subjects and in patients with type 2 diabetes.

Absorption

The absolute bioavailability of sitagliptin is approximately 87%. Because coadministration of a high-fat meal with JANUVIA had no effect on the pharmacokinetics, JANUVIA may be administered with or without food.

Distribution

The mean volume of distribution at steady state following a single 100 mg intravenous dose of sitagliptin to healthy subjects is approximately 198 liters. The fraction of sitagliptin reversibly bound to plasma proteins is low (38%).

$$CrCl = \frac{[140 - age\ (years)] \times weight\ (kg)}{[72 \times serum\ creatinine\ (mg/dL)]} \quad \{\times\ 0.85\ for\ female\ patients\}$$

Table 4: Glycemic Parameters in 18- and 24-Week Placebo-Controlled Studies of JANUVIA in Patients with Type 2 Diabetes*

	18-Week Study		24-Week Study	
	JANUVIA 100 mg	Placebo	JANUVIA 100 mg	Placebo
A1C (%)	N = 193	N = 103	N = 229	N = 244
Baseline (mean)	8.0	8.1	8.0	8.0
Change from baseline (adjusted mean[†])	-0.5	0.1	-0.6	0.2
Difference from placebo (adjusted mean[†])	-0.6[‡]		-0.8[‡]	
(95% CI)	(-0.8, -0.4)		(-1.0, -0.6)	
Patients (%) achieving A1C <7%	69 (36%)	16 (16%)	93 (41%)	41 (17%)
FPG (mg/dL)	N = 201	N = 107	N = 234	N = 247
Baseline (mean)	180	184	170	176
Change from baseline (adjusted mean[†])	-13	7	-12	5
Difference from placebo (adjusted mean[†])	-20[‡]		-17[‡]	
(95% CI)	(-31, -9)		(-24, -10)	
2-hour PPG (mg/dL)	[§]	[§]	N = 201	N = 204
Baseline (mean)			257	271
Change from baseline (adjusted mean[†])			-49	-2
Difference from placebo (adjusted mean[†])			-47[‡]	
(95% CI)			(-59, -34)	

* Intent-to-treat population using last observation on study prior to metformin rescue therapy.
† Least squares means adjusted for prior antihyperglycemic therapy status and baseline value.
‡ p<0.001 compared to placebo.
§ Data not available.

Metabolism
Approximately 79% of sitagliptin is excreted unchanged in the urine with metabolism being a minor pathway of elimination.
Following a [^{14}C]sitagliptin oral dose, approximately 16% of the radioactivity was excreted as metabolites of sitagliptin. Six metabolites were detected at trace levels and are not expected to contribute to the plasma DPP-4 inhibitory activity of sitagliptin. *In vitro* studies indicated that the primary enzyme responsible for the limited metabolism of sitagliptin was CYP3A4, with contribution from CYP2C8.
Excretion
Following administration of an oral [^{14}C]sitagliptin dose to healthy subjects, approximately 100% of the administered radioactivity was eliminated in feces (13%) or urine (87%) within one week of dosing. The apparent terminal $t_{1/2}$ following a 100 mg oral dose of sitagliptin was approximately 12.4 hours and renal clearance was approximately 350 mL/min.
Elimination of sitagliptin occurs primarily via renal excretion and involves active tubular secretion. Sitagliptin is a substrate for human organic anion transporter-3 (hOAT-3), which may be involved in the renal elimination of sitagliptin. The clinical relevance of hOAT-3 in sitagliptin transport has not been established. Sitagliptin is also a substrate for p-glycoprotein, which may also be involved in mediating the renal elimination of sitagliptin. However, cyclosporine, a p-glycoprotein inhibitor, did not reduce the renal clearance of sitagliptin.
Special Populations
Renal Insufficiency
A single-dose, open-label study was conducted to evaluate the pharmacokinetics of JANUVIA (50 mg dose) in patients with varying degrees of chronic renal insufficiency compared to normal healthy control subjects. The study included patients with renal insufficiency classified on the basis of creatinine clearance as mild (50 to <80 mL/min), moderate (30 to <50 mL/min), and severe (<30 mL/min), as well as patients with ESRD on hemodialysis. In addition, the effects of renal insufficiency on sitagliptin pharmacokinetics in patients with type 2 diabetes and mild or moderate renal insufficiency were assessed using population pharmacokinetic analyses. Creatinine clearance was measured by 24-hour urinary creatinine clearance measurements or estimated from serum creatinine based on the Cockcroft-Gault formula:
[See table above]
Compared to normal healthy control subjects, an approximate 1.1- to 1.6-fold increase in plasma AUC of sitagliptin was observed in patients with mild renal insufficiency. Because increases of this magnitude are not clinically relevant, dosage adjustment in patients with mild renal insufficiency is not necessary. Plasma AUC levels of sitagliptin were increased approximately 2-fold and 4-fold in patients with moderate renal insufficiency and in patients with se-

vere renal insufficiency, including patients with ESRD on hemodialysis, respectively. Sitagliptin was modestly removed by hemodialysis (13.5% over a 3- to 4-hour hemodialysis session starting 4 hours postdose). To achieve plasma concentrations of sitagliptin similar to those in patients with normal renal function, lower dosages are recommended in patients with moderate and severe renal insufficiency, as well as in ESRD patients requiring dialysis. *[See Dosage and Administration (2.2).]*
Hepatic Insufficiency
In patients with moderate hepatic insufficiency (Child-Pugh score 7 to 9), mean AUC and C_{max} of sitagliptin increased approximately 21% and 13%, respectively, compared to healthy matched controls following administration of a single 100 mg dose of JANUVIA. These differences are not considered to be clinically meaningful. No dosage adjustment for JANUVIA is necessary for patients with mild or moderate hepatic insufficiency.
There is no clinical experience in patients with severe hepatic insufficiency (Child-Pugh score >9).
Body Mass Index (BMI)
No dosage adjustment is necessary based on BMI. Body mass index had no clinically meaningful effect on the pharmacokinetics of sitagliptin based on a composite analysis of Phase I pharmacokinetic data and on a population pharmacokinetic analysis of Phase I and Phase II data.
Gender
No dosage adjustment is necessary based on gender. Gender had no clinically meaningful effect on the pharmacokinetics of sitagliptin based on a composite analysis of Phase I pharmacokinetic data and on a population pharmacokinetic analysis of Phase I and Phase II data.
Geriatric
No dosage adjustment is required based solely on age. When the effects of age on renal function are taken into account, age alone did not have a clinically meaningful impact on the pharmacokinetics of sitagliptin based on a population pharmacokinetic analysis. Elderly subjects (65 to 80 years) had approximately 19% higher plasma concentrations of sitagliptin compared to younger subjects.
Pediatric
Studies characterizing the pharmacokinetics of sitagliptin in pediatric patients have not been performed.
Race
No dosage adjustment is necessary based on race. Race had no clinically meaningful effect on the pharmacokinetics of sitagliptin based on a composite analysis of available pharmacokinetic data, including subjects of white, Hispanic, black, Asian, and other racial groups.
Drug Interactions
In Vitro Assessment of Drug Interactions
Sitagliptin is not an inhibitor of CYP isozymes CYP3A4, 2C8, 2C9, 2D6, 1A2, 2C19 or 2B6, and is not an inducer of CYP3A4. Sitagliptin is a p-glycoprotein substrate, but does not inhibit p-glycoprotein mediated transport of digoxin.

Based on these results, sitagliptin is considered unlikely to cause interactions with other drugs that utilize these pathways.
Sitagliptin is not extensively bound to plasma proteins. Therefore, the propensity of sitagliptin to be involved in clinically meaningful drug-drug interactions mediated by plasma protein binding displacement is very low.
In Vivo Assessment of Drug Interactions
Effects of Sitagliptin on Other Drugs
In clinical studies, as described below, sitagliptin did not meaningfully alter the pharmacokinetics of metformin, glyburide, simvastatin, rosiglitazone, warfarin, or oral contraceptives, providing *in vivo* evidence of a low propensity for causing drug interactions with substrates of CYP3A4, CYP2C8, CYP2C9, and organic cationic transporter (OCT).
Digoxin: Sitagliptin had a minimal effect on the pharmacokinetics of digoxin. Following administration of 0.25 mg digoxin concomitantly with 100 mg of JANUVIA daily for 10 days, the plasma AUC of digoxin was increased by 11%, and the plasma C_{max} by 18%.
Metformin: Co-administration of multiple twice-daily doses of sitagliptin with metformin, an OCT substrate, did not meaningfully alter the pharmacokinetics of metformin in patients with type 2 diabetes. Therefore, sitagliptin is not an inhibitor of OCT-mediated transport.
Sulfonylureas: Single-dose pharmacokinetics of glyburide, a CYP2C9 substrate, was not meaningfully altered in subjects receiving multiple doses of sitagliptin. Clinically meaningful interactions would not be expected with other sulfonylureas (e.g., glipizide, tolbutamide, and glimepiride) which, like glyburide, are primarily eliminated by CYP2C9.
Simvastatin: Single-dose pharmacokinetics of simvastatin, a CYP3A4 substrate, was not meaningfully altered in subjects receiving multiple daily doses of sitagliptin. Therefore, sitagliptin is not an inhibitor of CYP3A4-mediated metabolism.
Thiazolidinediones: Single-dose pharmacokinetics of rosiglitazone was not meaningfully altered in subjects receiving multiple daily doses of sitagliptin, indicating that JANUVIA is not an inhibitor of CYP2C8-mediated metabolism.
Warfarin: Multiple daily doses of sitagliptin did not meaningfully alter the pharmacokinetics, as assessed by measurement of S(-) or R(+) warfarin enantiomers, or pharmacodynamics (as assessed by measurement of prothrombin INR) of a single dose of warfarin. Because S(-) warfarin is primarily metabolized by CYP2C9, these data also support the conclusion that sitagliptin is not a CYP2C9 inhibitor.
Oral Contraceptives: Co-administration with sitagliptin did not meaningfully alter the steady-state pharmacokinetics of norethindrone or ethinyl estradiol.
Effects of Other Drugs on Sitagliptin
Clinical data described below suggest that sitagliptin is not susceptible to clinically meaningful interactions by co-administered medications.
Metformin: Co-administration of multiple twice-daily doses of metformin with sitagliptin did not meaningfully alter the pharmacokinetics of sitagliptin in patients with type 2 diabetes.
Cyclosporine: A study was conducted to assess the effect of cyclosporine, a potent inhibitor of p-glycoprotein, on the pharmacokinetics of sitagliptin. Co-administration of a single 100 mg oral dose of JANUVIA and a single 600 mg oral dose of cyclosporine increased the AUC and C_{max} of sitagliptin by approximately 29% and 68%, respectively. These modest changes in sitagliptin pharmacokinetics were not considered to be clinically meaningful. The renal clearance of sitagliptin was also not meaningfully altered. Therefore, meaningful interactions would not be expected with other p-glycoprotein inhibitors.

13   NONCLINICAL TOXICOLOGY
13.1   Carcinogenesis, Mutagenesis, Impairment of Fertility
A two-year carcinogenicity study was conducted in male and female rats given oral doses of sitagliptin of 50, 150, and 500 mg/kg/day. There was an increased incidence of combined liver adenoma/carcinoma in males and females and of liver carcinoma in females at 500 mg/kg. This dose results in exposures approximately 60 times the human exposure at the maximum recommended daily adult human dose (MRHD) of 100 mg/day based on AUC comparisons. Liver tumors were not observed at 150 mg/kg, approximately 20 times the human exposure at the MRHD. A two-year carcinogenicity study was conducted in male and female mice given oral doses of 50, 125, 250, and 500 mg/kg/day. There was no increase in the incidence of tumors in any organ up to 500 mg/kg, approximately 70 times human exposure at the MRHD. Sitagliptin was not mutagenic or clastogenic with or without metabolic activation in the Ames bacterial mutagenicity assay, a Chinese hamster ovary (CHO) chromosome aberration assay, an *in vitro* cytogenetics assay in CHO, an *in vitro* rat hepatocyte DNA alkaline elution assay, and an *in vivo* micronucleus assay.

In rat fertility studies with oral gavage doses of 125, 250, and 1000 mg/kg, males were treated for 4 weeks prior to mating, during mating, up to scheduled termination (approximately 8 weeks total) and females were treated 2 weeks prior to mating through gestation day 7. No adverse effect on fertility was observed at 125 mg/kg (approximately 12 times human exposure at the MRHD of 100 mg/day based on AUC comparisons). At higher doses, nondose-related increased resorptions in females were observed (approximately 25 and 100 times human exposure at the MRHD based on AUC comparison).

14 CLINICAL STUDIES

There were approximately 5200 patients with type 2 diabetes randomized in nine double-blind, placebo-controlled clinical safety and efficacy studies conducted to evaluate the effects of sitagliptin on glycemic control. In a pooled analysis of seven of these studies, the ethnic/racial distribution was approximately 59% white, 20% Hispanic, 10% Asian, 6% black, and 6% other groups. Patients had an overall mean age of approximately 55 years (range 18 to 87 years). In addition, an active (glipizide)-controlled study of 52-weeks duration was conducted in 1172 patients with type 2 diabetes who had inadequate glycemic control on metformin.

In patients with type 2 diabetes, treatment with JANUVIA produced clinically significant improvements in hemoglobin A1C, fasting plasma glucose (FPG) and 2-hour postprandial glucose (PPG) compared to placebo.

14.1 Monotherapy

A total of 1262 patients with type 2 diabetes participated in two double-blind, placebo-controlled studies, one of 18-week and another of 24-week duration, to evaluate the efficacy and safety of JANUVIA monotherapy. In both monotherapy studies, patients currently on an antihyperglycemic agent discontinued the agent, and underwent a diet, exercise, and drug washout period of about 7 weeks. Patients with inadequate glycemic control (A1C 7% to 10%) after the washout period were randomized after completing a 2-week single-blind placebo run-in period; patients not currently on antihyperglycemic agents (off therapy for at least 8 weeks) with inadequate glycemic control (A1C 7% to 10%) were randomized after completing the 2-week single-blind placebo run-in period. In the 18-week study, 521 patients were randomized to placebo, JANUVIA 100 mg, or JANUVIA 200 mg, and in the 24-week study 741 patients were randomized to placebo, JANUVIA 100 mg, or JANUVIA 200 mg. Patients who failed to meet specific glycemic goals during the studies were treated with metformin rescue, added on to placebo or JANUVIA.

Treatment with JANUVIA at 100 mg daily provided significant improvements in A1C, FPG, and 2-hour PPG compared to placebo (Table 4). In the 18-week study, 9% of patients receiving JANUVIA 100 mg and 17% who received placebo required rescue therapy. In the 24-week study, 9% of patients receiving JANUVIA 100 mg and 21% of patients receiving placebo required rescue therapy. The improvement in A1C compared to placebo was not affected by gender, age, race, prior antihyperglycemic therapy, or baseline BMI. As is typical for trials of agents to treat type 2 diabetes, the mean reduction in A1C with JANUVIA appears to be related to the degree of A1C elevation at baseline. In these 18- and 24-week studies, among patients who were not on an antihyperglycemic agent at study entry, the reductions from baseline in A1C were -0.7% and -0.8%, respectively, for those given JANUVIA, and -0.1% and -0.2%, respectively, for those given placebo. Overall, the 200 mg daily dose did not provide greater glycemic efficacy than the 100 mg daily dose. The effect of JANUVIA on lipid endpoints was similar to placebo. Body weight did not increase from baseline with JANUVIA therapy in either study, compared to a small reduction in patients given placebo.

[See table 4 at top of previous page]

Additional Monotherapy Study

A multinational, randomized, double-blind, placebo-controlled study was also conducted to assess the safety and tolerability of JANUVIA in 91 patients with type 2 diabetes and chronic renal insufficiency (creatinine clearance <50 mL/min). Patients with moderate renal insufficiency received 50 mg daily of JANUVIA and those with severe renal insufficiency or with ESRD on hemodialysis or peritoneal dialysis received 25 mg daily. In this study, the safety and tolerability of JANUVIA were generally similar to placebo. A small increase in serum creatinine was reported in patients with moderate renal insufficiency treated with JANUVIA relative to those on placebo. In addition, the reductions in A1C and FPG with JANUVIA compared to placebo were generally similar to those observed in other monotherapy studies. [See Clinical Pharmacology (12.3).]

14.2 Combination Therapy

Add-on Combination Therapy with Metformin

A total of 701 patients with type 2 diabetes participated in a 24-week, randomized, double-blind, placebo-controlled study designed to assess the efficacy of JANUVIA in combination with metformin. Patients already on metformin (N=431) at a dose of at least 1500 mg per day were randomized after completing a 2-week single-blind placebo run-in period. Patients on metformin and another antihyperglycemic agent (N=229) and patients not on any antihyperglycemic agents (off therapy for at least 8 weeks, N=41) were randomized after a run-in period of approximately 10 weeks on metformin (at a dose of at least 1500 mg per day) in monotherapy. Patients with inadequate glycemic control (A1C 7% to 10%) were randomized to the addition of either 100 mg of JANUVIA or placebo, administered once daily. Patients who failed to meet specific glycemic goals during the studies were treated with pioglitazone rescue.

In combination with metformin, JANUVIA provided significant improvements in A1C, FPG, and 2-hour PPG compared to placebo with metformin (Table 5). Rescue glycemic therapy was used in 5% of patients treated with JANUVIA 100 mg and 14% of patients treated with placebo. A similar decrease in body weight was observed for both treatment groups.

[See table 5 above]

Initial Combination Therapy with Metformin

A total of 1091 patients with type 2 diabetes and inadequate glycemic control on diet and exercise participated in a 24-week, randomized, double-blind, placebo-controlled factorial study designed to assess the efficacy of sitagliptin as initial therapy in combination with metformin. Patients on an antihyperglycemic agent (N=541) discontinued the agent, and underwent a diet, exercise, and drug washout period of up to 12 weeks duration. After the washout period, patients with inadequate glycemic control (A1C 7.5% to 11%) were randomized after completing a 2-week single-blind placebo run-in period. Patients not on antihyperglycemic agents at study entry (N=550) with inadequate glycemic control (A1C 7.5% to 11%) immediately entered the 2-week single-blind placebo run-in period and then were randomized. Approximately equal numbers of patients were randomized to receive initial therapy with placebo, 100 mg of JANUVIA once daily, 500 mg or 1000 mg of metformin twice daily, or 50 mg of sitagliptin twice daily in combination with 500 mg or 1000 mg of metformin twice daily. Patients who failed to meet specific glycemic goals during the study were treated with glyburide (glibenclamide) rescue.

Table 5: Glycemic Parameters at Final Visit (24-Week Study) for JANUVIA in Add-on Combination Therapy with Metformin*

	JANUVIA 100 mg + Metformin	Placebo + Metformin
A1C (%)	**N = 453**	**N = 224**
Baseline (mean)	8.0	8.0
Change from baseline (adjusted mean[†])	-0.7	-0.0
Difference from placebo + metformin (adjusted mean[†]) (95% CI)	-0.7[‡] (-0.8, -0.5)	
Patients (%) achieving A1C <7%	213 (47%)	41 (18%)
FPG (mg/dL)	**N = 454**	**N = 226**
Baseline (mean)	170	174
Change from baseline (adjusted mean[†])	-17	9
Difference from placebo + metformin (adjusted mean[†]) (95% CI)	-25[‡] (-31, -20)	
2-hour PPG (mg/dL)	**N = 387**	**N = 182**
Baseline (mean)	275	272
Change from baseline (adjusted mean[†])	-62	-11
Difference from placebo + metformin (adjusted mean[†]) (95% CI)	-51[‡] (-61, -41)	

* Intent-to-treat population using last observation on study prior to pioglitazone rescue therapy.
† Least squares means adjusted for prior antihyperglycemic therapy and baseline value.
‡ p<0.001 compared to placebo + metformin.

Table 6: Glycemic Parameters at Final Visit (24-Week Study) for Sitagliptin and Metformin, Alone and in Combination as Initial Therapy*

	Placebo	Sitagliptin (JANUVIA) 100 mg QD	Metformin 500 mg bid	Metformin 1000 mg bid	Sitagliptin 50 mg bid + Metformin 500 mg bid	Sitagliptin 50 mg bid + Metformin 1000 mg bid
A1C (%)	**N = 165**	**N = 175**	**N = 178**	**N = 177**	**N = 183**	**N = 178**
Baseline (mean)	8.7	8.9	8.9	8.7	8.8	8.8
Change from baseline (adjusted mean[†])	0.2	-0.7	-0.8	-1.1	-1.4	-1.9
Difference from placebo (adjusted mean[†]) (95% CI)		-0.8[‡] (-1.1, -0.6)	-1.0[‡] (-1.2, -0.8)	-1.3[‡] (-1.5, -1.1)	-1.6[‡] (-1.8, -1.3)	-2.1[‡] (-2.3, -1.8)
Patients (%) achieving A1C <7%	15 (9%)	35 (20%)	41 (23%)	68 (38%)	79 (43%)	118 (66%)
% Patients receiving rescue medication	32	21	17	12	8	2
FPG (mg/dL)	**N = 169**	**N = 178**	**N = 179**	**N = 179**	**N = 183**	**N = 180**
Baseline (mean)	196	201	205	197	204	197
Change from baseline (adjusted mean[†])	6	-17	-27	-29	-47	-64
Difference from placebo (adjusted mean[†]) (95% CI)		-23[‡] (-33, -14)	-33[‡] (-43, -24)	-35[‡] (-45, -26)	-53[‡] (-62, -43)	-70[‡] (-79, -60)
2-hour PPG (mg/dL)	**N = 129**	**N = 136**	**N = 141**	**N = 138**	**N = 147**	**N = 152**
Baseline (mean)	277	285	293	283	292	287
Change from baseline (adjusted mean[†])	0	-52	-53	-78	-93	-117
Difference from placebo (adjusted mean[†]) (95% CI)		-52[‡] (-67, -37)	-54[‡] (-69, -39)	-78[‡] (-93, -63)	-93[‡] (-107, -78)	-117[‡] (-131, -102)

* Intent-to-treat population using last observation on study prior to glyburide (glibenclamide) rescue therapy.
† Least squares means adjusted for prior antihyperglycemic therapy status and baseline value.
‡ p<0.001 compared to placebo.

Table 8: Glycemic Parameters at Final Visit (24-Week Study) for JANUVIA in Add-on Combination Therapy with Pioglitazone*

	JANUVIA 100 mg + Pioglitazone	Placebo + Pioglitazone
A1C (%)	N = 163	N = 174
Baseline (mean)	8.1	8.0
Change from baseline (adjusted mean[†])	-0.9	-0.2
Difference from placebo + pioglitazone (adjusted mean[†]) (95% CI)	-0.7[‡] (-0.9, -0.5)	
Patients (%) achieving A1C <7%	74 (45%)	40 (23%)
FPG (mg/dL)	N = 163	N = 174
Baseline (mean)	168	166
Change from baseline (adjusted mean[†])	-17	1
Difference from placebo + pioglitazone (adjusted mean[†]) (95% CI)	-18[‡] (-24, -11)	

* Intent-to-treat population using last observation on study prior to metformin rescue therapy.
† Least squares means adjusted for prior antihyperglycemic therapy status and baseline value.
‡ p<0.001 compared to placebo + pioglitazone.

Table 9: Glycemic Parameters at Final Visit (24-Week Study) for JANUVIA in Combination with Pioglitazone as Initial Therapy*

	JANUVIA 100 mg + Pioglitazone	Pioglitazone
A1C (%)	N = 251	N = 246
Baseline (mean)	9.5	9.4
Change from baseline (adjusted mean[†])	-2.4	-1.5
Difference from pioglitazone (adjusted mean[†]) (95% CI)	-0.9[‡] (-1.1, -0.7)	
Patients (%) achieving A1C <7%	151 (60%)	68 (28%)
FPG (mg/dL)	N = 256	N = 253
Baseline (mean)	203	201
Change from baseline (adjusted mean[†])	-63	-40
Difference from pioglitazone (adjusted mean[†]) (95% CI)	-23[‡] (-30, -15)	
2-hour PPG (mg/dL)	N = 216	N = 211
Baseline (mean)	283	284
Change from baseline (adjusted mean[†])	-114	-69
Difference from pioglitazone (adjusted mean[†]) (95% CI)	-45[‡] (-57, -32)	

* Intent-to-treat population using last observation on study.
† Least squares means adjusted for baseline value.
‡ p<0.001 compared to placebo + pioglitazone.

Initial therapy with the combination of JANUVIA and metformin provided significant improvements in A1C, FPG, and 2-hour PPG compared to placebo, to metformin alone, and to JANUVIA alone (Table 6, Figure 1). Mean reductions from baseline in A1C were generally greater for patients with higher baseline A1C values. For patients not on an antihyperglycemic agent at study entry, mean reductions from baseline in A1C were: JANUVIA 100 mg once daily, -1.1%; metformin 500 mg bid, -1.1%; metformin 1000 mg bid, -1.2%; sitagliptin 50 mg bid with metformin 500 mg bid, -1.6%; sitagliptin 50 mg bid with metformin 1000 mg bid, -1.9%; and for patients receiving placebo, -0.2%. Lipid effects were generally neutral. The decrease in body weight in the groups given sitagliptin in combination with metformin was similar to that in the groups given metformin alone or placebo.
[See table 6 on previous page]
[See figure 1 at top of next column]
Initial combination therapy or maintenance of combination therapy may not be appropriate for all patients. These management options are left to the discretion of the health care provider.
Active-Controlled Study vs Glipizide in Combination with Metformin
The efficacy of JANUVIA was evaluated in a 52-week, double-blind, glipizide-controlled noninferiority trial in patients with type 2 diabetes. Patients not on treatment or on other antihyperglycemic agents entered a run-in treatment period of up to 12 weeks duration with metformin monotherapy (dose of ≥1500 mg per day) which included washout of medications other than metformin, if applicable. After the run-in period, those with inadequate glycemic control (A1C 6.5% to 10%) were randomized 1:1 to the addition of JANUVIA 100 mg once daily or glipizide for 52 weeks. Patients receiving glipizide were given an initial dosage of

Figure 1: Mean Change from Baseline for A1C (%) over 24 Weeks with Sitagliptin and Metformin, Alone and in Combination as Initial Therapy in Patients with Type 2 Diabetes*

○ Placebo
● Sitagliptin 100 mg q.d.
◆ Metformin 500 mg b.i.d.
□ Metformin 1000 mg b.i.d.
✦ Sitagliptin 50 mg b.i.d. + Metformin 500 mg b.i.d.
■ Sitagliptin 50 mg b.i.d. + Metformin 1000 mg b.i.d.

* All Patients Treated Population: least squares means adjusted for prior antihyperglycemic therapy and baseline value.

5 mg/day and then electively titrated over the next 18 weeks to a maximum dosage of 20 mg/day as needed to optimize glycemic control. Thereafter, the glipizide dose was to be kept constant, except for down-titration to prevent hypoglycemia. The mean dose of glipizide after the titration period was 10 mg.
After 52 weeks, JANUVIA and glipizide had similar mean reductions from baseline in A1C in the intent-to-treat analysis (Table 7). These results were consistent with the per protocol analysis (Figure 2). A conclusion in favor of the non-

inferiority of JANUVIA to glipizide may be limited to patients with baseline A1C comparable to those included in the study (over 70% of patients had baseline A1C <8% and over 90% had A1C <9%).

Table 7: Glycemic Parameters in a 52-Week Study Comparing JANUVIA to Glipizide as Add-On Therapy in Patients Inadequately Controlled on Metformin (Intent-to-Treat Population)*

	JANUVIA 100 mg	Glipizide
A1C (%)	N = 576	N = 559
Baseline (mean)	7.7	7.6
Change from baseline (adjusted mean[†])	-0.5	-0.6
FPG (mg/dL)	N = 583	N = 568
Baseline (mean)	166	164
Change from baseline (adjusted mean[†])	-8	-8

* The intent-to-treat analysis used the patients' last observation in the study prior to discontinuation.
† Least squares means adjusted for prior antihyperglycemic therapy status and baseline A1C value.

Figure 2: Mean Change from Baseline for A1C (%) Over 52 Weeks in a Study Comparing JANUVIA to Glipizide as Add-On Therapy in Patients Inadequately Controlled on Metformin (Per Protocol Population)*

◆ Januvia 100 mg   ○ Glipizide

* The per protocol population (mean baseline A1C of 7.5%) included patients without major protocol violations who had observations at baseline and at Week 52.

The incidence of hypoglycemia in the JANUVIA group (4.9%) was significantly (p<0.001) lower than that in the glipizide group (32.0%). Patients treated with JANUVIA exhibited a significant mean decrease from baseline in body weight compared to a significant weight gain in patients administered glipizide (-1.5 kg vs +1.1 kg).
Add-on Combination Therapy with Pioglitazone
A total of 353 patients with type 2 diabetes participated in a 24-week, randomized, double-blind, placebo-controlled study designed to assess the efficacy of JANUVIA in combination with pioglitazone. Patients on any oral antihyperglycemic agent in monotherapy (N=212) or on a PPARγ agent in combination therapy (N=106) or not on an antihyperglycemic agent (off therapy for at least 8 weeks, N=34) were switched to monotherapy with pioglitazone (at a dose of 30-45 mg per day), and completed a run-in period of approximately 12 weeks in duration. After the run-in period on pioglitazone monotherapy, patients with inadequate glycemic control (A1C 7% to 10%) were randomized to the addition of either 100 mg of JANUVIA or placebo, administered once daily. Patients who failed to meet specific glycemic goals during the studies were treated with metformin rescue. Glycemic endpoints measured were A1C and fasting glucose.
In combination with pioglitazone, JANUVIA provided significant improvements in A1C and FPG compared to placebo with pioglitazone (Table 8). Rescue therapy was used in 7% of patients treated with JANUVIA 100 mg and 14% of patients treated with placebo. There was no significant difference between JANUVIA and placebo in body weight change.
[See table 8 above]
Initial Combination Therapy with Pioglitazone
A total of 520 patients with type 2 diabetes and inadequate glycemic control on diet and exercise participated in a 24-week, randomized, double-blind study designed to assess the efficacy of JANUVIA as initial therapy in combination

with pioglitazone. Patients not on antihyperglycemic agents at study entry (<4 weeks cumulative therapy over the past 2 years, and with no treatment over the prior 4 months) with inadequate glycemic control (A1C 8% to 12%) immediately entered the 2-week single-blind placebo run-in period and then were randomized. Approximately equal numbers of patients were randomized to receive initial therapy with 100 mg of JANUVIA in combination with 30 mg of pioglitazone once daily or 30 mg of pioglitazone once daily as monotherapy. There was no glycemic rescue therapy in this study. Initial therapy with the combination of JANUVIA and pioglitazone provided significant improvements in A1C, FPG, and 2-hour PPG compared to pioglitazone monotherapy (Table 9). The improvement in A1C was generally consistent across subgroups defined by gender, age, race, baseline BMI, baseline A1C, or duration of disease. In this study, patients treated with JANUVIA in combination with pioglitazone had a mean increase in body weight of 1.1 kg compared to pioglitazone alone (3.0 kg vs. 1.9 kg). Lipid effects were generally neutral.
[See table 9 at top of previous page]

Add-on Combination Therapy with Metformin and Rosiglitazone

A total of 278 patients with type 2 diabetes participated in a 54-week, randomized, double-blind, placebo-controlled study designed to assess the efficacy of JANUVIA in combination with metformin and rosiglitazone. Patients on dual therapy with metformin ≥1500 mg/day and rosiglitazone ≥4 mg/day or with metformin ≥1500 mg/day and pioglitazone ≥30 mg/day (switched to rosiglitazone ≥4 mg/day) entered a dose-stable run-in period of 6 weeks. Patients on other dual therapy were switched to metformin ≥1500 mg/day and rosiglitazone ≥4 mg/day in a dose titration/stabilization run-in period of up to 20 weeks in duration. After the run-in period, patients with inadequate glycemic control (A1C 7.5% to 11%) were randomized 2:1 to the addition of either 100 mg of JANUVIA or placebo, administered once daily. Patients who failed to meet specific glycemic goals during the study were treated with glipizide (or other sulfonylurea) rescue. The primary time point for evaluation of glycemic parameters was Week 18.

In combination with metformin and rosiglitazone, JANUVIA provided significant improvements in A1C, FPG, and 2-hour PPG compared to placebo with metformin and rosiglitazone (Table 10) at Week 18. At Week 54, mean reduction in A1C was -1.0% for patients treated with JANUVIA and -0.3% for patients treated with placebo in an analysis based on the intent-to-treat population. Rescue therapy was used in 18% of patients treated with JANUVIA 100 mg and 40% of patients treated with placebo. There was no significant difference between JANUVIA and placebo in body weight change.
[See table 10 above]

Add-on Combination Therapy with Glimepiride, with or without Metformin

A total of 441 patients with type 2 diabetes participated in a 24-week, randomized, double-blind, placebo-controlled study designed to assess the efficacy of JANUVIA in combination with glimepiride, with or without metformin. Patients entered a run-in treatment period on glimepiride (≥4 mg per day) alone or glimepiride in combination with metformin (≥1500 mg per day). After a dose-titration and dose-stable run-in period of up to 16 weeks and a 2-week placebo run-in period, patients with inadequate glycemic control (A1C 7.5% to 10.5%) were randomized to the addition of either 100 mg of JANUVIA or placebo, administered once daily. Patients who failed to meet specific glycemic goals during the studies were treated with pioglitazone rescue.

In combination with glimepiride, with or without metformin, JANUVIA provided significant improvements in A1C and FPG compared to placebo (Table 11). In the entire study population (patients on JANUVIA in combination with glimepiride and patients on JANUVIA in combination with glimepiride and metformin), a mean reduction from baseline relative to placebo in A1C of -0.7% and in FPG of -20 mg/dL was seen. Rescue therapy was used in 12% of patients treated with JANUVIA 100 mg and 27% of patients treated with placebo. In this study, patients treated with JANUVIA had a mean increase in body weight of 1.1 kg vs. placebo (+0.8 kg vs. -0.4 kg). In addition, there was an increased rate of hypoglycemia. *[See Warnings and Precautions (5.3); Adverse Reactions (6.1).]*
[See table 11 above]

Add-on Combination Therapy with Insulin (with or without Metformin)

A total of 641 patients with type 2 diabetes participated in a 24-week, randomized, double-blind, placebo-controlled study designed to assess the efficacy of JANUVIA as add-on to insulin therapy (with or without metformin). The racial distribution in this study was approximately 70% white, 18% Asian, 7% black, and 5% other groups. Approximately 14% of the patients in this study were Hispanic. Patients entered a 2-week, single-blind run-in treatment period on

Table 10: Glycemic Parameters at Week 18 for JANUVIA in Add-on Combination Therapy with Metformin and Rosiglitazone*

	JANUVIA 100 mg + Metformin + Rosiglitazone	Placebo + Metformin + Rosiglitazone
A1C (%)	**N = 176**	**N = 93**
Baseline (mean)	8.8	8.7
Change from baseline (adjusted mean†)	-1.0	-0.4
Difference from placebo + rosiglitazone + metformin (adjusted mean†) (95% CI)	-0.7‡ (-0.9, -0.4)	
Patients (%) achieving A1C <7%	39 (22%)	9 (10%)
FPG (mg/dL)	**N = 179**	**N = 94**
Baseline (mean)	181	182
Change from baseline (adjusted mean†)	-30	-11
Difference from placebo + rosiglitazone + metformin (adjusted mean†) (95% CI)	-18‡ (-26, -10)	
2-hour PPG (mg/dL)	**N = 152**	**N = 80**
Baseline (mean)	256	248
Change from baseline (adjusted mean†)	-59	-21
Difference from placebo + rosiglitazone + metformin (adjusted mean†) (95% CI)	-39‡ (-51, -26)	

* Intent-to-treat population using last observation on study prior to glipizide (or other sulfonylurea) rescue therapy.
† Least squares means adjusted for prior antihyperglycemic therapy status and baseline value.
‡ p<0.001 compared to placebo + metformin + rosiglitazone.

Table 11: Glycemic Parameters at Final Visit (24-Week Study) for JANUVIA as Add-On Combination Therapy with Glimepiride, with or without Metformin*

	JANUVIA 100 mg + Glimepiride	Placebo + Glimepiride	JANUVIA 100 mg + Glimepiride + Metformin	Placebo + Glimepiride + Metformin
A1C (%)	**N = 102**	**N = 103**	**N = 115**	**N = 105**
Baseline (mean)	8.4	8.5	8.3	8.3
Change from baseline (adjusted mean†)	-0.3	0.3	-0.6	0.3
Difference from placebo (adjusted mean†) (95% CI)	-0.6‡ (-0.8, -0.3)		-0.9‡ (-1.1, -0.7)	
Patients (%) achieving A1C <7%	11 (11%)	9 (9%)	26 (23%)	1 (1%)
FPG (mg/dL)	**N = 104**	**N = 104**	**N = 115**	**N = 109**
Baseline (mean)	183	185	179	179
Change from baseline (adjusted mean†)	-1	18	-8	13
Difference from placebo (adjusted mean†) (95% CI)	-19§ (-32, -7)		-21‡ (-32, -10)	

* Intent-to-treat population using last observation on study prior to pioglitazone rescue therapy.
† Least squares means adjusted for prior antihyperglycemic therapy status and baseline value.
‡ p<0.001 compared to placebo.
§ p<0.01 compared to placebo.

pre-mixed, long-acting, or intermediate-acting insulin, with or without metformin (≥1500 mg per day). Patients using short-acting insulins were excluded unless the short-acting insulin was administered as part of a pre-mixed insulin. After the run-in period, patients with inadequate glycemic control (A1C 7.5% to 11%) were randomized to the addition of either 100 mg of JANUVIA or placebo, administered once daily. Patients were on a stable dose of insulin prior to enrollment with no changes in insulin dose permitted during the run-in period. Patients who failed to meet specific glycemic goals during the double-blind treatment period were to have uptitration of the background insulin dose as rescue therapy.

The median daily insulin dose at baseline was 42 units in the patients treated with JANUVIA and 45 units in the placebo-treated patients. The median change from baseline in daily dose of insulin was zero for both groups at the end of the study. In combination with insulin (with or without metformin), JANUVIA provided significant improvements in A1C, FPG, and 2-hour PPG compared to placebo (Table 12). Both treatment groups had an adjusted mean increase in body weight of 0.1 kg from baseline to Week 24. There was an increased rate of hypoglycemia in patients treated with JANUVIA. *[See Warnings and Precautions (5.3); Adverse Reactions (6.1).]*
[See table 12 at top of next page]

16   HOW SUPPLIED/STORAGE AND HANDLING

No. 6737 — Tablets JANUVIA, 25 mg, are pink, round, film-coated tablets with "221" on one side. They are supplied as follows:
NDC 0006-0221-31 unit-of-use bottles of 30
NDC 0006-0221-54 unit-of-use bottles of 90
NDC 0006-0221-28 unit dose blister packages of 100.
No. 6738 — Tablets JANUVIA, 50 mg, are light beige, round, film-coated tablets with "112" on one side. They are supplied as follows:
NDC 0006-0112-31 unit-of-use bottles of 30
NDC 0006-0112-54 unit-of-use bottles of 90
NDC 0006-0112-28 unit dose blister packages of 100.
No. 6739 — Tablets JANUVIA, 100 mg, are beige, round, film-coated tablets with "277" on one side. They are supplied as follows:
NDC 0006-0277-31 unit-of-use bottles of 30
NDC 0006-0277-54 unit-of-use bottles of 90
NDC 0006-0277-33 unit-of-use blister calendar package of 30
NDC 0006-0277-28 unit dose blister packages of 100
NDC 0006-0277-82 bottles of 1000.
Storage
Store at 20-25°C (68-77°F), excursions permitted to 15-30°C (59-86°F). [See USP Controlled Room Temperature.]

17   PATIENT COUNSELING INFORMATION

See FDA-Approved Patient Labeling (Medication Guide).
17.1   Instructions
Patients should be informed of the potential risks and benefits of JANUVIA and of alternative modes of therapy. Patients should also be informed about the importance of adherence to dietary instructions, regular physical activity, periodic blood glucose monitoring and A1C testing, recognition and management of hypoglycemia and hyperglycemia, and assessment for diabetes complications. During periods of stress such as fever, trauma, infection, or surgery, medication requirements may change and patients should be advised to seek medical advice promptly.

Table 12: Glycemic Parameters at Final Visit (24-Week Study) for JANUVIA as Add-on Combination Therapy with Insulin*

	JANUVIA 100 mg + Insulin (+/- Metformin)	Placebo + Insulin (+/- Metformin)
A1C (%)	N = 305	N = 312
Baseline (mean)	8.7	8.6
Change from baseline (adjusted mean[†])	-0.6	-0.1
Difference from placebo (adjusted mean[†,‡]) (95% CI)	-0.6[§] (-0.7, -0.4)	
Patients (%) achieving A1C <7%	39 (12.8%)	16 (5.1%)
FPG (mg/dL)	N = 310	N = 313
Baseline (mean)	176	179
Change from baseline (adjusted mean[†])	-18	-4
Difference from placebo (adjusted mean[†]) (95% CI)	-15[§] (-23, -7)	
2-hour PPG (mg/dL)	N = 240	N = 257
Baseline (mean)	291	292
Change from baseline (adjusted mean[†])	-31	5
Difference from placebo (adjusted mean[†]) (95% CI)	-36[§] (-47, -25)	

* Intent-to-treat population using last observation on study prior to rescue therapy.
† Least squares means adjusted for metformin use at the screening visit (yes/no), type of insulin used at the screening visit (pre-mixed vs. non-pre-mixed [intermediate- or long-acting]), and baseline value.
‡ Treatment by stratum interaction was not significant (p>0.10) for metformin stratum and for insulin stratum.
§ p<0.001 compared to placebo.

Patients should be informed that acute pancreatitis has been reported during postmarketing use of JANUVIA. Patients should be informed that persistent severe abdominal pain, sometimes radiating to the back, which may or may not be accompanied by vomiting, is the hallmark symptom of acute pancreatitis. Patients should be instructed to promptly discontinue JANUVIA and contact their physician if persistent severe abdominal pain occurs [see Warnings and Precautions (5.1)].

Patients should be informed that the incidence of hypoglycemia is increased when JANUVIA is added to a sulfonylurea or insulin and that a lower dose of the sulfonylurea or insulin may be required to reduce the risk of hypoglycemia. Patients should be informed that allergic reactions have been reported during postmarketing use of JANUVIA. If symptoms of allergic reactions (including rash, hives, and swelling of the face, lips, tongue, and throat that may cause difficulty in breathing or swallowing) occur, patients must stop taking JANUVIA and seek medical advice promptly. Physicians should instruct their patients to read the Medication Guide before starting JANUVIA therapy and to re-read each time the prescription is renewed. Patients should be instructed to inform their doctor or pharmacist if they develop any unusual symptom, or if any known symptom persists or worsens.

17.2   Laboratory Tests
Patients should be informed that response to all diabetic therapies should be monitored by periodic measurements of blood glucose and A1C levels, with a goal of decreasing these levels towards the normal range. A1C is especially useful for evaluating long-term glycemic control. Patients should be informed of the potential need to adjust dose based on changes in renal function tests over time.
Distributed by: Merck Sharp & Dohme Corp., a subsidiary of
MERCK & CO., INC., Whitehouse Station, NJ 08889, USA
For patent information: www.merck.com/product/patent/home.html
Copyright © 2006, 2007, 2009, 2010 Merck Sharp & Dohme Corp., a subsidiary of **Merck & Co., Inc.**
All rights reserved.
uspi-mk0431-t-1402r013

Medication Guide
JANUVIA® (jah-NEW-vee-ah)
(sitagliptin)
Tablets
Read this Medication Guide carefully before you start taking JANUVIA and each time you get a refill. There may be new information. This information does not take the place of talking with your doctor about your medical condition or your treatment. If you have any questions about JANUVIA, ask your doctor or pharmacist.

What is the most important information I should know about JANUVIA?
Serious side effects can happen in people taking JANUVIA, including inflammation of the pancreas (pancreatitis) which may be severe and lead to death.

Certain medical problems make you more likely to get pancreatitis.
Before you start taking JANUVIA:
Tell your doctor if you have ever had
• pancreatitis
• stones in your gallbladder (gallstones)
• a history of alcoholism
• high blood triglyceride levels
• kidney problems
Stop taking JANUVIA and call your doctor right away if you have pain in your stomach area (abdomen) that is severe and will not go away. The pain may be felt going from your abdomen through to your back. The pain may happen with or without vomiting. These may be symptoms of pancreatitis.

What is JANUVIA?
• JANUVIA is a prescription medicine used along with diet and exercise to lower blood sugar in adults with type 2 diabetes.
• JANUVIA is not for people with type 1 diabetes.
• JANUVIA is not for people with diabetic ketoacidosis (increased ketones in your blood or urine).
• If you have had pancreatitis (inflammation of the pancreas) in the past, it is not known if you have a higher chance of getting pancreatitis while you take JANUVIA.
• It is not known if JANUVIA is safe and effective when used in children under 18 years of age.

Who should not take JANUVIA?
Do not take JANUVIA if:
• you are allergic to any of the ingredients in JANUVIA. See the end of this Medication Guide for a complete list of ingredients in JANUVIA.
Symptoms of a serious allergic reaction to JANUVIA may include:
• rash
• raised red patches on your skin (hives)
• swelling of the face, lips, tongue, and throat that may cause difficulty in breathing or swallowing

What should I tell my doctor before taking JANUVIA?
Before you take JANUVIA, tell your doctor if you:
• have or have had inflammation of your pancreas (pancreatitis).
• have kidney problems.
• have any other medical conditions.
• are pregnant or plan to become pregnant. It is not known if JANUVIA will harm your unborn baby. If you are pregnant, talk with your doctor about the best way to control your blood sugar while you are pregnant.
Pregnancy Registry: If you take JANUVIA at any time during your pregnancy, talk with your doctor about how you can join the JANUVIA pregnancy registry. The purpose of this registry is to collect information about the health of you and your baby. You can enroll in this registry by calling 1-800-986-8999.
• are breast-feeding or plan to breast-feed. It is not known if JANUVIA will pass into your breast milk. Talk with your doctor about the best way to feed your baby if you are taking JANUVIA.

Tell your doctor about all the medicines you take, including prescription and non-prescription medicines, vitamins, and herbal supplements.
Know the medicines you take. Keep a list of your medicines and show it to your doctor and pharmacist when you get a new medicine.
How should I take JANUVIA?
• Take JANUVIA 1 time each day exactly as your doctor tells you.
• You can take JANUVIA with or without food.
• Your doctor may do blood tests from time to time to see how well your kidneys are working. Your doctor may change your dose of JANUVIA based on the results of your blood tests.
• Your doctor may tell you to take JANUVIA along with other diabetes medicines. Low blood sugar can happen more often when JANUVIA is taken with certain other diabetes medicines. See "**What are the possible side effects of JANUVIA?**".
• If you miss a dose, take it as soon as you remember. If you do not remember until it is time for your next dose, skip the missed dose and go back to your regular schedule. Do not take two doses of JANUVIA at the same time.
• If you take too much JANUVIA, call your doctor or local Poison Control Center right away.
• When your body is under some types of stress, such as fever, trauma (such as a car accident), infection or surgery, the amount of diabetes medicine that you need may change. Tell your doctor right away if you have any of these conditions and follow your doctor's instructions.
• Check your blood sugar as your doctor tells you to.
• Stay on your prescribed diet and exercise program while taking JANUVIA.
• Talk to your doctor about how to prevent, recognize and manage low blood sugar (hypoglycemia), high blood sugar (hyperglycemia), and problems you have because of your diabetes.
• Your doctor will check your diabetes with regular blood tests, including your blood sugar levels and your hemoglobin A1C.

What are the possible side effects of JANUVIA?
Serious side effects have happened in people taking JANUVIA.
• See "**What is the most important information I should know about JANUVIA?**"
• **Low blood sugar (hypoglycemia).** If you take JANUVIA with another medicine that can cause low blood sugar, such as a sulfonylurea or insulin, your risk of getting low blood sugar is higher. The dose of your sulfonylurea medicine or insulin may need to be lowered while you use JANUVIA. Signs and symptoms of low blood sugar may include:

• headache	• irritability
• drowsiness	• hunger
• weakness	• fast heart beat
• dizziness	• sweating
• confusion	• feeling jittery

• **Serious allergic reactions.** If you have any symptoms of a serious allergic reaction, stop taking JANUVIA and call your doctor right away. See "**Who should not take JANUVIA?**". Your doctor may give you a medicine for your allergic reaction and prescribe a different medicine for your diabetes.
• **Kidney problems,** sometimes requiring dialysis
The most common side effects of JANUVIA include:
• upper respiratory infection
• stuffy or runny nose and sore throat
• headache
JANUVIA may have other side effects, including:
• stomach upset and diarrhea
• swelling of the hands or legs, when JANUVIA is used with rosiglitazone (Avandia®). Rosiglitazone is another type of diabetes medicine.
These are not all the possible side effects of JANUVIA. For more information, ask your doctor or pharmacist.
Tell your doctor if you have any side effect that bothers you, is unusual or does not go away.
Call your doctor for medical advice about side effects. You may report side effects to FDA at 1-800-FDA-1088.
How should I store JANUVIA?
Store JANUVIA at 68°F to 77°F (20°C to 25°C).
Keep JANUVIA and all medicines out of the reach of children.
General information about the use of JANUVIA
Medicines are sometimes prescribed for purposes that are not listed in Medication Guides. Do not use JANUVIA for a condition for which it was not prescribed. Do not give JANUVIA to other people, even if they have the same symptoms you have. It may harm them.

This Medication Guide summarizes the most important information about JANUVIA. If you would like to know more information, talk with your doctor. You can ask your doctor or pharmacist for additional information about JANUVIA that is written for health professionals. For more information, go to www.JANUVIA.com or call 1-800-622-4477.

What are the ingredients in JANUVIA?
Active ingredient: sitagliptin
Inactive ingredients: microcrystalline cellulose, anhydrous dibasic calcium phosphate, croscarmellose sodium, magnesium stearate, and sodium stearyl fumarate. The tablet film coating contains the following inactive ingredients: polyvinyl alcohol, polyethylene glycol, talc, titanium dioxide, red iron oxide, and yellow iron oxide.

What is type 2 diabetes?
Type 2 diabetes is a condition in which your body does not make enough insulin, and the insulin that your body produces does not work as well as it should. Your body can also make too much sugar. When this happens, sugar (glucose) builds up in the blood. This can lead to serious medical problems.
High blood sugar can be lowered by diet and exercise, and by certain medicines when necessary.
This Medication Guide has been approved by the U.S. Food and Drug Administration.
Distributed by: Merck Sharp & Dohme Corp., a subsidiary of
MERCK & CO., INC., Whitehouse Station, NJ 08889, USA
For patent information: www.merck.com/product/patent/home.html
The trademarks depicted herein are owned by their respective companies.
Copyright © 2010 Merck Sharp & Dohme Corp., a subsidiary of **Merck & Co., Inc.**
All rights reserved.
Revised: 02/2014
usmg-mk0431-t-1402r013
Shown in Product Identification Guide, page 308

KEYTRUDA® ℞
(pembrolizumab)
for injection, for intravenous use

HIGHLIGHTS OF PRESCRIBING INFORMATION
These highlights do not include all the information needed to use KEYTRUDA safely and effectively. See full prescribing information for KEYTRUDA.
KEYTRUDA® (pembrolizumab) for injection, for intravenous use
Initial U.S. Approval: 2014

————————INDICATIONS AND USAGE————————
KEYTRUDA is a human programmed death receptor-1 (PD-1)-blocking antibody indicated for the treatment of patients with unresectable or metastatic melanoma and disease progression following ipilimumab and, if BRAF V600 mutation positive, a BRAF inhibitor.
This indication is approved under accelerated approval based on tumor response rate and durability of response. An improvement in survival or disease-related symptoms has not yet been established. Continued approval for this indication may be contingent upon verification and description of clinical benefit in the confirmatory trials. (1)

————————DOSAGE AND ADMINISTRATION————————
• Administer 2 mg/kg as an intravenous infusion over 30 minutes every 3 weeks. (2.1)
• Reconstitute and dilute prior to intravenous infusion. (2.3)

————————DOSAGE FORMS AND STRENGTHS————————
For injection: 50 mg, lyophilized powder in single-use vial for reconstitution (3)

————————CONTRAINDICATIONS————————
None. (4)

————————WARNINGS AND PRECAUTIONS————————
• Immune-mediated adverse reactions: Administer corticosteroids based on the severity of the reaction. (5.1, 5.2, 5.3, 5.4, 5.5, 5.6)
  ◦ Immune-mediated pneumonitis: Withhold for moderate, and permanently discontinue for severe or life-threatening pneumonitis. (5.1)
  ◦ Immune-mediated colitis: Withhold for moderate or severe, and permanently discontinue for life-threatening colitis. (5.2)
  ◦ Immune-mediated hepatitis: Monitor for changes in hepatic function. Based on severity of liver enzyme elevations, withhold or discontinue. (5.3)
  ◦ Immune-mediated hypophysitis: Withhold for moderate, withhold or discontinue for severe, and permanently discontinue for life-threatening hypophysitis. (5.4)
  ◦ Immune-mediated nephritis: Monitor for changes in renal function. Withhold for moderate, and permanently discontinue for severe or life-threatening nephritis. (5.5)
  ◦ Immune-mediated hyperthyroidism and hypothyroidism: Monitor for changes in thyroid function. Withhold for severe and permanently discontinue for life-threatening hyperthyroidism. (5.6)

• Embryofetal Toxicity: KEYTRUDA may cause fetal harm. Advise females of reproductive potential of the potential risk to a fetus. (5.8)

————————ADVERSE REACTIONS————————
Most common adverse reactions (reported in ≥20% of patients) included fatigue, cough, nausea, pruritus, rash, decreased appetite, constipation, arthralgia, and diarrhea. (6.1)

To report SUSPECTED ADVERSE REACTIONS, contact Merck Sharp & Dohme Corp., a subsidiary of Merck & Co., Inc., at 1-877-888-4231 or FDA at 1-800-FDA-1088 or www.fda.gov/medwatch.

————————USE IN SPECIFIC POPULATIONS————————
Nursing mothers: Discontinue nursing or discontinue KEYTRUDA. (8.3)
See 17 for PATIENT COUNSELING INFORMATION and Medication Guide

Revised: 09/2014

FULL PRESCRIBING INFORMATION: CONTENTS*

FULL PRESCRIBING INFORMATION

1 INDICATIONS AND USAGE
KEYTRUDA® (pembrolizumab) is indicated for the treatment of patients with unresectable or metastatic melanoma and disease progression following ipilimumab and, if BRAF V600 mutation positive, a BRAF inhibitor *[see Clinical Studies (14)]*.
This indication is approved under accelerated approval based on tumor response rate and durability of response. An improvement in survival or disease-related symptoms has not yet been established. Continued approval for this indication may be contingent upon verification and description of clinical benefit in the confirmatory trials.

2 DOSAGE AND ADMINISTRATION
2.1 Recommended Dosing
The recommended dose of KEYTRUDA is 2 mg/kg administered as an intravenous infusion over 30 minutes every 3 weeks until disease progression or unacceptable toxicity.
2.2 Dose Modifications
Withhold KEYTRUDA for any of the following:
• Grade 2 pneumonitis *[see Warnings and Precautions (5.1)]*
• Grade 2 or 3 colitis *[see Warnings and Precautions (5.2)]*
• Symptomatic hypophysitis *[see Warnings and Precautions (5.4)]*
• Grade 2 nephritis *[see Warnings and Precautions (5.5)]*
• Grade 3 hyperthyroidism *[see Warnings and Precautions (5.6)]*

• Aspartate aminotransferase (AST) or alanine aminotransferase (ALT) greater than 3 and up to 5 times upper limit of normal (ULN) or total bilirubin greater than 1.5 and up to 3 times ULN
• Any other severe or Grade 3 treatment-related adverse reaction *[see Warnings and Precautions (5.7)]*
Resume KEYTRUDA in patients whose adverse reactions recover to Grade 0-1.
Permanently discontinue KEYTRUDA for any of the following:
• Any life-threatening adverse reaction
• Grade 3 or 4 pneumonitis *[see Warnings and Precautions (5.1)]*
• Grade 3 or 4 nephritis *[see Warnings and Precautions (5.5)]*
• AST or ALT greater than 5 times ULN or total bilirubin greater than 3 times ULN
  ◦ For patients with liver metastasis who begin treatment with Grade 2 AST or ALT, if AST or ALT increases by greater than or equal to 50% relative to baseline and lasts for at least 1 week
• Grade 3 or 4 infusion-related reactions
• Inability to reduce corticosteroid dose to 10 mg or less of prednisone or equivalent per day within 12 weeks
• Persistent Grade 2 or 3 adverse reactions that do not recover to Grade 0-1 within 12 weeks after last dose of KEYTRUDA
• Any severe or Grade 3 treatment-related adverse reaction that recurs *[see Warnings and Precautions (5.7)]*

2.3 Preparation and Administration
Preparation
• Add 2.3 mL of Sterile Water for Injection, USP by injecting the water along the walls of the vial and not directly on the lyophilized powder (resulting concentration 25 mg/mL).
• Slowly swirl the vial. Allow up to 5 minutes for the bubbles to clear. Do not shake the vial.
• Visually inspect the reconstituted solution for particulate matter and discoloration prior to administration. Reconstituted KEYTRUDA is a clear to slightly opalescent, colorless to slightly yellow solution. Discard reconstituted vial if extraneous particulate matter other than translucent to white proteinaceous particles is observed.
• Withdraw the required volume from the vial(s) of KEYTRUDA and transfer into an intravenous (IV) bag containing 0.9% Sodium Chloride Injection, USP. Mix diluted solution by gentle inversion. The final concentration of the diluted solution should be between 1 mg/mL to 10 mg/mL.
• Discard any unused portion left in the vial.
Storage of Reconstituted and Diluted Solutions
The product does not contain a preservative.
Store the reconstituted and diluted solutions of KEYTRUDA either:
• At room temperature for no more than 4 hours from the time of reconstitution. This includes room temperature storage of reconstituted vials, storage of the infusion solution in the IV bag, and the duration of infusion.
• Under refrigeration at 2°C to 8°C (36°F to 46°F) for no more than 24 hours from the time of reconstitution. If refrigerated, allow the diluted solution to come to room temperature prior to administration.
Do not freeze.
Administration
• Administer infusion solution intravenously over 30 minutes through an intravenous line containing a sterile, non-pyrogenic, low-protein binding 0.2 micron to 5 micron in-line or add-on filter.
• Do not co-administer other drugs through the same infusion line.

3 DOSAGE FORMS AND STRENGTHS
For injection: 50 mg lyophilized powder in a single-use vial for reconstitution

4 CONTRAINDICATIONS
None.

5 WARNINGS AND PRECAUTIONS
5.1 Immune-Mediated Pneumonitis
Pneumonitis occurred in 12 (2.9%) of 411 melanoma patients, including Grade 2 or 3 cases in 8 (1.9%) and 1 (0.2%) patients, respectively, receiving KEYTRUDA in Trial 1. The median time to development of pneumonitis was 5 months (range 0.3 weeks-9.9 months). The median duration was 4.9 months (range 1 week-14.4 months). Five of eight patients with Grade 2 and the one patient with Grade 3 pneumonitis required initial treatment with high-dose systemic corticosteroids (greater than or equal to 40 mg prednisone or equivalent per day) followed by a corticosteroid taper. The median initial dose of high-dose corticosteroid treatment was 63.4 mg/day of prednisone or equivalent with a median duration of treatment of 3 days (range 1-34) followed by a corticosteroid taper. Pneumonitis led to discontinuation of

KEYTRUDA in 3 (0.7%) patients. Pneumonitis completely resolved in seven of the nine patients with Grade 2-3 pneumonitis.

Monitor patients for signs and symptoms of pneumonitis. Evaluate patients with suspected pneumonitis with radiographic imaging and administer corticosteroids for Grade 2 or greater pneumonitis. Withhold KEYTRUDA for moderate (Grade 2) pneumonitis, and permanently discontinue KEYTRUDA for severe (Grade 3) or life-threatening (Grade 4) pneumonitis [see Dosage and Administration (2.2) and Adverse Reactions (6.1)].

5.2 Immune-Mediated Colitis
Colitis (including microscopic colitis) occurred in 4 (1%) of 411 patients, including Grade 2 or 3 cases in 1 (0.2%) and 2 (0.5%) patients, respectively, receiving KEYTRUDA in Trial 1. The median time to onset of colitis was 6.5 months (range 2.3-9.8). The median duration was 2.6 months (range 0.6 weeks-3.6 months). All three patients with Grade 2 or 3 colitis were treated with high-dose corticosteroids (greater than or equal to 40 mg prednisone or equivalent per day) with a median initial dose of 70 mg/day of prednisone or equivalent; the median duration of initial treatment was 7 days (range 4-41), followed by a corticosteroid taper. One patient (0.2%) required permanent discontinuation of KEYTRUDA due to colitis. All four patients with colitis experienced complete resolution of the event.

Monitor patients for signs and symptoms of colitis. Administer corticosteroids for Grade 2 or greater colitis. Withhold KEYTRUDA for moderate (Grade 2) or severe (Grade 3) colitis, and permanently discontinue KEYTRUDA for life-threatening (Grade 4) colitis [see Dosage and Administration (2.2) and Adverse Reactions (6.1)].

5.3 Immune-Mediated Hepatitis
Hepatitis (including autoimmune hepatitis) occurred in 2 (0.5%) of 411 patients, including a Grade 4 case in 1 (0.2%) patient, receiving KEYTRUDA in Trial 1. The time to onset was 22 days for the case of Grade 4 hepatitis which lasted 1.1 months. The patient with Grade 4 hepatitis permanently discontinued KEYTRUDA and was treated with high-dose (greater than or equal to 40 mg prednisone or equivalent per day) systemic corticosteroids followed by a corticosteroid taper. Both patients with hepatitis experienced complete resolution of the event.

Monitor patients for changes in liver function. Administer corticosteroids for Grade 2 or greater hepatitis and, based on severity of liver enzyme elevations, withhold or discontinue KEYTRUDA [see Dosage and Administration (2.2) and Adverse Reactions (6.1)].

5.4 Immune-Mediated Hypophysitis
Hypophysitis occurred in 2 (0.5%) of 411 patients, consisting of one Grade 2 and one Grade 4 case (0.2% each), in patients receiving KEYTRUDA in Trial 1. The time to onset was 1.7 months for the patient with Grade 4 hypophysitis and 1.3 months for the patient with Grade 2 hypophysitis. Both patients were treated with high-dose (greater than or equal to 40 mg prednisone or equivalent per day) corticosteroids followed by a corticosteroid taper and remained on a physiologic replacement dose.

Monitor for signs and symptoms of hypophysitis. Administer corticosteroids for Grade 2 or greater hypophysitis. Withhold KEYTRUDA for moderate (Grade 2) hypophysitis, withhold or discontinue KEYTRUDA for severe (Grade 3) hypophysitis, and permanently discontinue KEYTRUDA for life-threatening (Grade 4) hypophysitis [see Dosage and Administration (2.2) and Adverse Reactions (6.1)].

5.5 Renal Failure and Immune-Mediated Nephritis
Nephritis occurred in 3 (0.7%) patients, consisting of one case of Grade 2 autoimmune nephritis (0.2%) and two cases of interstitial nephritis with renal failure (0.5%), one Grade 3 and one Grade 4. The time to onset of autoimmune nephritis was 11.6 months after the first dose of KEYTRUDA (5 months after the last dose) and lasted 3.2 months; this patient did not have a biopsy. Acute interstitial nephritis was confirmed by renal biopsy in two patients with Grades 3-4 renal failure. All three patients fully recovered renal function with treatment with high-dose corticosteroids (greater than or equal to 40 mg prednisone or equivalent per day) followed by a corticosteroid taper.

Monitor patients for changes in renal function. Administer corticosteroids for Grade 2 or greater nephritis. Withhold KEYTRUDA for moderate (Grade 2) nephritis, and permanently discontinue KEYTRUDA for severe (Grade 3), or life-threatening (Grade 4) nephritis [see Dosage and Administration (2.2) and Adverse Reactions (6.1)].

5.6 Immune-Mediated Hyperthyroidism and Hypothyroidism
Hyperthyroidism occurred in 5 (1.2%) of 411 patients, including Grade 2 or 3 cases in 2 (0.5%) and 1 (0.2%) patients, respectively, receiving KEYTRUDA in Trial 1. The median time to onset was 1.5 months (range 0.5-2.1). The median duration was 2.8 months (range 0.9 to 6.1). One of two patients with Grade 2 and the one patient with Grade 3 hyperthyroidism required initial treatment with high-dose corticosteroids (greater than or equal to 40 mg prednisone or equivalent per day) followed by a corticosteroid taper. One patient (0.2%) required permanent discontinuation of KEYTRUDA due to hyperthyroidism. All five patients with hyperthyroidism experienced complete resolution of the event.

Hypothyroidism occurred in 34 (8.3%) of 411 patients, including a Grade 3 case in 1 (0.2%) patient, receiving KEYTRUDA in Trial 1. The median time to onset of hypothyroidism was 3.5 months (range 0.7 weeks-19 months). All but two of the patients with hypothyroidism were treated with long-term thyroid hormone replacement therapy. The other two patients only required short-term thyroid hormone replacement therapy. No patient received corticosteroids or discontinued KEYTRUDA for management of hypothyroidism.

Thyroid disorders can occur at any time during treatment. Monitor patients for changes in thyroid function (at the start of treatment, periodically during treatment, and as indicated based on clinical evaluation) and for clinical signs and symptoms of thyroid disorders.

Administer corticosteroids for Grade 3 or greater hyperthyroidism, withhold KEYTRUDA for severe (Grade 3) hyperthyroidism, and permanently discontinue KEYTRUDA for life-threatening (Grade 4) hyperthyroidism. Isolated hypothyroidism may be managed with replacement therapy without treatment interruption and without corticosteroids [see Dosage and Administration (2.2) and Adverse Reactions (6.1)].

5.7 Other Immune-Mediated Adverse Reactions
Other clinically important immune-mediated adverse reactions can occur.

The following clinically significant, immune-mediated adverse reactions occurred in less than 1% of patients treated with KEYTRUDA in Trial 1: exfoliative dermatitis, uveitis, arthritis, myositis, pancreatitis, hemolytic anemia, partial seizures arising in a patient with inflammatory foci in brain parenchyma, and adrenal insufficiency.

Across clinical studies with KEYTRUDA in approximately 2000 patients, the following additional clinically significant, immune-mediated adverse reactions were reported in less than 1% of patients: myasthenic syndrome, optic neuritis, and rhabdomyolysis.

For suspected immune-mediated adverse reactions, ensure adequate evaluation to confirm etiology or exclude other causes. Based on the severity of the adverse reaction, withhold KEYTRUDA and administer corticosteroids. Upon improvement to Grade 1 or less, initiate corticosteroid taper and continue to taper over at least 1 month. Restart KEYTRUDA if the adverse reaction remains at Grade 1 or less. Permanently discontinue KEYTRUDA for any severe or Grade 3 immune-mediated adverse reaction that recurs and for any life-threatening immune-mediated adverse reaction [see Dosage and Administration (2.2) and Adverse Reactions (6.1)].

5.8 Embryofetal Toxicity
Based on its mechanism of action, KEYTRUDA may cause fetal harm when administered to a pregnant woman. Animal models link the PD-1/PDL-1 signaling pathway with maintenance of pregnancy through induction of maternal immune tolerance to fetal tissue. If this drug is used during pregnancy, or if the patient becomes pregnant while taking this drug, apprise the patient of the potential hazard to a fetus. Advise females of reproductive potential to use highly effective contraception during treatment with KEYTRUDA and for 4 months after the last dose of KEYTRUDA [see Use in Specific Populations (8.1, 8.8)].

6 ADVERSE REACTIONS
The following adverse reactions are discussed in greater detail in other sections of the labeling.
- Immune-mediated pneumonitis [see Warnings and Precautions (5.1)].
- Immune-mediated colitis [see Warnings and Precautions (5.2)].
- Immune-mediated hepatitis [see Warnings and Precautions (5.3)].
- Immune-mediated hypophysitis [see Warnings and Precautions (5.4)].
- Renal failure and immune-mediated nephritis [see Warnings and Precautions (5.5)].
- Immune-mediated hyperthyroidism and hypothyroidism [see Warnings and Precautions (5.6)].
- Immune-mediated adverse reactions [see Warnings and Precautions (5.7)].

6.1 Clinical Trials Experience
Because clinical trials are conducted under widely varying conditions, adverse reaction rates observed in the clinical trials of a drug cannot be directly compared to rates in the clinical trials of another drug and may not reflect the rates observed in practice.

The data described in the WARNINGS and PRECAUTIONS section reflect exposure to KEYTRUDA in Trial 1, an uncontrolled, open-label, multiple cohort trial in which 411 patients with unresectable or metastatic melanoma received KEYTRUDA at either 2 mg/kg every 3 weeks or 10 mg/kg every 2 or 3 weeks. The median duration of exposure to KEYTRUDA was 6.2 months (range 1 day to 24.6 months) with a median of 10 doses (range 1 to 51). The study population characteristics were: median age of 61 years (range 18-94), 39% age 65 years or older, 60% male, 97% white, 73% with M1c disease, 8% with brain metastases, 35% with elevated LDH, 54% with prior exposure to ipilimumab, and 47% with two or more prior systemic therapies for advanced or metastatic disease.

KEYTRUDA was discontinued for adverse reactions in 9% of the 411 patients. Adverse reactions, reported in at least two patients, that led to discontinuation of KEYTRUDA were: pneumonitis, renal failure, and pain. Serious adverse reactions occurred in 36% of patients receiving KEYTRUDA. The most frequent serious adverse drug reactions reported in 2% or more of patients in Trial 1 were renal failure, dyspnea, pneumonia, and cellulitis.

Table 1 presents adverse reactions identified from analyses of the 89 patients with unresectable or metastatic melanoma who received KEYTRUDA 2 mg/kg every three weeks in one cohort of Trial 1. Patients had documented disease progression following treatment with ipilimumab and, if BRAF V600 mutation positive, a BRAF inhibitor. This cohort of Trial 1 excluded patients with severe immune-related toxicity related to ipilimumab, defined as any Grade 4 toxicity requiring treatment with corticosteroids or Grade 3 toxicity requiring corticosteroid treatment (greater than 10 mg/day prednisone or equivalent dose) for greater than 12 weeks; a medical condition that required systemic corticosteroids or other immunosuppressive medication; a history of pneumonitis or interstitial lung disease; or any active infection requiring therapy, including HIV or hepatitis B or C. Of the 89 patients in this cohort, the median age was 59 years (range 18-88), 33% were age 65 years or older, 53% were male, 98% were white, 44% had an elevated LDH, 84% had Stage M1c disease, 8% had brain metastases, and 70% received two or more prior therapies for advanced or metastatic disease. The median duration of exposure to KEYTRUDA was 6.2 months (range 1 day to 15.3 months) with a median of nine doses (range 1 to 23). Fifty-one percent of patients were exposed to KEYTRUDA for greater than 6 months and 21% for greater than 1 year.

KEYTRUDA was discontinued for adverse reactions in 6% of the 89 patients. The most common adverse reactions (reported in at least 20% of patients) were fatigue, cough, nausea, pruritus, rash, decreased appetite, constipation, arthralgia, and diarrhea.

Table 1: Adverse Reactions in ≥10% of Patients with Unresectable or Metastatic Melanoma

Adverse Reaction	KEYTRUDA 2 mg/kg every 3 weeks N=89	
	All Grades (%)	Grade 3* (%)
General Disorders and Administration Site Conditions		
Fatigue	47	7
Peripheral Edema	17	1
Chills	14	0
Pyrexia	11	0
Gastrointestinal Disorders		
Nausea	30	0
Constipation	21	0
Diarrhea	20	0
Vomiting	16	0
Abdominal pain	12	0
Respiratory, Thoracic And Mediastinal Disorders		
Cough	30	1
Dyspnea	18	2
Skin And Subcutaneous Tissue Disorders		
Pruritus	30	0
Rash	29	0

	11	0
Vitiligo	11	0
Metabolism and Nutrition Disorders		
Decreased appetite	26	0
Musculoskeletal and Connective Tissue Disorders		
Arthralgia	20	0
Pain in extremity	18	1
Myalgia	14	1
Back pain	12	0
Nervous System Disorders		
Headache	16	0
Dizziness	11	0
Blood and Lymphatic System Disorders		
Anemia	14	5
Psychiatric Disorders		
Insomnia	14	0
Infections and Infestations		
Upper respiratory tract infection	11	1

* There were no Grade 5 adverse reactions reported. Of the ≥10% adverse reactions, none was reported as Grade 4.

Other clinically important adverse reactions observed in up to 10% of patients treated with KEYTRUDA were:
Infections and infestations: sepsis

Table 2: Laboratory Abnormalities Increased from Baseline in ≥20% of Patients with Unresectable or Metastatic Melanoma

Laboratory Test	KEYTRUDA 2 mg/kg every 3 weeks N=89	
	All Grades %	Grades 3-4 %
Chemistry		
Hyperglycemia	40	2*
Hyponatremia	35	9
Hypoalbuminemia	34	0
Hypertriglyceridemia	25	0
Increased Aspartate Aminotransferase	24	2*
Hypocalcemia	24	1
Hematology		
Anemia	55	8*

* Grade 4 abnormalities in this table limited to hyperglycemia, increased aspartate aminotransferase, and anemia (one patient each)

6.2 Immunogenicity

As with all therapeutic proteins, there is the potential for immunogenicity. Because trough levels of pembrolizumab interfere with the electrochemiluminescent (ECL) assay results, a subset analysis was performed in the patients with a concentration of pembrolizumab below the drug tolerance level of the anti-product antibody assay. In this analysis, none of the 97 patients who were treated with 2 mg/kg every 3 weeks tested positive for treatment-emergent anti-pembrolizumab antibodies.

The detection of antibody formation is highly dependent on the sensitivity and specificity of the assay. Additionally, the observed incidence of antibody (including neutralizing antibody) positivity in an assay may be influenced by several factors including assay methodology, sample handling, tim-

ing of sample collection, concomitant medications, and underlying disease. For these reasons, comparison of incidence of antibodies to KEYTRUDA with the incidences of antibodies to other products may be misleading.

7 DRUG INTERACTIONS

No formal pharmacokinetic drug interaction studies have been conducted with KEYTRUDA.

8 USE IN SPECIFIC POPULATIONS
8.1 Pregnancy
Pregnancy Category D.
Risk Summary
Based on its mechanism of action, KEYTRUDA may cause fetal harm when administered to a pregnant woman. Animal models link the PD-1/PDL-1 signaling pathway with maintenance of pregnancy through induction of maternal immune tolerance to fetal tissue. If this drug is used during pregnancy, or if the patient becomes pregnant while taking this drug, apprise the patient of the potential hazard to a fetus.
Animal Data
Animal reproduction studies have not been conducted with KEYTRUDA to evaluate its effect on reproduction and fetal development, but an assessment of the effects on reproduction was provided. A central function of the PD-1/PD-L1 pathway is to preserve pregnancy by maintaining maternal immune tolerance to the fetus. Blockade of PD-L1 signaling has been shown in murine models of pregnancy to disrupt tolerance to the fetus and to result in an increase in fetal loss; therefore, potential risks of administering KEYTRUDA during pregnancy include increased rates of abortion or stillbirth. As reported in the literature, there were no malformations related to the blockade of PD-1 signaling in the offspring of these animals; however, immune-mediated disorders occurred in PD-1 knockout mice. Human IgG4 (immunoglobulins) are known to cross the placenta; therefore, pembrolizumab has the potential to be transmitted from the mother to the developing fetus. Based on its mechanism of action, fetal exposure to pembrolizumab may increase the risk of developing immune-mediated disorders or of altering the normal immune response.
8.3 Nursing Mothers
It is not known whether KEYTRUDA is excreted in human milk. No studies have been conducted to assess the impact of KEYTRUDA on milk production or its presence in breast milk. Because many drugs are excreted in human milk, instruct women to discontinue nursing during treatment with KEYTRUDA.
8.4 Pediatric Use
Safety and effectiveness of KEYTRUDA have not been established in pediatric patients.
8.5 Geriatric Use
Of the 411 patients treated with KEYTRUDA, 39% were 65 years and over. No overall differences in safety or efficacy were reported between elderly patients and younger patients.
8.6 Renal Impairment
Based on a population pharmacokinetic analysis, no dose adjustment is needed for patients with renal impairment *[see Clinical Pharmacology (12.3)].*
8.7 Hepatic Impairment
Based on a population pharmacokinetic analysis, no dose adjustment is needed for patients with mild hepatic impairment [total bilirubin (TB) less than or equal to ULN and AST greater than ULN or TB greater than 1 to 1.5 times ULN and any AST]. KEYTRUDA has not been studied in patients with moderate (TB greater than 1.5 to 3 times ULN and any AST) or severe (TB greater than 3 times ULN and any AST) hepatic impairment *[see Clinical Pharmacology (12.3)].*
8.8 Females and Males of Reproductive Potential
Based on its mechanism of action, KEYTRUDA may cause fetal harm when administered to a pregnant woman *[see Warnings and Precautions (5.8) and Use in Specific Populations (8.1)].* Advise females of reproductive potential to use highly effective contraception during treatment with KEYTRUDA and for at least 4 months following the last dose of pembrolizumab.

10 OVERDOSAGE

There is no information on overdosage with KEYTRUDA.

11 DESCRIPTION

Pembrolizumab is a humanized monoclonal antibody that blocks the interaction between PD-1 and its ligands, PD-L1 and PD-L2. Pembrolizumab is an IgG4 kappa immunoglobulin with an approximate molecular weight of 149 kDa. KEYTRUDA is a sterile, preservative-free, white to off-white lyophilized powder in single-use vials. Each vial is reconstituted and diluted for intravenous infusion. Each 2 mL of reconstituted solution contains 50 mg of pembrolizumab and is formulated in L-histidine (3.1 mg), polysorbate-80 (0.4 mg), sucrose (140 mg). May contain hydrochloric acid/sodium hydroxide to adjust pH to 5.5.

12 CLINICAL PHARMACOLOGY
12.1 Mechanism of Action
Binding of the PD-1 ligands, PD-L1 and PD-L2, to the PD-1 receptor found on T cells, inhibits T cell proliferation and cytokine production. Upregulation of PD-1 ligands occurs in some tumors and signaling through this pathway can contribute to inhibition of active T-cell immune surveillance of tumors. Pembrolizumab is a monoclonal antibody that binds to the PD-1 receptor and blocks its interaction with PD-L1 and PD-L2, releasing PD-1 pathway-mediated inhibition of the immune response, including the anti-tumor immune response. In syngeneic mouse tumor models, blocking PD-1 activity resulted in decreased tumor growth.
12.3 Pharmacokinetics
The pharmacokinetics of pembrolizumab was studied in 479 patients who received doses of 1 to 10 mg/kg every 2 weeks or 2 to 10 mg/kg every 3 weeks. Based on a population pharmacokinetic analysis, the mean [% coefficient of variation (CV%)] clearance (CL) is 0.22 L/day (28%) and the mean (CV%) elimination half-life ($t_{1/2}$) is 26 days (24%). Steady-state concentrations of pembrolizumab were reached by 18 weeks of repeated dosing with an every 3-week regimen and the systemic accumulation was 2.1-fold. The peak concentration (C_{max}), trough concentration (C_{min}), and area under the plasma concentration versus time curve at steady state (AUC_{ss}) of pembrolizumab increased dose proportionally in the dose range of 2 to 10 mg/kg every 3 weeks.
Specific Populations: The effects of various covariates on the pharmacokinetics of pembrolizumab were assessed in population pharmacokinetic analyses. The CL of pembrolizumab increased with increasing body weight; the resulting exposure differences were adequately addressed by the administration of a weight-based dose. The following factors had no clinically important effect on the CL of pembrolizumab: age (range 18-94 years), gender, renal impairment, mild hepatic impairment, and tumor burden. The effect of race could not be assessed due to limited data available in non-White patients.
Renal Impairment: The effect of renal impairment on the CL of pembrolizumab was evaluated by population pharmacokinetic analyses in patients with mild (eGFR 60 to 89 mL/min/1.73 m²; n=210), moderate (eGFR 30 to 59 mL/min/1.73m²; n=43), or severe (eGFR 15 to 29 mL/min/1.73m²; n=2) renal impairment compared to patients with normal (eGFR greater than or equal to 90 mL/min/1.73m²; n=221) renal function. No clinically important differences in the CL of pembrolizumab were found between patients with renal impairment and patients with normal renal function *[see Use in Specific Populations (8.6)].*
Hepatic Impairment: The effect of hepatic impairment on the CL of pembrolizumab was evaluated by population pharmacokinetic analyses in patients with mild hepatic impairment (TB less than or equal to ULN and AST greater than ULN or TB between 1 and 1.5 times ULN and any AST; n=59) compared to patients with normal hepatic function (TB and AST less than or equal to ULN; n=410). No clinically important differences in the CL of pembrolizumab were found between patients with mild hepatic impairment and normal hepatic function. KEYTRUDA has not been studied in patients with moderate (TB greater than 1.5 to 3 times ULN and any AST) or severe (TB greater than 3 times ULN and any AST) hepatic impairment *[see Use in Specific Populations (8.7)].*

13 NONCLINICAL TOXICOLOGY
13.1 Carcinogenesis, Mutagenesis, Impairment of Fertility
No studies have been performed to test the potential of pembrolizumab for carcinogenicity or genotoxicity.
Fertility studies have not been conducted with pembrolizumab. In 1-month and 6-month repeat-dose toxicology studies in monkeys, there were no notable effects in the male and female reproductive organs; however, most animals in these studies were not sexually mature.
13.2 Animal Toxicology and/or Pharmacology
In animal models, inhibition of PD-1 signaling resulted in an increased incidence of infections and enhanced inflammatory responses. M. tuberculosis-infected PD-1 knockout mice exhibit markedly decreased survival compared with wild-type controls, which correlated with increased bacterial proliferation and inflammatory responses in these animals. PD-1 knockout mice have also shown decreased survival following infection with lymphocytic choriomeningitis virus (LCMV). Administration of pembrolizumab in chimpanzees with naturally occurring chronic hepatitis B infection resulted in two out of four animals with significantly increased levels of serum ALT, AST, and GGT, which persisted for at least 1 month after discontinuation of pembrolizumab.

14 CLINICAL STUDIES

The efficacy of KEYTRUDA was investigated in a multicenter, open-label, randomized (1:1), dose-comparative, activity-estimating cohort of Trial 1. Key eligibility criteria were unresectable or metastatic melanoma with progression of disease; refractory to two or more doses of ipilimumab (3 mg/kg or higher) and, if BRAF V600 mutation-positive, a BRAF or MEK inhibitor; and disease progression within 24 weeks following the last dose of ipilimumab. The trial excluded patients with autoimmune disease; a medical condition that required immunosuppression; and a history of severe immune-mediated adverse reactions with ipilimumab, defined as any Grade 4 toxicity requiring treatment with corticosteroids or Grade 3 toxicity requiring corticosteroid treatment (greater than 10 mg/day prednisone or equivalent dose) for greater than 12 weeks. Patients were randomized to receive 2 mg/kg (n=89) or 10 mg/kg (n=84) of KEYTRUDA every 3 weeks until unacceptable toxicity or disease progression that was symptomatic, was rapidly progressive, required urgent intervention, occurred with a decline in performance status, or was confirmed at 4 to 6 weeks with repeat imaging. Assessment of tumor status was performed every 12 weeks. The major efficacy outcome measures were confirmed overall response rate (ORR) according to Response Evaluation Criteria in Solid Tumors (RECIST 1.1) as assessed by blinded independent central review and duration of response.

Among the 173 patients enrolled, the median age was 61 years (36% age 65 or older); 60% male; 97% White; and 66% and 34% with an ECOG performance status 0 and 1, respectively. Disease characteristics were BRAF V600 mutation (17%), elevated lactate dehydrogenase (39%), M1c (82%), brain metastases (9%), and two or more prior therapies for advanced or metastatic disease (73%).

The ORR was 24% (95% confidence interval: 15, 34) in the 2 mg/kg arm, consisting of 1 complete response and 20 partial responses. Among the 21 patients with an objective response, 3 (14%) had progression of disease 2.8, 2.9, and 8.2 months after initial response. The remaining 18 patients (86%) had ongoing responses with durations ranging from 1.4+ to 8.5+ months, which included 8 patients with ongoing responses of 6 months or longer. One additional patient developed two new asymptomatic lesions at the first tumor assessment concurrent with a 75% decrease in overall tumor burden; KEYTRUDA was continued and this reduction in tumor burden was durable for 5+ months.

There were objective responses in patients with and without BRAF V600 mutation-positive melanoma. Similar ORR results were observed in the 10 mg/kg arm.

16 HOW SUPPLIED/STORAGE AND HANDLING

KEYTRUDA is supplied in a carton containing one 50 mg single-use vial (NDC 0006-3029-02).
Store vials under refrigeration at 2°C to 8°C (36°F to 46°F).

17 PATIENT COUNSELING INFORMATION

Advise the patient to read the FDA-approved patient labeling (Medication Guide).
• Inform patients of the risk of immune-mediated adverse reactions that may require corticosteroid treatment and interruption or discontinuation of KEYTRUDA, including:
  • Pneumonitis: Advise patients to contact their healthcare provider immediately for new or worsening cough, chest pain, or shortness of breath *[see Warnings and Precautions (5.1)]*.
  • Colitis: Advise patients to contact their healthcare provider immediately for diarrhea or severe abdominal pain *[see Warnings and Precautions (5.2)]*.
  • Hepatitis: Advise patients to contact their healthcare provider immediately for jaundice, severe nausea or vomiting, or easy bruising or bleeding *[see Warnings and Precautions (5.3)]*.
  • Hypophysitis: Advise patients to contact their healthcare provider immediately for persistent or unusual headache, extreme weakness, dizziness or fainting, or vision changes *[see Warnings and Precautions (5.4)]*.
  • Nephritis: Advise patients to contact their healthcare provider immediately for signs or symptoms of nephritis *[see Warnings and Precautions (5.5)]*.
  • Hyperthyroidism and Hypothyroidism: Advise patients to contact their healthcare provider immediately for signs or symptoms of hyperthyroidism and hypothyroidism *[see Warnings and Precautions (5.6)]*.
• Advise patients of the importance of keeping scheduled appointments for blood work or other laboratory tests *[see Warnings and Precautions (5.3, 5.5, 5.6)]*.
• Advise women that KEYTRUDA may cause fetal harm. Instruct women of reproductive potential to use highly effective contraception during and for 4 months after the last dose of KEYTRUDA *[see Warnings and Precautions (5.8) and Use in Specific Populations (8.1, 8.8)]*.
• Advise nursing mothers not to breastfeed while taking KEYTRUDA *[see Use in Specific Populations (8.3)]*.

Manufactured by: Merck Sharp & Dohme Corp., a subsidiary of
MERCK & CO., INC., Whitehouse Station, NJ 08889, USA
U.S. License No. 0002
At:
Schering-Plough (Brinny) Co.,
County Cork, Ireland

For patent information:
www.merck.com/product/patent/home.html
Copyright © 2014 Merck Sharp & Dohme Corp., a subsidiary of **Merck & Co., Inc.**
All rights reserved.
uspi-mk3475-iv-1409r000

MEDICATION GUIDE

KEYTRUDA® (key-true-duh)
(pembrolizumab)
for injection

What is the most important information I should know about KEYTRUDA?
KEYTRUDA is a medicine that may treat your melanoma by working with your immune system. KEYTRUDA can cause your immune system to attack normal organs and tissues in many areas of your body and can affect the way they work. These problems can sometimes become serious or life-threatening.
Call or see your doctor right away if you develop any symptoms of the following problems or these symptoms get worse:
• **Lung problems (pneumonitis). Symptoms of pneumonitis may include:**
  • shortness of breath
  • chest pain
  • new or worse cough
• **Intestinal problems (colitis) that can lead to tears or holes in your intestine. Signs and symptoms of colitis may include:**
  • diarrhea or more bowel movements than usual
  • stools that are black, tarry, sticky, or have blood or mucus
  • severe stomach-area (abdomen) pain or tenderness
• **Liver problems (hepatitis). Signs and symptoms of hepatitis may include:**
  • yellowing of your skin or the whites of your eyes
  • dark urine
  • nausea or vomiting
  • feeling less hungry than usual
  • pain on the right side of your stomach area (abdomen)
  • bleeding or bruising more easily than normal
• **Hormone gland problems (especially the thyroid, pituitary, and adrenal glands). Signs and symptoms that your hormone glands are not working properly may include:**
  • rapid heart beat
  • weight loss
  • increased sweating
  • weight gain
  • hair loss
  • feeling cold
  • constipation
  • your voice gets deeper
  • muscle aches
  • dizziness or fainting
  • headaches that will not go away or unusual headache
• **Kidney problems, including nephritis and kidney failure. Signs of kidney problems may include:**
  • change in the amount or color of your urine
• **Problems in other organs. Signs of these problems may include:**
  • rash
  • changes in eyesight
  • severe or persistent muscle or joint pains
  • severe muscle weakness
Getting medical treatment right away may help keep these problems from becoming more serious.
Your doctor will check you for these problems during treatment with KEYTRUDA. Your doctor may treat you with corticosteroid medicines and delay or completely stop treatment with KEYTRUDA, if you have severe side effects.
What is KEYTRUDA?
KEYTRUDA is a prescription medicine used to treat a kind of skin cancer called melanoma. KEYTRUDA may be used when your melanoma:
• has spread or cannot be removed by surgery (advanced melanoma)
and,
• after you have tried a medicine called ipilimumab and it did not work or is no longer working
and,
• if your tumor has an abnormal "BRAF" gene, and you also have tried a different medicine called a BRAF inhibitor, and it did not work or is no longer working.
It is not known if KEYTRUDA is safe and effective in children less than 18 years of age.
What should I tell my doctor before receiving KEYTRUDA?
Before you receive KEYTRUDA, tell your doctor if you:
• have immune system problems such as Crohn's disease, ulcerative colitis, or lupus
• have had an organ transplant
• have lung or breathing problems
• have liver problems
• have any other medical problems

• are pregnant or plan to become pregnant.
  ◦ KEYTRUDA may harm your unborn baby.
  ◦ Females who are able to become pregnant should use an effective method of birth control during and for at least 4 months after the last dose of KEYTRUDA. Talk to your doctor about birth control methods that you can use during this time.
  ◦ Tell your doctor right away if you become pregnant during treatment with KEYTRUDA.
• are breastfeeding or plan to breastfeed.
  ◦ It is not known if KEYTRUDA passes into your breast milk.
  ◦ Do not breastfeed during treatment with KEYTRUDA.
Tell your doctor about all the medicines you take, including prescription and over-the-counter medicines, vitamins, and herbal supplements.
Know the medicines you take. Keep a list of them to show your doctor and pharmacist when you get a new medicine.
How will I receive KEYTRUDA?
• Your doctor will give you KEYTRUDA into your vein through an intravenous (IV) line over 30 minutes.
• KEYTRUDA is usually given every 3 weeks.
• Your doctor will decide how many treatments you need.
• Your doctor will do blood tests to check you for side effects.
• If you miss any appointments, call your doctor as soon as possible to reschedule your appointment.
What are the possible side effects of KEYTRUDA?
KEYTRUDA can cause serious side effects. See "What is the most important information I should know about KEYTRUDA?"
The most common side effects of KEYTRUDA include:
• feeling tired
• cough
• nausea
• itching
• rash
• decreased appetite
• constipation
• diarrhea
• joint pain
Tell your doctor if you have any side effect that bothers you or that does not go away.
These are not all the possible side effects of KEYTRUDA. For more information, ask your doctor or pharmacist.
Call your doctor for medical advice about side effects. You may report side effects to FDA at 1-800-FDA-1088.
General information about the safe and effective use of KEYTRUDA
Medicines are sometimes prescribed for purposes other than those listed in a Medication Guide. If you would like more information about KEYTRUDA, talk with your doctor. You can ask your doctor or nurse for information about KEYTRUDA that is written for healthcare professionals. For more information, go to www.keytruda.com.
What are the ingredients in KEYTRUDA?
Active ingredient: pembrolizumab
Inactive ingredients: L-histidine, polysorbate-80, sucrose. May contain hydrochloric acid/sodium hydroxide.
This Medication Guide has been approved by the U.S. Food and Drug Administration.
Manufactured by: Merck Sharp & Dohme Corp., a subsidiary of **MERCK & CO., INC.**, Whitehouse Station, NJ 08889, USA
U.S. License No. 0002
At:
Schering-Plough (Brinny) Co.,
County Cork, Ireland
Issued: September 2014
For patent information:
www.merck.com/product/patent/home.html
Copyright © 2014 Merck Sharp & Dohme Corp., a subsidiary of **Merck & Co., Inc.**
All rights reserved.
usmg-mk3475-iv-1409r000

LIPTRUZET™   ℞
[LIP-true-zett]
(ezetimibe and atorvastatin)
tablets for oral use

HIGHLIGHTS OF PRESCRIBING INFORMATION
These highlights do not include all the information needed to use LIPTRUZET safely and effectively. See full prescribing information for LIPTRUZET.
LIPTRUZET™ (ezetimibe and atorvastatin) tablets for oral use
Initial U.S. Approval: 2013

——————INDICATIONS AND USAGE——————
LIPTRUZET, which contains a cholesterol absorption inhibitor and an HMG-CoA reductase inhibitor (statin), is indicated as adjunctive therapy to diet to:

- reduce elevated total-C, LDL-C, Apo B, TG, and non-HDL-C, and to increase HDL-C in patients with primary (heterozygous familial and non-familial) hyperlipidemia or mixed hyperlipidemia. (1.1)
- reduce elevated total-C and LDL-C in patients with homozygous familial hypercholesterolemia (HoFH), as an adjunct to other lipid-lowering treatments. (1.2)

Limitations of Use
- No incremental benefit of LIPTRUZET on cardiovascular morbidity and mortality over and above that demonstrated for atorvastatin has been established. LIPTRUZET has not been studied in Fredrickson Type I, III, IV, and V dyslipidemias. (1.3)

———DOSAGE AND ADMINISTRATION———

- Dosage range is 10/10 mg/day through 10/80 mg/day. (2.1)
- Recommended starting dose is 10/10 mg/day or 10/20 mg/day. (2.1)
- Recommended starting dose is 10/40 mg/day for patients requiring a >55% reduction in LDL-C. (2.1)
- Dosing of LIPTRUZET should occur either ≥2 hours before or ≥4 hours after administration of a bile acid sequestrant. (2.3, 7.11)

———DOSAGE FORMS AND STRENGTHS———

- Tablets (ezetimibe mg/atorvastatin mg): 10/10, 10/20, 10/40, 10/80. (3)

———CONTRAINDICATIONS———

- Active liver disease or unexplained persistent elevations of hepatic transaminase levels. (4, 5.2)
- Hypersensitivity to any component of LIPTRUZET. (4, 6.2)
- Women who are pregnant or may become pregnant. (4, 8.1)
- Nursing mothers. (4, 8.3)

———WARNINGS AND PRECAUTIONS———

- Patients should be advised to report promptly any unexplained and/or persistent muscle pain, tenderness, or weakness. LIPTRUZET should be discontinued immediately if myopathy is diagnosed or suspected. (5.1)
- Skeletal muscle effects (e.g., myopathy and rhabdomyolysis): Risks increase with higher doses and concomitant use of certain CYP3A4 inhibitors, fibric acid derivatives, and cyclosporine. Predisposing factors include advanced age (>65), uncontrolled hypothyroidism, and renal impairment. Rare cases of rhabdomyolysis with acute renal failure secondary to myoglobinuria have been reported. (5.1, 8.5)
- Liver enzyme abnormalities: Persistent elevations in hepatic transaminase can occur. Check liver enzyme tests before initiating therapy and as clinically indicated thereafter. (5.2)

———ADVERSE REACTIONS———

- Common adverse reactions (incidence ≥2% and greater than placebo) are: increased ALT, increased AST, and musculoskeletal pain. (6.1)

To report SUSPECTED ADVERSE REACTIONS, contact Merck Sharp & Dohme Corp., a subsidiary of Merck & Co., Inc., at 1-877-888-4231 or FDA at 1-800-FDA-1088 or www.fda.gov/medwatch.

———DRUG INTERACTIONS———

Drug Interactions Associated with Increased Risk of Myopathy/Rhabdomyolysis with Atorvastatin (2.3, 5.1, 7, 12.3)

Interacting Agents	Prescribing Recommendations for LIPTRUZET
Cyclosporine, HIV protease inhibitors (tipranavir plus ritonavir), hepatitis C protease inhibitor (telaprevir), gemfibrozil	Avoid LIPTRUZET
HIV protease inhibitor (lopinavir plus ritonavir)	Use with caution and lowest dose necessary.
Clarithromycin, itraconazole, HIV protease inhibitors (saquinavir plus ritonavir, darunavir plus ritonavir, fosamprenavir, fosamprenavir plus ritonavir)	Do not exceed 10/20 mg LIPTRUZET daily.
HIV protease inhibitor (nelfinavir), hepatitis C protease inhibitor (boceprevir)	Do not exceed 10/40 mg LIPTRUZET daily.

- Other lipid-lowering medications: Use with fenofibrates or lipid-modifying doses (≥1 g/day) of niacin increases the risk of adverse skeletal muscle effects. Caution should be used when prescribing with LIPTRUZET. (7)
- Fenofibrates: Combination increases exposure of ezetimibe. If cholelithiasis is suspected in a patient receiving ezetimibe and a fenofibrate, gallbladder studies are indicated and alternative lipid-lowering therapy should be considered. (7.5, 12.3)
- Cholestyramine: Combination decreases exposure of ezetimibe. (2.3, 12.3)
- Digoxin: Patients should be monitored appropriately. (7.7)
- Oral contraceptives: Values for norethindrone and ethinyl estradiol may be increased. (7.8)
- Rifampin should be simultaneously coadministered with LIPTRUZET. (7.9)

———USE IN SPECIFIC POPULATIONS———

- Hepatic impairment: Plasma concentrations of atorvastatin are markedly increased in patients with chronic alcoholic liver disease. (8.6, 12.3)

See 17 for PATIENT COUNSELING INFORMATION and FDA-approved patient labeling

Revised: 09/2013

———

FULL PRESCRIBING INFORMATION: CONTENTS*

* Sections or subsections omitted from the full prescribing information are not listed

FULL PRESCRIBING INFORMATION

1 INDICATIONS AND USAGE

Therapy with lipid-altering agents should be only one component of multiple risk factor intervention in individuals at significantly increased risk for atherosclerotic vascular disease due to hypercholesterolemia. Drug therapy is indicated as an adjunct to diet when the response to a diet restricted in saturated fat and cholesterol and other nonpharmacologic measures alone has been inadequate.

1.1 Primary Hyperlipidemia

LIPTRUZET™ is indicated for the reduction of elevated total cholesterol (total-C), low-density lipoprotein cholesterol (LDL-C), apolipoprotein B (Apo B), triglycerides (TG), and non-high-density lipoprotein cholesterol (non-HDL-C), and to increase high-density lipoprotein cholesterol (HDL-C) in patients with primary (heterozygous familial and non-familial) hyperlipidemia or mixed hyperlipidemia.

1.2 Homozygous Familial Hypercholesterolemia (HoFH)

LIPTRUZET is indicated for the reduction of elevated total-C and LDL-C in patients with homozygous familial hypercholesterolemia, as an adjunct to other lipid-lowering treatments (e.g., LDL apheresis) or if such treatments are unavailable.

1.3 Limitations of Use

No incremental benefit of LIPTRUZET on cardiovascular morbidity and mortality over and above that demonstrated for atorvastatin has been established. LIPTRUZET has not been studied in Fredrickson type I, III, IV, and V dyslipidemias.

2 DOSAGE AND ADMINISTRATION

2.1 Recommended Dosing

The dosage range of LIPTRUZET is 10/10 mg/day to 10/80 mg/day. The recommended starting dose of LIPTRUZET is 10/10 mg/day or 10/20 mg/day. LIPTRUZET can be administered as a single dose at any time of the day, with or without food. The recommended starting dose for patients who require a larger reduction in LDL-C (greater than 55%) is 10/40 mg/day. After initiation and/or upon titration of LIPTRUZET, lipid levels should be analyzed within 2 or more weeks and dosage adjusted accordingly.

Patients should swallow LIPTRUZET tablets whole. Tablets should not be crushed, dissolved, or chewed.

2.2 Patients with Homozygous Familial Hypercholesterolemia

The dosage of LIPTRUZET in patients with homozygous familial hypercholesterolemia is 10/40 mg/day or 10/80 mg/day. LIPTRUZET should be used as an adjunct to other lipid-lowering treatments (e.g., LDL apheresis) in these patients or if such treatments are unavailable.

2.3 Coadministration with Other Drugs

Bile Acid Sequestrants

Dosing of LIPTRUZET should occur either ≥2 hours before or ≥4 hours after administration of a bile acid sequestrant *[see Drug Interactions (7.11)]*.

Cyclosporine, Clarithromycin, Itraconazole, or Certain Protease Inhibitors

In patients taking cyclosporine or the HIV protease inhibitors (tipranavir plus ritonavir) or the hepatitis C protease inhibitor (telaprevir), therapy with LIPTRUZET should be avoided. In patients with HIV taking lopinavir plus ritonavir, caution should be used when prescribing LIPTRUZET and the lowest dose necessary employed. In patients taking clarithromycin, itraconazole, or in patients with HIV taking a combination of saquinavir plus ritonavir, darunavir plus ritonavir, fosamprenavir, or fosamprenavir plus ritonavir, therapy with LIPTRUZET should be limited to 10/20 mg, and appropriate clinical assessment is recommended to ensure that the lowest dose necessary of LIPTRUZET is employed. In patients taking the HIV protease inhibitor nelfinavir or the hepatitis C protease inhibitor boceprevir, therapy with LIPTRUZET should be limited to 10/40 mg, and appropriate clinical assessment is recommended to ensure that the lowest dose necessary of LIPTRUZET is employed. *[See Warnings and Precautions (5.1) and Drug Interactions (7).]*

Other Concomitant Lipid-Lowering Therapy

The combination of LIPTRUZET and gemfibrozil is not recommended *[see Warnings and Precautions (5.1) and Drug Interactions (7.4)]*.

3 DOSAGE FORMS AND STRENGTHS

- LIPTRUZET™ 10 mg/10 mg (ezetimibe 10 mg/atorvastatin 10 mg) tablets are white to off-white capsule-shaped, biconvex film-coated tablets with code "320" on one side.
- LIPTRUZET™ 10 mg/20 mg (ezetimibe 10 mg/atorvastatin 20 mg) tablets are white to off-white round, biconvex film-coated tablets with code "321" on one side.
- LIPTRUZET™ 10 mg/40 mg (ezetimibe 10 mg/atorvastatin 40 mg) tablets are white to off-white oval, biconvex film-coated tablets with code "322" on one side.

• LIPTRUZET™ 10 mg/80 mg (ezetimibe 10 mg/atorvastatin 80 mg) tablets are white to off-white capsule-shaped, biconvex film-coated tablets with code "323" on one side.

4 CONTRAINDICATIONS

Active liver disease or unexplained persistent elevations of hepatic transaminase levels.

Hypersensitivity to any component of LIPTRUZET [see Adverse Reactions (6.2)].

Women who are pregnant or may become pregnant. LIPTRUZET may cause fetal harm when administered to a pregnant woman. Serum cholesterol and triglycerides increase during normal pregnancy, and cholesterol or cholesterol derivatives are essential for fetal development. Atherosclerosis is a chronic process and discontinuation of lipid-lowering drugs during pregnancy should have little impact on the outcome of long-term therapy of primary hypercholesterolemia. There are no adequate and well-controlled studies of LIPTRUZET use during pregnancy; however in rare reports, congenital anomalies were observed following intrauterine exposure to statins. In rat and rabbit animal reproduction studies, atorvastatin revealed no evidence of teratogenicity. LIPTRUZET should be administered to women of childbearing age only when such patients are highly unlikely to conceive and have been informed of the potential hazards. If the patient becomes pregnant while taking this drug, LIPTRUZET should be discontinued immediately, and the patient should be apprised of the potential hazard to the fetus [see Use in Specific Populations (8.1)].

Nursing mothers. It is not known whether atorvastatin is excreted into human milk; however, a small amount of another drug in this class does pass into breast milk. Because statins have the potential for serious adverse reactions in nursing infants, women who require LIPTRUZET treatment should not breast-feed their infants [see Use in Specific Populations (8.3)].

5 WARNINGS AND PRECAUTIONS

5.1 Myopathy/Rhabdomyolysis

Atorvastatin

Rare cases of rhabdomyolysis with acute renal failure secondary to myoglobinuria have been reported with atorvastatin and with other drugs in this class. A history of renal impairment may be a risk factor for the development of rhabdomyolysis. Such patients merit closer monitoring for skeletal muscle effects.

Atorvastatin, like other statins, occasionally causes myopathy, defined as muscle aches or muscle weakness in conjunction with increases in creatine phosphokinase (CPK) values >10 times upper limit of normal (ULN). The concomitant use of higher doses of atorvastatin with certain drugs such as cyclosporine and strong CYP3A4 inhibitors (e.g., clarithromycin, itraconazole, and HIV protease inhibitors) increases the risk of myopathy/rhabdomyolysis.

There have been rare reports of immune-mediated necrotizing myopathy (IMNM), an autoimmune myopathy, associated with statin use. IMNM is characterized by: proximal muscle weakness and elevated serum creatinine kinase, which persist despite discontinuation of statin treatment; muscle biopsy showing necrotizing myopathy without significant inflammation; improvement with immunosuppressive agents.

Myopathy should be considered in any patient with diffuse myalgias, muscle tenderness or weakness, and/or marked elevation of CPK. Patients should be advised to report promptly unexplained muscle pain, tenderness or weakness, particularly if accompanied by malaise or fever or if muscle signs and symptoms persist after discontinuing LIPTRUZET. LIPTRUZET therapy should be discontinued if markedly elevated CPK levels occur or myopathy is diagnosed or suspected.

The risk of myopathy during treatment with statins is increased with concurrent administration of cyclosporine, fibric acid derivatives, erythromycin, clarithromycin, the hepatitis C protease inhibitor telaprevir, combinations of HIV protease inhibitors, including saquinavir plus ritonavir, lopinavir plus ritonavir, tipranavir plus ritonavir, darunavir plus ritonavir, fosamprenavir, and fosamprenavir plus ritonavir, niacin, or azole antifungals. Physicians considering combined therapy with LIPTRUZET and fibric acid derivatives, erythromycin, clarithromycin, a combination of saquinavir plus ritonavir, lopinavir plus ritonavir, darunavir plus ritonavir, fosamprenavir, or fosamprenavir plus ritonavir, azole antifungals, or lipid-modifying doses of niacin should carefully weigh the potential benefits and risks and should carefully monitor patients for any signs or symptoms of muscle pain, tenderness, or weakness, particularly during the initial months of therapy and during any periods of upward dosage titration of either drug. Lower starting and maintenance doses of LIPTRUZET should be considered when taken concomitantly with the aforementioned drugs. [See Drug Interactions (7).] Periodic CPK determinations

may be considered in such situations, but there is no assurance that such monitoring will prevent the occurrence of severe myopathy.

Prescribing recommendations for interacting agents are summarized in Table 1 [see also Dosage and Administration (2.3), Drug Interactions (7), Clinical Pharmacology (12.3)].

Table 1: Drug Interactions Associated with Increased Risk of Myopathy/Rhabdomyolysis with Atorvastatin

Interacting Agents	Prescribing Recommendations for LIPTRUZET
Cyclosporine, HIV protease inhibitors (tipranavir plus ritonavir), hepatitis C protease inhibitor (telaprevir), gemfibrozil	Avoid LIPTRUZET.
HIV protease inhibitor (lopinavir plus ritonavir)	Use with caution and lowest dose necessary.
Clarithromycin, itraconazole, HIV protease inhibitors (saquinavir plus ritonavir*, darunavir plus ritonavir, fosamprenavir, fosamprenavir plus ritonavir)	Do not exceed 10/20 mg LIPTRUZET daily.
HIV protease inhibitor (nelfinavir), hepatitis C protease inhibitor (boceprevir)	Do not exceed 10/40 mg LIPTRUZET daily.

* Use with caution and with the lowest dose necessary [see Clinical Pharmacology (12.3)]

Cases of myopathy, including rhabdomyolysis, have been reported with atorvastatin coadministered with colchicine, and caution should be exercised when prescribing LIPTRUZET with colchicine [see Drug Interactions (7.10)]. **LIPTRUZET therapy should be temporarily withheld or discontinued in any patient with an acute, serious condition suggestive of a myopathy or having a risk factor predisposing to the development of renal failure secondary to rhabdomyolysis (e.g., severe acute infection, hypotension, major surgery, trauma, severe metabolic, endocrine and electrolyte disorders, and uncontrolled seizures).**

Ezetimibe

In clinical trials, there was no excess of myopathy or rhabdomyolysis associated with ezetimibe compared with the relevant control arm (placebo or statin alone). However, myopathy and rhabdomyolysis are known adverse reactions to statins and other lipid-lowering drugs. In clinical trials, the incidence of creatine phosphokinase (CPK) >10 times ULN was 0.2% for ezetimibe vs. 0.1% for placebo, and 0.1% for ezetimibe coadministered with a statin vs. 0.4% for statins alone. Risk for skeletal muscle toxicity increases with higher doses of statin, advanced age (>65), hypothyroidism, renal impairment, and depending on the statin used, concomitant use of other drugs.

In post-marketing experience with ezetimibe, cases of myopathy and rhabdomyolysis have been reported. Most patients who developed rhabdomyolysis were taking a statin prior to initiating ezetimibe. However, rhabdomyolysis has been reported with ezetimibe monotherapy and with the addition of ezetimibe to agents known to be associated with increased risk of rhabdomyolysis, such as fibric acid derivatives. LIPTRUZET and a fenofibrate, if taking concomitantly, should both be immediately discontinued if myopathy is diagnosed or suspected. The presence of muscle symptoms and a CPK level >10 times the ULN indicates myopathy.

5.2 Liver Enzymes

Atorvastatin

Statins, like some other lipid-lowering therapies, have been associated with biochemical abnormalities of liver function. Persistent elevations (>3 times ULN occurring on 2 or more occasions) in serum transaminases occurred in 0.7% of patients who received atorvastatin in clinical trials. The incidence of these abnormalities was 0.2%, 0.2%, 0.6%, and 2.3% for 10, 20, 40, and 80 mg atorvastatin, respectively. One patient in clinical trials of atorvastatin developed jaundice. Increases in liver function tests (LFT) in other patients were not associated with jaundice or other clinical signs or symptoms. Upon dose reduction, drug interruption, or discontinuation, transaminase levels returned to or near pretreatment levels without sequelae. Eighteen of 30 patients with persistent LFT elevations continued treatment with a reduced dose of atorvastatin.

Ezetimibe

In controlled clinical studies, the incidence of consecutive elevations (≥3 times ULN) in hepatic transaminase levels was similar between ezetimibe (0.5%) and placebo (0.3%).

In controlled clinical combination studies of ezetimibe coadministered with atorvastatin, the incidence of consecutive elevations (≥3 times ULN) in hepatic transaminase levels was 0.6% for patients treated with ezetimibe administered with atorvastatin. These elevations in transaminases were generally asymptomatic, not associated with cholestasis, and returned to baseline after discontinuation of therapy or with continued treatment.

LIPTRUZET

It is recommended that liver enzyme tests be obtained prior to initiating therapy with LIPTRUZET and repeated as clinically indicated. There have been rare postmarketing reports of fatal and non-fatal hepatic failure in patients taking statins, including atorvastatin. If serious liver injury with clinical symptoms and/or hyperbilirubinemia or jaundice occurs during treatment with LIPTRUZET, promptly interrupt therapy. If an alternate etiology is not found, do not restart LIPTRUZET.

LIPTRUZET should be used with caution in patients who consume substantial quantities of alcohol and/or have a history of liver disease. Active liver disease or unexplained persistent transaminase elevations are contraindications to the use of LIPTRUZET [see Contraindications (4)].

5.3 Endocrine Function

Increases in HbA1c and fasting serum glucose levels have been reported with HMG-CoA reductase inhibitors, including atorvastatin.

Statins interfere with cholesterol synthesis and theoretically might blunt adrenal and/or gonadal steroid production. Clinical studies have shown that atorvastatin does not reduce basal plasma cortisol concentration or impair adrenal reserve and that ezetimibe did not impair adrenocortical steroid hormone production. The effects of statins on male fertility have not been studied in adequate numbers of patients. The effects, if any, on the pituitary-gonadal axis in premenopausal women are unknown. Caution should be exercised if LIPTRUZET is administered concomitantly with drugs that may decrease the levels or activity of endogenous steroid hormones, such as ketoconazole, spironolactone, and cimetidine.

5.4 Use in Patients with Recent Stroke or TIA

In a post-hoc analysis of the Stroke Prevention by Aggressive Reduction in Cholesterol Levels (SPARCL) study where atorvastatin 80 mg vs. placebo was administered in 4,731 subjects without CHD who had a stroke or TIA within the preceding 6 months, a higher incidence of hemorrhagic stroke was seen in the atorvastatin 80 mg group compared to placebo (55, 2.3% atorvastatin vs. 33, 1.4% placebo; HR: 1.68, 95% CI: 1.09, 2.59; p=0.0168). The incidence of fatal hemorrhagic stroke was similar across treatment groups (17 vs. 18 for the atorvastatin and placebo groups, respectively). The incidence of nonfatal hemorrhagic stroke was significantly higher in the atorvastatin (38, 1.6%) group as compared to the placebo group (16, 0.7%). Some baseline characteristics, including hemorrhagic and lacunar stroke on study entry, were associated with a higher incidence of hemorrhagic stroke in the atorvastatin group.

5.5 CNS Toxicity

Atorvastatin

Brain hemorrhage was seen in a female dog treated for 3 months at 120 mg/kg/day. Brain hemorrhage and optic nerve vacuolation were seen in another female dog that was sacrificed in moribund condition after 11 weeks of escalating doses up to 280 mg/kg/day. The 120 mg/kg dose resulted in a systemic exposure approximately 16 times the human plasma area-under-the-curve (AUC, 0-24 hours) based on the maximum human dose of 80 mg/day. A single tonic convulsion was seen in each of 2 male dogs (one treated at 10 mg/kg/day and one at 120 mg/kg/day) in a 2-year study. No CNS lesions have been observed in mice after chronic treatment for up to 2 years at doses up to 400 mg/kg/day or in rats at doses up to 100 mg/kg/day. These doses were 6 to 11 times (mouse) and 8 to 16 times (rat) the human AUC$_{(0-24)}$ based on the maximum recommended human dose of 80 mg/day.

CNS vascular lesions, characterized by perivascular hemorrhages, edema, and mononuclear cell infiltration of perivascular spaces, have been observed in dogs treated with other members of this class. A chemically similar drug in this class produced optic nerve degeneration (Wallerian degeneration of retinogeniculate fibers) in clinically normal dogs in a dose-dependent fashion at a dose that produced plasma drug levels about 30 times higher than the mean drug level in humans taking the highest recommended dose.

6 ADVERSE REACTIONS

The following serious adverse reactions are discussed in greater detail in other sections of the label:
• Rhabdomyolysis and myopathy [see Warnings and Precautions (5.1)]
• Liver enzyme abnormalities [see Warnings and Precautions (5.2)]

6.1 Clinical Trials Experience

LIPTRUZET

Because clinical studies are conducted under widely varying conditions, adverse reaction rates observed in the clinical studies of a drug cannot be directly compared to rates in the clinical studies of another drug and may not reflect the rates observed in clinical practice.

In a LIPTRUZET (ezetimibe and atorvastatin) placebo-controlled clinical trial, 628 patients (age range 18-86 years, 59% women, 85% Caucasians, 6% Blacks, 5% Hispanics, 3% Asians) with a median treatment duration of 12 weeks, 6% of patients on LIPTRUZET and 5% of patients on placebo discontinued due to adverse reactions.

The most common adverse reactions in the group treated with LIPTRUZET that led to treatment discontinuation and occurred at a rate greater than placebo were:
- Myalgia (0.8%)
- Abdominal pain (0.8%)
- Increased hepatic enzymes (0.8%)

The most commonly reported adverse reactions (incidence ≥2% and greater than placebo) in this trial were: increased ALT (5%), increased AST (4%), and musculoskeletal pain (4%).

LIPTRUZET has been evaluated for safety in 2403 patients in 7 clinical trials (one placebo-controlled trial and six active-controlled trials).

Table 2 summarizes the frequency of clinical adverse reactions reported in ≥2% of patients treated with LIPTRUZET (n=255) and at an incidence greater than placebo, regardless of causality assessment, from the placebo-controlled trial.

[See table 2 above]

After completing the 12-week study, eligible patients were assigned to coadministered ezetimibe and atorvastatin equivalent to LIPTRUZET (10/10-10/80) or atorvastatin (10-80 mg/day) for an additional 48 weeks. The long-term coadministration of ezetimibe plus atorvastatin had an overall safety profile similar to that of atorvastatin alone.

Ezetimibe

In 10 double-blind, placebo-controlled clinical trials, 2396 patients with primary hyperlipidemia (age range 9-86 years, 50% women, 90% Caucasians, 5% Blacks, 3% Hispanics, 2% Asians) and elevated LDL-C were treated with ezetimibe 10 mg/day for a median treatment duration of 12 weeks (range 0 to 39 weeks).

Adverse reactions reported in ≥2% of patients treated with ezetimibe and at an incidence greater than placebo regardless of causality assessment are shown in Table 3.

Table 3: Clinical Adverse Reactions Occurring in ≥2% of Patients Treated with Ezetimibe and at an Incidence Greater than Placebo, Regardless of Causality

Body System/Organ Class Adverse Reaction	Ezetimibe 10 mg (%) n=2396	Placebo (%) n=1159
Gastrointestinal disorders		
Diarrhea	4.1	3.7
General disorders and administration site conditions		
Fatigue	2.4	1.5
Infections and infestations		
Influenza	2.0	1.5
Sinusitis	2.8	2.2
Upper respiratory tract infection	4.3	2.5
Musculoskeletal and connective tissue disorders		
Arthralgia	3.0	2.2
Pain in extremity	2.7	2.5

Atorvastatin

In an atorvastatin placebo-controlled clinical trial database of 16,066 patients (8755 atorvastatin vs. 7311 placebo; age range 10–93 years, 39% women, 91% Caucasians, 3% Blacks, 2% Asians, 4% other) with a median treatment duration of 53 weeks, 9.7% of patients on atorvastatin and 9.5% of the patients on placebo discontinued due to adverse reactions regardless of causality.

The most commonly reported adverse reactions (incidence ≥2% and greater than placebo) regardless of causality, in patients treated with atorvastatin in placebo controlled trials (n=8755) were: nasopharyngitis (8.3%), arthralgia (6.9%), diarrhea (6.8%), pain in extremity (6.0%), and urinary tract infection (5.7%).

Table 4 summarizes the frequency of clinical adverse reactions, regardless of causality, reported in ≥2% and at a rate greater than placebo in patients treated with atorvastatin (n=8755), from seventeen placebo-controlled trials.

Table 2*: Clinical and Selected Laboratory Adverse Reactions Occurring in ≥2% of Patients Treated with LIPTRUZET and at an Incidence Greater than Placebo, Regardless of Causality

Body System/Organ Class Adverse Reaction	Placebo (%) n=60	Ezetimibe 10 mg (%) n=65	Atorvastatin† (%) n=248	LIPTRUZET† (%) n=255
Nervous system disorders				
Dizziness	0	6	<1	2
Respiratory, thoracic, and mediastinal disorders				
Coughing	0	3	<1	2
Gastrointestinal disorders				
Abdominal pain	2	2	4	3
Nausea	0	2	5	2
Musculoskeletal and connective tissue disorders				
Arthralgia	0	5	6	3
Muscle weakness	0	2	0	2
Musculoskeletal pain	3	8	5	4
Metabolism and nutrition disorders				
Hyperkalemia	0	0	<1	2
Infections and infestations				
Bronchitis	0	2	2	2
Sinusitis	0	3	2	2
Vascular disorders				
Hot flushes	0	0	<1	2
Investigations				
ALT increased	0	0	2	5
AST increased	0	0	<1	4

* Placebo-controlled combination study in which the active ingredients equivalent to LIPTRUZET were coadministered.
† All doses.

Table 4: Clinical Adverse Reactions Occurring in > 2% in Patents Treated with any dose of Atorvastatin and at an Incidence Greater than Placebo Regardless of Causality (% of patients).

Adverse Reaction*	Any dose n=8755	Atorvastatin 10 mg n=3908	Atorvastatin 20 mg n=188	Atorvastatin 40 mg n=604	Atorvastatin 80 mg n=4055	Placebo n=7311
Nasopharyngitis	8.3	12.9	5.3	7.0	4.2	8.2
Arthralgia	6.9	8.9	11.7	10.6	4.3	6.5
Diarrhea	6.8	7.3	6.4	14.1	5.2	6.3
Pain in extremity	6.0	8.5	3.7	9.3	3.1	5.9
Urinary tract infection	5.7	6.9	6.4	8.0	4.1	5.6
Dyspepsia	4.7	5.9	3.2	6.0	3.3	4.3
Nausea	4.0	3.7	3.7	7.1	3.8	3.5
Musculoskeletal pain	3.8	5.2	3.2	5.1	2.3	3.6
Muscle spasms	3.6	4.6	4.8	5.1	2.4	3.0
Myalgia	3.5	3.6	5.9	8.4	2.7	3.1
Insomnia	3.0	2.8	1.1	5.3	2.8	2.9
Pharyngolaryngeal pain	2.3	3.9	1.6	2.8	0.7	2.1

* Adverse Reaction >2% in any dose greater than placebo

[See table 4 above]

6.2 Postmarketing Experience

Because the reactions below are reported voluntarily from a population of uncertain size, it is generally not possible to reliably estimate their frequency or establish a causal relationship to drug exposure.

The additional events described below have been identified during post-approval use of ezetimibe and/or atorvastatin.

Blood and lymphatic system disorders: thrombocytopenia

Nervous system disorders: headache; paresthesia; peripheral neuropathy

There have been rare postmarketing reports of cognitive impairment (e.g., memory loss, forgetfulness, amnesia, memory impairment, confusion) associated with statin use. These cognitive issues have been reported for all statins. The reports are generally nonserious, and reversible upon statin discontinuation, with variable times to symptom onset (1 day to years) and symptom resolution (median of 3 weeks).

Gastrointestinal disorders: pancreatitis

Skin and subcutaneous tissue disorders: angioedema; bullous rashes (including erythema multiforme, Stevens-Johnson syndrome, and toxic epidermal necrolysis); rash; urticaria

Musculoskeletal and connective tissue disorders: myopathy/rhabdomyolysis [see Warnings and Precautions (5.1)]

There have been rare reports of immune-mediated necrotizing myopathy associated with statin use [see Warnings and Precautions (5.1)].

Injury, poisoning and procedural complications: tendon rupture

Immune system disorders: anaphylaxis; hypersensitivity reactions

Hepatobiliary disorders: hepatitis; cholelithiasis; cholecystitis; fatal and nonfatal hepatic failure

Psychiatric disorders: depression

Laboratory abnormalities: elevated creatine phosphokinase

7 DRUG INTERACTIONS

[See Clinical Pharmacology (12.3).]

LIPTRUZET

The risk of myopathy during treatment with statins is increased with concurrent administration of fibric acid derivatives, lipid-modifying doses of niacin, cyclosporine, or strong CYP3A4 inhibitors (e.g., clarithromycin, HIV protease inhibitors, and itraconazole) [see Warnings and Precautions (5.1) and Clinical Pharmacology (12.3)].

7.1 Strong Inhibitors of Cytochrome P450 3A4

Atorvastatin is metabolized by cytochrome P450 3A4. Concomitant administration of atorvastatin with strong inhibitors of CYP3A4 can lead to increases in plasma concentrations of atorvastatin. The extent of interaction and potentiation of effects depend on the variability of effect on CYP3A4. Because LIPTRUZET contains atorvastatin, the risk of myopathy during treatment with LIPTRUZET is increased with concurrent administration of:

Clarithromycin: Atorvastatin AUC was significantly increased with concomitant administration of 80 mg atorvastatin with clarithromycin (500 mg twice daily) compared to that of atorvastatin alone [see Clinical Pharmacology (12.3)]. Therefore, in patients taking clarithromycin, caution should be used when the LIPTRUZET dose exceeds 10/20 mg [see Warnings and Precautions (5.1) and Dosage and Administration (2.3)].

Combination of Protease Inhibitors: Atorvastatin AUC was significantly increased with concomitant administration of atorvastatin with several combinations of HIV protease inhibitors, as well as with the hepatitis C protease inhibitor telaprevir, compared to that of atorvastatin alone [see Clinical Pharmacology (12.3)]. Therefore, in patients taking the HIV protease inhibitor tipranavir plus ritonavir, or the hepatitis C protease inhibitor telaprevir, concomitant use of LIPTRUZET should be avoided. In patients taking the HIV protease inhibitor lopinavir plus ritonavir, caution should be used when prescribing LIPTRUZET and the lowest dose necessary should be used. In patients taking the HIV protease inhibitors saquinavir plus ritonavir, darunavir plus ritonavir, fosamprenavir, or fosamprenavir plus ritonavir, the dose of LIPTRUZET should not exceed 10/20 mg and should be used with caution [see Warnings and Precautions (5.1) and Dosage and Administration (2.3)]. In patients taking the HIV protease inhibitor nelfinavir or the hepatitis C protease inhibitor boceprevir, the dose of LIPTRUZET should not exceed 10/40 mg daily and close clinical monitoring is recommended.

Itraconazole: Atorvastatin AUC was significantly increased with concomitant administration of atorvastatin 40 mg and itraconazole 200 mg [see Clinical Pharmacology (12.3)]. Therefore, in patients taking itraconazole, do not use a LIPTRUZET dose that exceeds 10/20 mg [see Warnings and Precautions (5.1) and Dosage and Administration (2.3)].

7.2 Cyclosporine

Atorvastatin and atorvastatin-metabolites are substrates of the OATP1B1 transporter. Inhibitors of the OATP1B1 (e.g., cyclosporine) can increase the bioavailability of atorvastatin. Atorvastatin AUC was significantly increased with concomitant administration of atorvastatin 10 mg and cyclosporine 5.2 mg/kg/day compared to that of atorvastatin alone [see Clinical Pharmacology (12.3)].

In addition, ezetimibe and cyclosporine used concomitantly can increase exposure to both ezetimibe and cyclosporine. The degree of increase in ezetimibe exposure may be greater in patients with severe renal impairment.

The coadministration of LIPTRUZET with cyclosporine should be avoided [see Warnings and Precautions (5.1)].

7.3 Grapefruit Juice

Grapefruit juice contains one or more components that inhibit CYP3A4 and can increase plasma concentrations of atorvastatin, especially with excessive grapefruit juice consumption (>1.2 liters per day).

7.4 Gemfibrozil

Due to an increased risk of myopathy/rhabdomyolysis when HMG-CoA reductase inhibitors are coadministered with gemfibrozil, concomitant administration of LIPTRUZET with gemfibrozil should be avoided [see Warnings and Precautions (5.1)].

7.5 Fenofibrates (e.g., fenofibrate and fenofibric acid)

Because it is known that the risk of myopathy during treatment with HMG-CoA reductase inhibitors is increased with concurrent administration of fenofibrates, LIPTRUZET should be administered with caution when used concomitantly with a fenofibrate [see Warnings and Precautions (5.1)].

Fenofibrates may increase cholesterol excretion into the bile, leading to cholelithiasis. If cholelithiasis is suspected in a patient receiving LIPTRUZET and a fenofibrate, gallbladder studies are indicated and alternative lipid-lowering therapy should be considered [see the product labeling for fenofibrate and fenofibric acid].

7.6 Niacin

The risk of skeletal muscle effects may be enhanced when LIPTRUZET is used in combination with niacin; a reduction in LIPTRUZET dosage should be considered in this setting [see Warnings and Precautions (5.1)].

7.7 Digoxin

When multiple doses of atorvastatin and digoxin were coadministered, steady state plasma digoxin concentrations increased by approximately 20%. Patients taking digoxin should be monitored appropriately.

7.8 Oral Contraceptives

Coadministration of atorvastatin and an oral contraceptive increased AUC values for norethindrone and ethinyl estradiol [see Clinical Pharmacology (12.3)]. These increases should be considered when selecting an oral contraceptive for a woman taking LIPTRUZET.

7.9 Rifampin or Other Inducers of Cytochrome P450 3A4

Concomitant administration of atorvastatin with inducers of cytochrome P450 3A4 (e.g., efavirenz, rifampin) can lead to variable reductions in plasma concentrations of atorvastatin. Due to the dual interaction mechanism of rifampin, simultaneous coadministration of LIPTRUZET with rifampin is recommended, as delayed administration of atorvastatin after administration of rifampin has been associated with a significant reduction in atorvastatin plasma concentrations.

7.10 Colchicine

Cases of myopathy, including rhabdomyolysis, have been reported with atorvastatin coadministered with colchicine, and caution should be exercised when prescribing LIPTRUZET with colchicine.

7.11 Cholestyramine

Concomitant cholestyramine administration decreased the mean area under the curve (AUC) of total ezetimibe approximately 55%. The incremental LDL-C reduction due to adding ezetimibe to cholestyramine may be reduced by this interaction.

7.12 Coumarin Anticoagulants

If LIPTRUZET is added to warfarin, a coumarin anticoagulant, the International Normalized Ratio (INR) should be appropriately monitored.

8 USE IN SPECIFIC POPULATIONS

8.1 Pregnancy

Pregnancy Category X.

[See Contraindications (4).]

LIPTRUZET

LIPTRUZET is contraindicated in women who are or may become pregnant. Serum cholesterol and triglycerides increase during normal pregnancy. Lipid-lowering drugs offer no benefit during pregnancy, because cholesterol and cholesterol derivatives are needed for normal fetal development. Atherosclerosis is a chronic process, and discontinuation of lipid-lowering drugs during pregnancy should have little impact on long-term outcomes of primary hypercholesterolemia therapy.

There are no adequate and well-controlled studies of LIPTRUZET use during pregnancy. There have been rare reports of congenital anomalies following intrauterine exposure to statins. In a review of about 100 prospectively followed pregnancies in women exposed to other statins, the incidences of congenital anomalies, spontaneous abortions, and fetal deaths/stillbirths did not exceed the rate expected in the general population. However, this study was only able to exclude a three-to-four-fold increased risk of congenital anomalies over background incidence. In 89% of these cases, drug treatment started before pregnancy and stopped during the first trimester when pregnancy was identified.

Statins may cause fetal harm when administered to a pregnant woman. Because LIPTRUZET contains atorvastatin, LIPTRUZET should be administered to women of childbearing potential only when such patients are highly unlikely to conceive and have been informed of the potential hazards. If the woman becomes pregnant while taking LIPTRUZET, it should be discontinued immediately and the patient advised again as to the potential hazards to the fetus and the lack of known clinical benefit with continued use during pregnancy.

Ezetimibe

In oral (gavage) embryo-fetal development studies of ezetimibe conducted in rats and rabbits during organogenesis, there was no evidence of embryolethal effects at the doses tested (250, 500, 1000 mg/kg/day). In rats, increased incidences of common fetal skeletal findings (extra pair of thoracic ribs, unossified cervical vertebral centra, shortened ribs) were observed at 1000 mg/kg/day (~10 times the human exposure at 10 mg daily based on AUC_{0-24hr} for total ezetimibe). In rabbits treated with ezetimibe, an increased incidence of extra thoracic ribs was observed at 1000 mg/kg/day (150 times the human exposure at 10 mg daily based on AUC_{0-24hr} for total ezetimibe). Ezetimibe crossed the placenta when pregnant rats and rabbits were given multiple oral doses.

Multiple-dose studies of ezetimibe given in combination with statins in rats and rabbits during organogenesis result in higher ezetimibe and statin exposures. Reproductive findings occur at lower doses in combination therapy compared to monotherapy.

Atorvastatin

Atorvastatin crosses the rat placenta and reaches a level in fetal liver equivalent to that of maternal plasma. Atorvastatin was not teratogenic in rats at doses up to 300 mg/kg/day or in rabbits at doses up to 100 mg/kg/day. These doses resulted in multiples of about 30 times (rat) or 20 times (rabbit) the human exposure based on surface area (mg/m^2).

In a study in rats given 20, 100, or 225 mg/kg/day, from gestation Day 7 through to lactation Day 21 (weaning), there was decreased pup survival at birth, neonate, weaning, and maturity in pups of mothers dosed at 225 mg/kg/day. Body weight was decreased on Days 4 and 21 in pups of mothers dosed at 100 mg/kg/day; pup body weight was decreased at birth and at Days 4, 21, and 91 at 225 mg/kg/day. Pup development was delayed (rotorod performance at 100 mg/kg/day and acoustic startle at 225 mg/kg/day; pinnae detachment and eye opening at 225 mg/kg/day). These doses correspond to 6 times (100 mg/kg) and 22 times (225 mg/kg) the human AUC at 80 mg/day. Rare reports of congenital anomalies have been received following intrauterine exposure to statin reductase inhibitors.

8.3 Nursing Mothers

In rat studies, exposure to total ezetimibe in nursing pups was up to half of that observed in maternal plasma. It is not known whether ezetimibe is excreted into human breast milk.

It is not known whether atorvastatin is excreted in human milk, but a small amount of another drug in this class does pass into breast milk. Nursing rat pups had plasma and liver atorvastatin levels of 50% and 40%, respectively, of that in their mother's milk. Because of the potential for adverse reactions in nursing infants, women taking LIPTRUZET should not breast-feed [see Contraindications (4)].

8.4 Pediatric Use

LIPTRUZET

Safety and effectiveness have not been established in pediatric patients.

Ezetimibe

Based on total ezetimibe (ezetimibe + ezetimibe-glucuronide) there are no pharmacokinetic differences between adolescents and adults. Pharmacokinetic data in the pediatric population <10 years of age are not available.

Atorvastatin

Pharmacokinetic data in the pediatric population are not available.

8.5 Geriatric Use

Of the patients who received ezetimibe coadministered with atorvastatin in clinical studies, 1166 were 65 and older (this included 291 who were 75 and older). The effectiveness and safety of LIPTRUZET were similar between these patients and younger subjects. Greater sensitivity of some older individuals cannot be ruled out. Since advanced age (≥65 years) is a predisposing factor for myopathy, LIPTRUZET should be prescribed with caution in the elderly. [See Clinical Pharmacology (12.3).]

In geriatric patients, no dosage adjustment of LIPTRUZET is necessary.

8.6 Hepatic Impairment

LIPTRUZET is contraindicated in patients with active liver disease or unexplained persistent elevations in hepatic transaminase levels [see Contraindications (4), Warnings and Precautions (5.2), and Clinical Pharmacology (12.3)].

8.7 Renal Impairment

A history of renal impairment may be a risk factor for statin-associated myopathy. These patients merit closer monitoring for skeletal muscle effects [see Warnings and Precautions (5.1)].

In patients with renal impairment, no dosage adjustment of LIPTRUZET is necessary.

10 OVERDOSAGE

LIPTRUZET

No specific treatment of overdosage with LIPTRUZET can be recommended. In the event of an overdose, the patient should be treated symptomatically, and supportive measures instituted as required.

Ezetimibe

In clinical studies, administration of ezetimibe, 50 mg/day to 15 healthy subjects for up to 14 days, 40 mg/day to 18 patients with primary hyperlipidemia for up to 56 days, and 40 mg/day to 27 patients with homozygous sitosterolemia for 26 weeks, was generally well tolerated. One female patient with homozygous sitosterolemia took an accidental overdose of ezetimibe 120 mg/day for 28 days with no reported clinical or laboratory adverse events.

Atorvastatin

Due to extensive drug binding to plasma proteins, hemodialysis is not expected to significantly enhance atorvastatin clearance.

11 DESCRIPTION

LIPTRUZET contains ezetimibe, a selective inhibitor of intestinal cholesterol and related phytosterol absorption, and atorvastatin, a 3-hydroxy-3-methylglutaryl-coenzyme A (HMG-CoA) reductase inhibitor.

The chemical name of ezetimibe is 1-(4-fluorophenyl)-3(R)-[3-(4-fluorophenyl)-3(S)-hydroxypropyl]-4(S)-(4-hydroxyphenyl)-2-azetidinone. The empirical formula is $C_{24}H_{21}F_2NO_3$. Its molecular weight is 409.4. Ezetimibe is a white, crystalline powder that is freely to very soluble in ethanol, methanol, and acetone and practically insoluble in water. Its structural formula is:

Atorvastatin is [R-(R*, R*)]-2-(4-fluorophenyl)-ß, δ-dihydroxy-5-(1-methylethyl)-3-phenyl-4-[(phenylamino) carbonyl]-1H-pyrrole-1-heptanoic acid, calcium salt (2:1). Atorvastatin calcium is a white to off-white amorphous powder that is very slightly soluble in water, insoluble in acetonitrile, and soluble in methanol. The empirical formula of atorvastatin calcium is $(C_{33}H_{34}FN_2O_5)_2Ca$. The molecular weight of atorvastatin calcium is 1155.37. Its structural formula is:

LIPTRUZET is available for oral use as tablets containing 10 mg of ezetimibe and: 10.34 mg of atorvastatin calcium, equivalent to 10 mg of atorvastatin (LIPTRUZET 10 mg/10 mg); 20.68 mg of atorvastatin calcium, equivalent to 20 mg of atorvastatin (LIPTRUZET 10 mg/20 mg); 41.37 mg of atorvastatin calcium, equivalent to 40 mg of atorvastatin (LIPTRUZET 10 mg/40 mg); or 82.73 mg of atorvastatin calcium, equivalent to 80 mg of atorvastatin (LIPTRUZET 10 mg/80 mg). Each film-coated tablet of LIPTRUZET contains the following inactive ingredients: lactose monohydrate, microcrystalline cellulose, croscarmellose sodium, povidone, sodium lauryl sulfate, magnesium stearate, lactose anhydrous, hydroxypropyl cellulose, and sodium bicarbonate. In addition, the film coating contains the following inactive ingredients: hydroxypropyl cellulose, hypromellose, titanium dioxide, and carnauba wax.

12 CLINICAL PHARMACOLOGY
12.1 Mechanism of Action
LIPTRUZET
Plasma cholesterol is derived from intestinal absorption and endogenous synthesis. LIPTRUZET contains ezetimibe and atorvastatin, two lipid-lowering compounds with complementary mechanisms of action.
Ezetimibe
Ezetimibe reduces blood cholesterol by inhibiting the absorption of cholesterol by the small intestine. The molecular target of ezetimibe has been shown to be the sterol transporter, Niemann-Pick C1-Like 1 (NPC1L1), which is involved in the intestinal uptake of cholesterol and phytosterols. In a 2-week clinical study in 18 hypercholesterolemic patients, ezetimibe inhibited intestinal cholesterol absorption by 54%, compared with placebo. Ezetimibe had no clinically meaningful effect on the plasma concentrations of the fat-soluble vitamins A, D, and E and did not impair adrenocortical steroid hormone production.
Ezetimibe does not inhibit cholesterol synthesis in the liver or increase bile acid excretion. Ezetimibe localizes at the brush border of the small intestine and inhibits the absorption of cholesterol, leading to a decrease in the delivery of intestinal cholesterol to the liver. This causes a reduction of hepatic cholesterol stores and an increase in clearance of cholesterol from the blood; this distinct mechanism is complementary to that of statins [see Clinical Studies (14)].
Atorvastatin
In animal models, atorvastatin lowers plasma cholesterol and lipoprotein levels by inhibiting HMG-CoA reductase and cholesterol synthesis in the liver and by increasing the number of hepatic LDL receptors on the cell-surface to enhance uptake and catabolism of LDL; atorvastatin also reduces LDL production and the number of LDL particles.

12.2 Pharmacodynamics
Clinical studies have demonstrated that elevated levels of total-C, LDL-C and Apo B, the major protein constituent of LDL, promote human atherosclerosis. In addition, decreased levels of HDL-C are associated with the development of atherosclerosis. Epidemiologic studies have established that cardiovascular morbidity and mortality vary directly with the level of total-C and LDL-C and inversely with the level of HDL-C. Like LDL, cholesterol-enriched triglyceride-rich lipoproteins, including very-low-density lipoproteins (VLDL), intermediate-density lipoproteins (IDL), and remnants, can also promote atherosclerosis. The independent effect of raising HDL-C or lowering TG on the risk of coronary and cardiovascular morbidity and mortality has not been determined.
Atorvastatin as well as some of its metabolites are pharmacologically active in humans. The liver is the primary site of action and the principal site of cholesterol synthesis and LDL clearance. Drug dosage, rather than systemic drug concentration, correlates better with LDL-C reduction. Individualization of drug dosage should be based on therapeutic response [see Dosage and Administration (2)].

12.3 Pharmacokinetics
LIPTRUZET
LIPTRUZET 10/10 and 10/80 tablets have been shown to be bioequivalent to coadministration of corresponding doses of ezetimibe and atorvastatin tablets. LIPTRUZET 10/20 and 10/40 tablets have been shown to be clinically equivalent in LDL-C response to the corresponding coadministered doses of ezetimibe and atorvastatin tablets. [See Clinical Studies (14.1).]

Absorption
Ezetimibe
After oral administration, ezetimibe is absorbed and extensively conjugated to a pharmacologically active phenolic glucuronide (ezetimibe-glucuronide).
Atorvastatin
Maximum plasma atorvastatin concentrations after oral administration occur within 1 to 2 hours. Extent of absorption increases in proportion to atorvastatin dose. The absolute bioavailability of atorvastatin (parent drug) is approximately 14% and the systemic availability of HMG-CoA reductase inhibitory activity is approximately 30%. The low systemic availability is attributed to presystemic clearance in gastrointestinal mucosa and/or hepatic first-pass metabolism. Plasma atorvastatin concentrations are lower (approximately 30% for C_{max} and AUC) following evening drug administration compared with morning. However, LDL-C reduction is the same regardless of the time of day of drug administration.

Effect of Food on Oral Absorption
LIPTRUZET
A high-fat meal decreased atorvastatin AUC and C_{max} 11% and 35%, respectively, of the LIPTRUZET 10/80 tablet. A high-fat meal decreased unconjugated ezetimibe AUC 2% and increased unconjugated ezetimibe C_{max} 10% of the LIPTRUZET 10/80 tablet.
LIPTRUZET can be taken with or without food [see Dosage and Administration (2.1)].

Distribution
Ezetimibe
Ezetimibe and ezetimibe-glucuronide are highly bound (>90%) to human plasma proteins.
Atorvastatin
Mean volume of distribution of atorvastatin is approximately 381 liters. Atorvastatin is ≥98% bound to plasma proteins. A blood/plasma ratio of approximately 0.25 indicates poor drug penetration into red blood cells. Based on observations in rats, atorvastatin is likely to be secreted in human milk [see Contraindications (4); Use in Specific Populations (8.3)].

Metabolism and Excretion
Ezetimibe
Ezetimibe is primarily metabolized in the small intestine and liver via glucuronide conjugation with subsequent biliary and renal excretion. Minimal oxidative metabolism has been observed in all species evaluated.
In humans, ezetimibe is rapidly metabolized to ezetimibe-glucuronide. Ezetimibe and ezetimibe-glucuronide are the major drug-derived compounds detected in plasma, constituting approximately 10 to 20% and 80 to 90% of the total drug in plasma, respectively. Both ezetimibe and ezetimibe-glucuronide are eliminated from plasma with a half-life of approximately 22 hours for both ezetimibe and ezetimibe-glucuronide. Plasma concentration-time profiles exhibit multiple peaks, suggesting enterohepatic recycling.
Following oral administration of ^{14}C-ezetimibe (20 mg) to human subjects, total ezetimibe (ezetimibe + ezetimibe-glucuronide) accounted for approximately 93% of the total radioactivity in plasma. After 48 hours, there were no detectable levels of radioactivity in the plasma.
Approximately 78% and 11% of the administered radioactivity were recovered in the feces and urine, respectively, over a 10-day collection period. Ezetimibe was the major component in feces and accounted for 69% of the administered dose, while ezetimibe-glucuronide was the major component in urine and accounted for 9% of the administered dose.
Atorvastatin
Atorvastatin is extensively metabolized to ortho- and para-hydroxylated derivatives and various beta-oxidation products. In vitro inhibition of HMG-CoA reductase by ortho- and parahydroxylated metabolites is equivalent to that of atorvastatin. Approximately 70% of circulating inhibitory activity for HMG-CoA reductase is attributed to active metabolites. In vitro studies suggest the importance of atorvastatin metabolism by cytochrome P450 3A4, consistent with increased plasma concentrations of atorvastatin in humans following coadministration with erythromycin, a known inhibitor of this isozyme [see Drug Interactions (7.1)]. In animals, the ortho-hydroxy metabolite undergoes further glucuronidation.
Atorvastatin and its metabolites are eliminated primarily in bile following hepatic and/or extra-hepatic metabolism; however, the drug does not appear to undergo enterohepatic recirculation. Mean plasma elimination half-life of atorvastatin in humans is approximately 14 hours, but the half-life of inhibitory activity for HMG-CoA reductase is 20 to 30 hours due to the contribution of active metabolites. Less than 2% of a dose of atorvastatin is recovered in urine following oral administration.

Specific Populations
Geriatric Patients
Ezetimibe
In a multiple-dose study with ezetimibe given 10 mg once daily for 10 days, plasma concentrations for total ezetimibe were about 2-fold higher in older (≥65 years) healthy subjects compared to younger subjects.
Atorvastatin
Plasma concentrations of atorvastatin are higher (approximately 40% for C_{max} and 30% for AUC) in healthy elderly subjects (age ≥65 years) than in young adults. Clinical data suggest a greater degree of LDL-lowering at any dose of drug in the elderly patient population compared to younger adults.
Pediatric Patients: [See Use in Specific Populations (8.4).]
Gender
Ezetimibe
In a multiple-dose study with ezetimibe given 10 mg once daily for 10 days, plasma concentrations for total ezetimibe were slightly higher (<20%) in women than in men.
Atorvastatin
Plasma concentrations of atorvastatin in women differ from those in men (approximately 20% higher for C_{max} and 10% lower for AUC); however, there is no clinically significant difference in LDL-C reduction with atorvastatin between men and women.
Race
Ezetimibe
Based on a meta-analysis of multiple-dose pharmacokinetic studies, there were no pharmacokinetic differences between Black and Caucasian subjects. Studies in Asian subjects indicated that the pharmacokinetics of ezetimibe were similar to those seen in Caucasian subjects.
Hepatic Impairment
Ezetimibe
After a single 10-mg dose of ezetimibe, the mean AUC for total ezetimibe was increased approximately 1.7-fold in patients with mild hepatic impairment (Child-Pugh score 5 to 6), compared to healthy subjects. The mean AUC values for total ezetimibe and ezetimibe increased approximately 3- to 4-fold and 5- to 6-fold, respectively, in patients with moderate (Child-Pugh score 7 to 9) or severe hepatic impairment (Child-Pugh score 10 to 15). In a 14-day, multiple-dose study (10 mg daily) in patients with moderate hepatic impairment, the mean AUC for total ezetimibe and ezetimibe increased approximately 4-fold on both Day 1 and Day 14 when compared to healthy subjects.
Atorvastatin
In patients with chronic alcoholic liver disease, plasma concentrations of atorvastatin are markedly increased. C_{max} and AUC are each 4-fold greater in patients with Child-Pugh A disease. C_{max} and AUC are approximately 16-fold and 11-fold increased, respectively, in patients with Child-Pugh B disease [see Contraindications (4)].
Renal Impairment
[See Warnings and Precautions (5.1), Use in Specific Populations (8.7)]
Ezetimibe
After a single 10-mg dose of ezetimibe in patients with severe renal disease (n=8; mean CrCl ≤30 mL/min/1.73 m²), the mean AUC values for total ezetimibe, ezetimibe-glucuronide, and ezetimibe were increased approximately 1.5-fold, compared to healthy subjects (n=9).
Atorvastatin
Renal disease has no influence on the plasma concentrations or LDL-C reduction of atorvastatin.
Hemodialysis
Atorvastatin
While studies have not been conducted in patients with end-stage renal disease, hemodialysis is not expected to significantly enhance clearance of atorvastatin since the drug is extensively bound to plasma proteins.
Drug Interactions [See also Drug Interactions (7).]
No clinically significant pharmacokinetic interaction was seen when ezetimibe was coadministered with atorvastatin. Specific pharmacokinetic drug interaction studies with LIPTRUZET have not been performed.
Cytochrome P450: Ezetimibe had no significant effect on a series of probe drugs (caffeine, dextromethorphan, tolbutamide, and IV midazolam) known to be metabolized by cytochrome P450 (1A2, 2D6, 2C8/9 and 3A4) in a "cocktail" study of twelve healthy adult males. This indicates that ezetimibe is neither an inhibitor nor an inducer of these cytochrome P450 isozymes, and it is unlikely that ezetimibe will affect the metabolism of drugs that are metabolized by these enzymes.
Atorvastatin is metabolized by cytochrome P450 3A4. Concomitant administration of LIPTRUZET with inhibitors of cytochrome P450 3A4 can lead to increases in plasma concentrations of the atorvastatin component of LIPTRUZET. The extent of interaction and potentiation of effects depends on the variability of effect on cytochrome P450 3A4.

Ezetimibe

Table 5: Effect of Coadministered Drugs on Total Ezetimibe

Coadministered Drug and Dosing Regimen	Total Ezetimibe*	
	Change in AUC	Change in C_{max}
Cyclosporine-stable dose required (75-150 mg BID)[†,‡]	↑240%	↑290%
Fenofibrate, 200 mg QD, 14 days[‡]	↑48%	↑64%
Gemfibrozil, 600 mg BID, 7 days[‡]	↑64%	↑91%
Cholestyramine, 4 g BID, 14 days[‡]	↓55%	↓4%
Aluminum & magnesium hydroxide combination antacid, single dose[§]	↓4%	↓30%
Cimetidine, 400 mg BID, 7 days	↑6%	↑22%
Glipizide, 10 mg, single dose	↑4%	↓8%
Statins		
Lovastatin 20 mg QD, 7 days	↑9%	↑3%
Pravastatin 20 mg QD, 14 days	↑7%	↑23%
Atorvastatin 10 mg QD, 14 days	↓2%	↑12%
Rosuvastatin 10 mg QD, 14 days	↑13%	↑18%
Fluvastatin 20 mg QD, 14 days	↓19%	↑7%

* Based on 10-mg dose of ezetimibe
† Post-renal transplant patients with mild impaired or normal renal function. In a different study, a renal transplant patient with severe renal impairment (creatinine clearance of 13.2 mL/min/1.73 m²) who was receiving multiple medications, including cyclosporine, demonstrated a 12-fold greater exposure to total ezetimibe compared to healthy subjects.
‡ *See Drug Interactions (7)*
§ Supralox®, 20 mL

[See table 6 above]
Atorvastatin
[See table 7 at top of next page]
[See table 8 at top of page 1552]

Table 6: Effect of Ezetimibe Coadministration on Systemic Exposure to Other Drugs

Coadministered Drug and its Dosage Regimen	Ezetimibe Dosage Regimen	Change in AUC of Coadministered Drug	Change in C_{max} of Coadministered Drug
Warfarin, 25 mg single dose on Day 7	10 mg QD, 11 days	↓2% (R-warfarin) ↓4% (S-warfarin)	↑3% (R-warfarin) ↑1% (S-warfarin)
Digoxin, 0.5 mg single dose	10 mg QD, 8 days	↑2%	↓7%
Gemfibrozil, 600 mg BID, 7 days*	10 mg QD, 7 days	↓1%	↓11%
Ethinyl estradiol & Levonorgestrel, QD, 21 days	10 mg QD, Days 8-14 of 21 d oral contraceptive cycle	Ethinyl estradiol 0% Levonorgestrel 0%	Ethinyl estradiol ↓9% Levonorgestrel ↓5%
Glipizide, 10 mg on Days 1 and 9	10 mg QD, Days 2-9	↓3%	↓5%
Fenofibrate, 200 mg QD, 14 days*	10 mg QD, 14 days	↑11%	↑7%
Cyclosporine, 100 mg single dose Day 7*	20 mg QD, 8 days	↑15%	↑10%
Statins			
Lovastatin 20 mg QD, 7 days	10 mg QD, 7 days	↑19%	↑3%
Pravastatin 20 mg QD, 14 days	10 mg QD, 14 days	↓20%	↓24%
Atorvastatin 10 mg QD, 14 days	10 mg QD, 14 days	↓4%	↑7%
Rosuvastatin 10 mg QD, 14 days	10 mg QD, 14 days	↑19%	↑17%
Fluvastatin 20 mg QD, 14 days	10 mg QD, 14 days	↓39%	↓27%

* *See Drug Interactions (7)*

13 NONCLINICAL TOXICOLOGY

13.1 Carcinogenesis, Mutagenesis, Impairment of Fertility

No animal carcinogenicity or fertility studies have been conducted with the combination of ezetimibe and atorvastatin. The combination of ezetimibe with atorvastatin did not show evidence of mutagenicity *in vitro* in a microbial mutagenicity (Ames) test with *Salmonella typhimurium* and *Escherichia coli* with or without metabolic activation. No evidence of clastogenicity was observed *in vitro* in a chromosomal aberration assay in human peripheral blood lymphocytes with ezetimibe and atorvastatin with or without metabolic activation. There was no evidence of genotoxicity at doses up to 250 mg/kg with the combination of ezetimibe and atorvastatin (1:1) in the *in vivo* mouse micronucleus test.

Ezetimibe
A 104-week dietary carcinogenicity study with ezetimibe was conducted in rats at doses up to 1500 mg/kg/day (males) and 500 mg/kg/day (females) (~20 times the human exposure at 10 mg daily based on AUC_{0-24hr} for total ezetimibe). A 104-week dietary carcinogenicity study with ezetimibe was also conducted in mice at doses up to 500 mg/kg/day (>150 times the human exposure at 10 mg daily based on AUC_{0-24hr} for total ezetimibe). There were no statistically significant increases in tumor incidences in drug-treated rats or mice.

No evidence of mutagenicity was observed *in vitro* in a microbial mutagenicity (Ames) test with *Salmonella typhimurium* and *Escherichia coli* with or without metabolic activation. No evidence of clastogenicity was observed *in vitro* in a chromosomal aberration assay in human peripheral blood lymphocytes with or without metabolic activation. In addition, there was no evidence of genotoxicity in the *in vivo* mouse micronucleus test.

In oral (gavage) fertility studies of ezetimibe conducted in rats, there was no evidence of reproductive toxicity at doses up to 1000 mg/kg/day in male or female rats (~7 times the human exposure at 10 mg daily based on AUC_{0-24hr} for total ezetimibe).

Atorvastatin
In a 2-year carcinogenicity study in rats at dose levels of 10, 30, and 100 mg/kg/day, 2 rare tumors were found in muscle in high-dose females: in one, there was a rhabdomyosarcoma and, in another, there was a fibrosarcoma. This dose represents a plasma AUC_{0-24hr} value of approximately 16 times the mean human plasma drug exposure after an 80-mg oral dose.

A 2-year carcinogenicity study in mice given 100, 200, or 400 mg/kg/day resulted in a significant increase in liver adenomas in high-dose males and liver carcinomas in high-dose females. These findings occurred at plasma AUC_{0-24hr} values of approximately 6 times the mean human plasma drug exposure after an 80-mg oral dose.

In vitro, atorvastatin was not mutagenic or clastogenic in the following tests with and without metabolic activation: the Ames test with *Salmonella typhimurium* and *Escherichia coli*, the HGPRT forward mutation assay in Chinese hamster lung cells, and the chromosomal aberration assay in Chinese hamster lung cells. Atorvastatin was negative in the *in vivo* mouse micronucleus test.

Studies in rats performed at doses up to 175 mg/kg (15 times the human exposure) produced no changes in fertility. There was aplasia and aspermia in the epididymis of 2 of 10 rats treated with 100 mg/kg/day of atorvastatin for 3 months (16 times the human AUC at the 80-mg dose); testis weights were significantly lower at 30 and 100 mg/kg and epididymal weight was lower at 100 mg/kg. Male rats given 100 mg/kg/day for 11 weeks prior to mating had decreased sperm motility, spermatid head concentration, and increased abnormal sperm. Atorvastatin caused no adverse effects on semen parameters, or reproductive organ histopathology in dogs given doses of 10, 40, or 120 mg/kg for two years.

13.2 Animal Toxicology and/or Pharmacology

Ezetimibe
In a rat model, where the glucuronide metabolite of ezetimibe (ezetimibe-glucuronide) was administered intraduodenally, the metabolite was as potent as ezetimibe in inhibiting the absorption of cholesterol, suggesting that the glucuronide metabolite had activity similar to the parent drug.

In 1-month studies in dogs given ezetimibe (0.03 to 300 mg/kg/day), the concentration of cholesterol in gallbladder bile increased ~2- to 4-fold. However, a dose of 300 mg/kg/day administered to dogs for one year did not result in gallstone formation or any other adverse hepatobiliary effects. In a 14-day study in mice given ezetimibe (0.3 to 5 mg/kg/day) and fed a low-fat or cholesterol-rich diet, the concentration of cholesterol in gallbladder bile was either unaffected or reduced to normal levels, respectively.

A series of acute preclinical studies was performed to determine the selectivity of ezetimibe for inhibiting cholesterol absorption. Ezetimibe inhibited the absorption of ¹⁴C-cholesterol with no effect on the absorption of triglycerides, fatty acids, bile acids, progesterone, ethinyl estradiol, or the fat-soluble vitamins A and D.

In 4- to 12-week toxicity studies in mice, ezetimibe did not induce cytochrome P450 drug metabolizing enzymes. In toxicity studies, a pharmacokinetic interaction of ezetimibe with statins (parents or their active hydroxy acid metabolites) was seen in rats, dogs, and rabbits.

14 CLINICAL STUDIES

14.1 Primary Hyperlipidemia

LIPTRUZET – Lipid Efficacy

LIPTRUZET reduces total-C, LDL-C, Apo B, TG, and non-HDL-C, and increases HDL-C in patients with hypercholesterolemia.

LIPTRUZET is effective in men and women with hyperlipidemia. Experience in non-Caucasians is limited and does not permit a precise estimate of the magnitude of the effects of LIPTRUZET.

In a multicenter, double-blind, placebo-controlled, clinical study in patients with hyperlipidemia, 628 patients were treated for up to 12 weeks and 246 for up to an additional 48 weeks. Patients were randomized to receive placebo, ezetimibe (10 mg), atorvastatin (10 mg, 20 mg, 40 mg, or 80 mg), or coadministered ezetimibe and atorvastatin equivalent to LIPTRUZET (10/10, 10/20, 10/40, and 10/80) in the 12-week study. After completing the 12-week study, patients who agreed to participate in the study extension were assigned to coadministered ezetimibe and atorvastatin equivalent to LIPTRUZET (10/10-10/80) or atorvastatin (10-80 mg/day) for an additional 48 weeks.

Table 7: Effect of Coadministered Drugs on the Pharmacokinetics of Atorvastatin

Coadministered Drug and Dosing Regimen	Atorvastatin		
	Dose (mg)	Change in AUC*	Change in C_{max}*
Cyclosporine 5.2 mg/kg/day, stable dose[†]	10 mg QD for 28 days	↑8.7 fold	↑10.7 fold
Tipranavir 500 mg BID/ritonavir 200 mg BID, 7 days[†]	10 mg, SD	↑9.4 fold	↑8.6 fold
Telaprevir 750 mg q8h, 10 days[†]	20 mg, SD	↑7.88 fold	↑10.6 fold
Saquinavir 400 mg BID/ritonavir 400 mg BID, 15 days[†,‡]	40 mg QD for 4 days	↑3.9 fold	↑4.3 fold
Clarithromycin 500 mg BID, 9 days[†]	80 mg QD for 8 days	↑4.4 fold	↑5.4 fold
Darunavir 300 mg BID/ritonavir 100 mg BID, 9 days[†]	10 mg QD for 4 days	↑3.4 fold	↑2.25 fold
Itraconazole 200 mg QD, 4 days[†]	40 mg, SD	↑3.3 fold	↑20%
Fosamprenavir 700 mg BID/ritonavir 100 mg BID, 14 days[†]	10 mg QD for 4 days	↑2.53 fold	↑2.84 fold
Fosamprenavir 1400 mg BID, 14 days[†]	10 mg QD for 4 days	↑2.3 fold	↑4.04 fold
Nelfinavir 1250 mg BID, 14 days[†]	10 mg QD for 28 days	↑74%	↑2.2 fold
Grapefruit Juice, 240 mL QD[†,§]	40 mg, SD	↑37%	↑16%
Diltiazem 240 mg QD, 28 days	40 mg, SD	↑51%	No change
Erythromycin 500 mg QID, 7 days	10 mg, SD	↑33%	↑38%
Amlodipine 10 mg, single dose	80 mg, SD	↑15%	↓12%
Cimetidine 300 mg QD, 4 weeks	10 mg QD for 2 weeks	↓Less than 1%	↓11%
Colestipol 10 mg BID, 28 weeks	40 mg QD for 28 weeks	Not determined	↓26%¶
Maalox TC® 30 mL QD, 17 days	10 mg QD for 15 days	↓33%	↓34%
Efavirenz 600 mg QD, 14 days	10 mg for 3 days	↓41%	↓1%
Rifampin 600 mg QD, 7 days (coadministered)[†,#]	40 mg, SD	↑30%	↑2.7 fold
Rifampin 600 mg QD, 5 days (doses separated)[†,#]	40 mg, SD	↓80%	↓40%
Gemfibrozil 600 mg BID, 7 days[†]	40 mg, SD	↑35%	↓Less than 1%
Fenofibrate 160 mg QD, 7 days[†]	40 mg, SD	↑3%	↑2%
Boceprevir 800 mg TID, 7 days	40 mg, SD	↑2.30 fold	↑2.66 fold

* Data given as x-fold change represent a simple ratio between coadministration and atorvastatin alone (i.e., 1-fold = no change). Data given as % change represent % difference relative to atorvastatin alone (i.e., 0% = no change).
† See Warnings and Precautions (5.1) and Drug Interactions (7) for clinical significance.
‡ The dose of saquinavir plus ritonavir in this study is not the clinically used dose. The increase in atorvastatin exposure when used clinically is likely to be higher than what was observed in this study. Therefore, caution should be applied and the lowest dose necessary should be used.
§ Greater increases in AUC (up to 2.5 fold) and/or C_{max} (up to 71%) have been reported with excessive grapefruit consumption (≥ 750 mL - 1.2 liters per day).
¶ Single sample taken 8-16 h post-dose.
# Due to the dual interaction mechanism of rifampin, simultaneous coadministration of atorvastatin with rifampin is recommended, as delayed administration of atorvastatin after administration of rifampin has been associated with a significant reduction in atorvastatin plasma concentrations.

The patient population was: 59% female; 85% Caucasian, 6% Black, 3% Asian, 5% Hispanic, 1% American Indian, <1% other; 18 to 86 years of age (mean age 57 years).
Patients receiving all doses of LIPTRUZET were compared to those receiving all doses of atorvastatin. LIPTRUZET lowered total-C, LDL-C, Apo B, TG, and non-HDL-C, and increased HDL-C significantly more than atorvastatin alone. (See Table 9.)
[See table 9 at top of next page]
The changes in lipid endpoints after an additional 48 weeks of treatment with LIPTRUZET (all doses) or with atorvastatin (all doses) were generally consistent with the 12-week data displayed above in the 245 subjects (out of the 576 who completed the 12-week study) who agreed to participate in the study extension.
A multicenter, double-blind, controlled, 14-week study was conducted in 621 patients with heterozygous familial hypercholesterolemia (HeFH), coronary heart disease (CHD), or multiple cardiovascular risk factors (≥2), adhering to an NCEP Step I or stricter diet. All patients received atorvastatin 10 mg for a minimum of 4 weeks prior to randomization. Patients were then randomized to receive either coadministered ezetimibe and atorvastatin (equivalent to LIPTRUZET 10/10) or atorvastatin 20 mg/day monotherapy. Patients who did not achieve their LDL-C target goal after 4 and/or 9 weeks of randomized treatment were titrated to double the atorvastatin dose.
The patient population was: 47% female; 91% Caucasian, 2% Black, 2% Asian, 5% Hispanic, <1% other; 18 to 82 years of age (mean age 61 years).
LIPTRUZET 10/10 was significantly more effective than doubling the dose of atorvastatin to 20 mg in further reducing total-C, LDL-C, TG, and non-HDL-C. Results for HDL-C between the two treatment groups were not significantly different. (See Table 10.) In addition, at Week 4 significantly more patients receiving LIPTRUZET 10/10 attained LDL-C <100 mg/dL (<2.6 mmol/L) compared to those receiving atorvastatin 20 mg, 12% vs. 2%. The baseline mean LDL-C levels for patients receiving LIPTRUZET 10/10 and atorvastatin 20 mg were 186 mg/dL and 187 mg/dL, respectively.
[See table 10 at top of page 1553]
The Titration of Atorvastatin Versus Ezetimibe Add-On to Atorvastatin in Patients with Hypercholesterolemia (TEMPO) study, a multicenter, double-blind, controlled, 6-week study, included 184 patients with an LDL-C level ≥100 mg/dL and ≤160 mg/dL (≥2.6 mmol/L and ≤4.1 mmol/L) and at moderate high risk for coronary heart disease (CHD). All patients received atorvastatin 20 mg for a minimum of 4 weeks prior to randomization. Patients not at the optional NCEP ATP III LDL-C level (<100 mg/dL [<2.6 mmol/L]) were randomized to receive either coadministered ezetimibe and atorvastatin (equivalent to LIPTRUZET 10/20) or atorvastatin 40 mg for 6 weeks.
The patient population was: 45% female; 60% Caucasian, 26% Multi-racial, 6% Black, 8% Asian, <1% American Indian or Alaska native; 24 to 78 years of age (mean age 58 years).
LIPTRUZET 10/20 was significantly more effective than doubling the dose of atorvastatin to 40 mg in further reducing total-C, LDL-C, Apo B and non-HDL-C. Results for HDL-C and TG between the two treatment groups were not significantly different. (See Table 11.) In addition, significantly more patients receiving LIPTRUZET 10/20 attained LDL-C <100 mg/dL (<2.6 mmol/L) compared to those receiving atorvastatin 40 mg, 84% vs. 49%.
[See table 11 at top of page 1553]
The Ezetimibe Plus Atorvastatin Versus Atorvastatin Titration in Achieving Lower LDL-C Targets in Hypercholesterolemic Patients (EZ-PATH) study, a multicenter, double-blind, controlled, 6-week study, included 556 patients with an LDL-C level ≥70 mg/dL and ≤160 mg/dL (≥1.8 mmol/L and ≤4.1 mmol/L) and at high risk for coronary heart disease (CHD). All patients received atorvastatin 40 mg for a minimum of 4 weeks prior to randomization. Patients not at the optional NCEP ATP III LDL-C level <70 mg/dL (<1.8 mmol/L) were randomized to receive either coadministered ezetimibe and atorvastatin (equivalent to LIPTRUZET 10/40) or atorvastatin 80 mg for 6 weeks.
The patient population was: 39% female; 81% Caucasian, 11% Black, 6% Multi-racial, 2% Asian; 31 to 80 years of age (mean age 52 years).
LIPTRUZET 10/40 was significantly more effective than doubling the dose of atorvastatin to 80 mg in further reducing total-C, LDL-C, Apo B, TG, and non-HDL-C. Results for HDL-C between the two treatment groups were not significantly different. (See Table 12.) In addition, significantly more patients receiving LIPTRUZET 10/40 attained LDL-C <70 mg/dL (<1.8 mmol/L) compared to those receiving atorvastatin 80 mg, 74% vs. 32%.
[See table 12 at top of page 1553]

Table 8: Effect of Atorvastatin on the Pharmacokinetics of Coadministered Drugs

Atorvastatin	Coadministered Drug and Dosing Regimen		
	Drug/Dose (mg)	Change in AUC	Change in C_{max}
80 mg QD for 15 days	Antipyrine, 600 mg SD	↑3%	↓11%
80 mg QD for 14 days	Digoxin 0.25 mg QD, 20 days*	↑15%	↑20%
40 mg QD for 22 days	Oral contraceptive QD, 2 months - norethindrone 1 mg - ethinyl estradiol 35 μg	↑28% ↑19%	↑23% ↑30%
10 mg, SD	Tipranavir 500 mg BID/ ritonavir 200 mg BID, 7 days	No change	No change
10 mg QD for 4 days	Fosamprenavir 1400 mg BID, 14 days	↓27%	↓18%
10 mg QD for 4 days	Fosamprenavir 700 mg BID/ritonavir 100 mg BID, 14 days	No change	No change

* *See Drug Interactions (7) for clinical significance.*

Table 9: Response to LIPTRUZET in Patients with Primary Hyperlipidemia (Mean* % Change from Untreated Baseline† at 12 weeks)

Treatment (Daily Dose)	N	Total-C [Baseline‡]	LDL-C [Baseline‡]	Apo B [Baseline‡]	TG* [Baseline‡]	HDL-C [Baseline‡]	Non-HDL-C [Baseline‡]
Pooled data (All LIPTRUZET doses)§	255	-41% [267]	-56% [182]	-45% [170]	-33% [165]	+7% [50.8]	-52% [217]
Pooled data (All atorvastatin doses)§	248	-32% [269]	-44% [181]	-36% [168]	-24% [155]	+4% [53.7]	-41% [215]
Ezetimibe 10 mg	65	-14% [259]	-20% [177]	-15% [167]	-5% [145]	+4% [50.6]	-18% [209]
Placebo	60	+4% [262]	+4% [180]	+3% [168]	-6% [143]	+4% [50.4]	+4% [212]
LIPTRUZET by dose							
10/10	65	-38% [262]	-53% [177]	-43% [165]	-31% [158]	+9% [51.9]	-49% [211]
10/20	62	-39% [269]	-54% [184]	-44% [174]	-30% [165]	+9% [49.3]	-50% [220]
10/40	65	-42% [271]	-56% [184]	-45% [173]	-34% [180]	+5% [51.1]	-52% [220]
10/80	63	-46% [267]	-61% [183]	-50% [169]	-40% [146]	+7% [50.9]	-58% [216]
Atorvastatin by dose							
10 mg	60	-26% [271]	-37% [185]	-28% [168]	-21% [153]	+6% [53.7]	-34% [217]
20 mg	60	-30% [267]	-42% [177]	-34% [164]	-23% [147]	+4% [55.5]	-39% [211]
40 mg	66	-32% [266]	-45% [180]	-37% [167]	-24% [159]	+4% [53.0]	-41% [213]
80 mg	62	-40% [270]	-54% [184]	-46% [171]	-31% [163]	+3% [52.7]	-51% [218]

* For triglycerides, median % change from baseline
† Baseline - on no lipid-lowering drug
‡ Baseline units: mg/dL; medians for TG, means for all other values
§ LIPTRUZET pooled (10/10-10/80) significantly reduced total-C, LDL-C, Apo B, TG, non-HDL-C, and significantly increased HDL-C compared to all doses of atorvastatin pooled (10-80 mg).

LIPTRUZET 10/20 and 10/40 - Clinical Equivalence to Coadministered Components
LIPTRUZET has been shown to be bioequivalent to coadministration of corresponding doses of its ezetimibe and atorvastatin components with the exception of slightly lower atorvastatin C_{max} for the 10/20 and 10/40 mg doses *[see Clinical Pharmacology (12.3)]*, which, in two separate studies, have been shown to be clinically equivalent in LDL-C response after six weeks of treatment to their corresponding coadministered components.
In these two multicenter, double-blind, controlled, crossover studies, patients with primary hypercholesterolemia and low, moderate, or moderately high cardiovascular risk re-

ceived LIPTRUZET 10/20-mg (Study 1) or 10/40-mg (Study 2) tablets or the corresponding coadministered components once daily for 6 weeks. They then crossed over, after a 6-week washout, to the coadministered components or LIPTRUZET at corresponding doses for an additional 6 weeks. From untreated baseline, mean changes in LDL-C for LIPTRUZET vs. the coadministered components, respectively, were -54.0% vs. -53.8% for 10/20-mg (Study 1), and -58.9% vs. -58.7% for 10/40-mg (Study 2). Mean changes for total-C, Apo B, non-HDL-C, and HDL-C were also similar between the two treatment groups and supported the conclusion of clinical equivalence.

14.2 Homozygous Familial Hypercholesterolemia (HoFH)

A double-blind, randomized, 12-week study was performed in patients with a clinical and/or genotypic diagnosis of HoFH. Data were analyzed from a subgroup of patients (n=36) receiving atorvastatin 40 mg at baseline. Increasing the dose of atorvastatin from 40 to 80 mg (n=12) produced a reduction of LDL-C of 2% from baseline on atorvastatin 40 mg. Coadministered ezetimibe and atorvastatin equivalent to LIPTRUZET (10/40 and 10/80 pooled, n=24), produced a reduction of LDL-C of 19% from baseline on atorvastatin 40 mg. In those patients coadministered ezetimibe and atorvastatin equivalent to LIPTRUZET (10/80, n=12), a reduction of LDL-C of 25% from baseline on atorvastatin 40 mg was produced.
After completing the 12-week study, eligible patients (n=35), who were receiving atorvastatin 40 mg at baseline, were assigned to coadministered ezetimibe and atorvastatin equivalent to LIPTRUZET 10/40 for up to an additional 24 months. Following at least 4 weeks of treatment, the atorvastatin dose could be doubled to a maximum dose of 80 mg.
At the end of the 24 months, LIPTRUZET (10/40 and 10/80 pooled) produced a reduction of LDL-C that was consistent with that seen in the 12-week study.

16 HOW SUPPLIED/STORAGE AND HANDLING

Tablets LIPTRUZET 10 mg/10 mg are white to off-white capsule-shaped, biconvex film-coated tablets with code "320" on one side.
They are supplied as follows:
NDC 66582-320-30 unit of use packages of 30 (three foil pouches each containing one 10-count blister card)
NDC 66582-320-54 unit of use packages of 90 (nine foil pouches each containing one 10-count blister card)
Tablets LIPTRUZET 10 mg/20 mg are white to off-white round, biconvex film-coated tablets with code "321" on one side.
They are supplied as follows:
NDC 66582-321-30 unit of use packages of 30 (three foil pouches each containing one 10-count blister card)
NDC 66582-321-54 unit of use packages of 90 (nine foil pouches each containing one 10-count blister card)
Tablets LIPTRUZET 10 mg/40 mg are white to off-white oval, biconvex film-coated tablets with code "322" on one side.
They are supplied as follows:
NDC 66582-322-30 unit of use packages of 30 (three foil pouches each containing one 10-count blister card)
NDC 66582-322-54 unit of use packages of 90 (nine foil pouches each containing one 10-count blister card)
Tablets LIPTRUZET 10 mg/80 mg are white to off-white capsule-shaped, biconvex film-coated tablets with code "323" on one side.
They are supplied as follows:
NDC 66582-323-30 unit of use packages of 30 (three foil pouches each containing one 10-count blister card)
NDC 66582-323-54 unit of use packages of 90 (nine foil pouches each containing one 10-count blister card)
Storage of Unit of Use Packages of 30 and 90
Store LIPTRUZET at 20-25°C (68-77°F), excursions permitted to 15-30°C (59-86°F) [see USP Controlled Room Temperature]. Store in the foil pouch until use. After the foil pouch is opened, protect LIPTRUZET from moisture and light. Once a tablet is removed, slide blister card back into case. Store the case in a dry place, and discard any unused tablets 30 days after the pouch is opened.

17 PATIENT COUNSELING INFORMATION

See FDA-Approved Patient Labeling (Patient Information).
Patients should be advised to adhere to their National Cholesterol Education Program (NCEP)-recommended diet, a regular exercise program, and periodic testing of a fasting lipid panel.

17.1 Muscle Pain

All patients starting therapy with LIPTRUZET should be advised of the risk of myopathy and told to report promptly any unexplained muscle pain, tenderness or weakness particularly if accompanied by malaise or fever or if these muscle signs or symptoms persist after discontinuing LIPTRUZET. The risk of this occurring is increased when taking certain types of medication or consuming larger quantities (>1 liter) of grapefruit juice. Patients should discuss all medication, both prescription and over-the-counter, with their physician.

17.2 Liver Enzymes

It is recommended that liver enzyme tests be performed before the initiation of LIPTRUZET and if signs or symptoms of liver injury occur. All patients treated with LIPTRUZET should be advised to report promptly any symptoms that may indicate liver injury, including fatigue, anorexia, right upper abdominal discomfort, dark urine, or jaundice.

17.3 Pregnancy

Women of childbearing age should be advised to use an effective method of birth control to prevent pregnancy while using LIPTRUZET. Discuss future pregnancy plans with your patients, and discuss when to stop taking LIPTRUZET if they are trying to conceive. Patients should be advised that if they become pregnant they should stop taking LIPTRUZET and call their healthcare professional.

17.4 Breast-Feeding

Women who are breast-feeding should be advised to not use LIPTRUZET. Patients who have a lipid disorder and are breast-feeding should be advised to discuss the options with their healthcare professionals.

17.5 Important Storage and Administration Instructions

Patients should be advised to store LIPTRUZET at room temperature, 20-25°C (68-77°F). They should also be advised:

- not to open a pouch until they are ready to use LIPTRUZET
- that after the foil pouch is opened, LIPTRUZET should be protected from moisture and light, and stored in a dry place
- that for packages containing a plastic case (unit of use packages of 30 and 90), once they remove a tablet from the blister card, they should slide the blister card back into the plastic case
- to discard any unused tablets 30 days after the pouch is opened

Tablets should be swallowed whole. Do not crush, dissolve, or chew tablets.

If a dose is missed, the patient should not take an extra dose. Just resume the usual schedule.

Manufactured by:
Merck Sharp & Dohme Corp., a subsidiary of
MERCK & CO., INC., Whitehouse Station, NJ 08889, USA
U.S. Patent Nos. 5,846,966 and RE37,721.
USPI-T-0653C1305R000

Patient Information
LIPTRUZET™ (LIP-true-zett)
(ezetimibe and atorvastatin)
Tablets
Generic name: ezetimibe and atorvastatin tablets

Read this information carefully before you start taking LIPTRUZET and each time you get more LIPTRUZET. There may be new information. This information does not take the place of talking with your doctor about your medical condition or your treatment. If you have any questions about LIPTRUZET, ask your doctor. Only your doctor can determine if LIPTRUZET is right for you.

What is LIPTRUZET?

LIPTRUZET contains 2 cholesterol-lowering medications, ezetimibe and atorvastatin.

LIPTRUZET is a prescription medicine used to lower levels of total cholesterol, LDL (bad) cholesterol and fatty substances called triglycerides in the blood. In addition, LIPTRUZET raises levels of HDL (good) cholesterol. LIPTRUZET is for patients who cannot control their cholesterol levels by diet and exercise alone. You should stay on a cholesterol-lowering diet while taking this medicine.

LIPTRUZET has not been shown to reduce heart attacks or strokes more than atorvastatin alone.

It is not known if LIPTRUZET is safe and effective in children.

Who should not take LIPTRUZET?

Do not take LIPTRUZET if you:

- have active liver problems or repeated blood tests showing possible liver problems.
- are allergic to ezetimibe or atorvastatin or any of the ingredients in LIPTRUZET. See the end of this leaflet for a complete list of ingredients in LIPTRUZET.
- are pregnant or plan to become pregnant. LIPTRUZET may harm your unborn baby. If you are a woman of childbearing age, you should use an effective method of birth control while taking LIPTRUZET. Stop taking LIPTRUZET and call your doctor right away if you get pregnant while taking LIPTRUZET.
- are breastfeeding or plan to breastfeed. LIPTRUZET can pass into your breast milk and may harm your baby. Talk to your doctor about the best way to feed your baby if you take LIPTRUZET. Do not breastfeed while taking LIPTRUZET.

What should I tell my doctor before taking LIPTRUZET?

Before you take LIPTRUZET, tell your doctor if you:

- have a thyroid problem
- have kidney problems
- have diabetes
- have unexplained muscle aches or weakness
- drink more than 2 glasses of alcohol daily or have or have had liver problems
- have any other medical conditions

Table 10: Response to LIPTRUZET after 4 Weeks in Patients with CHD or Multiple Cardiovascular Risk Factors and an LDL-C ≥130 mg/dL (Mean* % Change from Baseline†)

Treatment (Daily Dose)	N	Total-C [Baseline‡]	LDL-C [Baseline‡]	HDL-C [Baseline‡]	TG* [Baseline‡]	Non-HDL-C [Baseline‡]
LIPTRUZET 10/10	305	-17%§ [262]	-24%§ [186]	+2% [50.0]	-9%§ [117]	-22%§ [212]
Atorvastatin 20 mg	316	-6% [264]	-9% [187]	+1% [49.9]	-4% [119]	-8% [214]

* For triglycerides, median % change from baseline
† Patients on atorvastatin 10 mg, then switched to LIPTRUZET 10/10 or titrated to atorvastatin 20 mg
‡ Baseline units: mg/dL; medians for TG, means for all other values
§ p<0.05 for difference with atorvastatin

Table 11: Response to LIPTRUZET in Patients with Primary Hypercholesterolemia (Mean* % Change from Baseline†)

Treatment (Daily Dose)	N	Total-C [Baseline‡]	LDL-C [Baseline‡]	Apo B [Baseline‡]	HDL-C [Baseline‡]	TG* [Baseline‡]	Non-HDL-C [Baseline‡]
LIPTRUZET 10/20	92	-20%§ [203]	-31%§ [120]	-21%§ [123]	+3% [50.9]	-18% [155]	-27%§ [152]
Atorvastatin 40 mg	92	-7% [201]	-11% [118]	-8% [120]	+1% [52.1]	-6% [148]	-10% [149]

* For triglycerides, median % change from baseline
† Patients on atorvastatin 20 mg, then switched to LIPTRUZET 10/20 or titrated to atorvastatin 40 mg
‡ Baseline units: mg/dL; medians for TG, means for all other values
§ p<0.05 for difference with atorvastatin

Table 12: Response to LIPTRUZET in Patients with Primary Hypercholesterolemia (Mean* % Change from Baseline†)

Treatment (Daily Dose)	N	Total-C [Baseline‡]	LDL-C [Baseline‡]	Apo B [Baseline‡]	HDL-C [Baseline‡]	TG* [Baseline‡]	Non-HDL-C [Baseline‡]
LIPTRUZET 10/40	277	-17%§ [165]	-27%§ [89]	-18%§ [101]	0% [47.7]	-12%§ [131]	-23%§ [117]
Atorvastatin 80 mg	279	-7% [165]	-11% [90]	-8% [102]	-1% [46.9]	-6% [136]	-9% [118]

* For triglycerides, median % change from baseline
† Patients on atorvastatin 20 mg, then switched to LIPTRUZET 10/40 or titrated to atorvastatin 80 mg
‡ Baseline units: mg/dL; medians for TG, means for all other values
§ p<0.05 for difference with atorvastatin

Tell your doctor about all the medicines you take, including prescription and non-prescription medicines, vitamins, and herbal supplements.

Taking LIPTRUZET with certain other medicines or substances can increase the risk of muscle problems or other side effects.

Especially tell your doctor if you take medicines for:

- your immune system
- cholesterol
- infections
- birth control
- heart failure
- HIV or AIDS
- hepatitis C
- gout

Also tell your doctor if you drink large amounts of grapefruit juice.

How should I take LIPTRUZET?

- Take LIPTRUZET exactly as your doctor tells you to take it.
- Your doctor will tell you how much LIPTRUZET to take and when to take it.
- Your doctor may change your dose if needed.
- Do not open your LIPTRUZET pouch until you are ready to take LIPTRUZET.
- Take LIPTRUZET 1 time each day, with or without food. It may be easier to remember to take your dose if you do it at the same time every day, such as with breakfast, dinner, or at bedtime.
- Tablets should be swallowed whole. Do not crush, dissolve, or chew tablets.
- Keep taking LIPTRUZET unless your doctor tells you to stop. If you stop taking LIPTRUZET, your cholesterol may rise again.
- If you miss a dose, do not take an extra dose. Just resume your usual schedule.
- If you take too much LIPTRUZET, call your doctor or Poison Control Center at 1-800-222-1222 or go to the nearest hospital emergency room right away.
- See your doctor regularly to check your cholesterol level and to check for side effects. Your doctor may do blood tests to check your liver before you start taking LIPTRUZET and during treatment.

What should I avoid while taking LIPTRUZET?

- Do not start any new medicines before talking to your doctor. This includes prescription and non-prescription medicines, vitamins, and herbal supplements. LIPTRUZET and certain other medicines can interact causing serious side effects.
- Do not drink more than 2 glasses of alcohol daily.
- Do not get pregnant. If you get pregnant, stop taking LIPTRUZET right away and call your doctor.

What are the possible side effects of LIPTRUZET?

LIPTRUZET may cause serious side effects, including:

- **muscle problems.** LIPTRUZET can cause serious muscle problems that can lead to kidney problems, including kidney failure. You have a higher chance for muscle problems if you are taking certain other medicines with LIPTRUZET.

Tell your doctor right away if:

- **you have unexplained muscle pain, tenderness, or weakness, especially if you have a fever or feel more tired than usual, while you take LIPTRUZET.**
- you have muscle problems that do not go away even after your doctor has advised you to stop taking LIPTRUZET. Your doctor may do further tests to diagnose the cause of your muscle problems.

- **liver problems.** Your doctor should do blood tests to check your liver before you start taking LIPTRUZET and if you have symptoms of liver problems while you take LIPTRUZET. Call your doctor right away if you have the following symptoms of liver problems:
  - feel tired or weak
  - loss of appetite
  - upper belly pain
  - dark urine
  - yellowing of your skin or the whites of your eyes

Also call your doctor right away if you have:

- allergic reactions including swelling of the face, lips, tongue, and/or throat that may cause difficulty in breathing or swallowing which may require treatment right away
- nausea and vomiting
- passing brown or dark-colored urine
- you feel more tired than usual
- stomach pain
- allergic skin reactions

The most common side effects of LIPTRUZET include:
• muscle and body pain
• changes in your liver function tests
Additional side effects that have been reported in people taking LIPTRUZET, ezetimibe or atorvastatin in clinical studies or general use include: joint pain; diarrhea; tendon problems; memory loss; confusion; depression.
Tell your doctor if you have any side effect that bothers you or that does not go away.
These are not all the possible side effects of LIPTRUZET. For more information, ask your doctor or pharmacist.
Call your doctor for medical advice about side effects. You may report side effects to FDA at 1-800-FDA-1088.

How should I store LIPTRUZET?
• Store LIPTRUZET at room temperature between 68°F to 77°F (20°C to 25°C).
• Keep LIPTRUZET in the foil pouch until you are ready to take it.
• After you remove a LIPTRUZET tablet from the blister card, slide the blister card back into the case (where a case is provided) and store in a dry place.
• Write down the date the foil pouch was opened in the space provided.
• Keep LIPTRUZET tablets dry and out of the light.
• Safely throw away unused LIPTRUZET tablets **30 days** after the foil pouch is opened.
Keep LIPTRUZET and all medicines out of the reach of children.

General information about the safe and effective use of LIPTRUZET.
LIPTRUZET may help to reduce your cholesterol in 2 ways. It reduces the cholesterol absorbed in your digestive tract, as well as the cholesterol your body makes by itself. LIPTRUZET does not help you lose weight.
Medicines are sometimes prescribed for purposes other than those listed in the Patient Information leaflet. Do not use LIPTRUZET for a condition for which it was not prescribed. Do not give LIPTRUZET to other people, even if they have the same problem that you have. It may harm them.
This Patient Information leaflet summarizes the most important information about LIPTRUZET. If you would like more information, talk with your doctor. You can ask your pharmacist or doctor for information about LIPTRUZET that is written for health professionals.
For more information, go to www.LIPTRUZET.com or call 1-800-672-6372.

What are the ingredients in LIPTRUZET?
Active ingredients: ezetimibe and atorvastatin
Inactive ingredients: lactose monohydrate, microcrystalline cellulose, croscarmellose sodium, povidone, sodium lauryl sulfate, magnesium stearate, lactose anhydrous, hydroxypropyl cellulose, sodium bicarbonate. The tablet film coating contains the following inactive ingredients: hydroxypropyl cellulose, hypromellose, titanium dioxide, and carnauba wax
This Patient Information has been approved by the U.S. Food and Drug Administration
Manufactured by:
Merck Sharp & Dohme Corp., a subsidiary of
MERCK & CO., INC., Whitehouse Station, NJ 08889, USA
U.S. Patent Nos. 5,846,966 and RE37,721.
Issued: 05/2013
USPPI-T-0653C1305R000
Shown in Product Identification Guide, page 308

M-M-R® II
[em em ar too]
(MEASLES, MUMPS, and RUBELLA VIRUS VACCINE LIVE)

DESCRIPTION
M-M-R® II (Measles, Mumps, and Rubella Virus Vaccine Live) is a live virus vaccine for vaccination against measles (rubeola), mumps, and rubella (German measles).
M-M-R II is a sterile lyophilized preparation of (1) ATTENUVAX® (Measles Virus Vaccine Live), a more attenuated line of measles virus, derived from Enders' attenuated Edmonston strain and propagated in chick embryo cell culture; (2) MUMPSVAX® (Mumps Virus Vaccine Live), the Jeryl Lynn™ (B level) strain of mumps virus propagated in chick embryo cell culture; and (3) MERUVAX® II (Rubella Virus Vaccine Live), the Wistar RA 27/3 strain of live attenuated rubella virus propagated in WI-38 human diploid lung fibroblasts.[1,2]
The growth medium for measles and mumps is Medium 199 (a buffered salt solution containing vitamins and amino acids and supplemented with fetal bovine serum) containing SPGA (sucrose, phosphate, glutamate, and recombinant human albumin) as stabilizer and neomycin.
The growth medium for rubella is Minimum Essential Medium (MEM) [a buffered salt solution containing vitamins and amino acids and supplemented with fetal bovine serum]

containing recombinant human albumin and neomycin. Sorbitol and hydrolyzed gelatin stabilizer are added to the individual virus harvests.
The cells, virus pools, and fetal bovine serum are all screened for the absence of adventitious agents.
The reconstituted vaccine is for subcutaneous administration. Each 0.5 mL dose contains not less than 1,000 $TCID_{50}$ (tissue culture infectious doses) of measles virus; 12,500 $TCID_{50}$ of mumps virus; and 1,000 $TCID_{50}$ of rubella virus. Each dose of the vaccine is calculated to contain sorbitol (14.5 mg), sodium phosphate, sucrose (1.9 mg), sodium chloride, hydrolyzed gelatin (14.5 mg), recombinant human albumin (≤0.3 mg), fetal bovine serum (<1 ppm), other buffer and media ingredients and approximately 25 mcg of neomycin. The product contains no preservative.
Before reconstitution, the lyophilized vaccine is a light yellow compact crystalline plug. M-M-R II, when reconstituted as directed, is clear yellow.

CLINICAL PHARMACOLOGY
Measles, mumps, and rubella are three common childhood diseases, caused by measles virus, mumps virus (paramyxoviruses), and rubella virus (togavirus), respectively, that may be associated with serious complications and/or death. For example, pneumonia and encephalitis are caused by measles. Mumps is associated with aseptic meningitis, deafness and orchitis; and rubella during pregnancy may cause congenital rubella syndrome in the infants of infected mothers.
The impact of measles, mumps, and rubella vaccination on the natural history of each disease in the United States can be quantified by comparing the maximum number of measles, mumps, and rubella cases reported in a given year prior to vaccine use to the number of cases of each disease reported in 1995. For measles, 894,134 cases reported in 1941 compared to 288 cases reported in 1995 resulted in a 99.97% decrease in reported cases; for mumps, 152,209 cases reported in 1968 compared to 840 cases reported in 1995 resulted in a 99.45% decrease in reported cases; and for rubella, 57,686 cases reported in 1969 compared to 200 cases reported in 1995 resulted in a 99.65% decrease.[3]
Clinical studies of 284 triple seronegative children, 11 months to 7 years of age, demonstrated that M-M-R II is highly immunogenic and generally well tolerated. In these studies, a single injection of the vaccine induced measles hemagglutination-inhibition (HI) antibodies in 95%, mumps neutralizing antibodies in 96%, and rubella HI antibodies in 99% of susceptible persons. However, a small percentage (1-5%) of vaccinees may fail to seroconvert after the primary dose (see also INDICATIONS AND USAGE, Recommended Vaccination Schedule).
A study[4] of 6-month-old and 15-month-old infants born to vaccine-immunized mothers demonstrated that, following vaccination with ATTENUVAX, 74% of the 6-month-old infants developed detectable neutralizing antibody (NT) titers while 100% of the 15-month-old infants developed NT. This rate of seroconversion is higher than that previously reported for 6-month-old infants born to naturally immune mothers tested by HI assay. When the 6-month-old infants of immunized mothers were revaccinated at 15 months, they developed antibody titers equivalent to the 15-month-old vaccinees. The lower seroconversion rate in 6-month-olds has two possible explanations: 1) Due to the limit of the detection level of the assays (NT and enzyme immunoassay [EIA]), the presence of trace amounts of undetectable maternal antibody might interfere with the seroconversion of infants; or 2) The immune system of 6-month-olds is not always capable of mounting a response to measles vaccine as measured by the two antibody assays.
There is some evidence to suggest that infants who are born to mothers who had wild-type measles and who are vaccinated at less than one year of age may not develop sustained antibody levels when later revaccinated. The advantage of early protection must be weighed against the chance for failure to respond adequately on reimmunization.[5,6]
Efficacy of measles, mumps, and rubella vaccines was established in a series of double-blind controlled field trials which demonstrated a high degree of protective efficacy afforded by the individual vaccine components.[7-12] These studies also established that seroconversion in response to vaccination against measles, mumps, and rubella paralleled protection from these diseases.[13-15]
Following vaccination, antibodies associated with protection can be measured by neutralization assays, HI, or ELISA (enzyme linked immunosorbent assay) tests. Neutralizing and ELISA antibodies to measles, mumps, and rubella viruses are still detectable in most individuals 11 to 13 years after primary vaccination.[16-18] See INDICATIONS AND USAGE, Non-Pregnant Adolescent and Adult Females, for Rubella Susceptibility Testing.
The RA 27/3 rubella strain in M-M-R II elicits higher immediate post-vaccination HI, complement-fixing and neutralizing antibody levels than other strains of rubella vaccine[19-

25] and has been shown to induce a broader profile of circulating antibodies including anti-theta and anti-iota precipitating antibodies.[26,27] The RA 27/3 rubella strain immunologically simulates natural infection more closely than other rubella vaccine viruses.[27-29] The increased levels and broader profile of antibodies produced by RA 27/3 strain rubella virus vaccine appear to correlate with greater resistance to subclinical reinfection with the wild virus,[27,29-31] and provide greater confidence for lasting immunity.

INDICATIONS AND USAGE
Recommended Vaccination Schedule
M-M-R II is indicated for simultaneous vaccination against measles, mumps, and rubella in individuals 12 months of age or older.
Individuals first vaccinated at 12 months of age or older should be revaccinated prior to elementary school entry. Revaccination is intended to seroconvert those who do not respond to the first dose. The Advisory Committee on Immunization Practices (ACIP) recommends administration of the first dose of M-M-R II at 12 to 15 months of age and administration of the second dose of M-M-R II at 4 to 6 years of age.[32] In addition, some public health jurisdictions mandate the age for revaccination. Consult complete text of applicable guidelines regarding routine revaccination including that of high-risk adult populations.

Measles Outbreak Schedule
Infants Between 6 to 12 Months of Age
Local health authorities may recommend measles vaccination of infants between 6 to 12 months of age in outbreak situations. This population may fail to respond to the components of the vaccine. Safety and effectiveness of mumps and rubella vaccine in infants less than 12 months of age have not been established. The younger the infant, the lower the likelihood of seroconversion (see CLINICAL PHARMACOLOGY). Such infants should receive a second dose of M-M-R II between 12 to 15 months of age followed by revaccination at elementary school entry.[32]
Unnecessary doses of a vaccine are best avoided by ensuring that written documentation of vaccination is preserved and a copy given to each vaccinee's parent or guardian.

Other Vaccination Considerations
Non-Pregnant Adolescent and Adult Females
Immunization of susceptible non-pregnant adolescent and adult females of childbearing age with live attenuated rubella virus vaccine is indicated if certain precautions are observed (see below and PRECAUTIONS). Vaccinating susceptible postpubertal females confers individual protection against subsequently acquiring rubella infection during pregnancy, which in turn prevents infection of the fetus and consequent congenital rubella injury.[33]
Women of childbearing age should be advised not to become pregnant for 3 months after vaccination and should be informed of the reasons for this precaution.
The ACIP has stated "If it is practical and if reliable laboratory services are available, women of childbearing age who are potential candidates for vaccination can have serologic tests to determine susceptibility to rubella. However, with the exception of premarital and prenatal screening, routinely performing serologic tests for all women of childbearing age to determine susceptibility (so that vaccine is given only to proven susceptible women) can be effective but is expensive. Also, 2 visits to the health-care provider would be necessary — one for screening and one for vaccination. Accordingly, rubella vaccination of a woman who is not known to be pregnant and has no history of vaccination is justifiable without serologic testing — and may be preferable, particularly when costs of serology are high and follow-up of identified susceptible women for vaccination is not assured."[33]
Postpubertal females should be informed of the frequent occurrence of generally self-limited arthralgia and/or arthritis beginning 2 to 4 weeks after vaccination (see ADVERSE REACTIONS).
Postpartum Women
It has been found convenient in many instances to vaccinate rubella-susceptible women in the immediate postpartum period (see PRECAUTIONS, Nursing Mothers).
Other Populations
Previously unvaccinated children older than 12 months who are in contact with susceptible pregnant women should receive live attenuated rubella vaccine (such as that contained in monovalent rubella vaccine or in M-M-R II) to reduce the risk of exposure to the pregnant woman.
Individuals planning travel outside the United States, if not immune, can acquire measles, mumps, or rubella and import these diseases into the United States. Therefore, prior to international travel, individuals known to be susceptible to one or more of these diseases can either receive the indicated monovalent vaccine (measles, mumps, or rubella), or a combination vaccine as appropriate. However, M-M-R II is preferred for persons likely to be susceptible to mumps and rubella; and if monovalent measles vaccine is not readily available, travelers should receive M-M-R II regardless of their immune status to mumps or rubella.[34-36]

Vaccination is recommended for susceptible individuals in high-risk groups such as college students, health-care workers, and military personnel.[33,34,37]

According to ACIP recommendations, most persons born in 1956 or earlier are likely to have been infected with measles naturally and generally need not be considered susceptible. All children, adolescents, and adults born after 1956 are considered susceptible and should be vaccinated, if there are no contraindications. This includes persons who may be immune to measles but who lack adequate documentation of immunity such as: (1) physician-diagnosed measles, (2) laboratory evidence of measles immunity, or (3) adequate immunization with live measles vaccine on or after the first birthday.[34]

The ACIP recommends that "Persons vaccinated with inactivated vaccine followed within 3 months by live vaccine should be revaccinated with two doses of live vaccine. Revaccination is particularly important when the risk of exposure to wild-type measles virus is increased, as may occur during international travel."[34]

Post-Exposure Vaccination

Vaccination of individuals exposed to wild-type measles may provide some protection if the vaccine is administered within 72 hours of exposure. If, however, vaccine is given a few days before exposure, substantial protection may be afforded.[34,38,39] There is no conclusive evidence that vaccination of individuals recently exposed to wild-type mumps or wild-type rubella will provide protection.[33,37]

Use With Other Vaccines

See DOSAGE AND ADMINISTRATION, Use With Other Vaccines.

CONTRAINDICATIONS

Hypersensitivity to any component of the vaccine, including gelatin.[40]

Do not give M-M-R II to pregnant females; the possible effects of the vaccine on fetal development are unknown at this time. If vaccination of postpubertal females is undertaken, pregnancy should be avoided for three months following vaccination (see INDICATIONS AND USAGE, Non-Pregnant Adolescent and Adult Females and PRECAUTIONS, Pregnancy).

Anaphylactic or anaphylactoid reactions to neomycin (each dose of reconstituted vaccine contains approximately 25 mcg of neomycin).

Febrile respiratory illness or other active febrile infection. However, the ACIP has recommended that all vaccines can be administered to persons with minor illnesses such as diarrhea, mild upper respiratory infection with or without low-grade fever, or other low-grade febrile illness.[41]

Patients receiving immunosuppressive therapy. This contraindication does not apply to patients who are receiving corticosteroids as replacement therapy, e.g., for Addison's disease.

Individuals with blood dyscrasias, leukemia, lymphomas of any type, or other malignant neoplasms affecting the bone marrow or lymphatic systems.

Primary and acquired immunodeficiency states, including patients who are immunosuppressed in association with AIDS or other clinical manifestations of infection with human immunodeficiency viruses;[41-43] cellular immune deficiencies; and hypogammaglobulinemic and dysgammaglobulinemic states. Measles inclusion body encephalitis[44] (MIBE), pneumonitis[45] and death as a direct consequence of disseminated measles vaccine virus infection have been reported in immunocompromised individuals inadvertently vaccinated with measles-containing vaccine.

Individuals with a family history of congenital or hereditary immunodeficiency, until the immune competence of the potential vaccine recipient is demonstrated.

WARNINGS

Due caution should be employed in administration of M-M-R II to persons with a history of cerebral injury, individual or family histories of convulsions, or any other condition in which stress due to fever should be avoided. The physician should be alert to the temperature elevation which may occur following vaccination (see ADVERSE REACTIONS).

Hypersensitivity to Eggs

Live measles vaccine and live mumps vaccine are produced in chick embryo cell culture. Persons with a history of anaphylactic, anaphylactoid, or other immediate reactions (e.g., hives, swelling of the mouth and throat, difficulty breathing, hypotension, or shock) subsequent to egg ingestion may be at an enhanced risk of immediate-type hypersensitivity reactions after receiving vaccines containing traces of chick embryo antigen. The potential risk to benefit ratio should be carefully evaluated before considering vaccination in such cases. Such individuals may be vaccinated with extreme caution, having adequate treatment on hand should a reaction occur (see PRECAUTIONS).[46]

However, the AAP has stated, "Most children with a history of anaphylactic reactions to eggs have no untoward reac-

tions to measles or MMR vaccine. Persons are not at increased risk if they have egg allergies that are not anaphylactic, and they should be vaccinated in the usual manner. In addition, skin testing of egg-allergic children with vaccine has not been predictive of which children will have an immediate hypersensitivity reaction...Persons with allergies to chickens or chicken feathers are not at increased risk of reaction to the vaccine."[47]

Hypersensitivity to Neomycin

The AAP states, "Persons who have experienced anaphylactic reactions to topically or systemically administered neomycin should not receive measles vaccine. Most often, however, neomycin allergy manifests as a contact dermatitis, which is a delayed-type (cell-mediated) immune response rather than anaphylaxis. In such persons, an adverse reaction to neomycin in the vaccine would be an erythematous, pruritic nodule or papule, 48 to 96 hours after vaccination. A history of contact dermatitis to neomycin is not a contraindication to receiving measles vaccine."[47]

Thrombocytopenia

Individuals with current thrombocytopenia may develop more severe thrombocytopenia following vaccination. In addition, individuals who experienced thrombocytopenia with the first dose of M-M-R II (or its component vaccines) may develop thrombocytopenia with repeat doses. Serologic status may be evaluated to determine whether or not additional doses of vaccine are needed. The potential risk to benefit ratio should be carefully evaluated before considering vaccination in such cases (see ADVERSE REACTIONS).

PRECAUTIONS
General

Adequate treatment provisions, including epinephrine injection (1:1000), should be available for immediate use should an anaphylactic or anaphylactoid reaction occur.

Special care should be taken to ensure that the injection does not enter a blood vessel.

Children and young adults who are known to be infected with human immunodeficiency viruses and are not immunosuppressed may be vaccinated. However, vaccinees who are infected with HIV should be monitored closely for vaccine-preventable diseases because immunization may be less effective than for uninfected persons (see CONTRAINDICATIONS).[42,43]

Vaccination should be deferred for 3 months or longer following blood or plasma transfusions, or administration of immune globulin (human).[47]

Excretion of small amounts of the live attenuated rubella virus from the nose or throat has occurred in the majority of susceptible individuals 7 to 28 days after vaccination. There is no confirmed evidence to indicate that such virus is transmitted to susceptible persons who are in contact with the vaccinated individuals. Consequently, transmission through close personal contact, while accepted as a theoretical possibility, is not regarded as a significant risk.[33] However, transmission of the rubella vaccine virus to infants via breast milk has been documented (see Nursing Mothers).

There are no reports of transmission of live attenuated measles or mumps viruses from vaccinees to susceptible contacts.

It has been reported that live attenuated measles, mumps and rubella virus vaccines given individually may result in a temporary depression of tuberculin skin sensitivity. Therefore, if a tuberculin test is to be done, it should be administered either before or simultaneously with M-M-R II. Children under treatment for tuberculosis have not experienced exacerbation of the disease when immunized with live measles virus vaccine;[48] no studies have been reported to date of the effect of measles virus vaccines on untreated tuberculous children. However, individuals with active untreated tuberculosis should not be vaccinated.

As for any vaccine, vaccination with M-M-R II may not result in protection in 100% of vaccinees.

The health-care provider should determine the current health status and previous vaccination history of the vaccinee.

The health-care provider should question the patient, parent, or guardian about reactions to a previous dose of M-M-R II or other measles-, mumps-, or rubella-containing vaccines.

Information for Patients

The health-care provider should provide the vaccine information required to be given with each vaccination to the patient, parent, or guardian.

The health-care provider should inform the patient, parent, or guardian of the benefits and risks associated with vaccination. For risks associated with vaccination see WARNINGS, PRECAUTIONS, and ADVERSE REACTIONS.

Patients, parents, or guardians should be instructed to report any serious adverse reactions to their health-care provider who in turn should report such events to the U.S. Department of Health and Human Services through the Vaccine Adverse Event Reporting System (VAERS), 1-800-822-7967.[49]

Pregnancy should be avoided for 3 months following vaccination, and patients should be informed of the reasons for this precaution (see INDICATIONS AND USAGE, Non-Pregnant Adolescent and Adult Females, CONTRAINDICATIONS, and PRECAUTIONS, Pregnancy).

Laboratory Tests

See INDICATIONS AND USAGE, Non-Pregnant Adolescent and Adult Females, for Rubella Susceptibility Testing, and CLINICAL PHARMACOLOGY.

Drug Interactions

See DOSAGE AND ADMINISTRATION, Use With Other Vaccines.

Immunosuppressive Therapy

The immune status of patients about to undergo immunosuppressive therapy should be evaluated so that the physician can consider whether vaccination prior to the initiation of treatment is indicated (see CONTRAINDICATIONS and PRECAUTIONS).

The ACIP has stated that "patients with leukemia in remission who have not received chemotherapy for at least 3 months may receive live virus vaccines. Short-term (<2 weeks), low- to moderate-dose systemic corticosteroid therapy, topical steroid therapy (e.g. nasal, skin), long-term alternate-day treatment with low to moderate doses of short-acting systemic steroid, and intra-articular, bursal, or tendon injection of corticosteroids are not immunosuppressive in their usual doses and do not contraindicate the administration of [measles, mumps, or rubella vaccine]."[33,34,37]

Immune Globulin

Administration of immune globulins concurrently with M-M-R II may interfere with the expected immune response.[33,34,47]

See also PRECAUTIONS, General.

Carcinogenesis, Mutagenesis, Impairment of Fertility

M-M-R II has not been evaluated for carcinogenic or mutagenic potential, or potential to impair fertility.

Pregnancy

Pregnancy Category C

Animal reproduction studies have not been conducted with M-M-R II. It is also not known whether M-M-R II can cause fetal harm when administered to a pregnant woman or can affect reproduction capacity. Therefore, the vaccine should not be administered to pregnant females; furthermore, pregnancy should be avoided for 3 months following vaccination (see INDICATIONS AND USAGE, Non-Pregnant Adolescent and Adult Females and CONTRAINDICATIONS).

In counseling women who are inadvertently vaccinated when pregnant or who become pregnant within 3 months of vaccination, the physician should be aware of the following: (1) In a 10-year survey involving over 700 pregnant women who received rubella vaccine within 3 months before or after conception (of whom 189 received the Wistar RA 27/3 strain), none of the newborns had abnormalities compatible with congenital rubella syndrome;[50] (2) Mumps infection during the first trimester of pregnancy may increase the rate of spontaneous abortion. Although mumps vaccine virus has been shown to infect the placenta and fetus, there is no evidence that it causes congenital malformations in humans;[37] and (3) Reports have indicated that contracting wild-type measles during pregnancy enhances fetal risk. Increased rates of spontaneous abortion, stillbirth, congenital defects and prematurity have been observed subsequent to infection with wild-type measles during pregnancy.[51,52] There are no adequate studies of the attenuated (vaccine) strain of measles virus in pregnancy. However, it would be prudent to assume that the vaccine strain of virus is also capable of inducing adverse fetal effects.

Nursing Mothers

It is not known whether measles or mumps vaccine virus is secreted in human milk. Recent studies have shown that lactating postpartum women immunized with live attenuated rubella vaccine may secrete the virus in breast milk and transmit it to breast-fed infants.[53] In the infants with serological evidence of rubella infection, none exhibited severe disease; however, one exhibited mild clinical illness typical of acquired rubella.[54,55] Caution should be exercised when M-M-R II is administered to a nursing woman.

Pediatric Use

Safety and effectiveness of measles vaccine in infants below the age of 6 months have not been established (see also CLINICAL PHARMACOLOGY). Safety and effectiveness of mumps and rubella vaccine in infants less than 12 months of age have not been established.

Geriatric Use

Clinical studies of M-M-R II did not include sufficient numbers of seronegative subjects aged 65 and over to determine whether they respond differently from younger subjects. Other reported clinical experience has not identified differences in responses between the elderly and younger subjects.

ADVERSE REACTIONS

The following adverse reactions are listed in decreasing order of severity, without regard to causality, within each body system category and have been reported during clinical trials, with use of the marketed vaccine, or with use of monovalent or bivalent vaccine containing measles, mumps, or rubella:

Body as a Whole
Panniculitis; atypical measles; fever; syncope; headache; dizziness; malaise; irritability.

Cardiovascular System
Vasculitis.

Digestive System
Pancreatitis; diarrhea; vomiting; parotitis; nausea.

Endocrine System
Diabetes mellitus.

Hemic and Lymphatic System
Thrombocytopenia (see WARNINGS, Thrombocytopenia); purpura; regional lymphadenopathy; leukocytosis.

Immune System
Anaphylaxis and anaphylactoid reactions have been reported as well as related phenomena such as angioneurotic edema (including peripheral or facial edema) and bronchial spasm in individuals with or without an allergic history.

Musculoskeletal System
Arthritis; arthralgia; myalgia.
Arthralgia and/or arthritis (usually transient and rarely chronic), and polyneuritis are features of infection with wild-type rubella and vary in frequency and severity with age and sex, being greatest in adult females and least in prepubertal children. This type of involvement as well as myalgia and paresthesia, have also been reported following administration of MERUVAX II.
Chronic arthritis has been associated with wild-type rubella infection and has been related to persistent virus and/or viral antigen isolated from body tissues. Only rarely have vaccine recipients developed chronic joint symptoms.
Following vaccination in children, reactions in joints are uncommon and generally of brief duration. In women, incidence rates for arthritis and arthralgia are generally higher than those seen in children (children: 0-3%; women: 12-26%),[17,56,57] and the reactions tend to be more marked and of longer duration. Symptoms may persist for a matter of months or on rare occasions for years. In adolescent girls, the reactions appear to be intermediate in incidence between those seen in children and in adult women. Even in women older than 35 years, these reactions are generally well tolerated and rarely interfere with normal activities.

Nervous System
Encephalitis; encephalopathy; measles inclusion body encephalitis (MIBE) (see CONTRAINDICATIONS); subacute sclerosing panencephalitis (SSPE); Guillain-Barré Syndrome (GBS); acute disseminated encephalomyelitis (ADEM); transverse myelitis; febrile convulsions; afebrile convulsions or seizures; ataxia; polyneuritis; polyneuropathy; ocular palsies; paresthesia.
Experience from more than 80 million doses of all live measles vaccines given in the U.S. through 1975 indicates that significant central nervous system reactions such as encephalitis and encephalopathy, occurring within 30 days after vaccination, have been temporally associated with measles vaccine very rarely.[58] In no case has it been shown that reactions were actually caused by vaccine. The Centers for Disease Control and Prevention has pointed out that "a certain number of cases of encephalitis may be expected to occur in a large childhood population in a defined period of time even when no vaccines are administered". However, the data suggest the possibility that some of these cases may have been caused by measles vaccines. The risk of such serious neurological disorders following live measles virus vaccine administration remains far less than that for encephalitis and encephalopathy with wild-type measles (one per two thousand reported cases).
Post-marketing surveillance of the more than 200 million doses of M-M-R and M-M-R II that have been distributed worldwide over 25 years (1971 to 1996) indicates that serious adverse events such as encephalitis and encephalopathy continue to be rarely reported.[17]
There have been reports of subacute sclerosing panencephalitis (SSPE) in children who did not have a history of infection with wild-type measles but did receive measles vaccine. Some of these cases may have resulted from unrecognized measles in the first year of life or possibly from the measles vaccination. Based on estimated nationwide measles vaccine distribution, the association of SSPE cases to measles vaccination is about one case per million vaccine doses distributed. This is far less than the association with infection with wild-type measles, 6-22 cases of SSPE per million cases of measles. The results of a retrospective case-controlled study conducted by the Centers for Disease Control and Prevention suggest that the overall effect of measles vaccine has been to protect against SSPE by preventing measles with its inherent higher risk of SSPE.[59]
Cases of aseptic meningitis have been reported to VAERS following measles, mumps, and rubella vaccination. Although a causal relationship between the Urabe strain of

mumps vaccine and aseptic meningitis has been shown, there is no evidence to link Jeryl Lynn™ mumps vaccine to aseptic meningitis.

Respiratory System
Pneumonia; pneumonitis (see CONTRAINDICATIONS); sore throat; cough; rhinitis.

Skin
Stevens-Johnson syndrome; erythema multiforme; urticaria; rash; measles-like rash; pruritis.
Local reactions including burning/stinging at injection site; wheal and flare; redness (erythema); swelling; induration; tenderness; vesiculation at injection site.

Special Senses — Ear
Nerve deafness; otitis media.

Special Senses — Eye
Retinitis; optic neuritis; papillitis; retrobulbar neuritis; conjunctivitis.

Urogenital System
Epididymitis; orchitis.

Other
Death from various, and in some cases unknown, causes has been reported rarely following vaccination with measles, mumps, and rubella vaccines; however, a causal relationship has not been established in healthy individuals (see CONTRAINDICATIONS). No deaths or permanent sequelae were reported in a published post-marketing surveillance study in Finland involving 1.5 million children and adults who were vaccinated with M-M-R II during 1982 to 1993.[60]
Under the National Childhood Vaccine Injury Act of 1986, health-care providers and manufacturers are required to record and report certain suspected adverse events occurring within specific time periods after vaccination. However, the U.S. Department of Health and Human Services (DHHS) has established a Vaccine Adverse Event Reporting System (VAERS) which will accept all reports of suspected events.[49] A VAERS report form as well as information regarding reporting requirements can be obtained by calling VAERS 1-800-822-7967.

DOSAGE AND ADMINISTRATION

FOR SUBCUTANEOUS ADMINISTRATION
Do not inject intravascularly.
The dose for any age is 0.5 mL administered subcutaneously, preferably into the outer aspect of the upper arm.
The recommended age for primary vaccination is 12 to 15 months.
Revaccination with M-M-R II is recommended prior to elementary school entry. See also INDICATIONS AND USAGE, Recommended Vaccination Schedule.
Children first vaccinated when younger than 12 months of age should receive another dose between 12 to 15 months of age followed by revaccination prior to elementary school entry.[32] See also INDICATIONS AND USAGE, Measles Outbreak Schedule.
Immune Globulin (IG) is not to be given concurrently with M-M-R II (see PRECAUTIONS, General and PRECAUTIONS, Drug Interactions).
CAUTION: A sterile syringe free of preservatives, antiseptics, and detergents should be used for each injection and/or reconstitution of the vaccine because these substances may inactivate the live virus vaccine. A 25 gauge, 5/8" needle is recommended.
To reconstitute, use only the diluent supplied, since it is free of preservatives or other antiviral substances which might inactivate the vaccine.
Single Dose Vial — First withdraw the entire volume of diluent into the syringe to be used for reconstitution. Inject all the diluent in the syringe into the vial of lyophilized vaccine, and agitate to mix thoroughly. If the lyophilized vaccine cannot be dissolved, discard. Withdraw the entire contents into a syringe and inject the total volume of restored vaccine subcutaneously.
It is important to use a separate sterile syringe and needle for each individual patient to prevent transmission of hepatitis B and other infectious agents from one person to another.
Parenteral drug products should be inspected visually for particulate matter and discoloration prior to administration whenever solution and container permit. M-M-R II, when reconstituted, is clear yellow.

Use With Other Vaccines

M-M-R II should be given one month before or after administration of other live viral vaccines.
M-M-R II has been administered concurrently with VARIVAX® [Varicella Virus Vaccine Live (Oka/Merck)], and PedvaxHIB® [*Haemophilus b* Conjugate Vaccine (Meningococcal Protein Conjugate)] using separate injection sites and syringes. No impairment of immune response to individually tested vaccine antigens was demonstrated. The type, frequency, and severity of adverse experiences observed with M-M-R II were similar to those seen when each vaccine was given alone.

Routine administration of DTP (diphtheria, tetanus, pertussis) and/or OPV (oral poliovirus vaccine) concurrently with measles, mumps and rubella vaccines is not recommended because there are limited data relating to the simultaneous administration of these antigens.
However, other schedules have been used. The ACIP has stated "Although data are limited concerning the simultaneous administration of the entire recommended vaccine series (i.e., DTaP [or DTwP], IPV [or OPV], Hib with or without Hepatitis B vaccine, and varicella vaccine), data from numerous studies have indicated no interference between routinely recommended childhood vaccines (either live, attenuated, or killed). These findings support the simultaneous use of all vaccines as recommended."[61]

HOW SUPPLIED

No. 4681 — M-M-R II is supplied as follows: (1) a box of 10 single-dose vials of lyophilized vaccine (package A), NDC 0006-4681-00; and (2) a box of 10 vials of diluent (package B). To conserve refrigerator space, the diluent may be stored separately at room temperature.

Storage

To maintain potency, M-M-R II must be stored between -58°F and +46°F (-50°C to +8°C). Use of dry ice may subject M-M-R II to temperatures colder than -58°F (-50°C).
Protect the vaccine from light at all times, since such exposure may inactivate the viruses.
Before reconstitution, store the lyophilized vaccine at 36°F to 46°F (2°C to 8°C). The diluent may be stored in the refrigerator with the lyophilized vaccine or separately at room temperature. **Do not freeze the diluent.**
It is recommended that the vaccine be used as soon as possible after reconstitution. Store reconstituted vaccine in the vaccine vial in a dark place at 36°F to 46°F (2°C to 8°C) and discard if not used within 8 hours.
For information regarding stability under conditions other than those recommended, call 1-800-MERCK-90.

REFERENCES

1. Plotkin, S.A.; Cornfeld, D.; Ingalls, T.H.: Studies of immunization with living rubella virus: Trials in children with a strain cultured from an aborted fetus, Am. J. Dis. Child. *110:* 381-389, 1965.
2. Plotkin, S.A.; Farquhar, J.; Katz, M.; Ingalls, T.H.: A new attenuated rubella virus grown in human fibroblasts: Evidence for reduced nasopharyngeal excretion, Am. J. Epidemiol. *86:* 468-477, 1967.
3. Monthly Immunization Table, MMWR *45*(1): 24-25, January 12, 1996.
4. Johnson, C.E.; et al: Measles Vaccine Immunogenicity in 6- Versus 15-Month-Old Infants Born to Mothers in the Measles Vaccine Era, Pediatrics, *93*(6): 939-943, 1994.
5. Linneman, C.C.; et al: Measles Immunity After Vaccination: Results in Children Vaccinated Before 10 Months of Age, Pediatrics, *69*(3): 332-335, March 1982.
6. Stetler, H.C.; et al: Impact of Revaccinating Children Who Initially Received Measles Vaccine Before 10 Months of Age, Pediatrics *77*(4): 471-476, April 1986.
7. Hilleman, M.R.; Buynak, E.B.; Weibel, R.E.; et al: Development and Evaluation of the Moraten Measles Virus Vaccine, JAMA *206*(3): 587-590, 1968.
8. Weibel, R.E.; Stokes, J.; Buynak, E.B.; et al: Live, Attenuated Mumps Virus Vaccine 3. Clinical and Serologic Aspects in a Field Evaluation, N. Engl. J. Med. *276:* 245-251, 1967.
9. Hilleman, M.R.; Weibel, R.E.; Buynak, E.B.; et al: Live, Attenuated Mumps Virus Vaccine 4. Protective Efficacy as Measured in a Field Evaluation, N. Engl. J. Med. *276:* 252-258, 1967.
10. Cutts, F.T.; Henderson, R.H.; Clements, C.J.; et al: Principles of measles control, Bull WHO *69*(1): 1-7, 1991.
11. Weibel, R.E.; Buynak, E.B.; Stokes, J.; et al: Evaluation Of Live Attenuated Mumps Virus Vaccine, Strain Jeryl Lynn, First International Conference on Vaccines Against Viral and Rickettsial Diseases of Man, World Health Organization, No. 147, May 1967.
12. Leibhaber, H.; Ingalls, T.H.; LeBouvier, G.L.; et al: Vaccination With RA 27/3 Rubella Vaccine, Am. J. Dis. Child. *123:* 133-136, February 1972.
13. Rosen, L.: Hemagglutination and Hemagglutination-Inhibition with Measles Virus, Virology *13:* 139-141, January 1961.
14. Brown, G.C.; et al: Fluorescent-Antibody Marker for Vaccine-Induced Rubella Antibodies, Infection and Immunity *2*(4): 360-363, 1970.
15. Buynak, E.B.; et al: Live Attenuated Mumps Virus Vaccine 1. Vaccine Development, Proceedings of the Society for Experimental Biology and Medicine, *123:* 768-775, 1966.
16. Weibel, R.E.; Carlson, A.J.; Villarejos, V.M.; Buynak, E.B.; McLean, A.A.; Hilleman, M.R.: Clinical and Laboratory Studies of Combined Live Measles, Mumps, and Rubella Vaccines Using the RA 27/3 Rubella Virus, Proc. Soc. Exp. Biol. Med. *165:* 323-326, 1980.

17. Unpublished data from the files of Merck Research Laboratories.

18. Watson, J.C.; Pearson, J.S.; Erdman, D.D.; et al: An Evaluation of Measles Revaccination Among School-Entry Age Children, 31st Interscience Conference on Antimicrobial Agents and Chemotherapy, Abstract #268, 143, 1991.

19. Fogel, A.; Moshkowitz, A.; Rannon, L.; Gerichter, Ch.B.: Comparative trials of RA 27/3 and Cendehill rubella vaccines in adult and adolescent females, Am. J. Epidemiol. 93: 392-393, 1971.

20. Andzhaparidze, O.G.; Desyatskova, R.G.; Chervonski, G.I.; Pryanichnikova, L.V.: Immunogenicity and reactogenicity of live attenuated rubella virus vaccines, Am. J. Epidemiol. 91: 527-530, 1970.

21. Freestone, D.S.; Reynolds, G.M.; McKinnon, J.A.; Prydie, J.: Vaccination of schoolgirls against rubella. Assessment of serological status and a comparative trial of Wistar RA 27/3 and Cendehill strain live attenuated rubella vaccines in 13-year-old schoolgirls in Dudley, Br. J. Prev. Soc. Med. 29: 258-261, 1975.

22. Grillner, L.; Hedstrom, C.E.; Bergstrom, H.; Forssman, L.; Rigner, A.; Lycke, E.: Vaccination against rubella of newly delivered women, Scand. J. Infect. Dis. 5: 237-241, 1973.

23. Grillner, L.: Neutralizing antibodies after rubella vaccination of newly delivered women: a comparison between three vaccines, Scand. J. Infect. Dis. 7: 169-172, 1975.

24. Wallace, R.B.; Isacson, P.: Comparative trial of HPV-77, DE-5 and RA 27/3 live-attenuated rubella vaccines, Am. J. Dis. Child. 124: 536-538, 1972.

25. Lalla, M.; Vesikari, T.; Virolainen, M.: Lymphoblast proliferation and humoral antibody response after rubella vaccination, Clin. Exp. Immunol. 15: 193-202, 1973.

26. LeBouvier, G.L.; Plotkin, S.A.: Precipitin responses to rubella vaccine RA 27/3, J. Infect. Dis. 123: 220-223, 1971.

27. Horstmann, D.M.: Rubella: The challenge of its control, J. Infect. Dis. 123: 640-654, 1971.

28. Ogra, P.L.; Kerr-Grant, D.; Umana, G.; Dzierba, J.; Weintraub, D.: Antibody response in serum and nasopharynx after naturally acquired and vaccine-induced infection with rubella virus, N. Engl. J. Med. 285: 1333-1339, 1971.

29. Plotkin, S.A.; Farquhar, J.D.; Ogra, P.L.: Immunologic properties of RA 27/3 rubella virus vaccine, J. Am. Med. Assoc. 225: 585-590, 1973.

30. Liebhaber, H.; Ingalls, T.H.; LeBouvier, G.L.; Horstmann, D.M.: Vaccination with RA 27/3 rubella vaccine. Persistence of immunity and resistance to challenge after two years, Am. J. Dis. Child. 123: 133-136, 1972.

31. Farquhar, J.D.: Follow-up on rubella vaccinations and experience with subclinical reinfection, J. Pediatr. 81: 460-465, 1972.

32. Measles, Mumps, and Rubella — Vaccine Use and Strategies for Elimination of Measles, Rubella, and Congenital Rubella Syndrome and Control of Mumps: Recommendations of the Advisory Committee on Immunization Practices (ACIP), MMWR 47(RR-8): May 22, 1998.

33. Rubella Prevention: Recommendation of the Immunization Practices Advisory Committee (ACIP), MMWR 39(RR-15): 1-18, November 23, 1990.

34. Measles Prevention: Recommendations of the Immunization Practices Advisory Committee (ACIP), MMWR 38(S-9): 5-22, December 29, 1989.

35. Jong, E.C., The Travel and Tropical Medicine Manual, W.B. Saunders Company, p. 12-16, 1987.

36. Committee on Immunization Council of Medical Societies, American College of Physicians, Phila., PA, Guide for Adult Immunization, First Edition, 1985.

37. Recommendations of the Immunization Practices Advisory Committee (ACIP), Mumps Prevention, MMWR 38(22): 388-400, June 9, 1989.

38. King, G.E.; Markowitz, L.E.; Patriarca, P.A.; et al: Clinical Efficacy of Measles Vaccine During the 1990 Measles Epidemic, Pediatr. Infect. Dis. J. 10(12): 883-888, December 1991.

39. Krasinski, K.; Borkowsky, W.: Measles and Measles Immunity in Children Infected With Human Immunodeficiency Virus, JAMA 261(17): 2512-2516, 1989.

40. Kelso, J.M.; Jones, R.T.; Yunginger, J.W.: Anaphylaxis to measles, mumps, and rubella vaccine mediated by IgE to gelatin, J. Allergy Clin. Immunol. 91: 867-872, 1993.

41. General Recommendations on Immunization, Recommendations of the Advisory Committee on Immunization Practices, MMWR 43(RR-1): 1-38, January 28, 1994.

42. Center for Disease Control: Immunization of Children Infected with Human T-Lymphotropic Virus Type III/Lymphadenopathy-Associated Virus, Annals of Internal Medicine, 106: 75-78, 1987.

43. Krasinski, K.; Borkowsky, W.; Krugman, S.: Antibody following measles immunization in children infected with human T-cell lymphotropic virus-type III/lymphadenopathy associated virus (HTLV-III/LAV) [Abstract]. In: Program and abstracts of the International Conference on Acquired Immunodeficiency Syndrome, Paris, France, June 23-25, 1986.

44. Bitnum, A.; et al: Measles Inclusion Body Encephalitis Caused by the Vaccine Strain of Measles Virus. Clin. Infect. Dis. 29: 855-861, 1999.

45. Angel, J.B.; et al: Vaccine Associated Measles Pneumonitis in an Adult with AIDS. Annals of Internal Medicine, 129: 104-106, 1998.

46. Isaacs, D.; Menser, M.: Modern Vaccines, Measles, Mumps, Rubella, and Varicella, Lancet 335: 1384-1387, June 9, 1990.

47. Peter, G.; et al (eds): Report of the Committee on Infectious Diseases, Twenty-fourth Edition, American Academy of Pediatrics, 344-357, 1997.

48. Starr, S.; Berkovich, S.: The effect of measles, gamma globulin modified measles, and attenuated measles vaccine on the course of treated tuberculosis in children, Pediatrics 35: 97-102, January 1965.

49. Vaccine Adverse Event Reporting System — United States, MMWR 39(41): 730-733, October 19, 1990.

50. Rubella vaccination during pregnancy — United States, 1971-1981. MMWR 31(35): 477-481, September 10, 1982.

51. Eberhart-Phillips, J.E.; et al: Measles in pregnancy: a descriptive study of 58 cases. Obstetrics and Gynecology, 82(5): 797-801, November 1993.

52. Jespersen, C.S.; et al: Measles as a cause of fetal defects: A retrospective study of ten measles epidemics in Greenland. Acta Paediatr Scand. 66: 367-372, May 1977.

53. Losonsky, G.A.; Fishaut, J.M.; Strussenber, J.; Ogra, P.L.: Effect of immunization against rubella on lactation products. II. Maternal-neonatal interactions, J. Infect. Dis. 145: 661-666, 1982.

54. Landes, R.D.; Bass, J.W.; Millunchick, E.W.; Oetgen, W.J.: Neonatal rubella following postpartum maternal immunization, J. Pediatr. 97: 465-467, 1980.

55. Lerman, S.J.: Neonatal rubella following postpartum maternal immunization, J. Pediatr. 98: 668, 1981. (Letter)

56. Gershon, A.; et al: Live attenuated rubella virus vaccine: comparison of responses to HPV-77-DE5 and RA 27/3 strains, Am. J. Med. Sci. 279(2): 95-97, 1980.

57. Weibel, R.E.; et al: Clinical and laboratory studies of live attenuated RA 27/3 and HPV-77-DE rubella virus vaccines, Proc. Soc. Exp. Biol. Med. 165: 44-49, 1980.

58. CDC. Important Information about Measles, Mumps, and Rubella, and Measles, Mumps, and Rubella Vaccines. 1980. 1983.

59. CDC, Measles Surveillance, Report No. 11, p. 14, September 1982.

60. Peltola, H.; et al: The elimination of indigenous measles, mumps, and rubella from Finland by a 12-year, two dose vaccination program. N. Engl. J. Med. 331: 1397-1402, 1994.

61. Centers for Disease Control and Prevention. Recommended childhood immunization schedule — United States, January-June 1996, MMWR 44(51 & 52): 940-943, January 5, 1996.

Dist. by: Merck Sharp & Dohme Corp., a subsidiary of MERCK & CO., INC., Whitehouse Station, NJ 08889, USA
For patent information: www.merck.com/product/patent/home.html

Copyright © 2014 Merck Sharp & Dohme Corp., a subsidiary of Merck & Co., Inc.
All rights reserved.
Revised: 06/2014
uspi-v205c-i-1406r004

PATIENT PACKAGE INSERT

Patient Information about
M-M-R® II (pronounced "em em ar too")
Generic name: Measles, Mumps, and Rubella Virus Vaccine Live

This is a summary of information about M-M-R II®. You should read it before you or your child receives the vaccine. If you have any questions about the vaccine after reading this leaflet, you should ask your health care provider. This is a summary only. It does not take the place of talking about M-M-R II with your doctor, nurse, or other health care provider. Only your health care provider can decide if M-M-R II is right for you or your child.

What is M-M-R II and how does it work?

M-M-R II is also known as Measles, Mumps, and Rubella Virus Vaccine Live. It is a live virus vaccine that is given as a shot. This vaccine is usually given to people one year old or older. It is meant to help prevent measles (rubeola), mumps, and rubella (German measles).

M-M-R II contains weakened forms of measles virus, mumps virus, and rubella virus.

M-M-R II works by helping the immune system protect you or your child from getting measles, mumps, or rubella.

M-M-R II may not protect everyone who gets the vaccine. M-M-R II does not treat measles, mumps, or rubella once you or your child has them.

What do I need to know about measles, mumps, and rubella?

Measles is also known as rubeola. It is a serious illness. Measles virus can be passed to others if you have it. Measles can give you a high fever, cough, and a rash. The illness can last for 1 to 2 weeks. In rare cases, it can also cause an infection of the brain. This could lead to seizures, hearing loss, mental retardation, and even death.

Mumps can also be passed to others. This virus can cause fever and headache. It also makes the glands under your jaw swell and be painful. The illness often lasts for several days. Sometimes, mumps can make the testicles swell and be painful. In some cases, it can cause meningitis, which is a mild swelling of the coverings of the brain and spinal cord.

Rubella is also known as German measles. It is often a mild illness. Rubella virus can cause a mild fever, swollen glands in the neck, pain and swelling in the joints, and a rash that lasts for a short time. It can be very dangerous if a pregnant woman catches it. Women who catch German measles when they are pregnant can have babies who are stillborn. Also, the babies may be blind or deaf, or have heart disease or mental retardation.

Who should not get M-M-R II?

Do not get M-M-R II if you or your child:

• are allergic to any of its ingredients (This includes gelatin or neomycin. See the ingredient list at the end of this leaflet.);

• have a weakened immune system, such as an immune deficiency, an inherited immune disorder, leukemia, lymphoma, or HIV/AIDS;

• take high doses of steroids by mouth or in a shot;

• have a fever higher than 101.3°F (38.5°C);

• are pregnant or plan to get pregnant within the next three months.

What should you tell your health care provider before getting M-M-R II?

Tell your health care provider if you or your child:

• have or have had any medical problems;

• have a history of seizures or a brain injury;

• have received blood or plasma transfusions or human serum globulin;

• have active tuberculosis that is not treated;

• take any medicines (This includes non-prescription medicines and dietary supplements.);

• have any allergies (This includes allergies to neomycin or gelatin.);

• had an allergic reaction to any other vaccine;

• are pregnant or plan to become pregnant within the next three months;

• are breast-feeding;

• have or have had a low blood platelet count;

• are allergic to eggs.

How is M-M-R II given?

M-M-R II is given as a shot to people one year old or older. The dose of the vaccine is the same for everyone. If your child gets the shot when he or she is one year old or older, a second dose is recommended. Often, the second dose is given right before the child goes to elementary school (4 to 6 years of age). If your child is less than one year old when he or she first gets the shot, a second dose should be given when they are 12 to 15 months old. Then, a third dose should be given between 4 and 6 years of age. Your doctor will decide the best time and number of shots by using official recommendations.

If a dose is missed, your health care provider will let you know when you should have it.

Non-pregnant adolescent and adult females of childbearing age who are susceptible to rubella can be vaccinated with M-M-R II (or live attenuated rubella virus vaccine) if certain precautions are taken. In many cases, it is convenient to give the vaccine to women at risk for rubella right after they give birth.

What are the possible side effects of M-M-R II?

The most common side effect of vaccination with M-M-R II is burning and/or stinging at the site of the shot for a short time.

Other side effects may include:
• Fever
• Rash

Less common side effects may also include:
• Swelling of the testicles
• Joint pain and/or swelling

Some side effects are rare but may be serious. You should call your health care provider if you notice any of the following problems:

• Difficulty breathing, wheezing, hives, or a skin rash may be signs of an allergic reaction.

• Bleeding or bruising under the skin.

• Seizures, a severe headache, a change in behavior or consciousness, or difficulty walking.

Other side effects may also occur. Your doctor has a more complete list of side effects for M-M-R II.

Contact your doctor or health care provider if you or your child have any new or unusual symptoms after receiving M-M-R II.

You may also report any adverse reactions to your doctor or your child's health care provider or submit a report directly to the Vaccine Adverse Event Reporting System (VAERS). The VAERS toll-free number is 1-800-822-7967 or you may report online to www.vaers.hhs.gov.

What are the ingredients of M-M-R II?
Active Ingredients: weakened forms of the measles, mumps, and rubella viruses.
Inactive Ingredients: sorbitol, sodium phosphate, potassium phosphate, sucrose, sodium chloride, hydrolyzed gelatin, recombinant human albumin, fetal bovine serum, other buffer and media ingredients, neomycin.

What else should I know about M-M-R II?
If you get M-M-R II while you are pregnant, please call 1-800-986-8999. Or, you can have your health care provider call.

This leaflet summarizes important information about M-M-R II.

If you would like more information, talk to your health care provider or call 1-800-622-4477.

Dist. by: Merck Sharp & Dohme Corp., a subsidiary of **MERCK & CO., INC.**, Whitehouse Station, NJ 08889, USA
For patent information: www.merck.com/product/patent/home.html
Copyright © 2009 Merck Sharp & Dohme Corp., a subsidiary of **Merck & Co., Inc.**
All rights reserved.
Revised: 06/2014
usppi-v205c-i-1406r204
Rx Only

NASONEX®   ℞
[nā-sō-něks]
(mometasone furoate monohydrate)
Nasal Spray, 50 mcg†

HIGHLIGHTS OF PRESCRIBING INFORMATION
These highlights do not include all the information needed to use NASONEX safely and effectively. See full prescribing information for NASONEX.
NASONEX® (mometasone furoate monohydrate)
Nasal Spray, 50 mcg†
†calculated on the anhydrous basis
Initial U.S. Approval: 1997

————————INDICATIONS AND USAGE————————
NASONEX is a corticosteroid indicated for:
1. Treatment of Nasal Symptoms of Allergic Rhinitis in patients ≥2 years of age (1.1)
2. Treatment of Nasal Congestion Associated with Seasonal Allergic Rhinitis in patients ≥2 years of age (1.2)
3. Prophylaxis of Seasonal Allergic Rhinitis in patients ≥12 years of age (1.3)
4. Treatment of Nasal Polyps in patients ≥18 years of age (1.4)

————————DOSAGE AND ADMINISTRATION————————
For Intranasal Use Only
• Treatment of Nasal Symptoms of Allergic Rhinitis (2.1)
Adults & Adolescents (12 yrs. and older): 2 sprays in each nostril once daily
Children (2-11 yrs.): 1 spray in each nostril once daily
• Treatment of Nasal Congestion Associated with Seasonal Allergic Rhinitis (2.2)
Adults & Adolescents (12 yrs. and older): 2 sprays in each nostril once daily
Children (2-11 yrs.): 1 spray in each nostril once daily
• Prophylaxis of Seasonal Allergic Rhinitis (2.3)
Adults & Adolescents (12 yrs. and older): 2 sprays in each nostril once daily
• Treatment of Nasal Polyps (2.4)
Adults (18 yrs. and older): 2 sprays in each nostril twice daily. 2 sprays in each nostril once daily may also be effective in some patients.

————————DOSAGE FORMS AND STRENGTHS————————
Nasal Spray: 50 mcg of mometasone furoate in each 100-microliter spray (3)

————————CONTRAINDICATIONS————————
Patients with known hypersensitivity to mometasone furoate or any of the ingredients of NASONEX. (4)

————————WARNINGS AND PRECAUTIONS————————
• Epistaxis, nasal ulceration, *Candida albicans* infection, nasal septal perforation, impaired wound healing. Monitor patients periodically for signs of adverse effects on the nasal mucosa. Avoid use in patients with recent nasal ulcers, nasal surgery, or nasal trauma. (5.1)

• Development of glaucoma or cataracts. Monitor patients closely with a change in vision or with a history of increased intraocular pressure, glaucoma, and/or cataracts. (5.2)
• Potential worsening of existing tuberculosis; fungal, bacterial, viral, or parasitic infections; or ocular herpes simplex. More serious or even fatal course of chickenpox or measles in susceptible patients. Use caution in patients with the above because of the potential for worsening of these infections. (5.4)
• Hypercorticism and adrenal suppression with higher than recommended dosages or at the regular dosage in susceptible individuals. If such changes occur, discontinue NASONEX Nasal Spray slowly. (5.5)
• Potential reduction in growth velocity in children. Monitor growth routinely in pediatric patients receiving NASONEX Nasal Spray. (5.6, 8.4)

————————ADVERSE REACTIONS————————
The most common adverse reactions (≥5%) included headache, viral infection, pharyngitis, epistaxis and cough. (6)
To report SUSPECTED ADVERSE REACTIONS, contact Merck Sharp & Dohme Corp., a subsidiary of Merck & Co., Inc., at 1-877-888-4231 or FDA at 1-800-FDA-1088 or www.fda.gov/medwatch.
See 17 for PATIENT COUNSELING INFORMATION and FDA-approved patient labeling

Revised: 03/2013

FULL PRESCRIBING INFORMATION: CONTENTS*

* Sections or subsections omitted from the full prescribing information are not listed

FULL PRESCRIBING INFORMATION

1   INDICATIONS AND USAGE
1.1   Treatment of Allergic Rhinitis
NASONEX® Nasal Spray 50 mcg is indicated for the treatment of the nasal symptoms of seasonal allergic and perennial allergic rhinitis, in adults and pediatric patients 2 years of age and older.

1.2   Treatment of Nasal Congestion Associated with Seasonal Allergic Rhinitis
NASONEX Nasal Spray 50 mcg is indicated for the relief of nasal congestion associated with seasonal allergic rhinitis, in adults and pediatric patients 2 years of age and older.
1.3   Prophylaxis of Seasonal Allergic Rhinitis
NASONEX Nasal Spray 50 mcg is indicated for the prophylaxis of the nasal symptoms of seasonal allergic rhinitis in adult and adolescent patients 12 years of age and older.
1.4   Treatment of Nasal Polyps
NASONEX Nasal Spray 50 mcg is indicated for the treatment of nasal polyps in patients 18 years of age and older.

2   DOSAGE AND ADMINISTRATION
Administer NASONEX Nasal Spray 50 mcg by the intranasal route only. Prior to initial use of NASONEX Nasal Spray, 50 mcg, the pump must be primed by actuating ten times or until a fine spray appears. The pump may be stored unused for up to 1 week without repriming. If unused for more than 1 week, reprime by actuating two times, or until a fine spray appears.

2.1   Treatment of Allergic Rhinitis
Adults and Adolescents 12 Years of Age and Older:
The recommended dose for treatment of the nasal symptoms of seasonal allergic and perennial allergic rhinitis is 2 sprays (50 mcg of mometasone furoate in each spray) in each nostril once daily (total daily dose of 200 mcg).
Children 2 to 11 Years of Age:
The recommended dose for treatment of the nasal symptoms of seasonal allergic and perennial allergic rhinitis is 1 spray (50 mcg of mometasone furoate in each spray) in each nostril once daily (total daily dose of 100 mcg).
2.2   Treatment of Nasal Congestion Associated with Seasonal Allergic Rhinitis
Adults and Adolescents 12 Years of Age and Older:
The recommended dose for treatment of nasal congestion associated with seasonal allergic rhinitis is two sprays (50 mcg of mometasone furoate in each spray) in each nostril once daily (total daily dose of 200 mcg).
Children 2 to 11 Years of Age:
The recommended dose for treatment of nasal congestion associated with seasonal allergic rhinitis is one spray (50 mcg of mometasone furoate in each spray) in each nostril once daily (total daily dose of 100 mcg).
2.3   Prophylaxis of Seasonal Allergic Rhinitis
Adults and Adolescents 12 Years of Age and Older:
The recommended dose for prophylaxis treatment of nasal symptoms of seasonal allergic rhinitis is 2 sprays (50 mcg of mometasone furoate in each spray) in each nostril once daily (total daily dose of 200 mcg).
In patients with a known seasonal allergen that precipitates nasal symptoms of seasonal allergic rhinitis, prophylaxis with NASONEX Nasal Spray 50 mcg (200 mcg/day) is recommended 2 to 4 weeks prior to the anticipated start of the pollen season.
2.4   Treatment of Nasal Polyps
Adults 18 Years of Age and Older:
The recommended dose for the treatment of nasal polyps is 2 sprays (50 mcg of mometasone furoate in each spray) in each nostril twice daily (total daily dose of 400 mcg). A dose of 2 sprays (50 mcg of mometasone furoate in each spray) in each nostril once daily (total daily dose of 200 mcg) is also effective in some patients.

3   DOSAGE FORMS AND STRENGTHS
NASONEX Nasal Spray 50 mcg is a metered-dose, manual pump spray unit containing an aqueous suspension of mometasone furoate monohydrate equivalent to 0.05% w/w mometasone furoate calculated on the anhydrous basis.
After initial priming (10 actuations), each actuation of the pump delivers a metered spray containing 100 mg or 100 microliter of suspension containing mometasone furoate monohydrate equivalent to 50 mcg of mometasone furoate calculated on the anhydrous basis. Each bottle of NASONEX Nasal Spray 50 mcg provides 120 sprays.

4   CONTRAINDICATIONS
NASONEX Nasal Spray is contraindicated in patients with known hypersensitivity to mometasone furoate or any of its ingredients.

5   WARNINGS AND PRECAUTIONS
5.1   Local Nasal Effects
Epistaxis
In clinical studies, epistaxis was observed more frequently in patients with allergic rhinitis with NASONEX Nasal Spray than those who received placebo [see Adverse Reactions (6)].
Candida Infection
In clinical studies with NASONEX Nasal Spray 50 mcg, the development of localized infections of the nose and pharynx with *Candida albicans* has occurred. When such an infection develops, use of NASONEX Nasal Spray 50 mcg should be discontinued and appropriate local or systemic therapy instituted, if needed.

Nasal Septum Perforation
Instances of nasal septum perforation have been reported following the intranasal application of corticosteroids. As with any long-term topical treatment of the nasal cavity, patients using NASONEX Nasal Spray 50 mcg over several months or longer should be examined periodically for possible changes in the nasal mucosa.

Impaired Wound Healing
Because of the inhibitory effect of corticosteroids on wound healing, patients who have experienced recent nasal septum ulcers, nasal surgery, or nasal trauma should not use a nasal corticosteroid until healing has occurred.

5.2   Glaucoma and Cataracts
Nasal and inhaled corticosteroids may result in the development of glaucoma and/or cataracts. Therefore, close monitoring is warranted in patients with a change in vision or with a history of increased intraocular pressure, glaucoma, and/or cataracts.

Glaucoma and cataract formation was evaluated in one controlled study of 12 weeks' duration and one uncontrolled study of 12 months' duration in patients treated with NASONEX Nasal Spray, 50 mcg at 200 mcg/day, using intraocular pressure measurements and slit lamp examination. No significant change from baseline was noted in the mean intraocular pressure measurements for the 141 NASONEX-treated patients in the 12-week study, as compared with 141 placebo-treated patients. No individual NASONEX-treated patient was noted to have developed a significant elevation in intraocular pressure or cataracts in this 12-week study. Likewise, no significant change from baseline was noted in the mean intraocular pressure measurements for the 139 NASONEX-treated patients in the 12-month study and again, no cataracts were detected in these patients. Nonetheless, nasal and inhaled corticosteroids have been associated with the development of glaucoma and/or cataracts.

5.3   Hypersensitivity Reactions
Hypersensitivity reactions including instances of wheezing may occur after the intranasal administration of mometasone furoate monohydrate. Discontinue NASONEX Nasal Spray if such reactions occur [see Contraindications (4)].

5.4   Immunosuppression
Persons who are on drugs which suppress the immune system are more susceptible to infections than healthy individuals. Chickenpox and measles, for example, can have a more serious or even fatal course in nonimmune children or adults on corticosteroids. In such children or adults who have not had these diseases, particular care should be taken to avoid exposure. How the dose, route, and duration of corticosteroid administration affect the risk of developing a disseminated infection is not known. The contribution of the underlying disease and/or prior corticosteroid treatment to the risk is also not known. If exposed to chickenpox, prophylaxis with varicella zoster immune globin (VZIG) may be indicated. If exposed to measles, prophylaxis with pooled intramuscular immunoglobulin (IG) may be indicated. (See the respective package inserts for complete VZIG and IG prescribing information.) If chickenpox develops, treatment with antiviral agents may be considered.

Corticosteroids should be used with caution, if at all, in patients with active or quiescent tuberculous infection of the respiratory tract, or in untreated fungal, bacterial, systemic viral infections, or ocular herpes simplex because of the potential for worsening of these infections.

5.5   Hypothalamic-Pituitary-Adrenal Axis Effect
Hypercorticism and Adrenal Suppression
When intranasal steroids are used at higher than recommended dosages or in susceptible individuals at recommended dosages, systemic corticosteroid effects such as hypercorticism and adrenal suppression may appear. If such changes occur, the dosage of NASONEX Nasal Spray should be discontinued slowly, consistent with accepted procedures for discontinuing oral corticosteroid therapy.

5.6   Effect on Growth
Corticosteroids may cause a reduction in growth velocity when administered to pediatric patients. Monitor the growth routinely of pediatric patients receiving NASONEX Nasal Spray. To minimize the systemic effects of intranasal corticosteroids, including NASONEX Nasal Spray, titrate each patient's dose to the lowest dosage that effectively controls his/her symptoms [see Use in Specific Populations (8.4)].

6   ADVERSE REACTIONS
Systemic and local corticosteroid use may result in the following:
- Epistaxis, ulcerations, Candida albicans infection, impaired wound healing [see Warnings and Precautions (5.1)]
- Cataracts and glaucoma [see Warnings and Precautions (5.2)]
- Immunosuppression [see Warnings and Precautions (5.4)]
- Hypothalamic-pituitary-adrenal (HPA) axis effects, including growth reduction [see Warnings and Precautions (5.5, 5.6), Use in Specific Populations (8.4)]

6.1   Clinical Trials Experience
Because clinical trials are conducted under widely varying conditions, adverse reaction rates observed in the clinical trials of a drug cannot be directly compared to rates in the clinical trials of another drug and may not reflect the rates observed in practice.

Allergic Rhinitis
Adults and adolescents 12 years of age and older
In controlled US and international clinical studies, a total of 3210 adult and adolescent patients 12 years and older with allergic rhinitis received treatment with NASONEX Nasal Spray 50 mcg at doses of 50 to 800 mcg/day. The majority of patients (n=2103) were treated with 200 mcg/day. A total of 350 adult and adolescent patients have been treated for one year or longer. Adverse events did not differ significantly based on age, sex, or race. Four percent or less of patients in clinical trials discontinued treatment because of adverse events and the discontinuation rate was similar for the vehicle and active comparators.

All adverse events (regardless of relationship to treatment) reported by 5% or more of adult and adolescent patients ages 12 years and older who received NASONEX Nasal Spray 50 mcg, 200 mcg/day vs. placebo and that were more common with NASONEX Nasal Spray 50 mcg than placebo, are displayed in TABLE 1 below.

TABLE 1: ADULT AND ADOLESCENT PATIENTS 12 YEARS AND OLDER – ADVERSE EVENTS FROM CONTROLLED CLINICAL TRIALS IN SEASONAL ALLERGIC AND PERENNIAL ALLERGIC RHINITIS (PERCENT OF PATIENTS REPORTING)

	NASONEX 200 mcg (n=2103)	VEHICLE PLACEBO (n=1671)
Headache	26	22
Viral Infection	14	11
Pharyngitis	12	10
Epistaxis/Blood-Tinged Mucus	11	6
Coughing	7	6
Upper Respiratory Tract Infection	6	2
Dysmenorrhea	5	3
Musculoskeletal Pain	5	3
Sinusitis	5	3

Other adverse events which occurred in less than 5% but greater than or equal to 2% of adult and adolescent patients (ages 12 years and older) treated with NASONEX Nasal Spray 50 mcg, 200-mcg/day (regardless of relationship to treatment), and more frequently than in the placebo group included: arthralgia, asthma, bronchitis, chest pain, conjunctivitis, diarrhea, dyspepsia, earache, flu-like symptoms, myalgia, nausea, and rhinitis.

Pediatric patients <12 years of age
In controlled US and international studies, a total of 990 pediatric patients (ages 3 to 11 years) with allergic rhinitis received treatment with NASONEX Nasal Spray 50 mcg, at doses of 25 to 200 mcg/day. The majority of pediatric patients (n=720) were treated with 100 mcg/day. A total of 163 pediatric patients have been treated for one year or longer. Two percent or less of patients in clinical trials who received NASONEX Nasal Spray 50 mcg discontinued treatment because of adverse events and the discontinuation rate was similar for the placebo and active comparators.

Adverse events which occurred in ≥5% of pediatric patients (ages 3 to 11 years) treated with NASONEX Nasal Spray 50 mcg, 100 mcg/day vs. placebo (regardless of relationship to treatment) and more frequently than in the placebo group included upper respiratory tract infection (5% in NASONEX Nasal Spray 50 mcg group vs. 4% in placebo) and vomiting (5% in NASONEX Nasal Spray 50 mcg group vs. 4% in placebo).

Other adverse events which occurred in less than 5% but greater than or equal to 2% of pediatric patients (ages 3 to 11 years) treated with NASONEX Nasal Spray 50 mcg, 100 mcg/day vs. placebo (regardless of relationship to treatment) and more frequently than in the placebo group included: diarrhea, nasal irritation, otitis media, and wheezing.

The adverse event (regardless of relationship to treatment) reported by 5% of pediatric patients ages 2 to 5 years who received NASONEX Nasal Spray, 50 mcg, 100 mcg/day in a clinical trial vs. placebo including 56 subjects (28 each NASONEX Nasal Spray, 50 mcg and placebo) and that was more common with NASONEX Nasal Spray, 50 mcg than placebo, included: upper respiratory tract infection (7% vs. 0%, respectively). The other adverse event which occurred in less than 5% but greater than or equal to 2% of mometasone furoate pediatric patients ages 2 to 5 years treated with 100 mcg doses vs. placebo (regardless of relationship to treatment) and more frequently than in the placebo group included: skin trauma.

Nasal Polyps
Adults 18 years of age and older
In controlled clinical studies, the types of adverse events observed in patients with nasal polyps were similar to those observed for patients with allergic rhinitis. A total of 594 adult patients (ages 18 to 86 years) received NASONEX Nasal Spray 50 mcg at doses of 200 mcg once or twice daily for up to 4 months of treatment of nasal polyps. The overall incidence of adverse events for patients treated with NASONEX Nasal Spray 50 mcg was comparable to patients with the placebo except for epistaxis, which was 9% for 200 mcg once daily, 13% for 200 mcg twice daily, and 5% for the placebo.

Nasal ulcers and nasal and oral candidiasis were also reported in patients treated with NASONEX Nasal Spray 50 mcg primarily in patients treated for longer than 4 weeks.

Nasal Congestion Associated with Seasonal Allergic Rhinitis
A total of 1008 patients aged 12 years and older received NASONEX Nasal Spray 50 mcg 200 mcg/day (n=506) or placebo (n=502) for 15 days. Adverse events that occurred more frequently in patients treated with NASONEX Nasal Spray 50 mcg than in patients with the placebo included sinus headache (1.2% in NASONEX Nasal Spray 50 mcg group vs. 0.2% in placebo) and epistaxis (1% in NASONEX Nasal Spray 50 mcg group vs. 0.2% in placebo) and the overall adverse event profile was similar to that observed in the other allergic rhinitis trials.

6.2   Post-Marketing Experience
The following adverse reactions have been identified during the post-marketing period for NASONEX Nasal Spray 50 mcg: nasal burning and irritation, anaphylaxis and angioedema, disturbances in taste and smell and nasal septal perforation. Because these reactions are reported voluntarily from a population of uncertain size, it is not always possible to reliably estimate their frequency or establish a causal relationship to drug exposure.

7   DRUG INTERACTIONS
No formal drug-drug interaction studies have been conducted with NASONEX Nasal Spray 50 mcg.

Inhibitors of Cytochrome P450 3A4: Studies have shown that mometasone furoate is primarily and extensively metabolized in the liver of all species investigated and undergoes extensive metabolism to multiple metabolites. *In vitro* studies have confirmed the primary role of cytochrome CYP 3A4 in the metabolism of this compound. Coadministration with ketoconazole, a potent CYP 3A4 inhibitor, may increase the plasma concentrations of mometasone furoate [see Clinical Pharmacology (12.3)].

8   USE IN SPECIFIC POPULATIONS
8.1   Pregnancy
Teratogenic Effects: Pregnancy Category C: There are no adequate and well-controlled studies in pregnant women. NASONEX Nasal Spray 50 mcg, like other corticosteroids, should be used during pregnancy only if the potential benefits justify the potential risk to the fetus. Experience with oral corticosteroids since their introduction in pharmacologic, as opposed to physiologic, doses suggests that rodents are more prone to teratogenic effects from corticosteroids than humans. In addition, because there is a natural increase in corticosteroid production during pregnancy, most women will require a lower exogenous corticosteroid dose and many will not need corticosteroid treatment during pregnancy.

In mice, mometasone furoate caused cleft palate at subcutaneous doses (less than the MRDID in adults on a mcg/m^2 basis). Fetal survival was reduced at approximately 2 times the MRDID in adults on a mcg/m^2 basis. No toxicity was observed at less than the MRDID in adults on a mcg/m^2 basis.

In rats, mometasone furoate produced umbilical hernia at topical dermal doses approximately 10 times the MRDID in adults on a mcg/m^2 basis. A topical dermal dose approximately 6 times the MRDID in adults on a mcg/m^2 basis produced delays in ossification, but no malformations.

In rabbits, mometasone furoate caused multiple malformations (e.g., flexed front paws, gallbladder agenesis, umbilical hernia, and hydrocephaly) at topical dermal doses approximately 6 times the MRDID in adults on a mcg/m^2 basis. In an oral study, mometasone furoate increased resorptions and caused cleft palate and/or head malformations (hydrocephaly or domed head) at approximately 30 times the

MRDID in adults on a mcg/m² basis. At approximately 110 times the MRDID in adults on a mcg/m² basis, most litters were aborted or resorbed. No toxicity was observed at approximately 6 times the MRDID in adults on a mcg/m² basis.

When rats received subcutaneous doses of mometasone furoate throughout pregnancy or during the later stages of pregnancy, a dose less than the MRDID in adults on a mcg/m² basis caused prolonged and difficult labor and reduced the number of live births, birth weight, and early pup survival.

Nonteratogenic Effects: Hypoadrenalism may occur in infants born to women receiving corticosteroids during pregnancy. Such infants should be carefully monitored.

8.3 Nursing Mothers

It is not known if mometasone furoate is excreted in human milk. Because other corticosteroids are excreted in human milk, caution should be used when NASONEX Nasal Spray, 50 mcg is administered to nursing women.

8.4 Pediatric Use

The safety and effectiveness of NASONEX Nasal Spray 50 mcg for allergic rhinitis in children 12 years of age and older have been established [see Adverse Reactions (6.1) and Clinical Studies (14.1)]. Use of NASONEX Nasal Spray 50 mcg for allergic rhinitis in pediatric patients 2 to 11 years of age is supported by safety and efficacy data from clinical studies. Seven hundred and twenty (720) patients 3 to 11 years of age with allergic rhinitis were treated with mometasone furoate nasal spray 50 mcg (100 mcg total daily dose) in controlled clinical trials [see Adverse Reactions (6.1) and Clinical Studies (14.2)]. Twenty-eight (28) patients 2 to 5 years of age with allergic rhinitis were treated with mometasone furoate nasal spray 50 mcg (100 mcg total daily dose) in a controlled trial to evaluate safety [see Adverse Reactions (6.1)]. Safety and effectiveness of NASONEX Nasal Spray 50 mcg for allergic rhinitis in children less than 2 years of age have not been established. The safety and effectiveness of NASONEX Nasal Spray for the treatment of nasal polyps in children less than 18 years of age have not been established. One 4-month trial was conducted to evaluate the safety and efficacy of NASONEX in the treatment of nasal polyps in pediatric patients 6 to 17 years of age. The primary objective of the study was to evaluate safety; efficacy parameters were collected as secondary endpoints. A total of 127 patients with nasal polyps were randomized to placebo or NASONEX Nasal Spray 100 mcg once or twice daily (patients 6 to 11 years of age) or 200 mcg once or twice daily (patients 12 to 17 years of age). The results of this trial did not support the efficacy of NASONEX Nasal Spray in the treatment of nasal polyps in pediatric patients. The adverse events reported in this trial were similar to the adverse events reported in patients 18 years of age and older with nasal polyps.

Controlled clinical studies have shown intranasal corticosteroids may cause a reduction in growth velocity in pediatric patients. This effect has been observed in the absence of laboratory evidence of hypothalamic-pituitary-adrenal (HPA) axis suppression, suggesting that growth velocity is a more sensitive indicator of systemic corticosteroid exposure in pediatric patients than some commonly used tests of HPA axis function. The long-term effects of this reduction in growth velocity associated with intranasal corticosteroids, including the impact on final adult height, are unknown. The potential for "catch up" growth following discontinuation of treatment with intranasal corticosteroids has not been adequately studied. The growth of pediatric patients receiving intranasal corticosteroids, including NASONEX Nasal Spray, 50 mcg, should be monitored routinely (e.g., via stadiometry). The potential growth effects of prolonged treatment should be weighed against clinical benefits obtained and the availability of safe and effective noncorticosteroid treatment alternatives. To minimize the systemic effects of intranasal corticosteroids, including NASONEX Nasal Spray, 50 mcg, each patient should be titrated to his/her lowest effective dose.

A clinical study to assess the effect of NASONEX Nasal Spray 50 mcg (100 mcg total daily dose) on growth velocity has been conducted in pediatric patients 3 to 9 years of age with allergic rhinitis. No statistically significant effect on growth velocity was observed for NASONEX Nasal Spray 50 mcg compared to placebo following one year of treatment. No evidence of clinically relevant HPA axis suppression was observed following a 30-minute cosyntropin infusion.

The potential of NASONEX Nasal Spray 50 mcg to cause growth suppression in susceptible patients or when given at higher doses cannot be ruled out.

8.5 Geriatric Use

A total of 280 patients above 64 years of age with allergic rhinitis or nasal polyps (age range 64 to 86 years) have been treated with NASONEX Nasal Spray 50 mcg for up to 3 or 4 months, respectively. The adverse reactions reported in this population were similar in type and incidence to those reported by younger patients.

8.6 Hepatic Impairment

Concentrations of mometasone furoate appear to increase with severity of hepatic impairment [see Clinical Pharmacology (12.3)].

10 OVERDOSAGE

There are no data available on the effects of acute or chronic overdosage with NASONEX Nasal Spray 50 mcg. Because of low systemic bioavailability, and an absence of acute drug-related systemic findings in clinical studies, overdose is unlikely to require any therapy other than observation. Intranasal administration of 1600 mcg (4 times the recommended dose of NASONEX Nasal Spray 50 mcg for the treatment of nasal polyps in patients 18 years of age and older) daily for 29 days, to healthy human volunteers, showed no increased incidence of adverse events. Single intranasal doses up to 4000 mcg and oral inhalation doses up to 8000 mcg have been studied in human volunteers with no adverse effects reported. Chronic over dosage with any corticosteroid may result in signs or symptoms of hypercorticism [see Warnings and Precautions (5.4)]. Acute overdosage with this dosage form is unlikely since one bottle of NASONEX Nasal Spray 50 mcg contains approximately 8500 mcg of mometasone furoate.

11 DESCRIPTION

Mometasone furoate monohydrate, the active component of NASONEX Nasal Spray, 50 mcg, is an anti-inflammatory corticosteroid having the chemical name, 9,21-Dichloro-11β,17-dihydroxy-16α-methylpregna-1,4-diene-3,20-dione 17-(2 furoate) monohydrate, and the following chemical structure:

Mometasone furoate monohydrate is a white powder, with an empirical formula of $C_{27}H_{30}Cl_2O_6 \cdot H_2O$, and a molecular weight of 539.45. It is practically insoluble in water; slightly soluble in methanol, ethanol, and isopropanol; soluble in acetone and chloroform; and freely soluble in tetrahydrofuran. Its partition coefficient between octanol and water is greater than 5000.

NASONEX Nasal Spray 50 mcg is a metered-dose, manual pump spray unit containing an aqueous suspension of mometasone furoate monohydrate equivalent to 0.05% w/w mometasone furoate calculated on the anhydrous basis; in an aqueous medium containing glycerin, microcrystalline cellulose and carboxymethylcellulose sodium, sodium citrate, citric acid, benzalkonium chloride, and polysorbate 80. The pH is between 4.3 and 4.9.

12 CLINICAL PHARMACOLOGY

12.1 Mechanism of Action

NASONEX Nasal Spray 50 mcg is a corticosteroid demonstrating potent anti-inflammatory properties. The precise mechanism of corticosteroid action on allergic rhinitis is not known. Corticosteroids have been shown to have a wide range of effects on multiple cell types (e.g., mast cells, eosinophils, neutrophils, macrophages, and lymphocytes) and mediators (e.g., histamine, eicosanoids, leukotrienes, and cytokines) involved in inflammation.

In two clinical studies utilizing nasal antigen challenge, NASONEX Nasal Spray, 50 mcg decreased some markers of the early- and late-phase allergic response. These observations included decreases (vs. placebo) in histamine and eosinophil cationic protein levels, and reductions (vs. baseline) in eosinophils, neutrophils, and epithelial cell adhesion proteins. The clinical significance of these findings is not known.

The effect of NASONEX Nasal Spray, 50 mcg on nasal mucosa following 12 months of treatment was examined in 46 patients with allergic rhinitis. There was no evidence of atrophy and there was a marked reduction in intraepithelial eosinophilia and inflammatory cell infiltration (e.g., eosinophils, lymphocytes, monocytes, neutrophils, and plasma cells).

12.2 Pharmacodynamics

Adrenal Function in Adults: Four clinical pharmacology studies have been conducted in humans to assess the effect of NASONEX Nasal Spray, 50 mcg at various doses on adrenal function. In one study, daily doses of 200 and 400 mcg of NASONEX Nasal Spray, 50 mcg and 10 mg of prednisone were compared to placebo in 64 patients (22 to 44 years of age) with allergic rhinitis. Adrenal function before and after 36 consecutive days of treatment was assessed by measuring plasma cortisol levels following a 6-hour Cortrosyn (ACTH) infusion and by measuring 24-hour urinary free cortisol levels. NASONEX Nasal Spray, 50 mcg, at both the

200- and 400-mcg dose, was not associated with a statistically significant decrease in mean plasma cortisol levels post-Cortrosyn infusion or a statistically significant decrease in the 24-hour urinary free cortisol levels compared to placebo. A statistically significant decrease in the mean plasma cortisol levels post-Cortrosyn infusion and 24-hour urinary free cortisol levels was detected in the prednisone treatment group compared to placebo.

A second study assessed adrenal response to NASONEX Nasal Spray, 50 mcg (400 and 1600 mcg/day), prednisone (10 mg/day), and placebo, administered for 29 days in 48 male volunteers (21 to 40 years of age). The 24-hour plasma cortisol area under the curve (AUC_{0-24}), during and after an 8-hour Cortrosyn infusion and 24-hour urinary free cortisol levels were determined at baseline and after 29 days of treatment. No statistically significant differences in adrenal function were observed with NASONEX Nasal Spray, 50 mcg compared to placebo.

A third study evaluated single, rising doses of NASONEX Nasal Spray, 50 mcg (1000, 2000, and 4000 mcg/day), orally administered mometasone furoate (2000, 4000, and 8000 mcg/day), orally administered dexamethasone (200, 400, and 800 mcg/day), and placebo (administered at the end of each series of doses) in 24 male volunteers (22 to 39 years of age). Dose administrations were separated by at least 72 hours. Determination of serial plasma cortisol levels at 8 AM and for the 24-hour period following each treatment were used to calculate the plasma cortisol area under the curve (AUC_{0-24}). In addition, 24-hour urinary free cortisol levels were collected prior to initial treatment administration and during the period immediately following each dose. No statistically significant decreases in the plasma cortisol AUC, 8 AM cortisol levels, or 24-hour urinary free cortisol levels were observed in volunteers treated with either NASONEX Nasal Spray, 50 mcg or oral mometasone, as compared with placebo treatment. Conversely, nearly all volunteers treated with the three doses of dexamethasone demonstrated abnormal 8 AM cortisol levels (defined as a cortisol level <10 mcg/dL), reduced 24-hour plasma AUC values, and decreased 24-hour urinary free cortisol levels, as compared to placebo treatment.

In a fourth study, adrenal function was assessed in 213 patients (18 to 81 years of age) with nasal polyps before and after 4 months of treatment with either NASONEX Nasal Spray, 50 mcg, (200 mcg once or twice daily) or placebo by measuring 24-hour urinary free cortisol levels. NASONEX Nasal Spray, 50 mcg, at both doses (200 and 400 mcg/day), was not associated with statistically significant decreases in the 24-hour urinary free cortisol levels compared to placebo.

Three clinical pharmacology studies have been conducted in pediatric patients to assess the effect of mometasone furoate nasal spray on the adrenal function at daily doses of 50, 100, and 200 mcg vs. placebo. In one study, adrenal function before and after 7 consecutive days of treatment was assessed in 48 pediatric patients with allergic rhinitis (ages 6 to 11 years) by measuring morning plasma cortisol and 24-hour urinary free cortisol levels. Mometasone furoate nasal spray, at all three doses, was not associated with a statistically significant decrease in mean plasma cortisol levels or a statistically significant decrease in the 24-hour urinary free cortisol levels compared to placebo. In the second study, adrenal function before and after 14 consecutive days of treatment was assessed in 48 pediatric patients (ages 3 to 5 years) with allergic rhinitis by measuring plasma cortisol levels following a 30-minute Cortrosyn infusion. Mometasone furoate nasal spray, 50 mcg, at all three doses (50, 100, and 200 mcg/day), was not associated with a statistically significant decrease in mean plasma cortisol levels post-Cortrosyn infusion compared to placebo. All patients had a normal response to Cortrosyn. In the third study, adrenal function before and after up to 42 consecutive days of once-daily treatment was assessed in 52 patients with allergic rhinitis (ages 2 to 5 years), 28 of whom received mometasone furoate nasal spray, 50 mcg per nostril (total daily dose 100 mcg), by measuring morning plasma cortisol and 24-hour urinary free cortisol levels. Mometasone furoate nasal spray was not associated with a statistically significant decrease in mean plasma cortisol levels or a statistically significant decrease in the 24-hour urinary free cortisol levels compared to placebo.

12.3 Pharmacokinetics

Absorption:
Mometasone furoate monohydrate administered as a nasal spray suspension has very low bioavailability (<1%) in plasma using a sensitive assay with a lower quantitation limit (LOQ) of 0.25 pcg/mL.

Distribution:
The in vitro protein binding for mometasone furoate was reported to be 98% to 99% in concentration range of 5 to 500 ng/mL.

Metabolism:
Studies have shown that any portion of a mometasone furoate dose which is swallowed and absorbed undergoes extensive metabolism to multiple metabolites. There are no

major metabolites detectable in plasma. Upon *in vitro* incubation, one of the minor metabolites formed is 6ß-hydroxy-mometasone furoate. In human liver microsomes, formation of the metabolite is regulated by cytochrome P-450 3A4 (CYP3A4).

Elimination:

Following intravenous administration, the effective plasma elimination half-life of mometasone furoate is 5.8 hours. Any absorbed drug is excreted as metabolites mostly via the bile, and to a limited extent, into the urine.

Specific Populations:

Hepatic Impairment: Administration of a single inhaled dose of 400 mcg mometasone furoate to subjects with mild (n=4), moderate (n=4), and severe (n=4) hepatic impairment resulted in only 1 or 2 subjects in each group having detectable peak plasma concentrations of mometasone furoate (ranging from 50 to 105 pcg/mL). The observed peak plasma concentrations appear to increase with severity of hepatic impairment, however, the numbers of detectable levels were few.

Renal Impairment: The effects of renal impairment on mometasone furoate pharmacokinetics have not been adequately investigated.

Pediatric: Mometasone furoate pharmacokinetics have not been investigated in the pediatric population *[see Use in Specific Populations (8.4)].*

Gender: The effects of gender on mometasone furoate pharmacokinetics have not been adequately investigated.

Race: The effects of race on mometasone furoate pharmacokinetics have not been adequately investigated.

Drug-Drug Interactions:

Inhibitors of Cytochrome P450 3A4: In a drug interaction study, an inhaled dose of mometasone furoate 400 mcg was given to 24 healthy subjects twice daily for 9 days and ketoconazole 200 mg (as well as placebo) were given twice daily concomitantly on Days 4 to 9. Mometasone furoate plasma concentrations were <150 pcg/mL on Day 3 prior to coadministration of ketoconazole or placebo. Following concomitant administration of ketoconazole, 4 out of 12 subjects in the ketoconazole treatment group (n=12) had peak plasma concentrations of mometasone furoate >200 pcg/mL on Day 9 (211-324 pcg/mL).

13 NONCLINICAL TOXICOLOGY

13.1 Carcinogenesis, Mutagenesis, Impairment of Fertility

In a 2-year carcinogenicity study in Sprague Dawley rats, mometasone furoate demonstrated no statistically significant increase in the incidence of tumors at inhalation doses up to 67 mcg/kg (approximately 1 and 2 times the maximum recommended daily intranasal dose [MRDID] in adults [400 mcg] and children [100 mcg], respectively, on a mcg/m² basis). In a 19-month carcinogenicity study in Swiss CD-1 mice, mometasone furoate demonstrated no statistically significant increase in the incidence of tumors at inhalation doses up to 160 mcg/kg (approximately 2 times the MRDID in adults and children, respectively, on a mcg/m² basis).

Mometasone furoate increased chromosomal aberrations in an *in vitro* Chinese hamster ovary-cell assay, but did not increase chromosomal aberrations in an *in vitro* Chinese hamster lung cell assay. Mometasone furoate was not mutagenic in the Ames test or mouse-lymphoma assay, and was not clastogenic in an *in vivo* mouse micronucleus assay and a rat bone marrow chromosomal aberration assay or a mouse male germ-cell chromosomal aberration assay. Mometasone furoate also did not induce unscheduled DNA synthesis *in vivo* in rat hepatocytes.

In reproductive studies in rats, impairment of fertility was not produced by subcutaneous doses up to 15 mcg/kg (less than the MRDID in adults on a mcg/m² basis).

13.2 Animal Toxicology and/or Pharmacology

Reproduction Toxicology Studies

In mice, mometasone furoate caused cleft palate at subcutaneous doses of 60 mcg/kg and above (less than the MRDID in adults on a mcg/m² basis). Fetal survival was reduced at 180 mcg/kg (approximately 2 times the MRDID in adults on a mcg/m² basis). No toxicity was observed at 20 mcg/kg (less than the MRDID in adults on a mcg/m² basis).

In rats, mometasone furoate produced umbilical hernia at topical dermal doses of 600 mcg/kg and above (approximately 10 times the MRDID in adults on a mcg/m² basis). A dose of 300 mcg/kg (approximately 6 times the MRDID in adults on a mcg/m² basis) produced delays in ossification, but no malformations. In rabbits, mometasone furoate caused multiple malformations (e.g., flexed front paws, gallbladder agenesis, umbilical hernia, hydrocephaly) at topical dermal doses of 150 mcg/kg and above (approximately 6 times the MRDID in adults on a mcg/m² basis). In an oral study, mometasone furoate increased resorptions and caused cleft palate and/or head malformations (hydrocephaly or domed head) at 700 mcg/kg (approximately 30 times the MRDID in adults on a mcg/m² basis). At 2800 mcg/kg (approximately 110 times the MRDID in adults on a mcg/m²

basis), most litters were aborted or resorbed. No toxicity was observed at 140 mcg/kg (approximately 6 times the MRDID in adults on a mcg/m² basis).

When rats received subcutaneous doses of mometasone furoate throughout pregnancy or during the later stages of pregnancy, 15 mcg/kg (less than the MRDID in adults on a mcg/m² basis) caused prolonged and difficult labor and reduced the number of live births, birth weight, and early pup survival. Similar effects were not observed at 7.5 mcg/kg (less than the MRDID in adults on a mcg/m² basis).

14 CLINICAL STUDIES

14.1 Allergic Rhinitis in Adults and Adolescents

The efficacy and safety of NASONEX Nasal Spray, 50 mcg in the prophylaxis and treatment of seasonal allergic rhinitis and the treatment of perennial allergic rhinitis have been evaluated in 18 controlled trials, and one uncontrolled clinical trial, in approximately 3000 adults (ages 17 to 85 years) and adolescents (ages 12 to 16 years). Of the total number of patients, there were 1757 males and 1453 females, including a total of 283 adolescents (182 boys and 101 girls) with seasonal allergic or perennial allergic rhinitis. Patients were treated with NASONEX Nasal Spray 50 mcg at doses ranging from 50 to 800 mcg/day. The majority of patients were treated with 200 mcg/day. The allergic rhinitis trials evaluated the total nasal symptom scores that included stuffiness, rhinorrhea, itching, and sneezing. Patients treated with NASONEX Nasal Spray 50 mcg, 200 mcg/day had a statistically significant decrease in total nasal symptom scores compared to placebo-treated patients. No additional benefit was observed for mometasone furoate doses greater than 200 mcg/day. A total of 350 patients have been treated with NASONEX Nasal Spray 50 mcg for 1 year or longer.

In patients with seasonal allergic rhinitis, NASONEX Nasal Spray 50 mcg, demonstrated improvement in nasal symptoms (vs. placebo) within 11 hours after the first dose based on one single-dose, parallel-group study of patients in an outdoor "park" setting (park study) and one environmental exposure unit (EEU) study, and within 2 days in two randomized, double-blind, placebo-controlled, parallel-group seasonal allergic rhinitis studies. Maximum benefit is usually achieved within 1 to 2 weeks after initiation of dosing.

Prophylaxis of seasonal allergic rhinitis for patients 12 years of age and older with NASONEX Nasal Spray 50 mcg, given at a dose of 200 mcg/day, was evaluated in two clinical studies in 284 patients. These studies were designed such that patients received 4 weeks of prophylaxis with NASONEX Nasal Spray 50 mcg prior to the anticipated onset of the pollen season; however, some patients received only 2 to 3 weeks of prophylaxis. Patients receiving 2 to 4 weeks of prophylaxis with NASONEX Nasal Spray 50 mcg demonstrated a statistically significantly smaller mean increase in total nasal symptom scores with onset of the pollen season as compared to placebo patients.

TABLE 2: EFFECT OF NASONEX NASAL SPRAY IN TWO RANDOMIZED, PLACEBO-CONTROLLED TRIALS IN PATIENTS WITH NASAL POLYPS

	NASONEX 200 mcg qd	NASONEX 200 mcg bid	Placebo	P-value for NASONEX 200 mcg qd vs. placebo	P-value for NASONEX 200 mcg bid vs. placebo
Study 1	N=115	N=122	N=117		
Baseline bilateral polyp grade*	4.21	4.27	4.25		
Mean change from baseline in bilateral polyps grade	-1.15	-0.96	-0.50	<0.001	0.01
Baseline nasal congestion†	2.29	2.35	2.28		
Mean change from baseline in nasal congestion	-0.47	-0.61	-0.24	0.001	<0.001
Study 2	N=102	N=102	N=106		
Baseline bilateral polyp grade*	4.00	4.10	4.17		
Mean change from baseline in bilateral polyps grade	-0.78	-0.96	-0.62	0.33	0.04
Baseline nasal congestion†	2.23	2.20	2.18		
Mean change from baseline in nasal congestion	-0.42	-0.66	-0.23	0.01	<0.001

* polyps in each nasal fossa were graded by the investigator based on endoscopic visualization, using a scale of 0-3 where 0=no polyps; 1=polyps in the middle meatus, not reaching below the inferior border of the middle turbinate; 2=polyps reaching below the inferior border of the middle turbinate but not the inferior border of the inferior turbinate; 3=polyps reaching to or below the border of the inferior turbinate, or polyps medial to the middle turbinate (score reflects sum of left and right nasal fossa grades).

† nasal congestion/obstruction was scored daily by the patient using a 0-3 categorical scale where 0=no symptoms, 1=mild symptoms, 2=moderate symptoms and 3=severe symptoms.

14.2 Allergic Rhinitis in Pediatrics

The efficacy and safety of NASONEX Nasal Spray 50 mcg in the treatment of seasonal allergic and perennial allergic rhinitis in pediatric patients (ages 3 to 11 years) have been evaluated in four controlled trials. This included approximately 990 pediatric patients ages 3 to 11 years (606 males and 384 females) with seasonal allergic or perennial allergic rhinitis treated with mometasone furoate nasal spray at doses ranging from 25 to 200 mcg/day. Pediatric patients treated with NASONEX Nasal Spray 50 mcg (100 mcg total daily dose, 374 patients) had a significant decrease in total nasal symptom (nasal congestion, rhinorrhea, itching, and sneezing) scores, compared to placebo-treated patients. No additional benefit was observed for the 200-mcg mometasone furoate total daily dose in pediatric patients (ages 3 to 11 years). A total of 163 pediatric patients have been treated for 1 year.

14.3 Nasal Polyps in Adults 18 Years of Age and Older

Two studies were performed to evaluate the efficacy and safety of NASONEX Nasal Spray in the treatment of nasal polyps. These studies involved 664 patients with nasal polyps, 441 of whom received NASONEX Nasal Spray. These studies were randomized, double-blind, placebo-controlled, parallel-group, multicenter studies in patients 18 to 86 years of age with bilateral nasal polyps. Patients were randomized to receive NASONEX Nasal Spray 200 mcg once daily, 200 mcg twice daily or placebo for a period of 4 months. The co-primary efficacy endpoints were 1) change from baseline in nasal congestion/obstruction averaged over the first month of treatment; and 2) change from baseline to last assessment in bilateral polyp grade during the entire 4 months of treatment as assessed by endoscopy. Efficacy was demonstrated in both studies at a dose of 200 mcg twice daily and in one study at a dose of 200 mcg once a day (see TABLE 2 below).

[See table 2 above]

There were no clinically relevant differences in the effectiveness of NASONEX Nasal Spray, 50 mcg, in the studies evaluating treatment of nasal polyps across subgroups of patients defined by gender, age, or race.

14.4 Nasal Congestion Associated with Seasonal Allergic Rhinitis

The efficacy and safety of NASONEX Nasal Spray 50 mcg for nasal congestion associated with seasonal allergic rhinitis were evaluated in three randomized, placebo-controlled, double blind clinical trials of 15 days duration. The three trials included a total of 1008 patients 12 years of age and older with nasal congestion associated with seasonal allergic rhinitis, of whom 506 received NASONEX Nasal Spray 200 mcg daily and 502 received placebo. Of the 1008 patients, the majority 784 (78 %) were Caucasians. The majority of the patients were between 18 to < 65 years of age with a mean age of 38.8 years and were predominantly women (66%). The primary efficacy endpoint was the change from baseline in average morning and evening re-

TABLE 3: EFFECT OF NASONEX NASAL SPRAY IN TWO RANDOMIZED, PLACEBO-CONTROLLED TRIALS ON NASAL CONGESTION IN PATIENTS WITH SEASONAL ALLERGIC RHINITIS

Treatment (Patient Number)	Baseline * LS Mean †	Change from Baseline LS Mean †	Difference from Placebo LS Mean †	P-value for NASONEX 200 mcg qd vs. placebo
Study 1				
NASONEX 200 mcg qd (N=176)	2.63	-0.64	-0.15	0.006
Placebo (N=175)	2.62	-0.49		
Study 2				
NASONEX 200 mcg qd (N=168)	2.62	-0.71	-0.31	<0.001
Placebo (N=164)	2.60	-0.40		

* nasal congestion/obstruction was scored daily by the patient using a 0-3 categorical scale where 0=no symptoms, 1=mild symptoms, 2=moderate symptoms and 3=severe symptoms.
† LS Mean and p-value was from an ANCOVA model with treatment, baseline value, and center effects.

TABLE 4: EFFECT OF NASONEX NASAL SPRAY ON TNSS IN TWO RANDOMIZED, PLACEBO-CONTROLLED TRIALS IN PATIENTS WITH SEASONAL ALLERGIC RHINITIS

Treatment (Patient Number)	Baseline * LS Mean †	Change from Baseline LS Mean †	Difference from Placebo LS Mean †	P-value for NASONEX 200 mcg qd vs. placebo
Study 1				
NASONEX 200 mcg qd (N=176)	9.60	-2.68	-0.83	<0.001
Placebo (N=175)	9.66	-1.85		
Study 2				
NASONEX 200 mcg qd (N=168)	9.39	-3.00	-1.27	<0.001
Placebo (N=164)	9.50	-1.73		

* TNSS was the sum of four individual symptom scores: rhinorrhea, nasal congestion/stuffiness, nasal itching and sneezing. Each symptom was to be rated on a scale of 0=none, 1=mild, 2=moderate, 3=severe.
† LS Mean and p-value was from an ANCOVA model with treatment, baseline value, and center effects.

flective nasal congestion score over treatment day 1 to day 15. The key secondary efficacy endpoint was the change from baseline in average morning and evening reflective total nasal symptom score (TNSS=rhinorrhea [nasal discharge/runny nose or postnasal drip], nasal congestion/stuffiness, nasal itching, sneezing) averaged over treatment day 1 to 15. Two out of three studies demonstrated that treatment with NASONEX Nasal Spray significantly reduced the nasal congestion symptom score and the TNSS compared to placebo in patients 12 years of age and older with seasonal allergic rhinitis (see TABLE 3 and 4 below).
[See table 3 above]
[See table 4 above]
Based on results in other studies with NASONEX Nasal Spray in pediatric patients, effects on nasal congestion associated with seasonal allergic rhinitis in patients below 12 years of age is similar to those seen in adults and adolescents *[see Clinical Studies (14.2)]*.

16   HOW SUPPLIED/STORAGE AND HANDLING

NASONEX (mometasone furoate monohydrate) Nasal Spray, 50 mcg is supplied in a white, high-density, polyethylene bottle fitted with a white metered-dose, manual spray pump, and blue cap. It contains 17 g of product formulation, 120 sprays, each delivering 50 mcg of mometasone furoate per actuation.
(NDC 0085-1288-01).
Store at 25°C (77°F); excursions permitted to 15-30°C (59-86°F) [see USP Controlled Room Temperature]. Protect from light.
When NASONEX Nasal Spray, 50 mcg is removed from its cardboard container, prolonged exposure of the product to direct light should be avoided. Brief exposure to light, as with normal use, is acceptable.
SHAKE WELL BEFORE EACH USE.
Keep out of reach of children.

17   PATIENT COUNSELING INFORMATION
See FDA-approved labeling
17.1   Local Nasal Effect
Patients should be informed that treatment with NASONEX Nasal Spray 50 mcg may be associated with adverse reactions which include epistaxis (nose bleed) and nasal septum perforation. *Candida* infection may also occur. Because of the inhibitory effect of corticosteroids on wound healing, patients who have experienced recent nasal septum ulcers, nasal surgery, or nasal trauma should not use a nasal corticosteroid until healing has occurred *[see Warnings and Precautions (5.1)]*. Patients should be cautioned not to spray NASONEX Nasal Spray 50 mcg directly onto the nasal septum.
17.2   Glaucoma and Cataracts
Patients should be informed that nasal and inhaled corticosteroids may result in the development of glaucoma and/or cataracts. Therefore, close monitoring is warranted in patients with a change in vision or with a history of increased intraocular pressure, glaucoma, and/or cataracts. Patients should be cautioned not to spray NASONEX Nasal Spray 50 mcg into the eyes *[see Warnings and Precautions (5.2)]*.
17.3   Immunosuppression
Persons who are on immunosuppressant doses of corticosteroids should be warned to avoid exposure to chickenpox or measles, and patients should also be advised that if they are exposed, medical advice should be sought without delay *[see Warnings and Precautions (5.4)]*.
17.4   Use Regularly for Best Effect
Patients should use NASONEX Nasal Spray 50 mcg on a regular basis for optimal effect. Improvement in nasal symptoms of allergic rhinitis has been shown to occur within 1 to 2 days after initiation of dosing. Maximum ben-

efit is usually achieved within 1 to 2 weeks after initiation of dosing. Patients should not increase the prescribed dosage but should contact their physician if symptoms do not improve, or if the condition worsens. Administration to young children should be aided by an adult.
If a patient missed a dose, the patient should be advised to take the dose as soon as they remember. The patient should not take more than the recommended dose for the day.
Manufactured for: Merck Sharp & Dohme Corp., a subsidiary of **MERCK & CO., INC.**, Whitehouse Station, NJ 08889, USA
Manufactured by:
MSD International GmbH (Singapore Branch),
Singapore 638414, Singapore
U.S. Patent No. 6,127,353.
Copyright © 1997, 2010 Merck Sharp & Dohme Corp., a subsidiary of **Merck & Co., Inc.**
All rights reserved.
Revised: 03/2013
032088-NSX-NS-USPI.13
Patient Information
NASONEX®   [nā-zə-neks]   (mometasone furoate monohydrate) **Nasal Spray, 50 mcg**
FOR INTRANASAL USE ONLY
Read the Patient Information that comes with NASONEX before you start using it and each time you get a refill. There may be new information. This Patient Information does not take the place of talking to your healthcare provider about your medical condition or treatment. If you have any questions about NASONEX, ask your healthcare provider.
What is NASONEX?
NASONEX Nasal Spray is a man-made (synthetic) corticosteroid medicine that is used to:
• treat the nasal symptoms of seasonal and year-round allergic rhinitis (inflammation of the lining of the nose) in adults and children 2 years of age and older.
• treat nasal congestion that happens with seasonal allergic rhinitis in adults and children 2 years of age and older.
• prevent nasal symptoms of seasonal allergic rhinitis in people 12 years of age and older.
• treat nasal polyps in people 18 years and older.
The safety and effectiveness of NASONEX has not been shown:
• in children under 2 years of age to treat allergic rhinitis.
• in children under 18 years of age to treat nasal polyps.
Who should not use NASONEX?
Do not use NASONEX if you are allergic to any of the ingredients in NASONEX. See the end of this leaflet for a complete list of ingredients in NASONEX.
What should I tell my healthcare provider before using NASONEX?
Before you take NASONEX, tell your healthcare provider if you:
• have had recent nasal sores, nasal surgery, or nasal injury.
• have eye or vision problems, such as cataracts or glaucoma (increased pressure in your eye).
• have tuberculosis or any untreated fungal, bacterial, viral infections, or eye infections caused by herpes.
• have been near someone who has chickenpox or measles.
• are not feeling well or have any other symptoms that you do not understand.
• have any other medical conditions.
• **are pregnant or planning to become pregnant.** It is not known if NASONEX will harm your unborn baby. Talk to your doctor if you are pregnant or plan to become pregnant.
• **are breastfeeding or planning to breastfeed.** It is not known whether NASONEX passes into your breast milk.
Tell your healthcare provider about all the medicines you take including prescription and non-prescription medicines, vitamins, and herbal supplements.
NASONEX and other medicines may affect each other and cause side effects. NASONEX may affect the way other medicines work, and other medicines may affect how NASONEX works.
Know the list of medicine you take. Keep a list of your medications with you to show your healthcare provider and pharmacist when a new medication is prescribed.
How should I use NASONEX?
• Use NASONEX exactly as prescribed by your healthcare provider.
• This medicine is for use in the nose only. Do not spray it into your mouth or eyes.
• An adult should help a young child use this medicine.
• For best results, you should keep using NASONEX regularly each day without missing a dose. If you do miss a dose of NASONEX, take it as soon as you remember. However, do not take more than the daily dose prescribed by your doctor.
• Do not use NASONEX more often than prescribed. Ask your healthcare provider if you have any questions.

• For detailed instructions on how to use NASONEX Nasal Spray, see the **"Patient Instructions for Use"** at the end of this leaflet.

See your healthcare provider regularly to assess your symptoms while taking NASONEX and to check for side effects.

What should I avoid while taking NASONEX?

If you are taking other corticosteroid medicines for allergy, either by mouth or injection, your healthcare provider may advise you to stop taking them once you begin using NASONEX.

What are the possible side effects of NASONEX?

NASONEX may cause serious side effects, including:

• **Thrush** *(candida)*, **a fungal infection in your nose and throat.** Tell your doctor if you have any redness or white colored patches in your nose or throat.

• **Slow wound healing. Do not** use NASONEX until your nose has healed if you have a sore in your nose, if you have surgery on your nose, or if your nose has been injured.

• **Some people may have eye problems, including glaucoma and cataracts.** You should have regular eye exams.

• **Immune system problems that may increase your risk of infections.** You are more likely to get infections if you take medicines that weaken your immune system. Avoid contact with people who have contagious diseases such as chicken pox or measles while using NASONEX. Symptoms of infection may include: fever, pain, aches, chills, feeling tired, nausea and vomiting. Tell your doctor about any signs of infection while you are using NASONEX.

• **Adrenal insufficiency.** Adrenal insufficiency is a condition in which the adrenal glands do not make enough steroid hormones. Symptoms of adrenal insufficiency can include: tiredness, weakness, nausea and vomiting and low blood pressure.

The most common side effects of NASONEX include:

• headache
• viral infection
• sore throat
• nosebleeds
• cough

Tell your healthcare provider if you have any side effect that bothers you or that does not go away.

These are not all the possible side effects of NASONEX. For more information ask your healthcare provider or pharmacist.

Call your doctor for medical advice about side effects. You may report side effects to FDA at 1-800-FDA-1088.

How should I store NASONEX?

• Store NASONEX at room temperature between 59°F to 86°F (15°C to 30°C).

• Avoid prolonged exposure of NASONEX container to bright light.

• Shake well before each use.

Keep NASONEX and all medicines out of the reach of children.

General information about NASONEX

Medicines are sometimes prescribed for conditions that are not listed in a Patient Information leaflet. Do not use NASONEX for a condition for which it was not prescribed. Do not give NASONEX to other people even if they have the same symptoms you have. It may harm them.

This Patient Information leaflet provides a summary of the most important information about NASONEX. If you would like more information, talk with your healthcare provider. You can ask your healthcare provider or pharmacist for information about NASONEX that is written for health professionals.

For more information, go to www.NASONEX.com or call 1-800-622-4477.

What are the ingredients in NASONEX?

Active Ingredients: mometasone furoate monohydrate
Inactive Ingredients: glycerin, microcrystalline cellulose and carboxymethylcellulose sodium, sodium citrate, citric acid, benzalkonium chloride, and polysorbate 80.

Patient Instructions for Use

For use in your nose only.

Read the Patient Instructions for Use carefully before you start to use your NASONEX Nasal Spray. If you have any questions, ask your healthcare provider.

Shake the bottle well before each use.

1. Remove the plastic cap (**See** Figure 1).
[See figure 1 at top of next column]

2. Before you use NASONEX for the first time, prime the pump by pressing downward on the shoulders of the white nasal applicator using your index finger and middle finger while holding the base of the bottle with your thumb (**See** Figure 2). **Do Not** pierce the nasal applicator. Press down and release the pump 10 times or until a fine spray appears. **Do Not** spray into eyes. The pump is now ready to use. The pump may be stored unused for up to 1 week without repriming. If unused for more than 1 week, reprime by spraying 2 times or until a fine spray appears.
[See figure 2 at top of next column]

PLASTIC CAP

NASAL APPLICATOR

BOTTLE

Figure 1

Figure 2

3. Gently blow your nose to clear the nostrils. Close 1 nostril. Tilt your head forward slightly, keep the bottle upright, carefully insert the nasal applicator into the other nostril (**See** Figure 3). **Do Not** spray directly onto the nasal septum (the wall between the two nostrils).

Figure 3

4. For each spray, hold the spray bottle upright and press firmly downward 1 time on the shoulders of the white nasal applicator using your index and middle fingers while supporting the base of the bottle with your thumb. Breathe gently inward through the nostril (**See** Figure 4).

Figure 4

Note: It is important to keep the NASONEX unit in an upright orientation (as seen in Figure 4). Failure to do so may result in an incomplete or non-existent spray.

5. Then breathe out through the mouth.
6. Repeat in the other nostril.
7. Wipe the nasal applicator with a clean tissue and replace the plastic cap.

Each bottle of NASONEX Nasal Spray contains enough medicine for you to spray medicine from the bottle 120 times. Do not use the bottle of NASONEX Nasal Spray after 120 sprays. Additional sprays after the 120 sprays may not contain the right amount of medicine, **you should keep track of the number of sprays used from each bottle of NASONEX Nasal Spray,** and throw away the bottle even if it has medicine still left in. **Do not count any sprays used for priming the device.** Talk with your healthcare provider before your supply runs out to see if you should get a refill of your medicine.

Pediatric Use: Administration to young children should be done by an adult, Steps 1 through 7 from the **Patient Instructions for Use**, should be followed.

Cleaning: **Do not try to unblock the nasal applicator with a sharp object.** Please see **Patient Instructions for Cleaning Applicator.**

Patient Instructions for Cleaning Applicator

1. To clean the nasal applicator, remove the plastic cap (**See** Figure 5).

PLASTIC CAP

Figure 5

2. Pull gently upward on the white nasal applicator to remove (**See** Figure 6).

WHITE NASAL APPLICATOR

PUMP STEM

Figure 6

3. Soak the nasal applicator in cold tap water and rinse both ends of the nasal applicator under cold tap water and dry (**See** Figure 7). **Do not try to unblock the nasal applicator by inserting a pin or other sharp object as this will damage the applicator and cause you not to get the right dose of medicine.**

WHITE NASAL APPLICATOR

Figure 7

4. Rinse the plastic cap under cold water and dry (**See** Figure 8).
[See figure 8 at top of next column]

5. Put the nasal applicator back together making sure the pump stem is reinserted into the applicator's center hole (**See** Figure 9).
[See figure 9 at top of next column]

6. Reprime the pump by pressing downward on the shoulders of the white nasal applicator using your index and middle fingers while holding the base of the bottle with your thumb. Press down and release the pump 2 times or until a fine spray appears. **Do Not** spray into eyes. The pump is now ready to use. The pump may be stored un-

PLASTIC CAP —

Figure 8

CENTER HOLE

WHITE NASAL
APPLICATOR

PUMP STEM

Figure 9

used for up to 1 week without repriming. If unused for
more than 1 week, reprime by spraying 2 times or until a
fine spray appears (**See** Figure 10).

Figure 10

7. Replace the plastic cap (**See** Figure 11).

Figure 11

Manufactured for: Merck Sharp & Dohme Corp., a subsid-
iary of **MERCK & CO., INC.**, Whitehouse Station, NJ 08889,
USA
Manufactured by:
MSD International GmbH (Singapore Branch),
Singapore 638414, Singapore
U.S. Patent No. 6,127,353.
Copyright © 1997, 2010 Merck Sharp & Dohme Corp., a
subsidiary of **Merck & Co., Inc.**
All rights reserved.
Revised: 03/2013
032088-NSX-NS-PPI.8
Shown in Product Identification Guide, page 308

NEXPLANON®   ℞
(etonogestrel implant)
Radiopaque
Subdermal Use Only

HIGHLIGHTS OF PRESCRIBING INFORMATION
These highlights do not include all the information needed
to use NEXPLANON safely and effectively. See full prescrib-
ing information for NEXPLANON.
NEXPLANON®(etonogestrel implant)
Radiopaque
Subdermal Use Only
Initial U.S. Approval: 2001

───────**INDICATIONS AND USAGE**───────
NEXPLANON is a progestin indicated for use by women to
prevent pregnancy. (1)

───────**DOSAGE AND ADMINISTRATION**───────
Insert one NEXPLANON subdermally just under the skin
at the inner side of the non-dominant upper arm.
NEXPLANON must be removed no later than by the end of
the third year. (2)

───────**DOSAGE FORMS AND STRENGTHS**───────
NEXPLANON consists of a single, radiopaque, rod-shaped
implant, containing 68 mg etonogestrel, pre-loaded in the
needle of a disposable applicator. (3)

───────**CONTRAINDICATIONS**───────
• Known or suspected pregnancy. (4)
• Current or past history of thrombosis or thromboembolic
  disorders. (4, 5.4)
• Liver tumors, benign or malignant, or active liver disease.
  (4, 5.7)
• Undiagnosed abnormal genital bleeding. (4, 5.2)
• Known or suspected breast cancer, personal history of
  breast cancer, or other progestin-sensitive cancer, now or
  in the past. (4, 5.6)
• Allergic reaction to any of the components of
  NEXPLANON. (4, 6)

───────**WARNINGS AND PRECAUTIONS**───────
• Insertion and removal complications: Pain, paresthesias, bleeding, hematoma, scarring or infection may occur.
  (5.1)
• Menstrual bleeding pattern: Counsel women regarding
  changes in bleeding frequency, intensity, or duration. (5.2)
• Ectopic pregnancies: Be alert to the possibility of an ectopic pregnancy in women using NEXPLANON who become pregnant or complain of lower abdominal pain. (5.3)
• Thrombotic and other vascular events: The
  NEXPLANON implant should be removed in the event of
  a thrombosis. (5.4)
• Liver disease: Remove the NEXPLANON implant if
  jaundice occurs. (5.7)
• Elevated blood pressure: The NEXPLANON implant
  should be removed if blood pressure rises significantly and
  becomes uncontrolled. (5.9)
• Carbohydrate and lipid metabolic effects: Monitor prediabetic and diabetic women using NEXPLANON. (5.11)

───────**ADVERSE REACTIONS**───────
Most common (≥10%) adverse reactions reported in clinical
trials were change in menstrual bleeding pattern, headache, vaginitis, weight increase, acne, breast pain, abdominal pain, and pharyngitis. (6.1)
**To report SUSPECTED ADVERSE REACTIONS, contact
Merck Sharp & Dohme Corp., a subsidiary of Merck & Co.,
Inc., at 1-877-888-4231 or FDA at 1-800-FDA-1088 or
www.fda.gov/medwatch.**

───────**DRUG INTERACTIONS**───────
Drugs or herbal products that induce certain enzymes, such
as CYP3A4, may decrease the effectiveness of progestin hormonal contraceptives or increase breakthrough bleeding.
(7.1)

───────**USE IN SPECIFIC POPULATIONS**───────
• Pregnant women: NEXPLANON should be removed if
  maintaining a pregnancy. (8.1)

• Overweight women: NEXPLANON may become less effective in overweight women over time, especially in the
presence of other factors that decrease etonogestrel concentrations, such as concomitant use of hepatic enzyme inducers. (8.8)
**See 17 for PATIENT COUNSELING INFORMATION
and FDA-approved patient labeling**

Revised: 07/2014

FULL PRESCRIBING INFORMATION

1   INDICATIONS AND USAGE
NEXPLANON® is indicated for use by women to prevent
pregnancy.

2   DOSAGE AND ADMINISTRATION
The efficacy of NEXPLANON does not depend on daily,
weekly or monthly administration.
All healthcare providers should receive instruction and
training prior to performing insertion and/or removal of
NEXPLANON.
A single NEXPLANON implant is inserted subdermally in
the upper arm. To reduce the risk of neural or vascular injury, the implant should be inserted at the inner side of the
non-dominant upper arm about 8-10 cm (3-4 inches) above

the medial epicondyle of the humerus. The implant should be inserted subdermally just under the skin to avoid the large blood vessels and nerves that lie deeper in the subcutaneous tissues in the sulcus between the triceps and biceps muscles. NEXPLANON must be inserted by the expiration date stated on the packaging. NEXPLANON is a long-acting (up to 3 years), reversible, hormonal contraceptive method. The implant must be removed by the end of the third year and may be replaced by a new implant at the time of removal, if continued contraceptive protection is desired.

2.1 Initiating Contraception With NEXPLANON
IMPORTANT: Rule out pregnancy before inserting the implant.
Timing of insertion depends on the woman's recent contraceptive history, as follows:
• No preceding hormonal contraceptive use in the past month
NEXPLANON should be inserted between Day 1 (first day of menstrual bleeding) and Day 5 of the menstrual cycle, even if the woman is still bleeding.
If inserted as recommended, back-up contraception is not necessary. If deviating from the recommended timing of insertion, the woman should be advised to use a barrier method until 7 days after insertion. If intercourse has already occurred, pregnancy should be excluded.
• Switching contraceptive method to NEXPLANON
Combination hormonal contraceptives:
NEXPLANON should preferably be inserted on the day after the last active tablet of the previous combined oral contraceptive or on the day of removal of the vaginal ring or transdermal patch. At the latest, NEXPLANON should be inserted on the day following the usual tablet-free, ring-free, patch-free or placebo tablet interval of the previous combined hormonal contraceptive.
If inserted as recommended, back-up contraception is not necessary. If deviating from the recommended timing of insertion, the woman should be advised to use a barrier method until 7 days after insertion. If intercourse has already occurred, pregnancy should be excluded.
Progestin-only contraceptives:
There are several types of progestin-only methods. NEXPLANON should be inserted as follows:
• Injectable Contraceptives: Insert NEXPLANON on the day the next injection is due.
• Minipill: A woman may switch to NEXPLANON on any day of the month. NEXPLANON should be inserted within 24 hours after taking the last tablet.
• Contraceptive implant or intrauterine system (IUS): Insert NEXPLANON on the same day the previous contraceptive implant or IUS is removed.
If inserted as recommended, back-up contraception is not necessary. If deviating from the recommended timing of insertion, the woman should be advised to use a barrier method until 7 days after insertion. If intercourse has already occurred, pregnancy should be excluded.
• Following abortion or miscarriage
• First Trimester: NEXPLANON should be inserted within 5 days following a first trimester abortion or miscarriage.
• Second Trimester: Insert NEXPLANON between 21 to 28 days following second trimester abortion or miscarriage.
If inserted as recommended, back-up contraception is not necessary. If deviating from the recommended timing of insertion, the woman should be advised to use a barrier method until 7 days after insertion. If intercourse has already occurred, pregnancy should be excluded.
• Postpartum
• Not Breastfeeding: NEXPLANON should be inserted between 21 to 28 days postpartum. If inserted as recommended, back-up contraception is not necessary. If deviating from the recommended timing of insertion, the woman should be advised to use a barrier method until 7 days after insertion. If intercourse has already occurred, pregnancy should be excluded.
• Breastfeeding: NEXPLANON should be inserted after the fourth postpartum week [see Use in Specific Populations (8.3)]. The woman should be advised to use a barrier method until 7 days after insertion. If intercourse has already occurred, pregnancy should be excluded.

2.2 Insertion of NEXPLANON
The basis for successful use and subsequent removal of NEXPLANON is a correct and carefully performed subdermal insertion of the single, rod-shaped implant in accordance with the instructions. Both the healthcare provider and the woman should be able to feel the implant under the skin after placement.
All healthcare providers performing insertions and/or removals of NEXPLANON should receive instructions and training prior to inserting or removing the implant. Information concerning the insertion and removal of NEXPLANON will be sent upon request free of charge [1-877-467-5266].

Preparation
Prior to inserting NEXPLANON carefully read the instructions for insertion as well as the full prescribing information.
Before insertion of NEXPLANON, the healthcare provider should confirm that:
• The woman is not pregnant nor has any other contraindication for the use of NEXPLANON [see Contraindications (4)].
• The woman has had a medical history and physical examination, including a gynecologic examination, performed.
• The woman understands the benefits and risks of NEXPLANON.
• The woman has received a copy of the Patient Labeling included in packaging.
• The woman has reviewed and completed a consent form to be maintained with the woman's chart.
• The woman does not have allergies to the antiseptic and anesthetic to be used during insertion.
Insert NEXPLANON under aseptic conditions.
The following equipment is needed for the implant insertion:
• An examination table for the woman to lie on
• Sterile surgical drapes, sterile gloves, antiseptic solution, sterile marker (optional)
• Local anesthetic, needles, and syringe
• Sterile gauze, adhesive bandage, pressure bandage

Insertion Procedure
Step 1. Have the woman lie on her back on the examination table with her non-dominant arm flexed at the elbow and externally rotated so that her wrist is parallel to her ear or her hand is positioned next to her head (Figure 1).

Figure 1

Step 2. Identify the insertion site, which is at the inner side of the non-dominant upper arm about 8-10 cm (3-4 inches) above the medial epicondyle of the humerus (Figure 2). **The implant should be inserted subdermally just under the skin to avoid the large blood vessels and nerves that lie deeper in the subcutaneous tissue in the sulcus between the triceps and biceps muscles** [see Warnings and Precautions (5.1)].
Step 3. Make two marks with a sterile marker: first, mark the spot where the etonogestrel implant will be inserted, and second, mark a spot a few centimeters proximal to the first mark (Figure 2). This second mark will later serve as a direction guide during insertion.

Guiding Mark

8–10 cm

Medial Epicondyle

Insertion Site

Figure 2

Step 4. Clean the insertion site with an antiseptic solution.
Step 5. Anesthetize the insertion area (for example, with anesthetic spray or by injecting 2 mL of 1% lidocaine just under the skin along the planned insertion tunnel).
Step 6. Remove the sterile preloaded disposable NEXPLANON applicator carrying the implant from its blister. The applicator should not be used if sterility is in question.
Step 7. Hold the applicator just above the needle at the textured surface area. Remove the transparent protection cap by sliding it horizontally in the direction of the arrow away from the needle (Figure 3). If the cap does not come off easily, the applicator should not be used. You can see the white colored implant by looking into the tip of the needle. **Do not touch the purple slider until you have fully inserted the needle subdermally, as it will retract the needle and prematurely release the implant from the applicator.**

Purple Slider

Figure 3

Step 8. With your free hand, stretch the skin around the insertion site with thumb and index finger (Figure 4).

Figure 4

Step 9. Puncture the skin with the tip of the needle angled about 30° (Figure 5).

~30°

Figure 5

Step 10. Lower the applicator to a horizontal position. While lifting the skin with the tip of the needle (Figure 6), slide the needle to its full length. You may feel slight resistance but do not exert excessive force. **If the needle is not inserted to its full length, the implant will not be inserted properly. You can best see movement of the needle if you are seated and are looking at the applicator from the side and NOT from above. In this position, you can clearly see the insertion site and the movement of the needle just under the skin.**

Figure 6

Step 11. Keep the applicator in the same position with the needle inserted to its full length. If needed, you may use your free hand to keep the applicator in the same position during the following procedure. Unlock the purple slider by pushing it slightly down. Move the slider fully back until it stops (Figure 7). The implant is now in its final subdermal position, and the needle is locked inside the body of the applicator. The applicator can now be removed. **If the applicator is not kept in the same position during this procedure or if the purple slider is not completely moved to the back, the implant will not be inserted properly.**

Figure 7

Step 12. **Always verify the presence of the implant in the woman's arm immediately after insertion by palpation.** By palpating both ends of the implant, you should be able to confirm the presence of the 4 cm rod (Figure 8).
[See figure 8 at top of next column]
If you cannot feel the implant or are in doubt of its presence,
• Check the applicator. The needle should be fully retracted and only the purple tip of the obturator should be visible.

Figure 8

- Use other methods to confirm the presence of the implant. Suitable methods are: two-dimensional X-ray, X-ray computerized tomography (CT scan), ultrasound scanning (USS) with a high-frequency linear array transducer (10 MHz or greater) or magnetic resonance imaging (MRI). If these methods fail, call 1-877-467-5266 for information on the procedure for measuring etonogestrel blood levels. **Until the presence of the implant has been verified, the woman should be advised to use a non-hormonal contraceptive method, such as condoms.**

Step 13. Place a small adhesive bandage over the insertion site. Request that the woman palpate the implant.

Step 14. Apply a pressure bandage with sterile gauze to minimize bruising. The woman may remove the pressure bandage in 24 hours and the small bandage over the insertion site after 3 to 5 days.

Step 15. Complete the USER CARD and give it to the woman to keep. Also, complete the PATIENT CHART LABEL and affix it to the woman's medical record.

Step 16. The applicator is for single use only and should be disposed in accordance with the Center for Disease Control and Prevention guidelines for handling of hazardous waste.

2.3   Removal of NEXPLANON
Preparation

Before initiating the removal procedure, the healthcare provider should carefully read the instructions for removal and consult the USER CARD and/or the PATIENT CHART LABEL for the location of the implant. The exact location of the implant in the arm should be verified by palpation. If the implant is not palpable, two-dimensional X-ray can be performed to verify its presence.

A non-palpable implant should always be first located prior to removal. Suitable methods for localization include: two-dimensional X-ray, X-ray computer tomography (CT), ultrasound scanning (USS) with a high-frequency linear array transducer (10 MHz or greater) or magnetic resonance imaging (MRI). If these imaging methods fail to locate the implant, etonogestrel blood level determination can be used for verification of the presence of the implant. For details on etonogestrel blood level determination, call 1-877-467-5266 for further instructions.

After localization of a non-palpable implant, consider conducting removal with ultrasound guidance.

There have been occasional reports of migration of the implant; usually this involves minor movement relative to the original position. This may complicate localization of the implant by palpation, CT, USS and/or MRI, and removal may require a larger incision and more time.

Exploratory surgery without knowledge of the exact location of the implant is strongly discouraged. Removal of deeply inserted implants should be conducted with caution in order to prevent injury to deeper neural or vascular structures in the arm and be performed by healthcare providers familiar with the anatomy of the arm.

Before removal of the implant, the healthcare provider should confirm that:
- The woman does not have allergies to the antiseptic or anesthetic to be used.

Remove the implant under aseptic conditions.

The following equipment is needed for removal of the implant:
- An examination table for the woman to lie on
- Sterile surgical drapes, sterile gloves, antiseptic solution, sterile marker (optional)
- Local anesthetic, needles, and syringe
- Sterile scalpel, forceps (straight and curved mosquito)
- Skin closure, sterile gauze, adhesive bandage and pressure bandages

Removal Procedure

Step 1. Clean the site where the incision will be made and apply an antiseptic. Locate the implant by palpation and mark the distal end (end closest to the elbow), for example, with a sterile marker (Figure 9).
[See figure 9 at top of next column]

Step 2. Anesthetize the arm, for example, with 0.5 to 1 mL 1% lidocaine at the marked site where the incision will be made (Figure 10). Be sure to inject the local anesthetic under the implant to keep it close to the skin surface.
[See figure 10 at top of next column]

Step 3. Push down the proximal end of the implant (Figure 11) to stabilize it; a bulge may appear indicating the distal end of the implant. Starting at the distal tip of the implant, make a longitudinal incision of 2 mm towards the elbow.
[See figure 11 at top of next column]

Figure 9

Figure 10

Figure 11

Step 4. Gently push the implant towards the incision until the tip is visible. Grasp the implant with forceps (preferably curved mosquito forceps) and gently remove the implant (Figure 12).

Figure 12

Step 5. If the implant is encapsulated, make an incision into the tissue sheath and then remove the implant with the forceps (Figures 13 and 14).

Figure 13

Figure 14

Step 6. If the tip of the implant does not become visible in the incision, gently insert a forceps into the incision (Figure 15). Flip the forceps over into your other hand (Figure 16).

Figure 15

Figure 16

Step 7. With a second pair of forceps carefully dissect the tissue around the implant and grasp the implant (Figure 17). The implant can then be removed.
[See figure 17 at top of next column]

Step 8. Confirm that the entire implant, which is 4 cm long, has been removed by measuring its length. If a partial implant (less than 4 cm) is removed, the remaining piece should be removed by following the instructions in section 2.3. *[See Dosage and Administration (2.3).]* If the woman would like to continue using NEXPLANON, a new implant may be inserted immediately after the old implant is removed using the same incision *[see Dosage and Administration (2.4)].*

Figure 17

Step 9. After removing the implant, close the incision with a steri-strip and apply an adhesive bandage.

Step 10. Apply a pressure bandage with sterile gauze to minimize bruising. The woman may remove the pressure bandage in 24 hours and the small bandage in 3 to 5 days.

2.4   Replacing NEXPLANON

Immediate replacement can be done after removal of the previous implant and is similar to the insertion procedure described in section 2.2 Insertion of NEXPLANON.

The new implant may be inserted in the same arm, and through the same incision from which the previous implant was removed. If the same incision is being used to insert a new implant, anesthetize the insertion site [for example, 2 mL lidocaine (1%)] applying it just under the skin along the 'insertion canal.'

Follow the subsequent steps in the insertion instructions *[see Dosage and Administration (2.2)].*

3   DOSAGE FORMS AND STRENGTHS

Single, white/off-white, soft, radiopaque, flexible, ethylene vinyl acetate (EVA) copolymer implant, 4 cm in length and 2 mm in diameter containing 68 mg etonogestrel and 15 mg of barium sulfate.

Single, white/off-white, soft, radiopaque, flexible, ethylene vinyl acetate (EVA) copolymer implant, 4 cm in length and 2 mm in diameter containing 68 mg etonogestrel, 15 mg of barium sulfate and 0.1 mg of magnesium stearate.

4   CONTRAINDICATIONS

NEXPLANON should not be used in women who have
- Known or suspected pregnancy
- Current or past history of thrombosis or thromboembolic disorders
- Liver tumors, benign or malignant, or active liver disease
- Undiagnosed abnormal genital bleeding
- Known or suspected breast cancer, personal history of breast cancer, or other progestin-sensitive cancer, now or in the past
- Allergic reaction to any of the components of NEXPLANON *[see Adverse Reactions (6)]*

5   WARNINGS AND PRECAUTIONS

The following information is based on experience with either the non-radiopaque etonogestrel implant (IMPLANON), other progestin-only contraceptives, or experience with combination (estrogen plus progestin) oral contraceptives.

5.1   Complications of Insertion and Removal

NEXPLANON should be inserted subdermally so that it will be palpable after insertion, and this should be confirmed by palpation immediately after insertion. Failure to insert NEXPLANON properly may go unnoticed unless it is palpated immediately after insertion. Undetected failure to insert the implant may lead to an unintended pregnancy. Complications related to insertion and removal procedures, such as pain, paresthesias, bleeding, hematoma, scarring or infection, may occur.

If NEXPLANON is inserted too deeply (intramuscular or in the fascia), neural or vascular injury may occur. To reduce the risk of neural or vascular injury, NEXPLANON should be inserted at the inner side of the non-dominant upper arm about 8-10 cm (3-4 inches) above the medial epicondyle of the humerus. NEXPLANON should be inserted subdermally just under the skin to avoid the large blood vessels and nerves that lie deeper in the subcutaneous tissues in the sulcus between the triceps and biceps muscles. Deep insertions of the non-radiopaque etonogestrel implant (IMPLANON) have been associated with paraesthesia (due to neural injury) and migration of the implant (due to intramuscular or fascial insertion), and in a very few cases with intravascular insertion. If infection develops at the insertion site, start suitable treatment. If the infection persists, the implant should be removed. Incomplete insertions or infections may lead to expulsion.

Implant removal may be difficult or impossible if the implant is not inserted correctly, is inserted too deeply, not palpable, encased in fibrous tissue, or has migrated. Deep insertions may lead to difficult localization of the implant and may also result in the need for a surgical procedure in an operating room in order to remove the implant. Exploratory surgery without knowledge of the exact location of the implant is strongly discouraged. Removal of deeply inserted implants should be conducted with caution in order to prevent injury to deeper neural or vascular structures in the arm and be performed by healthcare providers familiar with the anatomy of the arm. Failure to remove the implant may result in continued effects of etonogestrel, such as compromised fertility, ectopic pregnancy, or persistence or occurrence of a drug-related adverse event.

5.2 Changes in Menstrual Bleeding Patterns

After starting NEXPLANON, women are likely to have a change from their normal menstrual bleeding pattern. These may include changes in bleeding frequency (absent, less, more frequent or continuous), intensity (reduced or increased) or duration. In clinical trials of the non-radiopaque etonogestrel implant (IMPLANON), bleeding patterns ranged from amenorrhea (1 in 5 women) to frequent and/or prolonged bleeding (1 in 5 women). The bleeding pattern experienced during the first three months of NEXPLANON use is broadly predictive of the future bleeding pattern for many women. Women should be counseled regarding the bleeding pattern changes they may experience so that they know what to expect. Abnormal bleeding should be evaluated as needed to exclude pathologic conditions or pregnancy.

In clinical studies of the non-radiopaque etonogestrel implant, reports of changes in bleeding pattern were the most common reason for stopping treatment (11.1%). Irregular bleeding (10.8%) was the single most common reason women stopped treatment, while amenorrhea (0.3%) was cited less frequently. In these studies, women had an average of 17.7 days of bleeding or spotting every 90 days (based on 3,315 intervals of 90 days recorded by 780 patients). The percentages of patients having 0, 1-7, 8-21, or >21 days of spotting or bleeding over a 90-day interval while using the non-radiopaque etonogestrel implant are shown in Table 1.

Table 1: Percentages of Patients With 0, 1-7, 8-21, or >21 Days of Spotting or Bleeding Over a 90-Day Interval While Using the Non-Radiopaque Etonogestrel Implant (IMPLANON)

Total Days of Spotting or Bleeding	Percentage of Patients		
	Treatment Days 91-180 (N = 745)	Treatment Days 271-360 (N = 657)	Treatment Days 631-720 (N = 547)
0 Days	19%	24%	17%
1-7 Days	15%	13%	12%
8-21 Days	30%	30%	37%
>21 Days	35%	33%	35%

Bleeding patterns observed with use of the non-radiopaque etonogestrel implant for up to 2 years, and the proportion of 90-day intervals with these bleeding patterns, are summarized in Table 2.

Table 2: Bleeding Patterns Using the Non-Radiopaque Etonogestrel Implant (IMPLANON) During the First 2 Years of Use*

BLEEDING PATTERNS	DEFINITIONS	%†
Infrequent	Less than three bleeding and/or spotting episodes in 90 days (excluding amenorrhea)	33.6
Amenorrhea	No bleeding and/or spotting in 90 days	22.2
Prolonged	Any bleeding and/or spotting episode lasting more than 14 days in 90 days	17.7
Frequent	More than 5 bleeding and/or spotting episodes in 90 days	6.7

* Based on 3315 recording periods of 90 days duration in 780 women, excluding the first 90 days after implant insertion
† % = Percentage of 90-day intervals with this pattern

In case of undiagnosed, persistent, or recurrent abnormal vaginal bleeding, appropriate measures should be conducted to rule out malignancy.

5.3 Ectopic Pregnancies

As with all progestin-only contraceptive products, be alert to the possibility of an ectopic pregnancy among women using NEXPLANON who become pregnant or complain of lower abdominal pain. Although ectopic pregnancies are uncommon among women using NEXPLANON, a pregnancy that occurs in a woman using NEXPLANON may be more likely to be ectopic than a pregnancy occurring in a woman using no contraception.

5.4 Thrombotic and Other Vascular Events

The use of combination hormonal contraceptives (progestin plus estrogen) increases the risk of vascular events, including arterial events (strokes and myocardial infarctions) or deep venous thrombotic events (venous thromboembolism, deep venous thrombosis, retinal vein thrombosis, and pulmonary embolism). NEXPLANON is a progestin-only contraceptive. It is unknown whether this increased risk is applicable to etonogestrel alone. It is recommended, however, that women with risk factors known to increase the risk of venous and arterial thromboembolism be carefully assessed.

There have been postmarketing reports of serious arterial and venous thromboembolic events, including cases of pulmonary emboli (some fatal), deep vein thrombosis, myocardial infarction, and strokes, in women using the non-radiopaque etonogestrel implant. NEXPLANON should be removed in the event of a thrombosis.

Due to the risk of thromboembolism associated with pregnancy and immediately following delivery, NEXPLANON should not be used prior to 21 days postpartum. Women with a history of thromboembolic disorders should be made aware of the possibility of a recurrence.

Evaluate for retinal vein thrombosis immediately if there is unexplained loss of vision, proptosis, diplopia, papilledema, or retinal vascular lesions.

Consider removal of the NEXPLANON implant in case of long-term immobilization due to surgery or illness.

5.5 Ovarian Cysts

If follicular development occurs, atresia of the follicle is sometimes delayed, and the follicle may continue to grow beyond the size it would attain in a normal cycle. Generally, these enlarged follicles disappear spontaneously. On rare occasion, surgery may be required.

5.6 Carcinoma of the Breast and Reproductive Organs

Women who currently have or have had breast cancer should not use hormonal contraception because breast cancer may be hormonally sensitive [see Contraindications (4)]. Some studies suggest that the use of combination hormonal contraceptives might increase the incidence of breast cancer; however, other studies have not confirmed such findings.

Some studies suggest that the use of combination hormonal contraceptives is associated with an increase in the risk of cervical cancer or intraepithelial neoplasia. However, there is controversy about the extent to which these findings are due to differences in sexual behavior and other factors.

Women with a family history of breast cancer or who develop breast nodules should be carefully monitored.

5.7 Liver Disease

Disturbances of liver function may necessitate the discontinuation of hormonal contraceptive use until markers of liver function return to normal. Remove NEXPLANON if jaundice develops.

Hepatic adenomas are associated with combination hormonal contraceptives use. An estimate of the attributable risk is 3.3 cases per 100,000 for combination hormonal contraceptives users. It is not known whether a similar risk exists with progestin-only methods like NEXPLANON.

The progestin in NEXPLANON may be poorly metabolized in women with liver impairment. Use of NEXPLANON in women with active liver disease or liver cancer is contraindicated [see Contraindications (4)].

5.8 Weight Gain

In clinical studies, mean weight gain in U.S. non-radiopaque etonogestrel implant (IMPLANON) users was 2.8 pounds after one year and 3.7 pounds after two years. How much of the weight gain was related to the non-radiopaque etonogestrel implant is unknown. In studies, 2.3% of the users reported weight gain as the reason for having the non-radiopaque etonogestrel implant removed.

5.9 Elevated Blood Pressure

Women with a history of hypertension-related diseases or renal disease should be discouraged from using hormonal contraception. For women with well-controlled hypertension, use of NEXPLANON can be considered. Women with hypertension using NEXPLANON should be closely monitored. If sustained hypertension develops during the use of NEXPLANON, or if a significant increase in blood pressure does not respond adequately to antihypertensive therapy, NEXPLANON should be removed.

5.10 Gallbladder Disease

Studies suggest a small increased relative risk of developing gallbladder disease among combination hormonal contraceptive users. It is not known whether a similar risk exists with progestin-only methods like NEXPLANON.

5.11 Carbohydrate and Lipid Metabolic Effects

Use of NEXPLANON may induce mild insulin resistance and small changes in glucose concentrations of unknown clinical significance. Carefully monitor prediabetic and diabetic women using NEXPLANON.

Women who are being treated for hyperlipidemia should be followed closely if they elect to use NEXPLANON. Some progestins may elevate LDL levels and may render the control of hyperlipidemia more difficult.

5.12 Depressed Mood

Women with a history of depressed mood should be carefully observed. Consideration should be given to removing NEXPLANON in patients who become significantly depressed.

5.13 Return to Ovulation

In clinical trials with the non-radiopaque etonogestrel implant (IMPLANON), the etonogestrel levels in blood decreased below sensitivity of the assay by one week after removal of the implant. In addition, pregnancies were observed to occur as early as 7 to 14 days after removal. Therefore, a woman should re-start contraception immediately after removal of the implant if continued contraceptive protection is desired.

5.14 Fluid Retention

Hormonal contraceptives may cause some degree of fluid retention. They should be prescribed with caution, and only with careful monitoring, in patients with conditions which might be aggravated by fluid retention. It is unknown if NEXPLANON causes fluid retention.

5.15 Contact Lenses

Contact lens wearers who develop visual changes or changes in lens tolerance should be assessed by an ophthalmologist.

5.16 Monitoring

A woman who is using NEXPLANON should have a yearly visit with her healthcare provider for a blood pressure check and for other indicated health care.

5.17 Drug-Laboratory Test Interactions

Sex hormone-binding globulin concentrations may be decreased for the first six months after NEXPLANON insertion followed by gradual recovery. Thyroxine concentrations may initially be slightly decreased followed by gradual recovery to baseline.

6 ADVERSE REACTIONS

The following adverse reactions reported with the use of hormonal contraception are discussed elsewhere in the labeling:
• Changes in Menstrual Bleeding Patterns [see Warnings and Precautions (5.2)]
• Ectopic Pregnancies [see Warnings and Precautions (5.3)]
• Thrombotic and Other Vascular Events [see Warnings and Precautions (5.4)]
• Liver Disease [see Warnings and Precautions (5.7)]

6.1 Clinical Trials Experience

Because clinical trials are conducted under widely varying conditions, adverse reaction rates observed in the clinical trials of a drug cannot be directly compared to rates in the clinical trials of another drug and may not reflect the rates observed in practice.

In clinical trials involving 942 women who were evaluated for safety, change in menstrual bleeding patterns (irregular menses) was the most common adverse reaction causing discontinuation of use of the non-radiopaque etonogestrel implant (IMPLANON) (11.1% of women).

Adverse reactions that resulted in a rate of discontinuation of ≥1% are shown in Table 3.

Table 3: Adverse Reactions Leading to Discontinuation of Treatment in 1% or More of Subjects in Clinical Trials of the Non-Radiopaque Etonogestrel Implant (IMPLANON)

Adverse Reactions	All Studies N = 942
Bleeding Irregularities*	11.1%
Emotional Lability†	2.3%
Weight Increase	2.3%
Headache	1.6%
Acne	1.3%
Depression‡	1.0%

* Includes "frequent", "heavy", "prolonged", "spotting", and other patterns of bleeding irregularity.
† Among US subjects (N=330), 6.1% experienced emotional lability that led to discontinuation.
‡ Among US subjects (N=330), 2.4% experienced depression that led to discontinuation.

Other adverse reactions that were reported by at least 5% of subjects in the non-radiopaque etonogestrel implant clinical trials are listed in Table 4.

Table 4: Common Adverse Reactions Reported by ≥5% of Subjects in Clinical Trials With the Non-Radiopaque Etonogestrel Implant (IMPLANON)

Adverse Reactions	All Studies N = 942
Headache	24.9%
Vaginitis	14.5%
Weight increase	13.7%
Acne	13.5%
Breast pain	12.8%
Abdominal pain	10.9%
Pharyngitis	10.5%
Leukorrhea	9.6%
Influenza-like symptoms	7.6%
Dizziness	7.2%
Dysmenorrhea	7.2%
Back pain	6.8%
Emotional lability	6.5%
Nausea	6.4%
Pain	5.6%
Nervousness	5.6%
Depression	5.5%
Hypersensitivity	5.4%
Insertion site pain	5.2%

In a clinical trial of NEXPLANON, in which investigators were asked to examine the implant site after insertion, implant site reactions were reported in 8.6% of women. Erythema was the most frequent implant site complication, reported during and/or shortly after insertion, occurring in 3.3% of subjects. Additionally, hematoma (3.0%), bruising (2.0%), pain (1.0%), and swelling (0.7%) were reported.

6.2 Postmarketing Experience

The following additional adverse reactions have been identified during post-approval use of the non-radiopaque etonogestrel implant (IMPLANON). Because these reactions are reported voluntarily from a population of uncertain size, it is not possible to reliably estimate their frequency or establish a causal relationship to drug exposure.

Gastrointestinal disorders: constipation, diarrhea, flatulence, vomiting.

General disorders and administration site conditions: edema, fatigue, implant site reaction, pyrexia.

Immune system disorders: anaphylactic reactions.

Infections and infestations: rhinitis, urinary tract infection.

Investigations: clinically relevant rise in blood pressure, weight decreased.

Metabolism and nutrition disorders: increased appetite.

Musculoskeletal and connective tissue disorders: arthralgia, musculoskeletal pain, myalgia.

Nervous system disorders: convulsions, migraine, somnolence.

Pregnancy, puerperium and perinatal conditions: ectopic pregnancy.

Psychiatric disorders: anxiety, insomnia, libido decreased.

Renal and urinary disorders: dysuria.

Reproductive system and breast disorders: breast discharge, breast enlargement, ovarian cyst, pruritus genital, vulvovaginal discomfort.

Skin and subcutaneous tissue disorders: angioedema, aggravation of angioedema and/or aggravation of hereditary angioedema, alopecia, chloasma, hypertrichosis, pruritus, rash, seborrhea, urticaria.

Vascular disorders: hot flush.

Complications related to insertion or removal of the non-radiopaque etonogestrel implant reported include: bruising, slight local irritation, pain or itching, fibrosis at the implant site, paresthesia or paresthesia-like events, scarring and abscess.

7 DRUG INTERACTIONS

7.1 Changes in Contraceptive Effectiveness Associated With Coadministration of Other Products

Drugs or herbal products that induce enzymes, including CYP3A4, that metabolize progestins may decrease the plasma concentrations of progestins, and may decrease the effectiveness of NEXPLANON. In women on long-term treatment with hepatic enzyme inducing drugs, it is recommended to remove the implant and to advise a contraceptive method that is unaffected by the interacting drug.

Some of these drugs or herbal products that induce enzymes, including CYP3A4, include:

- barbiturates
- bosentan
- carbamazepine
- felbamate
- griseofulvin
- oxcarbazepine
- phenytoin
- rifampin
- St. John's wort
- topiramate

HIV Antiretrovirals

Significant changes (increase or decrease) in the plasma levels of progestin have been noted in some cases of co-administration with HIV protease inhibitors or with non-nucleoside reverse transcriptase inhibitors. Consult the labeling of all concurrently-used drugs to obtain further information about interactions with hormonal contraceptives or the potential for enzyme alterations.

7.2 Increase in Plasma Concentrations of Etonogestrel Associated With Coadministered Drugs

CYP3A4 inhibitors such as itraconazole or ketoconazole may increase plasma concentrations of etonogestrel.

7.3 Changes in Plasma Concentrations of Coadministered Drugs

Hormonal contraceptives may affect the metabolism of other drugs. Consequently, plasma concentrations may either increase (for example, cyclosporin) or decrease (for example, lamotrigine). Consult the labeling of all concurrently-used drugs to obtain further information about interactions with hormonal contraceptives or the potential for enzyme alterations.

8 USE IN SPECIFIC POPULATIONS

8.1 Pregnancy

NEXPLANON is not indicated for use during pregnancy *[see Contraindications (4)].*

Teratology studies have been performed in rats and rabbits using oral administration up to 390 and 790 times the human etonogestrel dose (based upon body surface), respectively, and revealed no evidence of fetal harm due to etonogestrel exposure.

Studies have revealed no increased risk of birth defects in women who have used combination oral contraceptives before pregnancy or during early pregnancy. There is no evidence that the risk associated with etonogestrel is different from that of combination oral contraceptives.

NEXPLANON should be removed if maintaining a pregnancy.

8.3 Nursing Mothers

Based on limited clinical data, NEXPLANON may be used during breastfeeding after the fourth postpartum week. Use of NEXPLANON before the fourth postpartum week has not been studied. Small amounts of etonogestrel are excreted in breast milk. During the first months after insertion of NEXPLANON, when maternal blood levels of etonogestrel are highest, about 100 ng of etonogestrel may be ingested by the child per day based on an average daily milk ingestion of 658 mL. Based on daily milk ingestion of 150 mL/kg, the mean daily infant etonogestrel dose one month after insertion of the non-radiopaque etonogestrel implant (IMPLANON) is about 2.2% of the weight-adjusted maternal daily dose, or about 0.2% of the estimated absolute maternal daily dose. The health of breastfed infants whose mothers began using the non-radiopaque etonogestrel implant during the fourth to eighth week postpartum (n=38) was evaluated in a comparative study with infants of mothers using a non-hormonal IUD (n=33). They were breastfed for a mean duration of 14 months and followed up to 36 months of age. No significant effects and no differences between the groups were observed on the physical and psychomotor development of these infants. No differences between groups in the production or quality of breast milk were detected.

Healthcare providers should discuss both hormonal and non-hormonal contraceptive options, as steroids may not be the initial choice for these patients.

8.4 Pediatric Use

Safety and efficacy of NEXPLANON have been established in women of reproductive age. Safety and efficacy of NEXPLANON are expected to be the same for postpubertal adolescents. However, no clinical studies have been conducted in women less than 18 years of age. Use of this product before menarche is not indicated.

8.5 Geriatric Use

This product has not been studied in women over 65 years of age and is not indicated in this population.

8.6 Hepatic Impairment

No studies were conducted to evaluate the effect of hepatic disease on the disposition of NEXPLANON. The use of NEXPLANON in women with active liver disease is contraindicated *[see Contraindications (4)].*

8.7 Renal Impairment

No studies were conducted to evaluate the effect of renal disease on the disposition of NEXPLANON.

8.8 Overweight Women

The effectiveness of the etonogestrel implant in women who weighed more than 130% of their ideal body weight has not been defined because such women were not studied in clinical trials. Serum concentrations of etonogestrel are inversely related to body weight and decrease with time after implant insertion. It is therefore possible that NEXPLANON may be less effective in overweight women, especially in the presence of other factors that decrease serum etonogestrel concentrations such as concomitant use of hepatic enzyme inducers.

10 OVERDOSAGE

Overdosage may result if more than one implant is inserted. In case of suspected overdose, the implant should be removed.

11 DESCRIPTION

NEXPLANON is a radiopaque, progestin-only, soft, flexible implant preloaded in a sterile, disposable applicator for subdermal use. The implant is white/off-white, non-biodegradable and 4 cm in length with a diameter of 2 mm (see Figure 18). Each implant consists of an ethylene vinyl acetate (EVA) copolymer core, containing 68 mg of the synthetic progestin etonogestrel, barium sulfate (radiopaque ingredient), and may also contain magnesium stearate, surrounded by an EVA copolymer skin. Once inserted subdermally, the release rate is 60-70 mcg/day in week 5-6 and decreases to approximately 35-45 mcg/day at the end of the first year, to approximately 30-40 mcg/day at the end of the second year, and then to approximately 25-30 mcg/day at the end of the third year. NEXPLANON is a progestin-only contraceptive and does not contain estrogen. NEXPLANON does not contain latex.

2 mm

4 cm

Figure 18 (Not to scale)

Etonogestrel [13-Ethyl-17-hydroxy-11-methylene-18,19-dinor-17α-pregn-4-en-20-yn-3-one], structurally derived from 19-nortestosterone, is the synthetic biologically active metabolite of the synthetic progestin desogestrel. It has a molecular weight of 324.46 and the following structural formula (Figure 19).

H_2C HO   C≡CH

O $C_{22}H_{28}O_2$

Figure 19

12 CLINICAL PHARMACOLOGY

12.1 Mechanism of Action

The contraceptive effect of NEXPLANON is achieved by suppression of ovulation, increased viscosity of the cervical mucus, and alterations in the endometrium.

12.2 Pharmacodynamics

Exposure-response relationships of NEXPLANON are unknown.

12.3 Pharmacokinetics

Absorption

After subdermal insertion of the etonogestrel implant, etonogestrel is released into the circulation and is approximately 100% bioavailable.

In a three year clinical trial, NEXPLANON and the non-radiopaque etonogestrel implant (IMPLANON) yielded comparable systemic exposure to etonogestrel. For NEXPLANON, the mean (± SD) maximum serum etonogestrel concentrations were 1200 (± 604) pg/mL and were reached within the first two weeks after insertion (n=50). The mean (± SD) serum etonogestrel concentration decreased gradually over time, declining to 202 (± 55) pg/mL at 12 months (n=41), 164 (± 58) pg/mL at 24 months (n=37), and 138 (± 43) pg/mL at 36 months (n=32). For the non-radiopaque etonogestrel implant (IMPLANON), the mean (± SD) maximum serum etonogestrel concentrations were 1145 (± 577) pg/mL and were reached within the first two weeks after insertion (n=53). The mean (± SD) serum etonogestrel concentration decreased gradually over time, declining to 223 (± 73) pg/mL at 12 months (n=40), 172 (± 77) pg/mL at 24 months (n=32), and 153 (± 52) pg/mL at 36 months (n=30).

The pharmacokinetic profile of NEXPLANON is shown in Figure 20.

[See figure 20 above]

Distribution
The apparent volume of distribution averages about 201 L. Etonogestrel is approximately 32% bound to sex hormone binding globulin (SHBG) and 66% bound to albumin in blood.

Metabolism
In vitro data shows that etonogestrel is metabolized in liver microsomes by the cytochrome P450 3A4 isoenzyme. The biological activity of etonogestrel metabolites is unknown.

Excretion
The elimination half-life of etonogestrel is approximately 25 hours. Excretion of etonogestrel and its metabolites, either as free steroid or as conjugates, is mainly in urine and to a lesser extent in feces. After removal of the implant, etonogestrel concentrations decreased below sensitivity of the assay by one week.

13 NONCLINICAL TOXICOLOGY
13.1 Carcinogenesis, Mutagenesis, Impairment of Fertility
In a 24-month carcinogenicity study in rats with subdermal implants releasing 10 and 20 mcg etonogestrel per day (equal to approximately 1.8-3.6 times the systemic steady state exposure in women using NEXPLANON), no drug-related carcinogenic potential was observed. Etonogestrel was not genotoxic in the *in vitro* Ames/Salmonella reverse mutation assay, the chromosomal aberration assay in Chinese hamster ovary cells or in the *in vivo* mouse micronucleus test. Fertility in rats returned after withdrawal from treatment.

14 CLINICAL STUDIES
14.1 Pregnancy
In clinical trials of up to 3 years duration that involved 923 subjects, 18-40 years of age at entry, and 1756 women-years of use with the non-radiopaque etonogestrel implant (IMPLANON), the total exposures expressed as 28-day cycle equivalents by study year were:

Year 1: 10,866 cycles
Year 2: 8581 cycles
Year 3: 3442 cycles

The clinical trials excluded women who:
• Weighed more than 130% of their ideal body weight
• Were chronically taking medications that induce liver enzymes

In the subgroup of women, 18-35 years of age at entry, 6 pregnancies during 20,648 cycles of use were reported. Two pregnancies occurred in each of Years 1, 2, and 3. Each conception was likely to have occurred shortly before or within 2 weeks after removal of the non-radiopaque etonogestrel implant. With these 6 pregnancies, the cumulative Pearl Index was 0.38 pregnancies per 100 women-years of use.

14.2 Return to Ovulation
In clinical trials with the non-radiopaque etonogestrel implant (IMPLANON), the etonogestrel levels in blood decreased below sensitivity of the assay by one week after removal of the implant. In addition, pregnancies were observed to occur as early as 7 to 14 days after removal. Therefore, a woman should re-start contraception immediately after removal of the implant if continued contraceptive protection is desired.

14.3 Implant Insertion and Removal Characteristics
Out of 301 insertions of the NEXPLANON implant in a clinical trial, the mean insertion time (from the removal of the protection cap of the applicator until retraction of the needle from the arm) was 27.9 ± 29.3 seconds. After insertion, 300 out of 301 (99.7%) NEXPLANON implants were palpable. The single, non-palpable implant was not inserted according to the instructions.

For 112 out of 114 (98.2%) subjects in 2 clinical trials for whom insertion and removal data were available, NEXPLANON implants were clearly visible with use of two-dimensional x-ray after insertion. The two implants that were not clearly visible after insertion were clearly visible with two-dimensional x-ray before removal.

16 HOW SUPPLIED/STORAGE AND HANDLING
16.1 How Supplied
NEXPLANON is supplied as follows:
NDC 0052-0274-01
One NEXPLANON package consists of a single implant containing 68 mg etonogestrel and 15 mg of barium sulfate that is 4 cm in length and 2 mm in diameter, which is pre-loaded in the needle of a disposable applicator. The sterile applicator containing the implant is packed in a blister pack.
NDC 0052-4330-01
One NEXPLANON package consists of a single implant containing 68 mg etonogestrel, 15 mg of barium sulfate and 0.1 mg of magnesium stearate that is 4 cm in length and 2 mm in diameter, which is pre-loaded in the needle of a disposable applicator. The sterile applicator containing the implant is packed in a blister pack.

Figure 20: Mean (± SD) Serum Concentration-Time Profile of Etonogestrel After Insertion of NEXPLANON During 3 Years of Use

16.2 Storage and Handling
Store NEXPLANON (etonogestrel implant) Radiopaque at 25°C (77°F); excursions permitted to 15-30°C (59-86°F) [see USP Controlled Room Temperature]. Avoid storing NEXPLANON at temperatures above 30°C (86°F).

17 PATIENT COUNSELING INFORMATION
See FDA-Approved Patient Labeling.
Information for Patients
• Counsel women about the insertion and removal procedure of the NEXPLANON implant. Provide the woman with a copy of the Patient Labeling and ensure that she understands the information in the Patient Labeling before insertion and removal. A USER CARD and consent form are included in the packaging. Have the woman complete a consent form and retain it in your records. The USER CARD should be filled out and given to the woman after insertion of the NEXPLANON implant so that she will have a record of the location of the implant in the upper arm and when it should be removed.
• Counsel women that NEXPLANON does not protect against HIV infection (AIDS) or other sexually transmitted diseases.
• Counsel women that the use of NEXPLANON may be associated with changes in their normal menstrual bleeding patterns so that they know what to expect.

FDA-Approved Patient Labeling
See the full patient product information for NEXPLANON.
Manufactured for: Merck Sharp & Dohme Corp., a subsidiary of
MERCK & CO., INC., Whitehouse Station, NJ 08889, USA
Manufactured by: N.V. Organon, Oss, The Netherlands, a subsidiary of **Merck & Co., Inc.**, Whitehouse Station, NJ 08889, USA
For patent information:
www.merck.com/product/patent/home.html
Copyright © 2011 Merck Sharp & Dohme B.V., a subsidiary of Merck & Co., Inc.
All rights reserved.
Revised: 07/2014
uspi-mk8415-iptx-1407r014
FDA-Approved Patient Labeling
NEXPLANON® (etonogestrel implant)
Radiopaque
Subdermal Use Only
NEXPLANON® does not protect against HIV infection (the virus that causes AIDS) or other sexually transmitted diseases. Read this Patient Information leaflet carefully before you decide if NEXPLANON is right for you. This information does not take the place of talking with your healthcare provider. If you have any questions about NEXPLANON, ask your healthcare provider.

What is NEXPLANON?
NEXPLANON is a hormone-releasing birth control implant for use by women to prevent pregnancy for up to 3 years. The implant is a flexible plastic rod about the size of a matchstick that contains a progestin hormone called etonogestrel. It contains a small amount of barium sulfate so that the implant can be seen by X-ray, and may also contain magnesium stearate. Your healthcare provider will insert the implant just under the skin of the inner side of your upper arm. You can use a single NEXPLANON implant for up to 3 years. NEXPLANON does not contain estrogen.
[See figure at top of next column]

What if I need birth control for more than 3 years?
The NEXPLANON implant must be removed after 3 years. Your healthcare provider can insert a new implant under your skin after taking out the old one if you choose to continue using NEXPLANON for birth control.

What if I change my mind about birth control and want to stop using NEXPLANON before 3 years?
Your healthcare provider can remove the implant at any time. You may become pregnant as early as the first week after removal of the implant. If you do not want to get pregnant after your healthcare provider removes the NEXPLANON implant, you should start another birth control method right away.

How does NEXPLANON work?
NEXPLANON prevents pregnancy in several ways. The most important way is by stopping the release of an egg from your ovary. NEXPLANON also thickens the mucus in your cervix and this change may keep sperm from reaching the egg. NEXPLANON also changes the lining of your uterus.

How well does NEXPLANON work?
When the NEXPLANON implant is placed correctly, your chance of getting pregnant is very low (less than 1 pregnancy per 100 women who use NEXPLANON for 1 year). It is not known if NEXPLANON is as effective in very overweight women because studies did not include many overweight women.
The following chart shows the chance of getting pregnant for women who use different methods of birth control. Each box on the chart contains a list of birth control methods that are similar in effectiveness. The most effective methods are at the top of the chart. The box on the bottom of the chart shows the chance of getting pregnant for women who do not use birth control and are trying to get pregnant.
[See figure at top of next page]

Who should not use NEXPLANON?
Do not use NEXPLANON if you:
• Are pregnant or think you may be pregnant
• Have, or have had blood clots, such as blood clots in your legs (deep venous thrombosis), lungs (pulmonary embolism), eyes (total or partial blindness), heart (heart attack), or brain (stroke)
• Have liver disease or a liver tumor
• Have unexplained vaginal bleeding
• Have breast cancer or any other cancer that is sensitive to progestin (a female hormone), now or in the past
• Are allergic to anything in NEXPLANON
Tell your healthcare provider if you have or have had any of the conditions listed above. Your healthcare provider can suggest a different method of birth control.
In addition, talk to your healthcare provider about using NEXPLANON if you:
• Have diabetes
• Have high cholesterol or triglycerides
• Have headaches
• Have gallbladder or kidney problems
• Have a history of depressed mood
• Have high blood pressure
• Have an allergy to numbing medicines (anesthetics) or medicines used to clean your skin (antiseptics). These medicines will be used when the implant is placed into or removed from your arm.

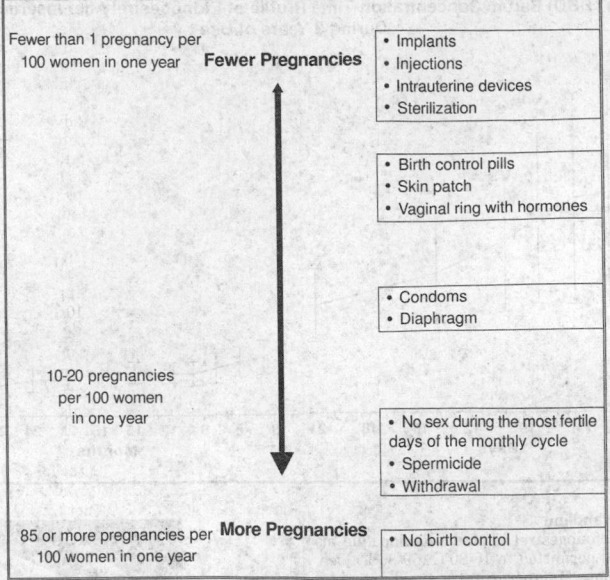

Fewer than 1 pregnancy per 100 women in one year **Fewer Pregnancies**
- Implants
- Injections
- Intrauterine devices
- Sterilization

- Birth control pills
- Skin patch
- Vaginal ring with hormones

- Condoms
- Diaphragm

10-20 pregnancies per 100 women in one year
- No sex during the most fertile days of the monthly cycle
- Spermicide
- Withdrawal

85 or more pregnancies per 100 women in one year **More Pregnancies**
- No birth control

- Scar tissue may form around the implant making it difficult to remove
- The implant may come out by itself. You may become pregnant if the implant comes out by itself. Use a back up birth control method and call your healthcare provider right away if the implant comes out.
- The need for surgery in the hospital to remove the implant
- Injury to nerves or blood vessels in your arm
- The implant breaks making removal difficult

- **Ectopic Pregnancy**
If you become pregnant while using NEXPLANON, you have a slightly higher chance that the pregnancy will be ectopic (occurring outside the womb) than do women who do not use birth control. Unusual vaginal bleeding or lower stomach (abdominal) pain may be a sign of ectopic pregnancy. Ectopic pregnancy is a medical emergency that often requires surgery. Ectopic pregnancies can cause serious internal bleeding, infertility, and even death. Call your healthcare provider right away if you think you are pregnant or have unexplained lower stomach (abdominal) pain.

- **Ovarian Cysts**
Cysts may develop on the ovaries and usually go away without treatment but sometimes surgery is needed to remove them.

- **Breast Cancer**
It is not known whether NEXPLANON use changes a woman's risk for breast cancer. If you have breast cancer now, or have had it in the past, do not use NEXPLANON because some breast cancers are sensitive to hormones.

- **Serious Blood Clots**
NEXPLANON may increase your chance of serious blood clots, especially if you have other risk factors such as smoking. It is possible to die from a problem caused by a blood clot, such as a heart attack or a stroke.
Some examples of serious blood clots are blood clots in the:
- Legs (deep vein thrombosis)
- Lungs (pulmonary embolism)
- Brain (stroke)
- Heart (heart attack)
- Eyes (total or partial blindness)
The risk of serious blood clots is increased in women who smoke. If you smoke and want to use NEXPLANON, you should quit. Your healthcare provider may be able to help. Tell your healthcare provider at least 4 weeks before if you are going to have surgery or will need to be on bed rest. You have an increased chance of getting blood clots during surgery or bed rest.

- **Other Risks**
A few women who use birth control that contains hormones may get:
- High blood pressure
- Gallbladder problems
- Rare cancerous or noncancerous liver tumors

When should I call my healthcare provider?
Call your healthcare provider right away if you have:
- Pain in your lower leg that does not go away
- Severe chest pain or heaviness in the chest
- Sudden shortness of breath, sharp chest pain, or coughing blood
- Symptoms of a severe allergic reaction, such as swollen face, tongue or throat; trouble breathing or swallowing
- Sudden severe headache unlike your usual headaches
- Weakness or numbness in your arm, leg, or trouble speaking
- Sudden partial or complete blindness
- Yellowing of your skin or whites of your eyes, especially with fever, tiredness, loss of appetite, dark colored urine, or light colored bowel movements
- Severe pain, swelling, or tenderness in the lower stomach (abdomen)
- Lump in your breast
- Problems sleeping, lack of energy, tiredness, or you feel very sad
- Heavy menstrual bleeding

What if I become pregnant while using NEXPLANON?
You should see your healthcare provider right away if you think that you may be pregnant. It is important to remove the implant and make sure that the pregnancy is not ectopic (occurring outside the womb). Based on experience with other hormonal contraceptives, NEXPLANON is not likely to cause birth defects.

Can I use NEXPLANON when I am breastfeeding?
If you are breastfeeding your child, you may use NEXPLANON if 4 weeks have passed since you had your baby. A small amount of the hormone contained in NEXPLANON passes into your breast milk. The health of breast-fed children whose mothers were using the implant has been studied up to 3 years of age in a small number of children. No effects on the growth and development of the children were seen. If you are breastfeeding and want to use NEXPLANON, talk with your healthcare provider for more information.

Additional Information
This Patient Information leaflet contains important information about NEXPLANON. If you would like more information, talk with your healthcare provider. You can ask your healthcare provider for information about NEXPLANON that is written for healthcare professionals. You may also call 1-877-467-5266 or visit www.NEXPLANON-USA.com.

Interaction with Other Medicines
Tell your healthcare provider about all the medicines you take, including prescription and non-prescription medicines, vitamins and herbal supplements. Certain medicines may make NEXPLANON less effective, including:
- barbiturates
- bosentan
- carbamazepine
- felbamate
- griseofulvin
- oxcarbazepine
- phenytoin
- rifampin
- St. John's wort
- topiramate
- HIV medicines

Ask your healthcare provider if you are not sure if your medicine is one listed above.
If there are medicines that you have been taking for a long time, that make NEXPLANON less effective, tell your healthcare provider. Your healthcare provider may remove the NEXPLANON implant and recommend a birth control method that can be used effectively with these medicines. When you are using NEXPLANON, tell all of your healthcare providers that you have NEXPLANON in place in your arm.

How is the NEXPLANON implant placed and removed?
Your healthcare provider will place and remove the NEXPLANON implant in a minor surgical procedure in his or her office. The implant is placed just under the skin on the inner side of your upper arm.
The timing of insertion is important. Your healthcare provider may:
- Perform a pregnancy test before inserting NEXPLANON
- Schedule the insertion at a specific time of your menstrual cycle (for example, within the first days of your regular menstrual bleeding)

Immediately after the NEXPLANON implant has been placed, you and your healthcare provider should check that the implant is in your arm by feeling for it.

If you and your healthcare provider cannot feel the NEXPLANON implant, use a non-hormonal birth control method (such as condoms) until your healthcare provider confirms that the implant is in place. You may need special tests to check that the implant is in place or to help find the implant when it is time to take it out.

Your healthcare provider will cover the site where NEXPLANON was placed with 2 bandages. Leave the top bandage on for 24 hours. Keep the smaller bandage clean, dry, and in place for 3 to 5 days.

You will be asked to review and sign a consent form prior to inserting the NEXPLANON implant. You will also get a USER CARD to keep at home with your health records. Your healthcare provider will fill out the USER CARD with the date the implant was inserted and the date the implant is to be removed. Keep track of the date the implant is to be removed. Schedule an appointment with your healthcare provider to remove the implant on or before the removal date.

Be sure to have checkups as advised by your healthcare provider.

What are the most common side effects I can expect while using NEXPLANON?

- **Changes in Menstrual Bleeding Patterns (menstrual periods)**
The most common side effect of NEXPLANON is a change in your normal menstrual bleeding pattern. In studies, one out of ten women stopped using the implant because of an unfavorable change in their bleeding pattern. You may experience longer or shorter bleeding during your periods or have no bleeding at all. The time between periods may vary, and in between periods you may also have spotting.
Tell your healthcare provider right away if:
- You think you may be pregnant
- Your menstrual bleeding is heavy and prolonged

Besides changes in menstrual bleeding patterns, other frequent side effects that caused women to stop using the implant include:
- Mood swings
- Weight gain
- Headache
- Acne
- Depressed mood

Other common side effects include:
- Headache
- Vaginitis (inflammation of the vagina)
- Weight gain
- Acne
- Breast pain
- Viral infections such as sore throats or flu-like symptoms
- Stomach pain
- Painful periods
- Mood swings, nervousness, or depressed mood
- Back pain
- Nausea
- Dizziness
- Pain
- Pain at the site of insertion

This is not a complete list of possible side effects. For more information, ask your healthcare provider for advice about any side effects that concern you. You may report side effects to the FDA at 1-800-FDA-1088.

What are the possible risks of using NEXPLANON?

- **Problems with Insertion and Removal**
The implant may not be placed in your arm at all due to a failed insertion. If this happens, you may become pregnant. Immediately after insertion, and with help from your healthcare provider, you should be able to feel the implant under your skin. If you can't feel the implant, tell your healthcare provider.

Removal of the implant may be very difficult or impossible because the implant is not where it should be. Special procedures, including surgery in the hospital, may be needed to remove the implant. If the implant is not removed, then the effects of NEXPLANON will continue for a longer period of time.

Other problems related to insertion and removal are:
- Pain, irritation, swelling, or bruising at the insertion site
- Scarring, including a thick scar called a keloid around the insertion site
- Infection

Manufactured for: Merck Sharp & Dohme Corp., a subsidiary of **MERCK & CO., INC.**, Whitehouse Station, NJ 08889, USA
Manufactured by: N.V. Organon, Oss, The Netherlands, a subsidiary of **Merck & Co., Inc.**, Whitehouse Station, NJ 08889, USA
For patent information:
www.merck.com/product/patent/home.html
Copyright © 2011 Merck Sharp & Dohme B.V., a subsidiary of **Merck & Co., Inc.**
All rights reserved.
Revised: 07/2014
usppi-mk8415-iptx-1407r014

NEXPLANON® (etonogestrel implant)
Radiopaque
Subdermal Use Only
PATIENT CONSENT FORM

I understand the Patient Labeling for NEXPLANON®. I have discussed NEXPLANON with my healthcare provider who answered all my questions. I understand that there are benefits as well as risks with using NEXPLANON. I understand that there are other birth control methods and that each has its own benefits and risks.

I also understand that this Patient Consent Form is important. I understand that I need to sign this form to show that I am making an informed and careful decision to use NEXPLANON, and that I have read and understand the following points:

- NEXPLANON helps to keep me from getting pregnant.
- No contraceptive method is 100% effective, including NEXPLANON.
- NEXPLANON has an implant that contains a hormone.
- It is important to have the NEXPLANON implant **placed in my arm** at the right time of my menstrual cycle.
- **After the implant is placed in my arm, I should check that it is in place by gently pressing my fingertips over the skin where the implant was placed. I should be able to feel the implant.**
- The implant must be removed at the end of three years. The implant can be removed sooner if I want.
- If I have trouble finding a healthcare provider to remove the implant, I can call 1-877-467-5266 for help.
- The implant is placed under the skin of my arm during a procedure done in my healthcare provider's office. There is a slight risk of getting a scar or an infection from this procedure.
- Removal is usually a minor procedure. Sometimes, removal may be more difficult. Special procedures, including surgery in the hospital, may be needed. Difficult removals may cause pain and scarring and may result in injury to nerves and blood vessels. If the implant is not removed, its effects may continue.
- **Most women have changes in their menstrual bleeding patterns while using NEXPLANON. I also will likely have changes in my menstrual bleeding pattern while using NEXPLANON. My bleeding may be irregular, lighter or heavier, or my bleeding may completely stop. If I think I am pregnant, I should contact my healthcare provider as soon as possible.**
- I understand the warning signs for problems with NEXPLANON. I should seek medical attention if any warning signs appear.
- I should tell all my healthcare providers that I am using NEXPLANON.
- I need to have a medical checkup regularly and at any time I am having problems.
- NEXPLANON does not protect me from HIV infection (AIDS) or any other sexually transmitted diseases.

After learning about NEXPLANON, I choose to use NEXPLANON.

_____
(Name of Healthcare Provider)

_____
(Patient Signature)   (Date)

WITNESSED BY:
The patient above has signed this consent in my presence after I counseled her and answered her questions.

_____
(Healthcare Provider Signature)   (Date)

I have provided an accurate translation of this information to the patient whose signature appears above. She has stated that she understands the information and has had an opportunity to have her questions answered.

_____
(Signature of Translator)   (Date)

Manufactured for: Merck Sharp & Dohme Corp., a subsidiary of **MERCK & CO., INC.**, Whitehouse Station, NJ 08889, USA

Manufactured by: N.V. Organon, Oss, The Netherlands, a subsidiary of **Merck & Co., Inc.**, Whitehouse Station, NJ 08889, USA
For patent information:
www.merck.com/product/patent/home.html
Copyright © 2011 Merck Sharp & Dohme B.V., a subsidiary of **Merck & Co., Inc.**
All rights reserved.
Revised: 09/2013
pcf-mk8415-ipt-1309r03

NITRO-DUR®   ℞
[nī-trō-dŭr]
(nitroglycerin)
Transdermal Infusion System

DESCRIPTION

Nitroglycerin is 1,2,3-propanetriol trinitrate, an organic nitrate whose structural formula is:

$$H_2CONO_2$$
$$|$$
$$HCONO_2$$
$$|$$
$$H_2CONO_2$$

and whose molecular weight is 227.09. The organic nitrates are vasodilators, active on both arteries and veins.
The NITRO-DUR® (nitroglycerin) Transdermal Infusion System is a flat unit designed to provide continuous controlled release of nitroglycerin through intact skin. The rate of release of nitroglycerin is linearly dependent upon the area of the applied system; each cm^2 of applied system delivers approximately 0.02 mg of nitroglycerin per hour. Thus, the 5-, 10-, 15-, 20-, 30-, and 40-cm^2 systems deliver approximately 0.1, 0.2, 0.3, 0.4, 0.6, and 0.8 mg of nitroglycerin per hour, respectively.
The remainder of the nitroglycerin in each system serves as a reservoir and is not delivered in normal use. After 12 hours, for example, each system has delivered approximately 6% of its original content of nitroglycerin.
The NITRO-DUR transdermal system contains nitroglycerin in acrylic-based polymer adhesives with a resinous cross-linking agent to provide a continuous source of active ingredient. Each unit is sealed in a paper polyethylene-foil pouch.
Cross section of the system.

Impermeable Backing — Nitroglycerin/Adhesive

CLINICAL PHARMACOLOGY

The principal pharmacological action of nitroglycerin is relaxation of vascular smooth muscle and consequent dilatation of peripheral arteries and veins, especially the latter. Dilatation of the veins promotes peripheral pooling of blood and decreases venous return to the heart, thereby reducing left ventricular end-diastolic pressure and pulmonary capillary wedge pressure (preload). Arteriolar relaxation reduces systemic vascular resistance, systolic arterial pressure, and mean arterial pressure (afterload). Dilatation of the coronary arteries also occurs. The relative importance of preload reduction, afterload reduction, and coronary dilatation remains undefined.
Dosing regimens for most chronically used drugs are designed to provide plasma concentrations that are continuously greater than a minimally effective concentration. This strategy is inappropriate for organic nitrates. Several well-controlled clinical trials have used exercise testing to assess the antianginal efficacy of continuously delivered nitrates. In the large majority of these trials, active agents were indistinguishable from placebo after 24 hours (or less) of continuous therapy. Attempts to overcome nitrate tolerance by dose escalation, even to doses far in excess of those used acutely, have consistently failed. Only after nitrates have been absent from the body for several hours has their antianginal efficacy been restored.

Pharmacokinetics

The volume of distribution of nitroglycerin is about 3 L/kg, and nitroglycerin is cleared from this volume at extremely rapid rates, with a resulting serum half-life of about 3 minutes. The observed clearance rates (close to 1 L/kg/min) greatly exceed hepatic blood flow; known sites of extrahepatic metabolism include red blood cells and vascular walls. The first products in the metabolism of nitroglycerin are inorganic nitrate and the 1,2- and 1,3-dinitroglycerols. The dinitrates are less effective vasodilators than nitroglycerin, but they are longer-lived in the serum, and their net contribution to the overall effect of chronic nitroglycerin regimens is not known. The dinitrates are further metabolized to (nonvasoactive) mononitrates and, ultimately, to glycerol and carbon dioxide.
To avoid development of tolerance to nitroglycerin, drug-free intervals of 10 to 12 hours are known to be sufficient;

shorter intervals have not been well studied. In one well-controlled clinical trial, subjects receiving nitroglycerin appeared to exhibit a rebound or withdrawal effect, so that their exercise tolerance at the end of the daily drug-free interval was less than that exhibited by the parallel group receiving placebo.
In healthy volunteers, steady-state plasma concentrations of nitroglycerin are reached by about 2 hours after application of a patch and are maintained for the duration of wearing the system (observations have been limited to 24 hours). Upon removal of the patch, the plasma concentration declines with a half-life of about an hour.

Clinical Trials

Regimens in which nitroglycerin patches were worn for 12 hours daily have been studied in well-controlled trials up to 4 weeks in duration. Starting about 2 hours after application and continuing until 10 to 12 hours after application, patches that deliver at least 0.4 mg of nitroglycerin per hour have consistently demonstrated greater antianginal activity than placebo. Lower-dose patches have not been as well studied, but in one large, well-controlled trial in which higher-dose patches were also studied, patches delivering 0.2 mg/hr had significantly less antianginal activity than placebo.
It is reasonable to believe that the rate of nitroglycerin absorption from patches may vary with the site of application, but this relationship has not been adequately studied.

INDICATIONS AND USAGE

Transdermal nitroglycerin is indicated for the prevention of angina pectoris due to coronary artery disease. The onset of action of transdermal nitroglycerin is not sufficiently rapid for this product to be useful in aborting an acute attack.

CONTRAINDICATIONS

Allergic reactions to organic nitrates are extremely rare, but they do occur. Nitroglycerin is contraindicated in patients who are allergic to it. Allergy to the adhesives used in nitroglycerin patches has also been reported, and it similarly constitutes a contraindication to the use of this product.

WARNINGS

Amplification of the vasodilatory effects of the NITRO-DUR patch by phosphodiesterase inhibitors, eg, sildenafil can result in severe hypotension. The time course and dose dependence of this interaction have not been studied. Appropriate supportive care has not been studied, but it seems reasonable to treat this as a nitrate overdose, with elevation of the extremities and with central volume expansion. The benefits of transdermal nitroglycerin in patients with acute myocardial infarction or congestive heart failure have not been established. If one elects to use nitroglycerin in these conditions, careful clinical or hemodynamic monitoring must be used to avoid the hazards of hypotension and tachycardia.
A cardioverter/defibrillator should not be discharged through a paddle electrode that overlies a NITRO-DUR patch. The arcing that may be seen in this situation is harmless in itself, but it may be associated with local current concentration that can cause damage to the paddles and burns to the patient.

PRECAUTIONS

General

Severe hypotension, particularly with upright posture, may occur with even small doses of nitroglycerin, particularly in the elderly. The NITRO-DUR Transdermal Infusion System should therefore be used with caution in elderly patients who may be volume-depleted, are on multiple medications, or who, for whatever reason, are already hypotensive. Hypotension induced by nitroglycerin may be accompanied by paradoxical bradycardia and increased angina pectoris.
Elderly patients may be more susceptible to hypotension and may be at greater risk of falling at the therapeutic doses of nitroglycerin.
Nitrate therapy may aggravate the angina caused by hypertrophic cardiomyopathy, particularly in the elderly.
In industrial workers who have had long-term exposure to unknown (presumably high) doses of organic nitrates, tolerance clearly occurs. Chest pain, acute myocardial infarction, and even sudden death have occurred during temporary withdrawal of nitrates from these workers, demonstrating the existence of true physical dependence.
Several clinical trials in patients with angina pectoris have evaluated nitroglycerin regimens which incorporated a 10- to 12-hour, nitrate-free interval. In some of these trials, an increase in the frequency of anginal attacks during the nitrate-free interval was observed in a small number of patients. In one trial, patients had decreased exercise tolerance at the end of the nitrate-free interval. Hemodynamic rebound has been observed only rarely; on the other hand, few studies were so designed that rebound, if it had occurred, would have been detected. The importance of these observations to the routine, clinical use of transdermal nitroglycerin is unknown.

Information for Patients

Daily headaches sometimes accompany treatment with nitroglycerin. In patients who get these headaches, the headaches may be a marker of the activity of the drug. Patients should resist the temptation to avoid headaches by altering the schedule of their treatment with nitroglycerin, since loss of headache may be associated with simultaneous loss of antianginal efficacy.

Treatment with nitroglycerin may be associated with lightheadedness on standing, especially just after rising from a recumbent or seated position. This effect may be more frequent in patients who have also consumed alcohol.

After normal use, there is enough residual nitroglycerin in discarded patches that they are a potential hazard to children and pets.

A patient leaflet is supplied with the systems.

Drug Interactions

The vasodilating effects of nitroglycerin may be additive with those of other vasodilators. Alcohol, in particular, has been found to exhibit additive effects of this variety.

Carcinogenesis, Mutagenesis, Impairment of Fertility

Animal carcinogenesis studies with topically applied nitroglycerin have not been performed.

Rats receiving up to 434 mg/kg/day of dietary nitroglycerin for 2 years developed dose-related fibrotic and neoplastic changes in liver, including carcinomas, and interstitial cell tumors in testes. At high dose, the incidences of hepatocellular carcinomas in both sexes were 52% vs 0% in controls, and incidences of testicular tumors were 52% vs 8% in controls. Lifetime dietary administration of up to 1058 mg/kg/day of nitroglycerin was not tumorigenic in mice.

Nitroglycerin was weakly mutagenic in Ames tests performed in two different laboratories. Nevertheless, there was no evidence of mutagenicity in an in vivo dominant lethal assay with male rats treated with doses up to about 363 mg/kg/day, po, or in in vitro cytogenetic tests in rat and dog tissues.

In a three-generation reproduction study, rats received dietary nitroglycerin at doses up to about 434 mg/kg/day for 6 months prior to mating of the F_0 generation with treatment continuing through successive F_1 and F_2 generations. The high dose was associated with decreased feed intake and body weight gain in both sexes at all matings. No specific effect on the fertility of the F_0 generation was seen. Infertility noted in subsequent generations, however, was attributed to increased interstitial cell tissue and aspermatogenesis in the high-dose males. In this three-generation study there was no clear evidence of teratogenicity.

Pregnancy

Pregnancy Category C

Animal teratology studies have not been conducted with nitroglycerin transdermal systems. Teratology studies in rats and rabbits, however, were conducted with topically applied nitroglycerin ointment at doses up to 80 mg/kg/day and 240 mg/kg/day, respectively. No toxic effects on dams or fetuses were seen at any dose tested. There are no adequate and well-controlled studies in pregnant women. Nitroglycerin should be given to a pregnant woman only if clearly needed.

Nursing Mothers

It is not known whether nitroglycerin is excreted in human milk. Because many drugs are excreted in human milk, caution should be exercised when nitroglycerin is administered to a nursing woman.

Pediatric Use

Safety and effectiveness in pediatric patients have not been established.

Geriatric Use

Clinical studies of NITRO-DUR Transdermal Infusion System did not include sufficient information to determine whether subjects 65 years and older respond differently from younger subjects. Additional clinical data from the published literature indicate that the elderly demonstrate increased sensitivity to nitrates, which may result in hypotension and increased risk of falling. In general, dose selection for an elderly patient should be cautious, usually starting at the low end of the dosing range, reflecting the greater frequency of the decreased hepatic, renal, or cardiac function, and of concomitant disease or other drug therapy.

ADVERSE REACTIONS

Adverse reactions to nitroglycerin are generally dose related, and almost all of these reactions are the result of nitroglycerin's activity as a vasodilator. Headache, which may be severe, is the most commonly reported side effect. Headache may be recurrent with each daily dose, especially at higher doses. Transient episodes of lightheadedness, occasionally related to blood pressure changes, may also occur. Hypotension occurs infrequently, but in some patients it may be severe enough to warrant discontinuation of therapy. Syncope, crescendo angina, and rebound hypertension have been reported but are uncommon.

Allergic reactions to nitroglycerin are also uncommon, and the great majority of those reported have been cases of contact dermatitis or fixed drug eruptions in patients receiving nitroglycerin in ointments or patches. There have been a few reports of genuine anaphylactoid reactions, and these reactions can probably occur in patients receiving nitroglycerin by any route.

Extremely rarely, ordinary doses of organic nitrates have caused methemoglobinemia in normal-seeming patients. Methemoglobinemia is so infrequent at these doses that further discussion of its diagnosis and treatment is deferred (see OVERDOSAGE).

Application-site irritation may occur but is rarely severe. In two placebo-controlled trials of intermittent therapy with nitroglycerin patches at 0.2 to 0.8 mg/hr, the most frequent adverse reactions among 307 subjects were as follows:

	Placebo	Patch
Headache	18%	63%
Lightheadedness	4%	6%
Hypotension, and/or Syncope	0%	4%
Increased Angina	2%	2%

OVERDOSAGE

Hemodynamic Effects

Nitroglycerin toxicity is generally mild. The estimated adult oral lethal dose of nitroglycerin is 200 mg to 1,200 mg. Infants may be more susceptible to toxicity from nitroglycerin. Consultation with a poison center should be considered. Laboratory determinations of serum levels of nitroglycerin and its metabolites are not widely available, and such determinations have, in any event, no established role in the management of nitroglycerin overdose.

No data are available to suggest physiological maneuvers (eg, maneuvers to change the pH of the urine) that might accelerate elimination of nitroglycerin and its active metabolites. Similarly, it is not known which – if any – of these substances can usefully be removed from the body by hemodialysis.

No specific antagonist to the vasodilator effects of nitroglycerin is known, and no intervention has been subject to controlled study as a therapy of nitroglycerin overdose. Because the hypotension associated with nitroglycerin overdose is the result of venodilatation and arterial hypovolemia, prudent therapy in this situation should be directed toward increase in central fluid volume. Passive elevation of the patient's legs may be sufficient, but intravenous infusion of normal saline or similar fluid may also be necessary. The use of epinephrine or other arterial vasoconstrictors in this setting is likely to do more harm than good.

In patients with renal disease or congestive heart failure, therapy resulting in central volume expansion is not without hazard. Treatment of nitroglycerin overdose in these patients may be subtle and difficult, and invasive monitoring may be required.

Methemoglobinemia

Nitrate ions liberated during metabolism of nitroglycerin can oxidize hemoglobin into methemoglobin. Even in patients totally without cytochrome b5 reductase activity, however, and even assuming that the nitrate moieties of nitroglycerin are quantitatively applied to oxidation of hemoglobin, about 1 mg/kg of nitroglycerin should be required before any of these patients manifests clinically significant (^{3}10%) methemoglobinemia. In patients with normal reductase function, significant production of methemoglobin should require even larger doses of nitroglycerin. In one study in which 36 patients received 2 to 4 weeks of continuous nitroglycerin therapy at 3.1 to 4.4 mg/hr, the average methemoglobin level measured was 0.2%; this was comparable to that observed in parallel patients who received placebo.

Notwithstanding these observations, there are case reports of significant methemoglobinemia in association with moderate overdoses of organic nitrates. None of the affected patients had been thought to be unusually susceptible.

Methemoglobin levels are available from most clinical laboratories. The diagnosis should be suspected in patients who exhibit signs of impaired oxygen delivery despite adequate cardiac output and adequate arterial PO_2. Classically, methemoglobinemic blood is described as chocolate brown, without color change on exposure to air.

Methemoglobinemia should be treated with methylene blue if the patient develops cardiac or CNS effects of hypoxia. The initial dose is 1 to 2 mg/kg infused intravenously over 5 minutes. Repeat methemoglobin levels should be obtained 30 minutes later and a repeat dose of 0.5 to 1.0 mg/kg may be used if the level remains elevated and the patient is still symptomatic. Relative contraindications for methylene blue include known NADH methemoglobin reductase deficiency or G-6-PD deficiency. Infants under the age of 4 months may not respond to methylene blue due to immature NADH methemoglobin reductase. Exchange transfusion has been used successfully in critically ill patients when methemoglobinemia is refractory to treatment.

DOSAGE AND ADMINISTRATION

The suggested starting dose is between 0.2 mg/hr[1] and 0.4 mg/hr[1]. Doses between 0.4 mg/hr[1] and 0.8 mg/hr[1] have shown continued effectiveness for 10 to 12 hours daily for at least 1 month (the longest period studied) of intermittent administration. Although the minimum nitrate-free interval has not been defined, data show that a nitrate-free interval of 10 to 12 hours is sufficient (see CLINICAL PHARMACOLOGY). Thus, an appropriate dosing schedule for nitroglycerin patches would include a daily patch-on period of 12 to 14 hours and a daily patch-off period of 10 to 12 hours.

Although some well-controlled clinical trials using exercise tolerance testing have shown maintenance of effectiveness when patches are worn continuously, the large majority of such controlled trials have shown the development of tolerance (ie, complete loss of effect) within the first 24 hours after therapy was initiated. Dose adjustment, even to levels much higher than generally used, did not restore efficacy.

[1] Release rates were formerly described in terms of drug delivered per 24 hours. In these terms, the supplied NITRO-DUR systems would be rated at 2.5 mg/24 hours (0.1 mg/hour), 5 mg/24 hours (0.2 mg/hour), 7.5 mg/24 hours (0.3 mg/hour), 10 mg/24 hours (0.4 mg/hour), and 15 mg/24 hours (0.6 mg/hour).

HOW SUPPLIED

NITRO-DUR System Rated Release In Vivo*	Total Nitroglycerin Content	System Size	Package Size
0.1 mg/hr	20 mg	5 cm^2	Unit Dose 30 (NDC 0085-3305-30) Institutional Package 30 (NDC 0085-3305-35)
0.2 mg/hr	40 mg	10 cm^2	Unit Dose 30 (NDC 0085-3310-30) Institutional Package 30 (NDC 0085-3310-35)
0.3 mg/hr	60 mg	15 cm^2	Unit Dose 30 (NDC 0085-3315-30) Institutional Package 30 (NDC 0085-3315-35)
0.4 mg/hr	80 mg	20 cm^2	Unit Dose 30 (NDC 0085-3320-30) Institutional Package 30 (NDC 0085-3320-35)
0.6 mg/hr	120 mg	30 cm^2	Unit Dose 30 (NDC 0085-3330-30) Institutional Package 30 (NDC 0085-3330-35)
0.8 mg/hr	160 mg	40 cm^2	Unit Dose 30 (NDC 0085-0819-30) Institutional Package 30 (NDC 0085-0819-35)

* Release rates were formerly described in terms of drug delivered per 24 hours. In these terms, the supplied NITRO-DUR systems would be rated at 2.5 mg/24 hours (0.1 mg/hour), 5 mg/24 hours (0.2 mg/hour), 7.5 mg/24 hours (0.3 mg/hour), 10 mg/24 hours (0.4 mg/hour), and 15 mg/24 hours (0.6 mg/hour).

Store at 25°C (77°F); excursions permitted to 15-30°C (59-86°F) [see USP Controlled Room Temperature]. Do not refrigerate.

Rx only

Merck Sharp & Dohme Corp., a subsidiary of **MERCK & CO., INC.**, Whitehouse Station, NJ 08889, USA
Copyright © 1987, 2012 Merck Sharp & Dohme Corp., a subsidiary of **Merck & Co., Inc.**
All rights reserved.

Revised: 05/2012
35208003T
Please read this instruction sheet carefully before using NITRO-DUR
Information for the Patient About—

Nitro-Dur®
(nitroglycerin)
Transdermal Infusion System

Summary
NITRO-DUR® is a unique method of administering nitroglycerin to the bloodstream. NITRO-DUR eliminates the swallowing of pills or the application of a messy ointment. Nitroglycerin is a medication your doctor has prescribed for you to help reduce the frequency and severity of angina attacks (chest pain).

How your NITRO-DUR Transdermal Infusion System works
Nitroglycerin causes the veins (vessels that return blood to the heart) to relax so that the work load of the heart is reduced. This lowers the heart's oxygen needs.

As a result, the heart muscle is well nourished and the frequency of angina attacks is reduced. NITRO-DUR is applied directly to the skin. The nitroglycerin passes from the adhesive surface through the skin—allowing medication to be absorbed directly into the bloodstream. This manner of delivering medicine to your bloodstream provides you with nitroglycerin with one daily application of a NITRO-DUR unit.

Instructions for use
Placement area
Select a reasonably hair-free application site. Avoid extremities below the knee or elbow, skin folds, scar tissue, burned or irritated areas.

Application
Wash hands before applying.

Hold the unit with brown lines facing you, in an up and down position.

Bend the sides of unit away from you, then toward you until you hear the "SNAP".
[See figure at top of next column]
Peel off one side of the plastic backing.
[See figure at top of next column]

Using the other half of the backing as a handle, apply the sticky side of the patch to the skin.

Press the sticky side on the skin, and smooth down.

Fold back the remaining side of the patch. Grasp the edge of the plastic applicator by the stripe, and pull it across the skin.

Wash hands to remove any drug.
Removal
[See figure at top of next column]
Press down on the center of the system to raise its outer edge away from the skin.
[See figure at top of next column]
Grasp the edge gently, and slowly peel the unit away from skin.
Wash skin area with soap and water. Towel dry. Wash hands. You may use a different application site every day.

Skin care
1. After you remove NITRO-DUR, your skin may feel warm and appear red. This is normal. The redness will disappear in a short time. If the area feels dry, you may apply a soothing lotion.
2. Any redness or rash that does not disappear should be called to your doctor's attention.

Cautions
If your doctor has prescribed "under-the-tongue" nitroglycerin tablets in addition to NITRO-DUR, you should sit down before taking the "under-the-tongue" tablet. If dizziness should occur, notify your doctor. This may be an indication that the "under-the-tongue" tablet dosage needs to be reduced.

Possible side effects
The most common side effect experienced by people taking nitroglycerin is headache. Your doctor may tell you to take a mild analgesic to relieve the headache.

Some people may experience dizziness. This is due to a slight decrease in blood pressure, which is usually experienced when a person changes position, from lying flat to sitting upright or from sitting to standing. If this occurs, sit down until the dizziness stops, then notify your doctor.

He or she may wish to reduce your NITRO-DUR dosage. In some people, nitroglycerin preparations may cause the skin to feel flushed or the heart to beat faster. If this should occur, notify your doctor; again, he or she may wish to change your NITRO-DUR dosage.

NITRO-DUR is a unique drug that depends on direct contact with the skin to work. For this reason, the skin should be reasonably hair-free, clean, and dry.

Other information
Allow NITRO-DUR to stay in place as directed by your doctor.

Showering is permitted with NITRO-DUR in place.

NITRO-DUR should be kept out of reach of children and pets.

Store at room temperature 77°F (25°C).

NITRO-DUR is boxed so that you have a 30-day supply. Be sure to check your supply periodically. Before it runs low, you should visit your pharmacist for a refill or ask your doctor to renew your NITRO-DUR prescription.

It is important that you do not miss a day of your NITRO-DUR therapy. If your schedule needs to be changed, your doctor will give you special instructions.

NITRO-DUR has been prescribed for you. Do not give your medication to anyone else.

NITRO-DUR is for prevention of angina; not for treatment of an acute angina attack.

Notify your doctor if angina attacks change for the worse.

> **You must consult your doctor for important information before using this drug.**

Merck Sharp & Dohme Corp., a subsidiary of
MERCK & CO.,INC., Whitehouse Station, NJ 08889, USA
Copyright © 1987, 2012 Merck Sharp & Dohme Corp., a subsidiary of **Merck & Co., Inc.**
All rights reserved.
Revised: 05/2012
35207902T

Shown in Product Identification Guide, page 308

Help Patients Save on Rx Drugs: PDR.net/PharmacyDiscountCard

NOXAFIL®
(posaconazole)
injection 18 mg/mL

NOXAFIL®
(posaconazole)
delayed-release tablets 100 mg

NOXAFIL®
(posaconazole)
oral suspension 40 mg/mL

Rx

HIGHLIGHTS OF PRESCRIBING INFORMATION
These highlights do not include all the information needed to use NOXAFIL safely and effectively. See full prescribing information for NOXAFIL.
Noxafil® (posaconazole) injection 18 mg/mL
Noxafil® (posaconazole) delayed-release tablets 100 mg
Noxafil® (posaconazole) oral suspension 40 mg/mL
Initial U.S. Approval: 2006 (oral suspension)

———RECENT MAJOR CHANGES———

Indications and Usage (1)	11/2013
Indications and Usage (1.1)	03/2014
Dosage and Administration (2)	11/2013
Dosage and Administration (2.1, 2.5)	03/2014
Dosage and Administration (2.4)	06/2014
Warnings and Precautions (5.1)	11/2013
Warnings and Precautions (5.4)	03/2014

———INDICATIONS AND USAGE———

Noxafil is an azole antifungal agent indicated for:
injection, delayed-release tablets, and oral suspension
• prophylaxis of invasive *Aspergillus* and *Candida* infections in patients who are at high risk of developing these infections due to being severely immunocompromised, such as HSCT recipients with GVHD or those with hematologic malignancies with prolonged neutropenia from chemotherapy. (1.1)
Oral suspension
• treatment of oropharyngeal candidiasis (OPC), including OPC refractory (rOPC) to itraconazole and/or fluconazole. (1.2)

———DOSAGE AND ADMINISTRATION———

Indication	Dose and Duration of Therapy
Prophylaxis of invasive *Aspergillus* and *Candida* infections	**Injection*:** Loading dose: 300 mg Noxafil injection intravenously twice a day on the first day. Maintenance dose: 300 mg Noxafil injection intravenously once a day thereafter. Duration of therapy is based on recovery from neutropenia or immunosuppression. (2.1) **Delayed-Release Tablets†:** Loading dose: 300 mg (three 100 mg delayed-release tablets) twice a day on the first day. Maintenance dose: 300 mg (three 100 mg delayed-release tablets) once a day, starting on the second day. Duration of therapy is based on recovery from neutropenia or immunosuppression. (2.2) **Oral Suspension‡:** 200 mg (5 mL) three times a day. Duration of therapy is based on recovery from neutropenia or immunosuppression. (2.3)
Oropharyngeal Candidiasis (OPC)	**Oral Suspension‡:** Loading dose: 100 mg (2.5 mL) twice a day on the first day. Maintenance dose: 100 mg (2.5 mL) once a day for 13 days. (2.3)
OPC Refractory (rOPC) to Itraconazole and/or Fluconazole	**Oral Suspension‡:** 400 mg (10 mL) twice a day. Duration of therapy is based on the severity of the patient's underlying disease and clinical response. (2.3)

* Noxafil injection must be administered through an in-line filter. Administer by intravenous infusion over approximately 90 minutes via a central venous line. Never give Noxafil injection as an intravenous bolus injection. (2)
† Noxafil delayed-release tablets should be taken with food. (2)
‡ Noxafil oral suspension should be taken with a full meal. (2)

———DOSAGE FORMS AND STRENGTHS———

• Noxafil injection: 300 mg per 16.7 mL (18 mg per mL) (3)
• Noxafil delayed-release tablet 100 mg (3)
• Noxafil oral suspension 40 mg per mL (3)

———CONTRAINDICATIONS———

• Do not administer to persons with known hypersensitivity to posaconazole or other azole antifungal agents. (4.1)
• Do not coadminister Noxafil with the following drugs; Noxafil increases concentrations of:
  ○ Sirolimus: can result in sirolimus toxicity (4.2, 7.1)
  ○ CYP3A4 substrates (pimozide, quinidine): can result in QTc interval prolongation and cases of TdP (4.3, 7.2)
  ○ HMG-CoA Reductase Inhibitors Primarily Metabolized Through CYP3A4: can lead to rhabdomyolysis (4.4, 7.3)
  ○ Ergot alkaloids: can result in ergotism (4.5, 7.4)

———WARNINGS AND PRECAUTIONS———

• Calcineurin Inhibitor Toxicity: Noxafil increases concentrations of cyclosporine or tacrolimus; reduce dose of cyclosporine and tacrolimus and monitor concentrations frequently. (5.1)
• Arrhythmias and QTc Prolongation: Noxafil has been shown to prolong the QTc interval and cause cases of TdP. Administer with caution to patients with potentially proarrhythmic conditions. Do not administer with drugs known to prolong QTc interval and metabolized through CYP3A4. Correct K^+, Mg^{++}, and Ca^{++} before starting Noxafil. (5.2)
• Hepatic Toxicity: Elevations in LFTs may occur. Discontinuation should be considered in patients who develop abnormal LFTs or monitor LFTs during treatment. (5.3)
• Noxafil injection should be avoided in patients with moderate or severe renal impairment (creatinine clearance <50 mL/min), unless an assessment of the benefit/risk to the patient justifies the use of Noxafil injection. (5.4, 8.6)
• Midazolam: Noxafil can prolong hypnotic/sedative effects. Monitor patients and benzodiazepine receptor antagonists should be available. (5.5, 7.5)

———ADVERSE REACTIONS———

• Common treatment-emergent adverse reactions in studies with posaconazole are diarrhea, nausea, fever, vomiting, headache, coughing, and hypokalemia. (6.2)
To report SUSPECTED ADVERSE REACTIONS, contact Merck Sharp & Dohme Corp., a subsidiary of Merck & Co., Inc., at 1-877-888-4231 or FDA at 1-800-FDA-1088 or www.fda.gov/medwatch.

———DRUG INTERACTIONS———

Interaction Drug	Interaction
Rifabutin, phenytoin, efavirenz, cimetidine, esomeprazole*	*Avoid coadministration unless the benefit outweighs the risks (7.6, 7.7, 7.8, 7.9)*
Other drugs metabolized by CYP3A4	*Consider dosage adjustment and monitor for adverse effects and toxicity (7.1, 7.10, 7.11)*
Digoxin	*Monitor digoxin plasma concentrations (7.12)*
Fosamprenavir, metoclopramide*	*Monitor for breakthrough fungal infections (7.6, 7.13)*

* The drug interactions with esomeprazole and metoclopramide do not apply to posaconazole tablets.

———USE IN SPECIFIC POPULATIONS———

• Pregnancy: Based on animal data, may cause fetal harm. (8.1)
• Nursing Mothers: Discontinue drug or nursing, taking in to consideration the importance of drug to the mother. (8.3)
• Severe renal impairment: Monitor closely for breakthrough fungal infections. (8.6)
See 17 for PATIENT COUNSELING INFORMATION and FDA-approved patient labeling

Revised: 06/2014

———FULL PRESCRIBING INFORMATION: CONTENTS*———

FULL PRESCRIBING INFORMATION

1 INDICATIONS AND USAGE

1.1 Prophylaxis of Invasive *Aspergillus* and *Candida* Infections

Noxafil® injection, delayed-release tablets, and oral suspension are indicated for prophylaxis of invasive *Aspergillus* and *Candida* infections in patients who are at high risk of developing these infections due to being severely immunocompromised, such as hematopoietic stem cell transplant (HSCT) recipients with graft-versus-host disease (GVHD) or those with hematologic malignancies with prolonged neutropenia from chemotherapy.

Noxafil injection is indicated in patients 18 years of age and older.

Noxafil delayed-release tablets and oral suspension are indicated in patients 13 years of age and older.

1.2 Treatment of Oropharyngeal Candidiasis Including Oropharyngeal Candidiasis Refractory to Itraconazole and/or Fluconazole

Noxafil oral suspension is indicated for the treatment of oropharyngeal candidiasis, including oropharyngeal candidiasis refractory to itraconazole and/or fluconazole.

2 DOSAGE AND ADMINISTRATION

General

The prescriber should follow the specific dosing instructions for each formulation.

Noxafil injection should be administered via a central venous line, including a central venous catheter or peripherally inserted central catheter (PICC), by slow intravenous infusion over approximately 90 minutes. If a central venous catheter is not available, Noxafil injection may be administered through a peripheral venous catheter by slow intravenous infusion over 30 minutes only as a single dose in advance of central venous line placement or to bridge the period during which a central venous line is replaced or is in use for other intravenous treatment. When multiple dosing is required, the infusion should be done via a central venous line. Never give Noxafil injection as an intravenous bolus injection.

The delayed-release tablet and oral suspension are not to be used interchangeably due to the differences in the dosing of each formulation.

Noxafil delayed-release tablets must be swallowed whole, and not be divided, crushed, or chewed. Noxafil delayed-release tablets should be taken with food [see Dosage and Administration (2.4) and Clinical Pharmacology (12.3)].

Noxafil oral suspension should be administered with a full meal or with a liquid nutritional supplement or an acidic carbonated beverage (e.g., ginger ale) in patients who cannot eat a full meal.

Coadministration of drugs that can decrease the plasma concentrations of posaconazole should generally be avoided unless the benefit outweighs the risk. If such drugs are necessary, patients should be monitored closely for breakthrough fungal infections [see Drug Interactions (7.6, 7.7, 7.8, 7.9, 7.13)].

Patients who have severe diarrhea or vomiting should be monitored closely for breakthrough fungal infections when receiving Noxafil delayed-release tablets or oral suspension.

2.1 Instructions for Use with Noxafil Injection

Dosing:

Table 1: Dosing for Noxafil Injection

Indication	Dose and Duration of Therapy
Prophylaxis of invasive *Aspergillus* and *Candida* infections	Loading dose: 300 mg Noxafil injection intravenously twice a day on the first day. Maintenance dose: 300 mg Noxafil injection intravenously once a day, starting on the second day. Duration of therapy is based on recovery from neutropenia or immunosuppression.

Preparation:

• Equilibrate the refrigerated vial of Noxafil (posaconazole) injection to room temperature.

• Aseptically transfer 16.7 mL of posaconazole solution to an intravenous bag (or bottle) containing approximately 150 mL of 5% dextrose in water or sodium chloride 0.9%. Noxafil injection should only be administered with these diluents. Use of other infusion solutions may result in particulate formation.

• Noxafil injection is a single dose sterile solution without preservatives. Once admixed, the product should be used immediately. If not used immediately, the solution can be stored up to 24 hours refrigerated 2-8°C (36-46°F). This medicinal product is for single use only and any unused solution should be discarded.

• Parenteral drug products should be inspected visually for particulate matter prior to administration, whenever solution and container permit. Once admixed, the solution of Noxafil ranges from colorless to yellow. Variations of color within this range do not affect the quality of the product.

Intravenous Line Compatibility:

A study was conducted to evaluate physical compatibility of Noxafil injection with injectable drug products and commonly used intravenous diluents during simulated Y-site infusion. Compatibility was determined through visual observations, measurement of particulate matter and turbidity. Based on the results of the study, the following drug products and diluents can be infused at the same time through

the same intravenous line (or cannula) as Noxafil injection. Co-administered drug products should be prepared in 5% dextrose in water or sodium chloride 0.9%. Co-administration of drug products prepared in other infusion solutions may result in particulate formation.

5% dextrose in water
Amikacin sulfate
Caspofungin
Ciprofloxacin
Daptomycin
Dobutamine hydrochloride
Famotidine
Filgrastim
Gentamicin sulfate
Hydromorphone hydrochloride
Levofloxacin
Lorazepam
Meropenem
Micafungin
Morphine sulfate
Norepinephrine bitartrate
Potassium chloride
Sodium chloride 0.9%
Vancomycin hydrochloride

Any products or diluents not listed in the table above should not be coadministered through the same intravenous line (or cannula).

Administration:

• Noxafil injection must be administered through a 0.22 micron polyethersulfone (PES) or polyvinylidene difluoride (PVDF) filter.

• Administer via a central venous line, including a central venous catheter or PICC by slow infusion over approximately 90 minutes. Noxafil injection is not for bolus administration.

If a central venous catheter is not available, Noxafil injection may be administered through a peripheral venous catheter only as a single dose in advance of central venous line placement or to bridge the period during which a central venous line is replaced or is in use for other treatment. When multiple dosing is required, the infusion should be done via a central venous line. When administered through a peripheral venous catheter, the infusion should be administered over approximately 30 minutes. Note: In clinical trials, multiple peripheral infusions given through the same vein resulted in infusion site reactions [see Adverse Reactions (6.2)].

2.2 Instructions for Use with Noxafil Delayed-Release Tablets

Table 2: Dosing for Noxafil Delayed-Release Tablets

Indication	Dose and Duration of Therapy
Prophylaxis of invasive *Aspergillus* and *Candida* infections	Loading dose: 300 mg (three 100 mg delayed-release tablets) twice a day on the first day. Maintenance dose: 300 mg (three 100 mg delayed-release tablets) once a day, starting on the second day. Duration of therapy is based on recovery from neutropenia or immunosuppression.

2.3 Instructions for Use with Noxafil Oral Suspension

Table 3: Dosing for Noxafil Oral Suspension

Indication	Dose and Duration of Therapy
Prophylaxis of invasive *Aspergillus* and *Candida* infections	200 mg (5 mL) three times a day. The duration of therapy is based on recovery from neutropenia or immunosuppression.
Oropharyngeal Candidiasis	Loading dose: 100 mg (2.5 mL) twice a day on the first day. Maintenance dose: 100 mg (2.5 mL) once a day for 13 days.
Oropharyngeal Candidiasis Refractory to Itraconazole and/or Fluconazole	400 mg (10 mL) twice a day. Duration of therapy should be based on the severity of the patient's underlying disease and clinical response.

Administration Instructions for Noxafil oral suspension

Shake Noxafil oral suspension well before use.

Figure 1: A measured dosing spoon is provided, marked for doses of 2.5 mL and 5 mL.

It is recommended that the spoon is rinsed with water after each administration and before storage.

2.4 Administration Information

Noxafil delayed-release tablets:

• Noxafil delayed-release tablets should be taken with food to enhance the oral absorption of posaconazole and optimize plasma concentrations.

• Noxafil delayed-release tablets should be used only for the prophylaxis indication.

• Noxafil delayed-release tablets generally provide higher plasma drug exposures than Noxafil oral suspension under both fed and fasted conditions, and therefore is the preferred oral formulation for the prophylaxis indication.

Noxafil oral suspension:

• Each dose of Noxafil oral suspension should be administered during or immediately (i.e., within 20 minutes) following a full meal to enhance the oral absorption of posaconazole and optimize plasma concentrations.

• In patients who cannot eat a full meal and for whom Noxafil delayed-release tablets or Noxafil injection are not options, each dose of Noxafil oral suspension should be administered with a liquid nutritional supplement or an acidic carbonated beverage.

• In patients who cannot eat a full meal or tolerate an oral nutritional supplement or an acidic carbonated beverage and who do not have the option of taking Noxafil delayed-release tablets or Noxafil injection, an alternative antifungal therapy should be considered or patients should be monitored closely for breakthrough fungal infections.

2.5 Use in Patients with Renal Impairment

The pharmacokinetics of Noxafil oral suspension are not significantly affected by renal impairment. Therefore, no adjustment is necessary for oral dosing in patients with mild to severe renal impairment.

Noxafil injection should be avoided in patients with moderate or severe renal impairment (eGFR <50 mL/min), unless an assessment of the benefit/risk to the patient justifies the use of Noxafil injection. In patients with moderate or severe renal impairment (estimated glomerular filtration rate (eGFR) <50 mL/min), receiving the Noxafil injection, accumulation of the intravenous vehicle, Betadex Sulfobutyl Ether Sodium (SBECD), is expected to occur. Serum creatinine levels should be closely monitored in these patients, and, if increases occur, consideration should be given to changing to oral Noxafil therapy.

3 DOSAGE FORMS AND STRENGTHS

Noxafil injection is available in Type I glass vials closed with bromobutyl rubber stopper and aluminum seal containing 300 mg per 16.7 mL of solution (18 mg of posaconazole per mL).

Noxafil 100 mg delayed-release tablets are available as yellow, coated, oblong tablets, debossed with "100" on one side.

Noxafil oral suspension is available in 4-ounce (123 mL) amber glass bottles with child-resistant closures containing 105 mL of suspension (40 mg of posaconazole per mL).

4 CONTRAINDICATIONS

4.1 Hypersensitivity

Noxafil is contraindicated in persons with known hypersensitivity to posaconazole or other azole antifungal agents.

4.2 Use with Sirolimus

Noxafil is contraindicated with sirolimus. Concomitant administration of Noxafil with sirolimus increases the sirolimus blood concentrations by approximately 9-fold and can result in sirolimus toxicity [see Drug Interactions (7.1) and Clinical Pharmacology (12.3)].

4.3 QT Prolongation with Concomitant Use with CYP3A4 Substrates

Noxafil is contraindicated with CYP3A4 substrates that prolong the QT interval. Concomitant administration of

Table 4: Posaconazole Injection Study 1: Number (%) of Subjects Treated with Posaconazole Injection 300 mg Daily Dose Reporting Treatment-Emergent Adverse Reactions: Frequency of at Least 10%

Body System Preferred Term	Posaconazole Injection Treatment Phase n=237 (%)*		Posaconazole Injection Treatment Phase or Subsequent Oral Suspension Treatment Phase n=237(%)†	
Subjects Reporting any Adverse Reaction	220	(93)	235	(99)
Blood and Lymphatic System Disorder				
Anemia	16	(7)	23	(10)
Thrombocytopenia	17	(7)	25	(11)
Gastrointestinal Disorders				
Abdominal Pain Upper	15	(6)	25	(11)
Abdominal Pain	30	(13)	41	(17)
Constipation	18	(8)	31	(13)
Diarrhea	75	(32)	93	(39)
Nausea	46	(19)	70	(30)
Vomiting	29	(12)	45	(19)
General Disorders and Administration Site Conditions				
Fatigue	19	(8)	24	(10)
Chills	28	(12)	38	(16)
Edema Peripheral	28	(12)	35	(15)
Pyrexia	49	(21)	73	(31)
Metabolism and Nutrition Disorders				
Decreased appetite	23	(10)	29	(12)
Hypokalemia	51	(22)	67	(28)
Hypomagnesemia	25	(11)	30	(13)
Nervous System Disorders				
Headache	33	(14)	49	(21)
Respiratory, Thoracic and Mediastinal Disorders				
Cough	21	(9)	31	(13)
Dyspnea	16	(7)	24	(10)
Epistaxis	34	(14)	40	(17)
Skin and Subcutaneous Tissue Disorders				
Petechiae	20	(8)	24	(10)
Rash	35	(15)	56	(24)
Vascular Disorders				
Hypertension	20	(8)	26	(11)

* Adverse reactions reported in patients with an onset during the posaconazole intravenous dosing phase of the study.
† Adverse reactions reported with an onset at any time during the study in patients who were treated for up to 28 days of posaconazole therapy.

Noxafil with the CYP3A4 substrates, pimozide and quinidine may result in increased plasma concentrations of these drugs, leading to QTc prolongation and cases of torsades de pointes [see Warnings and Precautions (5.2) and Drug Interactions (7.2)].

4.4 HMG-CoA Reductase Inhibitors Primarily Metabolized Through CYP3A4
Coadministration with the HMG-CoA reductase inhibitors that are primarily metabolized through CYP3A4 (e.g., atorvastatin, lovastatin, and simvastatin) is contraindicated since increased plasma concentration of these drugs can lead to rhabdomyolysis [see Drug Interactions (7.3) and Clinical Pharmacology (12.3)].

4.5 Use with Ergot Alkaloids
Posaconazole may increase the plasma concentrations of ergot alkaloids (ergotamine and dihydroergotamine) which may lead to ergotism [see Drug Interactions (7.4)].

5 WARNINGS AND PRECAUTIONS
5.1 Calcineurin-Inhibitor Drug Interactions
Concomitant administration of Noxafil with cyclosporine or tacrolimus increases the whole blood trough concentrations of these calcineurin-inhibitors [see Drug Interactions (7.1) and Clinical Pharmacology (12.3)]. Nephrotoxicity and leukoencephalopathy (including deaths) have been reported in clinical efficacy studies in patients with elevated cyclosporine or tacrolimus concentrations. Frequent monitoring of tacrolimus or cyclosporine whole blood trough concentrations should be performed during and at discontinuation of posaconazole treatment and the tacrolimus or cyclosporine dose adjusted accordingly.

5.2 Arrhythmias and QT Prolongation
Some azoles, including posaconazole, have been associated with prolongation of the QT interval on the electrocardiogram. In addition, cases of torsades de pointes have been reported in patients taking posaconazole.

Results from a multiple time-matched ECG analysis in healthy volunteers did not show any increase in the mean of the QTc interval. Multiple, time-matched ECGs collected over a 12-hour period were recorded at baseline and steady-state from 173 healthy male and female volunteers (18-85 years of age) administered posaconazole oral suspension 400 mg BID with a high-fat meal. In this pooled analysis, the mean QTc (Fridericia) interval change from baseline was −5 msec following administration of the recommended clinical dose. A decrease in the QTc(F) interval (−3 msec) was also observed in a small number of subjects (n=16) administered placebo. The placebo-adjusted maximum QTc(F) interval change from baseline was <0 msec (−8 msec). No healthy subject administered posaconazole had a QTc(F) interval ≥500 msec or an increase ≥60 msec in their QTc(F) interval from baseline.

Posaconazole should be administered with caution to patients with potentially proarrhythmic conditions. Do not administer with drugs that are known to prolong the QTc interval and are metabolized through CYP3A4 [see Contraindications (4.3) and Drug Interactions (7.2)]. Rigorous attempts to correct potassium, magnesium, and calcium should be made before starting posaconazole.

5.3 Hepatic Toxicity
Hepatic reactions (e.g., mild to moderate elevations in alanine aminotransferase (ALT), aspartate aminotransferase (AST), alkaline phosphatase, total bilirubin, and/or clinical hepatitis) have been reported in clinical trials. The elevations in liver function tests were generally reversible on discontinuation of therapy, and in some instances these tests normalized without drug interruption. Cases of more severe hepatic reactions including cholestasis or hepatic failure including deaths have been reported in patients with serious underlying medical conditions (e.g., hematologic malignancy) during treatment with posaconazole. These severe hepatic reactions were seen primarily in subjects receiving the posaconazole oral suspension 800 mg daily (400 mg BID or 200 mg QID) in clinical trials.

Liver function tests should be evaluated at the start of and during the course of posaconazole therapy. Patients who develop abnormal liver function tests during posaconazole therapy should be monitored for the development of more severe hepatic injury. Patient management should include laboratory evaluation of hepatic function (particularly liver function tests and bilirubin). Discontinuation of posaconazole must be considered if clinical signs and symptoms consistent with liver disease develop that may be attributable to posaconazole.

5.4 Renal Impairment
Due to the variability in exposure with Noxafil delayed-release tablets and oral suspension, patients with severe renal impairment should be monitored closely for breakthrough fungal infections [see Dosage and Administration (2.5) and Use in Specific Populations (8.6)].

Noxafil injection should be avoided in patients with moderate or severe renal impairment (eGFR <50 mL/min), unless an assessment of the benefit/risk to the patient justifies the use of Noxafil injection. In patients with moderate or severe renal impairment (eGFR <50 mL/min), receiving the Noxafil injection, accumulation of the intravenous vehicle, SBECD, is expected to occur. Serum creatinine levels should be closely monitored in these patients, and, if increases occur, consideration should be given to changing to oral Noxafil therapy [see Dosage and Administration (2.5) and Use in Specific Populations (8.6)].

5.5 Use with Midazolam
Concomitant administration of Noxafil with midazolam increases the midazolam plasma concentrations by approximately 5-fold. Increased plasma midazolam concentrations could potentiate and prolong hypnotic and sedative effects. Patients must be monitored closely for adverse effects associated with high plasma concentrations of midazolam and benzodiazepine receptor antagonists must be available to reverse these effects [see Drug Interactions (7.5) and Clinical Pharmacology (12.3)].

6 ADVERSE REACTIONS
6.1 Serious and Otherwise Important Adverse Reactions
The following serious and otherwise important adverse reactions are discussed in detail in another section of the labeling:
• Hypersensitivity [see Contraindications (4.1)]
• Arrhythmias and QT Prolongation [see Warnings and Precautions (5.2)]
• Hepatic Toxicity [see Warnings and Precautions (5.3)]

6.2 Clinical Trials Experience
Because clinical trials are conducted under widely varying conditions, adverse reaction rates observed in clinical trials of Noxafil cannot be directly compared to rates in the clinical trials of another drug and may not reflect the rates observed in practice. In clinical trials, the type of adverse reactions reported for posaconazole injection and posaconazole delayed-release tablets were generally similar to that reported in trials of posaconazole oral suspension.

Table 6: Posaconazole Oral Suspension Study 1 and Study 2. Number (%) of Randomized Subjects Reporting Treatment-Emergent Adverse Reactions: Frequency of at Least 10% in the Posaconazole Oral Suspension or Fluconazole Treatment Groups (Pooled Prophylaxis Safety Analysis)

Body System Preferred Term	Posaconazole (n=605)		Fluconazole (n=539)		Itraconazole (n=58)	
Subjects Reporting any Adverse Reaction	595	(98)	531	(99)	58	(100)
Body as a Whole - General Disorders						
Fever	274	(45)	254	(47)	32	(55)
Headache	171	(28)	141	(26)	23	(40)
Rigors	122	(20)	87	(16)	17	(29)
Fatigue	101	(17)	98	(18)	5	(9)
Edema Legs	93	(15)	67	(12)	11	(19)
Anorexia	92	(15)	94	(17)	16	(28)
Dizziness	64	(11)	56	(10)	5	(9)
Edema	54	(9)	68	(13)	8	(14)
Weakness	51	(8)	52	(10)	2	(3)
Cardiovascular Disorders, General						
Hypertension	106	(18)	88	(16)	3	(5)
Hypotension	83	(14)	79	(15)	10	(17)
Disorders of Blood and Lymphatic System						
Anemia	149	(25)	124	(23)	16	(28)
Neutropenia	141	(23)	122	(23)	23	(40)
Disorders of the Reproductive System and Breast						
Vaginal Hemorrhage*	24	(10)	20	(9)	3	(12)
Gastrointestinal System Disorders						
Diarrhea	256	(42)	212	(39)	35	(60)
Nausea	232	(38)	198	(37)	30	(52)
Vomiting	174	(29)	173	(32)	24	(41)
Abdominal Pain	161	(27)	147	(27)	21	(36)
Constipation	126	(21)	94	(17)	10	(17)
Dyspepsia	61	(10)	50	(9)	6	(10)
Heart Rate and Rhythm Disorders						
Tachycardia	72	(12)	75	(14)	3	(5)
Infection and Infestations						
Pharyngitis	71	(12)	60	(11)	12	(21)
Liver and Biliary System Disorders						
Bilirubinemia	59	(10)	51	(9)	11	(19)
Metabolic and Nutritional Disorders						
Hypokalemia	181	(30)	142	(26)	30	(52)
Hypomagnesemia	110	(18)	84	(16)	11	(19)
Hyperglycemia	68	(11)	76	(14)	2	(3)
Hypocalcemia	56	(9)	55	(10)	5	(9)

(Table continued on next page)

Clinical Trial Experience with Posaconazole Injection
Multiple doses of posaconazole injection administered via a peripheral venous catheter were associated with thrombophlebitis (60% incidence). Therefore, in subsequent studies, posaconazole injection was administered via central venous catheter.
The safety of posaconazole injection has been assessed in 268 patients in a clinical trial. Patients were enrolled in a non-comparative pharmacokinetic and safety trial of posaconazole injection when given as antifungal prophylaxis (Posaconazole Injection Study 1). Patients were immunocompromised with underlying conditions including hema-tological malignancy, neutropenia post-chemotherapy, GVHD, and post HSCT. This patient population was 55% male, had a mean age of 51 years (range 18-82 years, 19% of patients were ≥65 years of age), and were 95% white and 8% Hispanic. Ten patients received a single dose of 200 mg posaconazole injection, 21 patients received 200 mg daily dose for a median of 14 days, and 237 patients received 300 mg daily dose for a median of 9 days.
Table 4 presents treatment-emergent adverse reactions observed in patients treated with posaconazole injection 300 mg daily dose in the posaconazole injection study. Each patient received a loading dose, 300 mg twice on Day 1. Fol-lowing posaconazole intravenous therapy, patients received posaconazole oral suspension to complete 28 days of total posaconazole therapy.
[See table 4 at top of previous page]
The most frequently reported adverse reactions with an onset during the posaconazole intravenous phase of dosing with 300 mg once daily were diarrhea (32%), hypokalemia (22%), pyrexia (21%), and nausea (19%). These adverse reactions were consistent with those seen in studies with Noxafil oral suspension.

Clinical Trial Experience with Posaconazole Delayed-Release Tablets
The safety of posaconazole delayed-release tablets has been assessed in 230 patients in clinical trials. Patients were enrolled in a non-comparative pharmacokinetic and safety trial of posaconazole delayed-release tablets when given as antifungal prophylaxis (Delayed-Release Tablet Study 1). Patients were immunocompromised with underlying conditions including hematological malignancy, neutropenia post-chemotherapy, GVHD, and post HSCT. This patient population was 62% male, had a mean age of 51 years (range 19-78 years, 17% of patients were ≥65 years of age), and were 93% white and 16% Hispanic. Posaconazole therapy was given for a median duration of 28 days. Twenty patients received 200 mg daily dose and 210 patients received 300 mg daily dose (following twice daily dosing on Day 1 in each cohort). **Table 5** presents treatment-emergent adverse reactions observed in patients treated with 300 mg daily dose at an incidence of ≥10% in posaconazole delayed-release tablet study.

Table 5: Posaconazole Delayed-Release Tablet Study 1: Number (%) of Subjects Treated with 300 mg Daily Dose Reporting Treatment-Emergent Adverse Reactions: Frequency of at Least 10%

Body System Preferred Term	Posaconazole delayed-release tablet (300 mg) (n=210)	
Subjects Reporting any Adverse Reaction	201	(99)
Blood and Lymphatic System Disorder		
Anemia	22	(10)
Thrombocytopenia	29	(14)
Gastrointestinal Disorders		
Abdominal Pain	23	(11)
Constipation	20	(10)
Diarrhea	61	(29)
Nausea	56	(27)
Vomiting	28	(13)
General Disorders and Administration Site Conditions		
Asthenia	20	(10)
Chills	22	(10)
Mucosal Inflammation	29	(14)
Edema Peripheral	33	(16)
Pyrexia	59	(28)
Metabolism and Nutrition Disorders		
Hypokalemia	46	(22)
Hypomagnesemia	20	(10)
Nervous System Disorders		
Headache	30	(14)
Respiratory, Thoracic and Mediastinal Disorders		
Cough	35	(17)
Epistaxis	30	(14)
Skin and Subcutaneous Tissue Disorders		
Rash	34	(16)
Vascular Disorders		
Hypertension	23	(11)

Table 6 *(cont.)*: Posaconazole Oral Suspension Study 1 and Study 2. Number (%) of Randomized Subjects Reporting Treatment-Emergent Adverse Reactions: Frequency of at Least 10% in the Posaconazole Oral Suspension or Fluconazole Treatment Groups (Pooled Prophylaxis Safety Analysis)

Body System Preferred Term	Posaconazole (n=605)		Fluconazole (n=539)		Itraconazole (n=58)	
Subjects Reporting any Adverse Reaction	595	(98)	531	(99)	58	(100)
Musculoskeletal System Disorders						
Musculoskeletal Pain	95	(16)	82	(15)	9	(16)
Arthralgia	69	(11)	67	(12)	5	(9)
Back Pain	63	(10)	66	(12)	4	(7)
Platelet, Bleeding and Clotting Disorders						
Thrombocytopenia	175	(29)	146	(27)	20	(34)
Petechiae	64	(11)	54	(10)	9	(16)
Psychiatric Disorders						
Insomnia	103	(17)	92	(17)	11	(19)
Respiratory System Disorders						
Coughing	146	(24)	130	(24)	14	(24)
Dyspnea	121	(20)	116	(22)	15	(26)
Epistaxis	82	(14)	73	(14)	12	(21)
Skin and Subcutaneous Tissue Disorders						
Rash	113	(19)	96	(18)	25	(43)
Pruritus	69	(11)	62	(12)	11	(19)

* Percentages of sex-specific adverse reactions are based on the number of males/females.

The most frequently reported adverse reactions (>25%) with posaconazole delayed-release tablets 300 mg once daily were diarrhea, pyrexia, and nausea.

The most common adverse reaction leading to discontinuation of posaconazole delayed-release tablets 300 mg once daily was nausea (2%).

Clinical Trial Safety Experience with Posaconazole Oral Suspension

The safety of posaconazole oral suspension has been assessed in 1844 patients. This includes 605 patients in the active-controlled prophylaxis studies, 557 patients in the active-controlled OPC studies, 239 patients in refractory OPC studies, and 443 patients from other indications. This represents a heterogeneous population, including immunocompromised patients, e.g., patients with hematological malignancy, neutropenia post-chemotherapy, GVHD post HSCT, and HIV infection, as well as non-neutropenic patients. This patient population was 71% male, had a mean age of 42 years (range 8-84 years, 6% of patients were ≥65 years of age and 1% was <18 years of age), and were 64% white, 16% Hispanic, and 36% non-white (including 14% black). Posaconazole therapy was given to 171 patients for ≥6 months, with 58 patients receiving posaconazole therapy for ≥12 months. **Table 6** presents treatment-emergent adverse reactions observed at an incidence of >10% in posaconazole prophylaxis studies. **Table 7** presents treatment-emergent adverse reactions observed at an incidence of at least 10% in the OPC/rOPC studies.

Prophylaxis of Aspergillus and Candida: In the 2 randomized, comparative prophylaxis studies (Oral Suspension Studies 1 and 2), the safety of posaconazole oral suspension 200 mg three times a day was compared to fluconazole 400 mg once daily or itraconazole 200 mg twice a day in severely immunocompromised patients.

The most frequently reported adverse reactions (>30%) in the prophylaxis clinical trials were fever, diarrhea, and nausea.

The most common adverse reactions leading to discontinuation of posaconazole in the prophylaxis studies were associated with GI disorders, specifically, nausea (2%), vomiting (2%), and hepatic enzymes increased (2%).

[See table 6 on previous page and above]

HIV Infected Subjects with OPC: In 2 randomized comparative studies in OPC, the safety of posaconazole oral suspension at a dose of less than or equal to 400 mg QD in 557 HIV-infected patients was compared to the safety of fluconazole in 262 HIV-infected patients at a dose of 100 mg QD. An additional 239 HIV-infected patients with refractory OPC received posaconazole oral suspension in 2 non-comparative trials for refractory OPC (rOPC). Of these subjects, 149 received the 800-mg/day dose and the remainder received the less than or equal to 400-mg QD dose.

In the OPC/rOPC studies, the most common adverse reactions were fever, diarrhea, nausea, headache, vomiting, and coughing.

The most common adverse reactions that led to treatment discontinuation of posaconazole in the Controlled OPC Pool included respiratory impairment (1%) and pneumonia (1%). In the refractory OPC pool, the most common adverse reactions that led to treatment discontinuation of posaconazole were AIDS (7%) and respiratory impairment (3%).

[See table 7 at top of next page]

Adverse reactions were reported more frequently in the pool of patients with refractory OPC. Among these highly immunocompromised patients with advanced HIV disease, serious adverse reactions (SARs) were reported in 55% (132/239). The most commonly reported SARs were fever (13%) and neutropenia (10%).

Less Common Adverse Reactions: Clinically significant adverse reactions reported during clinical trials in prophylaxis, OPC/rOPC or other trials with posaconazole which occurred in less than 5% of patients are listed below:

- **Blood and lymphatic system disorders:** hemolytic uremic syndrome, thrombotic thrombocytopenic purpura, neutropenia aggravated
- **Endocrine disorders:** adrenal insufficiency
- **Nervous system disorders:** paresthesia
- **Immune system disorders:** allergic reaction *[see Contraindications (4.1)]*
- **Cardiac disorders:** Torsades de pointes *[see Warnings and Precautions (5.2)]*
- **Vascular disorders:** pulmonary embolism
- **Liver and Biliary System Disorders:** bilirubinemia, hepatic enzymes increased, hepatic function abnormal, hepatitis, hepatomegaly, jaundice, AST Increased, ALT Increased
- **Metabolic and Nutritional Disorders:** hypokalemia
- **Platelet, Bleeding, and Clotting Disorders:** thrombocytopenia
- **Renal & Urinary System Disorders:** renal failure acute

Clinical Laboratory Values: In healthy volunteers and patients, elevation of liver function test values did not appear to be associated with higher plasma concentrations of posaconazole.

For the prophylaxis studies, the number of patients with changes in liver function tests from Common Toxicity Criteria (CTC) Grade 0, 1, or 2 at baseline to Grade 3 or 4 during the study is presented in **Table 8**.

Table 8: Posaconazole Oral Suspension Study 1 and Study 2. Changes in Liver Function Test Results from CTC Grade 0, 1, or 2 at Baseline to Grade 3 or 4

Number (%) of Patients With Change*		
Oral Suspension Study 1		
Laboratory Parameter	Posaconazole n=301	Fluconazole n=299
AST	11/266 (4)	13/266 (5)
ALT	47/271 (17)	39/272 (14)
Bilirubin	24/271 (9)	20/275 (7)
Alkaline Phosphatase	9/271 (3)	8/271 (3)
Oral Suspension Study 2		
Laboratory Parameter	Posaconazole (n=304)	Fluconazole/ Itraconazole (n=298)
AST	9/286 (3)	5/280 (2)
ALT	18/289 (6)	13/284 (5)
Bilirubin	20/290 (7)	25/285 (9)
Alkaline Phosphatase	4/281 (1)	1/276 (<1)

CTC = Common Toxicity Criteria; AST= Aspartate Aminotransferase; ALT= Alanine Aminotransferase.
* Change from Grade 0 to 2 at baseline to Grade 3 or 4 during the study. These data are presented in the form X/Y, where X represents the number of patients who met the criterion as indicated, and Y represents the number of patients who had a baseline observation and at least one post-baseline observation.

The number of patients treated for OPC with clinically significant liver function test (LFT) abnormalities at any time during the studies is provided in **Table 9** (LFT abnormalities were present in some of these patients prior to initiation of the study drug).

[See table 9 at top of page 1580]

6.3　Postmarketing Experience

No clinically significant postmarketing adverse reactions were identified that have not previously been reported during clinical trials experience.

7　DRUG INTERACTIONS

Posaconazole is primarily metabolized via UDP glucuronosyltransferase and is a substrate of p-glycoprotein (P-gp) efflux. Therefore, inhibitors or inducers of these clearance pathways may affect posaconazole plasma concentrations. Coadministration of drugs that can decrease the plasma concentrations of posaconazole should generally be avoided unless the benefit outweighs the risk. If such drugs are necessary, patients should be monitored closely for breakthrough fungal infections.

Posaconazole is also a strong inhibitor of CYP3A4. Therefore, plasma concentrations of drugs predominantly metabolized by CYP3A4 may be increased by posaconazole *[see Clinical Pharmacology (12.3)]*.

The following information was derived from data with posaconazole oral suspension or early tablet formulation. All drug interactions with posaconazole oral suspension, except for those that affect the absorption of posaconazole (via gastric pH and motility) are considered relevant to posaconazole injection as well *[see Drug Interactions (7.9) and (7.13)]*.

7.1　Immunosuppressants Metabolized by CYP3A4

Sirolimus: Concomitant administration of posaconazole with sirolimus increases the sirolimus blood concentrations by approximately 9-fold and can result in sirolimus toxicity. Therefore, posaconazole is contraindicated with sirolimus *[see Contraindications (4.2) and Clinical Pharmacology (12.3)]*.

Tacrolimus: Posaconazole has been shown to significantly increase the C_{max} and AUC of tacrolimus. At initiation of posaconazole treatment, reduce the tacrolimus dose to approximately one-third of the original dose. Frequent monitoring of tacrolimus whole blood trough concentrations should be performed during and at discontinuation of posaconazole treatment and the tacrolimus dose adjusted accordingly *[see Warnings and Precautions (5.1) and Clinical Pharmacology (12.3)]*.

Cyclosporine: Posaconazole has been shown to increase cyclosporine whole blood concentrations in heart transplant patients upon initiation of posaconazole treatment. It is recommended to reduce cyclosporine dose to approximately three-fourths of the original dose upon initiation of posaconazole treatment. Frequent monitoring of cyclosporine whole blood trough concentrations should be performed during and at discontinuation of posaconazole treatment and the cyclosporine dose adjusted accordingly [see Warnings and Precautions (5.1) and Clinical Pharmacology (12.3)].

7.2 CYP3A4 Substrates

Concomitant administration of posaconazole with CYP3A4 substrates such as pimozide and quinidine may result in increased plasma concentrations of these drugs, leading to QTc prolongation and cases of torsades de pointes. Therefore, posaconazole is contraindicated with these drugs [see Contraindications (4.3) and Warnings and Precautions (5.2)].

7.3 HMG-CoA Reductase Inhibitors (Statins) Primarily Metabolized Through CYP3A4

Concomitant administration of posaconazole with simvastatin increases the simvastatin plasma concentrations by approximately 10-fold. Therefore, posaconazole is contraindicated with HMG-CoA reductase inhibitors primarily metabolized through CYP3A4 [see Contraindications (4.4) and Clinical Pharmacology (12.3)].

7.4 Ergot Alkaloids

Most of the ergot alkaloids are substrates of CYP3A4. Posaconazole may increase the plasma concentrations of ergot alkaloids (ergotamine and dihydroergotamine) which may lead to ergotism. Therefore, posaconazole is contraindicated with ergot alkaloids [see Contraindications (4.5)].

7.5 Benzodiazepines Metabolized by CYP3A4

Concomitant administration of posaconazole with midazolam increases the midazolam plasma concentrations by approximately 5-fold. Increased plasma midazolam concentrations could potentiate and prolong hypnotic and sedative effects. Concomitant use of posaconazole and other benzodiazepines metabolized by CYP3A4 (e.g., alprazolam, triazolam) could result in increased plasma concentrations of these benzodiazepines. Patients must be monitored closely for adverse effects associated with high plasma concentrations of benzodiazepines metabolized by CYP3A4 and benzodiazepine receptor antagonists must be available to reverse these effects [see Warnings and Precautions (5.5) and Clinical Pharmacology (12.3)].

7.6 Anti-HIV Drugs

Efavirenz: Efavirenz induces UDP-glucuronidase and significantly decreases posaconazole plasma concentrations [see Clinical Pharmacology (12.3)]. It is recommended to avoid concomitant use of efavirenz with posaconazole unless the benefit outweighs the risks.

Ritonavir and Atazanavir: Ritonavir and atazanavir are metabolized by CYP3A4 and posaconazole increases plasma concentrations of these drugs [see Clinical Pharmacology (12.3)]. Frequent monitoring of adverse effects and toxicity of ritonavir and atazanavir should be performed during coadministration with posaconazole.

Fosamprenavir: Combining fosamprenavir with posaconazole may lead to decreased posaconazole plasma concentrations. If concomitant administration is required, close monitoring for breakthrough fungal infections is recommended [see Clinical Pharmacology (12.3)].

7.7 Rifabutin

Rifabutin induces UDP-glucuronidase and decreases posaconazole plasma concentrations. Rifabutin is also metabolized by CYP3A4. Therefore, coadministration of rifabutin with posaconazole increases rifabutin plasma concentrations [see Clinical Pharmacology (12.3)]. Concomitant use of posaconazole and rifabutin should be avoided unless the benefit to the patient outweighs the risk. However, if concomitant administration is required, close monitoring for breakthrough fungal infections as well as frequent monitoring of full blood counts and adverse reactions due to increased rifabutin plasma concentrations (e.g., uveitis, leukopenia) are recommended.

7.8 Phenytoin

Phenytoin induces UDP-glucuronidase and decreases posaconazole plasma concentrations. Phenytoin is also metabolized by CYP3A4. Therefore, coadministration of phenytoin with posaconazole increases phenytoin plasma concentrations [see Clinical Pharmacology (12.3)]. Concomitant use of posaconazole and phenytoin should be avoided unless the benefit to the patient outweighs the risk. However, if concomitant administration is required, close monitoring for breakthrough fungal infections is recommended and frequent monitoring of phenytoin concentrations should be performed while coadministered with posaconazole and dose reduction of phenytoin should be *considered*.

7.9 Gastric Acid Suppressors/Neutralizers

Posaconazole Delayed-Release Tablet:
No clinically relevant effects on the pharmacokinetics of posaconazole were observed when posaconazole delayed-release tablets are concomitantly used with antacids, H$_2$-receptor antagonists and proton pump inhibitors [see Clinical Pharmacology (12.3)]. No dosage adjustment of posaconazole delayed-release tablets is required when posaconazole delayed-release tablets are concomitantly used with antacids, H$_2$-receptor antagonists and proton pump inhibitors.

Posaconazole Oral Suspension:
Cimetidine (an H$_2$-receptor antagonist) and esomeprazole (a proton pump inhibitor) when given with posaconazole oral

suspension results in decreased posaconazole plasma concentrations [see Clinical Pharmacology (12.3)]. It is recommended to avoid concomitant use of cimetidine and esomeprazole with posaconazole oral suspension unless the benefit outweighs the risks. However, if concomitant administration is required, close monitoring for breakthrough fungal infections is recommended.

No clinically relevant effects were observed when posaconazole oral suspension is concomitantly used with antacids and H$_2$-receptor antagonists other than cimetidine. No dosage adjustment of posaconazole oral suspension is required when posaconazole oral suspension is concomitantly used with antacids and H$_2$-receptor antagonists other than cimetidine.

7.10 Vinca Alkaloids

Most of the vinca alkaloids are substrates of CYP3A4. Posaconazole may increase the plasma concentrations of vinca alkaloids (e.g., vincristine and vinblastine) which may lead to neurotoxicity. Therefore, it is recommended that dose adjustment of the vinca alkaloid be considered.

7.11 Calcium Channel Blockers Metabolized by CYP3A4

Posaconazole may increase the plasma concentrations of calcium channel blockers metabolized by CYP3A4 (e.g., verapamil, diltiazem, nifedipine, nicardipine, felodipine). Frequent monitoring for adverse reactions and toxicity related to calcium channel blockers is recommended during coadministration. Dose reduction of calcium channel blockers may be needed.

7.12 Digoxin

Increased plasma concentrations of digoxin have been reported in patients receiving digoxin and posaconazole. Therefore, monitoring of digoxin plasma concentrations is recommended during coadministration.

Table 7: Treatment-Emergent Adverse Reactions with Frequency of at Least 10% in OPC Studies with Posaconazole Oral Suspension (Treated Population)

Body System Preferred Term	Number (%) of Subjects		
	Controlled OPC Pool		Refractory OPC Pool
	Posaconazole	Fluconazole	Posaconazole
	n=557	n=262	n=239
Subjects Reporting any Adverse Reaction*	356 (64)	175 (67)	221 (92)
Body as a Whole – General Disorders			
Fever	34 (6)	22 (8)	82 (34)
Headache	44 (8)	23 (9)	47 (20)
Anorexia	10 (2)	4 (2)	46 (19)
Fatigue	18 (3)	12 (5)	31 (13)
Asthenia	9 (2)	5 (2)	31 (13)
Rigors	2 (<1)	4 (2)	29 (12)
Pain	4 (1)	2 (1)	27 (11)
Disorders of Blood and Lymphatic System			
Neutropenia	21 (4)	8 (3)	39 (16)
Anemia	11 (2)	5 (2)	34 (14)
Gastrointestinal System Disorders			
Diarrhea	58 (10)	34 (13)	70 (29)
Nausea	48 (9)	30 (11)	70 (29)
Vomiting	37 (7)	18 (7)	67 (28)
Abdominal Pain	27 (5)	17 (6)	43 (18)
Infection and Infestations			
Candidiasis, Oral	3 (1)	1 (<1)	28 (12)
Herpes Simplex	16 (3)	8 (3)	26 (11)
Pneumonia	17 (3)	6 (2)	25 (10)
Metabolic and Nutritional Disorders			
Weight Decrease	4 (1)	2 (1)	33 (14)
Dehydration	4 (1)	7 (3)	27 (11)
Psychiatric Disorders			
Insomnia	8 (1)	3 (1)	39 (16)
Respiratory System Disorders			
Coughing	18 (3)	11 (4)	60 (25)
Dyspnea	8 (1)	8 (3)	28 (12)
Skin and Subcutaneous Tissue Disorders			
Rash	15 (3)	10 (4)	36 (15)
Sweating Increased	13 (2)	5 (2)	23 (10)

OPC=oropharyngeal candidiasis

* Number of subjects reporting treatment-emergent adverse reactions at least once during the study, without regard to relationship to treatment. Subjects may have reported more than 1 event.

Table 9: Posaconazole Oral Suspension Studies: Clinically Significant Laboratory Test Abnormalities without Regard to Baseline Value

	Controlled		Refractory
	Posaconazole	Fluconazole	Posaconazole
Laboratory Test	n=557(%)	n=262(%)	n=239(%)
ALT > 3.0 × ULN	16/537 (3)	13/254 (5)	25/226 (11)
AST > 3.0 × ULN	33/537 (6)	26/254 (10)	39/223 (17)
Total Bilirubin > 1.5 × ULN	15/536 (3)	5/254 (2)	9/197 (5)
Alkaline Phosphatase > 3.0 × ULN	17/535 (3)	15/253 (6)	24/190 (13)

ALT= Alanine Aminotransferase; AST= Aspartate Aminotransferase.

Table 10: Noxafil Oral Suspension Exposure Analysis (Cavg) in Prophylaxis Trials

	Prophylaxis in AML/MDS*		Prophylaxis in GVHD†	
	Cavg Range (ng/mL)	Treatment Failure‡ (%)	Cavg Range (ng/mL)	Treatment Failure‡ (%)
Quartile 1	90-322	54.7	22-557	44.4
Quartile 2	322-490	37.0	557-915	20.6
Quartile 3	490-734	46.8	915-1563	17.5
Quartile 4	734-2200	27.8	1563-3650	17.5

Cavg = the average posaconazole concentration when measured at steady state
* Neutropenic patients who were receiving cytotoxic chemotherapy for AML or MDS
† HSCT recipients with GVHD
‡ Defined as treatment discontinuation, use of empiric systemic antifungal therapy (SAF), or occurrence of breakthrough invasive fungal infections

7.13 Gastrointestinal Motility Agents
Posaconazole Delayed-Release Tablet:
Concomitant administration of metoclopramide with posaconazole delayed-release tablets did not affect the pharmacokinetics of posaconazole [see Clinical Pharmacology (12.3)]. No dosage adjustment of posaconazole delayed-release tablets is required when given concomitantly with metoclopramide.

Posaconazole Oral Suspension:
Metoclopramide, when given with posaconazole oral suspension, decreases posaconazole plasma concentrations [see Clinical Pharmacology (12.3)]. If metoclopramide is concomitantly administered with posaconazole oral suspension, it is recommended to closely monitor for breakthrough fungal infections.
Loperamide does not affect posaconazole plasma concentrations after posaconazole oral suspension administration [see Clinical Pharmacology (12.3)]. No dosage adjustment of posaconazole is required when loperamide and posaconazole are used concomitantly.

7.14 Glipizide
Although no dosage adjustment of glipizide is required, it is recommended to monitor glucose concentrations when posaconazole and glipizide are concomitantly used.

8 USE IN SPECIFIC POPULATIONS
8.1 Pregnancy
Pregnancy Category C: There are no adequate and well-controlled studies in pregnant women. Noxafil should be used in pregnancy only if the potential benefit outweighs the potential risk to the fetus.
Posaconazole has been shown to cause skeletal malformations (cranial malformations and missing ribs) in rats when given in doses ≥27 mg/kg (≥1.4 times the 400-mg BID oral suspension regimen based on steady-state plasma concentrations of drug in healthy volunteers). The no-effect dose for malformations in rats was 9 mg/kg, which is 0.7 times the exposure achieved with the 400-mg BID oral suspension regimen. No malformations were seen in rabbits at doses up to 80 mg/kg. In the rabbit, the no-effect dose was 20 mg/kg, while high doses of 40 mg/kg and 80 mg/kg, 2.9 or 5.2 times the exposure achieved with the 400-mg BID oral suspension regimen, caused an increase in resorptions. In rabbits dosed at 80 mg/kg, a reduction in body weight gain of females and a reduction in litter size were seen.

8.3 Nursing Mothers
Posaconazole is excreted in milk of lactating rats. It is not known whether Noxafil is excreted in human milk. Because of the potential for serious adverse reactions from Noxafil in nursing infants, a decision should be made whether to discontinue nursing or to discontinue the drug, taking into account the importance of the drug to the mother.

8.4 Pediatric Use
The safety and effectiveness of Noxafil injection in pediatric patients below the age of 18 years of age has not been established. Noxafil injection should not be used in pediatric patients because of nonclinical safety concerns [see Nonclinical Toxicology (13.2)].
The safety and effectiveness of posaconazole oral suspension and posaconazole delayed-release tablets have been established in the age groups 13 to 17 years of age. Use of posaconazole in these age groups is supported by evidence from adequate and well-controlled studies of posaconazole in adults. The safety and effectiveness of posaconazole in pediatric patients below the age of 13 years have not been established.
A total of 12 patients 13 to 17 years of age received 600 mg/day (200 mg three times a day) of posaconazole oral suspension for prophylaxis of invasive fungal infections. The safety profile in these patients <18 years of age appears similar to the safety profile observed in adults. Based on pharmacokinetic data in 10 of these pediatric patients, the mean steady-state average posaconazole concentration (Cavg) was similar between these patients and adults (≥18 years of age).
A total of 16 patients 8 to 17 years of age were treated with 800 mg/day (400 mg twice a day or 200 mg four times a day) of posaconazole oral suspension in a study for another indication. Based on pharmacokinetic data in 12 of these pediatric patients, the mean steady-state average posaconazole concentration (Cavg) was similar between these patients and adults (≥18 years of age).
In the prophylaxis studies, the mean steady-state posaconazole average concentration (Cavg) was similar among ten adolescents (13 to 17 years of age) and adults (≥18 years of age). This is consistent with pharmacokinetic data from another study in which mean steady-state posaconazole Cavg from 12 adolescent patients (8 to 17 years of age) was similar to that in the adults (≥18 years of age).

8.5 Geriatric Use
Of the 279 patients treated with posaconazole injection, 52 (19%) were greater than 65 years of age. The pharmacokinetics of posaconazole injection are comparable in young and elderly subjects. No overall differences in safety were observed between the geriatric patients and younger patients; therefore, no dosage adjustment is recommended for Noxafil injection in geriatric patients.
Of the 230 patients treated with posaconazole delayed-release tablets, 38 (17%) were greater than 65 years of age. The pharmacokinetics of posaconazole delayed-release tablets are comparable in young and elderly patients. No overall differences in safety were observed between the geriatric patients and younger patients; therefore, no dosage adjustment is recommended for geriatric patients.

Of the 605 patients randomized to posaconazole oral suspension in the prophylaxis clinical trials, 63 (10%) were ≥65 years of age. In addition, 48 patients treated with greater than or equal to 800-mg/day posaconazole in another indication were ≥65 years of age. No overall differences in safety were observed between the geriatric patients and younger patients.
The pharmacokinetics of posaconazole oral suspension are comparable in young and elderly subjects (≥65 years of age); therefore no adjustment in the dosage of Noxafil oral suspension is necessary in geriatric patients.
No overall differences in the pharmacokinetics and safety were observed between elderly and young subjects during clinical trials, but greater sensitivity of some older individuals cannot be ruled out.

8.6 Renal Impairment
Following single-dose administration of 400 mg of the oral suspension, there was no significant effect of mild (eGFR: 50-80 mL/min/1.73 m^2, n=6) or moderate (eGFR: 20-49 mL/min/1.73 m^2, n=6) renal impairment on posaconazole pharmacokinetics; therefore, no dose adjustment is required in patients with mild to moderate renal impairment. In subjects with severe renal impairment (eGFR: <20 mL/min/1.73 m^2), the mean plasma exposure (AUC) was similar to that in patients with normal renal function (eGFR: >80 mL/min/1.73 m^2); however, the range of the AUC estimates was highly variable (CV=96%) in these subjects with severe renal impairment as compared to that in the other renal impairment groups (CV<40%). Due to the variability in exposure, patients with severe renal impairment should be monitored closely for breakthrough fungal infections [see Dosage and Administration (2)]. Similar recommendations apply to posaconazole delayed-release tablets; however, a specific study has not been conducted with the delayed-release tablets.
Noxafil injection should be avoided in patients with moderate or severe renal impairment (eGFR <50 mL/min), unless an assessment of the benefit/risk to the patient justifies the use of Noxafil injection. In patients with moderate or severe renal impairment (eGFR <50 mL/min), receiving the Noxafil injection, accumulation of the intravenous vehicle, SBECD, is expected to occur. Serum creatinine levels should be closely monitored in these patients, and, if increases occur, consideration should be given to changing to oral Noxafil therapy [see Dosage and Administration (2.5) and Warnings and Precautions (5.4)].

8.7 Hepatic Impairment
After a single oral dose of posaconazole oral suspension 400 mg, the mean AUC was 43%, 27%, and 21% higher in subjects with mild (Child-Pugh Class A, N=6), moderate (Child-Pugh Class B, N=6), or severe (Child-Pugh Class C, N=6) hepatic impairment, respectively, compared to subjects with normal hepatic function (N=18). Compared to subjects with normal hepatic function, the mean C_{max} was 1% higher, 40% higher, and 34% lower in subjects with mild, moderate, or severe hepatic impairment, respectively. The mean apparent oral clearance (CL/F) was reduced by 18%, 36%, and 28% in subjects with mild, moderate, or severe hepatic impairment, respectively, compared to subjects with normal hepatic function. The elimination half-life ($t_{1/2}$) was 27 hours, 39 hours, 27 hours, and 43 hours in subjects with normal hepatic function and mild, moderate, or severe hepatic impairment, respectively.
It is recommended that no dose adjustment of Noxafil is needed in patients with mild to severe hepatic impairment (Child-Pugh Class A, B, or C) [see Dosage and Administration (2) and Warnings and Precautions (5.3)]. Similar recommendations apply to posaconazole delayed-release tablets; however, a specific study has not been conducted with the delayed-release tablets.
Similar recommendations apply to posaconazole injection; however, a specific study has not been conducted with the posaconazole injection.

8.8 Gender
The pharmacokinetics of posaconazole are comparable in men and women. No adjustment in the dosage of Noxafil is necessary based on gender.

8.9 Race
The pharmacokinetic profile of posaconazole is not significantly affected by race. No adjustment in the dosage of Noxafil is necessary based on race.

8.10 Weight
Pharmacokinetic modeling suggests that patients weighing greater than 120 kg may have lower posaconazole plasma drug exposure. It is, therefore, suggested to closely monitor for breakthrough fungal infections.

10 OVERDOSAGE
There is no experience with overdosage of posaconazole injection and delayed-release tablets.
During the clinical trials, some patients received posaconazole oral suspension up to 1600 mg/day with no adverse reactions noted that were different from the lower doses. In addition, accidental overdose was noted in one pa-

tient who took 1200 mg BID posaconazole oral suspension for 3 days. No related adverse reactions were noted by the investigator.

Posaconazole is not removed by hemodialysis.

11   DESCRIPTION

Noxafil is an azole antifungal agent available as concentrated solution to be diluted before intravenous administration, delayed-release tablet, or suspension for oral administration.

Posaconazole is designated chemically as 4-[4-[4-[4-[[(3R,5R)-5-(2,4-difluorophenyl)tetrahydro-5-(1H-1,2,4-triazol-1-ylmethyl)-3-furanyl]methoxy]phenyl]-1-piperazinyl]phenyl]-2-[(1S,2S)-1-ethyl-2-hydroxypropyl]-2,4-dihydro-3H-1,2,4-triazol-3-one with an empirical formula of $C_{37}H_{42}F_2N_8O_4$ and a molecular weight of 700.8. The chemical structure is:

Posaconazole is a white powder with a low aqueous solubility.

Noxafil injection is available as a clear colorless to yellow, sterile liquid essentially free of foreign matter. Each vial contains 300 mg of posaconazole and the following inactive ingredients: 6.68 g Betadex Sulfobutyl Ether Sodium (SBECD), 0.003 g edetate disodium, hydrochloric acid and sodium hydroxide to adjust the pH to 2.6, and water for injection.

Noxafil delayed-release tablet is a yellow, coated, oblong tablet containing 100 mg of posaconazole. Each delayed-release tablet contains the inactive ingredients: hypromellose acetate succinate, microcrystalline cellulose, hydroxypropylcellulose, silicon dioxide, croscarmellose sodium, magnesium stearate, and Opadry® II Yellow (consists of the following ingredients: polyvinyl alcohol partially hydrolyzed, Macrogol/PEG 3350, titanium dioxide, talc, and iron oxide yellow).

Noxafil oral suspension is a white, cherry-flavored immediate-release suspension containing 40 mg of posaconazole per mL and the following inactive ingredients: polysorbate 80, simethicone, sodium benzoate, sodium citrate dihydrate, citric acid monohydrate, glycerin, xanthan gum, liquid glucose, titanium dioxide, artificial cherry flavor, and purified water.

12   CLINICAL PHARMACOLOGY

12.1   Mechanism of Action

Posaconazole is an azole antifungal agent *[see Clinical Pharmacology (12.4)]*.

12.2   Pharmacodynamics

Exposure Response Relationship: In clinical studies of neutropenic patients who were receiving cytotoxic chemotherapy for acute myelogenous leukemia (AML) or myelodysplastic syndromes (MDS) or hematopoietic stem cell transplant (HSCT) recipients with Graft versus Host Disease (GVHD), a wide range of plasma exposures to posaconazole was noted following administration of Noxafil oral suspension. A pharmacokinetic-pharmacodynamic analysis of patient data revealed an apparent association between average posaconazole concentrations (Cavg) and prophylactic efficacy (**Table 10**). A lower Cavg may be associated with an increased risk of treatment failure, defined as treatment discontinuation, use of empiric systemic antifungal therapy (SAF), or occurrence of breakthrough invasive fungal infections.

[See table 10 at top of previous page]

12.3   Pharmacokinetics

General Pharmacokinetic Characteristics

Posaconazole Injection

Posaconazole injection exhibits dose proportional pharmacokinetics after single doses between 200 and 300 mg in healthy volunteers and patients. The mean pharmacokinetic parameters after single doses with posaconazole injection in healthy volunteers and patients are shown in **Table 11**.

[See table 11 above]

Table 12 displays the pharmacokinetic parameters of posaconazole in patients following administration of posaconazole injection 300 mg taken once a day for 10 or 14 days following BID dosing on Day 1.

[See table 12 above]

Posaconazole Delayed-Release Tablets

Noxafil delayed-release tablets exhibit dose proportional pharmacokinetics after single and multiple dosing up to 300 mg. The mean pharmacokinetic parameters of

posaconazole at steady state following administration of Noxafil delayed-release tablets 300 mg twice daily (BID) on Day 1, then 300 mg once daily (QD) thereafter in healthy volunteers and in neutropenic patients who are receiving cytotoxic chemotherapy for AML or MDS or HSCT recipients with GVHD are shown in **Table 13**.

[See table 13 above]

Posaconazole Oral Suspension

Dose-proportional increases in plasma exposure (AUC) to posaconazole oral suspension were observed following single oral doses from 50 mg to 800 mg and following multiple-

dose administration from 50 mg BID to 400 mg BID in healthy volunteers. No further increases in exposure were observed when the dose of the oral suspension increased from 400 mg BID to 600 mg BID in febrile neutropenic patients or those with refractory invasive fungal infections. The mean (%CV) [min-max] posaconazole oral suspension average steady-state plasma concentrations (Cavg) and steady-state pharmacokinetic parameters in patients following administration of 200 mg TID and 400 mg BID of the oral suspension are provided in **Table 14**.

[See table 14 above]

Table 11: Summary of Mean Pharmacokinetic Parameters (%CV) in Healthy Volunteers (30 minute infusion via peripheral venous line) and Patients (90 minute infusion via central venous line) after Dosing with Posaconazole Injection on Day 1

	Dose (mg)	n	$AUC_{0-\infty}$ (ng·hr/mL)	AUC_{0-12} (ng·hr/mL)	C_{max} (ng/mL)	$t_{1/2}$ (hr)	CL (L/hr)
Healthy Volunteers	200	9	35400 (50)	8840 (20)	2250 (29)	23.6 (23)	6.5 (32)
	300	9	46400 (26)	13000 (13)	2840 (30)	24.6 (20)	6.9 (27)
Patients	200	30	N/D	5570 (32)	954 (44)	N/D	N/D
	300	22	N/D	8240 (26)	1590 (62)	N/D	N/D

$AUC_{0-\infty}$ = Area under the plasma concentration-time curve from time zero to infinity; AUC_{0-12} = Area under the plasma concentration-time curve from time zero to 12 hr after the first dose on Day 1; C_{max} = maximum observed concentration; $t_{1/2}$ = terminal phase half-life; CL = total body clearance; N/D = Not Determined

---

Table 12: Arithmetic Mean (%CV) of PK Parameters in Serial PK-Evaluable Patients Following Dosing of Posaconazole Injection (300 mg)*

Day	N	C_{max} (ng/mL)	T_{max} † (hr)	AUC_{0-24} (ng*hr/mL)	Cav (ng/mL)	C_{min} (ng/mL)
10/14	49	3280 (74)	1.5 (0.98-4.0)	36100 (35)	1500 (35)	1090 (44)

AUC_{0-24} = area under the concentration-time curve over the dosing interval (i.e. 24 hours); Cav= time-averaged concentrations (i.e., $AUC_{0-24h}/24hr$); C_{min} = POS trough level immediately before a subject received the dose of POS on the day specified in the protocol; C_{max} = observed maximum plasma concentration; CV = coefficient of variation, expressed as a percent (%); Day = study day on treatment; T_{max} = time of observed maximum plasma concentration.

* 300 mg dose administered over 90 minutes once a day following BID dosing on Day 1

† Median (minimum-maximum)

Table 13: Arithmetic Mean (%CV) of Steady State PK Parameters in Healthy Volunteers and Patients Following Administration of Posaconazole Delayed-Release Tablets (300 mg)*

	N	$AUC_{0-24 hr}$ (ng·hr/mL)	Cav† (ng/mL)	C_{max} (ng/mL)	C_{min} (ng/mL)	T_{max} ‡ (hr)	$t_{1/2}$ (hr)	CL/F (L/hr)
Healthy Volunteers	12	51618 (25)	2151 (25)	2764 (21)	1785 (29)	4 (3-6)	31 (40)	7.5 (26)
Patients	50	37900 (42)	1580 (42)	2090 (38)	1310 (50)	4 (1.3-8.3)	-	9.39 (45)

CV = coefficient of variation expressed as a percentage (%CV); AUC_{0-T} = Area under the plasma concentration-time curve from time zero to 24 hr; C_{max} = maximum observed concentration; C_{min} = minimum observed plasma concentration; T_{max} = time of maximum observed concentration; $t_{1/2}$ = terminal phase half-life; CL /F = Apparent total body clearance

* 300 mg BID on Day 1, then 300 mg QD thereafter

† Cav = time-averaged concentrations (i.e., $AUC_{0-24 hr}/24hr$)

‡ Median (minimum-maximum)

Table 14: The Mean (%CV) [min-max] Posaconazole Steady-State Pharmacokinetic Parameters in Patients Following Oral Administration of Posaconazole Oral Suspension 200 mg TID and 400 mg BID

Dose*	Cavg (ng/mL)	AUC† (ng·hr/mL)	CL/F (L/hr)	V/F (L)	$t_{1/2}$ (hr)
200 mg TID‡ (n=252)	1103 (67) [21.5-3650]	ND§	ND§	ND§	ND§
200 mg TID¶ (n=215)	583 (65) [89.7-2200]	15,900 (62) [4100-56,100]	51.2 (54) [10.7-146]	2425 (39) [828-5702]	37.2 (39) [19.1-148]
400 mg BID# (n=23)	723 (86) [6.70-2256]	9093 (80) [1564-26,794]	76.1 (78) [14.9-256]	3088 (84) [407-13,140]	31.7 (42) [12.4-67.3]

Cavg = the average posaconazole concentration when measured at steady state

The variability in average plasma posaconazole concentrations in patients was relatively higher than that in healthy subjects.

* Oral suspension administration

† AUC $_{(0-24 hr)}$ for 200 mg TID and AUC $_{(0-12 hr)}$ for 400 mg BID

‡ HSCT recipients with GVHD

§ Not done

¶ Neutropenic patients who were receiving cytotoxic chemotherapy for acute myelogenous leukemia or myelodysplastic syndromes

Febrile neutropenic patients or patients with refractory invasive fungal infections, Cavg n=24

Table 15: Statistical Comparison of Plasma Pharmacokinetics of Posaconazole Following Single Oral Dose Administration of 300 mg Posaconazole Delayed-Release Tablet to Healthy Subjects under Fasting and Fed Conditions

Pharmacokinetic Parameter	Fasting Conditions		Fed Conditions (High Fat Meal)*		Fed/Fasting
	N	Mean (%CV)	N	Mean (%CV)	GMR (90% CI)
C_{max} (ng/mL)	14	935 (34)	16	1060 (25)	1.16 (0.96, 1.41)
AUC_{0-72hr} (hr•ng/mL)	14	26200 (28)	16	38400 (18)	1.51 (1.33, 1.72)
T_{max} † (hr)	14	5.00 (3.00, 8.00)	16	6.00 (5.00, 24.00)	N/A

GMR=Geometric least-squares mean ratio; CI=Confidence interval
* 48.5 g fat
† Median (Min, Max) reported for T_{max}

Table 16: The Effect of Concomitant Medications that Affect the Gastric pH and Gastric Motility on the Pharmacokinetics of Posaconazole Delayed-Release Tablets in Healthy Volunteers

Coadministered Drug	Administration Arms	Change in C_{max} (ratio estimate*; 90% CI of the ratio estimate)	Change in AUC_{0-last} (ratio estimate*; 90% CI of the ratio estimate)
Mylanta® Ultimate strength liquid (Increase in gastric pH)	25.4 meq/5 mL, 20 mL	↑6% (1.06; 0.90 -1.26)↑	↑4% (1.04; 0.90 -1.20)
Ranitidine (Zantac®) (Alteration in gastric pH)	150 mg (morning dose of 150 mg Ranitidine BID)	↑4% (1.04; 0.88 -1.23)↑	↓3% (0.97; 0.84 -1.12)
Esomeprazole (Nexium®) (Increase in gastric pH)	40 mg (QAM 5 days, day -4 to 1)	↑2% (1.02; 0.88-1.17)↑	↑5% (1.05; 0.89 -1.24)
Metoclopramide (Reglan®) (Increase in gastric motility)	15 mg four times daily during 2 days (Day -1 and 1)	↓14% (0.86, 0.73,1.02)	↓7% (0.93, 0.803,1.07)

* Ratio Estimate is the ratio of coadministered drug plus posaconazole to posaconazole alone for C_{max} or AUC_{0-last}.

Table 17: The Mean (%CV) [min-max] Posaconazole Pharmacokinetic Parameters Following Single-Dose Oral Suspension Administration of 200 mg and 400 mg Under Fed and Fasted Conditions

Dose (mg)	C_{max} (ng/mL)	T_{max}* (hr)	AUC (I) (ng·hr/mL)	CL/F (L/hr)	$t_{1/2}$ (hr)
200 mg fasted (n=20)†	132 (50) [45-267]	3.50 [1.5-36‡]	4179 (31) [2705-7269]	51 (25) [28-74]	23.5 (25) [15.3-33.7]
200 mg nonfat (n=20)†	378 (43) [131-834]	4 [3-5]	10,753 (35) [4579-17,092]	21 (39) [12-44]	22.2 (18) [17.4-28.7]
200 mg high fat (54 gm fat) (n=20)†	512 (34) [241-1016]	5 [4-5]	15,059 (26) [10,341-24,476]	14 (24) [8.2-19]	23.0 (19) [17.2-33.4]
400 mg fasted (n=23)§	121 (75) [27-366]	4 [2-12]	5258 (48) [2834-9567]	91 (40) [42-141]	27.3 (26) [16.8-38.9]
400 mg with liquid nutritional supplement (14 gm fat) (n=23)§	355 (43) [145-720]	5 [4-8]	11,295 (40) [3865-20,592]	43 (56) [19-103]	26.0 (19) [18.2-35.0]

* Median [min-max].
† n=15 for AUC (I), CL/F, and $t_{1/2}$
‡ The subject with T_{max} of 36 hrs had relatively constant plasma levels over 36 hrs (1.7 ng/mL difference between 4 hrs and 36 hrs).
§ n=10 for AUC (I), CL/F, and $t_{1/2}$

Absorption:
Posaconazole Delayed-Release Tablets
When given orally in healthy volunteers, posaconazole delayed-release tablets are absorbed with a median T_{max} of 4 to 5 hours. Steady-state plasma concentrations are attained by Day 6 at the 300 mg dose (QD after BID loading dose at Day 1). The absolute bioavailability of the oral delayed-release tablet is approximately 54% under fasted conditions. The C_{max} and AUC of posaconazole following administration of posaconazole delayed-release tablets is increased 16% and 51%, respectively, when given with a high fat meal compared to a fasted state (see **Table 15**). In order to enhance the oral absorption of posaconazole and optimize plasma concentrations, posaconazole delayed-release tablets should be administered with food.
[See table 15 above]
Concomitant administration of posaconazole delayed-release tablets with drugs affecting gastric pH or gastric motility did not demonstrate any significant effects on posaconazole pharmacokinetic exposure (see **Table 16**).

[See table 16 above]
Posaconazole Oral Suspension
Posaconazole oral suspension is absorbed with a median T_{max} of ~3 to 5 hours. Steady-state plasma concentrations are attained at 7 to 10 days following multiple-dose administration.
Following single-dose administration of 200 mg, the mean AUC and C_{max} of posaconazole are approximately 3-times higher when the oral suspension is administered with a nonfat meal and approximately 4-times higher when administered with a high-fat meal (~50 gm fat) relative to the fasted state. Following single-dose administration of posaconazole oral suspension 400 mg, the mean AUC and C_{max} of posaconazole are approximately 3-times higher when administered with a liquid nutritional supplement (14 gm fat) relative to the fasted state (see **Table 17**). In addition, the effects of varying gastric administration conditions on the C_{max} and AUC of posaconazole oral suspension in healthy volunteers have been investigated and are shown in **Table 18**.

In order to assure attainment of adequate plasma concentrations, it is recommended to administer Noxafil oral suspension during or immediately following a full meal. In patients who cannot eat a full meal, Noxafil oral suspension should be taken with a liquid nutritional supplement or an acidic carbonated beverage (e.g., ginger ale).
[See table 17 above]
[See table 18 at top of next page]
Concomitant administration of posaconazole oral suspension with drugs affecting gastric pH or gastric motility results in lower posaconazole exposure. (See **Table 19**.)
[See table 19 at top of next page]
Distribution:
The mean volume of distribution of posaconazole after intravenous solution administration was 261 L and ranged from 226-295 L between studies and dose levels.
Posaconazole is highly bound to human plasma proteins (>98%), predominantly to albumin.
Metabolism:
Posaconazole primarily circulates as the parent compound in plasma. Of the circulating metabolites, the majority are glucuronide conjugates formed via UDP glucuronidation (phase 2 enzymes). Posaconazole does not have any major circulating oxidative (CYP450 mediated) metabolites. The excreted metabolites in urine and feces account for ~17% of the administered radiolabeled dose.
Posaconazole is primarily metabolized via UDP glucuronidation (phase 2 enzymes) and is a substrate for p-glycoprotein (P-gp) efflux. Therefore, inhibitors or inducers of these clearance pathways may affect posaconazole plasma concentrations. A summary of drugs studied clinically with the oral suspension or an early tablet formulation, which affect posaconazole concentrations, is provided in **Table 20**.
[See table 20 at top of page 1584]
In vitro studies with human hepatic microsomes and clinical studies indicate that posaconazole is an inhibitor primarily of CYP3A4. A clinical study in healthy volunteers also indicates that posaconazole is a strong CYP3A4 inhibitor as evidenced by a >5-fold increase in midazolam AUC. Therefore, plasma concentrations of drugs predominantly metabolized by CYP3A4 may be increased by posaconazole. A summary of the drugs studied clinically, for which plasma concentrations were affected by posaconazole, is provided in **Table 21** *[see Contraindications (4) and Drug Interactions (7.1) including recommendations].*
[See table 21 at top of page 1585]
Additional clinical studies demonstrated that no clinically significant effects on zidovudine, lamivudine, indinavir, or caffeine were observed when administered with posaconazole 200 mg QD; therefore, no dose adjustments are required for these coadministered drugs when coadministered with posaconazole 200 mg QD.
Excretion:
Following administration of Noxafil oral suspension, posaconazole is predominantly eliminated in the feces (71% of the radiolabeled dose up to 120 hours) with the major component eliminated as parent drug (66% of the radiolabeled dose). Renal clearance is a minor elimination pathway, with 13% of the radiolabeled dose excreted in urine up to 120 hours (<0.2% of the radiolabeled dose is parent drug). Posaconazole injection is eliminated with a mean terminal half-life ($t_{1/2}$) of 27 hours and a total body clearance (CL) of 7.3 L/h.
Posaconazole delayed-release tablet is eliminated with a mean half-life ($t_{1/2}$) ranging between 26 to 31 hours.
Posaconazole oral suspension is eliminated with a mean half-life ($t_{1/2}$) of 35 hours (range: 20-66 hours).
12.4   Microbiology
Mechanism of Action:
Posaconazole blocks the synthesis of ergosterol, a key component of the fungal cell membrane, through the inhibition of cytochrome P-450 dependent enzyme lanosterol 14α-demethylase responsible for the conversion of lanosterol to ergosterol in the fungal cell membrane. This results in an accumulation of methylated sterol precursors and a depletion of ergosterol within the cell membrane thus weakening the structure and function of the fungal cell membrane. This may be responsible for the antifungal activity of posaconazole.
Activity in vitro:
Posaconazole has *in vitro* activity against *Aspergillus fumigatus* and *Candida albicans*, including *Candida albicans* isolates from patients refractory to itraconazole or fluconazole or both drugs *[see Clinical Studies (14), Indications and Usage (1) and Dosage and Administration (2)].* However, correlation between the results of susceptibility tests and clinical outcome has not been established. Posaconazole interpretive criteria (breakpoints) have not been established for any fungus.
Drug Resistance:
Clinical isolates of *Candida albicans* and *Candida glabrata* with decreased susceptibility to posaconazole were observed in oral swish samples taken during prophylaxis with

Table 18: The Effect of Varying Gastric Administration Conditions on the C_{max} and AUC of Posaconazole Oral Suspension in Healthy Volunteers*

Study Description	Administration Arms	Change in C_{max} (ratio estimate[†]; 90% CI of the ratio estimate)	Change in AUC (ratio estimate[†]; 90% CI of the ratio estimate)
400-mg single dose with a high-fat meal relative to fasted state (n=12)	5 minutes before high-fat meal	↑96% (1.96; 1.48-2.59)	↑111% (2.11; 1.60-2.78)
	During high-fat meal	↑339% (4.39; 3.32-5.80)	↑382% (4.82; 3.66-6.35)
	20 minutes after high-fat meal	↑333% (4.33; 3.28-5.73)	↑387% (4.87; 3.70-6.42)
400 mg BID and 200 mg QID for 7 days in fasted state and with liquid nutritional supplement (BOOST®) (n=12)	400 mg BID with BOOST	↑65% (1.65; 1.29-2.11)	↑66% (1.66; 1.30-2.13)
	200 mg QID with BOOST	No Effect	No Effect
Divided daily dose from 400 mg BID to 200 mg QID for 7 days regardless of fasted conditions or with BOOST (n=12)	Fasted state	↑136% (2.36; 1.84-3.02)	↑161% (2.61; 2.04-3.35)
	With BOOST	↑137% (2.37; 1.86-3.04)	↑157% (2.57; 2.00-3.30)
400-mg single dose with carbonated acidic beverage (ginger ale) and/or proton pump inhibitor (esomeprazole) (n=12)	Ginger ale	↑92% (1.92; 1.51-2.44)	↑70% (1.70; 1.43-2.03)
	Esomeprazole	↓32% (0.68; 0.53-0.86)	↓30% (0.70; 0.59-0.83)
400-mg single dose with a prokinetic agent (metoclopramide 10 mg TID for 2 days) + BOOST or an antikinetic agent (loperamide 4-mg single dose) + BOOST (n=12)	With metoclopramide + BOOST	↓21% (0.79; 0.72-0.87)	↓19% (0.81; 0.72-0.91)
	With loperamide + BOOST	↓3% (0.97; 0.88-1.07)	↑11% (1.11; 0.99-1.25)
400-mg single dose either orally with BOOST or via an NG tube with BOOST (n=16)	Via NG tube[‡]	↓19% (0.81; 0.71-0.91)	↓23% (0.77; 0.69-0.86)

* In 5 subjects, the C_{max} and AUC decreased substantially (range: -27% to -53% and -33% to -51%, respectively) when Noxafil was administered via an NG tube compared to when Noxafil was administered orally. It is recommended to closely monitor patients for breakthrough fungal infections when Noxafil is administered via an NG tube because a lower plasma exposure may be associated with an increased risk of treatment failure.
† Ratio Estimate is the ratio of coadministered drug plus posaconazole to coadministered drug alone for C_{max} or AUC.
‡ NG = nasogastric

Table 19: The Effect of Concomitant Medications that Affect the Gastric pH and Gastric Motility on the Pharmacokinetics of Posaconazole Oral Suspension in Healthy Volunteers

Coadministered Drug (Postulated Mechanism of Interaction)	Coadministered Drug Dose/Schedule	Posaconazole Dose/Schedule	Change in Mean C_{max} (ratio estimate*; 90% CI of the ratio estimate)	Change in Mean AUC (ratio estimate*; 90% CI of the ratio estimate)
Cimetidine (Alteration of gastric pH)	400 mg BID × 10 days	200 mg (tablets) QD × 10 days[†]	↓ 39% (0.61; 0.53-0.70)	↓ 39% (0.61; 0.54-0.69)
Esomeprazole (Increase in gastric pH)[‡]	40 mg QAM × 3 days	400 mg (oral suspension) single dose	↓ 46% (0.54; 0.43-0.69)	↓ 32% (0.68; 0.57-0.81)
Metoclopramide (Increase in gastric motility)[‡]	10 mg TID × 2 days	400 mg (oral suspension) single dose	↓ 21% (0.79; 0.72-0.87)	↓ 19% (0.81; 0.72-0.91)

* Ratio Estimate is the ratio of coadministered drug plus posaconazole to coadministered drug alone for C_{max} or AUC.
† The tablet refers to a non-commercial tablet formulation without polymer.
‡ The drug interactions associated with the oral suspension are also relevant for the delayed-release tablet with the exception of Esomeprazole and Metoclopramide.

posaconazole and fluconazole, suggesting a potential for development of resistance. These isolates also showed reduced susceptibility to other azoles, suggesting cross-resistance between azoles. The clinical significance of this finding is not known.

13 NONCLINICAL TOXICOLOGY

13.1 Carcinogenesis, Mutagenesis, Impairment of Fertility

No drug-related neoplasms were recorded in rats or mice treated with posaconazole for 2 years at doses higher than the clinical dose. In a 2-year carcinogenicity study, rats were given posaconazole orally at doses up to 20 mg/kg (females), or 30 mg/kg (males). These doses are equivalent to 3.9- or 3.5-times the exposure achieved with a 400-mg BID oral suspension regimen, respectively, based on steady-state AUC in healthy volunteers administered a high-fat meal (400-mg BID oral suspension regimen). In the mouse study, mice were treated at oral doses up to 60 mg/kg/day or 4.8-times the exposure achieved with a 400-mg BID oral suspension regimen.

Posaconazole was not genotoxic or clastogenic when evaluated in bacterial mutagenicity (Ames), a chromosome aberration study in human peripheral blood lymphocytes, a Chinese hamster ovary cell mutagenicity study, and a mouse bone marrow micronucleus study.

Posaconazole had no effect on fertility of male rats at a dose up to 180 mg/kg (1.7 × the 400-mg BID oral suspension regimen based on steady-state plasma concentrations in healthy volunteers) or female rats at a dose up to 45 mg/kg (2.2 × the 400-mg BID oral suspension regimen).

13.2 Animal Toxicology and/or Pharmacology

In a nonclinical study using intravenous administration of posaconazole in very young dogs (dosed from 2 to 8 weeks of age), an increase in the incidence of brain ventricle enlargement was observed in treated animals as compared with concurrent control animals. No difference in the incidence of brain ventricle enlargement between control and treated animals was observed following the subsequent 5-month treatment-free period. There were no neurologic, behavioral or developmental abnormalities in the dogs with this finding, and a similar brain finding was not seen with oral posaconazole administration to juvenile dogs (4 days to 9 months of age).

The clinical significance of this finding is unknown; therefore, the use of posaconazole injection to patients under 18 years of age is not recommended.

14 CLINICAL STUDIES

14.1 Prophylaxis of *Aspergillus* and *Candida* Infections with Posaconazole Oral Suspension

Two randomized, controlled studies were conducted using posaconazole as prophylaxis for the prevention of invasive fungal infections (IFIs) among patients at high risk due to severely compromised immune systems.

The first study (Oral Suspension Study 1) was a randomized, double-blind trial that compared posaconazole oral suspension (200 mg three times a day) with fluconazole capsules (400 mg once daily) as prophylaxis against invasive fungal infections in allogeneic hematopoietic stem cell transplant (HSCT) recipients with Graft versus Host Disease (GVHD). Efficacy of prophylaxis was evaluated using a composite endpoint of proven/probable IFIs, death, or treatment with systemic antifungal therapy (patients may have met more than one of these criteria). This assessed all patients while on study therapy plus 7 days and at 16 weeks post-randomization. The mean duration of therapy was comparable between the 2 treatment groups (80 days, posaconazole; 77 days, fluconazole). **Table 22** contains the results from Oral Suspension Study 1.

Table 22: Results from Blinded Clinical Study in Prophylaxis of IFI in All Randomized Patients with Hematopoietic Stem Cell Transplant (HSCT) and Graft-vs.-Host Disease (GVHD): Oral Suspension Study 1

	Posaconazole n=301	Fluconazole n=299
On therapy plus 7 days		
Clinical Failure*	50 (17%)	55 (18%)
Failure due to:		
Proven/Probable IFI	7 (2%)	22 (7%)
(*Aspergillus*)	3 (1%)	17 (6%)
(*Candida*)	1 (<1%)	3 (1%)
(Other)	3 (1%)	2 (1%)
All Deaths	22 (7%)	24 (8%)
Proven/probable fungal infection prior to death	2 (<1%)	6 (2%)
SAF[†]	27 (9%)	25 (8%)
Through 16 weeks		
Clinical Failure*,[‡]	99 (33%)	110 (37%)
Failure due to:		
Proven/Probable IFI	16 (5%)	27 (9%)
(*Aspergillus*)	7 (2%)	21 (7%)
(*Candida*)	4 (1%)	4 (1%)
(Other)	5 (2%)	2 (1%)
All Deaths	58 (19%)	59 (20%)
Proven/probable fungal infection prior to death	10 (3%)	16 (5%)
SAF[†]	26 (9%)	30 (10%)

Event free lost to follow-up§	24 (8%)	30 (10%)

* Patients may have met more than one criterion defining failure.
† Use of systemic antifungal therapy (SAF) criterion is based on protocol definitions (empiric/IFI usage >4 consecutive days).
‡ 95% confidence interval (posaconazole-fluconazole) = (-11.5%, +3.7%).
§ Patients who are lost to follow-up (not observed for 112 days), and who did not meet another clinical failure endpoint. These patients were considered failures.

The second study (Oral Suspension Study 2) was a randomized, open-label study that compared posaconazole oral suspension (200 mg 3 times a day) with fluconazole suspension (400 mg once daily) or itraconazole oral solution (200 mg twice a day) as prophylaxis against IFIs in neutropenic patients who were receiving cytotoxic chemotherapy for AML or MDS. As in Oral Suspension Study 1, efficacy of prophylaxis was evaluated using a composite endpoint of proven/probable IFIs, death, or treatment with systemic antifungal therapy (Patients might have met more than one of these criteria). This study assessed patients while on treatment plus 7 days and 100 days postrandomization. The mean duration of therapy was comparable between the 2 treatment groups (29 days, posaconazole; 25 days, fluconazole or itraconazole). **Table 23** contains the results from Oral Suspension Study 2.

Table 23: Results from Open-Label Clinical Study 2 in Prophylaxis of IFI in All Randomized Patients with Hematologic Malignancy and Prolonged Neutropenia: Oral Suspension Study 2

	Posaconazole n=304	Fluconazole/ Itraconazole n=298
On therapy plus 7 days		
Clinical Failure*,†	82 (27%)	126 (42%)
Failure due to:		
Proven/ Probable IFI	7 (2%)	25 (8%)
(*Aspergillus*)	2 (1%)	20 (7%)
(*Candida*)	3 (1%)	2 (1%)
(Other)	2 (1%)	3 (1%)
All Deaths Proven/probable fungal infection prior to death	17 (6%) 1 (<1%)	25 (8%) 2 (1%)
SAF‡	67 (22%)	98 (33%)
Through 100 days postrandomization		
Clinical Failure†	158 (52%)	191 (64%)
Failure due to:		
Proven/ Probable IFI	14 (5%)	33 (11%)
(*Aspergillus*)	2 (1%)	26 (9%)
(*Candida*)	10 (3%)	4 (1%)
(Other)	2 (1%)	3 (1%)
All Deaths Proven/probable fungal infection prior to death	44 (14%) 2 (1%)	64 (21%) 16 (5%)
SAF‡	98 (32%)	125 (42%)
Event free lost to follow-up§	34 (11%)	24 (8%)

* 95% confidence interval (posaconazole-fluconazole/ itraconazole) = (-22.9%, -7.8%).
† Patients may have met more than one criterion defining failure.

Table 20: Summary of the Effect of Coadministered Drugs on Posaconazole in Healthy Volunteers

Coadministered Drug (Postulated Mechanism of Interaction)	Coadministered Drug Dose/Schedule	Posaconazole Dose/ Schedule	Effect on Bioavailability of Posaconazole	
			Change in Mean C_{max} (ratio estimate*; 90% CI of the ratio estimate)	Change in Mean AUC (ratio estimate*; 90% CI of the ratio estimate)
Efavirenz (UDP-G Induction)	400 mg QD × 10 and 20 days	400 mg (oral suspension) BID × 10 and 20 days	↓45% (0.55; 0.47-0.66)	↓ 50% (0.50; 0.43-0.60)
Fosamprenavir (unknown mechanism)	700 mg BID × 10 days	200 mg QD on the 1st day, 200 mg BID on the 2nd day, then 400 mg BID × 8 Days	↓21% 0.79 (0.71-0.89)	↓23% 0.77 (0.68-0.87)
Rifabutin (UDP-G Induction)	300 mg QD × 17 days	200 mg (tablets) QD × 10 days†	↓ 43% (0.57; 0.43-0.75)	↓ 49% (0.51; 0.37-0.71)
Phenytoin (UDP-G Induction)	200 mg QD × 10 days	200 mg (tablets) QD × 10 days†	↓ 41% (0.59; 0.44-0.79)	↓ 50% (0.50; 0.36-0.71)

* Ratio Estimate is the ratio of coadministered drug plus posaconazole to posaconazole alone for C_{max} or AUC.
† The tablet refers to a non-commercial tablet formulation without polymer.

‡ Use of systemic antifungal therapy (SAF) criterion is based on protocol definitions (empiric/IFI usage >3 consecutive days).
§ Patients who are lost to follow-up (not observed for 100 days), and who did not meet another clinical failure endpoint. These patients were considered failures.

In summary, 2 clinical studies of prophylaxis were conducted with the posaconazole oral suspension. As seen in the accompanying tables (**Tables 22 and 23**), clinical failure represented a composite endpoint of breakthrough IFI, mortality and use of systemic antifungal therapy. In Oral Suspension Study 1 (**Table 22**), the clinical failure rate of posaconazole (33%) was similar to fluconazole (37%), (95% CI for the difference posaconazole–comparator -11.5% to 3.7%) while in Oral Suspension Study 2 (**Table 23**) clinical failure was lower for patients treated with posaconazole (27%) when compared to patients treated with fluconazole or itraconazole (42%), (95% CI for the difference posaconazole–comparator -22.9% to -7.8%).
All-cause mortality was similar at 16 weeks for both treatment arms in Oral Suspension Study 1 [POS 58/301 (19%) vs. FLU 59/299 (20%)]; all-cause mortality was lower at 100 days for posaconazole-treated patients in Oral Suspension Study 2 [POS 44/304 (14%) vs. FLU/ITZ 64/298 (21%)]. Both studies demonstrated substantially fewer breakthrough infections caused by *Aspergillus* species in patients receiving posaconazole prophylaxis when compared to patients receiving fluconazole or itraconazole.

14.2 Treatment of Oropharyngeal Candidiasis with Posaconazole Oral Suspension

Posaconazole Oral Suspension Study 3 was a randomized, controlled, evaluator-blinded study in HIV-infected patients with oropharyngeal candidiasis. Patients were treated with posaconazole or fluconazole oral suspension (both posaconazole and fluconazole were given as follows: 100 mg twice a day for 1 day followed by 100 mg once a day for 13 days).
Clinical and mycological outcomes were assessed after 14 days of treatment and at 4 weeks after the end of treatment. Patients who received at least 1 dose of study medication and had a positive oral swish culture of *Candida* species at baseline were included in the analyses (see **Table 24**). The majority of the subjects had *C. albicans* as the baseline pathogen.
Clinical success at Day 14 (complete or partial resolution of all ulcers and/or plaques and symptoms) and clinical relapse rates (recurrence of signs or symptoms after initial cure or improvement) 4 weeks after the end of treatment were similar between the treatment arms (see **Table 24**).
Mycologic eradication rates (absence of colony forming units in quantitative culture at the end of therapy, Day 14), as well as mycologic relapse rates (4 weeks after the end of treatment) were also similar between the treatment arms (see **Table 24**).

Table 24: Posaconazole Oral Suspension Clinical Success, Mycological Eradication, and Relapse Rates in Oropharyngeal Candidiasis

	Posaconazole	Fluconazole
Clinical Success at End of Therapy (Day 14)	155/169 (91.7%)	148/160 (92.5%)
Clinical Relapse (4 Weeks after End of Therapy)	45/155 (29.0%)	52/148 (35.1%)
Mycological Eradication (absence of CFU) at End of Therapy (Day 14)	88/169 (52.1%)	80/160 (50.0%)
Mycological Relapse (4 Weeks after End of Treatment)	49/88 (55.6%)	51/80 (63.7%)

Mycologic response rates, using a criterion for success as a posttreatment quantitative culture with ≤20 colony forming units (CFU/mL) were also similar between the two groups (posaconazole 68.0%, fluconazole 68.1%). The clinical significance of this finding is unknown.

14.3 Posaconazole Oral Suspension Treatment of Oropharyngeal Candidiasis Refractory to Treatment with Fluconazole or Itraconazole

Posaconazole Oral Suspension Study 4 was a noncomparative study of posaconazole oral suspension in HIV-infected subjects with OPC that was refractory to treatment with fluconazole or itraconazole. An episode of OPC was considered refractory if there was failure to improve or worsening of OPC after a standard course of therapy with fluconazole greater than or equal to 100 mg/day for at least 10 consecutive days or itraconazole 200 mg/day for at least 10 consecutive days and treatment with either fluconazole or itraconazole had not been discontinued for more than 14 days prior to treatment with posaconazole. Of the 199 subjects enrolled in this study, 89 subjects met these strict criteria for refractory infection.
Forty-five subjects with refractory OPC were treated with posaconazole oral suspension 400 mg BID for 3 days, followed by 400 mg QD for 25 days with an option for further treatment during a 3-month maintenance period. Following a dosing amendment, a further 44 subjects were treated with posaconazole 400 mg BID for 28 days. The efficacy of posaconazole was assessed by the clinical success (cure or improvement) rate after 4 weeks of treatment. The clinical success rate was 74.2% (66/89). The clinical success rates for both the original and the amended dosing regimens were similar (73.3% and 75.0%, respectively).

16 HOW SUPPLIED/STORAGE AND HANDLING

Injection
Noxafil injection is available in Type I glass vials closed with bromobutyl rubber stopper and aluminum seal (NDC 0085-4331-01) containing 300 mg per 16.7 mL of solution (18 mg of posaconazole per mL). Store refrigerated at 2-8°C (36-46°F).
Delayed-Release Tablets
Noxafil 100 mg delayed-release tablets; yellow, coated, oblong, debossed with "100" on one side. Bottles with child-resistant closures of 60 delayed-release tablets (NDC 0085-4324-02). Store at 20-25°C (68-77°F), excursions permitted to 15-30°C (59-86°F) [see USP Controlled Room Temperature].
Oral Suspension
Noxafil oral suspension is available in 4-ounce (123 mL) amber glass bottles with child-resistant closures (NDC 0085-1328-01) containing 105 mL of suspension (40 mg of posaconazole per mL).
Supplied with each oral suspension bottle is a plastic dosing spoon calibrated for measuring 2.5-mL and 5-mL doses. Store at 25°C (77°F); excursions permitted to 15-30°C (59-86°F) [see USP Controlled Room Temperature]. **DO NOT FREEZE.**

17 PATIENT COUNSELING INFORMATION

Advise the patient to read the FDA-approved patient labeling (Patient Information).

17.1 Administration

Noxafil Delayed-Release Tablets

Advise patients to take Noxafil delayed-release tablets with food.

Physicians should instruct their patients that if they miss a dose, they should take it as soon as they remember. If they do not remember until it is within 12 hours of the next dose, they should be instructed to skip the missed dose and go back to the regular schedule. Patients should not double their next dose or take more than the prescribed dose.

Noxafil Oral Suspension

Advise patients to take each dose of Noxafil oral suspension during or immediately (i.e., within 20 minutes) following a full meal. In patients who cannot eat a full meal, each dose of Noxafil oral suspension should be administered with a liquid nutritional supplement or an acidic carbonated beverage (e.g., ginger ale) in order to enhance absorption.

17.2 Drug Interactions

Patients should be advised to inform their physician immediately if they:

• develop severe diarrhea or vomiting.
• are currently taking drugs that are known to prolong the QTc interval and are metabolized through CYP3A4.
• are currently taking a cyclosporine or tacrolimus, or they notice swelling in an arm or leg or shortness of breath.
• are taking other drugs or before they begin taking other drugs as certain drugs can decrease or increase the plasma concentrations of posaconazole.

17.3 Serious and Potentially Serious Adverse Reactions

Patients should be advised to inform their physician immediately if they:

• notice a change in heart rate or heart rhythm, or have a heart condition or circulatory disease. Posaconazole can be administered with caution to patients with potentially proarrhythmic conditions.
• are pregnant, plan to become pregnant, or are nursing.
• have liver disease or develop itching, nausea or vomiting, their eyes or skin turn yellow, they feel more tired than usual or feel like they have the flu.
• have ever had an allergic reaction to other antifungal medicines such as ketoconazole, fluconazole, itraconazole, or voriconazole.

Manuf. for: Merck Sharp & Dohme Corp., a subsidiary of **MERCK & CO., INC.**, Whitehouse Station, NJ 08889, USA
Injection: Manuf. by: Schering-Plough (Brinny) Co., Brinny, Innishannon, County Cork, Ireland
Delayed-Release Tablets: Manuf. by: N. V. Organon, Kloosterstraat 6, 5349 AB Oss, Netherlands
Oral Suspension: Manuf. by: Patheon Inc., Whitby, Ontario, Canada L1N 5Z5
For patent information: www.merck.com/product/patent/home.html
The trademarks referenced herein are owned by their respective companies.

Copyright © 2006, 2010, 2013, 2014 Merck Sharp & Dohme Corp., a subsidiary of **Merck & Co., Inc.**
All rights reserved.

uspi-mk5592-mf-1406r032

Patient Information

Noxafil® (**NOX**-a-fil)
(posaconazole)
injection
Noxafil® (**NOX**-a-fil)
(posaconazole)
delayed-release tablets
Noxafil® (**NOX**-a-fil)
(posaconazole)
oral suspension

What is Noxafil?

Noxafil injection, delayed-release tablets, and oral suspension are prescription medicines used to help prevent fungal infections that can spread throughout your body (invasive fungal infections). These infections are caused by fungi called *Aspergillus* or *Candida*. Noxafil is used in people who have an increased chance of getting these infections due to a weak immune system. These include people who have:

• had a hematopoietic stem cell transplantation (bone marrow transplant) with graft versus host disease
• a low white blood cell count due to chemotherapy for blood cancers (hematologic malignancy)

Noxafil oral suspension is also used to treat a fungal infection called "thrush" caused by *Candida* in your mouth or throat area. Noxafil oral suspension can be used as the first treatment for thrush, or as another treatment for thrush after itraconazole or fluconazole treatment has not worked.

Noxafil injection is for adults over 18 years of age. It is not known if Noxafil injection is safe and effective in children under 18 years of age.

Noxafil delayed-release tablets and oral suspension are for adults and children over 13 years of age.

Table 21: Summary of the Effect of Posaconazole on Coadministered Drugs in Healthy Volunteers and Patients

Coadministered Drug (Postulated Mechanism of Interaction is Inhibition of CYP3A4 by posaconazole)	Coadministered Drug Dose/Schedule	Posaconazole Dose/ Schedule	Effect on Bioavailability of Coadministered Drugs	
			Change in Mean C_{max} (ratio estimate*; 90% CI of the ratio estimate)	Change in Mean AUC (ratio estimate*; 90% CI of the ratio estimate)
Sirolimus	2-mg single oral dose	400 mg (oral suspension) BID × 16 days	↑ 572% (6.72; 5.62-8.03)	↑ 788% (8.88; 7.26-10.9)
Cyclosporine	Stable maintenance dose in heart transplant recipients	200 mg (tablets) QD × 10 days†	↑ cyclosporine whole blood trough concentrations Cyclosporine dose reductions of up to 29% were required	
Tacrolimus	0.05-mg/kg single oral dose	400 mg (oral suspension) BID × 7 days	↑ 121% (2.21; 2.01-2.42)	↑ 358% (4.58; 4.03-5.19)
Simvastatin	40-mg single oral dose	100 mg (oral suspension) QD × 13 days	Simvastatin ↑ 841% (9.41, 7.13-12.44) Simvastatin Acid ↑ 817% (9.17, 7.36-11.43)	Simvastatin ↑ 931% (10.31, 8.40-12.67) Simvastatin Acid ↑634% (7.34, 5.82-9.25)
		200 mg (oral suspension) QD × 13 days	Simvastatin ↑ 1041% (11.41, 7.99-16.29) Simvastatin Acid ↑851% (9.51, 8.15-11.10)	Simvastatin ↑ 960% (10.60, 8.63-13.02) Simvastatin Acid ↑748% (8.48, 7.04-10.23)
Midazolam	0.4-mg single intravenous dose‡	200 mg (oral suspension) BID × 7 days	↑ 30% (1.3; 1.13-1.48)	↑ 362% (4.62; 4.02-5.3)
	0.4-mg single intravenous dose‡	400 mg (oral suspension) BID × 7 days	↑62% (1.62; 1.41-1.86)	↑524% (6.24; 5.43-7.16)
	2-mg single oral dose‡	200 mg (oral suspension) QD × 7 days	↑ 169% (2.69; 2.46-2.93)	↑ 470% (5.70; 4.82-6.74)
	2-mg single oral dose‡	400 mg (oral suspension) BID × 7 days	↑ 138% (2.38; 2.13-2.66)	↑ 397% (4.97; 4.46-5.54)
Rifabutin	300 mg QD × 17 days	200 mg (tablets) QD × 10 days†	↑31% (1.31; 1.10-1.57)	↑ 72% (1.72;1.51-1.95)
Phenytoin	200 mg QD PO × 10 days	200 mg (tablets) QD × 10 days†	↑ 16% (1.16; 0.85-1.57)	↑ 16% (1.16; 0.84-1.59)
Ritonavir	100 mg QD × 14 days	400 mg (oral suspension) BID × 7 days	↑ 49% (1.49; 1.04-2.15)	↑ 80% (1.8;1.39-2.31)
Atazanavir	300 mg QD × 14 days	400 mg (oral suspension) BID × 7 days	↑ 155% (2.55; 1.89-3.45)	↑ 268% (3.68; 2.89-4.70)
Atazanavir/ ritonavir boosted regimen	300 mg/100 mg QD × 14 days	400 mg (oral suspension) BID × 7 days	↑ 53% (1.53; 1.13-2.07)	↑ 146% (2.46; 1.93-3.13)

* Ratio Estimate is the ratio of coadministered drug plus posaconazole to coadministered drug alone for C_{max} or AUC.
† The tablet refers to a non-commercial tablet formulation without polymer.
‡ The mean terminal half-life of midazolam was increased from 3 hours to 7 to 11 hours during coadministration with posaconazole.

It is not known if Noxafil oral suspension and delayed-release tablets are safe and effective in children under 13 years of age.

Who should not take Noxafil?

Do not take Noxafil if you:

• are allergic to posaconazole, any of the ingredients in Noxafil, or other azole antifungal medicines. See the end of this leaflet for a complete list of ingredients in Noxafil.
• are taking any of the following medicines:
  ◦ sirolimus
  ◦ pimozide
  ◦ quinidine
  ◦ certain statin medicines that lower cholesterol (atorvastatin, lovastatin, simvastatin)
  ◦ ergot alkaloids (ergotamine, dihydroergotamine)

Ask your healthcare provider or pharmacist if you are not sure if you are taking any of these medicines.
Do not start taking a new medicine without talking to your healthcare provider or pharmacist.

What should I tell my healthcare provider before taking Noxafil?

Before you take Noxafil, tell your healthcare provider if you:

• are taking certain medicines that lower your immune system like cyclosporine or tacrolimus.
• are taking certain drugs for HIV infection, such as ritonavir, atazanavir, efavirenz, or fosamprenavir. Efavirenz and fosamprenavir can cause a decrease in the Noxafil levels in your body. Efavirenz and fosamprenavir should not be taken with Noxafil.
• are taking midazolam, a hypnotic and sedative medicine.
• have or had liver problems.
• have or had kidney problems.
• have or had an abnormal heart rate or rhythm, heart problems, or blood circulation problems.
• are pregnant or plan to become pregnant. It is not known if Noxafil will harm your unborn baby.
• are breastfeeding or plan to breastfeed. It is not known if Noxafil passes into your breast milk. You and your healthcare provider should decide if you will take Noxafil or breastfeed. You should not do both.

Tell your healthcare provider about all the medicines you take, including prescription and over-the-counter medicines, vitamins, and herbal supplements.
Especially tell your healthcare provider if you take:

• rifabutin or phenytoin. If you are taking these medicines, you should not take Noxafil delayed-release tablets or Noxafil oral suspension.
• cimetidine or esomeprazole. If you are taking these medicines, you should not take Noxafil oral suspension.

Ask your healthcare provider or pharmacist for a list of these medicines if you are not sure.
Know the medicines you take. Keep a list of them with you to show your healthcare provider or pharmacist when you get a new medicine.

How will I take Noxafil?

• Take Noxafil exactly as your healthcare provider tells you to take it.
• Your healthcare provider will tell you how much Noxafil to take and when to take it.

- Take Noxafil for as long as your healthcare provider tells you to take it.
- If you take too much Noxafil, call your healthcare provider or go to the nearest hospital emergency room right away.
- Noxafil injection is usually given over 30 to 90 minutes through a plastic tube placed in your vein.
- **Noxafil delayed-release tablets:**
  ○ Take Noxafil delayed-release tablets with food.
  ○ Take Noxafil delayed-release tablets whole. Do not break, crush, dissolve or chew Noxafil delayed-release tablets before swallowing. If you cannot swallow Noxafil delayed-release tablets whole, tell your healthcare provider. You may need a different medicine.
  ○ If you miss a dose, take it as soon as you remember and then take your next scheduled dose at its regular time. If, however, it is within 12 hours of your next dose, do not take the missed dose. Skip the missed dose and go back to your regular schedule. Do not double your next dose or take more than your prescribed dose.
- **Noxafil oral suspension:**
  ○ Shake Noxafil oral suspension well before use.
  ○ Take each dose of Noxafil oral suspension during or within 20 minutes after a full meal. If you cannot eat a full meal, take each dose of Noxafil oral suspension with a liquid nutritional supplement or an acidic carbonated beverage, like ginger ale.
  ○ A measured dosing spoon comes with your Noxafil oral suspension and is marked for doses of **2.5 mL** and **5 mL.** **See Figure A.**

Figure A

  ○ Rinse the spoon with water after each dose of Noxafil oral suspension and before you store it away.
Follow your doctor's instructions on how much Noxafil you should take and when to take it.

What are the possible side effects of Noxafil?
Noxafil may cause serious side effects, including:
- **drug interactions with cyclosporine or tacrolimus.** If you take Noxafil with cyclosporine or tacrolimus, your blood levels of cyclosporine or tacrolimus may increase. Serious side effects can happen in your kidney or brain if you have high levels of cyclosporine or tacrolimus in your blood. Your healthcare provider should do blood tests to check your levels of cyclosporine or tacrolimus if you are taking these medicines while taking Noxafil. Tell your healthcare provider right away if you have swelling in your arm or leg or shortness of breath.
- **problems with the electrical system of your heart (arrhythmias and QTc prolongation).** Certain medicines used to treat fungus called azoles, including posaconazole, the active ingredient in Noxafil, may cause heart rhythm problems. People who have certain heart problems or who take certain medicines have a higher chance for this problem. Tell your healthcare provider right away if your heartbeat becomes fast or irregular.
- **liver problems.** Some people who also have other serious medical problems may have severe liver problems that may lead to death, especially if you take certain doses of Noxafil. Your healthcare provider should do blood tests to check your liver while you are taking Noxafil. Call your healthcare provider right away if you have any of the following symptoms of liver problems:
  ○ itchy skin
  ○ nausea or vomiting
  ○ yellowing of your eyes
  ○ feeling very tired
  ○ flu-like symptoms
- **increased amounts of midazolam in your blood.** If you take Noxafil with midazolam, Noxafil increases the amount of midazolam in your blood. This can make your sleepiness last longer. Your healthcare provider should check you closely for side effects if you take midazolam with Noxafil.

The most common side effects of Noxafil include:
- diarrhea
- nausea
- headache
- vomiting
- fever
- low potassium levels in the blood
Tell your healthcare provider if you have any side effect that bothers you or that does not go away.
These are not all the possible side effects of Noxafil. For more information, ask your healthcare provider or pharmacist.
Call your doctor for medical advice about side effects. You may report side effects to FDA at 1-800-FDA-1088.

How should I store Noxafil?
- Store Noxafil injection refrigerated at 36°F to 46°F (2°C to 8°C).
- Store Noxafil delayed-release tablets and oral suspension at room temperature between 68°F to 77°F (20°C to 25°C).
- Keep Noxafil injection and delayed-release tablets in a tightly closed container.
- **Do not** freeze Noxafil injection or oral suspension.
- Safely throw away medicine that is out of date or no longer needed.
Keep Noxafil and all medicines out of the reach of children.
General information about the safe and effective use of Noxafil.
Medicines are sometimes prescribed for purposes other than those listed in a Patient Information leaflet. Do not use Noxafil for a condition for which it was not prescribed. Do not give Noxafil to other people, even if they have the same symptoms that you have. It may harm them.
This Patient Information leaflet summarizes the most important information about Noxafil. If you would like more information, talk to your healthcare provider. You can ask your pharmacist or healthcare provider for information about Noxafil that is written for healthcare professionals. For more information, go to www.noxafil.com or call 1-800-672-6372.
What are the ingredients in Noxafil?
Active ingredient: posaconazole
- **Noxafil injection:**
  Inactive ingredients: Betadex Sulfobutyl Ether Sodium (SBECD), edetate sodium, hydrochloric acid, sodium hydroxide, and water for injection.
- **Noxafil delayed-release tablets:**
  Inactive ingredients: hypromellose acetate succinate, microcrystalline cellulose, hydroxypropylcellulose, silicon dioxide, croscarmellose sodium, magnesium stearate, and Opadry® II Yellow (consists of the following ingredients: polyvinyl alcohol partially hydrolyzed, Macrogol/PEG 3350, titanium dioxide, talc, and iron oxide yellow)
- **Noxafil oral suspension:**
  Inactive ingredients: polysorbate 80, simethicone, sodium benzoate, sodium citrate dihydrate, citric acid monohydrate, glycerin, xanthan gum, liquid glucose, titanium dioxide, artificial cherry flavor, and purified water
This Patient Information has been approved by the U.S. Food and Drug Administration.
Manuf. for: Merck Sharp & Dohme Corp., a subsidiary of **MERCK & CO., INC.,** Whitehouse Station, NJ 08889, USA
Injection: Schering-Plough (Brinny) Co., Innishannon, County Cork, Ireland
Delayed-Release Tablets: Manuf. by: N. V. Organon, Kloosterstraat 6, 5349 AB Oss, Netherlands
Oral Suspension: Manuf. by: Patheon Inc., Whitby, Ontario, Canada L1N 5Z5
For patent information:
www.merck.com/product/patent/home.html
The trademarks depicted in this piece are owned by their respective companies.
Copyright © 2006, 2010, 2013, 2014 Merck Sharp & Dohme Corp., a subsidiary of **Merck & Co., Inc.**
All rights reserved.
Revised: 06/2014
usppi-mk5592-mf-1406r014

NUVARING®   ℞
(etonogestrel/ethinyl estradiol vaginal ring)

HIGHLIGHTS OF PRESCRIBING INFORMATION
These highlights do not include all the information needed to use NuvaRing safely and effectively. See full prescribing information for NuvaRing.
NuvaRing® (etonogestrel/ethinyl estradiol vaginal ring)
Initial U.S. Approval: 2001

> **WARNING: CIGARETTE SMOKING AND SERIOUS CARDIOVASCULAR EVENTS**
> *See full prescribing information for complete boxed warning.*
> - **Women over 35 years old who smoke should not use NuvaRing. (4)**
> - **Cigarette smoking increases the risk of serious cardiovascular events from combination hormonal contraceptive (CHC) use. (4)**

———RECENT MAJOR CHANGES———
Warnings and Precautions (5.1)   10/2013

———INDICATIONS AND USAGE———
NuvaRing is an estrogen/progestin combination hormonal contraceptive (CHC) indicated for use by women to prevent pregnancy. (1)

———DOSAGE AND ADMINISTRATION———
One NuvaRing is inserted in the vagina. The ring must remain in place continuously for three weeks, followed by a one-week ring-free interval. (2)

———DOSAGE FORMS AND STRENGTHS———
NuvaRing is a polymeric vaginal ring containing 11.7 mg etonogestrel and 2.7 mg ethinyl estradiol, which releases on average 0.12 mg/day of etonogestrel and 0.015 mg/day of ethinyl estradiol. (3)

———CONTRAINDICATIONS———
- A high risk of arterial or venous thrombotic diseases (4)
- Breast cancer or other estrogen- or progestin-sensitive cancer (4)
- Liver tumors or liver disease (4)
- Undiagnosed abnormal uterine bleeding (4)
- Pregnancy (4)
- Hypersensitivity to any of the components of NuvaRing (4)

———WARNINGS AND PRECAUTIONS———
- Vascular risks: Stop NuvaRing use if a thrombotic event occurs. Stop NuvaRing use at least 4 weeks before and through 2 weeks after major surgery. Start no earlier than 4 weeks after delivery, in women who are not breastfeeding. (5.1)
- Toxic Shock Syndrome (TSS): If patient exhibits signs or symptoms of TSS, consider the possibility of this diagnosis and initiate appropriate medical evaluation and treatment. (5.2)
- Liver disease: Discontinue NuvaRing use if jaundice develops. (5.3)
- High blood pressure: If used in women with well-controlled hypertension, monitor blood pressure and stop NuvaRing use if blood pressure rises significantly. (5.4)
- Carbohydrate and lipid metabolic effects: Monitor prediabetic and diabetic women. Consider an alternate contraceptive method for women with uncontrolled dyslipidemia. (5.7)
- Headache: Evaluate significant change in headaches and discontinue NuvaRing use if indicated. (5.8)
- Uterine bleeding: Evaluate irregular bleeding or amenorrhea. (5.9)

———ADVERSE REACTIONS———
The most common adverse reactions (≥2%) in clinical trials were: vaginitis, headache (including migraine), mood changes (e.g., depression, mood swings, mood altered, depressed mood, affect lability), device-related events (e.g., expulsion/discomfort/foreign body sensation), nausea/vomiting, vaginal discharge, increased weight, vaginal discomfort, breast pain/discomfort/tenderness, dysmenorrhea, abdominal pain, acne, and decreased libido. (6)
To report SUSPECTED ADVERSE REACTIONS, contact Merck, Sharp & Dohme Corp., a subsidiary of Merck & Co., Inc., at 1-877-888-4231 or FDA at 1-800-FDA-1088 or www.fda.gov/medwatch.

———DRUG INTERACTIONS———
Drugs or herbal products that induce certain enzymes, such as CYP3A4, may decrease the effectiveness of CHCs or increase breakthrough bleeding. Counsel patients to use a back-up or alternative method of contraception when enzyme inducers are used with CHCs. (7)

———USE IN SPECIFIC POPULATIONS———
- Nursing mothers: Not recommended; can decrease milk production. (8.3)
See 17 for PATIENT COUNSELING INFORMATION and FDA-approved patient labeling
                                                                            Revised: 12/2013

FULL PRESCRIBING INFORMATION: CONTENTS*
WARNING: CIGARETTE SMOKING AND SERIOUS CARDIOVASCULAR EVENTS

FULL PRESCRIBING INFORMATION

WARNING: CIGARETTE SMOKING AND SERIOUS CARDIOVASCULAR EVENTS

Cigarette smoking increases the risk of serious cardiovascular events from combination hormonal contraceptive (CHC) use. This risk increases with age, particularly in women over 35 years of age, and with the number of cigarettes smoked. For this reason, CHCs, including NuvaRing, should not be used by women who are over 35 years of age and smoke. *[See Contraindications (4).]*

1   INDICATIONS AND USAGE

FOR VAGINAL USE ONLY
NuvaRing® is indicated for use by females of reproductive age to prevent pregnancy.

2   DOSAGE AND ADMINISTRATION

2.1 How to Use NuvaRing

To achieve maximum contraceptive effectiveness, NuvaRing must be used as directed *[see Dosing and Administration (2.2)]*. One NuvaRing is inserted in the vagina. **The ring is to remain in place continuously for three weeks.** It is removed for a one-week break, during which a withdrawal bleed usually occurs. A new ring is inserted one week after the last ring was removed.

The user can choose the insertion position that is most comfortable to her, for example, standing with one leg up, squatting, or lying down. The ring is to be compressed and inserted into the vagina. The exact position of NuvaRing inside the vagina is not critical for its function. The vaginal ring must be inserted on the appropriate day and left in place for three consecutive weeks. This means that the ring should be removed three weeks later on the same day of the week as it was inserted and at about the same time. NuvaRing can be removed by hooking the index finger under the forward rim or by grasping the rim between the index and middle finger and pulling it out. The used ring should be placed in the sachet (foil pouch) and discarded in a waste receptacle out of the reach of children and pets (do not flush in toilet).

After a one-week break, during which a withdrawal bleed usually occurs, a new ring is inserted on the same day of the week as it was inserted in the previous cycle. The withdrawal bleed usually starts on Day 2-3 after removal of the ring and may not have finished before the next ring is inserted. In order to maintain contraceptive effectiveness, the new ring must be inserted exactly one week after the previous one was removed even if menstrual bleeding has not finished.

2.2 How to Start Using NuvaRing

IMPORTANT: Consider the possibility of ovulation and conception prior to the first use of NuvaRing.

No Hormonal Contraceptive Use in the Preceding Cycle:
The woman should insert NuvaRing on the first day of her menstrual bleeding. NuvaRing may also be started on Days 2-5 of the woman's cycle, but in this case a barrier method, such as male condoms with spermicide, should be used for the first seven days of NuvaRing use in the first cycle.

Changing From a CHC:
The woman may switch from her previous CHC on any day, but at the latest on the day following the usual hormone-free interval, if she has been using her hormonal method consistently and correctly, or if it is reasonably certain that she is not pregnant.

Changing From a Progestin-Only Method (progestin-only pill [POP], Implant, or Injection or a Progestin-Releasing Intrauterine System [IUS]):
The woman may switch from the POP on any day; instruct her to start using NuvaRing on the day after she took her last POP. She should switch from an implant or the IUS on the day of its removal, and from an injectable on the day when the next injection would be due. In all of these cases, the woman should use an additional barrier method such as a male condom with spermicide, for the first seven days.

Use after Abortion or Miscarriage
The woman may start using NuvaRing within the first five days following a complete first trimester abortion or miscarriage, and she does not need to use an additional method of contraception. If use of NuvaRing is not started within five days following a first trimester abortion or miscarriage, the woman should follow the instructions for "No Hormonal Contraceptive Use in the Preceding Cycle." In the meantime, she should be advised to use a non-hormonal contraceptive method.

Start NuvaRing no earlier than four weeks after a second trimester abortion or miscarriage, due to the increased risk of thromboembolism. *[See Contraindications (4), and Warnings and Precautions (5.1).]*

Following Childbirth
The use of NuvaRing may be initiated no sooner than four weeks postpartum in women who elect not to breastfeed, due to the increased risk of thromboembolism in the postpartum period. *[See Contraindications (4), and Warnings and Precautions (5.1).]*

Advise women who are breastfeeding not to use NuvaRing but to use other forms of contraception until the child is weaned.

If a woman begins using NuvaRing postpartum, instruct her to use an additional method of contraception, such as male condoms with spermicide, for the first seven days. If she has not yet had a period, consider the possibility of ovulation and conception occurring prior to initiation of NuvaRing.

2.3 Deviations from the Recommended Regimen

To prevent loss of contraceptive efficacy, advise women not to deviate from the recommended regimen. NuvaRing should be left in the vagina for a continuous period of three weeks.

Inadvertent Removal or Expulsion
NuvaRing can be accidentally expelled, for example, while removing a tampon, during intercourse, or with straining during a bowel movement. NuvaRing should be left in the vagina for a continuous period of three weeks. If the ring is accidentally expelled and is left outside of the vagina for less than three hours, contraceptive efficacy is not reduced. NuvaRing can be rinsed with cool to lukewarm (not hot) water and **reinserted as soon as possible**, but at the latest within three hours. If NuvaRing is lost, a new vaginal ring should be inserted and the regimen should be continued without alteration.

If NuvaRing is out of the vagina for more than three continuous hours:

During Weeks 1 and 2: Contraceptive efficacy may be reduced. The woman should reinsert the ring as soon as she remembers. A barrier method such as condoms with spermicides must be used until the ring has been used continuously for seven days.

During Week 3: The woman should discard that ring. One of the following two options should be chosen:
1. Insert a new ring immediately. Inserting a new ring will start the next three-week use period. The woman may not experience a withdrawal bleed from her previous cycle. However, breakthrough spotting or bleeding may occur.
2. Insert a new ring no later than seven days from the time the previous ring was removed or expelled, during which time she may have a withdrawal bleed. This option should only be chosen if the ring was used continuously for at least seven days prior to inadvertent removal/expulsion.

In either case, a barrier method such as condoms with spermicides must be used until the new ring has been used continuously for seven days.

Prolonged Ring-Free Interval
If the ring-free interval has been extended beyond one week, consider the possibility of pregnancy, and an additional method of contraception, such as male condoms with spermicide, **MUST** be used until NuvaRing has been used **continuously for seven days.**

Prolonged Use of NuvaRing
If NuvaRing has been left in place for up to one extra week (i.e., up to four weeks total), the woman will remain protected. NuvaRing should be removed and the woman should insert a new ring after a one-week ring-free interval.

If NuvaRing has been left in place for longer than four weeks, instruct the woman to remove the ring, and rule out pregnancy. If pregnancy is ruled out, NuvaRing may be restarted, and an additional method of contraception, such as male condoms with spermicide, **MUST** be used until a new NuvaRing has been used **continuously for seven days.**

Ring Breakage
There have been reported cases of NuvaRing disconnecting at the weld joint. This is not expected to affect the contraceptive effectiveness of NuvaRing. In the event of a disconnected ring, vaginal discomfort or expulsion (slipping out) is more likely to occur. If a woman discovers that her NuvaRing has disconnected, she should discard the ring and replace it with a new ring.

2.4 In the Event of a Missed Menstrual Period

1. If the woman has not adhered to the prescribed regimen (NuvaRing has been out of the vagina for more than three hours or the preceding ring-free interval was extended beyond one week), consider the possibility of pregnancy at the time of the first missed period and discontinue NuvaRing use if pregnancy is confirmed.
2. If the woman has adhered to the prescribed regimen and misses two consecutive periods, rule out pregnancy.
3. If the woman has retained one NuvaRing for longer than four weeks, rule out pregnancy.

2.5 Use with Other Vaginal Products

NuvaRing may interfere with the correct placement and position of a diaphragm. A diaphragm is therefore not recommended as a back-up method with NuvaRing use.

Pharmacokinetic data show that the use of tampons has no effect on the systemic absorption of the hormones released by NuvaRing.

3   DOSAGE FORMS AND STRENGTHS

NuvaRing (etonogestrel/ethinyl estradiol vaginal ring) is a non-biodegradable, flexible, transparent, colorless to almost colorless, combination contraceptive vaginal ring, with an outer diameter of 54 mm and a cross-sectional diameter of 4 mm. It is made of ethylene vinylacetate copolymers and magnesium stearate, and contains 11.7 mg etonogestrel and 2.7 mg ethinyl estradiol. When placed in the vagina, each ring releases on average 0.120 mg/day of etonogestrel and 0.015 mg/day of ethinyl estradiol over a three-week period of use. NuvaRing is not made with natural rubber latex.

4   CONTRAINDICATIONS

Do not prescribe NuvaRing to women who are known to have the following:
- A high risk of arterial or venous thrombotic diseases. Examples include women who are known to:
  - Smoke, if over age 35 *[see Boxed Warning and Warnings and Precautions (5.1)]*
  - Have deep vein thrombosis or pulmonary embolism, now or in the past *[see Warnings and Precautions (5.1)]*
  - Have cerebrovascular disease *[see Warnings and Precautions (5.1)]*
  - Have coronary artery disease *[see Warnings and Precautions (5.1)]*
  - Have thrombogenic valvular or thrombogenic rhythm diseases of the heart (for example, subacute bacterial endocarditis with valvular disease, or atrial fibrillation) *[see Warnings and Precautions (5.1)]*
  - Have inherited or acquired hypercoagulopathies *[see Warnings and Precautions (5.1)]*
  - Have uncontrolled hypertension *[see Warnings and Precautions (5.4)]*
  - Have diabetes mellitus with vascular disease *[see Warnings and Precautions (5.7)]*
  - Have headaches with focal neurological symptoms or migraine headaches with aura *[see Warnings and Precautions (5.8)]*
    - Women over age 35 with any migraine headaches *[see Warnings and Precautions (5.8)]*
- Liver tumors, benign or malignant or liver disease *[see Warnings and Precautions (5.3) and Use in Specific Populations (8.7)]*
- Undiagnosed abnormal uterine bleeding *[see Warnings and Precautions (5.9)]*
- Pregnancy, because there is no reason to use CHCs during pregnancy *[see Warnings and Precautions (5.8) and Use in Specific Populations (8.1)]*
- Breast cancer or other estrogen- or progestin-sensitive cancer, now or in the past *[see Warnings and Precautions (5.13)]*
- Hypersensitivity to any of the components of NuvaRing *[see Adverse Reactions (6)]*

5 WARNINGS AND PRECAUTIONS

5.1 Thromboembolic Disorders and Other Vascular Problems

Stop NuvaRing use if an arterial thrombotic or venous thromboembolic event (VTE) occurs. Stop NuvaRing use if there is unexplained loss of vision, proptosis, diplopia, papilledema, or retinal vascular lesions. Evaluate for retinal vein thrombosis immediately. *[See Adverse Reactions (6).]*

If feasible, stop NuvaRing at least four weeks before and through two weeks after major surgery or other surgeries known to have an elevated risk of thromboembolism, and during and following prolonged immobilization.

Start NuvaRing no earlier than 4 weeks after delivery, in women who are not breastfeeding. The risk of postpartum thromboembolism decreases after the third postpartum week, whereas the risk of ovulation increases after the third postpartum week.

The use of CHCs increases the risk of VTE. Known risk factors for VTE include smoking, obesity, and family history of VTE, in addition to other factors that contraindicate use of CHCs *[see Contraindications (4)].*

Two epidemiologic studies[1, 2, 3] that assessed the risk of VTE associated with the use of NuvaRing are described below. In these studies, which were required or sponsored by regulatory agencies, NuvaRing users had a risk of VTE similar to COC users (see Table 1 for adjusted hazard ratios). A large prospective, observational study, the Transatlantic Active Surveillance on Cardiovascular Safety of NuvaRing (TASC), investigated the risk of VTE for new users, and women who were switching to or restarting NuvaRing or COCs in a population that is representative of routine clinical users. The women were followed for 24 to 48 months. The results showed a similar risk of VTE among NuvaRing users (VTE incidence 8.3 per 10,000 WY) and women using COCs (VTE incidence 9.2 per 10,000 WY). For women using COCs that did not contain the progestins desogestrel (DSG) or gestodene (GSD), VTE incidence was 8.9 per 10,000 WY. A retrospective cohort study using data from 4 health plans in the US (FDA-funded Study in Kaiser Permanente and Medicaid databases) showed the VTE incidence for new users of NuvaRing to be 11.4 events per 10,000 WY, for new users of a levonorgestrel (LNG)-containing COC 9.2 events per 10,000 WY, and for users of other COCs available during the course of the study[1] 8.2 events per 10,000 WY.

Table 1: Estimates (Hazard Ratios) of Venous Thromboembolism Risk in Users of NuvaRing Compared to Users of Combined Oral Contraceptives (COCs)

Epidemiologic Study (Author, Year of Publication) Population Studied	Comparator Product(s)	Hazard Ratios (HR) (95% CI)
TASC (Dinger, 2012)		
Initiators, including new users, switchers and restarters	All COCs available during the course of the study *	HR[‡]: 0.8 (0.5-1.5)
	COCs available excluding DSG- or GSD-containing OCs	HR[†]: 0.8 (0.4-1.7)
FDA-funded Study in Kaiser Permanente and Medicaid databases (Sidney, 2011) First use of a combined hormonal contraceptive (CHC) during the study period	COCs available during the course of the study[‡]	HR[§]: 1.1 (0.6-2.2)
	LNG/0.03 mg ethinyl estradiol	HR[§]: 1.0 (0.5-2.0)

* Includes low-dose COCs containing the following progestins: chlormadinone acetate, cyproterone acetate, desogestrel, dienogest, drospirenone, ethynodiol diacetate, gestodene, levonorgestrel, norethindrone, norgestimate, or norgestrel

† Adjusted for age, BMI, duration of use, VTE history

‡ Includes low-dose COCs containing the following progestins: norgestimate, norethindrone, or levonorgestrel

§ Adjusted for age, site, year of entry into study

An increased risk of thromboembolic and thrombotic disease associated with the use of CHCs is well-established. Although the absolute VTE rates are increased for users of CHCs compared to non-users, the rates associated with pregnancy are even greater, especially during the postpartum period (see Figure 1).

The frequency of VTE in women using CHCs has been estimated to be 3 to 12 cases per 10,000 women-years.

The risk of VTE is highest during the first year of CHC use and after restarting a CHC following a break of at least four weeks. The risk of VTE due to CHCs gradually disappears after use is discontinued.

Figure 1 shows the risk of developing a VTE for women who are not pregnant and do not use CHCs, for women who use CHCs, for pregnant women, and for women in the postpartum period. To put the risk of developing a VTE into perspective: If 10,000 women who are not pregnant and do not use CHCs are followed for one year, between 1 and 5 of these women will develop a VTE.

Figure 1: Likelihood of Developing a VTE

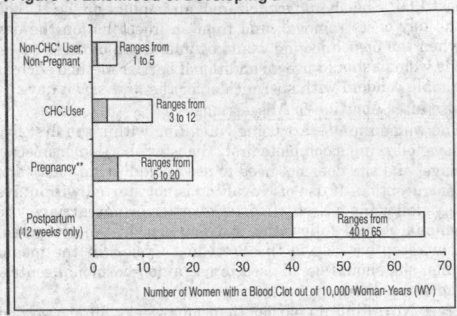

*CHC=combination hormonal contraception

**Pregnancy data based on actual duration of pregnancy in the reference studies. Based on a model assumption that pregnancy duration is nine months, the rate is 7 to 27 per 10,000 WY.

Several epidemiology studies indicate that third generation oral contraceptives, including those containing desogestrel (etonogestrel, the progestin in NuvaRing, is the biologically active metabolite of desogestrel), may be associated with a higher risk of VTE than oral contraceptives containing other progestins. Some of these studies indicate an approximate two-fold increased risk. However, data from other studies have not shown this two-fold increase in risk.

Use of CHCs also increases the risk of arterial thromboses such as strokes and myocardial infarctions, especially in women with other risk factors for these events. CHCs have been shown to increase both the relative and attributable risks of cerebrovascular events (thrombotic and hemorrhagic strokes). In general, the risk is greatest among older (>35 years of age), hypertensive women who also smoke. Use NuvaRing with caution in women with cardiovascular disease risk factors.

[1]Includes low-dose COCs containing the following progestins: norgestimate, norethindrone, or levonorgestrel.

5.2 Toxic Shock Syndrome (TSS)

Cases of TSS have been reported by NuvaRing users. TSS has been associated with tampons and certain barrier contraceptives, and, in some cases the NuvaRing users were also using tampons. A causal relationship between the use of NuvaRing and TSS has not been established. If a patient exhibits signs or symptoms of TSS, consider the possibility of this diagnosis and initiate appropriate medical evaluation and treatment.

5.3 Liver Disease

Impaired Liver Function

Do not use NuvaRing in women with liver disease such as acute viral hepatitis or severe (decompensated) cirrhosis of the liver *[see Contraindications (4)].* Acute or chronic disturbances of liver function may necessitate the discontinuation of CHC use until markers of liver function return to normal and CHC causation has been excluded *[see Use in Specific Populations (8.7)].* Discontinue NuvaRing use if jaundice develops.

Liver Tumors

NuvaRing is contraindicated in women with benign and malignant liver tumors *[see Contraindications (4)].* Hepatic adenomas are associated with CHC use. An estimate of the attributable risk is 3.3 cases per 100,000 CHC users. Rupture of hepatic adenomas may cause death through intra-abdominal hemorrhage.

Studies have shown an increased risk of developing hepatocellular carcinoma in long term (>8 years) CHC users. However, the attributable risk of liver cancers in CHC users is less than one case per million users.

5.4 High Blood Pressure

NuvaRing is contraindicated in women with uncontrolled hypertension or hypertension with vascular disease *[see

---

Contraindications (4)]. For women with well-controlled hypertension, monitor blood pressure and stop NuvaRing use if blood pressure rises significantly.

An increase in blood pressure has been reported in women using CHCs and this increase is more likely in older women and with extended duration of use. The incidence of hypertension increases with increasing concentrations of progestin.

5.5 Vaginal Use

NuvaRing may not be suitable for women with conditions that make the vagina more susceptible to vaginal irritation or ulceration. Vaginal/cervical erosion or ulceration in women using NuvaRing has been reported. In some cases, the ring adhered to vaginal tissue, necessitating removal by a healthcare provider.

Some women are aware of the ring on occasion during the 21 days of use or during intercourse, and sexual partners may feel NuvaRing in the vagina.

5.6 Gallbladder Disease

Studies suggest a small increased relative risk of developing gallbladder disease among CHC users. Use of CHCs may also worsen existing gallbladder disease.

A past history of CHC-related cholestasis predicts an increased risk with subsequent CHC use. Women with a history of pregnancy-related cholestasis may be at an increased risk for CHC-related cholestasis.

5.7 Carbohydrate and Lipid Metabolic Effects

Carefully monitor prediabetic and diabetic women who are using NuvaRing. CHCs may decrease glucose tolerance. Consider alternative contraception for women with uncontrolled dyslipidemia. Some women will have adverse lipid changes while on CHCs.

Women with hypertriglyceridemia, or a family history thereof, may be at an increased risk of pancreatitis when using CHCs.

5.8 Headache

If a woman using NuvaRing develops new headaches that are recurrent, persistent, or severe, evaluate the cause and discontinue NuvaRing if indicated.

Consider discontinuation of NuvaRing in the case of an increased frequency or severity of migraine during CHC use (which may be prodromal of a cerebrovascular event) *[see Contraindications (4)].*

5.9 Bleeding Irregularities and Amenorrhea

Unscheduled Bleeding and Spotting

Unscheduled bleeding (breakthrough or intracyclic) bleeding and spotting sometimes occur in women using CHCs, especially during the first three months of use. If bleeding persists or occurs after previously regular cycles, check for causes such as pregnancy or malignancy. If pathology and pregnancy are excluded, bleeding irregularities may resolve over time or with a change to a different CHC.

Bleeding patterns were evaluated in three large clinical studies. In the North American study (US and Canada, N=1,177), the percentages of subjects with breakthrough bleeding/spotting ranged from 7.2% to 11.7% during cycles 1-13. In the two non-US studies, the percentages of subjects with breakthrough bleeding/spotting ranged from 2.6% to 6.4% (Europe, N=1,145) and from 2.0% to 8.7% (Europe, Brazil, Chile, N=512).

Amenorrhea and Oligomenorrhea

If scheduled (withdrawal) bleeding does not occur, consider the possibility of pregnancy. If the patient has not adhered to the prescribed dosing schedule, consider the possibility of pregnancy at the time of the first missed period and take appropriate diagnostic measures.

Occasional missed periods may occur with the appropriate use of NuvaRing. In the clinical studies, the percent of women who did not have withdrawal bleeding in a given cycle ranged from 0.3% to 3.8%.

If the patient has adhered to the prescribed regimen and misses two consecutive periods, rule out pregnancy.

Some women may experience amenorrhea or oligomenorrhea after discontinuing CHC use, especially when such a condition was pre-existent.

5.10 Inadvertent Urinary Bladder Insertion

There have been reports of inadvertent insertions of NuvaRing into the urinary bladder, which required cystoscopic removal. Assess for ring insertion into the urinary bladder in NuvaRing users who present with persistent urinary symptoms and are unable to locate the ring.

5.11 CHC Use Before or During Early Pregnancy

Extensive epidemiological studies have revealed no increased risk of birth defects in women who have used oral contraceptives prior to pregnancy. Studies also do not suggest a teratogenic effect, particularly in so far as cardiac anomalies and limb reduction defects are concerned, when taken inadvertently during early pregnancy. Discontinue NuvaRing if pregnancy is confirmed.

5.12 Depression

Carefully observe women with a history of depression and discontinue NuvaRing use if depression recurs to a serious degree.

5.13 Carcinoma of the Breasts and Cervix

NuvaRing is contraindicated in women who currently have or have had breast cancer because breast cancer is a hormonally-sensitive tumor [see Contraindications (4)]. There is substantial evidence that CHCs do not increase the incidence of breast cancer. Although some past studies have suggested that CHCs might increase the incidence of breast cancer, more recent studies have not confirmed such findings.

Some studies suggest that CHCs are associated with an increase in the risk of cervical cancer or intraepithelial neoplasia. However, there is controversy about the extent to which these findings may be due to differences in sexual behavior and other factors.

5.14 Effect on Binding Globulins

The estrogen component of CHCs may raise the serum concentrations of thyroxine-binding globulin, sex hormone-binding globulin, and cortisol-binding globulin. The dose of replacement thyroid hormones or cortisol therapy may need to be increased.

5.15 Monitoring

A woman who is using NuvaRing should have a yearly visit with her healthcare provider for a blood pressure check and for other indicated healthcare.

5.16 Hereditary Angioedema

In women with hereditary angioedema, exogenous estrogens may induce or exacerbate symptoms of angioedema.

5.17 Chloasma

Chloasma may occasionally occur, especially in women with a history of chloasma gravidarum. Women with a tendency to chloasma should avoid exposure to the sun or ultraviolet radiation while using NuvaRing.

6 ADVERSE REACTIONS

The following serious adverse reactions with the use of CHCs are discussed elsewhere in the labeling.
• Serious cardiovascular events and stroke [see Boxed Warning and Warnings and Precautions (5.1)]
• Vascular events [see Warnings and Precautions (5.1)]
• Liver disease [see Warnings and Precautions (5.3)]
Adverse reactions commonly reported by CHC users are:
• Irregular uterine bleeding
• Nausea
• Breast tenderness
• Headache

6.1 Clinical Trials Experience

Because clinical trials are conducted under widely varying conditions, adverse reaction rates observed in the clinical trials of a drug cannot be directly compared to rates in the clinical trials of another drug and may not reflect the rates observed in practice.

Trials with a duration of 6 to 13 28-day cycles provided safety data. In total, 2,501 women, aged 18 to 41 contributed 24,520 cycles of exposure.

Common Adverse Reactions (≥ 2%): vaginitis (13.8%), headache (including migraine) (11.2%), mood changes (e.g., depression, mood swings, mood altered, depressed mood, affect lability) (6.4%), device-related events (e.g., expulsion/discomfort/foreign body sensation) (6.3%), nausea/vomiting (5.9%), vaginal discharge (5.7%), increased weight (4.9%), vaginal discomfort (4.0%), breast pain/discomfort/tenderness (3.8%), dysmenorrhea (3.5%), abdominal pain (3.2%), acne (2.4%), and decreased libido (2.0%).

Adverse Reactions (≥ 1%) Leading to Study Discontinuation: 13.0% of the women discontinued from the clinical trials due to an adverse reaction; the most common adverse reactions leading to discontinuation were device-related events (2.7%), mood changes (1.7%), headache (including migraine) (1.5%) and vaginal symptoms (1.2%).

Serious Adverse Reactions: deep vein thrombosis [see Warnings and Precautions (5.1)], anxiety, cholelithiasis, and vomiting.

6.2 Postmarketing Experience

The following adverse reactions have been identified during post-approval use of NuvaRing. Because these reactions are reported voluntarily from a population of uncertain size, it is not always possible to reliably estimate their frequency or establish a causal relationship to drug exposure.

Immune system disorders: hypersensitivity
Nervous system disorders: stroke/cerebrovascular accident
Vascular disorders: arterial events (including arterial thromboembolism and myocardial infarction), aggravation of varicose veins
Skin and subcutaneous tissue disorders: urticaria, chloasma
Reproductive system and breast disorders: penile disorders, including local reactions on penis (in male partners of women using NuvaRing), galactorrhea

7 DRUG INTERACTIONS

Consult the labeling of all concurrently-used drugs to obtain further information about interactions with hormonal contraceptives or the potential for enzyme alterations.

7.1 Effects of Other Drugs on CHCs

Substances decreasing the plasma concentrations of CHCs and potentially diminishing the effectiveness of CHCs

Drugs or herbal products that induce certain enzymes, including cytochrome P450 3A4 (CYP3A4), may decrease the plasma concentrations of CHCs and potentially diminish the effectiveness of CHCs or increase breakthrough bleeding. Some drugs or herbal products that may decrease the effectiveness of hormonal contraceptives include: phenytoin, barbiturates, carbamazepine, bosentan, felbamate, griseofulvin, oxcarbazepine, rifampicin, topiramate, rifabutin, rufinamide, aprepitant, and products containing St. John's wort. Interactions between CHCs and other drugs may lead to breakthrough bleeding and/or contraceptive failure. Counsel women to use an alternative method of contraception or a back-up method when enzyme inducers are used with NuvaRing, and to continue back-up contraception for 28 days after discontinuing the enzyme inducer to ensure contraceptive reliability.

The serum concentrations of etonogestrel and ethinyl estradiol were not affected by concomitant administration of oral amoxicillin or doxycycline in standard dosages during 10 days of antibiotic treatment. The effects of other antibiotics on etonogestrel or ethinyl estradiol concentrations have not been evaluated.

Substances increasing the plasma concentrations of CHCs

Co-administration of atorvastatin and certain CHCs containing ethinyl estradiol increase AUC values for ethinyl estradiol by approximately 20-25%. Ascorbic acid and acetaminophen may increase plasma ethinyl estradiol concentrations, possibly by inhibition of conjugation. CYP3A4 inhibitors such as itraconazole, voriconazole, fluconazole, grapefruit juice, or ketoconazole may increase plasma hormone concentrations. Co-administration of vaginal miconazole nitrate and NuvaRing increases the serum concentrations of etonogestrel and ethinyl estradiol by up to 40% [see Clinical Pharmacology (12.3)].

Human immunodeficiency virus (HIV)/ Hepatitis C Virus (HCV) protease inhibitors and non-nucleoside reverse transcriptase inhibitors:

Significant changes in the plasma concentrations of the estrogen and/or progestin have been noted in some cases of co-administration with HIV protease inhibitors (decrease [e.g., nelfinavir, ritonavir, darunavir/ritonavir, (fos)amprenavir/ritonavir, lopinavir/ritonavir, and tipranavir/ritonavir] or increase [e.g., indinavir and atazanavir/ritonavir]) /HCV protease inhibitors (decrease [e.g., boceprevir and telaprevir]) or with non-nucleoside reverse transcriptase inhibitors (decrease [e.g., nevirapine] or increase [e.g., etravirine]).

7.2 Effects of CHCs on Other Drugs

CHCs containing ethinyl estradiol may inhibit the metabolism of other compounds (e.g., cyclosporine, prednisolone, theophylline, tizanidine, and voriconazole) and increase their plasma concentrations. CHCs have been shown to decrease plasma concentrations of acetaminophen, clofibric acid, morphine, salicylic acid and temazepam. A significant decrease in the plasma concentrations of lamotrigine has been shown, likely due to induction of lamotrigine glucuronidation. This may reduce seizure control, therefore, dosage adjustments of lamotrigine may be necessary.

Women on thyroid hormone replacement therapy may need increased doses of thyroid hormone because serum concentrations of thyroid-binding globulin increase with use of CHCs.

7.3 Interference with Laboratory Tests

The use of contraceptive steroids may influence the results of certain laboratory tests, such as coagulation factors, lipids, glucose tolerance, and binding proteins.

8 USE IN SPECIFIC POPULATIONS

8.1 Pregnancy

There is little or no increased risk of birth defects in women who inadvertently use CHCs during early pregnancy. Epidemiologic studies and meta-analyses have not found an increased risk of genital or non-genital birth defects (including cardiac anomalies and limb-reduction defects) following exposure to low dose CHCs prior to conception or during early pregnancy.

The administration of CHCs to induce withdrawal bleeding should not be used as a test for pregnancy. CHCs should not be used during pregnancy to treat threatened or habitual abortion.

8.3 Nursing Mothers

The effects of NuvaRing in nursing mothers have not been evaluated and are unknown. When possible, advise the nursing mother to use other forms of contraception until she has completely weaned her child. CHCs can reduce milk production in breastfeeding mothers. This is less likely to occur once breastfeeding is well-established; however, it can occur at any time in some women. Small amounts of contraceptive steroids and/or metabolites are present in breast milk.

8.4 Pediatric Use

Safety and efficacy of NuvaRing have been established in women of reproductive age. Efficacy is expected to be the same for postpubertal adolescents under the age of 18 and for users 18 years and older. Use of this product before menarche is not indicated.

8.5 Geriatric Use

NuvaRing has not been studied in postmenopausal women and is not indicated in this population.

8.6 Hepatic Impairment

The effect of hepatic impairment on the pharmacokinetics of NuvaRing has not been studied. Steroid hormones may be poorly metabolized in patients with impaired liver function. Acute or chronic disturbances of liver function may necessitate the discontinuation of CHC use until markers of liver function return to normal. [See Contraindications (4) and Warnings and Precautions (5.3).]

8.7 Renal Impairment

The effect of renal impairment on the pharmacokinetics of NuvaRing has not been studied.

10 OVERDOSAGE

There have been no reports of serious ill effects from overdose of CHCs. Overdosage may cause withdrawal bleeding in females and nausea. If the ring breaks, it does not release a higher dose of hormones. In case of suspected overdose, all NuvaRing rings should be removed and symptomatic treatment given.

11 DESCRIPTION

NuvaRing (etonogestrel/ethinyl estradiol vaginal ring) is a non-biodegradable, flexible, transparent, colorless to almost colorless, combination contraceptive vaginal ring containing two active components, a progestin, etonogestrel (13-ethyl-17-hydroxy-11-methylene-18,19-dinor-17α-pregn-4-en-20-yn-3-one) and an estrogen, ethinyl estradiol (19-nor-17α-pregna-1,3,5(10)-trien-20-yne-3,17-diol). When placed in the vagina, each ring releases on average 0.120 mg/day of etonogestrel and 0.015 mg/day of ethinyl estradiol over a three-week period of use. NuvaRing is made of ethylene vinylacetate copolymers (28% and 9% vinylacetate) and magnesium stearate and contains 11.7 mg etonogestrel and 2.7 mg ethinyl estradiol. NuvaRing is not made with natural rubber latex. NuvaRing has an outer diameter of 54 mm and a cross-sectional diameter of 4 mm. The molecular weights for etonogestrel and ethinyl estradiol are 324.46 and 296.40, respectively.

The structural formulas are as follows:

ETONOGESTREL $C_{22}H_{28}O_2$

ETHINYL ESTRADIOL $C_{20}H_{24}O_2$

12 CLINICAL PHARMACOLOGY

12.1 Mechanism of Action

Combination hormonal contraceptives act by suppression of gonadotropins. Although the primary effect of this action is inhibition of ovulation, other alterations include changes in the cervical mucus (which increase the difficulty of sperm entry into the uterus) and the endometrium (which reduce the likelihood of implantation).

12.3 Pharmacokinetics

Absorption

Etonogestrel: Etonogestrel released by NuvaRing is rapidly absorbed. The bioavailability of etonogestrel after vaginal administration is approximately 100%. The serum etonogestrel and ethinyl estradiol concentrations observed during three weeks of NuvaRing use are summarized in Table 2.

Ethinyl estradiol: Ethinyl estradiol released by NuvaRing is rapidly absorbed. The bioavailability of ethinyl estradiol after vaginal administration is approximately 56%, which is comparable to that with oral administration of ethinyl estradiol. The serum ethinyl estradiol concentrations observed during three weeks of NuvaRing use are summarized in Table 2.

Table 2: Mean (SD) Serum Etonogestrel and Ethinyl Estradiol Concentrations (n=16)

	1 week	2 weeks	3 weeks
etonogestrel (pg/mL)	1578 (408)	1476 (362)	1374 (328)
ethinyl estradiol (pg/mL)	19.1 (4.5)	18.3 (4.3)	17.6 (4.3)

The pharmacokinetic profile of etonogestrel and ethinyl estradiol during use of NuvaRing is shown in Figure 2.

Table 3: Mean (SD) Pharmacokinetic Parameters of NuvaRing (n=16)

Hormone	C_{max} pg/mL	T_{max} hr	$t_{1/2}$ hr	CL L/hr
etonogestrel	1716 (445)	200.3 (69.6)	29.3 (6.1)	3.4 (0.8)
ethinyl estradiol	34.7 (17.5)	59.3 (67.5)	44.7 (28.8)	34.8 (11.6)

C_{max} - maximum serum drug concentration
T_{max} - time at which maximum serum drug concentration occurs
$t_{1/2}$ - elimination half-life, calculated by $0.693/K_{elim}$
CL - apparent clearance

Figure 2: Mean Serum Concentration-Time Profile of Etonogestrel and Ethinyl Estradiol during Three Weeks of NuvaRing Use

The pharmacokinetic parameters of etonogestrel and ethinyl estradiol were determined during one cycle of NuvaRing use in 16 healthy female subjects and are summarized in Table 3.
[See table 3 above]
Prolonged use of NuvaRing: The mean serum etonogestrel concentration at the end of the fourth week of continuous use of NuvaRing was 1272 ± 311 pg/mL compared to a mean concentration range of 1578 ± 408 to 1374 ± 328 pg/mL at the end of weeks one to three. The mean serum ethinyl estradiol concentration at the end of the fourth week of continuous use of NuvaRing was 16.8 ± 4.6 pg/mL compared to a mean concentration range of 19.1 ± 4.5 to 17.6 ± 4.3 pg/mL at the end of weeks one to three.
Distribution
Etonogestrel: Etonogestrel is approximately 32% bound to sex hormone-binding globulin (SHBG) and approximately 66% bound to albumin in blood.
Ethinyl estradiol: Ethinyl estradiol is highly but not specifically bound to serum albumin (98.5%) and induces an increase in the serum concentrations of SHBG.
Metabolism
In vitro data shows that both etonogestrel and ethinyl estradiol are metabolized in liver microsomes by the cytochrome P450 3A4 isoenzyme. Ethinyl estradiol is primarily metabolized by aromatic hydroxylation, but a wide variety of hydroxylated and methylated metabolites are formed. These are present as free metabolites and as sulfate and glucuronide conjugates. The hydroxylated ethinyl estradiol metabolites have weak estrogenic activity. The biological activity of etonogestrel metabolites is unknown.
Excretion
Etonogestrel and ethinyl estradiol are primarily eliminated in urine, bile and feces.
Drug Interactions
[See also Drug Interactions (7).]
The drug interactions of NuvaRing were evaluated in several studies.
A single-dose vaginal administration of an oil-based 1200-mg miconazole nitrate capsule increased the serum concentrations of etonogestrel and ethinyl estradiol by approximately 17% and 16%, respectively. Following multiple doses of 200 mg miconazole nitrate by vaginal suppository or vaginal cream, the mean serum concentrations of etonogestrel and ethinyl estradiol increased by up to 40%. A single-dose vaginal administration of 100-mg water-based nonoxynol-9 spermicide gel did not affect the serum concentrations of etonogestrel or ethinyl estradiol.
The serum concentrations of etonogestrel and ethinyl estradiol were not affected by concomitant administration of oral amoxicillin or doxycycline in standard dosages during 10 days of antibiotic treatment.
Tampon Use
The use of tampons had no effect on serum concentrations of etonogestrel and ethinyl estradiol during use of NuvaRing [see Dosage and Administration (2.5)].

13 NONCLINICAL TOXICOLOGY
13.1 Carcinogenesis, Mutagenesis, Impairment of Fertility
In a 24-month carcinogenicity study in rats with subdermal implants releasing 10 and 20 mcg etonogestrel per day, (approximately 0.3 and 0.6 times the systemic steady-state exposure of women using NuvaRing), no drug-related carcinogenic potential was observed. Etonogestrel was not genotoxic in the in vitro Ames/Salmonella reverse mutation assay, the chromosomal aberration assay in Chinese hamster ovary cells or in the in vivo mouse micronucleus test. Fertility returned in rats after withdrawal from treatment.

14 CLINICAL STUDIES
In three large one-year clinical trials enrolling 2,834 women aged 18-40 years, in North America, Europe, Brazil, and Chile, the racial distribution was 93% Caucasian, 5.0% Black, 0.8% Asian, and 1.2% Other. Women with BMI ≥ 30 kg/m^2 were excluded from these studies.
Based on pooled data from the three trials, 2,356 women aged < 35 years completed 23,515 evaluable cycles of NuvaRing use (cycles in which no back-up contraception was used). The pooled pregnancy rate (Pearl Index) was 1.28 (95% CI [0.8, 1.9]) per 100 women-years of NuvaRing use. In the US study, the Pearl Index was 2.02 (95% CI [1.1, 3.4]) per 100 women-years of NuvaRing use.

15 REFERENCES
1. Dinger, J et. al., Cardiovascular risk associated with the use of an etonogestrel-containing vaginal ring. Obstetrics & Gynecology 2013; 122(4): 800-808.
2. Sidney, S. et. al., Recent combined hormonal contraceptives (CHCs) and the risk of thromboembolism and other cardiovascular events in new users. Contraception 2013; 87: 93–100.
3. Combined hormonal contraceptives (CHCs) and the risk of cardiovascular endpoints. Sidney, S. (primary author) http://www.fda.gov/downloads/Drugs/DrugSafety/UCM277384.pdf, accessed 23-Aug-2013.

16 HOW SUPPLIED/STORAGE AND HANDLING
Each NuvaRing (etonogestrel/ethinyl estradiol vaginal ring) is individually packaged in a reclosable aluminum laminate sachet consisting of three layers, from outside to inside: polyester, aluminum foil, and low-density polyethylene. The ring should be replaced in this reclosable sachet after use and discarded in a waste receptacle out of the reach of children and pets. It should not be flushed down the toilet.

Box of 3 sachets   NDC 0052-0273-03
16.1 Storage
Prior to dispensing to the user, store refrigerated 2-8°C (36-46°F). After dispensing to the user, NuvaRing can be stored for up to 4 months at 25°C (77°F); excursions permitted to 15-30°C (59-86°F) [see USP Controlled Room Temperature].
Avoid storing NuvaRing in direct sunlight or at temperatures above 30°C (86°F).
For the Dispenser: When NuvaRing is dispensed to the user, place an expiration date on the label. The date should not exceed either 4 months from the date of dispensing or the expiration date, whichever comes first.

17 PATIENT COUNSELING INFORMATION
See FDA-approved patient labeling (Patient Information and Instructions for Use).
Counsel patients regarding the following:
• Cigarette smoking increases the risk of serious cardiovascular events from use of NuvaRing, and women who are over 35 years old and smoke should not use NuvaRing.
• The increased risk of VTE compared to non-users of CHCs is greatest after initially starting a CHC or restarting (following a 4-week or greater CHC-free interval) the same or a different CHC.
• NuvaRing does not protect against HIV infection (AIDS) and other sexually transmitted infections.
• The Warnings and Precautions associated with NuvaRing.
• NuvaRing is not to be used during pregnancy. If pregnancy is planned or occurs during treatment with NuvaRing, instruct the patient to discontinue NuvaRing use.
• The proper usage of NuvaRing and what to do if she does not comply with the labeled timing of insertion and removal.
• The need to use a barrier method of contraception when the ring is out for more than three continuous hours until NuvaRing has been used continuously for at least seven days.
• The proper disposal of a used NuvaRing.

• Use a back-up or alternative method of contraception when enzyme inducers are used with NuvaRing.
• CHCs may reduce breast milk production. This is less likely to occur if breastfeeding is well established.
• Women who start NuvaRing postpartum and have not yet had a normal period should use an additional non-hormonal method of contraception for the first seven days.
• Amenorrhea may occur. Rule out pregnancy in the event of amenorrhea if NuvaRing has been out of the vagina for more than three consecutive hours, if the ring-free interval was extended beyond one week, if the woman has missed a period for two or more consecutive cycles, and if the ring has been retained for longer than four weeks.

Manufactured for: Merck Sharp & Dohme Corp., a subsidiary of
MERCK & CO., INC., Whitehouse Station, NJ 08889, USA
Manufactured by: N.V. Organon, Oss, The Netherlands, a subsidiary of
Merck & Co., Inc., Whitehouse Station, NJ 08889, USA
For patent information: www.merck.com/product/patent/home.html
Copyright © 2001-2012 Merck Sharp & Dohme B.V., a subsidiary of **Merck & Co., Inc.**
All rights reserved.
Revised: 12/2013
uspi-mk8342a-rng-1312r05
Patient Information
NuvaRing® (NEW-vah-ring)
(etonogestrel/ethinyl estradiol vaginal ring)

> **What is the most important information I should know about NuvaRing?**
> Do not use NuvaRing if you smoke cigarettes and are over 35 years old. Smoking increases your risk of serious cardiovascular side effects (heart and blood vessel problems) from combination hormonal contraceptives (CHCs), including death from heart attack, blood clots or stroke. This risk increases with age and the number of cigarettes you smoke.

Hormonal birth control methods help to lower the chances of becoming pregnant. They do not protect against HIV infection (AIDS) and other sexually transmitted infections.
What is NuvaRing?
NuvaRing (NEW-vah-ring) is a flexible birth control vaginal ring used to prevent pregnancy.
NuvaRing contains a combination of a progestin and estrogen, 2 kinds of female hormones. Birth control methods that contain both an estrogen and a progestin are called combination hormonal contraceptives (CHCs).
How well does NuvaRing work?
Your chance of getting pregnant depends on how well you follow the directions for using NuvaRing. The better you follow the directions, the less chance you have of getting pregnant.
Based on the results of a US clinical study, approximately 1 to 3 women out of 100 women may get pregnant during the first year they use NuvaRing.
The following chart shows the chance of getting pregnant for women who use different methods of birth control. Each box on the chart contains a list of birth control methods that are similar in effectiveness. The most effective methods are at the top of the chart. The box on the bottom of the chart shows the chance of getting pregnant for women who do not use birth control and are trying to get pregnant.
[See figure at top of next column]
Who should not use NuvaRing?
Do not use NuvaRing if you:
• smoke and are over 35 years old
• have or have had blood clots in your arms, legs, eyes or lungs
• have an inherited problem with your blood that makes it clot more than normal
• have had a stroke
• have had a heart attack
• have certain heart valve problems or heart rhythm problems that can cause blood clots to form in the heart
• have high blood pressure that medicine can't control
• have diabetes with kidney, eye, nerve, or blood vessel damage
• have certain kinds of severe migraine headaches with aura, numbness, weakness, or changes in vision, or have any migraine headaches if you are over age 35
• have liver disease, including liver tumors
• have unexplained vaginal bleeding
• are pregnant or think you may be pregnant. NuvaRing is not for pregnant women.
• have or have had breast cancer or any cancer that is sensitive to female hormones
• are allergic to etonogestrel, ethinyl estradiol or any of the ingredients in NuvaRing. See the list of ingredients in NuvaRing at the end of this leaflet.
Hormonal birth control methods may not be a good choice for you if you have ever had jaundice (yellowing of the skin or eyes) caused by pregnancy or related to previous use of hormonal birth control.

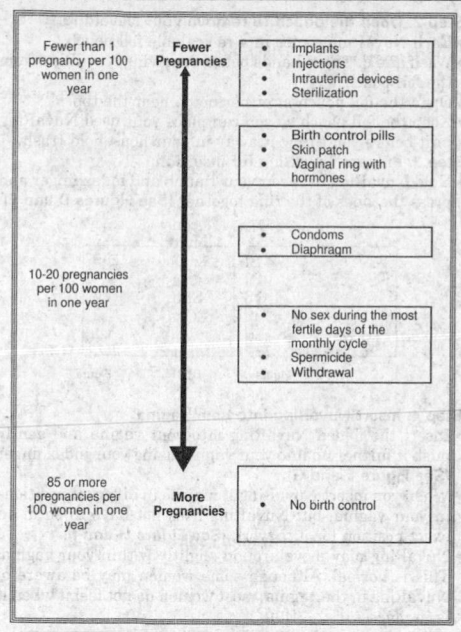

Tell your healthcare provider if you have ever had any of the conditions listed above. Your healthcare provider can suggest another method of birth control.

What should I tell my healthcare provider before using NuvaRing?

Before you use NuvaRing tell your healthcare provider if you:
• have any medical conditions
• smoke
• are pregnant or think you are pregnant
• recently had a baby
• recently had a miscarriage or abortion
• have a family history of breast cancer
• have or have had breast nodules, fibrocystic disease, an abnormal breast x-ray, or abnormal mammogram
• use tampons and have a history of toxic shock syndrome
• have been diagnosed with depression
• have had liver problems including jaundice during pregnancy
• have or have had elevated cholesterol or triglycerides
• have or have had gallbladder, liver, heart, or kidney disease
• have diabetes
• have a history of jaundice (yellowing of the skin or eyes) caused by pregnancy (also called cholestasis of pregnancy)
• have a history of scanty or irregular menstrual periods
• have any condition that makes the vagina become irritated easily
• have or have had high blood pressure
• have or have had migraines or other headaches or seizures
• are scheduled for surgery. NuvaRing may increase your risk of blood clots after surgery. You should stop using NuvaRing at least 4 weeks before you have surgery and not restart it until at least 2 weeks after your surgery.
• are scheduled for any laboratory tests. Certain blood tests may be affected by hormonal birth control methods.
• are breastfeeding or plan to breastfeed. Hormonal birth control methods that contain estrogen, like NuvaRing, may decrease the amount of milk you make. A small amount of hormones from NuvaRing may pass into your breast milk. Consider another non-hormonal method of birth control until you are ready to stop breastfeeding.

Tell your healthcare provider about all medicines and herbal products you take, including prescription and over-the-counter medicines, vitamins and herbal supplements.

Some medicines and herbal products may make hormonal birth control less effective, including, but not limited to:
• certain anti-seizure medicines (such as barbiturates, carbamazepine, felbamate, oxcarbazepine, phenytoin, rufinamide, topiramate)
• medicine to treat fungal infections (griseofulvin)
• certain combinations of HIV medicines, (such as nelfinavir, ritonavir, darunavir/ritonavir, (fos)amprenavir/ritonavir, lopinavir/ritonavir, and tipranavir/ritonavir)
• certain hepatitis C (HCV) medicines (such as boceprevir, telaprevir)
• non-nucleoside reverse transcriptase inhibitors (such as nevirapine)
• medicine to treat tuberculosis (such as rifampicin and rifabutin)
• medicine to treat high blood pressure in the vessels of the lung (bosentan)

• medicine to treat chemotherapy-induced nausea and vomiting (aprepitant)
• St John's wort

Use an additional birth control method (such as a male condom with spermicide) when you take medicines that may make NuvaRing less effective. Continue back-up birth control for 28 days after stopping the medicine to help prevent you from becoming pregnant.

Some medicines and grapefruit juice may increase the level of ethinyl estradiol in your blood if used together, including:
• the pain reliever acetaminophen
• ascorbic acid (vitamin C)
• medicines that affect how your liver breaks down other medicines (such as itraconazole, ketoconazole, voriconazole, and fluconazole)
• certain HIV medicines (atazanavir/ritonavir, indinavir)
• non-nucleoside reverse transcriptase inhibitors (such as etravirine)
• medicines to lower cholesterol such as atorvastatin and rosuvastatin

Hormonal birth control methods may interact with lamotrigine, a medicine used for seizures. This may increase the risk of seizures, so your healthcare provider may need to adjust your dose of lamotrigine.

Women on thyroid replacement therapy may need increased doses of thyroid hormone.

Ask your healthcare provider if you are not sure if you take any of the medicines listed above. Know the medicines you take. Keep a list of them to show your doctor and pharmacist when you get a new medicine.

• How should I use NuvaRing?
• Read the **Instructions for Use** at the end of this Patient Information that comes with your NuvaRing for information about the right way to use NuvaRing.
• Use NuvaRing exactly as your healthcare provider tells you to use it.
• NuvaRing is used in a 4 week cycle.
  ◦ Insert 1 NuvaRing in the vagina and keep it in place for 3 weeks (21 days).
  ◦ Remove the NuvaRing for a 1 week break (7 days). During the 1-week break (7 days), you will usually have your menstrual period.
    Note: Insert and remove NuvaRing on the same day of the week and at the same time:
    ◦ For example, if you insert your NuvaRing on a Monday at 8:00 am, you should remove it on the Monday 3 weeks later at 8:00 am.
    ◦ After your 1 week (7 days) break, you should insert a new NuvaRing on the next Monday at 8:00 am.
• While using NuvaRing, you should not use a vaginal diaphragm as your back-up method of birth control because NuvaRing may interfere with the correct placement and position of a diaphragm.
• Use of spermicides or vaginal yeast products will not make NuvaRing less effective at preventing pregnancy.
• Use of tampons will not make NuvaRing less effective or stop NuvaRing from working.
• If NuvaRing has been left inside your vagina for more than 4 weeks (28 days), you may not be protected from pregnancy and you should see your healthcare provider to be sure you are not pregnant. Until you know the results of your pregnancy test, you should use an extra method of birth control, such as male condoms with spermicide, until the new NuvaRing has been in place for 7 days in a row.
• Do not use more than 1 NuvaRing at a time. Too much hormonal birth control medicine in your body may cause nausea, vomiting, or vaginal bleeding.

Your healthcare provider should examine you at least 1 time a year to see if you have any signs of side effects from using NuvaRing.

What are the possible side effects of using NuvaRing?

See "What is the most important information I should know about NuvaRing?"

NuvaRing may cause serious side effects, including:

blood clots. Like pregnancy, combination hormonal birth control methods increase the risk of serious blood clots (see following graph), especially in women who have other risk factors, such as smoking, obesity, or age greater than 35. This increased risk is highest when you first start using a combination hormonal birth control method or when you restart the same or different combination hormonal birth control method after not using it for a month or more. Talk with your healthcare provider about your risk of getting a blood clot before using NuvaRing or before deciding which type of birth control is right for you.

In some studies of women who used NuvaRing, the risk of getting a blood clot was similar to the risk in women who used combination birth control pills.

Other studies have reported that the risk of blood clots was higher for women who use combination birth control pills containing desogestrel (a progestin similar to the progestin in NuvaRing) than for women who use combination birth control pills that do not contain desogestrel.

It is possible to die or be permanently disabled from a problem caused by a blood clot, such as heart attack or stroke. Some examples of serious blood clots are blood clots in the:
◦ legs (deep vein thrombosis)
◦ lungs (pulmonary embolus)
◦ eyes (loss of eyesight)
◦ heart (heart attack)
◦ brain (stroke)

To put the risk of developing a blood clot into perspective: If 10,000 women who are not pregnant and do not use hormonal birth control are followed for one year, between 1 and 5 of these women will develop a blood clot. The figure below shows the likelihood of developing a serious blood clot for women who are not pregnant and do not use hormonal birth control, for women who use hormonal birth control, for pregnant women, and for women in the first 12 weeks after delivering a baby.

Likelihood of Developing a Serious Blood Clot (Venous Thromboembolism [VTE])

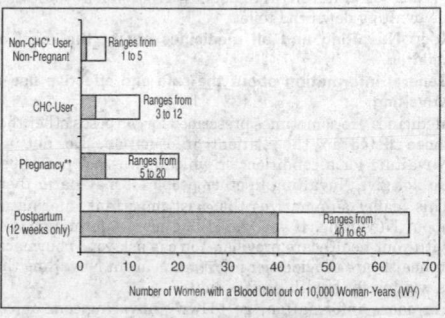

*CHC=combination hormonal contraception

**Pregnancy data based on actual duration of pregnancy in the reference studies. Based on a model assumption that pregnancy duration is nine months, the rate is 7 to 27 per 10,000 WY.

Call your healthcare provider right away if you have:
◦ leg pain that does not go away
◦ sudden shortness of breath
◦ sudden blindness, partial or complete
◦ severe pain or pressure in your chest
◦ sudden, severe headache unlike your usual headaches
◦ weakness or numbness in an arm or leg, or trouble speaking
◦ yellowing of the skin or eyeballs

Other serious risks include:
• Toxic Shock Syndrome (TSS). Some of the symptoms are much the same as the flu, but they can become serious very quickly. Call your healthcare provider or get emergency treatment right away if you have the following symptoms:
  ◦ sudden high fever   ◦ muscle aches
  ◦ vomiting   ◦ dizziness
  ◦ diarrhea   ◦ fainting or feeling faint
  ◦ a sunburn-like rash   when standing up
• liver problems, including liver tumors
• high blood pressure
• gallbladder problems
• accidental insertion into bladder
• symptoms of a problem called angioedema if you already have a family history of angioedema

The most common side effects of NuvaRing are:
• tissue irritation inside your vagina or on your cervix
• headache (including migraine)
• mood changes (including depression, especially if you had depression in the past). Call your healthcare provider immediately if you have any thoughts of harming yourself.
• NuvaRing problems, including the ring slipping out or causing discomfort
• nausea and vomiting
• vaginal discharge
• weight gain
• vaginal discomfort
• breast pain, discomfort, or tenderness
• painful menstrual periods
• abdominal pain
• acne
• less sexual desire

Some women have spotting or light bleeding during NuvaRing use. If these symptoms occur, do not stop using NuvaRing. The problem will usually go away. If it doesn't go away, check with your healthcare provider.

Other side effects seen with NuvaRing include allergic reaction, hives, breast discharge, and penis discomfort of the partner (such as irritation, rash, itching).

Less common side effects seen with combination hormonal birth control include:

- Blotchy darkening of your skin, especially on your face
- High blood sugar, especially in women who already have diabetes
- High fat (cholesterol, triglycerides) levels in the blood

Tell your healthcare provider about any side effect that bothers you or that does not go away. These are not all the possible side effects of NuvaRing. For more information, ask your healthcare provider or pharmacist. Call your healthcare provider for medical advice about side effects. You may report side effects to FDA at 1-800-FDA-1088.

How should I store NuvaRing and throw away used NuvaRings?

- Store NuvaRing at room temperature between 68°F to 77°F (20°C to 25°C).
- Store NuvaRing at room temperature for up to 4 months after you receive it. Throw NuvaRing away if the expiration date on the label has passed.
- Do not store NuvaRing above 86°F (30°C).
- Avoid direct sunlight
- Place the used NuvaRing in the re-closable foil pouch and properly throw it away in your household trash out of the reach of children and pets. Do not flush your used NuvaRing down the toilet.

Keep NuvaRing and all medicines out of the reach of children.

General information about the safe and effective use of NuvaRing

Medicines are sometimes prescribed for purposes other than those listed in the Patient Information. Do not use NuvaRing for a condition for which it was not prescribed. Do not give NuvaRing to other people. It may harm them. This leaflet summarizes the most important information about NuvaRing. If you would like more information, talk with your healthcare provider. You can ask your pharmacist or healthcare provider for information about NuvaRing that is written for health professionals.

For more information, go to www.nuvaring.com or call 1-877-NUVARING (1-877-688-2746).

What are the ingredients in NuvaRing?

Active ingredients: etonogestrel and ethinyl estradiol

Inactive ingredients: ethylene vinylacetate copolymers (28% and 9% vinylacetate) and magnesium stearate.

NuvaRing is not made with natural rubber latex.

Do Hormonal Birth Control Methods Cause Cancer?

Hormonal birth control methods do not seem to cause breast cancer. However, if you have breast cancer now or have had it in the past, do not use hormonal birth control, including NuvaRing, because some breast cancers are sensitive to hormones.

Women who use hormonal birth control methods may have a slightly higher chance of getting cervical cancer. However, this may be due to other reasons such as having more sexual partners.

What should I know about my period when using NuvaRing?

When you use NuvaRing you may have bleeding and spotting between periods, called unplanned bleeding. Unplanned bleeding may vary from slight staining between menstrual periods to breakthrough bleeding, which is a flow much like a regular period. Unplanned bleeding occurs most often during the first few months of NuvaRing use, but may also occur after you have been using NuvaRing for some time. Such bleeding may be temporary and usually does not indicate any serious problems. It is important to continue using the ring on schedule. If the unplanned bleeding or spotting is heavy or lasts for more than a few days, you should discuss this with your healthcare provider.

What if I miss my regular scheduled period when using NuvaRing?

Some women miss periods on hormonal birth control, even when they are not pregnant. Consider the possibility that you may be pregnant if:

1. you miss a period and NuvaRing was out of the vagina for more than 3 hours during the 3 weeks (21 days) of ring use
2. you miss a period and waited longer than 1 week to insert a new ring
3. you have followed the instructions and you miss 2 periods in a row
4. you have left NuvaRing in place for longer than 4 weeks (28 days)

What if I want to become pregnant?

You may stop using NuvaRing whenever you wish. Consider a visit with your healthcare provider for a pre-pregnancy checkup before you stop using NuvaRing.

Instructions for Use

NuvaRing (NEW-vah-ring)

(etonogestrel/ethinyl estradiol vaginal ring)

Read these Instructions for Use before you start using NuvaRing and each time you get a refill. There may be new information. This information does not take the place of talking to your healthcare provider about your treatment.

How should I start using NuvaRing?

If you are not currently using hormonal birth control, you have 2 ways to start using NuvaRing. Choose the best way for you:

- **First Day Start:** Insert NuvaRing on the first day of your menstrual period. You will not need to use another birth control method since you are using NuvaRing on the first day of your menstrual period.
- **Day 2 to Day 5 Cycle Start:** You may choose to start NuvaRing on days 2 to 5 of your menstrual period. Make sure you also use an extra method of birth control (barrier method), such as male condoms with spermicide for the first 7 days of NuvaRing use in the first cycle.

If you are changing from a birth control pill or patch to NuvaRing:

If you have been using your birth control method correctly and are certain that you are not pregnant, you can change to NuvaRing any day. Do not start NuvaRing any later than the day you would start your next birth control pill or apply your patch.

If you are changing from a progestin-only birth control method, such as a minipill, implant or injection or from an intrauterine system (IUS):

- You may switch from a minipill on any day. Start using NuvaRing on the day that you would have taken your next minipill.
- You should switch from an implant or the IUS and start using NuvaRing on the day that you remove the implant or IUS
- You should switch from an injectable and start using NuvaRing on the day when your next injection would be due.

If you are changing from a minipill, implant or injection or from an intrauterine system (IUS), you should use an extra method of birth control, such as a male condom with spermicide during the first 7 days of using NuvaRing.

If you start using NuvaRing after an abortion or miscarriage:

- **Following a first trimester abortion or miscarriage:** You may start NuvaRing within 5 days following a first trimester abortion or miscarriage (the first 12 weeks of pregnancy). You do not need to use an additional birth control method.
- If you do not start NuvaRing within 5 days after a first trimester abortion or miscarriage, use a non-hormonal birth control method, such as male condoms and spermicide, while you wait for your period to start. Begin NuvaRing at the time of your next menstrual period. Count the first day of your menstrual period as "Day 1" and start NuvaRing one of the following 2 ways below.
  ○ **First Day Start:** Insert NuvaRing on the first day of your menstrual period. You will not need to use another birth control method since you are using NuvaRing on the first day of your menstrual period.
  ○ **Day 2 to Day 5 Cycle Start:** You may choose to start NuvaRing on Days 2 to 5 of your menstrual period. Make sure you also use an extra method of birth control (barrier method), such as male condoms with spermicide for the first 7 days of NuvaRing use in the first cycle.
- **Following a second trimester abortion or miscarriage:** You may start using NuvaRing no sooner than 4 weeks (28 days) after a second trimester abortion (after the first 12 weeks of pregnancy).

If you are starting NuvaRing after childbirth:

- You may start using NuvaRing no sooner than 4 weeks (28 days) after having a baby if you are not breastfeeding.
- If you have not gotten your menstrual period after childbirth, you should talk to your healthcare provider. You may need a pregnancy test to make sure you are not pregnant before you start using NuvaRing.
- Use another birth control method such as male condoms with spermicide for the first 7 days in addition to NuvaRing.

If you are breastfeeding you should not use NuvaRing. Use other birth control methods until you are no longer breastfeeding.

Step 1. Choose a position for insertion of NuvaRing.

- Choose the position that is comfortable for you. For example, lying down, squatting, or standing with 1 leg up (See Figures A, B, and C).

Positions for NuvaRing insertion

Figure A   Figure B   Figure C

Step 2. Open the pouch to remove your NuvaRing.

- Each NuvaRing comes in a re-sealable foil pouch.
- Wash and dry your hands before removing NuvaRing from the foil pouch.
- Open the foil pouch at either notch near the top.
- Keep the foil pouch so you can place your used NuvaRing in it before you throw it away in your household trash.

Step 3. Prepare NuvaRing for insertion.

- Hold NuvaRing between your thumb and index finger and press the sides of the ring together (See Figures D and E).

Figure D   Figure E

Step 4. Insert NuvaRing into your vagina.

- Insert the folded NuvaRing into your vagina and gently push it further up into your vagina using your index finger (See Figure F and G).
- When you insert NuvaRing it may be in different positions in your vagina, but NuvaRing does not have to be in an exact position for it to work (See Figure H and I).
- NuvaRing may move around slightly within your vagina. This is normal. Although some women may be aware of NuvaRing in the vagina, most women do not feel it when it is in place.

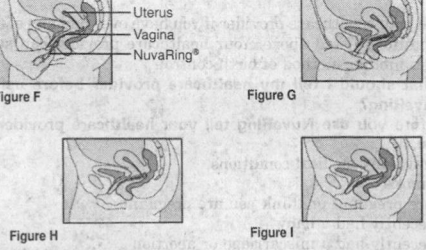

Uterus
Vagina
NuvaRing®

Figure F   Figure G

Figure H   Figure I

Inserting NuvaRing (**Figure F, Figure G**) and positioning NuvaRing (**Figure H, Figure I**)

Note:

- If the NuvaRing feels uncomfortable, you may not have pushed the ring into your vagina far enough. Use your finger to gently push the NuvaRing as far as you can into your vagina. There is no danger of NuvaRing being pushed too far up in the vagina or getting lost (See Figure G).
- Some women have accidently inserted NuvaRing into their bladder. If you have pain during or after insertion and you cannot find NuvaRing in your vagina, call your healthcare provider right away.

Step 5. How do I remove NuvaRing?

- Wash and dry your hands.
- Choose the position that is most comfortable for you (See Figures A, B, and C).
- Put your index finger into your vagina and hook it through the NuvaRing. Gently pull downward and forward to remove the NuvaRing and pull it out (See Figure J).

Figure J

Step 6. Throw away the used NuvaRing.

- Place the used NuvaRing in the re-sealable foil pouch and put it in a trash can out of the reach of children and pets.
- Do not throw NuvaRing in the toilet.

What else should I know about using NuvaRing?

What If I leave NuvaRing in too long?

- If you leave NuvaRing in your vagina for up to 4 weeks (28 days) you will still be getting pregnancy protection. Remove your old NuvaRing for 1 week (7 days) and insert a new NuvaRing 1 week (7 days) later (See Steps 1 through 4).
- If you leave NuvaRing in your vagina longer than 4 weeks (28 days), remove the ring and check to make sure you are not pregnant.

  If you are not pregnant, insert a new NuvaRing (See Steps 1 through 4). You must use another birth control method, such as male condoms with spermicide, until the new NuvaRing has been used for 7 days in a row.

What should I do if my NuvaRing comes out of my vagina?

NuvaRing can slip or accidentally come out (expelled) of your vagina during sexual intercourse, bowel movements, use of tampons, or if it breaks.

- NuvaRing may break causing the ring to lose its shape. If the ring stays in your vagina this should not lower NuvaRing's effectiveness at preventing pregnancy.
  - If NuvaRing breaks and slips out of your vagina, throw the broken ring in your household trash out of the reach of children and pets.
  - Insert a new NuvaRing (See Steps 1 through 4).
- You should pay attention when removing a tampon to be sure that your NuvaRing is not accidentally pulled out.
  - Be sure to insert NuvaRing before inserting a tampon.
  - If you accidentally pull out your NuvaRing while using tampons, rinse your NuvaRing in cool to lukewarm (not hot) water and insert it again right away.
- NuvaRing can be pushed out of (expelled from) your vagina during sexual intercourse or during a bowel movement.
  - If the expelled ring has been left out of your vagina for less than 3 hours, rinse the expelled NuvaRing in cool to lukewarm (not hot) water and insert it again right away.
  - If the expelled NuvaRing has been out of your vagina for more than 3 hours, insert a new NuvaRing as soon as you remember (See Step 1 thru Step 4).
    - During Weeks 1 and 2 after you have inserted your new NuvaRing, you may not be protected from pregnancy. You should use another birth control method, such as male condoms with spermicide, until the ring has been in place for 7 days in a row.
    - At the end of Week 3, you should remove the NuvaRing and throw it away in your household trash away from children and pets and follow one of the two options below:
    Option 1. Insert a new ring right away to start your 21 Day NuvaRing use cycle. You may not have your regular period but you may have spotting or vaginal bleeding.
    Option 2. Insert a new ring no later than 7 days, from the time the previous ring was removed or expelled. During this time, you may have your period.
    Note: You should only choose to do option 2 if you used NuvaRing for 7 days in a row, prior to the day that your previous NuvaRing was accidently removed or expelled. With either option 1 or 2, you should use another birth control method such as male condoms with spermicides until the new NuvaRing has been used for 7 days in a row.

This Patient Information and Instructions for Use have been approved by the U.S. Food and Drug Administration. Manufactured for: Merck Sharp & Dohme Corp., a subsidiary of
MERCK & CO., INC., Whitehouse Station, NJ 08889, USA
Manufactured by: N.V. Organon, Oss, The Netherlands, a subsidiary of
Merck & Co., Inc., Whitehouse Station, NJ 08889, USA
For patent information: www.merck.com/product/patent/home.html

Copyright © 2001-2012 Merck Sharp & Dohme B.V., a subsidiary of Merck & Co., Inc.
All rights reserved.
Revised: 12/2013
usppi-mk8342a-rng-1312r05
Shown in Product Identification Guide, page 308

PEDVAXHIB® LIQUID   ℞

[ped-vax-hib]
[Haemophilus b Conjugate Vaccine (Meningococcal Protein Conjugate)]

DESCRIPTION

PedvaxHIB® [Haemophilus b Conjugate Vaccine (Meningococcal Protein Conjugate)] is a highly purified capsular polysaccharide (polyribosylribitol phosphate or PRP) of *Haemophilus influenzae* type b (Haemophilus b, Ross strain) that is covalently bound to an outer membrane protein complex (OMPC) of the B11 strain of *Neisseria meningitidis* serogroup B. The covalent bonding of the PRP to the OMPC which is necessary for enhanced immunogenicity of the PRP is confirmed by quantitative analysis of the conjugate's components following chemical treatment which yields a unique amino acid. The potency of PedvaxHIB is determined by assay of PRP.

Haemophilus influenzae type b and *Neisseria meningitidis* serogroup B are grown in complex fermentation media. The PRP is purified from the culture broth by purification procedures which include ethanol fractionation, enzyme digestion, phenol extraction and diafiltration. The OMPC from *Neisseria meningitidis* is purified by detergent extraction, ultracentrifugation, diafiltration and sterile filtration.

Liquid PedvaxHIB is ready to use and does not require a diluent. Each 0.5 mL dose of Liquid PedvaxHIB is a sterile product formulated to contain: 7.5 mcg of Haemophilus b PRP, 125 mcg of *Neisseria meningitidis* OMPC and 225 mcg of aluminum as amorphous aluminum hydroxyphosphate sulfate (previously referred to as aluminum hydroxide), in

0.9% sodium chloride, but does not contain lactose or thimerosal. Liquid PedvaxHIB is a slightly opaque white suspension.
This vaccine is for intramuscular administration and not for intravenous injection. (See DOSAGE AND ADMINISTRATION.)

CLINICAL PHARMACOLOGY

Prior to the introduction of Haemophilus b Conjugate Vaccines, *Haemophilus influenzae* type b (Hib) was the most frequent cause of bacterial meningitis and a leading cause of serious, systemic bacterial disease in young children worldwide.[1,2,3,4]
Hib disease occurred primarily in children under 5 years of age in the United States prior to the initiation of a vaccine program and was estimated to account for nearly 20,000 cases of invasive infections annually, approximately 12,000 of which were meningitis. The mortality rate from Hib meningitis is about 5%. In addition, up to 35% of survivors develop neurologic sequelae including seizures, deafness, and mental retardation.[5,6] Other invasive diseases caused by this bacterium include cellulitis, epiglottitis, sepsis, pneumonia, septic arthritis, osteomyelitis and pericarditis.
Prior to the introduction of the vaccine, it was estimated that 17% of all cases of Hib disease occurred in infants less than 6 months of age.[7] The peak incidence of Hib meningitis occurs between 6 to 11 months of age. Forty-seven percent of all cases occur by one year of age with the remaining 53% of cases occurring over the next four years.[2,20]
Among children under 5 years of age, the risk of invasive Hib disease is increased in certain populations including the following:
- Daycare attendees[8,9]
- Lower socio-economic groups[10]
- Blacks[11] (especially those who lack the Km(1) immunoglobulin allotype)[12]
- Caucasians who lack the G2m(n or 23) immunoglobulin allotype[13]
- Native Americans[14,15,16]
- Household contacts of cases[17]
- Individuals with asplenia, sickle cell disease, or antibody deficiency syndromes[18,19]

An important virulence factor of the Hib bacterium is its polysaccharide capsule (PRP). Antibody to PRP (anti-PRP) has been shown to correlate with protection against Hib disease.[3,21] While the anti-PRP level associated with protection using conjugated vaccines has not yet been determined, the level of anti-PRP associated with protection in studies using bacterial polysaccharide immune globulin or nonconjugated PRP vaccines ranged from >0.15 to >1.0 mcg/mL.[22-28]
Nonconjugated PRP vaccines are capable of stimulating B-lymphocytes to produce antibody without the help of T-lymphocytes (T-independent). The responses to many other antigens are augmented by helper T-lymphocytes (T-dependent). PedvaxHIB is a PRP-conjugate vaccine in which the PRP is covalently bound to the OMPC carrier[29] producing an antigen which is postulated to convert the T-independent antigen (PRP alone) into a T-dependent antigen resulting in both an enhanced antibody response and immunologic memory.

Clinical Evaluation of PedvaxHIB

PedvaxHIB, in a lyophilized formulation (lyophilized PedvaxHIB), was initially evaluated in 3,486 Native American (Navajo) infants, who completed the primary two-dose regimen in a randomized, double-blind, placebo-controlled study (The Protective Efficacy Study). At the time of the study, this population had a much higher incidence of Hib disease than the United States population as a whole and also had a lower antibody response to Haemophilus b Conjugate Vaccines, including PedvaxHIB.[14,15,16,30,33]
Each infant in this study received two doses of either placebo or lyophilized PedvaxHIB with the first dose adminis-

tered at a mean of 8 weeks of age and the second administered approximately two months later; DTP and OPV were administered concomitantly. Antibody levels were measured in a subset of each group (TABLE 1).
[See table 1 above]

Most subjects were initially followed until 15 to 18 months of age. During this time, 22 cases of invasive Hib disease occurred in the placebo group (8 cases after the first dose and 14 cases after the second dose) and only 1 case in the vaccine group (none after the first dose and 1 after the second dose). Following the primary two-dose regimen, the protective efficacy of lyophilized PedvaxHIB was calculated to be 93% with a 95% confidence interval of 57%-98% (p=0.001, two-tailed). In the two months between the first and second doses, the difference in number of cases of disease between placebo and vaccine recipients (8 vs. 0 cases, respectively) was statistically significant (p=0.008, two-tailed); however, a primary two-dose regimen is required for infants 2-14 months of age.
At termination of the study, placebo recipients were offered vaccine. All original participants were then followed two years and nine months from termination of the study. During this extended follow-up, invasive Hib disease occurred in an additional seven of the original placebo recipients prior to receiving vaccine and in one of the original vaccine recipients (who had received only one dose of vaccine). No cases of invasive Hib disease were observed in placebo recipients after they received at least one dose of vaccine. Efficacy for this follow-up period, estimated from person-days at risk, was 96.6% (95 C.I., 72.2-99.9%) in children under 18 months of age and 100% (95 C.I., 23.5-100%) in children over 18 months of age.[33]
Since protective efficacy with lyophilized PedvaxHIB was demonstrated in such a high risk population, it would be expected to be predictive of efficacy in other populations.
The safety and immunogenicity of lyophilized PedvaxHIB were evaluated in infants and children in other clinical studies that were conducted in various locations throughout the United States. PedvaxHIB was highly immunogenic in all age groups studied.[31,32]
Lyophilized PedvaxHIB induced antibody levels greater than 1.0 mcg/mL in children who were poor responders to nonconjugated PRP vaccines. In a study involving such a subpopulation,[33,34] 34 children ranging in age from 27 to 61 months who developed invasive Hib disease despite previous vaccination with nonconjugated PRP vaccines were randomly assigned to 2 groups. One group (n=14) was vaccinated with lyophilized PedvaxHIB and the other group (n=20) with a nonconjugated PRP vaccine at a mean interval of approximately 12 months after recovery from disease. All 14 children vaccinated with lyophilized PedvaxHIB but only 6 of 20 children re-vaccinated with a nonconjugated PRP vaccine achieved an antibody level of >1.0 mcg/mL. The 14 children who had not responded to revaccination with the nonconjugated PRP vaccine were then vaccinated with a single dose of lyophilized PedvaxHIB; following this vaccination, all achieved antibody levels of >1.0 mcg/mL.
In addition, lyophilized PedvaxHIB has been studied in children at high risk of Hib disease because of genetically-related deficiencies [Blacks who were Km(1) allotype negative and Caucasians who were G2m(23) allotype negative] and are considered hyporesponsive to nonconjugated PRP vaccines on this basis.[35] The hyporesponsive children had anti-PRP responses comparable to those of allotype positive children of similar age range when vaccinated with lyophilized PedvaxHIB. All children achieved anti-PRP levels of >1.0 mcg/mL.
The safety and immunogenicity of Liquid PedvaxHIB were compared with those of lyophilized PedvaxHIB in a randomized clinical study involving 903 infants 2 to 6 months of age from the general U.S. population. DTP and OPV were administered concomitantly to most subjects. The antibody re-

TABLE 1: Antibody Responses in Navajo Infants

Vaccine	No. of Subjects	Time	% Subjects with >0.15 mcg/mL	% Subjects with >1.0 mcg/mL	Anti-PRP GMT (mcg/mL)
Lyophilized PedvaxHIB*	416[†]	Pre-Vaccination	44	10	0.16
	416	Post-Dose 1	88	52	0.95
	416	Post-Dose 2	91	60	1.43
Placebo*	461[†]	Pre-Vaccination	44	9	0.16
	461	Post-Dose 1	21	2	0.09
	461	Post-Dose 2	14	1	0.08
Lyophilized PedvaxHIB	27[‡]	Prebooster	70	33	0.51
	27	Postbooster[§]	100	89	8.39

* Post-Vaccination values obtained approximately 1–3 months after each dose.
† The Protective Efficacy Study
‡ Immunogenicity Trial[34]
§ Booster given at 12 months of age; Post-Vaccination values obtained 1 month after administration of booster dose.

TABLE 2: Antibody Responses to Liquid and Lyophilized PedvaxHIB in Infants From the General U.S. Population

Formulation	Age (Months)	Time	No. of Subjects	% Subjects with anti-PRP >0.15 mcg/mL	>1.0 mcg/mL	Anti-PRP GMT (mcg/mL)
Liquid PedvaxHIB (7.5 mcg PRP)	2-3	Pre-Vaccination	487	32	7	0.12
		Post-Dose 1*	480	94	64	1.55
		Post-Dose 2†	393	97	80	3.22
	12-15	Prebooster	284	80	30	0.49
		Postbooster†	284	99	95	10.23
	24‡	Persistence	94	97	55	1.29
Lyophilized PedvaxHIB (15 mcg PRP)	2-3	Pre-Vaccination	171	37	6	0.13
		Post-Dose 1*	169	97	72	1.88
		Post-Dose 2†	133	99	81	2.69
	12-15	Prebooster	87	71	28	0.39
		Postbooster†	87	99	91	7.64
	24‡	Persistence	37	97	54	1.10

* Approximately two months Post-Vaccination
† Approximately one month Post-Vaccination
‡ Approximately

TABLE 3: Antibody Responses* After Two Doses of Lyophilized PedvaxHIB Among Infants Initially Vaccinated at 2–3 Months of Age By Racial/Ethnic Group

Racial/Ethnic Groups	LYOPHILIZED No. of Subjects	% Subjects With Anti-PRP >0.15 mcg/mL	>1.0 mcg/mL	Anti-PRP GMT (mcg/mL)
Native American†	54	96	70	2.47
Caucasian	201	99	82	3.52
Hispanic	76	99	88	3.54
Black	23	100	96	5.40

* One month after the second dose
† Apache and Navajo

TABLE 4: Antibody Responses* After Two Doses of Liquid PedvaxHIB Among Infants Initially Vaccinated at 2–3 Months of Age By Racial/Ethnic Group

Racial/Ethnic Groups	LIQUID No. of Subjects	% Subjects With Anti-PRP >0.15 mcg/mL	>1.0 mcg/mL	Anti-PRP GMT (mcg/mL)
Native American†	90	97	78	2.76
Caucasian	143	94	72	2.16
Hispanic	184	98	85	4.34
Black	18	100	94	7.58

* One month after the second dose
† Apache and Navajo

sponses induced by each formulation of PedvaxHIB were similar. TABLE 2 shows antibody responses from this clinical study in subjects who received their first dose at 2 to 3 months of age.
[See table 2 above]
A booster dose of PedvaxHIB is required in infants who complete the primary two-dose regimen before 12 months of age. This booster dose will help maintain antibody levels during the first two years of life when children are at highest risk for invasive Hib disease. (See TABLE 2 and DOSAGE AND ADMINISTRATION.)
In four United States studies, antibody responses to lyophilized PedvaxHIB were evaluated in several subpopulations of infants initially vaccinated between 2 to 3 months of age. (See TABLE 3.)
[See table 3 above]
In two United States studies, antibody responses to Liquid PedvaxHIB were evaluated in several subpopulations of infants initially vaccinated between 2 to 3 months of age. (See TABLE 4.)
[See table 4 above]
Antibodies to the OMPC of *N. meningitidis* have been demonstrated in vaccinee sera, but the clinical relevance of these antibodies has not been established.[33]

Interchangeability of Licensed Haemophilus b Conjugate Vaccines and PedvaxHIB
Published studies have examined the interchangeability of other licensed Haemophilus b Conjugate Vaccines and PedvaxHIB.[42,43,44,45,52] According to the American Academy of Pediatrics, excellent immune responses have been achieved when different vaccines have been interchanged in the primary series. If PedvaxHIB is given in a series with one of the other products licensed for infants, the recommended number of doses to complete the series is determined by the other product and not by PedvaxHIB. PedvaxHIB may be interchanged with other licensed Haemophilus b Conjugate Vaccines for the booster dose.[52]

Use with Other Vaccines
Results from clinical studies indicate that Liquid PedvaxHIB can be administered concomitantly with DTP, OPV, eIPV (enhanced inactivated poliovirus vaccine), VARIVAX® [Varicella Virus Vaccine Live (Oka/Merck)], M-M-R® II (Measles, Mumps, and Rubella Virus Vaccine Live) or RECOMBIVAX HB® [Hepatitis B Vaccine (Recombinant)].[33] No impairment of immune response to individual tested vaccine antigens was demonstrated.
The type, frequency and severity of adverse experiences observed in these studies with PedvaxHIB were similar to those seen when the other vaccines were given alone.
In addition, a PRP-OMPC-containing product, COMVAX® [Haemophilus b Conjugate (Meningococcal Protein Conjugate) and Hepatitis B (Recombinant) Vaccine], was given concomitantly with a booster dose of DTaP [diphtheria, tetanus, acellular pertussis] at approximately 15 months of age, using separate sites and syringes for injectable vaccines. No impairment of immune response to these individually tested vaccine antigens was demonstrated. COMVAX has also been administered concomitantly with the primary series of DTaP to a limited number of infants. PRP antibody responses are satisfactory for COMVAX, but immune responses are currently unavailable for DTaP (see Manufacturer's Product Circular for COMVAX). No serious vaccine-related adverse events were reported.[33]

INDICATIONS AND USAGE
Liquid PedvaxHIB is indicated for routine vaccination against invasive disease caused by *Haemophilus influenzae* type b in infants and children 2 to 71 months of age.
Liquid PedvaxHIB will not protect against disease caused by *Haemophilus influenzae* other than type b or against other microorganisms that cause invasive disease such as meningitis or sepsis. As with any vaccine, vaccination with Liquid PedvaxHIB may not result in a protective antibody response in all individuals given the vaccine.

BECAUSE OF THE POTENTIAL FOR IMMUNE TOLERANCE, Liquid PedvaxHIB IS NOT RECOMMENDED FOR USE IN INFANTS YOUNGER THAN 6 WEEKS OF AGE. (See PRECAUTIONS.)

Revaccination
Infants completing the primary two-dose regimen before 12 months of age should receive a booster dose (see DOSAGE AND ADMINISTRATION).

CONTRAINDICATIONS
Hypersensitivity to any component of the vaccine or the diluent.
Persons who develop symptoms suggestive of hypersensitivity after an injection should not receive further injections of the vaccine.

PRECAUTIONS
General
As for any vaccine, adequate treatment provisions, including epinephrine, should be available for immediate use should an anaphylactoid reaction occur.
Use caution when vaccinating latex-sensitive individuals since the vial stopper contains dry natural latex rubber that may cause allergic reactions.
Special care should be taken to ensure that the injection does not enter a blood vessel.
It is important to use a separate sterile syringe and needle for each patient to prevent transmission of hepatitis B or other infectious agents from one person to another.
As with other vaccines, Liquid PedvaxHIB may not induce protective antibody levels immediately following vaccination.
As reported with Haemophilus b Polysaccharide Vaccine[36] and another Haemophilus b Conjugate Vaccine[37], cases of Hib disease may occur in the week after vaccination, prior to the onset of the protective effects of the vaccines.
There is insufficient evidence that Liquid PedvaxHIB given immediately after exposure to natural *Haemophilus influenzae* type b will prevent illness.
The decision to administer or delay vaccination because of current or recent febrile illness depends on the severity of symptoms and on the etiology of the disease. The Advisory Committee on Immunization Practices (ACIP) has recommended that vaccination should be delayed during the course of an acute febrile illness. All vaccines can be administered to persons with minor illnesses such as diarrhea, mild upper-respiratory infection with or without low-grade fever, or other low-grade febrile illness. Persons with moderate or severe febrile illness should be vaccinated as soon as they have recovered from the acute phase of the illness.[46]
If PedvaxHIB is used in persons with malignancies or those receiving immunosuppressive therapy or who are otherwise immunocompromised, the expected immune response may not be obtained.

Instructions to Healthcare Provider
The healthcare provider should determine the current health status and previous vaccination history of the vaccinee.
The healthcare provider should question the patient, parent, or guardian about reactions to a previous dose of PedvaxHIB or other Haemophilus b Conjugate Vaccines.

Information for Patients
The healthcare provider should provide the vaccine information required to be given with each vaccination to the patient, parent, or guardian.
The healthcare provider should inform the patient, parent, or guardian of the benefits and risks associated with vaccination. For risks associated with vaccination, see ADVERSE REACTIONS.
Patients, parents, and guardians should be instructed to report any serious adverse reactions to their healthcare provider who in turn should report such events to the U. S. Department of Health and Human Services through the Vaccine Adverse Event Reporting System (VAERS), 1-800-822-7967.[47]

Laboratory Test Interactions
Sensitive tests (e.g., Latex Agglutination Kits) may detect PRP derived from the vaccine in urine of some vaccinees for at least 30 days following vaccination with lyophilized PedvaxHIB;[38] in clinical studies with lyophilized PedvaxHIB, such children demonstrated normal immune response to the vaccine.

Carcinogenesis, Mutagenesis, Impairment of Fertility
Liquid PedvaxHIB has not been evaluated for carcinogenic or mutagenic potential, or potential to impair fertility.

Pregnancy
Pregnancy Category C
Animal reproduction studies have not been conducted with PedvaxHIB. Liquid PedvaxHIB is not recommended for use in individuals 6 years of age and older.

Pediatric Use
Safety and effectiveness in infants below the age of 2 months and in children 6 years of age and older have not

been established. In addition, Liquid PedvaxHIB should not be used in infants younger than 6 weeks of age because this will lead to a reduced anti-PRP response and may lead to immune tolerance (impaired ability to respond to subsequent exposure to the PRP antigen).[49-51] Liquid PedvaxHIB is not recommended for use in individuals 6 years of age and older because they are generally not at risk of Hib disease.

Geriatric Use
This vaccine is NOT recommended for use in adult populations.

ADVERSE REACTIONS

Liquid PedvaxHIB
In a multicenter clinical study (n=903) comparing the effects of Liquid PedvaxHIB with those of lyophilized PedvaxHIB, 1,699 doses of Liquid PedvaxHIB were administered to 678 healthy infants 2 to 6 months of age from the general U.S. population. DTP and OPV were administered concomitantly to most subjects. Both formulations of PedvaxHIB were generally well tolerated and no serious vaccine-related adverse reactions were reported.

During a three-day period following primary vaccination with Liquid PedvaxHIB in these infants, the most frequently reported (>1%) adverse reactions, without regard to causality, excluding those shown in TABLE 5, in decreasing order of frequency, were: irritability, sleepiness, injection site pain/soreness, injection site erythema (≤2.5 cm diameter, see also TABLE 5), injection site swelling/induration (≤2.5 cm diameter, see also TABLE 5), unusual high-pitched crying, prolonged crying (>4 hr), diarrhea, vomiting, crying, pain, otitis media, rash, and upper respiratory infection. Selected objective observations reported by parents over a 48-hour period in these infants following primary vaccination with Liquid PedvaxHIB are summarized in TABLE 5. [See table 5 above]

Adverse reactions during a three-day period following administration of the booster dose were generally similar in type and frequency to those seen following primary vaccination.

Lyophilized PedvaxHIB
In The Protective Efficacy Study (see CLINICAL PHARMACOLOGY), 4,459 healthy Navajo infants 6 to 12 weeks of age received lyophilized PedvaxHIB or placebo. Most of these infants received DTP/OPV concomitantly. No differences were seen in the type and frequency of serious health problems expected in this Navajo population or in serious adverse experiences reported among those who received lyophilized PedvaxHIB and those who received placebo, and none was reported to be related to lyophilized PedvaxHIB. Only one serious reaction (tracheitis) was reported as possibly related to lyophilized PedvaxHIB and only one (diarrhea) as possibly related to placebo. Seizures occurred infrequently in both groups (9 occurred in vaccine recipients, 8 of whom also received DTP; 8 occurred in placebo recipients, 7 of whom also received DTP) and were not reported to be related to lyophilized PedvaxHIB.

In early clinical studies involving the administration of 8,086 doses of lyophilized PedvaxHIB alone to 5,027 healthy infants and children 2 months to 71 months of age, lyophilized PedvaxHIB was generally well tolerated. No serious adverse reactions were reported. In a subset of these infants, urticaria was reported in two children, and thrombocytopenia was seen in one child. A cause and effect relationship between these side effects and the vaccination has not been established.

Potential Adverse Reactions
The use of Haemophilus b Polysaccharide Vaccines and another Haemophilus b Conjugate Vaccine has been associated with the following additional adverse effects: early onset Hib disease and Guillain-Barré syndrome. A cause and effect relationship between these side effects and the vaccination was not established.[36,37,39,40,41,49]

Post-Marketing Adverse Reactions
The following additional adverse reactions have been reported with the use of the lyophilized and liquid formulations of PedvaxHIB:

Hemic and Lymphatic System
Lymphadenopathy
Hypersensitivity
Rarely, angioedema
Nervous System
Febrile seizures
Skin
Sterile injection site abscess

DOSAGE AND ADMINISTRATION

Liquid PedvaxHIB
FOR INTRAMUSCULAR ADMINISTRATION
DO NOT INJECT INTRAVENOUSLY
If there is an interruption or delay between doses in the primary series, there is no need to repeat the series, but dosing should be continued at the next clinic visit. (See CONTRAINDICATIONS and PRECAUTIONS.)

TABLE 5: Fever or Local Reactions in Subjects First Vaccinated at 2 to 6 Months of Age with Liquid PedvaxHIB*

Reaction	No. of Subjects Evaluated	Post-Dose 1 (hr)			No. of Subjects Evaluated	Post-Dose 2 (hr)		
		6	24	48		6	24	48
		Percentage				Percentage		
Fever[†] >38.3°C (≥101°F) Rectal	222	18.1	4.4	0.5	206	14.1	9.4	2.8
Erythema >2.5 cm diameter	674	2.2	1.0	0.5	562	1.6	1.1	0.4
Swelling >2.5 cm diameter	674	2.5	1.9	0.9	562	0.9	0.9	1.3

* DTP and OPV were administered concomitantly to most subjects.
† Fever was also measured by another method or reported as normal for an additional 345 infants after dose 1 and for an additional 249 infants after dose 2; however, these data are not included in this table.

2 to 14 Months of Age
Infants 2 to 14 months of age should receive a 0.5 mL dose of vaccine ideally beginning at 2 months of age followed by a 0.5 mL dose 2 months later (or as soon as possible thereafter). When the primary two-dose regimen is completed before 12 months of age, a booster dose is required (see below and TABLE 6). Infants born prematurely, regardless of birth weight, should be vaccinated at the same chronological age and according to the same schedule and precautions as full-term infants and children.[46]

15 Months of Age and Older
Children 15 months of age and older previously unvaccinated against Hib disease should receive a single 0.5 mL dose of vaccine.

Booster Dose
In infants completing the primary two-dose regimen before 12 months of age, a booster dose (0.5 mL) should be administered at 12 to 15 months of age, but not earlier than 2 months after the second dose.
Vaccination regimens for Liquid PedvaxHIB by age group are outlined in TABLE 6.

TABLE 6: Vaccination Regimens for Liquid PedvaxHIB By Age Groups

Age (Months) at First Dose	Primary	Age (Months) at Booster Dose
2–10	2 doses, 2 mo. apart	12–15
11–14	2 doses, 2 mo. apart	—
15–71	1 dose	—

Interchangeability
PedvaxHIB may be interchanged with other licensed Haemophilus b Conjugate Vaccines for the primary and booster doses.[52] (See CLINICAL PHARMACOLOGY.)

Use with Other Vaccines
Results from clinical studies indicate that Liquid PedvaxHIB can be administered concomitantly with DTP, OPV, eIPV (enhanced inactivated poliovirus vaccine), VARIVAX [Varicella Virus Vaccine Live (Oka/Merck)], M-M-R II (Measles, Mumps, and Rubella Virus Vaccine Live) or RECOMBIVAX HB [Hepatitis B Vaccine (Recombinant)]. No impairment of immune response to these individually tested vaccine antigens was demonstrated.

The type, frequency and severity of adverse experiences observed in these studies with PedvaxHIB were similar to those seen with the other vaccines when given alone. (See CLINICAL PHARMACOLOGY.)

In addition, a PRP-OMPC-containing product, COMVAX [Haemophilus b Conjugate (Meningococcal Protein Conjugate) and Hepatitis B (Recombinant) Vaccine], was given concomitantly with a booster dose of DTaP [diphtheria, tetanus, acellular pertussis] at approximately 15 months of age, using separate sites and syringes for injectable vaccines. No impairment of immune response to these individually tested vaccine antigens was demonstrated. COMVAX has also been administered concomitantly with the primary series of DTaP to a limited number of infants. PRP antibody responses are satisfactory for COMVAX, but immune responses are currently unavailable for DTaP (see Manufacturer's Product Circular for COMVAX). No serious vaccine-related adverse events were reported.[33]

Parenteral drug products should be inspected visually for extraneous particulate matter and discoloration prior to administration whenever solution and container permit.

Liquid PedvaxHIB is a slightly opaque white suspension. (See DESCRIPTION.)

The vaccine should be used as supplied; no reconstitution is necessary.

Shake well before withdrawal and use. Thorough agitation is necessary to maintain suspension of the vaccine.

Inject 0.5 mL intramuscularly, preferably into the anterolateral thigh or the outer aspect of the upper arm. The but-

tocks should not be used for active vaccination of infants and children, because of the potential risk of injury to the sciatic nerve.

HOW SUPPLIED
Liquid PedvaxHIB is supplied as follows:
No. 4897 — A box of 10 single-dose vials of liquid vaccine, NDC 0006-4897-00.

Storage
Store vaccine at 2-8°C (36-46°F).
DO NOT FREEZE.

REFERENCES
1. Cochi, S. L., et al: Immunization of U.S. children with *Haemophilus influenzae* type b polysaccharide vaccine: A cost-effectiveness model of strategy assessment. JAMA 253: 521-529, 1985.
2. Schlech, W. F., III, et al: Bacterial meningitis in the United States, 1978 through 1981. The National Bacterial Meningitis Surveillance Study. JAMA 253: 1749-1754, 1985.
3. Peltola, H., et al: Prevention of *Haemophilus influenzae* type b bacteremic infections with the capsular polysaccharide vaccine. N Engl J Med 310: 1561-1566, 1984.
4. Cadoz, M., et al: Etude epidemiologique des cas de meningitis purulentes hospitalises a Dakar pendant la decemie 1970-1979. Bull WHO 59: 575-584, 1981.
5. Sell, S. H., et al: Long-term Sequelae of *Haemophilus influenzae* meningitis. Pediatr 49: 206-217, 1972.
6. Taylor, H. G., et al: Intellectual, neuropsychological, and achievement outcomes in children six to eight years after recovery from *Haemophilus influenzae* meningitis. Pediatr 74: 198-205, 1984.
7. Hay, J. W., et al: Cost-benefit analysis of two strategies for prevention of *Haemophilus influenzae* type b infection. Pediatr 80(3): 319-329, 1987.
8. Redmond, S. R., et al: *Haemophilus influenzae* type b disease: an epidemiologic study with special reference to daycare centers. JAMA 252: 2581-2584, 1984.
9. Istre, G. R., et al: Risk factors for primary invasive *Haemophilus influenzae* disease: increased risk from daycare attendance and school age household members. J Pediatr 106: 190-195, 1985.
10. Fraser, D.W., et al: Risk factors in bacterial meningitis: Charleston County, South Carolina. J Infect Dis 127: 271-277, 1973.
11. Tarr, P. I., et al: Demographic factors in the epidemiology of *Haemophilus influenzae* meningitis in young children. J Pediatr 92: 884-888, 1978.
12. Granoff, D. M., et al: Response to immunization with *Haemophilus influenzae* type b polysaccharide-pertussis vaccine and risk of Haemophilus meningitis in children with Km(1) immunoglobulin allotype. J Clin Invest 74: 1708-1714, 1984.
13. Ambrosino, D. M., et al: Correlation between G2m(n) immunoglobulin allotype and human antibody response and susceptibility to polysaccharide encapsulated bacteria. J Clin Invest 75: 1935-1942, 1985.
14. Coulehan, J. L., et al: Epidemiology of *Haemophilus influenzae* type b disease among Navajo Indians. Pub Health Rep 99: 404-409, 1984.
15. Losonsky, G. A., et al: *Haemophilus influenzae* disease in the White Mountain Apaches: molecular epidemiology of a high risk population. Pediatr Infect Dis J 3: 539-547, 1985.
16. Ward, J. I., et al: *Haemophilus influenzae* disease in Alaskan Eskimos: characteristics of a population with an unusual incidence of disease. Lancet 1: 1281-1285, 1981.
17. Ward, J. I., et al: *Haemophilus influenzae* meningitis: a national study of secondary spread in household contacts. N Engl J Med 301: 122-126, 1979.
18. Ward, J., et al: *Haemophilus influenzae* bacteremia in children with sickle cell disease. J Pediatr 88: 261-263, 1976.

19. Bartlett, A. V., et al: Unusual presentations of *Haemophilus influenzae* infections in immunocompromised patients. J Pediatr *102*: 55-58, 1983.
20. Recommendations of the Immunization Practices Advisory Committee. Polysaccharide vaccine for prevention of *Haemophilus influenzae* type b disease. MMWR *34*(15): 201-205, 1985.
21. Santosham, M., et al: Prevention of *Haemophilus influenzae* type b infections in high-risk infants treated with bacterial polysaccharide immune globulin. N Engl J Med *317*: 923-929, 1987.
22. Siber, G. R., et al: Preparation of human hyperimmune globulin to *Haemophilus influenzae* b, *Streptococcus pneumoniae*, and *Neisseria meningitidis*. Infect Immun *45*: 248-254, 1984.
23. Smith, D. H., et al: Responses of children immunized with the capsular polysaccharide of *Haemophilus influenzae* type b. Pediatr *52*: 637-645, 1973.
24. Robbins, J. B., et al: Quantitative measurement of 'natural' and immunization-induced *Haemophilus influenzae* type b capsular polysaccharide antibodies. Pediatr Res *7*: 103-110, 1973.
25. Kaythy, H., et al: The protective level of serum antibodies to the capsular polysaccharide of *Haemophilus influenzae* type b. J Infect Dis *147*: 1100, 1983.
26. Peltola, H., et al: *Haemophilus influenzae* type b capsular polysaccharide vaccine in children: a double-blind field study of 100,000 vaccinees 3 months to 5 years of age in Finland. Pediatr *60*: 730-737, 1977.
27. Ward, J. I., et al: *Haemophilus influenzae* type b vaccines: Lessons For the Future. Pediatr *81*: 886-893, 1988.
28. Daum, R. S., et al: *Haemophilus influenzae* type b vaccines: Lessons From the Past. Pediatr *81*: 893-897, 1988.
29. Marburg, S., et al: Bimolecular chemistry of macromolecules: Synthesis of bacterial polysaccharide conjugates with *Neisseria meningitidis* membrane protein. J Am Chem Soc *108*: 5282-5287, 1986.
30. Letson, G. W., et al: Comparison of active and combined passive/active immunization of Navajo children against *Haemophilus influenzae* type b. Pediatr Infect Dis J *7*(111): 747-752, 1988.
31. Einhorn, M. S., et al: Immunogenicity in infants of *Haemophilus influenzae* type b polysaccharide in a conjugate vaccine with *Neisseria meningitidis* outer-membrane protein. Lancet *2*: 299-302, 1986.
32. Ahonkhai, V.I., et al: *Haemophilus influenzae* type b Conjugate Vaccine (Meningococcal Protein Conjugate) (PedvaxHIB TM): Clinical Evaluation. Pediatr *85*(4): 676-681, 1990.
33. Data on file at Merck Research Laboratories.
34. Granoff, D. M., et al: Immunogenicity of *Haemophilus influenzae* type b polysaccharide—outer membrane protein conjugate vaccine in patients who acquired *Haemophilus* disease despite previous vaccination with type b polysaccharide vaccine. J. Pediatr. *114*(6): 925-933, June 1989.
35. Lenoir, A. A., et al: Response to *Haemophilus influenzae* type b (*H. influenzae* type b) polysaccharide *N. meningitidis* outer membrane protein (PS-OMP) conjugate vaccine in relation to Km(1) and G2m(23) allotypes. Twenty-sixth Interscience Conference on Antimicrobial Agents and Chemotherapy (Abstract #216) 133, 1986.
36. Mortimer, E. A.: Efficacy of Haemophilus b polysaccharide vaccine: An enigma. JAMA *260*: 1454, 1988.
37. Meekison, W., et al: Post-marketing surveillance of adverse effects following ProHIBiT vaccine. British Columbia Canada Diseases Weekly Report *15-28*: 143-145, 1989.
38. Goepp, J. G., et al: Persistent urinary antigen excretion in infants vaccinated with *Haemophilus influenzae* type b capsular polysaccharide conjugated with outer membrane protein from *Neisseria meningitidis*. Pediatr Infect Dis J *11*(1): 2-5, 1992.
39. Milstein, J. B., et al: Adverse reactions reported following receipt of *Haemophilus influenzae* type b vaccine: An analysis after one year of marketing. Pediatr *80*: 270, 1987.
40. Black, S., et al: b-CAPSA 1 *Haemophilus influenzae* type b capsular polysaccharide vaccine safety. Pediatr *79*: 321-325, 1987.
41. D'Cruz, O. F., et al: Acute inflammatory demyelinating polyradiculoneuropathy (Guillain-Barré syndrome) after immunization with *Haemophilus influenzae* type b Conjugate Vaccine. J Pediatr *115*: 743-746, 1989.
42. Recommendations of the Immunization Practices Advisory Committee. Recommendations for use of Haemophilus b Conjugate Vaccines and a combined diphtheria, tetanus, pertussis, and Haemophilus b vaccine. MMWR *42*(RR-13): 1-15, 1993.
43. Daum, R. S., et al: Interchangeability of *Haemophilus influenzae* type b vaccines for the primary series (mix and match): a preliminary analysis [Abstract 976]. Pediatr Res *33*: 166A, 1993.
44. Greenberg, D. P., et al: Enhanced antibody responses in infants given different sequences of heterogenous *Haemophilus influenzae* type b Conjugate Vaccines. J Pediatr *126*: 206-211, 1995.
45. Anderson, E. L., et al: Interchangeability of Conjugated *Haemophilus influenzae* type b Vaccines in Infants. JAMA *273*: 849-853, 1995.
46. Recommendations of the Immunization Practices Advisory Committee. General Recommendations on Immunization. MMWR *43*(RR-1), 1994.
47. Vaccine Adverse Event Reporting System - United States. MMWR *39*(41): 730-733, October 19, 1990.
48. Institute of Medicine Adverse Events Associated With Childhood Vaccines Evidence Bearing on Causality. National Academy Press, Washington, D.C., 260-261, 1994.
49. Keyserling, H.L., et al: Program and Abstracts of the 30th ICAAC, (Abstract #63), 1990.
50. Ward, J.I., et al: Program and Abstracts of the 32nd ICAAC, (Abstract #984), 1992.
51. Lieberman, J.M., et al: Infect Dis, (Abstract #1028), 1993.
52. American Academy of Pediatrics. Recommended Childhood Immunization Schedule - United States, January-December 1998. Pediatr *101*(1): 154-157, 1998.

Manuf. and Dist. by: Merck Sharp & Dohme Corp., a subsidiary of **MERCK & CO., INC.**, Whitehouse Station, NJ 08889, USA
Issued December 2010
Printed in USA
9877903
Copyright © 1998 Merck Sharp & Dohme Corp., a subsidiary of **Merck & Co., Inc.**
All rights reserved

PEGINTRON®   ℞
[pĕg-ĭn-trŏn]
(peginterferon alfa-2b)
injection, for subcutaneous use

HIGHLIGHTS OF PRESCRIBING INFORMATION
These highlights do not include all the information needed to use PEGINTRON safely and effectively. See full prescribing information for PEGINTRON.
PEGINTRON® (peginterferon alfa-2b) injection, for subcutaneous use
Initial U.S. Approval: 2001

> **WARNING: RISK OF SERIOUS DISORDERS AND RIBAVIRIN-ASSOCIATED EFFECTS**
> *See full prescribing information for complete boxed warning.*
> • **May cause or aggravate fatal or life-threatening neuropsychiatric, autoimmune, ischemic, and infectious disorders. Monitor closely and withdraw therapy with persistently severe or worsening signs or symptoms of the above disorders. (5.2)**
> **Use with Ribavirin**
> • **Ribavirin may cause birth defects and fetal death; avoid pregnancy in female patients and female partners of male patients. (5.1)**

——RECENT MAJOR CHANGES——

——INDICATIONS AND USAGE——
PegIntron is an antiviral indicated for treatment of Chronic Hepatitis C (CHC) in patients with compensated liver disease. (1.1)

——DOSAGE AND ADMINISTRATION——
• PegIntron is administered by subcutaneous injection. (2)
[See table below]
• Dose reduction is recommended in patients experiencing certain adverse reactions or renal dysfunction. (2.3, 2.5)

——DOSAGE FORMS AND STRENGTHS——
Injection: 50 mcg per 0.5 mL, 80 mcg per 0.5 mL, 120 mcg per 0.5 mL, 150 mcg per 0.5 mL in single-use vial (with 1.25 mL diluent) and single-use pre-filled pens (3)

——CONTRAINDICATIONS——
• Known hypersensitivity reactions, such as urticaria, angioedema, bronchoconstriction, anaphylaxis, Stevens-Johnson syndrome, and toxic epidermal necrolysis to interferon alpha or any other product component. (4)
• Autoimmune hepatitis. (4)
• Hepatic decompensation (Child-Pugh score greater than 6 [class B and C]) in cirrhotic CHC patients before or during treatment. (4)
Additional contraindications for combination therapy with ribavirin:
■ Pregnant women and men whose female partners are pregnant. (4, 8.1)
■ Hemoglobinopathies (e.g., thalassemia major, sickle-cell anemia). (4)
• Creatinine clearance less than 50 mL/min. (4)

——WARNINGS AND PRECAUTIONS——
• Birth defects and fetal death with ribavirin: Patients must have a negative pregnancy test prior to therapy, use at least 2 forms of contraception, and undergo monthly pregnancy tests. (5.1)
Patients exhibiting the following conditions should be closely monitored and may require dose reduction or discontinuation of therapy:
• Hemolytic anemia with ribavirin. (5.1)
• Neuropsychiatric events. (5.2)
• History of significant or unstable cardiac disease. (5.3)
• Hypothyroidism, hyperthyroidism, hyperglycemia, diabetes mellitus that cannot be effectively treated by medication. (5.4)
• New or worsening ophthalmologic disorders. (5.5)
• Ischemic and hemorrhagic cerebrovascular events. (5.6)
• Severe decreases in neutrophil or platelet counts. (5.7)
• History of autoimmune disorders. (5.8)
• Pancreatitis and ulcerative or hemorrhagic/ischemic colitis and pancreatitis. (5.9, 5.10)
• Pulmonary infiltrates or pulmonary function impairment. (5.11)
• Child-Pugh score greater than 6 (class B and C). (4, 5.12)
• Increased creatinine levels in patients with renal insufficiency. (5.13)
• Serious, acute hypersensitivity reactions and cutaneous eruptions. (5.14)
• Dental/periodontal disorders reported with combination therapy. (5.16)
• Hypertriglyceridemia may result in pancreatitis (e.g., triglycerides greater than 1000 mg/dL). (5.17)
• Weight loss and growth inhibition reported during combination therapy in pediatric patients. Long-term growth inhibition (height) reported in some patients. (5.18)
• Peripheral neuropathy when used in combination with telbivudine. (5.19)

——ADVERSE REACTIONS——
Most common adverse reactions (greater than 40%) in adult patients receiving either PegIntron or PegIntron/REBETOL are injection site inflammation/reaction, fatigue/asthenia, headache, rigors, fevers, nausea, myalgia and anxiety/emotional lability/irritability (6.1). Most common adverse reactions (greater than 25%) in pediatric patients receiving PegIntron/REBETOL are pyrexia, headache, neutropenia, fatigue, anorexia, injection-site erythema, vomiting (6.1).
To report SUSPECTED ADVERSE REACTIONS, contact Schering Corporation, a subsidiary of Merck & Co., Inc., at 1-800-526-4099 or FDA at 1-800-FDA-1088 or www.fda.gov/medwatch.

——DRUG INTERACTIONS——
• Drug metabolized by CYP450: Caution with drugs metabolized by CYP2C8/9 (e.g., warfarin, phenytoin) or CYP2D6 (e.g., flecainide). (7.1)
• Methadone: Monitor for increased narcotic effect. (7.2)
• Nucleoside analogues: Closely monitor for toxicities. Discontinue nucleoside reverse transcriptase inhibitors or reduce dose or discontinue interferon, ribavirin, or both with worsening toxicities. (7.3)

	PegIntron Dose (Adults)*	PegIntron Dose (Pediatric Patients)	REBETOL Dose* (Adults)	REBETOL Dose (Pediatric Patients)
PegIntron Combination Therapy (2.1)	1.5 mcg/kg/week	60 mcg/m²/week	800-1400 mg orally daily with food	15 mg/kg/day orally with food in 2 divided doses

* Refer to Tables 1-7 of the Full Prescribing Information.

- Didanosine: Concurrent use with REBETOL is not recommended. (7.3)

—————USE IN SPECIFIC POPULATIONS—————
- Ribavirin Pregnancy Registry (8.1)
- Pediatrics: safety and efficacy in pediatrics less than 3 years old have not been established. (8.4)
- Geriatrics: neuropsychiatric, cardiac, pulmonary, GI, and systemic (flu-like) adverse reactions may be more severe. (8.5)
- Organ transplant: safety and efficacy have not been studied. (8.6)
- HIV or HBV co-infection: safety and efficacy have not been established. (8.7)

See 17 for PATIENT COUNSELING INFORMATION and Medication Guide

Revised: 07/2014

FULL PRESCRIBING INFORMATION: CONTENTS*
WARNING: RISK OF SERIOUS DISORDERS AND RIBAVIRIN-ASSOCIATED EFFECTS

FULL PRESCRIBING INFORMATION

WARNING: RISK OF SERIOUS DISORDERS AND RIBAVIRIN-ASSOCIATED EFFECTS

Alpha interferons, including PegIntron, may cause or aggravate fatal or life-threatening neuropsychiatric, autoimmune, ischemic, and infectious disorders. Patients should be monitored closely with periodic clinical and laboratory evaluations. Patients with persistently severe or worsening signs or symptoms of these conditions should be withdrawn from therapy. In many, but not all cases, these disorders resolve after stopping PegIntron therapy [see Warnings and Precautions (5) and Adverse Reactions (6.1)].

Use with Ribavirin

Ribavirin may cause birth defects and death of the unborn child. Extreme care must be taken to avoid pregnancy in female patients and in female partners of male patients. Ribavirin causes hemolytic anemia. The anemia associated with ribavirin therapy may result in a worsening of cardiac disease. [See ribavirin labeling.]

1 INDICATIONS AND USAGE
1.1 Chronic Hepatitis C (CHC)

PegIntron®, as part of a combination regimen, is indicated for the treatment of Chronic Hepatitis C (CHC) in patients with compensated liver disease.

- PegIntron in combination with REBETOL® (ribavirin) and an approved Hepatitis C Virus (HCV) NS3/4A protease inhibitor is indicated in adult patients with HCV genotype 1 infection (see labeling of the specific HCV NS3/4A protease inhibitor for further information).
- PegIntron in combination with REBETOL is indicated in patients with genotypes other than 1, pediatric patients (3-17 years of age), or in patients with genotype 1 infection where use of an HCV NS3/4A protease inhibitor is not warranted based on tolerability, contraindications or other clinical factors.

PegIntron monotherapy should only be used in the treatment of CHC in patients with compensated liver disease if there are contraindications to or significant intolerance of REBETOL and is indicated for use only in previously untreated adult patients. Combination therapy provides substantially better response rates than monotherapy [see Clinical Studies (14.1, 14.2)].

2 DOSAGE AND ADMINISTRATION
2.1 PegIntron Combination Therapy
Adults
The recommended dose of PegIntron is 1.5 mcg/kg/week. The volume of PegIntron to be injected depends on the strength of PegIntron and patient's body weight (see Table 1).
The recommended dose of REBETOL for use with PegIntron is 800 to 1400 mg orally based on patient body weight.

Table 1: Recommended PegIntron Combination Therapy Dosing (Adults)

Body Weight kg (lbs)	PegIntron REDIPEN Pre-filled pen or Vial Strength to Use	Amount of PegIntron to Administer (mcg)	Volume* of PegIntron to Administer (mL)	REBETOL Daily Dose	REBETOL Number of Capsules
<40 (<88)	50 mcg per 0.5 mL	50	0.5	800 mg/day	2 × 200 mg capsules A.M. 2 × 200 mg capsules P.M.
40-50 (88-111)	80 mcg per 0.5 mL	64	0.4	800 mg/day	2 × 200 mg capsules A.M. 2 × 200 mg capsules P.M.
51-60 (112-133)	80 mcg per 0.5 mL	80	0.5	800 mg/day	2 × 200 mg capsules A.M. 2 × 200 mg capsules P.M.
61-65 (134-144)	120 mcg per 0.5 mL	96	0.4	800 mg/day	2 × 200 mg capsules A.M. 2 × 200 mg capsules P.M.
66-75 (145-166)	120 mcg per 0.5 mL	96	0.4	1000 mg/day	2 × 200 mg capsules A.M. 3 × 200 mg capsules P.M.
76-80 (167-177)	120 mcg per 0.5 mL	120	0.5	1000 mg/day	2 × 200 mg capsules A.M. 3 × 200 mg capsules P.M.
81-85 (178-187)	120 mcg per 0.5 mL	120	0.5	1200 mg/day	3 × 200 mg capsules A.M. 3 × 200 mg capsules P.M.
86-105 (188-231)	150 mcg per 0.5 mL	150	0.5	1200 mg/day	3 × 200 mg capsules A.M. 3 × 200 mg capsules P.M.
>105 (>231)	†	†	†	1400 mg/day	3 × 200 mg capsules A.M. 4 × 200 mg capsules P.M.

* When reconstituted as directed.
† For patients weighing greater than 105 kg (greater than 231 pounds), the PegIntron dose of 1.5 mcg/kg/week should be calculated based on the individual patient weight. This may require combinations of various PegIntron dose strengths and volumes.

REBETOL should be taken with food. REBETOL should not be used in patients with creatinine clearance less than 50 mL/min.
See labeling of the specific HCV NS3/4A protease inhibitor for information regarding dosing regimen and administration of the protease inhibitor in combination with PegIntron and ribavirin.
Duration of Treatment – Treatment with PegIntron/ REBETOL of Interferon Alpha-naive Patients
The treatment duration for patients with genotype 1 is 48 weeks. Discontinuation of therapy should be considered in patients who do not achieve at least a 2 log$_{10}$ drop or loss of HCV-RNA at 12 weeks, or if HCV-RNA remains detectable after 24 weeks of therapy. Patients with genotype 2 and 3 should be treated for 24 weeks.
Duration of Treatment – Re-treatment with PegIntron/ REBETOL of Prior Treatment Failures
For patients with genotype 1 infection, PegIntron and REBETOL without an HCV NS3/4A protease inhibitor should only be used if there are contraindications, significant intolerance or other clinical factors that would not warrant use of an HCV NS3/4A protease inhibitor. The treatment duration for patients who previously failed therapy is 48 weeks, regardless of HCV genotype. Re-treated patients who fail to achieve undetectable HCV-RNA at Week 12 of therapy, or whose HCV-RNA remains detectable after 24 weeks of therapy, are highly unlikely to achieve SVR and discontinuation of therapy should be considered [see Clinical Studies (14.1)].
[See table 1 above]
Pediatric Patients
Dosing for pediatric patients is determined by body surface area for PegIntron and by body weight for REBETOL. The recommended dose of PegIntron is 60 mcg/m²/week subcutaneously in combination with 15 mg/kg/day of REBETOL orally in 2 divided doses (see Table 2) for pediatric patients ages 3 to 17 years. Patients who reach their 18th birthday while receiving PegIntron/REBETOL should remain on the pediatric dosing regimen. The treatment duration for patients with genotype 1 is 48 weeks. Patients with genotype 2 and 3 should be treated for 24 weeks.

Table 2: Recommended REBETOL* Dosing in Combination Therapy (Pediatrics)

Body Weight kg (lbs)	REBETOL Daily Dose	REBETOL Number of Capsules
<47 (<103)	15 mg/kg/day	Use REBETOL oral solution†

47-59 (103-131)	800 mg/day	2 × 200 mg capsules A.M. 2 × 200 mg capsules P.M.
60-73 (132-162)	1000 mg/day	2 × 200 mg capsules A.M. 3 × 200 mg capsules P.M.
>73 (>162)	1200 mg/day	3 × 200 mg capsules A.M. 3 × 200 mg capsules P.M.

* REBETOL to be used in combination with PegIntron 60 mcg/m² weekly.
† REBETOL oral solution may be used for any patient regardless of body weight.

2.2 PegIntron Monotherapy

The recommended dose of PegIntron regimen is 1 mcg/kg/week subcutaneously for 1 year administered on the same day of the week. Discontinuation of therapy should be considered in patients who do not achieve at least a 2 $\log_{10}$ drop or loss of HCV-RNA at 12 weeks of therapy, or whose HCV-RNA levels remain detectable after 24 weeks of therapy. The volume of PegIntron to be injected depends on patient weight (see *Table 3*).

Table 3: Recommended PegIntron Monotherapy Dosing

Body Weight kg (lbs)	PegIntron REDIPEN Pre-filled pen or Vial Strength to Use	Amount of PegIntron to Administer (mcg)	Volume of PegIntron to Administer (mL)*
≤45 (≤100)	50 mcg per 0.5 mL	40	0.4
46-56 (101-124)	50 mcg per 0.5 mL	50	0.5
57-72 (125-159)	80 mcg per 0.5 mL	64	0.4
73-88 (160-195)	80 mcg per 0.5 mL	80	0.5
89-106 (196-234)	120 mcg per 0.5 mL	96	0.4
107-136 (235-300)	120 mcg per 0.5 mL	120	0.5
137-160 (301-353)	150 mcg per 0.5 mL	150	0.5

* When reconstituted as directed.

2.3 Dose Reduction

If a serious adverse reaction develops during the course of treatment discontinue or modify the dosage of PegIntron and REBETOL until the adverse event abates or decreases in severity [see *Warnings and Precautions (5)*]. If persistent or recurrent serious adverse events develop despite adequate dosage adjustment, discontinue treatment. For guidelines for dose modifications and discontinuation based on depression or laboratory parameters see **Tables 4** and **5**. Dose reduction of PegIntron in adult patients on PegIntron/REBETOL combination therapy is accomplished in a two-step process from the original starting dose of 1.5 mcg/kg/week, to 1 mcg/kg/week, then to 0.5 mcg/kg/week, if needed. Dose reduction in patients on PegIntron monotherapy is accomplished by reducing the original starting dose of 1 mcg/kg/week to 0.5 mcg/kg/week. Instructions for dose reductions in adults are outlined in **Tables 6** (Monotherapy: REDIPEN/Vial) and **7** (Combination therapy: REDIPEN/Vial).

In the adult combination therapy Study 2, dose reductions occurred in 42% of subjects receiving PegIntron 1.5 mcg/kg plus REBETOL 800 mg daily, including 57% of those subjects weighing 60 kg or less. In Study 4, 16% of subjects had a dose reduction of PegIntron to 1 mcg/kg in combination with REBETOL, with an additional 4% requiring the second dose reduction of PegIntron to 0.5 mcg/kg due to adverse events [see *Adverse Reactions (6.1)*].

Dose reduction in pediatric patients is accomplished by modifying the recommended dose in a 2-step process from the original starting dose of 60 mcg/m²/week, to 40 mcg/m²/week, then to 20 mcg/m²/week, if needed (see *Tables 4 and 5*). In the pediatric combination therapy trial, dose reductions occurred in 25% of subjects receiving PegIntron 60 mcg/m² weekly plus REBETOL 15 mg/kg daily.
[See table 4 above]
[See table 5 above]

Table 6: Reduced PegIntron Dose (0.5 mcg/kg) for (1 mcg/kg) Monotherapy in Adults

Body Weight kg (lbs)	PegIntron REDIPEN/Vial		
	Strength to Use	Amount to Administer (mcg)	Volume* to Administer (mL)
≤45 (≤100)	50 mcg per 0.5 mL†	20	0.2
46-56 (101-124)	50 mcg per 0.5 mL†	25	0.25
57-72 (125-159)	50 mcg per 0.5 mL	30	0.3
73-88 (160-195)	50 mcg per 0.5 mL	40	0.4
89-106 (196-234)	50 mcg per 0.5 mL	50	0.5
107-136 (235-300)	80 mcg per 0.5 mL	64	0.4
≥137 (≥301)	80 mcg per 0.5 mL	80	0.5

* When reconstituted as directed.

† Must use vial. Minimum delivery for REDIPEN 0.3 mL.

[See table 7 at top of next page]

Table 4: Guidelines for Modification or Discontinuation of PegIntron or PegIntron/REBETOL and for Scheduling Visits for Patients with Depression

Depression Severity*	Initial Management (4-8 weeks)		Depression Status		
	Dose Modification	Visit Schedule	Remains Stable	Improves	Worsens
Mild	No change	Evaluate once weekly by visit or phone	Continue weekly visit schedule	Resume normal visit schedule	See moderate or severe depression
Moderate	Adults: Adjust Dose* Pediatrics: Decrease dose to 40 mcg/m²/week, then to 20 mcg/m²/week, if needed	Evaluate once weekly (office visit at least every other week)	Consider psychiatric consultation. Continue reduced dosing	If symptoms improve and are stable for 4 weeks, may resume normal visit schedule. Continue reduced dosing or return to normal dose	See severe depression
Severe	Discontinue PegIntron/REBETOL permanently	Obtain immediate psychiatric consultation	Psychiatric therapy as necessary		

* See DSM-IV for definitions. For patients on PegIntron/REBETOL combination therapy: 1st dose reduction of PegIntron is to 1 mcg/kg/week, 2nd dose reduction (if needed) of PegIntron is to 0.5 mcg/kg/week. For patients on PegIntron monotherapy: decrease PegIntron dose to 0.5 mcg/kg/week.

Table 5: Guidelines for Dose Modification and Discontinuation of PegIntron or PegIntron/REBETOL Based on Laboratory Parameters in Adults and Pediatrics

Laboratory Parameters	Reduce PegIntron Dose (see note 1) if:	Reduce ribavirin Daily Dose (see note 2) if:	Discontinue Therapy if:
WBC	1.0 to <1.5 × 10⁹/L	N/A	<1.0 × 10⁹/L
Neutrophils	0.5 to <0.75 × 10⁹/L	N/A	<0.5 × 10⁹/L
Platelets	25 to <50 × 10⁹/L (adults) 50 to <70 × 10⁹/L (pediatrics)	N/A	<25 × 10⁹/L (adults) <50 × 10⁹/L (pediatrics)
Creatinine	N/A	N/A	>2 mg/dL (pediatrics)
Hemoglobin in patients without history of cardiac disease	N/A	8.5 to <10 g/dL	<8.5 g/dL
	Reduce PegIntron Dose by Half and the Ribavirin Dose by 200 mg/day if:		
Hemoglobin in patients with history of cardiac disease*†	≥2 g/dL decrease in hemoglobin during any four week period during treatment		<8.5 g/dL or <12 g/dL after four weeks of dose reduction

Note 1: *Adult patients on combination therapy*: 1st dose reduction of PegIntron is to 1 mcg/kg/week. If needed, 2nd dose reduction of PegIntron is to 0.5 mcg/kg/week.
Adult patients on PegIntron monotherapy: decrease PegIntron dose to 0.5 mcg/kg/week.
Pediatric patients: 1st dose reduction of PegIntron is to 40 mcg/m²/week, 2nd dose reduction of PegIntron is to 20 mcg/m²/week.
Note 2: *Adult patients*: 1st dose reduction of ribavirin is by 200 mg/day (except in patients receiving the 1400 mg, dose reduction should be by 400 mg/day). If needed, 2nd dose reduction of ribavirin is by an additional 200 mg/day. Patients whose dose of ribavirin is reduced to 600 mg daily receive one 200 mg capsule in the morning and two 200 mg capsules in the evening.
Pediatric patients: 1st dose reduction of ribavirin is to 12 mg/kg/day, 2nd dose reduction of ribavirin is to 8 mg/kg/day.
* Pediatric patients who have pre-existing cardiac conditions and experience a hemoglobin decrease greater than or equal to 2 g/dL during any 4-week period during treatment should have weekly evaluations and hematology testing.
† These guidelines are for patients with stable cardiac disease. Patients with a history of significant or unstable cardiac disease should not be treated with PegIntron/REBETOL combination therapy [see *Warnings and Precautions (5.3)*].

2.4 Discontinuation of Dosing

Adults

See labeling of the specific HCV NS3/4A protease inhibitor for information regarding discontinuation of dosing based on treatment futility.

In HCV genotype 1, interferon-alfa-naïve patients receiving PegIntron, alone or in combination with REBETOL, discontinuation of therapy is recommended if there is not at least a 2 $\log_{10}$ drop or loss of HCV-RNA at 12 weeks of therapy, or if HCV-RNA levels remain detectable after 24 weeks of therapy. Regardless of genotype, previously treated patients who have detectable HCV-RNA at Week 12 or 24, are highly unlikely to achieve SVR and discontinuation of therapy is recommended.

Pediatrics (3-17 years of age)

It is recommended that patients receiving PegIntron/REBETOL combination (excluding those with HCV genotype 2 and 3) be discontinued from therapy at 12 weeks if their treatment Week 12 HCV-RNA dropped less than 2 $\log_{10}$ compared to pretreatment or at 24 weeks if they have detectable HCV-RNA at treatment Week 24.

2.5 Renal Function

In patients with moderate renal dysfunction (creatinine clearance 30-50 mL/min), the PegIntron dose should be reduced by 25%. Patients with severe renal dysfunction (creatinine clearance 10-29 mL/min), including those on hemodialysis, should have the PegIntron dose reduced by 50%. If renal function decreases during treatment, PegIntron therapy should be discontinued. When PegIntron is administered in combination with REBETOL, subjects with impaired renal function or those over the age of 50 should be more carefully monitored with respect to the development of anemia. PegIntron/REBETOL should not be used in patients with creatinine clearance less than 50 mL/min.

2.6 Preparation and Administration

A patient should self-inject PegIntron only if the physician determines that it is appropriate and the patient agrees to medical follow-up as necessary and has been trained in proper injection technique *[see illustrated FDA-approved Medication Guide and Instructions for Use for directions on injection site preparation and injection instructions].*

The reconstituted solution should be visually inspected for discoloration and particulate matter prior to administration. Do not use the solution if it is discolored or not clear, or if particulates are present.

DO NOT REUSE THE VIAL OR PRE-FILLED PEN; DISCARD THE UNUSED PORTION. Pooling of unused portions of some medications has been linked to bacterial contamination and morbidity.

3 DOSAGE FORMS AND STRENGTHS

- Single-use vial: 1.25 mL diluent vial: 50 mcg per 0.5 mL, 80 mcg per 0.5 mL, 120 mcg per 0.5 mL, 150 mcg per 0.5 mL.
- REDIPEN® single-use pre-filled pen: 50 mcg per 0.5 mL, 80 mcg per 0.5 mL, 120 mcg per 0.5 mL, 150 mcg per 0.5 mL.

4 CONTRAINDICATIONS

PegIntron is contraindicated in patients with:

- known hypersensitivity reactions, such as urticaria, angioedema, bronchoconstriction, anaphylaxis, Stevens-Johnson syndrome, and toxic epidermal necrolysis to interferon alpha or any other component of the product
- autoimmune hepatitis
- hepatic decompensation (Child-Pugh score greater than 6 [class B and C]) in cirrhotic CHC patients before or during treatment

PegIntron/ribavirin combination therapy is additionally contraindicated in:

- women who are pregnant. Ribavirin may cause fetal harm when administered to a pregnant woman. Ribavirin is contraindicated in women who are or may become pregnant. If ribavirin is used during pregnancy, or if the patient becomes pregnant while taking ribavirin, the patient should be apprised of the potential hazard to her fetus *[see Use in Specific Populations (8.1)].*
- men whose female partners are pregnant
- patients with hemoglobinopathies (e.g., thalassemia major, sickle-cell anemia)
- patients with creatinine clearance less than 50 mL/min

5 WARNINGS AND PRECAUTIONS

Patients should be monitored for the following serious conditions, some of which may become life threatening. Patients with persistently severe or worsening signs or symptoms should be withdrawn from therapy.

5.1 Use with Ribavirin

Pregnancy

Ribavirin may cause birth defects and death of the unborn child. Ribavirin therapy should not be started until a report of a negative pregnancy test has been obtained immediately prior to planned initiation of therapy. Patients should use at least 2 forms of contraception and have monthly

Table 7: Two-Step Dose Reduction of PegIntron REDIPEN/Vial in Combination Therapy in Adults

First Dose Reduction to PegIntron 1 mcg/kg				Second Dose Reduction to PegIntron 0.5 mcg/kg			
Body weight kg (lbs)	PegIntron REDIPEN/Vial Strength to Use	Amount of PegIntron (mcg) to Administer	Volume (mL) * of PegIntron to Administer	Body weight kg (lbs)	PegIntron REDIPEN/Vial Strength to Use	Amount of PegIntron (mcg) to Administer	Volume (mL) * of PegIntron to Administer
<40 (<88)	50 mcg per 0.5 mL	35	0.35	<40 (<88)	50 mcg per 0.5 mL†	20	0.2
40-50 (88-111)		45	0.45	40-50 (88-111)		25	0.25
51-60 (112-133)		50	0.5	51-60 (112-133)		30	0.3
61-75 (134-166)	80 mcg per 0.5 mL	64	0.4	61-75 (134-166)	50 mcg per 0.5 mL	35	0.35
76-85 (167-187)		80	0.5	76-85 (167-187)		45	0.45
86-104 (188-230)	120 mcg per 0.5 mL	96	0.4	86-104 (188-230)		50	0.5
105-125 (231-275)		108	0.45	105-125 (231-275)	80 mcg per 0.5 mL	64	0.4
>125 (>275)	150 mcg per 0.5 mL	135	0.45	>125 (>275)		72	0.45

* When reconstituted as directed.
† Must use vial. Minimum delivery for REDIPEN 0.3 mL.

pregnancy tests during treatment and during the 6-month period after treatment has been stopped *[see Contraindications (4) and ribavirin labeling].*

Anemia

Ribavirin caused hemolytic anemia in 10% of PegIntron/REBETOL-treated subjects within 1 to 4 weeks of initiation of therapy. Complete blood counts should be obtained pretreatment and at Week 2 and Week 4 of therapy or more frequently if clinically indicated. Anemia associated with ribavirin therapy may result in a worsening of cardiac disease. Decrease in dosage or discontinuation of ribavirin may be necessary *[see Dosage and Administration (2.3) and ribavirin labeling].*

5.2 Neuropsychiatric Events

Life-threatening or fatal neuropsychiatric events, including suicide, suicidal and homicidal ideation, depression, relapse of drug addiction/overdose, and aggressive behavior sometimes directed towards others have occurred in patients with and without a previous psychiatric disorder during PegIntron treatment and follow-up. Psychoses, hallucinations, bipolar disorders, and mania have been observed in patients treated with interferon alpha.

PegIntron should be used with caution in patients with a history of psychiatric disorders. Treatment with interferons may be associated with exacerbated symptoms of psychiatric disorders in patients with co-occurring psychiatric and substance use disorders. If treatment with interferons is initiated in patients with prior history or existence of psychiatric condition or with a history of substance use disorders, treatment considerations should include the need for drug screening and periodic health evaluation, including psychiatric symptom monitoring. Early intervention for re-emergence or development of neuropsychiatric symptoms and substance use is recommended.

Patients should be advised to report immediately any symptoms of depression or suicidal ideation to their prescribing physicians. Physicians should monitor all patients for evidence of depression and other psychiatric symptoms. If patients develop psychiatric problems, including clinical depression, it is recommended that the patients be carefully monitored during treatment and in the 6-month follow-up period. If psychiatric symptoms persist or worsen, or suicidal ideation or aggressive behavior towards others is identified, it is recommended that treatment with PegIntron be discontinued, and the patient followed, with psychiatric intervention as appropriate. In severe cases, PegIntron should be stopped immediately and psychiatric intervention instituted *[see Dosage and Administration (2.3)].* Cases of encephalopathy have been observed in some patients, usually elderly, treated at higher doses of PegIntron.

5.3 Cardiovascular Events

Cardiovascular events, which include hypotension, arrhythmia, tachycardia, cardiomyopathy, angina pectoris, and myocardial infarction, have been observed in patients treated with PegIntron. PegIntron should be used cautiously in patients with cardiovascular disease. Patients

with a history of myocardial infarction and arrhythmic disorder who require PegIntron therapy should be closely monitored *[see Warnings and Precautions (5.15)].* Patients with a history of significant or unstable cardiac disease should not be treated with PegIntron/ribavirin combination therapy *[see ribavirin labeling].*

5.4 Endocrine Disorders

PegIntron causes or aggravates hypothyroidism and hyperthyroidism. Hyperglycemia has been observed in patients treated with PegIntron. Diabetes mellitus, including cases of new onset Type 1 diabetes, has been observed in patients treated with alpha interferons, including PegIntron. Patients with these conditions who cannot be effectively treated by medication should not begin PegIntron therapy. Patients who develop these conditions during treatment and cannot be controlled with medication should not continue PegIntron therapy.

5.5 Ophthalmologic Disorders

Decrease or loss of vision, retinopathy including macular edema, retinal artery or vein thrombosis, retinal hemorrhages and cotton wool spots, optic neuritis, papilledema, and serous retinal detachment may be induced or aggravated by treatment with peginterferon alfa-2b or other alpha interferons. All patients should receive an eye examination at baseline. Patients with preexisting ophthalmologic disorders (e.g., diabetic or hypertensive retinopathy) should receive periodic ophthalmologic exams during interferon alpha treatment. Any patient who develops ocular symptoms should receive a prompt and complete eye examination. Peginterferon alfa-2b treatment should be discontinued in patients who develop new or worsening ophthalmologic disorders.

5.6 Cerebrovascular Disorders

Ischemic and hemorrhagic cerebrovascular events have been observed in patients treated with interferon alfa-based therapies, including PegIntron. Events occurred in patients with few or no reported risk factors for stroke, including patients less than 45 years of age. Because these are spontaneous reports, estimates of frequency cannot be made, and a causal relationship between interferon alfa-based therapies and these events is difficult to establish.

5.7 Bone Marrow Toxicity

PegIntron suppresses bone marrow function, sometimes resulting in severe cytopenias. PegIntron should be discontinued in patients who develop severe decreases in neutrophil or platelet counts *[see Dosage and Administration (2.3)].* Ribavirin may potentiate the neutropenia induced by interferon alpha. Very rarely alpha interferons may be associated with aplastic anemia.

5.8 Autoimmune Disorders

Development or exacerbation of autoimmune disorders (e.g., thyroiditis, thrombotic thrombocytopenic purpura, idiopathic thrombocytopenic purpura, rheumatoid arthritis, interstitial nephritis, systemic lupus erythematosus, and psoriasis) has been observed in patients receiving PegIntron. PegIntron should be used with caution in patients with autoimmune disorders.

5.9 Pancreatitis
Fatal and nonfatal pancreatitis has been observed in patients treated with alpha interferon. PegIntron therapy should be suspended in patients with signs and symptoms suggestive of pancreatitis and discontinued in patients diagnosed with pancreatitis.

5.10 Colitis
Fatal and nonfatal ulcerative or hemorrhagic/ischemic colitis have been observed within 12 weeks of the start of alpha interferon treatment. Abdominal pain, bloody diarrhea, and fever are the typical manifestations. PegIntron treatment should be discontinued immediately in patients who develop these signs and symptoms. The colitis usually resolves within 1 to 3 weeks of discontinuation of alpha interferons.

5.11 Pulmonary Disorders
Dyspnea, pulmonary infiltrates, pneumonia, bronchiolitis obliterans, interstitial pneumonitis, pulmonary hypertension, and sarcoidosis, some resulting in respiratory failure or patient deaths, may be induced or aggravated by PegIntron or alpha interferon therapy. Recurrence of respiratory failure has been observed with interferon rechallenge. PegIntron combination treatment should be suspended in patients who develop pulmonary infiltrates or pulmonary function impairment. Patients who resume interferon treatment should be closely monitored.
Because of the fever and other "flu-like" symptoms associated with PegIntron administration, it should be used cautiously in patients with debilitating medical conditions, such as those with a history of pulmonary disease (e.g., chronic obstructive pulmonary disease).

5.12 Hepatic Failure
Chronic Hepatitis C (CHC) patients with cirrhosis may be at risk of hepatic decompensation and death when treated with alpha interferons, including PegIntron. Cirrhotic CHC patients co-infected with HIV receiving highly active antiretroviral therapy (HAART) and alpha interferons with or without ribavirin appear to be at increased risk for the development of hepatic decompensation compared to patients not receiving HAART. During treatment, patients' clinical status and hepatic function should be closely monitored, and PegIntron treatment should be immediately discontinued if decompensation (Child-Pugh score greater than 6) is observed [see Contraindications (4)].

5.13 Patients with Renal Insufficiency
Increases in serum creatinine levels have been observed in patients with renal insufficiency receiving interferon alpha products, including PegIntron. Patients with impaired renal function should be closely monitored for signs and symptoms of interferon toxicity, including increases in serum creatinine, and PegIntron dosing should be adjusted accordingly or discontinued [see Clinical Pharmacology (12.3) and Dosage and Administration (2.3)]. PegIntron monotherapy should be used with caution in patients with creatinine clearance less than 50 mL/min; the potential risks should be weighed against the potential benefits in these patients. Combination therapy with ribavirin must not be used in patients with creatinine clearance less than 50 mL/min [see ribavirin labeling].

5.14 Hypersensitivity
Serious, acute hypersensitivity reactions (e.g., urticaria, angioedema, bronchoconstriction, anaphylaxis) and cutaneous eruptions (Stevens-Johnson syndrome, toxic epidermal necrolysis) have been rarely observed during alpha interferon therapy. If such a reaction develops during treatment with PegIntron, discontinue treatment and institute appropriate medical therapy immediately. Transient rashes do not necessitate interruption of treatment.

5.15 Laboratory Tests
PegIntron alone or in combination with ribavirin may cause severe decreases in neutrophil and platelet counts, and hematologic, endocrine (e.g., TSH), and hepatic abnormalities. Transient elevations in ALT (2- to 5-fold above baseline) were observed in 10% of subjects treated with PegIntron, and were not associated with deterioration of other liver functions. Triglyceride levels are frequently elevated in patients receiving alpha interferon therapy including PegIntron and should be periodically monitored.
Patients on PegIntron or PegIntron/REBETOL combination therapy should have hematology and blood chemistry testing before the start of treatment and then periodically thereafter. In the adult clinical trial, complete blood counts (including hemoglobin, neutrophil, and platelet counts) and chemistries (including AST, ALT, bilirubin, and uric acid) were measured during the treatment period at Weeks 2, 4, 8, and 12, and then at 6-week intervals, or more frequently if abnormalities developed. In pediatric subjects, the same laboratory parameters were evaluated with additional assessment of hemoglobin at treatment Week 6. TSH levels were measured every 12 weeks during the treatment period. HCV-RNA should be measured periodically during treatment [see Dosage and Administration (2.1, 2.2, 2.4)].

Patients who have pre-existing cardiac abnormalities should have electrocardiograms done before treatment with PegIntron/ribavirin.

5.16 Dental and Periodontal Disorders
Dental and periodontal disorders have been reported in patients receiving PegIntron/REBETOL combination therapy.

Table 8: Adverse Reactions Occurring in Greater than 5% of Subjects

Adverse Reactions	Percentage of Subjects Reporting Adverse Reactions*			
	Study 1		Study 2	
	PegIntron 1 mcg/kg	INTRON A 3 MIU	PegIntron 1.5 mcg/kg/ REBETOL	INTRON A/ REBETOL
	(N=297)	(N=303)	(N=511)	(N=505)
Application Site				
Injection Site	47	20	75	49
Inflammation/Reaction				
Autonomic Nervous System				
Dry Mouth	6	7	12	8
Increased Sweating	6	7	11	7
Flushing	6	3	4	3
Body as a Whole				
Fatigue/Asthenia	52	54	66	63
Headache	56	52	62	58
Rigors	23	19	48	41
Fever	22	12	46	33
Weight Loss	11	13	29	20
Right Upper Quadrant Pain	8	8	12	6
Chest Pain	6	4	8	7
Malaise	7	6	4	6
Central/Peripheral Nervous System				
Dizziness	12	10	21	17
Endocrine				
Hypothyroidism	5	3	5	4
Gastrointestinal				
Nausea	26	20	43	33
Anorexia	20	17	32	27
Diarrhea	18	16	22	17
Vomiting	7	6	14	12
Abdominal Pain	15	11	13	13
Dyspepsia	6	7	9	8
Constipation	1	3	5	5
Hematologic Disorders				
Neutropenia	6	2	26	14
Anemia	0	0	12	17
Leukopenia	<1	0	6	5
Thrombocytopenia	7	<1	5	2
Liver and Biliary System				
Hepatomegaly	6	5	4	4
Musculoskeletal				
Myalgia	54	53	56	50
Arthralgia	23	27	34	28
Musculoskeletal Pain	28	22	21	19

(Table continued on next page)

In addition, dry mouth could have a damaging effect on teeth and mucous membranes of the mouth during long-term treatment with the combination of REBETOL and PegIntron. Patients should brush their teeth thoroughly twice daily and have regular dental examinations. If vomiting occurs, patients should be advised to rinse out their mouth thoroughly afterwards.

5.17 Triglycerides
Elevated triglyceride levels have been observed in patients treated with interferon alpha, including PegIntron therapy. Hypertriglyceridemia may result in pancreatitis [see Warnings and Precautions (5.9)]. Elevated triglyceride levels should be managed as clinically appropriate. Discontinuation of PegIntron therapy should be considered for patients with symptoms of potential pancreatitis, such as abdominal pain, nausea, or vomiting, and persistently elevated triglycerides (e.g., triglycerides greater than 1000 mg/dL).

5.18 Impact on Growth — Pediatric Use
Data on the effects of PegIntron plus REBETOL on growth come from an open-label trial in 107 subjects, 3 through 17 years of age, in which weight and height changes are compared to US normative population data. In general, the weight and height gain of pediatric subjects treated with PegIntron plus REBETOL lags behind that predicted by normative population data for the entire length of treatment. Severely inhibited growth velocity (less than 3rd percentile) was observed in 70% of the subjects while on treatment. Following treatment, rebound growth and weight gain occurred in most subjects. Long-term follow-up data in pediatric subjects, however, indicates that PegIntron in combination therapy with REBETOL may induce a growth inhibition that results in reduced adult height in some patients [see Adverse Reactions (6.1)].

5.19 Peripheral Neuropathy
Peripheral neuropathy has been reported when alpha interferons were given in combination with telbivudine. In one clinical trial, an increased risk and severity of peripheral neuropathy was observed with the combination use of telbivudine and pegylated interferon alfa-2a as compared to telbivudine alone. The safety and efficacy of telbivudine in combination with interferons for the treatment of chronic hepatitis B has not been demonstrated.

6 ADVERSE REACTIONS

6.1 Clinical Trials Experience
Because clinical trials are conducted under widely varying conditions, adverse reaction rates observed in the clinical trials of a drug cannot be directly compared to rates in the clinical trials of another drug and may not reflect the rates observed in clinical practice.

Clinical trials with PegIntron alone or in combination with REBETOL have been conducted in over 6900 subjects from 3 to 75 years of age.

Serious adverse reactions have occurred in approximately 12% of subjects in clinical trials with PegIntron with or without REBETOL [see Warnings and Precautions (5)]. The most common serious events occurring in subjects treated with PegIntron and REBETOL were depression and suicidal ideation [see Warnings and Precautions (5.2)], each occurring at a frequency of less than 1%. The most common fatal events occurring in subjects treated with PegIntron and REBETOL were cardiac arrest, suicidal ideation, and suicide attempt [see Warnings and Precautions (5.2, 5.3)], all occurring in less than 1% of subjects.

Greater than 96% of all subjects in clinical trials experienced one or more adverse events. The most commonly reported adverse reactions in adult subjects receiving either PegIntron or PegIntron/REBETOL were injection-site inflammation/reaction, fatigue/asthenia, headache, rigors, fevers, nausea, myalgia, and emotional lability/irritability. The most common adverse events in pediatric subjects, ages 3 and older, were pyrexia, headache, vomiting, neutropenia, fatigue, anorexia, injection-site erythema, and abdominal pain.

Adults
Study 1 compared PegIntron monotherapy with INTRON® A monotherapy. Study 2 compared combination therapy of PegIntron/REBETOL with combination therapy with INTRON A/REBETOL. In these clinical trials, nearly all subjects experienced one or more adverse reactions. Study 3 compared a PegIntron/weight-based REBETOL combination to a PegIntron/flat dose REBETOL regimen. Study 4 compared two PegIntron (1.5 mcg/kg/week and 1 mcg/kg/week) doses in combination with REBETOL and a third treatment group receiving Pegasys® (180 mcg/week)/Copegus® (1000-1200 mg/day).

Adverse reactions that occurred in Studies 1 and 2 at greater than 5% incidence are provided in **Table 8** by treatment group. Due to potential differences in ascertainment procedures, adverse reaction rate comparisons across trials should not be made. **Table 9** summarizes the treatment-related adverse reactions in Study 4 that occurred at a greater than or equal to 10% incidence.

[See table 8 on previous page and above]

Table 8 (cont.): Adverse Reactions Occurring in Greater than 5% of Subjects

Adverse Reactions	Percentage of Subjects Reporting Adverse Reactions*			
	Study 1		Study 2	
	PegIntron 1 mcg/kg (N=297)	INTRON A 3 MIU (N=303)	PegIntron 1.5 mcg/kg/ REBETOL (N=511)	INTRON A/ REBETOL (N=505)
Psychiatric				
Insomnia	23	23	40	41
Depression	29	25	31	34
Anxiety/Emotional Lability/Irritability	28	34	47	47
Concentration Impaired	10	8	17	21
Agitation	2	2	8	5
Nervousness	4	3	6	6
Reproductive, Female				
Menstrual Disorder	4	3	7	6
Resistance Mechanism				
Viral Infection	11	10	12	12
Fungal Infection	<1	3	6	1
Respiratory System				
Dyspnea	4	2	26	24
Coughing	8	5	23	16
Pharyngitis	10	7	12	13
Rhinitis	2	2	8	6
Sinusitis	7	7	6	5
Skin and Appendages				
Alopecia	22	22	36	32
Pruritus	12	8	29	28
Rash	6	7	24	23
Skin Dry	11	9	24	23
Special Senses, Other				
Taste Perversion	<1	2	9	4
Vision Disorders				
Vision Blurred	2	3	5	6
Conjunctivitis	4	2	4	5

* Subjects reporting one or more adverse reactions. A subject may have reported more than one adverse reaction within a body system/organ class category.

Table 9: Treatment-Related Adverse Reactions (Greater than or Equal to 10% Incidence) By Descending Frequency

Adverse Reactions	Percentage of Subjects Reporting Treatment-Related Adverse Reactions Study 4		
	PegIntron 1.5 mcg/kg with REBETOL (N=1019)	PegIntron 1 mcg/kg with REBETOL (N=1016)	Pegasys 180 mcg with Copegus (N=1035)
Fatigue	67	68	64
Headache	50	47	41
Nausea	40	35	34
Chills	39	36	23
Insomnia	38	37	41
Anemia	35	30	34
Pyrexia	35	32	21
Injection Site Reactions	34	35	23
Anorexia	29	25	21
Rash	29	25	34
Myalgia	27	26	22
Neutropenia	26	19	31
Irritability	25	25	25
Depression	25	19	20
Alopecia	23	20	17
Dyspnea	21	20	22
Arthralgia	21	22	22
Pruritus	18	15	19

Influenza-like Illness	16	15	15
Dizziness	16	14	13
Diarrhea	15	16	14
Cough	15	16	17
Weight Decreased	13	10	10
Vomiting	12	10	9
Unspecified Pain	12	13	9
Dry Skin	11	11	12
Anxiety	11	11	10
Abdominal Pain	10	10	10
Leukopenia	9	7	10

The adverse reaction profile in Study 3, which compared PegIntron/weight-based REBETOL combination to a PegIntron/flat-dose REBETOL regimen, revealed an increased rate of anemia with weight-based dosing (29% vs. 19% for weight-based vs. flat-dose regimens, respectively). However, the majority of cases of anemia were mild and responded to dose reductions.

The incidence of serious adverse reactions was comparable in all trials. In the PegIntron monotherapy trial (Study 1) the incidence of serious adverse reactions was similar (about 12%) in all treatment groups. In Study 2, the incidence of serious adverse reactions was 17% in the PegIntron/REBETOL groups compared to 14% in the INTRON A/REBETOL group. In Study 3, there was a similar incidence of serious adverse reactions reported for the weight-based REBETOL group (12%) and for the flat-dose REBETOL regimen.

In many but not all cases, adverse reactions resolved after dose reduction or discontinuation of therapy. Some subjects experienced ongoing or new serious adverse reactions during the 6-month follow-up period.

There have been 31 subject deaths that occurred during treatment or during follow-up in these clinical trials. In Study 1, there was 1 suicide in a subject receiving PegIntron monotherapy and 2 deaths among subjects receiving INTRON A monotherapy (1 murder/suicide and 1 sudden death). In Study 2, there was 1 suicide in a subject receiving PegIntron/REBETOL combination therapy, and 1 subject death in the INTRON A/REBETOL group (motor vehicle accident). In Study 3, there were 14 deaths, 2 of which were probable suicides, and 1 was an unexplained death in a person with a relevant medical history of depression. In Study 4, there were 12 deaths, 6 of which occurred in subjects receiving PegIntron/REBETOL combination therapy; 5 in the PegIntron 1.5 mcg/REBETOL arm (N=1019) and 1 in the PegIntron 1 mcg/REBETOL arm (n=1016); and 6 of which occurred in subjects receiving Pegasys/Copegus (N=1035). There were 3 suicides that occurred during the off-treatment follow-up period in subjects who received PegIntron (1.5 mcg/kg)/REBETOL combination therapy.

In Studies 1 and 2, 10% to 14% of subjects receiving PegIntron, alone or in combination with REBETOL, discontinued therapy compared with 6% treated with INTRON A alone and 13% treated with INTRON A in combination with REBETOL. Similarly in Study 3, 15% of subjects receiving PegIntron in combination with weight-based REBETOL and 14% of subjects receiving PegIntron and flat-dose REBETOL discontinued therapy due to an adverse reaction. The most common reasons for discontinuation of therapy were related to known interferon effects of psychiatric, systemic (e.g., fatigue, headache), or gastrointestinal adverse reactions. In Study 4, 13% of subjects in the PegIntron 1.5 mcg/REBETOL arm, 10% in the PegIntron 1 mcg/REBETOL arm, and 13% in the Pegasys 180 mcg/Copegus arm discontinued therapy due to adverse events.

In Study 2, dose reductions due to adverse reactions occurred in 42% of subjects receiving PegIntron (1.5 mcg/kg)/REBETOL and in 34% of those receiving INTRON A/REBETOL. The majority of subjects (57%) weighing 60 kg or less receiving PegIntron (1.5 mcg/kg)/REBETOL required dose reduction. Reduction of interferon was dose-related (PegIntron 1.5 mcg/kg more than PegIntron 0.5 mcg/kg or INTRON A), 40%, 27%, 28%, respectively. Dose reduction for REBETOL was similar across all three groups, 33% to 35%. The most common reasons for dose modifications were neutropenia (18%) or anemia (9%). Other common reasons included depression, fatigue, nausea, and thrombocytopenia. In Study 3, dose modifications due to adverse reactions occurred more frequently with weight-based dosing (WBD) compared to flat dosing (29%

and 23%, respectively). In Study 4, 16% of subjects had a dose reduction of PegIntron to 1 mcg/kg in combination with REBETOL, with an additional 4% requiring the second dose reduction of PegIntron to 0.5 mcg/kg due to adverse events, compared to 15% of subjects in the Pegasys/Copegus arm, who required a dose reduction to 135 mcg/week with Pegasys, with an additional 7% requiring a second dose reduction to 90 mcg/week with Pegasys.

In the PegIntron/REBETOL combination trials the most common adverse reactions were psychiatric, which occurred among 77% of subjects in Study 2 and 68% to 69% of subjects in Study 3. These psychiatric adverse reactions included most commonly depression, irritability, and insomnia, each reported by approximately 30% to 40% of subjects in all treatment groups. Suicidal behavior (ideation, attempts, and suicides) occurred in 2% of subjects during treatment or during follow-up after treatment cessation [see Warnings and Precautions (5.2)]. In Study 4, psychiatric adverse reactions occurred in 58% of subjects in the PegIntron 1.5 mcg/REBETOL arm, 55% of subjects in the PegIntron 1 mcg/REBETOL arm, and 57% of subjects in the Pegasys 180 mcg/Copegus arm.

PegIntron induced fatigue or headache in approximately two-thirds of subjects, with fever or rigors in approximately half of the subjects. The severity of some of these systemic symptoms (e.g., fever and headache) tended to decrease as treatment continued. In Studies 1 and 2, application site inflammation and reaction (e.g., bruise, itchiness, and irritation) occurred at approximately twice the incidence with PegIntron therapies (in up to 75% of subjects) compared with INTRON A. However, injection-site pain was infrequent (2-3%) in all groups. In Study 3, there was a 23% to 24% incidence overall for injection-site reactions or inflammation.

In Study 2, many subjects continued to experience adverse reactions several months after discontinuation of therapy. By the end of the 6-month follow-up period, the incidence of ongoing adverse reactions by body class in the PegIntron 1.5/REBETOL group was 33% (psychiatric), 20% (musculoskeletal), and 10% (for endocrine and for GI). In approximately 10% to 15% of subjects, weight loss, fatigue, and headache had not resolved.

Individual serious adverse reactions in Study 2 occurred at a frequency less than or equal to 1% and included suicide attempt, suicidal ideation, severe depression; psychosis, aggressive reaction, relapse of drug addiction/overdose; nerve palsy (facial, oculomotor); cardiomyopathy, myocardial infarction, angina, pericardial effusion, retinal ischemia, retinal artery or vein thrombosis, blindness, decreased visual acuity, optic neuritis, transient ischemic attack, supraventricular arrhythmias, loss of consciousness; neutropenia, infection (sepsis, pneumonia, abscess, cellulitis); emphysema, bronchiolitis obliterans, pleural effusion, gastroenteritis, pancreatitis, gout, hyperglycemia, hyperthyroidism and hypothyroidism, autoimmune thrombocytopenia with or without purpura, rheumatoid arthritis, interstitial nephritis, lupus-like syndrome, sarcoidosis, aggravated psoriasis; urticaria, injection-site necrosis, vasculitis, and phototoxicity. Subjects receiving PegIntron/REBETOL as re-treatment after failing a previous interferon combination regimen reported adverse reactions similar to those previously associated with this regimen during clinical trials of treatment-naïve subjects.

Pediatric Subjects
In general, the adverse-reaction profile in the pediatric population was similar to that observed in adults. In the pediatric trial, the most prevalent adverse reactions in all subjects were pyrexia (80%), headache (62%), neutropenia (33%), fatigue (30%), anorexia (29%), injection-site erythema (29%), and vomiting (27%). The majority of adverse reactions reported in the trial were mild or moderate in severity. Severe adverse reactions were reported in 7% (8/107) of all subjects and included injection-site pain (1%), pain in extremity (1%), headache (1%), neutropenia (1%), and pyrexia (4%). Important adverse reactions that occurred in this subject population were nervousness (7%; 7/107), aggression (3%; 3/107), anger (2%; 2/107), and depression (1%; 1/107). Five subjects received levothyroxine treatment; three with clinical hypothyroidism and two with asymptomatic TSH elevations. Weight and height gain of pediatric subjects treated with PegIntron plus REBETOL lagged behind that predicted by normative population data for the entire length of treatment. Severely inhibited growth velocity (less than 3rd percentile) was observed in 70% of the subjects while on treatment.

Dose modifications were required in 25% of subjects, most commonly for anemia, neutropenia, and weight loss. Two subjects (2%; 2/107) discontinued therapy as the result of an adverse reaction.

Adverse reactions that occurred with a greater than or equal to 10% incidence in the pediatric trial subjects are provided in Table 10.

Table 10: Percentage of Pediatric Subjects with Treatment-related Adverse Reactions (in At Least 10% of All Subjects)

System Organ Class Preferred Term	All Subjects N=107
Blood and Lymphatic System Disorders	
Neutropenia	33%
Anemia	11%
Leukopenia	10%
Gastrointestinal Disorders	
Abdominal Pain	21%
Abdominal Pain Upper	12%
Vomiting	27%
Nausea	18%
General Disorders and Administration Site Conditions	
Pyrexia	80%
Fatigue	30%
Injection-site Erythema	29%
Chills	21%
Asthenia	15%
Irritability	14%
Investigations	
Weight Decreased	19%
Metabolism and Nutrition Disorders	
Anorexia	29%
Decreased Appetite	22%
Musculoskeletal and Connective Tissue Disorders	
Arthralgia	17%
Myalgia	17%
Nervous System Disorders	
Headache	62%
Dizziness	14%
Skin and Subcutaneous Tissue Disorders	
Alopecia	17%

Ninety-four of 107 subjects enrolled in a 5 year long-term follow-up trial. The long-term effects on growth were less in those subjects treated for 24 weeks than those treated for 48 weeks. Twenty-four percent of subjects (11/46) treated for 24 weeks and 40% of subjects (19/48) treated for 48 weeks had a >15 percentile height-for-age decrease from pre-treatment to the end of the 5 year long-term follow-up compared to pre-treatment baseline percentiles. Eleven percent of subjects (5/46) treated for 24 weeks and 13% of subjects (6/48) treated for 48 weeks were observed to have a decrease from pre-treatment baseline of >30 height-for-age percentiles to the end of the 5 year long-term follow-up. While observed across all age groups, the highest risk for reduced height at the end of long-term follow-up appeared to correlate with initiation of combination therapy during the years of expected peak growth velocity [see Warnings and Precautions (5.18)].

Laboratory Values
Adults
Changes in selected laboratory values during treatment with PegIntron alone or in combination with REBETOL treatment are described below. **Decreases in hemoglobin, neutrophils, and platelets may require dose reduction or permanent discontinuation from therapy** [see Dosage and Administration (2.3) and Warnings and Precautions (5.1, 5.7)].

Hemoglobin. Hemoglobin levels decreased to less than 11 g/dL in about 30% of subjects in Study 2. In Study 3, 47% of subjects receiving WBD REBETOL and 33% on flat-dose REBETOL had decreases in hemoglobin levels less than 11 g/dL. Reductions in hemoglobin to less than 9 g/dL occurred more frequently in subjects receiving WBD compared to flat dosing (4% and 2%, respectively). In Study 2, dose modification was required in 9% and 13% of subjects in the PegIntron/REBETOL and INTRON A/REBETOL groups. In Study 4, subjects receiving PegIntron (1.5 mcg/kg)/REBETOL had decreases in hemoglobin levels to between 8.5 to less than 10 g/dL (28%) and to less than 8.5 g/dL (3%), whereas in subjects receiving Pegasys 180 mcg/Copegus these decreases occurred in 26% and 4% of subjects, respectively. Hemoglobin levels became stable by treatment Weeks 4 to 6 on average. The typical pattern observed was a decrease in hemoglobin levels by treatment Week 4 followed by stabilization and a plateau, which was maintained to the end of treatment. In the PegIntron monotherapy trial, hemoglobin decreases were generally mild and dose modifications were rarely necessary *[see Dosage and Administration (2.3)]*.

Neutrophils. Decreases in neutrophil counts were observed in a majority of subjects treated with PegIntron alone (70%) or as combination therapy with REBETOL in Study 2 (85%) and INTRON A/REBETOL (60%). Severe potentially life-threatening neutropenia (less than 0.5×10^9/L) occurred in 1% of subjects treated with PegIntron monotherapy, 2% of subjects treated with INTRON A/REBETOL, and approximately 4% of subjects treated with PegIntron/REBETOL in Study 2. Two percent of subjects receiving PegIntron monotherapy and 18% of subjects receiving PegIntron/REBETOL in Study 2 required modification of interferon dosage. Few subjects (less than 1%) required permanent discontinuation of treatment. Neutrophil counts generally returned to pretreatment levels 4 weeks after cessation of therapy *[see Dosage and Administration (2.3)]*.

Platelets. Platelet counts decreased to less than 100,000/mm³ in approximately 20% of subjects treated with PegIntron alone or with REBETOL and in 6% of subjects treated with INTRON A/REBETOL. Severe decreases in platelet counts (less than 50,000/mm³) occur in less than 4% of subjects. Patients may require discontinuation or dose modification as a result of platelet decreases *[see Dosage and Administration (2.3)]*. In Study 2, 1% or 3% of subjects required dose modification of INTRON A or PegIntron, respectively. Platelet counts generally returned to pretreatment levels 4 weeks after the cessation of therapy.

Triglycerides. Elevated triglyceride levels have been observed in patients treated with interferon alphas, including PegIntron *[see Warnings and Precautions (5.17)]*.

Thyroid Function. Development of TSH abnormalities, with or without clinical manifestations, is associated with interferon therapies. In Study 2, clinically apparent thyroid disorders occurred among subjects treated with either INTRON A or PegIntron (with or without REBETOL) at a similar incidence (5% for hypothyroidism and 3% for hyperthyroidism). Subjects developed new-onset TSH abnormalities while on treatment and during the follow-up period. At the end of the follow-up period, 7% of subjects still had abnormal TSH values *[see Warnings and Precautions (5.4)]*.

Bilirubin and Uric Acid. In Study 2, 10% to 14% of subjects developed hyperbilirubinemia and 33% to 38% developed hyperuricemia in association with hemolysis. Six subjects developed mild to moderate gout.

Pediatric Subjects

Decreases in hemoglobin, white blood cells, platelets, and neutrophils may require dose reduction or permanent discontinuation from therapy *[see Dosage and Administration (2.3)]*. Changes in selected laboratory values during treatment of 107 pediatric subjects with PegIntron/REBETOL combination therapy are described in **Table 11**. Most of the changes in laboratory values in this trial were mild or moderate.

Table 11: Selected Laboratory Abnormalities during Treatment Phase with PegIntron Plus REBETOL in Previously Untreated Pediatric Subjects

Laboratory Parameter*	All Subjects (N=107)
Hemoglobin (g/dL)	
9.5 to <11.0	30%
8.0 to <9.5	2%
WBC (× 10⁹/L)	
2.0-2.9	39%
1.5 to <2.0	3%

Platelets (× 10⁹/L)	
70-100	1%
50 to <70	—
25 to <50	1%
Neutrophils (× 10⁹/L)	
1.0-1.5	35%
0.75 to <1.0	26%
0.5 to <0.75	13%
<0.5	3%
Total Bilirubin	
1.26-2.59 × ULN†	7%
Evidence of Hepatic Failure	—

* The table summarizes the worst category observed within the period per subject per laboratory test. Only subjects with at least one treatment value for a given laboratory test are included.
† ULN=Upper limit of normal.

6.2 Immunogenicity

As with all therapeutic proteins, there is potential for immunogenicity. Approximately 2% of subjects receiving PegIntron (32/1759) or INTRON A (11/728) with or without REBETOL developed low-titer (less than or equal to 160) neutralizing antibodies to PegIntron or INTRON A. The clinical and pathological significance of the appearance of serum-neutralizing antibodies is unknown. The incidence of antibody formation is highly dependent on the sensitivity and specificity of the assay. Additionally, the observed incidence of antibody (including neutralizing antibody) positivity in an assay may be influenced by several factors, including assay methodology, sample handling, timing of sample collection, concomitant medications, and underlying disease. For these reasons, comparison of the incidence of antibodies to PegIntron with the incidence of antibodies to other products may be misleading.

6.3 Postmarketing Experience

The following adverse reactions have been identified during post-approval use of PegIntron therapy. Because these reactions are reported voluntarily from a population of uncertain size, it is not always possible to reliably estimate their frequency or establish a causal relationship to drug exposure.

Blood and Lymphatic System Disorders
Pure red cell aplasia, thrombotic thrombocytopenic purpura

Cardiac Disorders
Palpitations

Ear and Labyrinth Disorders
Hearing loss, vertigo, hearing impairment

Endocrine Disorders
Diabetic ketoacidosis, diabetes

Eye Disorders
Vogt-Koyanagi-Harada syndrome, serous retinal detachment

Gastrointestinal Disorders
Aphthous stomatitis

General Disorders and Administration Site Conditions
Asthenic conditions (including asthenia, malaise, fatigue)

Immune System Disorders
Cases of acute hypersensitivity reactions (including anaphylaxis, angioedema, urticaria); Stevens-Johnson syndrome, toxic epidermal necrolysis, systemic lupus erythematosus, erythema multiforme

Infections and Infestations
Bacterial infection including sepsis

Metabolism and Nutrition Disorders
Dehydration, hypertriglyceridemia

Musculoskeletal and Connective Tissue Disorders
Rhabdomyolysis, myositis

Nervous System Disorders
Seizures, memory loss, peripheral neuropathy, paraesthesia, migraine headache

Psychiatric Disorders
Homicidal ideation

Respiratory, Thoracic, and Mediastinal Disorders
Pulmonary hypertension

Renal and Urinary Disorders
Renal failure, renal insufficiency

Skin and Subcutaneous Tissue Disorders
Psoriasis

Vascular Disorders
Hypertension, hypotension

7 DRUG INTERACTIONS

7.1 Drugs Metabolized by Cytochrome P-450

When administering PegIntron with medications metabolized by CYP2C8/9 (e.g., warfarin and phenytoin) or CYP2D6 (e.g., flecainide), the therapeutic effect of these substrates may be decreased *[see Clinical Pharmacology (12.3)]*.

7.2 Methadone

PegIntron may increase methadone concentrations *[see Clinical Pharmacology (12.3)]*. The clinical significance of this finding is unknown; however, patients should be monitored for signs and symptoms of increased narcotic effect.

7.3 Use with Ribavirin (Nucleoside Analogues)

Hepatic decompensation (some fatal) has occurred in cirrhotic HIV/HCV co-infected patients receiving combination antiretroviral therapy for HIV and interferon alpha and ribavirin. Adding treatment with alpha interferons alone or in combination with ribavirin may increase the risk in this patient subset. Patients receiving interferon with ribavirin and nucleoside reverse transcriptase inhibitors (NRTIs) should be closely monitored for treatment-associated toxicities, especially hepatic decompensation and anemia. Discontinuation of NRTIs should be considered as medically appropriate *[see labeling for individual NRTI product]*. Dose reduction or discontinuation of interferon, ribavirin, or both should also be considered if worsening clinical toxicities are observed, including hepatic decompensation (e.g., Child-Pugh greater than 6).

Stavudine, Lamivudine, and Zidovudine

In vitro studies have shown ribavirin can reduce the phosphorylation of pyrimidine nucleoside analogues such as stavudine, lamivudine, and zidovudine. In a trial with another pegylated interferon alpha, no evidence of a pharmacokinetic or pharmacodynamic (e.g., loss of HIV/HCV virologic suppression) interaction was seen when ribavirin was co-administered with zidovudine, lamivudine, or stavudine in HIV/HCV co-infected subjects *[see Clinical Pharmacology (12.3)]*.

HIV/HCV co-infected subjects who were administered zidovudine in combination with pegylated interferon alpha and ribavirin developed severe neutropenia (ANC less than 500) and severe anemia (hemoglobin less than 8 g/dL) more frequently than similar subjects not receiving zidovudine.

Didanosine

Co-administration of ribavirin and didanosine is not recommended. Reports of fatal hepatic failure, as well as peripheral neuropathy, pancreatitis, and symptomatic hyperlactatemia/lactic acidosis have been reported in clinical trials *[see Clinical Pharmacology (12.3)]*.

8 USE IN SPECIFIC POPULATIONS

8.1 Pregnancy

PegIntron Monotherapy

Pregnancy Category C: Nonpegylated interferon alfa-2b has been shown to have abortifacient effects in *Macaca mulatta* (rhesus monkeys) at 15 and 30 million IU/kg (estimated human equivalent of 5 and 10 million IU/kg, based on body surface area adjustment for a 60-kg adult). PegIntron should be assumed to also have abortifacient potential. There are no adequate and well-controlled trials in pregnant women. PegIntron therapy is to be used during pregnancy only if the potential benefit justifies the potential risk to the fetus. Therefore, PegIntron is recommended for use in fertile women only when they are using effective contraception during the treatment period.

Use with Ribavirin

Pregnancy Category X: Significant teratogenic and/or embryocidal effects have been demonstrated in all animal species exposed to ribavirin. Ribavirin therapy is contraindicated in women who are pregnant and in the male partners of women who are pregnant *[see Contraindications (4) and ribavirin labeling]*.

A Ribavirin Pregnancy Registry has been established to monitor maternal-fetal outcomes of pregnancies in female patients and female partners of male patients exposed to ribavirin during treatment and for 6 months following cessation of treatment. Physicians and patients are encouraged to report such cases by calling 1-800-593-2214.

8.3 Nursing Mothers

It is not known whether the components of PegIntron and/or ribavirin are excreted in human milk. Studies in mice have shown that mouse interferons are excreted in breast milk. Because of the potential for adverse reactions from the drug in nursing infants, a decision must be made whether to discontinue nursing or discontinue the PegIntron and ribavirin treatment, taking into account the importance of the therapy to the mother.

8.4 Pediatric Use

Safety and effectiveness in pediatric patients below the age of 3 years have not been established. Clinical trials in pediatric subjects less than 3 years of age are not considered feasible due to the small proportion of patients in this age group requiring treatment for CHC.

Long-term follow-up data in pediatric subjects indicates that PegIntron in combination with REBETOL may induce a growth inhibition that results in reduced height in some patients [see Warnings and Precautions (5.18) and Adverse Reactions (6.1)].

8.5 Geriatric Use

In general, younger patients tend to respond better than older patients to interferon-based therapies. Clinical trials of PegIntron alone or in combination with REBETOL did not include sufficient numbers of subjects aged 65 and over to determine whether they respond differently than younger subjects. Treatment with alpha interferons, including PegIntron, is associated with neuropsychiatric, cardiac, pulmonary, GI, and systemic (flu-like) adverse effects. Because these adverse reactions may be more severe in the elderly, caution should be exercised in the use of PegIntron in this population. This drug is known to be substantially excreted by the kidney. Because elderly patients are more likely to have decreased renal function, the risk of toxic reactions to this drug may be greater in patients with impaired renal function [see Clinical Pharmacology (12.3)]. When using PegIntron/ribavirin therapy, refer also to the ribavirin labeling.

8.6 Organ Transplant Recipients

The safety and efficacy of PegIntron alone or in combination with ribavirin for the treatment of hepatitis C in liver or other organ transplant recipients have not been studied. In a small (n=16) single-center, uncontrolled case experience, renal failure in renal allograft recipients receiving interferon alpha and ribavirin combination therapy was more frequent than expected from the center's previous experience with renal allograft recipients not receiving combination therapy. The relationship of the renal failure to renal allograft rejection is not clear.

8.7 HIV or HBV Co-infection

The safety and efficacy of PegIntron/ribavirin for the treatment of patients with HCV co-infected with HIV or HBV have not been established.

10 OVERDOSAGE

There is limited experience with overdosage. In the clinical trials, a few subjects accidentally received a dose greater than that prescribed. There were no instances in which a participant in the monotherapy or combination therapy trials received more than 10.5 times the intended dose of PegIntron. The maximum dose received by any subject was 3.45 mcg/kg weekly over a period of approximately 12 weeks. The maximum known overdosage of ribavirin was an intentional ingestion of 10 g (fifty 200 mg capsules). There were no serious reactions attributed to these overdosages. In cases of overdosing, symptomatic treatment and close observation of the patient are recommended.

11 DESCRIPTION

PegIntron, peginterferon alfa-2b, is a covalent conjugate of recombinant alfa-2b interferon with monomethoxy polyethylene glycol (PEG). The average molecular weight of the PEG portion of the molecule is 12,000 daltons. The average molecular weight of the PegIntron molecule is approximately 31,000 daltons. The specific activity of peginterferon alfa-2b is approximately 0.7×10^8 IU/mg protein.

Interferon alfa-2b is a water-soluble protein with a molecular weight of 19,271 daltons produced by recombinant DNA techniques. It is obtained from the bacterial fermentation of a strain of Escherichia coli bearing a genetically engineered plasmid containing an interferon gene from human leukocytes.

PegIntron is supplied in both vials and the REDIPEN single-use pre-filled pen for subcutaneous use.

Vials

Each vial contains either 74 mcg, 118.4 mcg, 177.6 mcg, or 222 mcg of PegIntron as a white to off-white tablet-like solid that is whole/in pieces or as a loose powder, and 1.11 mg dibasic sodium phosphate anhydrous, 1.11 mg monobasic sodium phosphate dihydrate, 59.2 mg sucrose, and 0.074 mg polysorbate 80. Following reconstitution with 0.7 mL of the supplied Sterile Water for Injection USP, each vial contains PegIntron at strengths of either 50 mcg per 0.5 mL, 80 mcg per 0.5 mL, 120 mcg per 0.5 mL, or 150 mcg per 0.5 mL.

REDIPEN single-use pre-filled pen

REDIPEN pre-filled pen is a dual-chamber glass cartridge containing lyophilized PegIntron as a white to off-white tablet or powder that is whole or in pieces in the sterile active chamber and a second chamber containing Sterile Water for Injection USP. Each PegIntron REDIPEN pre-filled pen contains either 67.5 mcg, 108 mcg, 162 mcg, or 202.5 mcg of PegIntron, and 1.013 mg dibasic sodium phosphate anhydrous, 1.013 mg monobasic sodium phosphate dihydrate, 54 mg sucrose, and 0.0675 mg polysorbate 80. Each cartridge is reconstituted to allow for the administration of up to 0.5 mL of solution. Following reconstitution, each REDIPEN pre-filled pen contains PegIntron at strengths of either 50 mcg per 0.5 mL, 80 mcg per 0.5 mL, 120 mcg per 0.5 mL, or 150 mcg per 0.5 mL for a single use. Because a small volume of reconstituted solution is lost during preparation of PegIntron, each REDIPEN pre-filled pen contains an excess amount of PegIntron powder and diluent to ensure delivery of the labeled dose.

12 CLINICAL PHARMACOLOGY

12.1 Mechanism of Action

Pegylated recombinant human interferon alfa-2b is an inducer of the innate antiviral immune response [see Microbiology (12.4)].

12.2 Pharmacodynamics

The pharmacodynamic effects of peginterferon alfa-2b include inhibition of viral replication in virus-infected cells, the suppression of cell cycle progression/cell proliferation, induction of apoptosis, anti-angiogenic activities, and numerous immunomodulating activities, such as enhancement of the phagocytic activity of macrophages, activation of NK cells, stimulation of cytotoxic T-lymphocytes, and the up-regulation of the Th1 T-helper cell subset.

PegIntron raises concentrations of effector proteins such as serum neopterin and 2′5′ oligoadenylate synthetase, raises body temperature, and causes reversible decreases in leukocyte and platelet counts. The correlation between the in vitro and in vivo pharmacologic and pharmacodynamic and clinical effects is unknown.

12.3 Pharmacokinetics

Following a single subcutaneous dose of PegIntron, the mean absorption half-life (t ½ k$_a$) was 4.6 hours. Maximal serum concentrations (C$_{max}$) occur between 15 and 44 hours postdose, and are sustained for up to 48 to 72 hours. The C$_{max}$ and AUC measurements of PegIntron increase in a dose-related manner. After multiple dosing, there is an increase in bioavailability of PegIntron. Week 48 mean trough concentrations (320 pg/mL; range 0, 2960) are approximately 3-fold higher than Week 4 mean trough concentrations (94 pg/mL; range 0, 416). The mean PegIntron elimination half-life is approximately 40 hours (range 22-60 hours) in patients with HCV infection. The apparent clearance of PegIntron is estimated to be approximately 22 mL/hr•kg. Renal elimination accounts for 30% of the clearance.

Pegylation of interferon alfa-2b produces a product (PegIntron) whose clearance is lower than that of nonpegylated interferon alfa-2b. When compared to INTRON A, PegIntron (1 mcg/kg) has approximately a 7-fold lower mean apparent clearance and a 5-fold greater mean half-life, permitting a reduced dosing frequency. At effective therapeutic doses, PegIntron has approximately 10-fold greater C$_{max}$ and 50-fold greater AUC than interferon alfa-2b.

Renal Dysfunction

Following multiple dosing of PegIntron (1 mcg/kg subcutaneously given every week for 4 weeks) the clearance of PegIntron is reduced by a mean of 17% in subjects with moderate renal impairment (creatinine clearance 30-49 mL/min) and by a mean of 44% in subjects with severe renal impairment (creatinine clearance 10-29 mL/min) compared to subjects with normal renal function. Clearance was similar in subjects with severe renal impairment not on dialysis and subjects who are receiving hemodialysis. The dose of PegIntron for monotherapy should be reduced in patients with moderate or severe renal impairment [see Dosage and Administration (2.3) and REBETOL labeling]. REBETOL should not be used in patients with creatinine clearance less than 50 mL/min [see REBETOL labeling, WARNINGS].

Gender

During the 48-week treatment period with PegIntron, no differences in the pharmacokinetic profiles were observed between male and female subjects with chronic hepatitis C infection.

Geriatric Patients

The pharmacokinetics of geriatric subjects (65 years of age and older) treated with a single subcutaneous dose of 1 mcg/kg of PegIntron were similar in C$_{max}$, AUC, clearance, or elimination half-life as compared to younger subjects (28-44 years of age).

Pediatric Patients

Population pharmacokinetics for PegIntron and REBETOL (capsules and oral solution) were evaluated in pediatric subjects with chronic hepatitis C between 3 and 17 years of age. In pediatric patients receiving PegIntron 60 mcg/m²/week subcutaneously, exposure may be approximately 50% higher than observed in adults receiving 1.5 mcg/kg/week subcutaneously. The pharmacokinetics of REBETOL (dose-normalized) in this trial were similar to those reported in a prior trial of REBETOL in combination with INTRON A in pediatric subjects and in adults.

Effect of Food on Absorption of Ribavirin

Both AUC$_{tf}$ and C$_{max}$ increased by 70% when REBETOL capsules were administered with a high-fat meal (841 kcal, 53.8 g fat, 31.6 g protein, and 57.4 g carbohydrate) in a single-dose pharmacokinetic trial [see Dosage and Administration (2.1)].

Drug Interactions

Drugs Metabolized by Cytochrome P-450

The pharmacokinetics of representative drugs metabolized by CYP1A2 (caffeine), CYP2C8/9 (tolbutamide), CYP2D6 (dextromethorphan), CYP3A4 (midazolam), and N-acetyltransferase (dapsone) were studied in 22 subjects with chronic hepatitis C who received PegIntron (1.5 mcg/kg) once weekly for 4 weeks. PegIntron treatment resulted in a 28% (mean) increase in a measure of CYP2C8/9 activity. PegIntron treatment also resulted in a 66% (mean) increase in a measure of CYP2D6 activity; however, the effect was variable as 13 subjects had an increase, 5 subjects had a decrease, and 4 subjects had no significant change [see Drug Interactions (7.1)].

No significant effect was observed on the pharmacokinetics of representative drugs metabolized by CYP1A2, CYP3A4, or N-acetyltransferase. The effects of PegIntron on CYP2C19 activity were not assessed.

Methadone

The pharmacokinetics of concomitant administration of methadone and PegIntron were evaluated in 18 PegIntron-naïve chronic hepatitis C subjects receiving 1.5 mcg/kg PegIntron subcutaneously weekly. All subjects were on stable methadone maintenance therapy receiving greater than or equal to 40 mg/day prior to initiating PegIntron. Mean methadone AUC was approximately 16% higher after 4 weeks of PegIntron treatment as compared to baseline. In 2 subjects, methadone AUC was approximately double after 4 weeks of PegIntron treatment as compared to baseline [see Drug Interactions (7.2)].

Use with Ribavirin

Zidovudine, Lamivudine, and Stavudine

Ribavirin has been shown in vitro to inhibit phosphorylation of zidovudine, lamivudine, and stavudine. However, in a trial with another pegylated interferon in combination with ribavirin, no pharmacokinetic (e.g., plasma concentrations or intracellular triphosphorylated active metabolite concentrations) or pharmacodynamic (e.g., loss of HIV/HCV virologic suppression) interaction was observed when ribavirin and lamivudine (n=18), stavudine (n=10), or zidovudine (n=6) were co-administered as part of a multi-drug regimen to HIV/HCV co-infected subjects [see Drug Interactions (7.3)].

Didanosine

Exposure to didanosine or its active metabolite (dideoxyadenosine 5′-triphosphate) is increased when didanosine is co-administered with ribavirin, which could cause or worsen clinical toxicities [see Drug Interactions (7.3)].

12.4 Microbiology

Mechanism of Action

The biological activity of PegIntron is derived from its interferon alfa-2b moiety. Peginterferon alfa-2b binds to and activates the human type 1 interferon receptor. Upon binding, the receptor subunits dimerize, and activate multiple intracellular signal transduction pathways. Signal transduction is initially mediated by the JAK/STAT activation, which may occur in a wide variety of cells. Interferon receptor activation also activates NFkB in many cell types. Given the diversity of cell types that respond to interferon alfa-2b, and the multiplicity of potential intracellular responses to interferon receptor activation, peginterferon alfa-2b is expected to have pleiotropic biological effects in the body.

The mechanism by which ribavirin contributes to its antiviral efficacy in the clinic is not fully understood. Ribavirin has direct antiviral activity in tissue culture against many RNA viruses. Ribavirin increases the mutation frequency in the genomes of several viruses and ribavirin triphosphate inhibits HCV polymerase in a biochemical reaction.

Antiviral Activity

The anti-HCV activity of interferon was demonstrated in cell culture using self-replicating HCV-RNA (HCV replicon cells) or HCV infection and resulted in an effective concentration (EC$_{50}$) value of 1 to 10 IU/mL.

The antiviral activity of ribavirin in the HCV-replicon is not well understood and has not been defined because of the cellular toxicity of ribavirin.

Resistance

HCV genotypes show wide variability in their response to pegylated recombinant human interferon/ribavirin therapy. Genetic changes associated with the variable response have not been identified.

Cross-resistance

There is no reported cross-resistance between pegylated/ nonpegylated interferons and ribavirin.

12.5 Pharmacogenomics

A retrospective genome-wide association analysis[1,2] of 1671 subjects (1604 subjects from Study 4 [see Clinical Studies (14.1)] and 67 subjects from another clinical trial) was performed to identify human genetic contributions to anti-HCV treatment response in previously untreated HCV genotype 1 subjects. A single nucleotide polymorphism near the gene encoding interferon-lambda-3 (*IL28B rs12979860*) was associated with variable SVR rates. The *rs12979860* genotype was categorized as CC, CT and TT. In the pooled analysis of Caucasian, African-American, and Hispanic subjects from these trials (n=1587), SVR rates by *rs12979860* genotype were as follows: CC 66% vs. CT 30% vs. TT 22%. The genotype frequencies differed depending on racial/ethnic background, but the relationship of SVR to *IL28B* genotype was consistent across various racial/ethnic groups (see *Table 12*). Other variants near the *IL28B* gene (e.g., *rs8099917* and *rs8103142*) have been identified; however, they have not been shown to independently influence SVR rates during treatment with pegylated interferon alpha therapies combined with ribavirin.[1]

Table 12: SVR Rates by IL28B Genotype*

Population	CC	CT	TT
Caucasian	69% (301/436)	33% (196/596)	27% (38/139)
African-American	48% (20/42)	15% (22/146)	13% (15/112)
Hispanic	56% (19/34)	38% (21/56)	27% (7/26)

* The SVR rates are the overall rates for subjects treated with PegIntron 1.0 mcg/kg/REBETOL, PegIntron 1.5 mcg/kg/REBETOL and Pegasys 180 mcg/Copegus according to self-reported race/ethnicity.

13 NONCLINICAL TOXICOLOGY

13.1 Carcinogenesis, Mutagenesis, Impairment of Fertility

Carcinogenesis and Mutagenesis

PegIntron has not been tested for its carcinogenic potential. Neither PegIntron nor its components, interferon or methoxypolyethylene glycol, caused damage to DNA when tested in the standard battery of mutagenesis assays, in the presence and absence of metabolic activation.

Use with Ribavirin: See ribavirin labeling for additional warnings relevant to PegIntron therapy in combination with ribavirin.

Impairment of Fertility

PegIntron may impair human fertility. Irregular menstrual cycles were observed in female cynomolgus monkeys given subcutaneous injections of 4239 mcg/m² PegIntron alone every other day for 1 month (approximately 345 times the recommended weekly human dose based upon body surface area). These effects included transiently decreased serum levels of estradiol and progesterone, suggestive of anovulation. Normal menstrual cycles and serum hormone levels resumed in these animals 2 to 3 months following cessation of PegIntron treatment. Every other day dosing with 262 mcg/m² (approximately 21 times the weekly human dose) had no effects on cycle duration or reproductive hormone status. The effects of PegIntron on male fertility have not been studied.

14 CLINICAL STUDIES

14.1 Chronic Hepatitis C in Adults

PegIntron Monotherapy — Study 1

A randomized trial compared treatment with PegIntron (0.5, 1, or 1.5 mcg/kg once weekly subcutaneously) to treatment with INTRON A (3 million units 3 times weekly subcutaneously) in 1219 adults with chronic hepatitis from HCV infection. The subjects were not previously treated with interferon alpha, had compensated liver disease, detectable HCV-RNA, elevated ALT, and liver histopathology consistent with chronic hepatitis. Subjects were treated for 48 weeks and were followed for 24 weeks post-treatment.

Seventy percent of all subjects were infected with HCV genotype 1, and 74 percent of all subjects had high baseline levels of HCV-RNA (more than 2 million copies per mL of serum), two factors known to predict poor response to treatment.

Response to treatment was defined as undetectable HCV-RNA and normalization of ALT at 24 weeks post-treatment. The response rates to the 1 and 1.5 mcg/kg PegIntron doses were similar (approximately 24%) to each other and were both higher than the response rate to INTRON A (12%) (see *Table 13*).

[See table 13 above]

Subjects with both viral genotype 1 and high serum levels of HCV-RNA at baseline were less likely to respond to treatment with PegIntron. Among subjects with the two unfavorable prognostic variables, 8% (12/157) responded to PegIntron treatment and 2% (4/169) responded to INTRON A. Doses of PegIntron higher than the recommended dose did not result in higher response rates in these subjects. Subjects receiving PegIntron with viral genotype 1 had a response rate of 14% (28/199) while subjects with other viral genotypes had a 45% (43/96) response rate.

Table 13: Rates of Response to Treatment – Study 1

	A PegIntron 0.5 mcg/kg (N=315)	B PegIntron 1 mcg/kg (N=298)	C INTRON A 3 MIU three times weekly (N=307)	B - C (95% CI) Difference between PegIntron 1 mcg/kg and INTRON A
Treatment Response (Combined Virologic Response and ALT Normalization)	17%	24%	12%	11 (5, 18)
Virologic Response*	18%	25%	12%	12 (6, 19)
ALT Normalization	24%	29%	18%	11 (5, 18)

* Serum HCV is measured by a research-based quantitative polymerase chain reaction assay by a central laboratory.

Table 15: SVR Rates by Treatment and Baseline Weight – Study 3

| Treatment Group | Subject Baseline Weight | | | |
	<65 kg (<143 lb)	65-85 kg (143-188 lb)	>85-105 kg (>188-231 lb)	>105 kg (>231 lb)
WBD*	50% (173/348)	45% (449/994)	42% (351/835)	47% (138/292)
Flat	51% (173/342)	44% (443/1011)	39% (318/819)	33% (91/272)

* *P*=0.01, primary efficacy comparison (based on data from subjects weighing 65 kg or higher at baseline and utilizing a logistic regression analysis that includes treatment [WBD or Flat], genotype and presence/absence of advanced fibrosis, in the model).

Ninety-six percent of the responders in the PegIntron groups and 100% of responders in the INTRON A group first cleared their viral RNA by Week 24 of treatment [see *Dosage and Administration (2.1)*].

The treatment response rates were similar in men and women. Response rates were lower in African-American and Hispanic subjects and higher in Asians compared to Caucasians. Although African Americans had a higher proportion of poor prognostic factors compared to Caucasians, the number of non-Caucasians studied (9% of the total) was insufficient to allow meaningful conclusions about differences in response rates after adjusting for prognostic factors.

Liver biopsies were obtained before and after treatment in 60% of subjects. A modest reduction in inflammation compared to baseline that was similar in all 4 treatment groups was observed.

PegIntron/REBETOL Combination Therapy — Study 2

A randomized trial compared treatment with two PegIntron/REBETOL regimens [PegIntron 1.5 mcg/kg subcutaneously once weekly/REBETOL 800 mg orally daily (in divided doses); PegIntron 1.5 mcg/kg subcutaneously once weekly for 4 weeks then 0.5 mcg/kg subcutaneously once weekly for 44 weeks/REBETOL 1000 or 1200 mg orally daily (in divided doses)] with INTRON A [3 MIU subcutaneously thrice weekly/REBETOL 1000 or 1200 mg orally daily (in divided doses)] in 1530 adults with chronic hepatitis C. Interferon-naïve subjects were treated for 48 weeks and followed for 24 weeks post-treatment. Eligible subjects had compensated liver disease, detectable HCV-RNA, elevated ALT, and liver histopathology consistent with chronic hepatitis.

Response to treatment was defined as undetectable HCV-RNA at 24 weeks post-treatment. The response rate to the PegIntron 1.5 mcg/kg plus REBETOL 800 mg dose was higher than the response rate to INTRON A/REBETOL (see *Table 14*). The response rate to PegIntron 1.5→0.5 mcg/kg/REBETOL was essentially the same as the response to INTRON A/REBETOL (data not shown).

Table 14: Rates of Response to Treatment – Study 2

	PegIntron 1.5 mcg/kg once weekly REBETOL 800 mg daily	INTRON A 3 MIU three times weekly REBETOL 1000/ 1200 mg daily
Overall response *†	52% (264/511)	46% (231/505)
Genotype 1	41% (141/348)	33% (112/343)
Genotype 2-6	75% (123/163)	73% (119/162)

* Serum HCV-RNA is measured with a research-based quantitative polymerase chain reaction assay by a central laboratory.

† Difference in overall treatment response (PegIntron/ REBETOL vs. INTRON A/REBETOL) is 6% with 95% confidence interval of (0.18, 11.63) adjusted for viral genotype and presence of cirrhosis at baseline. Response to treatment was defined as undetectable HCV-RNA at 24 weeks post-treatment.

Subjects with viral genotype 1, regardless of viral load, had a lower response rate to PegIntron (1.5 mcg/kg)/REBETOL (800 mg) compared to subjects with other viral genotypes. Subjects with both poor prognostic factors (genotype 1 and high viral load) had a response rate of 30% (78/256) compared to a response rate of 29% (71/247) with INTRON A/REBETOL.

Subjects with lower body weight tended to have higher adverse reaction rates [see *Adverse Reactions (6.1)*] and higher response rates than subjects with higher body weights. Differences in response rates between treatment arms did not substantially vary with body weight.

Treatment response rates with PegIntron/REBETOL were 49% in men and 56% in women. Response rates were lower in African American and Hispanic subjects and higher in Asians compared to Caucasians. Although African Americans had a higher proportion of poor prognostic factors compared to Caucasians, the number of non-Caucasians studied (11% of the total) was insufficient to allow meaningful conclusions about differences in response rates after adjusting for prognostic factors in this trial.

Liver biopsies were obtained before and after treatment in 68% of subjects. Compared to baseline, approximately two-thirds of subjects in all treatment groups were observed to have a modest reduction in inflammation.

PegIntron/REBETOL Combination Therapy — Study 3

In a large United States community-based trial, 4913 subjects with chronic hepatitis C were randomized to receive PegIntron 1.5 mcg/kg subcutaneously once weekly in combination with a REBETOL dose of 800 to 1400 mg (weight-based dosing [WBD]) or 800 mg (flat) orally daily (in divided doses) for 24 or 48 weeks based on genotype. Response to treatment was defined as undetectable HCV-RNA (based on an assay with a lower limit of detection of 125 IU/mL) at 24 weeks post-treatment.

Treatment with PegIntron 1.5 mcg/kg and REBETOL 800 to 1400 mg resulted in a higher sustained virologic response compared to PegIntron in combination with a flat 800 mg daily dose of REBETOL. Subjects weighing greater than 105 kg obtained the greatest benefit with WBD, although a modest benefit was also observed in subjects weighing greater than 85 to 105 kg (see *Table 15*). The benefit of WBD in subjects weighing greater than 85 kg was observed with HCV genotypes 1-3. Insufficient data were available to reach conclusions regarding other genotypes. Use of WBD resulted in an increased incidence of anemia [see *Adverse Reactions (6.1)*].

[See table 15 above]

A total of 1552 subjects weighing greater than 65 kg in Study 3 had genotype 2 or 3 and were randomized to 24 or 48 weeks of therapy. No additional benefit was observed with the longer treatment duration.

PegIntron/REBETOL Combination Therapy — Study 4

A large randomized trial compared the safety and efficacy of treatment for 48 weeks with two PegIntron/REBETOL regimens [PegIntron 1.5 mcg/kg and 1 mcg/kg subcutaneously once weekly both in combination with REBETOL 800 to 1400 mg PO daily (in two divided doses)] and Pegasys

Table 17: SVR Rates by Baseline Characteristics of Prior Treatment Failures

HCV Genotype/ Metavir Fibrosis Score	Overall SVR by Previous Response and Treatment			
	Nonresponder		Relapser	
	alfa interferon/ ribavirin % (number of subjects)	peginterferon (2a and 2b combined)/ ribavirin % (number of subjects)	alfa interferon/ ribavirin % (number of subjects)	peginterferon (2a and 2b combined)/ ribavirin % (number of subjects)
Overall	18 (158/903)	6 (30/476)	43 (130/300)	35 (113/344)
HCV 1	13 (98/761)	4 (19/431)	32 (67/208)	23 (56/243)
F2	18 (36/202)	6 (7/117)	42 (33/79)	32 (23/72)
F3	16 (38/233)	4 (4/112)	28 (16/58)	21 (14/67)
F4	7 (24/325)	4 (8/202)	26 (18/70)	18 (19/104)
HCV 2/3	49 (53/109)	36 (10/28)	67 (54/81)	57 (52/92)
F2	68 (23/34)	56 (5/9)	76 (19/25)	61 (11/18)
F3	39 (11/28)	38 (3/8)	67 (18/27)	62 (18/29)
F4	40 (19/47)	18 (2/11)	59 (17/29)	51 (23/45)
HCV 4	17 (5/29)	7 (1/15)	88 (7/8)	50 (4/8)

180 mcg subcutaneously once weekly in combination with Copegus 1000 to 1200 mg PO daily (in two divided doses) in 3070 treatment-naïve adults with chronic hepatitis C genotype 1. In this trial, lack of early virologic response (undetectable HCV-RNA or greater than or equal to 2 $\log_{10}$ reduction from baseline) by treatment Week 12 was the criterion for discontinuation of treatment. SVR was defined as undetectable HCV-RNA (Roche COBAS TaqMan assay, a lower limit of quantitation of 27 IU/mL) at 24 weeks post-treatment (see **Table 16**).

Table 16: SVR Rates by Treatment – Study 4

	PegIntron 1.5 mcg/kg/ REBETOL	PegIntron 1 mcg/kg/ REBETOL	Pegasys 180 mcg/ Copegus
SVR	40% (406/ 1019)	38% (386/ 1016)	41% (423/ 1035)

Overall SVR rates were similar among the three treatment groups. Regardless of treatment group, SVR rates were lower in subjects with poor prognostic factors. Subjects with poor prognostic factors randomized to PegIntron (1.5 mcg/kg)/REBETOL or Pegasys/Copegus, however, achieved higher SVR rates compared to similar subjects randomized to PegIntron 1 mcg/kg/REBETOL. For the PegIntron 1.5 mcg/kg plus REBETOL dose, SVR rates for subjects with and without the following prognostic factors were as follows: cirrhosis (10% vs. 42%), normal ALT levels (32% vs. 42%), baseline viral load greater than 600,000 IU/mL (35% vs. 61%), 40 years of age and older (38% vs. 50%), and African American race (23% vs. 44%). In subjects with undetectable HCV-RNA at Week 12 who received PegIntron (1.5 mcg/kg)/REBETOL, the SVR rate was 81% (328/407).

PegIntron/REBETOL Combination Therapy in Prior Treatment Failures — Study 5
In a noncomparative trial, 2293 subjects with moderate to severe fibrosis who failed previous treatment with combination alpha interferon/ribavirin were re-treated with PegIntron, 1.5 mcg/kg subcutaneously, once weekly, in combination with weight adjusted ribavirin. Eligible subjects included prior nonresponders (subjects who were HCV-RNA positive at the end of a minimum 12 weeks of treatment) and prior relapsers (subjects who were HCV-RNA negative at the end of a minimum 12 weeks of treatment and subsequently relapsed after post-treatment follow-up). Subjects who were negative at Week 12 were treated for 48 weeks and followed for 24 weeks post-treatment. Response to treatment was defined as undetectable HCV-RNA at 24 weeks post-treatment (measured using a research-based test, limit of detection 125 IU/mL). The overall response rate was 22% (497/2293) (99% CI: 19.5, 23.9). Subjects with the following characteristics were less likely to benefit from re-treatment: previous nonresponse, previous pegylated interferon treatment, significant bridging fibrosis or cirrhosis, and genotype 1 infection.
The re-treatment sustained virologic response rates by baseline characteristics are summarized in **Table 17**.
[See table 17 above]

Achievement of an undetectable HCV-RNA at treatment Week 12 was a strong predictor of SVR. In this trial, 1470 (64%) subjects did not achieve an undetectable HCV-RNA at treatment Week 12, and were offered enrollment into long-term treatment trials, due to an inadequate treatment response. Of the 823 (36%) subjects who were HCV-RNA undetectable at treatment Week 12, those infected with genotype 1 had an SVR of 48% (245/507), with a range of responses by fibrosis scores (F4-F2) of 39-55%. Subjects infected with genotype 2/3 who were HCV-RNA undetectable at treatment Week 12 had an overall SVR of 70% (196/281), with a range of responses by fibrosis scores (F4-F2) of 60-83%. For all genotypes, higher fibrosis scores were associated with a decreased likelihood of achieving SVR.

14.2 Chronic Hepatitis C in Pediatrics
PegIntron/REBETOL Combination Therapy — Pediatric Trial
Previously untreated pediatric subjects 3 to 17 years of age with compensated chronic hepatitis C and detectable HCV-RNA were treated with REBETOL 15 mg/kg/day plus PegIntron 60 mcg/m² once weekly for 24 or 48 weeks based on HCV genotype and baseline viral load. All subjects were to be followed for 24 weeks post-treatment. A total of 107 subjects received treatment, of which 52% were female, 89% were Caucasian, and 67% were infected with HCV genotype 1. Subjects infected with genotype 1, 4 or genotype 3 with HCV-RNA greater than or equal to 600,000 IU/mL received 48 weeks of therapy while those infected with genotype 2 or genotype 3 with HCV-RNA less than 600,000 IU/mL received 24 weeks of therapy. The trial results are summarized in **Table 18**.

Table 18: SVR Rates by Genotype and Treatment Duration – Pediatric Trial

	All Subjects N=107	
	24 Weeks	48 Weeks
	Virologic Response N* † (%)	Virologic Response N* † (%)
Genotype		
All	26/27 (96.3)	44/80 (55.0)
1	—	38/72 (52.8)
2	14/15 (93.3)	—
3‡	12/12 (100)	2/3 (66.7)
4	—	4/5 (80.0)

* Response to treatment was defined as undetectable HCV-RNA at 24 weeks post-treatment.
† N = number of responders/number of subjects with given genotype, and assigned treatment duration.
‡ Subjects with genotype 3 low viral load (less than 600,000 IU/mL) were to receive 24 weeks of treatment while those with genotype 3 and high viral load were to receive 48 weeks of treatment.

15 REFERENCES

1. Ge, D., Fellay, J., Thompson, A.J., Simon, J.S., Shianna, K.V., Urban, T.J., Heinzen, E.L., Qiu, P., Bertelsen, A.H., Muir, A.J., Sulkowski, M., McHutchison, J.G., Goldstein, D.B., Genetic variation in IL28B predicts hepatitis C treatment-induced viral clearance, Nature 2009;461(7262):399-401.
2. Thompson, A.J., Muir, A.J., Sulkowski, M.S., Ge, D., Fellay, J., Shianna, K.V., Urban, T., Afdhal, N.H., Jacobson, I.M., Esteban, R., Poordad, F., Lawitz, E.J., McCone, J., Shiffman, M.L., Galler, G.W., Lee, W.M., Reindollar, R., King, J.W., Kwo, P.Y., Ghalib, R.H., Freilich, B., Nyberg, L.M., Zeuzem, S., Poynard, T., Vock, D.M., Pieper, K.S., Patel, K., Tillmann, H.L., Noviello, S., Koury, K., Pedicone, L.D., Brass, C.A., Albrecht, J.K., Goldstein, D.B., McHutchison, J.G., Interlukin-28B polymorphism improves viral kinetics and is the strongest pretreatment predictor of sustained virologic response in genotype 1 hepatitis C virus, Gastroenterology 2010;139:120-129.

16 HOW SUPPLIED/STORAGE AND HANDLING
PegIntron REDIPEN

Each PegIntron REDIPEN Package Contains:	
A box containing one 50 mcg per 0.5 mL PegIntron REDIPEN and 1 BD needle and 2 alcohol swabs.	(NDC 0085-1323-01)
A box containing one 80 mcg per 0.5 mL PegIntron REDIPEN and 1 BD needle and 2 alcohol swabs.	(NDC 0085-1316-01)
A box containing one 120 mcg per 0.5 mL PegIntron REDIPEN and 1 BD needle and 2 alcohol swabs.	(NDC 0085-1297-01)
A box containing one 150 mcg per 0.5 mL PegIntron REDIPEN and 1 BD needle and 2 alcohol swabs.	(NDC 0085-1370-01)

Each PegIntron REDIPEN PAK 4 Contains:	
A box containing four 50 mcg per 0.5 mL PegIntron REDIPEN Units, each containing 1 BD needle and 2 alcohol swabs.	(NDC 0085-1323-02)
A box containing four 80 mcg per 0.5 mL PegIntron REDIPEN Units, each containing 1 BD needle and 2 alcohol swabs.	(NDC 0085-1316-02)
A box containing four 120 mcg per 0.5 mL PegIntron REDIPEN Units, each containing 1 BD needle and 2 alcohol swabs.	(NDC 0085-1297-02)
A box containing four 150 mcg per 0.5 mL PegIntron REDIPEN Units, each containing 1 BD needle and 2 alcohol swabs.	(NDC 0085-1370-02)

PegIntron Vials

Each PegIntron Package Contains:	
A box containing one 50 mcg per 0.5 mL vial of PegIntron Powder for Injection and one 1.25 mL vial of Diluent (Sterile Water for Injection USP), 2 BD Safety Lok syringes with a safety sleeve and 2 alcohol swabs.	(NDC 0085-1368-01)
A box containing one 80 mcg per 0.5 mL vial of PegIntron Powder for Injection and one 1.25 mL vial of Diluent (Sterile Water for Injection USP), 2 BD Safety Lok syringes with a safety sleeve and 2 alcohol swabs.	(NDC 0085-1291-01)
A box containing one 120 mcg per 0.5 mL vial of PegIntron Powder for Injection and one 1.25 mL vial of Diluent (Sterile Water for Injection USP), 2 BD Safety Lok syringes with a safety sleeve and 2 alcohol swabs.	(NDC 0085-1304-01)

A box containing one 150 mcg per 0.5 mL vial of PegIntron Powder for Injection and one 1.25 mL vial of Diluent (Sterile Water for Injection USP), 2 BD Safety Lok syringes with a safety sleeve and 2 alcohol swabs.	(NDC 0085-1279-01)

Storage

PegIntron REDIPEN single-use pre-filled pen
PegIntron REDIPEN pre-filled pen should be stored at 2-8°C (36-46°F).
After reconstitution, the solution should be used immediately, but may be stored up to 24 hours at 2-8°C (36-46°F). The reconstituted solution contains no preservative, and is clear and colorless. **DO NOT FREEZE. Keep away from heat.**
PegIntron Vials
PegIntron should be stored at 25°C (77°F); excursions permitted to 15-30°C (59-86°F) [see USP Controlled Room Temperature]. After reconstitution with supplied diluent, the solution should be used immediately but may be stored up to 24 hours at 2-8°C (36-46°F). The reconstituted solution contains no preservative, and is clear and colorless. **DO NOT FREEZE. Keep away from heat.**

Disposal Instructions

Patients should be thoroughly instructed in the importance of proper disposal. After preparation and administration of PegIntron for Injection, patients should be advised to use a puncture-resistant container for the disposal of used syringes, needles, and the REDIPEN pre-filled pen. The full container should be disposed of in accordance with state and local laws. Patients should also be cautioned against reusing or sharing needles, syringes, or the REDIPEN pre-filled pen.

17   PATIENT COUNSELING INFORMATION

• Advise the patient to read the FDA-approved patient labeling (Medication Guide and Instructions for Use)
A patient who self-inject PegIntron only if it has been determined that it is appropriate, the patient agrees to medical follow-up as necessary, and training in proper injection technique has been given to him/her.

Pregnancy

Patients must be informed that REBETOL (ribavirin) may cause birth defects and death of the unborn child. Extreme care must be taken to avoid pregnancy in female patients and in female partners of male patients during treatment with combination PegIntron/ribavirin therapy and for 6 months post-therapy. Combination PegIntron/ribavirin therapy should not be initiated until a report of a negative pregnancy test has been obtained immediately prior to initiation of therapy. It is recommended that patients undergo monthly pregnancy tests during therapy and for 6 months post-therapy *[see Contraindications (4), Use in Specific Populations (8.1), and ribavirin labeling].*

HCV Transmission

Inform patients that there are no data regarding whether PegIntron therapy will prevent transmission of HCV infection to others. Also, it is not known if treatment with PegIntron will cure hepatitis C or prevent cirrhosis, liver failure, or liver cancer that may be the result of infection with the hepatitis C virus.

Laboratory Evaluations, Hydration, "Flu-like" Symptoms

Patients should be advised that laboratory evaluations are required before starting therapy and periodically thereafter *[see Warnings and Precautions (5.15)]*. It is advised that patients be well hydrated, especially during the initial stages of treatment. "Flu-like" symptoms associated with administration of PegIntron may be minimized by bedtime administration of PegIntron or by use of antipyretics.
Patients developing fever, cough, shortness of breath or other symptoms of a lung problem during treatment with PegIntron may need to have a chest X-ray or other tests to adequately treat them.

Instructions for Use

Patients receiving PegIntron should be directed in its appropriate preparation, handling, measurement, and injection, and referred to the Instructions for Use for PegIntron Powder for Solution and PegIntron REDIPEN Single-use Pre-filled pen.
Patients should be directed to store PegIntron before mixing as follows:
• PegIntron REDIPEN single-use pre-filled pens: store in the refrigerator between 36-46°F (2-8°C)
• PegIntron Powder for Solution: store at room temperature between 59-86°F (15-30°C)
Patients should be instructed on the importance of site selection for self-administering the injection, as well as the importance on rotating the injection sites.

Manufactured by: Schering Corporation, a subsidiary of
MERCK & CO., INC., Whitehouse Station, NJ 08889, USA
For patent information:
www.merck.com/product/patent/home.html

BD and Safety-Lok are registered trademarks of Becton, Dickinson and Company.
Copyright © 2001, 2013 Schering Corporation, a subsidiary of Merck & Co., Inc.
All rights reserved.
uspi-mk4031-mf-1407r077

MEDICATION GUIDE

PegIntron® (peg-In-tron)
(Peginterferon alfa-2b) for injection, for subcutaneous use
Read this Medication Guide before you start taking PegIntron®, and each time you get a refill. There may be new information. This information does not take the place of talking with your healthcare provider about your medical condition or your treatment.

If you are taking PegIntron with REBETOL (ribavirin) with or without an approved hepatitis C virus (HCV) protease inhibitor, also read the Medication Guides for those medicines.

PegIntron, by itself or in combination with other approved medicines, is a treatment for some people who are infected with hepatitis C virus.

What is the most important information I should know about PegIntron?

PegIntron can cause serious side effects that:
• **may cause death, or**
• **may worsen certain serious diseases that you may already have.**

Tell your healthcare provider right away if you have any of the symptoms listed below while taking PegIntron. If symptoms get worse, or become severe and continue, your healthcare provider may tell you to stop taking PegIntron permanently. In many, but not all, people, these symptoms go away after they stop taking PegIntron.

1. **Mental health problems and suicide.** PegIntron may cause you to develop mood or behavior problems that may get worse during treatment with PegIntron or after your last dose, including:
   • irritability (getting upset easily)
   • depression (feeling low, feeling bad about yourself, or feeling hopeless)
   • aggressive behavior
   • thoughts of hurting yourself or others, or suicide
   • former drug addicts may fall back into drug addiction or overdose
   If you have these symptoms, your healthcare provider should carefully monitor you during treatment with PegIntron and for 6 months after your last dose.

2. **Heart problems.** Some people who take PegIntron may get heart problems, including:
   • low blood pressure
   • fast heart rate or abnormal heart beat
   • trouble breathing or chest pain
   • heart attacks or heart muscle problems (cardiomyopathy)

3. **Stroke or symptoms of a stroke. Symptoms may include weakness, loss of coordination, and numbness.** Stroke or symptoms of a stroke may happen in people who have some risk factors **or** no known risk factors for a stroke.

4. **New or worsening autoimmune problems.** Some people taking PegIntron develop autoimmune problems (a condition where the body's immune cells attack other cells or organs in the body), including rheumatoid arthritis, systemic lupus erythematosus, and psoriasis. In some people who already have an autoimmune problem, it may get worse during your treatment with PegIntron.

5. **Infections.** Some people who take PegIntron may get an infection. Symptoms may include:
   • fever
   • chills
   • bloody diarrhea
   • burning or pain with urination
   • urinating often
   • coughing up mucus (phlegm) that is discolored (for example, yellow or pink)

PegIntron in combination with REBETOL (ribavirin) may cause birth defects or the death of your unborn baby. Do not take PegIntron and ribavirin combination therapy if you or your sexual partner is pregnant or plan to become pregnant. Do not become pregnant within 6 months after discontinuing PegIntron and ribavirin combination therapy. You must use 2 forms of birth control when you take PegIntron and ribavirin and for the 6 months after treatment.
• Females must have a pregnancy test before starting PegIntron and ribavirin combination therapy, every month while on the combination therapy, and every month for the 6 months after the last dose of combination therapy.
• If you or your female sexual partner becomes pregnant while taking PegIntron and ribavirin combination therapy or within 6 months after you stop taking the combination therapy, tell your healthcare provider right away. You or your healthcare provider should contact the Ribavirin pregnancy registry by calling 1-800-593-2214. The

Ribavirin pregnancy registry collects information about what happens to mothers and their babies if the mother takes ribavirin while she is pregnant.
While taking PegIntron, you should see a healthcare provider regularly for check-ups and blood tests to make sure that your treatment is working, and to check for side effects.

What is PegIntron?

PegIntron is a prescription medicine that is used:
• with REBETOL (ribavirin) and an approved hepatitis C virus (HCV) protease inhibitor to treat chronic (lasting a long time) hepatitis C infection in adults.
• with REBETOL (ribavirin) to treat chronic (lasting a long time) hepatitis C infection in people 3 years and older with stable liver problems.
• alone, sometimes to treat adults who have chronic (lasting a long time) hepatitis C infection with stable liver problems and who can not take REBETOL (ribavirin).
People with hepatitis C have the virus in their blood and in their liver. PegIntron reduces the amount of virus in the body and helps the body's immune system fight the virus. REBETOL (ribavirin) is a drug that helps to fight the viral infection but does not work when used by itself to treat chronic hepatitis C.
It is not known if PegIntron use for longer than 1 year is safe and will work.
It is not known if PegIntron use in children younger than 3 years old is safe and will work.

Who should not take PegIntron?

Do not take PegIntron:
• if you have had a serious allergic reaction to another alpha interferon or to any of the ingredients in PegIntron. See the end of this Medication Guide for a complete list of ingredients. Ask your healthcare provider if you are not sure.
• if you have certain types of hepatitis (autoimmune hepatitis).
• if you have certain other liver problems.
• with REBETOL (ribavirin) if you are pregnant, planning to get pregnant, or breastfeeding. See "What is the most important information I should know about PegIntron?"
Talk to your healthcare provider before taking PegIntron if you have any of these conditions.

What should I tell my healthcare provider before taking PegIntron?

Before you take PegIntron, see "What is the most important information I should know about PegIntron?", and tell your healthcare provider if you:
• are being treated for a mental illness or had treatment in the past for any mental illness, including depression and suicidal behavior
• have or ever had any problems with your heart, including heart attack or high blood pressure
• have any kind of autoimmune disease (where the body's immune system attacks the body's own cells), such as psoriasis, systemic lupus erythematosus, rheumatoid arthritis
• have or ever had bleeding problems or a blood clot
• have or ever had low blood cell counts
• have ever been addicted to drugs or alcohol
• have liver disease (other than hepatitis C infection)
• have or had lung disease such as chronic obstructive pulmonary disease (COPD)
• have thyroid problems
• have diabetes
• have colitis (inflammation of your intestine)
• have a condition that suppresses your immune system, such as cancer
• have hepatitis B infection
• have HIV infection
• have kidney problems
• have high blood triglyceride levels (fat in your blood)
• have an organ transplant and are taking medicine that keeps your body from rejecting your transplant (suppresses your immune system)
• have any other medical conditions
• are pregnant or plan to become pregnant. PegIntron may harm your unborn baby. You should use effective birth control during treatment with PegIntron. Talk to your healthcare provider about birth control choices for you during treatment with PegIntron. Tell your healthcare provider if you become pregnant during treatment with PegIntron.
• are breastfeeding or plan to breastfeed. It is not known if PegIntron passes into your breast milk. You and your healthcare provider should decide if you will use PegIntron or breastfeed.

Tell your healthcare provider about all the medicines you take, including prescription and non-prescription medicines, vitamins, and herbal supplements. PegIntron and certain other medicines may affect each other and cause side effects.

Especially tell your healthcare provider if you take the anti-hepatitis B medicine telbivudine (Tyzeka).
Know the medicines you take. Keep a list of them and show it to your healthcare provider and pharmacist when you get a new medicine.

How should I take PegIntron?

- Take PegIntron exactly as your healthcare provider tells you to. Your healthcare provider will tell you how much PegIntron to take and when to take it. Do not take more than your prescribed dose.
- Take your prescribed dose of PegIntron every week, on the same day of each week and at the same time.
- PegIntron is given as an injection under your skin (subcutaneous injection). Your healthcare provider should show you how to prepare and measure your dose of PegIntron, and how to inject yourself before you use PegIntron for the first time.
- You should not inject PegIntron until your healthcare provider has shown you how to use PegIntron the right way.
- PegIntron comes as a:
  - powder in a single-use vial
  - single-use REDIPEN

Your healthcare provider will prescribe the PegIntron that is right for you. See the Instructions for Use that comes with your PegIntron for detailed instructions for preparing and injecting a dose of PegIntron.
- If you miss a dose of PegIntron, take the missed dose as soon as possible during the same day or the next day, then continue on your regular dosing schedule. If several days go by after you miss a dose, check with your healthcare provider about what to do.
- Do not inject more than 1 dose of PegIntron in one week without talking to your healthcare provider.
- If you take too much PegIntron, call your healthcare provider right away. Your healthcare provider may examine you more closely, and do blood tests.
- Your healthcare provider should do regular blood tests before you start PegIntron, and during treatment to see how well the treatment is working and to check you for side effects.

What are the possible side effects of PegIntron?

PegIntron may cause serious side effects including:

See "What is the most important information I should know about PegIntron?"

- **Serious eye problems.** PegIntron may cause eye problems that may lead to vision loss or blindness. You should have an eye exam before you start taking PegIntron. If you have eye problems or have had them in the past, you may need eye exams while you are taking PegIntron. Tell your healthcare provider or eye doctor right away if you have any vision changes while taking PegIntron.
- **Blood problems.** PegIntron can affect your bone marrow and cause low white blood cell and platelet counts. In some people, these blood counts may fall to dangerously low levels. If your blood counts become very low, you can get infections, and problems with bleeding and bruising.
- **Swelling of your pancreas (pancreatitis) or intestines (colitis).**
  Symptoms may include:
  - severe stomach area (abdomen) pain
  - severe back pain
  - nausea and vomiting
  - bloody diarrhea
  - fever
- **Lung problems including:**
  - trouble breathing
  - pneumonia
  - inflammation of lung tissue
  - new or worse high blood pressure of the lungs (pulmonary hypertension). This can be severe and may lead to death.
  You may need to have a chest X-ray or other tests if you develop fever, cough, shortness of breath or other symptoms of a lung problem during treatment with PegIntron.
- **Severe liver problems, or worsening of liver problems, including liver failure and death.** Symptoms may include:
  - nausea
  - loss of appetite
  - tiredness
  - diarrhea
  - yellowing of your skin or the white part of your eyes
  - bleeding more easily than normal
  - swelling of your stomach area (abdomen)
  - confusion
  - sleepiness
  - you cannot be awakened (coma)
- **Thyroid problems.** Some people develop changes in their thyroid function. Symptoms of thyroid changes include:
  - problems concentrating
  - feeling cold or hot all of the time
  - weight changes
  - skin changes
- **Blood sugar problems.** Some people may develop high blood sugar or diabetes. If you have high blood sugar or diabetes that is not controlled before starting PegIntron, talk to your healthcare provider before you take PegIntron. If you develop high blood sugar or diabetes while taking PegIntron, your healthcare provider may tell you to stop PegIntron and prescribe a different medicine for you. Symptoms of high blood sugar or diabetes may include:

- increased thirst
- tiredness
- urinating more often than normal
- increased appetite
- weight loss
- your breath smells like fruit
- **Serious allergic reactions and skin reactions. Symptoms may include:**
  - itching
  - swelling of the face, eyes, lips, tongue, or throat
  - trouble breathing
  - anxiousness
  - chest pain
  - feeling faint
  - skin rash, hives, sores in your mouth, or your skin blisters and peels
- **Growth problems in children.** Weight loss and slowed growth are common in children during combination treatment with PegIntron and REBETOL. Most children will go through a growth spurt and gain weight after treatment stops. Some children may not reach the height that they were expected to have before treatment. Talk to your healthcare provider if you are concerned about your child's growth during treatment with PegIntron and REBETOL.
- **Nerve problems.** People who take PegIntron or other alpha interferon products with telbivudine (Tyzeka) can develop nerve problems such as continuing numbness, tingling, or burning sensation in the arms or legs (peripheral neuropathy). Call your healthcare provider if you have any of these symptoms.
- **Dental and gum problems.**

Tell your healthcare provider right away if you have any of the symptoms listed above.

The most common side effects of PegIntron include:

- **Flu-like symptoms.** Symptoms may include: headache, muscle aches, tiredness, and fever. Some of these symptoms may be decreased by injecting your PegIntron dose at bedtime. Talk to your healthcare provider about which over-the-counter medicines you can take to help prevent or decrease some of these symptoms.
- **Tiredness.** Many people become very tired during treatment with PegIntron.
- **Appetite problems.** Nausea, loss of appetite, and weight loss can happen with PegIntron.
- **Skin reactions.** Redness, swelling, and itching are common at the site of injection.
- **Hair thinning.**

Tell your healthcare provider if you have any side effect that bothers you or that does not go away.

These are not all of the possible side effects of PegIntron. For more information, ask your healthcare provider or pharmacist.

Call your doctor for medical advice about side effects. You may report side effects to FDA at 1–800–FDA–1088.

How should I store PegIntron?

- Before mixing, store PegIntron single-use REDIPEN in the refrigerator between 36°F to 46°F (2°C to 8°C).
- Before mixing, store PegIntron vials at room temperature between 68°F to 77°F (20°C to 25°C).
- Keep PegIntron away from heat.
- After mixing, use PegIntron right away or store it in the refrigerator for up to 24 hours between 36°F to 46°F (2°C to 8°C).
- Do not freeze PegIntron.
- **Keep PegIntron and all medicines out of the reach of children.**

General Information about PegIntron

Medicines are sometimes prescribed for purposes other than those listed in a Medication Guide. Do not use PegIntron for a condition for which it was not prescribed. Do not give PegIntron to other people, even if they have the same symptoms that you have. It may harm them.

This Medication Guide summarizes the most important information about PegIntron. If you would like more information, ask your healthcare provider. You can ask your healthcare provider or pharmacist for information about PegIntron that was written for healthcare professionals.

For more information, go to www.PegIntron.com or call 1-800-526-4099.

What are the ingredients in PegIntron?

Active ingredients: peginterferon alfa-2b

Inactive ingredients: dibasic sodium phosphate anhydrous, monobasic sodium phosphate dihydrate, sucrose, polysorbate 80. Sterile water for injection is supplied as a diluent.

This Medication Guide has been approved by the U.S. Food and Drug Administration.

Manufactured by: Schering Corporation, a subsidiary of **MERCK & CO., INC.**, Whitehouse Station, NJ 08889, USA.

Revised: 07/2014

For patent information:
www.merck.com/product/patent/home.html

Copyright © 2001, 2013 Schering Corporation, a subsidiary of **Merck & Co., Inc.**
All rights reserved.
usmg-mk4031-mf-1407r018

Instructions for Use

PegIntron® (peg-In-tron)
(Peginterferon alfa-2b)
REDIPEN® single-use pre-filled pen

This Instructions for Use is only for use with the REDIPEN single-use pre-filled pen. If your healthcare provider prescribes the Selectdose single-use pre-filled pen for you, use only those Instructions for Use.

Be sure that you read, understand, and follow these instructions before injecting PegIntron. Your healthcare provider should show you how to prepare and inject PegIntron properly using the REDIPEN single-use pre-filled pen before you use it for the first time. Ask your healthcare provider if you have any questions.

Important:
- Make sure that you have the correct strength of REDIPEN pre-filled pen prescribed by your healthcare provider.
- Throw away REDIPEN after you use it. **Do not re-use your pre-filled pen or needle.** See "Disposal of used needles and pre-filled pens" in this Instructions for Use.

Before starting, collect all of the supplies that you will need to use for preparing and injecting PegIntron. For each injection you will need a package that contains:
- 1 PegIntron REDIPEN single-use pre-filled pen
- 1 disposable needle
- 2 alcohol swabs
- dosing tray (the dosing tray is the bottom half of the REDIPEN package)
- You will need gauze or a cotton ball to press to the injection site after injecting. You will also need 1 sharps disposal container for throwing away your used pre-filled pen. See "Disposal of used needles and pre-filled pens" in this Instructions for Use.

The REDIPEN single-use pre-filled pen should only be used with the injection needle that comes in the package. If you use other needles, the pen may not work the right way.

- Figures A and B below show the different parts of the REDIPEN single-use pre-filled pen and the injection needle. Figure C below shows the dosing tray with the pre-filled pen. The parts of the pre-filled pen you need to know are:

PegIntron Redipen

Grip · Window · Dosing Tab · Rubber Membrane · Cartridge Holder · Pen Body · Dosing Button

Figure A

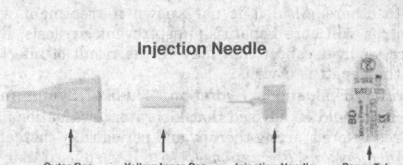

Injection Needle

Outer Cap · Yellow Inner Cap · Injection Needle · Paper Tab

Figure B

Figure C

How should I prepare a dose of PegIntron using the REDIPEN single-use pre-filled pen?

1. Find a clean, well-lit, flat work surface.
2. Take the pre-filled pen out of the refrigerator and allow the medicine to come to room temperature. Look at the date printed on the carton to make sure that the expiration date has not passed. Do not use if the expiration date has passed.

3. After taking the pre-filled pen out of the carton, look in the window of the pre-filled pen and make sure the PegIntron in the cartridge holder window is a white to off-white tablet that is whole, or in pieces, or powdered.
4. Wash your hands well with soap and water. It is important to keep your work area, your hands, and the injection site clean to decrease the risk of infection. See Figure D.

Figure D

Mix the PegIntron

5. **Place the pre-filled pen upright** in the dosing tray on a hard, flat, non-slip surface with the dosing button down. See Figure E. You may want to hold the pre-filled pen using the grip.

Figure E

6. To mix the powder and the liquid, keep the pre-filled pen upright in the dosing tray and press the top half of the pre-filled pen downward toward the hard, flat, non-slip surface **until you hear the "click" sound.** See Figure F. When you hear the click, you will notice in the window that both dark stoppers are now touching. The dosing button should be flat with the pen body.

Figure F

7. Wait several seconds for the powder to completely dissolve. Do not shake. If the solution does not dissolve, gently turn the pre-filled pen upside down two times. See Figure G.

Figure G

8. Keep the pre-filled pen **UPRIGHT**, with the dosing button down. Look through the pre-filled pen window to see that the mixed PegIntron solution is completely dissolved. The solution should be clear and colorless **before use**. It is normal to see some small bubbles in the pre-filled pen window, near the top of the solution. Do not use the REDIPEN pre-filled pen if the solution is discolored, or is not clear, or if it has particles in it.
9. Place the pre-filled pen back into the dosing tray provided in the packaging. See Figure H. The dosing button will be on the bottom.
[See figure H at top of next column]

Attach the Needle

10. Before you attach the needle to the pre-filled pen, wipe the rubber membrane of the pre-filled pen with an alcohol swab.
11. Remove the protective paper tab from the injection needle, but do not remove either the outer cap or the yellow inner cap from the injection needle.

Figure H

12. Keep the pre-filled pen upright in the dosing tray and push the injection needle straight into the pre-filled pen rubber membrane. Screw the needle onto the pre-filled pen by turning it in a clockwise direction. See Figure I.
   • Remember to leave the needle caps in place when you attach the needle to the pre-filled pen. Pushing the needle through the rubber membrane "primes" the needle and allows the extra liquid and air in the pen to be removed.

Figure I

NOTE: Some fluid will trickle out. This is **normal**. The dark stoppers move up and you will no longer see the fluid in the window once the needle is successfully primed.
   • Remove the outer clear needle cap on the pre-filled pen, but leave the yellow cap on. See Figure J.

Figure J

How should I set the dose prescribed by my healthcare provider?

Dial the Dose

13. Holding the pre-filled pen firmly, pull the dosing button out as far as it will go. See Figure K. You will see a dark band.
Do not push the dosing button in until you are ready to self-inject the PegIntron dose.

Figure K

14. Turn the dosing button until your prescribed dose is lined up with the dosing tab. See Figure L. The dosing button will turn freely. If you have trouble dialing your dose, check to make sure the dosing button has been pulled out **as far** as it will go. See Figure M.

Figure L   Figure M

15. Carefully lay the pre-filled pen down on the dosing tray or on a hard, flat, non-slip surface. Do not remove the yellow needle cap and do not push the dosing button in until you are ready to self-inject the PegIntron dose.

Choosing an Injection Site

The best sites for giving yourself an injection are those areas with a layer of fat between the skin and muscle, like your thigh, the outer surface of your upper arm, and abdomen. See Figure N. Do not inject yourself in the area near your belly-button (navel) or waistline. If you are very thin, you should only use the thigh or outer surface of the arm for injection.

Figure N

You should use a different site each time you inject PegIntron to avoid soreness at any one site. Do not inject PegIntron into an area where the skin is irritated, red, bruised, infected, or has scars, stretch marks, or lumps.

How should I Inject a dose of PegIntron?

16. Clean the skin where the injection is to be given with the second alcohol swab provided, and wait for the skin to dry.
17. There may be some liquid around the yellow inner needle cap. See Figure O. This is normal.

Figure O

18. Remove the **yellow** inner needle cap when the injection site is dry. See Figure P. You are now ready to inject.

Figure P

19. Hold the pre-filled pen with your fingers wrapped around the pen body barrel and your thumb on the dosing button. See Figure Q.

Figure Q

20. With your other hand, pinch the skin in the area you have cleaned for injection.
21. Insert the needle into the pinched skin at an angle of 45° to 90°. See Figure R.
[See figure at top of next column]
22. Press the dosing button down slowly and firmly until you can not push it any further. Keep your thumb pressed down on the dosing button for an additional 5 seconds to make sure that you get the complete dose.
23. Slowly release the dosing button and remove the needle from your skin.

Figure R

24. Gently press the injection site with a small bandage or sterile gauze if needed for a few seconds but do not massage the injection site. If there is bleeding, cover with an adhesive bandage. Do not recap the needle and do not reuse the pre-filled pen.

Disposal of the used needles and pre-filled pens

• Put your used needles and pre-filled pens in a FDA-cleared sharps disposal container right away after use. **Do not throw away (dispose of) loose needles and pre-filled pens in your household trash.**

• If you do not have a FDA-cleared sharps disposal container, you may use a household container that is:
  ◦ made of a heavy-duty plastic,
  ◦ can be closed with a tight-fitting, puncture-resistant lid, without sharps being able to come out,
  ◦ upright and stable during use,
  ◦ leak-resistant, and
  ◦ properly labeled to warn of hazardous waste inside the container.

• When your sharps disposal container is almost full, you will need to follow your community guidelines for the right way to dispose of your sharps disposal container. There may be state or local laws about how you should throw away used needles, syringes and pre-filled pens. For more information about safe sharps disposal, and for specific information about sharps disposal in the state that you live in, go to the FDA's website at: http://www.fda.gov/safesharpsdisposal.

• Do not dispose of your used sharps disposal container in your household trash unless your community guidelines permit this. Do not recycle your used sharps disposal container.

Always keep the sharps disposal container out of the reach of children.

How should I store PegIntron REDIPEN pre-filled pen?

• Before mixing, store PegIntron REDIPEN pre-filled pen in the refrigerator between 36°F to 46°F (2°C to 8°C).

• After mixing, use PegIntron right away or store it in the refrigerator for up to 24 hours between 36°F to 46°F (2°C to 8°C).

• Do not freeze PegIntron.

• Keep PegIntron away from heat.

Keep PegIntron and all medicines out of reach of children.
This Instructions for Use has been approved by the U.S. Food and Drug Administration.
Manufactured by: Schering Corporation, a subsidiary of **MERCK & CO., INC.**, Whitehouse Station, NJ 08889, USA.
Revised: 12/2013
Copyright © 2001, 2011 Schering Corporation, a subsidiary of **Merck & Co., Inc.** All rights reserved.
U.S. Patent Nos. 5,951,974; 6,180,096; and 6,610,830.
B-D is a registered trademark of Becton, Dickinson and Company.
usifu-mk4031-pwi-p-redipen-1312r002

Instructions for Use
PegIntron® (peg-In-tron)
(Peginterferon alfa-2b)
Powder for Injection
This Instructions for Use is only for use with the single-use vials of Powder for injection. If your healthcare provider prescribes the REDIPEN or Selectdose Pre-filled Pen for you, use only those Instructions for Use.
Be sure that you read, understand and follow these instructions before injecting PegIntron. Your healthcare provider should show you how to prepare, measure, and inject PegIntron properly using a vial before you use it for the first time. Ask your healthcare provider if you have any questions.
Important:
• Make sure that you have:
  ◦ the correct strength of PegIntron vial prescribed by your healthcare provider.
  ◦ the correct syringe and needle to use with PegIntron. Your healthcare provider should tell you what syringes and needles to use to inject PegIntron.
• Throw away the syringe and needle after you use it. Do not re-use your syringes and needles. See "Disposal of the used needles, syringes and vials" in this Instructions for Use.
• The vial of mixed PegIntron should be used right away. Do not mix more than 1 vial of PegIntron at a time. If you do not use the vial of the prepared solution right away, store it in a refrigerator and use within 24 hours. See the end of these Instructions for Use for information about "How should I store PegIntron?"

Before starting, collect all of the supplies that you will need to use for preparing and injecting PegIntron. For each injection you will need a PegIntron vial package that contains:
• 1 vial of PegIntron powder for injection
• 1 vial of sterile water for injection (diluent)
• 2 single-use disposable syringes (BD Safety Lok syringes with a safety sleeve)
• 2 alcohol swabs
You will also need:
• 1 cotton ball or gauze
• 1 sharps disposal container for throwing away your used syringes, needles, and vials.

How should I prepare a dose of PegIntron?
Before you inject PegIntron, the powder must be mixed with 0.7 mL of the sterile water for injection (diluent) that comes in the PegIntron vial package.

1. Find a clean, well-lit, flat work surface.
2. Get 1 of your PegIntron vial packages. Check the date printed on the PegIntron carton. Make sure that the expiration date has not passed. Do not use your PegIntron vial packages if the expiration date has passed. The medicine in the PegIntron vial should look like a white to off-white tablet that is whole, or in pieces, or powdered.
   If you have already mixed the PegIntron solution and stored it in the refrigerator, take it out of the refrigerator before use and allow the solution to come to room temperature. See the Medication Guide section "How should I store PegIntron?"
3. Wash your hands well with soap and water, rinse and towel dry (See Figure A). Keep your work area, your hands, and injection site clean to decrease the risk of infection.

Figure A

The disposable syringes have needles that are already attached and cannot be removed. Each syringe has a clear plastic safety sleeve that is pulled over the needle for disposal after use. The safety sleeve should remain tight against the flange while using the syringe and moved over the needle only when ready for disposal. (See Figure B)

FLANGES
GREEN STRIPE
SAFETY SLEEVE
RED STRIPE
PROTECTIVE CAP

Figure B

4. Remove the protective wrapper from one of the syringes provided. Use the syringe for steps 4 through 15. Make sure that the syringe safety sleeve is sitting against the flange. (See Figure B)
5. Remove the protective plastic cap from the tops of both the sterile water for injection (diluent) and the PegIntron vials (See Figure C). Clean the rubber stopper on the top of both vials with an alcohol swab.

Figure C

6. Carefully remove the protective cap straight off of the needle to avoid damaging the needle point.
7. Fill the syringe with air by pulling back on the plunger to 0.7 mL. (See Figure D)

Figure D

8. Hold the diluent vial upright. Do not touch the cleaned top of the vial with your hands.
   • Push the needle through the center of the rubber stopper of the diluent vial. (See Figure E)
   • Slowly inject all the air from the syringe into the air space above the diluent in the vial. (See Figure F)

Figure E   **Figure F**

9. Turn the vial upside down and make sure the tip of the needle is in the liquid.
10. Withdraw only 0.7 mL of diluent by pulling the plunger back to the 0.7 mL mark on the side of the syringe. (See Figure G)

Figure G

11. With the needle still inserted in the vial, check the syringe for air bubbles.
    ◦ If there are any air bubbles, gently tap the syringe with your finger until the air bubbles rise to the top of the syringe.
    ◦ Slowly push the plunger up to remove the air bubbles.
    ◦ If you push diluent back into the vial, slowly pull back on the plunger to draw the correct amount of diluent back into the syringe.
12. Remove the needle from the vial (See Figure H). Do not let the syringe touch anything.

Figure H

13. Throw away any diluent that is left over in the vial.
14. Insert the needle through the center of the rubber stopper of the PegIntron powder vial. Do not touch the cleaned rubber stopper.
    ◦ Place the needle tip, at an angle, against the side of the vial. (See Figure I)
    ◦ Slowly push the plunger down to inject the 0.7 mL diluent. The stream of diluent should run down the side of the vial.

○ To prevent bubbles from forming, do not aim the stream of diluent directly on the medicine in the bottom of the vial.

Figure I

15. Remove the needle from the vial.
    ○ Firmly grasp the safety sleeve and pull it over the exposed needle until you hear a click (See Figure J). The green stripe on the safety sleeve will completely cover the red stripe on the needle. Throw away the syringe, needle, and vial in the sharps disposal container (See "Disposal of the used needles, syringes, and vials").

Figure J

16. Gently swirl the vial in a gentle circular motion, until the PegIntron is completely dissolved (mixed together). (See Figure K)
    ○ Do not shake the vial. If any powder remains undissolved in the vial, gently turn the vial upside down until all of the powder is dissolved.
    • The solution may look cloudy or bubbly for a few minutes. If air bubbles form, wait until the solution settles and all bubbles rise to the top.

DO NOT SHAKE

Figure K

17. After the PegIntron completely dissolves, the solution should be clear, colorless and without particles. It is normal to see a ring of foam or bubbles on the surface.
    Do not use the mixed solution if you see particles in it, or it is not clear and colorless. Throw away the syringe, needle, and vial in the sharps disposal container (See the section "Disposal of the used needles, syringes, and vials"). Then, repeat steps 1 through 17 with a new vial of PegIntron and diluent to prepare a new syringe.
18. After the PegIntron powder completely dissolves, clean the rubber stopper again with an alcohol swab before you withdraw your dose.
19. Unwrap the second syringe provided. You will use it to give yourself the injection.
    ○ Carefully remove the protective cap from the needle. Fill the syringe with air by pulling the plunger to the number on the side of the syringe (mL) that matches your prescribed dose. (See Figure L)
    [See figure L at top of next column]
    ○ Hold the PegIntron vial upright. Do not touch the cleaned top of the vial with your hands. (See Figure M)
    [See figure M at top of next column]
    ○ Insert the needle into the vial containing the PegIntron solution. Inject the air into the center of the vial. (See Figure N)
    [See figure N at top of next column]
20. Turn the PegIntron vial upside down. Be sure the tip of the needle is in the PegIntron solution.
    ○ Hold the vial and syringe with one hand. Be sure the tip of the needle is in the PegIntron solution. With the other hand, slowly pull the plunger back to fill the syringe with the exact amount of PegIntron into the sy-

Figure L

Figure M

Figure N

ringe your healthcare provider told you to use. (See Figure O)

Figure O

21. Check for air bubbles in the syringe. If you see any air bubbles, hold the syringe with the needle pointing up. Gently tap the syringe until the air bubbles rise. Then, slowly push the plunger up to remove any air bubbles. If you push solution into the syringe, slowly pull back on the plunger again to draw the correct amount of PegIntron back into the syringe. When you are ready to inject the medicine, remove the needle from the vial. (See Figure P)

Figure P

How should I choose a site for injection?
The best sites for giving yourself an injection are those areas with a layer of fat between the skin and muscle, like your thigh, the outer surface of your upper arm, and abdomen (See Figure Q). Do not inject yourself in the area near your belly-button (navel) or waistline. If you are very thin, you should only use the thigh or outer surface of the arm for injection.
[See figure Q at top of next column]
You should use a different site each time you inject PegIntron to avoid soreness at any one site. **Do not inject PegIntron solution into an area where the skin is irritated, red, bruised, infected or has scars, stretch marks, or lumps.**

Figure Q

How should I inject a dose of PegIntron?
22. Clean the skin where the injection is to be given with an alcohol swab. Wait for the area to dry.
    ○ Make sure the safety sleeve of the syringe is pushed firmly against the syringe flange so that the needle is fully exposed.
23. With one hand, pinch a fold of skin. With your other hand, pick up the syringe and hold it like a pencil.
    ○ Insert the needle into the pinched skin at a 45- to 90-degree angle with a quick dart-like motion. (See Figure R)

90° angle
45° angle

Figure R

○ After the needle is inserted, remove the hand that you used to pinch your skin. Use it to hold the syringe barrel.
○ Pull the plunger of the syringe back very slightly.
○ **If no blood is present in the syringe**, inject the medicine by gently pressing the plunger all the way down the syringe barrel, until the syringe is empty.
○ **If blood comes into the syringe**, the needle has entered a blood vessel. Do not inject.
○ Withdraw the needle and throw away the syringe and needle in the sharps disposal container. (See "Disposal of the used needles, syringes, and vials")
○ Then, repeat steps 1 through 23 with a new vial of PegIntron and diluent to prepare a new syringe, and inject the medicine at a new site.
24. When the syringe is empty, pull the needle out of the skin.
    ○ Place a cotton ball or gauze over the injection site and press for several seconds. Do not massage the injection site.
    ○ If there is bleeding, cover it with a bandage.
25. After injecting your dose:
    ○ Firmly grasp the safety sleeve and pull it over the exposed needle until you hear a click, and the green stripe on the safety sleeve covers the red stripe on the needle. (See Figure S)

Figure S

Disposal of the used needles, syringes, and vials
• Put your used needles, syringes and vials in a FDA-cleared sharps disposal container right away after use. **Do not throw away (dispose of) loose needles, syringes and vials in your household trash.**
• If you do not have a FDA-cleared sharps disposal container, you may use a household container that is:
    ○ made of a heavy-duty plastic,
    ○ can be closed with a tight-fitting, puncture-resistant lid, without sharps being able to come out,
    ○ upright and stable during use,
    ○ leak-resistant, and
    ○ properly labeled to warn of hazardous waste inside the container.
• When your sharps disposal container is almost full, you will need to follow your community guidelines for the right way to dispose of your sharps disposal container. There may be state or local laws about how you

should throw away used syringes and needles. For more information about safe sharps disposal, and for specific information about sharps disposal in the state that you live in, go to the FDA's website at: http://www.fda.gov/safesharpsdisposal.

• Do not dispose of your used sharps disposal container in your household trash unless your community guidelines permit this. Do not recycle your used sharps disposal container.

Always keep the sharps disposal container out of the reach of children.

How should I store PegIntron?

• Before mixing, store PegIntron vials at room temperature, between 68°F to 77°F (20°C to 25°C).

• After mixing, use PegIntron right away or store it in the refrigerator for up to 24 hours between 36°F to 46°F (2°C to 8°C).

• Do not freeze PegIntron.

• Keep PegIntron away from heat.

Keep PegIntron and all medicines out of the reach of children.

This Instructions for Use has been approved by the U.S. Food and Drug Administration.

Manufactured by: Schering Corporation, a subsidiary of **MERCK & CO., INC.**, Whitehouse Station, NJ 08889, USA.

Revised 12/2013

Copyright © 2001, 2011 Schering Corporation, a subsidiary of **Merck & Co., Inc.** All rights reserved

U.S. Patent Nos. 5,951,974; 6,180,096; and 6,610,830.

B-D is a registered trademark of Becton, Dickinson and Company.

usifu-mk4031-pwi-1312r003

Shown in Product Identification Guide, page 309

PNEUMOVAX® 23   ℞
(pneumococcal vaccine polyvalent)
Sterile, Liquid Vaccine for Intramuscular or Subcutaneous Injection

HIGHLIGHTS OF PRESCRIBING INFORMATION
These highlights do not include all the information needed to use PNEUMOVAX 23 safely and effectively. See full prescribing information for PNEUMOVAX 23.
PNEUMOVAX® 23 (pneumococcal vaccine polyvalent)
Sterile, Liquid Vaccine for Intramuscular or Subcutaneous Injection
Initial U.S. Approval: 1983

———————RECENT MAJOR CHANGES———————
Dosage and Administration
Preparation (2.1)   05/2014
Administration (2.2)   05/2014

———————INDICATIONS AND USAGE———————
PNEUMOVAX 23 is a vaccine indicated for active immunization for the prevention of pneumococcal disease caused by the 23 serotypes contained in the vaccine (1, 2, 3, 4, 5, 6B, 7F, 8, 9N, 9V, 10A, 11A, 12F, 14, 15B, 17F, 18C, 19F, 19A, 20, 22F, 23F, and 33F). (1.1)
PNEUMOVAX 23 is approved for use in persons 50 years of age or older and persons aged ≥2 years who are at increased risk for pneumococcal disease. (1.1, 14.1)

———————DOSAGE AND ADMINISTRATION———————
Single 0.5-mL dose of PNEUMOVAX 23 administered intramuscularly or subcutaneously only. (2.2)

———————DOSAGE FORMS AND STRENGTHS———————
Clear, sterile solution supplied in a (0.5-mL dose) single-dose vial, a multidose (5-dose) vial, and a single-dose, prefilled syringe. (3)

———————CONTRAINDICATIONS———————
Severe allergic reaction (e.g., anaphylaxis) to any component of PNEUMOVAX 23. (4.1)

———————WARNINGS AND PRECAUTIONS———————
• Use caution and appropriate care for individuals with severely compromised cardiovascular and/or pulmonary function in whom a systemic reaction would pose a significant risk. (5.2)

———————ADVERSE REACTIONS———————
The most common adverse reactions, reported in >10% of subjects vaccinated with PNEUMOVAX 23 in clinical trials, were: injection-site pain/soreness/tenderness (60.0%), injection-site swelling/induration (20.3%), headache (17.6%), injection-site erythema (16.4%), asthenia and fatigue (13.2%), and myalgia (11.9%). (6.1)
To report SUSPECTED ADVERSE REACTIONS, contact Merck Sharp & Dohme Corp., a subsidiary of Merck & Co., Inc., at 1-877-888-4231 or VAERS at 1-800-822-7967 or www.vaers.hhs.gov.

———————DRUG INTERACTIONS———————
In a randomized clinical study, a reduced immune response to ZOSTAVAX® as measured by gpELISA was observed in individuals who received concurrent administration of PNEUMOVAX 23 and ZOSTAVAX compared with individuals who received these vaccines 4 weeks apart. Consider administration of the two vaccines separated by at least 4 weeks. (7.1, 14.3)

———————USE IN SPECIFIC POPULATIONS———————
Pregnancy: No human or animal data are available. Use only if clearly needed. (8.1)
Pediatrics: PNEUMOVAX 23 is not approved for use in children younger than 2 years of age because children in this age group do not develop an effective immune response to capsular types contained in the polysaccharide vaccine. (8.4)
Geriatrics: For subjects aged 65 years or older in a clinical study systemic adverse reactions, determined by the investigator to be vaccine-related, were higher following revaccination (33.1%) than following initial vaccination (21.7%). Routine revaccination of immunocompetent persons previously vaccinated with a 23-valent vaccine, is not recommended.{1} (8.5)
Immunocompromised Individuals: Response to vaccination may be diminished. (5.4, 8.6)

See 17 for PATIENT COUNSELING INFORMATION and FDA-approved patient labeling

Revised: 05/2014

FULL PRESCRIBING INFORMATION: CONTENTS*

FULL PRESCRIBING INFORMATION

1   INDICATIONS AND USAGE
1.1   Indications and Use
PNEUMOVAX® 23 is a vaccine indicated for active immunization for the prevention of pneumococcal disease caused by the 23 serotypes contained in the vaccine (1, 2, 3, 4, 5, 6B, 7F, 8, 9N, 9V, 10A, 11A, 12F, 14, 15B, 17F, 18C, 19F, 19A, 20, 22F, 23F, and 33F). PNEUMOVAX 23 is approved for use in persons 50 years of age or older and persons aged ≥2 years who are at increased risk for pneumococcal disease.
1.2   Limitations of Use
PNEUMOVAX 23 will not prevent disease caused by capsular types of pneumococcus other than those contained in the vaccine.

2   DOSAGE AND ADMINISTRATION
For intramuscular or subcutaneous injection only.
2.1   Preparation
• Parenteral drug products should be inspected visually for particulate matter and discoloration prior to administration. If either of these two conditions exists, the vaccine should not be administered.
• Do not mix PNEUMOVAX 23 with other vaccines in the same syringe or vial.
• Use a separate sterile syringe and needle for each individual patient to prevent transmission of infectious agents from one person to another.
Single-Dose and Multidose Vials
Withdraw 0.5 mL from the vial using a sterile needle and syringe free of preservatives, antiseptics, and detergents.
Single-Dose, Prefilled Syringe
The package does not contain a needle. Attach a sterile needle to the prefilled syringe by twisting in a clockwise direction until the needle fits securely on the syringe.
2.2   Administration
Administer PNEUMOVAX 23 intramuscularly or subcutaneously into the deltoid muscle or lateral mid-thigh. Do not inject intravascularly or intradermally.
Single-Dose and Multidose Vials
Administer a single 0.5-mL dose of PNEUMOVAX 23 using a sterile needle and syringe.
Single-Dose, Prefilled Syringe
Administer the entire contents of the single-dose, prefilled syringe per standard protocol using a sterile needle.
2.3   Revaccination
The Advisory Committee on Immunization Practices (ACIP) has recommendations for revaccination against pneumococcal disease for persons at high risk who were previously vaccinated with PNEUMOVAX 23. Routine revaccination of immunocompetent persons previously vaccinated with a 23-valent vaccine, is not recommended.{1,2}

3   DOSAGE FORMS AND STRENGTHS
PNEUMOVAX 23 is a clear, sterile solution supplied in a (0.5-mL dose) single-dose vial, a 5-dose vial, and a single-dose, prefilled syringe. *[See Description (11) and How Supplied/Storage and Handling (16).]*

4   CONTRAINDICATIONS
4.1   Hypersensitivity
Do not administer PNEUMOVAX 23 to individuals with a history of anaphylactic/anaphylactoid or severe allergic reaction to any component of the vaccine. *[See Description (11).]*

5   WARNINGS AND PRECAUTIONS
5.1   Persons with Moderate or Severe Acute Illness
Defer vaccination with PNEUMOVAX 23 in persons with moderate or severe acute illness.
5.2   Persons with Severely Compromised Cardiovascular or Pulmonary Function
Caution and appropriate care should be exercised in administering PNEUMOVAX 23 to individuals with severely compromised cardiovascular and/or pulmonary function in whom a systemic reaction would pose a significant risk.
5.3   Use of Antibiotic Prophylaxis
This vaccine does not replace the need for penicillin (or other antibiotic) prophylaxis against pneumococcal infection. In patients who require penicillin (or other antibiotic) prophylaxis against pneumococcal infection, such prophylaxis should not be discontinued after vaccination with PNEUMOVAX 23.
5.4   Persons with Altered Immunocompetence
Persons who are immunocompromised, including persons receiving immunosuppressive therapy, may have a diminished immune response to PNEUMOVAX 23. *[See Use in Specific Populations (8.6).]*
5.5   Persons with Chronic Cerebrospinal Fluid Leakage
PNEUMOVAX 23 may not be effective in preventing pneumococcal meningitis in patients who have chronic cerebrospinal fluid (CSF) leakage resulting from congenital lesions, skull fractures, or neurosurgical procedures.

6   ADVERSE REACTIONS
The most common adverse reactions, reported in >10% of subjects vaccinated with PNEUMOVAX 23 in clinical trials were: injection-site pain/soreness/tenderness (60.0%), injection-site swelling/induration (20.3%), headache (17.6%), injection-site erythema (16.4%), asthenia/fatigue (13.2%), and myalgia (11.9%). *[See Adverse Reactions (6.1).]*
6.1   Clinical Trials Experience
Because clinical trials are conducted under widely varying conditions, adverse reaction rates observed in the clinical trials of a vaccine cannot be directly compared to rates in the clinical trials of another vaccine and may not reflect the rates observed in practice.
In a randomized, double-blind, placebo-controlled crossover clinical trial, subjects were enrolled in four different cohorts defined by age (50-64 years of age and ≥65 years of age) and vaccination status (no pneumococcal vaccination or receipt of a pneumococcal polysaccharide vaccine 3-5 years prior to the study). Subjects in each cohort were randomized to re-

ceive intramuscular injections of PNEUMOVAX 23 followed by placebo (saline containing 0.25% phenol), or placebo followed by PNEUMOVAX 23, at 30-day (±7 days) intervals. The safety of an initial vaccination (first dose) was compared to revaccination (second dose) with PNEUMOVAX 23 for 14 days following each vaccination.

All 1008 subjects (average age, 67 years; 49% male and 51% female; 91% Caucasian, 4.7% African-American, 3.5% Hispanic, and 0.8% Other) received placebo injections.

Initial vaccination was evaluated in a total of 444 subjects (average age 65 years; 32% male and 68% female; 93% Caucasian, 3.2% African-American, 3.4% Hispanic, and 1.1% Other).

Revaccination was evaluated in 564 subjects (average age 69 years; 53% male and 47% female; 90% Caucasian, 3.5% Hispanic, 6.0% African-American, and 0.5% Other).

Serious Adverse Experiences

In this study, 10 subjects had serious adverse experiences within 14 days of vaccination: 6 who received PNEUMOVAX 23 and 4 who received placebo. Serious adverse experiences within 14 days after PNEUMOVAX 23 included angina pectoris, heart failure, chest pain, ulcerative colitis, depression, and headache/tremor/stiffness/sweating. Serious adverse experiences within 14 days after placebo included myocardial infarction complicated with heart failure, alcohol intoxication, angina pectoris, and edema/urinary retention/heart failure/diabetes.

Five subjects reported serious adverse experiences that occurred outside the 14-day follow-up window: 3 who received PNEUMOVAX 23 and 2 who received placebo. Serious adverse experiences after PNEUMOVAX 23 included cerebrovascular accident, lumbar radiculopathy, and pancreatitis/myocardial infarction resulting in death. Serious adverse experiences after placebo included heart failure and motor vehicle accident resulting in death.

Solicited and Unsolicited Reactions

Table 1 presents the adverse event rates for all solicited and unsolicited reactions reported in ≥1% in any group in this study, without regard to causality.

The most common local adverse reactions reported at the injection site after initial vaccination with PNEUMOVAX 23 were pain/tenderness/soreness (60.0%), swelling/induration (20.3%), and erythema (16.4%). The most common systemic adverse experiences were headache (17.6%), asthenia/fatigue (13.2%), and myalgia (11.9%).

The most common local adverse reactions reported at the injection site after revaccination with PNEUMOVAX 23 were pain/soreness/tenderness (77.2%), swelling (39.8%), and erythema (34.5%). The most common systemic adverse reactions with revaccination were headache (18.1%), asthenia/fatigue (17.9%), and myalgia (17.3%). All of these adverse reactions were reported at a rate lower than 10% after receiving a placebo injection.

[See table 1 above]

In this clinical study an increased rate of local reactions was observed with revaccination at 3-5 years following initial vaccination.

For subjects aged 65 years or older, injection-site adverse reaction rate was higher following revaccination (79.3%) than following initial vaccination (52.9%). The proportion of subjects reporting injection site discomfort that interfered with or prevented usual activity or injection site induration ≥4 inches was higher following revaccination (30.6%) than following initial vaccination (10.4%). Injection site reactions typically resolved by 5 days following vaccination.

For subjects aged 50-64 years, the injection-site adverse reaction rate for revaccinees and initial vaccinees was similar (79.6% and 72.8% respectively).

The rate of systemic adverse reactions was similar among both initial vaccinees and revaccinees within each age group. The rate of vaccine-related systemic adverse reactions was higher following revaccination (33.1%) than following initial vaccination (21.7%) in subjects 65 years of age or older, and was similar following revaccination (37.5%) and initial vaccination (35.5%) in subjects 50-64 years of age. The most common systemic adverse reactions reported after PNEUMOVAX 23 were as follows: asthenia/fatigue, myalgia and headache.

Regardless of age, the observed increase in post vaccination use of analgesics (≤13% in the revaccinees and ≤4% in the initial vaccinees) returned to baseline by day 5.

6.2   Post-Marketing Experience

The following list of adverse reactions includes those identified during post approval use of PNEUMOVAX 23. Because these reactions are reported voluntarily from a population of uncertain size, it is not always possible to reliably estimate their frequency or their causal relationship to product exposure.

General disorders and administration site conditions
   Cellulitis
   Malaise
   Fever (>102°F)
   Warmth at the injection site
   Decreased limb mobility
   Peripheral edema in the injected extremity
Digestive System
   Nausea
   Vomiting

Hematologic / Lymphatic
   Lymphadenitis
   Lymphadenopathy
   Thrombocytopenia in patients with stabilized idiopathic thrombocytopenic purpura{3}
   Hemolytic anemia in patients who have had other hematologic disorders
   Leukocytosis
Hypersensitivity reactions including
   Anaphylactoid reactions
   Serum Sickness
   Angioneurotic edema
Musculoskeletal System
   Arthralgia
   Arthritis
Nervous System
   Paresthesia
   Radiculoneuropathy
   Guillain-Barré syndrome
   Febrile convulsion
Skin
   Rash
   Urticaria
   Cellulitis-like reactions
   Erythema multiforme
Investigations
   Increased serum C-reactive protein

Table 1: Incidence of Injection-Site and Systemic Complaints in Adults ≥50 Years of Age Receiving Their First (Initial) or Second (Revaccination) Dose of PNEUMOVAX 23 (Pneumococcal Polysaccharide Vaccine, 23 Valent) or Placebo Occurring at ≥1% in Any Group

	PNEUMOVAX 23 Initial Vaccination N=444	PNEUMOVAX 23 Revaccination* N=564	Placebo Injection† N=1008
Number Followed for Safety	438	548	984‡
	AE Rate	AE Rate	AE Rate
Injection-Site Complaints			
Solicited Events			
Pain/Soreness/Tenderness	60.0%	77.2%	7.7%
Swelling/Induration	20.3%	39.8%	2.8%
Erythema	16.4%	34.5%	3.3%
Unsolicited Events			
Ecchymosis	0%	1.1%	0.3%
Pruritus	0.2%	1.6%	0.0%
Systemic Complaints			
Solicited Events			
Asthenia/Fatigue	13.2%	17.9%	6.7%
Chills	2.7%	7.8%	1.8%
Myalgia	11.9%	17.3%	3.3%
Headache	17.6%	18.1%	8.9%
Unsolicited Events			
Fever§	1.4%	2.0%	0.7%
Diarrhea	1.1%	0.7%	0.5%
Dyspepsia	1.1%	1.1%	0.9%
Nausea	1.8%	1.8%	0.9%
Back Pain	0.9%	0.9%	1.0%
Neck Pain	0.7%	1.5%	0.2%
Upper Respiratory Infection	1.8%	2.6%	1.8%
Pharyngitis	1.1%	0.4%	1.3%

* Subjects receiving their second dose of pneumococcal polysaccharide vaccine as PNEUMOVAX 23 approximately 3-5 years after their first dose.
† Subjects receiving placebo injection from this study combined over periods.
‡ The number of subjects receiving placebo followed for injection-site complaints. The corresponding number of subjects followed for systemic complaints was 981.
§ Fever events include subjects who felt feverish in addition to subjects with elevated temperature.

7   DRUG INTERACTIONS
7.1   Concomitant Administration with Other Vaccines
In a randomized clinical study, a reduced immune response to ZOSTAVAX® as measured by gpELISA was observed in individuals who received concurrent administration of PNEUMOVAX 23 and ZOSTAVAX compared with individuals who received these vaccines 4 weeks apart. Consider administration of the two vaccines separated by at least 4 weeks. [See Clinical Studies (14.3).]

Limited safety and immunogenicity data from clinical trials are available on the concurrent administration of PNEUMOVAX 23 and vaccines other than ZOSTAVAX.

8   USE IN SPECIFIC POPULATIONS
8.1   Pregnancy
Pregnancy Category C: Animal reproduction studies have not been conducted with PNEUMOVAX 23. It is also not known whether PNEUMOVAX 23 can cause fetal harm when administered to a pregnant woman or can affect reproduction capacity. PNEUMOVAX 23 should be given to a pregnant woman only if clearly needed.

8.3   Nursing Mothers
It is not known whether this drug is excreted in human milk. Because many drugs are excreted in human milk, caution should be exercised when PNEUMOVAX 23 is administered to a nursing woman.

8.4   Pediatric Use

PNEUMOVAX 23 is not approved for use in children less than 2 years of age. Children in this age group do not develop an effective immune response to the capsular types contained in this polysaccharide vaccine.

The ACIP has recommendations for use of PNEUMOVAX 23 in children 2 years of age or older, who have previously received pneumococcal vaccines, and who are at increased risk for pneumococcal disease.[2]

8.5   Geriatric Use

In one clinical trial of PNEUMOVAX 23, conducted post-licensure, a total of 629 subjects who were aged ≥65 years and 201 subjects who were aged ≥75 years were enrolled.

In this trial, the safety of PNEUMOVAX 23 in adults 65 years of age and older (N=629) was compared to the safety of PNEUMOVAX 23 in adults 50 to 64 years of age (N=379). The subjects in this study had underlying chronic illness but were in stable condition; at least 1 medical condition at enrollment was reported by 86.3% of subjects who were 50 to 64 years old, and by 96.7% of subjects who were 65 to 91 years old. The rate of vaccine-related systemic adverse experiences was higher following revaccination (33.1%) than following primary vaccination (21.7%) in subjects ≥65 years of age, and was similar following revaccination (37.5%) and primary vaccination (35.5%) in subjects 50 to 64 years of age.

Since elderly individuals may not tolerate medical interventions as well as younger individuals, a higher frequency and/or a greater severity of reactions in some older individuals cannot be ruled out.

Post-marketing reports have been received in which some elderly individuals had severe adverse experiences and a complicated clinical course following vaccination. Some individuals with underlying medical conditions of varying severity experienced local reactions and fever associated with clinical deterioration requiring hospital care.

8.6   Immunocompromised Individuals

Persons who are immunocompromised, including persons receiving immunosuppressive therapy, may have a diminished immune response to PNEUMOVAX 23.

11   DESCRIPTION

PNEUMOVAX 23 (Pneumococcal Vaccine Polyvalent) is a sterile, liquid vaccine consisting of a mixture of purified capsular polysaccharides from *Streptococcus pneumoniae* types (1, 2, 3, 4, 5, 6B, 7F, 8, 9N, 9V, 10A, 11A, 12F, 14, 15B, 17F, 18C, 19F, 19A, 20, 22F, 23F, and 33F).

PNEUMOVAX 23 is a clear, colorless solution. Each 0.5-mL dose of vaccine contains 25 micrograms of each polysaccharide type in isotonic saline solution containing 0.25% phenol as a preservative. The vaccine is used directly as supplied. No dilution or reconstitution is necessary.

12   CLINICAL PHARMACOLOGY

12.1   Mechanism of Action

PNEUMOVAX 23 induces type-specific antibodies that enhance opsonization, phagocytosis, and killing of pneumococci by leukocytes and other phagocytic cells. The levels of antibodies that correlate with protection against pneumococcal disease have not been clearly defined.

14   CLINICAL STUDIES

14.1   Effectiveness

The protective efficacy of pneumococcal vaccines containing six (types 1, 2, 4, 8, 12F, and 25) or twelve (types 1, 2, 3, 4, 6A, 8, 9N, 12F, 25, 7F, 18C, and 46) capsular polysaccharides was investigated in two controlled studies in South Africa in male novice gold miners ranging in age from 16 to 58 years, in whom there was a high attack rate for pneumococcal pneumonia and bacteremia.[4] In both studies, participants in the control groups received either meningococcal polysaccharide serogroup A vaccine or saline placebo. In both studies, attack rates for vaccine type pneumococcal pneumonia were observed for the period from 2 weeks through about 1 year after vaccination. Protective efficacy was 76% and 92%, respectively, for the 6- and 12-valent vaccines, for the capsular types represented.

Three similar studies in South African young adult male novice gold miners were carried out by Dr. R. Austrian and associates[5] using similar pneumococcal vaccines prepared for the National Institute of Allergy and Infectious Diseases, with pneumococcal vaccines containing a 6-valent formulation (types 1, 3, 4, 7, 8, and 12) or a 13-valent formulation (types 1, 2, 3, 4, 6, 7, 8, 9, 12, 14, 18, 19, and 25) capsular polysaccharides. The reduction in pneumococcal pneumonia caused by the capsular types contained in the vaccines was 79%. Reduction in type-specific pneumococcal bacteremia was 82%.

A prospective study in France found a pneumococcal vaccine containing fourteen (types 1, 2, 3, 4, 6A, 7F, 8, 9N, 12F, 14, 18C, 19F, 23F, and 25) capsular polysaccharides to be 77% (95%CI: 51% to 89%) effective in reducing the incidence of pneumonia among male and female nursing home residents with a mean age of 74 (standard deviation of 4 years).[6]

In a study using a pneumococcal vaccine containing eight (types 1, 3, 6, 7, 14, 18, 19, and 23) capsular polysaccharides, vaccinated children and young adults aged 2 to 25 years who had sickle cell disease, congenital asplenia, or undergone a splenectomy experienced significantly less bacteremic pneumococcal disease than patients who were not vaccinated.[7]

In the United States, one post-licensure randomized controlled trial, in the elderly or patients with chronic medical conditions who received a 14-valent pneumococcal polysaccharide vaccine (types 1, 2, 3, 4, 6A, 8, 9N, 12F, 14, 19F, 23F, 25, 7F, and 18C), did not support the efficacy of the vaccine for nonbacteremic pneumonia.[8]

A retrospective cohort analysis study based on the U.S. Centers for Disease Control and Prevention (CDC) pneumococcal surveillance system, showed 57% (95%CI: 45% to 66%) overall protective effectiveness against invasive infections caused by serotypes included in PNEUMOVAX 23 in persons ≥6 years of age, 65 to 84% effectiveness among specific patient groups (e.g., persons with diabetes mellitus, coronary vascular disease, congestive heart failure, chronic pulmonary disease, and anatomic asplenia) and 75% (95%CI: 57% to 85%) effectiveness in immunocompetent persons aged ≥65 years of age. Vaccine effectiveness could not be confirmed for certain groups of immunocompromised patients.[9]

14.2   Immunogenicity

The levels of antibodies that correlate with protection against pneumococcal disease have not been clearly defined. Antibody responses to most pneumococcal capsular types are generally low or inconsistent in children less than 2 years of age.

14.3   Concomitant Administration with Other Vaccines

In a double-blind, controlled clinical trial, 473 adults, 60 years of age or older, were randomized to receive ZOSTAVAX and PNEUMOVAX 23 concomitantly (N=237), or PNEUMOVAX 23 alone followed 4 weeks later by ZOSTAVAX alone (N=236). At four weeks postvaccination, the varicella-zoster virus (VZV) antibody levels following concomitant use were significantly lower than the VZV antibody levels following nonconcomitant administration (GMTs of 338 vs. 484 gpELISA units/mL, respectively; GMT ratio = 0.70 (95% CI: [0.61, 0.80]).

Limited safety and immunogenicity data from clinical trials are available on the concurrent administration of PNEUMOVAX 23 and vaccines other than ZOSTAVAX.

15   REFERENCES

1. Centers for Disease Control and Prevention. Prevention of Pneumococcal Disease. Recommendations of the Advisory Committee on Immunization Practices (ACIP). MMWR. 46(No. RR-8): 1-25, 1997. Available from: http://www.cdc.gov/mmwr/PDF/rr/rr4608.pdf
2. Centers for Disease Control and Prevention. Prevention of Pneumococcal Disease Among Infants and Children --- Use of 13-Valent Pneumococcal Conjugate Vaccine and 23-Valent Pneumococcal Polysaccharide Vaccine, MMWR 59(RR11): 1-18, 2010. http://www.cdc.gov/mmwr/preview/mmwrhtml/rr5911a1.htm?s_cid=rr5911a1_e
3. Kelton, J.G.: Vaccination-associated relapse of immune thrombocytopenia, JAMA. 245(4): 369-371, 1981.
4. Smit, P.; Oberholzer, D.; Hayden-Smith, S.; Koornhof, H.J.; Hilleman, M.R.: Protective efficacy of pneumococcal polysaccharide vaccines, JAMA. 238: 2613-2616, 1977.
5. Austrian, R.; Douglas, R.M.; Schiffman, G.; Coetzee, A.M.; Koornhof, H.J.; Hayden-Smith, S.; Reid, R.D.W.: Prevention of pneumococcal pneumonia by vaccination, Trans. Assoc. Am. Physicians. 89: 184-194, 1976.
6. Gaillat, J.; Zmirou, D.; Mallaret, M.R.: Essai clinique du vaccin antipneuomococcique chez des personnes agees vivant en institution, Rev. Epidemiol. Sante Publique. 33: 437-44, 1985.
7. Ammann, A.J.; Addiego, J.; Wara, D.W.; Lubin, B.; Smith, W.B.; Mentzer, W.C.: Polyvalent pneumococcal-polysaccharide immunization of patients with sickle-cell anemia and patients with splenectomy, N. Engl. J. Med. 297: 897-900, 1977.
8. Simberkoff, M.S.; Cross, A.P.; Al-Ibrahim, M.: Efficacy of pneumococcal vaccine in high risk patients: results of a Veterans Administration cooperative study, N. Engl. J. Med. 315: 1318-27, 1986.
9. Butler, J.C.; Breiman, R.F.; Campbell, J.F.; Lipman, H.B.; Broome, C.V.; Facklam, R.R.: Pneumococcal polysaccharide vaccine efficacy. An evaluation of current recommendations, JAMA. 270: 1826-31, 1993.
10. Vaccine Adverse Event Reporting System - United States, MMWR. 39(41): 730-33, October 19, 1990.

16   HOW SUPPLIED/STORAGE AND HANDLING

PNEUMOVAX 23 is supplied as follows:

NDC 0006-4739-00 — one 5-dose vial, color coded with a purple cap and stripe on the vial labels and cartons.

NDC 0006-4943-00 — a box of 10 single-dose vials, color coded with a purple cap and stripe on the vial labels and cartons.

NDC 0006-4837-03 — a box of 10 single-dose, pre-filled Luer-Lok™ syringes with tip caps, color coded with a violet plunger rod and purple stripe on the syringe labels and cartons.

Storage and Handling

• Store at 2-8°C (36-46°F).

• All vaccine must be discarded after the expiration date.

17   PATIENT COUNSELING INFORMATION

Advise the patient to read the FDA-approved patient labeling (Patient Information).

• Inform the patient, parent or guardian of the benefits and risks associated with vaccination.

• Tell the patient, parent or guardian that vaccination with PNEUMOVAX 23 may not offer 100% protection from pneumococcal infection.

• Provide the patient, parent or guardian with the vaccine information statements required by the National Childhood Vaccine Injury Act of 1986, with each immunization.

• Instruct the patient, parent or guardian to report any serious adverse reactions to their health care provider who in turn should report such events to the vaccine manufacturer or the U.S. Department of Health and Human Services through the Vaccine Adverse Event Reporting System (VAERS), 1-800-822-7967, or report online at www.vaers.hhs.gov. [10]

Manuf. and Dist. by: Merck Sharp & Dohme Corp., a subsidiary of

MERCK & CO., INC., Whitehouse Station, NJ 08889, USA For patent information: www.merck.com/product/patent/home.html

The trademarks depicted herein are owned by their respective companies.

Copyright © 1986, 2011 Merck Sharp & Dohme Corp., a subsidiary of Merck & Co., Inc.
All rights reserved.
uspi-v110-i-1405r039
Printed in USA

Patient Information about

PNEUMOVAX® 23 (pronounced "noo-mo-vax 23")

Generic Name: pneumococcal vaccine polyvalent

Read this leaflet before you or your child gets the vaccine called PNEUMOVAX 23. If you have any questions about the vaccine after you read this, you should ask your health care provider. This is a summary only. It does not take the place of talking to your doctor, nurse or other health care provider about the vaccine. Only your health care provider can decide if PNEUMOVAX 23 is right for you or your child.

What is PNEUMOVAX 23?

PNEUMOVAX 23 is a vaccine that is given as a shot. It helps protect you from infection by certain germs or bacteria which are called pneumococcus (pronounced "noo-mo-ca-cus"). PNEUMOVAX 23 is for people 50 years of age and older. It is also for people who are 2 years of age and older if they have certain medical conditions that put them at increased risk for infection.

Illnesses or health problems may allow these germs to spread into the blood, lungs, or brain where they can cause serious diseases such as:

• An infection in the blood

• A lung infection (pneumonia) that can also come with an infection in the blood

• An infection of the coverings of the brain and spinal cord (meningitis).

PNEUMOVAX 23 may not protect everyone who gets it. It will not protect against diseases that are caused by bacteria types that are not in the vaccine.

Who should not get PNEUMOVAX 23?

You should not get this vaccine if you (or your child):

• are allergic to any of its ingredients

• had an allergic reaction to PNEUMOVAX 23 in the past

• are less than 2 years old.

What should I tell my health care provider before getting PNEUMOVAX 23?

Tell your health care provider if you (or your child):

• are allergic to PNEUMOVAX 23

• have heart or lung problems

• have a fever

• have immune problems or are receiving radiation treatment for chemotherapy

• are pregnant or breast-feeding

How is PNEUMOVAX 23 given?

Most often, just one shot is given.

If you or your child is in a high-risk group for pneumococcal infection, then your health care provider will decide if it would be helpful to give a second shot of PNEUMOVAX 23 at a later time.

Can PNEUMOVAX 23 be given with other vaccines?
Talk to your health care provider if you plan to get ZOSTAVAX at the same time as PNEUMOVAX 23 because it may be better to get these vaccines at least 4 weeks apart. Talk to your health care provider if you plan to get PNEUMOVAX 23 at the same time as other vaccines.

What are the possible side effects of PNEUMOVAX 23?
The most common side effects are:
- pain, warmth, soreness, redness, swelling, and hardening at the injection site
- headache
- weakness, feeling tired
- muscle pain

Tell your health care provider or get emergency help right away if you get any of the following problems after vaccination because these may be signs of an allergic reaction or other serious conditions:
- difficulty breathing
- wheezing
- rash
- hives

Side effects at the site where you get the shot may be more common and may feel worse after a second shot than after the first shot.

Tell your health care provider if you or your child has a side effect that bothers you or that does not go away.

For a more complete list of side effects, ask your health care provider.

You may also report any side effect to your or your child's health care provider, or directly to the Vaccine Adverse Event Reporting System (VAERS). You may call the VAERS number 1-800-822-7967 at no charge, or report online to www.vaers.hhs.gov.

What are the ingredients of PNEUMOVAX 23?

Active Ingredients:	Bacterial sugars from 23 pneumococcal types: 1, 2, 3, 4, 5, 6B, 7F, 8, 9N, 9V, 10A, 11A, 12F, 14, 15B, 17F, 18C, 19F, 19A, 20, 22F, 23F, and 33F
Inactive Ingredients:	Phenol (a preservative)

What else should I know about PNEUMOVAX 23?
Some adults and children have problems with leakage of spinal fluid after the skull is cracked or injured or after medical operations and this may increase their risk for pneumococcal infection. PNEUMOVAX 23 may not be able to prevent all of these infections.

This leaflet is a summary of information about PNEUMOVAX 23. If you would like more information, talk to your health care provider. You can also call the Merck National Service Center at 1-800-622-4477.

Manuf. and Dist. by: Merck Sharp & Dohme Corp., a subsidiary of
MERCK & CO., INC., Whitehouse Station, NJ 08889, USA
Copyright © 2011 Merck Sharp & Dohme Corp., a subsidiary of **Merck & Co., Inc.**
All rights reserved.
Revised: 03/2013
USPPI-I-V1101303R038
Printed in USA
Rx Only

PREGNYL®
(chorionic gonadotropin for injection, USP)   ℞

DESCRIPTION
Human chorionic gonadotropin (HCG), a polypeptide hormone produced by the human placenta, is composed of an alpha and a beta subunit. The alpha sub-unit is essentially identical to the alpha subunits of the human pituitary gonadotropins, luteinizing hormone (LH) and follicle-stimulating hormone (FSH), as well as to the alpha subunit of human thyroid-stimulating hormone (TSH). The beta subunits of these hormones differ in amino acid sequence. PREGNYL® (chorionic gonadotropin for injection USP) is a highly purified pyrogen-free preparation obtained from the urine of pregnant females. It is standardized by a biological assay procedure. It is available for intramuscular injection in multiple dose vials containing 10,000 USP units of sterile dried powder with 5 mg monobasic sodium phosphate and 4.4 mg dibasic sodium phosphate. If required, pH is adjusted with sodium hydroxide and/or phosphoric acid. Each package also contains a 10-mL vial of solvent containing: water for injection with 0.56% sodium chloride and 0.9% BENZYL ALCOHOL, WHICH IS NOT FOR USE IN NEWBORNS. If required, pH is adjusted with sodium hydroxide and/or hydrochloric acid.

CLINICAL PHARMACOLOGY
The action of HCG is virtually identical to that of pituitary LH, although HCG appears to have a small degree of FSH

activity as well. It stimulates production of gonadal steroid hormones by stimulating the interstitial cells (Leydig cells) of the testis to produce androgens and the corpus luteum of the ovary to produce progesterone.

Androgen stimulation in the male leads to the development of secondary sex characteristics and may stimulate testicular descent when no anatomical impediment to descent is present. This descent is usually reversible when HCG is discontinued.

During the normal menstrual cycle, LH participates with FSH in the development and maturation of the normal ovarian follicle, and the mid-cycle LH surge triggers ovulation. HCG can substitute for LH in this function. During a normal pregnancy, HCG secreted by the placenta maintains the corpus luteum after LH secretion decreases, supporting continued secretion of estrogen and progesterone and preventing menstruation. HCG HAS NO KNOWN EFFECT ON FAT MOBILIZATION, APPETITE OR SENSE OF HUNGER, OR BODY FAT DISTRIBUTION.

INDICATIONS AND USAGE
HCG HAS NOT BEEN DEMONSTRATED TO BE EFFECTIVE ADJUNCTIVE THERAPY IN THE TREATMENT OF OBESITY. THERE IS NO SUBSTANTIAL EVIDENCE THAT IT INCREASES WEIGHT LOSS BEYOND THAT RESULTING FROM CALORIC RESTRICTION, THAT IT CAUSES A MORE ATTRACTIVE OR "NORMAL" DISTRIBUTION OF FAT, OR THAT IT DECREASES THE HUNGER AND DISCOMFORT ASSOCIATED WITH CALORIE-RESTRICTED DIETS.

1. Prepubertal cryptorchidism not due to anatomical obstruction. In general, HCG is thought to induce testicular descent in situations when descent would have occurred at puberty. HCG thus may help predict whether or not orchiopexy will be needed in the future. Although, in some cases, descent following HCG administration is permanent, in most cases, the response is temporary. Therapy is usually instituted in children between the ages of 4 and 9.
2. Selected cases of hypogonadotropic hypogonadism (hypogonadism secondary to a pituitary deficiency) in males.
3. Induction of ovulation and pregnancy in the anovulatory, infertile woman in whom the cause of anovulation is secondary and not due to primary ovarian failure, and who has been appropriately pretreated with human menotropins.

CONTRAINDICATIONS
Precocious puberty, prostatic carcinoma or other androgen-dependent neoplasm, prior allergic reaction to HCG.

WARNINGS
HCG should be used in conjunction with human menopausal gonadotropins only by physicians experienced with infertility problems who are familiar with the criteria for patient selection, contraindications, warnings, precautions, and adverse reactions described in the package insert for menotropins.

Anaphylaxis has been reported with urinary-derived HCG products.

The principal serious adverse reactions during this use are: (1) ovarian hyperstimulation, a syndrome of sudden ovarian enlargement, ascites with or without pain, and/or pleural effusion, (2) rupture of ovarian cysts with resultant hemoperitoneum, (3) multiple births, and (4) arterial thromboembolism.

PRECAUTIONS
General
Since androgens may cause fluid retention, HCG should be used with caution in patients with cardiac or renal disease, epilepsy, migraine, or asthma.
Pediatric Use
Induction of androgen secretion by HCG may induce precocious puberty in pediatric patients treated for cryptorchidism. Therapy should be discontinued if signs of precocious puberty occur.
Geriatric Use
Clinical studies of PREGNYL® (chorionic gonadotropin for injection USP) did not include subjects aged 65 and over.

ADVERSE REACTIONS
Headache, irritability, restlessness, depression, fatigue, edema, precocious puberty, gynecomastia, pain at the site of injection.

Hypersensitivity reactions, both localized and systemic in nature, have been reported.

DOSAGE AND ADMINISTRATION
For intramuscular use only. The dosage regimen employed in any particular case will depend upon the indication for the use, the age and weight of the patient, and the physician's preference. The following regimens have been advocated by various authorities:
Prepubertal cryptorchidism not due to anatomical obstruction. Therapy is usually instituted in children between the ages of 4 and 9.

1. 4000 USP units 3 times weekly for 3 weeks.
2. 5000 USP units every second day for 4 injections.
3. 15 injections for 500 to 1000 USP units over a period of 6 weeks.
4. 500 USP units 3 times weekly for 4 to 6 weeks. If this course of treatment is not successful, another series is begun 1 month later, giving 1000 USP units per injection.

Selected cases of hypogonadotropic hypogonadism in males.
1. 500 to 1000 USP units 3 times a week for 3 weeks, followed by the same dose twice a week for 3 weeks.
2. 4000 USP units 3 times weekly for 6 to 9 months, following which the dosage may be reduced to 2000 USP units 3 times weekly for an additional 3 months.

Induction of ovulation and pregnancy in the anovulatory, infertile woman in whom the cause of anovulation is secondary and not due to primary ovarian failure and who has been appropriately pretreated with human menotropins.
(See prescribing information for menotropins for dosage and administration for that drug product.)
5000 to 10,000 USP units 1 day following the last dose of menotropins. (A dosage of 10,000 USP units is recommended in the labeling for menotropins.)

Directions for Reconstitution
Two-vial package: Withdraw sterile air from lyophilized vial and inject into diluent vial. Remove 1–10 mL from diluent and add to lyophilized vial; agitate gently until powder is completely dissolved in solution.

Parenteral drug products should be inspected visually for particulate matter and discoloration prior to administration, whenever solution and container permit.

IMPORTANT: USE COMPLETELY AFTER RECONSTITUTION. RECONSTITUTED SOLUTION IS STABLE FOR 60 DAYS WHEN REFRIGERATED.

HOW SUPPLIED
Two-vial package containing:
1-10 mL lyophilized multiple dose vial containing: 10,000 USP units chorionic gonadotropin per vial, NDC 0052-0315-10.
1-10 mL vial of solvent containing: water for injection with sodium chloride 0.56% and benzyl alcohol 0.9%, NDC 0052-0325-10.
When reconstituted, each 10 mL vial contains:

Chorionic gonadotropin	10,000 USP Units
Monobasic sodium phosphate	5 mg
Dibasic sodium phosphate	4.4 mg
Sodium chloride	0.56%
Benzyl alcohol	0.9%

If required pH adjusted with sodium hydroxide and/or phosphoric acid.
Storage
Store at controlled room temperature 15–30°C (59–86°F). Reconstituted solution is stable for 60 days when refrigerated.

Manufactured for: Merck Sharp & Dohme Corp., a subsidiary of **MERCK & CO., INC.,** Whitehouse Station, NJ 08889, USA
Manufactured by: Baxter Pharmaceutical Solutions LLC, Bloomington, IN 47403, USA
For patient information:
www.merck.com/product/patent/home.html
Copyright © 1976, 2011 Merck Sharp & Dohme B.V., a subsidiary of **Merck & Co., Inc.**
All rights reserved.
Revised: 12/2013
uspi-mk8829-pwi-1312-r006
Rx only

PRIMAXIN® I.V.
(iMiPENEM AND CILASTATIN FOR INJECTION)   ℞

To reduce the development of drug-resistant bacteria and maintain the effectiveness of PRIMAXIN® I.V. and other antibacterial drugs, PRIMAXIN I.V. should be used only to treat or prevent infections that are proven or strongly suspected to be caused by bacteria.
For Intravenous Injection Only

DESCRIPTION
PRIMAXIN I.V. (Imipenem and Cilastatin for Injection) is a sterile formulation of imipenem (a thienamycin antibiotic) and cilastatin sodium (the inhibitor of the renal dipeptidase, dehydropeptidase l), with sodium bicarbonate added as a buffer. PRIMAXIN I.V. is a potent broad spectrum antibacterial agent for intravenous administration.

Imipenem (N-formimidoylthienamycin monohydrate) is a crystalline derivative of thienamycin, which is produced by *Streptomyces cattleya*. Its chemical name is (5R ,6S)-3-[[2-(formimidoylamino)ethyl]thio]-6-[(R)-1-hydroxyethyl]-7-oxo-1-azabicyclo[3.2.0]hept-2-ene-2-carboxylic acid monohydrate. It is an off-white, nonhygroscopic crystalline compound with a molecular weight of 317.37. It is sparingly

Table 1: Susceptibility Interpretive Criteria for Imipenem

Pathogen	Minimum Inhibitory Concentrations MIC (µg/mL)			Disk Diffusion Zone Diameter (mm)		
	S	I	R	S	I	R
Enterobacteriaceae	≤1.0	2.0	≥4.0	≥23	20-22	≤19
Pseudomonas aeruginosa	≤2	4	≥8	≥19	16-18	≤15
Acinetobacter spp.	≤4	8	≥16	≥16	14-15	≤13
Staphylococcus spp.*	≤4	8	≥16	≥16	14-15	≤13
Haemophilus influenzae and H. parainfluenzae†	≤4	-	-	≥16	-	-
Streptococcus pneumoniae‡	≤0.12	0.25-0.5	≥1	-	-	-
Anaerobes	≤4.0	8.0	≥16.0	-	-	-

* For oxacillin-susceptible S. aureus and coagulase negative staphylococci results for carbapenems, including imipenem, if tested, should be reported according to the results generated using routine interpretive criteria. For oxacillin-resistant S. aureus and coagulase negative staphylococci, other beta lactam agents, including carbapenems, may appear active in vitro but are not effective clinically. Results for beta lactam agents other than cephalosporins with anti-MRSA activity should be reported as resistant or should not be reported.

† For some organism/antimicrobial combinations, the absence or rare occurrence of resistant strains precludes defining any results categories other than "susceptible". For strains yielding results suggestive of a "non-susceptible" category, organism identification and antimicrobial susceptibility test results should be confirmed.

‡ For non-meningitis S. pneumoniae isolates, penicillin MICs ≤0.06 µg/mL (or oxacillin zones ≥20 mm) indicate susceptibility to imipenem.

soluble in water and slightly soluble in methanol. Its empirical formula is $C_{12}H_{17}N_3O_4S \cdot H_2O$, and its structural formula is:

Cilastatin sodium is the sodium salt of a derivatized heptenoic acid. Its chemical name is sodium (Z)-7[[(R)-2-amino-2-carboxyethyl]thio]-2-[(S)-2,2-dimethylcyclopropanecarboxamido]-2-heptenoate. It is an off-white to yellowish-white, hygroscopic, amorphous compound with a molecular weight of 380.43. It is very soluble in water and in methanol. Its empirical formula is $C_{16}H_{25}N_2O_5SNa$, and its structural formula is:

PRIMAXIN I.V. is buffered to provide solutions in the pH range of 6.5 to 8.5. There is no significant change in pH when solutions are prepared and used as directed. (See COMPATIBILITY AND STABILITY.) PRIMAXIN I.V. 250 contains 18.8 mg of sodium (0.8 mEq) and PRIMAXIN I.V. 500 contains 37.5 mg of sodium (1.6 mEq). Solutions of PRIMAXIN I.V. range from colorless to yellow. Variations of color within this range do not affect the potency of the product.

CLINICAL PHARMACOLOGY
Adults
Intravenous Administration
Intravenous infusion of PRIMAXIN I.V. over 20 minutes results in peak plasma levels of imipenem antimicrobial activity that range from 14 to 24 µg/mL for the 250 mg dose, from 21 to 58 µg/mL for the 500 mg dose, and from 41 to 83 µg/mL for the 1000 mg dose. At these doses, plasma levels of imipenem antimicrobial activity decline to below 1 µg/mL or less in 4 to 6 hours. Peak plasma levels of cilastatin following a 20-minute intravenous infusion of PRIMAXIN I.V. range from 15 to 25 µg/mL for the 250 mg dose, from 31 to 49 µg/mL for the 500 mg dose, and from 56 to 88 µg/mL for the 1000 mg dose.

The plasma half-life of each component is approximately 1 hour. The binding of imipenem to human serum proteins is approximately 20% and that of cilastatin is approximately 40%. Approximately 70% of the administered imipenem is recovered in the urine within 10 hours after which no further urinary excretion is detectable. Urine concentrations of imipenem in excess of 10 µg/mL can be maintained for up to 8 hours with PRIMAXIN I.V. at the 500-mg dose. Approximately 70% of the cilastatin sodium dose is recovered in the urine within 10 hours of administration of PRIMAXIN I.V. No accumulation of imipenem/cilastatin in plasma or urine is observed with regimens administered as frequently as every 6 hours in patients with normal renal function.

In healthy elderly volunteers (65 to 75 years of age with normal renal function for their age), the pharmacokinetics of a single dose of imipenem 500 mg and cilastatin 500 mg administered intravenously over 20 minutes are consistent with those expected in subjects with slight renal impairment for which no dosage alteration is considered necessary. The mean plasma half-lives of imipenem and cilastatin are 91 ± 7.0 minutes and 69 ± 15 minutes, respectively. Multiple dosing has no effect on the pharmacokinetics of either imipenem or cilastatin, and no accumulation of imipenem/cilastatin is observed.

Imipenem, when administered alone, is metabolized in the kidneys by dehydropeptidase I resulting in relatively low levels in urine. Cilastatin sodium, an inhibitor of this enzyme, effectively prevents renal metabolism of imipenem so that when imipenem and cilastatin sodium are given concomitantly, fully adequate antibacterial levels of imipenem are achieved in the urine.

After a 1 gram dose of PRIMAXIN I.V., the following average levels of imipenem were measured (usually at 1 hour post dose except where indicated) in the tissues and fluids listed:

Tissue or Fluid	N	Imipenem Level µg/mL or µg/g	Range
Vitreous Humor	3	3.4 (3.5 hours post dose)	2.88–3.6
Aqueous Humor	5	2.99 (2 hours post dose)	2.4–3.9
Lung Tissue	8	5.6 (median)	3.5–15.5
Sputum	1	2.1	—
Pleural	1	22.0	—
Peritoneal	12	23.9 S.D.±5.3 (2 hours post dose)	—
Bile	2	5.3 (2.25 hours post dose)	4.6–6.0
CSF (uninflamed)	5	1.0 (4 hours post dose)	0.26–2.0
CSF (inflamed)	7	2.6 (2 hours post dose)	0.5–5.5
Fallopian Tubes	1	13.6	—
Endometrium	1	11.1	—
Myometrium	1	5.0	—
Bone	10	2.6	0.4–5.4
Interstitial Fluid	12	16.4	10.0–22.6
Skin	12	4.4	NA
Fascia	12	4.4	NA

Imipenem-cilastatin sodium is hemodialyzable. However, usefulness of this procedure in the overdosage setting is questionable. (See OVERDOSAGE.)
Microbiology
The bactericidal activity of imipenem results from the inhibition of cell wall synthesis. Its greatest affinity is for penicillin binding proteins (PBPs) 1A, 1B, 2, 4, 5 and 6 of Escherichia coli, and 1A, 1B, 2, 4 and 5 of Pseudomonas aeruginosa. The lethal effect is related to binding to PBP 2 and PBP 1B.

Imipenem has a high degree of stability in the presence of beta-lactamases, both penicillinases and cephalosporinases produced by gram-negative and gram-positive bacteria. It is a potent inhibitor of beta-lactamases from certain gram-negative bacteria which are inherently resistant to most beta-lactam antibiotics, e.g., Pseudomonas aeruginosa, Serratia spp., and Enterobacter spp.

Imipenem has in vitro activity against a wide range of gram-positive and gram-negative organisms. Imipenem has been shown to be active against most strains of the following microorganisms, both in vitro and in clinical infections treated with the intravenous formulation of imipenem-cilastatin sodium as described in the INDICATIONS AND USAGE section.

Gram-positive aerobes:
Enterococcus faecalis (formerly S. faecalis)
(NOTE: Imipenem is inactive in vitro against Enterococcus faecium [formerly S. faecium].)
Staphylococcus aureus including penicillinase-producing strains
Staphylococcus epidermidis including penicillinase-producing strains
(NOTE: Methicillin-resistant staphylococci should be reported as resistant to imipenem.)
Streptococcus agalactiae (Group B streptococci)
Streptococcus pneumoniae
Streptococcus pyogenes
Gram-negative aerobes:
Acinetobacter spp.
Citrobacter spp.
Enterobacter spp.
Escherichia coli
Gardnerella vaginalis
Haemophilus influenzae
Haemophilus parainfluenzae
Klebsiella spp.
Morganella morganii
Proteus vulgaris
Providencia rettgeri
Pseudomonas aeruginosa
(NOTE: Imipenem is inactive in vitro against Stenotrophomonas [formerly Xanthomonas, formerly Pseudomonas] maltophilia and some strains of Burkholderia cepacia.)
Serratia spp., including S. marcescens
Gram-positive anaerobes:
Bifidobacterium spp.
Clostridium spp.
Eubacterium spp.
Peptococcus spp.
Peptostreptococcus spp.
Propionibacterium spp.
Gram-negative anaerobes:
Bacteroides spp., including B. fragilis
Fusobacterium spp.
The following in vitro data are available, **but their clinical significance is unknown.**

Imipenem exhibits in vitro minimum inhibitory concentrations (MICs) of 4 µg/mL or less against most (≥90%) strains of the following microorganisms; however, the safety and effectiveness of imipenem in treating clinical infections due to these microorganisms have not been established in adequate and well-controlled clinical trials.
Gram-positive aerobes:
Bacillus spp.
Listeria monocytogenes
Nocardia spp.
Staphylococcus saprophyticus
Group C streptococci
Group G streptococci
Viridans group streptococci
Gram-negative aerobes:
Aeromonas hydrophila
Alcaligenes spp.
Capnocytophaga spp.
Haemophilus ducreyi
Neisseria gonorrhoeae including penicillinase-producing strains
Pasteurella spp.
Providencia stuartii
Gram-negative anaerobes:
Prevotella bivia
Prevotella disiens
Prevotella melaninogenica
Veillonella spp.

In vitro tests show imipenem to act synergistically with aminoglycoside antibiotics against some isolates of Pseudomonas aeruginosa.
Susceptibility Test Methods
When available, the clinical microbiology laboratory should provide to the physician the results of in vitro susceptibility tests for antimicrobial drug products used in resident hospitals as periodic reports which describe the susceptibility profile of nosocomial and community-acquired pathogens. These reports should aid the physician in selecting the most effective antimicrobial.

Dilution Techniques

Quantitative methods are used to determine antimicrobial minimum inhibitory concentrations (MICs). These MICs provide estimates of the susceptibility of bacteria to antimicrobial compounds. The MICs should be determined using a standardized procedure. Standardized procedures are based on a broth dilution method[1,2] or equivalent with standardized inoculum concentrations and standardized concentrations of imipenem powder. The MIC values should be interpreted according to criteria provided in Table 1.

Diffusion Techniques

Quantitative methods that require measurement of zone diameters also provide reproducible estimates of the susceptibility of bacteria to antimicrobial compounds. One such standardized procedure requires the use of standardized inoculum concentrations [2,3]. This procedure uses paper disks impregnated with 10-µg imipenem to test the susceptibility of microorganisms to imipenem. The disk diffusion interpretive criteria should be interpreted according to criteria provided in Table 1.

Anaerobic Techniques

For anaerobic bacteria, the susceptibility to imipenem as MICs can be determined by standardized test methods.[2,4] The MIC values obtained should be interpreted according to criteria provided in Table 1.

The MIC and disk diffusion values obtained should be interpreted according to the following criteria:

[See table 1 at top of previous page]

A report of "Susceptible" indicates that the pathogen is likely to be inhibited if the antimicrobial compound at the infection site reaches the concentrations usually achievable. A report of "Intermediate" indicates that the result should be considered equivocal, and, if the microorganism is not fully susceptible to alternative, clinically feasible drugs, the test should be repeated. This category implies possible clinical applicability in body sites where the drug is physiologically concentrated or in situations where high dosage of drug can be used. This category also provides a buffer zone which prevents small uncontrolled technical factors from causing major discrepancies in interpretation. A report of "Resistant" indicates that the pathogen is not likely to be inhibited if the antimicrobial compound at the infection site reaches the concentrations usually achievable, and that other therapy should be selected.

Quality Control

Standardized susceptibility test procedures require the use of laboratory control microorganisms to ensure the accuracy and precision of supplies and reagents used in the assay, and the techniques of the individuals performing the test. Quality control microorganisms are specific strains of organisms with intrinsic biological properties. QC strains are very stable strains which will give a standard and repeatable susceptibility pattern. The specific strains used for microbiological quality control are not clinically significant. Standard imipenem powder should provide the following range of values noted in Table 2.[2]

[See table 2 above]

INDICATIONS AND USAGE

PRIMAXIN I.V. is indicated for the treatment of serious infections caused by susceptible strains of the designated microorganisms in the conditions listed below:

1. **Lower respiratory tract infections.** *Staphylococcus aureus* (penicillinase-producing strains), *Acinetobacter* species, *Enterobacter* species, *Escherichia coli*, *Haemophilus influenzae*, *Haemophilus parainfluenzae*[1], *Klebsiella* species, *Serratia marcescens*

2. **Urinary tract infections** (complicated and uncomplicated). *Enterococcus faecalis*, *Staphylococcus aureus* (penicillinase-producing strains)[1], *Enterobacter* species, *Escherichia coli*, *Klebsiella* species, *Morganella morganii*[1], *Proteus vulgaris*[1], *Providencia rettgeri*[1], *Pseudomonas aeruginosa*

3. **Intra-abdominal infections.** *Enterococcus faecalis*, *Staphylococcus aureus* (penicillinase-producing strains)[1], *Staphylococcus epidermidis*, *Citrobacter* species, *Enterobacter* species, *Escherichia coli*, *Klebsiella* species, *Morganella morganii*[1], *Proteus* species, *Pseudomonas aeruginosa*, *Bifidobacterium* species, *Clostridium* species, *Eubacterium* species, *Peptococcus* species, *Peptostreptococcus* species, *Propionibacterium* species[1], *Bacteroides* species including *B. fragilis*, *Fusobacterium* species

4. **Gynecologic infections.** *Enterococcus faecalis*, *Staphylococcus aureus* (penicillinase-producing strains)[1], *Staphylococcus epidermidis*, *Streptococcus agalactiae* (Group B streptococci), *Enterobacter* species[1], *Escherichia coli*, *Gardnerella vaginalis*, *Klebsiella* species[1], *Proteus* species, *Bifidobacterium* species[1], *Peptococcus* species[1], *Peptostreptococcus* species, *Propionibacterium* species[1], *Bacteroides* species including *B. fragilis*[1]

5. **Bacterial septicemia.** *Enterococcus faecalis*, *Staphylococcus aureus* (penicillinase-producing strains), *Enterobacter* species, *Escherichia coli*, *Klebsiella* species, *Pseudomonas aeruginosa*, *Serratia* species[1], *Bacteroides* species including *B. fragilis*[1]

Table 2: Acceptable Quality Control Ranges for Imipenem

Microorganism	Minimum Inhibitory Concentrations MIC Range (µg/mL)	Disk Diffusion Zone Diameter (mm)
Pseudomonas aeruginosa ATCC 27853	1-4	20-28
Escherichia coli ATCC 25922	0.06-0.25	26-32
Haemophilus influenzae ATCC 49247	-	21-29
Haemophilus influenzae ATCC 49766	0.25-1.0	-
Staphylococcus aureus ATCC 29213	0.015-0.06	-
Enterococcus faecalis ATCC 29212	0.5-2.0	-
Streptococcus pneumoniae ATCC 49619	0.03-0.12	-
Bacteroides fragilis ATCC 25285	0.03-0.25* 0.03-0.125†	-
Bacteroides thetaiotaomicron ATCC 29741	0.25-1.0* 0.125-0.5†	-
Eubacterium lentum ATCC 43055	0.25-2.0* 0.125-0.5†	-

* Quality control ranges for broth microdilution testing
† Quality control ranges for agar dilution testing

6. **Bone and joint infections.** *Enterococcus faecalis*, *Staphylococcus aureus* (penicillinase-producing strains), *Staphylococcus epidermidis*, *Enterobacter* species, *Pseudomonas aeruginosa*

7. **Skin and skin structure infections.** *Enterococcus faecalis*, *Staphylococcus aureus* (penicillinase-producing strains), *Staphylococcus epidermidis*, *Acinetobacter* species, *Citrobacter* species, *Enterobacter* species, *Escherichia coli*, *Klebsiella* species, *Morganella morganii*, *Proteus vulgaris*, *Providencia rettgeri*[1], *Pseudomonas aeruginosa*, *Serratia* species, *Peptococcus* species, *Peptostreptococcus* species, *Bacteroides* species including *B. fragilis*, *Fusobacterium* species[1]

8. **Endocarditis.** *Staphylococcus aureus* (penicillinase-producing strains)

9. **Polymicrobic infections.** PRIMAXIN I.V. is indicated for polymicrobic infections including those in which *S. pneumoniae* (pneumonia, septicemia), *S. pyogenes* (skin and skin structure), or nonpenicillinase-producing *S. aureus* is one of the causative organisms. However, monobacterial infections due to these organisms are usually treated with narrower spectrum antibiotics, such as penicillin G.

PRIMAXIN I.V. is not indicated in patients with meningitis because safety and efficacy have not been established.

For Pediatric Use information, see PRECAUTIONS, Pediatric Use, and DOSAGE AND ADMINISTRATION sections.

Because of its broad spectrum of bactericidal activity against gram-positive and gram-negative aerobic and anaerobic bacteria, PRIMAXIN I.V. is useful for the treatment of mixed infections and as presumptive therapy prior to the identification of the causative organisms.

Although clinical improvement has been observed in patients with cystic fibrosis, chronic pulmonary disease, and lower respiratory tract infections caused by *Pseudomonas aeruginosa*, bacterial eradication may not necessarily be achieved.

As with other beta-lactam antibiotics, some strains of *Pseudomonas aeruginosa* may develop resistance fairly rapidly during treatment with PRIMAXIN I.V. During therapy of *Pseudomonas aeruginosa* infections, periodic susceptibility testing should be done when clinically appropriate.

Infections resistant to other antibiotics, for example, cephalosporins, penicillin, and aminoglycosides, have been shown to respond to treatment with PRIMAXIN I.V.

To reduce the development of drug-resistant bacteria and maintain the effectiveness of PRIMAXIN I.V. and other antibacterial drugs, PRIMAXIN I.V. should be used only to treat or prevent infections that are proven or strongly suspected to be caused by susceptible bacteria. When culture and susceptibility information are available, they should be considered in selecting or modifying antibacterial therapy. In the absence of such data, local epidemiology and susceptibility patterns may contribute to the empiric selection of therapy.

[1] Efficacy for this organism in this organ system was studied in fewer than 10 infections.

CONTRAINDICATIONS

PRIMAXIN I.V. is contraindicated in patients who have shown hypersensitivity to any component of this product.

WARNINGS

SERIOUS AND OCCASIONALLY FATAL HYPERSENSITIVITY (ANAPHYLACTIC) REACTIONS HAVE BEEN REPORTED IN PATIENTS RECEIVING THERAPY WITH BETA-LACTAMS. THESE REACTIONS ARE MORE APT TO OCCUR IN PERSONS WITH A HISTORY OF SENSITIVITY TO MULTIPLE ALLERGENS.

THERE HAVE BEEN REPORTS OF PATIENTS WITH A HISTORY OF PENICILLIN HYPERSENSITIVITY WHO HAVE EXPERIENCED SEVERE HYPERSENSITIVITY REACTIONS WHEN TREATED WITH ANOTHER BETA-LACTAM. BEFORE INITIATING THERAPY WITH PRIMAXIN I.V., CAREFUL INQUIRY SHOULD BE MADE CONCERNING PREVIOUS HYPERSENSITIVITY REACTIONS TO PENICILLINS, CEPHALOSPORINS, OTHER BETA-LACTAMS, AND OTHER ALLERGENS. IF AN ALLERGIC REACTION OCCURS, PRIMAXIN SHOULD BE DISCONTINUED.

SERIOUS ANAPHYLACTIC REACTIONS REQUIRE IMMEDIATE EMERGENCY TREATMENT WITH EPINEPHRINE. OXYGEN, INTRAVENOUS STEROIDS, AND AIRWAY MANAGEMENT, INCLUDING INTUBATION, MAY ALSO BE ADMINISTERED AS INDICATED.

Seizure Potential

Seizures and other CNS adverse experiences, such as confusional states and myoclonic activity, have been reported during treatment with PRIMAXIN I.V. (See PRECAUTIONS and ADVERSE REACTIONS.)

Case reports in the literature have shown that co-administration of carbapenems, including imipenem, to patients receiving valproic acid or divalproex sodium results in a reduction in valproic acid concentrations. The valproic acid concentrations may drop below the therapeutic range as a result of this interaction, therefore increasing the risk of breakthrough seizures. Increasing the dose of valproic acid or divalproex sodium may not be sufficient to overcome this interaction. The concomitant use of imipenem and valproic acid/divalproex sodium is generally not recommended. Anti-bacterials other than carbapenems should be considered to treat infections in patients whose seizures are well controlled on valproic acid or divalproex sodium. If administration of PRIMAXIN I.V. is necessary, supplemental anticonvulsant therapy should be considered (see PRECAUTIONS, Drug Interactions).

Clostridium difficile associated diarrhea (CDAD) has been reported with use of nearly all antibacterial agents, including PRIMAXIN I.V., and may range in severity from mild diarrhea to fatal colitis. Treatment with antibacterial agents alters the normal flora of the colon leading to overgrowth of *C. difficile*.

C. difficile produces toxins A and B which contribute to the development of CDAD.

Hypertoxin producing strains of *C. difficile* cause increased morbidity and mortality, as these infections can be refractory to antimicrobial therapy and may require colectomy. CDAD must be considered in all patients who present with diarrhea following antibiotic use. Careful medical history is necessary since CDAD has been reported to occur over two months after the administration of antibacterial agents.

If CDAD is suspected or confirmed, ongoing antibiotic use not directed against *C. difficile* may need to be discontinued.

Appropriate fluid and electrolyte management, protein supplementation, antibiotic treatment of *C. difficile*, and surgical evaluation should be instituted as clinically indicated.

PRECAUTIONS
General
CNS adverse experiences such as confusional states, myoclonic activity, and seizures have been reported during treatment with PRIMAXIN I.V., especially when recommended dosages were exceeded. These experiences have occurred most commonly in patients with CNS disorders (e.g., brain lesions or history of seizures) and/or compromised renal function. However, there have been reports of CNS adverse experiences in patients who had no recognized or documented underlying CNS disorder or compromised renal function.

When recommended doses were exceeded, adult patients with creatinine clearances of ≤20 mL/min/1.73 m², whether or not undergoing hemodialysis, had a higher risk of seizure activity than those without impairment of renal function. Therefore, close adherence to the dosing guidelines for these patients is recommended. (See DOSAGE AND ADMINISTRATION.)

Patients with creatinine clearances of ≤5 mL/min/1.73 m² should not receive PRIMAXIN I.V. unless hemodialysis is instituted within 48 hours.

For patients on hemodialysis, PRIMAXIN I.V. is recommended only when the benefit outweighs the potential risk of seizures.

Close adherence to the recommended dosage and dosage schedules is urged, especially in patients with known factors that predispose to convulsive activity. Anticonvulsant therapy should be continued in patients with known seizure disorders. If focal tremors, myoclonus, or seizures occur, patients should be evaluated neurologically, placed on anticonvulsant therapy if not already instituted, and the dosage of PRIMAXIN I.V. re-examined to determine whether it should be decreased or the antibiotic discontinued.

As with other antibiotics, prolonged use of PRIMAXIN I.V. may result in overgrowth of nonsusceptible organisms. Repeated evaluation of the patient's condition is essential. If superinfection occurs during therapy, appropriate measures should be taken.

Prescribing PRIMAXIN I.V. in the absence of a proven or strongly suspected bacterial infection or a prophylactic indication is unlikely to provide benefit to the patient and increases the risk of the development of drug-resistant bacteria.

Information for Patients
Patients should be counseled to inform their physician if they are taking valproic acid or divalproex sodium. Valproic acid concentrations in the blood may drop below the therapeutic range upon co-administration with PRIMAXIN I.V. If treatment with PRIMAXIN I.V. is necessary and continued, alternative or supplemental anti-convulsant medication to prevent and/or treat seizures may be needed.

Patients should be counseled that antibacterial drugs including PRIMAXIN I.V. should only be used to treat bacterial infections. They do not treat viral infections (e.g., the common cold). When PRIMAXIN I.V. is prescribed to treat a bacterial infection, patients should be told that although it is common to feel better early in the course of therapy, the medication should be taken exactly as directed. Skipping doses or not completing the full course of therapy may (1) decrease the effectiveness of the immediate treatment and (2) increase the likelihood that bacteria will develop resistance and will not be treatable by PRIMAXIN I.V. or other antibacterial drugs in the future.

Diarrhea is a common problem caused by antibiotics, which usually ends when the antibiotic is discontinued. Sometimes after starting treatment with antibiotics, patients can develop watery and bloody stools (with or without stomach cramps and fever) even as late as two or more months after having taken the last dose of the antibiotic. If this occurs, patients should contact their physician as soon as possible.

Laboratory Tests
While PRIMAXIN I.V. possesses the characteristic low toxicity of the beta-lactam group of antibiotics, periodic assessment of organ system functions, including renal, hepatic, and hematopoietic, is advisable during prolonged therapy.

Drug Interactions
Generalized seizures have been reported in patients who received ganciclovir and PRIMAXIN. These drugs should not be used concomitantly unless the potential benefits outweigh the risks.

Since concomitant administration of PRIMAXIN and probenecid results in only minimal increases in plasma levels of imipenem and plasma half-life, it is not recommended that probenecid be given with PRIMAXIN.

PRIMAXIN should not be mixed with or physically added to other antibiotics. However, PRIMAXIN may be administered concomitantly with other antibiotics, such as aminoglycosides.

Case reports in the literature have shown that co-administration of carbapenems, including imipenem, to patients receiving valproic acid or divalproex sodium results in a reduction in valproic acid concentrations. The valproic acid concentrations may drop below the therapeutic range as a result of this interaction, therefore increasing the risk of breakthrough seizures. Although the mechanism of this interaction is unknown, data from *in vitro* and animal studies suggest that carbapenems may inhibit the hydrolysis of valproic acid's glucuronide metabolite (VPA-g) back to valproic acid, thus decreasing the serum concentrations of valproic acid (see WARNINGS, Seizure Potential).

Carcinogenesis, Mutagenesis, Impairment of Fertility
Long term studies in animals have not been performed to evaluate carcinogenic potential of imipenem-cilastatin. Genetic toxicity studies were performed in a variety of bacterial and mammalian tests *in vivo* and *in vitro*. The tests used were: V79 mammalian cell mutagenesis assay (imipenem-cilastatin sodium alone and imipenem alone), Ames test (cilastatin sodium alone and imipenem alone), unscheduled DNA synthesis assay (imipenem-cilastatin sodium) and *in vivo* mouse cytogenetics test (imipenem-cilastatin sodium). None of these tests showed any evidence of genetic alterations.

Reproductive tests in male and female rats were performed with imipenem-cilastatin sodium at intravenous doses up to 80 mg/kg/day and at a subcutaneous dose of 320 mg/kg/day, approximately equal to the highest recommended human dose of the intravenous formulation (on a mg/m² body surface area basis). Slight decreases in live fetal body weight were restricted to the highest dosage level. No other adverse effects were observed on fertility, reproductive performance, fetal viability, growth or postnatal development of pups.

Pregnancy
Teratogenic Effects
Pregnancy Category C:
Teratology studies with cilastatin sodium at doses of 30, 100, and 300 mg/kg/day administered intravenously to rabbits and 40, 200, and 1000 mg/kg/day administered subcutaneously to rats, up to approximately 1.9 and 3.2 times² the maximum recommended daily human dose (on a mg/m² body surface area basis) of the intravenous formulation of imipenem-cilastatin sodium (50 mg/kg/day) in the two species, respectively, showed no evidence of adverse effect on the fetus. No evidence of teratogenicity was observed in rabbits given imipenem at intravenous doses of 15, 30 or 60 mg/kg/day and rats given imipenem at intravenous doses of 225, 450, or 900 mg/kg/day, up to approximately 0.4 and 2.9 times² the maximum recommended daily human dose (on a mg/m² body surface area basis) in the two species, respectively.

Teratology studies with imipenem-cilastatin sodium at intravenous doses of 20 and 80, and a subcutaneous dose of 320 mg/kg/day, up to 0.5 times² (mice) to approximately equal to (rats) the highest recommended daily intravenous human dose (on a mg/m² body surface area basis) in pregnant rodents during the period of major organogenesis, revealed no evidence of teratogenicity.

Imipenem-cilastatin sodium, when administered subcutaneously to pregnant rabbits at dosages equivalent to the usual human dose of the intravenous formulation and higher (1000-4000 mg/day), caused body weight loss, diarrhea, and maternal deaths. When comparable doses of imipenem-cilastatin sodium were given to non-pregnant rabbits, body weight loss, diarrhea, and deaths were also observed. This intolerance is not unlike that seen with other beta-lactam antibiotics in this species and is probably due to alteration of gut flora.

A teratology study in pregnant cynomolgus monkeys given imipenem-cilastatin sodium at doses of 40 mg/kg/day (bolus intravenous injection) or 160 mg/kg/day (subcutaneous injection) resulted in maternal toxicity including emesis, inappetence, body weight loss, diarrhea, abortion, and death in some cases. In contrast, no significant toxicity was observed when non-pregnant cynomolgus monkeys were given doses of imipenem-cilastatin sodium up to 180 mg/kg/day (subcutaneous injection). When doses of imipenem-cilastatin sodium (approximately 100 mg/kg/day or approximately 0.6 times² the maximum recommended daily human dose of the intravenous formulation) were administered to pregnant cynomolgus monkeys at an intravenous infusion rate which mimics human clinical use, there was minimal maternal intolerance (occasional emesis), no maternal deaths, no evidence of teratogenicity, but an increase in embryonic loss relative to control groups.

No adverse effects on the fetus or on lactation were observed when imipenem-cilastatin sodium was administered subcutaneously to rats late in gestation at dosages up to 320 mg/kg/day, approximately equal to the highest recommended human dose (on a mg/m² body surface area basis).

There are, however, no adequate and well-controlled studies in pregnant women. PRIMAXIN I.V. should be used during pregnancy only if the potential benefit justifies the potential risk to the mother and fetus.

²Based on patient body surface area of 1.6 m² (weight of 60 kg).

Nursing Mothers
It is not known whether imipenem-cilastatin sodium is excreted in human milk. Because many drugs are excreted in human milk, caution should be exercised when PRIMAXIN I.V. is administered to a nursing woman.

Pediatric Use
Use of PRIMAXIN I.V. in pediatric patients, neonates to 16 years of age, is supported by evidence from adequate and well-controlled studies of PRIMAXIN I.V. in adults and by the following clinical studies and published literature in pediatric patients: Based on published studies of 178[3] pediatric patients ≥3 months of age (with non-CNS infections), the recommended dose of PRIMAXIN I.V. is 15-25 mg/kg/dose administered every six hours. Doses of 25 mg/kg/dose in patients 3 months to <3 years of age, and 15 mg/kg/dose in patients 3-12 years of age were associated with mean trough plasma concentrations of imipenem of 1.1±0.4 µg/mL and 0.6±0.2 µg/mL following multiple 60-minute infusions, respectively; trough urinary concentrations of imipenem were in excess of 10 µg/mL for both doses. These doses have provided adequate plasma and urine concentrations for the treatment of non-CNS infections. Based on studies in adults, the maximum daily dose for treatment of infections with fully susceptible organisms is 2.0 g per day, and of infections with moderately susceptible organisms (primarily some strains of *P. aeruginosa*) is 4.0 g/day. (See DOSAGE AND ADMINISTRATION, Table 3.) Higher doses (up to 90 mg/kg/day in older children) have been used in patients with cystic fibrosis. (See DOSAGE AND ADMINISTRATION.)

Based on studies of 135[4] pediatric patients ≤3 months of age (weighing ≥1,500 g), the following dosage schedule is recommended for non-CNS infections:

<1 wk of age: 25 mg/kg every 12 hrs
1-4 wks of age: 25 mg/kg every 8 hrs
4 wks-3 mos. of age: 25 mg/kg every 6 hrs.

In a published dose-ranging study of smaller premature infants (670-1,890 g) in the first week of life, a dose of 20 mg/kg q12h by 15-30 minutes infusion was associated with mean peak and trough plasma imipenem concentrations of 43 µg/mL and 1.7 µg/mL after multiple doses, respectively. However, moderate accumulation of cilastatin in neonates may occur following multiple doses of PRIMAXIN I.V. The safety of this accumulation is unknown.

PRIMAXIN I.V. is not recommended in pediatric patients with CNS infections because of the risk of seizures.

PRIMAXIN I.V. is not recommended in pediatric patients <30 kg with impaired renal function, as no data are available.

[3]Two patients were less than 3 months of age.
[4]One patient was greater than 3 months of age.

Geriatric Use
Of the approximately 3600 subjects ≥18 years of age in clinical studies of PRIMAXIN I.V., including postmarketing studies, approximately 2800 received PRIMAXIN I.V. Of the subjects who received PRIMAXIN I.V., data are available on approximately 800 subjects who were 65 and over, including approximately 300 subjects who were 75 and over. No overall differences in safety or effectiveness were observed between these subjects and younger subjects. Other reported clinical experience has not identified differences in responses between the elderly and younger patients, but greater sensitivity of some older individuals cannot be ruled out.

This drug is known to be substantially excreted by the kidney, and the risk of toxic reactions to this drug may be greater in patients with impaired renal function. Because elderly patients are more likely to have decreased renal function, care should be taken in dose selection, and it may be useful to monitor renal function.

No dosage adjustment is required based on age (see CLINICAL PHARMACOLOGY, Adults). Dosage adjustment in the case of renal impairment is necessary (see DOSAGE AND ADMINISTRATION, Reduced Intravenous Schedule for Adults with Impaired Renal Function and/or Body Weight <70 kg).

ADVERSE REACTIONS
Adults
PRIMAXIN I.V. is generally well tolerated. Many of the 1,723 patients treated in clinical trials were severely ill and had multiple background diseases and physiological impairments, making it difficult to determine causal relationship of adverse experiences to therapy with PRIMAXIN I.V.

Local Adverse Reactions
Adverse local clinical reactions that were reported as possibly, probably, or definitely related to therapy with PRIMAXIN I.V. were:
Phlebitis/thrombophlebitis — 3.1%
Pain at the injection site — 0.7%
Erythema at the injection site — 0.4%

Vein induration — 0.2%
Infused vein infection — 0.1%

Systemic Adverse Reactions
The most frequently reported systemic adverse clinical reactions that were reported as possibly, probably, or definitely related to PRIMAXIN I.V. were nausea (2.0%), diarrhea (1.8%), vomiting (1.5%), rash (0.9%), fever (0.5%), hypotension (0.4%), seizures (0.4%) (see PRECAUTIONS), dizziness (0.3%), pruritus (0.3%), urticaria (0.2%), somnolence (0.2%).

Additional adverse systemic clinical reactions reported as possibly, probably, or definitely drug related occurring in less than 0.2% of the patients or reported since the drug was marketed are listed within each body system in order of decreasing severity: *Gastrointestinal* — pseudomembranous colitis (the onset of pseudomembranous colitis symptoms may occur during or after antibacterial treatment, see WARNINGS), hemorrhagic colitis, hepatitis (including fulminant hepatitis), hepatic failure, jaundice, gastroenteritis, abdominal pain, glossitis, tongue papillar hypertrophy, staining of the teeth and/or tongue, heartburn, pharyngeal pain, increased salivation; *Hematologic* — pancytopenia, bone marrow depression, thrombocytopenia, neutropenia, leukopenia, hemolytic anemia; *CNS* — encephalopathy, tremor, confusion, myoclonus, paresthesia, vertigo, headache, psychic disturbances including hallucinations; *Special Senses* — hearing loss, tinnitus, taste perversion; *Respiratory* — chest discomfort, dyspnea, hyperventilation, thoracic spine pain; *Cardiovascular* — palpitations, tachycardia; *Skin* — Stevens-Johnson syndrome, toxic epidermal necrolysis, erythema multiforme, angioneurotic edema, flushing, cyanosis, hyperhidrosis, skin texture changes, candidiasis, pruritus vulvae; *Body as a whole* — polyarthralgia, asthenia/weakness, drug fever; *Renal* — acute renal failure, oliguria/anuria, polyuria, urine discoloration. The role of PRIMAXIN I.V. in changes in renal function is difficult to assess, since factors predisposing to pre-renal azotemia or to impaired renal function usually have been present.

Adverse Laboratory Changes
Adverse laboratory changes without regard to drug relationship that were reported during clinical trials or reported since the drug was marketed were:
Hepatic: Increased ALT (SGPT), AST (SGOT), alkaline phosphatase, bilirubin, and LDH
Hemic: Increased eosinophils, positive Coombs test, increased WBC, increased platelets, decreased hemoglobin and hematocrit, agranulocytosis, increased monocytes, abnormal prothrombin time, increased lymphocytes, increased basophils
Electrolytes: Decreased serum sodium, increased potassium, increased chloride
Renal: Increased BUN, creatinine
Urinalysis: Presence of urine protein, urine red blood cells, urine white blood cells, urine casts, urine bilirubin, and urine urobilinogen.

Pediatric Patients
In studies of 178 pediatric patients ≥3 months of age, the following adverse events were noted:

The Most Common Clinical Adverse Experiences Without Regard to Drug Relationship (Patient Incidence >1%)

Adverse Experience	No. of Patients (%)
Digestive System	
Diarrhea	7* (3.9)
Gastroenteritis	2 (1.1)
Vomiting	2* (1.1)
Skin	
Rash	4 (2.2)
Irritation, I.V. site	2 (1.1)
Urogenital System	
Urine discoloration	2 (1.1)
Cardiovascular System	
Phlebitis	4 (2.2)

*One patient had both vomiting and diarrhea and is counted in each category.

In studies of 135 patients (newborn to 3 months of age), the following adverse events were noted:

The Most Common Clinical Adverse Experiences Without Regard to Drug Relationship (Patient Incidence >1%)

Adverse Experience	No. of Patients (%)
Digestive System	
Diarrhea	4 (3.0%)
Oral Candidiasis	2 (1.5%)
Skin	
Rash	2 (1.5%)
Urogenital System	
Oliguria/anuria	3 (2.2%)

Patients (≥3 Months of Age) With Normal Pretherapy but Abnormal During Therapy Laboratory Values

Laboratory Parameter	Abnormality			No. of Patients With Abnormalities/No. of Patients With Lab Done (%)
Hemoglobin	Age	<5 mos.:	<10 gm %	19/129 (14.7)
		6 mos. – 12 yrs.:	<11.5 gm %	
Hematocrit	Age	<5 mos.:	<30 vol %	23/129 (17.8)
		6 mos. – 12 yrs.:	<34.5 vol %	
Neutrophils	≤1000/mm³ (absolute)			4/123 (3.3)
Eosinophils	≥7%			15/117 (12.8)
Platelet Count	≥500 ths/mm³			16/119 (13.4)
Urine Protein	≥1			8/97 (8.2)
Serum Creatinine	>1.2 mg/dL			0/105 (0)
BUN	>22 mg/dL			0/108 (0)
AST (SGOT)	>36 IU/L			14/78 (17.9)
ALT (SGPT)	>30 IU/L			10/93 (10.8)

Cardiovascular System	
Tachycardia	2 (1.5%)
Nervous System	
Convulsions	8 (5.9%)

[See table above]

Patients (<3 Months of Age) With Normal Pretherapy but Abnormal During Therapy Laboratory Values

Laboratory Parameter	No. of Patients With Abnormalities* (%)
Eosinophil Count↑	11 (9.0%)
Hematocrit↓	3 (2.0%)
Hematocrit↑	1 (1.0%)
Platelet Count↑	5 (4.0%)
Platelet Count↓	2 (2.0%)
Serum Creatinine↑	5 (5.0%)
Bilirubin↑	3 (3.0%)
Bilirubin↓	1 (1.0%)
AST (SGOT)↑	5 (6.0%)
ALT (SGPT)↑	3 (3.0%)
Serum Alkaline Phosphate↑	2 (3.0%)

* The denominator used for percentages was the number of patients for whom the test was performed during or post-treatment and, therefore, varies by test.

Examination of published literature and spontaneous adverse event reports suggested a similar spectrum of adverse events in adult and pediatric patients.

OVERDOSAGE
The acute intravenous toxicity of imipenem-cilastatin sodium in a ratio of 1:1 was studied in mice at doses of 751 to 1359 mg/kg. Following drug administration, ataxia was rapidly produced and clonic convulsions were noted in about 45 minutes. Deaths occurred within 4-56 minutes at all doses. The acute intravenous toxicity of imipenem-cilastatin sodium was produced within 5-10 minutes in rats at doses of 771 to 1583 mg/kg. In all dosage groups, females had decreased activity, bradypnea, and ptosis with clonic convulsions preceding death; in males, ptosis was seen at all dose levels while tremors and clonic convulsions were seen at all but the lowest dose (771 mg/kg). In another rat study, female rats showed ataxia, bradypnea, and decreased activity in all but the lowest dose (550 mg/kg); deaths were preceded by clonic convulsions. Male rats showed tremors at all doses and clonic convulsions and ptosis were seen at the two highest doses (1130 and 1734 mg/kg). Deaths occurred between 6 and 88 minutes with doses of 771 to 1734 mg/kg.
In the case of overdosage, discontinue PRIMAXIN I.V., treat symptomatically, and institute supportive measures as required. Imipenem-cilastatin sodium is hemodialyzable. However, usefulness of this procedure in the overdosage setting is questionable.

DOSAGE AND ADMINISTRATION
Adults
The dosage recommendations for PRIMAXIN I.V. represent the quantity of imipenem to be administered. An equivalent amount of cilastatin is also present in the solution. Each 125 mg, 250 mg, or 500 mg dose should be given by intravenous administration over 20 to 30 minutes. Each 750 mg or 1000 mg dose should be infused over 40 to 60 minutes. In patients who develop nausea during the infusion, the rate of infusion may be slowed.
The total daily dosage for PRIMAXIN I.V. should be based on the type or severity of infection and given in equally divided doses based on consideration of degree of susceptibility of the pathogen(s), renal function, and body weight. Adult patients with impaired renal function, as judged by creatinine clearance ≤70 mL/min/1.73 m², require adjustment of dosage as described in the succeeding section of these guidelines.
Intravenous Dosage Schedule for Adults with Normal Renal Function and Body Weight ≥70 kg
Doses cited in Table 3 are based on a patient with normal renal function and a body weight of 70 kg. These doses should be used for a patient with a creatinine clearance of ≥71 mL/min/1.73 m² and a body weight of ≥70 kg. A reduction in dose must be made for a patient with a creatinine clearance of ≤70 mL/min/1.73 m² and/or a body weight less than 70 kg. (See Tables 4 and 5.)
Dosage regimens in column A of Table 3 are recommended for infections caused by fully susceptible organisms which represent the majority of pathogenic species. Dosage regimens in column B of Table 3 are recommended for infections caused by organisms with moderate susceptibility to imipenem, primarily some strains of *P. aeruginosa*.

TABLE 3: INTRAVENOUS DOSAGE SCHEDULE FOR ADULTS WITH NORMAL RENAL FUNCTION AND BODY WEIGHT ≥70 kg

Type or Severity of Infection	A Fully susceptible organisms including gram-positive and gram-negative aerobes and anaerobes	B Moderately susceptible organisms, primarily some strains of P. aeruginosa
Mild	250 mg q6h (TOTAL DAILY DOSE = 1.0g)	500 mg q6h (TOTAL DAILY DOSE = 2.0g)
Moderate	500 mg q8h (TOTAL DAILY DOSE = 1.5g) or 500 mg q6h (TOTAL DAILY DOSE = 2.0g)	500 mg q6h (TOTAL DAILY DOSE = 2.0g) or 1 g q8h (TOTAL DAILY DOSE = 3.0g)
Severe, life threatening only	500 mg q6h (TOTAL DAILY DOSE = 2.0g)	1 g q8h (TOTAL DAILY DOSE = 3.0g) or 1 g q6h (TOTAL DAILY DOSE = 4.0g)
Uncomplicated urinary tract infection	250 mg q6h (TOTAL DAILY DOSE = 1.0g)	250 mg q6h (TOTAL DAILY DOSE = 1.0g)
Complicated urinary tract infection	500 mg q6h (TOTAL DAILY DOSE = 2.0g)	500 mg q6h (TOTAL DAILY DOSE = 2.0g)

Due to the high antimicrobial activity of PRIMAXIN I.V., it is recommended that the maximum total daily dosage not exceed 50 mg/kg/day or 4.0 g/day, whichever is lower. There is no evidence that higher doses provide greater efficacy. However, patients over twelve years of age with cystic fibrosis and normal renal function have been treated with PRIMAXIN I.V. at doses up to 90 mg/kg/day in divided doses, not exceeding 4.0 g/day.

TABLE 4: REDUCED INTRAVENOUS DOSAGE OF PRIMAXIN I.V. IN ADULT PATIENTS WITH IMPAIRED RENAL FUNCTION AND/OR BODY WEIGHT <70 kg

And Body Weight (kg) is:	If TOTAL DAILY DOSE from TABLE 3 is:											
	1.0 g/day				1.5 g/day				2.0 g/day			
	and creatinine clearance (mL/min/1.73 m²) is:				and creatinine clearance (mL/min/1.73 m²) is:				and creatinine clearance (mL/min/1.73 m²) is:			
	≥71	41-70	21-40	6-20	≥71	41-70	21-40	6-20	≥71	41-70	21-40	6-20
	then the reduced dosage regimen (mg) is:				then the reduced dosage regimen (mg) is:				then the reduced dosage regimen (mg) is:			
≥70	250 q6h	250 q8h	250 q12h	250 q12h	500 q8h	250 q6h	250 q8h	250 q12h	500 q6h	500 q8h	250 q6h	250 q12h
60	250 q8h	125 q6h	250 q12h	125 q12h	250 q6h	250 q8h	250 q8h	250 q12h	500 q8h	250 q6h	250 q8h	250 q12h
50	125 q6h	125 q6h	125 q8h	125 q12h	250 q6h	250 q8h	250 q12h	250 q12h	250 q6h	250 q8h	250 q8h	250 q12h
40	125 q6h	125 q8h	125 q12h	125 q12h	250 q8h	125 q6h	125 q8h	125 q12h	250 q6h	250 q8h	250 q12h	250 q12h
30	125 q8h	125 q8h	125 q12h	125 q12h	125 q6h	125 q8h	125 q8h	125 q12h	250 q8h	125 q6h	125 q8h	125 q12h

TABLE 5: REDUCED INTRAVENOUS DOSAGE OF PRIMAXIN I.V. IN ADULT PATIENTS WITH IMPAIRED RENAL FUNCTION AND/OR BODY WEIGHT <70 kg

And Body Weight (kg) is:	If TOTAL DAILY DOSE from TABLE 3 is:							
	3.0 g/day				4.0 g/day			
	and creatinine clearance (mL/min/1.73 m²) is:				and creatinine clearance (mL/min/1.73 m²) is:			
	≥71	41-70	21-40	6-20	≥71	41-70	21-40	6-20
	then the reduced dosage regimen (mg) is:				then the reduced dosage regimen (mg) is:			
≥70	1000 q8h	500 q6h	500 q8h	500 q12h	1000 q6h	750 q8h	500 q6h	500 q12h
60	750 q8h	500 q8h	500 q8h	500 q12h	1000 q8h	750 q8h	500 q8h	500 q12h
50	500 q6h	500 q8h	250 q6h	250 q12h	750 q8h	500 q8h	500 q8h	500 q12h
40	500 q8h	250 q6h	250 q8h	250 q12h	500 q6h	500 q8h	250 q6h	250 q12h
30	250 q6h	250 q8h	250 q8h	250 q12h	500 q8h	250 q6h	250 q8h	250 q12h

Reduced Intravenous Schedule for Adults with Impaired Renal Function and/or Body Weight <70 kg

Patients with creatinine clearance of ≤70 mL/min/1.73 m² and/or body weight less than 70 kg require dosage reduction of PRIMAXIN I.V. as indicated in the tables below. Creatinine clearance may be calculated from serum creatinine concentration by the following equation:

$$T_{cc} \text{ (Males)} = \frac{\text{(wt. in kg) (140 - age)}}{(72) \text{ (creatinine in mg/dL)}}$$

$$T_{cc} \text{ (Females)} = 0.85 \times \text{(above value)}$$

To determine the dose for adults with impaired renal function and/or reduced body weight:
1. Choose a total daily dose from Table 3 based on infection characteristics.
2. a) If the total daily dose is 1.0 g, 1.5 g, or 2.0 g, use the appropriate subsection of Table 4 and continue with step 3.
   b) If the total daily dose is 3.0 g or 4.0 g, use the appropriate subsection of Table 5 and continue with step 3.
3. From Table 4 or 5:
   a) Select the body weight on the far left which is closest to the patient's body weight (kg).
   b) Select the patient's creatinine clearance category.
   c) Where the row and column intersect is the reduced dosage regimen.
[See table 4 above]
[See table 5 above]

Patients with creatinine clearances of 6 to 20 mL/min/1.73 m² should be treated with PRIMAXIN I.V. 125 mg or 250 mg every 12 hours for most pathogens. There may be an increased risk of seizures when doses of 500 mg every 12 hours are administered to these patients.

Patients with creatinine clearance ≤5 mL/min/1.73 m² should not receive PRIMAXIN I.V. unless hemodialysis is instituted within 48 hours. There is inadequate information to recommend usage of PRIMAXIN I.V. for patients undergoing peritoneal dialysis.

Hemodialysis
When treating patients with creatinine clearances of ≤5 mL/min/1.73 m² who are undergoing hemodialysis, use the dosage recommendations for patients with creatinine clearances of 6-20 mL/min/1.73 m². (See Reduced Intravenous Dosage Schedule for Adults with Impaired Renal Function and/or Body Weight <70 kg.) Both imipenem and cilastatin are cleared from the circulation during hemodialysis. The patient should receive PRIMAXIN I.V. after hemodialysis and at 12 hour intervals timed from the end of that hemodialysis session. Dialysis patients, especially those with background CNS disease, should be carefully monitored; for patients on hemodialysis, PRIMAXIN I.V. is recommended only when the benefit outweighs the potential risk of seizures. (See PRECAUTIONS.)

Pediatric Patients
See PRECAUTIONS, Pediatric Patients.

For pediatric patients ≥3 months of age, the recommended dose for non-CNS infections is 15-25 mg/kg/dose administered every six hours. Based on studies in adults, the maximum daily dose for treatment of infections with fully susceptible organisms is 2.0 g per day, and of infections with moderately susceptible organisms (primarily some strains of P. aeruginosa) is 4.0 g/day. Higher doses (up to 90 mg/kg/day in older children) have been used in patients with cystic fibrosis.

For pediatric patients ≤3 months of age (weighing ≥1,500 g), the following dosage schedule is recommended for non-CNS infections:

<1 wk of age: 25 mg/kg every 12 hrs
1-4 wks of age: 25 mg/kg every 8 hrs
4 wks-3 mos. of age: 25 mg/kg every 6 hrs.

Doses less than or equal to 500 mg should be given by intravenous infusion over 15 to 30 minutes. Doses greater than 500 mg should be given by intravenous infusion over 40 to 60 minutes.

PRIMAXIN I.V. is not recommended in pediatric patients with CNS infections because of the risk of seizures.

PRIMAXIN I.V. is not recommended in pediatric patients <30 kg with impaired renal function, as no data are available.

PREPARATION OF SOLUTION

Vials
Contents of the vials must be suspended and transferred to 100 mL of an appropriate infusion solution.

A suggested procedure is to add approximately 10 mL from the appropriate infusion solution (see list of diluents under COMPATIBILITY AND STABILITY) to the vial. Shake well and transfer the resulting suspension to the infusion solution container.

Benzyl alcohol as a preservative has been associated with toxicity in neonates. While toxicity has not been demonstrated in pediatric patients greater than three months of age, small pediatric patients in this age range may also be at risk for benzyl alcohol toxicity. Therefore, diluents containing benzyl alcohol should not be used when PRIMAXIN I.V. is constituted for administration to pediatric patients in this age range.

CAUTION: THE SUSPENSION IS NOT FOR DIRECT INFUSION.

Repeat with an additional 10 mL of infusion solution to ensure complete transfer of vial contents to the infusion solution. **The resulting mixture should be agitated until clear.**

ADD-Vantage®5 Vials
See separate INSTRUCTIONS FOR USE OF 'PRIMAXIN I.V.' IN ADD-Vantage® VIALS. PRIMAXIN I.V. in ADD-Vantage® vials should be reconstituted with ADD-Vantage® diluent containers containing 100 mL of either 0.9% Sodium Chloride Injection or 100 mL 5% Dextrose Injection.

[5]Registered trademark of Abbott Laboratories, Inc.

COMPATIBILITY AND STABILITY
Before Reconstitution:
The dry powder should be stored at a temperature below 25°C (77°F).

Reconstituted Solutions:
Solutions of PRIMAXIN I.V. range from colorless to yellow. Variations of color within this range do not affect the potency of the product.

Vials
PRIMAXIN I.V., as supplied in single use vials and reconstituted with the following diluents (see PREPARATION OF SOLUTION), maintains satisfactory potency for 4 hours at room temperature or for 24 hours under refrigeration (5°C). Solutions of PRIMAXIN I.V. should not be frozen.
0.9% Sodium Chloride Injection
5% or 10% Dextrose Injection
5% Dextrose and 0.9% Sodium Chloride Injection
5% Dextrose Injection with 0.225% or 0.45% saline solution
5% Dextrose Injection with 0.15% potassium chloride solution
Mannitol 5% and 10%

ADD-Vantage® vials
PRIMAXIN I.V., as supplied in single dose ADD-Vantage® vials and reconstituted with the following diluents (see PREPARATION OF SOLUTION), maintains satisfactory potency for 4 hours at room temperature.
0.9% Sodium Chloride Injection
5% Dextrose Injection

PRIMAXIN I.V. should not be mixed with or physically added to other antibiotics. However, PRIMAXIN I.V. may be administered concomitantly with other antibiotics, such as aminoglycosides.

HOW SUPPLIED
PRIMAXIN I.V. is supplied as a sterile powder mixture in single dose containers including vials and ADD-Vantage® vials containing imipenem (anhydrous equivalent) and cilastatin sodium as follows:

No. 3514 — 250 mg imipenem equivalent and 250 mg cilastatin equivalent and 10 mg sodium bicarbonate as a buffer
NDC 0006-3514-58 in trays of 25 vials.
No. 3516 — 500 mg imipenem equivalent and 500 mg cilastatin equivalent and 20 mg sodium bicarbonate as a buffer
NDC 0006-3516-59 in trays of 25 vials.
No. 3551 — 250 mg imipenem equivalent and 250 mg cilastatin equivalent and 10 mg sodium bicarbonate as a buffer
NDC 0006-3551-58 in trays of 25 ADD-Vantage® vials.
No. 3552 — 500 mg imipenem equivalent and 500 mg cilastatin equivalent and 20 mg sodium bicarbonate as a buffer
NDC 0006-3552-59 in trays of 25 ADD-Vantage® vials.

REFERENCES
1. Clinical and Laboratory Standards Institute (CLSI). Methods for Dilution Antimicrobial Susceptibility Tests for Bacteria that Grow Aerobically; Approved Standard - 9th ed. CLSI document M07-A9. CLSI, 950 West Valley Rd., Suite 2500, Wayne, PA 19087, 2012.
2. CLSI. Performance Standards for Antimicrobial Susceptibility Testing; 22nd Informational Supplement. CLSI document M100-S22, 2012.
3. CLSI. Performance Standards for Antimicrobial Disk Susceptibility Tests; Approved Standard – 11th ed. CLSI document M02-A11, 2012.
4. CLSI. Methods for Antimicrobial Susceptibility Testing of Anaerobic Bacteria; Approved Standard – 8th ed. CLSI document M11-A8, 2012.

Merck Sharp & Dohme Corp., a subsidiary of **MERCK & CO., INC.**, Whitehouse Station, NJ 08889, USA
Copyright © 1987, 1994, 1998 Merck Sharp & Dohme Corp., a subsidiary of Merck & Co., Inc.
All rights reserved.
Revised: April 2012
USPI-IV-0787B1204R037

INSTRUCTIONS FOR USE OF PRIMAXIN® I.V.
(Imipenem and Cilastatin for Injection)
(Formerly called Imipenem-Cilastatin Sodium for Injection)
IN ADD-Vantage®5 VIALS
For IV Use Only.
INSTRUCTIONS FOR USE
To Open Diluent Container:
Peel overwrap from the corner and remove container. Some opacity of the plastic due to moisture absorption during the sterilization process may be observed. This is normal and does not affect the solution quality or safety. The opacity will diminish gradually.
To Assemble Vial and Flexible Diluent Container:
(Use Aseptic Technique)
1. Remove the protective covers from the top of the vial and the vial port on the diluent container as follows:
   a. To remove the breakaway vial cap, swing the pull ring over the top of the vial and pull down far enough to start the opening. (SEE FIGURE 1.) Pull the ring approximately half way around the cap and then pull straight up to remove the cap. (SEE FIGURE 2.) NOTE: DO NOT ACCESS VIAL WITH SYRINGE.

Fig. 1   Fig. 2

   b. To remove the vial port cover, grasp the tab on the pull ring, pull up to break the three tie strings, then pull back to remove the cover. (SEE FIGURE 3.)
2. Screw the vial into the vial port until it will go no further. THE VIAL MUST BE SCREWED IN TIGHTLY TO ASSURE A SEAL. This occurs approximately ½ turn (180°) after the first audible click. (SEE FIGURE 4.) The clicking sound does not assure a seal; the vial must be turned as far as it will go. NOTE: Once vial is seated, do not attempt to remove. (SEE FIGURE 4.)
3. Recheck the vial to assure that it is tight by trying to turn it further in the direction of assembly.
4. Label appropriately.

Fig. 3   Fig. 4

To Prepare Admixture:
1. Squeeze the bottom of the diluent container gently to inflate the portion of the container surrounding the end of the drug vial.
2. With the other hand, push the drug vial down into the container telescoping the walls of the container. Grasp the inner cap of the vial through the walls of the container. (SEE FIGURE 5.)
3. Pull the inner cap from the drug vial. (SEE FIGURE 6.) Verify that the rubber stopper has been pulled out, allowing the drug and diluent to mix.
4. Mix container contents thoroughly and use within the specified time.

Fig. 5   Fig. 6

Preparation for Administration:
(Use Aseptic Technique)
1. Confirm the activation and admixture of vial contents.
2. Check for leaks by squeezing container firmly. If leaks are found, discard unit as sterility may be impaired.
3. Close flow control clamp of administration set.
4. Remove cover from outlet port at bottom of container.
5. Insert piercing pin of administration set into port with a twisting motion until the pin is firmly seated. NOTE: See full directions on administration set carton.
6. Lift the free end of the hanger loop on the bottom of the vial, breaking the two tie strings. Bend the loop outward to lock it in the upright position, then suspend container from hanger.
7. Squeeze and release drip chamber to establish proper fluid level in chamber.
8. Open flow control clamp and clear air from set. Close clamp.
9. Attach set to venipuncture device. If device is not indwelling, prime and make venipuncture.
10. Regulate rate of administration with flow control clamp.
WARNING: Do not use flexible container in series connections.
Stability
PRIMAXIN I.V.[6] (Imipenem and Cilastatin for Injection) 250 or 500 single dose ADD-Vantage® vials should be prepared with ADD-Vantage® diluent containers containing 100 mL of either 0.9 percent Sodium Chloride Injection or 5 percent Dextrose Injection. When prepared with either of these diluents, PRIMAXIN I.V. (Imipenem and Cilastatin for Injection) maintains satisfactory potency for 4 hours at room temperature.
Before administering, see accompanying package circular for PRIMAXIN I.V. (Imipenem and Cilastatin for Injection).
Issued February 2010
Printed In USA
9805601

---

[6]Registered trademark of Merck Sharp & Dohme Corp., a subsidiary of **Merck & Co., Inc.**

PRINIVIL® TABLETS   ℞
[pri-ni-vil]
(LISINOPRIL)

WARNING: FETAL TOXICITY
• **When pregnancy is detected, discontinue PRINIVIL as soon as possible.**
• **Drugs that act directly on the renin-angiotensin system can cause injury and death to the developing fetus. See WARNINGS, Fetal Toxicity**

DESCRIPTION
PRINIVIL® (Lisinopril), a synthetic peptide derivative, is an oral long-acting angiotensin converting enzyme inhibitor. Lisinopril is chemically described as (S)-1-$[N^2$-(1-carboxy-3-phenylpropyl)-L-lysyl]-L-proline dihydrate. Its empirical formula is $C_{21}H_{31}N_3O_5 \cdot 2H_2O$ and its structural formula is:

$$\text{C}_6\text{H}_5\text{—CH}_2\text{CH}_2\text{—CH—N—CH—C—N} \quad \cdot 2\text{H}_2\text{O}$$

Lisinopril is a white to off-white, crystalline powder, with a molecular weight of 441.52. It is soluble in water and sparingly soluble in methanol and practically insoluble in ethanol.
PRINIVIL is supplied as 5 mg, 10 mg, and 20 mg tablets for oral administration. In addition to the active ingredient lisinopril, each tablet contains the following inactive ingredients: calcium phosphate, mannitol, magnesium stearate, and starch. The 10 mg and 20 mg tablets also contain iron oxide.

CLINICAL PHARMACOLOGY
Mechanism of Action
Lisinopril inhibits angiotensin converting enzyme (ACE) in human subjects and animals. ACE is a peptidyl dipeptidase that catalyzes the conversion of angiotensin I to the vasoconstrictor substance, angiotensin II. Angiotensin II also stimulates aldosterone secretion by the adrenal cortex. The beneficial effects of lisinopril in hypertension and heart failure appear to result primarily from suppression of the renin-angiotensin-aldosterone system. Inhibition of ACE results in decreased plasma angiotensin II which leads to decreased vasopressor activity and to decreased aldosterone secretion. The latter decrease may result in a small increase of serum potassium. In hypertensive patients with normal renal function treated with PRINIVIL alone for up to 24

weeks, the mean increase in serum potassium was approximately 0.1 mEq/L; however, approximately 15 percent of patients had increases greater than 0.5 mEq/L and approximately six percent had a decrease greater than 0.5 mEq/L. In the same study, patients treated with PRINIVIL and hydrochlorothiazide for up to 24 weeks had a mean decrease in serum potassium of 0.1 mEq/L; approximately 4 percent of patients had increases greater than 0.5 mEq/L and approximately 12 percent had a decrease greater than 0.5 mEq/L. (See PRECAUTIONS.) Removal of angiotensin II negative feedback on renin secretion leads to increased plasma renin activity.
ACE is identical to kininase, an enzyme that degrades bradykinin. Whether increased levels of bradykinin, a potent vasodepressor peptide, play a role in the therapeutic effects of PRINIVIL remains to be elucidated.
While the mechanism through which PRINIVIL lowers blood pressure is believed to be primarily suppression of the renin-angiotensin-aldosterone system, PRINIVIL is antihypertensive even in patients with low-renin hypertension. Although PRINIVIL was antihypertensive in all races studied, Black hypertensive patients (usually a low-renin hypertensive population) had a smaller average response to monotherapy than non-Black patients.
Concomitant administration of PRINIVIL and hydrochlorothiazide further reduced blood pressure in Black and non-Black patients and any racial difference in blood pressure response was no longer evident.
Pharmacokinetics and Metabolism
Adult Patients: Following oral administration of PRINIVIL, peak serum concentrations of lisinopril occur within about 7 hours, although there was a trend to a small delay in time taken to reach peak serum concentrations in acute myocardial infarction patients. Declining serum concentrations exhibit a prolonged terminal phase which does not contribute to drug accumulation. This terminal phase probably represents saturable binding to ACE and is not proportional to dose. Lisinopril does not appear to be bound to other serum proteins.
Lisinopril does not undergo metabolism and is excreted unchanged entirely in the urine. Based on urinary recovery, the mean extent of absorption of lisinopril is approximately 25 percent, with large inter-subject variability (6-60 percent) at all doses tested (5-80 mg). Lisinopril absorption is not influenced by the presence of food in the gastrointestinal tract. The absolute bioavailability of lisinopril is reduced to about 16 percent in patients with stable NYHA Class II-IV congestive heart failure, and the volume of distribution appears to be slightly smaller than that in normal subjects.
The oral bioavailability of lisinopril in patients with acute myocardial infarction is similar to that in healthy volunteers.
Upon multiple dosing, lisinopril exhibits an effective half-life of accumulation of 12 hours.
Impaired renal function decreases elimination of lisinopril, which is excreted principally through the kidneys, but this decrease becomes clinically important only when the glomerular filtration rate is below 30 mL/min. Above this glomerular filtration rate, the elimination half-life is little changed. With greater impairment, however, peak and trough lisinopril levels increase, time to peak concentration increases and time to attain steady state is prolonged. Older patients, on average, have (approximately doubled) higher blood levels and area under the plasma concentration time curve (AUC) than younger patients. (See DOSAGE AND ADMINISTRATION.) Lisinopril can be removed by hemodialysis.
Studies in rats indicate that lisinopril crosses the blood-brain barrier poorly. Multiple doses of lisinopril in rats do not result in accumulation in any tissues. Milk of lactating rats contains radioactivity following administration of ^{14}C lisinopril. By whole body autoradiography, radioactivity was found in the placenta following administration of labeled drug to pregnant rats, but none was found in the fetuses.
Pediatric Patients: The pharmacokinetics of lisinopril were studied in 29 pediatric hypertensive patients between 6 years and 16 years with glomerular filtration rate >30 mL/min/1.73 m². After doses of 0.1 to 0.2 mg/kg, steady state peak plasma concentrations of lisinopril occurred within 6 hours and the extent of absorption based on urinary recovery was about 28%. These values are similar to those obtained previously in adults. The typical value of lisinopril oral clearance (systemic clearance/absolute bioavailability) in a child weighing 30 kg is 10 L/h, which increases in proportion to renal function.
Pharmacodynamics and Clinical Effects
Hypertension:
Adult Patients: Administration of PRINIVIL to patients with hypertension results in a reduction of supine and standing blood pressure to about the same extent with no compensatory tachycardia. Symptomatic postural hypotension is usually not observed although it can occur and should be anticipated in volume and/or salt-depleted pa-

tients. (See WARNINGS.) When given together with thiazide-type diuretics, the blood pressure lowering effects of the two drugs are approximately additive.

In most patients studied, onset of antihypertensive activity was seen at one hour after oral administration of an individual dose of PRINIVIL, with peak reduction of blood pressure achieved by six hours. Although an antihypertensive effect was observed 24 hours after dosing with recommended single daily doses, the effect was more consistent and the mean effect was considerably larger in some studies with doses of 20 mg or more than with lower doses. However, at all doses studied, the mean antihypertensive effect was substantially smaller 24 hours after dosing than it was six hours after dosing.

In some patients achievement of optimal blood pressure reduction may require two to four weeks of therapy.

The antihypertensive effects of PRINIVIL are maintained during long-term therapy. Abrupt withdrawal of PRINIVIL has not been associated with a rapid increase in blood pressure or a significant increase in blood pressure compared to pretreatment levels.

Two dose-response studies utilizing a once daily regimen were conducted in 438 mild to moderate hypertensive patients not on a diuretic. Blood pressure was measured 24 hours after dosing. An antihypertensive effect of PRINIVIL was seen with 5 mg in some patients. However, in both studies blood pressure reduction occurred sooner and was greater in patients treated with 10, 20, or 80 mg of PRINIVIL. In controlled clinical studies, PRINIVIL 20-80 mg has been compared in patients with mild to moderate hypertension to hydrochlorothiazide 12.5-50 mg and with atenolol 50-500 mg; and in patients with moderate to severe hypertension to metoprolol 100-200 mg. It was superior to hydrochlorothiazide in effects on systolic and diastolic blood pressure in a population that was ¾ Caucasian. PRINIVIL was approximately equivalent to atenolol and metoprolol in effects on diastolic blood pressure and had somewhat greater effects on systolic blood pressure.

PRINIVIL had similar effectiveness and adverse effects in younger and older (>65 years) patients. It was less effective in Blacks than in Caucasians.

In hemodynamic studies in patients with essential hypertension, blood pressure reduction was accompanied by a reduction in peripheral arterial resistance with little or no change in cardiac output and in heart rate. In a study in nine hypertensive patients, following administration of PRINIVIL, there was an increase in mean renal blood flow that was not significant. Data from several small studies are inconsistent with respect to the effect of PRINIVIL on glomerular filtration rate in hypertensive patients with normal renal function, but suggest that changes, if any, are not large.

In patients with renovascular hypertension PRINIVIL has been shown to be well tolerated and effective in controlling blood pressure (see PRECAUTIONS).

Pediatric Patients: In a clinical study involving 115 hypertensive pediatric patients 6 to 16 years of age, patients who weighed <50 kg received either 0.625, 2.5, or 20 mg of lisinopril daily and patients who weighed ≥50 kg received either 1.25, 5, or 40 mg of lisinopril daily. At the end of 2 weeks, lisinopril administered once daily lowered trough blood pressure in a dose-dependent manner with consistent antihypertensive efficacy demonstrated at doses >1.25 mg (0.02 mg/kg). This effect was confirmed in a withdrawal phase, where the diastolic pressure rose by about 9 mmHg more in patients randomized to placebo than it did in patients who were randomized to remain on the middle and high doses of lisinopril. The dose-dependent antihypertensive effect of lisinopril was consistent across several demographic subgroups: age, Tanner stage, gender, race. In this study, lisinopril was generally well-tolerated.

In the above pediatric studies, lisinopril was given either as tablets or in a suspension for those children and infants who were unable to swallow tablets or who required a lower dose than is available in tablet form (see DOSAGE AND ADMINISTRATION, Preparation of Suspension).

Heart Failure:

During baseline-controlled clinical trials, in patients receiving digitalis and diuretics, single doses of PRINIVIL resulted in decreases in pulmonary capillary wedge pressure, systemic vascular resistance and blood pressure accompanied by an increase in cardiac output and no change in heart rate.

In two placebo-controlled, 12-week clinical studies using doses of PRINIVIL up to 20 mg, PRINIVIL as adjunctive therapy to digitalis and diuretics improved the following signs and symptoms due to congestive heart failure: edema, rales, paroxysmal nocturnal dyspnea and jugular venous distention. In one of the studies beneficial response was also noted for: orthopnea, presence of third heart sound and the number of patients classified as NYHA Class III and IV. Exercise tolerance was also improved in this study. The effect of lisinopril on mortality in patients with heart failure has not been evaluated.

The once daily dosing for the treatment of congestive heart failure was the only dosage regimen used during clinical trial development and was determined by the measurement of hemodynamic responses.

Acute Myocardial Infarction:

The Gruppo Italiano per lo Studio della Sopravvivenza nell'Infarto Miocardico (GISSI - 3) study was a multicenter, controlled, randomized, unblinded clinical trial conducted in 19,394 patients with acute myocardial infarction admitted to a coronary care unit. It was designed to examine the effects of short-term (6 week) treatment with lisinopril, nitrates, their combination, or no therapy on short-term (6 week) mortality and on long-term death and markedly impaired cardiac function. Patients presenting within 24 hours of the onset of symptoms who were hemodynamically stable were randomized, in a 2 × 2 factorial design, to six weeks of either

1. PRINIVIL alone (n=4841),
2. nitrates alone (n=4869),
3. PRINIVIL plus nitrates (n=4841), or
4. open control (n=4843).

All patients received routine therapies, including thrombolytics (72%), aspirin (84%), and a beta-blocker (31%), as appropriate, normally utilized in acute myocardial infarction (MI) patients.

The protocol excluded patients with hypotension (systolic blood pressure ≤100 mmHg), severe heart failure, cardiogenic shock and renal dysfunction (serum creatinine >2 mg/dL and/or proteinuria >500 mg/24 h). Doses of PRINIVIL were adjusted as necessary according to protocol. (See DOSAGE AND ADMINISTRATION.)

Study treatment was withdrawn at six weeks except where clinical conditions indicated continuation of treatment.

The primary outcomes of the trial were the overall mortality at six weeks and a combined endpoint at six months after the myocardial infarction, consisting of the number of patients who died, had late (day 4) clinical congestive heart failure, or had extensive left ventricular damage defined as ejection fraction ≤35%, or an akinetic-dyskinetic [A-D] score ≥45%. Patients receiving PRINIVIL (n=9646) alone or with nitrates, had an 11 percent lower risk of death (2p [two-tailed]=0.04) compared to patients receiving no PRINIVIL (n=9672) (6.4 percent versus 7.2 percent, respectively) at six weeks. Although patients randomized to receive PRINIVIL for up to six weeks also fared numerically better on the combined end-point at 6 months, the open nature of the assessment of heart failure, substantial loss to follow-up echocardiography, and substantial excess use of lisinopril between 6 weeks and 6 months in the group randomized to 6 weeks of lisinopril, preclude any conclusion about this endpoint.

Patients with acute myocardial infarction, treated with PRINIVIL had a higher (9.0 percent versus 3.7 percent, respectively) incidence of persistent hypotension (systolic blood pressure <90 mmHg for more than 1 hour) and renal dysfunction (2.4 percent versus 1.1 percent) in-hospital and at six weeks (increasing creatinine concentration to over 3 mg/dL or a doubling or more of the baseline serum creatinine concentration). (See ADVERSE REACTIONS, ACUTE MYOCARDIAL INFARCTION.)

INDICATIONS AND USAGE

Hypertension

PRINIVIL is indicated for the treatment of hypertension. It may be used alone as initial therapy or concomitantly with other classes of antihypertensive agents.

Heart Failure

PRINIVIL is indicated as adjunctive therapy in the management of heart failure in patients who are not responding adequately to diuretics and digitalis.

Acute Myocardial Infarction

PRINIVIL is indicated for the treatment of hemodynamically stable patients within 24 hours of acute myocardial infarction, to improve survival. Patients should receive, as appropriate, the standard recommended treatments such as thrombolytics, aspirin and beta-blockers.

In using PRINIVIL, consideration should be given to the fact that another angiotensin converting enzyme inhibitor, captopril, has caused agranulocytosis, particularly in patients with renal impairment or collagen vascular disease, and that available data are insufficient to show that PRINIVIL does not have a similar risk. (See WARNINGS.) In considering use of PRINIVIL, it should be noted that in controlled clinical trials ACE inhibitors have an effect on blood pressure that is less in Black patients than in non-Blacks. In addition, it should be noted that Black patients receiving ACE inhibitors have been reported to have a higher incidence of angioedema compared to non-Blacks (see WARNINGS, Anaphylactoid and Possibly Related Reactions, Head and Neck Angioedema).

CONTRAINDICATIONS

PRINIVIL is contraindicated in patients who are hypersensitive to this product and in patients with a history of angioedema related to previous treatment with an angiotensin converting enzyme inhibitor and in patients with hereditary or idiopathic angioedema.

Do not coadminister aliskiren with PRINIVIL in patients with diabetes.

WARNINGS

Anaphylactoid and Possibly Related Reactions

Presumably because angiotensin converting enzyme inhibitors affect the metabolism of eicosanoids and polypeptides, including endogenous bradykinin, patients receiving ACE inhibitors (including PRINIVIL) may be subject to a variety of adverse reactions, some of them serious.

Head and Neck Angioedema: Angioedema of the face, extremities, lips, tongue, glottis and/or larynx has been reported in patients treated with angiotensin converting enzyme inhibitors, including PRINIVIL. This may occur at any time during treatment. ACE inhibitors have been associated with a higher rate of angioedema in Black than in non-Black patients. In such cases PRINIVIL should be promptly discontinued and appropriate therapy and monitoring should be provided until complete and sustained resolution of signs and symptoms has occurred. Even in those instances where swelling of only the tongue is involved, without respiratory distress, patients may require prolonged observation since treatment with antihistamines and corticosteroids may not be sufficient. Very rarely, fatalities have been reported due to angioedema associated with laryngeal edema or tongue edema. Patients with involvement of the tongue, glottis or larynx are likely to experience airway obstruction, especially those with a history of airway surgery. **Where there is involvement of the tongue, glottis or larynx, likely to cause airway obstruction, appropriate therapy, e.g., subcutaneous epinephrine solution 1:1000 (0.3 mL to 0.5 mL) and/or measures necessary to ensure a patent airway, should be promptly provided.** (See ADVERSE REACTIONS.)

Patients with a history of angioedema unrelated to ACE inhibitor therapy may be at increased risk of angioedema while receiving an ACE inhibitor (see also INDICATIONS AND USAGE and CONTRAINDICATIONS).

Intestinal Angioedema: Intestinal angioedema has been reported in patients treated with ACE inhibitors. These patients presented with abdominal pain (with or without nausea or vomiting); in some cases there was no prior history of facial angioedema and C-1 esterase levels were normal. The angioedema was diagnosed by procedures including abdominal CT scan or ultrasound, or at surgery, and symptoms resolved after stopping the ACE inhibitor. Intestinal angioedema should be included in the differential diagnosis of patients on ACE inhibitors presenting with abdominal pain.

Anaphylactoid reactions during desensitization: Two patients undergoing desensitizing treatment with hymenoptera venom while receiving ACE inhibitors sustained life-threatening anaphylactoid reactions. In the same patients, these reactions were avoided when ACE inhibitors were temporarily withheld, but they reappeared upon inadvertent rechallenge.

Anaphylactoid reactions during membrane exposure: Sudden and potentially life-threatening anaphylactoid reactions have been reported in some patients dialyzed with high-flux membranes (e.g., AN69®) and treated concomitantly with an ACE inhibitor. In such patients, dialysis must be stopped immediately, and aggressive therapy for anaphylactoid reactions be initiated. Symptoms have not been relieved by antihistamines in these situations. In these patients, consideration should be given to using a different type of dialysis membrane or a different class of antihypertensive agent. Anaphylactoid reactions have also been reported in patients undergoing low-density lipoprotein apheresis with dextran sulfate absorption.

Hypotension

Excessive hypotension is rare in patients with uncomplicated hypertension treated with PRINIVIL alone.

Patients with heart failure given PRINIVIL commonly have some reduction in blood pressure with peak blood pressure reduction occurring 6 to 8 hours post dose, but discontinuation of therapy because of continuing symptomatic hypotension usually is not necessary when dosing instructions are followed; caution should be observed when initiating therapy. (See DOSAGE AND ADMINISTRATION.)

Patients at risk of excessive hypotension, sometimes associated with oliguria and/or progressive azotemia, and rarely with acute renal failure and/or death, include those with the following conditions or characteristics: heart failure with systolic blood pressure below 100 mmHg, hyponatremia, high-dose diuretic therapy, recent intensive diuresis or increase in diuretic dose, renal dialysis, or severe volume and/or salt depletion of any etiology. It may be advisable to eliminate the diuretic (except in patients with heart failure), reduce the diuretic dose or increase salt intake cautiously before initiating therapy with PRINIVIL in patients at risk for excessive hypotension who are able to tolerate such adjustments. (See PRECAUTIONS, Drug Interactions, and ADVERSE REACTIONS.)

Patients with acute myocardial infarction in the GISSI - 3 study had a higher (9.0 percent versus 3.7 percent) incidence of persistent hypotension (systolic blood pressure <90 mmHg for more than 1 hour) when treated with PRINIVIL. Treatment with PRINIVIL must not be initiated in acute myocardial infarction patients at risk of further serious hemodynamic deterioration after treatment with a vasodilator (e.g., systolic blood pressure of 100 mmHg or lower) or cardiogenic shock.

In patients at risk of excessive hypotension, therapy should be started under very close medical supervision and such patients should be followed closely for the first two weeks of treatment and whenever the dose of PRINIVIL and/or diuretic is increased. Similar considerations may apply to patients with ischemic heart or cerebrovascular disease, or in patients with acute myocardial infarction, in whom an excessive fall in blood pressure could result in a myocardial infarction or cerebrovascular accident.

If excessive hypotension occurs, the patient should be placed in the supine position and, if necessary, receive an intravenous infusion of normal saline. A transient hypotensive response is not a contraindication to further doses of PRINIVIL which usually can be given without difficulty once the blood pressure has stabilized. If symptomatic hypotension develops, a dose reduction or discontinuation of PRINIVIL or concomitant diuretic may be necessary.

Leukopenia/Neutropenia/Agranulocytosis

Another angiotensin converting enzyme inhibitor, captopril, has been shown to cause agranulocytosis and bone marrow depression, rarely in uncomplicated patients but more frequently in patients with renal impairment especially if they also have a collagen vascular disease. Available data from clinical trials of PRINIVIL are insufficient to show that PRINIVIL does not cause agranulocytosis at similar rates. Marketing experience has revealed rare cases of leukopenia/neutropenia and bone marrow depression in which a causal relationship to lisinopril cannot be excluded. Periodic monitoring of white blood cell counts in patients with collagen vascular disease and renal disease should be considered.

Hepatic Failure

Rarely, ACE inhibitors have been associated with a syndrome that starts with cholestatic jaundice or hepatitis and progresses to fulminant hepatic necrosis, and (sometimes) death. The mechanism of this syndrome is not understood. Patients receiving ACE inhibitors who develop jaundice or marked elevations of hepatic enzymes should discontinue the ACE inhibitor and receive appropriate medical follow-up.

Fetal Toxicity

Pregnancy Category D

Use of drugs that act on the renin-angiotensin system during the second and third trimesters of pregnancy reduces fetal renal function and increases fetal and neonatal morbidity and death. Resulting oligohydramnios can be associated with fetal lung hypoplasia and skeletal deformations. Potential neonatal adverse effects include skull hypoplasia, anuria, hypotension, renal failure, and death. When pregnancy is detected, discontinue PRINIVIL as soon as possible. These adverse outcomes are usually associated with the use of these drugs in the second and third trimester of pregnancy. Most epidemiologic studies examining fetal abnormalities after exposure to antihypertensive use in the first trimester have not distinguished drugs affecting the renin-angiotensin system from other antihypertensive agents. Appropriate management of maternal hypertension during pregnancy is important to optimize outcomes for both mother and fetus.

In the unusual case that there is no appropriate alternative therapy to drugs affecting the renin-angiotensin system for a particular patient, apprise the mother of the potential risk to the fetus. Perform serial ultrasound examinations to assess the intra-amniotic environment. If oligohydramnios is observed, discontinue PRINIVIL, unless it is considered lifesaving for the mother. Fetal testing may be appropriate, based on the week of pregnancy. Patients and physicians should be aware, however, that oligohydramnios may not appear until after the fetus has sustained irreversible injury. Closely observe infants with histories of *in utero* exposure to PRINIVIL for hypotension, oliguria, and hyperkalemia (see Precautions, Pediatric Use).

No teratogenic effects of lisinopril were seen in studies of pregnant mice, rats, and rabbits. On a body surface area basis, the doses used were 55 times, 33 times, and 0.15 times, respectively, the maximum recommended human daily dose (MRHDD).

PRECAUTIONS
General

Aortic Stenosis/Hypertrophic Cardiomyopathy: As with all vasodilators, lisinopril should be given with caution to patients with obstruction in the outflow tract of the left ventricle.

Impaired Renal Function: As a consequence of inhibiting the renin-angiotensin-aldosterone system, changes in renal function may be anticipated in susceptible individuals. In patients with severe congestive heart failure whose renal function may depend on the activity of the renin-angiotensin-aldosterone system, treatment with angiotensin converting enzyme inhibitors, including PRINIVIL, may be associated with oliguria and/or progressive azotemia and rarely with acute renal failure and/or death.

In hypertensive patients with unilateral or bilateral renal artery stenosis, increases in blood urea nitrogen and serum creatinine may occur. Experience with another angiotensin converting enzyme inhibitor suggests that these increases are usually reversible upon discontinuation of PRINIVIL and/or diuretic therapy. In such patients renal function should be monitored during the first few weeks of therapy. Some patients with hypertension or heart failure with no apparent pre-existing renal vascular disease have developed increases in blood urea nitrogen and serum creatinine, usually minor and transient, especially when PRINIVIL has been given concomitantly with a diuretic. This is more likely to occur in patients with pre-existing renal impairment. Dosage reduction and/or discontinuation of the diuretic and/or PRINIVIL may be required.

Patients with acute myocardial infarction in the GISSI - 3 study, treated with PRINIVIL, had a higher (2.4 percent versus 1.1 percent) incidence of renal dysfunction in-hospital and at six weeks (increasing creatinine concentration to over 3 mg/dL or a doubling or more of the baseline serum creatinine concentration). In acute myocardial infarction, treatment with PRINIVIL should be initiated with caution in patients with evidence of renal dysfunction, defined as serum creatinine concentration exceeding 2 mg/dL. If renal dysfunction develops during treatment with PRINIVIL (serum creatinine concentration exceeding 3 mg/dL or a doubling from the pre-treatment value) then the physician should consider withdrawal of PRINIVIL.

Evaluation of patients with hypertension, heart failure, or myocardial infarction should always include assessment of renal function. (See DOSAGE AND ADMINISTRATION.)

Hyperkalemia: In clinical trials hyperkalemia (serum potassium greater than 5.7 mEq/L) occurred in approximately 2.2 percent of hypertensive patients and 4.8 percent of patients with heart failure. In most cases these were isolated values which resolved despite continued therapy. Hyperkalemia was a cause of discontinuation of therapy in approximately 0.1 percent of hypertensive patients, 0.6 percent of patients with heart failure and 0.1 percent of patients with myocardial infarction. Risk factors for the development of hyperkalemia include renal insufficiency, diabetes mellitus, and the concomitant use of potassium-sparing diuretics, potassium supplements and/or potassium-containing salt substitutes. Hyperkalemia can cause serious, sometimes fatal, arrhythmias. PRINIVIL should be used cautiously, if at all, with these agents and with frequent monitoring of serum potassium. (See Drug Interactions.)

Cough: Presumably due to the inhibition of the degradation of endogenous bradykinin, persistent nonproductive cough has been reported with all ACE inhibitors, always resolving after discontinuation of therapy. ACE inhibitor-induced cough should be considered in the differential diagnosis of cough.

Surgery/Anesthesia: In patients undergoing major surgery or during anesthesia with agents that produce hypotension, PRINIVIL may block angiotensin II formation secondary to compensatory renin release. If hypotension occurs and is considered to be due to this mechanism, it can be corrected by volume expansion.

Information for Patients

Angioedema: Angioedema, including laryngeal edema, may occur at any time during treatment with angiotensin converting enzyme inhibitors, including lisinopril. Patients should be so advised and told to report immediately any signs or symptoms suggesting angioedema (swelling of face, extremities, eyes, lips, tongue, difficulty in swallowing or breathing) and to take no more drug until they have consulted with the prescribing physician.

Symptomatic Hypotension: Patients should be cautioned to report lightheadedness especially during the first few days of therapy. If actual syncope occurs, the patients should be told to discontinue the drug until they have consulted with the prescribing physician.

All patients should be cautioned that excessive perspiration and dehydration may lead to an excessive fall in blood pressure because of reduction in fluid volume. Other causes of volume depletion such as vomiting or diarrhea may also lead to a fall in blood pressure; patients should be advised to consult with their physician.

Hyperkalemia: Patients should be told not to use salt substitutes containing potassium without consulting their physician.

Hypoglycemia: Diabetic patients treated with oral antidiabetic agents or insulin starting an ACE inhibitor should be told to closely monitor for hypoglycemia, especially during the first month of combined use. (See Drug Interactions.)

Leukopenia/Neutropenia: Patients should be told to report promptly any indication of infection (e.g., sore throat, fever) which may be a sign of leukopenia/neutropenia.

Pregnancy: Female patients of childbearing age should be told about the consequences of exposure to PRINIVIL during pregnancy. Discuss treatment options with women planning to become pregnant. Patients should be asked to report pregnancies to their physicians as soon as possible.

Drug Interactions

Hypotension - Patients on Diuretic Therapy: Patients on diuretics, and especially those in whom diuretic therapy was recently instituted, may occasionally experience an excessive reduction of blood pressure after initiation of therapy with PRINIVIL. The possibility of hypotensive effects with PRINIVIL can be minimized by either discontinuing the diuretic or increasing the salt intake prior to initiation of treatment with PRINIVIL. If it is necessary to continue the diuretic, initiate therapy with PRINIVIL at a dose of 5 mg daily, and provide close medical supervision after the initial dose until blood pressure has stabilized. (See WARNINGS and DOSAGE AND ADMINISTRATION.) When a diuretic is added to the therapy of a patient receiving PRINIVIL, an additional antihypertensive effect is usually observed. Studies with ACE inhibitors in combination with diuretics indicate that the dose of the ACE inhibitor can be reduced when it is given with a diuretic. (See DOSAGE AND ADMINISTRATION.)

Antidiabetics: Epidemiological studies have suggested that concomitant administration of ACE inhibitors and antidiabetic medicines (insulins, oral hypoglycemic agents) may cause an increased blood-glucose-lowering effect with risk of hypoglycemia. This phenomenon appeared to be more likely to occur during the first weeks of combined treatment and in patients with renal impairment. In diabetic patients treated with oral antidiabetic agents or insulin, glycemic control should be closely monitored for hypoglycemia, especially during the first month of treatment with an ACE inhibitor.

Non-steroidal Anti-inflammatory Agents Including Selective Cyclooxygenase-2 (COX-2) Inhibitors: Reports suggest that NSAIDs including selective COX-2 inhibitors may diminish the antihypertensive effect of ACE inhibitors, including lisinopril. This interaction should be given consideration in patients taking NSAIDs or selective COX-2 inhibitors concomitantly with ACE inhibitors.

In a study in 36 patients with mild to moderate hypertension where the antihypertensive effects of PRINIVIL alone were compared to PRINIVIL given concomitantly with indomethacin, the use of indomethacin was associated with a reduced antihypertensive effect, although the difference between the two regimens was not significant.

In some patients with compromised renal function (e.g., elderly patients or patients who are volume-depleted including those on diuretic therapy) who are being treated with non-steroidal anti-inflammatory drugs, including selective COX-2 inhibitors, the co-administration of angiotensin II receptor antagonists or ACE inhibitors may result in a further deterioration of renal function, including possible acute renal failure. These effects are usually reversible.

These interactions should be considered in patients taking NSAIDS including selective COX-2 inhibitors concomitantly with diuretics and angiotensin II antagonists or ACE inhibitors. Therefore, monitor effects on blood pressure and renal function when administering the combination, especially in the elderly.

Dual Blockade of the Renin-angiotensin-aldosterone System: Dual blockade of the renin-angiotensin-aldosterone system (RAAS) with angiotensin receptor blockers, ACE inhibitors, or direct renin inhibitors (such as aliskiren) is associated with increased risks of hypotension, syncope, hyperkalemia, and changes in renal function (including acute renal failure) compared to monotherapy. Closely monitor blood pressure, renal function, and electrolytes in patients on PRINIVIL and other agents that affect the RAAS. Do not coadminister aliskiren with PRINIVIL in patients with diabetes. Avoid use of aliskiren with PRINIVIL in patients with renal impairment (GFR <60ml/min).

Other Agents: PRINIVIL has been used concomitantly with nitrates and/or digoxin without evidence of clinically significant adverse interactions. This included post myocardial infarction patients who were receiving intravenous or transdermal nitroglycerin. No clinically important pharmacokinetic interactions occurred when PRINIVIL was used concomitantly with propranolol or hydrochlorothiazide. The presence of food in the stomach does not alter the bioavailability of PRINIVIL.

Agents Increasing Serum Potassium: PRINIVIL attenuates potassium loss caused by thiazide-type diuretics. Use of PRINIVIL with potassium-sparing diuretics (e.g., spironolactone, eplerenone, triamterene, or amiloride), potassium supplements, or potassium-containing salt substitutes may lead to significant increases in serum potassium. Therefore, if concomitant use of these agents is indicated because of demonstrated hypokalemia, they should be used with caution and with frequent monitoring of serum potassium. Potassium-sparing agents should generally not be used in patients with heart failure who are receiving PRINIVIL.

Table 1: Percent of Patients in Controlled Studies

	PRINIVIL (n=1349) Incidence (discontinuation)	PRINIVIL/ Hydrochlorothiazide (n=629) Incidence (discontinuation)	Placebo (n=207) Incidence (discontinuation)
Body As A Whole			
Fatigue	2.5 (0.3)	4.0 (0.5)	1.0 (0.0)
Asthenia	1.3 (0.5)	2.1 (0.2)	1.0 (0.0)
Orthostatic Effects	1.2 (0.0)	3.5 (0.2)	1.0 (0.0)
Cardiovascular			
Hypotension	1.2 (0.5)	1.6 (0.3)	0.5 (0.5)
Digestive			
Diarrhea	2.7 (0.2)	2.7 (0.3)	2.4 (0.0)
Nausea	2.0 (0.4)	2.5 (0.2)	2.4 (0.0)
Vomiting	1.1 (0.2)	1.4 (0.1)	0.5 (0.0)
Dyspepsia	0.9 (0.0)	1.9 (0.0)	0.0 (0.0)
Musculoskeletal			
Muscle Cramps	0.5 (0.0)	2.9 (0.8)	0.5 (0.0)
Nervous/Psychiatric			
Headache	5.7 (0.2)	4.5 (0.5)	1.9 (0.0)
Dizziness	5.4 (0.4)	9.2 (1.0)	1.9 (0.0)
Paresthesia	0.8 (0.1)	2.1 (0.1)	0.0 (0.0)
Decreased Libido	0.4 (0.1)	1.3 (0.1)	0.0 (0.0)
Vertigo	0.2 (0.1)	1.1 (0.2)	0.0 (0.0)
Respiratory			
Cough	3.5 (0.7)	4.6 (0.8)	1.0 (0.0)
Upper Respiratory Infection	2.1 (0.1)	2.7 (0.1)	0.0 (0.0)
Common Cold	1.1 (0.1)	1.3 (0.1)	0.0 (0.0)
Nasal Congestion	0.4 (0.1)	1.3 (0.1)	0.0 (0.0)
Influenza	0.3 (0.1)	1.1 (0.1)	0.0 (0.0)
Skin			
Rash	1.3 (0.4)	1.6 (0.2)	0.5 (0.5)
Urogenital			
Impotence	1.0 (0.4)	1.6 (0.5)	0.0 (0.0)

Lithium: Lithium toxicity has been reported in patients receiving lithium concomitantly with drugs which cause elimination of sodium, including ACE inhibitors. Lithium toxicity was usually reversible upon discontinuation of lithium and the ACE inhibitor. It is recommended that serum lithium levels be monitored frequently if PRINIVIL is administered concomitantly with lithium.

Gold: Nitritoid reactions (symptoms include facial flushing, nausea, vomiting and hypotension) have been reported rarely in patients on therapy with injectable gold (sodium aurothiomalate) and concomitant ACE inhibitor therapy including PRINIVIL.

Carcinogenesis, Mutagenesis, Impairment of Fertility

There was no evidence of a tumorigenic effect when lisinopril was administered orally for 105 weeks to male and female rats at doses up to 90 mg/kg/day or for 92 weeks to male and female mice at doses up to 135 mg/kg/day. These doses are 10 times and 7 times, respectively, the maximum recommended human daily dose (MRHDD) when compared on a body surface area basis.

Lisinopril was not mutagenic in the Ames microbial mutagen test with or without metabolic activation. It was also negative in a forward mutation assay using Chinese hamster lung cells. Lisinopril did not produce single strand DNA breaks in an *in vitro* alkaline elution rat hepatocyte assay. In addition, lisinopril did not produce increases in chromosomal aberrations in an *in vitro* test in Chinese hamster ovary cells or in an *in vivo* study in mouse bone marrow.

There were no adverse effects on reproductive performance in male and female rats treated with up to 300 mg/kg/day of lisinopril (33 times the MRHDD when compared on a body surface area basis).

Nursing Mothers

Milk of lactating rats contains radioactivity following administration of ^{14}C lisinopril. It is not known whether this drug is secreted in human milk. Because many drugs are secreted in human milk, and because of the potential for serious adverse reactions in nursing infants from ACE inhibitors, a decision should be made whether to discontinue nursing or discontinue PRINIVIL, taking into account the importance of the drug to the mother.

Pediatric Use

Neonates with a history of *in utero* exposure to PRINIVIL: If oliguria or hypotension occurs, direct attention toward support of blood pressure and renal perfusion. Exchange transfusions or dialysis may be required as a means of reversing hypotension and/or substituting for disordered renal function. Lisinopril, which crosses the placenta, has been removed from neonatal circulation by peritoneal dialysis with some clinical benefit, and theoretically may be removed by exchange transfusion, although there is no experience with the latter procedure.

Antihypertensive effects of PRINIVIL have been established in hypertensive pediatric patients aged 6 to 16 years. There are no data on the effect of PRINIVIL on blood pressure in pediatric patients under the age of 6 or in pediatric patients with glomerular filtration rate <30 mL/min/1.73 m² (see CLINICAL PHARMACOLOGY, Pharmacokinetics and Metabolism and Pharmacodynamics and Clinical Effects, and DOSAGE AND ADMINISTRATION).

Geriatric Use

Clinical studies of PRINIVIL in patients with hypertension and congestive heart failure did not include sufficient numbers of subjects aged 65 and over to determine whether they respond differently from younger subjects. Other clinical experience in this population has not identified differences in responses between the elderly and younger patients. In general, dose selection for an elderly patient should be cautious, usually starting at the low end of the dosing range, reflecting the greater frequency of decreased hepatic, renal, or cardiac function, and of concomitant disease or other drug therapy.

In a clinical study of PRINIVIL in patients with myocardial infarctions 4413 (47 percent) were 65 and over, while 1656 (18 percent) were 75 and over. No overall differences in safety or efficacy were observed between elderly and younger patients.

Other reported clinical experience has not identified differences in responses between elderly and younger patients, but greater sensitivity of some older individuals cannot be ruled out.

Pharmacokinetic studies indicate that maximum blood levels and area under plasma concentration time curve (AUC) are doubled in elderly patients.

This drug is known to be substantially excreted by the kidney, and the risk of toxic reactions to this drug may be greater in patients with impaired renal function. Because elderly patients are more likely to have decreased renal function, care should be taken in dose selection. Evaluation of patients with hypertension, congestive heart failure, or myocardial infarction should always include assessment of renal function. (See DOSAGE AND ADMINISTRATION.)

ADVERSE REACTIONS

PRINIVIL has been found to be generally well tolerated in controlled clinical trials involving 1969 patients with hypertension or heart failure. For the most part, adverse experiences were mild and transient.

HYPERTENSION

In clinical trials in patients with hypertension treated with PRINIVIL, discontinuation of therapy due to clinical adverse experiences occurred in 5.7 percent of patients. The overall frequency of adverse experiences could not be related to total daily dosage within the recommended therapeutic dosage range.

For adverse experiences occurring in greater than one percent of patients with hypertension treated with PRINIVIL or PRINIVIL plus hydrochlorothiazide in controlled clinical trials and more frequently with PRINIVIL and/or PRINIVIL plus hydrochlorothiazide than placebo, comparative incidence data are listed in table 1 below:

[See table 1 above]

Chest pain and back pain were also seen but were more common on placebo than PRINIVIL.

HEART FAILURE

In patients with heart failure treated with PRINIVIL for up to four years, discontinuation of therapy due to clinical adverse experiences occurred in 11.0 percent of patients. In controlled studies in patients with heart failure, therapy was discontinued in 8.1 percent of patients treated with PRINIVIL for up to 12 weeks, compared to 7.7 percent of patients treated with placebo for 12 weeks.

The following table lists those adverse experiences which occurred in greater than one percent of patients with heart failure treated with PRINIVIL or placebo for up to 12 weeks in controlled clinical trials and more frequently on PRINIVIL than placebo.

Table 2: Controlled Trials

	PRINIVIL (n=407) Incidence (discontinuation) 12 weeks	Placebo (n=155) Incidence (discontinuation) 12 weeks
Body As A Whole		
Chest Pain	3.4 (0.2)	1.3 (0.0)
Abdominal Pain	2.2 (0.7)	1.9 (0.0)
Cardiovascular		
Hypotension	4.4 (1.7)	0.6 (0.6)
Digestive		
Diarrhea	3.7 (0.5)	1.9 (0.0)
Nervous/Psychiatric		
Dizziness	11.8 (1.2)	4.5 (1.3)
Headache	4.4 (0.2)	3.9 (0.0)
Respiratory		
Upper Respiratory Infection	1.5 (0.0)	1.3 (0.0)
Skin		
Rash	1.7 (0.5)	0.6 (0.6)

Also observed at >1% with PRINIVIL but more frequent or as frequent on placebo than PRINIVIL in controlled trials were asthenia, angina pectoris, nausea, dyspnea, cough and pruritus.

Worsening of heart failure, anorexia, increased salivation, muscle cramps, back pain, myalgia, depression, chest sound abnormalities and pulmonary edema were also seen in controlled clinical trials, but were more common on placebo than PRINIVIL.

ACUTE MYOCARDIAL INFARCTION

In the GISSI - 3 trial, in patients treated with PRINIVIL for six weeks following acute myocardial infarction, discontinuation of therapy occurred in 17.6 percent of patients.

Patients treated with PRINIVIL had a significantly higher incidence of hypotension and renal dysfunction compared with patients not taking PRINIVIL.

In the GISSI - 3 trial, hypotension (9.7 percent), renal dysfunction (2.0 percent), cough (0.5 percent), post-infarction angina (0.3 percent), skin rash and generalized edema (0.01 percent) and angioedema (0.01 percent) resulted in withdrawal of treatment. In elderly patients treated with PRINIVIL, discontinuation due to renal dysfunction was 4.2 percent.

Other clinical adverse experiences occurring in 0.3 to 1.0 percent of patients with hypertension or heart failure treated with PRINIVIL in controlled trials and rarer, serious, possibly drug-related events reported in uncontrolled studies or marketing experience are listed below, and within each category, are in order of decreasing severity:

Body as a Whole: Anaphylactoid reactions (see WARNINGS, Anaphylactoid and Possibly Related Reactions), syncope, orthostatic effects, chest discomfort, pain, pelvic pain, flank pain, edema, facial edema, virus infection, fever, chills, malaise.

Cardiovascular: Cardiac arrest; myocardial infarction or cerebrovascular accident, possibly secondary to excessive hypotension in high-risk patients (see WARNINGS, Hypotension); pulmonary embolism and infarction, arrhythmias (including ventricular tachycardia, atrial tachycardia, atrial fibrillation, bradycardia and premature ventricular contractions), palpitations, transient ischemic attacks, paroxysmal nocturnal dyspnea, orthostatic hypotension, decreased blood pressure, peripheral edema, vasculitis.

Digestive: Pancreatitis, hepatitis (hepatocellular or cholestatic jaundice) (see WARNINGS, Hepatic Failure), vomiting, gastritis, dyspepsia, heartburn, gastrointestinal cramps, constipation, flatulence, dry mouth.

Hematologic: Rare cases of bone marrow depression, hemolytic anemia, leukopenia/neutropenia, and thrombocytopenia.

Endocrine: Diabetes mellitus, syndrome of inappropriate antidiuretic hormone secretion (SIADH).

Metabolic: Weight loss, dehydration, fluid overload, gout, weight gain. Cases of hypoglycemia in diabetic patients on oral antidiabetic agents or insulin have been reported (see PRECAUTIONS, Drug Interactions).

Musculoskeletal: Arthritis, arthralgia, neck pain, hip pain, low back pain, joint pain, leg pain, knee pain, shoulder pain, arm pain, lumbago.

Nervous System/Psychiatric: Stroke, ataxia, memory impairment, tremor, peripheral neuropathy (e.g., dysesthesia), spasm, paresthesia, confusion, insomnia, somnolence, hypersomnia, irritability, and nervousness.

Respiratory System: Malignant lung neoplasms, hemoptysis, pulmonary infiltrates, eosinophilic pneumonitis, bronchospasm, asthma, pleural effusion, pneumonia, bronchitis, wheezing, orthopnea, painful respiration, epistaxis, laryngitis, sinusitis, pharyngeal pain, pharyngitis, rhinitis, rhinorrhea.

Skin: Urticaria, alopecia, herpes zoster, photosensitivity, skin lesions, skin infections, pemphigus, erythema, flushing, diaphoresis. Other severe skin reactions (including toxic epidermal necrolysis, Stevens-Johnson syndrome and cutaneous pseudolymphoma) have been reported rarely; causal relationship has not been established.

Special Senses: Visual loss, diplopia, blurred vision, tinnitus, photophobia, taste disturbances.

Urogenital System: Acute renal failure, oliguria, anuria, uremia, progressive azotemia, renal dysfunction (see PRECAUTIONS and DOSAGE AND ADMINISTRATION), pyelonephritis, dysuria, urinary tract infection, breast pain.

Miscellaneous: A symptom complex has been reported which may include a positive ANA, an elevated erythrocyte sedimentation rate, arthralgia/arthritis, myalgia, fever, vasculitis, eosinophilia and leukocytosis. Rash, photosensitivity or other dermatological manifestations may occur alone or in combination with these symptoms.

Angioedema: Angioedema has been reported in patients receiving PRINIVIL (0.1%) with an incidence higher in Black than in non-Black patients. Angioedema associated with laryngeal edema may be fatal. If angioedema of the face, extremities, lips, tongue, glottis and/or larynx occurs, treatment with PRINIVIL should be discontinued and appropriate therapy instituted immediately. In rare cases, intestinal angioedema has been reported with angiotensin converting enzyme inhibitors including lisinopril. (See WARNINGS.)

Hypotension: In hypertensive patients, hypotension occurred in 1.2 percent and syncope occurred in 0.1 percent of patients. Hypotension or syncope was a cause for discontinuation of therapy in 0.5 percent of hypertensive patients. In patients with heart failure, hypotension occurred in 5.3 percent and syncope occurred in 1.8 percent of patients. These adverse experiences were causes for discontinuation of therapy in 1.8 percent of these patients. In patients treated with PRINIVIL for six weeks after acute myocardial infarction, hypotension (systolic blood pressure ≤100 mmHg) resulted in discontinuation of therapy in 9.7 percent of the patients. (See WARNINGS.)

Fetal/Neonatal Morbidity and Mortality: See WARNINGS, Fetal/Neonatal Morbidity and Mortality.

Cough: See PRECAUTIONS, Cough.

Pediatric Patients: No relevant differences between the adverse experience profile for pediatric patients and that previously reported for adult patients were identified.

Clinical Laboratory Test Findings

Serum Electrolytes: Hyperkalemia (see PRECAUTIONS), hyponatremia.

Creatinine, Blood Urea Nitrogen: Minor increases in blood urea nitrogen and serum creatinine, reversible upon discontinuation of therapy, were observed in about 2.0 percent of patients with essential hypertension treated with PRINIVIL alone. Increases were more common in patients receiving concomitant diuretics and in patients with renal artery stenosis. (See PRECAUTIONS.) Reversible minor in-

creases in blood urea nitrogen and serum creatinine were observed in approximately 11.6 percent of patients with heart failure on concomitant diuretic therapy. Frequently, these abnormalities resolved when the dosage of the diuretic was decreased.

Hemoglobin and Hematocrit: Small decreases in hemoglobin and hematocrit (mean decreases of approximately 0.4 g percent and 1.3 vol percent, respectively) occurred frequently in patients treated with PRINIVIL but were rarely of clinical importance in patients without some other cause of anemia. In clinical trials, less than 0.1 percent of patients discontinued therapy due to anemia. Hemolytic anemia has been reported; a causal relationship to lisinopril cannot be excluded.

Liver Function Tests: Rarely, elevations of liver enzymes and/or serum bilirubin have occurred (see WARNINGS, Hepatic Failure).

In hypertensive patients, 2.0 percent discontinued therapy due to laboratory adverse experiences, principally elevations in blood urea nitrogen (0.6 percent), serum creatinine (0.5 percent) and serum potassium (0.4 percent). In the heart failure trials, 3.4 percent of patients discontinued therapy due to laboratory adverse experiences, 1.8 percent due to elevations in blood urea nitrogen and/or creatinine and 0.6 percent due to elevations in serum potassium. In the myocardial infarction trial, 2.0 percent of patients receiving PRINIVIL discontinued therapy due to renal dysfunction (increasing creatinine concentration to over 3 mg/dL or a doubling or more of the baseline serum creatinine concentration); less than 1.0 percent of patients discontinued therapy due to other laboratory adverse experiences: 0.1 percent with hyperkalemia and less than 0.1 percent with hepatic enzyme alterations.

OVERDOSAGE

Following a single oral dose of 20 g/kg, no lethality occurred in rats and death occurred in one of 20 mice receiving the same dose. The most likely manifestation of overdosage would be hypotension, for which the usual treatment would be intravenous infusion of normal saline solution.

Lisinopril can be removed by hemodialysis. (See WARNINGS, Anaphylactoid reactions during membrane exposure.)

DOSAGE AND ADMINISTRATION

Hypertension

Initial Therapy: In patients with uncomplicated essential hypertension not on diuretic therapy, the recommended initial dose is 10 mg once a day. Dosage should be adjusted according to blood pressure response. The usual dosage range is 20 to 40 mg per day administered in a single daily dose. The antihypertensive effect may diminish toward the end of the dosing interval regardless of the administered dose, but most commonly with a dose of 10 mg daily. This can be evaluated by measuring blood pressure just prior to dosing to determine whether satisfactory control is being maintained for 24 hours. If it is not, an increase in dose should be considered. Doses up to 80 mg have been used but do not appear to give a greater effect. If blood pressure is not controlled with PRINIVIL alone, a low dose of a diuretic may be added. Hydrochlorothiazide 12.5 mg has been shown to provide an additive effect. After the addition of a diuretic, it may be possible to reduce the dose of PRINIVIL.

Diuretic Treated Patients: In hypertensive patients who are currently being treated with a diuretic, symptomatic hypotension may occur occasionally following the initial dose of PRINIVIL. The diuretic should be discontinued, if possible, for two to three days before beginning therapy with PRINIVIL to reduce the likelihood of hypotension. (See WARNINGS.) The dosage of PRINIVIL should be adjusted according to blood pressure response. If the patient's blood pressure is not controlled with PRINIVIL alone, diuretic therapy may be resumed as described above.

If the diuretic cannot be discontinued, an initial dose of 5 mg should be used under medical supervision for at least two hours and until blood pressure has stabilized for at least an additional hour. (See WARNINGS and PRECAUTIONS, Drug Interactions.)

Concomitant administration of PRINIVIL with potassium supplements, potassium salt substitutes, or potassium-sparing diuretics may lead to increases of serum potassium (see PRECAUTIONS).

Dosage Adjustment in Renal Impairment: The usual dose of PRINIVIL (10 mg) is recommended for patients with a creatinine clearance greater than 30 mL/min (serum creatinine of up to approximately 3 mg/dL). For patients with creatinine clearance greater than or equal to 10 mL/min and less than or equal to 30 mL/min (serum creatinine greater than or equal to 3 mg/dL), the first dose is 5 mg once daily. For patients with creatinine clearance less than 10 mL/min (usually on hemodialysis) the recommended initial dose is 2.5 mg. The dosage may be titrated upward until blood pressure is controlled or to a maximum of 40 mg daily.

Table 3

Renal Status	Creatinine-Clearance mL/min	Initial Dose mg/day
Normal Renal Function to Mild Impairment	>30 mL/min	10 mg
Moderate to Severe Impairment	≥10 ≤30 mL/min	5 mg
Dialysis Patients*	<10 mL/min	2.5 mg†

* See WARNINGS, Anaphylactoid reactions during membrane exposure.

† Dosage or dosing interval should be adjusted depending on the blood pressure response.

Heart Failure

PRINIVIL is indicated as adjunctive therapy with diuretics and (usually) digitalis. The recommended starting dose is 5 mg once a day.

When initiating treatment with lisinopril in patients with heart failure, the initial dose should be administered under medical observation, especially in those patients with low blood pressure (systolic blood pressure below 100 mmHg). The mean peak blood pressure lowering occurs six to eight hours after dosing. Observation should continue until blood pressure is stable. The concomitant diuretic dose should be reduced, if possible, to help minimize hypovolemia which may contribute to hypotension. (See WARNINGS and PRECAUTIONS, Drug Interactions.) The appearance of hypotension after the initial dose of PRINIVIL does not preclude subsequent careful dose titration with the drug, following effective management of the hypotension.

The usual effective dosage range is 5 to 20 mg per day administered as a single daily dose.

Dosage Adjustment in Patients with Heart Failure and Renal Impairment or Hyponatremia: In patients with heart failure who have hyponatremia (serum sodium less than 130 mEq/L) or moderate to severe renal impairment (creatinine clearance less than or equal to 30 mL/min or serum creatinine greater than 3 mg/dL), therapy with PRINIVIL should be initiated at a dose of 2.5 mg once a day under close medical supervision. (See WARNINGS and PRECAUTIONS, Drug Interactions.)

Acute Myocardial Infarction

In hemodynamically stable patients within 24 hours of the onset of symptoms of acute myocardial infarction, the first dose of PRINIVIL is 5 mg given orally, followed by 5 mg after 24 hours, 10 mg after 48 hours and then 10 mg of PRINIVIL once daily. Dosing should continue for six weeks. Patients should receive, as appropriate, the standard recommended treatments such as thrombolytics, aspirin and beta-blockers. Patients with a low systolic blood pressure (less than or equal to 120 mmHg) when treatment is started or during the first 3 days after the infarct should be given a lower 2.5 mg oral dose of PRINIVIL (see WARNINGS). If hypotension occurs (systolic blood pressure less than or equal to 100 mmHg) a daily maintenance dose of 5 mg may be given with temporary reductions to 2.5 mg if needed. If prolonged hypotension occurs (systolic blood pressure less than 90 mmHg for more than 1 hour) PRINIVIL should be withdrawn. For patients who develop symptoms of heart failure, see DOSAGE AND ADMINISTRATION, Heart Failure.

Dosage Adjustment in Patients with Myocardial Infarction with Renal Impairment: In acute myocardial infarction, treatment with PRINIVIL should be initiated with caution in patients with evidence of renal dysfunction, defined as serum creatinine concentration exceeding 2 mg/dL. No evaluation of dosage adjustment in myocardial infarction patients with severe renal impairment has been performed.

Use in Elderly

In general, blood pressure response and adverse experiences were similar in younger and older patients given similar doses of PRINIVIL. Pharmacokinetic studies, however, indicate that maximum blood levels and area under the plasma concentration time curve (AUC) are doubled in older patients, so that dosage adjustments should be made with particular caution.

Pediatric Hypertensive Patients 6 years of age and older

The usual recommended starting dose is 0.07 mg/kg once daily (up to 5 mg total). Dosage should be adjusted according to blood pressure response. Doses above 0.61 mg/kg (or in excess of 40 mg) have not been studied in pediatric patients. (See CLINICAL PHARMACOLOGY, Pharmacokinetics and Metabolism and Pharmacodynamics and Clinical Effects.)

PRINIVIL is not recommended in pediatric patients younger than 6 years or in pediatric patients with glomerular filtration rate less than 30 mL/min/1.73 m² (see CLIN-

ICAL PHARMACOLOGY, Pharmacokinetics and Metabolism, Pharmacodynamics and Clinical Effects and PRECAUTIONS.]

Preparation of Suspension (for 200 mL of a 1.0 mg/mL suspension)

Add 10 mL of Purified Water USP to a polyethylene terephthalate (PET) bottle containing ten 20-mg tablets of PRINIVIL and shake for at least one minute. Add 30 mL of Bicitra® diluent and 160 mL of Ora-Sweet SF™ to the concentrate in the PET bottle and gently shake for several seconds to disperse the ingredients. The suspension should be stored at or below 25°C (77°F) and can be stored for up to four weeks. Shake the suspension before each use.

HOW SUPPLIED

No. 8110 — Tablets PRINIVIL, 5 mg, are white, oval shaped compressed tablets with code MSD 19 on one side and scored on the other side. They are supplied as follows:
NDC 0006-0019-54 unit of use bottles of 90.
No. 8111 — Tablets PRINIVIL, 10 mg, are light yellow, oval shaped compressed tablets with code MSD 106 on one side and scored on the other side. They are supplied as follows:
NDC 0006-0106-54 unit of use bottles of 90.
No. 8112 — Tablets PRINIVIL, 20 mg, are peach, oval shaped compressed tablets with code MSD 207 on one side and scored on the other side. They are supplied as follows:
NDC 0006-0207-54 unit of use bottles of 90.

Storage

Store at controlled room temperature, 15-30°C (59-86°F), and protect from moisture.
Dispense in a tight container, if product package is subdivided.
Manuf. for: Merck Sharp & Dohme Corp., a subsidiary of **MERCK & CO., INC.**, Whitehouse Station, NJ 08889, USA
Manufactured by:
MERCK SHARP & DOHME LTD.
Cramlington, Northumberland, UK NE23 3JU
Copyright © 1988, 1989, 1992, 1993, 1995, 2005, 2006, 2011, 2012 Merck Sharp & Dohme Corp., a subsidiary of **Merck & Co., Inc.**
All rights reserved.
Trademarks depicted herein are the property of their respective owners.
Revised: 12/2012
USPI-T-05211212R008
Shown in Product Identification Guide, page 309

PROPECIA®　　　　　℞

[Pro-pee-sha]
(finasteride)
tablets for oral use

HIGHLIGHTS OF PRESCRIBING INFORMATION
These highlights do not include all the information needed to use PROPECIA safely and effectively. See full prescribing information for PROPECIA.
PROPECIA® (finasteride) tablets for oral use
Initial U.S. Approval: 1992

—————INDICATIONS AND USAGE—————

• PROPECIA is a 5α-reductase inhibitor indicated for the treatment of male pattern hair loss (androgenetic alopecia) in **MEN ONLY** (1).
• PROPECIA is not indicated for use in women (1, 4, 5.1).

—————DOSAGE AND ADMINISTRATION—————

• PROPECIA may be administered with or without meals (2).
• One tablet (1 mg) taken once daily (2).
• In general, daily use for three months or more is necessary before benefit is observed (2).

—————DOSAGE FORMS AND STRENGTHS—————

1 mg tablets (3).

—————CONTRAINDICATIONS—————

• Pregnancy (4, 5.1, 8.1, 16).
• Hypersensitivity to any components of this product (4).

—————WARNINGS AND PRECAUTIONS—————

• PROPECIA is not indicated for use in women or pediatric patients (5.1, 5.4).
• Women should not handle crushed or broken PROPECIA tablets when they are pregnant or may potentially be pregnant due to potential risk to a male fetus (5.1, 8.1, 16).
• PROPECIA causes a decrease in serum PSA levels. Any confirmed increase in PSA while on PROPECIA may signal the presence of prostate cancer and should be evaluated, even if those values are still within the normal range for men not taking a 5α-reductase inhibitor (5.2).
• 5α-reductase inhibitors may increase the risk of high-grade prostate cancer (5.3, 6.1).

—————ADVERSE REACTIONS—————

The most common adverse reactions, reported in ≥1% of patients treated with PROPECIA and greater than in patients treated with placebo are: decreased libido, erectile dysfunction and ejaculation disorder (6.1).

To report SUSPECTED ADVERSE REACTIONS, contact Merck Sharp & Dohme Corp., a subsidiary of Merck & Co., Inc., at 1-877-888-4231 or FDA at 1-800-FDA-1088 or www.fda.gov/medwatch.
See 17 for PATIENT COUNSELING INFORMATION and FDA-approved patient labeling

Revised: 09/2013

FULL PRESCRIBING INFORMATION: CONTENTS*

FULL PRESCRIBING INFORMATION

1　INDICATIONS AND USAGE

PROPECIA® is indicated for the treatment of male pattern hair loss (androgenetic alopecia) in **MEN ONLY**.
Efficacy in bitemporal recession has not been established.
PROPECIA is not indicated for use in women.

2　DOSAGE AND ADMINISTRATION

PROPECIA may be administered with or without meals.
The recommended dose of PROPECIA is one tablet (1 mg) taken once daily.
In general, daily use for three months or more is necessary before benefit is observed. Continued use is recommended to sustain benefit, which should be re-evaluated periodically. Withdrawal of treatment leads to reversal of effect within 12 months.

3　DOSAGE FORMS AND STRENGTHS

PROPECIA tablets (1 mg) are tan, octagonal, film-coated convex tablets with "stylized P" logo on one side and PROPECIA on the other.

4　CONTRAINDICATIONS

PROPECIA is contraindicated in the following:
• Pregnancy. Finasteride use is contraindicated in women when they are or may potentially be pregnant. Because of the ability of Type II 5α-reductase inhibitors to inhibit the conversion of testosterone to 5α-dihydrotestosterone (DHT), finasteride may cause abnormalities of the external genitalia of a male fetus of a pregnant woman who receives finasteride. If this drug is used during pregnancy, or if pregnancy occurs while taking this drug, the pregnant woman should be apprised of the potential hazard to the male fetus. [See Warnings and Precautions (5.1), Use in

Specific Populations (8.1), How Supplied/Storage and Handling (16) and Patient Counseling Information (17.1).]
In female rats, low doses of finasteride administered during pregnancy have produced abnormalities of the external genitalia in male offspring.
• Hypersensitivity to any component of this medication.

5　WARNINGS AND PRECAUTIONS

5.1　Exposure of Women — Risk to Male Fetus

PROPECIA is not indicated for use in women. Women should not handle crushed or broken PROPECIA tablets when they are pregnant or may potentially be pregnant because of the possibility of absorption of finasteride and the subsequent potential risk to a male fetus. PROPECIA tablets are coated and will prevent contact with the active ingredient during normal handling, provided that the tablets have not been broken or crushed. [See Indications and Usage (1), Contraindications (4), Use in Specific Populations (8.1), How Supplied/Storage and Handling (16) and Patient Counseling Information (17.1).]

5.2　Effects on Prostate Specific Antigen (PSA)

In clinical studies with PROPECIA (finasteride, 1 mg) in men 18-41 years of age, the mean value of serum prostate specific antigen (PSA) decreased from 0.7 ng/mL at baseline to 0.5 ng/mL at Month 12. Further, in clinical studies with PROSCAR (finasteride, 5 mg) when used in older men who have benign prostatic hyperplasia (BPH), PSA levels are decreased by approximately 50%. Other studies with PROSCAR showed it may also cause decreases in serum PSA in the presence of prostate cancer. These findings should be taken into account for proper interpretation of serum PSA when evaluating men treated with finasteride. Any confirmed increase from the lowest PSA value while on PROPECIA may signal the presence of prostate cancer and should be evaluated, even if PSA levels are still within the normal range for men not taking a 5α-reductase inhibitor. Non-compliance to therapy with PROPECIA may also affect PSA test results.

5.3　Increased Risk of High-Grade Prostate Cancer with 5α-Reductase Inhibitors

Men aged 55 and over with a normal digital rectal examination and PSA ≤3.0 ng/mL at baseline taking finasteride 5 mg/day (5 times the dose of PROPECIA) in the 7-year Prostate Cancer Prevention Trial (PCPT) had an increased risk of Gleason score 8-10 prostate cancer (finasteride 1.8% vs placebo 1.1%). [See Adverse Reactions (6.1).] Similar results were observed in a 4-year placebo-controlled clinical trial with another 5α-reductase inhibitor (dutasteride, AVODART) (1% dutasteride vs 0.5% placebo). 5α-reductase inhibitors may increase the risk of development of high-grade prostate cancer. Whether the effect of 5α-reductase inhibitors to reduce prostate volume, or study-related factors, impacted the results of these studies has not been established.

5.4　Pediatric Patients

PROPECIA is not indicated for use in pediatric patients [see Use in Specific Populations (8.4)].

6　ADVERSE REACTIONS

6.1　Clinical Trials Experience

Because clinical trials are conducted under widely varying conditions, adverse reaction rates observed in the clinical trials of a drug cannot be directly compared to rates in the clinical trials of another drug and may not reflect the rates observed in clinical practice.

Clinical Studies for PROPECIA (finasteride 1 mg) in the Treatment of Male Pattern Hair Loss

In three controlled clinical trials for PROPECIA of 12-month duration, 1.4% of patients taking PROPECIA (n=945) were discontinued due to adverse experiences that were considered to be possibly, probably or definitely drug-related (1.6% for placebo; n=934).
Clinical adverse experiences that were reported as possibly, probably or definitely drug-related in ≥1% of patients treated with PROPECIA or placebo are presented in Table 1.

TABLE 1: Drug-Related Adverse Experiences for PROPECIA (finasteride 1 mg) in Year 1 (%) MALE PATTERN HAIR LOSS

	PROPECIA N=945	Placebo N=934
Decreased Libido	1.8	1.3
Erectile Dysfunction	1.3	0.7
Ejaculation Disorder *(Decreased Volume of Ejaculate)*	1.2 *(0.8)*	0.7 *(0.4)*
Discontinuation due to drug-related sexual adverse experiences	1.2	0.9

Integrated analysis of clinical adverse experiences showed that during treatment with PROPECIA, 36 (3.8%) of 945 men had reported one or more of these adverse experiences as compared to 20 (2.1%) of 934 men treated with placebo (p=0.04). Resolution occurred in men who discontinued therapy with PROPECIA due to these side effects and in most of those who continued therapy. The incidence of each of the above adverse experiences decreased to ≤0.3% by the fifth year of treatment with PROPECIA.

In a study of finasteride 1 mg daily in healthy men, a median decrease in ejaculate volume of 0.3 mL (-11%) compared with 0.2 mL (-8%) for placebo was observed after 48 weeks of treatment. Two other studies showed that finasteride at 5 times the dosage of PROPECIA (5 mg daily) produced significant median decreases of approximately 0.5 mL (-25%) compared to placebo in ejaculate volume, but this was reversible after discontinuation of treatment.

In the clinical studies with PROPECIA, the incidences for breast tenderness and enlargement, hypersensitivity reactions, and testicular pain in finasteride-treated patients were not different from those in patients treated with placebo.

Controlled Clinical Trials and Long-Term Open Extension Studies for PROSCAR® (finasteride 5 mg) and AVODART (dutasteride) in the Treatment of Benign Prostatic Hyperplasia

In the PROSCAR Long-Term Efficacy and Safety Study (PLESS), a 4-year controlled clinical study, 3040 patients between the ages of 45 and 78 with symptomatic BPH and an enlarged prostate were evaluated for safety over a period of 4 years (1524 on PROSCAR 5 mg/day and 1516 on placebo). 3.7% (57 patients) treated with PROSCAR 5 mg and 2.1% (32 patients) treated with placebo discontinued therapy as a result of adverse reactions related to sexual function, which are the most frequently reported adverse reactions.

Table 2 presents the only clinical adverse reactions considered possibly, probably or definitely drug related by the investigator, for which the incidence on PROSCAR was ≥1% and greater than placebo over the 4 years of the study. In years 2-4 of the study, there was no significant difference between treatment groups in the incidences of impotence, decreased libido and ejaculation disorder.

[See table 2 above]

The adverse experience profiles in the 1-year, placebo-controlled, Phase III BPH studies and the 5-year open extensions with PROSCAR 5 mg and PLESS were similar.

There is no evidence of increased sexual adverse experiences with increased duration of treatment with PROSCAR 5 mg. New reports of drug-related sexual adverse experiences decreased with duration of therapy.

During the 4- to 6-year placebo- and comparator-controlled Medical Therapy of Prostatic Symptoms (MTOPS) study that enrolled 3047 men, there were 4 cases of breast cancer in men treated with PROSCAR but no cases in men not treated with PROSCAR. During the 4-year placebo-controlled PLESS study that enrolled 3040 men, there were 2 cases of breast cancer in placebo-treated men, but no cases were reported in men treated with PROSCAR.

During the 7-year placebo-controlled Prostate Cancer Prevention Trial (PCPT) that enrolled 18,882 men, there was 1 case of breast cancer in men treated with PROSCAR, and 1 case of breast cancer in men treated with placebo. The relationship between long-term use of finasteride and male breast neoplasia is currently unknown.

The PCPT trial was a 7-year randomized, double-blind, placebo-controlled trial that enrolled 18,882 healthy men ≥55 years of age with a normal digital rectal examination and a PSA ≤3.0 ng/mL. Men received either PROSCAR (finasteride 5 mg) or placebo daily. Patients were evaluated annually with PSA and digital rectal exams. Biopsies were performed for elevated PSA, an abnormal digital rectal exam, or the end of study. The incidence of Gleason score 8-10 prostate cancer was higher in men treated with finasteride (1.8%) than in those treated with placebo (1.1%). In a 4-year placebo-controlled clinical trial with another 5α-reductase inhibitor [AVODART (dutasteride)], similar results for Gleason score 8-10 prostate cancer were observed (1% dutasteride vs 0.5% placebo). The clinical significance of these findings with respect to use of PROPECIA by men is unknown.

No clinical benefit has been demonstrated in patients with prostate cancer treated with PROSCAR. PROSCAR is not approved to reduce the risk of developing prostate cancer.

6.2   Postmarketing Experience

The following adverse reactions have been identified during post approval use of PROPECIA. Because these reactions are reported voluntarily from a population of uncertain size, it is not always possible to reliably estimate their frequency or establish a causal relationship to drug exposure:

Hypersensitivity Reaction: hypersensitivity reactions such as rash, pruritus, urticaria, and angioedema (including swelling of the lips, tongue, throat, and face);

Reproductive System: sexual dysfunction that continued after discontinuation of treatment, including erectile dysfunction, libido disorders, ejaculation disorders, and orgasm

TABLE 2: Drug-Related Adverse Experiences for PROSCAR (finasteride 5 mg) BENIGN PROSTATIC HYPERPLASIA

	Year 1 (%)		Years 2, 3 and 4* (%)	
	Finasteride, 5 mg	Placebo	Finasteride, 5 mg	Placebo
Impotence	8.1	3.7	5.1	5.1
Decreased Libido	6.4	3.4	2.6	2.6
Decreased Volume of Ejaculate	3.7	0.8	1.5	0.5
Ejaculation Disorder	0.8	0.1	0.2	0.1
Breast Enlargement	0.5	0.1	1.8	1.1
Breast Tenderness	0.4	0.1	0.7	0.3
Rash	0.5	0.2	0.5	0.1

N = 1524 and 1516, finasteride vs placebo, respectively
* Combined Years 2-4

disorders; male infertility and/or poor seminal quality (normalization or improvement of seminal quality has been reported after discontinuation of finasteride); testicular pain. *[See Adverse Reactions (6.1).]*

Neoplasms: male breast cancer;
Breast disorders: breast tenderness and enlargement;
Nervous System/Psychiatric: depression

7   DRUG INTERACTIONS

7.1   Cytochrome P450-Linked Drug Metabolizing Enzyme System

No drug interactions of clinical importance have been identified. Finasteride does not appear to affect the cytochrome P450-linked drug-metabolizing enzyme system. Compounds that have been tested in man include antipyrine, digoxin, propranolol, theophylline, and warfarin and no clinically meaningful interactions were found.

7.2   Other Concomitant Therapy

Although specific interaction studies were not performed, finasteride doses of 1 mg or more were concomitantly used in clinical studies with acetaminophen, acetylsalicylic acid, α-blockers, analgesics, angiotensin-converting enzyme (ACE) inhibitors, anticonvulsants, benzodiazepines, beta blockers, calcium-channel blockers, cardiac nitrates, diuretics, H_2 antagonists, HMG-CoA reductase inhibitors, prostaglandin synthetase inhibitors (also referred to as NSAIDs), and quinolone anti-infectives without evidence of clinically significant adverse interactions.

8   USE IN SPECIFIC POPULATIONS

8.1   Pregnancy

Pregnancy Category X *[see Contraindications (4)].* PROPECIA is contraindicated for use in women who are or may become pregnant. PROPECIA is a Type II 5α-reductase inhibitor that prevents conversion of testosterone to 5α-dihydrotestosterone (DHT), a hormone necessary for normal development of male genitalia. In animal studies, finasteride caused abnormal development of external genitalia in male fetuses. If this drug is used during pregnancy, or if the patient becomes pregnant while taking this drug, the patient should be apprised of the potential hazard to the male fetus.

Abnormal male genital development is an expected consequence when conversion of testosterone to 5α-dihydrotestosterone (DHT) is inhibited by 5α-reductase inhibitors. These outcomes are similar to those reported in male infants with genetic 5α-reductase deficiency. Women could be exposed to finasteride through contact with crushed or broken PROPECIA tablets or semen from a male partner taking PROPECIA. With regard to finasteride exposure through the skin, PROPECIA tablets are coated and will prevent skin contact with finasteride during normal handling if the tablets have not been crushed or broken. Women who are pregnant or may become pregnant should not handle crushed or broken PROPECIA tablets because of possible exposure of a male fetus. If a pregnant woman comes in contact with crushed or broken PROPECIA tablets, the contact area should be washed immediately with soap and water. With regard to potential finasteride exposure through semen, a study has been conducted in men receiving PROPECIA 1 mg/day that measured finasteride concentrations in semen *[see Clinical Pharmacology (12.3)].*

In an embryo-fetal development study, pregnant rats received finasteride during the period of major organogenesis (gestation days 6 to 17). At maternal doses of oral finasteride approximately 1 to 684 times the recommended human dose (RHD) of 1 mg/day (based on AUC at animal doses of 0.1 to 100 mg/kg/day) there was a dose-dependent increase in hypospadias that occurred in 3.6 to 100% of male offspring. Exposure multiples were estimated using data from nonpregnant rats. Days 16 to 17 of gestation is a crit-

ical period in male fetal rats for differentiation of the external genitalia. At oral maternal doses approximately 0.2 times the RHD (based on AUC at animal dose of 0.03 mg/kg/day), male offspring had decreased prostatic and seminal vesicular weights, delayed preputial separation and transient nipple development. Decreased anogenital distance occurred in male offspring of pregnant rats that received approximately 0.02 times the RHD (based on AUC at animal dose of 0.003 mg/kg/day). No abnormalities were observed in female offspring exposed to any dose of finasteride *in utero.*

No developmental abnormalities were observed in the offspring of untreated females mated with finasteride-treated male rats that received approximately 488 times the RHD (based on AUC at animal dose of 80 mg/kg/day). Slightly decreased fertility was observed in male offspring after administration of about 20 times the RHD (based on AUC at animal dose of 3 mg/kg/day) to female rats during late gestation and lactation. No effects on fertility were seen in female offspring under these conditions.

No evidence of male external genital malformations or other abnormalities were observed in rabbit fetuses exposed to finasteride during the period of major organogenesis (gestation days 6-18) at maternal doses up to 100 mg/kg/day (finasteride exposure levels were not measured in rabbits). However, this study may not have included the critical period for finasteride effects on development of male external genitalia in the rabbit.

The fetal effects of maternal finasteride exposure during the period of embryonic and fetal development were evaluated in the rhesus monkey (gestation days 20-100), in a species and development period more predictive of specific effects in humans than the studies in rats and rabbits. Intravenous administration of finasteride to pregnant monkeys at doses as high as 800 ng/day (estimated maximal blood concentration of 1.86 ng/mL or about 930 times the highest estimated exposure of pregnant women to finasteride from semen of men taking 1 mg/day) resulted in no abnormalities in male fetuses. In confirmation of the relevance of the rhesus model for human fetal development, oral administration of a dose of finasteride (2 mg/kg/day or approximately 120,000 times the highest estimated blood levels of finasteride from semen of men taking 1 mg/day) to pregnant monkeys resulted in external genital abnormalities in male fetuses. No other abnormalities were observed in male fetuses and no finasteride-related abnormalities were observed in female fetuses at any dose.

8.3   Nursing Mothers

PROPECIA is not indicated for use in women.

It is not known whether finasteride is excreted in human milk.

8.4   Pediatric Use

PROPECIA is not indicated for use in pediatric patients. Safety and effectiveness in pediatric patients have not been established.

8.5   Geriatric Use

Clinical efficacy studies with PROPECIA did not include subjects aged 65 and over. Based on the pharmacokinetics of finasteride 5 mg, no dosage adjustment is necessary in the elderly for PROPECIA *[see Clinical Pharmacology (12.3)].* However the efficacy of PROPECIA in the elderly has not been established.

8.6   Hepatic Impairment

Caution should be exercised in the administration of PROPECIA in those patients with liver function abnormalities, as finasteride is metabolized extensively in the liver *[see Clinical Pharmacology (12.3)].*

8.7   Renal Impairment

No dosage adjustment is necessary in patients with renal impairment *[see Clinical Pharmacology (12.3)].*

10 OVERDOSAGE

In clinical studies, single doses of finasteride up to 400 mg and multiple doses of finasteride up to 80 mg/day for three months did not result in adverse reactions. Until further experience is obtained, no specific treatment for an overdose with finasteride can be recommended.

Significant lethality was observed in male and female mice at single oral doses of 1500 mg/m^2 (500 mg/kg) and in female and male rats at single oral doses of 2360 mg/m^2 (400 mg/kg) and 5900 mg/m^2 (1000 mg/kg), respectively.

11 DESCRIPTION

PROPECIA (finasteride) tablets contain finasteride as the active ingredient. Finasteride, a synthetic 4-azasteroid compound, is a specific inhibitor of steroid Type II 5α-reductase, an intracellular enzyme that converts the androgen testosterone into 5α-dihydrotestosterone (DHT).

The chemical name of finasteride is *N-tert*-Butyl-3-oxo-4-aza-5α-androst-1-ene-17β-carboxamide. The empirical formula of finasteride is $C_{23}H_{36}N_2O_2$ and its molecular weight is 372.55. Its structural formula is:

Finasteride is a white crystalline powder with a melting point near 250°C. It is freely soluble in chloroform and in lower alcohol solvents but is practically insoluble in water. PROPECIA (finasteride) tablets are film-coated tablets for oral administration. Each tablet contains 1 mg of finasteride and the following inactive ingredients: lactose monohydrate, microcrystalline cellulose, pregelatinized starch, sodium starch glycolate, hydroxypropyl methylcellulose, hydroxypropyl cellulose, titanium dioxide, magnesium stearate, talc, docusate sodium, yellow ferric oxide, and red ferric oxide.

12 CLINICAL PHARMACOLOGY

12.1 Mechanism of Action

Finasteride is a competitive and specific inhibitor of Type II 5α-reductase, an intracellular enzyme that converts the androgen testosterone into DHT. Two distinct isozymes are found in mice, rats, monkeys, and humans: Type I and II. Each of these isozymes is differentially expressed in tissues and developmental stages. In humans, Type I 5α-reductase is predominant in the sebaceous glands of most regions of skin, including scalp, and liver. Type I 5α-reductase is responsible for approximately one-third of circulating DHT. The Type II 5α-reductase isozyme is primarily found in prostate, seminal vesicles, epididymides, and hair follicles as well as liver, and is responsible for two-thirds of circulating DHT.

In humans, the mechanism of action of finasteride is based on its preferential inhibition of the Type II isozyme. Using native tissues (scalp and prostate), *in vitro* binding studies examining the potential of finasteride to inhibit either isozyme revealed a 100-fold selectivity for the human Type II 5α-reductase over Type I isozyme (IC$_{50}$=500 and 4.2 nM for Type I and II, respectively). For both isozymes, the inhibition by finasteride is accompanied by reduction of the inhibitor to dihydrofinasteride and adduct formation with NADP+. The turnover for the enzyme complex is slow (t$_{1/2}$ approximately 30 days for the Type II enzyme complex and 14 days for the Type I complex). Inhibition of Type II 5α-reductase blocks the peripheral conversion of testosterone to DHT, resulting in significant decreases in serum and tissue DHT concentrations.

In men with male pattern hair loss (androgenetic alopecia), the balding scalp contains miniaturized hair follicles and increased amounts of DHT compared with hairy scalp. Administration of finasteride decreases scalp and serum DHT concentrations in these men. The relative contributions of these reductions to the treatment effect of finasteride have not been defined. By this mechanism, finasteride appears to interrupt a key factor in the development of androgenetic alopecia in those patients genetically predisposed.

12.2 Pharmacodynamics

Finasteride produces a rapid reduction in serum DHT concentration, reaching 65% suppression within 24 hours of oral dosing with a 1-mg tablet. Mean circulating levels of testosterone and estradiol were increased by approximately 15% as compared to baseline, but these remained within the physiologic range.

Finasteride has no affinity for the androgen receptor and has no androgenic, antiandrogenic, estrogenic, antiestrogenic, or progestational effects. In studies with finasteride, no clinically meaningful changes in luteinizing hormone (LH), follicle-stimulating hormone (FSH) or prolactin were detected. In healthy volunteers, treatment with finasteride did not alter the response of LH and FSH to gonadotropin-releasing hormone indicating that the hypothalamic-pituitary-testicular axis was not affected. Finasteride had no effect on circulating levels of cortisol, thyroid-stimulating hormone, or thyroxine, nor did it affect the plasma lipid profile (e.g., total cholesterol, low-density lipoproteins, high-density lipoproteins and triglycerides) or bone mineral density.

12.3 Pharmacokinetics

Absorption

In a study in 15 healthy young male subjects, the mean bioavailability of finasteride 1-mg tablets was 65% (range 26-170%), based on the ratio of area under the curve (AUC) relative to an intravenous (IV) reference dose. At steady state following dosing with 1 mg/day (n=12), maximum finasteride plasma concentration averaged 9.2 ng/mL (range, 4.9-13.7 ng/mL) and was reached 1 to 2 hours postdose; AUC$_{(0-24 \ hr)}$ was 53 ng•hr/mL (range, 20-154 ng•hr/mL). Bioavailability of finasteride was not affected by food.

Distribution

Mean steady-state volume of distribution was 76 liters (range, 44-96 liters; n=15). Approximately 90% of circulating finasteride is bound to plasma proteins. There is a slow accumulation phase for finasteride after multiple dosing.

Finasteride has been found to cross the blood-brain barrier. Semen levels have been measured in 35 men taking finasteride 1 mg/day for 6 weeks. In 60% (21 of 35) of the samples, finasteride levels were undetectable (<0.2 ng/mL). The mean finasteride level was 0.26 ng/mL and the highest level measured was 1.52 ng/mL. Using the highest semen level measured and assuming 100% absorption from a 5-mL ejaculate per day, human exposure through vaginal absorption would be up to 7.6 ng per day, which is 650-fold less than the dose of finasteride (5 μg) that had no effect on circulating DHT levels in men. *[See Use in Specific Populations (8.1).]*

Metabolism

Finasteride is extensively metabolized in the liver, primarily via the cytochrome P450 3A4 enzyme subfamily. Two metabolites, the t-butyl side chain monohydroxylated and monocarboxylic acid metabolites, have been identified that possess no more than 20% of the 5α-reductase inhibitory activity of finasteride.

Excretion

Following intravenous infusion in healthy young subjects (n=15), mean plasma clearance of finasteride was 165 mL/min (range, 70-279 mL/min). Mean terminal half-life in plasma was 4.5 hours (range, 3.3-13.4 hours; n=12). Following an oral dose of ^{14}C-finasteride in man (n=6), a mean of 39% (range, 32-46%) of the dose was excreted in the urine in the form of metabolites; 57% (range, 51-64%) was excreted in the feces.

Mean terminal half-life is approximately 5-6 hours in men 18-60 years of age and 8 hours in men more than 70 years of age.

TABLE 3: Mean (SD) Pharmacokinetic Parameters in Healthy Men (ages 18-26)

	Mean (± SD) n=15
Bioavailability	65% (26-170%)*
Clearance (mL/min)	165 (55)
Volume of Distribution (L)	76 (14)

* Range

TABLE 4: Mean (SD) Noncompartmental Pharmacokinetic Parameters After Multiple Doses of 1 mg/day in Healthy Men (ages 19-42)

	Mean (± SD) (n=12)
AUC (ng•hr/mL)	53 (33.8)
Peak Concentration (ng/mL)	9.2 (2.6)
Time to Peak (hours)	1.3 (0.5)
Half-Life (hours)*	4.5 (1.6)

* First-dose values; all other parameters are last-dose values

Renal Impairment

No dosage adjustment is necessary in patients with renal impairment. In patients with chronic renal impairment, with creatinine clearances ranging from 9.0 to 55 mL/min, AUC, maximum plasma concentration, half-life, and protein binding after a single dose of ^{14}C-finasteride were similar to those obtained in healthy volunteers. Urinary excretion of metabolites was decreased in patients with renal impairment. This decrease was associated with an increase in fecal excretion of metabolites. Plasma concentrations of metabolites were significantly higher in patients with renal impairment (based on a 60% increase in total radioactivity AUC). However, finasteride has been tolerated in men with normal renal function receiving up to 80 mg/day for 12 weeks where exposure of these patients to metabolites would presumably be much greater.

Hepatic Impairment

The effect of hepatic impairment on finasteride pharmacokinetics has not been studied. Caution should be used in the administration of PROPECIA in patients with liver function abnormalities, as finasteride is metabolized extensively in the liver.

13 NONCLINICAL TOXICOLOGY

13.1 Carcinogenesis, Mutagenesis, Impairment of Fertility

No evidence of a tumorigenic effect was observed in a 24-month study in Sprague-Dawley rats receiving doses of finasteride up to 160 mg/kg/day in males and 320 mg/kg/day in females. These doses produced respective systemic exposure in rats of 888 and 2192 times those observed in man receiving the recommended human dose of 1 mg/day. All exposure calculations were based on calculated AUC$_{(0-24 \ hr)}$ for animals and mean AUC$_{(0-24 \ hr)}$ for man (0.05 μg•hr/mL).

In a 19-month carcinogenicity study in CD-1 mice, a statistically significant (p≤0.05) increase in the incidence of testicular Leydig cell adenomas was observed at 1824 times the human exposure (250 mg/kg/day). In mice at 184 times the human exposure, estimated (25 mg/kg/day) and in rats at 312 times the human exposure (≥40 mg/kg/day) an increase in the incidence of Leydig cell hyperplasia was observed. A positive correlation between the proliferative changes in the Leydig cells and an increase in serum LH levels (2- to 3-fold above control) has been demonstrated in both rodent species treated with high doses of finasteride. No drug-related Leydig cell changes were seen in either rats or dogs treated with finasteride for 1 year at 240 and 2800 times (20 mg/kg/day and 45 mg/kg/day, respectively), or in mice treated for 19 months at 18.4 times the human exposure, estimated (2.5 mg/kg/day).

No evidence of mutagenicity was observed in an *in vitro* bacterial mutagenesis assay, a mammalian cell mutagenesis assay, or in an *in vitro* alkaline elution assay. In an *in vitro* chromosome aberration assay, using Chinese hamster ovary cells, there was a slight increase in chromosome aberrations. In an *in vivo* chromosome aberration assay in mice, no treatment-related increase in chromosome aberration was observed with finasteride at the maximum tolerated dose of 250 mg/kg/day (1824 times the human exposure) as determined in the carcinogenicity studies.

In sexually mature male rabbits treated with finasteride at 4344 times the human exposure (80 mg/kg/day) for up to 12 weeks, no effect on fertility, sperm count, or ejaculate volume was seen. In sexually mature male rats treated with 488 times the human exposure (80 mg/kg/day), there were no significant effects on fertility after 6 or 12 weeks of treatment; however, when treatment was continued for up to 24 or 30 weeks, there was an apparent decrease in fertility, fecundity, and an associated significant decrease in the weights of the seminal vesicles and prostate. All these effects were reversible within 6 weeks of discontinuation of treatment. No drug-related effect on testes or on mating performance has been seen in rats or rabbits. This decrease in fertility in finasteride-treated rats is secondary to its effect on accessory sex organs (prostate and seminal vesicles) resulting in failure to form a seminal plug. The seminal plug is essential for normal fertility in rats but is not relevant in man.

14 CLINICAL STUDIES

14.1 Studies in Men

The efficacy of PROPECIA was demonstrated in men (88% Caucasian) with mild to moderate androgenetic alopecia (male pattern hair loss) between 18 and 41 years of age. In order to prevent seborrheic dermatitis which might confound the assessment of hair growth in these studies, all men, whether treated with finasteride or placebo, were instructed to use a specified, medicated, tar-based shampoo (Neutrogena T/Gel® Shampoo) during the first 2 years of the studies.

There were three double-blind, randomized, placebo-controlled studies of 12-month duration. The two primary endpoints were hair count and patient self-assessment; the two secondary endpoints were investigator assessment and ratings of photographs. In addition, information was collected regarding sexual function (based on a self-administered questionnaire) and non-scalp body hair growth. The three studies were conducted in 1879 men with mild to moderate, but not complete, hair loss. Two of the studies enrolled men with predominantly mild to moderate vertex hair loss (n=1553). The third enrolled men having mild to moderate hair loss in the anterior mid-scalp area with or without vertex balding (n=326).

Studies in Men with Vertex Baldness

Of the men who completed the first 12 months of the two vertex baldness trials, 1215 elected to continue in double-blind, placebo-controlled, 12-month extension studies. There were 547 men receiving PROPECIA for both the initial study and first extension periods (up to 2 years of treatment) and 60 men receiving placebo for the same periods. The extension studies were continued for 3 additional years, with 323 men on PROPECIA and 23 on placebo entering the fifth year of the study.

In order to evaluate the effect of discontinuation of therapy, there were 65 men who received PROPECIA for the initial 12 months followed by placebo in the first 12-month extension period. Some of these men continued in additional extension studies and were switched back to treatment with PROPECIA, with 32 men entering the fifth year of the study. Lastly, there were 543 men who received placebo for the initial 12 months followed by PROPECIA in the first 12-month extension period. Some of these men continued in additional extension studies receiving PROPECIA, with 290 men entering the fifth year of the study (see Figure 1 below).

Hair counts were assessed by photographic enlargements of a representative area of active hair loss. In these two studies in men with vertex baldness, significant increases in hair count were demonstrated at 6 and 12 months in men treated with PROPECIA, while significant hair loss from baseline was demonstrated in those treated with placebo. At 12 months there was a 107-hair difference from placebo (p<0.001, PROPECIA [n=679] vs placebo [n=672]) within a 1-inch diameter circle (5.1 cm^2). Hair count was maintained in those men taking PROPECIA for up to 2 years, resulting in a 138-hair difference between treatment groups (p<0.001, PROPECIA [n=433] vs placebo [n=47]) within the same area. In men treated with PROPECIA, the maximum improvement in hair count compared to baseline was achieved during the first 2 years. Although the initial improvement was followed by a slow decline, hair count was maintained above baseline throughout the 5 years of the studies. Furthermore, because the decline in the placebo group was more rapid, the difference between treatment groups also continued to increase throughout the studies, resulting in a 277-hair difference (p<0.001, PROPECIA [n=219] vs placebo [n=15]) at 5 years (see Figure 1 below).

Patients who switched from placebo to PROPECIA (n=425) had a decrease in hair count at the end of the initial 12-month placebo period, followed by an increase in hair count after 1 year of treatment with PROPECIA. This increase in hair count was less (56 hairs above original baseline) than the increase (91 hairs above original baseline) observed after 1 year of treatment in men initially randomized to PROPECIA. Although the increase in hair count, relative to when therapy was initiated, was comparable between these two groups, a higher absolute hair count was achieved in patients who were started on treatment with PROPECIA in the initial study. This advantage was maintained through the remaining 3 years of the studies. A change of treatment from PROPECIA to placebo (n=48) at the end of the initial 12 months resulted in reversal of the increase in hair count 12 months later, at 24 months (see Figure 1 below).

At 12 months, 58% of men in the placebo group had further hair loss (defined as any decrease in hair count from baseline), compared with 14% of men treated with PROPECIA. In men treated for up to 2 years, 72% of men in the placebo group demonstrated hair loss, compared with 17% of men treated with PROPECIA. At 5 years, 100% of men in the placebo group demonstrated hair loss, compared with 35% of men treated with PROPECIA.

Figure 1

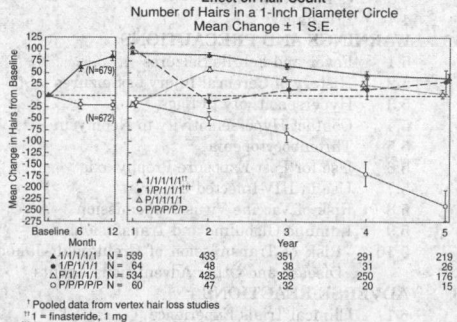

Effect on Hair Count[1]
Number of Hairs in a 1-Inch Diameter Circle
Mean Change ± 1 S.E.

	Baseline	6	12	1	2	3	4	5
▲ 1/1/1/1/1	N = 539			433	351	291	219
▲ 1/P/1/1/1	N = 64			48	38	31	26
△ P/1/1/1/1	N = 534			425	329	250	176
○ P/P/P/P/P	N = 60			47	32	20	15

[1] Pooled data from vertex hair loss studies
[1] 1 = finasteride, 1 mg
[1] P = placebo

Patient self-assessment was obtained at each clinic visit from a self-administered questionnaire, which included questions on their perception of hair growth, hair loss, and appearance. This self-assessment demonstrated an increase in amount of hair, a decrease in hair loss, and improvement in appearance in men treated with PROPECIA. Overall improvement compared with placebo was seen as early as 3 months (p<0.05), with improvement maintained over 5 years.

Investigator assessment was based on a 7-point scale evaluating increases or decreases in scalp hair at each patient visit. This assessment showed significantly greater increases in hair growth in men treated with PROPECIA compared with placebo as early as 3 months (p<0.001). At 12 months, the investigators rated 65% of men treated with PROPECIA as having increased hair growth compared with 37% in the placebo group. At 2 years, the investigators rated 80% of men treated with PROPECIA as having increased hair growth compared with 47% of men treated with placebo. At 5 years, the investigators rated 77% of men treated with PROPECIA as having increased hair growth, compared with 15% of men treated with placebo.

An independent panel rated standardized photographs of the head in a blinded fashion based on increases or decreases in scalp hair using the same 7-point scale as the investigator assessment. At 12 months, 48% of men treated with PROPECIA had an increase as compared with 7% of men treated with placebo. At 2 years, an increase in hair growth was demonstrated in 66% of men treated with PROPECIA, compared with 7% of men treated with placebo. At 5 years, 48% of men treated with PROPECIA demonstrated an increase in hair growth, 42% were rated as having no change (no further visible progression of hair loss from baseline) and 10% were rated as having lost hair when compared to baseline. In comparison, 6% of men treated with placebo demonstrated an increase in hair growth, 19% were rated as having no change and 75% were rated as having lost hair when compared to baseline.

A 48-week, placebo-controlled study designed to assess by phototrichogram the effect of PROPECIA on total and actively growing (anagen) scalp hairs in vertex baldness enrolled 212 men with androgenetic alopecia. At baseline and 48 weeks, total and anagen hair counts were obtained in a 1-cm^2 target area of the scalp. Men treated with PROPECIA showed increases from baseline in total and anagen hair counts of 7 hairs and 18 hairs, respectively, whereas men treated with placebo had decreases of 10 hairs and 9 hairs, respectively. These changes in hair counts resulted in a between-group difference of 17 hairs in total hair count (p<0.001) and 27 hairs in anagen hair count (p<0.001), and an improvement in the proportion of anagen hairs from 62% at baseline to 68% for men treated with PROPECIA.

Other Results in Vertex Baldness Studies

A sexual function questionnaire was self-administered by patients participating in the two vertex baldness trials to detect more subtle changes in sexual function. At Month 12, statistically significant differences in favor of placebo were found in 3 of 4 domains (sexual interest, erections, and perception of sexual problems). However, no significant difference was seen in the question on overall satisfaction with sex life.

In one of the two vertex baldness studies, patients were questioned on non-scalp body hair growth. PROPECIA did not appear to affect non-scalp body hair.

Study in Men with Hair Loss in the Anterior Mid-Scalp Area

A study of 12-month duration, designed to assess the efficacy of PROPECIA in men with hair loss in the anterior mid-scalp area, also demonstrated significant increases in hair count compared with placebo. Increases in hair count were accompanied by improvements in patient self-assessment, investigator assessment, and ratings based on standardized photographs. Hair counts were obtained in the anterior mid-scalp area, and did not include the area of bitemporal recession or the anterior hairline.

Summary of Clinical Studies in Men

Clinical studies were conducted in men aged 18 to 41 with mild to moderate degrees of androgenetic alopecia. All men treated with PROPECIA or placebo received a tar-based shampoo (Neutrogena T/Gel® Shampoo) during the first 2 years of the studies. Clinical improvement was seen as early as 3 months in the patients treated with PROPECIA and led to a net increase in scalp hair count and hair regrowth. In clinical studies for up to 5 years, treatment with PROPECIA slowed the further progression of hair loss observed in the placebo group. In general, the difference between treatment groups continued to increase throughout the 5 years of the studies.

Ethnic Analysis of Clinical Data from Men

In a combined analysis of the two studies on vertex baldness, mean hair count changes from baseline were 91 vs -19 hairs (PROPECIA vs placebo) among Caucasians (n=1185), 49 vs -27 hairs among Blacks (n=84), 53 vs -38 hairs among Asians (n=17), 67 vs 5 hairs among Hispanics (n=45) and 67 vs -15 hairs among other ethnic groups (n=20). Patient self-assessment showed improvement across racial groups with

PROPECIA treatment, except for satisfaction of the frontal hairline and vertex in Black men, who were satisfied overall.

14.2 Study in Women

In a study involving 137 postmenopausal women with androgenetic alopecia who were treated with PROPECIA (n=67) or placebo (n=70) for 12 months, effectiveness could not be demonstrated. There was no improvement in hair counts, patient self-assessment, investigator assessment, or ratings of standardized photographs in the women treated with PROPECIA when compared with the placebo group [see Indications and Usage (1)].

16   HOW SUPPLIED/STORAGE AND HANDLING

No. 6642 — PROPECIA tablets, 1 mg, are tan, octagonal, film-coated convex tablets with "stylized P" logo on one side and PROPECIA on the other. They are supplied as follows:
   NDC 0006-0071-31 bottles of 30 (with desiccant)
   NDC 0006-0071-54 PROPAK® bottles of 90 (with desiccant).

Storage and Handling
Store at room temperature, 15-30°C (59-86°F). Keep container closed and protect from moisture.

Women should not handle crushed or broken PROPECIA tablets when they are pregnant or may potentially be pregnant because of the possibility of absorption of finasteride and the subsequent potential risk to a male fetus. PROPECIA tablets are coated and will prevent contact with the active ingredient during normal handling, provided that the tablets are not broken or crushed [see Warnings and Precautions (5.1), Use in Specific Populations (8.1) and Patient Counseling Information (17.1)].

17   PATIENT COUNSELING INFORMATION

See FDA-approved patient labeling (Patient Information).

17.1   Exposure of Women — Risk to Male Fetus

Physicians should inform patients that women who are pregnant or may potentially be pregnant should not handle crushed or broken PROPECIA tablets because of the possibility of absorption of finasteride and the subsequent potential risk to a male fetus. PROPECIA tablets are coated and will prevent contact with the active ingredient during normal handling, provided that the tablets have not been broken or crushed. If a woman who is pregnant or may potentially be pregnant comes in contact with crushed or broken PROPECIA tablets, the contact area should be washed immediately with soap and water [see Contraindications (4), Warnings and Precautions (5.1), Use in Specific Populations (8.1) and How Supplied/Storage and Handling (16)].

17.2   Increased Risk of High-Grade Prostate Cancer

Patients should be informed that there was an increase in high-grade prostate cancer in men treated with 5α-reductase inhibitors indicated for BPH treatment, compared to those treated with placebo in studies looking at the use of these drugs to prevent prostate cancer [see Warnings and Precautions (5.3) and Adverse Reactions (6.1)].

17.3   Additional Instructions

Physicians should instruct their patients to promptly report any changes in their breasts such as lumps, pain or nipple discharge. Breast changes including breast enlargement, tenderness and neoplasm have been reported [see Adverse Reactions (6.1)].

Physicians should instruct their patients to read the patient package insert before starting therapy with PROPECIA and to read it again each time the prescription is renewed so that they are aware of current information for patients regarding PROPECIA.

Dist. by: Merck Sharp & Dohme Corp., a subsidiary of **MERCK & CO., INC., Whitehouse Station, NJ 08889, USA**
For patent information:
www.merck.com/product/patent/home.html
The trademarks depicted herein are owned by their respective companies.
Copyright © 1997 Merck Sharp & Dohme Corp., a subsidiary of **Merck & Co., Inc.**
All rights reserved.
uspi-mk0906-1t-1309r011

Patient Information

PROPECIA (Pro-pee-sha)
(finasteride)
Tablets

PROPECIA® is for use by **MEN ONLY** and should **NOT** be used by women or children.
Read this Patient Information before you start taking PROPECIA and each time you get a refill. There may be new information. This information does not take the place of talking with your healthcare provider about your medical condition or treatment.

What is PROPECIA?

PROPECIA is a prescription medicine used for the treatment of male pattern hair loss (androgenetic alopecia).

It is not known if PROPECIA works for a receding hairline on either side of and above your forehead (temporal area).

PROPECIA is not for use by women and children.

Who should not take PROPECIA?
Do not take PROPECIA if you:
- are pregnant or may become pregnant. PROPECIA may harm your unborn baby.
  - PROPECIA tablets are coated and will prevent contact with the medicine during handling, as long as the tablets are not broken or crushed. Females who are pregnant or who may become pregnant should not come in contact with broken or crushed PROPECIA tablets. If a pregnant woman comes in contact with crushed or broken PROPECIA tablets, wash the contact area right away with soap and water. If a woman who is pregnant comes into contact with the active ingredient in PROPECIA, a healthcare provider should be consulted.
  - If a woman who is pregnant with a male baby swallows or comes in contact with the medicine in PROPECIA, the male baby may be born with sex organs that are not normal.
- are allergic to any of the ingredients in PROPECIA. See the end of this leaflet for a complete list of ingredients in PROPECIA.

What should I tell my healthcare provider before taking PROPECIA?
Before taking PROPECIA, tell your healthcare provider if you:
- have any other medical conditions, including problems with your prostate or liver

Tell your healthcare provider about all the medicines you take, including prescription and non-prescription medicines, vitamins, and herbal supplements.
Know the medicines you take. Keep a list of them to show your healthcare provider and pharmacist when you get a new medicine.

How should I take PROPECIA?
- Take PROPECIA exactly as your healthcare provider tells you to take it.
- You may take PROPECIA with or without food.
- If you forget to take PROPECIA, do not take an extra tablet. Just take the next tablet as usual.
PROPECIA will not work faster or better if you take it more than once a day.

What are the possible side effects of PROPECIA?
- **decrease in your blood Prostate Specific Antigen (PSA) levels.** PROPECIA can affect a blood test called PSA (Prostate-Specific Antigen) for the screening of prostate cancer. If you have a PSA test done you should tell your healthcare provider that you are taking PROPECIA because PROPECIA decreases PSA levels. Changes in PSA levels will need to be evaluated by your healthcare provider. Any increase in follow-up PSA levels from their lowest point may signal the presence of prostate cancer and should be evaluated, even if the test results are still within the normal range for men not taking PROPECIA. You should also tell your healthcare provider if you have not been taking PROPECIA as prescribed because this may affect the PSA test results. For more information, talk to your healthcare provider.
- There may be an increased risk of a more serious form of prostate cancer in men taking finasteride at 5 times the dose of PROPECIA.

The most common side effects of PROPECIA include:
- decrease in sex drive
- trouble getting or keeping an erection
- a decrease in the amount of semen

The following have been reported in general use with PROPECIA:
- breast tenderness and enlargement. Tell your healthcare provider about any changes in your breasts such as lumps, pain or nipple discharge.
- depression;
- decrease in sex drive that continued after stopping the medication;
- allergic reactions including rash, itching, hives and swelling of the lips, tongue, throat, and face;
- problems with ejaculation that continued after stopping medication;
- testicular pain;
- difficulty in achieving an erection that continued after stopping the medication;
- male infertility and/or poor quality of semen.
- in rare cases, male breast cancer.
Tell your healthcare provider if you have any side effect that bothers you or that does not go away.
These are not all the possible side effects of PROPECIA. For more information, ask your healthcare provider or pharmacist.
Call your doctor for medical advice about side effects. You may report side effects to FDA at 1-800-FDA-1088.

How should I store PROPECIA?
- Store PROPECIA at room temperature between 59°F to 86°F (15°C to 30°C).
- Keep PROPECIA in a closed container and keep PROPECIA tablets dry (protect from moisture).

Keep PROPECIA and all medicines out of the reach of children.
General information about the safe and effective use of PROPECIA.
Medicines are sometimes prescribed for purposes other than those listed in this Patient Information leaflet. Do not use PROPECIA for a condition for which it was not prescribed. Do not give PROPECIA to other people, even if they have the same symptoms you have. It may harm them.
This Patient Information leaflet summarizes the most important information about PROPECIA. If you would like more information, talk with your healthcare provider. You can ask your pharmacist or healthcare provider for information about PROPECIA that is written for health professionals. For more information, **call 1-888-637-2522.**

What are the ingredients in PROPECIA?
Active ingredient: finasteride
Inactive ingredients: lactose monohydrate, microcrystalline cellulose, pregelatinized starch, sodium starch glycolate, hydroxypropyl methylcellulose, hydroxypropyl cellulose, titanium dioxide, magnesium stearate, talc, docusate sodium, yellow ferric oxide, and red ferric oxide.
This Patient Information has been approved by the U.S. Food and Drug Administration.
Dist. by: Merck Sharp & Dohme Corp., a subsidiary of **MERCK & CO., INC., Whitehouse Station, NJ 08889, USA**
For patent information:
www.merck.com/product/patent/home.html
Copyright © 1997 Merck Sharp & Dohme Corp., a subsidiary of **Merck & Co., Inc.**
All rights reserved.
Revised: 09/2013
usppi-mk0906-1t-1309r011
Shown in Product Identification Guide, page 309

PROQUAD®   ℞
[prō-kwăd]
Measles, Mumps, Rubella and Varicella Virus Vaccine Live
Lyophilized preparation for subcutaneous injection

HIGHLIGHTS OF PRESCRIBING INFORMATION
These highlights do not include all the information needed to use ProQuad safely and effectively. See full prescribing information for ProQuad.
ProQuad®
Measles, Mumps, Rubella and Varicella Virus Vaccine Live
Lyophilized preparation for subcutaneous injection
Initial U.S. Approval: 2005

——————**INDICATIONS AND USAGE**——————
ProQuad is a vaccine indicated for active immunization for the prevention of measles, mumps, rubella, and varicella in children 12 months through 12 years of age. (1)

——————**DOSAGE AND ADMINISTRATION**——————
A 0.5-mL dose for subcutaneous injection only. (2.1)
- The first dose is usually administered at 12 to 15 months of age. (2.1)
- A second dose, if needed, is usually administered at 4 to 6 years of age. (2.1)

——————**DOSAGE FORMS AND STRENGTHS**——————
Suspension for injection (0.5-mL dose) supplied as a lyophilized vaccine to be reconstituted using only accompanying sterile diluent. (2.2, 3)

——————**CONTRAINDICATIONS**——————
- History of anaphylactic reaction to neomycin or hypersensitivity to gelatin or any other component of the vaccine. (4.1)
- Primary or acquired immunodeficiency states. (4.2)
- Family history of congenital or hereditary immunodeficiency. (4.2)
- Immunosuppressive therapy. (4.2, 7.3)
- Active untreated tuberculosis or febrile illness (>101.3°F or >38.5°C). (4.3)
- Pregnancy. (4.4, 8.1, 17)

——————**WARNINGS AND PRECAUTIONS**——————
- Administration of ProQuad (dose 1) to children 12 to 23 months old who have not been previously vaccinated against measles, mumps, rubella, or varicella, nor had a history of the wild-type infections, is associated with higher rates of fever and febrile seizures at 5 to 12 days after vaccination when compared to children vaccinated with M-M-R® II and VARIVAX® administered separately. (5.1, 6.1, 6.3)

- Use caution when administering ProQuad to children with a history of cerebral injury or seizures or any other condition in which stress due to fever should be avoided. (5.2)
- Use caution when administering ProQuad to children with anaphylaxis or immediate hypersensitivity to eggs (5.3) or contact hypersensitivity to neomycin. (5.4)
- Use caution when administering ProQuad to children with thrombocytopenia. (5.5)
- Avoid close contact with high-risk individuals susceptible to varicella since transmission of varicella vaccine virus may occur between vaccinees and susceptible contacts. (5.8)
- Defer vaccination for at least 3 months following blood or plasma transfusions, or administration of immune globulins (IG). (5.9, 7.1)
- Avoid using salicylates for 6 weeks after vaccination with ProQuad. (6.1, 7.2, 17)
- Avoid pregnancy for 3 months following vaccination with measles, mumps, rubella, and/or varicella vaccines. (8.1, 17)

——————**ADVERSE REACTIONS**——————
- The most frequent vaccine-related adverse events reported in ≥5% of subjects vaccinated with ProQuad were:
  - injection-site reactions (pain/tenderness/soreness, erythema, and swelling)
  - fever
  - irritability. (6.1)
- Systemic vaccine-related adverse events that were reported at a significantly greater rate in recipients of ProQuad than in recipients of the component vaccines administered concomitantly were:
  - fever
  - measles-like rash. (6.1)

To report SUSPECTED ADVERSE REACTIONS or exposure during pregnancy or within three months prior to conception, contact Merck Sharp & Dohme Corp., a subsidiary of Merck & Co., Inc., at 1-877-888-4231 or VAERS at 1-800-822-7967 or www.vaers.hhs.gov.

——————**DRUG INTERACTIONS**——————
- Tuberculin testing should be administered anytime before, simultaneously with, or at least 4 to 6 weeks after ProQuad. (7.4)
- ProQuad may be administered concomitantly with *Haemophilus influenzae* type b conjugate vaccine and/or hepatitis B vaccine at separate injection sites. (7.5)
- ProQuad may be administered concomitantly with pneumococcal 7-valent conjugate vaccine and/or hepatitis A vaccine (inactivated) at separate injection sites. (7.5)

——————**USE IN SPECIFIC POPULATIONS**——————
Pregnancy: Do not administer ProQuad to females who are pregnant; the possible effects of the vaccine on fetal development are unknown at this time. (8.1)

See 17 for PATIENT COUNSELING INFORMATION
Revised: 03/2014

FULL PRESCRIBING INFORMATION

1 INDICATIONS AND USAGE

ProQuad® is a vaccine indicated for active immunization for the prevention of measles, mumps, rubella, and varicella in children 12 months through 12 years of age.

2 DOSAGE AND ADMINISTRATION

2.1 Recommended Dose and Schedule
FOR SUBCUTANEOUS ADMINISTRATION ONLY
Each 0.5-mL dose of ProQuad is administered subcutaneously.
The first dose is usually administered at 12 to 15 months of age but may be given anytime through 12 years of age.
If a second dose of measles, mumps, rubella, and varicella vaccine is needed, ProQuad may be used. This dose is usually administered at 4 to 6 years of age. At least 1 month should elapse between a dose of a measles-containing vaccine such as M-M-R® II (measles, mumps, and rubella virus vaccine live) and a dose of ProQuad. At least 3 months should elapse between a dose of varicella-containing vaccine and ProQuad.

2.2 Preparation for Administration
CAUTION: Preservatives, antiseptics, detergents, and other anti-viral substances may inactivate the vaccine. Use only sterile syringes that are free of preservatives, antiseptics, detergents, and other anti-viral substances for reconstitution and injection of ProQuad.
Withdraw the entire volume of the supplied diluent into a syringe. Use only the diluent supplied with the vaccine since it is free of preservatives or other anti-viral substances.
Inject the entire content of the syringe into the vial containing the powder. Gently agitate to dissolve completely.
Parenteral drug products should be inspected visually for particulate matter and discoloration prior to administration. Visually inspect the vaccine before and after reconstitution prior to administration. Before reconstitution, the lyophilized vaccine is a white to pale yellow compact crystalline plug. ProQuad, when reconstituted, is a clear pale yellow to light pink liquid.
Withdraw the entire amount of the reconstituted vaccine from the vial into the same syringe and inject the entire volume.
TO MINIMIZE LOSS OF POTENCY, THE VACCINE SHOULD BE ADMINISTERED IMMEDIATELY AFTER RECONSTITUTION. IF NOT USED IMMEDIATELY, THE RECONSTITUTED VACCINE MAY BE STORED AT ROOM TEMPERATURE, PROTECTED FROM LIGHT, FOR UP TO 30 MINUTES. DISCARD RECONSTITUTED VACCINE IF IT IS NOT USED WITHIN 30 MINUTES.

2.3 Method of Administration
Inject the vaccine subcutaneously into the outer aspect of the deltoid region of the upper arm or into the higher anterolateral area of the thigh.
Use With Other Vaccines
Use different injection sites to administer each vaccine if other vaccines are administered concomitantly. [See Drug Interactions (7.5).]

3 DOSAGE FORMS AND STRENGTHS

ProQuad is a suspension for injection supplied as a 0.5-mL single dose vial of lyophilized vaccine to be reconstituted using the sterile diluent supplied [see How Supplied/Storage and Handling (16)].

4 CONTRAINDICATIONS

4.1 Hypersensitivity
Do not administer ProQuad to individuals with a history of anaphylactic reactions to neomycin. If vaccination with ProQuad is medically necessary for such individuals, they are advised to consult an allergist or immunologist and should receive ProQuad only in settings where anaphylactic reactions can be appropriately managed.
Do not administer ProQuad to individuals with a history of hypersensitivity to gelatin or any other component of the vaccine or following previous vaccination with ProQuad, VARIVAX® (varicella virus vaccine live), or any measles-, mumps-, or rubella-containing vaccine [see Description (11) and Warnings and Precautions (5) for exceptions].

4.2 Immunosuppression
Do not administer ProQuad to individuals with blood dyscrasias, leukemia, lymphomas of any type, or other malignant neoplasms affecting the bone marrow or lymphatic system; or to individuals on immunosuppressive therapy (including high-dose systemic corticosteroids) [see Drug Interactions (7.3)]. Vaccination with a live, attenuated vaccine, such as varicella, can result in a more extensive vaccine-associated rash or disseminated disease in individuals on immunosuppressive drugs. ProQuad may be used by individuals who are receiving topical corticosteroids or low-dose corticosteroids, as are commonly used for asthma prophylaxis or in patients who are receiving corticosteroids as replacement therapy, e.g., for Addison's disease.
Do not administer ProQuad to individuals with primary and acquired immunodeficiency states, including AIDS or other clinical manifestations of infection with human immunodeficiency viruses; cellular immune deficiencies; and hypogammaglobulinemic and dysgammaglobulinemic states. Measles inclusion body encephalitis, pneumonitis, and death as a direct consequence of disseminated measles vaccine virus infection have been reported in severely immunocompromised individuals inadvertently vaccinated with measles-containing vaccine. In addition, disseminated varicella vaccine virus infection has been reported in children with underlying immunodeficiency disorders who were inadvertently vaccinated with a varicella-containing vaccine [1].
Do not administer ProQuad to individuals with a family history of congenital or hereditary immunodeficiency, unless the immune competence of the potential vaccine recipient is demonstrated.

4.3 Concurrent Illness
Do not administer ProQuad to individuals with active untreated tuberculosis or to individuals with an active febrile illness with fever >101.3°F (>38.5°C).

4.4 Pregnancy
Do not administer ProQuad to individuals who are pregnant; the possible effects of the vaccine on fetal development are unknown at this time [see Use in Specific Populations (8.1)].

5 WARNINGS AND PRECAUTIONS

5.1 Fever and Febrile Seizures
Administration of ProQuad (dose 1) to children 12 to 23 months old who have not been previously vaccinated against measles, mumps, rubella, or varicella, nor had a history of the wild-type infections, is associated with higher rates of fever and febrile seizures at 5 to 12 days after vaccination when compared to children vaccinated with dose 1 of both M-M-R II and VARIVAX administered separately [see Adverse Reactions (6.3)].

5.2 History of Cerebral Injury or Seizures
Exercise caution when administering ProQuad to persons with a history of cerebral injury, individual or family history of convulsions, or any other condition in which stress due to fever should be avoided. Healthcare providers should be alert to the temperature elevations that may occur following vaccination.

5.3 Hypersensitivity to Eggs
Live measles vaccine and live mumps vaccine are produced in chick embryo cell culture. Persons with a history of anaphylactic or other immediate hypersensitivity reactions (e.g., hives, swelling of the mouth and throat, difficulty breathing, hypotension, or shock) subsequent to egg ingestion may be at an enhanced risk of immediate-type hypersensitivity reactions after receiving vaccines containing traces of chick embryo antigen. Carefully evaluate the potential risk-to-benefit ratio before considering vaccination in such cases. Such individuals may be vaccinated with extreme caution; adequate treatment should be readily available should a reaction occur [see Contraindications (4.1) [2]. Children with egg allergy are at low risk for anaphylactic reactions to measles-containing vaccines (including M-M-R II), and skin testing of children allergic to eggs is not predictive of reactions to M-M-R II vaccine. Persons with allergies to chickens or feathers are not at increased risk of reaction to the vaccine [2].

5.4 Contact Hypersensitivity to Neomycin
Most often, neomycin allergy manifests as a contact dermatitis, which is not a contraindication to receiving measles-, mumps-, rubella-, or varicella-containing vaccine.

5.5 Thrombocytopenia
Carefully evaluate the potential risk-to-benefit ratio before considering vaccination with ProQuad in children with thrombocytopenia or in those who experienced thrombocytopenia after vaccination with a previous dose of measles, mumps, rubella, and/or varicella vaccine. No clinical data are available regarding the development or worsening of thrombocytopenia in individuals vaccinated with ProQuad. Cases of thrombocytopenia have been reported after primary vaccination with measles vaccine; measles, mumps, and rubella vaccine; after varicella vaccination; and following re-vaccination with measles vaccine or M-M-R II [see Adverse Reactions (6.2)].

5.6 Use for Post-Exposure Prophylaxis
The safety and efficacy of ProQuad for use after exposure to measles, mumps, rubella, or varicella have not been established.

5.7 Use in HIV-Infected Children
The safety and efficacy of ProQuad for use in children known to be infected with human immunodeficiency viruses have not been established.

5.8 Risk of Vaccine Virus Transmission
Post-licensing experience with VARIVAX suggests that transmission of varicella vaccine virus may occur between healthy vaccine recipients (who develop or do not develop a varicella-like rash) and contacts susceptible to varicella, as well as high-risk individuals susceptible to varicella.
High-risk individuals susceptible to varicella include:
• Immunocompromised individuals;
• Pregnant women without documented positive history of varicella (chickenpox) or laboratory evidence of prior infection;
• Newborn infants of mothers without documented positive history of varicella or laboratory evidence of prior infection and all newborn infants born at <28 weeks gestation regardless of maternal varicella immunity.
Vaccine recipients should attempt to avoid, to the extent possible, close association with high-risk individuals susceptible to varicella for up to 6 weeks following vaccination. In circumstances where contact with high-risk individuals susceptible to varicella is unavoidable, the potential risk of transmission of the varicella vaccine virus should be weighed against the risk of acquiring and transmitting wild-type varicella virus.
Excretion of small amounts of the live, attenuated rubella virus from the nose or throat has occurred in the majority of susceptible individuals 7 to 28 days after vaccination. There is no confirmed evidence to indicate that such virus is transmitted to susceptible persons who are in contact with the vaccinated individuals. Consequently, transmission through close personal contact, while accepted as a theoretical possibility, is not regarded as a significant risk. However, transmission of the rubella vaccine virus to infants via breast milk has been documented [see Use in Specific Populations (8.3)].
There are no reports of transmission of the more attenuated Enders' Edmonston strain of measles virus or the Jeryl Lynn™ strain of mumps virus from vaccine recipients to susceptible contacts.

5.9 Immune Globulins and Transfusions
Immune globulins (IG) administered concomitantly with ProQuad contain antibodies that may interfere with vaccine virus replication and decrease the expected immune response. Vaccination should be deferred for at least 3 months following blood or plasma transfusions, or administration of IG.
The appropriate suggested interval between transfusion or IG administration and vaccination will vary with the type of transfusion or indication for, and dose of, IG (e.g., 5 months for Varicella Zoster Immune Globulin [VZIG]) [2]. Following administration of ProQuad, any IG including VZIG should not be given for 1 month thereafter unless its use outweighs the benefits of vaccination [2]. [See Drug Interactions (7.1).]

5.10 Risk of Transmission of Creutzfeldt-Jakob Disease and Other Adventitious Agents
This product contains albumin, a derivative of human blood. Based on effective donor screening and product manufacturing processes, it carries an extremely remote risk for transmission of viral diseases. Although there is a theoretical risk for transmission of Creutzfeldt-Jakob disease (CJD), no cases of transmission of CJD or viral disease have ever been identified that were associated with the use of albumin. The cells, virus pools, bovine serum, and human albumin used

Table 3: Vaccine-Related Injection-Site and Systemic Adverse Reactions Reported in ≥1% of Children Previously Vaccinated with M-M-R II and VARIVAX Who Received ProQuad + Placebo, M-M-R II + Placebo, or M-M-R II + VARIVAX at 4 to 6 Years of Age (1 to 43 Days Postvaccination)

Adverse Reactions	ProQuad + Placebo (N=399) (n=397) %	M-M-R II + Placebo (N=205) (n=205) %	M-M-R II + VARIVAX (N=195) (n=193) %
Systemic			
Fever*,†	2.5	2.0	4.1
Cough	1.3	0.5	0.5
Irritability	1.0	0.5	1.0
Headache	0.8	1.5	1.6
Rhinorrhea	0.5	1.0	1.0
Nasopharyngitis	0.3	1.0	1.0
Vomiting	0.3	1.0	0.5
Upper respiratory infection	0.0	0.0	1.0

	ProQuad %	Placebo %	M-M-R II %	Placebo %	M-M-R II %	VARIVAX %
Injection-Site						
Pain*	41.1	34.5	36.6	34.1	35.2	36.8
Erythema*	24.4	13.4	15.6	14.1	14.5	15.5
Swelling*	15.6	8.1	10.2	8.8	7.8	10.9
Bruising	3.5	3.8	2.4	3.4	1.6	2.1
Rash	1.5	1.3	0.0	0.0	0.5	0.0
Pruritus	1.0	0.3	0.0	0.0	0.0	1.0
Nodule	0.0	0.0	0.0	0.0	0.0	1.0

N = number of subjects vaccinated.
n = number of subjects with safety follow-up.
* Designates a solicited adverse reaction. Injection-site adverse reactions were solicited only from Days 1 to 5 postvaccination.
† Temperature reported as elevated (≥102°F, oral equivalent) or abnormal.

in manufacturing are all evaluated and tested to provide assurance that the final product is free of potential adventitious agents [see Description (11)].

6 ADVERSE REACTIONS

6.1 Clinical Trials Experience

Because clinical trials are conducted under widely varying conditions, adverse reaction rates observed in the clinical trials of a vaccine cannot be directly compared to rates in the clinical trials of another vaccine and may not reflect the rates observed in clinical practice. Vaccine-related adverse reactions reported during clinical trials were assessed by the study investigators to be possibly, probably, or definitely vaccine-related and are summarized below.

Children 12 Through 23 Months of Age Who Received a Single Dose of ProQuad

ProQuad was administered to 4497 children 12 through 23 months of age involved in 4 randomized clinical trials without concomitant administration with other vaccines. The safety of ProQuad was compared with the safety of M-M-R II and VARIVAX given concomitantly (N=2038) at separate injection sites. The safety profile for ProQuad was similar to the component vaccines. Children in these studies were monitored for up to 42 days postvaccination using vaccination report card-aided surveillance. Safety follow-up was obtained for 98% of children in each group. Few subjects (<0.1%) who received ProQuad discontinued the study due to an adverse reaction. The race distribution of the study subjects across these studies following a first dose of ProQuad was as follows: 65.2% White; 13.1% African-American; 11.1% Hispanic; 5.8% Asian/Pacific; 4.5% other; and 0.2% American Indian. The racial distribution of the control group was similar to that of the group who received ProQuad. The gender distribution across the studies following a first dose of ProQuad was 52.5% male and 47.5% female. The gender distribution of the control group was similar to that of the group who received ProQuad. Vaccine-related injection-site and systemic adverse reactions observed among recipients of ProQuad or M-M-R II and VARIVAX at a rate of at least 1% are shown in Table 1. Systemic vaccine-related adverse reactions that were reported at a significantly greater rate in individuals who received a first dose of ProQuad than in individuals who received first doses of M-M-R II and VARIVAX concomitantly at separate injection sites were fever (≥102°F [≥38.9°C] oral equivalent or abnormal) (21.5% versus 14.9%, respectively, risk difference 6.6%, 95% CI: 4.6, 8.5), and measles-like rash (3.0% versus 2.1%, respectively, risk difference 1.0%, 95% CI: 0.1, 1.8). Both fever and measles-like rash usually occurred within 5 to 12 days following the vaccination, were of short duration, and resolved with no long-term sequelae. Pain/tenderness/soreness at the injection site was reported at a statistically lower rate in individuals who received ProQuad than in individuals who received M-M-R II and VARIVAX concomitantly at separate injection sites (22.0% versus 26.8%, respectively, risk difference -4.8%, 95% CI: -7.1, -2.5). The only vaccine-related injection-site adverse reaction that

was more frequent among recipients of ProQuad than recipients of M-M-R II and VARIVAX was rash at the injection site (2.4% versus 1.6%, respectively, risk difference 0.9%, 95% CI: 0.1, 1.5).

Table 1: Vaccine-Related Injection-Site and Systemic Adverse Reactions Reported in ≥1% of Children Who Received ProQuad Dose 1 or M-M-R II and VARIVAX at 12 to 23 Months of Age (0 to 42 Days Postvaccination)

Adverse Reactions	ProQuad (N=4497) (n=4424) %	M-M-R II and VARIVAX (N=2038) (n=1997) %
*Injection Site**		
Pain/tenderness/soreness†	22.0	26.7
Erythema†	14.4	15.8
Swelling†	8.4	9.8
Ecchymosis	1.5	2.3
Rash	2.3	1.5
Systemic		
Fever†,‡	21.5	14.9
Irritability	6.7	6.7
Measles-like rash†	3.0	2.1
Varicella-like rash†	2.1	2.2
Rash (not otherwise specified)	1.6	1.4
Upper respiratory infection	1.3	1.1
Viral exanthema	1.2	1.1
Diarrhea	1.2	1.3

N = number of subjects vaccinated.
n = number of subjects with safety follow-up.
* Injection-site adverse reactions for M-M-R II and VARIVAX are based on occurrence with either of the vaccines administered.
† Designates a solicited adverse reaction. Injection-site adverse reactions were solicited only from Days 0 to 4 postvaccination.
‡ Temperature reported as elevated (≥102°F, oral equivalent) or abnormal.

Rubella-like rashes were observed in <1% of subjects following a first dose of ProQuad.

In these clinical trials, two cases of herpes zoster were reported among 2108 healthy subjects 12 through 23 months of age who were vaccinated with their first dose of ProQuad

and followed for 1 year. Both cases were unremarkable and no sequelae were reported.

Children 15 to 31 Months of Age Who Received a Second Dose of ProQuad

In 5 clinical trials, 2780 healthy children were vaccinated with ProQuad (dose 1) at 12 to 23 months of age and then administered a second dose approximately 3 to 9 months later. The race distribution of the study subjects across these studies following a second dose of ProQuad was as follows: 64.4% White; 14.1% African-American; 12.0% Hispanic; 5.9% other; 3.5% Asian/Pacific; and 0.1% American Indian. The gender distribution across the studies following a second dose of ProQuad was 51.5% male and 48.5% female. Children in these open-label studies were monitored for at least 28 days postvaccination using vaccination report card-aided surveillance. Safety follow-up was obtained for approximately 97% of children overall. Vaccine-related injection-site and systemic adverse reactions observed after Dose 1 and 2 of ProQuad at a rate of at least 1% are shown in Table 2. In these trials, the overall rates of systemic adverse reactions after ProQuad (dose 2) were comparable to, or lower than, those seen with the first dose. In the subset of children who received both ProQuad dose 1 and dose 2 in these trials (N=2408) with follow-up for fever, fever ≥102.2°F (≥38.9°C) was observed significantly less frequently days 1 to 28 after the second dose (10.8%) than after the first dose (19.1%) (risk difference 8.3%, 95% CI: 6.4, 10.3). Fevers ≥102.2°F (≥38.9°C) days 5 to 12 after vaccinations were also reported significantly less frequently after dose 2 (3.9%) than after dose 1 (13.6%) (risk difference 9.7%, 95% CI: 8.1, 11.3). In the subset of children who received both doses and for whom injection-site reactions were reported (N=2679), injection-site erythema was noted significantly more frequently after ProQuad (dose 2) as compared to ProQuad (dose 1) (12.6% and 10.8%, respectively, risk difference -1.8, 95% CI: -3.3, -0.3); however, pain and tenderness at the injection site was significantly lower after dose 2 (16.1%) as compared with after dose 1 (21.9%) (risk difference, 5.8%, 95% CI: 4.1, 7.6). Two children had febrile seizures after ProQuad (dose 2); both febrile seizures were thought to be related to a concurrent viral illness [see Adverse Reactions (6.3) and Clinical Studies (14)]. These studies were not designed or statistically powered to detect a difference in rates of febrile seizure between recipients of ProQuad as compared to M-M-R II and VARIVAX. The risk of febrile seizure has not been evaluated in a clinical study comparing the incidence rate after ProQuad (dose 2) with the incidence rate after concomitant M-M-R II (dose 2) and VARIVAX (dose 2). [See Adverse Reactions (6.1), Children 4 to 6 Years of Age Who Received ProQuad After Primary Vaccination with M-M-R II and VARIVAX.]

Table 2: Vaccine-Related Injection-Site and Systemic Adverse Reactions Reported in ≥1% of Children Who Received ProQuad Dose 1 at 12 to 23 Months of Age and Dose 2 at 15 to 31 Months of Age (1 to 28 Days Postvaccination)

Adverse Reactions	ProQuad Dose 1 (N=3112) (n=3019) %	ProQuad Dose 2 (N=2780) (n=2695) %
Injection-Site		
Pain/tenderness/soreness*	21.4	15.9
Erythema*	10.7	12.4
Swelling*	8.0	8.5
Injection-site bruising	1.1	0.0
Systemic		
Fever*,†	20.4	8.3
Irritability	6.0	2.4
Measles-like/Rubella-like rash	4.3	0.9
Varicella-like/Vesicular rash	1.5	0.1
Diarrhea	1.3	0.6
Upper respiratory infection	1.3	1.4
Rash (not otherwise specified)	1.2	0.6
Rhinorrhea	1.1	1.0

N = number of subjects vaccinated.
n = number of subjects with safety follow-up.
* Designates a solicited adverse reaction. Injection-site adverse reactions were solicited only from Days 1 to 5 postvaccination.
† Temperature reported as elevated or abnormal.

Children 4 to 6 Years of Age Who Received ProQuad After Primary Vaccination with M-M-R II and VARIVAX

In a double-blind clinical trial, 799 healthy 4- to 6-year-old children who received M-M-R II and VARIVAX at least 1 month prior to study entry were randomized to receive ProQuad and placebo (N=399), M-M-R II and placebo concomitantly (N=205) at separate injection sites, or M-M-R II and VARIVAX (N=195) concomitantly at separate injection sites *[see Clinical Studies (14)]*. Children in these studies were monitored for up to 42 days postvaccination using vaccination report card-aided surveillance. Safety follow-up was obtained for >98% of children in each group. The race distribution of the study subjects following a dose of ProQuad was as follows: 78.4% White; 12.3% African-American; 3.8% Hispanic; 3.5% other; and 2.0% Asian/Pacific. The gender distribution following a dose of ProQuad was 52.1% male and 47.9% female. Injection-site and systemic adverse reactions observed after Dose 1 and 2 of ProQuad at a rate of at least 1% are shown in Table 3. *[See Clinical Studies (14).]*

[See table 3 at top of previous page]

Safety in Trials That Evaluated Concomitant Use with Other Vaccines

ProQuad Administered with Diphtheria and Tetanus Toxoids and Acellular Pertussis Vaccine Adsorbed (DTaP) and Haemophilus influenzae type b Conjugate (Meningococcal Protein Conjugate) and Hepatitis B (Recombinant) Vaccine

In an open-label clinical trial, 1434 children were randomized to receive ProQuad given with diphtheria and tetanus toxoids and acellular pertussis vaccine adsorbed (DTaP) and *Haemophilus influenzae* type b conjugate (meningococcal protein conjugate) and hepatitis B (recombinant) vaccine concomitantly (N=949) or non-concomitantly with ProQuad given first and the other vaccines 6 weeks later (N=485). No clinically significant differences in adverse events were reported between treatment groups *[see Clinical Studies (14)]*. The race distribution of the study subjects who received ProQuad was as follows: 70.7% White; 10.9% Asian/Pacific; 10.7% African-American; 4.5% Hispanic; 3.0% other; and 0.2% American Indian. The gender distribution of the study subjects who received ProQuad was 53.6% male and 46.4% female.

ProQuad Administered with Pneumococcal 7-valent Conjugate Vaccine and/or Hepatitis A Vaccine, Inactivated

In an open-label clinical trial, 1027 healthy children 12 to 23 months of age were randomized to receive ProQuad (dose 1) and pneumococcal 7-valent conjugate vaccine (dose 4) concomitantly (N=510) or non-concomitantly at different clinic visits (N=517). The race distribution of the study subjects was as follows: 65.2% White; 15.1% African-American; 10.0% Hispanic; 6.6% other; and 3.0% Asian/Pacific. The gender distribution of the study subjects was 54.5% male and 45.5% female. Injection-site and systemic adverse reactions observed among recipients of ProQuad administered concomitantly or non-concomitantly with pneumococcal 7-valent conjugate vaccine at a rate of at least 1% are shown in Table 4. No clinically significant differences in adverse reactions were reported between the concomitant and non-concomitant treatment groups *[see Clinical Studies (14)]*.

Table 4: Vaccine-Related Injection-Site and Systemic Adverse Reactions Reported in ≥1% of Children Who Received ProQuad (dose 1) Concomitantly or Non-Concomitantly with PCV7* (dose 4) at the First Visit (1 to 28 Days Postvaccination)

Adverse Reactions	ProQuad + PCV7 (N=510) (n=498) %	PCV7 (N=258) (n=250) %	ProQuad (N=259) (n=255) %
Injection-Site - ProQuad			
Pain[†]	24.9	N/A	24.7
Erythema[†]	12.4	N/A	11.0
Swelling[†]	10.8	N/A	7.5
Bruising	2.0	N/A	1.6
Injection-Site - PCV7			
Pain[†]	30.5	29.6	N/A
Erythema[†]	21.1	24.4	N/A
Swelling[†]	17.9	20.0	N/A
Bruising	1.6	1.2	N/A
Systemic			
Fever[†,‡]	15.5	10.0	15.3
Measles-like rash	4.4	0.8	5.1
Irritability	3.8	3.6	3.5
Upper respiratory infection	1.6	0.8	1.2
Varicella-like/ vesicular rash	1.6	0.0	1.2
Diarrhea	0.8	1.2	1.2
Vomiting	0.6	0.8	1.2
Rash	0.4	0.0	1.2
Somnolence	0.0	0.0	1.2

N/A = Not applicable.
N = number of subjects vaccinated.
n = number of subjects with safety follow-up.
* PCV7 = Pneumococcal 7-valent conjugate vaccine, dose 4.
† Designates a solicited adverse reaction. Injection-site adverse reactions were solicited only from Days 1 to 5 postvaccination.
‡ Temperature reported as elevated (≥102°F, oral equivalent) or abnormal.

In an open-label clinical trial, 699 healthy children 12 to 23 months of age were randomized to receive 2 doses of VAQTA® (hepatitis A vaccine, inactivated) (N=352) or 2 doses of VAQTA concomitantly with 2 doses of ProQuad (N=347) at least 6 months apart. An additional 1101 subjects received 2 doses of VAQTA alone at least 6 months apart (non-randomized), resulting in 1453 subjects receiving 2 doses of VAQTA alone (1101 non-randomized and 352 randomized) and 347 subjects receiving 2 doses of VAQTA concomitantly with ProQuad (all randomized). The race distribution of the study subjects following a dose of ProQuad was as follows: 47.3% White; 42.7% Hispanic; 5.5% other; 2.9% African-American; and 1.7% Asian/Pacific. The gender distribution of the study subjects following a dose of

Table 5: Vaccine-Related Injection-Site Adverse Reactions Reported in ≥1% of Children Who Received VAQTA or ProQuad Concomitantly with VAQTA 1 to 5 Days After Vaccination with VAQTA or VAQTA and ProQuad

Adverse Reactions	Dose 1		Dose 2	
	VAQTA (N=1453) (n=1412) %	ProQuad + VAQTA (N=347) (n=328) %	VAQTA (N=1301) (n=1254) %	ProQuad + VAQTA (N=292) (n=264) %
Injection-Site - VAQTA				
Pain/tenderness*	29.2	27.1	30.1	25.0
Erythema*	13.5	12.5	14.3	11.7
Swelling*	7.1	9.1	9.0	8.0
Injection-site bruising	1.9	2.4	1.0	0.8
Injection-Site - ProQuad				
Pain/tenderness*	N/A	30.5	N/A	26.2
Erythema*	N/A	13.4	N/A	12.9
Swelling*	N/A	6.7	N/A	6.5
Injection-site bruising	N/A	1.5	N/A	0.4

N/A = Not applicable.
N = number of subjects vaccinated.
n = number of subjects with safety follow-up.
* Designates a solicited adverse reaction. Injection-site adverse reactions were solicited only from Days 1 to 5 postvaccination.

Table 6: Vaccine-Related Systemic Adverse Reactions Reported in ≥1% of Children Who Received VAQTA* or ProQuad Concomitantly with VAQTA 1 to 14 Days After VAQTA or Vaccination with ProQuad and VAQTA and 1 to 28 Days After Vaccination with ProQuad and VAQTA

Adverse Reactions	Dose 1			Dose 2		
	Days 1 to 14		Days 1 to 28	Days 1 to 14		Days 1 to 28
	VAQTA[†] (N=1453) (n=1412) %	ProQuad + VAQTA[†] (N=347) (n=328) %	ProQuad + VAQTA (N=347) (n=328) %	VAQTA (N=1301) (n=1254) %	ProQuad + VAQTA[†] (N=292) (n=264) %	ProQuad + VAQTA[†] (N=291) (n=263) %
Fever[‡,§]	5.7	14.9	15.2	4.1	8.0	8.4
Irritability	5.8	7.0	7.3	3.5	5.3	5.3
Measles-like rash	0.0	3.4	3.4	0.0	1.1	1.1
Rhinorrhea	0.6	2.7	3.0	0.6	1.1	2.7
Diarrhea	1.5	1.8	2.4	1.7	0.4	0.8
Cough	0.6	2.1	2.1	0.2	0.8	1.5
Vomiting	1.1	0.3	0.9	0.6	0.8	1.1

N = number of subjects vaccinated.
n = number of subjects with safety follow-up.
* Systemic adverse events for subjects given VAQTA alone were collected for 14 days postvaccination.
† Safety follow-up for systemic adverse reactions was 14 days for VAQTA and 28 days for ProQuad + VAQTA.
‡ Designates a solicited adverse reaction.
§ Temperature reported as elevated or abnormal.

ProQuad was 49.3% male and 50.7% female. Vaccine-related injection-site adverse reactions (days 1 to 5 postvaccination) and systemic adverse events (days 1 to 14 post VAQTA and days 1 to 28 post ProQuad vaccination) observed among recipients of VAQTA and ProQuad administered concomitantly with VAQTA at a rate of at least 1% are shown in Tables 5 and 6, respectively. In addition, among the randomized cohort, in the 14 days after each vaccination, the rates of fever (including all vaccine- and non-vaccine-related reports) were significantly higher in subjects who received ProQuad with VAQTA concomitantly after dose 1 (22.0%) as compared to subjects given dose 1 of VAQTA without ProQuad (10.8%). However, rates of fever were not significantly higher in subjects who received ProQuad with VAQTA concomitantly after dose 2 (12.5%) as compared to subjects given dose 2 of VAQTA without ProQuad (9.4%). In post-hoc analyses, these rates were significantly different for dose 1 (relative risk (RR) 2.03 [95% CI: 1.42, 2.94]), but not dose 2 (RR 1.32 [95% CI: 0.82, 2.13]). Rates of injection-site adverse reactions and other systemic adverse events were lower following a second dose than following the first dose of both vaccines given concomitantly.

[See table 5 above]

[See table 6 above]

In an open-label clinical trial, 653 children 12 to 23 months of age were randomized to receive a first dose of ProQuad with VAQTA and pneumococcal 7-valent conjugate vaccine concomitantly (N=330) or a first dose of ProQuad and pneumococcal 7-valent conjugate vaccine concomitantly and then vaccinated with VAQTA 6 weeks later (N=323). Approximately 6 months later, subjects received either the second doses of ProQuad and VAQTA concomitantly or the second

Table 7: Vaccine-Related Injection-Site Adverse Reactions Reported in ≥1% of Children Who Received ProQuad + VAQTA + PCV7* Concomitantly or VAQTA Alone Followed by ProQuad + PCV7 Concomitantly (1 to 5 Days After a Dose of ProQuad)

Adverse Reactions	Dose 1		Dose 2	
	VAQTA + ProQuad + PCV7 (N=330) (n=311) %	VAQTA Alone Followed by ProQuad + PCV7 (N=323) (n=302) %	VAQTA + ProQuad (N=273) (n=265) %	VAQTA Alone Followed by ProQuad (N=240) (n=230) %
Injection-Site - ProQuad				
Pain/tenderness[†]	21.2	24.2	18.1	17.0
Erythema[†]	13.5	11.9	10.6	13.0
Swelling[†]	7.4	10.9	8.3	11.7
Bruising	1.9	1.3	0.8	0.4
Injection-Site - VAQTA				
Pain/tenderness[†]	20.6	15.3	17.5	20.3
Erythema[†]	9.6	11.7	9.1	12.7
Swelling[†]	6.8	9.5	6.1	7.6
Bruising	1.3	1.1	1.1	1.6
Rash	1.0	0.0	0.4	0.4
Injection-Site - PCV7				
Pain/tenderness[†]	25.4	27.6	N/A	N/A
Erythema[†]	16.4	16.6	N/A	N/A
Swelling[†]	13.2	14.3	N/A	N/A
Bruising	0.6	1.7	N/A	N/A

N/A = Not applicable.
N = number of subjects vaccinated.
n = number of subjects with safety follow-up.
* PCV7 = Pneumococcal 7-valent conjugate vaccine.
† Designates a solicited adverse reaction. Injection-site adverse reactions were solicited only from Days 1 to 5 postvaccination at each vaccine injection site.

Table 8: Vaccine-Related Systemic Adverse Reactions Reported in ≥1% of Children Who Received ProQuad + VAQTA + PCV7* Concomitantly, or VAQTA Alone Followed by ProQuad + PCV7 Concomitantly (1 to 28 Days After a Dose of ProQuad)

Adverse Reactions	Dose 1		Dose 2	
	VAQTA + ProQuad + PCV7 (N=330) (n=311) %	VAQTA Alone Followed by ProQuad + PCV7 (N=323) (n=302) %	VAQTA + ProQuad (N=273) (n=265) %	VAQTA Alone Followed by ProQuad (N=240) (n=230) %
Fever[†,‡]	26.4	27.2	9.1	9.6
Irritability	4.8	6.3	1.9	1.3
Measles-like rash[†]	2.3	4.0	0.0	0.0
Varicella-like rash[†]	1.0	1.7	0.0	0.0
Rash (not otherwise specified)	1.3	1.3	0.0	0.9
Diarrhea	1.3	1.3	0.4	1.3
Upper respiratory infection	1.0	1.3	1.1	0.9
Viral infection	1.0	0.7	0.0	0.0
Rhinorrhea	0.0	0.7	1.1	0.0

N = number of subjects vaccinated.
n = number of subjects with safety follow-up.
* PCV7 = Pneumococcal 7-valent conjugate vaccine.
† Designates a solicited adverse reaction.
‡ Temperature reported as elevated or abnormal.

Table 9: Confirmed Febrile Seizures Days 5 to 12 and 0 to 30 After Vaccination with ProQuad (dose 1) Compared to Concomitant Vaccination with M-M-R II and VARIVAX (dose 1) in Children 12 to 60 Months of Age

Time Period	ProQuad cohort (N=31,298)		MMR+V cohort (N=31,298)		Relative risk (95% CI)
	n	Incidence per 1000	n	Incidence per 1000	
5 to 12 Days	22	0.70	10	0.32	2.20 (1.04, 4.65)
0 to 30 Days	44	1.41	40	1.28	1.10 (0.72, 1.69)

doses of ProQuad and VAQTA separately. The race distribution of the study subjects was as follows: 60.3% White; 21.6% African-American; 9.5% Hispanic; 7.2% other; 1.1% Asian/Pacific; and 0.3% American Indian. The gender distribution of the study subjects was 50.7% male and 49.3% female. Vaccine-related injection-site and systemic adverse reactions observed among recipients of concomitant ProQuad, VAQTA, and pneumococcal 7-valent conjugate vaccine and ProQuad and pneumococcal 7-valent conjugate

vaccine at a rate of at least 1% are shown in Tables 7 and 8. In the 28 days after vaccination with the first dose of ProQuad, the rates of fever (including all vaccine- and non-vaccine-related reports) were comparable in subjects who received the 3 vaccines together (38.6%) as compared with subjects given ProQuad and pneumococcal 7-valent conjugate vaccine (42.7%). The rates of fever in the 28 days following the second dose of ProQuad were also comparable in subjects who received ProQuad and VAQTA together

(17.4%) as compared with subjects given ProQuad separately from VAQTA (17.0%). In a post-hoc analysis, these differences were not statistically significant after ProQuad (dose 1) (RR 0.90 [95% CI: 0.75, 1.09]) nor after dose 2 (RR 1.02 [95% CI: 0.70, 1.51]). No clinically significant differences in adverse reactions were reported among treatment groups *[see Clinical Studies (14)]*.

[See table 7 above]
[See table 8 above]

Reye syndrome following wild-type varicella infection has occurred in children and adolescents, the majority of whom had received salicylates. In all clinical studies of ProQuad or VARIVAX, the recommendation was made to avoid the use of salicylates for 6 weeks after vaccination. There were no reports of Reye syndrome in recipients of ProQuad or VARIVAX during these studies *[see Drug Interactions (7.2) and Patient Counseling Information (17)]*.

6.2   Post-Marketing Experience

The following adverse events have been identified during post-approval use of either the components of ProQuad or ProQuad. Because the reactions are in some cases described in the literature or reported voluntarily from a population of uncertain size, it is not always possible to reliably estimate their frequency or establish a causal relationship.

Post-Marketing Reports

Adverse events reported with post-marketing use of ProQuad and/or in clinical studies and/or post-marketing use of M-M-R II, the component vaccines, and VARIVAX without regard to causality or frequency are summarized below.

Infections and infestations
Atypical measles, candidiasis, cellulitis, herpes zoster, infection, influenza, measles, orchitis, parotitis, respiratory infection, skin infection, varicella (vaccine strain).

Blood and the lymphatic system disorders
Aplastic anemia, lymphadenitis, regional lymphadenopathy, thrombocytopenia.

Immune system disorders
Anaphylactoid reaction, anaphylaxis and related phenomena such as angioneurotic edema, facial edema, and peripheral edema, anaphylaxis in individuals with or without an allergic history.

Psychiatric disorders
Agitation, apathy, nervousness.

Nervous system disorders
Acute disseminated encephalomyelitis (ADEM), afebrile convulsions or seizures, aseptic meningitis (see below), ataxia, Bell's palsy, cerebrovascular accident, convulsion, dizziness, dream abnormality, encephalitis (see below), encephalopathy (see below), febrile seizure, Guillain-Barré syndrome, headache, hypersomnia, measles inclusion body encephalitis *[see Contraindications (4.2)]*, ocular palsies, paraesthesia, polyneuritis, polyneuropathy, subacute sclerosing panencephalitis (see below), syncope, transverse myelitis, tremor.

Eye disorders
Edema of the eyelid, irritation, necrotizing retinitis (in immunocompromised individuals), optic neuritis, retinitis, retrobulbar neuritis.

Ear and labyrinth disorders
Ear pain, nerve deafness.

Vascular disorders
Extravasation.

Respiratory, thoracic and mediastinal disorders
Bronchial spasm, bronchitis, epistaxis, pneumonitis *[see Contraindications (4.3)]*, pneumonia, pulmonary congestion, rhinitis, sinusitis, sneezing, sore throat, wheezing.

Gastrointestinal disorders
Abdominal pain, flatulence, hematochezia, mouth ulcer.

Skin and subcutaneous tissue disorders
Erythema multiforme, Henoch-Schönlein purpura, herpes simplex, impetigo, panniculitis, pruritus, purpura, skin induration, Stevens-Johnson syndrome, sunburn.

Musculoskeletal, connective tissue and bone disorders
Arthritis and/or arthralgia (usually transient and rarely chronic; see below); musculoskeletal pain; myalgia; pain of the hip, leg, or neck; swelling.

Reproductive system and breast disorders
Epididymitis.

General disorders and administration site conditions
Injection-site complaints (burning and/or stinging of short duration, eczema, edema/swelling, hive-like rash, discoloration, hematoma, induration, lump, vesicles, wheal and flare), inflammation, lip abnormality, papillitis, roughness/dryness, stiffness, trauma, varicella-like rash, venipuncture site hemorrhage, warm sensation, warm to touch.

Deaths have been reported following vaccination with measles, mumps, and rubella vaccines; however, a causal relationship has not been established in healthy individuals. Death as a direct consequence of disseminated measles vaccine virus infection has been reported in severely immunocompromised individuals in whom a measles-containing vaccine is contraindicated and who were inadvertently vaccinated. However, there were no deaths or permanent sequelae reported in a published post-marketing surveillance study in Finland involving 1.5 million children and adults who were vaccinated with M-M-R II during 1982 to 1993 {3}. Encephalitis and encephalopathy have been reported approximately once for every 3 million doses of the combination of measles, mumps, and rubella vaccine contained in M-M-R II. In no case has it been shown conclusively that reactions were actually caused by the vaccine; however, the data suggest the possibility that some of these cases may have been caused by measles vaccines. The risk of such serious neurological disorders following live measles virus vaccine administration remains far less than that for encephalitis and encephalopathy with wild-type measles (1 per 2000 reported cases).

Recipients of rubella vaccine may develop chronic joint symptoms. Arthralgia and/or arthritis, and polyneuritis after wild-type rubella virus infection vary in frequency and severity with age and gender, being greatest in adult females and least in pre-pubertal children. Following vaccination in children, reactions in joints are uncommon (0 to 3%) and of brief duration. In women, incidence rates for arthritis and arthralgia are higher than those seen in children (12 to 26%), and the reactions tend to be more marked and of longer duration (e.g., months or years). In adolescent girls, the reactions appear to be intermediate in incidence between those seen in children and adult women.

Chronic arthritis has been associated with wild-type rubella infection and has been related to persistent virus and/or viral antigen isolated from body tissues. Chronic joint symptoms have been reported following administration of rubella-containing vaccine.

There have been reports of subacute sclerosing panencephalitis (SSPE) in children who did not have a history of infection with wild-type measles but did receive measles vaccine. Some of these cases may have resulted from unrecognized measles in the first year of life or possibly from the measles vaccination. Based on estimated measles vaccine distribution in the United States (US), the association of SSPE cases to measles vaccination is about one case per million vaccine doses distributed. The association with wild-type measles virus infection is 6 to 22 cases of SSPE per million cases of measles. The results of a retrospective case-controlled study suggest that the overall effect of measles vaccine has been to protect against SSPE by preventing measles with its inherent higher risk of SSPE.

Cases of aseptic meningitis have been reported to Vaccine Adverse Event Reporting System (VAERS) following measles, mumps, and rubella vaccination. Although a causal relationship between other strains of mumps vaccine and aseptic meningitis has been shown, there is no evidence to link Jeryl Lynn™ mumps vaccine to aseptic meningitis. Cases of thrombocytopenia have been reported after use of measles vaccine; measles, mumps, and rubella vaccine; and after varicella vaccination. Post-marketing experience with live measles, mumps, and rubella vaccine indicates that individuals with current thrombocytopenia may develop more severe thrombocytopenia following vaccination. In addition, individuals who experienced thrombocytopenia following the first dose of a live measles, mumps, and rubella vaccine may develop thrombocytopenia with repeat doses. Serologic testing for antibody to measles, mumps, or rubella should be considered in order to determine if additional doses of vaccine are needed [see Warnings and Precautions (5.5)].

The reported rate of zoster in recipients of VARIVAX appears not to exceed that previously determined in a population-based study of healthy children who had experienced wild-type varicella {4}. In clinical trials, 8 cases of herpes zoster were reported in 9454 vaccinated individuals 12 months to 12 years of age during 42,556 person-years of follow-up. This resulted in a calculated incidence of at least 18.8 cases per 100,000 person-years. All 8 cases reported after VARIVAX were mild and no sequelae were reported. The long-term effect of VARIVAX on the incidence of herpes zoster is unknown at present.

6.3 Post-Marketing Observational Safety Surveillance Study

Safety was evaluated in an observational study that included 69,237 children vaccinated with ProQuad 12 months to 12 years old. A historical comparison group included 69,237 age-, gender-, and date-of-vaccination (day and month) matched subjects who were given M-M-R II and VARIVAX concomitantly. The primary objective was to assess the incidence of febrile seizures occurring within various time intervals after vaccination in 12- to 60-month-old children who had neither been vaccinated against measles, mumps, rubella, or varicella, nor had a history of the wild-type infections (N=31,298 vaccinated with ProQuad, including 31,043 who were 12 to 23 months old). The incidence of febrile seizures was also assessed in a historical control group of children who had received their first vaccination with M-M-R II and VARIVAX concomitantly (N=31,298, in-

cluding 31,019 who were 12 to 23 months old). The secondary objective was to assess the general safety of ProQuad in the 30-day period after vaccination in children 12 months to 12 years old.

In pre-licensure clinical studies, an increase in fever was observed 5 to 12 days after vaccination with ProQuad (dose 1) compared to M-M-R II and VARIVAX (dose 1) given concomitantly. In the post-marketing observational surveillance study, results from the primary safety analysis revealed an approximate two-fold increase in the risk of febrile seizures in the same 5 to 12 day timeframe after vaccination with ProQuad (dose 1). The incidence of febrile seizures 5 to 12 days after ProQuad (dose 1) (0.70 per 1000 children) was higher than that in children receiving M-M-R II and VARIVAX concomitantly (0.32 per 1000 children) [RR 2.20, 95% confidence interval (CI): 1.04, 4.65]. The incidence of

febrile seizures 0 to 30 days after ProQuad (dose 1) (1.41 per 1000 children) was similar to that observed in children receiving M-M-R II and VARIVAX concomitantly [RR 1.10 (95% CI: 0.72, 1.69)]. See Table 9. General safety analyses revealed that the risks of fever (RR=1.89; 95% CI: 1.67, 2.15) and skin eruption (RR=1.68; 95% CI: 1.07, 2.64) were significantly higher after ProQuad (dose 1) compared with those who received concomitant first doses of M-M-R II and VARIVAX, respectively. All medical events that resulted in hospitalization or emergency room visits were compared between the group given ProQuad and the historical comparison group, and no other safety concerns were identified in this study.

[See table 9 at top of previous page]

In this observational post-marketing study, no case of febrile seizure was observed during the 5 to 12 day post-

Table 10: Summary of Combined Immunogenicity Results 6 Weeks Following the Administration of a Single Dose of ProQuad (Varicella Virus Potency ≥3.97 log$_{10}$ PFU) or M-M-R II and VARIVAX (Per-Protocol Population)

Group	Antigen	n	Observed Response Rate (95% CI)	Observed GMT (95% CI)
ProQuad (N=5446*)	Varicella	4381	91.2% (90.3%, 92.0%)	15.5 (15.0, 15.9)
	Measles	4733	97.4% (96.9%, 97.9%)	3124.9 (3038.9, 3213.3)
	Mumps (OD cutoff)†	973	98.8% (97.9%, 99.4%)	105.3 (98.0, 113.1)
	Mumps (wild-type ELISA)†	3735	95.8% (95.1%, 96.4%)	93.1 (90.2, 96.0)
	Rubella	4773	98.5% (98.1%, 98.8%)	91.8 (89.6, 94.1)
M-M-R II + VARIVAX (N=2038*)	Varicella	1417	94.1% (92.8%, 95.3%)	16.6 (15.9, 17.4)
	Measles	1516	98.2% (97.4%, 98.8%)	2239.6 (2138.3, 2345.6)
	Mumps (OD cutoff)†	501	99.4% (98.3%, 99.9%)	87.5 (79.7, 96.0)
	Mumps (wild-type ELISA)†	1017	98.0% (97.0%, 98.8%)	90.8 (86.2, 95.7)
	Rubella	1528	98.5% (97.7%, 99.0%)	102.2 (97.8, 106.7)

n = Number of per-protocol subjects with evaluable serology.
CI = Confidence interval.
GMT = Geometric mean titer.
ELISA = Enzyme-linked immunosorbent assay.
PFU = Plaque-forming units.
OD = Optical density.
* Includes ProQuad + Placebo followed by ProQuad (Visit 1) (Protocol 009), ProQuad Middle and High Doses (Visit 1) (Protocol 011), ProQuad (Lot 1, Lot 2, Lot 3) (Protocol 012), both the Concomitant and Non-concomitant groups (Protocol 013).
† The mumps antibody response was assessed by a vaccine-strain ELISA in Protocols 009 and 011 and by a wild-type ELISA in Protocols 012 and 013. In the former assay, the serostatus was based on the OD cutoff of the assay. In the latter assay, 10 mumps ELISA units was used as the serostatus cutoff.

Table 11: Summary of Immune Response to a First and Second Dose of ProQuad in Subjects <3 Years of Age Who Received ProQuad with a Varicella Virus Dose ≥3.97 Log$_{10}$ PFU*

Antigen	Serostatus Cutoff/ Response Criteria	Dose 1 N=1097			Dose 2 N=1097		
		n	Observed Response Rate (95% CI)	Observed GMT (95% CI)	n	Observed Response Rate (95% CI)	Observed GMT (95% CI)
Measles	≥120 mIU/mL†	915	98.1% (97.0%, 98.9%)	2956.8 (2786.3, 3137.7)	915	99.5% (98.7%, 99.8%)	5958.0 (5518.9, 6432.1)
	≥255 mIU/mL	943	97.8% (96.6%, 98.6%)	2966.0 (2793.4, 3149.2)	943	99.4% (98.6%, 99.8%)	5919.3 (5486.2, 6386.6)
Mumps	≥OD Cutoff (ELISA antibody units)	920	98.7% (97.7%, 99.3%)	106.7 (99.1, 114.8)	920	99.9% (99.4%, 100%)	253.1 (237.9, 269.2)
Rubella	≥10 IU/mL	937	97.7% (96.5%, 98.5%)	91.1 (85.9, 96.6)	937	98.3% (97.2%, 99.0%)	158.8 (149.1, 169.2)

(Table continued on next page)

Table 11 (cont.): Summary of Immune Response to a First and Second Dose of ProQuad in Subjects <3 Years of Age Who Received ProQuad with a Varicella Virus Dose ≥3.97 Log$_{10}$ PFU*

Antigen	Serostatus Cutoff/ Response Criteria	Dose 1 N=1097				Dose 2 N=1097			
		n	Observed Response Rate (95% CI)	Observed GMT (95% CI)		n	Observed Response Rate (95% CI)	Observed GMT (95% CI)	
Varicella	<1.25 to ≥5 gpELISA units	864	86.6% (84.1%, 88.8%)	11.6 (10.9, 12.3)		864	99.4% (98.7%, 99.8%)	477.5 (437.8, 520.7)	
	≥OD Cutoff (gpELISA units)	695	87.2% (84.5%, 89.6%)	11.6 (10.9, 12.4)		695	99.4% (98.5%, 99.8%)	478.7 (434.8, 527.1)	

ProQuad (Middle Dose) = ProQuad containing a varicella virus dose of 3.97 log$_{10}$ PFU.
ProQuad (High Dose) = ProQuad containing a varicella virus dose of 4.25 log$_{10}$ PFU.
ELISA = Enzyme-linked immunosorbent assay.
gpELISA = Glycoprotein enzyme-linked immunosorbent assay.
N = Number vaccinated at baseline.
n = Number of subjects who were per-protocol Postdose 1 and Postdose 2 and satisfied the given prevaccination serostatus cutoff.
CI = Confidence interval.
GMT = Geometric mean titer.
PFU = Plaque-forming units.
* Includes the following treatment groups: ProQuad + Placebo followed by ProQuad (Visit 1) (Protocol 009) and ProQuad (Middle and High Dose) (Protocol 011).
† Samples from Protocols 009 and 011 were assayed in the legacy format Measles ELISA, which reported antibody titers in Measles ELISA units. To convert titers from ELISA units to mIU/mL, titers for these 2 protocols were divided by 0.1025. The lowest measurable titer postvaccination is 207.5 mIU/mL. The response rate for measles in the legacy format is the percent of subjects with a negative baseline measles antibody titer, as defined by the optical density (OD) cutoff, with a postvaccination measles antibody titer ≥207.5 mIU/mL.
Samples from Protocols 009 and 011 were assayed in the legacy format Rubella ELISA, which reported antibody titers in Rubella ELISA units. To convert titers from ELISA units to IU/mL, titers for these 2 protocols were divided by 1.28.

Table 12: Summary of Antibody Responses to Measles, Mumps, Rubella, and Varicella at 6 Weeks Postvaccination in Subjects 4 to 6 Years of Age Who Had Previously Received M-M-R II and VARIVAX (Per-Protocol Population)

Group Number (Description)	n	GMT (95% CI)	Seropositivity Rate (95% CI)	% ≥4-Fold Rise in Titer (95% CI)	Geometric Mean Fold Rise (95% CI)
		Measles*			
Group 1 (N=399) (ProQuad + placebo)	367	1985.9 (1817.6, 2169.9)	100% (99.0%, 100%)	4.9% (2.9%, 7.6%)	1.21 (1.13, 1.30)
Group 2 (N=205) (M-M-R II + placebo)	185	2046.9 (1815.2, 2308.2)	100% (98.0%, 100%)	4.3% (1.9%, 8.3%)	1.28 (1.17, 1.40)
Group 3 (N=195) (M-M-R II + VARIVAX)	171	2084.3 (1852.3, 2345.5)	99.4% (96.8%, 100%)	4.7% (2.0%, 9.0%)	1.31 (1.17, 1.46)
		Mumps†			
Group 1 (N=399) (ProQuad + placebo)	367	206.0 (188.2, 225.4)	99.5% (98.0%, 99.9%)	27.2% (22.8%, 32.1%)	2.43 (2.19, 2.69)
Group 2 (N=205) (M-M-R II + placebo)	185	308.5 (269.6, 352.9)	100% (98.0%, 100%)	41.1% (33.9%, 48.5%)	3.69 (3.14, 4.32)
Group 3 (N=195) (M-M-R II + VARIVAX)	171	295.9 (262.5, 333.5)	100% (97.9%, 100%)	41.5% (34.0%, 49.3%)	3.36 (2.84, 3.97)
		Rubella‡			
Group 1 (N=399) (ProQuad + placebo)	367	217.3 (200.1, 236.0)	100% (99.0%, 100%)	32.7% (27.9%, 37.8%)	3.00 (2.72, 3.31)
Group 2 (N=205) (M-M-R II + placebo)	185	174.0 (157.3, 192.6)	100% (98.0%, 100%)	31.9% (25.2%, 39.1%)	2.81 (2.41, 3.27)
Group 3 (N=195) (M-M-R II + VARIVAX)	171	154.1 (138.9, 170.9)	99.4% (96.8%, 100%)	26.9% (20.4%, 34.2%)	2.47 (2.17, 2.81)
		Varicella§			
Group 1 (N=399) (ProQuad + placebo)	367	322.2 (278.9, 372.2)	98.9% (97.2%, 99.7%)	80.7 (76.2%, 84.6%)	12.43 (10.63, 14.53)
Group 2 (N=205) (M-M-R II + placebo)	185	N/A	N/A	N/A	N/A
Group 3 (N=195) (M-M-R II + VARIVAX)	171	209.3 (171.2, 255.9)	99.4% (96.8%, 100%)	71.9% (64.6%, 78.5%)	8.50 (6.69, 10.81)

gpELISA = Glycoprotein enzyme-linked immunosorbent assay; ELISA = Enzyme-linked immunosorbent assay; CI = Confidence interval; GMT = Geometric mean titer; N/A = Not applicable; N = Number of subjects vaccinated; n = number of subjects in the per-protocol analysis.
* Measles GMTs are reported in mIU/mL; seropositivity corresponds to ≥120 mIU/mL.
† Mumps GMTs are reported in mumps Ab units/mL; seropositivity corresponds to ≥10 Ab units/mL.
‡ Rubella titers obtained by the legacy format were converted to their corresponding titers in the modified format. Rubella serostatus was determined after the conversion to IU/mL; seropositivity corresponds to ≥10 IU/mL.
§ Varicella GMTs are reported in gpELISA units/mL; seropositivity rate is reported by % of subjects with postvaccination antibody titers ≥5 gpELISA units/mL. Percentages are calculated as the number of subjects who met the criterion divided by the number of subjects contributing to the per-protocol analysis.

vaccination time period among 26,455 children who received ProQuad as a second dose of M-M-R II and VARIVAX. In addition, detailed general safety data were available from more than 25,000 children who received ProQuad as a second dose of M-M-R II and VARIVAX, most of them (95%) between 4 and 6 years of age, and an analysis of these data by an independent, external safety monitoring committee did not identify any specific safety concern.

7 DRUG INTERACTIONS

7.1 Immune Globulins and Transfusions
Immune globulins (IG) administered concomitantly with ProQuad contain antibodies that may interfere with vaccine virus replication and decrease the expected immune response. Vaccination should be deferred for at least 3 months following blood or plasma transfusions, or administration of IG.
The appropriate suggested interval between transfusion or IG administration and vaccination will vary with the type of transfusion or indication for, and dose of, IG (e.g., 5 months for Varicella Zoster Immune Globulin [VZIG]) [2]. Following administration of ProQuad, any IG including VZIG should not be given for 1 month thereafter unless its use outweighs the benefits of vaccination [2]. [See Warnings and Precautions (5.9).]

7.2 Salicylates
Reye syndrome has been reported following the use of salicylates during wild-type varicella infection. Vaccine recipients should avoid use of salicylates for 6 weeks after vaccination with ProQuad. [See Adverse Reactions (6.1) and Patient Counseling Information (17).]

7.3 Corticosteroids and Immunosuppressive Drugs
ProQuad may be used in individuals who are receiving topical corticosteroids or low-dose corticosteroids for asthma prophylaxis or replacement therapy, e.g., for Addison's disease. ProQuad should not be given to individuals receiving immunosuppressive doses of corticosteroids or other immunosuppressive drugs. Vaccination with a live, attenuated vaccine, such as varicella or measles, can result in a more extensive vaccine-associated rash or disseminated disease in individuals on immunosuppressive drugs [see Contraindications (4.2)].

7.4 Drug/Laboratory Test Interactions
Live, attenuated measles, mumps, and rubella virus vaccines given individually may result in a temporary depression of tuberculin skin sensitivity. Therefore, if a tuberculin test is to be done, it should be administered either any time before, simultaneously with, or at least 4 to 6 weeks after ProQuad.

7.5 Use With Other Vaccines
At least 1 month should elapse between a dose of a measles-containing vaccine such as M-M-R II and a dose of ProQuad, and at least 3 months should elapse between administration of 2 doses of ProQuad or varicella-containing vaccines.
ProQuad may be administered concomitantly with Haemophilus influenzae type b conjugate (meningococcal protein conjugate) and hepatitis B (recombinant). Additionally, ProQuad may be administered concomitantly with pneumococcal 7-valent conjugate vaccine, and/or hepatitis A (inactivated) vaccines. [See Clinical Studies (14).]
There are no data regarding the administration of ProQuad with inactivated poliovirus vaccine or with other live virus vaccines.
There are insufficient data to support concomitant vaccination with diphtheria and tetanus toxoids and acellular pertussis vaccine adsorbed. [See Clinical Studies (14).]
Children under treatment for tuberculosis have not experienced exacerbation of the disease when vaccinated with live measles virus vaccine; no studies have been reported to date of the effect of measles virus vaccines on children with untreated tuberculosis.

8 USE IN SPECIFIC POPULATIONS

8.1 Pregnancy
Pregnancy Category: Contraindication [see Contraindications (4.4)].
Do not administer ProQuad to pregnant females. It is also not known whether ProQuad can cause fetal harm when administered to a pregnant woman or can affect reproduction capacity. If vaccination of postpubertal females is undertaken, pregnancy should be avoided for 3 months following vaccination. [See Contraindications (4.4) and Patient Counseling Information (17).]
In counseling women who are inadvertently vaccinated when pregnant or who become pregnant within 3 months of vaccination, the healthcare provider should be aware of the following: (1) Reports have indicated that contracting wild-type measles during pregnancy enhances fetal risk. Increased rates of spontaneous abortion, stillbirth, congenital defects, and prematurity have been observed subsequent to wild-type measles during pregnancy. There are no adequate studies of the attenuated (vaccine) strain of measles virus in pregnancy. However, it would be prudent to assume that the vaccine strain of virus is also capable of inducing adverse fetal effects; (2) Mumps infection during the first trimester

of pregnancy may increase the rate of spontaneous abortion. Although mumps vaccine virus has been shown to infect the placenta and fetus, there is no evidence that it causes congenital malformations in humans {5}; (3) In a 10-year survey involving over 700 pregnant women who received rubella vaccine within 3 months before or after conception (of whom 189 received the Wistar RA 27/3 strain), none of the newborns had abnormalities compatible with congenital rubella syndrome {6}; and (4) Wild-type varicella can sometimes cause congenital varicella infection.

Pregnancy Registry

From 1995 to 2013, Merck Sharp & Dohme Corp., a subsidiary of Merck & Co., Inc., maintained a Pregnancy Registry to monitor fetal outcomes following inadvertent administration of VARIVAX during pregnancy or within three months prior to conception. In 2006, reports of exposure to two other varicella (Oka/Merck)-containing vaccines, ProQuad and ZOSTAVAX® (Zoster Vaccine Live), were added to the Registry. The Pregnancy Registry has been discontinued. As of March 2011, 811 women with pregnancy outcome information available for analysis were prospectively enrolled following vaccination with VARIVAX, within three months prior to conception or any time during pregnancy. Of these women, 170 were seronegative at the time of exposure and 627 women had an unknown serostatus. The remaining women were seropositive. Nine exposures to either ProQuad or ZOSTAVAX have been reported that met criteria for inclusion into the Registry.

None of the 820 women who received a varicella-containing vaccine delivered infants with abnormalities consistent with congenital varicella syndrome.

All exposures to VARIVAX, ProQuad, or ZOSTAVAX during pregnancy or within three months prior to conception should be reported as suspected adverse reactions by contacting Merck Sharp & Dohme Corp., a subsidiary of Merck & Co., Inc., at 1-877-888-4231 or VAERS at 1-800-822-7967 or www.vaers.hhs.gov.

8.3 Nursing Mothers

Do not administer ProQuad to nursing women. It is not known whether ProQuad is excreted in human milk. Because many drugs are excreted in human milk, caution should be exercised when ProQuad is administered to a nursing woman. The secretion of measles and mumps viruses in human milk has not been studied; however, studies have shown that lactating postpartum women vaccinated with live rubella vaccine may secrete the virus in breast milk and transmit it to breast-fed infants. Limited evidence in the literature suggests that virus, viral DNA, or viral antigen could not be detected in the breast milk of women who were vaccinated postpartum with the vaccine strain of varicella virus {7,8}. [See Warnings and Precautions (5.8).]

8.4 Pediatric Use

Do not administer ProQuad to infants younger than 12 months of age or to children 13 years and older. Safety and effectiveness of ProQuad in infants younger than 12 months of age and in children 13 years and older have not been studied. ProQuad is not approved for use in persons in these age groups. [See Adverse Reactions (6) and Clinical Studies (14).]

8.5 Geriatric Use

ProQuad is not indicated for use in the geriatric population (≥age 65).

11 DESCRIPTION

ProQuad (Measles, Mumps, Rubella and Varicella Virus Vaccine Live) is a combined, attenuated, live virus vaccine containing measles, mumps, rubella, and varicella viruses. ProQuad is a sterile lyophilized preparation of (1) the components of M-M-R II (Measles, Mumps, and Rubella Virus Vaccine Live): Measles Virus Vaccine Live, a more attenuated line of measles virus, derived from Enders' attenuated Edmonston strain and propagated in chick embryo cell culture; Mumps Virus Vaccine Live, the Jeryl Lynn™ (B level) strain of mumps virus propagated in chick embryo cell culture; Rubella Virus Vaccine Live, the Wistar RA 27/3 strain of live attenuated rubella virus propagated in WI-38 human diploid lung fibroblasts; and (2) Varicella Virus Vaccine Live (Oka/Merck), the Oka/Merck strain of varicella-zoster virus propagated in MRC-5 cells. The cells, virus pools, bovine serum, and human albumin used in manufacturing are all tested to provide assurance that the final product is free of potential adventitious agents.

ProQuad, when reconstituted as directed, is a sterile suspension for subcutaneous administration. Each 0.5-mL dose contains not less than 3.00 $\log_{10}$ TCID$_{50}$ of measles virus; 4.30 $\log_{10}$ TCID$_{50}$ of mumps virus; 3.00 $\log_{10}$ TCID$_{50}$ of rubella virus; and a minimum of 3.99 $\log_{10}$ PFU of Oka/Merck varicella virus.

Each 0.5-mL dose of the vaccine contains no more than 21 mg of sucrose, 11 mg of hydrolyzed gelatin, 2.4 mg of sodium chloride, 1.8 mg of sorbitol, 0.40 mg of monosodium L-glutamate, 0.34 mg of sodium phosphate dibasic, 0.31 mg of human albumin, 0.17 mg of sodium bicarbonate, 72 mcg of potassium phosphate monobasic, 60 mcg of potassium chloride; 36 mcg of potassium phosphate dibasic; residual components of MRC-5 cells including DNA and protein; <16 mcg of neomycin, bovine calf serum (0.5 mcg), and other buffer and media ingredients. The product contains no preservative.

12 CLINICAL PHARMACOLOGY

12.1 Mechanism of Action

ProQuad has been shown to induce measles-, mumps-, rubella-, and varicella-specific immunity, which is thought to be the mechanism by which it protects against these four childhood diseases.

The efficacy of ProQuad was established through the use of immunological correlates for protection against measles, mumps, rubella, and varicella. Results from efficacy studies or field effectiveness studies that were previously conducted for the component vaccines were used to define levels of serum antibodies that correlated with protection against measles, mumps, and rubella. Also, in previous studies with varicella vaccine, antibody responses against varicella virus ≥5 gpELISA units/mL in a glycoprotein enzyme-linked immunosorbent assay (gpELISA) (not commercially available) similarly correlated with long-term protection. In these efficacy studies, the clinical endpoint for measles and mumps was a clinical diagnosis of either disease confirmed by a 4-fold or greater rise in serum antibody titers between either postvaccination or acute and convalescent titers; for rubella, a 4-fold or greater rise in antibody titers with or without clinical symptoms of rubella; and for varicella, varicella-like rash that occurred >42 days postvaccination and for which varicella was not excluded by either viral cultures of the lesion or serological tests. Specific laboratory evidence of varicella either by serology or culture was not required to confirm the diagnosis of varicella. Clinical studies with a single dose of ProQuad have shown that vaccination elicited rates of antibody responses against measles,

Table 13: Statistical Analysis of Non-Inferiority in Antibody Response Rates to Measles, Mumps, Rubella, and Varicella at 6 Weeks Postvaccination for Subjects Initially Seronegative to Measles, Mumps, or Rubella, or With Varicella Antibody Titer <1.25 gpELISA units at Baseline in the ProQuad + PCV7* Treatment Group and the ProQuad Followed by PCV7 Control Group (Per-Protocol Analysis)

Assay Parameter	ProQuad + PCV7 (N=510)		ProQuad followed by PCV7 (N=259)		Difference (percentage points)[†,‡] (95% CI)
	n	Estimated Response[†]	n	Estimated Response[†]	
Measles % ≥255 mIU/mL	406	97.3%	204	99.5%	-2.2 (-4.6, 0.2)
Mumps % ≥10 Ab units/mL	403	96.6%	208	98.6%	-1.9 (-4.5, 1.0)
Rubella % ≥10 IU/mL	377	98.7%	195	97.9%	0.9 (-1.3, 4.1)
Varicella % ≥5 gpELISA units/mL	379	92.5%	192	87.9%	4.5 (-0.4, 10.4)

N = Number of subjects vaccinated in each treatment group.

n = Number of subjects with measles antibody titer <255 mIU/mL, mumps antibody titer <10 ELISA Ab units/mL, rubella antibody titer <10 IU/mL, or varicella antibody titer <1.25 gpELISA units/mL at baseline and with postvaccination serology contributing to the per-protocol analysis.

Ab = antibody; ELISA = Enzyme-linked immunosorbent assay; gpELISA = Glycoprotein enzyme-linked immunosorbent assay; CI = Confidence interval.

* PCV7 = Pneumococcal 7-valent conjugate vaccine.

Seronegative defined as baseline measles antibody titer <255 mIU/mL for measles, baseline mumps antibody titer <10 ELISA Ab units/mL for mumps, and baseline rubella antibody titer <10 IU/mL for rubella.

† Estimated responses and their differences were based on statistical analysis models adjusting for study center.

‡ ProQuad + PCV7 - ProQuad followed by PCV7.

The conclusion of non-inferiority is based on the lower bound of the 2-sided 95% CI on the risk difference being greater than -10 percentage points (i.e., excluding a decrease equal to or more than the prespecified criterion of 10.0 percentage points). This indicates that the difference is statistically significantly less than the prespecified clinically relevant decrease of 10.0 percentage points at the 1-sided alpha = 0.025 level.

Table 14: Statistical Analysis of Non-Inferiority in GMTs to S. pneumoniae Serotypes at 6 Weeks Postvaccination in the ProQuad + PCV7* Treatment Group and the PCV7 Followed by ProQuad Control Group (Per-Protocol Analysis)

Serotype	Parameter	Group 1 ProQuad + PCV7 (N=510)		Group 2 PCV7 followed by ProQuad (N=258)		Fold-Difference*,[‡] (95% CI)
		n	Estimated Response[†]	n	Estimated Response[†]	
4	GMT	410	1.5	193	1.3	1.2 (1.0, 1.4)
6B	GMT	410	8.9	192	8.4	1.1 (0.9, 1.2)
9V	GMT	409	2.9	193	2.5	1.2 (1.0, 1.3)
14	GMT	408	6.5	193	5.7	1.1 (1.0, 1.3)
18C	GMT	408	2.3	193	2.0	1.2 (1.0, 1.3)
19F	GMT	408	3.5	192	3.1	1.1 (1.0, 1.3)
23F	GMT	413	4.1	197	3.7	1.1 (1.0, 1.3)

N = Number of subjects vaccinated in each treatment group; n = Number of subjects contributing to the per-protocol analysis for the given serotype; GMT = geometric mean titer; CI = Confidence interval.

* PCV7 = Pneumococcal 7-valent conjugate vaccine.

† Estimated responses and their fold-difference were based on statistical analysis models adjusting for study center and prevaccination titer.

‡ ProQuad + PCV7 / PCV7 followed by ProQuad.

The conclusion of non-inferiority is based on the lower bound of the 2-sided 95% CI on the fold-difference being greater than 0.5, (i.e., excluding a decrease of 2-fold or more). This indicates that the fold-difference is statistically significantly less than the pre-specified clinically relevant 2-fold difference at the 1-sided alpha = 0.025 level.

Table 15: Statistical Analysis of Non-Inferiority of the Response Rate for Varicella Antibody at 6 Weeks Postvaccination Among Subjects Who Received VAQTA Concomitantly or Non-Concomitantly With ProQuad and PCV7* (Per-Protocol Analysis Set)

Parameter	Group 1: Concomitant VAQTA with ProQuad + PCV7 (N=330)		Group 2: Non-concomitant VAQTA separate from ProQuad + PCV7 (N=323)		Difference[†] (percentage points): Group 1 – Group 2 (95% CI)
	n	Estimated Response[†]	n	Estimated Response[†]	
% ≥5 gpELISA units/mL[‡]	225[§]	93.2%	232[§]	98.3%	-5.1 (-9.3, -1.4)

N = Number of subjects enrolled/randomized; n = Number of subjects contributing to the per-protocol analysis for varicella; CI = Confidence interval.
* PCV7 = Pneumococcal 7-valent conjugate vaccine.
† Estimated responses and their differences were based on a statistical analysis model adjusting for combined study center.
‡ 6 weeks following Dose 1.
§ Initial Serostatus <1.25 gpELISA units/ mL.
The conclusion of similarity (non-inferiority) was based on the lower bound of the 2-sided 95% CI on the risk difference excluding a decrease of 10 percentage points or more (lower bound >-10.0). This indicated that the risk difference was statistically significantly greater than the pre-specified clinically relevant difference of -10 percentage points at the 1-sided alpha = 0.025 level.

Table 16: Statistical Analysis of Non-Inferiority of the Seropositivity Rate (SPR) for Hepatitis A Antibody at 4 Weeks Postdose 2 of VAQTA Among Subjects Who Received VAQTA Concomitantly or Non-Concomitantly With ProQuad and PCV7* (Per-Protocol Analysis Set)

Parameter	Group 1: Concomitant VAQTA with ProQuad + PCV7 (N=330)		Group 2: Non-concomitant VAQTA separate from ProQuad + PCV7 (N=323)		Difference[†] (percentage points): Group 1 - Group 2 (95% CI)
	n	Estimated Response[†]	n	Estimated Response[†]	
% ≥10 mIU/mL[‡]	182[§]	100.0%	159[§]	99.3%	0.7 (-1.4, 3.8)

CI = Confidence interval; N = Number of subjects enrolled/randomized; n = Number of subjects contributing to the per-protocol analysis for hepatitis A.
* PCV7 = Pneumococcal 7-valent conjugate vaccine.
† Estimated responses and their differences were based on a statistical analysis model adjusting for combined study center.
‡ 4 weeks following receipt of 2 doses of VAQTA.
§ Regardless of initial serostatus.
The conclusion of non-inferiority was based on the lower bound of the 2-sided 95% CI on the risk difference being greater than -10 percentage points (i.e., excluding a decrease of 10 percentage points or more) (lower bound >-10.0). This indicated that the risk difference was statistically significantly greater than the pre-specified clinically relevant difference of -10 percentage points at the 1-sided alpha = 0.025 level.

mumps, and rubella that were similar to those observed after vaccination with a single dose of M-M-R II [see Clinical Studies (14)] and seroresponse rates for varicella virus were similar to those observed after vaccination with a single dose of VARIVAX [see Clinical Studies (14)]. The duration of protection from measles, mumps, rubella, and varicella infections after vaccination with ProQuad is unknown.

12.4 Persistence of Antibody Responses After Vaccination
The persistence of antibody at 1 year after vaccination was evaluated in a subset of 2107 children enrolled in the clinical trials. Antibody was detected in 98.9% (1722/1741) for measles, 96.7% (1676/1733) for mumps, 99.6% (1796/1804) for rubella, and 97.5% (1512/1550) for varicella (≥5 gpELISA units/mL) of vaccinees following a single dose of ProQuad.
Experience with M-M-R II demonstrates that antibodies to measles, mumps, and rubella viruses are still detectable in most individuals 11 to 13 years after primary vaccination (9). Varicella antibodies were present for up to ten years postvaccination in most of the individuals tested who received 1 dose of VARIVAX.

13 NONCLINICAL TOXICOLOGY
13.1 Carcinogenesis, Mutagenesis, Impairment of Fertility
ProQuad has not been evaluated for its carcinogenic, mutagenic, or teratogenic potential, or its potential to impair fertility.

14 CLINICAL STUDIES
Formal studies to evaluate the clinical efficacy of ProQuad have not been performed.
Efficacy of the measles, mumps, rubella, and varicella components of ProQuad was previously established in a series of clinical studies with the monovalent vaccines. A high degree of protection from infection was demonstrated in these studies [10-17].
Immunogenicity in Children 12 Months to 6 Years of Age
Prior to licensure, immunogenicity was studied in 5845 healthy children 12 months to 6 years of age with a negative clinical history of measles, mumps, rubella, and varicella who participated in 5 randomized clinical trials. The immu-

nogenicity of ProQuad was similar to that of its individual component vaccines (M-M-R II and VARIVAX), which are currently used in routine vaccination.
The presence of detectable antibody was assessed by an appropriately sensitive enzyme-linked immunosorbent assay (ELISA) for measles, mumps (wild-type and vaccine-type strains), and rubella, and by gpELISA for varicella. For evaluation of vaccine response rates, a positive result in the measles ELISA corresponded to measles antibody concentrations of ≥255 mIU/mL when compared to the WHO II (66/202) Reference Immunoglobulin for Measles.
Children were positive for mumps antibody if the antibody level was ≥10 ELISA units/mL. A positive result in the rubella ELISA corresponded to concentrations of ≥10 IU rubella antibody/mL when compared to the WHO International Reference Serum for Rubella; children with varicella antibody levels ≥5 gpELISA units/mL were considered to be seropositive since a response rate based on ≥5 gpELISA units/mL has been shown to be highly correlated with long-term protection.
Immunogenicity in Children 12 to 23 Months of Age After a Single Dose
In 4 randomized clinical trials, 5446 healthy children 12 to 23 months of age were administered ProQuad, and 2038 children were vaccinated with M-M-R II and VARIVAX given concomitantly at separate injection sites. Subjects enrolled in each of these trials had a negative clinical history, no known recent exposure, and no vaccination history for varicella, measles, mumps, and rubella. Children were excluded from study participation if they had an immune impairment or had a history of allergy to components of the vaccine(s). Except for in 1 trial [see ProQuad Administered with Diphtheria and Tetanus Toxoids and Acellular Pertussis Vaccine Adsorbed (DTaP) and Haemophilus influenzae type b Conjugate (Meningococcal Protein Conjugate) and Hepatitis B (Recombinant) Vaccine below], no concomitant vaccines were permitted during study participation. The race distribution of the study subjects across these studies following a first dose of ProQuad was as follows: 66.3% White; 12.7% African-American; 9.9% Hispanic; 6.7% Asian/Pacific; 4.2% other; and 0.2% American Indian. The gender distribution of the study subjects across these studies fol-

lowing a first dose of ProQuad was 52.6% male and 47.4% female. A summary of combined immunogenicity results 6 weeks following administration of a single dose of ProQuad or M-M-R II and VARIVAX is shown in Table 10. These results were similar to the immune response rates induced by concomitant administration of single doses of M-M-R II and VARIVAX at separate injection sites (lower bound of the 95% CI for the risk difference in measles, mumps, and rubella seroconversion rates were >-5.0 percentage points and the lower bound of the 95% CI for the risk difference in varicella seroprotection rates were either >-15 percentage points [one study] or >-10.0 percentage points [three studies]).
[See table 10 at top of page 1635]
Immunogenicity in Children 15 to 31 Months of Age After a Second Dose of ProQuad
In 2 of the 4 randomized clinical trials described above, a subgroup (N=1035) of the 5446 children administered a single dose of ProQuad were administered a second dose of ProQuad approximately 3 to 9 months after the first dose. Children were excluded from receiving a second dose of ProQuad if they were recently exposed to or developed varicella, measles, mumps, and/or rubella prior to receipt of the second dose. No concomitant vaccines were administered to these children. The race distribution across these studies following a second dose of ProQuad was as follows: 67.3% White; 14.3% African-American; 8.3% Hispanic; 5.4% Asian/Pacific; 4.4% other; 0.2% American Indian; and 0.10% mixed. The gender distribution of the study subjects across these studies following a second dose of ProQuad was 50.4% male and 49.6% female. A summary of immune responses following a second dose of ProQuad is presented in Table 11. Results from this study showed that 2 doses of ProQuad administered at least 3 months apart elicited a positive antibody response to all four antigens in greater than 98% of subjects. The geometric mean titers (GMTs) following the second dose of ProQuad increased approximately 2-fold each for measles, mumps, and rubella, and approximately 41-fold for varicella.
[See table 11 on pages 1635 and 1636]
Immunogenicity in Children 4 to 6 Years of Age Who Received a First Dose of ProQuad After Primary Vaccination With M-M-R II and VARIVAX
In a clinical trial, 799 healthy 4- to 6-year-old children who had received M-M-R II and VARIVAX at least 1 month prior to study entry were randomized to receive ProQuad and placebo (N=399), M-M-R II and placebo concomitantly at separate injection sites (N=205), or M-M-R II and VARIVAX concomitantly at separate injection sites (N=195). Children were eligible if they were previously administered primary doses of M-M-R II and VARIVAX, either concomitantly or non-concomitantly, at 12 months of age or older. Children were excluded if they were recently exposed to measles, mumps, rubella, and/or varicella, had an immune impairment, or had a history of allergy to components of the vaccine(s). No concomitant vaccines were permitted during study participation. [See Adverse Reactions (6.1) for ethnicity and gender information.]
A summary of antibody responses to measles, mumps, rubella, and varicella at 6 weeks postvaccination in subjects who had previously received M-M-R II and VARIVAX is shown in Table 12. Results from this study showed that a first dose of ProQuad after primary vaccination with M-M-R II and VARIVAX elicited a positive antibody response to all four antigens in greater than 98% of subjects. Postvaccination GMTs for recipients of ProQuad were similar to those following a second dose of M-M-R II and VARIVAX administered concomitantly at separate injection sites (the lower bound of the 95% CI around the fold difference in measles, mumps, rubella, and varicella GMTs excluded 0.5). Additionally, GMTs for measles, mumps, and rubella were similar to those following a second dose of M-M-R II given concomitantly with placebo (the lower bound of the 95% CI around the fold difference for the comparison of measles, mumps, and rubella GMTs excluded 0.5).
[See table 12 at bottom of page 1636]
Immunogenicity Following Concomitant Use with Other Vaccines
ProQuad with Pneumococcal 7-valent Conjugate Vaccine and/or VAQTA
In a clinical trial, 1027 healthy children 12 to 15 months of age were randomized to receive ProQuad and pneumococcal 7-valent conjugate vaccine concomitantly (N=510) at separate injection sites or ProQuad and pneumococcal 7-valent conjugate vaccine non-concomitantly (N=517) at separate clinic visits. [See Adverse Reactions (6.1) for ethnicity and gender information.] The statistical analysis of non-inferiority in antibody response rates to measles, mumps, rubella, and varicella at 6 weeks postvaccination for subjects are shown in Table 13. In the per-protocol population, seroconversion rates were not inferior in children given ProQuad and pneumococcal 7-valent conjugate vaccine concomitantly when compared to seroconversion rates seen in children given these vaccines non-concomitantly for

measles, mumps, and rubella. In children with baseline varicella antibody titers <1.25 gpELISA units/mL, the varicella seroprotection rates were not inferior when rates after concomitant and non-concomitant vaccination were compared 6 weeks postvaccination. Statistical analysis of non-inferiority in GMTs to *S. pneumoniae* serotypes at 6 weeks postvaccination are shown in Table 14. Geometric mean antibody titers (GMTs) for *S. pneumoniae* types 4, 6B, 9V, 14, 18C, 19F, and 23F were not inferior when antibody titers in the concomitant and non-concomitant groups were compared 6 weeks postvaccination.
[See table 13 at top of page 1637]
[See table 14 at top of page 1637]
In a clinical trial, 653 healthy children 12 to 15 months of age were randomized to receive VAQTA, ProQuad, and pneumococcal 7-valent conjugate vaccine concomitantly (N=330) or ProQuad and pneumococcal 7-valent conjugate vaccine concomitantly followed by VAQTA 6 weeks later (N=323). *[See Adverse Reactions (6.1) for ethnicity and gender information.]* Statistical analysis of non-inferiority of the response rate for varicella antibody at 6 weeks postvaccination among subjects who received VAQTA concomitantly or non-concomitantly with ProQuad and pneumococcal 7-valent conjugate vaccine is shown in Table 15. For the varicella component of ProQuad, in subjects with baseline antibody titers <1.25 gpELISA units/mL, the proportion with a titer ≥5 gpELISA units/mL 6 weeks after their first dose of ProQuad was non-inferior when ProQuad was administered with VAQTA and pneumococcal 7-valent conjugate vaccine as compared to the proportion with a titer ≥5 gpELISA units/mL when ProQuad was administered with pneumococcal 7-valent conjugate vaccine alone. Statistical analysis of non-inferiority of the seropositivity rate for hepatitis A antibody at 4 weeks postdose 2 of VAQTA among subjects who received VAQTA concomitantly or non-concomitantly with ProQuad and pneumococcal 7-valent conjugate vaccine is shown in Table 16. The seropositivity rate to hepatitis A 4 weeks after a second dose of VAQTA given concomitantly with ProQuad and pneumococcal 7-valent conjugate vaccine (defined as the percent of subjects with a titer ≥10 mIU/mL) was non-inferior to the seropositivity rate observed when VAQTA was administered separately from ProQuad and pneumococcal 7-valent conjugate vaccine. Statistical analysis of non-inferiority in GMT to *S. pneumoniae* serotypes at 6 weeks postvaccination among subjects who received VAQTA concomitantly or non-concomitantly with ProQuad and pneumococcal 7-valent conjugate vaccine is shown in Table 17. Additionally, the GMTs for *S. pneumoniae* types 4, 6B, 9V, 14, 18C, 19F, and 23F 6 weeks after vaccination with pneumococcal 7-valent conjugate vaccine administered concomitantly with ProQuad and VAQTA were non-inferior as compared to GMTs observed in the group given pneumococcal 7-valent conjugate vaccine with ProQuad alone. An earlier clinical study involving 617 healthy children provided data that indicated that the seroresponse rates 6 weeks post vaccination for measles, mumps, and rubella in those given M-M-R II and VAQTA concomitantly (N=309) were non-inferior as compared to historical controls.
[See table 15 at top of previous page]
[See table 16 at top of previous page]
[See table 17 above]
ProQuad Administered with Diphtheria and Tetanus Toxoids and Acellular Pertussis Vaccine Adsorbed (DTaP) and Haemophilus influenzae type b Conjugate (Meningococcal Protein Conjugate) and Hepatitis B (Recombinant) Vaccine
In a clinical trial, 1913 healthy children 12 to 15 months of age were randomized to receive ProQuad plus diphtheria and tetanus toxoids and acellular pertussis vaccine adsorbed (DTaP) and *Haemophilus influenzae* type b conjugate (meningococcal protein conjugate) and hepatitis B (recombinant) vaccine concomitantly at separate injection sites (N=949), ProQuad at the initial visit followed by DTaP and *Haemophilus* b conjugate and hepatitis B (recombinant) vaccine given concomitantly 6 weeks later (N=485), or M-M-R II and VARIVAX given concomitantly at separate injection sites (N=479) at the first visit. *[See Adverse Reactions (6.1) for ethnicity and gender information.]* Seroconversion rates and antibody titers for measles, mumps, rubella, varicella, anti-PRP, and hepatitis B were comparable between the 2 groups given ProQuad at approximately 6 weeks postvaccination indicating that ProQuad and *Haemophilus* b conjugate (meningococcal protein conjugate) and hepatitis B (recombinant) vaccine may be administered concomitantly at separate injection sites (see Table 18 below). Response rates for measles, mumps, rubella, varicella, *Haemophilus influenzae* type b, and hepatitis B were not inferior in children given ProQuad plus *Haemophilus influenzae* type b conjugate (meningococcal protein conjugate) and hepatitis B (recombinant) vaccines concomitantly when compared to ProQuad at the initial visit and *Haemophilus influenzae* type b conjugate (meningococcal protein conjugate) and hepatitis B (recombinant) vaccines given concomitantly 6 weeks later. There are insufficient data to support

concomitant vaccination with diphtheria and tetanus toxoids and acellular pertussis vaccine adsorbed (data not shown).
[See table 18 above]

15 REFERENCES

1. Levy O, et al. Disseminated varicella infection due to the vaccine strain of varicella-zoster virus, in a patient with a novel deficiency in natural killer T cells. *J Infect Dis.* 188(7):948-53, 2003.
2. Committee on Infectious Diseases, American Academy of Pediatrics. In: Pickering LK, Baker CJ, Overturf GD, et al., eds. Red Book: 2003 Report of the Committee on Infectious Diseases. 26th ed. Elk Grove Village, IL: American Academy of Pediatrics. 419-29, 2003.
3. Peltola H, et al. The elimination of indigenous measles, mumps, and rubella from Finland by a 12-year, two-dose vaccination program. *N Engl J Med.* 331(21):1397-1402, 1994.
4. Guess HA, et al. Population-based studies of varicella complications. *Pediatrics.* 78(4 Pt 2):723-727, 1986.
5. Recommendations of the Immunization Practices Advisory Committee (ACIP), Mumps Prevention. *MMWR.* 38(22):388-392, 397-400, 1989.
6. Rubella vaccination during pregnancy--United States, 1971-1986. *MMWR Morb Mortal Wkly Rep.* 36(28):457-61, 1987.
7. Bohlke K, Galil K, Jackson LA, et al. Postpartum varicella vaccination: Is the vaccine virus excreted in breast milk? *Obstetrics and Gynecology.* 102(5):970-977, 2003.
8. Dolbear GL, Moffat J, Falkner C and Wojtowycz M. A Pilot Study: Is attenuated varicella virus present in breast milk after postpartum immunization? *Obstetrics and Gynecology.* 101(4 Suppl.):47S-47S, 2003.
9. Weibel RE, et al. Clinical and laboratory studies of combined live measles, mumps, and rubella vaccines using the RA 27/3 rubella virus. *Proc Soc Exp Biol Med.* 165(2):323-326, 1980.
10. Hilleman MR, Stokes J, Jr., Buynak EB, Weibel R, Halenda R, Goldner H. Studies of live attenuated measles virus vaccine in man: II. appraisal of efficacy. *Am J Public Health.* 52(2):44-56, 1962.
11. Krugman S, Giles JP, Jacobs AM. Studies on an attenuated measles-virus vaccine: VI. clinical, antigenic and prophylactic effects of vaccine in institutionalized children. *N Engl J Med.* 263(4):174-7, 1960.

Table 17: Statistical Analysis of Non-Inferiority in Geometric Mean Titers (GMT) to S. pneumoniae Serotypes at 6 Weeks Postvaccination Among Subjects Who Received VAQTA Concomitantly or Non-Concomitantly With ProQuad and PCV7* (Per-Protocol Analysis Set)

Serotype	Group 1: Concomitant VAQTA with ProQuad + PCV7 (N=330)		Group 2: Non-concomitant VAQTA separate from ProQuad + PCV7 (N=323)		Fold-Difference[†] (95% CI)
	n	Estimated Response[†]	n	Estimated Response[†]	
4	246	1.9	247	1.7	1.1 (0.9, 1.3)
6B	246	9.9	246	9.9	1.0 (0.8, 1.2)
9V	247	3.7	247	4.2	0.9 (0.8, 1.0)
14	248	7.8	247	7.6	1.0 (0.9, 1.2)
18C	247	2.9	247	2.7	1.1 (0.9, 1.3)
19F	248	4.0	248	3.8	1.1 (0.9, 1.2)
23F	247	5.1	247	4.4	1.1 (1.0, 1.3)

CI = Confidence interval; GMT = Geometric mean titer; N = Number of subjects enrolled/randomized; n = Number of subjects contributing to the per-protocol analysis for *S. pneumoniae* serotypes.
* PCV7 = Pneumococcal 7-valent conjugate vaccine.
† Estimated responses and their fold-difference were based on statistical analysis models adjusting for combined study center and prevaccination titer.
The conclusion of non-inferiority was based on the lower bound of the 2-sided 95% CI on the fold-difference being greater than 0.5 (*i.e.*, excluding a decrease of 2-fold or more). This indicates that the fold-difference was statistically significantly less than the prespecified clinically relevant 2-fold difference at the 1-sided alpha = 0.025 level.

Table 18: Summary of the Comparison of the Immunogenicity Endpoints for Measles, Mumps, Rubella, Varicella, Haemophilus influenzae type b, and Hepatitis B Responses Following Vaccination with ProQuad, Haemophilus influenzae type b Conjugate (Meningococcal Protein Conjugate), and Hepatitis B (Recombinant) Vaccine and DTaP Administered Concomitantly Versus Non-Concomitant Vaccination with ProQuad Followed by These Vaccines

Vaccine Antigen	Parameter	Concomitant Group N=949 Response	Non-Concomitant Group N=485 Response	Risk Difference (95% CI)	Criterion for Non-inferiority
Measles	% ≥120 mIU/mL	97.8%	98.7%	-0.9 (-2.3, 0.6)	LB >-5.0
Mumps	% ≥10 ELISA Ab units/mL	95.4%	95.1%	0.3 (-1.7, 2.6)	LB >-5.0
Rubella	% ≥10 IU/mL	98.6%	99.3%	-0.7 (-1.8, 0.5)	LB >-5.0
Varicella	% ≥5 gpELISA units/mL	89.6%	90.8%	-1.2 (-4.1, 2.0)	LB >-10.0
HiB-PRP	% ≥1.0 mcg/mL	94.6%	96.5%	-1.9 (-4.1, 0.8)	LB >-10.0
HepB	% ≥10 mIU/mL	95.9%	98.8%	-2.8 (-4.8, -0.8)	LB >10.0

HiB-PRP = *Haemophilus influenzae* type b, polyribosyl phosphate; HepB = hepatitis B; LB = lower bound, limit for non-inferiority comparison.

12. Hilleman MR, Weibel RE, Buynak EB, Stokes J, Jr., Whitman JE, Jr. Live, attenuated mumps-virus vaccine. 4. Protective efficacy as measured in a field evaluation. *N Engl J Med.* 276(5):252-8, 1967.

13. Sugg WC, Finger JA, Levine RH, Pagano JS. Field evaluation of live virus mumps vaccine. *J Pediatr.* 72(4):461-6, 1968.

14. The Benevento and Compobasso Pediatricians Network for the Control of Vaccine-Preventable Diseases, D'Argenio P, Citarella A, Selvaggi MTM. Field evaluation of the clinical effectiveness of vaccines against pertussis, measles, rubella and mumps. *Vaccine.* 16(8):818-22, 1998.

15. Furukawa T, Miyata T, Kondo K, Kuno K, Isomura S, Takekoshi T. Rubella vaccination during an epidemic. *JAMA.* 213(6):987-90, 1970.

16. Vazquez M, et al. The effectiveness of the varicella vaccine in clinical practice. *N Engl J Med.* 344(13):955-960, 2001.

17. Kuter B, et al. Ten year follow-up of healthy children who received one or two injections of varicella vaccine. *Pediatr Infect Dis J.* 23(2):132-137, 2004.

16   HOW SUPPLIED/STORAGE AND HANDLING

No. 4999 — ProQuad is supplied as follows:
(1) a package of 10 single-dose vials of lyophilized vaccine, NDC 0006-4999-00 (package A)
(2) a separate package of 10 vials of sterile water diluent (package B).

Storage
To maintain potency, ProQuad must be stored frozen between -58°F and +5°F (-50°C to -15°C). Use of dry ice may subject ProQuad to temperatures colder than -58°F (-50°C).
Before reconstitution, store the lyophilized vaccine continuously in a reliably maintained freezer (*e.g.*, chest, frost-free) for up to 18 months.
ProQuad may be stored at refrigerator temperature (36° to 46°F, 2° to 8°C) for up to 72 hours prior to reconstitution. Discard any ProQuad vaccine stored at 36° to 46°F which is not used within 72 hours of removal from 5°F (-15°C) storage.
Protect the vaccine from light at all times since such exposure may inactivate the vaccine viruses.
IF NOT USED IMMEDIATELY, THE RECONSTITUTED VACCINE MAY BE STORED AT ROOM TEMPERATURE, PROTECTED FROM LIGHT, FOR UP TO 30 MINUTES. DISCARD RECONSTITUTED VACCINE IF IT IS NOT USED WITHIN 30 MINUTES.
DO NOT FREEZE RECONSTITUTED VACCINE.
Diluent should be stored separately at room temperature (68° to 77°F, 20° to 25°C), or in a refrigerator (36° to 46°F, 2° to 8°C).
For information regarding stability under conditions other than those recommended, call 1-800-MERCK-90.

17   PATIENT COUNSELING INFORMATION

Instructions
Provide the required vaccine information to the patient, parent, or guardian.
Inform the patient, parent, or guardian of the benefits and risks associated with vaccination.
Inform the patient, parent, or guardian that the vaccine recipient should avoid use of salicylates for 6 weeks after vaccination with ProQuad *[see Adverse Reactions (6.1) and Drug Interactions (7.2)].*
Instruct postpubertal females to avoid pregnancy for 3 months following vaccination *[see Indications and Usage (1) and Use In Specific Populations (8.1)].*
Inform patients, parents, or guardians that vaccination with ProQuad may not offer 100% protection from measles, mumps, rubella, and varicella infection.
Instruct patients, parents, or guardians to report any adverse reactions to their health care provider. The U.S. Department of Health and Human Services has established a Vaccine Adverse Event Reporting System (VAERS) to accept all reports of suspected adverse events after the administration of any vaccine, including but not limited to the reporting of events required by the National Childhood Vaccine Injury Act of 1986. For information or a copy of the vaccine reporting form, call the VAERS toll-free number at 1-800-822-7967, or report online at http://www.vaers.hhs.gov.
Dist. by: Merck Sharp & Dohme Corp., a subsidiary of **MERCK & CO., INC.,** Whitehouse Station, NJ 08889, USA
For patent information:
www.merck.com/product/patent/home.html
Copyright © 2014 Merck Sharp & Dohme Corp., a subsidiary of Merck & Co., Inc.
All rights reserved.
uspi-v221-i-fro-1403r909

PROSCAR®
(finasteride)
Tablets   ℞

HIGHLIGHTS OF PRESCRIBING INFORMATION
These highlights do not include all the information needed to use PROSCAR safely and effectively. See full prescribing information for PROSCAR.
PROSCAR® (finasteride) Tablets
Initial U.S. Approval: 1992

————INDICATIONS AND USAGE————
PROSCAR, is a 5α-reductase inhibitor, indicated for the treatment of symptomatic benign prostatic hyperplasia (BPH) in men with an enlarged prostate to (1.1):
• Improve symptoms
• Reduce the risk of acute urinary retention
• Reduce the risk of the need for surgery including transurethral resection of the prostate (TURP) and prostatectomy.
PROSCAR administered in combination with the alpha-blocker doxazosin is indicated to reduce the risk of symptomatic progression of BPH (a confirmed ≥4 point increase in American Urological Association (AUA) symptom score) (1.2).
Limitations of Use: PROSCAR is not approved for the prevention of prostate cancer (1.3).

———DOSAGE AND ADMINISTRATION———
PROSCAR may be administered with or without meals (2).
Monotherapy: One tablet (5 mg) taken once a day (2.1).
Combination with Doxazosin: One tablet (5 mg) taken once a day in combination with the alpha-blocker doxazosin (2.2).

———DOSAGE FORMS AND STRENGTHS———
5-mg film-coated tablets (3).

————————CONTRAINDICATIONS————————
Hypersensitivity to any components of this product (4).
Women who are or may potentially be pregnant (4, 5.4, 8.1, 16).

————WARNINGS AND PRECAUTIONS————
• PROSCAR reduces serum prostate specific antigen (PSA) levels by approximately 50%. However, any confirmed increase in PSA while on PROSCAR may signal the presence of prostate cancer and should be evaluated, even if those values are still within the normal range for men not taking a 5α-reductase inhibitor (5.1).
• PROSCAR may increase the risk of high-grade prostate cancer (5.2, 6.1).
• Women should not handle crushed or broken PROSCAR tablets when they are pregnant or may potentially be pregnant due to potential risk to a male fetus (5.3, 8.1, 16).
• PROSCAR is not indicated for use in pediatric patients or women (5.4, 8.1, 8.3, 8.4, 12.3).
• Prior to initiating treatment with PROSCAR for BPH, consideration should be given to other urological conditions that may cause similar symptoms (5.6).

————————ADVERSE REACTIONS————————
The drug-related adverse reactions, reported in ≥1% in patients treated with PROSCAR and greater than in patients treated with placebo over a 4-year study are: impotence, decreased libido, decreased volume of ejaculate, breast enlargement, breast tenderness and rash (6.1).
To report SUSPECTED ADVERSE REACTIONS, contact Merck Sharp & Dohme Corp., a subsidiary of Merck & Co., Inc., at 1-877-888-4231 or FDA at 1-800-FDA-1088 or www.fda.gov/medwatch.
See 17 for PATIENT COUNSELING INFORMATION and FDA-approved patient labeling
                                                    Revised: 09/2013

FULL PRESCRIBING INFORMATION

1   INDICATIONS AND USAGE
1.1   Monotherapy
PROSCAR® is indicated for the treatment of symptomatic benign prostatic hyperplasia (BPH) in men with an enlarged prostate to:
• Improve symptoms
• Reduce the risk of acute urinary retention
• Reduce the risk of the need for surgery including transurethral resection of the prostate (TURP) and prostatectomy.
1.2   Combination with Alpha-Blocker
PROSCAR administered in combination with the alpha-blocker doxazosin is indicated to reduce the risk of symptomatic progression of BPH (a confirmed ≥4 point increase in American Urological Association (AUA) symptom score).
1.3   Limitations of Use
PROSCAR is not approved for the prevention of prostate cancer.

2   DOSAGE AND ADMINISTRATION
PROSCAR may be administered with or without meals.
2.1   Monotherapy
The recommended dose of PROSCAR is one tablet (5 mg) taken once a day *[see Clinical Studies (14.1)].*
2.2   Combination with Alpha-Blocker
The recommended dose of PROSCAR is one tablet (5 mg) taken once a day in combination with the alpha-blocker doxazosin *[see Clinical Studies (14.2)].*

3   DOSAGE FORMS AND STRENGTHS
5-mg blue, modified apple-shaped, film-coated tablets, with the code MSD 72 on one side and PROSCAR on the other.

4   CONTRAINDICATIONS
PROSCAR is contraindicated in the following:
• Hypersensitivity to any component of this medication.
• Pregnancy. Finasteride use is contraindicated in women when they are or may potentially be pregnant. Because of the ability of Type II 5α-reductase inhibitors to inhibit the conversion of testosterone to 5α-dihydrotestosterone (DHT), finasteride may cause abnormalities of the external genitalia of a male fetus of a pregnant woman who receives finasteride. If this drug is used during pregnancy, or if pregnancy occurs while taking this drug, the pregnant woman should be apprised of the potential hazard to the male fetus. *[See also Warnings and Precautions (5.3), Use in Specific Populations (8.1), How Supplied/Storage and Handling (16) and Patient Counseling Information (17.2).]* In female rats, low doses of finasteride administered during pregnancy have produced abnormalities of the external genitalia in male offspring.

5   WARNINGS AND PRECAUTIONS
5.1   Effects on Prostate Specific Antigen (PSA) and the Use of PSA in Prostate Cancer Detection
In clinical studies, PROSCAR reduced serum PSA concentration by approximately 50% within six months of treat-

ment. This decrease is predictable over the entire range of PSA values in patients with symptomatic BPH, although it may vary in individuals.

For interpretation of serial PSAs in men taking PROSCAR, a new PSA baseline should be established at least six months after starting treatment and PSA monitored periodically thereafter. Any confirmed increase from the lowest PSA value while on PROSCAR may signal the presence of prostate cancer and should be evaluated, even if PSA levels are still within the normal range for men not taking a 5α-reductase inhibitor. Non-compliance with PROSCAR therapy may also affect PSA test results. To interpret an isolated PSA value in patients treated with PROSCAR for six months or more, PSA values should be doubled for comparison with normal ranges in untreated men. These adjustments preserve the utility of PSA to detect prostate cancer in men treated with PROSCAR.

PROSCAR may also cause decreases in serum PSA in the presence of prostate cancer.

The ratio of free to total PSA (percent free PSA) remains constant even under the influence of PROSCAR. If clinicians elect to use percent free PSA as an aid in the detection of prostate cancer in men undergoing finasteride therapy, no adjustment to its value appears necessary.

5.2 Increased Risk of High-Grade Prostate Cancer
Men aged 55 and over with a normal digital rectal examination and PSA ≤3.0 ng/mL at baseline taking finasteride 5 mg/day in the 7-year Prostate Cancer Prevention Trial (PCPT) had an increased risk of Gleason score 8-10 prostate cancer (finasteride 1.8% vs placebo 1.1%). [See Indications and Usage (1.3) and Adverse Reactions (6.1).] Similar results were observed in a 4-year placebo-controlled clinical trial with another 5α-reductase inhibitor (dutasteride, AVODART) (1% dutasteride vs 0.5% placebo). 5α-reductase inhibitors may increase the risk of development of high-grade prostate cancer. Whether the effect of 5α-reductase inhibitors to reduce prostate volume, or study-related factors, impacted the results of these studies has not been established.

5.3 Exposure of Women — Risk to Male Fetus
Women should not handle crushed or broken PROSCAR tablets when they are pregnant or may potentially be pregnant because of the possibility of absorption of finasteride and the subsequent potential risk to a male fetus. PROSCAR tablets are coated and will prevent contact with the active ingredient during normal handling, provided that the tablets have not been broken or crushed. [See Contraindications (4), Use in Specific Populations (8.1), Clinical Pharmacology (12.3), How Supplied/Storage and Handling (16) and Patient Counseling Information (17.2).]

5.4 Pediatric Patients and Women
PROSCAR is not indicated for use in pediatric patients [see Use in Specific Populations (8.4) and Clinical Pharmacology (12.3)] or women [see also Warnings and Precautions (5.3), Use in Specific Populations (8.1), Clinical Pharmacology (12.3), How Supplied/Storage and Handling (16) and Patient Counseling Information (17.2)].

5.5 Effect on Semen Characteristics
Treatment with PROSCAR for 24 weeks to evaluate semen parameters in healthy male volunteers revealed no clinically meaningful effects on sperm concentration, mobility, morphology, or pH. A 0.6 mL (22.1%) median decrease in ejaculate volume with a concomitant reduction in total sperm per ejaculate was observed. These parameters remained within the normal range and were reversible upon discontinuation of therapy with an average time to return to baseline of 84 weeks.

5.6 Consideration of Other Urological Conditions
Prior to initiating treatment with PROSCAR, consideration should be given to other urological conditions that may cause similar symptoms. In addition, prostate cancer and BPH may coexist.

Patients with large residual urinary volume and/or severely diminished urinary flow should be carefully monitored for obstructive uropathy. These patients may not be candidates for finasteride therapy.

6 ADVERSE REACTIONS
6.1 Clinical Trials Experience
PROSCAR is generally well tolerated; adverse reactions usually have been mild and transient.

4-Year Placebo-Controlled Study (PLESS)
In PLESS, 1524 patients treated with PROSCAR and 1516 patients treated with placebo were evaluated for safety over a period of 4 years. The most frequently reported adverse reactions were related to sexual function. 3.7% (57 patients) treated with PROSCAR and 2.1% (32 patients) treated with placebo discontinued therapy as a result of adverse reactions related to sexual function, which are the most frequently reported adverse reactions.

Table 1 presents the only clinical adverse reactions considered possibly, probably or definitely drug related by the investigator, for which the incidence on PROSCAR was ≥1% and greater than placebo over the 4 years of the study. In

years 2-4 of the study, there was no significant difference between treatment groups in the incidences of impotence, decreased libido and ejaculation disorder.
[See table 1 above]

Phase III Studies and 5-Year Open Extensions
The adverse experience profile in the 1-year, placebo-controlled, Phase III studies, the 5-year open extensions, and PLESS were similar.

Medical Therapy of Prostatic Symptoms (MTOPS) Study
In the MTOPS study, 3047 men with symptomatic BPH were randomized to receive PROSCAR 5 mg/day (n=768), doxazosin 4 or 8 mg/day (n=756), the combination of PROSCAR 5 mg/day and doxazosin 4 or 8 mg/day (n=786), or placebo (n=737) for 4 to 6 years. [See Clinical Studies (14.2).]

The incidence rates of drug-related adverse experiences reported by ≥2% of patients in any treatment group in the MTOPS Study are listed in Table 2.

The individual adverse effects which occurred more frequently in the combination group compared to either drug

alone were: asthenia, postural hypotension, peripheral edema, dizziness, decreased libido, rhinitis, abnormal ejaculation, impotence and abnormal sexual function (see Table 2). Of these, the incidence of abnormal ejaculation in patients receiving combination therapy was comparable to the sum of the incidences of this adverse experience reported for the two monotherapies.

Combination therapy with finasteride and doxazosin was associated with no new clinical adverse experience.

Four patients in MTOPS reported the adverse experience breast cancer. Three of these patients were on finasteride only and one was on combination therapy. [See Long-Term Data.]

The MTOPS Study was not specifically designed to make statistical comparisons between groups for reported adverse experiences. In addition, direct comparisons of safety data between the MTOPS study and previous studies of the single agents may not be appropriate based upon differences in patient population, dosage or dose regimen, and other procedural and study design elements.
[See table 2 above]

Table 1: Drug-Related Adverse Experiences

	Year 1 (%)		Years 2, 3 and 4* (%)	
	Finasteride	Placebo	Finasteride	Placebo
Impotence	8.1	3.7	5.1	5.1
Decreased Libido	6.4	3.4	2.6	2.6
Decreased Volume of Ejaculate	3.7	0.8	1.5	0.5
Ejaculation Disorder	0.8	0.1	0.2	0.1
Breast Enlargement	0.5	0.1	1.8	1.1
Breast Tenderness	0.4	0.1	0.7	0.3
Rash	0.5	0.2	0.5	0.1

N = 1524 and 1516, finasteride vs placebo, respectively
* Combined Years 2-4

Table 2: Incidence ≥2% in One or More Treatment Groups Drug-Related Clinical Adverse Experiences in MTOPS

Adverse Experience	Placebo (N=737) (%)	Doxazosin 4 mg or 8 mg* (N=756) (%)	Finasteride (N=768) (%)	Combination (N=786) (%)
Body as a whole				
Asthenia	7.1	15.7	5.3	16.8
Headache	2.3	4.1	2.0	2.3
Cardiovascular				
Hypotension	0.7	3.4	1.2	1.5
Postural Hypotension	8.0	16.7	9.1	17.8
Metabolic and Nutritional				
Peripheral Edema	0.9	2.6	1.3	3.3
Nervous				
Dizziness	8.1	17.7	7.4	23.2
Libido Decreased	5.7	7.0	10.0	11.6
Somnolence	1.5	3.7	1.7	3.1
Respiratory				
Dyspnea	0.7	2.1	0.7	1.9
Rhinitis	0.5	1.3	1.0	2.4
Urogenital				
Abnormal Ejaculation	2.3	4.5	7.2	14.1
Gynecomastia	0.7	1.1	2.2	1.5
Impotence	12.2	14.4	18.5	22.6
Sexual Function Abnormal	0.9	2.0	2.5	3.1

* Doxazosin dose was achieved by weekly titration (1 to 2 to 4 to 8 mg). The final tolerated dose (4 mg or 8 mg) was administered at end-Week 4. Only those patients tolerating at least 4 mg were kept on doxazosin. The majority of patients received the 8-mg dose over the duration of the study.

Long-Term Data

High-Grade Prostate Cancer

The PCPT trial was a 7-year randomized, double-blind, placebo-controlled trial that enrolled 18,882 men ≥55 years of age with a normal digital rectal examination and a PSA ≤3.0 ng/mL. Men received either PROSCAR (finasteride 5 mg) or placebo daily. Patients were evaluated annually with PSA and digital rectal exams. Biopsies were performed for elevated PSA, an abnormal digital rectal exam, or the end of study. The incidence of Gleason score 8-10 prostate cancer was higher in men treated with finasteride (1.8%) than in those treated with placebo (1.1%) *[see Indications and Usage (1.3) and Warnings and Precautions (5.2)]*. In a 4-year placebo-controlled clinical trial with another 5α-reductase inhibitor (dutasteride, AVODART), similar results for Gleason score 8-10 prostate cancer were observed (1% dutasteride vs 0.5% placebo).

No clinical benefit has been demonstrated in patients with prostate cancer treated with PROSCAR.

Breast Cancer

During the 4- to 6-year placebo- and comparator-controlled MTOPS study that enrolled 3047 men, there were 4 cases of breast cancer in men treated with finasteride but no cases in men not treated with finasteride. During the 4-year, placebo-controlled PLESS study that enrolled 3040 men, there were 2 cases of breast cancer in placebo-treated men but no cases in men treated with finasteride. During the 7-year placebo-controlled Prostate Cancer Prevention Trial (PCPT) that enrolled 18,882 men, there was 1 case of breast cancer in men treated with finasteride, and 1 case of breast cancer in men treated with placebo. The relationship between long-term use of finasteride and male breast neoplasia is currently unknown.

Sexual Function

There is no evidence of increased sexual adverse experiences with increased duration of treatment with PROSCAR. New reports of drug-related sexual adverse experiences decreased with duration of therapy.

6.2 Postmarketing Experience

The following additional adverse events have been reported in postmarketing experience with PROSCAR. Because these events are reported voluntarily from a population of uncertain size, it is not always possible to reliably estimate their frequency or establish a causal relationship to drug exposure:

- hypersensitivity reactions, such as pruritus, urticaria, and angioedema (including swelling of the lips, tongue, throat, and face)
- testicular pain
- sexual dysfunction that continued after discontinuation of treatment, including erectile dysfunction, decreased libido and ejaculation disorders (e.g. reduced ejaculate volume). These events were reported rarely in men taking PROSCAR for the treatment of BPH. Most men were older and were taking concomitant medications and/or had comorbid conditions. The independent role of PROSCAR in these events is unknown.
- male infertility and/or poor seminal quality were reported rarely in men taking PROSCAR for the treatment of BPH. Normalization or improvement of poor seminal quality has been reported after discontinuation of finasteride. The independent role of PROSCAR in these events is unknown.
- depression
- male breast cancer.

The following additional adverse event related to sexual dysfunction that continued after discontinuation of treatment has been reported in postmarketing experience with finasteride at lower doses used to treat male pattern baldness. Because the event is reported voluntarily from a population of uncertain size, it is not always possible to reliably estimate its frequency or establish a causal relationship to drug exposure:

- orgasm disorders

7 DRUG INTERACTIONS

7.1 Cytochrome P450-Linked Drug Metabolizing Enzyme System

No drug interactions of clinical importance have been identified. Finasteride does not appear to affect the cytochrome P450-linked drug metabolizing enzyme system. Compounds that have been tested in man have included antipyrine, digoxin, propranolol, theophylline, and warfarin and no clinically meaningful interactions were found.

7.2 Other Concomitant Therapy

Although specific interaction studies were not performed, PROSCAR was concomitantly used in clinical studies with acetaminophen, acetylsalicylic acid, α-blockers, angiotensin-converting enzyme (ACE) inhibitors, analgesics, anti-convulsants, beta-adrenergic blocking agents, diuretics, calcium channel blockers, cardiac nitrates, HMG-CoA reductase inhibitors, nonsteroidal anti-inflammatory drugs (NSAIDs), benzodiazepines, H₂ antagonists and quinolone anti-infectives without evidence of clinically significant adverse interactions.

8 USE IN SPECIFIC POPULATIONS

8.1 Pregnancy

Pregnancy Category X. *[See Contraindications (4).]*

PROSCAR is contraindicated for use in women who are or may become pregnant. PROSCAR is a Type II 5α-reductase inhibitor that prevents conversion of testosterone to 5α-dihydrotestosterone (DHT), a hormone necessary for normal development of male genitalia. In animal studies, finasteride caused abnormal development of external genitalia in male fetuses. If this drug is used during pregnancy, or if the patient becomes pregnant while taking this drug, the patient should be apprised of the potential hazard to the male fetus.

Abnormal male genital development is an expected consequence when conversion of testosterone to 5α-dihydrotestosterone (DHT) is inhibited by 5α-reductase inhibitors. These outcomes are similar to those reported in male infants with genetic 5α-reductase deficiency. Women could be exposed to finasteride through contact with crushed or broken PROSCAR tablets or semen from a male partner taking PROSCAR. With regard to finasteride exposure through the skin, PROSCAR tablets are coated and will prevent skin contact with finasteride during normal handling if the tablets have not been crushed or broken. Women who are pregnant or may become pregnant should not handle crushed or broken PROSCAR tablets because of possible exposure of a male fetus. If a pregnant woman comes in contact with crushed or broken PROSCAR tablets, the contact area should be washed immediately with soap and water. With regard to potential finasteride exposure through semen, two studies have been conducted in men receiving PROSCAR 5 mg/day that measured finasteride concentrations in semen *[see Clinical Pharmacology (12.3)]*.

In an embryo-fetal development study, pregnant rats received finasteride during the period of major organogenesis (gestation days 6 to 17). At maternal doses of oral finasteride approximately 0.1 to 86 times the maximum recommended human dose (MRHD) of 5 mg/day (based on AUC at animal doses of 0.1 to 100 mg/kg/day) there was a dose-dependent increase in hypospadias that occurred in 3.6 to 100% of male offspring. Exposure multiples were estimated using data from nonpregnant rats. Days 16 to 17 of gestation is a critical period in male fetal rats for differentiation of the external genitalia. At oral maternal doses approximately 0.03 times the MRHD (based on AUC at animal dose of 0.03 mg/kg/day), male offspring had decreased prostatic and seminal vesicular weights, delayed preputial separation and transient nipple development. Decreased anogenital distance occurred in male offspring of pregnant rats that received approximately 0.003 times the MRHD (based on AUC at animal dose of 0.003 mg/kg/day). No abnormalities were observed in female offspring at any maternal dose of finasteride.

No developmental abnormalities were observed in the offspring of untreated females mated with finasteride treated male rats that received approximately 61 times the MRHD (based on AUC at animal dose of 80 mg/kg/day). Slightly decreased fertility was observed in male offspring after administration of about 3 times the MRHD (based on AUC at animal dose of 3 mg/kg/day) to female rats during late gestation and lactation. No effects on fertility were seen in female offspring under these conditions.

No evidence of male external genital malformations or other abnormalities were observed in rabbit fetuses exposed to finasteride during the period of major organogenesis (gestation days 6-18) at maternal oral doses up to 100 mg/kg/day, (finasteride exposure levels were not measured in rabbits). However, this study may not have included the critical period for finasteride effects on development of male external genitalia in the rabbit.

The fetal effects of maternal finasteride exposure during the period of embryonic and fetal development were evaluated in the rhesus monkey (gestation days 20-100), in a species and development period more predictive of specific effects in humans than the studies in rats and rabbits. Intravenous administration of finasteride to pregnant monkeys at doses as high as 800 ng/day (estimated maximal blood concentration of 1.86 ng/mL or about 143 times the highest estimated exposure of pregnant women to finasteride from semen of men taking 5 mg/day) resulted in no abnormalities in male fetuses. In confirmation of the relevance of the rhesus model for human fetal development, oral administration of a dose of finasteride (2 mg/kg/day or approximately 18,000 times the highest estimated blood levels of finasteride from semen of men taking 5 mg/day) to pregnant monkeys resulted in external genital abnormalities in male fetuses. No other abnormalities were observed in male fetuses and no finasteride-related abnormalities were observed in female fetuses at any dose.

8.3 Nursing Mothers

PROSCAR is not indicated for use in women.

It is not known whether finasteride is excreted in human milk.

8.4 Pediatric Use

PROSCAR is not indicated for use in pediatric patients. Safety and effectiveness in pediatric patients have not been established.

8.5 Geriatric Use

Of the total number of subjects included in PLESS, 1480 and 105 subjects were 65 and over and 75 and over, respectively. No overall differences in safety or effectiveness were observed between these subjects and younger subjects, and other reported clinical experience has not identified differences in responses between the elderly and younger patients. No dosage adjustment is necessary in the elderly *[see Clinical Pharmacology (12.3) and Clinical Studies (14)]*.

8.6 Hepatic Impairment

Caution should be exercised in the administration of PROSCAR in those patients with liver function abnormalities, as finasteride is metabolized extensively in the liver *[see Clinical Pharmacology (12.3)]*.

8.7 Renal Impairment

No dosage adjustment is necessary in patients with renal impairment *[see Clinical Pharmacology (12.3)]*.

10 OVERDOSAGE

Patients have received single doses of PROSCAR up to 400 mg and multiple doses of PROSCAR up to 80 mg/day for three months without adverse effects. Until further experience is obtained, no specific treatment for an overdose with PROSCAR can be recommended.

Significant lethality was observed in male and female mice at single oral doses of 1500 mg/m² (500 mg/kg) and in female and male rats at single oral doses of 2360 mg/m² (400 mg/kg) and 5900 mg/m² (1000 mg/kg), respectively.

11 DESCRIPTION

PROSCAR (finasteride), a synthetic 4-azasteroid compound, is a specific inhibitor of steroid Type II 5α-reductase, an intracellular enzyme that converts the androgen testosterone into 5α-dihydrotestosterone (DHT).

Finasteride is 4-azaandrost-1-ene-17-carboxamide, N-(1,1-dimethylethyl)-3-oxo-,(5α,17β)-. The empirical formula of finasteride is $C_{23}H_{36}N_2O_2$ and its molecular weight is 372.55. Its structural formula is:

Finasteride is a white crystalline powder with a melting point near 250°C. It is freely soluble in chloroform and in lower alcohol solvents, but is practically insoluble in water. PROSCAR (finasteride) tablets for oral administration are film-coated tablets that contain 5 mg of finasteride and the following inactive ingredients: hydrous lactose, microcrystalline cellulose, pregelatinized starch, sodium starch glycolate, hydroxypropyl cellulose LF, hydroxypropyl methylcellulose, titanium dioxide, magnesium stearate, talc, docusate sodium, FD&C Blue 2 aluminum lake and yellow iron oxide.

12 CLINICAL PHARMACOLOGY

12.1 Mechanism of Action

The development and enlargement of the prostate gland is dependent on the potent androgen, 5α-dihydrotestosterone (DHT). Type II 5α-reductase metabolizes testosterone to DHT in the prostate gland, liver and skin. DHT induces androgenic effects by binding to androgen receptors in the cell nuclei of these organs.

Finasteride is a competitive and specific inhibitor of Type II 5α-reductase with which it slowly forms a stable enzyme complex. Turnover from this complex is extremely slow (t½ ~ 30 days). This has been demonstrated both *in vivo* and *in vitro*. Finasteride has no affinity for the androgen receptor. In man, the 5α-reduced steroid metabolites in blood and urine are decreased after administration of finasteride.

12.2 Pharmacodynamics

In man, a single 5-mg oral dose of PROSCAR produces a rapid reduction in serum DHT concentration, with the maximum effect observed 8 hours after the first dose. The suppression of DHT is maintained throughout the 24-hour dosing interval and with continued treatment. Daily dosing of PROSCAR at 5 mg/day for up to 4 years has been shown to reduce the serum DHT concentration by approximately 70%. The median circulating level of testosterone increased by approximately 10-20% but remained within the physiologic range. In a separate study in healthy men treated with finasteride 1 mg/day (n=82) or placebo (n=69), mean circulating levels of testosterone and estradiol were increased by approximately 15% as compared to baseline, but these remained within the physiologic range.

In patients receiving PROSCAR 5 mg/day, increases of about 10% were observed in luteinizing hormone (LH) and follicle-stimulating hormone (FSH), but levels remained within the normal range. In healthy volunteers, treatment with PROSCAR did not alter the response of LH and FSH to gonadotropin-releasing hormone indicating that the hypothalamic-pituitary-testicular axis was not affected.

In patients with BPH, PROSCAR has no effect on circulating levels of cortisol, prolactin, thyroid-stimulating hormone, or thyroxine. No clinically meaningful effect was observed on the plasma lipid profile (i.e., total cholesterol, low density lipoproteins, high density lipoproteins and triglycerides) or bone mineral density.

Adult males with genetically inherited Type II 5α-reductase deficiency also have decreased levels of DHT. Except for the associated urogenital defects present at birth, no other clinical abnormalities related to Type II 5α-reductase deficiency have been observed in these individuals. These individuals have a small prostate gland throughout life and do not develop BPH.

In patients with BPH treated with finasteride (1-100 mg/day) for 7-10 days prior to prostatectomy, an approximate 80% lower DHT content was measured in prostatic tissue removed at surgery, compared to placebo; testosterone tissue concentration was increased up to 10 times over pretreatment levels, relative to placebo. Intraprostatic content of PSA was also decreased.

In healthy male volunteers treated with PROSCAR for 14 days, discontinuation of therapy resulted in a return of DHT levels to pretreatment levels in approximately 2 weeks. In patients treated for three months, prostate volume, which declined by approximately 20%, returned to close to baseline value after approximately three months of discontinuation of therapy.

12.3 Pharmacokinetics

Absorption

In a study of 15 healthy young subjects, the mean bioavailability of finasteride 5-mg tablets was 63% (range 34-108%), based on the ratio of area under the curve (AUC) relative to an intravenous (IV) reference dose. Maximum finasteride plasma concentration averaged 37 ng/mL (range, 27-49 ng/mL) and was reached 1-2 hours postdose. Bioavailability of finasteride was not affected by food.

Distribution

Mean steady-state volume of distribution was 76 liters (range, 44-96 liters). Approximately 90% of circulating finasteride is bound to plasma proteins. There is a slow accumulation phase for finasteride after multiple dosing. After dosing with 5 mg/day of finasteride for 17 days, plasma concentrations of finasteride were 47 and 54% higher than after the first dose in men 45-60 years old (n=12) and ≥70 years old (n=12), respectively. Mean trough concentrations after 17 days of dosing were 6.2 ng/mL (range, 2.4-9.8 ng/mL) and 8.1 ng/mL (range, 1.8-19.7 ng/mL), respectively, in the two age groups. Although steady state was not reached in this study, mean trough plasma concentration in another study in patients with BPH (mean age, 65 years) receiving 5 mg/day was 9.4 ng/mL (range, 7.1-13.3 ng/mL; n=22) after over a year of dosing.

Finasteride has been shown to cross the blood brain barrier but does not appear to distribute preferentially to the CSF. In 2 studies of healthy subjects (n=69) receiving PROSCAR 5 mg/day for 6-24 weeks, finasteride concentrations in semen ranged from undetectable (<0.1 ng/mL) to 10.54 ng/mL. In an earlier study using a less sensitive assay, finasteride concentrations in the semen of 16 subjects receiving PROSCAR 5 mg/day ranged from undetectable (<1.0 ng/mL) to 21 ng/mL. Thus, based on a 5-mL ejaculate volume, the amount of finasteride in semen was estimated to be 50- to 100-fold less than the dose of finasteride (5 μg) that had no effect on circulating DHT levels in men [see also Use in Specific Populations (8.1)].

Metabolism

Finasteride is extensively metabolized in the liver, primarily via the cytochrome P450 3A4 enzyme subfamily. Two metabolites, the t-butyl side chain monohydroxylated and monocarboxylic acid metabolites, have been identified that possess no more than 20% of the 5α-reductase inhibitory activity of finasteride.

Excretion

In healthy young subjects (n=15), mean plasma clearance of finasteride was 165 mL/min (range, 70-279 mL/min) and mean elimination half-life in plasma was 6 hours (range, 3-16 hours). Following an oral dose of ^{14}C-finasteride in man (n=6), a mean of 39% (range, 32-46%) of the dose was excreted in the urine in the form of metabolites; 57% (range, 51-64%) was excreted in the feces.

The mean terminal half-life of finasteride in subjects ≥70 years of age was approximately 8 hours (range, 6-15 hours; n=12), compared with 6 hours (range, 4-12 hours; n=12) in subjects 45-60 years of age. As a result, mean $AUC_{(0-24\ hr)}$ after 17 days of dosing was 15% higher in subjects ≥70 years of age than in subjects 45-60 years of age (p=0.02).

Table 3: Mean (SD) Pharmacokinetic Parameters in Healthy Young Subjects (n=15)

	Mean (± SD)
Bioavailability	63% (34-108%)*
Clearance (mL/min)	165 (55)
Volume of Distribution (L)	76 (14)
Half-Life (hours)	6.2 (2.1)

* Range

Pediatric

Finasteride pharmacokinetics have not been investigated in patients <18 years of age.

Finasteride is not indicated for use in pediatric patients [see Warnings and Precautions (5.4), Use in Specific Populations (8.4)].

Gender

Finasteride is not indicated for use in women [see Contraindications (4), Warnings and Precautions (5.3 and 5.4), Use in Specific Populations (8.1), How Supplied/Storage and Handling (16) and Patient Counseling Information (17.2)].

Geriatric

No dosage adjustment is necessary in the elderly. Although the elimination rate of finasteride is decreased in the elderly, these findings are of no clinical significance. [See Clinical Pharmacology (12.3) and Use in Specific Populations (8.5).]

Table 4: Mean (SD) Noncompartmental Pharmacokinetic Parameters After Multiple Doses of 5 mg/day in Older Men

	Mean (± SD)	
	45-60 years old (n=12)	≥70 years old (n=12)
AUC (ng•hr/mL)	389 (98)	463 (186)
Peak Concentration (ng/mL)	46.2 (8.7)	48.4 (14.7)
Time to Peak (hours)	1.8 (0.7)	1.8 (0.6)
Half-Life (hours)*	6.0 (1.5)	8.2 (2.5)

* First-dose values; all other parameters are last-dose values

Race

The effect of race on finasteride pharmacokinetics has not been studied.

Hepatic Impairment

The effect of hepatic impairment on finasteride pharmacokinetics has not been studied. Caution should be exercised in the administration of PROSCAR in those patients with liver function abnormalities, as finasteride is metabolized extensively in the liver.

Renal Impairment

No dosage adjustment is necessary in patients with renal impairment. In patients with chronic renal impairment, with creatinine clearances ranging from 9.0 to 55 mL/min, AUC, maximum plasma concentration, half-life, and protein binding after a single dose of ^{14}C-finasteride were similar to values obtained in healthy volunteers. Urinary excretion of metabolites was decreased in patients with renal impairment. This decrease was associated with an increase in fecal excretion of metabolites. Plasma concentrations of metabolites were significantly higher in patients with renal impairment (based on a 60% increase in total radioactivity AUC). However, finasteride has been well tolerated in BPH patients with normal renal function receiving up to 80 mg/day for 12 weeks, where exposure of these patients to metabolites would presumably be much greater.

13 NONCLINICAL TOXICOLOGY

13.1 Carcinogenesis, Mutagenesis, Impairment of Fertility

No evidence of a tumorigenic effect was observed in a 24-month study in Sprague-Dawley rats receiving doses of finasteride up to 160 mg/kg/day in males and 320 mg/kg/day in females. These doses produced respective systemic exposure in rats of 111 and 274 times those observed in man receiving the recommended human dose of 5 mg/day. All exposure calculations were based on calculated $AUC_{(0-24\ hr)}$ for animals and mean $AUC_{(0-24\ hr)}$ for man (0.4 μg•hr/mL).

In a 19-month carcinogenicity study in CD-1 mice, a statistically significant (p≤0.05) increase in the incidence of testicular Leydig cell adenomas was observed at 228 times the human exposure (250 mg/kg/day). In mice at 23 times the human exposure, estimated (25 mg/kg/day) and in rats at 39 times the human exposure (40 mg/kg/day) an increase in the incidence of Leydig cell hyperplasia was observed. A positive correlation between the proliferative changes in the

---

Leydig cells and an increase in serum LH levels (2- to 3-fold above control) has been demonstrated in both rodent species treated with high doses of finasteride. No drug-related Leydig cell changes were seen in either rats or dogs treated with finasteride for 1 year at 30 and 350 times the human exposure (20 mg/kg/day and 45 mg/kg/day, respectively) or in mice treated for 19 months at 2.3 times the human exposure, estimated (2.5 mg/kg/day).

No evidence of mutagenicity was observed in an in vitro bacterial mutagenesis assay, a mammalian cell mutagenesis assay, or in an in vitro alkaline elution assay. In an in vitro chromosome aberration assay, using Chinese hamster ovary cells, there was a slight increase in chromosome aberrations. These concentrations correspond to 4000-5000 times the peak plasma levels in man given a total dose of 5 mg. In an in vivo chromosome aberration assay in mice, no treatment-related increase in chromosome aberration was observed with finasteride at the maximum tolerated dose of 250 mg/kg/day (228 times the human exposure) as determined in the carcinogenicity studies.

In sexually mature male rabbits treated with finasteride at 543 times the human exposure (80 mg/kg/day) for up to 12 weeks, no effect on fertility, sperm count, or ejaculate volume was seen. In sexually mature male rats treated with 61 times the human exposure (80 mg/kg/day), there were no significant effects on fertility after 6 or 12 weeks of treatment; however, when treatment was continued for up to 24 or 30 weeks, there was an apparent decrease in fertility, fecundity and an associated significant decrease in the weights of the seminal vesicles and prostate. All these effects were reversible within 6 weeks of discontinuation of treatment. No drug-related effect on testes or on mating performance has been seen in rats or rabbits. This decrease in fertility in finasteride-treated rats is secondary to its effect on accessory sex organs (prostate and seminal vesicles) resulting in failure to form a seminal plug. The seminal plug is essential for normal fertility in rats and is not relevant in man.

14 CLINICAL STUDIES

14.1 Monotherapy

PROSCAR 5 mg/day was initially evaluated in patients with symptoms of BPH and enlarged prostates by digital rectal examination in two 1-year, placebo-controlled, randomized, double-blind studies and their 5-year open extensions.

PROSCAR was further evaluated in the PROSCAR Long-Term Efficacy and Safety Study (PLESS), a double-blind, randomized, placebo-controlled, 4-year, multicenter study. 3040 patients between the ages of 45 and 78, with moderate to severe symptoms of BPH and an enlarged prostate upon digital rectal examination, were randomized into the study (1524 to finasteride, 1516 to placebo) and 3016 patients were evaluable for efficacy. 1883 patients completed the 4-year study (1000 in the finasteride group, 883 in the placebo group).

Effect on Symptom Score

Symptoms were quantified using a score similar to the American Urological Association Symptom Score, which evaluated both obstructive symptoms (impairment of size and force of stream, sensation of incomplete bladder emptying, delayed or interrupted urination) and irritative symptoms (nocturia, daytime frequency, need to strain or push the flow of urine) by rating on a 0 to 5 scale for six symptoms and a 0 to 4 scale for one symptom, for a total possible score of 34.

Patients in PLESS had moderate to severe symptoms at baseline (mean of approximately 15 points on a 0-34 point scale). Patients randomized to PROSCAR who remained on therapy for 4 years had a mean (± 1 SD) decrease in symptom score of 3.3 (± 5.8) points compared with 1.3 (± 5.6) points in the placebo group. (See Figure 1.) A statistically significant improvement in symptom score was evident at 1 year in patients treated with PROSCAR vs placebo (−2.3 vs −1.6), and this improvement continued through Year 4. [See figure 1 at top of next column]

Results seen in earlier studies were comparable to those seen in PLESS. Although an early improvement in urinary symptoms was seen in some patients, a therapeutic trial of at least 6 months was generally necessary to assess whether a beneficial response in symptom relief had been achieved. The improvement in BPH symptoms was seen during the first year and maintained throughout an additional 5 years of open extension studies.

Effect on Acute Urinary Retention and the Need for Surgery

In PLESS, efficacy was also assessed by evaluating treatment failures. Treatment failure was prospectively defined as BPH-related urological events or clinical deterioration, lack of improvement and/or the need for alternative therapy. BPH-related urological events were defined as urological surgical intervention and acute urinary retention requiring catheterization. Complete event information was available for 92% of the patients. The following table (Table 5) summarizes the results.

[See table 5 at top of next page]

Table 5: All Treatment Failures in PLESS

Event	Patients (%)*		Relative Risk†	95% CI	P Value†
	Placebo N=1503	Finasteride N=1513			
All Treatment Failures	37.1	26.2	0.68	(0.57 to 0.79)	<0.001
Surgical Interventions for BPH	10.1	4.6	0.45	(0.32 to 0.63)	<0.001
Acute Urinary Retention Requiring Catheterization	6.6	2.8	0.43	(0.28 to 0.66)	<0.001
Two consecutive symptom scores ≥20	9.2	6.7			
Bladder Stone	0.4	0.5			
Incontinence	2.1	1.7			
Renal Failure	0.5	0.6			
UTI	5.7	4.9			
Discontinuation due to worsening of BPH, lack of improvement, or to receive other medical treatment	21.8	13.3			

* patients with multiple events may be counted more than once for each type of event
† Hazard ratio based on log rank test

Figure 1: Symptom Score in PLESS

Compared with placebo, PROSCAR was associated with a significantly lower risk for acute urinary retention or the need for BPH-related surgery [13.2% for placebo vs 6.6% for PROSCAR; 51% reduction in risk, 95% CI: (34 to 63%)]. Compared with placebo, PROSCAR was associated with a significantly lower risk for surgery [10.1% for placebo vs 4.6% for PROSCAR; 55% reduction in risk, 95% CI: (37 to 68%)] and with a significantly lower risk of acute urinary retention [6.6% for placebo vs 2.8% for PROSCAR; 57% reduction in risk, 95% CI: (34 to 72%)]; see Figures 2 and 3.
[See figure 2 at top of next column]
[See figure 3 at top of next column]

Effect on Maximum Urinary Flow Rate
In the patients in PLESS who remained on therapy for the duration of the study and had evaluable urinary flow data, PROSCAR increased maximum urinary flow rate by 1.9 mL/sec compared with 0.2 mL/sec in the placebo group. There was a clear difference between treatment groups in maximum urinary flow rate in favor of PROSCAR by month 4 (1.0 vs 0.3 mL/sec) which was maintained throughout the study. In the earlier 1-year studies, increase in maximum urinary flow rate was comparable to PLESS and was maintained through the first year and throughout an additional 5 years of open extension studies.

Effect on Prostate Volume
In PLESS, prostate volume was assessed yearly by magnetic resonance imaging (MRI) in a subset of patients. In patients treated with PROSCAR who remained on therapy, prostate volume was reduced compared with both baseline and placebo throughout the 4-year study. PROSCAR decreased prostate volume by 17.9% (from 55.9 cc at baseline to 45.8 cc at 4 years) compared with an increase of 14.1% (from 51.3 cc to 58.5 cc) in the placebo group (p<0.001). (See Figure 4.)

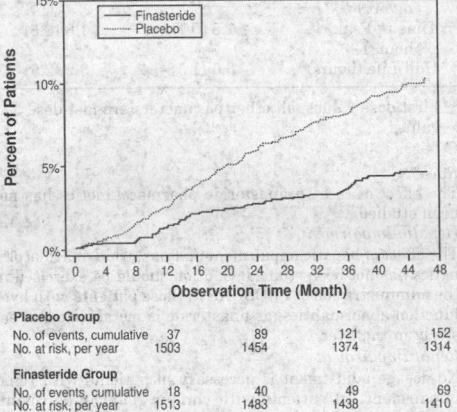

Figure 2: Percent of Patients Having Surgery for BPH, Including TURP

Placebo Group
No. of events, cumulative 37 89 121 152
No. at risk, per year 1503 1454 1374 1314

Finasteride Group
No. of events, cumulative 18 40 49 69
No. at risk, per year 1513 1483 1438 1410

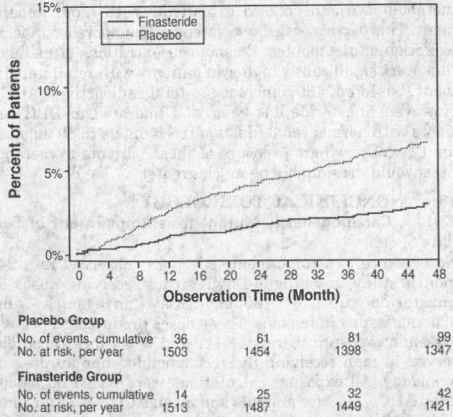

Figure 3: Percent of Patients Developing Acute Urinary Retention (Spontaneous and Precipitated)

Placebo Group
No. of events, cumulative 36 61 81 99
No. at risk, per year 1503 1454 1398 1347

Finasteride Group
No. of events, cumulative 14 25 32 42
No. at risk, per year 1513 1487 1449 1421

Results seen in earlier studies were comparable to those seen in PLESS. Mean prostate volume at baseline ranged between 40-50 cc. The reduction in prostate volume was seen during the first year and maintained throughout an additional five years of open extension studies.

Placebo (●) n = 155 136 119 98 85
Finasteride (■) n = 157 144 130 116 102

Figure 4: Prostate Volume in PLESS

Prostate Volume as a Predictor of Therapeutic Response
A meta-analysis combining 1-year data from seven double-blind, placebo-controlled studies of similar design, including 4491 patients with symptomatic BPH, demonstrated that, in patients treated with PROSCAR, the magnitude of symptom response and degree of improvement in maximum urinary flow rate were greater in patients with an enlarged prostate at baseline.

14.2   Combination with Alpha-Blocker Therapy
The Medical Therapy of Prostatic Symptoms (MTOPS) Trial was a double-blind, randomized, placebo-controlled, multi-center, 4- to 6-year study (average 5 years) in 3047 men with symptomatic BPH, who were randomized to receive PROSCAR 5 mg/day (n=768), doxazosin 4 or 8 mg/day (n=756), the combination of PROSCAR 5 mg/day and doxazosin 4 or 8 mg/day (n=786), or placebo (n=737). All participants underwent weekly titration of doxazosin (or its placebo) from 1 to 2 to 4 to 8 mg/day. Only those who tolerated the 4 or 8 mg dose level were kept on doxazosin (or its placebo) in the study. The participant's final tolerated dose (either 4 mg or 8 mg) was administered beginning at end-Week 4. The final doxazosin dose was administered once per day, at bedtime.
The mean patient age at randomization was 62.6 years (±7.3 years). Patients were Caucasian (82%), African American (9%), Hispanic (7%), Asian (1%) or Native American (<1%). The mean duration of BPH symptoms was 4.7 years (±4.6 years). Patients had moderate to severe BPH symptoms at baseline with a mean AUA symptom score of approximately 17 out of 35 points. Mean maximum urinary flow rate was 10.5 mL/sec (±2.6 mL/sec). The mean prostate volume as measured by transrectal ultrasound was 36.3 mL (±20.1 mL). Prostate volume was ≤20 mL in 16% of patients, ≥50 mL in 18% of patients and between 21 and 49 mL in 66% of patients.
The primary endpoint was a composite measure of the first occurrence of any of the following five outcomes: a ≥4 point confirmed increase from baseline in symptom score, acute urinary retention, BPH-related renal insufficiency (creatinine rise), recurrent urinary tract infections or urosepsis, or incontinence. Compared to placebo, treatment with PROSCAR, doxazosin, or combination therapy resulted in a reduction in the risk of experiencing one of these five outcome events by 34% (p=0.002), 39% (p<0.001), and 67% (p<0.001), respectively. Combination therapy resulted in a significant reduction in the risk of the primary endpoint compared to treatment with PROSCAR alone (49%; p≤0.001) or doxazosin alone (46%; p≤0.001). (See Table 6.)
[See table 6 at top of next page]
The majority of the events (274 out of 351; 78%) was a confirmed ≥4 point increase in symptom score, referred to as symptom score progression. The risk of symptom score progression was reduced by 30% (p=0.016), 46% (p<0.001), and 64% (p<0.001) in patients treated with PROSCAR, doxazosin, or the combination, respectively, compared to patients treated with placebo (see Figure 5). Combination therapy significantly reduced the risk of symptom score progression compared to the effect of PROSCAR alone (p<0.001) and compared to doxazosin alone (p=0.037).

Figure 5: Cumulative Incidence of a 4-Point Rise in AUA Symptom Score by Treatment Group

Treatment with PROSCAR, doxazosin or the combination of PROSCAR with doxazosin, reduced the mean symptom score from baseline at year 4. Table 7 provides the mean change from baseline for AUA symptom score by treatment group for patients who remained on therapy for four years. [See table 7 above]

The results of MTOPS are consistent with the findings of the 4-year, placebo-controlled study PLESS [see *Clinical Studies (14.1)]* in that treatment with PROSCAR reduces the risk of acute urinary retention and the need for BPH-related surgery. In MTOPS, the risk of developing acute urinary retention was reduced by 67% in patients treated with PROSCAR compared to patients treated with placebo (0.8% for PROSCAR and 2.4% for placebo). Also, the risk of requiring BPH-related invasive therapy was reduced by 64% in patients treated with PROSCAR compared to patients treated with placebo (2.0% for PROSCAR and 5.4% for placebo).

14.3 Summary of Clinical Studies

The data from these studies, showing improvement in BPH-related symptoms, reduction in treatment failure (BPH-related urological events), increased maximum urinary flow rates, and decreasing prostate volume, suggest that PROSCAR arrests the disease process of BPH in men with an enlarged prostate.

16 HOW SUPPLIED/STORAGE AND HANDLING

No. 3094 — PROSCAR tablets 5 mg are blue, modified apple-shaped, film-coated tablets, with the code MSD 72 on one side and PROSCAR on the other. They are supplied as follows:

NDC 0006-0072-31 unit of use bottles of 30
NDC 0006-0072-58 unit of use bottles of 100.
Storage and Handling
Store at room temperatures below 30°C (86°F). Protect from light and keep container tightly closed.
Women should not handle crushed or broken PROSCAR tablets when they are pregnant or may potentially be pregnant because of the possibility of absorption of finasteride and the subsequent potential risk to a male fetus [see *Warnings and Precautions (5.3), Use in Specific Populations (8.1) and Patient Counseling Information (17.2)].*

17 PATIENT COUNSELING INFORMATION

See FDA-Approved Patient Labeling (Patient Information).
17.1 Increased Risk of High-Grade Prostate Cancer
Patients should be informed that there was an increase in high-grade prostate cancer in men treated with 5α-reductase inhibitors indicated for BPH treatment, including PROSCAR, compared to those treated with placebo in studies looking at the use of these drugs to prevent prostate cancer [see *Indications and Usage (1.3), Warnings and Precautions (5.2), and Adverse Reactions (6.1)].*

17.2 Exposure of Women — Risk to Male Fetus
Physicians should inform patients that women who are pregnant or may potentially be pregnant should not handle crushed or broken PROSCAR tablets because of the possibility of absorption of finasteride and the subsequent potential risk to the male fetus. PROSCAR tablets are coated and will prevent contact with the active ingredient during normal handling, provided that the tablets have not been broken or crushed. If a woman who is pregnant or may potentially be pregnant comes in contact with crushed or broken PROSCAR tablets, the contact area should be washed immediately with soap and water [see *Contraindications (4), Warnings and Precautions (5.3), Use in Specific Populations (8.1) and How Supplied/Storage and Handling (16)].*

17.3 Additional Instructions
Physicians should inform patients that the volume of ejaculate may be decreased in some patients during treatment with PROSCAR. This decrease does not appear to interfere with normal sexual function. However, impotence and decreased libido may occur in patients treated with PROSCAR [see *Adverse Reactions (6.1)].*
Physicians should instruct their patients to promptly report any changes in their breasts such as lumps, pain or nipple discharge. Breast changes including breast enlargement, tenderness and neoplasm have been reported [see *Adverse Reactions (6.1)].*
Physicians should instruct their patients to read the patient package insert before starting therapy with PROSCAR and to reread it each time the prescription is renewed so that they are aware of current information for patients regarding PROSCAR.

Dist. by: Merck Sharp & Dohme Corp., a subsidiary of **MERCK & CO., INC.**,Whitehouse Station, NJ 08889, USA
For patent information:
www.merck.com/product/patent/home.html
Copyright © 1992, 1995, 1998, 2011 Merck Sharp & Dohme Corp., a subsidiary of **Merck & Co., Inc.**
All rights reserved.
uspi-mk0906-5t-1309r011

Table 6: Count and Percent Incidence of Primary Outcome Events by Treatment Group in MTOPS

Event	Treatment Group				
	Placebo N=737 N (%)	Doxazosin N=756 N (%)	Finasteride N=768 N (%)	Combination N=786 N (%)	Total N=3047 N (%)
AUA 4-point rise	100 (13.6)	59 (7.8)	74 (9.6)	41 (5.2)	274 (9.0)
Acute urinary retention	18 (2.4)	13 (1.7)	6 (0.8)	4 (0.5)	41 (1.3)
Incontinence	8 (1.1)	11 (1.5)	9 (1.2)	3 (0.4)	31 (1.0)
Recurrent UTI/urosepsis	2 (0.3)	2 (0.3)	0 (0.0)	1 (0.1)	5 (0.2)
Creatinine rise	0 (0.0)	0 (0.0)	0 (0.0)	0 (0.0)	0 (0.0)
Total Events	128 (17.4)	85 (11.2)	89 (11.6)	49 (6.2)	351 (11.5)

Table 7: Change From Baseline in AUA Symptom Score by Treatment Group at Year 4 in MTOPS

	Placebo N=534	Doxazosin N=582	Finasteride N=565	Combination N=598
Baseline Mean (SD)	16.8 (6.0)	17.0 (5.9)	17.1 (6.0)	16.8 (5.8)
Mean Change AUA Symptom Score (SD)	-4.9 (5.8)	-6.6 (6.1)	-5.6 (5.9)	-7.4 (6.3)
Comparison to Placebo (95% CI)		-1.8 (-2.5, -1.1)	-0.7 (-1.4, 0.0)	-2.5 (-3.2, -1.8)
Comparison to Doxazosin alone (95% CI)				-0.7 (-1.4, 0.0)
Comparison to Finasteride alone (95% CI)				-1.8 (-2.5, -1.1)

PROSCAR® (finasteride) Tablets
Patient Information about
PROSCAR®(Prahs-car)
Generic name: finasteride
(fin-AS-tur-eyed)
PROSCAR is for use by men only.
Please read this leaflet before you start taking PROSCAR. Also, read it each time you renew your prescription, just in case anything has changed. Remember, this leaflet does not take the place of careful discussions with your doctor. You and your doctor should discuss PROSCAR when you start taking your medication and at regular checkups.
What is PROSCAR?
PROSCAR is a medication used to treat symptoms of benign prostatic hyperplasia (BPH) in men with an enlarged prostate. PROSCAR may also be used to reduce the risk of a sudden inability to pass urine and the need for surgery related to BPH in men with an enlarged prostate.
PROSCAR may be prescribed along with another medicine, an alpha-blocker called doxazosin, to help you better manage your BPH symptoms.
Who should NOT take PROSCAR?
PROSCAR is for use by MEN only.
Do Not Take PROSCAR if you are:
• a woman who is pregnant or may potentially be pregnant. PROSCAR may harm your unborn baby. Do not touch or handle crushed or broken PROSCAR tablets (see **"A warning about PROSCAR and pregnancy"**).
• allergic to finasteride or any of the ingredients in PROSCAR. See the end of this leaflet for a complete list of ingredients in PROSCAR.
A warning about PROSCAR and pregnancy:
Women who are or may potentially be pregnant must not use PROSCAR. They should also not handle crushed or broken tablets of PROSCAR. PROSCAR tablets are coated and will prevent contact with the active ingredient during normal handling, provided that the tablets are not broken or crushed.
If a woman who is pregnant with a male baby absorbs the active ingredient in PROSCAR after oral use or through the skin, it may cause the male baby to be born with abnormalities of the sex organs. If a woman who is pregnant comes into contact with the active ingredient in PROSCAR, a doctor should be consulted.
How should I take PROSCAR?
Follow your doctor's instruction.
• Take one tablet by mouth each day. To avoid forgetting to take PROSCAR, you can take it at the same time every day.
• If you forget to take PROSCAR, do not take an extra tablet. Just take the next tablet as usual.
• You may take PROSCAR with or without food.
• Do not share PROSCAR with anyone else; it was prescribed only for you.
What are the possible side effects of PROSCAR?
PROSCAR may increase the chance of a more serious form of prostate cancer.
The most common side effects of PROSCAR include:
• trouble getting or keeping an erection (impotence)

• decrease in sex drive
• decreased volume of ejaculate
• ejaculation disorders
• enlarged or painful breast. You should promptly report to your doctor any changes in your breasts such as lumps, pain or nipple discharge.
The following have been reported in general use with PROSCAR and/or finasteride at lower doses:
• allergic reactions, including rash, itching, hives, and swelling of the lips, tongue, throat, and face
• rarely, some men may have testicular pain
• trouble getting or keeping an erection that continued after stopping the medication
• problems with ejaculation that continued after stopping the medication
• male infertility and/or poor quality of semen. Improvement in the quality of semen has been reported after stopping the medication.
• depression
• decrease in sex drive that continued after stopping the medication
• in rare cases, male breast cancer has been reported.
You should discuss side effects with your doctor before taking PROSCAR and anytime you think you are having a side effect. These are not all the possible side effects with PROSCAR. For more information, ask your doctor or pharmacist.
Call your doctor for medical advice about side effects. You may report side effects to FDA at: 1-800-FDA-1088.
What you need to know while taking PROSCAR:
• **You should see your doctor regularly while taking PROSCAR.** Follow your doctor's advice about when to have these checkups.
• **Checking for prostate cancer.** Your doctor has prescribed PROSCAR for BPH and not for treatment of prostate cancer — but a man can have BPH and prostate cancer at the same time. Your doctor may continue checking for prostate cancer while you take PROSCAR.
• **About Prostate-Specific Antigen (PSA).** Your doctor may have done a blood test called PSA for the screening of prostate cancer. Because PROSCAR decreases PSA levels, you should tell your doctor(s) that you are taking PROSCAR. Changes in PSA levels will need to be evaluated by your doctor(s). Any increase in follow-up PSA levels from their lowest point may signal the presence of prostate cancer and should be evaluated, even if the test results are still within the normal range. You should also tell your doctor if you have not been taking PROSCAR as prescribed because this may affect the PSA test results. For more information, talk to your doctor.
How should I store PROSCAR?
• Store PROSCAR tablets in a dry place at room temperature.
• Keep PROSCAR in the original container and keep the container closed.
PROSCAR tablets are coated and will prevent contact with the active ingredient during normal handling, provided that the tablets are not broken or crushed.
Keep PROSCAR and all medications out of the reach of children.

Do not give your PROSCAR tablets to anyone else. It has been prescribed only for you.

For more information call 1-800-622-4477.

What are the ingredients in PROSCAR?

Active ingredients: finasteride

Inactive ingredients: hydrous lactose, microcrystalline cellulose, pregelatinized starch, sodium starch glycolate, hydroxypropyl cellulose LF, hydroxypropyl methylcellulose, titanium dioxide, magnesium stearate, talc, docusate sodium, FD&C Blue 2 aluminum lake and yellow iron oxide.

What is BPH?

BPH is an enlargement of the prostate gland. The prostate is located below the bladder. As the prostate enlarges, it may slowly restrict the flow of urine. This can lead to symptoms such as:

• a weak or interrupted urinary stream
• a feeling that you cannot empty your bladder completely
• a feeling of delay or hesitation when you start to urinate
• a need to urinate often, especially at night
• a feeling that you must urinate right away.

In some men, BPH can lead to serious problems, including urinary tract infections, a sudden inability to pass urine (acute urinary retention), as well as the need for surgery.

What PROSCAR does:

PROSCAR lowers levels of a hormone called DHT (dihydrotestosterone), which is a cause of prostate growth. Lowering DHT leads to shrinkage of the enlarged prostate gland in most men. This can lead to gradual improvement in urine flow and symptoms over the next several months. PROSCAR will help reduce the risk of developing a sudden inability to pass urine and the need for surgery related to an enlarged prostate. However, since each case of BPH is different, you should know that:

• Even though the prostate shrinks, you may NOT notice an improvement in urine flow or symptoms.
• You may need to take PROSCAR for six (6) months or more to see whether it improves your symptoms.
• Therapy with PROSCAR may reduce your risk for a sudden inability to pass urine and the need for surgery for an enlarged prostate.

Dist. by: Merck Sharp & Dohme Corp., a subsidiary of **MERCK & CO., INC.,**Whitehouse Station, NJ 08889, USA

For patent information:
www.merck.com/product/patent/home.html

Copyright © 1992, 1995, 1998, 2011 Merck Sharp & Dohme Corp., a subsidiary of **Merck & Co., Inc.**

All rights reserved.

Revised: 09/2013

usppi-mk0906-5t-1309r011

Shown in Product Identification Guide, page 309

PROVENTIL® HFA ℞

[prō-věn-těl H-F-A]
(albuterol sulfate)
Inhalation Aerosol

FOR ORAL INHALATION ONLY
Prescribing Information

DESCRIPTION

The active component of PROVENTIL® HFA (albuterol sulfate) Inhalation Aerosol is albuterol sulfate, USP racemic α^1 [(*tert*-Butylamino)methyl]-4-hydroxy-*m*-xylene-α,α'-diol sulfate (2:1)(salt), a relatively selective beta$_2$-adrenergic bronchodilator having the following chemical structure:

$$\left[\text{(structure of albuterol)} \right]_2 \cdot SO_4$$

Albuterol sulfate is the official generic name in the United States. The World Health Organization recommended name for the drug is salbutamol sulfate. The molecular weight of albuterol sulfate is 576.7, and the empirical formula is (C13H21 NO3)2•H2SO4. Albuterol sulfate is a white to off-white crystalline solid. It is soluble in water and slightly soluble in ethanol. PROVENTIL HFA Inhalation Aerosol is a pressurized metered-dose aerosol unit for oral inhalation. It contains a microcrystalline suspension of albuterol sulfate in propellant HFA-134a (1,1,1,2-tetrafluoroethane), ethanol, and oleic acid.

Each actuation delivers 120 mcg albuterol sulfate, USP from the valve and 108 mcg albuterol sulfate, USP from the mouthpiece (equivalent to 90 mcg of albuterol base from the mouthpiece). Each canister provides 200 inhalations. It is recommended to prime the inhaler before using for the first time and in cases where the inhaler has not been used for more than 2 weeks by releasing four "test sprays" into the air, away from the face.

This product does not contain chlorofluorocarbons (CFCs) as the propellant.

CLINICAL PHARMACOLOGY

Mechanism of Action *In vitro* studies and *in vivo* pharmacologic studies have demonstrated that albuterol has a preferential effect on beta$_2$-adrenergic receptors compared with isoproterenol. While it is recognized that beta$_2$-adrenergic receptors are the predominant receptors on bronchial smooth muscle, data indicate that there is a population of beta$_2$-receptors in the human heart existing in a concentration between 10% and 50% of cardiac beta-adrenergic receptors. The precise function of these receptors has not been established. (See **WARNINGS, Cardiovascular Effects** section.)

Activation of beta$_2$-adrenergic receptors on airway smooth muscle leads to the activation of adenylcyclase and to an increase in the intracellular concentration of cyclic-3',5'-adenosine monophosphate (cyclic AMP). This increase of cyclic AMP leads to the activation of protein kinase A, which inhibits the phosphorylation of myosin and lowers intracellular ionic calcium concentrations, resulting in relaxation. Albuterol relaxes the smooth muscles of all airways, from the trachea to the terminal bronchioles. Albuterol acts as a functional antagonist to relax the airway irrespective of the spasmogen involved, thus protecting against all bronchoconstrictor challenges. Increased cyclic AMP concentrations are also associated with the inhibition of release of mediators from mast cells in the airway.

Albuterol has been shown in most clinical trials to have more effect on the respiratory tract, in the form of bronchial smooth muscle relaxation, than isoproterenol at comparable doses while producing fewer cardiovascular effects. Controlled clinical studies and other clinical experience have shown that inhaled albuterol, like other beta-adrenergic agonist drugs, can produce a significant cardiovascular effect in some patients, as measured by pulse rate, blood pressure, symptoms, and/or electrocardiographic changes.

Preclinical Intravenous studies in rats with albuterol sulfate have demonstrated that albuterol crosses the blood-brain barrier and reaches brain concentrations amounting to approximately 5% of the plasma concentrations. In structures outside the blood-brain barrier (pineal and pituitary glands), albuterol concentrations were found to be 100 times those in the whole brain.

Studies in laboratory animals (minipigs, rodents, and dogs) have demonstrated the occurrence of cardiac arrhythmias and sudden death (with histologic evidence of myocardial necrosis) when beta$_2$-agonist and methylxanthines were administered concurrently. The clinical significance of these findings is unknown.

Propellant HFA-134a is devoid of pharmacological activity except at very high doses in animals (380-1300 times the maximum human exposure based on comparisons of AUC values), primarily producing ataxia, tremors, dyspnea, or salivation. These are similar to effects produced by the structurally related chlorofluorocarbons (CFCs), which have been used extensively in metered dose inhalers.

In animals and humans, propellant HFA-134a was found to be rapidly absorbed and rapidly eliminated, with an elimination half-life of 3 to 27 minutes in animals and 5 to 7 minutes in humans. Time to maximum plasma concentration (Tmax) and mean residence time are both extremely short, leading to a transient appearance of HFA-134a in the blood with no evidence of accumulation.

Pharmacokinetics In a single-dose bioavailability study which enrolled six healthy, male volunteers, transient low albuterol levels (close to the lower limit of quantitation) were observed after administration of two puffs from both PROVENTIL® HFA Inhalation Aerosol and a CFC 11/12 propelled albuterol inhaler. No formal pharmacokinetic analyses were possible for either treatment, but systemic albuterol levels appeared similar.

Clinical Trials In a 12-week, randomized, double-blind, double-dummy, active- and placebo-controlled trial, 565 patients with asthma were evaluated for the bronchodilator efficacy of PROVENTIL HFA Inhalation Aerosol (193 patients) in comparison to a CFC 11/12 propelled albuterol inhaler (186 patients) and an HFA-134a placebo inhaler (186 patients).

Serial FEV1 measurements (shown below as percent change from test-day baseline) demonstrated that two inhalations of PROVENTIL HFA Inhalation Aerosol produced significantly greater improvement in pulmonary function than placebo and produced outcomes which were clinically comparable to a CFC 11/12 propelled albuterol inhaler.

The mean time to onset of a 15% increase in FEV1 was 6 minutes and the mean time to peak effect was 50 to 55 minutes. The mean duration of effect as measured by a 15% increase in FEV1 was 3 hours. In some patients, duration of effect was as long as 6 hours.

In another clinical study in adults, two inhalations of PROVENTIL HFA Inhalation Aerosol taken 30 minutes before exercise prevented exercise-induced bronchospasm as demonstrated by the maintenance of FEV1 within 80% of baseline values in the majority of patients.

In a 4-week, randomized, open-label trial, 63 children, 4 to 11 years of age, with asthma were evaluated for the bronchodilator efficacy of PROVENTIL HFA Inhalation Aerosol (33 pediatric patients) in comparison to a CFC 11/12 propelled albuterol inhaler (30 pediatric patients).

FEV₁ as Percent Change from Predose in a Large 12-Week Clinical Trial

Serial FEV1 measurements as percent change from test-day baseline demonstrated that two inhalations of PROVENTIL HFA Inhalation Aerosol produced outcomes which were clinically comparable to a CFC 11/12 propelled albuterol inhaler.

The mean time to onset of a 12% increase in FEV1 for PROVENTIL HFA Inhalation Aerosol was 7 minutes and the mean time to peak effect was approximately 50 minutes. The mean duration of effect as measured by a 12% increase in FEV1 was 2.3 hours. In some pediatric patients, duration of effect was as long as 6 hours.

In another clinical study in pediatric patients, two inhalations of PROVENTIL HFA Inhalation Aerosol taken 30 minutes before exercise provided comparable protection against exercise-induced bronchospasm as a CFC 11/12 propelled albuterol inhaler.

INDICATIONS AND USAGE

PROVENTIL® HFA Inhalation Aerosol is indicated in adults and children 4 years of age and older for the treatment or prevention of bronchospasm with reversible obstructive airway disease and for the prevention of exercise-induced bronchospasm.

CONTRAINDICATIONS

PROVENTIL® HFA Inhalation Aerosol is contraindicated in patients with a history of hypersensitivity to albuterol or any other PROVENTIL HFA components.

WARNINGS

1. **Paradoxical Bronchospasm:** Inhaled albuterol sulfate can produce paradoxical bronchospasm that may be life threatening. If paradoxical bronchospasm occurs, PROVENTIL® HFA Inhalation Aerosol should be discontinued immediately and alternative therapy instituted. It should be recognized that paradoxical bronchospasm, when associated with inhaled formulations, frequently occurs with the first use of a new canister.

2. **Deterioration of Asthma:** Asthma may deteriorate acutely over a period of hours or chronically over several days or longer. If the patient needs more doses of PROVENTIL HFA Inhalation Aerosol than usual, this may be a marker of destabilization of asthma and requires re-evaluation of the patient and treatment regimen, giving special consideration to the possible need for anti-inflammatory treatment, e.g., corticosteroids.

3. **Use of Anti-inflammatory Agents:** The use of beta-adrenergic-agonist bronchodilators alone may not be adequate to control asthma in many patients. Early consideration should be given to adding anti-inflammatory agents, e.g., corticosteroids, to the therapeutic regimen.

4. **Cardiovascular Effects:** PROVENTIL HFA Inhalation Aerosol, like other beta-adrenergic agonists, can produce clinically significant cardiovascular effects in some patients as measured by pulse rate, blood pressure, and/or symptoms. Although such effects are uncommon after administration of PROVENTIL HFA Inhalation Aerosol at recommended doses, if they occur, the drug may need to be discontinued. In addition, beta-agonists have been reported to produce ECG changes, such as flattening of the T wave, prolongation of the QTc interval, and ST segment depression. The clinical significance of these findings is unknown. Therefore, PROVENTIL HFA Inhalation Aerosol, like all sympathomimetic amines, should be used with caution in patients with cardiovascular disorders, especially coronary insufficiency, cardiac arrhythmias, and hypertension.

5. **Do Not Exceed Recommended Dose:** Fatalities have been reported in association with excessive use of inhaled sympathomimetic drugs in patients with asthma. The exact cause of death is unknown, but cardiac arrest following an unexpected development of a severe acute asthmatic crisis and subsequent hypoxia is suspected.

6. **Immediate Hypersensitivity Reactions:** Immediate hypersensitivity reactions may occur after administration of

albuterol sulfate, as demonstrated by rare cases of urticaria, angioedema, rash, bronchospasm, anaphylaxis, and oropharyngeal edema.

PRECAUTIONS

General Albuterol sulfate, as with all sympathomimetic amines, should be used with caution in patients with cardiovascular disorders, especially coronary insufficiency, cardiac arrhythmias, and hypertension; in patients with convulsive disorders, hyperthyroidism, or diabetes mellitus; and in patients who are unusually responsive to sympathomimetic amines. Clinically significant changes in systolic and diastolic blood pressure have been seen in individual patients and could be expected to occur in some patients after use of any beta-adrenergic bronchodilator.

Large doses of intravenous albuterol have been reported to aggravate preexisting diabetes mellitus and ketoacidosis. As with other beta-agonists, albuterol may produce significant hypokalemia in some patients, possibly through intracellular shunting, which has the potential to produce adverse cardiovascular effects. The decrease is usually transient, not requiring supplementation.

Information for Patients See illustrated Patient's Instructions for Use. SHAKE WELL BEFORE USING. Patients should be given the following information:

It is recommended to prime the inhaler before using for the first time and in cases where the inhaler has not been used for more than 2 weeks by releasing four "test sprays" into the air, away from the face.

KEEPING THE PLASTIC MOUTHPIECE CLEAN IS VERY IMPORTANT TO PREVENT MEDICATION BUILDUP AND BLOCKAGE. THE MOUTHPIECE SHOULD BE WASHED, SHAKEN TO REMOVE EXCESS WATER, AND AIR DRIED THOROUGHLY AT LEAST ONCE A WEEK. INHALER MAY CEASE TO DELIVER MEDICATION IF NOT PROPERLY CLEANED.

The mouthpiece should be cleaned (with the canister removed) by running warm water through the top and bottom for 30 seconds at least once a week. The mouthpiece must be shaken to remove excess water, then air dried thoroughly (such as overnight). Blockage from medication buildup or improper medication delivery may result from failure to thoroughly air dry the mouthpiece.

If the mouthpiece should become blocked (little or no medication coming out of the mouthpiece), the blockage may be removed by washing as described above.

If it is necessary to use the inhaler before it is completely dry, shake off excess water, replace canister, test spray away from face, and take the prescribed dose. After such use, the mouthpiece should be rewashed and allowed to air dry thoroughly.

The action of PROVENTIL® HFA Inhalation Aerosol should last up to 4 to 6 hours. PROVENTIL HFA Inhalation Aerosol should not be used more frequently than recommended. Do not increase the dose or frequency of doses of PROVENTIL HFA Inhalation Aerosol without consulting your physician. If you find that treatment with PROVENTIL HFA Inhalation Aerosol becomes less effective for symptomatic relief, your symptoms become worse, and/or you need to use the product more frequently than usual, medical attention should be sought immediately. While you are taking PROVENTIL HFA Inhalation Aerosol, other inhaled drugs and asthma medications should be taken only as directed by your physician.

Common adverse effects of treatment with inhaled albuterol include palpitations, chest pain, rapid heart rate, tremor, or nervousness. If you are pregnant or nursing, contact your physician about use of PROVENTIL HFA Inhalation Aerosol. Effective and safe use of PROVENTIL HFA Inhalation Aerosol includes an understanding of the way that it should be administered. Use PROVENTIL HFA Inhalation Aerosol only with the actuator supplied with the product. Discard the canister after 200 sprays have been used.

In general, the technique for administering PROVENTIL HFA Inhalation Aerosol to children is similar to that for adults. Children should use PROVENTIL HFA Inhalation Aerosol under adult supervision, as instructed by the patient's physician. (See Patient's Instructions for Use.)

Drug Interactions

1. **Beta-Blockers:** Beta-adrenergic-receptor blocking agents not only block the pulmonary effect of beta-agonists, such as PROVENTIL HFA Inhalation Aerosol, but may produce severe bronchospasm in asthmatic patients. Therefore, patients with asthma should not normally be treated with beta-blockers. However, under certain circumstances, e.g., as prophylaxis after myocardial infarction, there may be no acceptable alternatives to the use of beta-adrenergic blocking agents in patients with asthma. In this setting, cardioselective beta-blockers should be considered, although they should be administered with caution.

2. **Diuretics:** The ECG changes and/or hypokalemia which may result from the administration of nonpotassium-sparing diuretics (such as loop or thiazide diuretics) can

be acutely worsened by beta-agonists, especially when the recommended dose of the beta-agonist is exceeded. Although the clinical significance of these effects is not known, caution is advised in the coadministration of beta-agonists with nonpotassium-sparing diuretics.

3. **Albuterol-Digoxin:** Mean decreases of 16% and 22% in serum digoxin levels were demonstrated after single-dose intravenous and oral administration of albuterol, respectively, to normal volunteers who had received digoxin for 10 days. The clinical significance of these findings for patients with obstructive airway disease who are receiving albuterol and digoxin on a chronic basis is unclear; nevertheless, it would be prudent to carefully evaluate the serum digoxin levels in patients who are currently receiving digoxin and albuterol.

4. **Monoamine Oxidase Inhibitors or Tricyclic Antidepressants:** PROVENTIL HFA Inhalation Aerosol should be administered with extreme caution to patients being treated with monoamine oxidase inhibitors or tricyclic antidepressants, or within 2 weeks of discontinuation of such agents, because the action of albuterol on the cardiovascular system may be potentiated.

Carcinogenesis, Mutagenesis, and Impairment of Fertility

In a 2-year study in SPRAGUE-DAWLEY® rats, albuterol sulfate caused a dose-related increase in the incidence of benign leiomyomas of the mesovarium at the above dietary doses of 2 mg/kg (approximately 15 times the maximum recommended daily inhalation dose for adults on a mg/m² basis and approximately 6 times the maximum recommended daily inhalation dose for children on a mg/m² basis). In another study this effect was blocked by the coadministration of propranolol, a nonselective beta-adrenergic antagonist. In an 18-month study in CD-1 mice, albuterol sulfate showed no evidence of tumorigenicity at dietary doses of up to 500 mg/kg (approximately 1700 times the maximum recommended daily inhalation dose for adults on a mg/m² basis and approximately 800 times the maximum recommended daily inhalation dose for children on a mg/m² basis). In a 22-month study in Golden Hamsters, albuterol sulfate showed no evidence of tumorigenicity at dietary doses of up to 50 mg/kg (approximately 225 times the maximum recommended daily inhalation dose for adults on a mg/m² basis and approximately 110 times the maximum recommended daily inhalation dose for children on a mg/m² basis).

Albuterol sulfate was not mutagenic in the Ames test or a mutation test in yeast. Albuterol sulfate was not clastogenic in a human peripheral lymphocyte assay or in an AH1 strain mouse micronucleus assay.

Reproduction studies in rats demonstrated no evidence of impaired fertility at oral doses up to 50 mg/kg (approximately 340 times the maximum recommended daily inhalation dose for adults on a mg/m² basis).

Pregnancy *Teratogenic Effects* Pregnancy Category C

Albuterol sulfate has been shown to be teratogenic in mice. A study in CD-1 mice given albuterol sulfate subcutaneously showed cleft palate formation in 5 of 111 (4.5%) fetuses at 0.25 mg/kg (less than the maximum recommended daily inhalation dose for adults on a mg/m² basis) and in 10 of 108 (9.3%) fetuses at 2.5 mg/kg (approximately 8 times the maximum recommended daily inhalation dose for adults on a mg/m² basis). The drug did not induce cleft palate formation at a dose of 0.025 mg/kg (less than the maximum recommended daily inhalation dose for adults on a mg/m² basis). Cleft palate also occurred in 22 of 72 (30.5%) fetuses from females treated subcutaneously with 2.5 mg/kg of isoproterenol (positive control).

A reproduction study in Stride Dutch rabbits revealed cranioschisis in 7 of 19 (37%) fetuses when albuterol sulfate was administered orally at 50 mg/kg dose (approximately 680 times the maximum recommended daily inhalation dose for adults on a mg/m² basis).

In an inhalation reproduction study in SPRAGUE-DAWLEY rats, the albuterol sulfate/HFA-134a formulation did not exhibit any teratogenic effects at 10.5 mg/kg (approximately 70 times the maximum recommended daily inhalation dose for adults on a mg/m² basis).

A study in which pregnant rats were dosed with radiolabeled albuterol sulfate demonstrated that drug-related material is transferred from the maternal circulation to the fetus.

There are no adequate and well-controlled studies of PROVENTIL HFA Inhalation Aerosol or albuterol sulfate in pregnant women. PROVENTIL HFA Inhalation Aerosol should be used during pregnancy only if the potential benefit justifies the potential risk to the fetus.

During worldwide marketing experience, various congenital anomalies, including cleft palate and limb defects, have been reported in the offspring of patients being treated with albuterol. Some of the mothers were taking multiple medications during their pregnancies. Because no consistent pattern of defects can be discerned, a relationship between albuterol use and congenital anomalies has not been established.

Use in Labor and Delivery

Because of the potential for beta-agonist interference with uterine contractility, use of PROVENTIL HFA Inhalation Aerosol for relief of bronchospasm during labor should be restricted to those patients in whom the benefits clearly outweigh the risk.

Tocolysis: Albuterol has not been approved for the management of preterm labor. The benefit:risk ratio when albuterol is administered for tocolysis has not been established. Serious adverse reactions, including pulmonary edema, have been reported during or following treatment of premature labor with beta₂-agonists, including albuterol.

Nursing Mothers

Plasma levels of albuterol sulfate and HFA-134a after inhaled therapeutic doses are very low in humans, but it is

Adverse Experience Incidences (% of patients) in a Large 12-week Clinical Trial*

Body System/ Adverse Event (Preferred Term)		PROVENTIL® HFA Inhalation Aerosol (N=193)	CFC 11/12 Propelled Albuterol Inhaler (N=186)	HFA-134a Placebo Inhaler (N=186)
Application Site Disorders	Inhalation Site Sensation	6	9	2
	Inhalation Taste Sensation	4	3	3
Body as a Whole	Allergic Reaction/Symptoms	6	4	<1
	Back Pain	4	2	3
	Fever	6	2	5
Central and Peripheral Nervous System	Tremor	7	8	2
Gastrointestinal System	Nausea	10	9	5
	Vomiting	7	2	3
Heart Rate and Rhythm Disorder	Tachycardia	7	2	<1
Psychiatric Disorders	Nervousness	7	9	3
Respiratory System Disorders	Respiratory Disorder (unspecified)	6	4	5
	Rhinitis	16	22	14
	Upper Resp Tract Infection	21	20	18
Urinary System Disorder	Urinary Tract Infection	3	4	2

*This table includes all adverse events (whether considered by the investigator drug related or unrelated to drug) which occurred at an incidence rate of at least 3.0% in the PROVENTIL HFA Inhalation Aerosol group and more frequently in the PROVENTIL HFA Inhalation Aerosol group than in the HFA-134a placebo inhaler group.

not known whether the components of PROVENTIL HFA Inhalation Aerosol are excreted in human milk.

Because of the potential for tumorigenicity shown for albuterol in animal studies and lack of experience with the use of PROVENTIL HFA Inhalation Aerosol by nursing mothers, a decision should be made whether to discontinue nursing or to discontinue the drug, taking into account the importance of the drug to the mother. Caution should be exercised when albuterol sulfate is administered to a nursing woman.

Pediatrics

The safety and effectiveness of PROVENTIL HFA Inhalation Aerosol in pediatric patients below the age of 4 years have not been established.

Geriatrics

PROVENTIL HFA Inhalation Aerosol has not been studied in a geriatric population. As with other beta$_2$-agonists, special caution should be observed when using PROVENTIL HFA Inhalation Aerosol in elderly patients who have concomitant cardiovascular disease that could be adversely affected by this class of drug.

ADVERSE REACTIONS

Adverse reaction information concerning PROVENTIL® HFA Inhalation Aerosol is derived from a 12-week, double-blind, double-dummy study which compared PROVENTIL HFA Inhalation Aerosol, a CFC 11/12 propelled albuterol inhaler, and an HFA-134a placebo inhaler in 565 asthmatic patients. The following table lists the incidence of all adverse events (whether considered by the investigator drug related or unrelated to drug) from this study which occurred at a rate of 3% or greater in the PROVENTIL HFA Inhalation Aerosol treatment group and more frequently in the PROVENTIL HFA Inhalation Aerosol treatment group than in the placebo group. Overall, the incidence and nature of the adverse reactions reported for PROVENTIL HFA Inhalation Aerosol and a CFC 11/12 propelled albuterol inhaler were comparable.

[See table at top of previous page]

Adverse events reported by less than 3% of the patients receiving PROVENTIL HFA Inhalation Aerosol, and by a greater proportion of PROVENTIL HFA Inhalation Aerosol patients than placebo patients, which have the potential to be related to PROVENTIL HFA Inhalation Aerosol include: dysphonia, increased sweating, dry mouth, chest pain, edema, rigors, ataxia, leg cramps, hyperkinesia, eructation, flatulence, tinnitus, diabetes mellitus, anxiety, depression, somnolence, rash. Palpitation and dizziness have also been observed with PROVENTIL HFA Inhalation Aerosol.

Adverse events reported in a 4-week pediatric clinical trial comparing PROVENTIL HFA Inhalation Aerosol and a CFC 11/12 propelled albuterol inhaler occurred at a low incidence rate and were similar to those seen in the adult trials.

In small, cumulative dose studies, tremor, nervousness, and headache appeared to be dose related.

Rare cases of urticaria, angioedema, rash, bronchospasm, and oropharyngeal edema have been reported after the use of inhaled albuterol. In addition, albuterol, like other sympathomimetic agents, can cause adverse reactions such as hypertension, angina, vertigo, central nervous system stimulation, insomnia, headache, metabolic acidosis, and drying or irritation of the oropharynx.

OVERDOSAGE

The expected symptoms with overdosage are those of excessive beta-adrenergic stimulation and/or occurrence or exaggeration of any of the symptoms listed under **ADVERSE REACTIONS**, e.g., seizures, angina, hypertension or hypotension, tachycardia with rates up to 200 beats per minute, arrhythmias, nervousness, headache, tremor, dry mouth, palpitation, nausea, dizziness, fatigue, malaise, and insomnia.

Hypokalemia may also occur. As with all sympathomimetic medications, cardiac arrest and even death may be associated with abuse of PROVENTIL® HFA Inhalation Aerosol. Treatment consists of discontinuation of PROVENTIL HFA Inhalation Aerosol together with appropriate symptomatic therapy. The judicious use of a cardioselective beta-receptor blocker may be considered, bearing in mind that such medication can produce bronchospasm. There is insufficient evidence to determine if dialysis is beneficial for overdosage of PROVENTIL HFA Inhalation Aerosol.

The oral median lethal dose of albuterol sulfate in mice is greater than 2000 mg/kg (approximately 6800 times the maximum recommended daily inhalation dose for adults on a mg/m² basis and approximately 3200 times the maximum recommended daily inhalation dose for children on a mg/m² basis). In mature rats, the subcutaneous median lethal dose of albuterol sulfate is approximately 450 mg/kg (approximately 3000 times the maximum recommended daily inhalation dose for adults on a mg/m² basis and approximately 1400 times the maximum recommended daily inhalation dose for children on a mg/m² basis). In young rats, the subcutaneous median lethal dose is approximately 2000 mg/kg

(approximately 14,000 times the maximum recommended daily inhalation dose for adults on a mg/m² basis and approximately 6400 times the maximum recommended daily inhalation dose for children on a mg/m² basis). The inhalation median lethal dose has not been determined in animals.

DOSAGE AND ADMINISTRATION

For treatment of acute episodes of bronchospasm or prevention of asthmatic symptoms, the usual dosage for adults and children 4 years of age and older is two inhalations repeated every 4 to 6 hours. More frequent administration or a larger number of inhalations is not recommended. In some patients, one inhalation every 4 hours may be sufficient. Each actuation of PROVENTIL® HFA Inhalation Aerosol delivers 108 mcg of albuterol sulfate (equivalent to 90 mcg of albuterol base) from the mouthpiece. It is recommended to prime the inhaler before using for the first time and in cases where the inhaler has not been used for more than 2 weeks by releasing four "test sprays" into the air, away from the face.

Exercise Induced Bronchospasm Prevention: The usual dosage for adults and children 4 years of age and older is two inhalations 15 to 30 minutes before exercise.

To maintain proper use of this product, it is important that the mouthpiece be washed and dried thoroughly at least once a week. The inhaler may cease to deliver medication if not properly cleaned and dried thoroughly (see **PRECAUTIONS, Information for Patients** section). Keeping the plastic mouthpiece clean is very important to prevent medication buildup and blockage. The inhaler may cease to deliver medication if not properly cleaned and air dried thoroughly. If the mouthpiece becomes blocked, washing the mouthpiece will remove the blockage.

If a previously effective dose regimen fails to provide the usual response, this may be a marker of destabilization of asthma and requires reevaluation of the patient and the treatment regimen, giving special consideration to the possible need for anti-inflammatory treatment, e.g., corticosteroids.

HOW SUPPLIED

PROVENTIL® HFA (albuterol sulfate) Inhalation Aerosol is supplied as a pressurized aluminum canister with a yellow plastic actuator and orange dust cap each in boxes of one. Each actuation delivers 120 mcg of albuterol sulfate from the valve and 108 mcg of albuterol sulfate from the mouthpiece (equivalent to 90 mcg of albuterol base). Canisters with a labeled net weight of 6.7 g contain 200 inhalations (NDC 0085-1132-01).

Rx only. Store between 15°-25°C (59°-77°F). For best results, canister should be at room temperature before use. SHAKE WELL BEFORE USING.

The yellow actuator supplied with PROVENTIL HFA Inhalation Aerosol should not be used with any other product canisters, and actuator from other products should not be used with a PROVENTIL HFA Inhalation Aerosol canister. The correct amount of medication in each canister cannot be assured after 200 actuations, even though the canister is not completely empty. The canister should be discarded when the labeled number of actuations have been used.

WARNING: Avoid spraying in eyes. Contents under pressure. Do not puncture or incinerate. Exposure to temperatures above 120°F may cause bursting. Keep out of reach of children.

PROVENTIL® HFA Inhalation Aerosol does not contain chlorofluorocarbons (CFCs) as the propellant.

Developed and Manufactured by:
3M Health Care Limited
Loughborough UK
or
3M Drug Delivery Systems
Northridge, CA 91324, USA
Distributed by:
Schering Corporation, a subsidiary of
MERCK & CO., INC.
Whitehouse Station, NJ 08889, USA

Copyright © 1996, 2011, 2012 Schering Corporation U.S. Patent No. 5,605,674 a subsidiary of **Merck & Co., Inc.** All rights reserved.
The trademarks depicted in this piece are owned by their respective companies.

658000
Rev. 06/12

Attention Health Care Professional:
Detach Patient's Instructions for Use from package insert and dispense with the product.
PROVENTIL® HFA
(albuterol sulfate)
Inhalation Aerosol
FOR ORAL INHALATION ONLY

Patient's Instructions for Use

Figure 1

Figure 2

Before using your PROVENTIL® HFA (albuterol sulfate) Inhalation Aerosol, read complete instructions carefully. Children should use PROVENTIL HFA Inhalation Aerosol under adult supervision, as instructed by the patient's doctor

Please note that ⓒⓕⓒ indicates that this inhalation aerosol does not contain chlorofluorocarbons (CFCs) as the propellant.

1. SHAKE THE INHALER WELL immediately before each use. **Then remove the cap from the mouthpiece** (see Figure 1). **Check mouthpiece for foreign objects prior to use.** Make sure the canister is fully inserted into the actuator.

2. As with all aerosol medications, it is recommended to prime the inhaler before using for the first time and in cases where the inhaler has not been used for more than 2 weeks. Prime by releasing four "test sprays" into the air, away from your face.

3. BREATHE OUT FULLY THROUGH THE MOUTH, expelling as much air from your lungs as possible. Place the mouthpiece fully into the mouth, holding the inhaler in its upright position (see Figure 2) and closing the lips around it.

4. WHILE BREATHING IN DEEPLY AND SLOWLY THROUGH THE MOUTH, FULLY DEPRESS THE TOP OF THE METAL CANISTER with your index finger (see Figure 2).

5. HOLD YOUR BREATH AS LONG AS POSSIBLE, up to 10 seconds. Before breathing out, remove the inhaler from your mouth and release your finger from the canister.

6. If your physician has prescribed additional puffs, wait 1 minute, shake the inhaler again, and repeat steps 3 through 5. Replace the cap after use.

7. KEEPING THE PLASTIC MOUTHPIECE CLEAN IS EXTREMELY IMPORTANT TO PREVENT MEDICATION BUILDUP AND BLOCKAGE. THE MOUTHPIECE SHOULD BE WASHED, SHAKEN TO REMOVE EXCESS WATER, AND AIR DRIED THOROUGHLY AT LEAST ONCE A WEEK. INHALER MAY STOP SPRAYING IF NOT PROPERLY CLEANED.

   Routine cleaning instructions:
   Step 1. To clean, remove the canister and mouthpiece cap. Wash the mouthpiece through the top and bottom with warm running water for 30 seconds at least once a week (see Figure A). **Never immerse the metal canister in water.**

Figure A

Wash mouthpiece under warm running water.

Figure B

Allow mouthpiece to air dry, such as overnight.
[See figure C at top of next column]
When blocked, little or no medicine comes out.
Step 2. To dry, shake off excess water and let the mouthpiece air dry thoroughly, such as overnight (see Figure B). When the mouthpiece is dry, replace the canister

Figure C

and the mouthpiece cap. Blockage from medication buildup is more likely to occur if the mouthpiece is not allowed to air dry thoroughly.

IF YOUR INHALER HAS BECOME BLOCKED (little or no medication coming out of the mouthpiece, see Figure C), wash the mouthpiece as described in Step 1 and air dry thoroughly as described in Step 2.

IF YOU NEED TO USE YOUR INHALER BEFORE IT IS COMPLETELY DRY, SHAKE OFF EXCESS WATER, replace the canister, and test spray twice into the air, away from your face, to remove most of the water remaining in the mouthpiece. Then take your dose as prescribed. **After such use, rewash and air dry thoroughly as described in Steps 1 and 2.**

8. The correct amount of medication in each inhalation cannot be assured after 200 actuations, even though the canister is not completely empty. The canister should be discarded when the labeled number of actuations have been used. Before you reach the specific number of actuations, you should consult your physician to determine whether a refill is needed. Just as you should not take extra doses without consulting your physician, you also should not stop using PROVENTIL HFA Inhalation Aerosol without consulting your physician.

You may notice a slightly different taste or spray force than you are used to with PROVENTIL HFA Inhalation Aerosol, compared to other albuterol inhalation aerosol products.

DOSAGE:
Use only as directed by your physician.

WARNINGS:
The action of PROVENTIL® HFA Inhalation Aerosol should last up to 4 to 6 hours. PROVENTIL HFA Inhalation Aerosol should not be used more frequently than recommended. Do not increase the number of puffs or frequency of doses of PROVENTIL HFA Inhalation Aerosol without consulting your physician. If you find that treatment with PROVENTIL HFA Inhalation Aerosol becomes less effective for symptomatic relief, your symptoms become worse, and/or you need to use the product more frequently than usual, medical attention should be sought immediately. While you are taking PROVENTIL HFA Inhalation Aerosol, other inhaled drugs should be taken only as directed by your physician. If you are pregnant or nursing, contact your physician about the use of PROVENTIL HFA Inhalation Aerosol.

Common adverse effects of treatment with PROVENTIL HFA Inhalation Aerosol include palpitations, chest pain, rapid heart rate, tremor, or nervousness. Effective and safe use of PROVENTIL HFA Inhalation Aerosol includes an understanding of the way that it should be administered. Use PROVENTIL HFA Inhalation Aerosol only with the yellow actuator supplied with the product. The PROVENTIL HFA Inhalation Aerosol actuator should not be used with other aerosol medications.

For best results, use at room temperature. Avoid exposing product to extreme heat and cold.

Shake well before use.

Contents Under Pressure.
Do not puncture. Do not store near heat or open flame. Exposure to temperatures above 120°F may cause bursting. Never throw container into fire or incinerator. Store between 15° - 25°C (59° - 77°F). Avoid spraying in eyes. Keep out of reach of children.

Further Information: Your PROVENTIL® HFA (albuterol sulfate) Inhalation Aerosol does not contain chlorofluorocarbons (CFCs) as the propellant. Instead, the inhaler contains a hydrofluoroalkane (HFA-134a) as the propellant.
Developed and Manufactured by:
3M Health Care Limited
Loughborough UK
or
3M Drug Delivery Systems
Northridge, CA 91324, USA
Distributed by:
Schering Corporation, a subsidiary of
MERCK & CO., INC.
Whitehouse Station, NJ 08889, USA

Rev. 06/12   658000
Copyright © 1996, 2011, 2012 Schering Corporation, a subsidiary of **Merck & Co., Inc.**
All rights reserved.
U.S. Patent No. 5,605,674.

RAGWITEK™   ℞
(Short Ragweed Pollen Allergen Extract)
Tablet for Sublingual Use

HIGHLIGHTS OF PRESCRIBING INFORMATION
These highlights do not include all the information needed to use RAGWITEK safely and effectively. See full prescribing information for RAGWITEK.
RAGWITEK™ (Short Ragweed Pollen Allergen Extract)
Tablet for Sublingual Use
Initial U.S. Approval: 2014

> **WARNING: SEVERE ALLERGIC REACTIONS**
> *See full prescribing information for complete boxed warning.*
> - RAGWITEK can cause life-threatening allergic reactions such as anaphylaxis and severe laryngopharyngeal restriction. (5.1)
> - Do not administer RAGWITEK to patients with severe, unstable or uncontrolled asthma. (4)
> - Observe patients in the office for at least 30 minutes following the initial dose. (5.1)
> - Prescribe auto-injectable epinephrine, instruct and train patients on its appropriate use, and instruct patients to seek immediate medical care upon its use. (5.2)
> - RAGWITEK may not be suitable for patients with certain underlying medical conditions that may reduce their ability to survive a serious allergic reaction. (5.2)
> - RAGWITEK may not be suitable for patients who may be unresponsive to epinephrine or inhaled bronchodilators, such as those taking beta-blockers. (5.2)

——————**INDICATIONS AND USAGE**——————
RAGWITEK is an allergen extract indicated as immunotherapy for the treatment of short ragweed pollen-induced allergic rhinitis, with or without conjunctivitis, confirmed by positive skin test or *in vitro* testing for pollen-specific IgE antibodies for short ragweed pollen. RAGWITEK is approved for use in adults 18 through 65 years of age. (1)

—————**DOSAGE AND ADMINISTRATION**—————
For sublingual use only.
- One tablet daily. (2.1)
- Initiate treatment at least 12 weeks before the expected onset of ragweed pollen season and continue treatment throughout the season. (2.2)
- Place the tablet immediately under the tongue. Allow it to remain there until completely dissolved. Do not swallow for at least 1 minute. (2.2)
- Administer the first dose of RAGWITEK under the supervision of a physician with experience in the diagnosis and treatment of allergic diseases. Observe patients in the office for at least 30 minutes following the initial dose. (2.2)

—————**DOSAGE FORMS AND STRENGTHS**—————
- Tablet, 12 Amb a 1-Unit (Amb a 1-U) (3)

——————**CONTRAINDICATIONS**——————
- Severe, unstable or uncontrolled asthma. (4)
- History of any severe systemic allergic reaction or any severe local reaction to sublingual allergen immunotherapy. (4)
- A history of eosinophilic esophagitis. (4)
- Hypersensitivity to any of the inactive ingredients contained in this product. (4)

————**WARNINGS AND PRECAUTIONS**————
- Inform patients of the signs and symptoms of serious allergic reactions and instruct them to seek immediate medical care and discontinue therapy should any of these occur. (5.1)
- In case of oral inflammation or wounds, stop treatment with RAGWITEK to allow complete healing of the oral cavity. (5.7)

——————**ADVERSE REACTIONS**——————
- Adverse reactions reported in ≥5% of patients were: throat irritation, oral pruritus, ear pruritus, oral paraesthesia, mouth edema, and tongue pruritus. (6)

To report SUSPECTED ADVERSE REACTIONS, contact Merck Sharp & Dohme Corp., a subsidiary of Merck & Co., Inc., at 1-877-888-4231 or FDA at 1-800-FDA-1088 or www.fda.gov/medwatch

See 17 for PATIENT COUNSELING INFORMATION and Medication Guide

                                    Revised: 06/2014

FULL PRESCRIBING INFORMATION: CONTENTS*
WARNING: SEVERE ALLERGIC REACTIONS
* Sections or subsections omitted from the full prescribing information are not listed

FULL PRESCRIBING INFORMATION

> **WARNING: SEVERE ALLERGIC REACTIONS**
> - RAGWITEK can cause life-threatening allergic reactions such as anaphylaxis and severe laryngopharyngeal restriction. (5.1)
> - Do not administer RAGWITEK to patients with severe, unstable or uncontrolled asthma. (4)
> - Observe patients in the office for at least 30 minutes following the initial dose. (5.1)
> - Prescribe auto-injectable epinephrine, instruct and train patients on its appropriate use, and instruct patients to seek immediate medical care upon its use. (5.2)
> - RAGWITEK may not be suitable for patients with certain underlying medical conditions that may reduce their ability to survive a serious allergic reaction. (5.2)
> - RAGWITEK may not be suitable for patients who may be unresponsive to epinephrine or inhaled bronchodilators, such as those taking beta-blockers. (5.2)

1   INDICATIONS AND USAGE
RAGWITEK™ is an allergen extract indicated as immunotherapy for the treatment of short ragweed pollen-induced allergic rhinitis, with or without conjunctivitis, confirmed by positive skin test or *in vitro* testing for pollen-specific IgE antibodies for short ragweed pollen. RAGWITEK is approved for use in adults 18 through 65 years of age.
RAGWITEK is not indicated for the immediate relief of allergic symptoms.

2   DOSAGE AND ADMINISTRATION
For sublingual use only.
2.1   Dose
One RAGWITEK tablet daily.
2.2   Administration
Administer the first dose of RAGWITEK in a healthcare setting under the supervision of a physician with experience in the diagnosis and treatment of allergic diseases. After receiving the first dose of RAGWITEK, observe the patient for at least 30 minutes to monitor for signs or symptoms of a severe systemic or a severe local allergic reaction. If the patient tolerates the first dose, the patient may take subsequent doses at home.
Take the tablet from the blister unit after carefully removing the foil with dry hands.
Place the tablet immediately under the tongue. Allow it to remain there until completely dissolved. Do not swallow for at least 1 minute.
Wash hands after handling the tablet.
Do not take the tablet with food or beverage. Food or beverage should not be taken for the following 5 minutes after taking the tablet.
Initiate treatment at least 12 weeks before the expected onset of ragweed pollen season and continue treatment throughout the season. The safety and efficacy of initiating treatment in season have not been established.

Data regarding the safety of restarting treatment after missing a dose of RAGWITEK are limited. In the clinical trials, treatment interruptions for up to seven days were allowed.

Prescribe auto-injectable epinephrine to patients prescribed RAGWITEK and instruct them in the proper use of emergency self-injection of epinephrine [see Warnings and Precautions (5.2)].

3 DOSAGE FORMS AND STRENGTHS

RAGWITEK is available as 12 Amb a 1-Unit (Amb a 1-U) tablets that are white to off-white, circular with a debossed double hexagon on one side.

4 CONTRAINDICATIONS

RAGWITEK is contraindicated in patients with:
• Severe, unstable or uncontrolled asthma
• A history of any severe systemic allergic reaction
• A history of any severe local reaction after taking any sublingual allergen immunotherapy
• A history of eosinophilic esophagitis
• Hypersensitivity to any of the inactive ingredients [gelatin, mannitol, and sodium hydroxide] contained in this product [see Description (11)].

5 WARNINGS AND PRECAUTIONS

5.1 Severe Allergic Reactions

RAGWITEK can cause systemic allergic reactions including anaphylaxis which may be life-threatening. In addition, RAGWITEK can cause severe local reactions, including laryngopharyngeal swelling, which can compromise breathing and be life-threatening. Educate patients to recognize the signs and symptoms of these allergic reactions and instruct them to seek immediate medical care and discontinue therapy should any of these occur. Allergic reactions may require treatment with epinephrine. [See Warnings and Precautions (5.2).]

Administer the initial dose of RAGWITEK in a healthcare setting under the supervision of a physician with experience in the diagnosis and treatment of allergic diseases and prepared to manage a life-threatening systemic or local allergic reaction. Observe patients in the office for at least 30 minutes following the initial dose of RAGWITEK.

5.2 Epinephrine

Prescribe auto-injectable epinephrine to patients receiving RAGWITEK. Instruct patients to recognize the signs and symptoms of a severe allergic reaction and in the proper use of emergency auto-injectable epinephrine. Instruct patients to seek immediate medical care upon use of auto-injectable epinephrine and to stop treatment with RAGWITEK. [See Patient Counseling Information (17).]

See the epinephrine package insert for complete information.

RAGWITEK may not be suitable for patients with certain medical conditions that may reduce the ability to survive a serious allergic reaction or increase the risk of adverse reactions after epinephrine administration. Examples of these medical conditions include but are not limited to: markedly compromised lung function (either chronic or acute), unstable angina, recent myocardial infarction, significant arrhythmia, and uncontrolled hypertension.

RAGWITEK may not be suitable for patients who are taking medications that can potentiate or inhibit the effect of epinephrine. These medications include:

Beta-adrenergic blockers: Patients taking beta-adrenergic blockers may be unresponsive to the usual doses of epinephrine used to treat serious systemic reactions, including anaphylaxis. Specifically, beta-adrenergic blockers antagonize the cardiostimulating and bronchodilating effects of epinephrine.

Alpha-adrenergic blockers, ergot alkaloids: Patients taking alpha-adrenergic blockers may be unresponsive to the usual doses of epinephrine used to treat serious systemic reactions, including anaphylaxis. Specifically, alpha-adrenergic blockers antagonize the vasoconstricting and hypertensive effects of epinephrine. Similarly, ergot alkaloids may reverse the pressor effects of epinephrine.

Tricyclic antidepressants, levothyroxine sodium, monoamine oxidase inhibitors, and certain antihistamines: The adverse effects of epinephrine may be potentiated in patients taking tricyclic antidepressants, levothyroxine sodium, monoamine oxidase inhibitors, and the antihistamines chlorpheniramine, and diphenhydramine.

Cardiac glycosides, diuretics: Patients who receive epinephrine while taking cardiac glycosides or diuretics should be observed carefully for the development of cardiac arrhythmias.

5.3 Upper Airway Compromise

RAGWITEK can cause local reactions in the mouth or throat that could compromise the upper airway [see Adverse Reactions (6.1)]. Consider discontinuation of RAGWITEK in patients who experience persistent and escalating adverse reactions in the mouth or throat.

5.4 Eosinophilic Esophagitis

Eosinophilic esophagitis has been reported in association with sublingual tablet immunotherapy [see Contraindica-

tions (4)]. Discontinue RAGWITEK and consider a diagnosis of eosinophilic esophagitis in patients who experience severe or persistent gastro-esophageal symptoms including dysphagia or chest pain.

5.5 Asthma

Subjects with asthma who participated in clinical trials had asthma of a severity that required, at most, a daily low dose of an inhaled corticosteroid. RAGWITEK has not been studied in subjects with moderate or severe asthma.

Withhold immunotherapy with RAGWITEK if the patient is experiencing an acute asthma exacerbation. Reevaluate patients who have recurrent asthma exacerbations and consider discontinuation of RAGWITEK.

5.6 Concomitant Allergen Immunotherapy

RAGWITEK has not been studied in subjects who are receiving concomitant allergen immunotherapy. Concomitant dosing with other allergen immunotherapy may increase the likelihood of local or systemic adverse reactions to either subcutaneous or sublingual allergen immunotherapy.

5.7 Oral Inflammation

Stop treatment with RAGWITEK to allow complete healing of the oral cavity in patients with oral inflammation (e.g., oral lichen planus, mouth ulcers, or thrush) or oral wounds, such as those following oral surgery or dental extraction.

6 ADVERSE REACTIONS

Adverse reactions reported in ≥5% of patients were: throat irritation, oral pruritus, ear pruritus, oral paraesthesia, mouth edema, and tongue pruritus.

6.1 Clinical Trials Experience

Because clinical trials are conducted under widely varying conditions, adverse reaction rates observed in the clinical trials of a drug cannot be directly compared to rates in the clinical trials of another drug and may not reflect the rates observed in clinical practice.

In 4 placebo-controlled clinical trials, 1057 subjects 18 years of age and older with short ragweed pollen-induced rhinitis, with or without conjunctivitis, received at least one dose of RAGWITEK, of whom 327 (31%) completed at least 12 weeks of therapy. Of the subjects treated with RAGWITEK, 52% were male, 25% had mild asthma, and 82% were sensitized to other allergens in addition to ragweed pollen. The subject population was 83% White, 12% African American, and 2% Asian. Subject demographics in placebo-treated subjects were similar to the active group. The pooled analysis includes safety data from two 28-day safety studies and safety data from the first 28 days of two 52-week safety and efficacy studies. Adverse reactions reported in ≥1% of subjects in the 28-day pooled analysis treated with RAGWITEK are shown in Table 1.

The most common adverse reactions reported in subjects treated with RAGWITEK were throat irritation (16.6% vs 3.3% placebo), oral pruritus (10.9% vs 2.0%), ear pruritus (10.4% vs 1.1%), and oral paraesthesia (10.0% vs 4.0%). The percentage of subjects who discontinued from the clinical trials because of an adverse reaction while exposed to RAGWITEK or placebo was 4.4% and 0.8%, respectively. The most common adverse reactions that led to study discontinuation in subjects who were exposed to RAGWITEK were mouth edema, swollen tongue, and dysphagia.

One subject (1/1057; 0.1%) who received RAGWITEK experienced a treatment-related severe systemic allergic reaction that led to discontinuation of RAGWITEK. The subject had local reactions starting on Day 1 of treatment with RAGWITEK. On Day 6 symptoms progressed and included swelling of the throat, dyspnea, nausea, and lightheadedness. The subject fully recovered after treatment with epinephrine (self-administered), antihistamines, and oral corticosteroids.

Table 1: Adverse Reactions Reported in ≥1% of Subjects Treated with RAGWITEK (28-day pooled analysis)

Adverse Reaction	RAGWITEK (N=1057)	Placebo (N=757)
Ear and Labyrinth Disorders		
Ear pruritus	10.4%	1.1%
Respiratory, Thoracic and Mediastinal Disorders		
Throat irritation	16.6%	3.3%
Oropharyngeal pain	1.5%	0.7%
Throat tightness	1.3%	0.5%
Gastrointestinal Disorders		
Oral pruritus	10.9%	2.0%
Paraesthesia oral	10.0%	4.0%
Mouth edema	6.1%	0.5%
Tongue pruritus	5.1%	0.5%
Lip swelling	3.0%	0.4%
Swollen tongue	2.9%	0.5%
Lip pruritus	1.5%	0.1%
Dry mouth	1.4%	0.7%
Tongue edema	1.3%	0.5%
Nausea	1.1%	0.3%
Palatal edema	1.1%	0%
Dysphagia	1.0%	0%
Skin and Subcutaneous Tissue Disorders		
Pruritus	1.8%	1.3%
General Disorders and Administration Site Conditions		
Chest discomfort	1.0%	0%

The overall safety profile beyond Day 28 in the two 52-week trials was similar to that observed in the pooled 28-day analysis.

8 USE IN SPECIFIC POPULATIONS

8.1 Pregnancy

Pregnancy Category C:
Animal reproduction studies have not been performed with RAGWITEK. It is also not known whether RAGWITEK can cause fetal harm when administered to a pregnant woman or can affect reproduction capacity. RAGWITEK should be used during pregnancy only if clearly needed.

Because systemic and local adverse reactions with immunotherapy may be poorly tolerated during pregnancy, RAGWITEK should be used during pregnancy only if clearly needed.

8.3 Nursing Mothers

It is not known if RAGWITEK is excreted in human milk. Because many drugs are excreted in human milk, caution should be exercised when RAGWITEK is administered to a nursing woman.

8.4 Pediatric Use

RAGWITEK is not approved for use in pediatric patients because safety and efficacy have not been established.

8.5 Geriatric Use

RAGWITEK is not approved for use in patients over 65 years of age because safety and efficacy have not been established.

11 DESCRIPTION

RAGWITEK tablets contain pollen allergen extract from Short Ragweed (*Ambrosia artemisiifolia*). RAGWITEK is a sublingual orally disintegrating tablet that dissolves rapidly.

RAGWITEK is available as a tablet of 12 Amb a 1-U of short ragweed pollen allergen extract.

Inactive ingredients: gelatin NF (fish source), mannitol USP, and sodium hydroxide NF.

12 CLINICAL PHARMACOLOGY

12.1 Mechanism of Action

The precise mechanisms of action of allergen immunotherapy are not known.

13 NONCLINICAL TOXICOLOGY

13.1 Carcinogenesis, Mutagenesis, Impairment of Fertility

No studies have been performed in animals to evaluate the carcinogenic potential of RAGWITEK.

There were no positive findings in a combined *in vivo* Comet and micronucleus assay in rats using Short Ragweed (*Ambrosia artemisiifolia*) pollen allergen extract.

Fertility studies have not been performed with Short Ragweed pollen allergen extract.

14 CLINICAL STUDIES

The efficacy of RAGWITEK in the treatment of ragweed pollen-induced allergic rhinitis, with or without conjunctivitis, was investigated in two double-blind, placebo-controlled clinical trials in adults 18 through 50 years of age. Subjects received RAGWITEK or placebo for approximately 12 weeks prior to the start of the ragweed pollen season and throughout the ragweed pollen season.

The subject population was 86% White, 9% African American, and 3% Asian. The subject population was almost equally divided between males and females. Overall, the mean age of subjects was 36 years. Subjects with asthma who participated in clinical trials had asthma of a severity that required, at most, a daily low dose of an inhaled corticosteroid. Approximately 16% of subjects had mild asthma at baseline.

Efficacy was established by self-reporting of rhinoconjunctivitis daily symptom scores (DSS) and daily medication scores (DMS). Daily rhinoconjunctivitis symptoms included four nasal symptoms (runny nose, stuffy nose, sneezing, and itchy nose), and two ocular symptoms (gritty/itchy eyes and watery eyes). The rhinoconjunctivitis symptoms were measured on a scale of 0 (none) to 3 (severe). Subjects in clinical trials were allowed to take symptom-relieving medications (including systemic and topical antihistamines, and topical and oral corticosteroids) as needed. The daily medication score measured the use of standard open-label allergy medications. Predefined values were assigned to each class of medication. Generally, systemic and topical antihistamines were given the lowest score, topical steroids an intermediate score, and oral corticosteroids the highest score.

The sums of the DSS and DMS were combined into the Total Combined Score (TCS) which was averaged over the peak ragweed pollen season. Also, in each study, the average TCS over the entire ragweed season was assessed. Other endpoints in both studies included the average DSS during the peak and entire ragweed season, and the average DMS during the peak ragweed season.

Trial 1

The first study was a placebo-controlled trial which evaluated subjects 18 through 50 years of age comparing RAGWITEK (n=187) and placebo (n=188) administered as a sublingual tablet daily. In this trial, approximately 22% of subjects had mild asthma and 85% were sensitized to other allergens in addition to short ragweed. Subjects with asthma who participated in this trial had asthma of a severity that required, at most, a daily low dose of an inhaled corticosteroid. Subjects with a clinical history of symptomatic allergies to non-short ragweed pollen allergens that required treatment during the ragweed pollen season were excluded from the trial. The subject population was 78% White, 12% African American, and 8% Asian, and almost equally divided between males and females. The mean age of subjects in this study was 35.4 years. The two treatment groups were balanced with regard to baseline characteristics. The results of this study are shown in Table 2.

Trial 2

The second study was a placebo-controlled trial which evaluated subjects 18 through 50 years of age comparing RAGWITEK (n=194) and placebo (n=198) administered as a sublingual tablet daily. Approximately 17% of subjects had mild asthma and 78% were sensitized to other allergens in addition to short ragweed. Subjects with asthma who participated in this trial had asthma of a severity that required, at most, a daily low dose of an inhaled corticosteroid. Subjects with a clinical history of symptomatic allergies to non-short ragweed pollen allergens that required treatment during the ragweed pollen season were excluded from the trial. The subject population was 88% White, 8.9% African American, 2% Asian, and almost equally divided between males and females. The mean age of subjects in this study was 36.4 years. The two treatment groups were balanced with regard to baseline characteristics. The results of this study are shown in Table 3.

A decrease in TCS during the peak ragweed season for subjects treated with RAGWITEK compared to placebo-treated subjects was demonstrated in both trials. Subjects treated with RAGWITEK also showed a decrease in the average TCS from the start of and throughout the entire ragweed pollen season. Similar decreases were observed in subjects treated with RAGWITEK for other endpoints (see Tables 2 and 3).

[See table 2 above]
[See table 3 above]

16 HOW SUPPLIED/STORAGE AND HANDLING

RAGWITEK 12 Amb a 1-U tablets are white to off-white, circular sublingual tablets with a debossed double hexagon on one side.

RAGWITEK is supplied as follows:

3 blister packages of 10 tablets (30 tablets total). NDC 0006-5420-30

9 blister packages of 10 tablets (90 tablets total). NDC 0006-5420-54

Store at controlled room temperature, 20°C-25°C (68°F-77°F); excursions permitted between 15°C-30°C (59°F-86°F). Store in the original package until use to protect from moisture.

17 PATIENT COUNSELING INFORMATION

Advise patients to read the FDA-approved patient labeling (Medication Guide) and to keep RAGWITEK and all medicines out of the reach of children.

Severe Allergic Reactions

Advise patients that RAGWITEK may cause life-threatening systemic or local allergic reactions, including anaphylaxis. Educate patients about the signs and symptoms of these allergic reactions *[see Warnings and Precautions (5.1)]*. The signs and symptoms of a severe allergic reaction may include: syncope, dizziness, hypotension, tachycardia, dyspnea, wheezing, bronchospasm, chest discomfort, cough, abdominal pain, vomiting, diarrhea, rash, pruritus, flushing, and urticaria.

Ensure that patients have auto-injectable epinephrine and instruct patients in its proper use. Instruct patients who experience a severe allergic reaction to seek immediate medical care, discontinue RAGWITEK, and resume treatment only when advised by a physician to do so. *[See Warnings and Precautions (5.2).]*

Advise patients to read the patient information for epinephrine.

Table 2: Trial 1: Total Combined Scores (TCS), Rhinoconjunctivitis Daily Symptom Scores (DSS), and Daily Medication Scores (DMS) During the Ragweed Pollen Season

Endpoint*	RAGWITEK (N)[†] Score[‡]	Placebo (N)[†] Score[‡]	Treatment Difference (RAGWITEK – Placebo)	Difference Relative to Placebo[§] Estimate (95% CI)
TCS Peak Season[¶]	(159) 6.22	(164) 8.46	-2.24	-26% (-38.7, -14.6)
TCS Entire Season	(160) 5.21	(166) 7.01	-1.80	-26% (-37.6, -13.5)
DSS Peak Season	(159) 4.65	(164) 5.59	-0.94	-17% (-28.6, -4.6)
DSS Entire Season	(160) 4.05	(166) 4.87	-0.82	-17% (-28.5, -4.5)
DMS Peak Season	(159) 1.57	(164) 2.87	-1.30	-45% (-65.4, -27.0)

TCS=Total Combined Score (DSS + DMS); DSS=Daily Symptom Score; DMS=Daily Medication Score.
* Parametric analysis using analysis of variance model for all endpoints.
† Number of subjects in analyses.
‡ The estimated group means are reported and difference relative to placebo is based on estimated group means.
§ Difference relative to placebo computed as: (RAGWITEK - placebo)/placebo × 100.
¶ Peak ragweed season was defined as maximum 15 days with the highest moving average pollen counts during the ragweed season.

Table 3: Trial 2: Total Combined Scores (TCS), Rhinoconjunctivitis Daily Symptom Scores (DSS), and Daily Medication Scores (DMS) During the Ragweed Pollen Season

Endpoint*	RAGWITEK (N)[†] Score[‡]	Placebo (N)[†] Score[‡]	Treatment Difference (RAGWITEK – Placebo)	Difference Relative to Placebo[§] Estimate (95% CI)
TCS Peak Season[¶]	(152) 6.41	(169) 8.46	-2.04	-24% (-36.5, -11.3)
TCS Entire Season	(158) 5.18	(174) 7.09	-1.92	-27% (-38.8, -14.1)
DSS Peak Season	(152) 4.43	(169) 5.37	-0.94	-18% (-29.2, -4.5)
DSS Entire Season	(158) 3.62	(174) 4.58	-0.96	-21% (-31.6, -8.8)
DMS Peak Season	(152) 1.99	(169) 3.09	-1.10	-36% (-55.8, -14.6)

TCS=Total Combined Score (DSS + DMS); DSS=Daily Symptom Score; DMS=Daily Medication Score.
* Parametric analysis using analysis of variance model for all endpoints.
† Number of subjects in analyses.
‡ The estimated group means are reported and difference relative to placebo is based on estimated group means.
§ Difference relative to placebo computed as: (RAGWITEK - placebo)/placebo × 100.
¶ Peak ragweed season was defined as maximum 15 days with the highest moving average pollen counts during the ragweed season.

Inform patients that the first dose of RAGWITEK must be administered in a healthcare setting under the supervision of a physician and that they will be monitored for at least 30 minutes to watch for signs and symptoms of life-threatening systemic or local allergic reaction *[see Warnings and Precautions (5.1)]*.

Because of the risk of upper airway compromise, instruct patients with persistent and escalating adverse reactions in the mouth or throat to discontinue RAGWITEK and to contact their healthcare professional. *[See Warnings and Precautions (5.3).]*

Because of the risk of eosinophilic esophagitis, instruct patients with severe or persistent symptoms of esophagitis to discontinue RAGWITEK and to contact their healthcare professional. *[See Warnings and Precautions (5.4).]*

Asthma

Instruct patients with asthma that if they have difficulty breathing or if their asthma becomes difficult to control, they should stop taking RAGWITEK and contact their healthcare professional immediately *[see Warnings and Precautions (5.5)]*.

Administration Instructions

Instruct patients to carefully remove the foil from the blister unit with dry hands and then take the sublingual tablet immediately by placing it under the tongue where it will dissolve. Also instruct patients to wash their hands after handling the tablet, and to avoid food or beverages for 5 minutes after taking the tablet. *[See Dosage and Administration (2.2).]*

Manufactured for: Merck Sharp & Dohme Corp., a subsidiary of **MERCK & CO., INC.**, Whitehouse Station, NJ 08889, USA

Manufactured by:
Catalent Pharma Solutions Limited, Blagrove, Swindon, Wiltshire, SN5 8RU UK
For patent information:
www.merck.com/product/patent/home.html
Copyright © 2014 Merck Sharp & Dohme Corp., a subsidiary of **Merck & Co., Inc.**
All rights reserved.
uspi-mk3641-sb-1406r001

MEDICATION GUIDE
RAGWITEK™ (RAG-wi-tek)
(Short Ragweed Pollen Allergen Extract)

Carefully read this Medication Guide before you start taking RAGWITEK™ and each time you get a refill. This Medication Guide does not take the place of talking with your doctor about your medical condition or treatment. Talk with your doctor or pharmacist if there is something you do not understand or if you want to learn more about RAGWITEK.

What is the Most Important Information I Should Know about RAGWITEK?

RAGWITEK can cause severe allergic reactions that may be life-threatening. Stop taking RAGWITEK and get medical treatment right away if you have any of the following symptoms after taking RAGWITEK:

- Trouble breathing
- Throat tightness or swelling
- Trouble swallowing or speaking
- Dizziness or fainting
- Rapid or weak heartbeat
- Severe stomach cramps or pain, vomiting, or diarrhea
- Severe flushing or itching of the skin

For home administration of RAGWITEK, your doctor will prescribe auto-injectable epinephrine, a medicine you can inject if you have a severe allergic reaction after taking RAGWITEK. Your doctor will train and instruct you on the proper use of auto-injectable epinephrine.

Talk to your doctor or read the epinephrine patient information if you have any questions about the use of auto-injectable epinephrine.

What is RAGWITEK?

RAGWITEK is a prescription medicine used for sublingual (under the tongue) immunotherapy to treat ragweed pollen allergies that can cause sneezing, runny or itchy nose, stuffy or congested nose, or itchy and watery eyes. RAGWITEK may be prescribed for persons 18 through 65 years of age who are allergic to ragweed pollen.

RAGWITEK is taken for about 12 weeks before ragweed pollen season and throughout ragweed pollen season.

RAGWITEK is NOT a medication that gives immediate relief for symptoms of ragweed allergy.

Who Should Not Take RAGWITEK?

You should not take RAGWITEK if:

- You have severe, unstable or uncontrolled asthma
- You had a severe allergic reaction in the past that included any of these symptoms:
  - Trouble breathing
  - Dizziness or fainting
  - Rapid or weak heartbeat
- You have ever had difficulty with breathing due to swelling of the throat or upper airway after using any sublingual immunotherapy before.
- You have ever been diagnosed with eosinophilic esophagitis.
- You are allergic to any of the inactive ingredients contained in RAGWITEK. The inactive ingredients contained in RAGWITEK are: gelatin, mannitol, and sodium hydroxide.

What Should I Tell My Doctor Before Taking RAGWITEK?

Your doctor may decide that RAGWITEK is not the best treatment if:

- You have asthma, depending on how severe it is.
- You suffer from lung disease such as chronic obstructive pulmonary disease (COPD)
- You suffer from heart disease such as coronary artery disease, an irregular heart rhythm, or you have hypertension that is not well controlled.
- You are pregnant, plan to become pregnant during the time you will be taking RAGWITEK, or are breast-feeding.
- You are unable or unwilling to administer auto-injectable epinephrine to treat a severe allergic reaction to RAGWITEK.
- You are taking certain medicines that enhance the likelihood of a severe reaction, or interfere with the treatment of a severe reaction. These medicines include:
  - beta blockers and alpha-blockers (prescribed for high blood pressure)
  - cardiac glycosides (prescribed for heart failure or problems with heart rhythm)
  - diuretics (prescribed for heart conditions and high blood pressure)
  - ergot alkaloids (prescribed for migraine headache)
  - monoamine oxidase inhibitors or tricyclic antidepressants (prescribed for depression)
  - thyroid hormone (prescribed for low thyroid activity).

You should tell your doctor if you are taking or have recently taken any other medicines, including medicines obtained without a prescription and herbal supplements. Keep a list of them and show it to your doctor and pharmacist each time you get a new supply of RAGWITEK. Ask your doctor or pharmacist for advice before taking RAGWITEK.

RAGWITEK is not indicated for use in children under 18 years of age.

Are there any Reasons to Stop Taking RAGWITEK?

Stop RAGWITEK and contact your doctor if you have any of the following after taking RAGWITEK:

- Any type of a serious allergic reaction
- Throat tightness that worsens or swelling of the tongue or throat that causes trouble speaking, breathing, or swallowing
- Asthma or any other breathing condition that gets worse
- Dizziness or fainting
- Rapid or weak heartbeat
- Severe stomach cramps or pain, vomiting, or diarrhea
- Severe flushing or itching of the skin
- Heartburn, difficulty swallowing, pain with swallowing, or chest pain that does not go away or worsens

Also, stop taking RAGWITEK following: mouth surgery procedures (such as tooth removal), or if you develop any mouth infections, ulcers or cuts in the mouth or throat.

How Should I Take RAGWITEK?

Take RAGWITEK exactly as your doctor tells you.

RAGWITEK is a prescription medicine that is placed under the tongue.

- Take the tablet from the blister package after carefully removing the foil with dry hands.
- Place the tablet immediately under the tongue. Allow it to remain there until completely dissolved. Do not swallow for at least 1 minute.
- Do not take RAGWITEK with food or beverage. Food and beverage should not be taken for the following 5 minutes.
- Wash hands after taking the tablet.

Take the first tablet of RAGWITEK in your doctor's office. After taking the first tablet, you will be watched for at least 30 minutes for symptoms of a serious allergic reaction.

If you tolerate the first dose of RAGWITEK, you will continue RAGWITEK therapy at home by taking one tablet every day.

Take RAGWITEK as prescribed by your doctor until the end of the treatment course. If you forget to take RAGWITEK, do not take a double dose. Take the next dose at your normal scheduled time the next day. If you miss more than one dose of RAGWITEK, contact your healthcare provider before restarting.

What are the Possible Side Effects of RAGWITEK?

The most commonly reported side effects were itching of the mouth, lips, or tongue, swelling under the tongue, or throat irritation. These side effects, by themselves, were not dangerous or life-threatening.

RAGWITEK can cause severe allergic reactions that may be life-threatening. Symptoms of allergic reactions to RAGWITEK include:

- Trouble breathing
- Throat tightness or swelling
- Trouble swallowing or speaking
- Dizziness or fainting
- Rapid or weak heartbeat
- Severe stomach cramps or pain, vomiting, or diarrhea
- Severe flushing or itching of the skin

For additional information on the possible side effects of RAGWITEK talk with your doctor or pharmacist. You may report side effects to the U.S. Food and Drug Administration (FDA) at 1-800-FDA-1088 or www.fda.gov/medwatch.

How Should I Store RAGWITEK?

Keep RAGWITEK out of the reach of children.

Throw away any unused RAGWITEK after the expiration date which is stated on the carton and blister pack after "EXP."

Store RAGWITEK in a dry place at room temperature, 15°C to 30°C (59°F to 86°F), in the original package.

General Information about RAGWITEK

Medicines are sometimes prescribed for purposes other than those listed in a Medication Guide. Do not use RAGWITEK for a condition for which it was not prescribed. Do not give RAGWITEK to other people, even if they have the same symptoms. It may harm them.

This Medication Guide summarizes the most important information about RAGWITEK. If you would like more information, talk with your doctor. You can ask your doctor or pharmacist for information about RAGWITEK that was written for healthcare professionals. For more information, go to: www.ragwitek.com or call 1-800-622-4477 (toll-free).

This Medication Guide has been approved by the U.S. Food and Drug Administration.

Manufactured for: Merck Sharp & Dohme Corp., a subsidiary of **MERCK & CO., INC.**, Whitehouse Station, NJ 08889, USA

Manufactured by:
Catalent Pharma Solutions Limited, Blagrove, Swindon, Wiltshire, SN5 8RU UK

For patent information:
www.merck.com/product/patent/home.html

Copyright © 2014 Merck Sharp & Dohme Corp., a subsidiary of **Merck & Co., Inc.**

All rights reserved.

Revised: 04/2014

usmg-mk3641-sb-1404r000

Shown in Product Identification Guide, page 309

REBETOL®
[rē' bə-tōl]
(ribavirin USP)
capsules, for oral use

REBETOL®
(ribavirin USP)
oral solution

HIGHLIGHTS OF PRESCRIBING INFORMATION
These highlights do not include all the information needed to use REBETOL safely and effectively. See full prescribing information for REBETOL.

REBETOL® (ribavirin USP) capsules, for oral use
REBETOL® (ribavirin USP) oral solution
Initial U.S. Approval: 1998

WARNING: RISK OF SERIOUS DISORDERS AND RIBAVIRIN-ASSOCIATED EFFECTS
See full prescribing information for complete boxed warning.

- **REBETOL monotherapy is not effective for the treatment of chronic hepatitis C (5.10).**
- **The hemolytic anemia associated with REBETOL therapy may result in worsening of cardiac disease that has led to fatal and nonfatal myocardial infarctions. Patients with a history of significant or unstable cardiac disease should not be treated with REBETOL (2.4, 5.2, 6.1).**
- **Significant teratogenic and embryocidal effects have been demonstrated in all animal species exposed to ribavirin. Therefore, REBETOL therapy is contraindicated in women who are pregnant and in the male partners of women who are pregnant. Extreme care must be taken to avoid pregnancy during therapy and for 6 months after completion of treatment in both female patients and in female partners of male patients who are taking REBETOL therapy (4, 5.1, 8.1, 13.1, 17.2).**

RECENT MAJOR CHANGES

Dosage and Administration

REBETOL/PegIntron Combination Therapy (2.1)	05/2013
Dose Modifications (2.4)	05/2013

Warnings and Precautions

Impact on Growth – Pediatric Use (5.9)	11/2013

INDICATIONS AND USAGE

REBETOL is a nucleoside analogue indicated in combination with interferon alfa-2b (pegylated and nonpegylated) for the treatment of Chronic Hepatitis C (CHC) in patients 3 years of age or older with compensated liver disease. (1.1) Patients with the following characteristics are less likely to benefit from re-treatment after failing a course of therapy: previous nonresponse, previous pegylated interferon treatment, significant bridging fibrosis or cirrhosis, and genotype 1 infection.

DOSAGE AND ADMINISTRATION

REBETOL is administered according to body weight. (2.1, 2.2)

Dose reduction or discontinuation is recommended in patients experiencing certain adverse reactions or renal dysfunction. (2.4, 2.5, 12.3)

DOSAGE FORMS AND STRENGTHS

REBETOL Capsules 200 mg (3)
REBETOL Oral Solution 40 mg per mL (3)

CONTRAINDICATIONS

- Pregnant women and men whose female partners are pregnant (4, 8.1)
- Known hypersensitivity reactions such as Stevens-Johnson syndrome, toxic epidermal necrolysis, and erythema multiforme to ribavirin or any component of the product (4)
- Autoimmune hepatitis (4)
- Hemoglobinopathies (4)
- Creatinine clearance less than 50 mL/min (4)
- Coadministration with didanosine (4, 7.1)

WARNINGS AND PRECAUTIONS

- *Pregnancy Category X* (5.1, 8.1, 8.3)
  - Birth defects and fetal death with ribavirin: Patients must have a negative pregnancy test prior to therapy; use at least 2 forms of contraception and undergo monthly pregnancy tests.

Patients exhibiting the following conditions should be closely monitored and may require dose reduction or discontinuation of therapy:

- Monotherapy with ribavirin is not permitted. (5.10)
- Hemolytic anemia may occur with a significant initial drop in hemoglobin. (5.2)
- Pancreatitis. (5.3)
- Pulmonary infiltrates or pulmonary function impairment. (5.4)
- New or worsening ophthalmologic disorders. (5.5)
- Severe decreases in neutrophil and platelet counts, and hematologic, endocrine (e.g., TSH), and hepatic abnormalities. (5.6)
- Dental/periodontal disorders reported with combination therapy. (5.7)
- Concomitant administration of azathioprine. (5.8)
- Weight loss and growth inhibition reported during combination therapy in pediatric patients. Long-term growth inhibition (height) reported in some patients. (5.9)

ADVERSE REACTIONS

Hemolytic anemia. (6.1)

Most common adverse reactions (approximately 40%) in adult patients receiving REBETOL/PegIntron or INTRON A combination therapy are injection site reaction, fatigue/asthenia, headache, rigors, fevers, nausea, myalgia and anxiety/emotional lability/irritability. (6.1, 6.2) Most common adverse reactions (greater than 25%) in pediatric patients receiving REBETOL/PegIntron therapy are: pyrexia, headache, neutropenia, fatigue, anorexia, injection site erythema, and vomiting. (6.1)

To report SUSPECTED ADVERSE REACTIONS, contact Merck Sharp & Dohme Corp., a subsidiary of Merck & Co. Inc. at 1-877-888-4231 or FDA at 1-800-FDA-1088 or www.fda.gov/medwatch.

DRUG INTERACTIONS

Nucleoside analogues: Closely monitor for toxicities. Discontinue nucleoside reverse transcriptase inhibitors or reduce dose or discontinue interferon, ribavirin or both with worsening toxicities. (7.2)

USE IN SPECIFIC POPULATIONS

• Nursing mothers: Potential adverse reactions from the drug in nursing infants. (8.1, 8.3)
• Pediatrics: Safety and efficacy in patients less than 3 years old have not been established. (8.4)
• Organ transplant recipients: Safety and efficacy not studied. (8.6)
• Co-infected Patients: Safety and efficacy with HIV or HBV co-infection have not been established. (8.7)

See 17 for PATIENT COUNSELING INFORMATION and Medication Guide

Revised: 11/2013

FULL PRESCRIBING INFORMATION: CONTENTS*
WARNING: RISK OF SERIOUS DISORDERS AND RIBAVIRIN-ASSOCIATED EFFECTS

FULL PRESCRIBING INFORMATION

> **WARNING: RISK OF SERIOUS DISORDERS AND RIBAVIRIN-ASSOCIATED EFFECTS**
> • **REBETOL monotherapy is not effective for the treatment of chronic hepatitis C virus infection and should not be used alone for this indication [see Warnings and Precautions (5.10)].**
> • **The primary toxicity of ribavirin is hemolytic anemia. The anemia associated with REBETOL therapy may result in worsening of cardiac disease that has led to fatal and nonfatal myocardial infarctions. Patients with a history of significant or unstable cardiac disease should not be treated with REBETOL [see Dosage and Administration (2.4), Warnings and Precautions (5.2), and Adverse Reactions (6.1)].**
> • **Significant teratogenic and embryocidal effects have been demonstrated in all animal species exposed to ribavirin. In addition, ribavirin has a multiple-dose half-life of 12 days, and so it may persist in nonplasma compartments for as long as 6 months. Therefore, REBETOL therapy is contraindicated in women who are pregnant and in the male partners of women who are pregnant. Extreme care must be taken to avoid pregnancy during therapy and for 6 months after completion of treatment in both female patients and in female partners of male patients who are taking REBETOL therapy. At least two reliable forms of effective contraception must be utilized during treatment and during the 6-month post-treatment follow-up period [see Contraindications (4), Warnings and Precautions (5.1), Use in Specific Populations (8.1), Nonclinical Toxicology (13.1), and Patient Counseling Information (17.2)].**

---

1   INDICATIONS AND USAGE
1.1   Chronic Hepatitis C (CHC)

REBETOL® (ribavirin) in combination with interferon alfa-2b (pegylated and nonpegylated) is indicated for the treatment of Chronic Hepatitis C (CHC) in patients 3 years of age and older with compensated liver disease [see Warnings and Precautions (5.9, 5.10), and Use in Specific Populations (8.4)].

The following points should be considered when initiating REBETOL combination therapy with PegIntron® or INTRON A®:
• These indications are based on achieving undetectable HCV-RNA after treatment for 24 or 48 weeks and maintaining a Sustained Virologic Response (SVR) 24 after the last dose.
• Combination therapy with REBETOL/PegIntron is preferred over REBETOL/INTRON A as this combination provides substantially better response rates [see Clinical Studies (14)].
• Patients with the following characteristics are less likely to benefit from re-treatment after failing a course of therapy: previous nonresponse, previous pegylated interferon treatment, significant bridging fibrosis or cirrhosis, and genotype 1 infection [see Clinical Studies (14)].
• No safety and efficacy data are available for treatment of longer than one year.

2   DOSAGE AND ADMINISTRATION

Under no circumstances should REBETOL capsules be opened, crushed, or broken. REBETOL should be taken with food [see Clinical Pharmacology (12.3)]. REBETOL should not be used in patients with creatinine clearance less than 50 mL/min.

2.1   REBETOL/PegIntron Combination Therapy
Adult Patients

The recommended dose of PegIntron is 1.5 mcg/kg/week subcutaneously in combination with 800 to 1400 mg REBETOL capsules orally based on patient body weight (see **Table 1**). The volume of PegIntron to be injected depends on the strength of PegIntron and patient's body weight, refer to labeling for PegIntron for additional dosing information.

Duration of Treatment – Interferon Alpha-naïve Patients
The treatment duration for patients with genotype 1 is 48 weeks. Discontinuation of therapy should be considered in patients who do not achieve at least a 2 log₁₀ drop or loss of HCV-RNA at 12 weeks, or if HCV-RNA remains detectable after 24 weeks of therapy. Patients with genotype 2 and 3 should be treated for 24 weeks.

Duration of Treatment – Re-treatment with PegIntron/REBETOL of Prior Treatment Failures
The treatment duration for patients who previously failed therapy is 48 weeks, regardless of HCV genotype. Re-treated patients who fail to achieve undetectable HCV-RNA at Week 12 of therapy, or whose HCV-RNA remains detect-

able after 24 weeks of therapy, are highly unlikely to achieve SVR and discontinuation of therapy should be considered [see Clinical Studies (14.1)].

Table 1: Recommended Dosing for REBETOL in Combination Therapy with PegIntron (Adults)

Body Weight kg (lbs)	REBETOL Daily Dose	REBETOL Number of Capsules
<66 (<144)	800 mg/day	2 × 200-mg capsules A.M. 2 × 200-mg capsules P.M.
66-80 (145-177)	1000 mg/day	2 × 200-mg capsules A.M. 3 × 200-mg capsules P.M.
81-105 (178-231)	1200 mg/day	3 × 200-mg capsules A.M. 3 × 200-mg capsules P.M.
>105 (231)	1400 mg/day	3 × 200-mg capsules A.M. 4 × 200-mg capsules P.M.

Pediatric Patients
Dosing for pediatric patients is determined by body surface area for PegIntron and by body weight for REBETOL. The recommended dose of PegIntron is 60 mcg/m²/week subcutaneously in combination with 15 mg/kg/day of REBETOL orally in two divided doses (see **Table 2**) for pediatric patients ages 3-17 years. Patients who reach their 18th birthday while receiving PegIntron/REBETOL should remain on the pediatric dosing regimen. The treatment duration for patients with genotype 1 is 48 weeks. Patients with genotype 2 and 3 should be treated for 24 weeks.

Table 2: Recommended REBETOL* Dosing in Combination Therapy (Pediatrics)

Body Weight kg (lbs)	REBETOL Daily Dose	REBETOL Number of Capsules
<47 (<103)	15 mg/kg/day	Use REBETOL Oral Solution†
47-59 (103-131)	800 mg/day	2 × 200-mg capsules A.M. 2 × 200-mg capsules P.M.
60-73 (132-162)	1000 mg/day	2 × 200-mg capsules A.M. 3 × 200-mg capsules P.M.
>73 (>162)	1200 mg/day	3 × 200-mg capsules A.M. 3 × 200-mg capsules P.M.

* REBETOL to be used in combination with PegIntron 60 mcg/m² weekly.
† REBETOL Oral Solution may be used for any patient regardless of body weight.

2.2   REBETOL/INTRON A Combination Therapy
Adults
Duration of Treatment – Interferon Alpha-naïve Patients
The recommended dose of INTRON A is 3 million IU three times weekly subcutaneously. The recommended dose of REBETOL capsules depends on the patient's body weight (refer to **Table 3**). The recommended duration of treatment for patients previously untreated with interferon is 24 to 48 weeks. The duration of treatment should be individualized to the patient depending on baseline disease characteristics, response to therapy, and tolerability of the regimen [see Indications and Usage (1.1), Adverse Reactions (6.1), and Clinical Studies (14)]. After 24 weeks of treatment, virologic response should be assessed. Treatment discontinuation should be considered in any patient who has not achieved an HCV-RNA below the limit of detection of the assay by 24 weeks. There are no safety and efficacy data on treatment for longer than 48 weeks in the previously untreated patient population.

Duration of Treatment – Re-treatment with INTRON A/REBETOL in Relapse Patients
In patients who relapse following nonpegylated interferon monotherapy, the recommended duration of treatment is 24 weeks.

Table 3: Recommended Dosing

Body Weight	REBETOL Capsules
≤75 kg	2 × 200-mg capsules AM 3 × 200-mg capsules PM daily orally
>75 kg	3 × 200-mg capsules AM 3 × 200-mg capsules PM daily orally

Pediatrics The recommended dose of REBETOL is 15 mg/kg per day orally (divided dose AM and PM). Refer to **Table 2** for Pediatric Dosing of REBETOL in combination with INTRON A. INTRON A for Injection by body weight of 25 kg to 61 kg is 3 million IU/m^2 three times weekly subcutaneously. Refer to adult dosing table for greater than 61 kg body weight.

The recommended duration of treatment is 48 weeks for pediatric patients with genotype 1. After 24 weeks of treatment, virologic response should be assessed. Treatment discontinuation should be considered in any patient who has not achieved an HCV-RNA below the limit of detection of the assay by this time. The recommended duration of treatment for pediatric patients with genotype 2/3 is 24 weeks.

2.3 Laboratory Tests
The following laboratory tests are recommended for all patients treated with REBETOL, prior to beginning treatment and then periodically thereafter.
- Standard hematologic tests - including hemoglobin (pretreatment, Week 2 and Week 4 of therapy, and as clinically appropriate [see Warnings and Precautions (5.2, 5.7)], complete and differential white blood cell counts, and platelet count.
- Blood chemistries - liver function tests and TSH.
- Pregnancy - including monthly monitoring for women of childbearing potential.
- ECG [see Warnings and Precautions (5.2)].

2.4 Dose Modifications
If severe adverse reactions or laboratory abnormalities develop during combination REBETOL/INTRON A therapy or REBETOL/PegIntron therapy, modify, or discontinue the dose until the adverse reaction abates or decreases in severity [see Warnings and Precautions (5)]. If intolerance persists after dose adjustment, combination therapy should be discontinued. Dose reduction of PegIntron in adult patients on REBETOL/PegIntron combination therapy is accomplished in a two-step process from the original starting dose

of 1.5 mcg/kg/week, to 1 mcg/kg/week, then to 0.5 mcg/kg/week, if needed. Refer to labeling for PegIntron for additional information regarding dose reduction of PegIntron.
In the adult combination therapy Study 2, dose reductions occurred in 42% of subjects receiving PegIntron 1.5 mcg/kg and REBETOL 800 mg daily, including 57% of those subjects weighing 60 kg or less. In Study 4, 16% of subjects had a dose reduction of PegIntron to 1 mcg/kg in combination with REBETOL, with an additional 4% requiring the second dose reduction of PegIntron to 0.5 mcg/kg due to adverse events [see Adverse Reactions (6.1)].
Dose reduction in pediatric patients is accomplished by modifying the recommended PegIntron dose in a two-step process from the original starting dose of 60 mcg/m²/week, to 40 mcg/m²/week, then to 20 mcg/m²/week, if needed (see **Table 4**). In the pediatric combination therapy trial, dose reductions occurred in 25% of subjects receiving PegIntron 60 mcg/m² weekly and REBETOL 15 mg/kg daily. Dose reduction in pediatric patients is accomplished by modifying the recommended REBETOL dose from the original starting dose of 15 mg/kg daily in a two-step process to 12 mg/kg/day, then to 8 mg/kg/day, if needed (see **Table 4**).
REBETOL should not be used in patients with creatinine clearance less than 50 mL/min. Patients with impaired renal function and those over the age of 50 should be carefully monitored with respect to development of anemia [see Warnings and Precautions (5.2), Use in Specific Populations (8.5), and Clinical Pharmacology (12.3)].
REBETOL should be administered with caution to patients with pre-existing cardiac disease. Patients should be assessed before commencement of therapy and should be appropriately monitored during therapy. If there is any deterioration of cardiovascular status, therapy should be stopped [see Warnings and Precautions (5.2)].
For patients with a history of stable cardiovascular disease, a permanent dose reduction is required if the hemoglobin decreases by greater than or equal to 2 g/dL during any 4-week period. In addition, for these cardiac history patients, if the hemoglobin remains less than 12 g/dL after 4 weeks on a reduced dose, the patient should discontinue combination therapy.
It is recommended that a patient whose hemoglobin level falls below 10 g/dL have his/her REBETOL dose modified or discontinued per Table 4 [see Warnings and Precautions (5.2)].
[See table 4 below]
Refer to labeling for INTRON A or PegIntron for additional information about how to reduce an INTRON A or PegIntron dose.

2.5 Discontinuation of Dosing
Adults In HCV genotype 1, interferon-alfa-naïve patients receiving PegIntron in combination with ribavirin, discontinuation of therapy is recommended if there is not at least a 2 log₁₀ drop or loss of HCV-RNA at 12 weeks of therapy, or if HCV-RNA levels remain detectable after 24 weeks of therapy. Regardless of genotype, previously treated patients who have detectable HCV-RNA at Week 12 or 24 are highly unlikely to achieve SVR and discontinuation of therapy should be considered.
Pediatrics (3-17 years of age) It is recommended that patients receiving PegIntron/REBETOL combination (excluding HCV Genotype 2 and 3) be discontinued from therapy at 12 weeks if their treatment Week 12 HCV-RNA dropped less than 2 log₁₀ compared to a pretreatment or at 24 weeks if they have detectable HCV-RNA at treatment Week 24.

3 DOSAGE FORMS AND STRENGTHS
REBETOL Capsules 200 mg
REBETOL Oral Solution 40 mg per mL

4 CONTRAINDICATIONS
REBETOL combination therapy is contraindicated in:
- women who are pregnant. REBETOL may cause fetal harm when administered to a pregnant woman. REBETOL is contraindicated in women who are or may become pregnant. If REBETOL is used during pregnancy, or if the patient becomes pregnant while taking REBETOL, the patient should be apprised of the potential hazard to her fetus [see Warnings and Precautions (5.1), Use in Specific Populations (8.1), and Patient Counseling Information (17.2)]
- men whose female partners are pregnant
- patients with known hypersensitivity reactions such as Stevens-Johnson syndrome, toxic, epidermal necrolysis, and erythema multiforme to ribavirin or any component of the product
- patients with autoimmune hepatitis
- patients with hemoglobinopathies (e.g., thalassemia major, sickle-cell anemia)
- patients with creatinine clearance less than 50 mL/min. [see Use in Specific Populations (8.5) and Clinical Pharmacology (12.3)]
- Coadministration of REBETOL and didanosine is contraindicated because exposure to the active metabolite of didanosine (dideoxyadenosine 5'-triphosphate) is increased. Fatal hepatic failure, as well as peripheral neuropathy, pancreatitis, and symptomatic hyperlactatemia/lactic acidosis have been reported in patients receiving didanosine in combination with ribavirin [see Drug Interactions (7.1)].

5 WARNINGS AND PRECAUTIONS
5.1 Pregnancy
REBETOL capsules and oral solution may cause birth defects and death of the unborn child. REBETOL therapy should not be started until a report of a negative pregnancy test has been obtained immediately prior to planned initiation of therapy. Patients should use at least two forms of contraception and have monthly pregnancy tests during treatment and during the 6-month period after treatment has been stopped. Extreme care must be taken to avoid pregnancy in female patients and in female partners of male patients. REBETOL has demonstrated significant teratogenic and embryocidal effects in all animal species in which adequate studies have been conducted. These effects occurred at doses as low as one twentieth of the recommended human dose of ribavirin. REBETOL therapy should not be started until a report of a negative pregnancy test has been obtained immediately prior to planned initiation of therapy [see Boxed Warning, Contraindications (4), Use in Specific Populations (8.1), and Patient Counseling Information (17.2)].
5.2 Anemia
The primary toxicity of ribavirin is hemolytic anemia, which was observed in approximately 10% of REBETOL/INTRON A-treated subjects in clinical trials. The anemia associated with REBETOL capsules occurs within 1 to 2 weeks of initiation of therapy. Because the initial drop in hemoglobin may be significant, it is advised that hemoglobin or hematocrit be obtained before the start of treatment and at Week 2 and Week 4 of therapy, or more frequently if clinically indicated. Patients should then be followed as clinically appropriate [see Dosage and Administration (2.4, 2.5)].
Fatal and nonfatal myocardial infarctions have been reported in patients with anemia caused by REBETOL. Patients should be assessed for underlying cardiac disease before initiation of ribavirin therapy. Patients with pre-existing cardiac disease should have electrocardiograms administered before treatment, and should be appropriately monitored during therapy. If there is any deterioration of cardiovascular status, therapy should be suspended or discontinued [see Dosage and Administration (2.4, 2.5)]. Because cardiac disease may be worsened by drug-induced anemia, patients with a history of significant or unstable cardiac disease should not use REBETOL.

Table 4: Guidelines for Dose Modification and Discontinuation of REBETOL in combination with PegIntron or INTRON A Based on Laboratory Parameters in Adults and Pediatrics

Laboratory Parameters	Reduce REBETOL Daily Dose (see note 1) if:	Reduce PegIntron or INTRON A Dose (see note 2) if:	Discontinue Therapy if:
WBC	N/A	1.0 to <1.5 × 10⁹/L	<1.0 × 10⁹/L
Neutrophils	N/A	0.5 to <0.75 × 10⁹/L	<0.5 × 10⁹/L
Platelets	N/A	25 to < 50 × 10⁹/L (adults)	<25 × 10⁹/L (adults)
	N/A	50 to <70 × 10⁹/L (pediatrics)	<50 × 10⁹/L (pediatrics)
Creatinine	N/A	N/A	>2 mg/dL (pediatrics)
Hemoglobin in patients without history of cardiac disease	8.5 to <10 g/dL	N/A	<8.5 g/dL
Reduce REBETOL Dose by 200 mg/day and PegIntron or INTRON A Dose by Half if:			
Hemoglobin in patients with history of stable cardiac disease*†	≥2 g/dL decrease in hemoglobin during any four week period during treatment		<8.5 g/dL or <12 g/dL after four weeks of dose reduction

Note 1: *Adult patients:* 1st dose reduction of ribavirin is by 200 mg/day (except in patients receiving the 1,400 mg, dose reduction should be by 400 mg/day). If needed, 2nd dose reduction of ribavirin is by an additional 200 mg/day. Patients whose dose of ribavirin is reduced to 600 mg daily receive one 200 mg capsule in the morning and two 200 mg capsules in the evening.
Pediatric patients: 1st dose reduction of ribavirin is to 12 mg/kg/day, 2nd dose reduction of ribavirin is to 8 mg/kg/day.
Note 2: *Adult patients treated with REBETOL and PegIntron:* 1st dose reduction of PegIntron is to 1 mcg/kg/week. If needed, 2nd dose reduction of PegIntron is to 0.5 mcg/kg/week.
Pediatric patients treated with REBETOL and PegIntron: 1st dose reduction of PegIntron is to 40 mcg/m²/week, 2nd dose reduction of PegIntron is to 20 mcg/m²/week.
For patients on REBETOL/INTRON A combination therapy: reduce INTRON A dose by 50%.
* Pediatric patients who have pre-existing cardiac conditions and experience a hemoglobin decrease greater than or equal to 2 g/dL during any 4-week period during treatment should have weekly evaluations and hematology testing.
† These guidelines are for patients with stable cardiac disease. Patients with a history of significant or unstable cardiac disease should not be treated with PegIntron/REBETOL combination therapy [see Warnings and Precautions (5.2)].

5.3 Pancreatitis

REBETOL and INTRON A or PegIntron therapy should be suspended in patients with signs and symptoms of pancreatitis and discontinued in patients with confirmed pancreatitis.

5.4 Pulmonary Disorders

Pulmonary symptoms, including dyspnea, pulmonary infiltrates, pneumonitis, pulmonary hypertension, and pneumonia, have been reported during therapy with REBETOL with alpha interferon combination therapy; occasional cases of fatal pneumonia have occurred. In addition, sarcoidosis or the exacerbation of sarcoidosis has been reported. If there is evidence of pulmonary infiltrates or pulmonary function impairment, the patient should be closely monitored, and if appropriate, combination therapy should be discontinued.

5.5 Ophthalmologic Disorders

Ribavirin is used in combination therapy with alpha interferons. Decrease or loss of vision, retinopathy including macular edema, retinal artery or vein, thrombosis, retinal hemorrhages and cotton wool spots, optic neuritis, papilledema, and serous retinal detachment are induced or aggravated by treatment with alpha interferons. All patients should receive an eye examination at baseline. Patients with pre-existing ophthalmologic disorders (e.g., diabetic or hypertensive retinopathy) should receive periodic ophthalmologic exams during combination therapy with alpha interferon treatment. Any patient who develops ocular symptoms should receive a prompt and complete eye examination. Combination therapy with alpha interferons should be discontinued in patients who develop new or worsening ophthalmologic disorders.

5.6 Laboratory Tests

PegIntron in combination with ribavirin may cause severe decreases in neutrophil and platelet counts, and hematologic, endocrine (e.g., TSH), and hepatic abnormalities. Patients on PegIntron/REBETOL combination therapy should have hematology and blood chemistry testing before the start of treatment and then periodically thereafter. In the adult clinical trial, complete blood counts (including hemoglobin, neutrophil, and platelet counts) and chemistries (including AST, ALT, bilirubin, and uric acid) were measured during the treatment period at Weeks 2, 4, 8, 12, and then at 6-week intervals, or more frequently if abnormalities developed. In pediatric subjects, the same laboratory parameters were evaluated with additional assessment of hemoglobin at treatment Week 6. TSH levels were measured every 12 weeks during the treatment period. HCV-RNA should be measured periodically during treatment [see Dosage and Administration (2)].

5.7 Dental and Periodontal Disorders

Dental and periodontal disorders have been reported in patients receiving ribavirin and interferon or peginterferon combination therapy. In addition, dry mouth could have a damaging effect on teeth and mucous membranes of the mouth during long-term treatment with the combination of REBETOL and pegylated or nonpegylated interferon alfa-2b. Patients should brush their teeth thoroughly twice daily and have regular dental examinations. If vomiting occurs, they should be advised to rinse out their mouth thoroughly afterwards.

5.8 Concomitant Administration of Azathioprine

Pancytopenia (marked decreases in red blood cells, neutrophils, and platelets) and bone marrow suppression have been reported in the literature to occur within 3 to 7 weeks after the concomitant administration of pegylated interferon/ribavirin and azathioprine. In this limited number of patients (n=8), myelotoxicity was reversible within 4 to 6 weeks upon withdrawal of both HCV antiviral therapy and concomitant azathioprine and did not recur upon reintroduction of either treatment alone. PegIntron, REBETOL, and azathioprine should be discontinued for pancytopenia, and pegylated interferon/ribavirin should not be reintroduced with concomitant azathioprine [see Drug Interactions (7.4)].

5.9 Impact on Growth - Pediatric Use

Data on the effects of PegIntron and REBETOL on growth come from an open-label study in subjects 3 through 17 years of age, in which weight and height changes are compared to US normative population data. In general, the weight and height gain of pediatric subjects treated with PegIntron and REBETOL lags behind that predicted by normative population data for the entire length of treatment. Severely inhibited growth velocity (less than 3rd percentile) was observed in 70% of the subjects while on treatment. Following treatment, rebound growth and weight gain occurred in most subjects. Long-term follow-up data in pediatric subjects, however, indicates that PegIntron in combination therapy with REBETOL may induce a growth inhibition that results in reduced adult height in some patients [see Adverse Reactions (6.1)].

Similarly, an impact on growth was seen in subjects after treatment with REBETOL and INTRON A combination therapy for one year. In a long-term follow-up trial of a limited number of these subjects, combination therapy resulted in reduced final adult height in some subjects [see Adverse Reactions (6.2)].

5.10 Usage Safeguards

Based on results of clinical trials, ribavirin monotherapy is not effective for the treatment of chronic hepatitis C virus infection; therefore, REBETOL capsules or oral solution must not be used alone. The safety and efficacy of REBETOL capsules and oral solution have only been established when used together with INTRON A or PegIntron (not other interferons) as combination therapy.

The safety and efficacy of REBETOL/INTRON A and PegIntron therapy for the treatment of HIV infection, adenovirus, RSV, parainfluenza, or influenza infections have

Table 5: Adverse Reactions Occurring in Greater Than 5% of Adult Subjects

Adverse Reactions	Percentage of Subjects Reporting Adverse Reactions*		Adverse Reactions	Percentage of Subjects Reporting Adverse Reactions*	
	PegIntron 1.5 mcg/kg/ REBETOL (N=511)	INTRON A/ REBETOL (N=505)		PegIntron 1.5 mcg/kg/ REBETOL (N=511)	INTRON A/ REBETOL (N=505)
Application Site			**Musculoskeletal**		
Injection Site Inflammation	25	18	Myalgia	56	50
Injection Site Reaction	58	36	Arthralgia	34	28
Autonomic Nervous System			Musculoskeletal Pain	21	19
Dry Mouth	12	8	**Psychiatric**		
Increased Sweating	11	7	Insomnia	40	41
Flushing	4	3	Depression	31	34
Body as a Whole			Anxiety/Emotional Lability/Irritability	47	47
Fatigue/Asthenia	66	63	Concentration Impaired	17	21
Headache	62	58	Agitation	8	5
Rigors	48	41	Nervousness	6	6
Fever	46	33	**Reproductive, Female**		
Weight Loss	29	20	Menstrual Disorder	7	6
Right Upper Quadrant Pain	12	6	**Resistance Mechanism**		
Chest Pain	8	7	Viral Infection	12	12
Malaise	4	6	Fungal Infection	6	1
Central/Peripheral Nervous System			**Respiratory System**		
Dizziness	21	17	Dyspnea	26	24
Endocrine			Coughing	23	16
Hypothyroidism	5	4	Pharyngitis	12	13
Gastrointestinal			Rhinitis	8	6
Nausea	43	33	Sinusitis	6	5
Anorexia	32	27	**Skin and Appendages**		
Diarrhea	22	17	Alopecia	36	32
Vomiting	14	12	Pruritus	29	28
Abdominal Pain	13	13	Rash	24	23
Dyspepsia	9	8	Skin Dry	24	23
Constipation	5	5	**Special Senses, Other**		
Hematologic Disorders			Taste Perversion	9	4
Neutropenia	26	14	**Vision Disorders**		
Anemia	12	17	Vision Blurred	5	6
Leukopenia	6	5	Conjunctivitis	4	5
Thrombocytopenia	5	2			
Liver and Biliary System					
Hepatomegaly	4	4			

* A subject may have reported more than one adverse reaction within a body system/organ class category.

Table 6: Treatment-Related Adverse Reactions (Greater Than or Equal to 10% Incidence) By Descending Frequency

Study 4
Percentage of Subjects Reporting Treatment-Related Adverse Reactions

Adverse Reactions	PegIntron 1.5 mcg/kg with REBETOL (N=1019)	PegIntron 1 mcg/kg with REBETOL (N=1016)	Pegasys 180 mcg with Copegus (N=1035)
Fatigue	67	68	64
Headache	50	47	41
Nausea	40	35	34
Chills	39	36	23
Insomnia	38	37	41
Anemia	35	30	34
Pyrexia	35	32	21
Injection Site Reactions	34	35	23
Anorexia	29	25	21
Rash	29	25	34
Myalgia	27	26	22
Neutropenia	26	19	31
Irritability	25	25	25
Depression	25	19	20
Alopecia	23	20	17
Dyspnea	21	20	22
Arthralgia	21	22	22
Pruritus	18	15	19
Influenza-like Illness	16	15	15
Dizziness	16	14	13
Diarrhea	15	16	14
Cough	15	16	17
Weight Decreased	13	10	10
Vomiting	12	10	9
Unspecified Pain	12	13	9
Dry Skin	11	11	12
Anxiety	11	11	10
Abdominal Pain	10	10	10
Leukopenia	9	7	10

not been established. REBETOL capsules should not be used for these indications. Ribavirin for inhalation has separate labeling, which should be consulted if ribavirin inhalation therapy is being considered.

There are significant adverse reactions caused by REBETOL/INTRON A or PegIntron therapy, including severe depression and suicidal ideation, hemolytic anemia, suppression of bone marrow function, autoimmune and infectious disorders, pulmonary dysfunction, pancreatitis, and diabetes. Suicidal ideation or attempts occurred more frequently among pediatric patients, primarily adolescents, compared to adult patients (2.4% versus 1%) during treatment and off-therapy follow-up. Labeling for INTRON A and PegIntron should be reviewed in their entirety for additional safety information prior to initiation of combination treatment.

6   ADVERSE REACTIONS

Clinical trials with REBETOL in combination with PegIntron or INTRON A have been conducted in over 7800 subjects from 3 to 76 years of age.

The primary toxicity of ribavirin is hemolytic anemia. Reductions in hemoglobin levels occurred within the first 1 to 2 weeks of oral therapy. Cardiac and pulmonary reactions associated with anemia occurred in approximately 10% of patients *[see Warnings and Precautions (5.2)]*.

Greater than 96% of all subjects in clinical trials experienced one or more adverse reactions. The most commonly reported adverse reactions in adult subjects receiving PegIntron or INTRON A in combination with REBETOL were injection site inflammation/reaction, fatigue/asthenia, headache, rigors, fevers, nausea, myalgia and anxiety/emotional lability/irritability. The most common adverse reactions in pediatric subjects, ages 3 and older, receiving REBETOL in combination with PegIntron or INTRON A were pyrexia, headache, neutropenia, fatigue, anorexia, injection site erythema, and vomiting.

The Adverse Reactions section references the following clinical trials:
- REBETOL/PegIntron Combination therapy trials:
  - Clinical Study 1 – evaluated PegIntron monotherapy (not further described in this label; see labeling for PegIntron for information about this trial).
  - Study 2 – evaluated REBETOL 800 mg/day flat dose in combination with 1.5 mcg/kg/week PegIntron or with INTRON A.
  - Study 3 – evaluated PegIntron/weight-based REBETOL in combination with PegIntron/flat dose REBETOL regimen.
  - Study 4 – compared two PegIntron (1.5 mcg/kg/week and 1 mcg/kg/week) doses in combination with REBETOL and a third treatment group receiving Pegasys® (180 mcg/week)/Copegus® (1000-1200 mg/day).
  - Study 5 – evaluated PegIntron (1.5 mcg/kg/week) in combination with weight-based REBETOL in prior treatment failure subjects.

- PegIntron/REBETOL Combination Therapy in Pediatric Patients
- REBETOL/INTRON A Combination Therapy trials for adults and pediatrics

Serious adverse reactions have occurred in approximately 12% of subjects in clinical trials with PegIntron with or without REBETOL *[see BOXED WARNING, Warnings and Precautions (5)]*. The most common serious events occurring in subjects treated with PegIntron and REBETOL were depression and suicidal ideation *[see Warnings and Precautions (5.2)]*, each occurring at a frequency of less than 1%. Suicidal ideation or attempts occurred more frequently among pediatric patients, primarily adolescents, compared to adult patients (2.4% versus 1%) during treatment and off-therapy follow-up *[see Warnings and Precautions (5.10)]*. The most common fatal reaction occurring in subjects treated with PegIntron and REBETOL was cardiac arrest, suicide ideation, and suicide attempt *[see Warnings and Precautions (5.10)]*, all occurring in less than 1% of subjects. Because clinical trials are conducted under widely varying conditions, adverse reactions rates observed in the clinical trials of a drug cannot be directly compared to rates in the clinical trials of another drug and may not reflect the rates observed in clinical practice.

6.1   Clinical Trials Experience – REBETOL/PegIntron Combination Therapy
Adult Subjects

Adverse reactions that occurred in the clinical trial at greater than 5% incidence are provided by treatment group from the REBETOL/PegIntron Combination Therapy (Study 2) in **Table 5**.
[See table 5 at top of previous page]
Table 6 summarizes the treatment-related adverse reactions in Study 4 that occurred at a greater than or equal to 10% incidence.
[See table 6 above]
The incidence of serious adverse reactions was comparable in all trials. In Study 3, there was a similar incidence of serious adverse reactions reported for the weight-based REBETOL group (12%) and for the flat-dose REBETOL regimen. In Study 2, the incidence of serious adverse reactions was 17% in the PegIntron/REBETOL groups compared to 14% in the INTRON A/REBETOL group.

In many but not all cases, adverse reactions resolved after dose reduction or discontinuation of therapy. Some subjects experienced ongoing or new serious adverse reactions during the 6-month follow-up period. In Study 2, many subjects continued to experience adverse reactions several months after discontinuation of therapy. By the end of the 6-month follow-up period, the incidence of ongoing adverse reactions by body class in the PegIntron 1.5/REBETOL group was 33% (psychiatric), 20% (musculoskeletal), and 10% (for endocrine and for GI). In approximately 10 to 15% of subjects, weight loss, fatigue, and headache had not resolved.

There have been 31 subject deaths that occurred during treatment or during follow-up in these clinical trials. In Study 1, there was 1 suicide in a subject receiving PegIntron monotherapy and 2 deaths among subjects receiving INTRON A monotherapy (1 murder/suicide and 1 sudden death). In Study 2, there was 1 suicide in a subject receiving PegIntron/REBETOL combination therapy; and 1 subject death in the INTRON A/REBETOL group (motor vehicle accident). In Study 3, there were 14 deaths, 2 of which were probable suicides and 1 was an unexplained death in a person with a relevant medical history of depression. In Study 4, there were 12 deaths, 6 of which occurred in subjects who received PegIntron/REBETOL combination therapy, 5 in the PegIntron 1.5 mcg/REBETOL arm (N=1019) and 1 in the PegIntron 1 mcg/REBETOL arm (N=1016), and 6 of which occurred in subjects receiving Pegasys/Copegus (N=1035); there were 3 suicides that occurred during the off treatment follow-up period in subjects who received PegIntron (1.5 mcg/kg)/REBETOL combination therapy.

In Studies 1 and 2, 10 to 14% of subjects receiving PegIntron, alone or in combination with REBETOL, discontinued therapy compared with 6% treated with INTRON A alone and 13% treated with INTRON A in combination with REBETOL. Similarly in Study 3, 15% of subjects receiving PegIntron in combination with weight-based REBETOL and 14% of subjects receiving PegIntron and flat dose REBETOL discontinued therapy due to an adverse reaction. The most common reasons for discontinuation of therapy were related to known interferon effects of psychiatric, systemic (e.g., fatigue, headache), or gastrointestinal adverse reactions. In Study 4, 13% of subjects in the PegIntron 1.5 mcg/REBETOL arm, 10% in the PegIntron 1 mcg/REBETOL arm and 13% in the Pegasys 180 mcg/Copegus arm discontinued due to adverse events.

In Study 2, dose reductions due to adverse reactions occurred in 42% of subjects receiving PegIntron (1.5 mcg/kg)/REBETOL and in 34% of those receiving INTRON A/REBETOL. The majority of subjects (57%) weighing 60 kg or less receiving PegIntron (1.5 mcg/kg)/REBETOL required dose reduction. Reduction of interferon was dose-related (PegIntron 1.5 mcg/kg greater than PegIntron 0.5 mcg/kg or INTRON A), 40%, 27%, 28%, respectively. Dose reduction for REBETOL was similar across all three groups, 33 to 35%. The most common reasons for dose modifications were neutropenia (18%), or anemia (9%) (see **Laboratory Values**). Other common reasons included depression, fatigue, nausea, and thrombocytopenia. In Study 3, dose modifications due to adverse reactions occurred more frequently with weight-based dosing (WBD) compared to flat dosing (29% and 23%, respectively). In Study 4, 16% of subjects had a dose reduction of PegIntron to 1 mcg/kg in combination with REBETOL, with an additional 4% requiring the second dose reduction of PegIntron to 0.5 mcg/kg due to adverse events compared to 15% of subjects in the Pegasys/Copegus arm, who required a dose reduction to 135 mcg/week with Pegasys, with an additional 7% in the Pegasys/Copegus arm requiring second dose reduction to 90 mcg/week with Pegasys.

In the PegIntron/REBETOL combination trials the most common adverse reactions were psychiatric, which occurred among 77% of subjects in Study 2 and 68% to 69% of subjects in Study 3. These psychiatric adverse reactions included most commonly depression, irritability, and insomnia, each reported by approximately 30% to 40% of subjects in all treatment groups. Suicidal behavior (ideation, attempts, and suicides) occurred in 2% of all subjects during treatment or during follow-up after treatment cessation [see *Warnings and Precautions (5)*]. In Study 4, psychiatric adverse reactions occurred in 58% of subjects in the PegIntron 1.5 mcg/REBETOL arm, 55% of subjects in the PegIntron 1 mcg/REBETOL arm, and 57% of subjects in the Pegasys 180 mcg/Copegus arm.

PegIntron induced fatigue or headache in approximately two-thirds of subjects, with fever or rigors in approximately half of the subjects. The severity of some of these systemic symptoms (e.g., fever and headache) tended to decrease as treatment continued. In Studies 1 and 2, application site inflammation and reaction (e.g., bruise, itchiness, and irritation) occurred at approximately twice the incidence with PegIntron therapies (in up to 75% of subjects) compared with INTRON A. However, injection site pain was infrequent (2 to 3%) in all groups. In Study 3, there was a 23% to 24% incidence overall for injection site reactions or inflammation.

Subjects receiving REBETOL/PegIntron as re-treatment after failing a previous interferon combination regimen reported adverse reactions similar to those previously associated with this regimen during clinical trials of treatment-naïve subjects.

Pediatric Subjects
In general, the adverse-reaction profile in the pediatric population was similar to that observed in adults. In the pediatric trial, the most prevalent adverse reactions in all subjects were pyrexia (80%), headache (62%), neutropenia (33%), fatigue (30%), anorexia (29%), injection-site erythema (29%) and vomiting (27%). The majority of adverse reactions reported in the trial were mild or moderate in severity. Severe adverse reactions were reported in 7% (8/107) of all subjects and included injection site pain (1%), pain in extremity (1%), headache (1%), neutropenia (1%), and pyrexia (4%). Important adverse reactions that occurred in this subject population were nervousness (7%; 7/107), aggression (3%; 3/107), anger (2%; 2/107), and depression (1%; 1/107). Five subjects received levothyroxine treatment, three with clinical hypothyroidism and two with asymptomatic TSH elevations. Weight and height gain of pediatric subjects treated with PegIntron plus REBETOL lagged behind that predicted by normative population data for the entire length of treatment. Severely inhibited growth velocity (less than 3rd percentile) was observed in 70% of the subjects while on treatment.

Dose modifications of PegIntron and/or ribavirin were required in 25% of subjects due to treatment-related adverse reactions, most commonly for anemia, neutropenia and weight loss. Two subjects (2%; 2/107) discontinued therapy as the result of an adverse reaction.

Adverse reactions that occurred with a greater than or equal to 10% incidence in the pediatric trial subjects are provided in **Table 7**.

Table 7: Percentage of Pediatric Subjects with Treatment-Related Adverse Reactions (in At Least 10% of All Subjects)

System Organ Class Preferred Term	All Subjects (N=107)
Blood and Lymphatic System Disorders	
Neutropenia	33%
Anemia	11%
Leukopenia	10%

Gastrointestinal Disorders	
Abdominal Pain	21%
Abdominal Pain Upper	12%
Vomiting	27%
Nausea	18%
General Disorders and Administration Site Conditions	
Pyrexia	80%
Fatigue	30%
Injection-site Erythema	29%
Chills	21%
Asthenia	15%
Irritability	14%
Investigations	
Weight Loss	19%
Metabolism and Nutrition Disorders	
Anorexia	29%
Decreased Appetite	22%
Musculoskeletal and Connective Tissue Disorders	
Arthralgia	17%
Myalgia	17%
Nervous System Disorders	
Headache	62%
Dizziness	14%
Skin and Subcutaneous Tissue Disorders	
Alopecia	17%

Ninety-four of 107 subjects enrolled in a 5 year long-term follow-up trial. The long-term effects on growth were less in those subjects treated for 24 weeks than those treated for 48 weeks. Twenty-four percent of subjects (11/46) treated for 24 weeks and 40% of subjects (19/48) treated for 48 weeks had a >15 percentile height-for-age decrease from pre-treatment to the end of 5 year long-term follow-up compared to pre-treatment baseline percentiles. Eleven percent of subjects (5/46) treated for 24 weeks and 13% of subjects (6/48) treated for 48 weeks were observed to have a decrease from pre-treatment baseline of >30 height-for-age percentiles to the end of the 5 year long-term follow-up. While observed across all age groups, the highest risk for reduced height at the end of long-term follow-up appeared to correlate with initiation of combination therapy during the years of expected peak growth velocity. [See *Warnings and Precautions (5.9)*.]

Laboratory Values
Adult and Pediatric Subjects
The adverse reaction profile in Study 3, which compared PegIntron/weight-based REBETOL combination to a PegIntron/flat dose REBETOL regimen, revealed an increased rate of anemia with weight-based dosing (29% vs. 19% for weight-based vs. flat dose regimens, respectively). However, the majority of cases of anemia were mild and responded to dose reductions.

Changes in selected laboratory values during treatment in combination with REBETOL treatment are described below. **Decreases in hemoglobin, leukocytes, neutrophils, and platelets may require dose reduction or permanent discontinuation from therapy** [see *Dosage and Administration (2.4)*]. Changes in selected laboratory values during therapy are described in **Table 8**. Most of the changes in laboratory values in the PegIntron/REBETOL trial with pediatrics were mild or moderate.
[See table 8 at top of next page]
Hemoglobin. Hemoglobin levels decreased to less than 11 g/dL in about 30% of subjects in Study 2. In Study 3, 47% of subjects receiving WBD REBETOL and 33% on flat-dose REBETOL had decreases in hemoglobin levels less than 11 g/dL. Reductions in hemoglobin to less than 9 g/dL occurred more frequently in subjects receiving WBD compared to flat dosing (4% and 2%, respectively). In Study 2, dose modification was required in 9% and 13% of subjects in

the PegIntron/REBETOL and INTRON A/REBETOL groups. In Study 4, subjects receiving PegIntron (1.5 mcg/kg)/REBETOL had decreases in hemoglobin levels to between 8.5 to less than 10 g/dL (28%) and to less than 8.5 g/dL (3%), whereas in patients receiving Pegasys 180 mcg/Copegus these decreases occurred in 26% and 4% of subjects respectively. Hemoglobin levels became stable by treatment Weeks 4-6 on average. The typical pattern observed was a decrease in hemoglobin levels by treatment Week 4 followed by stabilization and a plateau, which was maintained to the end of treatment. In the PegIntron monotherapy trial, hemoglobin decreases were generally mild and dose modifications were rarely necessary [see *Dosage and Administration (2.4)*].
Neutrophils. Decreases in neutrophil counts were observed in a majority of adult subjects treated with combination therapy with REBETOL in Study 2 (85%) and INTRON A/REBETOL (60%). Severe potentially life-threatening neutropenia (less than 0.5×10^9/L) occurred in 2% of subjects treated with INTRON A/REBETOL and in approximately 4% of subjects treated with PegIntron/REBETOL in Study 2. Eighteen percent of subjects receiving PegIntron/REBETOL in Study 2 required modification of interferon dosage. Few subjects (less than 1%) required permanent discontinuation of treatment. Neutrophil counts generally returned to pre-treatment levels 4 weeks after cessation of therapy [see *Dosage and Administration (2.4)*].
Platelets. Platelet counts decreased to less than 100,000/mm^3 in approximately 20% of subjects treated with PegIntron alone or with REBETOL and in 6% of adult subjects treated with INTRON A/REBETOL. Severe decreases in platelet counts (less than 50,000/mm^3) occur in less than 4% of adult subjects. Patients may require discontinuation or dose modification as a result of platelet decreases [see *Dosage and Administration (2.4)*]. In Study 2, 1% or 3% of subjects required dose modification of INTRON A or PegIntron, respectively. Platelet counts generally returned to pretreatment levels 4 weeks after the cessation of therapy.
Thyroid Function. Development of TSH abnormalities, with or without clinical manifestations, is associated with interferon therapies. In Study 2, clinically apparent thyroid disorders occurred among subjects treated with either INTRON A or PegIntron (with or without REBETOL) at a similar incidence (5% for hypothyroidism and 3% for hyperthyroidism). Subjects developed new onset TSH abnormalities while on treatment and during the follow-up period. At the end of the follow-up period 7% of subjects still had abnormal TSH values.
Bilirubin and uric acid. In Study 2, 10 to 14% of subjects developed hyperbilirubinemia and 33 to 38% developed hyperuricemia in association with hemolysis. Six subjects developed mild to moderate gout.

6.2   Clinical Trials Experience – REBETOL/INTRON A Combination Therapy
Adult Subjects
In clinical trials, 19% and 6% of previously untreated and relapse subjects, respectively, discontinued therapy due to adverse reactions in the combination arms compared to 13% and 3% in the interferon arms. Selected treatment-related adverse reactions that occurred in the US trials with greater than or equal to 5% incidence are provided by treatment group (see **Table 9**). In general, the selected treatment-related adverse reactions were reported with lower incidence in the international trials as compared to the US trials, with the exception of asthenia, influenza-like symptoms, nervousness, and pruritus.
Pediatric Subjects
In clinical trials of 118 pediatric subjects 3 to 16 years of age, 6% discontinued therapy due to adverse reactions. Dose modifications were required in 30% of subjects, most commonly for anemia and neutropenia. In general, the adverse-reaction profile in the pediatric population was similar to that observed in adults. Injection site disorders, fever, anorexia, vomiting, and emotional lability occurred more frequently in pediatric subjects compared to adult subjects. Conversely, pediatric subjects experienced less fatigue, dyspepsia, arthralgia, insomnia, irritability, impaired concentration, dyspnea, and pruritus compared to adult subjects. Selected treatment-related adverse reactions that occurred with greater than or equal to 5% incidence among all pediatric subjects who received the recommended dose of REBETOL/INTRON A combination therapy are provided in **Table 9**.
[See table 9 on pages 1659 and 1660]
During a 48-week course of therapy there was a decrease in the rate of linear growth (mean percentile assignment decrease of 7%) and a decrease in the rate of weight gain (mean percentile assignment decrease of 9%). A general reversal of these trends was noted during the 24-week post-treatment period. Long-term data in a limited number of patients, however, suggests that combination therapy may induce a growth inhibition that results in reduced final adult height in some patients [see *Warnings and Precautions (5.9)*].

Laboratory Values
Changes in selected hematologic values (hemoglobin, white blood cells, neutrophils, and platelets) during therapy are described below (see **Table 10**).

Hemoglobin. Hemoglobin decreases among subjects receiving REBETOL therapy began at Week 1, with stabilization by Week 4. In previously untreated subjects treated for 48 weeks, the mean maximum decrease from baseline was 3.1 g/dL in the US trial and 2.9 g/dL in the international trial. In relapse subjects, the mean maximum decrease from baseline was 2.8 g/dL in the US trial and 2.6 g/dL in the international trial. Hemoglobin values returned to pretreatment levels within 4 to 8 weeks of cessation of therapy in most subjects.

Bilirubin and Uric Acid. Increases in both bilirubin and uric acid, associated with hemolysis, were noted in clinical trials. Most were moderate biochemical changes and were reversed within 4 weeks after treatment discontinuation. This observation occurred most frequently in subjects with a previous diagnosis of Gilbert's syndrome. This has not been associated with hepatic dysfunction or clinical morbidity. [See table 10 at top of page 1661]

6.3   Postmarketing Experiences
The following adverse reactions have been identified and reported during post approval use of REBETOL in combination with INTRON A or PegIntron. Because these reactions are reported voluntarily from a population of uncertain size, it is not always possible to reliably estimate their frequency or establish a causal relationship to drug exposure.
Blood and Lymphatic System disorders
    Pure red cell aplasia, aplastic anemia
Ear and Labyrinth disorders
    Hearing disorder, vertigo
Respiratory, Thoracic and Mediastinal disorders
    Pulmonary hypertension
Eye disorders
    Serous retinal detachment
Endocrine disorders
    Diabetes

7   DRUG INTERACTIONS
7.1   Didanosine
Exposure to didanosine or its active metabolite (dideoxyadenosine 5'-triphosphate) is increased when didanosine is coadministered with ribavirin, which could cause or worsen clinical toxicities; therefore, coadministration of REBETOL capsules or oral solution and didanosine is contraindicated. Reports of fatal hepatic failure, as well as peripheral neuropathy, pancreatitis, and symptomatic hyperlactatemia/lactic acidosis have been reported in clinical trials.
7.2   Nucleoside Analogues
Hepatic decompensation (some fatal) has occurred in cirrhotic HIV/HCV co-infected patients receiving combination antiretroviral therapy for HIV and interferon alpha and ribavirin. Adding treatment with alpha interferons alone or in combination with ribavirin may increase the risk in this patient population. Patients receiving interferon with ribavirin and nucleoside reverse transcriptase inhibitors (NRTIs) should be closely monitored for treatment-associated toxicities, especially hepatic decompensation and anemia. Discontinuation of NRTIs should be considered as medically appropriate *(see labeling for individual NRTI product)*. Dose reduction or discontinuation of interferon, ribavirin, or both should also be considered if worsening clinical toxicities are observed, including hepatic decompensation (e.g., Child-Pugh greater than 6).
Ribavirin may antagonize the cell culture antiviral activity of stavudine and zidovudine against HIV. Ribavirin has been shown in cell culture to inhibit phosphorylation of lamivudine, stavudine, and zidovudine, which could lead to decreased antiretroviral activity. However, in a study with another pegylated interferon in combination with ribavirin, no pharmacokinetic (e.g., plasma concentrations or intracellular triphosphorylated active metabolite concentrations) or pharmacodynamic (e.g., loss of HIV/HCV virologic suppress) interaction was observed when ribavirin and lamivudine (n=18), stavudine (n=10), or zidovudine (n=6) were coadministered as part of a multidrug regimen in HIV/HCV co-infected subjects. Therefore, concomitant use of ribavirin with either of these drugs should be used with caution.
7.3   Drugs Metabolized by Cytochrome P-450
Results of *in vitro* studies using both human and rat liver microsome preparations indicated little or no cytochrome P-450 enzyme-mediated metabolism of ribavirin, with minimal potential for P-450 enzyme-based drug interactions.
No pharmacokinetic interactions were noted between INTRON A and REBETOL capsules in a multiple-dose pharmacokinetic study.
7.4   Azathioprine
The use of ribavirin for the treatment of chronic hepatitis C in patients receiving azathioprine has been reported to induce severe pancytopenia and may increase the risk of azathioprine-related myelotoxicity. Inosine monophosphate dehydrogenase (IMDH) is required for one of the metabolic

Table 8: Selected Laboratory Abnormalities During Treatment with REBETOL and PegIntron or REBETOL and INTRON A in Previously Untreated Subjects

Laboratory Parameters*	Percentage of Subjects		
	Adults (Study 2)		Pediatrics
	PegIntron/REBETOL (N=511)	INTRON A/REBETOL (N=505)	PegIntron/REBETOL (N=107)*
Hemoglobin (g/dL)			
9.5 to <11.0	26	27	30
8.0 to <9.5	3	3	2
6.5-7.9	0.2	0.2	
Leukocytes (× 10⁹/L)			
2.0-2.9	46	41	39
1.5 to <2.0	24	8	3
1.0-1.4	5	1	-
Neutrophils (× 10⁹/L)			
1.0-1.5	33	37	35
0.75 to <1.0	25	13	26
0.5 to <0.75	18	7	13
<0.5	4	2	3
Platelets (× 10⁹/L)			
70-100	15	5	1
50 to <70	3	0.8	-
30-49	0.2	0.2	-
25 to <50	-	-	1
Total Bilirubin	**(mg/dL)**		**(µmole/L)**
1.5-3.0	10	13	
1.26-2.59 × ULN†	-	-	7
3.1-6.0	0.6	0.2	
2.6-5 × ULN†	-	-	-
6.1-12.0	0	0.2	
ALT (U/L)			
2 × Baseline	0.6	0.2	1
2.1-5 × Baseline	3	1	5
5.1-10 × Baseline	0	0	3

* The table summarizes the worst category observed within the period per subject per laboratory test. Only subjects with at least one treatment value for a given laboratory test are included.
† ULN=Upper limit of normal.

pathways of azathioprine. Ribavirin is known to inhibit IMDH, thereby leading to accumulation of an azathioprine metabolite, 6-methylthioinosine monophosphate (6-MTITP), which is associated with myelotoxicity (neutropenia, thrombocytopenia, and anemia). Patients receiving azathioprine with ribavirin should have complete blood counts, including platelet counts, monitored weekly for the first month, twice monthly for the second and third months of treatment, then monthly or more frequently if dosage or other therapy changes are necessary *[see Warnings and Precautions (5.8)]*.

8   USE IN SPECIFIC POPULATIONS
8.1   Pregnancy
Pregnancy Category X
[See Contraindications (4), Warnings and Precautions (5.1), and Nonclinical Toxicology (13.1)].
Treatment and Post-treatment:
Potential Risk to the Fetus:
Ribavirin is known to accumulate in intracellular components from where it is cleared very slowly. It is not known whether ribavirin contained in sperm will exert a potential teratogenic effect upon fertilization of the ova. In a study in rats, it was concluded that dominant lethality was not induced by ribavirin at doses up to 200 mg/kg for 5 days (estimated human equivalent doses of 7.14 to 28.6 mg/kg, based on body surface area adjustment for a 60 kg adult; up to 1.7 times the maximum recommended human dose of ribavirin). However, because of the potential human teratogenic effects of ribavirin, male patients should be advised to take every precaution to avoid risk of pregnancy for their female partners.
Women of childbearing potential should not receive REBETOL unless they are using effective contraception (two reliable forms) during the therapy period. In addition, effective contraception should be utilized for 6 months post-therapy based on a multiple-dose half-life (t₁/₂) of ribavirin of 12 days.
Male patients and their female partners must practice effective contraception (two reliable forms) during treatment with REBETOL and for the 6-month post-therapy period (e.g., 15 half-lives for ribavirin clearance from the body).
A Ribavirin Pregnancy Registry has been established to monitor maternal-fetal outcomes of pregnancies in female patients and female partners of male patients exposed to ribavirin during treatment and for 6 months following cessation of treatment. Physicians and patients are encouraged to report such cases by calling 1-800-593-2214.
8.3   Nursing Mothers
It is not known whether the REBETOL product is excreted in human milk. Because of the potential for serious adverse

reactions from the drug in nursing infants, a decision should be made whether to discontinue nursing or to delay or discontinue REBETOL.

8.4   Pediatric Use
Safety and effectiveness of REBETOL in combination with PegIntron has not been established in pediatric patients below the age of 3 years. For treatment with REBETOL/INTRON A, evidence of disease progression, such as hepatic inflammation and fibrosis, as well as prognostic factors for response, HCV genotype and viral load should be considered when deciding to treat a pediatric patient. The benefits of treatment should be weighed against the safety findings observed.

Long-term follow-up data in pediatric subjects indicates that REBETOL in combination with PegIntron or with INTRON A may induce a growth inhibition that results in reduced height in some patients [see Warnings and Precautions (5.9) and Adverse Reactions (6.1, 6.2)].

Suicidal ideation or attempts occurred more frequently among pediatric patients, primarily adolescents, compared to adult patients (2.4% vs. 1%) during treatment and off-therapy follow-up [see Warnings and Precautions (5.10)]. As in adult patients, pediatric patients experienced other psychiatric adverse reactions (e.g., depression, emotional lability, somnolence), anemia, and neutropenia [see Warnings and Precautions (5.2)].

8.5   Geriatric Use
Clinical trials of REBETOL/INTRON A or PegIntron therapy did not include sufficient numbers of subjects aged 65 and over to determine if they respond differently from younger subjects.

REBETOL is known to be substantially excreted by the kidney, and the risk of toxic reactions to this drug may be greater in patients with impaired renal function. Because elderly patients often have decreased renal function, care should be taken in dose selection. Renal function should be monitored and dosage adjustments should be made accordingly. REBETOL should not be used in patients with creatinine clearance less than 50 mL/min [see Contraindications (4)].

In general, REBETOL capsules should be administered to elderly patients cautiously, starting at the lower end of the dosing range, reflecting the greater frequency of decreased hepatic and cardiac function, and of concomitant disease or other drug therapy. In clinical trials, elderly subjects had a higher frequency of anemia (67%) than younger patients (28%) [see Warnings and Precautions (5.2)].

8.6   Organ Transplant Recipients
The safety and efficacy of INTRON A and PegIntron alone or in combination with REBETOL for the treatment of hepatitis C in liver or other organ transplant recipients have not been established. In a small (n=16) single-center, uncontrolled case experience, renal failure in renal allograft recipients receiving interferon alpha and ribavirin combination therapy was more frequent than expected from the center's previous experience with renal allograft recipients not receiving combination therapy. The relationship of the renal failure to renal allograft rejection is not clear.

8.7   HIV or HBV Co-infection
The safety and efficacy of PegIntron/REBETOL and INTRON A/REBETOL for the treatment of patients with HCV co-infected with HIV or HBV have not been established.

10   OVERDOSAGE

There is limited experience with overdosage. Acute ingestion of up to 20 g of REBETOL capsules, INTRON A ingestion of up to 120 million units, and subcutaneous doses of INTRON A up to 10 times the recommended doses have been reported. Primary effects that have been observed are increased incidence and severity of the adverse reactions related to the therapeutic use of INTRON A and REBETOL. However, hepatic enzyme abnormalities, renal failure, hemorrhage, and myocardial infarction have been reported with administration of single subcutaneous doses of INTRON A that exceed dosing recommendations.

There is no specific antidote for INTRON A or REBETOL overdose, and hemodialysis and peritoneal dialysis are not effective for treatment of overdose of these agents.

11   DESCRIPTION

REBETOL (ribavirin), is a synthetic nucleoside analogue (purine analogue). The chemical name of ribavirin is 1-β-D-ribofuranosyl-1H-1,2,4-triazole-3-carboxamide and has the following structural formula (see **Figure 1**).

[See figure 1 at top of next column]

Ribavirin is a white, crystalline powder. It is freely soluble in water and slightly soluble in anhydrous alcohol. The empirical formula is $C_8H_{12}N_4O_5$ and the molecular weight is 244.21.

REBETOL capsules consist of a white powder in a white, opaque, gelatin capsule. Each capsule contains 200 mg ribavirin and the inactive ingredients microcrystalline cel-

Table 9: Selected Treatment-Related Adverse Reactions: Previously Untreated and Relapse Adult Subjects and Previously Untreated Pediatric Subjects

Subjects Reporting Adverse Reactions*	Percentage of Subjects						
	US Previously Untreated Study				US Relapse Study		Pediatric Subjects
	24 weeks of treatment		48 weeks of treatment		24 weeks of treatment		48 weeks of treatment
	INTRON A/ REBETOL (N=228)	INTRON A/ Placebo (N=231)	INTRON A/ REBETOL (N=228)	INTRON A/ Placebo (N=225)	INTRON A/ REBETOL (N=77)	INTRON A/ Placebo (N=76)	INTRON A/ REBETOL (N=118)
Application Site Disorders							
Injection Site Inflammation	13	10	12	14	6	8	14
Injection Site Reaction	7	9	8	9	5	3	19
Body as a Whole - General Disorders							
Headache	63	63	66	67	66	68	69
Fatigue	68	62	70	72	60	53	58
Rigors	40	32	42	39	43	37	25
Fever	37	35	41	40	32	36	61
Influenza-like Symptoms	14	18	18	20	13	13	31
Asthenia	9	4	9	9	10	4	5
Chest Pain	5	4	9	8	6	7	5
Central & Peripheral Nervous System Disorders							
Dizziness	17	15	23	19	26	21	20
Gastrointestinal System Disorders							
Nausea	38	35	46	33	47	33	33
Anorexia	27	16	25	19	21	14	51
Dyspepsia	14	6	16	9	16	9	<1
Vomiting	11	10	9	13	12	8	42
Musculoskeletal System Disorders							
Myalgia	61	57	64	63	61	58	32
Arthralgia	30	27	33	36	29	29	15
Musculoskeletal Pain	20	26	28	32	22	28	21

(Table continued on next page)

Figure 1: Structural Formula

lulose, lactose monohydrate, croscarmellose sodium, and magnesium stearate. The capsule shell consists of gelatin, sodium lauryl sulfate, silicon dioxide, and titanium dioxide. The capsule is printed with edible blue pharmaceutical ink which is made of shellac, anhydrous ethyl alcohol, isopropyl alcohol, n-butyl alcohol, propylene glycol, ammonium hydroxide, and FD&C Blue #2 aluminum lake.

REBETOL oral solution is a clear, colorless to pale or light yellow bubble gum-flavored liquid. Each milliliter of the solution contains 40 mg of ribavirin and the inactive ingredients sucrose, glycerin, sorbitol, propylene glycol, sodium citrate, citric acid, sodium benzoate, natural and artificial flavor for bubble gum #15864, and water.

12   CLINICAL PHARMACOLOGY
12.1   Mechanism of Action
Ribavirin is an antiviral agent [see Microbiology (12.4)].

12.3   Pharmacokinetics
Single- and multiple-dose pharmacokinetic properties in adults are summarized in **Table 11**. Ribavirin was rapidly and extensively absorbed following oral administration. However, due to first-pass metabolism, the absolute bioavailability averaged 64% (44%). There was a linear relationship between dose and AUC_{tf} (AUC from time zero to last measurable concentration) following single doses of 200 to 1200 mg ribavirin. The relationship between dose and C_{max} was curvilinear, tending to asymptote above single doses of 400 to 600 mg.

Upon multiple oral dosing, based on AUC_{12hr}, a 6-fold accumulation of ribavirin was observed in plasma. Following oral dosing with 600 mg twice daily, steady-state was reached by approximately 4 weeks, with mean steady-state plasma concentrations of 2200 ng/mL (37%). Upon discontinuation of dosing, the mean half-life was 298 (30%) hours, which probably reflects slow elimination from nonplasma compartments.

Effect of Antacid on Absorption of Ribavirin:
Coadministration of REBETOL capsules with an antacid containing magnesium, aluminum, and simethicone resulted in a 14% decrease in mean ribavirin AUC_{tf}. The clinical relevance of results from this single-dose study is unknown.

[See table 11 at top of page 1662]

Tissue Distribution: Ribavirin transport into nonplasma compartments has been most extensively studied in red blood cells, and has been identified to be primarily via an e_s-type equilibrative nucleoside transporter. This type of

Table 9 (cont.): Selected Treatment-Related Adverse Reactions: Previously Untreated and Relapse Adult Subjects and Previously Untreated Pediatric Subjects

	Percentage of Subjects						
	US Previously Untreated Study				US Relapse Study		Pediatric Subjects
	24 weeks of treatment		48 weeks of treatment		24 weeks of treatment		48 weeks of treatment
Subjects Reporting Adverse Reactions*	INTRON A/ REBETOL (N=228)	INTRON A/ Placebo (N=231)	INTRON A/ REBETOL (N=228)	INTRON A/ Placebo (N=225)	INTRON A/ REBETOL (N=77)	INTRON A/ Placebo (N=76)	INTRON A/ REBETOL (N=118)
Psychiatric Disorders							
Insomnia	39	27	39	30	26	25	14
Irritability	23	19	32	27	25	20	10
Depression	32	25	36	37	23	14	13
Emotional Lability	7	6	11	8	12	8	16
Concentration Impaired	11	14	14	14	10	12	5
Nervousness	4	2	4	4	5	4	3
Respiratory System Disorders							
Dyspnea	19	9	18	10	17	12	5
Sinusitis	9	7	10	14	12	7	<1
Skin and Appendages Disorders							
Alopecia	28	27	32	28	27	26	23
Rash	20	9	28	8	21	5	17
Pruritus	21	9	19	8	13	4	12
Special Senses, Other Disorders							
Taste Perversion	7	4	8	4	6	5	<1

* Subjects reporting one or more adverse reactions. A subject may have reported more than one adverse reaction within a body system/organ class category.

transporter is present on virtually all cell types and may account for the extensive volume of distribution. Ribavirin does not bind to plasma proteins.

Metabolism and Excretion: Ribavirin has two pathways of metabolism: (i) a reversible phosphorylation pathway in nucleated cells; and (ii) a degradative pathway involving deribosylation and amide hydrolysis to yield a triazole carboxylic acid metabolite. Ribavirin and its triazole carboxamide and triazole carboxylic acid metabolites are excreted renally. After oral administration of 600 mg of ^{14}C-ribavirin, approximately 61% and 12% of the radioactivity was eliminated in the urine and feces, respectively, in 336 hours. Unchanged ribavirin accounted for 17% of the administered dose.

Special Populations:
Renal Dysfunction
The pharmacokinetics of ribavirin were assessed after administration of a single oral dose (400 mg) of ribavirin to non HCV-infected subjects with varying degrees of renal dysfunction. The mean AUC_{tf} value was threefold greater in subjects with creatinine clearance values between 10 to 30 mL/min when compared to control subjects (creatinine clearance greater than 90 mL/min). In subjects with creatinine clearance values between 30 to 60 mL/min, AUC_{tf} was twofold greater when compared to control subjects. The increased AUC_{tf} appears to be due to reduction of renal and nonrenal clearance in these subjects. Phase 3 efficacy trials included subjects with creatinine clearance values greater than 50 mL/min. The multiple-dose pharmacokinetics of ribavirin cannot be accurately predicted in patients with renal dysfunction. Ribavirin is not effectively removed by hemodialysis. Patients with creatinine clearance less than 50 mL/min should not be treated with REBETOL [see Contraindications (4)].

Hepatic Dysfunction
The effect of hepatic dysfunction was assessed after a single oral dose of ribavirin (600 mg). The mean AUC_{tf} values were not significantly different in subjects with mild, moderate, or severe hepatic dysfunction (Child-Pugh Classification A, B, or C) when compared to control subjects. However, the mean C_{max} values increased with severity of hepatic dysfunction and was twofold greater in subjects with severe hepatic dysfunction when compared to control subjects.

Elderly Patients
Pharmacokinetic evaluations in elderly subjects have not been performed.

Gender
There were no clinically significant pharmacokinetic differences noted in a single-dose trial of 18 male and 18 female subjects.

Pediatric Patients
Multiple-dose pharmacokinetic properties for REBETOL capsules and INTRON A in pediatric subjects with chronic hepatitis C between 5 and 16 years of age are summarized in **Table 12**. The pharmacokinetics of REBETOL and INTRON A (dose-normalized) are similar in adults and pediatric subjects.
Complete pharmacokinetic characteristics of REBETOL oral solution have not been determined in pediatric subjects. Ribavirin C_{min} values were similar following administration of REBETOL oral solution or REBETOL capsules during 48 weeks of therapy in pediatric subjects (3 to 16 years of age).

Table 12: Mean (% CV) Multiple-dose Pharmacokinetic Parameters for INTRON A and REBETOL Capsules When Administered to Pediatric Subjects with Chronic Hepatitis C

Parameter	REBETOL 15 mg/kg/day as 2 divided doses (N=17)	INTRON A 3 MIU/m² three times weekly (N=54)
T_{max} (hr)	1.9 (83)	5.9 (36)
C_{max} (ng/mL)	3275 (25)	51 (48)
AUC*	29,774 (26)	622 (48)

Apparent Clearance L/hr/kg	0.27 (27)	ND†

Note: numbers in parenthesis indicate % coefficient of variation.
* AUC_{12} (ng•hr/mL) for REBETOL; AUC_{0-24} (IU•hr/mL) for INTRON A.
† ND=not done.

A clinical trial in pediatric subjects with chronic hepatitis C between 3 and 17 years of age was conducted in which pharmacokinetics for PegIntron and REBETOL (capsules and oral solution) were evaluated. In pediatric subjects receiving body surface area-adjusted dosing of PegIntron at 60 mcg/m²/week, the log transformed ratio estimate of exposure during the dosing interval was predicted to be 58% [90% CI: 141%, 177%] higher than observed in adults receiving 1.5 mcg/kg/week. The pharmacokinetics of REBETOL (dose-normalized) in this trial were similar to those reported in a prior study of REBETOL in combination with INTRON A in pediatric subjects and in adults.
Effect of Food on Absorption of Ribavirin
Both AUC_{tf} and C_{max} increased by 70% when REBETOL capsules were administered with a high-fat meal (841 kcal, 53.8 g fat, 31.6 g protein, and 57.4 g carbohydrate) in a single-dose pharmacokinetic study [see Dosage and Administration (2)].

12.4   Microbiology
Mechanism of Action
The mechanism by which ribavirin contributes to its antiviral efficacy in the clinic is not fully understood. Ribavirin has direct antiviral activity in tissue culture against many RNA viruses. Ribavirin increases the mutation frequency in the genomes of several viruses and ribavirin triphosphate inhibits HCV polymerase in a biochemical reaction.
Antiviral Activity in Cell Culture
The antiviral activity of ribavirin in the HCV-replicon is not well understood and has not been defined because of the cellular toxicity of ribavirin. Direct antiviral activity has been observed in tissue culture of other RNA viruses. The anti-HCV activity of interferon was demonstrated in cell containing self-replicating HCV-RNS (HCV replicon cells) or HCV infection.
Resistance
HCV genotypes show wide variability in their response to pegylated recombinant human interferon/ribavirin therapy. Genetic changes associated with the variable response have not been identified.
Cross-resistance
There is no reported cross-resistance between pegylated/non-pegylated interferons and ribavirin.

13   NONCLINICAL TOXICOLOGY
13.1   Carcinogenesis, Mutagenesis, Impairment of Fertility
Carcinogenesis
Ribavirin did not cause an increase in any tumor type when administered for 6 months in the transgenic p53 deficient mouse model at doses up to 300 mg/kg (estimated human equivalent of 25 mg/kg based on body surface area adjustment for a 60 kg adult; approximately 1.9 times the maximum recommended human daily dose). Ribavirin was noncarcinogenic when administered for 2 years to rats at doses up to 40 mg/kg (estimated human equivalent of 5.71 mg/kg based on body surface area adjustment for a 60 kg adult).
Mutagenesis
Ribavirin demonstrated increased incidences of mutation and cell transformation in multiple genotoxicity assays. Ribavirin was active in the Balb/3T3 In Vitro Cell Transformation Assay. Mutagenic activity was observed in the mouse lymphoma assay, and at doses of 20 to 200 mg/kg (estimated human equivalent of 1.67 to 16.7 mg/kg, based on body surface area adjustment for a 60 kg adult; 0.1 to 1 times the maximum recommended human 24-hour dose of ribavirin) in a mouse micronucleus assay. A dominant lethal assay in rats was negative, indicating that if mutations occurred in rats they were not transmitted through male gametes.
Impairment of Fertility
Ribavirin demonstrated significant embryocidal and teratogenic effects at doses well below the recommended human dose in all animal species in which adequate studies have been conducted. Malformations of the skull, palate, eye, jaw, limbs, skeleton, and gastrointestinal tract were noted. The incidence and severity of teratogenic effects increased with escalation of the drug dose. Survival of fetuses and offspring was reduced. In conventional embryotoxicity/teratogenicity studies in rats and rabbits, observed no-effect dose levels were well below those for proposed clinical use (0.3 mg/kg/day for both the rat and rabbit; approximately 0.06 times the recommended human 24-hour dose of

Table 10: Selected Laboratory Abnormalities During Treatment With REBETOL and INTRON A: Previously Untreated and Relapse Adult Subjects and Previously Untreated Pediatric Subjects

	Percentage of Subjects						
	US Previously Untreated Study				US Relapse Study		Pediatric Subjects
	24 weeks of treatment		48 weeks of treatment		24 weeks of treatment		48 weeks of treatment
	INTRON A/ REBETOL (N=228)	INTRON A/ Placebo (N=231)	INTRON A/ REBETOL (N=228)	INTRON A/ Placebo (N=225)	INTRON A/ REBETOL (N=77)	INTRON A/ Placebo (N=76)	INTRON A/ REBETOL (N=118)
Hemoglobin (g/dL)							
9.5 to 10.9	24	1	32	1	21	3	24
8.0 to 9.4	5	0	4	0	4	0	3
6.5 to 7.9	0	0	0	0.4	0	0	0
<6.5	0	0	0	0	0	0	0
Leukocytes (× 10^9/L)							
2.0 to 2.9	40	20	38	23	45	26	35
1.5 to 1.9	4	1	9	2	5	3	8
1.0 to 1.4	0.9	0	2	0	0	0	0
<1.0	0	0	0	0	0	0	0
Neutrophils (× 10^9/L)							
1.0 to 1.49	30	32	31	44	42	34	37
0.75 to 0.99	14	15	14	11	16	18	15
0.5 to 0.74	9	9	14	7	8	4	16
<0.5	11	8	11	5	5	8	3
Platelets (× 10^9/L)							
70 to 99	9	11	11	14	6	12	0.8
50 to 69	2	3	2	3	0	5	2
30 to 49	0	0.4	0	0.4	0	0	0
<30	0.9	0	1	0.9	0	0	0
Total Bilirubin (mg/dL)							
1.5 to 3.0	27	13	32	13	21	7	2
3.1 to 6.0	0.9	0.4	2	0	3	0	0
6.1 to 12.0	0	0	0.4	0	0	0	0
>12.0	0	0	0	0	0	0	0

ribavirin). No maternal toxicity or effects on offspring were observed in a peri/postnatal toxicity study in rats dosed orally at up to 1 mg/kg/day (estimated human equivalent dose of 0.17 mg/kg based on body surface area adjustment for a 60 kg adult; approximately 0.01 times the maximum recommended human 24-hour dose of ribavirin) [see Contraindications (4), and Warnings and Precautions (5.1)].

Fertile women and partners of fertile women should not receive REBETOL unless the patient and his/her partner are using effective contraception (two reliable forms). Based on a multiple-dose half-life ($t_{1/2}$) of ribavirin of 12 days, effective contraception must be utilized for 6 months post-therapy (e.g., 15 half-lives of clearance for ribavirin).

REBETOL should be used with caution in fertile men. In studies in mice to evaluate the time course and reversibility of ribavirin-induced testicular degeneration at doses of 15 to 150 mg/kg/day (estimated human equivalent of 1.25 to 12.5 mg/kg/day, based on body surface area adjustment for a 60-kg adult; 0.1-0.8 times the maximum human 24-hour dose of ribavirin) administered for 3 or 6 months, abnormalities in sperm occurred. Upon cessation of treatment, essentially total recovery from ribavirin-induced testicular toxicity was apparent within 1 or 2 spermatogenesis cycles.

13.2   Animal Toxicology and Pharmacology
Long-term studies in the mouse and rat [18 to 24 months; doses of 20 to 75 and 10 to 40 mg/kg/day, respectively (esti-

mated human equivalent doses of 1.67 to 6.25 and 1.43 to 5.71 mg/kg/day, respectively, based on body surface area adjustment for a 60 kg adult; approximately 0.1 to 0.4 times the maximum human 24-hour dose of ribavirin)] have demonstrated a relationship between chronic ribavirin exposure and increased incidences of vascular lesions (microscopic hemorrhages) in mice. In rats, retinal degeneration occurred in controls, but the incidence was increased in ribavirin-treated rats.

In a study in which rat pups were dosed postnatally with ribavirin at doses of 10, 25, and 50 mg/kg/day, drug-related deaths occurred at 50 mg/kg (at rat pup plasma concentrations below human plasma concentrations at the human therapeutic dose) between study Days 13 and 48. Rat pups dosed from postnatal Days 7 through 63 demonstrated a minor, dose-related decrease in overall growth at all doses, which was subsequently manifested as slight decreases in body weight, crown-rump length, and bone length. These effects showed evidence of reversibility, and no histopathological effects on bone were observed. No ribavirin effects were observed regarding neurobehavioral or reproductive development.

14   CLINICAL STUDIES
Clinical Study 1 evaluated PegIntron monotherapy. See PegIntron labeling for information about this trial.

14.1   REBETOL/PegIntron Combination Therapy
Adult Subjects
Study 2
A randomized trial compared treatment with two PegIntron/REBETOL regimens [PegIntron 1.5 mcg/kg subcutaneously once weekly/REBETOL 800 mg orally daily (in divided doses); PegIntron 1.5 mcg/kg subcutaneously once weekly for 4 weeks then 0.5 mcg/kg subcutaneously once weekly for 44 weeks/REBETOL 1000 or 1200 mg orally daily (in divided doses)] with INTRON A [3 MIU subcutaneously three times weekly/REBETOL 1000 or 1200 mg orally daily (in divided doses)] in 1530 adults with chronic hepatitis C. Interferon-naïve subjects were treated for 48 weeks and followed for 24 weeks post-treatment. Eligible subjects had compensated liver disease, detectable HCV-RNA, elevated ALT, and liver histopathology consistent with chronic hepatitis.

Response to treatment was defined as undetectable HCV-RNA at 24 weeks post-treatment (see Table 13). The response rate to the PegIntron 1.5 mcg/kg and ribavirin 800 mg dose was higher than the response rate to INTRON A/REBETOL (see Table 13).The response rate to PegIntron 1.5→0.5 mcg/kg/REBETOL was essentially the same as the response to INTRON A/REBETOL (data not shown).

Table 13: Rates of Response to Combination Treatment – Study 2

	PegIntron 1.5 mcg/kg once weekly REBETOL 800 mg once daily	INTRON A 3 MIU three times weekly REBETOL 1000/ 1200 mg once daily
Overall response[*,†]	52% (264/511)	46% (231/505)
Genotype 1	41% (141/348)	33% (112/343)
Genotype 2-6	75% (123/163)	73% (119/162)

* Serum HCV-RNA was measured with a research-based quantitative polymerase chain reaction assay by a central laboratory.
† Difference in overall treatment response (PegIntron/ REBETOL vs. INTRON A/REBETOL) is 6% with 95% confidence interval of (0.18, 11.63) adjusted for viral genotype and presence of cirrhosis at baseline. Response to treatment was defined as undetectable HCV-RNA at 24 weeks post-treatment.

Subjects with viral genotype 1, regardless of viral load, had a lower response rate to PegIntron (1.5 mcg/kg)/REBETOL (800 mg) compared to subjects with other viral genotypes. Subjects with both poor prognostic factors (genotype 1 and high viral load) had a response rate of 30% (78/256) compared to a response rate of 29% (71/247) with INTRON A/REBETOL combination therapy.

Subjects with lower body weight tended to have higher adverse-reaction rates [see Adverse Reactions (6.1)] and higher response rates than subjects with higher body weights. Differences in response rates between treatment arms did not substantially vary with body weight.

Treatment response rates with PegIntron/REBETOL combination therapy were 49% in men and 56% in women. Response rates were lower in African American and Hispanic subjects and higher in Asians compared to Caucasians. Although African Americans had a higher proportion of poor prognostic factors compared to Caucasians, the number of non-Caucasians studied (11% of the total) was insufficient to allow meaningful conclusions about differences in response rates after adjusting for prognostic factors in this trial.

Liver biopsies were obtained before and after treatment in 68% of subjects. Compared to baseline, approximately two-thirds of subjects in all treatment groups were observed to have a modest reduction in inflammation.

Study 3
In a large United States community-based trial, 4913 subjects with chronic hepatitis C were randomized to receive PegIntron 1.5 mcg/kg subcutaneously once weekly in combination with a REBETOL dose of 800 to 1400 mg (weight-based dosing (WBD)) or 800 mg (flat) orally daily (in divided doses) for 24 or 48 weeks based on genotype. Response to treatment was defined as undetectable HCV-RNA (based on an assay with a lower limit of detection of 125 IU/mL) at 24 weeks post-treatment.

Treatment with PegIntron 1.5 mcg/kg and REBETOL 800 to 1400 mg resulted in a higher sustained virologic response compared to PegIntron in combination with a flat 800 mg daily dose of REBETOL. Subjects weighing greater than 105 kg obtained the greatest benefit with WBD, although a modest benefit was also observed in subjects weighing greater than 85 to 105 kg (see Table 14). The benefit of WBD

Table 11: Mean (% CV) Pharmacokinetic Parameters for REBETOL When Administered Individually to Adults

Parameter	REBETOL		
	Single-Dose 600 mg Oral Solution (N=14)	Single-Dose 600 mg Capsules (N=12)	Multiple-Dose 600 mg Capsules twice daily (N=12)
T_{max} (hr)	1.00 (34)	1.7 (46)*	3 (60)
C_{max} (ng/mL)	872 (42)	782 (37)	3680 (85)
AUC_{tf} (ng•hr/mL)	14,098 (38)	13,400 (48)	228,000 (25)
$T_{1/2}$ (hr)		43.6 (47)	298 (30)
Apparent Volume of Distribution (L)		2825 (9)[†]	
Apparent Clearance (L/hr)		38.2 (40)	
Absolute Bioavailability		64% (44)[‡]	

* N=11.
[†] Data obtained from a single-dose pharmacokinetic study using ^{14}C labeled ribavirin; N=5.
[‡] N=6.

Table 14: SVR Rate by Treatment and Baseline Weight - Study 3

Treatment Group	Subject Baseline Weight			
	<65 kg (<143 lb)	65-85 kg (143-188 lb)	>85-105 kg (>188-231 lb)	>105 kg (>231 lb)
WBD*	50% (173/348)	45% (449/994)	42% (351/835)	47% (138/292)
Flat	51% (173/342)	44% (443/1011)	39% (318/819)	33% (91/272)

* P=0.01, primary efficacy comparison (based on data from subjects weighing 65 kg or higher at baseline and utilizing a logistic regression analysis that includes treatment [WBD or Flat], genotype and presence/absence of advanced fibrosis, in the model).

in subjects weighing greater than 85 kg was observed with HCV genotypes 1-3. Insufficient data were available to reach conclusions regarding other genotypes. Use of WBD resulted in an increased incidence of anemia *[see Adverse Reactions (6.1)]*.
[See table 14 above]

A total of 1552 subjects weighing greater than 65 kg in Study 3 had genotype 2 or 3 and were randomized to 24 or 48 weeks of therapy. No additional benefit was observed with the longer treatment duration.

Study 4
A large randomized trial compared the safety and efficacy of treatment for 48 weeks with two PegIntron/REBETOL regimens [PegIntron 1.5 mcg/kg and 1 mcg/kg subcutaneously once weekly both in combination with REBETOL 800 to 1400 mg PO daily (in two divided doses)] and Pegasys 180 mcg subcutaneously once weekly in combination with Copegus 1000 to 1200 mg PO daily (in two divided doses) in 3070 treatment-naïve adults with chronic hepatitis C genotype 1. In this trial, lack of early virologic response (undetectable HCV-RNA or greater than or equal to 2 log_{10} reduction from baseline) by treatment Week 12 was the criterion for discontinuation of treatment. SVR was defined as undetectable HCV-RNA (Roche COBAS TaqMan assay, a lower limit of quantitation of 27 IU/mL) at 24 weeks post-treatment (see **Table 15**).

Table 15: SVR Rate by Treatment – Study 4

% (number) of Subjects		
PegIntron 1.5 mcg/kg/ REBETOL	PegIntron 1 mcg/ kg/REBETOL	Pegasys 180 mcg/Copegus
40 (406/1019)	38 (386/1016)	41 (423/1035)

Overall SVR rates were similar among the three treatment groups. Regardless of treatment group, SVR rates were lower in subjects with poor prognostic factors. Subjects with poor prognostic factors randomized to PegIntron (1.5 mcg/kg)/REBETOL or Pegasys/Copegus, however, achieved higher SVR rates compared to similar subjects randomized to PegIntron 1 mcg/kg/REBETOL. For the PegIntron 1.5 mcg/kg and REBETOL dose, SVR rates for subjects with and without the following prognostic factors were as follows: cirrhosis (10% vs. 42%), normal ALT levels (32% vs. 42%), baseline viral load greater than 600,000 IU/mL (35% vs. 61%), 40 years of age and older (38% vs. 50%), and African American race (23% vs. 44%). In

subjects with undetectable HCV-RNA at treatment Week 12 who received PegIntron (1.5 mcg/kg)/REBETOL, the SVR rate was 81% (328/407).

Study 5 - REBETOL/PegIntron Combination Therapy in Prior Treatment Failures
In a noncomparative trial, 2293 subjects with moderate to severe fibrosis who failed previous treatment with combination alpha interferon/ribavirin were re-treated with PegIntron, 1.5 mcg/kg subcutaneously, once weekly, in combination with weight adjusted ribavirin. Eligible subjects included prior nonresponders (subjects who were HCV-RNA positive at the end of a minimum 12 weeks of treatment) and prior relapsers (subjects who were HCV-RNA negative at the end of a minimum 12 weeks of treatment and subsequently relapsed after post-treatment follow-up). Subjects who were negative at Week 12 were treated for 48 weeks and followed for 24 weeks post-treatment. Response to treatment was defined as undetectable HCV-RNA at 24 weeks post-treatment (measured using a research-based test, limit of detection 125 IU/mL). The overall response rate was 22% (497/2293) (99% CI: 19.5, 23.9). Subjects with the following characteristics were less likely to benefit from re-treatment: previous nonresponse, previous pegylated interferon treatment, significant bridging fibrosis or cirrhosis, and genotype 1 infection.

The re-treatment sustained virologic response rates by baseline characteristics are summarized in **Table 16**.
[See table 16 at top of next page]

Achievement of an undetectable HCV-RNA at treatment Week 12 was a strong predictor of SVR. In this trial, 1470 (64%) subjects did not achieve an undetectable HCV-RNA at treatment Week 12, and were offered enrollment into long-term treatment trials, due to an inadequate treatment response. Of the 823 (36%) subjects who were HCV-RNA undetectable at treatment Week 12, those infected with genotype 1 had an SVR of 48% (245/507), with a range of responses by fibrosis scores (F4-F2) of 39-55%. Subjects infected with genotype 2/3 who were HCV-RNA undetectable at treatment Week 12 had an overall SVR of 70% (196/281), with a range of responses by fibrosis scores (F4-F2) of 60-83%. For all genotypes, higher fibrosis scores were associated with a decreased likelihood of achieving SVR.

Pediatric Subjects
Previously untreated pediatric subjects 3 to 17 years of age with compensated chronic hepatitis C and detectable HCV-RNA were treated with REBETOL 15 mg/kg per day and PegIntron 60 mcg/m² once weekly for 24 or 48 weeks based on HCV genotype and baseline viral load. All subjects were to be followed for 24 weeks post-treatment. A total of 107

subjects received treatment, of which 52% were female, 89% were Caucasian, and 67% were infected with HCV Genotype 1. Subjects infected with Genotypes 1, 4 or Genotype 3 with HCV-RNA greater than or equal to 600,000 IU/mL received 48 weeks of therapy while those infected with Genotype 2 or Genotype 3 with HCV-RNA less than 600,000 IU/mL received 24 weeks of therapy. The trial results are summarized in **Table 17**.

Table 17: Sustained Virologic Response Rates by Genotype and Assigned Treatment Duration – Pediatric Trial

	All Subjects N=107	
	24 Weeks	48 Weeks
Genotype	Virologic Response N*,[†] (%)	Virologic Response N*,[†] (%)
All	26/27 (96.3)	44/80 (55.0)
1	-	38/72 (52.8)
2	14/15 (93.3)	-
3[‡]	12/12 (100)	2/3 (66.7)
4	-	4/5 (80.0)

* Response to treatment was defined as undetectable HCV-RNA at 24 weeks post-treatment.
[†] N=number of responders/number of subjects with given genotype, and assigned treatment duration.
[‡] Subjects with genotype 3 low viral load (less than 600,000 IU/mL) were to receive 24 weeks of treatment while those with genotype 3 and high viral load were to receive 48 weeks of treatment.

14.2 REBETOL/INTRON A Combination Therapy
Adult Subjects
Previously Untreated Subjects
Adults with compensated chronic hepatitis C and detectable HCV-RNA (assessed by a central laboratory using a research-based RT-PCR assay) who were previously untreated with alpha interferon therapy were enrolled into two multicenter, double-blind trials (US and international) and randomized to receive REBETOL capsules 1200 mg/day (1000 mg/day for subjects weighing less than or equal to 75 kg) and INTRON A 3 MIU three times weekly or INTRON A and placebo for 24 or 48 weeks followed by 24 weeks of off-therapy follow-up. The international trial did not contain a 24-week INTRON A and placebo treatment arm. The US trial enrolled 912 subjects who, at baseline, were 67% male, 89% Caucasian with a mean HAI score (I+II+III) of 7.5, and 72% genotype 1. The international trial, conducted in Europe, Israel, Canada, and Australia, enrolled 799 subjects (65% male, 95% Caucasian, mean Knodell score 6.8, and 58% genotype 1).
Trial results are summarized in **Table 18**.
[See table 18 at top of next page]
Of subjects who had not achieved HCV-RNA below the limit of detection of the research-based assay by Week 24 of REBETOL/INTRON A treatment, less than 5% responded to an additional 24 weeks of combination treatment.
Among subjects with HCV Genotype 1 treated with REBETOL/INTRON A therapy who achieved HCV-RNA below the detection limit of the research-based assay by 24 weeks, those randomized to 48 weeks of treatment had higher virologic responses compared to those in the 24-week treatment group. There was no observed increase in response rates for subjects with HCV non-genotype 1 randomized to REBETOL/INTRON A therapy for 48 weeks compared to 24 weeks.
Relapse Subjects
Subjects with compensated chronic hepatitis C and detectable HCV-RNA (assessed by a central laboratory using a research-based RT-PCR assay) who had relapsed following one or two courses of interferon therapy (defined as abnormal serum ALT levels) were enrolled into two multicenter, double-blind trials (US and international) and randomized to receive REBETOL 1200 mg/day (1000 mg/day for subjects weighing ≤75 kg) and INTRON A 3 MIU three times weekly or INTRON A and placebo for 24 weeks followed by 24 weeks of off-therapy follow-up. The US trial enrolled 153 subjects who, at baseline, were 67% male, 92% Caucasian with a mean Knodell HAI score (I+II+III) of 6.8, and 58% genotype 1. The international trial, conducted in Europe, Israel, Canada, and Australia, enrolled 192 subjects (64% male, 95% Caucasian, mean Knodell score 6.6, and 56% genotype 1). Trial results are summarized in **Table 19**.
[See table 19 at top of page 1664]
Virologic and histologic responses were similar among male and female subjects in both the previously untreated and relapse trials.

Pediatric Subjects

Pediatric subjects 3 to 16 years of age with compensated chronic hepatitis C and detectable HCV-RNA (assessed by a central laboratory using a research-based RT-PCR assay) were treated with REBETOL 15 mg/kg per day and INTRON A 3 MIU/m^2 three times weekly for 48 weeks followed by 24 weeks of off-therapy follow-up. A total of 118 subjects received treatment, of which 57% were male, 80% Caucasian, and 78% genotype 1. Subjects less than 5 years of age received REBETOL oral solution and those 5 years of age or older received either REBETOL oral solution or capsules.

Trial results are summarized in **Table 20.**

Table 20: Virologic Response: Previously Untreated Pediatric Subjects*

	INTRON A 3 MIU/m^2 three times weekly/REBETOL 15 mg/kg/day
Overall Response† (N=118)	54 (46)
Genotype 1 (N=92)	33 (36)
Genotype non-1 (N=26)	21 (81)

* Number (%) of subjects.
† Defined as HCV-RNA below limit of detection using a research-based RT-PCR assay at end of treatment and during follow-up period.

Subjects with viral genotype 1, regardless of viral load, had a lower response rate to INTRON A/REBETOL combination therapy compared to subjects with genotype non-1, 36% vs. 81%. Subjects with both poor prognostic factors (genotype 1 and high viral load) had a response rate of 26% (13/50).

16 HOW SUPPLIED/STORAGE AND HANDLING

REBETOL 200 mg Capsules are white, opaque capsules with REBETOL, 200 mg, and the Schering Corporation logo imprinted on the capsule shell; the capsules are packaged in a bottle containing 56 capsules (NDC 0085-1351-05), 70 capsules (NDC 0085-1385-07), and 84 capsules (NDC 0085-1194-03).
REBETOL Oral Solution 40 mg per mL is a clear, colorless to pale or light yellow bubble gum-flavored liquid and it is packaged in 4-oz amber glass bottles (100 mL/bottle) with child-resistant closures (NDC 0085-1318-01).
The bottle of REBETOL Capsules should be stored at 25°C (77°F); excursions permitted to 15-30°C (59-86°F) [see USP Controlled Room Temperature].
REBETOL Oral Solution should be stored between 2-8°C (36-46°F) or at 25°C (77°F); excursions permitted to 15-30°C (59-86°F) [see USP Controlled Room Temperature].

17 PATIENT COUNSELING INFORMATION

Advise the patient to read the FDA-Approved Patient Labeling (Medication Guide).

Anemia

The most common adverse experience occurring with REBETOL capsules is anemia, which may be severe *[see Warnings and Precautions (5.2) and Adverse Reactions (6)]*. Patients should be advised that laboratory evaluations are required prior to starting therapy and periodically thereafter *[see Dosage and Administration (2.3)]*. It is advised that patients be well hydrated, especially during the initial stages of treatment.

Pregnancy

Patients must be informed that REBETOL capsules and oral solution may cause birth defects and death of the unborn child. REBETOL must not be used by women who are pregnant or by men whose female partners are pregnant. Extreme care must be taken to avoid pregnancy in female patients and in female partners of male patients taking REBETOL. REBETOL should not be initiated until a report of a negative pregnancy test has been obtained immediately prior to initiation of therapy. Patients must perform a pregnancy test monthly during therapy and for 6 months post therapy. Women of childbearing potential must be counseled about use of effective contraception (two reliable forms) prior to initiating therapy. Patients (male and female) must be advised of the teratogenic/embryocidal risks and must be instructed to practice effective contraception during REBETOL and for 6 months post therapy. Patients (male and female) should be advised to notify the physician immediately in the event of a pregnancy *[see Contraindications (4), Warnings and Precautions (5.1), and Use in Specific Populations (8.1)]*.

If pregnancy does occur during treatment or during 6 months post therapy, the patient must be advised of the teratogenic risk of REBETOL therapy to the fetus. Patients, or partners of patients, should immediately report any pregnancy that occurs during treatment or within 6 months after treatment cessation to their physician. Prescribers should report such cases by calling 1-800-593-2214.

Risks versus Benefits

Patients receiving REBETOL capsules should be informed of the benefits and risks associated with treatment, directed in its appropriate use, and referred to the patient **MEDICATION GUIDE**. Patients should be informed that the effect of treatment of hepatitis C infection on transmission is not known, and that appropriate precautions to prevent transmission of the hepatitis C virus should be taken.
Patients should be informed about what to do in the event they miss a dose of REBETOL; the missed dose should be taken as soon as possible during the same day. Patients should not double the next dose. Patients should be advised to contact their healthcare provider if they have questions.
REBETOL Oral Solution manufactured for:
Merck Sharp & Dohme Corp., a subsidiary of
MERCK & CO., INC.
Whitehouse Station, NJ 08889, USA

Manufactured by:
Schering-Plough Canada, Inc.
Pointe Claire, Quebec, Canada
REBETOL Capsules manufactured by:
Merck Sharp & Dohme Corp., a subsidiary of
MERCK & CO., INC.
Whitehouse Station, NJ 08889, USA
U.S. Patent No. 6,790,837.
Copyright © 2003, 2013 Merck Sharp & Dohme Corp., a subsidiary of **Merck & Co., Inc.**
All rights reserved.
Trademarks depicted herein are the property of their respective owners.
uspi-mk8908-mtl-1311r027
MEDICATION GUIDE
REBETOL® (REB-eh-tol)
(ribavirin)
Capsules and Oral Solution
Read this Medication Guide before you start taking REBETOL, and each time you get a refill. There may be new information. This information does not take the place of talking to your health care provider about your medical condition or your treatment.

Table 16: SVR Rates by Baseline Characteristics of Prior Treatment Failures - Study 5

HCV Genotype/ Metavir Fibrosis Score		Overall SVR by Previous Response and Treatment			
		Nonresponder		**Relapser**	
		interferon alfa/ribavirin % (number of subjects)	peginterferon (2a and 2b combined)/ribavirin % (number of subjects)	interferon alfa/ribavirin % (number of subjects)	peginterferon (2a and 2b combined)/ribavirin % (number of subjects)
Overall		18 (158/903)	6 (30/476)	43 (130/300)	35 (113/344)
HCV 1		13 (98/761)	4 (19/431)	32 (67/208)	23 (56/243)
	F2	18 (36/202)	6 (7/117)	42 (33/79)	32 (23/72)
	F3	16 (38/233)	4 (4/112)	28 (16/58)	21 (14/67)
	F4	7 (24/325)	4 (8/202)	26 (18/70)	18 (19/104)
HCV 2/3		49 (53/109)	36 (10/28)	67 (54/81)	57 (52/92)
	F2	68 (23/34)	56 (5/9)	76 (19/25)	61 (11/18)
	F3	39 (11/28)	38 (3/8)	67 (18/27)	62 (18/29)
	F4	40 (19/47)	18 (2/11)	59 (17/29)	51 (23/45)
HCV 4		17 (5/29)	7 (1/15)	88 (7/8)	50 (4/8)

Table 18: Virologic and Histologic Responses: Previously Untreated Subjects*

	US Trial				International Trial		
	24 weeks of treatment		**48 weeks of treatment**		**24 weeks of treatment**	**48 weeks of treatment**	
	INTRON A/ REBETOL (N=228)	INTRON A/ Placebo (N=231)	INTRON A/ REBETOL (N=228)	INTRON A/ Placebo (N=225)	INTRON A/ REBETOL (N=265)	INTRON A/ REBETOL (N=268)	INTRON A/ Placebo (N=266)
Virologic Response							
Responder†	65 (29)	13 (6)	85 (37)	27 (12)	86 (32)	113 (42)	46 (17)
Nonresponder	147 (64)	194 (84)	110 (48)	168 (75)	158 (60)	120 (45)	196 (74)
Missing Data	16 (7)	24 (10)	33 (14)	30 (13)	21 (8)	35 (13)	24 (9)
Histologic Response							
Improvement‡	102 (45)	77 (33)	96 (42)	65 (29)	103 (39)	102 (38)	69 (26)
No improvement	77 (34)	99 (43)	61 (27)	93 (41)	85 (32)	58 (22)	111 (41)
Missing Data	49 (21)	55 (24)	71 (31)	67 (30)	77 (29)	108 (40)	86 (32)

* Number (%) of subjects.
† Defined as HCV-RNA below limit of detection using a research-based RT-PCR assay at end of treatment and during follow-up period.
‡ Defined as post-treatment (end of follow-up) minus pretreatment liver biopsy Knodell HAI score (I+II+III) improvement of greater than or equal to 2 points.

Table 19: Virologic and Histologic Responses: Relapse Subjects*

	US Trial		International Trial	
	INTRON A/REBETOL (N=77)	INTRON A/Placebo (N=76)	INTRON A/REBETOL (N=96)	INTRON A/Placebo (N=96)
Virologic Response				
Responder[†]	33 (43)	3 (4)	46 (48)	5 (5)
Nonresponder	36 (47)	66 (87)	45 (47)	91 (95)
Missing Data	8 (10)	7 (9)	5 (5)	0 (0)
Histologic Response				
Improvement[‡]	38 (49)	27 (36)	49 (51)	30 (31)
No improvement	23 (30)	37 (49)	29 (30)	44 (46)
Missing Data	16 (21)	12 (16)	18 (19)	22 (23)

* Number (%) of subjects.
† Defined as HCV-RNA below limit of detection using a research-based RT-PCR assay at end of treatment and during follow-up period.
‡ Defined as post-treatment (end of follow-up) minus pretreatment liver biopsy Knodell HAI score (I+II+III) improvement of greater than or equal to 2 points.

What is the most important information I should know about REBETOL®?

1. **Do Not take REBETOL alone to treat chronic hepatitis C infection.** REBETOL should be used in combination with **either interferon alfa-2b (Intron® A) or peginterferon alfa-2b (PegIntron®)** to treat chronic hepatitis C infection.
2. **REBETOL may cause a significant drop in your red blood cell count and cause anemia in some cases.** Anemia has been associated with worsening of Heart Problems, and in rare cases can cause a Heart Attack and Death. Tell your health care provider if you have ever had any heart problems. REBETOL may not be right for you. **Seek medical attention right away if you experience chest pain.**
3. **REBETOL may cause Birth Defects or the Death of your unborn baby. Do Not Take REBETOL if you or your sexual partner is pregnant or plan to become pregnant. Do Not become Pregnant within 6 months after discontinuing REBETOL therapy.** You must use 2 forms of birth control when you take REBETOL and for the 6 months after treatment.
   - Females must have a pregnancy test before starting REBETOL, every month while taking REBETOL, and every month for the 6 months after the last dose of REBETOL.
   - If you or your female sexual partner becomes pregnant while taking REBETOL or within 6 months after you stop taking REBETOL, tell your health care provider right away. You or your health care provider should contact the REBETOL pregnancy registry by calling 1-800-593-2214. The REBETOL pregnancy registry collects information about what happens to mothers and their babies if the mother takes REBETOL while she is pregnant.

What is REBETOL®?

REBETOL is a medicine used with either interferon alfa-2b (Intron A) or peginterferon alfa-2b (PegIntron) to treat chronic (lasting a long time) hepatitis C infection in people 3 years and older with liver disease.

It is not known if REBETOL use for longer than 1 year is safe and will work.

It is not known if REBETOL use in children younger than 3 years old is safe and will work.

Who should not take REBETOL®?

See "What is the most important information I should know about REBETOL?"

Do not take REBETOL if you have:

- or ever had serious allergic reactions to the ingredients in REBETOL. See the end of this Medication Guide for a complete list of ingredients.
- certain types of hepatitis (autoimmune hepatitis).
- certain blood disorders (hemoglobinopathies).
- severe kidney disease.
- taken or currently take didanosine (VIDEX®).

Talk to your health care provider before taking REBETOL if you have any of these conditions.

What should I tell my health care provider before taking REBETOL®?

Before you take REBETOL, tell your health care provider if you have or ever had:

- treatment for hepatitis C that did not work for you.
- breathing problems. REBETOL may cause or worsen breathing problems you already have.
- vision problems. REBETOL may cause eye problems or worsen eye problems you already have. You should have an eye exam before you start treatment with REBETOL.

- certain blood disorders such as anemia (low red blood cell count).
- high blood pressure, heart problems, or have had a heart attack. Your health care provider should check your blood and heart before you start treatment with REBETOL.
- thyroid problems.
- liver problems other than hepatitis C infection.
- human immunodeficiency virus (HIV) or any immunity problems.
- mental health problems, including depression or thoughts of suicide.
- kidney problems.
- an organ transplant.
- diabetes. REBETOL may make your diabetes worse or harder to treat.
- any other medical condition.
- are breastfeeding. It is not known if REBETOL passes into your breast milk. You and your health care provider should decide if you will take REBETOL or breastfeed.

Tell your health care provider about all the medicines you take, including prescription medicines, vitamins, and herbal supplements. REBETOL may affect the way other medicines work.

Especially tell your health care provider if you take didanosine (VIDEX®) or azathioprine (Imuran and Azasan).

Know the medicines you take. Keep a list of them to show your health care provider or pharmacist when you get a new medicine.

How should I take REBETOL®?

- Take REBETOL exactly as your health care provider tells you. Your health care provider will tell you how much REBETOL to take and when to take it.
- Take REBETOL with food.
- Take REBETOL Capsules whole. Do not open, break, or crush REBETOL Capsules before swallowing. If you cannot swallow REBETOL Capsules whole, tell your health care provider.
- If you miss a dose of REBETOL, take the missed dose as soon as possible during the same day. Do not double the next dose. If you have questions about what to do, call your health care provider.
- If you take too much REBETOL, call your health care provider or Poison Control Center at 1-800-222-1222, or go to the nearest hospital emergency room right away.

What are the possible side effects of REBETOL®?

REBETOL may cause serious side effects, including:

See "What is the most important information I should know about REBETOL?"

- **Swelling and irritation of your pancreas (pancreatitis).** You may have stomach pain, nausea, vomiting, or diarrhea.
- **Serious breathing problems.** Difficulty breathing may be a sign of a serious lung infection (pneumonia) that can lead to death.
- **Serious eye problems** that may lead to vision loss or blindness.
- **Dental problems.** Your mouth may be very dry, which can lead to problems with your teeth and gums.
- **Severe depression.**
- **Suicidal thoughts and attempts.** Adults and children who take REBETOL, especially teenagers, are more likely to have suicidal thoughts or attempt to hurt themselves while taking REBETOL. Call your health care provider right away or go to the nearest hospital emergency room if you have new or worse depression or thoughts about suicide or dying.

- **Severe blood disorders.** An increased risk when used in combination with pegylated alpha interferons and azathioprine.
- **Growth problems in children.** Weight loss and slowed growth are common in children during combination treatment with PegIntron or INTRON A. Most children will go through a growth spurt and gain weight after treatment stops. Some children may not reach the height that they were expected to have before treatment. Talk to your healthcare provider if you are concerned about your child's growth during treatment with REBETOL and PegIntron or with REBETOL and INTRON A.

Tell your health care provider right away if you have any side effect that bothers you or that does not go away.

The most common side effects of REBETOL include:

- flu-like symptoms - feeling tired, headache, shaking along with high temperature (fever), nausea, and muscle aches.
- mood changes, feeling irritable.

The most common side effects of REBETOL in children include:

- a decrease in the blood cells that fight infection (neutropenia).
- a decrease in appetite.
- stomach pain and vomiting.

Tell your health care provider if you have any side effect that bothers you or that does not go away.

These are not all the possible side effects of REBETOL. For more information ask your health care provider or pharmacist.

Call your doctor for medical advice about side effects. You may report side effects to FDA at 1-800-FDA-1088.

How should I store REBETOL®?

- Store REBETOL Capsules between 59-86°F (15-30°C).
- Store REBETOL Oral Solution between 59-86°F (15-30°C) or in the refrigerator between 36-46°F (2-8°C).

Keep REBETOL and all medicines out of the reach of children.

GENERAL INFORMATION ABOUT THE SAFE AND EFFECTIVE USE OF REBETOL®.

It is not known if treatment with REBETOL will cure hepatitis C virus infections or prevent cirrhosis, liver failure, or liver cancer that can be caused by hepatitis C virus infections. It is not known if taking REBETOL will prevent you from infecting another person with the hepatitis C virus.

Medicines are sometimes prescribed for purposes other than those listed in a Medication Guide. Do not use REBETOL for a condition for which it was not prescribed. Do not give REBETOL to other people, even if they have the same symptoms that you have. It may harm them.

This Medication Guide summarizes the most important information about REBETOL. If you would like more information, talk with your health care provider. You can ask your pharmacist or health care provider for information about REBETOL that is written for health professionals.

What are the ingredients in REBETOL®?

Active ingredients: ribavirin

REBETOL Capsules

Inactive ingredients: microcrystalline cellulose, lactose monohydrate, croscarmellose sodium, and magnesium stearate. The capsule shell consists of gelatin, sodium lauryl sulfate, silicon dioxide, and titanium dioxide. The capsule is printed with edible blue pharmaceutical ink which is made of shellac, anhydrous ethyl alcohol, isopropyl alcohol, n-butyl alcohol, propylene glycol, ammonium hydroxide, and FD&C Blue #2 aluminum lake.

REBETOL Oral Solution

Inactive ingredients: sucrose, glycerin, sorbitol, propylene glycol, sodium citrate, citric acid, sodium benzoate, natural and artificial flavor for bubble gum # 15864, and water.

This Medication Guide has been approved by the U.S. Food and Drug Administration.

REBETOL Oral Solution manufactured for:
Merck Sharp & Dohme Corp., a subsidiary of
MERCK & CO., INC.
Whitehouse Station, NJ 08889, USA
Manufactured by: Schering-Plough Canada, Inc., Pointe Claire, Quebec, Canada
REBETOL Capsules manufactured by:
Merck Sharp & Dohme Corp., a subsidiary of
MERCK & CO., INC.
Whitehouse Station, NJ 08889, USA
VIDEX® is a registered trademark of Bristol-Myers Squibb Company.
Copyright © 2003, 2010 Merck Sharp & Dohme Corp., a subsidiary of **Merck & Co., Inc.**
All rights reserved.
Revised: 11/2013
mg-mk8908-mtl-1311r017
Shown in Product Identification Guide, page 309

RECOMBIVAX HB®
[re-com-biv-ax]
Hepatitis B Vaccine (Recombinant)
Suspension for intramuscular injection

℞

HIGHLIGHTS OF PRESCRIBING INFORMATION
These highlights do not include all the information needed to use RECOMBIVAX HB safely and effectively. See full prescribing information for RECOMBIVAX HB.
RECOMBIVAX HB® Hepatitis B Vaccine (Recombinant)
Suspension for intramuscular injection
Initial U.S. Approval: 1983

———INDICATIONS AND USAGE———

RECOMBIVAX HB is a vaccine indicated for prevention of infection caused by all known subtypes of hepatitis B virus. RECOMBIVAX HB is approved for use in individuals of all ages. RECOMBIVAX HB Dialysis Formulation is approved for use in predialysis and dialysis patients 18 years of age and older. (1)

———DOSAGE AND ADMINISTRATION———

RECOMBIVAX HB
• Persons from birth through 19 years of age: A series of 3 doses (0.5 mL each) given on a 0-, 1-, and 6-month schedule. (2.1)
• Adolescents 11 through 15 years of age: A series of either 3 doses (0.5 mL each) given on a 0-, 1-, and 6-month schedule or a series of 2 doses (1.0 mL) on a 0- and 4- to 6-month schedule. (2.1)
• Persons 20 years of age and older: A series of 3 doses (1.0 mL each) given on a 0-, 1-, and 6-month schedule. (2.1)

RECOMBIVAX HB Dialysis Formulation
• Adults on predialysis or dialysis: A series of 3 doses (1.0 mL each) given on a 0-, 1-, and 6-month schedule. (2.1)

———DOSAGE FORMS AND STRENGTHS———

RECOMBIVAX HB is a sterile suspension available in the following presentations:
• 0.5 mL (5 mcg) Pediatric/Adolescent Formulation single-dose vials and prefilled syringes (3, 11, 16)
• 1 mL (10 mcg) Adult Formulation single-dose vials and prefilled syringes (3, 11, 16)
RECOMBIVAX HB Dialysis Formulation is a sterile suspension available in the following presentation:
• 1 mL (40 mcg) single-dose vials (3, 11, 16)

———CONTRAINDICATIONS———

Severe allergic or hypersensitivity reactions (e.g., anaphylaxis) after a previous dose of any hepatitis B-containing vaccine, or to any component of RECOMBIVAX HB, including yeast. (4, 11)

———WARNINGS AND PRECAUTIONS———

The vial stopper, the syringe plunger stopper, and tip cap contain dry natural latex rubber which may cause allergic reactions in latex-sensitive individuals. (5.1)
Apnea following intramuscular vaccination has been observed in some infants born prematurely. Decisions about when to administer an intramuscular vaccine, including RECOMBIVAX HB, to infants born prematurely should be based on consideration of the individual infant's medical status and the potential benefits and possible risks of vaccination. (5.2)

———ADVERSE REACTIONS———

In healthy infants and children (up to 10 years of age), the most frequently reported systemic adverse reactions (>1% injections), in decreasing order of frequency, were irritability, fever, diarrhea, fatigue/weakness, diminished appetite, and rhinitis. (6.1)
In healthy adults, injection site reactions and systemic adverse reactions were reported following 17% and 15% of the injections, respectively. (6.1)

To report SUSPECTED ADVERSE REACTIONS, contact Merck Sharp & Dohme Corp., a subsidiary of Merck & Co., Inc., at 1-877-888-4231 or VAERS at 1-800-822-7967 or www.vaers.hhs.gov.

———DRUG INTERACTIONS———

Do not mix RECOMBIVAX HB with any other vaccine in the same syringe or vial. (7.1)

———USE IN SPECIFIC POPULATIONS———

Safety and effectiveness of RECOMBIVAX HB have not been established in pregnant women and nursing mothers. RECOMBIVAX HB should only be given to a pregnant woman if clearly needed. (8.1, 8.3)

See 17 for PATIENT COUNSELING INFORMATION

Revised: 05/2014

FULL PRESCRIBING INFORMATION

1   INDICATIONS AND USAGE

RECOMBIVAX HB® [Hepatitis B Vaccine, Recombinant] is indicated for prevention of infection caused by all known subtypes of hepatitis B virus. RECOMBIVAX HB is approved for use in individuals of all ages. RECOMBIVAX HB Dialysis Formulation is approved for use in adult predialysis and dialysis patients 18 years of age and older.

2   DOSAGE AND ADMINISTRATION

For intramuscular administration. See Section 2.2 for subcutaneous administration in persons with hemophilia.

2.1   Dosage and Schedule
RECOMBIVAX HB:
Persons from birth through 19 years of age: A series of 3 doses (0.5 mL each) given on a 0-, 1-, and 6-month schedule.
Adolescents 11 through 15 years of age: A series of 3 doses (0.5 mL each) given on a 0-, 1-, and 6-month schedule or a series of 2 doses (1.0 mL each) on a 0- and 4- to 6-month schedule.
Persons 20 years of age and older: A series of 3 doses (1.0 mL each) given on a 0-, 1-, and 6-month schedule.
RECOMBIVAX HB Dialysis Formulation:
Adults on predialysis and dialysis: A series of 3 doses (1.0 mL each) given on a 0-, 1-, and 6-month schedule.
Table 1 summarizes the dose and formulation of RECOMBIVAX HB for specific populations, regardless of the risk of infection with hepatitis B virus.

Table 1: RECOMBIVAX HB Recommended Dose and Administration Schedules

Group	Dose/Regimen
Infants*, Children and Adolescents 0-19 years of age (Pediatric/Adolescent Formulation)	5 mcg (0.5 mL) 3 doses at 0, 1, and 6 months
Adolescents† 11 through 15 years of age (Adult formulation)	10 mcg‡ (1.0 mL) 2 doses at 0 and 4-6 months
Adults ≥20 years of age (Adult formulation)	10 mcg‡ (1.0 mL) 3 doses at 0, 1, and 6 months
Predialysis and Dialysis Patients§ (Dialysis formulation)	40 mcg (1.0 mL) 3 doses at 0, 1, and 6 months

* For specific recommendations for infants see ACIP recommendations.{1}
† Adolescents (11 through 15 years of age) may receive either regimen: 3 × 5 mcg (Pediatric Formulation) or 2 × 10 mcg (Adult Formulation).
‡ If the suggested dose (10 mcg) is not available, the appropriate dosage can be achieved with two 5 mcg doses. However, the Dialysis Formulation may be used only for adult predialysis/dialysis patients.
§ See also recommendations for revaccination of predialysis and dialysis patients in [Dosage and Administration (2.4)].

2.2   Preparation and Administration
Shake the single-dose vial or single-dose prefilled syringe well to obtain a slightly opaque, white suspension before withdrawal and use. Parenteral drug products should be inspected visually for particulate matter and discoloration prior to administration, whenever solution and container permit. Discard if the suspension does not appear homogeneous or if extraneous particulate matter remains or if discoloration is observed.
For single-dose vials, withdraw and administer entire dose of RECOMBIVAX HB intramuscularly using a sterile needle and syringe.
For single-dose prefilled syringes, securely attach a needle by twisting in a clockwise direction and administer dose of RECOMBIVAX HB intramuscularly.
The deltoid muscle is the preferred site for intramuscular injection for adults, adolescents and children 1 year of age and older whose deltoid is large enough for intramuscular injection. The anterolateral aspect of the thigh is the preferred site for intramuscular injection for infants younger than 1 year of age. RECOMBIVAX HB should not be administered in the gluteal region, as injections given in the buttocks have resulted in lower seroconversion rates than expected.{2}
RECOMBIVAX HB may be administered subcutaneously to persons at risk for hemorrhage following intramuscular injections (e.g., hemophiliacs). However, hepatitis B vaccines are known to result in lower antibody response when administered subcutaneously.{3} Additionally, when other aluminum-adsorbed vaccines have been administered subcutaneously, an increased incidence of local reactions including subcutaneous nodules has been observed. Therefore, consider subcutaneous administration only in persons who are at risk of hemorrhage following intramuscular injections.
Do not administer intravenously or intradermally

2.3   Known or Presumed Exposure to Hepatitis B Virus
Known or Presumed Exposure to HBsAg
Refer to recommendations of the Advisory Committee on Immunization Practices (ACIP) and to the package insert for hepatitis B immune globulin (HBIG) for management of persons with known or presumed exposure to the hepatitis B virus (e.g., neonates born of infected mothers or persons who experienced percutaneous or permucosal exposure to the virus). When recommended, administer RECOMBIVAX HB and HBIG intramuscularly at separate sites (e.g., opposite anterolateral thighs for exposed neonates) as soon as possible after exposure. Administer additional doses of RECOMBIVAX HB (to complete a vaccination series) in accordance with ACIP recommendations.

2.4   Booster Vaccinations
The duration of the protective effect of RECOMBIVAX HB in healthy vaccinees is unknown at present and the need for booster doses is not yet defined. The ACIP provides recommendations for use of a booster dose or revaccination series in previously vaccinated individuals with known or presumed exposure to Hepatitis B Virus.
Consider a booster dose or revaccination with RECOMBIVAX HB Dialysis Formulation (blue color code) in predialysis/dialysis patients if the anti-HBs level is less than 10 mIU/mL at 1 to 2 months after the third dose. Assess the need for a booster dose annually by antibody testing, and give a booster dose when the anti-HBs level declines to less than 10 mIU/mL.{3}

3   DOSAGE FORMS AND STRENGTHS

RECOMBIVAX HB is a sterile suspension available in the following presentations:
• 0.5 mL (5 mcg) Pediatric/Adolescent Formulation single-dose vials and prefilled syringes
• 1 mL (10 mcg) Adult Formulation single-dose vials and prefilled syringes
RECOMBIVAX HB DIALYSIS FORMULATION is a sterile suspension available in the following presentation:
• 1 mL (40 mcg) single-dose vial [see Description (11) and How Supplied/Storage and Handling (16)]

4　CONTRAINDICATIONS

Do not administer RECOMBIVAX HB to individuals with a history of severe allergic or hypersensitivity reactions (e.g., anaphylaxis) after a previous dose of any hepatitis B-containing vaccine or to any component of RECOMBIVAX HB, including yeast [see Description (11)].

5　WARNINGS AND PRECAUTIONS

5.1　Hypersensitivity to Latex
The vial stopper and the syringe plunger stopper and tip cap contain dry natural latex rubber, which may cause allergic reactions in latex-sensitive individuals.

5.2　Apnea in Premature Infants
Apnea following intramuscular vaccination has been observed in some infants born prematurely. Decisions about when to administer an intramuscular vaccine, including RECOMBIVAX HB, to infants born prematurely should be based on consideration of the individual infant's medical status and the potential benefits and possible risks of vaccination. For RECOMBIVAX HB, this assessment should include consideration of the mother's hepatitis B antigen status and the high probability of maternal transmission of hepatitis B virus to infants born to mothers who are HBsAg positive if vaccination is delayed.

5.3　Infants Weighing Less Than 2000 g
Hepatitis B vaccination should be delayed until 1 month of age or hospital discharge in infants weighing <2000 g if the mother is documented to be HBsAg negative at the time of the infant's birth. Infants weighing <2000 g born to HBsAg positive or HBsAg unknown mothers should receive vaccine and hepatitis B immune globulin (HBIG) in accordance with ACIP recommendations{3} [see Dosage and Administration (2)].

5.4　Prevention and Management of Allergic Vaccine Reactions
Appropriate medical treatment and supervision must be available to manage possible anaphylactic reactions following administration [see Contraindications (4)].

5.5　Limitations of Vaccine Effectiveness
Hepatitis B virus has a long incubation period. RECOMBIVAX HB may not prevent hepatitis B infection in individuals who have an unrecognized hepatitis B infection at the time of vaccination. Additionally, vaccination with RECOMBIVAX HB may not protect all individuals.

6　ADVERSE REACTIONS

In healthy infants and children (up to 10 years of age), the most frequently reported systemic adverse reactions (>1% injections), in decreasing order of frequency, were irritability, fever, diarrhea, fatigue/weakness, diminished appetite, and rhinitis. In healthy adults, injection site reactions and systemic adverse reactions were reported following 17% and 15% of the injections, respectively.

6.1　Clinical Trials Experience
Because clinical trials are conducted under widely varying conditions, adverse reaction rates observed in the clinical trials of a vaccine cannot be directly compared to rates in the clinical trials of another vaccine and may not reflect the rates observed in practice.

In three clinical studies, 434 doses of RECOMBIVAX HB, 5 mcg, were administered to 147 healthy infants and children (up to 10 years of age) who were monitored for 5 days after each dose. Injection site reactions and systemic adverse reactions were reported following 0.2% and 10.4% of the injections, respectively. The most frequently reported systemic adverse reactions (>1% injections), in decreasing order of frequency, were irritability, fever (≥101°F oral equivalent), diarrhea, fatigue/weakness, diminished appetite, and rhinitis.

In a study that compared the three-dose regimen (5 mcg) with the two-dose regimen (10 mcg) of RECOMBIVAX HB in adolescents, the overall frequency of adverse reactions was generally similar.

In a group of studies, 3258 doses of RECOMBIVAX HB, 10 mcg, were administered to 1252 healthy adults who were monitored for 5 days after each dose. Injection site reactions and systemic adverse reactions were reported following 17% and 15% of the injections, respectively. The following adverse reactions were reported:

Incidence Equal To or Greater Than 1% of Injections
GENERAL DISORDERS AND ADMINISTRATION SITE CONDITIONS
Injection site reactions consisting principally of soreness, and including pain, tenderness, pruritus, erythema, ecchymosis, swelling, warmth, nodule formation.
The most frequent systemic complaints include fatigue/weakness; headache; fever (≥100°F); malaise.
GASTROINTESTINAL DISORDERS
Nausea; diarrhea
RESPIRATORY, THORACIC AND MEDIASTINAL DISORDERS
Pharyngitis; upper respiratory infection

Incidence Less Than 1% of Injections
GENERAL DISORDERS AND ADMINISTRATION SITE CONDITIONS
Sweating; achiness; sensation of warmth; lightheadedness; chills; flushing
GASTROINTESTINAL DISORDERS
Vomiting; abdominal pains/cramps; dyspepsia; diminished appetite
RESPIRATORY, THORACIC AND MEDIASTINAL DISORDERS
Rhinitis; influenza; cough
NERVOUS SYSTEM DISORDERS
Vertigo/dizziness; paresthesia
SKIN AND SUBCUTANEOUS TISSUE DISORDERS
Pruritus; rash (non-specified); angioedema; urticaria
MUSCULOSKELETAL AND CONNECTIVE TISSUE DISORDERS
Arthralgia including monoarticular; myalgia; back pain; neck pain; shoulder pain; neck stiffness
BLOOD AND LYMPHATIC DISORDERS
Lymphadenopathy
PSYCHIATRIC DISORDERS
Insomnia/disturbed sleep
EAR AND LABYRINTH DISORDERS
Earache
RENAL AND URINARY DISORDERS
Dysuria
CARDIAC DISORDERS
Hypotension

6.2　Post-Marketing Experience
The following additional adverse reactions have been reported with use of the marketed vaccine. Because these reactions are reported voluntarily from a population of uncertain size, it is not possible to reliably estimate their frequency or establish a causal relationship to a vaccine exposure.

Immune System Disorders
Hypersensitivity reactions including anaphylactic/anaphylactoid reactions, bronchospasm, and urticaria have been reported within the first few hours after vaccination. An apparent hypersensitivity syndrome (serum-sickness-like) of delayed onset has been reported days to weeks after vaccination, including: arthralgia/arthritis (usually transient), fever, and dermatologic reactions such as urticaria, erythema multiforme, ecchymoses and erythema nodosum [see Warnings and Precautions (5.1)]. Autoimmune diseases including systemic lupus erythematosus (SLE), lupus-like syndrome, vasculitis, and polyarteritis nodosa have also been reported.

Gastrointestinal Disorders
Elevation of liver enzymes; constipation
Nervous System Disorders
Guillain-Barré syndrome; multiple sclerosis; exacerbation of multiple sclerosis; myelitis including transverse myelitis; seizure; febrile seizure; peripheral neuropathy including Bell's Palsy; radiculopathy; herpes zoster; migraine; muscle weakness; hypesthesia; encephalitis
Skin and Subcutaneous Disorders
Stevens-Johnson syndrome; alopecia; petechiae; eczema
Musculoskeletal and Connective Tissue Disorders
Arthritis
Pain in extremity
Blood and Lymphatic System Disorders
Increased erythrocyte sedimentation rate; thrombocytopenia
Psychiatric Disorders
Irritability; agitation; somnolence
Eye Disorders
Optic neuritis; tinnitus; conjunctivitis; visual disturbances; uveitis
Cardiac Disorders
Syncope; tachycardia
The following adverse reaction has been reported with another Hepatitis B Vaccine (Recombinant) but not with RECOMBIVAX HB: keratitis.

7　DRUG INTERACTIONS

7.1　Concomitant Administration With Other Vaccines
Do not mix RECOMBIVAX HB with any other vaccine in the same syringe or vial. Use separate injection sites and syringes for each vaccine.

In clinical trials in children, RECOMBIVAX HB was concomitantly administered with one or more of the following US licensed vaccines: Diphtheria, Tetanus and whole cell Pertussis; oral Poliomyelitis vaccine; Measles, Mumps, and Rubella Virus Vaccine, Live; Haemophilus b Conjugate Vaccine (Meningococcal Protein Conjugate)] or a booster dose of Diphtheria, Tetanus, acellular Pertussis. Safety and immunogenicity were similar for concomitantly administered vaccines compared to separately administered vaccines.

In another clinical trial, a related HBsAg-containing product, COMVAX® [Haemophilus b Conjugate (Meningococcal Protein Conjugate) and Hepatitis B (Recombinant) Vaccine], was given concomitantly with eIPV (enhanced inactivated Poliovirus vaccine) or VARIVAX® [Varicella Virus Vaccine Live (Oka/Merck)], using separate sites and syringes for injectable vaccines. No serious vaccine-related adverse events were reported, and no impairment of immune response to these individually tested vaccine antigens was demonstrated.

COMVAX has also been administered concomitantly with the primary series of DTaP to a limited number of infants. No serious vaccine-related adverse events were reported.

7.2　Concomitant Administration with Immune Globulin
RECOMBIVAX HB may be administered concomitantly with HBIG. The first dose of RECOMBIVAX HB may be given at the same time as HBIG, but the injections should be administered at different sites.

8　USE IN SPECIFIC POPULATIONS

8.1　Pregnancy
Pregnancy Category C: Animal reproduction studies have not been conducted with the vaccine. It is also not known whether the vaccine can cause fetal harm when administered to a pregnant woman or can affect reproduction capacity. The vaccine should be given to a pregnant woman only if clearly needed.

8.3　Nursing Mothers
It is not known whether the vaccine is excreted in human milk. Because many drugs are excreted in human milk, caution should be exercised when the vaccine is administered to a nursing woman.

8.4　Pediatric Use
Safety and effectiveness of RECOMBIVAX HB have been established in all pediatric age groups. Maternally transferred antibodies do not interfere with the active immune response to the vaccine. [See Adverse Reactions (6.1) and Clinical Studies (14.1 and 14.2).] The safety and effectiveness of RECOMBIVAX HB Dialysis Formulation in children have not been established.

8.5　Geriatric Use
Clinical studies of RECOMBIVAX HB used for licensure did not include sufficient numbers of subjects 65 years of age and older to determine whether they respond differently from younger subjects. However, in later studies it has been shown that a diminished antibody response can be expected in persons older than 60 years of age.

11　DESCRIPTION

RECOMBIVAX HB Hepatitis B Vaccine (Recombinant) is a sterile suspension of non-infectious subunit viral vaccine derived from HBsAg produced in yeast cells. A portion of the hepatitis B virus gene, coding for HBsAg, is cloned into yeast, and the vaccine for hepatitis B is produced from cultures of this recombinant yeast strain according to methods developed in the Merck Research Laboratories.

The antigen is harvested and purified from fermentation cultures of a recombinant strain of the yeast *Saccharomyces cerevisiae* containing the gene for the *adw* subtype of HBsAg. The fermentation process involves growth of *Saccharomyces cerevisiae* on a complex fermentation medium which consists of an extract of yeast, soy peptone, dextrose, amino acids and mineral salts. The HBsAg protein is released from the yeast cells by cell disruption and purified by a series of physical and chemical methods. The purified protein is treated in phosphate buffer with formaldehyde and then coprecipitated with alum (potassium aluminum sulfate) to form bulk vaccine adjuvanted with amorphous aluminum hydroxyphosphate sulfate. Each dose contains less than 1% yeast protein. The vaccine produced by the Merck method has been shown to be comparable to the plasma-derived vaccine in terms of animal potency (mouse, monkey, and chimpanzee) and protective efficacy (chimpanzee and human).

The vaccine against hepatitis B, prepared from recombinant yeast cultures, is free of association with human blood or blood products.

RECOMBIVAX HB Hepatitis B Vaccine (Recombinant) is supplied in three formulations. [See How Supplied/Storage and Handling (16).]

Pediatric/Adolescent Formulation (Without Preservative), 10 mcg/mL: each 0.5 mL dose contains 5 mcg of hepatitis B surface antigen.

Adult Formulation (Without Preservative), 10 mcg/mL: each 1 mL dose contains 10 mcg of hepatitis B surface antigen.

Dialysis Formulation (Without Preservative), 40 mcg/mL: each 1 mL dose contains 40 mcg of hepatitis B surface antigen.

All formulations contain approximately 0.5 mg of aluminum (provided as amorphous aluminum hydroxyphosphate sulfate, previously referred to as aluminum hydroxide) per mL of vaccine. In each formulation, hepatitis B surface antigen is adsorbed onto approximately 0.5 mg of aluminum (provided as amorphous aluminum hydroxyphosphate sulfate) per mL of vaccine. The vaccine contains <15 mcg/mL residual formaldehyde. The vaccine is of the *adw* subtype.

12 CLINICAL PHARMACOLOGY

12.1 Mechanism of Action

RECOMBIVAX HB has been shown to elicit antibodies to hepatitis B virus as measured by ELISA.

Antibody concentrations ≥10mIU/mL against HBsAg are recognized as conferring protection against hepatitis B infection.[2]

Infection with hepatitis B virus can have serious consequences including acute massive hepatic necrosis and chronic active hepatitis. Chronically infected persons are at increased risk for cirrhosis and hepatocellular carcinoma.

13 NONCLINICAL TOXICOLOGY

13.1 Carcinogenesis, Mutagenesis, Impairment of Fertility

RECOMBIVAX HB has not been evaluated for its carcinogenic or mutagenic potential, or its potential to impair fertility.

14 CLINICAL STUDIES

14.1 Efficacy in Neonates with Peripartum Exposure to Hepatitis B

The protective efficacy of three 5 mcg doses of RECOMBIVAX HB has been demonstrated in neonates born of mothers positive for both HBsAg and HBeAg (a core-associated antigenic complex which correlates with high infectivity). In a clinical study of infants who received one dose of HBIG at birth followed by the recommended three-dose regimen of RECOMBIVAX HB, chronic infection had not occurred in 96% of 130 infants after nine months of follow-up.[4] The estimated efficacy in prevention of chronic hepatitis B infection was 95% as compared to the infection rate in untreated historical controls.[5] Significantly fewer neonates became chronically infected when given one dose of HBIG at birth followed by the recommended three-dose regimen of RECOMBIVAX HB when compared to historical controls who received only a single dose of HBIG.[6] As demonstrated in the above study, HBIG, when administered simultaneously with RECOMBIVAX HB at separate body sites, did not interfere with the induction of protective antibodies against hepatitis B virus elicited by the vaccine.[6]

14.2 Immunogenicity of a Three-Dose Regimen in Healthy Infants, Children, and Adolescents

Three 5 mcg doses of RECOMBIVAX HB induced a protective level of antibody in 100% of 92 infants, 99% of 129 children, and in 99% of 112 adolescents [see Dosage and Administration (2.3)].

14.3 Immunogenicity of a Two-Dose Regimen in Healthy Adolescents 11 through 15 Years of Age

For adolescents (11 through 15 years of age), the immunogenicity of a two-dose regimen (10 mcg at 0 and 4-6 months) was compared with that of the standard three-dose regimen (5 mcg at 0, 1, and 6 months) in an open, randomized, multicenter study. The proportion of adolescents receiving the two-dose regimen who developed a protective level of antibody one month after the last dose (99% of 255 subjects) appears similar to that among adolescents who received the three-dose regimen (98% of 121 subjects). After adolescents (11 through 15 years of age) received the first 10-mcg dose of the two-dose regimen, the proportion who developed a protective level of antibody was approximately 72%.

14.4 Immunogenicity in Healthy Adults

Clinical studies have shown that RECOMBIVAX HB when injected into the deltoid muscle induced protective levels of antibody in 96% of 1213 healthy adults who received the recommended three-dose regimen. Antibody responses varied with age; a protective level of antibody was induced in 98% of 787 young adults 20-29 years of age, 94% of 249 adults 30-39 years of age and in 89% of 177 adults ≥40 years of age.

14.5 Efficacy and Immunogenicity in Specific Populations

Chronic Hepatitis C Infection

In one published study, the seroprotection rates in individuals with chronic hepatitis C virus (HCV) infection given the standard regimen of RECOMBIVAX HB was approximately 70%.[7] In a second published study of intravenous drug users given an accelerated schedule of RECOMBIVAX HB, infection with HCV did not affect the response to RECOMBIVAX HB.[8]

Predialysis and Dialysis Adult Patients

Predialysis and dialysis adult patients respond less well to hepatitis B vaccines than do healthy individuals; however, vaccination of adult patients early in the course of their renal disease produces higher seroconversion rates than vaccination after dialysis has been initiated.[9] In addition, the responses to these vaccines may be lower if the vaccine is administered as a buttock injection. When 40 mcg of Hepatitis B Vaccine (Recombinant), was administered in the deltoid muscle, 89% of 28 participants developed anti-HBs with 86% achieving levels ≥10 mIU/mL. However, when the same dosage of this vaccine was administered inappropriately either in the buttock or a combination of buttock and deltoid, 62% of 47 participants developed anti-HBs with 55% achieving levels of ≥10 mIU/mL.

15 REFERENCES

1. CDC. A Comprehensive Strategy to Eliminate Transmission of Hepatitis B Virus Infection in the United States. Recommendations of the Advisory Committee on Immunization Practices (ACIP) Part I: Immunization of Infants, Children and Adolescents. MMWR Recommendations and Reports 2005; 54(RR16): 1-23. Appendix C - Postexposure Prophylaxis of Persons with Discrete Identifiable Exposures to Hepatitis B Virus (HBV) and http://www.cdc.gov/hepatitis/hbv/pdfs/correctedtable4.pdf
2. CDC. Suboptimal Response to Hepatitis B Vaccine given by Injection into the Buttock. MMWR Weekly Report 1985; 34: 105-8, 113.
3. Centers for Disease Control and Prevention. A Comprehensive Immunization Strategy to Eliminate Transmission of Hepatitis B Virus Infection in the United States. Recommendations of the Advisory Committee on Immunization Practices (ACIP). Part 2: Immunization of Adults, MMWR 2006, 55(RR-16): 1-25.
4. Stevens, C.E.; Taylor, P.E.; Tong, M.J., et al.: Prevention of Perinatal Hepatitis B Virus Infection with Hepatitis B Immune Globulin and Hepatitis B Vaccine, in Zuckerman, A.J. (ed.), "Viral Hepatitis and Liver Diseases", Alan R. Liss, 982-983, 1988.
5. Stevens, C.E.; Taylor, P.E.; Tong, M.J., et al.: Yeast-Recombinant Hepatitis B Vaccine, Efficacy with Hepatitis B Immune Globulin in Prevention of Perinatal Hepatitis B Virus Transmission, JAMA 257(19): 2612-2616, 1987.
6. Beasley, R.P.; Hwang, L.; Stevens, C.E.; Lin, C.; Hsieh, F.; Wang, K.; Sun, T.; Szmuness, W.: Efficacy of Hepatitis B Immune Globulin for Prevention of Perinatal Transmission of the Hepatitis B Virus Carrier State: Final Report of a Randomized Double-Blind, Placebo-Controlled Trial, Hepatology 3: 135-141, 1983.
7. Wiedmann, M.; Liebert, U.G.; Oesen, U.; Porst, H.; Wiese, M.; Schroeder, S.; Halm, U.; Mossner, J.; Berr, F.: Decreased Immunogenicity of Recombinant Hepatitis B Vaccine in Chronic Hepatitis C, Hepatology, 31: 230-234, 2000.
8. Minniti, F.; Baldo, V.; Trivello, R.; Bricolo, R.; Di Furia, L.; Renzulli, G.; Chiaramonte, M.: Response to HBV vaccine in Relation to anti-HCV and anti-HBc Positivity: a Study in Intravenous Drug Addicts, Vaccine, 17: 3083-3085, 1999.
9. Recommendations of the Advisory Committee on Immunization Practices (ACIP): Hepatitis B Virus Infection: A Comprehensive Strategy to Eliminate Transmission in the United States, 1996 update, MMWR (draft January 13, 1996).

16 HOW SUPPLIED/STORAGE AND HANDLING

RECOMBIVAX HB and RECOMBIVAX HB DIALYSIS FORMULATION are available in single-dose vials and pre-filled Luer-Lok® syringes.

Pediatric/Adolescent Formulation (PRESERVATIVE FREE)
0.5 mL (5 mcg) in single-dose vials and prefilled Luer-Lok® syringes

NDC 0006-4981-00 – box of ten 0.5-mL single-dose vials
Color coded with a yellow cap and stripe on the vial labels and cartons and an orange banner on the vial labels and cartons

NDC 0006-4093-02 – carton of 10 prefilled single-dose Luer-Lok® syringes with tip caps
Color coded with a yellow plunger rod

NDC 0006-4093-09 – carton of six 0.5-mL prefilled single-dose Luer-Lok® syringes with tip caps
Color coded with a yellow plunger rod and stripe

Adult Formulation *(PRESERVATIVE FREE)*
1 mL (10mcg) in single-dose vials and prefilled Luer-Lok® syringes

NDC 0006-4995-00 – 1-mL single dose vial
Color coded with a green cap and stripe

NDC 0006-4995-41 – box of ten 1-mL single-dose vials
Color coded with a green cap and stripe

NDC 0006-4094-02 – carton of 10 pre-filled single-dose syringes with tip caps
Color coded with a green plunger rod

NDC 0006-4094-09 – carton of six 1-mL prefilled single-dose Luer-Lok® syringes with tip caps
Color coded with a green plunger rod and stripe

RECOMBIVAX HB DIALYSIS FORMULATION
1 mL (40mcg) in single-dose vials

NDC 0006-4992-00 – 1-mL single-dose vial
Color coded with a blue cap and stripe

Store vials and syringes at 2-8°C (36-46°F). Storage above or below the recommended temperature may reduce potency.

Do not freeze since freezing destroys potency.

17 PATIENT COUNSELING INFORMATION

Information for Vaccine Recipients and Parents/Guardians
- Inform the patient, parent or guardian of the potential benefits and risks associated with vaccination, as well as the importance of completing the immunization series.
- Question the vaccine recipient, parent or guardian about the occurrence of any symptoms and/or signs of adverse reaction after a previous dose of hepatitis B vaccine.
- Tell the patient, parent or guardian to report adverse events to the physician or clinic where the vaccine was administered.
- Prior to vaccination, give the patient, parent or guardian the Vaccine Information Statements which are required by the National Vaccine Injury Act of 1986. The materials are available free of charge at the Centers for Disease Control and Prevention (CDC) website (www.cdc.gov/vaccines).
- Tell the patient, parent or guardian that the United States Department of Health and Human Services has established a Vaccine Adverse Event Reporting System (VAERS) to accept all reports of suspected adverse events after the administration of any vaccine, including but not limited to the reporting of events by the National Childhood Vaccine Injury Act of 1986. The VAERS toll-free number is 1-800-822-7967. Reporting forms may also be obtained at the VAERS website at (www.vaers.hhs.gov).

Manuf. and Dist. by: Merck Sharpe & Dohme Corp., a subsidiary of **MERCK & CO., INC.**, Whitehouse Station, NJ 08889, USA

For patent information:
www.merck.com/product/patent/home.htmI

The trademarks depicted herein are owned by their respective companies.

Copyright © 2014 Merck Sharp & Dohme Corp., a subsidiary of **Merck & Co., Inc.**
All rights reserved.
uspi-v232-i-1405r438

REMERON®
[rem-er-on]
(mirtazapine)
Tablets

℞

Suicidality and Antidepressant Drugs

Antidepressants increased the risk compared to placebo of suicidal thinking and behavior (suicidality) in children, adolescents, and young adults in short-term studies of major depressive disorder (MDD) and other psychiatric disorders. Anyone considering the use of REMERON® (mirtazapine) Tablets or any other antidepressant in a child, adolescent, or young adult must balance this risk with the clinical need. Short-term studies did not show an increase in the risk of suicidality with antidepressants compared to placebo in adults beyond age 24; there was a reduction in risk with antidepressants compared to placebo in adults aged 65 and older. Depression and certain other psychiatric disorders are themselves associated with increases in the risk of suicide. Patients of all ages who are started on antidepressant therapy should be monitored appropriately and observed closely for clinical worsening, suicidality, or unusual changes in behavior. Families and caregivers should be advised of the need for close observation and communication with the prescriber. REMERON is not approved for use in pediatric patients. (See WARNINGS: Clinical Worsening and Suicide Risk, PRECAUTIONS: Information for Patients, and PRECAUTIONS: Pediatric Use)

DESCRIPTION

REMERON® (mirtazapine) Tablets are an orally administered drug. Mirtazapine has a tetracyclic chemical structure and belongs to the piperazino-azepine group of compounds. It is designated 1,2,3,4,10,14b-hexahydro-2-methylpyrazino [2,1-a] pyrido [2,3-c] benzazepine and has the empirical formula of $C_{17}H_{19}N_3$. Its molecular weight is 265.36. The structural formula is the following and it is the racemic mixture:

Mirtazapine is a white to creamy white crystalline powder which is slightly soluble in water.

REMERON is supplied for oral administration as scored film-coated tablets containing 15 or 30 mg of mirtazapine, and unscored film-coated tablets containing 45 mg of mirtazapine. Each tablet also contains corn starch, hydroxypropyl cellulose, magnesium stearate, colloidal silicon dioxide, lactose, and other inactive ingredients.

CLINICAL PHARMACOLOGY

Pharmacodynamics

The mechanism of action of REMERON (mirtazapine) Tablets, as with other drugs effective in the treatment of major depressive disorder, is unknown.

Evidence gathered in preclinical studies suggests that mirtazapine enhances central noradrenergic and serotonergic activity. These studies have shown that mirtazapine acts as an antagonist at central presynaptic α_2–adrenergic inhibitory autoreceptors and heteroreceptors, an action that is postulated to result in an increase in central noradrenergic and serotonergic activity.

Mirtazapine is a potent antagonist of 5-HT$_2$ and 5-HT$_3$ receptors. Mirtazapine has no significant affinity for the 5-HT$_{1A}$ and 5-HT$_{1B}$ receptors.

Mirtazapine is a potent antagonist of histamine (H$_1$) receptors, a property that may explain its prominent sedative effects.

Mirtazapine is a moderate peripheral α_1–adrenergic antagonist, a property that may explain the occasional orthostatic hypotension reported in association with its use.

Mirtazapine is a moderate antagonist at muscarinic receptors, a property that may explain the relatively low incidence of anticholinergic side effects associated with its use.

Pharmacokinetics

REMERON (mirtazapine) Tablets are rapidly and completely absorbed following oral administration and have a half-life of about 20 to 40 hours. Peak plasma concentrations are reached within about 2 hours following an oral dose. The presence of food in the stomach has a minimal effect on both the rate and extent of absorption and does not require a dosage adjustment.

Mirtazapine is extensively metabolized after oral administration. Major pathways of biotransformation are demethylation and hydroxylation followed by glucuronide conjugation. *In vitro* data from human liver microsomes indicate that cytochrome 2D6 and 1A2 are involved in the formation of the 8-hydroxy metabolite of mirtazapine, whereas cytochrome 3A is considered to be responsible for the formation of the N-desmethyl and N-oxide metabolite. Mirtazapine has an absolute bioavailability of about 50%. It is eliminated predominantly via urine (75%) with 15% in feces. Several unconjugated metabolites possess pharmacological activity but are present in the plasma at very low levels. The (–) enantiomer has an elimination half-life that is approximately twice as long as the (+) enantiomer and therefore achieves plasma levels that are about 3 times as high as that of the (+) enantiomer.

Plasma levels are linearly related to dose over a dose range of 15 to 80 mg. The mean elimination half-life of mirtazapine after oral administration ranges from approximately 20 to 40 hours across age and gender subgroups, with females of all ages exhibiting significantly longer elimination half-lives than males (mean half-life of 37 hours for females vs. 26 hours for males). Steady state plasma levels of mirtazapine are attained within 5 days, with about 50% accumulation (accumulation ratio = 1.5).

Mirtazapine is approximately 85% bound to plasma proteins over a concentration range of 0.01 to 10 mcg/mL.

Special Populations

Geriatric

Following oral administration of REMERON (mirtazapine) Tablets 20 mg/day for 7 days to subjects of varying ages (range, 25–74), oral clearance of mirtazapine was reduced in the elderly compared to the younger subjects. The differences were most striking in males, with a 40% lower clearance in elderly males compared to younger males, while the clearance in elderly females was only 10% lower compared to younger females. Caution is indicated in administering REMERON to elderly patients (see PRECAUTIONS and DOSAGE AND ADMINISTRATION).

Pediatrics

Safety and effectiveness of mirtazapine in the pediatric population have not been established (see PRECAUTIONS).

Gender

The mean elimination half-life of mirtazapine after oral administration ranges from approximately 20 to 40 hours across age and gender subgroups, with females of all ages exhibiting significantly longer elimination half-lives than males (mean half-life of 37 hours for females vs. 26 hours for males) (see Pharmacokinetics).

Race

There have been no clinical studies to evaluate the effect of race on the pharmacokinetics of REMERON.

Renal Insufficiency

The disposition of mirtazapine was studied in patients with varying degrees of renal function. Elimination of mirtazapine is correlated with creatinine clearance. Total body clearance of mirtazapine was reduced approximately 30% in patients with moderate (Clcr=11–39 mL/min/1.73 m^2) and approximately 50% in patients with severe (Clcr=<10 mL/min/1.73 m^2) renal impairment when compared to normal subjects. Caution is indicated in admin-

istering REMERON to patients with compromised renal function (see PRECAUTIONS and DOSAGE AND ADMINISTRATION).

Hepatic Insufficiency

Following a single 15-mg oral dose of REMERON, the oral clearance of mirtazapine was decreased by approximately 30% in hepatically impaired patients compared to subjects with normal hepatic function. Caution is indicated in administering REMERON to patients with compromised hepatic function (see PRECAUTIONS and DOSAGE AND ADMINISTRATION).

Clinical Trials Showing Effectiveness

The efficacy of REMERON (mirtazapine) Tablets as a treatment for major depressive disorder was established in 4 placebo-controlled, 6-week trials in adult outpatients meeting DSM-III criteria for major depressive disorder. Patients were titrated with mirtazapine from a dose range of 5 mg up to 35 mg/day. Overall, these studies demonstrated mirtazapine to be superior to placebo on at least 3 of the following 4 measures: 21-Item Hamilton Depression Rating Scale (HDRS) total score; HDRS Depressed Mood Item; CGI Severity score; and Montgomery and Asberg Depression Rating Scale (MADRS). Superiority of mirtazapine over placebo was also found for certain factors of the HDRS, including anxiety/somatization factor and sleep disturbance factor. The mean mirtazapine dose for patients who completed these 4 studies ranged from 21 to 32 mg/day. A fifth study of similar design utilized a higher dose (up to 50 mg) per day and also showed effectiveness.

Examination of age and gender subsets of the population did not reveal any differential responsiveness on the basis of these subgroupings.

In a longer-term study, patients meeting (DSM-IV) criteria for major depressive disorder who had responded during an initial 8 to 12 weeks of acute treatment on REMERON were randomized to continuation of REMERON or placebo for up to 40 weeks of observation for relapse. Response during the open phase was defined as having achieved a HAM-D 17 total score of ≤8 and a CGI-Improvement score of 1 or 2 at 2 consecutive visits beginning with week 6 of the 8 to 12 weeks in the open-label phase of the study. Relapse during the double-blind phase was determined by the individual investigators. Patients receiving continued REMERON treatment experienced significantly lower relapse rates over the subsequent 40 weeks compared to those receiving placebo. This pattern was demonstrated in both male and female patients.

INDICATIONS AND USAGE

REMERON (mirtazapine) Tablets are indicated for the treatment of major depressive disorder.

The efficacy of REMERON in the treatment of major depressive disorder was established in 6-week controlled trials of outpatients whose diagnoses corresponded most closely to the Diagnostic and Statistical Manual of Mental Disorders – 3rd edition (DSM-III) category of major depressive disorder (see CLINICAL PHARMACOLOGY).

A major depressive episode (DSM-IV) implies a prominent and relatively persistent (nearly every day for at least 2 weeks) depressed or dysphoric mood that usually interferes with daily functioning, and includes at least 5 of the following 9 symptoms: depressed mood, loss of interest in usual activities, significant change in weight and/or appetite, insomnia or hypersomnia, psychomotor agitation or retardation, increased fatigue, feelings of guilt or worthlessness, slowed thinking or impaired concentration, a suicide attempt, or suicidal ideation.

The effectiveness of REMERON in hospitalized depressed patients has not been adequately studied.

The efficacy of REMERON in maintaining a response in patients with major depressive disorder for up to 40 weeks following 8 to 12 weeks of initial open-label treatment was demonstrated in a placebo-controlled trial. Nevertheless, the physician who elects to use REMERON for extended periods should periodically re-evaluate the long-term usefulness of the drug for the individual patient (see CLINICAL PHARMACOLOGY).

CONTRAINDICATIONS

Hypersensitivity

REMERON (mirtazapine) Tablets are contraindicated in patients with a known hypersensitivity to mirtazapine or to any of the excipients.

Monoamine Oxidase Inhibitors

The use of monoamine oxidase inhibitors (MAOIs) intended to treat psychiatric disorders with REMERON Tablets or within 14 days of stopping treatment with REMERON is contraindicated because of an increased risk of serotonin syndrome. The use of REMERON within 14 days of stopping an MAOI intended to treat psychiatric disorders is also contraindicated (see WARNINGS and DOSAGE AND ADMINISTRATION).

Starting REMERON in a patient who is being treated with MAOIs such as linezolid or intravenous methylene blue is

also contraindicated because of an increased risk of serotonin syndrome (see WARNINGS and DOSAGE AND ADMINISTRATION).

WARNINGS

Clinical Worsening and Suicide Risk

Patients with major depressive disorder (MDD), both adult and pediatric, may experience worsening of their depression and/or the emergence of suicidal ideation and behavior (suicidality) or unusual changes in behavior, whether or not they are taking antidepressant medications, and this risk may persist until significant remission occurs. Suicide is a known risk of depression and certain other psychiatric disorders, and these disorders themselves are the strongest predictors of suicide. There has been a long-standing concern, however, that antidepressants may have a role in inducing worsening of depression and the emergence of suicidality in certain patients during the early phases of treatment. Pooled analyses of short-term placebo-controlled trials of antidepressant drugs (SSRIs and others) showed that these drugs increase the risk of suicidal thinking and behavior (suicidality) in children, adolescents, and young adults (ages 18–24) with major depressive disorder (MDD) and other psychiatric disorders. Short-term studies did not show an increase in the risk of suicidality with antidepressants compared to placebo in adults beyond age 24; there was a reduction in risk with antidepressants compared to placebo in adults aged 65 and older.

The pooled analyses of placebo-controlled trials in children and adolescents with MDD, obsessive compulsive disorder (OCD), or other psychiatric disorders included a total of 24 short-term trials of 9 antidepressant drugs in over 4400 patients. The pooled analyses of placebo-controlled trials in adults with MDD or other psychiatric disorders included a total of 295 short-term trials (median duration of 2 months) of 11 antidepressant drugs in over 77,000 patients. There was considerable variation in risk of suicidality among drugs, but a tendency toward an increase in the younger patients for almost all drugs studied. There were differences in absolute risk of suicidality across different indications, with the highest incidence in MDD. The risk differences (drug vs. placebo), however, were relatively stable within age strata and across indications. These risk differences (drug-placebo difference in the number of cases of suicidality per 1000 patients treated) are provided in Table 1.

Table 1

Age Range	Drug-Placebo Difference in Number of Cases of Suicidality per 1000 Patients Treated
Increases Compared to Placebo	
<18	14 additional cases
18–24	5 additional cases
Decreases Compared to Placebo	
25–64	1 fewer case
≥65	6 fewer cases

No suicides occurred in any of the pediatric trials. There were suicides in the adult trials, but the number was not sufficient to reach any conclusion about drug effect on suicide.

It is unknown whether the suicidality risk extends to longer-term use, i.e., beyond several months. However, there is substantial evidence from placebo-controlled maintenance trials in adults with depression that the use of antidepressants can delay the recurrence of depression.

All patients being treated with antidepressants for any indication should be monitored appropriately and observed closely for clinical worsening, suicidality, and unusual changes in behavior, especially during the initial few months of a course of drug therapy, or at times of dose changes, either increases or decreases.

The following symptoms, anxiety, agitation, panic attacks, insomnia, irritability, hostility, aggressiveness, impulsivity, akathisia (psychomotor restlessness), hypomania, and mania, have been reported in adult and pediatric patients being treated with antidepressants for major depressive disorder as well as for other indications, both psychiatric and nonpsychiatric. Although a causal link between the emergence of such symptoms and either the worsening of depression and/or the emergence of suicidal impulses has not been established, there is concern that such symptoms may represent precursors to emerging suicidality.

Consideration should be given to changing the therapeutic regimen, including possibly discontinuing the medication, in patients whose depression is persistently worse, or who are experiencing emergent suicidality or symptoms that might be precursors to worsening depression or suicidality, especially if these symptoms are severe, abrupt in onset, or were not part of the patient's presenting symptoms.

Families and caregivers of patients being treated with antidepressants for major depressive disorder or other indications, both psychiatric and nonpsychiatric, should be alerted about the need to monitor patients for the emergence of agitation, irritability, unusual changes in behavior, and the other symptoms described above, as well as the emergence of suicidality, and to report such symptoms immediately to health care providers. Such monitoring should include daily observation by families and caregivers. Prescriptions for REMERON (mirtazapine) Tablets should be written for the smallest quantity of tablets consistent with good patient management, in order to reduce the risk of overdose.

Screening Patients for Bipolar Disorder

A major depressive episode may be the initial presentation of bipolar disorder. It is generally believed (though not established in controlled trials) that treating such an episode with an antidepressant alone may increase the likelihood of precipitation of a mixed/manic episode in patients at risk for bipolar disorder. Whether any of the symptoms described above represent such a conversion is unknown. However, prior to initiating treatment with an antidepressant, patients with depressive symptoms should be adequately screened to determine if they are at risk for bipolar disorder; such screening should include a detailed psychiatric history, including a family history of suicide, bipolar disorder, and depression. It should be noted that REMERON (mirtazapine) Tablets are not approved for use in treating bipolar depression.

Agranulocytosis

In premarketing clinical trials, 2 (1 with Sjögren's Syndrome) out of 2796 patients treated with REMERON (mirtazapine) Tablets developed agranulocytosis [absolute neutrophil count (ANC) <500/mm^3 with associated signs and symptoms, e.g., fever, infection, etc.] and a third patient developed severe neutropenia (ANC <500/mm^3 without any associated symptoms). For these 3 patients, onset of severe neutropenia was detected on days 61, 9, and 14 of treatment, respectively. All 3 patients recovered after REMERON was stopped. These 3 cases yield a crude incidence of severe neutropenia (with or without associated infection) of approximately 1.1 per thousand patients exposed, with a very wide 95% confidence interval, i.e., 2.2 cases per 10,000 to 3.1 cases per 1000. If a patient develops a sore throat, fever, stomatitis, or other signs of infection, along with a low WBC count, treatment with REMERON should be discontinued and the patient should be closely monitored.

Serotonin Syndrome

The development of a potentially life-threatening serotonin syndrome has been reported with SNRIs and SSRIs, including REMERON, alone but particularly with concomitant use of other serotonergic drugs (including triptans, tricyclic antidepressants, fentanyl, lithium, tramadol, tryptophan, buspirone, and St. John's wort), and with drugs that impair metabolism of serotonin (in particular, MAOIs, both those intended to treat psychiatric disorders and also others, such as linezolid and intravenous methylene blue).

Serotonin syndrome symptoms may include mental status changes (e.g., agitation, hallucinations, delirium, and coma), autonomic instability (e.g., tachycardia, labile blood pressure, dizziness, diaphoresis, flushing, hyperthermia), neuromuscular symptoms (e.g., tremor, rigidity, myoclonus, hyperreflexia, incoordination), seizures, and/or gastrointestinal symptoms (e.g., nausea, vomiting, diarrhea). Patients should be monitored for the emergence of serotonin syndrome.

The concomitant use of REMERON with MAOIs intended to treat psychiatric disorders is contraindicated. REMERON should also not be started in a patient who is being treated with MAOIs such as linezolid or intravenous methylene blue. All reports with methylene blue that provided information on the route of administration involved intravenous administration in the dose range of 1 mg/kg to 8 mg/kg. No reports involved the administration of methylene blue by other routes (such as oral tablets or local tissue injection) or at lower doses. There may be circumstances when it is necessary to initiate treatment with an MAOI such as linezolid or intravenous methylene blue in a patient taking REMERON. REMERON should be discontinued before initiating treatment with the MAOI (see CONTRAINDICATIONS and DOSAGE AND ADMINISTRATION).

If concomitant use of REMERON with other serotonergic drugs, including triptans, tricyclic antidepressants, fentanyl, lithium, tramadol, buspirone, tryptophan, and St. John's wort, is clinically warranted, be aware of a potential increased risk for serotonin syndrome, particularly during treatment initiation and dose increases.

Treatment with REMERON and any concomitant serotonergic agents should be discontinued immediately if the above events occur and supportive symptomatic treatment should be initiated.

Angle-Closure Glaucoma

The pupillary dilation that occurs following use of many antidepressant drugs including REMERON may trigger an angle-closure attack in a patient with anatomically narrow angles who does not have a patent iridectomy.

PRECAUTIONS
General
Discontinuation Symptoms

There have been reports of adverse reactions upon the discontinuation of REMERON (mirtazapine) Tablets (particularly when abrupt), including but not limited to the following: dizziness, abnormal dreams, sensory disturbances (including paresthesia and electric shock sensations), agitation, anxiety, fatigue, confusion, headache, tremor, nausea, vomiting, and sweating, or other symptoms which may be of clinical significance. The majority of the reported cases are mild and self-limiting. Even though these have been reported as adverse reactions, it should be realized that these symptoms may be related to underlying disease.

Patients currently taking REMERON should NOT discontinue treatment abruptly, due to risk of discontinuation symptoms. At the time that a medical decision is made to discontinue treatment with REMERON, a gradual reduction in the dose, rather than an abrupt cessation, is recommended.

Akathisia/Psychomotor Restlessness

The use of antidepressants has been associated with the development of akathisia, characterized by a subjectively unpleasant or distressing restlessness and need to move, often accompanied by an inability to sit or stand still. This is most likely to occur within the first few weeks of treatment. In patients who develop these symptoms, increasing the dose may be detrimental.

Hyponatremia

Hyponatremia has been reported very rarely with the use of mirtazapine. Caution should be exercised in patients at risk, such as elderly patients or patients concomitantly treated with medications known to cause hyponatremia.

Somnolence

In US controlled studies, somnolence was reported in 54% of patients treated with REMERON (mirtazapine) Tablets, compared to 18% for placebo and 60% for amitriptyline. In these studies, somnolence resulted in discontinuation for 10.4% of REMERON-treated patients, compared to 2.2% for placebo. It is unclear whether or not tolerance develops to the somnolent effects of REMERON. Because of the potentially significant effects of REMERON on impairment of performance, patients should be cautioned about engaging in activities requiring alertness until they have been able to assess the drug's effect on their own psychomotor performance (see PRECAUTIONS: Information for Patients).

Dizziness

In US controlled studies, dizziness was reported in 7% of patients treated with REMERON, compared to 3% for placebo and 14% for amitriptyline. It is unclear whether or not tolerance develops to the dizziness observed in association with the use of REMERON.

Increased Appetite/Weight Gain

In US controlled studies, appetite increase was reported in 17% of patients treated with REMERON, compared to 2% for placebo and 6% for amitriptyline. In these same trials, weight gain of ≥7% of body weight was reported in 7.5% of patients treated with mirtazapine, compared to 0% for placebo and 5.9% for amitriptyline. In a pool of premarketing US studies, including many patients for long-term, open-label treatment, 8% of patients receiving REMERON discontinued for weight gain. In an 8-week-long pediatric clinical trial of doses between 15 to 45 mg/day, 49% of REMERON-treated patients had a weight gain of at least 7%, compared to 5.7% of placebo-treated patients (see PRECAUTIONS: Pediatric Use).

Cholesterol/Triglycerides

In US controlled studies, nonfasting cholesterol increases to ≥20% above the upper limits of normal were observed in 15% of patients treated with REMERON, compared to 7% for placebo and 8% for amitriptyline. In these same studies, nonfasting triglyceride increases to ≥500 mg/dL were observed in 6% of patients treated with mirtazapine, compared to 3% for placebo and 3% for amitriptyline.

Transaminase Elevations

Clinically significant ALT (SGPT) elevations (≥3 times the upper limit of the normal range) were observed in 2.0% (8/424) of patients exposed to REMERON in a pool of short-term US controlled trials, compared to 0.3% (1/328) of placebo patients and 2.0% (3/181) of amitriptyline patients. Most of these patients with ALT increases did not develop signs or symptoms associated with compromised liver function. While some patients were discontinued for the ALT increases, in other cases, the enzyme levels returned to normal despite continued REMERON treatment. REMERON should be used with caution in patients with impaired hepatic function (see CLINICAL PHARMACOLOGY and DOSAGE AND ADMINISTRATION).

Activation of Mania/Hypomania

Mania/hypomania occurred in approximately 0.2% (3/1299 patients) of REMERON-treated patients in US studies. Although the incidence of mania/hypomania was very low during treatment with mirtazapine, it should be used carefully in patients with a history of mania/hypomania.

Seizure

In premarketing clinical trials, only 1 seizure was reported among the 2796 US and non-US patients treated with REMERON. However, no controlled studies have been carried out in patients with a history of seizures. Therefore, care should be exercised when mirtazapine is used in these patients.

Use in Patients with Concomitant Illness

Clinical experience with REMERON in patients with concomitant systemic illness is limited. Accordingly, care is advisable in prescribing mirtazapine for patients with diseases or conditions that affect metabolism or hemodynamic responses.

REMERON has not been systematically evaluated or used to any appreciable extent in patients with a recent history of myocardial infarction or other significant heart disease. REMERON was associated with significant orthostatic hypotension in early clinical pharmacology trials with normal volunteers. Orthostatic hypotension was infrequently observed in clinical trials with depressed patients. REMERON should be used with caution in patients with known cardiovascular or cerebrovascular disease that could be exacerbated by hypotension (history of myocardial infarction, angina, or ischemic stroke) and conditions that would predispose patients to hypotension (dehydration, hypovolemia, and treatment with antihypertensive medication).

Mirtazapine clearance is decreased in patients with moderate [glomerular filtration rate (GFR)=11–39 mL/min/1.73 m^2] and severe [GFR <10 mL/min/1.73 m^2] renal impairment, and also in patients with hepatic impairment. Caution is indicated in administering REMERON to such patients (see CLINICAL PHARMACOLOGY and DOSAGE AND ADMINISTRATION).

Information for Patients

Prescribers or other health professionals should inform patients, their families, and their caregivers about the benefits and risks associated with treatment with REMERON (mirtazapine) Tablets and should counsel them in its appropriate use. A patient Medication Guide about "Antidepressant Medicines, Depression and other Serious Mental Illnesses, and Suicidal Thoughts or Actions" is available for REMERON. The prescriber or health professional should instruct patients, their families, and their caregivers to read the Medication Guide and should assist them in understanding its contents. Patients should be given the opportunity to discuss the contents of the Medication Guide and to obtain answers to any questions they may have. The complete text of the Medication Guide is reprinted at the end of this document.

Patients should be advised of the following issues and asked to alert their prescriber if these occur while taking REMERON.

Clinical Worsening and Suicide Risk

Patients, their families, and their caregivers should be encouraged to be alert to the emergence of anxiety, agitation, panic attacks, insomnia, irritability, hostility, aggressiveness, impulsivity, akathisia (psychomotor restlessness), hypomania, mania, other unusual changes in behavior, worsening of depression, and suicidal ideation, especially early during antidepressant treatment and when the dose is adjusted up or down. Families and caregivers of patients should be advised to look for the emergence of such symptoms on a day-to-day basis, since changes may be abrupt. Such symptoms should be reported to the patient's prescriber or health professional, especially if they are severe, abrupt in onset, or were not part of the patient's presenting symptoms. Symptoms such as these may be associated with an increased risk for suicidal thinking and behavior and indicate a need for very close monitoring and possibly changes in the medication.

Agranulocytosis

Patients who are to receive REMERON should be warned about the risk of developing agranulocytosis. Patients should be advised to contact their physician if they experience any indication of infection such as fever, chills, sore throat, mucous membrane ulceration, or other possible signs of infection. Particular attention should be paid to any flu-like complaints or other symptoms that might suggest infection.

Interference with Cognitive and Motor Performance

REMERON may impair judgment, thinking, and particularly, motor skills, because of its prominent sedative effect. The drowsiness associated with mirtazapine use may impair a patient's ability to drive, use machines, or perform tasks that require alertness. Thus, patients should be cautioned about engaging in hazardous activities until they are reasonably certain that REMERON therapy does not adversely affect their ability to engage in such activities.

Completing Course of Therapy

While patients may notice improvement with REMERON therapy in 1 to 4 weeks, they should be advised to continue therapy as directed.

Concomitant Medication

Patients should be advised to inform their physician if they are taking, or intend to take, any prescription or over-the-counter drugs, since there is a potential for REMERON to interact with other drugs.

Patients should be made aware of a potential increased risk for serotonin syndrome if concomitant use of REMERON with other serotonergic drugs, including triptans, tricyclic antidepressants, fentanyl, lithium, tramadol, buspirone, tryptophan, and St. John's wort, is clinically warranted, particularly during treatment initiation and dose increases.

Alcohol

The impairment of cognitive and motor skills produced by REMERON has been shown to be additive with those produced by alcohol. Accordingly, patients should be advised to avoid alcohol while taking mirtazapine.

Pregnancy

Patients should be advised to notify their physician if they become pregnant or intend to become pregnant during REMERON therapy.

Nursing

Patients should be advised to notify their physician if they are breastfeeding an infant.

Laboratory Tests

There are no routine laboratory tests recommended.

Drug Interactions

As with other drugs, the potential for interaction by a variety of mechanisms (e.g., pharmacodynamic, pharmacokinetic inhibition or enhancement, etc.) is a possibility (see CLINICAL PHARMACOLOGY).

Monoamine Oxidase Inhibitors
(See CONTRAINDICATIONS, WARNINGS, and DOSAGE AND ADMINISTRATION.)

Serotonergic Drugs
(See CONTRAINDICATIONS and WARNINGS.)

Drugs Affecting Hepatic Metabolism
The metabolism and pharmacokinetics of REMERON (mirtazapine) may be affected by the induction or inhibition of drug-metabolizing enzymes.

Drugs that are Metabolized by and/or Inhibit Cytochrome P450 Enzymes

CYP Enzyme Inducers
(these studies used both drugs at steady state)

Phenytoin

In healthy male patients (n=18), phenytoin (200 mg daily) increased mirtazapine (30 mg daily) clearance about 2-fold, resulting in a decrease in average plasma mirtazapine concentrations of 45%. Mirtazapine did not significantly affect the pharmacokinetics of phenytoin.

Carbamazepine

In healthy male patients (n=24), carbamazepine (400 mg b.i.d.) increased mirtazapine (15 mg b.i.d.) clearance about 2-fold, resulting in a decrease in average plasma mirtazapine concentrations of 60%.

When phenytoin, carbamazepine, or another inducer of hepatic metabolism (such as rifampicin) is added to mirtazapine therapy, the mirtazapine dose may have to be increased. If treatment with such a medicinal product is discontinued, it may be necessary to reduce the mirtazapine dose.

CYP Enzyme Inhibitors

Cimetidine

In healthy male patients (n=12), when cimetidine, a weak inhibitor of CYP1A2, CYP2D6, and CYP3A4, given at 800 mg b.i.d. at steady state was coadministered with mirtazapine (30 mg daily) at steady state, the Area Under the Curve (AUC) of mirtazapine increased more than 50%. Mirtazapine did not cause relevant changes in the pharmacokinetics of cimetidine. The mirtazapine dose may have to be decreased when concomitant treatment with cimetidine is started, or increased when cimetidine treatment is discontinued.

Ketoconazole

In healthy, male, Caucasian patients (n=24), coadministration of the potent CYP3A4 inhibitor ketoconazole (200 mg b.i.d. for 6.5 days) increased the peak plasma levels and the AUC of a single 30-mg dose of mirtazapine by approximately 40% and 50%, respectively.

Caution should be exercised when coadministering mirtazapine with potent CYP3A4 inhibitors, HIV protease inhibitors, azole antifungals, erythromycin, or nefazodone.

Paroxetine

In an *in vivo* interaction study in healthy, CYP2D6 extensive metabolizer patients (n=24), mirtazapine (30 mg/day), at steady state, did not cause relevant changes in the pharmacokinetics of steady state paroxetine (40 mg/day), a CYP2D6 inhibitor.

Other Drug-Drug Interactions

Amitriptyline

In healthy, CYP2D6 extensive metabolizer patients (n=32), amitriptyline (75 mg daily), at steady state, did not cause relevant changes in the pharmacokinetics of steady state mirtazapine (30 mg daily); mirtazapine also did not cause relevant changes to the pharmacokinetics of amitriptyline.

Warfarin

In healthy male subjects (n=16), mirtazapine (30 mg daily), at steady state, caused a small (0.2) but statistically significant increase in the International Normalized Ratio (INR) in subjects treated with warfarin. As at a higher dose of

mirtazapine, a more pronounced effect can not be excluded, it is advisable to monitor the INR in case of concomitant treatment of warfarin with mirtazapine.

Lithium

No relevant clinical effects or significant changes in pharmacokinetics have been observed in healthy male subjects on concurrent treatment with subtherapeutic levels of lithium (600 mg/day for 10 days) at steady state and a single 30-mg dose of mirtazapine. The effects of higher doses of lithium on the pharmacokinetics of mirtazapine are unknown.

Risperidone

In an *in vivo*, nonrandomized, interaction study, subjects (n=6) in need of treatment with an antipsychotic and antidepressant drug, showed that mirtazapine (30 mg daily) at steady state did not influence the pharmacokinetics of risperidone (up to 3 mg b.i.d.).

Alcohol

Concomitant administration of alcohol (equivalent to 60 g) had a minimal effect on plasma levels of mirtazapine (15 mg) in 6 healthy male subjects. However, the impairment of cognitive and motor skills produced by REMERON were shown to be additive with those produced by alcohol. Accordingly, patients should be advised to avoid alcohol while taking REMERON.

Diazepam

Concomitant administration of diazepam (15 mg) had a minimal effect on plasma levels of mirtazapine (15 mg) in 12 healthy subjects. However, the impairment of motor skills produced by REMERON has been shown to be additive with those caused by diazepam. Accordingly, patients should be advised to avoid diazepam and other similar drugs while taking REMERON.

Carcinogenesis, Mutagenesis, Impairment of Fertility

Carcinogenesis

Carcinogenicity studies were conducted with mirtazapine given in the diet at doses of 2, 20, and 200 mg/kg/day to mice and 2, 20, and 60 mg/kg/day to rats. The highest doses used are approximately 20 and 12 times the maximum recommended human dose (MRHD) of 45 mg/day on an mg/m^2 basis in mice and rats, respectively. There was an increased incidence of hepatocellular adenoma and carcinoma in male mice at the high dose. In rats, there was an increase in hepatocellular adenoma in females at the mid and high doses and in hepatocellular tumors and thyroid follicular adenoma/cystadenoma and carcinoma in males at the high dose. The data suggest that the above effects could possibly be mediated by non-genotoxic mechanisms, the relevance of which to humans is not known.

The doses used in the mouse study may not have been high enough to fully characterize the carcinogenic potential of REMERON (mirtazapine) Tablets.

Mutagenesis

Mirtazapine was not mutagenic or clastogenic and did not induce general DNA damage as determined in several genotoxicity tests: Ames test, *in vitro* gene mutation assay in Chinese hamster V 79 cells, *in vitro* sister chromatid exchange assay in cultured rabbit lymphocytes, *in vivo* bone marrow micronucleus test in rats, and unscheduled DNA synthesis assay in HeLa cells.

Impairment of Fertility

In a fertility study in rats, mirtazapine was given at doses up to 100 mg/kg [20 times the maximum recommended human dose (MRHD) on an mg/m^2 basis]. Mating and conception were not affected by the drug, but estrous cycling was disrupted at doses that were 3 or more times the MRHD, and pre-implantation losses occurred at 20 times the MRHD.

Pregnancy

Teratogenic Effects

Pregnancy Category C

Reproduction studies in pregnant rats and rabbits at doses up to 100 mg/kg and 40 mg/kg, respectively [20 and 17 times the maximum recommended human dose (MRHD) on an mg/m^2 basis, respectively], have revealed no evidence of teratogenic effects. However, in rats, there was an increase in postimplantation losses in dams treated with mirtazapine. There was an increase in pup deaths during the first 3 days of lactation and a decrease in pup birth weights. The cause of these deaths is not known. The effects occurred at doses that were 20 times the MRHD, but not at 3 times the MRHD, on an mg/m^2 basis. There are no adequate and well-controlled studies in pregnant women. Because animal reproduction studies are not always predictive of human response, this drug should be used during pregnancy only if clearly needed.

Nursing Mothers

Because some REMERON may be excreted into breast milk, caution should be exercised when REMERON (mirtazapine) Tablets are administered to nursing women.

Pediatric Use

Safety and effectiveness in the pediatric population have not been established (see BOXED WARNING and WARNINGS: Clinical Worsening and Suicide Risk). Two placebo-

controlled trials in 258 pediatric patients with MDD have been conducted with REMERON (mirtazapine) Tablets, and the data were not sufficient to support a claim for use in pediatric patients. Anyone considering the use of REMERON in a child or adolescent must balance the potential risks with the clinical need.

In an 8-week-long pediatric clinical trial of doses between 15 to 45 mg/day, 49% of REMERON-treated patients had a weight gain of at least 7%, compared to 5.7% of placebo-treated patients. The mean increase in weight was 4 kg (2 kg SD) for REMERON-treated patients versus 1 kg (2 kg SD) for placebo-treated patients (see PRECAUTIONS: Increased Appetite/Weight Gain).

Geriatric Use

Approximately 190 elderly individuals (≥65 years of age) participated in clinical studies with REMERON (mirtazapine) Tablets. This drug is known to be substantially excreted by the kidney (75%), and the risk of decreased clearance of this drug is greater in patients with impaired renal function. Because elderly patients are more likely to have decreased renal function, care should be taken in dose selection. Sedating drugs may cause confusion and over-sedation in the elderly. No unusual adverse age-related phenomena were identified in this group. Pharmacokinetic studies revealed a decreased clearance in the elderly. Caution is indicated in administering REMERON to elderly patients (see CLINICAL PHARMACOLOGY and DOSAGE AND ADMINISTRATION).

ADVERSE REACTIONS

Associated with Discontinuation of Treatment

Approximately 16% of the 453 patients who received REMERON (mirtazapine) Tablets in US 6-week controlled clinical trials discontinued treatment due to an adverse experience, compared to 7% of the 361 placebo-treated patients in those studies. The most common events (≥1%) associated with discontinuation and considered to be drug related (i.e., those events associated with dropout at a rate at least twice that of placebo) are included in Table 2.

Table 2: Common Adverse Events Associated With Discontinuation of Treatment in 6-Week US REMERON Trials

Adverse Event	Percentage of Patients Discontinuing With Adverse Event	
	REMERON (n=453)	Placebo (n=361)
Somnolence	10.4%	2.2%
Nausea	1.5%	0%

Commonly Observed Adverse Events in US Controlled Clinical Trials

The most commonly observed adverse events associated with the use of REMERON (mirtazapine) Tablets (incidence of 5% or greater) and not observed at an equivalent incidence among placebo-treated patients (REMERON incidence at least twice that for placebo) are listed in Table 3.

Table 3: Common Treatment-Emergent Adverse Events Associated With the Use of REMERON in 6-Week US Trials

Adverse Event	Percentage of Patients Reporting Adverse Event	
	REMERON (n=453)	Placebo (n=361)
Somnolence	54%	18%
Increased Appetite	17%	2%
Weight Gain	12%	2%
Dizziness	7%	3%

Adverse Events Occurring at an Incidence of 1% or More Among REMERON-Treated Patients

Table 4 enumerates adverse events that occurred at an incidence of 1% or more, and were more frequent than in the placebo group, among REMERON (mirtazapine) Tablets-treated patients who participated in short-term US placebo-controlled trials in which patients were dosed in a range of 5 to 60 mg/day. This table shows the percentage of patients in each group who had at least 1 episode of an event at some time during their treatment. Reported adverse events were classified using a standard COSTART-based dictionary terminology.

The prescriber should be aware that these figures cannot be used to predict the incidence of side effects in the course of usual medical practice where patient characteristics and other factors differ from those which prevailed in the clinical trials. Similarly, the cited frequencies cannot be compared with figures obtained from other investigations involving different treatments, uses, and investigators. The cited figures, however, do provide the prescribing physician with some basis for estimating the relative contribution of drug and nondrug factors to the side-effect incidence rate in the population studied.

Table 4: Incidence of Adverse Clinical Experiences* (≥1%) in Short-Term US Controlled Studies

Body System Adverse Clinical Experience	REMERON (n=453)	Placebo (n=361)
Body as a Whole		
Asthenia	8%	5%
Flu Syndrome	5%	3%
Back Pain	2%	1%
Digestive System		
Dry Mouth	25%	15%
Increased Appetite	17%	2%
Constipation	13%	7%
Metabolic and Nutritional Disorders		
Weight Gain	12%	2%
Peripheral Edema	2%	1%
Edema	1%	0%
Musculoskeletal System		
Myalgia	2%	1%
Nervous System		
Somnolence	54%	18%
Dizziness	7%	3%
Abnormal Dreams	4%	1%
Thinking Abnormal	3%	1%
Tremor	2%	1%
Confusion	2%	0%
Respiratory System		
Dyspnea	1%	0%
Urogenital System		
Urinary Frequency	2%	1%

* Events reported by at least 1% of patients treated with REMERON are included, except the following events, which had an incidence on placebo greater than or equal to REMERON: headache, infection, pain, chest pain, palpitation, tachycardia, postural hypotension, nausea, dyspepsia, diarrhea, flatulence, insomnia, nervousness, libido decreased, hypertonia, pharyngitis, rhinitis, sweating, amblyopia, tinnitus, taste perversion.

ECG Changes
The electrocardiograms for 338 patients who received REMERON (mirtazapine) Tablets and 261 patients who received placebo in 6-week, placebo-controlled trials were analyzed. Prolongation in QTc ≥500 msec was not observed among mirtazapine-treated patients; mean change in QTc was +1.6 msec for mirtazapine and −3.1 msec for placebo. Mirtazapine was associated with a mean increase in heart rate of 3.4 bpm, compared to 0.8 bpm for placebo. The clinical significance of these changes is unknown.

Other Adverse Events Observed During the Premarketing Evaluation of REMERON
During its premarketing assessment, multiple doses of REMERON (mirtazapine) Tablets were administered to 2796 patients in clinical studies. The conditions and duration of exposure to mirtazapine varied greatly, and included (in overlapping categories) open and double-blind studies, uncontrolled and controlled studies, inpatient and outpatient studies, fixed-dose and titration studies. Untoward events associated with this exposure were recorded by clinical investigators using terminology of their own choosing. Consequently, it is not possible to provide a meaningful es-

timate of the proportion of individuals experiencing adverse events without first grouping similar types of untoward events into a smaller number of untoward event categories.

In the tabulations that follow, reported adverse events were classified using a standard COSTART-based dictionary terminology. The frequencies presented, therefore, represent the proportion of the 2796 patients exposed to multiple doses of REMERON who experienced an event of the type cited on at least 1 occasion while receiving REMERON. All reported events are included except those already listed in Table 4, those adverse experiences subsumed under COSTART terms that are either overly general or excessively specific so as to be uninformative, and those events for which a drug cause was very remote.

It is important to emphasize that, although the events reported occurred during treatment with REMERON, they were not necessarily caused by it.

Events are further categorized by body system and listed in order of decreasing frequency according to the following definitions: frequent adverse events are those occurring on 1 or more occasions in at least 1/100 patients; infrequent adverse events are those occurring in 1/100 to 1/1000 patients; rare events are those occurring in fewer than 1/1000 patients. Only those events not already listed in Table 4 appear in this listing. Events of major clinical importance are also described in the WARNINGS and PRECAUTIONS sections.

Body as a Whole: *frequent:* malaise, abdominal pain, abdominal syndrome acute; *infrequent:* chills, fever, face edema, ulcer, photosensitivity reaction, neck rigidity, neck pain, abdomen enlarged; *rare:* cellulitis, chest pain substernal.

Cardiovascular System: *frequent:* hypertension, vasodilatation; *infrequent:* angina pectoris, myocardial infarction, bradycardia, ventricular extrasystoles, syncope, migraine, hypotension; *rare:* atrial arrhythmia, bigeminy, vascular headache, pulmonary embolus, cerebral ischemia, cardiomegaly, phlebitis, left heart failure.

Digestive System: *frequent:* vomiting, anorexia; *infrequent:* eructation, glossitis, cholecystitis, nausea and vomiting, gum hemorrhage, stomatitis, colitis, liver function tests abnormal; *rare:* tongue discoloration, ulcerative stomatitis, salivary gland enlargement, increased salivation, intestinal obstruction, pancreatitis, aphthous stomatitis, cirrhosis of liver, gastritis, gastroenteritis, oral moniliasis, tongue edema.

Endocrine System: *rare:* goiter, hypothyroidism.

Hemic and Lymphatic System: *rare:* lymphadenopathy, leukopenia, petechia, anemia, thrombocytopenia, lymphocytosis, pancytopenia.

Metabolic and Nutritional Disorders: *frequent:* thirst; *infrequent:* dehydration, weight loss; *rare:* gout, SGOT increased, healing abnormal, acid phosphatase increased, SGPT increased, diabetes mellitus, hyponatremia.

Musculoskeletal System: *frequent:* myasthenia, arthralgia; *infrequent:* arthritis, tenosynovitis; *rare:* pathologic fracture, osteoporosis fracture, bone pain, myositis, tendon rupture, arthrosis, bursitis.

Nervous System: *frequent:* hypesthesia, apathy, depression, hypokinesia, vertigo, twitching, agitation, anxiety, amnesia, hyperkinesia, paresthesia; *infrequent:* ataxia, delirium, delusions, depersonalization, dyskinesia, extrapyramidal syndrome, libido increased, coordination abnormal, dysarthria, hallucinations, manic reaction, neurosis, dystonia, hostility, reflexes increased, emotional lability, euphoria, paranoid reaction; *rare:* aphasia, nystagmus, akathisia (psychomotor restlessness), stupor, dementia, diplopia, drug dependence, paralysis, grand mal convulsion, hypotonia, myoclonus, psychotic depression, withdrawal syndrome, serotonin syndrome.

Respiratory System: *frequent:* cough increased, sinusitis; *infrequent:* epistaxis, bronchitis, asthma, pneumonia; *rare:* asphyxia, laryngitis, pneumothorax, hiccup.

Skin and Appendages: *frequent:* pruritus, rash; *infrequent:* acne, exfoliative dermatitis, dry skin, herpes simplex, alopecia; *rare:* urticaria, herpes zoster, skin hypertrophy, seborrhea, skin ulcer.

Special Senses: *infrequent:* eye pain, abnormality of accommodation, conjunctivitis, deafness, keratoconjunctivitis, lacrimation disorder, angle-closure glaucoma, hyperacusis, ear pain; *rare:* blepharitis, partial transitory deafness, otitis media, taste loss, parosmia.

Urogenital System: *frequent:* urinary tract infection; *infrequent:* kidney calculus, cystitis, dysuria, urinary incontinence, urinary retention, vaginitis, hematuria, breast pain, amenorrhea, dysmenorrhea, leukorrhea, impotence; *rare:* polyuria, urethritis, metrorrhagia, menorrhagia, abnormal ejaculation, breast engorgement, breast enlargement, urinary urgency.

Other Adverse Events Observed During Postmarketing Evaluation of REMERON
Adverse events reported since market introduction, which were temporally (but not necessarily causally) related to

mirtazapine therapy, include 4 cases of the ventricular arrhythmia torsades de pointes. In 3 of the 4 cases, however, concomitant drugs were implicated. All patients recovered. Cases of severe skin reactions, including Stevens-Johnson syndrome, bullous dermatitis, erythema multiforme and toxic epidermal necrolysis have also been reported.

DRUG ABUSE AND DEPENDENCE
Controlled Substance Class
REMERON (mirtazapine) Tablets are not a controlled substance.

Physical and Psychologic Dependence
REMERON (mirtazapine) Tablets have not been systematically studied in animals or humans for its potential for abuse, tolerance, or physical dependence. While the clinical trials did not reveal any tendency for any drug-seeking behavior, these observations were not systematic and it is not possible to predict on the basis of this limited experience the extent to which a CNS-active drug will be misused, diverted and/or abused once marketed. Consequently, patients should be evaluated carefully for history of drug abuse, and such patients should be observed closely for signs of REMERON misuse or abuse (e.g., development of tolerance, incrementations of dose, drug-seeking behavior).

OVERDOSAGE
Human Experience
There is very limited experience with REMERON (mirtazapine) Tablets overdose. In premarketing clinical studies, there were 8 reports of REMERON overdose alone or in combination with other pharmacological agents. The only drug overdose death reported while taking REMERON was in combination with amitriptyline and chlorprothixene in a non-US clinical study. Based on plasma levels, the REMERON dose taken was 30 to 45 mg, while plasma levels of amitriptyline and chlorprothixene were found to be at toxic levels. All other premarketing overdose cases resulted in full recovery. Signs and symptoms reported in association with overdose included disorientation, drowsiness, impaired memory, and tachycardia. There were no reports of ECG abnormalities, coma, or convulsions following overdose with REMERON alone.

Overdose Management
Treatment should consist of those general measures employed in the management of overdose with any drug effective in the treatment of major depressive disorder. Ensure an adequate airway, oxygenation, and ventilation. Monitor cardiac rhythm and vital signs. General supportive and symptomatic measures are also recommended. Induction of emesis is not recommended. Gastric lavage with a large-bore orogastric tube with appropriate airway protection, if needed, may be indicated if performed soon after ingestion, or in symptomatic patients. Activated charcoal should be administered. There is no experience with the use of forced diuresis, dialysis, hemoperfusion, or exchange transfusion in the treatment of mirtazapine overdosage. No specific antidotes for mirtazapine are known.

In managing overdosage, consider the possibility of multiple-drug involvement. The physician should consider contacting a poison control center for additional information on the treatment of any overdose. Telephone numbers for certified poison control centers are listed in the *Physicians' Desk Reference* (PDR).

DOSAGE AND ADMINISTRATION
Initial Treatment
The recommended starting dose for REMERON (mirtazapine) Tablets is 15 mg/day, administered in a single dose, preferably in the evening prior to sleep. In the controlled clinical trials establishing the efficacy of REMERON in the treatment of major depressive disorder, the effective dose range was generally 15 to 45 mg/day. While the relationship between dose and satisfactory response in the treatment of major depressive disorder for REMERON has not been adequately explored, patients not responding to the initial 15-mg dose may benefit from dose increases up to a maximum of 45 mg/day. REMERON has an elimination half-life of approximately 20 to 40 hours; therefore, dose changes should not be made at intervals of less than 1 to 2 weeks in order to allow sufficient time for evaluation of the therapeutic response to a given dose.

Elderly and Patients with Renal or Hepatic Impairment
The clearance of mirtazapine is reduced in elderly patients and in patients with moderate to severe renal or hepatic impairment. Consequently, the prescriber should be aware that plasma mirtazapine levels may be increased in these patient groups, compared to levels observed in younger adults without renal or hepatic impairment (see PRECAUTIONS and CLINICAL PHARMACOLOGY).

Maintenance/Extended Treatment
It is generally agreed that acute episodes of depression require several months or longer of sustained pharmacological therapy beyond response to the acute episode. Systematic evaluation of REMERON (mirtazapine) Tablets has demonstrated that its efficacy in major depressive disorder

is maintained for periods of up to 40 weeks following 8 to 12 weeks of initial treatment at a dose of 15 to 45 mg/day (see CLINICAL PHARMACOLOGY). Based on these limited data, it is unknown whether or not the dose of REMERON needed for maintenance treatment is identical to the dose needed to achieve an initial response. Patients should be periodically reassessed to determine the need for maintenance treatment and the appropriate dose for such treatment.

Switching a Patient To or From a Monoamine Oxidase Inhibitor (MAOI) Intended to Treat Psychiatric Disorders

At least 14 days should elapse between discontinuation of an MAOI intended to treat psychiatric disorders and initiation of therapy with REMERON (mirtazapine) Tablets. Conversely, at least 14 days should be allowed after stopping REMERON before starting an MAOI intended to treat psychiatric disorders (see CONTRAINDICATIONS).

Use of REMERON With Other MAOIs, Such as Linezolid or Methylene Blue

Do not start REMERON in a patient who is being treated with linezolid or intravenous methylene blue because there is an increased risk of serotonin syndrome. In a patient who requires more urgent treatment of a psychiatric condition, other interventions, including hospitalization, should be considered (see CONTRAINDICATIONS).

In some cases, a patient already receiving therapy with REMERON may require urgent treatment with linezolid or intravenous methylene blue. If acceptable alternatives to linezolid or intravenous methylene blue treatment are not available and the potential benefits of linezolid or intravenous methylene blue treatment are judged to outweigh the risks of serotonin syndrome in a particular patient, REMERON should be stopped promptly, and linezolid or intravenous methylene blue can be administered. The patient should be monitored for symptoms of serotonin syndrome for 2 weeks or until 24 hours after the last dose of linezolid or intravenous methylene blue, whichever comes first. Therapy with REMERON may be resumed 24 hours after the last dose of linezolid or intravenous methylene blue (see WARNINGS).

The risk of administering methylene blue by non-intravenous routes (such as oral tablets or by local injection) or in intravenous doses much lower than 1 mg/kg with REMERON is unclear. The clinician should, nevertheless, be aware of the possibility of emergent symptoms of serotonin syndrome with such use (see WARNINGS).

Discontinuation of Remeron Treatment

Symptoms associated with the discontinuation or dose reduction of REMERON Tablets have been reported. Patients should be monitored for these and other symptoms when discontinuing treatment or during dosage reduction. A gradual reduction in the dose over several weeks, rather than abrupt cessation, is recommended whenever possible. If intolerable symptoms occur following a decrease in the dose or upon discontinuation of treatment, dose titration should be managed on the basis of the patient's clinical response (see PRECAUTIONS and ADVERSE REACTIONS).

Information for Patients

Patients should be advised that taking REMERON can cause mild pupillary dilation, which in susceptible individuals, can lead to an episode of angle-closure glaucoma. Preexisting glaucoma is almost always open-angle glaucoma because angle-closure glaucoma, when diagnosed, can be treated definitively with iridectomy. Open-angle glaucoma is not a risk factor for angle-closure glaucoma. Patients may wish to be examined to determine whether they are susceptible to angle-closure, and have a prophylactic procedure (e.g., iridectomy), if they are susceptible.

HOW SUPPLIED

REMERON (mirtazapine) Tablets are supplied as:

15 mg Tablets — oval, scored, yellow, coated, with "Organon" debossed on 1 side and "T₃Z" on the other side.

Bottles of 30   NDC 0052-0105-30

30 mg Tablets — oval, scored, red-brown, coated, with "Organon" debossed on 1 side and "T₅Z" on the other side.

Bottles of 30   NDC 0052-0107-30

45 mg Tablets — oval, white, coated, with "Organon" debossed on 1 side and "T₇Z" on the other side.

Bottles of 30   NDC 0052-0109-30

Storage

Store at 25°C (77°F); excursions permitted to 15-30°C (59-86°F) [see USP Controlled Room Temperature]. Protect from light and moisture.

Manufactured for: Merck Sharp & Dohme Corp., a subsidiary of

MERCK & CO., INC., Whitehouse Station, NJ 08889, USA

Manufactured by: N.V. Organon, Oss, The Netherlands, a subsidiary of

Merck & Co., Inc., Whitehouse Station, NJ 08889, USA

For patent information:

www.merck.com/product/patent/home.html

Copyright © 1996, 2010 Merck Sharp & Dohme B.V., a subsidiary of **Merck & Co., Inc.**

All rights reserved.

Revised: 08/2014
uspi-mk8246-t-1408r007
Rx only

Medication Guide

REMERON® (rĕm' - ĕ – rŏn)
(mirtazapine)
Tablets

Read the Medication Guide that comes with REMERON before you start taking it and each time you get a refill. There may be new information. This Medication Guide does not take the place of talking to your healthcare provider about your medical condition or treatment. If you have any questions about REMERON, talk to your healthcare provider.

What is the most important information I should know about REMERON®?

REMERON and other antidepressant medicines may cause serious side effects, including:

1. **Suicidal thoughts or actions:**
   - **REMERON and other antidepressant medicines may increase suicidal thoughts or actions in some children, teenagers, or young adults within the first few months of treatment or when the dose is changed.**
   - Depression or other serious mental illnesses are the most important causes of suicidal thoughts or actions.
   - Watch for these changes and call your healthcare provider right away if you notice:
     ○ New or sudden changes in mood, behavior, actions, thoughts, or feelings, especially if severe.
     ○ Pay particular attention to such changes when REMERON is started or when the dose is changed.

Keep all follow-up visits with your healthcare provider and call between visits if you are worried about symptoms.

Call your healthcare provider right away if you have any of the following symptoms, or call 911 if an emergency, especially if they are new, worse, or worry you:

- attempts to commit suicide
- acting on dangerous impulses
- acting aggressive or violent
- thoughts about suicide or dying
- new or worse depression
- new or worse anxiety or panic attacks
- feeling agitated, restless, angry or irritable
- trouble sleeping
- an increase in activity or talking more than what is normal for you
- other unusual changes in behavior or mood

Call your healthcare provider right away if you have any of the following symptoms, or call 911 if an emergency. REMERON may be associated with these serious side effects:

2. **Manic episodes:**
   - greatly increased energy
   - severe trouble sleeping
   - racing thoughts
   - reckless behavior
   - unusually grand ideas
   - excessive happiness or irritability
   - talking more or faster than usual

3. **Decreased White Blood Cells** called neutrophils, which are needed to fight infections. Tell your doctor if you have any indication of infection such as fever, chills, sore throat, or mouth or nose sores, especially symptoms which are flu-like.

4. **Serotonin Syndrome. This condition can be life-threatening and may include:**
   - agitation, hallucinations, coma or other changes in mental status
   - coordination problems or muscle twitching (overactive reflexes)
   - racing heartbeat, high or low blood pressure
   - sweating or fever
   - nausea, vomiting, or diarrhea
   - muscle rigidity

5. **Visual problems**
   - eye pain
   - changes in vision
   - swelling or redness in or around the eye
   Only some people are at risk for these problems. You may want to undergo an eye examination to see if you are at risk and receive preventative treatment if you are.

6. **Seizures**

7. **Low salt (sodium) levels in the blood.** Elderly people may be at greater risk for this. Symptoms may include:
   - headache
   - weakness or feeling unsteady
   - confusion, problems concentrating or thinking or memory problems

8. **Sleepiness.** It is best to take **REMERON** close to bedtime.

9. **Severe skin reactions:** Call your doctor right away if you have any or all of the following symptoms:
   - severe rash with skin swelling (including on the palms of the hands and soles of the feet)
   - painful reddening of the skin and/or blisters/ulcers on the body or in the mouth

---

10. **Severe allergic reactions: trouble breathing, swelling of the face, tongue, eyes or mouth**
    - rash, itchy welts (hives) or blisters, alone or with fever or joint pain

11. **Increases in appetite or weight.** Children and adolescents should have height and weight monitored during treatment.

12. **Increased cholesterol and triglyceride levels in your blood**

Do not stop REMERON without first talking to your healthcare provider. Stopping REMERON too quickly may cause potentially serious symptoms including:
- dizziness
- abnormal dreams
- agitation
- anxiety
- fatigue
- confusion
- headache
- shaking
- tingling sensation
- nausea, vomiting
- sweating

What is REMERON?

REMERON is a prescription medicine used to treat depression. It is important to talk with your healthcare provider about the risks of treating depression and also the risks of not treating it. You should discuss all treatment choices with your healthcare provider.

Talk to your healthcare provider if you do not think that your condition is getting better with REMERON treatment.

Who should not take REMERON?

Do not take REMERON:
- if you are allergic to mirtazapine or any of the ingredients in REMERON. See the end of this Medication Guide for a complete list of ingredients in REMERON.
- if you take a monoamine oxidase inhibitor (MAOI). Ask your healthcare provider or pharmacist if you are not sure if you take an MAOI, including the antibiotic linezolid.
- Do not take an MAOI within 2 weeks of stopping REMERON unless directed to do so by your physician.
- Do not start REMERON if you stopped taking an MAOI in the last 2 weeks unless directed to do so by your physician.

People who take REMERON close in time to an MAOI may have serious or even life-threatening side effects. Get medical help right away if you have any of these symptoms:
- high fever
- uncontrolled muscle spasms
- stiff muscles
- rapid changes in heart rate or blood pressure
- confusion
- loss of consciousness (pass out)

What should I tell my healthcare provider before taking REMERON?

Ask if you are not sure.

Before starting REMERON, tell your healthcare provider if you:
- Are taking certain drugs such as:
  ○ Triptans used to treat migraine headache
  ○ Medicines used to treat mood, anxiety, psychotic or thought disorders, including tricyclics, lithium, SSRIs, SNRIs, or antipsychotics
  ○ Tramadol used to treat pain
  ○ Over-the-counter supplements such as tryptophan or St. John's wort
  ○ Phenytoin, carbamazepine, or rifampicin (these drugs can decrease your blood level of REMERON)
  ○ Cimetidine or ketoconazole (these drugs can increase your blood level of REMERON)
- Have or had:
  ○ liver problems
  ○ kidney problems
  ○ heart problems
  ○ seizures or convulsions
  ○ bipolar disorder or mania
  ○ a tendency to get dizzy or faint
- are pregnant or plan to become pregnant. It is not known if REMERON will harm your unborn baby. Talk to your healthcare provider about the benefits and risks of treating depression during pregnancy
- are breastfeeding or plan to breastfeed. Some REMERON may pass into your breast milk. Talk to your healthcare provider about the best way to feed your baby while taking REMERON

Tell your healthcare provider about all the medicines that you take, including prescription and non-prescription medicines, vitamins, and herbal supplements. REMERON and some medicines may interact with each other, may not work as well, or may cause serious side effects.

Your healthcare provider or pharmacist can tell you if it is safe to take REMERON with your other medicines. Do not start or stop any medicine while taking REMERON without talking to your healthcare provider first.

If you take REMERON, you should not take any other medicines that contain mirtazapine including REMERONSolTab®.

How should I take REMERON?

- Take REMERON exactly as prescribed. Your healthcare provider may need to change the dose of REMERON until it is the right dose for you.
- Take REMERON at the same time each day, preferably in the evening at bedtime.
- Swallow REMERON as directed.
- It is common for antidepressant medicines such as REMERON to take up to a few weeks before you start to feel better. Do not stop taking REMERON if you do not feel results right away.
- Do not stop taking or change the dose of REMERON without first talking to your doctor, even if you feel better.
- REMERON may be taken with or without food.
- If you miss a dose of REMERON, take the missed dose as soon as you remember. If it is almost time for the next dose, skip the missed dose and take your next dose at the regular time. Do not take two doses of REMERON at the same time.
- If you take too much REMERON, call your healthcare provider or poison control center right away, or get emergency treatment.

What should I avoid while taking REMERON?

- REMERON can cause sleepiness or may affect your ability to make decisions, think clearly, or react quickly. You should not drive, operate heavy machinery, or do other dangerous activities until you know how REMERON affects you.
- Avoid drinking alcohol or taking diazepam (a medicine used for anxiety, insomnia and seizures, for example) or similar medicines while taking REMERON. If you are uncertain about whether certain medication can be taken with REMERON, please discuss with your doctor.

What are the possible side effects of REMERON?

REMERON may cause serious side effects, including all of those described in the section entitled "What is the most important information I should know about REMERON?"

Common possible side effects in people who take REMERON include:

- sleepiness
- increased appetite, weight gain
- dry mouth
- constipation
- dizziness
- abnormal dreams

Tell your healthcare provider if you have any side effect that bothers you or that does not go away. These are not all the possible side effects of REMERON. For more information, ask your healthcare provider or pharmacist.

CALL YOUR DOCTOR FOR MEDICAL ADVICE ABOUT SIDE EFFECTS. YOU MAY REPORT SIDE EFFECTS TO THE FDA AT 1-800-FDA-1088.

How should I store REMERON?

- Store REMERON at room temperature 25°C (77°F). Storage at 15°C-30°C (59°F-86°F) is permitted occasionally.
- Keep REMERON away from light.
- Keep REMERON bottle closed tightly.

Keep REMERON and all medicines out of the reach of children.

General information about REMERON

Medicines are sometimes prescribed for purposes other than those listed in a Medication Guide. Do not use REMERON for a condition for which it was not prescribed. Do not give REMERON to other people, even if they have the same condition. It may harm them.

This Medication Guide summarizes the most important information about REMERON. If you would like more information, talk with your healthcare provider. You may ask your healthcare provider or pharmacist for information about REMERON that is written for healthcare professionals.

For more information about REMERON call 1-800-526-4099 or go to www.REMERON.com.

What are the ingredients in REMERON?

Active ingredient: mirtazapine

Inactive ingredients:

- **15 mg tablets:** Starch (corn), hydroxypropyl cellulose, magnesium stearate, colloidal silicon dioxide, lactose, hypromellose, polyethylene glycol 8000, titanium dioxide, ferric oxide (yellow).
- **30 mg tablets:** Starch (corn), hydroxypropyl cellulose, magnesium stearate, colloidal silicon dioxide, lactose, hypromellose, polyethylene glycol 8000, titanium dioxide, ferric oxide (yellow), ferric oxide (red).
- **45 mg tablets:** Starch (corn), hydroxypropyl cellulose, magnesium stearate, colloidal silicon dioxide, lactose, hypromellose, polyethylene glycol 8000, titanium dioxide.

This Medication Guide has been approved by the U.S. Food and Drug Administration.

Manufactured for: Merck Sharp & Dohme Corp., a subsidiary of
MERCK & CO., INC., Whitehouse Station, NJ 08889, USA
Manufactured by: N.V. Organon, Oss, The Netherlands, a subsidiary of
Merck & Co., Inc., Whitehouse Station, NJ 08889, USA
For patent information:
www.merck.com/product/patent/home.html
Copyright © 2007, 2009 Merck Sharp & Dohme B.V., a subsidiary of **Merck & Co., Inc.**
All rights reserved.
Revised: 08/2014
usmg-mk8246-t-1408r007

Shown in Product Identification Guide, page 309

REMERONSolTab®
[rem-er-on]
(mirtazapine)
Orally Disintegrating Tablets
ONCE-A-DAY

℞

Suicidality and Antidepressant Drugs
Antidepressants increased the risk compared to placebo of suicidal thinking and behavior (suicidality) in children, adolescents, and young adults in short-term studies of major depressive disorder (MDD) and other psychiatric disorders. Anyone considering the use of REMERONSolTab® (mirtazapine) Orally Disintegrating Tablets or any other antidepressant in a child, adolescent, or young adult must balance this risk with the clinical need. Short-term studies did not show an increase in the risk of suicidality with antidepressants compared to placebo in adults beyond age 24; there was a reduction in risk with antidepressants compared to placebo in adults aged 65 and older. Depression and certain other psychiatric disorders are themselves associated with increases in the risk of suicide. Patients of all ages who are started on antidepressant therapy should be monitored appropriately and observed closely for clinical worsening, suicidality, or unusual changes in behavior. Families and caregivers should be advised of the need for close observation and communication with the prescriber. REMERONSolTab is not approved for use in pediatric patients. (See WARNINGS: Clinical Worsening and Suicide Risk, PRECAUTIONS: Information for Patients, and PRECAUTIONS: Pediatric Use.)

DESCRIPTION

REMERONSolTab® (mirtazapine) Orally Disintegrating Tablets are an orally administered drug. Mirtazapine has a tetracyclic chemical structure and belongs to the piperazino-azepine group of compounds. It is designated 1,2,3,4,10,14b-hexahydro-2-methylpyrazino [2,1-a] pyrido [2,3-c] benzazepine and has the empirical formula of

$C_{17}H_{19}N_3$. Its molecular weight is 265.36. The structural formula is the following and it is the racemic mixture: Mirtazapine is a white to creamy white crystalline powder which is slightly soluble in water. REMERONSolTab is available for oral administration as an orally disintegrating tablet containing 15, 30, or 45 mg of mirtazapine. It disintegrates in the mouth within seconds after placement on the tongue, allowing its contents to be subsequently swallowed with or without water. REMERONSolTab also contains the following inactive ingredients: aspartame, citric acid, crospovidone, hypromellose, magnesium stearate, mannitol, microcrystalline cellulose, natural and artificial orange flavor, polymethacrylate, povidone, sodium bicarbonate, starch, and sucrose.

CLINICAL PHARMACOLOGY
Pharmacodynamics

The mechanism of action of REMERONSolTab (mirtazapine) Orally Disintegrating Tablets, as with other drugs effective in the treatment of major depressive disorder, is unknown.

Evidence gathered in preclinical studies suggests that mirtazapine enhances central noradrenergic and serotonergic activity. These studies have shown that mirtazapine acts as an antagonist at central presynaptic α_2-adrenergic inhibitory autoreceptors and heteroreceptors, an action that is postulated to result in an increase in central noradrenergic and serotonergic activity.

Mirtazapine is a potent antagonist of 5-HT$_2$ and 5-HT$_3$ receptors. Mirtazapine has no significant affinity for the 5-HT$_{1A}$ and 5-HT$_{1B}$ receptors.

Mirtazapine is a potent antagonist of histamine (H$_1$) receptors, a property that may explain its prominent sedative effects.

Mirtazapine is a moderate peripheral α_1-adrenergic antagonist, a property that may explain the occasional orthostatic hypotension reported in association with its use.

Mirtazapine is a moderate antagonist at muscarinic receptors, a property that may explain the relatively low incidence of anticholinergic side effects associated with its use.

Pharmacokinetics

REMERONSolTab (mirtazapine) Orally Disintegrating Tablets are rapidly and completely absorbed following oral administration and have a half-life of about 20 to 40 hours. Peak plasma concentrations are reached within about 2 hours following an oral dose. The presence of food in the stomach has a minimal effect on both the rate and extent of absorption and does not require a dosage adjustment. REMERONSolTab Orally Disintegrating Tablets are bioequivalent to REMERON® (mirtazapine) Tablets.

Mirtazapine is extensively metabolized after oral administration. Major pathways of bio-transformation are demethylation and hydroxylation followed by glucuronide conjugation. *In vitro* data from human liver microsomes indicate that cytochrome 2D6 and 1A2 are involved in the formation of the 8-hydroxy metabolite of mirtazapine, whereas cytochrome 3A is considered to be responsible for the formation of the N-desmethyl and N-oxide metabolite. Mirtazapine has an absolute bioavailability of about 50%. It is eliminated predominantly via urine (75%) with 15% in feces. Several unconjugated metabolites possess pharmacological activity but are present in the plasma at very low levels. The (−) enantiomer has an elimination half-life that is approximately twice as long as the (+) enantiomer and therefore achieves plasma levels that are about 3 times as high as that of the (+) enantiomer.

Plasma levels are linearly related to dose over a dose range of 15 to 80 mg. The mean elimination half-life of mirtazapine after oral administration ranges from approximately 20 to 40 hours across age and gender subgroups, with females of all ages exhibiting significantly longer elimination half-lives than males (mean half-life of 37 hours for females vs. 26 hours for males). Steady state plasma levels of mirtazapine are attained within 5 days, with about 50% accumulation (accumulation ratio=1.5).

Mirtazapine is approximately 85% bound to plasma proteins over a concentration range of 0.01 to 10 mcg/mL.

Special Populations
Geriatric

Following oral administration of REMERON (mirtazapine) Tablets 20 mg/day for 7 days to subjects of varying ages (range, 25–74), oral clearance of mirtazapine was reduced in the elderly compared to the younger subjects. The differences were most striking in males, with a 40% lower clearance in elderly males compared to younger males, while the clearance in elderly females was only 10% lower compared to younger females. Caution is indicated in administering REMERONSolTab (mirtazapine) Orally Disintegrating Tablets to elderly patients (see PRECAUTIONS and DOSAGE AND ADMINISTRATION).

Pediatrics

Safety and effectiveness of mirtazapine in the pediatric population have not been established (see PRECAUTIONS).

Gender

The mean elimination half-life of mirtazapine after oral administration ranges from approximately 20 to 40 hours across age and gender subgroups, with females of all ages exhibiting significantly longer elimination half-lives than males (mean half-life of 37 hours for females vs. 26 hours for males) (see Pharmacokinetics).

Race

There have been no clinical studies to evaluate the effect of race on the pharmacokinetics of REMERONSolTab.

Renal Insufficiency

The disposition of mirtazapine was studied in patients with varying degrees of renal function. Elimination of mirtazapine is correlated with creatinine clearance. Total body clearance of mirtazapine was reduced approximately 30% in patients with moderate (Clcr=11–39 mL/min/1.73 m^2) and approximately 50% in patients with severe (Clcr=<10 mL/min/1.73 m^2) renal impairment when compared to normal subjects. Caution is indicated in administering REMERONSolTab to patients with compromised renal function (see PRECAUTIONS and DOSAGE AND ADMINISTRATION).

Hepatic Insufficiency

Following a single 15-mg oral dose of REMERON, the oral clearance of mirtazapine was decreased by approximately 30% in hepatically impaired patients compared to subjects with normal hepatic function. Caution is indicated in administering REMERONSolTab to patients with compromised hepatic function (see PRECAUTIONS and DOSAGE AND ADMINISTRATION).

Clinical Trials Showing Effectiveness

The efficacy of REMERON (mirtazapine) Tablets as a treatment for major depressive disorder was established in 4 placebo-controlled, 6-week trials in adult outpatients meeting DSM-III criteria for major depressive disorder. Patients were titrated with mirtazapine from a dose range of 5 mg up to 35 mg/day. Overall, these studies demonstrated mirtazapine to be superior to placebo on at least 3 of the following 4 measures: 21-Item Hamilton Depression Rating Scale (HDRS) total score; HDRS Depressed Mood Item; CGI Severity score; and Montgomery and Asberg Depression Rating Scale (MADRS). Superiority of mirtazapine over placebo was also found for certain factors of the HDRS, including anxiety/somatization factor and sleep disturbance factor. The mean mirtazapine dose for patients who completed these 4 studies ranged from 21 to 32 mg/day. A fifth study of similar design utilized a higher dose (up to 50 mg) per day and also showed effectiveness.

Examination of age and gender subsets of the population did not reveal any differential responsiveness on the basis of these subgroupings.

In a longer-term study, patients meeting (DSM-IV) criteria for major depressive disorder who had responded during an initial 8 to 12 weeks of acute treatment on REMERON were randomized to continuation of REMERON or placebo for up to 40 weeks of observation for relapse. Response during the open phase was defined as having achieved a HAM-D 17 total score of ≤8 and a CGI-Improvement score of 1 or 2 at 2 consecutive visits beginning with week 6 of the 8 to 12 weeks in the open-label phase of the study. Relapse during the double-blind phase was determined by the individual investigators. Patients receiving continued REMERON treatment experienced significantly lower relapse rates over the subsequent 40 weeks compared to those receiving placebo. This pattern was demonstrated in both male and female patients.

INDICATIONS AND USAGE

REMERONSolTab (mirtazapine) Orally Disintegrating Tablets are indicated for the treatment of major depressive disorder.

The efficacy of REMERON (mirtazapine) Tablets in the treatment of major depressive disorder was established in 6-week controlled trials of outpatients whose diagnoses corresponded most closely to the Diagnostic and Statistical Manual of Mental Disorders – 3rd edition (DSM-III) category of major depressive disorder (see CLINICAL PHARMACOLOGY).

A major depressive episode (DSM-IV) implies a prominent and relatively persistent (nearly every day for at least 2 weeks) depressed or dysphoric mood that usually interferes with daily functioning, and includes at least 5 of the following 9 symptoms: depressed mood, loss of interest in usual activities, significant change in weight and/or appetite, insomnia or hypersomnia, psychomotor agitation or retardation, increased fatigue, feelings of guilt or worthlessness, slowed thinking or impaired concentration, a suicide attempt, or suicidal ideation.

The effectiveness of REMERONSolTab in hospitalized depressed patients has not been adequately studied.

The efficacy of REMERON in maintaining a response in patients with major depressive disorder for up to 40 weeks following 8 to 12 weeks of initial open-label treatment was demonstrated in a placebo-controlled trial. Nevertheless, the physician who elects to use REMERON for extended periods should periodically re-evaluate the long-term usefulness of the drug for the individual patient (see CLINICAL PHARMACOLOGY).

CONTRAINDICATIONS

Hypersensitivity

REMERONSolTab (mirtazapine) Orally Disintegrating Tablets are contraindicated in patients with a known hypersensitivity to mirtazapine or to any of the excipients.

Monoamine Oxidase Inhibitors

The use of monoamine oxidase inhibitors (MAOIs) intended to treat psychiatric disorders with REMERONSolTab Orally Disintegrating Tablets or within 14 days of stopping treatment with REMERONSolTab is contraindicated because of an increased risk of serotonin syndrome. The use of REMERONSolTab within 14 days of stopping an MAOI intended to treat psychiatric disorders is also contraindicated (see WARNINGS and DOSAGE AND ADMINISTRATION). Starting REMERONSolTab in a patient who is being treated with MAOIs such as linezolid or intravenous methylene blue is also contraindicated because of an increased risk of serotonin syndrome (see WARNINGS and DOSAGE AND ADMINISTRATION).

WARNINGS

Clinical Worsening and Suicide Risk

Patients with major depressive disorder (MDD), both adult and pediatric, may experience worsening of their depression and/or the emergence of suicidal ideation and behavior (suicidality) or unusual changes in behavior, whether or not they are taking antidepressant medications, and this risk may persist until significant remission occurs. Suicide is a known risk of depression and certain other psychiatric disorders, and these disorders themselves are the strongest predictors of suicide. There has been a long-standing concern, however, that antidepressants may have a role in inducing worsening of depression and the emergence of suicidality in certain patients during the early phases of treatment. Pooled analyses of short-term placebo-controlled trials of antidepressant drugs (SSRIs and others) showed that these drugs increase the risk of suicidal thinking and behavior (suicidality) in children, adolescents, and young adults (ages 18–24) with major depressive disorder (MDD) and other psychiatric disorders. Short-term studies did not show an increase in the risk of suicidality with antidepressants compared to placebo in adults beyond age 24; there was a reduction in risk with antidepressants compared to placebo in adults aged 65 and older.

The pooled analyses of placebo-controlled trials in children and adolescents with MDD, obsessive compulsive disorder (OCD), or other psychiatric disorders included a total of 24 short-term trials of 9 antidepressant drugs in over 4400 patients. The pooled analyses of placebo-controlled trials in adults with MDD or other psychiatric disorders included a total of 295 short-term trials (median duration of 2 months) of 11 antidepressant drugs in over 77,000 patients. There was considerable variation in risk of suicidality among drugs, but a tendency toward an increase in the younger patients for almost all drugs studied. There were differences in absolute risk of suicidality across different indications, with the highest incidence in MDD. The risk differences (drug vs. placebo), however, were relatively stable within age strata and across indications. These risk differences (drug-placebo difference in the number of cases of suicidality per 1000 patients treated) are provided in Table 1.

Table 1

Age Range	Drug-Placebo Difference in Number of Cases of Suicidality per 1000 Patients Treated
Increases Compared to Placebo	
<18	14 additional cases
18–24	5 additional cases
Decreases Compared to Placebo	
25–64	1 fewer case
≥65	6 fewer cases

No suicides occurred in any of the pediatric trials. There were suicides in the adult trials, but the number was not sufficient to reach any conclusion about drug effect on suicide.

It is unknown whether the suicidality risk extends to longer-term use, i.e., beyond several months. However, there is substantial evidence from placebo-controlled maintenance trials in adults with depression that the use of antidepressants can delay the recurrence of depression.

All patients being treated with antidepressants for any indication should be monitored appropriately and observed closely for clinical worsening, suicidality, and unusual changes in behavior, especially during the initial few months of a course of drug therapy, or at times of dose changes, either increases or decreases.

The following symptoms, anxiety, agitation, panic attacks, insomnia, irritability, hostility, aggressiveness, impulsivity, akathisia (psychomotor restlessness), hypomania, and mania, have been reported in adult and pediatric patients being treated with antidepressants for major depressive disorder as well as for other indications, both psychiatric and nonpsychiatric. Although a causal link between the emergence of such symptoms and either the worsening of depression and/or the emergence of suicidal impulses has not been established, there is concern that such symptoms may represent precursors to emerging suicidality.

Consideration should be given to changing the therapeutic regimen, including possibly discontinuing the medication, in patients whose depression is persistently worse, or who are experiencing emergent suicidality or symptoms that might be precursors to worsening depression or suicidality, especially if these symptoms are severe, abrupt in onset, or were not part of the patient's presenting symptoms.

Families and caregivers of patients being treated with antidepressants for major depressive disorder or other indications, both psychiatric and nonpsychiatric, should be alerted about the need to monitor patients for the emergence of agitation, irritability, unusual changes in behavior, and the other symptoms described above, as well as the emergence of suicidality, and to report such symptoms immediately to health care providers. Such monitoring should include daily observation by families and caregivers. Prescriptions for REMERONSolTab (mirtazapine) Orally Disintegrating Tablets should be written for the smallest quantity of tablets consistent with good patient management, in order to reduce the risk of overdose.

Screening Patients for Bipolar Disorder

A major depressive episode may be the initial presentation of bipolar disorder. It is generally believed (though not established in controlled trials) that treating such an episode with an antidepressant alone may increase the likelihood of precipitation of a mixed/manic episode in patients at risk for bipolar disorder. Whether any of the symptoms described above represent such a conversion is unknown. However, prior to initiating treatment with an antidepressant, patients with depressive symptoms should be adequately screened to determine if they are at risk for bipolar disorder; such screening should include a detailed psychiatric history, including a family history of suicide, bipolar disorder, and depression. It should be noted that REMERONSolTab (mirtazapine) Orally Disintegrating Tablets are not approved for use in treating bipolar depression.

Agranulocytosis

In premarketing clinical trials, 2 (1 with Sjögren's Syndrome) out of 2796 patients treated with REMERON (mirtazapine) Tablets developed agranulocytosis [absolute neutrophil count (ANC) <500/mm³ with associated signs and symptoms, e.g., fever, infection, etc.] and a third patient developed severe neutropenia (ANC <500/mm³ without any associated symptoms). For these 3 patients, onset of severe neutropenia was detected on days 61, 9, and 14 of treatment, respectively. All 3 patients recovered after REMERON was stopped. These 3 cases yield a crude incidence of severe neutropenia (with or without associated infection) of approximately 1.1 per thousand patients exposed, with a very wide 95% confidence interval, i.e., 2.2 cases per 10,000 to 3.1 cases per 1000. If a patient develops a sore throat, fever, stomatitis, or other signs of infection, along with a low WBC count, treatment with REMERONSolTab (mirtazapine) Orally Disintegrating Tablets should be discontinued and the patient should be closely monitored.

Serotonin Syndrome

The development of a potentially life-threatening serotonin syndrome has been reported with SNRIs and SSRIs, including REMERONSolTab, alone but particularly with concomitant use of other serotonergic drugs (including triptans, tricyclic antidepressants, fentanyl, lithium, tramadol, tryptophan, buspirone, and St. John's wort) and with drugs that impair metabolism of serotonin (in particular, MAOIs, both those intended to treat psychiatric disorders and also others, such as linezolid and intravenous methylene blue). Serotonin syndrome symptoms may include mental status changes (e.g., agitation, hallucinations, delirium, and coma), autonomic instability (e.g., tachycardia, labile blood pressure, dizziness, diaphoresis, flushing, hyperthermia), neuromuscular symptoms (e.g., tremor, rigidity, myoclonus, hyperreflexia, incoordination), seizures, and/or gastrointestinal symptoms (e.g., nausea, vomiting, diarrhea). Patients should be monitored for the emergence of serotonin syndrome.

The concomitant use of REMERONSolTab with MAOIs intended to treat psychiatric disorders is contraindicated. REMERONSolTab should also not be started in a patient who is being treated with MAOIs such as linezolid or intravenous methylene blue. All reports with methylene blue that provided information on the route of administration involved intravenous administration in the dose range of 1 mg/kg to 8 mg/kg. No reports involved the administration of methylene blue by other routes (such as oral tablets or local tissue injection) or at lower doses. There may be circumstances when it is necessary to initiate treatment with an MAOI such as linezolid or intravenous methylene blue in a patient taking REMERONSolTab. REMERONSolTab should be discontinued before initiating treatment with the MAOI (see CONTRAINDICATIONS and DOSAGE AND ADMINISTRATION).

If concomitant use of REMERONSolTab with other serotonergic drugs, including triptans, tricyclic antidepressants, fentanyl, lithium, tramadol, buspirone, tryptophan, and St. John's wort, is clinically warranted, be aware of a potential increased risk for serotonin syndrome, particularly during treatment initiation and dose increases.

Treatment with REMERONSolTab and any concomitant serotonergic agents should be discontinued immediately if the above events occur and supportive symptomatic treatment should be initiated.

Angle-Closure Glaucoma

The pupillary dilation that occurs following use of many antidepressant drugs including REMERONSolTab may trigger an angle-closure attack in a patient with anatomically narrow angles who does not have a patent iridectomy.

PRECAUTIONS

General

Discontinuation Symptoms

There have been reports of adverse reactions upon the discontinuation of REMERON/REMERONSolTab (mirtazapine) Orally Disintegrating Tablets (particularly when abrupt), including but not limited to the following: dizziness, abnormal dreams, sensory disturbances (including paresthesia and electric shock sensations), agitation, anxiety, fatigue, confusion, headache, tremor, nausea, vomiting, and sweating, or other symptoms which may be of clinical significance. The majority of the reported cases are mild and self-limiting. Even though these have been reported as adverse reactions, it should be realized that these symptoms may be related to underlying disease.

Patients currently taking REMERONSolTab should NOT discontinue treatment abruptly, due to risk of discontinuation symptoms. At the time that a medical decision is made to discontinue treatment with REMERON, a gradual reduction in the dose, rather than an abrupt cessation, is recommended.

Akathisia/Psychomotor Restlessness

The use of antidepressants has been associated with the development of akathisia, characterized by a subjectively unpleasant or distressing restlessness and need to move, often accompanied by an inability to sit or stand still. This is most likely to occur within the first few weeks of treatment. In patients who develop these symptoms, increasing the dose may be detrimental.

Hyponatremia

Hyponatremia has been reported very rarely with the use of mirtazapine. Caution should be exercised in patients at risk, such as elderly patients or patients concomitantly treated with medications known to cause hyponatremia.

Somnolence

In US controlled studies, somnolence was reported in 54% of patients treated with REMERON (mirtazapine) Tablets, compared to 18% for placebo and 60% for amitriptyline. In these studies, somnolence resulted in discontinuation for 10.4% of REMERON-treated patients, compared to 2.2% for placebo. It is unclear whether or not tolerance develops to the somnolent effects of REMERON. Because of the potentially significant effects of REMERON on impairment of performance, patients should be cautioned about engaging in activities requiring alertness until they have been able to assess the drug's effect on their own psychomotor performance (see PRECAUTIONS: Information for Patients).

Dizziness

In US controlled studies, dizziness was reported in 7% of patients treated with REMERON, compared to 3% for placebo and 14% for amitriptyline. It is unclear whether or not tolerance develops to the dizziness observed in association with the use of REMERON.

Increased Appetite/Weight Gain

In US controlled studies, appetite increase was reported in 17% of patients treated with REMERON, compared to 2% for placebo and 6% for amitriptyline. In these same trials, weight gain of ≥7% of body weight was reported in 7.5% of patients treated with mirtazapine, compared to 0% for placebo and 5.9% for amitriptyline. In a pool of premarketing US studies, including many patients for long-term, open-label treatment, 8% of patients receiving REMERON discontinued for weight gain. In an 8-week-long pediatric clinical trial of doses between 15 to 45 mg/day, 49% of REMERON-treated patients had a weight gain of at least 7%, compared to 5.7% of placebo-treated patients (see PRECAUTIONS: Pediatric Use).

Cholesterol/Triglycerides

In US controlled studies, nonfasting cholesterol increases to ≥20% above the upper limits of normal were observed in 15% of patients treated with REMERON, compared to 7% for placebo and 8% for amitriptyline. In these same studies, nonfasting triglyceride increases to ≥500 mg/dL were observed in 6% of patients treated with mirtazapine, compared to 3% for placebo and 3% for amitriptyline.

Transaminase Elevations

Clinically significant ALT (SGPT) elevations (≥3 times the upper limit of the normal range) were observed in 2.0% (8/424) of patients exposed to REMERON in a pool of short-term US controlled trials, compared to 0.3% (1/328) of placebo patients and 2.0% (3/181) of amitriptyline patients. Most of these patients with ALT increases did not develop signs or symptoms associated with compromised liver function. While some patients were discontinued for the ALT increases, in other cases, the enzyme levels returned to normal despite continued REMERON treatment. REMERONSolTab (mirtazapine) Orally Disintegrating Tablets should be used with caution in patients with impaired hepatic function (see CLINICAL PHARMACOLOGY and DOSAGE AND ADMINISTRATION).

Activation of Mania/Hypomania

Mania/hypomania occurred in approximately 0.2% (3/1299 patients) of REMERON-treated patients in US studies. Although the incidence of mania/hypomania was very low during treatment with mirtazapine, it should be used carefully in patients with a history of mania/hypomania.

Seizure

In premarketing clinical trials, only 1 seizure was reported among the 2796 US and non-US patients treated with REMERON. However, no controlled studies have been carried out in patients with a history of seizures. Therefore, care should be exercised when mirtazapine is used in these patients.

Use in Patients with Concomitant Illness

Clinical experience with REMERONSolTab in patients with concomitant systemic illness is limited. Accordingly, care is advisable in prescribing mirtazapine for patients with diseases or conditions that affect metabolism or hemodynamic responses.

REMERONSolTab has not been systematically evaluated or used to any appreciable extent in patients with a recent history of myocardial infarction or other significant heart disease. REMERON was associated with significant orthostatic hypotension in early clinical pharmacology trials with normal volunteers. Orthostatic hypotension was infrequently observed in clinical trials with depressed patients. REMERONSolTab should be used with caution in patients with known cardiovascular or cerebrovascular disease that could be exacerbated by hypotension (history of myocardial infarction, angina, or ischemic stroke) and conditions that would predispose patients to hypotension (dehydration, hypovolemia, and treatment with antihypertensive medication).

Mirtazapine clearance is decreased in patients with moderate [glomerular filtration rate (GFR)=11–39 mL/min/1.73 m^2] and severe [GFR <10 mL/min/1.73 m^2] renal impairment, and also in patients with hepatic impairment. Caution is indicated in administering REMERONSolTab to such patients (see CLINICAL PHARMACOLOGY and DOSAGE AND ADMINISTRATION).

Information for Patients

Prescribers or other health professionals should inform patients, their families, and their caregivers about the benefits and risks associated with treatment with REMERONSolTab (mirtazapine) Orally Disintegrating Tablets and should counsel them in its appropriate use. A patient Medication Guide about "Antidepressant Medicines, Depression and other Serious Mental Illnesses, and Suicidal Thoughts or Actions" is available for REMERONSolTab. The prescriber or health professional should instruct patients, their families, and their caregivers to read the Medication Guide and should assist them in understanding its contents. Patients should be given the opportunity to discuss the contents of the Medication Guide and to obtain answers to any questions they may have. The complete text of the Medication Guide is reprinted at the end of this document.

Patients should be advised of the following issues and asked to alert their prescriber if these occur while taking REMERONSolTab.

Clinical Worsening and Suicide Risk

Patients, their families, and their caregivers should be encouraged to be alert to the emergence of anxiety, agitation, panic attacks, insomnia, irritability, hostility, aggressiveness, impulsivity, akathisia (psychomotor restlessness), hypomania, mania, other unusual changes in behavior, worsening of depression, and suicidal ideation, especially early during antidepressant treatment and when the dose is adjusted up or down. Families and caregivers of patients should be advised to look for the emergence of such symptoms on a day-to-day basis, since changes may be abrupt. Such symptoms should be reported to the patient's prescriber or health professional, especially if they are severe, abrupt in onset, or were not part of the patient's presenting symptoms. Symptoms such as these may be associated with an increased risk for suicidal thinking and behavior and indicate a need for very close monitoring and possibly changes in the medication.

Agranulocytosis

Patients who are to receive REMERONSolTab should be warned about the risk of developing agranulocytosis. Patients should be advised to contact their physician if they experience any indication of infection such as fever, chills, sore throat, mucous membrane ulceration, or other possible signs of infection. Particular attention should be paid to any flu-like complaints or other symptoms that might suggest infection.

Interference with Cognitive and Motor Performance

REMERONSolTab may impair judgment, thinking, and particularly, motor skills, because of its prominent sedative effect. The drowsiness associated with mirtazapine use may impair a patient's ability to drive, use machines, or perform tasks that require alertness. Thus, patients should be cautioned about engaging in hazardous activities until they are reasonably certain that REMERONSolTab therapy does not adversely affect their ability to engage in such activities.

Completing Course of Therapy

While patients may notice improvement with REMERONSolTab therapy in 1 to 4 weeks, they should be advised to continue therapy as directed.

Concomitant Medication

Patients should be advised to inform their physician if they are taking, or intend to take, any prescription or over-the-counter drugs, since there is a potential for REMERONSolTab to interact with other drugs.

Patients should be made aware of a potential increased risk for serotonin syndrome if concomitant use of REMERONSolTab with other serotonergic drugs, including triptans, tricyclic antidepressants, fentanyl, lithium, tramadol, buspirone, tryptophan, and St. John's wort, is clinically warranted, particularly during treatment initiation and dose increases.

Alcohol

The impairment of cognitive and motor skills produced by REMERON has been shown to be additive with those produced by alcohol. Accordingly, patients should be advised to avoid alcohol while taking any dosage form of mirtazapine.

Phenylalanine

Phenylketonuric patients should be informed that REMERONSolTab contains phenylalanine 2.6 mg per 15-mg tablet, 5.2 mg per 30-mg tablet, and 7.8 mg per 45-mg tablet.

Pregnancy

Patients should be advised to notify their physician if they become pregnant or intend to become pregnant during REMERONSolTab therapy.

Nursing

Patients should be advised to notify their physician if they are breastfeeding an infant.

Laboratory Tests

There are no routine laboratory tests recommended.

Drug Interactions

As with other drugs, the potential for interaction by a variety of mechanisms (e.g., pharmacodynamic, pharmacokinetic inhibition or enhancement, etc.) is a possibility (see CLINICAL PHARMACOLOGY).

Monoamine Oxidase Inhibitors

(See CONTRAINDICATIONS, WARNINGS, and DOSAGE AND ADMINISTRATION.)

Serotonergic Drugs

(See CONTRAINDICATIONS and WARNINGS.)

Drugs Affecting Hepatic Metabolism

The metabolism and pharmacokinetics of REMERONSolTab (mirtazapine) Orally Disintegrating Tablets may be affected by the induction or inhibition of drug-metabolizing enzymes.

Drugs that are Metabolized by and/or Inhibit Cytochrome P450 Enzymes

CYP Enzyme Inducers (these studies used both drugs at steady state)

Phenytoin

In healthy male patients (n=18), phenytoin (200 mg daily) increased mirtazapine (30 mg daily) clearance about 2-fold, resulting in a decrease in average plasma mirtazapine concentrations of 45%. Mirtazapine did not significantly affect the pharmacokinetics of phenytoin.

Carbamazepine

In healthy male patients (n=24), carbamazepine (400 mg b.i.d.) increased mirtazapine (15 mg b.i.d.) clearance about 2-fold, resulting in a decrease in average plasma mirtazapine concentrations of 60%.

When phenytoin, carbamazepine, or another inducer of hepatic metabolism (such as rifampicin) is added to mirtazapine therapy, the mirtazapine dose may have to be increased. If treatment with such a medicinal product is discontinued, it may be necessary to reduce the mirtazapine dose.

CYP Enzyme Inhibitors

Cimetidine

In healthy male patients (n=12), when cimetidine, a weak inhibitor of CYP1A2, CYP2D6, and CYP3A4, given at 800 mg b.i.d. at steady state was coadministered with mirtazapine (30 mg daily) at steady state, the Area Under the Curve (AUC) of mirtazapine increased more than 50%. Mirtazapine did not cause relevant changes in the pharmacokinetics of cimetidine. The mirtazapine dose may have to be decreased when concomitant treatment with cimetidine is started, or increased when cimetidine treatment is discontinued.

Ketoconazole

In healthy, male, Caucasian patients (n=24), coadministration of the potent CYP3A4 inhibitor ketoconazole (200 mg b.i.d. for 6.5 days) increased the peak plasma levels and the AUC of a single 30-mg dose of mirtazapine by approximately 40% and 50%, respectively.

Caution should be exercised when coadministering mirtazapine with potent CYP3A4 inhibitors, HIV protease inhibitors, azole antifungals, erythromycin, or nefazodone.

Paroxetine

In an *in vivo* interaction study in healthy, CYP2D6 extensive metabolizer patients (n=24), mirtazapine (30 mg/day), at steady state, did not cause relevant changes in the pharmacokinetics of steady state paroxetine (40 mg/day), a CYP2D6 inhibitor.

Other Drug-Drug Interactions

Amitriptyline

In healthy, CYP2D6 extensive metabolizer patients (n=32), amitriptyline (75 mg daily), at steady state, did not cause relevant changes to the pharmacokinetics of steady state mirtazapine (30 mg daily); mirtazapine also did not cause relevant changes to the pharmacokinetics of amitriptyline.

Warfarin
In healthy male subjects (n=16), mirtazapine (30 mg daily), at steady state, caused a small (0.2) but statistically significant increase in the International Normalized Ratio (INR) in subjects treated with warfarin. As at a higher dose of mirtazapine, a more pronounced effect can not be excluded, it is advisable to monitor the INR in case of concomitant treatment of warfarin with mirtazapine.

Lithium
No relevant clinical effects or significant changes in pharmacokinetics have been observed in healthy male subjects on concurrent treatment with subtherapeutic levels of lithium (600 mg/day for 10 days) at steady state and a single 30 mg dose of mirtazapine. The effects of higher doses of lithium on the pharmacokinetics of mirtazapine are unknown.

Risperidone
In an *in vivo*, nonrandomized, interaction study, subjects (n=6) in need of treatment with an antipsychotic and antidepressant drug, showed that mirtazapine (30 mg daily) at steady state did not influence the pharmacokinetics of risperidone (up to 3 mg b.i.d.).

Alcohol
Concomitant administration of alcohol (equivalent to 60 g) had a minimal effect on plasma levels of mirtazapine (15 mg) in 6 healthy male subjects. The impairment of cognitive and motor skills produced by REMERON were shown to be additive with those produced by alcohol. Accordingly, patients should be advised to avoid alcohol while taking REMERONSolTab.

Diazepam
Concomitant administration of diazepam (15 mg) had a minimal effect on plasma levels of mirtazapine (15 mg) in 12 healthy subjects. However, the impairment of motor skills produced by REMERON has been shown to be additive with those caused by diazepam. Accordingly, patients should be advised to avoid diazepam and other similar drugs while taking REMERONSolTab.

Carcinogenesis, Mutagenesis, Impairment of Fertility
Carcinogenesis
Carcinogenicity studies were conducted with mirtazapine given in the diet at doses of 2, 20, and 200 mg/kg/day to mice and 2, 20, and 60 mg/kg/day to rats. The highest doses used are approximately 20 and 12 times the maximum recommended human dose (MRHD) of 45 mg/day on an mg/m^2 basis in mice and rats, respectively. There was an increased incidence of hepatocellular adenoma and carcinoma in male mice at the high dose. In rats, there was an increase in hepatocellular adenoma in females at the mid and high doses and in hepatocellular tumors and thyroid follicular adenoma/cystadenoma and carcinoma in males at the high dose. The data suggest that the above effects could possibly be mediated by non-genotoxic mechanisms, the relevance of which to humans is not known.

The doses used in the mouse study may not have been high enough to fully characterize the carcinogenic potential of REMERON (mirtazapine) Tablets.

Mutagenesis
Mirtazapine was not mutagenic or clastogenic and did not induce general DNA damage as determined in several genotoxicity tests: Ames test, *in vitro* gene mutation assay in Chinese hamster V 79 cells, *in vitro* sister chromatid exchange assay in cultured rabbit lymphocytes, *in vivo* bone marrow micronucleus test in rats, and unscheduled DNA synthesis assay in HeLa cells.

Impairment of Fertility
In a fertility study in rats, mirtazapine was given at doses up to 100 mg/kg [20 times the maximum recommended human dose (MRHD) on an mg/m^2 basis]. Mating and conception were not affected by the drug, but estrous cycling was disrupted at doses that were 3 or more times the MRHD, and pre-implantation losses occurred at 20 times the MRHD.

Pregnancy
Teratogenic Effects
Pregnancy Category C
Reproduction studies in pregnant rats and rabbits at doses up to 100 mg/kg and 40 mg/kg, respectively [20 and 17 times the maximum recommended human dose (MRHD) on an mg/m^2 basis, respectively], have revealed no evidence of teratogenic effects. However, in rats, there was an increase in postimplantation losses in dams treated with mirtazapine. There was an increase in pup deaths during the first 3 days of lactation and a decrease in pup birth weights. The cause of these deaths is not known. The effects occurred at doses that were 20 times the MRHD, but not at 3 times the MRHD, on an mg/m^2 basis. There are no adequate and well-controlled studies in pregnant women. Because animal reproduction studies are not always predictive of human response, this drug should be used during pregnancy only if clearly needed.

Nursing Mothers
Because some REMERONSolTab may be excreted in breast milk, caution should be exercised when REMERONSolTab (mirtazapine) Orally Disintegrating Tablets are administered to nursing women.

Pediatric Use
Safety and effectiveness in the pediatric population have not been established (see BOXED WARNING and WARNINGS: Clinical Worsening and Suicide Risk). Two placebo-controlled trials in 258 pediatric patients with MDD have been conducted with REMERON (mirtazapine) Tablets, and the data were not sufficient to support a claim for use in pediatric patients. Anyone considering the use of REMERONSolTab (mirtazapine) Orally Disintegrating Tablets in a child or adolescent must balance the potential risks with the clinical need.

In an 8-week-long pediatric clinical trial of doses between 15 to 45 mg/day, 49% of REMERON-treated patients had a weight gain of at least 7%, compared to 5.7% of placebo-treated patients. The mean increase in weight was 4 kg (2 kg SD) for REMERON-treated patients versus 1 kg (2 kg SD) for placebo-treated patients (see PRECAUTIONS: Increased Appetite/Weight Gain).

Geriatric Use
Approximately 190 elderly individuals (≥65 years of age) participated in clinical studies with REMERON (mirtazapine) Tablets. This drug is known to be substantially excreted by the kidney (75%), and the risk of decreased clearance of this drug is greater in patients with impaired renal function. Because elderly patients are more likely to have decreased renal function, care should be taken in dose selection. Sedating drugs may cause confusion and over-sedation in the elderly. No unusual adverse age-related phenomena were identified in this group. Pharmacokinetic studies revealed a decreased clearance in the elderly. Caution is indicated in administering REMERONSolTab (mirtazapine) Orally Disintegrating Tablets to elderly patients (see CLINICAL PHARMACOLOGY and DOSAGE AND ADMINISTRATION).

ADVERSE REACTIONS
Associated with Discontinuation of Treatment
Approximately 16% of the 453 patients who received REMERON (mirtazapine) Tablets in US 6-week controlled clinical trials discontinued treatment due to an adverse experience, compared to 7% of the 361 placebo-treated patients in those studies. The most common events (≥1%) associated with discontinuation and considered to be drug related (i.e., those events associated with dropout at a rate at least twice that of placebo) are included in Table 2.

Table 2: Common Adverse Events Associated With Discontinuation of Treatment in 6-Week US REMERON Trials

	Percentage of Patients Discontinuing with Adverse Event	
Adverse Event	REMERON (n=453)	Placebo (n=361)
Somnolence	10.4%	2.2%
Nausea	1.5%	0%

Commonly Observed Adverse Events in US Controlled Clinical Trials
The most commonly observed adverse events associated with the use of REMERON (mirtazapine) Tablets (incidence of 5% or greater) and not observed at an equivalent incidence among placebo-treated patients (REMERON incidence at least twice that for placebo) are listed in Table 3.

Table 3: Common Treatment-Emergent Adverse Events Associated With the Use of REMERON in 6-Week US Trials

	Percentage of Patients Reporting Adverse Event	
Adverse Event	REMERON (n=453)	Placebo (n=361)
Somnolence	54%	18%
Increased Appetite	17%	2%
Weight Gain	12%	2%
Dizziness	7%	3%

Adverse Events Occurring at an Incidence of 1% or More Among REMERON-Treated Patients
Table 4 enumerates adverse events that occurred at an incidence of 1% or more, and were more frequent than in the placebo group, among REMERON (mirtazapine) Tablets-treated patients who participated in short-term US placebo-controlled trials in which patients were dosed in a range of 5 to 60 mg/day. This table shows the percentage of patients in each group who had at least 1 episode of an event at some time during their treatment. Reported adverse events were classified using a standard COSTART-based dictionary terminology.

The prescriber should be aware that these figures cannot be used to predict the incidence of side effects in the course of usual medical practice where patient characteristics and other factors differ from those which prevailed in the clinical trials. Similarly, the cited frequencies cannot be compared with figures obtained from other investigations involving different treatments, uses, and investigators. The cited figures, however, do provide the prescribing physician with some basis for estimating the relative contribution of drug and nondrug factors to the side-effect incidence rate in the population studied.

Table 4: Incidence of Adverse Clinical Experiences* (≥1%) in Short-Term US Controlled Studies

Body System Adverse Clinical Experience	REMERON (n=453)	Placebo (n=361)
Body as a Whole		
Asthenia	8%	5%
Flu Syndrome	5%	3%
Back Pain	2%	1%
Digestive System		
Dry Mouth	25%	15%
Increased Appetite	17%	2%
Constipation	13%	7%
Metabolic and Nutritional Disorders		
Weight Gain	12%	2%
Peripheral Edema	2%	1%
Edema	1%	0%
Musculoskeletal System		
Myalgia	2%	1%
Nervous System		
Somnolence	54%	18%
Dizziness	7%	3%
Abnormal Dreams	4%	1%
Thinking Abnormal	3%	1%
Tremor	2%	1%
Confusion	2%	0%
Respiratory System		
Dyspnea	1%	0%
Urogenital System		
Urinary Frequency	2%	1%

* Events reported by at least 1% of patients treated with REMERON are included, except the following events, which had an incidence on placebo greater than or equal to REMERON: headache, infection, pain, chest pain, palpitation, tachycardia, postural hypotension, nausea, dyspepsia, diarrhea, flatulence, insomnia, nervousness, libido decreased, hypertonia, pharyngitis, rhinitis, sweating, amblyopia, tinnitus, taste perversion.

ECG Changes
The electrocardiograms for 338 patients who received REMERON (mirtazapine) Tablets and 261 patients who received placebo in 6-week, placebo-controlled trials were analyzed. Prolongation in QTc ≥500 msec was not observed among mirtazapine-treated patients; mean change in QTc was +1.6 msec for mirtazapine and –3.1 msec for placebo. Mirtazapine was associated with a mean increase in heart rate of 3.4 bpm, compared to 0.8 bpm for placebo. The clinical significance of these changes is unknown.

Other Adverse Events Observed During the Premarketing Evaluation of REMERON

During its premarketing assessment, multiple doses of REMERON (mirtazapine) Tablets were administered to 2796 patients in clinical studies. The conditions and duration of exposure to mirtazapine varied greatly, and included (in overlapping categories) open and double-blind studies, uncontrolled and controlled studies, inpatient and outpatient studies, fixed-dose and titration studies. Untoward events associated with this exposure were recorded by clinical investigators using terminology of their own choosing. Consequently, it is not possible to provide a meaningful estimate of the proportion of individuals experiencing adverse events without first grouping similar types of untoward events into a smaller number of standardized event categories.

In the tabulations that follow, reported adverse events were classified using a standard COSTART-based dictionary terminology. The frequencies presented, therefore, represent the proportion of the 2796 patients exposed to multiple doses of REMERON who experienced an event of the type cited on at least 1 occasion while receiving REMERON. All reported events are included except those already listed in Table 4, those adverse experiences subsumed under COSTART terms that are either overly general or excessively specific so as to be uninformative, and those events for which a drug cause was very remote.

It is important to emphasize that, although the events reported occurred during treatment with REMERON, they were not necessarily caused by it.

Events are further categorized by body system and listed in order of decreasing frequency according to the following definitions: frequent adverse events are those occurring on 1 or more occasions in at least 1/100 patients; infrequent adverse events are those occurring in 1/100 to 1/1000 patients; rare events are those occurring in fewer than 1/1000 patients. Only those events not already listed in Table 4 appear in this listing. Events of major clinical importance are also described in the WARNINGS and PRECAUTIONS sections.

Body as a Whole: *frequent:* malaise, abdominal pain, abdominal syndrome acute; *infrequent:* chills, fever, face edema, ulcer, photosensitivity reaction, neck rigidity, neck pain, abdomen enlarged; *rare:* cellulitis, chest pain substernal.

Cardiovascular System: *frequent:* hypertension, vasodilatation; *infrequent:* angina pectoris, myocardial infarction, bradycardia, ventricular extrasystoles, syncope, migraine, hypotension; *rare:* atrial arrhythmia, bigeminy, vascular headache, pulmonary embolus, cerebral ischemia, cardiomegaly, phlebitis, left heart failure.

Digestive System: *frequent:* vomiting, anorexia; *infrequent:* eructation, glossitis, cholecystitis, nausea and vomiting, gum hemorrhage, stomatitis, colitis, liver function tests abnormal; *rare:* tongue discoloration, ulcerative stomatitis, salivary gland enlargement, increased salivation, intestinal obstruction, pancreatitis, aphthous stomatitis, cirrhosis of liver, gastritis, gastroenteritis, oral moniliasis, tongue edema.

Endocrine System: *rare:* goiter, hypothyroidism.

Hemic and Lymphatic System: *rare:* lymphadenopathy, leukopenia, petechia, anemia, thrombocytopenia, lymphocytosis, pancytopenia.

Metabolic and Nutritional Disorders: *frequent:* thirst; *infrequent:* dehydration, weight loss; *rare:* gout, SGOT increased, healing abnormal, acid phosphatase increased, SGPT increased, diabetes mellitus, hyponatremia.

Musculoskeletal System: *frequent:* myasthenia, arthralgia; *infrequent:* arthritis, tenosynovitis; *rare:* pathologic fracture, osteoporosis fracture, bone pain, myositis, tendon rupture, arthrosis, bursitis.

Nervous System: *frequent:* hypesthesia, apathy, depression, hypokinesia, vertigo, twitching, agitation, anxiety, amnesia, hyperkinesia, paresthesia; *infrequent:* ataxia, delirium, delusions, depersonalization, dyskinesia, extrapyramidal syndrome, libido increased, coordination abnormal, dysarthria, hallucinations, manic reaction, neurosis, dystonia, hostility, reflexes increased, emotional lability, euphoria, paranoid reaction; *rare:* aphasia, nystagmus, akathisia (psychomotor restlessness), stupor, dementia, diplopia, drug dependence, paralysis, grand mal convulsion, hypotonia, myoclonus, psychotic depression, withdrawal syndrome, serotonin syndrome.

Respiratory System: *frequent:* cough increased, sinusitis; *infrequent:* epistaxis, bronchitis, asthma, pneumonia; *rare:* asphyxia, laryngitis, pneumothorax, hiccup.

Skin and Appendages: *frequent:* pruritus, rash; *infrequent:* acne, exfoliative dermatitis, dry skin, herpes simplex, alopecia; *rare:* urticaria, herpes zoster, skin hypertrophy, seborrhea, skin ulcer.

Special Senses: *infrequent:* eye pain, abnormality of accommodation, conjunctivitis, deafness, keratoconjunctivitis, lacrimation disorder, angle-closure glaucoma, hyperacusis, ear pain; *rare:* blepharitis, partial transitory deafness, otitis media, taste loss, parosmia.

Urogenital System: *frequent:* urinary tract infection; *infrequent:* kidney calculus, cystitis, dysuria, urinary incontinence, urinary retention, vaginitis, hematuria, breast pain, amenorrhea, dysmenorrhea, leukorrhea, impotence; *rare:* polyuria, urethritis, metrorrhagia, menorrhagia, abnormal ejaculation, breast engorgement, breast enlargement, urinary urgency.

Other Adverse Events Observed During Postmarketing Evaluation of REMERON

Adverse events reported since market introduction, which were temporally (but not necessarily causally) related to mirtazapine therapy, include 4 cases of the ventricular arrhythmia torsades de pointes. In 3 of the 4 cases, however, concomitant drugs were implicated. All patients recovered. Cases of severe skin reactions, including Stevens-Johnson syndrome, bullous dermatitis, erythema multiforme and toxic epidermal necrolysis have also been reported.

DRUG ABUSE AND DEPENDENCE
Controlled Substance Class

REMERONSolTab (mirtazapine) Orally Disintegrating Tablets are not a controlled substance.

Physical and Psychologic Dependence

REMERONSolTab (mirtazapine) Orally Disintegrating Tablets have not been systematically studied in animals or humans for its potential for abuse, tolerance, or physical dependence. While the clinical trials did not reveal any tendency for any drug-seeking behavior, these observations were not systematic and it is not possible to predict on the basis of this limited experience the extent to which a CNS-active drug will be misused, diverted and/or abused once marketed. Consequently, patients should be evaluated carefully for history of drug abuse, and such patients should be observed closely for signs of REMERONSolTab misuse or abuse (e.g., development of tolerance, incrementations of dose, drug-seeking behavior).

OVERDOSAGE
Human Experience

There is very limited experience with REMERONSolTab (mirtazapine) Orally Disintegrating Tablets overdose. In premarketing clinical studies, there were 8 reports of REMERON overdose alone or in combination with other pharmacological agents. The only drug overdose death reported while taking REMERON was in combination with amitriptyline and chlorprothixene in a non-US clinical study. Based on plasma levels, the REMERON dose taken was 30 to 45 mg, while plasma levels of amitriptyline and chlorprothixene were found to be at toxic levels. All other premarketing overdose cases resulted in full recovery. Signs and symptoms reported in association with overdose included disorientation, drowsiness, impaired memory, and tachycardia. There were no reports of ECG abnormalities, coma, or convulsions following overdose with REMERON alone.

Overdose Management

Treatment should consist of those general measures employed in the management of overdose with any drug effective in the treatment of major depressive disorder. Ensure an adequate airway, oxygenation, and ventilation. Monitor cardiac rhythm and vital signs. General supportive and symptomatic measures are also recommended. Induction of emesis is not recommended. Gastric lavage with a large-bore orogastric tube with appropriate airway protection, if needed, may be indicated if performed soon after ingestion, or in symptomatic patients. Because of the rapid disintegration of REMERONSolTab (mirtazapine) Orally Disintegrating Tablets, pill fragments may not appear in gastric contents obtained with lavage. Activated charcoal should be administered. There is no experience with the use of forced diuresis, dialysis, hemoperfusion, or exchange transfusion in the treatment of mirtazapine overdosage. No specific antidotes for mirtazapine are known.

In managing overdosage, consider the possibility of multiple-drug involvement. The physician should consider contacting a poison control center for additional information on the treatment of any overdose. Telephone numbers for certified poison control centers are listed in the *Physicians' Desk Reference* (PDR).

DOSAGE AND ADMINISTRATION
Initial Treatment

The recommended starting dose for REMERONSolTab (mirtazapine) Orally Disintegrating Tablets is 15 mg/day, administered in a single dose, preferably in the evening prior to sleep. In the controlled clinical trials establishing the efficacy of REMERON in the treatment of major depressive disorder, the effective dose range was generally 15 to 45 mg/day. While the relationship between dose and satisfactory response in the treatment of major depressive disorder for REMERON has not been adequately explored, patients not responding to the initial 15-mg dose may benefit from dose increases up to a maximum of 45 mg/day. REMERON has an elimination half-life of approximately 20 to 40 hours; therefore, dose changes should not be made at intervals of less than 1 to 2 weeks in order to allow sufficient time for evaluation of the therapeutic response to a given dose.

Administration of REMERONSolTab (mirtazapine) Orally Disintegrating Tablets

Patients should be instructed to open tablet blister pack with dry hands and place the tablet on the tongue. The tablet should be used immediately after removal from its blister; once removed, it cannot be stored. REMERONSolTab (mirtazapine) Orally Disintegrating Tablets will disintegrate rapidly on the tongue and can be swallowed with saliva. No water is needed for taking the tablet. Patients should not attempt to split the tablet.

Elderly and Patients with Renal or Hepatic Impairment

The clearance of mirtazapine is reduced in elderly patients and in patients with moderate to severe renal or hepatic impairment. Consequently, the prescriber should be aware that plasma mirtazapine levels may be increased in these patient groups, compared to levels observed in younger adults without renal or hepatic impairment (see PRECAUTIONS and CLINICAL PHARMACOLOGY).

Maintenance/Extended Treatment

It is generally agreed that acute episodes of depression require several months or longer of sustained pharmacological therapy beyond response to the acute episode. Systematic evaluation of REMERON (mirtazapine) Tablets has demonstrated that its efficacy in major depressive disorder is maintained for periods of up to 40 weeks following 8 to 12 weeks of initial treatment at a dose of 15 to 45 mg/day (see CLINICAL PHARMACOLOGY). Based on these limited data, it is unknown whether or not the dose of REMERON needed for maintenance treatment is identical to the dose needed to achieve an initial response. Patients should be periodically reassessed to determine the need for maintenance treatment and the appropriate dose for such treatment.

Switching a Patient To or From a Monoamine Oxidase Inhibitor (MAOI) Intended to Treat Psychiatric Disorders

At least 14 days should elapse between discontinuation of an MAOI intended to treat psychiatric disorders and initiation of therapy with REMERONSolTab Orally Disintegrating Tablets. Conversely, at least 14 days should be allowed after stopping REMERONSolTab before starting an MAOI intended to treat psychiatric disorders (see CONTRAINDICATIONS).

Use of REMERONSolTab With Other MAOIs, Such as Linezolid or Methylene Blue

Do not start REMERONSolTab in a patient who is being treated with linezolid or intravenous methylene blue because there is an increased risk of serotonin syndrome. In a patient who requires more urgent treatment of a psychiatric condition, other interventions, including hospitalization, should be considered (see CONTRAINDICATIONS).

In some cases, a patient already receiving therapy with REMERONSolTab may require urgent treatment with linezolid or intravenous methylene blue. If acceptable alternatives to linezolid or intravenous methylene blue treatment are not available and the potential benefits of linezolid or intravenous methylene blue treatment are judged to outweigh the risks of serotonin syndrome in a particular patient, REMERONSolTab should be stopped promptly, and linezolid or intravenous methylene blue can be administered. The patient should be monitored for symptoms of serotonin syndrome for 2 weeks or until 24 hours after the last dose of linezolid or intravenous methylene blue, whichever comes first. Therapy with REMERONSolTab may be resumed 24 hours after the last dose of linezolid or intravenous methylene blue (see WARNINGS).

The risk of administering methylene blue by non-intravenous routes (such as oral tablets or by local injection) or in intravenous doses much lower than 1 mg/kg with REMERONSolTab is unclear. The clinician should, nevertheless, be aware of the possibility of emergent symptoms of serotonin syndrome with such use (see WARNINGS).

Discontinuation of Remeron Treatment

Symptoms associated with the discontinuation or dose reduction of REMERONSolTab Orally Disintegrating Tablets have been reported. Patients should be monitored for these and other symptoms when discontinuing treatment or during dosage reduction. A gradual reduction in the dose over several weeks, rather than abrupt cessation, is recommended whenever possible. If intolerable symptoms occur following a decrease in the dose or upon discontinuation of treatment, dose titration should be managed on the basis of the patient's clinical response (see PRECAUTIONS and ADVERSE REACTIONS).

Information for Patients

Patients should be advised that taking REMERONSolTab can cause mild pupillary dilation, which in susceptible individuals, can lead to an episode of angle-closure glaucoma. Pre-existing glaucoma is almost always open-angle glaucoma because angle-closure glaucoma, when diagnosed, can be treated definitively with iridectomy. Open-angle glaucoma is not a risk factor for angle-closure glaucoma. Patients may wish to be examined to determine whether they are susceptible to angle-closure, and have a prophylactic procedure (e.g., iridectomy), if they are susceptible.

HOW SUPPLIED
REMERONSolTab (mirtazapine) Orally Disintegrating Tablets are supplied as:

15 mg Tablets — round, white, with "T₁Z" debossed on 1 side.

Box of 30	5 × 6 Unit Dose Blisters	NDC 0052-0106-30

30 mg Tablets — round, white, with "T₂Z" debossed on 1 side.

Box of 30	5 × 6 Unit Dose Blisters	NDC 0052-0108-30

45 mg Tablets — round, white, with "T₄Z" debossed on 1 side.

Box of 30	5 × 6 Unit Dose Blisters	NDC 0052-0110-30

Storage
Store at 25°C (77°F); excursions permitted to 15-30°C (59-86°F) [see USP Controlled Room Temperature]. Protect from light and moisture. Use immediately upon opening individual tablet blister.
Manufactured for: Merck Sharp & Dohme Corp., a subsidiary of
MERCK & CO., INC., Whitehouse Station, NJ 08889, USA
Manufactured by:
Cephalon, Inc.
Salt Lake City, UT 84116, USA
For patent information:
www.merck.com/product/patent/home.html
Copyright © 2001, 2010 Merck Sharp & Dohme B.V., a subsidiary of **Merck & Co., Inc.**
All rights reserved.
Revised: 08/2014
uspi-mk8246-toc-1408r007
Rx only

Medication Guide
REMERONSolTab® (rĕm′- ĕ - rŏn - sŏl′ – tăb)
(mirtazapine)
Orally Disintegrating Tablets
Read the Medication Guide that comes with REMERONSolTab before you start taking it and each time you get a refill. There may be new information. This Medication Guide does not take the place of talking to your healthcare provider about your medical condition or treatment. If you have any questions about REMERONSolTab, talk to your healthcare provider.

What is the most important information I should know about REMERONSolTab?
REMERONSolTab and other antidepressant medicines may cause serious side effects, including:
1. Suicidal thoughts or actions:
- **REMERONSolTab and other antidepressant medicines may increase suicidal thoughts or actions in some children, teenagers, or young adults within the first few months of treatment or when the dose is changed.**
- Depression or other serious mental illnesses are the most important causes of suicidal thoughts or actions.
- Watch for these changes and call your healthcare provider right away if you notice:
  ○ New or sudden changes in mood, behavior, actions, thoughts, or feelings, especially if severe.
  ○ Pay particular attention to such changes when REMERONSolTab is started or when the dose is changed.
Keep all follow-up visits with your healthcare provider and call between visits if you are worried about symptoms.
Call your healthcare provider right away if you have any of the following symptoms, or call 911 if an emergency, especially if they are new, worse, or worry you:
- attempts to commit suicide
- acting on dangerous impulses
- acting aggressive or violent
- thoughts about suicide or dying
- new or worse depression
- new or worse anxiety or panic attacks
- feeling agitated, restless, angry or irritable
- trouble sleeping
- an increase in activity or talking more than what is normal for you
- other unusual changes in behavior or mood
Call your healthcare provider right away if you have any of the following symptoms, or call 911 if an emergency. REMERONSolTab may be associated with these serious side effects:

2. Manic episodes:
- greatly increased energy
- severe trouble sleeping
- racing thoughts
- reckless behavior
- unusually grand ideas
- excessive happiness or irritability
- talking more or faster than usual
3. Decreased White Blood Cells called neutrophils, which are needed to fight infections. Tell your doctor if you have any indication of infection such as fever, chills, sore throat, or mouth or nose sores, especially symptoms which are flu-like.
4. Serotonin Syndrome. This condition can be life-threatening and may include:
- agitation, hallucinations, coma or other changes in mental status
- coordination problems or muscle twitching (overactive reflexes)
- racing heartbeat, high or low blood pressure
- sweating or fever
- nausea, vomiting, or diarrhea
- muscle rigidity
5. Visual problems
- eye pain
- changes in vision
- swelling or redness in or around the eye
Only some people are at risk for these problems. You may want to undergo an eye examination to see if you are at risk and receive preventative treatment if you are.
6. Seizures
7. Low salt (sodium) levels in the blood. Elderly people may be at greater risk for this. Symptoms may include:
- headache
- weakness or feeling unsteady
- confusion, problems concentrating or thinking or memory problems
8. Sleepiness. It is best to take REMERONSolTab close to bedtime.
9. Severe skin reactions: Call your doctor right away if you have any or all of the following symptoms:
- severe rash with skin swelling (including on the palms of the hands and soles of the feet)
- painful reddening of the skin and/or blisters/ulcers on the body or in the mouth
10. Severe allergic reactions: trouble breathing, swelling of the face, tongue, eyes or mouth
- rash, itchy welts (hives) or blisters, alone or with fever or joint pain
11. Increases in appetite or weight. Children and adolescents should have height and weight monitored during treatment.
12. Increased cholesterol and triglyceride levels in your blood
Do not stop REMERONSolTab without first talking to your healthcare provider. Stopping REMERONSolTab too quickly may cause potentially serious symptoms including:
- dizziness
- abnormal dreams
- agitation
- anxiety
- fatigue
- confusion
- headache
- shaking
- tingling sensation
- nausea, vomiting
- sweating

What is REMERONSolTab?
REMERONSolTab is a prescription medicine used to treat depression. It is important to talk with your healthcare provider about the risks of treating depression and also the risks of not treating it. You should discuss all treatment choices with your healthcare provider.
Talk to your healthcare provider if you do not think that your condition is getting better with REMERONSolTab treatment.
Who should not take REMERONSolTab?
Do not take REMERONSolTab:
- if you are allergic to mirtazapine or any of the ingredients in REMERONSolTab. See the end of this Medication Guide for a complete list of ingredients in REMERONSolTab.
- if you take a monoamine oxidase inhibitor (MAOI). Ask your healthcare provider or pharmacist if you are not sure if you take an MAOI, including the antibiotic linezolid.
- Do not take an MAOI within 2 weeks of stopping REMERONSolTab unless directed to do so by your physician.
- Do not start REMERONSolTab if you stopped taking an MAOI in the last 2 weeks unless directed to do so by your physician.

People who take REMERONSolTab close in time to an MAOI may have serious or even life-threatening side effects. Get medical help right away if you have any of these symptoms:
- high fever
- uncontrolled muscle spasms
- stiff muscles
- rapid changes in heart rate or blood pressure
- confusion
- loss of consciousness (pass out)
What should I tell my healthcare provider before taking REMERONSolTab?
Ask if you are not sure.
Before starting REMERONSolTab, tell your healthcare provider if you:
- are taking certain drugs such as:
  ○ Triptans used to treat migraine headache
  ○ Medicines used to treat mood, anxiety, psychotic or thought disorders, including tricyclics, lithium, SSRIs, SNRIs, or antipsychotics
  ○ Tramadol used to treat pain
  ○ Over-the-counter supplements such as tryptophan or St. John's wort
  ○ Phenytoin, carbamazepine, or rifampicin (these drugs can decrease your blood level of REMERONSolTab)
  ○ Cimetidine or ketoconazole (these drugs can increase your blood level of REMERONSolTab)
- Have or had:
  ○ liver problems
  ○ kidney problems
  ○ heart problems
  ○ seizures or convulsions
  ○ bipolar disorder or mania
  ○ a tendency to get dizzy or faint
- are pregnant or plan to become pregnant. It is not known if REMERONSolTab will harm your unborn baby. Talk to your healthcare provider about the benefits and risks of treating depression during pregnancy
- are breastfeeding or plan to breastfeed. Some REMERONSolTab may pass into your breast milk. Talk to your healthcare provider about the best way to feed your baby while taking REMERONSolTab
Tell your healthcare provider about all the medicines that you take, including prescription and non-prescription medicines, vitamins, and herbal supplements. REMERONSolTab and some medicines may interact with each other, may not work as well, or may cause serious side effects.
Your healthcare provider or pharmacist can tell you if it is safe to take REMERONSolTab with your other medicines. Do not start or stop any medicine while taking REMERONSolTab without talking to your healthcare provider first.

> If you take REMERONSolTab, you should not take any other medicines that contain mirtazapine including REMERON® Tablets.

How should I take REMERONSolTab?
- Take REMERONSolTab exactly as prescribed. Your healthcare provider may need to change the dose of REMERONSolTab until it is the right dose for you.
- Take REMERONSolTab at the same time each day, preferably in the evening at bedtime.
- Open the tablet blister pack with dry hands and place the tablet whole on the tongue, immediately after removal from the blister pack.
- REMERONSolTab will disintegrate rapidly on the tongue and can be swallowed with saliva. No water is needed for taking it.
- Do not attempt to split the REMERONSolTab.
- It is common for antidepressant medicines such as REMERONSolTab to take up to a few weeks before you start to feel better. Do not stop taking REMERONSolTab if you do not feel results right away.
- Do not stop taking or change the dose of REMERONSolTab without first talking to your doctor, even if you feel better.
- REMERONSolTab may be taken with or without food.
- If you miss a dose of REMERONSolTab, take the missed dose as soon as you remember. If it is almost time for the next dose, skip the missed dose and take your next dose at the regular time. Do not take two doses of REMERONSolTab at the same time.
- If you take too much REMERONSolTab, call your healthcare provider or poison control center right away, or get emergency treatment.

What should I avoid while taking REMERONSolTab?

- REMERONSolTab can cause sleepiness or may affect your ability to make decisions, think clearly, or react quickly. You should not drive, operate heavy machinery, or do other dangerous activities until you know how REMERONSolTab affects you.
- Avoid drinking alcohol or taking diazepam (a medicine used for anxiety, insomnia and seizures, for example) or similar medicines while taking REMERONSolTab. If you are uncertain about whether certain medication can be taken with REMERONSolTab, please discuss with your doctor.

What are the possible side effects of REMERONSolTab?

REMERONSolTab may cause serious side effects, including all of those described in the section entitled "What is the most important information I should know about REMERONSolTab?"

Common possible side effects in people who take REMERONSolTab include:

- sleepiness
- increased appetite, weight gain
- dry mouth
- constipation
- dizziness
- abnormal dreams

Tell your healthcare provider if you have any side effect that bothers you or that does not go away. These are not all the possible side effects of REMERONSolTab. For more information, ask your healthcare provider or pharmacist.

CALL YOUR DOCTOR FOR MEDICAL ADVICE ABOUT SIDE EFFECTS. YOU MAY REPORT SIDE EFFECTS TO THE FDA AT 1-800-FDA-1088.

How should I store REMERONSolTab?

- Store REMERONSolTab at room temperature 25°C (77°F). Storage at 15°C-30°C (59°F-86°F) is permitted occasionally.
- Keep REMERONSolTab away from light and moisture.
- Use immediately upon opening individual tablet blister.

Keep REMERONSolTab and all medicines out of the reach of children.

General information about REMERONSolTab

Medicines are sometimes prescribed for purposes other than those listed in a Medication Guide. Do not use REMERONSolTab for a condition for which it was not prescribed. Do not give REMERONSolTab to other people, even if they have the same condition. It may harm them.

This Medication Guide summarizes the most important information about REMERONSolTab. If you would like more information, talk with your healthcare provider. You may ask your healthcare provider or pharmacist for information about REMERONSolTab that is written for healthcare professionals.

For more information about REMERONSolTab call 1-800-526-4099 or go to www.REMERONSolTab.com.

What are the ingredients in REMERONSolTab?

Active ingredient: mirtazapine

Inactive ingredients 15mg, 30mg and 45mg tablets: Aspartame, citric acid anhydrous, crospovidone, magnesium stearate, mannitol, microcrystalline cellulose, natural and artificial orange flavor, sodium bicarbonate, hypromellose, povidone, sugar spheres, Eudragit E100.

This Medication Guide has been approved by the U.S. Food and Drug Administration.

Manufactured for: Merck Sharp & Dohme Corp., a subsidiary of
MERCK & Co., INC., Whitehouse Station, NJ 08889, USA
Manufactured by:
Cephalon, Inc.
Salt Lake City, UT 84116, USA
For patent information:
www.merck.com/product/patent/home.html
Copyright © 2007, 2009 Merck Sharp & Dohme B.V., a subsidiary of **Merck & Co., Inc.**
All rights reserved.
Revised: 08/2014
usmg-mk8246-tod-1408r007

Shown in Product Identification Guide, page 309

ROTATEQ ℞

[Row-ta-tech]
(Rotavirus Vaccine, Live, Oral, Pentavalent)
Oral Solution

HIGHLIGHTS OF PRESCRIBING INFORMATION
These highlights do not include all the information needed to use RotaTeq safely and effectively. See full prescribing information for RotaTeq.
RotaTeq (Rotavirus Vaccine, Live, Oral, Pentavalent) Oral Solution
Initial U.S. Approval: 2006

———RECENT MAJOR CHANGES———

Warnings and Precautions
 Managing Allergic Reactions (5.1)   12/2012
 Intussusception (5.3)   06/2013

———INDICATIONS AND USAGE———

RotaTeq® is indicated for the prevention of rotavirus gastroenteritis caused by the G1, G2, G3 and G4 serotypes contained in the vaccine. (1)
RotaTeq is approved for use in infants 6 weeks to 32 weeks of age.

———DOSAGE AND ADMINISTRATION———

- FOR ORAL USE ONLY. NOT FOR INJECTION. (2)
- The vaccination series consists of three ready-to-use liquid doses of RotaTeq administered orally starting at 6 to 12 weeks of age, with the subsequent doses administered at 4- to 10-week intervals. The third dose should not be given after 32 weeks of age. (2)

———DOSAGE FORMS AND STRENGTHS———

2 mL solution for oral administration of 5 live human-bovine reassortant rotaviruses which contains a minimum of $2.0 - 2.8 \times 10^6$ infectious units (IU) per reassortant dose, depending on the serotype, and not greater than 116×10^6 IU per aggregate dose. (3)

———CONTRAINDICATIONS———

- A demonstrated history of hypersensitivity to the vaccine or any component of the vaccine. (4.1)
- History of Severe Combined Immunodeficiency Disease (SCID). (4.2) (6.2)
- History of intussusception. (4.3)

———WARNINGS AND PRECAUTIONS———

- No safety or efficacy data are available from clinical trials regarding the administration of RotaTeq to infants who are potentially immunocompromised (e.g., HIV/AIDS). (5.2)
- In a post-marketing study, cases of intussusception were observed in temporal association within 21 days following the first dose of RotaTeq, with a clustering of cases in the first 7 days. (5.3, 6.2)
- No safety or efficacy data are available for the administration of RotaTeq to infants with a history of gastrointestinal disorders (e.g., active acute gastrointestinal illness, chronic diarrhea, failure to thrive, history of congenital abdominal disorders, and abdominal surgery). (5.4)
- Vaccine virus transmission from vaccine recipient to non-vaccinated contacts has been reported. Caution is advised when considering whether to administer RotaTeq to individuals with immunodeficient contacts. (5.5)

———ADVERSE REACTIONS———

Most common adverse events included diarrhea, vomiting, irritability, otitis media, nasopharyngitis, and bronchospasm. (6.1)

To report SUSPECTED ADVERSE REACTIONS, contact Merck Sharp & Dohme Corp., a subsidiary of Merck & Co., Inc., at 1-877-888-4231 or VAERS at 1-800-822-7967 or www.vaers.hhs.gov{4}.

———USE IN SPECIFIC POPULATIONS———

Pediatric Use: Safety and efficacy have not been established in infants less than 6 weeks of age or greater than 32 weeks of age. Data are available from clinical studies to support the use of RotaTeq in:

- Pre-term infants according to their age in weeks since birth
- Infants with controlled gastroesophageal reflux disease. (8.4)

See 17 for PATIENT COUNSELING INFORMATION and FDA-approved patient labeling

                    Revised: 06/2013

FULL PRESCRIBING INFORMATION

1   INDICATIONS AND USAGE

RotaTeq® is indicated for the prevention of rotavirus gastroenteritis in infants and children caused by the serotypes G1, G2, G3, and G4 when administered as a 3-dose series to infants between the ages of 6 to 32 weeks. The first dose of RotaTeq should be administered between 6 and 12 weeks of age *[see Dosage and Administration (2)]*.

2   DOSAGE AND ADMINISTRATION

FOR ORAL USE ONLY. NOT FOR INJECTION.

The vaccination series consists of three ready-to-use liquid doses of RotaTeq administered orally starting at 6 to 12 weeks of age, with the subsequent doses administered at 4- to 10-week intervals. The third dose should not be given after 32 weeks of age *[see Clinical Studies (14)]*.

There are no restrictions on the infant's consumption of food or liquid, including breast milk, either before or after vaccination with RotaTeq.

Do not mix the RotaTeq vaccine with any other vaccines or solutions. Do not reconstitute or dilute *[see Dosage and Administration (2.2)]*.

For storage instructions *[see How Supplied/Storage and Handling (16.1)]*.

Each dose is supplied in a container consisting of a squeezable plastic dosing tube with a twist-off cap, allowing for direct oral administration. The dosing tube is contained in a pouch *[see Dosage and Administration (2.2)]*.

2.1   Use with Other Vaccines

In clinical trials, RotaTeq was administered concomitantly with other licensed pediatric vaccines *[see Adverse Reactions (6.1), Drug Interactions (7.1), and Clinical Studies (14)]*.

2.2   Instructions for Use

To administer the vaccine:

Tear open the pouch and remove the dosing tube.

Clear the fluid from the dispensing tip by holding tube vertically and tapping cap.

Help Patients Save on Rx Drugs: PDR.net/PharmacyDiscountCard

Open the dosing tube in 2 easy motions:

1. Puncture the dispensing tip by screwing cap *clockwise* until it becomes tight.

2. Remove cap by turning it *counterclockwise.*

Administer dose by gently squeezing liquid into infant's mouth toward the inner cheek until dosing tube is empty. (A residual drop may remain in the tip of the tube.)

If for any reason an incomplete dose is administered (e.g., infant spits or regurgitates the vaccine), a replacement dose is not recommended, since such dosing was not studied in the clinical trials. The infant should continue to receive any remaining doses in the recommended series.

Discard the empty tube and cap in approved biological waste containers according to local regulations.

3 DOSAGE FORMS AND STRENGTHS

RotaTeq, 2 mL for oral use, is a ready-to-use solution of live reassortant rotaviruses, containing G1, G2, G3, G4 and P1A[8] which contains a minimum of $2.0 - 2.8 \times 10^6$ infectious units (IU) per individual reassortant dose, depending on the serotype, and not greater than 116×10^6 IU per aggregate dose.

Each dose is supplied in a container consisting of a squeezable plastic dosing tube with a twist-off cap, allowing for direct oral administration. The dosing tube is contained in a pouch.

4 CONTRAINDICATIONS

4.1 Hypersensitivity

A demonstrated history of hypersensitivity to any component of the vaccine.

Infants who develop symptoms suggestive of hypersensitivity after receiving a dose of RotaTeq should not receive further doses of RotaTeq.

4.2 Severe Combined Immunodeficiency Disease

Infants with Severe Combined Immunodeficiency Disease (SCID) should not receive RotaTeq. Post-marketing reports of gastroenteritis, including severe diarrhea and prolonged

shedding of vaccine virus, have been reported in infants who were administered RotaTeq and later identified as having SCID [see Adverse Reactions (6.2)].

4.3 History of Intussusception

Infants with a history of intussusception should not receive RotaTeq.

5 WARNINGS AND PRECAUTIONS

5.1 Managing Allergic Reactions

Appropriate medical treatment and supervision must be available to manage possible anaphylactic reactions following administration of the vaccine.

5.2 Immunocompromised Populations

No safety or efficacy data are available from clinical trials regarding the administration of RotaTeq to infants who are potentially immunocompromised including:

- Infants with blood dyscrasias, leukemia, lymphomas of any type, or other malignant neoplasms affecting the bone marrow or lymphatic system.
- Infants on immunosuppressive therapy (including high-dose systemic corticosteroids). RotaTeq may be administered to infants who are being treated with topical corticosteroids or inhaled steroids.
- Infants with primary and acquired immunodeficiency states, including HIV/AIDS or other clinical manifestations of infection with human immunodeficiency viruses; cellular immune deficiencies; and hypogammaglobulinemic and dysgammaglobulinemic states. There are insufficient data from the clinical trials to support administration of RotaTeq to infants with indeterminate HIV status who are born to mothers with HIV/AIDS.
- Infants who have received a blood transfusion or blood products, including immunoglobulins within 42 days.

Vaccine virus transmission from vaccine recipient to non-vaccinated contacts has been reported [see Warnings and Precautions (5.5)].

5.3 Intussusception

Following administration of a previously licensed live rhesus rotavirus reassortant vaccine, an increased risk of intussusception was observed.{1}

In a post-marketing observational study in the US cases of intussusception were observed within 21 days following the first dose of RotaTeq, with a clustering of cases in the first 7 days. [See Adverse Reactions (6.2)]

In worldwide passive post-marketing surveillance, cases of intussusception have been reported in temporal association with RotaTeq. [See Adverse Reactions (6.2)]

5.4 Gastrointestinal Illness

No safety or efficacy data are available for administration of RotaTeq to infants with a history of gastrointestinal disorders including infants with active acute gastrointestinal illness, infants with chronic diarrhea and failure to thrive, and infants with a history of congenital abdominal disorders, and abdominal surgery. Caution is advised when considering administration of RotaTeq to these infants.

5.5 Shedding and Transmission

Shedding of vaccine virus was evaluated among a subset of subjects in the Rotavirus Efficacy and Safety Trial (REST) 4 to 6 days after each dose and among all subjects who submitted a stool antigen rotavirus positive sample at any time. RotaTeq was shed in the stools of 32 of 360 [8.9%, 95% CI (6.2%, 12.3%)] vaccine recipients tested after dose 1; 0 of 249 [0.0%, 95% CI (0.0%, 1.5%)] vaccine recipients tested after dose 2; and in 1 of 385 [0.3%, 95% CI (<0.1%, 1.4%)] vaccine recipients after dose 3. In phase 3 studies, shedding was observed as early as 1 day and as late as 15 days after a dose. Transmission of vaccine virus was not evaluated in phase 3 studies.

Transmission of vaccine virus strains from vaccinees to non-vaccinated contacts has been observed post-marketing.

The potential risk of transmission of vaccine virus should be weighed against the risk of acquiring and transmitting natural rotavirus.

Caution is advised when considering whether to administer RotaTeq to individuals with immunodeficient close contacts such as:

- Individuals with malignancies or who are otherwise immunocompromised;

- Individuals with primary immunodeficiency; or
- Individuals receiving immunosuppressive therapy.

5.6 Febrile Illness

Febrile illness may be reason for delaying use of RotaTeq except when, in the opinion of the physician, withholding the vaccine entails a greater risk. Low-grade fever (<100.5°F [38.1°C]) itself and mild upper respiratory infection do not preclude vaccination with RotaTeq.

5.7 Incomplete Regimen

The clinical studies were not designed to assess the level of protection provided by only one or two doses of RotaTeq.

5.8 Limitations of Vaccine Effectiveness

RotaTeq may not protect all vaccine recipients against rotavirus.

5.9 Post-Exposure Prophylaxis

No clinical data are available for RotaTeq when administered after exposure to rotavirus.

6 ADVERSE REACTIONS

6.1 Clinical Studies Experience

71,725 infants were evaluated in 3 placebo-controlled clinical trials including 36,165 infants in the group that received RotaTeq and 35,560 infants in the group that received placebo. Parents/guardians were contacted on days 7, 14, and 42 after each dose regarding intussusception and any other serious adverse events. The racial distribution was as follows: White (69% in both groups); Hispanic-American (14% in both groups); Black (8% in both groups); Multiracial (5% in both groups); Asian (2% in both groups); Native American (RotaTeq 2%, placebo 1%); and Other (<1% in both groups). The gender distribution was 51% male and 49% female in both vaccination groups.

Because clinical trials are conducted under conditions that may not be typical of those observed in clinical practice, the adverse reaction rates presented below may not be reflective of those observed in clinical practice.

Serious Adverse Events

Serious adverse events occurred in 2.4% of recipients of RotaTeq when compared to 2.6% of placebo recipients within the 42-day period of a dose in the phase 3 clinical studies of RotaTeq. The most frequently reported serious adverse events for RotaTeq compared to placebo were:

bronchiolitis	(0.6% RotaTeq vs. 0.7% Placebo),
gastroenteritis	(0.2% RotaTeq vs. 0.3% Placebo),
pneumonia	(0.2% RotaTeq vs. 0.2% Placebo),
fever	(0.1% RotaTeq vs. 0.1% Placebo), and
urinary tract infection	(0.1% RotaTeq vs. 0.1% Placebo).

Deaths

Across the clinical studies, 52 deaths were reported. There were 25 deaths in the RotaTeq recipients compared to 27 deaths in the placebo recipients. The most commonly reported cause of death was sudden infant death syndrome, which was observed in 8 recipients of RotaTeq and 9 placebo recipients.

Intussusception

In REST, 34,837 vaccine recipients and 34,788 placebo recipients were monitored by active surveillance to identify potential cases of intussusception at 7, 14, and 42 days after each dose, and every 6 weeks thereafter for 1 year after the first dose.

For the primary safety outcome, cases of intussusception occurring within 42 days of any dose, there were 6 cases among RotaTeq recipients and 5 cases among placebo recipients (see Table 1). The data did not suggest an increased risk of intussusception relative to placebo.

Table 1: Confirmed cases of intussusception in recipients of RotaTeq as compared with placebo recipients during REST

	RotaTeq (n=34,837)	Placebo (n=34,788)
Confirmed intussusception cases within 42 days of any dose	6	5
Relative risk (95% CI) *	1.6 (0.4, 6.4)	
Confirmed intussusception cases within 365 days of dose 1	13	15
Relative risk (95% CI)	0.9 (0.4, 1.9)	

* Relative risk and 95% confidence interval based upon group sequential design stopping criteria employed in REST.

Among vaccine recipients, there were no confirmed cases of intussusception within the 42-day period after the first dose, which was the period of highest risk for the rhesus rotavirus-based product (see Table 2).

[See table 2 below]

All of the children who developed intussusception recovered without sequelae with the exception of a 9-month-old male who developed intussusception 98 days after dose 3 and

Table 2: Intussusception cases by day range in relation to dose in REST

Day Range	Dose 1 RotaTeq	Dose 1 Placebo	Dose 2 RotaTeq	Dose 2 Placebo	Dose 3 RotaTeq	Dose 3 Placebo	Any Dose RotaTeq	Any Dose Placebo
1-7	0	0	1	0	0	0	1	0
1-14	0	0	1	0	0	1	1	1
1-21	0	0	3	0	0	1	3	1
1-42	0	1	4	1	2	3	6	5

died of post-operative sepsis. There was a single case of in-tussusception among 2,470 recipients of RotaTeq in a 7-month-old male in the phase 1 and 2 studies (716 placebo recipients).

Hematochezia

Hematochezia reported as an adverse experience occurred in 0.6% (39/6,130) of vaccine and 0.6% (34/5,560) of placebo recipients within 42 days of any dose. Hematochezia reported as a serious adverse experience occurred in <0.1% (4/36,150) of vaccine and <0.1% (7/35,536) of placebo recipients within 42 days of any dose.

Seizures

All seizures reported in the phase 3 trials of RotaTeq (by vaccination group and interval after dose) are shown in Table 3.

Table 3: Seizures reported by day range in relation to any dose in the phase 3 trials of RotaTeq

Day range	1-7	1-14	1-42
RotaTeq	10	15	33
Placebo	5	8	24

Seizures reported as serious adverse experiences occurred in <0.1% (27/36,150) of vaccine and <0.1% (18/35,536) of placebo recipients (not significant). Ten febrile seizures were reported as serious adverse experiences, 5 were observed in vaccine recipients and 5 in placebo recipients.

Kawasaki Disease

In the phase 3 clinical trials, infants were followed for up to 42 days of vaccine dose. Kawasaki disease was reported in 5 of 36,150 vaccine recipients and in 1 of 35,536 placebo recipients with unadjusted relative risk 4.9 (95% CI 0.6, 239.1).

Most Common Adverse Events

Solicited Adverse Events

Detailed safety information was collected from 11,711 infants (6,138 recipients of RotaTeq) which included a subset of subjects in REST and all subjects from Studies 007 and 009 (Detailed Safety Cohort). A Vaccination Report Card was used by parents/guardians to record the child's temperature and any episodes of diarrhea and vomiting on a daily basis during the first week following each vaccination. Table 4 summarizes the frequencies of these adverse events and irritability.

[See table 4 above]

Other Adverse Events

Parents/guardians of the 11,711 infants were also asked to report the presence of other events on the Vaccination Report Card for 42 days after each dose.

Fever was observed at similar rates in vaccine (N=6,138) and placebo (N=5,573) recipients (42.6% vs. 42.8%). Adverse events that occurred at a statistically higher incidence (i.e., 2-sided p-value <0.05) within the 42 days of any dose among recipients of RotaTeq as compared with placebo recipients are shown in Table 5.

Table 5: Adverse events that occurred at a statistically higher incidence within 42 days of any dose among recipients of RotaTeq as compared with placebo recipients

Adverse event	RotaTeq N=6,138	Placebo N=5,573
	n (%)	n (%)
Diarrhea	1,479 (24.1%)	1,186 (21.3%)
Vomiting	929 (15.2%)	758 (13.6%)
Otitis media	887 (14.5%)	724 (13.0%)
Nasopharyngitis	422 (6.9%)	325 (5.8%)
Bronchospasm	66 (1.1%)	40 (0.7%)

Safety in Pre-Term Infants

RotaTeq or placebo was administered to 2,070 pre-term infants (25 to 36 weeks gestational age, median 34 weeks) according to their age in weeks since birth in REST. All pre-term infants were followed for serious adverse experiences; a subset of 308 infants was monitored for all adverse experiences. There were 4 deaths throughout the study, 2 among vaccine recipients (1 SIDS and 1 motor vehicle accident) and 2 among placebo recipients (1 SIDS and 1 unknown cause). No cases of intussusception were reported. Serious adverse experiences occurred in 5.5% of vaccine and 5.8% of placebo recipients. The most common serious adverse experience was bronchiolitis, which occurred in 1.4% of vaccine and 2.0% of placebo recipients. Parents/guardians were asked to record the child's temperature and any episodes of vomiting and diarrhea daily for the first week following vaccination. The frequencies of these adverse experiences and irritability within the week after dose 1 are summarized in Table 6.

[See table 6 above]

Table 4: Solicited adverse experiences within the first week after doses 1, 2, and 3 (Detailed Safety Cohort)

Adverse experience	Dose 1		Dose 2		Dose 3	
	RotaTeq	Placebo	RotaTeq	Placebo	RotaTeq	Placebo
Elevated temperature*	n=5,616 17.1%	n=5,077 16.2%	n=5,215 20.0%	n=4,725 19.4%	n=4,865 18.2%	n=4,382 17.6%
	n=6,130	n=5,560	n=5,703	n=5,173	n=5,496	n=4,989
Vomiting	6.7%	5.4%	5.0%	4.4%	3.6%	3.2%
Diarrhea	10.4%	9.1%	8.6%	6.4%	6.1%	5.4%
Irritability	7.1%	7.1%	6.0%	6.5%	4.3%	4.5%

* Temperature ≥100.5°F [38.1°C] rectal equivalent obtained by adding 1 degree F to otic and oral temperatures and 2 degrees F to axillary temperatures

Table 6: Solicited adverse experiences within the first week of doses 1, 2, and 3 among pre-term infants

Adverse event	Dose 1		Dose 2		Dose 3	
	RotaTeq	Placebo	RotaTeq	Placebo	RotaTeq	Placebo
Elevated temperature*	N=127 18.1%	N=133 17.3%	N=124 25.0%	N=121 28.1%	N=115 14.8%	N=108 20.4%
	N=154	N=154	N=137	N=137	N=135	N=129
Vomiting	5.8%	7.8%	2.9%	2.2%	4.4%	4.7%
Diarrhea	6.5%	5.8%	7.3%	7.3%	3.7%	3.9%
Irritability	3.9%	5.2%	2.9%	4.4%	8.1%	5.4%

* Temperature ≥100.5°F [38.1°C] rectal equivalent obtained by adding 1 degree F to otic and oral temperatures and 2 degrees F to axillary temperatures

6.2 Post-Marketing Experience

The following adverse events have been identified during post-approval use of RotaTeq from reports to the Vaccine Adverse Event Reporting System (VAERS).

Reporting of adverse events following immunization to VAERS is voluntary, and the number of doses of vaccine administered is not known; therefore, it is not always possible to reliably estimate the adverse event frequency or establish a causal relationship to vaccine exposure using VAERS data.

In post-marketing experience, the following adverse events have been reported following the use of RotaTeq:

Immune system disorders:
Anaphylactic reaction

Gastrointestinal disorders:
Intussusception (including death)
Hematochezia
Gastroenteritis with vaccine viral shedding in infants with Severe Combined Immunodeficiency Disease (SCID)

Skin and subcutaneous tissue disorders:
Urticaria
Angioedema

Infections and infestations:
Kawasaki disease
Transmission of vaccine virus strains from vaccine recipient to non-vaccinated contacts.

Post-Marketing Observational Safety Surveillance Studies

The temporal association between vaccination with RotaTeq and intussusception was evaluated in the Post-licensure Rapid Immunization Safety Monitoring (PRISM) program [2], an electronic active surveillance program comprised of 3 US health insurance plans.

More than 1.2 million RotaTeq vaccinations (507,000 of which were first doses) administered to infants 5 through 36 weeks of age were evaluated. From 2004 through 2011, potential cases of intussusception in either the inpatient or emergency department setting and vaccine exposures were identified through electronic procedure and diagnosis codes. Medical records were reviewed to confirm intussusception and rotavirus vaccination status.

The risk of intussusception was assessed using self-controlled risk interval and cohort designs, with adjustment for age. Risk windows of 1-7 and 1-21 days were evaluated. Cases of intussusception were observed in temporal association within 21 days following the first dose of RotaTeq, with a clustering of cases in the first 7 days. Based on the results, approximately 1 to 1.5 excess cases of intussusception occur per 100,000 vaccinated US infants within 21 days following the first dose of RotaTeq. In the first year of life, the background rate of intussusception hospitalizations in the US has been estimated to be approximately 34 per 100,000 infants.[3]

In an earlier prospective post-marketing observational cohort study conducted using a large US medical claims database, the risks of intussusception or Kawasaki disease resulting in emergency department visits or hospitalizations during the 30 days following any dose of vaccine were analyzed among 85,150 infants receiving one or more doses of RotaTeq from February 2006 through March 2009. Medical

charts were reviewed to confirm these diagnoses. Evaluation included concurrent (n = 62,617) and historical (n=100,000 from 2001-2005) control groups of infants who received diphtheria, tetanus and acellular pertussis vaccine (DTaP) but not RotaTeq.

Confirmed intussusception cases in the RotaTeq group were compared with those in the concurrent DTaP control group and in the historical control group. The data were analyzed post-dose 1 and post any dose, in both 7 day and 30 day risk windows. A statistically significant increased risk of intussusception after RotaTeq vaccination was not observed.

One confirmed case of Kawasaki disease (23 days post-dose 3) was identified among infants vaccinated with RotaTeq and one confirmed case of Kawasaki disease (22 days post-dose 2) was identified among concurrent DTaP controls (relative risk = 0.7; 95% CI: 0.01-55.56).

In addition, general safety was monitored by electronic search of the automated records database for all emergency department visits and hospitalizations in the 30-day period after each dose of RotaTeq compared with: 1) days 31-60 after each dose of RotaTeq (self-matched controls) and 2) the 30-day period after each dose of DTaP vaccine (historical control subset from 2004-2005, n=40,000). In safety analyses which evaluated multiple follow-up windows after vaccination (days: 0-7, 1-7, 8-14 and 0-30), no safety concerns were identified for infants vaccinated with RotaTeq when compared with self-matched controls and the historical control subset.

Reporting Adverse Events

Parents or guardians should be instructed to report any adverse reactions to their health care provider.

Health care providers should report all adverse events to the U.S. Department of Health and Human Services' Vaccine Adverse Events Reporting System (VAERS).

VAERS accepts all reports of suspected adverse events after the administration of any vaccine, including but not limited to the reporting of events required by the National Childhood Vaccine Injury Act of 1986. For information or a copy of the vaccine reporting form, call the VAERS toll-free number at 1-800-822-7967 or report on line to www.vaers.hhs.gov.[4]

7 DRUG INTERACTIONS

Immunosuppressive therapies including irradiation, antimetabolites, alkylating agents, cytotoxic drugs and corticosteroids (used in greater than physiologic doses), may reduce the immune response to vaccines.

7.1 Concomitant Vaccine Administration

In clinical trials, RotaTeq was administered concomitantly with diphtheria and tetanus toxoids and acellular pertussis (DTaP), inactivated poliovirus vaccine (IPV), H. influenzae type b conjugate (Hib), hepatitis B vaccine, and pneumococcal conjugate vaccine *[see Clinical Studies (14)]*. The safety data available are in the ADVERSE REACTIONS section *[see Adverse Reactions (6.1)]*. There was no evidence for reduced antibody responses to the vaccines that were concomitantly administered with RotaTeq.

8 USE IN SPECIFIC POPULATIONS

8.1 Pregnancy

Pregnancy Category C: Animal reproduction studies have not been conducted with RotaTeq. It is also not known

Table 7

Name of Reassortant	Human Rotavirus Parent Strains and Outer Surface Protein Compositions	Bovine Rotavirus Parent Strain and Outer Surface Protein Composition	Reassortant Outer Surface Protein Composition (Human Rotavirus Component in Bold)	Minimum Dose Levels (10^6 infectious units)
G1	WI79 – G1P1A[8]		**G1**P7[5]	2.2
G2	SC2 – G2P2[6]		**G2**P7[5]	2.8
G3	WI78 – G3P1A[8]	WC3 - G6, P7[5]	**G3**P7[5]	2.2
G4	BrB – G4P2[6]		**G4**P7[5]	2.0
P1A[8]	WI79 – G1P1A[8]		G6**P1A[8]**	2.3

Table 8: Efficacy of RotaTeq against any grade of severity of and severe* G1-4 rotavirus gastroenteritis through the first rotavirus season postvaccination in REST

	Per Protocol		Intent-to-Treat[†]	
	RotaTeq	Placebo	RotaTeq	Placebo
Subjects vaccinated	2,834	2,839	2,834	2,839
Gastroenteritis cases				
Any grade of severity	82	315	150	371
Severe*	1	51	2	55

	Efficacy estimate % and (95% confidence interval)	
Any grade of severity	74.0 (66.8, 79.9)	60.0 (51.5, 67.1)
Severe*	98.0 (88.3, 100.0)	96.4 (86.2, 99.6)

* Severe gastroenteritis defined by a clinical scoring system based on the intensity and duration of symptoms of fever, vomiting, diarrhea, and behavioral changes
† ITT analysis includes all subjects in the efficacy cohort who received at least one dose of vaccine.

Table 9: Efficacy of RotaTeq in reducing G1-4 rotavirus-related hospitalizations in REST

	Per Protocol		Intent-to-Treat*	
	RotaTeq	Placebo	RotaTeq	Placebo
Subjects vaccinated	34,035	34,003	34,035	34,003
Number of hospitalizations	6	144	10	187
Efficacy estimate % and (95% confidence interval)	95.8 (90.5, 98.2)		94.7 (89.3, 97.3)	

* ITT analysis includes all subjects who received at least one dose of vaccine.

whether RotaTeq can cause fetal harm when administered to a pregnant woman or can affect reproduction capacity. RotaTeq is not indicated in women of child-bearing age and should not be administered to pregnant females.

8.4 Pediatric Use

Safety and efficacy have not been established in infants less than 6 weeks of age or greater than 32 weeks of age.

Data are available from clinical studies to support the use of RotaTeq in pre-term infants according to their age in weeks since birth [see Adverse Reactions (6.1)].

Data are available from clinical studies to support the use of RotaTeq in infants with controlled gastroesophageal reflux disease.

10 OVERDOSAGE

There have been post-marketing reports of infants who received more than one dose or a replacement dose of RotaTeq after regurgitation [see Dosage and Administration (2.2)]. In limited post-marketing experience of reported overdosage, the adverse events reported after incorrect administration of higher than recommended doses of RotaTeq were similar to adverse events observed with the approved dosage and schedule.

11 DESCRIPTION

RotaTeq is a live, oral pentavalent vaccine that contains 5 live reassortant rotaviruses. The rotavirus parent strains of the reassortants were isolated from human and bovine hosts. Four reassortant rotaviruses express one of the outer capsid proteins (G1, G2, G3, or G4) from the human rotavirus parent strain and the attachment protein (serotype P7) from the bovine rotavirus parent strain. The fifth reassortant virus expresses the attachment protein, P1A (genotype P[8]), herein referred to as serotype P1A[8], from the human rotavirus parent strain and the outer capsid protein of serotype G6 from the bovine rotavirus parent strain (see Table 7).
[See table 7 above]

The reassortants are propagated in Vero cells using standard cell culture techniques in the absence of antifungal agents.

The reassortants are suspended in a buffered stabilizer solution. Each vaccine dose contains sucrose, sodium citrate, sodium phosphate monobasic monohydrate, sodium hydroxide, polysorbate 80, cell culture media, and trace amounts of fetal bovine serum. RotaTeq contains no preservatives.

In the manufacturing process for RotaTeq, a porcine-derived material is used. DNA from porcine circoviruses (PCV) 1 and 2 has been detected in RotaTeq. PCV-1 and PCV-2 are not known to cause disease in humans.

RotaTeq is a pale yellow clear liquid that may have a pink tint.

The plastic dosing tube and cap do not contain latex.

12 CLINICAL PHARMACOLOGY

Rotavirus is a leading cause of severe acute gastroenteritis in infants and young children, with over 95% of these children infected by the time they are 5 years old.[5] The most severe cases occur among infants and young children between 6 months and 24 months of age.[6]

12.1 Mechanism of Action

The exact immunologic mechanism by which RotaTeq protects against rotavirus gastroenteritis is unknown [see Clinical Studies (14.6)]. RotaTeq is a live viral vaccine that replicates in the small intestine and induces immunity.

13 NONCLINICAL TOXICOLOGY

13.1 Carcinogenesis, Mutagenesis, Impairment of Fertility

RotaTeq has not been evaluated for its carcinogenic or mutagenic potential or its potential to impair fertility.

14 CLINICAL STUDIES

Overall, 72,324 infants were randomized in 3 placebo-controlled, phase 3 studies conducted in 11 countries on 3 continents. The data demonstrating the efficacy of RotaTeq in preventing rotavirus gastroenteritis come from 6,983 of these infants from the US (including Navajo and White Mountain Apache Nations) and Finland who were enrolled in 2 of these studies: REST and Study 007. The third trial, Study 009, provided clinical evidence supporting the consistency of manufacture and contributed data to the overall safety evaluation.

The racial distribution of the efficacy subset was as follows: White (RotaTeq 68%, placebo 69%); Hispanic-American (RotaTeq 10%, placebo 9%); Black (2% in both groups); Multiracial (RotaTeq 4%, placebo 5%); Asian (<1% in both groups); Native American (RotaTeq 15%, placebo 14%); and Other (<1% in both groups). The gender distribution was 52% male and 48% female in both vaccination groups.

The efficacy evaluations in these studies included: 1) Prevention of any grade of severity of rotavirus gastroenteritis; 2) Prevention of severe rotavirus gastroenteritis, as defined by a clinical scoring system; and 3) Reduction in hospitalizations due to rotavirus gastroenteritis.

The vaccine was given as a three-dose series to healthy infants with the first dose administered between 6 and 12 weeks of age and followed by two additional doses administered at 4- to 10-week intervals. The age of infants receiving the third dose was 32 weeks of age or less. Oral polio vaccine administration was not permitted; however, other childhood vaccines could be concomitantly administered. Breast-feeding was permitted in all studies.

The case definition for rotavirus gastroenteritis used to determine vaccine efficacy required that a subject meet both of the following clinical and laboratory criteria: (1) greater than or equal to 3 watery or looser-than-normal stools within a 24-hour period and/or forceful vomiting; and (2) rotavirus antigen detection by enzyme immunoassay (EIA) in a stool specimen taken within 14 days of onset of symptoms. The severity of rotavirus acute gastroenteritis was determined by a clinical scoring system that took into account the intensity and duration of symptoms of fever, vomiting, diarrhea, and behavioral changes.

The primary efficacy analyses included cases of rotavirus gastroenteritis caused by serotypes G1, G2, G3, and G4 that occurred at least 14 days after the third dose through the first rotavirus season post vaccination.

Analyses were also done to evaluate the efficacy of RotaTeq against rotavirus gastroenteritis caused by serotypes G1, G2, G3, and G4 at any time following the first dose through the first rotavirus season postvaccination among infants who received at least one vaccination (Intent-to-treat, ITT).

14.1 Rotavirus Efficacy and Safety Trial

Primary efficacy against any grade of severity of rotavirus gastroenteritis caused by naturally occurring serotypes G1, G2, G3, or G4 through the first rotavirus season after vaccination was 74.0% (95% CI: 66.8, 79.9) and the ITT efficacy was 60.0% (95% CI: 51.5, 67.1). Primary efficacy against severe rotavirus gastroenteritis caused by naturally occurring serotypes G1, G2, G3, or G4 through the first rotavirus season after vaccination was 98.0% (95% CI: 88.3, 100.0), and ITT efficacy was 96.4% (95% CI: 86.2, 99.6). See Table 8.
[See table 8 above]

The efficacy of RotaTeq against severe disease was also demonstrated by a reduction in hospitalizations for rotavirus gastroenteritis among all subjects enrolled in REST. RotaTeq reduced hospitalizations for rotavirus gastroenteritis caused by serotypes G1, G2, G3, and G4 through the first two years after the third dose by 95.8% (95% CI: 90.5, 98.2). The ITT efficacy in reducing hospitalizations was 94.7% (95% CI: 89.3, 97.3) as shown in Table 9.
[See table 9 above]

14.2 Study 007

Primary efficacy against any grade of severity of rotavirus gastroenteritis caused by naturally occurring serotypes G1, G2, G3, or G4 through the first rotavirus season after vaccination was 72.5% (95% CI: 50.6, 85.6) and the ITT efficacy was 58.4% (95% CI: 33.8, 74.5). Primary efficacy against severe rotavirus gastroenteritis caused by naturally occurring serotypes G1, G2, G3, or G4 through the first rotavirus season after vaccination was 100% (95% CI: 13.0, 100.0) and ITT efficacy against severe rotavirus disease was 100% (95% CI: 30.2, 100.0) as shown in Table 10.
[See table 10 at top of next page]

14.3 Multiple Rotavirus Seasons

The efficacy of RotaTeq through a second rotavirus season was evaluated in a single study (REST). Efficacy against any grade of severity of rotavirus gastroenteritis caused by rotavirus serotypes G1, G2, G3, and G4 through the two rotavirus seasons after vaccination was 71.3% (95% CI: 64.7, 76.9). The efficacy of RotaTeq in preventing cases occurring only during the second rotavirus season postvaccination was 62.6% (95% CI: 44.3, 75.4). The efficacy of RotaTeq beyond the second season postvaccination was not evaluated.

14.4 Rotavirus Gastroenteritis Regardless of Serotype

The rotavirus serotypes identified in the efficacy subset of REST and Study 007 were G1P1A[8]; G2P1[4]; G3P1A[8]; G4P1A[8]; and G9P1A[8].

In REST, the efficacy of RotaTeq against any grade of severity of naturally occurring rotavirus gastroenteritis regardless of serotype was 71.8% (95% CI: 64.5, 77.8) and efficacy against severe rotavirus disease was 98.0% (95% CI: 88.3, 99.9). The ITT efficacy starting at dose 1 was 50.9% (95% CI: 41.6, 58.9) for any grade of severity of rotavirus disease and was 96.4% (95% CI: 86.3, 99.6) for severe rotavirus disease.

In Study 007, the primary efficacy of RotaTeq against any grade of severity of rotavirus gastroenteritis regardless of serotype was 72.7% (95% CI: 51.9, 85.4) and efficacy against severe rotavirus disease was 100% (95% CI: 12.7, 100). The ITT efficacy starting at dose 1 was 48.0% (95% CI: 21.6, 66.1) for any grade of severity of rotavirus disease and was 100% (95% CI: 30.4, 100.0) for severe rotavirus disease.

14.5 Rotavirus Gastroenteritis by Serotype

The efficacy against any grade of severity of rotavirus gastroenteritis by serotype in the REST efficacy cohort is shown in Table 11.

[See table 11 above]

In a separate post hoc analysis of health care utilization data from 68,038 infants (RotaTeq 34,035 and placebo 34,003) in REST, using a case definition that included culture confirmation, hospitalization and emergency departments visits due to G9P1A[8] rotavirus gastroenteritis were reduced (RotaTeq 0 cases: placebo 14 cases) by 100% (95% CI: 69.6%, 100.0%).

14.6 Immunogenicity

A relationship between antibody responses to RotaTeq and protection against rotavirus gastroenteritis has not been established. In phase 3 studies, 92.9% to 100% of 439 recipients of RotaTeq achieved a 3-fold or more rise in serum anti-rotavirus IgA after a three-dose regimen when compared to 12.3%-20.0% of 397 placebo recipients.

15 REFERENCES

1. Murphy TV, Gargiullo PM, Massoudi MS et al. Intussusception among infants given an oral rotavirus vaccine. N Engl J Med 2001;344:564-572.
2. Yih WK, Lieu TA, Kulldorff M, et al. Intussusception risk after rotavirus vaccination in US infants. Mini-Sentinel. www.mini-sentinel.org.
3. Tate JE, Simonsen L, Viboud C, et al. Trends in intussusception hospitalizations among US infants, 1993-2004: implications for monitoring the safety of the new rotavirus vaccination program. Pediatrics 2008;121(5):e1125-e1132.
4. Centers for Disease Control and Prevention. General recommendations on immunization: recommendations of the Advisory Committee on Immunization Practices (ACIP) and the American Academy of Family Physicians (AAFP). MMWR 2002;51(RR-2):1-35.
5. Parashar UD et al. Global illness and deaths caused by rotavirus disease in children. Emerg Infect Dis 2003;9(5):565-572.
6. Parashar UD, Holman RC, Clarke MJ, Bresee JS, Glass RI. Hospitalizations associated with rotavirus diarrhea in the United States, 1993 through 1995: surveillance based on the new ICD-9-CM rotavirus-specific diagnostic code. J Infect Dis 1998;177:13-7.

16 HOW SUPPLIED/STORAGE AND HANDLING

RotaTeq, 2 mL, a solution for oral use, is a pale yellow clear liquid that may have a pink tint. It is supplied as follows:

NDC 0006-4047-41 package of 10 individually pouched single-dose tubes.

NDC 0006-4047-20 package of 25 individually pouched single-dose tubes.

The plastic dosing tube and cap do not contain latex.

16.1 Storage and Handling

Store and transport refrigerated at 2-8°C (36-46°F). RotaTeq should be administered as soon as possible after being removed from refrigeration. For information regarding stability under conditions other than those recommended, call 1-800-MERCK-90.

Protect from light.

RotaTeq should be discarded in approved biological waste containers according to local regulations.

The product must be used before the expiration date.

17 PATIENT COUNSELING INFORMATION

See FDA-Approved Patient Labeling (Patient Information). Parents or guardians should be given a copy of the required vaccine information and be given the "Patient Information" appended to this insert. Parents and/or guardians should be encouraged to read the patient information that describes the benefits and risks associated with the vaccine and ask any questions they may have during the visit *[see Warnings and Precautions (5) and Patient Information]*.

Manuf. and Dist. by: Merck Sharp & Dohme Corp., a subsidiary of **MERCK & CO., INC.**, Whitehouse Station, NJ 08889, USA

Table 10: Efficacy of RotaTeq against any grade of severity of and severe* G1-4 rotavirus gastroenteritis through the first rotavirus season postvaccination in Study 007

	Per Protocol		Intent-to-Treat[†]	
	RotaTeq	Placebo	RotaTeq	Placebo
Subjects vaccinated	650	660	650	660
Gastroenteritis cases				
Any grade of severity	15	54	27	64
Severe*	0	6	0	7

Efficacy estimate % and (95% confidence interval)

	Per Protocol		Intent-to-Treat	
Any grade of severity	72.5 (50.6, 85.6)		58.4 (33.8, 74.5)	
Severe*	100.0 (13.0, 100.0)		100.0 (30.2, 100.0)	

* Severe gastroenteritis defined by a clinical scoring system based on the intensity and duration of symptoms of fever, vomiting, diarrhea, and behavioral change
† ITT analysis includes all subjects in the efficacy cohort who received at least one dose of vaccine.

Table 11: Serotype-specific efficacy of RotaTeq against any grade of severity of rotavirus gastroenteritis among infants in the REST efficacy cohort through the first rotavirus season postvaccination (Per Protocol)

	Number of cases		
Serotype identified by PCR	RotaTeq (N=2,834)	Placebo (N=2,839)	% Efficacy (95% Confidence Interval)
Serotypes present in RotaTeq			
G1P1A[8]	72	286	74.9 (67.3, 80.9)
G2P1[4]	6	17	63.4 (2.6, 88.2)
G3P1A[8]	1	6	NS
G4P1A[8]	3	6	NS
Serotypes not present in RotaTeq			
G9P1A[8]	1	3	NS
Unidentified*	11	15	NS

N=number vaccinated
NS=not significant

* Includes rotavirus antigen-positive samples in which the specific serotype could not be identified by PCR

Copyright © 2006, 2007, 2011 Merck Sharp & Dohme Corp., a subsidiary of **Merck & Co., Inc.**
All rights reserved.
Revised: 06/2013
Printed in USA
USPI-OS-V2601306R020

Patient Information

RotaTeq® (pronounced "RŌ-tuh-tek")
rotavirus vaccine, live, oral, pentavalent

Read this information carefully before your child receives each dose of RotaTeq® in case any information about the vaccine changes. Your child will need 3 doses of the vaccine over the course of a few months. This leaflet is a summary of certain information about RotaTeq and does not take the place of talking with your child's doctor, who can give you more complete information written for health care professionals.

What is RotaTeq?

RotaTeq is an oral vaccine used to help prevent rotavirus infection in children. Rotavirus infection can cause fever, vomiting, and diarrhea that can be severe and can lead to loss of body fluids (dehydration), hospitalization and even death in some children. RotaTeq may not fully protect all children that get the vaccine, and if your child already has the virus it will not help them.

Who should not receive RotaTeq?

Your child should not get RotaTeq if:
- He or she had an allergic reaction after getting a dose of this vaccine.
- He or she is allergic to any of the ingredients of the vaccine. A list of ingredients can be found at the end of this leaflet.
- He or she has Severe Combined Immunodeficiency Disease (SCID).
- He or she has ever had intussusception, a form of blockage of the intestines.

What should I tell the doctor before my child gets RotaTeq?

Tell your doctor if your child:
- Has illness with fever. A mild fever or cold by itself is not reason to delay taking the vaccine.
- Has diarrhea or has been vomiting.
- Has not been gaining weight or is not growing as expected.
- Has a blood disorder.
- Has any type of cancer.
- Has a weak immune system because of a disease (this includes HIV/AIDS).
- Gets treatment or takes medicines that may weaken the immune system (such as high doses of steroids) or has received a blood transfusion or blood products within the past 42 days.
- Was born with gastrointestinal problems, or has had a blockage or abdominal surgery.
- Has regular close contact with a member of family or household who has a weak immune system such as someone with cancer or someone taking medicines that weaken their immune system.

What are the possible side effects of RotaTeq?

The most common side effects reported after taking RotaTeq were diarrhea, vomiting, fever, runny nose and sore throat, wheezing or coughing, and ear infection.

Call your child's doctor or go to the emergency department right away if your child has any of the following problems after getting RotaTeq, even if it has been several weeks since the last dose because these may be signs of a serious problem called intussusception:
- bad vomiting
- bad diarrhea
- severe stomach pain
- blood in the stool.

Intussusception happens when a part of the intestine gets blocked or twisted.

Since FDA approval, reports of infants with intussusception following RotaTeq have been received by the Vaccine Adverse Event Reporting System (VAERS). Intussusception occurred days and sometimes weeks after vaccination. Some infants needed hospitalization, surgery on their intestines, or a special enema to treat this problem. Death due to intussusception has occurred.

A study conducted after approval of RotaTeq showed an increased risk of intussusception in the 21 days after the first dose of RotaTeq, but especially in the first 7 days.

Other reported side effects include:
- allergic reactions, which may be severe and may include face and mouth swelling, difficulty breathing, wheezing, hives, and/or skin rash; and

- Kawasaki disease (a serious condition that can affect the heart; symptoms may include fever, rash, red eyes, red mouth, swollen glands, swollen hands and feet and, if not treated, death can occur).

Call your doctor right away if your child has any side effects that concern you or seem to get worse.

These are NOT all the possible side effects of RotaTeq. You can ask your doctor for a more complete list.

You, as a parent or guardian, may also report any adverse reactions to your child's doctor or directly to VAERS. The VAERS toll-free number is 1-800-822-7967 or report online to www.vaers.hhs.gov.

Events that have been identified or reported as side effects following RotaTeq can happen when no vaccine has been given.

What other important information should I know?
Since FDA approval, the spread of vaccine virus to non-vaccinated contacts has been reported. Tell your doctor if you have someone in your household who has a weak immune system, cancer or is taking medications that can weaken the immune system so that your doctor can provide further advice. Hand washing is recommended after diaper changes to help prevent the spread of vaccine virus.

Can RotaTeq be given with other vaccines?
Your child may get RotaTeq at the same time as other childhood vaccines.

How is RotaTeq given?
The vaccine is given by mouth. Your child will receive 3 doses of the vaccine. The first dose is given when your child is 6 to 12 weeks of age, the second dose is given 4 to 10 weeks later and the third dose is given 4 to 10 weeks after the second dose. The last (third) dose should be given to your child by 32 weeks of age.

Your doctor will gently squeeze the vaccine into your child's mouth (see Figure 1). Your infant may spit out some or all of it. If this happens, the dose does not need to be given again during that visit.

Figure 1

What do I do if my child misses a dose of RotaTeq?
All 3 doses of the vaccine should be given to your child by 32 weeks of age. Your doctor will tell you when your child should come for the follow-up doses. It is important to keep those appointments. If you forget or are not able to go back at the planned time, ask your doctor for advice.

What else should I know about RotaTeq?
This leaflet gives a summary of certain information about the vaccine. If you have any questions or concerns about RotaTeq, talk to your doctor.

What are the ingredients in RotaTeq?
5 live rotavirus strains (G1, G2, G3, G4, and P1).
Sucrose, sodium citrate, sodium phosphate monobasic monohydrate, sodium hydroxide, polysorbate 80 and also fetal bovine serum.
Parts of porcine circovirus (a virus that infects pigs) types 1 and 2 have been found in RotaTeq. Porcine circovirus type 1 (PCV-1) and porcine circovirus type 2 (PCV-2) are not known to cause disease in humans.

Rx only
Manuf. and Dist. by: Merck Sharp & Dohme Corp., a subsidiary of
MERCK & CO., INC., Whitehouse Station, NJ 08889, USA
Copyright © 2008, 2009 Merck Sharp & Dohme Corp., a subsidiary of **Merck & Co., Inc.**
All rights reserved.
Revised: 06/2013
USPPI-OS-V2601306R019

SAPHRIS®
[sa-ph-ris]
(asenapine)
sublingual tablets
℞

HIGHLIGHTS OF PRESCRIBING INFORMATION
These highlights do not include all the information needed to use SAPHRIS (asenapine) safely and effectively. See full prescribing information for SAPHRIS.
SAPHRIS® (asenapine) sublingual tablets
Initial U.S. Approval: 2009

WARNING: INCREASED MORTALITY IN ELDERLY PATIENTS WITH DEMENTIA-RELATED PSYCHOSIS
See full prescribing information for complete boxed warning.
Elderly patients with dementia-related psychosis treated with antipsychotic drugs are at an increased

---

	Starting Dose	Recommended Dose	Maximum Dose
Schizophrenia – acute treatment in adults (2.2)	5 mg sublingually twice daily	5 mg sublingually twice daily	10 mg sublingually twice daily
Schizophrenia – maintenance treatment in adults (2.2)	5 mg sublingually twice daily for one week	10 mg sublingually twice daily	10 mg sublingually twice daily
Bipolar mania – adults: monotherapy (2.3)	10 mg sublingually twice daily	5–10 mg sublingually twice daily	10 mg sublingually twice daily
Bipolar mania – adults: as an adjunct to lithium or valproate (2.3)	5 mg sublingually twice daily	5–10 mg sublingually twice daily	10 mg sublingually twice daily

risk of death. SAPHRIS is not approved for the treatment of patients with dementia-related psychosis. (5.1)

---INDICATIONS AND USAGE---
SAPHRIS is an atypical antipsychotic indicated for:
- Treatment of schizophrenia. (1.1)
  Efficacy was established in two 6-week clinical trials and one maintenance trial in patients with schizophrenia in adults. (14.1)
- Acute treatment, as monotherapy or adjunctive therapy, of manic or mixed episodes associated with bipolar I disorder. (1.2)
  Efficacy was established in two 3-week monotherapy trials and in one 3-week adjunctive trial in patients with manic or mixed episodes associated with bipolar I disorder in adults. (14.2)

---DOSAGE AND ADMINISTRATION---
[See table above]
Administration: Do not swallow tablet. SAPHRIS sublingual tablets should be placed under the tongue and left to dissolve completely. The tablet will dissolve in saliva within seconds. Eating and drinking should be avoided for 10 minutes after administration. (2.1, 17.1)

---DOSAGE FORMS AND STRENGTHS---
Sublingual tablets: 5 mg and 10 mg (3)
Sublingual tablets, black cherry flavor: 5 mg and 10 mg (3)

---CONTRAINDICATIONS---
Known hypersensitivity to SAPHRIS (asenapine), or to any components in the formulation. (4, 5.7, 17.3)

---WARNINGS AND PRECAUTIONS---
- *Cerebrovascular Adverse Events:* An increased incidence of cerebrovascular adverse events (e.g., stroke, transient ischemic attack) has been seen in elderly patients with dementia-related psychoses treated with atypical antipsychotic drugs. (5.2)
- *Neuroleptic Malignant Syndrome:* Manage with immediate discontinuation and close monitoring. (5.3)
- *Tardive Dyskinesia:* Discontinue if clinically appropriate. (5.4)
- *Hyperglycemia and Diabetes Mellitus:* Monitor patients for symptoms of hyperglycemia including polydipsia, polyuria, polyphagia, and weakness. Monitor glucose regularly in patients with, and at risk for, diabetes. (5.5)
- *Weight Gain:* Patients should receive regular monitoring of weight. (5.6)
- *Hypersensitivity Reactions:* Hypersensitivity reactions, including anaphylaxis and angioedema, have been observed. (5.7)
- *Orthostatic Hypotension and Syncope:* Dizziness, tachycardia or bradycardia, and syncope may occur, especially early in treatment. Use with caution in patients with known cardiovascular or cerebrovascular disease, and in antipsychotic-naïve patients. (5.8)
- *Leukopenia, Neutropenia, and Agranulocytosis* have been reported with antipsychotics. Patients with a pre-existing low white blood cell count (WBC) or a history of leukopenia/neutropenia should have their complete blood count (CBC) monitored frequently during the first few months of therapy and SAPHRIS should be discontinued at the first sign of a decline in WBC in the absence of other causative factors. (5.9)
- *QT Prolongation:* Increases in QT interval; avoid use with drugs that also increase the QT interval and in patients with risk factors for prolonged QT interval. (5.10)
- *Seizures:* Use cautiously in patients with a history of seizures or with conditions that lower the seizure threshold. (5.12)
- *Potential for Cognitive and Motor Impairment:* Use caution when operating machinery. (5.13)
- *Suicide:* The possibility of a suicide attempt is inherent in schizophrenia and bipolar disorder. Closely supervise high-risk patients. (5.15)

---ADVERSE REACTIONS---
Commonly observed adverse reactions (incidence ≥5% and at least twice that for placebo) were (6.1):
- Schizophrenia: akathisia, oral hypoesthesia, and somnolence.
- Bipolar Disorder (Monotherapy): somnolence, dizziness, extrapyramidal symptoms other than akathisia, and weight increased.
- Bipolar Disorder (Adjunctive): somnolence and oral hypoesthesia.

To report SUSPECTED ADVERSE REACTIONS, contact Merck Sharp & Dohme Corp., a subsidiary of Merck & Co., Inc., at 1-877-888-4231 or FDA at 1-800-FDA-1088 or www.fda.gov/medwatch.

---DRUG INTERACTIONS---
- *Fluvoxamine (strong CYP1A2 inhibitor) and Paroxetine (CYP2D6 substrate and inhibitor):* cautiously approach coadministration with SAPHRIS. (7.1, 7.2)

---USE IN SPECIFIC POPULATIONS---
- *Pregnancy:* Use SAPHRIS during pregnancy only if the potential benefit justifies the potential risk. (8.1)
- *Nursing Mothers:* Breast feeding is not recommended. (8.3)
- *Pediatric Use:* Safety and effectiveness have not been established. (8.4)
- *Renal Impairment:* No dose adjustment needed. (8.6)
- *Hepatic Impairment:* SAPHRIS is not recommended in patients with severe hepatic impairment (Child-Pugh C). (2.4, 8.7, 12.3)

See 17 for PATIENT COUNSELING INFORMATION
Revised: 03/2013

FULL PRESCRIBING INFORMATION: CONTENTS*
WARNING: INCREASED MORTALITY IN ELDERLY PATIENTS WITH DEMENTIA-RELATED PSYCHOSIS

FULL PRESCRIBING INFORMATION

> **WARNING: INCREASED MORTALITY IN ELDERLY PATIENTS WITH DEMENTIA-RELATED PSYCHOSIS**
>
> Elderly patients with dementia-related psychosis treated with antipsychotic drugs are at an increased risk of death. Analyses of 17 placebo-controlled trials (modal duration of 10 weeks), largely in patients taking atypical antipsychotic drugs, revealed a risk of death in the drug-treated patients of between 1.6 to 1.7 times that seen in placebo-treated patients. Over the course of a typical 10-week controlled trial, the rate of death in drug-treated patients was about 4.5%, compared to a rate of about 2.6% in the placebo group. Although the causes of death were varied, most of the deaths appeared to be either cardiovascular (e.g., heart failure, sudden death) or infectious (e.g., pneumonia) in nature. Observational studies suggest that, similar to atypical antipsychotic drugs, treatment with conventional antipsychotic drugs may increase mortality. The extent to which the findings of increased mortality in observational studies may be attributed to the antipsychotic drug as opposed to some characteristic(s) of the patients is not clear. SAPHRIS® (asenapine) is not approved for the treatment of patients with dementia-related psychosis *[see Warnings and Precautions (5.1)].*

1 INDICATIONS AND USAGE

1.1 Schizophrenia

SAPHRIS is indicated for the treatment of schizophrenia. The efficacy of SAPHRIS was established in two 6-week trials and one maintenance trial in adults *[see Clinical Studies (14.1)].*

1.2 Bipolar Disorder

Monotherapy: SAPHRIS is indicated for the acute treatment of manic or mixed episodes associated with bipolar I disorder. Efficacy was established in two 3-week monotherapy trials in adults *[see Clinical Studies (14.2)].*

Adjunctive Therapy: SAPHRIS is indicated as adjunctive therapy with either lithium or valproate for the acute treatment of manic or mixed episodes associated with bipolar I disorder. Efficacy was established in one 3-week adjunctive trial in adults *[see Clinical Studies (14.2)].*

2 DOSAGE AND ADMINISTRATION

2.1 Administration Instructions

SAPHRIS is a sublingual tablet. To ensure optimal absorption, patients should be instructed to place the tablet under the tongue and allow it to dissolve completely. The tablet will dissolve in saliva within seconds. SAPHRIS sublingual tablets should not be crushed, chewed, or swallowed *[see Clinical Pharmacology (12.3)].* Patients should be instructed to not eat or drink for 10 minutes after administration *[see Clinical Pharmacology (12.3) and Patient Counseling Information (17.1)].*

2.2 Schizophrenia

Usual Dose for Acute Treatment in Adults: The recommended starting and target dose of SAPHRIS is 5 mg given twice daily. In short term controlled trials, there was no suggestion of added benefit with a 10 mg twice daily dose, but there was a clear increase in certain adverse reactions. The safety of doses above 10 mg twice daily has not been evaluated in clinical studies.

Maintenance Treatment: Efficacy was demonstrated with SAPHRIS in a maintenance trial in patients with schizophrenia. The starting dose in this study was 5 mg twice daily with an increase up to 10 mg twice daily after 1 week based on tolerability *[see Clinical Studies (14.1)].* While there is no body of evidence available to answer the question of how long the schizophrenic patient should remain on SAPHRIS, patients should be periodically reassessed to determine the need for maintenance treatment.

2.3 Bipolar Disorder

Usual Dose for Acute Treatment of Manic or Mixed Episodes Associated with Bipolar I Disorder in Adults:

Monotherapy: The recommended starting dose of SAPHRIS, and the dose maintained by 90% of the patients studied, is 10 mg twice daily. The dose can be decreased to 5 mg twice daily if warranted by adverse effects or based on individual tolerability.

In controlled monotherapy trials, the starting dose for SAPHRIS was 10 mg twice daily. On the second and subsequent days of the trials, the dose could be lowered to 5 mg twice daily, based on tolerability, but less than 10% of patients had their dose reduced. The safety of doses above 10 mg twice daily has not been evaluated in clinical trials.

Adjunctive Therapy: The recommended starting dose of SAPHRIS is 5 mg twice daily when administered as adjunctive therapy with either lithium or valproate. Depending on the clinical response and tolerability in the individual patient, the dose can be increased to 10 mg twice daily. The safety of doses above 10 mg twice daily as adjunctive therapy with lithium or valproate has not been evaluated in clinical trials.

Maintenance Treatment: While there is no body of evidence available to answer the question of how long the bipolar patient should remain on SAPHRIS, whether used as monotherapy or as adjunctive therapy with lithium or valproate, it is generally recommended that responding patients be continued beyond the acute response. If SAPHRIS is used for extended periods in bipolar disorder, the physician should periodically re-evaluate the long-term risks and benefits of the drug for the individual patient.

2.4 Dosage in Special Populations

In a study of subjects with hepatic impairment who were treated with a single dose of SAPHRIS 5 mg, there were increases in asenapine exposures (compared to subjects with normal hepatic function), that correlated with the degree of hepatic impairment. While the results indicated that no dosage adjustments are required in patients with mild (Child-Pugh A) or moderate (Child-Pugh B) hepatic impairment, there was a 7-fold increase (on average) in asenapine concentrations in subjects with severe hepatic impairment (Child-Pugh C) compared to the concentrations of those in subjects with normal hepatic function. Therefore, SAPHRIS is not recommended in patients with severe hepatic impairment *[see Use in Special Populations (8.7)].* Dosage adjustments are not routinely required on the basis of age, gender, race, or renal impairment status *[see Use in Specific Populations (8.4, 8.5, 8.6) and Clinical Pharmacology (12.3)].*

2.5 Switching from Other Antipsychotics

There are no systematically collected data to specifically address switching patients with schizophrenia or bipolar mania from other antipsychotics to SAPHRIS or concerning concomitant administration with other antipsychotics. While immediate discontinuation of the previous antipsychotic treatment may be acceptable for some patients with schizophrenia, more gradual discontinuation may be most appropriate for others. In all cases, the period of overlapping antipsychotic administration should be minimized.

3 DOSAGE FORMS AND STRENGTHS

- SAPHRIS 5-mg tablets are round, white to off-white sublingual tablets, with "5" on one side.
- SAPHRIS 10-mg tablets are round, white to off-white sublingual tablets, with "10" on one side.
- SAPHRIS 5-mg tablets, black cherry flavor, are round, white to off-white sublingual tablets, with "5" on one side within a circle.
- SAPHRIS 10-mg tablets, black cherry flavor, are round, white to off-white sublingual tablets, with "10" on one side within a circle.

4 CONTRAINDICATIONS

Hypersensitivity reactions, including anaphylaxis and angioedema, have been observed in patients treated with asenapine. Therefore, SAPHRIS is contraindicated in patients with a known hypersensitivity to the product *[see Warnings and Precautions (5.7), Adverse Reactions (6) and Patient Counseling Information (17.3)].*

5 WARNINGS AND PRECAUTIONS

5.1 Increased Mortality in Elderly Patients with Dementia-Related Psychosis

Elderly patients with dementia-related psychosis treated with antipsychotic drugs are at an increased risk of death. SAPHRIS is not approved for the treatment of patients with dementia-related psychosis *[see Boxed Warning].*

5.2 Cerebrovascular Adverse Events, Including Stroke, In Elderly Patients with Dementia-Related Psychosis

In placebo-controlled trials with risperidone, aripiprazole, and olanzapine in elderly subjects with dementia, there was a higher incidence of cerebrovascular adverse reactions (cerebrovascular accidents and transient ischemic attacks) including fatalities compared to placebo-treated subjects. SAPHRIS is not approved for the treatment of patients with dementia-related psychosis *[see also Boxed Warning and Warnings and Precautions (5.1)].*

5.3 Neuroleptic Malignant Syndrome

A potentially fatal symptom complex sometimes referred to as Neuroleptic Malignant Syndrome (NMS) has been reported in association with administration of antipsychotic drugs, including SAPHRIS. Clinical manifestations of NMS are hyperpyrexia, muscle rigidity, altered mental status, and evidence of autonomic instability (irregular pulse or blood pressure, tachycardia, diaphoresis, and cardiac dysrhythmia). Additional signs may include elevated creatine phosphokinase, myoglobinuria (rhabdomyolysis), and acute renal failure.

The diagnostic evaluation of patients with this syndrome is complicated. It is important to exclude cases where the clinical presentation includes both serious medical illness (e.g. pneumonia, systemic infection) and untreated or inadequately treated extrapyramidal signs and symptoms (EPS). Other important considerations in the differential diagnosis include central anticholinergic toxicity, heat stroke, drug fever, and primary central nervous system pathology.

The management of NMS should include: 1) immediate discontinuation of antipsychotic drugs and other drugs not essential to concurrent therapy; 2) intensive symptomatic treatment and medical monitoring; and 3) treatment of any concomitant serious medical problems for which specific treatments are available. There is no general agreement about specific pharmacological treatment regimens for NMS.

If a patient requires antipsychotic drug treatment after recovery from NMS, the potential reintroduction of drug therapy should be carefully considered. The patient should be carefully monitored, since recurrences of NMS have been reported.

5.4 Tardive Dyskinesia

A syndrome of potentially irreversible, involuntary, dyskinetic movements can develop in patients treated with antipsychotic drugs. Although the prevalence of the syndrome appears to be highest among the elderly, especially elderly women, it is impossible to rely upon prevalence estimates to predict, at the inception of antipsychotic treatment, which patients are likely to develop the syndrome. Whether antipsychotic drug products differ in their potential to cause Tardive Dyskinesia (TD) is unknown.

The risk of developing TD and the likelihood that it will become irreversible are believed to increase as the duration of treatment and the total cumulative dose of antipsychotic drugs administered to the patient increase. However, the syndrome can develop, although much less commonly, after relatively brief treatment periods at low doses.

There is no known treatment for established cases of TD, although the syndrome may remit, partially or completely, if antipsychotic treatment is withdrawn. Antipsychotic treatment, itself, however, may suppress (or partially suppress) the signs and symptoms of the syndrome and thereby may possibly mask the underlying process. The effect that symptomatic suppression has upon the long-term course of the syndrome is unknown.

Given these considerations, SAPHRIS should be prescribed in a manner that is most likely to minimize the occurrence of TD. Chronic antipsychotic treatment should generally be reserved for patients who suffer from a chronic illness that (1) is known to respond to antipsychotic drugs, and (2) for whom alternative, equally effective, but potentially less harmful treatments are not available or appropriate. In patients who do require chronic treatment, the smallest dose and the shortest duration of treatment producing a satisfactory clinical response should be sought. The need for continued treatment should be reassessed periodically.

If signs and symptoms of TD appear in a patient on SAPHRIS, drug discontinuation should be considered. However, some patients may require treatment with SAPHRIS despite the presence of the syndrome.

5.5 Hyperglycemia and Diabetes Mellitus

Hyperglycemia, in some cases extreme and associated with ketoacidosis or hyperosmolar coma or death, has been reported in patients treated with atypical antipsychotics. Assessment of the relationship between atypical antipsychotic use and glucose abnormalities is complicated by the possibility of an increased background risk of diabetes mellitus in patients with schizophrenia and the increasing incidence of diabetes mellitus in the general population. Given these confounders, the relationship between atypical antipsychotic use and hyperglycemia-related adverse reactions is not completely understood. However, epidemiological studies suggest an increased risk of treatment-emergent hyperglycemia-related adverse events in patients treated with the atypical antipsychotics included in these studies. Because SAPHRIS was not marketed at the time these studies were performed, it is not known if SAPHRIS is associated with this increased risk. Precise risk estimates for hyperglycemia-related adverse events in patients treated with atypical antipsychotics are not available.

Patients with an established diagnosis of diabetes mellitus who are started on atypical antipsychotics should be monitored regularly for worsening of glucose control. Patients with risk factors for diabetes mellitus (e.g., obesity, family history of diabetes) who are starting treatment with atypical antipsychotics should undergo fasting blood glucose testing at the beginning of treatment and periodically during treatment. Any patient treated with atypical antipsychotics should be monitored for symptoms of hyperglycemia including polydipsia, polyuria, polyphagia, and weakness. Patients who develop symptoms of hyperglycemia during treatment with atypical antipsychotics should undergo fasting blood glucose testing. In some cases, hyperglycemia has resolved when the atypical antipsychotic was discontinued; however, some patients required continuation of antidiabetic treatment despite discontinuation of the antipsychotic drug.

5.6 Weight Gain

Increases in weight have been observed in pre-marketing clinical trials with SAPHRIS. Patients receiving SAPHRIS should receive regular monitoring of weight [see Patient Counseling Information (17.7)].

In short-term schizophrenia and bipolar mania trials, there were differences in mean weight gain between SAPHRIS-treated and placebo-treated patients. In short-term, placebo-controlled schizophrenia trials, the mean weight gain was 1.1 kg for SAPHRIS-treated patients compared to 0.1 kg for placebo-treated patients. The proportion of patients with a ≥7% increase in body weight (at Endpoint) was 4.9% for SAPHRIS-treated patients versus 2% for placebo-treated patients. In short-term, placebo-controlled bipolar mania trials, the mean weight gain for SAPHRIS-treated patients was 1.3 kg compared to 0.2 kg for placebo-treated patients. The proportion of patients with a ≥7% increase in body weight (at Endpoint) was 5.8% for SAPHRIS-treated patients versus 0.5% for placebo-treated patients.

In a 52-week, double-blind, comparator-controlled trial of patients with schizophrenia or schizoaffective disorder, the mean weight gain from baseline was 0.9 kg. The proportion of patients with a ≥7% increase in body weight (at Endpoint) was 14.7%. **Table 1** provides the mean weight change from baseline and the proportion of patients with a weight gain of ≥7% categorized by Body Mass Index (BMI) at baseline:

Table 1: Weight Change Results Categorized by BMI at Baseline: Comparator-Controlled 52-Week Study in Schizophrenia

	BMI <23 SAPHRIS N=295	BMI 23 - ≤27 SAPHRIS N=290	BMI >27 SAPHRIS N=302
Mean change from Baseline (kg)	1.7	1	0
% with ≥7% increase in body weight	22%	13%	9%

5.7 Hypersensitivity Reactions

Hypersensitivity reactions, including anaphylaxis and angioedema, have been observed in patients treated with asenapine. In several cases, these reactions occurred after the first dose. These hypersensitivity reactions included: anaphylaxis, angioedema, hypotension, tachycardia, swollen tongue, dyspnea, wheezing and rash.

5.8 Orthostatic Hypotension, Syncope, and Other Hemodynamic Effects

SAPHRIS may induce orthostatic hypotension and syncope in some patients, especially early in treatment, because of its α1-adrenergic antagonist activity. In short-term schizophrenia trials, syncope was reported in 0.2% (1/572) of patients treated with therapeutic doses (5 mg or 10 mg twice daily) of SAPHRIS, compared to 0.3% (1/378) of patients treated with placebo. In short-term bipolar mania trials, syncope was reported in 0.3% (1/379) of patients treated with therapeutic doses (5 mg or 10 mg twice daily) of SAPHRIS, compared to 0% (0/203) of patients treated with placebo. During pre-marketing clinical trials with SAPHRIS, including long-term trials without comparison to placebo, syncope was reported in 0.6% (11/1953) of patients treated with SAPHRIS.

Four normal volunteers in clinical pharmacology studies treated with either intravenous, oral, or sublingual SAPHRIS experienced hypotension, bradycardia, and sinus pauses. These spontaneously resolved in 3 cases, but the fourth subject received external cardiac massage. The risk of this sequence of hypotension, bradycardia, and sinus pause might be greater in nonpsychiatric patients compared to psychiatric patients who are possibly more adapted to certain effects of psychotropic drugs.

Patients should be instructed about nonpharmacologic interventions that help to reduce the occurrence of orthostatic hypotension (e.g., sitting on the edge of the bed for several minutes before attempting to stand in the morning and slowly rising from a seated position). SAPHRIS should be used with caution in (1) patients with known cardiovascular disease (history of myocardial infarction or ischemic heart disease, heart failure or conduction abnormalities), cerebrovascular disease, or conditions which would predispose patients to hypotension (dehydration, hypovolemia, and treatment with antihypertensive medications); and (2) in the elderly. SAPHRIS should be used cautiously when treating patients who receive treatment with other drugs that can induce hypotension, bradycardia, respiratory or central nervous system depression [see Drug Interactions (7)]. Monitoring of orthostatic vital signs should be considered in all such patients, and a dose reduction should be considered if hypotension occurs.

5.9 Leukopenia, Neutropenia, and Agranulocytosis

In clinical trial and postmarketing experience, events of leukopenia/neutropenia have been reported temporally related to antipsychotic agents, including SAPHRIS. Agranulocytosis (including fatal cases) has been reported with other agents in the class.

Possible risk factors for leukopenia/neutropenia include pre-existing low white blood cell count (WBC) and history of drug induced leukopenia/neutropenia. Patients with a pre-existing low WBC or a history of drug induced leukopenia/neutropenia should have their complete blood count (CBC) monitored frequently during the first few months of therapy and SAPHRIS should be discontinued at the first sign of decline in WBC in the absence of other causative factors.

Patients with neutropenia should be carefully monitored for fever or other symptoms or signs of infection and treated promptly if such symptoms or signs occur. Patients with severe neutropenia (absolute neutrophil count <1000/mm³) should discontinue SAPHRIS and have their WBC followed until recovery.

5.10 QT Prolongation

The effects of SAPHRIS on the QT/QTc interval were evaluated in a dedicated QT study. This trial involved SAPHRIS doses of 5 mg, 10 mg, 15 mg, and 20 mg twice daily, and placebo, and was conducted in 151 clinically stable patients with schizophrenia, with electrocardiographic assessments throughout the dosing interval at baseline and steady state. At these doses, SAPHRIS was associated with increases in QTc interval ranging from 2 to 5 msec compared to placebo. No patients treated with SAPHRIS experienced QTc increases ≥60 msec from baseline measurements, nor did any patient experience a QTc of ≥500 msec.

Electrocardiogram (ECG) measurements were taken at various time points during the SAPHRIS clinical trial program (5-mg or 10-mg twice daily doses). Post-baseline QT prolongations exceeding 500 msec were reported at comparable rates for SAPHRIS and placebo in these short-term trials. There were no reports of Torsade de Pointes or any other adverse reactions associated with delayed ventricular repolarization.

The use of SAPHRIS should be avoided in combination with other drugs known to prolong QTc including Class 1A antiarrhythmics (e.g., quinidine, procainamide) or Class 3 antiarrhythmics (e.g., amiodarone, sotalol), antipsychotic medications (e.g., ziprasidone, chlorpromazine, thioridazine), and antibiotics (e.g., gatifloxacin, moxifloxacin). SAPHRIS should also be avoided in patients with a history of cardiac arrhythmias and in other circumstances that may increase the risk of the occurrence of torsade de pointes and/or sudden death in association with the use of drugs that prolong the QT interval, including bradycardia; hypokalemia or hypomagnesemia; and presence of congenital prolongation of the QT interval.

5.11 Hyperprolactinemia

Like other drugs that antagonize dopamine D2 receptors, SAPHRIS can elevate prolactin levels, and the elevation can persist during chronic administration. Hyperprolactinemia may suppress hypothalamic GnRH, resulting in reduced pituitary gonadotropin secretion. This, in turn, may inhibit reproductive function by impairing gonadal steroidogenesis in both female and male patients. Galactorrhea, amenorrhea, gynecomastia, and impotence have been reported in patients receiving prolactin-elevating compounds. Longstanding hyperprolactinemia when associated with hypogonadism may lead to decreased bone density in both female and male subjects. In SAPHRIS clinical trials, the incidences of adverse events related to abnormal prolactin levels were 0.4% versus 0% for placebo [see Adverse Reactions (6.1)].

Tissue culture experiments indicate that approximately one-third of human breast cancers are prolactin-dependent in vitro, a factor of potential importance if the prescription of these drugs is considered in a patient with previously-detected breast cancer. Neither clinical studies nor epidemiologic studies conducted to date have shown an association between chronic administration of this class of drugs and tumorigenesis in humans, but the available evidence is too limited to be conclusive.

5.12 Seizures

Seizures were reported in 0% and 0.3% (0/572, 1/379) of patients treated with doses of 5 mg and 10 mg twice daily of SAPHRIS, respectively, compared to 0% (0/503, 0/203) of patients treated with placebo in short-term schizophrenia and bipolar mania trials, respectively. During pre-marketing clinical trials with SAPHRIS, including long-term trials without comparison to placebo, seizures were reported in 0.3% (5/1953) of patients treated with SAPHRIS. As with other antipsychotic drugs, SAPHRIS should be used with caution in patients with a history of seizures or with conditions that potentially lower the seizure threshold, e.g., Alzheimer's dementia. Conditions that lower the seizure threshold may be more prevalent in patients 65 years or older.

5.13 Potential for Cognitive and Motor Impairment

Somnolence was reported in patients treated with SAPHRIS. It was usually transient with the highest incidence reported during the first week of treatment. In short-term, fixed-dose, placebo-controlled schizophrenia trials, somnolence was reported in 15% (41/274) of patients on SAPHRIS 5 mg twice daily and in 13% (26/208) of patients on SAPHRIS 10 mg twice daily compared to 7% (26/378) of placebo patients. In short-term, placebo-controlled bipolar mania trials of therapeutic doses (5-10 mg twice daily), somnolence was reported in 24% (90/379) of patients on SAPHRIS compared to 6% (13/203) of placebo patients. During pre-marketing clinical trials with SAPHRIS, including long-term trials without comparison to placebo, somnolence was reported in 18% (358/1953) of patients treated with SAPHRIS. Somnolence (including sedation) led to discontinuation in 0.6% (12/1953) of patients in short-term, placebo-controlled trials.

Patients should be cautioned about performing activities requiring mental alertness, such as operating hazardous machinery or operating a motor vehicle, until they are reasonably certain that SAPHRIS therapy does not affect them adversely.

5.14 Body Temperature Regulation

Disruption of the body's ability to reduce core body temperature has been attributed to antipsychotic agents. In the short-term placebo-controlled trials for both schizophrenia and acute bipolar disorder, the incidence of adverse reactions suggestive of body temperature increases was low (≤1%) and comparable to placebo. During pre-marketing clinical trials with SAPHRIS, including long-term trials without comparison to placebo, the incidence of adverse reactions suggestive of body temperature increases (pyrexia and feeling hot) was ≤1%. Appropriate care is advised when prescribing SAPHRIS for patients who will be experiencing conditions that may contribute to an elevation in core body temperature, e.g., exercising strenuously, exposure to extreme heat, receiving concomitant medication with anticholinergic activity, or being subject to dehydration.

5.15 Suicide

The possibility of a suicide attempt is inherent in psychotic illnesses and bipolar disorder, and close supervision of high-risk patients should accompany drug therapy. Prescriptions for SAPHRIS should be written for the smallest quantity of tablets consistent with good patient management in order to reduce the risk of overdose.

5.16 Dysphagia

Esophageal dysmotility and aspiration have been associated with antipsychotic drug use. Dysphagia was reported in 0.2% and 0% (1/572, 0/379) of patients treated with therapeutic doses (5-10 mg twice daily) of SAPHRIS as compared to 0% (0/378, 0/203) of patients treated with placebo in short-term schizophrenia and bipolar mania trials, respectively. During pre-marketing clinical trials with SAPHRIS, including long-term trials without comparison to placebo, dysphagia was reported in 0.1% (2/1953) of patients treated with SAPHRIS.

Aspiration pneumonia is a common cause of morbidity and mortality in elderly patients, in particular those with advanced Alzheimer's dementia. SAPHRIS is not indicated for the treatment of dementia-related psychosis, and should not be used in patients at risk for aspiration pneumonia *[see also Warnings and Precautions (5.1)]*.

5.17   Use in Patients with Concomitant Illness

Clinical experience with SAPHRIS in patients with certain concomitant systemic illnesses is limited *[see Clinical Pharmacology (12.3)]*.

SAPHRIS has not been evaluated in patients with a recent history of myocardial infarction or unstable heart disease. Patients with these diagnoses were excluded from pre-marketing clinical trials. Because of the risk of orthostatic hypotension with SAPHRIS, caution should be observed in cardiac patients *[see Warnings and Precautions (5.6)]*.

6   ADVERSE REACTIONS

The following adverse reactions are discussed in more detail in other sections of the labeling:

- Use in Elderly Patients with Dementia-Related Psychosis *[see Boxed Warning and Warnings and Precautions (5.1 and 5.2)]*
- Neuroleptic Malignant Syndrome *[see Warnings and Precautions (5.3)]*
- Tardive Dyskinesia *[see Warnings and Precautions (5.4)]*
- Hyperglycemia and Diabetes Mellitus *[see Warnings and Precautions (5.5)]*
- Weight Gain *[see Warnings and Precautions (5.6)]*
- Hypersensitivity Reactions *[see Warnings and Precautions (5.7) and Patient Counseling Information (17.3)]*
- Application site reactions including oral ulcers, blisters, peeling/sloughing and inflammation *[see Adverse Reactions (6.2)]*
- Orthostatic Hypotension, Syncope, and other Hemodynamic Effects *[see Warnings and Precautions (5.8)]*
- Leukopenia, Neutropenia, and Agranulocytosis *[see Warnings and Precautions (5.9)]*
- QT Interval Prolongation *[see Warnings and Precautions (5.10)]*
- Hyperprolactinemia *[see Warnings and Precautions (5.11)]*
- Seizures *[see Warnings and Precautions (5.12)]*
- Potential for Cognitive and Motor Impairment *[see Warnings and Precautions (5.13)]*
- Body Temperature Regulation *[see Warnings and Precautions (5.14)]*
- Suicide *[see Warnings and Precautions (5.15)]*
- Dysphagia *[see Warnings and Precautions (5.16)]*
- Use in Patients with Concomitant Illness *[see Warnings and Precautions (5.17)]*

The most common adverse reactions (≥5% and at least twice the rate of placebo) reported with acute treatment in schizophrenia were akathisia, oral hypoesthesia, and somnolence. The safety profile of SAPHRIS in the maintenance treatment of schizophrenia was similar to that seen with acute treatment.

The most common adverse reactions (≥5% and at least twice the rate of placebo) reported with acute monotherapy treatment of manic or mixed episodes associated with bipolar I disorder were somnolence, dizziness, extrapyramidal symptoms other than akathisia, and weight increased and during the adjunctive therapy trial in bipolar disorder were somnolence and oral hypoesthesia.

The information below is derived from a clinical trial database for SAPHRIS consisting of over 4565 patients and/or normal subjects exposed to one or more sublingual doses of SAPHRIS. A total of 1314 SAPHRIS-treated patients were treated for at least 24 weeks and 785 SAPHRIS-treated patients had at least 52 weeks of exposure at therapeutic doses.

The stated frequencies of adverse reactions represent the proportion of individuals who experienced a treatment-emergent adverse event of the type listed. A reaction was considered treatment emergent if it occurred for the first time or worsened while receiving therapy following baseline evaluation.

The figures in the tables and tabulations cannot be used to predict the incidence of side effects in the course of usual medical practice where patient characteristics and other factors differ from those that prevailed in the clinical trials. Similarly, the cited frequencies cannot be compared with figures obtained from other clinical investigations involving different treatment, uses, and investigators. The cited figures, however, do provide the prescriber with some basis for estimating the relative contribution of drug and nondrug factors to the adverse reaction incidence in the population studied.

Table 2: Adverse Reactions Reported in 2% or More of Subjects in One of the SAPHRIS Dose Groups and Which Occurred at Greater Incidence Than in the Placebo Group in 6-Week Schizophrenia Trials

System Organ Class/ Preferred Term	Placebo N=378	SAPHRIS 5 mg twice daily N=274	SAPHRIS 10 mg twice daily N=208	All SAPHRIS* 5 mg or 10 mg twice daily N=572
Gastrointestinal disorders				
Constipation	6%	7%	4%	5%
Dry mouth	1%	3%	1%	2%
Oral hypoesthesia	1%	6%	7%	5%
Salivary hypersecretion	0%	<1%	4%	2%
Stomach discomfort	1%	<1%	3%	2%
Vomiting	5%	4%	7%	5%
General disorders				
Fatigue	3%	4%	3%	3%
Irritability	<1%	2%	1%	2%
Investigations				
Weight increased	<1%	2%	2%	3%
Metabolism disorders				
Increased appetite	<1%	3%	0%	2%
Nervous system disorders				
Akathisia†	3%	4%	11%	6%
Dizziness	4%	7%	3%	5%
Extrapyramidal symptoms (excluding akathisia)‡	7%	9%	12%	10%
Somnolence§	7%	15%	13%	13%
Psychiatric disorders				
Insomnia	13%	16%	15%	15%
Vascular disorders				
Hypertension	2%	2%	3%	2%

* Also includes the Flexible-dose trial (N=90).
† Akathisia includes: akathisia and hyperkinesia.
‡ Extrapyramidal symptoms included dystonia, oculogyration, dyskinesia, tardive dyskinesia, muscle rigidity, parkinsonism, tremor, and extrapyramidal disorder (excluding akathisia).
§ Somnolence includes the following events: somnolence, sedation, and hypersomnia.

6.1   Clinical Studies Experience

Adult Patients with Schizophrenia: The following findings are based on the short-term placebo-controlled pre-marketing trials for schizophrenia (a pool of three 6-week fixed-dose trials and one 6-week flexible-dose trial) in which sublingual SAPHRIS was administered in doses ranging from 5 to 10 mg twice daily.

Adverse Reactions Associated with Discontinuation of Treatment: A total of 9% of SAPHRIS-treated subjects and 10% of placebo subjects discontinued due to adverse reactions. There were no drug-related adverse reactions associated with discontinuation in subjects treated with SAPHRIS at the rate of at least 1% and at least twice the placebo rate.

Adverse Reactions Occurring at an Incidence of 2% or More in SAPHRIS-Treated Schizophrenic Patients: Adverse reactions associated with the use of SAPHRIS (incidence of 2% or greater, rounded to the nearest percent, and SAPHRIS incidence greater than placebo) that occurred during acute therapy (up to 6-weeks in patients with schizophrenia) are shown in **Table 2**.

[See table 2 above]

Dose-Related Adverse Reactions: Of all the adverse reactions listed in **Table 2**, the only apparent dose-related adverse reaction was akathisia.

Monotherapy in Adult Patients with Bipolar Mania: The following findings are based on the short-term placebo-controlled trials for bipolar mania (a pool of two 3-week flexible-dose trials) in which sublingual SAPHRIS was administered in doses of 5 mg or 10 mg twice daily.

Adverse Reactions Associated with Discontinuation of Treatment: Approximately 10% (38/379) of SAPHRIS-treated patients in short-term, placebo-controlled trials discontinued treatment due to an adverse reaction, compared with about 6% (12/203) on placebo. The most common adverse reactions associated with discontinuation in subjects treated with SAPHRIS (rates at least 1% and at least twice the placebo rate) were anxiety (1.1%) and oral hypoesthesia (1.1%) compared to placebo (0%).

Adverse Reactions Occurring at an Incidence of 2% or More Among SAPHRIS-Treated (Monotherapy) Bipolar Patients: Adverse reactions associated with the use of SAPHRIS (incidence of 2% or greater, rounded to the nearest percent, and SAPHRIS incidence greater than placebo) that occurred during acute monotherapy (up to 3-weeks in patients with bipolar mania) are shown in **Table 3**.

Table 3: Adverse Reactions Reported in 2% or More of Subjects in One of the SAPHRIS Dose Groups and Which Occurred at Greater Incidence Than in the Placebo Group in 3-Week Bipolar Mania Trials

System Organ Class/ Preferred Term	Placebo N=203	SAPHRIS 5 mg or 10 mg twice daily* N=379
Gastrointestinal disorders		
Dry mouth	1%	3%
Dyspepsia	2%	4%
Oral hypoesthesia	<1%	4%
Toothache	2%	3%

General disorders

Fatigue	2%	4%

Investigations

Weight increased	<1%	5%

Metabolism disorders

Increased appetite	1%	4%

Musculoskeletal and connective tissue disorders

Arthralgia	1%	3%
Pain in extremity	<1%	2%

Nervous system disorders

Akathisia	2%	4%
Dizziness	3%	11%
Dysgeusia	<1%	3%
Headache	11%	12%
Other extrapyramidal symptoms (excluding akathisia)[†]	2%	7%
Somnolence[‡]	6%	24%

Psychiatric disorders

Anxiety	2%	4%
Depression	1%	2%
Insomnia	5%	6%

* SAPHRIS 5 mg to 10 mg twice daily with flexible dosing.
† Extrapyramidal symptoms included: dystonia, blepharospasm, torticollis, dyskinesia, tardive dyskinesia, muscle rigidity, parkinsonism, gait disturbance, masked facies, and tremor (excluding akathisia).
‡ Somnolence includes the following events: somnolence, sedation, and hypersomnia.

Adjunctive Therapy in Adult Patients with Bipolar Mania: The following findings are based on a 12 week placebo-controlled trial (with a 3 week efficacy endpoint) in adult patients with bipolar mania in which sublingual SAPHRIS was administered in doses of 5 mg or 10 mg twice daily as adjunctive therapy with lithium or valproate.
Adverse Reactions Associated with Discontinuation of Treatment: Approximately 16% (25/158) of SAPHRIS-treated patients discontinued treatment due to an adverse reaction, compared with about 11% (18/166) on placebo. The most common adverse reactions associated with discontinuation in subjects treated with SAPHRIS (rates at least 1% and at least twice the placebo rate) were depression (2.5%), suicidal ideation (2.5%), bipolar 1 disorder (1.9%), insomnia (1.9%) and depressive symptoms (1.3%).
Adverse Reactions Occurring at an Incidence of 2% or More Among SAPHRIS-Treated (Adjunctive) Bipolar Patients: Adverse reactions associated with the use of SAPHRIS (incidence of 2% or greater, rounded to the nearest percent, and SAPHRIS incidence greater than placebo) that occurred during acute adjunctive therapy at 3 weeks, a time when most of the patients were still participating in the trial, are shown in **Table 4.**

Table 4: Adverse Reactions Reported in 2% or More Among SAPHRIS-Treated (Adjunctive) Bipolar Mania Patients and Which Occurred at Greater Incidence Than in the Placebo Group at 3 Weeks

System Organ Class/ Preferred Term	Placebo N=166	SAPHRIS 5 mg or 10 mg twice daily* N=158
Gastrointestinal disorders		
Dyspepsia	2%	3%
Oral hypoesthesia	0%	5%
General disorders		
Fatigue	2%	4%
Edema peripheral	<1%	3%
Investigations		
Weight increased	0%	3%
Nervous system disorders		
Dizziness	2%	4%
Other extrapyramidal symptoms (excluding akathisia)[†]	5%	6%
Somnolence[‡]	10%	22%
Psychiatric disorders		
Insomnia	8%	10%
Vascular disorders		
Hypertension	<1%	3%

* SAPHRIS 5 mg to 10 mg twice daily with flexible dosing.
† Extrapyramidal symptoms included: dystonia, parkinsonism, oculogyration, and tremor (excluding akathisia).
‡ Somnolence includes the following events: somnolence and sedation.

Dystonia: *Antipsychotic Class Effect:* Symptoms of dystonia, prolonged abnormal contractions of muscle groups, may occur in susceptible individuals during the first few days of treatment. Dystonic symptoms include: spasm of the neck muscles, sometimes progressing to tightness of the throat, swallowing difficulty, difficulty breathing, and/or protrusion of the tongue. While these symptoms can occur at low doses, they occur more frequently and with greater severity with high potency and at higher doses of first generation antipsychotic drugs. An elevated risk of acute dystonia is observed in males and younger age groups.
Extrapyramidal Symptoms: In the short-term, placebo-controlled schizophrenia and bipolar mania trials, data was objectively collected on the Simpson Angus Rating Scale for extrapyramidal symptoms (EPS), the Barnes Akathisia Scale (for akathisia) and the Assessments of Involuntary Movement Scales (for dyskinesias). The mean change from baseline for the all-SAPHRIS 5 mg or 10 mg twice daily treated group was comparable to placebo in each of the rating scale scores.
In the short-term, placebo-controlled schizophrenia trials, the incidence of reported EPS-related events, excluding events related to akathisia, for SAPHRIS-treated patients was 10% versus 7% for placebo; and the incidence of akathisia-related events for SAPHRIS-treated patients was 6% versus 3% for placebo. In short-term placebo-controlled bipolar mania trials, the incidence of EPS-related events, excluding events related to akathisia, for SAPHRIS-treated patients was 7% versus 2% for placebo; and the incidence of akathisia-related events for SAPHRIS-treated patients was 4% versus 2% for placebo.
Other Findings: Oral hypoesthesia and/or oral paraesthesia may occur directly after administration of asenapine and usually resolves within 1 hour.
Laboratory Test Abnormalities:
Glucose: The effects on fasting serum glucose levels in the short-term schizophrenia and bipolar mania trials revealed no clinically relevant mean changes *[see also Warnings and Precautions (5.5)]*. In the short-term placebo-controlled schizophrenia trials, the mean increase in fasting glucose levels for SAPHRIS-treated patients was 3.2 mg/dL compared to a decrease of 1.6 mg/dL for placebo-treated patients. The proportion of patients with fasting glucose elevations ≥126 mg/dL (at Endpoint), was 7.4% for SAPHRIS-treated patients versus 6% for placebo-treated patients. In the short-term, placebo-controlled bipolar mania trials, the mean decreases in fasting glucose levels for both SAPHRIS-treated and placebo-treated patients were 0.6 mg/dL. The proportion of patients with fasting glucose elevations ≥126 mg/dL (at Endpoint), was 4.9% for SAPHRIS-treated patients versus 2.2% for placebo-treated patients. In a 52-week, double-blind, comparator-controlled trial of patients with schizophrenia and schizoaffective disorder, the mean increase from baseline of fasting glucose was 2.4 mg/dL.
Lipids: The effects on total cholesterol and fasting triglycerides in the short-term schizophrenia and bipolar mania trials revealed no clinically relevant mean changes. In short-term, placebo-controlled schizophrenia trials, the mean increase in total cholesterol levels for SAPHRIS-treated patients was 0.4 mg/dL compared to a decrease of

3.6 mg/dL for placebo-treated patients. The proportion of patients with total cholesterol elevations ≥240 mg/dL (at Endpoint) was 8.3% for SAPHRIS-treated patients versus 7% for placebo-treated patients. In short-term, placebo-controlled bipolar mania trials, the mean increase in total cholesterol levels for SAPHRIS-treated patients was 1.1 mg/dL compared to a decrease of 1.5 mg/dL in placebo-treated patients. The proportion of patients with total cholesterol elevations ≥240 mg/dL (at Endpoint) was 8.7% for SAPHRIS-treated patients versus 8.6% for placebo-treated patients. In short-term, placebo-controlled schizophrenia trials, the mean increase in triglyceride levels for SAPHRIS-treated patients was 3.8 mg/dL compared to a decrease of 13.5 mg/dL for placebo-treated patients. The proportion of patients with elevations in triglycerides ≥200 mg/dL (at Endpoint) was 13.2% for SAPHRIS-treated patients versus 10.5% for placebo-treated patients. In short-term, placebo-controlled bipolar mania trials, the mean decrease in triglyceride levels for SAPHRIS-treated patients was 3.5 mg/dL versus 17.9 mg/dL for placebo-treated subjects. The proportion of patients with elevations in triglycerides ≥200 mg/dL (at Endpoint) was 15.2% for SAPHRIS-treated patients versus 11.4% for placebo-treated patients. In a 52-week, double-blind, comparator-controlled trial of patients with schizophrenia and schizoaffective disorder, the mean decrease from baseline of total cholesterol was 6 mg/dL and the mean decrease from baseline of fasting triglycerides was 9.8 mg/dL.
Transaminases: Transient elevations in serum transaminases (primarily ALT) in the short-term schizophrenia and bipolar mania trials were more common in treated patients but mean changes were not clinically relevant. In short-term, placebo-controlled schizophrenia trials, the mean increase in transaminase levels for SAPHRIS-treated patients was 1.6 units/L compared to a decrease of 0.4 units/L for placebo-treated patients. The proportion of patients with transaminase elevations ≥3 times ULN (at Endpoint) was 0.9% for SAPHRIS-treated patients versus 1.3% for placebo-treated patients. In short-term, placebo-controlled bipolar mania trials, the mean increase in transaminase levels for SAPHRIS-treated patients was 8.9 units/L compared to a decrease of 4.9 units/L in placebo-treated patients. The proportion of patients with transaminase elevations ≥3 times upper limit of normal (ULN) (at Endpoint) was 2.5% for SAPHRIS-treated patients versus 0.6% for placebo-treated patients. No cases of more severe liver injury were seen.
In a 52-week, double-blind, comparator-controlled trial of patients with schizophrenia and schizoaffective disorder, the mean increase from baseline of ALT was 1.7 units/L.
Prolactin: The effects on prolactin levels in the short-term schizophrenia and bipolar mania trials revealed no clinically relevant mean changes in baseline. In short-term, placebo-controlled schizophrenia trials, the mean decreases in prolactin levels were 6.5 ng/mL for SAPHRIS-treated patients compared to 10.7 ng/mL for placebo-treated patients. The proportion of patients with prolactin elevations ≥4 times ULN (at Endpoint) were 2.6% for SAPHRIS-treated patients versus 0.6% for placebo-treated patients. In short-term, placebo-controlled bipolar mania trials, the mean increase in prolactin levels was 4.9 ng/mL for SAPHRIS-treated patients compared to a decrease of 0.2 ng/mL for placebo-treated patients. The proportion of patients with prolactin elevations ≥4 times ULN (at Endpoint) were 2.3% for SAPHRIS-treated patients versus 0.7% for placebo-treated patients.
In a long-term (52-week), double-blind, comparator-controlled trial of patients with schizophrenia and schizoaffective disorder, the mean decrease in prolactin from baseline for SAPHRIS-treated patients was 26.9 ng/mL.
Creatine Kinase (CK): The proportion of patients with CK elevations >3 times ULN at any time were 6.4% and 11.1% for patients treated with SAPHRIS 5 mg bid and 10 mg bid, respectively, as compared to 6.7% for placebo-treated patients in short-term, fixed-dose trials in schizophrenia and bipolar mania. The clinical relevance of this finding is unknown.
Other Adverse Reactions Observed During the Premarketing Evaluation of SAPHRIS: Following is a list of MedDRA terms that reflect adverse reactions reported by patients treated with sublingual SAPHRIS at multiple doses of ≥5 mg twice daily during any phase of a trial within the database of adult patients. The reactions listed are those that could be of clinical importance, as well as reactions that are plausibly drug-related on pharmacologic or other grounds. Reactions already listed in other parts of *Adverse Reactions (6),* or those considered in *Warnings and Precautions (5)* or *Overdosage (10)* are not included. Although the reactions reported occurred during treatment with SAPHRIS, they were not necessarily caused by it. Reactions are further categorized by MedDRA system organ class and listed in order of decreasing frequency according to the following definitions: those occurring in at least 1/100 patients (only those not already listed in the tabulated results from placebo-controlled trials appear in this listing); those occurring in 1/100 to 1/1000 patients; and those occurring in fewer than 1/1000 patients.

Blood and lymphatic disorders: <1/1000 patients: thrombocytopenia; ≥1/1000 patients and <1/100 patients: anemia
Cardiac disorders: ≥1/1000 patients and <1/100 patients: tachycardia, temporary bundle branch block
Eye disorders: ≥1/1000 patients and <1/100 patients: accommodation disorder
Gastrointestinal disorders: ≥1/1000 patients and <1/100 patients: oral paraesthesia, glossodynia, swollen tongue
General disorders: <1/1000 patients: idiosyncratic drug reaction
Investigations: ≥1/1000 patients and <1/100 patients: hyponatremia
Nervous system disorders: ≥1/1000 patients and <1/100 patients: dysarthria

6.2 Postmarketing Experience

The following adverse reactions have been identified during post-approval use of SAPHRIS. Application site reactions, primarily in the sublingual area, have been reported. These application site reactions included oral ulcers, blisters, peeling/sloughing, and inflammation. In many cases, the occurrence of these application site reactions led to discontinuation of therapy.

7 DRUG INTERACTIONS

The risks of using SAPHRIS in combination with other drugs have not been extensively evaluated. Given the primary CNS effects of SAPHRIS, caution should be used when it is taken in combination with other centrally acting drugs or alcohol.

Because of its α_1-adrenergic antagonism with potential for inducing hypotension, SAPHRIS may enhance the effects of certain antihypertensive agents.

7.1 Potential for Other Drugs to Affect SAPHRIS

Asenapine is cleared primarily through direct glucuronidation by UGT1A4 and oxidative metabolism by cytochrome P450 isoenzymes (predominantly CYP1A2). The potential effects of inhibitors of several of these enzyme pathways on asenapine clearance were studied.

[See table 5 above]

A population pharmacokinetic analysis indicated that the concomitant administration of lithium had no effect on the pharmacokinetics of asenapine.

7.2 Potential for SAPHRIS to Affect Other Drugs

Coadministration with CYP2D6 Substrates: In vitro studies indicate that asenapine weakly inhibits CYP2D6.

Following coadministration of dextromethorphan and SAPHRIS in healthy subjects, the ratio of dextrorphan/dextromethorphan (DX/DM) as a marker of CYP2D6 activity was measured. Indicative of CYP2D6 inhibition, treatment with SAPHRIS 5 mg twice daily decreased the DX/DM ratio to 0.43. In the same study, treatment with paroxetine 20 mg daily decreased the DX/DM ratio to 0.032. In a separate study, coadministration of a single 75-mg dose of imipramine with a single 5-mg dose of SAPHRIS did not affect the plasma concentrations of the metabolite desipramine (a CYP2D6 substrate). Thus, *in vivo*, SAPHRIS appears to be at most a weak inhibitor of CYP2D6. Coadministration of a single 20-mg dose of paroxetine (a CYP2D6 substrate and inhibitor) during treatment with 5 mg SAPHRIS twice daily in 15 healthy male subjects resulted in an almost 2-fold increase in paroxetine exposure. Asenapine may enhance the inhibitory effects of paroxetine on its own metabolism.

SAPHRIS should be coadministered cautiously with drugs that are both substrates and inhibitors for CYP2D6.

Valproic acid and lithium pre-dose serum concentrations collected from an adjunctive therapy study were comparable between asenapine treated patients and placebo treated patients indicating a lack of effect of asenapine on valproic and lithium plasma levels.

8 USE IN SPECIFIC POPULATIONS

8.1 Pregnancy

Pregnancy Category C: There are no adequate and well-controlled studies of SAPHRIS in pregnant women.

In animal studies, asenapine increased post-implantation loss and decreased pup weight and survival at doses similar to or less than recommended clinical doses. In these studies there was no increase in the incidence of structural abnormalities caused by asenapine.

Asenapine was not teratogenic in reproduction studies in rats and rabbits at intravenous doses up to 1.5 mg/kg in rats and 0.44 mg/kg in rabbits. These doses are 0.7 and 0.4 times, respectively, the maximum recommended human dose (MRHD) of 10 mg twice daily given sublingually on a mg/m² basis. Plasma levels of asenapine were measured in the rabbit study, and the area under the curve (AUC) at the highest dose tested was 2 times that in humans receiving the MRHD.

In a study in which rats were treated from day 6 of gestation through day 21 postpartum with intravenous doses of asenapine of 0.3, 0.9, and 1.5 mg/kg/day (0.15, 0.4, and 0.7 times the MRHD of 10 mg twice daily given sublingually on a mg/m² basis), increases in post-implantation loss and early pup deaths were seen at all doses, and decreases in subsequent pup survival and weight gain were seen at the two higher doses. A cross-fostering study indicated that the decreases in pup survival were largely due to prenatal drug effects. Increases in post-implantation loss and decreases in pup weight and survival were also seen when pregnant rats were dosed orally with asenapine.

Non-teratogenic Effects

Neonates exposed to antipsychotic drugs during the third trimester of pregnancy are at risk for extrapyramidal and/or withdrawal symptoms following delivery. There have been reports of agitation, hypertonia, hypotonia, tremor, somnolence, respiratory distress and feeding disorder in these neonates. These complications have varied in severity; while in some cases symptoms have been self-limited, in other cases neonates have required intensive care unit support and prolonged hospitalization. SAPHRIS (asenapine) should be used during pregnancy only if the potential benefit justifies the potential risk to the fetus.

8.2 Labor and Delivery

The effect of SAPHRIS on labor and delivery in humans is unknown.

8.3 Nursing Mothers

Asenapine is excreted in milk of rats during lactation. It is not known whether asenapine or its metabolites are excreted in human milk. Because many drugs are excreted in human milk, caution should be exercised when SAPHRIS is administered to a nursing woman. It is recommended that women receiving SAPHRIS should not breast feed.

8.4 Pediatric Use

Safety and effectiveness in pediatric patients have not been established.

8.5 Geriatric Use

Clinical studies of SAPHRIS in the treatment of schizophrenia and bipolar mania did not include sufficient numbers of patients aged 65 and over to determine whether or not they respond differently than younger patients. Of the approximately 2250 patients in pre-marketing clinical studies of SAPHRIS, 1.1% (25) were 65 years of age or over. Multiple factors that might increase the pharmacodynamic response to SAPHRIS, causing poorer tolerance or orthostasis, could be present in elderly patients, and these patients should be monitored carefully.

In elderly patients with psychosis, asenapine exposure (AUC) was on average 40% higher compared to younger adult patients [see Clinical Pharmacology (12.3)].

Elderly patients with dementia-related psychosis treated with SAPHRIS are at an increased risk of death compared to placebo. SAPHRIS is not approved for the treatment of patients with dementia-related psychosis [see Boxed Warning].

8.6 Renal Impairment

The exposure of asenapine following a single dose of 5 mg was similar among subjects with varying degrees of renal impairment and subjects with normal renal function [see Clinical Pharmacology (12.3)].

8.7 Hepatic Impairment

In subjects with severe hepatic impairment who were treated with a single dose of SAPHRIS 5 mg, asenapine exposures (on average), were 7-fold higher than the exposures observed in subjects with normal hepatic function. Thus, SAPHRIS is not recommended in patients with severe hepatic impairment (Child-Pugh C) [see Dosage and Administration (2.4) and Clinical Pharmacology (12.3)].

9 DRUG ABUSE AND DEPENDENCE

9.1 Controlled Substance

SAPHRIS is not a controlled substance.

9.2 Abuse

SAPHRIS has not been systematically studied in animals or humans for its abuse potential or its ability to induce tolerance or physical dependence. Thus, it is not possible to predict the extent to which a CNS-active drug will be misused, diverted and/or abused once it is marketed. Patients should be evaluated carefully for a history of drug abuse, and such patients should be observed carefully for signs that they are misusing or abusing SAPHRIS (e.g., drug-seeking behavior, increases in dose).

10 OVERDOSAGE

Human Experience: In pre-marketing clinical studies involving more than 3350 patients and/or healthy subjects, accidental or intentional acute overdosage of SAPHRIS was identified in 3 patients. Among these few reported cases of overdose, the highest estimated ingestion of SAPHRIS was 400 mg. Reported adverse reactions at the highest dosage included agitation and confusion.

Management of Overdosage: There is no specific antidote to SAPHRIS. The possibility of multiple drug involvement should be considered. An electrocardiogram should be obtained and management of overdose should concentrate on supportive therapy, maintaining an adequate airway, oxygenation and ventilation, and management of symptoms. Hypotension and circulatory collapse should be treated with appropriate measures, such as intravenous fluids and/or sympathomimetic agents (epinephrine and dopamine should not be used, since beta stimulation may worsen hypotension in the setting of SAPHRIS-induced alpha blockade). In case of severe extrapyramidal symptoms, anticholinergic medication should be administered. Close medical supervision and monitoring should continue until the patient recovers.

11 DESCRIPTION

SAPHRIS is a psychotropic agent that is available for sublingual administration. Asenapine belongs to the class dibenzo-oxepino pyrroles. The chemical designation is (3aRS,12bRS)-5-Chloro-2-methyl-2,3,3a,12b-tetrahydro-1Hdibenzo[2,3:6,7]oxepino[4,5-c]pyrrole (2Z)-2-butene-dioate (1:1). Its molecular formula is $C_{17}H_{16}ClNO \bullet C_4H_4O_4$ and its molecular weight is 401.84 (free base: 285.8). The chemical structure is:

Table 5: Summary of Effect of Coadministered Drugs on Exposure to Asenapine in Healthy Volunteers

Coadministered drug (Postulated effect on CYP450/UGT)	Dose schedules		Effect on asenapine pharmacokinetics		Recommendation
	Coadministered drug	Asenapine	C_{max}	$AUC_{0-\infty}$	
Fluvoxamine (CYP1A2 inhibitor)	25 mg twice daily for 8 days	5-mg Single Dose	+13%	+29%	Coadminister with caution*
Paroxetine (CYP2D6 inhibitor)	20 mg once daily for 9 days	5-mg Single Dose	–13%	–9%	No SAPHRIS dose adjustment required [see Drug Interactions (7.2)]
Imipramine (CYP1A2/2C19/3A4 inhibitor)	75-mg Single Dose	5-mg Single Dose	+17%	+10%	No SAPHRIS dose adjustment required
Cimetidine (CYP3A4/2D6/1A2 inhibitor)	800 mg twice daily for 8 days	5-mg Single Dose	–13%	+1%	No SAPHRIS dose adjustment required
Carbamazepine (CYP3A4 inducer)	400 mg twice daily for 15 days	5-mg Single Dose	–16%	–16%	No SAPHRIS dose adjustment required
Valproate (UGT1A4 inhibitor)	500 mg twice daily for 9 days	5-mg Single Dose	2%	–1%	No SAPHRIS dose adjustment required

* The full therapeutic dose of fluvoxamine would be expected to cause a greater increase in asenapine plasma concentrations. AUC: Area under the curve.

Asenapine is a white to off-white powder.

SAPHRIS is supplied for sublingual administration in tablets containing 5-mg or 10-mg asenapine; inactive ingredients include gelatin and mannitol.

SAPHRIS, black cherry flavor, is supplied for sublingual administration in tablets containing 5-mg or 10-mg asenapine; inactive ingredients include gelatin, mannitol, sucralose, and black cherry flavor.

12 CLINICAL PHARMACOLOGY

12.1 Mechanism of Action

The mechanism of action of asenapine, as with other drugs having efficacy in schizophrenia and bipolar disorder, is unknown. It has been suggested that the efficacy of asenapine in schizophrenia is mediated through a combination of antagonist activity at D_2 and $5-HT_{2A}$ receptors.

12.2 Pharmacodynamics

Asenapine exhibits high affinity for serotonin $5-HT_{1A}$, $5-HT_{1B}$, $5-HT_{2A}$, $5-HT_{2B}$, $5-HT_{2C}$, $5-HT_5$, $5-HT_6$ and $5-HT_7$ receptors (Ki values of 2.5, 4.0, 0.06, 0.16, 0.03, 1.6, 0.25, and 0.13 nM), dopamine D_2, D_3, D_4, and D_1 receptors (Ki values of 1.3, 0.42, 1.1, and 1.4 nM), α_1 and α_2-adrenergic receptors (Ki values of 1.2 and 1.2 nM), and histamine H_1 receptors (Ki value 1.0 nM), and moderate affinity for H_2 receptors (Ki value of 6.2 nM). In in vitro assays asenapine acts as an antagonist at these receptors. Asenapine has no appreciable affinity for muscarinic cholinergic receptors (e.g., Ki value of 8128 nM for M_1).

12.3 Pharmacokinetics

Following a single 5-mg dose of SAPHRIS, the mean C_{max} was approximately 4 ng/mL and was observed at a mean t_{max} of 1 hour. Elimination of asenapine is primarily through direct glucuronidation by UGT1A4 and oxidative metabolism by cytochrome P450 isoenzymes (predominantly CYP1A2). Following an initial more rapid distribution phase, the mean terminal half-life is approximately 24 hrs. With multiple-dose twice-daily dosing, steady-state is attained within 3 days. Overall, steady-state asenapine pharmacokinetics are similar to single-dose pharmacokinetics.

Absorption: Following sublingual administration, asenapine is rapidly absorbed with peak plasma concentrations occurring within 0.5 to 1.5 hours. The absolute bioavailability of sublingual asenapine at 5 mg is 35%. Increasing the dose from 5 mg to 10 mg twice daily (a two-fold increase) results in less than linear (1.7 times) increases in both the extent of exposure and maximum concentration. The absolute bioavailability of asenapine when swallowed is low (<2% with an oral tablet formulation).

The intake of water several (2 or 5) minutes after asenapine administration resulted in decreased asenapine exposure. Therefore, eating and drinking should be avoided for 10 minutes after administration *[see Dosage and Administration (2.1)]*.

Distribution: Asenapine is rapidly distributed and has a large volume of distribution (approximately 20 - 25 L/kg), indicating extensive extravascular distribution. Asenapine is highly bound (95%) to plasma proteins, including albumin and α_1-acid glycoprotein.

Metabolism and Elimination: Direct glucuronidation by UGT1A4 and oxidative metabolism by cytochrome P450 isoenzymes (predominantly CYP1A2) are the primary metabolic pathways for asenapine.

Asenapine is a high clearance drug with a clearance after intravenous administration of 52 L/h. In this circumstance, hepatic clearance is influenced primarily by changes in liver blood flow rather than by changes in the intrinsic clearance, i.e., the metabolizing enzymatic activity. Following an initial more rapid distribution phase, the terminal half life of asenapine is approximately 24 hours. Steady-state concentrations of asenapine are reached within 3 days of twice daily dosing.

After administration of a single dose of $[^{14}C]$-labeled asenapine, about 90% of the dose was recovered; approximately 50% was recovered in urine, and 40% recovered in feces. About 50% of the circulating species in plasma have been identified. The predominant species was asenapine N^+-glucuronide; others included N-desmethylasenapine, N-desmethylasenapine N-carbamoyl glucuronide, and unchanged asenapine in smaller amounts. SAPHRIS activity is primarily due to the parent drug.

In vitro studies indicate that asenapine is a substrate for UGT1A4, CYP1A2 and to a lesser extent CYP3A4 and CYP2D6. Asenapine is a weak inhibitor of CYP2D6. Asenapine does not cause induction of CYP1A2 or CYP3A4 activities in cultured human hepatocytes. Coadministration of asenapine with known inhibitors, inducers or substrates of these metabolic pathways has been studied in a number of drug-drug interaction studies *[see Drug Interactions (7)]*.

Smoking: A population pharmacokinetic analysis indicated that smoking, which induces CYP1A2, had no effect on the clearance of asenapine in smokers. In a crossover study in which 24 healthy male subjects (who were smok-

ers) were administered a single 5-mg sublingual dose, concomitant smoking had no effect on the pharmacokinetics of asenapine.

Food: A crossover study in 26 healthy male subjects was performed to evaluate the effect of food on the pharmacokinetics of a single 5-mg dose of asenapine. Consumption of food immediately prior to sublingual administration decreased asenapine exposure by 20%; consumption of food 4 hours after sublingual administration decreased asenapine exposure by about 10%. These effects are probably due to increased hepatic blood flow.

In clinical trials establishing the efficacy and safety of SAPHRIS, patients were instructed to avoid eating for 10 minutes following sublingual dosing. There were no other restrictions with regard to the timing of meals in these trials *[see Dosage and Administration (2.1) and Patient Counseling Information (17.1)]*.

Water: In clinical trials establishing the efficacy and safety of SAPHRIS, patients were instructed to avoid drinking for 10 minutes following sublingual dosing. The effect of water administration following 10-mg sublingual SAPHRIS dosing was studied at different time points of 2, 5, 10, and 30 minutes in 15 healthy male subjects. The exposure of asenapine following administration of water 10 minutes after sublingual dosing was equivalent to that when water was administered 30 minutes after dosing. Reduced exposure to asenapine was observed following water administration at 2 minutes (19% decrease) and 5 minutes (10% decrease) *[see Dosage and Administration (2.1) and Patient Counseling Information (17.1)]*.

Special Populations:

Hepatic Impairment: The effect of decreased hepatic function on the pharmacokinetics of asenapine, administered as a single 5-mg sublingual dose, was studied in 30 subjects (8 each in those with normal hepatic function and Child-Pugh A and B groups, and 6 in the Child-Pugh C group). In subjects with mild or moderate hepatic impairment (Child-Pugh A or B), asenapine exposure was 12% higher than that in subjects with normal hepatic function, indicating that dosage adjustment is not required for these subjects. In subjects with severe hepatic impairment, asenapine exposures were on average 7 times higher than the exposures of those in subjects with normal hepatic function. Thus, SAPHRIS is not recommended in patients with severe hepatic impairment (Child-Pugh C) *[see Dosage in Specific Populations (2.4) and Use in Specific Populations (8.7) and Warnings and Precautions (5.14)]*.

Renal Impairment: The effect of decreased renal function on the pharmacokinetics of asenapine was studied in subjects with mildly (creatinine clearance (CrCl) 51 to 80 mL/min; N=8), moderately (CrCl 30 to 50 mL/min; N=8), and severely (CrCl less than 30 mL/min but not on dialysis; N=8) impaired renal function and compared to normal subjects (CrCl greater than 80 mL/min; N=8). The exposure of asenapine following a single dose of 5 mg was similar among subjects with varying degrees of renal impairment and subjects with normal renal function. Dosage adjustment based upon degree of renal impairment is not required. The effect of renal function on the excretion of other metabolites and the effect of dialysis on the pharmacokinetics of asenapine has not been studied *[see Use in Specific Populations (8.6)]*.

Geriatric Patients: In elderly patients (N=96) with psychosis (65-85 years of age), asenapine exposure (AUC) was on average 40% higher compared to younger adult patients. No dosage adjustment is necessary. In a population pharmacokinetic analysis, a decrease in clearance with increasing age was observed, implying a 30% higher exposure in elderly as compared to adult patients *[see Use in Specific Populations (8.5)]*.

Gender: The potential difference in asenapine pharmacokinetics between males and females was not studied in a dedicated trial. In a population pharmacokinetic analysis, no significant differences between genders were observed.

Race: In a population pharmacokinetic analysis, no effect of race on asenapine concentrations was observed. In a dedicated study, the pharmacokinetics of SAPHRIS were similar in Caucasian and Japanese subjects.

13 NONCLINICAL TOXICOLOGY

13.1 Carcinogenesis, Mutagenesis, Impairment of Fertility

Carcinogenesis: In a lifetime carcinogenicity study in CD-1 mice asenapine was administered subcutaneously at doses up to those resulting in plasma levels (AUC) estimated to be 5 times those in humans receiving the MRHD of 10 mg twice daily. The incidence of malignant lymphomas was increased in female mice, with a no-effect dose resulting in plasma levels estimated to be 1.5 times those in humans receiving the MRHD. The mouse strain used has a high and variable incidence of malignant lymphomas, and the significance of these results to humans is unknown. There were no increases in other tumor types in female mice. In male mice, there were no increases in any tumor type.

In a lifetime carcinogenicity study in Sprague-Dawley rats, asenapine did not cause any increases in tumors when administered subcutaneously at doses up to those resulting in plasma levels (AUC) estimated to be 5 times those in humans receiving the MRHD.

Mutagenesis: No evidence for genotoxic potential of asenapine was found in the in vitro bacterial reverse mutation assay, the in vitro forward gene mutation assay in mouse lymphoma cells, the in vitro chromosomal aberration assays in human lymphocytes, the in vitro sister chromatid exchange assay in rabbit lymphocytes, or the in vivo micronucleus assay in rats.

Impairment of Fertility: Asenapine did not impair fertility in rats when tested at doses up to 11 mg/kg twice daily given orally. This dose is 10 times the maximum recommended human dose of 10 mg twice daily given sublingually on a mg/m² basis.

14 CLINICAL STUDIES

14.1 Schizophrenia

The efficacy of SAPHRIS in the treatment of schizophrenia in adults was evaluated in three fixed-dose, short-term (6 week) randomized, double-blind, placebo-controlled, and active-controlled (haloperidol, risperidone, and olanzapine) trials of adult patients who met DSM-IV criteria for schizophrenia and were having an acute exacerbation of their schizophrenic illness. In two of the three trials SAPHRIS demonstrated superior efficacy to placebo. In a third trial, SAPHRIS could not be distinguished from placebo; however, an active control in that trial was superior to placebo.

In the two positive trials for SAPHRIS, the primary efficacy rating scale was the Positive and Negative Syndrome Scale (PANSS), which assesses the symptoms of schizophrenia. The primary endpoint was change from baseline to endpoint on the PANSS total score. The results of the SAPHRIS trials in schizophrenia follow:

In trial 1, a 6-week trial (n=174), comparing SAPHRIS (5 mg twice daily) to placebo, SAPHRIS 5 mg twice daily was statistically superior to placebo on the PANSS total score.

In trial 2, a 6-week trial (n=448), comparing two fixed doses of SAPHRIS (5 mg and 10 mg twice daily) to placebo, SAPHRIS 5 mg twice daily was statistically superior to placebo on the PANSS total score. SAPHRIS 10 mg twice daily showed no added benefit compared to 5 mg twice daily and was not significantly different from placebo.

An examination of population subgroups did not reveal any clear evidence of differential responsiveness on the basis of age, gender or race.

Maintenance of efficacy has been demonstrated in a placebo-controlled, double-blind, multicenter, flexible dose (5 mg or 10 mg twice daily based on tolerability) clinical trial with a randomized withdrawal design. A total of 700 patients entered open-label treatment with SAPHRIS for a period of 26 weeks. Of these, a total of 386 patients who met pre-specified criteria for continued stability (mean length of stabilization was 22 weeks) were randomized to a double-blind, placebo-controlled, randomized withdrawal phase. SAPHRIS was statistically superior to placebo in time to relapse or impending relapse defined as increase in PANSS ≥20% from baseline and a Clinical Global Impression–Severity of Illness (CGI-S) score ≥4 (at least 2 days within 1 week) or PANSS score ≥5 on "hostility" or "uncooperativeness" items and CGI-S score ≥4 (≥2 days within a week), or PANSS score ≥5 on any two of the following items: "unusual thought content," "conceptual disorganization," or "hallucinatory behavior" items, and CGI-S score ≥4 (≥2 days within 1 week) or investigator judgment of worsening symptoms or increased risk of violence to self (including suicide) or other persons. The Kaplan-Meier curves of the time to relapse or impending relapse during the double-blind, placebo-controlled, randomized withdrawal phase of this trial for SAPHRIS and placebo are shown in Figure 1.

Figure 1: Kaplan-Meier Estimation of Percent Relapse/Impending Relapse for SAPHRIS and placebo

Time(days) represents the number of days from randomization to the first date of achieving relapse/impending relapse status.
The product limit estimators are based on the Kaplan-Meier distribution with censoring at last double-blind dose date.

14.2 Bipolar Disorder

Monotherapy: The efficacy of SAPHRIS in the treatment of acute mania was established in two similarly designed 3-week, randomized, double-blind, placebo-controlled, and active-controlled (olanzapine) trials of adult patients who met DSM-IV criteria for Bipolar I Disorder with an acute manic or mixed episode with or without psychotic features.

The primary rating instrument used for assessing manic symptoms in these trials was the Young Mania Rating Scale (YMRS). Patients were also assessed on the Clinical Global Impression – Bipolar (CGI-BP) scale. In both trials, all patients randomized to SAPHRIS were initially administered 10 mg twice daily, and the dose could be adjusted within the dose range of 5 to 10 mg twice daily from Day 2 onward based on efficacy and tolerability. Ninety percent of patients remained on the 10-mg twice daily dose. SAPHRIS was statistically superior to placebo on the YMRS total score and the CGI-BP Severity of Illness score (mania) in both studies. An examination of subgroups did not reveal any clear evidence of differential responsiveness on the basis of age, gender or race.

Adjunctive Therapy: The efficacy of SAPHRIS as an adjunctive therapy in acute mania was established in a 12-week, placebo-controlled trial with a 3-week primary efficacy endpoint involving 326 patients with a manic or mixed episode of Bipolar I Disorder, with or without psychotic features, who were partially responsive to lithium or valproate monotherapy after at least 2 weeks of treatment. SAPHRIS was statistically superior to placebo in the reduction of manic symptoms (measured by the YMRS total score) as an adjunctive therapy to lithium or valproate monotherapy at week 3.

16 HOW SUPPLIED/STORAGE AND HANDLING

SAPHRIS (asenapine) sublingual tablets are supplied as:

5-mg Tablets
Round, white to off-white sublingual tablets, with "5" on one side.
Child-resistant packaging

Box of 60	6 blisters with 10 tablets	NDC 0052-0118-06
Hospital Unit Dose		
Box of 100	10 blisters with 10 tablets	NDC 0052-0118-90

10-mg Tablets
Round, white to off-white sublingual tablets, with "10" on one side.
Child-resistant packaging

Box of 60	6 blisters with 10 tablets	NDC 0052-0119-06
Hospital Unit Dose		
Box of 100	10 blisters with 10 tablets	NDC 0052-0119-90

5-mg Tablets, black cherry flavor
Round, white to off-white sublingual tablets, with "5" on one side within a circle.
Child-resistant packaging

Box of 60	6 blisters with 10 tablets	NDC 0052-2139-03
Hospital Unit Dose		
Box of 100	10 blisters with 10 tablets	NDC 0052-2139-04

10-mg Tablets, black cherry flavor
Round, white to off-white sublingual tablets, with "10" on one side within a circle.
Child-resistant packaging

Box of 60	6 blisters with 10 tablets	NDC 0052-2142-03
Hospital Unit Dose		
Box of 100	10 blisters with 10 tablets	NDC 0052-2142-04

Storage
Store at 15°-30°C (59°-86°F) [see USP Controlled Room Temperature].

17 PATIENT COUNSELING INFORMATION

17.1 Tablet Administration
IMPORTANT:
• **Do not remove tablet until ready to administer.**
• **Use dry hands when handling tablet.**

Step 1. Firmly press and hold thumb button, then pull out tablet pack.
Do not push tablet through tablet pack.
Do not cut or tear tablet pack.

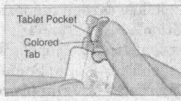

Step 2. Peel back colored tab.

Step 3. Gently remove tablet.
Do not crush tablet.

Step 4. Place tablet **under** tongue and allow it to dissolve completely.

Do not chew or swallow tablet.
Do not eat or drink for 10 minutes.

Step 5. Slide tablet pack into case until it clicks.
[see Drug Interactions (7) and Clinical Pharmacology (12.3)].

17.2 Increased Mortality in Elderly Patients with Dementia-Related Psychosis
Patients and caregivers should be advised that elderly patients with dementia-related psychoses treated with atypical antipsychotic drugs are at increased risk of death compared with placebo. SAPHRIS is not approved for elderly patients with dementia-related psychosis *[see Warnings and Precautions (5.1)].*

17.3 Hypersensitivity Reactions
Patients should be informed of the signs and symptoms of a serious allergic reaction (e.g., difficulty breathing, itching, swelling of the face, tongue or throat, feeling lightheaded etc.). Patients should be instructed to seek immediate emergency assistance if they develop any of these signs and symptoms *[see Warnings and Precautions (5.7) and Adverse Reactions (6)].*

17.4 Application Site Reactions
Inform patients that application site reactions including oral ulcers, blisters, peeling/sloughing and inflammation have been reported. Instruct patients to monitor for these reactions *[see Adverse Reactions (6.2)].*

17.5 Neuroleptic Malignant Syndrome
Patients and caregivers should be counseled that a potentially fatal symptom complex sometimes referred to as Neuroleptic Malignant Syndrome (NMS) has been reported in association with administration of antipsychotic drugs. Signs and symptoms of NMS include hyperpyrexia, muscle rigidity, altered mental status, and evidence of autonomic instability (irregular pulse or blood pressure, tachycardia, diaphoresis, and cardiac dysrhythmia) *[see Warnings and Precautions (5.3)].*

17.6 Hyperglycemia and Diabetes Mellitus
Patients should be aware of the symptoms of hyperglycemia (high blood sugar) and diabetes mellitus. Patients who are diagnosed with diabetes, those with risk factors for diabetes, or those that develop these symptoms during treatment should have their blood glucose monitored at the beginning of and periodically during treatment *[see Warnings and Precautions (5.5)].*

17.7 Weight Gain
Patients should be advised that they may experience weight gain. Patients should have their weight monitored regularly *[see Warnings and Precautions (5.6)].*

17.8 Orthostatic Hypotension
Patients should be advised of the risk of orthostatic hypotension (symptoms include feeling dizzy or lightheaded upon standing) especially early in treatment, and also at times of re-initiating treatment or increases in dose *[see Warnings and Precautions (5.8)].*

17.9 Leukopenia/Neutropenia
Patients with a pre-existing low WBC or a history of drug induced leukopenia/neutropenia should be advised that they should have their CBC monitored while taking SAPHRIS *[see Warnings and Precautions (5.9)].*

17.10 Interference with Cognitive and Motor Performance
Patients should be cautioned about performing activities requiring mental alertness, such as operating hazardous machinery or operating a motor vehicle, until they are reasonably certain that SAPHRIS therapy does not affect them adversely *[see Warnings and Precautions (5.13)].*

17.11 Heat Exposure and Dehydration
Patients should be advised regarding appropriate care in avoiding overheating and dehydration *[see Warnings and Precautions (5.14)].*

17.12 Concomitant Medication and Alcohol
Patients should be advised to inform their physicians if they are taking, or plan to take, any prescription or over-the-counter medications since there is a potential for interactions. Patients should be advised to avoid alcohol while taking SAPHRIS *[see Drug Interactions (7)].*

17.13 Pregnancy and Nursing
Patients should be advised to notify their physician if they become pregnant or intend to become pregnant during therapy with SAPHRIS. Patients should be advised not to breast feed if they are taking SAPHRIS *[see Use in Special Populations (8.1, 8.3)].*

Manufactured for: Merck Sharp & Dohme Corp., a subsidiary of
MERCK & CO., INC., Whitehouse Station, NJ 08889, USA
Manufactured by: Catalent UK Swindon Zydis Ltd., Blagrove, Swindon, Wiltshire, SN5 8RU, UK
U.S. Patent Nos. 5,763,476 and 7,741,358.
Copyright © 2009, 2011 MSD Oss B.V., a subsidiary of
Merck & Co., Inc.
All rights reserved.
Revised: 03/2013
900274-ASP-TB-USPI.25

Shown in Product Identification Guide, page 309

SINEMET®   ℞
(carbidopa-levodopa)
Tablets

DESCRIPTION

SINEMET® (carbidopa levodopa) is a combination of carbidopa and levodopa for the treatment of Parkinson's disease and syndrome.

Carbidopa, an inhibitor of aromatic amino acid decarboxylation, is a white, crystalline compound, slightly soluble in water, with a molecular weight of 244.3. It is designated chemically as (—)-L-α-hydrazino-α-methyl-β-(3,4-dihydroxybenzene) propanoic acid monohydrate. Its empirical formula is $C_{10}H_{14}N_2O_4 \cdot H_2O$, and its structural formula is:

$$\text{HO} \underset{\text{OH}}{\bigcirc} \text{CH}_2 \underset{\text{CH}_3}{\overset{}{\text{CCOOH}}} \cdot H_2O$$
$$\text{NHNH}_2$$

Tablet content is expressed in terms of anhydrous carbidopa which has a molecular weight of 226.3.

Levodopa, an aromatic amino acid, is a white, crystalline compound, slightly soluble in water, with a molecular weight of 197.2. It is designated chemically as (—)-L-α-amino-β-(3,4-dihydroxybenzene) propanoic acid. Its empirical formula is $C_9H_{11}NO_4$, and its structural formula is:

SINEMET is supplied as tablets in three strengths:
SINEMET 25-100, containing 25 mg of carbidopa and 100 mg of levodopa.
SINEMET 10-100, containing 10 mg of carbidopa and 100 mg of levodopa.
SINEMET 25-250, containing 25 mg of carbidopa and 250 mg of levodopa.
Inactive ingredients are hydroxypropyl cellulose, pregelatinized starch, crospovidone, microcrystalline cellulose, and magnesium stearate. SINEMET 10-100 and 25-250 Tablets also contain FD&C Blue #2/Indigo Carmine AL. SINEMET 25-100 Tablets also contain D&C Yellow #10 Lake.

CLINICAL PHARMACOLOGY
Mechanism of Action
Parkinson's disease is a progressive, neurodegenerative disorder of the extrapyramidal nervous system affecting the mobility and control of the skeletal muscular system. Its characteristic features include resting tremor, rigidity, and bradykinetic movements. Symptomatic treatments, such as levodopa therapies, may permit the patient better mobility. Current evidence indicates that symptoms of Parkinson's disease are related to depletion of dopamine in the corpus striatum. Administration of dopamine is ineffective in the treatment of Parkinson's disease apparently because it does not cross the blood-brain barrier. However, levodopa, the metabolic precursor of dopamine, does cross the blood-brain barrier, and presumably is converted to dopamine in the brain. This is thought to be the mechanism whereby levodopa relieves symptoms of Parkinson's disease.

Pharmacodynamics
When levodopa is administered orally, it is rapidly decarboxylated to dopamine in extracerebral tissues so that only a small portion of a given dose is transported unchanged to the central nervous system. For this reason, large doses of levodopa are required for adequate therapeutic effect, and these may often be accompanied by nausea and other adverse reactions, some of which are attributable to dopamine formed in extracerebral tissues.
Since levodopa competes with certain amino acids for transport across the gut wall, the absorption of levodopa may be impaired in some patients on a high protein diet.
Carbidopa inhibits decarboxylation of peripheral levodopa. It does not cross the blood-brain barrier and does not affect the metabolism of levodopa within the central nervous system.
The incidence of levodopa-induced nausea and vomiting is less with SINEMET than with levodopa. In many patients, this reduction in nausea and vomiting will permit more rapid dosage titration.
Since its decarboxylase inhibiting activity is limited to extracerebral tissues, administration of carbidopa with levodopa makes more levodopa available for transport to the brain.

Pharmacokinetics
Carbidopa reduces the amount of levodopa required to produce a given response by about 75% and, when administered with levodopa, increases both plasma levels and the plasma half-life of levodopa, and decreases plasma and urinary dopamine and homovanillic acid.
The plasma half-life of levodopa is about 50 minutes, without carbidopa. When carbidopa and levodopa are administered together, the half-life of levodopa is increased to about 1.5 hours. At steady state, the bioavailability of carbidopa from SINEMET tablets is approximately 99% relative to the concomitant administration of carbidopa and levodopa.
In clinical pharmacologic studies, simultaneous administration of carbidopa and levodopa produced greater urinary excretion of levodopa in proportion to the excretion of dopamine than administration of the two drugs at separate times.
Pyridoxine hydrochloride (vitamin B_6), in oral doses of 10 mg to 25 mg, may reverse the effects of levodopa by increasing the rate of aromatic amino acid decarboxylation. Carbidopa inhibits this action of pyridoxine; therefore, SINEMET can be given to patients receiving supplemental pyridoxine (vitamin B_6).

Special Populations
Geriatric
A study in eight young healthy subjects (21-22 yr) and eight elderly healthy subjects (69-76 yr) showed that the absolute bioavailability of levodopa was similar between young and elderly subjects following oral administration of levodopa and carbidopa. However, the systemic exposure (AUC) of levodopa was increased by 55% in elderly subjects compared to young subjects. Based on another study in forty patients with Parkinson's disease, there was a correlation between age of patients and the increase of AUC of levodopa following administration of levodopa and an inhibitor of peripheral dopa decarboxylase. AUC of levodopa was increased by 28% in elderly patients (≥ 65 yr) compared to young patients (< 65 yr). Additionally, mean value of Cmax for levodopa was increased by 24% in elderly patients (≥ 65 yr) compared to young patients (< 65 yr) (see PRECAUTIONS, Geriatric Use).
The AUC of carbidopa was increased in elderly subjects (n=10, 65-76 yr) by 29% compared to young subjects (n=24, 23-64 yr) following IV administration of 50 mg levodopa with carbidopa (50 mg). This increase is not considered a clinically significant impact.

INDICATIONS AND USAGE
SINEMET is indicated in the treatment of Parkinson's disease, post-encephalitic parkinsonism, and symptomatic parkinsonism that may follow carbon monoxide intoxication or manganese intoxication.
Carbidopa allows patients treated for Parkinson's disease to use much lower doses of levodopa. Some patients who responded poorly to levodopa have improved on SINEMET. This is most likely due to decreased peripheral decarboxylation of levodopa caused by administration of carbidopa rather than by a primary effect of carbidopa on the nervous system. Carbidopa has not been shown to enhance the intrinsic efficacy of levodopa.
Carbidopa may also reduce nausea and vomiting and permit more rapid titration of levodopa.

CONTRAINDICATIONS
Nonselective monoamine oxidase (MAO) inhibitors are contraindicated for use with SINEMET. These inhibitors must be discontinued at least two weeks prior to initiating therapy with SINEMET. SINEMET may be administered concomitantly with the manufacturer's recommended dose of an MAO inhibitor with selectivity for MAO type B (e.g., selegiline HCl) (see PRECAUTIONS, Drug Interactions).
SINEMET is contraindicated in patients with known hypersensitivity to any component of this drug, and in patients with narrow-angle glaucoma.

WARNINGS
When SINEMET is to be given to patients who are being treated with levodopa, levodopa must be discontinued at least twelve hours before therapy with SINEMET is started. In order to reduce adverse reactions, it is necessary to individualize therapy. See DOSAGE AND ADMINISTRATION section before initiating therapy.
The addition of carbidopa with levodopa in the form of SINEMET reduces the peripheral effects (nausea, vomiting) due to decarboxylation of levodopa; however, carbidopa does not decrease the adverse reactions due to the central effects of levodopa. Because carbidopa permits more levodopa to reach the brain and more dopamine to be formed, certain adverse central nervous system (CNS) effects, e.g., dyskinesias (involuntary movements), may occur at lower dosages and sooner with SINEMET than with levodopa alone.
All patients should be observed carefully for the development of depression with concomitant suicidal tendencies. SINEMET should be administered cautiously to patients with severe cardiovascular or pulmonary disease, bronchial asthma, renal, hepatic or endocrine disease.
As with levodopa, care should be exercised in administering SINEMET to patients with a history of myocardial infarction who have residual atrial, nodal, or ventricular arrhythmias. In such patients, cardiac function should be monitored with particular care during the period of initial dosage adjustment, in a facility with provisions for intensive cardiac care.
As with levodopa, treatment with SINEMET may increase the possibility of upper gastrointestinal hemorrhage in patients with a history of peptic ulcer.

Falling Asleep During Activities of Daily Living and Somnolence
Patients taking SINEMET alone or with other dopaminergic drugs have reported suddenly falling asleep without prior warning of sleepiness while engaged in activities of daily living (includes operation of motor vehicles). Road traffic accidents attributed to sudden sleep onset have been reported. Although many patients reported somnolence while on dopaminergic medications, there have been reports of road traffic accidents attributed to sudden onset of sleep in which the patient did not perceive any warning signs, such as excessive drowsiness, and believed that they were alert immediately prior to the event. Sudden onset of sleep has been reported to occur as long as one year after the initiation of treatment.
Falling asleep while engaged in activities of daily living usually occurs in patients experiencing pre-existing somnolence, although some patients may not give such a history. For this reason, prescribers should reassess patients for drowsiness or sleepiness especially since some of the events occur well after the start of treatment. Prescribers should be aware that patients may not acknowledge drowsiness or sleepiness until directly questioned about drowsiness or sleepiness during specific activities. Patients should be advised to exercise caution while driving or operating machines during treatment with SINEMET. Patients who have already experienced somnolence or an episode of sudden sleep onset should not participate in these activities during treatment with SINEMET.
Before initiating treatment with SINEMET, advise patients about the potential to develop drowsiness and ask specifically about factors that may increase the risk for somnolence with SINEMET such as the use of concomitant sedating medications and the presence of sleep disorders. Consider discontinuing SINEMET in patients who report significant daytime sleepiness or episodes of falling asleep during activities that require active participation (e.g., conversations, eating, etc.). If treatment with SINEMET continues, patients should be advised not to drive and to avoid other potentially dangerous activities that might result in harm if the patients become somnolent. There is insufficient information to establish that dose reduction will eliminate episodes of falling asleep while engaged in activities of daily living.

Hyperpyrexia and Confusion
Sporadic cases of a symptom complex resembling neuroleptic malignant syndrome (NMS) have been reported in association with dose reductions or withdrawal of certain antiparkinsonian agents such as levodopa, carbidopa levodopa, or carbidopa levodopa extended release. Therefore, patients should be observed carefully when the dosage of levodopa is reduced abruptly or discontinued, especially if the patient is receiving neuroleptics.
NMS is an uncommon but life-threatening syndrome characterized by fever or hyperthermia. Neurological findings, including muscle rigidity, involuntary movements, altered consciousness, mental status changes; other disturbances, such as autonomic dysfunction, tachycardia, tachypnea, sweating, hyper- or hypotension; laboratory findings, such as creatine phosphokinase elevation, leukocytosis, myoglobinuria, and increased serum myoglobin have been reported.
The early diagnosis of this condition is important for the appropriate management of these patients. Considering NMS as a possible diagnosis and ruling out other acute illnesses (e.g., pneumonia, systemic infection, etc.) is essential. This may be especially complex if the clinical presentation includes both serious medical illness and untreated or inadequately treated extrapyramidal signs and symptoms (EPS). Other important considerations in the differential diagnosis include central anticholinergic toxicity, heat stroke, drug fever, and primary central nervous system (CNS) pathology. The management of NMS should include: 1) intensive symptomatic treatment and medical monitoring and 2) treatment of any concomitant serious medical problems for which specific treatments are available. Dopamine agonists, such as bromocriptine, and muscle relaxants, such as dantrolene, are often used in the treatment of NMS; however, their effectiveness has not been demonstrated in controlled studies.

PRECAUTIONS
General
As with levodopa, periodic evaluations of hepatic, hematopoietic, cardiovascular, and renal function are recommended during extended therapy.
Patients with chronic wide-angle glaucoma may be treated cautiously with SINEMET provided the intraocular pressure is well-controlled and the patient is monitored carefully for changes in intraocular pressure during therapy.
Dyskinesia
Levodopa alone, as well as SINEMET, is associated with dyskinesias. The occurrence of dyskinesias may require dosage reduction.
Hallucinations / Psychotic-Like Behavior
Hallucinations and psychotic-like behavior have been reported with dopaminergic medications. In general, hallucinations present shortly after the initiation of therapy and may be responsive to dose reduction in levodopa. Hallucinations may be accompanied by confusion and to a lesser extent sleep disorder (insomnia) and excessive dreaming. SINEMET may have similar effects on thinking and behavior. This abnormal thinking and behavior may present with one or more symptoms, including paranoid ideation, delusions, hallucinations, confusion, psychotic-like behavior, disorientation, aggressive behavior, agitation, and delirium. Ordinarily, patients with a major psychotic disorder should not be treated with SINEMET, because of the risk of exacerbating psychosis. In addition, certain medications used to treat psychosis may exacerbate the symptoms of Parkinson's disease and may decrease the effectiveness of SINEMET.
Impulse Control / Compulsive Behaviors
Reports of patients taking dopaminergic medications (medications that increase central dopaminergic tone), suggest

that patients may experience an intense urge to gamble, increased sexual urges, intense urges to spend money, binge eating, and/or other intense urges, and the inability to control these urges. In some cases, although not all, these urges were reported to have stopped when the dose was reduced or the medication was discontinued. Because patients may not recognize these behaviors as abnormal, it is important for prescribers to specifically ask patients or the caregivers about the development of new or increased gambling urges, sexual urges, uncontrolled spending or other urges while being treated with SINEMET. Physicians should consider dose reduction or stopping the medication if a patient develops such urges while taking SINEMET [see *Information for Patients*].

Melanoma
Epidemiological studies have shown that patients with Parkinson's disease have a higher risk (2- to approximately 6-fold higher) of developing melanoma than the general population. Whether the increased risk observed was due to Parkinson's disease or other factors, such as drugs used to treat Parkinson's disease, is unclear.

For the reasons stated above, patients and providers are advised to monitor for melanomas frequently and on a regular basis when using SINEMET for any indication. Ideally, periodic skin examinations should be performed by appropriately qualified individuals (e.g., dermatologists).

Information for Patients
The patient should be informed that SINEMET is an immediate-release formulation of carbidopa levodopa that is designed to begin release of ingredients within 30 minutes. It is important that SINEMET be taken at regular intervals according to the schedule outlined by the physician. The patient should be cautioned not to change the prescribed dosage regimen and not to add any additional antiparkinson medications, including other carbidopa levodopa preparations, without first consulting the physician.

Patients should be advised that sometimes a 'wearing-off' effect may occur at the end of the dosing interval. The physician should be notified if such response poses a problem to lifestyle.

Patients should be advised that occasionally, dark color (red, brown, or black) may appear in saliva, urine, or sweat after ingestion of SINEMET. Although the color appears to be clinically insignificant, garments may become discolored.

The patient should be advised that a change in diet to foods that are high in protein may delay the absorption of levodopa and may reduce the amount taken up in the circulation. Excessive acidity also delays stomach emptying, thus delaying the absorption of levodopa. Iron salts (such as in multivitamin tablets) may also reduce the amount of levodopa available to the body. The above factors may reduce the clinical effectiveness of the levodopa or carbidopa levodopa therapy.

Patients should be alerted to the possibility of sudden onset of sleep during daily activities, in some cases without awareness or warning signs, when they are taking dopaminergic agents, including levodopa. Patients should be advised to exercise caution while driving or operating machinery and that if they have experienced somnolence and/or sudden sleep onset, they must refrain from these activities. (See WARNINGS, Falling Asleep During Activities of Daily Living and Somnolence.)

There have been reports of patients experiencing intense urges to gamble, increased sexual urges, and other intense urges, and the inability to control these urges while taking one or more of the medications that increase central dopaminergic tone and that are generally used for the treatment of Parkinson's disease, including SINEMET. Although it is not proven that the medications caused these events, these urges were reported to have stopped in some cases when the dose was reduced or the medication was stopped. Prescribers should ask patients about the development of new or increased gambling urges, sexual urges or other urges while being treated with SINEMET. Patients should inform their physician if they experience new or increased gambling urges, increased sexual urges, or other intense urges while taking SINEMET. Physicians should consider dose reduction or stopping the medication if a patient develops such urges while taking SINEMET (See PRECAUTIONS, Impulse Control / Compulsive Behaviors).

Laboratory Tests
Abnormalities in laboratory tests may include elevations of liver function tests such as alkaline phosphatase, SGOT (AST), SGPT (ALT), lactic dehydrogenase (LDH), and bilirubin. Abnormalities in blood urea nitrogen (BUN) and positive Coombs test have also been reported. Commonly, levels of blood urea nitrogen, creatinine, and uric acid are lower during administration of SINEMET than with levodopa. SINEMET may cause a false-positive reaction for urinary ketone bodies when a test tape is used for determination of ketonuria. This reaction will not be altered by boiling the urine specimen. False-negative tests may result with the use of glucose-oxidase methods of testing for glucosuria.

Cases of falsely diagnosed pheochromocytoma in patients on carbidopa levodopa therapy have been reported very rarely. Caution should be exercised when interpreting the plasma and urine levels of catecholamines and their metabolites in patients on levodopa or carbidopa levodopa therapy.

Drug Interactions
Caution should be exercised when the following drugs are administered concomitantly with SINEMET.
Symptomatic postural hypotension occurred when SINEMET was added to the treatment of a patient receiving antihypertensive drugs. Therefore, when therapy with SINEMET is started, dosage adjustment of the antihypertensive drug may be required.

For patients receiving MAO inhibitors (Type A or B), see CONTRAINDICATIONS. Concomitant therapy with selegiline and carbidopa levodopa may be associated with severe orthostatic hypotension not attributable to carbidopa levodopa alone (see CONTRAINDICATIONS).

There have been rare reports of adverse reactions, including hypertension and dyskinesia, resulting from the concomitant use of tricyclic antidepressants and SINEMET.

Dopamine D_2 receptor antagonists (e.g., phenothiazines, butyrophenones, risperidone) and isoniazid may reduce the therapeutic effects of levodopa. In addition, the beneficial effects of levodopa in Parkinson's disease have been reported to be reversed by phenytoin and papaverine. Patients taking these drugs with SINEMET should be carefully observed for loss of therapeutic response.

Use of SINEMET with dopamine-depleting agents (e.g., reserpine and tetrabenazine) or other drugs known to deplete monoamine stores is not recommended.

SINEMET and iron salts or multivitamins containing iron salts should be coadministered with caution. Iron salts can form chelates with levodopa and carbidopa and consequently reduce the bioavailability of carbidopa and levodopa.

Although metoclopramide may increase the bioavailability of levodopa by increasing gastric emptying, metoclopramide may also adversely affect disease control by its dopamine receptor antagonistic properties.

Carcinogenesis, Mutagenesis, Impairment of Fertility
In a two-year bioassay of SINEMET, no evidence of carcinogenicity was found in rats receiving doses of approximately two times the maximum daily human dose of carbidopa and four times the maximum daily human dose of levodopa.

In reproduction studies with SINEMET, no effects on fertility were found in rats receiving doses of approximately two times the maximum daily human dose of carbidopa and four times the maximum daily human dose of levodopa.

Pregnancy
Pregnancy Category C
No teratogenic effects were observed in a study in mice receiving up to 20 times the maximum recommended human dose of SINEMET. There was a decrease in the number of live pups delivered by rats receiving approximately two times the maximum recommended human dose of carbidopa and approximately five times the maximum recommended human dose of levodopa during organogenesis. SINEMET caused both visceral and skeletal malformations in rabbits at all doses and ratios of carbidopa/levodopa tested, which ranged from 10 times/5 times the maximum recommended human dose of carbidopa/levodopa to 20 times/10 times the maximum recommended human dose of carbidopa/levodopa. There are no adequate or well-controlled studies in pregnant women. It has been reported from individual cases that levodopa crosses the human placental barrier, enters the fetus, and is metabolized. Carbidopa concentrations in fetal tissue appeared to be minimal. Use of SINEMET in women of childbearing potential requires that the anticipated benefits of the drug be weighed against possible hazards to mother and child.

Nursing Mothers
Levodopa has been detected in human milk. Caution should be exercised when SINEMET is administered to a nursing woman.

Pediatric Use
Safety and effectiveness in pediatric patients have not been established. Use of the drug in patients below the age of 18 is not recommended.

Geriatric Use
In the clinical efficacy trials for SINEMET, almost half of the patients were older than 65, but few were older than 75. No overall meaningful differences in safety or effectiveness were observed between these subjects and younger subjects, but greater sensitivity of some older individuals to adverse drug reactions such as hallucinations cannot be ruled out. There is no specific dosing recommendation based upon clinical pharmacology data as SINEMET is titrated as tolerated for clinical effect.

ADVERSE REACTIONS
The most common adverse reactions reported with SINEMET have included dyskinesias, such as choreiform, dystonic, and other involuntary movements, and nausea.

The following other adverse reactions have been reported with SINEMET:
Body as a Whole
Chest pain, asthenia.
Cardiovascular
Cardiac irregularities, hypotension, orthostatic effects including orthostatic hypotension, hypertension, syncope, phlebitis, palpitation.
Gastrointestinal
Dark saliva, gastrointestinal bleeding, development of duodenal ulcer, anorexia, vomiting, diarrhea, constipation, dyspepsia, dry mouth, taste alterations.
Hematologic
Agranulocytosis, hemolytic and non-hemolytic anemia, thrombocytopenia, leukopenia.
Hypersensitivity
Angioedema, urticaria, pruritus, Henoch-Schönlein purpura, bullous lesions (including pemphigus-like reactions).
Musculoskeletal
Back pain, shoulder pain, muscle cramps.
Nervous System / Psychiatric
Psychotic episodes including delusions, hallucinations, and paranoid ideation, bradykinetic episodes ("on-off" phenomenon), confusion, agitation, dizziness, somnolence, dream abnormalities including nightmares, insomnia, paresthesia, headache, depression with or without development of suicidal tendencies, dementia, pathological gambling, increased libido including hypersexuality, impulse control symptoms. Convulsions also have occurred; however, a causal relationship with SINEMET has not been established.
Respiratory
Dyspnea, upper respiratory infection.
Skin
Rash, increased sweating, alopecia, dark sweat.
Urogenital
Urinary tract infection, urinary frequency, dark urine.
Laboratory Tests
Decreased hemoglobin and hematocrit; abnormalities in alkaline phosphatase, SGOT (AST), SGPT (ALT), LDH, bilirubin, BUN, Coombs test; elevated serum glucose; white blood cells, bacteria, and blood in the urine.

Other adverse reactions that have been reported with levodopa alone and with various carbidopa levodopa formulations, and may occur with SINEMET are:
Body as a Whole
Abdominal pain and distress, fatigue.
Cardiovascular
Myocardial infarction.
Gastrointestinal
Gastrointestinal pain, dysphagia, sialorrhea, flatulence, bruxism, burning sensation of the tongue, heartburn, hiccups.
Metabolic
Edema, weight gain, weight loss.
Musculoskeletal
Leg pain.
Nervous System / Psychiatric
Ataxia, extrapyramidal disorder, falling, anxiety, gait abnormalities, nervousness, decreased mental acuity, memory impairment, disorientation, euphoria, blepharospasm (which may be taken as an early sign of excess dosage; consideration of dosage reduction may be made at this time), trismus, increased tremor, numbness, muscle twitching, activation of latent Horner's syndrome, peripheral neuropathy.
Respiratory
Pharyngeal pain, cough.
Skin
Malignant melanoma (see also CONTRAINDICATIONS), flushing.
Special Senses
Oculogyric crises, diplopia, blurred vision, dilated pupils.
Urogenital
Urinary retention, urinary incontinence, priapism.
Miscellaneous
Bizarre breathing patterns, faintness, hoarseness, malaise, hot flashes, sense of stimulation.
Laboratory Tests
Decreased white blood cell count and serum potassium; increased serum creatinine and uric acid; protein and glucose in urine.

OVERDOSAGE
Management of acute overdosage with SINEMET is the same as management of acute overdosage with levodopa. Pyridoxine is not effective in reversing the actions of SINEMET.

General supportive measures should be employed, along with immediate gastric lavage. Intravenous fluids should be administered judiciously and an adequate airway maintained. Electrocardiographic monitoring should be instituted and the patient carefully observed for the development of arrhythmias; if required, appropriate antiarrhythmic therapy should be given. The possibility that the patient may have taken other drugs as well as SINEMET should be taken into consideration. To date, no experience has been reported with dialysis; hence, its value in overdosage is not known.

Based on studies in which high doses of levodopa and/or carbidopa were administered, a significant proportion of rats and mice given single oral doses of levodopa of approximately 1500-2000 mg/kg are expected to die. A significant proportion of infant rats of both sexes are expected to die at a dose of 800 mg/kg. A significant proportion of rats are expected to die after treatment with similar doses of carbidopa. The addition of carbidopa in a 1:10 ratio with levodopa increases the dose at which a significant proportion of mice are expected to die to 3360 mg/kg.

DOSAGE AND ADMINISTRATION

The optimum daily dosage of SINEMET must be determined by careful titration in each patient. SINEMET tablets are available in a 1:4 ratio of carbidopa to levodopa (SINEMET 25-100) as well as 1:10 ratio (SINEMET 25-250 and SINEMET 10-100). Tablets of the two ratios may be given separately or combined as needed to provide the optimum dosage.

Studies show that peripheral dopa decarboxylase is saturated by carbidopa at approximately 70 to 100 mg a day. Patients receiving less than this amount of carbidopa are more likely to experience nausea and vomiting.

Usual Initial Dosage

Dosage is best initiated with one tablet of SINEMET 25-100 three times a day. This dosage schedule provides 75 mg of carbidopa per day. Dosage may be increased by one tablet every day or every other day, as necessary, until a dosage of eight tablets of SINEMET 25-100 a day is reached.

If SINEMET 10-100 is used, dosage may be initiated with one tablet three or four times a day. However, this will not provide an adequate amount of carbidopa for many patients. Dosage may be increased by one tablet every day or every other day until a total of eight tablets (2 tablets q.i.d.) is reached.

How to Transfer Patients from Levodopa

Levodopa **must be discontinued at least twelve hours before starting SINEMET.** A daily dosage of SINEMET should be chosen that will provide approximately 25% of the previous levodopa dosage. Patients who are taking less than 1500 mg of levodopa a day should be started on one tablet of SINEMET 25-100 three or four times a day. The suggested starting dosage for most patients taking more than 1500 mg of levodopa is one tablet of SINEMET 25-250 three or four times a day.

Maintenance

Therapy should be individualized and adjusted according to the desired therapeutic response. At least 70 to 100 mg of carbidopa per day should be provided. When a greater proportion of carbidopa is required, one tablet of SINEMET 25-100 may be substituted for each tablet of SINEMET 10-100. When more levodopa is required, SINEMET 25-250 should be substituted for SINEMET 25-100 or SINEMET 10-100. If necessary, the dosage of carbidopa levodopa 25-250 may be increased by one-half or one tablet every day or every other day to a maximum of eight tablets a day. Experience with total daily dosages of carbidopa greater than 200 mg is limited.

Because both therapeutic and adverse responses occur more rapidly with SINEMET than with levodopa alone, patients should be monitored closely during the dose adjustment period. Specifically, involuntary movements will occur more rapidly with SINEMET than with levodopa. The occurrence of involuntary movements may require dosage reduction. Blepharospasm may be a useful early sign of excess dosage in some patients.

Addition of Other Antiparkinsonian Medications

Standard drugs for Parkinson's disease, other than levodopa without a decarboxylase inhibitor, may be used concomitantly while SINEMET is being administered, although dosage adjustments may be required.

Interruption of Therapy

Sporadic cases of hyperpyrexia and confusion have been associated with dose reductions and withdrawal of SINEMET. Patients should be observed carefully if abrupt reduction or discontinuation of SINEMET is required, especially if the patient is receiving neuroleptics. (See WARNINGS.)

If general anesthesia is required, SINEMET may be continued as long as the patient is permitted to take fluids and medication by mouth. If therapy is interrupted temporarily, the patient should be observed for symptoms resembling NMS, and the usual daily dosage may be administered as soon as the patient is able to take oral medication.

HOW SUPPLIED

No. 3916A — SINEMET 25-100 Tablets are yellow, round, uncoated tablets, that are coded "650" on one side and plain on the other. They are supplied as follows: **NDC** 0006-3916-68 bottles of 100.

No. 3915 — SINEMET 10-100 Tablets are light dapple-blue, round, uncoated tablets, that are coded "647" on one side and plain on the other. They are supplied as follows: **NDC** 0006-3915-68 bottles of 100.

No. 3917 — SINEMET 25-250 Tablets are light dapple-blue, round, uncoated tablets, that are coded "654" on one side and plain on the other. They are supplied as follows: **NDC** 0006-3917-68 bottles of 100.

Storage and Handling

Store at 25°C (77°F), excursions permitted to 15-30°C (59-86°F) [see USP Controlled Room Temperature]. Store in a tightly closed container, protected from light and moisture.

Dispense in a tightly closed, light-resistant container.

Manufactured for: Merck Sharp & Dohme Corp., a subsidiary of

MERCK & CO., INC., Whitehouse Station, NJ 08889, USA

Manufactured by:

Mylan Pharmaceuticals, Inc.

Morgantown, WV 26505, USA

Copyright © 1996-2014 Merck Sharp & Dohme Corp., a subsidiary of **Merck & Co., Inc.**

All rights reserved.

Revised: 07/2014

uspi-mk0295b-t-1407r003

Rx Only

SINEMET® CR   ℞
(carbidopa levodopa)
Sustained-Release Tablets

DESCRIPTION

SINEMET® CR (carbidopa levodopa) is a sustained-release combination of carbidopa and levodopa for the treatment of Parkinson's disease and syndrome.

Carbidopa, an inhibitor of aromatic amino acid decarboxylation, is a white, crystalline compound, slightly soluble in water, with a molecular weight of 244.3. It is designated chemically as $(-)$-L-α-hydrazino-α-methyl-β-(3,4-dihydroxybenzene) propanoic acid monohydrate. Its empirical formula is $C_{10}H_{14}N_2O_4 \bullet H_2O$, and its structural formula is:

Tablet content is expressed in terms of anhydrous carbidopa, which has a molecular weight of 226.3.

Levodopa, an aromatic amino acid, is a white, crystalline compound, slightly soluble in water, with a molecular weight of 197.2. It is designated chemically as $(-)$-L-α-amino-β-(3,4-dihydroxybenzene) propanoic acid. Its empirical formula is $C_9H_{11}NO_4$, and its structural formula is:

SINEMET CR is supplied as sustained-release tablets containing either 50 mg of carbidopa and 200 mg of levodopa, or 25 mg of carbidopa and 100 mg of levodopa. Inactive ingredients are hydroxypropyl cellulose, magnesium stearate, and hypromellose. SINEMET CR 25-100 and SINEMET CR 50-200 also contain FD&C Blue #2/Indigo Carmine AL and FD&C Red #40/Allura Red AC AL.

The 50-200 tablet is supplied as an oval, compressed tablet that is dappled-purple in color and is coded "521" on one side and plain on the other. The 25-100 tablet is supplied as an oval, compressed tablet that is dappled-purple in color and is coded "601" on one side and plain on the other. The SINEMET CR tablet is a polymeric-based drug delivery system that controls the release of carbidopa and levodopa as it slowly erodes. SINEMET CR 25-100 is available to facilitate titration when 100 mg steps are required.

CLINICAL PHARMACOLOGY

Mechanism of Action

Parkinson's disease is a progressive, neurodegenerative disorder of the extrapyramidal nervous system affecting the mobility and control of the skeletal muscular system. Its characteristic features include resting tremor, rigidity, and bradykinetic movements. Symptomatic treatments, such as levodopa therapies, may permit the patient better mobility. Current evidence indicates that symptoms of Parkinson's disease are related to depletion of dopamine in the corpus striatum. Administration of dopamine is ineffective in the treatment of Parkinson's disease apparently because it does not cross the blood-brain barrier. However, levodopa, the metabolic precursor of dopamine, does cross the blood-brain

barrier, and presumably is converted to dopamine in the brain. This is thought to be the mechanism whereby levodopa relieves symptoms of Parkinson's disease.

Pharmacodynamics

When levodopa is administered orally, it is rapidly decarboxylated to dopamine in extracerebral tissues so that only a small portion of a given dose is transported unchanged to the central nervous system. For this reason, large doses of levodopa are required for adequate therapeutic effect, and these may often be accompanied by nausea and other adverse reactions, some of which are attributable to dopamine formed in extracerebral tissues.

Since levodopa competes with certain amino acids for transport across the gut wall, the absorption of levodopa may be impaired in some patients on a high protein diet.

Carbidopa inhibits decarboxylation of peripheral levodopa. It does not cross the blood-brain barrier and does not affect the metabolism of levodopa within the central nervous system.

Since its decarboxylase inhibiting activity is limited to extracerebral tissues, administration of carbidopa with levodopa makes more levodopa available for transport to the brain.

Patients treated with levodopa therapy for Parkinson's disease may develop motor fluctuations characterized by end-of-dose failure, peak dose dyskinesia, and akinesia. The advanced form of motor fluctuations ('on-off' phenomenon) is characterized by unpredictable swings from mobility to immobility. Although the causes of the motor fluctuations are not completely understood, in some patients they may be attenuated by treatment regimens that produce steady plasma levels of levodopa.

SINEMET CR contains either 50 mg of carbidopa and 200 mg of levodopa, or 25 mg of carbidopa and 100 mg of levodopa in a sustained-release dosage form designed to release these ingredients over a 4- to 6-hour period. With SINEMET CR there is less variation in plasma levodopa levels than with SINEMET® (carbidopa levodopa) immediate release tablets, the conventional formulation. *However, SINEMET CR is less systemically bioavailable than SINEMET and may require increased daily doses to achieve the same level of symptomatic relief as provided by SINEMET.*

In clinical trials, patients with moderate to severe motor fluctuations who received SINEMET CR *did not experience quantitatively significant reductions* in 'off' time when compared to SINEMET. However, global ratings of improvement as assessed by both patient and physician were better during therapy with SINEMET CR than with SINEMET. In patients without motor fluctuations, SINEMET CR, under controlled conditions, provided the same therapeutic benefit with less frequent dosing when compared to SINEMET.

Pharmacokinetics

Carbidopa reduces the amount of levodopa required to produce a given response by about 75% and, when administered with levodopa, increases both plasma levels and the plasma half-life of levodopa, and decreases plasma and urinary dopamine and homovanillic acid.

Elimination half-life of levodopa in the presence of carbidopa is about 1.5 hours. Following SINEMET CR, the apparent half-life of levodopa may be prolonged because of continuous absorption.

In healthy elderly subjects (56-67 years old) the mean time-to-peak concentration of levodopa after a single dose of SINEMET CR 50-200 was about 2 hours as compared to 0.5 hours after standard SINEMET. The maximum concentration of levodopa after a single dose of SINEMET CR was about 35% of the standard SINEMET (1151 vs. 3256 ng/mL). The extent of availability of levodopa from SINEMET CR was about 70-75% relative to intravenous levodopa or standard SINEMET in the elderly. The absolute bioavailability of levodopa from SINEMET CR (relative to I.V.) in young subjects was shown to be only about 44%. The extent of availability and the peak concentrations of levodopa were comparable in the elderly after a single dose and at steady state after t.i.d. administration of SINEMET CR 50-200. In elderly subjects, the average trough levels of levodopa at steady state after the CR tablet were about 2 fold higher than after the standard SINEMET (163 vs. 74 ng/mL).

In these studies, using similar total daily doses of levodopa, plasma levodopa concentrations with SINEMET CR fluctuated in a narrower range than with SINEMET. Because the bioavailability of levodopa from SINEMET CR relative to SINEMET is approximately 70-75%, the daily dosage of levodopa necessary to produce a given clinical response with the sustained-release formulation will usually be higher.

The extent of availability and peak concentrations of levodopa after a single dose of SINEMET CR 50-200 increased by about 50% and 25%, respectively, when administered with food.

At steady state, the bioavailability of carbidopa from SINEMET Tablets is approximately 99% relative to the concomitant administration of carbidopa and levodopa. At steady state, carbidopa bioavailability from SINEMET CR 50-200 is approximately 58% relative to that from SINEMET.

Pyridoxine hydrochloride (vitamin B$_6$), in oral doses of 10 mg to 25 mg, may reverse the effects of levodopa by increasing the rate of aromatic amino acid decarboxylation. Carbidopa inhibits this action of pyridoxine.

Special Populations

Geriatric

A study in eight young healthy subjects (21-22 yr) and eight elderly healthy subjects (69-76 yr) showed that the absolute bioavailability of levodopa was similar between young and elderly subjects following oral administration of levodopa and carbidopa. However, the systemic exposure (AUC) of levodopa was increased by 55% in elderly subjects compared to young subjects. Based on another study in forty patients with Parkinson's disease, there was a correlation between age of patients and the increase of AUC of levodopa following administration of levodopa and an inhibitor of peripheral dopa decarboxylase. AUC of levodopa was increased by 28% in elderly patients ($\geq$ 65 yr) compared to young patients ($<$ 65 yr). Additionally, mean value of Cmax for levodopa was increased by 24% in elderly patients ($\geq$ 65 yr) compared to young patients ($<$ 65 yr) (see PRECAUTIONS, Geriatric Use).

The AUC of carbidopa was increased in elderly subjects (n=10, 65-76 yr) by 29% compared to young subjects (n=24, 23-64 yr) following IV administration of 50 mg levodopa with carbidopa (50 mg). This increase is not considered a clinically significant impact.

INDICATIONS AND USAGE

SINEMET CR is indicated in the treatment of Parkinson's disease, post-encephalitic parkinsonism, and symptomatic parkinsonism that may follow carbon monoxide intoxication or manganese intoxication.

CONTRAINDICATIONS

Nonselective monoamine oxidase (MAO) inhibitors are contraindicated for use with SINEMET CR. These inhibitors must be discontinued at least two weeks prior to initiating therapy with SINEMET CR. SINEMET CR may be administered concomitantly with the manufacturer's recommended dose of an MAO inhibitor with selectivity for MAO type B (e.g., selegiline HCl) (see PRECAUTIONS, Drug Interactions).

SINEMET CR is contraindicated in patients with known hypersensitivity to any component of this drug, and in patients with narrow-angle glaucoma.

WARNINGS

When patients are receiving levodopa without a decarboxylase inhibitor, levodopa must be discontinued at least twelve hours before SINEMET CR is started. In order to reduce adverse reactions, it is necessary to individualize therapy. See DOSAGE AND ADMINISTRATION section before initiating therapy.

SINEMET CR should be substituted at a dosage that will provide approximately 25% of the previous levodopa dosage (see DOSAGE AND ADMINISTRATION).

Carbidopa does not decrease adverse reactions due to central effects of levodopa. By permitting more levodopa to reach the brain, particularly when nausea and vomiting is not a dose-limiting factor, certain adverse central nervous system (CNS) effects, e.g., dyskinesias, will occur at lower dosages and sooner during therapy with SINEMET CR than with levodopa alone.

Patients receiving SINEMET CR may develop increased dyskinesias compared to SINEMET. Dyskinesias are a common side effect of carbidopa levodopa treatment. The occurrence of dyskinesias may require dosage reduction.

All patients should be observed carefully for the development of depression with concomitant suicidal tendencies.

SINEMET CR should be administered cautiously to patients with severe cardiovascular or pulmonary disease, bronchial asthma, renal, hepatic or endocrine disease.

As with levodopa, care should be exercised in administering SINEMET CR to patients with a history of myocardial infarction who have residual atrial, nodal, or ventricular arrhythmias. In such patients, cardiac function should be monitored with particular care during the period of initial dosage adjustment, in a facility with provisions for intensive cardiac care.

As with levodopa, treatment with SINEMET CR may increase the possibility of upper gastrointestinal hemorrhage in patients with a history of peptic ulcer.

Falling Asleep During Activities of Daily Living and Somnolence

Patients taking SINEMET CR alone or with other dopaminergic drugs have reported suddenly falling asleep without prior warning of sleepiness while engaged in activities of daily living (includes operation of motor vehicles). Road traffic accidents attributed to sudden sleep onset have been reported. Although many patients reported somnolence while on dopaminergic medications, there have been reports of road traffic accidents attributed to sudden onset of sleep in which the patient did not perceive any warning signs, such as excessive drowsiness, and believed that they were

alert immediately prior to the event. Sudden onset of sleep has been reported to occur as long as one year after the initiation of treatment.

Falling asleep while engaged in activities of daily living usually occurs in patients experiencing pre-existing somnolence, although some patients may not give such a history. For this reason, prescribers should reassess patients for drowsiness or sleepiness especially since some of the events occur well after the start of treatment. Prescribers should be aware that patients may not acknowledge drowsiness or sleepiness until directly questioned about drowsiness or sleepiness during specific activities. Patients should be advised to exercise caution while driving or operating machines during treatment with SINEMET CR. Patients who have already experienced somnolence or an episode of sudden sleep onset should not participate in these activities during treatment with SINEMET CR.

Before initiating treatment with SINEMET CR, advise patients about the potential to develop drowsiness and ask specifically about factors that may increase the risk for somnolence with SINEMET CR such as the use of concomitant sedating medications and the presence of sleep disorders. Consider discontinuing SINEMET CR in patients who report significant daytime sleepiness or episodes of falling asleep during activities that require active participation (e.g., conversations, eating, etc.). If treatment with SINEMET CR continues, patients should be advised not to drive and to avoid other potentially dangerous activities that might result in harm if the patients become somnolent. There is insufficient information to establish that dose reduction will eliminate episodes of falling asleep while engaged in activities of daily living.

Hyperpyrexia and Confusion

Sporadic cases of a symptom complex resembling neuroleptic malignant syndrome (NMS) have been reported in association with dose reductions or withdrawal of certain antiparkinsonian agents such as levodopa, carbidopa levodopa and carbidopa levodopa extended release. Therefore, patients should be observed carefully when the dosage of levodopa is reduced abruptly or discontinued, especially if the patient is receiving neuroleptics.

NMS is an uncommon but life-threatening syndrome characterized by fever or hyperthermia. Neurological findings, including muscle rigidity, involuntary movements, altered consciousness, mental status changes; other disturbances, such as autonomic dysfunction, tachycardia, tachypnea, sweating, hyper- or hypotension; laboratory findings, such as creatine phosphokinase elevation, leukocytosis, myoglobinuria, and increased serum myoglobin have been reported.

The early diagnosis of this condition is important for the appropriate management of these patients. Considering NMS as a possible diagnosis and ruling out other acute illnesses (e.g., pneumonia, systemic infection, etc.) is essential. This may be especially complex if the clinical presentation includes both serious medical illness and untreated or inadequately treated extrapyramidal signs and symptoms (EPS). Other important considerations in the differential diagnosis include central anticholinergic toxicity, heat stroke, drug fever, and primary central nervous system (CNS) pathology. The management of NMS should include: 1) intensive symptomatic treatment and medical monitoring and 2) treatment of any concomitant serious medical problems for which specific treatments are available. Dopamine agonists, such as bromocriptine, and muscle relaxants, such as dantrolene, are often used in the treatment of NMS; however, their effectiveness has not been demonstrated in controlled studies.

PRECAUTIONS

General

As with levodopa, periodic evaluations of hepatic, hematopoietic, cardiovascular, and renal function are recommended during extended therapy.

Patients with chronic wide-angle glaucoma may be treated cautiously with SINEMET CR provided the intraocular pressure is well-controlled and the patient is monitored carefully for changes in intraocular pressure during therapy.

Dyskinesia

Levodopa alone, as well as SINEMET CR, is associated with dyskinesias. The occurrence of dyskinesias may require dosage reduction.

Hallucinations / Psychotic-Like Behavior

Hallucinations and psychotic-like behavior have been reported with dopaminergic medications. In general, hallucinations present shortly after the initiation of therapy and may be responsive to dose reduction in levodopa. Hallucinations may be accompanied by confusion and to a lesser extent sleep disorder (insomnia) and excessive dreaming. SINEMET CR may have similar effects on thinking and behavior. This abnormal thinking and behavior may present with one or more symptoms, including paranoid ideation, delusions, hallucinations, confusion, psychotic-like behavior, disorientation, aggressive behavior, agitation, and delirium.

Ordinarily, patients with a major psychotic disorder should not be treated with SINEMET CR, because of the risk of exacerbating psychosis. In addition, certain medications used to treat psychosis may exacerbate the symptoms of Parkinson's disease and may decrease the effectiveness of SINEMET CR.

Impulse Control / Compulsive Behaviors

Reports of patients taking dopaminergic medications (medications that increase central dopaminergic tone), suggest that patients may experience an intense urge to gamble, increased sexual urges, intense urges to spend money, binge eating, and/or other intense urges, and the inability to control these urges. In some cases, although not all, these urges were reported to have stopped when the dose was reduced or the medication was discontinued. Because patients may not recognize these behaviors as abnormal, it is important for prescribers to specifically ask patients or the caregivers about the development of new or increased gambling urges, sexual urges, uncontrolled spending or other urges while being treated with SINEMET CR. Physicians should consider dose reduction or stopping the medication if a patient develops such urges while taking SINEMET CR [see Information for Patients].

Melanoma

Epidemiological studies have shown that patients with Parkinson's disease have a higher risk (2- to approximately 6-fold higher) of developing melanoma than the general population. Whether the increased risk observed was due to Parkinson's disease or other factors, such as drugs used to treat Parkinson's disease, is unclear.

For the reasons stated above, patients and providers are advised to monitor for melanomas frequently and on a regular basis when using SINEMET CR for any indication. Ideally, periodic skin examinations should be performed by appropriately qualified individuals (e.g., dermatologists).

Information for Patients

The patient should be informed that SINEMET CR is a sustained-release formulation of carbidopa levodopa which releases these ingredients over a 4- to 6-hour period. It is important that SINEMET CR be taken at regular intervals according to the schedule outlined by the physician. The patient should be cautioned not to change the prescribed dosage regimen and not to add any additional antiparkinson medications, including other carbidopa levodopa preparations, without first consulting the physician.

If abnormal involuntary movements appear or get worse during treatment with SINEMET CR, the physician should be notified, as dosage adjustment may be necessary.

Patients should be advised that sometimes the onset of effect of the first morning dose of SINEMET CR may be delayed for up to 1 hour compared with the response usually obtained from the first morning dose of SINEMET. The physician should be notified if such delayed responses pose a problem in treatment.

Patients should be advised that, occasionally, dark color (red, brown, or black) may appear in saliva, urine, or sweat after ingestion of SINEMET CR. Although the color appears to be clinically insignificant, garments may become discolored.

The patient should be informed that a change in diet to foods that are high in protein may delay the absorption of levodopa and may reduce the amount taken up in the circulation. Excessive acidity also delays stomach emptying, thus delaying the absorption of levodopa. Iron salts (such as in multivitamin tablets) may also reduce the amount of levodopa available to the body. The above factors may reduce the clinical effectiveness of the levodopa or carbidopa levodopa therapy.

Patients must be advised that the whole or half tablet should be swallowed without chewing or crushing.

Patients should be alerted to the possibility of sudden onset of sleep during daily activities, in some cases without awareness or warning signs, when they are taking dopaminergic agents, including levodopa. Patients should be advised to exercise caution while driving or operating machinery and that if they have experienced somnolence and/or sudden sleep onset, they must refrain from these activities. (See WARNINGS, Falling Asleep During Activities of Daily Living and Somnolence.)

There have been reports of patients experiencing intense urges to gamble, increased sexual urges, and other intense urges, and the inability to control these urges while taking one or more of the medications that increase central dopaminergic tone and that are generally used for the treatment of Parkinson's disease, including SINEMET CR. Although it is not proven that the medications caused these events, these urges were reported to have stopped in some cases when the dose was reduced or the medication was stopped. Prescribers should ask patients about the development of new or increased gambling urges, sexual urges or other urges while being treated with SINEMET CR. Patients should inform their physician if they experience new or increased gambling urges, increased sexual urges, or other intense urges while taking SINEMET CR. Physicians should consider dose reduction or stopping the medication if a patient develops such urges while taking SINEMET CR. (See PRECAUTIONS, Impulse Control / Compulsive Behaviors).

Laboratory Tests

Abnormalities in laboratory tests may include elevations of liver function tests such as alkaline phosphatase, SGOT (AST), SGPT (ALT), lactic dehydrogenase (LDH), and bilirubin. Abnormalities in blood urea nitrogen (BUN) and positive Coombs test have also been reported. Commonly, levels of blood urea nitrogen, creatinine, and uric acid are lower during administration of carbidopa levodopa preparations than with levodopa.

Carbidopa levodopa preparations, such as SINEMET and SINEMET CR, may cause a false-positive reaction for urinary ketone bodies when a test tape is used for determination of ketonuria. This reaction will not be altered by boiling the urine specimen. False-negative tests may result with the use of glucose-oxidase methods of testing for glucosuria. Cases of falsely diagnosed pheochromocytoma in patients on carbidopa levodopa therapy have been reported very rarely. Caution should be exercised when interpreting the plasma and urine levels of catecholamines and their metabolites in patients on levodopa or carbidopa levodopa therapy.

Drug Interactions

Caution should be exercised when the following drugs are administered concomitantly with SINEMET CR.

Symptomatic postural hypotension has occurred when carbidopa levodopa preparations were added to the treatment of patients receiving some antihypertensive drugs. Therefore, when therapy with SINEMET CR is started, dosage adjustment of the antihypertensive drug may be required.

For patients receiving MAO inhibitors (Type A or B), see CONTRAINDICATIONS. Concomitant therapy with selegiline and carbidopa levodopa may be associated with severe orthostatic hypotension not attributable to carbidopa levodopa alone (see CONTRAINDICATIONS).

There have been rare reports of adverse reactions, including hypertension and dyskinesia, resulting from the concomitant use of tricyclic antidepressants and carbidopa levodopa preparations.

Dopamine D_2 receptor antagonists (e.g., phenothiazines, butyrophenones, risperidone) and isoniazid may reduce the therapeutic effects of levodopa. In addition, the beneficial effects of levodopa in Parkinson's disease have been reported to be reversed by phenytoin and papaverine. Patients taking these drugs with SINEMET CR should be carefully observed for loss of therapeutic response.

Use of SINEMET CR with dopamine-depleting agents (e.g., reserpine and tetrabenazine) or other drugs known to deplete monoamine stores is not recommended.

SINEMET CR and iron salts or multivitamins containing iron salts should be coadministered with caution. Iron salts can form chelates with levodopa and carbidopa and consequently reduce the bioavailability of carbidopa and levodopa.

Although metoclopramide may increase the bioavailability of levodopa by increasing gastric emptying, metoclopramide may also adversely affect disease control by its dopamine receptor antagonistic properties.

Carcinogenesis, Mutagenesis, Impairment of Fertility

In a two-year bioassay of SINEMET, no evidence of carcinogenicity was found in rats receiving doses of approximately two times the maximum daily human dose of carbidopa and four times the maximum daily human dose of levodopa (equivalent to 8 SINEMET CR tablets).

In reproduction studies with SINEMET, no effects on fertility were found in rats receiving doses of approximately two times the maximum daily human dose of carbidopa and four times the maximum daily human dose of levodopa (equivalent to 8 SINEMET CR tablets).

Pregnancy

Pregnancy Category C. No teratogenic effects were observed in a study in mice receiving up to 20 times the maximum recommended human dose. There was a decrease in the number of live pups delivered by rats receiving approximately two times the maximum recommended human dose of carbidopa and approximately five times the maximum recommended human dose of levodopa during organogenesis. SINEMET caused both visceral and skeletal malformations in rabbits at all doses and ratios of carbidopa/levodopa tested, which ranged from 10 times/5 times the maximum recommended human dose of carbidopa/levodopa to 20 times/10 times the maximum recommended human dose of carbidopa/levodopa.

There are no adequate or well-controlled studies in pregnant women. It has been reported from individual cases that levodopa crosses the human placental barrier, enters the fetus, and is metabolized. Carbidopa concentrations in fetal tissue appeared to be minimal. Use of SINEMET CR in women of childbearing potential requires that the anticipated benefits of the drug be weighed against possible hazards to mother and child.

Nursing Mothers

Levodopa has been detected in human milk. Caution should be exercised when SINEMET CR is administered to a nursing woman.

Pediatric Use

Safety and effectiveness in pediatric patients have not been established. Use of the drug in patients below the age of 18 is not recommended.

Geriatric Use

In the clinical efficacy trials for SINEMET, almost half of the patients were older than 65, but few were older than 75. No overall meaningful differences in safety or effectiveness were observed between these subjects and younger subjects, but greater sensitivity of some older individuals to adverse drug reactions such as hallucinations cannot be ruled out. There is no specific dosing recommendation based upon clinical pharmacology data as SINEMET and SINEMET CR are titrated as tolerated for clinical effect.

ADVERSE REACTIONS

In controlled clinical trials, patients predominantly with moderate to severe motor fluctuations while on SINEMET were randomized to therapy with either SINEMET or SINEMET CR. The adverse experience frequency profile of SINEMET CR did not differ substantially from that of SINEMET, as shown in Table 1.

Table 1: Clinical Adverse Experiences Occurring in 1% or Greater of Patients

Adverse Experience	SINEMET CR n=491 %	SINEMET n=524 %
Dyskinesia	16.5	12.2
Nausea	5.5	5.7
Hallucinations	3.9	3.2
Confusion	3.7	2.3
Dizziness	2.9	2.3
Depression	2.2	1.3
Urinary tract infection	2.2	2.3
Headache	2.0	1.9
Dream abnormalities	1.8	0.8
Dystonia	1.8	0.8
Vomiting	1.8	1.9
Upper respiratory infection	1.8	1.0
Dyspnea	1.6	0.4
'On-Off' phenomena	1.6	1.1
Back pain	1.6	0.6
Dry mouth	1.4	1.1
Anorexia	1.2	1.1
Diarrhea	1.2	0.6
Insomnia	1.2	1.0
Orthostatic hypotension	1.0	1.1
Shoulder pain	1.0	0.6
Chest pain	1.0	0.8
Muscle cramps	0.8	1.0
Paresthesia	0.8	1.1
Urinary frequency	0.8	1.1
Dyspepsia	0.6	1.1
Constipation	0.2	1.5

Abnormal laboratory findings occurring at a frequency of 1% or greater in approximately 443 patients who received SINEMET CR and 475 who received SINEMET during controlled clinical trials included: decreased hemoglobin and hematocrit; elevated serum glucose; white blood cells, bacteria and blood in the urine.

The adverse experiences observed in patients in uncontrolled studies were similar to those seen in controlled clinical studies.

Other adverse experiences reported overall in clinical trials in 748 patients treated with SINEMET CR, listed by body system in order of decreasing frequency, include:

Body as a Whole
Asthenia, fatigue, abdominal pain, orthostatic effects.
Cardiovascular
Palpitation, hypertension, hypotension, myocardial infarction.
Gastrointestinal
Gastrointestinal pain, dysphagia, heartburn.
Metabolic
Weight loss.
Musculoskeletal
Leg pain.
Nervous System / Psychiatric
Chorea, somnolence, falling, anxiety, disorientation, decreased mental acuity, gait abnormalities, extrapyramidal disorder, agitation, nervousness, sleep disorders, memory impairment.
Respiratory
Cough, pharyngeal pain, common cold.
Skin
Rash.

Special Senses
Blurred vision.
Urogenital
Urinary incontinence.
Laboratory Tests
Decreased white blood cell count and serum potassium; increased BUN, serum creatinine and serum LDH; protein and glucose in the urine.

The following adverse experiences have been reported in postmarketing experience with SINEMET CR:
Cardiovascular
Cardiac irregularities, syncope.
Gastrointestinal
Taste alterations, dark saliva.
Hypersensitivity
Angioedema, urticaria, pruritus, bullous lesions (including pemphigus-like reactions).
Nervous System / Psychiatric
Increased tremor, peripheral neuropathy, psychotic episodes including delusions and paranoid ideation, pathological gambling, increased libido including hypersexuality, impulse control symptoms.
Skin
Alopecia, flushing, dark sweat.
Urogenital
Dark urine.

Other adverse reactions that have been reported with levodopa alone and with various carbidopa levodopa formulations and may occur with SINEMET CR are:
Cardiovascular
Phlebitis.
Gastrointestinal
Gastrointestinal bleeding, development of duodenal ulcer, sialorrhea, bruxism, hiccups, flatulence, burning sensation of tongue.
Hematologic
Hemolytic and non-hemolytic anemia, thrombocytopenia, leukopenia, agranulocytosis.
Hypersensitivity
Henoch-Schönlein purpura.
Metabolic
Weight gain, edema.
Nervous System / Psychiatric
Ataxia, depression with suicidal tendencies, dementia, euphoria, convulsions (however, a causal relationship has not been established); bradykinetic episodes, numbness, muscle twitching, blepharospasm (which may be taken as an early sign of excess dosage; consideration of dosage reduction may be made at this time); trismus, activation of latent Horner's syndrome, nightmares.
Skin
Malignant melanoma (see also CONTRAINDICATIONS), increased sweating.
Special Senses
Oculogyric crises, mydriasis, diplopia.
Urogenital
Urinary retention, priapism.
Miscellaneous
Faintness, hoarseness, malaise, hot flashes, sense of stimulation, bizarre breathing patterns.
Laboratory Tests
Abnormalities in alkaline phosphatase, SGOT (AST), SGPT (ALT), bilirubin, Coombs test, uric acid.

OVERDOSAGE

Management of acute overdosage with SINEMET CR is the same as with levodopa. Pyridoxine is not effective in reversing the actions of SINEMET CR.

General supportive measures should be employed, along with immediate gastric lavage. Intravenous fluids should be administered judiciously and an adequate airway maintained. Electrocardiographic monitoring should be instituted and the patient carefully observed for the development of arrhythmias; if required, appropriate antiarrhythmic therapy should be given. The possibility that the patient may have taken other drugs as well as SINEMET CR should be taken into consideration. To date, no experience has been reported with dialysis; hence, its value in overdosage is not known.

Based on studies in which high doses of levodopa and/or carbidopa were administered, a significant proportion of rats and mice given single oral doses of levodopa of approximately 1500-2000 mg/kg are expected to die. A significant proportion of infant rats of both sexes are expected to die at a dose of 800 mg/kg. A significant proportion of rats are expected to die after treatment with similar doses of carbidopa. The addition of carbidopa in a 1:10 ratio with levodopa increases the dose at which a significant proportion of mice are expected to die to 3360 mg/kg.

DOSAGE AND ADMINISTRATION

SINEMET CR contains carbidopa and levodopa in a 1:4 ratio as either the 50-200 tablet or the 25-100 tablet. The daily dosage of SINEMET CR must be determined by careful ti-

Table 2: Approximate Bioavailabilities at Steady State*

Tablet	Amount of Levodopa (mg) in Each Tablet	Approximate Bioavailability	Approximate Amount of Bioavailable Levodopa (mg) in Each Tablet
SINEMET CR 50-200	200	0.70-0.75[†]	140-150
SINEMET 25-100	100	0.99[‡]	99

* This table is only a guide to bioavailabilities since other factors such as food, drugs, and inter-patient variabilities may affect the bioavailability of carbidopa and levodopa.

† The extent of availability of levodopa from SINEMET CR was about 70-75% relative to intravenous levodopa or standard SINEMET in the elderly.

‡ The extent of availability of levodopa from SINEMET was 99% relative to intravenous levodopa in the healthy elderly.

tration. Patients should be monitored closely during the dose adjustment period, particularly with regard to appearance or worsening of involuntary movements, dyskinesias or nausea. SINEMET CR should not be chewed or crushed. Standard drugs for Parkinson's disease, other than levodopa without a decarboxylase inhibitor, may be used concomitantly while SINEMET CR is being administered, although their dosage may have to be adjusted.

Since carbidopa prevents the reversal of levodopa effects caused by pyridoxine, SINEMET CR can be given to patients receiving supplemental pyridoxine (vitamin B_6).

Initial Dosage

Patients currently treated with conventional carbidopa levodopa preparations: Studies show that peripheral dopa-decarboxylase is saturated by the bioavailable carbidopa at doses of 70 mg a day and greater. Because the bioavailabilities of carbidopa and levodopa in SINEMET and SINEMET CR are different, appropriate adjustments should be made, as shown in Table 2.

[See table 2 above]

Dosage with SINEMET CR should be substituted at an amount that provides approximately 10% more levodopa per day, although this may need to be increased to a dosage that provides up to 30% more levodopa per day depending on clinical response (see DOSAGE AND ADMINISTRATION, Titration with SINEMET CR). The interval between doses of SINEMET CR should be 4-8 hours during the waking day. (See CLINICAL PHARMACOLOGY, Pharmacodynamics.)

A guideline for initiation of SINEMET CR is shown in Table 3.

Table 3: Guidelines for Initial Conversion from SINEMET to SINEMET CR

SINEMET Total Daily Dose* Levodopa (mg)	SINEMET CR Suggested Dosage Regimen
300-400	200 mg b.i.d.
500-600	300 mg b.i.d. or 200 mg t.i.d.
700-800	A total of 800 mg in 3 or more divided doses (e.g., 300 mg a.m., 300 mg early p.m., and 200 mg later p.m.)
900-1000	A total of 1000 mg in 3 or more divided doses (e.g., 400 mg a.m., 400 mg early p.m., and 200 mg later p.m.)

* For dosing ranges not shown in the table see DOSAGE AND ADMINISTRATION, Initial Dosage — *Patients currently treated with conventional carbidopa levodopa preparations.*

Patients currently treated with levodopa without a decarboxylase inhibitor: Levodopa must be discontinued at least twelve hours before therapy with SINEMET CR is started. SINEMET CR should be substituted at a dosage that will provide approximately 25% of the previous levodopa dosage. In patients with mild to moderate disease, the initial dose is usually 1 tablet of SINEMET CR 50-200 b.i.d.

Patients not receiving levodopa: In patients with mild to moderate disease, the initial recommended dose is 1 tablet of SINEMET CR 50-200 b.i.d. Initial dosage should not be given at intervals of less than 6 hours.

Titration with SINEMET CR

Following initiation of therapy, doses and dosing intervals may be increased or decreased depending upon therapeutic response. Most patients have been adequately treated with doses of SINEMET CR that provide 400 to 1600 mg of levodopa per day, administered as divided doses at intervals ranging from 4 to 8 hours during the waking day. Higher

doses of SINEMET CR (2400 mg or more of levodopa per day) and shorter intervals (less than 4 hours) have been used, but are not usually recommended.

When doses of SINEMET CR are given at intervals of less than 4 hours, and/or if the divided doses are not equal, it is recommended that the smaller doses be given at the end of the day.

An interval of at least 3 days between dosage adjustments is recommended.

Maintenance

Because Parkinson's disease is progressive, periodic clinical evaluations are recommended; adjustment of the dosage regimen of SINEMET CR may be required.

Addition of Other Antiparkinson Medications

Anticholinergic agents, dopamine agonists, and amantadine can be given with SINEMET CR. Dosage adjustment of SINEMET CR may be necessary when these agents are added.

A dose of carbidopa levodopa immediate release 25-100 or 10-100 (one half or a whole tablet) can be added to the dosage regimen of SINEMET CR in selected patients with advanced disease who need additional immediate-release levodopa for a brief time during daytime hours.

Interruption of Therapy

Sporadic cases of hyperpyrexia and confusion have been associated with dose reductions and withdrawal of SINEMET or SINEMET CR.

Patients should be observed carefully if abrupt reduction or discontinuation of SINEMET CR is required, especially if the patient is receiving neuroleptics. (See WARNINGS.)

If general anesthesia is required, SINEMET CR may be continued as long as the patient is permitted to take oral medication. If therapy is interrupted temporarily, the patient should be observed for symptoms resembling NMS, and the usual dosage should be administered as soon as the patient is able to take oral medication.

HOW SUPPLIED

No. 3919 — SINEMET CR 50-200 (carbidopa levodopa) Sustained-Release Tablets containing 50 mg of carbidopa and 200 mg of levodopa, are dappled-purple in color, oval, compressed tablets, that are coded "521" on one side and plain on the other. They are supplied as follows:

NDC 0006-3919-68 bottles of 100.

No. 3918 — SINEMET CR 25-100 (carbidopa levodopa) Sustained-Release Tablets containing 25 mg of carbidopa and 100 mg of levodopa, are dappled-purple in color, oval, compressed tablets, that are coded "601" on one side and plain on the other. They are supplied as follows:

NDC 0006-3918-68 bottles of 100.

Storage and Handling

Store at 25°C (77°F), excursions permitted to 15-30°C (59-86°F) [see USP Controlled Room Temperature]. Store in a tightly closed container, protected from light and moisture.

Dispense in a tightly closed, light-resistant container.

Manufactured for: Merck Sharp & Dohme Corp., a subsidiary of

MERCK & CO., INC., Whitehouse Station, NJ 08889, USA

Manufactured by:

Mylan Pharmaceuticals, Inc.

Morgantown, WV 26505, USA

Copyright © 1996-2014 Merck Sharp & Dohme Corp., a subsidiary of Merck & Co., Inc.

All rights reserved.

Revised: 07/2014

uspi-mk0295b-txr-1407r003

Rx Only

STROMECTOL®

[*stro-mec-tol*]

(ivermectin)

Tablets

℞

DESCRIPTION

STROMECTOL[1] (Ivermectin) is a semisynthetic, anthelmintic agent for oral administration. Ivermectin is derived

from the avermectins, a class of highly active broad-spectrum, anti-parasitic agents isolated from the fermentation products of *Streptomyces avermitilis*. Ivermectin is a mixture containing at least 90% 5-*O*-demethyl-22,23-dihydroavermectin A_{1a} and less than 10% 5-*O*-demethyl-25-de(1-methylpropyl)-22,23-dihydro-25-(1-methylethyl)avermectin A_{1a}, generally referred to as 22,23-dihydroavermectin B_{1a} and B_{1b}, or H_2B_{1a} and H_2B_{1b}, respectively. The respective empirical formulas are $C_{48}H_{74}O_{14}$ and $C_{47}H_{72}O_{14}$, with molecular weights of 875.10 and 861.07, respectively. The structural formulas are:

Component B_{1a}, R = C_2H_5 Component B_{1b}, R = CH_3

Ivermectin is a white to yellowish-white, nonhygroscopic, crystalline powder with a melting point of about 155°C. It is insoluble in water but is freely soluble in methanol and soluble in 95% ethanol.

STROMECTOL is available in 3-mg tablets containing the following inactive ingredients: microcrystalline cellulose, pregelatinized starch, magnesium stearate, butylated hydroxyanisole, and citric acid powder (anhydrous).

---

[1]Registered trademark of Merck Sharp & Dohme Corp., a subsidiary of **Merck & Co., Inc.**

Copyright © 1996, 2007 Merck Sharp & Dohme Corp., a subsidiary of **Merck & Co., Inc.**

All rights reserved

CLINICAL PHARMACOLOGY

Pharmacokinetics

Following oral administration of ivermectin, plasma concentrations are approximately proportional to the dose. In two studies, after single 12-mg doses of STROMECTOL in fasting healthy volunteers (representing a mean dose of 165 mcg/kg), the mean peak plasma concentrations of the major component (H_2B_{1a}) were 46.6 (±21.9) (range: 16.4-101.1) and 30.6 (±15.6) (range: 13.9-68.4) ng/mL, respectively, at approximately 4 hours after dosing. Ivermectin is metabolized in the liver, and ivermectin and/or its metabolites are excreted almost exclusively in the feces over an estimated 12 days, with less than 1% of the administered dose excreted in the urine. The plasma half-life of ivermectin in man is approximately 18 hours following oral administration.

The safety and pharmacokinetic properties of ivermectin were further assessed in a multiple-dose clinical pharmacokinetic study involving healthy volunteers. Subjects received oral doses of 30 to 120 mg (333 to 2000 mcg/kg) ivermectin in a fasted state or 30 mg (333 to 600 mcg/kg) ivermectin following a standard high-fat (48.6 g of fat) meal. Administration of 30 mg ivermectin following a high-fat meal resulted in an approximate 2.5-fold increase in bioavailability relative to administration of 30 mg ivermectin in the fasted state.

In vitro studies using human liver microsomes and recombinant CYP450 enzymes have shown that ivermectin is primarily metabolized by CYP3A4. Depending on the *in vitro* method used, CYP2D6 and CYP2E1 were also shown to be involved in the metabolism of ivermectin but to a significantly lower extent compared to CYP3A4. The findings of *in vitro* studies using human liver microsomes suggest that clinically relevant concentrations of ivermectin do not significantly inhibit the metabolizing activities of CYP3A4, CYP2D6, CYP2C9, CYP1A2, and CYP2E1.

Microbiology

Ivermectin is a member of the avermectin class of broad-spectrum antiparasitic agents which have a unique mode of action. Compounds of the class bind selectively and with high affinity to glutamate-gated chloride ion channels which occur in invertebrate nerve and muscle cells. This leads to an increase in the permeability of the cell membrane to chloride ions with hyperpolarization of the nerve or muscle cell, resulting in paralysis and death of the parasite. Compounds of this class may also interact with other ligand-gated chloride channels, such as those gated by the neurotransmitter gamma-aminobutyric acid (GABA).

The selective activity of compounds of this class is attributable to the facts that some mammals do not have glutamate-gated chloride channels and that the avermectins have a low affinity for mammalian ligand-gated chloride channels. In addition, ivermectin does not readily cross the blood-brain barrier in humans.

Ivermectin is active against various life-cycle stages of many but not all nematodes. It is active against the tissue microfilariae of *Onchocerca volvulus* but not against the adult form. Its activity against *Strongyloides stercoralis* is limited to the intestinal stages.

Clinical Studies

Strongyloidiasis

Two controlled clinical studies using albendazole as the comparative agent were carried out in international sites where albendazole is approved for the treatment of strongyloidiasis of the gastrointestinal tract, and three controlled studies were carried out in the U.S. and internationally using thiabendazole as the comparative agent. Efficacy, as measured by cure rate, was defined as the absence of larvae in at least two follow-up stool examinations 3 to 4 weeks post-therapy. Based on this criterion, efficacy was significantly greater for STROMECTOL (a single dose of 170 to 200 mcg/kg) than for albendazole (200 mg b.i.d. for 3 days). STROMECTOL administered as a single dose of 200 mcg/kg for 1 day was as efficacious as thiabendazole administered at 25 mg/kg b.i.d. for 3 days.

Summary of Cure Rates for Ivermectin Versus Comparative Agents in the Treatment of Strongyloidiasis

| | Cure Rate* (%) | |
	Ivermectin[†]	Comparative Agent
Albendazole[‡] Comparative		
International Study	24/26 (92)	12/22 (55)
WHO Study	126/152 (83)	67/149 (45)
Thiabendazole[§] Comparative		
International Study	9/14 (64)	13/15 (87)
US Studies	14/14 (100)	16/17 (94)

* Number and % of evaluable patients
[†] 170-200 mcg/kg
[‡] 200 mg b.i.d. for 3 days
[§] 25 mg/kg b.i.d. for 3 days

In one study conducted in France, a non-endemic area where there was no possibility of reinfection, several patients were observed to have recrudescence of *Strongyloides* larvae in their stool as long as 106 days following ivermectin therapy. Therefore, at least three stool examinations should be conducted over the three months following treatment to ensure eradication. If recrudescence of larvae is observed, retreatment with ivermectin is indicated. Concentration techniques (such as using a Baermann apparatus) should be employed when performing these stool examinations, as the number of *Strongyloides* larvae per gram of feces may be very low.

Onchocerciasis

The evaluation of STROMECTOL in the treatment of onchocerciasis is based on the results of clinical studies involving 1278 patients. In a double-blind, placebo-controlled study involving adult patients with moderate to severe onchocercal infection, patients who received a single dose of 150 mcg/kg STROMECTOL experienced an 83.2% and 99.5% decrease in skin microfilariae count (geometric mean) 3 days and 3 months after the dose, respectively. A marked reduction of >90% was maintained for up to 12 months after the single dose. As with other microfilaricidal drugs, there was an increase in the microfilariae count in the anterior chamber of the eye at day 3 after treatment in some patients. However, at 3 and 6 months after the dose, a significantly greater percentage of patients treated with STROMECTOL had decreases in microfilariae count in the anterior chamber than patients treated with placebo.

In a separate open study involving pediatric patients ages 6 to 13 (n=103; weight range: 17-41 kg), similar decreases in skin microfilariae counts were observed for up to 12 months after dosing.

INDICATIONS AND USAGE

STROMECTOL is indicated for the treatment of the following infections:

Strongyloidiasis of the intestinal tract. STROMECTOL is indicated for the treatment of intestinal (i.e., nondisseminated) strongyloidiasis due to the nematode parasite *Strongyloides stercoralis*.

This indication is based on clinical studies of both comparative and open-label designs, in which 64-100% of infected patients were cured following a single 200-mcg/kg dose of ivermectin. (See CLINICAL PHARMACOLOGY, Clinical Studies.)

Onchocerciasis. STROMECTOL is indicated for the treatment of onchocerciasis due to the nematode parasite *Onchocerca volvulus*.

This indication is based on randomized, double-blind, placebo-controlled and comparative studies conducted in 1427 patients in onchocerciasis-endemic areas of West Africa. The comparative studies used diethylcarbamazine citrate (DEC-C).

NOTE: STROMECTOL has no activity against adult *Onchocerca volvulus* parasites. The adult parasites reside in subcutaneous nodules which are infrequently palpable. Surgical excision of these nodules (nodulectomy) may be considered in the management of patients with onchocerciasis, since this procedure will eliminate the microfilariae-producing adult parasites.

CONTRAINDICATIONS

STROMECTOL is contraindicated in patients who are hypersensitive to any component of this product.

WARNINGS

Historical data have shown that microfilaricidal drugs, such as diethylcarbamazine citrate (DEC-C), might cause cutaneous and/or systemic reactions of varying severity (the Mazzotti reaction) and ophthalmological reactions in patients with onchocerciasis. These reactions are probably due to allergic and inflammatory responses to the death of microfilariae. Patients treated with STROMECTOL for onchocerciasis may experience these reactions in addition to clinical adverse reactions possibly, probably, or definitely related to the drug itself. (See ADVERSE REACTIONS, Onchocerciasis.)

The treatment of severe Mazzotti reactions has not been subjected to controlled clinical trials. Oral hydration, recumbency, intravenous normal saline, and/or parenteral corticosteroids have been used to treat postural hypotension. Antihistamines and/or aspirin have been used for most mild to moderate cases.

PRECAUTIONS

General

After treatment with microfilaricidal drugs, patients with hyperreactive onchodermatitis (sowda) may be more likely than others to experience severe adverse reactions, especially edema and aggravation of onchodermatitis.

Rarely, patients with onchocerciasis who are also heavily infected with *Loa loa* may develop a serious or even fatal encephalopathy either spontaneously or following treatment with an effective microfilaricide. In these patients, the following adverse experiences have also been reported: pain (including neck and back pain), red eye, conjunctival hemorrhage, dyspnea, urinary and/or fecal incontinence, difficulty in standing/walking, mental status changes, confusion, lethargy, stupor, seizures, or coma. This syndrome has been seen very rarely following the use of ivermectin. In individuals who warrant treatment with ivermectin for any reason and have had significant exposure to *Loa loa*-endemic areas of West or Central Africa, pretreatment assessment for loiasis and careful post-treatment follow-up should be implemented.

Information for Patients

STROMECTOL should be taken on an empty stomach with water. (See CLINICAL PHARMACOLOGY, Pharmacokinetics.)

Strongyloidiasis: The patient should be reminded of the need for repeated stool examinations to document clearance of infection with *Strongyloides stercoralis.*

Onchocerciasis: The patient should be reminded that treatment with STROMECTOL does not kill the adult *Onchocerca* parasites, and therefore repeated follow-up and retreatment is usually required.

Drug Interactions

Post-marketing reports of increased INR (International Normalized Ratio) have been rarely reported when ivermectin was co-administered with warfarin.

Carcinogenesis, Mutagenesis, Impairment of Fertility

Long-term studies in animals have not been performed to evaluate the carcinogenic potential of ivermectin.

Ivermectin was not genotoxic *in vitro* in the Ames microbial mutagenicity assay of *Salmonella typhimurium* strains TA1535, TA1537, TA98, and TA100 with and without rat liver enzyme activation, the Mouse Lymphoma Cell Line L5178Y (cytotoxicity and mutagenicity) assays, or the unscheduled DNA synthesis assay in human fibroblasts.

Ivermectin had no adverse effects on the fertility in rats in studies at repeated doses of up to 3 times the maximum recommended human dose of 200 mcg/kg (on a mg/m²/day basis).

Pregnancy

Teratogenic Effects

Pregnancy Category C

Ivermectin has been shown to be teratogenic in mice, rats, and rabbits when given in repeated doses of 0.2, 8.1, and 4.5 times the maximum recommended human dose, respectively (on a mg/m²/day basis). Teratogenicity was character-

ized in the three species tested by cleft palate; clubbed forepaws were additionally observed in rabbits. These developmental effects were found only at or near doses that were maternotoxic to the pregnant female. Therefore, ivermectin does not appear to be selectively fetotoxic to the developing fetus. There are, however, no adequate and well-controlled studies in pregnant women. Ivermectin should not be used during pregnancy since safety in pregnancy has not been established.

Nursing Mothers

STROMECTOL is excreted in human milk in low concentrations. Treatment of mothers who intend to breast-feed should only be undertaken when the risk of delayed treatment to the mother outweighs the possible risk to the newborn.

Pediatric Use

Safety and effectiveness in pediatric patients weighing less than 15 kg have not been established.

Geriatric Use

Clinical studies of STROMECTOL did not include sufficient numbers of subjects aged 65 and over to determine whether they respond differently from younger subjects. Other reported clinical experience has not identified differences in responses between the elderly and younger patients. In general, treatment of an elderly patient should be cautious, reflecting the greater frequency of decreased hepatic, renal, or cardiac function, and of concomitant disease or other drug therapy.

Strongyloidiasis in Immunocompromised Hosts

In immunocompromised (including HIV-infected) patients being treated for intestinal strongyloidiasis, repeated courses of therapy may be required. Adequate and well-controlled clinical studies have not been conducted in such patients to determine the optimal dosing regimen. Several treatments, i.e., at 2-week intervals, may be required, and cure may not be achievable. Control of extra-intestinal strongyloidiasis in these patients is difficult, and suppressive therapy, i.e., once per month, may be helpful.

ADVERSE REACTIONS

Strongyloidiasis

In four clinical studies involving a total of 109 patients given either one or two doses of 170 to 200 mcg/kg of STROMECTOL, the following adverse reactions were reported as possibly, probably, or definitely related to STROMECTOL:

Body as a Whole: asthenia/fatigue (0.9%), abdominal pain (0.9%)

Gastrointestinal: anorexia (0.9%), constipation (0.9%), diarrhea (1.8%), nausea (1.8%), vomiting (0.9%)

Nervous System/Psychiatric: dizziness (2.8%), somnolence (0.9%), vertigo (0.9%), tremor (0.9%)

Skin: pruritus (2.8%), rash (0.9%), and urticaria (0.9%).

In comparative trials, patients treated with STROMECTOL experienced more abdominal distention and chest discomfort than patients treated with albendazole. However, STROMECTOL was better tolerated than thiabendazole in comparative studies involving 37 patients treated with thiabendazole.

The Mazzotti-type and ophthalmologic reactions associated with the treatment of onchocerciasis or the disease itself would not be expected to occur in strongyloidiasis patients treated with STROMECTOL. (See ADVERSE REACTIONS, Onchocerciasis.)

Laboratory Test Findings

In clinical trials involving 109 patients given either one or two doses of 170 to 200 mcg/kg STROMECTOL, the following laboratory abnormalities were seen regardless of drug relationship: elevation in ALT and/or AST (2%), decrease in leukocyte count (3%). Leukopenia and anemia were seen in one patient.

Onchocerciasis

In clinical trials involving 963 adult patients treated with 100 to 200 mcg/kg STROMECTOL, worsening of the following Mazzotti reactions during the first 4 days post-treatment were reported: arthralgia/synovitis (9.3%), axillary lymph node enlargement and tenderness (11.0% and 4.4%, respectively), cervical lymph node enlargement and tenderness (5.3% and 1.2%, respectively), inguinal lymph node enlargement and tenderness (12.6% and 13.9%, respectively), other lymph node enlargement and tenderness (3.0% and 1.9%, respectively), pruritus (27.5%), skin involvement including edema, papular and pustular or frank urticarial rash (22.7%), and fever (22.6%). (See WARNINGS.)

In clinical trials, ophthalmological conditions were examined in 963 adult patients before treatment, at day 3, and months 3 and 6 after treatment with 100 to 200 mcg/kg STROMECTOL. Changes observed were primarily deterioration from baseline 3 days post-treatment. Most changes either returned to baseline condition or improved over baseline severity at the month 3 and 6 visits. The percentages of patients with worsening of the following conditions at day 3, month 3 and 6, respectively, were: limbitis: 5.5%, 4.8%, and

3.5% and punctate opacity: 1.8%, 1.8%, and 1.4%. The corresponding percentages for patients treated with placebo were: limbitis: 6.2%, 9.9%, and 9.4% and punctate opacity: 2.0%, 6.4%, and 7.2%. (See WARNINGS.)

In clinical trials involving 963 adult patients who received 100 to 200 mcg/kg STROMECTOL, the following clinical adverse reactions were reported as possibly, probably, or definitely related to the drug in ≥1% of the patients: facial edema (1.2%), peripheral edema (3.2%), orthostatic hypotension (1.1%), and tachycardia (3.5%). Drug-related headache and myalgia occurred in <1% of patients (0.2% and 0.4%, respectively). However, these were the most common adverse experiences reported overall during these trials regardless of causality (22.3% and 19.7%, respectively).

A similar safety profile was observed in an open study in pediatric patients ages 6 to 13.

The following ophthalmological side effects do occur due to the disease itself but have also been reported after treatment with STROMECTOL: abnormal sensation in the eyes, eyelid edema, anterior uveitis, conjunctivitis, limbitis, keratitis, and chorioretinitis or choroiditis. These have rarely been severe or associated with loss of vision and have generally resolved without corticosteroid treatment.

Laboratory Test Findings

In controlled clinical trials, the following laboratory adverse experiences were reported as possibly, probably, or definitely related to the drug in ≥1% of the patients: eosinophil-ia (3%) and hemoglobin increase (1%).

Post-Marketing Experience

The following adverse reactions have been reported since the drug was registered overseas:

Onchocerciasis
Conjunctival hemorrhage
All Indications

Hypotension (mainly orthostatic hypotension), worsening of bronchial asthma, toxic epidermal necrolysis, Stevens-Johnson syndrome, seizures, hepatitis, elevation of liver enzymes, and elevation of bilirubin.

OVERDOSAGE

Significant lethality was observed in mice and rats after single oral doses of 25 to 50 mg/kg and 40 to 50 mg/kg, respectively. No significant lethality was observed in dogs after single oral doses of up to 10 mg/kg. At these doses, the treatment-related signs that were observed in these animals include ataxia, bradypnea, tremors, ptosis, decreased activity, emesis, and mydriasis.

In accidental intoxication with, or significant exposure to, unknown quantities of veterinary formulations of ivermectin in humans, either by ingestion, inhalation, injection, or exposure to body surfaces, the following adverse effects have been reported most frequently: rash, edema, headache, dizziness, asthenia, nausea, vomiting, and diarrhea. Other adverse effects that have been reported include: seizure, ataxia, dyspnea, abdominal pain, paresthesia, urticaria, and contact dermatitis.

In case of accidental poisoning, supportive therapy, if indicated, should include parenteral fluids and electrolytes, respiratory support (oxygen and mechanical ventilation if necessary) and pressor agents if clinically significant hypotension is present. Induction of emesis and/or gastric lavage as soon as possible, followed by purgatives and other routine anti-poison measures, may be indicated if needed to prevent absorption of ingested material.

DOSAGE AND ADMINISTRATION

Strongyloidiasis

The recommended dosage of STROMECTOL for the treatment of strongyloidiasis is a single oral dose designed to provide approximately 200 mcg of ivermectin per kg of body weight. See Table 1 for dosage guidelines. Patients should take tablets on an empty stomach with water. (See CLINICAL PHARMACOLOGY, Pharmacokinetics.) In general, additional doses are not necessary. However, follow-up stool examinations should be performed to verify eradication of infection. (See CLINICAL PHARMACOLOGY, Clinical Studies.)

Table 1: Dosage Guidelines for STROMECTOL for Strongyloidiasis

Body Weight (kg)	Single Oral Dose Number of 3-mg Tablets
15-24	1 tablet
25-35	2 tablets
36-50	3 tablets
51-65	4 tablets
66-79	5 tablets
≥80	200 mcg/kg

Onchocerciasis

The recommended dosage of STROMECTOL for the treatment of onchocerciasis is a single oral dose designed to provide approximately 150 mcg of ivermectin per kg of body weight. See Table 2 for dosage guidelines. Patients should take tablets on an empty stomach with water. (See CLINICAL PHARMACOLOGY, Pharmacokinetics.) In mass distribution campaigns in international treatment programs, the most commonly used dose interval is 12 months. For the treatment of individual patients, retreatment may be considered at intervals as short as 3 months.

Table 2: Dosage Guidelines for STROMECTOL for Onchocerciasis

Body Weight (kg)	Single Oral Dose Number of 3-mg Tablets
15-25	1 tablet
26-44	2 tablets
45-64	3 tablets
65-84	4 tablets
≥85	150 mcg/kg

HOW SUPPLIED

No. 8495 — Tablets STROMECTOL 3 mg are white, round, flat, bevel-edged tablets coded MSD on one side and 32 on the other side. They are supplied as follows:
NDC 0006-0032-20 unit dose packages of 20.
Storage
Store at temperatures below 30°C (86°F).
Dist. by: Merck Sharp & Dohme Corp., a subsidiary of **MERCK & CO., INC.,** Whitehouse Station, NJ 08889, USA
Manufactured by:
Merck Sharp & Dohme BV
Waarderweg 39
2031 BN Haarlem
Netherlands
Issued May 2010
Printed in the Netherlands
9032319
87447/080610
8495
Shown in Product Identification Guide, page 309

SYLATRON™
(peginterferon alfa-2b)
for injection, for subcutaneous use
℞

HIGHLIGHTS OF PRESCRIBING INFORMATION
These highlights do not include all the information needed to use SYLATRON safely and effectively. See full prescribing information for SYLATRON.
SYLATRON™ (peginterferon alfa-2b)
for injection, for subcutaneous use
Initial U.S. Approval: 2011

WARNING: DEPRESSION AND OTHER NEUROPSYCHIATRIC DISORDERS
See full prescribing information for complete boxed warning.
The risk of serious depression, with suicidal ideation and completed suicides, and other serious neuropsychiatric disorders are increased with alpha interferons, including SYLATRON. Permanently discontinue SYLATRON in patients with persistently severe or worsening signs or symptoms of depression, psychosis, or encephalopathy. These disorders may not resolve after stopping SYLATRON *[see Warnings and Precautions (5.1) and Adverse Reactions (6.1)].*

———RECENT MAJOR CHANGES———

Dosage and Administration,
    Recommended Dosing (2.1)   08/2014

———INDICATIONS AND USAGE———

SYLATRON is an alpha interferon indicated for the adjuvant treatment of melanoma with microscopic or gross nodal involvement within 84 days of definitive surgical resection including complete lymphadenectomy. (1)

———DOSAGE AND ADMINISTRATION———

• 6 mcg/kg/week subcutaneously for 8 doses followed by;
• 3 mcg/kg/week subcutaneously for up to 5 years. (2.1)

———DOSAGE FORMS AND STRENGTHS———

• 200 mcg of deliverable lyophilized powder per single-use vial (3)
• 300 mcg of deliverable lyophilized powder per single-use vial (3)
• 600 mcg of deliverable lyophilized powder per single-use vial (3)

———CONTRAINDICATIONS———

• Known serious hypersensitivity reactions to peginterferon alfa-2b or interferon alfa-2b. (4)
• Autoimmune hepatitis. (4)
• Hepatic decompensation (Child-Pugh score >6 [class B and C]). (4)

———WARNINGS AND PRECAUTIONS———

• Depression and other serious neuropsychiatric adverse reactions. (5.1)
• History of significant or unstable cardiac disease. (5.2)
• Retinal disorders. (5.3)
• Child-Pugh score >6 (class B and C). (4, 5.4)
• Hypothyroidism, hyperthyroidism, hyperglycemia, diabetes mellitus that cannot be effectively treated by medication. (4, 5.5)

———ADVERSE REACTIONS———

Most common adverse reactions (>60%) are: fatigue, increased ALT, increased AST, pyrexia, headache, anorexia, myalgia, nausea, chills, and injection site reaction. (6.1)
To report SUSPECTED ADVERSE REACTIONS, contact Schering Corporation at 1-800-526-4099 or FDA at 1-800-FDA-1088 or www.fda.gov/medwatch.

———DRUG INTERACTIONS———

• Drug metabolized by cytochrome P-450 (CYP) enzymes: Monitor closely when used in combination with drugs metabolized by CYP2C9 or CYP2D6. (7)

———USE IN SPECIFIC POPULATIONS———

• Pregnancy: Based on animal data, may cause fetal harm. (8.1)
• Pediatrics: Safety and efficacy in patients <18 years old have not been established. (8.4)
• Renal Impairment: Reduce the dose of SYLATRON by 25% in patients with moderate renal impairment and 50% in patients with severe renal impairment or end-stage renal disease (ESRD) requiring dialysis. (2.1, 8.7)

See 17 for PATIENT COUNSELING INFORMATION and Medication Guide

Revised: 08/2014

FULL PRESCRIBING INFORMATION: CONTENTS*
WARNING: DEPRESSION AND OTHER NEUROPSYCHIATRIC DISORDERS

FULL PRESCRIBING INFORMATION

WARNING: DEPRESSION AND OTHER NEUROPSYCHIATRIC DISORDERS

The risk of serious depression, with suicidal ideation and completed suicides, and other serious neuropsychiatric disorders are increased with alpha interferons, including SYLATRON. Permanently discontinue

Table 1: Recommended Starting Dose for Moderate and Severe Renal Impairment and End-Stage Renal Disease

Degree of Renal Impairment	Creatinine Clearance (mL/min/1.73m²)	Initial doses for 8 weeks	Follow-up doses for 5 years
Moderate	30 – 50	4.5 mcg/kg/week	2.25 mcg/kg/week
Severe	<30	3 mcg/kg/week	1.5 mcg/kg/week
End-Stage Renal Disease	On dialysis	3 mcg/kg/week	1.5 mcg/kg/week

Table 3: Reconstitution of SYLATRON Single-Use Vials

SYLATRON Single-Use Vial		Diluent (Sterile Water for Injection, USP)		Deliverable Product and Volume	Final Concentration
200 mcg*	add	0.7 mL	=	200 mcg in 0.5 mL	40 mcg/0.1 mL
300 mcg‡	add	0.7 mL	=	300 mcg in 0.5 mL	60 mcg/0.1 mL
600 mcg‡	add	0.7 mL	=	600 mcg in 0.5 mL	120 mcg/0.1 mL

* Total vial content of SYLATRON is 296 mcg.
† Total vial content of SYLATRON is 444 mcg.
‡ Total vial content of SYLATRON is 888 mcg.

SYLATRON in patients with persistently severe or worsening signs or symptoms of depression, psychosis, or encephalopathy. These disorders may not resolve after stopping SYLATRON *[see Warnings and Precautions (5.1) and Adverse Reactions (6.1)]*.

1 INDICATIONS AND USAGE

SYLATRON™ is an alpha interferon indicated for the adjuvant treatment of melanoma with microscopic or gross nodal involvement within 84 days of definitive surgical resection including complete lymphadenectomy.

2 DOSAGE AND ADMINISTRATION
2.1 Recommended Dosing
• The recommended starting dose is 6 mcg/kg/week subcutaneously for 8 doses, followed by 3 mcg/kg/week subcutaneously for up to 5 years.
• Premedicate with acetaminophen 500 to 1000 mg orally 30 minutes prior to the first dose of SYLATRON and as needed for subsequent doses.
• The recommended starting doses of SYLATRON in patients with moderate or severe renal impairment or end-stage renal disease (ESRD) are listed in Table 1 *[see Use in Specific Populations (8.7)]*. No dose adjustment is needed for patients with a creatinine clearance (CLcr) > 50 mL/min/1.73m².
[See table 1 above]

2.2 Dose Modification Guidelines
Guidelines for Dose Modification provided below are based on the National Cancer Institute Common Terminology Criteria for Adverse Events (NCI-CTCAE Version 2.0).
• Permanently discontinue SYLATRON for:
  ◦ Persistent or worsening severe neuropsychiatric disorders
  ◦ Grade 4 non-hematologic toxicity
  ◦ Inability to tolerate a dose of 1 mcg/kg/wk
  ◦ New or worsening retinopathy
• Withhold SYLATRON dose for any of the following:
  ◦ Absolute Neutrophil Count (ANC) less than 0.5×10⁹/L
  ◦ Platelet Count (PLT) less than 50×10⁹/L
  ◦ ECOG PS greater than or equal to 2
  ◦ Non-hematologic toxicity greater than or equal to Grade 3
• Resume dosing at a reduced dose (see Table 1) when all of the following are present:
  ◦ Absolute Neutrophil Count (ANC) greater than or equal to 0.5×10⁹/L
  ◦ Platelet Count (PLT) greater than or equal to 50×10⁹/L
  ◦ ECOG PS 0–1
  ◦ Non-hematologic toxicity has completely resolved or improved to Grade 1

Table 2: SYLATRON Dose Modifications

Starting Dose	Dose Modifications for Doses 1 to 8
6 mcg/kg/week	First Dose Modification: 3 mcg/kg/week
	Second Dose Modification: 2 mcg/kg/week
	Third Dose Modification: 1 mcg/kg/week
	Permanently discontinue if unable to tolerate 1 mcg/kg/week

Starting Dose	Dose Modifications for Doses 9 to 260
3 mcg/kg/week	First Dose Modification: 2 mcg/kg/week
	Second Dose Modification: 1 mcg/kg/week
	Permanently discontinue if unable to tolerate 1 mcg/kg/week

2.3 Preparation and Administration
Reconstitute SYLATRON with 0.7 mL of Sterile Water for Injection, USP.
[See table 3 above]
• Swirl gently to dissolve the lyophilized powder. **DO NOT SHAKE.**
• Visually inspect the solution for particulate matter and discoloration prior to administration. Discard if solution is discolored, cloudy, or if particulates are present.
• Do not withdraw more than 0.5 mL of reconstituted solution from each vial.
• Administer SYLATRON subcutaneously. Rotate injection sites.
• If reconstituted solution is not used immediately, store at 2°–8°C (36°–46°F) for no more than 24 hours. Discard reconstituted solution after 24 hours. **DO NOT FREEZE.**
• For single-use only. **DISCARD ANY UNUSED PORTION.**

3 DOSAGE FORMS AND STRENGTHS
• 200 mcg of deliverable lyophilized powder per single-use vial
• 300 mcg of deliverable lyophilized powder per single-use vial
• 600 mcg of deliverable lyophilized powder per single-use vial

4 CONTRAINDICATIONS
SYLATRON is contraindicated in patients with:
• A history of anaphylaxis to peginterferon alfa-2b or interferon alfa-2b
• autoimmune hepatitis
• hepatic decompensation (Child-Pugh score >6 [class B and C])

5 WARNINGS AND PRECAUTIONS
5.1 Depression and Other Serious Neuropsychiatric Adverse Reactions
Peginterferon alfa-2b can cause life-threatening or fatal neuropsychiatric reactions. These include suicide, suicidal and homicidal ideation, depression, and an increased risk of relapse of recovering drug addicts. In the clinical trial, depression occurred in 59% of SYLATRON-treated patients and 24% of patients in the observation group. Depression was severe or life threatening in 7% of SYLATRON-treated patients compared with <1% of patients in the observation arm.
In post-marketing experience, neuropsychiatric adverse reactions have been reported up to 6 months after discontinuation of peginterferon alfa-2b. Based on post-marketing experience with peginterferon alfa-2b and interferon alfa-2b, treatment may also result in aggressive behavior, psychoses, hallucinations, bipolar disorders, mania, and encephalopathy.
Advise patients and their caregivers to immediately report any symptoms of depression or suicidal ideation to their healthcare provider. Monitor and evaluate patients for signs and symptoms of depression and other psychiatric symptoms every 3 weeks during the first 8 weeks of treatment and every 6 months thereafter. Monitor patients during treatment and for at least 6 months after the last dose of SYLATRON. Permanently discontinue SYLATRON for persistent severe or worsening psychiatric symptoms or behaviors and refer for psychiatric evaluation.

5.2 Cardiovascular Adverse Reactions
In the clinical trial, cardiac adverse reactions, including myocardial infarction, bundle-branch block, ventricular tachycardia, and supraventricular arrhythmia occurred in 4% of SYLATRON-treated patients compared with 2% of patients in the observation group. In post-marketing experience, hypotension, cardiomyopathy, and angina pectoris have occurred in patients treated with peginterferon alfa-2b. Permanently discontinue SYLATRON for new onset of ventricular arrhythmia or cardiovascular decompensation.

5.3 Retinopathy and Other Serious Ocular Adverse Reactions
Peginterferon alfa-2b can cause decrease in visual acuity or blindness due to retinopathy. Retinal and ocular changes include macular edema, retinal artery or vein thrombosis, retinal hemorrhages and cotton wool spots, optic neuritis, papilledema, and serous retinal detachment may be induced or aggravated by treatment with peginterferon alfa-2b or other alpha interferons. In the clinical study, two SYLATRON-treated patients developed partial loss of vision due to retinal thrombosis (n=1) or retinopathy (n=1). The overall incidence of serious retinal disorders, visual disturbances, blurred vision, and reduction in visual acuity was <1% in both SYLATRON-treated patients and the observation group.
Perform an eye examination that includes assessment of visual acuity and indirect ophthalmoscopy or fundus photography at baseline in patients with preexisting retinopathy and at any time during SYLATRON treatment in patients who experience changes in vision. Permanently discontinue SYLATRON in patients who develop new or worsening retinopathy.

5.4 Hepatic Failure
Peginterferon alfa-2b, increases the risk of hepatic decompensation and death in patients with cirrhosis. Monitor hepatic function with serum bilirubin, ALT, AST, alkaline phosphatase, and LDH at 2 and 8 weeks, and 2 and 3 months following initiation of SYLATRON, then every 6 months while receiving SYLATRON. Permanently discontinue SYLATRON for evidence of severe (Grade 3) hepatic injury or hepatic decompensation (Child-Pugh score >6 [class B and C]) *[see Contraindications (4)]*.

5.5 Endocrinopathies
Peginterferon alfa-2b can cause new onset or worsening of hypothyroidism, hyperthyroidism, and diabetes mellitus. In the clinical study, 1% of patients developed hypothyroidism; the overall incidence of endocrine disorders was 2% in SYLATRON-treated patients compared to <1% for patients in the observation group.
Obtain TSH levels within 4 weeks prior to initiation of SYLATRON, at 3 and 6 months following initiation, then every 6 months thereafter while receiving SYLATRON. Permanently discontinue SYLATRON in patients who develop hypothyroidism, hyperthyroidism or diabetes mellitus that cannot be effectively managed.

6 ADVERSE REACTIONS
The following serious adverse reactions are discussed in greater detail in other sections of the labeling:
• Depression and Other Neuropsychiatric Adverse Reactions *[see Warnings and Precautions (5.1)]*
• Cardiovascular Adverse Reactions *[see Warnings and Precautions (5.2)]*
• Retinopathy and Other Serious Ocular Adverse Reactions *[see Warnings and Precautions (5.3)]*
• Hepatic Failure *[see Warnings and Precautions (5.4)]*
• Endocrinopathies *[see Warnings and Precautions (5.5)]*
6.1 Clinical Trials Experience
Because clinical trials are conducted under widely varying conditions, adverse reaction rates observed in the clinical trials of a drug cannot be directly compared to rates in the clinical trials of another drug and may not reflect the rates observed in clinical practice.
The data described below reflect exposure to SYLATRON in 608 patients with surgically resected, AJCC Stage III melanoma. SYLATRON was studied in an open label, multicenter, randomized, observation controlled trial. The median age of the population was 50 years with 10% of patients 65 years or older, and 42% were female. Fourteen percent of patients completed the 5 year treatment schedule.
Patients randomized to SYLATRON were to receive total doses of 48 mcg/kg (6 mcg/kg subcutaneous once weekly for 8 doses) and 780 mcg/kg (3 mcg/kg subcutaneous once weekly until disease recurrence or for up to 5 years), as tolerated. The median total dose received was 42 mcg/kg (range: 6 to 78 mcg/kg) for the first 8 doses, and 136 mcg/kg (range: 1 to 774 mcg/kg) for doses 9 to 260.

Serious adverse events were reported in 199 (33%) patients who received SYLATRON and 94 (15%) patients in the observation group.

The most common adverse reactions experienced by SYLATRON-treated patients were fatigue (94%), increased ALT (77%), increased AST (77%), pyrexia (75%), headache (70%), anorexia (69%), myalgia (68%), nausea (64%), chills (63%), and injection site reaction (62%). The most common serious adverse reactions were fatigue (7%), increased ALT (3%), increased AST (3%), and pyrexia (3%) in the SYLATRON-treated group vs. <1% in the observation group for these reactions.

Thirty three percent of patients receiving SYLATRON discontinued treatment due to adverse reactions. The most common adverse reactions present at the time of treatment discontinuation were fatigue (27%), depression (17%), anorexia (15%), increased ALT (14%), increased AST (14%), myalgia (13%), nausea (13%), headache (13%), and pyrexia (11%). Adverse events that occurred in the clinical study at ≥ 5% incidence in the SYLATRON-treated group and with a greater incidence in patients receiving SYLATRON as compared to the observation group are presented in **Table 4**.
[See table 4 above]

6.2 Immunogenicity
As with all therapeutic proteins, there is potential for immunogenicity. In a clinical study conducted in patients with melanoma, the incidence of binding antibodies to peg-interferon alfa-2b was approximately 35% (50/144 patients). Among the patients who tested positive for binding antibodies, one patient developed neutralizing antibodies. The impact of antibody formation on pharmacokinetics, safety and efficacy of peg-interferon alfa-2b could not be assessed based on limited available data.

The incidence of antibody formation is highly dependent on the sensitivity and specificity of the assay. Additionally, the observed incidence of antibody (including neutralizing antibody) positivity in an assay may be influenced by several factors, including assay methodology, sample handling, timing of sample collection, concomitant medications, and underlying disease. For these reasons, comparison of the incidence of antibodies to SYLATRON with the incidence of antibodies to other products may be misleading.

6.3 Postmarketing Experience
The following adverse reactions have been identified during post-approval use of peginterferon alfa-2b as monotherapy and in combination with ribavirin in chronic hepatitis C (CHC) patients. Because these reactions are reported voluntarily from a population of uncertain size, it is not always possible to reliably estimate their frequency or establish a causal relationship to drug exposure.

Blood and Lymphatic System Disorders
pure red cell aplasia, thrombotic thrombocytopenic purpura

Ear and Labyrinth Disorders
hearing loss, vertigo, hearing impairment

Endocrine Disorders
diabetic ketoacidosis

Eye Disorders
Vogt-Koyanagi-Harada syndrome

Gastrointestinal Disorders
aphthous stomatitis, pancreatitis, colitis

Infusion reactions
angioedema, urticaria, bronchoconstriction

Immune System Disorders
systemic lupus erythematosus, erythema multiforme, thyroiditis, thrombotic thrombocytopenic purpura, idiopathic thrombocytopenic purpura, rheumatoid arthritis, interstitial nephritis, and systemic lupus erythematosus

Infections
sepsis

Metabolism and Nutrition Disorders
hypertriglyceridemia

Musculoskeletal and Connective Tissue Disorders
rhabdomyolysis, myositis

Nervous System Disorders
seizures, memory loss, peripheral neuropathy, paraesthesia, migraine headache

Respiratory, Thoracic and Mediastinal Disorders
dyspnea, pulmonary infiltrates, pneumonia, bronchiolitis obliterans, interstitial pneumonitis, sarcoidosis and pulmonary hypertension

Skin and Subcutaneous Tissue Disorders
Stevens-Johnson syndrome, toxic epidermal necrolysis, psoriasis

Vascular Disorders
hypertension, hypotension, stroke

7 DRUG INTERACTIONS

In healthy subjects who were administered peginterferon alfa-2b subcutaneously at 1 mcg/kg once weekly for four weeks with probe drugs of metabolic enzymes administered before the first dose and after the fourth dose, a measure of CYP2C9 activity increased to 125% of baseline, whereas a

Table 4: Incidence of Adverse Reactions[*] Occurring in ≥ 5% of Melanoma Patients Treated with SYLATRON and with a Greater Incidence as Compared to Observation

Adverse Reaction	SYLATRON N=608		Observation N=628	
	All Grades (%)	Grade 3 and 4 (%)	All Grades (%)	Grade 3 and 4 (%)
Any Adverse Reaction	100	51	82	18
General Disorders and Administrative Site Conditions				
Fatigue	94	16	41	1
Pyrexia	75	4	9	0
Chills	63	1	6	0
Injection Site Reaction	62	1.8	0	0
Metabolic/Laboratory				
ALT or AST Increased	77	11	26	1
Blood Alkaline Phosphatase Increased	23	0	11	<1
Weight Decreased	11	<1	1	<1
GGT Increased	8	4	1	<1
Proteinuria	7	0	3	0
Anemia	6	<1	2	<1
Nervous System Disorders				
Headache	70	4	19	1
Dysgeusia	38	0	1	0
Dizziness	35	2	11	<1
Olfactory Nerve Disorder	23	0	1	0
Paraesthesia	21	<1	14	<1
Metabolism and Nutrition Disorders				
Anorexia	69	3	13	0
Musculoskeletal and Connective Tissue Disorders				
Myalgia	68	4	23	<1
Arthralgia	51	3	22	1
Gastrointestinal Disorders				
Nausea	64	3	11	<1
Diarrhea	37	1	8	<1
Vomiting	26	1	4	0
Psychiatric Disorders				
Depression	59	7	24	<1
Skin and Subcutaneous Tissue Disorders				
Exfoliative Rash	36	1	4	0
Alopecia	34	0	1	0
Respiratory, Thoracic and Mediastinal Disorders				
Dyspnea	6	1	2	1
Cough	5	<1	2	0

* Adverse reactions were graded using NCI CTCAE, V.2.0.

measure of CYP2D6 activity decreased to 51% of baseline *[see Clinical Pharmacology (12.3)]*. When administering SYLATRON with medications metabolized by CYP2C9 or CYP2D6, the therapeutic effect of these drugs may be altered.

The effects of pegylated interferon alfa-2b on the pharmacokinetics of drugs metabolized by cytochrome P-450 enzymes have not been studied at the higher clinical doses for patients with melanoma (3 mcg/kg/week and 6 mcg/kg/week).

8 USE IN SPECIFIC POPULATIONS
8.1 Pregnancy
Pregnancy Category C:
There are no adequate and well-controlled studies of SYLATRON in pregnant women. Nonpegylated interferon alfa-2b was an abortifacient in *Macaca mulatta* (rhesus monkeys) at 15 and 30 million international units (IU)/kg (estimated human equivalent of 5 and 10 million IU/kg, based on body surface area adjustment for a 60-kg adult). The estimated Intron A human equivalent dose of 5 to

10 million IU/kg daily is approximately equal to a human equivalent dose of 79 to 158 mcg/kg/week of SYLATRON. Use SYLATRON during pregnancy only if the potential benefit justifies the potential risk to the fetus.

8.3 Nursing Mothers
It is not known whether the components of SYLATRON are excreted in human milk. Studies in mice have shown that mouse interferons are excreted in breast milk. Because of the potential for adverse reactions from the drug in nursing infants, a decision must be made whether to discontinue nursing or discontinue the SYLATRON treatment, taking into account the importance of the therapy to the mother.

8.4 Pediatric Use
Safety and effectiveness in patients below the age of 18 years have not been established.

8.5 Geriatric Use
Clinical studies of SYLATRON did not include sufficient numbers of subjects aged 65 and over to determine whether they respond differently from younger subjects.

8.6 Hepatic Impairment
SYLATRON has not been studied in patients with melanoma who have hepatic impairment. In patients treated for viral hepatitis, peginterferon alfa-2b treatment is contraindicated in those with moderate or severe hepatic impairment (Child-Pugh scores >6). Discontinue SYLATRON if hepatic decompensation (Child-Pugh scores >6) occurs during treatment. [See Contraindications (4) and Warnings and Precautions (5.4).]

8.7 Renal Impairment
Reduce the dose of SYLATRON by 25% in patients with moderate renal impairment (CLcr 30 to 50 mL/min/1.73m^2) and 50% in patients with severe renal impairment (CLcr < 30 mL/min/1.73m^2) or ESRD requiring dialysis [see Dosage and Administration (2.1)]. A study in subjects with varying degrees of renal impairment showed that the mean exposure (AUC) to peginterferon alfa-2b increased in subjects with moderate and severe renal impairment or ESRD requiring dialysis, as compared to subjects with normal renal function (CLcr > 80 mL/min/1.73m^2) following a single 4.5 mcg/kg dose of peginterferon alfa-2b [See Clinical Pharmacology (12.3)].

10   OVERDOSAGE
The experience with overdose of SYLATRON is limited. Patients who were over dosed experienced the following adverse reactions: severe fatigue, headache, myalgia, neutropenia, and thrombocytopenia. The highest single dose administered was 14 mcg/kg.

11   DESCRIPTION
SYLATRON, peginterferon alfa-2b, is a covalent conjugate of recombinant alfa-2b interferon with monomethoxy polyethylene glycol (PEG). The average molecular weight of the PEG portion of the molecule is 12,000 daltons. The average molecular weight of the SYLATRON molecule is approximately 31,000 daltons. The specific activity of pegylated interferon alfa-2b is approximately 0.7×10^8 international units/mg protein.
Interferon alfa-2b is a protein with a molecular weight of 19,271 daltons produced by recombinant DNA techniques. It is obtained from the bacterial fermentation of a strain of Escherichia coli bearing a genetically engineered plasmid containing an interferon gene from human leukocytes.
Each vial contains either 296 mcg, 444 mcg or 888 mcg of peginterferon alfa-2b as a sterile, white to off-white lyophilized powder, and dibasic sodium phosphate anhydrous (1.11 mg), monobasic sodium phosphate dihydrate (1.11 mg), polysorbate 80 (0.074 mg), and sucrose (59.2 mg).

12   CLINICAL PHARMACOLOGY
12.1   Mechanism of Action
Peginterferon alfa-2b is a pleiotropic cytokine; the mechanism by which it exerts its effects in patients with melanoma is unknown.

12.3   Pharmacokinetics
The pharmacokinetics were studied in 32 patients receiving adjuvant therapy for melanoma with SYLATRON according to the recommended dose and schedule (6 mcg/kg/week for 8 doses, followed by 3 mcg/kg/week thereafter). At a dose of 6 mcg/kg/week once weekly, the geometric mean C_{max} was 4.4 ng/mL (CV 51%) and the geometric mean $AUC_{(tau)}$ was 430 ng•hr/mL (CV 35%) at week 8. The mean terminal half-life was approximately 51 hours (CV 18%). The mean accumulation from week 1 to week 8 was 1.7. After administration of 3 mcg/kg/week once weekly, the mean geometric C_{max} was 2.5 ng/mL (CV 33%) and the geometric mean $AUC_{(tau)}$ was 228 ng•hr/mL (CV 24%) at week 4. The mean terminal half-life was approximately 43 hours (CV 19%).

Renal Impairment:
Renal clearance accounts for approximately 30% of total peginterferon alfa-2b clearance. The effect of renal impairment on the pharmacokinetics of peginterferon alfa-2b was studied in 24 subjects with normal or impaired renal function after a single 4.5 mcg/kg dose. Compared to subjects with normal renal function (CLcr > 80 mL/min/1.73 m^2), the

geometric mean exposure (AUC$_{last}$) to peginterferon alfa-2b increased by 1.4-fold in subjects with moderate renal impairment (CLcr 30 to 50 mL/min/1.73m^2) and 2.1-fold in subjects with severe renal impairment (CLcr < 30 mL/min/1.73m^2) or ESRD requiring dialysis [see Use in Specific Populations (8.7)].
No clinically meaningful amounts of peginterferon alfa-2b were removed during hemodialysis following a single 1 mcg/kg dose in subjects with renal impairment.

Drug Interactions:
In a two-way crossover trial, 12 healthy subjects were administered probe drugs of metabolic enzymes: caffeine (CYP1A2), tolbutamide (CYP2C9), dextromethorphan (CYP2D6), midazolam (CYP3A4), and dapsone (N-acetyltransferase, NAT), with or without a single subcutaneous (SC) dose of peginterferon alfa-2b at 1 mcg/kg. The results suggest that single doses of peginterferon alfa-2b do not affect activities of CYP1A2, CYP2C9, CYP2D6, CYP3A4 and NAT enzymes.
In 24 healthy subjects, the effect of subcutaneous doses of peginterferon alfa-2b at 1 mcg/kg/week for 4 weeks on the pharmacokinetics of caffeine, tolbutamide, dextromethorphan and midazolam were studied. A measure of CYP2C9 activity increased to 125% (90% CI: 116% to 135%) of baseline, whereas a measure of CYP2D6 activity decreased to 51% (90% CI: 38% to 67%) of baseline when coadministered with peginterferon alfa-2b at week 4, indicating that peginterferon alfa-2b may affect the metabolism of CYP2C9 and CYP2D6 drugs. A measure of CYP1A2 and CYP3A4 activity did not show clinically meaningful changes.
When patients are administered SYLATRON with medications metabolized by CYP2C9 or CYP2D6, the therapeutic effect of these drugs may be altered.
The effects of peginterferon alfa-2b at the clinical doses for melanoma (3 mcg/kg/week and 6 mcg/kg/week) on the systemic exposure of drugs metabolized by cytochrome P-450 enzymes have not been studied [see Drug Interactions (7)].

13   NONCLINICAL TOXICOLOGY
13.1   Carcinogenesis, Mutagenesis, Impairment of Fertility
Carcinogenesis and Mutagenesis:
SYLATRON has not been tested for its carcinogenic potential. Neither peginterferon alfa-2b nor its components, interferon or methoxypolyethylene glycol, caused damage to DNA when tested in the standard battery of mutagenesis assays, in the presence and absence of metabolic activation.
Impairment of Fertility:
SYLATRON may impair human fertility. Irregular menstrual cycles were observed in female cynomolgus monkeys given subcutaneous injections of 4239 mcg/m^2 peginterferon alfa-2b alone every other day for 1 month (approximately 72 to 144 times the recommended weekly human dose based upon body surface area). These effects included transiently decreased serum levels of estradiol and progesterone, suggestive of anovulation. Normal menstrual cycles and serum hormone levels resumed in these animals 2 to 3 months following cessation of peginterferon alfa-2b treatment. Every other day dosing with 262 mcg/m^2 (approximately 3.5 to 7 times the recommended weekly human dose) had no effects on cycle duration or reproductive hormone status. The effects of SYLATRON on male fertility have not been studied.

14   CLINICAL STUDIES
The safety and effectiveness of SYLATRON were evaluated in an open-label, multicenter, randomized (1:1) study conducted in 1256 patients with surgically resected, AJCC Stage III melanoma within 84 days of regional lymph node dissection. Patients were randomized to observation (no therapy) (n=629) or to SYLATRON (n=627) at a dose of 6 mcg/kg by subcutaneous injection once weekly for 8 doses followed by a 3 mcg/kg subcutaneous injection once weekly for a period of up to 5 years total treatment. The dose of SYLATRON was adjusted to maintain an ECOG Performance Status of 0 to 1.
The median age of the population was 50 years with 11% of patients 65 years or older, and 42% were female. Forty percent of the study population had microscopic, nonpalpable nodal involvement and 59% had clinically palpable nodes prior to lymphadenectomy. A total of 54% of subjects had one pathologically positive lymph node, 34% had 2 to 4 positive nodes, and 12% had 5 or more. Most subjects had no second primary lesion (98%). Ulceration of the primary lesion was present in 30% of subjects (52% had no ulceration of the primary lesion, and the status was missing/unknown for 18% of subjects). The most common sites were the trunk (43%) or the leg (32%). Eighty-four percent had an International Prognostic Index (IPI) score of 0 and 16% had an IPI score of 1. The main outcome measure was relapse-free survival (RFS), defined as the time from randomization to the earliest date of any relapse (local, regional, in-transit, or distant), or death from any cause. Secondary outcome measures included overall survival.
Patients in the SYLATRON arm received 6 mcg/kg/week for a median of 8.0 weeks. Less than 1% of patients took longer

than 9 weeks to complete the 6 mcg/kg/week dosing regimen. Approximately one-third (36%) of patients required dose reductions and 29% of patients required a dose delay, with an average delay of 1.2 weeks, during the initial 8 weeks of SYLATRON. Ninety-four patients (16%) did not continue on to the 3 mcg/kg/week dosing regimen.
Patients who continued on SYLATRON after the initial 8 doses, received 3 mcg/kg/week for a median duration of treatment of 14.3 months. Approximately half (52%) of the patients underwent dose reductions and 70% required dose delays (average delay 2.2 weeks).
Based on 696 RFS events, determined by the Independent Review Committee, median RFS was 34.8 months (95% CI: 26.1, 47.4) and 25.5 months (95% CI: 19.6, 30.8) in the SYLATRON and observation arms, respectively. The estimated hazard ratio for RFS was 0.82 (95% CI: 0.71, 0.96; unstratified log-rank p =0.011) in favor of SYLATRON. Figure 1 shows the Kaplan-Meier curves of RFS.

FIGURE 1: Kaplan-Meier Curves for Relapse-Free Survival

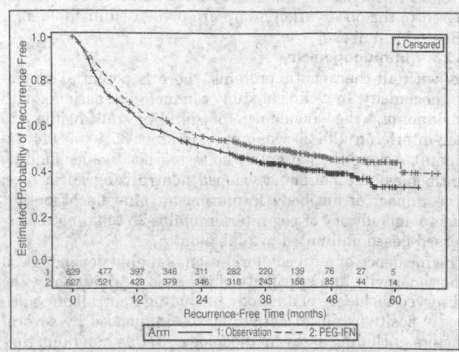

There was no statistically significant difference in survival between the SYLATRON and the observation arms. Based on 525 deaths, the estimated hazard ratio of SYLATRON versus observation was 0.98 (95% CI: 0.82, 1.16).

16   HOW SUPPLIED/STORAGE AND HANDLING

Each SYLATRON Package Contains:

A box containing one 200 mcg per vial of SYLATRON powder and one 1.25 mL vial of Sterile Water for Injection, USP, 2 B-D Safety Lok syringes with a safety sleeve and 2 alcohol swabs.	(NDC 0085-1388-01)
A box containing one 300 mcg per vial of SYLATRON powder and one 1.25 mL vial of Sterile Water for Injection, USP, 2 B-D Safety Lok syringes with a safety sleeve and 2 alcohol swabs.	(NDC 0085-1287-02)
A box containing one 600 mcg per vial of SYLATRON powder and one 1.25 mL vial of Sterile Water for Injection, USP, 2 B-D Safety Lok syringes with a safety sleeve and 2 alcohol swabs.	(NDC 0085-1312-01)

Each SYLATRON PACK 4 Contains:

A box containing four 200 mcg per vial of SYLATRON powder and four 1.25 mL vials of Sterile Water for Injection, USP, 8 B-D Safety Lok syringes with a safety sleeve and 8 alcohol swabs.	(NDC 0085-1388-02)
A box containing four 300 mcg per vial of SYLATRON powder and four 1.25 mL vials of Sterile Water for Injection, USP, 8 B-D Safety Lok syringes with a safety sleeve and 8 alcohol swabs.	(NDC 0085-1287-03)

Storage:
SYLATRON should be stored at 25°C (77°F); excursions permitted to 15°-30°C (59–86°F) [see USP Controlled Room Temperature]. **DO NOT FREEZE.**

17   PATIENT COUNSELING INFORMATION
See FDA-approved patient labeling (Instructions for Use and Medication Guide).
• Advise patients that SYLATRON may be administered with antipyretics at bedtime to minimize common "flu-like" symptoms (including chills, fever, muscle aches, joint pain, headaches, tiredness).

- Advise patients to maintain hydration if experiencing "flu-like" symptoms.
- Advise patients and their caregivers to immediately report any symptoms of depression or suicidal ideation to their healthcare provider during treatment and up to 6 months after the last dose.
- Use SYLATRON during pregnancy only if the potential benefit justifies the potential risk to the fetus [see Use in Specific Populations (8.1)].
- Instruct patients to not re-use or share syringes and needles.
- Instruct patients on proper disposal of vials, syringes and needles.

Manufactured by: Schering Corporation, a subsidiary of **MERCK & CO., INC.,** Whitehouse Station, NJ 08889, USA
Revised: 08/2014
For patent information:
www.merck.com/product/patent/home.html.
BD and Safety-Lok are registered trademarks of Becton, Dickinson and Company.
Copyright © 2011 Merck Sharp & Dohme Corp., a subsidiary of **Merck & Co., Inc.**
All rights reserved.
uspi-mk4031-pwi-1408r023

Instructions for Use

SYLATRON™ (SY-LA-TRON)
(peginterferon alfa-2b)
for injection
Powder for Injection
Be sure that you read, understand and follow these instructions before injecting SYLATRON. Your healthcare provider should show you how to prepare, measure, and inject SYLATRON properly before you use it for the first time. Ask your healthcare provider if you have any questions.
Before starting, collect all of the supplies that you will need to use for preparing and injecting SYLATRON. For each injection you will need a SYLATRON vial package that contains:
- 1 vial of SYLATRON powder
- 1 vial of sterile water for injection (diluent)
- 2 single-use disposable syringes (BD Safety Lok syringes with a safety sleeve)
- 2 alcohol swabs
You will also need:
- 1 cotton ball or gauze
- 1 sharps disposal container to throw away (dispose of) used syringes, needles, and vials. See "How should I dispose of used syringes, needles, and vials" at the end of this Instructions for Use.

Important:
- **Do not re-use or share syringes and needles.**
- The vial of mixed SYLATRON should be used right away. Do not mix more than 1 vial of SYLATRON at a time. If you do not use the vial of the prepared solution right away, store it in a refrigerator and use within 24 hours. See the end of this Instructions for Use for information about "How should I store SYLATRON?"
- Make sure you have the right syringe and needle to use with SYLATRON. Your healthcare provider should tell you what syringes and needles to use to inject SYLATRON.

How should I prepare a dose of SYLATRON?
Before you inject SYLATRON, the powder must be mixed with 0.7 mL of the sterile water for injection (diluent) that comes in the SYLATRON vial package.
1. Find a clean, well-lit, flat work surface.
2. Get 1 of your SYLATRON vial packages. Check the date printed on the SYLATRON carton. Make sure that the expiration date has not passed. Do not use your SYLATRON vial packages if the expiration date has passed. The medicine in the SYLATRON vial should look like a white to off-white tablet that is whole, or in pieces, or powdered.
   If you have already mixed the SYLATRON solution and stored it in the refrigerator, take it out of the refrigerator before use and allow the solution to come to room temperature.
3. Wash your hands well with soap and water, rinse and towel dry (See Figure A). Keep your work area, your hands, and injection site clean to decrease the risk of infection.
   [See figure A at top of next column]
   The disposable syringes have needles that are already attached and cannot be removed. Each syringe has a clear plastic safety sleeve that is pulled over the needle for disposal after use. The safety sleeve should remain tight against the flange while using the syringe and moved over the needle only when ready for disposal. (See Figure B)
   [See figure B at top of next column]
4. Remove the protective wrapper from one of the syringes provided. Use the syringe for steps 4 through 15. Make sure that the syringe safety sleeve is sitting against the flange. (See Figure B)

Figure A

FLANGES
GREEN STRIPE
SAFETY SLEEVE
RED STRIPE
PROTECTIVE CAP

Figure B

5. Remove the protective plastic cap from the tops of both the sterile water for injection (diluent) and the SYLATRON vials (See Figure C). Clean the rubber stopper on the top of both vials with an alcohol swab.

Figure C

6. Carefully remove the protective cap straight off of the needle to avoid damaging the needle point.
7. Fill the syringe with air by pulling back on the plunger to 0.7 mL. (See Figure D)

Figure D

8. Hold the diluent vial upright. Do not touch the cleaned top of the vial with your hands.
   - Push the needle through the center of the rubber stopper of the diluent vial. (See Figure E)
   - Slowly inject all the air from the syringe into the air space above the diluent in the vial. (See Figure F)

Figure E   **Figure F**

9. Turn the vial upside down and make sure the tip of the needle is in the liquid.
10. Withdraw only 0.7 mL of diluent by pulling the plunger back to the 0.7 mL mark on the side of the syringe. (See Figure G)

Figure G

11. With the needle still inserted in the vial, check the syringe for air bubbles.
    - If there are any air bubbles, gently tap the syringe with your finger until the air bubbles rise to the top of the syringe.
    - Slowly push the plunger up to remove the air bubbles.
    - If you push diluent back into the vial, slowly pull back on the plunger to draw the correct amount of diluent back into the syringe.
12. Remove the needle from the vial (See Figure H). Do not let the syringe touch anything.

Figure H

13. Throw away the diluent vial.
14. Insert the needle through the center of the rubber stopper of the SYLATRON powder vial. Do not touch the cleaned rubber stopper.
    - Place the needle tip, at an angle, against the side of the vial. (See Figure I)
    - Slowly push the plunger down to inject the 0.7 mL diluent. The stream of diluent should run down the side of the vial.
    - To prevent bubbles from forming, do not aim the stream of diluent directly on the medicine in the bottom of the vial.

Figure I

15. Remove the needle from the vial.
    - Firmly grasp the safety sleeve and pull it over the exposed needle until you hear a click (See Figure J). The green stripe on the safety sleeve will completely cover the red stripe on the needle. Dispose of the syringe, needle, and vial in the sharps disposal container. See "How should I dispose of used syringes, needles, and vials?" at the end of this Instructions for Use.

Figure J

16. Gently swirl the vial in a gentle circular motion, until the SYLATRON is completely dissolved (mixed together). (See Figure K)
    - Do not shake the vial. If any powder remains undissolved in the vial, gently turn the vial upside down until all of the powder is dissolved.
    - The solution may look cloudy or bubbly for a few minutes. If air bubbles form, wait until the solution settles and all bubbles rise to the top.

DO NOT SHAKE

Figure K

17. After the SYLATRON completely dissolves, the solution should be clear, colorless and without particles. It is normal to see a ring of foam or bubbles on the surface.
    - Do not use the mixed solution if you see particles in it, or it is not clear and colorless. Dispose of the syringe and needle in the sharps disposal container. See the section "How should I dispose of used syringes, needles, and vials?" at the end of this Instructions for Use. Then, repeat steps 1 through 17 with a new vial of SYLATRON and diluent to prepare a new syringe.
18. After the SYLATRON powder completely dissolves, clean the rubber stopper again with an alcohol swab before you withdraw your dose.
19. Unwrap the second syringe provided. You will use it to give yourself the injection.
    - Carefully remove the protective cap from the needle. Fill the syringe with air by pulling the plunger to the number on the side of the syringe (mL) that matches your prescribed dose. (See Figure L)

Figure L

- Hold the SYLATRON vial upright. Do not touch the cleaned top of the vial with your hands. (See Figure M)

Figure M

- Insert the needle into the vial containing the SYLATRON solution. Inject the air into the center of the vial. (See Figure N)
  [See figure N at top of next column]
20. Turn the SYLATRON vial upside down. Be sure the tip of the needle is in the SYLATRON solution.
    - Hold the vial and syringe with one hand. Be sure the tip of the needle is in the SYLATRON solution. With the other hand, slowly pull the plunger back to fill the syringe with the exact amount of SYLATRON into the syringe your healthcare provider told you to use. (See Figure O)

Figure N

Figure O

21. Check for air bubbles in the syringe. If you see any air bubbles, hold the syringe with the needle pointing up. Gently tap the syringe until the air bubbles rise. Then, slowly push the plunger up to remove any air bubbles. If you push solution into the vial, slowly pull back on the plunger again to draw the correct amount of SYLATRON back into the syringe. When you are ready to inject the medicine, remove the needle from the vial. (See Figure P)

Figure P

How should I choose a site for injection?
The best sites for giving yourself an injection are those areas with a layer of fat between the skin and muscle, like your thigh, the outer surface of your upper arm, and abdomen (See Figure Q). Do not inject yourself in the area near your navel or waistline. If you are very thin, you should only use the thigh or outer surface of the arm for injection.

Figure Q

You should use a different site each time you inject SYLATRON to help avoid soreness at any one site. Do not inject SYLATRON solution into an area where the skin is irritated, red, bruised, infected or has scars, stretch marks, or lumps.
How should I inject a dose of SYLATRON?
22. Clean the skin where the injection is to be given with an alcohol swab. Wait for the area to dry.
    - Make sure the safety sleeve of the syringe is pushed firmly against the syringe flange so that the needle is fully exposed. (See Figure B)
23. With one hand, pinch a fold of skin. With your other hand, pick up the syringe and hold it like a pencil.
    - Insert the needle into the pinched skin at a 45- to 90-degree angle with a quick dart-like motion. (See Figure R)
      [See figure R at top of next column]
    - After the needle is inserted, remove the hand that you used to pinch your skin. Use it to hold the syringe barrel.
    - Pull the plunger of the syringe back very slightly.

90° angle
45° angle

Figure R

- **If no blood is present in the syringe**, inject the medicine by gently pressing the plunger all the way down the syringe barrel, until the syringe is empty.
- **If blood comes into the syringe**, the needle has entered a blood vessel. Do not inject.
  - Withdraw the needle and dispose of the syringe and needle in the sharps disposal container. (See the section "How should I dispose of used syringes, needles, and vials?" at the end of this Instructions for Use.)
  - If there is bleeding, cover the injection site with a bandage.
  - Then, repeat steps 1 through 23 with a new vial of SYLATRON and diluent to prepare a new syringe, and inject the medicine at a new site.
24. When the syringe is empty, pull the needle out of the skin.
    - Place a cotton ball or gauze over the injection site and press for several seconds. Do not massage the injection site.
    - If there is bleeding, cover it with a bandage.
25. After injecting your dose:
    - Firmly grasp the safety sleeve and pull it over the exposed needle until you hear a click, and the green stripe on the safety sleeve covers the red stripe on the needle. (See Figure S)

Figure S

26. Dispose of the used syringes, needles, and vials in the sharps disposal container. (See "How should I dispose of used syringes, needles, and vials?" below.)
How should I dispose of used syringes, needles, and vials?
- Put your used syringes and needles in a FDA-cleared sharps disposal container right away after use. **Do not throw away (dispose of) loose syringes and needles in your household trash.**
- If you do not have a FDA-cleared sharps disposal container, you may use a household container that is:
  - made of a heavy-duty plastic,
  - can be closed with a tight-fitting, puncture-resistant lid, without sharps being able to come out,
  - upright and stable during use,
  - leak resistant, and
  - properly labeled to warn of hazardous waste inside the container.
- When your sharps disposal container is almost full, you will need to follow your community guidelines for the right way to dispose of your sharps disposal container. There may be state or local laws about how you should throw away used syringes and needles. For more information about safe sharps disposal, and for specific information about sharps disposal in the state that you live in, go to FDA's website at: http://www.fda.gov/safesharpsdisposal.
- Do not dispose of your used sharps disposal container in your household trash unless your community guidelines permit this. Do not recycle your used sharps disposal container.
Always keep the sharps disposal container out of the reach of children.
How should I store SYLATRON?
- Before mixing, store SYLATRON vials at 59°F to 86°F (15°C to 30°C).
- After mixing, use SYLATRON right away or store it in the refrigerator for up to 24 hours between 36°F to 46°F (2°C to 8°C). Throw away any mixed SYLATRON that is not used within 24 hours.
- Do not freeze SYLATRON.
- Keep SYLATRON away from heat.
Keep SYLATRON and all medicines out of the reach of children.

This Instructions for Use has been approved by the U.S. Food and Drug Administration.
Manufactured by: Schering Corporation, a subsidiary of **MERCK & CO., INC.**, Whitehouse Station, NJ 08889, USA
Revised: August 2014
For patent information:
www.merck.com/product/patent/home.html
Copyright © 2011 Merck Sharp & Dohme Corp., a subsidiary of **Merck & Co., Inc.**
All rights reserved.
usifu-mk4031-pwi-1408r009

MEDICATION GUIDE
SYLATRON™ (SY-LA-TRON)
(Peginterferon alfa-2b)
Read this Medication Guide before you start taking SYLATRON, and each time you get a refill. There may be new information. This Medication Guide does not take the place of talking with your healthcare provider about your medical condition or your treatment.

What is the most important information I should know about SYLATRON?
SYLATRON can cause serious mental health problems which can lead to suicide.
SYLATRON may cause you to develop mood or behavior problems that may get worse during treatment with SYLATRON or after your last dose. Call your healthcare provider right away if you, your family, or caregiver notice any of the following:
• irritability (getting upset easily)
• depression (feeling low, feeling bad about yourself, or feeling hopeless)
• aggressive behavior
• thoughts of hurting yourself or others, or thoughts of suicide
Former drug addicts may fall back into drug addiction or overdose.
If you have these symptoms, your healthcare provider should carefully monitor you during treatment with SYLATRON and for 6 months after your last dose.
If symptoms get worse or become severe and continue, your healthcare provider may tell you to stop taking SYLATRON permanently. These signs or symptoms may not go away after you stop taking SYLATRON.
See "**What are the possible side effects of SYLATRON?**" for more information about side effects.

What is SYLATRON?
SYLATRON is a prescription medicine that is used to prevent malignant melanoma (a kind of skin cancer) from coming back after it has been removed by surgery. SYLATRON should be started within 84 days of surgery to remove lymph nodes containing cancer.
It is not known if SYLATRON is safe and effective in children less than 18 years of age.

Who should not take SYLATRON?
Do not take SYLATRON:
• if you have had a serious allergic reaction to peginterferon alfa-2b or to interferon alfa-2b
• if you have certain types of hepatitis
• if you have severe liver damage

What should I tell my healthcare provider before taking SYLATRON?
Before you take SYLATRON, tell your healthcare provider about all of your health problems, including if you:
• are being treated for a mental illness or had treatment in the past for mental illness, including depression or thoughts of suicide or suicide attempts. See "**What is the most important information I should know about SYLATRON?**"
• have liver damage from drugs or disease
• have kidney problems or are receiving kidney dialysis treatment
• have ever been addicted to drugs or alcohol
• have or had an overactive or underactive thyroid gland
• have diabetes
• have any other medical problem(s)
• are pregnant or plan to become pregnant. It is not known if SYLATRON will harm your unborn baby.
• are breastfeeding or plan to breastfeed. You and your healthcare provider should decide if you should use SYLATRON or breastfeed. You should not do both.
Tell your healthcare provider about all the medicines you take, including prescription and non-prescription medicines, vitamins, and herbal supplements.
SYLATRON and certain other medicines may affect each other and cause side effects.
Know the medicines you take. Keep a list of them to show your healthcare providers and pharmacists each time you get a new medicine.

You should not start a new medicine before your talk with the healthcare provider who prescribes you SYLATRON.
How should I take SYLATRON?
• Take SYLATRON exactly as your healthcare provider tells you to. Your healthcare provider will tell you how much SYLATRON to take and when to take it.
• Do not take more than your prescribed dose. Call your healthcare provider right away if you take too much SYLATRON.
• Inject SYLATRON one time each week unless instructed differently by your healthcare provider. Call your healthcare provider for instructions if you miss a dose.
• SYLATRON is given as an injection under your skin (subcutaneous injection). Your healthcare provider should show you how to prepare and measure your dose of SYLATRON, and how to inject yourself before you use SYLATRON for the first time.
• Expect to get "flu-like" symptoms when taking SYLATRON. To help reduce flu-like symptoms:
  ○ You should take 500 mg to 1,000 mg of acetaminophen 30 minutes before your first dose of SYLATRON.
  ○ Follow your healthcare provider's instructions about taking acetaminophen before future doses of SYLATRON.
  ○ Inject SYLATRON at bedtime to help reduce flu-like symptoms.
  ○ Drink plenty of fluids.
Your healthcare provider should do blood tests before starting and during treatment with SYLATRON.
Your healthcare provider will monitor you while taking SYLATRON. Based on this monitoring, your healthcare provider may:
• Keep your prescribed dose the same;
• Reduce your prescribed dose;
• Tell you to skip a dose or doses; or
• Tell you to stop taking SYLATRON permanently.

What are the possible side effects of SYLATRON?
SYLATRON can cause serious side effects or worsen existing problems, including:
See "**What is the most important information I should know about SYLATRON?**".
• **Heart problems.** Signs and symptoms can include:
  ○ fast heart rate or abnormal heart beat
  ○ trouble breathing or chest pain
• **Serious eye problems.** Symptoms can include:
  ○ decrease in vision
  ○ blurred vision
• **Severe or worsening liver problems.** Symptoms can include:
  ○ yellowing of your skin or the white part of your eyes
  ○ swelling of your stomach area (abdomen)
• **Thyroid problems.** Signs and symptoms can include:
  ○ problems concentrating
  ○ feeling cold or hot all of the time
  ○ weight changes
• **High blood sugar (diabetes).** Signs and symptoms can include:
  ○ increased thirst
  ○ urinating more often than normal
  ○ weight loss
  ○ your breath smells like fruit
Call your healthcare provider right away if you have any of these serious side effects.
The most common side effects of SYLATRON include:
• flu-like symptoms, which may include fever, headache, tiredness, muscle or joint aches, chills, nausea, or loss of appetite
• feeling sad or depressed
• redness, swelling, or itching around the injection site
• changes in blood tests measuring how your liver works
These are not all of the possible side effects of SYLATRON. For more information, ask your healthcare provider.
Call your doctor for medical advice about side effects. You may report side effects to FDA at 1-800-FDA-1088.
You may also report side effects to Schering Corporation at 1-800-526-4099.
How should I store SYLATRON?
• Store SYLATRON vials in the carton at 59°F to 86°F (15°C to 30°C).
• After mixing, use SYLATRON right away or store it in the refrigerator for no longer than 24 hours at 36°F to 46°F (2°C to 8°C).
• Do not freeze SYLATRON.
Keep SYLATRON and all medicines out of the reach of children.
General information about the safe and effective use of SYLATRON
Medicines are sometimes prescribed for purposes other than those listed in a Medication Guide. Do not use SYLATRON for a condition for which it was not prescribed. Do not give SYLATRON to other people, even if they have the same symptoms that you have. It may harm them.

This Medication Guide summarizes the most important information about SYLATRON. If you would like more information, talk with your healthcare provider. You can ask your healthcare provider for information about SYLATRON that is written for healthcare professionals.
For more information, go to www.SYLATRON.com or call 1-800-526-4099.
What are the ingredients in SYLATRON?
Active ingredient: peginterferon alfa-2b
Inactive ingredients: dibasic sodium phosphate anhydrous, monobasic sodium phosphate dihydrate, polysorbate 80, sucrose, sterile water for injection is supplied as a diluent.
The Medication Guide has been approved by the U.S. Food and Drug Administration.
Manufactured by: Schering Corporation, a subsidiary of **MERCK & CO., INC.**, Whitehouse Station, NJ 08889, USA
Revised: August 2014
For patent information:
www.merck.com/product/patent/home.html
Copyright © 2011 Merck Sharp & Dohme Corp., a subsidiary of **Merck & Co., Inc.**
All rights reserved.
usmg-mk4031-pwi-1408r010

TEMODAR®   ℞
[těm-ō-dăr]
(temozolomide)
Capsules

TEMODAR®
(temozolomide)
for Injection administered via intravenous infusion

HIGHLIGHTS OF PRESCRIBING INFORMATION
These highlights do not include all the information needed to use TEMODAR safely and effectively. See full prescribing information for TEMODAR.
TEMODAR® (temozolomide) Capsules
TEMODAR® (temozolomide) for Injection administered via intravenous infusion
Initial U.S. Approval: 1999

————————**RECENT MAJOR CHANGES**————————
Warnings and Precautions, Hepatotoxicity (5.5)   05/2014

————————**INDICATIONS AND USAGE**————————
TEMODAR is an alkylating drug indicated for the treatment of adult patients with:
• Newly diagnosed glioblastoma multiforme (GBM) concomitantly with radiotherapy and then as maintenance treatment. (1.1)
• Refractory anaplastic astrocytoma patients who have experienced disease progression on a drug regimen containing nitrosourea and procarbazine. (1.2)

————————**DOSAGE AND ADMINISTRATION**————————
• Newly Diagnosed GBM: 75 mg/m^2 for 42 days concomitant with focal radiotherapy followed by initial maintenance dose of 150 mg/m^2 once daily for Days 1–5 of a 28-day cycle of TEMODAR for 6 cycles. (2.1)
• Refractory Anaplastic Astrocytoma: Initial dose 150 mg/m^2 once daily for 5 consecutive days per 28-day treatment cycle. (2.1)
• The recommended dose for TEMODAR as an intravenous infusion over 90 minutes is the same as the dose for the oral capsule formulation. Bioequivalence has been established only when TEMODAR for Injection was given over 90 minutes. (2.1, 12.3)

————————**DOSAGE FORMS AND STRENGTHS**————————
• 5-mg, 20-mg, 100-mg, 140-mg, 180-mg, and 250-mg capsules. (3)
• 100-mg powder for injection. (3)

————————**CONTRAINDICATIONS**————————
• Known hypersensitivity to any TEMODAR component or to dacarbazine (DTIC). (4.1)

————————**WARNINGS AND PRECAUTIONS**————————
• Myelosuppression — monitor Absolute Neutrophil Count (ANC) and platelet count prior to dosing and throughout treatment. Geriatric patients and women have a higher risk of developing myelosuppression. (5.1)
• Cases of myelodysplastic syndrome and secondary malignancies, including myeloid leukemia, have been observed. (5.2)
• *Pneumocystis* pneumonia (PCP) – PCP prophylaxis required for all patients receiving concomitant TEMODAR and radiotherapy for the 42-day regimen for the treatment of newly diagnosed glioblastoma multiforme. (5.3)

- All patients, particularly those receiving steroids, should be observed closely for the development of lymphopenia and PCP. (5.4)
- Complete blood counts should be obtained throughout the treatment course as specified. (5.4)
- Hepatotoxicity – fatal and severe hepatotoxicity have been reported. Perform liver function tests at baseline, midway through the first cycle, prior to each subsequent cycle, and approximately two to four weeks after the last dose of TEMODAR. (5.5)
- Fetal harm can occur when administered to a pregnant woman. Women should be advised to avoid becoming pregnant when receiving TEMODAR. (5.6)
- As bioequivalence has been established only when given over 90 minutes, infusion over a shorter or longer period of time may result in suboptimal dosing; the possibility of an increase in infusion-related adverse reactions cannot be ruled out. (5.7)

──────────ADVERSE REACTIONS──────────

- The most common adverse reactions (≥10% incidence) are: alopecia, fatigue, nausea, vomiting, headache, constipation, anorexia, convulsions, rash, hemiparesis, diarrhea, asthenia, fever, dizziness, coordination abnormal, viral infection, amnesia, and insomnia. (6.1)
- The most common Grade 3 to 4 hematologic laboratory abnormalities (≥10% incidence) that have developed during treatment with temozolomide are: lymphopenia, thrombocytopenia, neutropenia, and leukopenia. (6.1)
- Allergic reactions have also been reported. (6)

To report SUSPECTED ADVERSE REACTIONS, contact Merck Sharp & Dohme Corp., a subsidiary of Merck & Co., Inc., at 1-877-888-4231 or FDA at 1-800-FDA-1088 or www.fda.gov/medwatch.

──────────DRUG INTERACTIONS──────────

- Valproic acid: decreases oral clearance of temozolomide. (7.1)

──────USE IN SPECIFIC POPULATIONS──────

- Nursing mothers: Not recommended. (8.3)
- Pediatric use: No established use. (8.4)
- Hepatic/Renal Impairment: Caution should be exercised when TEMODAR is administered to patients with severe renal or hepatic impairment. (8.6, 8.7)

See 17 for PATIENT COUNSELING INFORMATION and FDA-approved patient labeling

Revised: 05/2014

FULL PRESCRIBING INFORMATION: CONTENTS*

* Sections or subsections omitted from the full prescribing information are not listed

FULL PRESCRIBING INFORMATION

1   INDICATIONS AND USAGE

1.1   Newly Diagnosed Glioblastoma Multiforme

TEMODAR® (temozolomide) is indicated for the treatment of adult patients with newly diagnosed glioblastoma multiforme concomitantly with radiotherapy and then as maintenance treatment.

1.2   Refractory Anaplastic Astrocytoma

TEMODAR is indicated for the treatment of adult patients with refractory anaplastic astrocytoma, i.e., patients who have experienced disease progression on a drug regimen containing nitrosourea and procarbazine.

2   DOSAGE AND ADMINISTRATION

2.1   Recommended Dosing and Dose Modification Guidelines

The recommended dose for TEMODAR as an intravenous infusion over 90 minutes is the same as the dose for the oral capsule formulation. Bioequivalence has been established only when TEMODAR for Injection was given over 90 minutes *[see Clinical Pharmacology (12.3)]*. Dosage of TEMODAR must be adjusted according to nadir neutrophil and platelet counts in the previous cycle and the neutrophil and platelet counts at the time of initiating the next cycle. For TEMODAR dosage calculations based on body surface area (BSA) see **Table 5**. For suggested capsule combinations on a daily dose see **Table 6**.

Patients with Newly Diagnosed High Grade Glioma:
Concomitant Phase:
TEMODAR is administered at 75 mg/m² daily for 42 days concomitant with focal radiotherapy (60 Gy administered in 30 fractions) followed by maintenance TEMODAR for 6 cycles. Focal RT includes the tumor bed or resection site with a 2- to 3-cm margin. No dose reductions are recommended during the concomitant phase; however, dose interruptions or discontinuation may occur based on toxicity. The TEMODAR dose should be continued throughout the 42-day concomitant period up to 49 days if all of the following conditions are met: absolute neutrophil count greater than or equal to 1.5 × 10⁹/L, platelet count greater than or equal to 100 × 10⁹/L, common toxicity criteria (CTC) nonhematological toxicity less than or equal to Grade 1 (except for alopecia, nausea, and vomiting). During treatment a complete blood count should be obtained weekly. Temozolomide dosing should be interrupted or discontinued during concomitant phase according to the hematological and non-hematological toxicity criteria as noted in **Table 1**. *Pneumocystis* pneumonia (PCP) prophylaxis is required during the concomitant administration of TEMODAR and radiotherapy, and should be continued in patients who develop lymphocytopenia until recovery from lymphocytopenia (CTC Grade less than or equal to 1).

TABLE 1: Temozolomide Dosing Interruption or Discontinuation During Concomitant Radiotherapy and Temozolomide

Toxicity	TMZ Interruption*	TMZ Discontinuation
Absolute Neutrophil Count	greater than or equal to 0.5 and less than 1.5 × 10⁹/L	less than 0.5 × 10⁹/L
Platelet Count	greater than or equal to 10 and less than 100 × 10⁹/L	less than 10 × 10⁹/L
CTC Nonhematological Toxicity (except for alopecia, nausea, vomiting)	CTC Grade 2	CTC Grade 3 or 4

TMZ=temozolomide; CTC=Common Toxicity Criteria.

* Treatment with concomitant TMZ could be continued when all of the following conditions were met: absolute neutrophil count greater than or equal to 1.5 × 10⁹/L; platelet count greater than or equal to 100 × 10⁹/L; CTC nonhematological toxicity less than or equal to Grade 1 (except for alopecia, nausea, vomiting).

Maintenance Phase:
Cycle 1:
Four weeks after completing the TEMODAR+RT phase, TEMODAR is administered for an additional 6 cycles of maintenance treatment. Dosage in Cycle 1 (maintenance) is 150 mg/m² once daily for 5 days followed by 23 days without treatment.
Cycles 2–6:
At the start of Cycle 2, the dose can be escalated to 200 mg/m², if the CTC nonhematologic toxicity for Cycle 1 is Grade less than or equal to 2 (except for alopecia, nausea, and vomiting), absolute neutrophil count (ANC) is greater than or equal to 1.5 × 10⁹/L, and the platelet count is greater than or equal to 100 × 10⁹/L. The dose remains at 200 mg/m² per day for the first 5 days of each subsequent cycle except if toxicity occurs. If the dose was not escalated at Cycle 2, escalation should not be done in subsequent cycles.
Dose Reduction or Discontinuation During Maintenance:
Dose reductions during the maintenance phase should be applied according to **Tables 2** and **3**.
During treatment, a complete blood count should be obtained on Day 22 (21 days after the first dose of TEMODAR) or within 48 hours of that day, and weekly until the ANC is above 1.5 × 10⁹/L and the platelet count exceeds 100 × 10⁹/L (100,000/µL). The next cycle of TEMODAR should not be started until the ANC and platelet count exceed these levels. Dose reductions during the next cycle should be based on the lowest blood counts and worst nonhematologic toxicity during the previous cycle. Dose reductions or discontinuations during the maintenance phase should be applied according to **Tables 2** and **3**.

TABLE 2: Temozolomide Dose Levels for Maintenance Treatment

Dose Level	Dose (mg/m²/day)	Remarks
−1	100	Reduction for prior toxicity
0	150	Dose during Cycle 1
1	200	Dose during Cycles 2–6 in absence of toxicity

TABLE 3: Temozolomide Dose Reduction or Discontinuation During Maintenance Treatment

Toxicity	Reduce TMZ by 1 Dose Level*	Discontinue TMZ
Absolute Neutrophil Count	less than 1.0 × 10⁹/L	See footnote†
Platelet Count	less than 50 × 10⁹/L	See footnote†
CTC Nonhematological Toxicity (except for alopecia, nausea, vomiting)	CTC Grade 3	CTC Grade 4†

TMZ=temozolomide; CTC=Common Toxicity Criteria.

* TMZ dose levels are listed in **Table 2**.

† TMZ is to be discontinued if dose reduction to less than 100 mg/m² is required or if the same Grade 3 nonhematological toxicity (except for alopecia, nausea, vomiting) recurs after dose reduction.

Patients with Refractory Anaplastic Astrocytoma:
For adults the initial dose is 150 mg/m² once daily for 5 consecutive days per 28-day treatment cycle. For adult patients, if both the nadir and day of dosing (Day 29, Day 1 of next cycle) ANC are greater than or equal to 1.5 × 10⁹/L (1500/µL) and both the nadir and Day 29, Day 1 of next cycle platelet counts are greater than or equal to 100 × 10⁹/L (100,000/µL), the TEMODAR dose may be increased to 200 mg/m²/day for 5 consecutive days per 28-day treatment cycle. During treatment, a complete blood count should be obtained on Day 22 (21 days after the first dose) or within 48 hours of that day, and weekly until the ANC is above 1.5 × 10⁹/L (1500/µL) and the platelet count exceeds 100 × 10⁹/L (100,000/µL). The next cycle of TEMODAR should not be started until the ANC and platelet count exceed these levels. If the ANC falls to less than 1.0 × 10⁹/L (1000/µL) or the platelet count is less than 50 × 10⁹/L (50,000/µL) during any cycle, the next cycle should be reduced by 50 mg/m², but not below 100 mg/m², the lowest recommended dose (see **Table 4**). TEMODAR therapy can be continued until disease progression. In the clinical trial, treatment could be continued for a maximum of 2 years, but the optimum duration of therapy is not known.

TABLE 4: Dosing Modification Table

TABLE 5: Daily Dose Calculations by Body Surface Area (BSA)

Total BSA (m²)	75 mg/m² (mg daily)	150 mg/m² (mg daily)	200 mg/m² (mg daily)
1.0	75	150	200
1.1	82.5	165	220
1.2	90	180	240
1.3	97.5	195	260
1.4	105	210	280
1.5	112.5	225	300
1.6	120	240	320
1.7	127.5	255	340
1.8	135	270	360
1.9	142.5	285	380
2.0	150	300	400
2.1	157.5	315	420
2.2	165	330	440
2.3	172.5	345	460
2.4	180	360	480
2.5	187.5	375	500

[See table 6 above]

2.2 Preparation and Administration

TEMODAR Capsules:

In clinical trials, TEMODAR was administered under both fasting and nonfasting conditions; however, absorption is affected by food *[see Clinical Pharmacology (12.3)]*, and consistency of administration with respect to food is recommended. There are no dietary restrictions with TEMODAR. To reduce nausea and vomiting, TEMODAR should be taken on an empty stomach. Bedtime administration may be advised. Antiemetic therapy may be administered prior to and/or following administration of TEMODAR.

TEMODAR (temozolomide) Capsules should not be opened or chewed. They should be swallowed whole with a glass of water.

If capsules are accidentally opened or damaged, precautions should be taken to avoid inhalation or contact with the skin or mucous membranes *[see How Supplied/Storage and Handling (16.1)]*.

TEMODAR for Injection:

Each vial of TEMODAR for Injection contains sterile and pyrogen-free temozolomide lyophilized powder. When reconstituted with 41 mL Sterile Water for Injection, the resulting solution will contain 2.5 mg/mL temozolomide. Bring the vial to room temperature prior to reconstitution with

TABLE 6: Suggested Capsule Combinations Based on Daily Dose in Adults

Total Daily Dose (mg)	Number of Daily Capsules by Strength (mg)					
	250 mg	180 mg	140 mg	100 mg	20 mg	5 mg
75	0	0	0	0	3	3
82.5	0	0	0	0	4	0
90	0	0	0	0	4	2
97.5	0	0	0	1	0	2
105	0	0	0	1	0	1
112.5	0	0	0	1	0	2
120	0	0	0	1	1	0
127.5	0	0	0	1	1	1
135	0	0	0	1	1	3
142.5	0	0	1	0	0	0
150	0	0	1	0	0	2
157.5	0	0	1	0	0	0
165	0	0	1	0	1	1
172.5	0	0	1	0	1	2
180	0	1	0	0	0	0
187.5	0	1	0	0	0	1
195	0	1	0	0	0	3
200	0	1	0	0	0	0
210	0	0	0	2	0	2
220	0	0	0	2	1	0
225	0	0	0	2	1	1
240	0	0	1	1	0	0
255	1	0	0	0	0	1
260	1	0	0	0	0	2
270	1	0	0	0	1	0
280	0	0	2	0	0	0
285	0	0	2	0	0	1
300	0	0	0	3	0	0
315	0	0	0	3	0	3
320	0	1	1	0	0	0
330	0	1	1	0	0	2
340	0	1	1	0	1	0
345	0	1	1	0	1	1
360	0	2	0	0	0	0
375	0	2	0	0	0	3
380	0	1	0	2	0	0
400	0	0	0	4	0	0
420	0	0	3	0	0	0
440	0	0	3	0	1	0
460	0	2	0	1	0	0
480	0	1	0	3	0	0
500	2	0	0	0	0	0

Sterile Water for Injection. The vials should be gently swirled and not shaken. Vials should be inspected, and any vial containing visible particulate matter should not be used. Do not further dilute the reconstituted solution. After reconstitution, store at room temperature (25°C [77°F]). Reconstituted product must be used within 14 hours, including infusion time.

Using aseptic technique, withdraw up to 40 mL from each vial to make up the total dose based on **Table 5** above and transfer into an empty 250 mL infusion bag [2]. TEMODAR for Injection should be infused intravenously using a pump over a period of 90 minutes. TEMODAR for Injection should be administered only by intravenous infusion. Flush the lines before and after each TEMODAR infusion.

TEMODAR for Injection may be administered in the same intravenous line with 0.9% Sodium Chloride injection only. Because no data are available on the compatibility of TEMODAR for Injection with other intravenous substances or additives, other medications should not be infused simultaneously through the same intravenous line.

3   DOSAGE FORMS AND STRENGTHS

- TEMODAR (temozolomide) Capsules for oral administration
  - 5-mg capsules have opaque white bodies with green caps. The capsule body is imprinted with two stripes, the dosage strength, and the Schering-Plough logo. The cap is imprinted with "TEMODAR."
  - 20-mg capsules have opaque white bodies with yellow caps. The capsule body is imprinted with two stripes, the dosage strength, and the Schering-Plough logo. The cap is imprinted with "TEMODAR."
  - 100-mg capsules have opaque white bodies with pink caps. The capsule body is imprinted with two stripes, the dosage strength, and the Schering-Plough logo. The cap is imprinted with "TEMODAR."
  - 140-mg capsules have opaque white bodies with blue caps. The capsule body is imprinted with two stripes, the dosage strength, and the Schering-Plough logo. The cap is imprinted with "TEMODAR."
  - 180-mg capsules have opaque white bodies with orange caps. The capsule body is imprinted with two stripes, the dosage strength, and the Schering-Plough logo. The cap is imprinted with "TEMODAR."
  - 250-mg capsules have opaque white bodies with white caps. The capsule body is imprinted with two stripes, the dosage strength, and the Schering-Plough logo. The cap is imprinted with "TEMODAR."
- TEMODAR (temozolomide) is available as 100-mg/vial powder for injection. The lyophilized powder is white to light tan/light pink.

4   CONTRAINDICATIONS

4.1   Hypersensitivity

TEMODAR (temozolomide) is contraindicated in patients who have a history of hypersensitivity reaction (such as urticaria, allergic reaction including anaphylaxis, toxic epidermal necrolysis, and Stevens-Johnson syndrome) to any of its components. TEMODAR is also contraindicated in patients who have a history of hypersensitivity to dacarbazine (DTIC), since both drugs are metabolized to 5-(3-methyltriazen-1-yl)-imidazole-4-carboxamide (MTIC).

5   WARNINGS AND PRECAUTIONS

5.1   Myelosuppression

Patients treated with TEMODAR may experience myelosuppression, including prolonged pancytopenia, which may result in aplastic anemia, which in some cases has resulted in a fatal outcome. In some cases, exposure to concomitant medications associated with aplastic anemia, including carbamazepine, phenytoin, and sulfamethoxazole/trimethoprim, complicates assessment. Prior to dosing, patients must have an absolute neutrophil count (ANC) greater than or equal to 1.5×10^9/L and a platelet count greater than or equal to 100×10^9/L. A complete blood count should be obtained on Day 22 (21 days after the first dose) or within 48 hours of that day, and weekly until the ANC is above 1.5×10^9/L and platelet count exceeds 100×10^9/L. Geriatric patients and women have been shown in clinical trials to have a higher risk of developing myelosuppression.

5.2   Myelodysplastic Syndrome

Cases of myelodysplastic syndrome and secondary malignancies, including myeloid leukemia, have been observed.

5.3   *Pneumocystis* Pneumonia

For treatment of newly diagnosed glioblastoma multiforme: Prophylaxis against *Pneumocystis* pneumonia (PCP) is required for all patients receiving concomitant TEMODAR and radiotherapy for the 42-day regimen. There may be a higher occurrence of PCP when temozolomide is administered during a longer dosing regi-

TABLE 7: Number (%) of Patients with Adverse Reactions: All and Severe/Life Threatening (Incidence of 5% or Greater)

	Concomitant Phase RT Alone (n=285)				Concomitant Phase RT+TMZ (n=288)*				Maintenance Phase TMZ (n=224)			
	All		Grade ≥3		All		Grade ≥3		All		Grade ≥3	
Subjects Reporting any Adverse Reaction	258	(91)	74	(26)	266	(92)	80	(28)	206	(92)	82	(37)
Body as a Whole — General Disorders												
Anorexia	25	(9)	1	(<1)	56	(19)	2	(1)	61	(27)	3	(1)
Dizziness	10	(4)	0		12	(4)	2	(1)	12	(5)	0	
Fatigue	139	(49)	15	(5)	156	(54)	19	(7)	137	(61)	20	(9)
Headache	49	(17)	11	(4)	56	(19)	5	(2)	51	(23)	9	(4)
Weakness	9	(3)	3	(1)	10	(3)	5	(2)	16	(7)	4	(2)
Central and Peripheral Nervous System Disorders												
Confusion	12	(4)	6	(2)	11	(4)	4	(1)	12	(5)	4	(2)
Convulsions	20	(7)	9	(3)	17	(6)	10	(3)	25	(11)	7	(3)
Memory Impairment	12	(4)	1	(<1)	8	(3)	1	(<1)	16	(7)	2	(1)
Disorders of the Eye												
Vision Blurred	25	(9)	4	(1)	26	(9)	2	(1)	17	(8)	0	
Disorders of the Immune System												
Allergic Reaction	7	(2)	1	(<1)	13	(5)	0		6	(3)	0	
Gastrointestinal System Disorders												
Abdominal Pain	2	(1)	0		7	(2)	1	(<1)	11	(5)	1	(<1)
Constipation	18	(6)	0		53	(18)	3	(1)	49	(22)	0	
Diarrhea	9	(3)	0		18	(6)	0		23	(10)	2	(1)
Nausea	45	(16)	1	(<1)	105	(36)	2	(1)	110	(49)	3	(1)
Stomatitis	14	(5)	1	(<1)	19	(7)	0		20	(9)	3	(1)
Vomiting	16	(6)	1	(<1)	57	(20)	1	(<1)	66	(29)	4	(2)
Injury and Poisoning												
Radiation Injury NOS	11	(4)	1	(<1)	20	(7)	0		5	(2)	0	
Musculoskeletal System Disorders												
Arthralgia	2	(1)	0		7	(2)	1	(<1)	14	(6)	0	
Platelet, Bleeding and Clotting Disorders												
Thrombocytopenia	3	(1)	0		11	(4)	8	(3)	19	(8)	8	(4)
Psychiatric Disorders												
Insomnia	9	(3)	1	(<1)	14	(5)	0		9	(4)	0	
Respiratory System Disorders												
Coughing	3	(1)	0		15	(5)	2	(1)	19	(8)	1	(<1)
Dyspnea	9	(3)	4	(1)	11	(4)	5	(2)	12	(5)	1	(<1)
Skin and Subcutaneous Tissue Disorders												
Alopecia	179	(63)	0		199	(69)	0		124	(55)	0	
Dry Skin	6	(2)	0		7	(2)	0		11	(5)	1	(<1)
Erythema	15	(5)	0		14	(5)	0		2	(1)	0	
Pruritus	4	(1)	0		11	(4)	0		11	(5)	0	
Rash	42	(15)	0		56	(19)	3	(1)	29	(13)	3	(1)
Special Senses Other, Disorders												
Taste Perversion	6	(2)	0		18	(6)	0		11	(5)	0	

RT+TMZ=radiotherapy plus temozolomide; NOS=not otherwise specified.
Note: Grade 5 (fatal) adverse reactions are included in the Grade ≥3 column.
* One patient who was randomized to RT only arm received RT+temozolomide.

men. However, all patients receiving temozolomide, particularly patients receiving steroids, should be observed closely for the development of PCP regardless of the regimen.

5.4   Laboratory Tests
For the concomitant treatment phase with RT, a complete blood count should be obtained prior to initiation of treatment and weekly during treatment.
For the 28-day treatment cycles, a complete blood count should be obtained prior to treatment on Day 1 and on Day 22 (21 days after the first dose) of each cycle. Blood counts should be performed weekly until recovery if the ANC falls below 1.5×10^9/L and the platelet count falls below 100×10^9/L [see Recommended Dosing and Dose Modification Guidelines (2.1)].

5.5   Hepatotoxicity
Fatal and severe hepatotoxicity have been reported in patients receiving TEMODAR. Perform liver function tests at baseline, midway through the first cycle, prior to each subsequent cycle, and approximately two to four weeks after the last dose of TEMODAR.

5.6   Use in Pregnancy
TEMODAR can cause fetal harm when administered to a pregnant woman. Administration of TEMODAR to rats and rabbits during organogenesis at 0.38 and 0.75 times the maximum recommended human dose (75 and 150 mg/m^2, respectively, caused numerous fetal malformations of the external organs, soft tissues, and skeleton in both species [see Use in Specific Populations (8.1)].

5.7   Infusion Time
As bioequivalence has been established only when TEMODAR for Injection was given over 90 minutes, infusion over a shorter or longer period of time may result in suboptimal dosing. Additionally, the possibility of an increase in infusion-related adverse reactions cannot be ruled out.

6   ADVERSE REACTIONS
6.1   Clinical Trials Experience
Because clinical trials are conducted under widely varying conditions, adverse reaction rates observed in the clinical trials of a drug cannot be directly compared to rates in the clinical trials of another drug and may not reflect the rates observed in practice.
Newly Diagnosed Glioblastoma Multiforme:
During the concomitant phase (TEMODAR+radiotherapy), adverse reactions including thrombocytopenia, nausea, vomiting, anorexia, and constipation were more frequent in the TEMODAR+RT arm. The incidence of other adverse reactions was comparable in the two arms. The most common adverse reactions across the cumulative TEMODAR experience were alopecia, nausea, vomiting, anorexia, headache, and constipation (see **Table 7**). Forty-nine percent (49%) of patients treated with TEMODAR reported one or more severe or life-threatening reactions, most commonly fatigue (13%), convulsions (6%), headache (5%), and thrombocytopenia (5%). Overall, the pattern of reactions during the maintenance phase was consistent with the known safety profile of TEMODAR.

[See table 7 above]
Myelosuppression (neutropenia and thrombocytopenia), which is a known dose-limiting toxicity for most cytotoxic agents, including TEMODAR, was observed. When laboratory abnormalities and adverse reactions were combined, Grade 3 or Grade 4 neutrophil abnormalities including neutropenic reactions were observed in 8% of the patients, and Grade 3 or Grade 4 platelet abnormalities, including thrombocytopenic reactions, were observed in 14% of the patients treated with TEMODAR.

Refractory Anaplastic Astrocytoma:
Tables 8 and 9 show the incidence of adverse reactions in the 158 patients in the anaplastic astrocytoma study for whom data are available. In the absence of a control group, it is not clear in many cases whether these reactions should be attributed to temozolomide or the patients' underlying conditions, but nausea, vomiting, fatigue, and hematologic effects appear to be clearly drug-related. The most frequently occurring adverse reactions were nausea, vomiting, headache, and fatigue. The adverse reactions were usually NCI Common Toxicity Criteria (CTC) Grade 1 or 2 (mild to moderate in severity) and were self-limiting, with nausea and vomiting readily controlled with antiemetics. The incidence of severe nausea and vomiting (CTC Grade 3 or 4) was 10% and 6%, respectively. Myelosuppression (thrombocytopenia and neutropenia) was the dose-limiting adverse reaction. It usually occurred within the first few cycles of therapy and was not cumulative.
Myelosuppression occurred late in the treatment cycle and returned to normal, on average, within 14 days of nadir counts. The median nadirs occurred at 26 days for platelets (range: 21–40 days) and 28 days for neutrophils (range: 1–44 days). Only 14% (22/158) of patients had a neutrophil nadir and 20% (32/158) of patients had a platelet nadir, which may have delayed the start of the next cycle. Less than 10% of patients required hospitalization, blood transfusion, or discontinuation of therapy due to myelosuppression.
In clinical trial experience with 110 to 111 women and 169 to 174 men (depending on measurements), there were higher rates of Grade 4 neutropenia (ANC less than 500 cells/µL) and thrombocytopenia (less than 20,000 cells/µL) in women than men in the first cycle of therapy (12% vs. 5% and 9% vs. 3%, respectively).
In the entire safety database for which hematologic data exist (N=932), 7% (4/61) and 9.5% (6/63) of patients over age 70 experienced Grade 4 neutropenia or thrombocytopenia in the first cycle, respectively. For patients less than or equal to age 70, 7% (62/871) and 5.5% (48/879) experienced Grade 4 neutropenia or thrombocytopenia in the first cycle, respectively. Pancytopenia, leukopenia, and anemia have also been reported.

TABLE 8: Adverse Reactions in the Anaplastic Astrocytoma Trial in Adults (≥5%)

	No. (%) of TEMODAR Patients (N=158)	
	All Reactions	**Grade 3/4**
Any Adverse Reaction	153 (97)	79 (50)
Body as a Whole		
Headache	65 (41)	10 (6)
Fatigue	54 (34)	7 (4)
Asthenia	20 (13)	9 (6)
Fever	21 (13)	3 (2)
Back pain	12 (8)	4 (3)
Cardiovascular		
Edema peripheral	17 (11)	1 (1)
Central and Peripheral Nervous System		
Convulsions	36 (23)	8 (5)
Hemiparesis	29 (18)	10 (6)
Dizziness	19 (12)	1 (1)
Coordination abnormal	17 (11)	2 (1)
Amnesia	16 (10)	6 (4)
Insomnia	16 (10)	0
Paresthesia	15 (9)	1 (1)
Somnolence	15 (9)	5 (3)
Paresis	13 (8)	4 (3)
Urinary incontinence	13 (8)	3 (2)
Ataxia	12 (8)	3 (2)
Dysphasia	11 (7)	1 (1)
Convulsions local	9 (6)	0
Gait abnormal	9 (6)	1 (1)
Confusion	8 (5)	0

Neutropenia	62 (51)	24 (20)

Endocrine		
Adrenal hypercorticism	13 (8)	0
Gastrointestinal System		
Nausea	84 (53)	16 (10)
Vomiting	66 (42)	10 (6)
Constipation	52 (33)	1 (1)
Diarrhea	25 (16)	3 (2)
Abdominal pain	14 (9)	2 (1)
Anorexia	14 (9)	1 (1)
Metabolic		
Weight increase	8 (5)	0
Musculoskeletal System		
Myalgia	8 (5)	0
Psychiatric Disorders		
Anxiety	11 (7)	1 (1)
Depression	10 (6)	0
Reproductive Disorders		
Breast pain, female	4 (6)	
Resistance Mechanism Disorders		
Infection viral	17 (11)	0
Respiratory System		
Upper respiratory tract infection	13 (8)	0
Pharyngitis	12 (8)	0
Sinusitis	10 (6)	0
Coughing	8 (5)	0
Skin and Appendages		
Rash	13 (8)	0
Pruritus	12 (8)	2 (1)
Urinary System		
Urinary tract infection	12 (8)	0
Micturition increased frequency	9 (6)	0
Vision		
Diplopia	8 (5)	0
Vision abnormal*	8 (5)	

* Blurred vision; visual deficit; vision changes; vision troubles

TABLE 9: Adverse Hematologic Effects (Grade 3 to 4) in the Anaplastic Astrocytoma Trial in Adults

	TEMODAR*
Hemoglobin	7/158 (4%)
Lymphopenia	83/152 (55%)
Neutrophils	20/142 (14%)
Platelets	29/156 (19%)
WBC	18/158 (11%)

* Change from Grade 0 to 2 at baseline to Grade 3 or 4 during treatment.

TEMODAR for injection delivers equivalent temozolomide dose and exposure to both temozolomide and 5-(3-methyltriazen-1-yl)-imidazole-4-carboxamide (MTIC) as the corresponding TEMODAR capsules. Adverse reactions probably related to treatment that were reported from the 2 studies with the intravenous formulation (n=35) that were not reported in studies using the TEMODAR capsules were: pain, irritation, pruritus, warmth, swelling, and erythema at infusion site as well as the following adverse reactions: petechiae and hematoma.

6.2 Postmarketing Experience

The following adverse reactions have been identified during postapproval use of TEMODAR. Because these reactions are reported voluntarily from a population of uncertain size, it is not always possible to reliably estimate their frequency or establish a causal relationship to the drug exposure.

Dermatologic disorders: Toxic epidermal necrolysis and Stevens-Johnson syndrome

Immune system disorders: Allergic reactions, including anaphylaxis. Erythema multiforme, which resolved after discontinuation of TEMODAR and, in some cases, recurred upon rechallenge.

Hematopoietic disorders: Prolonged pancytopenia, which may result in aplastic anemia and fatal outcomes *[see Warnings and Precautions (5.2)]*.

Hepatobiliary disorders: Fatal and severe hepatotoxicity, elevation of liver enzymes, hyperbilirubinemia, cholestasis, and hepatitis *[see Warnings and Precautions (5.5)]*.

Infections and infestations: Opportunistic infections including *Pneumocystis* pneumonia (PCP) *[see Warnings and Precautions (5.3)]*.

Pulmonary disorders: Interstitial pneumonitis, pneumonitis, alveolitis, and pulmonary fibrosis.

7 DRUG INTERACTIONS

7.1 Valproic Acid

Administration of valproic acid decreases oral clearance of temozolomide by about 5%. The clinical implication of this effect is not known *[see Clinical Pharmacology (12.3)]*.

8 USE IN SPECIFIC POPULATIONS

8.1 Pregnancy

Pregnancy Category D. See Warnings and Precautions section.

TEMODAR can cause fetal harm when administered to a pregnant woman. Five consecutive days of oral temozolomide administration of 0.38 and 0.75 times the highest recommended human dose (75 and 150 mg/m² in rats and rabbits, respectively, during the period of organogenesis caused numerous malformations of the external and internal soft tissues and skeleton in both species. Doses equivalent to 0.75 times the highest recommended human dose (150 mg/m²) caused embryolethality in rats and rabbits as indicated by increased resorptions. There are no adequate and well-controlled studies in pregnant women. If this drug is used during pregnancy, or if the patient becomes pregnant while taking this drug, the patient should be apprised of the potential hazard to a fetus. Women of childbearing potential should be advised to avoid becoming pregnant during therapy with TEMODAR.

8.3 Nursing Mothers

It is not known whether this drug is excreted in human milk. Because many drugs are excreted in human milk and because of the potential for serious adverse reactions in nursing infants and tumorigenicity shown for temozolomide in animal studies, a decision should be made whether to discontinue nursing or to discontinue the drug, taking into account the importance of TEMODAR to the mother.

8.4 Pediatric Use

Safety and effectiveness in pediatric patients have not been established. TEMODAR Capsules have been studied in 2 open-label studies in pediatric patients (aged 3–18 years) at a dose of 160 to 200 mg/m² daily for 5 days every 28 days. In one trial, 29 patients with recurrent brain stem glioma and 34 patients with recurrent high grade astrocytoma were enrolled. All patients had recurrence following surgery and radiation therapy, while 31% also had disease progression following chemotherapy. In a second study conducted by the Children's Oncology Group (COG), 122 patients were enrolled, including patients with medulloblastoma/PNET (29), high grade astrocytoma (23), low grade astrocytoma (22), brain stem glioma (16), ependymoma (14), other CNS tumors (9), and non-CNS tumors (9). The TEMODAR toxicity profile in pediatric patients is similar to adults. **Table 10** shows the adverse reactions in 122 children in the COG study.

TABLE 10: Adverse Reactions Reported in the Pediatric Cooperative Group Trial (≥10%)

Body System/Organ Class Adverse Reaction	No. (%) of TEMODAR Patients (N=122)*	
	All Reactions	Grade 3/4
Subjects Reporting an AE Body as a Whole	107 (88)	69 (57)
Central and Peripheral Nervous System		
Central cerebral CNS cortex	22 (18)	13 (11)
Gastrointestinal System		
Nausea	56 (46)	5 (4)
Vomiting	62 (51)	4 (3)
Platelet, Bleeding and Clotting		
Thrombocytopenia	71 (58)	31 (25)
Red Blood Cell Disorders		
Decreased Hemoglobin	62 (51)	7 (6)
White Cell and RES Disorders		
Decreased WBC	71 (58)	21 (17)
Lymphopenia	73 (60)	48 (39)

* These various tumors included the following: PNET-medulloblastoma, glioblastoma, low grade astrocytoma, brain stem tumor, ependymoma, mixed glioma, oligodendroglioma, neuroblastoma, Ewing's sarcoma, pineoblastoma, alveolar soft part sarcoma, neurofibrosarcoma, optic glioma, and osteosarcoma.

8.5 Geriatric Use

Clinical studies of temozolomide did not include sufficient numbers of subjects aged 65 and over to determine whether they responded differently from younger subjects. Other reported clinical experience has not identified differences in responses between the elderly and younger patients. In general, dose selection for an elderly patient should be cautious, reflecting the greater frequency of decreased hepatic, renal, or cardiac function, and of concomitant disease or other drug therapy.

In the anaplastic astrocytoma study population, patients 70 years of age or older had a higher incidence of Grade 4 neutropenia and Grade 4 thrombocytopenia (2/8; 25%, P=0.31 and 2/10; 20%, P=0.09, respectively) in the first cycle of therapy than patients under 70 years of age *[see Warnings and Precautions (5.1) and Adverse Reactions (6.1)]*.

In newly diagnosed patients with glioblastoma multiforme, the adverse reaction profile was similar in younger patients (<65 years) vs. older (≥65 years).

8.6 Renal Impairment

Caution should be exercised when TEMODAR is administered to patients with severe renal impairment *[see Clinical Pharmacology (12.3)]*.

8.7 Hepatic Impairment

Caution should be exercised when TEMODAR is administered to patients with severe hepatic impairment *[see Clinical Pharmacology (12.3)]*.

10 OVERDOSAGE

Doses of 500, 750, 1000, and 1250 mg/m² (total dose per cycle over 5 days) have been evaluated clinically in patients. Dose-limiting toxicity was hematologic and was reported with any dose but is expected to be more severe at higher doses. An overdose of 2000 mg per day for 5 days was taken by one patient and the adverse reactions reported were pancytopenia, pyrexia, multi-organ failure, and death. There are reports of patients who have taken more than 5 days of treatment (up to 64 days), with adverse reactions reported including bone marrow suppression, which in some cases was severe and prolonged, and infections and resulted in death. In the event of an overdose, hematologic evaluation is needed. Supportive measures should be provided as necessary.

11 DESCRIPTION

TEMODAR contains temozolomide, an imidazotetrazine derivative. The chemical name of temozolomide is 3,4-dihydro-3-methyl-4-oxoimidazo[5,1-d]-*as*-tetrazine-8-carboxamide. The structural formula is:

The material is a white to light tan/light pink powder with a molecular formula of $C_6H_6N_6O_2$ and a molecular weight of 194.15. The molecule is stable at acidic pH (<5) and labile at pH >7; hence TEMODAR can be administered orally and intravenously. The prodrug, temozolomide, is rapidly hydrolyzed to the active 5-(3-methyltriazen-1-yl) imidazole-4-carboxamide (MTIC) at neutral and alkaline pH values, with hydrolysis taking place even faster at alkaline pH.

TEMODAR Capsules:
Each capsule for oral use contains either 5 mg, 20 mg, 100 mg, 140 mg, 180 mg, or 250 mg of temozolomide.
The inactive ingredients for TEMODAR Capsules are as follows:

TEMODAR 5 mg: lactose anhydrous (132.8 mg), colloidal silicon dioxide (0.2 mg), sodium starch glycolate (7.5 mg), tartaric acid (1.5 mg), and stearic acid (3 mg).
TEMODAR 20 mg: lactose anhydrous (182.2 mg), colloidal silicon dioxide (0.2 mg), sodium starch glycolate (11 mg), tartaric acid (2.2 mg), and stearic acid (4.4 mg).
TEMODAR 100 mg: lactose anhydrous (175.7 mg), colloidal silicon dioxide (0.3 mg), sodium starch glycolate (15 mg), tartaric acid (3 mg), and stearic acid (6 mg).
TEMODAR 140 mg: lactose anhydrous (246 mg), colloidal silicon dioxide (0.4 mg), sodium starch glycolate (21 mg), tartaric acid (4.2 mg), and stearic acid (8.4 mg).
TEMODAR 180 mg: lactose anhydrous (316.3 mg), colloidal silicon dioxide (0.5 mg), sodium starch glycolate (27 mg), tartaric acid (5.4 mg), and stearic acid (10.8 mg).

TEMODAR 250 mg: lactose anhydrous (154.3 mg), colloidal silicon dioxide (0.7 mg), sodium starch glycolate (22.5 mg), tartaric acid (9 mg), and stearic acid (13.5 mg). The body of the capsules is made of gelatin, and is opaque white. The cap is also made of gelatin, and the colors vary based on the dosage strength. The capsule body and cap are imprinted with pharmaceutical branding ink, which contains shellac, dehydrated alcohol, isopropyl alcohol, butyl alcohol, propylene glycol, purified water, strong ammonia solution, potassium hydroxide, and ferric oxide.

TEMODAR 5 mg: The green cap contains gelatin, titanium dioxide, iron oxide yellow, sodium lauryl sulfate, and FD&C Blue #2.

TEMODAR 20 mg: The yellow cap contains gelatin, sodium lauryl sulfate, and iron oxide yellow.

TEMODAR 100 mg: The pink cap contains gelatin, titanium dioxide, sodium lauryl sulfate, and iron oxide red.

TEMODAR 140 mg: The blue cap contains gelatin, sodium lauryl sulfate, and FD&C Blue #2.

TEMODAR 180 mg: The orange cap contains gelatin, iron oxide red, iron oxide yellow, titanium dioxide, and sodium lauryl sulfate.

TEMODAR 250 mg: The white cap contains gelatin, titanium dioxide, and sodium lauryl sulfate.

TEMODAR for Injection:
Each vial contains 100 mg of sterile and pyrogen-free temozolomide lyophilized powder for intravenous injection. The inactive ingredients are: mannitol (600 mg), L-threonine (160 mg), polysorbate 80 (120 mg), sodium citrate dihydrate (235 mg), and hydrochloric acid (160 mg).

12 CLINICAL PHARMACOLOGY
12.1 Mechanism of Action
Temozolomide is not directly active but undergoes rapid nonenzymatic conversion at physiologic pH to the reactive compound 5-(3-methyltriazen-1-yl)-imidazole-4-carboxamide (MTIC). The cytotoxicity of MTIC is thought to be primarily due to alkylation of DNA. Alkylation (methylation) occurs mainly at the O^6 and N^7 positions of guanine.

12.3 Pharmacokinetics
Absorption:
Temozolomide is rapidly and completely absorbed after oral administration with a peak plasma concentration (C_{max}) achieved in a median T_{max} of 1 hour. Food reduces the rate and extent of temozolomide absorption. Mean peak plasma concentration and AUC decreased by 32% and 9%, respectively, and median T_{max} increased by 2-fold (from 1–2.25 hours) when temozolomide was administered after a modified high-fat breakfast.

A pharmacokinetic study comparing oral and intravenous temozolomide in 19 patients with primary CNS malignancies showed that 150 mg/m² TEMODAR for injection administered over 90 minutes is bioequivalent to 150 mg/m² TEMODAR oral capsules with respect to both C_{max} and AUC of temozolomide and MTIC. Following a single 90-minute intravenous infusion of 150 mg/m², the geometric mean C_{max} values for temozolomide and MTIC were 7.3 mcg/mL and 276 ng/mL, respectively. Following a single oral dose of 150 mg/m², the geometric mean C_{max} values for temozolomide and MTIC were 7.5 mcg/mL and 282 ng/mL, respectively. Following a single 90-minute intravenous infusion of 150 mg/m², the geometric mean AUC values for temozolomide and MTIC were 24.6 mcg•hr/mL and 891 ng•hr/mL, respectively. Following a single oral dose of 150 mg/m², the geometric mean AUC values for temozolomide and MTIC were 23.4 mcg•hr/mL and 864 ng•hr/mL, respectively.

Distribution:
Temozolomide has a mean apparent volume of distribution of 0.4 L/kg (%CV=13%). It is weakly bound to human plasma proteins; the mean percent bound of drug-related total radioactivity is 15%.

Metabolism and Elimination:
Temozolomide is spontaneously hydrolyzed at physiologic pH to the active species, MTIC and to temozolomide acid metabolite. MTIC is further hydrolyzed to 5-amino-imidazole-4-carboxamide (AIC), which is known to be an intermediate in purine and nucleic acid biosynthesis, and to methylhydrazine, which is believed to be the active alkylating species. Cytochrome P450 enzymes play only a minor role in the metabolism of temozolomide and MTIC. Relative to the AUC of temozolomide, the exposure to MTIC and AIC is 2.4% and 23%, respectively.

Excretion:
About 38% of the administered temozolomide total radioactive dose is recovered over 7 days: 37.7% in urine and 0.8% in feces. The majority of the recovery of radioactivity in urine is unchanged temozolomide (5.6%), AIC (12%), temozolomide acid metabolite (2.3%), and unidentified polar metabolite(s) (17%). Overall clearance of temozolomide is about 5.5 L/hr/m². Temozolomide is rapidly eliminated, with a mean elimination half-life of 1.8 hours, and exhibits linear kinetics over the therapeutic dosing range of 75 to 250 mg/m²/day.

Effect of Age:
A population pharmacokinetic analysis indicated that age (range: 19–78 years) has no influence on the pharmacokinetics of temozolomide.

Effect of Gender:
A population pharmacokinetic analysis indicated that women have an approximately 5% lower clearance (adjusted for body surface area) for temozolomide than men.

Effect of Race:
The effect of race on the pharmacokinetics of temozolomide has not been studied.

Tobacco Use:
A population pharmacokinetic analysis indicated that the oral clearance of temozolomide is similar in smokers and nonsmokers.

Effect of Renal Impairment:
A population pharmacokinetic analysis indicated that creatinine clearance over the range of 36 to 130 mL/min/m² has no effect on the clearance of temozolomide after oral administration. The pharmacokinetics of temozolomide have not been studied in patients with severely impaired renal function (CLcr <36 mL/min/m²). Caution should be exercised when TEMODAR is administered to patients with severe renal impairment *[see Use in Special Populations (8.6)]*. TEMODAR has not been studied in patients on dialysis.

Effect of Hepatic Impairment:
A study showed that the pharmacokinetics of temozolomide in patients with mild-to-moderate hepatic impairment (Child-Pugh Class I – II) were similar to those observed in patients with normal hepatic function. Caution should be exercised when temozolomide is administered to patients with severe hepatic impairment *[see Use in Specific Populations (8.7)]*.

Effect of Other Drugs on Temozolomide Pharmacokinetics:
In a multiple-dose study, administration of TEMODAR Capsules with ranitidine did not change the C_{max} or AUC values for temozolomide or MTIC.

A population analysis indicated that administration of valproic acid decreases the clearance of temozolomide by about 5% *[see Drug Interactions (7.1)]*.

A population analysis did not demonstrate any influence of coadministered dexamethasone, prochlorperazine, phenytoin, carbamazepine, ondansetron, H_2-receptor antagonists, or phenobarbital on the clearance of orally administered temozolomide.

13 NONCLINICAL TOXICOLOGY
13.1 Carcinogenesis, Mutagenesis, Impairment of Fertility
Temozolomide is carcinogenic in rats at doses less than the maximum recommended human dose. Temozolomide induced mammary carcinomas in both males and females at doses 0.13 to 0.63 times the maximum human dose (25–125 mg/m²) when administered orally on 5 consecutive days every 28 days for 6 cycles. Temozolomide also induced fibrosarcomas of the heart, eye, seminal vesicles, salivary glands, abdominal cavity, uterus, and prostate, carcinomas of the seminal vesicles, schwannomas of the heart, optic nerve, and harderian gland, and adenomas of the skin, lung, pituitary, and thyroid at doses 0.5 times the maximum daily dose. Mammary tumors were also induced following 3 cycles of temozolomide at the maximum recommended daily dose. Temozolomide is a mutagen and a clastogen. In a reverse bacterial mutagenesis assay (Ames assay), temozolomide increased revertant frequency in the absence and presence of metabolic activation. Temozolomide was clastogenic in human lymphocytes in the presence and absence of metabolic activation.

Temozolomide impairs male fertility. Temozolomide caused syncytial cells/immature sperm formation at 0.25 and 0.63 times the maximum recommended human dose (50 and 125 mg/m²) in rats and dogs, respectively, and testicular atrophy in dogs at 0.63 times the maximum recommended human dose (125 mg/m²).

13.2 Animal Toxicology and/or Pharmacology
Toxicology studies in rats and dogs identified a low incidence of hemorrhage, degeneration, and necrosis of the retina at temozolomide doses equal to or greater than 0.63 times the maximum recommended human dose (125 mg/m²). These changes were most commonly seen at doses where mortality was observed.

14 CLINICAL STUDIES
14.1 Newly Diagnosed Glioblastoma Multiforme
Five hundred and seventy-three patients were randomized to receive either TEMODAR (TMZ)+Radiotherapy (RT) (n=287) or RT alone (n=286). Patients in the TEMODAR+RT arm received concomitant TEMODAR (75 mg/m²) once daily, starting the first day of RT until the last day of RT, for 42 days (with a maximum of 49 days). This was followed by 6 cycles of TEMODAR alone (150 or 200 mg/m²) on Days 1 to 5 of every 28-day cycle, starting 4 weeks after the end of RT. Patients in the control arm received RT only. In both arms, focal radiation therapy was delivered as 60 Gy/30 fractions. Focal RT includes the tumor bed or resection site with a 2- to 3-cm margin. *Pneumocystis* pneumonia (PCP) prophylaxis was required during the TMZ+RT, regardless of lymphocyte count, and was to continue until recovery of lymphocyte count to less than or equal to Grade 1.

At the time of disease progression, TEMODAR was administered as salvage therapy in 161 patients of the 282 (57%) in the RT alone arm, and 62 patients of the 277 (22%) in the TEMODAR+RT arm.

The addition of concomitant and maintenance TEMODAR to radiotherapy in the treatment of patients with newly diagnosed GBM showed a statistically significant improvement in overall survival compared to radiotherapy alone (**Figure 1**). The hazard ratio (HR) for overall survival was 0.63 (95% CI for HR=0.52-0.75) with a log-rank *P*<0.0001 in favor of the TEMODAR arm. The median survival was increased by 2.5 months in the TEMODAR arm.

FIGURE 1: Kaplan-Meier Curves for Overall Survival (ITT Population)

14.2 Refractory Anaplastic Astrocytoma
A single-arm, multicenter study was conducted in 162 patients who had anaplastic astrocytoma at first relapse and who had a baseline Karnofsky performance status of 70 or greater. Patients had previously received radiation therapy and may also have previously received a nitrosourea with or without other chemotherapy. Fifty-four patients had disease progression on prior therapy with both a nitrosourea and procarbazine, and their malignancy was considered refractory to chemotherapy (refractory anaplastic astrocytoma population). Median age of this subgroup of 54 patients was 42 years (19–76). Sixty-five percent were male. Seventy-two percent of patients had a KPS of >80. Sixty-three percent of patients had surgery other than a biopsy at the time of initial diagnosis. Of those patients undergoing resection, 73% underwent a subtotal resection and 27% underwent a gross total resection. Eighteen percent of patients had surgery at the time of first relapse. The median time from initial diagnosis to first relapse was 13.8 months (4.2–75.4).

TEMODAR Capsules were given for the first 5 consecutive days of a 28-day cycle at a starting dose of 150 mg/m²/day. If the nadir and day of dosing (Day 29, Day 1 of next cycle) absolute neutrophil count was greater than or equal to 1.5×10^9/L (1500/µL) and the nadir and Day 29, Day 1 of next cycle platelet count was greater than or equal to 100×10^9/L (100,000/µL), the TEMODAR dose was increased to 200 mg/m²/day for the first 5 consecutive days of a 28-day cycle.

In the refractory anaplastic astrocytoma population, the overall tumor response rate (CR+PR) was 22% (12/54 patients) and the complete response rate was 9% (5/54 patients). The median duration of all responses was 50 weeks (range: 16–114 weeks) and the median duration of complete responses was 64 weeks (range: 52–114 weeks). In this population, progression-free survival at 6 months was 45% (95% CI: 31%–58%) and progression-free survival at 12 months was 29% (95% CI: 16%–42%). Median progression-free survival was 4.4 months. Overall survival at 6 months was 74% (95% CI: 62%–86%) and 12-month overall survival was 65% (95% CI: 52%–78%). Median overall survival was 15.9 months.

15 REFERENCES
1. OSHA Technical Manual, TED 1-0.15A, Section VI: Chapter 2. Controlling Occupational Exposure to Hazardous Drugs. OSHA, 1999.
2. American Society of Health-System Pharmacists. ASHP guidelines on handling hazardous drugs. *Am J Health-Syst Pharm.* 2006; 63:1172–1193.
3. NIOSH Alert: Preventing occupational exposures to antineoplastic and other hazardous drugs in healthcare settings. 2004. U.S. Department of Health and Human Services, Public Health Service, Centers for Disease Control and Prevention, National Institute for Occupational Safety and Health, DHHS (NIOSH) Publication No. 2004-165.[3]
4. Polovich, M., White, J. M., & Kelleher, L.O. (eds.) 2005. Chemotherapy and biotherapy guidelines and recommendations for practice (2nd. ed.) Pittsburgh, PA: Oncology.

16 HOW SUPPLIED/STORAGE AND HANDLING

16.1 Safe Handling and Disposal

Care should be exercised in the handling and preparation of TEMODAR. Vials and capsules should not be opened. If vials or capsules are accidentally opened or damaged, rigorous precautions should be taken with the contents to avoid inhalation or contact with the skin or mucous membranes. The use of gloves and safety glasses is recommended to avoid exposure in case of breakage of the vial or capsules. Procedures for proper handling and disposal of anticancer drugs should be considered {1–4}. Several guidelines on this subject have been published.

16.2 How Supplied

TEMODAR Capsules:

TEMODAR (temozolomide) Capsules are supplied in amber glass bottles with child-resistant polypropylene caps or child-resistant sachets containing the following capsule strengths:

TEMODAR Capsules 5 mg: have opaque white bodies with green caps. The capsule body is imprinted with two stripes, the dosage strength, and the Schering-Plough logo. The cap is imprinted with "TEMODAR".
They are supplied as follows:

Bottles:
  5-count – NDC 0085-3004-02
  14-count – NDC 0085-3004-01
Sachets:
  5-count – NDC 0085-3004-03
  14-count – NDC 0085-3004-04

TEMODAR Capsules 20 mg: have opaque white bodies with yellow caps. The capsule body is imprinted with two stripes, the dosage strength, and the Schering-Plough logo. The cap is imprinted with "TEMODAR".
They are supplied as follows:

Bottles:
  5-count – NDC 0085-1519-02
  14-count – NDC 0085-1519-01
Sachets:
  5-count – NDC 0085-1519-03
  14-count – NDC 0085-1519-04

TEMODAR Capsules 100 mg: have opaque white bodies with pink caps. The capsule body is imprinted with two stripes, the dosage strength, and the Schering-Plough logo. The cap is imprinted with "TEMODAR".
They are supplied as follows:

Bottles:
  5-count – NDC 0085-1366-02
  14-count – NDC 0085-1366-01
Sachets:
  5-count – NDC 0085-1366-03
  14-count – NDC 0085-1366-04

TEMODAR Capsules 140 mg: have opaque white bodies with blue caps. The capsule body is imprinted with two stripes, the dosage strength, and the Schering-Plough logo. The cap is imprinted with "TEMODAR".
They are supplied as follows:

Bottles:
  5-count – NDC 0085-1425-01
  14-count – NDC 0085-1425-02
Sachets:
  5-count – NDC 0085-1425-03
  14-count – NDC 0085-1425-04

TEMODAR Capsules 180 mg: have opaque white bodies with orange caps. The capsule body is imprinted with two stripes, the dosage strength, and the Schering-Plough logo. The cap is imprinted with "TEMODAR".
They are supplied as follows:

Bottles:
  5-count – NDC 0085-1430-01
  14-count – NDC 0085-1430-02
Sachets:
  5-count – NDC 0085-1430-03
  14-count – NDC 0085-1430-04

TEMODAR Capsules 250 mg: have opaque white bodies with white caps. The capsule body is imprinted with two stripes, the dosage strength, and the Schering-Plough logo. The cap is imprinted with "TEMODAR".
They are supplied as follows:

Bottles:
  5-count – NDC 0085-1417-01
Sachets:
  5-count – NDC 0085-1417-02

TEMODAR for Injection:

TEMODAR (temozolomide) for Injection is supplied in single-use glass vials containing 100 mg temozolomide. The lyophilized powder is white to light tan/light pink.

TEMODAR for Injection 100 mg:
  NDC 0085-1381-01

16.3 Storage

Store TEMODAR Capsules at 25°C (77°F); excursions permitted to 15–30°C (59–86°F) [see USP Controlled Room Temperature].

Store TEMODAR for Injection refrigerated at 2–8°C (36–46°F). After reconstitution, store reconstituted product at room temperature (25°C [77°F]). Reconstituted product must be used within 14 hours, including infusion time.

17 PATIENT COUNSELING INFORMATION

See FDA-Approved Patient Labeling (Patient Information).

17.1 Information for the Patient

Physicians should discuss the following with their patients:

- Nausea and vomiting are the most frequently occurring adverse reactions. Nausea and vomiting are usually either self-limiting or readily controlled with standard antiemetic therapy.
- Capsules should not be opened. If capsules are accidentally opened or damaged, rigorous precautions should be taken with the capsule contents to avoid inhalation or contact with the skin or mucous membranes.
- The medication should be kept away from children and pets.

Distributed by: Merck Sharp & Dohme Corp., a subsidiary of **MERCK & CO., INC.**, Whitehouse Station, NJ 08889, USA
For patent information:
www.merck.com/product/patent/home.html
Copyright © 1999, 2008 Merck Sharp & Dohme Corp., a subsidiary of **Merck & Co., Inc.**
All rights reserved.
Revised: 05/2014
uspi-mk7365-mtl-1405r016

Patient Information
TEMODAR® (tĕm-ō-där)
(temozolomide)
Capsules
TEMODAR® (tĕm-ō-där)
(temozolomide)
for Injection

What is the most important information I should know about TEMODAR?

- **TEMODAR may cause birth defects.** Male and female patients who take TEMODAR should use effective birth control. Female patients and female partners of male patients should avoid becoming pregnant while taking TEMODAR.

See the section "What are the possible side effects of TEMODAR?" for more information about side effects.

What is TEMODAR?

TEMODAR (temozolomide) is a prescription medicine used to treat adults with certain brain cancer tumors. TEMODAR blocks cell growth, especially cells that grow fast, such as cancer cells. TEMODAR may decrease the size of certain brain tumors in some patients.

It is not known if TEMODAR is safe and effective in children.

Who should not take TEMODAR?

Do not take TEMODAR if you:

- have had an allergic reaction to dacarbazine (DTIC), another cancer medicine.
- have had a red itchy rash, or a severe allergic reaction, such as trouble breathing, swelling of the face, throat, or tongue, or severe skin reaction to TEMODAR or any of the ingredients in TEMODAR. If you are not sure, ask your doctor. See the end of the leaflet for a list of ingredients in TEMODAR.

What should I tell my doctor before taking TEMODAR?

Tell your doctor about all your medical conditions, including if you:

- are allergic to dacarbazine (DTIC) or have had a severe allergic reaction to TEMODAR. See "Who should not take TEMODAR?"
- have kidney problems
- have liver problems
- are pregnant. See "What is the most important information I should know about TEMODAR?"
- are breast-feeding. It is not known whether TEMODAR passes into breast milk. You and your doctor should decide if you will breast-feed or take TEMODAR. You should not do both without talking with your doctor.

Tell your doctor about all the medicines you take, including prescription and non-prescription medicines, vitamins, and herbal supplements. Especially tell your doctor if you take a medicine that contains valproic acid (Stavzor®, Depakene®). Know the medicines you take. Keep a list of them and show it to your doctor and pharmacist when you get a new medicine.

How should I take TEMODAR?

TEMODAR may be taken by mouth as a capsule at home, or you may receive TEMODAR by injection into a vein (intravenous). Your doctor will decide the best way for you to take TEMODAR.

There are two common dosing schedules for taking TEMODAR.

- Some people take TEMODAR for 42 days in a row (possibly 49 days depending on side effects) with radiation treatment. This is one cycle of treatment. After this, you may have "maintenance" treatment. Your doctor may prescribe 6 more cycles of TEMODAR. For each of these cycles, you

take TEMODAR one time each day for 5 days in a row and then you stop taking it for the next 23 days. This is a 28-day maintenance treatment cycle.

- Another way to take TEMODAR is to take it one time each day for 5 days in a row only, and then you stop taking it for the next 23 days. This is one cycle of treatment (28 days). Your doctor will watch your progress on TEMODAR and decide how long you should take it. You might take TEMODAR until your tumor gets worse or for possibly up to 2 years.
- Your dose is based on your height and weight, and the number of treatment cycles will depend on how you respond to and tolerate this treatment.
- Your doctor may modify your schedule based on how you tolerate the treatment.
- If your doctor prescribes a treatment regimen that is different from the information in this leaflet, make sure you follow the specific instructions given to you by your doctor.

TEMODAR Capsules:

- Take TEMODAR Capsules exactly as prescribed.
- TEMODAR Capsules come in different strengths. Each strength has a different color cap. Your doctor may prescribe more than one strength of TEMODAR Capsules for you, so it is important that you understand how to take your medicine the right way. Be sure that you understand exactly how many capsules you need to take on each day of your treatment, and what strengths to take. This may be different whenever you start a new cycle.
- Talk to your doctor before you take your dose if you are not sure how much to take. This will help to prevent taking too much TEMODAR and decrease your chances of getting serious side effects.
- Take each day's dose of TEMODAR Capsules at one time, with a full glass of water.
- **Swallow TEMODAR Capsules whole. Do not chew, open, or split the capsules.**
- If TEMODAR Capsules are accidentally opened or damaged, be careful not to breathe in (inhale) the powder from the capsules or get the powder on your skin or mucous membranes (for example, in your nose or mouth). If contact with any of these areas happens, flush the area with water.
- If you vomit TEMODAR Capsules, do not take any more capsules. Wait and take your next planned dose.
- The medicine is used best by your body if you take it at the same time every day in relation to a meal.
- To lessen nausea, try to take TEMODAR on an empty stomach or at bedtime. Your doctor may prescribe medicine to prevent or treat nausea, or other medicines to lessen side effects with TEMODAR.
- See your doctor regularly to check your progress. Your doctor will check you for side effects that you might not notice.
- If you miss a dose of TEMODAR, talk with your doctor for instructions about when to take your next dose of TEMODAR.
- Call your doctor right away if you take more than the prescribed amount of TEMODAR. It is important that you do not take more than the amount of TEMODAR prescribed for you.

TEMODAR for Injection:

- You will receive TEMODAR as an infusion directly into your vein. Your treatment will take about 90 minutes.
- Your doctor may prescribe medicine to prevent or treat nausea, or other medicines to relieve side effects with TEMODAR.

What should I avoid while taking TEMODAR?

- Female patients and female partners of male patients should avoid becoming pregnant while taking TEMODAR. See "What is the most important information I should know about TEMODAR?"

What are the possible side effects of TEMODAR?
TEMODAR can cause serious side effects.

- See "What is the most important information I should know about TEMODAR?"
- **Decreased blood cells.** TEMODAR affects cells that grow rapidly, including bone marrow cells. This can cause you to have a decrease in blood cells. Your doctor can monitor your blood for these effects.
  - White blood cells are needed to fight infections. Neutrophils are a type of white blood cell that help prevent bacterial infections. Decreased neutrophils can lead to serious infections that can lead to death. Other white blood cells called lymphocytes may also be decreased.
  - Platelets are blood cells needed for normal blood clotting. Low platelet counts can lead to bleeding. Tell your doctor about any unusual bruising or bleeding.

Your doctor will check your blood regularly while you are taking TEMODAR to see if these side effects are happening. Your doctor may need to change the dose of TEMODAR or when you get it depending on your blood cell counts. People who are age 70 or older and women may be more likely to have their blood cells affected.

- *Pneumocystis* **pneumonia (PCP).** PCP is an infection that people can get when their immune system is weak.

TEMODAR decreases white blood cells, which makes your immune system weaker and can increase your risk of getting PCP. **All patients** taking TEMODAR will be watched carefully by their doctor for this infection, especially patients who take steroids. Tell your doctor if you have any of the following signs and symptoms of PCP infection: shortness of breath and/or fever, chills, dry cough.

• **Secondary cancers.** Blood problems such as myelodysplastic syndrome and secondary cancers, such as a certain kind of leukemia, can happen in people who take TEMODAR. Your doctor will watch you for this.
• **Convulsions.** Convulsions may be severe or life-threatening in people who take TEMODAR.
• **Liver side effects** have been reported, which very rarely included death.

Common side effects with TEMODAR include:

• nausea and vomiting. Your doctor can prescribe medicines that may help reduce these symptoms.
• headache
• feeling tired
• loss of appetite
• hair loss
• constipation
• bruising
• rash
• paralysis on one side of the body
• diarrhea
• weakness
• fever
• dizziness
• coordination problems
• viral infection
• sleep problems
• memory loss
• pain, irritation, itching, warmth, swelling or redness at the site of infusion
• bruising or small red or purple spots under the skin

Tell your doctor about any side effect that bothers you or that does not go away.

These are not all the possible side effects with TEMODAR. For more information, ask your doctor or pharmacist.

Call your doctor for medical advice about side effects. You may report side effects to FDA at 1-800-FDA-1088.

How should I store TEMODAR Capsules?

• Store TEMODAR Capsules at 77°F (controlled room temperature). Storage at 59°F to 86°F (15°C to 30°C) is permitted occasionally.
• **Keep TEMODAR Capsules out of the reach of children and pets.**

General information about TEMODAR.

Medicines are sometimes prescribed for purposes other than those listed in the Patient Information leaflet. Do not use TEMODAR for a condition for which it was not prescribed. Do not give TEMODAR to other people, even if they have the same symptoms that you have. It may harm them.

This leaflet summarizes the most important information about TEMODAR. If you would like more information, talk with your doctor. You can ask your pharmacist or doctor for information about TEMODAR that is written for health professionals.

For more information, go to www.TEMODAR.com or call 1-877-888-4231.

How are TEMODAR Capsules supplied?

TEMODAR Capsules contain a white capsule body with a color cap and the colors vary based on the dosage strength. The capsules are available in six different strengths.

TEMODAR Capsule Strength	Color
5 mg	Green Cap
20 mg	Yellow Cap
100 mg	Pink Cap
140 mg	Blue Cap
180 mg	Orange Cap
250 mg	White Cap

What are the ingredients in TEMODAR?
TEMODAR Capsules:

Active ingredient: temozolomide.
Inactive ingredients: lactose anhydrous, colloidal silicon dioxide, sodium starch glycolate, tartaric acid, stearic acid.
The body of the capsules is made of gelatin and is opaque white. The cap is also made of gelatin, and the colors vary based on the dosage strength. The capsule body and cap are imprinted with pharmaceutical branding ink, which contains shellac, dehydrated alcohol, isopropyl alcohol, butyl alcohol, propylene glycol, purified water, strong ammonia, potassium hydroxide, and ferric oxide.
TEMODAR 5 mg: The green cap contains gelatin, titanium dioxide, iron oxide yellow, sodium lauryl sulfate, and FD&C Blue #2.

TEMODAR 20 mg: The yellow cap contains gelatin, sodium lauryl sulfate, and iron oxide yellow.
TEMODAR 100 mg: The pink cap contains gelatin, titanium dioxide, sodium lauryl sulfate, and iron oxide red.
TEMODAR 140 mg: The blue cap contains gelatin, sodium lauryl sulfate, and FD&C Blue #2.
TEMODAR 180 mg: The orange cap contains gelatin, iron oxide red, iron oxide yellow, titanium dioxide, and sodium lauryl sulfate.
TEMODAR 250 mg: The white cap contains gelatin, titanium dioxide, and sodium lauryl sulfate.

TEMODAR for Injection:

Active ingredient: temozolomide.
Inactive ingredients: mannitol, L-threonine, polysorbate 80, sodium citrate dihydrate, and hydrochloric acid.
Distributed by: Merck Sharp & Dohme Corp., a subsidiary of **MERCK & CO., INC.,** Whitehouse Station, NJ 08889, USA
For patent information:
www.merck.com/product/patent/home.html
The trademarks depicted herein are owned by their respective companies.
Copyright © 1999, 2008 Merck Sharp & Dohme Corp., a subsidiary of **Merck & Co., Inc.**
All rights reserved.
Revised: 05/2014
usppi-mk7365-mtl-1405r008

TEMODAR® (temozolomide) for Injection
PHARMACIST:
Dispense enclosed Patient Package Insert to each patient.

PHARMACIST INFORMATION SHEET

What is TEMODAR? *[See Full Prescribing Information, Indications and Usage (1)].*

TEMODAR® (temozolomide) is an alkylating drug for the treatment of adult patients with newly diagnosed glioblastoma multiforme and refractory anaplastic astrocytoma.

How is TEMODAR dosed? *[See Full Prescribing Information, Recommended Dosing and Dose Modification Guidelines (2.1)].*

The daily dose of TEMODAR for a given patient is calculated by the physician, based on the patient's body surface area (BSA) *[see* **Table 5** *in the Full Prescribing Information, Recommended Dosing and Dose Modification Guidelines (2.1).* The recommended dose for TEMODAR as an intravenous infusion over 90 minutes is the same as the dose for the oral capsule formulation. Bioequivalence has been established only when TEMODAR for Injection was given over 90 minutes. The dose for subsequent cycles may be adjusted according to nadir neutrophil and platelet counts in the previous cycle and at the time of initiating the next cycle.

Dosing for Patients with Refractory Anaplastic Astrocytoma *[See Full Prescribing Information, Recommended Dosing and Dose Modification Guidelines, Patients with Refractory Anaplastic Astrocytoma (2.1)].*

Dosage of TEMODAR must be adjusted according to nadir neutrophil and platelet counts in the previous cycle and neutrophil and platelet counts at the time of initiating the next cycle. The initial dose is 150 mg/m² orally once daily for 5 consecutive days per 28-day treatment cycle. If both the nadir and day of dosing (Day 29, Day 1 of next cycle) absolute neutrophil counts (ANC) are greater than or equal to 1.5×10^9/L (1500/µL) and both the nadir and Day 29, Day 1 of next cycle platelet counts are greater than or equal to 100 $\times 10^9$/L (100,000/µL), the TEMODAR dose may be increased to 200 mg/m²/day for 5 consecutive days per 28-day treatment cycle. During treatment, a complete blood count should be obtained on Day 22 (21 days after the first dose) or within 48 hours of that day, and weekly until the ANC is above 1.5×10^9/L (1500/µL) and the platelet count exceeds 100 $\times 10^9$/L (100,000/µL). The next cycle of TEMODAR should not be started until the ANC and platelet count exceed these levels. If the ANC falls to less than 1.0×10^9/L (1000/µL) or the platelet count is less than 50 $\times 10^9$/L (50,000/µL) during any cycle, the next cycle should be reduced by 50 mg/m², but not below 100 mg/m², the lowest recommended dose *[see* **Table 4** *in the Full Prescribing Information, Recommended Dosing and Dose Modification Guidelines (2.1)].*

Patients should continue to receive TEMODAR until their physician determines that their disease has progressed, or until unacceptable side effects or toxicities occur. Physicians may alter the treatment regimen for a given patient.

Dosing for Patients with Newly Diagnosed Glioblastoma Multiforme *[See Full Prescribing Information, Recommended Dosing and Dose Modification Guidelines, Patients with Newly Diagnosed High Grade Glioma (2.1)].*

Concomitant Phase Treatment Schedule

TEMODAR is administered at 75 mg/m² daily for 42 days concomitant with focal radiotherapy (60 Gy administered in 30 fractions), followed by maintenance TEMODAR for 6 cycles. No dose reductions are recommended; however, dose

interruptions may occur based on patient tolerance. The TEMODAR dose can be continued throughout the 42-day concomitant period up to 49 days if all of the following conditions are met: absolute neutrophil count greater than or equal to 1.5×10^9/L, platelet count greater than or equal to 100 $\times 10^9$/L, common toxicity criteria (CTC) non-hematological toxicity less than or equal to Grade 1 (except for alopecia, nausea, and vomiting). During treatment a complete blood count should be obtained weekly. Temozolomide dosing should be interrupted or discontinued during concomitant phase according to the hematological and non-hematological toxicity criteria as noted in **Table 1** of the Full Prescribing Information under 2.1 Recommended Dosing and Dose Modification Guidelines. *Pneumocystis* pneumonia (PCP) prophylaxis is required during the concomitant administration of TEMODAR and radiotherapy, and should be continued in patients who develop lymphocytopenia until recovery from lymphocytopenia (CTC Grade less than or equal to 1).

Maintenance Phase Treatment Schedule

Four weeks after completing the TEMODAR + RT phase, TEMODAR is administered for an additional 6 cycles of maintenance treatment. Dosage in Cycle 1 (maintenance) is 150 mg/m² once daily for 5 days followed by 23 days without treatment. At the start of Cycle 2, the dose can be escalated to 200 mg/m², if the CTC non-hematologic toxicity for Cycle 1 is Grade less than or equal to 2 (except for alopecia, nausea, and vomiting), absolute neutrophil count (ANC) is greater than or equal to 1.5×10^9/L, and the platelet count is greater than or equal to 100 $\times 10^9$/L. If the dose was not escalated at Cycle 2, escalation should not be done in subsequent cycles. The dose remains at 200 mg/m² per day for the first 5 days of each subsequent cycle except if toxicity occurs.

During treatment a complete blood count should be obtained on Day 22 (21 days after the first dose) or within 48 hours of that day, and weekly until the ANC is above 1.5×10^9/L (1500/µL) and the platelet count exceeds 100 $\times 10^9$/L (100,000/µL). The next cycle of TEMODAR should not be started until the ANC and platelet count exceed these levels. Dose reductions during the next cycle should be based on the lowest blood counts and worst nonhematologic toxicity during the previous cycle. Dose reductions or discontinuations during the maintenance phase should be applied according to **Tables 2** and **3** in the Full Prescribing Information under 2.1 Recommended Dosing and Dose Modification Guidelines.

How is TEMODAR for Injection prepared? *[See Full Prescribing Information, Preparation and Administration, TEMODAR for Injection (2.2)].*

Care should be exercised in the handling and preparation of TEMODAR. Vials should not be opened. If vials are accidentally opened or damaged, rigorous precautions should be taken with the contents to avoid inhalation or contact with the skin or mucous membranes. The use of gloves and safety glasses is recommended to avoid exposure in case of breakage of the vial. Procedures for proper handling and disposal of anticancer drugs should be considered [1-4]. Several guidelines on this subject have been published.

1. TEMODAR for Injection vials should be stored refrigerated at 2°–8°C (36°–46°F).
2. Bring the vial to room temperature prior to reconstitution with Sterile Water for Injection.
3. Using aseptic technique, reconstitute each vial with 41 mL Sterile Water for Injection. The resulting solution will contain 2.5 mg/mL temozolomide.
4. Vial should be gently swirled and not shaken. Inspect vials, and any vial containing visible particulate matter should not be used. Do not further dilute the reconstituted solution. Upon reconstitution, store at room temperature for up to 14 hours, including infusion time.
5. Using aseptic technique, withdraw up to 40 mL from each vial to make up the total dose and transfer into an empty 250 mL infusion bag.
6. Attach the pump tubing to the bag, purge the tubing and then cap.

How is TEMODAR for Injection administered? *[See Full Prescribing Information, Preparation and Administration, TEMODAR for Injection (2.2)].*

TEMODAR for Injection is administered as an intravenous infusion over 90 minutes. Bioequivalence has been established only when TEMODAR for Injection was given over 90 minutes. TEMODAR for Injection should be administered only by intravenous infusion. Flush the lines before and after each TEMODAR infusion.

TEMODAR for Injection may be administered in the same intravenous line with 0.9% Sodium Chloride injection only. Because no data are available on the compatibility of TEMODAR for Injection with other intravenous substances or additives, other medications should not be infused simultaneously through the same intravenous line.

What should the patient avoid during treatment with TEMODAR? *[See Full Prescribing Information, Use in Specific Populations, Pregnancy (8.1) and Nursing Mothers (8.3)].*

There are no dietary restrictions for patients taking TEMODAR. TEMODAR may affect testicular function, so male patients should exercise adequate birth control measures. TEMODAR may cause birth defects. Female patients should avoid becoming pregnant while receiving this drug. It is not known whether TEMODAR is excreted into breast milk. Because many drugs are excreted in human milk, and because of the potential for serious adverse reactions in nursing infants and tumorigenicity shown for temozolomide in animal studies, a decision should be made whether to discontinue nursing or to discontinue the drug, taking into account the importance of TEMODAR to the mother.

What are the side effects of TEMODAR? *[See Full Prescribing Information, Adverse Reactions (6)].*

Nausea and vomiting are the most common side effects associated with TEMODAR. Noncumulative myelosuppression is the dose-limiting toxicity. Patients should be evaluated periodically by their physician to monitor blood counts.

Other commonly reported side effects reported by patients taking TEMODAR are fatigue, constipation, alopecia, anorexia, headache, and bruising, as well as pain, irritation, itching, warmth, swelling, and redness at the site of infusion.

How is TEMODAR supplied? *[See Full Prescribing Information, How Supplied/Storage and Handling (16)].*

TEMODAR for Injection is supplied in single-use glass vials containing 100 mg temozolomide. TEMODAR is also available as capsules in 5-mg, 20-mg, 100-mg, 140-mg, 180-mg, and 250-mg strengths.

1. OSHA Technical Manual, TED 1-0.15A, Section VI: Chapter 2. Controlling Occupational Exposure to Hazardous Drugs. OSHA, 1999.
2. American Society of Health-System Pharmacists. ASHP guidelines on handling hazardous drugs. *Am J Health-Syst Pharm.* 2006; 63:1172–1193.
3. NIOSH Alert: Preventing occupational exposures to antineoplastic and other hazardous drugs in healthcare settings. 2004. U.S. Department of Health and Human Services, Public Health Service, Centers for Disease Control and Prevention, National Institute for Occupational Safety and Health, DHHS (NIOSH) Publication No. 2004-165.[3]
4. Polovich, M., White, J. M., & Kelleher, L.O. (eds.) 2005. Chemotherapy and biotherapy guidelines and recommendations for practice (2nd. ed.) Pittsburgh, PA: Oncology.

Distributed by: Merck Sharp & Dohme Corp., a subsidiary of **MERCK & CO., INC.,** Whitehouse Station, NJ 08889, USA
For patent information:
www.merck.com/product/patent/home.html
Copyright © 2008 Merck Sharp & Dohme Corp., a subsidiary of **Merck & Co., Inc.**
All rights reserved.
Revised: 05/2014
usphi-mk7365-pwi-1405r014
TEMODAR® (temozolomide) Capsules
PHARMACIST:
Dispense enclosed Patient Package Insert to each patient.
PHARMACIST INFORMATION SHEET

IMPORTANT DISPENSING INFORMATION
For every patient, TEMODAR must be dispensed in a separate vial or in its original package making sure each container lists the strength per capsule and that patients take the appropriate number of capsules from each package or vial.
Please see the dispensing instructions below for more information.

What is TEMODAR?
TEMODAR® (temozolomide) is an oral alkylating agent for the treatment of newly diagnosed glioblastoma multiforme and refractory anaplastic astrocytoma.

How is TEMODAR dosed?
The daily dose of TEMODAR Capsules for a given patient is calculated by the physician, based on the patient's body surface area (BSA). The resulting dose is then rounded off to the nearest 5 mg. An example of the dosing may be as follows: the initial daily dose of TEMODAR in milligrams is the BSA multiplied by $mg/m^2/day$, (a patient with a BSA of 1.84 is 1.84×75 mg = 138, or 140 mg/day). The dose for subsequent cycles may be adjusted according to nadir neutrophil and platelet counts in the previous cycle and at the time of initiating the next cycle.

How might the dose of TEMODAR be modified for Refractory Anaplastic Astrocytoma?
Dosage of TEMODAR must be adjusted according to nadir neutrophil and platelet counts in the previous cycle and neutrophil and platelet counts at the time of initiating the next cycle. The initial dose is 150 mg/m² orally once daily for

---

5 consecutive days per 28-day treatment cycle. If both the nadir and day of dosing (Day 29, Day 1 of next cycle) absolute neutrophil counts (ANC) are greater than or equal to 1.5×10^9/L (1500/µL) and both the nadir and Day 29, Day 1 of next cycle platelet counts are greater than or equal to 100×10^9/L (100,000/µL), the TEMODAR dose may be increased to 200 mg/m²/day for 5 consecutive days per 28-day treatment cycle. During treatment, a complete blood count should be obtained on Day 22 (21 days after the first dose) or within 48 hours of that day, and weekly until the ANC is above 1.5×10^9/L (1500/µL) and the platelet count exceeds 100×10^9/L (100,000/µL). The next cycle of TEMODAR should not be started until the ANC and platelet count exceed these levels. If the ANC falls to less than 1.0×10^9/L (1000/µL) or the platelet count is less than 50×10^9/L (50,000/µL) during any cycle, the next cycle should be reduced by 50 mg/m², but not below 100 mg/m², the lowest recommended dose (see **Table 1** below).

TABLE 1: Dosing Modification Table for Refractory Anaplastic Astrocytoma

What is the TEMODAR Capsules treatment regimen?
TEMODAR is given for 5 consecutive days on a 28-day cycle. Patients should continue taking TEMODAR until their physician determines that their disease has progressed, up to 2 years, or until unacceptable side effects or toxicities occur. Physicians may alter the treatment regimen for a given patient.

Newly Diagnosed Concomitant Phase Treatment Schedule
TEMODAR is administered orally at 75 mg/m² daily for 42 days concomitant with focal radiotherapy (60 Gy administered in 30 fractions), followed by maintenance TEMODAR for 6 cycles. No dose reductions are recommended; however, dose interruptions may occur based on patient tolerance. The TEMODAR dose can be continued throughout the 42-day concomitant period up to 49 days if all of the following conditions are met: absolute neutrophil count greater than or equal to 1.5×10^9/L, platelet count greater than or equal to 100×10^9/L, common toxicity criteria (CTC) nonhematological toxicity less than or equal to Grade 1 (except for alopecia, nausea and vomiting). During treatment a complete blood count should be obtained weekly. Temozolomide dosing should be interrupted or discontinued during concomitant phase according to the hematological and nonhematological toxicity criteria as noted in **Table 2**. *Pneumocystis* pneumonia (PCP) prophylaxis is required during the concomitant administration of TEMODAR and radiotherapy, and should be continued in patients who develop lymphocytopenia until recovery from lymphocytopenia (CTC grade less than or equal to 1).

TABLE 2: Temozolomide Dosing Interruption or Discontinuation During Concomitant Radiotherapy and Temozolomide

Toxicity	TMZ Interruption*	TMZ Discontinuation
Absolute Neutrophil Count	greater than or equal to 0.5 and less than 1.5 × 10^9/L	less than 0.5 × 10^9/L
Platelet Count	greater than or equal to 10 and less than 100 × 10^9/L	less than 10 × 10^9/L

CTC Nonhematological Toxicity (except for alopecia, nausea, vomiting)	CTC Grade 2	CTC Grade 3 or 4

TMZ = temozolomide; CTC = Common Toxicity Criteria.
* Treatment with concomitant TMZ could be continued when all of the following conditions were met: absolute neutrophil count greater than or equal to 1.5×10^9/L; platelet count greater than or equal to 100×10^9/L; CTC nonhematological toxicity less than or equal to Grade 1 (except for alopecia, nausea, vomiting).

Maintenance Phase Treatment Schedule
Four weeks after completing the TEMODAR + RT phase, TEMODAR is administered for an additional 6 cycles of maintenance treatment. Dosage in Cycle 1 (maintenance) is 150 mg/m² once daily for 5 days followed by 23 days without treatment. At the start of Cycle 2, the dose is escalated to 200 mg/m², if the CTC nonhematologic toxicity for Cycle 1 is Grade less than or equal to 2 (except for alopecia, nausea and vomiting), absolute neutrophil count (ANC) is greater than or equal to 1.5×10^9/L, and the platelet count is greater than or equal to 100×10^9/L. If the dose was not escalated at Cycle 2, escalation should not be done in subsequent cycles. The dose remains at 200 mg/m² per day for the first 5 days of each subsequent cycle except if toxicity occurs.

During treatment a complete blood count should be obtained on Day 22 (21 days after the first dose) or within 48 hours of that day, and weekly until the ANC is above 1.5×10^9/L (1500/µL) and the platelet count exceeds 100×10^9/L (100,000/µL). The next cycle of TEMODAR should not be started until the ANC and platelet count exceed these levels. Dose reductions during the next cycle should be based on the lowest blood counts and worst nonhematologic toxicity during the previous cycle. Dose reductions or discontinuations during the maintenance phase should be applied according to **Tables 3** and **4**.

TABLE 3: Temozolomide Dose Levels for Maintenance Treatment

Dose Level	Dose (mg/m²/day)	Remarks
−1	100	Reduction for prior toxicity
0	150	Dose during Cycle 1
1	200	Dose during Cycles 2–6 in absence of toxicity

TABLE 4: Temozolomide Dose Reduction or Discontinuation During Maintenance Treatment

Toxicity	Reduce TMZ by 1 Dose Level*	Discontinue TMZ
Absolute Neutrophil Count	less than 1.0 × 10^9/L	See footnote†
Platelet Count	less than 50 × 10^9/L	See footnote†
CTC Nonhematological Toxicity (except for alopecia, nausea, vomiting)	CTC Grade 3	CTC Grade 4†

TMZ = temozolomide; CTC = Common Toxicity Criteria.
* TMZ dose levels are listed in **Table 3**.
† TMZ is to be discontinued if dose reduction to less than 100 mg/m² is required or if the same Grade 3 nonhematological toxicity (except for alopecia, nausea, vomiting) recurs after dose reduction.

How is TEMODAR taken?
Patients should take each day's dose with a full glass of water at the same time each day. Taking the medication on an empty stomach or at bedtime may help ease nausea. If patients are also taking antinausea or other medications to relieve the side effects associated with TEMODAR, they should be advised to take these medications 30 minutes before they take TEMODAR. Temozolomide causes the rapid appearance of malignant tumors in rats. Patients **SHOULD NOT** open or split the capsules. If capsules are accidentally opened or damaged, rigorous precautions should be taken with the capsule contents to avoid inhalation or contact with the skin or mucous membranes. The medication should be kept away from children and pets. The TEMODAR capsules should be swallowed whole and **NEVER CHEWED**.

What should the patient avoid during treatment with TEMODAR?

There are no dietary restrictions for patients taking TEMODAR. TEMODAR may affect testicular function, so male patients should exercise adequate birth control measures. TEMODAR may cause birth defects. Female patients should avoid becoming pregnant while receiving this drug. Women who are nursing prior to receiving TEMODAR should discontinue nursing. It is not known whether TEMODAR is excreted into breast milk.

Because many drugs are excreted in human milk, and because of the potential for serious adverse reactions in nursing infants and tumorigenicity shown for temozolomide in animal studies, a decision should be made whether to discontinue nursing or to discontinue the drug, taking into account the importance of TEMODAR to the mother.

What are the side effects of TEMODAR?

Nausea and vomiting are the most common side effects associated with TEMODAR. Noncumulative myelosuppression is the dose-limiting toxicity. Patients should be evaluated periodically by their physician to monitor blood counts. Other commonly reported side effects reported by patients taking TEMODAR are fatigue, constipation, alopecia, anorexia, and headache.

How is TEMODAR supplied?

TEMODAR Capsules are available in 5-mg, 20-mg, 100-mg, 140-mg, 180-mg, and 250-mg strengths. The capsules contain a white capsule body with a color cap, and the colors vary based on the dosage strength.

TEMODAR Capsule Strength	Color
5 mg	Green Cap
20 mg	Yellow Cap
100 mg	Pink Cap
140 mg	Blue Cap
180 mg	Orange Cap
250 mg	White Cap

The 5-mg, 20-mg, 100-mg, 140-mg, and 180-mg capsule strengths are available in 5-count and 14-count packages. The 250-mg capsule strength is available in a 5-count package.

How is TEMODAR dispensed?

Each strength of TEMODAR must be dispensed in a separate vial or in its original package (one strength per one container). Follow the instructions below:

Based on the dose prescribed, determine the number of each strength of TEMODAR capsules needed for the full 42- or 5-day cycle as prescribed by the physician. For example, in a 5-day cycle, 275 mg/day would be dispensed as five 250-mg capsules, five 20-mg capsules and five 5-mg capsules. Label each container with the appropriate number of capsules to be taken each day. Dispense to the patient, making sure each container lists the strength (mg) per capsule and that he or she understands to take the appropriate number of capsules of TEMODAR from each package or vial to equal the total daily dose prescribed by the physician.

How can TEMODAR be ordered?

TEMODAR can be ordered from your wholesaler. It is important to understand if TEMODAR is being used as part of a 42-day regimen or as part of a 5-day course. Remember to order enough TEMODAR for the appropriate cycle.

For example:

• a 5-day course of 360 mg/day would require the following to be ordered: two 5-count packages of 180-mg capsules.

• a 42-day course of 140 mg/day would require the following to be ordered: three 14-count packages of 140-mg capsules.

For examples of other dosing regimens, please refer to the full **Prescribing Information (Table 6)**.

TEMODAR Product	NDC Number
Bottles:	
5-mg capsules (5 count)	0085-3004-02
5-mg capsules (14 count)	0085-3004-01
20-mg capsules (5 count)	0085-1519-01
20-mg capsules (14 count)	0085-1519-01
100-mg capsules (5 count)	0085-1366-02
100-mg capsules (14 count)	0085-1366-01
140-mg capsules (5 count)	0085-1425-01
140-mg capsules (14 count)	0085-1425-02
180-mg capsules (5 count)	0085-1430-01
180-mg capsules (14 count)	0085-1430-02
250-mg capsules (5 count)	0085-1417-01
Sachets:	
5-mg capsules (5 count)	0085-3004-03
5-mg capsules (14 count)	0085-3004-04
20-mg capsules (5 count)	0085-1519-03
20-mg capsules (14 count)	0085-1519-04
100-mg capsules (5 count)	0085-1366-03
100-mg capsules (14 count)	0085-1366-04
140-mg capsules (5 count)	0085-1425-03
140-mg capsules (14 count)	0085-1425-04
180-mg capsules (5 count)	0085-1430-03
180-mg capsules (14 count)	0085-1430-04
250-mg capsules (5 count)	0085-1417-02

Distributed by: Merck Sharp & Dohme Corp., a subsidiary of **MERCK & CO., INC.**, Whitehouse Station, NJ 08889, USA

For patent information:
www.merck.com/product/patent/home.html

Copyright © 2005 Merck Sharp & Dohme Corp., a subsidiary of **Merck & Co., Inc.**

All rights reserved.

Revised: 05/2014

usphi-mk7365-cp-1405r010

Shown in Product Identification Guide, page 309

TRUSOPT®　　　　　　　　　　　　　　　　℞
(dorzolamide hydrochloride ophthalmic solution) 2%

HIGHLIGHTS OF PRESCRIBING INFORMATION

These highlights do not include all the information needed to use TRUSOPT safely and effectively. See full prescribing information for TRUSOPT.

TRUSOPT® **(dorzolamide hydrochloride ophthalmic solution) 2%**

Initial U.S. Approval: 1994

————**INDICATIONS AND USAGE**————

TRUSOPT is a carbonic anhydrase inhibitor indicated in the treatment of elevated intraocular pressure in patients with ocular hypertension or open-angle glaucoma. (1)

————**DOSAGE AND ADMINISTRATION**————

The dose is one drop of TRUSOPT in the affected eye(s) three times daily. TRUSOPT may be used concomitantly with other topical ophthalmic drug products to lower intraocular pressure. (2)

————**DOSAGE FORMS AND STRENGTHS**————

Solution containing 20 mg/mL dorzolamide. (3)

————**CONTRAINDICATIONS**————

TRUSOPT is contraindicated in patients who are hypersensitive to any component of this product. (4, 5.1)

————**WARNINGS AND PRECAUTIONS**————

• Sulfonamide Hypersensitivity (5.1)
• Bacterial Keratitis (5.2)
• Corneal Endothelium (5.3)
• Allergic Reactions (5.4)
• Acute Angle-Closure Glaucoma (5.5)

————**ADVERSE REACTIONS**————

The most frequently reported adverse reactions associated with TRUSOPT were ocular burning, stinging, or discomfort immediately following ocular administration (approximately one-third of patients). Approximately one-quarter of patients noted a bitter taste following administration. Superficial punctate keratitis occurred in 10 to 15% of patients and signs and symptoms of ocular allergic reaction in approximately 10%. (6)

To report SUSPECTED ADVERSE REACTIONS, contact Merck Sharp & Dohme Corp., a subsidiary of Merck & Co., Inc., at 1-877-888-4231 or FDA at 1-800-FDA-1088 or www.fda.gov/medwatch

————**DRUG INTERACTIONS**————

• Potential additive effect of oral carbonic anhydrase inhibitor with TRUSOPT. (7.1)

• Potential acid-base and electrolyte disturbances. (7.2)

See 17 for PATIENT COUNSELING INFORMATION and FDA-approved patient labeling

　　　　　　　　　　　　　　　　Revised: 02/2014

FULL PRESCRIBING INFORMATION: CONTENTS*

1　**INDICATIONS AND USAGE**
2　**DOSAGE AND ADMINISTRATION**
3　**DOSAGE FORMS AND STRENGTHS**
4　**CONTRAINDICATIONS**
5　**WARNINGS AND PRECAUTIONS**
　　5.1　Sulfonamide Hypersensitivity
　　5.2　Bacterial Keratitis
　　5.3　Corneal Endothelium
　　5.4　Allergic Reactions
　　5.5　Acute Angle-Closure Glaucoma
6　**ADVERSE REACTIONS**
　　6.1　Clinical Studies Experience
　　6.2　Post-Marketing Experience
7　**DRUG INTERACTIONS**
　　7.1　Oral Carbonic Anhydrase Inhibitors
　　7.2　High-Dose Salicylate Therapy

8　**USE IN SPECIFIC POPULATIONS**
　　8.1　Pregnancy
　　8.3　Nursing Mothers
　　8.4　Pediatric Use
　　8.5　Geriatric Use
　　8.6　Renal and Hepatic Impairment
10　**OVERDOSAGE**
11　**DESCRIPTION**
12　**CLINICAL PHARMACOLOGY**
　　12.1　Mechanism of Action
　　12.3　Pharmacokinetics
13　**NONCLINICAL TOXICOLOGY**
　　13.1　Carcinogenesis, Mutagenesis, Impairment of Fertility
14　**CLINICAL STUDIES**
16　**HOW SUPPLIED/STORAGE AND HANDLING**
17　**PATIENT COUNSELING INFORMATION**
　　17.1　Sulfonamide Reactions
　　17.2　Intercurrent Ocular Conditions
　　17.3　Handling Ophthalmic Solutions
　　17.4　Concomitant Topical Ocular Therapy
　　17.5　Contact Lens Use
　　17.6　Patient Instructions

* Sections or subsections omitted from the full prescribing information are not listed

---

FULL PRESCRIBING INFORMATION

1　INDICATIONS AND USAGE

TRUSOPT® Ophthalmic Solution is indicated in the treatment of elevated intraocular pressure in patients with ocular hypertension or open-angle glaucoma.

2　DOSAGE AND ADMINISTRATION

The dose is one drop of TRUSOPT Ophthalmic Solution in the affected eye(s) three times daily.

TRUSOPT may be used concomitantly with other topical ophthalmic drug products to lower intraocular pressure. If more than one topical ophthalmic drug is being used, the drugs should be administered at least five minutes apart.

3　DOSAGE FORMS AND STRENGTHS

Solution containing 20 mg/mL dorzolamide (22.3 mg of dorzolamide hydrochloride).

4　CONTRAINDICATIONS

TRUSOPT is contraindicated in patients who are hypersensitive to any component of this product *[see Warnings and Precautions (5.1)]*.

5　WARNINGS AND PRECAUTIONS

5.1　Sulfonamide Hypersensitivity

TRUSOPT contains dorzolamide, a sulfonamide; and although administered topically, it is absorbed systemically. Therefore, the same types of adverse reactions that are attributable to sulfonamides may occur with topical administration of TRUSOPT. Fatalities have occurred, although rarely, due to severe reactions to sulfonamides including Stevens-Johnson syndrome, toxic epidermal necrolysis, fulminant hepatic necrosis, agranulocytosis, aplastic anemia, and other blood dyscrasias. Sensitization may recur when a sulfonamide is readministered irrespective of the route of administration. If signs of serious reactions or hypersensitivity occur, discontinue the use of this preparation *[see Contraindications (4) and Patient Counseling Information (17.3)]*.

5.2　Bacterial Keratitis

There have been reports of bacterial keratitis associated with the use of multiple-dose containers of topical ophthalmic products. These containers had been inadvertently contaminated by patients who, in most cases, had a concurrent corneal disease or a disruption of the ocular epithelial surface.

5.3　Corneal Endothelium

Carbonic anhydrase activity has been observed in both the cytoplasm and around the plasma membranes of the corneal endothelium. There is an increased potential for developing corneal edema in patients with low endothelial cell counts. Caution should be used when prescribing TRUSOPT to this group of patients.

5.4　Allergic Reactions

In clinical studies, local ocular adverse effects, primarily conjunctivitis and lid reactions, were reported with chronic administration of TRUSOPT. Many of these reactions had the clinical appearance and course of an allergic-type reaction that resolved upon discontinuation of drug therapy. If such reactions are observed, TRUSOPT should be discontinued and the patient evaluated before considering restarting the drug *[see Adverse Reactions (6)]*.

5.5　Acute Angle-Closure Glaucoma

The management of patients with acute angle-closure glaucoma requires therapeutic interventions in addition to ocular hypotensive agents.

6　ADVERSE REACTIONS

6.1　Clinical Studies Experience

Because clinical trials are conducted under widely varying conditions, adverse reaction rates observed in the clinical

trials of a drug cannot be directly compared to rates in the clinical trials of another drug and may not reflect the rates observed in practice.

Controlled clinical trials: The most frequent adverse reactions associated with TRUSOPT were ocular burning, stinging, or discomfort immediately following ocular administration (approximately one-third of patients). Approximately one-quarter of patients noted a bitter taste following administration. Superficial punctate keratitis occurred in 10 to 15% of patients and signs and symptoms of ocular allergic reaction in approximately 10%. Reactions occurring in approximately 1 to 5% of patients were conjunctivitis and lid reactions *[see Warnings and Precautions (5.5)]*, blurred vision, eye redness, tearing, dryness, and photophobia. Other ocular reactions and systemic reactions were reported infrequently, including headache, nausea, asthenia/fatigue; and, rarely, skin rashes, urolithiasis and iridocyclitis.

In a 3-month, double-masked, active-treatment-controlled, multicenter study in pediatric patients, the adverse reactions profile of TRUSOPT was comparable to that seen in adult patients.

6.2 Post-Marketing Experience

The following adverse reactions have been identified during post-approval use of TRUSOPT. Because these reactions are reported voluntarily from a population of uncertain size, it is not always possible to reliably estimate their frequency or establish a causal relationship to drug exposure: signs and symptoms of systemic allergic reactions including angioedema, bronchospasm, pruritus, and urticaria; Stevens-Johnson syndrome and toxic epidermal necrolysis; dizziness, paresthesia; ocular pain, transient myopia, choroidal detachment following filtration surgery, eyelid crusting; dyspnea; contact dermatitis, epistaxis, dry mouth and throat irritation.

7 DRUG INTERACTIONS

7.1 Oral Carbonic Anhydrase Inhibitors

There is a potential for an additive effect on the known systemic effects of carbonic anhydrase inhibition in patients receiving an oral carbonic anhydrase inhibitor and TRUSOPT. The concomitant administration of TRUSOPT and oral carbonic anhydrase inhibitors is not recommended.

7.2 High-Dose Salicylate Therapy

Although acid-base and electrolyte disturbances were not reported in the clinical trials with dorzolamide hydrochloride ophthalmic solution, these disturbances have been reported with oral carbonic anhydrase inhibitors and have, in some instances, resulted in drug interactions (e.g., toxicity associated with high-dose salicylate therapy). Therefore, the potential for such drug interactions should be considered in patients receiving TRUSOPT.

8 USE IN SPECIFIC POPULATIONS

8.1 Pregnancy

Teratogenic Effects. Pregnancy Category C. Developmental toxicity studies with dorzolamide hydrochloride in rabbits at oral doses of ≥ 2.5 mg/kg/day revealed malformations of the vertebral bodies. These malformations occurred at doses that caused metabolic acidosis with decreased body weight gain in dams and decreased fetal weights. No treatment-related malformations were seen at 1 mg/kg/day. These doses represent estimated plasma C_{max} levels in rabbits, 37 and 15 times higher than the lower limit of detection in human plasma following ocular administration, respectively. There are no adequate and well-controlled studies in pregnant women. TRUSOPT should be used during pregnancy only if the potential benefit justifies the potential risk to the fetus.

8.3 Nursing Mothers

In a study of dorzolamide hydrochloride in lactating rats, decreases in body weight gain of 5 to 7% in offspring at an oral dose of 7.5 mg/kg/day were seen during lactation. A slight delay in postnatal development (incisor eruption, vaginal canalization and eye openings), secondary to lower fetal body weight, was noted. This dose represents an estimated plasma C_{max} level in rats, 52 times higher than the lower limit of detection in human plasma following ocular administration.

It is not known whether this drug is excreted in human milk. Because many drugs are excreted in human milk and because of the potential for serious adverse reactions in nursing infants from TRUSOPT, a decision should be made whether to discontinue nursing or to discontinue the drug, taking into account the importance of the drug to the mother.

8.4 Pediatric Use

Safety and effectiveness of TRUSOPT have been demonstrated in pediatric patients in a 3-month, multicenter, double-masked, active-treatment-controlled trial.

8.5 Geriatric Use

No overall differences in safety or effectiveness have been observed between elderly and younger patients.

8.6 Renal and Hepatic Impairment

Dorzolamide has not been studied in patients with severe renal impairment (CrCl < 30 mL/min). Because

dorzolamide and its metabolite are excreted predominantly by the kidney, TRUSOPT is not recommended in such patients.

Dorzolamide has not been studied in patients with hepatic impairment and should therefore be used with caution in such patients.

10 OVERDOSAGE

Electrolyte imbalance, development of an acidotic state, and possible central nervous system effects may occur. Serum electrolyte levels (particularly potassium) and blood pH levels should be monitored.

11 DESCRIPTION

TRUSOPT® (dorzolamide hydrochloride ophthalmic solution) is a carbonic anhydrase inhibitor formulated for topical ophthalmic use.

Dorzolamide hydrochloride is described chemically as: (4S-*trans*)-4-(ethylamino)-5,6-dihydro-6-methyl-4H-thieno[2,3-b]thiopyran-2-sulfonamide 7,7-dioxide monohydrochloride. Dorzolamide hydrochloride is optically active. The specific rotation is

$$[\alpha]_{405}^{25^\circ} \quad (C=1, water) = \sim -17^\circ.$$

Its empirical formula is $C_{10}H_{16}N_2O_4S_3 \cdot HCl$ and its structural formula is:

Dorzolamide hydrochloride has a molecular weight of 360.9 and a melting point of about 264°C. It is a white to off-white, crystalline powder, which is soluble in water and slightly soluble in methanol and ethanol.

TRUSOPT Sterile Ophthalmic Solution is supplied as a sterile, isotonic, buffered, slightly viscous, aqueous solution of dorzolamide hydrochloride. The pH of the solution is approximately 5.6, and the osmolarity is 260-330 mOsM. Each mL of TRUSOPT 2% contains 20 mg dorzolamide (22.3 mg of dorzolamide hydrochloride). Inactive ingredients are hydroxyethyl cellulose, mannitol, sodium citrate dihydrate, sodium hydroxide (to adjust pH) and water for injection. Benzalkonium chloride 0.0075% is added as a preservative.

12 CLINICAL PHARMACOLOGY

12.1 Mechanism of Action

Carbonic anhydrase (CA) is an enzyme found in many tissues of the body including the eye. It catalyzes the reversible reaction involving the hydration of carbon dioxide and the dehydration of carbonic acid. In humans, carbonic anhydrase exists as a number of isoenzymes, the most active being carbonic anhydrase II (CA-II), found primarily in red blood cells (RBCs), but also in other tissues. Inhibition of carbonic anhydrase in the ciliary processes of the eye decreases aqueous humor secretion, presumably by slowing the formation of bicarbonate ions with subsequent reduction in sodium and fluid transport. The result is a reduction in intraocular pressure (IOP).

TRUSOPT Ophthalmic Solution contains dorzolamide hydrochloride, an inhibitor of human carbonic anhydrase II. Following topical ocular administration, TRUSOPT reduces elevated intraocular pressure. Elevated intraocular pressure is a major risk factor in the pathogenesis of optic nerve damage and glaucomatous visual field loss.

12.3 Pharmacokinetics

When topically applied, dorzolamide reaches the systemic circulation. To assess the potential for systemic carbonic anhydrase inhibition following topical administration, drug and metabolite concentrations in RBCs and plasma and carbonic anhydrase inhibition in RBCs were measured.

Dorzolamide accumulates in RBCs during chronic dosing as a result of binding to CA-II. The parent drug forms a single N-desethyl metabolite, which inhibits CA-II less potently than the parent drug but also inhibits CA-I. The metabolite also accumulates in RBCs where it binds primarily to CA-I. Plasma concentrations of dorzolamide and metabolite are generally below the assay limit of quantitation (15nM). Dorzolamide binds moderately to plasma proteins (approximately 33%).

Dorzolamide is primarily excreted unchanged in the urine; the metabolite also is excreted in urine. After dosing is stopped, dorzolamide washes out of RBCs nonlinearly, resulting in a rapid decline of drug concentration initially, followed by a slower elimination phase with a half-life of about four months.

To simulate the systemic exposure after long-term topical ocular administration, dorzolamide was given orally to eight healthy subjects for up to 20 weeks. The oral dose of 2 mg twice daily closely approximates the amount of drug delivered by topical ocular administration of dorzolamide 2% three times daily. Steady state was reached within 8 weeks. The inhibition of CA-II and total carbonic anhydrase

activities was below the degree of inhibition anticipated to be necessary for a pharmacological effect on renal function and respiration in healthy individuals.

13 NONCLINICAL TOXICOLOGY

13.1 Carcinogenesis, Mutagenesis, Impairment of Fertility

In a two-year study of dorzolamide hydrochloride administered orally to male and female Sprague-Dawley rats, urinary bladder papillomas were seen in male rats in the highest dosage group of 20 mg/kg/day. Papillomas were not seen in rats given oral doses of 1 mg/kg/day. These doses represent estimated plasma C_{max} levels in rats, 138 and 7 times higher than the lower limit of detection in human plasma following ocular administration, respectively.

No treatment-related tumors were seen in a 21-month study in female and male mice given oral doses up to 75 mg/kg/day. This dose represents an estimated plasma C_{max} level in mice, 582 times higher than the lower limit of detection in human plasma following ocular administration. The increased incidence of urinary bladder papillomas seen in the high-dose male rats is a class-effect of carbonic anhydrase inhibitors in rats. Rats are particularly prone to developing papillomas in response to foreign bodies, compounds causing crystalluria, and diverse sodium salts.

No changes in bladder urothelium were seen in dogs given oral dorzolamide hydrochloride for one year at 2 mg/kg/day or monkeys dosed topically to the eye for one year. An oral dose of 2 mg/kg/day in dogs represents an estimated plasma C_{max} level, 137 times higher than the lower limit of detection in human plasma following ocular administration. The topical ophthalmic dose in monkeys was approximately equivalent to the human topical ophthalmic dose.

The following tests for mutagenic potential were negative: (1) *in vivo* (mouse) cytogenetic assay; (2) *in vitro* chromosomal aberration assay; (3) alkaline elution assay; (4) V-79 assay; and (5) Ames test.

In reproduction studies of dorzolamide hydrochloride in rats, there were no adverse effects on the reproductive capacity of males or females at doses of 15 and 7.5 mg/kg/day, respectively. These doses represent estimated plasma C_{max} levels in rats, 104 and 52 times higher than the lower limit of detection in human plasma following ocular administration, respectively.

14 CLINICAL STUDIES

The efficacy of TRUSOPT was demonstrated in clinical studies in the treatment of elevated intraocular pressure in patients with glaucoma or ocular hypertension (baseline IOP ≥ 23 mmHg). The IOP-lowering effect of TRUSOPT was approximately 3 to 5 mmHg throughout the day and this was consistent in clinical studies of up to one year duration. The efficacy of TRUSOPT when dosed less frequently than three times a day (alone or in combination with other products) has not been established.

In a one year clinical study, the effect of TRUSOPT 2% three times daily on the corneal endothelium was compared to that of betaxolol ophthalmic solution twice daily and timolol maleate ophthalmic solution 0.5% twice daily. There were no statistically significant differences between groups in corneal endothelial cell counts or in corneal thickness measurements. There was a mean loss of approximately 4% in the endothelial cell counts for each group over the one year period.

16 HOW SUPPLIED/STORAGE AND HANDLING

TRUSOPT is supplied in an OCUMETER® PLUS container, a white, translucent, HDPE plastic ophthalmic dispenser with a controlled drop tip and a white polystyrene cap with orange label as follows:

NDC 0006-3519-36, 10 mL, in an 18 mL capacity bottle.

Storage

Store TRUSOPT Ophthalmic Solution at 15-30°C (59-86°F). Protect from light.

17 PATIENT COUNSELING INFORMATION

See FDA-approved patient labeling (Instructions for Use).

17.1 Sulfonamide Reactions

TRUSOPT is a sulfonamide and although administered topically is absorbed systemically. Therefore the same types of adverse reactions that are attributable to sulfonamides may occur with topical administration. Advise patients that if serious or unusual reactions including severe skin reactions or signs of hypersensitivity occur, they should discontinue the use of the product *[see Warnings and Precautions (5.1)]*.

17.2 Intercurrent Ocular Conditions

Advise patients that if they have ocular surgery or develop an intercurrent ocular condition (e.g., trauma or infection), they should immediately seek their physician's advice concerning the continued use of the present multidose container.

17.3 Handling Ophthalmic Solutions

Instruct patients that ocular solutions, if handled improperly or if the tip of the dispensing container contacts the eye or surrounding structures, can become contaminated by common bacteria known to cause ocular infections. Serious damage to the eye and subsequent loss of vision may result from using contaminated solutions.

17.4   Concomitant Topical Ocular Therapy
If more than one topical ophthalmic drug is being used, the drugs should be administered at least five minutes apart.

17.5   Contact Lens Use
Advise patients that TRUSOPT contains benzalkonium chloride which may be absorbed by soft contact lenses. Contact lenses should be removed prior to administration of the solution. Lenses may be reinserted 15 minutes following TRUSOPT administration.

17.6   Patient Instructions
Advise patients that if they develop any ocular reactions, particularly conjunctivitis and lid reactions, they should discontinue use and seek their physician's advice.

Instruct patients to avoid allowing the tip of the dispensing container to contact the eye or surrounding structures.

Manuf. for: Merck Sharp & Dohme Corp., a subsidiary of **MERCK & CO., INC.,** Whitehouse Station, NJ 08889, USA
By: Laboratoires Merck Sharp & Dohme-Chibret
Clermont Ferrand Cedex 9, 63963, France
Copyright © 1994, 2014 Merck Sharp & Dohme Corp., a subsidiary of **Merck & Co., Inc.**
All rights reserved.
Revised: 02/2014
uspi-mk0507-os-1402r013

INSTRUCTIONS FOR USE
TRUSOPT® ("TRU-sopt")
(dorzolamide hydrochloride ophthalmic solution) 2%

Before using your TRUSOPT
Before using your TRUSOPT for the first time, make sure the safety strip on the front of the bottle is unbroken. A gap between the bottle and the cap is normal for an unopened bottle. (See Figure A).

Opening Arrows ▸
Safety Strip ▸

Figure A

Step 1. Wash your hands.
Step 2. Tear off the safety strip to break the seal. See Figure B.

Gap ▸

Figure B

Step 3. Unscrew the cap by turning in the direction of the arrows on the top of the cap. **Do not** pull the cap directly up and away from the bottle. Pulling the cap directly up will keep your TRUSOPT dispenser from working the right way. See Figure C.
[See figure C at top of next column]

Giving your TRUSOPT drops
Step 4. Tilt your head back and pull your lower eyelid down slightly to form a pocket between your eyelid and your eye. See Figure D.
[See figure D at top of next column]

Step 5. Turn your TRUSOPT dispenser upside down and press lightly with your thumb or index finger over the "Finger Push Area" until a single drop is placed in your eye.

Finger Push Area ▸

Figure C

Figure D

Do not touch your eye or eyelid with the dropper tip. See Figure E.

Finger Push Area ▸

Figure E

Step 6. If the medicine does not drop easily from the TRUSOPT dispenser after you open it for the first time, replace the cap on the bottle and tighten. **Do not** over tighten. Remove the cap by turning the cap in the direction of the arrows on the top of the cap. See Figure F. This should make the hole on the dispenser tip larger. **Do not** try to make the hole of the dispenser tip larger in any other way. The dispenser tip is made to provide a single drop. Repeat Steps 4 and 5 to give your TRUSOPT drop.

Replace cap ▸   Remove cap ▸

Figure F

Step 7. If your doctor has told you to use TRUSOPT drops in both eyes, repeat Steps 4 and 5.

After using your TRUSOPT
Step 8. Replace the cap by turning it until it is firmly touching your TRUSOPT dispenser. The arrow on the left side of the cap must be lined up with the arrow on the left side of the TRUSOPT dispenser label for it to be closed correctly. **Do not** over tighten or you may damage the TRUSOPT dispenser and cap. See Figure G.
[See figure G at top of next column]
After you have used all of your TRUSOPT doses, there will be some TRUSOPT medicine left in the dispenser. **Do not** try to remove the extra medicine from the TRUSOPT dispenser. Throw away your TRUSOPT dispenser in your household trash.

How should I store TRUSOPT?
• Store TRUSOPT between 59°F to 86°F (15°C to 30°C)
• Protect from light
• Safely throw away medicine that is out of date or no longer needed.

Keep TRUSOPT and all medicines out of the reach of children.

Figure G

Important information about using TRUSOPT
• If you have any eye or skin reactions, especially conjunctivitis or eyelid reactions to TRUSOPT, stop using it and call your doctor right away.
• If you have eye surgery or have a problem such as trauma or infection of your eye while using TRUSOPT, call your doctor right away.
• If you do not handle eye medicines the right way the medicine can become contaminated. If the tip of the dispenser touches your eye or areas around your eye, the tip can become contaminated with bacteria which can cause an eye infection and other serious problems including loss of eyesight.
• If you use other eye medicines dropped onto the eye like TRUSOPT, use the medicines at least 5 minutes before or after you use TRUSOPT.
• TRUSOPT contains benzalkonium chloride which may be absorbed by soft contact lenses. If you wear contact lenses, remove them before you use your TRUSOPT. You can place your contact lenses back into your eyes 15 minutes after using your TRUSOPT.

This Instructions for Use has been approved by the U.S. Food and Drug Administration.

Manuf. for: Merck Sharp & Dohme Corp., a subsidiary of **MERCK & CO., Inc.,** Whitehouse Station, NJ 08889, USA
By: Laboratoires Merck Sharp & Dohme-Chibret
Clermont Ferrand Cedex 9, 63963, France
Copyright © 2000, 2014 Merck Sharp & Dohme Corp., a subsidiary of **Merck & Co., Inc.**
All rights reserved.
Revised: 02/2014
ifu-mk0507-os-1402r013

VAQTA®   ℞
[va-q-ta]
(Hepatitis A Vaccine, Inactivated)
Suspension for Intramuscular Injection

HIGHLIGHTS OF PRESCRIBING INFORMATION
These highlights do not include all the information needed to use VAQTA safely and effectively. See full prescribing information for VAQTA.
VAQTA® (Hepatitis A Vaccine, Inactivated)
Suspension for Intramuscular Injection
Initial U.S. Approval: 1996

————INDICATIONS AND USAGE————
VAQTA is a vaccine indicated for the prevention of disease caused by hepatitis A virus (HAV) in persons 12 months of age and older. The primary dose should be given at least 2 weeks prior to expected exposure to HAV. (1.1)

————DOSAGE AND ADMINISTRATION————
• For intramuscular administration only. (2)
• Children/Adolescents: vaccination consists of a 0.5-mL primary dose administered intramuscularly, and a 0.5-mL booster dose administered intramuscularly 6 to 18 months later. (2.1)
• Adults: vaccination consists of a 1-mL primary dose administered intramuscularly, and a 1-mL booster dose administered intramuscularly 6 to 18 months later. (2.1)

————DOSAGE FORMS AND STRENGTHS————
Suspension supplied in four presentations:
• 0.5-mL pediatric dose in single-dose vials and prefilled syringes. (3, 11, 16)
• 1-mL adult dose in single-dose vials and prefilled syringes. (3, 11, 16)

————CONTRAINDICATIONS————
Do not administer VAQTA to individuals with a history of immediate and/or severe allergic or hypersensitivity reactions (e.g., anaphylaxis) after a previous dose of any hepatitis A vaccine or with an anaphylactic reaction to neomycin. (4, 11)

—WARNINGS AND PRECAUTIONS—

- Appropriate medical treatment and supervision must be available to manage possible anaphylactic reactions following administration of the vaccine. (5.1)
- The vial stopper and the syringe plunger stopper and tip cap contain dry natural latex rubber that may cause allergic reactions in latex-sensitive individuals. (5.2)

—ADVERSE REACTIONS—

The most common local adverse reactions and systemic adverse events (≥15%) reported in different clinical trials across different age groups when VAQTA was administered alone or concomitantly were:
- Children — 12 through 23 months of age: injection-site pain/tenderness (37.0%), injection-site erythema (21.2%), fever (16.4% when administered alone, and 27.0% when administered concomitantly) (6.1)
- Children/Adolescents — 2 through 18 years of age: injection-site pain (18.7%) (6.1)
- Adults — 19 years of age and older: injection-site pain, tenderness, or soreness (67.0%), injection-site warmth (18.2%) and headache (16.1%) (6.1)

To report SUSPECTED ADVERSE REACTIONS, contact Merck Sharp & Dohme Corp., a subsidiary of Merck & Co., Inc., at 1-877-888-4231 or VAERS at 1-800-822-7967 or www.vaers.hhs.gov.

—DRUG INTERACTIONS—

- Do not mix VAQTA with any other vaccine in the same syringe or vial. (7.1)

—USE IN SPECIFIC POPULATIONS—

- Pregnancy: No human or animal studies have been conducted. Use only if clearly indicated. (8.1)
- Safety and effectiveness of VAQTA have not been established in children less than 12 months of age. (8.4)

See 17 for PATIENT COUNSELING INFORMATION

Revised: 02/2014

FULL PRESCRIBING INFORMATION: CONTENTS*

* Sections or subsections omitted from the full prescribing information are not listed

FULL PRESCRIBING INFORMATION

1 INDICATIONS AND USAGE

1.1 Indications and Use

VAQTA® [Hepatitis A Vaccine, Inactivated] is indicated for the prevention of disease caused by hepatitis A virus (HAV) in persons 12 months of age and older. The primary dose should be given at least 2 weeks prior to expected exposure to HAV.

2 DOSAGE AND ADMINISTRATION

FOR INTRAMUSCULAR ADMINISTRATION ONLY.

2.1 Dosage and Schedule

Children/Adolescents (12 months through 18 years of age): The vaccination schedule consists of a primary 0.5-mL dose administered intramuscularly, and a 0.5-mL booster dose administered intramuscularly 6 to 18 months later.

Adults (19 years of age and older): The vaccination schedule consists of a primary 1-mL dose administered intramuscularly, and a 1-mL booster dose administered intramuscularly 6 to 18 months later.

Booster Immunization Following Another Manufacturer's Hepatitis A Vaccine: A booster dose of VAQTA may be given at 6 to 12 months following a primary dose of HAVRIX [see Clinical Studies (14.6)].

2.2 Preparation and Administration

Shake the single-dose vial or single-dose prefilled syringe well to obtain a slightly opaque, white suspension before withdrawal and use. Parenteral drug products should be inspected visually for particulate matter and discoloration prior to administration, whenever solution and container permit. Discard if the suspension does not appear homogenous or if extraneous particulate matter remains or discoloration is observed.

For single-dose vials, withdraw and administer entire dose of VAQTA intramuscularly using a sterile needle and syringe.

For single-dose prefilled syringes, securely attach a needle by twisting in a clockwise direction and administer dose of VAQTA intramuscularly.

For adults, adolescents, and children older than 2 years of age, the deltoid muscle is the preferred site for intramuscular injection. For children 12 through 23 months of age, the anterolateral area of the thigh is the preferred site for intramuscular injection.

3 DOSAGE FORMS AND STRENGTHS

Suspension for injection available in four presentations:
- 0.5-mL pediatric dose in single-dose vials and prefilled syringes
- 1-mL adult dose in single-dose vials and prefilled syringes

[See Description (11) for listing of vaccine components and How Supplied/Storage and Handling (16).]

4 CONTRAINDICATIONS

Do not administer VAQTA to individuals with a history of immediate and/or severe allergic or hypersensitivity reactions (e.g., anaphylaxis) after a previous dose of any hepatitis A vaccine, or to individuals who have had an anaphylactic reaction to any component of VAQTA, including neomycin [see Description (11)].

5 WARNINGS AND PRECAUTIONS

5.1 Prevention and Management of Allergic Vaccine Reactions

Appropriate medical treatment and supervision must be available to manage possible anaphylactic reactions following administration of the vaccine [see Contraindications (4)].

5.2 Hypersensitivity to Latex

The vial stopper and the syringe plunger stopper and tip cap contain dry natural latex rubber that may cause allergic reactions in latex-sensitive individuals [see How Supplied/Storage and Handling (16)].

5.3 Altered Immunocompetence

Immunocompromised persons, including individuals receiving immunosuppressive therapy, may have a diminished immune response to VAQTA and may not be protected against HAV infection after vaccination [see Use in Specific Populations (8.6)].

5.4 Limitations of Vaccine Effectiveness

Hepatitis A virus has a relatively long incubation period (approximately 20 to 50 days). VAQTA may not prevent hepatitis A infection in individuals who have an unrecognized hepatitis A infection at the time of vaccination. Vaccination with VAQTA may not result in a protective response in all susceptible vaccinees.

6 ADVERSE REACTIONS

6.1 Clinical Trials Experience

Because clinical trials are conducted under widely varying conditions, adverse reaction rates observed in the clinical trials of a vaccine cannot be directly compared to rates in the clinical trials of another vaccine and may not reflect the rates observed in practice.

The safety of VAQTA has been evaluated in over 10,000 subjects 1 year to 85 years of age. Subjects were given one or two doses of the vaccine. The second (booster dose) was given 6 months or more after the first dose.

The most common local adverse reactions and systemic adverse events (≥15%) reported in different clinical trials across different age groups when VAQTA was administered alone or concomitantly were:
- Children — 12 through 23 months of age: injection-site pain/tenderness (37.0%), injection-site erythema (21.2%), fever (16.4% when administered alone, and 27.0% when administered concomitantly)
- Children/Adolescents — 2 through 18 years of age: injection-site pain (18.7%)
- Adults — 19 years of age and older: injection-site pain, tenderness, or soreness (67.0%), injection-site warmth (18.2%) and headache (16.1%)

Allergic Reactions

Local and/or systemic allergic reactions that occurred in <1% of over 10,000 children/adolescents or adults in clinical trials regardless of causality included: injection-site pruritus and/or rash; bronchial constriction; asthma; wheezing; edema/swelling; rash; generalized erythema; urticaria; pruritus; eye irritation/itching; dermatitis [see Contraindications (4) and Warnings and Precautions (5.1)].

Children — 12 through 23 Months of Age

Across five clinical trials, 4374 children 12 to 23 months of age received one or two 25U doses of VAQTA, including 3885 children who received 2 doses of VAQTA and 1250 children who received VAQTA concomitantly with one or more other vaccines, including Measles, Mumps, and Rubella Virus Vaccine, Live (M-M-R II®), Varicella Vaccine, Live (VARIVAX®), Diphtheria and Tetanus Toxoids and Acellular Pertussis Vaccine, Adsorbed (Tripedia or INFANRIX), Measles, Mumps, Rubella, and Varicella Vaccine, Live (ProQuad®), Pneumococcal 7-valent Conjugate Vaccine (Diphtheria CRM$_{197}$, Prevnar), or Haemophilus B Conjugate

Table 1: Incidences of Solicited Local Adverse Reactions at the VAQTA Injection Site and Elevated Temperatures Following Each Dose of VAQTA in Healthy Children 12-23 Months of Age Receiving VAQTA Alone or Concomitantly With ProQuad and PREVNAR*

Adverse reaction: Days 1-5 unless noted	Dose 1		Dose 2	
	VAQTA alone	VAQTA + ProQuad + Prevnar concomitantly	VAQTA alone	VAQTA + ProQuad concomitantly
Injection site adverse reactions	N=274	N=311	N=251	N=263
Injection site erythema	11.7%	9.6%	12.7%	9.5%
Injection site pain/tenderness	15.3%	20.9%	20.3%	17.5%
Injection site swelling	9.5%	6.8%	7.6%	6.1%
Temperature > 98.6°F or feverish (Days 1-14)	12.4%	35.7%	10.8%	10.3%
	N=243	N=285	N=221	N=237
Temperature ≥ 100.4°F	10.3%	16.8%	10%	4.2%
Temperature ≥ 102.2 °F	2.1%	3.5%	2.3%	2.5%

N=number of subjects for whom data are available.
* Pneumococcal 7-valent Conjugate Vaccine

Table 2: Incidences of Unsolicited Systemic Adverse Events ≥5% in Any Group Following Each Dose of VAQTA in Healthy Children 12-23 Months of Age Receiving VAQTA Alone or Concomitantly With ProQuad and PREVNAR*

Adverse Event: Days 1-14	Dose 1		Dose 2	
	VAQTA alone	VAQTA + ProQuad + PREVNAR concomitantly	VAQTA alone	VAQTA + ProQuad concomitantly
	N=274	N=311	N=251	N=263
General Disorders and Administration Site Conditions				
Irritability	3.6%	6.1%	2.8%	2.7%
Infections and Infestations				
Upper respiratory tract infection	3.3%	6.1%	4.8%	5.7%
Skin and Subcutaneous Tissue Disorders				
Dermatitis diaper	1.1%	6.1%	2.4%	3.4%

* Pneumococcal 7-valent Conjugate Vaccine

Table 3: Incidences of Solicited Local Adverse Reactions at the VAQTA Injection Site and Elevated Temperatures Following Each Dose of VAQTA in Healthy Children 12-23 Months of Age Receiving VAQTA Alone or Concomitantly with PedvaxHIB With or Without INFANRIX (Stage I) and those Receiving VAQTA Alone at Both Doses (Stage II)

Adverse Reaction: Days 1-5 unless noted	Stage I			Stage II	
	Dose 1		Dose 2	Dose 1	Dose 2
	VAQTA alone	VAQTA + PedvaxHIB and Infanrix or VAQTA + PedvaxHIB concomitantly	VAQTA alone	VAQTA alone	VAQTA alone
Injection site adverse reactions	N=256	N=302	N=503	N=647	N=599
Injection site erythema	18.0%	19.9%	21.5%	11.7%	16.2%
Injection site pain/tenderness	21.9%	36.4%	27.4%	20.1%	22.9%
Injection site swelling	10.2%	14.2%	10.1%	7.1%	7.0%
Temperature > 98.6°F or feverish (Days 1-14)	10.2%	17.2%	10.7%	10.0%	8.2%
	N=234	N=290	N=473	N=631	N=591
Temperature ≥ 100.4°F	9.0%	16.9%	9.1%	9.4%	8.6%
Temperature ≥ 102.2 °F	3.8%	3.1%	3.2%	2.9%	2.4%

N= number of subjects for whom data is available

Vaccine (Meningococcal Protein Conjugate, PedvaxHIB®). Overall, the race distribution of study subjects was as follows: 64.7% Caucasian; 15.7% Hispanic-American; 12.3% Black; 4.8% other; 1.4% Asian; and 1.1% Native American. The distribution of subjects by gender was 51.8% male and 48.2% female.

In an open-label clinical trial, 653 children 12 to 23 months of age were randomized to receive a first dose of VAQTA with ProQuad and Prevnar concomitantly (N=330) or a first dose of ProQuad and pneumococcal 7-valent conjugate vaccine concomitantly, followed by a first dose of VAQTA 6 weeks later (N=323). Approximately 6 months later, subjects received either the second doses of ProQuad and VAQTA concomitantly or the second doses of ProQuad and VAQTA separately. The race distribution of the study subjects was as follows: 60.3% Caucasian, 21.6% African-American; 9.5% Hispanic-American; 7.2% other; 1.1% Asian; and 0.3% Native American. The distribution of subjects by gender was 50.7% male and 49.3% female.

Table 1 presents rates of solicited local reactions at the VAQTA injection site and rates of elevated temperatures (≥100.4°F and ≥102.2°F) that occurred within 5 days following each dose of VAQTA and elevated temperatures >98.6°F for a total of 14 days after vaccination; occurrences of these events were recorded daily on diary cards. Table 2 presents rates of unsolicited systemic adverse events that occurred within 14 days at ≥5% in any group following each dose of VAQTA.

[See table 1 at top of previous page]
[See table 2 above]

In Stage I of an open, multicenter, randomized study, children 15 months of age were randomized to receive the first dose of VAQTA alone (N=151) or concomitantly with PedvaxHIB and INFANRIX (N=155); another group of children 15 months of age were randomized to receive the first dose of VAQTA alone (N=152) or concomitantly with PedvaxHIB (N=159). All groups received the second dose of VAQTA alone at least 6 months following the first dose. The race distribution of Stage I study subjects was: 63.9% Caucasian; 17.5% Hispanic-American; 14.7% Black; 2.6% other; and 1.3% Asian. The distribution of subjects by gender was 54.0% male and 46.0% female. In Stage II of this study, an additional 654 children 12-17 months of age received the first dose of VAQTA alone followed by the second dose of VAQTA 6 months later. The race distribution of Stage II of the study subjects was: 66.1% Caucasian; 10.6% Hispanic-American; 16.8% Black; 4.7% other; and 1.5% Asian. The distribution of subjects by gender was 51.2% male and 48.8% female.

Table 3 presents rates of solicited local reactions at the VAQTA injection-site and rates of elevated temperatures (≥100.4°F and ≥102.2°F) that occurred within 5 days following each dose of VAQTA and elevated temperatures >98.6°F for a total of 14 days following each dose of VAQTA. Occurrences of these events were recorded daily on diary cards. Table 4 presents rates of unsolicited systemic adverse events that occurred within 14 days at ≥5% following each dose of VAQTA.

[See table 3 above]
[See table 4 at top of next page]

Data presented in Tables 1 through 4 on solicited local reactions, and solicited and unsolicited systemic adverse events with incidence ≥5% following each dose of VAQTA are representative of other clinical trials of VAQTA in children 12 through 23 months of age. Across the five studies conducted in children 12-23 months of age, ≥39.9% of subjects experienced local adverse reactions and ≥55.7% of subjects experienced systemic adverse events. The majority of local and systemic adverse events were mild to moderate in intensity.

The following additional unsolicited local adverse reactions and systemic adverse events were observed at a common frequency of ≥1% to <10% in any individual clinical study. This listing includes only the adverse reactions not reported elsewhere in the label. These local adverse reactions and systemic adverse events occurred among recipients of VAQTA alone or VAQTA given concomitantly within 14 days following any dose of VAQTA across four clinical studies.

Eye disorders: Conjunctivitis
Gastrointestinal disorders: Constipation; vomiting
General disorders and administration site conditions: Injection-site bruising; injection-site ecchymosis
Infections and infestations: Otitis media; nasopharyngitis; rhinitis; viral infection; croup; pharyngitis streptococcal; laryngotracheobronchitis; viral exanthema; gastroenteritis viral; roseola
Metabolism and nutrition disorders: Anorexia
Psychiatric disorders: Insomnia; crying
Respiratory, thoracic and mediastinal disorders: Cough; nasal congestion; respiratory congestion
Skin and subcutaneous tissue disorders: Rash vesicular; measles-like/rubella-like rash; varicella-like rash; rash morbilliform

Serious Adverse Events (Children 12 through 23 Months of Age): Across the five studies conducted in subjects 12-23 months of age, 0.7% (32/4374) of subjects reported a serious adverse event following any dose of VAQTA, and 0.1% (5/4374) of subjects reported a serious adverse event judged to be vaccine related by the study investigator. The serious adverse events were collected over the period defined in each protocol (14, 28, or 42 days). Vaccine-related serious adverse events which occurred following any dose of VAQTA with or without concomitant vaccines included febrile seizure (0.05%), dehydration (0.02%), gastroenteritis (0.02%), and cellulitis (0.02%).

Children / Adolescents — 2 Years through 18 Years of Age
In 11 clinical trials, 2615 healthy children 2 years through 18 years of age received at least one dose of VAQTA. These studies included administration of VAQTA in varying doses and regimens (1377 children received one or more 25U doses). The race distribution of the study subjects who received at least one dose of VAQTA in these studies was as follows: 84.7% Caucasian; 10.6% American Indian; 2.3% African-American; 1.5% Hispanic-American; 0.6% other; 0.2% Oriental. The distribution of subjects by gender was 51.2% male and 48.8% female.

In a double-blind, placebo-controlled efficacy trial (i.e. The Monroe Efficacy Study), 1037 healthy children and adolescents 2 through 16 years of age were randomized to receive a primary dose of 25U of VAQTA and a booster dose of VAQTA 6, 12, or 18 months later, or placebo (alum diluent). All study subjects were Caucasian: 51.5% were male and 48.5% were female. Subjects were followed days 1 to 5 postvaccination for fever and local adverse reactions and days 1 to 14 for systemic adverse events. The most common adverse events/reactions were injection site reactions, reported by 6.4% of subjects. Table 5 summarizes local adverse reactions and systemic adverse events reported in ≥1% of subjects. There were no significant differences in the rates of any adverse events or adverse reactions between vaccine and placebo recipients after Dose 1.

Table 5: Local Adverse Reactions and Systemic Adverse Events (≥1%) in Healthy Children and Adolescents from the Monroe Efficacy Study

Adverse Event	VAQTA (N=519)		Placebo (Alum Diluent)*,†,‡ (N=518) Rate (Percent)
	Dose 1* Rate (Percent)	Booster Rate (Percent)	
Injection Site§	n=515	n=475	n=510
Pain	6.4%	3.4%	6.3%
Tenderness	4.9%	1.7%	6.1%
Erythema	1.9%	0.8%	1.8%
Swelling	1.7%	1.5%	1.6%
Warmth	1.7%	0.6%	1.6%

Table 4: Incidences of Unsolicited Systemic Adverse Events ≥5% in Any Group Following Each Dose of VAQTA in Healthy Children 12-23 Months of Age Receiving VAQTA Alone or Concomitantly with PedvaxHIB With or Without INFANRIX (Stage I) and Those Receiving VAQTA Alone at Both Doses (Stage II)

Adverse Event: Days 1-14	Stage I			Stage II	
	Dose 1		Dose 2	Dose 1	Dose 2
	VAQTA alone	VAQTA + PedvaxHIB and Infanrix or VAQTA + PedvaxHIB concomitantly	VAQTA alone	VAQTA alone	VAQTA alone
	N=256	N=302	N=503	N=647	N=599
Gastrointestinal Disorders					
Diarrhea	3.9%	8.3%	3.8%	4.6%	3.8%
Teething	3.1%	2.3%	1.4%	5.7%	4.3%
General Disorders and Administration Site Conditions					
Irritability	6.3%	9.6%	4.0%	8.8%	6.5%
Infections and Infestations					
Upper respiratory tract infection	2.3%	3.3%	3.0%	4.9%	5.2%
Respiratory, Thoracic and Mediastinal Disorders					
Rhinorrhea	2.0%	4.0%	3.8%	6.2%	3.8%

Systemic[¶]	n=519	n=475	n=518
Abdominal pain	1.2%	1.1%	1.0%
Pharyngitis	1.2%	0%	0.8%
Headache	0.4%	0.8%	1.0%

N=Number of subjects enrolled/randomized.
Percent=percentage of subjects for whom data are available with adverse event
n=number of subjects for whom adverse events available
* No statistically significant differences between the two groups.
† Second injection of placebo not administered because code for the trial was broken.
‡ Placebo (Alum diluent) = amorphous aluminum hydroxyphosphate sulfate.
§ Adverse Reactions at the injection site (VAQTA) Days 1-5 after vaccination with VAQTA
¶ Systemic adverse events reported Days 1-15 after vaccination, regardless of causality.

Adults — 19 Years of Age and Older
In an open-label clinical trial, 240 healthy adults 18 to 54 years of age were randomized to receive either VAQTA (50U/1-mL) with Typhim Vi (Typhoid Vi polysaccharide vaccine) and YF-Vax (yellow fever vaccine) concomitantly (N=80), typhoid Vi polysaccharide and yellow fever vaccines concomitantly (N=80), or VAQTA alone (N=80). Approximately 6 months later, subjects who received VAQTA were administered a second dose of VAQTA. The race distribution of the study subjects who received VAQTA with or without typhoid Vi polysaccharide and yellow fever vaccine was as follows: 78.3% Caucasian; 14.2% Oriental; 3.3% other; 2.1% African-American; 1.7% Indian; 0.4% Hispanic-American. The distribution of subjects by gender was 40.8% male and 59.2% female. Subjects were monitored for local adverse reactions and fever for 5 days and systemic adverse events for 14 days after each vaccination. In the 14 days after the first dose of VAQTA, the proportion of subjects with adverse events was similar between recipients of VAQTA given concomitantly with typhoid Vi polysaccharide and yellow fever vaccines compared to recipients of typhoid Vi polysaccharide and yellow fever vaccines without VAQTA. Table 6 summarizes solicited local adverse reactions and Table 7 summarizes unsolicited systemic adverse events reported in ≥5% in adults who received one or two doses of VAQTA alone and for subjects who received VAQTA concomitantly with typhoid Vi polysaccharide and yellow fever vaccines. There were no solicited systemic complaints reported at a rate ≥5%. Fever ≥101°F occurred in 1.3% of subjects in each group.

Table 6: Incidences of Solicited Local Adverse Reactions in Healthy Adults ≥19 Years of Age Occurring at ≥5% After Any Dose

Adverse Event	VAQTA administered alone (N=80)	VAQTA + ViCPS* and Yellow Fever vaccines administered concomitantly[†] (N=80)
	Rate (Percent)	
Injection-site[‡]		
Pain/tenderness/soreness	78.8%	70.3%
Warmth	23.7%	23.7%
Swelling	16.2%	8.8%
Erythema	17.5%	6.3%

N=Number of subjects enrolled/randomized.
Percent=percentage of subjects with adverse event.
* ViCPS=Typhoid Vi polysaccharide vaccine.
† VAQTA administered concomitantly with typhoid Vi polysaccharide (ViCPS) and yellow fever vaccines.
‡ Adverse Reactions at the injection site (VAQTA) Days 1-5 after vaccination

Table 7: Incidences of Unsolicited Systemic Adverse Events in Adults ≥19 Years of Age Occurring at ≥5% After Any Dose

Body System Adverse Event	VAQTA administered alone (N=80)	VAQTA + ViCPS* and Yellow Fever vaccines administered concomitantly[†] (N=80)
	Rate (Percent)	
General disorders and administration site reactions[‡]		
Asthenia/fatigue	7.5%	11.3%
Chills	1.3%	7.5%
Gastrointestinal disorders[‡]		
Nausea	7.5%	12.5%

Musculoskeletal and connective tissue disorders[‡]

Myalgia	5.0%	10.0%
Arm pain	0.0%	6.3%

Nervous system disorders[‡]

Headache	23.8%	26.3%

Infections and infestations[‡]

Upper respiratory infection	7.5%	3.8%
Pharyngitis	2.5%	6.3%

N=Number of subjects enrolled/randomized with data available.
Percent=percentage of subjects with adverse event for whom data are available.
* ViCPS=Typhoid Vi polysaccharide vaccine.
† VAQTA administered concomitantly with typhoid Vi polysaccharide (ViCPS) and yellow fever vaccines.
‡ Systemic Adverse Events reported Days 1-15 after vaccination, regardless of causality.

In four clinical trials involving 1645 healthy adults 19 years of age and older who received one or more 50U doses of hepatitis A vaccine, subjects were followed for fever and local adverse reactions 1 to 5 days postvaccination and for systemic adverse events 1 to 14 days postvaccination. One single-blind study evaluated doses of VAQTA with varying amounts of viral antigen and/or alum content in healthy adults ≥170 pounds and ≥30 years of age (N=210 adults administered 50U/1-mL). One open-label study evaluated VAQTA given with immune globulin (IG) or alone (N=164 adults who received VAQTA alone). A third study was single-blind and evaluated 3 different lots of VAQTA (N=1112). The fourth study that was also single-blind evaluated doses of VAQTA with varying amounts of viral antigen in healthy adults ≥170 pounds and ≥30 years of age (N=159 adults administered the 50U/1-mL dose). Overall, the race distribution of the study subjects who received at least one dose of VAQTA was as follows: 94.2% Caucasian; 2.2% Black; 1.5% Hispanic; 1.5% Oriental; 0.4% other; 0.2% American Indian. 47.6% of subjects were male and 52.4% were female. The most common adverse event/reaction was injection-site pain/soreness/tenderness reported by 67.0% of subjects. Of all reported injection-site reactions 99.8% were mild (*i.e.*, easily tolerated with no medical intervention) or moderate (*i.e.*, minimally interfered with usual activity possibly requiring little medical intervention). Listed below in Table 8 are the local adverse reactions and systemic adverse events reported by ≥5% of subjects, in decreasing order of frequency within each body system.

Table 8: Incidences of Local Adverse Reactions and Systemic Adverse Events ≥5% in Adults 19 Years of Age and Older

Body System Adverse Events	VAQTA (Any Dose) (N=1645) Rate (n/total n)
Nervous system disorders*	n=1641
Headache	16.1%
General disorders and administration site reactions[†]	n=1640
Injection-site pain/tenderness/soreness	67.0%
Injection-site warmth	18.2%
Injection-site swelling	14.7%
Injection-site erythema	13.7%

N=Number of subjects enrolled/randomized.
n=Number of subjects in each category with data available.
Percent=percentage of subjects for whom data are available with adverse event.
* Systemic Adverse Events reported Days 1 to 14 after vaccination, regardless of causality.
† Adverse Reactions at the injection site (VAQTA) and measured fever Days 1 to 5 after vaccination.

The following additional unsolicited systemic adverse events were observed among recipients of VAQTA that occurred within 14 days at a common frequency of ≥1% to

<10% following any dose not reported elsewhere in the label. These adverse reactions have been reported across 4 clinical studies.

Musculoskeletal and connective tissue disorders: Back pain; stiffness

Reproductive system and breast disorders: Menstruation disorders

6.2 Post-Marketing Experience

The following additional adverse events have been reported with use of the marketed vaccine. Because these reactions are reported voluntarily from a population of uncertain size, it is not possible to reliably estimate their frequency or establish a causal relationship to a vaccine exposure.

Blood and lymphatic disorders: Thrombocytopenia.

Nervous system disorders: Guillain-Barré syndrome; cerebellar ataxia; encephalitis.

Post-Marketing Observational Safety Study

In a post-marketing, 60-day safety surveillance study, conducted at a large health maintenance organization in the United States, a total of 42,110 individuals ≥2 years of age received 1 or 2 doses of VAQTA (13,735 children/adolescents and 28,375 adult subjects). Safety was passively monitored by electronic search of the automated medical records database for emergency room and outpatient visits, hospitalizations, and deaths. Medical charts were reviewed when an event was considered to be possibly vaccine-related by the investigator. None of the serious adverse events identified were assessed as being related to vaccine by the investigator. Diarrhea/gastroenteritis, resulting in outpatient visits, was determined by the investigator to be the only vaccine-related nonserious adverse reaction in the study. There was no vaccine-related adverse reaction identified that had not been reported in earlier clinical trials with VAQTA.

7 DRUG INTERACTIONS
7.1 Use with Other Vaccines

Do not mix VAQTA with any other vaccine in the same syringe or vial. Use separate injection sites and syringes for each vaccine. Please refer to package inserts of coadministered vaccines.

In clinical trials in children, VAQTA was concomitantly administered with one or more of the following US licensed vaccines: Measles, Mumps, and Rubella Virus Vaccine, Live; Varicella Vaccine, Live; Diphtheria and Tetanus Toxoids and Acellular Pertussis Vaccine, Adsorbed; Measles, Mumps, Rubella, and Varicella Vaccine, Live; Pneumococcal 7-valent Conjugate Vaccine (Diphtheria CRM$_{197}$); and Haemophilus B Conjugate Vaccine (Meningococcal Protein Conjugate). Safety and immunogenicity were similar for concomitantly administered vaccines compared to separately administered vaccines.

In clinical trials in adults, VAQTA was concomitantly administered with typhoid Vi polysaccharide and yellow fever vaccines *[see Adverse Reactions (6.1) and Clinical Studies (14.2, 14.7)]*. Safety and immunogenicity were similar for concomitantly administered vaccines compared to separately administered vaccines.

7.2 Use with Immune Globulin

VAQTA may be administered concomitantly with Immune Globulin, human, using separate sites and syringes. The recommended vaccination regimen for VAQTA should be followed. Consult the manufacturer's product circular for the appropriate dosage of Immune Globulin. A booster dose of VAQTA should be administered at the appropriate time as outlined in the recommended regimen for VAQTA *[see Clinical Studies (14.5)]*.

7.3 Immunosuppressive Therapy

If VAQTA is administered to a person receiving immunosuppressive therapy, an adequate immunologic response may not be obtained.

8 USE IN SPECIFIC POPULATIONS
8.1 Pregnancy

Pregnancy Category C: Animal reproduction studies have not been conducted with VAQTA. It is also not known whether VAQTA can cause fetal harm when administered to a pregnant woman or can affect reproduction capacity. VAQTA should be given to a pregnant woman only if clearly needed.

8.3 Nursing Mothers

It is not known whether VAQTA is excreted in human milk. Because many drugs are excreted in human milk, caution should be exercised when VAQTA is administered to a nursing woman.

8.4 Pediatric Use

The safety of VAQTA has been evaluated in 4374 children 12 through 23 months of age, and 2615 children/adolescents 2 through 18 years of age who received at least one 25U dose of VAQTA *[see Adverse Reactions (6) and Dosage and Administration (2)]*.

Safety and effectiveness in infants below 12 months of age have not been established.

8.5 Geriatric Use

In the post-marketing observational safety study which included 42,110 persons who received VAQTA *[see Adverse Re-*

actions (6.2)], 4769 persons were 65 years of age or older and 1073 persons were 75 years of age or older. There were no adverse events judged by the investigator to be vaccine-related in the geriatric study population. In other clinical studies, 68 subjects 65 years of age or older were vaccinated with VAQTA, 10 of whom were 75 years of age or older. No overall differences in safety and immunogenicity were observed between these subjects and younger subjects; however, greater sensitivity of some older individuals cannot be ruled out. Other reported clinical experience has not identified differences in responses between the elderly and younger subjects.

8.6 Immunocompromised Individuals

Immunocompromised persons may have a diminished immune response to VAQTA and may not be protected against HAV infection.

11 DESCRIPTION

VAQTA is an inactivated whole virus vaccine derived from hepatitis A virus grown in cell culture in human MRC-5 diploid fibroblasts. It contains inactivated virus of a strain which was originally derived by further serial passage of a proven attenuated strain. The virus is grown, harvested, purified by a combination of physical and high performance liquid chromatographic techniques developed at the Merck Research Laboratories, formalin inactivated, and then adsorbed onto amorphous aluminum hydroxyphosphate sulfate.

VAQTA is a sterile suspension for intramuscular injection. One milliliter of the vaccine contains approximately 50U of hepatitis A virus antigen, which is purified and formulated without a preservative. Within the limits of current assay variability, the 50U dose of VAQTA contains less than 0.1 mcg of non-viral protein, less than 4×10^{-6} mcg of DNA, less than 10^{-4} mcg of bovine albumin, and less than 0.8 mcg of formaldehyde. Other process chemical residuals are less than 10 parts per billion (ppb), including neomycin.

Each 0.5-mL pediatric dose contains 25U of hepatitis A virus antigen and adsorbed onto approximately 0.225 mg of aluminum provided as amorphous aluminum hydroxyphosphate sulfate, and 35 mcg of sodium borate as a pH stabilizer, in 0.9% sodium chloride.

Each 1-mL adult dose contains 50U of hepatitis A virus antigen and adsorbed onto approximately 0.45 mg of aluminum provided as amorphous aluminum hydroxyphosphate sulfate, and 70 mcg of sodium borate as a pH stabilizer, in 0.9% sodium chloride.

12 CLINICAL PHARMACOLOGY
12.1 Mechanism of Action

VAQTA has been shown to elicit antibodies to hepatitis A as measured by ELISA.

Protection from hepatitis A disease has been shown to be related to the presence of antibody. However, the lowest titer needed to confer protection has not been determined.

13 NONCLINICAL TOXICOLOGY
13.1 Carcinogenesis, Mutagenesis, Impairment of Fertility

VAQTA has not been evaluated for its carcinogenic or mutagenic potential, or its potential to impair fertility.

14 CLINICAL STUDIES
14.1 Efficacy of VAQTA: The Monroe Clinical Study

The immunogenicity and protective efficacy of VAQTA were evaluated in a randomized, double-blind, placebo-controlled study involving 1037 susceptible healthy children and adolescents 2 through 16 years of age in a U.S. community with recurrent outbreaks of hepatitis A (The Monroe Efficacy Study). All of these children were Caucasian, and there were 51.5% male and 48.5% female. Each child received an intramuscular dose of VAQTA (25U) (N=519) or placebo (alum diluent) (N=518). Among those individuals who were initially seronegative (measured by a modification of the HAVAB radioimmunoassay[1] [RIA]), seroconversion was achieved in >99% of vaccine recipients within 4 weeks after vaccination. The onset of seroconversion following a single dose of VAQTA was shown to parallel the onset of protection against clinical hepatitis A disease.

Because of the long incubation period of the disease (approximately 20 to 50 days, or longer in children), clinical efficacy was based on confirmed cases[1] of hepatitis A occurring ≥50 days after vaccination in order to exclude any children incubating the infection before vaccination. In subjects who were initially seronegative, the protective efficacy of a single dose of VAQTA was observed to be 100% with 21 cases of clinically confirmed hepatitis A occurring in the placebo group and none in the vaccine group (p<0.001). The number of clinically confirmed cases of hepatitis A ≥30 days after vaccination were also compared. In this analysis, 28 cases of clinically confirmed hepatitis A occurred in the placebo group while none occurred in the vaccine group ≥30 days after vaccination. In addition, it was observed in this trial that no cases of clinically confirmed hepatitis A occurred in the vaccine group after day 16.[2] Following demonstration of

protection with a single dose and termination of the study, a booster dose was administered to a subset of vaccinees 6, 12, or 18 months after the primary dose.

No cases of clinically confirmed hepatitis A disease ≥50 days after vaccination have occurred in those vaccinees from The Monroe Efficacy Study monitored for up to 9 years.

---

[1] The clinical case definition included all of the following occurring at the same time: 1) one or more typical clinical signs or symptoms of hepatitis A (*e.g.*, jaundice, malaise, fever ≥38.3°C); 2) elevation of hepatitis A IgM antibody (HAVAB-M); 3) elevation of alanine transferase (ALT) ≥2 times the upper limit of normal.

[2] One vaccinee did not meet the pre-defined criteria for clinically confirmed hepatitis A but did have positive hepatitis A IgM and borderline liver enzyme (ALT) elevations on days 34, 50, and 58 after vaccination with mild clinical symptoms observed on days 49 and 50.

14.2 Other Clinical Studies

The efficacy of VAQTA in other age groups was based upon immunogenicity measured 4 to 6 weeks following vaccination. VAQTA was found to be immunogenic in all age groups.

Children — 12 through 23 Months of Age

In a clinical trial, children 12 through 23 months of age were randomized to receive the first dose of VAQTA with or without M-M-R II and VARIVAX (N=617) and the second dose of VAQTA with or without Tripedia and optionally either oral poliovirus vaccine (no longer licensed in the US) or IPOL (N=555). The race distribution of study subjects who received at least one dose of VAQTA was as follows: 56.7% Caucasian; 17.5% Hispanic-American; 14.3% African-American; 7.0% Native American; 3.4% other; 0.8% Oriental; 0.2% Asian; and 0.2% Indian. The distribution of subjects by gender was 53.6% male and 46.4% female. In the analysis population, there were 471 initially seronegative children 12 through 23 months of age, who received the first dose of VAQTA with (N=237) or without (N=234) M-M-R II and VARIVAX of whom 96% (95% CI: 93.7%, 97.5%) seroconverted (defined as having an anti-HAV titer ≥10 mIU/mL) post dose 1 with an anti-HAV geometric mean titer (GMT) of 48 mIU/mL (95% CI: 44.7, 51.6). There were 343 children in the analysis population who received the second dose of VAQTA with (N=168) or without (N=175) Tripedia and optional oral poliovirus vaccine or IPOL of whom 100% (95% CI: 99.3%, 100%) seroconverted post dose 2 with an anti-HAV GMT of 6920 mIU/mL (95% CI: 6136, 7801). Of children who received only VAQTA at both visits, 100% (n=97) seroconverted after the second dose of VAQTA.

In a clinical trial involving 653 healthy children 12 to 15 months of age, 330 were randomized to receive VAQTA, ProQuad, and pneumococcal 7-valent conjugate vaccine concomitantly, and 323 were randomized to receive ProQuad and pneumococcal 7-valent conjugate vaccine concomitantly followed by VAQTA 6 weeks later. The race distribution of the study subjects was as follows: 60.3% Caucasian; 21.6% African-American; 9.5% Hispanic-American; 7.2% other; 1.1% Asian/Pacific; and 0.3% Native American. The distribution of subjects by gender was 50.7% male and 49.3% female. In the analysis population, the seropositivity rate for hepatitis A antibody (defined as the percent of subjects with an anti-HAV titer ≥10 mIU/mL) was 100% (n=182; 95% CI: 98.0%, 100%) post dose 2 with an anti-HAV GMT of 4977 mIU/mL (95% CI: 4068, 6089) when VAQTA was given with ProQuad and pneumococcal 7-valent conjugate vaccine and 99.4% (n=159, 95% CI: 96.5%, 100%) post dose 2 with an anti-HAV GMT of 6123 mIU/mL (95% CI: 4826, 7770) when VAQTA alone was given. These seropositivity rates were similar whether VAQTA was administered with or without ProQuad and pneumococcal 7-valent conjugate vaccine.

In an open, multicenter, randomized study involving 617 children 15 months of age, 306 were randomized to receive VAQTA with or without PedvaxHIB and INFANRIX, and 311 were randomized to receive VAQTA with or without PedvaxHIB. The race distribution of the study subjects was as follows: 63.9% Caucasian; 17.5% Hispanic-American; 14.7% Black; 2.6% other; and 1.3% Asian. The distribution of subjects by gender was 54.0% male and 46.0% female. The seropositivity rate for hepatitis A antibody (defined as the percent of subjects with an anti-HAV titer ≥ 10 mIU/mL) 4 weeks post dose 2 was 100% (n=208, 95% CI: 98.2%, 100.0%) in those who received VAQTA concomitantly with PedvaxHIB and INFANRIX or concomitantly with PedvaxHIB. In those subjects who received VAQTA alone, the seropositivity rate for hepatitis A antibody was 100% (n=183, 95% CI: 98.0%, 100.0%), regardless of baseline hepatitis A serostatus. Overall, the anti-HAV GMT in the concomitant groups was 3616.5 mIU/mL (95% CI: 3084.5, 4240.2). The anti-HAV GMT in the nonconcomitant groups was 4712.6 mIU/mL (95% CI: 3996.8, 5556.8). Comparable responses were observed in both the initially seronegative and seropositive subjects.

In three combined clinical studies 1022 initially seronegative subjects received 2 doses of VAQTA alone or concomitantly with other vaccines. Of the seronegative subjects, 99.9% achieved an anti-HAV titer ≥10 mIU/mL (95% CI: 99.5%, 100%) and an anti-HAV GMT of 5392.1 mIU/mL (95% CI: 4996.5, 5819.0) 4 weeks following dose 2 of VAQTA.

Children/Adolescents — 2 Years through 18 Years of Age
Immunogenicity data were combined from eleven randomized clinical studies in children and adolescents 2 through 18 years of age who received VAQTA (25U/0.5 mL). These included administration of VAQTA in varying doses and regimens (N=404 received 25U/0.5 mL), the Monroe Efficacy Study (N=973), and comparison studies for process and formulation changes (N=1238). The race distribution of the study subjects who received at least one dose of VAQTA in these studies was as follows: 84.8% Caucasian; 10.6% American Indian; 2.3% African-American; 1.5% Hispanic-American; 0.6% other; 0.2% Oriental. The distribution of subjects by gender was 51.2% male and 48.8% female. The proportions of subjects who seroconverted 4 weeks after the first and second doses administered 6 months apart were 97% (n=1230; 95% CI: 96%, 98%) and 100% (n=1057; 95% CI: 99.5%, 100%) of subjects with anti-HAV GMTs of 43 mIU/mL (95% CI: 40, 45) and 10,077 mIU/mL (95% CI: 9394, 10,810), respectively.

Adults — 19 Years of Age and Older
Immunogenicity data were combined from five randomized clinical studies in adults 19 years of age and older who received VAQTA (50U/1-mL). One single-blind study evaluated doses of VAQTA with varying amounts of viral antigen and/or alum content in healthy adults ≥170 pounds and ≥30 years of age (N=208 adults administered 50U/1-mL dose). One open-label study evaluated VAQTA given with immune globulin or alone (N=164 adults who received VAQTA alone). A third study was single-blind and evaluated 3 different lots of VAQTA (N=1112). The fourth study was single-blind and evaluated doses of VAQTA with varying amounts of viral antigen in healthy adults ≥170 pounds and ≥30 years of age (N=159 adults administered the 50U/1-mL dose). The fifth study was an open-label study to evaluate various regimens for time of administration of the booster dose of VAQTA (6, 12, and 18 months post dose 1, N=354). The race distribution of the study subjects who received at least one dose of VAQTA in these studies was as follows: 93.2% Caucasian; 2.5% African-American; 2.1% Hispanic-American; 1.4% Oriental; 0.5% other; 0.3% American Indian. The distribution of subjects by gender was 44.8% male and 55.2% female. The proportion of subjects who seroconverted 4 weeks after the first and second doses administered 6 months apart was 95% (n=1411; 95% CI: 94%, 96%) and 99.9% (n=1244; 95% CI: 99.4%, 100%) with GMTs of 37 mIU/mL (95% CI: 35, 38) and 6013 mIU/mL (95% CI: 5592, 6467), respectively. Furthermore, at 2 weeks postvaccination, 69.2% (n=744; 95% CI: 65.7%, 72.5%) of adults seroconverted with an anti-HAV GMT of 16 mIU/mL after a single dose of VAQTA.

14.3 Timing of Booster Dose Administration
Children/Adolescents — 2 through 18 Years of Age
In the Monroe Efficacy Study, children were administered a second dose of VAQTA (25U/0.5 mL) 6, 12, or 18 months following the initial dose. For subjects who received both doses of VAQTA, the GMTs and proportions of subjects who seroconverted 4 weeks after the booster dose administered 6, 12, and 18 months after the first dose are presented in Table 9. [See table 9 above]

Adults — 19 years of age and older
Among the 5 randomized clinical studies in adults 19 years of age and older described in Section 14.2, there were additional data in which a booster dose of VAQTA (50U/1-mL) was administered 12 or 18 months after the first dose. For subjects in these studies who received both doses of VAQTA, the proportions who seroconverted 4 weeks after the booster dose administered 6, 12, and 18 months after the first dose were 100% of 1201 subjects, 98% of 91 subjects, and 100% of 84 subjects, respectively. GMTs in mIU/mL one month after the subjects received the booster dose at 6, 12, or 18 months after the primary dose were 5987 mIU/mL (95% CI: 5561, 6445), 4896 mIU/mL (95% CI: 3589, 6679), and 6043 mIU/mL (95% CI: 4687, 7793), respectively.

14.4 Duration of Immune Response
In follow-up of subjects in The Monroe Efficacy Study, in children (≥2 years of age) and adolescents who received two doses (25U) of VAQTA, detectable levels of anti-HAV antibodies (≥10 mIU/mL) were present in 100% of subjects for at least 10 years postvaccination. In subjects who received VAQTA at 0 and 6 months, the GMT was 819 mIU/mL (n=175) at 2.5 to 3.5 years and 505 mIU/mL (n=174) at 5 to 6 years, and 574 mIU/mL (n=114) at 10 years postvaccination. In subjects who received VAQTA at 0 and 12 months, the GMT was 2224 mIU/mL (n=49) at 2.5 to 3.5 years, 1191 mIU/mL (n=47) at 5 to 6 years, and 1005 mIU/mL (n=36) at 10 years postvaccination. In subjects who received VAQTA at 0 and 18 months, the GMT was 2501 mIU/mL (n=53) at 2.5 to 3.5 years, 1614 mIU/mL (n=56) at 5 to 6 years, and 1507 mIU/mL (n=41) at 10 years postvaccination.

Table 9: Children/Adolescents from the Monroe Efficacy Study Seroconversion Rates (%) and Geometric Mean Titers (GMT) for Cohorts of Initially Seronegative Vaccinees at the Time of the Booster(25U) and 4 Weeks Later

Months Following Initial 25U Dose	Cohort* (n=960) 0 and 6 Months	Cohort* (n=35) 0 and 12 Months	Cohort* (n=39) 0 and 18 Months
	Seroconversion Rate GMT (mIU/mL) (95% CI)		
6	97% 107 (98, 117)	—	—
7	100% 10433 (9681, 11243)	—	—
12	—	91% 48 (33, 71)	—
13	—	100% 12308 (9337, 16226)	—
18	—	—	90% 50 (28, 89)
19	—	—	100% 9591 (7613, 12082)

* Blood samples were taken at prebooster and postbooster time points.

In adults that were administered VAQTA at 0 and 6 months, the hepatitis A antibody response to date has been shown to persist at least 6 years. Detectable levels of anti-HAV antibodies (≥10 mIU/mL) were present in 100% (378/378) of subjects with a GMT of 1734 mIU/mL at 1 year, 99.2% (252/254) of subjects with a GMT of 687 mIU/mL at 2 to 3 years, 99.1% (219/221) of subjects with a GMT of 605 mIU/mL at 4 years, and 99.4% (170/171) of subjects with a GMT of 684 mIU/mL at 6 years postvaccination.

The total duration of the protective effect of VAQTA in healthy vaccinees is unknown at present.

14.5 Concomitant Administration of VAQTA and Immune Globulin
The concurrent use of VAQTA (50U) and immune globulin (IG, 0.06 mL/kg) was evaluated in an open-label, randomized clinical study involving 294 healthy adults 18 to 39 years of age. Adults were randomized to receive 2 doses of VAQTA 24 weeks apart (N=129), the first dose of VAQTA concomitant with a dose of IG followed by the second dose of VAQTA alone 24 weeks later (N=135), or IG alone (N=30). The race distribution of the study subjects who received at least one dose of VAQTA or IG in this study was as follows: 92.3% Caucasian; 4.0% Hispanic-American; 3.0% African-American; 0.3% Native American; 0.3% Asian/Pacific. The distribution of subjects by gender was 28.7% male and 71.3% female. Table 10 provides seroconversion rates and GMTs at 4 and 24 weeks after the first dose in each treatment group and at one month after a booster dose of VAQTA (administered at 24 weeks) *[see Drug Interactions (7.2)]*.

Table 10: Seroconversion Rates (%) and Geometric Mean Titers (GMT) After Vaccination with VAQTA Plus IG, VAQTA Alone, and IG Alone

Weeks	VAQTA plus IG	VAQTA	IG
	Seroconversion Rate GMT (mIU/mL) (95% CI)		
4	100% 42 (39, 45) (n=129)	96% 38 (33, 42) (n=135)	87% 19 (15, 23) (n=30)
24	92% 83 (65, 105) (n=125)	97%* 137*(112, 169) (n=132)	0% Undetectable† (n=28)
28	100% 4872 (3716, 6388) (n=114)	100% 6498 (5111, 8261) (n=128)	N/A

N/A = Not Applicable.
* The seroconversion rate and the GMT in the group receiving VAQTA alone were significantly higher than in the group receiving VAQTA plus IG (p=0.05, p<0.001, respectively).
† Undetectable is defined as <10mIU/mL.

14.6 Interchangeability of the Booster Dose
A randomized, double-blind clinical study in 537 healthy adults, 18 to 83 years of age, evaluated the immune response to a booster dose of VAQTA and HAVRIX given at 6 or 12 months following an initial dose of HAVRIX. Subjects

were randomized to receive VAQTA (50U) as a booster dose 6 months (N=232) or 12 months (N=124) following an initial dose of HAVRIX or HAVRIX (1440 EL. U) as a booster dose 6 months (N=118) or 12 months (N=63) following an initial dose of HAVRIX. The race distribution of the study subjects who received the booster dose of VAQTA or HAVRIX in this study was as follows: 87.2% Caucasian; 8.0% African-American; 1.9% Hispanic-American; 1.3% Oriental; 0.9% Asian; 0.4% Indian; 0.4% other. The distribution of subjects by gender was 44.9% male and 55.1% female. When VAQTA was given as a booster dose following HAVRIX, the vaccine produced an adequate immune response (see Table 11) *[see Dosage and Administration (2.1)]*.

[See table 11 at top of next page]

14.7 Immune Response to Concomitantly Administered Vaccines
Clinical Studies of VAQTA with M-M-R II, VARIVAX, and Tripedia
In the clinical trial in which children 12 months of age received the first dose of VAQTA concomitantly with M-M-R II and VARIVAX described in Section 14.2, rates of seroprotection to hepatitis A were similar between the two groups who received VAQTA with or without M-M-R II and VARIVAX. Measles, mumps, and rubella immune responses were tested in 241 subjects, 263 subjects, and 270 subjects, respectively. Seropositivity rates were 98.8% [95% CI: 96.4%, 99.7%] for measles, 99.6% [95% CI: 97.9%, 100%] for mumps, and 100% [95% CI: 98.6%, 100%] for rubella, which were similar to observed historical rates (seropositivity rates 99% for all three antigens, with lower bound of the 95% CI >89%) following vaccination with a first dose of M-M-R II in this age group. Data from this study were insufficient to adequately assess the immune response to VARIVAX administered concomitantly with VAQTA. In this same study, the second dose of VAQTA at 18 months of age was given with or without Tripedia (DTaP). Seropositivity rates for diphtheria and tetanus were similar to those in historical controls. However, data from this study were insufficient to assess the pertussis response of DTaP when administered with VAQTA. Rates of seroprotection to hepatitis A were similar between the two groups who received VAQTA with or without M-M-R II and VARIVAX, and between the two groups who received VAQTA with or without DTaP.

Clinical Studies of VAQTA with ProQuad and Prevnar
In the clinical trial of concomitant use of VAQTA with ProQuad and pneumococcal 7-valent conjugate vaccine in children 12 to 15 months of age described in Section 14.2, the antibody GMTs for *S. pneumoniae* types 4, 6B, 9V, 14, 18C, 19F, and 23F 6 weeks after vaccination with pneumococcal 7-valent conjugate vaccine administered concomitantly with ProQuad and VAQTA were non-inferior as compared to GMTs observed in the group given pneumococcal 7-valent conjugate vaccine with ProQuad alone (the lower bounds of the 95% CI around the fold-difference for the 7 serotypes excluded 0.5). For the varicella component of ProQuad, in subjects with baseline antibody titers <1.25 gpELISA units/mL, the proportion with a titer ≥5 gpELISA units/mL 6 weeks after their first dose of ProQuad was non-inferior (defined as -10 percentage point change) when ProQuad was administered with VAQTA and pneumococcal 7-valent conjugate vaccine as compared to the proportion with a titer ≥5 gpELISA units/mL when ProQuad was administered with pneumococcal 7-valent conjugate vaccine alone (differ-

Table 11: Seropositivity Rate, Booster Response Rate* and Geometric Mean Titer 4 Weeks Following a Booster Dose of VAQTA or HAVRIX Administered 6 to 12 Months After First Dose of HAVRIX[†]

First Dose	Booster Dose	Seropositivity Rate	Booster Response Rate*	Geometric Mean Titer
HAVRIX 1440 EL.U.	VAQTA 50 U	99.7% (n=313)	86.1% (n=310)	3272 (n=313)
HAVRIX 1440 EL.U.	HAVRIX 1440 EL.U.	99.3% (n=151)	80.1% (n=151)	2423 (n=151)

* Booster Response Rate is defined as greater than or equal to a tenfold rise from prebooster to postbooster titer and postbooster titer ≥100 mIU/mL.
† Study conducted in adults 18 years of age and older.

ence in seroprotection rate -5.1% [95% CI: -9.3, -1.4%]). Hepatitis A responses were similar when compared between the two groups who received VAQTA with or without ProQuad and pneumococcal 7-valent conjugate vaccine. Seroconversion rates and antibody titers for varicella and *S. pneumoniae* types 4, 6B, 9V, 14, 18C, 19F, and 23F were similar between groups at 6 weeks postvaccination.

Clinical Studies of VAQTA with INFANRIX and PedvaxHIB
In the clinical trial of concomitant administration of VAQTA with INFANRIX and PedvaxHIB in children 15 months of age, described in Section 14.2, when the first dose of VAQTA was administered concomitantly with either INFANRIX and PedvaxHIB or PedvaxHIB, there was no interference in immune response to hepatitis A as measured by seropositivity rates after dose 2 of VAQTA compared to administration of both doses of VAQTA alone. When dose 1 of VAQTA was administered concomitantly with either PedvaxHIB and INFANRIX or PedvaxHIB, there was no interference in immune response to *Haemophilus influenzae b* (as measured by the proportion of subjects who attained an anti-polyribosylribitol phosphate antibody titer >1.0 mcg/mL at 4 weeks after vaccination), compared to subjects receiving either PedvaxHIB and INFANRIX or PedvaxHIB. When VAQTA was administered concomitantly with INFANRIX and PedvaxHIB, there was no interference in immune responses at 4 weeks after vaccination to the pertussis antigens (PT, FHA, or pertactin, as measured by GMTs) and no interference in immune responses to diphtheria toxoid or tetanus toxoid (as measured by the proportion of subjects achieving an antibody titer >0.1 IU/mL) compared to administration of INFANRIX and PedvaxHIB.

Clinical Studies of VAQTA with Typhoid Vi Polysaccharide Vaccine and Yellow Fever Vaccine, Live Attenuated
In the clinical trial of concomitant use of VAQTA with typhoid Vi polysaccharide and yellow fever vaccines in adults 18-54 years of age described in Section 6.1, the antibody response rates for typhoid Vi polysaccharide and yellow fever were adequate when typhoid Vi polysaccharide and yellow fever vaccines were administered concomitantly with (N=80) and nonconcomitantly without VAQTA (N=80). The seropositivity rate for hepatitis A when VAQTA, typhoid Vi polysaccharide, and yellow fever vaccines were administered concomitantly was generally similar to when VAQTA was given alone *[see Drug Interactions (7.1)]*.
Data are insufficient to assess the immune response to VAQTA and poliovirus vaccine when administered concomitantly.

16   HOW SUPPLIED/STORAGE AND HANDLING

VAQTA is available in single-dose vials and prefilled Luer-Lok® syringes.
Pediatric/Adolescent Formulations
25U/0.5 mL in single-dose vials and prefilled Luer-Lok® syringes.
NDC 0006-4831-41 – box of ten 0.5-mL single dose vials.
NDC 0006-4095-02 – carton of ten 0.5-mL prefilled single-dose Luer-Lok® syringes with tip caps.
NDC 0006-4095-09 – carton of six 0.5-mL prefilled single-dose Luer-Lok® syringes with tip caps.
Adult Formulations
50U/1-mL in single-dose vials and prefilled Luer-Lok® syringes.
NDC 0006-4841-00 – 1-mL single dose vial.
NDC 0006-4841-41 – box of ten 1-mL single dose vials.
NDC 0006-4096-02 – carton of ten 1-mL prefilled single-dose Luer-Lok® syringes with tip caps.
NDC 0006-4096-09 – carton of six 1-mL prefilled single-dose Luer-Lok® syringes with tip caps.
Store vaccine at 2-8°C (36-46°F).
DO NOT FREEZE since freezing destroys potency.

17   PATIENT COUNSELING INFORMATION

Information for Vaccine Recipients and Parents or Guardians
• Inform the patient, parent or guardian of the potential benefits and risks of the vaccine.

• Question the vaccine recipient, parent, or guardian about the occurrence of any symptoms and/or signs of an adverse reaction after a previous dose of hepatitis A vaccine.
• Inform the patient, parent, or guardian about the potential for adverse events that have been temporally associated with administration of VAQTA.
• Tell the patient, parent, or guardian accompanying the recipient, to report adverse events to the physician or clinic where the vaccine was administered.
• Prior to vaccination, give the patient, parent, or guardian the Vaccine Information Statements which are required by the National Childhood Vaccine Injury Act of 1986. These materials are available free of charge at the Centers for Disease Control and Prevention (CDC) website (www.cdc.gov/vaccines).
• Tell the patient, parent, or guardian that the United States Department of Health and Human Services has established a Vaccine Adverse Event Reporting System (VAERS) to accept all reports of suspected adverse events after the administration of any vaccine, including but not limited to the reporting of events required by the National Childhood Vaccine Injury Act of 1986. The VAERS toll-free number is 1-800-822-7967. Reporting forms may also be obtained at the VAERS website at (www.vaers.hhs.gov).

Manuf. and Dist. by: Merck Sharp & Dohme Corp., a subsidiary of
MERCK & CO., INC., Whitehouse Station, NJ 08889, USA
For patent information:
www.merck.com/product/patent/home.html
The trademarks depicted herein are owned by their respective companies.
Copyright ©1996-2014 Merck Sharp & Dohme Corp., a subsidiary of Merck & Co., Inc.
All rights reserved.
uspi-v251-i-1402r016
Printed in USA

VARIVAX®   ℞
[*var-i-vax*]
Varicella Virus Vaccine Live
Suspension for subcutaneous injection

HIGHLIGHTS OF PRESCRIBING INFORMATION
These highlights do not include all the information needed to use VARIVAX safely and effectively. See full prescribing information for VARIVAX.
VARIVAX®
Varicella Virus Vaccine Live
Suspension for subcutaneous injection
Initial U.S. Approval: 1995

INDICATIONS AND USAGE

VARIVAX is a vaccine indicated for active immunization for the prevention of varicella in individuals 12 months of age and older. (1)

DOSAGE AND ADMINISTRATION

Each dose is approximately 0.5 mL after reconstitution and is administered by subcutaneous injection. (2.1)
Children (12 months to 12 years of age)
• If a second dose is administered, there should be a minimum interval of 3 months between doses. (2.1)
Adolescents (≥13 years of age) and Adults
• Two doses, to be administered a minimum of 4 weeks apart. (2.1)

DOSAGE FORMS AND STRENGTHS

Suspension for injection (approximately 0.5-mL dose) supplied as a lyophilized vaccine to be reconstituted using the accompanying sterile diluent. (2.2, 3, 16)

CONTRAINDICATIONS

• History of severe allergic reaction to any component of the vaccine (including neomycin and gelatin) or to a previous dose of varicella vaccine. (4.1)
• Primary or acquired immunodeficiency states. (4.2)

• Any febrile illness or active infection, including untreated tuberculosis. (4.3)
• Pregnancy. (4.4, 8.1, 17)

WARNINGS AND PRECAUTIONS

• Evaluate individuals for immune competence prior to administration of VARIVAX if there is a family history of congenital or hereditary immunodeficiency. (5.2)
• Avoid contact with high-risk individuals susceptible to varicella because of possible transmission of varicella vaccine virus. (5.4)
• Defer vaccination for at least 5 months following blood or plasma transfusions, or administration of immune globulins (IG). (5.5, 7.2)
• Avoid use of salicylates for 6 weeks following administration of VARIVAX to children and adolescents. (5.6, 7.1)

ADVERSE REACTIONS

• Frequently reported (≥10%) adverse reactions in children ages 1 to 12 years include:
  ◦ fever ≥102.0°F (38.9°C) oral: 14.7%
  ◦ injection-site complaints: 19.3% (6.1)
• Frequently reported (≥10%) adverse reactions in adolescents and adults ages 13 years and older include:
  ◦ fever ≥100.0°F (37.8°C) oral: 10.2%
  ◦ injection-site complaints: 24.4% (6.1)
• Other reported adverse reactions in all age groups include:
  ◦ varicella-like rash (injection site)
  ◦ varicella-like rash (generalized) (6.1)
To report SUSPECTED ADVERSE REACTIONS or exposure during pregnancy or within three months prior to conception, contact Merck Sharp & Dohme Corp., a subsidiary of Merck & Co., Inc., at 1-877-888-4231 or VAERS at 1-800-822-7967 or www.vaers.hhs.gov.

DRUG INTERACTIONS

• Reye syndrome has been reported in children and adolescents following the use of salicylates during wild-type varicella infection. (5.6, 7.1)
• Passively acquired antibodies from blood, plasma, or immunoglobulin potentially may inhibit the response to varicella vaccination. (5.5, 7.2)
• Tuberculin skin testing may be performed before VARIVAX is administered or on the same day, or six weeks following vaccination with VARIVAX. (7.3)

USE IN SPECIFIC POPULATIONS

Pregnancy: Do not administer VARIVAX to females who are pregnant; the possible effects of the vaccine on fetal development are unknown. Pregnancy should be avoided for 3 months following vaccination with VARIVAX. (4.4, 8.1, 17)
See 17 for PATIENT COUNSELING INFORMATION and FDA-approved patient labeling
                                                  Revised: 07/2014

FULL PRESCRIBING INFORMATION

1 INDICATIONS AND USAGE

VARIVAX® is a vaccine indicated for active immunization for the prevention of varicella in individuals 12 months of age and older.

2 DOSAGE AND ADMINISTRATION

Subcutaneous administration only

2.1 Recommended Dose and Schedule

VARIVAX is administered as an approximately 0.5-mL dose by subcutaneous injection into the outer aspect of the upper arm (deltoid region) or the anterolateral thigh.

Do not administer this product intravascularly or intramuscularly.

Children (12 months to 12 years of age)

If a second dose is administered, there should be a minimum interval of 3 months between doses *[see Clinical Studies (14.1)]*.

Adolescents (≥13 years of age) and Adults

Two doses of vaccine, to be administered with a minimum interval of 4 weeks between doses *[see Clinical Studies (14.1)]*.

2.2 Reconstitution Instructions

When reconstituting the vaccine, use only the sterile diluent supplied with VARIVAX. The sterile diluent does not contain preservatives or other anti-viral substances which might inactivate the vaccine virus.

Use a sterile syringe free of preservatives, antiseptics, and detergents for each reconstitution and injection of VARIVAX because these substances may inactivate the vaccine virus.

To reconstitute the vaccine, first withdraw the total volume of provided sterile diluent into a syringe. Inject all of the withdrawn diluent into the vial of lyophilized vaccine and gently agitate to mix thoroughly. Withdraw the entire contents into the syringe and inject the total volume (approximately 0.5 mL) of reconstituted vaccine subcutaneously. VARIVAX, when reconstituted, is a clear, colorless to pale yellow liquid.

Parenteral drug products should be inspected visually for particulate matter and discoloration prior to administration, whenever solution and container permit. Do not use the product if particulates are present or if it appears discolored.

To minimize loss of potency, administer VARIVAX immediately after reconstitution. Discard if reconstituted vaccine is not used within 30 minutes.

Do not freeze reconstituted vaccine.

Do not combine VARIVAX with any other vaccine through reconstitution or mixing.

3 DOSAGE FORMS AND STRENGTHS

VARIVAX is a suspension for injection supplied as a single-dose vial of lyophilized vaccine to be reconstituted using the accompanying sterile diluent *[see Dosage and Administration (2.2) and How Supplied/Storage and Handling (16)]*. A single dose after reconstitution is approximately 0.5 mL.

4 CONTRAINDICATIONS

4.1 Severe Allergic Reaction

Do not administer VARIVAX to individuals with a history of anaphylactic or severe allergic reaction to any component of the vaccine (including neomycin and gelatin) or to a previous dose of a varicella-containing vaccine.

4.2 Immunosuppression

Do not administer VARIVAX to immunosuppressed or immunodeficient individuals, including those with a history of primary or acquired immunodeficiency states, leukemia, lymphoma or other malignant neoplasms affecting the bone marrow or lymphatic system, AIDS, or other clinical manifestations of infection with human immunodeficiency virus (HIV).

Do not administer VARIVAX to individuals receiving immunosuppressive therapy, including individuals receiving immunosuppressive doses of corticosteroids.

VARIVAX is a live, attenuated varicella-zoster vaccine (VZV) and may cause an extensive vaccine-associated rash or disseminated disease in individuals who are immunosuppressed or immunodeficient.

4.3 Concurrent Illness

Do not administer VARIVAX to individuals with any febrile illness. Do not administer VARIVAX to individuals with active, untreated tuberculosis.

4.4 Pregnancy

Do not administer VARIVAX to individuals who are pregnant because the effects of the vaccine on fetal development are unknown. Wild-type varicella (natural infection) is known to sometimes cause fetal harm. If vaccination of postpubertal females is undertaken, pregnancy should be avoided for three months following vaccination *[see Use in Specific Populations (8.1) and Patient Counseling Information (17)]*.

Table 1: Fever, Local Reactions, and Rashes (%) in Children 1 to 12 Years of Age 0 to 42 Days After Receipt of a Single Dose of VARIVAX

Reaction	N	% Experiencing Reaction	Peak Occurrence During Postvaccination Days
Fever ≥102.0°F (38.9°C) Oral	8827	14.7%	0 to 42
Injection-site complaints	8916	19.3%	0 to 2
(pain/soreness, swelling and/or erythema, rash, pruritus, hematoma, induration, stiffness)			
Varicella-like rash (injection site) Median number of lesions	8916	3.4% 2	8 to 19
Varicella-like rash (generalized) Median number of lesions	8916	3.8% 5	5 to 26

Table 2: Fever, Local Reactions, and Rashes (%) in Adolescents and Adults 0 to 42 Days After Receipt of VARIVAX

Reaction	N	% Post Dose 1	Peak Occurrence in Postvaccination Days	N	% Post Dose 2	Peak Occurrence in Postvaccination Days
Fever ≥100.0°F (37.8°C) Oral	1584	10.2%	14 to 27	956	9.5%	0 to 42
Injection-site complaints	1606	24.4%	0 to 2	955	32.5%	0 to 2
(soreness, erythema, swelling, rash, pruritus, pyrexia, hematoma, induration, numbness)						
Varicella-like rash (injection site) Median number of lesions	1606	3% 2	6 to 20	955	1% 2	0 to 6
Varicella-like rash (generalized) Median number of lesions	1606	5.5% 5	7 to 21	955	0.9% 5.5	0 to 23

---

5 WARNINGS AND PRECAUTIONS

5.1 Management of Allergic Reactions

Adequate treatment provisions, including epinephrine injection (1:1000), should be available for immediate use should anaphylaxis occur.

5.2 Family History of Immunodeficiency

Vaccination should be deferred in patients with a family history of congenital or hereditary immunodeficiency until the patient's immune status has been evaluated and the patient has been found to be immunocompetent.

5.3 Use in HIV-Infected Individuals

The Advisory Committee for Immunization Practices (ACIP) has recommendations on the use of varicella vaccine in HIV-infected individuals.

5.4 Risk of Vaccine Virus Transmission

Post-marketing experience suggests that transmission of vaccine virus may occur rarely between healthy vaccinees who develop a varicella-like rash and healthy susceptible contacts. Transmission of vaccine virus from a mother who did not develop a varicella-like rash to her newborn infant has been reported.

Due to the concern for transmission of vaccine virus, vaccine recipients should attempt to avoid whenever possible close association with susceptible high-risk individuals for up to six weeks following vaccination with VARIVAX. Susceptible high-risk individuals include:

- Immunocompromised individuals;
- Pregnant women without documented history of varicella or laboratory evidence of prior infection;
- Newborn infants of mothers without documented history of varicella or laboratory evidence of prior infection and all newborn infants born at <28 weeks gestation regardless of maternal varicella immunity.

5.5 Immune Globulins and Transfusions

Immunoglobulins should not be given concomitantly with VARIVAX. Vaccination should be deferred for at least 5 months following blood or plasma transfusions, or administration of immune globulin(s) [1].

Following administration of VARIVAX, immune globulin(s) should not be given for 2 months thereafter unless its use outweighs the benefits of vaccination [1]. *[See Drug Interactions (7.2).]*

5.6 Salicylate Therapy

Avoid use of salicylates (aspirin) or salicylate-containing products in children and adolescents 12 months through 17 years of age for six weeks following vaccination with VARIVAX because of the association of Reye syndrome with aspirin therapy and wild-type varicella infection. *[See Drug Interactions (7.1).]*

6 ADVERSE REACTIONS

6.1 Clinical Trials Experience

Because clinical trials are conducted under widely varying conditions, adverse reaction rates observed in the clinical trials of a vaccine cannot be directly compared to rates in the clinical trials of another vaccine and may not reflect the rates observed in clinical practice. Vaccine-related adverse reactions reported during clinical trials were assessed by the study investigators to be possibly, probably, or definitely vaccine-related and are summarized below.

In clinical trials [2-9], VARIVAX was administered to over 11,000 healthy children, adolescents, and adults.

In a double-blind, placebo-controlled study among 914 healthy children and adolescents who were serologically confirmed to be susceptible to varicella, the only adverse reactions that occurred at a significantly (p<0.05) greater rate in vaccine recipients than in placebo recipients were pain and redness at the injection site [2].

Children 1 to 12 Years of Age
One-Dose Regimen in Children

In clinical trials involving healthy children monitored for up to 42 days after a single dose of VARIVAX, the frequency of fever, injection-site complaints, or rashes were reported as shown in Table 1:

[See table 1 above]

In addition, adverse events occurring at a rate of ≥1% are listed in decreasing order of frequency: upper respiratory illness, cough, irritability/nervousness, fatigue, disturbed sleep, diarrhea, loss of appetite, vomiting, otitis, diaper rash/contact rash, headache, teething, malaise, abdominal pain, other rash, nausea, eye complaints, chills, lymphadenopathy, myalgia, lower respiratory illness, allergic reactions (including allergic rash, hives), stiff neck, heat rash/prickly heat, arthralgia, eczema/dry skin/dermatitis, constipation, itching.

Pneumonitis has been reported rarely (<1%) in children vaccinated with VARIVAX.

Febrile seizures have occurred at a rate of <0.1% in children vaccinated with VARIVAX.

Two-Dose Regimen in Children

Nine hundred eighty-one (981) subjects in a clinical trial received 2 doses of VARIVAX 3 months apart and were actively followed for 42 days after each dose. The 2-dose regimen of varicella vaccine had a safety profile comparable to that of the 1-dose regimen. The overall incidence of injection-site clinical complaints (primarily erythema and swelling) observed in the first 4 days following vaccination was 25.4% Postdose 2 and 21.7% Postdose 1, whereas the overall incidence of systemic clinical complaints in the 42-day follow-up period was lower Postdose 2 (66.3%) than Postdose 1 (85.8%).

Adolescents (13 Years of Age and Older) and Adults

In clinical trials involving healthy adolescents and adults, the majority of whom received two doses of VARIVAX and were monitored for up to 42 days after any dose, the frequencies of fever, injection-site complaints, or rashes are shown in Table 2.

[See table 2 above]

In addition, adverse events reported at a rate of ≥1% are listed in decreasing order of frequency: upper respiratory illness, headache, fatigue, cough, myalgia, disturbed sleep, nausea, malaise, diarrhea, stiff neck, irritability/nervousness, lymphadenopathy, chills, eye complaints, abdominal pain, loss of appetite, arthralgia, otitis, itching, vomiting, other rashes, constipation, lower respiratory illness, allergic reactions (including allergic rash, hives), contact rash, cold/canker sore.

6.2 Post-Marketing Experience

Broad use of VARIVAX could reveal adverse events not observed in clinical trials.

The following additional adverse events, regardless of causality, have been reported during post-marketing use of VARIVAX:

Body as a Whole

Anaphylaxis (including anaphylactic shock) and related phenomena such as angioneurotic edema, facial edema, and peripheral edema.

Eye Disorders

Necrotizing retinitis (in immunocompromised individuals).

Hemic and Lymphatic System

Aplastic anemia; thrombocytopenia (including idiopathic thrombocytopenic purpura (ITP)).

Infections and Infestations

Varicella (vaccine strain).

Nervous/Psychiatric

Encephalitis; cerebrovascular accident; transverse myelitis; Guillain-Barré syndrome; Bell's palsy; ataxia; non-febrile seizures; aseptic meningitis; dizziness; paresthesia.

Respiratory

Pharyngitis; pneumonia/pneumonitis.

Skin

Stevens-Johnson syndrome; erythema multiforme; Henoch-Schönlein purpura; secondary bacterial infections of skin and soft tissue, including impetigo and cellulitis; herpes zoster.

7 DRUG INTERACTIONS

7.1 Salicylates

No cases of Reye syndrome have been observed following vaccination with VARIVAX. Vaccine recipients should avoid use of salicylates for 6 weeks after vaccination with VARIVAX, as Reye syndrome has been reported following the use of salicylates during wild-type varicella infection *[see Warnings and Precautions (5.6)].*

7.2 Immune Globulins and Transfusions

Blood, plasma, and immune globulins contain antibodies that may interfere with vaccine virus replication and decrease the immune response to VARIVAX. Vaccination should be deferred for at least 5 months following blood or plasma transfusions, or administration of immune globulin(s) [1].

Following administration of VARIVAX, immune globulin(s) should not be given for 2 months thereafter unless its use outweighs the benefits of vaccination [1]. *[See Warnings and Precautions (5.5).]*

7.3 Tuberculin Skin Testing

Tuberculin skin testing, with tuberculin purified protein derivative (PPD), may be performed before VARIVAX is administered or on the same day, or at least 4 weeks following vaccination with VARIVAX, as other live virus vaccines may cause a temporary depression of tuberculin skin test sensitivity leading to false negative results.

8 USE IN SPECIFIC POPULATIONS

8.1 Pregnancy

Pregnancy Category: Contraindication *[see Contraindications (4.4)].* VARIVAX should not be administered to pregnant females since wild-type varicella can sometimes cause congenital varicella infection. Pregnancy should be avoided for three months following vaccination with VARIVAX *[see Contraindications (4.4) and Patient Counseling Information (17)].*

Pregnancy Registry

From 1995 to 2013, Merck Sharp & Dohme Corp., a subsidiary of Merck & Co., Inc., maintained a Pregnancy Registry to monitor fetal outcomes following inadvertent administration of VARIVAX during pregnancy or within three months prior to conception. In 2006, reports of exposure to two other varicella (Oka/Merck)-containing vaccines, ProQuad® (Measles, Mumps, Rubella and Varicella Virus Vaccine Live) and ZOSTAVAX® (Zoster Vaccine Live), were added to the Registry. The Pregnancy Registry has been discontinued. As of March 2011, 811 women with pregnancy outcome information available for analysis were prospectively enrolled following vaccination with VARIVAX, within three months prior to conception or any time during pregnancy. Of these women, 170 were seronegative at the time of exposure and 627 women had an unknown serostatus. The remaining women were seropositive. Nine exposures to either ProQuad or ZOSTAVAX have been reported that met criteria for inclusion into the Registry.

None of the 820 women who received a varicella-containing vaccine delivered infants with abnormalities consistent with congenital varicella syndrome.

All exposures to VARIVAX, ProQuad, or ZOSTAVAX during pregnancy or within three months prior to conception should be reported as suspected adverse reactions by contacting Merck Sharp & Dohme Corp., a subsidiary of Merck & Co., Inc., at 1-877-888-4231 or VAERS at 1-800-822-7967 or www.vaers.hhs.gov.

8.3 Nursing Mothers

It is not known whether varicella vaccine virus is excreted in human milk. Therefore, because some viruses are excreted in human milk, caution should be exercised if VARIVAX is administered to a nursing woman. *[See Warnings and Precautions (5.4).]*

8.4 Pediatric Use

No clinical data are available on safety or efficacy of VARIVAX in children less than 12 months of age.

8.5 Geriatric Use

Clinical studies of VARIVAX did not include sufficient numbers of seronegative subjects aged 65 and over to determine whether they respond differently from younger subjects.

11 DESCRIPTION

VARIVAX [Varicella Virus Vaccine Live] is a preparation of the Oka/Merck strain of live, attenuated varicella virus. The virus was initially obtained from a child with wild-type varicella, then introduced into human embryonic lung cell cultures, adapted to and propagated in embryonic guinea pig cell cultures and finally propagated in human diploid cell cultures (WI-38). Further passage of the virus for varicella vaccine was performed at Merck Research Laboratories (MRL) in human diploid cell cultures (MRC-5) that were free of adventitious agents. This live, attenuated varicella vaccine is a lyophilized preparation containing sucrose, phosphate, glutamate, and processed gelatin as stabilizers.

VARIVAX, when reconstituted as directed, is a sterile preparation for subcutaneous injection. Each approximately 0.5-mL dose contains a minimum of 1350 plaque-forming units (PFU) of Oka/Merck varicella virus when reconstituted and stored at room temperature for a maximum of 30 minutes. Each 0.5-mL dose also contains approximately 25 mg of sucrose, 12.5 mg hydrolyzed gelatin, 3.2 mg of sodium chloride, 0.5 mg of monosodium L-glutamate, 0.45 mg of sodium phosphate dibasic, 0.08 mg of potassium phosphate monobasic, and 0.08 mg of potassium chloride. The product also contains residual components of MRC-5 cells including DNA and protein and trace quantities of sodium phosphate monobasic, EDTA, neomycin and fetal bovine serum. The product contains no preservative.

12 CLINICAL PHARMACOLOGY

12.1 Mechanism of Action

VARIVAX induces both cell-mediated and humoral immune responses to varicella-zoster virus. The relative contributions of humoral immunity and cell-mediated immunity to protection from varicella are unknown.

12.2 Pharmacodynamics

Transmission

In the placebo-controlled efficacy trial, transmission of vaccine virus was assessed in household settings (during the 8-week postvaccination period) in 416 susceptible placebo recipients who were household contacts of 445 vaccine recipients. Of the 416 placebo recipients, three developed varicella and seroconverted, nine reported a varicella-like rash and did not seroconvert, and six had no rash but seroconverted. If vaccine virus transmission occurred, it did so at a very low rate and possibly without recognizable clinical disease in contacts. These cases may represent either wild-type varicella from community contacts or a low incidence of transmission of vaccine virus from vaccinated contacts *[see Warnings and Precautions (5.4)]* [2,10]. Post-marketing experience suggests that transmission of vaccine virus may occur rarely between healthy vaccinees who develop a varicella-like rash and healthy susceptible contacts. Transmission of vaccine virus from a mother who did not develop a varicella-like rash to her newborn infant has also been reported.

Herpes Zoster

Overall, 9454 healthy children (12 months to 12 years of age) and 1648 adolescents and adults (13 years of age and older) have been vaccinated with VARIVAX in clinical trials. Eight cases of herpes zoster have been reported in children during 42,556 person-years of follow-up in clinical trials, resulting in a calculated incidence of at least 18.8 cases per 100,000 person-years. The completeness of this reporting has not been determined. One case of herpes zoster has been reported in the adolescent and adult age group during 5410 person-years of follow-up in clinical trials, resulting in a calculated incidence of 18.5 cases per 100,000 person-years. All 9 cases were mild and without sequelae. Two cultures (one child and one adult) obtained from vesicles were positive for wild-type VZV as confirmed by restriction endo-

nuclease analysis [11]. The long-term effect of VARIVAX on the incidence of herpes zoster, particularly in those vaccinees exposed to wild-type varicella, is unknown at present. In children, the reported rate of herpes zoster in vaccine recipients appears not to exceed that previously determined in a population-based study of healthy children who had experienced wild-type varicella [12]. The incidence of herpes zoster in adults who have had wild-type varicella infection is higher than that in children.

12.4 Duration of Protection

The duration of protection of VARIVAX is unknown; however, long-term efficacy studies have demonstrated continued protection up to 10 years after vaccination [13] *[see Clinical Studies (14.1)].* A boost in antibody levels has been observed in vaccinees following exposure to wild-type varicella which could account for the apparent long-term protection after vaccination in these studies.

14 CLINICAL STUDIES

14.1 Clinical Efficacy

The protective efficacy of VARIVAX was established by: (1) a placebo-controlled, double-blind clinical trial, (2) comparing varicella rates in vaccinees versus historical controls, and (3) assessing protection from disease following household exposure.

Clinical Data in Children

One-Dose Regimen in Children

Although no placebo-controlled trial was carried out with VARIVAX using the current vaccine, a placebo-controlled trial was conducted using a formulation containing 17,000 PFU per dose [2,14]. In this trial, a single dose of VARIVAX protected 96 to 100% of children against varicella over a two-year period. The study enrolled healthy individuals 1 to 14 years of age (n=491 vaccine, n=465 placebo). In the first year, 8.5% of placebo recipients contracted varicella, while no vaccine recipient did, for a calculated protection rate of 100% during the first varicella season. In the second year, when only a subset of individuals agreed to remain in the blinded study (n=163 vaccine, n=161 placebo), 96% protective efficacy was calculated for the vaccine group as compared to placebo.

In early clinical trials, a total of 4240 children 1 to 12 years of age received 1000 to 1625 PFU of attenuated virus per dose of VARIVAX and have been followed for up to nine years post single-dose vaccination. In this group there was considerable variation in varicella rates among studies and study sites, and much of the reported data were acquired by passive follow-up. It was observed that 0.3 to 3.8% of vaccinees per year reported varicella (called breakthrough cases). This represents an approximate 83% (95% confidence interval [CI], 82%, 84%) decrease from the age-adjusted expected incidence rates in susceptible subjects over this same period [12]. In those who developed breakthrough varicella postvaccination, the majority experienced mild disease (median of the maximum number of lesions <50). In one study, a total of 47% (27/58) of breakthrough cases had <50 lesions compared with 8% (7/92) in unvaccinated individuals, and 7% (4/58) of breakthrough cases had >300 lesions compared with 50% (46/92) in unvaccinated individuals [15].

Among a subset of vaccinees who were actively followed in these early trials for up to nine years postvaccination, 179 individuals had household exposure to varicella. There were no reports of breakthrough varicella in 84% (150/179) of exposed children, while 16% (29/179) reported a mild form of varicella (38% [11/29] of the cases with a maximum total number of <50 lesions; no individuals with >300 lesions). This represents an 81% reduction in the expected number of varicella cases utilizing the historical attack rate of 87% following household exposure to varicella in unvaccinated individuals in the calculation of efficacy.

In later clinical trials, a total of 1114 children 1 to 12 years of age received 2900 to 9000 PFU of attenuated virus per dose of VARIVAX and have been actively followed for up to 10 years post single-dose vaccination. It was observed that 0.2% to 2.3% of vaccinees per year reported breakthrough varicella for up to 10 years post single-dose vaccination. This represents an estimated efficacy of 94% (95% CI, 93%, 96%), compared with the age-adjusted expected incidence rates in susceptible subjects over the same period [2,12,16]. In those who developed breakthrough varicella postvaccination, the majority experienced mild disease, with the median of the maximum total number of lesions <50. The severity of reported breakthrough varicella, as measured by number of lesions and maximum temperature, appeared not to increase with time since vaccination.

Among a subset of vaccinees who were actively followed in these later trials for up to 10 years postvaccination, 95 individuals were exposed to an unvaccinated individual with wild-type varicella in a household setting. There were no reports of breakthrough varicella in 92% (87/95) of exposed children, while 8% (8/95) reported a mild form of varicella (maximum total number of lesions <50; observed range, 10 to 34). This represents an estimated efficacy of 90% (95% CI,

82%, 96%) based on the historical attack rate of 87% following household exposure to varicella in unvaccinated individuals in the calculation of efficacy.

Two-Dose Regimen in Children

In a clinical trial, a total of 2216 children 12 months to 12 years of age with a negative history of varicella were randomized to receive either 1 dose of VARIVAX (n=1114) or 2 doses of VARIVAX (n=1102) given 3 months apart. Subjects were actively followed for varicella, any varicella-like illness, or herpes zoster and any exposures to varicella or herpes zoster on an annual basis for 10 years after vaccination. Persistence of VZV antibody was measured annually for 9 years. Most cases of varicella reported in recipients of 1 dose or 2 doses of vaccine were mild [13]. The estimated vaccine efficacy for the 10-year observation period was 94% for 1 dose and 98% for 2 doses (p<0.001). This translates to a 3.4-fold lower risk of developing varicella >42 days postvaccination during the 10-year observation period in children who received 2 doses than in those who received 1 dose (2.2% vs. 7.5%, respectively).

Clinical Data in Adolescents and Adults

Two-Dose Regimen in Adolescents and Adults

In early clinical trials, a total of 796 adolescents and adults received 905 to 1230 PFU of attenuated virus per dose of VARIVAX and have been followed for up to six years following 2-dose vaccination. A total of 50 clinical varicella cases were reported >42 days following 2-dose vaccination. Based on passive follow-up, the annual varicella breakthrough event rate ranged from <0.1 to 1.9%. The median of the maximum total number of lesions ranged from 15 to 42 per year.

Although no placebo-controlled trial was carried out in adolescents and adults, the protective efficacy of VARIVAX was determined by evaluation of protection when vaccinees received 2 doses of VARIVAX 4 or 8 weeks apart and were subsequently exposed to varicella in a household setting. Among the subset of vaccinees who were actively followed in these early trials for up to six years, 76 individuals had household exposure to varicella. There were no reports of breakthrough varicella in 83% (63/76) of exposed vaccinees, while 17% (13/76) reported a mild form of varicella. Among 13 vaccinated individuals who developed breakthrough varicella after a household exposure, 62% (8/13) of the cases reported maximum total number of lesions <50, while no individual reported >75 lesions. The attack rate of unvaccinated adults exposed to a single contact in a household has not been previously studied. Utilizing the previously reported historical attack rate of 87% for wild-type varicella following household exposure to varicella among unvaccinated children in the calculation of efficacy, this represents an approximate 80% reduction in the expected number of cases in the household setting.

In later clinical trials, a total of 220 adolescents and adults received 3315 to 9000 PFU of attenuated virus per dose of VARIVAX and have been actively followed for up to six years following 2-dose vaccination. A total of 3 clinical varicella cases were reported >42 days following 2-dose vaccination. Two cases reported <50 lesions and none reported >75. The annual varicella breakthrough event rate ranged from 0 to 1.2%. Among the subset of vaccinees who were actively followed in these later trials for up to five years, 16 individuals were exposed to an unvaccinated individual with wild-type varicella in a household setting. There were no reports of breakthrough varicella among the exposed vaccinees.

There are insufficient data to assess the rate of protective efficacy of VARIVAX against the serious complications of varicella in adults (*e.g.*, encephalitis, hepatitis, pneumonitis) and during pregnancy (congenital varicella syndrome).

14.2   Immunogenicity

In clinical trials, varicella antibodies have been evaluated following vaccination with formulations of VARIVAX containing attenuated virus ranging from 1000 to 50,000 PFU per dose in healthy individuals ranging from 12 months to 55 years of age [2,9].

One-Dose Regimen in Children

In prelicensure efficacy studies, seroconversion was observed in 97% of vaccinees at approximately 4 to 6 weeks postvaccination in 6889 susceptible children 12 months to 12 years of age. Titers ≥5 gpELISA units/mL were induced in approximately 76% of children vaccinated with a single dose of vaccine at 1000 to 17,000 PFU per dose. Rates of breakthrough disease were significantly lower among children with VZV antibody titers ≥5 gpELISA units/mL compared with children with titers <5 gpELISA units/mL.

Two-Dose Regimen in Children

In a multicenter study, 2216 healthy children 12 months to 12 years of age received either 1 dose of VARIVAX or 2 doses administered 3 months apart. The immunogenicity results are shown in Table 3.

[See table 3 above]

The results from this study and other studies in which a second dose of VARIVAX was administered 3 to 6 years after the initial dose demonstrate significant boosting of the VZV

Table 3: Summary of VZV Antibody Responses at 6 Weeks Postdose 1 and 6 Weeks Postdose 2 in Initially Seronegative Children 12 Months to 12 Years of Age (Vaccinations 3 Months Apart)

	VARIVAX 1-Dose Regimen (N=1114)	VARIVAX 2-Dose Regimen (3 months apart) (N=1102)	
	6 Weeks Postvaccination (n=892)	6 Weeks Postdose 1 (n=851)	6 Weeks Postdose 2 (n=769)
Seroconversion Rate	98.9%	99.5%	99.9%
Percent with VZV Antibody Titer ≥5 gpELISA units/mL	84.9%	87.3%	99.5%
Geometric mean titers in gpELISA units/mL (95% CI)	12.0 (11.2, 12.8)	12.8 (11.9, 13.7)	141.5 (132.3, 151.3)

N = Number of subjects vaccinated.
n = Number of subjects included in immunogenicity analysis.

antibodies with a second dose. VZV antibody levels after 2 doses given 3 to 6 years apart are comparable to those obtained when the 2 doses are given 3 months apart.

Two-Dose Regimen in Adolescents and Adults

In a multicenter study involving susceptible adolescents and adults 13 years of age and older, 2 doses of VARIVAX administered 4 to 8 weeks apart induced a seroconversion rate of approximately 75% in 539 individuals 4 weeks after the first dose and 99% in 479 individuals 4 weeks after the second dose. The average antibody response in vaccinees who received the second dose 8 weeks after the first dose was higher than that in vaccinees who received the second dose 4 weeks after the first dose. In another multicenter study involving adolescents and adults, 2 doses of VARIVAX administered 8 weeks apart induced a seroconversion rate of 94% in 142 individuals 6 weeks after the first dose and 99% in 122 individuals 6 weeks after the second dose.

14.3   Persistence of Immune Response

One-Dose Regimen in Children

In clinical studies involving healthy children who received 1 dose of vaccine, detectable VZV antibodies were present in 99.0% (3886/3926) at 1 year, 99.3% (1555/1566) at 2 years, 98.6% (1106/1122) at 3 years, 99.4% (1168/1175) at 4 years, 99.2% (737/743) at 5 years, 100% (142/142) at 6 years, 97.4% (38/39) at 7 years, 100% (34/34) at 8 years, and 100% (16/16) at 10 years postvaccination.

Two-Dose Regimen in Children

In recipients of 1 dose of VARIVAX over 9 years of follow-up, the geometric mean titers (GMTs) and the percent of subjects with VZV antibody titers ≥5 gpELISA units/mL generally increased. The GMTs and percent of subjects with VZV antibody titers ≥5 gpELISA units/mL in the 2-dose recipients were higher than those in the 1-dose recipients for the first year of follow-up and generally comparable thereafter. The cumulative rate of VZV antibody persistence with both regimens remained very high at year 9 (99.0% for the 1-dose group and 98.8% for the 2-dose group).

Two-Dose Regimen in Adolescents and Adults

In clinical studies involving healthy adolescents and adults who received 2 doses of vaccine, detectable VZV antibodies were present in 97.9% (568/580) at 1 year, 97.1% (34/35) at 2 years, 100% (144/144) at 3 years, 97.0% (98/101) at 4 years, 97.4% (76/78) at 5 years, and 100% (34/34) at 6 years postvaccination.

A boost in antibody levels has been observed in vaccinees following exposure to wild-type varicella, which could account for the apparent long-term persistence of antibody levels in these studies.

14.4   Studies with Other Vaccines

Concomitant Administration with M-M-R II

In combined clinical studies involving 1080 children 12 to 36 months of age, 653 received VARIVAX and M-M-R II concomitantly at separate injection sites and 427 received the vaccines six weeks apart. Seroconversion rates and antibody levels to measles, mumps, rubella, and varicella were comparable between the two groups at approximately six weeks post-vaccination.

Concomitant Administration with Diphtheria and Tetanus Toxoids and Acellular Pertussis Vaccine Adsorbed (DTaP) and Oral Poliovirus Vaccine (OPV)

In a clinical study involving 318 children 12 months to 42 months of age, 160 received an investigational varicella-containing vaccine (a formulation combining measles, mumps, rubella, and varicella in one syringe) concomitantly with booster doses of DTaP and OPV (no longer licensed in the United States). The comparator group of 144 children received M-M-R II concomitantly with booster doses of DTaP and OPV followed by VARIVAX six weeks later. At six weeks postvaccination, seroconversion rates for measles, mumps, rubella, and VZV and the percentage of vaccinees whose titers were boosted for diphtheria, tetanus, pertussis, and polio were comparable between the two groups. Anti-

VZV levels were decreased when the investigational vaccine containing varicella was administered concomitantly with DTaP [17]. No clinically significant differences were noted in adverse reactions between the two groups.

Concomitant Administration with PedvaxHIB®

In a clinical study involving 307 children 12 to 18 months of age, 150 received an investigational varicella-containing vaccine (a formulation combining measles, mumps, rubella, and varicella in one syringe) concomitantly with a booster dose of PedvaxHIB [Haemophilus b Conjugate Vaccine (Meningococcal Protein Conjugate)], while 130 received M-M-R II concomitantly with a booster dose of PedvaxHIB followed by VARIVAX 6 weeks later. At six weeks postvaccination, seroconversion rates for measles, mumps, rubella, and VZV, and GMTs for PedvaxHIB were comparable between the two groups. Anti-VZV levels were decreased when the investigational vaccine containing varicella was administered concomitantly with PedvaxHIB [18]. No clinically significant differences in adverse reactions were seen between the two groups.

Concomitant Administration with M-M-R II and COMVAX

In a clinical study involving 822 children 12 to 15 months of age, 410 received COMVAX, M-M-R II, and VARIVAX concomitantly at separate injection sites, and 412 received COMVAX followed by M-M-R II and VARIVAX given concomitantly at separate injection sites, 6 weeks later. At 6 weeks postvaccination, the immune responses for the subjects who received the concomitant doses of COMVAX, M-M-R II, and VARIVAX were similar to those of the subjects who received COMVAX followed 6 weeks later by M-M-R II and VARIVAX with respect to all antigens administered. There were no clinically important differences in reaction rates when the three vaccines were administered concomitantly versus six weeks apart.

15   REFERENCES

1. CDC: General Recommendations on Immunization: Recommendations of the Advisory Committee on Immunization Practices (ACIP). MMWR. 55(No. RR-15): 1-47, 2006.

2. Weibel, R.E.; et al.: Live Attenuated Varicella Virus Vaccine. Efficacy Trial in Healthy Children. N Engl J Med. 310(22): 1409-1415, 1984.

3. Arbeter, A.M.; et al.: Varicella Vaccine Trials in Healthy Children. A Summary of Comparative and Follow-up Studies. Am J Dis Child. 138: 434-438, 1984.

4. Weibel, R.E.; et al.: Live Oka/Merck Varicella Vaccine in Healthy Children. Further Clinical and Laboratory Assessment. JAMA. 254(17): 2435-2439, 1985.

5. Chartrand, D.M.; et al.: New Varicella Vaccine Production Lots in Healthy Children and Adolescents. Abstracts of the 1988 Inter-Science Conference Antimicrobial Agents and Chemotherapy: 237(Abstract #731).

6. Johnson, C.E.; et al.: Live Attenuated Varicella Vaccine in Healthy 12- to 24-Month-Old Children. Pediatrics. 81(4): 512-518, 1988.

7. Gershon, A.A.; et al.: Immunization of Healthy Adults with Live Attenuated Varicella Vaccine. J Infect Dis. 158(1): 132-137, 1988.

8. Gershon, A.A.; et al.: Live Attenuated Varicella Vaccine: Protection in Healthy Adults Compared with Leukemic Children. J Infect Dis. 161: 661-666, 1990.

9. White, C.J.; et al.: Varicella Vaccine (VARIVAX) in Healthy Children and Adolescents: Results From Clinical Trials, 1987 to 1989. Pediatrics. 87(5): 604-610, 1991.

10. Galea, S.; et al.: The Safety Profile of Varicella Vaccine: A 10-Year Review. J Infect Dis. 197(S2): 165-169, 2008.

11. Hammerschlag, M.R.; et al.: Herpes Zoster in an Adult Recipient of Live Attenuated Varicella Vaccine. J Infect Dis. 160(3): 535-537, 1989.

12. Guess, H.A.; et al.: Population-Based Studies of Varicella Complications. Pediatrics. 78(suppl): 723-727, 1986.

13. Kuter, B.J.; et al.: Ten Year Follow-up of Healthy Children who Received One or Two Injections of Varicella Vaccine. Pediatr Infect Dis J. 23: 132-37, 2004.

14. Kuter, B.J.; et al.: Oka/Merck Varicella Vaccine in Healthy Children: Final Report of a 2-Year Efficacy Study and 7-Year Follow-up Studies. Vaccine. 9: 643-647, 1991.

15. Bernstein, H.H.; et al.: Clinical Survey of Natural Varicella Compared with Breakthrough Varicella After Immunization with Live Attenuated Oka/Merck Varicella Vaccine. Pediatrics. 92(6): 833-837, 1993.

16. Wharton, M.: The Epidemiology of Varicella-zoster Virus Infections. Infect Dis Clin North Am. 10(3):571-581, 1996.

17. White, C.J. et al.: Measles, Mumps, Rubella, and Varicella Combination Vaccine: Safety and Immunogenicity Alone and in Combination with Other Vaccines Given to Children. Clin Infect Dis. 24(5): 925-931, 1997.

18. Reuman, P.D.; et al.: Safety and Immunogenicity of Concurrent Administration of Measles-Mumps-Rubella-Varicella Vaccine and PedvaxHIB® Vaccines in Healthy Children Twelve to Eighteen Months Old. Pediatr Infect Dis J. 16(7): 662-667, 1997.

16   HOW SUPPLIED/STORAGE AND HANDLING

No. 4826/4309 —VARIVAX is supplied as follows:
(1) a single-dose vial of lyophilized vaccine (package A), NDC 0006-4826-00
(2) a box of 10 vials of diluent (package B).
No. 4827/4309 —VARIVAX is supplied as follows:
(1) a box of 10 single-dose vials of lyophilized vaccine (package A), NDC 0006-4827-00
(2) a box of 10 vials of diluent (package B).

Storage
Vaccine Vial
During shipment, maintain the vaccine at a temperature between –58°F and +5°F (–50°C and –15°C). Use of dry ice may subject VARIVAX to temperatures colder than –58°F (–50°C).
Before reconstitution, store the lyophilized vaccine in a freezer at a temperature between –58°F and +5°F (–50°C and –15°C). Any freezer (*e.g.*, chest, frost-free) that reliably maintains a temperature between –58°F and +5°F (–50°C and –15°C) and has a separate sealed freezer door is acceptable for storing VARIVAX. VARIVAX may be stored at refrigerator temperature (36°F to 46°F, 2°C to 8°C) for up to 72 continuous hours prior to reconstitution. Vaccine stored at 2°C to 8°C which is not used within 72 hours of removal from +5°F (–15°C) storage should be discarded.
Before reconstitution, protect from light.
DISCARD IF RECONSTITUTED VACCINE IS NOT USED WITHIN 30 MINUTES.
Diluent Vial
The vial of diluent should be stored separately at room temperature (68°F to 77°F, 20°C to 25°C), or in the refrigerator.
For further product information, call 1-800-9-VARIVAX (1-800-982-7482).

17   PATIENT COUNSELING INFORMATION

See FDA-Approved Patient Labeling (Patient Information). Discuss the following with the patient:
• Question the patient, parent, or guardian about reactions to previous vaccines.
• Provide a copy of the patient information (PPI) located at the end of this insert and discuss any questions or concerns.
• Inform patient, parent, or guardian that vaccination with VARIVAX may not result in protection of all healthy, susceptible children, adolescents, and adults.
• Inform female patients to avoid pregnancy for three months following vaccination.
• Inform patient, parent, or guardian of the benefits and risks of VARIVAX.
• Instruct patient, parent, or guardian to report any adverse reactions or any symptoms of concern to their healthcare professional.
The U.S. Department of Health and Human Services has established a Vaccine Adverse Event Reporting System (VAERS) to accept all reports of suspected adverse events after the administration of any vaccine. For information or a copy of the vaccine reporting form, call the VAERS toll-free number at 1-800-822-7967, or report online at http://www.vaers.hhs.gov.
Dist. by: Merck Sharp & Dohme Corp., a subsidiary of **MERCK & CO., INC.**, Whitehouse Station, NJ 08889, USA
For patent information: www.merck.com/product/patent/home.html
Copyright © 2013 Merck Sharp & Dohme Corp., a subsidiary of **Merck & Co., Inc.**
All rights reserved.
uspi-v210-i-fro-1407r710

Patient Information about
VARIVAX®(pronounced "VAR ih vax")
Generic name: Varicella Virus Vaccine Live
This is a summary of information about VARIVAX®. You should read it before you or your child get the vaccine. If you have any questions about the vaccine after reading this leaflet, you should ask your healthcare professional. This is a summary only. It does not take the place of talking about VARIVAX with your doctor, nurse, or other healthcare professional. Only your healthcare professional can decide if VARIVAX is right for you or your child.

What is VARIVAX and how does it work?
VARIVAX is also known as Varicella Virus Vaccine Live. It is a live virus vaccine that is given as a shot. It is meant to help prevent chickenpox. Chickenpox is sometimes called varicella (pronounced VAR ih sell a).
VARIVAX contains a weakened form of chickenpox virus.
VARIVAX works by helping the immune system protect you or your child from getting chickenpox.
VARIVAX may not protect everyone who gets it.
VARIVAX does not treat chickenpox once you or your child have it.

What do I need to know about chickenpox?
Chickenpox is an illness that occurs most often in children who are 5 to 9 years old. It can be passed to others. The illness can include headache, fever, and general discomfort. Then an itchy rash occurs, which can turn into blisters. The most common complication is that the blisters can get infected. Less common but very serious complications can occur. These include pneumonia, inflammation of the brain, Reye syndrome (which affects the liver and the brain), and death. Severe disease and serious complications are more likely to occur in adolescents and adults.

Who should not get VARIVAX?
Do not get VARIVAX if you or your child:
• are allergic to any of its ingredients. (This includes gelatin or neomycin. See the ingredient list at the end of this leaflet.)
• have a weakened immune system, such as an immune deficiency, an inherited immune disorder, leukemia, lymphoma, or HIV/AIDS.
• take high doses of steroids by mouth or in a shot.
• have active tuberculosis that is not treated.
• have a fever.
• are pregnant or plan to get pregnant within the next three months.

What should I tell my healthcare professional before getting VARIVAX?
Tell your healthcare professional if you or your child:
• have or have had any medical problems.
• have received blood or plasma transfusions or human serum globulin within the last 5 months.
• take any medicines. (This includes non-prescription medicines and dietary supplements.)
• have any allergies. (This includes allergies to neomycin or gelatin.)
• had an allergic reaction to any other vaccine.
• are pregnant or plan to become pregnant within the next three months.
• are breast-feeding.

How is VARIVAX given?
VARIVAX is given as a shot to people who are 12 months old or older. If your child is 12 months to 12 years old and your doctor gives a second dose, the second dose must be given at least 3 months after the first shot.
A second dose should be given to those who first get the vaccine when they are 13 years old or older. This second dose should be given 4 to 8 weeks after the first dose.
Your doctor or healthcare professional will use the official recommendations to decide the number of shots needed and when to get them.
If a dose is missed, your healthcare professional will let you know when you should have it.

What should you or your child avoid when getting VARIVAX?
Do not take aspirin or aspirin-containing products for 6 weeks after getting VARIVAX.
It is rare, but possible, that once you have the vaccine, you could spread the chickenpox virus to others. Whenever possible, try to avoid contact with certain groups of people for up to six weeks after receiving the vaccine. This is because the disease for these groups may be quite serious. These groups include:
• people who have a weakened immune system.
• pregnant women who have never had chickenpox.
• newborn babies whose mothers have never had chickenpox.
• newborn babies born at less than 28 weeks of pregnancy.
Tell your doctor or healthcare professional if you or your child expect to have contact with someone who falls into one of these groups.

What are the possible side effects of VARIVAX?
The most common side effects reported after taking VARIVAX are:

• Fever
• Pain, swelling, itching, or redness at the site of the shot
• Chickenpox-like rash on the body or at the site of the shot
• Irritability
Other less common side effects have also been reported.
• Tingling of the skin
• Shingles
Tell your healthcare professional if you have any of the following problems within a short time after getting VARIVAX because they may be signs of an allergic reaction:
• Shortness of breath or wheezing
• Rash or hives
Other side effects have been reported. Some of them were serious. These include bruising more easily than normal; red or purple, flat, pinhead spots under the skin; severe paleness; difficulty walking; severe skin disorders; skin infection; and chickenpox. Rarely, swelling of the brain, stroke, inflammation of the lungs (known as pneumonia or pneumonitis), and seizures with or without a fever have been reported. It is not known if these rare side effects are related to the vaccine.
Your doctor has a more complete list of side effects for VARIVAX.
Tell your doctor or healthcare professional if you or your child have any new or unusual symptoms after getting VARIVAX.
Report the following to your doctor or your child's doctor:
• any adverse reactions following vaccination
• exposure to VARIVAX during pregnancy
• exposure to VARIVAX during the 3 months before getting pregnant.
You may also report these events to Merck Sharp & Dohme Corp., a subsidiary of Merck & Co., Inc., at 1-877-888-4231, or directly to the Vaccine Adverse Event Reporting System (VAERS). The VAERS toll-free number is 1-800-822-7967 or report online at www.vaers.hhs.gov.

What are the ingredients of VARIVAX?
Active Ingredient: a weakened form of chickenpox virus.
Inactive Ingredients: sucrose, hydrolyzed gelatin, sodium chloride, monosodium L-glutamate, sodium phosphate dibasic, potassium phosphate monobasic, potassium chloride, residual components of MRC-5 cells including DNA and protein, sodium phosphate monobasic, EDTA, neomycin, fetal bovine serum.

What else should I know about VARIVAX?
This leaflet summarizes important information about VARIVAX.
If you would like more information, talk to your healthcare professional, visit the web site at www.merckvaccines.com, or call 1-800-Merck-90.
Rx Only
Dist by: Merck Sharp & Dohme Corp., a subsidiary of **MERCK & CO., INC.**, Whitehouse Station, NJ 08889, USA
For patent information: www.merck.com/product/patent/home.html
Copyright © 2013 Merck Sharp & Dohme Corp., a subsidiary of **Merck & Co., Inc.**
All rights reserved.
usppi-v210-i-fro-1309r707

VICTRELIS®   ℞
[*vĭc-TRĚL-ĭs*]
(boceprevir)
capsules for oral use

HIGHLIGHTS OF PRESCRIBING INFORMATION
These highlights do not include all the information needed to use VICTRELIS safely and effectively. See full prescribing information for VICTRELIS.
VICTRELIS® (boceprevir) capsules, for oral use
Initial U.S. Approval: 2011

————RECENT MAJOR CHANGES————

Dosage and Administration (2.1, 2.4)	02/2014
Dosage and Administration (2.2)	07/2014
Contraindications (4)	01/2014
Warnings and Precautions	
Pancytopenia (5.4)	02/2014
Laboratory Tests (5.7)	07/2014

————INDICATIONS AND USAGE————

VICTRELIS is a hepatitis C virus (HCV) NS3/4A protease inhibitor indicated for the treatment of chronic hepatitis C (CHC) genotype 1 infection, in combination with peginterferon alfa and ribavirin, in adult patients with compensated liver disease, including cirrhosis, who are previously untreated or who have failed previous interferon and ribavirin therapy, including prior null responders, partial responders, and relapsers. (1)
• VICTRELIS must not be used as a monotherapy and should only be used in combination with peginterferon alfa and ribavirin. (1)
• The efficacy of VICTRELIS has not been studied in patients who have previously failed therapy with a treatment regimen that includes VICTRELIS or other HCV NS3/4A protease inhibitors. (1)

DOSAGE AND ADMINISTRATION

- 800 mg administered orally three times daily (every 7 to 9 hours) with food (a meal or light snack). (2)
- VICTRELIS must be administered in combination with peginterferon alfa and ribavirin. Initiate therapy with peginterferon alfa and ribavirin for 4 weeks, then add VICTRELIS to peginterferon alfa and ribavirin regimen. The duration of treatment is based on viral response, prior response status and presence of cirrhosis. (2)
- Refer to the prescribing information for peginterferon alfa and ribavirin for specific dosing instructions. (2)

DOSAGE FORMS AND STRENGTHS

Capsules: 200 mg (3)

CONTRAINDICATIONS

- **All contraindications to peginterferon alfa and ribavirin also apply since VICTRELIS must be administered with peginterferon alfa and ribavirin. (4)**
- Because ribavirin may cause birth defects and fetal death, boceprevir in combination with peginterferon alfa and ribavirin is contraindicated in pregnant women and in men whose female partners are pregnant. (4)
- Contraindicated in patients with a history of a hypersensitivity reaction to boceprevir. (4)
- Coadministration with drugs that are highly dependent on CYP3A4/5 for clearance, and for which elevated plasma concentrations are associated with serious and/or life-threatening events is contraindicated. (4)
- Coadministration with potent CYP3A4/5 inducers where significantly reduced boceprevir plasma concentrations may be associated with reduced efficacy is contraindicated. (4)

WARNINGS AND PRECAUTIONS

Use of VICTRELIS with Ribavirin and Peginterferon alfa:

- **Embryofetal Toxicity (Use with Ribavirin and Peginterferon Alfa):** Ribavirin may cause birth defects and fetal death; avoid pregnancy in female patients and female partners of male patients. Patients must have a negative pregnancy test prior to therapy; use two or more forms of contraception, and have monthly pregnancy tests. (5.1)
- Anemia - The addition of VICTRELIS to peginterferon alfa and ribavirin is associated with an additional decrease in hemoglobin concentrations compared with peginterferon alfa and ribavirin alone. (5.2)
- Neutropenia - The addition of VICTRELIS to peginterferon alfa and ribavirin may result in worsening of neutropenia associated with peginterferon alfa and ribavirin therapy alone. (5.3)
- Hypersensitivity – Serious acute hypersensitivity reactions (e.g., urticaria, angioedema) have been observed during combination therapy with VICTRELIS, peginterferon alfa and ribavirin. (5.5)

ADVERSE REACTIONS

The most commonly reported adverse reactions (greater than 35% of subjects) in clinical trials in adult subjects receiving the combination of VICTRELIS with PegIntron and REBETOL were fatigue, anemia, nausea, headache and dysgeusia. (6.1)

To report SUSPECTED ADVERSE REACTIONS, contact Merck Sharp & Dohme Corp., a subsidiary of Merck & Co., Inc., at 1-877-888-4231 or FDA at 1-800-FDA-1088 or www.fda.gov/medwatch.

DRUG INTERACTIONS

- VICTRELIS is a strong inhibitor of CYP3A4/5 and is partly metabolized by CYP3A4/5. The potential for drug-drug interactions must be considered prior to and during therapy. (4, 7, 12.3)

USE IN SPECIFIC POPULATIONS

- Safety and efficacy have not been studied in the following populations:
  ○ Patients with decompensated cirrhosis (8.7); and
  ○ Organ transplant recipients (8.8)

See 17 for PATIENT COUNSELING INFORMATION and Medication Guide

Revised: 07/2014

FULL PRESCRIBING INFORMATION: CONTENTS*

1 **INDICATIONS AND USAGE**
2 **DOSAGE AND ADMINISTRATION**
   2.1 VICTRELIS/Peginterferon alfa/Ribavirin Combination Therapy: Patients Without Cirrhosis Who Are Previously Untreated or Who Previously Failed Interferon and Ribavirin Therapy
   2.2 VICTRELIS/Peginterferon alfa/Ribavirin Combination Therapy: Patients with Cirrhosis
   2.3 Dose Modification
   2.4 Discontinuation of Dosing Based on Treatment Futility
3 **DOSAGE FORMS AND STRENGTHS**
4 **CONTRAINDICATIONS**
5 **WARNINGS AND PRECAUTIONS**
   5.1 Embryofetal Toxicity (Use with Ribavirin and Peginterferon Alfa)
   5.2 Anemia (Use with Ribavirin and Peginterferon Alfa)
   5.3 Neutropenia (Use with Ribavirin and Peginterferon Alfa)
   5.4 Pancytopenia (Use with Ribavirin and Peginterferon Alfa)
   5.5 Hypersensitivity
   5.6 Drug Interactions
   5.7 Laboratory Tests
6 **ADVERSE REACTIONS**
   6.1 Clinical Trials Experience
   6.2 Postmarketing Experience
7 **DRUG INTERACTIONS**
   7.1 Potential for VICTRELIS to Affect Other Drugs
   7.2 Potential for Other Drugs to Affect VICTRELIS
   7.3 Established and Other Potential Significant Drug Interactions
8 **USE IN SPECIFIC POPULATIONS**
   8.1 Pregnancy
   8.3 Nursing Mothers
   8.4 Pediatric Use
   8.5 Geriatric Use
   8.6 Renal Impairment
   8.7 Hepatic Impairment
   8.8 Organ Transplantation
10 **OVERDOSAGE**
11 **DESCRIPTION**
12 **CLINICAL PHARMACOLOGY**
   12.1 Mechanism of Action
   12.2 Pharmacodynamics
   12.3 Pharmacokinetics
   12.4 Microbiology
   12.5 Pharmacogenomics
13 **NONCLINICAL TOXICOLOGY**
   13.1 Carcinogenesis, Mutagenesis, Impairment of Fertility
14 **CLINICAL STUDIES**
16 **HOW SUPPLIED/STORAGE AND HANDLING**
   16.1 How Supplied
   16.2 Storage and Handling
17 **PATIENT COUNSELING INFORMATION**
* Sections or subsections omitted from the full prescribing information are not listed

---

FULL PRESCRIBING INFORMATION

1 INDICATIONS AND USAGE

VICTRELIS® (boceprevir) is indicated for the treatment of chronic hepatitis C genotype 1 infection, in combination with peginterferon alfa and ribavirin, in adult patients with compensated liver disease, including cirrhosis, who are previously untreated or who have failed previous interferon and ribavirin therapy, including prior null responders, partial responders, and relapsers [see Clinical Studies (14)].

The following points should be considered when initiating VICTRELIS for treatment of chronic hepatitis C infection:

- VICTRELIS must not be used as monotherapy and should only be used in combination with peginterferon alfa and ribavirin.
- The efficacy of VICTRELIS has not been studied in patients who have previously failed therapy with a treatment regimen that includes VICTRELIS or other HCV NS3/4A protease inhibitors.
- Poorly interferon responsive patients who were treated with VICTRELIS in combination with peginterferon alfa and ribavirin have a lower likelihood of achieving a sustained virologic response (SVR), and a higher rate of detection of resistance-associated substitutions upon treatment failure, compared to patients with a greater response to peginterferon alfa and ribavirin [see Microbiology (12.4) and Clinical Studies (14)].

2 DOSAGE AND ADMINISTRATION

VICTRELIS must be administered in combination with peginterferon alfa and ribavirin. The dose of VICTRELIS is 800 mg (four 200-mg capsules) three times daily (every 7 to 9 hours) with food [a meal or light snack] (see Table 1). Refer to the prescribing information for peginterferon alfa and ribavirin for instructions on dosing.

The following dosing recommendations differ for some subgroups from the dosing studied in the Phase 3 trials [see Clinical Studies (14)]. Response-Guided Therapy (RGT) is recommended for most individuals, but longer dosing is recommended in targeted subgroups (e.g., patients with cirrhosis).

2.1 VICTRELIS/Peginterferon alfa/Ribavirin Combination Therapy: Patients Without Cirrhosis Who Are Previously Untreated or Who Previously Failed Interferon and Ribavirin Therapy

- Initiate therapy with peginterferon alfa and ribavirin for 4 weeks (Treatment Weeks 1–4).
- Add VICTRELIS 800 mg (four 200-mg capsules) orally three times daily (every 7 to 9 hours) to peginterferon alfa and ribavirin regimen after 4 weeks of treatment. Based on the patient's HCV-RNA at Treatment Week (TW) 8, TW12 and TW24, use the following guidelines to determine duration of treatment (see Table 1).

[See table 1 above]

Consideration should be given to treating previously untreated patients who are poorly interferon responsive (as determined at TW4) with 4 weeks peginterferon alfa and ribavirin followed by 44 weeks of VICTRELIS 800 mg orally three times daily (every 7 to 9 hours) in combination with peginterferon alfa and ribavirin in order to maximize rates of SVR.

Table 1 Duration of Therapy in Patients Without Cirrhosis Who Are Previously Untreated or Who Previously Failed Interferon and Ribavirin Therapy

	ASSESSMENT* (HCV-RNA Results†)		RECOMMENDATION
	At Treatment Week 8	**At Treatment Week 24**	
Previously Untreated Patients	Not Detected	Not Detected	Complete three-medicine regimen at TW28.
	Detected	Not Detected	1. Continue all three medicines and finish through TW36; and then 2. Administer peginterferon alfa and ribavirin and finish through TW48.
Previous Partial Responders or Relapsers‡	Not Detected	Not Detected	Complete three-medicine regimen at TW36.
	Detected	Not Detected	1. Continue all three medicines and finish through TW36; and then 2. Administer peginterferon alfa and ribavirin and finish through TW48.
Previous Null Responders‡	Detected or Not Detected	Not Detected	Continue all three medicines and finish through TW48.

*TREATMENT FUTILITY

If the patient has HCV-RNA results greater than or equal to 1000 IU/mL at TW8, then discontinue three-medicine regimen.

If the patient has HCV-RNA results greater than or equal to 100 IU/mL at TW12, then discontinue three-medicine regimen.

If the patient has confirmed, detectable HCV-RNA at TW24, then discontinue three-medicine regimen.

†"Not Detected" refers to HCV-RNA assay results reported as "Target Not Detected" or "HCV-RNA Not Detected". In clinical trials, HCV-RNA in plasma was measured using a Roche COBAS® TaqMan® assay with a lower limit of quantification of 25 IU/mL and a limit of detection of 9.3 IU/mL. See Warnings and Precautions (5.7) for a description of HCV-RNA assay recommendations.

‡See Clinical Studies (14) for definitions of previous response to interferon and ribavirin therapy.

Table 2 Drugs that are contraindicated with VICTRELIS

Drug Class	Drugs Within Class that are Contraindicated With VICTRELIS	Clinical Comments
Alpha 1-Adrenoreceptor antagonists	Alfuzosin, doxazosin, silodosin, tamsulosin	Potential for alpha 1-adrenoreceptor antagonist-associated adverse events, such as hypotension and priapism
Anticonvulsants	Carbamazepine, phenobarbital, phenytoin	May lead to loss of virologic response to VICTRELIS
Antimycobacterial Agents	Rifampin	May lead to loss of virologic response to VICTRELIS.
Ergot Derivatives	Dihydroergotamine, ergonovine, ergotamine, methylergonovine	Potential for acute ergot toxicity characterized by peripheral vasospasm and ischemia of the extremities and other tissues.
GI Motility Agent	Cisapride	Potential for cardiac arrhythmias.
Herbal Products	St. John's wort (Hypericum perforatum)	May lead to loss of virologic response to VICTRELIS.
HMG-CoA Reductase Inhibitors	Lovastatin, simvastatin	Potential for myopathy, including rhabdomyolysis.
Oral Contraceptives	Drospirenone	Potential for hyperkalemia.
PDE5 enzyme Inhibitor	REVATIO® (sildenafil) or ADCIRCA® (tadalafil) when used for the treatment of pulmonary arterial hypertension*	Potential for PDE5 inhibitor-associated adverse events, including visual abnormalities, hypotension, prolonged erection, and syncope.
Neuroleptic	Pimozide	Potential for cardiac arrhythmias.
Sedative/Hypnotics	Triazolam; orally administered midazolam†	Prolonged or increased sedation or respiratory depression.

*See *Drug Interactions*, *Table 5* for coadministration of sildenafil and tadalafil when dosed for erectile dysfunction.
†See *Drug Interactions*, *Table 5* for parenterally administered midazolam.

2.2 VICTRELIS/Peginterferon alfa/Ribavirin Combination Therapy: Patients with Cirrhosis

Prior to initiating therapy in patients with compensated cirrhosis, see Use in Specific Populations (8.7) for additional information.

Patients with compensated cirrhosis should receive 4 weeks peginterferon alfa and ribavirin followed by 44 weeks VICTRELIS 800 mg (four 200-mg capsules) three times daily (every 7 to 9 hours) in combination with peginterferon alfa and ribavirin.

2.3 Dose Modification

Dose reduction of VICTRELIS is not recommended.

If a patient has a serious adverse reaction potentially related to peginterferon alfa and/or ribavirin, the peginterferon alfa and/or ribavirin dose should be reduced or discontinued. Refer to the prescribing information for peginterferon alfa and ribavirin for additional information about how to reduce and/or discontinue the peginterferon alfa and/or ribavirin dose. VICTRELIS must not be administered in the absence of peginterferon alfa and ribavirin. If peginterferon alfa or ribavirin is permanently discontinued, VICTRELIS must also be discontinued.

2.4 Discontinuation of Dosing Based on Treatment Futility

Discontinuation of therapy is recommended in all patients with 1) HCV-RNA levels of greater than or equal to 1000 IU per mL at TW8; or 2) HCV-RNA levels of greater than or equal to 100 IU per mL at TW12; or 3) confirmed detectable HCV-RNA levels at TW24.

3 DOSAGE FORMS AND STRENGTHS

VICTRELIS 200 mg Capsules, red-colored cap with the Merck logo printed in yellow ink, and a yellow-colored body with "314" printed in red ink.

4 CONTRAINDICATIONS

Contraindications to peginterferon alfa and ribavirin also apply to VICTRELIS combination treatment. Refer to the respective prescribing information for a list of the contraindications for peginterferon alfa and ribavirin.

VICTRELIS in combination with peginterferon alfa and ribavirin is contraindicated in:
- Pregnant women and men whose female partners are pregnant because of the risks for birth defects and fetal death associated with ribavirin [see Warnings and Precautions (5.1) and Use in Specific Populations (8.1)].
- Patients with a history of a hypersensitivity reaction to boceprevir [see Warnings and Precautions (5.5)].

Coadministration with drugs that are highly dependent on CYP3A4/5 for clearance, and for which elevated plasma concentrations are associated with serious and/or life-threatening events, including those in Table 2, is contraindicated [see Drug Interactions (7)].

Coadministration with potent CYP3A4/5 inducers, where significantly reduced boceprevir plasma concentrations may be associated with reduced efficacy, including those in Table 2, is contraindicated [see Drug Interactions (7)].

[See table 2 above]

5 WARNINGS AND PRECAUTIONS

5.1 Embryofetal Toxicity (Use with Ribavirin and Peginterferon Alfa)

Ribavirin may cause birth defects and/or death of the exposed fetus. Extreme care must be taken to avoid pregnancy in female patients and in female partners of male patients. Ribavirin therapy should not be started unless a report of a negative pregnancy test has been obtained immediately prior to initiation of therapy. Refer to the prescribing information for ribavirin for additional information.

Women of childbearing potential and men must use at least two forms of effective contraception during treatment and for at least 6 months after treatment has concluded. One of these forms of contraception can be a combined oral contraceptive product containing at least 1 mg of norethindrone. Oral contraceptives containing lower doses of norethindrone and other forms of hormonal contraception have not been studied or are contraindicated. Routine monthly pregnancy tests must be performed during this time [see Contraindications (4) and Drug Interactions (7)].

5.2 Anemia (Use with Ribavirin and Peginterferon Alfa)

Anemia has been reported with peginterferon alfa and ribavirin therapy. The addition of VICTRELIS to peginterferon alfa and ribavirin is associated with an additional decrease in hemoglobin concentrations. Complete blood counts (with white blood cell differential counts) should be obtained pretreatment, and at Treatment Weeks 2, 4, 8, and 12, and should be monitored closely at other time points, as clinically appropriate. If hemoglobin is less than 10 g per dL, a decrease in dosage of ribavirin is recommended; and if hemoglobin is less than 8.5 g per dL, discontinuation of ribavirin is recommended [see Adverse Reactions (6.1) and Clinical Studies (14)]. If ribavirin is permanently discontinued for management of anemia, then peginterferon alfa and VICTRELIS must also be discontinued [see Dosage and Administration (2.3)].

Refer to the prescribing information for ribavirin for additional information regarding dose reduction and/or discontinuation.

In clinical trials with VICTRELIS, the proportion of subjects who experienced hemoglobin values less than 10 g per dL and less than 8.5 g per dL was higher in subjects treated with the combination of VICTRELIS with PegIntron®/REBETOL® than in those treated with PegIntron/REBETOL alone (see Table 4). With the interventions used for anemia management in the clinical trials, the average additional decrease of hemoglobin was approximately 1 g per dL.

In clinical trials, the median time to onset of hemoglobin less than 10 g per dL from the initiation of therapy was similar among subjects treated with the combination of VICTRELIS and PegIntron/REBETOL (71 days with a range of 15-337 days), compared to those who received PegIntron/REBETOL (71 days with a range of 8-337 days). Certain adverse reactions consistent with symptoms of anemia, such as dyspnea, exertional dyspnea, dizziness and syncope were reported more frequently in subjects who received the combination of VICTRELIS with PegIntron/REBETOL than in those treated with PegIntron/REBETOL alone [see Adverse Reactions (6.1)].

In clinical trials with VICTRELIS, dose modifications (generally of PegIntron/REBETOL) due to anemia occurred twice as often in subjects treated with the combination of VICTRELIS with PegIntron/REBETOL (26%) compared to PegIntron/REBETOL (13%). The proportion of subjects who discontinued study drug due to anemia was 1% in subjects treated with the combination of VICTRELIS with PegIntron/REBETOL and 1% in subjects who received PegIntron/REBETOL. The use of erythropoiesis stimulating agents (ESAs) was permitted for management of anemia, at the investigator's discretion, with or without ribavirin dose reduction in the Phase 2 and 3 clinical trials. The proportion of subjects who received an ESA was 43% in those treated with the combination of VICTRELIS with PegIntron/REBETOL compared to 24% in those treated with PegIntron/REBETOL alone. The proportion of subjects who received a transfusion for the management of anemia was 3% of subjects treated with the combination of VICTRELIS with PegIntron/REBETOL compared to less than 1% in subjects who received PegIntron/REBETOL alone.

Thromboembolic events have been associated with ESA use in other disease states; and have also been reported with peginterferon alfa use in hepatitis C patients. Thromboembolic events were reported in clinical trials with VICTRELIS among subjects receiving the combination of VICTRELIS with PegIntron/REBETOL, and among those receiving PegIntron/REBETOL alone, regardless of ESA use. No definite causality assessment or benefit risk assessment could be made for these events due to the presence of confounding factors and lack of randomization of ESA use. A randomized, parallel-arm, open-label clinical trial was conducted in previously untreated CHC subjects with genotype 1 infection to compare use of an ESA versus ribavirin dose reduction for initial management of anemia during therapy with VICTRELIS in combination with peginterferon alfa-2b and ribavirin. Similar SVR rates were reported in subjects who were randomized to receive ribavirin dose reduction compared to subjects who were randomized to receive an ESA. In this trial, use of ESAs was associated with an increased risk of thromboembolic events including pulmonary embolism, acute myocardial infarction, cerebrovascular accident, and deep vein thrombosis compared to ribavirin dose reduction alone. The treatment discontinuation rate due to anemia was similar in subjects randomized to receive ribavirin dose reduction compared to subjects randomized to receive ESA (2% in each group). The transfusion rate was 4% in subjects randomized to receive ribavirin dose reduction and 2% in subjects randomized to receive ESA. Ribavirin dose reduction is recommended for the initial management of anemia.

5.3 Neutropenia (Use with Ribavirin and Peginterferon Alfa)

In Phase 2 and 3 clinical trials, seven percent of subjects receiving the combination of VICTRELIS with PegIntron/REBETOL had neutrophil counts of less than 0.5 × 10⁹ per L compared to 4% of subjects receiving PegIntron/REBETOL alone (see Table 4). Three subjects experienced severe or life-threatening infections associated with neutropenia, and two subjects experienced life-threatening neutropenia while receiving the combination of VICTRELIS with PegIntron/REBETOL. Complete blood counts (with white blood cell differential counts) should be obtained at pretreatment, and at Treatment Weeks 2, 4, 8, and 12, and should be monitored closely at other time points, as clinically appropriate. Decreases in neutrophil counts may require dose reduction or discontinuation of peginterferon alfa and ribavirin. If peginterferon alfa and ribavirin are permanently discontinued, then VICTRELIS must also be discontinued [see Dosage and Administration (2.3)].

Refer to the prescribing information for peginterferon alfa and ribavirin for additional information regarding dose reduction or discontinuation.

5.4 Pancytopenia (Use with Ribavirin and Peginterferon Alfa)

Serious cases of pancytopenia have been reported postmarketing in patients receiving VICTRELIS in combination with peginterferon alfa and ribavirin. Complete blood counts (with white blood cell differential counts) should be obtained at pretreatment, and at Treatment Weeks 2, 4, 8, and 12, and should be monitored closely at other time points, as clinically appropriate.

Refer to the prescribing information for ribavirin and peginterferon alfa for guidelines for discontinuation of therapy based on laboratory parameters.

5.5 Hypersensitivity

Serious acute hypersensitivity reactions (e.g., urticaria, angioedema) have been observed during combination therapy with VICTRELIS, peginterferon alfa and ribavirin. If such an acute reaction occurs, combination therapy should be discontinued and appropriate medical therapy immediately instituted [see Contraindications (4) and Adverse Reactions (6.2)].

5.6 Drug Interactions

See Table 2 for a listing of drugs that are contraindicated for use with VICTRELIS due to potentially life-threatening adverse events, significant drug interactions or loss of virologic activity [see Contraindications (4)]. Please refer to Table 5 for established and other potentially significant drug interactions [see Drug Interactions (7.3)].

5.7 Laboratory Tests

HCV-RNA levels should be monitored at Treatment Weeks 4, 8, 12, and 24, at the end of treatment, during treatment follow-up, and for other time points as clinically indicated. Use of a sensitive real-time reverse-transcription polymerase chain reaction (RT-PCR) assay for monitoring HCV-RNA levels during treatment is recommended. The assay should have a lower limit of HCV-RNA quantification of equal to or less than 25 IU per mL, and a limit of HCV-RNA detection of approximately 10 to 15 IU per mL. For the purposes of assessing Response-Guided Therapy milestones, a confirmed "detectable but below limit of quantification" HCV-RNA result should not be considered equivalent to an "undetectable" HCV-RNA result (reported as "Target Not Detected" or "HCV-RNA Not Detected").

Complete blood count (with white blood cell differential counts) should be obtained at pretreatment, and at Treatment Weeks 2, 4, 8, and 12, and should be monitored closely at other time points, as clinically appropriate.

Refer to the prescribing information for peginterferon alfa and ribavirin for pre-treatment, on-treatment and post-treatment laboratory testing recommendations including hematology, biochemistry (including hepatic function tests), and pregnancy testing requirements.

6 ADVERSE REACTIONS

See the peginterferon alfa and ribavirin prescribing information for description of adverse reactions associated with their use.

6.1 Clinical Trials Experience

Because clinical trials are conducted under widely varying conditions, adverse reaction rates observed in clinical trials of VICTRELIS cannot be directly compared to rates in the clinical trials of another drug and may not reflect the rates observed in practice.

The following serious and otherwise important adverse drug reactions (ADRs) are discussed in detail in another section of the labeling:
• Anemia [see Warnings and Precautions (5.2)]
• Neutropenia [see Warnings and Precautions (5.3)]
• Pancytopenia [see Warnings and Precautions (5.4)]
• Hypersensitivity [see Contraindications (4) and Warnings and Precautions (5.5)]

The most commonly reported adverse reactions (more than 35% of subjects regardless of investigator's causality assessment) in adult subjects were fatigue, anemia, nausea, headache, and dysgeusia when VICTRELIS was used in combination with PegIntron and REBETOL.

The safety of the combination of VICTRELIS 800 mg three times daily with PegIntron/REBETOL was assessed in 2095 subjects with chronic hepatitis C in one Phase 2, open-label trial and two Phase 3, randomized, double-blind, placebo-controlled clinical trials. SPRINT-1 (subjects who were previously untreated) evaluated the use of VICTRELIS in combination with PegIntron/REBETOL with or without a four-week lead-in period with PegIntron/REBETOL compared to PegIntron/REBETOL alone. SPRINT-2 (subjects who were previously untreated) and RESPOND-2 (subjects who had failed previous therapy) evaluated the use of VICTRELIS 800 mg three times daily in combination with PegIntron/REBETOL with a four-week lead-in period with PegIntron/REBETOL compared to PegIntron/REBETOL alone [see Clinical Studies (14)]. The population studied had a mean age of 49 years (3% of subjects were older than 65 years of age), 39% were female, 82% were white and 15% were black.

During the four week lead-in period with PegIntron/REBETOL in subjects treated with the combination of VICTRELIS with PegIntron/REBETOL, 28/1263 (2%) subjects experienced adverse reactions leading to discontinuation of treatment. During the entire course of treat-

ment, the proportion of subjects who discontinued treatment due to adverse reactions was 13% for subjects receiving the combination of VICTRELIS with PegIntron/REBETOL and 12% for subjects receiving PegIntron/REBETOL alone. Events resulting in discontinuation were similar to those seen in previous studies with PegIntron/REBETOL. Only anemia and fatigue were reported as events that led to discontinuation in more than 1% of subjects in any arm.

Adverse reactions that led to dose modifications of any drug (primarily PegIntron and REBETOL) occurred in 39% of subjects receiving the combination of VICTRELIS with PegIntron/REBETOL compared to 24% of subjects receiving PegIntron/REBETOL alone. The most common reason for dose reduction was anemia, which occurred more frequently in subjects receiving the combination of VICTRELIS with PegIntron/REBETOL than in subjects receiving PegIntron/REBETOL alone.

Serious adverse events were reported in 11% of subjects receiving the combination of VICTRELIS with PegIntron/REBETOL and in 8% of subjects receiving PegIntron/REBETOL.

Adverse events (regardless of investigator's causality assessment) reported in greater than or equal to 10% of subjects receiving the combination of VICTRELIS with PegIntron/REBETOL and reported at a rate of greater than or equal to 5% than PegIntron/REBETOL alone in SPRINT-1, SPRINT-2, and RESPOND-2 are presented in Table 3.

[See table 3 above]

Other Important Adverse Reactions Reported in Clinical Trials

Among subjects (previously untreated subjects or those who failed previous therapy) who received VICTRELIS in combination with peginterferon alfa and ribavirin, the following adverse drug reactions were reported. These events are notable because of their seriousness, severity, or increased frequency in subjects who received VICTRELIS in combination with peginterferon alfa and ribavirin compared with subjects who received only peginterferon alfa and ribavirin.

Gastrointestinal Disorders

Dysgeusia (alteration of taste) was an adverse event reported at an increased frequency in subjects receiving VICTRELIS in combination with peginterferon alfa and ri-

Table 3 Adverse Events Reported in ≥10% of Subjects Receiving the Combination of VICTRELIS with PegIntron/REBETOL and Reported at a Rate of ≥5% than PegIntron/REBETOL alone

Adverse Events	Previously Untreated (SPRINT-1 and SPRINT-2)		Previous Treatment Failures (RESPOND-2)	
	Percentage of Subjects Reporting Adverse Events		Percentage of Subjects Reporting Adverse Events	
Body System Organ Class	VICTRELIS + PegIntron + REBETOL (n=1225)	PegIntron + REBETOL (n=467)	VICTRELIS + PegIntron + REBETOL (n=323)	PegIntron + REBETOL (n=80)
Median Exposure (days)	197	216	253	104
Blood and Lymphatic System Disorders				
Anemia	50	30	45	20
Neutropenia	25	19	14	10
Gastrointestinal Disorders				
Nausea	46	42	43	38
Dysgeusia	35	16	44	11
Diarrhea	25	22	24	16
Vomiting	20	13	15	8
Dry Mouth	11	10	15	9
General Disorders and Administration Site Conditions				
Fatigue	58	59	55	50
Chills	34	29	33	30
Asthenia	15	18	21	16
Metabolism and Nutrition Disorders				
Decreased Appetite	25	24	26	16
Musculoskeletal and Connective Tissue Disorders				
Arthralgia	19	19	23	16
Nervous System Disorders				
Dizziness	19	16	16	10
Psychiatric Disorders				
Insomnia	34	34	30	24
Irritability	22	23	21	13
Respiratory, Thoracic, and Mediastinal Disorders				
Dyspnea Exertional	8	8	11	5
Skin and Subcutaneous Tissue Disorders				
Alopecia	27	27	22	16
Dry Skin	18	18	22	9
Rash	17	19	16	6

Table 4 Selected Hematological Parameters

Hematological Parameters	Previously Untreated (SPRINT-1 and SPRINT-2)		Previous Treatment Failures (RESPOND-2)	
	Percentage of Subjects Reporting Selected Hematological Parameters		Percentage of Subjects Reporting Selected Hematological Parameters	
	VICTRELIS + PegIntron + REBETOL (n=1225)	PegIntron + REBETOL (n=467)	VICTRELIS + PegIntron + REBETOL (n=323)	PegIntron + REBETOL (n=80)
Hemoglobin (g/dL)				
<10	49	29	49	25
<8.5	6	3	10	1
Neutrophils ($\times 10^9$/L)				
<0.75	31	18	26	13
<0.5	8	4	7	4
Platelets ($\times 10^9$/L)				
<50	3	1	4	0
<25	<1	0	0	0

bavirin compared with subjects receiving peginterferon alfa and ribavirin alone (Table 3). Adverse events such as dry mouth, nausea, vomiting and diarrhea were also reported at an increased frequency in subjects receiving VICTRELIS in combination with peginterferon alfa and ribavirin.

Laboratory Values
Changes in selected hematological parameters during treatment of adult subjects with the combination of VICTRELIS with PegIntron and REBETOL are described in Table 4.

Hemoglobin
Decreases in hemoglobin may require a decrease in dosage or discontinuation of ribavirin *[see Warnings and Precautions (5.2) and Clinical Studies (14)] [see prescribing information for ribavirin]*. If ribavirin is permanently discontinued, then peginterferon alfa and VICTRELIS must also be discontinued *[see Dosage and Administration (2.3)]*.

Neutrophils and Platelets
The proportion of subjects with decreased neutrophil and platelet counts was higher in subjects treated with VICTRELIS in combination with PegIntron/REBETOL compared to subjects receiving PegIntron/REBETOL alone. Three percent of subjects receiving the combination of VICTRELIS with PegIntron/REBETOL had platelet counts of less than 50×10^9 per L compared to 1% of subjects receiving PegIntron/REBETOL alone. Decreases in neutrophils or platelets may require a decrease in dosage or interruption of peginterferon alfa, or discontinuation of therapy *[see prescribing information for peginterferon alfa and ribavirin]*. If peginterferon alfa is permanently discontinued, then ribavirin and VICTRELIS must also be discontinued *[see Dosage and Administration (2.3)]*.
[See table 4 above]

6.2   Postmarketing Experience
The following adverse reactions have been identified during post-approval use of VICTRELIS in combination with peginterferon alfa and ribavirin. Because these reactions are reported voluntarily from a population of uncertain size, it is not always possible to reliably estimate their frequency or establish a causal relationship to drug exposure.
Blood and Lymphatic System Disorders: agranulocytosis, pancytopenia, thrombocytopenia *[see Warnings and Precautions (5.4)]*
Gastrointestinal Disorders: mouth ulceration, stomatitis
Infections and Infestations: pneumonia, sepsis
Skin and Subcutaneous Tissue Disorders: angioedema, urticaria *[see Warnings and Precautions (5.5)]*; drug rash with eosinophilia and systemic symptoms (DRESS) syndrome, exfoliative rash, exfoliative dermatitis, Stevens-Johnson syndrome, toxic skin eruption, toxicoderma

7   DRUG INTERACTIONS
[See Contraindications (4), Warnings and Precautions (5.6), and Clinical Pharmacology (12.3).]
7.1   Potential for VICTRELIS to Affect Other Drugs
Boceprevir is a strong inhibitor of CYP3A4/5. Drugs metabolized primarily by CYP3A4/5 may have increased exposure when administered with VICTRELIS, which could increase or prolong their therapeutic and adverse effects. Boceprevir does not inhibit CYP1A2, CYP2A6, CYP2B6, CYP2C8, CYP2C9, CYP2C19, CYP2D6 or CYP2E1 *in vitro*. In addition, boceprevir does not induce CYP1A2, CYP2B6, CYP2C8, CYP2C9, CYP2C19 or CYP3A4/5 *in vitro*.

Boceprevir is a potential inhibitor of p-glycoprotein (P-gp) based on *in vitro* studies. In a drug interaction trial conducted with digoxin, VICTRELIS had limited p-glycoprotein inhibitory potential at clinically relevant concentrations.

7.2   Potential for Other Drugs to Affect VICTRELIS
Boceprevir is primarily metabolized by aldo-ketoreductase (AKR). In drug interaction trials conducted with AKR inhibitors diflunisal and ibuprofen, boceprevir exposure did not increase to a clinically significant extent. VICTRELIS may be coadministered with AKR inhibitors.
Boceprevir is partly metabolized by CYP3A4/5. It is also a substrate for p-glycoprotein. Coadministration of VICTRELIS with drugs that induce or inhibit CYP3A4/5 could decrease or increase exposure to boceprevir.

7.3   Established and Other Potential Significant Drug Interactions
Table 5 provides recommendations based on established or potentially clinically significant drug interactions. VICTRELIS is contraindicated with drugs that are potent inducers of CYP3A4/5 and drugs that are highly dependent on CYP3A4/5 for clearance, and for which elevated plasma concentrations are associated with serious and/or life-threatening events *[see Contraindications (4)]*.
[See table 5 on pages 1731 through 1733]

8   USE IN SPECIFIC POPULATIONS
8.1   Pregnancy
VICTRELIS must be administered in combination with peginterferon alfa and ribavirin *[see Dosage and Administration (2)]*.

Pregnancy Category X: Use with Ribavirin and Peginterferon Alfa
Significant teratogenic and/or embryocidal effects have been demonstrated in all animal species exposed to ribavirin; and therefore ribavirin is contraindicated in women who are pregnant and in the male partners of women who are pregnant *[see Contraindications (4) and Warnings and Precautions (5.1)] [see prescribing information for ribavirin]*. Interferons have abortifacient effects in animals and should be assumed to have abortifacient potential in humans *[see prescribing information for peginterferon alfa]*.
Extreme caution must be taken to avoid pregnancy in female patients and female partners of male patients while taking this combination. Women of childbearing potential and their male partners should not receive ribavirin unless they are using effective contraception (two reliable forms) during treatment with ribavirin and for 6 months after treatment. One of these reliable forms of contraception can be a combined oral contraceptive product containing at least 1 mg of norethindrone. Oral contraceptives containing lower doses of norethindrone and other forms of hormonal contraception have not been studied or are contraindicated *[see Contraindications (4) and Warnings and Precautions (5.1)]*.
In case of exposure during pregnancy, a Ribavirin Pregnancy Registry has been established to monitor maternal-fetal outcomes of pregnancies in female patients and female partners of male patients exposed to ribavirin during treatment and for 6 months following cessation of treatment. Physicians and patients are encouraged to report such cases by calling 1-800-593-2214.

Pregnancy Category B: VICTRELIS
VICTRELIS must not be used as a monotherapy *[see Indications and Usage (1)]*. There are no adequate and well-controlled studies with VICTRELIS in pregnant women. No effects on fetal development have been observed in rats and rabbits at boceprevir AUC exposures approximately 11.8- and 2.0-fold higher, respectively, than those in humans at the recommended dose of 800 mg three times daily *[see Nonclinical Toxicology (13.1)]*.
8.3   Nursing Mothers
It is not known whether VICTRELIS is excreted into human breast milk. Levels of boceprevir and/or metabolites in the milk of lactating rats were slightly higher than levels observed in maternal blood. Peak blood concentrations of boceprevir and/or metabolites in nursing pups were less than 1% of those of maternal blood concentrations. Because of the potential for adverse reactions from the drug in nursing infants, a decision must be made whether to discontinue nursing or discontinue treatment with VICTRELIS, taking into account the importance of the therapy to the mother.
8.4   Pediatric Use
The safety, efficacy, and pharmacokinetic profile of VICTRELIS in pediatric patients have not been studied.
8.5   Geriatric Use
Clinical studies of VICTRELIS did not include sufficient numbers of subjects aged 65 and over to determine whether they respond differently from younger subjects. In general, caution should be exercised in the administration and monitoring of VICTRELIS in geriatric patients due to the greater frequency of decreased hepatic function, concomitant diseases and other drug therapy *[see Clinical Pharmacology (12.3)]*.
8.6   Renal Impairment
No dosage adjustment of VICTRELIS is required for patients with any degree of renal impairment *[see Clinical Pharmacology (12.3)]*.
8.7   Hepatic Impairment
No dose adjustment of VICTRELIS is required for patients with mild, moderate or severe hepatic impairment *[see Clinical Pharmacology (12.3)]*. Safety and efficacy of VICTRELIS have not been studied in patients with decompensated cirrhosis.
In published observational studies of patients with compensated cirrhosis treated with first generation HCV protease inhibitors, including boceprevir, in combination with peginterferon alfa and ribavirin, platelet count < 100,000/mm^3 and serum albumin < 3.5 g/dL were baseline characteristics that were identified as predictors of death or serious complications (severe infection or hepatic decompensation) during therapy.
The potential risks and benefits of VICTRELIS in combination with peginterferon alfa and ribavirin should be carefully considered before initiating therapy in patients with compensated cirrhosis who have platelet count < 100,000/mm^3 and serum albumin < 3.5 g/dL at baseline. If therapy is initiated, close monitoring for signs of infections and worsening liver function is warranted.
[See the prescribing information for peginterferon alfa for use in patients with hepatic decompensation.]
8.8   Organ Transplantation
The safety and efficacy of VICTRELIS alone or in combination with peginterferon alfa and ribavirin for the treatment of chronic hepatitis C genotype 1 infection in liver or other organ transplant recipients have not been studied. For data regarding drug-drug interactions with immunosuppressants, see *Drug Interactions (7.3)* and *Clinical Pharmacology (12.3)*.

10   OVERDOSAGE
Daily doses of 3600 mg have been taken by healthy volunteers for 5 days without untoward symptomatic effects.
There is no specific antidote for overdose with VICTRELIS. Treatment of overdosage with VICTRELIS should consist of general supportive measures, including monitoring of vital signs, and observation of the patient's clinical status.

11   DESCRIPTION
VICTRELIS (boceprevir) is an inhibitor of the hepatitis C virus (HCV) non-structural protein 3 (NS3) serine protease. Boceprevir has the following chemical name: (1R,5S)-N-[3-Amino-1-(cyclobutylmethyl)-2,3-dioxopropyl]-3-[2(S)-[[[(1,1-dimethylethyl)amino]carbonyl]amino]-3,3-dimethyl-1-oxobutyl]-6,6-dimethyl-3-azabicyclo[3.1.0]hexan-2(S)-carboxamide. The molecular formula is $C_{27}H_{45}N_5O_5$ and its molecular weight is 519.7. Boceprevir has the following structural formula:

Boceprevir is manufactured as an approximately equal mixture of two diastereomers. Boceprevir is a white to off-white amorphous powder. It is freely soluble in methanol, ethanol and isopropanol and slightly soluble in water.

VICTRELIS 200 mg capsules are available as hard gelatin capsules for oral administration. Each capsule contains 200 mg of boceprevir and the following inactive ingredients: sodium lauryl sulfate, microcrystalline cellulose, lactose monohydrate, croscarmellose sodium, pre-gelatinized starch, and magnesium stearate. The red capsule cap consists of gelatin, titanium dioxide, D&C Yellow #10, FD&C Blue #1, and FD&C Red #40. The yellow capsule body contains gelatin, titanium dioxide, D&C Yellow #10, FD&C Red #40, and FD&C Yellow #6. The capsule is printed with red and yellow ink. The red ink contains shellac and red iron oxide, while the yellow ink consists of shellac, titanium dioxide, povidone and D&C Yellow #10 Aluminum Lake.

12 CLINICAL PHARMACOLOGY

12.1 Mechanism of Action

VICTRELIS is a direct acting antiviral drug against the hepatitis C virus [see Microbiology (12.4)].

12.2 Pharmacodynamics

Evaluation of Effect of VICTRELIS on QTc Interval

The effect of boceprevir 800 mg and 1200 mg on QTc interval was evaluated in a randomized, multiple-dose, placebo-, and active-controlled (moxifloxacin 400 mg) 4-way crossover thorough QT study in 36 healthy subjects. In the study with demonstrated ability to detect small effects, the upper bound of the one-sided 95% confidence interval for the largest placebo-adjusted, baseline-corrected QTc based on individual correction method (QTcI) was below 10 ms, the threshold for regulatory concern. The dose of 1200 mg yields a boceprevir maximum exposure increase of approximately 15% which may not cover exposures due to coadministration with strong CYP3A4 inhibitors or use in patients with severe hepatic impairment. However, at the doses studied in the thorough QT study, no apparent concentration-QT relationship was identified. Thus, there is no expectation of a QTc effect under a higher exposure scenario.

12.3 Pharmacokinetics

VICTRELIS capsules contain a 1:1 mixture of two diastereomers, SCH534128 and SCH534129. In plasma the diastereomer ratio changes to 2:1, favoring the active diastereomer, SCH534128. Plasma concentrations of boceprevir described below consist of both diastereomers SCH534128 and SCH534129, unless otherwise specified.

In healthy subjects who received 800 mg three times daily alone, boceprevir drug exposure was characterized by $AUC(\tau)$ of 5408 ng × hr per mL (n=71), C_{max} of 1723 ng per mL (n=71), and C_{min} of 88 ng per mL (n=71). Pharmacokinetic results were similar between healthy subjects and HCV-infected subjects.

Absorption

Boceprevir was absorbed following oral administration with a median T_{max} of 2 hours. Steady state AUC, C_{max}, and C_{min} increased in a less-than-dose-proportional manner and individual exposures overlapped substantially at 800 mg and 1200 mg, suggesting diminished absorption at higher doses. Accumulation is minimal (0.8- to 1.5-fold) and pharmacokinetic steady state is achieved after approximately 1 day of three times daily dosing.

The absolute bioavailability of boceprevir has not been studied.

Effects of Food on Oral Absorption

VICTRELIS should be administered with food. Food enhanced the exposure of boceprevir by up to 65% at the 800 mg three times daily dose, relative to the fasting state. The bioavailability of boceprevir was similar regardless of meal type (e.g., high-fat vs. low-fat) or whether taken 5 minutes prior to eating, during a meal, or immediately following completion of the meal. Therefore, VICTRELIS may be taken without regard to either meal type or timing of the meal.

Distribution

Boceprevir has a mean apparent volume of distribution (Vd/F) of approximately 772 L at steady state in healthy subjects. Human plasma protein binding is approximately 75% following a single dose of boceprevir 800 mg. Boceprevir is administered as an approximately equal mixture of two diastereomers, SCH534128 and SCH534129, which rapidly interconvert in plasma. The predominant diastereomer, SCH534128, is pharmacologically active and the other diastereomer is inactive.

Metabolism

Studies in vitro indicate that boceprevir primarily undergoes metabolism through the aldo-keto reductase (AKR)-mediated pathway to ketone-reduced metabolites that are inactive against HCV. After a single 800-mg oral dose of ^{14}C-boceprevir, the most abundant circulating metabolites were a diastereomeric mixture of ketone-reduced metabolites with a mean exposure approximately 4-fold greater than that of boceprevir. Boceprevir also undergoes, to a lesser extent, oxidative metabolism mediated by CYP3A4/5.

Table 5 Established and Other Potentially Significant Drug Interactions

Concomitant Drug Class: Drug Name	Effect on Concentration of Boceprevir or Concomitant Drug	Recommendations
Antiarrhythmics: amiodarone, bepridil, propafenone, quinidine	↑ antiarrhythmics	Coadministration with VICTRELIS has the potential to produce serious and/or life-threatening adverse events and has not been studied. Caution is warranted and therapeutic concentration monitoring of these drugs is recommended if they are used concomitantly with VICTRELIS.
digoxin*	↑ digoxin	Digoxin concentrations increased when administered with VICTRELIS [see Clinical Pharmacology (12.3)]. Measure serum digoxin concentrations before initiating VICTRELIS. Continue monitoring digoxin concentrations; consult the digoxin prescribing information for information on titrating the digoxin dose.
Anticoagulant: warfarin	↑ or ↓ warfarin	Concentrations of warfarin may be altered when co-administered with VICTRELIS. Monitor INR closely.
Antidepressants: trazodone, desipramine	↑ trazodone ↑ desipramine	Plasma concentrations of trazodone and desipramine may increase when administered with VICTRELIS, resulting in adverse events such as dizziness, hypotension and syncope. Use with caution and consider a lower dose of trazodone or desipramine.
escitalopram*	↓escitalopram	Exposure of escitalopram was slightly decreased when coadministered with VICTRELIS. Selective serotonin reuptake inhibitors such as escitalopram have a wide therapeutic index, but doses may need to be adjusted when combined with VICTRELIS.
Antifungals: ketoconazole*, itraconazole, posaconazole, voriconazole	↑ boceprevir ↑ itraconazole ↑ ketoconazole ↑ posaconazole ↑ voriconazole	Plasma concentrations of ketoconazole, itraconazole, voriconazole or posaconazole may be increased with VICTRELIS. When coadministration is required, doses of ketoconazole and itraconazole should not exceed 200 mg/day.
Anti-gout: colchicine	↑ colchicine	Significant increases in colchicine levels are expected; fatal colchicine toxicity has been reported with other strong CYP3A4 inhibitors. Patients with renal or hepatic impairment should not be given colchicine with VICTRELIS. Treatment of gout flares (during treatment with VICTRELIS): 0.6 mg (1 tablet) × 1 dose, followed by 0.3 mg (half tablet) 1 hour later. Dose to be repeated no earlier than 3 days. Prophylaxis of gout flares (during treatment with VICTRELIS): If the original regimen was 0.6 mg twice a day, reduce dose to 0.3 mg once a day. If the original regimen was 0.6 mg once a day, reduce the dose to 0.3 mg once every other day. Treatment of familial Mediterranean fever (FMF) (during treatment with VICTRELIS): Maximum daily dose of 0.6 mg (may be given as 0.3 mg twice a day).
Anti-infective: clarithromycin	↑ clarithromycin	Concentrations of clarithromycin may be increased with VICTRELIS; however, no dosage adjustment is necessary for patients with normal renal function.
Antimycobacterial: rifabutin	↓ boceprevir ↑ rifabutin	Increases in rifabutin exposure are anticipated, while exposure of boceprevir may be decreased. Doses have not been established for the 2 drugs when used in combination. Concomitant use is not recommended.
Calcium Channel Blockers such as: amlodipine, diltiazem, felodipine, nifedipine, nicardipine, nisoldipine, verapamil	↑ calcium channel blockers	Plasma concentrations of calcium channel blockers may increase when administered with VICTRELIS. Caution is warranted and clinical monitoring is recommended.
Corticosteroid, systemic: dexamethasone	↓ boceprevir	Coadministration of VICTRELIS with CYP3A4/5 inducers may decrease plasma concentrations of boceprevir, which may result in loss of therapeutic effect. Therefore, this combination should be avoided if possible and used with caution if necessary.
prednisone*	↑ prednisone	Concentrations of prednisone and its active metabolite, prednisolone, increased when administered with VICTRELIS [see Clinical Pharmacology (12.3)]. No dose adjustment of prednisone is necessary when co-administered with VICTRELIS. Patients receiving prednisone and VICTRELIS should be monitored appropriately.

(Table continued on next page)

Drug Interactions

Drug interaction studies were performed with boceprevir and drugs likely to be coadministered or drugs commonly used as probes for pharmacokinetic interactions. The effects of coadministration of boceprevir on AUC, C_{max} and C_{min} are summarized in Table 6 (effects of coadministered drugs on boceprevir) and Table 7 (effects of boceprevir on coadministered drugs).

[See table 6 on pages 1734 and 1735]
[See table 7 on pages 1736 and 1737]

Table 5 *(cont.)* **Established and Other Potentially Significant Drug Interactions**

Concomitant Drug Class: Drug Name	Effect on Concentration of Boceprevir or Concomitant Drug	Recommendations
Corticosteroid, inhaled: budesonide, fluticasone	↑ budesonide ↑ fluticasone	Concomitant use of inhaled budesonide or fluticasone with VICTRELIS may result in increased plasma concentrations of budesonide or fluticasone, resulting in significantly reduced serum cortisol concentrations. Avoid coadministration if possible, particularly for extended durations.
Endothelin Receptor Antagonist: bosentan	↑ bosentan	Concentrations of bosentan may be increased when coadministered with VICTRELIS. Use with caution and monitor closely.
HIV Integrase Inhibitor: raltegravir*	↔ raltegravir	No dose adjustment required for VICTRELIS or raltegravir.
HIV Non-Nucleoside Reverse Transcriptase Inhibitors: efavirenz*	↓ boceprevir	Plasma trough concentrations of boceprevir were decreased when VICTRELIS was coadministered with efavirenz, which may result in loss of therapeutic effect. Avoid combination.
etravirine*	↓ etravirine	Concentrations of etravirine decreased when coadministered with VICTRELIS. The clinical significance of the reductions in etravirine pharmacokinetic parameters has not been directly assessed.
rilpivirine*	↑ rilpivirine	Concomitant administration of rilpivirine with VICTRELIS increased the exposure to rilpivirine. No dose adjustment of VICTRELIS or rilpivirine is recommended.
HIV Protease Inhibitors: atazanavir/ritonavir*	↓ atazanavir ↓ ritonavir	Concomitant administration of boceprevir and atazanavir/ritonavir resulted in reduced steady-state exposures to atazanavir and ritonavir. Coadministration of atazanavir/ritonavir and boceprevir is not recommended.
darunavir/ritonavir*	↓ darunavir ↓ ritonavir ↓ boceprevir	Concomitant administration of boceprevir and darunavir/ritonavir resulted in reduced steady-state exposures to boceprevir, darunavir and ritonavir. Coadministration of darunavir/ritonavir and boceprevir is not recommended.
lopinavir/ritonavir*	↓ lopinavir ↓ ritonavir ↓ boceprevir	Concomitant administration of boceprevir and lopinavir/ritonavir resulted in reduced steady-state exposures to boceprevir, lopinavir and ritonavir. Coadministration of lopinavir/ritonavir and boceprevir is not recommended.
ritonavir*	↓ boceprevir	When boceprevir is administered with ritonavir alone, boceprevir concentrations are decreased.
HMG-CoA Reductase Inhibitors: atorvastatin*	↑ atorvastatin	Exposure to atorvastatin was increased when administered with VICTRELIS. Use the lowest effective dose of atorvastatin, but do not exceed a daily dose of 40 mg when coadministered with VICTRELIS.
pravastatin*	↑ pravastatin	Concomitant administration of pravastatin with VICTRELIS increased exposure to pravastatin. Treatment with pravastatin can be initiated at the recommended dose when coadministered with VICTRELIS. Close clinical monitoring is warranted.
Immunosuppressants: cyclosporine* tacrolimus* sirolimus	↑cyclosporine	Dose adjustments of cyclosporine should be anticipated when administered with VICTRELIS and should be guided by close monitoring of cyclosporine blood concentrations, and frequent assessments of renal function and cyclosporine-related side effects.
tacrolimus*	↑tacrolimus	Concomitant administration of VICTRELIS with tacrolimus requires significant dose reduction and prolongation of the dosing interval for tacrolimus, with close monitoring of tacrolimus blood concentrations and frequent assessments of renal function and tacrolimus-related side effects.
sirolimus*	↑sirolimus	Concomitant administration of VICTRELIS with sirolimus requires significant dose reduction and prolongation of the dosing interval for sirolimus, with close monitoring of sirolimus blood concentrations and frequent assessments of renal function and sirolimus-related side effects.

(Table continued on next page)

Elimination

Boceprevir is eliminated with a mean plasma half-life (t½) of approximately 3.4 hours. Boceprevir has a mean total body clearance (CL/F) of approximately 161 L per hr. Following a single 800 mg oral dose of ^{14}C-boceprevir, approximately 79% and 9% of the dose was excreted in feces and urine, respectively, with approximately 8% and 3% of the dosed radiocarbon eliminated as boceprevir in feces and urine. The data indicate that boceprevir is eliminated primarily by the liver.

Special Populations

Hepatic Impairment

The pharmacokinetics of boceprevir was studied in adult non-HCV infected subjects with normal, mild (Child-Pugh score 5 to 6), moderate (Child-Pugh score 7 to 9), and severe (Child-Pugh score 10 to 12) hepatic impairment following a single 400 mg dose of VICTRELIS. The mean AUC of the active diastereomer of boceprevir (SCH534128) was 32% and 45% higher in subjects with moderate and severe hepatic impairment, respectively, relative to subjects with normal hepatic function. Mean C_{max} values for SCH534128 were 28% and 62% higher in moderate and severe hepatic impairment, respectively. Subjects with mild hepatic impairment had similar SCH534128 exposure as subjects with normal hepatic function. A similar magnitude of effect is anticipated for boceprevir. No dosage adjustment of VICTRELIS is recommended for patients with hepatic impairment. For additional information in patients with compensated cirrhosis, see Use in Specific Populations (8.7).

[See the prescribing information for peginterferon alfa for use in patients with hepatic decompensation.]

Renal Impairment

The pharmacokinetics of boceprevir was studied in non-HCV-infected subjects with end-stage renal disease (ESRD) requiring hemodialysis following a single 800 mg dose of VICTRELIS. The mean AUC of boceprevir was 10% lower in subjects with ESRD requiring hemodialysis relative to subjects with normal renal function. Hemodialysis removed less than 1% of the boceprevir dose. No dosage adjustment of VICTRELIS is required in patients with any degree of renal impairment.

Gender

Population pharmacokinetic analysis of VICTRELIS indicated that gender had no apparent effect on exposure.

Race

Population pharmacokinetic analysis of VICTRELIS indicated that race had no apparent effect on exposure.

Age

Population pharmacokinetic analysis of VICTRELIS showed that boceprevir exposure was not different across subjects 19 to 65 years old.

12.4   Microbiology

Mechanism of Action

Boceprevir is an inhibitor of the HCV NS3/4A protease that is necessary for the proteolytic cleavage of the HCV encoded polyprotein into mature forms of the NS4A, NS4B, NS5A and NS5B proteins. Boceprevir covalently, yet reversibly, binds to the NS3 protease active site serine (S139) through an (alpha)-ketoamide functional group to inhibit viral replication in HCV-infected host cells. In a biochemical assay, boceprevir inhibited the activity of recombinant HCV genotype 1a and 1b NS3/4A protease enzymes, with K_i values of 14 nM for each subtype.

Activity in Cell Culture

The EC_{50} and EC_{90} values for boceprevir against an HCV replicon constructed from a single genotype 1b isolate were approximately 200 nM and 400 nM, respectively, in a 72-hour cell culture assay. Boceprevir cell culture anti-HCV activity was approximately 2-fold lower for an HCV replicon derived from a single genotype 1a isolate, relative to the 1b isolate-derived replicon. In replicon assays, boceprevir had approximately 2-fold reduced activity against a genotype 2a isolate relative to genotype 1a and 1b replicon isolates. In a biochemical assay, boceprevir had approximately 3- and 2-fold reduced activity against NS3/4A proteases derived from single isolates representative of HCV genotypes 2 and 3a, respectively, relative to a genotype 1b-derived NS3/4A protease. The presence of 50% human serum reduced the cell culture anti-HCV activity of boceprevir by approximately 3-fold.

Evaluation of varying combinations of boceprevir and interferon alfa-2b that produced 90% suppression of replicon RNA in cell culture showed additivity of effect without evidence of antagonism.

Resistance

In HCV Replicon Cell Culture and Biochemical Studies

The activity of boceprevir against the HCV genotype 1a replicon was reduced (2- to 6-fold) by the following amino acid substitutions in the NS3 protease domain: V36A/L/M, Q41R, T54A/S, V55A, R155K and V158I. A greater than 10-fold reduction in boceprevir susceptibility was conferred by the amino acid substitutions R155T and A156S. The V55I and D168N single substitutions did not reduce sensitivity to boceprevir. The following double amino acid substitutions conferred more than 10-fold reduced sensitivity to boceprevir: V55A+I170V, T54S+R155K, R155K+D168N, R155T+D168N and V36M+R155K.

The activity of boceprevir against the HCV genotype 1b replicon was reduced (2- to 8-fold) by the following amino acid substitutions in the NS3 protease domain: V36A/M, Q41R, F43S, T54A/G/S, V55A/I, R155K, V158I, V170M and M175L. A greater than 10-fold reduction in boceprevir susceptibility was conferred by the amino acid substitutions A156S/T/V, V170A and V36M+R155K. The D168V single substitution did not reduce sensitivity to boceprevir.

Additional NS3 protease domain substitutions that have not been evaluated in the HCV replicon but have been shown to reduce boceprevir activity against the HCV NS3/4A protease in a biochemical assay include F43C and R155G/I/M/Q.

Resistance-associated amino acid substitutions for HCV genotype 1a and 1b observed in clinical trials are presented in Table 8.

In Clinical Studies

An as-treated, pooled genotypic resistance analysis was conducted for subjects who received four weeks of PegIntron/REBETOL followed by VICTRELIS 800 mg three times daily in combination with PegIntron/REBETOL in two Phase 3 studies, SPRINT-2 and RESPOND-2. Among subjects treated with VICTRELIS who did not achieve a sustained virologic response, and for whom samples were analyzed, 53% had one or more specific post-baseline, treatment-emergent NS3 protease domain amino acid substitutions detected by a population-based sequencing assay

(Table 8). Similar patterns of treatment-emergent substitutions were observed in P06086, a Phase 3 clinical trial in previously untreated CHC subjects with genotype 1 infection comparing the use of ESA to ribavirin dose reduction for initial management of anemia during therapy with VICTRELIS in combination with PegIntron/REBETOL. Nearly all of these substitutions have been shown to reduce boceprevir anti-HCV activity in cell culture or biochemical assays. Among subjects treated with VICTRELIS in SPRINT-2 and RESPOND-2 who did not achieve SVR and for whom post-baseline samples were analyzed, 31% of PegIntron/REBETOL-responsive subjects, as defined by greater than or equal to 1-log$_{10}$ decline in viral load at Treatment Week 4 (end of 4-week PegIntron/REBETOL lead-in period), had detectable treatment-emergent substitutions, compared to 68% of subjects with less than 1-log$_{10}$ decline in viral load at Treatment Week 4. Clear patterns of boceprevir treatment-emergent substitutions in the NS3 helicase domain or NS4A coding regions of the HCV genome were not observed.

Table 8 Treatment-Emergent NS3 Protease Domain Amino Acid Substitutions Detected Among Subjects treated with VICTRELIS in SPRINT-2, RESPOND-2 and P06086 Who Did Not Achieve a Sustained Virologic Response (SVR)

	Subjects Infected with HCV Genotype 1a	Subjects Infected with HCV Genotype 1b
>10% of subjects treated with VICTRELIS who did not achieve SVR	V36M, T54S, R155K	T54A, T54S, V55A, A156S, V170A
<1% to 10% of subjects treated with VICTRELIS who did not achieve SVR	V36A, T54A, V55A, V55I, V107I, R155T, A156S, A156T, V158I, D168N, I170F, I170T, I170V	V36A, V36M, T54C, T54G, V107I, R155C, R155K, A156T, A156V, V158I, I/V170T, M175L

Persistence of Resistance-Associated Substitutions
Data from an ongoing, long-term follow-up study of subjects who did not achieve SVR in Phase 2 trials with VICTRELIS, with a median duration of follow-up of approximately 2 years, indicate that HCV populations harboring certain post-baseline, treatment-emergent substitutions may decline in relative abundance over time. However, among those subjects with available data, one or more treatment-emergent substitutions remained detectable with a population-based sequencing assay in 25% of subjects after 2.5 years of follow-up. The most common NS3 substitutions detected after 2.5 years of follow-up were T54S and R155K. The lack of detection of a substitution based on a population-based assay does not necessarily indicate that viral populations carrying that substitution have declined to a background level that may have existed prior to treatment. The long-term clinical impact of the emergence or persistence of boceprevir-resistance-associated substitutions is unknown. No data are available regarding the efficacy of VICTRELIS among subjects who were previously exposed to VICTRELIS, or who previously failed treatment with a regimen containing VICTRELIS.

Effect of Baseline HCV Polymorphisms on Treatment Response
A pooled analysis was conducted to explore the association between the detection of baseline NS3/4A amino acid polymorphisms and treatment outcome in the two Phase 3 studies, SPRINT-2 and RESPOND-2.
Baseline resistance associated polymorphisms were detected in 7% of subjects by a population-based sequencing method. Overall, the presence of these polymorphisms alone did not impact SVR rates in subjects treated with VICTRELIS. However, among subjects with a relatively poor response to PegIntron/REBETOL during the 4-week lead-in period, the efficacy of VICTRELIS appeared to be reduced for those who had V36M, T54A, T54S, V55A or R155K detected at baseline. Subjects with these baseline polymorphisms and reduced response to PegIntron/REBETOL represented approximately 1% of the total number of subjects treated with VICTRELIS.

Cross-Resistance
Many of the treatment-emergent NS3 amino acid substitutions detected in subjects treated with VICTRELIS who did not achieve SVR in the Phase 3 clinical trials have been demonstrated to reduce the anti-HCV activity of other HCV NS3/4A protease inhibitors. The impact of prior exposure to VICTRELIS or treatment failure on the efficacy of other HCV NS3/4A protease inhibitors has not been studied. The efficacy of VICTRELIS has not been established for patients with a history of exposure to other NS3/4A protease inhibitors. Cross-resistance is not expected between VICTRELIS and interferons, or VICTRELIS and ribavirin.

12.5 Pharmacogenomics
A genetic variant near the gene encoding interferon-lambda-3 (IL28B rs12979860, a C to T change) is a strong predictor of response to PegIntron/REBETOL. IL28B rs12979860 was genotyped in 653 of 1048 (62%) subjects in SPRINT-2 (previously untreated) and 259 of 394 (66%) subjects in RESPOND-2 (previous partial responders and relapsers) [see Clinical Studies (14) for trial descriptions]. Among subjects that received at least one dose of placebo or VICTRELIS (Modified-Intent-to-Treat population), SVR rates tended to be lower in subjects with the C/T and T/T genotypes compared to those with the C/C genotype, particularly among previously untreated subjects receiving 48 weeks of PegIntron and REBETOL (see Table 9). Among previous treatment failures, subjects of all genotypes appeared to have higher SVR rates with regimens containing VICTRELIS. The results of this retrospective subgroup analysis should be viewed with caution because of the small sample size and potential differences in demographic or clinical characteristics of the substudy population relative to the overall trial population.
[See table 9 at bottom of page 1737]

Table 5 (cont.) Established and Other Potentially Significant Drug Interactions

Concomitant Drug Class: Drug Name	Effect on Concentration of Boceprevir or Concomitant Drug	Recommendations
Inhaled beta-agonist: salmeterol	↑ salmeterol	Concurrent use of inhaled salmeterol and VICTRELIS is not recommended due to the risk of cardiovascular events associated with salmeterol.
Narcotic Analgesic/Opioid Dependence: methadone*	↓ R-methadone	Plasma concentrations of R-methadone decreased when coadministered with VICTRELIS [see Clinical Pharmacology (12.3)]. The observed changes are not considered clinically relevant. No dose adjustment of methadone or VICTRELIS is recommended. Individual patients may require additional titration of their methadone dosage when VICTRELIS is started or stopped to ensure clinical effect of methadone.
buprenorphine/naloxone*	↑ buprenorphine/ naloxone	Plasma concentrations of buprenorphine and naloxone increased when coadministered with VICTRELIS [see Clinical Pharmacology (12.3)]. The observed changes are not considered clinically relevant. No dose adjustment of buprenorphine/naloxone or VICTRELIS is recommended.
Oral hormonal contraceptives: drospirenone/ethinyl estradiol*	↑ drospirenone ↓ ethinyl estradiol	Concentrations of drospirenone increased in the presence of boceprevir. Thus, the use of drospirenone-containing products is contraindicated during treatment with VICTRELIS due to potential for hyperkalemia [see Contraindications (4)].
norethindrone/ethinyl estradiol*	↓ ethinyl estradiol ↔ norethindrone	Concentrations of ethinyl estradiol decreased in the presence of boceprevir. Norethindrone C$_{max}$ decreased 17% in the presence of boceprevir [see Clinical Pharmacology (12.3)]. Coadministration of VICTRELIS with a combined oral contraceptive containing ethinyl estradiol and at least 1 mg of norethindrone is not likely to alter the effectiveness of this combined oral contraceptive [see Use in Specific Populations (8.1)]. Patients using estrogens as hormone replacement therapy should be clinically monitored for signs of estrogen deficiency.
PDE5 inhibitors: sildenafil, tadalafil, vardenafil	↑ sildenafil ↑ tadalafil ↑ vardenafil	Increases in PDE5 inhibitor concentrations are expected, and may result in an increase in adverse events, including hypotension, syncope, visual disturbances, and priapism. Use of REVATIO® (sildenafil) or ADCIRCA® (tadalafil) for the treatment of pulmonary arterial hypertension (PAH) is contraindicated with VICTRELIS [see Contraindications (4)]. Use of PDE5 inhibitors for erectile dysfunction: Use with caution in combination with VICTRELIS with increased monitoring for PDE5 inhibitor-associated adverse events. Do not exceed the following doses: Sildenafil: 25 mg every 48 hours Tadalafil: 10 mg every 72 hours Vardenafil: 2.5 mg every 24 hours
Proton Pump Inhibitor: omeprazole*	↔ omeprazole	No dose adjustment of omeprazole or VICTRELIS is recommended.
Sedative/hypnotics: alprazolam; IV midazolam	↑ midazolam ↑ alprazolam	Close clinical monitoring for respiratory depression and/or prolonged sedation should be exercised during coadministration of VICTRELIS. A lower dose of IV midazolam or alprazolam should be considered.

*These combinations have been studied; see Clinical Pharmacology (12.3) for magnitude of interaction.

13 NONCLINICAL TOXICOLOGY
13.1 Carcinogenesis, Mutagenesis, Impairment of Fertility
Carcinogenesis and Mutagenesis
Use with Ribavirin and Peginterferon alfa: Ribavirin is genotoxic in in vitro and in vivo assays. Ribavirin was not oncogenic in mouse and rat carcinogenicity studies at doses less than the maximum recommended daily human dose. Please refer to the prescribing information for ribavirin for additional information.
Two-year carcinogenicity studies in mice and rats were conducted with boceprevir. Mice were administered doses of up to 500 mg per kg in males and 650 mg per kg in females, and rats were administered doses of up to 125 mg per kg in males and 100 mg per kg in females. In mice, no significant increases in the incidence of drug-related neoplasms were observed at the highest doses tested resulting in boceprevir AUC exposures approximately 2.3- and 6.0-fold higher in males and females, respectively, than those in humans at the recommended dose of 800 mg three times daily. In rats, no increases in the incidence of drug-related neoplasms were observed at the highest doses tested resulting in boceprevir AUC exposures similar to those in humans at the recommended dose of 800 mg three times daily.

Table 6 Summary of the Effect of Co-administered Drugs on Boceprevir in Healthy Subjects or HCV Positive Genotype-1 Subjects

Co-administered Drug	Co-administered Drug Dose/Schedule	Boceprevir Dose/Schedule	Ratio Estimate of Boceprevir Pharmacokinetic Parameters (in Combination vs. Alone) (90% CI of the Ratio Estimate) *		
			Change in mean C_{max}	Change in mean AUC	Change in mean C_{min}
Atazanavir/Ritonavir	300 mg/100 mg daily × 22 days	800 mg three times daily × 6 days	0.93 (0.80-1.08)	0.95 (0.87-1.05)	0.82 (0.68-0.98)
Atorvastatin	40 mg single dose	800 mg three times daily × 7 days	1.04 (0.89-1.21)	0.95 (0.90-1.01)	N/A
Buprenorphine/Naloxone	Buprenorphine: 8-24 mg + Naloxone: 2-6 mg daily × 6 days	800 mg three times daily × 6 days	0.82 (0.71-0.94)	0.88 (0.76-1.02)	0.95 (0.70-1.28)
Cyclosporine	100 mg single dose	800 mg single dose	1.08 (0.97-1.20)	1.16 (1.06-1.26)	N/A
Darunavir/Ritonavir	600 mg/100 mg two times daily × 22 days	800 mg three times daily × 6 days	0.75 (0.67-0.85)	0.68 (0.65-0.72)	0.65 (0.56-0.76)
Diflunisal	250 mg two times daily × 7 days	800 mg three times daily × 12 days	0.86 (0.56-1.32)	0.96 (0.79-1.17)	1.31 (1.04-1.65)
Efavirenz	600 mg daily × 16 days	800 mg three times daily × 6 days	0.92 (0.78-1.08)	0.81 (0.75-0.89)	0.56 (0.42-0.74)
Escitalopram	10 mg single dose	800 mg three times daily × 11 days	0.91 (0.81-1.02)	1.02 (0.96-1.08)	N/A
Etravirine	200 mg two times daily × 11-14 days	800 mg three times daily × 11-14 days	1.10 (0.94-1.29)	1.10 (0.94-1.28)	0.88[†] (0.66-1.17)
Ibuprofen	600 mg three times daily × 6 days	400 mg single oral dose	0.94 (0.67-1.32)	1.04 (0.90-1.20)	N/A
Ketoconazole	400 mg two times daily × 6 days	400 mg single oral dose	1.41 (1.00-1.97)	2.31 (2.00-2.67)	N/A
Lopinavir/Ritonavir	400 mg/100 mg two times daily × 22 days	800 mg three times daily × 6 days	0.50 (0.45-0.55)	0.55 (0.49-0.61)	0.43 (0.36-0.53)
Methadone	20-150 mg daily × 6 days	800 mg three times daily × 6 days	0.62 (0.53-0.72)	0.80 (0.69-0.93)	1.03 (0.75-1.42)

(Table continued on next page)

Boceprevir was not genotoxic in a battery of *in vitro* or *in vivo* assays, including bacterial mutagenicity, chromosomal aberration in human peripheral blood lymphocytes and mouse micronucleus assays.

Impairment of Fertility
Use with Ribavirin and Peginterferon alfa: In fertility studies in male animals, ribavirin induced reversible testicular toxicity; while peginterferon alfa may impair fertility in females. Please refer to the prescribing information for ribavirin and peginterferon alfa for additional information. Boceprevir-induced reversible effects on fertility and early embryonic development in female rats, with no effects observed at a 75 mg per kg dose level. At this dose, boceprevir AUC exposures are approximately 1.3-fold higher than those in humans at the recommended dose of 800 mg three times daily. Decreased fertility was also observed in male rats, most likely as a consequence of testicular degeneration. No testicular degeneration was observed at a 15 mg per kg dose level resulting in boceprevir AUC exposures of less than those in humans at the recommended dose of 800 mg three times daily. Testicular degeneration was not observed in mice or monkeys administered boceprevir for 3 months at doses of up to 900 or 1000 mg per kg, respectively. At these doses, boceprevir AUC exposures are approximately 6.8- and 4.4-fold higher in mice and monkeys, respectively, than those in humans at the recommended dose of 800 mg three times daily. Additionally, limited clinical monitoring has revealed no evidence of testicular toxicity in human subjects.

14 CLINICAL STUDIES

The efficacy of VICTRELIS as a treatment for chronic hepatitis C (genotype 1) infection was assessed in approximately 1500 adult subjects who were previously untreated (SPRINT-2) or who had failed previous peginterferon alfa and ribavirin therapy (RESPOND-2) in Phase 3 clinical studies.

Previously Untreated Subjects
SPRINT-2 was a randomized, double-blind, placebo-controlled study comparing two therapeutic regimens of VICTRELIS 800 mg orally three times daily in combination with PR [PegIntron 1.5 micrograms per kg per week subcutaneously and weight-based dosing with REBETOL (600–1400 mg per day orally divided twice daily)] to PR alone in adult subjects who had chronic hepatitis C (HCV genotype 1) infection with detectable levels of HCV-RNA and were not previously treated with interferon alfa therapy. Subjects were randomized in a 1:1:1 ratio within two separate cohorts (Cohort 1/non-Black and Cohort 2/Black) and were stratified by HCV genotype (1a or 1b) and by HCV-RNA viral load (less than or equal to 400,000 IU per mL vs. more than 400,000 IU per mL) to one of the following three treatment arms:
• PegIntron + REBETOL for 48 weeks (PR48).
• PegIntron + REBETOL for four weeks followed by VICTRELIS 800 mg three times daily + PegIntron + REBETOL for 24 weeks. The subjects were then continued on different regimens based on Treatment Week (TW) 8

through TW24 response-guided therapy (boceprevir-RGT). All subjects in this treatment arm were limited to 24 weeks of therapy with VICTRELIS.
  ◦ Subjects with undetectable HCV-RNA (Target Not Detected) at TW8 (early responders) and remained undetectable through TW24 discontinued therapy and entered follow-up at the TW28 visit.
  ◦ Subjects with detectable HCV-RNA at TW8 or any subsequent treatment week but subsequently achieving undetectable HCV-RNA (Target Not Detected) at TW24 (late responders) were changed in a blinded fashion to placebo at the TW28 visit and continued therapy with PegIntron + REBETOL for an additional 20 weeks, for a total treatment duration of 48 weeks.
• PegIntron + REBETOL for four weeks followed by VICTRELIS 800 mg three times daily + PegIntron + REBETOL for 44 weeks (boceprevir-PR48).
All subjects with detectable HCV-RNA in plasma at TW24 were discontinued from treatment. Sustained Virologic Response (SVR) was defined as plasma HCV-RNA less than 25 IU/mL at Follow-up Week 24. Plasma HCV-RNA results at Follow-up Week 12 were used if plasma HCV-RNA results at Follow-up Week 24 were missing.
Mean age of subjects randomized was 49 years. The racial distribution of subjects was as follows: 82% White, 14% Black, and 4% others. The distribution of subjects by gender was 60% men and 40% women.
The addition of VICTRELIS to PegIntron and REBETOL significantly increased the SVR rates compared to PegIntron and REBETOL alone in the combined cohort (63% to 66% in arms containing VICTRELIS vs. 38% PR48 control) for randomized subjects who received at least one dose of any study medication (Full-Analysis-Set population). SVR rates for Blacks who received the combination of VICTRELIS with PegIntron and REBETOL were 42% to 53% in a predefined analysis (see Table 10).
[See table 10 at top of page 1738]
In subjects with cirrhosis at baseline, sustained virologic response was higher in those who received treatment with the combination of VICTRELIS with PegIntron and REBETOL for 44 weeks after lead-in therapy with PegIntron and REBETOL (10/24, 42%) compared to those who received RGT (5/16 , 31%).
Sustained Virologic Response (SVR) Based on TW8 HCV-RNA Results
Table 11 presents sustained virologic response based on TW8 HCV-RNA results in previously untreated subjects. Fifty-seven percent (208/368) of subjects in the boceprevir-RGT arm and 56% (204/366) of subjects in the boceprevir-PR48 arm had undetectable HCV-RNA (Target Not Detected) at TW8 (early responders) compared with 17% (60/363) of subjects in the PR48 arm.
[See table 11 at top of page 1738]
Among subjects with detectable HCV-RNA at TW8 who had attained undetectable HCV-RNA (Target Not Detected) at TW24 and completed at least 28 weeks of treatment, the SVR rates were 66% (45/68) in boceprevir-RGT arm (4 weeks of PegIntron and REBETOL then 24 weeks of VICTRELIS with PegIntron and REBETOL followed by 20 weeks of PegIntron and REBETOL alone) and 75% (55/73) in boceprevir-PR48 arms (4 weeks of PegIntron and REBETOL then 44 weeks of VICTRELIS with PegIntron and REBETOL).

Previous Partial Responders and Relapsers to Interferon and Ribavirin Therapy
RESPOND-2 was a randomized, parallel-group, double-blind study comparing two therapeutic regimens of VICTRELIS 800 mg orally three times daily in combination with PR [PegIntron 1.5 micrograms per kg per week subcutaneously and weight-based ribavirin (600–1400 mg per day orally divided twice daily)] compared to PR alone in adult subjects with chronic hepatitis C (HCV genotype 1) infection with demonstrated interferon responsiveness (as defined historically by a decrease in HCV viral load greater than or equal to 2-log₁₀ by Week 12, but never achieved SVR [partial responders] or undetectable HCV-RNA at end of prior treatment with a subsequent detectable HCV-RNA in plasma [relapsers]). Subjects with less than 2-log₁₀ decrease in HCV-RNA by week 12 of previous treatment (prior null responders) were not eligible for enrollment in this trial. Subjects were randomized in a 1:2:2 ratio and stratified based on response to their previous qualifying regimen (relapsers vs. partial responders) and by HCV subtype (1a vs. 1b) to one of the following treatment arms:
• PegIntron + REBETOL for 48 weeks (PR48)
• PegIntron + REBETOL for 4 weeks followed by VICTRELIS 800 mg three times daily + PegIntron + REBETOL for 32 weeks. The subjects were then continued on different treatment regimens based on TW8 and TW12 response-guided therapy (boceprevir-RGT). All subjects in this treatment arm were limited to 32 weeks of VICTRELIS.
  ◦ Subjects with undetectable HCV-RNA (Target Not Detected) at TW8 (early responders) and TW12 completed therapy at TW36 visit.
  ◦ Subjects with a detectable HCV-RNA at TW8 but subsequently undetectable (Target Not Detected) at TW12 (late responders) were changed in a blinded fashion to

placebo at the TW36 visit and continued treatment with PegIntron + REBETOL for an additional 12 weeks, for a total treatment duration of 48 weeks.

• PegIntron + REBETOL for 4 weeks followed by VICTRELIS 800 mg three times daily + PegIntron + REBETOL for 44 weeks (boceprevir-PR48).

All subjects with detectable HCV-RNA in plasma at TW12 were discontinued from treatment. Sustained Virologic Response (SVR) was defined as plasma HCV-RNA less than 25 IU/mL at Follow-up Week 24. Plasma HCV-RNA results at Follow-up Week 12 were used if plasma HCV-RNA results at Follow-up Week 24 were missing.

Mean age of subjects randomized was 53 years. The racial distribution of subjects was as follows: 85% White, 12% Black, and 3% others. The distribution of subjects by gender was 67% men and 33% women.

The addition of VICTRELIS to the PegIntron and REBETOL therapy significantly increased the SVR rates compared to PegIntron/REBETOL alone (59% to 66% in arms containing VICTRELIS vs. 23% PR48 control) for randomized subjects who received at least one dose of any study medication (Full-Analysis-Set population) (see Table 12).
[See table 12 at bottom of page 1738]

In subjects with cirrhosis at baseline, sustained virologic response was higher in those who received treatment with the combination of VICTRELIS with PegIntron and REBETOL for 44 weeks after 4 weeks of lead-in therapy with PegIntron and REBETOL (17/22, 77%) compared to those who received RGT (6/17, 35%).

Sustained Virologic Response (SVR) Based on TW8 HCV-RNA Results
Table 13 presents sustained virologic response based on TW8 HCV-RNA results in subjects who were relapsers or partial responders to previous interferon and ribavirin therapy. Forty-six percent (74/162) of subjects in the boceprevir-RGT arm and 52% (84/161) in the boceprevir-PR48 had undetectable HCV-RNA (Target Not Detected) at TW8 (early responders) compared with 9% (7/80) in the PR48 arm.
[See table 13 at top of page 1739]

Among subjects with detectable HCV-RNA at TW8 who attained an undetectable HCV-RNA (Target Not Detected) at TW12 and completed at least 36 weeks of treatment, the SVR rates were 79% (27/34) in boceprevir-RGT arm (4 weeks of PegIntron and REBETOL then 32 weeks of VICTRELIS with PegIntron and REBETOL followed by 12 weeks of PegIntron and REBETOL alone) and 72% (29/40) in boceprevir-PR48 arm (4 weeks of PegIntron and REBETOL then 44 weeks of VICTRELIS with PegIntron and REBETOL).

Interferon Responsiveness during Lead-in Therapy with Peginterferon alfa and Ribavirin
Previously Untreated Subjects
In previously untreated subjects evaluated in SPRINT-2, interferon-responsiveness (defined as greater than or equal to 1-$\log_{10}$ decline in viral load at TW4) was predictive of SVR. Subjects treated with VICTRELIS who demonstrated interferon responsiveness at TW4 achieved SVR rates of 81% (203/252) in boceprevir-RGT arm and 79% (200/254) in boceprevir-PR48 arm, compared to 52% (134/260) in subjects treated with PegIntron/REBETOL.

Subjects treated with VICTRELIS who demonstrated poor interferon responsiveness (defined as less than 1-$\log_{10}$ decline in viral load at TW4), achieved SVR rates of 28% (27/97) in boceprevir-RGT arm and 38% (36/95) in boceprevir-PR48 arm, compared to 4% (3/83) in subjects treated with PegIntron/REBETOL. Subjects with less than a 0.5-$\log_{10}$ decline in viral load at TW4 achieved SVR rates of 28% (13/47) in boceprevir-RGT arm and 30% (11/37) in boceprevir-PR48 arm, compared to 0% (0/25) in subjects treated with PegIntron/REBETOL. Subjects with less than a 0.5-$\log_{10}$ decline in viral load at TW4 with peginterferon alfa plus ribavirin therapy alone are predicted to have a null response (less than 2-$\log_{10}$ viral load decline at TW12) to peginterferon alfa and ribavirin.

Previous Partial Responders and Relapsers to Interferon and Ribavirin Therapy
In subjects who were previous relapsers and partial responders evaluated in RESPOND-2, interferon-responsiveness (defined as greater than or equal to 1-$\log_{10}$ decline in viral load at TW4) was predictive of SVR. Subjects treated with VICTRELIS who demonstrated interferon responsiveness at TW4 achieved SVR rates of 74% (81/110) in boceprevir-RGT arm and 79% (90/114) in boceprevir-PR48 arm, compared to 27% (18/67) in subjects treated with PegIntron/REBETOL. Subjects treated with VICTRELIS who demonstrated poor interferon responsiveness (defined as less than 1-$\log_{10}$ decline in viral load at TW4) achieved SVR rates of 33% (15/46) in boceprevir-RGT arm and 34% (15/44) in boceprevir-PR48 arm, compared to 0% (0/12) in subjects treated with PegIntron/REBETOL.

Prior Null Responders to Interferon and Ribavirin Therapy
PROVIDE was an open-label, single-arm trial of VICTRELIS 800 mg orally three times daily in combination with peginterferon alfa-2b 1.5 micrograms per kg per week

subcutaneously and weight-based ribavirin (600 – 1,400 mg per day orally divided twice daily) in adult subjects with chronic hepatitis C (HCV) genotype 1 infection who did not achieve SVR while in the peginterferon alfa/ribavirin control arms of previous Phase 2 and 3 trials of combination therapy with VICTRELIS. Subjects who enrolled in PROVIDE within 2 weeks after the last dose of peginterferon alfa/ribavirin in the prior trial received VICTRELIS 800 mg three times daily + peginterferon alfa-2b + ribavirin for 44 weeks. Subjects who were not able to enroll in this trial within 2 weeks received PegIntron/REBETOL lead-in for 4 weeks followed by VICTRELIS 800 mg three times daily + peginterferon alfa-2b + ribavirin for 44 weeks.

Among subjects who were null responders in the peginterferon alfa/ribavirin control arm of the prior trial, SVR (reported as plasma HCV-RNA <25 IU/mL at follow-up week 24) was 38% (20/52) and the relapse rate was 13% (3/23).

Use of Ribavirin Dose Reduction versus Erythropoiesis Stimulating Agent (ESA) in the Management of Anemia in Previously Untreated Subjects
A randomized, parallel-arm, open-label study was conducted to compare two strategies for the management of anemia (use of ESA versus ribavirin dose reduction) in 687 subjects with previously untreated CHC genotype 1 infection who became anemic during therapy with VICTRELIS 800 mg orally three times daily plus peginterferon alfa-2b 1.5 micrograms per kg per week subcutaneously and weight-based ribavirin (600 – 1,400 mg per day divided twice daily). The study enrolled subjects with serum hemoglobin concentrations of less than 15 g per dL. Subjects were treated for 4 weeks with peginterferon alfa-2b and ribavirin followed by up to 44 weeks of VICTRELIS plus peginterferon alfa-2b and ribavirin. If a subject became anemic (serum hemoglobin of approximately less than or equal to 10 g per dL within the treatment period), the subject was randomized in a 1:1 ratio to either ribavirin dose reduction (N=249) or use of erythropoietin 40,000 units subcutaneously once weekly for the management of the anemia (N=251). If serum hemoglobin concentrations continued to decrease to less than or equal to 8.5 g per dL, subjects could be treated with additional anemia interventions, including the addition of erythropoietin (18% of those in the ribavirin dose reduction arm) or ribavirin dose reduction (37% of those in the ESA arm).

Mean age of subjects randomized was 49 years. The racial distribution of subjects was as follows: 77% White, 19% Black, and 4% other. The distribution of subjects by gender was 37% men and 63% women.

The overall intent-to-treat SVR rate for all enrolled subjects (including those subjects who were not randomized to RBV dose reduction or ESA for the management of anemia) was 63% (431/687). The SVR rate in subjects randomized who received ribavirin dose reduction was 71% (178/249), similar to the SVR rate of 71% (178/251) in subjects randomized to receive an ESA. The relapse rates in subjects randomized to receive ribavirin dose reduction or an ESA were 10% (19/196) and 10% (19/197), respectively.

16 HOW SUPPLIED/STORAGE AND HANDLING
16.1 How Supplied
VICTRELIS 200 mg capsules are comprised of a red-colored cap with the Merck logo printed in yellow ink, and a yellow-colored body with "314" printed in red ink. The capsules are packaged into a carton with 28 bottles containing 12 capsules (NDC 0085-0314-02).
16.2 Storage and Handling
VICTRELIS Capsules should be refrigerated at 2–8°C (36–46°F) until dispensed. Avoid exposure to excessive heat. For patient use, refrigerated capsules of VICTRELIS can remain stable until the expiration date printed on the label. VICTRELIS can also be stored at room temperature up to 25°C (77°F) for 3 months. Keep container tightly closed.

17 PATIENT COUNSELING INFORMATION
• Advise the patient to read the FDA-approved patient labeling (Medication Guide)
VICTRELIS must be used in combination with peginterferon alfa and ribavirin, and thus all contraindications and warnings for peginterferon alfa and ribavirin also apply. If peginterferon alfa or ribavirin is permanently discontinued, VICTRELIS must also be discontinued *[see Dosage and Administration (2.3)]*.
Pregnancy
Ribavirin must not be used by women who are pregnant or by men whose female partners are pregnant. Ribavirin therapy should not be initiated until a report of a negative pregnancy test has been obtained immediately before starting therapy. Female patients of childbearing potential and male patients with female partners of childbearing potential must be advised of the teratogenic/embryocidal risks of ri-

Table 6 (cont.) Summary of the Effect of Co-administered Drugs on Boceprevir in Healthy Subjects or HCV Positive Genotype-1 Subjects

Co-administered Drug	Co-administered Drug Dose/ Schedule	Boceprevir Dose/ Schedule	Ratio Estimate of Boceprevir Pharmacokinetic Parameters (in Combination vs. Alone) (90% CI of the Ratio Estimate) *		
			Change in mean C_{max}	Change in mean AUC	Change in mean C_{min}
Omeprazole	40 mg daily × 5 days	800 mg three times daily × 5 days	0.94 (0.86-1.02)	0.92 (0.87-0.97)	1.17[†] (0.97-1.42)
Peginterferon alfa-2b	1.5 mcg/kg subcutaneous weekly × 2 weeks	400 mg three times daily × 1 week	0.88 (0.66-1.18)	1.00* (0.89-1.13)	N/A
Pravastatin	40 mg single dose	800 mg three times daily × 6 days	0.93 (0.83-1.04)	0.94 (0.88-1.01)	N/A
Raltegravir	400 mg every 12 hours × 6 days	800 mg every 8 hours × 6 days	0.96 (0.88, 1.05)	0.98[‡] (0.90, 1.08)	0.74[†] (0.47, 1.16)
Rilpivirine	25 mg every 24 hours × 11 days	800 mg three times daily × 11 days	0.98 (0.89, 1.08)	0.94[‡] (0.88, 1.00)	1.04[†] (0.93, 1.16)
Ritonavir	100 mg daily × 12 days	400 mg three times daily × 15 days	0.73 (0.57-0.93)	0.81 (0.73-0.91)	1.04 (0.62-1.75)
Sirolimus	2 mg single dose	800 mg three times daily × 9 days	0.94 (0.82, 1.07)	0.95[‡] (0.89, 1.01)	1.21[†] (1.00, 1.47)
Tacrolimus	0.5 mg single dose	800 mg single dose	0.97 (0.84-1.13)	1.00* (0.95-1.06)	N/A
Tenofovir	300 mg daily × 7 days	800 mg three times daily × 7 days	1.05 (0.98-1.12)	1.08 (1.02-1.14)	1.08 (0.97-1.20)

N/A = not available
*No effect = 1.00
[†]$C_{8\ hours}$
[‡]AUC_{0-last}

Table 7 Summary of the Effect of Boceprevir on Co-administered Drugs in Healthy Subjects or HCV Positive Genotype-1 Subjects

Co-administered Drug	Co-administered Drug Dose/ Schedule	Boceprevir Dose/ Schedule	Ratio Estimate of Co-administered Pharmacokinetic Parameters (in Combination vs. Alone) (90% CI of the Ratio Estimate) *		
			Change in mean C_{max}	Change in mean $AUC(\tau)$	Change in mean C_{min}
Atazanavir/Ritonavir	300 mg/100 mg daily × 22 days	800 mg three times daily × 6 days	Atazanavir: 0.75 (0.64-0.88) Ritonavir: 0.73 (0.64-0.83)	Atazanavir: 0.65[†] (0.55-0.78) Ritonavir: 0.64 (0.58-0.72)	Atazanavir: 0.51 (0.44-0.61) Ritonavir: 0.55 (0.45-0.67)
Atorvastatin	40 mg single dose	800 mg three times daily × 7 days	2.66 (1.81-3.90)	2.30[‡] (1.84-2.88)	N/A
Buprenorphine/ Naloxone	Buprenorphine: 8-24 mg + Naloxone: 2-6 mg daily × 6 days	800 mg three times daily × 6 days	Buprenorphine: 1.18 (0.93-1.50) Naloxone: 1.09 (0.79-1.51)	Buprenorphine: 1.19 (0.91-1.57) Naloxone: 1.33 (0.90-1.98)	Buprenorphine: 1.31 (0.95-1.79) Naloxone: N/A
Cyclosporine	100 mg single dose	800 mg three times daily × 7 days	2.01 (1.69-2.40)	2.68[‡] (2.38-3.03)	N/A
Darunavir/Ritonavir	600 mg/100 mg two times daily × 22 days	800 mg three times daily × 6 days	Darunavir: 0.64 (0.58-0.71) Ritonavir: 0.87 (0.76-1.00)	Darunavir: 0.56[†] (0.51-0.61) Ritonavir: 0.73 (0.68-0.79)	Darunavir: 0.41 (0.38-0.45) Ritonavir: 0.55 (0.52-0.59)
Digoxin	0.25 mg single dose	800 mg three times daily × 10 days	1.18 (1.07-1.31)	1.19[‡] (1.12-1.27)	N/A
Drospirenone/Ethinyl estradiol	Drospirenone: 3 mg + Ethinyl estradiol: 0.02 mg daily × 14 days	800 mg three times daily × 7 days	Drospirenone: 1.57 (1.46-1.70) Ethinyl estradiol: 1.00 (0.91-1.10)	Drospirenone: 1.99 (1.87-2.11) Ethinyl estradiol: 0.76 (0.73-0.79)	N/A
Efavirenz	600 mg daily × 16 days	800 mg three times daily × 6 days	1.11 (1.02-1.20)	1.20 (1.15-1.26)	N/A
Escitalopram	10 mg single dose	800 mg three times daily × 11 days	0.81 (0.76-0.87)	0.79[‡] (0.71-0.87)	N/A
Etravirine	200 mg two times daily × 11-14 days	800 mg three times daily × 11-14 days	0.76 (0.68-0.85)	0.77 (0.66-0.91)	0.71 (0.54-0.95)
Lopinavir/Ritonavir	400 mg/100 mg two times daily × 22 days	800 mg three times daily × 6 days	Lopinavir: 0.70 (0.65-0.77) Ritonavir: 0.88 (0.72-1.07)	Lopinavir: 0.66[†] (0.60-0.72) Ritonavir: 0.78 (0.71-0.87)	Lopinavir: 0.57 (0.49-0.65) Ritonavir: 0.58 (0.52-0.65)
Methadone	20-150 mg daily × 6 days	800 mg three times daily × 6 days	R-methadone: 0.90 (0.71-1.13) S-methadone: 0.83 (0.64-1.09)	R-methadone: 0.85 (0.74-0.96) S-methadone: 0.78 (0.66-0.93)	R-methadone: 0.81 (0.66-1.00) S-methadone: 0.74 (0.58-0.95)

(Table continued on next page)

bavirin and must be instructed to practice effective contraception during therapy and for 6 months post-therapy. Patients should be advised to notify the healthcare provider immediately in the event of a pregnancy *[see Contraindications (4) and Warnings and Precautions (5.1)].*

Women of childbearing potential and men must use at least two forms of effective contraception during treatment and for at least 6 months after treatment has been stopped; routine monthly pregnancy tests must be performed during this time. One of these reliable forms of contraception can be a combined oral contraceptive product containing at least 1 mg of norethindrone. Oral contraceptives containing lower doses of norethindrone and other forms of hormonal contraception have not been studied or are contraindicated *[see Contraindications (4) and Warnings and Precautions (5.1)].* To monitor maternal and fetal outcomes of pregnant women exposed to ribavirin, the Ribavirin Pregnancy Registry has been established. Patients should be encouraged to register by calling 1-800-593-2214.

Anemia
Patients should be informed that anemia may be increased when VICTRELIS is administered with peginterferon alfa

and ribavirin *[see Warnings and Precautions (5.2) and Adverse Reactions (6.1)].* Patients should be advised that laboratory evaluations are required prior to starting therapy and periodically thereafter *[see Warnings and Precautions (5.7)].*

Neutropenia
Patients should be informed that neutropenia may be increased when VICTRELIS is administered with peginterferon alfa and ribavirin *[see Warnings and Precautions (5.3) and Adverse Reactions (6.1)].* Patients should be advised that laboratory evaluations are required prior to starting therapy and periodically thereafter *[see Warnings and Precautions (5.7)].*

Pancytopenia
Patients should be informed that serious cases of pancytopenia have been reported during postmarketing when VICTRELIS was administered with peginterferon alfa and ribavirin *[see Warnings and Precautions (5.4) and Adverse Reactions (6.2)].* Patients should be advised that laboratory evaluations are required prior to starting therapy and periodically thereafter *[see Warnings and Precautions (5.7)].*

Hypersensitivity
Patients should be informed that serious acute hypersensitivity reactions have been observed during combination therapy with VICTRELIS, peginterferon alfa, and ribavirin therapy *[see Contraindications (4) and Warnings and Precautions (5.5)].* If symptoms of acute hypersensitivity reactions (e.g., itching; hives; swelling of the face, eyes, lips, tongue, or throat; trouble breathing or swallowing) occur, patients should seek medical advice promptly.

Usage Safeguards
Patients should be advised that VICTRELIS must not be used alone due to the high probability of resistance without combination anti-HCV therapies *[see Indications and Usage (1)].* See the prescribing information for peginterferon alfa and ribavirin for additional patient counseling information on the use of these drugs in combination with VICTRELIS. Patients should be informed of the potential for serious drug interactions with VICTRELIS, and that some drugs should not be taken with VICTRELIS *[see Contraindications (4), Warnings and Precautions (5.6), Drug Interactions (7), and Clinical Pharmacology (12.3)].*
Patients should be advised that the total daily dose of VICTRELIS is packaged into a single bottle containing 12-capsules and the patient should take four capsules three times daily with food.

Missed VICTRELIS Doses
If a patient misses a dose and it is less than 2 hours before the next dose is due, the missed dose should be skipped. If a patient misses a dose and it is 2 or more hours before the next dose is due, the patient should take the missed dose with food and resume the normal dosing schedule.

Hepatitis C Virus Transmission
Patients should be informed that the effect of treatment of hepatitis C infection on transmission is not known, and that appropriate precautions to prevent transmission of the hepatitis C virus should be taken.

Manufactured for:
Merck Sharp & Dohme Corp., a subsidiary of **Merck & Co., Inc.**, Whitehouse Station, NJ 08889, USA
Manufactured by:
MSD International GmbH (Singapore Branch) Singapore 638414, Singapore
For patent information:
www.merck.com/product/patent/home.html
Trademarks depicted herein are the property of their respective owners.
Copyright © 2011, 2013 Merck Sharp & Dohme Corp., a subsidiary of **Merck & Co., Inc.** All rights reserved.
uspi-mk3034-c-1407r068

MEDICATION GUIDE
VICTRELIS® (vic-TREL-is)
(boceprevir)
capsules
Read this Medication Guide before you start taking VICTRELIS and each time you get a refill. There may be new information. This information does not take the place of talking with your healthcare provider about your medical condition or treatment.
VICTRELIS is taken along with peginterferon alfa and ribavirin. You should also read those Medication Guides.

What is the most important information I should know about VICTRELIS?
VICTRELIS, in combination with peginterferon alfa and ribavirin, may cause birth defects or death of your unborn baby. If you are pregnant or your sexual partner is pregnant or plans to become pregnant, do not take these medicines. You or your sexual partner should not become pregnant while taking VICTRELIS, peginterferon alfa, and ribavirin combination therapy and for 6 months after treatment is over.

- **Females and males must use 2 effective forms of birth control during treatment and for 6 months after treatment with VICTRELIS, peginterferon alfa, and ribavirin combination therapy.** Hormonal forms of birth control such as implants, injections, vaginal rings, and some birth control pills may not work during treatment with VICTRELIS. The use of certain types of birth control pills may be acceptable. Talk to your healthcare provider about forms of birth control that may be used during this time.
- Females must have a pregnancy test before starting treatment with VICTRELIS, peginterferon alfa, and ribavirin combination therapy, every month while being treated, and every month for 6 months after treatment with VICTRELIS, peginterferon alfa, and ribavirin combination therapy is over.
- If you or your female sexual partner becomes pregnant while taking VICTRELIS, peginterferon alfa, and ribavirin combination therapy or within 6 months after you stop taking these medicines, tell your healthcare provider right away. You or your healthcare provider should contact the Ribavirin Pregnancy Registry by calling 1-800-593-2214. The Ribavirin Pregnancy Registry collects information about what happens to mothers and their babies if the mother takes ribavirin while she is pregnant.

Table 7 (cont.) Summary of the Effect of Boceprevir on Co-administered Drugs in Healthy Subjects or HCV Positive Genotype-1 Subjects

Co-administered Drug	Co-administered Drug Dose/ Schedule	Boceprevir Dose/ Schedule	Ratio Estimate of Co-administered Pharmacokinetic Parameters (in Combination vs. Alone) (90% CI of the Ratio Estimate) *		
			Change in mean C_{max}	Change in mean $AUC_{(\tau)}$	Change in mean C_{min}
Midazolam	4 mg single oral dose	800 mg three times daily × 6 days	2.77 (2.36-3.25)	5.30 (4.66-6.03)	N/A
Norethindrone/Ethinyl estradiol	Norethindrone: 1 mg + Ethinyl estradiol : 0.035 mg daily × 21 days	800 mg three times daily × 28 days	Norethindrone: 0.83 (0.76-0.90) Ethinyl estradiol: 0.79 (0.75 -0.84)	Norethindrone: 0.96 (0.87-1.06) Ethinyl estradiol: 0.74 (0.68-0.80)	N/A
Omeprazole	40 mg daily × 5 days	800 mg three times daily × 5 days	1.03 (0.85-1.26)	1.06 (0.90-1.25)	1.12 § (0.75-1.67)
Peginterferon alfa-2b	1.5 mcg/kg subcutaneous weekly × 2 weeks	200 mg or 400 mg three times daily × 1 week	N/A	0.99¶,# (0.83-1.17)	N/A
Pravastatin	40 mg single dose	800 mg three times daily × 6 days	1.49 (1.03-2.14)	1.63‡ (1.01-2.62)	N/A
Prednisone	40 mg single dose	800 mg three times daily × 6 days	Prednisone: 0.99 (0.94-1.04) Prednisolone: 1.16 (1.09-1.24)	Prednisone: 1.22 (1.16-1.28) Prednisolone: 1.37 (1.31-1.44)	Prednisone: N/A Prednisolone: N/A
Raltegravir	400 mg single dose	800 mg three times daily × 10 days	1.11 (0.91-1.36)	1.04 (0.88-1.22)	0.75þ (0.45-1.23)
Rilpivirine	25 mg every 24 hours × 11 days	800 mg three times daily × 11 days	1.15 (1.04, 1.28)	1.39† (1.27, 1.52)	1.51 (1.36, 1.68)
Sirolimus	2 mg single dose	800 mg every 8 hours × 9 days	4.84 (3.99, 5.88)	8.12‡ (7.08, 9.32)	N/A
Tacrolimus	0.5 mg single dose	800 mg three times daily × 11 days	9.90 (7.96-12.3)	17.1‡ (14.0-20.8)	N/A
Tenofovir	300 mg daily × 7 days	800 mg three times daily × 7 days	1.32 (1.19-1.45)	1.05 (1.01-1.09)	N/A

N/A = not available
*No effect = 1.00
†AUC_{0-last}
‡AUC_{0-inf}
§$C_{8\ hours}$
¶0-168 hours
#Reported AUC is 200 mg and 400 mg cohorts combined.
þ$C_{12\ hours}$

Table 9 Sustained Virologic Response (SVR) Rates by IL28B rs12979860 Genotype

Clinical Study	IL28B rs12979860 Genotype	SVR, % (n/N)		
		PR48*	Boceprevir-RGT*	Boceprevir-PR48*
SPRINT-2 (Previously Untreated Subjects)				
	C/C	78 (50/64)	82 (63/77)	80 (44/55)
	C/T	28 (33/116)	65 (67/103)	71 (82/115)
	T/T	27 (10/37)	55 (23/42)	59 (26/44)
RESPOND-2 (Previous Partial Responders and Relapsers)				
	C/C	46 (6/13)	79 (22/28)	77 (17/22)
	C/T	17 (5/29)	61 (38/62)	73 (48/66)
	T/T	50 (5/10)	55 (6/11)	72 (13/18)

*For description of each treatment arm, see *Clinical Studies (14)*.

- Do not take VICTRELIS alone to treat chronic hepatitis C infection. VICTRELIS must be used with peginterferon alfa and ribavirin to treat chronic hepatitis C infection.

What is VICTRELIS?
VICTRELIS is a prescription medicine used with the medicines peginterferon alfa and ribavirin to treat long-lasting (chronic) hepatitis C genotype 1 infection in adults with stable (compensated) liver disease who have not been treated before or who have failed previous treatment.
It is not known if VICTRELIS is safe and effective in children under 18 years of age.

Who should not take VICTRELIS?
See "What is the most important information I should know about VICTRELIS?"

Do not take VICTRELIS if you:
- have had an allergic reaction to boceprevir or any of the ingredients in VICTRELIS. See the end of this Medication Guide for a complete list of ingredients in VICTRELIS.
- take certain medicines. VICTRELIS may cause serious side effects when taken with certain medicines. Read the section "What should I tell my healthcare provider before taking VICTRELIS?"
Talk to your healthcare provider before taking VICTRELIS if you have any of the conditions listed below.

What should I tell my healthcare provider before taking VICTRELIS?
Before and while you take VICTRELIS, tell your healthcare provider if you:
- have certain blood disorders such as low red blood cell count (anemia), a certain type of low white blood cell count (neutropenia) or combination of low platelet, red and white blood cell counts (pancytopenia)
- have liver failure
- have liver problems other than hepatitis C infection
- have had a liver or other organ transplant
- plan to have surgery
- have any other medical condition
- are breastfeeding. It is not known if VICTRELIS passes into breast milk. You and your healthcare provider should decide if you will take VICTRELIS or breastfeed. You should not do both.

Tell your healthcare provider about all the medicines you take, including prescription and non-prescription medicines, vitamins, and herbal supplements.
VICTRELIS and other medicines may affect each other. This can cause you to have too much or not enough VICTRELIS or your other medicines in your body, affecting the way VICTRELIS and your other medicines work, or causing side effects that can be serious or life-threatening. Do not start taking a new medicine without telling your healthcare provider or pharmacist.

Do not take VICTRELIS if you take a medicine that contains:
- alfuzosin hydrochloride (UROXATRAL®)
- anti-seizure medicines:
  ○ carbamazepine (CARBATROL®, EPITOL®, EQUETRO®, TEGRETOL®, TEGRETOL® XR, TERIL™)
  ○ phenobarbital
  ○ phenytoin (DILANTIN®)
- cisapride (PROPULSID®)
- drospirenone-containing birth control medicines, including:
  ○ YAZ®, YASMIN®, ZARAH®, OCELLA®, GIANVI®, BEYAZ®, ANGELIQ®, LORYNA®, SYEDA®, SAFYRAL®
- doxazosin (CARDURA®, CARDURA® XL)
- ergot-containing medicines, including:
  ○ dihydroergotamine mesylate (D.H.E. 45®, MIGRANAL®)
  ○ ergonovine and methylergonovine (ERGOTRATE®, METHERGINE®)
  ○ ergotamine tartrate (CAFERGOT®, MIGERGOT®, ERGOMAR®, ERGOSTAT, MEDIHALER ERGOTAMINE, WIGRAINE, WIGRETTES)
- lovastatin (ADVICOR®, ALTOPREV®, MEVACOR®)
- midazolam, when taken by mouth
- pimozide (ORAP®)
- rifampin (RIFADIN®, RIFAMATE®, RIFATER®, RIMACTANE)
- sildenafil (REVATIO®), when used for treating lung problems
- silodosin (RAPAFLO®)
- simvastatin (SIMCOR®, VYTORIN®, JUVISYNC®, ZOCOR®)
- St. John's Wort (*Hypericum perforatum*) or products containing St. John's Wort
- tadalafil (ADCIRCA®), when used for treating lung problems
- tamsulosin (FLOMAX®, JALYN®)
- triazolam (HALCION®)

Tell your healthcare provider if you are taking or starting to take any of these medicines:
- atazanavir (REYATAZ®)
- clarithromycin (BIAXIN®, BIAXIN® XL, PREVPAC®)
- darunavir (PREZISTA®)
- dexamethasone

- efavirenz (SUSTIVA®, ATRIPLA®)
- etravirine (INTELENCE®)
- itraconazole (ONMEL®,SPORANOX®)
- ketoconazole (NIZORAL®)
- lopinavir (KALETRA®)
- posaconazole (NOXAFIL®)
- rifabutin (MYCOBUTIN®)
- ritonavir (NORVIR®, KALETRA®)
- voriconazole (VFEND®)

Your healthcare provider may need to monitor your therapy more closely if you take VICTRELIS with the following medicines. Talk to your healthcare provider if you are taking or starting to take a medicine that contains:

- alprazolam (XANAX®)
- amiodarone (CORDARONE®, NEXTERONE®, PACERONE®)
- amlodipine (AMTURNIDE®, NORVASC®, TEKAMLO®)
- atorvastatin (LIPITOR®)
- bepridil (VASCOR®)
- bosentan (TRACLEER®)
- budesonide (PULMICORT®, PULMICORT FLEXHALER®, RHINOCORT®, PULMICORT RESPULES®, SYMBICORT®)
- buprenorphine (BUTRANS®, BUPRENEX®, SUBOXONE®, SUBUTEX®)
- cyclosporine (GENGRAF®, NEORAL®, SANDIMMUNE®)
- desipramine (NORPRAMIN®)
- digoxin (LANOXIN®)
- diltiazem (CARDIZEM®, CARDIZEM® CD, CARDIZEM® LA, CARTIA XT®, DILACOR XR®, DILT-CD, DILTZAC, TIAZAC®, TAZTIA XT®)
- escitalopram (LEXAPRO®)
- felodipine (PLENDIL®)
- fluticasone (VERAMYST®, FLOVENT® HFA, FLOVENT® DISKUS, ADVAIR® HFA, ADVAIR DISKUS®)
- hormonal forms of birth control, including birth control pills, vaginal rings, implants and injections
- hormone replacement therapy
- methadone (METHADOSE®,DOLOPHINE®)
- naloxone
- nifedipine (PROCARDIA®, ADALAT® CC, PROCARDIA XL®, AFEDITAB® CR)
- nicardipine (CARDENE® SR, CARDENE®)
- nisoldipine (SULAR®)
- omeprazole
- prednisone
- oral and IV prednisolone
- pravastatin (PRAVACHOL®)
- propafenone (RYTHMOL®, RYTHMOL® SR)
- quinidine
- raltegravir (ISENTRESS®)
- salmeterol (ADVAIR® HFA, ADVAIR DISKUS®, SEREVENT®)
- sildenafil (VIAGRA®), when used for treating erectile dysfunction
- sirolimus (RAPAMUNE®)
- tacrolimus (PROGRAF®)
- tadalafil (CIALIS®), when used for treating erectile dysfunction
- colchicine (COLCRYS®, Probenecid and Colchicine, COL-Probenecid)
- trazodone (OLEPTRO ®)
- vardenafil (STAXYN®, LEVITRA®), when used for treating erectile dysfunction
- verapamil (CALAN®, CALAN® SR, COVERA-HS®, TARKA®, VERELAN®, VERELAN® PM
- warfarin (COUMADIN®, JANTOVEN®)

Know the medicines you take. Keep a list of them to show your healthcare provider and pharmacist when you get a new medicine.

How should I take VICTRELIS?

- Take VICTRELIS exactly as your healthcare provider tells you to take it.
- Your healthcare provider will tell you how much to take and when to take it.
- Take VICTRELIS with food (a meal or light snack).
- VICTRELIS is packaged into single daily-use bottles. Each bottle has your entire day's worth of medicine. Make sure you are taking the correct amount of medicine each time.
- If you miss a dose of VICTRELIS and it is less than 2 hours before the next dose, the missed dose should be skipped.
- If you miss a dose of VICTRELIS and it is 2 or more hours before the next dose, take the missed dose with food. Take your next dose at your normal time and continue the normal dosing schedule.
- Do not double the next dose. If you have questions about what to do, call your healthcare provider.
- Your healthcare provider should do blood tests before you start treatment, at weeks 2, 4, 8, 12 and 24, and at other times as needed during treatment, to see how well the medicines are working and to check for side effects.
- If you take too much VICTRELIS, call your healthcare provider or go to the nearest hospital emergency room right away.

Table 10 Sustained Virologic Response (SVR)*, † and Relapse Rates‡ for Previously Untreated Subjects

Study Cohorts	Boceprevir-RGT	Boceprevir-PR48	PR48
Cohort 1 Plus Cohort 2 (all subjects)	n=368	n=366	n=363
SVR† %	63	66	38
Relapse‡ % (n/N)	9 (24/257)	9 (24/265)	22 (39/176)
Cohort 1 Plus Cohort 2 (subjects without cirrhosis)	n=352	n=342	n=350
SVR†,§ % (n/N)	65 (228/352)	68 (232/342)	38 (132/350)
Cohort 1 (non-Black)	n=316	n=311	n=311
SVR† %	67	68	40
Relapse‡ % (n/N)	9 (21/232)	8 (18/230)	23 (37/162)
Cohort 2 (Black)	n=52	n=55	n=52
SVR† %	42	53	23
Relapse‡ % (n/N)	12 (3/25)	17 (6/35)	14 (2/14)

*The Full Analysis Set (FAS) consisted of all randomized subjects (N=1097) who received at least one dose of any study medication (PegIntron, REBETOL, or VICTRELIS).
†Sustained Virologic Response (SVR): reported as plasma HCV-RNA <25 IU/mL at follow-up week (FW) 24. If other HCV-RNA values were available after FW24, the last available HCV-RNA value in the period after FW24 was used. If HCV-RNA values at and after FW24 were missing, the FW12 value was used.
‡Relapse rate was the proportion of subjects with undetectable HCV-RNA (Target Not Detected) at End of Treatment (EOT) and HCV-RNA ≥25 IU/mL at End of Follow-up (EOF) among subjects who were undetectable at EOT and not missing End of Follow-up (EOF) data.
§Includes subjects with missing baseline data regarding cirrhosis as diagnosed by liver biopsy.

Table 11 Sustained Virologic Response (SVR) by HCV-RNA Detectability at TW8 in Previously Untreated Subjects in the Combined Cohort

	Boceprevir-RGT	Boceprevir-PR48	PR48
SVR by TW8 Detectability, % (n/N)*	N=337	N=335	N=331
Undetectable (Target Not Detected)	88 (184/208)	90 (184/204)	85 (51/60)
Detectable	36 (46/129)	40 (52/131)	30 (82/271)

*Denominator included only subjects with HCV-RNA results at TW8.

Table 12 Sustained Virologic Response (SVR)*, † and Relapse‡ Rates for Subjects Who have Failed Previous Therapy with Peginterferon Alfa and Ribavirin (Previous Partial Responders and Relapsers)

		Boceprevir-RGT	Boceprevir-PR48	PR48
		N=162	N=161	N=80
SVR‡ %		59	66	23
Relapse‡ % (n/N)		14 (16/111)	12 (14/121)	28 (7/25)
SVR (subjects without cirrhosis) § (n/N)		62 (90/145)	65 (90/139)	26 (18/70)
SVR by Response to Previous Peginterferon and Ribavirin Therapy				
Previous Response	Relapser, % (n/N)	70 (73/105)	75 (77/103)	31 (16/51)
	Partial responder, % (n/N)	40 (23/57)	52 (30/58)	7 (2/29)

Previous Partial Responder = subject who failed to achieve SVR after at least 12 weeks of previous treatment with peginterferon alfa and ribavirin, but demonstrated a ≥2-log$_{10}$ reduction in HCV-RNA by Week 12 and had detectable HCV-RNA at End of Treatment (EOT).
Previous Relapser = subject who failed to achieve SVR after at least 12 weeks of previous treatment with peginterferon alfa and ribavirin, but had undetectable HCV-RNA at the end of treatment.
*The Full Analysis Set (FAS) consisted of all randomized subjects (N=403) who received at least one dose of any study medication (PegIntron, REBETOL, or VICTRELIS).
†Sustained Virologic Response (SVR): reported as plasma HCV-RNA <25 IU/mL at follow-up week (FW) 24. If other HCV-RNA values were available after FW24, the last available HCV-RNA value in the period after FW24 was used. If HCV-RNA values at and after FW24 were missing, the FW12 value was used.
‡Relapse rate was the proportion of subjects with undetectable HCV-RNA (Target Not Detected) at End of Treatment (EOT) and HCV-RNA ≥25 IU/mL at End of Follow-up (EOF) among subjects who were undetectable at EOT and not missing End of Follow-up (EOF) data.
§Includes subjects with missing baseline data regarding cirrhosis as diagnosed by liver biopsy.

Table 13 Sustained Virologic Response (SVR) by HCV-RNA Detectability at TW8 in Subjects Who Have Failed Previous Therapy (Previous Partial Responders and Relapsers)

	Boceprevir-RGT	Boceprevir-PR48	PR48
SVR by TW8 Detectability, % (n/N)*	N=146	N=154	N=72
Undetectable (Target Not Detected)	88 (65/74)	88 (74/84)	100 (7/7)
Detectable	40 (29/72)	43 (30/70)	14 (9/65)

*Denominator included only subjects with HCV-RNA results at TW8.

What are the possible side effects of VICTRELIS?
VICTRELIS may cause serious side effects, including:
See "What is the most important information I should know about VICTRELIS?"
Serious allergic reactions. Serious allergic reactions can happen and may become severe requiring treatment in a hospital. Tell your healthcare provider right away if you have any of these symptoms:
• itching
• hives
• swelling of your face, eyes, lips, tongue, or throat
• trouble breathing or swallowing
Blood problems. VICTRELIS can affect your bone marrow and cause low red blood cell, low white blood cell, and low platelet counts. In some people, these blood counts may fall to dangerously low levels. If your blood cell counts become very low, you can get anemia, infections, or bleed easily.
The most common side effects of VICTRELIS in combination with peginterferon alfa and ribavirin include:
• tiredness
• nausea
• headache
• change in taste
Additionally, while the medicine has been on the market, serious skin reactions, including blistering or peeling of the skin, and infections of the blood and pneumonia have been reported. Tell your healthcare provider about any side effect that bothers you or that does not go away.
These are not all the possible side effects of VICTRELIS. For more information, ask your healthcare provider or pharmacist.
Call your doctor for medical advice about side effects. You may report side effects to FDA at 1-800-FDA-1088.
How should I store VICTRELIS?
• Store VICTRELIS capsules in a refrigerator at 36 to 46°F (2 to 8°C). Safely throw away refrigerated VICTRELIS after the expiration date.
• VICTRELIS capsules may also be stored at room temperature up to 77°F (25°C) for 3 months.
• Keep VICTRELIS in a tightly closed container and away from heat.
Keep VICTRELIS and all medicines out of the reach of children.
General information about the safe and effective use of VICTRELIS.
It is not known if treatment with VICTRELIS will prevent you from infecting another person with the hepatitis C virus during your treatment. Talk with your healthcare provider about ways to prevent spreading the hepatitis C virus.
Medicines are sometimes prescribed for purposes other than those listed in a Medication Guide.
Do not use VICTRELIS for a condition for which it was not prescribed. Do not give VICTRELIS to other people, even if they have the same symptoms that you have. It may harm them.
This Medication Guide summarizes the most important information about VICTRELIS. If you would like more information, talk with your healthcare provider. You can ask your pharmacist or healthcare provider for information about VICTRELIS that is written for health professionals.
For more information, go to www.victrelis.com or call 1-877-888-4231.
What are the ingredients in VICTRELIS?
Active ingredients: boceprevir
Inactive ingredients: sodium lauryl sulfate, microcrystalline cellulose, lactose monohydrate, croscarmellose sodium, pre-gelatinized starch, and magnesium stearate.
Red capsule shell: gelatin, titanium dioxide, D&C Yellow #10, FD&C Blue #1, FD&C Red #40.
Yellow capsule shell: gelatin, titanium dioxide, D&C Yellow #10, FD&C Red #40, FD&C Yellow #6.
Red printing ink: shellac, red iron oxide. **Yellow printing ink:** shellac, titanium dioxide, povidone, D&C Yellow #10 Aluminum Lake.
This Medication Guide has been approved by the U.S. Food and Drug Administration.

Manufactured for:
Merck Sharp & Dohme Corp., a subsidiary of **Merck & Co., Inc.**, Whitehouse Station, NJ 08889, USA
Manufactured by:
MSD International GmbH (Singapore Branch) Singapore 638414, Singapore
Revised: 07/2014
For patent information:
www.merck.com/product/patent/home.html
Trademarks depicted herein are the property of their respective owners.
Copyright © 2011, 2012 Merck Sharp & Dohme Corp., a subsidiary of **Merck & Co., Inc.** All rights reserved.
usmg-mk3034-c-1407r038
Shown in Product Identification Guide, page 309

VYTORIN®   ℞
[vĭ-tŏr-in]
(ezetimibe/simvastatin)
Tablets

HIGHLIGHTS OF PRESCRIBING INFORMATION
These highlights do not include all the information needed to use VYTORIN safely and effectively. See full prescribing information for VYTORIN.
VYTORIN® (ezetimibe/simvastatin) Tablets
Initial U.S. Approval: 2004

—————**RECENT MAJOR CHANGES**—————

Dosage and Administration	
Patients with Homozygous Familial Hypercholesterolemia (2.4)	10/2013
Patients with Hepatic Impairment (2.5)	removal 02/2014
Contraindications (4)	02/2014
Warnings and Precautions	
Myopathy/Rhabdomyolysis (5.1)	02/2014
Hepatic Impairment (5.3)	removal 02/2014

—————**INDICATIONS AND USAGE**—————

VYTORIN, which contains a cholesterol absorption inhibitor and an HMG-CoA reductase inhibitor (statin), is indicated as adjunctive therapy to diet to:
• reduce elevated total-C, LDL-C, Apo B, TG, and non-HDL-C, and to increase HDL-C in patients with primary (heterozygous familial and non-familial) hyperlipidemia or mixed hyperlipidemia. (1.1)
• reduce elevated total-C and LDL-C in patients with homozygous familial hypercholesterolemia (HoFH), as an adjunct to other lipid-lowering treatments. (1.2)
Limitations of Use (1.3)
• No incremental benefit of VYTORIN on cardiovascular morbidity and mortality over and above that demonstrated for simvastatin has been established.
• VYTORIN has not been studied in Fredrickson Type I, III, IV, and V dyslipidemias.

—————**DOSAGE AND ADMINISTRATION**—————

• Dose range is 10/10 mg/day to 10/40 mg/day. (2.1)
• Recommended usual starting dose is 10/10 or 10/20 mg/day. (2.1)
• Due to the increased risk of myopathy, including rhabdomyolysis, use of the 10/80-mg dose of VYTORIN should be restricted to patients who have been taking VYTORIN 10/80 mg chronically (e.g., for 12 months or more) without evidence of muscle toxicity. (2.2)
• Patients who are currently tolerating the 10/80-mg dose of VYTORIN who need to be initiated on an interacting drug that is contraindicated or is associated with a dose cap for simvastatin should be switched to an alternative statin or statin-based regimen with less potential for the drug-drug interaction. (2.2)
• Due to the increased risk of myopathy, including rhabdomyolysis, associated with the 10/80-mg dose of VYTORIN, patients unable to achieve their LDL-C goal utilizing the 10/40-mg dose of VYTORIN should not be titrated to the 10/80-mg dose, but should be placed on alternative LDL-C-lowering treatment(s) that provides greater LDL-C lowering. (2.2)
• Dosing of VYTORIN should occur either ≥2 hours before or ≥4 hours after administration of a bile acid sequestrant. (2.3, 7.5)

—————**DOSAGE FORMS AND STRENGTHS**—————

• Tablets (ezetimibe mg/simvastatin mg): 10/10, 10/20, 10/40, 10/80 (3)

—————**CONTRAINDICATIONS**—————

• Concomitant administration of strong CYP3A4 inhibitors. (4, 5.1)
• Concomitant administration of gemfibrozil, cyclosporine, or danazol. (4, 5.1)
• Hypersensitivity to any component of this medication (4, 6.2)
• Active liver disease or unexplained persistent elevations of hepatic transaminase levels (4, 5.2)
• Women who are pregnant or may become pregnant (4, 8.1)
• Nursing mothers (4, 8.3)

—————**WARNINGS AND PRECAUTIONS**—————

• Patients should be advised of the increased risk of myopathy, including rhabdomyolysis, with the 10/80-mg dose. (5.1)
• Patients should be advised to report promptly any unexplained and/or persistent muscle pain, tenderness, or weakness. VYTORIN should be discontinued immediately if myopathy is diagnosed or suspected. (5.1)
• Skeletal muscle effects (e.g., myopathy and rhabdomyolysis): Risks increase with higher doses and concomitant use of certain medicines. Predisposing factors include advanced age (≥65), female gender, uncontrolled hypothyroidism, and renal impairment. Rare cases of rhabdomyolysis with acute renal failure secondary to myoglobinuria have been reported. (4, 5.1, 8.5, 8.6)
• Liver enzyme abnormalities: Persistent elevations in hepatic transaminases can occur. Check liver enzyme tests before initiating therapy and as clinically indicated thereafter. (5.2)

—————**ADVERSE REACTIONS**—————

• Common (incidence ≥2% and greater than placebo) adverse reactions in clinical trials: headache, increased ALT, myalgia, upper respiratory tract infection, and diarrhea. (6.1)

To report SUSPECTED ADVERSE REACTIONS, contact Merck Sharp & Dohme Corp., a subsidiary of Merck & Co., Inc., at 1-877-888-4231 or FDA at 1-800-FDA-1088 or www.fda.gov/medwatch.

—————**DRUG INTERACTIONS**—————

Drug Interactions Associated with Increased Risk of Myopathy/Rhabdomyolysis (2.3, 2.4, 4, 5.1, 7.1, 7.2, 7.3, 7.6, 7.8, 12.3)

Interacting Agents	Prescribing Recommendations
Strong CYP3A4 Inhibitors, (e.g., itraconazole, ketoconazole, posaconazole, voriconazole, erythromycin, clarithromycin, telithromycin, HIV protease inhibitors, boceprevir, telaprevir, nefazodone, cobicistat-containing products), gemfibrozil, cyclosporine, danazol	Contraindicated with VYTORIN
Verapamil, diltiazem, dronedarone	Do not exceed 10/10 mg VYTORIN daily
Amiodarone, amlodipine, ranolazine	Do not exceed 10/20 mg VYTORIN daily
Lomitapide	For patients with HoFH, do not exceed 10/20 mg VYTORIN daily*
Grapefruit juice	Avoid grapefruit juice

* For patients with HoFH who have been taking 80 mg simvastatin chronically (e.g., for 12 months or more) without evidence of muscle toxicity, do not exceed 10/40 mg VYTORIN when taking lomitapide.

• Coumarin anticoagulants: simvastatin prolongs INR. Achieve stable INR prior to starting VYTORIN. Monitor INR frequently until stable upon initiation or alteration of VYTORIN therapy. (7.8)
• Cholestyramine: Combination decreases exposure of ezetimibe. (2.3, 7.5)

- Other Lipid-lowering Medications: Use with fenofibrates or lipid-modifying doses (≥1 g/day) of niacin increases the risk of adverse skeletal muscle effects. Caution should be used when prescribing with VYTORIN. (5.1, 7.2, 7.4)
- Fenofibrates: Combination increases exposure of ezetimibe. If cholelithiasis is suspected in a patient receiving ezetimibe and a fenofibrate, gallbladder studies are indicated and alternative lipid-lowering therapy should be considered. (7.2, 7.7 12.3)

---USE IN SPECIFIC POPULATIONS---

- Moderate to severe renal impairment: Doses exceeding 10/20 mg/day should be used with caution and close monitoring (2.5, 8.6).

See 17 for PATIENT COUNSELING INFORMATION and FDA-approved patient labeling

Revised: 02/2014

FULL PRESCRIBING INFORMATION

1 INDICATIONS AND USAGE

Therapy with lipid-altering agents should be only one component of multiple risk factor intervention in individuals at significantly increased risk for atherosclerotic vascular disease due to hypercholesterolemia. Drug therapy is indicated as an adjunct to diet when the response to a diet restricted in saturated fat and cholesterol and other nonpharmacologic measures alone has been inadequate.

1.1 Primary Hyperlipidemia

VYTORIN® is indicated for the reduction of elevated total cholesterol (total-C), low-density lipoprotein cholesterol (LDL-C), apolipoprotein B (Apo B), triglycerides (TG), and non-high-density lipoprotein cholesterol (non-HDL-C), and to increase high-density lipoprotein cholesterol (HDL-C) in patients with primary (heterozygous familial and non-familial) hyperlipidemia or mixed hyperlipidemia.

1.2 Homozygous Familial Hypercholesterolemia (HoFH)

VYTORIN is indicated for the reduction of elevated total-C and LDL-C in patients with homozygous familial hypercholesterolemia, as an adjunct to other lipid-lowering treatments (e.g., LDL apheresis) or if such treatments are unavailable.

1.3 Limitations of Use

No incremental benefit of VYTORIN on cardiovascular morbidity and mortality over and above that demonstrated for simvastatin has been established.

VYTORIN has not been studied in Fredrickson type I, III, IV, and V dyslipidemias.

2 DOSAGE AND ADMINISTRATION

2.1 Recommended Dosing

The usual dosage range is 10/10 mg/day to 10/40 mg/day. The recommended usual starting dose is 10/10 mg/day or 10/20 mg/day. VYTORIN should be taken as a single daily dose in the evening, with or without food. Patients who require a larger reduction in LDL-C (greater than 55%) may be started at 10/40 mg/day in the absence of moderate or severe renal impairment (estimated glomerular filtration rate <60 mL/min/1.73 m^2). After initiation or titration of VYTORIN, lipid levels may be analyzed after 2 or more weeks and dosage adjusted, if needed.

2.2 Restricted Dosing for 10/80 mg

Due to the increased risk of myopathy, including rhabdomyolysis, particularly during the first year of treatment, use of the 10/80-mg dose of VYTORIN should be restricted to patients who have been taking VYTORIN 10/80 mg chronically (e.g., for 12 months or more) without evidence of muscle toxicity [see Warnings and Precautions (5.1)].

Patients who are currently tolerating the 10/80-mg dose of VYTORIN who need to be initiated on an interacting drug that is contraindicated or is associated with a dose cap for simvastatin should be switched to an alternative statin or statin-based regimen with less potential for the drug-drug interaction.

Due to the increased risk of myopathy, including rhabdomyolysis, associated with the 10/80-mg dose of VYTORIN, patients unable to achieve their LDL-C goal utilizing the 10/40-mg dose of VYTORIN should not be titrated to the 10/80-mg dose, but should be placed on alternative LDL-C-lowering treatment(s) that provides greater LDL-C lowering.

2.3 Coadministration with Other Drugs

Patients taking Verapamil, Diltiazem, or Dronedarone
- The dose of VYTORIN should not exceed 10/10 mg/day [see Warnings and Precautions (5.1), Drug Interactions (7.3), and Clinical Pharmacology (12.3)].

Patients taking Amiodarone, Amlodipine or Ranolazine
- The dose of VYTORIN should not exceed 10/20 mg/day [see Warnings and Precautions (5.1), Drug Interactions (7.3), and Clinical Pharmacology (12.3)].

Patients taking Bile Acid Sequestrants
- Dosing of VYTORIN should occur either greater than or equal to 2 hours before or greater than or equal to 4 hours after administration of a bile acid sequestrant [see Drug Interactions (7.5)].

2.4 Patients with Homozygous Familial Hypercholesterolemia

The recommended dosage for patients with homozygous familial hypercholesterolemia is VYTORIN 10/40 mg/day in the evening [see Dosage and Administration, Restricted Dosing for 10/80 mg (2.2)]. VYTORIN should be used as an adjunct to other lipid-lowering treatments (e.g., LDL apheresis) in these patients or if such treatments are unavailable.

Simvastatin exposure is approximately doubled with concomitant use of lomitapide; therefore, the dose of VYTORIN should be reduced by 50% if initiating lomitapide. VYTORIN dosage should not exceed 10/20 mg/day (or 10/40 mg/day for patients who have previously taken simvastatin 80 mg/day chronically, e.g., for 12 months or more, without evidence of muscle toxicity) while taking lomitapide.

2.5 Patients with Renal Impairment/Chronic Kidney Disease

In patients with mild renal impairment (estimated GFR greater than or equal to 60 mL/min/1.73 m^2), no dosage adjustment is necessary. In patients with chronic kidney disease and estimated glomerular filtration rate less than 60 mL/min/1.73 m^2, the dose of VYTORIN is 10/20 mg/day in the evening. In such patients, higher doses should be used with caution and close monitoring [see Warnings and Precautions (5.1); Clinical Pharmacology (12.3)].

2.6 Geriatric Patients

No dosage adjustment is necessary in geriatric patients [see Clinical Pharmacology (12.3)].

2.7 Chinese Patients Taking Lipid-Modifying Doses (greater than or equal to 1 g/day Niacin) of Niacin-Containing Products

Because of an increased risk for myopathy in Chinese patients taking simvastatin 40 mg coadministered with lipid-modifying doses (greater than or equal to 1 g/day niacin) of niacin-containing products, caution should be used when treating Chinese patients with VYTORIN doses exceeding 10/20 mg/day coadministered with lipid-modifying doses (greater than or equal to 1 g/day niacin) of niacin-containing products. Because the risk for myopathy is dose-related, Chinese patients should not receive VYTORIN 10/80 mg coadministered with lipid-modifying doses of niacin-containing products. The cause of the increased risk of myopathy is not known. It is also unknown if the risk for myopathy with coadministration of simvastatin with lipid-modifying doses of niacin-containing products observed in Chinese patients applies to other Asian patients. [See Warnings and Precautions (5.1).]

3 DOSAGE FORMS AND STRENGTHS

- VYTORIN® 10/10, (ezetimibe 10 mg/simvastatin 10 mg tablets) are white to off-white capsule-shaped tablets with code "311" on one side.
- VYTORIN® 10/20, (ezetimibe 10 mg/simvastatin 20 mg tablets) are white to off-white capsule-shaped tablets with code "312" on one side.
- VYTORIN® 10/40, (ezetimibe 10 mg/simvastatin 40 mg tablets) are white to off-white capsule-shaped tablets with code "313" on one side.
- VYTORIN® 10/80, (ezetimibe 10 mg/simvastatin 80 mg tablets) are white to off-white capsule-shaped tablets with code "315" on one side.

4 CONTRAINDICATIONS

VYTORIN is contraindicated in the following conditions:
- Concomitant administration of strong CYP3A4 inhibitors (e.g., itraconazole, ketoconazole, posaconazole, voriconazole, HIV protease inhibitors, boceprevir, telaprevir, erythromycin, clarithromycin, telithromycin, nefazodone, and cobicistat-containing products) [see Warnings and Precautions (5.1)].
- Concomitant administration of gemfibrozil, cyclosporine, or danazol [see Warnings and Precautions (5.1)].
- Hypersensitivity to any component of this medication [see Adverse Reactions (6.2)].
- Active liver disease or unexplained persistent elevations in hepatic transaminase levels [see Warnings and Precautions (5.2)].
- Women who are pregnant or may become pregnant. Serum cholesterol and triglycerides increase during normal pregnancy, and cholesterol or cholesterol derivatives are essential for fetal development. Because HMG-CoA reductase inhibitors (statins), such as simvastatin, decrease cholesterol synthesis and possibly the synthesis of other biologically active substances derived from cholesterol, VYTORIN may cause fetal harm when administered to a pregnant woman. Atherosclerosis is a chronic process and the discontinuation of lipid-lowering drugs during pregnancy should have little impact on the outcome of long-term therapy of primary hypercholesterolemia. There are no adequate and well-controlled studies of VYTORIN use during pregnancy; however, in rare reports congenital anomalies were observed following intrauterine exposure to statins. In rat and rabbit animal reproduction studies, simvastatin revealed no evidence of teratogenicity. **VYTORIN should be administered to women of childbearing age only when such patients are highly unlikely to conceive.** If the patient becomes pregnant while taking this drug, VYTORIN should be discontinued immediately and the patient should be apprised of the potential hazard to the fetus [see Use in Specific Populations (8.1)].
- Nursing mothers. It is not known whether simvastatin is excreted into human milk; however, a small amount of another drug in this class does pass into breast milk. Because statins have the potential for serious adverse reactions in nursing infants, women who require VYTORIN treatment should not breastfeed their infants [see Use in Specific Populations (8.3)].

5 WARNINGS AND PRECAUTIONS

5.1 Myopathy/Rhabdomyolysis

Simvastatin occasionally causes myopathy manifested as muscle pain, tenderness or weakness with creatine kinase above ten times the upper limit of normal (ULN). Myopathy sometimes takes the form of rhabdomyolysis with or without acute renal failure secondary to myoglobinuria, and rare fatalities have occurred. The risk of myopathy is increased by high levels of statin activity in plasma. Predisposing factors for myopathy include advanced age (≥65 years), female gender, uncontrolled hypothyroidism, and renal impairment.

The risk of myopathy, including rhabdomyolysis, is dose related. In a clinical trial database in which 41,413 patients were treated with simvastatin, 24,747 (approximately 60%) of whom were enrolled in studies with a median follow-up of at least 4 years, the incidence of myopathy was approximately 0.03% and 0.08% at 20 and 40 mg/day, respectively. The incidence of myopathy with 80 mg (0.61%) was disproportionately higher than that observed at the lower doses. In these trials, patients were carefully monitored and some interacting medicinal products were excluded.

In a clinical trial in which 12,064 patients with a history of myocardial infarction were treated with simvastatin (mean follow-up 6.7 years), the incidence of myopathy (defined as unexplained muscle weakness or pain with a serum creatine kinase [CK] >10 times upper limit of normal [ULN]) in patients on 80 mg/day was approximately 0.9% compared with 0.02% for patients on 20 mg/day. The incidence of rhabdomyolysis (defined as myopathy with a CK >40 times ULN) in patients on 80 mg/day was approximately 0.4% compared with 0% for patients on 20 mg/day. The incidence of myopathy, including rhabdomyolysis, was highest during the first year and then notably decreased during the subsequent years of treatment. In this trial, patients were carefully monitored and some interacting medicinal products were excluded.

The risk of myopathy, including rhabdomyolysis, is greater in patients on simvastatin 80 mg compared with other statin therapies with similar or greater LDL-C-lowering efficacy and compared with lower doses of simvastatin. Therefore, the 10/80-mg dose of VYTORIN should be used only in patients who have been taking VYTORIN 10/80 mg chronically (e.g., for 12 months or more) without evidence of muscle toxicity [see Dosage and Administration, Restricted Dosing for 10/80 mg (2.2)]. If, however, a patient who is currently tolerating the 10/80-mg dose of VYTORIN needs to be initiated on an interacting drug that is contraindicated or is associated with a dose cap for simvastatin, that patient should be switched to an alternative statin or statin-based regimen with less potential for the drug-drug interaction. Patients should be advised of the increased risk of myopathy, including rhabdomyolysis, and to report promptly any unexplained muscle pain, tenderness or weakness. If symptoms occur, treatment should be discontinued immediately [see Warnings and Precautions (5.2)].

In the Study of Heart and Renal Protection (SHARP), 9270 patients with chronic kidney disease were allocated to receive VYTORIN 10/20 mg daily (n=4650) or placebo (n=4620). During a median follow-up period of 4.9 years, the incidence of myopathy (defined as unexplained muscle weakness or pain with a serum creatine kinase [CK] >10 times upper limit of normal [ULN]) was 0.2% for VYTORIN and 0.1% for placebo: the incidence of rhabdomyolysis (defined as myopathy with a CK > 40 times ULN) was 0.09% for VYTORIN and 0.02% for placebo.

In postmarketing experience with ezetimibe, cases of myopathy and rhabdomyolysis have been reported. Most patients who developed rhabdomyolysis were taking a statin prior to initiating ezetimibe. However, rhabdomyolysis has been reported with ezetimibe monotherapy and with the addition of ezetimibe to agents known to be associated with increased risk of rhabdomyolysis, such as fibric acid derivatives. VYTORIN and a fenofibrate, if taking concomitantly, should both be immediately discontinued if myopathy is diagnosed or suspected.

There have been rare reports of immune-mediated necrotizing myopathy (IMNM), an autoimmune myopathy, associated with statin use. IMNM is characterized by: proximal muscle weakness and elevated serum creatine kinase, which persist despite discontinuation of statin treatment; muscle biopsy showing necrotizing myopathy without significant inflammation; improvement with immunosuppressive agents.

All patients starting therapy with VYTORIN or whose dose of VYTORIN is being increased should be advised of the risk of myopathy, including rhabdomyolysis, and told to report promptly any unexplained muscle pain, tenderness or weakness particularly if accompanied by malaise or fever or if muscle signs and symptoms persist after discontinuing VYTORIN. VYTORIN therapy should be discontinued immediately if myopathy is diagnosed or suspected. In most cases, muscle symptoms and CK increases resolved when simvastatin treatment was promptly discontinued. Periodic CK determinations may be considered in patients starting therapy with VYTORIN or whose dose is being increased, but there is no assurance that such monitoring will prevent myopathy.

Many of the patients who have developed rhabdomyolysis on therapy with simvastatin have had complicated medical histories, including renal insufficiency usually as a consequence of long-standing diabetes mellitus. Such patients taking VYTORIN merit closer monitoring.

VYTORIN therapy should be discontinued if markedly elevated CPK levels occur or myopathy is diagnosed or suspected. VYTORIN therapy should also be temporarily withheld in any patient experiencing an acute or serious condition predisposing to the development of renal failure secondary to rhabdomyolysis, e.g., sepsis; hypotension; major surgery; trauma; severe metabolic, endocrine, or electrolyte disorders; or uncontrolled epilepsy.

Drug Interactions

The risk of myopathy and rhabdomyolysis is increased by high levels of statin activity in plasma. Simvastatin is metabolized by the cytochrome P450 isoform 3A4. Certain drugs that inhibit this metabolic pathway can raise the plasma levels of simvastatin and may increase the risk of myopathy. These include itraconazole, ketoconazole, posaconazole, and voriconazole, the macrolide antibiotics erythromycin and clarithromycin, and the ketolide antibiotic telithromycin, HIV protease inhibitors, boceprevir, telaprevir, the antidepressant nefazodone, cobicistat-containing products, or grapefruit juice. [See Clinical Pharmacology (12.3).] Combination of these drugs with VYTORIN is contraindicated. If short-term treatment with strong CYP3A4 inhibitors is unavoidable, therapy with VYTORIN must be suspended during the course of treatment. [See Contraindications (4) and Drug Interactions (7).]

The combined use of VYTORIN with gemfibrozil, cyclosporine, or danazol is contraindicated [see Contraindications (4) and Drug Interactions (7.1 and 7.2)].

Caution should be used when prescribing fenofibrates with VYTORIN, as these agents can cause myopathy when given alone and the risk is increased when they are coadministered [see Drug Interactions (7.2, 7.7)].

Cases of myopathy, including rhabdomyolysis, have been reported with simvastatin coadministered with colchicine, and caution should be exercised when prescribing VYTORIN with colchicine [see Drug Interactions (7.9)].

The benefits of the combined use of VYTORIN with the following drugs should be carefully weighed against the potential risks of combinations: other lipid-lowering drugs (fenofibrates, ≥1 g/day of niacin, or, for patients with HoFH, lomitapide), amiodarone, dronedarone, verapamil, diltiazem, amlodipine, or ranolazine [see Drug Interactions (7.3) and Table 6 in Clinical Pharmacology (12.3)] [also see Dosage and Administration, Patients with Homozygous Familial Hypercholesterolemia (2.4)].

Cases of myopathy, including rhabdomyolysis, have been observed with simvastatin coadministered with lipid-modifying doses (≥1 g/day niacin) of niacin-containing products. In an ongoing, double-blind, randomized cardiovascular outcomes trial, an independent safety monitoring committee identified that the incidence of myopathy is higher in Chinese compared with non-Chinese patients taking simvastatin 40 mg or ezetimibe/simvastatin 10/40 mg coadministered with lipid-modifying doses of a niacin-containing product. Caution should be used when treating Chinese patients with VYTORIN in doses exceeding 10/20 mg/day coadministered with lipid-modifying doses of niacin-containing products. Because the risk for myopathy is dose-related, Chinese patients should not receive VYTORIN 10/80 mg coadministered with lipid-modifying doses of niacin-containing products. It is unknown if the risk for myopathy with coadministration of simvastatin with lipid-modifying doses of niacin-containing products observed in Chinese patients applies to other Asian patients [see Drug Interactions (7.4)].

Prescribing recommendations for interacting agents are summarized in Table 1 [see also Dosage and Administration (2.3, 2.4), Drug Interactions (7), and Clinical Pharmacology (12.3)].

Table 1: Drug Interactions Associated with Increased Risk of Myopathy/Rhabdomyolysis

Interacting Agents	Prescribing Recommendations
Strong CYP3A4 Inhibitors, e.g.: Itraconazole Ketoconazole Posaconazole Voriconazole Erythromycin Clarithromycin Telithromycin HIV protease inhibitors Boceprevir Telaprevir Nefazodone Cobicistat-containing products Gemfibrozil Cyclosporine Danazol	Contraindicated with VYTORIN
Verapamil Diltiazem Dronedarone	Do not exceed 10/10 mg VYTORIN daily
Amiodarone Amlodipine Ranolazine	Do not exceed 10/20 mg VYTORIN daily
Lomitapide	For patients with HoFH, do not exceed 10/20 mg VYTORIN daily*
Grapefruit juice	Avoid grapefruit juice

* For patients with HoFH who have been taking 80 mg simvastatin chronically (e.g., for 12 months or more) without evidence of muscle toxicity, do not exceed 10/40 mg VYTORIN when taking lomitapide.

5.2   Liver Enzymes

In three placebo-controlled, 12-week trials, the incidence of consecutive elevations (≥3 × ULN) in serum transaminases was 1.7% overall for patients treated with VYTORIN and appeared to be dose-related with an incidence of 2.6% for patients treated with VYTORIN 10/80. In controlled long-term (48-week) extensions, which included both newly-treated and previously-treated patients, the incidence of consecutive elevations (≥3 × ULN) in serum transaminases was 1.8% overall and 3.6% for patients treated with VYTORIN 10/80. These elevations in transaminases were generally asymptomatic, not associated with cholestasis, and returned to baseline after discontinuation of therapy or with continued treatment.

In SHARP, 9270 patients with chronic kidney disease were allocated to receive VYTORIN 10/20 mg daily (n=4650), or placebo (n=4620). During a median follow-up period of 4.9 years, the incidence of consecutive elevations of transaminases (>3 × ULN) was 0.7% for VYTORIN and 0.6% for placebo.

It is recommended that liver function tests be performed before the initiation of treatment with VYTORIN, and thereafter when clinically indicated. There have been rare postmarketing reports of fatal and non-fatal hepatic failure in patients taking statins, including simvastatin. If serious liver injury with clinical symptoms and/or hyperbilirubinemia or jaundice occurs during treatment with VYTORIN, promptly interrupt therapy. If an alternate etiology is not found do not restart VYTORIN. Note that ALT may emanate from muscle, therefore ALT rising with CK may indicate myopathy [see Warnings and Precautions (5.1)].

VYTORIN should be used with caution in patients who consume substantial quantities of alcohol and/or have a past history of liver disease. Active liver diseases or unexplained persistent transaminase elevations are contraindications to the use of VYTORIN.

5.3   Endocrine Function

Increases in HbA1c and fasting serum glucose levels have been reported with HMG-CoA reductase inhibitors, including simvastatin.

6   ADVERSE REACTIONS

The following serious adverse reactions are discussed in greater detail in other sections of the label:
• Rhabdomyolysis and myopathy [see Warnings and Precautions (5.1)]
• Liver enzyme abnormalities [see Warnings and Precautions (5.2)]

6.1   Clinical Trials Experience

VYTORIN

Because clinical studies are conducted under widely varying conditions, adverse reaction rates observed in the clinical studies of a drug cannot be directly compared to rates in the clinical studies of another drug and may not reflect the rates observed in practice.

In the VYTORIN (ezetimibe/simvastatin) placebo-controlled clinical trials database of 1420 patients (age range 20-83 years, 52% women, 87% Caucasians, 3% Blacks, 5% Hispanics, 3% Asians) with a median treatment duration of 27 weeks, 5% of patients on VYTORIN and 2.2% of patients on placebo discontinued due to adverse reactions.

The most common adverse reactions in the group treated with VYTORIN that led to treatment discontinuation and occurred at a rate greater than placebo were:
• Increased ALT (0.9%)
• Myalgia (0.6%)
• Increased AST (0.4%)
• Back pain (0.4%)

The most commonly reported adverse reactions (incidence ≥2% and greater than placebo) in controlled clinical trials were: headache (5.8%), increased ALT (3.7%), myalgia (3.6%), upper respiratory tract infection (3.6%), and diarrhea (2.8%).

VYTORIN has been evaluated for safety in more than 10,189 patients in clinical trials.

Table 2*: Clinical Adverse Reactions Occurring in ≥2% of Patients Treated with VYTORIN and at an Incidence Greater than Placebo, Regardless of Causality

Body System/Organ Class Adverse Reaction	Placebo (%) n=371	Ezetimibe 10 mg (%) n=302	Simvastatin† (%) n=1234	VYTORIN† (%) n=1420
Body as a whole – general disorders				
Headache	5.4	6.0	5.9	5.8
Gastrointestinal system disorders				
Diarrhea	2.2	5.0	3.7	2.8
Infections and infestations				
Influenza	0.8	1.0	1.9	2.3
Upper respiratory tract infection	2.7	5.0	5.0	3.6
Musculoskeletal and connective tissue disorders				
Myalgia	2.4	2.3	2.6	3.6
Pain in extremity	1.3	3.0	2.0	2.3

* Includes two placebo-controlled combination studies in which the active ingredients equivalent to VYTORIN were coadministered and two placebo-controlled studies in which VYTORIN was administered.
† All doses.

Table 2 summarizes the frequency of clinical adverse reactions reported in ≥2% of patients treated with VYTORIN (n=1420) and at an incidence greater than placebo, regardless of causality assessment, from four placebo-controlled trials.

[See table 2 above]

Study of Heart and Renal Protection
In SHARP, 9270 patients were allocated to VYTORIN 10/20 mg daily (n=4650) or placebo (n=4620) for a median follow-up period of 4.9 years. The proportion of patients who permanently discontinued study treatment as a result of either an adverse event or abnormal safety blood result was 10.4% vs. 9.8% among patients allocated to VYTORIN and placebo, respectively. Comparing those allocated to VYTORIN vs. placebo, the incidence of myopathy (defined as unexplained muscle weakness or pain with a serum CK >10 times ULN) was 0.2% vs. 0.1% and the incidence of rhabdomyolysis (defined as myopathy with a CK >40 times ULN) was 0.09% vs. 0.02%, respectively. Consecutive elevations of transaminases (>3 × ULN) occurred in 0.7% vs. 0.6%, respectively. Patients were asked about the occurrence of unexplained muscle pain or weakness at each study visit: 21.5% vs. 20.9% patients ever reported muscle symptoms in the VYTORIN and placebo groups, respectively. Cancer was diagnosed during the trial in 9.4% vs. 9.5% of patients assigned to VYTORIN and placebo, respectively.

Ezetimibe
Other adverse reactions reported with ezetimibe in placebo-controlled studies, regardless of causality assessment: *Musculoskeletal system disorders:* arthralgia; *Infections and infestations:* sinusitis; *Body as a whole – general disorders:* fatigue.

Simvastatin
In a clinical trial in which 12,064 patients with a history of myocardial infarction were treated with simvastatin (mean follow-up 6.7 years), the incidence of myopathy (defined as unexplained muscle weakness or pain with a serum creatine kinase [CK] >10 times upper limit of normal [ULN]) in patients on 80 mg/day was approximately 0.9% compared with 0.02% for patients on 20 mg/day. The incidence of rhabdomyolysis (defined as myopathy with a CK >40 times ULN) in patients on 80 mg/day was approximately 0.4% compared with 0% for patients on 20 mg/day. The incidence of myopathy, including rhabdomyolysis, was highest during the first year and then notably decreased during the subsequent years of treatment. In this trial, patients were carefully monitored and some interacting medicinal products were excluded.

Other adverse reactions reported with simvastatin in placebo-controlled clinical studies, regardless of causality assessment: *Cardiac disorders:* atrial fibrillation; *Ear and labyrinth disorders:* vertigo; *Gastrointestinal disorders:* abdominal pain, constipation, dyspepsia, flatulence, gastritis; *Skin and subcutaneous tissue disorders:* eczema, rash; *Endocrine disorders:* diabetes mellitus; *Infections and infestations:* bronchitis, sinusitis, urinary tract infections; *Body as a whole – general disorders:* asthenia, edema/swelling; *Psychiatric disorders:* insomnia.

Laboratory Tests
Marked persistent increases of hepatic serum transaminases have been noted *[see Warnings and Precautions (5.2)]*. Elevated alkaline phosphatase and γ-glutamyl transpeptidase have been reported. About 5% of patients taking simvastatin had elevations of CK levels of 3 or more times the normal value on one or more occasions. This was attributable to the noncardiac fraction of CK *[see Warnings and Precautions (5.1)]*.

6.2   Postmarketing Experience
Because the below reactions are reported voluntarily from a population of uncertain size, it is generally not possible to reliably estimate their frequency or establish a causal relationship to drug exposure.
The following adverse reactions have been reported in postmarketing experience for VYTORIN or ezetimibe or simvastatin: pruritus; alopecia; erythema multiforme; a variety of skin changes (e.g., nodules, discoloration, dryness of skin/mucous membranes, changes to hair/nails); dizziness; muscle cramps; myalgia; arthralgia; pancreatitis; paresthesia; peripheral neuropathy; vomiting; nausea; anemia; erectile dysfunction; interstitial lung disease; myopathy/rhabdomyolysis *[see Warnings and Precautions (5.1)]*; hepatitis/jaundice; fatal and non-fatal hepatic failure; depression; cholelithiasis; cholecystitis; thrombocytopenia; elevations in liver transaminases; elevated creatine phosphokinase.
There have been rare reports of immune-mediated necrotizing myopathy associated with statin use. *[see Warnings and Precautions (5.1)]*.
Hypersensitivity reactions, including anaphylaxis, angioedema, rash, and urticaria have been reported.
In addition, an apparent hypersensitivity syndrome has been reported rarely that has included one or more of the following features: anaphylaxis, angioedema, lupus erythematous-like syndrome, polymyalgia rheumatica, dermatomyositis, vasculitis, purpura, thrombocytopenia, leukopenia, hemolytic anemia, positive ANA, ESR increase, eosinophilia, arthritis, arthralgia, urticaria, asthenia, photosensitivity, fever, chills, flushing, malaise, dyspnea, toxic epidermal necrolysis, erythema multiforme, including Stevens-Johnson syndrome.
There have been rare postmarketing reports of cognitive impairment (e.g., memory loss, forgetfulness, amnesia, memory impairment, confusion) associated with statin use. These cognitive issues have been reported for all statins. The reports are generally nonserious, and reversible upon statin discontinuation, with variable times to symptom onset (1 day to years) and symptom resolution (median of 3 weeks).

7   DRUG INTERACTIONS
[See Clinical Pharmacology (12.3).]
VYTORIN
7.1   Strong CYP3A4 Inhibitors, Cyclosporine, or Danazol
Strong CYP3A4 inhibitors: The risk of myopathy is increased by reducing the elimination of the simvastatin component of VYTORIN. Hence when VYTORIN is used with an inhibitor of CYP3A4 (e.g., as listed below), elevated plasma levels of HMG-CoA reductase inhibitory activity increases the risk of myopathy and rhabdomyolysis, particularly with higher doses of VYTORIN. *[See Warnings and Precautions (5.1) and Clinical Pharmacology (12.3).]* Concomitant use of drugs labeled as having a strong inhibitory effect on CYP3A4 is contraindicated *[see Contraindications (4)]*. If treatment with itraconazole, ketoconazole, posaconazole, voriconazole, erythromycin, clarithromycin or telithromycin is unavoidable, therapy with VYTORIN must be suspended during the course of treatment.
Cyclosporine or Danazol: The risk of myopathy, including rhabdomyolysis is increased by concomitant administration of cyclosporine or danazol. Therefore, concomitant use of these drugs is contraindicated *[see Contraindications (4), Warnings and Precautions (5.1) and Clinical Pharmacology (12.3)]*.
7.2   Lipid-Lowering Drugs That Can Cause Myopathy When Given Alone
Gemfibrozil: Contraindicated with VYTORIN *[see Contraindications (4) and Warnings and Precautions (5.1)]*.

Fenofibrates (e.g., fenofibrate and fenofibric acid): Caution should be used when prescribing with VYTORIN *[see Warnings and Precautions (5.1) and Drug Interactions (7.7)]*.
7.3   Amiodarone, Dronedarone, Ranolazine, or Calcium Channel Blockers
The risk of myopathy, including rhabdomyolysis, is increased by concomitant administration of amiodarone, dronedarone, ranolazine, or calcium channel blockers such as verapamil, diltiazem or amlodipine *[see Dosage and Administration (2.3) and Warnings and Precautions (5.1) and Table 6 in Clinical Pharmacology (12.3)]*.
7.4   Niacin
Cases of myopathy/rhabdomyolysis have been observed with simvastatin coadministered with lipid-modifying doses (≥1 g/day niacin) of niacin-containing products. The benefits of the combined use of VYTORIN with niacin should be carefully weighed against the potential risks of myopathy/rhabdomyolysis. In particular, caution should be used when treating Chinese patients with VYTORIN doses exceeding 10/20 mg/day coadministered with lipid-modifying doses of niacin-containing products. Because the risk for myopathy is dose-related, Chinese patients should not receive VYTORIN 10/80 mg coadministered with lipid-modifying doses of niacin-containing products. *[See Warnings and Precautions (5.1).]*
7.5   Cholestyramine
Concomitant cholestyramine administration decreased the mean AUC of total ezetimibe approximately 55%. The incremental LDL-C reduction due to adding VYTORIN to cholestyramine may be reduced by this interaction.
7.6   Digoxin
In one study, concomitant administration of digoxin with simvastatin resulted in a slight elevation in plasma digoxin concentrations. Patients taking digoxin should be monitored appropriately when VYTORIN is initiated.
7.7   Fenofibrates (e.g., fenofibrate and fenofibric acid)
The safety and effectiveness of VYTORIN administered with fibrates have not been established. Because it is known that the risk of myopathy during treatment with HMG-CoA reductase inhibitors is increased with concurrent administration of fenofibrates, VYTORIN should be administered with caution when used concomitantly with a fenofibrate *[see Warnings and Precautions (5.1)]*.
Fenofibrates may increase cholesterol excretion into the bile, leading to cholelithiasis. In a preclinical study in dogs, ezetimibe increased cholesterol in the gallbladder bile *[see Animal Toxicology and/or Pharmacology (13.2)]*. If cholelithiasis is suspected in a patient receiving VYTORIN and a fenofibrate, gallbladder studies are indicated and alternative lipid-lowering therapy should be considered *[see the product labeling for fenofibrate and fenofibric acid]*.
7.8   Coumarin Anticoagulants
Simvastatin 20-40 mg/day modestly potentiated the effect of coumarin anticoagulants: the prothrombin time, reported as International Normalized Ratio (INR), increased from a baseline of 1.7 to 1.8 and from 2.6 to 3.4 in a normal volunteer study and in a hypercholesterolemic patient study, respectively. With other statins, clinically evident bleeding and/or increased prothrombin time has been reported in a few patients taking coumarin anticoagulants concomitantly. In such patients, prothrombin time should be determined before starting VYTORIN and frequently enough during early therapy to ensure that no significant alteration of prothrombin time occurs. Once a stable prothrombin time has been documented, prothrombin times can be monitored at the intervals usually recommended for patients on coumarin anticoagulants. If the dose of VYTORIN is changed or discontinued, the same procedure should be repeated. Simvastatin therapy has not been associated with bleeding or with changes in prothrombin time in patients not taking anticoagulants.
Concomitant administration of ezetimibe (10 mg once daily) had no significant effect on bioavailability of warfarin and prothrombin time in a study of twelve healthy adult males. There have been postmarketing reports of increased INR in patients who had ezetimibe added to warfarin. Most of these patients were also on other medications.
The effect of VYTORIN on the prothrombin time has not been studied.
7.9   Colchicine
Cases of myopathy, including rhabdomyolysis, have been reported with simvastatin coadministered with colchicine, and caution should be exercised when prescribing VYTORIN with colchicine.

8   USE IN SPECIFIC POPULATIONS
8.1   Pregnancy
Pregnancy Category X.
[See Contraindications (4).]
VYTORIN
VYTORIN is contraindicated in women who are or may become pregnant. Lipid-lowering drugs offer no benefit during pregnancy, because cholesterol and cholesterol derivatives are needed for normal fetal development. Atherosclerosis is

a chronic process, and discontinuation of lipid-lowering drugs during pregnancy should have little impact on long-term outcomes of primary hypercholesterolemia therapy. There are no adequate and well-controlled studies of VYTORIN use during pregnancy; however, there are rare reports of congenital anomalies in infants exposed to statins in utero. Animal reproduction studies of simvastatin in rats and rabbits showed no evidence of teratogenicity. Serum cholesterol and triglycerides increase during normal pregnancy, and cholesterol or cholesterol derivatives are essential for fetal development. Because statins, such as simvastatin, decrease cholesterol synthesis and possibly the synthesis of other biologically active substances derived from cholesterol, VYTORIN may cause fetal harm when administered to a pregnant woman. If VYTORIN is used during pregnancy or if the patient becomes pregnant while taking this drug, the patient should be apprised of the potential hazard to the fetus.

Women of childbearing potential, who require VYTORIN treatment for a lipid disorder, should be advised to use effective contraception. For women trying to conceive, discontinuation of VYTORIN should be considered. If pregnancy occurs, VYTORIN should be immediately discontinued.

Ezetimibe
In oral (gavage) embryo-fetal development studies of ezetimibe conducted in rats and rabbits during organogenesis, there was no evidence of embryolethal effects at the doses tested (250, 500, 1000 mg/kg/day). In rats, increased incidences of common fetal skeletal findings (extra pair of thoracic ribs, unossified cervical vertebral centra, shortened ribs) were observed at 1000 mg/kg/day (~10 times the human exposure at 10 mg daily based on AUC_{0-24hr} for total ezetimibe). In rabbits treated with ezetimibe, an increased incidence of extra thoracic ribs was observed at 1000 mg/kg/day (150 times the human exposure at 10 mg daily based on AUC_{0-24hr} for total ezetimibe). Ezetimibe crossed the placenta when pregnant rats and rabbits were given multiple oral doses.

Multiple-dose studies of ezetimibe coadministered with statins in rats and rabbits during organogenesis result in higher ezetimibe and statin exposures. Reproductive findings occur at lower doses in coadministration therapy compared to monotherapy.

Simvastatin
Simvastatin was not teratogenic in rats or rabbits at doses (25, 10 mg/kg/day, respectively) that resulted in 3 times the human exposure based on mg/m² surface area. However, in studies with another structurally-related statin, skeletal malformations were observed in rats and mice.

There are rare reports of congenital anomalies following intrauterine exposure to statins. In a review[1] of approximately 100 prospectively followed pregnancies in women exposed to simvastatin or another structurally-related statin, the incidences of congenital anomalies, spontaneous abortions and fetal deaths/stillbirths did not exceed what would be expected in the general population. The number of cases is adequate only to exclude a 3- to 4-fold increase in congenital anomalies over the background incidence. In 89% of the prospectively followed pregnancies, drug treatment was initiated prior to pregnancy and was discontinued at some point in the first trimester when pregnancy was identified.

---

[1] Manson, J.M., Freyssinges, C., Ducrocq, M.B., Stephenson, W.P., Postmarketing Surveillance of Lovastatin and Simvastatin Exposure During Pregnancy, *Reproductive Toxicology*, 10(6):439-446, 1996.

8.3 Nursing Mothers
It is not known whether simvastatin is excreted in human milk. Because a small amount of another drug in this class is excreted in human milk and because of the potential for serious adverse reactions in nursing infants, women taking simvastatin should not nurse their infants. A decision should be made whether to discontinue nursing or discontinue drug, taking into account the importance of the drug to the mother *[see Contraindications (4)]*.

In rat studies, exposure to ezetimibe in nursing pups was up to half of that observed in maternal plasma. It is not known whether ezetimibe or simvastatin are excreted into human breast milk. Because a small amount of another drug in the same class as simvastatin is excreted in human milk and because of the potential for serious adverse reactions in nursing infants, women who are nursing should not take VYTORIN *[see Contraindications (4)]*.

8.4 Pediatric Use
The effects of ezetimibe coadministered with simvastatin (n=126) compared to simvastatin monotherapy (n=122) have been evaluated in adolescent boys and girls with heterozygous familial hypercholesterolemia (HeFH). In a multicenter, double-blind, controlled study followed by an open-label phase, 142 boys and 106 postmenarchal girls, 10 to 17 years of age (mean age 14.2 years, 43% females, 82% Caucasians, 4% Asian, 2% Blacks, 13% multiracial) with HeFH were randomized to receive either ezetimibe coadministered with simvastatin or simvastatin monotherapy. Inclusion in

the study required 1) a baseline LDL-C level between 160 and 400 mg/dL and 2) a medical history and clinical presentation consistent with HeFH. The mean baseline LDL-C value was 225 mg/dL (range: 161-351 mg/dL) in the ezetimibe coadministered with simvastatin group compared to 219 mg/dL (range: 149-336 mg/dL) in the simvastatin monotherapy group. The patients received coadministered ezetimibe and simvastatin (10 mg, 20 mg, or 40 mg) or simvastatin monotherapy (10 mg, 20 mg, or 40 mg) for 6 weeks, coadministered ezetimibe and 40 mg simvastatin or 40 mg simvastatin monotherapy for the next 27 weeks, and open-label coadministered ezetimibe and simvastatin (10 mg, 20 mg, or 40 mg) for 20 weeks thereafter.

The results of the study at Week 6 are summarized in Table 3. Results at Week 33 were consistent with those at Week 6. [See table 3 above]

From the start of the trial to the end of Week 33, discontinuations due to an adverse reaction occurred in 7 (6%) patients in the ezetimibe coadministered with simvastatin group and in 2 (2%) patients in the simvastatin monotherapy group.

During the trial, hepatic transaminase elevations (two consecutive measurements for ALT and/or AST ≥3 × ULN) occurred in four (3%) individuals in the ezetimibe coadministered with simvastatin group and in two (2%) individuals in the simvastatin monotherapy group. Elevations of CPK (≥10 × ULN) occurred in two (2%) individuals in the ezetimibe coadministered with simvastatin group and in zero individuals in the simvastatin monotherapy group.

In this limited controlled study, there was no significant effect on growth or sexual maturation in the adolescent boys or girls, or on menstrual cycle length in girls.

Coadministration of ezetimibe with simvastatin at doses greater than 40 mg/day has not been studied in adolescents. Also, VYTORIN has not been studied in patients younger than 10 years of age or in pre-menarchal girls.

Ezetimibe
Based on total ezetimibe (ezetimibe + ezetimibe-glucuronide) there are no pharmacokinetic differences between adolescents and adults. Pharmacokinetic data in the pediatric population <10 years of age are not available.

Simvastatin
The pharmacokinetics of simvastatin has not been studied in the pediatric population.

8.5 Geriatric Use
Of the 10,189 patients who received VYTORIN in clinical studies, 3242 (32%) were 65 and older (this included 844 (8%) who were 75 and older). No overall differences in safety or effectiveness were observed between these subjects and younger subjects, and other reported clinical experience has not identified differences in responses between the elderly and younger patients but greater sensitivity of some older individuals cannot be ruled out. Since advanced age (≥65 years) is a predisposing factor for myopathy, VYTORIN should be prescribed with caution in the elderly. *[See Clinical Pharmacology (12.3).]*

Because advanced age (≥65 years) is a predisposing factor for myopathy, including rhabdomyolysis, VYTORIN should be prescribed with caution in the elderly. In a clinical trial of patients treated with simvastatin 80 mg/day, patients ≥65 years of age had an increased risk of myopathy, including rhabdomyolysis, compared to patients <65 years of age. *[See Warnings and Precautions (5.1) and Clinical Pharmacology (12.3).]*

8.6 Renal Impairment
In the SHARP trial of 9270 patients with moderate to severe renal impairment (6247 non-dialysis patients with median serum creatinine 2.5 mg/dL and median estimated glomerular filtration rate 25.6 mL/min/1.73 m², and 3023 dialysis patients), the incidence of serious adverse events, adverse events leading to discontinuation of study treatment, or adverse events of special interest (musculoskeletal adverse events, liver enzyme abnormalities, incident cancer) was similar between patients ever assigned to VYTORIN 10/20 mg (n=4650) or placebo (n=4620) during a median follow-up of 4.9 years. However, because renal impairment is a risk factor for statin-associated myopathy, doses of VYTORIN exceeding 10/20 mg should be used with caution and close monitoring in patients with moderate to severe renal impairment. *[See Dosage and Administration (2.5), Adverse Reactions (6.1), and Clinical Studies (14.3).]*

8.7 Hepatic Impairment
VYTORIN is contraindicated in patients with active liver disease or unexplained persistent elevations in hepatic transaminases. *[See Contraindications (4) and Warnings and Precautions (5.2).]*

10 OVERDOSAGE
VYTORIN
No specific treatment of overdosage with VYTORIN can be recommended. In the event of an overdose, symptomatic and supportive measures should be employed.

Ezetimibe
In clinical studies, administration of ezetimibe, 50 mg/day to 15 healthy subjects for up to 14 days, or 40 mg/day to 18 patients with primary hyperlipidemia for up to 56 days, was generally well tolerated.

A few cases of overdosage have been reported; most have not been associated with adverse experiences. Reported adverse experiences have not been serious.

Simvastatin
Significant lethality was observed in mice after a single oral dose of 9 g/m². No evidence of lethality was observed in rats or dogs treated with doses of 30 and 100 g/m², respectively. No specific diagnostic signs were observed in rodents. At these doses the only signs seen in dogs were emesis and mucoid stools.

A few cases of overdosage with simvastatin have been reported; the maximum dose taken was 3.6 g. All patients recovered without sequelae.

The dialyzability of simvastatin and its metabolites in man is not known at present.

11 DESCRIPTION
VYTORIN contains ezetimibe, a selective inhibitor of intestinal cholesterol and related phytosterol absorption, and simvastatin, an HMG-CoA reductase inhibitor.

The chemical name of ezetimibe is 1-(4-fluorophenyl)-3 (R)-[3-(4-fluorophenyl)-3(S)-hydroxypropyl]-4(S)-(4-hydroxyphenyl)-2-azetidinone. The empirical formula is $C_{24}H_{21}F_2NO_3$ and its molecular weight is 409.4.

Ezetimibe is a white, crystalline powder that is freely to very soluble in ethanol, methanol, and acetone and practically insoluble in water. Its structural formula is:

Simvastatin, an inactive lactone, is hydrolyzed to the corresponding β-hydroxyacid form, which is an inhibitor of HMG-CoA reductase. Simvastatin is butanoic acid, 2,2-dimethyl-,1,2,3,7,8,8a-hexahydro-3,7-dimethyl-8-[2-(tetrahydro-4-hydroxy-6-oxo-2H-pyran-2-yl)-ethyl]-1-naphthalenyl ester, [1S-[1α,3α,7β,8β(2S*,4S*),-8aβ]]. The empirical formula of simvastatin is $C_{25}H_{38}O_5$ and its molecular weight is 418.57.

Simvastatin is a white to off-white, nonhygroscopic, crystalline powder that is practically insoluble in water and freely soluble in chloroform, methanol and ethanol. Its structural formula is:

VYTORIN is available for oral use as tablets containing 10 mg of ezetimibe, and 10 mg of simvastatin (VYTORIN 10/10), 20 mg of simvastatin (VYTORIN 10/20), 40 mg of simvastatin (VYTORIN 10/40), or 80 mg of simvastatin

Table 3: Mean Percent Difference at Week 6 Between the Pooled Ezetimibe Coadministered with Simvastatin Group and the Pooled Simvastatin Monotherapy Group in Adolescent Patients with Heterozygous Familial Hypercholesterolemia

	Total-C	LDL-C	Apo B	Non-HDL-C	TG*	HDL-C
Mean percent difference between treatment groups	-12%	-15%	-12%	-14%	-2%	+0.1%
95% Confidence Interval	(-15%, -9%)	(-18%, -12%)	(-15%, -9%)	(-17%, -11%)	(-9, +4)	(-3, +3)

* For triglycerides, median % change from baseline.

Table 4: Effect of Coadministered Drugs on Total Ezetimibe

Coadministered Drug and Dosing Regimen	Total Ezetimibe*	
	Change in AUC	Change in C_{max}
Cyclosporine-stable dose required (75-150 mg BID)[†,‡]	↑240%	↑290%
Fenofibrate, 200 mg QD, 14 days[‡]	↑48%	↑64%
Gemfibrozil, 600 mg BID, 7 days[‡]	↑64%	↑91%
Cholestyramine, 4 g BID, 14 days[‡]	↓55%	↓4%
Aluminum & magnesium hydroxide combination antacid, single dose[§]	↓4%	↓30%
Cimetidine, 400 mg BID, 7 days	↑6%	↑22%
Glipizide, 10 mg, single dose	↑4%	↓8%
Statins		
Lovastatin 20 mg QD, 7 days	↑9%	↑3%
Pravastatin 20 mg QD, 14 days	↑7%	↑23%
Atorvastatin 10 mg QD, 14 days	↓2%	↑12%
Rosuvastatin 10 mg QD, 14 days	↑13%	↑18%
Fluvastatin 20 mg QD, 14 days	↓19%	↑7%

* Based on 10 mg-dose of ezetimibe.
† Post-renal transplant patients with mild impaired or normal renal function. In a different study, a renal transplant patient with severe renal insufficiency (creatinine clearance of 13.2 mL/min/1.73 m^2) who was receiving multiple medications, including cyclosporine, demonstrated a 12-fold greater exposure to total ezetimibe compared to healthy subjects.
‡ See 7. Drug Interactions.
§ Supralox, 20 mL.

(VYTORIN 10/80). Each tablet contains the following inactive ingredients: butylated hydroxyanisole NF, citric acid monohydrate USP, croscarmellose sodium NF, hypromellose USP, lactose monohydrate NF, magnesium stearate NF, microcrystalline cellulose NF, and propyl gallate NF.

12 CLINICAL PHARMACOLOGY
12.1 Mechanism of Action
VYTORIN
Plasma cholesterol is derived from intestinal absorption and endogenous synthesis. VYTORIN contains ezetimibe and simvastatin, two lipid-lowering compounds with complementary mechanisms of action. VYTORIN reduces elevated total-C, LDL-C, Apo B, TG, and non-HDL-C, and increases HDL-C through dual inhibition of cholesterol absorption and synthesis.
Ezetimibe
Ezetimibe reduces blood cholesterol by inhibiting the absorption of cholesterol by the small intestine. The molecular target of ezetimibe has been shown to be the sterol transporter, Niemann-Pick C1-Like 1 (NPC1L1), which is involved in the intestinal uptake of cholesterol and phytosterols. In a 2-week clinical study in 18 hypercholesterolemic patients, ezetimibe inhibited intestinal cholesterol absorption by 54%, compared with placebo. Ezetimibe had no clinically meaningful effect on the plasma concentrations of the fat-soluble vitamins A, D, and E and did not impair adrenocortical steroid hormone production.
Ezetimibe localizes at the brush border of the small intestine and inhibits the absorption of cholesterol, leading to a decrease in the delivery of intestinal cholesterol to the liver. This causes a reduction of hepatic cholesterol stores and an increase in clearance of cholesterol from the blood; this distinct mechanism is complementary to that of statins [see Clinical Studies (14)].
Simvastatin
Simvastatin is a prodrug and is hydrolyzed to its active β-hydroxyacid form, simvastatin acid, after administration. Simvastatin is a specific inhibitor of 3-hydroxy-3-methylglutaryl-coenzyme A (HMG-CoA) reductase, the enzyme that catalyzes the conversion of HMG-CoA to mevalonate, an early and rate limiting step in the biosynthetic pathway for cholesterol. In addition, simvastatin reduces very-low-density lipoproteins (VLDL) and TG and increases HDL-C.

12.2 Pharmacodynamics
Clinical studies have demonstrated that elevated levels of total-C, LDL-C and Apo B, the major protein constituent of LDL, promote human atherosclerosis. In addition, decreased levels of HDL-C are associated with the development of atherosclerosis. Epidemiologic studies have established that cardiovascular morbidity and mortality vary directly with the level of total-C and LDL-C and inversely with the level of HDL-C. Like LDL, cholesterol-enriched triglyceride-rich lipoproteins, including VLDL, intermediate-density lipoproteins (IDL), and remnants, can also promote atherosclerosis. The independent effect of raising HDL-C or lowering TG on the risk of coronary and cardiovascular morbidity and mortality has not been determined.

12.3 Pharmacokinetics
The results of a bioequivalence study in healthy subjects demonstrated that the VYTORIN (ezetimibe/simvastatin) 10 mg/10 mg to 10 mg/80 mg combination tablets are bioequivalent to coadministration of corresponding doses of ezetimibe (ZETIA®) and simvastatin (ZOCOR®) as individual tablets.
Absorption
Ezetimibe
After oral administration, ezetimibe is absorbed and extensively conjugated to a pharmacologically active phenolic glucuronide (ezetimibe-glucuronide).
Simvastatin
The availability of the β-hydroxyacid to the systemic circulation following an oral dose of simvastatin was found to be less than 5% of the dose, consistent with extensive hepatic first-pass extraction.
Effect of Food on Oral Absorption
Ezetimibe
Concomitant food administration (high-fat or non-fat meals) had no effect on the extent of absorption of ezetimibe when administered as 10-mg tablets. The C_{max} value of ezetimibe was increased by 38% with consumption of high-fat meals.
Simvastatin
Relative to the fasting state, the plasma profiles of both active and total inhibitors of HMG-CoA reductase were not affected when simvastatin was administered immediately before an American Heart Association recommended low-fat meal.
Distribution
Ezetimibe
Ezetimibe and ezetimibe-glucuronide are highly bound (>90%) to human plasma proteins.
Simvastatin
Both simvastatin and its β-hydroxyacid metabolite are highly bound (approximately 95%) to human plasma proteins. When radiolabeled simvastatin was administered to rats, simvastatin-derived radioactivity crossed the blood-brain barrier.
Metabolism and Excretion
Ezetimibe
Ezetimibe is primarily metabolized in the small intestine and liver via glucuronide conjugation with subsequent biliary and renal excretion. Minimal oxidative metabolism has been observed in all species evaluated.
In humans, ezetimibe is rapidly metabolized to ezetimibe-glucuronide. Ezetimibe and ezetimibe-glucuronide are the major drug-derived compounds detected in plasma, constituting approximately 10 to 20% and 80 to 90% of the total

drug in plasma, respectively. Both ezetimibe and ezetimibe-glucuronide are eliminated from plasma with a half-life of approximately 22 hours for both ezetimibe and ezetimibe-glucuronide. Plasma concentration-time profiles exhibit multiple peaks, suggesting enterohepatic recycling.
Following oral administration of ^{14}C-ezetimibe (20 mg) to human subjects, total ezetimibe (ezetimibe + ezetimibe-glucuronide) accounted for approximately 93% of the total radioactivity in plasma. After 48 hours, there were no detectable levels of radioactivity in the plasma.
Approximately 78% and 11% of the administered radioactivity were recovered in the feces and urine, respectively, over a 10-day collection period. Ezetimibe was the major component in feces and accounted for 69% of the administered dose, while ezetimibe-glucuronide was the major component in urine and accounted for 9% of the administered dose.
Simvastatin
Simvastatin is a lactone that is readily hydrolyzed in vivo to the corresponding β-hydroxyacid, a potent inhibitor of HMG-CoA reductase. Inhibition of HMG-CoA reductase is a basis for an assay in pharmacokinetic studies of the β-hydroxyacid metabolites (active inhibitors) and, following base hydrolysis, active plus latent inhibitors (total inhibitors) in plasma following administration of simvastatin. The major active metabolites of simvastatin present in human plasma are the β-hydroxyacid of simvastatin and its 6'-hydroxy, 6'-hydroxymethyl, and 6'-exomethylene derivatives.
Following an oral dose of ^{14}C-labeled simvastatin in man, 13% of the dose was excreted in urine and 60% in feces. Plasma concentrations of total radioactivity (simvastatin plus ^{14}C-metabolites) peaked at 4 hours and declined rapidly to about 10% of peak by 12 hours postdose.
Specific Populations
Geriatric Patients
Ezetimibe
In a multiple-dose study with ezetimibe given 10 mg once daily for 10 days, plasma concentrations for total ezetimibe were about 2-fold higher in older (≥65 years) healthy subjects compared to younger subjects.
Simvastatin
In a study including 16 elderly patients between 70 and 78 years of age who received simvastatin 40 mg/day, the mean plasma level of HMG-CoA reductase inhibitory activity was increased approximately 45% compared with 18 patients between 18-30 years of age.
Pediatric Patients: [See Pediatric Use (8.4).]
Gender
Ezetimibe
In a multiple-dose study with ezetimibe given 10 mg once daily for 10 days, plasma concentrations for total ezetimibe were slightly higher (<20%) in women than in men.
Race
Ezetimibe
Based on a meta-analysis of multiple-dose pharmacokinetic studies, there were no pharmacokinetic differences between Black and Caucasian subjects. Studies in Asian subjects indicated that the pharmacokinetics of ezetimibe was similar to those seen in Caucasian subjects.
Hepatic Impairment
Ezetimibe
After a single 10-mg dose of ezetimibe, the mean exposure (based on area under the curve [AUC]) to total ezetimibe was increased approximately 1.7-fold in patients with mild hepatic impairment (Child-Pugh score 5 to 6), compared to healthy subjects. The mean AUC values for total ezetimibe and ezetimibe increased approximately 3- to 4-fold and 5- to 6-fold, respectively, in patients with moderate (Child-Pugh score 7 to 9) or severe hepatic impairment (Child-Pugh score 10 to 15). In a 14-day, multiple-dose study (10 mg daily) in patients with moderate hepatic impairment, the mean AUC for total ezetimibe and ezetimibe increased approximately 4-fold compared to healthy subjects.
Renal Impairment
Ezetimibe
After a single 10-mg dose of ezetimibe in patients with severe renal disease (n=8; mean CrCl ≤30 mL/min/1.73 m^2), the mean AUC for total ezetimibe and ezetimibe increased approximately 1.5-fold, compared to healthy subjects (n=9).
Simvastatin
Pharmacokinetic studies with another statin having a similar principal route of elimination to that of simvastatin have suggested that for a given dose level higher systemic exposure may be achieved in patients with severe renal impairment (as measured by creatinine clearance).
Drug Interactions [See also Drug Interactions (7).]
No clinically significant pharmacokinetic interaction was seen when ezetimibe was coadministered with simvastatin. No specific pharmacokinetic drug interaction studies with VYTORIN have been conducted other than the following study with NIASPAN (Niacin extended-release tablets).
Niacin: The effect of VYTORIN (10/20 mg daily for 7 days) on the pharmacokinetics of NIASPAN extended-release tablets (1000 mg for 2 days and 2000 mg for 5 days following a

low-fat breakfast) was studied in healthy subjects. The mean C_{max} and AUC of niacin increased 9% and 22%, respectively. The mean C_{max} and AUC of nicotinuric acid increased 10% and 19%, respectively (N=13). In the same study, the effect of NIASPAN on the pharmacokinetics of VYTORIN was evaluated (N=15). While concomitant NIASPAN decreased the mean C_{max} of total ezetimibe (1%), and simvastatin (2%), it increased the mean C_{max} of simvastatin acid (18%). In addition, concomitant NIASPAN increased the mean AUC of total ezetimibe (26%), simvastatin (20%), and simvastatin acid (35%).

Cases of myopathy/rhabdomyolysis have been observed with simvastatin coadministered with lipid-modifying doses (≥1 g/day niacin) of niacin-containing products. [See Warnings and Precautions (5.1) and Drug Interactions (7.4).]

Cytochrome P450: Ezetimibe had no significant effect on a series of probe drugs (caffeine, dextromethorphan, tolbutamide, and IV midazolam) known to be metabolized by cytochrome P450 (1A2, 2D6, 2C8/9 and 3A4) in a "cocktail" study of twelve healthy adult males. No evidence that ezetimibe is neither an inhibitor nor an inducer of these cytochrome P450 isozymes, and it is unlikely that ezetimibe will affect the metabolism of drugs that are metabolized by these enzymes.

In a study of 12 healthy volunteers, simvastatin at the 80-mg dose had no effect on the metabolism of the probe cytochrome P450 isoform 3A4 (CYP3A4) substrates midazolam and erythromycin. This indicates that simvastatin is not an inhibitor of CYP3A4 and, therefore, is not expected to affect the plasma levels of other drugs metabolized by CYP3A4.

Although the mechanism is not fully understood, cyclosporine has been shown to increase the AUC of statins. The increase in AUC for simvastatin acid is presumably due, in part, to inhibition of CYP3A4.

Simvastatin is a substrate for CYP3A4. Inhibitors of CYP3A4 can raise the plasma levels of HMG-CoA reductase inhibitory activity and increase the risk of myopathy. [See Warnings and Precautions (5.1); Drug Interactions (7.1).]

Ezetimibe

[See table 4 at top of previous page]

[See table 5 above]

Simvastatin

[See table 6 on next page]

13 NONCLINICAL TOXICOLOGY

13.1 Carcinogenesis, Mutagenesis, Impairment of Fertility

VYTORIN

No animal carcinogenicity or fertility studies have been conducted with the combination of ezetimibe and simvastatin. The combination of ezetimibe with simvastatin did not show evidence of mutagenicity in vitro in a microbial mutagenicity (Ames) test with *Salmonella typhimurium* and *Escherichia coli* with or without metabolic activation. No evidence of clastogenicity was observed in vitro in a chromosomal aberration assay in human peripheral blood lymphocytes with ezetimibe and simvastatin with or without metabolic activation. There was no evidence of genotoxicity at doses up to 600 mg/kg with the combination of ezetimibe and simvastatin (1:1) in the in vivo mouse micronucleus test.

Ezetimibe

A 104-week dietary carcinogenicity study with ezetimibe was conducted in rats at doses up to 1500 mg/kg/day (males) and 500 mg/kg/day (females) (~20 times the human exposure at 10 mg daily based on AUC_{0-24hr} for total ezetimibe). A 104-week dietary carcinogenicity study with ezetimibe was also conducted in mice at doses up to 500 mg/kg/day (>150 times the human exposure at 10 mg daily based on AUC_{0-24hr} for total ezetimibe). There were no statistically significant increases in tumor incidences in drug-treated rats or mice.

No evidence of mutagenicity was observed in vitro in a microbial mutagenicity (Ames) test with *Salmonella typhimurium* and *Escherichia coli* with or without metabolic activation. No evidence of clastogenicity was observed in vitro in a chromosomal aberration assay in human peripheral blood lymphocytes with or without metabolic activation. In addition, there was no evidence of genotoxicity in the in vivo mouse micronucleus test.

In oral (gavage) fertility studies of ezetimibe conducted in rats, there was no evidence of reproductive toxicity at doses up to 1000 mg/kg/day in male or female rats (~7 times the human exposure at 10 mg daily based on AUC_{0-24hr} for total ezetimibe).

Simvastatin

In a 72-week carcinogenicity study, mice were administered daily doses of simvastatin of 25, 100, and 400 mg/kg body weight, which resulted in mean plasma drug levels approximately 1, 4, and 8 times higher than the mean human plasma drug level, respectively, (as total inhibitory activity based on AUC) after an 80-mg oral dose. Liver carcinomas were significantly increased in high-dose females and mid- and high-dose males with a maximum incidence of 90% in

males. The incidence of adenomas of the liver was significantly increased in mid- and high-dose females. Drug treatment also significantly increased the incidence of lung adenomas in mid- and high-dose males and females. Adenomas of the Harderian gland (a gland of the eye of rodents) were significantly higher in high-dose mice than in controls. No evidence of a tumorigenic effect was observed at 25 mg/kg/day.

In a separate 92-week carcinogenicity study in mice at doses up to 25 mg/kg/day, no evidence of a tumorigenic effect was observed (mean plasma drug levels were 1 times higher than humans given 80 mg simvastatin as measured by AUC).

In a two-year study in rats at 25 mg/kg/day, there was a statistically significant increase in the incidence of thyroid follicular adenomas in female rats exposed to approximately 11 times higher levels of simvastatin than in humans given 80 mg simvastatin (as measured by AUC).

A second two-year rat carcinogenicity study with doses of 50 and 100 mg/kg/day produced hepatocellular adenomas and carcinomas (in female rats at both doses and in males at 100 mg/kg/day). Thyroid follicular cell adenomas were increased in males and females at both doses; thyroid follicular cell carcinomas were increased in females at 100 mg/kg/day. The increased incidence of thyroid neoplasms appears to be consistent with findings from other statins. These treatment levels represented plasma drug levels (AUC) of approximately 7 and 15 times (males) and 22 and 25 times (females) the mean human plasma drug exposure after an 80-mg daily dose.

No evidence of mutagenicity was observed in a microbial mutagenicity (Ames) test with or without rat or mouse liver metabolic activation. In addition, no evidence of damage to genetic material was noted in an in vitro alkaline elution assay using rat hepatocytes, a V-79 mammalian cell forward mutation study, an in vitro chromosome aberration study in CHO cells, or an in vivo chromosomal aberration assay in mouse bone marrow.

There was decreased fertility in male rats treated with simvastatin for 34 weeks at 25 mg/kg body weight (4 times the maximum human exposure level, based on AUC, in patients receiving 80 mg/day); however, this effect was not observed during a subsequent fertility study in which simvastatin was administered at this same dose level to male rats for 11 weeks (the entire cycle of spermatogenesis including epididymal maturation). No microscopic changes were observed in the testes of rats from either study. At 180 mg/kg/day (which produces exposure levels 22 times higher than those in humans taking 80 mg/day based on surface area, mg/m²), seminiferous tubule degeneration (necrosis and loss of spermatogenic epithelium) was observed. In dogs, there was drug-related testicular atrophy, decreased spermatogenesis, spermatocytic degeneration and giant cell formation at 10 mg/kg/day (approximately 2 times the human exposure, based on AUC, at 80 mg/day). The clinical significance of these findings is unclear.

13.2 Animal Toxicology and/or Pharmacology

CNS Toxicity

Optic nerve degeneration was seen in clinically normal dogs treated with simvastatin for 14 weeks at 180 mg/kg/day, a dose that produced mean plasma drug levels about 12 times higher than the mean plasma drug level in humans taking 80 mg/day.

A chemically similar drug in this class also produced optic nerve degeneration (Wallerian degeneration of retinogeniculate fibers) in clinically normal dogs in a dose-dependent fashion starting at 60 mg/kg/day, a dose that produced mean plasma drug levels about 30 times higher than the mean plasma drug level in humans taking the highest recommended dose (as measured by total enzyme inhibitory activity). This same drug also produced vestibulocochlear Wallerian-like degeneration and retinal ganglion cell chromatolysis in dogs treated for 14 weeks at 180 mg/kg/day, a dose that resulted in a mean plasma drug level similar to that seen with the 60 mg/kg/day dose.

CNS vascular lesions, characterized by perivascular hemorrhage and edema, mononuclear cell infiltration of perivascular spaces, perivascular fibrin deposits and necrosis of small vessels, were seen in dogs treated with simvastatin at a dose of 360 mg/kg/day, a dose that produced mean plasma drug levels that were about 14 times higher than the mean plasma drug levels in humans taking 80 mg/day. Similar CNS vascular lesions have been observed with several other drugs of this class.

There were cataracts in female rats after two years of treatment with 50 and 100 mg/kg/day (22 and 25 times the human AUC at 80 mg/day, respectively) and in dogs after three months at 90 mg/kg/day (19 times) and at two years at 50 mg/kg/day (5 times).

Ezetimibe

The hypocholesterolemic effect of ezetimibe was evaluated in cholesterol-fed Rhesus monkeys, dogs, rats, and mouse models of human cholesterol metabolism. Ezetimibe was found to have an ED_{50} value of 0.5 μg/kg/day for inhibiting the rise in plasma cholesterol levels in monkeys. The ED_{50} values in dogs, rats, and mice were 7, 30, and 700 μg/kg/day, respectively. These results are consistent with ezetimibe being a potent cholesterol absorption inhibitor.

In a rat model, where the glucuronide metabolite of ezetimibe (ezetimibe-glucuronide) was administered intraduodenally, the metabolite was as potent as ezetimibe in inhibiting the absorption of cholesterol, suggesting that the glucuronide metabolite had activity similar to the parent drug.

In 1-month studies in dogs given ezetimibe (0.03 to 300 mg/kg/day), the concentration of cholesterol in gallbladder bile increased ~2- to 4-fold. However, a dose of 300 mg/kg/day administered to dogs for one year did not result in gallstone formation or any other adverse hepatobiliary effects. In a 14-day study in mice given ezetimibe (0.3 to 5 mg/kg/day) and fed a low-fat or cholesterol-rich diet, the concentration of cholesterol in gallbladder bile was either unaffected or reduced to normal levels, respectively.

Table 5: Effect of Ezetimibe Coadministration on Systemic Exposure to Other Drugs

Coadministered Drug and its Dosage Regimen	Ezetimibe Dosage Regimen	Change in AUC of Coadministered Drug	Change in C_{max} of Coadministered Drug
Warfarin, 25 mg single dose on Day 7	10 mg QD, 11 days	↓2% (R-warfarin) ↓4% (S-warfarin)	↑3% (R-warfarin) ↑1% (S-warfarin)
Digoxin, 0.5 mg single dose	10 mg QD, 8 days	↑2%	↓7%
Gemfibrozil, 600 mg BID, 7 days*	10 mg QD, 7 days	↓1%	↓11%
Ethinyl estradiol & Levonorgestrel, QD, 21 days	10 mg QD, Days 8-14 of 21 day oral contraceptive cycle	Ethinyl estradiol 0% Levonorgestrel 0%	Ethinyl estradiol ↓9% Levonorgestrel ↓5%
Glipizide, 10 mg on Days 1 and 9	10 mg QD, Days 2-9	↓3%	↓5%
Fenofibrate, 200 mg QD, 14 days*	10 mg QD, 14 days	↑11%	↑7%
Cyclosporine, 100 mg single dose Day 7*	20 mg QD, 8 days	↑15%	↑10%
Statins			
Lovastatin 20 mg QD, 7 days	10 mg QD, 7 days	↑19%	↑3%
Pravastatin 20 mg QD, 14 days	10 mg QD, 14 days	↓20%	↓24%
Atorvastatin 10 mg QD, 14 days	10 mg QD, 14 days	↓4%	↑7%
Rosuvastatin 10 mg QD, 14 days	10 mg QD, 14 days	↑19%	↑17%
Fluvastatin 20 mg QD, 14 days	10 mg QD, 14 days	↓39%	↓27%

* See 7. Drug Interactions.

A series of acute preclinical studies was performed to determine the selectivity of ezetimibe for inhibiting cholesterol absorption. Ezetimibe inhibited the absorption of ^{14}C-cholesterol with no effect on the absorption of triglycerides, fatty acids, bile acids, progesterone, ethinyl estradiol, or the fat-soluble vitamins A and D.

In 4- to 12-week toxicity studies in mice, ezetimibe did not induce cytochrome P450 drug-metabolizing enzymes. In toxicity studies, a pharmacokinetic interaction of ezetimibe with statins (parents or their active hydroxy acid metabolites) was seen in rats, dogs, and rabbits.

14 CLINICAL STUDIES
14.1 Primary Hyperlipidemia
VYTORIN

VYTORIN reduces total-C, LDL-C, Apo B, TG, and non-HDL-C, and increases HDL-C in patients with hyperlipidemia. Maximal to near maximal response is generally achieved within 2 weeks and maintained during chronic therapy.

VYTORIN is effective in men and women with hyperlipidemia. Experience in non-Caucasians is limited and does not permit a precise estimate of the magnitude of the effects of VYTORIN.

Five multicenter, double-blind studies conducted with either VYTORIN or coadministered ezetimibe and simvastatin equivalent to VYTORIN in patients with primary hyperlipidemia are reported: two were comparisons with simvastatin, two were comparisons with atorvastatin, and one was a comparison with rosuvastatin.

In a multicenter, double-blind, placebo-controlled, 12-week trial, 1528 hyperlipidemic patients were randomized to one of ten treatment groups: placebo, ezetimibe (10 mg), simvastatin (10 mg, 20 mg, 40 mg, or 80 mg), or VYTORIN (10/10, 10/20, 10/40, or 10/80).

When patients receiving VYTORIN were compared to those receiving all doses of simvastatin, VYTORIN significantly lowered total-C, LDL-C, Apo B, TG, and non-HDL-C. The effects of VYTORIN on HDL-C were similar to the effects seen with simvastatin. Further analysis showed VYTORIN significantly increased HDL-C compared with placebo. (See Table 7.) The lipid response to VYTORIN was similar in patients with TG levels greater than or less than 200 mg/dL. [See table 7 at top of next page]

In a multicenter, double-blind, controlled, 23-week study, 710 patients with known CHD or CHD risk equivalents, as defined by the NCEP ATP III guidelines, and an LDL-C ≥130 mg/dL were randomized to one of four treatment groups: coadministered ezetimibe and simvastatin equivalent to VYTORIN (10/10, 10/20, and 10/40) or simvastatin 20 mg. Patients not reaching an LDL-C <100 mg/dL had their simvastatin dose titrated at 6-week intervals to a maximal dose of 80 mg.

At Week 5, the LDL-C reductions with VYTORIN 10/10, 10/20, or 10/40 were significantly larger than with simvastatin 20 mg (see Table 8).
[See table 8 at top of next page]

In a multicenter, double-blind, 6-week study, 1902 patients with primary hyperlipidemia, who had not met their NCEP ATP III target LDL-C goal, were randomized to one of eight treatment groups: VYTORIN (10/10, 10/20, 10/40, or 10/80) or atorvastatin (10 mg, 20 mg, 40 mg, or 80 mg).

Across the dosage range, when patients receiving VYTORIN were compared to those receiving milligram-equivalent statin doses of atorvastatin, VYTORIN lowered total-C, LDL-C, Apo B, and non-HDL-C significantly more than atorvastatin. Only the 10/40 mg and 10/80 mg VYTORIN doses increased HDL-C significantly more than the corresponding milligram-equivalent statin dose of atorvastatin. The effects of VYTORIN on TG were similar to the effects seen with atorvastatin. (See Table 9.)
[See table 9 at top of next page]

In a multicenter, double-blind, 24-week, forced-titration study, 788 patients with primary hyperlipidemia, who had not met their NCEP ATP III target LDL-C goal, were randomized to receive coadministered ezetimibe and simvastatin equivalent to VYTORIN (10/10 and 10/20) or atorvastatin 10 mg. For all three treatment groups, the dose of the statin was titrated at 6-week intervals to 80 mg. At each pre-specified dose comparison, VYTORIN lowered LDL-C to a greater degree than atorvastatin (see Table 10).
[See table 10 at top of page 1748]

In a multicenter, double-blind, 6-week study, 2959 patients with primary hyperlipidemia, who had not met their NCEP ATP III target LDL-C goal, were randomized to one of six treatment groups: VYTORIN (10/20, 10/40, or 10/80) or rosuvastatin (10 mg, 20 mg, or 40 mg).

The effects of VYTORIN and rosuvastatin on total-C, LDL-C, Apo B, TG, non-HDL-C and HDL-C are shown in Table 11.
[See table 11 at top of page 1748]

In a multicenter, double-blind, 24-week trial, 214 patients with type 2 diabetes mellitus treated with thiazolidinediones (rosiglitazone or pioglitazone) for a minimum of 3

Table 6: Effect of Coadministered Drugs or Grapefruit Juice on Simvastatin Systemic Exposure

Coadministered Drug or Grapefruit Juice	Dosing of Coadministered Drug or Grapefruit Juice	Dosing of Simvastatin		Geometric Mean Ratio (Ratio* with / without coadministered drug) No Effect = 1.00	
				AUC	C_{max}
Contraindicated with VYTORIN *[see Contraindications (4) and Warnings and Precautions (5.1)]*					
Telithromycin[†]	200 mg QD for 4 days	80 mg	simvastatin acid[‡]	12	15
			simvastatin	8.9	5.3
Nelfinavir[†]	1250 mg BID for 14 days	20 mg QD for 28 days	simvastatin acid[‡]		
			simvastatin	6	6.2
Itraconazole[†]	200 mg QD for 4 days	80 mg	simvastatin acid[‡]		13.1
			simvastatin		13.1
Posaconazole	100 mg (oral suspension) QD for 13 days	40 mg	simvastatin acid[‡]	7.3	9.2
			simvastatin	10.3	9.4
	200 mg (oral suspension) QD for 13 days	40 mg	simvastatin acid[‡]	8.5	9.5
			simvastatin	10.6	11.4
Gemfibrozil	600 mg BID for 3 days	40 mg	simvastatin acid[‡]	2.85	2.18
			simvastatin	1.35	0.91
Avoid grapefruit juice with VYTORIN *[see Warnings and Precautions (5.1)]*					
Grapefruit Juice[§] (high dose)	200 mL of double-strength TID[¶]	60 mg single dose	simvastatin acid	7	
			simvastatin	16	
Grapefruit Juice[§] (low dose)	8 oz (about 237 mL) of single-strength[#]	20 mg single dose	simvastatin acid	1.3	
			simvastatin	1.9	
Avoid taking with >10/10 mg VYTORIN, based on clinical and/or postmarketing simvastatin experience *[see Warnings and Precautions (5.1)]*					
Verapamil SR	240 mg QD Days 1-7 then 240 mg BID on Days 8-10	80 mg on Day 10	simvastatin acid	2.3	2.4
			simvastatin	2.5	2.1
Diltiazem	120 mg BID for 10 days	80 mg on Day 10	simvastatin acid	2.69	2.69
			simvastatin	3.10	2.88
Diltiazem	120 mg BID for 14 days	20 mg on Day 14	simvastatin	4.6	3.6
Dronedarone	400 mg BID for 14 days	40 mg QD for 14 days	simvastatin acid	1.96	2.14
			simvastatin	3.90	3.75
Avoid taking with >10/20 mg VYTORIN, based on clinical and/or postmarketing simvastatin experience *[see Warnings and Precautions (5.1)]*					
Amiodarone	400 mg QD for 3 days	40 mg on Day 3	simvastatin acid	1.75	1.72
			simvastatin	1.76	1.79
Amlodipine	10 mg QD for 10 days	80 mg on Day 10	simvastatin acid	1.58	1.56
			simvastatin	1.77	1.47
Ranolazine SR	1000 mg BID for 7 days	80 mg on Day 1 and Days 6-9	simvastatin acid	2.26	2.28
			simvastatin	1.86	1.75
Avoid taking with >10/20 mg VYTORIN (or 10/40 mg for patients who have previously taken 80 mg simvastatin chronically, e.g., for 12 months or more, without evidence of muscle toxicity), based on clinical experience					
Lomitapide	60 mg QD for 7 days	40 mg single dose	simvastatin acid	1.7	1.6
			simvastatin	2	2
Lomitapide	10 mg QD for 7 days	20 mg single dose	simvastatin acid	1.4	1.4
			simvastatin	1.6	1.7
No dosing adjustments required for the following:					
Fenofibrate	160 mg QD for 14 days	80 mg QD on Days 8-14	simvastatin acid	0.64	0.89
			simvastatin	0.89	0.83
Propranolol	80 mg single dose	80 mg single dose	total inhibitor	0.79	↓ from 33.6 to 21.1 ng·eq/mL
			active inhibitor	0.79	↓ from 7.0 to 4.7 ng·eq/mL

* Results based on a chemical assay except results with propranolol as indicated.
† Results could be representative of the following CYP3A4 inhibitors: ketoconazole, erythromycin, clarithromycin, HIV protease inhibitors, and nefazodone.
‡ Simvastatin acid refers to the β-hydroxyacid of simvastatin.
§ The effect of amounts of grapefruit juice between those used in these two studies on simvastatin pharmacokinetics has not been studied.
¶ Double-strength: one can of frozen concentrate diluted with one can of water. Grapefruit juice was administered TID for 2 days, and 200 mL together with single dose simvastatin and 30 and 90 minutes following single dose simvastatin on Day 3.
# Single-strength: one can of frozen concentrate diluted with 3 cans of water. Grapefruit juice was administered with breakfast for 3 days, and simvastatin was administered in the evening on Day 3.

Table 7: Response to VYTORIN in Patients with Primary Hyperlipidemia (Mean* % Change from Untreated Baseline[†])

Treatment (Daily Dose)	N	Total-C	LDL-C	Apo B	HDL-C	TG*	Non-HDL-C
Pooled data (All VYTORIN doses)[‡]	609	-38	-53	-42	+7	-24	-49
Pooled data (All simvastatin doses)[‡]	622	-28	-39	-32	+7	-21	-36
Ezetimibe 10 mg	149	-13	-19	-15	+5	-11	-18
Placebo	148	-1	-2	0	0	-2	-2
VYTORIN by dose							
10/10	152	-31	-45	-35	+8	-23	-41
10/20	156	-36	-52	-41	+10	-24	-47
10/40	147	-39	-55	-44	+6	-23	-51
10/80	154	-43	-60	-49	+6	-31	-56
Simvastatin by dose							
10 mg	158	-23	-33	-26	+5	-17	-30
20 mg	150	-24	-34	-28	+7	-18	-32
40 mg	156	-29	-41	-33	+8	-21	-38
80 mg	158	-35	-49	-39	+7	-27	-45

* For triglycerides, median % change from baseline.
† Baseline - on no lipid-lowering drug.
‡ VYTORIN doses pooled (10/10-10/80) significantly reduced total-C, LDL-C, Apo B, TG, and non-HDL-C compared to simvastatin and significantly increased HDL-C compared to placebo.

Table 8: Response to VYTORIN after 5 Weeks in Patients with CHD or CHD Risk Equivalents and an LDL-C ≥130 mg/dL

	Simvastatin 20 mg	VYTORIN 10/10	VYTORIN 10/20	VYTORIN 10/40
N	253	251	109	97
Mean baseline LDL-C	174	165	167	171
Percent change LDL-C	-38	-47	-53	-59

Table 9: Response to VYTORIN and Atorvastatin in Patients with Primary Hyperlipidemia (Mean* % Change from Untreated Baseline[†])

Treatment (Daily Dose)	N	Total-C[‡]	LDL-C[‡]	Apo B[‡]	HDL-C	TG*	Non-HDL-C[‡]
VYTORIN by dose							
10/10	230	-34[§]	-47[§]	-37[§]	+8	-26	-43[§]
10/20	233	-37[§]	-51[§]	-40[§]	+7	-25	-46[§]
10/40	236	-41[§]	-57[§]	-46[§]	+9[§]	-27	-52[§]
10/80	224	-43[§]	-59[§]	-48[§]	+8[§]	-31	-54[§]
Atorvastatin by dose							
10 mg	235	-27	-36	-31	+7	-21	-34
20 mg	230	-32	-44	-37	+5	-25	-41
40 mg	232	-36	-48	-40	+4	-24	-45
80 mg	230	-40	-53	-44	+1	-32	-50

* For triglycerides, median % change from baseline.
† Baseline - on no lipid-lowering drug.
‡ VYTORIN doses pooled (10/10-10/80) provided significantly greater reductions in total-C, LDL-C, Apo B, and non-HDL-C compared to atorvastatin doses pooled (10-80).
§ p<0.05 for difference with atorvastatin at equal mg doses of the simvastatin component.

months and simvastatin 20 mg for a minimum of 6 weeks were randomized to receive either simvastatin 40 mg or the coadministered active ingredients equivalent to VYTORIN 10/20. The median LDL-C and HbA1c levels at baseline were 89 mg/dL and 7.1%, respectively.
VYTORIN 10/20 was significantly more effective than doubling the dose of simvastatin to 40 mg. The median percent changes from baseline for VYTORIN vs. simvastatin were: LDL-C -25% and -5%; total-C -16% and -5%; Apo B -19% and -5%; and non-HDL-C -23% and -5%. Results for HDL-C and TG between the two treatment groups were not significantly different.
Ezetimibe
In two multicenter, double-blind, placebo-controlled, 12-week studies in 1719 patients with primary hyperlipidemia, ezetimibe significantly lowered total-C (-13%), LDL-C (-19%), Apo B (-14%), and TG (-8%), and increased HDL-C (+3%) compared to placebo. Reduction in LDL-C was consistent across age, sex, and baseline LDL-C.
Simvastatin
In two large, placebo-controlled clinical trials, the Scandinavian Simvastatin Survival Study (N=4,444 patients) and the Heart Protection Study (N=20,536 patients), the effects of treatment with simvastatin were assessed in patients at high risk of coronary events because of existing coronary heart disease, diabetes, peripheral vessel disease, history of stroke or other cerebrovascular disease. Simvastatin was proven to reduce: the risk of total mortality by reducing CHD deaths; the risk of non-fatal myocardial infarction and stroke; and the need for coronary and non-coronary revascularization procedures.
No incremental benefit of VYTORIN on cardiovascular morbidity and mortality over and above that demonstrated for simvastatin has been established.

14.2 Homozygous Familial Hypercholesterolemia (HoFH)
A double-blind, randomized, 12-week study was performed in patients with a clinical and/or genotypic diagnosis of HoFH. Data were analyzed from a subgroup of patients (n=14) receiving simvastatin 40 mg at baseline. Increasing the dose of simvastatin from 40 to 80 mg (n=5) produced a reduction of LDL-C of 13% from baseline on simvastatin 40 mg. Coadministered ezetimibe and simvastatin equivalent to VYTORIN (10/40 and 10/80 pooled, n=9), produced a reduction of LDL-C of 23% from baseline on simvastatin 40 mg. In those patients coadministered ezetimibe and simvastatin equivalent to VYTORIN (10/80, n=5), a reduction of LDL-C of 29% from baseline on simvastatin 40 mg was produced.

14.3 Chronic Kidney Disease (CKD)
The Study of Heart and Renal Protection (SHARP) was a multinational, randomized, placebo-controlled, double-blind trial that investigated the effect of VYTORIN on the time to a first major vascular event (MVE) among 9438 patients with moderate to severe chronic kidney disease (approximately one-third on dialysis at baseline) who did not have a history of myocardial infarction or coronary revascularization. An MVE was defined as nonfatal MI, cardiac death, stroke, or any revascularization procedure. Patients were allocated to treatment using a method that took into account the distribution of 8 important baseline characteristics of patients already enrolled and minimized the imbalance of those characteristics across the groups.
For the first year, 9438 patients were allocated 4:4:1, to VYTORIN 10/20, placebo, or simvastatin 20 mg daily, respectively. The 1-year simvastatin arm enabled the comparison of VYTORIN to simvastatin with regard to safety and effect on lipid levels. At 1 year the simvastatin-only arm was re-allocated 1:1 to VYTORIN 10/20 or placebo. A total of 9270 patients were ever allocated to VYTORIN 10/20 (n=4650) or placebo (n=4620) during the trial. The median follow-up duration was 4.9 years. Patients had a mean age of 61 years; 63% were male, 72% were Caucasian, and 23% were diabetic; and, for those not on dialysis at baseline, the median serum creatinine was 2.5 mg/dL and the median estimated glomerular filtration rate (eGFR) was 25.6 mL/min/1.73 m², with 94% of patients having an eGFR < 45 mL/min/1.73m². Eligibility did not depend on lipid levels. Mean LDL-C at baseline was 108 mg/dL. At 1 year, the mean LDL-C was 26% lower in the simvastatin arm and 38% lower in the VYTORIN arm relative to placebo. At the midpoint of the study (2.5 years), the mean LDL-C was 32% lower for VYTORIN relative to placebo. Patients no longer taking study medication were included in all lipid measurements.
In the primary intent-to-treat analysis, 639 (15.2%) of 4193 patients initially allocated to VYTORIN and 749 (17.9%) of 4191 patients initially allocated to placebo experienced an MVE. This corresponded to a relative risk reduction of 16% (p=0.001) (see Figure 1). Similarly, 526 (11.3%) of 4650 patients ever allocated to VYTORIN and 619 (13.4%) of 4620 patients ever allocated to placebo experienced a major atherosclerotic event (MAE; a subset of the MVE composite that excluded non-coronary cardiac deaths and hemorrhagic stroke), corresponding to a relative risk reduction of 17% (p=0.002). The trial demonstrated that treatment with VYTORIN 10/20 mg versus placebo reduced the risk for MVE and MAE in this CKD population. The study design precluded drawing conclusions regarding the independent contribution of either ezetimibe or simvastatin to the observed effect.
The treatment effect of VYTORIN on MVE was attenuated among patients on dialysis at baseline compared with those not on dialysis at baseline. Among 3023 patients on dialysis at baseline, VYTORIN reduced the risk of MVE by 6% (RR 0.94: 95% CI 0.80-1.09) compared with 22% (RR 0.78: 95% CI 0.69-0.89) among 6247 patients not on dialysis at baseline (interaction P=0.08).

Figure 1: Effect of VYTORIN on the Primary Endpoint of Risk of Major Vascular Events

At risk						
Pbo	4191	3807	3495	3177	2419	1239
VYT	4193	3868	3567	3273	2501	1232

The individual components of MVE in all patients ever allocated to VYTORIN or placebo are presented in Table 12. [See table 12 at top of next page]

Among patients not on dialysis at baseline, VYTORIN did not reduce the risk of progressing to end-stage renal disease compared with placebo (RR 0.97; 95% CI 0.89-1.05).

16 HOW SUPPLIED/STORAGE AND HANDLING

No. 3873 — Tablets VYTORIN 10/10 are white to off-white capsule-shaped tablets with code "311" on one side.
They are supplied as follows:
NDC 66582-311-31 bottles of 30
NDC 66582-311-54 bottles of 90
NDC 66582-311-82 bottles of 1000 (If repackaged in blisters, then opaque or light-resistant blisters should be used.)
NDC 66582-311-87 bottles of 10,000 (If repackaged in blisters, then opaque or light-resistant blisters should be used.)
NDC 66582-311-28 unit dose packages of 100.
No. 3874 — Tablets VYTORIN 10/20 are white to off-white capsule-shaped tablets with code "312" on one side.
They are supplied as follows:
NDC 66582-312-31 bottles of 30
NDC 66582-312-54 bottles of 90
NDC 66582-312-82 bottles of 1000 (If repackaged in blisters, then opaque or light-resistant blisters should be used.)
NDC 66582-312-87 bottles of 10,000 (If repackaged in blisters, then opaque or light-resistant blisters should be used.)
NDC 66582-312-28 unit dose packages of 100.
No. 3875 — Tablets VYTORIN 10/40 are white to off-white capsule-shaped tablets with code "313" on one side.
They are supplied as follows:
NDC 66582-313-31 bottles of 30
NDC 66582-313-54 bottles of 90
NDC 66582-313-74 bottles of 500 (If repackaged in blisters, then opaque or light-resistant blisters should be used.)
NDC 66582-313-86 bottles of 5000 (If repackaged in blisters, then opaque or light-resistant blisters should be used.)
NDC 66582-313-52 unit dose packages of 50.
No. 3876 — Tablets VYTORIN 10/80 are white to off-white capsule-shaped tablets with code "315" on one side.
They are supplied as follows:
NDC 66582-315-31 bottles of 30
NDC 66582-315-54 bottles of 90
NDC 66582-315-74 bottles of 500 (If repackaged in blisters, then opaque or light-resistant blisters should be used.)
NDC 66582-315-66 bottles of 2500 (If repackaged in blisters, then opaque or light-resistant blisters should be used.)
NDC 66582-315-52 unit dose packages of 50.

Storage
Store at 20-25°C (68-77°F). [See USP Controlled Room Temperature.] Keep container tightly closed.

Storage of 10,000, 5000, and 2500 count bottles
Store bottle of 10,000 VYTORIN 10/10 and 10/20, 5000 VYTORIN 10/40, and 2500 VYTORIN 10/80 capsule-shaped tablets at 20-25°C (68-77°F). [See USP Controlled Room Temperature.] Store in original container until time of use. When product container is subdivided, repackage into a tightly-closed, light-resistant container. Entire contents must be repackaged immediately upon opening.

17 PATIENT COUNSELING INFORMATION
See FDA-Approved Patient Labeling (Patient Information). Patients should be advised to adhere to their National Cholesterol Education Program (NCEP)-recommended diet, a regular exercise program, and periodic testing of a fasting lipid panel.

Patients should be advised about substances they should not take concomitantly with VYTORIN *[see Contraindications (4) and Warnings and Precautions (5.1)].* **Patients should also be advised to inform other healthcare profes-**

Table 10: Response to VYTORIN and Atorvastatin in Patients with Primary Hyperlipidemia (Mean* % Change from Untreated Baseline†)

Treatment	N	Total-C	LDL-C	Apo B	HDL-C	TG*	Non-HDL-C
Week 6							
Atorvastatin 10 mg‡	262	-28	-37	-32	+5	-23	-35
VYTORIN 10/10§	263	-34¶	-46¶	-38¶	+8¶	-26	-43¶
VYTORIN 10/20#	263	-36¶	-50¶	-41¶	+10¶	-25	-46¶
Week 12							
Atorvastatin 20 mg	246	-33	-44	-38	+7	-28	-42
VYTORIN 10/20	250	-37¶	-50¶	-41¶	+9	-28	-46¶
VYTORIN 10/40	252	-39¶	-54¶	-45¶	+12¶	-31	-50¶
Week 18							
Atorvastatin 40 mg	237	-37	-49	-42	+8	-31	-47
VYTORIN 10/40Þ	482	-40¶	-56¶	-45¶	+11¶	-32	-52¶
Week 24							
Atorvastatin 80 mg	228	-40	-53	-45	+6	-35	-50
VYTORIN 10/80Þ	459	-43¶	-59¶	-49¶	+12¶	-35	-55¶

* For triglycerides, median % change from baseline.
† Baseline - on no lipid-lowering drug.
‡ Atorvastatin: 10 mg start dose titrated to 20 mg, 40 mg, and 80 mg through Weeks 6, 12, 18, and 24.
§ VYTORIN: 10/10 start dose titrated to 10/20, 10/40, and 10/80 through Weeks 6, 12, 18, and 24.
¶ p≤0.05 for difference with atorvastatin in the specified week.
# VYTORIN: 10/20 start dose titrated to 10/40, 10/40, and 10/80 through Weeks 6, 12, 18, and 24.
Þ Data pooled for common doses of VYTORIN at Weeks 18 and 24.

Table 11: Response to VYTORIN and Rosuvastatin in Patients with Primary Hyperlipidemia (Mean* % Change from Untreated Baseline†)

Treatment (Daily Dose)	N	Total-C‡	LDL-C‡	Apo B‡	HDL-C	TG*	Non-HDL-C‡
VYTORIN by dose							
10/20	476	-37§	-52§	-42§	+7	-23§	-47§
10/40	477	-39¶	-55¶	-44¶	+8	-27	-50¶
10/80	474	-44#	-61#	-50#	+8	-30#	-56#
Rosuvastatin by dose							
10 mg	475	-32	-46	-37	+7	-20	-42
20 mg	478	-37	-52	-43	+8	-26	-48
40 mg	475	-41	-57	-47	+8	-28	-52

* For triglycerides, median % change from baseline.
† Baseline - on no lipid-lowering drug.
‡ VYTORIN doses pooled (10/20-10/80) provided significantly greater reductions in total-C, LDL-C, Apo B, and non-HDL-C compared to rosuvastatin doses pooled (10-40 mg).
§ p<0.05 vs. rosuvastatin 10 mg.
¶ p<0.05 vs. rosuvastatin 20 mg.
# p<0.05 vs. rosuvastatin 40 mg.

---

sionals prescribing a new medication or increasing the dose of an existing medication that they are taking **VYTORIN.**

17.1 Muscle Pain
All patients starting therapy with VYTORIN should be advised of the risk of myopathy, including rhabdomyolysis, and told to report promptly any unexplained muscle pain, tenderness or weakness particularly if accompanied by malaise or fever or if these muscle signs or symptoms persist after discontinuing VYTORIN. **Patients using the 10/80-mg dose should be informed that the risk of myopathy, including rhabdomyolysis, is increased with the use of the 10/80-mg dose.** The risk of myopathy, including rhabdomyolysis, occurring with use of VYTORIN is increased when taking certain types of medication or consuming grapefruit juice. Patients should discuss all medication, both prescription and over the counter, with their healthcare professional.

17.2 Liver Enzymes
It is recommended that liver function tests be performed before the initiation of VYTORIN, and thereafter when clinically indicated. All patients treated with VYTORIN should be advised to report promptly any symptoms that may indicate liver injury, including fatigue, anorexia, right upper abdominal discomfort, dark urine or jaundice.

17.3 Pregnancy
Women of childbearing age should be advised to use an effective method of birth control to prevent pregnancy while using VYTORIN. Discuss future pregnancy plans with your patients, and discuss when to stop taking VYTORIN if they are trying to conceive. Patients should be advised that if they become pregnant they should stop taking VYTORIN and call their healthcare professional.

17.4 Breastfeeding
Women who are breastfeeding should be advised to not use VYTORIN. Patients who have a lipid disorder and are breastfeeding should be advised to discuss the options with their healthcare professional.

Manufactured for: Merck Sharp & Dohme Corp., a subsidiary of
MERCK & CO., INC., Whitehouse Station, NJ 08889, USA
Manufactured by:
MSD International GmbH (Singapore Branch)
Singapore 637766

Or
Merck Sharp & Dohme (Italia) S.p.A.
Via Emilia 21,
Pavia 27100, Italy
Or
Merck Sharp & Dohme Ltd.
Cramlington, Northumberland NE23 3JU, UK
Or
Jointly manufactured by:
Merck Sharp & Dohme (Italia) S.p.A.
Via Emilia 21,
Pavia 27100, Italy
and
MSD International GmbH (Singapore Branch)
Singapore 637766
For patent information: www.merck.com/product/patent/home.html
Copyright © 2004-2012 MSD International GmbH, a subsidiary of **Merck & Co., Inc.**
All rights reserved.
uspi-mk0653a-t-1402r029

Patient Information
VYTORIN® (VI-tor-in)
(ezetimibe/simvastatin)
Tablets
Read this Patient Information carefully before you start taking VYTORIN® and each time you get a refill. There may be new information. This information does not take the place of talking with your doctor about your medical condition or your treatment. If you have any questions about VYTORIN, ask your doctor. Only your doctor can determine if VYTORIN is right for you.

What is VYTORIN?
VYTORIN is a prescription medicine that contains 2 cholesterol lowering medicines, ezetimibe and simvastatin. VYTORIN is used along with diet to:
• lower the level of your "bad" cholesterol (LDL)
• increase the level of your "good" cholesterol (HDL)
• lower the level of fat in your blood (triglycerides)
VYTORIN is for patients who cannot control their cholesterol levels by diet and exercise alone.
VYTORIN has not been shown to reduce heart attacks or strokes more than simvastatin alone.
It is not known if VYTORIN is safe and effective in children under 10 years of age or in girls who have not started their period (menses).
The usual dose of VYTORIN is 10/10 mg to 10/40 mg 1 time each day.
VYTORIN 10/80 mg increases your chance of developing muscle damage. The 10/80 mg dose should only be used by people who:
• have been taking VYTORIN 10/80 mg chronically (such as 12 months or more) without having muscle damage
• do not need to take certain other medicines with VYTORIN that would increase your chance of getting muscle damage.
If you are unable to reach your LDL-cholesterol goal using VYTORIN 10/40 mg, your doctor should switch you to another cholesterol-lowering medicine.

Who should not take VYTORIN?
Do not take VYTORIN if you take:
• Certain anti-fungal medicines including:
  ◦ itraconazole
  ◦ ketoconazole
  ◦ posaconazole
  ◦ voriconazole
• HIV protease inhibitors (indinavir, nelfinavir, ritonavir, saquinavir, tipranavir, or atazanavir)
• Certain hepatitis C virus protease inhibitors (such as boceprevir or telaprevir)
• Certain antibiotics, including:
  ◦ erythromycin
  ◦ clarithromycin
  ◦ telithromycin
• nefazodone
• medicines containing cobicistat
• A fibric acid medicine for lowering cholesterol called gemfibrozil
• cyclosporine
• danazol
Ask your doctor or pharmacist for a list of these medicines if you are not sure.

Also do not take VYTORIN if you:
• are allergic to ezetimibe or simvastatin or any of the ingredients in VYTORIN. See the end of this leaflet for a complete list of ingredients in VYTORIN.
• have liver problems.
• are pregnant or plan to become pregnant. VYTORIN may harm your unborn baby. If you are a woman of childbearing age, you should use an effective method of birth control to prevent pregnancy while using VYTORIN. If you become pregnant while taking VYTORIN, stop taking VYTORIN and call your doctor.

• are breastfeeding or plan to breastfeed. It is not known if VYTORIN passes into your breast milk. You and your doctor should decide the best way to feed your baby if you take VYTORIN.

What should I tell my doctor before and while taking VYTORIN?
Tell your doctor if you:
• have unexplained muscle aches or weakness
• have kidney problems
• have or have had liver problems or drink more than 2 glasses of alcohol daily
• have thyroid problems
• are 65 years of age or older
Also see "What are the possible side effects of VYTORIN?"
Tell your doctor about all the medicines you take, including prescription and over-the-counter medicines, vitamins, and herbal supplements.
Tell your doctor who prescribes VYTORIN if another doctor increases the dose of another medicine you are taking.
Talk to your doctor before you start taking any new medicines.
Taking VYTORIN with certain other medicines may affect each other causing side effects. VYTORIN may affect the way other medicines work, and other medicines may affect how VYTORIN works.
Taking VYTORIN with certain substances can increase the risk of muscle problems. It is especially important to tell your doctor if you take:
• fibric acid derivatives (such as fenofibrate)
• amiodarone or dronedarone (drugs used to treat an irregular heartbeat)
• verapamil, diltiazem, amlodipine, or ranolazine (drugs used to treat high blood pressure, chest pain associated with heart disease, or other heart conditions)
• grapefruit juice (which should be avoided while taking VYTORIN)
• colchicine (a medicine used to treat gout)
• lomitapide (a medicine used to treat a serious and rare genetic cholesterol condition)
• large doses of niacin or nicotinic acid
Tell your doctor if you are taking niacin or a niacin-containing product, as this may increase your risk of muscle problems, especially if you are Chinese.
It is also important to tell your doctor if you are taking coumarin anticoagulants (drugs that prevent blood clots, such as warfarin).
Tell your doctor about all the medicines you take, including any prescription and nonprescription medicines, vitamins, and herbal supplements.

How should I take VYTORIN?
• Take VYTORIN exactly as your doctor tells you to take it.
• Do not change your dose or stop taking VYTORIN without talking to your doctor.
• Take VYTORIN 1 time each day in the evening.
• Take VYTORIN with or without food.
• While taking VYTORIN, continue to follow your cholesterol-lowering diet and to exercise as your doctor told you to.
• If you miss a dose, do not take an extra dose. Just resume your usual schedule.
• Your doctor should do fasting blood tests to check your cholesterol while you take VYTORIN. Your doctor may change your dose of VYTORIN if needed.
• If you take too much VYTORIN, call your doctor or Poison Control Center at 1-800-222-1222 or go to the nearest hospital emergency room right away.

What are the possible side effects of VYTORIN?
VYTORIN may cause serious side effects, including:
• **Muscle pain, tenderness and weakness (myopathy)** Muscle problems, including muscle breakdown, can be serious in some people and rarely cause kidney damage that can lead to death.

Tell your doctor right away if:
◦ **you have unexplained muscle pain, tenderness, or weakness, especially if you have a fever or feel more tired than usual, while you take VYTORIN.**
◦ you have muscle problems that do not go away even after your doctor has advised you to stop taking VYTORIN. Your doctor may do further tests to diagnose the cause of your muscle problems.
Your chances of getting muscle problems are higher if you:
◦ are taking certain other medicines while you take VYTORIN
◦ are 65 years of age or older
◦ are female
◦ have thyroid problems (hypothyroidism) that are not controlled
◦ have kidney problems
◦ are taking higher doses of VYTORIN, particularly the 10/80 mg dose
• **Liver problems.** Your doctor should do blood tests to check your liver before you start taking VYTORIN and if you have any symptoms of liver problems while you take VYTORIN. Call your doctor right away if you have the following symptoms of liver problems:
◦ loss of appetite
◦ upper belly pain
◦ dark urine
◦ yellowing of your skin or the whites of your eyes
◦ feel tired or weak
The most common side effects of VYTORIN include:
• headache
• increased liver enzyme levels
• muscle pain
• upper respiratory infection
• diarrhea
Additional side effects that have been reported in general use with VYTORIN or with ezetimibe or simvastatin tablets (tablets that contain the active ingredients of VYTORIN) include:
• allergic reactions including swelling of the face, lips, tongue, and/or throat that may cause difficulty in breathing or swallowing (which may require treatment right away), rash, hives; joint pain; inflammation of the pancreas; nausea; dizziness; tingling sensation; depression; gallstones; trouble sleeping; poor memory; memory loss; confusion; erectile dysfunction; breathing problems including persistent cough and/or shortness of breath or fever.
Tell your doctor if you have any side effect that bothers you or does not go away.
These are not all the possible side effects of VYTORIN. For more information, ask your doctor or pharmacist.
Call your doctor for medical advice about side effects. You may report side effects to FDA at 1-800-FDA-1088.

How should I store VYTORIN?
• Store VYTORIN at room temperature between 68°F to 77°F (20°C to 25°C).
• Keep VYTORIN in its original container until you use it.
• Keep VYTORIN in a tightly closed container, and keep VYTORIN out of light.
Keep VYTORIN and all medicines out of the reach of children.

General Information about the safe and effective use of VYTORIN.
VYTORIN works to reduce your cholesterol in two ways. It reduces the cholesterol absorbed in your digestive tract, as well as the cholesterol your body makes by itself. VYTORIN does not help you lose weight.
Medicines are sometimes prescribed for purposes other than those listed in a Patient Information leaflet. Do not use VYTORIN for a condition for which it was not prescribed. Do not give VYTORIN to other people, even if they have the same condition that you have. It may harm them.

Table 12: Number of First Events for Each Component of the Major Vascular Event Composite Endpoint in SHARP*

Outcome	VYTORIN 10/20 (N=4650)	Placebo (N=4620)	Risk Ratio (95% CI)	P-value
Major Vascular Events	701 (15.1%)	814 (17.6%)	0.85 (0.77-0.94)	0.001
Nonfatal MI	134 (2.9%)	159 (3.4%)	0.84 (0.66-1.05)	0.12
Cardiac Death	253 (5.4%)	272 (5.9%)	0.93 (0.78-1.10)	0.38
Any Stroke	171 (3.7%)	210 (4.5%)	0.81 (0.66-0.99)	0.038
Non-hemorrhagic Stroke	131 (2.8%)	174 (3.8%)	0.75 (0.60-0.94)	0.011
Hemorrhagic Stroke	45 (1.0%)	37 (0.8%)	1.21 (0.78-1.86)	0.40
Any Revascularization	284 (6.1%)	352 (7.6%)	0.79 (0.68-0.93)	0.004

* Intention-to-treat analysis on all SHARP patients ever allocated to VYTORIN or placebo.

This Patient Information summarizes the most important information about VYTORIN. If you would like more information, talk with your doctor. You can ask your pharmacist or doctor for information about VYTORIN that is written for health professionals.

For more information, go to www.VYTORIN.com, or call 1-800-672-6372.

What are the ingredients in VYTORIN?
Active Ingredients: ezetimibe and simvastatin
Inactive ingredients: butylated hydroxyanisole NF, citric acid monohydrate USP, croscarmellose sodium NF, hypromellose USP, lactose monohydrate NF, magnesium stearate NF, microcrystalline cellulose NF, and propyl gallate NF.

This Patient Information has been approved by the U.S. Food and Drug Administration.
Manufactured for: Merck Sharp & Dohme Corp., a subsidiary of
MERCK & CO., INC., Whitehouse Station, NJ 08889, USA
Copyright © 2004-2012 MSD International GmbH, a subsidiary of Merck & Co., Inc.
All rights reserved.
Revised: 02/2014
usppi-mk0653a-t-1402r027
Shown in Product Identification Guide, page 309

ZEMURON®   ℞
(rocuronium bromide)
Injection solution for intravenous use

HIGHLIGHTS OF PRESCRIBING INFORMATION
These highlights do not include all the information needed to use ZEMURON safely and effectively. See full prescribing information for ZEMURON.
ZEMURON® (rocuronium bromide) injection solution for intravenous use
Initial U.S. Approval: 1994

—————INDICATIONS AND USAGE—————
ZEMURON is a nondepolarizing neuromuscular blocking agent indicated as an adjunct to general anesthesia to facilitate both rapid sequence and routine tracheal intubation, and to provide skeletal muscle relaxation during surgery or mechanical ventilation. (1)

—————DOSAGE AND ADMINISTRATION—————
To be administered only by experienced clinicians or adequately trained individuals supervised by an experienced clinician familiar with the use, actions, characteristics, and complications of neuromuscular blocking agents. (2)
• Individualize the dose for each patient. (2)
• Peripheral nerve stimulator recommended for determination of drug response and need for additional doses, and to evaluate recovery. (2)
• Tracheal intubation: Recommended initial dose is 0.6 mg/kg. (2.1)
• Rapid sequence intubation: 0.6 to 1.2 mg/kg. (2.2)
• Maintenance doses: Guided by response to prior dose, not administered until recovery is evident. (2.3)
• Continuous infusion: Initial rate of 10 to 12 mcg/kg/min. Start only after early evidence of spontaneous recovery from an intubating dose. (2.4)

—————DOSAGE FORMS AND STRENGTHS—————
• 5 mL multiple dose vials containing 50 mg rocuronium bromide injection (10 mg/mL). (3)

—————CONTRAINDICATIONS—————
• Hypersensitivity (e.g., anaphylaxis) to rocuronium bromide or other neuromuscular blocking agents. (4)

—————WARNINGS AND PRECAUTIONS—————
• Appropriate Administration and Monitoring: Use only if facilities for intubation, mechanical ventilation, oxygen therapy, and an antagonist are immediately available. (5.1)
• Anaphylaxis: Severe anaphylaxis has been reported. Consider cross-reactivity among neuromuscular blocking agents. (5.2)
• Need for Adequate Anesthesia: Must be accompanied by adequate anesthesia or sedation. (5.3)
• Residual Paralysis: Consider using a reversal agent in cases where residual paralysis is more likely to occur. (5.4)

—————ADVERSE REACTIONS—————
Most common adverse reactions (2%) are transient hypotension and hypertension. (6.1)
To report SUSPECTED ADVERSE REACTIONS, contact Merck Sharp & Dohme Corp., a subsidiary of Merck & Co., Inc., at 1-877-888-4231 or FDA at 1-800-FDA-1088 or www.fda.gov/medwatch.

—————DRUG INTERACTIONS—————
• Succinylcholine: Use before succinylcholine has not been studied. (7.11)

• Nondepolarizing muscle relaxants: Interactions have been observed. (7.7)
• Enhanced ZEMURON activity possible: Inhalation anesthetics (7.3), certain antibiotics (7.1), quinidine (7.10), magnesium (7.6), lithium (7.4), local anesthetics (7.5), procainamide (7.8)
• Reduced ZEMURON activity possible: Anticonvulsants. (7.2)

—————USE IN SPECIFIC POPULATIONS—————
• Labor and Delivery: Not recommended for rapid sequence induction in patients undergoing Cesarean section. (8.2)
• Pediatric Use: Onset time and duration will vary with dose, age, and anesthetic technique. Not recommended for rapid sequence intubation in pediatric patients. (8.4)
See 17 for PATIENT COUNSELING INFORMATION
Revised: 10/2013

FULL PRESCRIBING INFORMATION

1   INDICATIONS AND USAGE
ZEMURON® (rocuronium bromide) Injection is indicated for inpatients and outpatients as an adjunct to general anesthesia to facilitate both rapid sequence and routine tracheal intubation, and to provide skeletal muscle relaxation during surgery or mechanical ventilation.

2   DOSAGE AND ADMINISTRATION
ZEMURON is for intravenous use only. **This drug should only be administered by experienced clinicians or trained individuals supervised by an experienced clinician familiar with the use, actions, characteristics, and complications of neuromuscular blocking agents. Doses of ZEMURON injection should be individualized and a peripheral nerve stimulator should be used to monitor drug effect, need for additional doses, adequacy of spontaneous recovery or antagonism, and to decrease the complications of overdosage if additional doses are administered.**
The dosage information which follows is derived from studies based upon units of drug per unit of body weight. It is intended to serve as an initial guide to clinicians familiar with other neuromuscular blocking agents to acquire experience with ZEMURON.
In patients in whom potentiation of, or resistance to, neuromuscular block is anticipated, a dose adjustment should be considered *[see Dosage and Administration (2.5), Warnings and Precautions (5.9, 5.12), Drug Interactions (7.2, 7.3, 7.4, 7.5, 7.6, 7.8, 7.10), and Use in Specific Populations (8.6)]*.

2.1   Dose for Tracheal Intubation
The recommended initial dose of ZEMURON, regardless of anesthetic technique, is 0.6 mg/kg. Neuromuscular block sufficient for intubation (80% block or greater) is attained in a median (range) time of 1 (0.4-6) minute(s) and most patients have intubation completed within 2 minutes. Maximum blockade is achieved in most patients in less than 3 minutes. This dose may be expected to provide 31 (15-85) minutes of clinical relaxation under opioid/nitrous oxide/oxygen anesthesia. Under halothane, isoflurane, and enflurane anesthesia, some extension of the period of clinical relaxation should be expected *[see Drug Interactions (7.3)]*.
A lower dose of ZEMURON (0.45 mg/kg) may be used. Neuromuscular block sufficient for intubation (80% block or greater) is attained in a median (range) time of 1.3 (0.8-6.2) minute(s), and most patients have intubation completed within 2 minutes. Maximum blockade is achieved in most patients in less than 4 minutes. This dose may be expected to provide 22 (12-31) minutes of clinical relaxation under opioid/nitrous oxide/oxygen anesthesia. Patients receiving this low dose of 0.45 mg/kg who achieve less than 90% block (about 16% of these patients) may have a more rapid time to 25% recovery, 12 to 15 minutes.
A large bolus dose of 0.9 or 1.2 mg/kg can be administered under opioid/nitrous oxide/oxygen anesthesia without adverse effects to the cardiovascular system *[see Clinical Pharmacology (12.2)]*.

2.2   Rapid Sequence Intubation
In appropriately premedicated and adequately anesthetized patients, ZEMURON 0.6 to 1.2 mg/kg will provide excellent or good intubating conditions in most patients in less than 2 minutes *[see Clinical Studies (14.1)]*.

2.3   Maintenance Dosing
Maintenance doses of 0.1, 0.15, and 0.2 mg/kg ZEMURON, administered at 25% recovery of control T_1 (defined as 3 twitches of train-of-four), provide a median (range) of 12 (2-31), 17 (6-50), and 24 (7-69) minutes of clinical duration under opioid/nitrous oxide/oxygen anesthesia *[see Clinical Pharmacology (12.2)]*. In all cases, dosing should be guided based on the clinical duration following initial dose or prior maintenance dose and not administered until recovery of neuromuscular function is evident. A clinically insignificant cumulation of effect with repetitive maintenance dosing has been observed *[see Clinical Pharmacology (12.2)]*.

2.4   Use by Continuous Infusion
Infusion at an initial rate of 10 to 12 mcg/kg/min of ZEMURON should be initiated only after early evidence of spontaneous recovery from an intubating dose. Due to rapid redistribution *[see Clinical Pharmacology (12.3)]* and the associated rapid spontaneous recovery, initiation of the infusion after substantial return of neuromuscular function (more than 10% of control T_1) may necessitate additional bolus doses to maintain adequate block for surgery.
Upon reaching the desired level of neuromuscular block, the infusion of ZEMURON must be individualized for each patient. The rate of administration should be adjusted according to the patient's twitch response as monitored with the use of a peripheral nerve stimulator. In clinical trials, infusion rates have ranged from 4 to 16 mcg/kg/min.
Inhalation anesthetics, particularly enflurane and isoflurane, may enhance the neuromuscular blocking action of nondepolarizing muscle relaxants. In the presence of steady-state concentrations of enflurane or isoflurane, it may be necessary to reduce the rate of infusion by 30% to 50%, at 45 to 60 minutes after the intubating dose.
Spontaneous recovery and reversal of neuromuscular blockade following discontinuation of ZEMURON infusion may be expected to proceed at rates comparable to that following comparable total doses administered by repetitive bolus injections *[see Clinical Pharmacology (12.2)]*.
Infusion solutions of ZEMURON can be prepared by mixing ZEMURON with an appropriate infusion solution such as

5% glucose in water or lactated Ringers *[see Dosage and Administration (2.6)]*. These infusion solutions should be used within 24 hours of mixing. Unused portions of infusion solutions should be discarded.

Infusion rates of ZEMURON can be individualized for each patient using the following tables for 3 different concentrations of ZEMURON solution as guidelines:

[See table 1 above]

[See table 2 above]

[See table 3 at top of next page]

2.5 Dosage in Specific Populations

Pediatric Patients: The recommended initial intubation dose of ZEMURON is 0.6 mg/kg; however, a lower dose of 0.45 mg/kg may be used depending on anesthetic technique and the age of the patient.

For sevoflurane (induction) ZEMURON doses of 0.45 mg/kg and 0.6 mg/kg in general produce excellent to good intubating conditions within 75 seconds. When halothane is used, a 0.6 mg/kg dose of ZEMURON resulted in excellent to good intubating conditions within 60 seconds.

The time to maximum block for an intubating dose was shortest in infants (28 days up to 3 months) and longest in neonates (birth to less than 28 days). The duration of clinical relaxation following an intubating dose is shortest in children (greater than 2 years up to 11 years) and longest in infants.

When sevoflurane is used for induction and isoflurane/nitrous oxide for maintenance of general anesthesia, maintenance dosing of ZEMURON can be administered as bolus doses of 0.15 mg/kg at reappearance of T_3 in all pediatric age groups. Maintenance dosing can also be administered at the reappearance of T_2 at a rate of 7 to 10 mcg/kg/min, with the lowest dose requirement for neonates (birth to less than 28 days) and the highest dose requirement for children (greater than 2 years up to 11 years).

When halothane is used for general anesthesia, patients ranging from 3 months old through adolescence can be administered ZEMURON maintenance doses of 0.075 to 0.125 mg/kg upon return of T_1 to 0.25% to provide clinical relaxation for 7 to 10 minutes. Alternatively, a continuous infusion of ZEMURON initiated at a rate of 12 mcg/kg/min upon return of T_1 to 10% (one twitch present in train-of-four) may also be used to maintain neuromuscular blockade in pediatric patients.

Additional information for administration to pediatric patients of all age groups is presented elsewhere in the label *[see Clinical Pharmacology (12.2)]*.

The infusion of ZEMURON must be individualized for each patient. The rate of administration should be adjusted according to the patient's twitch response as monitored with the use of a peripheral nerve stimulator. Spontaneous recovery and reversal of neuromuscular blockade following discontinuation of ZEMURON infusion may be expected to proceed at rates comparable to that following similar total exposure to single bolus doses *[see Clinical Pharmacology (12.2)]*.

ZEMURON is not recommended for rapid sequence intubation in pediatric patients.

Geriatric Patients: Geriatric patients (65 years or older) exhibited a slightly prolonged median (range) clinical duration of 46 (22-73), 62 (49-75), and 94 (64-138) minutes under opioid/nitrous oxide/oxygen anesthesia following doses of 0.6, 0.9, and 1.2 mg/kg, respectively. No differences in duration of neuromuscular blockade following maintenance doses of ZEMURON were observed between these subjects and younger subjects, and other reported clinical experience has not identified differences in response between elderly and younger patients, but greater sensitivity of some older individuals cannot be ruled out *[see Clinical Pharmacology (12.2, 12.3)]*.

Patients with Renal or Hepatic Impairment: No differences from patients with normal hepatic and kidney function were observed for onset time at a dose of 0.6 mg/kg ZEMURON. When compared to patients with normal renal and hepatic function, the mean clinical duration is similar in patients with end-stage renal disease undergoing renal transplant, and is about 1.5 times longer in patients with hepatic disease. Patients with renal failure may have a greater variation in duration of effect *[see Use in Specific Populations (8.6, 8.7) and Clinical Pharmacology (12.3)]*.

Obese Patients: In obese patients, the initial dose of ZEMURON 0.6 mg/kg should be based upon the patient's actual body weight *[see Clinical Studies (14.1)]*.

An analysis across all US controlled clinical studies indicates that the pharmacodynamics of ZEMURON are not different between obese and nonobese patients when dosed based upon their actual body weight.

Patients with Reduced Plasma Cholinesterase Activity: Rocuronium metabolism does not depend on plasma cholinesterase so dosing adjustments are not needed in patients with reduced plasma cholinesterase activity.

Table 1: Infusion Rates Using ZEMURON Injection (0.5 mg/mL)*

Patient Weight		Drug Delivery Rate (mcg/kg/min)									
		4	5	6	7	8	9	10	12	14	16
(kg)	(lbs)	Infusion Delivery Rate (mL/hr)									
10	22	4.8	6	7.2	8.4	9.6	10.8	12	14.4	16.8	19.2
15	33	7.2	9	10.8	12.6	14.4	16.2	18	21.6	25.2	28.8
20	44	9.6	12	14.4	16.8	19.2	21.6	24	28.8	33.6	38.4
25	55	12	15	18	21	24	27	30	36	42	48
35	77	16.8	21	25.2	29.4	33.6	37.8	42	50.4	58.8	67.2
50	110	24	30	36	42	48	54	60	72	84	96
60	132	28.8	36	43.2	50.4	57.6	64.8	72	86.4	100.8	115.2
70	154	33.6	42	50.4	58.8	67.2	75.6	84	100.8	117.6	134.4
80	176	38.4	48	57.6	67.2	76.8	86.4	96	115.2	134.4	153.6
90	198	43.2	54	64.8	75.6	86.4	97.2	108	129.6	151.2	172.8
100	220	48	60	72	84	96	108	120	144	168	192

* 50 mg ZEMURON in 100 mL solution.

Table 2: Infusion Rates Using ZEMURON Injection (1 mg/mL)*

Patient Weight		Drug Delivery Rate (mcg/kg/min)									
		4	5	6	7	8	9	10	12	14	16
(kg)	(lbs)	Infusion Delivery Rate (mL/hr)									
10	22	2.4	3	3.6	4.2	4.8	5.4	6	7.2	8.4	9.6
15	33	3.6	4.5	5.4	6.3	7.2	8.1	9	10.8	12.6	14.4
20	44	4.8	6	7.2	8.4	9.6	10.8	12	14.4	16.8	19.2
25	55	6	7.5	9	10.5	12	13.5	15	18	21	24
35	77	8.4	10.5	12.6	14.7	16.8	18.9	21	25.2	29.4	33.6
50	110	12	15	18	21	24	27	30	36	42	48
60	132	14.4	18	21.6	25.2	28.8	32.4	36	43.2	50.4	57.6
70	154	16.8	21	25.2	29.4	33.6	37.8	42	50.4	58.8	67.2
80	176	19.2	24	28.8	33.6	38.4	43.2	48	57.6	67.2	76.8
90	198	21.6	27	32.4	37.8	43.2	48.6	54	64.8	75.6	86.4
100	220	24	30	36	42	48	54	60	72	84	96

* 100 mg ZEMURON in 100 mL solution.

Patients with Prolonged Circulation Time: Because higher doses of ZEMURON produce a longer duration of action, the initial dosage should usually not be increased in these patients to reduce onset time; instead, in these situations, when feasible, more time should be allowed for the drug to achieve onset of effect *[see Warnings and Precautions (5.7)]*.

Patients with Drugs or Conditions Causing Potentiation of Neuromuscular Block: The neuromuscular blocking action of ZEMURON is potentiated by isoflurane and enflurane anesthesia. Potentiation is minimal when administration of the recommended dose of ZEMURON occurs prior to the administration of these potent inhalation agents. The median clinical duration of a dose of 0.57 to 0.85 mg/kg was 34, 38, and 42 minutes under opioid/nitrous oxide/oxygen, enflurane and isoflurane maintenance anesthesia, respectively. During 1 to 2 hours of infusion, the infusion rate of ZEMURON required to maintain about 95% block was decreased by as much as 40% under enflurane and isoflurane anesthesia *[see Drug Interactions (7.3)]*.

2.6 Preparation for Administration of ZEMURON

Diluent Compatibility: ZEMURON is compatible in solution with:

0.9% NaCl solution	sterile water for injection
5% glucose in water	lactated Ringers
5% glucose in saline	

ZEMURON is compatible in the above solutions at concentrations up to 5 mg/mL for 24 hours at room temperature in plastic bags, glass bottles, and plastic syringe pumps.

Drug Admixture Incompatibility: ZEMURON is physically incompatible when mixed with the following drugs:

amphotericin	hydrocortisone sodium succinate
amoxicillin	insulin
azathioprine	Intralipid
cefazolin	ketorolac
cloxacillin	lorazepam
dexamethasone	methohexital
diazepam	methylprednisolone
erythromycin	thiopental
famotidine	trimethoprim
furosemide	vancomycin

If ZEMURON is administered via the same infusion line that is also used for other drugs, it is important that this infusion line is adequately flushed between administration of ZEMURON and drugs for which incompatibility with ZEMURON has been demonstrated or for which compatibility with ZEMURON has not been established.

Infusion solutions should be used within 24 hours of mixing. Unused portions of infusion solutions should be discarded. ZEMURON should not be mixed with alkaline solutions *[see Warnings and Precautions (5.10)]*.

Visual Inspection: Parenteral drug products should be inspected visually for particulate matter and clarity prior to administration whenever solution and container permit. Do not use solution if particulate matter is present.

3 DOSAGE FORMS AND STRENGTHS

ZEMURON (rocuronium bromide) injection is available as
• 5 mL multiple dose vials containing 50 mg rocuronium bromide injection (10 mg/mL)

Table 3: Infusion Rates Using ZEMURON Injection (5 mg/mL)*

Patient Weight		Drug Delivery Rate (mcg/kg/min)									
		4	5	6	7	8	9	10	12	14	16
(kg)	(lbs)	Infusion Delivery Rate (mL/hr)									
10	22	0.5	0.6	0.7	0.8	1	1.1	1.2	1.4	1.7	1.9
15	33	0.7	0.9	1.1	1.3	1.4	1.6	1.8	2.2	2.5	2.9
20	44	1	1.2	1.4	1.7	1.9	2.2	2.4	2.9	3.4	3.8
25	55	1.2	1.5	1.8	2.1	2.4	2.7	3	3.6	4.2	4.8
35	77	1.7	2.1	2.5	2.9	3.4	3.8	4.2	5	5.9	6.7
50	110	2.4	3	3.6	4.2	4.8	5.4	6	7.2	8.4	9.6
60	132	2.9	3.6	4.3	5	5.8	6.5	7.2	8.6	10.1	11.5
70	154	3.4	4.2	5	5.9	6.7	7.6	8.4	10.1	11.8	13.4
80	176	3.8	4.8	5.8	6.7	7.7	8.6	9.6	11.5	13.4	15.4
90	198	4.3	5.4	6.5	7.6	8.6	9.7	10.8	13	15.1	17.3
100	220	4.8	6	7.2	8.4	9.6	10.8	12	14.4	16.8	19.2

* 500 mg ZEMURON in 100 mL solution.

4   CONTRAINDICATIONS

ZEMURON is contraindicated in patients known to have hypersensitivity (e.g., anaphylaxis) to rocuronium bromide or other neuromuscular blocking agents [see Warnings and Precautions (5.2)].

5   WARNINGS AND PRECAUTIONS

5.1   Appropriate Administration and Monitoring

ZEMURON should be administered in carefully adjusted dosages by or under the supervision of experienced clinicians who are familiar with the drug's actions and the possible complications of its use. The drug should not be administered unless facilities for intubation, mechanical ventilation, oxygen therapy, and an antagonist are immediately available. It is recommended that clinicians administering neuromuscular blocking agents such as ZEMURON employ a peripheral nerve stimulator to monitor drug effect, need for additional doses, adequacy of spontaneous recovery or antagonism, and to decrease the complications of overdosage if additional doses are administered.

5.2   Anaphylaxis

Severe anaphylactic reactions to neuromuscular blocking agents, including ZEMURON, have been reported. These reactions have, in some cases (including cases with ZEMURON), been life threatening and fatal. Due to the potential severity of these reactions, the necessary precautions, such as the immediate availability of appropriate emergency treatment, should be taken. Precautions should also be taken in those patients who have had previous anaphylactic reactions to other neuromuscular blocking agents, since cross-reactivity between neuromuscular blocking agents, both depolarizing and nondepolarizing, has been reported.

5.3   Need for Adequate Anesthesia

ZEMURON has no known effect on consciousness, pain threshold, or cerebration. Therefore, its administration must be accompanied by adequate anesthesia or sedation.

5.4   Residual Paralysis

In order to prevent complications resulting from residual paralysis, it is recommended to extubate only after the patient has recovered sufficiently from neuromuscular block. Other factors which could cause residual paralysis after extubation in the post-operative phase (such as drug interactions or patient condition) should also be considered. If not used as part of standard clinical practice the use of a reversal agent should be considered, especially in those cases where residual paralysis is more likely to occur.

5.5   Long-Term Use in an Intensive Care Unit

ZEMURON has not been studied for long-term use in the intensive care unit (ICU). As with other nondepolarizing neuromuscular blocking drugs, apparent tolerance to ZEMURON may develop during chronic administration in the ICU. While the mechanism for development of this resistance is not known, receptor up-regulation may be a contributing factor. **It is strongly recommended that neuromuscular transmission be monitored continuously during administration and recovery with the help of a nerve stimulator. Additional doses of ZEMURON or any other neuromuscular blocking agent should not be given until there is a definite response (one twitch of the train-of-four) to nerve stimulation.** Prolonged paralysis and/or skeletal mus-

cle weakness may be noted during initial attempts to wean from the ventilator patients who have chronically received neuromuscular blocking drugs in the ICU.

Myopathy after long-term administration of other nondepolarizing neuromuscular blocking agents in the ICU alone or in combination with corticosteroid therapy has been reported. Therefore, for patients receiving both neuromuscular blocking agents and corticosteroids, the period of use of the neuromuscular blocking agent should be limited as much as possible and only used in the setting where in the opinion of the prescribing physician, the specific advantages of the drug outweigh the risk.

5.6   Malignant Hyperthermia (MH)

ZEMURON has not been studied in MH-susceptible patients. Because ZEMURON is always used with other agents, and the occurrence of malignant hyperthermia during anesthesia is possible even in the absence of known triggering agents, clinicians should be familiar with early signs, confirmatory diagnosis, and treatment of malignant hyperthermia prior to the start of any anesthetic.

In an animal study in MH-susceptible swine, the administration of ZEMURON Injection did not appear to trigger malignant hyperthermia.

5.7   Prolonged Circulation Time

Conditions associated with an increased circulatory delayed time, e.g., cardiovascular disease or advanced age, may be associated with a delay in onset time [see Dosage and Administration (2.5)].

5.8   QT Interval Prolongation

The overall analysis of ECG data in pediatric patients indicates that the concomitant use of ZEMURON with general anesthetic agents can prolong the QTc interval [see Clinical Studies (14.3)].

5.9   Conditions/Drugs Causing Potentiation of, or Resistance to, Neuromuscular Block

Potentiation: Nondepolarizing neuromuscular blocking agents have been found to exhibit profound neuromuscular blocking effects in cachectic or debilitated patients, patients with neuromuscular diseases, and patients with carcinomatosis.

Certain inhalation anesthetics, particularly enflurane and isoflurane, antibiotics, magnesium salts, lithium, local anesthetics, procainamide, and quinidine have been shown to increase the duration of neuromuscular block and decrease infusion requirements of neuromuscular blocking agents [see Drug Interactions (7.3)].

In these or other patients in whom potentiation of neuromuscular block or difficulty with reversal may be anticipated, a decrease from the recommended initial dose of ZEMURON should be considered [see Dosage and Administration (2.5)].

Resistance: Resistance to nondepolarizing agents, consistent with up-regulation of skeletal muscle acetylcholine receptors, is associated with burns, disuse atrophy, denervation, and direct muscle trauma. Receptor up-regulation may also contribute to the resistance to nondepolarizing muscle relaxants which sometimes develops in patients with cerebral palsy, patients chronically receiving anticonvulsant agents such as carbamazepine or phenytoin, or with chronic exposure to nondepolarizing agents. When ZEMURON is

administered to these patients, shorter durations of neuromuscular block may occur, and infusion rates may be higher due to the development of resistance to nondepolarizing muscle relaxants.

Potentiation or Resistance: Severe acid-base and/or electrolyte abnormalities may potentiate or cause resistance to the neuromuscular blocking action of ZEMURON. No data are available in such patients and no dosing recommendations can be made.

ZEMURON-induced neuromuscular blockade was modified by alkalosis and acidosis in experimental pigs. Both respiratory and metabolic acidosis prolonged the recovery time. The potency of ZEMURON was significantly enhanced in metabolic acidosis and alkalosis, but was reduced in respiratory alkalosis. In addition, experience with other drugs has suggested that acute (e.g., diarrhea) or chronic (e.g., adrenocortical insufficiency) electrolyte imbalance may alter neuromuscular blockade. Since electrolyte imbalance and acid-base imbalance are usually mixed, either enhancement or inhibition may occur.

5.10   Incompatibility with Alkaline Solutions

ZEMURON, which has an acid pH, should not be mixed with alkaline solutions (e.g., barbiturate solutions) in the same syringe or administered simultaneously during intravenous infusion through the same needle.

5.11   Increase in Pulmonary Vascular Resistance

ZEMURON may be associated with increased pulmonary vascular resistance, so caution is appropriate in patients with pulmonary hypertension or valvular heart disease [see Clinical Studies (14.1)].

5.12   Use In Patients with Myasthenia

In patients with myasthenia gravis or myasthenic (Eaton-Lambert) syndrome, small doses of nondepolarizing neuromuscular blocking agents may have profound effects. In such patients, a peripheral nerve stimulator and use of a small test dose may be of value in monitoring the response to administration of muscle relaxants.

5.13   Extravasation

If extravasation occurs, it may be associated with signs or symptoms of local irritation. The injection or infusion should be terminated immediately and restarted in another vein.

6   ADVERSE REACTIONS

In clinical trials, the most common adverse reactions (2%) are transient hypotension and hypertension.

The following adverse reactions are described, or described in greater detail, in other sections:

• Anaphylaxis [see Warnings and Precautions (5.2)]
• Residual paralysis [see Warnings and Precautions (5.4)]
• Myopathy [see Warnings and Precautions (5.5)]
• Increased pulmonary vascular resistance [see Warnings and Precautions (5.11)]

6.1   Clinical Trials Experience

Because clinical trials are conducted under widely varying conditions, adverse reaction rates observed in the clinical trials of a drug cannot be directly compared to rates in the clinical trials of another drug and may not reflect the rates observed in practice.

Clinical studies in the US (n=1137) and Europe (n=1394) totaled 2531 patients. The patients exposed in the US clinical studies provide the basis for calculation of adverse reaction rates. The following adverse reactions were reported in patients administered ZEMURON (all events judged by investigators during the clinical trials to have a possible causal relationship):

Adverse reactions in greater than 1% of patients: None
Adverse reactions in less than 1% of patients (probably related or relationship unknown):

 Cardiovascular: arrhythmia, abnormal electrocardiogram, tachycardia
 Digestive: nausea, vomiting
 Respiratory: asthma (bronchospasm, wheezing, or rhonchi), hiccup
 Skin and Appendages: rash, injection site edema, pruritus

In the European studies, the most commonly reported reactions were transient hypotension (2%) and hypertension (2%); these are in greater frequency than the US studies (0.1% and 0.1%). Changes in heart rate and blood pressure were defined differently from in the US studies in which changes in cardiovascular parameters were not considered as adverse events unless judged by the investigator as unexpected, clinically significant, or thought to be histamine related.

In a clinical study in patients with clinically significant cardiovascular disease undergoing coronary artery bypass graft, hypertension and tachycardia were reported in some patients, but these occurrences were less frequent in patients receiving beta or calcium channel-blocking drugs. In some patients, ZEMURON was associated with transient increases (30% or greater) in pulmonary vascular resistance. In another clinical study of patients undergoing abdominal aortic surgery, transient increases (30% or greater) in pulmonary vascular resistance were observed in about 24% of patients receiving ZEMURON 0.6 or 0.9 mg/kg.

In pediatric patient studies worldwide (n=704), tachycardia occurred at an incidence of 5.3% (n=37), and it was judged by the investigator as related in 10 cases (1.4%).

6.2 Postmarketing Experience

In clinical practice, there have been reports of severe allergic reactions (anaphylactic and anaphylactoid reactions and shock) with ZEMURON, including some that have been life-threatening and fatal [see Warnings and Precautions (5.2)]. Because these reactions were reported voluntarily from a population of uncertain size, it is not possible to reliably estimate their frequency.

7 DRUG INTERACTIONS

7.1 Antibiotics

Drugs which may enhance the neuromuscular blocking action of nondepolarizing agents such as ZEMURON include certain antibiotics (e.g., aminoglycosides; vancomycin; tetracyclines; bacitracin; polymyxins; colistin; and sodium colistimethate). If these antibiotics are used in conjunction with ZEMURON, prolongation of neuromuscular block may occur.

7.2 Anticonvulsants

In 2 of 4 patients receiving chronic anticonvulsant therapy, apparent resistance to the effects of ZEMURON was observed in the form of diminished magnitude of neuromuscular block, or shortened clinical duration. As with other nondepolarizing neuromuscular blocking drugs, if ZEMURON is administered to patients chronically receiving anticonvulsant agents such as carbamazepine or phenytoin, shorter durations of neuromuscular block may occur and infusion rates may be higher due to the development of resistance to nondepolarizing muscle relaxants. While the mechanism for development of this resistance is not known, receptor up-regulation may be a contributing factor [see Warnings and Precautions (5.9)].

7.3 Inhalation Anesthetics

Use of inhalation anesthetics has been shown to enhance the activity of other neuromuscular blocking agents (enflurane > isoflurane > halothane).

Isoflurane and enflurane may also prolong the duration of action of initial and maintenance doses of ZEMURON and decrease the average infusion requirement of ZEMURON by 40% compared to opioid/nitrous oxide/oxygen anesthesia. No definite interaction between ZEMURON and halothane has been demonstrated. In one study, use of enflurane in 10 patients resulted in a 20% increase in mean clinical duration of the initial intubating dose, and a 37% increase in the duration of subsequent maintenance doses, when compared in the same study to 10 patients under opioid/nitrous oxide/oxygen anesthesia. The clinical duration of initial doses of ZEMURON of 0.57 to 0.85 mg/kg under enflurane or isoflurane anesthesia, as used clinically, was increased by 11% and 23%, respectively. The duration of maintenance doses was affected to a greater extent, increasing by 30% to 50% under either enflurane or isoflurane anesthesia.

Potentiation by these agents is also observed with respect to the infusion rates of ZEMURON required to maintain approximately 95% neuromuscular block. Under isoflurane and enflurane anesthesia, the infusion rates are decreased by approximately 40% compared to opioid/nitrous oxide/oxygen anesthesia. The median spontaneous recovery time (from 25% to 75% of control T_1) is not affected by halothane, but is prolonged by enflurane (15% longer) and isoflurane (62% longer). Reversal-induced recovery of ZEMURON neuromuscular block is minimally affected by anesthetic technique [see Dosage and Administration (2.5) and Warnings and Precautions (5.9)].

7.4 Lithium Carbonate

Lithium has been shown to increase the duration of neuromuscular block and decrease infusion requirements of neuromuscular blocking agents [see Warnings and Precautions (5.9)].

7.5 Local Anesthetics

Local anesthetics have been shown to increase the duration of neuromuscular block and decrease infusion requirements of neuromuscular blocking agents [see Warnings and Precautions (5.9)].

7.6 Magnesium

Magnesium salts administered for the management of toxemia of pregnancy may enhance neuromuscular blockade [see Warnings and Precautions (5.9)].

7.7 Nondepolarizing Muscle Relaxants

There are no controlled studies documenting the use of ZEMURON before or after other nondepolarizing muscle relaxants. Interactions have been observed when other nondepolarizing muscle relaxants have been administered in succession.

7.8 Procainamide

Procainamide has been shown to increase the duration of neuromuscular block and decrease infusion requirements of neuromuscular blocking agents [see Warnings and Precautions (5.9)].

7.9 Propofol

The use of propofol for induction and maintenance of anesthesia does not alter the clinical duration or recovery characteristics following recommended doses of ZEMURON.

7.10 Quinidine

Injection of quinidine during recovery from use of muscle relaxants is associated with recurrent paralysis. This possibility must also be considered for ZEMURON [see Warnings and Precautions (5.9)].

7.11 Succinylcholine

The use of ZEMURON before succinylcholine, for the purpose of attenuating some of the side effects of succinylcholine, has not been studied.

If ZEMURON is administered following administration of succinylcholine, it should not be given until recovery from succinylcholine has been observed. The median duration of action of ZEMURON 0.6 mg/kg administered after a 1 mg/kg dose of succinylcholine when T_1 returned to 75% of control was 36 minutes (range: 14-57, n=12) vs. 28 minutes (range: 17-51, n=12) without succinylcholine.

8 USE IN SPECIFIC POPULATIONS

8.1 Pregnancy

Pregnancy Category C: Developmental toxicology studies have been performed with rocuronium bromide in pregnant, conscious, nonventilated rabbits and rats. Inhibition of neuromuscular function was the endpoint for high-dose selection. The maximum tolerated dose served as the high dose and was administered intravenously 3 times a day to rats (0.3 mg/kg, 15%-30% of human intubation dose of 0.6-1.2 mg/kg based on the body surface unit of mg/m²) from Day 6 to 17 and to rabbits (0.02 mg/kg, 25% human dose) from Day 6 to 18 of pregnancy. High-dose treatment caused acute symptoms of respiratory dysfunction due to the pharmacological activity of the drug. Teratogenicity was not observed in these animal species. The incidence of late embryonic death was increased at the high dose in rats, most likely due to oxygen deficiency. Therefore, this finding probably has no relevance for humans because immediate mechanical ventilation of the intubated patient will effectively prevent embryo-fetal hypoxia. However, there are no adequate and well-controlled studies in pregnant women. ZEMURON should be used during pregnancy only if the potential benefit justifies the potential risk to the fetus.

8.2 Labor and Delivery

The use of ZEMURON in Cesarean section has been studied in a limited number of patients [see Clinical Studies (14.1)]. ZEMURON is not recommended for rapid sequence induction in Cesarean section patients.

8.4 Pediatric Use

The use of ZEMURON has been studied in pediatric patients 3 months to 14 years of age under halothane anesthesia. Of the pediatric patients anesthetized with halothane who did not receive atropine for induction, about 80% experienced a transient increase (30% or greater) in heart rate after intubation. One of the 19 infants anesthetized with halothane and fentanyl who received atropine for induction experienced this magnitude of change [see Dosage and Administration (2.5) and Clinical Studies (14.3)].

ZEMURON was also studied in pediatric patients up to 17 years of age, including neonates, under sevoflurane (induction) and isoflurane/nitrous oxide (maintenance) anesthesia. Onset time and clinical duration varied with dose, the age of the patient, and anesthetic technique. The overall analysis of ECG data in pediatric patients indicates that the concomitant use of ZEMURON with general anesthetic agents can prolong the QTc interval. The data also suggest that ZEMURON may increase heart rate. However, it was not possible to conclusively identify an effect of ZEMURON independent of that of anesthesia and other factors. Additionally, when examining plasma levels of ZEMURON in correlation to QTc interval prolongation, no relationship was observed [see Dosage and Administration (2.5), Warnings and Precautions (5.8), and Clinical Studies (14.3)].

ZEMURON is not recommended for rapid sequence intubation in pediatric patients. Recommendations for use in pediatric patients are discussed in other sections [see Dosage and Administration (2.5) and Clinical Pharmacology (12.2)].

8.5 Geriatric Use

ZEMURON was administered to 140 geriatric patients (65 years or greater) in US clinical trials and 128 geriatric patients in European clinical trials. The observed pharmacokinetic profile for geriatric patients (n=20) was similar to that for other adult surgical patients [see Clinical Pharmacology (12.3)]. Onset time and duration of action were slightly longer for geriatric patients (n=43) in clinical trials. Clinical experiences and recommendations for use in geriatric patients are discussed in other sections [see Dosage and Administration (2.5), Clinical Pharmacology (12.2), and Clinical Studies (14.2)].

8.6 Patients with Hepatic Impairment

Since ZEMURON is primarily excreted by the liver, it should be used with caution in patients with clinically significant hepatic impairment. ZEMURON 0.6 mg/kg has been studied in a limited number of patients (n=9) with clinically significant hepatic impairment under steady-state isoflurane anesthesia. After ZEMURON 0.6 mg/kg, the median (range) clinical duration of 60 (35-166) minutes was moderately prolonged compared to 42 minutes in patients with normal hepatic function. The median recovery time of 53 minutes was also prolonged in patients with cirrhosis compared to 20 minutes in patients with normal hepatic function. Four of 8 patients with cirrhosis, who received ZEMURON 0.6 mg/kg under opioid/nitrous oxide/oxygen anesthesia, did not achieve complete block. These findings are consistent with the increase in volume of distribution at steady state observed in patients with significant hepatic impairment [see Clinical Pharmacology (12.3)]. If used for rapid sequence induction in patients with ascites, an increased initial dosage may be necessary to assure complete block. Duration will be prolonged in these cases. The use of doses higher than 0.6 mg/kg has not been studied [see Dosage and Administration (2.5)].

8.7 Patients with Renal Impairment

Due to the limited role of the kidney in the excretion of ZEMURON, usual dosing guidelines should be followed. In patients with renal dysfunction, the duration of neuromuscular blockade was not prolonged; however, there was substantial individual variability (range: 22-90 minutes) [see Clinical Pharmacology (12.3)].

10 OVERDOSAGE

Overdosage with neuromuscular blocking agents may result in neuromuscular block beyond the time needed for surgery and anesthesia. The primary treatment is maintenance of a patent airway, controlled ventilation, and adequate sedation until recovery of normal neuromuscular function is assured. Once evidence of recovery from neuromuscular block is observed, further recovery may be facilitated by administration of an anticholinesterase agent in conjunction with an appropriate anticholinergic agent.

Reversal of Neuromuscular Blockade: **Anticholinesterase agents should not be administered prior to the demonstration of some spontaneous recovery from neuromuscular blockade. The use of a nerve stimulator to document recovery is recommended.**

Patients should be evaluated for adequate clinical evidence of neuromuscular recovery, e.g., 5-second head lift, adequate phonation, ventilation, and upper airway patency. Ventilation must be supported while patients exhibit any signs of muscle weakness.

Recovery may be delayed in the presence of debilitation, carcinomatosis, and concomitant use of certain drugs which enhance neuromuscular blockade or separately cause respiratory depression. Under such circumstances the management is the same as that of prolonged neuromuscular blockade.

11 DESCRIPTION

ZEMURON (rocuronium bromide) injection is a nondepolarizing neuromuscular blocking agent with a rapid to intermediate onset depending on dose and intermediate duration. Rocuronium bromide is chemically designated as 1-[17β-(acetyloxy)-3α-hydroxy-2β-(4-morpholinyl)-5α-androstan-16β-yl]-1-(2-propenyl)pyrrolidinium bromide. The structural formula is:

The chemical formula is $C_{32}H_{53}BrN_2O_4$ with a molecular weight of 609.70. The partition coefficient of rocuronium bromide in n-octanol/water is 0.5 at 20°C.

ZEMURON is supplied as a sterile, nonpyrogenic, isotonic solution that is clear, colorless to yellow/orange, for intravenous injection only. Each mL contains 10 mg rocuronium bromide and 2 mg sodium acetate. The aqueous solution is adjusted to isotonicity with sodium chloride and to a pH of 4 with acetic acid and/or sodium hydroxide.

12 CLINICAL PHARMACOLOGY

12.1 Mechanism of Action

ZEMURON is a nondepolarizing neuromuscular blocking agent with a rapid to intermediate onset depending on dose and intermediate duration. It acts by competing for cholinergic receptors at the motor end-plate. This action is antagonized by acetylcholinesterase inhibitors, such as neostigmine and edrophonium.

12.2 Pharmacodynamics

The ED_{95} (dose required to produce 95% suppression of the first [T_1] mechanomyographic [MMG] response of the adductor pollicis muscle [thumb] to indirect supramaximal train-of-four stimulation of the ulnar nerve) during opioid/nitrous oxide/oxygen anesthesia is approximately 0.3 mg/kg. Patient variability around the ED_{95} dose suggests that 50% of patients will exhibit T_1 depression of 91% to 97%.

Table 4 presents intubating conditions in patients with intubation initiated at 60 to 70 seconds.

Table 4: Percent of Excellent or Good Intubating Conditions and Median (Range) Time to Completion of Intubation in Patients with Intubation Initiated at 60 to 70 Seconds

ZEMURON Dose (mg/kg) Administered Over 5 sec	Percent of Patients with Excellent or Good Intubating Conditions	Time to Completion of Intubation (min)
Adults* 18 to 64 yrs		
0.45 (n=43)	86%	1.6 (1.0-7.0)
0.6 (n=51)	96%	1.6 (1.0-3.2)
Infants† 3 mo to 1 yr		
0.6 (n=18)	100%	1.0 (1.0-1.5)
Pediatric† 1 to 12 yrs		
0.6 (n=12)	100%	1.0 (0.5-2.3)

Excellent intubating conditions=jaw relaxed, vocal cords apart and immobile, no diaphragmatic movement.
Good intubating conditions=same as excellent but with some diaphragmatic movement.
* Excludes patients undergoing Cesarean section.
† Pediatric patients were under halothane anesthesia.

Table 5 presents the time to onset and clinical duration for the initial dose of ZEMURON (rocuronium bromide) injection under opioid/nitrous oxide/oxygen anesthesia in adults and geriatric patients, and under halothane anesthesia in pediatric patients.
[See table 5 above]

Table 6 presents the time to onset and clinical duration for the initial dose of ZEMURON (rocuronium bromide) Injection under sevoflurane (induction) and isoflurane/nitrous oxide (maintenance) anesthesia in pediatric patients.

Table 6: Median (Range) Time to Onset and Clinical Duration Following Initial (Intubating) Dose During Sevoflurane (induction) and Isoflurane/Nitrous Oxide (maintenance) Anesthesia (Pediatric Patients)

ZEMURON Dose (mg/kg) Administered Over 5 sec	Time to Maximum Block (min)	Time to Reappearance T_3 (min)
Neonates birth to <28 days		
0.45 (n=5)	1.1 (0.6-2.2)	40.3 (32.5-62.6)
0.6 (n=10)	1.0 (0.2-2.1)	49.7 (16.6-119.0)
1 (n=6)	0.6 (0.3-1.8)	114.4 (92.6-136.3)
Infants 28 days to ≤3 mo		
0.45 (n=9)	0.5 (0.4-1.3)	49.1 (13.5-79.9)
0.6 (n=11)	0.4 (0.2-0.8)	59.8 (32.3-87.8)
1 (n=5)	0.3 (0.2-0.7)	103.3 (90.8-155.4)
Toddlers >3 mo to ≤2 yrs		
0.45 (n=17)	0.8 (0.3-1.9)	39.2 (16.9-59.4)
0.6 (n=29)	0.6 (0.2-1.6)	44.2 (18.9-68.8)
1 (n=15)	0.5 (0.2-1.5)	72.0 (36.2-128.2)
Children >2 yrs to ≤11 yrs		
0.45 (n=14)	0.9 (0.4-1.9)	21.5 (17.5-38.0)
0.6 (n=37)	0.8 (0.3-1.7)	36.7 (20.1-65.9)
1 (n=16)	0.7 (0.4-1.2)	53.1 (31.2-89.9)
Adolescents >11 to ≤17 yrs		
0.45 (n=18)	1.0 (0.5-1.7)	37.5 (18.3-65.7)
0.6 (n=31)	0.9 (0.2-2.1)	41.4 (16.3-91.2)
1 (n=14)	0.7 (0.5-1.2)	67.1 (25.6-93.8)

n=the number of patients with the highest number of observations for time to maximum block or reappearance T_3.

The time to 80% or greater block and clinical duration as a function of dose are presented in **Figures 1** and **2**.

Table 5: Median (Range) Time to Onset and Clinical Duration Following Initial (Intubating) Dose During Opioid/Nitrous Oxide/Oxygen Anesthesia (Adults) and Halothane Anesthesia (Pediatric Patients)

ZEMURON Dose (mg/kg) Administered Over 5 sec	Time to ≥80% Block (min)	Time to Maximum Block (min)	Clinical Duration (min)
Adults 18 to 64 yrs			
0.45 (n=50)	1.3 (0.8-6.2)	3.0 (1.3-8.2)	22 (12-31)
0.6 (n=142)	1.0 (0.4-6.0)	1.8 (0.6-13.0)	31 (15-85)
0.9 (n=20)	1.1 (0.3-3.8)	1.4 (0.8-6.2)	58 (27-111)
1.2 (n=18)	0.7 (0.4-1.7)	1.0 (0.6-4.7)	67 (38-160)
Geriatric ≥65 yrs			
0.6 (n=31)	2.3 (1.0-8.3)	3.7 (1.3-11.3)	46 (22-73)
0.9 (n=5)	2.0 (1.0-3.0)	2.5 (1.2-5.0)	62 (49-75)
1.2 (n=7)	1.0 (0.8-3.5)	1.3 (1.2-4.7)	94 (64-138)
Infants 3 mo to 1 yr			
0.6 (n=17)	—	0.8 (0.3-3.0)	41 (24-68)
0.8 (n=9)	—	0.7 (0.5-0.8)	40 (27-70)
Pediatric 1 to 12 yrs			
0.6 (n=27)	0.8 (0.4-2.0)	1.0 (0.5-3.3)	26 (17-39)
0.8 (n=18)	—	0.5 (0.3-1.0)	30 (17-56)

n=the number of patients who had time to maximum block recorded.
Clinical duration=time until return to 25% of control T_1. Patients receiving doses of 0.45 mg/kg who achieved less than 90% block (16% of these patients) had about 12 to 15 minutes to 25% recovery.

Figure 1: Time to 80% or Greater Block vs. Initial Dose of ZEMURON by Age Group (Median, 25th and 75th Percentile, and Individual Values)

Figure 2: Duration of Clinical Effect vs. Initial Dose of ZEMURON by Age Group (Median, 25th and 75th Percentile, and Individual Values)

The clinical durations for the first 5 maintenance doses, in patients receiving 5 or more maintenance doses are represented in **Figure 3** [see Dosage and Administration (2.3)].

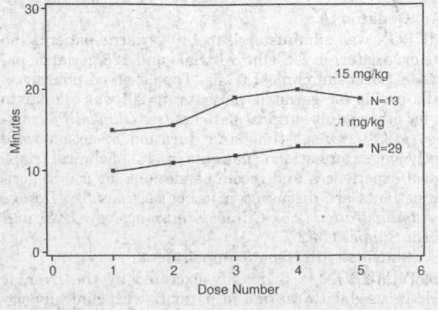

Figure 3: Duration of Clinical Effect vs. Number of ZEMURON Maintenance Doses, by Dose

Once spontaneous recovery has reached 25% of control T_1, the neuromuscular block produced by ZEMURON is readily reversed with anticholinesterase agents, e.g., edrophonium or neostigmine.

The median spontaneous recovery from 25% to 75% T_1 was 13 minutes in adult patients. When neuromuscular block was reversed in 36 adults at a T_1 of 22% to 27%, recovery to a T_1 of 89 (50-132)% and T_4/T_1 of 69 (38-92)% was achieved within 5 minutes. Only 5 of 320 adults reversed received an additional dose of reversal agent. The median (range) dose of neostigmine was 0.04 (0.01-0.09) mg/kg and the median (range) dose of edrophonium was 0.5 (0.3-1.0) mg/kg.

In geriatric patients (n=51) reversed with neostigmine, the median T_4/T_1 increased from 40% to 88% in 5 minutes.

In clinical trials with halothane, pediatric patients (n=27) who received 0.5 mg/kg edrophonium had increases in the median T_4/T_1 from 37% at reversal to 93% after 2 minutes. Pediatric patients (n=58) who received 1 mg/kg edrophonium had increases in the median T_4/T_1 from 72% at reversal to 100% after 2 minutes. Infants (n=10) who were reversed with 0.03 mg/kg neostigmine recovered from 25% to 75% T_1 within 4 minutes.

There were no reports of less than satisfactory clinical recovery of neuromuscular function.

The neuromuscular blocking action of ZEMURON may be enhanced in the presence of potent inhalation anesthetics [see Drug Interactions (7.3)].

Hemodynamics: There were no dose-related effects on the incidence of changes from baseline (30% or greater) in mean arterial blood pressure (MAP) or heart rate associated with ZEMURON administration over the dose range of 0.12 to 1.2 mg/kg ($4 \times ED_{95}$) within 5 minutes after ZEMURON administration and prior to intubation. Increases or decreases in MAP were observed in 2% to 5% of geriatric and other adult patients, and in about 1% of pediatric patients. Heart rate changes (30% or greater) occurred in 0% to 2% of geriatric and other adult patients. Tachycardia (30% or greater) occurred in 12 of 127 pediatric patients. Most of the pediatric patients developing tachycardia were from a single study where the patients were anesthetized with halothane and who did not receive atropine for induction [see Clinical Studies (14.3)]. In US studies, laryngoscopy and tracheal intubation following ZEMURON administration were accompanied by transient tachycardia (30% or greater increases) in about one-third of adult patients under opioid/nitrous oxide/oxygen anesthesia. Animal studies have indicated that the ratio of vagal:neuromuscular block following ZEMURON administration is less than vecuronium but greater than pancuronium. The tachycardia observed in some patients may result from this vagal blocking activity.

Histamine Release: In studies of histamine release, clinically significant concentrations of plasma histamine occurred in 1 of 88 patients. Clinical signs of histamine release (flushing, rash, or bronchospasm) associated with the administration of ZEMURON were assessed in clinical trials and reported in 9 of 1137 (0.8%) patients.

12.3 Pharmacokinetics

Adult and Geriatric Patients: In an effort to maximize the information gathered in the in vivo pharmacokinetic studies, the data from the studies was used to develop population estimates of the parameters for the subpopulations represented (e.g., geriatric, pediatric, renal, and hepatic impairment). These population-based estimates and a measure of the estimate variability are contained in the following section.

Following intravenous administration of ZEMURON, plasma levels of rocuronium follow a three-compartment open model. The rapid distribution half-life is 1 to 2 minutes and the slower distribution half-life is 14 to 18 minutes. Rocuronium is approximately 30% bound to human plasma proteins. In geriatric and other adult surgical patients undergoing either opioid/nitrous oxide/oxygen or inhalational anesthesia, the observed pharmacokinetic profile was essentially unchanged.

Table 7: Mean (SD) Pharmacokinetic Parameters in Adults (n=22; ages 27 to 58 yrs) and Geriatric (n=20; 65 yrs or greater) During Opioid/Nitrous Oxide/Oxygen Anesthesia

PK Parameters	Adults (Ages 27-58 yrs)	Geriatrics (≥65 yrs)
Clearance (L/kg/hr)	0.25 (0.08)	0.21 (0.06)
Volume of Distribution at Steady State (L/kg)	0.25 (0.04)	0.22 (0.03)
$t_{1/2}$ β Elimination (hr)	1.4 (0.4)	1.5 (0.4)

In general, studies with normal adult subjects did not reveal any differences in the pharmacokinetics of rocuronium due to gender.

Studies of distribution, metabolism, and excretion in cats and dogs indicate that rocuronium is eliminated primarily by the liver. The rocuronium analog 17-desacetyl-rocuronium, a metabolite, has been rarely observed in the plasma or urine of humans administered single doses of 0.5 to 1 mg/kg with or without a subsequent infusion (for up to 12 hr) of rocuronium. In the cat, 17-desacetyl-rocuronium has approximately one-twentieth the neuromuscular blocking potency of rocuronium. The effects of renal failure and hepatic disease on the pharmacokinetics and pharmacodynamics of rocuronium in humans are consistent with these findings.

In general, patients undergoing cadaver kidney transplant have a small reduction in clearance which is offset pharmacokinetically by a corresponding increase in volume, such that the net effect is an unchanged plasma half-life. Patients with demonstrated liver cirrhosis have a marked increase in their volume of distribution resulting in a plasma half-life approximately twice that of patients with normal hepatic function. **Table 8** shows the pharmacokinetic parameters in subjects with either impaired renal or hepatic function.

[See table 8 above]

The net result of these findings is that subjects with renal failure have clinical durations that are similar to but somewhat more variable than the duration that one would expect in subjects with normal renal function. Hepatically impaired patients, due to the large increase in volume, may demonstrate clinical durations approaching 1.5 times that of subjects with normal hepatic function. In both populations the clinician should individualize the dose to the needs of the patient [see Dosage and Administration (2.5)].

Tissue redistribution accounts for most (about 80%) of the initial amount of rocuronium administered. As tissue compartments fill with continued dosing (4-8 hours), less drug is redistributed away from the site of action and, for an infusion-only dose, the rate to maintain neuromuscular blockade falls to about 20% of the initial infusion rate. The use of a loading dose and a smaller infusion rate reduces the need for adjustment of dose.

Pediatric Patients: Under halothane anesthesia, the clinical duration of effects of ZEMURON did not vary with age in patients 4 months to 8 years of age. The terminal half-life and other pharmacokinetic parameters of rocuronium in these pediatric patients are presented in **Table 9.**

Table 9: Mean (SD) Pharmacokinetic Parameters of Rocuronium in Pediatric Patients (ages 3 to less than 12 mos, n=6; 1 to less than 3 yrs, n=5; 3 to less than 8 yrs, n=7) During Halothane Anesthesia

PK Parameters	Patient Age Range		
	3 to <12 mos	1 to <3 yrs	3 to <8 yrs
Clearance (L/kg/hr)	0.35 (0.08)	0.32 (0.07)	0.44 (0.16)
Volume of Distribution at Steady State (L/kg)	0.30 (0.04)	0.26 (0.06)	0.21 (0.03)
$t_{1/2}$ β Elimination (hr)	1.3 (0.5)	1.1 (0.7)	0.8 (0.3)

Table 8: Mean (SD) Pharmacokinetic Parameters in Adults with Normal Renal and Hepatic Function (n=10, ages 23 to 65), Renal Transplant Patients (n=10, ages 21 to 45), and Hepatic Dysfunction Patients (n=9, ages 31 to 67) During Isoflurane Anesthesia

PK Parameters	Normal Renal and Hepatic Function	Renal Transplant Patients	Hepatic Dysfunction Patients
Clearance (L/kg/hr)	0.16 (0.05)*	0.13 (0.04)	0.13 (0.06)
Volume of Distribution at Steady State (L/kg)	0.26 (0.03)	0.34 (0.11)	0.53 (0.14)
$t_{1/2}$ β Elimination (hr)	2.4 (0.8)*	2.4 (1.1)	4.3 (2.6)

* Differences in the calculated $t_{1/2}$ β and Cl between this study and the study in young adults vs. geriatrics (≥65 years) is related to the different sample populations and anesthetic techniques.

Table 10: Mean (SD) Pharmacokinetic Parameters of Rocuronium in Pediatric Patients During Sevoflurane (induction) and Isoflurane/Nitrous Oxide (maintenance) Anesthesia

PK Parameters	Patient Age Range				
	Birth to <28 days	28 days to ≤3 mos	3 mos to ≤2 yrs	2 to ≤11 yrs	11 to ≤17 yrs
CL (L/kg/hr)	0.31 (0.07)	0.30 (0.08)	0.33 (0.10)	0.35 (0.09)	0.29 (0.14)
Volume of Distribution (L/kg)	0.42 (0.06)	0.31 (0.03)	0.23 (0.03)	0.18 (0.02)	0.18 (0.01)
$t_{1/2}$ β (hr)	1.1 (0.2)	0.9 (0.3)	0.8 (0.2)	0.7 (0.2)	0.8 (0.3)

Pharmacokinetics of ZEMURON were evaluated using a population analysis of the pooled pharmacokinetic datasets from 2 trials under sevoflurane (induction) and isoflurane/nitrous oxide (maintenance) anesthesia. All pharmacokinetic parameters were found to be linearly proportional to body weight. In patients under the age of 18 years clearance (CL) and volume of distribution (Vss) increase with body-weight (kg) and age (years). As a result the terminal half-life of ZEMURON decreases with increasing age from 1.1 hour to 0.7-0.8 hour. **Table 10** presents the pharmacokinetic parameters in the different age groups in the studies with sevoflurane (induction) and isoflurane/nitrous oxide (maintenance) anesthesia.

[See table 10 above]

13   NONCLINICAL TOXICOLOGY

13.1   Carcinogenesis, Mutagenesis, Impairment of Fertility

Studies in animals have not been performed with rocuronium bromide to evaluate carcinogenic potential or impairment of fertility. Mutagenicity studies (Ames test, analysis of chromosomal aberrations in mammalian cells, and micronucleus test) conducted with rocuronium bromide did not suggest mutagenic potential.

14   CLINICAL STUDIES

In US clinical studies, a total of 1137 patients received ZEMURON, including 176 pediatric, 140 geriatric, 55 obstetric, and 766 other adults. Most patients (90%) were ASA physical status I or II, about 9% were ASA III, and 10 patients (undergoing coronary artery bypass grafting or valvular surgery) were ASA IV. In European clinical studies, a total of 1394 patients received ZEMURON, including 52 pediatric, 128 geriatric (65 years or greater), and 1214 other adults.

14.1   Adult Patients

Intubation using doses of ZEMURON 0.6 to 0.85 mg/kg was evaluated in 203 adults in 11 clinical studies. Excellent to good intubating conditions were generally achieved within 2 minutes and maximum block occurred within 3 minutes in most patients. Doses within this range provide clinical relaxation for a median (range) time of 33 (14-85) minutes under opioid/nitrous oxide/oxygen anesthesia. Larger doses (0.9 and 1.2 mg/kg) were evaluated in 2 studies with 19 and 16 patients under opioid/nitrous oxide/oxygen anesthesia and provided 58 (27-111) and 67 (38-160) minutes of clinical relaxation, respectively.

Cardiovascular Disease: In 1 clinical study, 10 patients with clinically significant cardiovascular disease undergoing coronary artery bypass graft received an initial dose of 0.6 mg/kg ZEMURON. Neuromuscular block was maintained during surgery with bolus maintenance doses of 0.3 mg/kg. Following induction, continuous 8 mcg/kg/min infusion of ZEMURON produced relaxation sufficient to support mechanical ventilation for 6 to 12 hours in the surgical intensive care unit (SICU) while the patients were recovering from surgery.

Rapid Sequence Intubation: Intubating conditions were assessed in 230 patients in 6 clinical studies where anesthesia was induced with either thiopental (3-6 mg/kg) or propofol (1.5-2.5 mg/kg) in combination with either fentanyl (2-5 mcg/kg) or alfentanil (1 mg). Most of the patients also received a premedication such as midazolam or temazepam. Most patients had intubation attempted within 60 to 90 seconds of administration of ZEMURON 0.6 mg/kg or succinylcholine 1 to 1.5 mg/kg. Excellent or good intubating conditions were achieved in 119/120 (99% [95% confidence interval: 95%-99.9%]) patients receiving ZEMURON and in 108/110 (98% [94%-99.8%]) patients receiving succinylcholine. The duration of action of ZEMURON 0.6 mg/kg is longer than succinylcholine and at this dose is approximately equivalent to the duration of other intermediate-acting neuromuscular blocking drugs.

Obese Patients: ZEMURON was dosed according to actual body weight (ABW) in most clinical studies. The administration of ZEMURON in the 47 of 330 (14%) patients who were at least 30% or more above their ideal body weight (IBW) was not associated with clinically significant differences in the onset, duration, recovery, or reversal of ZEMURON-induced neuromuscular block.

In 1 clinical study in obese patients, ZEMURON 0.6 mg/kg was dosed according to ABW (n=12) or IBW (n=11). Obese patients dosed according to IBW had a longer time to maximum block, a shorter median (range) clinical duration of 25 (14-29) minutes, and did not achieve intubating conditions comparable to those dosed based on ABW. These results support the recommendation that obese patients be dosed based on actual body weight [see Dosage and Administration (2.5)].

Obstetric Patients: ZEMURON 0.6 mg/kg was administered with thiopental, 3 to 4 mg/kg (n=13) or 4 to 6 mg/kg (n=42), for rapid sequence induction of anesthesia for Cesarean section. No neonate had APGAR scores greater than 7 at 5 minutes. The umbilical venous plasma concentrations were 18% of maternal concentrations at delivery. Intubating conditions were poor or inadequate in 5 of 13 women receiving 3 to 4 mg/kg thiopental when intubation was attempted 60 seconds after drug injection. Therefore, ZEMURON is not recommended for rapid sequence induction in Cesarean section patients.

14.2   Geriatric Patients

ZEMURON was evaluated in 55 geriatric patients (ages 65-80 years) in 6 clinical studies. Doses of 0.6 mg/kg provided excellent to good intubating conditions in a median (range) time of 2.3 (1-8) minutes. Recovery times from 25% to 75% after these doses were not prolonged in geriatric patients compared to other adult patients [see Dosage and Administration (2.5) and Use in Specific Populations (8.5)].

14.3   Pediatric Patients

ZEMURON 0.45, 0.6, or 1 mg/kg was evaluated under sevoflurane (induction) and isoflurane/nitrous oxide (maintenance) anesthesia for intubation in 326 patients in 2 studies. In 1 of these studies maintenance bolus and infusion requirements were evaluated in 137 patients. In all age groups, doses of 0.6 mg/kg provided time to maximum block in about 1 minute. Across all age groups, median (range) time to reappearance of T_3 for doses of 0.6 mg/kg was shortest in the children [36.7 (20.1-65.9) minutes] and longest in infants [59.8 (32.3-87.8) minutes]. For pediatric patients older than 3 months, the time to recovery was shorter when compared with bolus maintenance [see Dosage and Administration (2.5) and Use in Specific Populations (8.4)].

ZEMURON 0.6 or 0.8 mg/kg was evaluated for intubation in 75 pediatric patients (n=28; age 3-12 months, n=47; age 1-12 years) in 3 studies using halothane (1%-5%) and nitrous oxide (60%-70%) in oxygen. Doses of 0.6 mg/kg provided a median (range) time to maximum block of 1 (0.5-3.3) minute(s). This dose provided a median (range) time of clinical relaxation of 41 (24-68) minutes in 3-month to 1-year-old infants and 26 (17-39) minutes in 1- to 12-year-old pediatric patients [see Dosage and Administration (2.5) and Use in Specific Populations (8.4)].

16 HOW SUPPLIED/STORAGE AND HANDLING

ZEMURON (rocuronium bromide) injection is available in the following:

- ZEMURON 5 mL multiple dose vials containing 50 mg rocuronium bromide injection (10 mg/mL)
  Box of 10   NDC 0052-0450-15

The packaging of this product contains **no** natural rubber (latex).

ZEMURON should be stored in a refrigerator, 2-8°C (36-46°F). DO NOT FREEZE. Upon removal from refrigeration to room temperature storage conditions (25°C/77°F), use ZEMURON within 60 days. Use opened vials of ZEMURON within 30 days.

Safety and Handling: There is no specific work exposure limit for ZEMURON. In case of eye contact, flush with water for at least 10 minutes.

17 PATIENT COUNSELING INFORMATION

Obtain information about your patient's medical history, current medications, any history of hypersensitivity to rocuronium bromide or other neuromuscular blocking agents. If applicable, inform your patients that certain medical conditions and medications might influence how ZEMURON works.

In addition, inform your patient that severe anaphylactic reactions to neuromuscular blocking agents, including ZEMURON, have been reported. Since allergic cross-reactivity has been reported in this class, request information from your patients about previous anaphylactic reactions to other neuromuscular blocking agents.

Manuf. for: Merck Sharp & Dohme Corp., a subsidiary of **MERCK & CO., INC.**, Whitehouse Station, NJ 08889, USA
Manufactured by: Organon (Ireland) Ltd., Swords, Co. Dublin, Ireland, a subsidiary of **Merck & Co., Inc.**, Whitehouse Station, NJ 08889, USA.
For patent information:
www.merck.com/product/patent/home.html
Copyright © 1994, 2010 Merck Sharp & Dohme B.V., a subsidiary of **Merck & Co., Inc.**
All rights reserved.
Revised: 09/2013
uspi-mk8085-i-1309r004

Shown in Product Identification Guide, page 309

ZETIA®

[zĕt'-ē-ă]
(ezetimibe)
Tablets

℞

HIGHLIGHTS OF PRESCRIBING INFORMATION
These highlights do not include all the information needed to use ZETIA safely and effectively. See full prescribing information for ZETIA.
ZETIA® (ezetimibe) Tablets
Initial U.S. Approval: 2002

INDICATIONS AND USAGE

ZETIA is an inhibitor of intestinal cholesterol (and related phytosterol) absorption, indicated as an adjunct to diet to:
- Reduce elevated total-C, LDL-C, Apo B, and non-HDL-C in patients with primary hyperlipidemia, alone or in combination with an HMG-CoA reductase inhibitor (statin) (1.1)
- Reduce elevated total-C, LDL-C, Apo B, and non-HDL-C in patients with mixed hyperlipidemia in combination with fenofibrate (1.1)
- Reduce elevated total-C and LDL-C in patients with homozygous familial hypercholesterolemia (HoFH), in combination with atorvastatin or simvastatin (1.2)
- Reduce elevated sitosterol and campesterol in patients with homozygous sitosterolemia (phytosterolemia) (1.3)
Limitations of Use (1.4)
- The effect of ZETIA on cardiovascular morbidity and mortality has not been determined.
- ZETIA has not been studied in Fredrickson Type I, III, IV, and V dyslipidemias.

DOSAGE AND ADMINISTRATION

- One 10-mg tablet once daily, with or without food (2.1)
- Dosing of ZETIA should occur either ≥2 hours before or ≥4 hours after administration of a bile acid sequestrant. (2.3, 7.4)

DOSAGE FORMS AND STRENGTHS

- Tablets: 10 mg (3)

CONTRAINDICATIONS

- Statin contraindications apply when ZETIA is used with a statin:
  ◦ Active liver disease, which may include unexplained persistent elevations in hepatic transaminase levels (4, 5.2)
  ◦ Women who are pregnant or may become pregnant (4, 8.1)
  ◦ Nursing mothers (4, 8.3)
- Known hypersensitivity to product components (4, 6.2)

WARNINGS AND PRECAUTIONS

- ZETIA is not recommended in patients with moderate or severe hepatic impairment. (5.4, 8.7, 12.3)
- Liver enzyme abnormalities and monitoring: Persistent elevations in hepatic transaminase can occur when ZETIA is added to a statin. Therefore, when ZETIA is added to statin therapy, monitor hepatic transaminase levels before and during treatment according to the recommendations for the individual statin used. (5.2)
- Skeletal muscle effects (e.g., myopathy and rhabdomyolysis):
  ◦ Cases of myopathy and rhabdomyolysis have been reported in patients treated with ZETIA coadministered with a statin and with ZETIA administered alone. Risk for skeletal muscle toxicity increases with higher doses of statin, advanced age (>65), hypothyroidism, renal impairment, and depending on the statin used, concomitant use of other drugs. (5.3, 6.2)

ADVERSE REACTIONS

- Common adverse reactions in clinical trials:
  ◦ ZETIA coadministered with a statin (incidence ≥2% and greater than statin alone):
    ■ nasopharyngitis, myalgia, upper respiratory tract infection, arthralgia, and diarrhea (6)
  ◦ ZETIA administered alone (incidence ≥2% and greater than placebo):
    ■ upper respiratory tract infection, diarrhea, arthralgia, sinusitis, and pain in extremity (6)

To report SUSPECTED ADVERSE REACTIONS, contact Merck Sharp & Dohme Corp., a subsidiary of Merck & Co., Inc., at 1-877-888-4231 or FDA at 1-800-FDA-1088 or www.fda.gov/medwatch.

DRUG INTERACTIONS

- Cyclosporine: Combination increases exposure of ZETIA and cyclosporine. Cyclosporine concentrations should be monitored in patients taking ZETIA concomitantly. (7.1, 12.3)
- Fenofibrate: Combination increases exposure of ZETIA. If cholelithiasis is suspected in a patient receiving ZETIA and fenofibrate, gallbladder studies are indicated and alternative lipid-lowering therapy should be considered. (6.1, 7.3)
- Fibrates: Coadministration of ZETIA with fibrates other than fenofibrate is not recommended until use in patients is adequately studied. (7.2)
- Cholestyramine: Combination decreases exposure of ZETIA. (2.3, 7.4, 12.3)

See 17 for PATIENT COUNSELING INFORMATION and FDA-approved patient labeling

Revised: 08/2013

FULL PRESCRIBING INFORMATION

1 INDICATIONS AND USAGE

Therapy with lipid-altering agents should be only one component of multiple risk factor intervention in individuals at significantly increased risk for atherosclerotic vascular disease due to hypercholesterolemia. Drug therapy is indicated as an adjunct to diet when the response to a diet restricted in saturated fat and cholesterol and other nonpharmacologic measures alone has been inadequate.

1.1 Primary Hyperlipidemia

Monotherapy
ZETIA®, administered alone, is indicated as adjunctive therapy to diet for the reduction of elevated total cholesterol (total-C), low-density lipoprotein cholesterol (LDL-C), apolipoprotein B (Apo B), and non-high-density lipoprotein cholesterol (non-HDL-C) in patients with primary (heterozygous familial and non-familial) hyperlipidemia.

Combination Therapy with HMG-CoA Reductase Inhibitors (Statins)
ZETIA, administered in combination with a 3-hydroxy-3-methylglutaryl-coenzyme A (HMG-CoA) reductase inhibitor (statin), is indicated as adjunctive therapy to diet for the reduction of elevated total-C, LDL-C, Apo B, and non-HDL-C in patients with primary (heterozygous familial and non-familial) hyperlipidemia.

Combination Therapy with Fenofibrate
ZETIA, administered in combination with fenofibrate, is indicated as adjunctive therapy to diet for the reduction of elevated total-C, LDL-C, Apo B, and non-HDL-C in adult patients with mixed hyperlipidemia.

1.2 Homozygous Familial Hypercholesterolemia (HoFH)

The combination of ZETIA and atorvastatin or simvastatin is indicated for the reduction of elevated total-C and LDL-C levels in patients with HoFH, as an adjunct to other lipid-lowering treatments (e.g., LDL apheresis) or if such treatments are unavailable.

1.3 Homozygous Sitosterolemia

ZETIA is indicated as adjunctive therapy to diet for the reduction of elevated sitosterol and campesterol levels in patients with homozygous familial sitosterolemia.

1.4 Limitations of Use

The effect of ZETIA on cardiovascular morbidity and mortality has not been determined.

ZETIA has not been studied in Fredrickson Type I, III, IV, and V dyslipidemias.

2 DOSAGE AND ADMINISTRATION

2.1 General Dosing Information

The recommended dose of ZETIA is 10 mg once daily.
ZETIA can be administered with or without food.

2.2 Concomitant Lipid-Lowering Therapy

ZETIA may be administered with a statin (in patients with primary hyperlipidemia) or with fenofibrate (in patients with mixed hyperlipidemia) for incremental effect. For convenience, the daily dose of ZETIA may be taken at the same time as the statin or fenofibrate, according to the dosing recommendations for the respective medications.

2.3 Coadministration with Bile Acid Sequestrants

Dosing of ZETIA should occur either ≥2 hours before or ≥4 hours after administration of a bile acid sequestrant *[see Drug Interactions (7.4)]*.

2.4 Patients with Hepatic Impairment

No dosage adjustment is necessary in patients with mild hepatic impairment *[see Warnings and Precautions (5.4)]*.

2.5 Patients with Renal Impairment

No dosage adjustment is necessary in patients with renal impairment *[see Clinical Pharmacology (12.3)]*. When given with simvastatin in patients with moderate to severe renal impairment (estimated glomerular filtration rate <60 mL/min/1.73 m²), doses of simvastatin exceeding 20 mg should be used with caution and close monitoring *[see Use in Specific Populations (8.6)]*.

2.6 Geriatric Patients

No dosage adjustment is necessary in geriatric patients *[see Clinical Pharmacology (12.3)]*.

3 DOSAGE FORMS AND STRENGTHS

10-mg tablets are white to off-white, capsule-shaped tablets debossed with "414" on one side.

4 CONTRAINDICATIONS

ZETIA is contraindicated in the following conditions:

• The combination of ZETIA with a statin is contraindicated in patients with active liver disease or unexplained persistent elevations in hepatic transaminase levels.

• Women who are pregnant or may become pregnant. Because statins decrease cholesterol synthesis and possibly the synthesis of other biologically active substances derived from cholesterol, ZETIA in combination with a statin may cause fetal harm when administered to pregnant women. Additionally, there is no apparent benefit to therapy during pregnancy, and safety in pregnant women has not been established. If the patient becomes pregnant while taking this drug, the patient should be apprised of the potential hazard to the fetus and the lack of known clinical benefit with continued use during pregnancy. *[See Use in Specific Populations (8.1).]*

• Nursing mothers. Because statins may pass into breast milk, and because statins have the potential to cause serious adverse reactions in nursing infants, women who require ZETIA treatment in combination with a statin should be advised not to nurse their infants *[see Use in Specific Populations (8.3)]*.

• Patients with a known hypersensitivity to any component of this product. Hypersensitivity reactions including anaphylaxis, angioedema, rash and urticaria have been reported with ZETIA *[see Adverse Reactions (6.2)]*.

5 WARNINGS AND PRECAUTIONS

5.1 Use with Statins or Fenofibrate

Concurrent administration of ZETIA with a specific statin or fenofibrate should be in accordance with the product labeling for that medication.

5.2 Liver Enzymes

In controlled clinical monotherapy studies, the incidence of consecutive elevations (≥3 × the upper limit of normal [ULN]) in hepatic transaminase levels was similar between ZETIA (0.5%) and placebo (0.3%).

In controlled clinical combination studies of ZETIA initiated concurrently with a statin, the incidence of consecutive elevations (≥3 × ULN) in hepatic transaminase levels was 1.3% for patients treated with ZETIA administered with statins and 0.4% for patients treated with statins alone. These elevations in transaminases were generally asymptomatic, not associated with cholestasis, and returned to baseline after discontinuation of therapy or with continued treatment. When ZETIA is coadministered with a statin, liver tests should be performed at initiation of therapy and according to the recommendations of the statin. Should an increase in ALT or AST ≥3 × ULN persist, consider withdrawal of ZETIA and/or the statin.

5.3 Myopathy/Rhabdomyolysis

In clinical trials, there was no excess of myopathy or rhabdomyolysis associated with ZETIA compared with the relevant control arm (placebo or a statin alone). However, myopathy and rhabdomyolysis are known adverse reactions to statins and other lipid-lowering drugs. In clinical trials, the incidence of creatine phosphokinase (CPK) >10 × ULN was 0.2% for ZETIA vs. 0.1% for placebo, and 0.1% for ZETIA coadministered with a statin vs. 0.4% for statins alone. Risk for skeletal muscle toxicity increases with higher doses of statin, advanced age (>65), hypothyroidism, renal impairment, and depending on the statin used, concomitant use of other drugs.

In post-marketing experience with ZETIA, cases of myopathy and rhabdomyolysis have been reported. Most patients who developed rhabdomyolysis were taking a statin prior to initiating ZETIA. However, rhabdomyolysis has been reported with ZETIA monotherapy and with the addition of ZETIA to agents known to be associated with increased risk of rhabdomyolysis, such as fibrates. ZETIA and any statin or fibrate that the patient is taking concomitantly should be

immediately discontinued if myopathy is diagnosed or suspected. The presence of muscle symptoms and a CPK level >10 × the ULN indicates myopathy.

5.4 Hepatic Impairment

Due to the unknown effects of the increased exposure to ezetimibe in patients with moderate to severe hepatic impairment, ZETIA is not recommended in these patients. *[See Clinical Pharmacology (12.3).]*

6 ADVERSE REACTIONS

The following serious adverse reactions are discussed in greater detail in other sections of the label:

• Liver enzyme abnormalities *[see Warnings and Precautions (5.2)]*

• Rhabdomyolysis and myopathy *[see Warnings and Precautions (5.3)]*

Monotherapy Studies: In the ZETIA controlled clinical trials database (placebo-controlled) of 2396 patients with a median treatment duration of 12 weeks (range 0 to 39 weeks), 3.3% of patients on ZETIA and 2.9% of patients on placebo discontinued due to adverse reactions. The most common adverse reactions in the group of patients treated with ZETIA that led to treatment discontinuation and occurred at a rate greater than placebo were:

• Arthralgia (0.3%)

• Dizziness (0.2%)

• Gamma-glutamyltransferase increased (0.2%)

The most commonly reported adverse reactions (incidence ≥2% and greater than placebo) in the ZETIA monotherapy controlled clinical trial database of 2396 patients were: upper respiratory tract infection (4.3%), diarrhea (4.1%), arthralgia (3.0%), sinusitis (2.8%), and pain in extremity (2.7%).

Statin Coadministration Studies: In the ZETIA + statin controlled clinical trials database of 11,308 patients with a median treatment duration of 8 weeks (range 0 to 112 weeks), 4.0% of patients on ZETIA + statin and 3.3% of patients on statin alone discontinued due to adverse reactions. The most common adverse reactions in the group of patients treated with ZETIA + statin that led to treatment discontinuation and occurred at a rate greater than statin alone were:

• Alanine aminotransferase increased (0.6%)

• Myalgia (0.5%)

• Fatigue, aspartate aminotransferase increased, headache, and pain in extremity (each at 0.2%)

The most commonly reported adverse reactions (incidence ≥2% and greater than statin alone) in the ZETIA + statin controlled clinical trial database of 11,308 patients were: nasopharyngitis (3.7%), myalgia (3.2%), upper respiratory tract infection (2.9%), arthralgia (2.6%) and diarrhea (2.5%).

6.1 Clinical Trials Experience

Because clinical studies are conducted under widely varying conditions, adverse reaction rates observed in the clinical studies of a drug cannot be directly compared to rates in the clinical studies of another drug and may not reflect the rates observed in clinical practice.

Monotherapy

In 10 double-blind, placebo-controlled clinical trials, 2396 patients with primary hyperlipidemia (age range 9–86 years, 50% women, 90% Caucasians, 5% Blacks, 3% Hispanics, 2% Asians) and elevated LDL-C were treated with ZETIA 10 mg/day for a median treatment duration of 12 weeks (range 0 to 39 weeks).

Adverse reactions reported in ≥2% of patients treated with ZETIA and at an incidence greater than placebo in placebo-controlled studies of ZETIA, regardless of causality assessment, are shown in **Table 1**.

TABLE 1: Clinical Adverse Reactions Occurring in ≥2% of Patients Treated with ZETIA and at an Incidence Greater than Placebo, Regardless of Causality

Body System/Organ Class Adverse Reaction	ZETIA 10 mg (%) n = 2396	Placebo (%) n = 1159
Gastrointestinal disorders		
Diarrhea	4.1	3.7
General disorders and administration site conditions		
Fatigue	2.4	1.5
Infections and infestations		
Influenza	2.0	1.5
Sinusitis	2.8	2.2
Upper respiratory tract infection	4.3	2.5
Musculoskeletal and connective tissue disorders		
Arthralgia	3.0	2.2
Pain in extremity	2.7	2.5

The frequency of less common adverse reactions was comparable between ZETIA and placebo.

Combination with a Statin

In 28 double-blind, controlled (placebo or active-controlled) clinical trials, 11,308 patients with primary hyperlipidemia (age range 10–93 years, 48% women, 85% Caucasians, 7% Blacks, 4% Hispanics, 3% Asians) and elevated LDL-C were treated with ZETIA 10 mg/day concurrently with or added to on-going statin therapy for a median treatment duration of 8 weeks (range 0 to 112 weeks).

The incidence of consecutive increased transaminases (≥3 × ULN) was higher in patients receiving ZETIA administered with statins (1.3%) than in patients treated with statins alone (0.4%). *[See Warnings and Precautions (5.2).]*

Clinical adverse reactions reported in ≥2% of patients treated with ZETIA + statin and at an incidence greater than statin, regardless of causality assessment, are shown in **Table 2**.

TABLE 2: Clinical Adverse Reactions Occurring in ≥2% of Patients Treated with ZETIA Coadministered with a Statin and at an Incidence Greater than Statin, Regardless of Causality

Body System/Organ Class Adverse Reaction	All Statins* (%) n = 9361	ZETIA + All Statins* (%) n = 11,308
Gastrointestinal disorders		
Diarrhea	2.2	2.5
General disorders and administration site conditions		
Fatigue	1.6	2.0
Infections and infestations		
Influenza	2.1	2.2
Nasopharyngitis	3.3	3.7
Upper respiratory tract infection	2.8	2.9
Musculoskeletal and connective tissue disorders		
Arthralgia	2.4	2.6
Back pain	2.3	2.4
Myalgia	2.7	3.2
Pain in extremity	1.9	2.1

* All Statins = all doses of all statins

Combination with Fenofibrate

This clinical study involving 625 patients with mixed dyslipidemia (age range 20–76 years, 44% women, 79% Caucasians, 0.1% Blacks, 11% Hispanics, 5% Asians) treated for up to 12 weeks and 576 patients treated for up to an additional 48 weeks evaluated coadministration of ZETIA and fenofibrate. This study was not designed to compare treatment groups for infrequent events. Incidence rates (95% CI) for clinically important elevations (≥3 × ULN, consecutive) in hepatic transaminase levels were 4.5% (1.9, 8.8) and 2.7% (1.2, 5.4) for fenofibrate monotherapy (n=188) and ZETIA coadministered with fenofibrate (n=183), respectively, adjusted for treatment exposure. Corresponding incidence rates for cholecystectomy were 0.6% (95% CI: 0.0%, 3.1%) and 1.7% (95% CI: 0.6%, 4.0%) for fenofibrate monotherapy and ZETIA coadministered with fenofibrate, respectively *[see Drug Interactions (7.3)]*. The numbers of patients exposed to coadministration therapy as well as fenofibrate and ezetimibe monotherapy were inadequate to assess gallbladder disease risk. There were no CPK elevations >10 × ULN in any of the treatment groups.

6.2 Post-Marketing Experience

Because the reactions below are reported voluntarily from a population of uncertain size, it is generally not possible to reliably estimate their frequency or establish a causal relationship to drug exposure.

The following additional adverse reactions have been identified during post-approval use of ZETIA:

Hypersensitivity reactions, including anaphylaxis, angioedema, rash, and urticaria; erythema multiforme; arthralgia; myalgia; elevated creatine phosphokinase; myopathy/ rhabdomyolysis *[see Warnings and Precautions (5.3)]*; elevations in liver transaminases; hepatitis; abdominal pain; thrombocytopenia; pancreatitis; nausea; dizziness; paresthesia; depression; headache; cholelithiasis; cholecystitis.

7 DRUG INTERACTIONS

[See Clinical Pharmacology (12.3).]

7.1 Cyclosporine

Caution should be exercised when using ZETIA and cyclosporine concomitantly due to increased exposure to both ezetimibe and cyclosporine. Cyclosporine concentrations should be monitored in patients receiving ZETIA and cyclosporine.

The degree of increase in ezetimibe exposure may be greater in patients with severe renal insufficiency. In patients

TABLE 3: Mean Percent Difference at Week 6 Between the Pooled ZETIA Coadministered with Simvastatin Group and the Pooled Simvastatin Monotherapy Group in Adolescent Patients with Heterozygous Familial Hypercholesterolemia

	Total-C	LDL-C	Apo B	Non-HDL-C	TG*	HDL-C
Mean percent difference between treatment groups	-12%	-15%	-12%	-14%	-2%	+0.1%
95% Confidence Interval	(-15%, -9%)	(-18%, -12%)	(-15%, -9%)	(-17%, -11%)	(-9%, +4%)	(-3%, +3%)

* For triglycerides, median % change from baseline.

treated with cyclosporine, the potential effects of the increased exposure to ezetimibe from concomitant use should be carefully weighed against the benefits of alterations in lipid levels provided by ezetimibe.

7.2 Fibrates

The efficacy and safety of coadministration of ezetimibe with fibrates other than fenofibrate have not been studied. Fibrates may increase cholesterol excretion into the bile, leading to cholelithiasis. In a preclinical study in dogs, ezetimibe increased cholesterol in the gallbladder bile *[see Nonclinical Toxicology (13.2)]*. Coadministration of ZETIA with fibrates other than fenofibrate is not recommended until use in patients is adequately studied.

7.3 Fenofibrate

If cholelithiasis is suspected in a patient receiving ZETIA and fenofibrate, gallbladder studies are indicated and alternative lipid-lowering therapy should be considered *[see Adverse Reactions (6.1) and the product labeling for fenofibrate]*.

7.4 Cholestyramine

Concomitant cholestyramine administration decreased the mean area under the curve (AUC) of total ezetimibe approximately 55%. The incremental LDL-C reduction due to adding ezetimibe to cholestyramine may be reduced by this interaction.

7.5 Coumarin Anticoagulants

If ezetimibe is added to warfarin, a coumarin anticoagulant, the International Normalized Ratio (INR) should be appropriately monitored.

8 USE IN SPECIFIC POPULATIONS

8.1 Pregnancy

Pregnancy Category C:

There are no adequate and well-controlled studies of ezetimibe in pregnant women. Ezetimibe should be used during pregnancy only if the potential benefit justifies the risk to the fetus.

In oral (gavage) embryo-fetal development studies of ezetimibe conducted in rats and rabbits during organogenesis, there was no evidence of embryolethal effects at the doses tested (250, 500, 1000 mg/kg/day). In rats, increased incidences of common fetal skeletal findings (extra pair of thoracic ribs, unossified cervical vertebral centra, shortened ribs) were observed at 1000 mg/kg/day (~10 × the human exposure at 10 mg daily based on AUC_{0-24hr} for total ezetimibe). In rabbits treated with ezetimibe, an increased incidence of extra thoracic ribs was observed at 1000 mg/kg/day (150 × the human exposure at 10 mg daily based on AUC_{0-24hr} for total ezetimibe). Ezetimibe crossed the placenta when pregnant rats and rabbits were given multiple oral doses.

Multiple-dose studies of ezetimibe given in combination with statins in rats and rabbits during organogenesis result in higher ezetimibe and statin exposures. Reproductive findings occur at lower doses in combination therapy compared to monotherapy.

All statins are contraindicated in pregnant and nursing women. When ZETIA is administered with a statin in a woman of childbearing potential, refer to the pregnancy category and product labeling for the statin. [See Contraindications (4).]

8.3 Nursing Mothers

It is not known whether ezetimibe is excreted into human breast milk. In rat studies, exposure to total ezetimibe in nursing pups was up to half of that observed in maternal plasma. Because many drugs are excreted in human milk, caution should be exercised when ZETIA is administered to a nursing woman. ZETIA should not be used in nursing mothers unless the potential benefit justifies the potential risk to the infant.

8.4 Pediatric Use

The effects of ZETIA coadministered with simvastatin (n=126) compared to simvastatin monotherapy (n=122) have been evaluated in adolescent boys and girls with heterozygous familial hypercholesterolemia (HeFH). In a multicenter, double-blind, controlled study followed by an open-label phase, 142 boys and 106 postmenarchal girls, 10 to 17 years of age (mean age 14.2 years, 43% females, 82% Caucasians, 4% Asian, 2% Blacks, 13% multi-racial) with HeFH were randomized to receive either ZETIA coadministered with simvastatin or simvastatin monotherapy. Inclusion in the study required 1) a baseline LDL-C level

between 160 and 400 mg/dL and 2) a medical history and clinical presentation consistent with HeFH. The mean baseline LDL-C value was 225 mg/dL (range: 161–351 mg/dL) in the ZETIA coadministered with simvastatin group compared to 219 mg/dL (range: 149–336 mg/dL) in the simvastatin monotherapy group. The patients received coadministered ZETIA and simvastatin (10 mg, 20 mg, or 40 mg) or simvastatin monotherapy (10 mg, 20 mg, or 40 mg) for 6 weeks, coadministered ZETIA and 40-mg simvastatin or 40-mg simvastatin monotherapy for the next 27 weeks, and open-label coadministered ZETIA and simvastatin (10 mg, 20 mg, or 40 mg) for 20 weeks thereafter.

The results of the study at Week 6 are summarized in **Table 3**. Results at Week 33 were consistent with those at Week 6. [See table 3 above]

From the start of the trial to the end of Week 33, discontinuations due to an adverse reaction occurred in 7 (6%) patients in the ZETIA coadministered with simvastatin group and in 2 (2%) patients in the simvastatin monotherapy group.

During the trial, hepatic transaminase elevations (two consecutive measurements for ALT and/or AST ≥3 × ULN) occurred in four (3%) individuals in the ZETIA coadministered with simvastatin group and in two (2%) individuals in the simvastatin monotherapy group. Elevations of CPK (≥10 × ULN) occurred in two (2%) individuals in the ZETIA coadministered with simvastatin group and in zero individuals in the simvastatin monotherapy group.

In this limited controlled study, there was no significant effect on growth or sexual maturation in the adolescent boys or girls, or on menstrual cycle length in girls.

Coadministration of ZETIA with simvastatin at doses greater than 40 mg/day has not been studied in adolescents. Also, ZETIA has not been studied in patients younger than 10 years of age or in pre-menarchal girls.

Based on total ezetimibe (ezetimibe + ezetimibe-glucuronide), there are no pharmacokinetic differences between adolescents and adults. Pharmacokinetic data in the pediatric population <10 years of age are not available.

8.5 Geriatric Use

Monotherapy Studies

Of the 2396 patients who received ZETIA in clinical studies, 669 (28%) were 65 and older, and 111 (5%) were 75 and older.

Statin Coadministration Studies

Of the 11,308 patients who received ZETIA + statin in clinical studies, 3587 (32%) were 65 and older, and 924 (8%) were 75 and older.

No overall differences in safety and effectiveness were observed between these patients and younger patients, and other reported clinical experience has not identified differences in responses between the elderly and younger patients, but greater sensitivity of some older individuals cannot be ruled out *[see Clinical Pharmacology (12.3)]*.

8.6 Renal Impairment

When used as monotherapy, no dosage adjustment of ZETIA is necessary.

In the Study of Heart and Renal Protection (SHARP) trial of 9270 patients with moderate to severe renal impairment (6247 non-dialysis patients with median serum creatinine 2.5 mg/dL and median estimated glomerular filtration rate 25.6 mL/min/1.73 m², and 3023 dialysis patients), the incidence of serious adverse events, adverse events leading to discontinuation of study treatment, or adverse events of special interest (musculoskeletal adverse events, liver enzyme abnormalities, incident cancer) was similar between patients ever assigned to ezetimibe 10 mg plus simvastatin 20 mg (n=4650) or placebo (n=4620) during a median follow-up of 4.9 years. However, because renal impairment is a risk factor for statin-associated myopathy, doses of simvastatin exceeding 20 mg should be used with caution and close monitoring when administered concomitantly with ZETIA in patients with moderate to severe renal impairment.

8.7 Hepatic Impairment

ZETIA is not recommended in patients with moderate to severe hepatic impairment *[see Warnings and Precautions (5.4) and Clinical Pharmacology (12.3)]*.

ZETIA given concomitantly with a statin is contraindicated in patients with active liver disease or unexplained persis-

tent elevations of hepatic transaminase levels *[see Contraindications (4); Warnings and Precautions (5.2) and Clinical Pharmacology (12.3)]*.

10 OVERDOSAGE

In clinical studies, administration of ezetimibe, 50 mg/day to 15 healthy subjects for up to 14 days, 40 mg/day to 18 patients with primary hyperlipidemia for up to 56 days, and 40 mg/day to 27 patients with homozygous sitosterolemia for 26 weeks was generally well tolerated. One female patient with homozygous sitosterolemia took an accidental overdose of ezetimibe 120 mg/day for 28 days with no reported clinical or laboratory adverse events.

In the event of an overdose, symptomatic and supportive measures should be employed.

11 DESCRIPTION

ZETIA (ezetimibe) is in a class of lipid-lowering compounds that selectively inhibits the intestinal absorption of cholesterol and related phytosterols. The chemical name of ezetimibe is 1-(4-fluorophenyl)-3(R)-[3-(4-fluorophenyl)-3(S)-hydroxypropyl]-4(S)-(4-hydroxyphenyl)-2-azetidinone. The empirical formula is $C_{24}H_{21}F_2NO_3$. Its molecular weight is 409.4 and its structural formula is:

Ezetimibe is a white, crystalline powder that is freely to very soluble in ethanol, methanol, and acetone and practically insoluble in water. Ezetimibe has a melting point of about 163°C and is stable at ambient temperature. ZETIA is available as a tablet for oral administration containing 10 mg of ezetimibe and the following inactive ingredients: croscarmellose sodium NF, lactose monohydrate NF, magnesium stearate NF, microcrystalline cellulose NF, povidone USP, and sodium lauryl sulfate NF.

12 CLINICAL PHARMACOLOGY

12.1 Mechanism of Action

Ezetimibe reduces blood cholesterol by inhibiting the absorption of cholesterol by the small intestine. In a 2-week clinical study in 18 hypercholesterolemic patients, ZETIA inhibited intestinal cholesterol absorption by 54%, compared with placebo. ZETIA had no clinically meaningful effect on the plasma concentrations of the fat-soluble vitamins A, D, and E (in a study of 113 patients), and did not impair adrenocortical steroid hormone production (in a study of 118 patients).

The cholesterol content of the liver is derived predominantly from three sources. The liver can synthesize cholesterol, take up cholesterol from the blood from circulating lipoproteins, or take up cholesterol absorbed by the small intestine. Intestinal cholesterol is derived primarily from cholesterol secreted in the bile and from dietary cholesterol. Ezetimibe has a mechanism of action that differs from those of other classes of cholesterol-reducing compounds (statins, bile acid sequestrants [resins], fibric acid derivatives, and plant stanols). The molecular target of ezetimibe has been shown to be the sterol transporter, Niemann-Pick C1-Like 1 (NPC1L1), which is involved in the intestinal uptake of cholesterol and phytosterols.

Ezetimibe does not inhibit cholesterol synthesis in the liver, or increase bile acid excretion. Instead, ezetimibe localizes at the brush border of the small intestine and inhibits the absorption of cholesterol, leading to a decrease in the delivery of intestinal cholesterol to the liver. This causes a reduction of hepatic cholesterol stores and an increase in clearance of cholesterol from the blood; this distinct mechanism is complementary to that of statins and of fenofibrate *[see Clinical Studies (14.1)]*.

12.2 Pharmacodynamics

Clinical studies have demonstrated that elevated levels of total-C, LDL-C and Apo B, the major protein constituent of LDL, promote human atherosclerosis. In addition, decreased levels of HDL-C are associated with the development of atherosclerosis. Epidemiologic studies have established that cardiovascular morbidity and mortality vary directly with the level of total-C and LDL-C and inversely with the level of HDL-C. Like LDL, cholesterol-enriched triglyceride-rich lipoproteins, including very-low-density lipoproteins (VLDL), intermediate-density lipoproteins (IDL), and remnants, can also promote atherosclerosis. The independent effect of raising HDL-C or lowering TG on the risk of coronary and cardiovascular morbidity and mortality has not been determined.

ZETIA reduces total-C, LDL-C, Apo B, non-HDL-C, and TG, and increases HDL-C in patients with hyperlipidemia. Administration of ZETIA with a statin is effective in improving serum total-C, LDL-C, Apo B, non-HDL-C, TG, and HDL-C beyond either treatment alone. Administration of ZETIA with fenofibrate is effective in improving serum total-C, LDL-C, Apo B, and non-HDL-C in patients with mixed hyperlipidemia as compared to either treatment alone. The effects of ezetimibe given either alone or in addition to a statin or fenofibrate on cardiovascular morbidity and mortality have not been established.

12.3 Pharmacokinetics

Absorption

After oral administration, ezetimibe is absorbed and extensively conjugated to a pharmacologically active phenolic glucuronide (ezetimibe-glucuronide). After a single 10-mg dose of ZETIA to fasted adults, mean ezetimibe peak plasma concentrations (C_{max}) of 3.4 to 5.5 ng/mL were attained within 4 to 12 hours (T_{max}). Ezetimibe-glucuronide mean C_{max} values of 45 to 71 ng/mL were achieved between 1 and 2 hours (T_{max}). There was no substantial deviation from dose proportionality between 5 and 20 mg. The absolute bioavailability of ezetimibe cannot be determined, as the compound is virtually insoluble in aqueous media suitable for injection.

Effect of Food on Oral Absorption

Concomitant food administration (high-fat or non-fat meals) had no effect on the extent of absorption of ezetimibe when administered as ZETIA 10-mg tablets. The C_{max} value of ezetimibe was increased by 38% with consumption of high-fat meals. ZETIA can be administered with or without food.

Distribution

Ezetimibe and ezetimibe-glucuronide are highly bound (>90%) to human plasma proteins.

Metabolism and Excretion

Ezetimibe is primarily metabolized in the small intestine and liver via glucuronide conjugation (a phase II reaction) with subsequent biliary and renal excretion. Minimal oxidative metabolism (a phase I reaction) has been observed in all species evaluated.

In humans, ezetimibe is rapidly metabolized to ezetimibe-glucuronide. Ezetimibe and ezetimibe-glucuronide are the major drug-derived compounds detected in plasma, constituting approximately 10 to 20% and 80 to 90% of the total drug in plasma, respectively. Both ezetimibe and ezetimibe-glucuronide are eliminated from plasma with a half-life of approximately 22 hours for both ezetimibe and ezetimibe-glucuronide. Plasma concentration-time profiles exhibit multiple peaks, suggesting enterohepatic recycling.

Following oral administration of ^{14}C-ezetimibe (20 mg) to human subjects, total ezetimibe (ezetimibe + ezetimibe-glucuronide) accounted for approximately 93% of the total radioactivity in plasma. After 48 hours, there were no detectable levels of radioactivity in the plasma.

Approximately 78% and 11% of the administered radioactivity were recovered in the feces and urine, respectively, over a 10-day collection period. Ezetimibe was the major component in feces and accounted for 69% of the administered dose, while ezetimibe-glucuronide was the major component in urine and accounted for 9% of the administered dose.

Specific Populations

Geriatric Patients: In a multiple-dose study with ezetimibe given 10 mg once daily for 10 days, plasma concentrations for total ezetimibe were about 2-fold higher in older (≥65 years) healthy subjects compared to younger subjects.

Pediatric Patients: *[See Use in Specific Populations (8.4).]*

Gender: In a multiple-dose study with ezetimibe given 10 mg once daily for 10 days, plasma concentrations for total ezetimibe were slightly higher (<20%) in women than in men.

Race: Based on a meta-analysis of multiple-dose pharmacokinetic studies, there were no pharmacokinetic differences between Black and Caucasian subjects. Studies in Asian subjects indicated that the pharmacokinetics of ezetimibe were similar to those seen in Caucasian subjects.

Hepatic Impairment: After a single 10-mg dose of ezetimibe, the mean AUC for total ezetimibe was increased approximately 1.7-fold in patients with mild hepatic impairment (Child-Pugh score 5 to 6), compared to healthy subjects. The mean AUC values for total ezetimibe and ezetimibe were increased approximately 3- to 4-fold and 5- to 6-fold, respectively, in patients with moderate (Child-Pugh score 7 to 9) or severe hepatic impairment (Child-Pugh score 10 to 15). In a 14-day, multiple-dose study (10 mg daily) in patients with moderate hepatic impairment, the mean AUC values for total ezetimibe and ezetimibe were increased approximately 4-fold on Day 1 and Day 14 compared to healthy subjects. Due to the unknown effects of the increased exposure to ezetimibe in patients with moderate or severe hepatic impairment, ZETIA is not recommended in these patients *[see Warnings and Precautions (5.4)].*

Renal Impairment: After a single 10-mg dose of ezetimibe in patients with severe renal disease (n=8; mean CrCl ≤30 mL/min/1.73 m²), the mean AUC values for total

ezetimibe, ezetimibe-glucuronide, and ezetimibe were increased approximately 1.5-fold, compared to healthy subjects (n=9).

Drug Interactions [See also Drug Interactions (7)]

ZETIA had no significant effect on a series of probe drugs (caffeine, dextromethorphan, tolbutamide, and IV midazolam) known to be metabolized by cytochrome P450 (1A2, 2D6, 2C8/9 and 3A4) in a "cocktail" study of twelve healthy adult males. This indicates that ezetimibe is neither an inhibitor nor an inducer of these cytochrome P450 isozymes, and it is unlikely that ezetimibe will affect the metabolism of drugs that are metabolized by these enzymes.

TABLE 4: Effect of Coadministered Drugs on Total Ezetimibe

Coadministered Drug and Dosing Regimen	Total Ezetimibe *	
	Change in AUC	Change in C_{max}
Cyclosporine-stable dose required (75–150 mg BID)[†,‡]	↑240%	↑290%
Fenofibrate, 200 mg QD, 14 days[‡]	↑48%	↑64%
Gemfibrozil, 600 mg BID, 7 days[‡]	↑64%	↑91%
Cholestyramine, 4 g BID, 14 days[‡]	↓55%	↓4%
Aluminum & magnesium hydroxide combination antacid, single dose[§]	↓4%	↓30%
Cimetidine, 400 mg BID, 7 days	↑6%	↑22%
Glipizide, 10 mg, single dose	↑4%	↓8%
Statins		
Lovastatin 20 mg QD, 7 days	↓9%	↑3%
Pravastatin 20 mg QD, 14 days	↑7%	↑23%
Atorvastatin 10 mg QD, 14 days	↓2%	↑12%
Rosuvastatin 10 mg QD, 14 days	↑13%	↑18%
Fluvastatin 20 mg QD, 14 days	↓19%	↑7%

* Based on 10-mg dose of ezetimibe.
† Post-renal transplant patients with mild impaired or normal renal function. In a different study, a renal transplant patient with severe renal insufficiency (creatinine clearance of 13.2 mL/min/1.73 m²) who was receiving multiple medications, including cyclosporine, demonstrated a 12-fold greater exposure to total ezetimibe compared to healthy subjects.
‡ See Drug Interactions (7).
§ Supralox, 20 mL.

[See table 5 above]

13 NONCLINICAL TOXICOLOGY

13.1 Carcinogenesis, Mutagenesis, Impairment of Fertility

A 104-week dietary carcinogenicity study with ezetimibe was conducted in rats at doses up to 1500 mg/kg/day (males) and 500 mg/kg/day (females) (~20 × the human exposure at 10 mg daily based on AUC_{0-24hr} for total ezetimibe). A 104-week dietary carcinogenicity study with ezetimibe was also conducted in mice at doses up to 500 mg/kg/day (>150 × the human exposure at 10 mg daily based on AUC_{0-24hr} for total ezetimibe). There were no statistically significant increases in tumor incidences in drug-treated rats or mice.

No evidence of mutagenicity was observed *in vitro* in a microbial mutagenicity (Ames) test with *Salmonella typhimurium* and *Escherichia coli* with or without metabolic activation. No evidence of clastogenicity was observed *in vitro* in a chromosomal aberration assay in human peripheral blood lymphocytes with or without metabolic activation. In addition, there was no evidence of genotoxicity in the *in vivo* mouse micronucleus test.

In oral (gavage) fertility studies of ezetimibe conducted in rats, there was no evidence of reproductive toxicity at doses

TABLE 5: Effect of Ezetimibe Coadministration on Systemic Exposure to Other Drugs

Coadministered Drug and its Dosage Regimen	Ezetimibe Dosage Regimen	Change in AUC of Coadministered Drug	Change in C_{max} of Coadministered Drug
Warfarin, 25-mg single dose on Day 7	10 mg QD, 11 days	↓2% (R-warfarin) ↓4% (S-warfarin)	↑3% (R-warfarin) ↑1% (S-warfarin)
Digoxin, 0.5-mg single dose	10 mg QD, 8 days	↑2%	↓7%
Gemfibrozil, 600 mg BID, 7 days*	10 mg QD, 7 days	↓1%	↓11%
Ethinyl estradiol & Levonorgestrel, QD, 21 days	10 mg QD, days 8–14 of 21d oral contraceptive cycle	Ethinyl estradiol 0% Levonorgestrel 0%	Ethinyl estradiol ↓9% Levonorgestrel ↓5%
Glipizide, 10 mg on Days 1 and 9	10 mg QD, days 2–9	↓3%	↓5%
Fenofibrate, 200 mg QD, 14 days*	10 mg QD, 14 days	↑11%	↑7%
Cyclosporine, 100-mg single dose Day 7*	20 mg QD, 8 days	↑15%	↑10%
Statins			
Lovastatin 20 mg QD, 7 days	10 mg QD, 7 days	↑19%	↑3%
Pravastatin 20 mg QD, 14 days	10 mg QD, 14 days	↓20%	↓24%
Atorvastatin 10 mg QD, 14 days	10 mg QD, 14 days	↓4%	↑7%
Rosuvastatin 10 mg QD, 14 days	10 mg QD, 14 days	↑19%	↑17%
Fluvastatin 20 mg QD, 14 days	10 mg QD, 14 days	↓39%	↓27%

* See Drug Interactions (7).

TABLE 6: Response to ZETIA in Patients with Primary Hyperlipidemia (Mean* % Change from Untreated Baseline[†])

Treatment Group		N	Total-C	LDL-C	Apo B	Non-HDL-C	TG*	HDL-C
Study 1[‡]	Placebo	205	+1	+1	-1	+1	-1	-1
	Ezetimibe	622	-12	-18	-15	-16	-7	+1
Study 2[‡]	Placebo	226	+1	+1	-1	+2	+2	-2
	Ezetimibe	666	-12	-18	-16	-16	-9	+1
Pooled Data[‡] (Studies 1 & 2)	Placebo	431	0	+1	-2	+1	0	-2
	Ezetimibe	1288	-13	-18	-16	-16	-8	+1

* For triglycerides, median % change from baseline.
† Baseline - on no lipid-lowering drug.
‡ ZETIA significantly reduced total-C, LDL-C, Apo B, non-HDL-C, and TG, and increased HDL-C compared to placebo.

TABLE 7: Response to Addition of ZETIA to On-Going Statin Therapy* in Patients with Hyperlipidemia (Mean[†] % Change from Treated Baseline[‡])

Treatment (Daily Dose)	N	Total-C	LDL-C	Apo B	Non-HDL-C	TG[†]	HDL-C
On-going Statin + Placebo[§]	390	-2	-4	-3	-3	-3	+1
On-going Statin + ZETIA[§]	379	-17	-25	-19	-23	-14	+3

* Patients receiving each statin: 40% atorvastatin, 31% simvastatin, 29% others (pravastatin, fluvastatin, cerivastatin, lovastatin).
† For triglycerides, median % change from baseline.
‡ Baseline - on a statin alone.
§ ZETIA + statin significantly reduced total-C, LDL-C, Apo B, non-HDL-C, and TG, and increased HDL-C compared to statin alone.

TABLE 8: Response to ZETIA and Atorvastatin Initiated Concurrently in Patients with Primary Hyperlipidemia (Mean* % Change from Untreated Baseline[†])

Treatment (Daily Dose)	N	Total-C	LDL-C	Apo B	Non-HDL-C	TG*	HDL-C
Placebo	60	+4	+4	+3	+4	-6	+4
ZETIA	65	-14	-20	-15	-18	-5	+4
Atorvastatin 10 mg	60	-26	-37	-28	-34	-21	+6
ZETIA + Atorvastatin 10 mg	65	-38	-53	-43	-49	-31	+9
Atorvastatin 20 mg	60	-30	-42	-34	-39	-23	+4
ZETIA + Atorvastatin 20 mg	62	-39	-54	-44	-50	-30	+9
Atorvastatin 40 mg	66	-32	-45	-37	-41	-24	+4
ZETIA + Atorvastatin 40 mg	65	-42	-56	-45	-52	-34	+5
Atorvastatin 80 mg	62	-40	-54	-46	-51	-31	+3
ZETIA + Atorvastatin 80 mg	63	-46	-61	-50	-58	-40	+7
Pooled data (All Atorvastatin Doses)[‡]	248	-32	-44	-36	-41	-24	+4
Pooled data (All ZETIA + Atorvastatin Doses)[‡]	255	-41	-56	-45	-52	-33	+7

* For triglycerides, median % change from baseline.
† Baseline - on no lipid-lowering drug.
‡ ZETIA + all doses of atorvastatin pooled (10–80 mg) significantly reduced total-C, LDL-C, Apo B, non-HDL-C, and TG, and increased HDL-C compared to all doses of atorvastatin pooled (10–80 mg).

up to 1000 mg/kg/day in male or female rats (~7 × the human exposure at 10 mg daily based on AUC_{0-24hr} for total ezetimibe).

13.2   Animal Toxicology and/or Pharmacology
The hypocholesterolemic effect of ezetimibe was evaluated in cholesterol-fed Rhesus monkeys, dogs, rats, and mouse models of human cholesterol metabolism. Ezetimibe was found to have an ED_{50} value of 0.5 µg/kg/day for inhibiting the rise in plasma cholesterol levels in monkeys. The ED_{50} values in dogs, rats, and mice were 7, 30, and 700 µg/kg/day, respectively. These results are consistent with ZETIA being a potent cholesterol absorption inhibitor.

In a rat model, where the glucuronide metabolite of ezetimibe (SCH 60663) was administered intraduodenally, the metabolite was as potent as the parent compound (SCH 58235) in inhibiting the absorption of cholesterol, suggesting that the glucuronide metabolite had activity similar to the parent drug.
In 1-month studies in dogs given ezetimibe (0.03 to 300 mg/kg/day), the concentration of cholesterol in gallbladder bile increased ~2- to 4-fold. However, a dose of 300 mg/kg/day administered to dogs for one year did not result in gallstone formation or any other adverse hepatobiliary effects. In a 14-day study in mice given ezetimibe (0.3 to

5 mg/kg/day) and fed a low-fat or cholesterol-rich diet, the concentration of cholesterol in gallbladder bile was either unaffected or reduced to normal levels, respectively.
A series of acute preclinical studies was performed to determine the selectivity of ZETIA for inhibiting cholesterol absorption. Ezetimibe inhibited the absorption of ^{14}C-cholesterol with no effect on the absorption of triglycerides, fatty acids, bile acids, progesterone, ethinyl estradiol, or the fat-soluble vitamins A and D.
In 4- to 12-week toxicity studies in mice, ezetimibe did not induce cytochrome P450 drug metabolizing enzymes. In toxicity studies, a pharmacokinetic interaction of ezetimibe with statins (parents or their active hydroxy acid metabolites) was seen in rats, dogs, and rabbits.

14   CLINICAL STUDIES
14.1   Primary Hyperlipidemia
ZETIA reduces total-C, LDL-C, Apo B, non-HDL-C, and TG, and increases HDL-C in patients with hyperlipidemia. Maximal to near maximal response is generally achieved within 2 weeks and maintained during chronic therapy.
Monotherapy
In two multicenter, double-blind, placebo-controlled, 12-week studies in 1719 patients with primary hyperlipidemia, ZETIA significantly lowered total-C, LDL-C, Apo B, non-HDL-C, and TG, and increased HDL-C compared to placebo (see **Table 6**). Reduction in LDL-C was consistent across age, sex, and baseline LDL-C.
[See table 6 above]
Combination with Statins
ZETIA Added to On-going Statin Therapy
In a multicenter, double-blind, placebo-controlled, 8-week study, 769 patients with primary hyperlipidemia, known coronary heart disease or multiple cardiovascular risk factors who were already receiving statin monotherapy, but who had not met their NCEP ATP II target LDL-C goal were randomized to receive either ZETIA or placebo in addition to their on-going statin.
ZETIA, added to on-going statin therapy, significantly lowered total-C, LDL-C, Apo B, non-HDL-C, and TG, and increased HDL-C compared with a statin administered alone (see **Table 7**). LDL-C reductions induced by ZETIA were generally consistent across all statins.
[See table 7 above]
ZETIA Initiated Concurrently with a Statin
In four multicenter, double-blind, placebo-controlled, 12-week trials, in 2382 hyperlipidemic patients, ZETIA or placebo was administered alone or with various doses of atorvastatin, simvastatin, pravastatin, or lovastatin.
When all patients receiving ZETIA with a statin were compared to all those receiving the corresponding statin alone, ZETIA significantly lowered total-C, LDL-C, Apo B, non-HDL-C, and TG, and, with the exception of pravastatin, increased HDL-C compared to the statin administered alone. LDL-C reductions induced by ZETIA were generally consistent across all statins. (See footnote [‡], **Tables 8 to 11**.)
[See table 8 above]
[See table 9 at top of next page]
[See table 10 at top of next page]
[See table 11 at top of page 1762]
Combination with Fenofibrate
In a multicenter, double-blind, placebo-controlled, clinical study in patients with mixed hyperlipidemia, 625 patients were treated for up to 12 weeks and 576 for up to an additional 48 weeks. Patients were randomized to receive placebo, ZETIA alone, 160-mg fenofibrate alone, or ZETIA and 160-mg fenofibrate in the 12-week study. After completing the 12-week study, eligible patients were assigned to ZETIA coadministered with fenofibrate or fenofibrate monotherapy for an additional 48 weeks.
ZETIA coadministered with fenofibrate significantly lowered total-C, LDL-C, Apo B, and non-HDL-C compared to fenofibrate administered alone. The percent decrease in TG and percent increase in HDL-C for ZETIA coadministered with fenofibrate were comparable to those for fenofibrate administered alone (see **Table 12**).
[See table 12 at top of page 1762]
The changes in lipid endpoints after an additional 48 weeks of treatment with ZETIA coadministered with fenofibrate or with fenofibrate alone were consistent with the 12-week data displayed above.
14.2   Homozygous   Familial   Hypercholesterolemia (HoFH)
A study was conducted to assess the efficacy of ZETIA in the treatment of HoFH. This double-blind, randomized, 12-week study enrolled 50 patients with a clinical and/or genotypic diagnosis of HoFH, with or without concomitant LDL apheresis, already receiving atorvastatin or simvastatin (40 mg). Patients were randomized to one of three treatment groups, atorvastatin or simvastatin (80 mg), ZETIA administered with atorvastatin or simvastatin (40 mg) or ZETIA administered with atorvastatin or simvastatin (80 mg). Due to decreased bioavailability of ezetimibe in patients concomitantly receiving cholestyramine [*see Drug In-*

teractions (7.4)], ezetimibe was dosed at least 4 hours before or after administration of resins. Mean baseline LDL-C was 341 mg/dL in those patients randomized to atorvastatin 80 mg or simvastatin 80 mg alone and 316 mg/dL in the group randomized to ZETIA plus atorvastatin 40 or 80 mg or simvastatin 40 or 80 mg. ZETIA, administered with atorvastatin or simvastatin (40- and 80-mg statin groups, pooled), significantly reduced LDL-C (21%) compared with increasing the dose of simvastatin or atorvastatin monotherapy from 40 to 80 mg (7%). In those treated with ZETIA plus 80-mg atorvastatin or with ZETIA plus 80-mg simvastatin, LDL-C was reduced by 27%.

14.3 Homozygous Sitosterolemia (Phytosterolemia)

A study was conducted to assess the efficacy of ZETIA in the treatment of homozygous sitosterolemia. In this multicenter, double-blind, placebo-controlled, 8-week trial, 37 patients with homozygous sitosterolemia with elevated plasma sitosterol levels (>5 mg/dL) on their current therapeutic regimen (diet, bile-acid-binding resins, statins, ileal bypass surgery and/or LDL apheresis), were randomized to receive ZETIA (n=30) or placebo (n=7). Due to decreased bioavailability of ezetimibe in patients concomitantly receiving cholestyramine *[see Drug Interactions (7.4)]*, ezetimibe was dosed at least 2 hours before or 4 hours after resins were administered. Excluding the one subject receiving LDL apheresis, ZETIA significantly lowered plasma sitosterol and campesterol, by 21% and 24% from baseline, respectively. In contrast, patients who received placebo had increases in sitosterol and campesterol of 4% and 3% from baseline, respectively. For patients treated with ZETIA, mean plasma levels of plant sterols were reduced progressively over the course of the study. The effects of reducing plasma sitosterol and campesterol on reducing the risks of cardiovascular morbidity and mortality have not been established.

Reductions in sitosterol and campesterol were consistent between patients taking ZETIA concomitantly with bile acid sequestrants (n=8) and patients not on concomitant bile acid sequestrant therapy (n=21).

Limitations of Use

The effect of ZETIA on cardiovascular morbidity and mortality has not been determined.

16 HOW SUPPLIED/STORAGE AND HANDLING

No. 3861 — Tablets ZETIA, 10 mg, are white to off-white, capsule-shaped tablets debossed with "414" on one side. They are supplied as follows:

NDC 66582-414-31 bottles of 30
NDC 66582-414-54 bottles of 90
NDC 66582-414-74 bottles of 500
NDC 66582-414-76 bottles of 5000
NDC 66582-414-28 unit dose packages of 100.

Storage

Store at 25°C (77°F); excursions permitted to 15–30°C (59–86°F). [See USP Controlled Room Temperature.] Protect from moisture.

17 PATIENT COUNSELING INFORMATION

See FDA-Approved Patient Labeling (Patient Information). Patients should be advised to adhere to their National Cholesterol Education Program (NCEP)-recommended diet, a regular exercise program, and periodic testing of a fasting lipid panel.

17.1 Muscle Pain

All patients starting therapy with ezetimibe should be advised of the risk of myopathy and told to report promptly any unexplained muscle pain, tenderness or weakness. The risk of this occurring is increased when taking certain types of medication. Patients should discuss all medication, both prescription and over-the-counter, with their physician.

17.2 Liver Enzymes

Liver tests should be performed when ZETIA is added to statin therapy and according to statin recommendations.

17.3 Pregnancy

Women of childbearing age should be advised to use an effective method of birth control to prevent pregnancy while using ZETIA added to statin therapy. Discuss future pregnancy plans with your patients, and discuss when to stop combination ZETIA and statin therapy if they are trying to conceive. Patients should be advised that if they become pregnant they should stop taking combination ZETIA and statin therapy and call their healthcare professional.

17.4 Breastfeeding

Women who are breastfeeding should be advised to not use ZETIA added to statin therapy. Patients who have a lipid disorder and are breastfeeding should be advised to discuss the options with their healthcare professionals.

Merck Sharp & Dohme Corp., a subsidiary of **MERCK & CO., INC.**, Whitehouse Station, NJ 08889, USA
For patent information:
www.merck.com/product/patent/home.html
Copyright © 2001-2012 MSD International GmbH, a subsidiary of **Merck & Co., Inc.**

TABLE 9: Response to ZETIA and Simvastatin Initiated Concurrently in Patients with Primary Hyperlipidemia (Mean* % Change from Untreated Baseline†)

Treatment (Daily Dose)	N	Total-C	LDL-C	Apo B	Non-HDL-C	TG*	HDL-C
Placebo	70	-1	-1	0	-1	+2	+1
ZETIA	61	-13	-19	-14	-17	-11	+5
Simvastatin 10 mg	70	-18	-27	-21	-25	-14	+8
ZETIA + Simvastatin 10 mg	67	-32	-46	-35	-42	-26	+9
Simvastatin 20 mg	61	-26	-36	-29	-33	-18	+6
ZETIA + Simvastatin 20 mg	69	-33	-46	-36	-42	-25	+9
Simvastatin 40 mg	65	-27	-38	-32	-35	-24	+6
ZETIA + Simvastatin 40 mg	73	-40	-56	-45	-51	-32	+11
Simvastatin 80 mg	67	-32	-45	-37	-41	-23	+8
ZETIA + Simvastatin 80 mg	65	-41	-58	-47	-53	-31	+8
Pooled data (All Simvastatin Doses)‡	263	-26	-36	-30	-34	-20	+7
Pooled data (All ZETIA + Simvastatin Doses)‡	274	-37	-51	-41	-47	-29	+9

* For triglycerides, median % change from baseline.
† Baseline - on no lipid-lowering drug.
‡ ZETIA + all doses of simvastatin pooled (10–80 mg) significantly reduced total-C, LDL-C, Apo B, non-HDL-C, and TG, and increased HDL-C compared to all doses of simvastatin pooled (10–80 mg).

TABLE 10: Response to ZETIA and Pravastatin Initiated Concurrently in Patients with Primary Hyperlipidemia (Mean* % Change from Untreated Baseline†)

Treatment (Daily Dose)	N	Total-C	LDL-C	Apo B	Non-HDL-C	TG*	HDL-C
Placebo	65	0	-1	-2	0	-1	+2
ZETIA	64	-13	-20	-15	-17	-5	+4
Pravastatin 10 mg	66	-15	-21	-16	-20	-14	+6
ZETIA + Pravastatin 10 mg	71	-24	-34	-27	-32	-23	+8
Pravastatin 20 mg	69	-15	-23	-18	-20	-8	+8
ZETIA + Pravastatin 20 mg	66	-27	-40	-31	-36	-21	+8
Pravastatin 40 mg	70	-22	-31	-26	-28	-19	+6
ZETIA + Pravastatin 40 mg	67	-30	-42	-32	-39	-21	+8
Pooled data (All Pravastatin Doses)‡	205	-17	-25	-20	-23	-14	+7
Pooled data (All ZETIA + Pravastatin Doses)‡	204	-27	-39	-30	-36	-21	+8

* For triglycerides, median % change from baseline.
† Baseline - on no lipid-lowering drug.
‡ ZETIA + all doses of pravastatin pooled (10–40 mg) significantly reduced total-C, LDL-C, Apo B, non-HDL-C, and TG compared to all doses of pravastatin pooled (10–40 mg).

All rights reserved.
uspi-mk0653-t-1308r026

ZETIA® (ezetimibe) Tablets
Patient Information about ZETIA (zĕt´-ē-ă)
Generic name: ezetimibe (ĕ-zĕt´-ĕ-mĭb)
Read this information carefully before you start taking ZETIA® and each time you get more ZETIA. There may be new information. This information does not take the place of talking with your doctor about your medical condition or your treatment. If you have any questions about ZETIA, ask your doctor. Only your doctor can determine if ZETIA is right for you.

What is ZETIA?
ZETIA is a medicine used to lower levels of total cholesterol and LDL (bad) cholesterol in the blood. ZETIA is for patients who cannot control their cholesterol levels by diet and exercise alone. It can be used by itself or with other medicines to treat high cholesterol. You should stay on a cholesterol-lowering diet while taking this medicine.
ZETIA works to reduce the amount of cholesterol your body absorbs. ZETIA does not help you lose weight. ZETIA has not been shown to prevent heart disease or heart attacks.

For more information about cholesterol, see the "What should I know about high cholesterol?" section that follows.

Who should not take ZETIA?
• Do not take ZETIA if you are allergic to ezetimibe, the active ingredient in ZETIA, or to the inactive ingredients. For a list of inactive ingredients, see the "Inactive ingredients" section that follows.
• If you have active liver disease, do not take ZETIA while taking cholesterol-lowering medicines called statins.
• If you are pregnant or breastfeeding, do not take ZETIA while taking a statin.
• If you are a woman of childbearing age, you should use an effective method of birth control to prevent pregnancy while using ZETIA added to statin therapy.
ZETIA has not been studied in children under age 10.

What should I tell my doctor before and while taking ZETIA?
Tell your doctor about any prescription and nonprescription medicines you are taking or plan to take, including natural or herbal remedies.
Tell your doctor about all your medical conditions including allergies.

TABLE 11: Response to ZETIA and Lovastatin Initiated Concurrently in Patients with Primary Hyperlipidemia (Mean* % Change from Untreated Baseline[†])

Treatment (Daily Dose)	N	Total-C	LDL-C	Apo B	Non-HDL-C	TG*	HDL-C
Placebo	64	+1	0	+1	+1	+6	0
ZETIA	72	-13	-19	-14	-16	-5	+3
Lovastatin 10 mg	73	-15	-20	-17	-19	-11	+5
ZETIA + Lovastatin 10 mg	65	-24	-34	-27	-31	-19	+8
Lovastatin 20 mg	74	-19	-26	-21	-24	-12	+3
ZETIA + Lovastatin 20 mg	62	-29	-41	-34	-39	-27	+9
Lovastatin 40 mg	73	-21	-30	-25	-27	-15	+5
ZETIA + Lovastatin 40 mg	65	-33	-46	-38	-43	-27	+9
Pooled data (All Lovastatin Doses)[‡]	220	-18	-25	-21	-23	-12	+4
Pooled data (All ZETIA + Lovastatin Doses)[‡]	192	-29	-40	-33	-38	-25	+9

* For triglycerides, median % change from baseline.
† Baseline - on no lipid-lowering drug.
‡ ZETIA + all doses of lovastatin pooled (10–40 mg) significantly reduced total-C, LDL-C, Apo B, non-HDL-C, and TG, and increased HDL-C compared to all doses of lovastatin pooled (10–40 mg).

TABLE 12: Response to ZETIA and Fenofibrate Initiated Concurrently in Patients with Mixed Hyperlipidemia (Mean* % Change from Untreated Baseline[†] at 12 weeks)

Treatment (Daily Dose)	N	Total-C	LDL-C	Apo B	TG*	HDL-C	Non-HDL-C
Placebo	63	0	0	-1	-9	+3	0
ZETIA	185	-12	-13	-11	-11	+4	-15
Fenofibrate 160 mg	188	-11	-6	-15	-43	+19	-16
ZETIA + Fenofibrate 160 mg	183	-22	-20	-26	-44	+19	-30

* For triglycerides, median % change from baseline.
† Baseline - on no lipid-lowering drug.

Tell your doctor if you:
• ever had liver problems. ZETIA may not be right for you.
• are pregnant or plan to become pregnant. Your doctor will discuss with you whether ZETIA is right for you.
• are breastfeeding. We do not know if ZETIA can pass to your baby through your milk. Your doctor will discuss with you whether ZETIA is right for you.
• experience unexplained muscle pain, tenderness, or weakness.

How should I take ZETIA?
• Take ZETIA once a day, with or without food. It may be easier to remember to take your dose if you do it at the same time every day, such as with breakfast, dinner, or at bedtime. If you also take another medicine to reduce your cholesterol, ask your doctor if you can take them at the same time.
• If you forget to take ZETIA, take it as soon as you remember. However, do not take more than one dose of ZETIA a day.
• Continue to follow a cholesterol-lowering diet while taking ZETIA. Ask your doctor if you need diet information.
• Keep taking ZETIA unless your doctor tells you to stop. It is important that you keep taking ZETIA even if you do not feel sick.
See your doctor regularly to check your cholesterol level and to check for side effects. Your doctor may do blood tests to check your liver before you start taking ZETIA with a statin and during treatment.

What are the possible side effects of ZETIA?
In clinical studies patients reported few side effects while taking ZETIA. These included diarrhea, joint pains, and feeling tired.
Patients have experienced severe muscle problems while taking ZETIA, usually when ZETIA was added to a statin drug. If you experience unexplained muscle pain, tenderness, or weakness while taking ZETIA, contact your doctor immediately. You need to do this promptly, because on rare occasions, these muscle problems can be serious, with muscle breakdown resulting in kidney damage.
Additionally, the following side effects have been reported in general use: allergic reactions (which may require treatment right away) including swelling of the face, lips, tongue,

and/or throat that may cause difficulty in breathing or swallowing, rash, and hives; raised red rash, sometimes with target-shaped lesions; joint pain; muscle aches; alterations in some laboratory blood tests; liver problems; stomach pain; inflammation of the pancreas; nausea; dizziness; tingling sensation; depression; headache; gallstones; inflammation of the gallbladder.
Tell your doctor if you are having these or any other medical problems while on ZETIA. For a complete list of side effects, ask your doctor or pharmacist.

What should I know about high cholesterol?
Cholesterol is a type of fat found in your blood. Your total cholesterol is made up of LDL and HDL cholesterol.
LDL cholesterol is called "bad" cholesterol because it can build up in the wall of your arteries and form plaque. Over time, plaque build-up can cause a narrowing of the arteries. This narrowing can slow or block blood flow to your heart, brain, and other organs. High LDL cholesterol is a major cause of heart disease and one of the causes for stroke.
HDL cholesterol is called "good" cholesterol because it keeps the bad cholesterol from building up in the arteries.
Triglycerides also are fats found in your blood.

General information about ZETIA
Medicines are sometimes prescribed for conditions that are not mentioned in patient information leaflets. Do not use ZETIA for a condition for which it was not prescribed. Do not give ZETIA to other people, even if they have the same condition you have. It may harm them.
This summarizes the most important information about ZETIA. If you would like more information, talk with your doctor. You can ask your pharmacist or doctor for information about ZETIA that is written for health professionals.

Inactive ingredients:
Croscarmellose sodium, lactose monohydrate, magnesium stearate, microcrystalline cellulose, povidone, and sodium lauryl sulfate.
Merck Sharp & Dohme Corp., a subsidiary of
MERCK & CO., INC., Whitehouse Station, NJ 08889, USA
For patent information:
www.merck.com/product/patent/home.html
Copyright © 2001-2012 MSD International GmbH, a subsidiary of **Merck & Co., Inc.**
All rights reserved.

Revised: 08/2013
usppi-mk0653-t-1308r026
Shown in Product Identification Guide, page 309

ZIOPTAN™   ℞
(tafluprost ophthalmic solution)
0.0015%

HIGHLIGHTS OF PRESCRIBING INFORMATION
These highlights do not include all the information needed to use ZIOPTAN (tafluprost ophthalmic solution) 0.0015% safely and effectively. See full prescribing information for ZIOPTAN.
ZIOPTAN™ (tafluprost ophthalmic solution) 0.0015%
Initial U.S. Approval: 2012

───INDICATIONS AND USAGE───
• ZIOPTAN (tafluprost ophthalmic solution) 0.0015% is a prostaglandin analog indicated for reducing elevated intraocular pressure in patients with open-angle glaucoma or ocular hypertension. (1)

───DOSAGE AND ADMINISTRATION───
• One drop in the affected eye(s) once daily in the evening. (2)

───DOSAGE FORMS AND STRENGTHS───
• Ophthalmic solution containing tafluprost 0.015 mg/mL. (3)

───CONTRAINDICATIONS───
• None. (4)

───WARNINGS AND PRECAUTIONS───
• Pigmentation
Pigmentation of the iris, periorbital tissue (eyelid) and eyelashes can occur. Iris pigmentation is likely to be permanent. (5.1)
• Eyelash Changes
Gradual changes to eyelashes including increased length, thickness and number of lashes. Usually reversible. (5.2)

───ADVERSE REACTIONS───
• Most common ocular adverse reaction is conjunctival hyperemia (range 4% – 20%). (6.1)
To report SUSPECTED ADVERSE REACTIONS, contact Merck Sharp & Dohme Corp., a subsidiary of Merck & Co., Inc., at 1-877-888-4231 or FDA at 1-800-FDA-1088 or www.fda.gov/medwatch

───USE IN SPECIFIC POPULATIONS───
• Use in pediatric patients is not recommended because of potential safety concerns related to increased pigmentation following long-term chronic use. (8.4)
See 17 for PATIENT COUNSELING INFORMATION and FDA-approved patient labeling

Revised: 08/2013

FULL PRESCRIBING INFORMATION

1 INDICATIONS AND USAGE

ZIOPTAN™ (tafluprost ophthalmic solution) 0.0015% is indicated for reducing elevated intraocular pressure in patients with open-angle glaucoma or ocular hypertension.

2 DOSAGE AND ADMINISTRATION

The recommended dose is one drop of ZIOPTAN in the conjunctival sac of the affected eye(s) once daily in the evening. The dose should not exceed once daily since it has been shown that more frequent administration of prostaglandin analogs may lessen the intraocular pressure lowering effect. Reduction of the intraocular pressure starts approximately 2 to 4 hours after the first administration with the maximum effect reached after 12 hours.

ZIOPTAN may be used concomitantly with other topical ophthalmic drug products to lower intraocular pressure. If more than one topical ophthalmic product is being used, each one should be administered at least 5 minutes apart. The solution from one individual unit is to be used immediately after opening for administration to one or both eyes. Since sterility cannot be maintained after the individual unit is opened, the remaining contents should be discarded immediately after administration.

3 DOSAGE FORMS AND STRENGTHS

Ophthalmic solution containing tafluprost 0.015 mg/mL.

4 CONTRAINDICATIONS

None.

5 WARNINGS AND PRECAUTIONS

5.1 Pigmentation

Tafluprost ophthalmic solution has been reported to cause changes to pigmented tissues. The most frequently reported changes have been increased pigmentation of the iris, periorbital tissue (eyelid) and eyelashes. Pigmentation is expected to increase as long as tafluprost is administered. The pigmentation change is due to increased melanin content in the melanocytes rather than to an increase in the number of melanocytes. After discontinuation of tafluprost, pigmentation of the iris is likely to be permanent, while pigmentation of the periorbital tissue and eyelash changes have been reported to be reversible in some patients. Patients who receive treatment should be informed of the possibility of increased pigmentation. The long term effects of increased pigmentation are not known.

Iris color change may not be noticeable for several months to years. Typically, the brown pigmentation around the pupil spreads concentrically towards the periphery of the iris and the entire iris or parts of the iris become more brownish. Neither nevi nor freckles of the iris appear to be affected by treatment. While treatment with ZIOPTAN can be continued in patients who develop noticeably increased iris pigmentation, these patients should be examined regularly. [See Patient Counseling Information (17.3).]

5.2 Eyelash Changes

ZIOPTAN may gradually change eyelashes and vellus hair in the treated eye. These changes include increased length, color, thickness, shape and number of lashes. Eyelash changes are usually reversible upon discontinuation of treatment.

5.3 Intraocular Inflammation

ZIOPTAN should be used with caution in patients with active intraocular inflammation (e.g., iritis/uveitis) because the inflammation may be exacerbated.

5.4 Macular Edema

Macular edema, including cystoid macular edema, has been reported during treatment with prostaglandin F2α analogs. ZIOPTAN should be used with caution in aphakic patients, in pseudophakic patients with a torn posterior lens capsule, or in patients with known risk factors for macular edema.

6 ADVERSE REACTIONS

6.1 Clinical Studies Experience

Because clinical studies are conducted under widely varying conditions, adverse reaction rates observed in the clinical studies of a drug cannot be directly compared to rates in the clinical studies of another drug and may not reflect the rates observed in practice.

Preservative-containing or preservative-free tafluprost 0.0015% was evaluated in 905 patients in five controlled clinical studies of up to 24-months duration. The most common adverse reaction observed in patients treated with tafluprost was conjunctival hyperemia which was reported in a range of 4% – 20% of patients. Approximately 1% of patients discontinued therapy due to ocular adverse reactions.

Ocular adverse reactions reported at an incidence of ≥2% in these clinical studies included ocular stinging/irritation (7%), ocular pruritus including allergic conjunctivitis (5%), cataract (3%), dry eye (3%), ocular pain (3%), eyelash darkening (2%), growth of eyelashes (2%) and vision blurred (2%).

Nonocular adverse reactions reported at an incidence of 2% – 6% in these clinical studies in patients treated with tafluprost 0.0015% were headache (6%), common cold (4%), cough (3%) and urinary tract infection (2%).

6.2 Postmarketing Experience

The following adverse reactions have been identified during postapproval use of tafluprost. Because postapproval adverse reactions are reported voluntarily from a population of uncertain size, it is not always possible to reliably estimate their frequency or establish a causal relationship to drug exposure.

Respiratory disorders: exacerbation of asthma, dyspnea
Eye disorders: iritis/uveitis

In postmarketing use with prostaglandin analogs, periorbital and lid changes including deepening of the eyelid sulcus have been observed.

8 USE IN SPECIFIC POPULATIONS

8.1 Pregnancy

Pregnancy Category C.

Teratogenic effects: In embryo-fetal development studies in rats and rabbits, tafluprost administered intravenously was teratogenic. Tafluprost caused increases in postimplantation losses in rats and rabbits and reductions in fetal body weights in rats. Tafluprost also increased the incidence of vertebral skeletal abnormalities in rats and the incidence of skull, brain and spine malformations in rabbits. In rats, there were no adverse effects on embryo-fetal development at a dose of 3 mcg/kg/day corresponding to maternal plasma levels of tafluprost acid that were 343 times the maximum clinical exposure based on C_{max}. In rabbits, effects were seen at a tafluprost dose of 0.03 mcg/kg/day corresponding to maternal plasma levels of tafluprost acid during organogenesis that were approximately 5 times higher than the clinical exposure based on C_{max}. At the no-effect dose in rabbits (0.01 mcg/kg/day), maternal plasma levels of tafluprost acid were below the lower level of quantification (20 pg/mL).

In a pre- and postnatal development study in rats, increased mortality of newborns, decreased body weights and delayed pinna unfolding were observed in offsprings. The no observed adverse effect level was at a tafluprost intravenous dose of 0.3 mcg/kg/day which is greater than 3 times the maximum recommended clinical dose based on body surface area comparison.

There are no adequate and well-controlled studies in pregnant woman. Although animal reproduction studies are not always predictive of human response, ZIOPTAN should not be used during pregnancy unless the potential benefit justifies the potential risk to the fetus.

Women of childbearing age/potential should have adequate contraceptive measures in place.

8.3 Nursing Mothers

A study in lactating rats demonstrated that radio-labeled tafluprost and/or its metabolites were excreted in milk. It is not known whether this drug or its metabolites are excreted in human milk. Because many drugs are excreted in human milk, caution should be exercised when ZIOPTAN is administered to a nursing woman.

8.4 Pediatric Use

Use in pediatric patients is not recommended because of potential safety concerns related to increased pigmentation following long-term chronic use.

8.5 Geriatric Use

No overall clinical differences in safety or effectiveness have been observed between elderly and other adult patients.

11 DESCRIPTION

Tafluprost is a fluorinated analog of prostaglandin F2α. The chemical name for tafluprost is 1-methylethyl (5Z)-7-[(1R, 2R, 3R, 5S)-2-[(1E)-3,3-difluoro-4-phenoxy-1-butenyl]-3,5-dihydroxycyclopentyl]-5-heptenoate. The molecular formula of tafluprost is $C_{25}H_{34}F_2O_5$ and its molecular weight is 452.53.

Its structural formula is:

Tafluprost is a colorless to light yellow viscous liquid that is practically insoluble in water.

ZIOPTAN (tafluprost ophthalmic solution) 0.0015% is supplied as a sterile solution of tafluprost with a pH range of 5.5 – 6.7 and an Osmolality range of 260 – 300 mOsmol/kg. ZIOPTAN contains Active: tafluprost 0.015 mg/mL; Inactives: glycerol, sodium dihydrogen phosphate dihydrate, disodium edetate, polysorbate 80, hydrochloric acid and/or sodium hydroxide (to adjust pH) and Water for Injection. ZIOPTAN does not contain a preservative.

12 CLINICAL PHARMACOLOGY

12.1 Mechanism of Action

Tafluprost acid, a prostaglandin analog is a selective FP prostanoid receptor agonist which is believed to reduce intraocular pressure by increasing uveoscleral outflow. The exact mechanism of action is unknown at this time.

12.3 Pharmacokinetics

Absorption

Following instillation, tafluprost is absorbed through the cornea and is hydrolyzed to the biologically active acid metabolite, tafluprost acid. Following instillation of one drop of the 0.0015% solution once daily into each eye of healthy volunteers, the plasma concentrations of tafluprost acid peaked at a median time of 10 minutes on both Days 1 and 8. The mean plasma C_{max} of tafluprost acid were 26 pg/mL and 27 pg/mL on Day 1, and Day 8, respectively. The mean plasma AUC estimates of tafluprost acid were 394 pg*min/mL and 432 pg*min/mL on Day 1 and 8, respectively.

Metabolism

Tafluprost, an ester prodrug, is hydrolyzed to its biologically active acid metabolite in the eye. The acid metabolite is further metabolized via fatty acid β-oxidation and phase II conjugation.

Elimination

Mean plasma tafluprost acid concentrations were below the limit of quantification of the bioanalytical assay (10 pg/mL) at 30 minutes following topical ocular administration of tafluprost 0.0015% ophthalmic solution.

13 NONCLINICAL TOXICOLOGY

13.1 Carcinogenesis, Mutagenesis, Impairment of Fertility

Tafluprost was not carcinogenic when administered subcutaneously daily for 24 months at doses up to 30 mcg/kg/day in rats and for 18 months at doses up to 100 mcg/kg/day in mice (over 1600 and 1300 times, respectively, the maximum clinical exposure based on plasma AUC).

Tafluprost was not mutagenic or clastogenic in a battery of genetic toxicology studies, including an *in vitro* microbial mutagenesis assay, an *in vitro* chromosomal aberration assay in Chinese hamster lung cells, and an *in vivo* mouse micronucleus assay in bone marrow.

In rats, no adverse effects on mating performance or fertility were observed with intravenous dosing of tafluprost at a dose of 100 mcg/kg/day (over 14000 times the maximum clinical exposure based on plasma C_{max} or over 3600 times based on plasma AUC).

14 CLINICAL STUDIES

In clinical studies up to 24 months in duration, patients with open-angle glaucoma or ocular hypertension and baseline pressure of 23–26 mm Hg who were treated with ZIOPTAN dosed once daily in the evening demonstrated reductions in intraocular pressure at 3 and 6 months of 6–8 mmHg and 5–8 mmHg, respectively.

16 HOW SUPPLIED/STORAGE AND HANDLING

ZIOPTAN (tafluprost ophthalmic solution) 0.0015% is supplied as a sterile solution in translucent low density polyethylene single-use containers packaged in foil pouches (10 single-use containers per pouch). Each single-use container has 0.3 mL solution corresponding to 0.0045 mg tafluprost.
NDC 0006-3931-30; Unit-of-Use Carton of 30.
NDC 0006-3931-54; Unit-of-Use Carton of 90.

Storage:

Store refrigerated at 2–8°C (36–46°F). Store in the original pouch. After the pouch is opened, the single-use containers may be stored in the opened foil pouch for up to 28 days at room temperature: 20–25°C (68–77°F). Protect from moisture. Write down the date you open the foil pouch in the space provided on the pouch. Discard any unused containers 28 days after first opening the pouch.

17 PATIENT COUNSELING INFORMATION

See FDA-Approved Patient Labeling (Patient Information).

17.1 Nightly Application

Advise patients to not exceed once daily dosing since more frequent administration may decrease the intraocular pressure lowering effect of ZIOPTAN.

17.2 Handling the Single-Use Container

Advise patients that ZIOPTAN is a sterile solution that does not contain a preservative. The solution from one individual unit is to be used immediately after opening for administration to one or both eyes. Since sterility cannot be maintained after the individual unit is opened, the remaining contents should be discarded immediately after administration.

17.3 Potential for Pigmentation

Advise patients about the potential for increased brown pigmentation of the iris, which may be permanent. Also inform patients about the possibility of eyelid skin darkening, which may be reversible after discontinuation of ZIOPTAN.

17.4 Potential for Eyelash Changes

Inform patients of the possibility of eyelash and vellus hair changes in the treated eye during treatment with ZIOPTAN. These changes may result in a disparity between eyes in length, thickness, pigmentation, number of eyelashes or vellus hairs, and/or direction of eyelash growth. Eyelash changes are usually reversible upon discontinuation of treatment.

17.5 When to Seek Physician Advice

Advise patients that if they develop a new ocular condition (e.g., trauma or infection), experience a sudden decrease in visual acuity, have ocular surgery, or develop any ocular reactions, particularly conjunctivitis and eyelid reactions, they should immediately seek their physician's advice concerning the continued use of ZIOPTAN.

17.6 Use with Other Ophthalmic Drugs

If more than one topical ophthalmic drug is being used, the drugs should be administered at least five (5) minutes between applications.

17.7 Storage Information

Instruct patients on proper storage of cartons, unopened foil pouches, and opened foil pouches *[see How Supplied/Storage and Handling (16)]*. Recommended storage for cartons and unopened foil pouches is to store refrigerated at 2–8°C (36–46°F). After the pouch is opened, the single-use containers may be stored in the opened foil pouch for up to 28 days at room temperature: 20–25°C (68–77°F). Protect from moisture.

Manufactured for: Merck Sharp & Dohme Corp., a subsidiary of
MERCK & CO., INC., Whitehouse Station, NJ 08889, USA
Manufactured by:
Laboratoire Unither
ZI de la Guerie
F-50211 COUTANCES Cedex
France
For patent information: www.merck.com/product/patent/home.html
Copyright © 2012 Merck Sharp & Dohme Corp., a subsidiary of **Merck & Co., Inc.**
All rights reserved.
USPI-PF-24521308R005

PATIENT INFORMATION
ZIOPTAN™ (zye OP tan)
(tafluprost ophthalmic solution) 0.0015%
Read this Patient Information before you start using ZIOPTAN™ and each time you get a refill. There may be new information. This information does not take the place of talking to your doctor about your medical condition or your treatment.

What is ZIOPTAN?
ZIOPTAN is a prescription sterile eye drop solution. ZIOPTAN is used to lower the pressure in the eye (intraocular pressure) in people with open-angle glaucoma or ocular hypertension when their eye pressure is too high. ZIOPTAN belongs to a group of medicines called prostaglandin analogs.
ZIOPTAN is not for use in children.

What should I tell my doctor before using ZIOPTAN?
Before you use ZIOPTAN, tell your doctor if you:
• have or have had eye problems including any surgery on your eye or eyes
• are using any other eye medicines
• have any other medical problems
• are pregnant or plan to become pregnant. It is not known if ZIOPTAN will harm your unborn baby. You should use an effective method of birth control while you use ZIOPTAN. If you become pregnant while using ZIOPTAN talk to your doctor right away.
• are breastfeeding or plan to breastfeed. It is not known if ZIOPTAN passes into your breast milk. Talk to your doctor about the best way to feed your baby if you use ZIOPTAN.
Tell your doctor about all the medicines you take, including prescription and non-prescription medicines, vitamins, and herbal supplements.
Know the medicines you take. Keep a list of them to show your doctor and pharmacist when you get a new medicine.
How should I take ZIOPTAN?
Read the Instructions for Use at the end of this Patient Information leaflet for additional instructions about the right way to use ZIOPTAN.
• **Use 1 drop of ZIOPTAN in your eye (or eyes) each evening.** Talk to your doctor or pharmacist if you are not sure how to use ZIOPTAN.
• Your ZIOPTAN may not work as well if you use it more than 1 time each evening.
• If you use other medicines in your eye, wait at least 5 minutes between using ZIOPTAN and your other eye medicines.

• Use your ZIOPTAN right away after opening. Each ZIOPTAN single-use container is sterile and is to be used 1 time then thrown away. Do not save any ZIOPTAN that may be left over after you use your medicine. Using ZIOPTAN that is not sterile may cause other eye problems.
What are the possible side effects of ZIOPTAN?
ZIOPTAN may cause serious side effects including:
• **changes in the color of your eye (iris).** Your iris may become more brown in color while using ZIOPTAN. This color change may not go away when you stop using ZIOPTAN. If ZIOPTAN is used in 1 eye only, the color of that eye may always be a different color from the color of your other eye.
• **darkening of the color of the skin around your eye (eyelid).** These skin changes usually go away when you stop using ZIOPTAN.
• **increasing the length, thickness, color, or number of your eyelashes.** These eyelash changes usually go away when you stop using ZIOPTAN.
• **hair growth on your eyelids.** This hair growth usually goes away when you stop using ZIOPTAN.
The most common side effects of ZIOPTAN include:
• redness, stinging or itching of your eye
• cataract formation
• dry eye
• eye pain
• blurred vision
• headache
• common cold
• cough
• urinary tract infection
Tell your doctor if you have any new eye problems while using ZIOPTAN including:
• an eye injury
• an eye infection
• a sudden loss of vision
• eye surgery
• swelling and redness of and around your eye (conjunctivitis)
• problems with your eyelids
Additionally, the following side effects have been reported in general use:
• worsening of asthma
• shortness of breath
Tell your doctor if you have any other side effects that bother you.
These are not all the possible side effects of ZIOPTAN. For more information, ask your doctor or pharmacist.
Call your doctor for medical advice about side effects. You may report side effects to FDA at 1-800-FDA-1088.
How should I store ZIOPTAN?
Keep the foil pouches and ZIOPTAN single-use containers dry.
Before opening the foil pouches:
• Store the unopened foil pouches in a refrigerator between 36°F to 46°F (2°C to 8°C).
• Do not open the pouch containing ZIOPTAN until you are ready to use the eye drops.
After opening the foil pouch:
• Store the opened foil pouch at room temperature, between 68°F to 77°F (20°C to 25°C), for up to 28 days.
• Throw away all unused ZIOPTAN single-use containers in the opened foil pouch after 28 days.
• Keep the ZIOPTAN single-use containers in their original foil pouch.
• After opening the foil pouch, refrigeration is not required.
Keep ZIOPTAN and all medicines out of the reach of children.
General information about the safe and effective use of ZIOPTAN.
Do not use ZIOPTAN for a condition for which it was not prescribed. Do not give ZIOPTAN to other people, even if they have the same symptoms that you have. It may harm them.
This Patient Information leaflet summarizes the most important information about ZIOPTAN. If you would like more information, talk with your doctor. You can ask your pharmacist or doctor for information about ZIOPTAN that is written for health professionals.
What are the ingredients in ZIOPTAN?
Active ingredients: tafluprost
Inactive ingredients: glycerol, sodium dihydrogen phosphate dihydrate, disodium edetate, and polysorbate 80, hydrochloric acid and/or sodium hydroxide, and water
Instructions for Use
Read these Instructions for Use before using your ZIOPTAN and each time you get a refill. There may be new information. This leaflet does not take the place of talking with your doctor about your medical condition or your treatment.
Important:
• **ZIOPTAN is for the eye only. Do not swallow ZIOPTAN.**
• ZIOPTAN single-use containers are packaged in a foil pouch.

• **Do not** use the ZIOPTAN single-use containers if the foil pouch is opened.
• Write down the date you open the foil pouch in the space provided on the pouch.
Every time you use ZIOPTAN:

Step	Instruction	
Step 1.	Wash your hands.	
Step 2.	Take the strip of single-use containers from the foil pouch.	
Step 3.	Pull off one single-use container from the strip.	
Step 4.	Put the remaining strip of single-use containers back in the foil pouch and fold the edge to close the pouch.	
Step 5.	Hold the single-use container upright. Make sure that your ZIOPTAN medicine is in the bottom part of the single-use container. See Figure A.	Figure A
Step 6.	Open the single-use container by twisting off the tab. See Figure B.	Figure B
Step 7.	Tilt your head backwards. If you are unable to tilt your head, lie down.	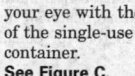
Step 8.	Place the tip of the single-use container close to your eye. Be careful not to touch your eye with the tip of the single-use container. See Figure C.	Figure C
Step 9.	Pull your lower eyelid downwards and look up.	
Step 10.	Gently squeeze the container and let 1 drop of ZIOPTAN fall into the space between your lower eyelid and your eye. If a drop misses your eye, try again. See Figure D.	Figure D

• If your doctor has told you to use ZIOPTAN drops in both eyes, repeat Steps 7 to 10 for your other eye.
• There is enough ZIOPTAN in one single-use container for both of your eyes.

- Throw away the opened single-use container with any remaining ZIOPTAN right away.

This Patient Information and Instructions for Use have been approved by the U.S. Food and Drug Administration.

Rx only

Manufactured for: Merck Sharp & Dohme Corp., a subsidiary of

MERCK & CO., INC., Whitehouse Station, NJ 08889, USA

Manufactured by:

Laboratoire Unither

ZI de la Guerie

F-50211 COUTANCES Cedex

France

For patent information: www.merck.com/product/patent/home.html

Copyright © 2012 Merck Sharp & Dohme Corp., a subsidiary of **Merck & Co., Inc.**

All rights reserved.

Revised: 08/2013

USPPI-PF-24521308R005

Shown in Product Identification Guide, page 309

ZOCOR ℞

(simvastatin)

Tablets

HIGHLIGHTS OF PRESCRIBING INFORMATION

These highlights do not include all the information needed to use ZOCOR safely and effectively. See full prescribing information for ZOCOR.

ZOCOR (simvastatin) Tablets

Initial U.S. Approval: 1991

---RECENT MAJOR CHANGES---

Dosage and Administration	
Patients with Homozygous Familial Hypercholesterolemia (2.4)	10/2013
Contraindications (4)	02/2014
Warnings and Precautions	
Myopathy/Rhabdomyolysis (5.1)	02/2014

---INDICATIONS AND USAGE---

ZOCOR® is an HMG-CoA reductase inhibitor (statin) indicated as an adjunctive therapy to diet to:

- Reduce the risk of total mortality by reducing CHD deaths and reduce the risk of non-fatal myocardial infarction, stroke, and the need for revascularization procedures in patients at high risk of coronary events. (1.1)
- Reduce elevated total-C, LDL-C, Apo B, TG and increase HDL-C in patients with primary hyperlipidemia (heterozygous familial and nonfamilial) and mixed dyslipidemia. (1.2)
- Reduce elevated TG in patients with hypertriglyceridemia and reduce TG and VLDL-C in patients with primary dysbetalipoproteinemia. (1.2)
- Reduce total-C and LDL-C in adult patients with homozygous familial hypercholesterolemia. (1.2)
- Reduce elevated total-C, LDL-C, and Apo B in boys and postmenarchal girls, 10 to 17 years of age with heterozygous familial hypercholesterolemia after failing an adequate trial of diet therapy. (1.2, 1.3)

Limitations of Use

ZOCOR has not been studied in Fredrickson Types I and V dyslipidemias. (1.4)

---DOSAGE AND ADMINISTRATION---

- Dose range is 5 to 40 mg/day. (2.1)
- Recommended usual starting dose is 10 or 20 mg once a day in the evening. (2.1)
- Recommended starting dose for patients at high risk of CHD is 40 mg/day. (2.1)
- Due to the increased risk of myopathy, including rhabdomyolysis, use of the 80-mg dose of ZOCOR should be restricted to patients who have been taking simvastatin 80 mg chronically (e.g., for 12 months or more) without evidence of muscle toxicity. (2.2)
- Patients who are currently tolerating the 80-mg dose of ZOCOR who need to be initiated on an interacting drug that is contraindicated or is associated with a dose cap for simvastatin should be switched to an alternative statin with less potential for the drug-drug interaction. (2.2)
- Due to the increased risk of myopathy, including rhabdomyolysis, associated with the 80-mg dose of ZOCOR, patients unable to achieve their LDL-C goal utilizing the 40-mg dose of ZOCOR should not be titrated to the 80-mg dose, but should be placed on alternative LDL-C-lowering treatment(s) that provides greater LDL-C lowering. (2.2)
- Adolescents (10-17 years of age) with HeFH: starting dose is 10 mg/day; maximum recommended dose is 40 mg/day. (2.5)

---DOSAGE FORMS AND STRENGTHS---

Tablets: 5 mg; 10 mg; 20 mg; 40 mg; 80 mg (3)

---CONTRAINDICATIONS---

- Concomitant administration of strong CYP3A4 inhibitors. (4, 5.1)
- Concomitant administration of gemfibrozil, cyclosporine, or danazol. (4, 5.1)
- Hypersensitivity to any component of this medication. (4, 6.2)
- Active liver disease, which may include unexplained persistent elevations in hepatic transaminase levels. (4, 5.2)
- Women who are pregnant or may become pregnant. (4, 8.1)
- Nursing mothers. (4, 8.3)

---WARNINGS AND PRECAUTIONS---

- Patients should be advised of the increased risk of myopathy including rhabdomyolysis with the 80-mg dose. (5.1)
- Skeletal muscle effects (e.g., myopathy and rhabdomyolysis): Risks increase with higher doses and concomitant use of certain medicines. Predisposing factors include advanced age (≥65), female gender, uncontrolled hypothyroidism, and renal impairment. Rare cases of rhabdomyolysis with acute renal failure secondary to myoglobinuria have been reported. (4, 5.1, 8.5, 8.6)
- Patients should be advised to report promptly any unexplained and/or persistent muscle pain, tenderness, or weakness. ZOCOR therapy should be discontinued immediately if myopathy is diagnosed or suspected. See Drug Interaction table. (5.1)
- Liver enzyme abnormalities: Persistent elevations in hepatic transaminases can occur. Check liver enzyme tests before initiating therapy and as clinically indicated thereafter. (5.2)

---ADVERSE REACTIONS---

Most common adverse reactions (incidence ≥5.0%) are: upper respiratory infection, headache, abdominal pain, constipation, and nausea. (6.1)

To report SUSPECTED ADVERSE REACTIONS, contact Merck Sharp & Dohme Corp., a subsidiary of Merck & Co., Inc., at 1-877-888-4231 or FDA at 1-800-FDA-1088 or www.fda.gov/medwatch.

---DRUG INTERACTIONS---

Drug Interactions Associated with Increased Risk of Myopathy/Rhabdomyolysis (2.3, 2.4, 4, 5.1, 7.1, 7.2, 7.3, 12.3)

Interacting Agents	Prescribing Recommendations
Strong CYP3A4 inhibitors (e.g., itraconazole, ketoconazole, posaconazole, voriconazole, erythromycin, clarithromycin, telithromycin, HIV protease inhibitors, boceprevir, telaprevir, nefazodone, cobicistat-containing products), gemfibrozil, cyclosporine, danazol	Contraindicated with simvastatin
Verapamil, diltiazem, dronedarone	Do not exceed 10 mg simvastatin daily
Amiodarone, amlodipine, ranolazine	Do not exceed 20 mg simvastatin daily
Lomitapide	For patients with HoFH, do not exceed 20 mg simvastatin daily*
Grapefruit juice	Avoid grapefruit juice

* For patients with HoFH who have been taking 80 mg simvastatin chronically (e.g., for 12 months or more) without evidence of muscle toxicity, do not exceed 40 mg simvastatin when taking lomitapide.

- Other Lipid-lowering Medications: Use with other fibrate products or lipid-modifying doses (≥1 g/day) of niacin increases the risk of adverse skeletal muscle effects. Caution should be used when prescribing with simvastatin. (5.1, 7.2, 7.4)
- Coumarin anticoagulants: Concomitant use with ZOCOR prolongs INR. Achieve stable INR prior to starting ZOCOR. Monitor INR frequently until stable upon initiation or alteration of ZOCOR therapy. (7.6)

---USE IN SPECIFIC POPULATIONS---

- Severe renal impairment: patients should be started at 5 mg/day and be closely monitored. (2.6, 8.6)

See 17 for PATIENT COUNSELING INFORMATION

Revised: 02/2014

FULL PRESCRIBING INFORMATION

1 INDICATIONS AND USAGE

Therapy with lipid-altering agents should be only one component of multiple risk factor intervention in individuals at significantly increased risk for atherosclerotic vascular disease due to hypercholesterolemia. Drug therapy is indicated as an adjunct to diet when the response to a diet restricted in saturated fat and cholesterol and other nonpharmacologic measures alone has been inadequate. In patients with coronary heart disease (CHD) or at high risk of CHD, ZOCOR® can be started simultaneously with diet.

1.1 Reductions in Risk of CHD Mortality and Cardiovascular Events

In patients at high risk of coronary events because of existing coronary heart disease, diabetes, peripheral vessel disease, history of stroke or other cerebrovascular disease, ZOCOR is indicated to:

- Reduce the risk of total mortality by reducing CHD deaths.
- Reduce the risk of non-fatal myocardial infarction and stroke.
- Reduce the need for coronary and non-coronary revascularization procedures.

1.2 Hyperlipidemia

ZOCOR is indicated to:

- Reduce elevated total cholesterol (total-C), low-density lipoprotein cholesterol (LDL-C), apolipoprotein B (Apo B), and triglycerides (TG), and to increase high-density lipoprotein cholesterol (HDL-C) in patients with primary hy-

perlipidemia (Fredrickson type IIa, heterozygous familial and nonfamilial) or mixed dyslipidemia (Fredrickson type IIb).
• Reduce elevated TG in patients with hypertriglyceridemia (Fredrickson type IV hyperlipidemia).
• Reduce elevated TG and VLDL-C in patients with primary dysbetalipoproteinemia (Fredrickson type III hyperlipidemia).
• Reduce total-C and LDL-C in patients with homozygous familial hypercholesterolemia (HoFH) as an adjunct to other lipid-lowering treatments (e.g., LDL apheresis) or if such treatments are unavailable.

1.3 Adolescent Patients with Heterozygous Familial Hypercholesterolemia (HeFH)

ZOCOR is indicated as an adjunct to diet to reduce total-C, LDL-C, and Apo B levels in adolescent boys and girls who are at least one year post-menarche, 10-17 years of age, with HeFH, if after an adequate trial of diet therapy the following findings are present:
1. LDL cholesterol remains ≥190 mg/dL; or
2. LDL cholesterol remains ≥160 mg/dL and
• There is a positive family history of premature cardiovascular disease (CVD) or
• Two or more other CVD risk factors are present in the adolescent patient.

The minimum goal of treatment in pediatric and adolescent patients is to achieve a mean LDL-C <130 mg/dL. The optimal age at which to initiate lipid-lowering therapy to decrease the risk of symptomatic adulthood CAD has not been determined.

1.4 Limitations of Use

ZOCOR has not been studied in conditions where the major abnormality is elevation of chylomicrons (i.e., hyperlipidemia Fredrickson types I and V).

2 DOSAGE AND ADMINISTRATION

2.1 Recommended Dosing

The usual dosage range is 5 to 40 mg/day. In patients with CHD or at high risk of CHD, ZOCOR can be started simultaneously with diet. The recommended usual starting dose is 10 or 20 mg once a day in the evening. For patients at high risk for a CHD event due to existing CHD, diabetes, peripheral vessel disease, history of stroke or other cerebrovascular disease, the recommended starting dose is 40 mg/day. Lipid determinations should be performed after 4 weeks of therapy and periodically thereafter.

2.2 Restricted Dosing for 80 mg

Due to the increased risk of myopathy, including rhabdomyolysis, particularly during the first year of treatment, use of the 80-mg dose of ZOCOR should be restricted to patients who have been taking simvastatin 80 mg chronically (e.g., for 12 months or more) without evidence of muscle toxicity *[see Warnings and Precautions (5.1)]*.

Patients who are currently tolerating the 80-mg dose of ZOCOR who need to be initiated on an interacting drug that is contraindicated or is associated with a dose cap for simvastatin should be switched to an alternative statin with less potential for the drug-drug interaction.

Due to the increased risk of myopathy, including rhabdomyolysis, associated with the 80-mg dose of ZOCOR, patients unable to achieve their LDL-C goal utilizing the 40-mg dose of ZOCOR should not be titrated to the 80-mg dose, but should be placed on alternative LDL-C-lowering treatment(s) that provides greater LDL-C lowering.

2.3 Coadministration with Other Drugs

Patients taking Verapamil, Diltiazem, or Dronedarone
• The dose of ZOCOR should not exceed 10 mg/day *[see Warnings and Precautions (5.1), Drug Interactions (7.3), and Clinical Pharmacology (12.3)]*.

Patients taking Amiodarone, Amlodipine or Ranolazine
• The dose of ZOCOR should not exceed 20 mg/day *[see Warnings and Precautions (5.1), Drug Interactions (7.3), and Clinical Pharmacology (12.3)]*.

2.4 Patients with Homozygous Familial Hypercholesterolemia

The recommended dosage is 40 mg/day in the evening *[see Dosage and Administration, Restricted Dosing for 80 mg (2.2)]*. ZOCOR should be used as an adjunct to other lipid-lowering treatments (e.g., LDL apheresis) in these patients or if such treatments are unavailable.

Simvastatin exposure is approximately doubled with concomitant use of lomitapide; therefore, the dose of ZOCOR should be reduced by 50% if initiating lomitapide. ZOCOR dosage should not exceed 20 mg/day (or 40 mg/day for patients who have previously taken ZOCOR 80 mg/day chronically, e.g., for 12 months or more, without evidence of muscle toxicity) while taking lomitapide.

2.5 Adolescents (10-17 years of age) with Heterozygous Familial Hypercholesterolemia

The recommended usual starting dose is 10 mg once a day in the evening. The recommended dosing range is 10 to 40 mg/day; the maximum recommended dose is 40 mg/day. Doses should be individualized according to the recommended goal of therapy *[see NCEP Pediatric Panel Guidelines[1] and Clinical Studies (14.2)]*. Adjustments should be made at intervals of 4 weeks or more.

[1] National Cholesterol Education Program (NCEP): Highlights of the Report of the Expert Panel on Blood Cholesterol Levels in Children and Adolescents. *Pediatrics*. 89(3):495-501. 1992.

2.6 Patients with Renal Impairment

Because ZOCOR does not undergo significant renal excretion, modification of dosage should not be necessary in patients with mild to moderate renal impairment. However, caution should be exercised when ZOCOR is administered to patients with severe renal impairment; such patients should be started at 5 mg/day and be closely monitored *[see Warnings and Precautions (5.1) and Clinical Pharmacology (12.3)]*.

2.7 Chinese Patients Taking Lipid-Modifying Doses (greater than or equal to 1 g/day Niacin) of Niacin-Containing Products

Because of an increased risk for myopathy in Chinese patients taking simvastatin 40 mg coadministered with lipid-modifying doses (greater than or equal to 1 g/day niacin) of niacin-containing products, caution should be used when treating Chinese patients with simvastatin doses exceeding 20 mg/day coadministered with lipid-modifying doses of niacin-containing products. Because the risk for myopathy is dose-related, Chinese patients should not receive simvastatin 80 mg coadministered with lipid-modifying doses of niacin-containing products. The cause of the increased risk of myopathy is not known. It is also unknown if the risk for myopathy with coadministration of simvastatin with lipid-modifying doses of niacin-containing products observed in Chinese patients applies to other Asian patients. *[See Warnings and Precautions (5.1).]*

3 DOSAGE FORMS AND STRENGTHS

• Tablets ZOCOR 5 mg are buff, oval, film-coated tablets, coded MSD 726 on one side and ZOCOR 5 on the other.
• Tablets ZOCOR 10 mg are peach, oval, film-coated tablets, coded MSD 735 on one side and plain on the other.
• Tablets ZOCOR 20 mg are tan, oval, film-coated tablets, coded MSD 740 on one side and plain on the other.
• Tablets ZOCOR 40 mg are brick red, oval, film-coated tablets, coded MSD 749 on one side and plain on the other.
• Tablets ZOCOR 80 mg are brick red, capsule-shaped, film-coated tablets, coded 543 on one side and 80 on the other.

4 CONTRAINDICATIONS

ZOCOR is contraindicated in the following conditions:
• Concomitant administration of strong CYP3A4 inhibitors (e.g., itraconazole, ketoconazole, posaconazole, voriconazole, HIV protease inhibitors, boceprevir, telaprevir, erythromycin, clarithromycin, telithromycin, nefazodone, and cobicistat-containing products) *[see Warnings and Precautions (5.1)]*.
• Concomitant administration of gemfibrozil, cyclosporine, or danazol *[see Warnings and Precautions (5.1)]*.
• Hypersensitivity to any component of this medication *[see Adverse Reactions (6.2)]*.
• Active liver disease, which may include unexplained persistent elevations in hepatic transaminase levels *[see Warnings and Precautions (5.2)]*.
• Women who are pregnant or may become pregnant. Serum cholesterol and triglycerides increase during normal pregnancy, and cholesterol or cholesterol derivatives are essential for fetal development. Because HMG-CoA reductase inhibitors (statins) decrease cholesterol synthesis and possibly the synthesis of other biologically active substances derived from cholesterol, ZOCOR may cause fetal harm when administered to a pregnant woman. Atherosclerosis is a chronic process and the discontinuation of lipid-lowering drugs during pregnancy should have little impact on the outcome of long-term therapy of primary hypercholesterolemia. There are no adequate and well-controlled studies of use with ZOCOR during pregnancy; however, in rare reports congenital anomalies were observed following intrauterine exposure to statins. In rat and rabbit animal reproduction studies, simvastatin revealed no evidence of teratogenicity. **ZOCOR should be administered to women of childbearing age only when such patients are highly unlikely to conceive.** If the patient becomes pregnant while taking this drug, ZOCOR should be discontinued immediately and the patient should be apprised of the potential hazard to the fetus *[see Use in Specific Populations (8.1)]*.
• Nursing mothers. It is not known whether simvastatin is excreted into human milk; however, a small amount of another drug in this class does pass into breast milk. Because statins have the potential for serious adverse reactions in nursing infants, women who require treatment with ZOCOR should not breastfeed their infants *[see Use in Specific Populations (8.3)]*.

5 WARNINGS AND PRECAUTIONS

5.1 Myopathy/Rhabdomyolysis

Simvastatin occasionally causes myopathy manifested as muscle pain, tenderness or weakness with creatine kinase (CK) above ten times the upper limit of normal (ULN). Myopathy sometimes takes the form of rhabdomyolysis with or without acute renal failure secondary to myoglobinuria, and rare fatalities have occurred. The risk of myopathy is increased by high levels of statin activity in plasma. Predisposing factors for myopathy include advanced age (≥65 years), female gender, uncontrolled hypothyroidism, and renal impairment.

The risk of myopathy, including rhabdomyolysis, is dose related. In a clinical trial database in which 41,413 patients were treated with ZOCOR, 24,747 (approximately 60%) of whom were enrolled in studies with a median follow-up of at least 4 years, the incidence of myopathy was approximately 0.03% and 0.08% at 20 and 40 mg/day, respectively. The incidence of myopathy with 80 mg (0.61%) was disproportionately higher than that observed at the lower doses. In these trials, patients were carefully monitored and some interacting medicinal products were excluded.

In a clinical trial in which 12,064 patients with a history of myocardial infarction were treated with ZOCOR (mean follow-up 6.7 years), the incidence of myopathy (defined as unexplained muscle weakness or pain with a serum creatine kinase [CK] >10 times upper limit of normal [ULN]) in patients on 80 mg/day was approximately 0.9% compared with 0.02% for patients on 20 mg/day. The incidence of rhabdomyolysis (defined as myopathy with a CK >40 times ULN) in patients on 80 mg/day was approximately 0.4% compared with 0% for patients on 20 mg/day. The incidence of myopathy, including rhabdomyolysis, was highest during the first year and then notably decreased during the subsequent years of treatment. In this trial, patients were carefully monitored and some interacting medicinal products were excluded.

**The risk of myopathy, including rhabdomyolysis, is greater in patients on simvastatin 80 mg compared with other statin therapies with similar or greater LDL-C-lowering efficacy and compared with lower doses of simvastatin. Therefore, the 80-mg dose of ZOCOR should be used only in patients who have been taking simvastatin 80 mg chronically (e.g., for 12 months or more) without evidence of muscle toxicity *[see Dosage and Administration, Restricted Dosing for 80 mg (2.2)]*. If, however, a patient who is currently tolerating the 80-mg dose of ZOCOR needs to be initiated on an interacting drug that is contraindicated or is associated with a dose cap for simvastatin, that patient should be switched to an alternative statin with less potential for the drug-drug interaction. Patients should be advised of the increased risk of myopathy, including rhabdomyolysis, and to report promptly any unexplained muscle pain, tenderness or weakness. If symptoms occur, treatment should be discontinued immediately. *[See Warnings and Precautions (5.2).]*

There have been rare reports of immune-mediated necrotizing myopathy (IMNM), an autoimmune myopathy, associated with statin use. IMNM is characterized by: proximal muscle weakness and elevated serum creatine kinase, which persist despite discontinuation of statin treatment; muscle biopsy showing necrotizing myopathy without significant inflammation; improvement with immunosuppressive agents.

All patients starting therapy with ZOCOR, or whose dose of ZOCOR is being increased, should be advised of the risk of myopathy, including rhabdomyolysis, and told to report promptly any unexplained muscle pain, tenderness or weakness particularly if accompanied by malaise or fever or if muscle signs and symptoms persist after discontinuing ZOCOR. ZOCOR therapy should be discontinued immediately if myopathy is diagnosed or suspected. In most cases, muscle symptoms and CK increases resolved when treatment was promptly discontinued. Periodic CK determinations may be considered in patients starting therapy with ZOCOR or whose dose is being increased, but there is no assurance that such monitoring will prevent myopathy.

Many of the patients who have developed rhabdomyolysis on therapy with simvastatin have had complicated medical histories, including renal insufficiency usually as a consequence of long-standing diabetes mellitus. Such patients merit closer monitoring. ZOCOR therapy should be discontinued if markedly elevated CPK levels occur or myopathy is diagnosed or suspected. ZOCOR therapy should also be temporarily withheld in any patient experiencing an acute or serious condition predisposing to the development of renal failure secondary to rhabdomyolysis, e.g., sepsis; hypotension; major surgery; trauma; severe metabolic, endocrine, or electrolyte disorders; or uncontrolled epilepsy.

Drug Interactions
The risk of myopathy and rhabdomyolysis is increased by high levels of statin activity in plasma. Simvastatin is metabolized by the cytochrome P450 isoform 3A4. Certain drugs which inhibit this metabolic pathway can raise the plasma levels of simvastatin and may increase the risk of myopathy. These include itraconazole, ketoconazole, posaconazole, voriconazole, the macrolide antibiotics erythromycin and clarithromycin, and the ketolide antibiotic telithro-

mycin, HIV protease inhibitors, boceprevir, telaprevir, the antidepressant nefazodone, cobicistat-containing products, or grapefruit juice *[see Clinical Pharmacology (12.3)]*. Combination of these drugs with simvastatin is contraindicated. If short-term treatment with strong CYP3A4 inhibitors is unavoidable, therapy with simvastatin must be suspended during the course of treatment. *[See Contraindications (4) and Drug Interactions (7.1).]*

The combined use of simvastatin with gemfibrozil, cyclosporine, or danazol is contraindicated *[see Contraindications (4) and Drug Interactions (7.1 and 7.2)]*.

Caution should be used when prescribing other fibrates with simvastatin, as these agents can cause myopathy when given alone and the risk is increased when they are co-administered *[see Drug Interactions (7.2)]*.

Cases of myopathy, including rhabdomyolysis, have been reported with simvastatin coadministered with colchicine, and caution should be exercised when prescribing simvastatin with colchicine *[see Drug Interactions (7.7)]*.

The benefits of the combined use of simvastatin with the following drugs should be carefully weighed against the potential risks of combinations: other lipid-lowering drugs (other fibrates, ≥1 g/day of niacin, or, for patients with HoFH, lomitapide), amiodarone, dronedarone, verapamil, diltiazem, amlodipine, or ranolazine *[see Drug Interactions (7.3) and Table 3 in Clinical Pharmacology (12.3)] [also see Dosage and Administration, Patients with Homozygous Familial Hypercholesterolemia (2.4)]*.

Cases of myopathy, including rhabdomyolysis, have been observed with simvastatin coadministered with lipid-modifying doses (≥1 g/day niacin) of niacin-containing products. In an ongoing, double-blind, randomized cardiovascular outcomes trial, an independent safety monitoring committee identified that the incidence of myopathy is higher in Chinese compared with non-Chinese patients taking simvastatin 40 mg coadministered with lipid-modifying doses of a niacin-containing product. Caution should be used when treating Chinese patients with simvastatin in doses exceeding 20 mg/day coadministered with lipid-modifying doses of niacin-containing products. Because the risk for myopathy is dose-related, Chinese patients should not receive simvastatin 80 mg coadministered with lipid-modifying doses of niacin-containing products. It is unknown if the risk for myopathy with coadministration of simvastatin with lipid-modifying doses of niacin-containing products observed in Chinese patients applies to other Asian patients *[see Drug Interactions (7.4)]*.

Prescribing recommendations for interacting agents are summarized in Table 1 *[see also Dosage and Administration (2.3, 2.4), Drug Interactions (7), Clinical Pharmacology (12.3)]*.

Table 1: Drug Interactions Associated with Increased Risk of Myopathy/Rhabdomyolysis

Interacting Agents	Prescribing Recommendations
Strong CYP3A4 Inhibitors, e.g.: Itraconazole Ketoconazole Posaconazole Voriconazole Erythromycin Clarithromycin Telithromycin HIV protease inhibitors Boceprevir Telaprevir Nefazodone Cobicistat-containing products Gemfibrozil Cyclosporine Danazol	Contraindicated with simvastatin
Verapamil Diltiazem Dronedarone	Do not exceed 10 mg simvastatin daily
Amiodarone Amlodipine Ranolazine	Do not exceed 20 mg simvastatin daily
Lomitapide	For patients with HoFH, do not exceed 20 mg simvastatin daily*
Grapefruit juice	Avoid grapefruit juice

* For patients with HoFH who have been taking 80 mg simvastatin chronically (e.g., for 12 months or more) without evidence of muscle toxicity, do not exceed 40 mg simvastatin when taking lomitapide.

5.2 Liver Dysfunction

Persistent increases (to more than 3X the ULN) in serum transaminases have occurred in approximately 1% of patients who received simvastatin in clinical studies. When drug treatment was interrupted or discontinued in these patients, the transaminase levels usually fell slowly to pretreatment levels. The increases were not associated with jaundice or other clinical signs or symptoms. There was no evidence of hypersensitivity.

In the Scandinavian Simvastatin Survival Study (4S) *[see Clinical Studies (14.1)]*, the number of patients with more than one transaminase elevation to >3X ULN, over the course of the study, was not significantly different between the simvastatin and placebo groups (14 [0.7%] vs. 12 [0.6%]). Elevated transaminases resulted in the discontinuation of 8 patients from therapy in the simvastatin group (n=2,221) and 5 in the placebo group (n=2,223). Of the 1,986 simvastatin treated patients in 4S with normal liver function tests (LFTs) at baseline, 8 (0.4%) developed consecutive LFT elevations to >3X ULN and/or were discontinued due to transaminase elevations during the 5.4 years (median follow-up) of the study. Among these 8 patients, 5 initially developed these abnormalities within the first year. All of the patients in this study received a starting dose of 20 mg of simvastatin; 37% were titrated to 40 mg.

In 2 controlled clinical studies in 1,105 patients, the 12-month incidence of persistent hepatic transaminase elevation without regard to drug relationship was 0.9% and 2.1% at the 40- and 80-mg dose, respectively. No patients developed persistent liver function abnormalities following the initial 6 months of treatment at a given dose.

It is recommended that liver function tests be performed before the initiation of treatment, and thereafter when clinically indicated. There have been rare postmarketing reports of fatal and non-fatal hepatic failure in patients taking statins, including simvastatin. If serious liver injury with clinical symptoms and/or hyperbilirubinemia or jaundice occurs during treatment with ZOCOR, promptly interrupt therapy. If an alternate etiology is not found do not restart ZOCOR. Note that ALT may emanate from muscle, therefore ALT rising with CK may indicate myopathy *[see Warnings and Precautions (5.1)]*.

The drug should be used with caution in patients who consume substantial quantities of alcohol and/or have a past history of liver disease. Active liver diseases or unexplained transaminase elevations are contraindications to the use of simvastatin.

Moderate (less than 3X ULN) elevations of serum transaminases have been reported following therapy with simvastatin. These changes appeared soon after initiation of therapy with simvastatin, were often transient, were not accompanied by any symptoms and did not require interruption of treatment.

5.3 Endocrine Function

Increases in HbA1c and fasting serum glucose levels have been reported with HMG-CoA reductase inhibitors, including ZOCOR.

6 ADVERSE REACTIONS

6.1 Clinical Trials Experience

Because clinical studies are conducted under widely varying conditions, adverse reaction rates observed in the clinical studies of a drug cannot be directly compared to rates in the clinical studies of another drug and may not reflect the rates observed in practice.

In the pre-marketing controlled clinical studies and their open extensions (2,423 patients with median duration of follow-up of approximately 18 months), 1.4% of patients were discontinued due to adverse reactions. The most common adverse reactions that led to treatment discontinuation were: gastrointestinal disorders (0.5%), myalgia (0.1%), and arthralgia (0.1%). The most commonly reported adverse reactions (incidence ≥5%) in simvastatin controlled clinical trials were: upper respiratory infections (9.0%), headache (7.4%), abdominal pain (7.3%), constipation (6.6%), and nausea (5.4%).

Scandinavian Simvastatin Survival Study

In 4S involving 4,444 (age range 35-71 years, 19% women, 100% Caucasians) treated with 20-40 mg/day of ZOCOR (n=2,221) or placebo (n=2,223) over a median of 5.4 years, adverse reactions reported in ≥2% of patients and at a rate greater than placebo are shown in Table 2.

Table 2: Adverse Reactions Reported Regardless of Causality by ≥2% of Patients Treated with ZOCOR and Greater than Placebo in 4S

	ZOCOR (N = 2,221) %	Placebo (N = 2,223) %
Body as a Whole		
Edema/swelling	2.7	2.3
Abdominal pain	5.9	5.8
Cardiovascular System Disorders		
Atrial fibrillation	5.7	5.1
Digestive System Disorders		
Constipation	2.2	1.6
Gastritis	4.9	3.9
Endocrine Disorders		
Diabetes mellitus	4.2	3.6
Musculoskeletal Disorders		
Myalgia	3.7	3.2
Nervous System / Psychiatric Disorders		
Headache	2.5	2.1
Insomnia	4.0	3.8
Vertigo	4.5	4.2
Respiratory System Disorders		
Bronchitis	6.6	6.3
Sinusitis	2.3	1.8
Skin / Skin Appendage Disorders		
Eczema	4.5	3.0
Urogenital System Disorders		
Infection, urinary tract	3.2	3.1

Heart Protection Study

In the Heart Protection Study (HPS), involving 20,536 patients (age range 40-80 years, 25% women, 97% Caucasians, 3% other races) treated with ZOCOR 40 mg/day (n=10,269) or placebo (n=10,267) over a mean of 5 years, only serious adverse reactions and discontinuations due to any adverse reactions were recorded. Discontinuation rates due to adverse reactions were 4.8% in patients treated with ZOCOR compared with 5.1% in patients treated with placebo. The incidence of myopathy/rhabdomyolysis was <0.1% in patients treated with ZOCOR.

Other Clinical Studies

In a clinical trial in which 12,064 patients with a history of myocardial infarction were treated with ZOCOR (mean follow-up 6.7 years), the incidence of myopathy (defined as unexplained muscle weakness or pain with a serum creatine kinase [CK] >10 times upper limit of normal [ULN]) in patients on 80 mg/day was approximately 0.9% compared with 0.02% for patients on 20 mg/day. The incidence of rhabdomyolysis (defined as myopathy with a CK >40 times ULN) in patients on 80 mg/day was approximately 0.4% compared with 0% for patients on 20 mg/day. The incidence of myopathy, including rhabdomyolysis, was highest during the first year and then notably decreased during the subsequent years of treatment. In this trial, patients were carefully monitored and some interacting medicinal products were excluded.

Other adverse reactions reported in clinical trials were: diarrhea, rash, dyspepsia, flatulence, and asthenia.

Laboratory Tests

Marked persistent increases of hepatic transaminases have been noted *[see Warnings and Precautions (5.2)]*. Elevated alkaline phosphatase and γ-glutamyl transpeptidase have also been reported. About 5% of patients had elevations of CK levels of 3 or more times the normal value on one or more occasions. This was attributable to the noncardiac fraction of CK. *[See Warnings and Precautions (5.1).]*

Adolescent Patients (ages 10-17 years)

In a 48-week, controlled study in adolescent boys and girls who were at least 1 year post-menarche, 10-17 years of age (43.4% female, 97.7% Caucasians, 1.7% Hispanics, 0.6% Multiracial) with heterozygous familial hypercholesterolemia (n=175), treated with placebo or ZOCOR (10-40 mg daily), the most common adverse reactions observed in both groups were upper respiratory infection, headache, abdominal pain, and nausea *[see Use in Specific Populations (8.4) and Clinical Studies (14.2)]*.

6.2 Postmarketing Experience

Because the below reactions are reported voluntarily from a population of uncertain size, it is generally not possible to reliably estimate their frequency or establish a causal relationship to drug exposure. The following additional adverse reactions have been identified during postapproval use of simvastatin: pruritus, alopecia, a variety of skin changes (e.g., nodules, discoloration, dryness of skin/mucous membranes, changes to hair/nails), dizziness, muscle cramps, myalgia, pancreatitis, paresthesia, peripheral neuropathy, vomiting, anemia, erectile dysfunction, interstitial lung disease, rhabdomyolysis, hepatitis/jaundice, fatal and non-fatal hepatic failure, and depression.

There have been rare reports of immune-mediated necrotizing myopathy associated with statin use *[see Warnings and Precautions (5.1)]*.

An apparent hypersensitivity syndrome has been reported rarely which has included some of the following features: anaphylaxis, angioedema, lupus erythematous-like syndrome, polymyalgia rheumatica, dermatomyositis, vasculitis, purpura, thrombocytopenia, leukopenia, hemolytic anemia, positive ANA, ESR increase, eosinophilia, arthritis, arthralgia, urticaria, asthenia, photosensitivity, fever, chills, flushing, malaise, dyspnea, toxic epidermal necrolysis, erythema multiforme, including Stevens-Johnson syndrome.

There have been rare postmarketing reports of cognitive impairment (e.g., memory loss, forgetfulness, amnesia, memory impairment, confusion) associated with statin use. These cognitive issues have been reported for all statins. The reports are generally nonserious, and reversible upon statin discontinuation, with variable times to symptom onset (1 day to years) and symptom resolution (median of 3 weeks).

7 DRUG INTERACTIONS

7.1 Strong CYP3A4 Inhibitors, Cyclosporine, or Danazol

Strong CYP3A4 inhibitors: Simvastatin, like several other inhibitors of HMG-CoA reductase, is a substrate of CYP3A4. Simvastatin is metabolized by CYP3A4 but has no CYP3A4 inhibitory activity; therefore it is not expected to affect the plasma concentrations of other drugs metabolized by CYP3A4.

Elevated plasma levels of HMG-CoA reductase inhibitory activity increases the risk of myopathy and rhabdomyolysis, particularly with higher doses of simvastatin. [See Warnings and Precautions (5.1) and Clinical Pharmacology (12.3).] Concomitant use of drugs labeled as having a strong inhibitory effect on CYP3A4 is contraindicated [see Contraindications (4)]. If treatment with itraconazole, ketoconazole, posaconazole, voriconazole, erythromycin, clarithromycin or telithromycin is unavoidable, therapy with simvastatin must be suspended during the course of treatment.

Cyclosporine or Danazol: The risk of myopathy, including rhabdomyolysis, is increased by concomitant administration of cyclosporine or danazol. Therefore, concomitant use of these drugs is contraindicated [see Contraindications (4), Warnings and Precautions (5.1) and Clinical Pharmacology (12.3)].

7.2 Lipid-Lowering Drugs That Can Cause Myopathy When Given Alone

Gemfibrozil: Contraindicated with simvastatin [see Contraindications (4) and Warnings and Precautions (5.1)]. Other fibrates: Caution should be used when prescribing with simvastatin [see Warnings and Precautions (5.1)].

7.3 Amiodarone, Dronedarone, Ranolazine, or Calcium Channel Blockers

The risk of myopathy, including rhabdomyolysis, is increased by concomitant administration of amiodarone, dronedarone, ranolazine, or calcium channel blockers such as verapamil, diltiazem, or amlodipine [see Dosage and Administration (2.3) and Warnings and Precautions (5.1), and Table 3 in Clinical Pharmacology (12.3)].

7.4 Niacin

Cases of myopathy/rhabdomyolysis have been observed with simvastatin coadministered with lipid-modifying doses (≥1 g/day niacin) of niacin-containing products. In particular, caution should be used when treating Chinese patients with simvastatin doses exceeding 20 mg/day coadministered with lipid-modifying doses of niacin-containing products. Because the risk for myopathy is dose-related, Chinese patients should not receive simvastatin 80 mg coadministered with lipid-modifying doses of niacin-containing products. [See Warnings and Precautions (5.1) and Clinical Pharmacology (12.3).]

7.5 Digoxin

In one study, concomitant administration of digoxin with simvastatin resulted in a slight elevation in digoxin concentrations in plasma. Patients taking digoxin should be monitored appropriately when simvastatin is initiated [see Clinical Pharmacology (12.3)].

7.6 Coumarin Anticoagulants

In two clinical studies, one in normal volunteers and the other in hypercholesterolemic patients, simvastatin 20-40 mg/day modestly potentiated the effect of coumarin anticoagulants: the prothrombin time, reported as International Normalized Ratio (INR), increased from a baseline of 1.7 to 1.8 and from 2.6 to 3.4 in the volunteer and patient studies, respectively. With other statins, clinically evident bleeding and/or increased prothrombin time has been reported in a few patients taking coumarin anticoagulants concomitantly. In such patients, prothrombin time should be determined before starting simvastatin and frequently enough during early therapy to ensure that no significant alteration of prothrombin time occurs. Once a stable prothrombin time has been documented, prothrombin times can be monitored at the intervals usually recommended for patients on coumarin anticoagulants. If the dose of simvastatin is changed or discontinued, the same procedure should be repeated. Simvastatin therapy has not been associated with bleeding or with changes in prothrombin time in patients not taking anticoagulants.

7.7 Colchicine

Cases of myopathy, including rhabdomyolysis, have been reported with simvastatin coadministered with colchicine, and caution should be exercised when prescribing simvastatin with colchicine.

8 USE IN SPECIFIC POPULATIONS

8.1 Pregnancy

Pregnancy Category X [See Contraindications (4).]

ZOCOR is contraindicated in women who are or may become pregnant. Lipid lowering drugs offer no benefit during pregnancy, because cholesterol and cholesterol derivatives are needed for normal fetal development. Atherosclerosis is a chronic process, and discontinuation of lipid-lowering drugs during pregnancy should have little impact on long-term outcomes of primary hypercholesterolemia therapy. There are no adequate and well-controlled studies of use with ZOCOR during pregnancy; however, there are rare reports of congenital anomalies in infants exposed to statins in utero. Animal reproduction studies of simvastatin in rats and rabbits showed no evidence of teratogenicity. Serum cholesterol and triglycerides increase during normal pregnancy, and cholesterol or cholesterol derivatives are essential for fetal development. Because statins decrease cholesterol synthesis and possibly the synthesis of other biologically active substances derived from cholesterol, ZOCOR may cause fetal harm when administered to a pregnant woman. If ZOCOR is used during pregnancy or if the patient becomes pregnant while taking this drug, the patient should be apprised of the potential hazard to the fetus. There are rare reports of congenital anomalies following intrauterine exposure to statins. In a review[2] of approximately 100 prospectively followed pregnancies in women exposed to simvastatin or another structurally related statin, the incidences of congenital anomalies, spontaneous abortions, and fetal deaths/stillbirths did not exceed those expected in the general population. However, the study was only able to exclude a 3- to 4-fold increased risk of congenital anomalies over the background rate. In 89% of these cases, drug treatment was initiated prior to pregnancy and was discontinued during the first trimester when pregnancy was identified.

Simvastatin was not teratogenic in rats or rabbits at doses (25, 10 mg/kg/day, respectively) that resulted in 3 times the human exposure based on mg/m² surface area. However, in studies with another structurally-related statin, skeletal malformations were observed in rats and mice.

Women of childbearing potential, who require treatment with ZOCOR for a lipid disorder, should be advised to use effective contraception. For women trying to conceive, discontinuation of ZOCOR should be considered. If pregnancy occurs, ZOCOR should be immediately discontinued.

[2] Manson, J.M., Freyssinges, C., Ducrocq, M.B., Stephenson, W.P., Postmarketing Surveillance of Lovastatin and Simvastatin Exposure During Pregnancy, Reproductive Toxicology, 10(6):439-446, 1996.

8.3 Nursing Mothers

It is not known whether simvastatin is excreted in human milk. Because a small amount of another drug in this class is excreted in human milk and because of the potential for serious adverse reactions in nursing infants, women taking simvastatin should not nurse their infants. A decision should be made whether to discontinue nursing or discontinue drug, taking into account the importance of the drug to the mother [see Contraindications (4)].

8.4 Pediatric Use

Safety and effectiveness of simvastatin in patients 10-17 years of age with heterozygous familial hypercholesterolemia have been evaluated in a controlled clinical trial in adolescent boys and in girls who were at least 1 year postmenarche. Patients treated with simvastatin had an adverse reaction profile similar to that of patients treated with placebo. **Doses greater than 40 mg have not been studied in this population.** In this limited controlled study, there was no significant effect on growth or sexual maturation in the adolescent boys or girls, or on menstrual cycle length in girls. [See Dosage and Administration (2.5), Adverse Reactions (6.1), Clinical Studies (14.2).] Adolescent females should be counseled on appropriate contraceptive methods while on simvastatin therapy [see Contraindications (4) and Use in Specific Populations (8.1)]. Simvastatin has not been studied in patients younger than 10 years of age, nor in pre-menarchal girls.

8.5 Geriatric Use

Of the 2,423 patients who received ZOCOR in Phase III clinical studies and the 10,269 patients in the Heart Protection Study who received ZOCOR, 363 (15%) and 5,366 (52%), respectively were ≥65 years old. In HPS, 615 (6%) were ≥75 years old. No overall differences in safety or effectiveness were observed between these subjects and younger subjects, and other reported clinical experience has not identified differences in responses between the elderly and younger patients, but greater sensitivity of some older individuals cannot be ruled out. Since advanced age (≥65 years) is a predisposing factor for myopathy, ZOCOR should be prescribed with caution in the elderly. [See Clinical Pharmacology (12.3).]

A pharmacokinetic study with simvastatin showed the mean plasma level of statin activity to be approximately

45% higher in elderly patients between 70-78 years of age compared with patients between 18-30 years of age. In 4S, 1,021 (23%) of 4,444 patients were 65 or older. Lipid-lowering efficacy was at least as great in elderly patients compared with younger patients, and ZOCOR significantly reduced total mortality and CHD mortality in elderly patients with a history of CHD. In HPS, 52% of patients were elderly (4,891 patients 65-69 years and 5,806 patients 70 years or older). The relative risk reductions of CHD death, non-fatal MI, coronary and non-coronary revascularization procedures, and stroke were similar in older and younger patients [see Clinical Studies (14.1)]. In HPS, among 32,145 patients entering the active run-in period, there were 2 cases of myopathy/rhabdomyolysis; these patients were aged 67 and 73. Of the 7 cases of myopathy/rhabdomyolysis among 10,269 patients allocated to simvastatin, 4 were aged 65 or more (at baseline), of whom one was over 75. There were no overall differences in safety between older and younger patients in either 4S or HPS.

Because advanced age (≥65 years) is a predisposing factor for myopathy, including rhabdomyolysis, ZOCOR should be prescribed with caution in the elderly. In a clinical trial of patients treated with simvastatin 80 mg/day, patients ≥65 years of age had an increased risk of myopathy, including rhabdomyolysis, compared to patients <65 years of age. [See Warnings and Precautions (5.1) and Clinical Pharmacology (12.3).]

8.6 Renal Impairment

Caution should be exercised when ZOCOR is administered to patients with severe renal impairment. [See Dosage and Administration (2.6).]

8.7 Hepatic Impairment

ZOCOR is contraindicated in patients with active liver disease which may include unexplained persistent elevations in hepatic transaminase levels [see Contraindications (4) and Warnings and Precautions (5.2)].

10 OVERDOSAGE

Significant lethality was observed in mice after a single oral dose of 9 g/m². No evidence of lethality was observed in rats or dogs treated with doses of 30 and 100 g/m², respectively. No specific diagnostic signs were observed in rodents. At these doses the only signs seen in dogs were emesis and mucoid stools.

A few cases of overdosage with ZOCOR have been reported; the maximum dose taken was 3.6 g. All patients recovered without sequelae. Supportive measures should be taken in the event of an overdose. The dialyzability of simvastatin and its metabolites in man is not known at present.

11 DESCRIPTION

ZOCOR (simvastatin) is a lipid-lowering agent that is derived synthetically from a fermentation product of Aspergillus terreus. After oral ingestion, simvastatin, which is an inactive lactone, is hydrolyzed to the corresponding β-hydroxyacid form. This is an inhibitor of 3-hydroxy-3-methylglutaryl-coenzyme A (HMG-CoA) reductase. This enzyme catalyzes the conversion of HMG-CoA to mevalonate, which is an early and rate-limiting step in the biosynthesis of cholesterol.

Simvastatin is butanoic acid, 2,2-dimethyl-,1,2,3,7,8,8a-hexahydro-3,7-dimethyl-8-[2-(tetrahydro-4-hydroxy-6-oxo-2H-pyran-2-yl)-ethyl]-1-naphthalenyl ester, [1S-[1α,3α,7β,8β(2S*,4S*),-8aβ]]. The empirical formula of simvastatin is $C_{25}H_{38}O_5$ and its molecular weight is 418.57. Its structural formula is:

Simvastatin is a white to off-white, nonhygroscopic, crystalline powder that is practically insoluble in water, and freely soluble in chloroform, methanol and ethanol.

Tablets ZOCOR for oral administration contain either 5 mg, 10 mg, 20 mg, 40 mg or 80 mg of simvastatin and the following inactive ingredients: ascorbic acid, citric acid, hydroxypropyl cellulose, hypromellose, iron oxides, lactose, magnesium stearate, microcrystalline cellulose, starch, talc, and titanium dioxide. Butylated hydroxyanisole is added as a preservative.

12 CLINICAL PHARMACOLOGY

12.1 Mechanism of Action

Simvastatin is a prodrug and is hydrolyzed to its active β-hydroxyacid form, simvastatin acid, after administration.

Simvastatin is a specific inhibitor of 3-hydroxy-3-methylglutaryl-coenzyme A (HMG-CoA) reductase, the enzyme that catalyzes the conversion of HMG-CoA to mevalonate, an early and rate limiting step in the biosynthetic pathway for cholesterol. In addition, simvastatin reduces VLDL and TG and increases HDL-C.

12.2 Pharmacodynamics

Epidemiological studies have demonstrated that elevated levels of total-C, LDL-C, as well as decreased levels of HDL-C are associated with the development of atherosclerosis and increased cardiovascular risk. Lowering LDL-C decreases this risk. However, the independent effect of raising HDL-C or lowering TG on the risk of coronary and cardiovascular morbidity and mortality has not been determined.

12.3 Pharmacokinetics

Simvastatin is a lactone that is readily hydrolyzed in vivo to the corresponding β-hydroxyacid, a potent inhibitor of HMG-CoA reductase. Inhibition of HMG-CoA reductase is the basis for an assay in pharmacokinetic studies of the β-hydroxyacid metabolites (active inhibitors) and, following base hydrolysis, active plus latent inhibitors (total inhibitors) in plasma following administration of simvastatin.

Following an oral dose of ^{14}C-labeled simvastatin in man, 13% of the dose was excreted in urine and 60% in feces. Plasma concentrations of total radioactivity (simvastatin plus ^{14}C-metabolites) peaked at 4 hours and declined rapidly to about 10% of peak by 12 hours postdose. Since simvastatin undergoes extensive first-pass extraction in the liver, the availability of the drug to the general circulation is low (<5%).

Both simvastatin and its β-hydroxyacid metabolite are highly bound (approximately 95%) to human plasma proteins. Rat studies indicate that when radiolabeled simvastatin was administered, simvastatin-derived radioactivity crossed the blood-brain barrier.

The major active metabolites of simvastatin present in human plasma are the β-hydroxyacid of simvastatin and its 6'-hydroxy, 6'-hydroxymethyl, and 6'-exomethylene derivatives. Peak plasma concentrations of both active and total inhibitors were attained within 1.3 to 2.4 hours postdose. While the recommended therapeutic dose range is 5 to 40 mg/day, there was no substantial deviation from linearity of AUC of inhibitors in the general circulation with an increase in dose to as high as 120 mg. Relative to the fasting state, the plasma profile of inhibitors was not affected when simvastatin was administered immediately before an American Heart Association recommended low-fat meal.

In a study including 16 elderly patients between 70 and 78 years of age who received ZOCOR 40 mg/day, the mean plasma level of HMG-CoA reductase inhibitory activity was increased approximately 45% compared with 18 patients between 18-30 years of age. Clinical study experience in the elderly (n=1522), suggests that there were no overall differences in safety between elderly and younger patients [see Use in Specific Populations (8.5)].

Kinetic studies with another statin, having a similar principal route of elimination, have suggested that for a given dose level higher systemic exposure may be achieved in patients with severe renal insufficiency (as measured by creatinine clearance).

Although the mechanism is not fully understood, cyclosporine has been shown to increase the AUC of statins. The increase in AUC for simvastatin acid is presumably due, in part, to inhibition of CYP3A4.

The risk of myopathy is increased by high levels of HMG-CoA reductase inhibitory activity in plasma. Inhibitors of CYP3A4 can raise the plasma levels of HMG-CoA reductase inhibitory activity and increase the risk of myopathy [see Warnings and Precautions (5.1) and Drug Interactions (7.1)].

[See table 3 above and on next page]

In a study of 12 healthy volunteers, simvastatin at the 80-mg dose had no effect on the metabolism of the probe cytochrome P450 isoform 3A4 (CYP3A4) substrates midazolam and erythromycin. This indicates that simvastatin is not an inhibitor of CYP3A4, and, therefore, is not expected to affect the plasma levels of other drugs metabolized by CYP3A4.

Coadministration of simvastatin (40 mg QD for 10 days) resulted in an increase in the maximum levels of cardioactive digoxin (given as a single 0.4 mg dose on day 10) by approximately 0.3 ng/mL.

13 NONCLINICAL TOXICOLOGY

13.1 Carcinogenesis, Mutagenesis, Impairment of Fertility

In a 72-week carcinogenicity study, mice were administered daily doses of simvastatin of 25, 100, and 400 mg/kg body weight, which resulted in mean plasma drug levels approximately 1, 4, and 8 times higher than the mean human plasma drug level, respectively (as total inhibitory activity based on AUC) after an 80-mg oral dose. Liver carcinomas were significantly increased in high-dose females and mid-

Table 3: Effect of Coadministered Drugs or Grapefruit Juice on Simvastatin Systemic Exposure

Coadministered Drug or Grapefruit Juice	Dosing of Coadministered Drug or Grapefruit Juice	Dosing of Simvastatin	Geometric Mean Ratio (Ratio*with / without coadministered drug) No Effect = 1.00		
				AUC	C_{max}
Contraindicated with simvastatin [see Contraindications (4) and Warnings and Precautions (5.1)]					
Telithromycin[†]	200 mg QD for 4 days	80 mg	simvastatin acid[‡] simvastatin	12 8.9	15 5.3
Nelfinavir[†]	1250 mg BID for 14 days	20 mg QD for 28 days	simvastatin acid[‡] simvastatin	6	6.2
Itraconazole[†]	200 mg QD for 4 days	80 mg	simvastatin acid[‡] simvastatin	13.1	13.1
Posaconazole	100 mg (oral suspension) QD for 13 days 200 mg (oral suspension) QD for 13 days	40 mg 40 mg	simvastatin acid simvastatin simvastatin acid simvastatin	7.3 10.3 8.5 10.6	9.2 9.4 9.5 11.4
Gemfibrozil	600 mg BID for 3 days	40 mg	simvastatin acid simvastatin	2.85 1.35	2.18 0.91
Avoid grapefruit juice with simvastatin [see Warnings and Precautions (5.1)]					
Grapefruit Juice[§] (high dose)	200 mL of double-strength TID[¶]	60 mg single dose	simvastatin acid simvastatin	7 16	
Grapefruit Juice[§] (low dose)	8 oz (about 237mL) of single-strength[#]	20 mg single dose	simvastatin acid simvastatin	1.3 1.9	
Avoid taking with >10 mg simvastatin, based on clinical and/or postmarketing experience [see Warnings and Precautions (5.1)]					
Verapamil SR	240 mg QD Days 1-7 then 240 mg BID on Days 8-10	80 mg on Day 10	simvastatin acid simvastatin	2.3 2.5	2.4 2.1
Diltiazem	120 mg BID for 10 days	80 mg on Day 10	simvastatin acid simvastatin	2.69 3.10	2.69 2.88
Diltiazem	120 mg BID for 14 days	20 mg on Day 14	simvastatin	4.6	3.6
Dronedarone	400 mg BID for 14 days	40 mg QD for 14 days	simvastatin acid simvastatin	1.96 3.90	2.14 3.75
Avoid taking with >20 mg simvastatin, based on clinical and/or postmarketing experience [see Warnings and Precautions (5.1)]					
Amiodarone	400 mg QD for 3 days	40 mg on Day 3	simvastatin acid simvastatin	1.75 1.76	1.72 1.79
Amlodipine	10 mg QD × 10 days	80 mg on Day 10	simvastatin acid simvastatin	1.58 1.77	1.56 1.47
Ranolazine SR	1000 mg BID for 7 days	80 mg on Day 1 and Days 6-9	simvastatin acid simvastatin	2.26 1.86	2.28 1.75

(Table continued on next page)

and high-dose males with a maximum incidence of 90% in males. The incidence of adenomas of the liver was significantly increased in mid- and high-dose females. Drug treatment also significantly increased the incidence of lung adenomas in mid- and high-dose males and females. Adenomas of the Harderian gland (a gland of the eye of rodents) were significantly higher in high-dose mice than in controls. No evidence of a tumorigenic effect was observed at 25 mg/kg/day.

In a separate 92-week carcinogenicity study in mice at doses up to 25 mg/kg/day, no evidence of a tumorigenic effect was observed (mean plasma drug levels were 1 times higher than humans given 80 mg simvastatin as measured by AUC).

In a two-year study in rats at 25 mg/kg/day, there was a statistically significant increase in the incidence of thyroid follicular adenomas in female rats exposed to approximately 11 times higher levels of simvastatin than in humans given 80 mg simvastatin (as measured by AUC).

A second two-year rat carcinogenicity study with doses of 50 and 100 mg/kg/day produced hepatocellular adenomas and carcinomas (in female rats at both doses and in males at 100 mg/kg/day). Thyroid follicular cell adenomas were increased in males and females at both doses; thyroid follicular cell carcinomas were increased in females at

100 mg/kg/day. The increased incidence of thyroid neoplasms appears to be consistent with findings from other statins. These treatment levels represented plasma drug levels (AUC) of approximately 7 and 15 times (males) and 22 and 25 times (females) the mean human plasma drug exposure after an 80 milligram daily dose.

No evidence of mutagenicity was observed in a microbial mutagenicity (Ames) test with or without rat or mouse liver metabolic activation. In addition, no evidence of damage to genetic material was noted in an in vitro alkaline elution assay using rat hepatocytes, a V-79 mammalian cell forward mutation study, an in vitro chromosome aberration study in CHO cells, or an in vivo chromosomal aberration assay in mouse bone marrow.

There was decreased fertility in male rats treated with simvastatin for 34 weeks at 25 mg/kg body weight (4 times the maximum human exposure level, based on AUC, in patients receiving 80 mg/day); however, this effect was not observed during a subsequent fertility study in which simvastatin was administered at this same dose level to male rats for 11 weeks (the entire cycle of spermatogenesis including epididymal maturation). No microscopic changes were observed in the testes of rats from either study. At 180 mg/kg/day, (which produces exposure levels 22 times higher than those in humans taking 80 mg/day based on

Table 3 *(cont.)*: Effect of Coadministered Drugs or Grapefruit Juice on Simvastatin Systemic Exposure

Coadministered Drug or Grapefruit Juice	Dosing of Coadministered Drug or Grapefruit Juice	Dosing of Simvastatin		Geometric Mean Ratio (Ratio*with / without coadministered drug) No Effect = 1.00	
				AUC	C_{max}
Avoid taking with >20 mg simvastatin (or 40 mg for patients who have previously taken 80 mg simvastatin chronically, e.g., for 12 months or more, without evidence of muscle toxicity), based on clinical experience					
Lomitapide	60 mg QD for 7 days	40 mg single dose	simvastatin acid simvastatin	1.7 2	1.6 2
Lomitapide	10 mg QD for 7 days	20 mg single dose	simvastatin acid simvastatin	1.4 1.6	1.4 1.7
No dosing adjustments required for the following:					
Fenofibrate	160 mg QD X 14 days	80 mg QD on Days 8-14	simvastatin acid simvastatin	0.64 0.89	0.89 0.83
Niacin extended-release[b]	2 g single dose	20 mg single dose	simvastatin acid simvastatin	1.6 1.4	1.84 1.08
Propranolol	80 mg single dose	80 mg single dose	total inhibitor active inhibitor	0.79 0.79	↓ from 33.6 to 21.1 ng·eq/mL ↓ from 7.0 to 4.7 ng·eq/mL

* Results based on a chemical assay except results with propranolol as indicated.
† Results could be representative of the following CYP3A4 inhibitors: ketoconazole, erythromycin, clarithromycin, HIV protease inhibitors, and nefazodone.
‡ Simvastatin acid refers to the β-hydroxyacid of simvastatin.
§ The effect of amounts of grapefruit juice between those used in these two studies on simvastatin pharmacokinetics has not been studied.
¶ Double-strength: one can of frozen concentrate diluted with one can of water. Grapefruit juice was administered TID for 2 days, and 200 mL together with single dose simvastatin and 30 and 90 minutes following single dose simvastatin on Day 3.
\# Single-strength: one can of frozen concentrate diluted with 3 cans of water. Grapefruit juice was administered with breakfast for 3 days, and simvastatin was administered in the evening on Day 3.
Þ Because Chinese patients have an increased risk for myopathy with simvastatin coadministered with lipid-modifying doses (≥1 gram/day niacin) of niacin-containing products, and the risk is dose-related, Chinese patients should not receive simvastatin 80 mg coadministered with lipid-modifying doses of niacin-containing products *[see Warnings and Precautions (5.1) and Drug Interactions (7.4)]*.

Table 4: Summary of Heart Protection Study Results

Endpoint	ZOCOR (N=10,269) n (%)*	Placebo (N=10,267) n (%)*	Risk Reduction (%) (95% CI)	p-Value
Primary				
Mortality	1,328 (12.9)	1,507 (14.7)	13 (6-19)	p=0.0003
CHD mortality	587 (5.7)	707 (6.9)	18 (8-26)	p=0.0005
Secondary				
Non-fatal MI	357 (3.5)	574 (5.6)	38 (30-46)	p<0.0001
Stroke	444 (4.3)	585 (5.7)	25 (15-34)	p<0.0001
Tertiary				
Coronary revascularization	513 (5)	725 (7.1)	30 (22-38)	p<0.0001
Peripheral and other non-coronary revascularization	450 (4.4)	532 (5.2)	16 (5-26)	p=0.006

* n = number of patients with indicated event

surface area, mg/m²), seminiferous tubule degeneration (necrosis and loss of spermatogenic epithelium) was observed. In dogs, there was drug-related testicular atrophy, decreased spermatogenesis, spermatocytic degeneration and giant cell formation at 10 mg/kg/day, (approximately 2 times the human exposure, based on AUC, at 80 mg/day). The clinical significance of these findings is unclear.

13.2 Animal Toxicology and/or Pharmacology
CNS Toxicity
Optic nerve degeneration was seen in clinically normal dogs treated with simvastatin for 14 weeks at 180 mg/kg/day, a dose that produced mean plasma drug levels about 12 times higher than the mean plasma drug level in humans taking 80 mg/day.
A chemically similar drug in this class also produced optic nerve degeneration (Wallerian degeneration of retinogeniculate fibers) in clinically normal dogs in a dose-dependent fashion starting at 60 mg/kg/day, a dose that produced mean plasma drug levels about 30 times higher than the mean plasma drug level in humans taking the highest recommended dose (as measured by total enzyme inhibitory activity). This same drug also produced vestibulocochlear Wallerian-like degeneration and retinal ganglion cell chro-

matolysis in dogs treated for 14 weeks at 180 mg/kg/day, a dose that resulted in a mean plasma drug level similar to that seen with the 60 mg/kg/day dose.
CNS vascular lesions, characterized by perivascular hemorrhage and edema, mononuclear cell infiltration of perivascular spaces, perivascular fibrin deposits and necrosis of small vessels were seen in dogs treated with simvastatin at a dose of 360 mg/kg/day, a dose that produced mean plasma drug levels that were about 14 times higher than the mean plasma drug levels in humans taking 80 mg/day. Similar CNS vascular lesions have been observed with several other drugs of this class.
There were cataracts in female rats after two years of treatment with 50 and 100 mg/kg/day (22 and 25 times the human AUC at 80 mg/day, respectively) and in dogs after three months at 90 mg/kg/day (19 times) and at two years at 50 mg/kg/day (5 times).

14 CLINICAL STUDIES
14.1 Clinical Studies in Adults
Reductions in Risk of CHD Mortality and Cardiovascular Events
In 4S, the effect of therapy with ZOCOR on total mortality was assessed in 4,444 patients with CHD and baseline total

cholesterol 212-309 mg/dL (5.5-8.0 mmol/L). In this multicenter, randomized, double-blind, placebo-controlled study, patients were treated with standard care, including diet, and either ZOCOR 20-40 mg/day (n=2,221) or placebo (n=2,223) for a median duration of 5.4 years. Over the course of the study, treatment with ZOCOR led to mean reductions in total-C, LDL-C and TG of 25%, 35%, and 10%, respectively, and a mean increase in HDL-C of 8%. ZOCOR significantly reduced the risk of mortality by 30% (p=0.0003, 182 deaths in the ZOCOR group vs 256 deaths in the placebo group). The risk of CHD mortality was significantly reduced by 42% (p=0.00001, 111 vs 189 deaths). There was no statistically significant difference between groups in non-cardiovascular mortality. ZOCOR significantly decreased the risk of having major coronary events (CHD mortality plus hospital-verified and silent non-fatal myocardial infarction [MI]) by 34% (p<0.00001, 431 vs 622 patients with one or more events). The risk of having a hospital-verified non-fatal MI was reduced by 37%. ZOCOR significantly reduced the risk for undergoing myocardial revascularization procedures (coronary artery bypass grafting or percutaneous transluminal coronary angioplasty) by 37% (p<0.00001, 252 vs 383 patients). ZOCOR significantly reduced the risk of fatal plus non-fatal cerebrovascular events (combined stroke and transient ischemic attacks) by 28% (p=0.033, 75 vs 102 patients). ZOCOR reduced the risk of major coronary events to a similar extent across the range of baseline total and LDL cholesterol levels. Because there were only 53 female deaths, the effect of ZOCOR on mortality in women could not be adequately assessed. However, ZOCOR significantly lessened the risk of having major coronary events by 34% (60 vs 91 women with one or more event). The randomization was stratified by angina alone (21% of each treatment group) or a previous MI. Because there were only 57 deaths among the patients with angina alone at baseline, the effect of ZOCOR on mortality in this subgroup could not be adequately assessed. However, trends in reduced coronary mortality, major coronary events and revascularization procedures were consistent between this group and the total study cohort. Additionally, ZOCOR resulted in similar decreases in relative risk for total mortality, CHD mortality, and major coronary events in elderly patients (≥65 years), compared with younger patients.
The Heart Protection Study (HPS) was a large, multicenter, placebo-controlled, double-blind study with a mean duration of 5 years conducted in 20,536 patients (10,269 on ZOCOR 40 mg and 10,267 on placebo). Patients were allocated to treatment using a covariate adaptive method[3] which took into account the distribution of 10 important baseline characteristics of patients already enrolled and minimized the imbalance of those characteristics across the groups. Patients had a mean age of 64 years (range 40-80 years), were 97% Caucasian and were at high risk of developing a major coronary event because of existing CHD (65%), diabetes (Type 2, 26%; Type 1, 3%), history of stroke or other cerebrovascular disease (16%), peripheral vessel disease (33%), or hypertension in males ≥65 years (6%). At baseline, 3,421 patients (17%) had LDL-C levels below 100 mg/dL, of whom 953 (5%) had LDL-C levels below 80 mg/dL; 7,068 patients (34%) had levels between 100 and 130 mg/dL; and 10,047 patients (49%) had levels greater than 130 mg/dL.
The HPS results showed that ZOCOR 40 mg/day significantly reduced: total and CHD mortality; non-fatal MI, stroke, and revascularization procedures (coronary and non-coronary) (see Table 4).
[See table 4 above]
Two composite endpoints were defined in order to have sufficient events to assess relative risk reductions across a range of baseline characteristics (see Figure 1). A composite of major coronary events (MCE) was comprised of CHD mortality and non-fatal MI (analyzed by time-to-first event; 898 patients treated with ZOCOR had events and 1,212 patients on placebo had events). A composite of major vascular events (MVE) was comprised of MCE, stroke and revascularization procedures including coronary, peripheral and other non-coronary procedures (analyzed by time-to-first event; 2,033 patients treated with ZOCOR had events and 2,585 patients on placebo had events). Significant relative risk reductions were observed for both composite endpoints (27% for MCE and 24% for MVE, p<0.0001). Treatment with ZOCOR produced significant relative risk reductions for all components of the composite endpoints. The risk reductions produced by ZOCOR in both MCE and MVE were evident and consistent regardless of cardiovascular disease related medical history at study entry (i.e., CHD alone; or peripheral vascular disease, cerebrovascular disease, diabetes or treated hypertension, with or without CHD), gender, age, creatinine levels up to the entry limit of 2.3 mg/dL, baseline levels of LDL-C, HDL-C, apolipoprotein B and A-1, baseline concomitant cardiovascular medications (i.e., aspirin, beta blockers, or calcium channel blockers), smoking status, alcohol intake, or obesity. Diabetics showed risk reductions for MCE and MVE due to ZOCOR treatment regardless of baseline HbA1c levels or obesity with the greatest effects seen for diabetics without CHD.

[See figure 1 above]

Angiographic Studies

In the Multicenter Anti-Atheroma Study, the effect of simvastatin on atherosclerosis was assessed by quantitative coronary angiography in hypercholesterolemic patients with CHD. In this randomized, double-blind, controlled study, patients were treated with simvastatin 20 mg/day or placebo. Angiograms were evaluated at baseline, two and four years. The co-primary study endpoints were mean change per-patient in minimum and mean lumen diameters, indicating focal and diffuse disease, respectively. ZOCOR significantly slowed the progression of lesions as measured in the Year 4 angiogram by both parameters, as well as by change in percent diameter stenosis. In addition, simvastatin significantly decreased the proportion of patients with new lesions and with new total occlusions.

Modifications of Lipid Profiles

Primary Hyperlipidemia (Fredrickson type lla and llb)

ZOCOR has been shown to be effective in reducing total-C and LDL-C in heterozygous familial and non-familial forms of hyperlipidemia and in mixed hyperlipidemia. Maximal to near maximal response is generally achieved within 4-6 weeks and maintained during chronic therapy. ZOCOR significantly decreased total-C, LDL-C, total-C/HDL-C ratio, and LDL-C/HDL-C ratio; ZOCOR also decreased TG and increased HDL-C (see Table 5).

[See table 5 above]

Hypertriglyceridemia (Fredrickson type IV)

The results of a subgroup analysis in 74 patients with type IV hyperlipidemia from a 130-patient, double-blind, placebo-controlled, 3-period crossover study are presented in Table 6.

[See table 6 at top of next page]

Dysbetalipoproteinemia (Fredrickson type lll)

The results of a subgroup analysis in 7 patients with type lll hyperlipidemia (dysbetalipoproteinemia) (apo E2/2) (VLDL-C/TG>0.25) from a 130-patient, double-blind, placebo-controlled, 3-period crossover study are presented in Table 7.

[See table 7 at top of next page]

Homozygous Familial Hypercholesterolemia

In a controlled clinical study, 12 patients 15-39 years of age with homozygous familial hypercholesterolemia received simvastatin 40 mg/day in a single dose or in 3 divided doses, or 80 mg/day in 3 divided doses. In 11 patients with reductions in LDL-C, the mean LDL-C changes for the 40- and 80-mg doses were 14% (range 8% to 23%, median 12%) and 30% (range 14% to 46%, median 29%), respectively. One patient had an increase of 15% in LDL-C. Another patient with absent LDL-C receptor function had an LDL-C reduction of 41% with the 80-mg dose.

Endocrine Function

In clinical studies, simvastatin did not impair adrenal reserve or significantly reduce basal plasma cortisol concentration. Small reductions from baseline in basal plasma testosterone in men were observed in clinical studies with simvastatin, an effect also observed with other statins and the bile acid sequestrant cholestyramine. There was no effect on plasma gonadotropin levels. In a placebo-controlled, 12-week study there was no significant effect of simvastatin 80 mg on the plasma testosterone response to human chorionic gonadotropin. In another 24-week study, simvastatin 20-40 mg had no detectable effect on spermatogenesis. In 4S, in which 4,444 patients were randomized to simvastatin 20-40 mg/day or placebo for a median duration of 5.4 years, the incidence of male sexual adverse events in the two treatment groups was not significantly different. Because of these factors, the small changes in plasma testosterone are unlikely to be clinically significant. The effects, if any, on the pituitary-gonadal axis in pre-menopausal women are unknown.

[3] D.R. Taves, Minimization: a new method of assigning patients to treatment and control groups. Clin. Pharmacol. Ther. 15 (1974), pp. 443-453.

14.2   Clinical Studies in Adolescents

In a double-blind, placebo-controlled study, 175 patients (99 adolescent boys and 76 post-menarchal girls) 10-17 years of age (mean age 14.1 years) with heterozygous familial hypercholesterolemia (HeFH) were randomized to simvastatin (n=106) or placebo (n=67) for 24 weeks (base study). Inclusion in the study required a baseline LDL-C level between 160 and 400 mg/dL and at least one parent with an LDL-C level >189 mg/dL. The dosage of simvastatin (once daily in the evening) was 10 mg for the first 8 weeks, 20 mg for the second 8 weeks, and 40 mg thereafter. In a 24-week extension, 144 patients elected to continue therapy with simvastatin 40 mg or placebo.

ZOCOR significantly decreased plasma levels of total-C, LDL-C, and Apo B (see Table 8). Results from the extension at 48 weeks were comparable to those observed in the base study.

[See table 8 at top of next page]

Baseline Characteristics	N	Major Vascular Events				Major Coronary Events			
		Incidence (%) ZOCOR	Placebo	Favors ZOCOR	Favors Placebo	Incidence (%) ZOCOR	Placebo	Favors ZOCOR	Favors Placebo
All patients	20,536	19.8	25.2			8.7	11.8		
Without CHD	7,150	16.1	20.8			5.1	8.0		
With CHD	13,386	21.8	27.5			10.7	14.0		
Diabetes mellitus	5,963	20.2	25.1			9.4	12.6		
Without CHD	3,982	13.8	18.6			5.5	8.4		
With CHD	1,981	33.4	37.8			17.4	21.0		
Without diabetes mellitus	14,573	19.6	25.2			8.5	11.5		
Peripheral vascular disease	6,748	26.4	32.7			10.9	13.8		
Without CHD	2,701	24.7	30.5			7.0	10.1		
With CHD	4,047	27.6	34.3			13.4	16.4		
Cerebrovascular disease	3,280	24.7	29.8			10.4	13.3		
Without CHD	1,820	18.7	23.6			5.9	8.7		
With CHD	1,460	32.4	37.4			16.2	19.0		
Gender									
Female	5,082	14.4	17.7			5.2	7.8		
Male	15,454	21.6	27.6			9.9	13.1		
Age (years)									
≥ 40 to < 65	9,839	16.9	22.1			6.2	9.2		
≥ 65 to < 70	4,891	20.9	27.2			9.5	13.1		
≥ 70	5,806	23.6	28.7			12.4	15.2		
LDL-cholesterol (mg/dL)									
< 100	3,421	16.4	21.0			7.5	9.8		
≥ 100 to < 130	7,068	18.9	24.7			7.9	11.9		
≥ 130	10,047	21.6	26.9			9.7	12.4		
HDL-cholesterol (mg/dL)									
< 35	7,176	22.6	29.9			10.2	14.4		
≥ 35 to < 43	5,666	20.0	25.1			8.9	11.7		
≥ 43	7,694	17.0	20.9			7.3	9.4		
		0.4 0.6 0.8 1.0 1.2				0.4 0.6 0.8 1.0 1.2			
		Risk Ratio (95% CI)				Risk Ratio (95% CI)			

N = number of patients in each subgroup. The inverted triangles are point estimates of the relative risk, with their 95% confidence intervals represented as a line. The area of a triangle is proportional to the number of patients with MVE or MCE in the subgroup relative to the number with MVE or MCE, respectively, in the entire study population. The vertical solid line represents a relative risk of one. The vertical dashed line represents the point estimate of relative risk in the entire study population.

Figure 1: The Effects of Treatment with ZOCOR on Major Vascular Events and Major Coronary Events in HPS

Table 5: Mean Response in Patients with Primary Hyperlipidemia and Combined (mixed) Hyperlipidemia (Mean Percent Change from Baseline After 6 to 24 Weeks)

TREATMENT	N	TOTAL-C	LDL-C	HDL-C	TG*
Lower Dose Comparative Study[†] (Mean % Change at Week 6)					
ZOCOR 5 mg q.p.m.	109	-19	-26	10	-12
ZOCOR 10 mg q.p.m.	110	-23	-30	12	-15
Scandinavian Simvastatin Survival Study[‡] (Mean % Change at Week 6)					
Placebo	2223	-1	-1	0	-2
ZOCOR 20 mg q.p.m.	2221	-28	-38	8	-19
Upper Dose Comparative Study[§] (Mean % Change Averaged at Weeks 18 and 24)					
ZOCOR 40 mg q.p.m.	433	-31	-41	9	-18
ZOCOR 80 mg q.p.m.[¶]	664	-36	-47	8	-24
Multi-Center Combined Hyperlipidemia Study[#] (Mean % Change at Week 6)					
Placebo	125	1	2	3	-4
ZOCOR 40 mg q.p.m.	123	-25	-29	13	-28
ZOCOR 80 mg q.p.m.	124	-31	-36	16	-33

* median percent change
† mean baseline LDL-C 244 mg/dL and median baseline TG 168 mg/dL
‡ mean baseline LDL-C 188 mg/dL and median baseline TG 128 mg/dL
§ mean baseline LDL-C 226 mg/dL and median baseline TG 156 mg/dL
¶ 21% and 36% median reduction in TG in patients with TG ≤200 mg/dL and TG >200 mg/dL, respectively. Patients with TG >350 mg/dL were excluded
# mean baseline LDL-C 156 mg/dL and median baseline TG 391 mg/dL.

After 24 weeks of treatment, the mean achieved LDL-C value was 124.9 mg/dL (range: 64.0-289.0 mg/dL) in the ZOCOR 40 mg group compared to 207.8 mg/dL (range: 128.0-334.0 mg/dL) in the placebo group.

The safety and efficacy of doses above 40 mg daily have not been studied in children with HeFH. The long-term efficacy of simvastatin therapy in childhood to reduce morbidity and mortality in adulthood has not been established.

16   HOW SUPPLIED/STORAGE AND HANDLING

No. 8360 — Tablets ZOCOR 5 mg are buff, oval, film-coated tablets, coded MSD 726 on one side and ZOCOR 5 on the other. They are supplied as follows:
NDC 0006-0726-31 unit of use bottles of 30.

No. 8146 — Tablets ZOCOR 10 mg are peach, oval, film-coated tablets, coded MSD 735 on one side and plain on the other. They are supplied as follows:
NDC 0006-0735-31 unit of use bottles of 30

NDC 0006-0735-54 unit of use bottles of 90.

No. 8147 — Tablets ZOCOR 20 mg are tan, oval, film-coated tablets, coded MSD 740 on one side and plain on the other. They are supplied as follows:
NDC 0006-0740-31 unit of use bottles of 30
NDC 0006-0740-54 unit of use bottles of 90.

No. 8148 — Tablets ZOCOR 40 mg are brick red, oval, film-coated tablets, coded MSD 749 on one side and plain on the other. They are supplied as follows:
NDC 0006-0749-31 unit of use bottles of 30
NDC 0006-0749-54 unit of use bottles of 90.

No. 6577 — Tablets ZOCOR 80 mg are brick red, capsule-shaped, film-coated tablets, coded 543 on one side and 80 on the other. They are supplied as follows:
NDC 0006-0543-31 unit of use bottles of 30
NDC 0006-0543-54 unit of use bottles of 90.

Table 6: Six-week, Lipid-lowering Effects of Simvastatin in Type IV Hyperlipidemia Median Percent Change (25th and 75th percentile) from Baseline*

TREATMENT	N	Total-C	LDL-C	HDL-C	TG	VLDL-C	Non-HDL-C
Placebo	74	+2 (-7, +7)	+1 (-8, +14)	+3 (-3, +10)	-9 (-25, +13)	-7 (-25, +11)	+1 (-9, +8)
ZOCOR 40 mg/day	74	-25 (-34, -19)	-28 (-40, -17)	+11 (+5, +23)	-29 (-43, -16)	-37 (-54, -23)	-32 (-42, -23)
ZOCOR 80 mg/day	74	-32 (-38, -24)	-37 (-46, -26)	+15 (+5, +23)	-34 (-45, -18)	-41 (-57, -28)	-38 (-49, -32)

* The median baseline values (mg/dL) for the patients in this study were: total-C = 254, LDL-C = 135, HDL-C = 36, TG = 404, VLDL-C = 83, and non-HDL-C = 215.

Table 7: Six-week, Lipid-lowering Effects of Simvastatin in Type III Hyperlipidemia Median Percent Change (min, max) from Baseline*

TREATMENT	N	Total-C	LDL-C + IDL	HDL-C	TG	VLDL-C+IDL	Non-HDL-C
Placebo	7	-8 (-24, +34)	-8 (-27, +23)	-2 (-21, +16)	+4 (-22, +90)	-4 (-28, +78)	-8 (-26, -39)
ZOCOR 40 mg/day	7	-50 (-66, -39)	-50 (-60, -31)	+7 (-8, +23)	-41 (-74, -16)	-58 (-90, -37)	-57 (-72, -44)
ZOCOR 80 mg/day	7	-52 (-55, -41)	-51 (-57, -28)	+7 (-5, +29)	-38 (-58, +2)	-60 (-72, -39)	-59 (-61, -46)

* The median baseline values (mg/dL) were: total-C = 324, LDL-C = 121, HDL-C = 31, TG = 411, VLDL-C = 170, and non-HDL-C = 291.

Table 8: Lipid-Lowering Effects of Simvastatin in Adolescent Patients with Heterozygous Familial Hypercholesterolemia (Mean Percent Change from Baseline)

Dosage	Duration	N		Total-C	LDL-C	HDL-C	TG*	Apo B
Placebo	24 Weeks	67	% Change from Baseline (95% CI)	1.6 (-2.2, 5.3)	1.1 (-3.4, 5.5)	3.6 (-0.7, 8.0)	-3.2 (-11.8, 5.4)	-0.5 (-4.7, 3.6)
			Mean baseline, mg/dL (SD)	278.6 (51.8)	211.9 (49.0)	46.9 (11.9)	90.0 (50.7)	186.3 (38.1)
ZOCOR	24 Weeks	106	% Change from Baseline (95% CI)	-26.5 (-29.6, -23.3)	-36.8 (-40.5, -33.0)	8.3 (4.6, 11.9)	-7.9 (-15.8, 0.0)	-32.4 (-35.9, -29.0)
			Mean baseline, mg/dL (SD)	270.2 (44.0)	203.8 (41.5)	47.7 (9.0)	78.3 (46.0)	179.9 (33.8)

* median percent change

Storage
Store between 5-30°C (41-86°F).

17   PATIENT COUNSELING INFORMATION

Patients should be advised to adhere to their National Cholesterol Education Program (NCEP)-recommended diet, a regular exercise program, and periodic testing of a fasting lipid panel.

Patients should be advised about substances they should not take concomitantly with simvastatin [see Contraindications (4) and Warnings and Precautions (5.1)]. Patients should also be advised to inform other healthcare professionals prescribing a new medication or increasing the dose of an existing medication that they are taking ZOCOR.

17.1   Muscle Pain

All patients starting therapy with ZOCOR should be advised of the risk of myopathy, including rhabdomyolysis, and told to report promptly any unexplained muscle pain, tenderness or weakness particularly if accompanied by malaise or fever or if these muscle signs or symptoms persist after discontinuing ZOCOR. **Patients using the 80-mg dose should be informed that the risk of myopathy, including rhabdomyolysis, is increased with use of the 80-mg dose.** The risk of myopathy, including rhabdomyolysis, occurring with use of ZOCOR is increased when taking certain types of medication or consuming grapefruit juice. Patients should discuss all medication, both prescription and over the counter, with their healthcare professional.

17.2   Liver Enzymes

It is recommended that liver function tests be performed before the initiation of ZOCOR, and thereafter when clinically indicated. All patients treated with ZOCOR should be advised to report promptly any symptoms that may indicate liver injury, including fatigue, anorexia, right upper abdominal discomfort, dark urine or jaundice.

17.3   Pregnancy

Women of childbearing age should be advised to use an effective method of birth control to prevent pregnancy while using ZOCOR. Discuss future pregnancy plans with your patients, and discuss when to stop taking ZOCOR if they are trying to conceive. Patients should be advised that if they become pregnant they should stop taking ZOCOR and call their healthcare professional.

17.4   Breastfeeding

Women who are breastfeeding should not use ZOCOR. Patients who have a lipid disorder and are breastfeeding should be advised to discuss the options with their healthcare professional.

Manuf. for: Merck Sharp & Dohme Corp., a subsidiary of **MERCK & CO., INC.**,Whitehouse Station, NJ 08889, USA
By:
MERCK SHARP & DOHME LTD.
Cramlington, Northumberland, UK NE23 3JU
For patent information:
www.merck.com/product/patent/home.html
Copyright © 1999-2014 Merck Sharp & Dohme Corp., a subsidiary of **Merck & Co., Inc.**
All rights reserved.
uspi-mk0733-t-1402r063
Shown in Product Identification Guide, page 309

ZOLINZA®   ℞

[zō-linz'-α]
(vorinostat)
Capsules

HIGHLIGHTS OF PRESCRIBING INFORMATION

These highlights do not include all the information needed to use ZOLINZA safely and effectively. See full prescribing information for ZOLINZA.
ZOLINZA® (vorinostat) Capsules
Initial U.S. Approval: 2006

——————RECENT MAJOR CHANGES——————

Dosage and Administration
Dose Modifications (2.2)   04/2013

——————INDICATIONS AND USAGE——————

ZOLINZA is a histone deacetylase (HDAC) inhibitor indicated for the treatment of cutaneous manifestations in patients with cutaneous T-cell lymphoma (CTCL) who have progressive, persistent or recurrent disease on or following two systemic therapies. (1)

——————DOSAGE AND ADMINISTRATION——————

- 400 mg orally once daily with food. (2.1)
- If patient is intolerant to therapy, reduce the dose to 300 mg orally once daily with food. If necessary, reduce the dose further to 300 mg once daily with food for 5 consecutive days each week. (2.2, 5)
- Reduce dose in patients with mild or moderate hepatic impairment. (2.2)

——————DOSAGE FORMS AND STRENGTHS——————

- Capsules: 100 mg (3)

——————CONTRAINDICATIONS——————

- None (4)

——————WARNINGS AND PRECAUTIONS——————

- Pulmonary embolism and deep vein thrombosis: Monitor for pertinent signs and symptoms. (5.1)
- Thrombocytopenia and anemia: May require dose modification or discontinuation. Monitor blood counts every 2 weeks during the first 2 months of therapy and monthly thereafter. (2.2, 5.2, 6)
- Gastrointestinal Toxicity: Nausea, vomiting and diarrhea; patients may require antiemetics, antidiarrheals, and fluid and electrolyte replacement to prevent dehydration. (5.3, 6, 17.1)
- Hyperglycemia: Monitor blood glucose every 2 weeks during the first 2 months of therapy and monthly thereafter. (5.4)
- Clinical chemistry abnormalities: Measure and correct abnormal electrolytes, creatinine, magnesium and calcium at baseline. Monitor every 2 weeks during the first 2 months of therapy and at least monthly during treatment. (5.5)
- Severe thrombocytopenia with gastrointestinal bleeding has been reported with concomitant use of ZOLINZA and other HDAC inhibitors (e.g., valproic acid). Monitor platelet counts more frequently. (5.6, 7.2)
- Fetal harm can occur when administered to a pregnant woman. Women should be apprised of the potential harm to the fetus. (5.7)

——————ADVERSE REACTIONS——————

- The most common adverse reactions (incidence ≥20%) are diarrhea, fatigue, nausea, thrombocytopenia, anorexia and dysgeusia. (6)

To report SUSPECTED ADVERSE REACTIONS, contact Merck Sharp & Dohme Corp., a subsidiary of Merck & Co., Inc., at 1-877-888-4231 or FDA at 1-800-FDA-1088 or www.fda.gov/medwatch.

——————DRUG INTERACTIONS——————

- Coumarin-derivative anticoagulants: Prolongation of prothrombin time and International Normalized Ratio (INR) have been observed with concomitant use. Monitor INR frequently. (7.1)

See 17 for PATIENT COUNSELING INFORMATION and FDA-approved patient labeling

Revised: 04/2013

FULL PRESCRIBING INFORMATION: CONTENTS*

FULL PRESCRIBING INFORMATION

1   INDICATIONS AND USAGE

ZOLINZA® is indicated for the treatment of cutaneous manifestations in patients with cutaneous T-cell lymphoma who have progressive, persistent or recurrent disease on or following two systemic therapies.

2   DOSAGE AND ADMINISTRATION

2.1   Dosing Information

The recommended dose is 400 mg orally once daily with food.

Treatment may be continued as long as there is no evidence of progressive disease or unacceptable toxicity.

ZOLINZA capsules should not be opened or crushed *[see How Supplied/Storage and Handling (16)].*

2.2   Dose Modifications

If a patient is intolerant to therapy, the dose may be reduced to 300 mg orally once daily with food. The dose may be further reduced to 300 mg once daily with food for 5 consecutive days each week, as necessary.

Hepatic Impairment

Reduce the starting dose to 300 mg orally once daily with food in patients with mild to moderate hepatic impairment (bilirubin 1 to 3 × ULN or AST > ULN). There is insufficient evidence to recommend a starting dose for patients with severe hepatic impairment (bilirubin > 3 × ULN). *[see Use in Specific Populations (8.6) and Clinical Pharmacology (12.3)].*

3   DOSAGE FORMS AND STRENGTHS

100 mg white, opaque, hard gelatin capsules with "568" over "100 mg" printed within radial bar in black ink on the capsule body.

4   CONTRAINDICATIONS

None.

5   WARNINGS AND PRECAUTIONS

5.1   Thromboembolism

Pulmonary embolism occurred in 5% (4/86) of patients receiving ZOLINZA, and deep vein thrombosis has also been reported. Monitor for signs and symptoms of these events, particularly in patients with a prior history of thromboembolic events *[see Adverse Reactions (6)].*

5.2   Myelosuppression

Treatment with ZOLINZA can cause dose-related thrombocytopenia and anemia. Monitor blood counts every 2 weeks during the first 2 months of therapy and monthly thereafter. Adjust dosage or discontinue treatment with ZOLINZA as clinically appropriate. *[See Dosage and Administration (2.2), Warnings and Precautions (5.6) and Adverse Reactions (6).]*

5.3   Gastrointestinal Toxicity

Gastrointestinal disturbances, including nausea, vomiting and diarrhea, have been reported *[see Adverse Reactions (6)]* and may require the use of antiemetic and antidiarrheal medications. Fluid and electrolytes should be replaced to prevent dehydration *[see Adverse Reactions (6.1)].* Pre-existing nausea, vomiting, and diarrhea should be adequately controlled before beginning therapy with ZOLINZA.

5.4   Hyperglycemia

Hyperglycemia has been observed in patients receiving ZOLINZA and was severe in 5% (4/86) of patients *[see Adverse Reactions (6.1)].* Monitor serum glucose every 2 weeks during the first 2 months of therapy and monthly thereafter.

5.5   Clinical Chemistry Abnormalities

Obtain chemistry tests, including serum electrolytes, creatinine, magnesium, and calcium, every 2 weeks during the first 2 months of therapy and monthly thereafter. Correct hypokalemia and hypomagnesemia prior to administration of ZOLINZA. Monitor potassium and magnesium more frequently in symptomatic patients (e.g., patients with nausea, vomiting, diarrhea, fluid imbalance or cardiac symptoms).

5.6   Severe thrombocytopenia when combined with other Histone Deacetylase (HDAC) Inhibitors

Severe thrombocytopenia leading to gastrointestinal bleeding has been reported with concomitant use of ZOLINZA and other HDAC inhibitors (e.g., valproic acid). Monitor platelet counts more frequently. *[See Drug Interactions (7.2)].*

5.7   Pregnancy

Pregnancy Category D

ZOLINZA can cause fetal harm when administered to a pregnant woman. There are no adequate and well-controlled studies of ZOLINZA in pregnant women. Results of animal studies indicate that vorinostat crosses the placenta and is found in fetal plasma at levels up to 50% of maternal concentrations. Doses up to 50 and 150 mg/kg/day were tested in rats and rabbits, respectively (~0.5 times the human exposure based on $AUC_{0-24\ hours}$). Treatment-related, developmental effects including decreased mean live fetal weights, incomplete ossifications of the skull, thoracic vertebra, sternebra, and skeletal variations (cervical ribs, supernumerary ribs, vertebral count and sacral arch variations) in rats at the highest dose of vorinostat tested. Reductions in mean live fetal weight and an elevated incidence of incomplete ossification of the metacarpals were seen in rabbits dosed at 150 mg/kg/day. The no observed effect levels (NOELs) for these findings were 15 and 50 mg/kg/day (<0.1 times the human exposure based on AUC) in rats and rabbits, respectively. A dose-related increase in the incidence of malformations of the gall bladder was noted in all drug treatment groups in rabbits versus the concurrent control. If this drug is used during pregnancy, or if the patient becomes pregnant while taking this drug, the patient should be apprised of the potential hazard to the fetus.

6   ADVERSE REACTIONS

The following serious adverse reactions have been associated with ZOLINZA in clinical trials and are discussed in greater detail in other sections of the label *[see Warnings and Precautions (5)].*

Thromboembolism *[see Warnings and Precautions (5.1)]*

Myelosuppression *[see Warnings and Precautions (5.2)]*

Gastrointestinal Toxicity *[see Warnings and Precautions (5.3)]*

Hyperglycemia *[see Warnings and Precautions (5.4)]*

Clinical Chemistry Abnormalities *[see Warnings and Precautions (5.5)]*

Severe thrombocytopenia when combined with other Histone Deacetylase (HDAC) Inhibitors *[see Warnings and Precautions (5.6)]*

The most common drug-related adverse reactions can be classified into 4 symptom complexes: gastrointestinal symptoms (diarrhea, nausea, anorexia, weight decrease, vomiting, constipation), constitutional symptoms (fatigue, chills), hematologic abnormalities (thrombocytopenia, anemia), and taste disorders (dysgeusia, dry mouth). The most common serious drug-related adverse reactions were pulmonary embolism and anemia.

6.1   Clinical Trials Experience

Because clinical trials are conducted under widely varying conditions, adverse reaction rates observed in the clinical trials of a drug cannot be directly compared to rates in the clinical trials of another drug and may not reflect the rates observed in practice.

The safety of ZOLINZA was evaluated in 107 CTCL patients in two single arm clinical studies in which 86 patients received 400 mg once daily.

The data described below reflect exposure to ZOLINZA 400 mg once daily in the 86 patients for a median number of 97.5 days on therapy (range 2 to 480+ days). Seventeen (19.8%) patients were exposed beyond 24 weeks and 8 (9.3%) patients were exposed beyond 1 year. The population of CTCL patients studied were 37 to 83 years of age, 47.7% female, 52.3% male, and 81.4% white, 16.3% black, and 1.2% Asian or multi-racial.

Common Adverse Reactions

Table 1 summarizes the frequency of CTCL patients with specific adverse reactions, using the National Cancer Institute-Common Terminology Criteria for Adverse Events (NCI-CTCAE, version 3.0).

Table 1: Clinical or Laboratory Adverse Reactions Occurring in CTCL Patients (Incidence ≥10% of patients)

Adverse Reactions	ZOLINZA 400 mg once daily (N=86)			
	All Grades		Grades 3-5*	
	n	%	n	%
Fatigue	45	52.3	3	3.5
Diarrhea	45	52.3	0	0.0
Nausea	35	40.7	3	3.5
Dysgeusia	24	27.9	0	0.0
Thrombocytopenia	22	25.6	5	5.8
Anorexia	21	24.4	2	2.3
Weight Decreased	18	20.9	1	1.2
Muscle Spasms	17	19.8	2	2.3
Alopecia	16	18.6	0	0.0
Dry Mouth	14	16.3	0	0.0
Blood Creatinine Increased	14	16.3	0	0.0
Chills	14	16.3	1	1.2
Vomiting	13	15.1	1	1.2
Constipation	13	15.1	0	0.0
Dizziness	13	15.1	1	1.2
Anemia	12	14.0	2	2.3
Decreased Appetite	12	14.0	1	1.2
Peripheral Edema	11	12.8	0	0.0
Headache	10	11.6	0	0.0
Pruritus	10	11.6	1	1.2
Cough	9	10.5	0	0.0
Upper Respiratory Infection	9	10.5	0	0.0
Pyrexia	9	10.5	1	1.2

* No Grade 5 reactions were reported.

The frequencies of more severe thrombocytopenia, anemia *[see Warnings and Precautions (5.2)]* and fatigue were increased at doses higher than 400 mg once daily of ZOLINZA.

Serious Adverse Reactions

The most common serious adverse reactions in the 86 CTCL patients in two clinical trials were pulmonary embolism reported in 4.7% (4/86) of patients, squamous cell carcinoma reported in 3.5% (3/86) of patients and anemia reported in 2.3% (2/86) of patients. There were single events of cholecystitis, death (of unknown cause), deep vein thrombosis, enterococcal infection, exfoliative dermatitis, gastrointestinal hemorrhage, infection, lobar pneumonia, myocardial infarction, ischemic stroke, pelviureteric obstruction, sepsis, spinal cord injury, streptococcal bacteremia, syncope, T-cell lymphoma, thrombocytopenia and ureteric obstruction.

Discontinuations

Of the CTCL patients who received the 400-mg once daily dose, 9.3% (8/86) of patients discontinued ZOLINZA due to adverse reactions. These adverse reactions, regardless of causality, included anemia, angioneurotic edema, asthenia, chest pain, exfoliative dermatitis, death, deep vein thrombosis, ischemic stroke, lethargy, pulmonary embolism, and spinal cord injury.

Dose Modifications

Of the CTCL patients who received the 400-mg once daily dose, 10.5% (9/86) of patients required a dose modification of ZOLINZA due to adverse reactions. These adverse reactions included increased serum creatinine, decreased appetite, hypokalemia, leukopenia, nausea, neutropenia, thrombocytopenia and vomiting. The median time to the first adverse reactions resulting in dose reduction was 42 days (range 17 to 263 days).

Laboratory Abnormalities

Laboratory abnormalities were reported in all of the 86 CTCL patients who received the 400-mg once-daily dose.

Increased serum glucose was reported as a laboratory abnormality in 69% (59/86) of CTCL patients who received the 400-mg once daily dose; only 4 of these abnormalities were severe (Grade 3). Increased serum glucose was reported as an adverse reaction in 8.1% (7/86) of CTCL patients who received the 400-mg once daily dose. *[See Warnings and Precautions (5.4).]*

Transient increases in serum creatinine were detected in 46.5% (40/86) of CTCL patients who received the 400-mg once daily dose. Of these laboratory abnormalities, 34 were NCI CTCAE Grade 1, 5 were Grade 2, and 1 was Grade 3. Proteinuria was detected as a laboratory abnormality (51.4%) in 38 of 74 patients tested. The clinical significance of this finding is unknown.

Dehydration

Based on reports of dehydration as a serious drug-related adverse reaction in clinical trials, patients were instructed to drink at least 2 L/day of fluids for adequate hydration. *[See Warnings and Precautions (5.3, 5.5).]*

Adverse Reactions in Non-CTCL Patients

The frequencies of individual adverse reactions were substantially higher in the non-CTCL population. Drug-related serious adverse reactions reported in the non-CTCL population which were not observed in the CTCL population included single events of blurred vision, asthenia, hyponatremia, tumor hemorrhage, Guillain-Barré syndrome, renal failure, urinary retention, cough, hemoptysis, hypertension, and vasculitis.

In patients recovering from bowel surgery and treated perioperatively with ZOLINZA, anastomotic healing complications including fistulas, perforations, and abscess formation have occurred.

7 DRUG INTERACTIONS

7.1 Coumarin-Derivative Anticoagulants
Prolongation of prothrombin time (PT) and International Normalized Ratio (INR) were observed in patients receiving ZOLINZA concomitantly with coumarin-derivative anticoagulants. Physicians should monitor PT and INR more frequently in patients concurrently administered ZOLINZA and coumarin derivatives.

7.2 Other HDAC Inhibitors
Severe thrombocytopenia and gastrointestinal bleeding have been reported with concomitant use of ZOLINZA and other HDAC inhibitors (e.g., valproic acid). Monitor platelet count every 2 weeks for the first 2 months. *[See Warnings and Precautions (5.6).]*

8 USE IN SPECIFIC POPULATIONS

8.1 Pregnancy
Pregnancy Category D [See Warnings and Precautions (5.7)]

8.3 Nursing Mothers
It is not known whether this drug is excreted in human milk. Because many drugs are excreted in human milk and because of the potential for serious adverse reactions in nursing infants from ZOLINZA, a decision should be made whether to discontinue nursing or discontinue the drug, taking into account the importance of the drug to the mother.

8.4 Pediatric Use
The safety and effectiveness of ZOLINZA in pediatric patients have not been established.

8.5 Geriatric Use
Of the total number of patients with CTCL in trials (N=107), 46 % were 65 years of age and over, while 15 % were 75 years of age and over. No overall differences in safety or effectiveness were observed between these subjects and younger subjects, and other reported clinical experience has not identified differences in responses between the elderly and younger patients, but greater sensitivity of some older individuals should be considered, reflecting the greater frequency of decreased hepatic, renal, or cardiac function, and of concomitant disease or other drug therapy.

8.6 Use in Patients with Hepatic Impairment
ZOLINZA was studied in 42 patients with non-CTCL cancer and varying degrees of hepatic impairment after single and multiple-dose administration. Compared to patients with normal liver function, AUC increases of 50 to 66% were observed in patients with hepatic impairment. The incidence of Grade 3 or 4 thrombocytopenia increased in patients with mild (bilirubin of 1 to $1.5 \times$ ULN and AST < ULN, or bilirubin $\leq$ ULN and AST > ULN) and moderate (bilirubin 1.5 to $\leq 3 \times$ ULN) hepatic impairment treated daily at doses of 300 and 200 mg respectively.

Patients with severe hepatic impairment (bilirubin > $3 \times$ ULN) have not been treated at doses greater than 200 mg a day. Reduce the initial dose of ZOLINZA in patients with bilirubin 1 to $3 \times$ ULN or AST > ULN. *[See Dosage and Administration (2.2) and Clinical Pharmacology (12.3).]*

8.7 Use in Patients with Renal Impairment
Vorinostat was not evaluated in patients with renal impairment. However, renal excretion does not play a role in the elimination of vorinostat. Patients with pre-existing renal impairment should be treated with caution. *[See Clinical Pharmacology (12.3).]*

10 OVERDOSAGE
No specific information is available on the treatment of overdosage of ZOLINZA.

In the event of overdose, it is reasonable to employ the usual supportive measures, e.g., remove unabsorbed material from the gastrointestinal tract, employ clinical monitoring, and institute supportive therapy, if required. It is not known if vorinostat is dialyzable.

11 DESCRIPTION
ZOLINZA contains vorinostat, which is described chemically as *N*-hydroxy-*N'*-phenyloctanediamide.

The empirical formula is $C_{14}H_{20}N_2O_3$. The molecular weight is 264.32 and the structural formula is:

Vorinostat is a white to light orange powder. It is very slightly soluble in water, slightly soluble in ethanol, isopro-

panol and acetone, freely soluble in dimethyl sulfoxide and insoluble in methylene chloride. It has no chiral centers and is non-hygroscopic. The differential scanning calorimetry ranged from 161.7 (endotherm) to 163.9°C. The pH of saturated water solutions of vorinostat drug substance was 6.6. The pKa of vorinostat was determined to be 9.2.

Each 100 mg ZOLINZA capsule for oral administration contains 100 mg vorinostat and the following inactive ingredients: microcrystalline cellulose, sodium croscarmellose and magnesium stearate. The capsule shell excipients are titanium dioxide, gelatin and sodium lauryl sulfate.

12 CLINICAL PHARMACOLOGY

12.1 Mechanism of Action
Vorinostat inhibits the enzymatic activity of histone deacetylases HDAC1, HDAC2 and HDAC3 (Class I) and HDAC6 (Class II) at nanomolar concentrations (IC_{50}<86 nM). These enzymes catalyze the removal of acetyl groups from the lysine residues of proteins, including histones and transcription factors. In some cancer cells, there is an overexpression of HDACs, or an aberrant recruitment of HDACs to oncogenic transcription factors causing hypoacetylation of core nucleosomal histones. Hypoacetylation of histones is associated with a condensed chromatin structure and repression of gene transcription. Inhibition of HDAC activity allows for the accumulation of acetyl groups on the histone lysine residues resulting in an open chromatin structure and transcriptional activation. *In vitro*, vorinostat causes the accumulation of acetylated histones and induces cell cycle arrest and/or apoptosis of some transformed cells. The mechanism of the antineoplastic effect of vorinostat has not been fully characterized.

12.2 Pharmacodynamics
Cardiac Electrophysiology
A randomized, partially-blind, placebo-controlled, 2-period crossover study was performed to assess the effects of a single 800-mg dose of vorinostat on the QTc interval in 24 patients with advanced cancer. This study was conducted to assess the impact of vorinostat on ventricular repolarization. The upper bound of the 90% confidence interval of the placebo-adjusted mean QTc interval change-from-baseline was less than 10 msec at every time point through 24 hours. Based on these study results, administration of a single supratherapeutic 800-mg dose of vorinostat does not appear to prolong the QTc interval in patients with advanced cancer; however the study did not include a positive control to demonstrate assay sensitivity. In the fasted state, oral administration of a single 800-mg dose of vorinostat resulted in a mean AUC and C_{max} and median T_{max} of 8.6±5.7 µM•hr and 1.7±0.67 µM and 2.1 (0.5-6) hours, respectively.

In clinical studies in patients with CTCL, three of 86 CTCL patients exposed to 400 mg once daily had Grade 1 (>450-470 msec) or 2 (>470-500 msec or increase of >60 msec above baseline) clinical adverse reactions of QTc prolongation. In a retrospective analysis of three Phase 1 and two Phase 2 studies, 116 patients had a baseline and at least one follow-up ECG. Four patients had Grade 2 (>470-500 msec or increase of >60 msec above baseline) and 1 patient had Grade 3 (>500 msec) QTc prolongation. In 49 non-CTCL patients from 3 clinical trials who had complete evaluation of QT interval, 2 had QTc measurements of >500 msec and 1 had a QTc prolongation of >60 msec.

12.3 Pharmacokinetics
Absorption
The pharmacokinetics of vorinostat were evaluated in 23 patients with relapsed or refractory advanced cancer. After oral administration of a single 400-mg dose of vorinostat with a high-fat meal, the mean ± standard deviation area under the curve (AUC) and peak serum concentration (C_{max}) and the median (range) time to maximum concentration (T_{max}) were 5.5±1.8 µM•hr, 1.2±0.62 µM and 4 (2-10) hours, respectively.

In the fasted state, oral administration of a single 400-mg dose of vorinostat resulted in a mean AUC and C_{max} and median T_{max} of 4.2±1.9 µM•hr and 1.2±0.35 µM and 1.5 (0.5-10) hours, respectively. Therefore, oral administration of vorinostat with a high-fat meal resulted in an increase (33%) in the extent of absorption and a modest decrease in the rate of absorption (T_{max} delayed 2.5 hours) compared to the fasted state. However, these small effects are not expected to be clinically meaningful. In clinical trials of patients with CTCL, vorinostat was taken with food. At steady state in the fed-state, oral administration of multiple 400-mg doses of vorinostat resulted in a mean AUC and C_{max} and a median T_{max} of 6.0±2.0 µM•hr, 1.2±0.53 µM and 4 (0.5-14) hours, respectively.

Distribution
Vorinostat is approximately 71% bound to human plasma proteins over the range of concentrations of 0.5 to 50 µg/mL.

Metabolism
The major pathways of vorinostat metabolism involve glucuronidation and hydrolysis followed by β-oxidation. Human serum levels of two metabolites, *O*-glucuronide of vorinostat

and 4-anilino-4-oxobutanoic acid were measured. Both metabolites are pharmacologically inactive. Compared to vorinostat, the mean steady state serum exposures in humans of the *O*-glucuronide of vorinostat and 4-anilino-4-oxobutanoic acid were 4-fold and 13-fold higher, respectively.

In vitro studies using human liver microsomes indicate negligible biotransformation by cytochromes P450 (CYP).

Excretion
Vorinostat is eliminated predominantly through metabolism with less than 1% of the dose recovered as unchanged drug in urine, indicating that renal excretion does not play a role in the elimination of vorinostat. The mean urinary recovery of two pharmacologically inactive metabolites at steady state was 16±5.8% of vorinostat dose as the *O*-glucuronide of vorinostat, and 36±8.6% of vorinostat dose as 4-anilino-4-oxobutanoic acid. Total urinary recovery of vorinostat and these two metabolites averaged 52±13.3% of vorinostat dose. The mean terminal half-life ($t_{\frac{1}{2}}$) was ~2.0 hours for both vorinostat and the *O*-glucuronide metabolite, while that of the 4-anilino-4-oxobutanoic acid metabolite was 11 hours.

Specific Populations
Gender, Race & Age
Based upon an exploratory analysis of limited data, gender, race and age do not appear to have meaningful effects on the pharmacokinetics of vorinostat.
Pediatric
Vorinostat was not evaluated in patients <18 years of age.
Hepatic Impairment
The single dose pharmacokinetics of a 400 mg ZOLINZA dose was evaluated in patients with non-CTCL cancers with varying degrees of hepatic impairment. The mean AUC of vorinostat in patients with mild (bilirubin > 1 to $1.5 \times$ ULN or AST > ULN but bilirubin ≤ ULN) and moderate (bilirubin 1.5 to ≤ $3 \times$ ULN) hepatic impairment increased by 50% compared to the AUC of vorinostat in patients with normal hepatic function. The mean vorinostat AUC in patients with severe hepatic impairment (bilirubin > $3 \times$ ULN) increased by 66% compared to the AUC of patients with normal hepatic function.

The safety of multiple daily doses of ZOLINZA was also evaluated in patients with non-CTCL cancers with varying degrees of hepatic impairment. The highest dose studied in mild, moderate and severe hepatic impairment was 400, 300 and 200 mg daily respectively. The incidence of Grade 3 or 4 adverse reactions was similar among the hepatic function groups. The most common Grade 3 or 4 adverse reaction was thrombocytopenia.

Reduce the dose in patients with mild to moderate hepatic impairment. There is not enough data in patients with severe hepatic impairment to recommend a dose modification. *[See Dosage and Administration (2.2) and Use in Specific Populations (8.6).]*
Renal Insufficiency
Vorinostat was not evaluated in patients with renal impairment. However, renal excretion does not play a role in the elimination of vorinostat. *[See Use in Specific Populations (8.7).]*

Pharmacokinetic effects of vorinostat with other agents
Vorinostat is not an inhibitor of CYP drug metabolizing enzymes in human liver microsomes at steady state C_{max} of the 400 mg dose (C_{max} of 1.2 µM vs IC_{50} of >75 µM). Gene expression studies in human hepatocytes detected some potential for suppression of CYP2C9 and CYP3A4 activities by vorinostat at concentrations higher (≥10 µM) than pharmacologically relevant. Thus, vorinostat is not expected to affect the pharmacokinetics of other agents. As vorinostat is not eliminated via the CYP pathways, it is anticipated that vorinostat will not be subject to drug-drug interactions when co-administered with drugs that are known CYP inhibitors or inducers. However, no formal clinical studies have been conducted to evaluate drug interactions with vorinostat.

In vitro studies indicate that vorinostat is not a substrate of human P-glycoprotein (P-gp). In addition, vorinostat has no inhibitory effect on human P-gp-mediated transport of vinblastine (a marker P-gp substrate) at concentrations of up to 100 µM. Thus, vorinostat is not likely to inhibit P-gp at the pharmacologically relevant serum concentration of 2 µM (C_{max}) in humans.

13 NONCLINICAL TOXICOLOGY

13.1 Carcinogenesis, Mutagenesis, Impairment of Fertility
Carcinogenicity studies have not been performed with vorinostat.

Vorinostat was mutagenic *in vitro* in the bacterial reverse mutation assays (Ames test), caused chromosomal aberrations *in vitro* in Chinese hamster ovary (CHO) cells and increased the incidence of micro-nucleated erythrocytes when administered to mice (Mouse Micronucleus Assay).

Effects on the female reproductive system were identified in the oral fertility study when females were dosed for 14 days prior to mating through gestational day 7. Doses of 15, 50 and 150 mg/kg/day to rats resulted in approximate exposures of 0.15, 0.36 and 0.70 times the expected clinical exposure based on AUC. Dose dependent increases in corpora lutea were noted at ≥15 mg/kg/day, which resulted in increased peri-implantation losses were noted at ≥50 mg/kg/day. At 150 mg/kg/day, there were increases in the incidences of dead fetuses and in resorptions.

No effects on reproductive performance were observed in male rats dosed (20, 50, 150 mg/kg/day; approximate exposures of 0.15, 0.36 and 0.70 times the expected clinical exposure based on AUC), for 70 days prior to mating with untreated females. [See Warnings and Precautions (5.7).]

14 CLINICAL STUDIES

Cutaneous T-cell Lymphoma

In two open-label clinical studies, patients with refractory CTCL have been evaluated to determine their response rate to oral ZOLINZA. One study was a single-arm clinical study and the other assessed several dosing regimens. In both studies, patients were treated until disease progression or intolerable toxicity.

Study 1

In an open-label, single-arm, multicenter non-randomized study, 74 patients with advanced CTCL were treated with ZOLINZA at a dose of 400 mg once daily. The primary endpoint was response rate to oral ZOLINZA in the treatment of skin disease in patients with advanced CTCL (Stage IIB and higher) who had progressive, persistent, or recurrent disease on or following two systemic therapies. Enrolled patients should have received, been intolerant to or not a candidate for bexarotene. Extent of skin disease was quantitatively assessed by investigators using a modified Severity Weighted Assessment Tool (SWAT). The investigator measured the percentage total body surface area (%TBSA) involvement separately for patches, plaques, and tumors within 12 body regions using the patient's palm as a "ruler". The total %TBSA for each lesion type was multiplied by a severity weighting factor (1=patch, 2=plaque and 4=tumor) and summed to derive the SWAT score. Efficacy was measured as either a Complete Clinical Response (CCR) defined as no evidence of disease, or Partial Response (PR) defined as a ≥50% decrease in SWAT skin assessment score compared to baseline. Both CCR and PR had to be maintained for at least 4 weeks.

Secondary efficacy endpoints included response duration, time to progression, and time to objective response.

The population had been exposed to a median of three prior therapies (range 1 to 12).

Table 2 summarizes the demographic and disease characteristics of the Study 1 population.

Table 2: Baseline Patient Characteristics (All Patients As Treated)

Characteristics	Vorinostat (N=74)
Age (year)	
Mean (SD)	61.2 (11.3)
Median (Range)	60.0 (39.0, 83.0)
Gender, n (%)	
Male	38 (51.4%)
Female	36 (48.6%)
CTCL stage, n (%)	
IB	11 (14.9%)
IIA	2 (2.7%)
IIB	19 (25.7%)
III	22 (29.7%)
IVA	16 (21.6%)
IVB	4 (5.4%)
Racial Origin, n (%)	
Asian	1 (1.4%)
Black	11 (14.9%)
Other	1 (1.4%)
White	61 (82.4%)
Time from Initial CTCL Diagnosis (year)	
Median (Range)	2.6 (0.0, 27.3)
Clinical Characteristics	
Number of prior systemic treatments, median (range)	3.0 (1.0, 12.0)

The overall objective response rate was 29.7% (22/74, 95% CI [19.7 to 41.5%]) in all patients treated with ZOLINZA. In patients with Stage IIB and higher CTCL, the overall objective response rate was 29.5% (18/61). One patient with Stage IIB CTCL achieved a CCR. Median times to response were 55 and 56 days (range 28 to 171 days), respectively in the overall population and in patients with Stage IIB and higher CTCL. However, in rare cases it took up to 6 months for patients to achieve an objective response to ZOLINZA. The median response duration was not reached since the majority of responses continued at the time of analysis, but was estimated to exceed 6 months for both the overall population and in patients with Stage IIB and higher CTCL. When end of response was defined as a 50% increase in SWAT score from the nadir, the estimated median response duration was 168 days and the median time to tumor progression was 202 days.

Using a 25% increase in SWAT score from the nadir as criterion for tumor progression, the estimated median time-to-progression was 148 days for the overall population and 169 days in the 61 patients with Stage IIB and higher CTCL. Response to any previous systemic therapy does not appear to be predictive of response to ZOLINZA.

Study 2

In an open-label, non-randomized study, ZOLINZA was evaluated to determine the response rate for patients with CTCL who were refractory or intolerant to at least one treatment. In this study, 33 patients were assigned to one of 3 cohorts: Cohort 1, 400 mg once daily; Cohort 2, 300 mg twice daily 3 days/week; or Cohort 3, 300 mg twice daily for 14 days followed by a 7-day rest (induction). In Cohort 3, if at least a partial response was not observed then patients were dosed with a maintenance regimen of 200 mg twice daily. The primary efficacy endpoint, objective response, was measured by the 7-point Physician's Global Assessment (PGA) scale. The investigator assessed improvement or worsening in overall disease compared to baseline based on overall clinical impression. Index and non-index cutaneous lesions as well as cutaneous tumors, lymph nodes and all other disease manifestations were also assessed and included in the overall clinical impression. CCR required 100% clearing of all findings, and PR required at least 50% improvement in disease findings.

The median age was 67.0 years (range 26.0 to 82.0). Fifty-five percent of patients were male, and 45% of patients were female. Fifteen percent of patients had Stage IA, IB, or IIA CTCL and 85% of patients had Stage IIB, III, IVA, or IVB CTCL. The median number of prior systemic therapies was 4 (range 0.0 to 11.0).

In all patients treated, the objective response was 24.2% (8/33) in the overall population, 25% (7/28) in patients with Stage IIB or higher disease and 36.4% (4/11) in patients with Sezary syndrome. The overall response rates were 30.8%, 9.1% and 33.3% in Cohort 1, Cohort 2 and Cohort 3, respectively. The 300 mg twice daily regimen had higher toxicity with no additional clinical benefit over the 400 mg once daily regimen. No CCR was observed.

Among the 8 patients who responded to study treatment, the median time to response was 83.5 days (range 25 to 153 days). The median response duration was 106 days (range 66 to 136 days). Median time to progression was 211.5 days (range 94 to 255 days).

15 REFERENCES

1. OSHA Hazardous Drugs. *OSHA.* [http://www.osha.gov/SLTC/hazardousdrugs/index.html]

16 HOW SUPPLIED/STORAGE AND HANDLING

ZOLINZA capsules, 100 mg, are white, opaque hard gelatin capsules with "568" over "100 mg" printed within the radial bar in black ink on the capsule body. They are supplied as follows:

NDC 0006-0568-40.

Each bottle contains 120 capsules.

Storage and Handling

Store at 20-25°C (68-77°F), excursions permitted between 15-30°C (59-86°F). [See USP Controlled Room Temperature.]

Procedures for proper handling and disposal of anticancer drugs should be considered. Several guidelines on this subject have been published.[1] There is no general agreement that all of the procedures recommended in the guidelines are necessary or appropriate.

ZOLINZA (vorinostat) capsules should not be opened or crushed. Direct contact of the powder in ZOLINZA capsules with the skin or mucous membranes should be avoided. If such contact occurs, wash thoroughly as outlined in the references. Personnel should avoid exposure to crushed and/or broken capsules [see Nonclinical Toxicology (13.1)].

17 PATIENT COUNSELING INFORMATION

See FDA-Approved Patient Labeling (Patient Information)

17.1 Instructions

Patients should be instructed to drink at least 2 L/day of fluid to prevent dehydration and should promptly report excessive vomiting or diarrhea to their physician. Patients should be instructed about the signs of deep vein thrombosis and should consult their physician should any evidence of deep vein thrombosis develop. Patients receiving ZOLINZA should seek immediate medical attention if unusual bleeding occurs. ZOLINZA capsules should not be opened or crushed.

Patients should be instructed to read the patient insert carefully.

Manuf. for: Merck Sharp & Dohme Corp., a subsidiary of **MERCK & CO., INC.**, Whitehouse Station, NJ 08889, USA

Manufactured by:

Patheon, Inc.

Mississauga, Ontario, Canada L5N 7K9

U.S. Patent Nos. RE 38,506 E; 6,087,367

Copyright © 2006, 2008, 2009, 2011, 2013 Merck Sharp & Dohme Corp., a subsidiary of **Merck & Co., Inc.**

All rights reserved.

Revised: 04/2013

USPI-C-0683-1304R006

Patient Information

ZOLINZA® (zo LINZ ah)

(vorinostat)

Capsules

Read the patient information that comes with ZOLINZA before you start taking it and each time you get a refill. There may be new information. This leaflet is a summary of the information for patients. Your doctor or pharmacist can give you additional information. This leaflet does not take the place of talking with your doctor about your medical condition or your treatment.

What is ZOLINZA?

ZOLINZA is a prescription medicine used to treat a type of cancer called cutaneous T-cell lymphoma (CTCL) in patients when the CTCL gets worse, does not go away, or comes back after treatment with other medicines.

ZOLINZA has not been studied in children under the age of 18.

What should I tell my doctor before taking ZOLINZA?

Tell your doctor about all of your medical conditions, including if you:

• Have any allergies

• Have had a blood clot in your lung (pulmonary embolus)

• Have had a blood clot in a vein (a blood vessel) anywhere in your body (deep vein thrombosis)

• Have nausea, vomiting, or diarrhea

• Have liver disease

• Have high blood sugar or diabetes

• Are pregnant or plan to become pregnant. ZOLINZA may harm your unborn baby. ZOLINZA has not been studied in pregnant women. If you use ZOLINZA during pregnancy, tell your doctor immediately.

• Are breastfeeding or plan to breastfeed. It is not known if ZOLINZA will pass into your breast milk. Talk to your doctor about the best way to feed your baby while you are taking ZOLINZA.

Tell your doctor about all of the medicines you take, including prescription and non-prescription medicines, vitamins and herbal supplements. Some medicines may affect how ZOLINZA works, or ZOLINZA may affect how your other medicines work. **Especially tell your doctor if you take:**

• **Valproic acid:** a medicine used to treat seizures. Your doctor will decide if you should continue to take valproic acid and may want to test your blood more frequently.

• **COUMADIN®: (warfarin) or any other blood thinner.** Ask your doctor if you are not sure if you are taking a blood thinner. Your doctor may want to test your blood more frequently.

Know the medicines you take. Keep a list of your medicines and show it to your doctor and pharmacist when you get a new medicine.

How should I take ZOLINZA?

• Take ZOLINZA exactly as your doctor tells you to.

• Your doctor will tell you how many ZOLINZA capsules to take and when to take them.

• Swallow each capsule whole. Do not chew or break open the capsule. If you can't swallow ZOLINZA capsules whole, tell your doctor. You may need a different medicine.

• Take ZOLINZA with food.

• If ZOLINZA capsules are accidentally opened or crushed, do not touch the capsules or the powder contents of the capsules. If the powder from an open or crushed capsule gets on your skin or in your eyes, wash the contacted area well with plenty of plain water.

• **Drink at least eight 8-ounce glasses of liquids every day while taking ZOLINZA.** Drinking enough fluids may help to decrease the chances of losing too much fluid from your body (dehydration) especially if you are having symptoms such as nausea, vomiting or diarrhea while taking ZOLINZA.

• If you miss a dose, take it as soon as you remember. If you do not remember until it is almost time for your next dose, just skip the missed dose. Just take the next dose at your regular time. Do not take two doses of ZOLINZA at the same time.

- If you take too much ZOLINZA, call your doctor, local emergency room, or poison control center right away.
- Your doctor will check your blood cell counts, blood sugar, blood electrolytes, and other chemistries every two weeks for the first two months of your treatment with ZOLINZA and then monthly. Your doctor may decide to do other tests to check your health as needed.
- If you have high blood sugar (hyperglycemia) or diabetes, continue to monitor your blood sugar as your doctor tells you to. Your doctor may need to change your diet or medicine to help control your blood sugar while you take ZOLINZA. Be sure to tell your doctor if you are unable to eat or drink normally due to nausea, vomiting or diarrhea.

What are the possible side effects of ZOLINZA?
ZOLINZA may cause **serious side effects.** Tell your doctor right away if you have any of the following symptoms:
- **Blood clots in the legs (deep vein thrombosis)**
  ◦ sudden swelling in a leg
  ◦ pain or tenderness in the leg. The pain may only be felt when standing or walking.
  ◦ increased warmth in the area where the swelling is.
  ◦ skin redness or change in skin color
- **Blood clots that travel to the lungs (pulmonary embolus)**
  • sudden sharp chest pain • rapid pulse
  • shortness of breath • fainting
  • cough with bloody secretions • feeling anxious
  • sweating
- **Dehydration** (loss of too much fluid from the body). This can happen if you are having nausea, vomiting or diarrhea and can not drink fluids well.
- **Changes in blood tests:** Your doctor will periodically do blood tests to check your blood counts and electrolytes.
  ◦ **Low red blood cells.** Low red blood cells may make you feel tired and get tired easily. You may look pale, and feel short of breath.
  ◦ **Low platelets.** Low platelets can cause unusual bleeding or bruising under the skin. Talk to your doctor right away if this happens.
- **High blood sugar** (blood glucose). If you have high blood sugar or diabetes, monitor your blood sugar frequently as directed by your doctor. Tell your doctor right away if your blood sugar is higher than normal.

In addition, the most common side effects with ZOLINZA include:
- **Stomach and intestinal problems,** including diarrhea, nausea, vomiting, loss of appetite, constipation and weight loss
- **Tiredness**
- **Dizziness**
- **Headache**
- **Changes in the way things taste and dry mouth**
- **Muscle aches**
- **Hair loss**
- **Chills**
- **Fever**
- **Upper respiratory infection**
- **Cough**
- **Increase in blood creatinine**
- **Swelling in the foot, ankle, and leg**
- **Itching**

Tell your doctor if you have any side effect that bothers you or that does not go away.

These are not all the possible side effects of ZOLINZA. For more information, ask your doctor or pharmacist.

General information about ZOLINZA
Medicines are sometimes prescribed for conditions that are not mentioned in patient information leaflets. Do not use ZOLINZA for a condition for which it was not prescribed. Do not give ZOLINZA to other people, even if they have the same symptoms you have. It may harm them.

Keep ZOLINZA and all medicines out of the reach of children.

This leaflet summarizes the most important information about ZOLINZA. If you would like to know more information, talk to your doctor. You can ask your doctor or pharmacist for information about ZOLINZA that is written for health professionals.

What are the ingredients in ZOLINZA?
Active ingredient: vorinostat
Inactive ingredients: microcrystalline cellulose, sodium croscarmellose and magnesium stearate. The inactive ingredients in the capsule shell are titanium dioxide, gelatin, and sodium lauryl sulfate.

How should I store ZOLINZA?
Store ZOLINZA at room temperature, 68°F-77°F (20°C-25°C).

Merck Sharp & Dohme Corp., a subsidiary of
MERCK & CO., INC., Whitehouse Station, NJ 08889, USA
Manufactured by:
Patheon, Inc.
Mississauga, Ontario, Canada L5N 7K9
U.S. Patent Nos. RE 38,506 E; 6,087,367

Copyright © 2006, 2009, 2011, 2013 Merck Sharp & Dohme Corp., a subsidiary of **Merck & Co., Inc.**
All rights reserved.
Revised: 04/2013
USPPI-C-0683-1304R006
Shown in Product Identification Guide, page 309

ZONTIVITY™ ℞
(vorapaxar)
Tablets 2.08 mg*, for oral use
*Equivalent to 2.5 mg vorapaxar sulfate

HIGHLIGHTS OF PRESCRIBING INFORMATION
These highlights do not include all the information needed to use ZONTIVITY safely and effectively. See full prescribing information for ZONTIVITY.
ZONTIVITY™ (vorapaxar) Tablets 2.08 mg*, for oral use
*Equivalent to 2.5 mg vorapaxar sulfate
Initial U.S. Approval: 2014

> **WARNING: BLEEDING RISK**
> *See full prescribing information for complete boxed warning.*
> - Do not use ZONTIVITY in patients with a history of stroke, transient ischemic attack (TIA), or intracranial hemorrhage (ICH); or active pathological bleeding. (4.1, 4.2)
> - Antiplatelet agents, including ZONTIVITY, increase the risk of bleeding, including ICH and fatal bleeding. (5.1)

——INDICATIONS AND USAGE——
ZONTIVITY is a protease-activated receptor-1 (PAR-1) antagonist indicated for the reduction of thrombotic cardiovascular events in patients with a history of myocardial infarction (MI) or with peripheral arterial disease (PAD). ZONTIVITY has been shown to reduce the rate of a combined endpoint of cardiovascular death, MI, stroke, and urgent coronary revascularization. (1.1)

——DOSAGE AND ADMINISTRATION——
- One tablet of ZONTIVITY orally once daily. (2.1)
- Use with aspirin and/or clopidogrel according to their indications or standard of care. There is limited clinical experience with other antiplatelet drugs or with ZONTIVITY as the only antiplatelet agent. (2.2)

——DOSAGE FORMS AND STRENGTHS——
Tablets: 2.08 mg vorapaxar. (3)

——CONTRAINDICATIONS——
- History of stroke, TIA, or ICH. (4.1)
- Active pathologic bleeding. (4.2)

——WARNINGS AND PRECAUTIONS——
- Like other antiplatelet agents, ZONTIVITY increases the risk of bleeding. (5.1)
- Avoid use with strong CYP3A inhibitors or inducers. (5.2)

——ADVERSE REACTIONS——
- Bleeding, including life-threatening and fatal bleeding, is the most commonly reported adverse reaction. (6.1)

To report SUSPECTED ADVERSE REACTIONS, contact Merck Sharp & Dohme Corp., a subsidiary of Merck & Co., Inc., at 1-877-888-4231 or FDA at 1-800-FDA-1088 or www.fda.gov/medwatch.
See 17 for PATIENT COUNSELING INFORMATION and Medication Guide.

Revised: 05/2014

FULL PRESCRIBING INFORMATION: CONTENTS*
WARNING: BLEEDING RISK

FULL PRESCRIBING INFORMATION

> **WARNING: BLEEDING RISK**
> - Do not use ZONTIVITY in patients with a history of stroke, transient ischemic attack (TIA), or intracranial hemorrhage (ICH); or active pathological bleeding *[see CONTRAINDICATIONS (4.1, 4.2)].*
> - Antiplatelet agents, including ZONTIVITY, increase the risk of bleeding, including ICH and fatal bleeding *[see Warnings and Precautions (5.1)].*

1 INDICATIONS AND USAGE
1.1 Patients with History of Myocardial Infarction (MI) or with Peripheral Arterial Disease (PAD)
ZONTIVITY™ is indicated for the reduction of thrombotic cardiovascular events in patients with a history of myocardial infarction (MI) or with peripheral arterial disease (PAD). ZONTIVITY has been shown to reduce the rate of a combined endpoint of cardiovascular death, MI, stroke, and urgent coronary revascularization (UCR).

2 DOSAGE AND ADMINISTRATION
2.1 General Dosing Information
Take one tablet of ZONTIVITY 2.08 mg orally once daily, with or without food.
2.2 Coadministration with Other Antiplatelet Drugs
There is no experience with use of ZONTIVITY alone as the only administered antiplatelet agent. ZONTIVITY has been studied only as an addition to aspirin and/or clopidogrel. Use ZONTIVITY with aspirin and/or clopidogrel according to their indications or standard of care *[see Clinical Studies (14)].* There is limited clinical experience with other antiplatelet drugs.

3 DOSAGE FORMS AND STRENGTHS
ZONTIVITY tablets, 2.08 mg vorapaxar, are yellow, oval-shaped, film-coated tablets with "351" on one side and the Merck logo on the other side.

4 CONTRAINDICATIONS
4.1 History of Stroke, Transient Ischemic Attack (TIA), or Intracranial Hemorrhage (ICH)
ZONTIVITY is contraindicated in patients with a history of stroke, TIA, or ICH because of an increased risk of ICH in this population *[see Adverse Reactions (6)].*
Discontinue ZONTIVITY in patients who experience a stroke, TIA, or ICH *[see Adverse Reactions (6.1) and Clinical Studies (14)].*
4.2 Active Pathologic Bleeding
ZONTIVITY is contraindicated in patients with active pathological bleeding such as ICH or peptic ulcer *[see Warnings and Precautions (5.1) and Adverse Reactions (6.1)].*

5 WARNINGS AND PRECAUTIONS
5.1 General Risk of Bleeding
Antiplatelet agents, including ZONTIVITY, increase the risk of bleeding, including ICH and fatal bleeding *[see Adverse Reactions (6.1)].*
ZONTIVITY increases the risk of bleeding in proportion to the patient's underlying bleeding risk. Consider the underlying risk of bleeding before initiating ZONTIVITY. General risk factors for bleeding include older age, low body weight, reduced renal or hepatic function, history of bleeding disorders, and use of certain concomitant medications (e.g., anticoagulants, fibrinolytic therapy, chronic nonsteroidal anti-inflammatory drugs [NSAIDS], selective serotonin reuptake inhibitors, serotonin norepinephrine reuptake inhibitors) increases the risk of bleeding *[see Use in Specific Populations (8.7) and Clinical Pharmacology (12.3)].* Avoid concomitant use of warfarin or other anticoagulants.
Suspect bleeding in any patient who is hypotensive and has recently undergone coronary angiography, percutaneous coronary intervention (PCI), coronary artery bypass graft surgery (CABG), or other surgical procedures.

Withholding ZONTIVITY for a brief period will not be useful in managing an acute bleeding event because of its long half-life. There is no known treatment to reverse the antiplatelet effect of ZONTIVITY. Significant inhibition of platelet aggregation remains 4 weeks after discontinuation [see Overdosage (10) and Clinical Pharmacology (12.2, 12.3)].

5.2 Strong CYP3A Inhibitors or Inducers

Strong CYP3A inhibitors increase and inducers decrease ZONTIVITY exposure. Avoid concomitant use of ZONTIVITY with strong CYP3A inhibitors or inducers [see Drug Interactions (7.1) and Clinical Pharmacology (12.3)].

6 ADVERSE REACTIONS

The following serious adverse reaction is also discussed elsewhere in the labeling:
• Bleeding [see Boxed Warning and Warnings and Precautions (5.1)].

6.1 Clinical Trials Experience

Because clinical trials are conducted under widely varying conditions, adverse reaction rates observed in the clinical trials of a drug cannot be directly compared to rates in the clinical trials of another drug and may not reflect the rates observed in clinical practice.

ZONTIVITY was evaluated for safety in 13,186 patients, including 2,187 patients treated for more than 3 years, in the Phase 3 study TRA 2°P TIMI 50 (Thrombin Receptor Antagonist in Secondary Prevention of Atherothrombotic Ischemic Events). The overall study population, patients who had evidence or a history of atherosclerosis involving the coronary (post-MI), cerebral (ischemic stroke), or peripheral vascular (documented history of PAD) systems, was treated once a day with ZONTIVITY (n=13,186) or placebo (n=13,166). Patients randomized to ZONTIVITY received treatment for a median of 2.3 years.

The adverse events in the ZONTIVITY-treated (n=10,059) and placebo-treated (n=10,049) post-MI or PAD patients with no history of stroke or TIA are shown below [see Contraindications (4)].

Bleeding

GUSTO severe bleeding was defined as fatal, intracranial, or bleeding with hemodynamic compromise requiring intervention; GUSTO moderate bleeding was defined as bleeding requiring transfusion of whole blood or packed red blood cells without hemodynamic compromise. (GUSTO: Global Utilization of Streptokinase and Tissue Plasminogen Activator for Occluded Arteries.)

The results for the bleeding endpoints in the post-MI or PAD patients without a history of stroke or TIA are shown in Table 1. ZONTIVITY increased GUSTO moderate or severe bleeding by 55%.

[See table 1 above]

The effects of ZONTIVITY on bleeding were examined in a number of subsets based on demographic and other baseline characteristics. Many of these are shown in Figure 1. Such analyses must be interpreted cautiously, as differences can reflect the play of chance among a large number of analyses.

[See figure 1 at top of next page]

In TRA 2°P, 367 post-MI or PAD patients without a history of stroke or TIA underwent CABG surgery. Study investigators were encouraged not to discontinue treatment with study drug (i.e., ZONTIVITY or placebo) prior to surgery. Approximately 12.3% of patients discontinued ZONTIVITY more than 30 days prior to CABG. The relative risk for GUSTO moderate or severe bleeding was approximately 1.2 on ZONTIVITY vs. placebo.

Bleeding events that occurred on ZONTIVITY were treated in the same manner as for other antiplatelet agents.

Use in Patients with History of Stroke, TIA, or ICH

In the TRA 2°P study, patients with a history of ischemic stroke had a higher rate for ICH on ZONTIVITY than on placebo. ZONTIVITY is contraindicated in patients with a history of stroke, TIA, or ICH [see Contraindications (4)].

Other Adverse Reactions

Adverse reactions other than bleeding were evaluated in 19,632 patients treated with ZONTIVITY [13,186 patients in the TRA 2°P study and 6,446 patients in the TRA•CER (Thrombin Receptor Antagonist for Clinical Event Reduction in Acute Coronary Syndrome) study]. Adverse events other than bleeding that occurred at a rate that was at least 2% in the ZONTIVITY group and also 10% greater than the rate in the placebo group are shown in Table 2.

Table 2: TRA 2°P / TRA•CER - Percentage of Patients Reporting Non-hemorrhagic Adverse Reactions at a Rate at Least 2% in the ZONTIVITY Group and at Least 10% Greater than Placebo

	ZONTIVITY N=19,632	Placebo N=19,607
	n (%)	n (%)
Anemia	982 (5.0)	783 (4.0)
Depression	477 (2.4)	405 (2.1)
Rashes, Eruptions, and Exanthemas	439 (2.2)	395 (2.0)

The following adverse reactions occurred at a rate less than 2% in the ZONTIVITY group but at least 40% greater than placebo. In descending order of rate in the ZONTIVITY group: iron deficiency, retinopathy or retinal disorder, and diplopia/oculomotor disturbances.

An increased rate of diplopia and related oculomotor disturbances was observed with ZONTIVITY treatment (30 subjects, 0.2%) vs. placebo (10 subjects, 0.06%). While some cases resolved during continued treatment, information on resolution of symptoms was not available for some cases.

7 DRUG INTERACTIONS

7.1 Effects of Other Drugs on ZONTIVITY

Vorapaxar is eliminated primarily by metabolism, with contributions from CYP3A4 and CYP2J2.

Strong CYP3A Inhibitors

Avoid concomitant use of ZONTIVITY with strong inhibitors of CYP3A (e.g., ketoconazole, itraconazole, posaconazole, clarithromycin, nefazodone, ritonavir, saquinavir, nelfinavir, indinavir, boceprevir, telaprevir, telithromycin and conivaptan) [see Warnings and Precautions (5.2) and Clinical Pharmacology (12.3)].

Strong CYP3A Inducers

Avoid concomitant use of ZONTIVITY with strong inducers of CYP3A (e.g., rifampin, carbamazepine, St. John's Wort and phenytoin) [see Warnings and Precautions (5.2) and Clinical Pharmacology (12.3)].

8 USE IN SPECIFIC POPULATIONS

8.1 Pregnancy

Pregnancy Category B

There are no adequate and well-controlled studies of ZONTIVITY use in pregnant women.

Risk Summary

Based on data in rats and rabbits, ZONTIVITY is predicted to have a low probability of increasing the risk of adverse developmental outcomes above background. No embryo/fetal toxicities, malformations or maternal toxicities were observed in rats exposed during gestation to 56 times the human systemic exposure at the recommended human dose (RHD). No embryo/fetal toxicities, malformations or maternal toxicities were observed in rabbits exposed during gestation to 26 times the human systemic exposure at the RHD. The No Adverse Effect Level (NOAEL) for decreased perinatal survival and body weight in off-spring exposed in utero and during lactation was 31 times the human systemic exposure at the RHD. Both male and female pups displayed transient effects on sensory function and neurobehavioral development at weaning at 67 times the human exposure at the RHD, whereas female pups displayed decreased memory at 31 times the human exposure at the RHD. However, animal studies are not always predictive of a human response. ZONTIVITY should be used during pregnancy only if the potential benefit to the mother justifies the potential risk to the fetus.

Animal Data

In the rat embryo/fetal developmental toxicity study, pregnant rats received daily oral doses of vorapaxar at 0, 5, 25, and 75 mg/kg from implantation to closure of the fetal hard palate (6th to 17th day of gestation). Maternal systemic exposures were approximately 0, 7, 56, and 285 times greater than exposures in women treated at the RHD based on AUC. No embryo/fetal toxicities, malformations, or maternal toxicities were observed in rats receiving exposures up to 56 times the human systemic exposure at the RHD.

In the rabbit embryo/fetal developmental toxicity study, pregnant rabbits received daily oral doses of vorapaxar at 0, 2, 10, or 20 mg/kg from implantation to closure of the fetal hard palate (7th to 19th day of gestation). The NOAEL for maternal and fetal toxicity was equal to or above the highest dose tested. However, an overall increase in the number of litters with any malformation was observed at the highest dose, where systemic exposures were 89-fold higher than the human exposure at RHD.

The effects of vorapaxar on prenatal and postnatal development were assessed in pregnant rats dosed at 0, 5, 25, or 50 mg/kg/day from implantation through the end of lactation. Rat pups had decreased survival and body weight gain from birth to postnatal day 4 and decreased body weight gain for the overall pre-weaning period at exposures 67 times the human exposure at the RHD. Both male and female pups displayed effects on sensory function (acoustic startle) and neurobehavioral (locomotor assay) development on post-natal day (PND) 20 and 21, but not later (PND 60, 61) in development, whereas decreased memory was observed in female pups on PND 27 at 31 times the human exposure at the RHD. In utero and lactational exposure did not affect fertility or reproductive behavior of offspring at exposures up to 67 times the RHD.

8.3 Nursing Mothers

It is unknown whether vorapaxar or its metabolites are excreted in human milk, but it is actively secreted in milk of rats. Because many drugs are excreted in human milk, and because of the potential for serious adverse reactions in nursing infants from ZONTIVITY, discontinue nursing or discontinue ZONTIVITY.

8.4 Pediatric Use

The safety and effectiveness of ZONTIVITY in pediatric patients have not been established.

8.5 Geriatric Use

In TRA 2°P, in post-MI or PAD patients without a history of stroke or TIA, 33% of patients were ≥65 years of age and 9% were ≥75 years of age. The relative risk of bleeding (ZONTIVITY compared with placebo) was similar across age groups. No overall differences in safety or effectiveness were observed between these patients and younger patients. ZONTIVITY increases the risk of bleeding in proportion to a patient's underlying risk. Because older patients are generally at a higher risk of bleeding, consider patient age before initiating ZONTIVITY [see Adverse Reactions (6.1)].

8.6 Renal Impairment

No dose adjustment is required in patients with renal impairment [see Clinical Pharmacology (12.3)].

8.7 Hepatic Impairment

No dose adjustment is required in patients with mild and moderate hepatic impairment. Based on the increased in-

Table 1: Non-CABG-Related Bleeds in Post-MI or PAD Patients without a History of Stroke or TIA (First Dose to Last Dose + 30 Days) in the TRA 2°P Study

Endpoints	Placebo (n=10,049) Patients with events (%)	K-M %‡	ZONTIVITY (n=10,059) Patients with events (%)	K-M %‡	Hazard Ratio*,† (95% CI)
GUSTO Bleeding Categories					
Severe	82 (0.8%)	1.0%	100 (1.0%)	1.3%	1.24 (0.92 - 1.66)
Moderate or Severe	199 (2.0%)	2.4%	303 (3.0%)	3.7%	1.55 (1.30 - 1.86)
Any GUSTO Bleeding (Severe/Moderate/Mild)	1769 (17.6%)	19.8%	2518 (25.0%)	27.7%	1.52 (1.43 - 1.61)
Fatal Bleeding	14 (0.1%)	0.2%	16 (0.2%)	0.2%	1.15 (0.56 - 2.36)
Intracranial Hemorrhage (ICH)	31 (0.3%)	0.4%	45 (0.4%)	0.6%	1.46 (0.92-2.31)
Clinically Significant Bleeding*	950 (9.5%)	10.9%	1349 (13.4%)	15.5%	1.47 (1.35 - 1.60)
Gastrointestinal Bleeding	297 (3.0%)	3.5%	400 (4.0%)	4.7%	1.37 (1.18-1.59)

* Clinically significant bleeding includes any bleeding requiring medical attention including ICH, or clinically significant overt signs of hemorrhage associated with a drop in hemoglobin (Hgb) of ≥3 g/dL (or, when Hgb is not available, an absolute drop in hematocrit (Hct) of ≥15% or a fall in Hct of 9 to <15%).
† Hazard ratio is ZONTIVITY group vs. placebo group.
‡ K-M estimate at 1,080 days.

herent risk of bleeding in patients with severe hepatic impairment, ZONTIVITY is not recommended in such patients [see Warnings and Precautions (5.1) and Clinical Pharmacology (12.3)].

10 OVERDOSAGE

There is no known treatment to reverse the antiplatelet effect of ZONTIVITY, and neither dialysis nor platelet transfusion can be expected to be beneficial if bleeding occurs after overdose. Inhibition of platelet aggregation can be expected for weeks after discontinuation of normal dosing [see Clinical Pharmacology (12.2)]. There is no standard test available to assess the risk of bleeding in an overdose situation.

11 DESCRIPTION

ZONTIVITY contains vorapaxar sulfate, a tricyclic himbacine-derived selective inhibitor of platelet aggregation mediated by PAR-1.

The chemical name of vorapaxar sulfate is ethyl [(1R,3aR,4aR,6R,8aR,9S,9aS)-9-[(1E)-2-[5-(3-fluorophenyl)pyridin-2-yl]ethen-1-yl]-1-methyl-3-oxododecahydronaphtho[2,3-c]furan-6-yl]carbamate sulfate. The empirical formula is $C_{29}H_{33}FN_2O_4 \cdot H_2SO_4$, and its molecular weight is 590.7. The structural formula is:

Vorapaxar sulfate is a white to off-white solid. Vorapaxar sulfate is freely soluble in methanol and slightly soluble in ethanol, acetone, 2-propanol, and acetonitrile. In aqueous solution, it is slightly soluble in pH 1; its solubility decreases with increasing pH. ZONTIVITY tablets are formulated with vorapaxar sulfate, but during manufacture and storage, partial conversion from vorapaxar sulfate to vorapaxar free base may occur.

ZONTIVITY is available for oral use as tablets containing 2.08 mg of vorapaxar, which is equivalent to 2.5 mg of vorapaxar sulfate.

Each film-coated tablet of ZONTIVITY contains the following inactive ingredients: lactose monohydrate, microcrystalline cellulose, croscarmellose sodium, povidone, and magnesium stearate. In addition, the film coating contains the following inactive ingredients: lactose monohydrate, hypromellose, titanium dioxide, triacetin (glycerol triacetate), and iron oxide yellow.

12 CLINICAL PHARMACOLOGY

12.1 Mechanism of Action

Vorapaxar is a reversible antagonist of the protease-activated receptor-1 (PAR-1) expressed on platelets, but its long half-life makes it effectively irreversible. Vorapaxar inhibits thrombin-induced and thrombin receptor agonist peptide (TRAP)-induced platelet aggregation in in vitro studies. Vorapaxar does not inhibit platelet aggregation induced by adenosine diphosphate (ADP), collagen or a thromboxane mimetic and does not affect coagulation parameters ex vivo. PAR-1 receptors are also expressed in a wide variety of cell types, including endothelial cells, neurons, and smooth muscle cells, but the pharmacodynamic effects of vorapaxar in these cell types have not been assessed.

12.2 Pharmacodynamics

At the recommended dose, ZONTIVITY achieves ≥80% inhibition of TRAP-induced platelet aggregation within one week of initiation of treatment. The duration of platelet inhibition is dose- and concentration-dependent. Inhibition of TRAP-induced platelet aggregation at a level of 50% can be expected at 4 weeks after discontinuation of daily doses of ZONTIVITY 2.08 mg, consistent with the terminal elimination half-life of vorapaxar [see Clinical Pharmacology (12.3)].

In healthy volunteer studies, no changes in platelet P-selectin and soluble CD40 ligand (sCD40L) expression or coagulation test parameters (TT, PT, aPTT, ACT, ECT) occurred after single- or multiple- dose (28 days) administration of vorapaxar. No meaningful changes in P-selectin, sCD40L, or hs-CRP concentrations were observed in patients treated with vorapaxar in the phase 2/3 clinical trials.

Evaluation of Vorapaxar on QTc Interval

The effect of vorapaxar on the QTc interval was evaluated in a thorough QT study and in other studies. Vorapaxar had no effect on the QTc interval at single doses up to 48 times the recommended dose.

Figure 1: Subgroup Analyses (GUSTO Moderate or Severe Bleeding) in Post-MI or PAD Patients without a History of Stroke or TIA in the TRA 2°P Study (First Dose to Last Dose + 30 Days)

Subgroup	Hazard Ratio (95% CI)	Total Patients	No. of Events (% per year) Z	No. of Events (% per year) P	HR (95% CI)
All		20108	303 (1.3)	199 (0.8)	1.55 (1.30, 1.86)
Sex					
Male		15764	221 (1.2)	150 (0.8)	1.51 (1.22, 1.85)
Female		4344	82 (1.7)	49 (1.0)	1.73 (1.21, 2.46)
Age					
<65 yrs		13399	138 (0.9)	85 (0.5)	1.68 (1.29, 2.21)
>= 65 yrs		6709	165 (2.1)	114 (1.5)	1.42 (1.12, 1.81)
<75 yrs		18265	241 (1.1)	158 (0.7)	1.55 (1.27, 1.90)
>= 75 yrs		1843	62 (3.1)	41 (2.0)	1.56 (1.05, 2.32)
Race					
White		17805	276 (1.3)	179 (0.9)	1.57 (1.30, 1.90)
Non-white		2293	27 (1.0)	20 (0.7)	1.43 (0.80, 2.54)
Asian		685	8 (1.0)	3 (0.4)	3.34 (0.88,12.65)
African-American		466	6 (1.2)	8 (1.6)	0.75 (0.26, 2.15)
Body Weight					
< 60 kg		1171	30 (2.3)	17 (1.3)	1.72 (0.95, 3.12)
>= 60 kg		18908	273 (1.2)	182 (0.8)	1.53 (1.27, 1.85)
Weight Quartiles					
<72 kg		4787	83 (1.5)	61 (1.1)	1.37 (0.98, 1.90)
>=72 kg to <82 kg		4999	85 (1.5)	49 (0.8)	1.79 (1.26, 2.55)
>=82 kg to <94 kg		5401	77 (1.2)	49 (0.8)	1.53 (1.07, 2.19)
>=94 kg		4892	58 (1.1)	40 (0.7)	1.56 (1.05, 2.34)
Primary Enrollment Stratum					
Post-MI		16856	212 (1.1)	139 (0.7)	1.54 (1.24, 1.90)
PAD		3252	91 (2.3)	60 (1.5)	1.60 (1.15, 2.21)
Renal Insufficiency					
eGFR <60 ml/min/1.73 m*m		2846	96 (2.9)	56 (1.8)	1.70 (1.22, 2.37)
eGFR >= 60 ml/min/1.73 m*m		17037	206 (1.1)	140 (0.7)	1.51 (1.22, 1.87)
Geographic Region					
US		4907	135 (2.4)	77 (1.4)	1.81 (1.37, 2.40)
Non-US		15201	168 (1.0)	122 (0.7)	1.40 (1.11, 1.76)
History of Diabetes Mellitus					
Yes		4745	93 (1.7)	61 (1.1)	1.56 (1.13, 2.15)
No		15362	210 (1.2)	138 (0.8)	1.55 (1.25, 1.92)
History of Heart Failure					
Yes		1722	49 (2.7)	24 (1.3)	2.12 (1.30, 3.46)
No		18385	254 (1.2)	175 (0.8)	1.48 (1.22, 1.79)
Thienopyridine Use at Baseline					
Yes		14353	220 (1.4)	153 (0.9)	1.48 (1.20, 1.82)
No		5755	83 (1.2)	46 (0.7)	1.80 (1.25, 2.57)
Aspirin Use at Baseline					
Yes		19446	292 (1.3)	188 (0.8)	1.59 (1.32, 1.90)
No		662	11 (1.5)	11 (1.4)	1.03 (0.45, 2.37)
<=100 mg		15011	219 (1.3)	135 (0.8)	1.65 (1.33, 2.05)
>100 mg to <300 mg		1821	17 (0.8)	11 (0.5)	1.64 (0.77, 3.51)
>=300 mg		2612	56 (1.9)	42 (1.4)	1.33 (0.89, 1.99)

0.125 0.25 0.5 1 2 4 8
← ZONTIVITY (Z) Better   Placebo (P) Better →

12.3 Pharmacokinetics

Vorapaxar exposure increases in an approximately dose-proportional manner following single doses up to 16 times the recommended dose. Vorapaxar pharmacokinetics are similar in healthy subjects and patients.

Absorption

After oral administration of a single ZONTIVITY 2.08 mg dose under fasted conditions, peak concentrations (C_{max}) occur at 1 hour post-dose (range: 1 to 2 h). The mean absolute bioavailability as determined from a microdosing study is approximately 100%.

Ingestion of vorapaxar with a high-fat meal resulted in no meaningful change in AUC with a small (21%) decrease in C_{max} and delayed time to peak concentration (45 minutes). ZONTIVITY may be taken with or without food.

Distribution

The mean volume of distribution of vorapaxar is approximately 424 liters (95% CI: 351-512). Vorapaxar and the major circulating active metabolite, M20, are extensively bound (≥99%) to human plasma proteins. Vorapaxar is highly bound to human serum albumin and does not preferentially distribute into red blood cells.

Metabolism

Vorapaxar is eliminated by metabolism via CYP3A4 and CYP2J2. The major active circulating metabolite is M20 (monohydroxy metabolite) and the predominant metabolite identified in excreta is M19 (amine metabolite). The systemic exposure of M20 is ~20% of the exposure to vorapaxar.

Excretion

The primary route of elimination is through the feces. In a 6-week study, 84% of the administered radiolabeled dose was recovered as total radioactivity with 58% collected in feces and 25% in urine. Vorapaxar is eliminated primarily in the form of metabolites, with no unchanged vorapaxar detected in urine.

Vorapaxar exhibits multi-exponential disposition with an effective half-life of 3-4 days and an apparent terminal elimination half-life of 8 days. Steady-state is achieved by 21 days following once-daily dosing with an accumulation of 5- to 6-fold. The apparent terminal elimination half-life for vorapaxar is approximately 8 days (range 5-13 days) and is similar for the active metabolite. The terminal elimination half-life is important to determine the time to offset the pharmacodynamic effect [see Clinical Pharmacology (12.2)].

Specific Populations

The effects of intrinsic factors on the pharmacokinetics of vorapaxar are presented in Figure 2 [see Use in Specific Populations (8.5, 8.6, 8.7)].

In general, effects on the exposure of vorapaxar based on age, race, gender, weight, and moderate renal insufficiency were modest (20-40%; see Figure 2). No dose adjustments are necessary based upon these factors. Because of the inherent bleeding risks in patients with severe hepatic impairment, ZONTIVITY is not recommended in such patients [see Warnings and Precautions (5.1) and Use in Specific Populations (8.7)].

Figure 2: Effect of Intrinsic Factors on the Pharmacokinetics of Vorapaxar

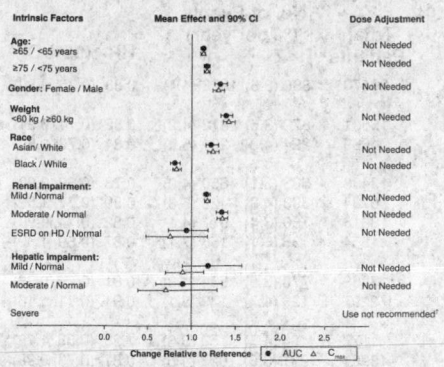

† See Warnings and Precautions. (5.1) and Use in Specific Populations. (8.7)

Drug Interactions [see also Drug Interactions (7)]

Anticoagulants and Antiplatelet Agents

An interaction study with vorapaxar and warfarin in healthy subjects did not demonstrate a clinically significant pharmacokinetic or pharmacodynamic interaction *[see Warnings and Precautions (5.1) and Figure 4]*.

Vorapaxar did not affect prasugrel pharmacokinetics and prasugrel did not affect vorapaxar pharmacokinetics following multiple-dose administration at steady-state *[see Warnings and Precautions (5.1) and Figures 3 and 4]*. The pharmacokinetic interaction between vorapaxar and clopidogrel has not been evaluated. However, the use of vorapaxar on a background of clopidogrel is supported by the clinical data from TRA 2°P and TRA•CER *[see Adverse Reactions (6.1) and Clinical Studies (14)]*.

Effects of Other Drugs on Vorapaxar

The effects of other drugs on the pharmacokinetics of vorapaxar are presented in Figure 3 as change relative to vorapaxar administered alone (test/reference). Phase 3 data suggest that coadministration of a weak or moderate CYP3A inhibitor with vorapaxar does not increase bleeding risk or alter the efficacy of vorapaxar. No dose adjustment for ZONTIVITY is required in patients taking weak to moderate inhibitors of CYP3A.

Figure 3: Effects of Other Drugs on the Pharmacokinetics of Vorapaxar

† See Warnings and Precautions. (5.2) and Drug Interactions. (7.1)
§ See Dosage and Administration. (2.2)

Effects of Vorapaxar on Other Drugs

In vitro metabolism studies demonstrate that vorapaxar or M20 is unlikely to cause clinically significant inhibition or induction of major CYP isoforms or inhibition of OATP1B1, OATP1B3, BCRP, OAT1, OAT3, and OCT2 transporters. Specific *in vivo* effects on the pharmacokinetics of digoxin, warfarin, rosiglitazone and prasugrel are presented in Figure 4 as a change relative to the interacting drug administered alone (test/reference). Vorapaxar is a weak inhibitor of the intestinal P-glycoprotein (P-gp) transporter. No dosage adjustment of digoxin or ZONTIVITY is required.

Figure 4: Effects of Vorapaxar on the Pharmacokinetics of Other Drugs

† See Warnings and Precautions. (5.1)
§ See Dosage and Administration. (2.2)

Table 3: TRA 2°P: Time to First Event in Post-MI or PAD Patients without a History of Stroke or TIA

Endpoints	Placebo (n=10,090)		ZONTIVITY (n=10,080)		Hazard Ratio‡,§ (95% CI)	p-value§
	Patients with events* (%)	K-M %†	Patients with events* (%)	K-M %†		
Primary Composite Efficacy Endpoint (CV death/MI/stroke/UCR)*,§	1073 (10.6%)	11.8%	896 (8.9%)	10.1%	0.83 (0.76-0.90)	<0.001
Secondary Composite Efficacy Endpoint (CV death/MI/stroke)*,§	851 (8.4%)	9.5%	688 (6.8%)	7.9%	0.80 (0.73-0.89)	<0.001
Other Secondary Efficacy Endpoints (first occurrences of specified event at any time) ¶						
CV Death	239 (2.4%)	2.8%	205 (2.0%)	2.4%	0.86 (0.71-1.03)	
MI	569 (5.6%)	6.4%	470 (4.7%)	5.4%	0.82 (0.73-0.93)	
Stroke	145 (1.4%)	1.6%	98 (1.0%)	1.2%	0.67 (0.52-0.87)	
UCR	283 (2.8%)	3.0%	249 (2.5%)	2.8%	0.88 (0.74-1.04)	

* Each patient was counted only once (first component event) in the component summary that contributed to the primary efficacy endpoint.
† K-M estimate at 1,080 days.
‡ Hazard ratio is ZONTIVITY group versus placebo group.
§ Cox proportional hazard model with covariates treatment and stratification factors (qualifying atherosclerotic disease and planned thienopyridine use).
¶ Including patients who could have had other non-fatal events or subsequently died.

13 NONCLINICAL TOXICOLOGY

13.1 Carcinogenesis, Mutagenesis, Impairment of Fertility

Carcinogenesis

Carcinogenicity studies were conducted in rats and mice dosed orally with vorapaxar for two years. Male and female rats dosed at 0, 3, 10 or 30 mg/kg/day showed no carcinogenic potential at systemic exposures (AUC) in males and females that were 9- and 29-fold, respectively, the human systemic exposure at the RHD. In male and female mice dosed at 0, 1, 5, and 15 mg/kg/day, vorapaxar showed no carcinogenic potential at systemic exposures (AUC) that were up to 30-fold the human systemic exposure.

Mutagenesis

Vorapaxar was not mutagenic in the Ames bacterial reverse mutation assay and not clastogenic in an *in vitro* human peripheral blood lymphocyte assay or an *in vivo* mouse micronucleus assay after intraperitoneal administration.

Impairment of Fertility

Fertility studies in rats showed that vorapaxar had no effect on either male or female fertility at doses up to 50 mg/kg/day, a dose resulting in systemic exposures (AUC) in male and female rats that are 40 and 67 times, respectively, the human systemic exposure at the RHD.

13.2 Animal Pharmacology

Vorapaxar did not increase bleeding time in non-human primates when administered alone. Bleeding time was prolonged slightly with administration of aspirin or aspirin plus vorapaxar. The combination of aspirin, vorapaxar, and clopidogrel produced significant prolongation of bleeding time. Transfusion of human platelet rich plasma normalized bleeding times with partial recovery of *ex vivo* platelet aggregation induced with arachidonic acid, but not induced with ADP or TRAP. Platelet poor plasma had no effect on bleeding times or platelet aggregation *[see Warnings and Precautions (5.1)]*.

14 CLINICAL STUDIES

The clinical evidence for the effectiveness of ZONTIVITY is supported by TRA 2°P - TIMI 50. TRA 2°P was a multicenter, randomized, double-blind, placebo-controlled study conducted in patients who had evidence or a history of atherosclerosis involving the coronary (spontaneous MI ≥2 weeks but ≤12 months prior), cerebral (ischemic stroke), or peripheral vascular (documented peripheral arterial disease [PAD]) systems. Patients were randomized to receive daily treatment with ZONTIVITY (n=13,225) or placebo (n=13,224) in addition to standard of care. The study's primary endpoint was the composite of cardiovascular death, MI, stroke, and urgent coronary revascularization (UCR). The composite of cardiovascular death, MI, and stroke was assessed as key secondary endpoint. The median follow-up was 2.5 years (up to 4 years).

The findings in all randomized patients for the primary efficacy composite endpoint show a 3-year K-M event rate of 11.2% in the ZONTIVITY group compared to 12.4% in the placebo group (hazard ratio [HR]: 0.88; 95% confidence interval [CI]: 0.82 to 0.95; p=0.001).

The findings for the key secondary efficacy endpoint show a 3-year Kaplan-Meier (K-M) event rate of 9.3% in the ZONTIVITY group compared to 10.5% in placebo group (HR 0.87; 95% CI, 0.80 to 0.94; p<0.001).

Although TRA 2°P was not designed to evaluate the relative benefits and risks of ZONTIVITY in individual patient subgroups, patients with a history of stroke or TIA showed an increased risk of ICH. Of the patients who comprised the post-MI and PAD strata and had no baseline history of stroke or TIA,10,080 were randomized to treatment with ZONTIVITY and 10,090 to placebo. These patients were 89% Caucasian, 22% female, and 33% ≥65 years of age, with a median age of 60 years. The population included patients with diabetes (24%) and patients with hypertension (65%). Of the patients who qualified for the trial with MI without a history of stroke or TIA, 98% were receiving aspirin, 78% were receiving a thienopyridine, and 77% were receiving both aspirin and a thienopyridine when they enrolled in the trial. Of the patients who qualified for the trial with PAD without a history of stroke or TIA, 88% were receiving aspirin, 35% were receiving a thienopyridine, and 27% were receiving both aspirin and a thienopyridine when they enrolled.

In post-MI or PAD patients without a history of stroke or TIA the 3-year K-M event rate for the primary efficacy endpoint (composite of time to first CV death, MI, stroke, or UCR) was of 10.1% in the ZONTIVITY group compared to 11.8% in the placebo group (HR 0.83; 95% CI, 0.76 to 0.90; p<0.001) (see Figure 5 and Table 3).

The results for the key secondary efficacy endpoint (composite of time to first CV death, MI, or stroke) show a 3-year K-M event rate of 7.9% in the ZONTIVITY group compared to 9.5% in the placebo group (HR 0.80; 95% CI, 0.73 to 0.89; p<0.001) (see Table 3).

The effect of chronic dosing with ZONTIVITY on the primary and key secondary endpoints was maintained for the duration of the trial (median follow up 2.5 years, up to 4 years).

[See figure 5 at top of next column]

[See table 3 above]

In post-MI or PAD patients who survived an on-study efficacy event, the incidence of subsequent events was lower with ZONTIVITY.

The time from the prior MI to randomization had no relationship to the treatment benefit for the primary study outcome.

A range of demographic, concurrent baseline medications, and other treatment differences were examined for their influence on outcomes as shown in Figure 6. Such analyses must be interpreted cautiously, as differences can reflect the play of chance among a large number of analyses.

[See figure 6 at top of next page]

16 HOW SUPPLIED/STORAGE AND HANDLING

ZONTIVITY tablets, 2.08 mg vorapaxar, are yellow, oval-shaped, film-coated tablets with "351" on one side and the Merck logo on the other side.

Figure 5: Time to First Occurrence of the Composite Endpoint of CV Death, MI, Stroke or UCR in Post-MI or PAD Patients without a History of Stroke or TIA in TRA 2°P

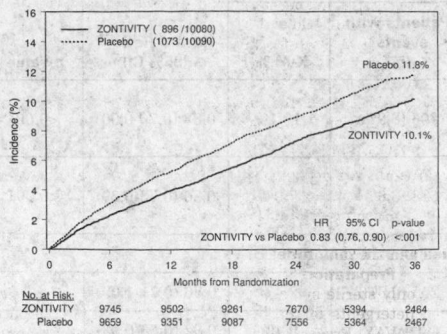

They are supplied as follows:
- NDC 0006-0351-31 bottles of 30 tablets
- NDC 0006-0351-54 bottles of 90 tablets
- NDC 0006-0351-48 unit dose packages of 100 tablets (one carton containing 10 10-count blister cards)

Storage of bottles
Store at 20-25°C (68-77°F), excursions permitted between 15-30°C (between 59-86°F). [See USP Controlled Room Temperature.] Store tablets in the original package with the bottle tightly closed. Keep the desiccant in the bottle to protect from moisture.

Storage of blisters
Store at 20-25°C (68-77°F), excursions permitted between 15-30°C (between 59-86°F). [See USP Controlled Room Temperature.] Store in the original package until use.

17 PATIENT COUNSELING INFORMATION

Advise the patient to read the FDA-approved Patient Labeling (Medication Guide).

Benefits and Risks
- Summarize the benefits and potential side effects of ZONTIVITY.
- Tell patients to take ZONTIVITY exactly as prescribed.
- Inform patients not to discontinue ZONTIVITY without discussing it with the prescribing physician.
- Tell patients to read the Medication Guide.

Bleeding
Inform patients that they:
- May bleed and bruise more easily.
- Should report any unanticipated, prolonged or excessive bleeding, or blood in their stool or urine.

Invasive Procedures
Instruct patients to:
- Inform physicians and dentists that they are taking ZONTIVITY before any surgery or dental procedure.
- Tell the doctor performing any surgery or dental procedure to talk to the prescribing physician before stopping ZONTIVITY.

Concomitant Medications
Tell patients to list all prescription medications, over-the-counter medications, or dietary supplements they are taking or plan to take so that the physician knows about other treatments that may affect bleeding risk.

Manufactured for: Merck Sharp & Dohme Corp., a subsidiary of
MERCK & CO., INC., Whitehouse Station, NJ 08889, USA
Manufactured by: MSD International GmbH (Singapore Branch),
Singapore 638414, Singapore
For patent information:
www.merck.com/product/patent/home.html
The trademarks depicted herein are owned by their respective companies.

Copyright © 2013 Merck Sharp & Dohme Corp., a subsidiary of Merck & Co., Inc.
All rights reserved.
uspi-mk5348-t-1405r000

Medication Guide
ZONTIVITY™ (zon-TIV-iti)
(vorapaxar)
Tablets
Read this Medication Guide before you start taking ZONTIVITY and each time you get a refill. There may be new information. This information does not take the place of talking with your doctor about your medical condition or your treatment.

What is the most important information I should know about ZONTIVITY?
ZONTIVITY is used to lower your chance of having another serious problem with your heart or blood vessels, **but ZONTIVITY (and similar drugs) can cause bleeding that can be serious and lead to death.**

Figure 6: Subgroup Analyses (Primary Endpoints) of the TRA 2°P Post-MI or PAD Patients without a History of Stroke or TIA

Subgroup	Hazard Ratio (95% CI)	Total Patients	No. of Events (% per year) Z	P	HR (95% CI)
All		20170	896 (3.6)	1073 (4.4)	0.83 (0.76, 0.90)
Sex					
Male		15801	672 (3.5)	812 (4.2)	0.82 (0.74, 0.91)
Female		4369	224 (4.2)	261 (5.0)	0.84 (0.70, 1.00)
Age					
<65 yrs		13436	503 (3.1)	650 (4.0)	0.78 (0.69, 0.88)
>= 65 yrs		6734	393 (4.7)	423 (5.3)	0.89 (0.77, 1.02)
<75 yrs		18316	760 (3.4)	917 (4.1)	0.82 (0.74, 0.90)
>= 75 yrs		1854	136 (6.1)	156 (7.1)	0.87 (0.69, 1.09)
Race					
White		17863	770 (3.5)	934 (4.3)	0.81 (0.74, 0.90)
Non-white		2297	126 (4.7)	139 (5.1)	0.91 (0.71, 1.16)
Body Weight					
< 60 kg		1177	64 (4.5)	50 (3.6)	1.23 (0.85, 1.78)
>= 60 kg		18961	831 (3.6)	1023 (4.5)	0.81 (0.73, 0.88)
Weight Quartiles					
<72 kg		4814	227 (3.9)	251 (4.4)	0.88 (0.74, 1.05)
>=72 kg to <82 kg		5008	204 (3.3)	234 (3.8)	0.87 (0.72, 1.05)
>=82 kg to <94 kg		5416	225 (3.3)	274 (4.3)	0.77 (0.65, 0.92)
>=94 kg		4900	239 (4.2)	314 (5.2)	0.80 (0.68, 0.95)
Primary Enrollment Stratum					
Post-MI		16897	719 (3.6)	867 (4.4)	0.82 (0.74, 0.90)
PAD		3273	177 (4.0)	206 (4.6)	0.87 (0.71, 1.06)
Thienopyridine Use at Baseline					
Yes		14392	656 (3.8)	789 (4.6)	0.83 (0.75, 0.92)
No		5778	240 (3.2)	284 (4.0)	0.82 (0.69, 0.98)
Aspirin Use at Baseline					
Yes		19502	857 (3.6)	1027 (4.4)	0.83 (0.75, 0.90)
No		668	39 (4.5)	46 (5.5)	0.82 (0.53, 1.25)
<=100 mg		15054	611 (3.3)	754 (4.2)	0.80 (0.72, 0.89)
>100 mg to <300 mg		1826	71 (3.3)	102 (4.6)	0.71 (0.52, 0.96)
>=300 mg		2620	175 (5.5)	171 (5.5)	0.99 (0.80, 1.22)
Renal Insufficiency					
eGFR <60 ml/min/1.73 m*m		2859	224 (6.1)	234 (7.0)	0.86 (0.72, 1.04)
eGFR >= 60 ml/min/1.73 m*m		17073	663 (3.2)	829 (4.0)	0.80 (0.73, 0.89)
Geographic Region					
US		4921	326 (5.4)	364 (6.1)	0.88 (0.76, 1.02)
Non-US		15249	570 (3.1)	709 (3.9)	0.80 (0.71, 0.89)
History of Diabetes Mellitus					
Yes		4762	316 (5.6)	391 (7.1)	0.79 (0.68, 0.91)
No		15407	580 (3.1)	682 (3.6)	0.85 (0.76, 0.94)
History of Prior ACS					
Yes		18183	808 (3.7)	972 (4.5)	0.82 (0.75, 0.90)
No		1985	88 (3.2)	101 (3.8)	0.85 (0.64, 1.13)
Stent at Baseline					
Yes		13306	587 (3.7)	731 (4.6)	0.80 (0.72, 0.89)
No		6864	309 (3.6)	342 (4.0)	0.89 (0.76, 1.04)
History of Tobacco Use					
Never Used		5411	242 (3.7)	268 (4.2)	0.88 (0.74, 1.05)
History of Use		10402	451 (3.5)	557 (4.4)	0.80 (0.71, 0.90)
Current User		4357	203 (3.9)	248 (4.7)	0.83 (0.69, 1.00)
Taking a Statin at Baseline					
Yes		18787	802 (3.5)	986 (4.3)	0.81 (0.74, 0.89)
No		1383	94 (5.1)	87 (5.6)	0.91 (0.68, 1.22)

Hazard Ratio axis: 0.25   0.5   1   2   4
ZONTIVITY (Z) Better ← → Placebo (P) Better

Call your doctor right away if you have any of these signs or symptoms of bleeding while taking ZONTIVITY:
- bleeding that is severe or that you cannot control
- pink, red, or brown urine
- vomiting blood or your vomit looks like "coffee grounds"
- red or black stools (looks like tar)
- coughing up blood or blood clots.

While you take ZONTIVITY and for about 4 weeks after your treatment with ZONTIVITY is stopped:
- you may bruise and bleed more easily (nose bleeds may be common)
- it will take longer than usual for any bleeding to stop.

Do not take ZONTIVITY if you:
- have had a stroke or "mini stroke" (also known as transient ischemic attack or TIA)
- have had bleeding in your brain
- currently have unusual bleeding, such as bleeding in your head, stomach or intestines (an ulcer).

If you have a stroke, TIA, or bleeding in your brain while taking ZONTIVITY your doctor should stop your treatment with ZONTIVITY. Follow your doctor's instructions about stopping ZONTIVITY.
Do not stop taking ZONTIVITY without talking to the doctor who prescribed it for you.

What is ZONTIVITY?
ZONTIVITY is a prescription medicine used to treat people who have

- had a heart attack or
- reduced blood flow in their legs (peripheral arterial disease).

ZONTIVITY is used with aspirin and/or clopidogrel to lower your chance of having another serious problem with your heart or blood vessels, such as heart attack, stroke, or death.
It is not known if ZONTIVITY is safe and effective in children.

What should I tell my doctor before taking ZONTIVITY?
Before you take ZONTIVITY, tell your doctor if you:
- have had bleeding problems or history of stomach ulcers
- have had a stroke or "mini-stroke" (also known as transient ischemic attack or TIA)
- have had any recent serious injury or surgery
- plan to have surgery or a dental procedure
- have severe liver problems
- are pregnant or plan to become pregnant. It is not known if ZONTIVITY will harm your unborn baby.
- are breastfeeding or plan to breastfeed. It is not known if ZONTIVITY passes into your breast milk. You and your doctor should decide if you will take ZONTIVITY or breastfeed. You should not do both.

Tell all of your doctors and dentists that you are taking ZONTIVITY. They should talk to the doctor who prescribed ZONTIVITY for you before you have any surgery or dental procedure.

Tell your doctor about all the medicines you take, including prescription and over-the-counter medicines, vitamins, dietary or herbal supplements. Taking ZONTIVITY with certain other medicines may increase your risk of bleeding and may affect how ZONTIVITY works.

Know the medicines you take. Keep a list of them to show your doctor and pharmacist when you get a new medicine.

How should I take ZONTIVITY?

Take ZONTIVITY exactly as prescribed by your doctor.

• Take ZONTIVITY 1 time each day.
• Take ZONTIVITY with or without food.
• Take ZONTIVITY with aspirin and/or clopidogrel as prescribed by your doctor.
• Do not stop taking ZONTIVITY without first talking to the doctor who prescribed it for you.
• If you take too much ZONTIVITY, call your doctor, or go to the nearest emergency room right away.

What are the possible side effects of ZONTIVITY?

• See "What is the most important information I should know about ZONTIVITY?"
• Anemia (low level of red blood cells)
• Depression
• Rash

These are not all the possible side effects of ZONTIVITY. Call your doctor for medical advice about side effects. You may report side effects to FDA at 1-800-FDA-1088.

How should I store ZONTIVITY?

• Store ZONTIVITY at room temperature between 68°F to 77°F (20°C to 25°C).
• Keep ZONTIVITY in the bottle it comes in.
• Keep the bottle tightly closed.
• The ZONTIVITY bottle contains a desiccant packet to help keep your medicine dry (protect it from moisture). Keep the desiccant packet in the bottle. Do not throw away the desiccant packet.
• Store blister packs of ZONTIVITY in the original package it comes in.

Keep ZONTIVITY and all medicines out of the reach of children.

You can ask your doctor or pharmacist for information about ZONTIVITY that is written for health professionals.

For more information, go to www.zontivity.com or call 1-800-622-4477.

What are the ingredients in ZONTIVITY?

Active ingredient: vorapaxar sulfate

Inactive ingredients:

Tablet: lactose monohydrate, microcrystalline cellulose, croscarmellose sodium, povidone, and magnesium stearate

Film coating: lactose monohydrate, hypromellose, titanium dioxide, triacetin (glycerol triacetate), and iron oxide yellow

This Medication Guide has been approved by the U.S. Food and Drug Administration.

Manufactured for: Merck Sharp & Dohme Corp., a subsidiary of

MERCK & CO., INC., Whitehouse Station, NJ 08889, USA

Manufactured by: MSD International GmbH (Singapore Branch),

Singapore 638414, Singapore

Issued: 05/2014

For patent information:

www.merck.com/product/patent/home.html

Copyright © 2013 Merck Sharp & Dohme Corp., a subsidiary of **Merck & Co., Inc.**

All rights reserved.

usmg-mk5348-t-1405r000

Shown in Product Identification Guide, page 309

ZOSTAVAX®

[ZOS tah vax]

(Zoster Vaccine Live)

Suspension for subcutaneous injection

℞

HIGHLIGHTS OF PRESCRIBING INFORMATION

These highlights do not include all the information needed to use ZOSTAVAX safely and effectively. See full prescribing information for ZOSTAVAX.

ZOSTAVAX® (Zoster Vaccine Live)

Suspension for subcutaneous injection

Initial U.S. Approval: 2006

——————INDICATIONS AND USAGE——————

ZOSTAVAX is a live attenuated virus vaccine indicated for prevention of herpes zoster (shingles) in individuals 50 years of age and older. (1)

Limitations of Use of ZOSTAVAX:

• ZOSTAVAX is not indicated for the treatment of zoster or postherpetic neuralgia (PHN) (1)
• ZOSTAVAX is not indicated for prevention of primary varicella infection (Chickenpox) (1)

————DOSAGE AND ADMINISTRATION————

Single 0.65 mL subcutaneous injection (2.1)

————DOSAGE FORMS AND STRENGTHS————

Single dose vials with not less than 19,400 plaque-forming units [PFU] per 0.65 mL dose when reconstituted to a suspension. (2.1, 3, 16)

——————CONTRAINDICATIONS——————

• History of anaphylactic/anaphylactoid reaction to gelatin, neomycin, or any other component of the vaccine. (4.1)
• Immunosuppression or Immunodeficiency. (4.2)
• Pregnancy. (4.3, 8.1)

————WARNINGS AND PRECAUTIONS————

• Hypersensitivity reactions including anaphylaxis have occurred with ZOSTAVAX (5.1)
• Transmission of vaccine virus may occur between vaccinees and susceptible contacts (5.2)
• Deferral should be considered in acute illness (for example, in the presence of fever) or in patients with active untreated tuberculosis (5.3)
• Avoid pregnancy for 3 months following vaccination with ZOSTAVAX (8.1)

——————ADVERSE REACTIONS——————

The most frequent adverse reactions, reported in ≥1% of subjects vaccinated with ZOSTAVAX, were headache and injection-site reactions. (6)

To report SUSPECTED ADVERSE REACTIONS or exposure during pregnancy or within three months prior to conception, contact Merck Sharp & Dohme Corp., a subsidiary of Merck & Co., Inc., at 1-877-888-4231 or VAERS at 1-800-822-7967 or www.vaers.hhs.gov.

——————DRUG INTERACTIONS——————

In a randomized clinical study, a reduced immune response to ZOSTAVAX as measured by gpELISA was observed in individuals who received concurrent administration of PNEUMOVAX® 23 and ZOSTAVAX compared with individuals who received these vaccines 4 weeks apart. Consider administration of the two vaccines separated by at least 4 weeks. (7.1, 14.3)

————USE IN SPECIFIC POPULATIONS————

Pregnancy: Do not administer ZOSTAVAX to females who are pregnant. Animal reproduction studies have not been conducted. It is not known whether ZOSTAVAX can cause fetal harm. (4.3, 8.1)

See 17 for PATIENT COUNSELING INFORMATION and FDA-approved patient labeling

Revised: 02/2014

FULL PRESCRIBING INFORMATION

1 INDICATIONS AND USAGE

ZOSTAVAX® is a live attenuated virus vaccine indicated for prevention of herpes zoster (shingles) in individuals 50 years of age and older.

Limitations of Use of ZOSTAVAX:

• ZOSTAVAX is not indicated for the treatment of zoster or postherpetic neuralgia (PHN).
• ZOSTAVAX is not indicated for prevention of primary varicella infection (Chickenpox).

2 DOSAGE AND ADMINISTRATION

Subcutaneous administration only. Do not inject intravascularly or intramuscularly.

2.1 Recommended Dose and Schedule

Administer ZOSTAVAX as a single 0.65-mL dose subcutaneously in the deltoid region of the upper arm.

2.2 Preparation for Administration

Use only sterile syringes free of preservatives, antiseptics, and detergents for each injection and/or reconstitution of ZOSTAVAX. Preservatives, antiseptics and detergents may inactivate the vaccine virus.

ZOSTAVAX is stored frozen and should be reconstituted immediately upon removal from the freezer.

When reconstituted, ZOSTAVAX is a semi-hazy to translucent, off-white to pale yellow liquid.

Reconstitution:

• Use only the diluent supplied.
• Withdraw the entire contents of the diluent into a syringe.
• To avoid excessive foaming, slowly inject all of the diluent in the syringe into the vial of lyophilized vaccine and gently agitate to mix thoroughly.
• Withdraw the entire contents of reconstituted vaccine into a syringe and inject the total volume subcutaneously.
• **ADMINISTER IMMEDIATELY AFTER RECONSTITUTION** to minimize loss of potency. Discard reconstituted vaccine if not used within 30 minutes. Do not freeze reconstituted vaccine.

3 DOSAGE FORMS AND STRENGTHS

ZOSTAVAX is a lyophilized preparation of live, attenuated varicella-zoster virus (Oka/Merck) to be reconstituted with sterile diluent to give a single dose suspension with a minimum of 19,400 PFU (plaque forming units) when stored at room temperature for up to 30 minutes.

4 CONTRAINDICATIONS

4.1 Hypersensitivity

Do not administer ZOSTAVAX to individuals with a history of anaphylactic/anaphylactoid reaction to gelatin, neomycin or any other component of the vaccine. Neomycin allergy manifested as contact dermatitis is not a contraindication to receiving this vaccine. (1)

4.2 Immunosuppression

ZOSTAVAX is a live, attenuated varicella-zoster vaccine and administration may result in disseminated disease in individuals who are immunosuppressed or immunodeficient. Do not administer ZOSTAVAX to immunosuppressed or immunodeficient individuals including those with a history of primary or acquired immunodeficiency states, leukemia, lymphoma or other malignant neoplasms affecting the bone marrow or lymphatic system, AIDS or other clinical manifestations of infection with human immunodeficiency viruses, and those on immunosuppressive therapy.

4.3 Pregnancy

Do not administer ZOSTAVAX to pregnant women. It is not known whether ZOSTAVAX can cause fetal harm when administered to a pregnant woman or can affect reproduction capacity. However, naturally occurring varicella-zoster virus (VZV) infection is known to sometimes cause fetal harm. Therefore, ZOSTAVAX should not be administered to pregnant women, and pregnancy should be avoided for 3 months following administration of ZOSTAVAX.

5 WARNINGS AND PRECAUTIONS

5.1 Hypersensitivity Reactions

Serious adverse reactions, including anaphylaxis, have occurred with ZOSTAVAX. Adequate treatment provisions, including epinephrine injection (1:1,000), should be available for immediate use should an anaphylactic/anaphylactoid reaction occur.

5.2 Transmission of Vaccine Virus

Transmission of vaccine virus may occur between vaccinees and susceptible contacts.

5.3 Concurrent Illness

Deferral should be considered in acute illness (for example, in the presence of fever) or in patients with active untreated tuberculosis.

5.4 Limitations of Vaccine Effectiveness

Vaccination with ZOSTAVAX does not result in protection of all vaccine recipients.

The duration of protection beyond 4 years after vaccination with ZOSTAVAX is unknown. The need for revaccination has not been defined.

6   ADVERSE REACTIONS

The most frequent adverse reactions, reported in ≥1% of subjects vaccinated with ZOSTAVAX, were headache and injection-site reactions.

6.1   Clinical Trials Experience

Because clinical trials are conducted under widely varying conditions, rates of adverse reactions observed in the clinical trials of a vaccine cannot be directly compared to rates in the clinical trials of another vaccine and may not reflect the rates observed in practice.

ZOSTAVAX Efficacy and Safety Trial (ZEST) in Subjects 50 to 59 Years of Age

In the ZEST study, subjects received a single dose of either ZOSTAVAX (N=11,184) or placebo (N=11,212). The racial distribution across both vaccination groups was similar: White (94.4%); Black (4.2%); Hispanic (3.3%) and Other (1.4%) in both vaccination groups. The gender distribution was 38% male and 62% female in both vaccination groups. The age distribution of subjects enrolled, 50 to 59 years, was similar in both vaccination groups. All subjects received a vaccination report card (VRC) to record adverse events occurring from Days 1 to 42 postvaccination.

In the ZEST study, serious adverse events occurred at a similar rate in subjects vaccinated with ZOSTAVAX (0.6%) or placebo (0.5%) from Days 1 to 42 postvaccination.

In the ZEST study, all subjects were monitored for adverse reactions. An anaphylactic reaction was reported for one subject vaccinated with ZOSTAVAX.

Most Common Adverse Reactions and Experiences in the ZEST Study

The overall incidence of vaccine-related injection-site adverse reactions within 5 days post-vaccination was greater for subjects vaccinated with ZOSTAVAX as compared to subjects who received placebo (63.6% for ZOSTAVAX and 14.0% for placebo). Injection-site adverse reactions occurring at an incidence ≥1% within 5 days post-vaccination are shown in Table 1.

Table 1: Injection-Site Adverse Reactions Reported in ≥1% of Adults Who Received ZOSTAVAX or Placebo Within 5 Days Post-Vaccination in the ZOSTAVAX Efficacy and Safety Trial

Injection-Site Adverse Reaction	ZOSTAVAX (N = 11094) %	Placebo (N = 11116) %
*Solicited**		
Pain	53.9	9.0
Erythema	48.1	4.3
Swelling	40.4	2.8
Unsolicited		
Pruritis	11.3	0.7
Warmth	3.7	0.2
Hematoma	1.6	1.6
Induration	1.1	0.0

* Solicited on the Vaccination Report Card

Systemic adverse reactions and experiences reported during Days 1-42 at an incidence of ≥1% in either vaccination group were headache (ZOSTAVAX 9.4%, placebo 8.2%) and pain in the extremity (ZOSTAVAX 1.3%, placebo 0.8%), respectively.

The overall incidence of systemic adverse experiences reported during Days 1-42 was higher for ZOSTAVAX (35.4%) than for placebo (33.5%).

Shingles Prevention Study (SPS) in Subjects 60 Years of Age and Older

In the SPS, the largest clinical trial of ZOSTAVAX, subjects received a single dose of either ZOSTAVAX (n=19,270) or placebo (n=19,276). The racial distribution across both vaccination groups was similar: White (95%); Black (2.0%); Hispanic (1.0%) and Other (1.0%) in both vaccination groups. The gender distribution was 59% male and 41% female in both vaccination groups. The age distribution of subjects enrolled, 59-99 years, was similar in both vaccination groups. The Adverse Event Monitoring Substudy of the SPS, designed to provide detailed data on the safety profile of the zoster vaccine (n=3,345 received ZOSTAVAX and n=3,271 received placebo) used vaccination report cards (VRC) to record adverse events occurring from Days 0 to 42 postvaccination (97% of subjects completed VRC in both vaccination groups). In addition, monthly surveillance for hospitalization was conducted through the end of the study, 2 to 5 years postvaccination.

The remainder of subjects in the SPS (n=15,925 received ZOSTAVAX and n=16,005 received placebo) were actively followed for safety outcomes through Day 42 postvaccination and passively followed for safety after Day 42.

Serious Adverse Events Occurring 0-42 Days Postvaccination

In the overall SPS study population, serious adverse events occurred at a similar rate (1.4%) in subjects vaccinated with ZOSTAVAX or placebo.

In the AE Monitoring Substudy, the rate of SAEs was increased in the group of subjects who received ZOSTAVAX as compared to the group of subjects who received placebo (Table 2).

[See table 2 below]

Among reported serious adverse events in the SPS (Days 0 to 42 postvaccination), serious cardiovascular events occurred more frequently in subjects who received ZOSTAVAX (20 [0.6%]) than in subjects who received placebo (12 [0.4%]) in the AE Monitoring Substudy. The frequencies of serious cardiovascular events were similar in subjects who received ZOSTAVAX (81 [0.4%]) and in subjects who received placebo (72 [0.4%]) in the entire study cohort (Days 0 to 42 postvaccination).

Serious Adverse Events Occurring Over the Entire Course of the Study

Rates of hospitalization were similar among subjects who received ZOSTAVAX and subjects who received placebo in the AE Monitoring Substudy, throughout the entire study. Fifty-one individuals (1.5%) receiving ZOSTAVAX were reported to have congestive heart failure (CHF) or pulmonary edema compared to 39 individuals (1.2%) receiving placebo in the AE Monitoring Substudy; 58 individuals (0.3%) receiving ZOSTAVAX were reported to have congestive heart failure (CHF) or pulmonary edema compared to 45 (0.2%) individuals receiving placebo in the overall study.

In the SPS, all subjects were monitored for vaccine-related SAEs. Investigator-determined, vaccine-related serious adverse experiences were reported for 2 subjects vaccinated with ZOSTAVAX (asthma exacerbation and polymyalgia rheumatica) and 3 subjects who received placebo (Goodpasture's syndrome, anaphylactic reaction, and polymyalgia rheumatica).

Deaths

The incidence of death was similar in the groups receiving ZOSTAVAX or placebo during the Days 0-42 postvaccination period; 14 deaths occurred in the group of subjects who received ZOSTAVAX and 16 deaths occurred in the group of subjects who received placebo. The most common reported cause of death was cardiovascular disease (10 in the group of subjects who received ZOSTAVAX, 8 in the group of subjects who received placebo). The overall incidence of death occurring at any time during the study was similar between vaccination groups: 793 deaths (4.1%) occurred in subjects who received ZOSTAVAX and 795 deaths (4.1%) in subjects who received placebo.

Most Common Adverse Reactions and Experiences in the AE Monitoring Substudy of the SPS

Injection-site adverse reactions reported at an incidence ≥1% are shown in Table 3. Most of these adverse reactions were reported as mild in intensity. The overall incidence of vaccine-related injection-site adverse reactions was significantly greater for subjects vaccinated with ZOSTAVAX versus subjects who received placebo (48% for ZOSTAVAX and 17% for placebo).

Table 3: Injection-Site Adverse Reactions* in ≥1% of Adults Who Received ZOSTAVAX or Placebo Within 5 Days Postvaccination from the AE Monitoring Substudy of the Shingles Prevention Study

Adverse Reaction	ZOSTAVAX (N = 3345) %	Placebo (N = 3271) %
Solicited†		
Erythema	35.6	6.9
Pain/Tenderness	34.3	8.3
Swelling	26.1	4.5
Unsolicited		
Hematoma	1.6	1.4
Pruritis	6.9	1.0
Warmth	1.6	0.3

* Patients instructed to report adverse experiences on a Vaccination Report Card
† Solicited on the Vaccination Report Card

Headache was the only systemic adverse reaction reported on the vaccine report card between Days 0-42 by ≥1% of subjects in the AE Monitoring Substudy in either vaccination group (ZOSTAVAX 1.4%, placebo 0.8%).

The numbers of subjects with elevated temperature (≥38.3°C [≥101.0°F]) within 42 days postvaccination were similar in the ZOSTAVAX and the placebo vaccination groups [27 (0.8%) vs. 27 (0.9%), respectively].

The following adverse experiences in the AE Monitoring Substudy of the SPS (Days 0 to 42 postvaccination) were reported at an incidence ≥1% and greater in subjects who received ZOSTAVAX than in subjects who received placebo, respectively: respiratory infection (65 [1.9%] vs. 55 [1.7%]), fever (59 [1.8%] vs. 53 [1.6%]), flu syndrome (57 [1.7%] vs. 52 [1.6%]), diarrhea (51 [1.5%] vs. 41 [1.3%]), rhinitis (46 [1.4%] vs. 36 [1.1%]), skin disorder (35 [1.1%] vs. 31 [1.0%]), respiratory disorder (35 [1.1%] vs. 27 [0.8%]), asthenia (32 [1.0%] vs. 14 [0.4%]).

6.2   VZV Rashes Following Vaccination

Within the 42-day postvaccination reporting period in the ZEST, noninjection-site zoster-like rashes were reported by 34 subjects (19 for ZOSTAVAX and 15 for placebo). Of 24 specimens that were adequate for Polymerase Chain Reaction (PCR) testing, wild-type VZV was detected in 10 (3 for ZOSTAVAX, 7 for placebo) of these specimens. The Oka/Merck strain of VZV was not detected from any of these specimens. Of reported varicella-like rashes (n=124, 69 for ZOSTAVAX and 55 for placebo), 23 had specimens that were available and adequate for PCR testing. VZV was detected in one of these specimens in the ZOSTAVAX group; however, the virus strain (wild-type or Oka/Merck strain) could not be determined.

Within the 42-day postvaccination reporting period in the SPS, noninjection-site zoster-like rashes were reported by 53 subjects (17 for ZOSTAVAX and 36 for placebo). Of 41 specimens that were adequate for Polymerase Chain Reaction (PCR) testing, wild-type VZV was detected in 25 (5 for ZOSTAVAX, 20 for placebo) of these specimens. The Oka/Merck strain of VZV was not detected from any of these specimens.

Of reported varicella-like rashes (n=59), 10 had specimens that were available and adequate for PCR testing. VZV was not detected in any of these specimens.

Table 2: Number of Subjects with ≥1 Serious Adverse Events (0-42 Days Postvaccination) in the Shingles Prevention Study

Cohort	ZOSTAVAX n/N %	Placebo n/N %	Relative Risk (95% CI)
Overall Study Cohort (60 years of age and older)	255/18671 1.4%	254/18717 1.4%	1.01 (0.85, 1.20)
60-69 years old	113/10100 1.1%	101/10095 1.0%	1.12 (0.86, 1.46)
70-79 years old	115/7351 1.6%	132/7333 1.8%	0.87 (0.68, 1.11)
≥80 years old	27/1220 2.2%	21/1289 1.6%	1.36 (0.78, 2.37)
AE Monitoring Substudy Cohort (60 years of age and older)	64/3326 1.9%	41/3249 1.3%	1.53 (1.04, 2.25)
60-69 years old	22/1726 1.3%	18/1709 1.1%	1.21 (0.66, 2.23)
70-79 years old	31/1383 2.2%	19/1367 1.4%	1.61 (0.92, 2.82)
≥80 years old	11/217 5.1%	4/173 2.3%	2.19 (0.75, 6.45)

N=number of subjects in cohort with safety follow-up
n=number of subjects reporting an SAE 0-42 Days postvaccination

In clinical trials in support of the initial licensure of the frozen formulation of ZOSTAVAX, the reported rates of noninjection-site zoster-like and varicella-like rashes within 42 days postvaccination were also low in both zoster vaccine and placebo recipients. Of 17 reported varicella-like rashes and non-injection site zoster-like rashes, 10 specimens were available and adequate for PCR testing, and 2 subjects had varicella (onset Day 8 and 17) confirmed to be Oka/Merck strain.

6.3 Postmarketing Experience

The following additional adverse reactions have been identified during postmarketing use of ZOSTAVAX. Because these reactions are reported voluntarily from a population of uncertain size, it is generally not possible to reliably estimate their frequency or establish a causal relationship to the vaccine.

Gastrointestinal disorders: nausea

Infections and infestations: herpes zoster (vaccine strain)

Skin and subcutaneous tissue disorders: rash

Musculoskeletal and connective tissue disorders: arthralgia; myalgia

General disorders and administration site conditions: injection-site rash; pyrexia; injection-site urticaria; transient injection-site lymphadenopathy

Immune system disorders: hypersensitivity reactions including anaphylactic reactions

Reporting Adverse Events

The U.S. Department of Health and Human Services has established a Vaccine Adverse Event Reporting System (VAERS) to accept all reports of suspected adverse events after the administration of any vaccine. For information or a copy of the vaccine reporting form, call the VAERS toll-free number at 1-800-822-7967 or report online to www.vaers.hhs.gov. [2]

7 DRUG INTERACTIONS

7.1 Concomitant Administration with Other Vaccines

In a randomized clinical study, a reduced immune response to ZOSTAVAX as measured by gpELISA was observed in individuals who received concurrent administration of PNEUMOVAX® 23 and ZOSTAVAX compared with individuals who received these vaccines 4 weeks apart. Consider administration of the two vaccines separated by at least 4 weeks [see Clinical Studies (14.3)].

For concomitant administration of ZOSTAVAX with trivalent inactivated influenza vaccine, [see Clinical Studies (14.3)].

7.2 Antiviral Medications

Concurrent administration of ZOSTAVAX and antiviral medications known to be effective against VZV has not been evaluated.

8 USE IN SPECIFIC POPULATIONS

8.1 Pregnancy

Pregnancy Category: Contraindication [see Contraindications (4.3)].

ZOSTAVAX should not be administered to pregnant females since wild-type varicella can sometimes cause congenital varicella infection. Pregnancy should be avoided for three months following vaccination with ZOSTAVAX [see Contraindications (4.3) and Patient Counseling Information (17)].

Pregnancy Registry

From 1995 to 2013, Merck Sharp & Dohme Corp., a subsidiary of Merck & Co., Inc., maintained a Pregnancy Registry to monitor fetal outcomes following inadvertent administration of VARIVAX® during pregnancy or within three months prior to conception. In 2006, reports of exposure to two other varicella (Oka/Merck)-containing vaccines, ProQuad® (Measles, Mumps, Rubella and Varicella Virus Vaccine Live) and ZOSTAVAX, were added to the Registry. The Pregnancy Registry has been discontinued. As of March 2011, 811 women with pregnancy outcome information available for analysis were prospectively enrolled following vaccination with VARIVAX, within three months prior to conception or any time during pregnancy. Of these women, 170 were seronegative at the time of exposure and 627 women had an unknown serostatus. The remaining women were seropositive. Nine exposures to either ProQuad or ZOSTAVAX have been reported that met criteria for inclusion into the Registry.

None of the 820 women who received a varicella-containing vaccine delivered infants with abnormalities consistent with congenital varicella syndrome.

All exposures to VARIVAX, ProQuad, or ZOSTAVAX during pregnancy or within three months prior to conception should be reported as suspected adverse reactions by contacting Merck Sharp & Dohme Corp., a subsidiary of Merck & Co., Inc., at 1-877-888-4231 or VAERS at 1-800-822-7967 or www.vaers.hhs.gov.

8.3 Nursing Mothers

ZOSTAVAX is not indicated in women who are nursing. It is not known whether VZV is secreted in human milk. Therefore, because some viruses are secreted in human milk, caution should be exercised if ZOSTAVAX is administered to a nursing woman.

8.4 Pediatric Use

ZOSTAVAX is not indicated for prevention of primary varicella infection (Chickenpox) and should not be used in children and adolescents.

8.5 Geriatric Use

The median age of subjects enrolled in the largest (N=38,546) clinical study of ZOSTAVAX was 69 years (range 59-99 years). Of the 19,270 subjects who received ZOSTAVAX, 10,378 were 60-69 years of age, 7,629 were 70-79 years of age, and 1,263 were 80 years of age or older.

11 DESCRIPTION

ZOSTAVAX is a lyophilized preparation of the Oka/Merck strain of live, attenuated varicella-zoster virus (VZV). ZOSTAVAX, when reconstituted as directed, is a sterile suspension for subcutaneous administration. Each 0.65-mL dose contains a minimum of 19,400 PFU (plaque-forming units) of Oka/Merck strain of VZV when reconstituted and stored at room temperature for up to 30 minutes.

Each dose contains 31.16 mg of sucrose, 15.58 mg of hydrolyzed porcine gelatin, 3.99 mg of sodium chloride, 0.62 mg of monosodium L-glutamate, 0.57 mg of sodium phosphate dibasic, 0.10 mg of potassium phosphate monobasic, 0.10 mg of potassium chloride; residual components of MRC-5 cells including DNA and protein; and trace quantities of neomycin and bovine calf serum. The product contains no preservatives.

12 CLINICAL PHARMACOLOGY

12.1 Mechanism of Action

The risk of developing zoster appears to be related to a decline in VZV-specific immunity. ZOSTAVAX was shown to boost VZV-specific immunity, which is thought to be the mechanism by which it protects against zoster and its complications. [See Clinical Studies (14).]

Herpes zoster (HZ), commonly known as shingles or zoster, is a manifestation of the reactivation of varicella zoster virus (VZV), which, as a primary infection, produces chickenpox (varicella). Following initial infection, the virus remains latent in the dorsal root or cranial sensory ganglia until it reactivates, producing zoster. Zoster is characterized by a unilateral, painful, vesicular cutaneous eruption with a dermatomal distribution.

Pain associated with zoster may occur during the prodrome, the acute eruptive phase, and the postherpetic phase of the infection. Pain occurring in the postherpetic phase of infection is commonly referred to as postherpetic neuralgia (PHN).

Serious complications, such as PHN, scarring, bacterial superinfection, allodynia, cranial and motor neuron palsies, pneumonia, encephalitis, visual impairment, hearing loss, and death can occur as the result of zoster.

13 NONCLINICAL TOXICOLOGY

13.1 Carcinogenesis, Mutagenesis, Impairment of Fertility

ZOSTAVAX has not been evaluated for its carcinogenic or mutagenic potential, or its potential to impair fertility.

14 CLINICAL STUDIES

In two large clinical trials (ZEST and SPS), ZOSTAVAX significantly reduced the risk of developing zoster when compared with placebo (see Table 4 and Table 5).

14.1 ZOSTAVAX Efficacy and Safety Trial (ZEST) in Subjects 50 to 59 Years of Age

Efficacy of ZOSTAVAX was evaluated in the ZOSTAVAX Efficacy and Safety Trial (ZEST), a placebo-controlled, double-blind clinical trial in which 22,439 subjects 50 to 59 years of age were randomized to receive a single dose of either ZOSTAVAX (n=11,211) or placebo (n=11,228). Subjects were followed for the development of zoster for a median of 1.3 years (range 0 to 2 years). Confirmed zoster cases were determined by Polymerase Chain Reaction (PCR) [86%] or, in the absence of virus detection, by a Clinical Evaluation Committee [14%]. The primary efficacy analysis included all subjects randomized in the study (intent-to-treat [ITT] analysis).

Compared with placebo, ZOSTAVAX significantly reduced the risk of developing zoster by 69.8% (95% CI [54.1, 80.6%]) in subjects 50 to 59 years of age (Table 4).

[See table 4 above]

Immune responses to vaccination were evaluated in a random 10% subcohort (n=1,136 for ZOSTAVAX and n=1,133 for placebo) of the subjects enrolled in the ZEST study. VZV antibody levels (Geometric Mean Titers, GMT), as measured by glycoprotein enzyme-linked immunosorbent assay (gpELISA) 6 weeks postvaccination, were increased 2.3-fold [95% CI (2.2, 2.4)] in the group of subjects who received ZOSTAVAX compared to subjects who received placebo; the specific antibody level that correlates with protection from zoster has not been established.

14.2 Shingles Prevention Study (SPS) in Subjects 60 Years of Age and Older

Efficacy of ZOSTAVAX was evaluated in the Shingles Prevention Study (SPS), a placebo-controlled, double-blind clinical trial in which 38,546 subjects 60 years of age or older were randomized to receive a single dose of either ZOSTAVAX (n=19,270) or placebo (n=19,276). Subjects were followed for the development of zoster for a median of 3.1 years (range 31 days to 4.90 years). The study excluded people who were immunocompromised or using corticosteroids on a regular basis, anyone with a previous history of HZ, and those with conditions that might interfere with study evaluations, including people with cognitive impairment, severe hearing loss, those who were non-ambulatory, and those whose survival was not considered to be at least 5 years. Randomization was stratified by age, 60-69 and ≥70 years of age. Suspected zoster cases were confirmed by Polymerase Chain Reaction (PCR) [93%], viral culture [1%], or in the absence of virus detection, as determined by a Clinical Evaluation Committee [6%]. Individuals in both vaccination groups who developed zoster were given famciclovir and, as necessary, pain medications. The primary efficacy analysis included all subjects randomized in the study who were followed for at least 30 days postvaccination and did not develop an evaluable case of HZ within the first 30 days postvaccination (Modified Intent-To-Treat [MITT] analysis). ZOSTAVAX significantly reduced the risk of developing zoster when compared with placebo (Table 5). In the SPS, vaccine efficacy for the prevention of HZ was highest for those subjects 60-69 years of age and declined with increasing age.

[See table 5 above]

Forty-five subjects were excluded from the MITT analysis (16 in the group of subjects who received ZOSTAVAX and 29

Table 4: Efficacy of ZOSTAVAX on HZ Incidence Compared with Placebo in the ZOSTAVAX Efficacy and Safety Trial*

Age group (yrs.)	ZOSTAVAX			Placebo			Vaccine Efficacy (95% CI)
	# subjects	# HZ cases	Incidence rate of HZ per 1000 person-yrs.	# subjects	# HZ cases	Incidence rate of HZ per 1000 person-yrs.	
50-59	11211	30	1.994	11228	99	6.596	69.8% (54.1%, 80.6%)

* The analysis was performed on the intent-to-treat (ITT) population that included all subjects randomized in the ZEST study.

Table 5: Efficacy of ZOSTAVAX on HZ Incidence Compared with Placebo in the Shingles Prevention Study*

Age group† (yrs.)	ZOSTAVAX			Placebo			Vaccine Efficacy (95% CI)
	# subjects	# HZ cases	Incidence rate of HZ per 1000 person-yrs.	# subjects	# HZ cases	Incidence rate of HZ per 1000 person-yrs.	
Overall	19254	315	5.4	19247	642	11.1	51% (44%, 58%)
60-69	10370	122	3.9	10356	334	10.8	64% (56%, 71%)
70-79	7621	156	6.7	7559	261	11.4	41% (28%, 52%)
≥80	1263	37	9.9	1332	47	12.2	18% (-29%, 48%)

* The analysis was performed on the Modified Intent-To-Treat (MITT) population that included all subjects randomized in the study who were followed for at least 30 days postvaccination and did not develop an evaluable case of HZ within the first 30 days postvaccination.

† Age strata at randomization were 60-69 and ≥70 years of age.

Table 6: Postherpetic Neuralgia (PHN)* in the Shingles Prevention Study[†]

Age group (yrs.)[‡]	ZOSTAVAX					Placebo					Vaccine efficacy against PHN in subjects who develop HZ postvaccination (95% CI)
	# subjects	# HZ cases	# PHN cases	Incidence rate of PHN per 1,000 person-yrs.	% HZ cases with PHN	# subjects	# HZ cases	# PHN cases	Incidence rate of PHN per 1,000 person-yrs.	% HZ cases with PHN	
Overall	19254	315	27	0.5	8.6%	19247	642	80	1.4	12.5%	39%[§] (7%, 59%)
60-69	10370	122	8	0.3	6.6%	10356	334	23	0.7	6.9%	5% (-107%, 56%)
70-79	7621	156	12	0.5	7.7%	7559	261	45	2.0	17.2%	55% (18%, 76%)
≥80	1263	37	7	1.9	18.9%	1332	47	12	3.1	25.5%	26% (-69%, 68%)

* PHN was defined as HZ-associated pain rated as ≥3 (on a 0-10 scale), persisting or appearing more than 90 days after onset of HZ rash using Zoster Brief Pain Inventory (ZBPI). {3}
[†] The table is based on the Modified Intent-To-Treat (MITT) population that included all subjects randomized in the study who were followed for at least 30 days postvaccination and did not develop an evaluable case of HZ within the first 30 days postvaccination.
[‡] Age strata at randomization were 60-69 and ≥70 years of age.
[§] Age-adjusted estimate based on the age strata (60-69 and ≥70 years of age) at randomization.

in the group of subjects who received placebo), including 24 subjects with evaluable HZ cases that occurred in the first 30 days postvaccination (6 evaluable HZ cases in the group of subjects who received ZOSTAVAX and 18 evaluable HZ cases in the group of subjects who received placebo).

Suspected HZ cases were followed prospectively for the development of HZ-related complications. Table 6 compares the rates of PHN defined as HZ-associated pain (rated as 3 or greater on a 10-point scale by the study subject and occurring or persisting at least 90 days) following the onset of rash in evaluable cases of HZ.
[See table 6 above]

The median duration of clinically significant pain (defined as ≥3 on a 0-10 point scale) among HZ cases in the group of subjects who received ZOSTAVAX as compared to the group of subjects who received placebo was 20 days vs. 22 days based on the confirmed HZ cases.

Overall, the benefit of ZOSTAVAX in the prevention of PHN can be primarily attributed to the effect of the vaccine on the prevention of herpes zoster. Vaccination with ZOSTAVAX in the SPS reduced the incidence of PHN in individuals 70 years of age and older who developed zoster postvaccination. Other prespecified zoster-related complications were reported less frequently in subjects who received ZOSTAVAX compared to subjects who received placebo. Among HZ cases, zoster-related complications were reported at similar rates in both vaccination groups (Table 7).
[See table 7 below]

Visceral complications reported by fewer than 1% of subjects with zoster included 3 cases of pneumonitis and 1 case of hepatitis in the placebo group, and 1 case of meningoencephalitis in the vaccine group.

Immune responses to vaccination were evaluated in a subset of subjects enrolled in the Shingles Prevention Study (N=1,395). VZV antibody levels (Geometric Mean Titers, GMT), as measured by glycoprotein enzyme-linked immunosorbent assay (gpELISA) 6 weeks postvaccination, were increased 1.7-fold (95% CI: [1.6 to 1.8]) in the group of subjects who received ZOSTAVAX compared to subjects who received placebo; the specific antibody level that correlates with protection from zoster has not been established.

14.3 Concomitant Use Studies

In a double-blind, controlled substudy, 374 adults in the US, 60 years of age and older (median age = 66 years), were randomized to receive trivalent inactivated influenza vaccine (TIV) and ZOSTAVAX concurrently (N=188), or TIV alone followed 4 weeks later by ZOSTAVAX alone (N=186). The antibody responses to both vaccines at 4 weeks postvaccination were similar in both groups.

In a double-blind, controlled clinical trial, 473 adults, 60 years of age or older, were randomized to receive ZOSTAVAX and PNEUMOVAX 23 concomitantly (N=237), or PNEUMOVAX 23 alone followed 4 weeks later by ZOSTAVAX alone (N=236). At 4 weeks postvaccination, the VZV antibody levels following concomitant use were significantly lower than the VZV antibody levels following nonconcomitant administration (GMTs of 338 vs. 484 gpELISA units/mL, respectively; GMT ratio = 0.70 (95% CI: [0.61, 0.80]).

15 REFERENCES

1. Reitschel RL, Bernier R. Neomycin sensitivity and the MMR vaccine. JAMA 1981;245(6):571.
2. Atkinson WL, Pickering LK, Schwartz B, Weniger BG, Iskander JK, Watson JC. General recommendations on immunization: Recommendations of the Advisory Committee on Immunization Practices (ACIP) and the American Academy of Family Physicians (AAFP). MMWR 2002;51(RR02):1-36.
3. Coplan PM, Schmader K, Nikas A, Chan ISF, Choo P, Levin MJ, et al. Development of a measure of the burden of pain due to herpes zoster and postherpetic neuralgia for prevention trials: Adaptation of the brief pain inventory. J Pain 2004;5(6):344-56.

16 HOW SUPPLIED/STORAGE AND HANDLING

No. 4963-00 — ZOSTAVAX is supplied as follows: (1) a package of 1 single-dose vial of lyophilized vaccine, **NDC** 0006-4963-00 (package A); and (2) a separate package of 10 vials of diluent (package B).

No. 4963-41 — ZOSTAVAX is supplied as follows: (1) a package of 10 single-dose vials of lyophilized vaccine, **NDC** 0006-4963-41 (package A); and (2) a separate package of 10 vials of diluent (package B).

Storage

To maintain potency, ZOSTAVAX must be stored frozen between -58°F and +5°F (-50°C and -15°C). Use of dry ice may subject ZOSTAVAX to temperatures colder than -58°F (-50°C).

Before reconstitution, ZOSTAVAX SHOULD BE STORED FROZEN at a temperature between -58°F and +5°F (-50°C and -15°C) until it is reconstituted for injection. Any freezer, including frost-free, that has a separate sealed freezer door and reliably maintains a temperature between -58°F and +5°F (-50°C and -15°C) is acceptable for storing ZOSTAVAX. ZOSTAVAX may be stored and/or transported at refrigerator temperature between 36°F and 46°F (2°C to 8°C) for up to 72 continuous hours prior to reconstitution. Vaccine stored between 36°F and 46°F (2°C to 8°C) that is not used within 72 hours of removal from +5°F (-15°C) storage should be discarded. ZOSTAVAX should be reconstituted immediately upon removal from the freezer. The diluent should be stored separately at room temperature (68°F to 77°F, 20°C to 25°C), or in the refrigerator (36°F to 46°F, 2°C to 8°C).

For further product information call 1-800-MERCK-90.
Before reconstitution, protect from light.
DO NOT FREEZE RECONSTITUTED VACCINE.

17 PATIENT COUNSELING INFORMATION

Advise the patient to read the FDA-approved patient labeling (Patient Information).

• Question the patient about reactions to previous vaccines.
• Provide a copy of the patient information (PPI) located at the end of this insert and discuss any questions or concerns.
• Inform patient of the benefits and risks of ZOSTAVAX, including the potential risk of transmitting the vaccine virus to susceptible individuals, such as immunosuppressed or immunodeficient individuals or pregnant women who have not had chickenpox.
• Instruct patient to report any adverse reactions or any symptoms of concern to their healthcare professional.

Dist. by: Merck Sharp & Dohme Corp., a subsidiary of **MERCK & CO., INC.**, Whitehouse Station, NJ 08889, USA
For patent information:
www.merck.com/product/patent/home.html
Copyright © 2006, 2014 Merck Sharp & Dohme Corp., a subsidiary of **Merck & Co., Inc.**
All rights reserved.
uspi-v211-i-fro-1402r018
Printed in USA
Rx only

Patient Information about
ZOSTAVAX® (pronounced "ZOS tah vax")
Generic name: Zoster Vaccine Live

You should read this summary of information about ZOSTAVAX before you are vaccinated. If you have any questions about ZOSTAVAX after reading this leaflet, you should ask your health care provider. This information does not take the place of talking about ZOSTAVAX with your doctor, nurse, or other health care provider. Only your health care provider can decide if ZOSTAVAX is right for you.

What is ZOSTAVAX and how does it work?

ZOSTAVAX is a vaccine that is used for adults 50 years of age or older to prevent shingles (also known as zoster). ZOSTAVAX contains a weakened chickenpox virus (varicella-zoster virus).

Table 7: Specific complications* of zoster among HZ cases in the Shingles Prevention Study

Complication	ZOSTAVAX (N = 19270)		Placebo (N = 19276)	
	(n = 321)	% Among Zoster Cases	(n = 659)	% Among Zoster Cases
Allodynia	135	42.1	310	47.0
Bacterial Superinfection	3	0.9	7	1.1
Dissemination	5	1.6	11	1.7
Impaired Vision	2	0.6	9	1.4
Ophthalmic Zoster	35	10.9	69	10.5
Peripheral Nerve Palsies (motor)	5	1.6	12	1.8
Ptosis	2	0.6	9	1.4
Scarring	24	7.5	57	8.6
Sensory Loss	7	2.2	12	1.8

N=number of subjects randomized
n=number of zoster cases, including those cases occurring within 30 days postvaccination, with these data available
* Complications reported at a frequency of ≥1% in at least one vaccination group among subjects with zoster

ZOSTAVAX works by helping your immune system protect you from getting shingles.

If you do get shingles even though you have been vaccinated, ZOSTAVAX may help prevent the nerve pain that can follow shingles in some people. ZOSTAVAX does not protect everyone, so some people who get the vaccine may still get shingles.

ZOSTAVAX cannot be used to treat shingles, or the nerve pain that may follow shingles, once you have it.

What do I need to know about shingles and the virus that causes it?

Shingles is caused by the same virus that causes chickenpox. Once you have had chickenpox, the virus can stay in your nervous system for many years. For reasons that are not fully understood, the virus may become active again and give you shingles. Age and problems with the immune system may increase your chances of getting shingles.

Shingles is a rash that is usually on one side of the body. The rash begins as a cluster of small red spots that often blister. The rash can be painful. Shingles rashes usually last up to 30 days and, for most people, the pain associated with the rash lessens as it heals.

Who should not get ZOSTAVAX?

You should not get ZOSTAVAX if you:
• are allergic to any of its ingredients.
• are allergic to gelatin or neomycin.
• have a weakened immune system (for example, an immune deficiency, leukemia, lymphoma, or HIV/AIDS).
• take high doses of steroids by injection or by mouth.
• are pregnant or plan to get pregnant.

You should not get ZOSTAVAX to prevent chickenpox.

Children should not get ZOSTAVAX.

How is ZOSTAVAX given?

ZOSTAVAX is given as a single dose by injection under the skin.

What should I tell my health care provider before I get ZOSTAVAX?

You should tell your health care provider if you:
• have or have had any medical problems.
• take any medicines, including non-prescription medicines, and dietary supplements.
• have any allergies, including allergies to neomycin or gelatin.
• had an allergic reaction to another vaccine.
• are pregnant or plan to become pregnant.
• are breast-feeding.

Tell your health care provider if you expect to be in close contact (including household contact) with newborn infants, someone who may be pregnant and has not had chickenpox or been vaccinated against chickenpox, or someone who has problems with their immune system. Your health care provider can tell you what situations you may need to avoid.

Can I get ZOSTAVAX with other vaccines?

Talk to your health care provider if you plan to get ZOSTAVAX at the same time as the flu vaccine.

Talk to your health care provider if you plan to get ZOSTAVAX at the same time as PNEUMOVAX® 23 because it may be better to get these vaccines at least 4 weeks apart.

What are the possible side effects of ZOSTAVAX?

The most common side effects that people in the clinical studies reported after receiving the vaccine include:
• redness, pain, itching, swelling, hard lump, warmth, or bruising where the shot was given.
• headache

The following additional side effects have been reported with ZOSTAVAX:
• allergic reactions, which may be serious and may include difficulty in breathing or swallowing. If you have an allergic reaction, call your doctor right away.
• chickenpox
• fever
• hives at the injection site
• joint pain
• muscle pain
• nausea
• rash
• rash at the injection site
• shingles
• swollen glands near the injection site (that may last a few days to a few weeks)

Tell your healthcare provider if you have any new or unusual symptoms after you receive ZOSTAVAX. For a complete list of side effects, ask your health care provider.

Report the following to your doctor or your child's doctor:
• any adverse reactions following vaccination
• exposure to ZOSTAVAX during pregnancy
• exposure to ZOSTAVAX during the 3 months before getting pregnant.

You may also report these events to Merck Sharp & Dohme Corp., a subsidiary of Merck & Co., Inc., at 1-877-888-4231, or directly to the Vaccine Adverse Event Reporting System (VAERS). The VAERS toll free number is 1-800-822-7967 or report online to www.vaers.hhs.gov.

What are the ingredients of ZOSTAVAX?

Active Ingredient: a weakened form of the varicella-zoster virus.

Inactive Ingredients: sucrose, hydrolyzed porcine gelatin, sodium chloride, monosodium L-glutamate, sodium phosphate dibasic, potassium phosphate monobasic, potassium chloride.

This leaflet summarizes important information about ZOSTAVAX. If you would like more information, talk to your health care provider or visit the website at www.ZOSTAVAX.com or call 1-800-622-4477.

Dist. by: Merck Sharp & Dohme Corp., a subsidiary of MERCK & CO., INC., Whitehouse Station, NJ 08889, USA

For patent information:

www.merck.com/product/patent/home.html

Copyright © 2006, 2014 Merck Sharp & Dohme Corp., a subsidiary of Merck & Co., Inc.

All rights reserved.

Revised: 02/2014

usppi-v211-i-fro-1402r017

Printed in USA

Rx Only

Merck Sharp & Dohme Corp.,

for product information, please see Merck

Mission Pharmacal Company

10999 IH 10 WEST, SUITE 1000
SAN ANTONIO, TX 78230-1355

Direct All Inquiries to:
PO Box 786099
San Antonio, TX 78278-6099
TOLL FREE: (800) 292-7364
Customer Service (M–W 7A–5:30P Central Time
Th 7:30A–5P Central Time)
(210) 696-8400; FAX: (210) 696-6010

BINOSTO®   ℞
(alendronate sodium)
effervescent tablets for oral solution

HIGHLIGHTS OF PRESCRIBING INFORMATION

These highlights do not include all the information needed to use BINOSTO® safely and effectively. See full prescribing information for BINOSTO.

BINOSTO (alendronate sodium) effervescent tablets for oral solution

Initial US Approval: 1995

——————RECENT MAJOR CHANGES——————

Indications and Usage (1.3)	04/2013
Warnings and Precautions (5.4)	04/2013

——————INDICATIONS AND USAGE——————

BINOSTO is a bisphosphonate indicated for:
• Treatment of osteoporosis in postmenopausal women (1.1)
• Treatment to increase bone mass in men with osteoporosis (1.2)

Limitation of use: Optimal duration of use has not been determined. For patients at low-risk for fracture, consider drug discontinuation after 3 to 5 years of use (1.3)

——————DOSAGE AND ADMINISTRATION——————

• 70 mg BINOSTO effervescent tablet once weekly (2.1, 2.2)
• Instruct patients to: (2.3)
  ○ Dissolve one tablet of BINOSTO in approximately half a glass of plain room temperature water (4 oz). Wait at least 5 minutes after the effervescence stops, stir the solution for approximately 10 seconds and consume contents.
  ○ Swallow solution *at least* 30 minutes before the first food, beverage, or medication of the day.
  ○ Avoid lying down for at least 30 minutes after taking BINOSTO and until after the first food of the day.

——————DOSAGE FORMS AND STRENGTHS——————

Effervescent tablets, 70 mg (3)

——————CONTRAINDICATIONS——————

• Abnormalities of the esophagus which delay emptying such as stricture or achalasia (4, 5.1)
• Inability to stand/sit upright for at least 30 minutes (4, 5.1)
• Increased risk of aspiration (4)

• Hypocalcemia (4, 5.2)
• Hypersensitivity to any component of this product (4, 6.2)

——————WARNINGS AND PRECAUTIONS——————

• *Upper Gastrointestinal Adverse Reactions* can occur. Instruct patients to follow dosing instructions. Discontinue if new or worsening symptoms occur. (5.1)
• *Hypocalcemia* can worsen and must be corrected prior to use. (5.2)
• *Severe Bone, Joint, Muscle Pain* may occur. Discontinue use if severe symptoms develop. (5.3)
• *Osteonecrosis of the Jaw* has been reported. (5.4)
• *Atypical Femur Fractures* have been reported. Patients with new thigh or groin pain should be evaluated to rule out a femoral fracture. (5.5)
• *Sodium Content:* Each tablet contains 650 mg sodium, equivalent to 1650 mg NaCl. Use caution in patients on sodium restriction. (5.7)

——————ADVERSE REACTIONS——————

The most common adverse reactions (incidence greater than or equal to 3%) are abdominal pain, acid regurgitation, constipation, diarrhea, dyspepsia, musculoskeletal pain, and nausea. (6.1)

To report SUSPECTED ADVERSE REACTIONS, contact Mission Pharmacal Company at 1-855-778-0177 or FDA at 1-800-FDA-1088 or www.fda.gov/medwatch

——————DRUG INTERACTIONS——————

• Calcium supplements, antacids or oral medications containing multivalent cations interfere with absorption of alendronate. (7.1)
• Use caution when co-prescribing aspirin/nonsteroidal anti-inflammatory drugs that may worsen gastrointestinal irritation. (7.2, 7.3)

——————USE IN SPECIFIC POPULATIONS——————

• BINOSTO is not indicated for use in pediatric patients. (8.4)
• BINOSTO is not recommended in patients with renal impairment (creatinine clearance less than 35 mL/min). (5.6, 8.6)

See 17 for PATIENT COUNSELING INFORMATION and Medication Guide

Revised: 08/2013

FULL PRESCRIBING INFORMATION: CONTENTS*

1   **INDICATIONS AND USAGE**
  1.1   Treatment of Osteoporosis in Postmenopausal Women
  1.2   Treatment to Increase Bone Mass in Men With Osteoporosis
  1.3   Important Limitations of Use
2   **DOSAGE AND ADMINISTRATION**
  2.1   Treatment of Osteoporosis in Postmenopausal Women
  2.2   Treatment to Increase Bone Mass in Men With Osteoporosis
  2.3   Important Administration Instructions
  2.4   Recommendations for Calcium and Vitamin D Supplementation
  2.5   Administration Instructions for Missed Doses
3   **DOSAGE FORMS AND STRENGTHS**
4   **CONTRAINDICATIONS**
5   **WARNINGS AND PRECAUTIONS**
  5.1   Upper Gastrointestinal Adverse Reactions
  5.2   Mineral Metabolism
  5.3   Musculoskeletal Pain
  5.4   Osteonecrosis of the Jaw
  5.5   Atypical Subtrochanteric and Diaphyseal Femoral Fractures
  5.6   Renal Impairment
  5.7   Patients Sensitive to High Sodium Intake
6   **ADVERSE REACTIONS**
  6.1   Clinical Trials Experience
  6.2   Post-Marketing Experience
7   **DRUG INTERACTIONS**
  7.1   Calcium Supplements/Antacids
  7.2   Aspirin
  7.3   Nonsteroidal Anti-inflammatory Drugs (NSAIDs)
8   **USE IN SPECIFIC POPULATIONS**
  8.1   Pregnancy
  8.3   Nursing Mothers
  8.4   Pediatric Use
  8.5   Geriatric Use
  8.6   Renal Impairment
  8.7   Hepatic Impairment
10   **OVERDOSAGE**
11   **DESCRIPTION**
12   **CLINICAL PHARMACOLOGY**
  12.1   Mechanism of Action
  12.2   Pharmacodynamics
  12.3   Pharmacokinetics

FULL PRESCRIBING INFORMATION

1 INDICATIONS AND USAGE

1.1 Treatment of Osteoporosis in Postmenopausal Women

BINOSTO effervescent tablet 70 mg is indicated for the treatment of osteoporosis in postmenopausal women. For the treatment of osteoporosis, alendronate sodium increases bone mass and reduces the incidence of fractures, including those of the hip and spine (vertebral compression fractures). [See Clinical Studies (14.1).]

1.2 Treatment to Increase Bone Mass in Men With Osteoporosis

BINOSTO is indicated for treatment to increase bone mass in men with osteoporosis [see Clinical Studies (14.2)].

1.3 Important Limitations of Use

The optimal duration of use has not been determined. The safety and effectiveness of BINOSTO for the treatment of osteoporosis are based on clinical data of four years duration. All patients on bisphosphonate therapy should have the need for continued therapy re-evaluated on a periodic basis. Patients at low risk for fracture should be considered for drug discontinuation after 3 to 5 years of use. Patients who discontinue therapy should have their risk for fracture re-evaluated periodically.

2 DOSAGE AND ADMINISTRATION

2.1 Treatment of Osteoporosis in Postmenopausal Women

The recommended dosage is one 70 mg effervescent tablet once weekly.

2.2 Treatment to Increase Bone Mass in Men With Osteoporosis

The recommended dosage is one 70 mg effervescent tablet once weekly.

2.3 Important Administration Instructions

Instruct patients to do the following to assure adequate drug absorption and to decrease the risk of esophageal adverse reactions: Waiting less than 30 minutes, or taking BINOSTO with food, beverages (other than plain water) or other medications will lessen the effect of BINOSTO by decreasing its absorption into the body [see Drug Interactions (7.1)].

- Take BINOSTO upon arising for the day and at least 30 minutes before the first food, beverage, or medication of the day.
- Dissolve the effervescent tablet in 4 ounces room temperature plain water only (not mineral water or flavored water).
- Wait at least 5 minutes after the effervescence stops and then stir the solution for approximately 10 seconds and ingest.
- Avoid lying down for at least 30 minutes after taking BINOSTO and until after their first food of the day.
- Do not take BINOSTO at bedtime or before arising for the day.
- Failure to follow these instructions may increase the risk of esophageal adverse reactions [see Warnings and Precautions (5.1)].

2.4 Recommendations for Calcium and Vitamin D Supplementation

Instruct patients to take supplemental calcium and vitamin D if dietary intake is inadequate [see Warnings and Precautions (5.2)]. Patients at increased risk for vitamin D insufficiency (e.g., over the age of 70 years, nursing home-bound, or chronically ill) may need vitamin D supplementation. Patients with gastrointestinal malabsorption syndromes may require higher doses of vitamin D supplementation and measurement of 25-hydroxyvitamin D should be considered.

2.5 Administration Instructions for Missed Doses

If the once-weekly dose is missed, instruct patients to take one dose on the morning after they remember. They should not take 2 doses on the same day but should return to taking one dose once a week, as originally scheduled on their chosen day.

3 DOSAGE FORMS AND STRENGTHS

BINOSTO effervescent tablets are round, flat-faced, white to off-white tablets, 25 mm in diameter, with beveled edges,

Table 1 Osteoporosis Treatment Studies in Postmenopausal Women
Adverse Reactions Considered Possibly, Probably, or Definitely Drug Related by the Investigators and Reported in Greater Than or Equal to 1% of Patients

	United States/Multinational Studies		Fracture Intervention Trial	
	Alendronate Sodium* % (N=196)	Placebo % (N=397)	Alendronate Sodium** % (N=3236)	Placebo % (N=3223)
Gastrointestinal				
Abdominal pain	6.6	4.8	1.5	1.5
Nausea	3.6	4.0	1.1	1.5
Dyspepsia	3.6	3.5	1.1	1.2
Constipation	3.1	1.8	0.0	0.2
Diarrhea	3.1	1.8	0.6	0.3
Flatulence	2.6	0.5	0.2	0.3
Acid regurgitation	2.0	4.3	1.1	0.9
Esophageal ulcer	1.5	0.0	0.1	0.1
Vomiting	1.0	1.5	0.2	0.3
Dysphagia	1.0	0.0	0.1	0.1
Abdominal distention	1.0	0.8	0.0	0.0
Gastritis	0.5	1.3	0.6	0.7
Musculoskeletal				
Musculoskeletal (bone, muscle or joint) pain	4.1	2.5	0.4	0.3
Muscle cramp	0.0	1.0	0.2	0.1
Nervous system/psychiatric				
Headache	2.6	1.5	0.2	0.2
Dizziness	0.0	1.0	0.0	0.1
Special senses				
Taste perversion	0.5	1.0	0.1	0.0

* 10 mg/day for three years
** 5 mg/day for 2 years and 10 mg/day for either 1 or 2 additional years

with "M" debossed on one side, containing 91.37 mg of alendronate sodium, which is equivalent to 70 mg of free alendronic acid.

4 CONTRAINDICATIONS

BINOSTO is contraindicated in patients with the following conditions:
- Abnormalities of the esophagus which delay esophageal emptying such as stricture or achalasia [see Warnings and Precautions (5.1)]
- Inability to stand or sit upright for at least 30 minutes [see Dosage and Administration (2.3); Warnings and Precautions (5.1)]

Do not administer BINOSTO to patients at increased risk of aspiration
- Hypocalcemia [see Warnings and Precautions (5.2)]
- Hypersensitivity to any component of this product. Hypersensitivity reactions including urticaria and angioedema have been reported [see Adverse Reactions (6.2)].

5 WARNINGS AND PRECAUTIONS

5.1 Upper Gastrointestinal Adverse Reactions

BINOSTO, like other bisphosphonates administered orally, may cause local irritation of the upper gastrointestinal mucosa. Because of these possible irritant effects and a potential for worsening of the underlying disease, caution should be used when BINOSTO is given to patients with active upper gastrointestinal problems (such as known Barrett's esophagus, dysphagia, other esophageal diseases, gastritis, duodenitis, or ulcers).

Esophageal adverse experiences, such as esophagitis, esophageal ulcers and esophageal erosions, occasionally with bleeding and rarely followed by esophageal stricture or perforation, have been reported in patients receiving treatment with oral bisphosphonates including alendronate sodium. In some cases these have been severe and required hospitalization. Physicians should therefore be alert to any signs or symptoms signaling a possible esophageal reaction and patients should be instructed to discontinue BINOSTO and seek medical attention if they develop dysphagia, odynophagia, retrosternal pain or new or worsening heartburn. The risk of severe esophageal adverse experiences appears to be greater in patients who lie down after taking oral bisphosphonates including alendronate sodium, and/or who continue to take oral bisphosphonates including alendronate sodium after developing symptoms suggestive of esophageal irritation. Therefore, it is very important that the full dosing instructions are provided to, and understood by, the patient [see Dosage and Administration (2.3)]. In patients who cannot comply with dosing instructions due to mental disability, therapy with BINOSTO should be used under appropriate supervision.

There have been post-marketing reports of gastric and duodenal ulcers with oral bisphosphonate use, some severe and with complications, although no increased risk was observed in controlled clinical trials [see Adverse Reactions (6.2)].

5.2 Mineral Metabolism

Hypocalcemia must be corrected before initiating therapy with BINOSTO [see Contraindications (4)]. Other disorders affecting mineral metabolism (such as vitamin D deficiency) should also be effectively treated. In patients with these conditions, serum calcium and symptoms of hypocalcemia should be monitored during therapy with BINOSTO. Presumably due to the effects of BINOSTO on increasing bone mineral, small, asymptomatic decreases in serum calcium and phosphate may occur. Patients should receive adequate calcium and vitamin D intake.

5.3 Musculoskeletal Pain

In post marketing experience, severe and occasionally incapacitating bone, joint, and/or muscle pain has been reported in patients taking bisphosphonates that are approved for the treatment of osteoporosis [see Adverse Reactions (6.2)]. This category of drugs includes BINOSTO. Most of the patients were postmenopausal women. The time to onset of symptoms varied from one day to several months after starting the drug. Discontinue use if severe symptoms develop. Most patients had relief of symptoms after stopping. A subset had recurrence of symptoms when rechallenged with the same drug or another bisphosphonate.

In placebo-controlled clinical studies of alendronate sodium, the percentages of patients with these symptoms were similar in the alendronate sodium and placebo groups.

5.4 Osteonecrosis of the Jaw

Osteonecrosis of the jaw (ONJ), which can occur spontaneously, is generally associated with tooth extraction and/or local infection with delayed healing, and has been reported in patients taking bisphosphonates, including alendronate sodium. Known risk factors for osteonecrosis of the jaw include invasive dental procedures (e.g., tooth extraction, dental implants, boney surgery), diagnosis of cancer, concomitant therapies (e.g., chemotherapy, corticosteroids), poor oral hygiene, and co-morbid disorders (e.g., periodontal and/or other pre-existing dental disease, anemia, coagulopathy, infection, ill-fitting dentures). The risk of ONJ may increase with duration of exposure to bisphosphonates.

For patients requiring invasive dental procedures, discontinuation of bisphosphonate treatment may reduce the risk for ONJ. Clinical judgment of the treating physician and/or oral surgeon should guide the management plan of each patient based on individual benefit/risk assessment.

Patients who develop osteonecrosis of the jaw while on bisphosphonate therapy should receive care by an oral surgeon. In these patients, extensive dental surgery to treat ONJ may exacerbate the condition. Discontinuation of bisphosphonate therapy should be considered based on individual benefit/risk assessment.

5.5 Atypical Subtrochanteric and Diaphyseal Femoral Fractures

Atypical, low-energy, or low trauma fractures of the femoral shaft have been reported in bisphosphonate-treated patients. These fractures can occur anywhere in the femoral shaft from just below the lesser trochanter to above the supracondylar flare and are transverse or short oblique in orientation without evidence of comminution. Causality has not been established as these fractures also occur in osteoporotic patients who have not been treated with bisphosphonates.

Atypical femur fractures most commonly occur with minimal or no trauma to the affected area. They may be bilateral and many patients report prodromal pain in the affected area, usually presenting as dull, aching thigh pain, weeks to months before a complete fracture occurs. A number of reports note that patients were also receiving treatment with glucocorticoids (e.g., prednisone) at the time of fracture.

Any patient with a history of bisphosphonate exposure who presents with thigh or groin pain should be suspected of having an atypical fracture and should be evaluated to rule out an incomplete femur fracture. Patients presenting with an atypical fracture should also be assessed for symptoms and signs of fracture in the contralateral limb. Interruption of bisphosphonate therapy should be considered, pending a risk/benefit assessment, on an individual basis.

5.6 Renal Impairment
BINOSTO is not recommended for patients with creatinine clearance < 35 mL/min.

5.7 Patients Sensitive to High Sodium Intake
Each BINOSTO effervescent tablet contains 650 mg of sodium, equivalent to approximately 1650 mg of salt (NaCl). Use caution in patients who must restrict their sodium intake, including some patients with a history of heart failure, hypertension, or other cardiovascular diseases *[see Patient Counseling Information (17.3)]*.

6 ADVERSE REACTIONS
6.1 Clinical Trials Experience
Because clinical trials are conducted under widely varying conditions, adverse reaction rates observed in the clinical trials of a drug cannot be directly compared to rates in the clinical trials of another drug and may not reflect the rates observed in clinical practice.

The safety of BINOSTO (alendronate sodium) effervescent tablet 70 mg is based on clinical trial data of alendronate sodium 10 mg daily and alendronate sodium 70 mg weekly.

Treatment of Osteoporosis in Postmenopausal Women
Daily Dosing
The safety of alendronate sodium 10 mg daily in the treatment of postmenopausal osteoporosis was assessed in four clinical trials that enrolled 7453 women aged 44-84 years. Study 1 and Study 2 were identically designed, three-year, placebo-controlled, double-blind, multicenter studies (United States and Multinational n=994); Study 3 was the three year vertebral fracture cohort of the Fracture Intervention Trial [FIT] (n=2027) and Study 4 was the four-year clinical fracture cohort of FIT (n=4432). Overall, 3620 patients were exposed to placebo and 3432 patients exposed to alendronate. Patients with pre-existing gastrointestinal disease and concomitant use of non-steroidal anti-inflammatory drugs were included in these clinical trials. In Study 1 and Study 2 all women received 500 mg elemental calcium as carbonate. In Study 3 and Study 4 all women with dietary calcium intake less than 1000 mg per day received 500 mg calcium and 250 IU Vitamin D per day.

Among patients treated with alendronate 10 mg or placebo in Study 1 and Study 2, and all patients in Study 3 and Study 4, the incidence of all-cause mortality was 1.8% in the placebo group and 1.8% in the alendronate group. The incidence of serious adverse events was 30.7% in the placebo group and 30.9% in the alendronate group. The percentage of patients who discontinued the study due to any clinical adverse event was 9.5% in the placebo group and 8.9% in the alendronate group. Adverse reactions from these studies considered by the investigators as possibly, probably, or definitely drug related in greater than or equal to 1% of patients treated with either alendronate or placebo are presented in Table 1.

[See table 1 at top of previous page]
Rarely, rash and erythema have occurred.

Gastrointestinal Adverse Reactions: One patient treated with alendronate sodium (10 mg/day), who had a history of peptic ulcer disease and gastrectomy and who was taking concomitant aspirin developed an anastomotic ulcer with mild hemorrhage, which was considered drug related. Aspirin and alendronate sodium were discontinued and the patient recovered. In the Study 1 and Study 2 populations, 49-54% had a history of gastrointestinal disorders at baseline and 54-89% used nonsteroidal anti-inflammatory drugs or aspirin at some time during the studies *[see Warnings and Precautions (5.1)]*.

Laboratory Test Findings: In double-blind, multicenter, controlled studies, asymptomatic, mild, and transient decreases in serum calcium and phosphate were observed in approximately 18% and 10%, respectively, of patients taking alendronate versus approximately 12% and 3% of those taking placebo. However, the incidences of decreases in serum calcium to less than 8.0 mg/dL (2.0 mM) and serum phosphate to less than or equal to 2.0 mg/dL (0.65 mM) were similar in both treatment groups.

Weekly Dosing
The safety of alendronate sodium 70 mg once weekly for the treatment of postmenopausal osteoporosis was assessed in a one-year, double-blind, multicenter study comparing alendronate 70 mg once weekly and alendronate 10 mg daily. The overall safety and tolerability profiles of once weekly alendronate 70 mg and alendronate 10 mg daily were similar. The adverse reactions considered by the investigators as possibly, probably, or definitely drug related in greater than or equal to 1% of patients in either treatment group are presented in Table 2.

Table 2 Osteoporosis Treatment Studies in Postmenopausal Women
Adverse Reactions Considered Possibly, Probably, or Definitely Drug Related by the Investigators and Reported in Greater Than or Equal to 1% of Patients

	Once Weekly Alendronate Sodium 70 mg % (N=519)	Once Daily Alendronate Sodium 10 mg % (N=370)
Gastrointestinal		
Abdominal pain	3.7	3.0
Dyspepsia	2.7	2.2
Acid regurgitation	1.9	2.4
Nausea	1.9	2.4
Abdominal distention	1.0	1.4
Constipation	0.8	1.6
Flatulence	0.4	1.6
Gastritis	0.2	1.1
Gastric ulcer	0.0	1.1
Musculoskeletal		
Musculoskeletal (bone, muscle, joint) pain	2.9	3.2
Muscle cramp	0.2	1.1

Osteoporosis in Men
In two placebo-controlled, double-blind, multicenter studies in men (a two-year study of alendronate sodium 10 mg/day and a one-year study of once weekly alendronate sodium 70 mg) the rates of discontinuation of therapy due to any clinical adverse event were 2.7% for alendronate 10 mg/day vs. 10.5% for placebo, and 6.4% for once weekly alendronate 70 mg vs. 8.6% for placebo. The adverse reactions considered by the investigators as possibly, probably, or definitely drug related in greater than or equal to 2% of patients treated with either alendronate or placebo are presented in the following table.

[See table 3 above]

6.2 Post-Marketing Experience
The following adverse reactions have been identified during post-approval use of alendronate sodium. Because these reactions are reported voluntarily from a population of uncertain size, it is not always possible to reliably estimate their frequency or establish a causal relationship to drug exposure.

Body as a Whole: hypersensitivity reactions including urticaria and angioedema. Transient symptoms of myalgia, malaise, asthenia and fever have been reported with alendronate, typically in association with initiation of treatment. Symptomatic hypocalcemia has occurred, generally in association with predisposing conditions. Peripheral edema.

Gastrointestinal: esophagitis, esophageal erosions, esophageal ulcers, esophageal stricture or perforation, and oropharyngeal ulceration. Gastric or duodenal ulcers, some severe and with complications have also been reported *[see Dosage and Administration (2.3); Warnings and Precautions (5.1)]*.

Dental: Localized osteonecrosis of the jaw, generally associated with tooth extraction and/or local infection with delayed healing, has been reported *[see Warnings and Precautions (5.4)]*.

Musculoskeletal: bone, joint, and/or muscle pain, occasionally severe and incapacitating *[see Warnings and Precautions (5.3)]*; joint swelling; low-energy femoral shaft and subtrochanteric fractures *[see Warnings and Precautions (5.5)]*.

Nervous system: dizziness and vertigo.
Pulmonary: asthma exacerbations.
Skin: rash (occasionally with photosensitivity), pruritus, alopecia, severe skin reactions, including Stevens-Johnson syndrome and toxic epidermal necrolysis.
Special Senses: uveitis, scleritis or episcleritis.

7 DRUG INTERACTIONS
7.1 Calcium Supplements/Antacids
Co-administration of BINOSTO and calcium, antacids, or oral medications containing multivalent cations will interfere with absorption of BINOSTO. Therefore, instruct patients to wait at least one-half hour after taking BINOSTO before taking any other oral medications.

7.2 Aspirin
In clinical studies, the incidence of upper gastrointestinal adverse events was increased in patients receiving concomitant therapy with daily doses of alendronate sodium greater than 10 mg and aspirin-containing products.

7.3 Nonsteroidal Anti-inflammatory Drugs (NSAIDs)
BINOSTO may be administered to patients taking NSAIDs. In a 3-year, controlled, clinical study (n=2027) during which a majority of patients received concomitant NSAIDs, the incidence of upper gastrointestinal adverse events was similar in patients taking alendronate sodium 5 or 10 mg/day compared to those taking placebo. However, since NSAID use is associated with gastrointestinal irritation, caution should be used during concomitant use with BINOSTO.

8 USE IN SPECIFIC POPULATIONS
8.1 Pregnancy
Pregnancy Category C:
There are no studies in pregnant women. BINOSTO should be used during pregnancy only if the potential benefit justifies the potential risk to the mother and fetus.

Bisphosphonates are incorporated into the bone matrix, from which they are gradually released over a period of years. The amount of bisphosphonate incorporated into adult bone, and hence, the amount available for release back into the systemic circulation, is directly related to the dose and duration of bisphosphonate use. There are no data on fetal risk in humans. However, there is a theoretical risk of fetal harm, predominantly skeletal, if a woman becomes pregnant after completing a course of bisphosphonate therapy. The impact of variables such as time between cessation of bisphosphonate therapy to conception, the particular bisphosphonate used, and the route of administration (intravenous versus oral) on the risk has not been studied.

Reproduction studies in rats showed decreased postimplantation survival and decreased body weight gain in normal pups at doses less than half of the recommended clinical dose. Sites of incomplete fetal ossification were statistically significantly increased in rats beginning at approximately 3 times the clinical dose in vertebral (cervical, thoracic, and lumbar), skull, and sternebral bones. No similar fetal effects were seen when pregnant rabbits were treated with doses approximately 10 times the clinical dose.

Both total and ionized calcium decreased in pregnant rats at approximately 4 times the clinical dose resulting in delays and failures of delivery. Protracted parturition due to maternal hypocalcemia occurred in rats at doses as low as one tenth the clinical dose when rats were treated from before mating through gestation. Maternotoxicity (late preg-

Table 3 Osteoporosis Studies in Men
Adverse Reactions Considered Possibly, Probably, or Definitely Drug Related by the Investigators and Reported in Greater Than or Equal to 2% of Patients

	Two-Year Study Once Daily Alendronate Sodium 10 mg % (N=146)	Placebo % (N=95)	One-Year Study Once Weekly Alendronate Sodium 70 mg % (N=109)	Placebo % (N=58)
Gastrointestinal				
Acid regurgitation	4.1	3.2	0.0	0.0
Flatulence	4.1	1.1	0.0	0.0
Gastroesophageal reflux disease	0.7	3.2	2.8	0.0
Dyspepsia	3.4	0.0	2.8	1.7
Diarrhea	1.4	1.1	2.8	0.0
Abdominal pain	2.1	1.1	0.9	3.4
Nausea	2.1	0.0	0.0	0.0

nancy deaths) also occurred in the female rats treated at approximately 4 times the clinical dose for varying periods of time ranging from treatment only during pre-mating to treatment only during early, middle, or late gestation; these deaths were lessened but not eliminated by cessation of treatment. Calcium supplementation either in the drinking water or by minipump could not ameliorate the hypocalcemia or prevent maternal and neonatal deaths due to delays in delivery; intravenous calcium supplementation prevented maternal, but not fetal deaths.

Exposure multiples based on surface area, mg/m^2, were calculated using a 40-mg human daily dose. Animal dose ranged between 1 and 15 mg/kg/day in rats and up to 40 mg/kg/day in rabbits.

8.3 Nursing Mothers

It is not known whether alendronate is excreted in human milk. Because many drugs are excreted in human milk, caution should be exercised when BINOSTO is administered to nursing women.

8.4 Pediatric Use

BINOSTO is not indicated for use in pediatric patients.
The safety and efficacy of alendronate sodium were examined in a randomized, double-blind, placebo-controlled two-year study of 139 pediatric patients, aged 4-18 years, with severe osteogenesis imperfecta (OI). One-hundred-and-nine patients were randomized to 5 mg alendronate sodium daily (weight less than 40 kg) or 10 mg alendronate sodium daily (weight greater than or equal to 40 kg) and 30 patients to placebo. The mean baseline lumbar spine BMD Z-score of the patients was -4.5. The mean change in lumbar spine BMD Z-score from baseline to Month 24 was 1.3 in the alendronate-treated patients and 0.1 in the placebo-treated patients. Treatment with alendronate sodium did not reduce the risk of fracture. Sixteen percent of the alendronate-treated patients who sustained a radiologically-confirmed fracture by Month 12 of the study had delayed fracture healing (callus remodeling) or fracture non-union when assessed radiographically at Month 24 compared with 9% of the placebo-treated patients. In alendronate-treated patients, bone histomorphometry data obtained at Month 24 demonstrated decreased bone turnover and delayed mineralization time; however, there were no mineralization defects. There were no statistically significant differences between the alendronate sodium and placebo groups in reduction of bone pain. The oral bioavailability in children was similar to that observed in adults.

The overall safety profile of alendronate sodium in osteogenesis imperfecta patients treated for up to 24 months was generally similar to that of adults with osteoporosis treated with alendronate sodium. However, there was an increased occurrence of vomiting in osteogenesis imperfecta patients treated with alendronate sodium compared to placebo. During the 24-month treatment period, vomiting was observed in 32 of 109 (29.4%) patients treated with alendronate sodium and 3 of 30 (10%) patients treated with placebo.

In a pharmacokinetic study, 6 of 24 pediatric osteogenesis imperfecta patients who received a single oral dose of alendronate sodium 35 or 70 mg developed fever, flu-like symptoms, and/or mild lymphocytopenia within 24 to 48 hours after administration. These events, lasting no more than 2 to 3 days and responding to acetaminophen, are consistent with an acute-phase response that has been reported in patients receiving bisphosphonates, including alendronate sodium. [See Adverse Reactions (6.2).]

8.5 Geriatric Use

Of the patients receiving alendronate sodium in the Fracture Intervention Trial (FIT), 71% (n=2302) were greater than or equal to 65 years of age and 17% (n=550) were greater than or equal to 75 years of age. Of the patients receiving alendronate sodium in the United States and Multinational osteoporosis treatment studies in women and osteoporosis studies in men, [see Clinical Studies (14.1), (14.2)], 45% and 54%, respectively, were 65 years of age or over. No overall differences in efficacy or safety were observed between these patients and younger patients, but greater sensitivity of some older individuals cannot be ruled out.

8.6 Renal Impairment

BINOSTO is not recommended for patients with creatinine clearance less than 35 mL/min. No dosage adjustment is necessary in patients with creatinine clearance values between 35-60 mL/min [see Clinical Pharmacology (12.3)].

8.7 Hepatic Impairment

As there is evidence that alendronate is not metabolized or excreted in the bile, no studies were conducted in patients with hepatic impairment. No dosage adjustment is necessary [see Clinical Pharmacology (12.3)].

10 OVERDOSAGE

Significant lethality after single oral doses was seen in female rats and mice at 552 mg/kg ($3256 mg/m^2$) and 966 mg/kg ($2898 mg/m^2$), respectively. In males, these values were slightly higher, 626 and 1280 mg/kg, respectively. There was no lethality in dogs at oral doses up to 200 mg/kg ($4000 mg/m^2$).

No specific information is available on the treatment of overdosage with BINOSTO. Hypocalcemia, hypophosphatemia, and upper gastrointestinal adverse events, such as upset stomach, heartburn, esophagitis, gastritis, or ulcer, may result from oral overdosage. Milk or antacids should be given to bind alendronate. Due to the risk of esophageal irritation, vomiting should not be induced and the patient should remain fully upright.
Dialysis would not be beneficial.

11 DESCRIPTION

BINOSTO (alendronate sodium) is a bisphosphonate that acts as a specific inhibitor of osteoclast-mediated bone resorption. Bisphosphonates are synthetic analogs of pyrophosphate that bind to the hydroxyapatite found in bone. Alendronate sodium is chemically described as (4 amino-1-hydroxybutylidene) bisphosphonic acid, monosodium salt, trihydrate. The molecular formula of alendronate sodium is $C_4H_{12}NNaO_7P_2 \cdot 3H_2O$ and its molecular weight is 325.12. The structural formula of alendronate sodium is

Alendronate sodium is a white or almost white crystalline powder that is soluble in water, very slightly soluble in methanol, and practically insoluble in methylene chloride. BINOSTO for oral administration is an effervescent tablet formulation that must be dissolved in water before use. Each individual tablet contains 91.37 mg of alendronate sodium, which is equivalent to 70 mg of free alendronic acid. Each tablet also contains the following inactive ingredients: monosodium citrate anhydrous, citric acid anhydrous, sodium hydrogen carbonate, and sodium carbonate anhydrous as buffering agents, strawberry flavor, acesulfame potassium, and sucralose.

Once the effervescent tablet is dissolved in water, the alendronate sodium is present in a citrate-buffered solution.

12 CLINICAL PHARMACOLOGY

12.1 Mechanism of Action

Animal studies have indicated the following mode of action. At the cellular level, alendronate shows preferential localization to sites of bone resorption, specifically under osteoclasts. The osteoclasts adhere normally to the bone surface but lack the ruffled border that is indicative of active resorption. Alendronate does not interfere with osteoclast recruitment or attachment, but it does inhibit osteoclast activity. Studies in mice on the localization of radioactive [^{3}H]alendronate in bone showed about 10-fold higher uptake on osteoclast surfaces than on osteoblast surfaces. Bones examined 6 and 49 days after [^{3}H]alendronate administration in rats and mice, respectively, showed that normal bone was formed on top of the alendronate, which was incorporated inside the matrix. While incorporated in bone matrix, alendronate is not pharmacologically active. Thus, alendronate must be continuously administered to suppress osteoclasts on newly formed resorption surfaces. Histomorphometry in baboons and rats showed that alendronate treatment reduces bone turnover (i.e., the number of sites at which bone is remodeled). In addition, bone formation exceeds bone resorption at these remodeling sites, leading to progressive gains in bone mass.

12.2 Pharmacodynamics

Alendronate is a bisphosphonate that binds to bone hydroxyapatite and specifically inhibits the activity of osteoclasts, the bone-resorbing cells. Alendronate reduces bone resorption with no direct effect on bone formation, although the latter process is ultimately reduced because bone resorption and formation are coupled during bone turnover.

Osteoporosis in Postmenopausal Women
Osteoporosis is characterized by low bone mass that leads to an increased risk of fracture. The diagnosis can be confirmed by the finding of low bone mass, evidence of fracture on x-ray, a history of osteoporotic fracture, or height loss or kyphosis, indicative of vertebral (spinal) fracture. Osteoporosis occurs in both males and females but is most common among women following the menopause, when bone turnover increases and the rate of bone resorption exceeds that of bone formation. These changes result in progressive bone loss and lead to osteoporosis in a significant proportion of women over age 50. Fractures, usually of the spine, hip, and wrist, are the common consequences. From age 50 to age 90, the risk of hip fracture in white women increases 50-fold and the risk of vertebral fracture 15- to 30-fold. It is estimated that approximately 40% of 50-year-old women will

sustain one or more osteoporosis-related fractures of the spine, hip, or wrist during their remaining lifetimes. Hip fractures, in particular, are associated with substantial morbidity, disability, and mortality.

Daily oral doses of alendronate sodium (5, 20, and 40 mg for six weeks) in postmenopausal women produced biochemical changes indicative of dose-dependent inhibition of bone resorption, including decreases in urinary calcium and urinary markers of bone collagen degradation (such as deoxypyridinoline and cross-linked N-telopeptides of type I collagen). These biochemical changes tended to return toward baseline values as early as 3 weeks following the discontinuation of therapy with alendronate and did not differ from placebo after 7 months.

Long-term treatment of osteoporosis with alendronate sodium 10 mg/day (for up to five years) reduced urinary excretion of markers of bone resorption, deoxypyridinoline and cross-linked N-telopeptides of type I collagen, by approximately 50% and 70%, respectively, to reach levels similar to those seen in healthy premenopausal women. Similar decreases were seen in patients in osteoporosis prevention studies who received alendronate sodium 5 mg/day. The decrease in the rate of bone resorption indicated by these markers was evident as early as 1 month and at 3 to 6 months reached a plateau that was maintained for the entire duration of treatment with alendronate sodium. In osteoporosis treatment studies alendronate sodium 10 mg/day decreased the markers of bone formation, osteocalcin and bone specific alkaline phosphatase by approximately 50%, and total serum alkaline phosphatase by approximately 25 to 30% to reach a plateau at 6 to 12 months. In osteoporosis prevention studies alendronate sodium 5 mg/day decreased osteocalcin and total serum alkaline phosphatase by approximately 40% and 15%, respectively. Similar reductions in the rate of bone turnover were observed in postmenopausal women during one-year studies with once weekly alendronate sodium 70 mg for the treatment of osteoporosis and once weekly alendronate sodium 35 mg for the prevention of osteoporosis. These data indicate that the rate of bone turnover reached a new steady state, despite the progressive increase in the total amount of alendronate deposited within bone.

As a result of inhibition of bone resorption, asymptomatic reductions in serum calcium and phosphate concentrations were also observed following treatment with alendronate sodium. In the long-term studies, reductions from baseline in serum calcium (approximately 2%) and phosphate (approximately 4 to 6%) were evident the first month after the initiation of alendronate sodium 10 mg. No further decreases in serum calcium were observed for the five-year duration of treatment; however, serum phosphate returned toward prestudy levels during years three through five. Similar reductions were observed with alendronate sodium 5 mg/day. In one-year studies with once weekly alendronate sodium 35 and 70 mg, similar reductions were observed at 6 and 12 months. The reduction in serum phosphate may reflect not only the positive bone mineral balance due to alendronate sodium but also a decrease in renal phosphate reabsorption.

Osteoporosis in Men
Treatment of men with osteoporosis with alendronate sodium 10 mg/day for two years reduced urinary excretion of cross-linked N-telopeptides of type I collagen by approximately 60% and bone-specific alkaline phosphatase by approximately 40%. Similar reductions were observed in a one-year study in men with osteoporosis receiving once weekly alendronate sodium 70 mg.

12.3 Pharmacokinetics

Absorption
Relative to an intravenous (IV) reference dose, the mean oral bioavailability of alendronate in women was 0.64% for doses ranging from 5 to 70 mg when administered after an overnight fast and two hours before a standardized breakfast. Oral bioavailability of the 10 mg tablet in men (0.59%) was similar to that in women when administered after an overnight fast and 2 hours before breakfast.

BINOSTO 70 mg effervescent tablet and alendronate sodium 70 mg tablet are bioequivalent.

A study evaluating the effect of food on the bioavailability of BINOSTO was performed in 119 healthy women. Bioavailability was decreased (by approximately 50%) when 70 mg alendronate sodium was administered 15 minutes before a standardized breakfast, when compared to dosing 4 hours before eating.

In studies of treatment and prevention of osteoporosis, alendronate was effective when administered at least 30 minutes before breakfast.

Bioavailability was negligible whether alendronate sodium was administered with or up to 2 hours after a standardized breakfast. Concomitant administration of alendronate with coffee or orange juice reduced bioavailability by approximately 60%.

Distribution
Preclinical studies (in male rats) show that alendronate sodium transiently distributes to soft tissues following

1 mg/kg IV administration but is then rapidly redistributed to bone or excreted in the urine. The mean steady-state volume of distribution, exclusive of bone, is at least 28 L in humans. Concentrations of drug in plasma following therapeutic oral doses are too low (less than 5 ng/mL) for analytical detection. Protein binding in human plasma is approximately 78%.

Metabolism
There is no evidence that alendronate sodium is metabolized in animals or humans.

Excretion
Following a single IV dose of [^{14}C]alendronate, approximately 50% of the radioactivity was excreted in the urine within 72 hours and little or no radioactivity was recovered in the feces. Following a single 10 mg IV dose, the renal clearance of alendronate was 71 mL/min (64, 78; 90% confidence interval [CI]), and systemic clearance did not exceed 200 mL/min. Plasma concentrations fell by more than 95% within 6 hours following IV administration. The terminal half-life in humans is estimated to exceed 10 years, probably reflecting release of alendronate from the skeleton. Based on the above, it is estimated that after 10 years of oral treatment with alendronate sodium (10 mg daily) the amount of alendronate released daily from the skeleton is approximately 25% of that absorbed from the gastrointestinal tract.

Specific Populations
Gender: Bioavailability and the fraction of an intravenous dose excreted in urine were similar in men and women.
Geriatric: Bioavailability and disposition (urinary excretion) were similar in elderly and younger patients. No dosage adjustment is necessary in elderly patients.
Race: Pharmacokinetic differences due to race have not been studied.
Renal Impairment: Preclinical studies show that, in rats with kidney failure, increasing amounts of drug are present in plasma, kidney, spleen, and tibia. In healthy controls, drug that is not deposited in bone is rapidly excreted in the urine. No evidence of saturation of bone uptake was found after 3 weeks dosing with cumulative intravenous doses of 35 mg/kg in young male rats. Although no formal renal impairment pharmacokinetic study has been conducted in patients, it is likely that, as in animals, elimination of alendronate via the kidney will be reduced in patients with impaired renal function. Therefore, somewhat greater accumulation of alendronate in bone might be expected in patients with impaired renal function.
No dosage adjustment is necessary for patients with creatinine clearance 35 to 60 mL/min. BINOSTO is not recommended for patients with creatinine clearance less than 35 mL/min due to lack of experience with alendronate in renal failure.
Hepatic Impairment: As there is evidence that alendronate is not metabolized or excreted in the bile, no studies were conducted in patients with hepatic impairment. No dosage adjustment is necessary.

Drug Interactions
Intravenous ranitidine was shown to double the bioavailability of oral alendronate. The clinical significance of this increased bioavailability and whether similar increases will occur in patients given oral H$_2$-antagonists is unknown.
In healthy subjects, oral prednisone (20 mg three times daily for five days) did not produce a clinically meaningful change in the oral bioavailability of alendronate (a mean increase ranging from 20 to 44%).
Products containing calcium and other multivalent cations are likely to interfere with absorption of alendronate.

13 NONCLINICAL TOXICOLOGY
13.1 Carcinogenesis, Mutagenesis, Impairment of Fertility
Harderian gland (a retro-orbital gland not present in humans) adenomas were increased in high-dose female mice (p=0.003) in a 92-week oral carcinogenicity study at doses of alendronate of 1, 3, and 10 mg/kg/day (males) or 1, 2, and 5 mg/kg/day (females). These doses are equivalent to 0.12 to 1.2 times a maximum recommended daily dose of 40 mg, based on surface area, mg/m². The relevance of this finding to humans is unknown.
Parafollicular cell (thyroid) adenomas were increased in high-dose male rats (p=0.003) in a 2-year oral carcinogenicity study at doses of 1 and 3.75 mg/kg body weight. These doses are equivalent to 0.26 and 1 times a 40 mg human daily dose based on surface area, mg/m². The relevance of this finding to humans is unknown.
Alendronate sodium was not genotoxic in the in vitro microbial mutagenesis assay with and without metabolic activation, in an in vitro mammalian cell mutagenesis assay, in an in vitro alkaline elution assay in rat hepatocytes, and in an in vivo chromosomal aberration assay in mice. In an in vitro chromosomal aberration assay in Chinese hamster ovary cells, however, alendronate gave equivocal results.
Alendronate sodium had no effect on fertility (male or female) in rats at oral doses up to 5 mg/kg/day (1.3 times a 40 mg human daily dose based on surface area, mg/m²).

13.2 Animal Toxicology and/or Pharmacology
The relative inhibitory activities on bone resorption and mineralization of alendronate and etidronate were compared in the Schenk assay, which is based on histological examination of the epiphyses of growing rats. In this assay, the lowest dose of alendronate that interfered with bone mineralization (leading to osteomalacia) was 6000-fold the antiresorptive dose. The corresponding ratio for etidronate was one to one. These data suggest that alendronate administered in therapeutic doses is highly unlikely to induce osteomalacia.

14 CLINICAL STUDIES
14.1 Treatment of Osteoporosis in Postmenopausal Women
BINOSTO (alendronate sodium) effervescent tablet 70 mg is bioequivalent to alendronate sodium tablet 70 mg. The fracture reduction efficacy and bone mineral density changes attributed to BINOSTO are based on clinical trial data of alendronate sodium 10 mg daily and alendronate sodium 70 mg weekly.
Daily Dosing
The efficacy of alendronate sodium 10 mg daily was assessed in four clinical trials. Study 1, a three-year, multicenter double-blind, placebo-controlled, US clinical study enrolled 478 patients with a BMD T-score at or below minus 2.5 with or without a prior vertebral fracture; Study 2, a three-year, multicenter double blind placebo controlled Multinational clinical study enrolled 516 patients with a BMD T-score at or below minus 2.5 with or without a prior vertebral fracture; Study 3, the Three-Year Study of the Fracture Intervention Trial (FIT) a study which enrolled 2027 postmenopausal patients with at least one baseline vertebral fracture; and Study 4, the Four-Year Study of FIT: a study which enrolled 4432 postmenopausal patients with low bone mass but without a baseline vertebral fracture.
Effect on Fracture Incidence
To assess the effects of alendronate sodium on the incidence of vertebral fractures (detected by digitized radiography; approximately one third of these were clinically symptomatic), the U.S. and Multinational studies were combined in an analysis that compared placebo to the pooled dosage groups of alendronate sodium (5 or 10 mg for three years or 20 mg for two years followed by 5 mg for one year). There was a statistically significant reduction in the proportion of patients treated with alendronate experiencing one or more new vertebral fractures relative to those treated with placebo (3.2% vs. 6.2%; a 48% relative risk reduction). A reduction in the total number of new vertebral fractures (4.2 vs. 11.3 per 100 patients) was also observed. In the pooled analysis, patients who received alendronate had a loss in stature that was statistically significantly less than was observed in those who received placebo (-3.0 mm vs. -4.6 mm).
The Fracture Intervention Trial (FIT) consisted of two studies in postmenopausal women: the Three-Year Study of patients who had at least one baseline radiographic vertebral fracture and the Four-Year Study of patients with low bone mass but without a baseline vertebral fracture. In both studies of FIT, 96% of randomized patients completed the studies (i.e., had a closeout visit at the scheduled end of the study); approximately 80% of patients were still taking study medication upon completion.
Fracture Intervention Trial: Three-Year Study (patients with at least one baseline radiographic vertebral fracture)
This randomized, double-blind, placebo-controlled, 2027-patient study (alendronate, n=1022; placebo, n=1005) demonstrated that treatment with alendronate sodium resulted in statistically significant reductions in fracture incidence at three years as shown in Table 4.
[See table 4 above]

Furthermore, in this population of patients with baseline vertebral fracture, treatment with alendronate sodium significantly reduced the incidence of hospitalizations (25.0% vs. 30.7%).
In the Three-Year Study of FIT, fractures of the hip occurred in 22 (2.2%) of 1005 patients on placebo and 11 (1.1%) of 1022 patients on alendronate sodium, p=0.047. Figure 1 displays the cumulative incidence of hip fractures in this study.

Figure 1   Cumulative Incidence of Hip Fractures in the Three-Year Study of FIT (Patients With Radiographic Vertebral Fracture at Baseline)

Fracture Intervention Trial: Four-Year Study (patients with low bone mass but without a baseline radiographic vertebral fracture)
This randomized, double-blind, placebo-controlled, 4432-patient study (alendronate, n=2214; placebo, n=2218) further investigated the reduction in fracture incidence due to alendronate sodium. The intent of the study was to recruit women with osteoporosis, defined as a baseline femoral neck BMD at least two standard deviations below the mean for young adult women. However, due to subsequent revisions to the normative values for femoral neck BMD, 31% of patients were found not to meet this entry criterion and thus this study included both osteoporotic and non-osteoporotic women. The results are shown in Table 5 for the patients with osteoporosis.
[See table 5 at top of next page]
Fracture Results Across Studies
In the Three-Year Study of FIT, alendronate sodium reduced the percentage of women experiencing at least one new radiographic vertebral fracture from 15.0% to 7.9% (47% relative risk reduction, p<0.001); in the Four-Year Study of FIT, the percentage was reduced from 3.8% to 2.1% (44% relative risk reduction, p=0.001); and in the combined U.S./Multinational studies, from 6.2% to 3.2% (48% relative risk reduction, p=0.034).
Alendronate sodium reduced the percentage of women experiencing multiple (two or more) new vertebral fractures from 4.2% to 0.6% (87% relative risk reduction, p<0.001) in the combined U.S./Multinational studies and from 4.9% to 0.5% (90% relative risk reduction, p<0.001) in the Three-Year Study of FIT. In the Four-Year Study of FIT, alendronate sodium reduced the percentage of osteoporotic women experiencing multiple vertebral fractures from 0.6% to 0.1% (78% relative risk reduction, p=0.035).
Thus, alendronate sodium reduced the incidence of radiographic vertebral fractures in osteoporotic women whether or not they had a previous radiographic vertebral fracture.
Effect on Bone Mineral Density
The bone mineral density efficacy of alendronate sodium 10 mg once daily in postmenopausal women, 44 to 84 years of age, with osteoporosis (lumbar spine bone mineral density [BMD] of at least 2 standard deviations below the premenopausal mean) was demonstrated in 4 double-blind, placebo-controlled clinical studies of 2 or 3 years' duration.

Table 4 Effect of Alendronate Sodium on Fracture Incidence in the Three-Year Study of FIT (Patients With Vertebral Fracture at Baseline)

| | Percent of Patients | | | |
	Alendronate Sodium (n=1022)	Placebo (n=1005)	Absolute Reduction in Fracture Incidence	Relative Reduction in Fracture Risk %
Patients with:				
Vertebral fractures (diagnosed by X-ray)*				
≥1 new vertebral fracture	7.9	15.0	7.1	47[†]
≥2 new vertebral fractures	0.5	4.9	4.4	90[†]
Clinical (symptomatic) fractures				
Any clinical (symptomatic) fracture	13.8	18.1	4.3	26[‡]
≥1 clinical (symptomatic) vertebral fracture	2.3	5.0	2.7	54[§]
Hip fracture	1.1	2.2	1.1	51[¶]
Wrist (forearm) fracture	2.2	4.1	1.9	48[¶]

*Number evaluable for vertebral fractures: alendronate, n=984; placebo, n=966
[†]p<0.001, [‡]p=0.007, [§]p<0.01, [¶]p<0.05

Table 5 Effect of Alendronate on Fracture Incidence in Osteoporotic* Patients in the Four-Year Study of FIT (Patients Without Vertebral Fracture at Baseline)

	Percent of Patients			
	Alendronate Sodium (n=1545)	Placebo (n=1521)	Absolute Reduction in Fracture Incidence	Relative Reduction in Fracture Risk (%)
Patients with:				
Vertebral fractures (diagnosed by X-ray)[†]				
≥1 new vertebral fracture	2.5	4.8	2.3	48[‡]
≥2 new vertebral fractures	0.1	0.6	0.5	78[§]
Clinical (symptomatic) fractures				
Any clinical (symptomatic) fracture	12.9	16.2	3.3	22[¶]
≥1 clinical (symptomatic) vertebral fracture	1.0	1.6	0.6	41 (NS)[#]
Hip fracture	1.0	1.4	0.4	29 (NS)[#]
Wrist (forearm) fracture	3.9	3.8	-0.1	NS[#]

*Baseline femoral neck BMD at least 2 SD below the mean for young adult women
[†]Number evaluable for vertebral fractures: alendronate, n=1426; placebo, n=1428
[‡]p<0.001, [§]p=0.035, [¶]p=0.01
[#]Not significant. This study was not powered to detect differences at these sites.

Figure 3   Osteoporosis Treatment in Studies in Postmenopausal Women Time Course Effect of Alendronate Sodium 10 mg/day Versus Placebo: Lumbar Spine BMD Percent Change From Baseline

Figure 2 shows the mean increases in BMD of the lumbar spine, femoral neck, and trochanter in patients receiving alendronate sodium 10 mg/day relative to placebo-treated patients at three years for each of these studies.

Figure 2   Osteoporosis Treatment Studies in Postmenopausal Women Increase in BMD Alendronate Sodium 10 mg/day at Three Years

At 3 years significant increases in BMD, relative both to baseline and placebo, were seen at each measurement site in each study in patients who received alendronate 10 mg/day. Total body BMD also increased significantly in each study, suggesting that the increases in bone mass of the spine and hip did not occur at the expense of other skeletal sites. Increases in BMD were evident as early as 3 months and continued throughout the 3 years of treatment. (See figures below for lumbar spine results.) In the 2-year extension of these studies, treatment of 147 patients with alendronate sodium 10 mg/day resulted in continued increases in BMD at the lumbar spine and trochanter (absolute additional increases between years 3 and 5: lumbar spine, 0.94%; trochanter, 0.88%). BMD at the femoral neck, forearm and total body were maintained. Alendronate sodium was similarly effective regardless of age, race, baseline rate of bone turnover, and baseline BMD in the range studied (at least 2 standard deviations below the premenopausal mean).

[See figure 3 above]

In patients with postmenopausal osteoporosis treated with alendronate sodium 10 mg/day for one or two years, the effects of treatment withdrawal were assessed. Following discontinuation, there were no further increases in bone mass and the rates of bone loss were similar to those of the placebo groups.

Bone Histology

Bone histology in 270 postmenopausal patients with osteoporosis treated with alendronate sodium at doses ranging from 1 to 20 mg/day for one, two, or three years revealed normal mineralization and structure, as well as the expected decrease in bone turnover relative to placebo. These data, together with the normal bone histology and increased bone strength observed in rats and baboons exposed to long-term alendronate treatment, support the conclusion that bone formed during therapy with alendronate sodium is of normal quality.

Effect on height

Alendronate sodium, over a three- or four-year period, was associated with statistically significant reductions in loss of height vs. placebo in patients with and without baseline radiographic vertebral fractures. At the end of the FIT studies the between-treatment group differences were 3.2 mm in the Three-Year Study and 1.3 mm in the Four-Year Study.

Weekly dosing

The therapeutic equivalence of once weekly alendronate sodium 70 mg (n=519) and alendronate sodium 10 mg daily (n=370) was demonstrated in a one-year, double-blind, multicenter study of postmenopausal women with osteoporosis. In the primary analysis of completers, the mean increases from baseline in lumbar spine BMD at 1 year were 5.1% (4.8, 5.4%; 95% CI) in the 70 mg once-weekly group (n=440) and 5.4% (5.0, 5.8%; 95% CI) in the 10 mg daily group (n=330). The 2 treatment groups were also similar with regard to BMD increases at other skeletal sites. The results of the intention-to-treat analysis were consistent with the primary analysis of completers.

14.2   Treatment to Increase Bone Mass in Men with Osteoporosis

The efficacy of alendronate sodium in men with hypogonadal or idiopathic osteoporosis was demonstrated in two clinical studies.

Daily Dosing

A two-year, double-blind, placebo-controlled, multicenter study of alendronate sodium 10 mg once daily enrolled a total of 241 men between the ages of 31 and 87 (mean, 63). All patients in the trial had either: 1) a BMD T-score less than or equal to -2 at the lumbar spine and less than or equal to -1 at the lumbar spine, or 2) a baseline osteoporotic fracture and a BMD T-score less than or equal to -1 at the femoral neck. At two years, the mean increases relative to placebo in BMD in men receiving alendronate sodium 10 mg/day were significant at the following sites: lumbar spine, 5.3%; femoral neck, 2.6%; trochanter, 3.1%; and total body, 1.6%. Treatment with alendronate sodium also reduced height loss (alendronate, -0.6 mm vs. placebo, -2.4 mm).

Weekly dosing

A one-year, double-blind, placebo-controlled, multicenter study of once weekly alendronate sodium 70 mg enrolled a total of 167 men between the ages of 38 and 91 (mean, 66). Patients in the study had either: 1) a BMD T-score less than or equal to -2 at the femoral neck and less than or equal to -1 at the lumbar spine, 2) a BMD T-score less than or equal to -2 at the lumbar spine and less than or equal to -1 at the femoral neck, or 3) a baseline osteoporotic fracture and a BMD T-score less than or equal to -1 at the femoral neck. At one year, the mean increases relative to placebo in BMD in men receiving alendronate sodium 70 mg once weekly were significant at the following sites: lumbar spine, 2.8%; femoral neck, 1.9%; trochanter, 2.0%; and total body, 1.2%. These increases in BMD were similar to those seen at one year in the alendronate sodium 10 mg once-daily study.

In both studies, BMD responses were similar regardless of age (greater than or equal to 65 years vs. less than 65 years), gonadal function (baseline testosterone less than 9 ng/dL vs. greater than or equal to 9 ng/dL), or baseline BMD (femoral neck and lumbar spine T-score less than or equal to -2.5 vs. greater than -2.5).

16   HOW SUPPLIED/STORAGE AND HANDLING

BINOSTO effervescent tablets are round, flat faced, white to off-white tablets with beveled edges and "M" debossed on one side. BINOSTO effervescent tablets, 70 mg are provided in blisters made of aluminum foil composite, as follows:
NDC 0178-0101-02 carton containing 4 units of use blisters
NDC 0178-0101-03 carton containing 12 units of use blisters
Store at 20°C to 25°C (68°F to 77°F), excursions permitted to 15°C to 30°C (59°F to 86°F), [See USP Controlled Room Temperature.] Protect from moisture. Store tablets in original blister package until use.

17   PATIENT COUNSELING INFORMATION

See FDA-approved patient labeling (Medication Guide).
Instruct patients to read the Medication Guide before starting therapy with BINOSTO and to reread it each time the prescription is renewed.
17.1   Osteoporosis Recommendations, Including Calcium and Vitamin D Supplementation
Instruct patients to take supplemental calcium and vitamin D, if daily dietary intake is inadequate. Weight-bearing exercise should be considered along with the modification of certain behavioral factors, such as cigarette smoking and/or excessive alcohol consumption, if these factors exist.
17.2   Dosing Instructions
Instruct patients that it is necessary to follow all dosing instructions for BINOSTO:
• BINOSTO should only be taken upon arising for the day and must be taken at least 30 minutes before the first food, beverage, or medication of the day.
• Instruct patients not to attempt to swallow, chew, or suck on the tablet because of a potential for oropharyngeal ulceration.
• Instruct patients to dissolve the effervescent tablet in 4 ounces room temperature plain water only (not mineral water or flavored water).
• Instruct patients to wait at least 5 minutes after the effervescence stops and then stir the solution for approximately 10 seconds and then consume the contents.
• Instruct patients to avoid lying down for at least 30 minutes after taking BINOSTO and until after their first food of the day.
• Instruct patients not to take BINOSTO at bedtime or before arising for the day.
• Instruct patients that waiting less than 30 minutes, or taking BINOSTO with food, beverages (other than plain water) or other medications will lessen the effect of BINOSTO by decreasing its absorption into the body [see Drug Interactions (7.1)]. Even dosing with orange juice or coffee has been shown to markedly reduce the absorption of BINOSTO [see Clinical Pharmacology (12.3)].
• Inform patients that failure to follow these instructions may increase their risk of esophageal problems. [see Warnings and Precautions (5.1)].
Instruct patients that if they develop symptoms of esophageal disease (such as difficulty or pain upon swallowing, retrosternal pain or new or worsening heartburn) they should stop taking BINOSTO and consult their physician. [see Warnings and Precautions (5.1)].
Instruct patients that if they miss a dose of once weekly BINOSTO, they should take one dose on the morning after they remember. They should not take 2 doses on the same day but should return to taking one dose once a week, as originally scheduled on their chosen day.

17.3   Patients on Sodium Restriction

Inform patients who are prescribed sodium restricted diets that BINOSTO contains 650 mg of sodium which is equivalent to approximately 1650 mg NaCl per tablet.

Mission® Pharmacal
Manufactured for: Mission Pharmacal Company, San Antonio, TX 78230-1355
Rev 0813

CITRANATAL ASSURE®   ℞
Rx Prenatal Vitamin Tablet and 300 mg DHA capsule

DESCRIPTION

CitraNatal Assure® is a prescription prenatal/postnatal multivitamin/mineral tablet with Ferr-Ease®, a patented dual-iron delivery comprising both a quick release and slow release iron, and a capsule of an essential fatty acid. The prenatal vitamin is a white, coated, oval multivitamin/mineral tablet. The tablet is debossed "0891" on one side and is blank on the other. The essential fatty acid DHA capsule is caramel colored and contains a light yellow to orange semisolid mixture.

Each prenatal tablet contains:

Vitamin C (Ascorbic acid)	120 mg
Calcium (Calcium citrate)	124 mg
Iron (Carbonyl iron, ferrous gluconate)	35 mg
Vitamin D_3 (Cholecalciferol)	400 IU
Vitamin E (dl-alpha tocopheryl acetate)	30 IU
Thiamin (Vitamin B_1)	3 mg
Riboflavin (Vitamin B_2)	3.4 mg
Niacinamide (Vitamin B_3)	20 mg
Vitamin B_6 (Pyridoxine HCl)	25 mg
Folic Acid	1 mg
Iodine (Potassium iodide)	150 mcg
Zinc (Zinc oxide)	25 mg
Copper (Cupric oxide)	2 mg
Docusate Sodium	50 mg

Each DHA gelatin capsule contains:

Docosahexaenoic Acid (DHA, 40% from 750 mg Algal Oil)	300 mg
Eicosapentaenoic Acid (EPA)	Not more than 0.750 mg

Other ingredients in DHA gelatin capsule: Gelatin, sunflower oil, glycerin, caramel color, sunflower lecithin, rosemary extract, tocopherols, ascorbyl palmitate.

INDICATIONS

CitraNatal Assure® is a multivitamin/mineral prescription drug indicated for use in improving the nutritional status of women prior to conception, throughout pregnancy, and in the postnatal period for both lactating and nonlactating mothers.

CONTRAINDICATIONS

This product is contraindicated in patients with a known hypersensitivity to any of the ingredients.

> **WARNING:** Accidental overdose of **iron-containing** products is a leading cause of fatal poisoning in children under 6. KEEP THIS PRODUCT OUT OF THE REACH OF CHILDREN. In case of accidental overdose, call a doctor or poison control center immediately.

WARNING

Ingestion of more than 3 grams of omega-3 fatty acids per day has been shown to have potential antithrombotic effects, including an increased bleeding time and INR. Administration of omega-3 fatty acids should be avoided in patients on anticoagulants and in those known to have an inherited or acquired bleeding diathesis.

WARNING

Folic acid alone is improper therapy in the treatment of pernicious anemia and other megaloblastic anemias where vitamin B_{12} is deficient.

PRECAUTIONS

Folic acid in doses above 0.1 mg daily may obscure pernicious anemia in that hematologic remission can occur while neurological manifestations progress.

ADVERSE REACTIONS

Allergic sensitization has been reported following both oral and parenteral administration of folic acid.

DOSAGE AND ADMINISTRATION

One tablet and one capsule daily or as directed by a physician.
STORAGE: Store at 20-25°C (68-77°F).
NOTICE: Contact with moisture can discolor or erode the tablet.

HOW SUPPLIED

Six child-resistant blister packs of 5 tablets and 5 capsules each - **NDC** 0178-0891-30
To report a serious adverse event or obtain product information, call (210) 696-8400.
Please consult your health care provider with any dietary concerns.
CitraNatal Assure® contains Ferr-Ease®.
Dual-iron delivery
Trademark of Mission Pharmacal Company
U.S. Patent No. 6,521,247
CitraNatal Assure® contains *life'sDHA®*.
life'sDHA® is a trademark of DSM.
U.S. Patent No. 7,579,174
U.S. Patent No. 8,129,172
U.S. Patent No. 8,124,384
U.S. Patent No. 8,288,135
U.S. Patent No. 8,669,090
DHA capsules manufactured for:
MISSION PHARMACAL COMPANY
San Antonio, TX USA 78230 1355
Prenatal tablets manufactured by:
MISSION PHARMACAL COMPANY
San Antonio, TX USA 78230 1355
Copyright © 2014 Mission Pharmacal Company. All rights reserved.
Rev 0614

CITRANATAL B-CALM®   ℞
Rx Prenatal Vitamin and two 25 mg each Vitamin B₆ tablets

DESCRIPTION

CitraNatal B-Calm® is a prescription prenatal multivitamin/mineral tablet with B_6, along with two vitamin B_6 tablets. The prenatal tablet contains Ferr-Ease®, a patented dual-iron delivery comprising both a quick release and slow release iron. The prenatal tablet is white, coated, modified oval, and is debossed with "0832" on one side and is blank on the other. The B_6 25 mg tablets are white to off-white, uncoated, round, and are debossed with "B" on one side and "6" on the other.

Each prenatal tablet contains:

Vitamin C (Ascorbic acid)	120 mg
Calcium (Calcium citrate)	120 mg
Iron (Carbonyl iron, ferrous gluconate)	20 mg
Vitamin D_3 (Cholecalciferol)	400 IU
Vitamin B_6 (Pyridoxine HCl)	25 mg
Folic Acid	1 mg

Each vitamin B₆ tablet contains:

Vitamin B_6 (Pyridoxine HCl)	25 mg

INDICATIONS

CitraNatal B-Calm® is a multivitamin/mineral prescription drug indicated for use in improving the nutritional status of women prior to conception, throughout pregnancy, and in the postnatal period for both lactating and nonlactating mothers. CitraNatal B-Calm® may be used in conjunction with a physician prescribed regimen to help minimize pregnancy related nausea and vomiting.

CONTRAINDICATIONS

This product is contraindicated in patients with a known hypersensitivity to any of the ingredients.

> **WARNING:** Accidental overdose of **iron-containing** products is a leading cause of fatal poisoning in children under 6. KEEP THIS AND ALL DRUGS OUT OF THE REACH OF CHILDREN. In case of accidental overdose, call a doctor or poison control center immediately.

WARNING

Folic acid alone is improper therapy in the treatment of pernicious anemia and other megaloblastic anemias where vitamin B_{12} is deficient.

PRECAUTION

Folic acid in doses above 0.1 mg daily may obscure pernicious anemia, in that hematologic remission can occur while neurological manifestations remain progressive.

ADVERSE REACTIONS

Allergic sensitization has been reported following both oral and parenteral administration of folic acid.

DOSAGE AND ADMINISTRATION

One tablet every eight hours, beginning with "Tablet 1", or as directed by a physician.
STORAGE
Store at 20-25°C (68-77°F)

NOTICE: Contact with moisture can discolor or erode tablets.

HOW SUPPLIED

Six child-resistant blister packs of 5 multivitamin/multimineral tablets and 10 vitamin B_6 tablets each - **NDC** 0178-0832-30.
To report a serious adverse event or obtain product information, call (210) 696-8400.
Please consult your health care provider with any dietary concerns.
CitraNatal B-Calm® contains Ferr-Ease®.
Dual-iron delivery
Trademark of Mission Pharmacal Company
U.S. Patent No. 6,521,247
Prenatal tablets manufactured by:
MISSION PHARMACAL COMPANY
San Antonio, TX USA 78230 1355
Copyright © 2014 Mission Pharmacal Company. All rights reserved.
Rev 0614

CITRANATAL® 90 DHA   ℞
Rx Prenatal Vitamin Tablet and 300 mg DHA Capsule

DESCRIPTION

CitraNatal® 90 90 DHA is a prescription prenatal/postnatal multivitamin/mineral tablet with Ferr-Ease®, a patented dual-iron delivery comprising both a quick release and slow release iron, and a capsule of an essential fatty acid. The prenatal vitamin is a scored, white, oval multivitamin/mineral tablet. The tablet is debossed "CN 90" on one side and "0821" on the other. The essential fatty acid DHA capsule is caramel colored and contains a light yellow to orange semisolid mixture.

Each prenatal tablet contains:

Vitamin C (Ascorbic acid)	120 mg
Calcium (Calcium citrate)	159 mg
Iron (Carbonyl iron, ferrous gluconate)	90 mg
Vitamin D_3 (Cholecalciferol)	400 IU
Vitamin E (dl-alpha tocopheryl acetate)	30 IU
Thiamin (Vitamin B_1)	3 mg
Riboflavin (Vitamin B_2)	3.4 mg
Niacinamide (Vitamin B_3)	20 mg
Vitamin B_6 (Pyridoxine HCl)	20 mg
Folic Acid	1 mg
Iodine (Potassium iodide)	150 mcg
Zinc (Zinc oxide)	25 mg
Copper (Cupric oxide)	2 mg
Docusate Sodium	50 mg

Each DHA gelatin capsule contains:

Docosahexaenoic Acid (DHA, 40% from 750 mg Algal Oil)	300 mg
Eicosapentaenoic Acid (EPA)	Not more than 0.750 mg

Other ingredients in DHA gelatin capsule: Gelatin, sunflower oil, glycerin, caramel color, sunflower lecithin, rosemary extract, tocopherols, ascorbyl palmitate.

INDICATIONS

CitraNatal® 90 DHA is a multivitamin/mineral prescription drug indicated for use in improving the nutritional status of women prior to conception, throughout pregnancy, and in the postnatal period for both lactating and nonlactating mothers.

CONTRAINDICATIONS

This product is contraindicated in patients with a known hypersensitivity to any of the ingredients.

> **WARNING**
> Accidental overdose of **iron-containing** products is a leading cause of fatal poisoning in children under 6. KEEP THIS PRODUCT OUT OF THE REACH OF CHILDREN. In case of accidental overdose, call a doctor or poison control center immediately.

WARNING

Ingestion of more than 3 grams of omega-3 fatty acids per day has been shown to have potential antithrombotic effects, including an increased bleeding time and INR. Administration of omega-3 fatty acids should be avoided in patients on anticoagulants and in those known to have an inherited or acquired bleeding diathesis.

WARNING

Folic acid alone is improper therapy in the treatment of pernicious anemia and other megaloblastic anemias where vitamin B_{12} is deficient.

PRECAUTIONS

Folic acid in doses above 0.1 mg daily may obscure pernicious anemia in that hematologic remission can occur while neurological manifestations progress.

ADVERSE REACTIONS

Allergic sensitization has been reported following both oral and parenteral administration of folic acid.

DOSAGE AND ADMINISTRATION

One tablet and one capsule daily or as directed by a physician.

STORAGE: Store at 20-25°C (68-77°F).

NOTICE: Contact with moisture can discolor or erode the tablet.

HOW SUPPLIED

Six child-resistant blister packs of 5 tablets and 5 capsules each - NDC 0178-0821-30

To report a serious adverse event or obtain product information, call (210) 696-8400.

Please consult your health care provider with any dietary concerns.

CitraNatal® 90DHA contains Ferr-Ease®.
Dual-iron delivery
Trademark of Mission Pharmacal Company
U.S. Patent No. 6,521,247
CitraNatal® 90DHA contains *life'sDHA*®.
*life's*DHA® is a trademark of DSM.
U.S. Patent No. 7,579,174
U.S. Patent No. 8,129,172
U.S. Patent No. 8,124,384
U.S. Patent No. 8,288,135
U.S. Patent No. 8,669,090
DHA capsules manufactured for:
MISSION PHARMACAL COMPANY
San Antonio, TX USA 78230 1355
Prenatal tablets manufactured by:
MISSION PHARMACAL COMPANY
San Antonio, TX USA 78230 1355
Copyright © 2014 Mission Pharmacal
Company. All rights reserved.
Rev 0614

CITRANATAL HARMONY® ℞
Rx Prenatal Vitamin Gel Cap

DESCRIPTION

CitraNatal Harmony® is a prescription prenatal/postnatal multivitamin/mineral soft gelatin capsule. The prenatal vitamin is a purple, opaque soft gelatin capsule containing a greenish-gray liquid to semi-solid fill. The capsule is printed "0796" in white ink.

Each prenatal capsule contains:

Calcium (Calcium citrate)	104 mg
Iron (Ferrous fumarate, carbonyl iron)	27 mg
Vitamin D₃ (Cholecalciferol)	400 IU
Vitamin E (dl-alpha tocopheryl acetate)	30 IU
Vitamin B₆ (Pyridoxine HCl)	25 mg
Folic Acid	1 mg
Docusate Sodium	50 mg
Docosahexaenoic Acid (DHA 40% from 650 mg Algal Oil)	260 mg

INDICATIONS

CitraNatal Harmony® is a multivitamin/mineral prescription drug indicated for use in improving the nutritional status of women prior to conception, throughout pregnancy, and in the postnatal period for both lactating and nonlactating mothers.

CONTRAINDICATIONS

This product is contraindicated in patients with a known hypersensitivity to any of the ingredients.

> **WARNING**
> Accidental overdose of **iron-containing** products is a leading cause of fatal poisoning in children under 6. KEEP THIS PRODUCT OUT OF THE REACH OF CHILDREN. In case of accidental overdose, call a doctor or poison control center immediately.

WARNING

Ingestion of more than 3 grams of omega-3 fatty acids per day has been shown to have potential antithrombotic effects, including an increased bleeding time and INR. Administration of omega-3 fatty acids should be avoided in patients on anticoagulants and in those known to have an inherited or acquired bleeding diathesis.

WARNING

Folic acid alone is improper therapy in the treatment of pernicious anemia and other megaloblastic anemias where vitamin B₁₂ is deficient.

PRECAUTIONS

Folic acid in doses above 0.1 mg daily may obscure pernicious anemia in that hematologic remission can occur while neurological manifestations progress.

ADVERSE REACTIONS

Allergic sensitization has been reported following both oral and parenteral administration of folic acid.

CAUTION: Exercise caution to ensure that the prescribed dosage of DHA does not exceed 1 gram (1000 mg) per day.

DOSAGE AND ADMINISTRATION

One capsule daily or as directed by a physician.
Store at controlled room temperature.

NOTICE: Contact with moisture can discolor or erode the capsule.

HOW SUPPLIED

Bottles of 30 capsules each - NDC 0178-0796-30.

To report a serious adverse event or obtain product information, call (210) 696-8400.

Please consult your health care provider with any dietary concerns.

CitraNatal Harmony® contains Ferr-Ease®
Dual-iron delivery
Trademark of Mission Pharmacal Company
U.S. Patent No. 6,521,247
CitraNatal Harmony®:
Capsules are MADE IN CANADA
CitraNatal Harmony® contains *life'sDHA*®.
*life's*DHA® is a trademark of DSM.
U.S. Patent No. 7,163,811
U.S. Patent No. 7,824,892
U.S. Patent No. 8,669,090
Copyright © 2014 Mission Pharmacal
Company. All rights reserved.
Rev 0614

FERRALET® 90 ℞
Carbonyl Iron/ferrous gluconate tablet

Rx Only

DESCRIPTION:

Each green film-coated tablet for oral administration contains:

Iron (Carbonyl iron, ferrous gluconate)	90 mg
Folic Acid	1 mg
Vitamin B₁₂ (Cyanocobalamin)	12 mcg
Vitamin C (Ascorbic acid)	120 mg
Docusate sodium	50 mg

Inactive Ingredients: Povidone, croscarmellose sodium, acrylic resin, color added, magnesium stearate, FD&C Yellow No. 5, magnesium silicate, FD&C Blue No. 1, polyethylene glycol, vitamin A palmitate, ethyl vanillin.

CLINICAL PHARMACOLOGY:

Oral iron is absorbed most efficiently when administered between meals. Iron is critical for normal hemoglobin synthesis to maintain oxygen transport for energy production and proper function of cells. Adequate amounts of iron are necessary for effective erythropoiesis. Iron also serves as a cofactor of several essential enzymes, including cytochromes, which are involved in electron transport.
Folic acid is required for nucleoprotein synthesis and the maintenance of normal erythropoiesis. Folic acid is the precursor of tetrahydrofolic acid, which is involved as a cofactor for transformylation reactions in the biosynthesis of purines and thymidylates of nucleic acids. Deficiency of folic acid may account for the defective deoxyribonucleic acid (DNA) synthesis that leads to megaloblast formation and megaloblastic macrocytic anemias. Vitamin B₁₂ is essential to growth, cell reproduction, hematopoiesis, nucleic acid, and myelin synthesis. Deficiency may result in megaloblastic anemia or pernicious anemia.

INDICATIONS AND USAGE:

Ferralet® 90 is indicated for the treatment of all anemias that are responsive to oral iron therapy. These include: hypochromic anemia associated with pregnancy, chronic and/or acute blood loss, metabolic disease, postsurgical convalescence, and dietary needs.

CONTRAINDICATIONS:

Hypersensitivity to any of the ingredients. Hemolytic anemia, hemochromatosis, and hemosiderosis are contraindications to iron therapy.

WARNING:

Folic acid alone is improper therapy in the treatment of pernicious anemia and other megaloblastic anemias where vitamin B₁₂ is deficient.

> **WARNING:** Accidental overdose of **iron-containing** products is a leading cause of fatal poisoning in children under 6. KEEP THIS PRODUCT OUT OF THE REACH OF CHILDREN. In case of accidental overdose, call a doctor or poison control center immediately.

PRECAUTIONS:

General: Take 2 hours after meals. Do not exceed recommended dose. Discontinue use if symptoms of intolerance appear. The type of anemia and underlying cause or causes should be determined before starting therapy with Ferralet® 90 tablets. Ensure Hgb, Hct, and reticulocyte counts are determined before starting therapy and periodically thereafter during prolonged treatment. Periodically review therapy to determine if it needs to be continued without change or if a dose change is indicated.
This product contains FD&C Yellow No. 5 (tartrazine) which may cause allergic-type reactions (including bronchial asthma) in certain susceptible persons. Although the overall incidence of FD&C Yellow No. 5 (tartrazine) sensitivity in the general population is low, it is frequently seen in patients who also have aspirin hypersensitivity.

Folic Acid: Folic acid in doses above 0.1 mg daily may obscure pernicious anemia in that hematologic remission can occur while neurological manifestations remain progressive. Pernicious anemia should be excluded before using these products since folic acid may mask the symptoms of pernicious anemia.

Pediatric Use: Safety and effectiveness in pediatric patients have not been established.

Geriatric Use: Dosing for elderly patients should be administered with caution. Due to the greater frequency of decreased hepatic, renal, or cardiac function, and of concomitant disease or other drug therapy, dosing should start at the lower end of the dosing range.

ADVERSE REACTIONS:

Adverse reactions with iron therapy may include GI irritation, constipation, diarrhea, nausea, vomiting, and dark stools. Adverse reactions with iron therapy are usually transient. Allergic sensitization has been reported following both oral and parenteral administration of folic acid.

DRUG INTERACTIONS: Prescriber should be aware of a number of iron/drug interactions, including antacids, tetracyclines, or fluoroquinolones.

OVERDOSAGE:

Symptoms: abdominal pain, metabolic acidosis, anuria, CNS damage, coma, convulsions, death, dehydration, diffuse vascular congestion, hepatic cirrhosis, hypotension, hypothermia, lethargy, nausea, vomiting, diarrhea, tarry stools, melena, hematemesis, tachycardia, hyperglycemia, drowsiness, pallor, cyanosis, lassitude, seizures, and shock.

DOSAGE AND ADMINISTRATION:

One tablet daily or as directed by a physician. Do not chew tablet.

STORAGE:

Store at 25°C (77°F). Excursions permitted to 15°-30°C (59°-86°F). (See USP Controlled Room Temperature.)

NOTICE: Contact with moisture can discolor or erode the tablet.

HOW SUPPLIED:

Ferralet® 90 (**NDC** 0178-0089-90) is a green, modified rectangle shaped, film-coated tablet, debossed with "F6" on one side and blank on the other, and packaged in bottles of 90.

To report a serious adverse event or obtain product information, call (210) 696-8400.

Ferralet® 90 contains Ferr-Ease®.
Dual-iron delivery
Trademark of Mission Pharmacal Company
U.S. Patent No. 6,521,247
MISSION PHARMACAL COMPANY
San Antonio, TX USA 78230 1355
Copyright © 2013 Mission Pharmacal Company. All rights reserved.
Rev 1213

LITHOSTAT® ℞
(Acetohydroxamic Acid)
Tablets

DESCRIPTION: Acetohydroxamic acid (AHA) is a stable, synthetic compound derived from hydroxylamine and ethyl acetate. Its molecular structure is similar to urea:

ACETOHYDROXAMIC ACID

AHA is weakly acidic, highly soluble in water, and chelates metals - notably iron. The molecular weight is 75.068. AHA has a pKa of 9.32 and a melting point of 89-91° C. AHA is a urease inhibitor. Available as 250 mg tablets.

CLINICAL PHARMACOLOGY: AHA reversibly inhibits the bacterial enzyme urease, thereby inhibiting the hydrolysis of urea and production of ammonia in urine infected with urea-splitting organisms. The reduced ammonia levels and decreased pH enhance the effectiveness of antimicrobial agents and allow an increased cure rate of these infections. AHA is well absorbed from the gastrointestinal tract after oral administration; peak blood levels occur from 0.25 to 1 hour after dosing. The compound is distributed throughout body water, and there is no known binding to any tissue. AHA chelates with dietary iron within the gut. This reaction may interfere with absorption of AHA and with iron. Concomitant hypochromic anemia should be treated with intramuscular iron.

In rodents, the metabolic fate of AHA is well known; 55% is excreted unchanged in urine, 25% is excreted as acetamide or acetate and 7% is excreted by the lungs as carbon dioxide. Less than 1% is excreted in the feces. Approximately 5% of the administered dose is unaccounted for. In rodents, AHA shows a dose-related change in pharmacokinetics; with increasing dose, there is an increase in the half-life and an increase in the percent of the administered dose recovered in urine as unchanged AHA.

Pharmacokinetics in man are generally similar to rodents including the dose-related increase in half-life, but they are not as well characterized as in the rodent. Thirty-six to sixty-five percent (36-65%) of the oral dosage is excreted unchanged in the urine. It is unaltered AHA in the urine that provides the therapeutic effect, but the precise concentration of AHA in urine that is necessary to inhibit urease is incompletely delineated. Therapeutic benefit may be obtained from concentrations as low as 8 mcg/ml; higher concentrations (i.e., 30 mcg/ml) are expected to provide more complete inhibition of urease. The plasma half-life of AHA is approximately 5-10 hours in subjects with normal renal function and is prolonged in patients with reduced renal function.

Acetohydroxamic acid has been evaluated clinically in patients with urea-splitting urinary infections, often accompanied by struvite stone disease, that were recalcitrant to other forms of medical and surgical management. In these clinical trials, AHA reduced the pathologically elevated urinary ammonia and pH levels that result from the hydrolysis of urea by the enzyme, urease.

AHA does not acidify urine directly nor does it have a direct antibacterial effect. The usefulness of reducing ammonia levels and decreasing urinary pH is suggested by single (not yet replicated) clinical trials in which urease inhibition 1) allowed successful antibiotic treatment of urea-splitting Proteus infections after surgical removal of struvite stones in patients not cured by 3 months of antibacterial treatment alone, and 2) reduced the rate of stone growth in patients who were not candidates for surgical removal of stones.

INDICATIONS AND USAGE: Acetohydroxamic acid is indicated as adjunctive therapy in patients with chronic urea-splitting urinary infection. AHA is intended to decrease urinary ammonia and alkalinity, but it should not be used in lieu of curative surgical treatment (for patients with stones) or antimicrobial treatment. Long-term treatment with AHA may be warranted to maintain urease inhibition as long as urea-splitting infection is present. Experience with AHA does not go beyond 7 years. A patient package insert should be distributed to each patient who receives AHA.

CONTRAINDICATIONS: Acetohydroxamic acid should not be used in:

a. patients whose physical state and disease are amenable to definitive surgery and appropriate antimicrobial agents
b. patients whose urine is infected by non-urease producing organisms
c. patients whose urinary infections can be controlled by culture-specific oral antimicrobial agents
d. patients whose renal function is poor (i.e., serum creatinine more than 2.5 mg/dl and/or creatinine clearance less than 20 ml/min)
e. female patients who do not evidence a satisfactory method of contraception
f. patients who are pregnant

Acetohydroxamic acid may cause fetal harm when administered to a pregnant woman. AHA was teratogenic (retarded and/or clubbed rear leg at 750 mg/kg and above and exencephaly and encephalocele at 1,500 mg/kg) when given intraperitoneally to rats. AHA is contraindicated in women who are or may become pregnant. If this drug is used during pregnancy, or if the patient becomes pregnant while taking this drug, the patient should be informed of the potential hazard to the fetus.

WARNINGS: A Coombs negative hemolytic anemia has occurred in patients receiving AHA. Gastrointestinal upset characterized by nausea, vomiting, anorexia and generalized malaise have accompanied the most severe forms of hemolytic anemia. Approximately 15% of patients receiving AHA have had only laboratory findings of an anemia. However, most patients developed a mild reticulocytosis. The

untoward reactions have reverted to normal following cessation of treatment. A complete blood count, including a reticulocyte count, is recommended after two weeks of treatment. If the reticulocyte count exceeds 6%, a reduced dosage should be entertained. A CBC and reticulocyte count are recommended at 3-month intervals for the duration of treatment .

PRECAUTIONS: GENERAL: Hematologic Effects: Bone marrow depression (leukopenia, anemia, and thrombocytopenia) has occurred in experimental animals receiving large doses of AHA, but has not been seen in man to date. AHA is a known inhibitor of DNA synthesis and also chelates metals - notably iron. Its bone marrow suppressant effect is probably related to its ability to inhibit DNA synthesis, but anemia could also be related to depletion of iron stores. To date, the only clinical effect noted has been hemolysis, with a decrease in the circulating red blood cells, hemoglobin and hematocrit. Abnormalities in platelet or white blood cell count have not been noted. However, clinical monitoring of the platelet and white cell count is recommended.

Monitoring Liver Function: Abnormalities of liver function have not been reported to date. However, a chlorobenzene derivative of acetohydroxamic acid caused significant liver dysfunction in an unrelated study. Therefore, close monitoring of liver function is recommended. (See Carcinogenesis for discussion of possible hepatic carcinogenesis.)

Use In Patients With Renal Impairment: Since AHA is eliminated primarily by the kidneys, patients with significantly impaired renal function should be closely monitored, and a reduction of daily dose may be needed to avoid excessive drug accumulation. (See Dosage and Administration.)

DRUG INTERACTIONS: AHA has been used concomitantly with insulin, oral and parenteral antibiotics, and progestational agents. No clinically significant interactions have been noted, but until wider clinical experience is obtained, AHA should be used with caution in patients receiving other therapeutic agents.

AHA taken in association with alcoholic beverages has resulted in a rash. (See Adverse Reactions.)

AHA chelates heavy metals-notably iron. The absorption of iron and AHA from the intestinal lumen may be reduced when both drugs are taken concomitantly. When iron administration is indicated, intramuscular iron is probably the product of choice.

CARCINOGENESIS, MUTAGENESIS, IMPAIRMENT OF FERTILITY: Well controlled, long-term animal studies that identify the carcinogenic potential of AHA treatment have not been conducted. Acetamide, a metabolite of AHA, has been shown to cause hepatocellular carcinoma in rats at oral doses 1,500 times the human dose. AHA is cytotoxic and was positive for mutagenicity in the Ames test.

PREGNANCY: Pregnancy Category X. (See Contraindications.)

NURSING MOTHERS: It is not known whether AHA is secreted in human milk. Because many drugs are excreted in human milk; and because of the potential for serious adverse reactions in nursing infants from AHA, a decision should be made to discontinue nursing or the drug, taking into account the significance of the drug to the mother's well being.

PEDIATRIC USE: Children with chronic, recalcitrant, urea-splitting urinary infection may benefit from treatment with AHA. However, detailed studies involving dosage and dose intervals in children have not been established. Children have tolerated a dose of 10 mg/kg/day, taken in two or three divided doses, satisfactorily for periods up to one year. Close monitoring of such patients is mandatory.

ADVERSE REACTIONS: Experience with AHA is limited. About 150 patients have been treated, most for periods of more than a year.

Adverse reactions have occurred in up to thirty percent (30%) of the patients receiving AHA. In some instances the reactions were symptomatic; in others only changes in laboratory parameters were noted. Adverse reactions seem to be more prevalent in patients with preexisting thrombophlebitis or phlebothrombosis and/or in patients with advanced degrees of renal insufficiency. The risk of adverse reactions is highest during the first year of treatment. Chronic treatment does not seem to increase the risk nor the severity of adverse reactions.

The following reactions have been reported:

NEUROLOGICAL: Mild headaches are commonly reported (about 30%) during the first 48 hours of treatment. These headaches are mild, responsive to oral salicylate-type analgesics, and usually disappear spontaneously. The headaches have not been associated with vertigo, tinnitus, or visual or auditory abnormalities. Tremulousness and nervousness have also been reported.

GASTROINTESTINAL: Gastrointestinal symptoms, nausea, vomiting, anorexia, and malaise have occurred in 20-25% of patients. In most patients the symptoms were mild, transitory, and did not result in interruption of treatment.

Approximately 3% of patients developed a hemolytic anemia of sufficient magnitude to warrant interruption in treatment; several of these patients also had symptoms of gastrointestinal upset.

HEMATOLOGICAL: Approximately 15% of patients have had laboratory findings characteristic of a hemolytic anemia. A mild reticulocytosis (5- 6%) without anemia, is even more prevalent. The laboratory findings are occasionally accompanied by systemic symptoms such as malaise, lethargy and fatigue, and gastrointestinal symptoms. Symptoms and laboratory findings have invariably improved following cessation of treatment with AHA. The hematological abnormalities are more prevalent in patients with advanced renal failure.

DERMATOLOGICAL: A nonpruritic, macular skin rash has occurred in the upper extremities and on the face of several patients taking AHA on a long-term basis, usually when AHA has been taken concomitantly with alcoholic beverages, but in a few patients in the absence of alcohol consumption. The rash commonly appears 30-45 minutes after ingestion of alcoholic beverages; it characteristically disappears spontaneously in 30-60 minutes. The rash may be associated with a general sensation of warmth. In some patients the rash is sufficiently severe to warrant discontinuation of treatment, but most patients have continued treatment, avoiding alcohol or using smaller quantities of it. Alopecia has also been reported in patients taking AHA.

CARDIOVASCULAR: Superficial phlebitis involving the lower extremities has occurred in several patients on AHA during the early (Phase II) clinical trials. Several of the affected patients had had phlebitic episodes prior to treatment. One patient developed deep vein thrombosis of the lower extremities. The patient with phlebothrombosis had an associated traumatic injury to the groin. It is unclear whether the phlebitis was related to or exacerbated by treatment with AHA. No patient in the three (3) year controlled (Phase III) clinical trial developed phlebitis. In all instances these vascular abnormalities returned to normal following appropriate medical therapy. Embolic phenomena have been reported in three patients taking AHA in the Phase II trial. The phlebitis and emboli resolved following discontinuation of AHA and implementation of appropriate medical therapy. Several patients have resumed treatment with AHA without ill effect. Palpitations have also been reported in patients taking AHA.

RESPIRATORY: No symptoms have been reported. Radiographic evidence of small pulmonary emboli has been seen in three patients with phlebitis in their lower legs.

PSYCHIATRIC: Depression, anxiety, nervousness, and tremulousness have been observed in approximately 20% of patients taking AHA. In most patients the symptoms were mild and transitory, but in about 6% of patients the symptoms were sufficiently distressing to warrant interruption or discontinuation of treatment.

OVERDOSAGE: Acute deliberate overdosage in man has not occurred, but would be expected to induce the following symptoms: anorexia, malaise, lethargy, diminished sense of well being, tremulousness, anxiety, nausea and vomiting. Laboratory findings are likely to include an elevated reticulocyte count and a severe hemolytic reaction requiring hospitalization, symptomatic treatment, and possibly blood transfusions. Concomitant reduction in platelets and/or white blood cells should be anticipated.

Milder overdosages resulting in hemolysis have occurred in an occasional patient with reduced renal function after several weeks or months of continuous treatment.

The acute LD 50 of AHA in animals (rats) is 4.8 gm/kg.

Recommended treatment for an overdosage reaction consists of (1) cessation of treatment, (2) close monitoring of hematologic status, (3) symptomatic treatment, and (4) blood transfusions as required by the clinical circumstances. The drug is probably dialyzable, but this property has not been tested clinically.

DOSAGE AND ADMINISTRATION: AHA should be administered orally, one tablet 3-4 times a day in a total daily dose of 10-15 mg/kg/day. The recommended starting dose is 12 mg/kg/day, administered at 6-8 hour intervals at a time when the stomach is empty. The maximum daily dose should be no more than 1.5 grams, regardless of body weight.

The dosage should be reduced in patients with reduced renal function. Patients whose serum creatinine is greater than 1.8 mg/dl should take no more than 1.0 gm/day; such patients should be dosed at q-12-h intervals. Further reductions in dosage to prevent the accumulation of toxic concentrations in the blood may also be desirable. Insufficient data exists to accurately characterize the optimum dose and/or dose interval in patients with moderate degrees of renal insufficiency.

Patients with advanced renal insufficiency (i.e., serum creatinine more than 2.5 mg/dl) should not be treated with AHA. The risk of accumulation of toxic blood levels of AHA seems to be greater than the chances for a beneficial effect in such patients.

In children an initial dose of 10 mg/kg/day is recommended. Close monitoring of the patient's clinical condition and hematologic status is recommended. Titration of the dose to higher or lower levels may be required to obtain an optimum therapeutic effect and/or to reduce the risk of side effects.

HOW SUPPLIED: LITHOSTAT®, NDC 0178-0500-01, is available for oral administration as 250 mg white, round tablets, in unit of use packages of 100 tablets. Each Lithostat® tablet is debossed MPC 500 on one side and blank on the other side. LITHOSTAT® should be stored in a dry place at room temperature, 15° - 30°C (59° - 86°F). Container should be closed tightly.

C08 Rev 010060

PATIENT INFORMATION

PLEASE READ THIS INFORMATION BEFORE USING THIS DRUG.

GENERAL INFORMATION: It has been known for many years that urinary infection may cause the formation of urinary stones. As these stones form, bacteria are trapped within the stones. The trapped bacteria cause the stones to grow, and the stones protect the bacteria from antibiotics. Surgical removal of the stone attempts to break this vicious cycle - many times successfully. However, if infection persists or if a small stone fragment persists, then there is an increased risk of stone recurrence. Multiple operations to remove kidney stones may result in damage and scarring of the kidney. In some situations removal of the kidney may be necessary.

In some instances stones may form initially as a result of non-infectious (i.e., metabolic) causes. If a metabolic stone becomes infected, then an "infection stone" may grow onto the "metabolic stone." Stone analysis and/or biochemical tests will usually determine which factors are present.

Experimental investigations have identified an enzyme called urease which is made by some (but not all) bacteria. Urease reacts with urine to make ammonia. Ammonia changes the acidity of the urine and the change in acidity encourages stone formation. LITHOSTAT® (acetohydroxamic acid) inhibits urease and thereby reduces urinary ammonia. In some instances, LITHOSTAT® enhances the effectiveness of antibiotics and thereby makes urinary infection easier to control.

WHAT IS LITHOSTAT®? LITHOSTAT® is a drug which prevents the excessive buildup of ammonia in your urine, which controls the acidity and alkalinity (pH) of your urine. The cause of excessive ammonia and alkalinity in your urine is a bacterial infection.

WHAT CAN LITHOSTAT® DO? Treatment with LITHOSTAT® is prescribed to decrease urinary ammonia. This may increase the chance of controlling your infection with antibiotics and may help the treatment of your kidney stones. Dissolution of existing stones is unlikely. LITHOSTAT® should not be used in place of surgical treatment. Surgical removal of all stones and elimination of all infection with antibiotics offers the possibility of curative treatment. LITHOSTAT® is likely to be more effective after large stones or obstructing stones have been removed.

WHAT ARE THE PROBLEMS OR SIDE EFFECTS WITH LITHOSTAT®? The complete spectrum of side effects induced by LITHOSTAT® (acetohydroxamic acid) is unknown. However, some side effects which have been reported to date have been headaches, abdominal discomfort, nausea, loss of hair, shakiness, and anemia. Lifethreatening problems (blood clot in the legs) occurred in several patients with advanced disease in early investigation. In more extensive later investigations, this problem has not occurred. No patient has died as a consequence of taking LITHOSTAT®. The most serious side effects seem to occur in patients with poor kidney function and/or in patients with a previous history of these conditions.

Problems related to LITHOSTAT® have disappeared following cessation of the drug and initiation of appropriate medical treatment. Most patients have resumed treatment without ill effect.

A flushing skin reaction (i.e., redness, warmth, and tingling) has occurred in several patients who consumed alcohol during treatment with LITHOSTAT®. The reaction persisted approximately 30 minutes and disappeared without treatment. The cause and significance of this reaction are unknown. Consequently, patients are encouraged to abstain from consumption of alcoholic beverages while being treated with LITHOSTAT®.

In animal studies doses of LITHOSTAT® about 20 times the maximum human dose have caused fetal abnormalities (birth defects) indicating a potential for such an adverse effect in an exposed human fetus. Therefore, LITHOSTAT® should not be given to pregnant women or to any sexually active woman of child-baring age, not using a highly effective method of contraception (oral contraceptive or IUD).

An acceptable long-term study of the cancer causing potential of LITHOSTAT® has not been conducted, but a known metabolite of LITHOSTAT®, acetamide, is carcinogenic

(cancer-causing) to the liver in rats at doses about 80 times the maximum human dose of LITHOSTAT®. LITHOSTAT® thus must be considered a potential human carcinogen. LITHOSTAT® kills tissue cells grown in tissue culture and alters genetic material in cells grown in culture.

LITHOSTAT® may induce other adverse reactions which have not yet been recognized.

Unusual symptoms should be reported to your physician. Mild symptoms usually do not warrant discontinuation of treatment. Severe symptoms may necessitate temporary cessation of treatment and/or alteration of dosage.

WHAT ABOUT TAKING OTHER DRUGS WITH LITHOSTAT®? Only take those drugs prescribed by your physician. Do not take prescription drugs or over the counter preparations without your physician's specific prescription or recommendation. Drugs that contain iron should not be taken at the same time as LITHOSTAT®, (acetohydroxamic acid). LITHOSTAT® reacts with iron, and may not be absorbed into the bloodstream. Both the iron you take and the LITHOSTAT® you take may be ineffective if both drugs are taken together.

HOW IMPORTANT IS MY DAILY DOSAGE OF LITHOSTAT®? If you fail to follow your daily dosage schedule with LITHOSTAT® you will probably suffer a setback in treatment effectiveness and new kidney stone formation is likely. LITHOSTAT® plus antibiotic therapy must be taken exactly as your physician prescribes it for optimum effectiveness.

IN CONCLUSION: Your daily dosage of LITHOSTAT® (acetohydroxamic acid) is important to the proper treatment of your condition. Any unusual side effects should be reported to your physician at once.

Rx only.

Rev 1006

THIOLA®
(Tiopronin)
Tablets

℞

DESCRIPTION

THIOLA® (Tiopronin) is a reducing and complexing thiol compound. Tiopronin is N-(2-Mercaptopropionyl) glycine and has the following structure:

$$CH_3\text{-}CH\text{-}CONHCH_2\text{-}COOH$$
$$|$$
$$SH$$

Tiopronin has the empirical formula $C_5H_9NO_3S$ and a molecular weight of 163.20. In this drug product tiopronin exists as a dl racemic mixture.

Tiopronin is a white crystalline powder which is freely soluble in water.

THIOLA® tablets are white, sugar coated tablets, each containing 100 mg. of Tiopronin and are taken orally.

Inactive ingredients: Calcium carbonate, carnauba wax, ethyl cellulose, Eudragit E 100, hydroxy-propyl cellulose, lactose, magnesium stearate, povidone, sugar, talc, titanium dioxide.

CLINICAL PHARMACOLOGY

THIOLA® is an active reducing agent which undergoes thiol-disulfide exchange with cystine to form a mixed disulfide of Thiola-cysteine.

$$2R\text{-}SH + R'\text{-}S\text{-}S\text{-}R' \rightleftharpoons 2R\text{-}S\text{-}S\text{-}R' + 2H^+$$

Thiola Cystine ⇌ Thiola-cysteine

From this reaction, a water-soluble mixed disulfide is formed and the amount of sparingly soluble cystine is reduced. When THIOLA® is given orally, up to 48% of dose appears in urine during the first 4 hours and up to 78% by 72 hours. Thus, in patients with cystinuria, sufficient amount of THIOLA® or its active metabolites could appear in urine to react with cystine, lowering cystine excretion. The decrement in urinary cystine produced by THIOLA® is generally proportional to the dose. A reduction in urinary cystine of 250-350 mg/day at a THIOLA® dosage of 1 g/day, and a decline of approximately 500 mg/day at a dosage of 2 g/day, might be expected. THIOLA® causes a sustained reduction in cystine excretion without apparent loss of effectiveness. THIOLA® has a rapid onset and offset of action, showing a fall in cystine excretion on the first day of administration and a rise on the first day of drug withdrawal.

INDICATIONS AND USAGE

THIOLA® is indicated for the prevention of cystine (kidney) stone formation in patients with severe homozygous cystinuria with urinary cystine greater than 500 mg/day, who are resistant to treatment with conservative measures of high fluid intake, alkali and diet modification, or who have adverse reactions to d-penicillamine.

Cystine stones typically occur in approximately 10,000 persons in the United States who are homozygous for cystinuria. These persons excrete abnormal amounts of cystine in

urine of over 250 mg/g creatinine, as well as excessive amounts of other dibasic amino acids (lysine, arginine and ornithine). In addition, they show varying intestinal transport defects for these same amino acids. The stone formation is the result of poor aqueous solubility of cystine.

Since there are no known inhibitors of the crystallization of cystine, the stone formation is determined primarily by the urinary supersaturation of cystine. Thus, cystine stones could theoretically form whenever urinary cystine concentration exceeds the solubility limit. Cystine solubility in urine is pH-dependent, and ranges from 170-300 mg/liter at pH 5, 190-400 mg/liter at pH 7 and 220-500 mg/liter at pH 7.5.

The goal of therapy is to reduce urinary cystine concentration below its solubility limit. It may be accomplished by dietary means aimed at reducing cystine synthesis and by a high fluid intake in order to increase urine volume and thereby lower cystine concentration.

Unfortunately, the above conservative measures alone may be ineffective in controlling cystine stone formation in some homozygous patients with severe cystinuria (urinary cystine exceeding 500 mg/day). In such patients, d-penicillamine has been used as an additional therapy. Like THIOLA™, dpenicillamine undergoes thiol-disulfide exchange with cystine, thereby lowering the amount of sparingly soluble cystine in urine.

However, d-penicillamine treatment is frequently accompanied by adverse reactions, such as dermatologic complications, hypersensitivity reactions, hematologic abnormalities and renal disturbances. THIOLA® may have a particular therapeutic role in such patients.

CONTRAINDICATIONS

The use of THIOLA® during pregnancy is contraindicated, except in those with severe cystinuria where the anticipated benefit of inhibited stone formation clearly outweighs possible hazards of treatment (see PRECAUTIONS).

THIOLA® should not be begun again in patients with a prior history of developing agranulocytosis, aplastic anemia or thrombocytopenia on this medication.

Mothers maintained on THIOLA® treatment should not nurse their infants.

WARNINGS

Despite apparent lower toxicity of THIOLA™, THIOLA® may potentially cause all the serious adverse reactions reported for d-penicillamine. Thus, although no death has been reported to result directly from THIOLA® treatment, a fatal outcome from THIOLA® is possible, as has been reported with d-penicillamine therapy from such complications as aplastic anemia, agranulocytosis, thrombocytopenia, Goodpasture's syndrome or myasthenia gravis.

Leukopenia of the granulocytic series may develop without eosinophilia. Thrombocytopenia may be immunologic in origin or occur on an idiosyncratic basis. The reduction in peripheral blood white count to less than 3500/cubic mm or in platelet count to below 100,000 cubic mm mandates cessation of therapy. Patients should be instructed to report promptly the occurrence of any symptom or sign of these hematological abnormalities, such as fever, sore throat, chills, bleeding or easy bruisability.

Proteinuria, sometimes sufficiently severe to cause nephrotic syndrome, may develop from membranous glomerulopathy. A close observation of affected patients is mandatory.

The following complications, though rare, have been reported during d-penicillamine therapy and could occur during THIOLA® treatment. When there are abnormal urinary findings associated with hemoptysis and pulmonary infiltrates suggestive of Goodpasture's syndrome, THIOLA® treatment should be stopped. Appearance of myasthenic syndrome or myasthenia gravis requires cessation of treatment. When pemphigus-type reactions develop, THIOLA® therapy should be stopped. Steroid treatment may be necessary.

PRECAUTIONS

Patients should be advised of the potential development of complications and to report promptly the occurrence of any symptom or sign of them.

To help monitor potential complications, the following tests are recommended: peripheral blood counts, direct platelet count, hemoglobin, serum albumin, liver function tests, 24-hour urinary protein and routine urinalysis at 3-6 month intervals during treatment. In order to assess effect on stone disease, urinary cystine analysis should be monitored frequently during the first 6 months when the optimum dose schedule is being determined, and at 6-month intervals thereafter. Abdominal roentgenogram (KUB) is advised on a yearly basis to monitor the size and appearance/disappearance of stone(s).

CARCINOGENESIS, MUTAGENESIS, IMPAIRMENT OF FERTILITY: Long-term carcino-genicity studies in animals have not been performed. High doses of THIOLA® in experimental animals have been shown to interfere with maintenance of pregnancy and viability of the fetus.

USE IN PREGNANCY: Pregnancy category C. D-penicillamine has been shown to cause skeletal defects and cleft palates in the fetus when given to pregnant rats at 10 times the dose recommended for human use. A similar teratogenicity might be expected for THIOLA® although no such findings could be related to the drug in studies in mice and rats at doses up to 10 times the highest recommended human dose.

There are no adequate and well-controlled studies in pregnant women. THIOLA® should be used during pregnancy only if the potential benefit justifies potential risk to the fetus.

NURSING MOTHERS: Because THIOLA® may be excreted in milk and because of the potential serious adverse reactions of nursing infants from THIOLA®, mothers taking THIOLA® should not nurse their infants.

PEDIATRIC USE: Safety and effectiveness below the age of 9 have not been established.

ADVERSE REACTIONS

Some patients may develop drug fever, usually during the first month of therapy. THIOLA® treatment should be discontinued until the fever subsides. It may be reinstated at a small dose, with a gradual increase in dosage until the desired level is achieved.

A generalized rash (erythematous, maculopapular or morbilliform) accompanied by pruritis may develop during the first few months of treatment. It may be controlled by antihistamine therapy, typically recedes when THIOLA® treatment is discontinued, and seldom recurs when THIOLA® treatment is restarted at a lower dosage. Less commonly, rash may appear late in the course of treatment (of more than 6 months). Located usually in the trunk, the late rash is associated with intense pruritis, recedes slowly after discontinuing treatment, and usually recurs upon resumption of treatment.

A drug reaction simulating lupus erythematous, manifested by fever, arthralgia and lymphadenopathy may develop. It may be associated with a positive antinuclear antibody test, but not necessarily with nephropathy. It may require discontinuance of THIOLA® treatment.

A reduction in taste perception may develop. It is believed to be the result of chelation of trace metals by THIOLA™. Hypogeusia is often self-limiting.

Unlike with d-penicillamine therapy, vitamin B$_6$ deficiency is uncommonly associated with THIOLA® treatment. Some patients may complain of wrinkling and friability of skin. This complication usually occurs after long-term treatment, and is believed to result from the effect of THIOLA® on collagen.

A multiclinic trial involving 66 cystinuric patients in the United States indicated that THIOLA® is associated with fewer or less severe adverse reactions than d-penicillamine. Among those who had to stop taking d-penicillamine due to toxicity, 64.7% could take THIOLA®. In those without prior history of d-penicillamine treatment, only 5.9% developed reactions of sufficient severity to require THIOLA® withdrawal. A review of available literature supports the findings from this trial.

Despite this apparent reduced toxicity to THIOLA® relative to d-penicillamine, THIOLA® treatment may potentially be associated with all the adverse reactions reported with d-penicillamine. They include:

Gastrointestinal side-effects (nausea, emesis, diarrhea or softstools, anorexia, abdominal pain, bloating or flatus) in about 1 in 6 patients;

Impairment in taste and smell in about 1 in 25 patients;

Dermatologic complications (pharyngitis, oral ulcers, rash, ecchymosis, prurites, uritcaria, warts, skin wrinkling, pemphigus, elastosis perforans serpiginosa) in about 1 in 6 patients;

Hypersensitivity reactions (laryngeal edema, dyspnea, respiratory distress, fever, chills, arthralgia, weakness, fatigue, myalgia, adenopathy) in about 1 in 25 patients;

Hematologic abnormalities (increased bleeding, anemia, leukopenia, thrombocytopenia, eosinophilia) in about 1 in 25 patients;

Renal complications (proteinuria, nephrotic syndrome, hematuria) in about 1 in 20 patients;

Pulmonary manifestations (bronchiolitis, hemoptysis, pulmonary infiltrates, dyspnea) in about 1 in 50 patients;

Neurologic complications (myasthenic syndrome) in about 1 in 50 patients.

These reactions are more likely to develop during THIOLA® therapy among patients who had previously shown toxicity to d-penicillamine.

In patients who had previously manifested adverse reactions to d-penicillamine, adverse reactions to THIOLA® are more likely to occur than in patients who took THIOLA® for the first time. A close supervision with a careful monitoring of potential side effects is mandatory during THIOLA®

treatment. Patients should be told to report promptly any symptoms suggesting toxicity. The treatment with THIOLA® should be stopped if severe toxicity develops. Jaundice and abnormal liver function tests have been reported during THIOLA® therapy for non-cystinuric conditions. A direct cause and effect relationship, based upon these foreign reports, has not been established. Although such complications were not encountered in the small multicenter trials in the United States, patients should be carefully monitored and if any abnormalities are noted, the drug should be discontinued and the patient treated by appropriate measures.

DOSAGE AND ADMINISTRATION

It is recommended that a conservative treatment program should be attempted first. At least 3 liters of fluid (10-10 oz. glassfuls) should be provided, including two glasses with each meal and at bedtime. The patients should be expected to awake at night to urinate; they should drink two more glasses of fluids before returning to bed. Additional fluids should be consumed if there is excessive sweating or intestinal fluid loss. A minimum urine output of 2 liters/day on a consistent basis should be sought. A modest amount of alkali should be provided in order to maintain urinary pH at a high normal range (6.5-7.0). Potassium alkali are advantageous over sodium alkali, because they do not cause hypercalciuria and are less likely to cause the complication of calcium stones.

Excessive alkali therapy is not advisable. When urinary pH increases above 7.0 with alkali therapy, the complication of calcium phosphate nephrolithiasis may ensue because of the enhanced urinary supersaturation of hydroxyapatite in an alkaline environment.

In patients who continue to form cystine stones on the above conservative program, THIOLA® may be added to the treatment program. THIOLA® may also be substituted for d-penicillamine in patients who have developed toxicity to the latter drug. In both situations, the conservative treatment program should be continued.

The dose of THIOLA® should not be arbitrary but should be based on that amount required to reduce urinary cystine concentration to below its solubility limit (generally <250 mg/liter). The extent of the decline in cystine excretion is generally dependent on the THIOLA® dosage.

THIOLA® may be begun at a dosage of 800 mg/day in adult patients with cystine stones. In a multiclinic trial, average dose of THIOLA® was about 1000 mg/day. However, some patients require a smaller dose. In children, initial dosage may be based on 15 mg/kg/day. Urinary cystine should be measured at 1 month after THIOLA® treatment, and every 3 months thereafter. THIOLA® dosage should be readjusted depending on the urinary cystine value. Whenever possible, THIOLA® should be given in divided doses 3 times/day at least one hour before or 2 hours after meals.

In patients who had shown severe toxicity to d-penicillamine, THIOLA® might be begun at a lower dosage.

HOW SUPPLIED

THIOLA® (NDC 0178-0900-01), is available for oral administration as 100 mg. round, white, sugar coated tablets in bottles of 100 tablets each. Each tablet is imprinted in red with "M" on one side and blank on the other. Store at 25°C (77°F); excursions permitted to 15-30°C (59-86°F) [see USP Controlled Room Temperature].

Rx only.

Rev 1006

TINDAMAX®   ℞

[tin-da-max]
(tinidazole)

HIGHLIGHTS OF PRESCRIBING INFORMATION
These highlights do not include all the information needed to use Tindamax® safely and effectively. See full prescribing information for Tindamax®.
Tindamax® (tinidazole) tablets for oral use
Initial U.S. Approval: 2004

To reduce the development of drug-resistant bacteria and maintain the effectiveness of Tindamax and other antibacterial drugs, Tindamax should be used only to treat or prevent infections that are proven or strongly suspected to be caused by bacteria.

WARNING: POTENTIAL RISK FOR CARCINOGENIC-ITY

See full prescribing information for complete boxed warning.

Carcinogenicity has been seen in mice and rats treated chronically with metronidazole, another nitroimidazole agent *(13.1).* **Although such data have not been reported for tinidazole, the two drugs are**

structurally related and have similar biologic effects. Use should be limited to approved indications only.

---RECENT MAJOR CHANGES---

Indications and Usage, Bacterial Vaginosis *(1.4)* 5/2007
Dosage and Administration, Bacterial Vaginosis *(2.6)* 5/2007

---INDICATIONS AND USAGE---

Tindamax is a nitroimidazole antimicrobial indicated for:
• Trichomoniasis *(1.1)*
• Giardiasis: in patients age 3 and older *(1.2)*
• Amebiasis: in patients age 3 and older *(1.3)*
• Bacterial Vaginosis: in non-pregnant, adult women *(1.4, 8.1)*

---DOSAGE AND ADMINISTRATION---

• Trichomoniasis: a single 2 g oral dose taken with food. Treat sexual partners with the same dose and at the same time *(2.3)*
• Giardiasis: Adults: a single 2 g dose taken with food. Pediatric patients older than three years of age: a single dose of 50 mg/kg (up to 2 g) with food *(2.4)*
• Amebiasis, *Intestinal:* Adults: 2 g per day for 3 days with food. Pediatric patients older than three years of age: 50 mg/kg/day (up to 2 g per day) for 3 days with food *(2.5)*. *Amebic liver abscess:* Adults: 2 g per day for 3-5 days with food. Pediatric patients older than three years of age: 50 mg/kg/day (up to 2 g per day) for 3-5 days with food *(2.5)*
• Bacterial vaginosis: Non-pregnant, adult women: 2 g once daily for 2 days taken with food, or 1 g once daily for 5 days taken with food *(2.6)*

---DOSAGE FORMS AND STRENGTHS---

Tablets: 250 mg and 500 mg *(3)*

---CONTRAINDICATIONS---

• Prior history of hypersensitivity to tinidazole or other nitroimidazole derivatives *(4, 6.1, 6.2)*
• First trimester of pregnancy *(4, 8.1)*
• Nursing mothers, unless breast-feeding is interrupted during tinidazole therapy and for 3 days following the last dose *(4, 8.3)*

---WARNINGS AND PRECAUTIONS---

• Seizures and neuropathy have been reported. Discontinue Tindamax if abnormal neurologic signs develop *(5.1)*
• Vaginal candidiasis may develop with Tindamax and require treatment with an antifungal agent *(5.2)*
• Use Tindamax with caution in patients with blood dyscrasias. Tindamax may produce transient leukopenia and neutropenia *(5.3, 7.3)*

---ADVERSE REACTIONS---

Most common adverse reactions for a single 2 g dose of tinidazole (incidence >1%) are metallic/bitter taste, nausea, weakness/fatigue/malaise, dyspepsia/ cramps/epigastric discomfort, vomiting, anorexia, headache, dizziness and constipation *(6.1)*

To report SUSPECTED ADVERSE REACTIONS, contact Mission Pharmacal Company at 1-800-298-1087 or FDA at 1-800-FDA-1088 or www.fda.gov/medwatch

---DRUG INTERACTIONS---

The following drug interactions were reported for metronidazole, a chemically-related nitroimidazole and may therefore occur with tinidazole:
• Warfarin and other oral coumarin anticoagulants: Anticoagulant dosage may need adjustment during and up to 8 days after tinidazole therapy *(7.1)*
• Alcohol-containing beverages/preparations: Avoid during and up to 3 days after tinidazole therapy *(7.1)*
• Lithium: Monitor serum lithium concentrations *(7.1)*
• Cyclosporine, tacrolimus: Monitor for toxicities of these immunosuppressive drugs *(7.1)*
• Fluorouracil: Monitor for fluorouracil-associated toxicities *(7.1)*
• Phenytoin, fosphenytoin: Adjustment of anticonvulsant and/or tinidazole dose(s) may be needed *(7.1, 7.2)*
• CYP3A4 inducers/inhibitors: Monitor for decreased tinidazole effect or increased adverse reactions *(7.2)*

---USE IN SPECIFIC POPULATIONS---

• Pediatric Use: Data on tinidazole use in children is limited to treatment of giardiasis and amebiasis in patients age 3 and older *(8.4)*
• Hemodialysis patients: If tinidazole is administered the same day and prior to hemodialysis, administer an additional ½ dose after end of hemodialysis *(8.6, 12.3)*

See 17 for PATIENT COUNSELING INFORMATION
Revised: 08/2007

FULL PRESCRIBING INFORMATION: CONTENTS*
WARNING: POTENTIAL RISK FOR CARCINOGE-NICITY
1   INDICATIONS AND USAGE
    1.1   Trichomoniasis
    1.2   Giardiasis

FULL PRESCRIBING INFORMATION

WARNING: POTENTIAL RISK FOR CARCINOGENICITY

Carcinogenicity has been seen in mice and rats treated chronically with metronidazole, another nitroimidazole agent *(13.1)*. Although such data have not been reported for tinidazole, the two drugs are structurally related and have similar biologic effects. **Its use should be reserved for the conditions described in INDICATIONS AND USAGE** *(1)*.

---

1 INDICATIONS AND USAGE

1.1 Trichomoniasis
Tinidazole is indicated for the treatment of trichomoniasis caused by *Trichomonas vaginalis*. The organism should be identified by appropriate diagnostic procedures. Because trichomoniasis is a sexually transmitted disease with potentially serious sequelae, partners of infected patients should be treated simultaneously in order to prevent re-infection *[see Clinical Studies (14.1)]*.

1.2 Giardiasis
Tinidazole is indicated for the treatment of giardiasis caused by *Giardia duodenalis* (also termed *G. lamblia*) in both adults and pediatric patients older than three years of age *[see Clinical Studies (14.2)]*.

1.3 Amebiasis
Tinidazole is indicated for the treatment of intestinal amebiasis and amebic liver abscess caused by *Entamoeba histolytica* in both adults and pediatric patients older than three years of age. It is not indicated in the treatment of asymptomatic cyst passage *[see Clinical Studies (14.3, 14.4)]*.

1.4 Bacterial Vaginosis
Tinidazole is indicated for the treatment of bacterial vaginosis (formerly referred to as *Haemophilus* vaginitis, *Gardnerella* vaginitis, nonspecific vaginitis, or anaerobic vaginosis) in non-pregnant women *[see Use in Specific Populations (8.1) and Clinical Studies (14.5)]*.

Other pathogens commonly associated with vulvovaginitis such as *Trichomonas vaginalis, Chlamydia trachomatis, Neisseria gonorrhoeae, Candida albicans* and *Herpes simplex* virus should be ruled out.

To reduce the development of drug-resistant bacteria and maintain the effectiveness of Tindamax and other antibacterial drugs, Tindamax should be used only to treat or prevent infections that are proven or strongly suspected to be caused by susceptible bacteria. When culture and susceptibility information are available, they should be considered in selecting or modifying antibacterial therapy. In the absence of such data, local epidemiology and susceptibility patterns may contribute to the empiric selection of therapy.

2 DOSAGE AND ADMINISTRATION

2.1 Dosing Instructions
It is advisable to take tinidazole with food to minimize the incidence of epigastric discomfort and other gastrointestinal side-effects. Food does not affect the oral bioavailability of tinidazole *[see Clinical Pharmacology (12.3)]*.

Alcoholic beverages should be avoided when taking tinidazole and for 3 days afterwards *[see Drug Interactions (7.1)]*.

2.2 Compounding of the Oral Suspension
For those unable to swallow tablets, tinidazole tablets may be crushed in artificial cherry syrup to be taken with food. *Procedure for Extemporaneous Pharmacy Compounding of the Oral Suspension:* Pulverize four 500 mg oral tablets with a mortar and pestle. Add approximately 10 mL of cherry syrup to the powder and mix until smooth. Transfer the suspension to a graduated amber container. Use several small rinses of cherry syrup to transfer any remaining drug in the mortar to the final suspension for a final volume of 30 mL. The suspension of crushed tablets in artificial cherry syrup is stable for 7 days at room temperature. When this suspension is used, it should be shaken well before each administration.

2.3 Trichomoniasis
The recommended dose in both females and males is a single 2 g oral dose taken with food. Since trichomoniasis is a sexually transmitted disease, sexual partners should be treated with the same dose and at the same time.

2.4 Giardiasis
The recommended dose in adults is a single 2 g dose taken with food. In pediatric patients older than three years of age, the recommended dose is a single dose of 50 mg/kg (up to 2 g) with food.

2.5 Amebiasis
Intestinal: The recommended dose in adults is a 2 g dose per day for 3 days taken with food. In pediatric patients older than three years of age, the recommended dose is 50 mg/kg/day (up to 2 g per day) for 3 days with food.

Amebic Liver Abscess: The recommended dose in adults is a 2 g dose per day for 3-5 days taken with food. In pediatric patients older than three years of age, the recommended dose is 50 mg/kg/day (up to 2 g per day) for 3-5 days with food. There are limited pediatric data on durations of therapy exceeding 3 days, although a small number of children were treated for 5 days without additional reported adverse reactions. Children should be closely monitored when treatment durations exceed 3 days.

2.6 Bacterial Vaginosis
The recommended dose in non-pregnant females is a 2 g oral dose once daily for 2 days taken with food or a 1 g oral dose once daily for 5 days taken with food. The use of tinidazole in pregnant patients has not been studied for bacterial vaginosis.

3 DOSAGE FORMS AND STRENGTHS
- 250 mg tablets are pink, round, scored tablets, with TM debossed on one side and 250 on the other
- 500 mg tablets are pink, oval, scored tablets, with TM debossed on one side and 500 on the other

4 CONTRAINDICATIONS
The use of tinidazole is contraindicated:
- In patients with a previous history of hypersensitivity to tinidazole or other nitroimidazole derivatives. Reported reactions have ranged in severity from urticaria to Stevens-Johnson syndrome *[see Adverse Reactions (6.1, 6.2)]*.
- During first trimester of pregnancy *[see Use in Specific Populations (8.1)]*.
- In nursing mothers: Interruption of breast-feeding is recommended during tinidazole therapy and for 3 days following the last dose *[see Use in Specific Populations (8.3)]*.

5 WARNINGS AND PRECAUTIONS

5.1 Neurological Adverse Reactions
Convulsive seizures and peripheral neuropathy, the latter characterized mainly by numbness or paresthesia of an extremity, have been reported in patients treated with tinidazole. The appearance of abnormal neurologic signs demands the prompt discontinuation of tinidazole therapy.

5.2 Vaginal Candidiasis
The use of tinidazole may result in *Candida* vaginitis. In a clinical study of 235 women who received tinidazole for bacterial vaginosis, a vaginal fungal infection developed in 11 (4.7%) of all study subjects *[see Clinical Studies (14.5)]*.

5.3 Blood Dyscrasia
Tinidazole should be used with caution in patients with evidence of or history of blood dyscrasia *[see Drug Interactions (7.3)]*.

5.4 Drug Resistance
Prescribing Tindamax in the absence of a proven or strongly suspected bacterial infection or a prophylactic indication is unlikely to provide benefit to the patient and increases the risk of the development of drug-resistant bacteria.

6 ADVERSE REACTIONS

6.1 Clinical Studies Experience
Because clinical trials are conducted under widely varying conditions, adverse reaction rates observed in the clinical trials of a drug cannot be directly compared to rates in the clinical trials of another drug and may not reflect the rates observed in practice.

Among 3669 patients treated with a single 2 g dose of tinidazole, in both controlled and uncontrolled trichomoniasis and giardiasis clinical studies, adverse reactions were reported by 11.0% of patients. For multi-day dosing in controlled and uncontrolled amebiasis studies, adverse reactions were reported by 13.8% of 1765 patients. The most common (≥ 1% incidence) adverse reactions reported by body system are as follows. (Note: Data described in Table 1 below are pooled from studies with variable designs and safety evaluations.)

Other adverse reactions reported with tinidazole include:
Central Nervous System: Two serious adverse reactions reported include convulsions and transient peripheral neuropathy including numbness and paresthesia *[see Warnings and Precautions (5.1)]*. Other CNS reports include vertigo, ataxia, giddiness, insomnia, drowsiness.
Gastrointestinal: tongue discoloration, stomatitis, diarrhea
Hypersensitivity: urticaria, pruritus, rash, flushing, sweating, dryness of mouth, fever, burning sensation, thirst, salivation, angioedema

Table 1. Adverse Reactions Summary of Published Reports

	2 g single dose	Multi-day dose
GI: Metallic/bitter taste	3.7%	6.3%
Nausea	3.2%	4.5%
Anorexia	1.5%	2.5%
Dyspepsia/cramps/epigastric discomfort	1.8%	1.4%
Vomiting	1.5%	0.9%
Constipation	0.4%	1.4%
CNS: Weakness/fatigue/malaise	2.1%	1.1%
Dizziness	1.1%	0.5%
Other: Headache	1.3%	0.7%
Total patients with adverse reactions	11.0% (403/3669)	13.8% (244/1765)

Renal: darkened urine
Cardiovascular: palpitations
Hematopoietic: transient neutropenia, transient leukopenia
Other: *Candida* overgrowth, increased vaginal discharge, oral candidiasis, hepatic abnormalities including raised transaminase level, arthralgias, myalgias, and arthritis. [See table 1 at top of previous page]
Rare reported adverse reactions include bronchospasm, dyspnea, coma, confusion, depression, furry tongue, pharyngitis and reversible thrombocytopenia.
Adverse Reactions in Pediatric Patients: In pooled pediatric studies, adverse reactions reported in pediatric patients taking tinidazole were similar in nature and frequency to adult findings including nausea, vomiting, diarrhea, taste change, anorexia, and abdominal pain.
Bacterial vaginosis: The most common adverse reactions in treated patients (incidence >2%), which were not identified in the trichomoniasis, giardiasis and amebiasis studies, are gastrointestinal: decreased appetite, and flatulence; renal: urinary tract infection, painful urination, and urine abnormality; and other reactions including pelvic pain, vulvovaginal discomfort, vaginal odor, menorrhagia, and upper respiratory tract infection *[See Clinical Studies (14.5)].*

6.2 Postmarketing Experience
The following adverse reactions have been identified and reported during post-approval use of Tindamax. Because the reports of these reactions are voluntary and the population is of uncertain size, it is not always possible to reliably estimate the frequency of the reaction or establish a causal relationship to drug exposure.
Severe acute hypersensitivity reactions have been reported on initial or subsequent exposure to tinidazole. Hypersensitivity reactions may include urticaria, pruritus, angioedema, Stevens-Johnson syndrome and erythema multiforme.

7 DRUG INTERACTIONS
Although not specifically identified in studies with tinidazole, the following drug interactions were reported for metronidazole, a chemically-related nitroimidazole. Therefore, these drug interactions may occur with tinidazole.

7.1 Potential Effects of Tinidazole on Other Drugs
Warfarin and Other Oral Coumarin Anticoagulants: As with metronidazole, tinidazole may enhance the effect of warfarin and other coumarin anticoagulants, resulting in a prolongation of prothrombin time. The dosage of oral anticoagulants may need to be adjusted during tinidazole coadministration and up to 8 days after discontinuation.
Alcohols, Disulfiram: Alcoholic beverages and preparations containing ethanol or propylene glycol should be avoided during tinidazole therapy and for 3 days afterward because abdominal cramps, nausea, vomiting, headaches, and flushing may occur. Psychotic reactions have been reported in alcoholic patients using metronidazole and disulfiram concurrently. Though no similar reactions have been reported with tinidazole, tinidazole should not be given to patients who have taken disulfiram within the last two weeks.
Lithium: Metronidazole has been reported to elevate serum lithium levels. It is not known if tinidazole shares this property with metronidazole, but consideration should be given to measuring serum lithium and creatinine levels after several days of simultaneous lithium and tinidazole treatment to detect potential lithium intoxication.
Phenytoin, Fosphenytoin: Concomitant administration of oral metronidazole and intravenous phenytoin was reported to result in prolongation of the half-life and reduction in the clearance of phenytoin. Metronidazole did not significantly affect the pharmacokinetics of orally-administered phenytoin.
Cyclosporine, Tacrolimus: There are several case reports suggesting that metronidazole has the potential to increase the levels of cyclosporine and tacrolimus. During tinidazole co-administration with either of these drugs, the patient should be monitored for signs of calcineurin-inhibitor associated toxicities.
Fluorouracil: Metronidazole was shown to decrease the clearance of fluorouracil, resulting in an increase in side-effects without an increase in therapeutic benefits. If the concomitant use of tinidazole and fluorouracil cannot be avoided, the patient should be monitored for fluorouracil-associated toxicities.

7.2 Potential Effects of Other Drugs on Tinidazole
CYP3A4 Inducers and Inhibitors: Simultaneous administration of tinidazole with drugs that induce liver microsomal enzymes, i.e., CYP3A4 inducers such as *phenobarbital, rifampin, phenytoin,* and *fosphenytoin* (a pro-drug of phenytoin), may accelerate the elimination of tinidazole, decreasing the plasma level of tinidazole. Simultaneous administration of drugs that inhibit the activity of liver microsomal enzymes, i.e., CYP3A4 inhibitors such as *cimetidine* and *ketoconazole,* may prolong the half-life and decrease the plasma clearance of tinidazole, increasing the plasma concentrations of tinidazole.

Cholestyramine: Cholestyramine was shown to decrease the oral bioavailability of metronidazole by 21%. Thus, it is advisable to separate dosing of cholestyramine and tinidazole to minimize any potential effect on the oral bioavailability of tinidazole.
Oxytetracycline: Oxytetracycline was reported to antagonize the therapeutic effect of metronidazole.

7.3 Laboratory Test Interactions
Tinidazole, like metronidazole, may interfere with certain types of determinations of serum chemistry values, such as aspartate aminotransferase (AST, SGOT), alanine aminotransferase (ALT, SGPT), lactate dehydrogenase (LDH), triglycerides, and hexokinase glucose. Values of zero may be observed. All of the assays in which interference has been reported involve enzymatic coupling of the assay to oxidation-reduction of nicotinamide adenine dinucleotide (NAD $^+$ ↔ NADH). Potential interference is due to the similarity of absorbance peaks of NADH and tinidazole.
Tinidazole, like metronidazole, may produce transient leukopenia and neutropenia; however, no persistent hematological abnormalities attributable to tinidazole have been observed in clinical studies. Total and differential leukocyte counts are recommended if re-treatment is necessary.

8 USE IN SPECIFIC POPULATIONS
8.1 Pregnancy
Teratogenic effects: Pregnancy Category C
The use of tinidazole in pregnant patients has not been studied. Since tinidazole crosses the placental barrier and enters fetal circulation it should not be administered to pregnant patients in the first trimester.
Embryo-fetal developmental toxicity studies in pregnant mice indicated no embryo-fetal toxicity or malformations at the highest dose level of 2,500 mg/kg (approximately 6.3-fold the highest human therapeutic dose based upon body surface area conversions). In a study with pregnant rats a slightly higher incidence of fetal mortality was observed at a maternal dose of 500 mg/kg (2.5-fold the highest human therapeutic dose based upon body surface area conversions). No biologically relevant neonatal developmental effects were observed in rat neonates following maternal doses as high as 600 mg/kg (3-fold the highest human therapeutic dose based upon body surface area conversions). Although there is some evidence of mutagenic potential and animal reproduction studies are not always predictive of human response, the use of tinidazole after the first trimester of pregnancy requires that the potential benefits of the drug be weighed against the possible risks to both the mother and the fetus.

8.3 Nursing Mothers
Tinidazole is excreted in breast milk in concentrations similar to those seen in serum. Tinidazole can be detected in breast milk for up to 72 hours following administration. Interruption of breast-feeding is recommended during tinidazole therapy and for 3 days following the last dose.

8.4 Pediatric Use
Other than for use in the treatment of giardiasis and amebiasis in pediatric patients older than three years of age, safety and effectiveness of tinidazole in pediatric patients have not been established.
Pediatric Administration: For those unable to swallow tablets, tinidazole tablets may be crushed in artificial cherry syrup, to be taken with food *[see Dosage and Administration (2.2)].*

8.5 Geriatric Use
Clinical studies of tinidazole did not include sufficient numbers of subjects aged 65 and over to determine whether they respond differently from younger subjects. In general, dose selection for an elderly patient should be cautious, reflecting the greater frequency of decreased hepatic, renal, or cardiac function, and of concomitant disease or other drug therapy.

8.6 Renal Impairment
Because the pharmacokinetics of tinidazole in patients with severe renal impairment (CrCL < 22 mL/min) are not significantly different from those in healthy subjects, no dose adjustments are necessary in these patients.
Patients undergoing hemodialysis: If tinidazole is administered on the same day as and prior to hemodialysis, it is recommended that an additional dose of tinidazole equivalent to one-half of the recommended dose be administered after the end of the hemodialysis *[see Clinical Pharmacology (12.3)].*

8.7 Hepatic Impairment
There are no data on tinidazole pharmacokinetics in patients with impaired hepatic function. Reduced elimination of metronidazole, a chemically-related nitroimidazole, has been reported in this population. Usual recommended doses of tinidazole should be administered cautiously in patients with hepatic dysfunction *[see Clinical Pharmacology (12.3)].*

10 OVERDOSAGE
There are no reported overdoses with tinidazole in humans.
Treatment of Overdosage: There is no specific antidote for the treatment of overdosage with tinidazole; therefore,

treatment should be symptomatic and supportive. Gastric lavage may be helpful. Hemodialysis can be considered because approximately 43% of the amount present in the body is eliminated during a 6-hour hemodialysis session.

11 DESCRIPTION
Tinidazole is a synthetic antiprotozoal and antibacterial agent. It is 1-(2-ethylsulfonylethyl)-2-methyl-5-nitroimidazole, a second-generation 2-methyl-5-nitroimidazole, which has the following chemical structure:

Tindamax pink oral tablets contain 250 mg or 500 mg of tinidazole. Inactive ingredients include croscarmellose sodium, FD&C Red 40 lake, FD&C Yellow 6 lake, hypromellose, magnesium stearate, microcrystalline cellulose, polydextrose, polyethylene glycol, pregelatinized corn starch, titanium dioxide, and triacetin.

12 CLINICAL PHARMACOLOGY
12.1 Mechanism of Action
Tinidazole is an antiprotozoal, antibacterial agent. *[See Clinical Pharmacology (12.4)].*
12.3 Pharmacokinetics
Absorption: After oral administration, tinidazole is rapidly and completely absorbed. A bioavailability study of Tindamax tablets was conducted in adult healthy volunteers. All subjects received a single oral dose of 2 g (four 500 mg tablets) of Tindamax following an overnight fast. Oral administration of four 500 mg tablets of Tindamax under fasted conditions produced a mean peak plasma concentration (C_{max}) of 47.7 (±7.5) µg/mL with a mean time to peak concentration (T_{max}) of 1.6 (±0.7) hours, and a mean area under the plasma concentration-time curve (AUC, 0-∞) of 901.6 (± 126.5) µg.hr/mL at 72 hours. The elimination half-life ($T_{1/2}$) was 13.2 (±1.4) hours. Mean plasma levels decreased to 14.3 µg/mL at 24 hours, 3.8 µg/mL at 48 hours and 0.8 µg/mL at 72 hours following administration. Steady-state conditions are reached in 2½-3 days of multiday dosing.
Administration of Tindamax tablets with food resulted in a delay in T_{max} of approximately 2 hours and a decline in C_{max} of approximately 10%, compared to fasted conditions. However, administration of Tindamax with food did not affect AUC or $T_{1/2}$ in this study.
In healthy volunteers, administration of crushed Tindamax tablets in artificial cherry syrup, [prepared as described in *Dosage and Administration (2.2)*] after an overnight fast had no effect on any pharmacokinetic parameter as compared to tablets swallowed whole under fasted conditions.
Distribution: Tinidazole is distributed into virtually all tissues and body fluids and also crosses the blood-brain barrier. The apparent volume of distribution is about 50 liters. Plasma protein binding of tinidazole is 12%. Tinidazole crosses the placental barrier and is secreted in breast milk.
Metabolism: Tinidazole is significantly metabolized in humans prior to excretion. Tinidazole is partly metabolized by oxidation, hydroxylation, and conjugation. Tinidazole is the major drug-related constituent in plasma after human treatment, along with a small amount of the 2-hydroxymethyl metabolite.
Tinidazole is biotransformed mainly by CYP3A4. In an *in vitro* metabolic drug interaction study, tinidazole concentrations of up to 75 µg/mL did not inhibit the enzyme activities of CYP1A2, CYP2B6, CYP2C9, CYP2D6, CYP2E1, and CYP3A4.
The potential of tinidazole to induce the metabolism of other drugs has not been evaluated.
Elimination: The plasma half-life of tinidazole is approximately 12-14 hours. Tinidazole is excreted by the liver and the kidneys. Tinidazole is excreted in the urine mainly as unchanged drug (approximately 20-25% of the administered dose). Approximately 12% of the drug is excreted in the feces.
Patients with impaired renal function: The pharmacokinetics of tinidazole in patients with severe renal impairment (CrCL < 22 mL/min) are not significantly different from the pharmacokinetics seen in healthy subjects. However, during hemodialysis, clearance of tinidazole is significantly increased; the half-life is reduced from 12.0 hours to 4.9 hours. Approximately 43% of the amount present in the body is eliminated during a 6-hour hemodialysis session *[see Use in Specific Populations (8.6)].* The pharmacokinetics of tinidazole in patients undergoing routine continuous peritoneal dialysis have not been investigated.
Patients with impaired hepatic function: There are no data on tinidazole pharmacokinetics in patients with impaired hepatic function. Reduction of metabolic elimination of metronidazole, a chemically-related nitroimidazole, in patients with hepatic dysfunction has been reported in several studies *[see Use in Specific Populations (8.7)].*

Table 2. Efficacy of Tindamax in the Treatment of Bacterial Vaginosis in a Randomized, Double-Blind, Double-Dummy, Placebo-Controlled Trial: Modified Intent-to-Treat Population[1] (n=227)

Outcome	Tindamax 1 g × 5 days (n=76)	Tindamax 2 g × 2 days (n=73)	Placebo (n=78)
	% Cure	% Cure	% Cure
Therapeutic Cure	36.8	27.4	5.1
Difference[2]	31.7	22.3	
97.5% CI[3]	(16.8, 46.6)	(8.0, 36.6)	
Clinical Cure	51.3	35.6	11.5
Difference[2]	39.8	24.1	
97.5% CI[3]	(23.3, 56.3)	(7.8, 40.3)	
Nugent Score Cure	38.2	27.4	5.1
Difference[2]	33.1	22.3	
97.5% CI[3]	(18.1, 48.0)	(8.0, 36.6)	

[1] Modified Intent-to-Treat defined as all patients randomized with a baseline Nugent score of at least 4
[2] Difference in cure rates (Tindamax-placebo)
[3] CI: confidence interval
p-values for both Tindamax regimens vs. placebo for therapeutic, clinical and Nugent score cure rates for both 2 and 5 days <0.001

12.4 Microbiology

Mechanism of Action: Tinidazole is an antiprotozoal, antibacterial agent. The nitro-group of tinidazole is reduced by cell extracts of *Trichomonas*. The free nitro-radical generated as a result of this reduction may be responsible for the antiprotozoal activity. Chemically reduced tinidazole was shown to release nitrites and cause damage to purified bacterial DNA *in vitro*. Additionally, the drug caused DNA base changes in bacterial cells and DNA strand breakage in mammalian cells. The mechanism by which tinidazole exhibits activity against *Giardia* and *Entamoeba* species is not known.

Antibacterial: Culture and sensitivity testing of bacteria are not routinely performed to establish the diagnosis of bacterial vaginosis *[see Indications and Usage (1.4)]*; standard methodology for the susceptibility testing of potential bacterial pathogens, *Gardnerella vaginalis*, *Mobiluncus spp.* or *Mycoplasma hominis*, has not been defined. The following *in vitro* data are available, but their clinical significance is unknown. Tinidazole is active *in vitro* against most strains of the following organisms that have been reported to be associated with bacterial vaginosis:
• *Bacteroides spp.*
• *Gardnerella vaginalis*
• *Prevotella spp.*
Tinidazole does not appear to have activity against most strains of vaginal lactobacilli.

Antiprotozoal: Tinidazole demonstrates activity both *in vitro* and in clinical infections against the following protozoa: *Trichomonas vaginalis*; *Giardia duodenalis* (also termed *G. lamblia*); and *Entamoeba histolytica*.
For protozoal parasites, standardized susceptibility tests do not exist for use in clinical microbiology laboratories.

Drug Resistance: The development of resistance to tinidazole by *G. duodenalis*, *E. histolytica*, or bacteria associated with bacterial vaginosis has not been examined.

Cross-resistance: Approximately 38% of *T. vaginalis* isolates exhibiting reduced susceptibility to metronidazole also show reduced susceptibility to tinidazole *in vitro*. The clinical significance of such an effect is not known.

13 NONCLINICAL TOXICOLOGY
13.1 Carcinogenesis, Mutagenesis, Impairment of Fertility

Metronidazole, a chemically-related nitroimidazole, has been reported to be carcinogenic in mice and rats but not hamsters. In several studies metronidazole showed evidence of pulmonary, hepatic, and lymphatic tumorigenesis in mice and mammary and hepatic tumors in female rats. Tinidazole carcinogenicity studies in rats, mice or hamsters have not been reported.

Tinidazole was mutagenic in the TA 100, *S. typhimurium* tester strain both with and without the metabolic activation system and was negative for mutagenicity in the TA 98 strain. Mutagenicity results were mixed (positive and negative) in the TA 1535, 1537, and 1538 strains. Tinidazole was also mutagenic in a tester strain of *Klebsiella pneumonia*. Tinidazole was negative for mutagenicity in a mammalian cell culture system utilizing Chinese hamster lung V79 cells (HGPRT test system) and negative for genotoxicity in the Chinese hamster ovary (CHO) sister chromatid exchange assay. Tinidazole was positive for *in vivo* genotoxicity in the mouse micronucleus assay.

In a 60-day fertility study, tinidazole reduced fertility and produced testicular histopathology in male rats at a 600 mg/kg/day dose level (approximately 3-fold the highest human

therapeutic dose based upon body surface area conversions). Spermatogenic effects resulted from 300 and 600 mg/kg/day dose levels. The no observed adverse reaction level for testicular and spermatogenic effects was 100 mg/kg/day (approximately 0.5-fold the highest human therapeutic dose based upon body surface area conversions). This effect is characteristic of agents in the 5-nitroimidazole class.

13.2 Animal Toxicology and/or Pharmacology

In acute studies with mice and rats, the LD_{50} for mice was generally > 3,600 mg/kg for oral administration and was > 2,300 mg/kg for intraperitoneal administration. In rats, the LD_{50} was > 2,000 mg/kg for both oral and intraperitoneal administration.

A repeated-dose toxicology study has been performed in beagle dogs using oral dosing of tinidazole at 100 mg/kg/day, 300 mg/kg/day, and 1000 mg/kg/day for 28-days. On Day 18 of the study, the highest dose was lowered to 600 mg/kg/day due to severe clinical symptoms. The two compound-related effects observed in the dogs treated with tinidazole were increased atrophy of the thymus in both sexes at the middle and high doses, and atrophy of the prostate at all doses in the males. A no-adverse-effect level (NOAEL) of 100 mg/kg/day for females was determined. There was no NOAEL identified for males because of minimal atrophy of the prostate at 100 mg/kg/day (approximately 0.9-fold the highest human dose based upon plasma AUC comparisons).

14 CLINICAL STUDIES
14.1 Trichomoniasis

Tinidazole (2 g single oral dose) use in trichomoniasis has been well documented in 34 published reports from the world literature involving over 2,800 patients treated with tinidazole. In four published, blinded, randomized, comparative studies of the 2 g tinidazole single oral dose where efficacy was assessed by culture at time points post-treatment ranging from one week to one month, reported cure rates ranged from 92% (37/40) to 100% (65/65) (n=172 total subjects). In four published, blinded, randomized, comparative studies where efficacy was assessed by wet mount between 7-14 days post-treatment, reported cure rates ranged from 80% (8/10) to 100% (16/16) (n=116 total subjects). In these studies, tinidazole was superior to placebo and comparable to other anti-trichomonal drugs. The single oral 2 g tinidazole dose was also assessed in four open-label trials in men (one comparative to metronidazole and 3 single-arm studies). Parasitological evaluation of the urine was performed both pre- and post-treatment and reported cure rates ranged from 83% (25/30) to 100% (80/80) (n=142 total subjects).

14.2 Giardiasis

Tinidazole (2 g single dose) use in giardiasis has been documented in 19 published reports from the world literature involving over 1,600 patients (adults and pediatric patients). In eight controlled studies involving a total of 619 subjects of whom 299 were given the 2 g × 1 day (50 mg/kg × 1 day in pediatric patients) oral dose of tinidazole, reported cure rates ranged from 80% (40/50) to 100% (15/15). In three of these trials where the comparator was 2 to 3 days of various doses of metronidazole, reported cure rates for metronidazole were 76% (19/25) to 93% (14/15). Data comparing a single 2 g dose of tinidazole to usually recommended 5-7 days of metronidazole are limited.

14.3 Intestinal Amebiasis

Tinidazole use in intestinal amebiasis has been documented in 26 published reports from the world literature involving over 1,400 patients. Most reports utilized tinidazole 2 g/day

× 3 days. In four published, randomized, controlled studies (1 investigator single- and, 3 open-label) of the 2 g/day × 3 days oral dose of tinidazole, reported cure rates after 3 days of therapy among a total of 220 subjects ranged from 86% (25/29) to 93% (25/27).

14.4 Amebic Liver Abscess

Tinidazole use in amebic liver abscess has been documented in 18 published reports from the world literature involving over 470 patients. Most reports utilized tinidazole 2 g/day × 2-5 days. In seven published, randomized, controlled studies (1 double-blind, 1 single-blind, 5 open-label) of the 2 g/day × 2-5 days oral dose of tinidazole accompanied by aspiration of the liver abscess when clinically necessary, reported cure rates among 133 subjects ranged from 81% (17/21) to 100% (16/16). Four of these studies utilized at least 3 days of tinidazole.

14.5 Bacterial Vaginosis

A randomized, double-blind, placebo-controlled clinical trial in 235 non-pregnant women was conducted to evaluate the efficacy of tinidazole for the treatment of bacterial vaginosis. A clinical diagnosis of bacterial vaginosis was based on Amsel's criteria and defined by the presence of an abnormal homogeneous vaginal discharge that (a) has a pH of greater than 4.5, (b) emits a "fishy" amine odor when mixed with a 10% KOH solution, and (c) contains ≥20% clue cells on microscopic examination. Clinical cure required a return to normal vaginal discharge and resolution of all Amsel's criteria. A microbiologic diagnosis of bacterial vaginosis was based on Gram stain of the vaginal smear demonstrating (a) markedly reduced or absent *Lactobacillus* morphology, (b) predominance of *Gardnerella* morphotype, and (c) absent or few white blood cells, with quantification of these bacterial morphotypes to determine the Nugent score, where a score ≥4 was required for study inclusion and a score of 0-3 considered a microbiologic cure. Therapeutic cure was a composite endpoint, consisting of both a clinical cure and microbiologic cure. In patients with all four Amsel's criteria and with a baseline Nugent score ≥4, tinidazole oral tablets given as either 2 g once daily for 2 days or 1 g once daily for 5 days demonstrated superior efficacy over placebo tablets as measured by therapeutic cure, clinical cure, and a microbiologic cure.

[See table 2 above]

The therapeutic cure rates reported in this clinical study conducted with Tindamax were based on resolution of 4 out of 4 Amsel's criteria and a Nugent score of <4. The cure rates for previous clinical studies with other products approved for bacterial vaginosis were based on resolution of either 2 or 3 out of 4 Amsel's criteria. At the time of approval for other products for bacterial vaginosis, there was no requirement for a Nugent score on Gram stain, resulting in higher reported rates of cure for bacterial vaginosis for those products than for those reported here for tinidazole.

16 HOW SUPPLIED/STORAGE AND HANDLING

Tindamax 250 mg tablets are pink, round, scored tablets, with TM debossed on one side and 250 on the other, supplied in bottles with child-resistant caps as:
NDC 0178-8250-40   Bottle of 40
Tindamax 500 mg tablets are pink, oval, scored tablets, with TM debossed on one side and 500 on the other, supplied in bottles with child-resistant caps as:
NDC 0178-8500-60   Bottle of 60
NDC 0178-8500-20   Bottle of 20
Professional Samples:
NDC 0178-8500-02   Bottle of 2
Storage: Store at controlled room temperature 20-25° C (68-77° F); excursions permitted to 15-30° C (59-86° F) [see USP]. Protect contents from light.

17 PATIENT COUNSELING INFORMATION
17.1 Administration of Drug

Patients should be told to take Tindamax with food to minimize the incidence of epigastric discomfort and other gastrointestinal side-effects. Food does not affect the oral bioavailability of tinidazole.

17.2 Alcohol Avoidance

Patients should be told to avoid alcoholic beverages and preparations containing ethanol or propylene glycol during Tindamax therapy and for 3 days afterward because abdominal cramps, nausea, vomiting, headaches, and flushing may occur.

17.3 Drug Resistance

Patients should be counseled that antibacterial drugs including Tindamax should only be used to treat bacterial infections. They do not treat viral infections (e.g., the common cold). When Tindamax is prescribed to treat a bacterial infection, patients should be told that although it is common to feel better early in the course of therapy, the medication should be taken exactly as directed. Skipping doses or not completing the full course of therapy may (1) decrease the effectiveness of the immediate treatment and (2) increase the likelihood that bacteria will develop resistance and will not be treatable by Tindamax or other antibacterial drugs in the future.
Rev 0907

UROCIT®-K R

[yu 'ro-cit kay]
(Potassium Citrate)
Extended-release tablets for oral use

HIGHLIGHTS OF PRESCRIBING INFORMATION

These highlights do not include all the information needed to use Urocit®-K safely and effectively. See full prescribing information for Urocit®-K.

Urocit®-K (Potassium Citrate) Extended-release tablets for oral use

Initial U.S. Approval: 1985

RECENT MAJOR CHANGES

Dosage and Administration, Urocit®-K 15 mEq (2.2, 2.3)	12/2009
Dosage Forms and Strengths, Urocit®-K 15 mEq (3)	12/2009
Description, Urocit®-K 15 mEq (11)	12/2009
Clinical Studies (14)	12/2009
How Supplied/Storage and Handling, Urocit®-K 15 mEq (16)	12/2009

INDICATIONS AND USAGE

Urocit®-K is a citrate salt of potassium indicated for the management of:
• Renal tubular acidosis (RTA) with calcium stones (1.1)
• Hypocitraturic calcium oxalate nephrolithiasis of any etiology (1.2)
• Uric acid lithiasis with or without calcium stones (1.3)

DOSAGE AND ADMINISTRATION

Objective: To restore normal urinary citrate (greater than 320 mg/day and as close to the normal mean of 640 mg/day as possible), and to increase urinary pH to a level of 6.0 to 7.0.
• Severe hypocitraturia (urinary citrate < 150 mg/day): therapy should be initiated at 60 mEq per day; a dose of 30 mEq two times per day or 20 mEq three times per day with meals or within 30 minutes after meals or bedtime snack (2.2)
• Mild to moderate hypocitraturia (urinary citrate >150 mg/day): therapy should be initiated at 30 mEq per day; a dose of 15 mEq two times per day or 10 mEq three times per day with meals or within 30 minutes after meals or bedtime snack (2.3)

DOSAGE FORMS AND STRENGTHS

Tablets: 5 mEq, 10 mEq and 15 mEq (3)

CONTRAINDICATIONS

• Patients with hyperkalemia (or who have conditions predisposing them to hyperkalemia). Such conditions include chronic renal failure, uncontrolled diabetes mellitus, acute dehydration, strenuous physical exercise in unconditioned individuals, adrenal insufficiency, extensive tissue breakdown (4)
• Patients for whom there is cause for arrest or delay in tablet passage through the gastrointestinal tract such as those suffering from delayed gastric emptying, esophageal compression, intestinal obstruction or stricture (4)
• Patients with peptic ulcer disease (4)
• Patients with active urinary tract infection (4)
• Patients with renal insufficiency (glomerular filtration rate of less than 0.7 ml/kg/min) (4)

WARNINGS AND PRECAUTIONS

• Hyperkalemia: In patients with impaired mechanisms for excreting potassium, Urocit®-K administration can produce hyperkalemia and cardiac arrest. Potentially fatal hyperkalemia can develop rapidly and be asymptomatic. The use of Urocit®-K in patients with chronic renal failure, or any other condition which impairs potassium excretion such as severe myocardial damage or heart failure, should be avoided (5.1)
• Gastrointestinal lesions: if there is severe vomiting, abdominal pain or gastrointestinal bleeding, Urocit®-K should be discontinued immediately and the possibility of bowel perforation or obstruction investigated (5.2)

ADVERSE REACTIONS

Some patients may develop minor gastrointestinal complaints such as abdominal discomfort, vomiting, diarrhea, loose bowel movements or nausea. These may be alleviated by taking the dose with meals or snacks or by reducing the dosage (6.1)

To report SUSPECTED ADVERSE REACTIONS, contact Mission Pharmacal Company at 1-800-298-1087 or FDA at 1-800-FDA-1088 or www.fda.gov/medwatch

DRUG INTERACTIONS

The following drug interactions may occur with potassium citrate:
• Potassium-sparing diuretics: concomitant administration should be avoided since the simultaneous administration of these agents can produce severe hyperkalemia (7.1)

• Drugs that slow gastrointestinal transit time: These agents (such as anticholinergics) can be expected to increase the gastrointestinal irritation produced by potassium salts (7.2)

USE IN SPECIFIC POPULATIONS

• Pregnant women: Pregnancy Category C; animal reproduction studies have not been conducted. It is not known whether Urocit®-K can cause fetal harm when administered to a pregnant woman or can affect reproduction capacity. Urocit®-K should be given to a pregnant woman only if clearly needed (8.1)
• Nursing mothers: The normal potassium ion content of human milk is about 13 mEq/L. It is not known if Urocit®-K has an effect on this content. Urocit®-K should be given to a woman who is breast feeding only if clearly needed (8.3)
• Pediatric Use: Safety and effectiveness in children have not been established (8.4)

See 17 for PATIENT COUNSELING INFORMATION

Revised: 04/2010

FULL PRESCRIBING INFORMATION: CONTENTS*

* Sections or subsections omitted from the full prescribing information are not listed

FULL PRESCRIBING INFORMATION

1 INDICATIONS AND USAGE

1.1 Renal tubular acidosis (RTA) with calcium stones
Potassium citrate is indicated for the management of renal tubular acidosis [see Clinical Studies (14.1)].

1.2 Hypocitraturic calcium oxalate nephrolithiasis of any etiology
Potassium citrate is indicated for the management of Hypocitraturic calcium oxalate nephrolithiasis [see Clinical Studies (14.2)].

1.3 Uric acid lithiasis with or without calcium stones
Potassium citrate is indicated for the management of Uric acid lithiasis with or without calcium stones [see Clinical Studies (14.3)].

2 DOSAGE AND ADMINISTRATION

2.1 Dosing Instructions
Treatment with extended release potassium citrate should be added to a regimen that limits salt intake (avoidance of foods with high salt content and of added salt at the table) and encourages high fluid intake (urine volume should be at least two liters per day). The objective of treatment with Urocit®-K is to provide Urocit®-K in sufficient dosage to restore normal urinary citrate (greater than 320 mg/day and as close to the normal mean of 640 mg/day as possible), and to increase urinary pH to a level of 6.0 or 7.0.

Monitor serum electrolytes (sodium, potassium, chloride and carbon dioxide), serum creatinine and complete blood counts every four months and more frequently in patients with cardiac disease, renal disease or acidosis. Perform electrocardiograms periodically. Treatment should be discontinued if there is hyperkalemia, a significant rise in serum creatinine or a significant fall in blood hemocrit or hemoglobin.

2.2 Severe Hypocitraturia
In patients with severe hypocitraturia (urinary citrate < 150 mg/day), therapy should be initiated at a dosage of 60 mEq/day (30 mEq two times/day or 20 mEq three times/day with meals or within 30 minutes after meals or bedtime snack). Twenty-four hour urinary citrate and/or urinary pH measurements should be used to determine the adequacy of the initial dosage and to evaluate the effectiveness of any dosage change. In addition, urinary citrate and/or pH should be measured every four months. Doses of Urocit®-K greater than 100 mEq/day have not been studied and should be avoided.

2.3 Mild to Moderate Hypocitraturia
In patients with mild to moderate hypocitraturia (urinary citrate > 150 mg/day) therapy should be initiated at 30 mEq/day (15 mEq two times/day or 10 mEq three times/day within 30 minutes after meals or bedtime snack). Twenty-four hour urinary citrate and/or urinary pH measurements should be used to determine the adequacy of the initial dosage and to evaluate the effectiveness of any dosage change. Doses of Urocit®-K greater than 100 mEq/day have not been studied and should be avoided.

3 DOSAGE FORMS AND STRENGTHS

• 5 mEq tablets are uncoated, tan to yellowish in color, modified ball shaped, with MPC 600 debossed on one side and blank on the other
• 10 mEq tablets are uncoated, tan to yellowish in color, elliptical shaped, with 610 debossed on one side and MISSION on the other
• 15 mEq tablets are uncoated, tan to yellowish in color, modified rectangle shaped, with M15 debossed on one side and blank on the other

4 CONTRAINDICATIONS

Urocit®-K is contraindicated:
• In patients with hyperkalemia (or who have conditions pre-disposing them to hyperkalemia), as a further rise in serum potassium concentration may produce cardiac arrest. Such conditions include: chronic renal failure, uncontrolled diabetes mellitus, acute dehydration, strenuous physical exercise in unconditioned individuals, adrenal insufficiency, extensive tissue breakdown or the administration of a potassium-sparing agent (such as triamterene, spironolactone or amiloride).
• In patients in whom there is cause for arrest or delay in tablet passage through the gastrointestinal tract, such as those suffering from delayed gastric emptying, esophageal compression, intestinal obstruction or stricture, or those taking anticholinergic medication.
• In patients with peptic ulcer disease because of its ulcerogenic potential.
• In patients with active urinary tract infection (with either urea-splitting or other organisms, in association with either calcium or struvite stones). The ability of Urocit®-K to increase urinary citrate may be attenuated by bacterial enzymatic degradation of citrate. Moreover, the rise in urinary pH resulting from Urocit®-K therapy might promote further bacterial growth.
• In patients with renal insufficiency (glomerular filtration rate of less than 0.7 ml/kg/min), because of the danger of soft tissue calcification and increased risk for the development of hyperkalemia.

5 WARNINGS AND PRECAUTIONS

5.1 Hyperkalemia
In patients with impaired mechanisms for excreting potassium, Urocit®-K administration can produce hyperkalemia and cardiac arrest. Potentially fatal hyperkalemia can develop rapidly and be asymptomatic. The use of Urocit®-K in patients with chronic renal failure, or any other condition which impairs potassium excretion such as severe myocardial damage or heart failure, should be avoided. Closely monitor for signs of hyperkalemia with periodic blood tests and ECGs.

5.2 Gastrointestinal Lesions
Because of reports of upper gastrointestinal mucosal lesions following administration of potassium chloride (wax-matrix), an endoscopic examination of the upper gastrointestinal mucosa was performed in 30 normal volunteers after they had taken glycopyrrolate 2 mg p.o. t.i.d., Urocit®-K 95 mEq/day, wax-matrix potassium chloride 96 mEq/day or wax-matrix placebo, in thrice daily schedule in the fasting state for one week. Urocit®-K and the wax-matrix formula-

Table 1. Effect of Urocit®-K In Patients With Calcium Oxalate Nephrolithiasis.

Group	Stones Formed Per Year			
	Baseline	On Treatment	Remission*	Any Decrease
I (n=19)	12 ± 30	0.9 ± 1.3	58%	95%
II (n=37)	1.2 ± 2	0.4 ± 1.5	89%	97%
III (n=15)	4.2 ± 7	0.7 ± 2	67%	100%
IV (n=18)	3.4 ± 8	0.5 ± 2	94%	100%
Total (n=89)	4.3 ±15	0.6 ± 2	80%	98%

*Remission defined as "the percentage of patients remaining free of newly formed stones during treatment".

tion of potassium chloride were indistinguishable but both were significantly more irritating than the wax-matrix placebo. In a subsequent, similar study, lesions were less severe when glycopyrrolate was omitted.

Solid dosage forms of potassium chlorides have produced stenotic and/or ulcerative lesions of the small bowel and deaths. These lesions are caused by a high local concentration of potassium ions in the region of the dissolving tablets, which injured the bowel. In addition, perhaps because wax-matrix preparations are not enteric-coated and release some of their potassium content in the stomach, there have been reports of upper gastrointestinal bleeding associated with these products. The frequency of gastrointestinal lesions with wax-matrix potassium chloride products is estimated at one per 100,000 patient-years. Experience with Urocit®-K is limited, but a similar frequency of gastrointestinal lesions should be anticipated.

If there is severe vomiting, abdominal pain or gastrointestinal bleeding, Urocit®-K should be discontinued immediately and the possibility of bowel perforation or obstruction investigated.

6   ADVERSE REACTIONS
6.1   Postmarketing Experience
Some patients may develop minor gastrointestinal complaints during Urocit®-K therapy, such as abdominal discomfort, vomiting, diarrhea, loose bowel movements or nausea. These symptoms are due to the irritation of the gastrointestinal tract, and may be alleviated by taking the dose with meals or snacks, or by reducing the dosage. Patients may find intact matrices in their feces.

7   DRUG INTERACTIONS
7.1   Potential Effects of Potassium citrate on Other Drugs
Potassium-sparing Diuretics: Concomitant administration of Urocit®-K and a potassium-sparing diuretic (such as triamterene, spironolactone or amiloride) should be avoided since the simultaneous administration of these agents can produce severe hyperkalemia.
7.2   Potential Effects of Other Drugs on Potassium citrate
Drugs that slow gastrointestinal transit time: These agents (such as anticholinergics) can be expected to increase the gastrointestinal irritation produced by potassium salts.

8   USE IN SPECIFIC POPULATIONS
8.1   Pregnancy
Pregnancy Category C
Animal reproduction studies have not been conducted. It is also not known whether Urocit®-K can cause fetal harm when administered to a pregnant woman or can affect reproduction capacity. Urocit®-K should be given to a pregnant woman only if clearly needed.
8.3   Nursing Mothers
The normal potassium ion content of human milk is about 13 mEq/L. It is not known if Urocit®-K has an effect on this content. Urocit®-K should be given to a woman who is breast feeding only if clearly needed.
8.4   Pediatric Use
Safety and effectiveness in children have not been established.

10   OVERDOSAGE
Treatment of Overdosage: The administration of potassium salts to persons without predisposing conditions for hyperkalemia rarely causes serious hyperkalemia at recommended dosages. It is important to recognize that hyperkalemia is usually asymptomatic and may be manifested only by an increased serum potassium concentration and characteristic electrocardiographic changes (peaking of T-wave, loss of P-wave, depression of S-T segment and prolongation of the QT interval). Late manifestations include muscle paralysis and cardiovascular collapse from cardiac arrest. Treatment measures for hyperkalemia include the following:

1. Patients should be closely monitored for arrhythmias and electrolyte changes.
2. Elimination of medications containing potassium and of agents with potassium-sparing properties such as potassium-sparing diuretics, ARBs, ACE inhibitors, NSAIDs, certain nutritional supplements and many others.
3. Elimination of foods containing high levels of potassium such as almonds, apricots, bananas, beans (lima, pinto, white), cantaloupe, carrot juice (canned), figs, grapefruit juice, halibut, milk, oat bran, potato (with skin), salmon, spinach, tuna and many others.
4. Intravenous calcium gluconate if the patient is at no risk or low risk of developing digitalis toxicity.
5. Intravenous administration of 300-500 mL/hr of 10% dextrose solution containing 10-20 units of crystalline insulin per 1,000 mL.
6. Correction of acidosis, if present, with intravenous sodium bicarbonate.
7. Hemodialysis or peritoneal dialysis.
8. Exchange resins may be used. However, this measure alone is not sufficient for the acute treatment of hyperkalemia.

Lowering potassium levels too rapidly in patients taking digitalis can produce digitalis toxicity.

11   DESCRIPTION
Urocit®-K is a citrate salt of potassium. Its empirical formula is $K_3C_6H_5O_7 \cdot H_2O$, and it has the following chemical structure:

$$HO - \overset{\displaystyle CH_2 - COOK}{\underset{\displaystyle CH_2 - COOK}{C - COOK}} \cdot H_2O$$

Urocit®-K yellowish to tan, oral wax-matrix tablets, contain 5 mEq (540 mg) potassium citrate, 10 mEq (1080 mg) potassium citrate and 15 mEq (1620 mg) potassium citrate each. Inactive ingredients include carnauba wax and magnesium stearate.

12   CLINICAL PHARMACOLOGY
12.1   Mechanism of Action
When Urocit®-K is given orally, the metabolism of absorbed citrate produces an alkaline load. The induced alkaline load in turn increases urinary pH and raises urinary citrate by augmenting citrate clearance without measurably altering ultrafilterable serum citrate. Thus, Urocit®-K therapy appears to increase urinary citrate principally by modifying the renal handling of citrate, rather than by increasing the filtered load of citrate. The increased filtered load of citrate may play some role, however, as in small comparisons of oral citrate and oral bicarbonate, citrate had a greater effect on urinary citrate.

In addition to raising urinary pH and citrate, Urocit®-K increases urinary potassium by approximately the amount contained in the medication. In some patients, Urocit®-K causes a transient reduction in urinary calcium.

The changes induced by Urocit®-K produce urine that is less conducive to the crystallization of stone-forming salts (calcium oxalate, calcium phosphate and uric acid). Increased citrate in the urine, by complexing with calcium, decreases calcium ion activity and thus the saturation of calcium oxalate. Citrate also inhibits the spontaneous nucleation of calcium oxalate and calcium phosphate (brushite).

The increase in urinary pH also decreases calcium ion activity by increasing calcium complexation to dissociated anions. The rise in urinary pH also increases the ionization of uric acid to the more soluble urate ion.

Urocit®-K therapy does not alter the urinary saturation of calcium phosphate, since the effect of increased citrate complexation of calcium is opposed by the rise in pH-dependent dissociation of phosphate. Calcium phosphate stones are more stable in alkaline urine.

In the setting of normal renal function, the rise in urinary citrate following a single dose begins by the first hour and lasts for 12 hours. With multiple doses the rise in citrate excretion reaches its peak by the third day and averts the normally wide circadian fluctuation in urinary citrate, thus maintaining urinary citrate at a higher, more constant level throughout the day. When the treatment is withdrawn, urinary citrate begins to decline toward the pre-treatment level on the first day.

The rise in citrate excretion is directly dependent on the Urocit®-K dosage. Following long-term treatment, Urocit®-K at a dosage of 60 mEq/day raises urinary citrate by approximately 400 mg/day and increases urinary pH by approximately 0.7 units.

In patients with severe renal tubular acidosis or chronic diarrheal syndrome where urinary citrate may be very low (<100 mg/day), Urocit®-K may be relatively ineffective in raising urinary citrate. A higher dose of Urocit®-K may therefore be required to produce a satisfactory citraturic response. In patients with renal tubular acidosis in whom urinary pH may be high, Urocit®-K produces a relatively small rise in urinary pH.

14   CLINICAL STUDIES
The pivotal Urocit®-K trials were non-randomized and non-placebo controlled where dietary management may have changed coincidentally with pharmacological treatment. Therefore, the results as presented in the following sections may overstate the effectiveness of the product.
14.1   Renal tubular acidosis (RTA) with calcium stones
The effect of oral potassium citrate therapy in a non-randomized, non-placebo controlled clinical study of five men and four women with calcium oxalate/calcium phosphate nephrolithiasis and documented incomplete distal renal tubular acidosis was examined. The main inclusion criterion was a history of stone passage or surgical removal of stones during the 3 years prior to initiation of potassium citrate therapy. All patients began alkali treatment with 60-80 mEq potassium citrate daily in 3 or 4 divided doses. Throughout treatment, patients were instructed to stay on a sodium restricted diet (100 mEq/day) and to reduce oxalate intake (limited intake of nuts, dark roughage, chocolate and tea). A moderate calcium restriction (400-800 mg/day) was imposed on patients with hypercalciuria.

X-rays of the urinary tract, available in all patients, were reviewed to determine presence of pre-existing stones, appearance of new stones, or change in the number of stones. Potassium citrate therapy was associated with inhibition of new stone formation in patients with distal tubular acidosis. Three of the nine patients continued to pass stones during the on-treatment phase. While it is likely that these patients passed pre-existing stones during therapy, the most conservative assumption is that the passed stones were newly formed. Using this assumption, the stone-passage remission rate was 67%. All patients had a reduced stone formation rate. Over the first 2 years of treatment, the on-treatment stone formation rate was reduced from 13±27 to 1±2 per year.
14.2   Hypocitraturic calcium oxalate nephrolithiasis of any etiology
Eighty-nine patients with hypocitraturic calcium nephrolithiasis or uric acid lithiasis with or without calcium nephrolithiasis participated in this non-randomized, non-placebo controlled clinical study. Four groups of patients were treated with potassium citrate: Group 1 was comprised of 19 patients, 10 with renal tubular acidosis and 9 with chronic diarrheal syndrome, Group 2 was comprised of 37 patients, 5 with uric acid stones alone, 6 with uric acid lithiasis and calcium stones, 3 with type 1 absorptive hypercalciuria, 9 with type 2 absorptive hypercalciuria and 14 with hypocitraturia. Group 3 was comprised of 15 patients with history of relapse on other therapy and Group 4 was comprised of 18 patients, 9 with type 1 absorptive hypercalciuria and calcium stones, 1 with type 2 absorptive hypercalciuria and calcium stones, 2 with hyperuricosuric calcium oxalate nephrolithiasis, 4 with uric acid lithiasis accompanied by calcium stones and 2 with hypocitraturia and hyperuricemia accompanied by calcium stones. The dose of potassium citrate ranged from 30 to 100 mEq per day, and usually was 20 mEq administered orally 3 times daily. Patients were followed in an outpatient setting every 4 months during treatment and were studied over a period from 1 to 4.33 years. A three-year retrospective pre-study history for stone passage or removal was obtained and corroborated by medical records. Concomitant therapy (with thiazide or allopurinol) was allowed if patients had hypercalciuria, hyperuricosuria or hyperuricemia. Group 2 was treated with potassium citrate alone.

In all groups, treatment that included potassium citrate was associated with a sustained increase in urinary citrate excretion from subnormal values to normal values (400 to 700 mg/day), and a sustained increase in urinary pH from 5.6-6.0 to approximately 6.5. The stone formation rate was reduced in all groups as shown in **Table 1**.
[See table 1 above]

14.3   Uric acid lithiasis with or without calcium stones

A long-term non-randomized, non-placebo controlled clinical trial with eighteen adult patients with uric acid lithiasis participated in the study. Six patients formed only uric acid stones, and the remaining 12 patients formed mixed stones containing both uric acid and calcium salts or formed both uric acid stones (without calcium salts) and calcium stones (without uric acid) on separate occasions.

Eleven of the 18 patients received potassium citrate alone. Six of the 7 other patients also received allopurinol for hyperuricemia with gouty arthritis, symptomatic hyperuricemia, or hyperuricosuria. One patient also received hydrochlorothiazide because of unclassified hypercalciuria. The main inclusion criterion was a history of stone passage or surgical removal of stones during the 3 years prior to initiation of potassium citrate therapy. All patients received potassium citrate at a dosage of 30-80 mEq/day in three-to-four divided doses and were followed every four months for up to 5 years.

While on potassium citrate treatment, urinary pH rose significantly from a low value of 5.3 ± 0.3 to within normal limits (6.2 to 6.5). Urinary citrate which was low before treatment rose to the high normal range and only one stone was formed in the entire group of 18 patients.

15   REFERENCES

1. Pak, C. (1987). Citrate and Renal Calculi. *Mineral and Electrolyte Metabolism* 13, 257-266.
2. Pak, C. (1985). Long-Term Treatment of Calcium Nephrolithiasis with Potassium Citrate. *The Journal of Urology* 134, 11-19.
3. Preminger, G.M., K. Sakhaee, C. Skurla and C.Y.C. Pak. (1985). Prevention of Recurrent Calcium Stone Formation with Potassium Citrate Therapy in Patients with Distal Renal Tubular Acidosis. *The Journal of Urology* 134, 20-23.
4. Pak, C.Y.C., K. Sakhaee and C. Fuller. (1986). Successful Management of Uric Acid Nephrolithiasis with Potassium Citrate. *Kidney International* 30, 422-428.
5. Hollander-Rodriguez, J et al. (2006). Hyperkalemia, *American Family Physician*, Vol. 73/No. 2.
6. Greenberg, A et al. (1998). Hyperkalemia: treatment options. *Semen Nephrol.* Jan; 18 (1): 46-57.

16   HOW SUPPLIED/STORAGE AND HANDLING

Urocit®-K 5 mEq tablets are uncoated, tan to yellowish in color, modified ball shaped, with MPC 600 debossed on one side and blank on the other, supplied in bottles as:
NDC 0178-0600-01   Bottle of 100
Urocit®-K 10 mEq tablets are uncoated, tan to yellowish in color, elliptical shaped, with 610 debossed on one side and MISSION on the other, supplied in bottles as:
NDC 0178-0610-01   Bottle of 100
Urocit®-K 15 mEq tablets are uncoated, tan to yellowish in color, modified rectangle shaped, with M15 debossed on one side and blank on the other, supplied in bottles as:
NDC 0178-0615-01   Bottle of 100
Storage: Store in a tight container.

17   PATIENT COUNSELING INFORMATION

17.1   Administration of Drug

Tell patients to take each dose without crushing, chewing or sucking the tablet.

Tell patients to take this medicine only as directed. This is especially important if the patient is also taking both diuretics and digitalis preparations.

Tell patients to check with the doctor if there is trouble swallowing tablets or if the tablet seems to stick in the throat.

Tell patients to check with the doctor at once if tarry stools or other evidence of gastrointestinal bleeding is noticed.

Tell patients that their doctor will perform regular blood tests and electrocardiograms to ensure safety.

Rev 0410

Help your patients save on prescription drugs with the PDR® Pharmacy Discount Card. For more, visit PDR.net/PharmacyDiscountCard.

MSD International GmbH,
for product information, please see Merck

MSD Oss B.V.,
for product information, please see Merck

Novartis Pharmaceuticals Corporation

ONE HEALTH PLAZA
EAST HANOVER, NJ 07936
(for branded products)

For Information Contact (branded products):
Customer Interaction Center
(888) NOW-NOVA [888-669-6682]
www.pharma.us.novartis.com

AFINITOR R
[a-fin-it-or]
(everolimus)
tablets for oral administration
AFINITOR DISPERZ
(everolimus tablets for oral suspension)

The following prescribing information is based on official labeling in effect July 2014.

HIGHLIGHTS OF PRESCRIBING INFORMATION
These highlights do not include all the information needed to use AFINITOR safely and effectively. See full prescribing information for AFINITOR.
AFINITOR® (everolimus) tablets for oral administration
AFINITOR® DISPERZ (everolimus tablets for oral suspension)
Initial U.S. Approval: 2009

RECENT MAJOR CHANGES

Indications and Usage (1.2)	11/2013
Dosage and Administration (2.2, 2.3, 2.5, 2.6, 2.7)	2/2014
Warnings and Precautions, Non-infectious Pneumonitis (5.1)	7/2014
Warnings and Precautions, Infections (5.2)	7/2014
Warnings and Precautions, Oral Ulceration (5.3)	2/2014
Warnings and Precautions, Impaired Wound Healing (5.5)	2/2014
Warnings and Precautions, Lab Tests and Monitoring (5.7)	2/2014
Warnings and Precautions, Embryo-fetal Toxicity (5.11)	2/2014

INDICATIONS AND USAGE

AFINITOR is a kinase inhibitor indicated for the treatment of:

- postmenopausal women with advanced hormone receptor-positive, HER2-negative breast cancer (advanced HR+ BC) in combination with exemestane after failure of treatment with letrozole or anastrozole. (1.1)
- adults with progressive neuroendocrine tumors of pancreatic origin (PNET) that are unresectable, locally advanced or metastatic. AFINITOR is not indicated for the treatment of patients with functional carcinoid tumors. (1.2)
- adults with advanced renal cell carcinoma (RCC) after failure of treatment with sunitinib or sorafenib. (1.3)
- adults with renal angiomyolipoma and tuberous sclerosis complex (TSC), not requiring immediate surgery. The effectiveness of AFINITOR in the treatment of renal angiomyolipoma is based on an analysis of durable objective responses in patients treated for a median of 8.3 months. Further follow-up of patients is required to determine long-term outcomes. (1.4)

AFINITOR and AFINITOR DISPERZ are kinase inhibitors indicated for the treatment of:

- pediatric and adult patients with tuberous sclerosis complex (TSC) who have subependymal giant cell astrocytoma (SEGA) that requires therapeutic intervention but cannot be curatively resected. The effectiveness is based on demonstration of durable objective response, as evidenced by reduction in SEGA tumor volume. Improvement in disease-related symptoms and overall survival in patients with SEGA and TSC has not been demonstrated. (1.5)

DOSAGE AND ADMINISTRATION

Advanced HR+ BC, advanced PNET, advanced RCC, or renal angiomyolipoma with TSC:

- 10 mg once daily with or without food. (2.1)
- For patients with hepatic impairment, reduce the AFINITOR dose. (2.2)
- If moderate inhibitors of CYP3A4 /P-glycoprotein (PgP) are required, reduce the AFINITOR dose to 2.5 mg once daily; if tolerated, consider increasing to 5 mg once daily. (2.2)
- If strong inducers of CYP3A4 are required, consider doubling the daily dose of AFINITOR using increments of 5 mg or less. (2.2)

SEGA with TSC:
- 4.5 mg/m^2 once daily; adjust dose to attain trough concentrations of 5-15 ng/mL. (2.3)
- Assess trough concentrations approximately 2 weeks after initiation of treatment, a change in dose, a change in co-administration of CYP3A4/PgP inducers or inhibitors, a change in hepatic function, or a change in dosage form between AFINITOR Tablets and AFINITOR DISPERZ. (2.3, 2.4)
- For patients with severe hepatic impairment reduce the starting dose of AFINITOR Tablets or AFINITOR DISPERZ. (2.3, 2.5)
- If concomitant use of moderate inhibitors of CYP3A4/PgP is required, reduce the dose of AFINITOR Tablets or AFINITOR DISPERZ by 50%. (2.3, 2.5)
- If concomitant use of strong inducers of CYP3A4/PgP is required, double the dose of AFINITOR Tablets or AFINITOR DISPERZ. (2.3, 2.5)

DOSAGE FORMS AND STRENGTHS

AFINITOR Tablets: 2.5 mg, 5 mg, 7.5 mg, and 10 mg tablets with no score (3.1)
AFINITOR DISPERZ (everolimus tablets for oral suspension):   2 mg, 3 mg, and 5 mg tablets for oral suspension with no score (3.2)

CONTRAINDICATIONS

Hypersensitivity to everolimus, to other rapamycin derivatives, or to any of the excipients (4)

WARNINGS AND PRECAUTIONS

- Non-infectious pneumonitis: Monitor for clinical symptoms or radiological changes; fatal cases have occurred. Manage by dose reduction or discontinuation until symptoms resolve, and consider use of corticosteroids. (5.1)
- Infections: Increased risk of infections, some fatal. Monitor for signs and symptoms, and treat promptly. (5.2)
- Oral ulceration: Mouth ulcers, stomatitis, and oral mucositis are common. Management includes mouthwashes and topical treatments. (5.3)
- Renal failure: Cases of renal failure (including acute renal failure), some with a fatal outcome, have been observed. (5.4)
- Impaired wound healing: Increased risk of wound-related complications. Monitor signs and symptoms. Exercise caution in the peri-surgical period. (5.5)
- Laboratory test alterations: Elevations of serum creatinine, urinary protein, blood glucose, and lipids may occur. Decreases in hemoglobin, neutrophils, and platelets may also occur. Monitor renal function, blood glucose, lipids, and hematologic parameters prior to treatment and periodically thereafter. (5.7)
- Vaccinations: Avoid live vaccines and close contact with those who have received live vaccines. (5.10)
- Embryo-fetal toxicity: Fetal harm can occur when administered to a pregnant woman. Apprise women of potential harm to the fetus. (5.11, 8.1)

ADVERSE REACTIONS

Advanced HR+ BC, advanced PNET, advanced RCC: Most common adverse reactions (incidence ≥30%) include stomatitis, infections, rash, fatigue, diarrhea, edema, abdominal pain, nausea, fever, asthenia, cough, headache and decreased appetite. (6.1, 6.2, 6.3)
Renal angiomyolipoma with TSC: Most common adverse reaction (incidence ≥ 30%) is stomatitis. (6.4)
SEGA with TSC: Most common adverse reactions (incidence ≥ 30%) are stomatitis and respiratory tract infection. (6.5)

To report SUSPECTED ADVERSE REACTIONS, contact Novartis Pharmaceuticals Corporation at 1-888-669-6682 or FDA at 1-800-FDA-1088 or www.fda.gov/medwatch.

DRUG INTERACTIONS

- Strong CYP3A4/PgP inhibitors: Avoid concomitant use. (2.2, 2.5, 5.8, 7.1)
- Moderate CYP3A4/PgP inhibitors: If combination is required, use caution and reduce dose of AFINITOR. (2.2, 2.3, 2.5, 5.8, 7.1)
- Strong CYP3A4/PgP inducers: Avoid concomitant use. If combination cannot be avoided, increase dose of AFINITOR. (2.2, 2.3, 2.5, 5.8, 7.2)

USE IN SPECIFIC POPULATIONS

- Nursing mothers: Discontinue drug or nursing, taking into consideration the importance of drug to the mother. (8.3)
- Hepatic impairment: For advanced HR+ BC, advanced PNET, advanced RCC, or renal angiomyolipoma with TSC patients with hepatic impairment, reduce AFINITOR

dose. For SEGA patients with severe hepatic impairment, reduce the starting dose of AFINITOR Tablets or AFINITOR DISPERZ. (2.2, 2.3, 2.5, 5.9, 8.8)

See 17 for PATIENT COUNSELING INFORMATION and FDA-approved patient labeling

Revised: 7/2014

FULL PRESCRIBING INFORMATION

1 INDICATIONS AND USAGE

1.1 Advanced Hormone Receptor-Positive, HER2-Negative Breast Cancer (Advanced HR+ BC)
AFINITOR® is indicated for the treatment of postmenopausal women with advanced hormone receptor-positive, HER2-negative breast cancer (advanced HR+ BC) in combination with exemestane, after failure of treatment with letrozole or anastrozole.

1.2 Advanced Neuroendocrine Tumors of Pancreatic Origin (PNET)
AFINITOR® is indicated for the treatment of adult patients with progressive neuroendocrine tumors of pancreatic origin (PNET) with unresectable, locally advanced or metastatic disease.

AFINITOR® is not indicated for the treatment of patients with functional carcinoid tumors.

1.3 Advanced Renal Cell Carcinoma (RCC)
AFINITOR® is indicated for the treatment of adult patients with advanced renal cell carcinoma (RCC) after failure of treatment with sunitinib or sorafenib.

1.4 Renal Angiomyolipoma with Tuberous Sclerosis Complex (TSC)
AFINITOR® is indicated for the treatment of adult patients with renal angiomyolipoma and tuberous sclerosis complex (TSC), not requiring immediate surgery.
The effectiveness of AFINITOR in the treatment of renal angiomyolipoma is based on an analysis of durable objective responses in patients treated for a median of 8.3 months. Further follow-up of patients is required to determine long-term outcomes.

1.5 Subependymal Giant Cell Astrocytoma (SEGA) with Tuberous Sclerosis Complex (TSC)
AFINITOR® Tablets and AFINITOR® DISPERZ are indicated in pediatric and adult patients with tuberous sclerosis complex (TSC) for the treatment of subependymal giant cell astrocytoma (SEGA) that requires therapeutic intervention but cannot be curatively resected.
The effectiveness of AFINITOR Tablets and AFINITOR DISPERZ is based on demonstration of durable objective response, as evidenced by reduction in SEGA tumor volume. Improvement in disease-related symptoms and overall survival in patients with SEGA and TSC has not been demonstrated [see Clinical Studies (14.5)].

2 DOSAGE AND ADMINISTRATION

AFINITOR is available in two dosage forms: tablets (AFINITOR Tablets) and tablets for oral suspension (AFINITOR DISPERZ).

• AFINITOR Tablets may be used for all approved indications.
• AFINITOR DISPERZ is approved for the treatment of patients with subependymal giant cell astrocytoma (SEGA) and tuberous sclerosis complex (TSC).

2.1 Recommended Dose in Advanced Hormone Receptor-Positive, HER2-Negative Breast Cancer, Advanced PNET, Advanced RCC, and Renal Angiomyolipoma with TSC
The recommended dose of AFINITOR Tablets is 10 mg, to be taken once daily at the same time every day. Administer either consistently with food or consistently without food [see Clinical Pharmacology (12.3)]. AFINITOR Tablets should be swallowed whole with a glass of water. Do not break or crush tablets.
Continue treatment until disease progression or unacceptable toxicity occurs.

2.2 Dose Modifications in Advanced Hormone Receptor-Positive, HER2-Negative Breast Cancer, Advanced PNET, Advanced RCC, and Renal Angiomyolipoma with TSC
Adverse Reactions
Management of severe or intolerable adverse reactions may require temporary dose interruption (with or without a dose reduction of AFINITOR therapy). If dose reduction is required, the suggested dose is approximately 50% lower than the daily dose previously administered [see Warnings and Precautions (5)].

Table 1 summarizes recommendations for dose reduction, interruption or discontinuation of AFINITOR in the management of adverse reactions. General management recommendations are also provided as applicable. Clinical judgment of the treating physician should guide the management plan of each patient based on individual benefit/risk assessment.
[See table 1 at top of next page]

Hepatic Impairment
Hepatic impairment will increase the exposure to everolimus [see Warnings and Precautions (5.9) and Use in Specific Populations (8.8)]. Dose adjustments are recommended:

• Mild hepatic impairment (Child-Pugh class A) – The recommended dose is 7.5 mg daily; the dose may be decreased to 5 mg if not well tolerated.
• Moderate hepatic impairment (Child-Pugh class B) – The recommended dose is 5 mg daily; the dose may be decreased to 2.5 mg if not well tolerated.
• Severe hepatic impairment (Child-Pugh class C) – If the desired benefit outweighs the risk, a dose of 2.5 mg daily may be used but must not be exceeded.

Dose adjustments should be made if a patient's hepatic (Child-Pugh) status changes during treatment.

CYP3A4/P-glycoprotein (PgP) Inhibitors
Avoid the use of strong CYP3A4/PgP inhibitors (e.g., ketoconazole, itraconazole, clarithromycin, atazanavir, nefazodone, saquinavir, telithromycin, ritonavir, indinavir, nelfinavir, voriconazole) [see Warnings and Precautions (5.8) and Drug Interactions (7.1)].
Use caution when co-administered with moderate CYP3A4/PgP inhibitors (e.g., amprenavir, fosamprenavir, aprepitant, erythromycin, fluconazole, verapamil, diltiazem). If patients require co-administration of a moderate CYP3A4/PgP inhibitor, reduce the AFINITOR dose to 2.5 mg daily. The reduced dose of AFINITOR is predicted to adjust the area under the curve (AUC) to the range observed without inhibitors. An AFINITOR dose increase from 2.5 mg to 5 mg may be considered based on patient tolerance. If the moderate inhibitor is discontinued, a washout period of approximately 2 to 3 days should be allowed before the AFINITOR dose is increased. If the moderate inhibitor is discontinued, the AFINITOR dose should be returned to the dose used prior to initiation of the moderate CYP3A4/PgP inhibitor.
Grapefruit, grapefruit juice, and other foods that are known to inhibit cytochrome P450 and PgP activity may increase everolimus exposures and should be avoided during treatment.

Strong CYP3A4/PgP Inducers
Avoid the use of concomitant strong CYP3A4/PgP inducers (e.g., phenytoin, carbamazepine, rifampin, rifabutin, rifapentine, phenobarbital). If patients require co-administration of a strong CYP3A4/PgP inducer, consider doubling the daily dose of AFINITOR using increments of 5 mg or less. This dose of AFINITOR is predicted, based on pharmacokinetic data, to adjust the AUC to the range observed without inducers. However, there are no clinical data with this dose adjustment in patients receiving strong CYP3A4/PgP inducers. If the strong inducer is discontinued, consider a washout period of 3 to 5 days, before the AFINITOR dose is returned to the dose used prior to initiation of the strong CYP3A4/PgP inducer [see Warnings and Precautions (5.8) and Drug Interactions (7.2)].
St. John's Wort (*Hypericum perforatum*) may decrease everolimus exposure unpredictably and should be avoided.

2.3 Recommended Dose in SEGA with TSC
The recommended starting dose is 4.5 mg/m², once daily. The recommended starting dose for patients with severe hepatic impairment (Child-Pugh class C) or requiring moderate CYP3A4/PgP inhibitors is 2.5 mg/m², once daily [see Dosage and Administration (2.5)]. The recommended starting dose for patients requiring a concomitant strong CYP3A4 inducer is 9 mg/m², once daily [see Dosage and Administration (2.5)]. Round dose to the nearest strength of either AFINITOR Tablets or AFINITOR DISPERZ.
Do not combine AFINITOR Tablets and AFINITOR DISPERZ to achieve the desired total dose.
Use therapeutic drug monitoring to guide subsequent dosing [see Dosage and Administration (2.4)]. Adjust dose at 2 week intervals as needed to achieve and maintain trough concentrations of 5 to 15 ng/mL [see Dosage and Administration (2.4, 2.5)].
Continue treatment until disease progression or unacceptable toxicity occurs. The optimal duration of therapy is unknown.

2.4 Therapeutic Drug Monitoring in SEGA with TSC
Monitor everolimus whole blood trough levels routinely in all patients. When possible, use the same assay and labora-

tory for therapeutic drug monitoring throughout treatment. Assess trough concentrations approximately 2 weeks after initiation of treatment, a change in dose, a change in co-administration of CYP3A4/PgP inducers and/or inhibitors, a change in hepatic function, or a change in dosage form between AFINITOR Tablets and AFINITOR DISPERZ. Once a stable dose is attained, monitor trough concentrations every 3 to 6 months in patients with changing body surface area or every 6 to 12 months in patients with stable body surface area for the duration of treatment.

Titrate the dose to attain trough concentrations of 5 to 15 ng/mL.

- For trough concentrations less than 5 ng/mL, increase the daily dose by 2.5 mg (in patients taking AFINITOR Tablets) or 2 mg (in patients taking AFINITOR DISPERZ).
- For trough concentrations greater than 15 ng/mL, reduce the daily dose by 2.5 mg (in patients taking AFINITOR Tablets) or 2 mg (in patients taking AFINITOR DISPERZ).
- If dose reduction is required for patients receiving the lowest available strength, administer every other day.

2.5   Dose Modifications in SEGA with TSC

Adverse Reactions

Temporarily interrupt or permanently discontinue AFINITOR Tablets or AFINITOR DISPERZ for severe or intolerable adverse reactions. If dose reduction is required when reinitiating therapy, reduce the dose by approximately 50% *[see Dosage and Administration (2.2) and Warnings and Precautions (5)]*. If dose reduction is required for patients receiving the lowest available strength, administer every other day.

Hepatic Impairment

- Reduce the starting dose of AFINITOR Tablets or AFINITOR DISPERZ by approximately 50% in patients with SEGA who have severe hepatic impairment (Child-Pugh class C) *[see Dosage and Administration (2.3)]*. Adjustment to the starting dose for patients with SEGA who have mild (Child-Pugh class A) or moderate (Child-Pugh class B) hepatic impairment may not be needed. Subsequent dosing should be based on therapeutic drug monitoring.
- Assess everolimus trough concentrations approximately 2 weeks after commencing treatment, a change in dose, or any change in hepatic function *[see Dosage and Administration (2.3, 2.4)]*.

CYP3A4/P-glycoprotein (PgP) Inhibitors

Avoid the use of concomitant strong CYP3A4/PgP inhibitors (e.g., ketoconazole, itraconazole, clarithromycin, atazanavir, nefazodone, saquinavir, telithromycin, ritonavir, indinavir, nelfinavir, voriconazole) in patients receiving AFINITOR Tablets or AFINITOR DISPERZ *[see Warnings and Precautions (5.8) and Drug Interactions (7.1)]*.

For patients who require treatment with moderate CYP3A4/PgP inhibitors (e.g., amprenavir, fosamprenavir, aprepitant, erythromycin, fluconazole, verapamil, diltiazem):

- Reduce the AFINITOR Tablets or AFINITOR DISPERZ dose by approximately 50%. Administer every other day if dose reduction is required for patients receiving the lowest available strength and maintain trough concentrations of 5 to 15 ng/mL *[see Dosage and Administration (2.3, 2.4)]*.
- Assess everolimus trough concentrations approximately 2 weeks after dose reduction *[see Dosage and Administration (2.3, 2.4)]*.
- Resume the dose that was used prior to initiating the CYP3A4/PgP inhibitor 2 to 3 days after discontinuation of a moderate inhibitor. Assess the everolimus trough concentration approximately 2 weeks later *[see Dosage and Administration (2.3, 2.4)]*.

Do not ingest foods or nutritional supplements (e.g., grapefruit, grapefruit juice) that are known to inhibit cytochrome P450 or PgP activity.

Strong CYP3A4/PgP Inducers

Avoid the use of concomitant strong CYP3A4/PgP inducers (e.g., phenytoin, carbamazepine, rifampin, rifabutin, rifapentine, phenobarbital) if alternative therapy is available *[see Warnings and Precautions (5.8) and Drug Interactions (7.2)]*. For patients who require treatment with a strong CYP3A4/PgP inducer:

- Double the dose of AFINITOR Tablets or AFINITOR DISPERZ and assess tolerability *[see Dosage and Administration (2.3)]*.
- Assess the everolimus trough concentration 2 weeks after doubling the dose and adjust dose if necessary to maintain a trough concentration of 5 to 15 ng/mL *[see Dosage and Administration (2.3, 2.4)]*.
- Return the AFINITOR Tablets or AFINITOR DISPERZ dose to that used prior to initiating the strong CYP3A4/PgP inducer if the strong inducer is discontinued, and as-

sess the everolimus trough concentrations approximately 2 weeks later *[see Dosage and Administration (2.3, 2.4)]*. Do not ingest foods or nutritional supplements (e.g., St. John's Wort (*Hypericum perforatum*)) that are known to induce cytochrome P450 activity.

Table 1: AFINITOR Dose Adjustment and Management Recommendation for Adverse Reactions

Adverse Reaction	Severity[a]	AFINITOR Dose Adjustment[b] and Management Recommendations
Non-infectious pneumonitis	Grade 1 Asymptomatic, radiographic findings only	No dose adjustment required. Initiate appropriate monitoring.
	Grade 2 Symptomatic, not interfering with ADL[c]	Consider interruption of therapy, rule out infection and consider treatment with corticosteroids until symptoms improve to ≤ Grade 1. Re-initiate AFINITOR at a lower dose. Discontinue treatment if failure to recover within 4 weeks.
	Grade 3 Symptomatic, interfering with ADL[c]; O2 indicated	Interrupt AFINITOR until symptoms resolve to ≤ Grade 1. Rule out infection, and consider treatment with corticosteroids. Consider re-initiating AFINITOR at a lower dose. If toxicity recurs at Grade 3, consider discontinuation.
	Grade 4 Life-threatening, ventilatory support indicated	Discontinue AFINITOR, rule out infection, and consider treatment with corticosteroids.
Stomatitis	Grade 1 Minimal symptoms, normal diet	No dose adjustment required. Manage with non-alcoholic or salt water (0.9%) mouth wash several times a day.
	Grade 2 Symptomatic but can eat and swallow modified diet	Temporary dose interruption until recovery to Grade ≤1. Re-initiate AFINITOR at the same dose. If stomatitis recurs at Grade 2, interrupt dose until recovery to Grade ≤1. Re-initiate AFINITOR at a lower dose. Manage with topical analgesic mouth treatments (e.g., benzocaine, butyl aminobenzoate, tetracaine hydrochloride, menthol or phenol) with or without topical corticosteroids (i.e., triamcinolone oral paste).[d]
	Grade 3 Symptomatic and unable to adequately aliment or hydrate orally	Temporary dose interruption until recovery to Grade ≤1. Re-initiate AFINITOR at a lower dose. Manage with topical analgesic mouth treatments (i.e., benzocaine, butyl aminobenzoate, tetracaine hydrochloride, menthol or phenol) with or without topical corticosteroids (i.e., triamcinolone oral paste).[d]
	Grade 4 Symptoms associated with life-threatening consequences	Discontinue AFINITOR and treat with appropriate medical therapy.
Other non-hematologic toxicities (excluding metabolic events)	Grade 1	If toxicity is tolerable, no dose adjustment required. Initiate appropriate medical therapy and monitor.
	Grade 2	If toxicity is tolerable, no dose adjustment required. Initiate appropriate medical therapy and monitor. If toxicity becomes intolerable, temporary dose interruption until recovery to Grade ≤1. Reinitiate AFINITOR at the same dose. If toxicity recurs at Grade 2, interrupt AFINITOR until recovery to Grade ≤1. Reinitiate AFINITOR at a lower dose.
	Grade 3	Temporary dose interruption until recovery to Grade ≤1. Initiate appropriate medical therapy and monitor. Consider reinitiating AFINITOR at a lower dose. If toxicity recurs at Grade 3, consider discontinuation.
	Grade 4	Discontinue AFINITOR and treat with appropriate medical therapy.
Metabolic events (e.g. hyperglycemia, dyslipidemia)	Grade 1	No dose adjustment required. Initiate appropriate medical therapy and monitor.
	Grade 2	No dose adjustment required. Manage with appropriate medical therapy and monitor.
	Grade 3	Temporary dose interruption. Re-initiate AFINITOR at a lower dose. Manage with appropriate medical therapy and monitor.
	Grade 4	Discontinue AFINITOR and treat with appropriate medical therapy.

[a] Severity grade description: 1 = mild symptoms; 2 = moderate symptoms; 3 = severe symptoms; 4 = life-threatening symptoms.
[b] If dose reduction is required, the suggested dose is approximately 50% lower than the dose previously administered.
[c] Activities of daily living (ADL)
[d] Avoid using agents containing alcohol, hydrogen peroxide, iodine, and thyme derivatives in management of stomatitis as they may worsen mouth ulcers.

2.6   Administration of AFINITOR Tablets in SEGA with TSC

Do not combine the 2 dosage forms (AFINITOR Tablets and AFINITOR DISPERZ) to achieve the desired total dose. Use one dosage form or the other.

Table 2: Adverse Reactions Reported ≥ 10% of Patients with Advanced HR+ BC*

	AFINITOR (10 mg/day) + exemestane[a] N=482			Placebo + exemestane[a] N=238		
	All grades %	Grade 3 %	Grade 4 %	All grades %	Grade 3 %	Grade 4 %
Any adverse reaction	100	41	9	90	22	5
Gastrointestinal disorders						
Stomatitis[b]	67	8	0	11	0.8	0
Diarrhea	33	2	0.2	18	0.8	0
Nausea	29	0.2	0.2	28	1	0
Vomiting	17	0.8	0.2	12	0.8	0
Constipation	14	0.4	0	13	0.4	0
Dry mouth	11	0	0	7	0	0
General disorders and administration site conditions						
Fatigue	36	4	0.4	27	1	0
Edema peripheral	19	1	0	6	0.4	0
Pyrexia	15	0.2	0	7	0.4	0
Asthenia	13	2	0.2	4	0	0
Infections and infestations						
Infections[c]	50	4	1	25	2	0
Investigations						
Weight decreased	25	1	0	6	0	0
Metabolism and nutrition disorders						
Decreased appetite	30	1	0	12	0.4	0
Hyperglycemia	14	5	0.4	2	0.4	0
Musculoskeletal and connective tissue disorders						
Arthralgia	20	0.8	0	17	0	0
Back pain	14	0.2	0	10	0.8	0
Pain in extremity	9	0.4	0	11	2	0
Nervous system disorders						
Dysgeusia	22	0.2	0	6	0	0
Headache	21	0.4	0	14	0	0
Psychiatric disorders						
Insomnia	13	0.2	0	8	0	0
Respiratory, thoracic and mediastinal disorders						
Cough	24	0.6	0	12	0	0
Dyspnea	21	4	0.2	11	0.8	0.4
Epistaxis	17	0	0	1	0	0
Pneumonitis[d]	19	4	0.2	0.4	0	0
Skin and subcutaneous tissue disorders						
Rash	39	1	0	6	0	0
Pruritus	13	0.2	0	5	0	0
Alopecia	10	0	0	5	0	0
Vascular disorders						
Hot flush	6	0	0	14	0	0
Median duration of treatment[e]	23.9 weeks			13.4 weeks		

Grading according to CTCAE Version 3.0
* 160 patients (33.2%) were exposed to AFINITOR therapy for a period of ≥ 32 weeks)
[a] Exemestane (25 mg/day)
[b] Includes stomatitis, mouth ulceration, aphthous stomatitis, glossodynia, gingival pain, glossitis and lip ulceration
[c] Includes all preferred terms within the 'infections and infestations' system organ class, the most common being nasopharyngitis (10%), urinary tract infection (10%), upper respiratory tract infection (5%), pneumonia (4%), bronchitis (4%), cystitis (3%), sinusitis (3%), and also including candidiasis (<1%), and sepsis (<1%), and hepatitis C (<1%).
[d] Includes pneumonitis, interstitial lung disease, lung infiltration, and pulmonary fibrosis
[e] Exposure to AFINITOR or placebo

Administer AFINITOR Tablets orally once daily at the same time every day. Administer either consistently with food or consistently without food [see Clinical Pharmacology (12.3)].
AFINITOR Tablets should be swallowed whole with a glass of water. Do not break or crush tablets.

2.7 Administration and Preparation of AFINITOR DISPERZ in SEGA with TSC
Wear gloves to avoid possible contact with everolimus when preparing suspensions of AFINITOR DISPERZ for another person.
Do not combine the 2 dosage forms (AFINITOR Tablets and AFINITOR DISPERZ) to achieve the desired total dose. Use one dosage form or the other.
Administer AFINITOR DISPERZ (everolimus tablets for oral suspension) as a suspension only.
Administer AFINITOR DISPERZ orally once daily at the same time every day. Administer either consistently with food or consistently without food [see Clinical Pharmacology (12.3)].
Administer suspension immediately after preparation. Discard suspension if not administered within 60 minutes after preparation.
Prepare suspension in water only.
Using an oral syringe:
• Place the prescribed dose of AFINITOR DISPERZ into a 10-mL syringe. Do not exceed a total of 10 mg per syringe. If higher doses are required, prepare an additional syringe. Do not break or crush tablets.
• Draw approximately 5 mL of water and 4 mL of air into the syringe.

• Place the filled syringe into a container (tip up) for 3 minutes, until the AFINITOR DISPERZ tablets are in suspension.
• Gently invert the syringe 5 times immediately prior to administration.
• After administration of the prepared suspension, draw approximately 5 mL of water and 4 mL of air into the same syringe, and swirl the contents to suspend remaining particles. Administer the entire contents of the syringe.
Using a small drinking glass:
• Place the prescribed dose of AFINITOR DISPERZ into a small drinking glass (maximum size 100 mL) containing approximately 25 mL of water. Do not exceed a total of 10 mg of AFINITOR DISPERZ per glass. If higher doses are required, prepare an additional glass. Do not break or crush tablets.
• Allow 3 minutes for suspension to occur.
• Stir the contents gently with a spoon, immediately prior to drinking.
• After administration of the prepared suspension, add 25 mL of water and stir with the same spoon to re-suspend remaining particles. Administer the entire contents of the glass.

3 DOSAGE FORMS AND STRENGTHS
3.1 AFINITOR (everolimus) Tablets
2.5 mg tablet
White to slightly yellow, elongated tablets with a bevelled edge and no score, engraved with "LCL" on one side and "NVR" on the other.

5 mg tablet
White to slightly yellow, elongated tablets with a bevelled edge and no score, engraved with "5" on one side and "NVR" on the other.
7.5 mg tablet
White to slightly yellow, elongated tablets with a bevelled edge and no score, engraved with "7P5" on one side and "NVR" on the other.
10 mg tablet
White to slightly yellow, elongated tablets with a bevelled edge and no score, engraved with "UHE" on one side and "NVR" on the other.

3.2 AFINITOR DISPERZ (everolimus tablets for oral suspension)
2 mg tablet for oral suspension
White to slightly yellowish, round, flat tablets with a bevelled edge and no score, engraved with "D2" on one side and "NVR" on the other.
3 mg tablet for oral suspension
White to slightly yellowish, round, flat tablets with a bevelled edge and no score, engraved with "D3" on one side and "NVR" on the other.
5 mg tablet for oral suspension
White to slightly yellowish, round, flat tablets with a bevelled edge and no score, engraved with "D5" on one side and "NVR" on the other.

4 CONTRAINDICATIONS
AFINITOR is contraindicated in patients with hypersensitivity to the active substance, to other rapamycin derivatives, or to any of the excipients. Hypersensitivity reactions manifested by symptoms including, but not limited to, anaphylaxis, dyspnea, flushing, chest pain, or angioedema (e.g., swelling of the airways or tongue, with or without respiratory impairment) have been observed with everolimus and other rapamycin derivatives.

5 WARNINGS AND PRECAUTIONS
5.1 Non-infectious Pneumonitis
Non-infectious pneumonitis is a class effect of rapamycin derivatives, including AFINITOR. Non-infectious pneumonitis was reported in up to 19% of patients treated with AFINITOR in clinical trials. The incidence of Common Terminology Criteria (CTC) Grade 3 and 4 non-infectious pneumonitis was up to 4.0% and up to 0.2%, respectively [see Adverse Reactions (6.1, 6.2, 6.3, 6.4, 6.5)]. Fatal outcomes have been observed.
Consider a diagnosis of non-infectious pneumonitis in patients presenting with non-specific respiratory signs and symptoms such as hypoxia, pleural effusion, cough, or dyspnea, and in whom infectious, neoplastic, and other causes have been excluded by means of appropriate investigations. Opportunistic infections such as pneumocystis jiroveci pneumonia (PJP) should be considered in the differential diagnosis. Advise patients to report promptly any new or worsening respiratory symptoms.
Patients who develop radiological changes suggestive of non-infectious pneumonitis and have few or no symptoms may continue AFINITOR therapy without dose alteration. Imaging appears to overestimate the incidence of clinical pneumonitis.
If symptoms are moderate, consider interrupting therapy until symptoms improve. The use of corticosteroids may be indicated. AFINITOR may be reintroduced at a daily dose approximately 50% lower than the dose previously administered [see Table 1 in Dosage and Administration (2.2)].
For cases of Grade 3 non-infectious pneumonitis interrupt AFINITOR until resolution to less than or equal to Grade 1. AFINITOR may be re-introduced at a daily dose approximately 50% lower than the dose previously administered depending on the individual clinical circumstances [see Dosage and Administration (2.2)]. If toxicity recurs at Grade 3, consider discontinuation of AFINITOR. For cases of Grade 4 non-infectious pneumonitis, discontinue AFINITOR. Corticosteroids may be indicated until clinical symptoms resolve. For patients who require use of corticosteroids for treatment of non-infectious pneumonitis, prophylaxis for PJP may be considered. The development of pneumonitis has been reported even at a reduced dose.
5.2 Infections
AFINITOR has immunosuppressive properties and may predispose patients to bacterial, fungal, viral, or protozoal infections, including infections with opportunistic pathogens [see Adverse Reactions (6.1, 6.2, 6.3, 6.4, 6.5)]. Localized and systemic infections, including pneumonia, mycobacterial infections, other bacterial infections, invasive fungal infections, such as aspergillosis, candidiasis, or pneumocystis jiroveci pneumonia (PJP) and viral infections including reactivation of hepatitis B virus have occurred in patients taking AFINITOR. Some of these infections have been severe (e.g., leading to sepsis, respiratory or hepatic failure) or fatal. Physicians and patients should be aware of the increased risk of infection with AFINITOR. Complete treatment of pre-existing invasive fungal infections prior to starting treatment with AFINITOR. While taking

AFINITOR, be vigilant for signs and symptoms of infection; if a diagnosis of an infection is made, institute appropriate treatment promptly and consider interruption or discontinuation of AFINITOR. If a diagnosis of invasive systemic fungal infection is made, discontinue AFINITOR and treat with appropriate antifungal therapy.

Pneumocystis jiroveci pneumonia, some with a fatal outcome, has been reported in patients who received everolimus. This may be associated with concomitant use of corticosteroids or other immunosuppressive agents. Prophylaxis for PJP should be considered when concomitant use of corticosteroids or other immunosuppressive agents are required.

5.3 Oral Ulceration

Mouth ulcers, stomatitis, and oral mucositis have occurred in patients treated with AFINITOR at an incidence ranging from 44%-78% across the clinical trial experience. Grade 3 or 4 stomatitis was reported in 4%-9% of patients [see Adverse Reactions (6.1, 6.2, 6.3, 6.4, 6.5)]. In such cases, topical treatments are recommended, but alcohol-, hydrogen peroxide-, iodine-, or thyme- containing mouthwashes should be avoided as they may exacerbate the condition. Antifungal agents should not be used unless fungal infection has been diagnosed [see Drug Interactions (7.1)].

5.4 Renal Failure

Cases of renal failure (including acute renal failure), some with a fatal outcome, have been observed in patients treated with AFINITOR [see Laboratory Tests and Monitoring (5.7)].

5.5 Impaired Wound Healing

Everolimus delays wound healing and increases the occurrence of wound-related complications like wound dehiscence, wound infection, incisional hernia, lymphocele, and seroma. These wound-related complications may require surgical intervention. Exercise caution with the use of AFINITOR in the peri-surgical period.

5.6 Geriatric Patients

In the randomized advanced hormone receptor-positive, HER2-negative breast cancer study, the incidence of deaths due to any cause within 28 days of the last AFINITOR dose was 6% in patients ≥ 65 years of age compared to 2% in patients < 65 years of age. Adverse reactions leading to permanent treatment discontinuation occurred in 33% of patients ≥ 65 years of age compared to 17% in patients < 65 years of age. Careful monitoring and appropriate dose adjustments for adverse reactions are recommended [see Dosage and Administration (2.2), Use in Specific Populations (8.5)].

5.7 Laboratory Tests and Monitoring

Renal Function

Elevations of serum creatinine and proteinuria have been reported in patients taking AFINITOR [see Adverse Reactions (6.1, 6.2, 6.3, 6.4, 6.5)]. Monitoring of renal function, including measurement of blood urea nitrogen (BUN), urinary protein, or serum creatinine, is recommended prior to the start of AFINITOR therapy and periodically thereafter. Renal function of patients should be monitored particularly where patients have additional risk factors that may further impair renal function.

Blood Glucose and Lipids

Hyperglycemia, hyperlipidemia, and hypertriglyceridemia have been reported in patients taking AFINITOR [see Adverse Reactions (6.1, 6.2, 6.3, 6.4, 6.5)]. Monitoring of fasting serum glucose and lipid profile is recommended prior to the start of AFINITOR therapy and periodically thereafter as well as management with appropriate medical therapy. More frequent monitoring is recommended when AFINITOR is co-administered with other drugs that may induce hyperglycemia. When possible, optimal glucose and lipid control should be achieved before starting a patient on AFINITOR.

Hematologic Parameters

Decreased hemoglobin, lymphocytes, neutrophils, and platelets have been reported in patients taking AFINITOR [see Adverse Reactions (6.1, 6.2, 6.3, 6.4, 6.5)]. Monitoring of complete blood count is recommended prior to the start of AFINITOR therapy and periodically thereafter.

5.8 Drug-drug Interactions

Due to significant increases in exposure of everolimus, co-administration with strong CYP3A4/PgP inhibitors should be avoided [see Dosage and Administration (2.2, 2.5) and Drug Interactions (7.1)].

A reduction of the AFINITOR dose is recommended when co-administered with a moderate CYP3A4/PgP inhibitor [see Dosage and Administration (2.2, 2.5) and Drug Interactions (7.1)].

An increase in the AFINITOR dose is recommended when co-administered with a strong CYP3A4/PgP inducer [see Dosage and Administration (2.2, 2.5) and Drug Interactions (7.2)].

5.9 Hepatic Impairment

Exposure to everolimus was increased in patients with hepatic impairment [see Clinical Pharmacology (12.3)].

Table 3: Key Laboratory Abnormalities Reported in ≥ 10% of Patients with Advanced HR+ BC

Laboratory parameter	AFINITOR (10 mg/day) + exemestane[a] N=482			Placebo + exemestane[a] N=238		
	All grades %	Grade 3 %	Grade 4 %	All grades %	Grade 3 %	Grade 4 %
Hematology[b]						
Hemoglobin decreased	68	6	0.6	40	0.8	0.4
WBC decreased	58	1	0	28	5	0.8
Platelets decreased	54	3	0.2	5	0	0.4
Lymphocytes decreased	54	11	0.6	37	5	0.8
Neutrophils decreased	31	2	0	11	0.8	0.8
Clinical chemistry						
Glucose increased	69	9	0.4	44	0.8	0.4
Cholesterol increased	70	0.6	0.2	38	0.8	0.8
Aspartate transaminase (AST) increased	69	4	0.2	45	3	0.4
Alanine transaminase (ALT) increased	51	4	0.2	29	5	0
Triglycerides increased	50	0.8	0	26	0	0
Albumin decreased	33	0.8	0	16	0.8	0
Potassium decreased	29	4	0.2	7	1	0
Creatinine increased	24	2	0.2	13	0	0

Grading according to CTCAE Version 3.0
[a] Exemestane (25 mg/day)
[b] Reflects corresponding adverse drug reaction reports of anemia, leukopenia, lymphopenia, neutropenia, and thrombocytopenia (collectively as pancytopenia), which occurred at lower frequency.

For advanced HR+ BC, advanced PNET, advanced RCC, and renal angiomyolipoma with TSC patients with severe hepatic impairment (Child-Pugh class C), AFINITOR may be used at a reduced dose if the desired benefit outweighs the risk. For patients with mild (Child-Pugh class A) or moderate (Child-Pugh class B) hepatic impairment, a dose reduction is recommended [see Dosage and Administration (2.2) and Clinical Pharmacology (12.3)].

For patients with SEGA and mild or moderate hepatic impairment, adjust the dose of AFINITOR Tablets or AFINITOR DISPERZ based on therapeutic drug monitoring. For patients with SEGA and severe hepatic impairment, reduce the starting dose of AFINITOR Tablets or AFINITOR DISPERZ by approximately 50% and adjust subsequent doses based on therapeutic drug monitoring [see Dosage and Administration (2.4, 2.5)].

5.10 Vaccinations

During AFINITOR treatment, avoid the use of live vaccines and avoid close contact with individuals who have received live vaccines (e.g., intranasal influenza, measles, mumps, rubella, oral polio, BCG, yellow fever, varicella, and TY21a typhoid vaccines).

For pediatric patients with SEGA that do not require immediate treatment, complete the recommended childhood series of live virus vaccinations according to American Council on Immunization Practices (ACIP) guidelines prior to the start of therapy. An accelerated vaccination schedule may be appropriate.

5.11 Embryo-fetal Toxicity

Based on the mechanism of action, AFINITOR can cause fetal harm. Everolimus caused embryo-fetal toxicities in animals at maternal exposures that were lower than human exposures. If this drug is used during pregnancy or if the patient becomes pregnant while taking this drug, the patient should be apprised of the potential hazard to a fetus [see Use in Specific Populations (8.1)].

Advise female patients of reproductive potential to avoid becoming pregnant and to use highly effective contraception while using AFINITOR and for up to 8 weeks after ending treatment [see Use in Specific Populations (8.6)].

6 ADVERSE REACTIONS

The following serious adverse reactions are discussed in greater detail in another section of the label [see Warnings and Precautions (5)]:

- Non-infectious pneumonitis [see Warnings and Precautions (5.1)].
- Infections [see Warnings and Precautions (5.2)].
- Oral ulceration [see Warnings and Precautions (5.3)].
- Renal failure [see Warnings and Precautions (5.4)].
- Impaired wound healing [see Warnings and Precautions (5.5)].

Because clinical trials are conducted under widely varying conditions, the adverse reaction rates observed cannot be directly compared to rates in other trials and may not reflect the rates observed in clinical practice.

6.1 Clinical Study Experience in Advanced Hormone Receptor-Positive, HER2-Negative Breast Cancer

The efficacy and safety of AFINITOR (10 mg/day) plus exemestane (25 mg/day) (n=485) versus placebo plus exemestane (25 mg/day) (n=239) was evaluated in a randomized, controlled trial in patients with advanced or metastatic hormone receptor-positive, HER2-negative breast cancer. The median age of patients was 61 years (range 28-93 years), and 75% were Caucasian. Safety results are based on a median follow-up of approximately 13 months.

The most common adverse reactions (incidence ≥ 30%) were stomatitis, infections, rash, fatigue, diarrhea, and decreased appetite. The most common Grade 3/4 adverse reactions (incidence ≥ 2%) were stomatitis, infections, hyperglycemia, fatigue, dyspnea, pneumonitis, and diarrhea. The most common laboratory abnormalities (incidence ≥ 50%) were hypercholesterolemia, hyperglycemia, increased aspartate transaminase (AST), anemia, leukopenia, thrombocytopenia, lymphopenia, increased alanine transaminase (ALT), and hypertriglyceridemia. The most common Grade 3/4 laboratory abnormalities (incidence ≥ 3%) were lymphopenia, hyperglycemia, anemia, decreased potassium, increased AST, increased ALT, and thrombocytopenia.

Fatal adverse reactions occurred more frequently in patients who received AFINITOR plus exemestane (2%) compared to patients on the placebo plus exemestane arm (0.4%). The rates of treatment-emergent adverse events resulting in permanent discontinuation were 24% and 5% for the AFINITOR plus exemestane and placebo plus exemestane treatment groups, respectively. Dose adjustments (interruptions or reductions) were more frequent among patients in the AFINITOR plus exemestane arm than in the placebo plus exemestane arm (63% versus 14%).

Table 2 compares the incidence of treatment-emergent adverse reactions reported with an incidence of ≥10% for patients receiving AFINITOR 10 mg daily versus placebo.

[See table 2 at top of previous page]

Key observed laboratory abnormalities are presented in Table 3.

[See table 3 above]

6.2 Clinical Study Experience in Advanced Pancreatic Neuroendocrine Tumors

In a randomized, controlled trial of AFINITOR (n=204) versus placebo (n=203) in patients with advanced PNET the median age of patients was 58 years (range 20-87), 79% were Caucasian, and 55% were male. Patients on the placebo arm could cross over to open-label AFINITOR upon disease progression.

The most common adverse reactions (incidence ≥ 30%) were stomatitis, rash, diarrhea, fatigue, edema, abdominal pain, nausea, fever, and headache. The most common Grade 3-4 adverse reactions (incidence ≥ 5%) were stomatitis and diarrhea. The most common laboratory abnormalities (incidence ≥ 50%) were decreased hemoglobin, hyperglycemia, alkaline phosphatase increased, hypercholesterolemia, bicarbonate decreased, and increased aspartate transaminase (AST). The most common Grade 3-4 laboratory abnormalities (incidence ≥ 3%) were hyperglycemia, lymphopenia, decreased hemoglobin, hypophosphatemia, increased alkaline phosphatase, neutropenia, increased aspartate transaminase (AST), potassium decreased, and thrombocytopenia. Deaths during double-blind treatment where an adverse event was the primary cause occurred in seven patients on AFINITOR and one patient on placebo. Causes of death on the AFINITOR arm included one case of each of the following: acute renal failure, acute respiratory distress, cardiac arrest, death (cause unknown), hepatic failure, pneumonia,

Table 4: Adverse Reactions Reported ≥ 10% of Patients with Advanced PNET

	AFINITOR N=204			Placebo N=203		
	All grades %	Grade 3 %	Grade 4 %	All grades %	Grade 3 %	Grade 4 %
Any adverse reaction	100	49	13	98	32	8
Gastrointestinal disorders						
Stomatitis[a]	70	7	0	20	0	0
Diarrhea[b]	50	5	0.5	25	3	0
Abdominal pain	36	4	0	32	6	1
Nausea	32	2	0	33	2	0
Vomiting	29	1	0	21	2	0
Constipation	14	0	0	13	0.5	0
Dry mouth	11	0	0	4	0	0
General disorders and administration site conditions						
Fatigue/malaise	45	3	0.5	27	2	0.5
Edema (general and peripheral)	39	1	0.5	12	1	0
Fever	31	0.5	0.5	13	0.5	0
Asthenia	19	3	0	20	3	0
Infections and infestations						
Nasopharyngitis/rhinitis/URI	25	0	0	13	0	0
Urinary tract infection	16	0	0	6	0.5	0
Investigations						
Weight decreased	28	0.5	0	11	0	0
Metabolism and nutrition disorders						
Decreased appetite	30	1	0	18	1	0
Diabetes mellitus	10	2	0	0.5	0	0
Musculoskeletal and connective tissue disorders						
Arthralgia	15	1	0.5	7	0.5	0
Back pain	15	1	0	11	1	0
Pain in extremity	14	0.5	0	6	1	0
Muscle spasms	10	0	0	4	0	0
Nervous system disorders						
Headache/migraine	30	0.5	0	15	1	0
Dysgeusia	19	0	0	5	0	0
Dizziness	12	0.5	0	7	0	0
Psychiatric disorders						
Insomnia	14	0	0	8	0	0
Respiratory, thoracic and mediastinal disorders						
Cough/productive cough	25	0.5	0	13	0	0
Epistaxis	22	0	0	1	0	0
Dyspnea/dyspnea exertional	20	2	0.5	7	0.5	0
Pneumonitis[c]	17	3	0.5	0	0	0
Oropharyngeal pain	11	0	0	6	0	0
Skin and subcutaneous disorders						
Rash	59	0.5	0	19	0	0
Nail disorders	22	0.5	0	2	0	0
Pruritus/pruritus generalized	21	0	0	13	0	0
Dry skin/xeroderma	13	0	0	6	0	0
Vascular disorders						
Hypertension	13	1	0	6	1	0
Median duration of treatment (wks)	37			16		

Grading according to CTCAE Version 3.0
[a] Includes stomatitis, aphthous stomatitis, gingival pain/swelling/ulceration, glossitis, glossodynia, lip ulceration, mouth ulceration, tongue ulceration, and mucosal inflammation.
[b] Includes diarrhea, enteritis, enterocolitis, colitis, defecation urgency, and steatorrhea.
[c] Includes pneumonitis, interstitial lung disease, pulmonary fibrosis and restrictive pulmonary disease.

and sepsis. There was one death due to pulmonary embolism on the placebo arm. After cross-over to open-label AFINITOR, there were three additional deaths, one due to hypoglycemia and cardiac arrest in a patient with insulinoma, one due to myocardial infarction with congestive heart failure, and the other due to sudden death. The rates of treatment-emergent adverse events resulting in permanent discontinuation were 20% and 6% for the AFINITOR and placebo treatment groups, respectively. Dose delay or reduction was necessary in 61% of everolimus patients and 29% of placebo patients. Grade 3-4 renal failure occurred in six patients in the everolimus arm and three patients in the placebo arm. Thrombotic events included five patients with pulmonary embolus in the everolimus arm and one in the placebo arm as well as three patients with thrombosis in the everolimus arm and two in the placebo arm.
Table 4 compares the incidence of treatment-emergent adverse reactions reported with an incidence of ≥ 10% for patients receiving AFINITOR 10 mg daily versus placebo.
[See table 4 above]
In female patients aged 18 to 55 years, irregular menstruation occurred in 5 of 46 (11%) AFINITOR-treated females and none of the 33 females in the placebo group.
Key observed laboratory abnormalities are presented in Table 5.
[See table 5 at top of next page]

6.3 Clinical Study Experience in Advanced Renal Cell Carcinoma

The data described below reflect exposure to AFINITOR (n=274) and placebo (n=137) in a randomized, controlled trial in patients with metastatic renal cell carcinoma who received prior treatment with sunitinib and/or sorafenib. The median age of patients was 61 years (range 27-85), 88% were Caucasian, and 78% were male. The median duration of blinded study treatment was 141 days (range 19-451 days) for patients receiving AFINITOR and 60 days (range 21-295 days) for those receiving placebo.
The most common adverse reactions (incidence ≥ 30%) were stomatitis, infections, asthenia, fatigue, cough, and diarrhea. The most common Grade 3-4 adverse reactions (incidence ≥ 3%) were infections, dyspnea, fatigue, stomatitis, dehydration, pneumonitis, abdominal pain, and asthenia. The most common laboratory abnormalities (incidence ≥ 50%) were anemia, hypercholesterolemia, hypertriglyceridemia, hyperglycemia, lymphopenia, and increased creatinine. The most common Grade 3-4 laboratory abnormalities (incidence ≥ 3%) were lymphopenia, hyperglycemia, anemia, hypophosphatemia, and hypercholesterolemia. Deaths due to acute respiratory failure (0.7%), infection (0.7%), and acute renal failure (0.4%) were observed on the AFINITOR arm but none on the placebo arm. The rates of treatment-emergent adverse events (irrespective of causality) resulting in permanent discontinuation were 14% and 3% for the AFINITOR and placebo treatment groups, respectively. The most common adverse reactions (irrespective of causality) leading to treatment discontinuation were pneumonitis and dyspnea. Infections, stomatitis, and pneumonitis were the most common reasons for treatment delay or dose reduction. The most common medical interventions required during AFINITOR treatment were for infections, anemia, and stomatitis.
Table 6 compares the incidence of treatment-emergent adverse reactions reported with an incidence of ≥ 10% for patients receiving AFINITOR 10 mg daily versus placebo. Within each MedDRA system organ class, the adverse reactions are presented in order of decreasing frequency.
[See table 6 at top of next page]
Other notable adverse reactions occurring more frequently with AFINITOR than with placebo, but with an incidence of < 10% include:
Gastrointestinal disorders: Abdominal pain (9%), dry mouth (8%), hemorrhoids (5%), dysphagia (4%)
General disorders and administration site conditions: Weight decreased (9%), chest pain (5%), chills (4%), impaired wound healing (< 1%)
Respiratory, thoracic and mediastinal disorders: Pleural effusion (7%), pharyngolaryngeal pain (4%), rhinorrhea (3%)
Skin and subcutaneous tissue disorders: Hand-foot syndrome (reported as palmar-plantar erythrodysesthesia syndrome) (5%), nail disorder (5%), erythema (4%), onychoclasis (4%), skin lesion (4%), acneiform dermatitis (3%)
Metabolism and nutrition disorders: Exacerbation of pre-existing diabetes mellitus (2%), new onset of diabetes mellitus (< 1%)
Psychiatric disorders: Insomnia (9%)
Nervous system disorders: Dizziness (7%), paresthesia (5%)
Eye disorders: Eyelid edema (4%), conjunctivitis (2%)
Vascular disorders: Hypertension (4%), deep vein thrombosis (< 1%)
Renal and urinary disorders: Renal failure (3%)
Cardiac disorders: Tachycardia (3%), congestive cardiac failure (1%)
Musculoskeletal and connective tissue disorders: Jaw pain (3%)
Hematologic disorders: Hemorrhage (3%)
Key laboratory abnormalities are presented in Table 7.
[See table 7 at top of page 1808]

6.4 Clinical Study Experience in Renal Angiomyolipoma with Tuberous Sclerosis Complex

The data described below are based on a randomized (2:1), double-blind, placebo-controlled trial of AFINITOR in 118 patients with renal angiomyolipoma as a feature of TSC (n=113) or sporadic lymphangioleiomyomatosis (n=5). The median age of patients was 31 years (range 18 to 61 years), 89% were Caucasian, and 34% were male. The median duration of blinded study treatment was 48 weeks (range 2 to 115 weeks) for patients receiving AFINITOR and 45 weeks (range 9 to 115 weeks) for those receiving placebo.
The most common adverse reaction reported for AFINITOR (incidence ≥ 30%) was stomatitis. The most common Grade 3-4 adverse reactions (incidence ≥ 2%) were stomatitis and amenorrhea. The most common laboratory abnormalities (incidence ≥ 50%) were hypercholesterolemia, hypertriglyceridemia, and anemia. The most common Grade 3-4 laboratory abnormality (incidence ≥ 3%) was hypophosphatemia. The rate of adverse reactions resulting in permanent discontinuation was 3.8% in the AFINITOR-treated patients. Adverse reactions leading to permanent discontinuation in the AFINITOR arm were hypersensitivity/angioedema/bronchospasm, convulsion, and hypophosphatemia. Dose adjustments (interruptions or reductions) due to adverse reactions occurred in 52% of AFINITOR-treated patients. The most common adverse reaction leading to AFINITOR dose adjustment was stomatitis.
Table 8 compares the incidence of adverse reactions reported with an incidence of ≥ 10% for patients receiving AFINITOR and occurring more frequently with AFINITOR than with placebo. Laboratory abnormalities are described separately in Table 9.
[See table 8 at top of page 1808]
Amenorrhea occurred in 15% of AFINITOR-treated females (8 of 52) and 4% (1 of 26) of females in the placebo group. Other adverse reactions involving the female reproductive system were menorrhagia (10%), menstrual irregularities (10%), and vaginal hemorrhage (8%).
The following additional adverse reactions occurred in less than 10% of Afinitor-treated patients: epistaxis (9%), decreased appetite (6%), otitis media (6%), depression (5%), abnormal taste (5%), increased blood luteinizing hormone (LH) levels (4%), increased blood follicle stimulating hormone (FSH) levels (3%), hypersensitivity (3%), and pneumonitis (1%).
[See table 9 at top of page 1808]

6.5 Clinical Study Experience in Subependymal Giant Cell Astrocytoma with Tuberous Sclerosis Complex

The data described below are based on a randomized (2:1), double-blind, placebo-controlled trial (Study 1) of AFINITOR in 117 patients with subependymal giant cell astrocytoma (SEGA) and tuberous sclerosis complex (TSC). The median age of patients was 9.5 years (range 0.8 to 26 years), 93% were Caucasian, and 57% were male. The median duration of blinded study treatment was 52 weeks (range 24 to 89 weeks) for patients receiving AFINITOR and 47 weeks (range 14 to 88 weeks) for those receiving placebo.
The most common adverse reactions reported for AFINITOR (incidence ≥ 30%) were stomatitis and respiratory tract infection. The most common Grade 3-4 adverse

reactions (incidence ≥ 2%) were stomatitis, pyrexia, pneumonia, gastroenteritis, aggression, agitation, and amenorrhea. The most common key laboratory abnormalities (incidence ≥ 50%) were hypercholesterolemia and elevated partial thromboplastin time. The most common Grade 3-4 laboratory abnormality (incidence ≥ 3%) was neutropenia. There were no adverse reactions resulting in permanent discontinuation. Dose adjustments (interruptions or reductions) due to adverse reactions occurred in 55% of AFINITOR-treated patients. The most common adverse reaction leading to AFINITOR dose adjustment was stomatitis.

Table 10 compares the incidence of adverse reactions reported with an incidence of ≥ 10% for patients receiving AFINITOR and occurring more frequently with AFINITOR than with placebo. Laboratory abnormalities are described separately in Table 11.

[See table 10 at top of page 1809]

Amenorrhea occurred in 17% of AFINITOR-treated females aged 10 to 55 years (3 of 18) and none of the females in the placebo group. For this same group of AFINITOR-treated females, the following menstrual abnormalities were reported: dysmenorrhea (6%), menorrhagia (6%), metrorrhagia (6%), and unspecified menstrual irregularity (6%).

The following additional adverse reactions occurred in less than 10% of AFINITOR-treated patients: nausea (8%), pain in extremity (8%), insomnia (6%), pneumonia (6%), epistaxis (5%), hypersensitivity (3%), increased blood luteinizing hormone (LH) levels (1%) and pneumonitis (1%).

[See table 11 at top of page 1809]

Longer-term follow-up of 34.2 months (range 4.7 to 47.1 months) from a non-randomized, open-label, 28-patient trial resulted in the following additional notable adverse reactions and key laboratory abnormalities: cellulitis (29%), hyperglycemia (25%), and elevated creatinine (14%).

6.6 Postmarketing Experience

The following adverse reactions have been identified during post approval use of AFINITOR. Because these reactions are reported voluntarily from a population of uncertain size, it is not always possible to reliably estimate frequency or establish a causal relationship to drug exposure: acute pancreatitis, cholecystitis, cholelithiasis, arterial thrombotic events and reflex sympathetic dystrophy.

7 DRUG INTERACTIONS

Everolimus is a substrate of CYP3A4, and also a substrate and moderate inhibitor of the multidrug efflux pump PgP. *In vitro*, everolimus is a competitive inhibitor of CYP3A4 and a mixed inhibitor of CYP2D6.

7.1 Agents That May Increase Everolimus Blood Concentrations

CYP3A4 Inhibitors and PgP Inhibitors

In healthy subjects, compared to AFINITOR treatment alone there were significant increases in everolimus exposure when AFINITOR was coadministered with:

- ketoconazole (a strong CYP3A4 inhibitor and a PgP inhibitor) - C_{max} and AUC increased by 3.9- and 15.0-fold, respectively.
- erythromycin (a moderate CYP3A4 inhibitor and a PgP inhibitor) - C_{max} and AUC increased by 2.0- and 4.4-fold, respectively.
- verapamil (a moderate CYP3A4 inhibitor and a PgP inhibitor) - C_{max} and AUC increased by 2.3- and 3.5-fold, respectively.

Concomitant strong inhibitors of CYP3A4/PgP should not be used [see Dosage and Administration (2.2, 2.5) and Warnings and Precautions (5.8)].

Use caution when AFINITOR is used in combination with moderate CYP3A4/PgP inhibitors. If alternative treatment cannot be administered reduce the AFINITOR dose [see Dosage and Administration (2.2, 2.5) and Warnings and Precautions (5.8)].

7.2 Agents That May Decrease Everolimus Blood Concentrations

CYP3A4/PgP Inducers

In healthy subjects, co-administration of AFINITOR with rifampin, a strong inducer of CYP3A4 and an inducer of PgP, decreased everolimus AUC and C_{max} by 63% and 58% respectively, compared to everolimus treatment alone. Consider a dose increase of AFINITOR when co-administered with strong CYP3A4/PgP inducers if alternative treatment cannot be administered. St. John's Wort may decrease everolimus exposure unpredictably and should be avoided [see Dosage and Administration (2.2, 2.5)].

7.3 Drugs That May Have Their Plasma Concentrations Altered by Everolimus

Studies in healthy subjects indicate that there are no clinically significant pharmacokinetic interactions between AFINITOR and the HMG-CoA reductase inhibitors atorvastatin (a CYP3A4 substrate) and pravastatin (a non-CYP3A4 substrate) and population pharmacokinetic analyses also detected no influence of simvastatin (a CYP3A4 substrate) on the clearance of AFINITOR.

A study in healthy subjects demonstrated that co-administration of an oral dose of midazolam (sensitive CYP3A4 substrate) with everolimus resulted in a 25% increase in midazolam C_{max} and a 30% increase in midazolam $AUC_{(0-inf)}$.

Coadministration of everolimus and exemestane increased exemestane C_{min} by 45% and C_{2h} by 64%. However, the corresponding estradiol levels at steady state (4 weeks) were not different between the 2 treatment arms. No increase in adverse events related to exemestane was observed in patients with hormone receptor-positive, HER2-negative advanced breast cancer receiving the combination.

Coadmiministration of everolimus and depot octreotide increased octreotide C_{min} by approximately 50%.

8 USE IN SPECIFIC POPULATIONS

8.1 Pregnancy

Pregnancy Category D

Risk Summary

Based on the mechanism of action, AFINITOR can cause fetal harm when administered to a pregnant woman. Everolimus caused embryo-fetal toxicities in animals at maternal exposures that were lower than human exposures. If this drug is used during pregnancy or if the patient becomes

Table 5: Key Laboratory Abnormalities Reported in ≥ 10% of Patients with Advanced PNET

Laboratory parameter	AFINITOR N=204		Placebo N=203	
	All grades %	Grade 3-4 %	All grades %	Grade 3-4 %
Hematology				
Hemoglobin decreased	86	15	63	1
Lymphocytes decreased	45	16	22	4
Platelets decreased	45	3	11	0
WBC decreased	43	2	13	0
Neutrophils decreased	30	4	17	2
Clinical chemistry				
Alkaline phosphatase increased	74	8	66	8
Glucose (fasting) increased	75	17	53	6
Cholesterol increased	66	0.5	22	0
Bicarbonate decreased	56	0	40	0
Aspartate transaminase (AST) increased	56	4	41	4
Alanine transaminase (ALT) increased	48	2	35	2
Phosphate decreased	40	10	14	3
Triglycerides increased	39	0	10	0
Calcium decreased	37	0.5	12	0
Potassium decreased	23	4	5	0
Creatinine increased	19	2	14	0
Sodium decreased	16	1	16	1
Albumin decreased	13	1	8	0
Bilirubin increased	10	1	14	2
Potassium increased	7	0	10	0.5

Grading according to CTCAE Version 3.0

Table 6: Adverse Reactions Reported in at Least 10% of Patients with RCC and at a Higher Rate in the AFINITOR Arm than in the Placebo Arm

	AFINITOR 10 mg/day N=274			Placebo N=137		
	All grades %	Grade 3 %	Grade 4 %	All grades %	Grade 3 %	Grade 4 %
Any adverse reaction	97	52	13	93	23	5
Gastrointestinal disorders						
Stomatitis[a]	44	4	<1	8	0	0
Diarrhea	30	1	0	7	0	0
Nausea	26	1	0	19	0	0
Vomiting	20	2	0	12	0	0
Infections and infestations[b]	37	7	3	18	1	0
General disorders and administration site conditions						
Asthenia	33	3	<1	23	4	0
Fatigue	31	5	0	27	3	<1
Edema peripheral	25	<1	0	8	<1	0
Pyrexia	20	<1	0	9	0	0
Mucosal inflammation	19	1	0	1	0	0
Respiratory, thoracic and mediastinal disorders						
Cough	30	<1	0	16	0	0
Dyspnea	24	6	1	15	3	0
Epistaxis	18	0	0	0	0	0
Pneumonitis[c]	14	4	0	0	0	0
Skin and subcutaneous tissue disorders						
Rash	29	1	0	7	0	0
Pruritus	14	<1	0	7	0	0
Dry skin	13	<1	0	5	0	0
Metabolism and nutrition disorders						
Anorexia	25	1	0	14	<1	0
Nervous system disorders						
Headache	19	<1	<1	9	<1	0
Dysgeusia	10	0	0	2	0	0
Musculoskeletal and connective tissue disorders						
Pain in extremity	10	1	0	7	0	0
Median duration of treatment (d)	141			60		

Grading according to CTCAE Version 3.0
[a] Stomatitis (including aphthous stomatitis), and mouth and tongue ulceration.
[b] Includes all preferred terms within the 'infections and infestations' system organ class, the most common being nasopharyngitis (6%), pneumonia (6%), urinary tract infection (5%), bronchitis (4%), and sinusitis (3%), and also including aspergillosis (<1%), candidiasis (<1%), and sepsis (<1%).
[c] Includes pneumonitis, interstitial lung disease, lung infiltration, pulmonary alveolar hemorrhage, pulmonary toxicity, and alveolitis.

pregnant while taking the drug, apprise the patient of the potential hazard to the fetus [see Warnings and Precautions (5.11)].

Animal Data

In animal reproductive studies, oral administration of everolimus to female rats before mating and through organogenesis induced embryo-fetal toxicities, including increased resorption, pre-implantation and post-implantation loss, decreased numbers of live fetuses, malformation (e.g., sternal cleft), and retarded skeletal development. These effects occurred in the absence of maternal toxicities. Embryofetal toxicities in rats occurred at doses ≥ 0.1 mg/kg (0.6 mg/m²) with resulting exposures of approximately 4% of the exposure (AUC_{0-24h}) achieved in patients receiving the 10 mg daily dose of everolimus. In rabbits, embryotoxicity evident as an increase in resorptions occurred at an oral dose of 0.8 mg/kg (9.6 mg/m²), approximately 1.6 times either the 10 mg daily dose or the median dose administered to SEGA patients on a body surface area basis. The effect in rabbits occurred in the presence of maternal toxicities.

In a pre- and post-natal development study in rats, animals were dosed from implantation through lactation. At the dose of 0.1 mg/kg (0.6 mg/m²), there were no adverse effects on delivery and lactation or signs of maternal toxicity; however, there were reductions in body weight (up to 9% reduction from the control) and in survival of offspring (~5% died or missing). There were no drug-related effects on the developmental parameters (morphological development, motor activity, learning, or fertility assessment) in the offspring.

8.3   Nursing Mothers

It is not known whether everolimus is excreted in human milk. Everolimus and/or its metabolites passed into the milk of lactating rats at a concentration 3.5 times higher than in maternal serum. Because many drugs are excreted in human milk and because of the potential for serious adverse reactions in nursing infants from everolimus, a decision should be made whether to discontinue nursing or to discontinue the drug, taking into account the importance of the drug to the mother.

8.4   Pediatric Use

Pediatric use of AFINITOR Tablets and AFINITOR DISPERZ is recommended for patients 1 year of age and older with TSC for the treatment of SEGA that requires therapeutic intervention but cannot be curatively resected. The safety and effectiveness of AFINITOR Tablets and AFINITOR DISPERZ have not been established in pediatric patients with renal angiomyolipoma with TSC in the absence of SEGA.

The effectiveness of AFINITOR in pediatric patients with SEGA was demonstrated in two clinical trials based on demonstration of durable objective response, as evidenced by reduction in SEGA tumor volume [see Clinical Studies (14.5)]. Improvement in disease-related symptoms and overall survival in pediatric patients with SEGA has not been demonstrated. The long term effects of AFINITOR on growth and pubertal development are unknown.

Study 1 was a randomized, double-blind, multicenter trial comparing AFINITOR (n=78) to placebo (n=39) in pediatric and adult patients. The median age was 9.5 years (range 0.8 to 26 years). At the time of randomization, a total of 20 patients were < 3 years of age, 54 patients were 3 to < 12 years of age, 27 patients were 12 to < 18 years of age, and 16 patients were ≥ 18 years of age. The overall nature, type, and frequency of adverse reactions across the age groups evaluated were similar, with the exception of a higher per patient incidence of infectious serious adverse events in patients < 3 years of age. A total of 6 of 13 patients (46%) < 3 years of age had at least 1 serious adverse event due to infection, compared to 2 of 7 patients (29%) treated with placebo. No patient in any age group discontinued AFINITOR due to infection [see Adverse Reactions (6.5)]. Subgroup analyses showed reduction in SEGA volume with AFINITOR treatment in all pediatric age subgroups.

Study 2 was an open-label, single-arm, single-center trial of AFINITOR (N=28) in patients aged ≥ 3 years; median age was 11 years (range 3 to 34 years). A total of 16 patients were 3 to < 12 years, 6 patients were 12 to < 18 years, and 6 patients were ≥ 18 years. The frequency of adverse reactions across the age groups was generally similar [see Adverse Reactions (6.5)]. Subgroup analyses showed reductions in SEGA volume with AFINITOR treatment in all pediatric age subgroups.

Everolimus clearance normalized to body surface area was higher in pediatric patients than in adults with SEGA [see Clinical Pharmacology (12.3)]. The recommended starting dose and subsequent requirement for therapeutic drug monitoring to achieve and maintain trough concentrations of 5 to 15 ng/mL are the same for adult and pediatric patients with SEGA [see Dosage and Administration (2.3, 2.4)].

8.5   Geriatric Use

In the randomized advanced hormone receptor positive, HER2-negative breast cancer study, 40% of AFINITOR-treated patients were ≥ 65 years of age, while 15% were 75

years and over. No overall differences in effectiveness were observed between elderly and younger patients. The incidence of deaths due to any cause within 28 days of the last AFINITOR dose was 6% in patients ≥ 65 years of age compared to 2% in patients < 65 years of age. Adverse reactions leading to permanent treatment discontinuation occurred in 33% of patients ≥ 65 years of age compared to 17% in patients < 65 years of age [see Warnings and Precautions (5.6)].

In two other randomized trials (advanced renal cell carcinoma and advanced neuroendocrine tumors of pancreatic origin), no overall differences in safety or effectiveness were observed between elderly and younger patients. In the randomized advanced RCC study, 41% of AFINITOR treated patients were ≥ 65 years of age, while 7% were 75 years and over. In the randomized advanced PNET study, 30% of AFINITOR-treated patients were ≥ 65 years of age, while 7% were 75 years and over.

Table 7: Key Laboratory Abnormalities Reported in Patients with RCC at a Higher Rate in the AFINITOR Arm than the Placebo Arm

Laboratory parameter	AFINITOR 10 mg/day N=274			Placebo N=137		
	All grades %	Grade 3 %	Grade 4 %	All grades %	Grade 3 %	Grade 4 %
Hematology[a]						
Hemoglobin decreased	92	12	1	79	5	<1
Lymphocytes decreased	51	16	2	28	5	0
Platelets decreased	23	1	0	2	0	<1
Neutrophils decreased	14	0	<1	4	0	0
Clinical chemistry						
Cholesterol increased	77	4	0	35	0	0
Triglycerides increased	73	<1	0	34	0	0
Glucose increased	57	15	<1	25	1	0
Creatinine increased	50	1	0	34	0	0
Phosphate decreased	37	6	0	8	0	0
Aspartate transaminase (AST) increased	25	<1	<1	7	0	0
Alanine transaminase (ALT) increased	21	1	0	4	0	0
Bilirubin increased	3	<1	<1	2	0	0

Grading according to CTCAE Version 3.0
[a] Reflects corresponding adverse drug reaction reports of anemia, leukopenia, lymphopenia, neutropenia, and thrombocytopenia (collectively pancytopenia), which occurred at lower frequency.

Table 8: Adverse Reactions Reported in ≥ 10% of AFINITOR-treated Patients with Renal Angiomyolipoma

	AFINITOR N=79			Placebo N=39		
	All grades %	Grade 3 %	Grade 4 %	All grades %	Grade 3 %	Grade 4 %
Any adverse reaction	100	25	5	97	8	5
Gastrointestinal disorders						
Stomatitis[a]	78	6	0	23	0	0
Vomiting	15	0	0	5	0	0
Diarrhea	14	0	0	5	0	0
General disorders and administration site conditions						
Peripheral edema	13	0	0	8	0	0
Infections and infestations						
Upper respiratory tract infection	11	0	0	5	0	0
Musculoskeletal and connective tissue disorders						
Arthralgia	13	0	0	5	0	0
Respiratory, thoracic and mediastinal disorders						
Cough	20	0	0	13	0	0
Skin and subcutaneous tissue disorders						
Acne	22	0	0	5	0	0

Grading according to CTCAE Version 3.0
[a] Includes stomatitis, aphthous stomatitis, mouth ulceration, gingival pain, glossitis, and glossodynia.

Table 9: Key Laboratory Abnormalities Reported in AFINITOR-treated Patients with Renal Angiomyolipoma

	AFINITOR N=79			Placebo N=39		
	All grades %	Grade 3 %	Grade 4 %	All grades %	Grade 3 %	Grade 4 %
Hematology						
Anemia	61	0	0	49	0	0
Leucopenia	37	0	0	21	0	0
Neutropenia	25	0	1	26	0	0
Lymphopenia	20	1	0	8	0	0
Thrombocytopenia	19	0	0	3	0	0
Clinical chemistry						
Hypercholesterolemia	85	1	0	46	0	0
Hypertriglyceridemia	52	0	0	10	0	0
Hypophosphatemia	49	5	0	15	0	0
Alkaline phosphatase increased	32	1	0	10	0	0
Elevated aspartate transaminase (AST)	23	1	0	8	0	0
Elevated alanine transaminase (ALT)	20	1	0	15	0	0
Fasting hyperglycemia	14	0	0	8	0	0

Grading according to CTCAE Version 3.0

Other reported clinical experience has not identified differences in response between the elderly and younger patients, but greater sensitivity of some older individuals cannot be ruled out *[see Clinical Pharmacology (12.3)]*.

No dosage adjustment in initial dosing is required in elderly patients, but close monitoring and appropriate dose adjustments for adverse reactions is recommended *[see Dosage and Administration (2.2), Clinical Pharmacology (12.3)]*.

8.6 Females and Males of Reproductive Potential
Contraception
Females

AFINITOR can cause fetal harm when administered to a pregnant woman. Advise female patients of reproductive potential to use highly effective contraception while receiving AFINITOR and for up to 8 weeks after ending treatment *[see Use in Specific Populations (8.1)]*.

Infertility
Females

Menstrual irregularities, secondary amenorrhea, and increases in luteinizing hormone (LH) and follicle stimulating hormone (FSH) occurred in female patients taking AFINITOR. Based on these clinical findings and findings in animals, female fertility may be compromised by treatment with AFINITOR *[see Adverse Reactions (6.2, 6.4, 6.5) and Nonclinical Toxicology (13.1)]*.

Males

AFINITOR treatment may impair fertility in male patients based on animal findings *[see Nonclinical Toxicology (13.1)]*.

8.7 Renal Impairment

No clinical studies were conducted with AFINITOR in patients with decreased renal function. Renal impairment is not expected to influence drug exposure and no dosage adjustment of everolimus is recommended in patients with renal impairment *[see Clinical Pharmacology (12.3)]*.

8.8 Hepatic Impairment

The safety, tolerability and pharmacokinetics of AFINITOR were evaluated in a 34 subject single oral dose study of everolimus in subjects with impaired hepatic function relative to subjects with normal hepatic function. Exposure was increased in patients with mild (Child-Pugh class A), moderate (Child-Pugh class B), and severe (Child-Pugh class C) hepatic impairment *[see Clinical Pharmacology (12.3)]*.

For advanced HR+ BC, advanced PNET, advanced RCC, and renal angiomyolipoma with TSC patients with severe hepatic impairment, AFINITOR may be used at a reduced dose if the desired benefit outweighs the risk. For patients with mild (Child-Pugh class A) or moderate (Child-Pugh class B) hepatic impairment, a dose reduction is recommended *[see Dosage and Administration (2.2)]*.

For patients with SEGA who have severe hepatic impairment (Child-Pugh class C), reduce the starting dose of AFINITOR Tablets or AFINITOR DISPERZ by approximately 50%. For patients with SEGA who have mild (Child-Pugh class A) or moderate (Child-Pugh class B) hepatic impairment, adjustment to the starting dose may not be needed. Subsequent dosing should be based on therapeutic drug monitoring *[see Dosage and Administration (2.4, 2.5)]*.

10 OVERDOSAGE

In animal studies, everolimus showed a low acute toxic potential. No lethality or severe toxicity was observed in either mice or rats given single oral doses of 2000 mg/kg (limit test).

Reported experience with overdose in humans is very limited. Single doses of up to 70 mg have been administered. The acute toxicity profile observed with the 70 mg dose was consistent with that for the 10 mg dose.

11 DESCRIPTION

AFINITOR (everolimus), an inhibitor of mammalian target of rapamycin (mTOR), an antineoplastic agent.

The chemical name of everolimus is (1R,9S,12S, 15R,16E,18R,19R,21R,23S,24E,26E,28E,30S,32S,35R)-1, 18- dihydroxy-12-[(1R)-2-[(1S,3R,4R)-4-(2-hydroxyethoxy)-3-methoxycyclohexyl]-1-methylethyl]-19,30-dimethoxy-15,17,21,23,29,35-hexamethyl-11,36-dioxa-4-aza-tricyclo[30. 3.1.0⁴,⁹]hexatriaconta-16,24,26,28-tetraene-2,3,10,14,20-pentaone.

The molecular formula is $C_{53}H_{83}NO_{14}$ and the molecular weight is 958.2. The structural formula is:

[See chemical structure at top of next column]

AFINITOR Tablets are supplied for oral administration and contain 2.5 mg, 5 mg, 7.5 mg, or 10 mg of everolimus. The tablets also contain anhydrous lactose, butylated hydroxytoluene, crospovidone, hypromellose, lactose monohydrate, and magnesium stearate as inactive ingredients.

AFINITOR DISPERZ (everolimus tablets for oral suspension) is supplied for oral administration and contains 2 mg, 3 mg, or 5 mg of everolimus. The tablets for oral suspension also contain butylated hydroxytoluene, colloidal silicon dioxide, crospovidone, hypromellose, lactose monohydrate, magnesium stearate, mannitol, and microcrystalline cellulose as inactive ingredients.

Table 10: Adverse Reactions Reported in ≥10% of AFINITOR-treated Patients with SEGA in Study 1

	AFINITOR N=78			Placebo N=39		
	All grades %	Grade 3 %	Grade 4 %	All grades %	Grade 3 %	Grade 4 %
Any adverse reaction	97	36	3	92	23	3
Gastrointestinal disorders						
Stomatitis[a]	62	9	0	26	3	0
Vomiting	22	1	0	13	0	0
Diarrhea	17	0	0	5	0	0
Constipation	10	0	0	3	0	0
Infections and infestations						
Respiratory tract infection[b]	31	1	1	23	0	0
Gastroenteritis[c]	10	4	1	3	0	0
Pharyngitis streptococcal	10	0	0	3	0	0
General disorders and administration site conditions						
Pyrexia	23	6	0	18	3	0
Fatigue	14	0	0	3	0	0
Psychiatric disorders						
Anxiety, aggression or other behavioral disturbance[d]	21	5	0	3	0	0
Skin and subcutaneous tissue disorders						
Rash[e]	21	0	0	8	0	0
Acne	10	0	0	5	0	0

Grading according to CTCAE Version 3.0
[a] Includes mouth ulceration, stomatitis, and lip ulceration
[b] Includes respiratory tract infection, upper respiratory tract infection, and respiratory tract infection viral
[c] Includes gastroenteritis, gastroenteritis viral, and gastrointestinal infection
[d] Includes agitation, anxiety, panic attack, aggression, abnormal behavior, and obsessive compulsive disorder
[e] Includes rash, rash generalized, rash macular, rash maculo-papular, rash papular, dermatitis allergic, and urticaria

Table 11: Key Laboratory Abnormalities Reported in AFINITOR-treated Patients with SEGA in Study 1

	AFINITOR N=78			Placebo N=39		
	All grades %	Grade 3 %	Grade 4 %	All grades %	Grade 3 %	Grade 4 %
Hematology						
Elevated partial thromboplastin time	72	3	0	44	5	0
Neutropenia	46	9	0	41	3	0
Anemia	41	0	0	21	0	0
Clinical chemistry						
Hypercholesterolemia	81	0	0	39	0	0
Elevated aspartate transaminase (AST)	33	0	0	0	0	0
Hypertriglyceridemia	27	0	0	15	0	0
Elevated alanine transaminase (ALT)	18	0	0	3	0	0
Hypophosphatemia	9	1	0	3	0	0

Grading according to CTCAE Version 3.0

12 CLINICAL PHARMACOLOGY

12.1 Mechanism of Action

Everolimus is an inhibitor of mammalian target of rapamycin (mTOR), a serine-threonine kinase, downstream of the PI3K/AKT pathway. The mTOR pathway is dysregulated in several human cancers. Everolimus binds to an intracellular protein, FKBP-12, resulting in an inhibitory complex formation with mTOR complex 1 (mTORC1) and thus inhibition of mTOR kinase activity. Everolimus reduced the activity of S6 ribosomal protein kinase (S6K1) and eukaryotic elongation factor 4E-binding protein (4E-BP1), downstream effectors of mTOR, involved in protein synthesis. S6K1 is a substrate of mTORC1 and phosphorylates the activation domain 1 of the estrogen receptor which results in ligand-independent activation of the receptor. In addition, everolimus inhibited the expression of hypoxia-inducible factor (e.g., HIF-1) and reduced the expression of vascular endothelial growth factor (VEGF). Inhibition of mTOR by everolimus has been shown to reduce cell proliferation, angiogenesis, and glucose uptake in *in vitro* and/or *in vivo* studies.

Constitutive activation of the PI3K/Akt/mTOR pathway can contribute to endocrine resistance in breast cancer. *In vitro* studies show that estrogen-dependent and HER2+ breast cancer cells are sensitive to the inhibitory effects of everolimus, and that combination treatment with everolimus and Akt, HER2, or aromatase inhibitors enhances the anti-tumor activity of everolimus in a synergistic manner.

Two regulators of mTORC1 signaling are the oncogene suppressors tuberin-sclerosis complexes 1 and 2 (*TSC1, TSC2*). Loss or inactivation of either *TSC1* or *TSC2* leads to activation of downstream signaling. In TSC, a genetic disorder, inactivating mutations in either the *TSC1* or the *TSC2* gene lead to hamartoma formation throughout the body.

12.2 Pharmacodynamics
Exposure Response Relationships

Markers of protein synthesis show that inhibition of mTOR is complete after a 10 mg daily dose.

In patients with SEGA, higher everolimus trough concentrations appear to be associated with larger reductions in SEGA volume. However, as responses have been observed at trough concentrations as low as 5 ng/mL, once acceptable efficacy has been achieved, additional dose increase may not be necessary.

12.3 Pharmacokinetics
Absorption

After administration of AFINITOR tablets in patients with advanced solid tumors, peak everolimus concentrations are reached 1 to 2 hours after administration of oral doses ranging from 5 mg to 70 mg. Following single doses, C_{max} is dose-proportional with daily dosing between 5 mg and 10 mg. With single doses of 20 mg and higher, the increase in C_{max} is less than dose-proportional, however AUC shows dose-proportionality over the 5 mg to 70 mg dose range. Steady-state was achieved within 2 weeks following once-daily dosing.

Dose Proportionality in Patients with SEGA and TSC: In patients with SEGA and TSC, everolimus C_{min} was approximately dose-proportional within the dose range from 1.35 mg/m² to 14.4 mg/m².

Table 12: Progression-free Survival Results

Analysis	AFINITOR + exemestane[a] N = 485	Placebo + exemestane[a] N = 239	Hazard ratio	P-value
Median progression-free survival (months, 95% CI)				
Investigator radiological review	7.8 (6.9 to 8.5)	3.2 (2.8 to 4.1)	0.45[b] (0.38 to 0.54)	<0.0001[c]
Independent radiological review	11.0 (9.7 to 15.0)	4.1 (2.9 to 5.6)	0.38[b] (0.3 to 0.5)	<0.0001[c]
Best overall response (%, 95% CI)				
Objective response rate (ORR)[d]	12.6% (9.8 to 15.9)	1.7% (0.5 to 4.2)	n/a[e]	

[a] Exemestane (25 mg/day)
[b] Hazard ratio is obtained from the stratified Cox proportional-hazards model by sensitivity to prior hormonal therapy and presence of visceral metastasis
[c] p-value is obtained from the one-sided log-rank test stratified by sensitivity to prior hormonal therapy and presence of visceral metastasis
[d] Objective response rate = proportion of patients with CR or PR
[e] not applicable

Food effect: In healthy subjects, high-fat meals reduced systemic exposure to AFINITOR 10 mg tablet (as measured by AUC) by 22% and the peak blood concentration C_{max} by 54%. Light-fat meals reduced AUC by 32% and C_{max} by 42%. Food, however, had no apparent effect on the post absorption phase concentration-time profile.

Relative bioavailability of AFINITOR DISPERZ (everolimus tablets for oral suspension): The $AUC_{0-\infty}$ of AFINITOR DISPERZ was equivalent to that of AFINITOR Tablets; the C_{max} of this dosage form was 20%-36% lower than that of AFINITOR Tablets. The predicted trough concentrations at steady-state were similar after daily administration.

Distribution
The blood-to-plasma ratio of everolimus, which is concentration-dependent over the range of 5 to 5000 ng/mL, is 17% to 73%. The amount of everolimus confined to the plasma is approximately 20% at blood concentrations observed in cancer patients given AFINITOR 10 mg/day. Plasma protein binding is approximately 74% both in healthy subjects and in patients with moderate hepatic impairment.

Metabolism
Everolimus is a substrate of CYP3A4 and PgP. Following oral administration, everolimus is the main circulating component in human blood. Six main metabolites of everolimus have been detected in human blood, including three mono-hydroxylated metabolites, two hydrolytic ring-opened products, and a phosphatidylcholine conjugate of everolimus. These metabolites were also identified in animal species used in toxicity studies, and showed approximately 100-times less activity than everolimus itself.
In vitro, everolimus competitively inhibited the metabolism of CYP3A4 and was a mixed inhibitor of the CYP2D6 substrate dextromethorphan.

Elimination
No specific elimination studies have been undertaken in cancer patients. Following the administration of a 3 mg single dose of radiolabeled everolimus in patients who were receiving cyclosporine, 80% of the radioactivity was recovered from the feces, while 5% was excreted in the urine. The parent substance was not detected in urine or feces. The mean elimination half-life of everolimus is approximately 30 hours.

Patients with Renal Impairment
Approximately 5% of total radioactivity was excreted in the urine following a 3 mg dose of [14C]-labeled everolimus. In a population pharmacokinetic analysis which included 170 patients with advanced cancer, no significant influence of creatinine clearance (25–178 mL/min) was detected on oral clearance (CL/F) of everolimus *[see Use in Specific Populations (8.7)]*.

Patients with Hepatic Impairment
The safety, tolerability and pharmacokinetics of AFINITOR were evaluated in a single oral dose study of everolimus in subjects with impaired hepatic function relative to subjects with normal hepatic function. Compared to normal subjects (N=13), there was a 1.8-fold, 3.2-fold, and 3.6-fold increase in exposure (i.e. AUC) for subjects with mild (Child-Pugh class A, n=6), moderate (Child-Pugh class B, n=9), and severe (Child-Pugh class C, n=6) hepatic impairment, respectively. In another study, the average AUC of everolimus in eight subjects with moderate hepatic impairment (Child-Pugh class B) was twice that found in eight subjects with normal hepatic function.
For advanced HR+ BC, advanced PNET, advanced RCC, and renal angiomyolipoma with TSC patients with severe

hepatic impairment, AFINITOR may be used at a reduced dose if the desired benefit outweighs the risk. For patients with moderate or mild hepatic impairment, a dose reduction is recommended *[see Dosage and Administration (2.2)]*.
For patients with SEGA and mild or moderate hepatic impairment, adjust the dose of AFINITOR Tablets or AFINITOR DISPERZ based on therapeutic drug monitoring. For patients with SEGA and severe hepatic impairment, reduce the starting dose of AFINITOR Tablets or AFINITOR DISPERZ by approximately 50% and adjust subsequent doses based on therapeutic drug monitoring *[see Dosage and Administration (2.4, 2.5)]*.

Effects of Age and Gender
In a population pharmacokinetic evaluation in cancer patients, no relationship was apparent between oral clearance and patient age or gender.
In patients with SEGA, the geometric mean C_{min} values normalized to mg/m² dose in patients aged < 10 years and 10 to 18 years were lower by 54% and 40%, respectively, than those observed in adults (> 18 years of age), suggesting that everolimus clearance normalized to body surface area was higher in pediatric patients as compared to adults.

Ethnicity
Based on a cross-study comparison, Japanese patients (n=6) had on average exposures that were higher than non-Japanese patients receiving the same dose.
Based on analysis of population pharmacokinetics, oral clearance (CL/F) is on average 20% higher in black patients than in Caucasians.
The significance of these differences on the safety and efficacy of everolimus in Japanese or black patients has not been established.

12.6 QT/QTc Prolongation Potential
In a randomized, placebo-controlled, cross-over study, 59 healthy subjects were administered a single oral dose of AFINITOR (20 mg and 50 mg) and placebo. There is no indication of a QT/QTc prolonging effect of AFINITOR in single doses up to 50 mg.

13 NONCLINICAL TOXICOLOGY
13.1 Carcinogenesis, Mutagenesis, Impairment of Fertility
Administration of everolimus for up to 2 years did not indicate oncogenic potential in mice and rats up to the highest doses tested (0.9 mg/kg) corresponding respectively to 3.9 and 0.2 times the estimated clinical exposure (AUC_{0-24h}) at the 10 mg daily human dose.
Everolimus was not genotoxic in a battery of *in vitro* assays (Ames mutation test in *Salmonella*, mutation test in L5178Y mouse lymphoma cells, and chromosome aberration assay in V79 Chinese hamster cells). Everolimus was not genotoxic in an *in vivo* mouse bone marrow micronucleus test at doses up to 500 mg/kg/day (1500 mg/m²/day, approximately 255-fold the 10 mg daily human dose, and 103-fold the maximum dose administered to patients with SEGA, based on the body surface area), administered as 2 doses, 24 hours apart.
Based on non-clinical findings, male fertility may be compromised by treatment with AFINITOR. In a 13-week male fertility study in rats, testicular morphology was affected at 0.5 mg/kg and above. Sperm motility, sperm count, and plasma testosterone levels were diminished in rats treated with 5 mg/kg. These doses result in exposures which are within the range of therapeutic exposure (52 ng•hr/mL and 414 ng•hr/mL respectively compared to 560 ng•hr/mL human exposure at 10 mg/day), and resulted in infertility in the rats at 5 mg/kg. Effects on male fertility occurred at the

AUC_{0-24h} values below that of therapeutic exposure (approximately 10%-81% of the AUC_{0-24h} in patients receiving the 10 mg daily dose). After a 10-13 week non-treatment period, the fertility index increased from zero (infertility) to 60% (12/20 mated females were pregnant).
Oral doses of everolimus in female rats at ≥0.1 mg/kg (approximately 4% the AUC_{0-24h} in patients receiving the 10 mg daily dose) resulted in increased incidence of pre-implantation loss, suggesting that the drug may reduce female fertility.

13.2 Animal Toxicology and/or Pharmacology
In juvenile rat toxicity studies, dose-related delayed attainment of developmental landmarks including delayed eye-opening, delayed reproductive development in males and females and increased latency time during the learning and memory phases were observed at doses as low as 0.15 mg/kg/day.

14 CLINICAL STUDIES
14.1 Advanced Hormone Receptor-Positive, HER2-Negative Breast Cancer
A randomized, double-blind, multicenter study of AFINITOR plus exemestane versus placebo plus exemestane was conducted in 724 postmenopausal women with estrogen receptor-positive, HER 2/neu-negative advanced breast cancer with recurrence or progression following prior therapy with letrozole or anastrozole. Randomization was stratified by documented sensitivity to prior hormonal therapy (yes versus no) and by the presence of visceral metastasis (yes versus no). Sensitivity to prior hormonal therapy was defined as either (1) documented clinical benefit (complete response [CR], partial response [PR], stable disease ≥ 24 weeks) to at least one prior hormonal therapy in the advanced setting or (2) at least 24 months of adjuvant hormonal therapy prior to recurrence. Patients were permitted to have received 0-1 prior lines of chemotherapy for advanced disease.
The primary endpoint for the trial was progression-free survival (PFS) evaluated by Response Evaluation Criteria In Solid Tumors (RECIST), based on investigator (local radiology) assessment. Other endpoints included overall survival (OS), objective response rate (ORR), and safety.
Patients were randomly allocated in a 2:1 ratio to AFINITOR 10 mg/day plus exemestane 25 mg/day (n = 485) or to placebo plus exemestane 25 mg/day (n = 239). The two treatment groups were generally balanced with respect to baseline demographics and disease characteristics. Patients were not permitted to cross over to AFINITOR at the time of disease progression.
The median progression-free survival by investigator assessment at the time of the final PFS analysis was 7.8 and 3.2 months in the AFINITOR and placebo arms, respectively [HR = 0.45 (95% CI: 0.38, 0.54), one-sided log-rank p < 0.0001] (see Table 12 and Figure 1). The results of the PFS analysis based on independent central radiological assessment were consistent with the investigator assessment. PFS results were also consistent across the subgroups of age, race, presence and extent of visceral metastases, and sensitivity to prior hormonal therapy.
Objective response rate was 12.6% (95% CI: 9.8, 15.9) in the AFINITOR plus exemestane arm versus 1.7% (95% CI: 0.5, 4.2) in the placebo plus exemestane arm. There were 3 complete responses (0.6%) and 58 partial responses (12.0%) in the AFINITOR plus exemestane arm. There were no complete responses and 4 partial responses (1.7%) in the placebo plus exemestane arm.
The overall survival results were not mature at the time of the interim analysis, and no statistically significant treatment-related difference in OS was noted [HR=0.77 (95% CI: 0.57, 1.04)].
[See table 12 above]

Figure 1: Kaplan-Meier Progression-free Survival Curves (Investigator Radiological Review)

14.2 Advanced Neuroendocrine Tumors
Locally Advanced or Metastatic Advanced Pancreatic Neuroendocrine Tumors (PNET)
A randomized, double-blind, multi-center trial of AFINITOR plus best supportive care (BSC) versus placebo plus BSC was conducted in patients with locally advanced or metastatic advanced pancreatic neuroendocrine tumors (PNET) and disease progression within the prior 12 months. Patients were stratified by prior cytotoxic chemotherapy (yes versus no) and by WHO performance status (0 versus 1

and 2). Treatment with somatostatin analogs was allowed as part of BSC. The primary endpoint for the trial was progression-free survival (PFS) evaluated by RECIST (Response Evaluation Criteria in Solid Tumors). After documented radiological progression, patients could be unblinded by the investigator; those randomized to placebo were then able to receive open-label AFINITOR. Other endpoints included safety, objective response rate [ORR (complete response (CR) or partial response (PR)], response duration, and overall survival.

Patients were randomized 1:1 to receive either AFINITOR 10 mg/day (n=207) or placebo (n=203). Demographics were well balanced (median age 58 years, 55% male, 79% Caucasian). Cross-over from placebo to open-label AFINITOR occurred in 73% (148/203) of patients.

The trial demonstrated a statistically significant improvement in PFS (median 11.0 months versus 4.6 months), resulting in a 65% risk reduction in investigator-determined PFS (HR 0.35; 95%CI: 0.27 to 0.45; p<0.001) (see Table 13 and Figure 2). PFS improvement was observed across all patient subgroups, irrespective of prior somatostatin analog use. The PFS results by investigator radiological review, central radiological review and adjudicated radiological review are shown below in Table 13.

[See table 13 above]

Table 13: Progression-free Survival Results

Analysis	N	AFINITOR N=207	Placebo N=203	Hazard Ratio (95%CI)	p-value
	410	Median progression-free survival (months) (95% CI)			
Investigator radiological review		11.0 (8.4 to 13.9)	4.6 (3.1 to 5.4)	0.35 (0.27 to 0.45)	<0.001
Central radiological review		13.7 (11.2 to 18.8)	5.7 (5.4 to 8.3)	0.38 (0.28 to 0.51)	<0.001
Adjudicated radiological review[a]		11.4 (10.8 to 14.8)	5.4 (4.3 to 5.6)	0.34 (0.26 to 0.44)	<0.001

[a] includes adjudication for discrepant assessments between investigator radiological review and central radiological review

Table 14: Efficacy Results by Central Radiologic Review

	AFINITOR N=277	Placebo N=139	Hazard Ratio (95% CI)	p-value [a]
Median Progression-free Survival (95% CI)	4.9 months (4.0 to 5.5)	1.9 months (1.8 to 1.9)	0.33 (0.25 to 0.43)	<0.0001
Objective Response Rate	2%	0%	n/a [b]	n/a [b]

[a] Log-rank test stratified by prognostic score.
[b] Not applicable.

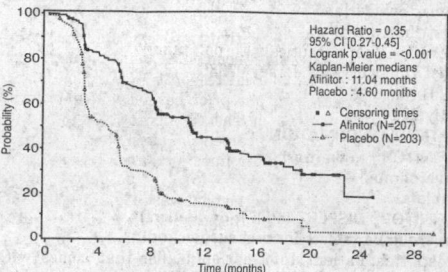

Figure 2: Kaplan-Meier Investigator-Determined Progression-free Survival Curves

Investigator-determined response rate was low (4.8%) in the AFINITOR arm and there were no complete responses. The overall survival results are not yet mature and no statistically significant treatment-related difference in OS was noted [HR=1.05 (95% CI: 0.71 to 1.55)].

Lack of Efficacy in Locally Advanced or Metastatic Functional Carcinoid Tumors

The safety and effectiveness of AFINITOR in patients with locally advanced or metastatic functional carcinoid tumors have not been demonstrated. In a randomized (1:1), double-blind, multi-center trial in 429 patients with carcinoid tumors, AFINITOR plus depot octreotide (Sandostatin LAR®) was compared to placebo plus depot octreotide. After documented radiological progression, patients on the placebo arm could receive AFINITOR; of those randomized to placebo, 143 (67%) patients received open-label AFINITOR plus depot octreotide. The study did not meet its primary efficacy endpoint of a statistically significant improvement in PFS and the final analysis of OS favored the placebo plus depot octreotide arm.

14.3   Advanced Renal Cell Carcinoma

An international, multi-center, randomized, double-blind trial comparing AFINITOR 10 mg daily and placebo, both in conjunction with best supportive care, was conducted in patients with metastatic RCC whose disease had progressed despite prior treatment with sunitinib, sorafenib, or both sequentially. Prior therapy with bevacizumab, interleukin 2, or interferon-α was also permitted. Randomization was stratified according to prognostic score[1] and prior anticancer therapy.

Progression-free survival (PFS), documented using Response Evaluation Criteria in Solid Tumors (RECIST) was assessed via a blinded, independent, central radiologic review. After documented radiological progression, patients could be unblinded by the investigator: those randomized to placebo were then able to receive open-label AFINITOR 10 mg daily.

In total, 416 patients were randomized 2:1 to receive AFINITOR (n=277) or placebo (n=139). Demographics were well balanced between the 2 arms (median age 61 years; 77% male, 88% Caucasian, 74% received prior sunitinib or sorafenib, and 26% received both sequentially).

AFINITOR was superior to placebo for PFS (see Table 14 and Figure 3). The treatment effect was similar across prognostic scores and prior sorafenib and/or sunitinib. Final overall survival (OS) results yield a hazard ratio of 0.90 (95% CI: 0.71 to 1.14), with no statistically significant difference between the 2 treatment groups. Planned cross-over from placebo due to disease progression to open label AFINITOR occurred in 111 of the 139 patients (79.9%) and may have confounded the OS benefit.

[See table 14 above]

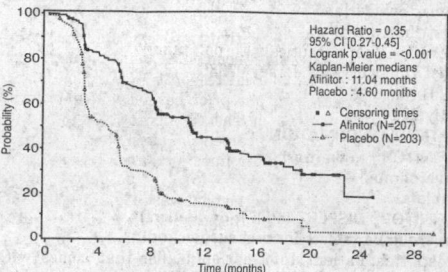

Figure 3: Kaplan-Meier Progression-free Survival Curves

14.4   Renal Angiomyolipoma with Tuberous Sclerosis Complex

A randomized (2:1), double-blind, placebo-controlled trial of AFINITOR was conducted in 118 patients with renal angiomyolipoma as a feature of TSC (n=113) or sporadic lymphangioleiomyomatosis (n=5).

The key eligibility requirements for this trial were at least one angiomyolipoma of ≥ 3 cm in longest diameter on CT/MRI based on local radiology assessment, no immediate indication for surgery, and age ≥ 18 years. Patients received daily oral AFINITOR 10 mg or matching placebo until disease progression or unacceptable toxicity. CT or MRI scans for disease assessment were obtained at baseline, 12, 24, and 48 weeks and annually thereafter. Clinical and photographic assessment of skin lesions were conducted at baseline and every 12 weeks thereafter until treatment discontinuation. The major efficacy outcome measure was angiomyolipoma response rate based on independent central radiology review, which was defined as a ≥ 50% reduction in angiomyolipoma volume, absence of new angiomyolipoma lesion ≥ 1 cm, absence of kidney volume increase ≥ 20%, and no angiomyolipoma related bleeding of ≥ Grade 2. Key supportive efficacy outcome measures were time to angiomyolipoma progression and skin lesion response rate. Analyses of efficacy outcome measures were limited to the blinded treatment period which ended 6 months after the last patient was randomized. The comparative angiomyolipoma response rate analysis was stratified by use of enzyme-inducing antiepileptic drugs (EIAEDs) at randomization (yes versus no).

Of the 118 patients enrolled, 79 were randomized to AFINITOR and 39 to placebo. The median age was 31 years (range 18 to 61 years), 34% were male, and 89% were Caucasian. At baseline, 17% of patients were receiving EIAEDs. On central radiology review at baseline, 92% of patients had at least 1 angiomyolipoma of ≥ 3 cm in longest diameter, 29% had angiomyolipomas ≥ 8 cm, 78% had bilateral angiomyolipomas, and 97% had skin lesions. The median values for the sum of all target renal angiomyolipoma lesions at baseline were 85 cm³ (range 9 to 1612 cm³) and 120 cm³ (range 3 to 4520 cm³) in the AFINITOR and placebo arms respectively. Forty-six (39%) patients had prior renal embolization or nephrectomy. The median duration of follow-up was 8.3 months (range 0.7 to 24.8 months).

The renal angiomyolipoma response rate was statistically significantly higher in AFINITOR-treated patients; there were 33 (41.8%) patients with angiomyolipoma responses in the AFINITOR arm as compared to none in the placebo arm. Results are displayed in Table 15. The median response duration was 5.3+ months (range 2.3+ to 19.6+ months).

Table 15: Angiomyolipoma Response

	AFINITOR N=79	Placebo N=39	p-value
Primary analysis Angiomyolipoma response rate[a] - % 95% CI	41.8 (30.8, 53.4)	0 (0.0, 9.0)	<0.0001

[a] Per independent central radiology review

There were 3 patients in the AFINITOR arm and 8 patients in the placebo arm with documented angiomyolipoma progression by central radiologic review. The time to angiomyolipoma progression was statistically significantly longer in the AFINITOR arm (HR 0.08 [95% CI: 0.02, 0.37]; p <0.0001).

Skin lesion response rates were assessed by local investigators in 77 patients in the AFINITOR arm and 37 patients in the placebo arm with skin lesions at study entry. The skin lesion response rate was statistically significantly higher in the AFINITOR arm (26% versus 0, p=0.0011); all skin lesion responses were partial responses, defined as visual improvement in 50%-99% skin lesions, considering all skin lesions, durable for at least 8 weeks (Physician's Global Assessment of Clinical Condition).

14.5   Subependymal Giant Cell Astrocytoma with Tuberous Sclerosis Complex

Study 1 was a randomized (2:1), double-blind, placebo-controlled trial of AFINITOR Tablets conducted in 117 pediatric and adult patients with subependymal giant cell astrocytoma (SEGA) and tuberous sclerosis complex (TSC). Eligible patients had at least one SEGA lesion ≥ 1.0 cm in longest diameter on MRI based on local radiology assessment and one or more of the following: serial radiological evidence of SEGA growth, a new SEGA lesion ≥ 1 cm in longest diameter, or new or worsening hydrocephalus. Patients randomized to the treatment arm received AFINITOR Tablets at a starting dose of 4.5 mg/m² daily, with subsequent dose adjustments as needed to achieve and maintain everolimus trough concentrations of 5 to 15 ng/mL as tolerated. AFINITOR/matched placebo treatment continued until disease progression or unacceptable toxicity. MRI scans for disease assessment were obtained at baseline, 12, 24, and 48 weeks, and annually thereafter.

The main efficacy outcome measure was SEGA response rate based on independent central radiology review. SEGA response was defined as a ≥ 50% reduction in the sum of SEGA volume relative to baseline, in the absence of unequivocal worsening of non-target SEGA lesions, a new SEGA lesion ≥ 1 cm, and new or worsening hydrocephalus. Analysis of SEGA response rate was limited to the blinded treatment period which ended 6 months after the last patient was randomized. The analysis of SEGA response rate was stratified by use of enzyme-inducing antiepileptic drugs (EIAEDs) at randomization (yes versus no).

Of the 117 patients enrolled, 78 were randomized to AFINITOR and 39 to placebo. The median age was 9.5 years (range 0.8 to 26 years; 69% were 3 to < 18 years at enrollment; 17% were < 3 years at enrollment, 57% were male, and 93% were Caucasian. At baseline, 18% of patients were receiving EIAEDs. Based on central radiology review at baseline, 98% of patients had at least one SEGA lesion ≥ 1.0 cm in longest diameter, 79% had bilateral SEGAs, 43% had ≥ 2 target SEGA lesions, 26% had growth in or into the inferior surface of the ventricle, 9% had evidence of growth beyond the subependymal tissue adjacent to the ventricle, and 7% had radiographic evidence of hydrocephalus. The median values for the sum of all target SEGA lesions at baseline were 1.63 cm^3 (range 0.18 to 25.15 cm^3) and 1.30 cm^3 (range 0.32 to 9.75 cm^3) in the AFINITOR and placebo arms respectively. Eight (7%) patients had prior SEGA-related surgery. The median duration of follow-up was 8.4 months (range 4.6 to 17.2 months).

The SEGA response rate was statistically significantly higher in AFINITOR-treated patients. There were 27 (35%) patients with SEGA responses in the AFINITOR arm and no SEGA responses in the placebo arm. Results are displayed in Table 16. At the time of the final analysis, all SEGA responses were ongoing and the median duration of response was 5.3 months (range 2.1 to 8.4 months). No patient in either treatment arm required surgical intervention during the course of Study 1.

Table 16: SEGA Response

	AFINITOR N=78	Placebo N=39	p-value
Final analysis			
SEGA response rate[a] - (%)	35	0	<0.0001
95% CI	24, 46	0, 9	

[a] Per independent central radiology review

With a median follow-up of 8.4 months, SEGA progression was detected in 6 of 39 (15.4%) patients randomized to receive placebo and none of the 78 patients randomized to receive AFINITOR.

Study 2 was an open-label, single-arm trial conducted to evaluate the safety and efficacy of AFINITOR in patients with SEGA and TSC. Serial radiological evidence of SEGA growth was required for entry. Change in SEGA volume at the end of the core 6-month treatment phase was assessed via independent central radiology review. In total, 28 patients received treatment with AFINITOR; median age was 11 years (range 3-34), 61% male, 86% Caucasian. Four patients had surgical resection of their SEGA lesions with subsequent re-growth prior to receiving AFINITOR treatment. After the core treatment phase, patients could continue to receive AFINITOR treatment as part of an extension treatment phase where SEGA volume was assessed every 6 months. The median duration of treatment was 34.2 months (range 4.7-47.1 months).

At 6 months, nine of 28 patients (32%, 95% CI: 16% to 52%) had a ≥ 50% reduction in the tumor volume of their largest SEGA lesion. The median duration of response for these nine patients was 11.8 months (range 3.2 to 39.1 months). Seven of these nine patients had an ongoing volumetric reduction of ≥ 50% at the data cutoff.

Three of four patients who had prior surgery experienced a ≥ 50% reduction in the tumor volume of their largest SEGA lesion. One of these three patients responded by month 6. No patient developed new lesions.

15 REFERENCES

1. Motzer RJ, Bacik J, Schwartz LH, et al. Prognostic factors for survival in previously treated patients with metastatic renal cell cancer. J Clin Oncol (2004) 22:454-63.
2. OSHA Hazardous Drugs. *OSHA.* http://www.osha.gov/SLTC/hazardousdrugs/index.html.

16 HOW SUPPLIED/STORAGE AND HANDLING

AFINITOR (everolimus) Tablets
2.5 mg tablets
White to slightly yellow, elongated tablets with a bevelled edge and no score, engraved with "LCL" on one side and "NVR" on the other; available in:

Blisters of 28 tablets ....NDC 0078-0594-51
Each carton contains 4 blister cards of 7 tablets each

5 mg tablets
White to slightly yellow, elongated tablets with a bevelled edge and no score, engraved with "5" on one side and "NVR" on the other; available in:

Blisters of 28 tablets ....NDC 0078-0566-51
Each carton contains 4 blister cards of 7 tablets each

7.5 mg tablets
White to slightly yellow, elongated tablets with a bevelled edge and no score, engraved with "7P5" on one side and "NVR" on the other; available in:

Blisters of 28 tablets ....NDC 0078-0620-51
Each carton contains 4 blister cards of 7 tablets each

10 mg tablets
White to slightly yellow, elongated tablets with a bevelled edge and no score, engraved with "UHE" on one side and "NVR" on the other; available in:

Blisters of 28 tablets ....NDC 0078-0567-51
Each carton contains 4 blister cards of 7 tablets each

AFINITOR DISPERZ (everolimus tablets for oral suspension)
2 mg tablets for oral suspension
White to slightly yellow, round, flat tablets with a bevelled edge and no score, engraved with "D2" on one side and "NVR" on the other; available in:

Blisters of 28 tablets ....NDC 0078-0626-51
Each carton contains 4 blister cards of 7 tablets each

3 mg tablets for oral suspension
White to slightly yellowish, round, flat tablets with a bevelled edge and no score, engraved with "D3" on one side and "NVR" on the other; available in:

Blisters of 28 tablets ....NDC 0078-0627-51
Each carton contains 4 blister cards of 7 tablets each

5 mg tablets for oral suspension
White to slightly yellowish, round, flat tablets with a bevelled edge and no score, engraved with "D5" on one side and "NVR" on the other; available in:

Blisters of 28 tablets ....NDC 0078-0628-51
Each carton contains 4 blister cards of 7 tablets each
Store AFINITOR (everolimus) Tablets and AFINITOR DISPERZ (everolimus tablets for oral suspension) at 25°C (77°F); excursions permitted between 15°-30°C (59°-86°F). See USP Controlled Room Temperature. Store in the original container, protect from light and moisture. Keep this and all drugs out of the reach of children.
Follow special handling and disposal procedures for anticancer pharmaceuticals.[2]
AFINITOR Tablets and AFINITOR DISPERZ should not be crushed. Do not take tablets which are crushed or broken.

17 PATIENT COUNSELING INFORMATION

Advise the patient to read the FDA-approved patient labeling (Patient Information and Instructions for Use)

Non-infectious Pneumonitis
Warn patients of the possibility of developing non-infectious pneumonitis. In clinical studies, some non-infectious pneumonitis cases have been severe and occasionally fatal. Advise patients to report promptly any new or worsening respiratory symptoms *[see Warnings and Precautions (5.1)].*

Infections
Inform patients that they are more susceptible to infections while being treated with AFINITOR and that cases of hepatitis B reactivation have been associated with AFINITOR treatment. In clinical studies, some of these infections have been severe (e.g., leading to sepsis, respiratory or hepatic failure) and occasionally fatal. Patients should be aware of the signs and symptoms of infection and should report any such signs or symptoms promptly to their physician *[see Warnings and Precautions (5.2)].*

Oral Ulceration
Inform patients of the possibility of developing mouth ulcers, stomatitis, and oral mucositis. In such cases, mouthwashes and/or topical treatments are recommended, but these should not contain alcohol, peroxide, iodine, or thyme *[see Warnings and Precautions (5.3)].*

Renal Failure
Inform patients of the possibility of developing kidney failure. In some cases kidney failure has been severe and occasionally fatal. Inform patients of the need for the healthcare provider to monitor kidney function, especially in patients with risk factors that may impair kidney function *[see Warnings and Precautions (5.4)].*

Impaired Wound Healing
Inform patients of the possibility of impaired wound healing or dehiscence while being treated with AFINITOR *[see Warnings and Precautions (5.5)].*

Laboratory Tests and Monitoring
Inform patients of the need to monitor blood chemistry and hematology prior to the start of AFINITOR therapy and periodically thereafter *[see Warnings and Precautions (5.7)].*

Drug-drug Interactions
Advise patients to inform their healthcare providers of all concomitant medications, including over-the-counter medications and dietary supplements. Advise patients to avoid concomitant administration of strong CYP3A4/PgP inhibitors or inducers while on AFINITOR treatment *[see Dosage and Administration (2.2, 2.5), Warnings and Precautions (5.8), and Drug Interactions (7.1, 7.2)].*

Vaccinations
Advise patients to avoid the use of live vaccines and close contact with those who have received live vaccines *[see Warnings and Precautions (5.10)].*

Embryo-fetal Toxicity
Advise female patients of childbearing potential that AFINITOR may cause fetal harm and that a highly effective method of contraception should be used during therapy with AFINITOR and for up to 8 weeks after ending treatment *[see Warnings and Precautions (5.11)].*

Safe Handling Practices for AFINITOR DISPERZ
Advise patients and their caregivers to read and carefully follow the FDA approved AFINITOR DISPERZ "Instructions for Use".

Dosing Instructions
Inform patients to take AFINITOR Tablets orally once daily at the same time every day, either consistently with food or consistently without food. Inform patients that AFINITOR Tablets should be swallowed whole with a glass of water.
Inform patients to take AFINITOR DISPERZ orally once daily at the same time every day as a suspension. Refer patients to the "Instructions for Use" pamphlet for additional information regarding these procedures.
Instruct patients that if they miss a dose of AFINITOR, they may still take it up to 6 hours after the time they would normally take it. If more than 6 hours have elapsed, they should be instructed to skip the dose for that day. The next day, they should take AFINITOR at the usual time. Warn patients to not take 2 doses to make up for the one that they missed.

Manufactured by:
Novartis Pharma Stein AG
Stein, Switzerland
Distributed by:
Novartis Pharmaceuticals Corporation
East Hanover, New Jersey 07936
T2014-66
July 2014

PATIENT INFORMATION
AFINITOR® (a-fin-it-or)
(everolimus)
Tablets
AFINITOR® DISPERZ (a-fin-it-or dis-perz)
(everolimus tablets for oral suspension)
Read this Patient Information leaflet that comes with AFINITOR or AFINITOR DISPERZ before you start taking it and each time you get a refill. There may be new information. This information does not take the place of talking to your healthcare provider about your medical condition or treatment.

What is the most important information I should know about AFINITOR and AFINITOR DISPERZ?
AFINITOR and AFINITOR DISPERZ can cause serious side effects. These serious side effects include:
1. You may develop lung or breathing problems. In some people lung or breathing problems may be severe, and can even lead to death. Tell your healthcare provider right away if you have any of these symptoms:
• New or worsening cough
• Shortness of breath
• Chest pain
• Difficulty breathing or wheezing

2. You may be more likely to develop an infection, such as pneumonia, or a bacterial, fungal or viral infection. Viral infections may include active hepatitis B in people who have had hepatitis B in the past (reactivation). In some people these infections may be severe, and can even lead to death. You may need to be treated as soon as possible.
Tell your healthcare provider right away if you have a temperature of 100.5°F or above, chills, or do not feel well.
Symptoms of hepatitis B or infection may include the following:
• Fever
• Chills
• Skin rash
• Joint pain and inflammation
• Tiredness
• Loss of appetite
• Nausea
• Pale stools or dark urine
• Yellowing of the skin
• Pain in the upper right side of the stomach

3. You may develop kidney failure. In some people this may be severe and can even lead to death. Your healthcare provider should do tests to check your kidney function before and during your treatment with AFINITOR or AFINITOR DISPERZ.
If you have any of the serious side effects listed above, you may need to stop taking AFINITOR or AFINITOR DISPERZ for a while or use a lower dose. Follow your healthcare provider's instructions.

What is AFINITOR?
AFINITOR is a prescription medicine used to treat:
○ advanced hormone receptor-positive, HER2-negative breast cancer, along with the medicine exemestane, in postmenopausal women who have already deceived certain other medicines for their cancer.
○ adults with a type of pancreatic cancer known as pancreatic neuroendocrine tumor (PNET), that has progressed

and cannot be treated with surgery.

AFINITOR is not for use in people with carcinoid tumors that actively produce hormones.

○ adults with advanced kidney cancer (renal cell carcinoma or RCC) when certain other medicines have not worked.

○ people with the following types of tumors that are seen with a genetic condition called tuberous sclerosis complex (TSC):
  ○ adults with a kidney tumor called angiomyolipoma, when their kidney tumor does not require surgery right away.
  ○ adults and children with a brain tumor called subependymal giant cell astrocytoma (SEGA) when the tumor cannot be removed completely by surgery.

What is AFINITOR DISPERZ?

AFINITOR DISPERZ is a prescription medicine used to treat:

○ adults and children with a genetic condition called tuberous sclerosis complex (TSC) who have a brain tumor called subependymal giant cell astrocytoma (SEGA) when the tumor cannot be removed completely by surgery.

Who should not take AFINITOR or AFINITOR DISPERZ?

Do not take AFINITOR or AFINITOR DISPERZ if you are allergic to everolimus or to any of the ingredients in AFINITOR or AFINITOR DISPERZ. See the end of this leaflet for a complete list of ingredients in AFINITOR and AFINITOR DISPERZ.

Talk to your healthcare provider before taking this medicine if you are allergic to:

• sirolimus (Rapamune®)
• temsirolimus (Torisel®)

Ask your healthcare provider if you do not know.

What should I tell my healthcare provider before taking AFINITOR or AFINITOR DISPERZ?

Before taking AFINITOR or AFINITOR DISPERZ, tell your healthcare provider about all of your medical conditions, including if you:

• Have or have had kidney problems
• Have or have had liver problems
• Have diabetes or high blood sugar
• Have high blood cholesterol levels
• Have any infections
• Previously had hepatitis B
• Are scheduled to receive any vaccinations. You should not receive a "live vaccine" or be around people who have recently received a "live vaccine" during your treatment with AFINITOR or AFINITOR DISPERZ. If you are not sure about the type of immunization or vaccine, ask your healthcare provider.
• Have other medical conditions
• Are pregnant, or could become pregnant. AFINITOR or AFINITOR DISPERZ can cause harm to your unborn baby. You should use effective birth control while using AFINITOR or AFINITOR DISPERZ and for 8 weeks after stopping treatment. Talk to your healthcare provider about birth control options while taking AFINITOR or AFINITOR DISPERZ.
• Are breastfeeding or plan to breastfeed. It is not known if AFINITOR or AFINITOR DISPERZ passes into your breast milk. You and your healthcare provider should decide if you will take AFINITOR or AFINITOR DISPERZ, or breastfeed. You should not do both.

Tell your healthcare provider about all of the medicines you take, including prescription and non-prescription medicines, vitamins, and herbal supplements.

AFINITOR or AFINITOR DISPERZ may affect the way other medicines work, and other medicines can affect how AFINITOR or AFINITOR DISPERZ work. Using AFINITOR or AFINITOR DISPERZ with other medicines can cause serious side effects.

Know the medicines you take. Keep a list of them and show it to your healthcare provider and pharmacist when you get a new medicine. Especially tell your healthcare provider if you take:

• St. John's Wort (Hypericum perforatum)
• Medicine for:
  ○ Fungal infections
  ○ Bacterial infections
  ○ Tuberculosis
  ○ Seizures
  ○ HIV-AIDS
  ○ Heart conditions or high blood pressure
• Medicines that weaken your immune system (your body's ability to fight infections and other problems)

Ask your healthcare provider or pharmacist if you are not sure if your medicine is one of those taken for the conditions listed above. If you are taking any medicines for the conditions listed above, your healthcare provider might need to prescribe a different medicine or your dose of AFINITOR or AFINITOR DISPERZ may need to be changed. You should also tell your healthcare provider before you start taking any new medicine.

How should I take AFINITOR or AFINITOR DISPERZ?

• Your healthcare provider will prescribe the dose of AFINITOR or AFINITOR DISPERZ that is right for you.

• Take AFINITOR or AFINITOR DISPERZ exactly as your healthcare provider tells you to.
• Your healthcare provider may change your dose of AFINITOR or AFINITOR DISPERZ or tell you to temporarily interrupt dosing, if needed.
• Use scissors to open the blister pack.

AFINITOR:

• Swallow AFINITOR tablets whole with a glass of water. Do not take any tablet that is broken or crushed.

AFINITOR DISPERZ:

• If your healthcare provider prescribes AFINITOR DISPERZ for you, see the "Instructions for Use" that come with your medicine for instructions on how to prepare and take your dose.
• Each dose of AFINITOR DISPERZ must be prepared as a suspension before it is given.
• AFINITOR DISPERZ can cause harm to an unborn baby. When possible, the suspension should be prepared by an adult who is not pregnant or planning to become pregnant.
• Anyone who prepares suspensions of AFINITOR DISPERZ for another person should wear gloves to avoid possible contact with the medicine.
• Take AFINITOR or AFINITOR DISPERZ 1 time each day at about the same time.
• Take AFINITOR or AFINITOR DISPERZ the same way each time, either with food or without food.
• If you take too much AFINITOR or AFINITOR DISPERZ contact your healthcare provider or go to the nearest hospital emergency room right away. Take the pack of AFINITOR or AFINITOR DISPERZ with you.
• If you miss a dose of AFINITOR or AFINITOR DISPERZ, you may still take it up to 6 hours after the time you normally take it. If it is more than 6 hours after you normally take your AFINITOR or AFINITOR DISPERZ, skip the dose for that day. The next day, take AFINITOR or AFINITOR DISPERZ at your usual time. Do not take 2 doses to make up for a missed dose. If you are not sure about what to do, call your healthcare provider.
• You should have blood tests before you start AFINITOR or AFINITOR DISPERZ and as needed during your treatment. These will include tests to check your blood cell count, kidney and liver function, cholesterol, and blood sugar levels.
• If you take AFINITOR or AFINITOR DISPERZ to treat SEGA, you will also need to have blood tests regularly to measure how much medicine is in your blood. This will help your healthcare provider decide how much AFINITOR or AFINITOR DISPERZ you need to take.

What should I avoid while taking AFINITOR or AFINITOR DISPERZ?

You should not drink grapefruit juice or eat grapefruit during your treatment with AFINITOR or AFINITOR DISPERZ. It may make the amount of AFINITOR in your blood increase to a harmful level.

What are the possible side effects of AFINITOR or AFINITOR DISPERZ?

AFINITOR and AFINITOR DISPERZ can cause serious side effects.

• See "What is the most important information I should know about AFINITOR and AFINITOR DISPERZ?" for more information.
• **Delayed wound healing.** AFINITOR can cause incisions to heal slowly or not heal well. Call your healthcare provider right away if you have any of the following symptoms:
  ○ your incision is red, warm or painful
  ○ blood, fluid, or pus in your incision
  ○ your incision opens up
  ○ swelling of your incision

Common side effects of AFINITOR in people with advanced hormone receptor-positive, HER 2-negative breast cancer, advanced pancreatic neuroendocrine tumors, and advanced kidney cancer include:

• Mouth ulcers. AFINITOR can cause mouth ulcers and sores. Tell your healthcare provider if you have pain, discomfort, or open sores in your mouth. Your healthcare provider may tell you to use a special mouthwash or mouth gel that does not contain alcohol, peroxide, iodine, or thyme.
• Infections
• Feeling weak or tired
• Cough, shortness of breath
• Diarrhea and constipation
• Rash, dry skin, and itching
• Nausea and vomiting
• Fever
• Loss of appetite, weight loss
• Swelling of arms, hands, feet, ankles, face or other parts of the body
• Abnormal taste
• Dry mouth
• Inflammation of lining of the digestive system
• Headache
• Nose bleeds
• Pain in arms and legs, mouth and throat, back or joints

• High blood glucose
• High blood pressure
• Difficulty sleeping
• Hair loss
• Muscle spasms
• Feeling dizzy
• Nail disorders

Common side effects of AFINITOR and AFINITOR DISPERZ in people who have SEGA or renal angiomyolipoma with TSC include:

• Mouth ulcers. AFINITOR can cause mouth ulcers and sores. Tell your healthcare provider if you have pain, discomfort, or open sores in your mouth. Your healthcare provider may tell you to use a special mouthwash or mouth gel that does not contain alcohol, peroxide iodine, or thyme.
• Infections
• Nausea and vomiting
• Diarrhea and constipation
• Swelling of your hands, arms, legs, and feet
• Joint pain
• Cough
• Skin problems (such as rash, acne, or dry skin)
• Fever
• Feeling tired
• Anxiety, aggression, and other abnormal behaviors
• Absence of menstrual periods (menstruation). You may miss 1 or more menstrual periods. Tell your healthcare provider if this happens.
• Low red blood cells, white blood cells or platelets
• Increased blood cholesterol level and certain other blood tests
• Increased blood sugar levels
• Decreased blood phosphate levels

Tell your healthcare provider if you have any side effect that bothers you or does not go away.

These are not all the possible side effects of AFINITOR and AFINITOR DISPERZ. For more information, ask your healthcare provider or pharmacist.

Call your doctor for medical advice about side effects. You may report side effects to FDA at 1-800-FDA-1088.

How should I store AFINITOR or AFINITOR DISPERZ?

• Store AFINITOR or AFINITOR DISPERZ at room temperature, between 68°F to 77°F (20°C to 25°C).
• Keep AFINITOR or AFINITOR DISPERZ in the pack it comes in.
• Open the blister pack just before taking AFINITOR or AFINITOR DISPERZ.
• Keep AFINITOR or AFINITOR DISPERZ dry and away from light.
• Do not use AFINITOR or AFINITOR DISPERZ that is out of date or no longer needed.

Keep AFINITOR or AFINITOR DISPERZ and all medicines out of the reach of children.

General information about AFINITOR and AFINITOR DISPERZ

Medicines are sometimes prescribed for purposes other than those listed in a Patient Information leaflet. Do not use AFINITOR or AFINITOR DISPERZ for a condition for which it was not prescribed. Do not give AFINITOR or AFINITOR DISPERZ to other people, even if they have the same problem you have. It may harm them.

This leaflet summarizes the most important information about AFINITOR and AFINITOR DISPERZ. If you would like more information, talk with your healthcare provider. You can ask your healthcare provider or pharmacist for information written for healthcare professionals.

For more information call 1-888-423-4648 or go to www.AFINITOR.com.

What are the ingredients in AFINITOR?

Active ingredient: everolimus.

Inactive ingredients: anhydrous lactose, butylated hydroxytoluene, crospovidone, hypromellose, lactose monohydrate, and magnesium stearate.

What are the ingredients in AFINITOR DISPERZ?

Active ingredient: everolimus.

Inactive ingredients: butylated hydroxytoluene, colloidal silicon dioxide, crospovidone, hypromellose, lactose monohydrate, magnesium stearate, mannitol, and microcrystalline cellulose.

This Patient Information has been approved by the U.S. Food and Drug Administration.

Manufactured by:
Novartis Pharma Stein AG
Stein, Switzerland

Distributed by:
Novartis Pharmaceuticals Corporation
East Hanover, New Jersey 07936

Revised Feb 2014

The brands listed are the trademarks or register marks of their respective owners and are not trademarks or register marks of Novartis.

© Novartis
T2014-17
February 2014

Instructions For Use
AFINITOR® (a-fin-it-or) DISPERZ™ (dis-perz)
(everolimus tablets for oral suspension)

Read these Instructions for Use for AFINITOR DISPERZ before you start taking it and each time you get a refill. There may be new information. This information does not take the place of talking to your healthcare provider about your medical condition or treatment.

Important Information:
- **Take AFINITOR DISPERZ as a suspension only.** AFINITOR DISPERZ is prepared as a suspension of un-dissolved medicine that is mixed with water, and then it is taken by mouth. Do not chew, crush, or swallow AFINITOR DISPERZ whole.
- **AFINITOR DISPERZ can cause harm to an unborn baby.** When possible, the suspension should be prepared by an adult who is not pregnant or planning to become pregnant.
- Keep AFINITOR DISPERZ and the prepared suspension out of the reach of children.
- Anyone who prepares suspensions of AFINITOR DISPERZ for another person should wear gloves to avoid possible contact with the drug.
- Only use water with AFINITOR DISPERZ to prepare the suspension. Do not prepare the suspension with juice or any other liquids.
- The suspension must be given right away. If you do not give the dose within 60 minutes after it has been prepared, throw away the dose and prepare a new dose of AFINITOR DISPERZ.
- Before starting to prepare the suspension, collect all of the supplies that you will need to prepare and take the suspension. Do not use any of these supplies for purposes other than preparing and taking the AFINITOR DISPERZ suspension.

Supplies needed to prepare the suspension in an oral syringe:
- Blister card with AFINITOR DISPERZ
- Scissors to open the blister card
- Disposable gloves (for one time use)
- 2 clean drinking glasses
- Approximately 30 mL of water
- 10 mL oral syringe (for one time use) (see Figure A)
- Paper towels

Figure A

Supplies needed to prepare the suspension in a small drinking glass:
- Blister card with AFINITOR DISPERZ
- Scissors to open the blister card
- Disposable gloves (for one time use)
- 30 mL dose cup for measuring water (you can ask your pharmacist for this)
- 1 clean drinking glass (maximum size 100 mL)
- Water to prepare the suspension
- Spoon for stirring
- Paper towels

Preparing a dose of AFINITOR DISPERZ suspension using an oral syringe:
Step 1: Prepare a clean, flat work surface that is away from where you prepare and eat food. Place a clean paper towel on the work surface. Place the needed supplies on the paper towel.
Step 2: Wash and dry your hands well before preparing the medicine (see Figure B).

Figure B

Step 3: If preparing the AFINITOR DISPERZ suspension for another person, put on disposable gloves (see Figure C).

Figure C

Step 4: Take a 10 mL oral syringe and pull back on the plunger. Remove the plunger from the barrel of the syringe (see Figure D).

Figure D

Step 5: Use scissors to open the blister card along the dotted line (see Figure E) and remove the prescribed number of AFINITOR DISPERZ tablets for oral suspension from the blister card. Place them into the barrel of the oral syringe (see Figure F).

Figure E

Figure F

- Doses of up to 10 mg can be prepared with the oral syringe. **If your total prescribed dose is more than 10 mg, you will need to split the dose. Follow steps 4 through 17 for the first half of the dose. Then repeat steps 4 through 17 for the second half of the dose. Do not prepare a dose of more than 10 mg in one syringe.** Ask your pharmacist or healthcare provider if you are not sure what to do.
Step 6: Re-insert the plunger into the barrel of the oral syringe (see Figure G) and push the plunger in until it comes into contact with the AFINITOR DISPERZ tablets for oral suspension (see Figure H).
[See figure G at top of next column]
[See figure H at top of next column]
Step 7: Fill a small drinking glass with about 30 mL of water. Insert the tip of the oral syringe into the water. Then slowly pull back on the plunger until the syringe is about half full of water and all the tablets are covered by water (see Figure I).
[See figure I at top of next column]
Step 8: Hold the oral syringe with the tip pointing up. Pull back on the plunger to draw back about 4 mL of air (see Figure J).
[See figure J at top of next column]

Figure G

Figure H

Figure I

Figure J

Step 9: Place the filled oral syringe in the clean, empty glass with the tip pointing up. Wait **3 minutes** to allow AFINITOR DISPERZ to break apart (see Figure K).

Figure K

Step 10: Slowly turn the oral syringe up and down five times just before giving the dose (see Figure L). **Do not shake** the syringe.

Figure L

Step 11: Hold the oral syringe in an upright position (with the tip up). Carefully remove most of the air by pushing up gently on the plunger (see Figure M).

Figure M

Step 12: Give the full contents of the oral syringe slowly and gently into the mouth right away, within 60 minutes of preparing it (see Figure N). Carefully remove the syringe from the mouth. Continue with steps 13 through 17 to make sure that the entire dose of medicine is given.

Figure N

Step 13: Insert the tip of the oral syringe into the drinking glass that is filled with water, and pull up about 5 mL of water by slowly pulling back on the plunger (see Figure O).

Figure O

Step 14: Hold the oral syringe with the tip pointing up and use the plunger to draw back about 4 mL of air (see Figure P).

Air

Figure P

Step 15: With the tip of the syringe still pointing up, swirl the contents by gently rotating the syringe in a circular motion (see Figure Q).

Figure Q

Step 16: Hold the oral syringe in an upright position (with the tip up). Carefully remove most of the air by pushing up gently on the plunger (see Figure R).

Figure R

Step 17: Give the full contents of the oral syringe slowly and gently into the mouth by pushing on the plunger (see Figure S). Carefully remove the syringe from the mouth.

Figure S

If the total prescribed dose is more than 10 mg, repeat steps 4 through 17 to finish giving the dose.
Step 18: Throw away the oral syringe, paper towel, and used gloves in your household trash.
Step 19: Wash your hands.
Preparing a dose of AFINITOR DISPERZ suspension using a small drinking glass:
Step 1: Prepare a clean, flat work surface that is away from where you prepare and eat food. Place a clean paper towel on the work surface. Place the needed supplies on the paper towel.
Step 2: Wash and dry your hands before preparing the medicine (See Figure T).

Figure T

Step 3: If preparing the AFINITOR DISPERZ suspension for another person, put on disposable gloves (see Figure U).

Figure U

Step 4: Add about 25 mL of water to the 30 mL dose cup. The amount of water added does not need to be exact (see Figure V).
[See figure V at top of next column]
Step 5: Pour the water from the dose cup into a small drinking glass (maximum size 100 mL) (see Figure W).
[See figure at top of next column]
• Doses up to 10 mg can be prepared in the small drinking glass. If your total prescribed dose is more than 10 mg you will need to split the dose. **Follow steps 4 through 10 for the first half of the dose. Then repeat steps 4 through 10**

30 ml
20 ml
10 ml
5 ml

25 mL of water

Figure V

Figure W

for the second half of the dose. Ask your pharmacist or healthcare provider if you are not sure what to do.
Step 6: Use scissors to open the blister card along the dotted line (see Figure X) and remove the prescribed number of AFINITOR DISPERZ tablets for oral suspension from the blister card.

Figure X

Step 7: Add the prescribed number of AFINITOR DISPERZ tablets for oral suspension into the water (see Figure Y).

Figure Y

Step 8: Wait **3 minutes** to allow AFINITOR DISPERZ tablets for oral suspension to break apart (see Figure Z).

3 Min

Figure Z

Step 9: Gently stir the contents of the glass with a spoon and place the spoon back on the paper towel (see Figure AA). Drink the full amount of the suspension right away, within 60 minutes of preparing it (see Figure BB).
[See figure AA at top of next column]
[See figure BB at top of next column]
Step 10: Refill the glass with the same amount of water (about 25 mL). Stir the contents with the same spoon and place the spoon back on the paper towel (see Figure CC).

Figure AA

Figure BB

Drink the full amount right away so that you take any remaining medicine (see Figure DD).

Figure CC

Figure DD

If your total prescribed dose is more than 10 mg, repeat steps 4 through 10 to finish taking your dose.

Step 11: Wash the glass and the spoon thoroughly with water. Wipe the glass and spoon with a clean paper towel and store them in a dry and clean place until your next dose of AFINITOR DISPERZ (see Figure EE).

Figure EE

Step 12: Throw away the used paper towel and gloves in your household trash.

Step 13: Wash your hands.

How should I store AFINITOR DISPERZ?

• Store AFINITOR at room temperature, between 68°F to 77°F (20°C to 25°C).

• Keep AFINITOR DISPERZ in the pack it comes in.

• Open the blister pack just before taking AFINITOR DISPERZ.

• Keep AFINITOR DISPERZ dry and away from light.

• Do not use AFINITOR DISPERZ that is out of date or no longer needed.

Keep AFINITOR DISPERZ and all medicines out of the reach of children.

This Instructions for Use has been approved by the U.S. Food and Drug Administration.

Manufactured by:
Novartis Pharma Stein AG
Stein, Switzerland
Distributed by:
Novartis Pharmaceuticals Corporation
East Hanover, New Jersey 07936
T2012-157
August 2012

Shown in Product Identification Guide, page 309

AMTURNIDE ℞
(aliskiren, amlodipine and hydrochlorothiazide) tablets, for oral use

The following prescribing information is based on official labeling in effect July 2014.

HIGHLIGHTS OF PRESCRIBING INFORMATION

These highlights do not include all the information needed to use AMTURNIDE safely and effectively. See full prescribing information for AMTURNIDE.

Amturnide (aliskiren, amlodipine and hydrochlorothiazide) tablets, for oral use

Initial U.S. Approval: 2010

> **WARNING: FETAL TOXICITY**
> *See full prescribing information for complete boxed warning.*
> • **When pregnancy is detected, discontinue Amturnide as soon as possible. (5.1)**
> • **Drugs that act directly on the renin-angiotensin system can cause injury and death to the developing fetus. (5.1)**

---RECENT MAJOR CHANGES---

Warnings and Precautions (5.4)   11/2013

---INDICATIONS AND USAGE---

Amturnide is a combination of aliskiren, a renin inhibitor, amlodipine besylate, a dihydropyridine calcium channel blocker, and hydrochlorothiazide (HCTZ), a thiazide diuretic. Amturnide is indicated for the treatment of hypertension, to lower blood pressure. Lowering blood pressure reduces the risk of fatal and nonfatal cardiovascular events, primarily strokes and myocardial infarctions:

• Not indicated for initial therapy. (1)

---DOSAGE AND ADMINISTRATION---

• Dose once-daily. Titrate as needed up to a maximum dose of 300/10/25 mg.

• Amturnide may be used as add-on/switch therapy for patients not adequately controlled on any two of the following: aliskiren, dihydropyridine calcium channel blockers, and thiazide diuretics. (2.2)

• Amturnide may be substituted for its individually titrated aliskiren, amlodipine and HCTZ. (2.3)

---DOSAGE FORMS AND STRENGTHS---

Tablets (aliskiren/ amlodipine/ HCTZ): 150/5/12.5, 300/5/12.5, 300/5/25, 300/10/12.5, 300/10/25 mg. (3)

---CONTRAINDICATIONS---

• Do not use with angiotensin receptor blockers (ARBs) or ACE inhibitors (ACEI) in patients with diabetes (4)

• Anuria (4)

• Hypersensitivity to sulfonamide-derived drugs or to any of the components (4)

---WARNINGS AND PRECAUTIONS---

• Avoid concomitant use with ARBs or ACEIs in patients with renal impairment (GFR<60 mL/min) (5.2)

• Anaphylactic Reactions and Head and Neck Angioedema: Discontinue Amturnide and monitor until signs and symptoms resolve. (5.3)

• Hypotension in volume and/or salt depleted patients or with combined use of other agents acting on RAAS : Correct imbalances before initiating therapy with Amturnide. (5.4)

• Increased angina or myocardial infarction may occur upon dosage initiation or increase in amlodipine. (5.5)

• Impaired renal function: Monitor serum creatinine periodically. (5.6)

• HCTZ may exacerbate or activate systemic lupus erythematosus. (5.8)

• Hyperkalemia: Monitor potassium levels periodically. (5.10)

• Acute myopia and secondary angle closure glaucoma: Discontinue HCTZ. (5.12)

• Hypersensitivity Reactions: May occur from HCTZ component. (5.7)

---ADVERSE REACTIONS---

The most common adverse events (incidence ≥2%) are: peripheral edema, dizziness, headache and nasopharyngitis. (6.1)

To report SUSPECTED ADVERSE REACTIONS, contact Novartis Pharmaceuticals Corporation at 1-888-669-6682 or FDA at 1-800-FDA-1088 or www.fda.gov/medwatch.

---DRUG INTERACTIONS---

• Cyclosporine: Avoid concomitant use (7, 12.3)

• Itraconazole: Avoid concomitant use (7, 12.3)

• NSAIDs use may lead to increased risk of renal impairment and loss of antihypertensive effect (7)

• If simvastatin is co-administered with amlodipine, do not exceed doses greater than 20 mg daily of simvastatin (7)

• Antidiabetic Drugs: Antidiabetic dosage adjustment may be required. (7)

• Cholestyramine and Colestipol: Reduce absorption of thiazides. (7)

• Lithium: Increased risk of lithium toxicity when used with diuretics. Monitor serum lithium concentrations during concurrent use. (7)

---USE IN SPECIFIC POPULATIONS---

Nursing Mothers: Discontinue drug or nursing. (8.3)

See 17 for PATIENT COUNSELING INFORMATION and FDA-approved patient labeling

Revised: 3/2014

FULL PRESCRIBING INFORMATION: CONTENTS*

WARNING: FETAL TOXICITY

1 INDICATIONS AND USAGE

2 DOSAGE AND ADMINISTRATION
  2.1 General Considerations
  2.2 Add-on/Switch Therapy
  2.3 Replacement Therapy
  2.4 Relationship to Meals

3 DOSAGE FORMS AND STRENGTHS

4 CONTRAINDICATIONS

5 WARNINGS AND PRECAUTIONS
  5.1 Fetal Toxicity
  5.2 Renal Impairment/Hyperkalemia/Hypotension when Amturnide is given in combination with ARBs or ACEIs
  5.3 Anaphylactic Reactions and Head and Neck Angioedema
  5.4 Hypotension
  5.5 Risk of Myocardial Infarction or Increased Angina
  5.6 Impaired Renal Function
  5.7 Hypersensitivity Reactions
  5.8 Systemic Lupus Erythematosus
  5.9 Lithium Interaction
  5.10 Serum Electrolyte Abnormalities
  5.11 Cyclosporine or Itraconazole
  5.12 Acute Myopia and Secondary Angle-Closure Glaucoma
  5.13 Metabolic Disturbances

6 ADVERSE REACTIONS
  6.1 Clinical Studies Experience
  6.2 Postmarketing Experience

7 DRUG INTERACTIONS

8 USE IN SPECIFIC POPULATIONS
  8.1 Pregnancy
  8.3 Nursing Mothers
  8.4 Pediatric Use
  8.5 Geriatric Use
  8.6 Hepatic Impairment
  8.7 Renal Impairment

10 OVERDOSAGE

11 DESCRIPTION

12 CLINICAL PHARMACOLOGY
  12.1 Mechanism of Action
  12.2 Pharmacodynamics
  12.3 Pharmacokinetics

13 NONCLINICAL TOXICOLOGY
  13.1 Carcinogenesis, Mutagenesis, Impairment of Fertility
  13.2 Animal Toxicology and/or Pharmacology

14 CLINICAL STUDIES
  14.1 Amturnide
  14.2 Aliskiren in Patients with Diabetes treated with ARB or ACEI (ALTITUDE study)

16 HOW SUPPLIED/STORAGE AND HANDLING

17 PATIENT COUNSELING INFORMATION

* Sections or subsections omitted from the full prescribing information are not listed

---

FULL PRESCRIBING INFORMATION

> **WARNING: FETAL TOXICITY**
> • **When pregnancy is detected, discontinue Amturnide as soon as possible. (5.1)**
> • **Drugs that act directly on the renin-angiotensin system can cause injury and death to the developing fetus. (5.1)**

1 INDICATIONS AND USAGE

Amturnide is indicated for the treatment of hypertension, to lower blood pressure. Lowering blood pressure reduces the risk of fatal and nonfatal cardiovascular events, primarily strokes and myocardial infarctions. These benefits have been seen in controlled trials of antihypertensive drugs from a wide variety of pharmacologic classes, including amlodipine and hydrochlorothiazide. There are no controlled trials demonstrating risk reduction with Amturnide.

Control of high blood pressure should be part of comprehensive cardiovascular risk management, including, as appropriate, lipid control, diabetes management, antithrombotic therapy, smoking cessation, exercise, and limited sodium intake. Many patients will require more than one drug to achieve blood pressure goals. For specific advice on goals and management, see published guidelines, such as those of the National High Blood Pressure Education Program's Joint National Committee on Prevention, Detection, Evaluation, and Treatment of High Blood Pressure (JNC).

Numerous antihypertensive drugs, from a variety of pharmacologic classes and with different mechanisms of action, have been shown in randomized controlled trials to reduce cardiovascular morbidity and mortality, and it can be concluded that it is blood pressure reduction, and not some other pharmacologic property of the drugs, that is largely responsible for those benefits. The largest and most consistent cardiovascular outcome benefit has been a reduction in the risk of stroke, but reductions in myocardial infarction and cardiovascular mortality also have been seen regularly. Elevated systolic or diastolic pressure causes increased cardiovascular risk, and the absolute risk increase per mmHg is greater at higher blood pressures, so that even modest reductions of severe hypertension can provide substantial benefit. Relative risk reduction from blood pressure reduction is similar across populations with varying absolute risk, so the absolute benefit is greater in patients who are at higher risk independent of their hypertension (for example, patients with diabetes or hyperlipidemia), and such patients would be expected to benefit from more aggressive treatment to a lower blood pressure goal.

Some antihypertensive drugs have smaller blood pressure effects (as monotherapy) in black patients, and many antihypertensive drugs have additional approved indications and effects (e.g., on angina, heart failure, or diabetic kidney disease). These considerations may guide selection of therapy.

This fixed combination drug is not indicated for initial therapy of hypertension.

2 DOSAGE AND ADMINISTRATION

2.1 General Considerations

Dose once-daily. The dosage may be increased after 2 weeks of therapy. The maximum recommended dose of Amturnide is 300/10/25 mg.

2.2 Add-on/Switch Therapy

Use Amturnide for patients not adequately controlled with any two of the following: aliskiren, dihydropyridine calcium channel blockers, and thiazide diuretics.

Switch a patient who experiences dose-limiting adverse reactions attributed to an individual component—while on any dual combination of the components of Amturnide—to Amturnide at a lower dose of that component to achieve similar blood pressure reductions.

2.3 Replacement Therapy

For patients receiving aliskiren, amlodipine and HCTZ from separate tablets, substitute Amturnide containing the same component doses.

2.4 Relationship to Meals

Patients should establish a routine pattern for taking Amturnide, either with or without a meal. High-fat meals decrease absorption of aliskiren substantially [see Clinical Pharmacology (12.3)].

3 DOSAGE FORMS AND STRENGTHS

Tablets are convex ovaloid with a beveled edge, film-coated, and unscored, in the following strengths:

Aliskiren/ Amlodipine/HCTZ (mg)	Color	Embossing Side 1/side 2
150/5/12.5	Violet white	YIY/NVR
300/5/12.5	Light pink	LIL/NVR
300/5/25	Pale orange brown	OIO/NVR
300/10/12.5	Light red	UIU/NVR
300/10/25	Brown	VIV/NVR

4 CONTRAINDICATIONS

Do not use aliskiren with ARBs or ACEIs in patients with diabetes [see Warnings and Precautions (5.2), Clinical Studies (14.2)].

Amturnide is contraindicated in patients with anuria or hypersensitivity to sulfonamide-derived drugs like HCTZ or to any of the components [see Warnings and Precautions (5.8) and Adverse Reactions (6.1)]. Hypersensitivity reactions may range from urticaria to anaphylaxis.

5 WARNINGS AND PRECAUTIONS

5.1 Fetal Toxicity

Pregnancy Category D

Use of drugs that act on the renin-angiotensin system during the second and third trimesters of pregnancy reduces fetal renal function and increases fetal and neonatal morbidity and death. Resulting oligohydramnios can be associated with fetal lung hypoplasia and skeletal deformations. Potential neonatal adverse effects include skull hypoplasia, anuria, hypotension, renal failure, and death. When pregnancy is detected, discontinue Amturnide as soon as possible [see Use in Specific Populations (8.1)].

5.2 Renal Impairment/Hyperkalemia/Hypotension when Amturnide is given in combination with ARBs or ACEIs

Amturnide is contraindicated in patients with diabetes who are receiving ARBs or ACEIs because of the increased risk of renal impairment, hyperkalemia, and hypotension [see Contraindications (4) and Clinical Studies (14.2)].

Avoid use of Amturnide with ARBs or ACEI in patients with moderate renal impairment (GFR <60 ml/min).

5.3 Anaphylactic Reactions and Head and Neck Angioedema

Aliskiren

Hypersensitivity reactions such as anaphylactic reactions and angioedema of the face, extremities, lips, tongue, glottis and/or larynx have been reported in patients treated with aliskiren and has necessitated hospitalization and intubation. This may occur at any time during treatment and has occurred in patients with and without a history of angioedema with ACE inhibitors or angiotensin receptor antagonists. Anaphylactic reactions have been reported from postmarketing experience with unknown frequency. If angioedema involves the throat, tongue, glottis or larynx, or if the patient has a history of upper respiratory surgery, airway obstruction may occur and be fatal. Patients who experience these effects, even without respiratory distress, require prolonged observation and appropriate monitoring measures since treatment with antihistamines and corticosteroids may not be sufficient to prevent respiratory involvement. Prompt administration of subcutaneous epinephrine solution 1:1000 (0.3 to 0.5 mL) and measures to ensure a patent airway may be necessary.

Discontinue Amturnide immediately in patients who develop anaphylactic reactions or angioedema, and do not re-administer.

5.4 Hypotension

Symptomatic hypotension may occur after initiation of treatment with Amturnide in patients with marked volume depletion, patients with salt depletion, or with combined use of aliskiren and other agents acting on the renin-angiotensin-aldosterone system. The volume or salt depletion should be corrected prior to administration of Amturnide, or the treatment should start under close medical supervision.

A transient hypotensive response is not a contraindication to further treatment, which usually can be continued without difficulty once the blood pressure has stabilized.

Amlodipine besylate

Symptomatic hypotension is possible, particularly in patients with severe aortic stenosis. Because of the gradual onset of action, acute hypotension is unlikely.

5.5 Risk of Myocardial Infarction or Increased Angina

Worsening angina and acute myocardial infarction can develop after starting or increasing the dose of amlodipine, particularly with severe obstructive coronary artery disease.

5.6 Impaired Renal Function

Monitor renal function periodically in patients treated with Amturnide. Changes in renal function, including acute renal failure, can be caused by drugs that affect the renin-angiotensin-aldosterone system and by diuretics. Patients whose renal function may depend in part on the activity of the renin-angiotensin-aldosterone system (e.g., patients with renal artery stenosis, severe heart failure, post-myocardial infarction or volume depletion) or patients receiving ARB, ACEI or non-steroidal anti-inflammatory (NSAID) therapy may be at particular risk of developing acute renal failure on Amturnide [see Contraindications (4), Warnings and Precautions (5.2), Clinical Studies (14.2)]. Consider withholding or discontinuing therapy in patients who develop a clinically significant decrease in renal function on Amturnide.

5.7 Hypersensitivity Reactions

Hydrochlorothiazide

Hypersensitivity reactions to HCTZ may occur in patients with or without a history of allergy or bronchial asthma, but are more likely in patients with such a history.

5.8 Systemic Lupus Erythematosus

Thiazide diuretics have been reported to cause exacerbation or activation of systemic lupus erythematosus.

5.9 Lithium Interaction

Lithium generally should not be given with thiazides [see Drug Interactions (7)].

5.10 Serum Electrolyte Abnormalities

Amturnide

In a short-term controlled trial the incidence of patients with hypertension not concomitantly treated with an ARB or ACEI who developed hypokalemia (serum potassium <3.5 mEq/L) was 11.0% of Amturnide-treated patients compared to 19.0% of amlodipine/HCTZ patients, 4.4% of aliskiren/HCTZ patients, and 2.1% of aliskiren/amlodipine patients; the incidence of hyperkalemia (serum potassium >5.5 mEq/L) was 3.0% compared to 2.0% of amlodipine/HCTZ patients, 0.7% of aliskiren/HCTZ patients, and 0.7% of aliskiren/amlodipine patients. No Amturnide-treated patients discontinued due to increase or decrease of serum potassium.

Aliskiren

Monitor serum potassium periodically in patients receiving aliskiren. Drugs that affect the renin-angiotensin-aldosterone system can cause hyperkalemia. Risk factors for the development of hyperkalemia include renal insufficiency, diabetes, combination use with ARBs or ACEI [see Contraindications (4), Warnings and Precautions (5.2), and Clinical Studies (14.2)], NSAIDs, or potassium supplements or potassium sparing diuretics.

Hydrochlorothiazide

Hydrochlorothiazide can cause hypokalemia and hyponatremia. Hypomagnesemia can result in hypokalemia which appears difficult to treat despite potassium repletion.

If hypokalemia is accompanied by clinical signs (e.g., muscular weakness, paresis, or ECG alterations), Amturnide should be discontinued. Correction of hypokalemia and any coexisting hypomagnesemia is recommended prior to the initiation of thiazides.

5.11 Cyclosporine or Itraconazole

When aliskiren was given with cyclosporine or itraconazole, the blood concentrations of aliskiren were significantly increased. Avoid concomitant use of Amturnide with cyclosporine or itraconazole [see Drug Interactions (7)].

5.12 Acute Myopia and Secondary Angle-Closure Glaucoma

Hydrochlorothiazide, a sulfonamide, can cause an idiosyncratic reaction, resulting in transient myopia and acute angle-closure glaucoma. Symptoms include acute onset of decreased visual acuity or ocular pain and typically occur within hours to weeks of drug initiation. Untreated acute angle-closure glaucoma can lead to permanent vision loss. The primary treatment is to discontinue hydrochlorothiazide as rapidly as possible. Prompt medical or surgical treatments may need to be considered if the intraocular pressure remains uncontrolled. Risk factors for developing acute angle-closure glaucoma may include a history of sulfonamide or penicillin allergy.

5.13 Metabolic Disturbances

Hydrochlorothiazide

Hydrochlorothiazide may alter glucose tolerance and raise serum levels of cholesterol and triglycerides.

Hydrochlorothiazide may raise the serum uric acid level due to reduced clearance of uric acid and may cause or exacerbate hyperuricemia and precipitate gout in susceptible patients.

Hydrochlorothiazide decreases urinary calcium excretion and may cause elevation of serum calcium. Monitor calcium levels in patients with hypercalcemia receiving Amturnide.

6 ADVERSE REACTIONS

6.1 Clinical Studies Experience

The following serious adverse reactions are discussed in greater detail in other sections of the label:

- Risk of fetal/neonatal morbidity and mortality [see Warnings and Precautions (5.1)]
- Head and neck angioedema [see Warnings and Precautions (5.3)]
- Hypotension [see Warnings and Precautions (5.4)]

Because clinical trials are conducted under widely varying conditions, adverse reaction rates observed in the clinical trials of a drug cannot be directly compared to rates in clinical trials of another drug and may not reflect the rates observed in practice.

Amturnide

Amturnide has been evaluated for safety in 1155 patients treated with Amturnide, including 182 patients for over 1 year.

In a short-term controlled trial, there were 60.5% males, 84.1% Caucasians, 10% Blacks, 6.4% Hispanics, and 19.1% who were ≥ 65 years of age. In this study, the overall incidence of adverse events on therapy with Amturnide was similar to that observed with the individual components. The overall frequency of adverse events was similar between men and women and Black and White patients. Discontinuation of therapy because of a clinical adverse event in this study occurred in 3.6% of patients treated with Amturnide versus 2.4% in aliskiren/amlodipine, 0.7% in aliskiren/HCTZ, and 2.7% in amlodipine/HCTZ.

Table 1. Adverse events in a short-term controlled trial that occurred in at least 2% of patients treated with Amturnide

	Amturnide	Ali/ amlo	Ali/ HCTZ	Amlo/ HCTZ
Edema peripheral	7.1%	8.0%	2.0%	4.1%
Dizziness	3.6%	2.4%	3.4%	1.7%
Headache	3.6%	3.1%	4.0%	5.1%
Nasopharyngitis	2.6%	0.7%	2.0%	3.4%

In a long-term safety trial, the safety profile was similar to that seen in the short-term controlled trial.

Aliskiren
Aliskiren has been evaluated for safety in 6460 patients, including 1740 treated for longer than 6 months, and 1250 for longer than 1 year. In placebo-controlled clinical trials, discontinuation of therapy because of a clinical adverse event, including uncontrolled hypertension, occurred in 2.2% of patients treated with aliskiren, versus 3.5% of patients given placebo. These data do not include information from the ALTITUDE study which evaluated the use of aliskiren in combination with ARBs or ACEI [see Contraindications (4), Warnings and Precautions (5.2), and Clinical Studies (14.2)].

Two cases of angioedema with respiratory symptoms were reported with aliskiren use in the clinical studies. Two other cases of periorbital edema without respiratory symptoms were reported as possible angioedema and resulted in discontinuation. The rate of these angioedema cases in the completed studies was 0.06%.

In addition, 26 other cases of edema involving the face, hands, or whole body were reported with aliskiren use, including 4 leading to discontinuation.

In the placebo-controlled studies, however, the incidence of edema involving the face, hands, or whole body was 0.4% with aliskiren compared with 0.5% with placebo. In a long-term active-controlled study with aliskiren and HCTZ arms, the incidence of edema involving the face, hands, or whole body was 0.4% in both treatment arms.

Aliskiren produces dose-related gastrointestinal (GI) adverse reactions. Diarrhea was reported by 2.3% of patients at 300 mg, compared to 1.2% in placebo patients. In women and the elderly (age ≥65) increases in diarrhea rates are evident starting at a dose of 150 mg daily, with rates for these subgroups at 150 mg similar to those seen at 300 mg for men or younger patients (all rates about 2%). Other GI symptoms included abdominal pain, dyspepsia, and gastroesophageal reflux, although increased rates for abdominal pain and dyspepsia were distinguished from placebo only at 600 mg daily. Diarrhea and other GI symptoms were typically mild and rarely led to discontinuation.

Aliskiren was associated with a slight increase in cough in the placebo-controlled studies (1.1% for any aliskiren use versus 0.6% for placebo). In active-controlled trials with ACE inhibitor (ramipril, lisinopril) arms, the rates of cough for the aliskiren arms were about one-third to one-half the rates in the ACE inhibitor arms.

Other adverse reactions with increased rates for aliskiren compared to placebo included rash (1% versus 0.3%), and renal stones (0.2% versus 0%).

Single episodes of tonic-clonic seizures with loss of consciousness were reported in 2 patients treated with aliskiren in the clinical trials. One patient had predisposing causes for seizures and had a negative electroencephalogram (EEG) and cerebral imaging following the seizures; for the other patient, EEG and imaging results were not reported. Aliskiren was discontinued and there was no rechallenge in either case.

No clinically meaningful changes in vital signs or in ECG (including QTc interval) were observed in patients treated with aliskiren.

Amlodipine
Amlodipine (Norvasc®) has been evaluated for safety in more than 11,000 patients in U.S. and foreign clinical trials. Other adverse events that have been reported at <1% but >0.1% of patients in controlled clinical trials or under conditions of open trials or marketing experience where a causal relationship is uncertain were:

Cardiovascular: arrhythmia (including ventricular tachycardia and atrial fibrillation), bradycardia, chest pain, peripheral ischemia, syncope, postural hypotension, vasculitis

Central and Peripheral Nervous System: neuropathy peripheral, paresthesia, tremor, vertigo

Gastrointestinal: anorexia, constipation, dyspepsia,** dysphagia, diarrhea, flatulence, pancreatitis, vomiting, gingival hyperplasia

General: allergic reaction, asthenia,** back pain, hot flushes, malaise, pain, rigors, weight gain, weight decrease

Musculoskeletal System: arthralgia, arthrosis, muscle cramps,** myalgia

Psychiatric: sexual dysfunction (male** and female), insomnia, nervousness, depression, abnormal dreams, anxiety, depersonalization

Respiratory System: dyspnea, epistaxis

Skin and Appendages: angioedema, erythema multiforme, pruritus,** rash,** rash erythematous, rash maculopapular

**These events occurred in less than 1% in placebo-controlled trials, but the incidence of these side effects was between 1% and 2% in all multiple dose studies.

Special Senses: abnormal vision, conjunctivitis, diplopia, eye pain, tinnitus

Urinary System: micturition frequency, micturition disorder, nocturia

Autonomic Nervous System: dry mouth, sweating increased

Metabolic and Nutritional: hyperglycemia, thirst

Hemopoietic: leukopenia, purpura, thrombocytopenia

Other events reported with amlodipine at a frequency of ≤0.1% of patients include: cardiac failure, pulse irregularity, extrasystoles, skin discoloration, urticaria, skin dryness, alopecia, dermatitis, muscle weakness, twitching, ataxia, hypertonia, migraine, cold and clammy skin, apathy, agitation, amnesia, gastritis, increased appetite, loose stools, rhinitis, dysuria, polyuria, parosmia, taste perversion, abnormal visual accommodation, and xerophthalmia. Other reactions occurred sporadically and cannot be distinguished from medications or concurrent disease states such as myocardial infarction and angina.

HCTZ
Other adverse reactions not listed above that have been reported with HCTZ, without regard to causality, are listed below:

Body as a Whole: weakness

Digestive: pancreatitis, jaundice (intrahepatic cholestatic jaundice), sialadenitis, cramping, gastric irritation

Hematologic: aplastic anemia, agranulocytosis, hemolytic anemia

Hypersensitivity: photosensitivity, urticaria, necrotizing angiitis (vasculitis and cutaneous vasculitis), fever, respiratory distress including pneumonitis and pulmonary edema, anaphylactic reactions

Musculoskeletal: muscle spasm

Nervous System/Psychiatric: restlessness

Renal: renal failure, renal dysfunction, interstitial nephritis

Skin: erythema multiforme including Stevens-Johnson syndrome, exfoliative dermatitis including toxic epidermal necrolysis

Special Senses: transient blurred vision, xanthopsia

Clinical Laboratory Test Abnormalities
Clinical laboratory findings for Amturnide in patients with hypertension not concomitantly treated with an ARB or ACEI were obtained in a controlled trial of Amturnide administered at the maximal dose of 300/10/25 mg compared to maximal doses of dual therapies, i.e., aliskiren/amlodipine 300/10 mg, aliskiren/HCTZ 300/25 mg and amlodipine/HCTZ 10/25 mg.

RBC Count, Hemoglobin and Hematocrit
Small mean changes from baseline were seen in RBC count, hemoglobin and hematocrit in patients treated with Amturnide. This effect is also seen with other agents acting on the renin angiotensin system. In aliskiren monotherapy trials these decreases led to slight increases in rates of anemia compared to placebo (0.1% for any aliskiren use, 0.3% for aliskiren 600 mg daily, versus 0% for placebo). No patients discontinued Amturnide because of anemia.

Blood Urea Nitrogen (BUN)/Creatinine
No patients with hypertension not concomitantly treated with an ARB or ACEI treated with Amturnide had elevations in BUN >40 mg/dL or creatinine >2.0 mg/dL.

Liver Function Tests
Occasional elevations (greater than 150% from baseline) in ALT (SGPT) were observed in 2.7% of patients treated with Amturnide, compared with 1.7-2.7% in patients treated with the dual combinations. No patients were discontinued due to abnormal liver function tests.

6.2 Postmarketing Experience
The following adverse reactions have been identified during post-approval use of either aliskiren, amlodipine or hydrochlorothiazide. Because these reactions are reported voluntarily from a population of uncertain size, it is not always possible to estimate their frequency or establish a causal relationship to drug exposure:

Aliskiren:
Hypersensitivity: anaphylactic reactions and angioedema requiring airway management and hospitalization.

Peripheral edema, severe cutaneous adverse reactions, including Stevens-Johnson syndrome and toxic epidermal necrolysis, urticaria, hepatic enzyme increase with clinical symptoms of hepatic dysfunction, pruritus, erythema.

Amlodipine: The following postmarketing event has been reported infrequently where a causal relationship is uncertain: gynecomastia. In postmarketing experience, jaundice and hepatic enzyme elevations (mostly consistent with cholestasis or hepatitis), in some cases severe enough to require hospitalization, have been reported in association with use of amlodipine.

Hydrochlorothiazide:
Acute renal failure, renal disorder, aplastic anemia, erythema multiforme, pyrexia, muscle spasm, asthenia, acute angle-closure glaucoma, bone marrow failure, worsening of diabetes control, hypokalemia, blood lipids increased, hyponatremia, hypomagnesemia, hypercalcemia, hyperchloremic alkalosis, impotence, visual impairment.

Pathological changes in the parathyroid gland of patients with hypercalcemia and hypophosphatemia have been observed in a few patients on prolonged thiazide therapy. If hypercalcemia occurs, further diagnostic evaluation is necessary.

7   DRUG INTERACTIONS

No drug interaction studies have been conducted between Amturnide and other drugs. In a phase III sub-study, there was no clinically relevant change in the exposure of aliskiren, amlodipine, and HCTZ observed with Amturnide compared to the dual combinations of aliskiren and amlodipine, amlodipine and HCTZ, and aliskiren and HCTZ. Studies with the individual aliskiren, amlodipine, and HCTZ components are described below.

Aliskiren
Cyclosporine: Avoid co-administration of cyclosporine with aliskiren.

Itraconazole: Avoid co-administration of itraconazole with aliskiren [see Clinical Pharmacology (12.3)].

Non-Steroidal Anti-Inflammatory Agents (NSAIDs) including selective Cyclooxygenase-2 inhibitors (COX-2 inhibitors): In patients who are elderly, volume-depleted (including those on diuretic therapy), or with compromised renal function, co-administration of NSAIDs, including selective COX-2 inhibitors with agents that affect the renin-angiotensin-aldosterone system, including aliskiren, may result in deterioration of renal function, including possible acute renal failure. These effects are usually reversible. Monitor renal function periodically in patients receiving aliskiren and NSAID therapy.
The antihypertensive effect of aliskiren may be attenuated by NSAIDs.

Dual Blockade of the renin-angiotensin-aldosterone system: The concomitant use of aliskiren with other agents acting on the renin-angiotensin-aldosterone system such as ACEIs or ARBs is associated with an increased risk of hypotension, hyperkalemia, and changes in renal function (including acute renal failure) compared to monotherapy. Monitor blood pressure, renal function, and electrolytes in patients on aliskiren and other agents that affect the renin-angiotensin-aldosterone system [see Warnings and Precautions (5.4, 5.6, 5.10)].
The concomitant use of aliskiren with an ARB or an ACEI in diabetic patients is contraindicated and should be avoided in patients with moderate renal impairment [see Contraindications (4) and Warnings and Precautions (5.2)].

Furosemide: Oral co-administration of aliskiren and furosemide reduced exposure to furosemide. Monitor diuretic effects when furosemide is co-administered with aliskiren.

Amlodipine
Simvastatin: Co-administration of simvastatin with amlodipine increases the systemic exposure of simvastatin. Limit the dose of simvastatin in patients on amlodipine to 20 mg daily.

CYP3A4 Inhibitors: Co-administration with CYP3A inhibitors (moderate and strong) result in increased systemic exposure to amlodipine warranting dose reduction. Monitor for symptoms of hypotension and edema when amlodipine is co-administered with CYP3A4 inhibitors to determine the need for dose adjustment.

CYP3A4 Inducers: No information is available on the quantitative effects of CYP3A4 inducers on amlodipine. Blood pressure should be monitored when amlodipine is co-administered with CYP3A4 inducers.

HCTZ
When administered concurrently, the following drugs may interact with thiazide diuretics.

Antidiabetic drugs (oral agents and insulin): Dosage adjustment of the antidiabetic drug may be required.

Lithium: Diuretic agents increase the risk of lithium toxicity. Refer to the package insert for lithium before use of such preparation with Amturnide. Monitoring of serum lithium concentrations is recommended during concurrent use.

Nonsteroidal anti-inflammatory drugs (NSAIDs) and COX-2 selective agents: When Amturnide and nonsteroidal anti-inflammatory agents are used concomitantly, observe the patient to determine if the desired effect of the diuretic is obtained.

Ion exchange resins: Staggering the dosage of hydrochlorothiazide and resin (e.g., cholestyramine, colestipol) such that hydrochlorothiazide is administered at least 4 hours before or 4-6 hours after the administration of resins would potentially minimize the interaction *[see Clinical Pharmacology (12.3)].*

8 USE IN SPECIFIC POPULATIONS

8.1 Pregnancy

Pregnancy Category D

Use of drugs that act on the renin-angiotensin system during the second and third trimesters of pregnancy reduces fetal renal function and increases fetal and neonatal morbidity and death. Resulting oligohydramnios can be associated with fetal lung hypoplasia and skeletal deformations. Potential neonatal adverse effects include skull hypoplasia, anuria, hypotension, renal failure, and death. When pregnancy is detected, discontinue Amturnide as soon as possible. These adverse outcomes are usually associated with use of drugs in the second and third trimesters of pregnancy. Most epidemiologic studies examining fetal abnormalities after exposure to antihypertensive use in the first trimester have not distinguished drugs affecting the renin-angiotensin system from other antihypertensive agents. Appropriate management of maternal hypertension during pregnancy is important to optimize outcomes for both mother and fetus. In the unusual case that there is no appropriate alternative to therapy with drugs affecting the renin-angiotensin system for a particular patient, apprise the mother of the potential risk to the fetus. Perform serial ultrasound examinations to assess the intra-amniotic environment. If oligohydramnios is observed, discontinue Amturnide, unless it is considered lifesaving for the mother. Fetal testing may be appropriate, based on the week of pregnancy. Patients and physicians should be aware, however, that oligohydramnios may not appear until after the fetus has sustained irreversible injury. Closely observe infants with histories of in utero exposure to Amturnide for hypotension, oliguria, and hyperkalemia *[see use in Specific Populations (8.4)].*

Animal Data

No reproductive toxicity studies have been conducted with the combination of aliskiren, amlodipine besylate and HCTZ. However, these studies have been conducted for aliskiren, amlodipine besylate and HCTZ alone.

Aliskiren

In developmental toxicity studies, pregnant rats and rabbits received oral aliskiren hemifumarate during organogenesis at doses up to 20 and 7 times the maximum recommended human dose (MRHD) based on body surface area (mg/m²), respectively, in rats and rabbits. (Actual animal doses were up to 600 mg/kg/day in rats and up to 100 mg/kg/day in rabbits.) No teratogenicity was observed; however, fetal birth weight was decreased in rabbits at doses 3.2 times the MRHD based on body surface area (mg/m²). Aliskiren was present in placentas, amniotic fluid and fetuses of pregnant rabbits.

Amlodipine

No evidence of teratogenicity or embryo/fetal toxicity was found when pregnant rats and rabbits were treated orally with amlodipine maleate at doses up to 10 mg amlodipine/kg/day during their respective periods of major organogenesis. However, litter size was significantly decreased (by about 50%) and the number of intrauterine deaths was significantly increased (about 5-fold). Amlodipine has been shown to prolong both the gestation period and the duration of labor in rats at this dose.

HCTZ

When pregnant mice and rats were given HCTZ at doses up to 3000 and 1000 mg/kg/day, respectively (about 600 and 400 times the MRHD), during their respective periods of major organogenesis, there was no evidence of fetal harm. Thiazides can cross the placenta, and concentrations reached in the umbilical vein approach those in the maternal plasma. Hydrochlorothiazide, like other diuretics, can cause placental hypoperfusion. It accumulates in the amniotic fluid, with reported concentrations up to 19 times higher than in umbilical vein plasma. Use of thiazides during pregnancy is associated with a risk of fetal or neonatal jaundice or thrombocytopenia. Since they do not prevent or alter the course of EPH (Edema, Proteinuria, Hypertension) gestosis (pre eclampsia), these drugs should not be used to treat hypertension in pregnant women. The use of hydrochlorothiazide for other indications (e.g. heart disease) in pregnancy should be avoided.

8.3 Nursing Mothers

It is not known whether aliskiren or amlodipine is excreted in human milk, but thiazides are excreted in human milk. Both aliskiren and amlodipine are secreted in the milk of lactating rats. Because of the potential for serious adverse reactions in human milk-fed infants from Amturnide, a de-

cision should be made whether to discontinue nursing or discontinue Amturnide, taking into account the importance of the drug to the mother.

8.4 Pediatric Use

Safety and effectiveness of Amturnide in pediatric patients have not been established.

Neonates with a history of in utero exposure to Amturnide: If oliguria or hypotension occurs, direct attention towards support of blood pressure and renal perfusion. Exchange transfusions or dialysis may be required as a means of reversing hypotension and/or substituting for disordered renal function.

8.5 Geriatric Use

As individual components, exposure to aliskiren, amlodipine and hydrochlorothiazide is increased in elderly patients, thus consider lower initial doses of Amturnide *[see Clinical Pharmacology (12.3)].*

In the short-term controlled clinical trial of Amturnide, 19% of patients treated with Amturnide were ≥ 65 years. No overall differences in safety or effectiveness were observed between these subjects and younger subjects. Other reported clinical experience has not identified differences in responses between the elderly and younger patients, but greater sensitivity of some older individuals cannot be ruled out.

8.6 Hepatic Impairment

Exposure to amlodipine is increased in patients with hepatic insufficiency, thus consider using lower doses of Amturnide *[see Clinical Pharmacology (12.3)].*

Hydrochlorothiazide

Minor alterations of fluid and electrolyte balance may precipitate hepatic coma in patients with impaired hepatic function or progressive liver disease.

8.7 Renal Impairment

Exposure to hydrochlorothiazide increases in patients with renal insufficiency, thus consider using lower doses of Amturnide *[see Clinical Pharmacology (12.3)].*

Safety and effectiveness of Amturnide in patients with severe renal impairment (creatinine clearance <30 mL/min) have not been established as these patients were excluded in clinical trials *[see Warnings and Precautions (5.6), Clinical Pharmacology (12.3) and Clinical Studies (14)].*

10 OVERDOSAGE

Aliskiren

Limited data are available related to overdosage in humans. The most likely manifestation of overdosage would be hypotension. If symptomatic hypotension occurs, provide supportive treatment.

Aliskiren is poorly dialyzed. Therefore, hemodialysis is not adequate to treat aliskiren overexposure *[see Clinical Pharmacology (12.3)].*

Amlodipine

Overdosage might be expected to cause excessive peripheral vasodilation with marked hypotension and possibly a reflex tachycardia. Marked and potentially prolonged systemic hypotension up to and including shock with fatal outcome have been reported. In humans, experience with intentional overdosage of amlodipine is limited.

Single oral doses of amlodipine maleate equivalent to 40 mg amlodipine/kg and 100 mg amlodipine/kg in mice and rats, respectively, caused deaths. Single oral amlodipine maleate doses equivalent to 4 or more mg amlodipine/kg or higher in dogs (11 or more times the maximum recommended human dose on a mg/m2 basis) caused a marked peripheral vasodilation and hypotension.

If massive overdose occurs, initiate active cardiac and respiratory monitoring. Frequent blood pressure measurements are essential. If hypotension occurs, provide cardiovascular support including elevation of the extremities and the judicious administration of fluids. If hypotension remains unresponsive to these conservative measures, consider administration of vasopressors (such as phenylephrine), with attention to circulating volume and urine output. As amlodipine is highly protein bound, hemodialysis is not likely to be of benefit. Administration of activated charcoal to healthy volunteers immediately or up to two hours after ingestion of amlodipine has been shown to significantly decrease amlodipine absorption.

HCTZ

The most common signs and symptoms of overdose observed in humans are those caused by electrolyte depletion (hypokalemia, hypochloremia, hyponatremia) and dehydration resulting from excessive diuresis. If digitalis has also been administered, hypokalemia may accentuate cardiac arrhythmias. The degree to which HCTZ is removed by hemodialysis has not been established. The oral LD_{50} of HCTZ is greater than 10 g/kg in both mice and rats. These doses are 1946 and 3892 times, respectively, the MRHD of 25 mg/day, when based on a mg/m² basis of a 60-kg individual.

11 DESCRIPTION

Amturnide is a single tablet for oral administration of aliskiren hemifumarate (an orally active, nonpeptide, po-

tent direct renin inhibitor), amlodipine besylate (a dihydropyridine calcium channel blocker) and HCTZ (a diuretic).

Aliskiren hemifumarate

Aliskiren hemifumarate is chemically described as (2S,4S,5S,7S)-N-(2-carbamoyl-2-methylpropyl)-5-amino-4-hydroxy-2,7-diisopropyl-8-[4-methoxy-3-(3-methoxypropoxy)phenyl]-octanamide hemifumarate, and its structural formula is

Molecular formula: $C_{30}H_{53}N_3O_6 \cdot 0.5\ C_4H_4O_4$

Aliskiren hemifumarate is a white to slightly yellowish powder with a molecular weight of 609.8 (free base- 551.8). It is highly soluble in water, and freely soluble in methanol, ethanol and isopropanol.

Amlodipine

Amlodipine besylate, USP is chemically described as 3-ethyl 5-methyl (±)-2-[(2-aminoethoxy)methyl]-4-(o-chlorophenyl)-1,4-dihydro-6-methyl-3,5-pyridinedicarboxylate, monobenzenesulfonate and its structural formula is

Molecular formula: $C_{20}H_{25}ClN_2O_5 \cdot C_6H_6O_3S$

Amlodipine besylate is a white to pale yellow crystalline powder with a molecular weight of 567.1. It is slightly soluble in water and sparingly soluble in ethanol.

HCTZ

HCTZ, USP is a white, or practically white, practically odorless, crystalline powder. It is slightly soluble in water; freely soluble in sodium hydroxide solution, in *n*-butylamine, and in dimethylformamide; sparingly soluble in methanol; and insoluble in ether, in chloroform, and in dilute mineral acids. HCTZ is chemically described as 6-chloro-3,4-dihydro-2H-1,2,4-benzothiadiazine-7-sulfonamide 1,1-dioxide. HCTZ is a thiazide diuretic. Its empirical formula is $C_7H_8ClN_3O_4S_2$, its molecular weight is 297.73, and its structural formula is

The inactive ingredients for all strengths of the tablets may contain colloidal silicon dioxide, crospovidone, hypromellose, iron oxide red, iron oxide yellow, iron oxide black, magnesium stearate, microcrystalline cellulose, polyethylene glycol, povidone, talc, and titanium dioxide.

12 CLINICAL PHARMACOLOGY

12.1 Mechanism of Action

Amturnide

The effects of combined treatment of aliskiren, amlodipine and HCTZ arise from the actions of these three agents on different but complementary mechanisms that regulate blood pressure. Together, inhibition of the renin-angiotensin-aldosterone system (RAAS), inhibition of calcium channel-mediated vasoconstriction, and increase of sodium chloride excretion lowers blood pressure to a greater degree than the individual components.

Aliskiren

Renin is secreted by the kidney in response to decreases in blood volume and renal perfusion. Renin cleaves angiotensinogen to form the inactive decapeptide angiotensin I (Ang I). Ang I is converted to the active octapeptide angiotensin II (Ang II) by angiotensin-converting enzyme (ACE) and non-ACE pathways. Ang II is a powerful vasoconstrictor and leads to the release of catecholamines from the adrenal medulla and prejunctional nerve endings. It also promotes aldosterone secretion and sodium reabsorption. Together, these effects increase blood pressure. Ang II also inhibits renin release, thus providing a negative feedback to the system. This cycle, from renin through angiotensin to aldosterone and its associated negative feedback loop, is known as the renin-angiotensin-aldosterone system (RAAS). Aliskiren is a direct renin inhibitor, decreasing plasma renin activity (PRA) and inhibiting the conversion of

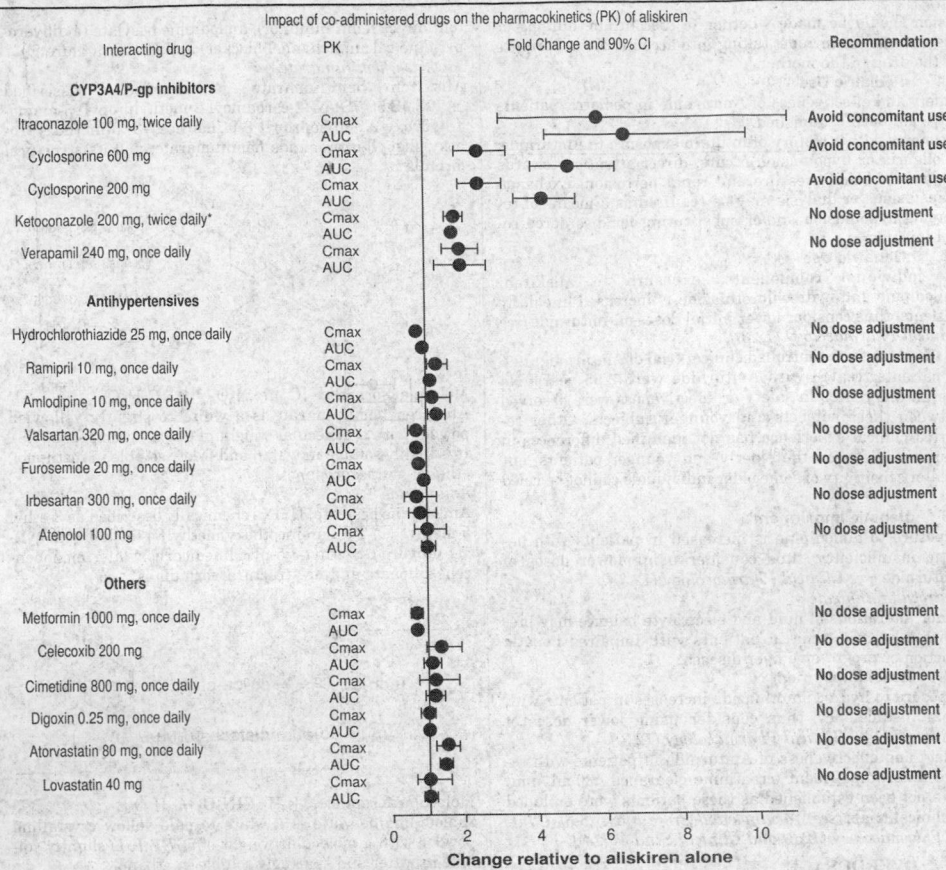

Figure 1: The impact of co-administered drugs on the pharmacokinetics of aliskiren.

The figure shows "Impact of co-administered drugs on the pharmacokinetics (PK) of aliskiren" with columns: Interacting drug | PK | Fold Change and 90% CI | Recommendation. X-axis "Change relative to aliskiren alone" (0, 2, 4, 6, 8, 10).

CYP3A4/P-gp inhibitors

Interacting drug	PK	Recommendation
Itraconazole 100 mg, twice daily	Cmax / AUC	Avoid concomitant use
Cyclosporine 600 mg	Cmax / AUC	Avoid concomitant use
Cyclosporine 200 mg	Cmax / AUC	Avoid concomitant use
Ketoconazole 200 mg, twice daily*	Cmax / AUC	No dose adjustment
Verapamil 240 mg, once daily	Cmax / AUC	No dose adjustment

Antihypertensives

Interacting drug	PK	Recommendation
Hydrochlorothiazide 25 mg, once daily	Cmax / AUC	No dose adjustment
Ramipril 10 mg, once daily	Cmax / AUC	No dose adjustment
Amlodipine 10 mg, once daily	Cmax / AUC	No dose adjustment
Valsartan 320 mg, once daily	Cmax / AUC	No dose adjustment
Furosemide 20 mg, once daily	Cmax / AUC	No dose adjustment
Irbesartan 300 mg, once daily	Cmax / AUC	No dose adjustment
Atenolol 100 mg	Cmax / AUC	No dose adjustment

Others

Interacting drug	PK	Recommendation
Metformin 1000 mg, once daily	Cmax / AUC	No dose adjustment
Celecoxib 200 mg	Cmax / AUC	No dose adjustment
Cimetidine 800 mg, once daily	Cmax / AUC	No dose adjustment
Digoxin 0.25 mg, once daily	Cmax / AUC	No dose adjustment
Atorvastatin 80 mg, once daily	Cmax / AUC	No dose adjustment
Lovastatin 40 mg	Cmax / AUC	No dose adjustment

*A 400 mg once daily dose was not studied, but would be expected to increase aliskiren blood levels further.

angiotensinogen to Ang I. Whether aliskiren affects other RAAS components, e.g., ACE or non-ACE pathways, is not known.

All agents that inhibit the RAAS, including renin inhibitors, suppress the negative feedback loop, leading to a compensatory rise in plasma renin concentration. When this rise occurs during treatment with ACE inhibitors and ARBs, the result is increased levels of PRA. During treatment with aliskiren, however, the effect of increased renin levels is blocked, so that PRA, Ang I and Ang II are all reduced, whether aliskiren is used as monotherapy or in combination with other antihypertensive agents.

Amlodipine
Amlodipine is a dihydropyridine calcium channel blocker that inhibits the transmembrane influx of calcium ions into vascular smooth muscle and cardiac muscle. Experimental data suggest that amlodipine binds to both dihydropyridine and nondihydropyridine binding sites. The contractile processes of cardiac muscle and vascular smooth muscle are dependent upon the movement of extracellular calcium ions into these cells through specific ion channels. Amlodipine inhibits calcium ion influx across cell membranes selectively, with a greater effect on vascular smooth muscle cells than on cardiac muscle cells. Negative inotropic effects can be detected *in vitro* but such effects have not been seen in intact animals at therapeutic doses. Serum calcium concentration is not affected by amlodipine. Within the physiologic pH range, amlodipine is an ionized compound (pKa=8.6), and its kinetic interaction with the calcium channel receptor is characterized by a gradual rate of association and dissociation with the receptor binding site, resulting in a gradual onset of effect.

Amlodipine is a peripheral arterial vasodilator that acts directly on vascular smooth muscle to cause a reduction in peripheral vascular resistance and reduction in blood pressure.

HCTZ
The mechanism of action of the antihypertensive effect of thiazides is unknown.

HCTZ is a thiazide diuretic. Thiazides affect the renal tubular mechanisms of electrolyte reabsorption, directly increasing excretion of sodium and chloride in approximately equivalent amounts. Indirectly, the diuretic action of HCTZ reduces plasma volume, with consequent increases in plasma renin activity, increases in aldosterone secretion, increases in urinary potassium loss, and decreases in serum potassium. The renin-aldosterone link is mediated by angiotensin II, so coadministration of agents that block the production or function of angiotensin II tends to reverse the potassium loss associated with these diuretics.

12.2   Pharmacodynamics
Amturnide
In an active-controlled trial which established the clinical efficacy of Amturnide in hypertensive patients, Amturnide was associated with a 34% reduction in PRA compared to a 63% reduction with aliskiren/amlodipine, 64% reduction with aliskiren/HCTZ and a 170% elevation with amlodipine/HCTZ.

Aliskiren
PRA reductions in clinical trials ranged from approximately 50% to 80%, were not dose-related and did not correlate with blood pressure reductions. The clinical implications of the differences in effect on PRA are not known.

Amlodipine
Following administration of therapeutic doses to patients with hypertension, amlodipine produces vasodilation resulting in a reduction of supine and standing blood pressures. These decreases in blood pressure are not accompanied by a significant change in heart rate or plasma catecholamine levels with chronic dosing. Although the acute intravenous administration of amlodipine decreases arterial blood pressure and increases heart rate in hemodynamic studies of patients with chronic stable angina, chronic oral administration of amlodipine in clinical trials did not lead to clinically significant changes in heart rate or blood pressures in normotensive patients with angina.

With chronic once-daily administration, antihypertensive effectiveness is maintained for at least 24 hours. Plasma concentrations correlate with effect in both young and elderly patients. The magnitude of reduction in blood pressure with amlodipine is also correlated with the height of pretreatment elevation; thus, individuals with moderate hypertension (diastolic pressure 105-114 mmHg) had about 50% greater response than patients with mild hypertension (diastolic pressure 90-104 mmHg). Normotensive subjects experienced no clinically significant change in blood pressure (+1/-2 mmHg).

In hypertensive patients with normal renal function, therapeutic doses of amlodipine resulted in a decrease in renal vascular resistance and an increase in glomerular filtration rate and effective renal plasma flow without change in filtration fraction or proteinuria.

As with other calcium channel blockers, hemodynamic measurements of cardiac function at rest and during exercise (or pacing) in patients with normal ventricular function treated with amlodipine have generally demonstrated a small increase in cardiac index without significant influence on dP/dt or on left ventricular end diastolic pressure or volume. In hemodynamic studies, amlodipine has not been associated with a negative inotropic effect when administered in therapeutic dose range to intact animals and man, even when co-administered with beta-blockers to man. Similar findings, however, have been observed in normal or well-compensated patients with heart failure with agents possessing significant negative inotropic effects.

Amlodipine does not change sinoatrial nodal function or atrioventricular conduction in intact animals or man. In patients with chronic stable angina, intravenous administration of 10 mg did not significantly alter A-H and H-V conduction and sinus node recovery time after pacing. Similar results were obtained in patients receiving amlodipine and concomitant beta-blockers. In clinical studies in which amlodipine was administered in combination with beta-blockers to patients with either hypertension or angina, no adverse effects of electrocardiographic parameters were observed. In clinical trials with angina patients alone, amlodipine therapy did not alter electrocardiographic intervals or produce higher degrees of AV blocks.

Amlodipine has indications other than hypertension, which can be found in the Norvasc® package insert.

HCTZ
After oral administration of HCTZ, diuresis begins within 2 hours, peaks in about 4 hours, and lasts about 6 to 12 hours.

Drug Interactions
Hydrochlorothiazide
Alcohol, barbiturates, or narcotics: Potentiation of orthostatic hypotension may occur.
Skeletal muscle relaxants: Possible increased responsiveness to muscle relaxants such as curare derivatives.
Digitalis glycosides: Thiazide-induced hypokalemia or hypomagnesemia may predispose the patient to digoxin toxicity.

12.3   Pharmacokinetics
Absorption and Distribution
Amturnide
Following oral administration of the fixed combination of aliskiren, amlodipine, and HCTZ, peak concentrations were achieved within 1-2 hours, 6-12 hours, and 1-4 hours for aliskiren, amlodipine and HCTZ, respectively. The rate and extent of absorption of aliskiren, amlodipine, and HCTZ following administration of the fixed combination are similar to when they are administered as individual dosage forms. When Amturnide is taken with food, mean AUC and Cmax of aliskiren are decreased by 78% and 89%, respectively. There is no impact of food on the exposures of amlodipine and HCTZ.

Aliskiren
Aliskiren is poorly absorbed (bioavailability about 2.5%). Following oral administration, peak plasma concentrations of aliskiren are reached within 1 to 3 hours. When taken with a high fat meal, mean AUC and Cmax of aliskiren are decreased by 71% and 85% respectively. In the clinical trials of aliskiren, it was administered without requiring a fixed relation of administration to meals.

Amlodipine
Peak plasma concentrations of amlodipine are reached 6-12 hours after an oral administration of amlodipine. Absolute bioavailability has been estimated to be between 64% and 90%. The bioavailability of amlodipine is not altered by the presence of food.

The apparent volume of distribution of amlodipine is about 21 L/kg. Approximately 93% of circulating amlodipine is bound to plasma proteins in hypertensive patients.

HCTZ
The estimated absolute bioavailability of hydrochlorothiazide after oral administration is about 70%. Peak plasma hydrochlorothiazide concentrations (Cmax) are reached within 2 to 5 hours after oral administration. There is no clinically significant effect of food on the bioavailability of hydrochlorothiazide.

Hydrochlorothiazide binds to albumin (40 to 70%) and distributes into erythrocytes. Following oral administration, plasma hydrochlorothiazide concentrations decline biexponentially, with a mean distribution half-life of about 2 hours and an elimination half-life of about 10 hours.

Metabolism and Elimination
Aliskiren
The effective half-life for aliskiren is 24 hours. Steady state blood levels are reached in about 7 – 8 days. About one-fourth of the absorbed dose appears in the urine as parent drug. How much of the absorbed dose is metabolized is unknown. Based on the *in vitro* studies, the major enzyme responsible for aliskiren metabolism appears to be CYP 3A4. Aliskiren does not inhibit the CYP450 isoenzymes (CYP 1A2, 2C8, 2C9, 2C19, 2D6, 2E1, and 3A) or induce CYP 3A4.

Transporters: Pgp (MDR1/Mdr1a/1b) was found to be the major efflux system involved in absorption and disposition of aliskiren in preclinical studies. The potential for drug interactions at the Pgp site will likely depend on the degree of inhibition of this transporter.

Amlodipine
Amlodipine is extensively (about 90%) converted to inactive metabolites via hepatic metabolism, with 10% of the parent compound and 60% of the metabolites excreted in the urine. Elimination of amlodipine from the plasma is biphasic, with a terminal elimination half-life of about 30-50 hours. Steady state plasma levels are reached after once-daily dosing for 7-8 days.

HCTZ
About 70% of an orally administered dose of hydrochlorothiazide is eliminated in the urine as unchanged drug.

Drug interactions:

Aliskiren
The effects of co-administered drugs on the pharmacokinetics of aliskiren, and vice versa, were studied in several single and multiple dose studies. Pharmacokinetic measures indicating the magnitude of these interactions are presented in Figure 1 (impact of co-administered drugs on aliskiren) and Figure 2 (impact on co-administered drugs).
[See figure 1 at top of previous page]
Warfarin: There was no clinically significant effect of a single dose of warfarin 25 mg on the pharmacokinetics of aliskiren.
[See figure 2 above]
Furosemide: In patients with heart failure, co-administration of aliskiren (300 mg/day) reduced plasma AUC and C_{max} of oral furosemide (60 mg/day) by 17% and 27%, respectively, and reduced 24 hour urinary furosemide excretion by 29%. This change in exposure did not result in statistically significant difference in total urine volume and urinary sodium excretion over 24 hours. However, a transient decrease in urinary sodium excretion and urine volume effects up to 12 hours were observed when furosemide was co-administered with aliskiren 300 mg/day.

Amlodipine
In vitro data in human plasma indicate that amlodipine has no effect on the protein binding of digoxin, phenytoin, warfarin, and indomethacin.
Cimetidine: Co-administration of amlodipine with cimetidine did not alter the pharmacokinetics of amlodipine.
Grapefruit juice: Co-administration of 240 mL of grapefruit juice with a single oral dose of amlodipine 10 mg in 20 healthy volunteers had no significant effect on the pharmacokinetics of amlodipine.
Maalox® (antacid): Co-administration of the antacid Maalox with a single dose of amlodipine had no significant effect on the pharmacokinetics of amlodipine.
Sildenafil: A single 100 mg dose of sildenafil in subjects with essential hypertension had no effect on the pharmacokinetic parameters of amlodipine. When amlodipine and sildenafil were used in combination, each agent independently exerted its own blood pressure lowering effect.
Atorvastatin: Co-administration of multiple 10 mg doses of amlodipine with 80 mg of atorvastatin resulted in no significant change in the steady-state pharmacokinetic parameters of atorvastatin.
Digoxin: Co-administration of amlodipine with digoxin did not change serum digoxin levels or digoxin renal clearance in normal volunteers.
Ethanol (alcohol): Single and multiple 10 mg doses of amlodipine had no significant effect on the pharmacokinetics of ethanol.
Warfarin: Co-administration of amlodipine with warfarin did not change the warfarin prothrombin response time.
Simvastatin: Co-administration of multiple doses of 10 mg of amlodipine with 80 mg simvastatin resulted in a 77% increase in exposure to simvastatin compared to simvastatin alone.
CYP3A inhibitors: Co-administration of a 180 mg daily dose of diltiazem with 5 mg amlodipine in elderly hypertensive patients resulted in a 60% increase in amlodipine systemic exposure. Erythromycin co-administration in healthy volunteers did not significantly change amlodipine systemic exposure. However, strong inhibitors of CYP3A4 (e.g. ketoconazole, itraconazole, ritonavir) may increase the plasma concentrations of amlodipine to a greater extent.

Hydrochlorothiazide
Drugs that alter gastrointestinal motility: The bioavailability of thiazide-type diuretics may be increased by anticholinergic agents (e.g. atropine, biperiden), apparently due to a decrease in gastrointestinal motility and the stomach emptying rate. Conversely, pro-kinetic drugs may decrease the bioavailability of thiazide diuretics.
Cholestyramine: In a dedicated drug interaction study, administration of cholestyramine 2 hours before hydrochlorothiazide resulted in a 70% reduction in exposure

to hydrochlorothiazide. Further, administration of hydrochlorothiazide 2 hours before cholestyramine, resulted in 35% reduction in exposure to hydrochlorothiazide.
Antineoplastic agents (e.g. cyclophosphamide, methotrexate): Concomitant use of thiazide diuretics may reduce renal excretion of cytotoxic agents and enhance their myelosuppressive effects.

Special Populations
Pediatric Patients
The pharmacokinetics of Amturnide have not been investigated in patients <18 years of age.
Geriatric Patients
Impact of aging on aliskiren pharmacokinetics has been assessed. When compared to young adults (18-40 years), aliskiren mean AUC and C_{max} in elderly subjects (> 65 years) are increased by 57% and 28%, respectively. In the elderly, clearance of amlodipine is decreased with resulting increases in peak plasma levels, elimination half-life and area-under-the-plasma-concentration curve. Limited data suggest that the systemic clearance of hydrochlorothiazide is reduced in both healthy and hypertensive elderly subjects compared to young healthy volunteers *[see Use in Specific Populations (8.5)].*
Race
With Amturnide, pharmacokinetic differences due to race have not been studied. The pharmacokinetic differences among Blacks, Caucasians, and Japanese are minimal with aliskiren therapy.
Hepatic Impairment
The pharmacokinetics of aliskiren is not significantly affected in patients with mild-to-severe liver disease. Patients with hepatic insufficiency have decreased clearance of amlodipine with resulting increase in AUC of approximately 40%-60% *[see Warnings and Precautions (5.6) and Use in Specific Populations (8.6)].*
Renal Impairment
The pharmacokinetics of aliskiren were evaluated in patients with varying degrees of renal impairment. Rate and extent of exposure (AUC and C_{max}) of aliskiren in subjects with renal impairment did not show a consistent correlation with the severity of renal impairment.
The pharmacokinetics of aliskiren following administration of a single oral dose of 300 mg was evaluated in patients with End Stage Renal Disease (ESRD) undergoing hemodialysis. When compared to matched healthy subjects, changes in the rate and extent of aliskiren exposure (C_{max} and AUC) in ESRD patients undergoing hemodialysis was not clinically significant. Timing of hemodialysis did not significantly alter the pharmacokinetics of aliskiren in ESRD patients.
The pharmacokinetics of amlodipine is not significantly influenced by renal impairment.
In a study in individuals with impaired renal function, the mean elimination half-life of hydrochlorothiazide was doubled in individuals with mild/moderate renal impairment

(30 < CLcr < 90 mL/min) and tripled in severe renal impairment (≤ 30 mL/min), compared to individuals with normal renal function (CLcr > 90 mL/min) *[see Warnings and Precautions (5.7) and Use in Specific Populations (8.7)].*

13   NONCLINICAL TOXICOLOGY
13.1   Carcinogenesis, Mutagenesis, Impairment of Fertility
Studies with Aliskiren hemifumarate, Amlodipine besylate and HCTZ
No carcinogenicity, mutagenicity or fertility studies have been conducted with the combination of aliskiren hemifumarate, amlodipine besylate and HCTZ. However, these studies have been conducted for aliskiren hemifumarate, amlodipine besylate and HCTZ alone.
Studies with Aliskiren hemifumarate
Carcinogenic potential was assessed in a 2-year rat study and a 6-month transgenic (rasH2) mouse study with aliskiren hemifumarate at oral doses of up to 1500 mg aliskiren/kg/day. Although there were no statistically significant increases in tumor incidence associated with exposure to aliskiren, mucosal epithelial hyperplasia (with or without erosion/ulceration) was observed in the lower gastrointestinal tract at doses of 750 or more mg/kg/day in both species, with a colonic adenoma identified in one rat and a cecal adenocarcinoma identified in another, rare tumors in the strain of rat studied. On a systemic exposure (AUC_{0-24h}) basis, 1500 mg/kg/day in the rat is about 4 times and in the mouse about 1.5 times the maximum recommended human dose (300 mg aliskiren/day). Mucosal hyperplasia in the cecum or colon of rats was also observed at doses of 250 mg/kg/day (the lowest tested dose) as well as at higher doses in 4- and 13-week studies.
Aliskiren hemifumarate was devoid of genotoxic potential in the Ames reverse mutation assay with *S. typhimurium* and *E. coli,* the *in vitro* Chinese hamster ovary cell chromosomal aberration assay, the *in vitro* Chinese hamster V79 cell gene mutation test and the *in vivo* rat bone marrow micronucleus assay.
Fertility of male and female rats was unaffected at doses of up to aliskiren 250 mg/kg/day (8 times the maximum recommended human dose of aliskiren 300 mg/60 kg on a mg/m² basis).
Studies with Amlodipine besylate
Rats and mice treated with amlodipine maleate in the diet for up to two years, at concentrations calculated to provide daily dosage levels of 0.5, 1.25, and 2.5 mg amlodipine/kg/day, showed no evidence of a carcinogenic effect of the drug. For the mouse, the highest dose was, on mg/m² basis, similar to the maximum recommended human dose (MRHD) of 10 mg amlodipine/day. For the rat, the highest dose was, on a mg/m² basis, about twice the MRHD.
Mutagenicity studies conducted with amlodipine maleate revealed no drug-related effects at either the gene or chromosome level.

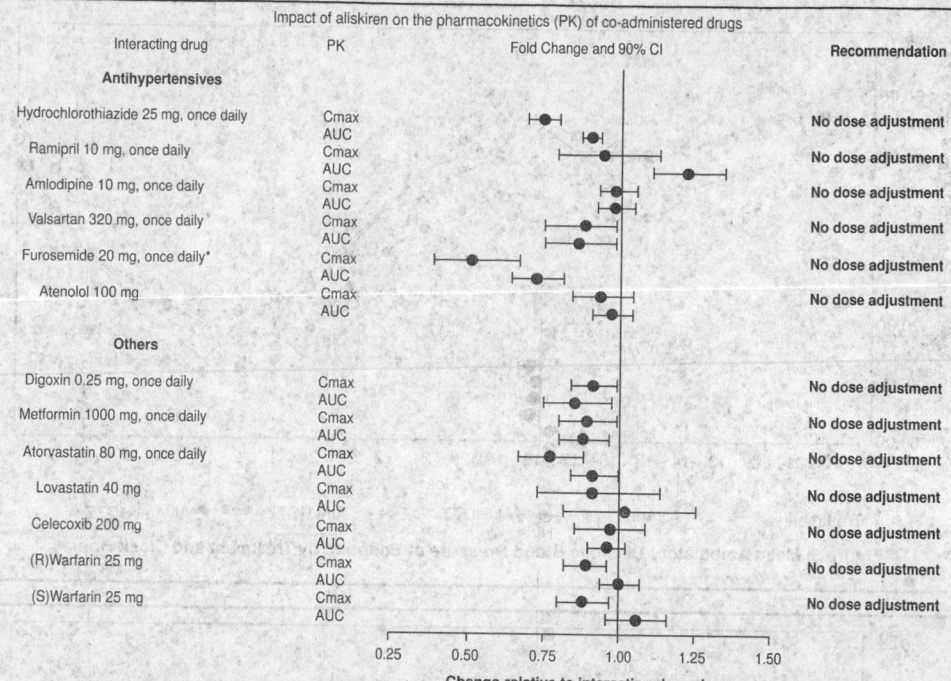

Impact of aliskiren on the pharmacokinetics (PK) of co-administered drugs

Interacting drug	PK	Fold Change and 90% CI	Recommendation
Antihypertensives			
Hydrochlorothiazide 25 mg, once daily	Cmax / AUC		No dose adjustment
Ramipril 10 mg, once daily	Cmax / AUC		No dose adjustment
Amlodipine 10 mg, once daily	Cmax / AUC		No dose adjustment
Valsartan 320 mg, once daily	Cmax / AUC		No dose adjustment
Furosemide 20 mg, once daily*	Cmax / AUC		No dose adjustment
Atenolol 100 mg	Cmax / AUC		No dose adjustment
Others			
Digoxin 0.25 mg, once daily	Cmax / AUC		No dose adjustment
Metformin 1000 mg, once daily	Cmax / AUC		No dose adjustment
Atorvastatin 80 mg, once daily	Cmax / AUC		No dose adjustment
Lovastatin 40 mg	Cmax / AUC		No dose adjustment
Celecoxib 200 mg	Cmax / AUC		No dose adjustment
(R)Warfarin 25 mg	Cmax / AUC		No dose adjustment
(S)Warfarin 25 mg	Cmax / AUC		No dose adjustment

Change relative to interacting drug alone

*Patients receiving furosemide could find its effect diminished after starting aliskiren.

Figure 2: The impact of aliskiren on the pharmacokinetics of co-administered drugs.

Figure 5. Mean Ambulatory Diastolic Blood Pressure at Endpoint by Treatment and Clock Hour

Figure 6. Mean Ambulatory Systolic Blood Pressure at Endpoint by Treatment and Clock Hour

The reductions in systolic/diastolic blood pressure with Amturnide were 9.9/6.3 mmHg greater than with aliskiren/HCTZ, 7.2/3.6 mmHg greater than with amlodipine/HCTZ, and 6.6/2.6 mmHg greater than with aliskiren/amlodipine. In the severe hypertensive patients, Amturnide produced greater reductions in blood pressure than each of the 3 dual combination treatments ($p < 0.001$ for both diastolic and systolic blood pressure reductions). The reductions in systolic/diastolic blood pressure with Amturnide were 16.3/8.2 mmHg greater than with aliskiren/HCTZ, 9.6/4.8 mmHg greater than with amlodipine/HCTZ, and 11.4/4.9 mmHg greater than with aliskiren/amlodipine.

The distribution of reductions in blood pressure on each treatment are shown in Figure 3 for diastolic blood pressure and in Figure 4 for systolic blood pressure. For example, Figure 3 shows that 50% of patients on Amturnide had more than 20.2 mmHg reduction in diastolic blood pressure compared to 18.7 mmHg on aliskiren/amlodipine combination, 12.7 mmHg on aliskiren/HCTZ combination, and 15.3 mmHg on amlodipine/HCTZ combination. Similarly, Figure 4 shows that 50% of patients on Amturnide had more than 36.3 mmHg reduction in systolic blood pressure compared to 30.8 mmHg on aliskiren/amlodipine combination, 28.3 mmHg on aliskiren/HCTZ combination, and 31.0 mmHg on amlodipine/HCTZ combination. The time course over which blood pressure effects developed is shown in Figures 5 and 6. As the trial had no placebo control, the treatment effects shown in Figures 3-6 include a placebo effect of unknown size.

The antihypertensive effect of Amturnide was similar in patients with and without diabetes, obese and non-obese patients, in patients ≥65 years of age and <65 years of age, and in women and men.

Figure 3. Distribution of diastolic blood pressure responses on Amturnide and combinations of two drugs.

Figure 4. Distribution of systolic blood pressure responses on Amturnide and combinations of two drugs.

[See figure 5 above]
[See figure 6 above]
There are no trials of the Amturnide triple combination tablet demonstrating reductions in cardiovascular risk in patients with hypertension, but two of the components, amlodipine and hydrochlorothiazide, have demonstrated such benefits.

14.2   Aliskiren in Patients with Diabetes treated with ARB or ACEI (ALTITUDE study)
Patients with diabetes with renal disease (defined either by the presence of albuminuria or reduced GFR) were randomized to aliskiren 300 mg daily (n=4296) or placebo (n=4310).

There was no effect on the fertility of rats treated orally with amlodipine maleate (males for 64 days and females for 14 days prior to mating) at doses of up to 10 mg amlodipine/kg/day (about 8 times the MRHD of 10 mg/day on a mg/m² basis). These doses in mice and rats are about 117 and 1300 mcg/mL, respectively. These doses in mice and rats represent 19 and 1.5 times, respectively, the maximum recommended human dose on a mg/m² basis. (Calculations assume an oral dose of 25 mg/day and a 60-kg patient.)

13.2   Animal Toxicology and/or Pharmacology
Reproductive Toxicology Studies
[See Use in Specific Populations (8.1).]

14   CLINICAL STUDIES
14.1   Amturnide
Amturnide was studied in a double-blind, active-controlled study in 1181 treated hypertensive patients, of whom 773 were classified as moderately hypertensive (SBP 160-180 mmHg) and 408 as severely hypertensive (SBP 180-200 mmHg) at baseline. The mean baseline systolic/diastolic blood pressure for all randomized patients was approximately 173/105 mmHg. A total of 61% of patients were male, 19% were 65 years or older, 84% were Caucasian, and 10% were Black.

At study initiation, patients assigned to the dual combination treatments received lower doses of their treatment combination (aliskiren 150 mg plus amlodipine 5 mg, aliskiren 150 mg plus HCTZ 12.5 mg, or amlodipine 5 mg plus HCTZ 12.5 mg), while patients assigned to the Amturnide arm received aliskiren/HCTZ 150/12.5 mg. After 3 days, Amturnide patients were titrated to aliskiren/amlodipine/HCTZ 150/5/12.5 mg, while all other patients continued receiving their initial doses. After 4 weeks, all patients were titrated to their full target doses of aliskiren/amlodipine/HCTZ 300/10/25 mg, aliskiren/amlodipine 300/10, aliskiren/HCTZ 300/25 mg, or amlodipine/HCTZ 10/25 mg.

Amturnide produced greater reductions in blood pressure than did any of the 3 dual combination treatments ($p < 0.001$ for both diastolic and systolic blood pressure reductions).

Studies with HCTZ
Two-year feeding studies in mice and rats conducted under the auspices of the National Toxicology Program (NTP) uncovered no evidence of a carcinogenic potential of HCTZ in female mice (at doses of up to approximately 600 mg/kg/day) or in male and female rats (at doses of up to approximately 100 mg/kg/day). These doses in mice and rats are about 117 and 39 times, respectively, the MRHD of 25 mg/day, when based on a mg/m² basis of a 60 kg individual. The NTP, however, found equivocal evidence for hepatocarcinogenicity in male mice.

HCTZ was not genotoxic *in vitro* in the Ames mutagenicity assay of *S. typhimurium* strains TA 98, TA 100, TA 1535, TA 1537, and TA 1538 and in the Chinese Hamster Ovary (CHO) test for chromosomal aberrations, or *in vivo* in assays using mouse germinal cell chromosomes, Chinese hamster bone marrow chromosomes, and the Drosophila sex-linked recessive lethal trait gene. Positive test results were obtained only in the *in vitro* CHO Sister Chromatid Exchange (clastogenicity) and in the Mouse Lymphoma Cell (mutagenicity) assays, using concentrations of HCTZ from 43 to 1300 mcg/mL, and in the *Aspergillus Nidulans* nondisjunction assay at an unspecified concentration.

HCTZ was not teratogenic and had no adverse effects on the fertility of mice and rats of either sex in studies wherein these species were exposed, via their diet, to doses of up to 100 and 4 mg/kg, respectively, prior to mating and throughout gestation. These doses of HCTZ in mice and rats represent

All patients were receiving background therapy with an ARB or ACEI. The primary efficacy outcome was the time to the first event of the primary composite endpoint consisting of cardiovascular death, resuscitated sudden death, non-fatal myocardial infarction, non-fatal stroke, unplanned hospitalization for heart failure, onset of end stage renal disease, renal death, and doubling of serum creatinine concentration from baseline sustained for at least one month. After a median follow up of about 32 months, the trial was terminated early for lack of efficacy. Higher risk of renal impairment, hypotension and hyperkalemia was observed in aliskiren compared to placebo treated patients, as shown in the table below.
[See table 2 above]
The risk of stroke (3.4% aliskiren vs 2.7% placebo) and death (8.4% aliskiren vs. 8.0% placebo) were also numerically higher in aliskiren treated patients.

16   HOW SUPPLIED/STORAGE AND HANDLING

Tablets are convex ovaloid with a beveled edge, film-coated, and unscored, in the following strengths and packages:
[See second table above]

Storage
Store at 25°C (77°F); excursions permitted to 15-30°C (59-86°F) in original container.
Protect from heat and moisture.
Dispense in original container.

17   PATIENT COUNSELING INFORMATION

See FDA-Approved Patient Labeling (Patient Information) Instruct patients to read the Patient Package Insert before starting Amturnide and to reread each time the prescription is renewed. Instruct patients to inform their doctor or pharmacist if they develop any unusual symptom, or if any known symptom persists or worsens.

Pregnancy
Female patients of childbearing age should be told about the consequences of exposure to Amturnide during pregnancy. Discuss treatment options with women planning to become pregnant. Patients should be asked to report pregnancies to their physicians as soon as possible.

Symptomatic Hypotension
Caution patients receiving Amturnide that lightheadedness can occur, especially during the first days of therapy, and that it should be reported to the prescribing physician. Tell patients that if syncope occurs, discontinue Amturnide until the physician has been consulted.
Caution all patients that inadequate fluid intake, excessive perspiration, diarrhea, or vomiting can lead to an excessive fall in blood pressure, with the same consequences of lightheadedness and possible syncope.

Anaphylactic Reactions and Angioedema
Advise patients to report immediately any signs or symptoms suggesting a severe allergic reaction (difficulty breathing or swallowing, tightness of the chest, hives, general rash, swelling, itching, dizziness, vomiting, or abdominal pain) or angioedema (swelling of face, extremities, eyes, lips, tongue, difficulty in swallowing or breathing) and to take no more drug until they have consulted with the prescribing physician. Angioedema, including laryngeal edema, may occur at any time during treatment with Amturnide.

Potassium Supplements
Tell patients receiving Amturnide not to use potassium supplements or salt substitutes containing potassium without consulting the prescribing physician.

Relationship to Meals
Patient should establish a routine pattern for taking Amturnide either with or without a meal. High-fat meals decrease absorption substantially.
T2014-21
March 2014
FDA-Approved Patient Labeling
Patient Information
Amturnide™ (AM-turn-ide)
Amturnide
(aliskiren, amlodipine and hydrochlorothiazide)
Tablets
Read the Patient Information leaflet that comes with Amturnide before you start taking it and each time you get a refill. There may be new information. This leaflet does not take the place of talking with your doctor about your medical condition and treatment. If you have any questions about Amturnide, ask your doctor or pharmacist.
What is the most important information I should know about Amturnide?
Amturnide can cause harm or death to an unborn baby. Talk to your doctor about other ways to lower your blood pressure if you plan to become pregnant. If you get pregnant while taking Amturnide, tell your doctor right away.
What is Amturnide?
Amturnide is a prescription medicine used to lower blood pressure (hypertension). Amturnide is not for use as the first medicine to treat your high blood pressure.
Amturnide contains 3 different prescription medicines:

Table 2: Incidence of Selected Adverse Events During the Treatment Phase in ALTITUDE

	Aliskiren N=4272		Placebo N=4285	
	Serious Adverse Events* (%)	Adverse Events (%)	Serious Adverse Events* (%)	Adverse Events (%)
Renal impairment †	5.7	14.5	4.3	12.4
Hypotension ††	2.3	19.9	1.9	16.3
Hyperkalemia †††	1.0	38.9	0.5	28.8

†renal failure, renal failure acute, renal failure chronic, renal impairment
††dizziness, dizziness postural, hypotension, orthostatic hypotension, presyncope, syncope
††† Given the variable baseline potassium levels of patients with renal insufficiency on dual RAAS therapy, the reporting of adverse event of hyperkalemia was at the discretion of the investigator.
* A Serious Adverse Event (SAE) is defined as: an event which is fatal or life-threatening, results in persistent or significant disability/incapacity, constitutes a congenital anomaly/birth defect, requires inpatient hospitalization or prolongation of existing hospitalization, or is medically significant (i.e. defined as an event that jeopardizes the patient or may require medical or surgical intervention to prevent one of the outcomes previously listed).

Aliskiren/Amlodipine/HCTZ (mg)	Color	Embossing Side 1/side 2	NDC 0078-XXXX-XX		
			Bottle/30	Bottle/90	Blister/100
150/5/12.5	Violet white	YIY/NVR	0610-15	0610-34	0610-35
300/5/12.5	Light pink	LIL/NVR	0611-15	0611-34	0611-35
300/5/25	Pale orange brown	OIO/NVR	0612-15	0612-34	0612-35
300/10/12.5	Light red	UIU/NVR	0613-15	0613-34	0613-35
300/10/25	Brown	VIV/NVR	0614-15	0614-34	0614-35

- aliskiren, a direct renin inhibitor (DRI)
- amlodipine, a calcium channel blocker (CCB) and
- hydrochlorothiazide (HCTZ), a diuretic (water pill)
It is not known if Amturnide is safe and works in children under 18 years of age.
Who should not take Amturnide?
Do not take Amturnide if you:
- If you get pregnant, stop taking Amturnide and call your doctor right away. If you plan to become pregnant, talk to your doctor about other treatment options for your high blood pressure.
- have diabetes and are taking a kind of medicine called an angiotensin-receptor-blocker or angiotensin-converting-enzyme-inhibitor.
- have low or no urine output
- are allergic to any ingredients in Amturnide or other medicines that contain sulfonamide. See the end of this leaflet for a complete list of ingredients in Amturnide.
What should I tell my doctor before taking Amturnide?
Before taking Amturnide, tell your doctor if you:
- have kidney problems
- have liver problems
- have lupus
- have had an allergic reaction to another blood pressure medicine. Symptoms may include: swelling of the face, lips, tongue, throat, arms and legs, and trouble breathing
- suffer from heart disorders or if you experienced a heart attack
- have any other medical problems
- are pregnant or planning to become pregnant. **See "What is the most important information I should know about Amturnide?"**
- are breast-feeding. It is not known if Amturnide passes into your breast milk and if it can harm your baby. You and your doctor should decide if you will take Amturnide or breastfeed. You should not do both.
Tell your doctor about all the medicines you take including prescription and nonprescription medicines, vitamins and herbal supplements. Amturnide and certain other medicines may affect each other and cause side effects.
Especially tell your doctor if you are taking:
- a kind of medicine called angiotensin receptor blocker or angiotensin converting enzyme inhibitor
- water pills (also called "diuretics")
- medicines for treating fungus or fungal infections
- cyclosporine (Gengraf®, Neoral, Sandimmune), a medicine used to suppress the immune system
- potassium-containing medicines, potassium supplements, or salt substitutes containing potassium
- cholesterol lowering medicines
  ○ simvastatin (Zocor®) or atorvastatin (Lipitor®)

  ○ cholestyramine (Questran, Questran Light, Cholestyramine Light, Locholest Light, Locholest, Prevalite)
  ○ colestipol (Colestipol hydrochloride, Colestid, Flavored Colestid)
- medicines used to treat diabetes, including insulin
- lithium, a medicine used to treat some types of depression. You should not take Amturnide if you are taking lithium.
- nonsteroidal anti-inflammatory (NSAIDs) medicines. Ask your doctor if you are not sure if you are taking one of these medicines.
- sleeping pills and anti-seizure medicines called barbiturates
- medicines used to treat AIDS or HIV infections (such as ritonavir, indinavir)
- narcotic pain medicines
Ask your doctor if you are not sure whether you are taking one of the medicines listed above.
Know the medicines you take. Keep a list of them to show your doctor or pharmacist when you get a new medicine. Your doctor or pharmacist will know what medicines are safe to take together.
How should I take Amturnide?
- Take Amturnide exactly as prescribed by your doctor. It is important to take Amturnide every day to control your blood pressure.
- Take Amturnide one time a day, at about the same time each day.
- Take Amturnide the same way every day, either with or without a meal.
- Your doctor may change your dose of Amturnide if needed. Do not change the amount of Amturnide you take without talking to your doctor.
- If you miss a dose of Amturnide, take it as soon as you remember. If it is close to your next dose, do not take the missed dose. Just take the next dose at your regular time.
- If you take too much Amturnide, call your doctor or a Poison Control Center, or go to the nearest hospital emergency room.
What should I avoid while taking Amturnide?
Drinking alcohol. Drinking alcohol during treatment with Amturnide can cause you to have low blood pressure. **See "What are the possible side effects of Amturnide?"**
What are the possible side effects of Amturnide?
Amturnide may cause serious side effects, including:
- **Harm to an unborn baby causing injury or death. See "What is the most important information I should know about Amturnide?"**
- **Severe Allergic Reactions and Angioedema.** Aliskiren, one of the medicines in Amturnide, can cause difficulty breathing or swallowing, tightness of the chest, hives, gen-

eral rash, swelling, itching, dizziness, vomiting, or abdominal pain (signs of a severe allergic reaction). Aliskiren can also cause swelling of your face, lips, tongue, throat, arms and legs, or the whole body (signs of angioedema). Get medical help right away and tell your doctor if you get any one or more of these symptoms. Serious allergic reactions can happen at any time while you are taking Amturnide.

• **Low blood pressure (hypotension).** Your blood pressure may get too low if you also take water pills, are on a low-salt diet, have dialysis treatments, have heart problems, or get sick with vomiting or diarrhea. Drinking alcohol and taking certain medicines (barbiturates or narcotics) can cause low blood pressure to get worse. Lie down if you feel faint or dizzy, and call your doctor right away.

• **Worsening chest pain or heart attack.** When you first start taking Amturnide or increase your dose, you may have a heart attack or your angina may get worse. If that happens, call your doctor right away or go directly to the nearest hospital emergency room.

• **Allergic reactions.** Hydrochlorothiazide, one of the medicines in Amturnide, can cause allergic reactions.

• **Worsening of lupus.** One of the medicines in Amturnide may cause your lupus to become active or get worse. Tell your doctor if your lupus gets worse or becomes active while taking Amturnide.

• **Low potassium level (hypokalemia).** Your doctor will do blood tests to check your potassium levels.

• **Eye problems.** One of the medicines in Amturnide can cause eye problems that may lead to vision loss. Symptoms of eye problems can happen within hours to weeks of starting Amturnide. Tell your doctor right away if you have:
  ◦ decrease in vision
  ◦ eye pain

• **Renal impairment or failure.** Aliskiren, one of the medicines in Amturnide, may cause renal disorder with symptoms such as severely decreased urine output or decreased urine output (signs of renal impairment or failure).

The most common side effects of Amturnide include:
• swelling of your ankles, feet, and hands
• dizziness
• headache
• stuffy or runny nose and sore throat

Common side effects of Amturnide include:
• diarrhea
• cough
• tiredness
• high levels of potassium in the blood (hyperkalemia)

Less common side effects include rash, severe skin reactions (signs may include severe blistering of the lips, eyes or mouth, rash with fever and skin peeling) and liver disorder (signs may include nausea, loss of appetite, dark colored urine or yellowing of skin and eyes).

Tell your doctor if you have any side effect that bothers you or that does not go away. These are not all of the possible side effects of Amturnide. For more information ask your doctor or pharmacist.

Call your doctor for medical advice about side effects. You may report side effects to FDA at 1-800-FDA-1088.

How should I store Amturnide?
• Store Amturnide tablets at room temperature between 59°F to 86°F (15°C to 30°C).
• Keep Amturnide in the original container.
• Protect Amturnide from heat and moisture.

Keep Amturnide and all medicines out of the reach of children.

General information about Amturnide
Medicines are sometimes prescribed for conditions not listed in the patient information leaflet. Do not take Amturnide for a condition for which it was not prescribed. Do not give Amturnide to other people, even if they have the same condition or symptoms you have. It may harm them. This leaflet summarizes the most important information about Amturnide. If you have questions about Amturnide, talk with your doctor. You can ask your doctor or pharmacist for information that is written for healthcare professionals.

For more information about Amturnide, visit www.Amturnide.com, or call 1-888-NOW-NOVA (1-888-669-6682).

What are the ingredients in Amturnide?
Active ingredients: Aliskiren hemifumarate, amlodipine besylate, and HCTZ.
Inactive ingredients: colloidal silicon dioxide, crospovidone, hypromellose, iron oxide red, iron oxide yellow, iron oxide black, magnesium stearate, microcrystalline cellulose, polyethylene glycol, povidone, talc, and titanium dioxide.

What is high blood pressure (hypertension)?
Blood pressure is the force of blood in your blood vessels when your heart beats and when your heart rests. You have high blood pressure when the force is too much.

High blood pressure makes the heart work harder to pump blood through the body and causes damage to blood vessels. Amturnide can help your blood vessels relax so your blood

pressure is lower. Medicines that lower your blood pressure may lower your chance of having a stroke or heart attack.
Distributed by:
Novartis Pharmaceuticals Corporation
East Hanover, New Jersey 07936
© Novartis
T2013-107
November 2013
Shown in Product Identification Guide, page 309

ARCAPTA™ NEOHALER™   ℞
[ar-CAP-ta]
(indacaterol inhalation powder)

The following prescribing information is based on official labeling in effect July 2013.
HIGHLIGHTS OF PRESCRIBING INFORMATION
These highlights do not include all the information needed to use ARCAPTA NEOHALER safely and effectively. See full prescribing information for ARCAPTA NEOHALER.
ARCAPTA™ NEOHALER™ (indacaterol inhalation powder)
Initial U.S. Approval: 2011

> **WARNING: ASTHMA-RELATED DEATH**
> *See full prescribing information for complete boxed warning*
> • Long-acting beta₂-adrenergic agonists (LABA) increase the risk of asthma-related death (5.1).
> • A placebo-controlled study with another long-acting beta₂-adrenergic agonist (salmeterol) showed an increase in asthma-related deaths in patients receiving salmeterol. (5.1)
> • This finding of an increased risk of asthma-related death with salmeterol is considered a class effect of LABA, including indacaterol, the active ingredient in ARCAPTA NEOHALER. The safety and efficacy of ARCAPTA NEOHALER in patients with asthma have not been established. ARCAPTA NEOHALER is not indicated for the treatment of asthma. (4, 5.1)

———————RECENT MAJOR CHANGES———————

Contraindications (4)	09/2012
Warnings and Precautions, Immediate Hypersensitivity Reactions (5.4)	09/2012

——————INDICATIONS AND USAGE——————
ARCAPTA NEOHALER is a long-acting beta₂-adrenergic agonist indicated for:
The long term, once-daily maintenance bronchodilator treatment of airflow obstruction in patients with chronic obstructive pulmonary disease (COPD), including chronic bronchitis and/or emphysema. (1.1)
Important limitations:
• ARCAPTA NEOHALER is NOT indicated to treat acute deteriorations of chronic obstructive pulmonary disease. (1.2)
• ARCAPTA NEOHALER is NOT indicated for asthma. (1.2)

————DOSAGE AND ADMINISTRATION————
For oral inhalation only. DO NOT swallow ARCAPTA capsule. ARCAPTA capsules should **always** be used with the NEOHALER inhaler **only**.
75 mcg inhaled every day (once-daily). (2)

————DOSAGE FORMS AND STRENGTHS————
Inhalation powder hard capsules: 75 mcg. (3)

——————CONTRAINDICATIONS——————
• All LABA are contraindicated in patients with asthma without use of a long-term asthma control medication. (4) ARCAPTA NEOHALER is not indicated for the treatment of asthma.
• ARCAPTA NEOHALER is contraindicated in patients with a history of hypersensitivity to indacaterol or to any of the ingredients. (4)

——————WARNINGS AND PRECAUTIONS——————
• Do not initiate in acutely deteriorating COPD patients (5.2)
• Do not use for relief of acute symptoms. Concomitant short-acting beta₂-agonists can be used as needed for acute relief (5.2)
• Do not exceed the recommended dose. Excessive use or use in conjunction with other medications containing LABA can result in clinically significant cardiovascular effects and may be fatal (5.3)
• Immediate hypersensitivity reactions may occur. Discontinue immediately. (5.4)
• Life-threatening paradoxical bronchospasm can occur. Discontinue immediately. (5.5)
• Use with caution in patients with cardiovascular or convulsive disorders, thyrotoxicosis or sensitivity to sympathomimetic drugs. (5.6, 5.7)

——————ADVERSE REACTIONS——————
Most common adverse reactions (>2% and more common than placebo) are cough, oropharyngeal pain, nasopharyngitis, headache and nausea. (6)

To report SUSPECTED ADVERSE REACTIONS, contact Novartis Pharmaceuticals Corporation at 1-888-669-6682 or FDA at 1-800-FDA-1088 or www.fda.gov/medwatch.

——————DRUG INTERACTIONS——————
• Other adrenergic drugs may potentiate effect: Use with caution. (5.3, 7.1)
• Xanthine derivatives, steroids, diuretics or non-potassium sparing diuretics may potentiate hypokalemia or ECG changes. Use with caution. (7.2, 7.3)
• MAO inhibitors, tricyclic antidepressants, and drugs that prolong QTc interval may potentiate effect on cardiovascular system. Use with extreme caution. (7.4)
• Beta-blockers may decrease effectiveness: Use with caution and only when medically necessary. (7.5)

See 17 for PATIENT COUNSELING INFORMATION and Medication Guide

Revised: 9/2012

FULL PRESCRIBING INFORMATION: CONTENTS*
WARNING: ASTHMA-RELATED DEATH
1 INDICATIONS AND USAGE
  1.1 Maintenance Treatment of COPD
  1.2 Important Limitations of Use
2 DOSAGE AND ADMINISTRATION
3 DOSAGE FORMS AND STRENGTHS
4 CONTRAINDICATIONS
5 WARNINGS AND PRECAUTIONS
  5.1 Asthma-Related Death *[See Boxed Warning]*
  5.2 Deterioration of Disease and Acute Episodes
  5.3 Excessive Use of ARCAPTA NEOHALER and Use with Other Long-Acting Beta₂-Agonists
  5.4 Immediate Hypersensitivity Reactions
  5.5 Paradoxical Bronchospasm
  5.6 Cardiovascular Effects
  5.7 Coexisting Conditions
  5.8 Hypokalemia and Hyperglycemia
6 ADVERSE REACTIONS
  6.1 Clinical Trials Experience in Chronic Obstructive Pulmonary Disease
  6.2 Clinical Trials Experience in Asthma
  6.3 Postmarketing Experience
7 DRUG INTERACTIONS
  7.1 Adrenergic Drugs
  7.2 Xanthine Derivatives, Steroids, or Diuretics
  7.3 Non-Potassium Sparing Diuretics
  7.4 Monoamine Oxidase Inhibitors, Tricyclic Antidepressants, QTc Prolonging Drugs
  7.5 Beta-Blockers
  7.6 Inhibitors of Cytochrome P450 3A4 and P-gp Efflux Transporter
8 USE IN SPECIFIC POPULATIONS
  8.1 Pregnancy
  8.2 Labor and Delivery
  8.3 Nursing Mothers
  8.4 Pediatric Use
  8.5 Geriatric Use
  8.6 Hepatic Impairment
  8.7 Renal Impairment
10 OVERDOSAGE
  10.1 Human Experience
11 DESCRIPTION
12 CLINICAL PHARMACOLOGY
  12.1 Mechanism of Action
  12.2 Pharmacodynamics
  12.3 Pharmacokinetics
  12.4 Pharmacogenomics
13 NONCLINICAL TOXICOLOGY
  13.1 Carcinogenesis, Mutagenesis, Impairment of Fertility
14 CLINICAL STUDIES
16 HOW SUPPLIED/STORAGE AND HANDLING
  16.1 How Supplied
  16.2 Storage and Handling
17 PATIENT COUNSELING INFORMATION
  17.1 Asthma-Related Death
  17.2 Instructions for Administering ARCAPTA NEOHALER
  17.3 Not for Acute Symptoms
  17.4 Do Not Use Additional Long-Acting Beta₂-Agonists
  17.5 Risks Associated With Beta-Agonist Therapy
* Sections or subsections omitted from the full prescribing information are not listed

---

FULL PRESCRIBING INFORMATION

> **WARNING: ASTHMA-RELATED DEATH**
> **Long-acting beta₂-adrenergic agonists (LABA) increase the risk of asthma-related death. Data from a large placebo-controlled US study that compared the safety of another long-acting beta₂-adrenergic agonist (salmeterol) or placebo added to usual asthma therapy in patients receiving salmeterol. This finding with sal-**

meterol is considered a class effect of LABA, including indacaterol, the active ingredient in ARCAPTA NEOHALER. The safety and efficacy of ARCAPTA NEOHALER in patients with asthma have not been established. ARCAPTA NEOHALER is not indicated for the treatment of asthma. [See *Contraindications (4), Warnings and Precautions (5.1)*].

1   INDICATIONS AND USAGE
1.1   Maintenance Treatment of COPD
ARCAPTA NEOHALER is a long-acting beta$_2$-agonist indicated for long-term, once-daily maintenance bronchodilator treatment of airflow obstruction in patients with chronic obstructive pulmonary disease (COPD), including chronic bronchitis and/or emphysema.
1.2   Important Limitations of Use
ARCAPTA NEOHALER is not indicated to treat acute deteriorations of chronic obstructive pulmonary disease [*see Warnings and Precautions (5.2)*].

ARCAPTA NEOHALER is not indicated to treat asthma. The safety and effectiveness of ARCAPTA NEOHALER in asthma have not been established.

2   DOSAGE AND ADMINISTRATION
DO NOT SWALLOW ARCAPTA CAPSULES
FOR USE WITH NEOHALER DEVICE ONLY
FOR ORAL INHALATION ONLY
ARCAPTA capsules must not be swallowed as the intended effects on the lungs will not be obtained. The contents of ARCAPTA capsules are only for oral inhalation and should only be used with the NEOHALER device.

The recommended dosage of ARCAPTA NEOHALER is the once-daily inhalation of the contents of one 75 mcg ARCAPTA capsule using the NEOHALER inhaler.

ARCAPTA NEOHALER should be administered once daily every day at the same time of the day by the orally inhaled route only. If a dose is missed, the next dose should be taken as soon as it is remembered. Do not use ARCAPTA NEOHALER more than one time every 24 hours.

ARCAPTA capsules must always be stored in the blister, and only removed IMMEDIATELY BEFORE USE.

No dosage adjustment is required for geriatric patients, patients with mild and moderate hepatic impairment, or renally impaired patients. No data are available for subjects with severe hepatic impairment [*see Clinical Pharmacology (12.3)*].

3   DOSAGE FORMS AND STRENGTHS
Inhalation powder:
75 mcg: hard gelatin capsule with black product code "IDL 75" above a bar printed on one side of the capsule and the logo "⁄." printed on the other side.

4   CONTRAINDICATIONS
All LABA are contraindicated in patients with asthma without use of a long-term asthma control medication. [*see Warnings and Precautions (5.1)*]. ARCAPTA NEOHALER is not indicated for the treatment of asthma.

ARCAPTA NEOHALER is contraindicated in patients with a history of hypersensitivity to indacaterol or to any of the ingredients. [*see Warnings and Precautions (5.4)*].

5   WARNINGS AND PRECAUTIONS
5.1   Asthma-Related Death [See Boxed Warning]
• Data from a large placebo-controlled study in asthma patients showed that long-acting beta$_2$-adrenergic agonists may increase the risk of asthma-related death. Data are not available to determine whether the rate of death in patients with COPD is increased by long-acting beta$_2$-adrenergic agonists.
• A 28-week, placebo-controlled US study comparing the safety of another long-acting beta$_2$-adrenergic agonist (salmeterol) with placebo, each added to usual asthma therapy, showed an increase in asthma-related deaths in patients receiving salmeterol (13/13,176 in patients treated with salmeterol vs. 3/13,179 in patients treated with placebo; RR 4.37, 95% CI 1.25, 15.34). The increased risk of asthma-related death is considered a class effect of the long-acting beta$_2$-adrenergic agonists, including ARCAPTA NEOHALER. No study adequate to determine whether the rate of asthma-related death is increased in patients treated with ARCAPTA NEOHALER has been conducted. The safety and efficacy of ARCAPTA NEOHALER in patients with asthma have not been established. ARCAPTA NEOHALER is not indicated for the treatment of asthma. [*see Contraindications (4)*].
• Serious asthma-related events, including death, were reported in clinical studies with ARCAPTA NEOHALER. The sizes of these studies were not adequate to precisely quantify the differences in serious asthma exacerbation rates between treatment groups. [*see Adverse Reactions (6.2)*].
5.2   Deterioration of Disease and Acute Episodes
ARCAPTA NEOHALER should not be initiated in patients with acutely deteriorating COPD, which may be a life-threatening condition. ARCAPTA NEOHALER has not been studied in patients with acutely deteriorating COPD. The use of ARCAPTA NEOHALER in this setting is inappropriate.

ARCAPTA NEOHALER should not be used for the relief of acute symptoms, i.e. as rescue therapy for the treatment of acute episodes of bronchospasm. ARCAPTA NEOHALER has not been studied in the relief of acute symptoms and extra doses should not be used for that purpose. Acute symptoms should be treated with an inhaled short-acting beta$_2$-agonist.

When beginning ARCAPTA NEOHALER, patients who have been taking inhaled, short-acting beta$_2$-agonists on a regular basis (e.g., four times a day) should be instructed to discontinue the regular use of these drugs and use them only for symptomatic relief of acute respiratory symptoms. When prescribing ARCAPTA NEOHALER, the healthcare provider should also prescribe an inhaled, short-acting beta$_2$-agonist and instruct the patient on how it should be used. Increasing inhaled beta$_2$-agonist use is a signal of deteriorating disease for which prompt medical attention is indicated.

COPD may deteriorate acutely over a period of hours or chronically over several days or longer. If ARCAPTA NEOHALER no longer controls the symptoms of bronchoconstriction, or the patient's inhaled, short-acting beta$_2$-agonist becomes less effective or the patient needs more inhalation of short-acting beta$_2$-agonist than usual, these may be markers of deterioration of disease. In this setting, a re-evaluation of the patient and the COPD treatment regimen should be undertaken at once. Increasing the daily dosage of ARCAPTA NEOHALER beyond the recommended dose is not appropriate in this situation.
5.3   Excessive Use of ARCAPTA NEOHALER and Use with Other Long-Acting Beta$_2$-Agonists
As with other inhaled beta$_2$-adrenergic drugs, ARCAPTA NEOHALER should not be used more often, at higher doses than recommended, or in conjunction with other medications containing long-acting beta$_2$-agonists, as an overdose may result. Clinically significant cardiovascular effects and fatalities have been reported in association with excessive use of inhaled sympathomimetic drugs.
5.4   Immediate Hypersensitivity Reactions
Immediate hypersensitivity reactions may occur after administration of ARCAPTA NEOHALER. If signs suggesting allergic reactions (in particular, difficulties in breathing or swallowing, swelling of tongue, lips and face, urticaria, skin rash) occur, ARCAPTA NEOHALER should be discontinued immediately and alternative therapy instituted.
5.5   Paradoxical Bronchospasm
As with other inhaled beta$_2$-agonists, ARCAPTA NEOHALER may produce paradoxical bronchospasm that may be life-threatening. If paradoxical bronchospasm occurs, ARCAPTA NEOHALER should be discontinued immediately and alternative therapy instituted.
5.6   Cardiovascular Effects
ARCAPTA NEOHALER, like other beta$_2$-agonists, can produce a clinically significant cardiovascular effect in some patients as measured by increases in pulse rate, systolic or diastolic blood pressure, or symptoms. If such effects occur, ARCAPTA NEOHALER may need to be discontinued. In addition, beta-agonists have been reported to produce ECG changes, such as flattening of the T wave, prolongation of the QTc interval, and ST segment depression, although the clinical significance of these findings is unknown. Therefore, ARCAPTA NEOHALER, like other sympathomimetic amines, should be used with caution in patients with cardiovascular disorders, especially coronary insufficiency, cardiac arrhythmias, and hypertension.
5.7   Coexisting Conditions
ARCAPTA NEOHALER, like other sympathomimetic amines, should be used with caution in patients with convulsive disorders or thyrotoxicosis, and in patients who are unusually responsive to sympathomimetic amines. Doses of the related beta$_2$-agonist albuterol, when administered intravenously, have been reported to aggravate pre-existing diabetes mellitus and ketoacidosis.
5.8   Hypokalemia and Hyperglycemia
Beta$_2$-agonist medications may produce significant hypokalemia in some patients, possibly through intracellular shunting, which has the potential to produce adverse cardiovascular effects [*see Clinical Pharmacology (12.2)*]. The decrease in serum potassium is usually transient, not requiring supplementation. Inhalation of high doses of beta$_2$-adrenergic agonists may produce increases in plasma glucose.

Clinically notable decreases in serum potassium or changes in blood glucose were infrequent during clinical studies with long-term administration of ARCAPTA NEOHALER with the rates similar to those for placebo controls. ARCAPTA NEOHALER has not been investigated in patients whose diabetes mellitus is not well controlled.

6   ADVERSE REACTIONS
Long-acting beta$_2$-adrenergic agonists, such as ARCAPTA NEOHALER, increase the risk of asthma-related death.

ARCAPTA NEOHALER is not indicated for the treatment of asthma [*See Boxed Warning* and *Warning and Precautions (5.1)*].
6.1   Clinical Trials Experience in Chronic Obstructive Pulmonary Disease
Because clinical trials are conducted under widely varying conditions, adverse reaction rates observed in the clinical trials of a drug cannot be directly compared to rates in the clinical trials of another drug and may not reflect the rates observed in practice.

The ARCAPTA NEOHALER safety database reflects exposure of 2516 patients to ARCAPTA NEOHALER at doses of 75 mcg or greater for at least 12 weeks in six confirmatory randomized, double-blind, placebo and active-controlled clinical trials (see Section 14). In these trials, 449 patients were exposed to the recommended dose of 75 mcg for up to 3 months, and 144, 583 and 425 COPD patients were exposed to a dose of 150, 300 or 600 mcg for one year, respectively. Overall, patients had a mean pre-bronchodilator forced expiratory volume in one second (FEV$_1$) percent predicted of 54%. The mean age of patients was 64 years, with 47% of patients aged 65 years or older, and the majority (88%) was Caucasian.

In these six clinical trials, 48% of patients treated with any dose of ARCAPTA NEOHALER reported an adverse reaction compared with 43% of patients treated with placebo. The proportion of patients who discontinued treatment due to adverse reaction was 5% for ARCAPTA NEOHALER-treated patients and 5% for placebo-treated patients. The most common adverse reactions that lead to discontinuation of ARCAPTA NEOHALER were COPD and dyspnea.

The most common serious adverse reactions were COPD exacerbation, pneumonia, angina pectoris, and atrial fibrillation, which occurred at similar rates across treatment groups.

Table 1 displays adverse drug reactions reported by at least 2% of patients (and higher than placebo) during a 3 month exposure at the recommended 75 mcg once daily dose. Adverse drug reactions are listed according to MedDRA (version 13.0) system organ class and sorted in descending order of frequency.

Table 1: Number and frequency of adverse drug reactions greater than 2% (and higher than placebo) in COPD patients exposed to ARCAPTA NEOHALER 75 mcg for up to 3 months in multiple dose, controlled trials

	Indacaterol 75 mcg once daily	Placebo
	n=449	n=445
	n (%)	n (%)
Respiratory, thoracic and mediastinal disorders		
- Cough	29 (6.5)	20 (4.5)
- Oropharyngeal pain	10 (2.2)	3 (0.7)
Infections and infestations		
- Nasopharyngitis	24 (5.3)	12 (2.7)
Nervous system disorders		
- Headache	23 (5.1)	11 (2.5)
Gastrointestinal disorders		
- Nausea	11 (2.4)	4 (0.9)

In these trials the overall frequency of all cardiovascular adverse reactions was 2.5% for ARCAPTA NEOHALER 75 mcg and 1.6% for placebo during a 3 month exposure. There were no frequently occurring specific cardiovascular adverse reactions for ARCAPTA NEOHALER 75 mcg (frequency at least 1% and greater than placebo).

Additional adverse drug reactions reported in greater than 2% (and higher than placebo) in patients dosed with 150, 300 or 600 mcg for up to 12 months were as follows:
• Musculoskeletal and connective tissue disorders: muscle spasm, musculoskeletal pain
• General disorders and administration site conditions: edema peripheral
• Metabolism and nutrition disorder: diabetes mellitus, hyperglycemia
• Infections and infestations: sinusitis, upper respiratory tract infection
Cough experienced post-inhalation
In the clinical trials, health care providers observed during clinic visits that an average of 24% of patients experienced a cough on at least 20% of visits following inhalation of the recommended 75 mcg dose of ARCAPTA NEOHALER com-

pared to 7% of patients receiving placebo. The cough usually occurred within 15 seconds following inhalation and lasted for no more than 15 seconds. Cough following inhalation in clinical trials was not associated with bronchospasm, exacerbations, deteriorations of disease or loss of efficacy.

6.2 Clinical Trials Experience in Asthma
In a 6-month randomized, active controlled asthma safety trial, 805 adult patients with moderate to severe persistent asthma were treated with ARCAPTA NEOHALER 300 mcg (n=268), ARCAPTA NEOHALER 600 mcg (n=268), and salmeterol (n=269), all concomitant with inhaled corticosteroids, which were not co-randomized. Of these patients, there were 2 respiratory-related deaths in the ARCAPTA NEOHALER 300 mcg dose group. There were no deaths in the ARCAPTA NEOHALER 600 mcg dose group or in the salmeterol active control group. Serious adverse reactions related to asthma exacerbation were reported for 2 patients in the indacaterol 300 mcg group, 3 patients in the indacaterol 600 mcg group, and no patients in the salmeterol active control group.

In addition, a two-week dose-ranging trial was conducted in 511 adult patients with mild persistent asthma taking inhaled corticosteroids. No deaths, intubations, or serious adverse reactions related to asthma exacerbation were reported in this trial.

6.3 Postmarketing Experience
The following adverse reactions have been identified during worldwide post-approval use of indacaterol, the active ingredient in ARCAPTA NEOHALER. Because these reactions are reported voluntarily from a population of uncertain size, it is not always possible to reliably estimate their frequency or establish a causal relationship to drug exposure. These adverse reactions are: hypersensitivity reactions, paradoxical bronchospasm, tachycardia/heart rate increase/palpitations, pruritus/rash and dizziness.

7 DRUG INTERACTIONS
7.1 Adrenergic Drugs
If additional adrenergic drugs are to be administered by any route, they should be used with caution because the sympathetic effects of ARCAPTA NEOHALER may be potentiated [see Warnings and Precautions (5.3, 5.6, 5.7, 5.8)].

7.2 Xanthine Derivatives, Steroids, or Diuretics
Concomitant treatment with xanthine derivatives, steroids, or diuretics may potentiate any hypokalemic effect of ARCAPTA NEOHALER [see Warnings and Precautions (5.8)].

7.3 Non-Potassium Sparing Diuretics
The ECG changes or hypokalemia that may result from the administration of non-potassium sparing diuretics (such as loop or thiazide diuretics) can be acutely worsened by beta-agonists, especially when the recommended dose of the beta-agonist is exceeded. Although the clinical relevance of these effects is not known, caution is advised in the co-administration of ARCAPTA NEOHALER with non-potassium-sparing diuretics.

7.4 Monoamine Oxidase Inhibitors, Tricyclic Antidepressants, QTc Prolonging Drugs
Indacaterol, as with other beta-agonists, should be administered with extreme caution to patients being treated with monoamine oxidase inhibitors, tricyclic antidepressants, or other drugs known to prolong the QTc interval because the action of adrenergic agonists on the cardiovascular system may be potentiated by these agents. Drugs that are known to prolong the QTc interval may have an increased risk of ventricular arrhythmias.

7.5 Beta-Blockers
Beta-adrenergic receptor antagonists (beta-blockers) and ARCAPTA NEOHALER may interfere with the effect of each other when administered concurrently. Beta-blockers not only block the therapeutic effects of beta-agonists, but may produce severe bronchospasm in COPD patients. Therefore, patients with COPD should not normally be treated with beta-blockers. However, under certain circumstances, e.g. as prophylaxis after myocardial infarction, there may be no acceptable alternatives to the use of beta-blockers in patients with COPD. In this setting, cardioselective beta-blockers could be considered, although they should be administered with caution.

7.6 Inhibitors of Cytochrome P450 3A4 and P-gp Efflux Transporter
Drug interaction studies were carried out using potent and specific inhibitors of CYP3A4 and P-gp (i.e., ketoconazole, erythromycin, verapamil and ritonavir). The data suggest that systemic clearance is influenced by modulation of both P-gp and CYP3A4 activities and that the 1.9-fold AUC_{0-24} increase caused by the strong dual inhibitor ketoconazole reflects the impact of maximal combined inhibition. ARCAPTA NEOHALER was evaluated in clinical trials for up to one year at doses up to 600 mcg. No dose adjustment is warranted at the 75 mcg dose. [See Drug-drug Interaction (12.3)]

8 USE IN SPECIFIC POPULATIONS
8.1 Pregnancy
Teratogenic Effects: Pregnancy Category C.
There are no adequate and well-controlled studies with ARCAPTA NEOHALER in pregnant women. ARCAPTA

NEOHALER should be used during pregnancy only if the potential benefit justifies the potential risk to the fetus. Indacaterol was not teratogenic following subcutaneous administration to rats and rabbits at doses up to 1 mg/kg, approximately 130 and 260 times, respectively, the 75 mcg dose on a mg/m² basis.

8.2 Labor and Delivery
There are no adequate and well-controlled human studies that have investigated effects of ARCAPTA NEOHALER on preterm labor or labor at term. Because of the potential for beta-agonist interference with uterine contractility, use of ARCAPTA NEOHALER during labor should be restricted to those patients in whom the benefits clearly outweigh the risks.

8.3 Nursing Mothers
It is not known that the active component of ARCAPTA NEOHALER, indacaterol, is excreted in human milk. Because many drugs are excreted in human milk and because indacaterol has been detected in the milk of lactating rats, caution should be exercised when ARCAPTA NEOHALER is administered to nursing women.

8.4 Pediatric Use
ARCAPTA NEOHALER is not indicated for use in children. The safety and effectiveness of ARCAPTA NEOHALER in pediatric patients have not been established.

8.5 Geriatric Use
Based on available data, no adjustment of ARCAPTA NEOHALER dosage in geriatric patients is warranted. Of the total number of patients who received ARCAPTA NEOHALER at the recommended dose of 75 mcg once daily in the clinical studies from the pooled 3-month database, 239 were <65 years, 153 were 65–74 years and 57 were ≥75 years of age.

No overall differences in effectiveness were observed, and in the 3-month pooled data, the adverse drug reaction profile was similar in the older population compared to the patient population overall. When treated at higher doses (300 mcg and 600 mcg) over the course of a year, the adverse drug reaction profiles for patients >65 years was similar to that of the general patient population.

8.6 Hepatic Impairment
Patients with mild and moderate hepatic impairment showed no relevant changes in C_{max} or AUC, nor did protein binding differ between mild and moderate hepatically impaired subjects and their healthy controls. Studies in subjects with severe hepatic impairment were not performed.

8.7 Renal Impairment
Due to the very low contribution of the urinary pathway to total body elimination, a study in renally impaired subjects was not performed.

10 OVERDOSAGE
10.1 Human Experience
In COPD patients single doses of 40 times the 75 mcg dose were associated with moderate increases in pulse rate, systolic blood pressure and QTc interval.

The expected signs and symptoms associated with overdosage of ARCAPTA NEOHALER are those of excessive beta-adrenergic stimulation and occurrence or exaggeration of any of the signs and symptoms, e.g., angina, hypertension or hypotension, tachycardia, with rates up to 200 bpm, arrhythmias, nervousness, headache, tremor, dry mouth, palpitation, muscle cramps, nausea, dizziness, fatigue, malaise, hypokalemia, hyperglycemia, metabolic acidosis and insomnia. As with all inhaled sympathomimetic medications, cardiac arrest and even death may be associated with an overdose of ARCAPTA NEOHALER.

Treatment of overdosage consists of discontinuation of ARCAPTA NEOHALER together with institution of appropriate symptomatic and supportive therapy. The judicious use of a cardioselective beta-receptor blocker may be considered, bearing in mind that such medication can produce bronchospasm. There is insufficient evidence to determine if dialysis is beneficial for overdosage of ARCAPTA NEOHALER. Cardiac monitoring is recommended in cases of overdosage.

11 DESCRIPTION
ARCAPTA NEOHALER consists of a dry powder formulation of indacaterol maleate for oral inhalation only with the NEOHALER inhaler. The inhalation powder is packaged in clear gelatin capsules.

Each clear, hard gelatin capsule contains a dry powder blend of 75 mcg of indacaterol (equivalent to 97 mcg of indacaterol maleate) with approximately 25 mg of lactose monohydrate (which contains trace levels of milk protein) as the carrier.

The active component of ARCAPTA NEOHALER is indacaterol maleate, a (R) enantiomer. Indacaterol maleate is a selective beta₂-adrenergic agonist. Its chemical name is (R)-5-[2-(5,6-Diethylindan-2-ylamino)-1-hydroxyethyl]-8-hydroxy-1H-quinolin-2-one maleate; its structural formula is

Indacaterol maleate has a molecular weight of 508.56, and its empirical formula is $C_{24}H_{28}N_2O_3 \cdot C_4H_4O_4$. Indacaterol maleate is a white to very slightly grayish or very slightly yellowish powder. Indacaterol maleate is freely soluble in N-methylpyrrolidone and dimethylformamide, slightly soluble in methanol, ethanol, propylene glycol and polyethylene glycol 400, very slightly soluble in water, isopropyl alcohol and practically insoluble in 0.9% sodium chloride in water, ethyl acetate and n-octanol.

The NEOHALER inhaler is a plastic device used for inhaling ARCAPTA. The amount of drug delivered to the lung will depend on patient factors, such as inspiratory flow rate and inspiratory time. Under standardized *in vitro* testing at a fixed flow rate of 60 L/min for 2 seconds, the NEOHALER inhaler delivered 57 mcg for the 75 mcg dose strength (equivalent to 73.9 mcg of indacaterol maleate) from the mouthpiece. Peak inspiratory flow rates (PIFR) achievable through the NEOHALER inhaler were evaluated in 26 adult patients with COPD of varying severity. Mean PIFR was 95 L/min (range 52-133 L/min) for adult patients. Approximately ninety-five percent of the population studied generated a PIFR through the device exceeding 60 L/min.

12 CLINICAL PHARMACOLOGY
12.1 Mechanism of Action
Indacaterol is a long-acting beta₂-adrenergic agonist. When inhaled, indacaterol acts locally in the lung as a bronchodilator. Although beta₂-receptors are the predominant adrenergic receptors in bronchial smooth muscle and beta₁-receptors are the predominant receptors in the heart, there are also beta₂-adrenergic receptors in the human heart comprising 10%-50% of the total adrenergic receptors. The precise function of these receptors is not known, but their presence raises the possibility that even highly selective beta₂-adrenergic agonists may have cardiac effects.

The pharmacological effects of beta₂-adrenoceptor agonist drugs, including indacaterol, are at least in part attributable to stimulation of intracellular adenyl cyclase, the enzyme that catalyzes the conversion of adenosine triphosphate (ATP) to cyclic-3′, 5′-adenosine monophosphate (cyclic monophosphate). Increased cyclic AMP levels cause relaxation of bronchial smooth muscle. *In vitro* studies have shown that indacaterol has more than 24-fold greater agonist activity at beta₂-receptors compared to beta₁-receptors and 20-fold greater agonist activity compared to beta₃-receptors. This selectivity profile is similar to formoterol. The clinical significance of these findings is unknown.

12.2 Pharmacodynamics
Systemic Safety
The major adverse effects of inhaled beta₂-adrenergic agonists occur as a result of excessive activation of systemic beta-adrenergic receptors. The most common adverse effects in adults include skeletal muscle tremor and cramps, insomnia, tachycardia, decreases in serum potassium and increases in plasma glucose.

Changes in serum potassium and plasma glucose were evaluated in COPD patients in double-blind Phase III studies. In pooled data, at the recommended 75 mcg dose, at 1 hour post-dose at week 12, there was no change compared to placebo in serum potassium, and change in mean plasma glucose was 0.07 mmol/L.

Electrophysiology
The effect of ARCAPTA NEOHALER on the QT interval was evaluated in a double-blind, placebo- and active-(moxifloxacin)-controlled study following multiple doses of indacaterol 150 mcg, 300 mcg or 600 mcg once-daily for 2 weeks in 404 healthy volunteers. Fridericia's method for heart rate correction was employed to derive the corrected QT interval (QTcF). Maximum mean prolongation of QTcF intervals were <5 ms, and the upper limit of the 90% confidence interval was below 10 ms for all time-matched comparisons versus placebo. During these studies, there were no clinically meaningful QT-interval prolongations. There was no evidence of a clinically relevant concentration-delta QTc relationship in the range of doses evaluated.

The effect of 150 mcg and 300 mcg once daily of ARCAPTA NEOHALER on heart rate and rhythm was assessed using continuous 24-hour ECG recording (Holter monitoring) in a subset of 605 patients with COPD from a 26-week, double-blind, placebo-controlled Phase III study. Holter monitoring occurred once at baseline and up to 3 times during the 26-week treatment period (at weeks 2, 12 and 26). A comparison of the mean heart rate over 24 hours showed no increase from baseline. The hourly heart rate analysis was similar compared to placebo. The pattern of diurnal variation over 24 hours was maintained and was similar to placebo. No difference from placebo was seen in the rates of atrial fibrillation, time spent in atrial fibrillation and also the maximum ventricular rate of atrial fibrillation. No clear patterns in the rates of single ectopic beats, couplets or runs were seen across visits. Because the summary data on rates of ventricular ectopic beats can be difficult to interpret, specific pro-arrhythmic criteria were analyzed. In this analysis, baseline occurrence of ventricular ectopic beats was compared to change from baseline, setting certain parameters for the change to describe the pro-arrhythmic response. The number of patients with a documented pro-arrhythmic response was very similar compared to placebo. Overall, there was no clinically relevant difference in the development of arrhythmic events in patients receiving indacaterol treatment over those patients who received placebo.

Tachyphylaxis/Tolerance
Tolerance to the effects of inhaled beta-agonists can occur with regularly-scheduled, chronic use. In two 12-week clinical efficacy trials in 323 and 318 adult patients with COPD, ARCAPTA NEOHALER improvement in lung function (as measured by the forced expiratory volume in one second, FEV_1) observed at Week 4 with ARCAPTA NEOHALER was consistently maintained over the 12-week treatment period in both trials.

12.3 Pharmacokinetics
Absorption
The median time to reach peak serum concentrations of indacaterol was approximately 15 minutes after single or repeated inhaled doses. Systemic exposure to indacaterol increased with increasing dose (150 mcg to 600 mcg) in a dose proportional manner, and was about dose-proportional in the dose range of 75 mcg to 150 mcg. Absolute bioavailability of indacaterol after an inhaled dose was on average 43-45%. Systemic exposure results from a composite of pulmonary and intestinal absorption.
Indacaterol serum concentrations increased with repeated once-daily administration. Steady-state was achieved within 12 to 15 days. The mean accumulation ratio of indacaterol, i.e. AUC over the 24-hour dosing interval on day 14 or day 15 compared to day 1, was in the range of 2.9 to 3.8 for once-daily inhaled doses between 75 mcg and 600 mcg.

Distribution
After intravenous infusion the volume of distribution (Vz) of indacaterol was 2,361 L to 2,557 L indicating an extensive distribution. The *in vitro* human serum and plasma protein binding was 94.1-95.3% and 95.1-96.2%, respectively.

Metabolism
After oral administration of radiolabeled indacaterol in the human ADME (absorption, distribution, metabolism, excretion) study unchanged indacaterol was the main component in serum, accounting for about one third of total drug-related AUC over 24 hours. A hydroxylated derivative was the most prominent metabolite in serum. Phenolic O-glucuronides of indacaterol and hydroxylated indacaterol were further prominent metabolites. A diastereomer of the hydroxylated derivative, a N-glucuronide of indacaterol, and C- and N-dealkylated products were further metabolites identified.
In vitro investigations indicated that UGT1A1 was the only UGT isoform that metabolized indacaterol to the phenolic O-glucuronide. The oxidative metabolites were found in incubations with recombinant CYP1A1, CYP2D6, and CYP3A4. CYP3A4 is concluded to be the predominant isoenzyme responsible for hydroxylation of indacaterol.
In vitro investigations indicated that indacaterol is a low affinity substrate for the efflux pump P-gp.
In vitro investigations indicated that indacaterol has negligible potential to cause metabolic interactions with medications (by inhibition or induction of cytochrome P450 enzymes, or induction of UGT1A1) at the systemic exposure levels achieved in clinical practice. *In vitro* investigation furthermore indicated that, *in vivo*, indacaterol is unlikely to significantly inhibit transporter proteins such as P-gp, MRP2, BCRP, the cationic substrate transporters hOCT1 and hOCT2, and the human multidrug and toxin extrusion transporters hMATE1 and hMATE2K, and that indacaterol has negligible potential to induce P-gp or MRP2.

Elimination
In clinical studies which included urine collection the amount of indacaterol excreted unchanged *via* urine was generally lower than 2% of the dose. Renal clearance of indacaterol was, on average, between 0.46 and 1.2 L/h. When compared with the serum clearance of indacaterol of 18.8 L/h to 23.3 L/h, it is evident that renal clearance plays a minor role (about 2 to 6% of systemic clearance) in the elimination of systemically available indacaterol.
In a human ADME study where indacaterol was given orally, the fecal route of excretion was dominant over the urinary route. Indacaterol was excreted into human feces primarily as unchanged parent drug (54% of the dose) and, to a lesser extent, hydroxylated indacaterol metabolites (23% of the dose). Mass balance was complete with ≥90% of the dose recovered in the excreta.

Indacaterol serum concentrations declined in a multi-phasic manner with an average terminal half-life ranging from 45.5 to 126 hours. The effective half-life, calculated from the accumulation of indacaterol after repeated dosing with once daily doses between 75 mcg and 600 mcg ranged from 40 to 56 hours which is consistent with the observed time-to-steady state of approximately 12-15 days.

Special Populations
A population pharmacokinetic analysis was performed for indacaterol utilizing data from 3 controlled clinical trials that included 1,844 patients with COPD aged 40 to 88 years who received treatment with ARCAPTA NEOHALER.
The population analysis showed that no dose adjustment is warranted based on the effect of age, gender and weight on systemic exposure in COPD patients after inhalation of ARCAPTA NEOHALER. The population pharmacokinetic analysis did not suggest any difference between ethnic subgroups in this population.

Hepatic Impairment
Patients with mild and moderate hepatic impairment showed no relevant changes in C_{max} or AUC of indacaterol, nor did protein binding differ between mild and moderate hepatically impaired subjects and their healthy controls. Studies in subjects with severe hepatic impairment were not performed.

Renal Impairment
Due to the very low contribution of the urinary pathway to total body elimination, a study in renally impaired subjects was not performed.

Drug-drug Interaction
Drug interaction studies were carried out using potent and specific inhibitors of CYP3A4 and P-gp (i.e., ketoconazole, erythromycin, verapamil and ritonavir).
Verapamil: Co-administration of indacaterol 300 mcg (single dose) with verapamil (80 mg t.i.d for 4 days) showed 2-fold increase in indacaterol AUC_{0-24}, and 1.5-fold increase in indacaterol C_{max}.
Erythromycin: Co-administration of indacaterol inhalation powder 300 mcg (single dose) with erythromycin (400 mg q.i.d for 7 days) showed a 1.4-fold increase in indacaterol AUC_{0-24}, and 1.2-fold increase in indacaterol C_{max}.
Ketoconazole: Co-administration of indacaterol inhalation powder 300 mcg (single dose) with ketoconazole (200 mg b.i.d for 7 days) caused a 1.9-fold increase in indacaterol AUC_{0-24}, and 1.3-fold increase in indacaterol C_{max}.
Ritonavir: Co-administration of indacaterol 300 mcg (single dose) with ritonavir (300 mg b.i.d for 7.5 days) resulted in a 1.7-fold increase in indacaterol AUC_{0-24} whereas indacaterol C_{max} was unaffected. *[See Drug Interactions (7.6)]*.

12.4 Pharmacogenomics
The pharmacokinetics of indacaterol were prospectively investigated in subjects with the $UGT1A1$ $(TA)_7/(TA)_7$ genotype (low UGT1A1 expression; also referred to as *28) and the $(TA)_6$, $(TA)_6$ genotype. Steady-state AUC and C_{max} of indacaterol were 1.2-fold higher in the $[(TA)_7, (TA)_7]$ genotype, suggesting no relevant effect of UGT1A1 genotype of indacaterol exposure.

13 NONCLINICAL TOXICOLOGY
13.1 Carcinogenesis, Mutagenesis, Impairment of Fertility
Long-term studies were conducted in transgenic mice using oral administration and in rats using inhalation administration to evaluate the carcinogenic potential of indacaterol maleate. Indacaterol did not show a statistically significant increase in tumor formation in mice or rats.
Lifetime treatment of rats resulted in increased incidences of benign ovarian leiomyoma and focal hyperplasia of ovarian smooth muscle in females at doses approximately 270-times the dose of 75 mcg once-daily for humans (on a mg/m² basis).
A 26-week oral (gavage) study in CB6F1/TgrasH2 hemizygous mice with indacaterol did not show any evidence of tumorigenicity at doses approximately 39,000-times the dose of 75 mcg once-daily for humans (on a mg/m² basis).
Increases in leiomyomas of the female rat genital tract have been similarly demonstrated with other beta₂-adrenergic agonist drugs. The relevance of these findings to human use is unknown.
Indacaterol was not mutagenic or clastogenic in Ames test, chromosome aberration test in V79 Chinese hamster cells, and bone marrow micronucleus test in rats.
Indacaterol did not impair fertility of rats in reproduction studies.

14 CLINICAL STUDIES
The ARCAPTA NEOHALER COPD clinical development program included three dose-ranging trials and six confirmatory trials (Trial 3, a 26-week seamless adaptive design trial that included an initial 2 week dose ranging phase; Trials 4, 5, and 6, 12-week trials; Trial 7, a 26-week trial; and Trial 8, a 52 week trial).

Dose-ranging trials:
Dose selection for ARCAPTA NEOHALER for COPD was based on three dose-ranging trials (Trial 1, a 2-week dose-ranging trial in an asthma population; Trial 2, a 2-week dose-ranging trial in a COPD population; and Trial 3, a 26-week adaptive seamless design trial that included an initial 2-week dose ranging phase). Although ARCAPTA NEOHALER is not indicated for asthma, dose selection was primarily based upon the results from the dose-ranging trial in asthma patients (Trial 1) as an asthma population is the most responsive to beta-agonist bronchodilation and is most likely to demonstrate a dose response. Dose-ranging in COPD patients (Trials 2 and 3) provided supportive information.

Dose-ranging in asthma
ARCAPTA NEOHALER is not indicated for asthma.
Trial 1 was a 2-week, randomized, double-blinded, placebo-controlled design that enrolled 511 patients with persistent asthma 18 years of age and older. All enrolled patients were required to be taking inhaled corticosteroids, had a forced expiratory volume in one second (FEV_1) of ≥ 50% and ≤ 90% predicted, and FEV_1 reversibility after albuterol of at least 12% and at least 200 mL. Trial 1 included ARCAPTA NEOHALER doses of 18.75, 37.5, 75, and 150 mcg once daily, a salmeterol active control group, and placebo. The trial showed that the effect on FEV_1 in patients treated with ARCAPTA NEOHALER 18.75 and 37.5 mcg doses was lower compared to patients treated with other ARCAPTA NEOHALER doses, particularly after the first dose. The effect did not clearly differ between the 75 and 150 mcg doses. Results of the ARCAPTA NEOHALER and placebo treatment arms are as follows. After the first dose (Day 1), the peak (4 hour) FEV_1 was 2.58L in the placebo group, with a treatment difference of 0.04L (95% CI -0.01, 0.09) in the 18.75 mcg ARCAPTA NEOHALER group, 0.04L (-0.01, 0.09) in the 37.5 mcg group, 0.12L (0.07, 0.17) in the 75 mcg group, and 0.15L (0.10, 0.20) in the 150 mcg group. The Day 2 trough FEV_1 was 2.45L in the placebo group, with a treatment difference of 0.02L (95% CI -0.05, 0.08), 0.08L (0.01, 0.15), 0.09L (0.03, 0.16) and 0.16L (0.09, 0.22) in the ARCAPTA NEOHALER groups, respectively. At Day 14, the peak (4 hour) FEV_1 was 2.55L in the placebo group, with a treatment difference of 0.12L (95% CI 0.05, 0.20) in the 18.75 mcg ARCAPTA NEOHALER group, 0.14L (0.06, 0.21) in the 37.5 mcg group, 0.23L (0.15, 0.30) in the 75 mcg group, and 0.20L (0.13, 0.27) in the 150 mcg group. The Day 15 FEV_1 (primary endpoint) was 2.42L in the placebo group, with a treatment difference of 0.09L (95% CI 0.00, 0.17), 0.11L (0.02, 0.19), 0.17L (0.08, 0.26), and 0.12L (0.04, 0.21) in the ARCAPTA NEOHALER groups, respectively.

Dose-ranging in COPD
Trial 2 was a 2-week, randomized, double-blinded, placebo-controlled design that enrolled 552 patients with a clinical diagnosis of COPD, who were 40 years or older, had a smoking history of at least 10 pack years, had a post-bronchodilator FEV_1 less than 80% and at least 30% of the predicated normal value and a post-bronchodilator ratio of FEV_1 over forced vital capacity (FEV_1/FVC) of less than 70%. Trial 2 included ARCAPTA NEOHALER doses of 18.75, 37.5, 75 and 150 mcg once daily, a salmeterol active control group, and placebo. Results of the ARCAPTA NEOHALER and placebo arms are shown in Figure 1. The trial showed that the effect on FEV_1 in patients treated with ARCAPTA NEOHALER 18.75 mcg dose was lower compared to patients treated with other ARCAPTA NEOHALER doses. Although a dose-response relationship was observed at Day 1, the effect did not clearly differ among the 37.5, 75 and 150 mcg doses by Day 15.
[See figure 1 at top of next column]
The 2-week dose ranging phase of Trial 3 included ARCAPTA NEOHALER doses of 75, 150, 300, and 600 mcg once daily, placebo, and two active comparators. Although a dose-response relationship was observed at week 2, the effect did not clearly differ among the ARCAPTA NEOHALER doses.

Confirmatory Trials:
The ARCAPTA NEOHALER COPD development program included six confirmatory trials that were randomized, double-blinded placebo and active-controlled in design (Trial 3, a 26-week seamless adaptive design trial that included an initial 2 week dose-ranging phase; Trials 4, 5, and 6, 12-week trials; Trial 7, a 26-week trial; and Trial 8, a 52 week trial). After the initial 2-week dose-ranging portion of the design, Trial 3 was conducted with ARCAPTA NEOHALER doses of 150 mcg and 300 mcg once daily, placebo, and an active comparator. Trials 4 and 5 were conducted with ARCAPTA NEOHALER dose of 75 mcg once daily, and placebo. Trial 6 was conducted with ARCAPTA NEOHALER dose of 150 mcg once daily and placebo. Trial 7 was conducted with ARCAPTA NEOHALER dose of 150 mcg once daily, an active comparator, and placebo. Trial 8 was conducted with ARCAPTA NEOHALER doses of 300 mcg and 600 mcg once daily, an active comparator, and placebo.

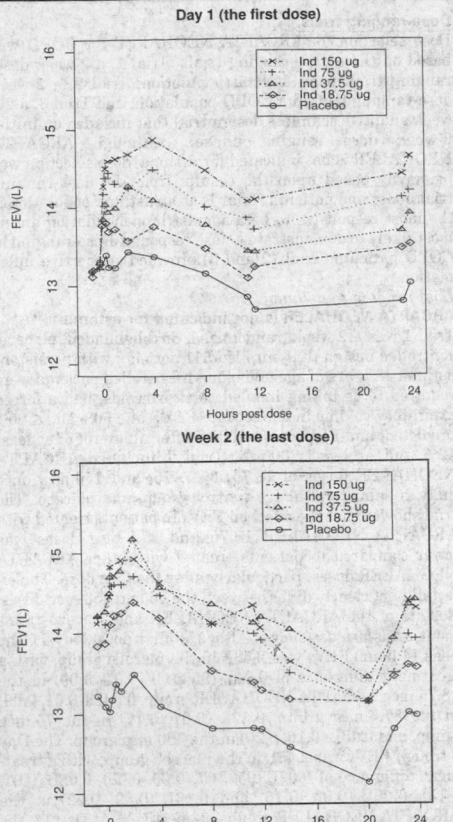

Figure 1: LS Mean FEV1 time profile curve over 24 hours after ARCAPTA NEOHALER Day 1 and Week 2 in Trial 2 (COPD dose ranging)

As Trials 3, 6, 7, and 8 were conducted with doses of ARCAPTA NEOHALER higher than 75 mcg, the results of Trials 4 and 5, which included ARCAPTA NEOHALER 75 mcg are the focus of this section.

These six trials enrolled 5474 patients with a clinical diagnosis of COPD, who were 40 years or older, had a smoking history of at least 10 pack years, had a post-bronchodilator FEV_1 less than 80% and at least 30% of the predicted normal value and a post-bronchodilator ratio of FEV_1 over FVC of less than 70%.

Assessment of efficacy in these six COPD trials was based on FEV_1. The primary efficacy endpoint was 24-hour post-dose trough FEV_1 (defined as the average of two FEV_1 measurements taken after 23 hours 10 minutes and 23 hours and 45 minutes after the previous dose) after 12 weeks of treatment in all 6 trials. Other efficacy variables included other FEV_1 and FVC time points, rescue medication use, symptoms, and health-related quality of life measured using the St. George's Respiratory Questionnaire (SGRQ).

In all six confirmatory COPD trials, all doses of ARCAPTA NEOHALER tested (75 mcg, 150 mcg, 300 mcg, and 600 mcg) showed significantly greater 24-hour post-dose trough FEV_1 compared to placebo at 12 weeks. Results of Trials 4 and 5, which compared ARCAPTA NEOHALER at the dose of 75 mcg once daily to placebo are shown in Table 2.

Table 2: LS Mean for trough FEV_1 at 12 weeks

Treatment	Trough FEV_1 at Week 12 (liters)	Treatment Difference LS Mean (95% CI)
Trial 4 (N=323)		
Indacaterol 75 mcg	1.38	0.12 (0.08, 0.15)
Placebo	1.26	
Trial 5 (N=318)		
Indacaterol 75 mcg	1.49	0.14 (0.10, 0.18)
Placebo	1.35	

In addition, serial FEV_1 measurements in patients treated with ARCAPTA NEOHALER demonstrated a bronchodilatory treatment effect after the first dose compared to placebo at 5 minutes post dose of 0.09 L (Trial 4) and 0.10 L (Trial 5). The mean peak improvement relative to baseline

within the first 4 hours after the first dose (Day 1) was 0.19 L (Trial 4) and 0.22 L (Trial 5) and was 0.24 L (Trial 4) and 0.27 L (Trial 5) after 12 weeks. Improvement in lung function observed at week 4 was consistently maintained over the 12-week treatment period in both trials. In Trial 5, 24-hour spirometry was assessed in a subset of 239 patients. See Figure 2.

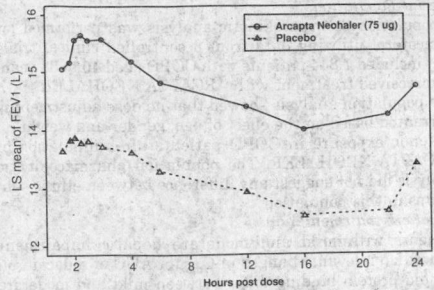

Figure 2: LS Mean FEV1 time profile curve over 24 hours at Week 12 in Trial 5

In both COPD clinical trials including the 75 mcg dose (Trials 4 and 5), patients treated with ARCAPTA NEOHALER used less daily rescue albuterol during the trial compared to patients treated with placebo.

Health-related quality of life was measured using the St. George's Respiratory Questionnaire (SGRQ) in all six confirmatory COPD clinical trials. SGRQ is a disease-specific patient reported instrument which measures symptoms, activities, and its impact on daily life. At week 12, pooled data from these trials demonstrated an improvement over placebo in SGRQ total score of -3.8 with a 95% CI of (-5.3, -2.3) for the ARCAPTA NEOHALER 75 mcg dose, -4.6 with a 95% CI of (-5.5, -3.6) for 150 mcg, and -3.8 with a 95% CI of (-4.9, -2.8) for 300 mcg. The confidence intervals for this change are widely overlapping with no dose ordering. Results from individual studies were variable, but are generally consistent with the pooled data results.

16 HOW SUPPLIED/STORAGE AND HANDLING
16.1 How Supplied
75 mcg ARCAPTA NEOHALER contains ARCAPTA (indacaterol inhalation powder) capsules packaged in aluminum blister cards, one NEOHALER inhaler, and an FDA approved Medication Guide.
Unit Dose (blister pack), Box of 30 (5 blister cards with 6 capsules each)   NDC 0078-0619-15
The NEOHALER inhaler consists of a white protective cap and a base with mouthpiece, capsule chamber and two translucent red push buttons.
16.2 Storage and Handling
Store in a dry place at 25°C (77°F); excursions permitted to 15-30°C (59-86° F) [see USP Controlled Room Temperature].
75 mcg: Protect capsule from light and moisture.
• ARCAPTA capsules should be used with the NEOHALER inhaler only. The NEOHALER inhaler should not be used with any other capsules.
• Capsules should always be stored in the blister and only removed from the blister immediately before use.
• Always use the new NEOHALER inhaler provided with each new prescription.
Keep out of the reach of children.

17 PATIENT COUNSELING INFORMATION
See FDA-approved patient labeling (Medication Guide)
17.1 Asthma-Related Death
Patients should be informed that LABA, such as ARCAPTA NEOHALER, increase the risk of asthma-related death. ARCAPTA NEOHALER is not indicated for the treatment of asthma.
17.2 Instructions for Administering ARCAPTA NEOHALER
It is important for patients to understand how to correctly administer ARCAPTA capsules using the NEOHALER device [*see Instructions for Use at the end of the Medication Guide*]. Patients should be instructed that ARCAPTA capsules should only be administered via the NEOHALER device and the NEOHALER device should not be used for administering other medications. **The contents of ARCAPTA capsules are for oral inhalation only and must not be swallowed.**
ARCAPTA capsules should always be stored in sealed blisters. Only one ARCAPTA capsule should be removed immediately before use, or its effectiveness may be reduced. Additional ARCAPTA capsules that are exposed to air (i.e. not intended for immediate use) should be discarded.
17.3 Not for Acute Symptoms
ARCAPTA NEOHALER is not meant to relieve acute symptoms or exacerbations of COPD and extra doses should not be used for that purpose. Acute symptoms should be treated

with an inhaled, short-acting beta2-agonist such as albuterol. (The healthcare provider should provide the patient with such medication and instruct the patient in how it should be used.)
Patients should be instructed to notify their physician immediately if they experience any of the following:
• Worsening of symptoms
• Decreasing effectiveness of inhaled, short-acting beta2-agonists
• Need for more inhalations than usual of inhaled, short-acting beta2-agonists
• Significant decrease in lung function as outlined by the physician.
Patients should not stop therapy with ARCAPTA NEOHALER without physician/provider guidance since symptoms may recur after discontinuation.
17.4 Do Not Use Additional Long-Acting Beta2-Agonists
Patients who have been taking inhaled, short-acting beta2-agonists on a regular basis should be instructed to discontinue the regular use of these products and use them only for the symptomatic relief of acute symptoms.
When patients are prescribed ARCAPTA NEOHALER, other inhaled medications containing long-acting beta2-agonists should not be used. Patients should not use more than the recommended once daily dose of ARCAPTA NEOHALER. Excessive use of sympathomimetics may cause significant cardiovascular effects, and may be fatal.
17.5 Risks Associated With Beta-Agonist Therapy
Patients should be informed of adverse effects associated with beta2-agonists, such as palpitations, chest pain, rapid heart rate, tremor, or nervousness.
T2012-174
September 2012
Medication Guide
ARCAPTA™ (ar-CAP-ta) NEOHALER™
(indacaterol inhalation powder)

Important: Do not swallow ARCAPTA capsules. ARCAPTA capsules are used only with the NEOHALER inhaler that comes with ARCAPTA NEOHALER. Never place a capsule in the mouthpiece of the NEOHALER inhaler.

Read the Medication Guide that comes with ARCAPTA NEOHALER before you start using it and each time you get a refill. There may be new information. This Medication Guide does not take the place of talking to your health care provider about your medical condition or treatment.
What is the most important information I should know about ARCAPTA NEOHALER?
ARCAPTA NEOHALER has been approved for COPD only. Therefore, ARCAPTA NEOHALER is NOT to be used in asthma.
ARCAPTA NEOHALER can cause serious side effects, including:
• **People with asthma who take long-acting beta2 adrenergic-agonist (LABA) medicines, such as ARCAPTA NEOHALER, have an increased risk of death from asthma problems.**
• **It is not known if LABA medicines, such as ARCAPTA NEOHALER, increase the risk of death in people with chronic obstructive pulmonary disease (COPD).**
• Get emergency medical care if:
  • breathing problems worsen quickly
  • you use your rescue inhaler medicine, but it does not relieve your breathing problems.
What is ARCAPTA NEOHALER?
ARCAPTA NEOHALER is used long term, 1 time each day, in controlling symptoms of chronic obstructive pulmonary disease (COPD) in adults with COPD.
LABA medicines such as ARCAPTA NEOHALER help the muscles around the airways in your lungs stay relaxed to prevent symptoms, such as wheezing, cough, chest tightness and shortness of breath.
ARCAPTA NEOHALER is not for use to treat sudden symptoms of COPD. Always have a short-acting beta2-agonist medicine with you to treat sudden symptoms. If you do not have an inhaled, short-acting bronchodilator, contact your healthcare provider to have one prescribed for you.
It is not known if ARCAPTA NEOHALER is safe and effective in people with asthma.
ARCAPTA NEOHALER should not be used in children. It is not known if ARCAPTA NEOHALER is safe and effective in children.
Who should not use ARCAPTA NEOHALER?
Do not use ARCAPTA NEOHALER if you:
• **have asthma.**
• **have had an allergic reaction to indacaterol or any of the ingredients in ARCAPTA NEOHALER. Ask your healthcare provider if you are not sure. See the end of the Medication Guide for a list of ingredients in ARCAPTA NEOHALER.**

What should I tell my healthcare provider before using ARCAPTA NEOHALER?

Tell your healthcare provider about all of your health conditions, including if you:

- have heart problems
- have high blood pressure
- have seizures
- have thyroid problems
- have diabetes
- are pregnant or planning to become pregnant. It is not known if ARCAPTA NEOHALER can harm your unborn baby.
- are breastfeeding. It is not known if ARCAPTA NEOHALER passes into your milk and if it can harm your baby.
- are allergic to ARCAPTA NEOHALER or any of its ingredients, any other medicines, or food products.

ARCAPTA NEOHALER contains lactose (milk sugar) and a small amount of milk proteins. It is possible that allergic reactions may happen in patients who have a severe milk protein allergy.

Tell your doctor about all the medicines you take, including prescription and non-prescription medicines, vitamins, and herbal supplements. ARCAPTA NEOHALER and certain other medicines may interact with each other. This may cause serious side effects.

Know the medicines you take. Keep a list of your medicines with you to show your healthcare provider and pharmacist each time you get a new medicine.

How should I use ARCAPTA NEOHALER?

- **Read the step-by-step instructions for using ARCAPTA NEOHALER at the end of this Medication Guide.**
- **Use ARCAPTA NEOHALER 1 time each day at the same time of the day.**
- If you miss a dose of ARCAPTA NEOHALER, take it as soon as you remember. Do not take more than one dose in 24 hours.
- **Do not swallow ARCAPTA capsules.** ARCAPTA capsules should always be used with the NEOHALER inhaler only.
- Always use the new NEOHALER inhaler that is provided with each new prescription.
- **ARCAPTA NEOHALER does not relieve sudden symptoms of COPD.** Always have a rescue inhaler medicine with you to treat sudden symptoms. If you do not have a rescue inhaler medicine, call your healthcare provider to have one prescribed for you.
- Do not stop using ARCAPTA NEOHALER or other medicines to control or treat your COPD unless told to do so by your healthcare provider because your symptoms might get worse. Your healthcare provider will change your medicines as needed.
- **Do not use ARCAPTA NEOHALER:**
  - more often than prescribed
  - more medicine than prescribed for you, or
  - with other LABA medicines
- **Call your health care provider or get emergency medical care right away if:**
  - your breathing problems worsen with ARCAPTA NEOHALER
  - you need to use your rescue medicine more often than usual
  - your rescue inhaler medicine does not work as well for you at relieving your symptoms

What are the possible side effects with ARCAPTA NEOHALER?

ARCAPTA NEOHALER can cause serious side effects, including:

- **See "What is the most important information I should know about ARCAPTA NEOHALER?"**
- If your COPD symptoms worsen over time do not increase your dose of ARCAPTA NEOHALER, instead call your healthcare provider.
- serious allergic reactions including rash, hives, swelling of the tongue, lips and face, difficulties in breathing or swallowing. Call your healthcare provider or get emergency medical care if you get any symptoms of a serious allergic reaction.
- sudden shortness of breath that may be life-threatening
- fast or irregular heartbeat (palpitations)
- increased blood pressure
- chest pain
- low blood potassium (which may cause symptoms of muscle spasm, muscle weakness or abnormal heart rhythm)
- high blood sugar

Common side effects of ARCAPTA NEOHALER include:

- runny nose
- cough
- sore throat
- headache
- nausea

Tell your healthcare provider about any side effect that bothers you or that does not go away.

These are not all the side effects with ARCAPTA NEOHALER. Ask your healthcare provider or pharmacist for more information.

Call your doctor for medical advice about side effects. You may report side effects to FDA at 1-800-FDA-1088.

How should I store ARCAPTA NEOHALER?

- Store ARCAPTA NEOHALER (inhaler and blister-packaged capsules) in a dry place 59° F to 86° F (15°C to 30°C). Protect ARCAPTA NEOHALER (inhaler and blister-packaged capsules) from moisture.
- Do not remove ARCAPTA capsules from their foil package until just before use.
- Keep ARCAPTA capsules out of the light.
- Do not store ARCAPTA capsules in the NEOHALER inhaler.
- **Keep ARCAPTA NEOHALER and all medicines out of the reach of children.**

General Information about ARCAPTA NEOHALER

Medicines are sometimes prescribed for purposes other than those listed in a Medication Guide. Do not use ARCAPTA NEOHALER for a condition for which it was not prescribed. Do not give ARCAPTA NEOHALER to other people, even if they have the same condition. It may harm them.

This Medication Guide summarizes the most important information about ARCAPTA NEOHALER. If you would like more information, talk with your healthcare provider. You can ask your healthcare provider or pharmacist for information about ARCAPTA NEOHALER that was written for healthcare professionals.

For more information, go to www.arcapta.com or call 1-888-669-6682.

Active ingredient: indacaterol

Inactive ingredients: lactose monohydrate (contains trace levels of milk protein)

T2012-175

Revised September 2012

Instructions for Use

ARCAPTA™ (ar-CAP-ta) NEOHALER™

(indacaterol inhalation powder)

Do not swallow ARCAPTA capsules.

Follow the instructions below for using ARCAPTA NEOHALER. You will breathe-in (inhale) the medicine in the ARCAPTA capsules from the NEOHALER inhaler. If you have any questions, ask your healthcare provider or pharmacist.

ARCAPTA NEOHALER

Cap — Mouthpiece

Base — Blisters — Screen — Button — Capsule chamber

Inhaler · Blister card · Inhaler base

ARCAPTA NEOHALER consists of both the inhaler and the blister-packaged capsules. Each package contains ARCAPTA capsules and a NEOHALER inhaler.

- ARCAPTA capsules come in blister cards (see figure above).
- NEOHALER inhaler consists of a cap and a base (see figure above).

Your inhaler is made to give you the medicine contained in the capsules.

Do not use ARCAPTA capsules with any other capsule inhaler, and **do not** use NEOHALER inhaler to take any other capsule medicine.

How to use your inhaler
Figure A

Step 1. Pull off cap. See Figure A.

Figure B

Step 2. Open inhaler: See Figure B
Hold the base of the inhaler firmly and tilt the mouthpiece to open the inhaler.

Figure C

Step 3. Prepare capsule: See Figure C
Separate one of the blisters from the blister card by tearing along the perforation.
Take one blister and peel away the protective backing to expose the foil.

Figure D

Step 4. Remove an ARCAPTA capsule: See Figure D
Capsules should always be stored in the blister and only removed immediately before use.
With dry hands, remove one capsule from the blister by pushing the ARCAPTA capsule through the foil.
Do not swallow ARCAPTA capsule.

Figure E

Step 5. Insert capsule: See Figure E
Place the capsule into the capsule chamber.
Do not place a capsule directly into the mouthpiece.

Figure F

Step 6. Close the inhaler: See Figure F
Close the inhaler fully. You should hear a 'click' as it fully closes.

Figure G

Step 7. Pierce the capsule: See Figure G
Hold the inhaler upright.
Press both buttons fully one time.
You should hear a 'click' as the capsule is being pierced.
Do not press the piercing buttons more than one time.

Figure H

Step 8. Release the buttons fully. See Figure H

Figure I

Step 9. Breathe out: See Figure I
Before placing the mouthpiece in your mouth, breathe out fully.
Never blow into the mouthpiece.

Figure J

Step 10. Inhale the medicine: See Figure J

Before breathing in, place the mouthpiece in your mouth and close your lips around the mouthpiece. Hold the inhaler with the buttons to the left and right (not up and down). Breathe in rapidly and steadily, as deeply as you can. **Do not press the piercing buttons.**

Note: See Figure K

Figure K

As you breathe in through the inhaler, the capsule spins around in the chamber and you should hear a whirring noise.

If you do not hear a whirring noise, the capsule may be stuck in the capsule cavity. If this occurs, open the inhaler and carefully loosen the capsule by tapping the base of the device. Do not press the piercing buttons to loosen the capsule. **(Repeat steps 9 and 10 if needed).**

Step 11. Hold breath: See Figure L

Figure L

Continue to hold your breath as long as comfortably possible while removing the inhaler from your mouth. Then breathe out.

Open the inhaler to see if any powder is left in the capsule. **If there is powder left in the capsule, close the inhaler and repeat steps 9 to 12.** Most people are able to empty the capsule in one or two inhalations.

Some people may cough soon after inhaling the medicine. If you do, don't worry, as long as the capsule is empty, you have received the full dose.

Figure M

Step 12. Remove capsule: See Figure M

After you have finished taking your daily dose of the ARCAPTA NEOHALER, open the mouthpiece again, remove the empty capsule by tipping it out, and discard it. Close the inhaler and replace the cap.

Do not store the capsules in the NEOHALER device.

Additional Information

Occasionally, very small pieces of the capsule can get past the screen and enter your mouth. If this happens, you may be able to feel these pieces on your tongue. It is not harmful if these pieces are swallowed or inhaled. **The chances of the capsule shattering will be increased if the capsule is pierced more than once (Step 7).** Therefore it is recommended that you follow the storage directions, remove the capsule from the blister immediately before use and pierce each capsule only once.

How to clean your inhaler

Cleaning the device is not necessary, however, if desired, a clean, dry lint-free cloth, or a clean, dry soft brush may be used to wipe the inhaler between uses.

Remember:

- ARCAPTA capsules should be stored in the blister, and only removed immediately before use.
- Do not breathe into the NEOHALER inhaler.
- Do not place the ARCAPTA capsule directly into the mouthpiece of the NEOHALER inhaler.
- Do not store the ARCAPTA capsule in the NEOHALER inhaler chamber.
- Always release the push buttons prior to inhalation
- Do not wash the NEOHALER inhaler. **Keep it dry.**
- Always keep the NEOHALER inhaler and ARCAPTA capsules in a dry place.
- Always use the new NEOHALER inhaler that comes with your refill.
- Do not use ARCAPTA capsules with inhalers from other medicines.
- Keep this and all drugs out of the reach of children.

This Medication Guide has been approved by the U.S. Food and Drug Administration.

Manufactured by:
Novartis Pharma Stein AG
Stein, Switzerland
Distributed by:
Novartis Pharmaceuticals Corporation
East Hanover, New Jersey 07936

© Novartis
T2012-179
Revised September 2012
Shown in Product Identification Guide, page 309

CLOZARIL®
(clozapine)
tablets, for oral use   ℞

The following prescribing information is based on official labeling in effect July 2014.

HIGHLIGHTS OF PRESCRIBING INFORMATION

These highlights do not include all the information needed to use CLOZARIL safely and effectively. See full prescribing information for CLOZARIL.

CLOZARIL® (clozapine) tablets, for oral use
Initial U.S. Approval: 1989

WARNING: AGRANULOCYTOSIS; ORTHOSTATIC HYPOTENSION, BRADYCARDIA, AND SYNCOPE; SEIZURE; MYOCARDITIS AND CARDIOMYOPATHY; INCREASED MORTALITY IN ELDERLY PATIENTS WITH DEMENTIA-RELATED PSYCHOSIS

See full prescribing information for complete boxed warning.

- **Agranulocytosis:** Can lead to serious infection and death. Monitor white blood cell count and absolute neutrophil count prior to and during treatment. Monitor for symptoms of agranulocytosis and infection. (2.1, 5.1)
- **Because of risk of agranulocytosis, CLOZARIL is available only through a restricted program called the CLOZARIL National Registry. Prescribers, patients, and pharmacies must enroll in the program. (5.2)**
- **Orthostatic Hypotension, Bradycardia, and Syncope:** Risk is dose-related. Starting dose is 12.5 mg. Titrate gradually and use divided dosages. (2.2, 2.5, 5.3)
- **Seizure:** Risk is dose-related. Titrate gradually and use divided doses. Use with caution in patients with history of seizure or risk factors for seizure. (2.2, 5.4)
- **Myocarditis and Cardiomyopathy:** Can be fatal. Discontinue and obtain cardiac evaluation if findings suggest these cardiac reactions. (5.5)
- **Increased Mortality in Elderly Patients with Dementia-Related Psychosis:** CLOZARIL is not approved for this condition. (5.6)

RECENT MAJOR CHANGES

Dosage and Administration (2.1, 2.6, 2.7)   07/2013
Contraindications (4)   07/2013
Warnings and Precautions (5.2, 5.3)   07/2013

INDICATIONS AND USAGE

CLOZARIL is an atypical antipsychotic indicated for:
- Treatment-resistant schizophrenia. Efficacy was established in an active-controlled study. (1.1, 14.1)
- Reducing suicidal behavior in patients with schizophrenia or schizoaffective disorder. Efficacy was established in an active-controlled study. (1.2, 14.2)

DOSAGE AND ADMINISTRATION

- Starting Dose: 12.5 mg once daily or twice daily. (2.2)
- Use cautious titration and divided dosage schedule. (2.2, 5.3)
- Titration: increase the total daily dosage in increments of 25 mg to 50 mg per day, if well-tolerated. (2.2)
- Target dose: 300 mg to 450 mg per day, in divided doses, by the end of 2 weeks. (2.2)
- Subsequent increases: increase in increments of 100 mg or less, once or twice weekly. (2.2)
- Maximum daily dose: 900 mg (2.2)

DOSAGE FORMS AND STRENGTHS

25 mg and 100 mg tablets with a facilitated score on one side (3)

CONTRAINDICATIONS

- History of clozapine-induced agranulocytosis or severe Granulocytopenia. (4)
- Known hypersensitivity to clozapine or any other component of CLOZARIL. (4)

WARNINGS AND PRECAUTIONS

- *Eosinophilia:* Assess for organ involvement (e.g., myocarditis, pancreatitis, hepatitis, colitis, nephritis). Discontinue if these occur. (5.7)
- *QT Interval Prolongation:* Can be fatal. Consider additional risk factors for prolonged QT interval (disorders and drugs). (5.8)
- *Metabolic Changes:* Atypical antipsychotic drugs have been associated with metabolic changes that may increase cardiovascular/cerebrovascular risk.
  These metabolic changes include:
  ○ *Hyperglycemia and Diabetes Mellitus:* Monitor for symptoms of hyperglycemia including polydipsia, poly-

---

uria, polyphagia, and weakness. Monitor glucose regularly in patients with diabetes or at risk for diabetes. (5.9)
○ *Dyslipidemia:* Undesirable alterations in lipids have occurred in patients treated with atypical antipsychotics. (5.9)
○ *Weight Gain:* Significant weight gain has occurred. Monitor weight gain. (5.9)
- *Neuroleptic Malignant Syndrome (NMS):* Immediately discontinue and monitor closely. Assess for co-morbid conditions. (5.10)
- *Fever:* Evaluate for infection, agranulocytosis, NMS. (5.11)
- *Pulmonary Embolism (PE):* Consider PE if respiratory distress, chest pain, or deep vein thrombosis occur. (5.12)
- *Anticholinergic Toxicity:* Use cautiously in presence of specific conditions (e.g., narrow angle glaucoma, use of anticholinergic drugs). (5.13)
- *Interference with Cognitive and Motor Performance:* Advise caution when operating machinery, including automobiles. (5.14)

ADVERSE REACTIONS

Most common adverse reactions (≥5%) were: CNS reactions (sedation, dizziness/vertigo, headache, and tremor); cardiovascular reactions (tachycardia, hypotension, and syncope); autonomic nervous system reactions (hypersalivation, sweating, dry mouth, and visual disturbances); gastrointestinal reactions (constipation and nausea); and fever. (6.1)

To report SUSPECTED ADVERSE REACTIONS, contact Novartis Pharmaceuticals Corporation at 1-888-669-6682 or FDA at 1-800-FDA-1088 or www.fda.gov/medwatch.

DRUG INTERACTIONS

- *Concomitant use of Strong CYP1A2 Inhibitors:* Reduce CLOZARIL dose to one-third when coadministered with strong CYP1A2 inhibitors (e.g., fluvoxamine, ciprofloxacin, enoxacin). (2.6, 7.1)
- Concomitant use of *Strong CYP3A4 Inducers* is not recommended. (2.6, 7.1)
- *Discontinuation of CYP1A2 or CYP3A4 Inducers:* Consider reducing CLOZARIL dose when CYP1A2 (e.g., tobacco smoke) or CYP3A4 inducers (e.g., carbamazepine) are discontinued. (2.6, 7.1)

USE IN SPECIFIC POPULATIONS

- *Nursing Mothers:* Discontinue drug or discontinue nursing, taking into consideration importance of drug to mother. (8.3)

See 17 for PATIENT COUNSELING INFORMATION
Revised: 11/2013

FULL PRESCRIBING INFORMATION: CONTENTS*
WARNING: AGRANULOCYTOSIS; ORTHOSTATIC HYPOTENSION, BRADYCARDIA, AND SYNCOPE; SEIZURE; MYOCARDITIS AND CARDIOMYOPATHY; INCREASED MORTALITY IN ELDERLY PATIENTS WITH DEMENTIA-RELATED PSYCHOSIS

1   INDICATIONS AND USAGE
    1.1   Treatment Resistant Schizophrenia
    1.2   Reduction in the Risk of Recurrent Suicidal Behavior in Schizophrenia or Schizoaffective Disorder
2   DOSAGE AND ADMINISTRATION
    2.1   Required Laboratory Testing Prior to Initiation and During Therapy
    2.2   Dosing Information
    2.3   Maintenance Treatment
    2.4   Discontinuation of Treatment
    2.5   Re-Initiation of Treatment
    2.6   Dosage Adjustments with Concomitant use of CYP1A2, CYP2D6, CYP3A4 Inhibitors or CYP1A2, CYP3A4 Inducers
    2.7   Renal or Hepatic Impairment or CYP2D6 Poor Metabolizers
3   DOSAGE FORMS AND STRENGTHS
4   CONTRAINDICATIONS
5   WARNINGS AND PRECAUTIONS
    5.1   Agranulocytosis
    5.2   CLOZARIL National Registry Because of the Risk of Agranulocytosis
    5.3   Orthostatic Hypotension, Bradycardia, and Syncope
    5.4   Seizures
    5.5   Myocarditis and Cardiomyopathy
    5.6   Increased Mortality in Elderly Patients with Dementia-Related Psychosis
    5.7   Eosinophilia
    5.8   QT Interval Prolongation
    5.9   Metabolic Changes
    5.10 Neuroleptic Malignant Syndrome
    5.11 Fever
    5.12 Pulmonary Embolism
    5.13 Anticholinergic Toxicity
    5.14 Interference with Cognitive and Motor Performance

FULL PRESCRIBING INFORMATION

WARNING: AGRANULOCYTOSIS; ORTHOSTATIC HYPOTENSION, BRADYCARDIA, AND SYNCOPE; SEIZURE; MYOCARDITIS AND CARDIOMYOPATHY; INCREASED MORTALITY IN ELDERLY PATIENTS WITH DEMENTIA-RELATED PSYCHOSIS

Agranulocytosis
CLOZARIL treatment has caused agranulocytosis, defined as an absolute neutrophil count (ANC) less than 500/mm³. Agranulocytosis can lead to serious infection and death. Prior to initiating treatment with CLOZARIL, obtain a baseline white blood cell (WBC) count and ANC. The ANC must be greater than or equal to 2000/mm³ and the WBC must be greater than or equal to 3500/mm³ for a patient to begin treatment with CLOZARIL. During treatment, patients must have regular monitoring of ANC and WBC. Discontinue CLOZARIL and do not rechallenge if the ANC is less than 1000/mm³ or the WBC is less than 2000/mm³. Advise patients to immediately report symptoms consistent with agranulocytosis or infection (e.g., fever, weakness, lethargy, or sore throat) *[see Dosage and Administration (2.1) and Warnings and Precautions (5.1)].*

Because of the risk of agranulocytosis, CLOZARIL is available only through a restricted program called the CLOZARIL National Registry. Under the CLOZARIL National Registry, prescribers, patients, and pharmacies must enroll in the program *[see Warnings and Precautions (5.2)].*

Orthostatic Hypotension, Bradycardia, Syncope
Orthostatic hypotension, bradycardia, syncope, and cardiac arrest have occurred with CLOZARIL treatment. The risk is highest during the initial titration period, particularly with rapid dose escalation. These reactions can occur with the first dose, with doses as low as 12.5 mg per day. Initiate treatment at 12.5 mg once or twice daily; titrate slowly; and use divided dosages. Use CLOZARIL cautiously in patients with cardiovascular or cerebrovascular disease or conditions predisposing to hypotension (e.g., dehydration, use of antihypertensive medications) *[see Dosage and Administration (2.2, and 2.5) and Warnings and Precautions (5.3)].*

Seizures
Seizures have occurred with CLOZARIL treatment. The risk is dose-related. Initiate treatment at 12.5 mg, titrate gradually, and use divided dosing. Use caution when administering CLOZARIL to patients with a history of seizures or other predisposing risk factors for seizure (CNS pathology, medications that lower the seizure threshold, alcohol abuse). Caution patients about engaging in any activity where sudden loss of

consciousness could cause serious risk to themselves or others *[see Dosage and Administration (2.2), Warnings and Precautions (5.4)].*

Myocarditis and Cardiomyopathy
Fatal myocarditis and cardiomyopathy have occurred with CLOZARIL treatment. Discontinue CLOZARIL and obtain a cardiac evaluation upon suspicion of these reactions. Generally, patients with CLOZARIL-related myocarditis or cardiomyopathy should not be rechallenged with CLOZARIL. Consider the possibility of myocarditis or cardiomyopathy if chest pain, tachycardia, palpitations, dyspnea, fever, flu-like symptoms, hypotension, or ECG changes occur *[see Warnings and Precautions (5.5)].*

Increased Mortality in Elderly Patients with Dementia-Related Psychosis
Elderly patients with dementia-related psychosis treated with antipsychotic drugs are at an increased risk of death. CLOZARIL is not approved for use in patients with dementia-related psychosis *[see Warnings and Precautions (5.6)].*

---

1 INDICATIONS AND USAGE

1.1 Treatment Resistant Schizophrenia
CLOZARIL is indicated for the treatment of severely ill patients with schizophrenia who fail to respond adequately to standard antipsychotic treatment. Because of the significant risk of agranulocytosis and seizure associated with its use, CLOZARIL should be used only in patients who have failed to respond adequately to standard antipsychotic treatment *[see Warnings and Precautions (5.1, 5.4)].*
The effectiveness of CLOZARIL in treatment-resistant schizophrenia was demonstrated in a 6-week, randomized, double-blind, active-controlled study comparing CLOZARIL and chlorpromazine in patients who had failed other antipsychotics *[see Clinical Studies (14.1)].*

1.2 Reduction in the Risk of Recurrent Suicidal Behavior in Schizophrenia or Schizoaffective Disorder
CLOZARIL is indicated for reducing the risk of recurrent suicidal behavior in patients with schizophrenia or schizoaffective disorder who are judged to be at chronic risk for re-experiencing suicidal behavior, based on history and recent clinical state. Suicidal behavior refers to actions by a patient that put him/herself at risk for death.
The effectiveness of CLOZARIL in reducing the risk of recurrent suicidal behavior was demonstrated over a 2-year treatment period in the InterSePT™ trial *[see Clinical Studies (14.2)].*

2 DOSAGE AND ADMINISTRATION

2.1 Required Laboratory Testing Prior to Initiation and During Therapy
Prior to initiating treatment with CLOZARIL, obtain a complete blood count (CBC) with differential. The absolute neutrophil count (ANC) must be greater than or equal to 2000/mm³ and the WBC must be greater than or equal to 3500 mm³ in order to initiate treatment. To continue treatment, the ANC and WBC must be monitored regularly *[see Warnings and Precautions (5.1)].*

2.2 Dosing Information
The starting dose is 12.5 mg once daily or twice daily. The total daily dose can be increased in increments of 25 mg to 50 mg per day, if well-tolerated, to achieve a target dose of 300 mg to 450 mg per day (administered in divided doses) by the end of 2 weeks. Subsequently, the dose can be in-

creased once weekly or twice weekly, in increments of up to 100 mg. The maximum dose is 900 mg per day. To minimize the risk of orthostatic hypotension, bradycardia, and syncope, it is necessary to use this low starting dose, gradual titration schedule, and divided dosages *[see Warnings and Precautions (5.3)].*
CLOZARIL can be taken with or without food *[see Pharmacokinetics (12.3)].*

2.3 Maintenance Treatment
Generally, it is recommended that patients responding to CLOZARIL continue maintenance treatment on their effective dose beyond the acute episode.

2.4 Discontinuation of Treatment
In the event of planned termination of CLOZARIL therapy, reduce the dose gradually over a period of 1 to 2 weeks. If abrupt discontinuation is necessary (because of agranulocytosis or another medical condition, for example), monitor carefully for the recurrence of psychotic symptoms and symptoms related to cholinergic rebound such as profuse sweating, headache, nausea, vomiting, and diarrhea.

2.5 Re-Initiation of Treatment
When restarting CLOZARIL in patients who have discontinued CLOZARIL (i.e., 2 days or more since the last dose), re-initiate with 12.5-mg once daily or twice daily. This is necessary to minimize the risk of hypotension, bradycardia, and syncope *[see Warnings and Precautions (5.3)].* If that dose is well tolerated, the dose may be increased to the previously therapeutic dose more quickly than recommended for initial treatment.

2.6 Dosage Adjustments with Concomitant use of CYP1A2, CYP2D6, CYP3A4 Inhibitors or CYP1A2, CYP3A4 Inducers
Dose adjustments may be necessary in patients with concomitant use of: strong CYP1A2 inhibitors (e.g., fluvoxamine, ciprofloxacin, or enoxacin); moderate or weak CYP1A2 inhibitors (e.g., oral contraceptives, or caffeine); CYP2D6 or CYP3A4 inhibitors (e.g., cimetidine, escitalopram, erythromycin, paroxetine, bupropion, fluoxetine, quinidine, duloxetine, terbinafine, or sertraline); CYP3A4 inducers (e.g., phenytoin, carbamazepine, St. John's wort, and rifampin); or CYP1A2 inducers (e.g., tobacco smoking) (Table 1) *[see Drug Interactions (7)].*
[See table 1 above]

2.7 Renal or Hepatic Impairment or CYP2D6 Poor Metabolizers
It may be necessary to reduce the CLOZARIL dose in patients with significant renal or hepatic impairment, or in CYP2D6 poor metabolizers *[see Use in Specific Populations (8.6, 8.7)].*

3 DOSAGE FORMS AND STRENGTHS
CLOZARIL (clozapine) is available as 25 mg and 100 mg round, pale-yellow, uncoated tablets with a facilitated score on one side.

4 CONTRAINDICATIONS
• **History of Clozapine-induced Agranulocytosis or Severe Granulocytopenia**
CLOZARIL is contraindicated in patients with a history of clozapine-induced agranulocytosis or severe granulocytopenia *[see Warnings and Precautions (5.1)].*
• **Hypersensitivity**
CLOZARIL is contraindicated in patients with a history of hypersensitivity to clozapine (e.g., photosensitivity, vasculitis, erythema multiforme, or Stevens-Johnson syndrome) or any other component of CLOZARIL *[see Adverse Reactions (6.2)].*

Table 1. Dose Adjustment in Patients Taking Concomitant Medications

Comedications	Scenarios		
	Initiating CLOZARIL while taking a comedication	Adding a comedication while taking CLOZARIL	Discontinuing a comedication while continuing CLOZARIL
Strong CYP1A2 Inhibitors	Use one-third of the CLOZARIL dose.		Increase CLOZARIL dose based on clinical response.
Moderate or Weak CYP1A2 Inhibitors	Monitor for adverse reactions. Consider reducing the CLOZARIL dose if necessary.		Monitor for lack of effectiveness. Consider increasing CLOZARIL dose if necessary.
CYP2D6 or CYP3A4 Inhibitors			
Strong CYP3A4 Inducers	Concomitant use is not recommended. However, if the inducer is necessary, it may be necessary to increase the CLOZARIL dose. Monitor for decreased effectiveness.		Reduce CLOZARIL dose based on clinical response.
Moderate or weak CYP1A2 or CYP3A4 Inducers	Monitor for decreased effectiveness. Consider increasing the CLOZARIL dose if necessary.		Monitor for adverse reactions. Consider reducing the CLOZARIL dose if necessary.

Help Patients Save on Rx Drugs: PDR.net/PharmacyDiscountCard

Table 2. Frequency of Monitoring Based on Stage of Therapy or Results from WBC Count and ANC Monitoring Tests

Situation	Hematological Values for Monitoring	Frequency of WBC Count and ANC Monitoring
Initiation of therapy	WBC count≥3500/mm³ and ANC≥2000/mm³ Note: Do not initiate in patients with a history of clozapine-induced agranulocytosis or severe granulocytopenia.	Weekly for 6 months
6 to 12 months of therapy	WBC ≥3500/mm³ and ANC ≥2000/mm³	Every 2 weeks for 6 months
12 months of therapy	WBC ≥3500/mm³ and ANC ≥2000/mm³	Every 4 weeks ad infinitum
Immature forms present	N/A	Repeat WBC and ANC
Discontinuation of therapy	N/A	Weekly for at least 4 weeks from day of discontinuation or until WBC ≥3500/mm³ and ANC ≥2000/mm³
Substantial drop in WBC or ANC	Single drop or cumulative drop within 3 weeks of: WBC ≥3000/mm³ or ANC ≥1500/mm³	1. Repeat WBC and ANC 2. If repeat values are: WBC 3000/mm³ to 3500 and ANC >2000/mm³, then monitor twice weekly
Mild leukopenia and/or Mild granulocytopenia	If WBC 3000 mm³ to <3500/mm³ and/or ANC 1500/mm³ to <2000/mm³	Twice weekly until WBC >3500/mm³ and ANC >2000/mm³ then return to previous monitoring frequency
Moderate leukopenia and/or Moderate granulocytopenia	WBC 2000/mm³ to <3000/mm³ and/or ANC 1000/mm³ to <1500/mm³	1. Interrupt therapy 2. Daily until WBC >3000/mm³ and ANC >1500/mm³ 3. Twice weekly until WBC >3500/mm³ and ANC >2000/mm³ 4. May rechallenge when WBC >3500/mm³ and ANC >2000/mm³ 5. If rechallenged, monitor weekly for 1 year before returning to the usual monitoring schedule of every 2 weeks for 6 months and then every 4 weeks ad infinitum
Severe leukopenia and/or Severe granulocytopenia	WBC count <2000/mm³ and/or ANC <1000/mm³	1. Discontinue treatment and do not rechallenge patient 2. Monitor until normal and for at least 4 weeks from day of discontinuation as follows: ○ Daily until WBC >3000/mm³ and ANC >1500/mm³ ○ Twice weekly until WBC >3500/mm³ and ANC >2000/mm³ ○ Weekly after WBC >3500/mm³
Agranulocytosis	ANC <500/mm³	1. Discontinue treatment and do not rechallenge patient 2. Monitor until normal and for at least 4 weeks from day of discontinuation as follows: ○ Daily until WBC >3000/mm³ and ANC >1500/mm³ ○ Twice weekly until WBC >3500/mm³ and ANC >2000/mm³ ○ Weekly after WBC >3500/mm³

WBC=White blood cell
ANC=Absolute neutrophil count

5   WARNINGS AND PRECAUTIONS
5.1   Agranulocytosis
Background
Agranulocytosis, defined as an ANC of less than 500/mm³, has been estimated to occur in association with clozapine use at a cumulative incidence at 1 year of approximately 1.3%, based on the occurrence of 15 US cases out of 1743 patients exposed to CLOZARIL during its clinical testing prior to domestic marketing. All of these cases occurred at a time when the need for close monitoring of WBC counts was already recognized. A hematologic risk analysis was conducted based upon the available information in the CLOZARIL National Registry for US patients. Based upon a cut-off date of April 30, 1995, the incidence rates of agranulocytosis based upon a weekly monitoring schedule rose steeply during the first 2 months of therapy, peaking in the third month. Among clozapine patients who continued the drug beyond the third month, the weekly incidence of agranulocytosis fell a substantial degree. After 6 months,

the weekly incidence of agranulocytosis declines still further; however, it never reaches zero. It should be noted that any type of reduction in the frequency of monitoring WBC counts may result in an increased incidence of agranulocytosis.
Risk Factors
Experience from clinical development, as well as from examples in the medical literature, suggests that patients who have developed agranulocytosis during clozapine therapy are at increased risk of subsequent episodes of agranulocytosis. Analysis of WBC count data from the CLOZARIL National Registry also suggests that patients who have an initial episode of moderate leukopenia (3000/mm³>WBC count ≥2000/mm³) are at an increased risk of subsequent episodes of agranulocytosis. Except for bone-marrow suppression during initial clozapine therapy, there are no other established risk factors based on worldwide experience for the development of agranulocytosis in association with clozapine use. However, a disproportionate number of the

US cases of agranulocytosis occurred in patients of Jewish background compared to the overall proportion of such patients exposed during domestic development of clozapine. Most of the US cases of agranulocytosis occurred within 4–10 weeks of exposure, but neither dose nor duration is a reliable predictor of this problem. Agranulocytosis associated with other antipsychotic drugs has been reported to occur with a greater frequency in women, the elderly, and in patients who are cachectic or have serious underlying medical illness; such patients may also be at particular risk with clozapine, although this has not been definitively demonstrated.
WBC Count and ANC Clinical Monitoring Schedule
CLOZARIL is available only through a distribution system that ensures monitoring of WBC count and ANC according to the schedule described below prior to delivery of the next supply of medication.
As described in Table 2, patients who are being treated with CLOZARIL must have a baseline WBC count and ANC before initiation of treatment, and a WBC count and ANC every week for the first 6 months. Thereafter, if acceptable WBC counts and ANCs (WBC count ≥3500/mm³ and ANC ≥2000/mm³) have been maintained during the first 6 months of continuous therapy, WBC counts and ANCs can be monitored every 2 weeks for the next 6 months. Thereafter, if acceptable WBC counts and ANCs (WBC count ≥3500/mm³ and ANC ≥2000/mm³) have been maintained during the second 6 months of continuous therapy, WBC count and ANC can be monitored every 4 weeks.
When treatment with CLOZARIL is discontinued (regardless of the reason), WBC count and ANC must be monitored weekly for at least 4 weeks from the day of discontinuation or until WBC count ≥3500/mm³ and ANC ≥2000/mm³.
Table 2 provides a summary of the frequency of monitoring that should occur based on various stages of therapy (e.g., initiation of therapy) or results from WBC count and ANC monitoring tests (e.g., moderate leukopenia). The text that follows should be consulted for additional details regarding the treatment of patients under the various conditions (e.g., severe leukopenia).
Advise patients to immediately report the appearance of signs/symptoms consistent with agranulocytosis or infection (e.g., fever, weakness, lethargy, or sore throat) at any time during CLOZARIL therapy. Such patients should have a WBC count and an ANC performed promptly.
[See table 2 above]
Decrements in WBC Count and/or ANC
Consult Table 2 above to determine how to monitor patients who experience decrements in WBC count and/or ANC at any point during treatment. Additionally, patients should be carefully monitored for flu-like symptoms or other symptoms suggestive of infection.
Nonrechallengeable Patients
If the total WBC count falls below 2000/mm³ or the ANC falls below 1000/mm³, bone-marrow aspiration should be considered to ascertain granulopoietic status and patients should not be rechallenged with clozapine. Protective isolation with close observation may be indicated if granulopoiesis is determined to be deficient. Should evidence of infection develop, the patient should have appropriate cultures performed and an appropriate antibiotic regimen instituted. Patients discontinued from clozapine therapy due to significant granulopoietic suppression have been found to develop agranulocytosis upon rechallenge, often with a shorter latency on re-exposure. To reduce the chances of rechallenge occurring in patients who have experienced significant bone-marrow suppression during clozapine therapy, a single, national master file (i.e., Nonrechallengeable Database) is confidentially maintained.
Treatment of Rechallengeable Patients
Patients may be rechallenged with clozapine if their WBC count does not fall below 2000/mm³ and the ANC does not fall below 1000/mm³. However, analysis of the data from the CLOZARIL National Registry suggests that patients who have an initial episode of moderate leukopenia (3000/mm³>WBC count ≥2000/mm³) have up to a 12-fold increased risk of having a subsequent episode of agranulocytosis when rechallenged as compared to the full cohort of patients treated with clozapine. Although CLOZARIL therapy may be resumed if no symptoms of infection develop and when the WBC count rises above 3500/mm³ and the ANC rises above 2000/mm³, prescribers are strongly advised to consider whether the benefit of continuing CLOZARIL treatment outweighs the increased risk of agranulocytosis.
Analyses of the CLOZARIL National Registry have shown an increased risk of having a subsequent episode of granulopoietic suppression up to a year after recovery from the initial episode. Therefore, as noted in Table 2, patients must undergo weekly WBC count and ANC monitoring for 1 year following recovery from an episode of moderate leukopenia and/or moderate granulocytopenia regardless of when the episode develops. If acceptable WBC counts and ANC (WBC count ≥3500/mm³ and ANC ≥2000/mm³) have been maintained during the year of weekly monitoring, WBC counts can be monitored every 2 weeks for the next 6 months. If

acceptable WBC counts and ANC (WBC count ≥3500/mm³ and ANC ≥2000/mm³) continue to be maintained during the 6 months of every 2-week monitoring, WBC counts can be monitored every 4 weeks thereafter, ad infinitum.

Interruptions in Therapy

Figure 1 provides instructions regarding re-initiating therapy and subsequently the frequency of WBC count and ANC monitoring after a period of interruption.

[See figure 1 above]

5.2 CLOZARIL National Registry Because of the Risk of Agranulocytosis

Because of the risk of agranulocytosis, CLOZARIL is available only through a restricted program called the CLOZARIL National Registry. Under the CLOZARIL National Registry, prescribers, patients, pharmacies, and distributors must enroll in the program.

Required components of the CLOZARIL National Registry are:

• Healthcare professionals who prescribe CLOZARIL must enroll in the program and comply with the Registry requirements.

• Pharmacies that dispense CLOZARIL must enroll in the program and comply with the Registry requirements.

• Routine monitoring and submission of laboratory results (WBC and ANC) is required during treatment with CLOZARIL [see Warnings and Precautions (5.1)].

• Patients who receive CLOZARIL must be enrolled in a registry.

Further information is available at http://www.clozarilregistry.com or 1-888-669-6682.

5.3 Orthostatic Hypotension, Bradycardia, and Syncope

Hypotension, bradycardia, syncope, and cardiac arrest have occurred with clozapine treatment. The risk is highest during the initial titration period, particularly with rapid dose-escalation. These reactions can occur with the first dose, at doses as low as 12.5 mg. These reactions can be fatal. The syndrome is consistent with neurally mediated reflex bradycardia (NMRB).

Treatment must begin at a maximum dose of 12.5 mg once daily or twice daily. The total daily dose can be increased in increments of 25 mg to 50 mg per day, if well-tolerated, to a target dose of 300 mg to 450 mg per day (administered in divided doses) by the end of 2 weeks. Subsequently, the dose can be increased weekly or twice weekly, in increments of up to 100 mg. The maximum dose is 900 mg per day. Use cautious titration and a divided dosage schedule to minimize the risk of serious cardiovascular reactions [see Dosage and Administration (2.2)]. Consider reducing the dose if hypotension occurs. When restarting patients who have had even a brief interval off CLOZARIL (i.e., 2 days or more since the last dose), re-initiate treatment at 12.5 mg once daily or twice daily [see Dosage and Administration (2.5)]. Use CLOZARIL cautiously in patients with cardiovascular disease (history of myocardial infarction or ischemia, heart failure, or conduction abnormalities), cerebrovascular disease, and conditions which would predispose patients to hypotension (e.g., concomitant use of antihypertensives, dehydration and hypovolemia).

5.4 Seizures

Seizure has been estimated to occur in association with clozapine use at a cumulative incidence at 1 year of approximately 5%, based on the occurrence of 1 or more seizures in 61 of 1743 patients exposed to clozapine during its clinical testing prior to domestic marketing (i.e., a crude rate of 3.5%). The risk of seizure is dose-related. Initiate treatment with a low dose (12.5 mg), titrate slowly, and use divided dosing.

Use caution when administering CLOZARIL to patients with a history of seizures or other predisposing risk factors for seizure (e.g., head trauma or other CNS pathology, use of medications that lower the seizure threshold, or alcohol abuse). Because of the substantial risk of seizure associated with CLOZARIL use, caution patients about engaging in any activity where sudden loss of consciousness could cause serious risk to themselves or others (e.g., driving an automobile, operating complex machinery, swimming, climbing).

5.5 Myocarditis and Cardiomyopathy

Myocarditis and cardiomyopathy have occurred with the use of CLOZARIL. These reactions can be fatal. Discontinue CLOZARIL and obtain a cardiac evaluation upon suspicion of myocarditis or cardiomyopathy. Generally, patients with a history of clozapine-associated myocarditis or cardiomyopathy should not be rechallenged with CLOZARIL. However, if the benefit of CLOZARIL treatment is judged to outweigh the potential risks of recurrent myocarditis or cardiomyopathy, the clinician may consider rechallenge with CLOZARIL in consultation with a cardiologist, after a complete cardiac evaluation, and under close monitoring.

Consider the possibility of myocarditis or cardiomyopathy in patients receiving CLOZARIL who present with chest pain, dyspnea, persistent tachycardia at rest, palpitations, fever, flu-like symptoms, hypotension, other signs or symptoms of heart failure, or electrocardiographic findings (low voltages, ST-T abnormalities, arrhythmias, right axis deviation, and

Figure 1. Resuming Monitoring Frequency after Interruption of Therapy

*Transitions to reduce frequency of monitoring only permitted if all WBC counts ≥3500/mm³ and ANCs ≥2000/mm³.

poor R wave progression). Myocarditis most frequently presents within the first 2 months of clozapine treatment. Symptoms of cardiomyopathy generally occur later than clozapine-associated myocarditis and usually after 8 weeks of treatment. However, myocarditis and cardiomyopathy can occur at any period during treatment with CLOZARIL. It is common for nonspecific flu-like symptoms such as malaise, myalgia, pleuritic chest pain, and low-grade fevers to precede more overt signs of heart failure. Typical laboratory findings include elevated troponin I or T, elevated creatinine kinase-MB, peripheral eosinophilia, and elevated C-reactive protein (CRP). Chest roentgenogram may demonstrate cardiac silhouette enlargement, and cardiac imaging (echocardiogram, radionucleotide studies, or cardiac catheterization) may reveal evidence of left ventricular dysfunction.

5.6 Increased Mortality in Elderly Patients with Dementia-Related Psychosis

Elderly patients with dementia-related psychosis treated with antipsychotic drugs are at an increased risk of death. Analyses of 17 placebo-controlled trials (modal duration of 10 weeks), largely in patients taking atypical antipsychotic drugs, revealed a risk of death in drug-treated patients of between 1.6 to 1.7 times the risk of death in placebo-treated patients. Over the course of a typical 10-week controlled trial, the rate of death in drug-treated patients was about 4.5%, compared to a rate of about 2.6% in the placebo group. Although the causes of death were varied, most of the deaths appeared to be either cardiovascular (e.g., heart failure, sudden death) or infectious (e.g., pneumonia) in nature. Observational studies suggest that, similar to atypical antipsychotic drugs, treatment with conventional antipsychotic drugs may increase mortality in this population. The extent to which the findings of increased mortality in observational studies may be attributed to the antipsychotic drug as opposed to some characteristic(s) of the patients is not clear. CLOZARIL is not approved for the treatment of patients with dementia-related psychosis [see Boxed Warning].

5.7 Eosinophilia

Eosinophilia, defined as a blood eosinophil count of greater than 700/mm³, has occurred with CLOZARIL treatment. In clinical trials, approximately 1% of patients developed eosinophilia. Clozapine-related eosinophilia usually occurs during the first month of treatment. In some patients, it has been associated with myocarditis, pancreatitis, hepatitis, colitis, and nephritis. Such organ involvement could be consistent with a drug reaction with eosinophilia and systemic symptoms (DRESS) syndrome, also known as drug induced hypersensitivity syndrome (DIHS). If eosinophilia develops during CLOZARIL treatment, evaluate promptly for signs and symptoms of systemic reactions, such as rash or other allergic symptoms, myocarditis, or other organ-specific disease associated with eosinophilia. If CLOZARIL-related systemic disease is suspected, discontinue CLOZARIL immediately.

If a cause of eosinophilia unrelated to CLOZARIL is identified (e.g., asthma, allergies, collagen vascular disease, parasitic infections, and specific neoplasms), treat the underlying cause and continue CLOZARIL.

Clozapine-related eosinophilia has also occurred in the absence of organ involvement and can resolve without intervention. There are reports of successful rechallenge after

discontinuation of clozapine, without recurrence of eosinophilia. In the absence of organ involvement, continue CLOZARIL under careful monitoring. If the total eosinophil count continues to increase over several weeks in the absence of systemic disease, the decision to interrupt CLOZARIL therapy and rechallenge after the eosinophil count decreases should be based on the overall clinical assessment, in consultation with an internist or hematologist.

5.8 QT Interval Prolongation

QT prolongation, Torsades de Pointes and other life-threatening ventricular arrhythmias, cardiac arrest, and sudden death have occurred with CLOZARIL treatment. When prescribing CLOZARIL, consider the presence of additional risk factors for QT prolongation and serious cardiovascular reactions. Conditions that increase these risks include the following: history of QT prolongation, long QT syndrome, family history of long QT syndrome or sudden cardiac death, significant cardiac arrhythmia, recent myocardial infarction, uncompensated heart failure, treatment with other medications that cause QT prolongation, treatment with medications that inhibit the metabolism of clozapine, and electrolyte abnormalities.

Prior to initiating treatment with CLOZARIL, perform a careful physical examination, medical history, and concomitant medication history. Consider obtaining a baseline ECG and serum chemistry panel. Correct electrolyte abnormalities. Discontinue CLOZARIL if the QTc interval exceeds 500 msec. If patients experience symptoms consistent with Torsades de Pointes, or other arrhythmias, (e.g., syncope, presyncope, dizziness, or palpitations), obtain a cardiac evaluation and discontinue CLOZARIL.

Use caution when administering concomitant medications that prolong the QT interval or inhibit the metabolism of CLOZARIL. Drugs that cause QT prolongation include: specific antipsychotics (e.g., ziprasidone, iloperidone, chlorpromazine, thioridazine, mesoridazine, droperidol, pimozide), specific antibiotics (e.g., erythromycin, gatifloxacin, moxifloxacin, sparfloxacin), Class 1A antiarrhythmic medications (e.g., quinidine, procainamide) or Class III antiarrhythmics (e.g., amiodarone, sotalol), and others (e.g., pentamidine, levomethadyl acetate, methadone, halofantrine, mefloquine, dolasetron mesylate, probucol or tacrolimus). Clozapine is primarily metabolized by CYP isoenzymes 1A2, 2D6, and 3A4. Concomitant treatment with inhibitors of these enzymes can increase the concentration of CLOZARIL [see Drug Interactions (7.1) and Clinical Pharmacology (12.3)].

Hypokalemia and hypomagnesemia increase the risk of QT prolongation. Hypokalemia can result from diuretic therapy, diarrhea, and other causes. Use caution when treating patients at risk for significant electrolyte disturbance, particularly hypokalemia. Obtain baseline measurements of serum potassium and magnesium levels, and periodically monitor electrolytes. Correct electrolyte abnormalities before initiating treatment with CLOZARIL.

5.9 Metabolic Changes

Atypical antipsychotic drugs, including CLOZARIL have been associated with metabolic changes that can increase cardiovascular and cerebrovascular risk. These metabolic changes include hyperglycemia, dyslipidemia, and body weight gain. While atypical antipsychotic drugs may produce some metabolic changes, each drug in the class has its own specific risk profile.

Table 3. Categorical Changes in Fasting Glucose Level in Studies in Adult Subjects with Schizophrenia

Laboratory Parameter	Category Change (at least once) from baseline	Treatment Arm	N	n (%)
Fasting Glucose	Normal (<100 mg/dL) to High (≥126 mg/dL)	CLOZARIL	198	53 (27)
		Chlorpromazine	135	14 (10)
	Borderline (100 to 125 mg/dL) to High (≥126 mg/dL)	CLOZARIL	57	24 (42)
		Chlorpromazine	43	12 (28)

Table 5. Categorical Changes in Lipid Concentrations in Studies in Adult Subjects with Schizophrenia

Laboratory Parameter	Category Change (at least once) from baseline	Treatment Arm	N	n (%)
Total Cholesterol (random or fasting)	Increase by ≥40 mg/dL	CLOZARIL	334	111 (33)
		Chlorpromazine	185	46 (25)
	Normal (<200 mg/dL) to High (≥240 mg/dL)	CLOZARIL	222	18 (8)
		Chlorpromazine	132	3 (2)
	Borderline (200-239 mg/dL) to High (≥240 mg/dL)	CLOZARIL	79	30 (38)
		Chlorpromazine	34	14 (41)
Triglycerides (fasting)	Increase by ≥50 mg/dL	CLOZARIL	6	3 (50)
		Chlorpromazine	7	3 (43)
	Normal (<150 mg/dL) to High (≥200 mg/dL)	CLOZARIL	4	0 (0)
		Chlorpromazine	6	2 (33)
	Borderline (≥150 mg/dL and <200 mg/dL) to High (≥200 mg/dL)	CLOZARIL	1	1 (100)
		Chlorpromazine	1	0 (0)

Table 6. Mean Change in Body Weight (kg) by duration of exposure from studies in adult subjects with schizophrenia

Metabolic parameter	Exposure duration	CLOZARIL (N=669)		Olanzapine (N=442)		Chlorpromazine (N=155)	
		n	Mean	n	Mean	n	Mean
Weight change from baseline	2 weeks (Day 11–17)	6	+0.9	3	+0.7	2	-0.5
	4 weeks (Day 21–35)	23	+0.7	8	+0.8	17	+0.6
	8 weeks (Day 49–63)	12	+1.9	13	+1.8	16	+0.9
	12 weeks (Day 70–98)	17	+2.8	5	+3.1	0	0
	24 weeks (154–182)	42	- 0.6	12	+5.7	0	0
	48 weeks (Day 322–350)	3	+3.7	3	+13.7	0	0

Clinical monitoring, including baseline and periodic follow-up lipid evaluations in patients using CLOZARIL, is recommended.

In a pooled data analysis of 10 studies in adult subjects with schizophrenia, CLOZARIL treatment was associated with increases in serum total cholesterol. No data were collected on LDL and HDL cholesterol. The mean increase in total cholesterol was 13 mg/dL in the CLOZARIL group and 15 mg/dL in the chlorpromazine group. In a pooled data analysis of 2 studies in adult subjects with schizophrenia, CLOZARIL treatment was associated with increases in fasting serum triglyceride. The mean increase in fasting triglyceride was 71 mg/dL (54%) in the CLOZARIL group and 39 mg/dL (35%) in the chlorpromazine group (Table 4). In addition, CLOZARIL treatment was associated with categorical increases in serum total cholesterol and triglyceride, as illustrated in Table 5. The proportion of patients with categorical increases in total cholesterol or fasting triglyceride increased with the duration of exposure. The median duration of CLOZARIL and chlorpromazine exposure was 45 days and 38 days, respectively. The CLOZARIL dose range was 100 mg to 900 mg daily; the maximum chlorpromazine dose was 1800 mg daily.

Table 4. Mean Changes in Total Cholesterol and Triglyceride Concentration in Studies in Adult Subjects with Schizophrenia

Treatment Arm	Baseline total cholesterol concentration (mg/dL)	Change from baseline mg/dL (%)
CLOZARIL (N=334)	184	+13 (7)
Chlorpromazine (185)	182	+15 (8)
	Baseline triglyceride concentration (mg/dL)	**Change from baseline mg/dL (%)**
CLOZARIL (N=6)	130	+71 (54)
Chlorpromazine (N=7)	110	+39 (35)

[See table 5 above]

Weight Gain
Weight gain has occurred with the use of antipsychotics, including CLOZARIL. Monitor weight during treatment with CLOZARIL. Table 6 summarizes the data on weight gain by the duration of exposure pooled from 11 studies with CLOZARIL and active comparators. The median duration of exposure was 609, 728, and 42 days, in the CLOZARIL, olanzapine, and chlorpromazine group, respectively.

[See table 6 above]

Table 7 summarizes pooled data from 11 studies in adult subjects with schizophrenia demonstrating weight gain ≥7% of body weight relative to baseline. The median duration of exposure was 609, 728, and 42 days, in the CLOZARIL, olanzapine, and chlorpromazine group, respectively.

Table 7. Proportion of Adult Subjects in Schizophrenia Studies with Weight Gain ≥7% Relative to Baseline Body Weight

Weight change	CLOZARIL	Olanzapine	Chlorpromazine
N	669	442	155
≥7% (inclusive)	236 (35%)	203 (46%)	13 (8%)

5.10   Neuroleptic Malignant Syndrome
Antipsychotic drugs including CLOZARIL can cause a potentially fatal symptom complex referred to as Neuroleptic Malignant Syndrome (NMS). Clinical manifestations of NMS include hyperpyrexia, muscle rigidity, altered mental status, and autonomic instability (irregular pulse or blood pressure, tachycardia, diaphoresis, and cardiac dysrhythmias). Associated findings can include elevated creatine phosphokinase (CPK), myoglobinuria, rhabdomyolysis, and acute renal failure.

The diagnostic evaluation of patients with this syndrome is complicated. It is important to consider the presence of other serious medical conditions (e.g., agranulocytosis, infection, heat stroke, primary CNS pathology, central anticholinergic toxicity, extrapyramidal symptoms, and drug fever).

Hyperglycemia and Diabetes Mellitus
Hyperglycemia, in some cases extreme and associated with ketoacidosis or hyperosmolar coma or death, has been reported in patients treated with atypical antipsychotics including CLOZARIL. Assessment of the relationship between atypical antipsychotic use and glucose abnormalities is complicated by the possibility of an increased background risk of diabetes mellitus in patients with schizophrenia and the increasing incidence of diabetes mellitus in the general population. Given these confounders, the relationship between atypical antipsychotic use and hyperglycemia-related adverse reactions is not completely understood. However, epidemiological studies suggest an increased risk of treatment-emergent, hyperglycemia-related adverse reactions in patients treated with the atypical antipsychotics. Precise risk estimates for hyperglycemia-related adverse reactions in patients treated with atypical antipsychotics are not available.

Patients with an established diagnosis of diabetes mellitus who are started on CLOZARIL should be monitored regularly for worsening of glucose control. Patients with risk factors for diabetes mellitus (e.g., obesity, family history of diabetes) who are starting treatment with atypical antipsychotics should undergo fasting blood glucose testing at the beginning of treatment and periodically during treatment.

Any patient treated with atypical antipsychotics should be monitored for symptoms of hyperglycemia including polydipsia, polyuria, polyphagia, and weakness. Patients who develop symptoms of hyperglycemia during treatment with atypical antipsychotics should undergo fasting blood glucose testing. In some cases, hyperglycemia has resolved when the atypical antipsychotic was discontinued; however, some patients required continuation of anti-diabetic treatment despite discontinuation of the suspect drug.

In a pooled data analysis of 8 studies in adult subjects with schizophrenia, the mean changes in fasting glucose concentration in the CLOZARIL and chlorpromazine groups were +11 mg/dL and +4 mg/dL respectively. A higher proportion of the CLOZARIL group demonstrated categorical increases from baseline in fasting glucose concentrations, compared to the chlorpromazine group (Table 3). The CLOZARIL doses were 100–900 mg per day (mean modal dose: 512 mg per day). The maximum chlorpromazine dose was 1800 mg per day (mean modal dose: 1029 mg per day). The median duration of exposure was 42 days for CLOZARIL and chlorpromazine.

[See table 3 above]

Dyslipidemia
Undesirable alterations in lipids have occurred in patients treated with atypical antipsychotics, including CLOZARIL.

The management of NMS should include (1) immediate discontinuation of antipsychotic drugs and other drugs not essential to concurrent therapy, (2) intensive symptomatic treatment and medical monitoring, and (3) treatment of comorbid medical conditions. There is no general agreement about specific pharmacological treatments for NMS.

If a patient requires antipsychotic drug treatment after recovery from NMS, the potential reintroduction of drug therapy should be carefully considered. NMS can recur. Monitor closely if treatment with antipsychotics.

NMS has occurred with CLOZARIL monotherapy and with concomitant CNS-active medications, including lithium.

5.11 Fever

During clozapine therapy, patients have experienced transient, clozapine-related fever. The peak incidence is within the first 3 weeks of treatment. While this fever is generally benign and self-limited, it may necessitate discontinuing treatment. The fever can be associated with an increase or decrease in WBC count. Carefully evaluate patients with fever to rule out agranulocytosis or infection. Consider the possibility of NMS [see Warnings and Precautions (5.10)].

5.12 Pulmonary Embolism

Pulmonary embolism and deep vein thrombosis have occurred in patients treated with CLOZARIL. Consider the possibility of pulmonary embolism in patients who present with deep-vein thrombosis, acute dyspnea, chest pain, or with other respiratory signs and symptoms. Whether pulmonary embolus and deep vein thrombosis can be attributed to clozapine or some characteristic(s) of patients is not clear.

5.13 Anticholinergic Toxicity

CLOZARIL has potent anticholinergic effects. Treatment with CLOZARIL can result in CNS and peripheral anticholinergic toxicity. Use with caution in the presence of narrow-angle glaucoma, concomitant anticholinergic medications, prostatic hypertrophy, or other conditions in which anticholinergic effects can lead to significant adverse reactions.

Treatment with CLOZARIL can result in gastrointestinal adverse reactions, including constipation, intestinal obstruction, fecal impaction, and paralytic ileus. Such reactions can be fatal. Constipation should be initially treated by ensuring adequate hydration and use of ancillary therapy such as bulk laxatives. Consultation with a gastroenterologist is advisable in more serious cases.

5.14 Interference with Cognitive and Motor Performance

CLOZARIL can cause sedation and impairment of cognitive and motor performance. Caution patients about operating hazardous machinery, including automobiles, until they are reasonably certain that CLOZARIL does not affect them adversely. These reactions may be dose-related. Consider reducing the dose if they occur.

5.15 Tardive Dyskinesia

Tardive dyskinesia (TD) has occurred in patients treated with antipsychotic drugs, including CLOZARIL. The syndrome consists of potentially irreversible, involuntary, dyskinetic movements. The risk of TD and the likelihood that it will become irreversible are believed to increase with greater durations of treatment and higher total cumulative doses. However, the syndrome can develop after relatively brief treatment periods at low doses. Prescribe CLOZARIL in a manner that is most likely to minimize the risk of developing TD. Use the lowest effective dose and the shortest duration necessary to control symptoms. Periodically assess the need for continued treatment. Consider discontinuing treatment if TD occurs. However, some patients may require treatment with CLOZARIL despite the presence of the syndrome.

There is no known treatment for TD. However, the syndrome may remit partially or completely if treatment is discontinued. Antipsychotic treatment, itself, may suppress (or partially suppress) the signs and symptoms, and it has the potential to mask the underlying process. The effect of symptom suppression on the long-term course of TD is unknown.

5.16 Cerebrovascular Adverse Reactions

In controlled trials, elderly patients with dementia-related psychosis treated with some atypical antipsychotics had an increased risk (compared to placebo) of cerebrovascular adverse reactions (e.g., stroke, transient ischemic attack), including fatalities. The mechanism for this increased risk is not known. An increased risk cannot be excluded for CLOZARIL or other antipsychotics or other patient populations. CLOZARIL should be used with caution in patients with risk factors for cerebrovascular adverse reactions.

5.17 Recurrence of Psychosis and Cholinergic Rebound after Abrupt Discontinuation of CLOZARIL

If abrupt discontinuation of CLOZARIL is necessary (because of agranulocytosis or another medical condition, for example), monitor carefully for the recurrence of psychotic symptoms and adverse reactions related to cholinergic rebound, such as profuse sweating, headache, nausea, vomiting and diarrhea.

6 ADVERSE REACTIONS

The following adverse reactions are discussed in more detail in other sections of the labeling:
- Agranulocytosis [see Warnings and Precautions (5.1)].
- Orthostatic Hypotension, Bradycardia, and Syncope [see Warnings and Precautions (5.3)].
- Seizures [see Warnings and Precautions (5.4)].
- Myocarditis and Cardiomyopathy [see Warnings and Precautions (5.5)].
- Increased Mortality in Elderly Patients with Dementia-Related Psychosis [see Warnings and Precautions (5.6)].
- Eosinophilia [see Warnings and Precautions (5.7)].
- QT Interval Prolongation [see Warnings and Precautions (5.8)].
- Metabolic Changes (Hyperglycemia and Diabetes Mellitus, Dyslipidemia, and Weight Gain) [see Warnings and Precautions (5.9)].
- Neuroleptic Malignant Syndrome [see Warnings and Precautions (5.10)].
- Fever [see Warnings and Precautions (5.11)].
- Pulmonary Embolism [see Warnings and Precautions (5.12)].
- Anticholinergic Toxicity [see Warnings and Precautions (5.13)].
- Interference with Cognitive and Motor Performance [see Warnings and Precautions (5.14)].
- Tardive Dyskinesia [see Warnings and Precautions (5.15)].
- Cerebrovascular Adverse Reactions [see Warnings and Precautions (5.16)].
- Recurrence of Psychosis and Cholinergic Rebound after Abrupt Discontinuation [see Warnings and Precautions (5.17)].

6.1 Clinical Trials Experience

Because clinical trials are conducted under widely varying conditions, adverse reaction rates observed in the clinical trials of a drug cannot be directly compared to rates in the clinical trials of another drug and may not reflect the rates observed in clinical practice.

The most commonly reported adverse reactions (>5%) across CLOZARIL clinical trials were: CNS reactions, including sedation, dizziness/vertigo, headache, and tremor; cardiovascular reactions, including tachycardia, hypotension, and syncope; autonomic nervous system reactions, including hypersalivation, sweating, dry mouth, and visual disturbances; gastrointestinal reactions, including constipation and nausea; and fever. Table 8 summarizes the most commonly reported adverse reactions (>5%) in CLOZARIL-treated patients (compared to chlorpromazine-treated patients) in the pivotal, 6-week, controlled trial in treatment-resistant schizophrenia.

Table 8. Common Adverse Reactions (≥5%) in the 6-Week, Randomized, Chlorpromazine-controlled Trial in Treatment-Resistant Schizophrenia

Adverse Reaction	CLOZARIL (N=126) (%)	Chlorpromazine (N=142) (%)
Sedation	21	13
Tachycardia	17	11
Constipation	16	12
Dizziness	14	16
Hypotension	13	38
Fever (hyperthermia)	13	4
Hypersalivation	13	1
Hypertension	12	5
Headache	10	10
Nausea/vomiting	10	12
Dry mouth	5	20

Table 9 summarizes the adverse reactions reported in CLOZARIL-treated patients at a frequency of 2% or greater across all CLOZARIL studies (excluding the 2-year InterSePT™ Study). These rates are not adjusted for duration of exposure.

Table 9. Adverse Reactions (≥2%) Reported in CLOZARIL-treated Patients (N=842) Across all CLOZARIL Studies (excluding the 2-year InterSePT™ Study)

Body System Adverse Reaction*	CLOZARIL N=842 Percentage of Patients
Central Nervous System	
Drowsiness/Sedation	39
Dizziness/Vertigo	19
Headache	7
Tremor	6
Syncope	6
Disturbed Sleep/Nightmares	4
Restlessness	4
Hypokinesia/Akinesia	4
Agitation	4
Seizures (convulsions)	3†
Rigidity	3
Akathisia	3
Confusion	3
Fatigue	2
Insomnia	2
Cardiovascular	
Tachycardia	25†
Hypotension	9
Hypertension	4
Gastrointestinal	
Constipation	14
Nausea	5
Abdominal Discomfort/ Heartburn	4
Nausea/Vomiting	3
Vomiting	3
Diarrhea	2
Urogenital	
Urinary Abnormalities	2
Autonomic Nervous System	
Salivation	31
Sweating	6
Dry Mouth	6
Visual Disturbances	5
Skin	
Rash	2
Hemic/Lymphatic	
Leukopenia/Decreased WBC/ Neutropenia	3
Miscellaneous	
Fever	5
Weight Gain	4

† Rate based on population of approximately 1700 exposed during premarket clinical evaluation of CLOZARIL.

Table 10 summarizes the most commonly reported adverse reactions (>10% of the CLOZARIL or olanzapine group) in the InterSePT™ Study. This was an adequate and well-controlled, 2-year study evaluating the efficacy of CLOZARIL relative to olanzapine in reducing the risk of suicidal behavior in patients with schizophrenia or schizoaffective disorder. The rates are not adjusted for duration of exposure.

Table 10. Incidence of Adverse Reactions in Patients Treated with CLOZARIL or Olanzapine in the InterSePT™ Study (>10% in the CLOZARIL or olanzapine group)

Adverse Reactions	CLOZARIL N=479 % Reporting	Olanzapine N=477 % Reporting
Salivary hypersecretion	48	6
Somnolence	46	25
Weight increased	31	56
Dizziness (excluding vertigo)	27	12
Constipation	25	10
Insomnia	20	33
Nausea	17	10
Vomiting	17	9
Dyspepsia	14	8

Dystonia

Class effect: Symptoms of dystonia, prolonged abnormal contractions of muscle groups, may occur in susceptible individuals during the first few days of treatment. Dystonic symptoms include: spasm of the neck muscles, sometimes progressing to tightness of the throat, swallowing difficulty, difficulty breathing, and/or protrusion of the tongue. While these symptoms can occur at low doses, they occur more frequently and with greater severity with high potency and at higher doses of first generation antipsychotic drugs. An elevated risk of acute dystonia is observed in males and younger age groups.

6.2 Postmarketing Experience

The following adverse reactions have been identified during post-approval use of clozapine. Because these reactions are reported voluntarily from a population of uncertain size, it is not always possible to reliably estimate their frequency or establish a causal relationship to drug exposure.

Central Nervous System
Delirium, EEG abnormal, myoclonus, paresthesia, possible cataplexy, status epilepticus, obsessive compulsive symptoms, and post-discontinuation cholinergic rebound adverse reactions.

Cardiovascular System
Atrial or ventricular fibrillation, ventricular tachycardia, QT interval prolongation, Torsades de Pointes, myocardial infarction, cardiac arrest, and periorbital edema.

Gastrointestinal System
Acute pancreatitis, dysphagia, salivary gland swelling.

Hepatobiliary System
Cholestasis, hepatitis, jaundice, hepatotoxicity, hepatic steatosis, hepatic necrosis, hepatic fibrosis, hepatic cirrhosis, liver injury (hepatic, cholestatic, and mixed), and liver failure.

Urogenital System
Acute interstitial nephritis, nocturnal enuresis, priapism, and renal failure.

Skin
Hypersensitivity reactions: photosensitivity, vasculitis, erythema multiforme, and Stevens-Johnson Syndrome.

Musculoskeletal System
Myasthenic syndrome and rhabdomyolysis.

Respiratory System
Aspiration, pleural effusion, pneumonia, lower respiratory tract infection.

Hemic and Lymphatic System
Deep-vein thrombosis, elevated hemoglobin/hematocrit, erythrocyte sedimentation rate (ESR) increased, sepsis, thrombocytosis, and thrombocytopenia.

Vision Disorders
Narrow-angle glaucoma.

Miscellaneous
Creatine phosphokinase elevation, hyperuricemia, hyponatremia, and weight loss.

7 DRUG INTERACTIONS

7.1 Potential for Other Drugs to Affect CLOZARIL
Clozapine is a substrate for many cytochrome P450 isozymes, in particular CYP1A2, CYP3A4, and CYP2D6. Use caution when administering CLOZARIL concomitantly with drugs that are inducers or inhibitors of these enzymes.

CYP1A2 Inhibitors
Concomitant use of CLOZARIL and CYP1A2 inhibitors can increase plasma levels of clozapine, potentially resulting in adverse reactions. Reduce the CLOZARIL dose to one-third of the original dose when CLOZARIL is coadministered with strong CYP1A2 inhibitors (e.g., fluvoxamine, ciprofloxacin, or enoxacin). The CLOZARIL dose should be increased to the original dose when coadministration of strong CYP1A2 inhibitors is discontinued *[see Dosage and Administration (2.6), Clinical Pharmacology (12.3)]*.

Moderate or weak CYP1A2 inhibitors include oral contraceptives and caffeine. Monitor patients closely when CLOZARIL is coadministered with these inhibitors. Consider reducing the CLOZARIL dosage if necessary *[see Dosage and Administration (2.6)]*.

CYP2D6 and CYP3A4 Inhibitors
Concomitant treatment with CLOZARIL and CYP2D6 or CYP3A4 inhibitors (e.g., cimetidine, escitalopram, erythromycin, paroxetine, bupropion, fluoxetine, quinidine, duloxetine, terbinafine, or sertraline) can increase clozapine levels and lead to adverse reactions *[see Clinical Pharmacology (12.3)]*. Use caution and monitor patients closely when using such inhibitors. Consider reducing the CLOZARIL dose *[see Dosage and Administration (2.6)]*.

CYP1A2 and CYP3A4 Inducers
Concomitant treatment with drugs that induce CYP1A2 or CYP3A4 can decrease the plasma concentration of clozapine, resulting in decreased effectiveness of CLOZARIL. Tobacco smoke is a moderate inducer of CYP1A2. Strong CYP3A4 inducers include carbamazepine, phenytoin, St. John's wort, and rifampin. It may be necessary to increase the CLOZARIL dose if used concomitantly with inducers of these enzymes. However, concomitant use of CLOZARIL and strong CYP3A4 inducers is not recommended *[see Dosage and Administration (2.6)]*.

Consider reducing the CLOZARIL dosage when discontinuing coadministered enzyme inducers; because discontinuation of inducers can result in increased clozapine plasma levels and an increased risk of adverse reactions *[see Dosage and Administration (2.6)]*.

Drugs that Cause QT Interval Prolongation
Use caution when administering concomitant medications that prolong the QT interval or inhibit the metabolism of clozapine. Drugs that cause QT prolongation include: specific antipsychotics (e.g., ziprasidone, iloperidone, chlorpromazine, thioridazine, mesoridazine, droperidol, and pimozide), specific antibiotics (e.g., erythromycin, gatifloxacin, moxifloxacin, sparfloxacin), Class 1A antiarrhythmics (e.g., quinidine, procainamide) or Class III antiarrhythmics (e.g., amiodarone, sotalol), and others (e.g., pentamidine, levomethadyl acetate, methadone, halofantrine, mefloquine, dolasetron mesylate, probucol or tacrolimus) *[see Warnings and Precautions (5.8)]*.

7.2 Potential for CLOZARIL to Affect Other Drugs
Concomitant use of CLOZARIL with other drugs metabolized by CYP2D6 can increase levels of these CYPD26 substrates. Use caution when coadministering CLOZARIL with other drugs that are metabolized by CYP2D6. It may be necessary to use lower doses of such drugs than usually prescribed. Such drugs include specific antidepressants, phenothiazines, carbamazepine, and Type 1C antiarrhythmics (e.g., propafenone, flecainide, and encainide).

8 USE IN SPECIFIC POPULATIONS

8.1 Pregnancy
Pregnancy Category B
Risk Summary
There are no adequate or well-controlled studies of clozapine in pregnant women.

Reproduction studies have been performed in rats and rabbits at doses up to 0.4 and 0.9 times, respectively, the maximum recommended human dose (MRHD) of 900 mg/day on a mg/m^2 body surface area basis. The studies revealed no evidence of impaired fertility or harm to the fetus due to clozapine. Because animal reproduction studies are not always predictive of human response, CLOZARIL should be used during pregnancy only if clearly needed.

Clinical Considerations
Consider the risk of exacerbation of psychosis when discontinuing or changing treatment with antipsychotic medications during pregnancy and postpartum. Consider early screening for gestational diabetes for patients treated with antipsychotic medications *[see Warnings and Precautions (5.9)]*. Neonates exposed to antipsychotic drugs during the third trimester of pregnancy are at risk for extrapyramidal and/or withdrawal symptoms following delivery. Monitor neonates for symptoms of agitation, hypertonia, hypotonia, tremor, somnolence, respiratory distress, and feeding difficulties. The severity of complications can vary from self-limited symptoms to some neonates requiring intensive care unit support and prolonged hospitalization.

Animal Data
In embryofetal developmental studies, clozapine had no effects on maternal parameters, litter sizes, or fetal parameters when administered orally to pregnant rats and rabbits during the period of organogenesis at doses up to 0.4 and 0.9 times, respectively, the MRHD of 900 mg/day on a mg/m^2 body surface area basis.

In peri/postnatal developmental studies, pregnant female rats were administered clozapine over the last third of pregnancy and until day 21 postpartum. Observations were made on fetuses at birth and during the postnatal period; the offspring were allowed to reach sexual maturity and mated. Clozapine caused a decrease in maternal body weight but had no effects on litter size or body weights of either F1 or F2 generations at doses up to 0.4 times the MRHD of 900 mg/day on a mg/m^2 body surface area basis.

8.3 Nursing Mothers
CLOZARIL is present in human milk. Because of the potential for serious adverse reactions in nursing infants from CLOZARIL, a decision should be made whether to discontinue nursing or to discontinue the drug, taking into account the importance of the drug to the mother.

8.4 Pediatric Use
Safety and effectiveness in pediatric patients have not been established.

8.5 Geriatric Use
There have not been sufficient numbers of geriatric patients in clinical studies utilizing CLOZARIL to determine whether those over 65 years of age differ from younger subjects in their response to CLOZARIL.

Orthostatic hypotension and tachycardia can occur with CLOZARIL treatment *[see Boxed Warning and Warnings and Precautions (5.3)]*. Elderly patients, particularly those with compromised cardiovascular functioning, may be more susceptible to these effects.

Elderly patients may be particularly susceptible to the anticholinergic effects of CLOZARIL, such as urinary retention and constipation *[see Warnings and Precautions (5.13)]*.

Carefully select CLOZARIL doses in elderly patients, taking into consideration their greater frequency of decreased hepatic, renal, or cardiac function, as well as other concomitant disease and other drug therapy. Clinical experience suggests that the prevalence of tardive dyskinesia appears to be highest among the elderly; especially elderly women *[see Warnings and Precautions (5.15)]*.

8.6 Patients with Renal or Hepatic Impairment
Dose reduction may be necessary in patients with significant impairment of renal or hepatic function. Clozapine concentrations may be increased in these patients, because clozapine is almost completely metabolized and then excreted *[see Dosage and Administration (2.7), Clinical Pharmacology (12.3)]*.

8.7 CYP2D6 Poor Metabolizers
Dose reduction may be necessary in patients who are CYP2D6 poor metabolizers. Clozapine concentrations may be increased in these patients, because clozapine is almost completely metabolized and then excreted *[see Dosage and Administration (2.7), Clinical Pharmacology (12.3)]*.

10 OVERDOSAGE

10.1 Overdosage Experience
The most commonly reported signs and symptoms associated with clozapine overdose are: sedation, delirium, coma, tachycardia, hypotension, respiratory depression or failure; and hypersalivation. There are reports of aspiration pneumonia, cardiac arrhythmias, and seizure. Fatal overdoses have been reported with clozapine, generally at doses above 2500 mg. There have also been reports of patients recovering from overdoses well in excess of 4 g.

10.2 Management of Overdosage
For the most up-to-date information on the management of CLOZARIL overdosage, contact a certified Regional Poison Control Center (1-800-222-1222). Telephone numbers of certified Regional Poison Control Centers are listed in the **Physicians' Desk Reference®*, a registered trademark of Thomson PDR. Establish and maintain an airway; ensure adequate oxygenation and ventilation. Monitor cardiac status and vital signs. Use general symptomatic and supportive measures. There are no specific antidotes for CLOZARIL.

In managing overdosage, consider the possibility of multiple-drug involvement.

**Trademark of Thomson Healthcare, Inc.

11 DESCRIPTION
CLOZARIL® (clozapine), an atypical antipsychotic drug, is a tricyclic dibenzodiazepine derivative, 8-chloro-11-(4-methyl-1-piperazinyl)-5H-dibenzo [b,e] [1,4] diazepine. The structural formula is:

$C_{18}H_{19}ClN_4$ Mol. wt. 326.83

CLOZARIL is available in pale yellow tablets of 25 mg and 100 mg for oral administration.
Active Ingredient: clozapine
Inactive Ingredients: colloidal silicon dioxide, lactose, magnesium stearate, povidone, starch (corn), and talc.

12 CLINICAL PHARMACOLOGY

12.1 Mechanism of Action
The mechanism of action of clozapine is unknown. However, it has been proposed that the therapeutic efficacy of clozapine in schizophrenia is mediated through antagonism of the dopamine type 2 (D_2) and the serotonin type 2A ($5\text{-}HT_{2A}$) receptors. CLOZARIL also acts as an antagonist at adrenergic, cholinergic, histaminergic and other dopaminergic and serotonergic receptors.

12.2 Pharmacodynamics
Clozapine demonstrated binding affinity to the following receptors: histamine H_1 (K_i 1.1 nM), adrenergic α_{1A} (K_i 1.6 nM), serotonin $5\text{-}HT_6$ (K_i 4 nM), serotonin $5\text{-}HT_{2A}$ (K_i 5.4 nM), muscarinic M_1 (K_i 6.2 nM), serotonin $5\text{-}HT_7$ (K_i 6.3 nM), serotonin $5\text{-}HT_{2C}$ (K_i 9.4 nM), dopamine D_4 (K_i 24 nM), adrenergic α_{2A} (K_i 90 nM), serotonin $5\text{-}HT_3$ (K_i 95 nM), serotonin $5\text{-}HT_{1A}$ (K_i 120 nM), dopamine D_2 (K_i 160 nM), dopamine D_1 (K_i 270 nM), dopamine D_5 (K_i 454 nM), and dopamine D_3 (K_i 555 nM).

Clozapine causes little or no prolactin elevation.

Clinical electroencephalogram (EEG) studies demonstrated that clozapine increases delta and theta activity and slows dominant alpha frequencies. Enhanced synchronization occurs. Sharp wave activity and spike and wave complexes may also develop. Patients have reported an intensification of dream activity during clozapine therapy. REM sleep was found to be increased to 85% of the total sleep time. In these patients, the onset of REM sleep occurred almost immediately after falling asleep.

12.3 Pharmacokinetics
Absorption
In man, CLOZARIL tablets (25 mg and 100 mg) are equally bioavailable relative to a CLOZARIL solution. Following oral administration of CLOZARIL 100 mg twice daily, the average steady-state peak plasma concentration was 319 ng/mL (range: 102 to 771 ng/mL), occurring at the average of 2.5 hours (range: 1 to 6 hours) after dosing. The average minimum concentration at steady state was 122 ng/mL (range: 41 to 343 ng/mL), after 100 mg twice

daily dosing. Food does not appear to affect the systemic bioavailability of CLOZARIL. Thus, CLOZARIL may be administered with or without food.

Distribution

Clozapine is approximately 97% bound to serum proteins. The interaction between clozapine and other highly protein-bound drugs has not been fully evaluated but may be important *[see Drug Interactions (7)]*.

Metabolism and Excretion

Clozapine is almost completely metabolized prior to excretion, and only trace amounts of unchanged drug are detected in the urine and feces. Clozapine is a substrate for many cytochrome P450 isozymes, in particular CYP1A2, CYP2D6, and CYP3A4. Approximately 50% of the administered dose is excreted in the urine and 30% in the feces. The demethylated, hydroxylated, and N-oxide derivatives are components in both urine and feces. Pharmacological testing has shown the desmethyl metabolite (norclozapine) to have only limited activity, while the hydroxylated and N- oxide derivatives were inactive. The mean elimination half-life of clozapine after a single 75 mg dose was 8 hours (range: 4 to 12 hours), compared to a mean elimination half-life of 12 hours (range: 4 to 66 hours), after achieving steady state with 100mg twice daily dosing.

A comparison of single-dose and multiple-dose administration of clozapine demonstrated that the elimination half-life increased significantly after multiple dosing relative to that after single-dose administration, suggesting the possibility of concentration-dependent pharmacokinetics. However, at steady state, approximately dose-proportional changes with respect to area under the curve (AUC), peak, and minimum clozapine plasma concentrations were observed after administration of 37.5, 75, and 150 mg twice daily.

Drug-Drug Interaction Studies

Fluvoxamine

A pharmacokinetic study was conducted in 16 schizophrenic patients who received clozapine under steady-state conditions. After coadministration of fluvoxamine for 14 days, mean trough concentrations of clozapine and its metabolites, N-desmethylclozapine and clozapine N-oxide, were elevated about 3-fold compared to baseline steady-state concentrations.

Paroxetine, Fluoxetine, and Sertraline

In a study of schizophrenic patients (n=14) who received clozapine under steady-state conditions, coadministration of paroxetine produced only minor changes in the levels of clozapine and its metabolites. However, other published reports describe modest elevations (less than 2-fold) of clozapine and metabolite concentrations when clozapine was taken with paroxetine, fluoxetine, and sertraline.

Specific Population Studies

Renal or Hepatic Impairment

No specific pharmacokinetic studies were conducted to investigate the effects of renal or hepatic impairment on the pharmacokinetics of clozapine. Higher clozapine plasma concentrations are likely in patients with significant renal or hepatic impairment when given usual doses.

CYP2D6 Poor Metabolizers

A subset (3%–10%) of the population has reduced activity of CYP2D6 (CYP2D6 poor metabolizers). These individuals may develop higher than expected plasma concentrations of clozapine when given usual doses.

13   NONCLINICAL TOXICOLOGY

13.1   Carcinogenesis, Mutagenesis, Impairment of Fertility

Carcinogenesis

No carcinogenic potential was demonstrated in long-term studies in mice and rats at doses up to 0.3 times and 0.4 times, respectively, the maximum recommended human dose (MRHD) of 900 mg/day on a mg/m^2 body surface area basis.

Mutagenesis

Clozapine was not genotoxic when tested in the following gene mutation and chromosomal aberration tests: the bacterial Ames test, the *in vitro* mammalian V79 in Chinese hamster cells, the *in vitro* unscheduled DNA synthesis in rat hepatocytes or the *in vivo* micronucleus assay in mice.

Impairment of Fertility

Clozapine had no effect on any parameters of fertility, pregnancy, fetal weight or postnatal development when administered orally to male rats 70 days before mating and to female rats for 14 days before mating at doses up to 0.4 times the MRHD of 900 mg/day on a mg/m^2 body surface area basis.

14   CLINICAL STUDIES

14.1   Treatment Resistant Schizophrenia

The efficacy of CLOZARIL in treatment-resistant schizophrenia was established in a multicenter, randomized, double-blind, active-controlled (chlorpromazine) study in patients with a DSM-III diagnosis of schizophrenia who had inadequate responses to at least 3 different antipsychotics (from at least 2 different chemical classes) during the preceding 5 years. The antipsychotic trials must have been

judged adequate; the antipsychotic dosages must have been equivalent to or greater than 1000 mg per day of chlorpromazine for a period of at least 6 weeks, each without significant reduction of symptoms. There must have been no period of good functioning within the preceding 5 years. Patients must have had a baseline score of at least 45 on the investigator-rated Brief Psychiatric Rating Scale (BPRS). On the 18-item BPRS, 1 indicates the absence of symptoms, and 7 indicates severe symptoms; the maximum potential total BPRS score is 126. At baseline, the mean BPRS score was 61. In addition, patients must have had a score of at least 4 on at least 2 of the following 4 individual BPRS items: conceptual disorganization, suspiciousness, hallucinatory behavior, and unusual thought content. Patients must have had a Clinical Global Impressions–Severity Scale score of at least 4 (moderately ill).

In the prospective, lead-in phase of the trial, all patients (N=305) initially received single-blind treatment with haloperidol (the mean dose was 61 mg per day) for 6 weeks. More than 80% of patients completed the 6-week trial. Patients with an inadequate response to haloperidol (n=268) were randomized to double-blind treatment with CLOZARIL (N=126) or chlorpromazine (N=142). The maximum daily CLOZARIL dose was 900 mg; the mean daily dose was >600 mg. The maximum daily chlorpromazine dose was 1800 mg; the mean daily dose was >1200 mg.

The primary endpoint was treatment response, predefined as a decrease in BPRS score of at least 20% and either (1) a CGI-S score of <3 (mildly ill), or (2) a BPRS score of <35, at the end of 6 weeks of treatment. Approximately 88% of patients from the CLOZARIL and chlorpromazine groups completed the 6-week trial. At the end of 6 weeks, 30% of the CLOZARIL group responded to treatment, and 4% of the chlorpromazine group responded to treatment. The difference was statistically significant (p <0.001). The mean change in total BPRS score was -16 and -5 in the CLOZARIL and chlorpromazine group, respectively; the mean change in the 4 key BPRS item scores was -5 and -2 in the CLOZARIL and chlorpromazine group, respectively; and the mean change in CGI-S score was -1.2 and -0.4, in the CLOZARIL and chlorpromazine group, respectively. These changes in the CLOZARIL group were statistically significantly greater than in the chlorpromazine group (p<0.001 in each analysis).

14.2   Recurrent Suicidal Behavior in Schizophrenia or Schizoaffective Disorder

The effectiveness of CLOZARIL in reducing the risk of recurrent suicidal behavior was assessed in the International Suicide Prevention Trial (InterSePT™, a trademark of Novartis Pharmaceuticals Corporation). This was a prospective, randomized, open-label, active-controlled, multicenter, international, parallel-group comparison of CLOZARIL versus olanzapine (*Zyprexa®, a registered trademark of Eli Lilly and Company) in 956 patients with schizophrenia or schizoaffective disorder (DSM-IV) who were judged to be at risk for recurrent suicidal behavior. Only about one-fourth of these patients (27%) were considered resistant to standard antipsychotic drug treatment. To enter the trial, patients must have met 1 of the following criteria:

- They had attempted suicide within the 3 years prior to their baseline evaluation.
- They had been hospitalized to prevent a suicide attempt within the 3 years prior to their baseline evaluation.
- They demonstrated moderate-to-severe suicidal ideation with a depressive component within 1 week prior to their baseline evaluation.
- They demonstrated moderate-to-severe suicidal ideation accompanied by command hallucinations to do self-harm within 1 week prior to their baseline evaluation.

Dosing regimens for each treatment group were determined by individual investigators and were individualized by patient. Dosing was flexible, with a dose range of 200–900 mg/day for CLOZARIL and 5–20 mg/day for olanzapine. For the 956 patients who received CLOZARIL or olanzapine in this study, there was extensive use of concomitant psychotropics: 84% with antipsychotics, 65% with anxiolytics, 53% with antidepressants, and 28% with mood stabilizers. There was significantly greater use of concomitant psychotropic medications among the patients in the olanzapine group.

The primary efficacy measure was time to (1) a significant suicide attempt, including a completed suicide; (2) hospitalization due to imminent suicide risk, including increased level of surveillance for suicidality for patients already hospitalized; or (3) worsening of suicidality severity as demonstrated by "much worsening" or "very much worsening" from baseline in the Clinical Global Impression of Severity of Suicidality as assessed by the Blinded Psychiatrist (CGI-SS-BP) scale. A determination of whether or not a reported event met criterion 1 or 2 above was made by the Suicide Monitoring Board (SMB), a group of experts blinded to patient data.

A total of 980 patients were randomized to the study and 956 received study medication. Sixty-two percent of the pa-

tients were diagnosed with schizophrenia, and the remainder (38%) were diagnosed with schizoaffective disorder. Only about one-fourth of the total patient population (27%) was identified as "treatment-resistant" at baseline. There were more males than females in the study (61% of all patients were male). The mean age of patients entering the study was 37 years of age (range 18–69). Most patients were Caucasian (71%), 15% were black, 1% were Asian, and 13% were classified as being of "other" races.

Patients treated with CLOZARIL had a statistically significant longer delay in the time to recurrent suicidal behavior in comparison with olanzapine. This result should be interpreted only as evidence of the effectiveness of CLOZARIL in delaying time to recurrent suicidal behavior and not a demonstration of the superior efficacy of CLOZARIL over olanzapine.

The probability of experiencing (1) a significant suicide attempt, including a completed suicide, or (2) hospitalization because of imminent suicide risk, including increased level of surveillance for suicidality for patients already hospitalized, was lower for CLOZARIL patients than for olanzapine patients at Week 104: CLOZARIL 24% versus olanzapine 32%; 95% CI of the difference: 2%, 14% (Figure 2).

Figure 2. Cumulative Probability of a Significant Suicide Attempt or Hospitalization to Prevent Suicide in Patients with Schizophrenia or Schizoaffective Disorder at High Risk of Suicidality

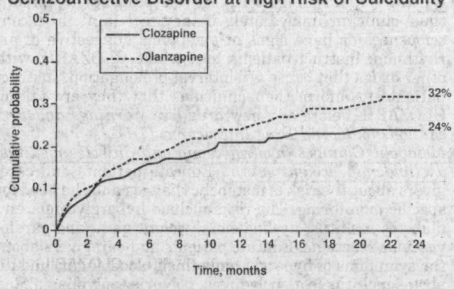

*Zyprexa® (olanzapine) is a registered trademark of Eli Lilly and Company.

16   HOW SUPPLIED/STORAGE AND HANDLING

16.1   How Supplied

CLOZARIL® (clozapine) is available as 25 mg and 100 mg round, pale-yellow, uncoated tablets with a facilitated score on one side.

CLOZARIL® (clozapine) Tablets

25 mg

Engraved with "CLOZARIL" once on the periphery of one side.
Engraved with a facilitated score and "25" once on the other side.

Bottle of 100	NDC 0078-0126-05
Bottle of 500	NDC 0078-0126-08
Unit dose packages of 100: 2 × 5 strips, 10 blisters per strip	NDC 0078-0126-06

100 mg

Engraved with "CLOZARIL" once on the periphery of one side.
Engraved with a facilitated score and "100" once on the other side.

Bottle of 100	NDC 0078-0127-05
Bottle of 500	NDC 0078-0127-08
Unit dose packages of 100: 2 × 5 strips, 10 blisters per strip	NDC 0078-0127-06

16.2   Storage and Handling

Storage temperature should not exceed 30°C (86°F). Keep out of reach of children.

17   PATIENT COUNSELING INFORMATION

Discuss the following issues with patients and caregivers:

- *Agranulocytosis:* Prior to initiating treatment, educate patients and caregivers about the significant risk of developing agranulocytosis. Advise them to immediately report the appearance of signs or symptoms consistent with agranulocytosis or infection (e.g., fever; mucus membrane ulcers; skin, pharyngeal, vaginal, urinary, or pulmonary infection; or extreme weakness or lethargy) at any time during CLOZARIL therapy *[see Boxed Warning and Warnings and Precautions (5.1)]*.
- Inform patients and caregivers that CLOZARIL will be made available only through a special program (CLOZARIL National Registry) designed to ensure the required blood monitoring, in order to reduce the risk of

developing agranulocytosis. Inform patients and caregivers the WBC count and ANC will be monitored as follows:

- Weekly blood tests are required for the first 6 months.
- If acceptable WBC counts and ANCs (WBC count ≥3500/mm³ and ANC ≥2000/mm³) have been maintained during the first 6 months of continuous therapy, then WBC counts and ANCs can be monitored every 2 weeks for the next 6 months.
- Thereafter, if acceptable WBC counts and ANCs have been maintained during the second 6 months of continuous therapy, WBC counts and ANCs can be monitored every 4 weeks.

- *Orthostatic Hypotension, Bradycardia, and Syncope:* Inform patients and caregivers about the risk of orthostatic hypotension and syncope, especially during the period of initial dose titration. Instruct them to strictly follow the clinician's instructions for dosage and administration. Advise patients to consult their clinician immediately if they feel faint, lose consciousness or have signs or symptoms suggestive of bradycardia or arrhythmia [see *Dosage and Administration (2.2) and Warnings and Precautions (5.3)*].
- *Seizures:* Inform patients and caregivers about the significant risk of seizure during CLOZARIL treatment. Caution them about driving and any other potentially hazardous activity while taking CLOZARIL [see *Warnings and Precautions (5.4)*].
- *QT Interval Prolongation:* Advise patients to consult their clinician immediately if they feel faint, lose consciousness or have signs or symptoms suggestive of arrhythmia. Instruct patients to not take CLOZARIL with other drugs that cause QT interval prolongation. Instruct patients to inform their clinicians that they are taking CLOZARIL before any new drug [see *Warnings and Precautions (5.8.) and Drug Interactions (7.1)*].
- *Metabolic Changes (hyperglycemia and diabetes mellitus, dyslipidemia, weight gain):* Educate patients and caregivers about the risk of metabolic changes and the need for specific monitoring. The risks include hyperglycemia and diabetes mellitus, dyslipidemia, weight gain, and cardiovascular reactions. Educate patients and caregivers about the symptoms of hyperglycemia (high blood sugar) and diabetes mellitus (e.g., polydipsia, polyuria, polyphagia, and weakness). Monitor all patients for these symptoms. Patients who are diagnosed with diabetes or have risk factors for diabetes (obesity, family history of diabetes) should have their fasting blood glucose monitored before beginning treatment and periodically during treatment. Patients who develop symptoms of hyperglycemia should have assessments of fasting glucose. Clinical monitoring of weight is recommended [see *Warnings and Precautions (5.9)*].
- *Interference with Cognitive and Motor Performance:* Because CLOZARIL may have the potential to impair judgment, thinking, or motor skills, patients should be cautioned about operating hazardous machinery, including automobiles, until they are reasonably certain that CLOZARIL therapy does not affect them adversely [see *Warnings and Precautions (5.14)*].
- *Missed Doses and Re-initiating Treatment:* Inform patients and caregivers that if the patient misses taking CLOZARIL for more than 2 days, they should not restart their medication at the same dosage but should contact their physician for dosing instructions adversely [see *Dosage and Administration (2.5) and Warnings and Precautions (5.3)*].
- *Pregnancy:* Patients and caregivers should notify the clinician if the patient becomes pregnant or intends to become pregnant during therapy [see *Use in Specific Populations (8.1)*].
- *Nursing:* Advice patients and caregivers that the patient should not breast feed an infant if they are taking CLOZARIL [see Use in Specific Populations (8.3)].
- *Concomitant Medication:* Advise patients to inform their health care provider if they are taking, or plan to take, any prescription or over-the-counter drugs; there is a potential for significant drug-drug interactions [see *Dosage and Administrations (2.6) and Drug Interactions (7.1)*].

CLOZARIL® is a registered trademark of Novartis Pharmaceuticals Corporation.

Novartis Pharmaceuticals Corporation
East Hanover, New Jersey 07936
© Novartis
T2013-114
November 2013

COARTEM ℞

[co-*AR*-tem]
(artemether/lumefantrine)
Tablets

The following prescribing information is based on official labeling in effect July 2013.

HIGHLIGHTS OF PRESCRIBING INFORMATION

These highlights do not include all the information needed to use Coartem Tablets safely and effectively. See full prescribing information for Coartem Tablets.

Coartem (artemether/lumefantrine) Tablets
Initial U.S. Approval: 2009

---RECENT MAJOR CHANGES---

Contraindications (4.2)	08/2012
Warnings and Precautions (5.1)	04/2013
Warnings and Precautions (5.2)	04/2013
Warnings and Precautions (5.3)	08/2012

---INDICATIONS AND USAGE---

- Coartem (artemether and lumefantrine) Tablets are indicated for treatment of acute, uncomplicated malaria infections due to *Plasmodium falciparum* in patients of 5 kg bodyweight and above. (1)
- Coartem Tablets have been shown to be effective in geographical regions where resistance to chloroquine has been reported. (1)
- Coartem Tablets should not be used to treat severe malaria or to prevent malaria. (1)

---DOSAGE AND ADMINISTRATION---

- Coartem Tablets should be taken with food. (2.1, 5.2)
- Tablets may be crushed and mixed with one to two teaspoons of water immediately prior to administration to patients, including children. (2.1)
- Coartem Tablets should be administered over 3-days for a total of 6 doses: an initial dose, second dose after 8 hours and then twice daily (morning and evening) for the following two days. (2.2, 2.3)
- The adult dosage for patients with bodyweight of 35 kg and above is 4 tablets per dose for a total of 6 doses. (2.2)
- The number of tablets per dose for children is determined by bodyweight, as shown in the chart below. (2.3)

Tablets per dose by bodyweight; total of 6 doses over 3 days

5 to <15 kg	1 tablet
15 to <25 kg	2 tablets
25 to <35 kg	3 tablets
35 kg and over	4 tablets

---DOSAGE FORMS AND STRENGTHS---

Tablets are scored and contain 20 mg artemether and 120 mg lumefantrine. (3)

---CONTRAINDICATIONS---

- Known hypersensitivity to artemether, lumefantrine, or to any of the excipients. (4.1)
- Co-administration of strong inducers of CYP3A4 such as rifampin, carbamazepine, phenytoin and St. John's wort with Coartem Tablets. (4.2, 7.1, 12.3)

---WARNINGS AND PRECAUTIONS---

- Avoid use in patients with known QT prolongation, those with hypokalemia or hypomagnesemia, and those taking other drugs that prolong the QT interval. (5.1, 12.6)
- Halofantrine and Coartem Tablets should not be administered within one month of each other due to potential additive effects on the QT interval. (5.1, 5.2, 12.3)
- Antimalarials should not be given concomitantly, unless there is no other treatment option, due to limited safety data. (5.2)
- QT prolonging drugs, including quinine and quinidine, should be used cautiously following Coartem Tablets. (5.1, 5.2, 7.7, 12.3)
- Substrates, inhibitors, or inducers of CYP3A4, including antiretroviral medications, should be used cautiously with Coartem Tablets, due to a potential loss of efficacy of the concomitant drug or additive QT prolongation. (5.3, 7.2, 7.3)

---ADVERSE REACTIONS---

The most common adverse reactions in adults (>30%) are headache, anorexia, dizziness, asthenia, arthralgia and myalgia. The most common adverse reactions in children (>12%) are pyrexia, cough, vomiting, anorexia and headache. (6.2)

To report SUSPECTED ADVERSE REACTIONS, contact Novartis Pharmaceuticals Corporation at 1-888-669-6682 or FDA at 1-800-FDA-1088 or www.fda.gov/medwatch

---DRUG INTERACTIONS---

- CYP3A4 Inducers: Potential for loss of antimalarial efficacy. (4.2, 5.3, 7.1, 12.3)
- CYP3A4 Inhibitors: Use cautiously due to potential for QT prolongation. (5.3, 7.2, 12.3)
- Antiretrovirals: Use cautiously due to potential for QT prolongation, loss of antiviral efficacy, or loss of antimalarial efficacy of Coartem Tablets. (5.3, 7.3, 12.3)
- Mefloquine: If used immediately before treatment, monitor for decreased efficacy of Coartem Tablets and encourage food consumption. (2.1, 7.4, 12.3)
- Hormonal Contraceptives: Effectiveness may be reduced; use an additional method of birth control. (5.3, 7.5, 12.3)
- CYP2D6 Substrates: Monitor for adverse reactions and potential QT prolongation. (5.1, 5.4, 7.6)

---USE IN SPECIFIC POPULATIONS---

- Pregnancy: Based on animal data, may increase fetal loss. (8.1)
- Nursing Mothers: Use caution when administering to a nursing woman. (8.3)
- Pediatric Use: Studied in children 2 months of age and older with a bodyweight of 5 kg and greater. (8.4)
- Geriatric Use: Not studied in geriatric patients. (8.5)

See 17 for PATIENT COUNSELING INFORMATION and FDA-approved patient labeling

Revised: 4/2013

FULL PRESCRIBING INFORMATION: CONTENTS*

* Sections or subsections omitted from the full prescribing information are not listed

---

FULL PRESCRIBING INFORMATION

1 INDICATIONS AND USAGE

Coartem (artemether/lumefantrine) Tablets are indicated for treatment of acute, uncomplicated malaria infections due to *Plasmodium falciparum* in patients of 5 kg bodyweight and above. Coartem Tablets have been shown to be effective in geographical regions where resistance to chloroquine has been reported [see *Clinical Studies (14.1)*].

Limitations of Use:
- Coartem Tablets are not approved for patients with severe or complicated *P. falciparum* malaria.
- Coartem Tablets are not approved for the prevention of malaria.

2 DOSAGE AND ADMINISTRATION

2.1 Administration Instructions

Coartem Tablets should be taken with food. Patients with acute malaria are frequently averse to food. Patients should be encouraged to resume normal eating as soon as food can be tolerated since this improves absorption of artemether and lumefantrine.

For patients who are unable to swallow the tablets such as infants and children, Coartem Tablets may be crushed and mixed with a small amount of water (one to two teaspoons) in a clean container for administration immediately prior to use. The container can be rinsed with more water and the contents swallowed by the patient. The crushed tablet preparation should be followed whenever possible by food/drink (e.g., milk, formula, pudding, broth, and porridge).

In the event of vomiting within 1 to 2 hours of administration, a repeat dose should be taken. If the repeat dose is vomited, the patient should be given an alternative antimalarial for treatment.

2.2 Dosage in Adult Patients (>16 years of age)

A 3-day treatment schedule with a total of 6 doses is recommended for adult patients with a bodyweight of 35 kg and above:

Four tablets as a single initial dose, 4 tablets again after 8 hours and then 4 tablets twice daily (morning and evening) for the following two days (total course of 24 tablets).

For patients weighing less than 35 kg, see Dosage in Pediatric Patients (2.3).

2.3 Dosage in Pediatric Patients

A 3-day treatment schedule with a total of 6 doses is recommended as below:

5 kg to less than 15 kg bodyweight: One tablet as an initial dose, 1 tablet again after 8 hours and then 1 tablet twice daily (morning and evening) for the following two days (total course of 6 tablets).

15 kg to less than 25 kg bodyweight: Two tablets as an initial dose, 2 tablets again after 8 hours and then 2 tablets twice daily (morning and evening) for the following two days (total course of 12 tablets).

25 kg to less than 35 kg bodyweight: Three tablets as an initial dose, 3 tablets again after 8 hours and then 3 tablets twice daily (morning and evening) for the following two days (total course of 18 tablets).

35 kg bodyweight and above: Four tablets as a single initial dose, 4 tablets again after 8 hours and then 4 tablets twice daily (morning and evening) for the following two days (total course of 24 tablets).

2.4 Dosage in Patients with Hepatic or Renal Impairment

No specific pharmacokinetic studies have been carried out in patients with hepatic or renal impairment. Most patients with acute malaria present with some degree of related hepatic and/or renal impairment. In clinical studies, the adverse event profile did not differ in patients with mild or moderate hepatic impairment compared to patients with normal hepatic function. No specific dose adjustments are needed for patients with mild or moderate hepatic impairment.

In clinical studies, the adverse event profile did not differ in patients with mild or moderate renal impairment compared to patients with normal renal function. There were few patients with severe renal impairment in clinical studies. There is no significant renal excretion of lumefantrine, artemether and dihydroartemisinin (DHA) in healthy volunteers and while clinical experience in this population is limited, no dose adjustment is recommended.

Caution should be exercised when administering Coartem Tablets in patients with severe hepatic or renal impairment [see Warnings and Precautions (5.6)].

3 DOSAGE FORMS AND STRENGTHS

Coartem Tablets contain 20 mg of artemether and 120 mg of lumefantrine. Coartem Tablets are supplied as yellow, round, flat tablets with beveled edges and scored on one side. Tablets are imprinted with N/C on one side and CG on the other side.

4 CONTRAINDICATIONS

4.1 Hypersensitivity

• Known hypersensitivity to artemether, lumefantrine, or to any of the excipients of Coartem Tablets [see Adverse Reactions (6.3)].

4.2 Strong CYP3A4 Inducers

• Co-administration of strong inducers of CYP3A4 such as rifampin, carbamazepine, phenytoin and St. John's wort with Coartem Tablets can result in decreased concentrations of artemether and/or lumefantrine and loss of antimalarial efficacy [see Warnings and Precautions (5.3), Drug Interactions (7.1), and Clinical Pharmacology (12.3)].

5 WARNINGS AND PRECAUTIONS

5.1 Prolongation of the QT Interval

Some antimalarials (e.g., halofantrine, quinine, quinidine) including Coartem Tablets have been associated with prolongation of the QT interval on the electrocardiogram.

Coartem Tablets should be avoided in patients:

• with congenital prolongation of the QT interval (e.g., long QT syndrome) or any other clinical condition known to prolong the QTc interval such as patients with a history of symptomatic cardiac arrhythmias, with clinically relevant bradycardia or with severe cardiac disease.

Table 1: Adverse Reactions Occurring in 3% or More of Adult Patients Treated in Clinical Trials with the 6-dose Regimen of Coartem Tablets

System Organ Class	Preferred Term	Adults* N=647 (%)
Nervous system disorders	Headache	360 (56)
	Dizziness	253 (39)
Metabolism and nutrition disorders	Anorexia	260 (40)
General disorders and administration site conditions	Asthenia	243 (38)
	Pyrexia	159 (25)
	Chills	147 (23)
	Fatigue	111 (17)
	Malaise	20 (3)
Musculoskeletal and connective tissue disorders	Arthralgia	219 (34)
	Myalgia	206 (32)
Gastrointestinal disorders	Nausea	169 (26)
	Vomiting	113 (17)
	Abdominal pain	112 (17)
	Diarrhea	46 (7)
Psychiatric disorders	Sleep disorder	144 (22)
	Insomnia	32 (5)
Cardiac disorders	Palpitations	115 (18)
Hepatobiliary disorders	Hepatomegaly	59 (9)
Blood and lymphatic system disorders	Splenomegaly	57 (9)
	Anemia	23 (4)
Respiratory, thoracic and mediastinal disorders	Cough	37 (6)
Skin and subcutaneous tissue disorders	Pruritus	24 (4)
	Rash	21 (3)
Ear and labyrinth disorders	Vertigo	21 (3)
Infections and infestations	Malaria	18 (3)
	Nasopharyngitis	17 (3)

* Adult patients defined as >16 years of age

• with a family history of congenital prolongation of the QT interval or sudden death.

• with known disturbances of electrolyte balance, e.g., hypokalemia or hypomagnesemia.

• receiving other medications that prolong the QT interval, such as class IA (quinidine, procainamide, disopyramide), or class III (amiodarone, sotalol) antiarrhythmic agents; antipsychotics (pimozide, ziprasidone); antidepressants; certain antibiotics (macrolide antibiotics, fluoroquinolone antibiotics, imidazole, and triazole antifungal agents) [see Clinical Pharmacology (12.6)].

• receiving medications that are metabolized by the cytochrome enzyme CYP2D6 which also have cardiac effects (e.g., flecainide, imipramine, amitriptyline, clomipramine) [see Warnings and Precautions (5.4), Drug Interactions (7.6), and Clinical Pharmacology (12.3)].

5.2 Use of QT Prolonging Drugs and Other Antimalarials

Halofantrine and Coartem Tablets should not be administered within one month of each other due to the long elimination half-life of lumefantrine (3-6 days) and potential additive effects on the QT interval [see Warnings and Precautions (5.1) and Clinical Pharmacology (12.3)].

Antimalarials should not be given concomitantly with Coartem Tablets, unless there is no other treatment option, due to limited safety data.

Drugs that prolong the QT interval, including antimalarials such as quinine and quinidine, should be used cautiously following Coartem Tablets, due to the long elimination half-life of lumefantrine (3-6 days) and the potential for additive effects on the QT interval; ECG monitoring is advised if use of drugs that prolong the QT interval is medically required [see Warnings and Precautions (5.1), Drug Interactions (7.7), and Clinical Pharmacology (12.3)].

If mefloquine is administered immediately prior to Coartem Tablets there may be a decreased exposure to lumefantrine, possibly due to a mefloquine-induced decrease in bile production. Therefore, patients should be monitored for decreased efficacy and food consumption should be encouraged while taking Coartem Tablets [see Dosage and Administration (2.1), Drug Interactions (7.4), and Clinical Pharmacology (12.3)].

5.3 Drug Interactions with CYP3A4

When Coartem Tablets are co-administered with substrates of CYP3A4 it may result in decreased concentrations of the substrate and potential loss of substrate efficacy. When Coartem Tablets are co-administered with an inhibitor of CYP3A4, including grapefruit juice it may result in increased concentrations of artemether and/or lumefantrine and potentiate QT prolongation. When Coartem Tablets are co-administered with inducers of CYP3A4 it may result in decreased concentrations of artemether and/or lumefantrine and loss of antimalarial efficacy [see Contraindications (4.2) and Drug Interactions (7)].

Drugs that have a mixed effect on CYP3A4, especially antiretroviral drugs such as HIV protease inhibitors and nonnucleoside reverse transcriptase inhibitors, and those that have an effect on the QT interval should be used with caution in patients taking Coartem Tablets [see Drug Interactions (7.3, 7.7)].

Coartem Tablets may reduce the effectiveness of hormonal contraceptives. Therefore, patients using oral, transdermal patch, or other systemic hormonal contraceptives should be advised to use an additional non-hormonal method of birth control [see Drug Interactions (7.5)].

5.4 Drug Interactions with CYP2D6

Administration of Coartem Tablets with drugs that are metabolized by CYP2D6 may significantly increase plasma concentrations of the co-administered drug and increase the risk of adverse effects. Many of the drugs metabolized by CYP2D6 can prolong the QT interval and should not be administered with Coartem Tablets due to the potential additive effect on the QT interval (e.g., flecainide, imipramine, amitriptyline, clomipramine) [see Warnings and Precautions (5.1), Drug Interactions (7.6), and Clinical Pharmacology (12.3)].

5.5 Recrudescence

Food enhances absorption of artemether and lumefantrine following administration of Coartem Tablets. Patients who remain averse to food during treatment should be closely monitored as the risk of recrudescence may be greater [see Dosage and Administration (2.1)].

In the event of recrudescent P. falciparum infection after treatment with Coartem Tablets, patients should be treated with a different antimalarial drug.

5.6 Hepatic and Renal Impairment

Coartem Tablets have not been studied for efficacy and safety in patients with severe hepatic and/or renal impairment [see Dosage and Administration (2.4)].

5.7 Plasmodium vivax Infection

Coartem Tablets have been shown in limited data (43 patients) to be effective in treating the erythrocytic stage of P. vivax infection. However, relapsing malaria caused by P. vivax requires additional treatment with other antimalarial agents to achieve radical cure i.e., eradicate any hypnozoites forms that may remain dormant in the liver.

Table 2: Adverse Reactions Occurring in 3% or More of Pediatric Patients Treated in Clinical Trials with the 6-dose Regimen of Coartem Tablets

System Organ Class	Preferred Term	Children* N=1,332 (%)
General disorders and administration site conditions	Pyrexia	381 (29)
	Chills	72 (5)
	Asthenia	63 (5)
	Fatigue	46 (3)
Respiratory, thoracic and mediastinal disorders	Cough	302 (23)
Gastrointestinal disorders	Vomiting	242 (18)
	Abdominal pain	112 (8)
	Diarrhea	100 (8)
	Nausea	61 (5)
Infections and infestations	*Plasmodium falciparum* infection	224 (17)
	Rhinitis	51 (4)
Metabolism and nutrition disorders	Anorexia	175 (13)
Nervous system disorders	Headache	168 (13)
	Dizziness	56 (4)
Blood and lymphatic system disorders	Splenomegaly	124 (9)
	Anemia	115 (9)
Hepatobiliary disorders	Hepatomegaly	75 (6)
Investigations	Aspartate aminotransferase increased	51 (4)
Musculoskeletal and connective tissue disorders	Arthralgia	39 (3)
	Myalgia	39 (3)
Skin and subcutaneous tissue disorders	Rash	38 (3)

* Children defined as patients ≤16 years of age

6 ADVERSE REACTIONS

6.1 Serious Adverse Reactions

The following serious and otherwise important adverse reactions are discussed in greater detail in other sections of labeling:

• Hypersensitivity Reactions [see *Contraindications (4.1)* and *Postmarketing Experience (6.3)*].

6.2 Clinical Studies Experience

Because clinical trials are conducted under widely varying conditions, adverse reaction rates observed in the clinical trials of a drug cannot be directly compared to rates in the clinical trials of another drug and may not reflect the rate observed in practice.

The data described below reflect exposure to a 6-dose regimen of Coartem Tablets in 1,979 patients including 647 adults (older than 16 years) and 1,332 children (16 years and younger). For the 6-dose regimen, Coartem Tablets was studied in active-controlled (366 patients) and non-controlled, open-label trials (1,613 patients). The 6-dose Coartem Tablets population was patients with malaria between ages 2 months and 71 years: 67% (1,332) were 16 years and younger and 33% (647) were older than 16 years. Males represented 73% and 53% of the adult and pediatric populations, respectively. The majority of adult patients were enrolled in studies in Thailand, while the majority of pediatric patients were enrolled in Africa.

Tables 1 and 2 show the most frequently reported adverse reactions (≥3%) in adults and children respectively who received the 6-dose regimen of Coartem Tablets. Adverse reactions collected in clinical trials included signs and symptoms at baseline but only treatment emergent adverse events, defined as events that appeared or worsened after the start of treatment, are presented below. In adults, the most frequently reported adverse reactions were headache, anorexia, dizziness, and asthenia. In children, the adverse reactions were pyrexia, cough, vomiting, anorexia, and headache. Most adverse reactions were mild, did not lead to discontinuation of study medication, and resolved.

In limited comparative studies, the adverse reaction profile of Coartem Tablets appeared similar to that of another antimalarial regimen.

Discontinuation of Coartem Tablets due to adverse drug reactions occurred in 1.1% of patients treated with the 6-dose regimen overall: 0.2% (1/647) in adults and 1.6% (21/1,332) in children.

[See table 1 at top of previous page]
[See table 2 above]

Clinically significant adverse reactions reported in adults and/or children treated with the 6-dose regimen of Coartem Tablets which occurred in clinical studies at <3% regardless of causality are listed below:

Blood and lymphatic system disorders: eosinophilia
Ear and labyrinth disorders: tinnitus
Eye disorders: conjunctivitis
Gastrointestinal disorders: constipation, dyspepsia, dysphagia, peptic ulcer
General disorders: gait disturbance
Infections and infestations: abscess, acrodermatitis, bronchitis, ear infection, gastroenteritis, helminthic infection, hookworm infection, impetigo, influenza, lower respiratory tract infection, malaria, nasopharyngitis, oral herpes, pneumonia, respiratory tract infection, subcutaneous abscess, upper respiratory tract infection, urinary tract infection
Investigations: alanine aminotransferase increased, aspartate aminotransferase increased, hematocrit decreased, lymphocyte morphology abnormal, platelet count decreased, platelet count increased, white blood cell count decreased, white blood cell count increased
Metabolism and nutrition disorders: hypokalemia
Musculoskeletal and connective tissue disorders: back pain
Nervous system disorders: ataxia, clonus, fine motor delay, hyperreflexia, hypoaesthesia, nystagmus, tremor
Psychiatric disorders: agitation, mood swings
Renal and urinary disorders: hematuria, proteinuria
Respiratory, thoracic and mediastinal disorders: asthma, pharyngo-laryngeal pain
Skin and subcutaneous tissue disorders: urticaria

6.3 Postmarketing Experience

The following adverse reactions have been identified during post-approval use of Coartem Tablets. Because these events are reported voluntarily from a population of uncertain size, it is not always possible to reliably estimate their frequency or establish a causal relationship to drug exposure.

• Hypersensitivity reactions including urticaria and angioedema. Serious skin reactions (bullous eruption) have been rarely reported.

7 DRUG INTERACTIONS

7.1 Rifampin

Oral administration of rifampin, a strong CYP3A4 inducer, with Coartem Tablets resulted in significant decreases in exposure to artemether, dihydroartemisinin (DHA, metabolite of artemether) and lumefantrine by 89%, 85% and 68%, respectively, when compared to exposure values after Coartem Tablets alone. Concomitant use of strong inducers of CYP3A4 such as rifampin, carbamazepine, phenytoin and St. John's wort is contraindicated with Coartem Tablets [see *Contraindications (4.2)* and *Clinical Pharmacology (12.3)*].

7.2 Ketoconazole

Concurrent oral administration of ketoconazole, a potent CYP3A4 inhibitor, with a single dose of Coartem Tablets resulted in a moderate increase in exposure to artemether, DHA, and lumefantrine in a study of 15 healthy subjects. No dose adjustment of Coartem Tablets is necessary when administered with ketoconazole or other potent CYP3A4 inhibitors. However, due to the potential for increased concen-

trations of lumefantrine which could lead to QT prolongation, Coartem Tablets should be used cautiously with drugs that inhibit CYP3A4 [see *Warnings and Precautions (5.1, 5.3)* and *Clinical Pharmacology (12.3)*].

7.3 Antiretroviral Drugs

Both artemether and lumefantrine are metabolized by CYP3A4. Antiretroviral drugs, such as protease inhibitors and non-nucleoside reverse transcriptase inhibitors, are known to have variable patterns of inhibition, induction or competition for CYP3A4. Therefore, the effects of antiretroviral drugs on the exposure to artemether, DHA, and lumefantrine are also variable [see *Clinical Pharmacology (12.3)*]. Coartem Tablets should be used cautiously in patients on antiretroviral drugs because decreased artemether, DHA, and/or lumefantrine concentrations may result in a decrease of antimalarial efficacy of Coartem Tablets, and increased lumefantrine concentrations may cause QT prolongation [see *Warnings and Precautions (5.3)*].

7.4 Prior Use of Mefloquine

Administration of three doses of mefloquine followed 12 hours later by a 6-dose regimen of Coartem Tablets in 14 healthy volunteers demonstrated no effect of mefloquine on plasma concentrations of artemether or the artemether/DHA ratio. However, exposure to lumefantrine was reduced, possibly due to lower absorption secondary to a mefloquine-induced decrease in bile production. Patients should be monitored for decreased efficacy and food consumption should be encouraged with administration of Coartem Tablets [see *Warnings and Precautions (5.2)* and *Clinical Pharmacology (12.3)*].

7.5 Hormonal Contraceptives

In vitro, the metabolism of ethinyl estradiol and levonorgestrel was not induced by artemether, DHA, or lumefantrine. However, artemether has been reported to weakly induce, in humans, the activity of CYP2C19, CYP2B6, and CYP3A. Therefore, Coartem Tablets may potentially reduce the effectiveness of hormonal contraceptives. Patients using oral, transdermal patch, or other systemic hormonal contraceptives should be advised to use an additional non-hormonal method of birth control [see *Warnings and Precautions (5.3)* and *Clinical Pharmacology (12.3)*].

7.6 CYP2D6 Substrates

Lumefantrine inhibits CYP2D6 *in vitro*. Administration of Coartem Tablets with drugs that are metabolized by CYP2D6 may significantly increase plasma concentrations of the co-administered drug and increase the risk of adverse effects. Many of the drugs metabolized by CYP2D6 can prolong the QT interval and should not be administered with Coartem Tablets due to the potential additive effect on the QT interval (e.g., flecainide, imipramine, amitriptyline, clomipramine) [see *Warnings and Precautions (5.1, 5.4)* and *Clinical Pharmacology (12.3)*].

7.7 Sequential Use of Quinine

A single dose of intravenous quinine (10 mg/kg bodyweight) concurrent with the final dose of a 6-dose regimen of Coartem Tablets demonstrated no effect of intravenous quinine on the systemic exposure of DHA or lumefantrine. Quinine exposure was also not altered. Exposure to artemether was decreased. This decrease in artemether exposure is not thought to be clinically significant. However, quinine and other drugs that prolong the QT interval should be used cautiously following treatment with Coartem Tablets due to the long elimination half-life of lumefantrine and the potential for additive QT effects; ECG monitoring is advised if use of drugs that prolong the QT interval is medically required [see *Warnings and Precautions (5.2)* and *Clinical Pharmacology (12.3)*].

7.8 Interaction with Drugs that are Known to Prolong the QT Interval

Coartem is to be used with caution when co-administered with drugs that may cause prolonged QT interval such as antiarrhythmics of classes IA and III, neuroleptics and antidepressant agents, certain antibiotics including some agents of the following classes: macrolides, fluoroquinolones, imidazole, and triazole antifungal agents [see *Warnings and Precautions (5.1, 5.2)*].

8 USE IN SPECIFIC POPULATIONS

8.1 Pregnancy

Pregnancy Category C

Safety data from an observational pregnancy study of approximately 500 pregnant women who were exposed to Coartem Tablets (including a third of patients who were exposed in the first trimester), and published data of over 1,000 pregnant patients who were exposed to artemisinin derivatives, did not show an increase in adverse pregnancy outcomes or teratogenic effects over background rate.

The efficacy of Coartem Tablets in the treatment of acute, uncomplicated malaria in pregnant women has not been established.

Coartem Tablets should be used during pregnancy only if the potential benefit justifies the potential risk to the fetus. Pregnant rats dosed during the period of organogenesis at or higher than a dose of about half the highest clinical dose of 1120 mg artemether-lumefantrine per day (based on body surface area comparisons), showed increases in fetal loss, early resorptions and post implantation loss. No adverse effects were observed in animals dosed at about one-third the highest clinical dose. Similarly, dosing in pregnant rabbits at about three times the clinical dose (based on body surface area comparisons) resulted in abortions, preimplantation loss, post implantation loss and decreases in the number of live fetuses. No adverse reproductive effects were detected in rabbits at two times the clinical dose. Embryo-fetal loss is a significant reproductive toxicity. Other artemisinins are known to be embryotoxic in animals. However, because metabolic profiles in animals and humans are dissimilar, artemether exposures in animals may not be predictive of human exposures [*see Nonclinical Toxicology (13.2)*]. These data cannot rule out an increased risk for early pregnancy loss or fetal defects in humans.

8.3 Nursing Mothers

It is not known whether artemether or lumefantrine is excreted in human milk. Because many drugs are excreted in human milk, caution should be exercised when Coartem Tablets are administered to a nursing woman. Animal data suggest both artemether and lumefantrine are excreted into breast milk. The benefits of breastfeeding to mother and infant should be weighed against potential risk from infant exposure to artemether and lumefantrine through breast milk.

8.4 Pediatric Use

The safety and effectiveness of Coartem Tablets have been established for the treatment of acute, uncomplicated malaria in studies involving pediatric patients weighing 5 kg or more [*see Clinical Studies (14.1)*]. The safety and efficacy have not been established in pediatric patients who weigh less than 5 kg. Children from non-endemic countries were not included in clinical trials.

8.5 Geriatric Use

Clinical studies of Coartem Tablets did not include sufficient numbers of subjects aged 65 years and over to determine they respond differently from younger subjects. In general, the greater frequency of decreased hepatic, renal, or cardiac function, and of concomitant disease or other drug therapy in elderly patients should be considered when prescribing Coartem Tablets.

8.6 Hepatic and Renal Impairment

No specific pharmacokinetic studies have been performed in patients with either hepatic or renal impairment. Coartem Tablets have not been studied for efficacy and safety in patients with severe hepatic and/or renal impairment. Based on the pharmacokinetic data in 16 healthy subjects showing no or insignificant renal excretion of lumefantrine, artemether and DHA, no dose adjustment for the use of Coartem in patients with renal impairment is advised. No dosage adjustment is necessary in patients with mild to moderate hepatic impairment [*see Dosage and Administration (2.4) and Warnings and Precautions (5.6)*].

10 OVERDOSAGE

There is no information on overdoses of Coartem Tablets higher than the doses recommended for treatment.
In cases of suspected overdosage, symptomatic and supportive therapy, which would include ECG and blood electrolyte monitoring, should be given as appropriate.

11 DESCRIPTION

Coartem Tablets contain a fixed combination of two antimalarial active ingredients, artemether, an artemisinin derivative, and lumefantrine. Both components are blood schizontocides. The chemical name of artemether is (3R,5aS,6R,8aS,9R,10S,12R,12aR)-10-methoxy-3,6,9-trimethyldecahydro-3,12-epoxypyrano[4,3-j]-1,2-benzodioxepine. Artemether is a white, crystalline powder that is freely soluble in acetone, soluble in methanol and ethanol, and practically insoluble in water. It has the empirical formula $C_{16}H_{26}O_5$ with a molecular weight of 298.4, and the following structural formula:

The chemical name of lumefantrine is (1RS)-2-(dibutylamino)-1-[(9Z)-2,7-dichloro-9-[(4-chlorophenyl) methylene]-9H-fluorene-4-yl]ethanol. Lumefantrine is a yellow, crystalline powder that is freely soluble in N,N-dimethylformamide, chloroform, and ethyl acetate; soluble in dichloromethane; slightly soluble in ethanol and methanol; and insoluble in water. It has the empirical formula $C_{30}H_{32}Cl_3NO$ with a molecular weight of 528.9, and the following structural formula:

Coartem Tablets are for oral administration. Each Coartem Tablet contains 20 mg of artemether and 120 mg lumefantrine. The inactive ingredients are colloidal silicon dioxide, croscarmellose sodium, hypromellose, magnesium stearate, microcrystalline cellulose, and polysorbate 80.

12 CLINICAL PHARMACOLOGY

12.1 Mechanism of Action

Coartem Tablets, a fixed dose combination of artemether and lumefantrine in the ratio of 1:6, is an antimalarial agent [*see Clinical Pharmacology (12.4)*].

12.3 Pharmacokinetics

Absorption

Following administration of Coartem Tablets to healthy volunteers and patients with malaria, artemether is absorbed with peak plasma concentrations reached about 2 hours after dosing. Absorption of lumefantrine, a highly lipophilic compound, starts after a lag-time of up to 2 hours, with peak plasma concentrations about 6 to 8 hours after administration. The single dose (4 tablets) pharmacokinetic parameters for artemether, dihydroartemisinin (DHA), an active antimalarial metabolite of artemether, and lumefantrine in adult Caucasian healthy volunteers are given in Table 3. Multiple dose data after the 6-dose regimen of Coartem Tablets in adult malaria patients are given in Table 4.

Table 3: Single Dose Pharmacokinetic Parameters[a] for Artemether, Dihydroartemisinin (DHA), and Lumefantrine under Fed Conditions

	Study 2102 (n=50)	Study 2104 (n=48)
Artemether		
C_{max} (ng/mL)	60.0 ± 32.5	83.8 ± 59.7
t_{max} (h)	1.50	2.00
AUC_{last} (ng•h/mL)	146 ± 72.2	259 ± 150
$t_{1/2}$ (h)	1.6 ± 0.7	2.2 ± 1.9
DHA		
C_{max} (ng/mL)	104 ± 35.3	90.4 ± 48.9
t_{max} (h)	1.76	2.00
AUC_{last} (ng•h/mL)	284 ± 83.8	285 ± 98.0
$t_{1/2}$ (h)	1.6 ± 0.6	2.2 ± 1.5
Lumefantrine		
C_{max} (µg/mL)	7.38 ± 3.19	9.80 ± 4.20
t_{max} (h)	6.01	8.00
AUC_{last} (µg•h/mL)	158 ± 70.1	243 ± 117
$t_{1/2}$ (h)	101 ± 35.6	119 ± 51.0

[a]Mean ± SD C_{max}, AUC_{last}, $t_{1/2}$ and Median t_{max}

Food enhances the absorption of both artemether and lumefantrine. In healthy volunteers, the relative bioavailability of artemether was increased between two- to three-fold, and that of lumefantrine sixteen-fold when Coartem Tablets were taken after a high-fat meal compared under fasted conditions. Patients should be encouraged to take Coartem Tablets with a meal as soon as food can be tolerated [*see Dosage and Administration (2.1)*].

Distribution

Artemether and lumefantrine are both highly bound to human serum proteins in vitro (95.4% and 99.7%, respectively). Dihydroartemisinin is also bound to human serum proteins (47% to 76%). Protein binding to human plasma proteins is linear.

Biotransformation

In human liver microsomes and recombinant CYP450 enzymes, the metabolism of artemether was catalyzed predominantly by CYP3A4/5. Dihydroartemisinin (DHA) is an active metabolite of artemether. The metabolism of artemether was also catalyzed to a lesser extent by CYP2B6, CYP2C9 and CYP2C19. In vitro studies with artemether at therapeutic concentrations revealed no significant inhibition of the metabolic activities of CYP1A2, CYP2A6, CYP2C9, CYP2C19, CYP2D6, CYP2E1, CYP3A4/5, and CYP4A9/11. In vitro studies with artemether, DHA, and lumefantrine at therapeutic concentrations revealed no significant induction of the metabolic activities of CYP1A1, CYP1A2, CYP2B6, CYP2C8, CYP2C9, CYP2C19, CYP3A4, or CYP3A5.

During repeated administration of Coartem Tablets, systemic exposure of artemether decreased significantly, while concentrations of DHA increased, although not to a statistically significant degree. The artemether/DHA AUC ratio is

1.2 after a single dose and 0.3 after 6 doses given over 3 days. This suggests that there was induction of enzymes responsible for the metabolism of artemether.
In human liver microsomes and in recombinant CYP450 enzymes, lumefantrine was metabolized mainly by CYP3A4 to desbutyl-lumefantrine. The systemic exposure to the metabolite desbutyl-lumefantrine was less than 1% of the exposure to the parent compound. In vitro, lumefantrine significantly inhibits the activity of CYP2D6 at therapeutic plasma concentrations.
Caution is recommended when combining Coartem Tablets with substrates, inhibitors, or inducers of CYP3A4, especially antiretroviral drugs and those that prolong the QT interval (e.g., macrolide antibiotics, pimozide) [*see Contraindications (4.2), Warnings and Precautions (5.1, 5.2, 5.3), and Drug Interactions (7)*].
Co-administration of Coartem Tablets with CYP2D6 substrates may result in increased plasma concentrations of the CYP2D6 substrate and increase the risk of adverse reactions. In addition, many of the drugs metabolized by CYP2D6 can prolong the QT interval and should not be administered with Coartem Tablets due to the potential additive effect on the QT interval (e.g., flecainide, imipramine, amitriptyline, clomipramine) [*see Warnings and Precautions (5.1, 5.4) and Drug Interactions (7.6)*].

Elimination

Artemether and DHA are cleared from plasma with an elimination half-life of about 2 hours. Lumefantrine is eliminated more slowly, with an elimination half-life of 3-6 days in healthy volunteers and in patients with *falciparum* malaria. Demographic characteristics such as sex and weight appear to have no clinically relevant effects on the pharmacokinetics of artemether and lumefantrine.
In 16 healthy volunteers, neither lumefantrine nor artemether was found in the urine after administration of Coartem, and urinary excretion of DHA amounted to less than 0.01% of the artemether dose.

Hepatic and Renal Impairment

No specific pharmacokinetic studies have been performed in patients with either hepatic or renal impairment. There is no significant renal excretion of lumefantrine, artemether and DHA in healthy volunteers and while clinical experience in this population is limited, no dose adjustment in renal impairment is recommended [*see Dosage and Administration (2.4)*].

Pediatric Patients

The PK of artemether, DHA, and lumefantrine were obtained in two pediatric studies by sparse sampling using a population based approach. PK estimates derived from a composite plasma concentration profile for artemether, DHA, and lumefantrine are provided in Table 4.
Systemic exposure to artemether, DHA, and lumefantrine, when dosed on a mg/kg body weight basis in pediatric patients (≥5 to <35 kg body weight), is comparable to that of the recommended dosing regimen in adult patients.
[See table 4 at top of next page]

Geriatric Patients

No specific pharmacokinetic studies have been performed in patients older than 65 years of age.

Drug Interactions

Rifampin (strong CYP3A4 inducer)

Oral administration of rifampin (600 mg daily), a strong CYP3A4 inducer, with Coartem Tablets (6-dose regimen over 3 days) in six HIV-1 and tuberculosis co-infected adults without malaria resulted in significant decreases in exposure, in terms of AUC, to artemether, DHA and lumefantrine by 89%, 85% and 68%, respectively, when compared to exposure values after Coartem Tablets alone. Concomitant use of strong inducers of CYP3A4 such as rifampin, carbamazepine, phenytoin and St. John's wort is contraindicated with Coartem Tablets [*see Contraindications (4.2)*].

Ketoconazole (potent CYP3A4 inhibitor)

Concurrent oral administration of ketoconazole (400 mg on Day 1 followed by 200 mg on days 2, 3, 4 and 5) with Coartem Tablets (single dose of 4 tablets of 20 mg artemether/120 mg lumefantrine per tablet) with a meal led to an increase in exposure, in terms of area under the curve (AUC), of artemether (2.3-fold), DHA (1.5-fold), and lumefantrine (1.6-fold) in 13 healthy subjects. The pharmacokinetics of ketoconazole were not evaluated. Based on this study, dose adjustment of Coartem Tablets is considered unnecessary when administered with ketoconazole or other CYP3A4 inhibitors. However, due to the potential for increased concentrations of lumefantrine which could lead to QT prolongation, Coartem Tablets should be used cautiously with other drugs that inhibit CYP3A4 (e.g., antiretroviral drugs, macrolide antibiotics, antidepressants, imidazole antifungal agents) [*see Warnings and Precautions (5.1, 5.3)*].

Antimalarials

The oral administration of mefloquine in 14 healthy volunteers administered as three doses of 500 mg, 250 mg and 250 mg, followed 12 hours later by Coartem Tablets (6 doses

Table 4: Summary of Pharmacokinetic Parameters for Lumefantrine, Artemether and DHA in Pediatric and Adult Patients with Malaria Following Administration of a 6-dose Regimen of Coartem Tablets

Drug	Adults[1]	Pediatric patients (body weight, kg)[2]		
		5 - <15	15 - <25	25 - <35
Lumefantrine				
Mean C_{max}, range (µg/mL)	5.60 - 9.0	4.71 – 12.6		Not Available
Mean AUC_{last}, range (µg•h/mL)	410 - 561	372 – 699		Not Available
Artemether				
Mean C_{max} ± SD (ng/mL)	186 ± 125	223 ± 309	198 ± 179	174 ± 145
Dihydroartemisinin				
Mean C_{max} ± SD (ng/mL)	101 ± 58	54.7 ± 58.9	79.8 ± 80.5	65.3 ± 23.6

[1] There are a total of 181 adults for lumefantrine pharmacokinetic parameters and a total of 25 adults for artemether and dihydroartemisinin pharmacokinetic parameters.
[2] There are 477 children for the lumefantrine pharmacokinetic parameters; for artemether and dihydroartemisinin pharmacokinetic parameters there are 55, 29, and 8 children for the 5 to <15, 15 to <25 and the 25 to <35 kg groups, respectively.

Table 5: Clinical Efficacy of Coartem Tablets versus Components (mITT Population)[1]

Study No. Region/patient ages	28-day cure rate[2] n/N (%) patients	Median FCT[3] [25th,75th percentile]	Median PCT [25th,75th percentile]
Study 1			
China, ages 13 - 57 years			
Coartem Tablets	50/51 (98.0)	24 hours [9, 48]	30 hours [24, 36]
Artemether[4]	24/52 (46.2)	21 hours [12, 30]	30 hours [24, 33]
Lumefantrine[5]	47/52 (90.4)	60 hours [36, 78]	54 hours [45, 66]
Study 2			
China, ages 12 - 65 years			
Coartem Tablets	50/52 (96.2)	21 hours [6, 33]	30 hours [24, 36]
Lumefantrine[6]	45/51 (88.2)	36 hours [12, 60]	48 hours [42, 60]

[1]In mITT analysis, patients whose status was uncertain were classified as treatment failures.
[2]Efficacy cure rate based on blood smear microscopy.
[3]For patients who had a body temperature >37.5°C at baseline only
[4]95% CI (Coartem Tablets – artemether) on 28-day cure rate: 37.8%, 66.0%
[5]P-value comparing Coartem Tablets to lumefantrine on parasite clearance time (PCT) and fever clearance time (FCT): <0.001
[6]P-value comparing Coartem Tablets to lumefantrine on parasite clearance time (PCT): <0.001 and on fever clearance time (FCT): <0.05

of 4 tablets of 20 mg artemether/120 mg lumefantrine per tablet), had no effect on plasma concentrations of artemether or the artemether/DHA ratio. In the same study, there was a 30% reduction in C_{max} and 40% reduction in AUC of lumefantrine, possibly due to lower absorption secondary to a mefloquine-induced decrease in bile production.

Intravenous administration of a single dose of quinine (10 mg/kg bodyweight) concurrent with the last dose of a 6-dose regimen of Coartem Tablets had no effect on systemic exposure of DHA, lumefantrine or quinine in 14 healthy volunteers. Mean AUC of artemether were 46% lower when administered with quinine compared to Coartem Tablets alone. This decrease in artemether exposure is not thought to be clinically significant. However, quinine should be used cautiously in patients following treatment with Coartem Tablets due to the long elimination half-life of lumefantrine and the potential for additive effects on the QT interval; ECG monitoring is advised if use of quinine is medically required [see Warnings and Precautions (5.2)].

Antiretroviral Drugs
The oral administration of lopinavir/ritonavir (400 mg/100 mg twice daily for 26 days) in 10 healthy volunteers co-administered with Coartem Tablets (6-dose regimen over 3 days), resulted in a decrease in systemic exposures, in terms of AUC, to artemether and DHA by approximately 40%, but an increase in exposure to lumefantrine by approximately 2.3-fold. The oral administration of efavirenz (600 mg once daily for 26 days) in 12 healthy volunteers co-administered with Coartem Tablets (6-dose regimen over 3 days), resulted in a decrease in exposures to artemether, DHA, and lumefantrine by approximately 50%, 45%, and 20%, respectively. Exposures to lopinavir/ritonavir and efavirenz were not significantly affected by concomitant use of Coartem Tablets. Coartem Tablets should be used cautiously in patients on antiretroviral drugs such as HIV protease inhibitors and non-nucleoside reverse transcriptase inhibitors because decreased artemether, DHA, and/or lumefantrine concentrations may result in a decrease of antimalarial efficacy of Coartem Tablets, and increased lumefantrine concentrations may cause QT prolongation [see Warnings and Precautions (5.3) and Drug Interactions (7.3)].

Hormonal Contraceptives
No clinical drug-drug interaction studies between Coartem Tablets and hormonal contraceptives have been performed. *In vitro* studies revealed that the metabolism of ethinyl estradiol and levonorgestrel was not induced by artemether, DHA or lumefantrine. However, artemether has been reported to weakly induce, in humans, the activity of CYP2C19, CYP2B6, and CYP3A. Therefore, co-administration of Coartem Tablets may potentially reduce the effectiveness of hormonal contraceptives [see Warnings and Precautions (5.3) and Drug Interactions (7.5)].

12.4   Microbiology
Mechanism of Action
Coartem Tablets, a fixed ratio of 1:6 parts of artemether and lumefantrine, respectively, is an antimalarial agent. Artemether is rapidly metabolized into an active metabolite dihydroartemisinin (DHA). The antimalarial activity of artemether and DHA has been attributed to endoperoxide moiety. The exact mechanism by which lumefantrine, exerts its antimalarial effect is not well defined. Available data suggest lumefantrine inhibits the formation of β-hematin by forming a complex with hemin. Both artemether and lumefantrine were shown to inhibit nucleic acid and protein synthesis.

Activity In Vitro and In Vivo
Artemether and lumefantrine are active against the erythrocytic stages of *Plasmodium falciparum*.

Drug Resistance
Strains of *P. falciparum* with a moderate decrease in susceptibility to artemether or lumefantrine alone can be selected *in vitro* or *in vivo*, but not maintained in the case of artemether. The clinical relevance of such an effect is not known.

12.6   Effects on the Electrocardiogram
In a healthy adult volunteer parallel group study including a placebo and moxifloxacin control group (n=42 per group), the administration of the 6-dose regimen of Coartem Tablets was associated with prolongation of QTcF (Fridericia). Following administration of a 6-dose regimen of Coartem Tablets consisting of 4 tablets per dose (total of 4 tablets of 80 mg artemether/480 mg lumefantrine) taken with food, the maximum mean change from baseline and placebo adjusted QTcF was 7.5 msec (1-sided 95% Upper CI: 11 msec). There was a concentration-dependent increase in QTcF for lumefantrine.
In clinical trials conducted in children, no patient had QTcF >500 msec. Over 5% of patients had an increase in QTcF of over 60 msec.
In clinical trials conducted in adults, QTcF prolongation of >500 msec was reported in 3 (0.3%) of patients. Over 6% of adults had a QTcF increase of over 60 msec from baseline.

13   NONCLINICAL TOXICOLOGY
13.1   Carcinogenesis, Mutagenesis, Impairment of Fertility
Carcinogenesis
Carcinogenicity studies were not conducted.
Mutagenesis
No evidence of mutagenicity was detected. The artemether:lumefantrine combination was evaluated using the *Salmonella* and *Escherichia*/mammalian-microsome mutagenicity test, the gene mutation test with Chinese hamster cells V79, the cytogenetic test on Chinese hamster cells *in vitro*, and the rat micronucleus test, *in vivo*.
Impairment of Fertility
Pregnancy rates were reduced by about one half in female rats dosed for 2 to 4 weeks with the artemether-lumefantrine combination at 1000 mg/kg (about 9 times the clinical dose based on body surface area comparisons). Male rats dosed for 70 days showed increases in abnormal sperm (87% abnormal) and increased testes weights at 30 mg/kg doses (about one third the clinical dose). Higher doses (about 9 times the clinical dose) resulted in decreased sperm motility and 100% abnormal sperm cells.

13.2   Animal Toxicology and/or Pharmacology
Neonatal rats (7-21 days old) were more sensitive to the toxic effects of artemether (a component of Coartem) than older juvenile rats or adults. Mortality and severe clinical signs were observed in neonatal rats at doses which were well tolerated in pups above 22 days old.

14   CLINICAL STUDIES
14.1   Treatment of Acute, Uncomplicated *P. falciparum* Malaria
The efficacy of Coartem Tablets was evaluated for the treatment of acute, uncomplicated malaria caused by *P. falciparum* in HIV negative patients in 8 clinical studies. Uncomplicated malaria was defined as symptomatic *P. falciparum* malaria without signs and symptoms of severe malaria or evidence of vital organ dysfunction. Baseline parasite density ranged from 500/µL - 200,000/µL (0.01% to 4% parasitemia) in the majority of patients. Studies were conducted in partially immune and non-immune adults and children (≥5kg body weight) with uncomplicated malaria in China, Thailand, sub-Saharan Africa, Europe, and South America. Patients who had clinical features of severe malaria, severe cardiac, renal, or hepatic impairment were excluded.
The studies include two 4-dose studies assessing the efficacy of the components of the regimen, a study comparing a 4-dose versus a 6-dose regimen, and 5 additional 6-dose regimen studies.
Coartem Tablets were administered at 0, 8, 24, and 48 hours in the 4-dose regimen, and at 0, 8, 24, 36, 48, and 60 hours in the 6-dose regimen. Efficacy endpoints consisted of:
• 28 day cure rate, defined as clearance of asexual parasites (the erythrocytic stage) within 7 days without recrudescence by day 28
• parasite clearance time (PCT), defined as time from first dose until first total and continued disappearance of asexual parasite which continues for a further 48 hours
• fever clearance time (FCT), defined as time from first dose until the first time body temperature fell below 37.5°C and remained below 37.5°C for at least a further 48 hours (only for patients with temperature >37.5°C at baseline)
The modified intent to treat (mITT) population includes all patients with malaria diagnosis confirmation who received at least one dose of study drug. Evaluable patients generally are all patients who had a day 7 and a day 28 parasitological assessment or experienced treatment failure by day 28.

Studies 1 and 2:   The two studies which assessed the efficacy of Coartem Tablets (4 doses of 4 tablets of 20 mg artemether/120 mg lumefantrine) compared to each component alone were randomized, double-blind, comparative, single center, conducted in China. The efficacy results (Table 5) support that the combination of artemether and lumefantrine in Coartem Tablets had a significantly higher 28-day cure rate compared to artemether and had a significantly faster parasite clearance time (PCT) and fever clearance time (FCT) compared to lumefantrine.
[See table 5 above]
Results of 4-dose studies conducted in areas with high resistance such as Thailand during 1995-96 showed lower efficacy results than the above studies. Therefore, Study 3 was conducted.
Study 3:   Study 3 was a randomized, double-blind, two-center study conducted in Thailand in adults and children (aged ≥2 years), which compared the 4-dose regimen (administered over 48 hours) of Coartem Tablets to a 6-dose regimen (administered over 60 hours). Twenty-eight day cure rate in mITT subjects was 81% (96/118) for the Coartem Tablets 6-dose arm as compared to 71% (85/120) in the 4-dose arm.

Studies 4, 5, 6, 7, and 8: In these studies, Coartem Tablets were administered as the 6-dose regimen.

In study 4, a total of 150 adults and children aged ≥2 years received Coartem Tablets. In study 5, a total 164 adults and children ≥12 years received Coartem Tablets. Both studies were conducted in Thailand.

Study 6 was a study of 165 non-immune adults residing in regions non-endemic for malaria (Europe and Colombia) who contracted acute uncomplicated *falciparum* malaria when traveling in endemic regions.

Study 7 was conducted in Africa in 310 infants and children aged 2 months to 9 years, weighing 5 kg to 25 kg, with an axillary temperature ≥37.5°C.

Study 8 was conducted in Africa in 452 infants and children, aged 3 months to 12 years, weighing 5 kg to <35 kg, with fever (≥37.5°C axillary or ≥38°C rectally) or history of fever in the preceding 24 hours.

Results of 28-day cure rate, median parasite clearance time (PCT), and fever clearance time (FCT) for Studies 3 to 8 are reported in Table 6.

[See table 6 above]

In all studies, patients' signs and symptoms of malaria resolved when parasites were cleared.

In studies conducted in areas with high transmission rates, such as Africa, reappearance of *P. falciparum* parasites may be due to recrudescence or a new infection.

The efficacy by body weight category for studies 7 and 8 is summarized in Table 7.

[See table 7 above]

The efficacy of Coartem Tablets for the treatment *P. falciparum* infections mixed with *P. vivax* was assessed in a small number of patients. Coartem Tablets are only active against the erythrocytic phase of *P. vivax* malaria. Of the 43 patients with mixed infections at baseline, all cleared their parasitemia within 48 hours. However, parasite relapse occurred commonly (14/43; 33%). Relapsing malaria caused by *P. vivax* requires additional treatment with other antimalarial agents to achieve radical cure i.e., eradicate any hypnozoite forms that may remain dormant in the liver.

16   HOW SUPPLIED/STORAGE AND HANDLING

Coartem (artemether/lumefantrine) Tablets

20 mg/120 mg Tablets - yellow, round flat tablets with beveled edges and scored on one side. Tablets are imprinted with N/C on one side and CG on the other.

Bottle of 24   NDC 0078-0568-45

Store at 25°C (77°F); excursions permitted to 15-30°C (59-86°F) [see *USP Controlled Room Temperature*].

Dispense in tight container (USP).

17   PATIENT COUNSELING INFORMATION

See FDA-Approved Patient Labeling.

Information for Safe Use

- Instruct patients to take Coartem Tablets with food. Patients who do not have an adequate intake of food are at risk for recrudescence of malaria.
- Patients with known hypersensitivity to artemether, lumefantrine, or to any of the excipients should not receive Coartem Tablets.
- Instruct patients to inform their physician of any personal or family history of QT prolongation or proarrhythmic conditions such as hypokalemia, bradycardia, or recent myocardial ischemia.
- Instruct patients to inform their physician if they are taking any other medications that prolong the QT interval, such as class IA (quinidine, procainamide, disopyramide), or class III (amiodarone, sotalol) antiarrhythmic agents; antipsychotics (pimozide, ziprasidone); antidepressants; certain antibiotics (macrolide antibiotics, fluoroquinolone antibiotics, imidazole, and triazole antifungal agents).
- Instruct patients to notify their physicians if they have any symptoms of prolongation of the QT interval, including prolonged heart palpitations or a loss of consciousness.
- Instruct patients to avoid medications that are metabolized by the cytochrome enzyme CYP2D6 while receiving Coartem Tablets since these drugs also have cardiac effects (e.g., flecainide, imipramine, amitriptyline, clomipramine).
- Inform patients that based on animal data, Coartem Tablets administered during pregnancy may result in fetal loss. Fetal defects have been reported when artemisinins are administered to animals.
- Halofantrine and Coartem Tablets should not be administered within one month of each other due to potential additive effects on the QT interval.
- Antimalarials should not be given concomitantly with Coartem Tablets, unless there is no other treatment option, due to limited safety data.
- QT prolonging drugs, including quinine and quinidine, should be used cautiously following Coartem Tablets due to the long elimination half-life of lumefantrine and the potential for additive effects on the QT interval. ECG monitoring is advised if use of drugs that prolong the QT interval is medically required.
- Closely monitor food intake in patients who received mefloquine immediately prior to treatment with Coartem Tablets.
- Use Coartem Tablets cautiously in patients receiving other drugs that are substrates, inhibitors or inducers of CYP3A4, including grapefruit juice, especially those that prolong the QT interval or are antiretroviral drugs.
- Co-administration of strong inducers of CYP3A4 such as rifampin, carbamazepine, phenytoin and St. John's wort is contraindicated with Coartem Tablets.
- Coartem Tablets may reduce the effectiveness of hormonal contraceptives. Therefore, patients using oral, transdermal patch, or other systemic hormonal contraceptives should be advised to use an additional non-hormonal method of birth control.
- Inform patients that Coartem Tablets can cause hypersensitivity reactions. Instruct patients to discontinue the drug at the first sign of a skin rash, hives or other skin reactions, a rapid heartbeat, difficulty in swallowing or breathing, any swelling suggesting angioedema (e.g.,

Table 6: Clinical Efficacy of 6-dose Regimen of Coartem Tablets

Study No. Region/ages	28-day cure rate[1] n/N (%) patients		Median FCT[2] [25th, 75th percentile]	Median PCT [25th, 75th percentile]
	mITT[3]	Evaluable		
Study 3 Thailand, ages 3 – 62 years	96/118 (81.4)	93/96 (96.9)	35 hours [20, 46]	44 hours [22, 47]
Early failure[4]	0	0		
Late failure[5]	4 (3.4)	3 (3.1)		
Lost to follow up	18 (15.3)			
Other[6]	0			
Study 4 Thailand, ages 2 – 63 years	130/149 (87.2)	130/134 (97.0)	22 hours [19, 44]	NA
Early failure[4]	0	0		
Late failure[5]	4 (2.7)	4 (3.0)		
Lost to follow up	13 (8.7)			
Other[6]	2 (1.3)			
Study 5 Thailand, ages 12 – 71 years	148/164 (90.2)	148/155 (95.5)	29 hours [8, 51]	29 hours [18, 40]
Early failure[4]	0	0		
Late failure[5]	7 (4.3)	7 (4.5)		
Lost to follow up	9 (5.5)			
Other[6]	0			
Study 6 Europe/Columbia, ages 16 – 66 years	120/162 (74.1)	119/124 (96.0)	37 hours [18, 44]	42 hours [34, 63]
Early failure[4]	6 (3.7)	1 (0.8)		
Late failure[5]	3 (1.9)	3 (2.4)		
Lost to follow up	17 (10.5)			
Other[6]	16 (9.9)	1 (0.8)		
Study 7 Africa, ages 2 months – 9 years	268/310 (86.5)	267/300 (89.0)	8 hours [8, 24]	24 hours [24, 36]
Early failure[4]	2 (0.6)	0		
Late failure[5]	34 (11.0)	33 (11.0)		
Lost to follow up	2 (0.6)			
Other[6]	4 (1.3)			
Study 8 Africa, ages 3 months – 12 years	374/452 (82.7)	370/419 (88.3)	8 hours [8, 23]	35 hours [24, 36]
Early failure[4]	13 (2.9)	0		
Late failure[5]	49 (10.8)	49 (11.7)		
Lost to follow up	6 (1.3)			
Other[6]	10 (2.2)			

[1] Efficacy cure rate based on blood smear microscopy
[2] For patients who had a body temperature >37.5°C at baseline only
[3] In mITT analysis, patients whose status was uncertain were classified as treatment failures.
[4] Early failures were usually defined as patients withdrawn for unsatisfactory therapeutic effect within the first 7 days or because they received another antimalarial medication within the first 7 days
[5] Late failures were defined as patients achieving parasite clearance within 7 days but having parasite reappearance including recrudescence or new infection during the 28 day follow-up period
[6] Other includes withdrawn due to protocol violation or non-compliance, received additional medication after day 7, withdrew consent, missing day 7 or 28 assessment

Table 7: Clinical Efficacy by Weight for Pediatric Studies

Study No. Age category	Coartem Tablets 6-dose Regimen		
	mITT population[1]		Evaluable population
	Median PCT [25th,75th percentile]	28-day cure rate[2] n/N (%) patients	28-day cure rate[2] n/N (%) patients
Study 7			
5 - <10 kg	24 [24, 36]	133/154 (86.4)	133/149 (89.3)
10 - <15 kg	35 [24, 36]	94/110 (85.5)	94/107 (87.9)
15 -25 kg	24 [24, 36]	41/46 (89.1)	40/44 (90.9)
Study 8[3]			
5 - <10 kg	36 [24, 36]	61/83 (73.5)	61/69 (88.4)
10 - <15 kg	35 [24, 36]	160/190 (84.2)	157/179 (87.7)
15 - <25 kg	35 [24, 36]	123/145 (84.8)	123/140 (87.9)
25 - <35 kg	26 [24, 36]	30/34 (88.2)	29/31 (93.5)

[1] In mITT analysis, patients whose status was uncertain were classified as treatment failures.
[2] Efficacy cure rate based on blood smear microscopy
[3] Coartem Tablets administered as crushed tablets

swelling of the lips, tongue, face, tightness of the throat, hoarseness), or other symptoms of an allergic reaction.
T2013-42
April 2013
FDA-APPROVED PATIENT LABELING
Patient Information
Coartem®
(co-AR-tem)
(artemether and lumefantrine)
Tablets
Read this patient information before you start taking Coartem. There may be new information. This information does not take the place of talking to your healthcare provider about your medical condition or your treatment.
What is Coartem?
Coartem is a prescription medicine used to treat uncomplicated malaria in adults and children who weigh at least 11 pounds (5 kg).
Who should not take Coartem?
Do not take Coartem if you are allergic to any of the ingredients. See the end of this leaflet for a complete list of ingredients in Coartem.
Do not take Coartem if you are taking rifampin (medicine to treat leprosy or tuberculosis), certain medicines used to treat epilepsy (such as carbamazepine, phenytoin), or St. John's wort (*Hypericum perforatum*, a medicinal plant or extract of this medicinal plant).
What should I tell my healthcare provider before taking Coartem?
Before you take Coartem, tell your healthcare provider about all your medical conditions including if you have:
• heart disease or a family history of heart problems or heart disease
• liver or kidney problems
• recently taken other medicines used to treat malaria
• if you are pregnant or are planning to become pregnant. Coartem may increase your risk for loss of pregnancy. Fetal defects have been reported when artemisinins are administered to animals. Talk to your healthcare provider before taking Coartem.
• if you are breast-feeding. It is not known if Coartem passes into your breast milk. You and your doctor will decide the best way to feed your baby if you take Coartem.
Tell your doctor about all the medicines you take, including prescription and non-prescription medicines, vitamins, and herbal supplements. Coartem and other medicines may affect each other causing side effects. Coartem may affect the way other medicines work and other medicines may affect how Coartem works.
Especially tell your doctor if you take:
• any other medicines to treat or prevent malaria
• medicines for your heart
• antipsychotic medicines
• antidepressants
• medicines for seizures or trigeminal neuralgia (facial nerve pain)
• antibiotics (including medicines to treat tuberculosis)
• medicines to treat HIV-infection
• hormonal methods of birth control (for example, birth control pills or patch). If you are taking a hormonal birth control medicine, you should also use an additional method of birth control.
Ask your healthcare provider if you are not sure if your medicine is one that is listed above. Know the medicines you take. Keep a list of your medicines with you to show your healthcare providers when you get a new medicine.
How should I take Coartem?
• Take Coartem exactly as prescribed.
• If you weigh 77 pounds (35 kg) or more, one dose of Coartem is 4 tablets.
• If you weigh less than 77 pounds (35 kg), your healthcare provider will tell you how many tablets to take for each dose.
• A full course of treatment is 6 doses of Coartem taken over 3 days:
Day 1: take 1 dose; 8 hours later take 1 dose
Day 2: take 1 dose in the morning, 1 dose in the evening
Day 3: take 1 dose in the morning, 1 dose in the evening
Take Coartem for 3 days even if you are feeling better.
• Every dose of Coartem should be taken with food, such as milk, infant formula, pudding, porridge, or broth. It is important for you to eat as soon as you can so that your malaria will go away and not get worse.
• Do not drink grapefruit juice while you take Coartem. Drinking grapefruit juice during treatment with Coartem can cause you to have too much medicine in your blood.
• Coartem may be crushed and mixed with one to two teaspoons of water in a clean container.
• If you vomit within 1 hour of taking Coartem you should take another dose of Coartem. If you vomit the second dose, tell your healthcare provider. A different medicine may need to be prescribed for you.
Tell your healthcare provider right away if:
• your malaria does not get better
• you vomited any of your doses of Coartem

• you are not able to eat
• you get flu-like symptoms (chills, fever, muscle pains, or headaches) again after you have finished your treatment with Coartem.
• you have any change in the way your heart beats or a loss of consciousness (fainting).
What are the possible side effects of Coartem?
Coartem can cause serious side effects including:
• **A heart problem called QT prolongation** that can cause an abnormal heartbeat can happen in people who take Coartem. The chance of this happening is higher in people with a family history of prolonged QT interval, low potassium (hypokalemia), and in people who take medicines to control heartbeats.
• **Allergic reactions.** Symptoms of an allergic reaction include: rash, hives, fast heartbeat, trouble swallowing or breathing, swelling of lips, tongue, face, tightness of the throat, or trouble speaking. If you have a serious allergic reaction, stop taking Coartem and get emergency medical help right away.
The most common side effects in adults are:
• headache
• feeling dizzy
• feeling weak
• loss of appetite
• muscle and joint pain or stiffness
• feeling tired
• chills
• fever
The most common side effects in children are:
• fever
• cough
• vomiting
• headache
• loss of appetite
These are not all the possible side effects of Coartem. For more information, ask your doctor or pharmacist. Call your doctor for medical advice about side effects. You may report side effects to FDA at 1-800-FDA-1088.
How should I store Coartem?
Store Coartem between 59°F to 86°F (15°C to 30°C).
Keep Coartem and all medicines out of the reach of children.
General information about the safe and effective use of Coartem.
Medicines are sometimes prescribed for purposes other than those listed in patient information leaflets. Do not use Coartem for a condition for which it was not prescribed. Do not give Coartem to other people, even if they have the same symptoms that you have. It may harm them.
This patient information leaflet summarizes the most important information about Coartem. If you would like more information about Coartem talk with your healthcare provider. You can ask your healthcare provider or pharmacist for information about Coartem that is written for health professionals. For more information call 1-888-294-6287.
What are the ingredients in Coartem?
Active ingredients include: artemether, lumefantrine
Inactive ingredients include: colloidal silicon dioxide, croscarmellose sodium, hypromellose, magnesium stearate, microcrystalline cellulose, polysorbate 80
Distributed by:
Novartis Pharmaceuticals Corporation
East Hanover, New Jersey 07936
© Novartis
T2013-43
April 2013
Shown in Product Identification Guide, page 309

DIOVAN ℞
[DYE'-o-van]
(valsartan)
Tablets

The following prescribing information is based on official labeling in effect July 2014.
HIGHLIGHTS OF PRESCRIBING INFORMATION
These highlights do not include all the information needed to use Diovan safely and effectively. See full prescribing information for Diovan.
Diovan (valsartan) Tablets
Initial U.S. Approval: 1996

┌───┐
WARNING: FETAL TOXICITY
See full prescribing information for complete boxed warning.
• **When pregnancy is detected, discontinue Diovan as soon as possible. (5.1)**
• **Drugs that act directly on the renin-angiotensin system can cause injury and death to the developing fetus. (5.1)**
└───┘

────────**INDICATIONS AND USAGE**────────
Diovan is an angiotensin II receptor blocker (ARB) indicated for:
• Treatment of **hypertension**, to lower blood pressure. Lowering blood pressure reduces the risk of fatal and nonfatal cardiovascular events, primarily strokes and myocardial infarctions (1.1)
• Treatment of **heart failure** (NYHA class II-IV); Diovan significantly reduced hospitalization for heart failure (1.2)
• Reduction of cardiovascular mortality in clinically stable patients with left ventricular failure or left ventricular dysfunction **following myocardial infarction** (1.3)
────**DOSAGE AND ADMINISTRATION**────
[See table at top of next page]
────**DOSAGE FORMS AND STRENGTHS**────
Tablets (mg): 40 (scored), 80, 160, 320 (3)
────────**CONTRAINDICATIONS**────────
Known hypersensitivity to any component; Do not coadminister aliskiren with Diovan in patients with diabetes (4)
────**WARNINGS AND PRECAUTIONS**────
• Observe for signs and symptoms of hypotension (5.2)
• Monitor renal function and potassium in susceptible patients (5.3, 5.4)
────────**ADVERSE REACTIONS**────────
Hypertension: Most common adverse reactions are headache, dizziness, viral infection, fatigue and abdominal pain (6.1)
Heart Failure: Most common adverse reactions are dizziness, hypotension, diarrhea, arthralgia, back pain, fatigue and hyperkalemia (6.1)
Post-Myocardial Infarction: Most common adverse reactions which caused patients to discontinue therapy are hypotension, cough and increased blood creatinine (6.1)
To report SUSPECTED ADVERSE REACTIONS, contact Novartis Pharmaceuticals Corporation at 1-888-669-6682 or FDA at 1-800-FDA-1088 or www.fda.gov/medwatch.
────────**DRUG INTERACTIONS**────────
• Potassium sparing diuretics, potassium supplements or salt substitutes may lead to increases in serum potassium, and in heart failure patients, increases in serum creatinine (7)
• NSAID use may lead to increased risk of renal impairment and loss of antihypertensive effect (7)
• Dual inhibition of the renin-angiotensin system: Increased risk of renal impairment, hypotension, and hyperkalemia (7)
• Lithium: Increases in serum lithium concentrations and lithium toxicity (7)
────**USE IN SPECIFIC POPULATIONS**────
Nursing Mothers: Nursing or drug should be discontinued (8.3);
Pediatrics: Efficacy and safety data support use in 6-16 year old patients; use is not recommended in patients <6 years old (6.1, 8.4)
See 17 for PATIENT COUNSELING INFORMATION and FDA-approved patient labeling
Revised: 3/2014

FULL PRESCRIBING INFORMATION: CONTENTS*
WARNING: FETAL TOXICITY
1 INDICATIONS AND USAGE
  1.1 Hypertension
  1.2 Heart Failure
  1.3 Post-Myocardial Infarction
2 DOSAGE AND ADMINISTRATION
  2.1 Adult Hypertension
  2.2 Pediatric Hypertension 6 to 16 Years of Age
  2.3 Heart Failure
  2.4 Post-Myocardial Infarction
3 DOSAGE FORMS AND STRENGTHS
4 CONTRAINDICATIONS
5 WARNINGS AND PRECAUTIONS
  5.1 Fetal Toxicity
  5.2 Hypotension
  5.3 Impaired Renal Function
  5.4 Hyperkalemia
6 ADVERSE REACTIONS
  6.1 Clinical Studies Experience
  6.2 Postmarketing Experience
7 DRUG INTERACTIONS
  7.1 Clinical Laboratory Test Findings
8 USE IN SPECIFIC POPULATIONS
  8.1 Pregnancy
  8.3 Nursing Mothers
  8.4 Pediatric Use
  8.5 Geriatric Use
  8.6 Renal Impairment
  8.7 Hepatic Impairment
10 OVERDOSAGE
11 DESCRIPTION
12 CLINICAL PHARMACOLOGY
  12.1 Mechanism of Action
  12.2 Pharmacodynamics
  12.3 Pharmacokinetics

13 NONCLINICAL TOXICOLOGY
   13.1 Carcinogenesis, Mutagenesis, Impairment of Fertility
   13.2 Animal Toxicology and/or Pharmacology
14 CLINICAL STUDIES
   14.1 Hypertension
   14.2 Heart Failure
   14.3 Post-Myocardial Infarction
16 HOW SUPPLIED/STORAGE AND HANDLING
17 PATIENT COUNSELING INFORMATION
* Sections or subsections omitted from the full prescribing information are not listed

Indication	Starting Dose	Dose Range	Target Maintenance Dose*
Adult Hypertension (2.1)	80 or 160 mg once daily	80-320 mg once daily	---
Pediatric Hypertension (6-16 years) (2.2)	1.3 mg/kg once daily (up to 40 mg total)	1.3-2.7 mg/kg once daily (up to 40-160 mg total)	---
Heart Failure (2.3)	40 mg twice daily	40-160 mg twice daily	160 mg twice daily
Post-Myocardial Infarction (2.4)	20 mg twice daily	20-160 mg twice daily	160 mg twice daily

* as tolerated by patient

FULL PRESCRIBING INFORMATION

> **WARNING: FETAL TOXICITY**
> - When pregnancy is detected, discontinue Diovan as soon as possible. (5.1)
> - Drugs that act directly on the renin-angiotensin system can cause injury and death to the developing fetus. (5.1)

1 INDICATIONS AND USAGE

1.1 Hypertension

Diovan® (valsartan) is indicated for the treatment of hypertension, to lower blood pressure. Lowering blood pressure reduces the risk of fatal and nonfatal cardiovascular events, primarily strokes and myocardial infarctions. These benefits have been seen in controlled trials of antihypertensive drugs from a wide variety of pharmacologic classes including the class to which valsartan principally belongs. There are no controlled trials in hypertensive patients demonstrating risk reduction with Diovan.

Control of high blood pressure should be part of comprehensive cardiovascular risk management, including, as appropriate, lipid control, diabetes management, antithrombotic therapy, smoking cessation, exercise, and limited sodium intake. Many patients will require more than one drug to achieve blood pressure goals. For specific advice on goals and management, see published guidelines, such as those of the National High Blood Pressure Education Program's Joint National Committee on Prevention, Detection, Evaluation, and Treatment of High Blood Pressure (JNC).

Numerous antihypertensive drugs, from a variety of pharmacologic classes and with different mechanisms of action, have been shown in randomized controlled trials to reduce cardiovascular morbidity and mortality, and it can be concluded that it is blood pressure reduction, and not some other pharmacologic property of the drugs, that is largely responsible for those benefits. The largest and most consistent cardiovascular outcome benefit has been a reduction in the risk of stroke, but reductions in myocardial infarction and cardiovascular mortality also have been seen regularly. Elevated systolic or diastolic pressure causes increased cardiovascular risk, and the absolute risk increase per mmHg is greater at higher blood pressures, so that even modest reductions of severe hypertension can provide substantial benefit. Relative risk reduction from blood pressure reduction is similar across populations with varying absolute risk, so the absolute benefit is greater in patients who are at higher risk independent of their hypertension (e.g., patients with diabetes or hyperlipidemia), and such patients would be expected to benefit from more aggressive treatment to a lower blood pressure goal.

Some antihypertensive drugs have smaller blood pressure effects (as monotherapy) in black patients, and many antihypertensive drugs have additional approved indications and effects (e.g., on angina, heart failure, or diabetic kidney disease). These considerations may guide selection of therapy.

Diovan may be used alone or in combination with other antihypertensive agents.

1.2 Heart Failure

Diovan is indicated for the treatment of heart failure (NYHA class II-IV). In a controlled clinical trial, Diovan significantly reduced hospitalizations for heart failure. There is no evidence that Diovan provides added benefits when it is used with an adequate dose of an ACE inhibitor [see Clinical Studies (14.2)].

1.3 Post-Myocardial Infarction

In clinically stable patients with left ventricular failure or left ventricular dysfunction following myocardial infarction, Diovan is indicated to reduce cardiovascular mortality [see Clinical Studies (14.3)].

2 DOSAGE AND ADMINISTRATION

2.1 Adult Hypertension

The recommended starting dose of Diovan (valsartan) is 80 mg or 160 mg once daily when used as monotherapy in patients who are not volume-depleted. Patients requiring greater reductions may be started at the higher dose. Diovan may be used over a dose range of 80 mg to 320 mg daily, administered once a day.

The antihypertensive effect is substantially present within 2 weeks and maximal reduction is generally attained after 4 weeks. If additional antihypertensive effect is required over the starting dose range, the dose may be increased to a maximum of 320 mg or a diuretic may be added. Addition of a diuretic has a greater effect than dose increases beyond 80 mg.

No initial dosage adjustment is required for elderly patients, for patients with mild or moderate renal impairment, or for patients with mild or moderate liver insufficiency. Care should be exercised with dosing of Diovan in patients with hepatic or severe renal impairment.

Diovan may be administered with other antihypertensive agents.

Diovan may be administered with or without food.

2.2 Pediatric Hypertension 6 to 16 Years of Age

For children who can swallow tablets, the usual recommended starting dose is 1.3 mg/kg once daily (up to 40 mg total). The dosage should be adjusted according to blood pressure response. Doses higher than 2.7 mg/kg (up to 160 mg) once daily have not been studied in pediatric patients 6 to 16 years old.

For children who cannot swallow tablets, or children for whom the calculated dosage (mg/kg) does not correspond to the available tablet strengths of Diovan, the use of a suspension is recommended. Follow the suspension preparation instructions below (see **Preparation of Suspension**) to administer valsartan as a suspension. When the suspension is replaced by a tablet, the dose of valsartan may have to be increased. The exposure to valsartan with the suspension is 1.6 times greater than with the tablet.

No data are available in pediatric patients either undergoing dialysis or with a glomerular filtration rate <30 mL/min/1.73 m^2 [see Pediatric Use (8.4)].

Diovan is not recommended for patients <6 years old [see Adverse Reactions (6.1), Clinical Studies (14.1)].

Preparation of Suspension (for 160 mL of a 4 mg/mL suspension)

Add 80 mL of Ora-Plus®* oral suspending vehicle to an amber glass bottle containing 8 Diovan 80 mg tablets, and shake for a minimum of 2 minutes. Allow the suspension to stand for a minimum of 1 hour. After the standing time, shake the suspension for a minimum of 1 additional minute. Add 80 mL of Ora-Sweet SF®* oral sweetening vehicle to the bottle and shake the suspension for at least 10 seconds to disperse the ingredients. The suspension is homogenous and can be stored for either up to 30 days at room temperature (below 30°C/86°F) or up to 75 days at refrigerated conditions (2-8°C/35-46°F) in the glass bottle with a child-resistant screw-cap closure. Shake the bottle well (at least 10 seconds) prior to dispensing the suspension.

*Ora-Sweet SF® and Ora-Plus® are registered trademarks of Paddock Laboratories, Inc.

2.3 Heart Failure

The recommended starting dose of Diovan is 40 mg twice daily. Uptitration to 80 mg and 160 mg twice daily should be done to the highest dose, as tolerated by the patient. Consideration should be given to reducing the dose of concomitant diuretics. The maximum daily dose administered in clinical trials is 320 mg in divided doses.

2.4 Post-Myocardial Infarction

Diovan may be initiated as early as 12 hours after a myocardial infarction. The recommended starting dose of Diovan is 20 mg twice daily. Patients may be uptitrated within 7 days to 40 mg twice daily, with subsequent titrations to a target maintenance dose of 160 mg twice daily, as tolerated by the patient. If symptomatic hypotension or renal dysfunction occurs, consideration should be given to a dosage reduction. Diovan may be given with other standard post-myocardial infarction treatment, including thrombolytics, aspirin, beta-blockers, and statins.

3 DOSAGE FORMS AND STRENGTHS

40 mg are scored yellow ovaloid tablets with beveled edges, imprinted NVR/DO (Side 1/Side 2)
80 mg are pale red almond-shaped tablets with beveled edges, imprinted NVR/DV
160 mg are grey-orange almond-shaped tablets with beveled edges, imprinted NVR/DX

320 mg are dark grey-violet almond-shaped tablets with beveled edges, imprinted NVR/DXL

4 CONTRAINDICATIONS

Do not use in patients with known hypersensitivity to any component.

Do not coadminister aliskiren with Diovan in patients with diabetes [see Drug Interactions (7)].

5 WARNINGS AND PRECAUTIONS

5.1 Fetal Toxicity

Pregnancy Category D

Use of drugs that act on the renin-angiotensin system during the second and third trimesters of pregnancy reduces fetal renal function and increases fetal and neonatal morbidity and death. Resulting oligohydramnios can be associated with fetal lung hypoplasia and skeletal deformations. Potential neonatal adverse effects include skull hypoplasia, anuria, hypotension, renal failure, and death. When pregnancy is detected, discontinue Diovan as soon as possible. [see Use in Specific Populations (8.1)].

5.2 Hypotension

Excessive hypotension was rarely seen (0.1%) in patients with uncomplicated hypertension treated with Diovan alone. In patients with an activated renin-angiotensin system, such as volume- and/or salt-depleted patients receiving high doses of diuretics, symptomatic hypotension may occur. This condition should be corrected prior to administration of Diovan, or the treatment should start under close medical supervision.

Caution should be observed when initiating therapy in patients with heart failure or post-myocardial infarction patients. Patients with heart failure or post-myocardial infarction patients given Diovan commonly have some reduction in blood pressure, but discontinuation of therapy because of continuing symptomatic hypotension usually is not necessary when dosing instructions are followed. In controlled trials in heart failure patients, the incidence of hypotension in valsartan-treated patients was 5.5% compared to 1.8% in placebo-treated patients. In the Valsartan in Acute Myocardial Infarction Trial (VALIANT), hypotension in post-myocardial infarction patients led to permanent discontinuation of therapy in 1.4% of valsartan-treated patients and 0.8% of captopril-treated patients.

If excessive hypotension occurs, the patient should be placed in the supine position and, if necessary, given an intravenous infusion of normal saline. A transient hypotensive response is not a contraindication to further treatment, which usually can be continued without difficulty once the blood pressure has stabilized.

5.3 Impaired Renal Function

Changes in renal function including acute renal failure can be caused by drugs that inhibit the renin-angiotensin system and by diuretics. Patients whose renal function may depend in part on the activity of the renin-angiotensin system (e.g., patients with renal artery stenosis, chronic kidney disease, severe congestive heart failure, or volume depletion) may be at particular risk of developing acute renal failure on Diovan. Monitor renal function periodically in these patients. Consider withholding or discontinuing therapy in patients who develop a clinically significant decrease in renal function on Diovan [see Drug Interactions (7)].

5.4 Hyperkalemia

Some patients with heart failure have developed increases in potassium. These effects are usually minor and transient, and they are more likely to occur in patients with pre-existing renal impairment. Dosage reduction and/or discontinuation of Diovan may be required [see Adverse Reactions (6.1)].

6 ADVERSE REACTIONS

6.1 Clinical Studies Experience

Because clinical studies are conducted under widely varying conditions, adverse reaction rates observed in the clinical studies of a drug cannot be directly compared to rates in the clinical studies of another drug and may not reflect the rates observed in practice.

Adult Hypertension

Diovan (valsartan) has been evaluated for safety in more than 4,000 patients, including over 400 treated for over 6 months, and more than 160 for over 1 year. Adverse reactions have generally been mild and transient in nature and have only infrequently required discontinuation of therapy. The overall incidence of adverse reactions with Diovan was similar to placebo.

The overall frequency of adverse reactions was neither dose-related nor related to gender, age, race, or regimen. Discontinuation of therapy due to side effects was required in 2.3% of valsartan patients and 2.0% of placebo patients. The most common reasons for discontinuation of therapy with Diovan were headache and dizziness.

The adverse reactions that occurred in placebo-controlled clinical trials in at least 1% of patients treated with Diovan and at a higher incidence in valsartan (n=2,316) than placebo (n=888) patients included viral infection (3% vs. 2%), fatigue (2% vs. 1%), and abdominal pain (2% vs. 1%).

Headache, dizziness, upper respiratory infection, cough, diarrhea, rhinitis, sinusitis, nausea, pharyngitis, edema, and arthralgia occurred at a more than 1% rate but at about the same incidence in placebo and valsartan patients.

In trials in which valsartan was compared to an ACE inhibitor with or without placebo, the incidence of dry cough was significantly greater in the ACE-inhibitor group (7.9%) than in the groups who received valsartan (2.6%) or placebo (1.5%). In a 129-patient trial limited to patients who had had dry cough when they had previously received ACE inhibitors, the incidences of cough in patients who received valsartan, HCTZ, or lisinopril were 20%, 19%, and 69% respectively (p <0.001).

Dose-related orthostatic effects were seen in less than 1% of patients. An increase in the incidence of dizziness was observed in patients treated with Diovan 320 mg (8%) compared to 10 to 160 mg (2% to 4%).

Diovan has been used concomitantly with hydrochlorothiazide without evidence of clinically important adverse interactions.

Other adverse reactions that occurred in controlled clinical trials of patients treated with Diovan (>0.2% of valsartan patients) are listed below. It cannot be determined whether these events were causally related to Diovan.

Body as a Whole: Allergic reaction and asthenia
Cardiovascular: Palpitations
Dermatologic: Pruritus and rash
Digestive: Constipation, dry mouth, dyspepsia, and flatulence
Musculoskeletal: Back pain, muscle cramps, and myalgia
Neurologic and Psychiatric: Anxiety, insomnia, paresthesia, and somnolence
Respiratory: Dyspnea
Special Senses: Vertigo
Urogenital: Impotence

Other reported events seen less frequently in clinical trials included chest pain, syncope, anorexia, vomiting, and angioedema.

Pediatric Hypertension
Diovan has been evaluated for safety in over 400 pediatric patients aged 6 to 17 years and more than 160 pediatric patients aged 6 months to 5 years. No relevant differences were identified between the adverse experience profile for pediatric patients aged 6 to 16 years and that previously reported for adult patients. Headache and hyperkalemia were the most common adverse events suspected to be study drug-related in older children (6 to 17 years old) and younger children (6 months to 5 years old), respectively. Hyperkalemia was mainly observed in children with underlying renal disease. Neurocognitive and developmental assessment of pediatric patients aged 6 to 16 years revealed no overall clinically relevant adverse impact after treatment with Diovan for up to 1 year.

Diovan is not recommended for pediatric patients under 6 years of age. In a study (n=90) of pediatric patients (1 to 5 years), two deaths and three cases of on-treatment transaminase elevations were seen in the one-year open-label extension phase. These 5 events occurred in a study population in which patients frequently had significant comorbidities. A causal relationship to Diovan has not been established. In a second study in which 75 children aged 1 to 6 years were randomized, no deaths and one case of marked liver transaminase elevations occurred during a 1 year open-label extension.

Heart Failure
The adverse experience profile of Diovan in heart failure patients was consistent with the pharmacology of the drug and the health status of the patients. In the Valsartan Heart Failure Trial, comparing valsartan in total daily doses up to 320 mg (n=2,506) to placebo (n=2,494), 10% of valsartan patients discontinued for adverse reactions vs. 7% of placebo patients.

The table shows adverse reactions in double-blind short-term heart failure trials, including the first 4 months of the Valsartan Heart Failure Trial, with an incidence of at least 2% that were more frequent in valsartan-treated patients than in placebo-treated patients. All patients received standard drug therapy for heart failure, frequently as multiple medications, which could include diuretics, digitalis, beta-blockers. About 93% of patients received concomitant ACE inhibitors.

	Valsartan (n=3,282)	Placebo (n=2,740)
Dizziness	17%	9%
Hypotension	7%	2%
Diarrhea	5%	4%
Arthralgia	3%	2%
Fatigue	3%	2%
Back Pain	3%	2%
Dizziness, postural	2%	1%
Hyperkalemia	2%	1%
Hypotension, postural	2%	1%

Discontinuations occurred in 0.5% of valsartan-treated patients and 0.1% of placebo patients for each of the following: elevations in creatinine and elevations in potassium.

Other adverse reactions with an incidence greater than 1% and greater than placebo included headache NOS, nausea, renal impairment NOS, syncope, blurred vision, upper abdominal pain and vertigo. (NOS = not otherwise specified). From the long-term data in the Valsartan Heart Failure Trial, there did not appear to be any significant adverse reactions not previously identified.

Post-Myocardial Infarction
The safety profile of Diovan was consistent with the pharmacology of the drug and the background diseases, cardiovascular risk factors, and clinical course of patients treated in the post-myocardial infarction setting. The table shows the percentage of patients discontinued in the valsartan and captopril-treated groups in the Valsartan in Acute Myocardial Infarction Trial (VALIANT) with a rate of at least 0.5% in either of the treatment groups.

Discontinuations due to renal dysfunction occurred in 1.1% of valsartan-treated patients and 0.8% of captopril-treated patients.

	Valsartan (n=4,885)	Captopril (n=4,879)
Discontinuation for adverse reaction	5.8%	7.7%
Adverse reactions		
Hypotension NOS	1.4%	0.8%
Cough	0.6%	2.5%
Blood creatinine increased	0.6%	0.4%
Rash NOS	0.2%	0.6%

6.2 Postmarketing Experience
The following additional adverse reactions have been reported in postmarketing experience:

Hypersensitivity: There are rare reports of angioedema. Some of these patients previously experienced angioedema with other drugs including ACE inhibitors. Diovan should not be re-administered to patients who have had angioedema.
Digestive: Elevated liver enzymes and very rare reports of hepatitis
Renal: Impaired renal function, renal failure
Clinical Laboratory Tests: Hyperkalemia
Dermatologic: Alopecia, bullous dermatitis
Blood and Lymphatic: There are very rare reports of thrombocytopenia
Vascular: Vasculitis
Rare cases of rhabdomyolysis have been reported in patients receiving angiotensin II receptor blockers.
Because these reactions are reported voluntarily from a population of uncertain size, it is not always possible to reliably estimate their frequency or establish a causal relationship to drug exposure.

7 DRUG INTERACTIONS

No clinically significant pharmacokinetic interactions were observed when Diovan (valsartan) was coadministered with amlodipine, atenolol, cimetidine, digoxin, furosemide, glyburide, hydrochlorothiazide, or indomethacin. The valsartan-atenolol combination was more antihypertensive than either component, but it did not lower the heart rate more than atenolol alone.

Coadministration of valsartan and warfarin did not change the pharmacokinetics of valsartan or the time-course of the anticoagulant properties of warfarin.

CYP 450 Interactions: In vitro metabolism studies indicate that CYP 450 mediated drug interactions between valsartan and coadministered drugs are unlikely because of the low extent of metabolism [see Clinical Pharmacology (12.3)].

Transporters: The results from an in vitro study with human liver tissue indicate that valsartan is a substrate of the hepatic uptake transporter OATP1B1 and the hepatic efflux transporter MRP2. Coadministration of inhibitors of the uptake transporter (rifampin, cyclosporine) or efflux transporter (ritonavir) may increase the systemic exposure to valsartan.

Potassium: Concomitant use of valsartan with other agents that block the renin-angiotensin system, potassium sparing diuretics (e.g. spironolactone, triamterene, amiloride), potassium supplements, or salt substitutes containing potassium may lead to increases in serum potassium and in heart failure patients to increases in serum creatinine. If co-medication is considered necessary, monitoring of serum potassium is advisable.

Non-Steroidal Anti-Inflammatory Agents including Selective Cyclooxygenase-2 Inhibitors (COX-2 Inhibitors): In patients who are elderly, volume-depleted (including those on diuretic therapy), or with compromised renal function, coadministration of NSAIDs, including selective COX-2 inhibitors, with angiotensin II receptor antagonists, including valsartan, may result in deterioration of renal function, including possible acute renal failure. These effects are usually reversible. Monitor renal function periodically in patients receiving valsartan and NSAID therapy.

The antihypertensive effect of angiotensin II receptor antagonists, including valsartan may be attenuated by NSAIDs including selective COX-2 inhibitors.

Dual Blockade of the Renin-Angiotensin System (RAS): Dual blockade of the RAS with angiotensin receptor blockers, ACE inhibitors, or aliskiren is associated with increased risks of hypotension, hyperkalemia, and changes in renal function (including acute renal failure) compared to monotherapy. Closely monitor blood pressure, renal function and electrolytes in patients on Diovan and other agents that affect the RAS.

Do not coadminister aliskiren with Diovan in patients with diabetes. Avoid use of aliskiren with Diovan in patients with renal impairment (GFR <60 mL/min).

Lithium: Increases in serum lithium concentrations and lithium toxicity have been reported during concomitant administration of lithium with angiotensin II receptor antagonists, including Diovan. Monitor serum lithium levels during concomitant use.

7.1 Clinical Laboratory Test Findings
In controlled clinical trials, clinically important changes in standard laboratory parameters were rarely associated with administration of Diovan.

Creatinine: Minor elevations in creatinine occurred in 0.8% of patients taking Diovan and 0.6% given placebo in controlled clinical trials of hypertensive patients. In heart failure trials, greater than 50% increases in creatinine were observed in 3.9% of Diovan-treated patients compared to 0.9% of placebo-treated patients. In post-myocardial infarction patients, doubling of serum creatinine was observed in 4.2% of valsartan-treated patients and 3.4% of captopril-treated patients.

Hemoglobin and Hematocrit: Greater than 20% decreases in hemoglobin and hematocrit were observed in 0.4% and 0.8%, respectively, of Diovan patients, compared with 0.1% and 0.1% in placebo-treated patients. One valsartan patient discontinued treatment for microcytic anemia.

Liver Function Tests: Occasional elevations (greater than 150%) of liver chemistries occurred in Diovan-treated patients. Three patients (< 0.1%) treated with valsartan discontinued treatment for elevated liver chemistries.

Neutropenia: Neutropenia was observed in 1.9% of patients treated with Diovan and 0.8% of patients treated with placebo.

Serum Potassium: In hypertensive patients, greater than 20% increases in serum potassium were observed in 4.4% of Diovan-treated patients compared to 2.9% of placebo-treated patients. In heart failure patients, greater than 20% increases in serum potassium were observed in 10.0% of Diovan-treated patients compared to 5.1% of placebo-treated patients.

Blood Urea Nitrogen (BUN): In heart failure trials, greater than 50% increases in BUN were observed in 16.6% of Diovan-treated patients compared to 6.3% of placebo-treated patients.

8 USE IN SPECIFIC POPULATIONS

8.1 Pregnancy

Pregnancy Category D

Use of drugs that act on the renin-angiotensin system during the second and third trimesters of pregnancy reduces fetal renal function and increases fetal and neonatal morbidity and death. Resulting oligohydramnios can be associated with fetal lung hypoplasia and skeletal deformations. Potential neonatal adverse effects include skull hypoplasia, anuria, hypotension, renal failure, and death. When pregnancy is detected, discontinue Diovan as soon as possible. These adverse outcomes are usually associated with use of these drugs in the second and third trimesters of pregnancy. Most epidemiologic studies examining fetal abnormalities after exposure to antihypertensive use in the first trimester have not distinguished drugs affecting the renin-angiotensin system from other antihypertensive agents. Appropriate management of maternal hypertension during pregnancy is important to optimize outcomes for both mother and fetus.

In the unusual case that there is no appropriate alternative to therapy with drugs affecting the renin-angiotensin system for a particular patient, apprise the mother of the potential risk to the fetus. Perform serial ultrasound examinations to assess the intra-amniotic environment. If oligohydramnios is observed, discontinue Diovan, unless it is considered lifesaving for the mother. Fetal testing may be appropriate, based on the week of pregnancy. Patients and physicians should be aware, however, that oligohydramnios may not appear until after the fetus has sustained irreversible injury. Closely observe infants with histories of in utero exposure to Diovan for hypotension, oliguria, and hyperkalemia [see Use in Specific Populations (8.4)].

8.3 Nursing Mothers

It is not known whether Diovan is excreted in human milk. Diovan was excreted in the milk of lactating rats; however, animal breast milk drug levels may not accurately reflect human breast milk levels. Because many drugs are excreted into human milk and because of the potential for adverse reactions in nursing infants from Diovan, a decision should be made whether to discontinue nursing or discontinue the drug, taking into account the importance of the drug to the mother.

8.4 Pediatric Use

The antihypertensive effects of Diovan have been evaluated in two randomized, double-blind clinical studies in pediatric patients from 1-5 and 6-16 years of age [see Clinical Studies(14.1)]. The pharmacokinetics of Diovan have been evaluated in pediatric patients 1 to 16 years of age [see Pharmacokinetics, Special Populations, Pediatric (12.3)]. Diovan was generally well tolerated in children 6-16 years and the adverse experience profile was similar to that described for adults.

In children and adolescents with hypertension where underlying renal abnormalities may be more common, renal function and serum potassium should be closely monitored as clinically indicated.

Diovan is not recommended for pediatric patients under 6 years of age due to safety findings for which a relationship to treatment could not be excluded [see Adverse Reactions, Pediatric Hypertension (6.1)].

No data are available in pediatric patients either undergoing dialysis or with a glomerular filtration rate <30 mL/min/1.73 m^2.

There is limited clinical experience with Diovan in pediatric patients with mild to moderate hepatic impairment [see Warnings and Precautions (5.3)].

Daily oral dosing of neonatal/juvenile rats with valsartan at doses as low as 1 mg/kg/day (about 10% of the maximum recommended pediatric dose on a mg/m^2 basis) from postnatal day 7 to postnatal day 70 produced persistent, irreversible kidney damage. These kidney effects in neonatal rats represent expected exaggerated pharmacological effects that are observed if rats are treated during the first 13 days of life. Since this period coincides with up to 44 weeks after conception in humans, it is not considered to point toward an increased safety concern in 6 to 16 year old children.

Neonates with a history of in utero exposure to Diovan:
If oliguria or hypotension occurs, direct attention toward support of blood pressure and renal perfusion. Exchange transfusions or dialysis may be required as a means of reversing hypotension and/or substituting for disordered renal function.

8.5 Geriatric Use

In the controlled clinical trials of valsartan, 1,214 (36.2%) hypertensive patients treated with valsartan were ≥65 years and 265 (7.9%) were ≥75 years. No overall difference in the efficacy or safety of valsartan was observed in this patient population, but greater sensitivity of some older individuals cannot be ruled out.

Of the 2,511 patients with heart failure randomized to valsartan in the Valsartan Heart Failure Trial, 45% (1,141) were 65 years of age or older. In the Valsartan in Acute Myocardial Infarction Trial (VALIANT), 53% (2,596) of the 4,909 patients treated with valsartan and 51% (2,515) of the 4,885 patients treated with valsartan + captopril were 65 years of age or older. There were no notable differences in efficacy or safety between older and younger patients in either trial.

8.6 Renal Impairment

Safety and effectiveness of Diovan in patients with severe renal impairment (CrCl ≤30 mL/min) have not been established. No dose adjustment is required in patients with mild (CrCl 60 to 90 mL/min) or moderate (CrCl 30 to 60 mL/min) renal impairment.

8.7 Hepatic Impairment

No dose adjustment is necessary for patients with mild-to-moderate liver disease. No dosing recommendations can be provided for patients with severe liver disease.

10 OVERDOSAGE

Limited data are available related to overdosage in humans. The most likely manifestations of overdosage would be hypotension and tachycardia; bradycardia could occur from parasympathetic (vagal) stimulation. Depressed level of consciousness, circulatory collapse and shock have been reported. If symptomatic hypotension should occur, supportive treatment should be instituted.

Diovan (valsartan) is not removed from the plasma by hemodialysis.

Valsartan was without grossly observable adverse effects at single oral doses up to 2000 mg/kg in rats and up to 1000 mg/kg in marmosets, except for salivation and diarrhea in the rat and vomiting in the marmoset at the highest dose (60 and 31 times, respectively, the maximum recommended human dose on a mg/m^2 basis). (Calculations assume an oral dose of 320 mg/day and a 60-kg patient.)

11 DESCRIPTION

Diovan (valsartan) is a nonpeptide, orally active, and specific angiotensin II receptor blocker acting on the AT$_1$ receptor subtype.

Valsartan is chemically described as N-(1-oxopentyl)-N-[[2'-(1H-tetrazol-5-yl) [1,1'-biphenyl]-4-yl]methyl]-L-valine. Its empirical formula is $C_{24}H_{29}N_5O_3$, its molecular weight is 435.5, and its structural formula is:

Valsartan is a white to practically white fine powder. It is soluble in ethanol and methanol and slightly soluble in water.

Diovan is available as tablets for oral administration, containing 40 mg, 80 mg, 160 mg or 320 mg of valsartan. The inactive ingredients of the tablets are colloidal silicon dioxide, crospovidone, hydroxypropyl methylcellulose, iron oxides (yellow, black and/or red), magnesium stearate, microcrystalline cellulose, polyethylene glycol 8000, and titanium dioxide.

12 CLINICAL PHARMACOLOGY

12.1 Mechanism of Action

Angiotensin II is formed from angiotensin I in a reaction catalyzed by angiotensin-converting enzyme (ACE, kininase II). Angiotensin II is the principal pressor agent of the renin-angiotensin system, with effects that include vasoconstriction, stimulation of synthesis and release of aldosterone, cardiac stimulation, and renal reabsorption of sodium. Diovan (valsartan) blocks the vasoconstrictor and aldosterone-secreting effects of angiotensin II by selectively blocking the binding of angiotensin II to the AT$_1$ receptor in many tissues, such as vascular smooth muscle and the adrenal gland. Its action is therefore independent of the pathways for angiotensin II synthesis.

There is also an AT$_2$ receptor found in many tissues, but AT$_2$ is not known to be associated with cardiovascular homeostasis. Valsartan has much greater affinity (about 20,000-fold) for the AT$_1$ receptor than for the AT$_2$ receptor. The increased plasma levels of angiotensin II following AT$_1$ receptor blockade with valsartan may stimulate the unblocked AT$_2$ receptor. The primary metabolite of valsartan is essentially inactive with an affinity for the AT$_1$ receptor about one-200th that of valsartan itself.

Blockade of the renin-angiotensin system with ACE inhibitors, which inhibit the biosynthesis of angiotensin II from angiotensin I, is widely used in the treatment of hypertension. ACE inhibitors also inhibit the degradation of bradykinin, a reaction also catalyzed by ACE. Because valsartan does not inhibit ACE (kininase II), it does not affect the response to bradykinin. Whether this difference has clinical relevance is not yet known. Valsartan does not bind to or block other hormone receptors or ion channels known to be important in cardiovascular regulation.

Blockade of the angiotensin II receptor inhibits the negative regulatory feedback of angiotensin II on renin secretion, but the resulting increased plasma renin activity and angiotensin II circulating levels do not overcome the effect of valsartan on blood pressure.

12.2 Pharmacodynamics

Valsartan inhibits the pressor effect of angiotensin II infusions. An oral dose of 80 mg inhibits the pressor effect by about 80% at peak with approximately 30% inhibition persisting for 24 hours. No information on the effect of larger doses is available.

Removal of the negative feedback of angiotensin II causes a 2- to 3-fold rise in plasma renin and consequent rise in angiotensin II plasma concentration in hypertensive patients. Minimal decreases in plasma aldosterone were observed after administration of valsartan; very little effect on serum potassium was observed.

In multiple-dose studies in hypertensive patients with stable renal insufficiency and patients with renovascular hypertension, valsartan had no clinically significant effects on glomerular filtration rate, filtration fraction, creatinine clearance, or renal plasma flow.

In multiple-dose studies in hypertensive patients, valsartan had no notable effects on total cholesterol, fasting triglycerides, fasting serum glucose, or uric acid.

12.3 Pharmacokinetics

Valsartan peak plasma concentration is reached 2 to 4 hours after dosing. Valsartan shows bi-exponential decay kinetics following intravenous administration, with an average elimination half-life of about 6 hours. Absolute bioavailability for Diovan is about 25% (range 10% to 35%). The bioavailability of the suspension [see Dosage and Administration; Pediatric Hypertension (2.2)] is 1.6 times greater than with the tablet. With the tablet, food decreases the exposure (as measured by AUC) to valsartan by about 40% and peak plasma concentration (C$_{max}$) by about 50%. AUC and C$_{max}$ values of valsartan increase approximately linearly with increasing dose over the clinical dosing range. Valsartan does not accumulate appreciably in plasma following repeated administration.

Metabolism and Elimination: Valsartan, when administered as an oral solution, is primarily recovered in feces (about 83% of dose) and urine (about 13% of dose). The recovery is mainly as unchanged drug, with only about 20% of dose recovered as metabolites. The primary metabolite, accounting for about 9% of dose, is valeryl 4-hydroxy valsartan. In vitro metabolism studies involving recombinant CYP 450 enzymes indicated that the CYP 2C9 isoenzyme is responsible for the formation of valeryl-4-hydroxy valsartan. Valsartan does not inhibit CYP 450 isozymes at clinically relevant concentrations. CYP 450 mediated drug interaction between valsartan and coadministered drugs are unlikely because of the low extent of metabolism.

Following intravenous administration, plasma clearance of valsartan is about 2 L/h and its renal clearance is 0.62 L/h (about 30% of total clearance).

Distribution: The steady state volume of distribution of valsartan after intravenous administration is small (17 L), indicating that valsartan does not distribute into tissues extensively. Valsartan is highly bound to serum proteins (95%), mainly serum albumin.

Special Populations:

Pediatric: In a study of pediatric hypertensive patients (n=26, 1 to 16 years of age) given single doses of a suspension of Diovan (mean: 0.9 to 2 mg/kg), the clearance (L/h/kg) of valsartan for children was similar to that of adults receiving the same formulation.

Geriatric: Exposure (measured by AUC) to valsartan is higher by 70% and the half-life is longer by 35% in the elderly than in the young. No dosage adjustment is necessary [see Dosage and Administration (2.1)].

Gender: Pharmacokinetics of valsartan does not differ significantly between males and females.

Heart Failure: The average time to peak concentration and elimination half-life of valsartan in heart failure patients are similar to those observed in healthy volunteers. AUC and C$_{max}$ values of valsartan increase linearly and are almost proportional with increasing dose over the clinical dosing range (40 to 160 mg twice a day). The average accumulation factor is about 1.7. The apparent clearance of valsartan following oral administration is approximately 4.5 L/h. Age does not affect the apparent clearance in heart failure patients.

Renal Insufficiency: There is no apparent correlation between renal function (measured by creatinine clearance) and exposure (measured by AUC) to valsartan in patients with different degrees of renal impairment. Consequently, dose adjustment is not required in patients with mild-to-moderate renal dysfunction. No studies have been performed in patients with severe impairment of renal function (creatinine clearance <10 mL/min). Valsartan is not re-

	Placebo (N=2,499)	Valsartan (N=2,511)	Hazard Ratio (95% CI*)	Nominal p-value
All-cause mortality	484 (19.4%)	495 (19.7%)	1.02 (0.90-1.15)	0.8
HF morbidity	801 (32.1%)	723 (28.8%)	0.87 (0.79-0.97)	0.009

* CI = Confidence Interval

	Without ACE Inhibitor		With ACE Inhibitor	
	Placebo (N=181)	Valsartan (N=185)	Placebo (N=2,318)	Valsartan (N=2,326)
Events (%)	77 (42.5%)	46 (24.9%)	724 (31.2%)	677 (29.1%)
Hazard ratio (95% CI)	0.51 (0.35, 0.73)		0.92 (0.82, 1.02)	
p-value	0.0002		0.0965	

	Placebo (N=181)	Valsartan (N=185)	Hazard Ratio (95% CI)
Components of HF morbidity			
All-cause mortality	49 (27.1%)	32 (17.3%)	0.59 (0.37, 0.91)
Sudden death with resuscitation	2 (1.1%)	1 (0.5%)	0.47 (0.04, 5.20)
CHF therapy	1 (0.6%)	0 (0.0%)	–
CHF hospitalization	48 (26.5%)	24 (13.0%)	0.43 (0.27, 0.71)
Cardiovascular mortality	40 (22.1%)	29 (15.7%)	0.65 (0.40, 1.05)
Non-fatal morbidity	49 (27.1%)	24 (13.0%)	0.42 (0.26, 0.69)

moved from the plasma by hemodialysis. In the case of severe renal disease, exercise care with dosing of valsartan [see Dosage and Administration (2.1)].

Hepatic Insufficiency: On average, patients with mild-to-moderate chronic liver disease have twice the exposure (measured by AUC values) to valsartan of healthy volunteers (matched by age, sex, and weight). In general, no dosage adjustment is needed in patients with mild-to-moderate liver disease. Care should be exercised in patients with liver disease [see Dosage and Administration (2.1)].

13 NONCLINICAL TOXICOLOGY

13.1 Carcinogenesis, Mutagenesis, Impairment of Fertility

There was no evidence of carcinogenicity when valsartan was administered in the diet to mice and rats for up to 2 years at doses up to 160 and 200 mg/kg/day, respectively. These doses in mice and rats are about 2.6 and 6 times, respectively, the maximum recommended human dose on a mg/m² basis. (Calculations assume an oral dose of 320 mg/day and a 60-kg patient.)

Mutagenicity assays did not reveal any valsartan-related effects at either the gene or chromosome level. These assays included bacterial mutagenicity tests with Salmonella (Ames) and E coli; a gene mutation test with Chinese hamster V79 cells; a cytogenetic test with Chinese hamster ovary cells; and a rat micronucleus test.

Valsartan had no adverse effects on the reproductive performance of male or female rats at oral doses up to 200 mg/kg/day. This dose is 6 times the maximum recommended human dose on a mg/m² basis. (Calculations assume an oral dose of 320 mg/day and a 60-kg patient.)

13.2 Animal Toxicology and/or Pharmacology

Reproductive Toxicology Studies

No teratogenic effects were observed when valsartan was administered to pregnant mice and rats at oral doses up to 600 mg/kg/day and to pregnant rabbits at oral doses up to 10 mg/kg/day. However, significant decreases in fetal weight, pup birth weight, pup survival rate, and slight delays in developmental milestones were observed in studies in which parental rats were treated with valsartan at oral, maternally toxic (reduction in body weight gain and food consumption) doses of 600 mg/kg/day during organogenesis or late gestation and lactation. In rabbits, fetotoxicity (i.e., resorptions, litter loss, abortions, and low body weight) associated with maternal toxicity (mortality) was observed at doses of 5 and 10 mg/kg/day. The no observed adverse effect doses of 600, 200, and 2 mg/kg/day in mice, rats and rabbits represent 9, 6, and 0.1 times, respectively, the maximum recommended human dose on a mg/m² basis. Calculations assume an oral dose of 320 mg/day and a 60-kg patient.

14 CLINICAL STUDIES

14.1 Hypertension

Adult Hypertension

The antihypertensive effects of Diovan (valsartan) were demonstrated principally in 7 placebo-controlled, 4- to 12-week trials (1 in patients over 65 years) of dosages from 10 to 320 mg/day in patients with baseline diastolic blood pressures of 95-115 mmHg. The studies allowed comparison of once-daily and twice-daily regimens of 160 mg/day; comparison of peak and trough effects; comparison (in pooled data) of response by gender, age, and race; and evaluation of incremental effects of hydrochlorothiazide.

Administration of valsartan to patients with essential hypertension results in a significant reduction of sitting, supine, and standing systolic and diastolic blood pressure, usually with little or no orthostatic change.

In most patients, after administration of a single oral dose, onset of antihypertensive activity occurs at approximately 2 hours, and maximum reduction of blood pressure is achieved within 6 hours. The antihypertensive effect persists for 24 hours after dosing, but there is a decrease from peak effect at lower doses (40 mg) presumably reflecting loss of inhibition of angiotensin II. At higher doses, however (160 mg), there is little difference in peak and trough effect. During repeated dosing, the reduction in blood pressure with any dose is substantially present within 2 weeks, and maximal reduction is generally attained after 4 weeks. In long-term follow-up studies (without placebo control), the effect of valsartan appeared to be maintained for up to 2 years. The antihypertensive effect is independent of age, gender or race. The latter finding regarding race is based on pooled data and should be viewed with caution, because antihypertensive drugs that affect the renin-angiotensin system (that is, ACE inhibitors and angiotensin-II blockers) have generally been found to be less effective in low-renin hypertensives (frequently blacks) than in high-renin hypertensives (frequently whites). In pooled, randomized, controlled trials of Diovan that included a total of 140 blacks and 830 whites, valsartan and an ACE-inhibitor control were generally at least as effective in blacks as whites. The explanation for this difference from previous findings is unclear.

Abrupt withdrawal of valsartan has not been associated with a rapid increase in blood pressure.

The blood pressure lowering effect of valsartan and thiazide-type diuretics are approximately additive.

The 7 studies of valsartan monotherapy included over 2,000 patients randomized to various doses of valsartan and about 800 patients randomized to placebo. Doses below 80 mg were not consistently distinguished from those of placebo at trough, but doses of 80, 160 and 320 mg produced dose-related decreases in systolic and diastolic blood pressure, with the difference from placebo of approximately 6-9/3-5 mmHg at 80 to 160 mg and 9/6 mmHg at 320 mg. In a controlled trial the addition of HCTZ to valsartan 80 mg resulted in additional lowering of systolic and diastolic blood pressure by approximately 6/3 and 12/5 mmHg for 12.5 and 25 mg of HCTZ, respectively, compared to valsartan 80 mg alone.

Patients with an inadequate response to 80 mg once daily were titrated to either 160 mg once daily or 80 mg twice daily, which resulted in a comparable response in both groups.

In controlled trials, the antihypertensive effect of once-daily valsartan 80 mg was similar to that of once-daily enalapril 20 mg or once-daily lisinopril 10 mg.

There are no trials of Diovan demonstrating reductions in cardiovascular risk in patients with hypertension, but at least one pharmacologically similar drug has demonstrated such benefits.

There was essentially no change in heart rate in valsartan-treated patients in controlled trials.

Pediatric Hypertension

The antihypertensive effects of Diovan were evaluated in two randomized, double-blind clinical studies.

In a clinical study involving 261 hypertensive pediatric patients 6 to 16 years of age, patients who weighed <35 kg received 10, 40 or 80 mg of valsartan daily (low, medium and high doses), and patients who weighed ≥35 kg received 20, 80, and 160 mg of valsartan daily (low, medium and high doses). Renal and urinary disorders, and essential hypertension with or without obesity were the most common underlying causes of hypertension in children enrolled in this study. At the end of 2 weeks, valsartan reduced both systolic and diastolic blood pressure in a dose-dependent manner. Overall, the three dose levels of valsartan (low, medium and high) significantly reduced systolic blood pressure by -8, -10, -12 mm Hg from the baseline, respectively. Patients were re-randomized to either continue receiving the same dose of valsartan or were switched to placebo. In patients who continued to receive the medium and high doses of valsartan, systolic blood pressure at trough was -4 and -7 mm Hg lower than patients who received the placebo treatment. In patients receiving the low dose of valsartan, systolic blood pressure at trough was similar to that of patients who received the placebo treatment. Overall, the dose-dependent antihypertensive effect of valsartan was consistent across all the demographic subgroups.

In a clinical study involving 90 hypertensive pediatric patients 1 to 5 years of age with a similar study design, there was some evidence of effectiveness, but safety findings for which a relationship to treatment could not be excluded mitigate against recommending use in this age group [see Adverse Reactions (6.1)].

14.2 Heart Failure

The Valsartan Heart Failure Trial (Val-HeFT) was a multinational, double-blind study in which 5,010 patients with NYHA class II (62%) to IV (2%) heart failure and LVEF <40%, on baseline therapy chosen by their physicians, were randomized to placebo or valsartan (titrated from 40 mg twice daily to the highest tolerated dose or 160 mg twice daily) and followed for a mean of about 2 years. Although Val-HeFT's primary goal was to examine the effect of valsartan when added to an ACE inhibitor, about 7% were not receiving an ACE inhibitor. Other background therapy included diuretics (86%), digoxin (67%), and beta-blockers (36%). The population studied was 80% male, 46% 65 years or older and 89% Caucasian. At the end of the trial, patients in the valsartan group had a blood pressure that was 4 mmHg systolic and 2 mmHg diastolic lower than the placebo group. There were two primary end points, both assessed as time to first event: all-cause mortality and heart failure morbidity, the latter defined as all-cause mortality, sudden death with resuscitation, hospitalization for heart failure, and the need for intravenous inotropic or vasodilatory drugs for at least 4 hours. These results are summarized in the following table.

[See first table above]

Although the overall morbidity result favored valsartan, this result was largely driven by the 7% of patients not receiving an ACE inhibitor, as shown in the following table.

[See second table above]

The modest favorable trend in the group receiving an ACE inhibitor was largely driven by the patients receiving less than the recommended dose of ACE inhibitor. Thus, there is little evidence of further clinical benefit when valsartan is added to an adequate dose of ACE inhibitor.

Secondary end points in the subgroup not receiving ACE inhibitors were as follows.

[See third table above]

In patients not receiving an ACE inhibitor, valsartan-treated patients had an increase in ejection fraction and reduction in left ventricular internal diastolic diameter (LVIDD).

Effects were generally consistent across subgroups defined by age and gender for the population of patients not receiving an ACE inhibitor. The number of black patients was small and does not permit a meaningful assessment in this subset of patients.

14.3 Post-Myocardial Infarction

The VALsartan In Acute myocardial iNfarcTion trial (VALIANT) was a randomized, controlled, multinational, double-blind study in 14,703 patients with acute myocardial infarction and either heart failure (signs, symptoms or radiological evidence) or left ventricular systolic dysfunction (ejection fraction ≤40% by radionuclide ventriculography or ≤35% by echocardiography or ventricular contrast angiography). Patients were randomized within 12 hours to 10 days after the onset of myocardial infarction symptoms to one of three treatment groups: valsartan (titrated from 20 or 40 mg twice daily to the highest tolerated dose up to a maximum of 160 mg twice daily), the ACE inhibitor, captopril (titrated from 6.25 mg three times daily to the highest tolerated dose up to a maximum of 50 mg three times daily), or the combination of valsartan plus captopril. In the combination group, the dose of valsartan was titrated from 20 mg twice daily to the highest tolerated dose up to a maximum of 80 mg twice daily; the dose of captopril was the same as for monotherapy. The population studied was 69% male, 94% Caucasian, and 53% were 65 years of age or older. Baseline therapy included aspirin (91%), beta-blockers (70%), ACE inhibitors (40%), thrombolytics (35%) and statins (34%). The mean treatment duration was 2 years. The mean daily dose of Diovan in the monotherapy group was 217 mg.

The primary endpoint was time to all-cause mortality. Secondary endpoints included (1) time to cardiovascular (CV) mortality, and (2) time to the first event of cardiovascular mortality, reinfarction, or hospitalization for heart failure. The results are summarized in the following table. [See first table above]

There was no difference in overall mortality among the three treatment groups. There was thus no evidence that combining the ACE inhibitor captopril and the angiotensin II blocker valsartan was of value.

The data were assessed to see whether the effectiveness of valsartan could be demonstrated by showing in a non-inferiority analysis that it preserved a fraction of the effect of captopril, a drug with a demonstrated survival effect in this setting. A conservative estimate of the effect of captopril (based on a pooled analysis of 3 post-infarction studies of captopril and 2 other ACE inhibitors) was a 14% to 16% reduction in mortality compared to placebo. Valsartan would be considered effective if it preserved a meaningful fraction of that effect and unequivocally preserved some of that effect. As shown in the table, the upper bound of the CI for the hazard ratio (valsartan/captopril) for overall or CV mortality is 1.09 to 1.11, a difference of about 9% to 11%, thus making it unlikely that valsartan has less than about half of the estimated effect of captopril and clearly demonstrating an effect of valsartan. The other secondary endpoints were consistent with this conclusion.

Effects on Mortality Amongst Subgroups in VALIANT

Subgroups	Patient (%)
All Patients	100.0
< 65 y	47.0
≥ 65 y	53.0
Male	68.6
Female	31.4
Caucasian	93.7
Non-Caucasian	6.3
US	27.0
Non-US	73.0
Beta-blocker	70.4
Beta-blocker (No)	29.6

There were no clear differences in all-cause mortality based on age, gender, race, or baseline therapies, as shown in the figure above.

16 HOW SUPPLIED/STORAGE AND HANDLING

Diovan (valsartan) is available as tablets containing valsartan 40 mg, 80 mg, 160 mg, or 320 mg. All strengths are packaged in bottles and unit dose blister packages (10 strips of 10 tablets) as described below.

40 mg tablets are scored on one side and ovaloid with bevelled edges. 80 mg, 160 mg, and 320 mg tablets are unscored and almond-shaped with bevelled edges.
[See second table above]

Store at 25°C (77°F); excursions permitted to 15-30°C (59 - 86°F) [see USP Controlled Room Temperature].
Protect from moisture.
Dispense in tight container (USP).

Tablet	Color		Deboss		NDC 0078-####-##					
		Side 1	Side 2		Bottle of					Blister
					30	90	3500	7000	14000	Packages of 100
40 mg	Yellow	NVR	DO		0423-15	–	–	–	–	0423-06
80 mg	Pale red	NVR	DV		–	0358-34	–	–	0358-33	0358-06
160 mg	Grey-orange	NVR	DX		–	0359-34	–	0359-17	–	0359-06
320 mg	Dark grey-violet	NVR	DXL		–	0360-34	0360-11	–	–	0360-06

	Valsartan vs. Captopril (N=4,909) (N=4,909)			Valsartan + Captopril vs. Captopril (N=4,885) (N=4,909)		
	No. of Deaths Valsartan/Captopril	Hazard Ratio CI	p-value	No. of Deaths Comb/Captopril	Hazard Ratio CI	p-value
All-cause mortality	979 (19.9%)/ 958 (19.5%)	1.001 (0.902, 1.111)	0.98	941 (19.3%)/ 958 (19.5%)	0.984 (0.886, 1.093)	0.73
CV mortality	827 (16.8%)/ 830 (16.9%)	0.976 (0.875, 1.090)				
CV mortality, hospitalization for HF, and recurrent non-fatal MI	1,529 (31.1%)/ 1,567 (31.9%)	0.955 (0.881, 1.035)				

17 PATIENT COUNSELING INFORMATION

Information for Patients

Pregnancy: Female patients of childbearing age should be told about the consequences of exposure to Diovan during pregnancy. Discuss treatment options with women planning to become pregnant. Patients should be asked to report pregnancies to their physicians as soon as possible.
T2014-28
March 2014
DIOVAN (DYE'-o-van)
(valsartan) Tablets
Read the Patient Information that comes with DIOVAN before you take it and each time you get a refill. There may be new information. This leaflet does not take the place of talking with your doctor about your medical condition or treatment. If you have any questions about DIOVAN, ask your doctor or pharmacist.
What is the most important information I should know about DIOVAN?
DIOVAN can cause harm or death to an unborn baby. Talk to your doctor about other ways to lower your blood pressure if you plan to become pregnant. If you get pregnant while taking DIOVAN, tell your doctor right away.
What is DIOVAN?
DIOVAN is a prescription medicine called an angiotensin receptor blocker (ARB). It is used in adults to:
• lower high blood pressure (hypertension) in adults and children, 6 to 16 years of age.
• treat heart failure in adults. In these patients, DIOVAN may lower the need for hospitalization that happens from heart failure.
• improve the chance of living longer after a heart attack (myocardial infarction) in adults.
DIOVAN is not for children under 6 years of age or children with certain kidney problems.
High Blood Pressure (Hypertension). Blood pressure is the force in your blood vessels when your heart beats and when your heart rests. You have high blood pressure when the force is too much. DIOVAN can help your blood vessels relax so your blood pressure is lower. Medicines that lower your blood pressure lower your chance of having a stroke or heart attack.
High blood pressure makes the heart work harder to pump blood throughout the body and causes damage to the blood vessels. If high blood pressure is not treated, it can lead to stroke, heart attack, heart failure, kidney failure and vision problems.
Heart Failure occurs when the heart is weak and cannot pump enough blood to your lungs and the rest of your body. Just walking or moving can make you short of breath, so you may have to rest a lot.
Heart Attack (Myocardial Infarction): A heart attack is caused by a blocked artery that results in damage to the heart muscle.
What should I tell my doctor before taking DIOVAN?
Tell your doctor about all your medical conditions including whether you:
• have any allergies. See the end of this leaflet for a complete list of ingredients in DIOVAN.

• have a heart condition
• have liver problems
• have kidney problems
• **are pregnant or planning to become pregnant. See "What is the most important information I should know about DIOVAN?"**
• are breastfeeding. It is not known if DIOVAN passes into your breast milk. You and your doctor should decide if you will take DIOVAN or breastfeed, but not both. Talk with your doctor about the best way to feed your baby if you take DIOVAN.
• have ever had a reaction called angioedema, to another blood pressure medicine. Angioedema causes swelling of the face, lips, tongue and/or throat, and may cause difficulty breathing.
Tell your doctor about all the medicines you take including prescription and nonprescription medicines, vitamins and herbal supplements. Especially tell your doctor if you take:
• other medicines for high blood pressure or a heart problem
• water pills (also called "diuretics")
• potassium supplements. Your doctor may check the amount of potassium in your blood periodically
• a salt substitute. Your doctor may check the amount of potassium in your blood periodically
• Nonsteroidal anti-inflammatory drugs (like ibuprofen or naproxen)
• certain antibiotics (rifamycin group), a drug used to protect against transplant rejection (cyclosporin) or an antiretroviral drug used to treat HIV/AIDS infection (ritonavir). These drugs may increase the effect of valsartan.
• Lithium, a medicine used in some types of depression
Know the medicines you take. Keep a list of your medicines with you to show to your doctor and pharmacist when a new medicine is prescribed. Talk to your doctor or pharmacist before you start taking any new medicine. Your doctor or pharmacist will know what medicines are safe to take together.
How should I take DIOVAN?
• Take DIOVAN exactly as prescribed by your doctor.
• For treatment of high blood pressure, take DIOVAN one time each day, at the same time each day.
• If your child cannot swallow tablets, or if tablets are not available in the prescribed strength, your pharmacist will mix DIOVAN as a liquid suspension for your child. If your child switches between taking the tablet and the suspension, your doctor will adjust the dose as needed. Shake the bottle of suspension well for at least 10 seconds before pouring the dose of medicine to give to your child.
• For adult patients with heart failure or who have had a heart attack, take DIOVAN two times each day, at the same time each day. Your doctor may start you on a low dose of DIOVAN and may increase the dose during your treatment.
• DIOVAN can be taken with or without food.
• If you miss a dose, take it as soon as you remember. If it is close to your next dose, do not take the missed dose. Take the next dose at your regular time.
• If you take too much DIOVAN, call your doctor or Poison Control Center, or go to the nearest hospital emergency room.

What are the possible side effects of DIOVAN?
DIOVAN may cause the following serious side effects:
Injury or death to an unborn baby. See "What is the most important information I should know about DIOVAN?"
Low Blood Pressure (Hypotension). Low blood pressure is most likely to happen if you also take water pills, are on a low-salt diet, get dialysis treatments, have heart problems, or get sick with vomiting or diarrhea. Lie down, if you feel faint or dizzy. Call your doctor right away.
Kidney problems. Kidney problems may get worse if you already have kidney disease. Some patients will have changes on blood tests for kidney function and may need a lower dose of DIOVAN. Call your doctor if you get swelling in your feet, ankles, or hands, or unexplained weight gain. If you have heart failure, your doctor should check your kidney function before prescribing DIOVAN.
The most common side effects of DIOVAN used to treat people with high blood pressure include:
• headache
• dizziness
• flu symptoms
• tiredness
• stomach (abdominal) pain
Side effects are generally mild and brief. They generally have not caused patients to stop taking DIOVAN.
The most common side effects of DIOVAN used to treat people with heart failure include:
• dizziness
• low blood pressure
• diarrhea
• joint and back pain
• tiredness
• high blood potassium
Common side effects of DIOVAN used to treat people after a heart attack which caused them to stop taking the drug include:
• low blood pressure
• cough
• high blood creatinine (decreased kidney function)
• rash
Tell your doctor if you get any side effect that bothers you or that does not go away.
These are not all the possible side effects of DIOVAN. For a complete list, ask your doctor or pharmacist.
How do I store DIOVAN?
• Store DIOVAN tablets at room temperature between 59° to 86°F (15°C to 30°C).
• Keep DIOVAN tablets in a closed container in a dry place.
• Store bottles of DIOVAN suspension at room temperature less than 86°F (30°C) for up to 30 days, or refrigerate between 35°F - 46°F (2°C - 8°C) for up to 75 days.
• Keep DIOVAN and all medicines out of the reach of children.
General information about DIOVAN
Medicines are sometimes prescribed for conditions that are not mentioned in patient information leaflets. Do not use DIOVAN for a condition for which it was not prescribed. Do not give DIOVAN to other people, even if they have the same symptoms you have. It may harm them.
This leaflet summarizes the most important information about DIOVAN. If you would like more information, talk with your doctor. You can ask your doctor or pharmacist for information about DIOVAN that is written for health professionals.
For more information about DIOVAN, ask your pharmacist or doctor, visit www.DIOVAN.com on the Internet, or call **1-866-404-6361.**
What are the ingredients in DIOVAN?
Active ingredient: valsartan
Inactive ingredients: colloidal silicon dioxide, crospovidone, hydroxypropyl methylcellulose, iron oxides (yellow, black and/or red), magnesium stearate, microcrystalline cellulose, polyethylene glycol 8000, and titanium dioxide
Distributed by:
Novartis Pharmaceuticals Corp.
East Hanover, NJ 07936
© Novartis
T2014-29
March 2014
Shown in Product Identification Guide, page 310

DIOVAN HCT®   ℞
[DYE'-o-van HCT]
(valsartan and hydrochlorothiazide USP)
Tablets

The following prescribing information is based on official labeling in effect July 2014.
HIGHLIGHTS OF PRESCRIBING INFORMATION
These highlights do not include all the information needed to use Diovan HCT safely and effectively. See full prescribing information for Diovan HCT.

Diovan HCT® (valsartan and hydrochlorothiazide USP)
Tablets
Initial U.S. Approval: 1998

┌──┐
WARNING: FETAL TOXICITY
See full prescribing information for complete boxed warning.
• **When pregnancy is detected, discontinue Diovan HCT as soon as possible. (5.1)**
• **Drugs that act directly on the renin-angiotensin system can cause injury and death to the developing fetus. (5.1)**
└──┘

————————INDICATIONS AND USAGE————————
Diovan HCT is the combination tablet of valsartan (Diovan), an angiotensin II receptor blocker (ARB) and hydrochlorothiazide (HCTZ), a diuretic. Diovan HCT is indicated for the treatment of hypertension, to lower blood pressure:
• In patients not adequately controlled with monotherapy (1)
• As initial therapy in patients likely to need multiple drugs to achieve their blood pressure goals (1)
Lowering blood pressure reduces the risk of fatal and nonfatal cardiovascular events, primarily strokes and myocardial infarctions.

————DOSAGE AND ADMINISTRATION————
• Dose once daily. Titrate as needed to a maximum dose of 320/25mg (2)
• May be used as add-on/switch therapy for patients not adequately controlled on any of the components (valsartan or HCTZ) (2)
• May be substituted for titrated components (2.3)

————DOSAGE FORMS AND STRENGTHS————
Tablets (valsartan/HCTZ mg): 80/12.5, 160/12.5, 160/25, 320/12.5, 320/25 (3)

————————CONTRAINDICATIONS————————
Anuria; Hypersensitivity to any sulfonamide-derived drugs or any component; Do not coadminister aliskiren with Diovan HCT in patients with diabetes (4)

————WARNINGS AND PRECAUTIONS————
• Hypotension: Correct volume depletion prior to initiation (5.2)
• Observe for signs of fluid or electrolyte imbalance (5.9)
• Monitor renal function and potassium in susceptible patients (5.3, 5.7)
• Exacerbation or activation of systemic lupus erythematosus (5.5)
• Acute angle-closure glaucoma (5.8)

————————ADVERSE REACTIONS————————
The most common reasons for discontinuation of therapy with Diovan HCT were headache and dizziness. The only adverse experience that occurred in ≥2% of patients treated with Diovan HCT and at a higher incidence than placebo was nasopharyngitis (2.4% vs. 1.9%). (6.1)
To report SUSPECTED ADVERSE REACTIONS, contact Novartis Pharmaceuticals Corporation at 1-888-669-6682 or FDA at 1-800-FDA-1088 or www.fda.gov/medwatch.

————————DRUG INTERACTIONS————————
• Antidiabetic drugs: Dosage adjustment of antidiabetic may be required (7)
• Cholestyramine and colestipol: Reduced absorption of thiazides (12.3)
• Lithium: Increased risk of lithium toxicity. Monitor serum lithium concentrations during concurrent use. (7)
• Non-Steroidal Anti-Inflammatory Drugs (NSAIDs): May increase risk of renal impairment. Can reduce diuretic, natriuretic and antihypertensive effects of diuretics. (7)
• Dual inhibition of the renin-angiotensin system: Increased risk of renal impairment, hypotension, and hyperkalemia (7)

————USE IN SPECIFIC POPULATIONS————
Nursing Mothers: Nursing or drug should be discontinued (8.3)
See 17 for PATIENT COUNSELING INFORMATION and FDA-approved patient labeling
                                        Revised: 3/2014

FULL PRESCRIBING INFORMATION

┌──┐
WARNING: FETAL TOXICITY
• **When pregnancy is detected, discontinue Diovan HCT as soon as possible. (5.1)**
• **Drugs that act directly on the renin-angiotensin system can cause injury and death to the developing fetus. (5.1)**
└──┘

1   INDICATIONS AND USAGE
Diovan HCT (valsartan and hydrochlorothiazide, USP) is indicated for the treatment of hypertension, to lower blood pressure. Lowering blood pressure reduces the risk of fatal and nonfatal cardiovascular events, primarily strokes and myocardial infarctions. These benefits have been seen in controlled trials of antihypertensive drugs from a wide variety of pharmacologic classes, including hydrochlorothiazide and the ARB class to which valsartan principally belongs. There are no controlled trials demonstrating risk reduction with Diovan HCT.
Control of high blood pressure should be part of comprehensive cardiovascular risk management, including, as appropriate, lipid control, diabetes management, antithrombotic therapy, smoking cessation, exercise, and limited sodium intake. Many patients will require more than 1 drug to achieve blood pressure goals. For specific advice on goals and management, see published guidelines, such as those of the National High Blood Pressure Education Program's Joint National Committee on Prevention, Detection, Evaluation, and Treatment of High Blood Pressure (JNC).
Numerous antihypertensive drugs, from a variety of pharmacologic classes and with different mechanisms of action, have been shown in randomized controlled trials to reduce cardiovascular morbidity and mortality, and it can be concluded that it is blood pressure reduction, and not some other pharmacologic property of the drugs, that is largely responsible for those benefits. The largest and most consistent cardiovascular outcome benefit has been a reduction in the risk of stroke, but reductions in myocardial infarction and cardiovascular mortality have also been seen regularly. Elevated systolic or diastolic pressure causes increased cardiovascular risk, and the absolute risk increase per mmHg is greater at higher blood pressures, so that even modest reductions of severe hypertension can provide substantial benefit. Relative risk reduction from blood pressure reduction is similar across populations with varying absolute risk, so the absolute benefit is greater in patients who are at higher risk independent of their hypertension (e.g., patients with diabetes or hyperlipidemia), and such patients would be expected to benefit from more aggressive treatment to a lower blood pressure goal.
Some antihypertensive drugs have smaller blood pressure effects (as monotherapy) in black patients, and many antihypertensive drugs have additional approved indications and effects (e.g., on angina, heart failure, or diabetic kidney disease). These considerations may guide selection of therapy.

Add-On Therapy
Diovan HCT may be used in patients whose blood pressure is not adequately controlled on monotherapy.
Replacement Therapy
Diovan HCT may be substituted for the titrated components.
Initial Therapy
Diovan HCT may be used as initial therapy in patients who are likely to need multiple drugs to achieve blood pressure goals.
The choice of Diovan HCT as initial therapy for hypertension should be based on an assessment of potential benefits and risks.
Patients with stage 2 hypertension are at a relatively high risk for cardiovascular events (such as strokes, heart attacks, and heart failure), kidney failure, and vision problems, so prompt treatment is clinically relevant. The decision to use a combination as initial therapy should be individualized and should be shaped by considerations such as baseline blood pressure, the target goal, and the incremental likelihood of achieving goal with a combination compared to monotherapy. Individual blood pressure goals may vary based upon the patient's risk.
Data from the high dose multifactorial trial *[see Clinical Studies (14.1)]* provides estimates of the probability of reaching a target blood pressure with Diovan HCT compared to valsartan or hydrochlorothiazide monotherapy. The figures below provide estimates of the likelihood of achieving systolic or diastolic blood pressure control with Diovan HCT 320/25 mg, based upon baseline systolic or diastolic blood pressure. The curve of each treatment group was estimated by logistic regression modeling. The estimated likelihood at the right tail of each curve is less reliable due to small numbers of subjects with high baseline blood pressures.
[See figures 1-4 above]
For example, a patient with a baseline blood pressure of 160/100 mmHg has about a 41% likelihood of achieving a goal of <140 mmHg (systolic) and 60% likelihood of achieving <90 mmHg (diastolic) on valsartan alone and the likelihood of achieving these goals on HCTZ alone is about 50% (systolic) or 57% (diastolic). The likelihood of achieving these goals on Diovan HCT rises to about 84% (systolic) or 80% (diastolic). The likelihood of achieving these goals on placebo is about 23% (systolic) or 36% (diastolic).

2 DOSAGE AND ADMINISTRATION
2.1 General Considerations
The usual starting dose is Diovan HCT 160/12.5 mg once daily. The dosage can be increased after 1 to 2 weeks of therapy to a maximum of one 320/25 tablet once daily as needed to control blood pressure *[see Clinical Studies (14.2)]*. Maximum antihypertensive effects are attained within 2 to 4 weeks after a change in dose.
2.2 Add-On Therapy
A patient whose blood pressure is not adequately controlled with valsartan (or another ARB) alone or hydrochlorothiazide alone may be switched to combination therapy with Diovan HCT.
A patient who experiences dose-limiting adverse reactions on either component alone may be switched to Diovan HCT containing a lower dose of that component in combination with the other to achieve similar blood pressure reductions. The clinical response to Diovan HCT should be subsequently evaluated and if blood pressure remains uncontrolled after 3 to 4 weeks of therapy, the dose may be titrated up to a maximum of 320/25 mg.
2.3 Replacement Therapy
Diovan HCT may be substituted for the titrated components.
2.4 Initial Therapy
Diovan HCT is not recommended as initial therapy in patients with intravascular volume depletion *[see Warnings and Precautions (5.2)]*.
2.5 Use with Other Antihypertensive Drugs
Diovan HCT may be administered with other antihypertensive agents.

3 DOSAGE FORMS AND STRENGTHS
80/12.5 mg tablets, imprinted CG/HGH (Side 1/Side 2)
160/12.5 mg tablets, imprinted CG/HHH
160/25 mg tablets, imprinted NVR/HXH
320/12.5 mg tablets, imprinted NVR/HIL
320/25 mg tablets, imprinted NVR/CTI

4 CONTRAINDICATIONS
Diovan HCT (valsartan and hydrochlorothiazide, USP) is contraindicated in patients who are hypersensitive to any component of this product.
Because of the hydrochlorothiazide component, this product is contraindicated in patients with anuria or hypersensitivity to other sulfonamide-derived drugs.
Do not coadminister aliskiren with Diovan HCT in patients with diabetes *[see Drug Interactions (7)]*.

Figure 1: Probability of Achieving Systolic Blood Pressure <140 mmHg at Week 8

Figure 2: Probability of Achieving Diastolic Blood Pressure <90 mmHg at Week 8

Figure 3: Probability of Achieving Systolic Blood Pressure <130 mmHg at Week 8

Figure 4: Probability of Achieving Diastolic Blood Pressure <80 mmHg at Week 8

5 WARNINGS AND PRECAUTIONS
5.1 Fetal Toxicity
Pregnancy Category D
Use of drugs that act on the renin-angiotensin system during the second and third trimesters of pregnancy reduces fetal renal function and increases fetal and neonatal morbidity and death. Resulting oligohydramnios can be associated with fetal lung hypoplasia and skeletal deformations. Potential neonatal adverse effects include skull hypoplasia, anuria, hypotension, renal failure, and death. When pregnancy is detected, discontinue Diovan HCT as soon as possible *[see Use in Specific Populations (8.1)]*.
Intrauterine exposure to thiazide diuretics is associated with fetal or neonatal jaundice, thrombocytopenia, and possibly other adverse reactions that have occurred in adults.
5.2 Hypotension in Volume- and/or Salt-Depleted Patients
Excessive reduction of blood pressure was rarely seen (0.7%) in patients with uncomplicated hypertension treated with Diovan HCT in controlled trials. In patients with an activated renin-angiotensin system, such as volume- and/or salt-depleted patients receiving high doses of diuretics, symptomatic hypotension may occur. This condition should be corrected prior to administration of Diovan HCT, or the treatment should start under close medical supervision.
If hypotension occurs, the patient should be placed in the supine position and, if necessary, given an intravenous infusion of normal saline. A transient hypotensive response is not a contraindication to further treatment, which usually can be continued without difficulty once the blood pressure has stabilized.
5.3 Impaired Renal Function
Changes in renal function including acute renal failure can be caused by drugs that inhibit the renin-angiotensin system and by diuretics. Patients whose renal function may depend in part on the activity of the renin-angiotensin system (e.g., patients with renal artery stenosis, chronic kidney disease, severe congestive heart failure, or volume depletion) may be at particular risk of developing acute renal failure on Diovan HCT. Monitor renal function periodically in these patients. Consider withholding or discontinuing therapy in patients who develop a clinically significant decrease in renal function on Diovan HCT *[see Drug Interactions (7)]*.
5.4 Hypersensitivity Reaction
Hydrochlorothiazide: Hypersensitivity reactions to hydrochlorothiazide may occur in patients with or without a history of allergy or bronchial asthma, but are more likely in patients with such a history.

5.5 Systemic Lupus Erythematosus
Hydrochlorothiazide: Thiazide diuretics have been reported to cause exacerbation or activation of systemic lupus erythematosus.
5.6 Lithium Interaction
Increases in serum lithium concentrations and lithium toxicity have been reported with concomitant use of valsartan or thiazide diuretics. Monitor lithium levels in patients receiving Diovan HCT and lithium. *[see Drug Interactions (7)]*.
5.7 Potassium Abnormalities
Valsartan–Hydrochlorothiazide: In the controlled trials of various doses of Diovan HCT the incidence of hypertensive patients who developed hypokalemia (serum potassium <3.5 mEq/L) was 3.0%; the incidence of hyperkalemia (serum potassium >5.7 mEq/L) was 0.4%.
Hydrochlorothiazide can cause hypokalemia and hyponatremia. Hypomagnesemia can result in hypokalemia which appears difficult to treat despite potassium repletion. Drugs that inhibit the renin-angiotensin system can cause hyperkalemia. Monitor serum electrolytes periodically.
If hypokalemia is accompanied by clinical signs (e.g., muscular weakness, paresis, or ECG alterations), Diovan HCT should be discontinued. Correction of hypokalemia and any coexisting hypomagnesemia is recommended prior to the initiation of thiazides.
Some patients with heart failure have developed increases in potassium with Diovan therapy. These effects are usually minor and transient, and they are more likely to occur in patients with pre-existing renal impairment. Dosage reduction and/or discontinuation of the diuretic and/or Diovan may be required *[see Adverse Reactions (6.1)]*.
5.8 Acute Myopia and Secondary Angle-Closure Glaucoma
Hydrochlorothiazide, a sulfonamide, can cause an idiosyncratic reaction, resulting in acute transient myopia and acute angle-closure glaucoma. Symptoms include acute onset of decreased visual acuity or ocular pain and typically occur within hours to weeks of drug initiation. Untreated acute angle-closure glaucoma can lead to permanent vision loss. The primary treatment is to discontinue hydrochlorothiazide as rapidly as possible. Prompt medical or surgical treatments may need to be considered if the intraocular pressure remains uncontrolled. Risk factors for developing acute angle-closure glaucoma may include a history of sulfonamide or penicillin allergy.

5.9 Metabolic Disturbances

Hydrochlorothiazide

Hydrochlorothiazide may alter glucose tolerance and raise serum levels of cholesterol and triglycerides.

Hydrochlorothiazide may raise the serum uric acid level due to reduced clearance of uric acid and may cause or exacerbate hyperuricemia and precipitate gout in susceptible patients.

Hydrochlorothiazide decreases urinary calcium excretion and may cause elevations of serum calcium. Monitor calcium levels in patients with hypercalcemia receiving Diovan HCT.

6 ADVERSE REACTIONS

6.1 Clinical Trials Experience

Because clinical studies are conducted under widely varying conditions, adverse reactions rates observed in the clinical studies of a drug cannot be directly compared to rates in the clinical studies of another drug and may not reflect the rates observed in practice. The adverse reaction information from clinical trials does, however, provide a basis for identifying the adverse events that appear to be related to drug use and for approximating rates.

Hypertension

Diovan HCT (valsartan and hydrochlorothiazide, USP) has been evaluated for safety in more than 5700 patients, including over 990 treated for over 6 months, and over 370 for over 1 year. Adverse experiences have generally been mild and transient in nature and have only infrequently required discontinuation of therapy. The overall incidence of adverse reactions with Diovan HCT was comparable to placebo.

The overall frequency of adverse reactions was neither dose-related nor related to gender, age, or race. In controlled clinical trials, discontinuation of therapy due to side effects was required in 2.3% of valsartan-hydrochlorothiazide patients and 3.1% of placebo patients. The most common reasons for discontinuation of therapy with Diovan HCT were headache and dizziness.

The only adverse reaction that occurred in controlled clinical trials in at least 2% of patients treated with Diovan HCT and at a higher incidence in valsartan-hydrochlorothiazide (n=4372) than placebo (n=262) patients was nasopharyngitis (2.4% vs. 1.9%).

Dose-related orthostatic effects were seen in fewer than 1% of patients. In individual trials, a dose-related increase in the incidence of dizziness was observed in patients treated with Diovan HCT.

Other adverse reactions that have been reported with valsartan-hydrochlorothiazide (>0.2% of valsartan-hydrochlorothiazide patients in controlled clinical trials) without regard to causality, are listed below:

Cardiovascular: Palpitations and tachycardia

Ear and Labyrinth: Tinnitus and vertigo

Gastrointestinal: Dyspepsia, diarrhea, flatulence, dry mouth, nausea, abdominal pain, abdominal pain upper, and vomiting

General and Administration Site Conditions: Asthenia, chest pain, fatigue, peripheral edema and pyrexia

Infections and Infestations: Bronchitis, bronchitis acute, influenza, gastroenteritis, sinusitis, upper respiratory tract infection, and urinary tract infection

Investigations: Blood urea increased

Musculoskeletal: Arthralgia, back pain, muscle cramps, myalgia, and pain in extremity

Nervous System: Dizziness postural, paresthesia, and somnolence

Psychiatric: Anxiety and insomnia

Renal and Urinary: Pollakiuria

Reproductive System: Erectile dysfunction

Respiratory, Thoracic and Mediastinal: Dyspnea, cough, nasal congestion, pharyngolaryngeal pain, and sinus congestion

Skin and Subcutaneous Tissue: Hyperhidrosis and rash

Vascular: Hypotension

Other reported reactions seen less frequently in clinical trials included abnormal vision, anaphylaxis, bronchospasm, constipation, depression, dehydration, decreased libido, dysuria, epistaxis, flushing, gout, increased appetite, muscle weakness, pharyngitis, pruritus, sunburn, syncope, and viral infection.

Initial Therapy-Hypertension

In a clinical study in patients with severe hypertension (diastolic blood pressure ≥110 mmHg and systolic blood pressure ≥140 mmHg), the overall pattern of adverse reactions reported through 6 weeks of follow-up was similar in patients treated with Diovan HCT as initial therapy and in patients treated with valsartan as initial therapy. Comparing the groups treated with Diovan HCT (force-titrated to 320/25 mg) and valsartan (force-titrated to 320 mg), dizziness was observed in 6% and 2% of patients, respectively. Hypotension was observed in 1% of those patients receiving Diovan HCT and 0% of patients receiving valsartan. There were no reported cases of syncope in either treatment group. Laboratory changes with Diovan HCT as initial ther-

apy in patients with severe hypertension were similar to those reported with Diovan HCT in patients with less severe hypertension [see Clinical Studies (14.2) and Drug Interactions (7)].

Valsartan: In trials in which valsartan was compared to an ACE inhibitor with or without placebo, the incidence of dry cough was significantly greater in the ACE inhibitor group (7.9%) than in the groups who received valsartan (2.6%) or placebo (1.5%). In a 129-patient trial limited to patients who had had dry cough when they had previously received ACE inhibitors, the incidences of cough in patients who received valsartan, hydrochlorothiazide, or lisinopril were 20%, 19%, 69% respectively (p <0.001).

Other reported reactions seen less frequently in clinical trials included chest pain, syncope, anorexia, vomiting, and angioedema.

Hydrochlorothiazide: Other adverse reactions not listed above that have been reported with hydrochlorothiazide, without regard to causality, are listed below:

Body As A Whole: weakness

Digestive: pancreatitis, jaundice (intrahepatic cholestatic jaundice), sialadenitis, cramping, gastric irritation

Hematologic: aplastic anemia, agranulocytosis, leukopenia, hemolytic anemia, thrombocytopenia

Hypersensitivity: purpura, photosensitivity, urticaria, necrotizing angiitis (vasculitis and cutaneous vasculitis), fever, respiratory distress including pneumonitis and pulmonary edema, anaphylactic reactions

Metabolic: hyperglycemia, glycosuria, hyperuricemia

Musculoskeletal: muscle spasm

Nervous System/Psychiatric: restlessness

Renal: renal failure, renal dysfunction, interstitial nephritis

Skin: erythema multiforme including Stevens-Johnson syndrome, exfoliative dermatitis including toxic epidermal necrolysis

Special Senses: transient blurred vision, xanthopsia

Clinical Laboratory Test Findings

In controlled clinical trials, clinically important changes in standard laboratory parameters were rarely associated with administration of Diovan HCT.

Creatinine/Blood Urea Nitrogen (BUN): Minor elevations in creatinine and BUN occurred in 2% and 15% respectively, of patients taking Diovan HCT and 0.4% and 6% respectively, given placebo in controlled clinical trials

Hemoglobin and Hematocrit: Greater than 20% decreases in hemoglobin and hematocrit were observed in less than 0.1% of Diovan HCT patients, compared with 0% in placebo-treated patients

Liver Function Tests: Occasional elevations (greater than 150%) of liver chemistries occurred in Diovan HCT-treated patients

Neutropenia: Neutropenia was observed in 0.1% of patients treated with Diovan HCT and 0.4% of patients treated with placebo

6.2 Postmarketing Experience

The following additional adverse reactions have been reported in valsartan or valsartan/hydrochlorothiazide postmarketing experience. Because these reactions are reported voluntarily from a population of uncertain size, it is not always possible to reliably estimate their frequency or establish a causal relationship to drug exposure.

Hypersensitivity: There are rare reports of angioedema. Some of these patients previously experienced angioedema with other drugs including ACE inhibitors. Diovan HCT should not be re-administered to patients who have had angioedema.

Digestive: Elevated liver enzymes and very rare reports of hepatitis

Renal: Impaired renal function

Clinical Laboratory Tests: Hyperkalemia

Dermatologic: Alopecia, bullous dermatitis

Vascular: Vasculitis

Nervous System: Syncope

Rare cases of rhabdomyolysis have been reported in patients receiving angiotensin II receptor blockers.

Hydrochlorothiazide:

The following additional adverse reactions have been reported in post-marketing experience with hydrochlorothiazide:

Acute renal failure, renal disorder, aplastic anemia, erythema multiforme, pyrexia, muscle spasm, asthenia, acute angle-closure glaucoma, bone marrow failure, worsening of diabetes control, hypokalemia, blood lipids increased, hyponatremia, hypomagnesemia, hypercalcemia, hypochloremic alkalosis, impotence, and visual impairment.

Pathological changes in the parathyroid gland of patients with hypercalcemia and hypophosphatemia have been observed in a few patients on prolonged thiazide therapy. If hypercalcemia occurs, further diagnostic evaluation is necessary.

7 DRUG INTERACTIONS

Valsartan-Hydrochlorothiazide:

Lithium: Increases in serum lithium concentrations and lithium toxicity have been reported during concomitant administration of lithium with angiotensin II receptor antagonists or thiazides. Monitor lithium levels in patients taking Diovan HCT.

Valsartan: No clinically significant pharmacokinetic interactions were observed when valsartan was coadministered with amlodipine, atenolol, cimetidine, digoxin, furosemide, glyburide, hydrochlorothiazide, or indomethacin. The valsartan-atenolol combination was more antihypertensive than either component, but it did not lower the heart rate more than atenolol alone.

Coadministration of valsartan and warfarin did not change the pharmacokinetics of valsartan or the time-course of the anticoagulant properties of warfarin.

CYP 450 Interactions: In vitro metabolism studies indicate that CYP 450 mediated drug interactions between valsartan and coadministered drugs are unlikely because of the low extent of metabolism [see Clinical Pharmacology (12.3)].

Transporters: The results from an in vitro study with human liver tissue indicate that valsartan is a substrate of the hepatic uptake transporter OATP1B1 and the hepatic efflux transporter MRP2. Coadministration of inhibitors of the uptake transporter (rifampin, cyclosporine) or efflux transporter (ritonavir) may increase the systemic exposure to valsartan.

Non-Steroidal Anti-Inflammatory Agents including Selective Cyclooxygenase-2 Inhibitors (COX-2 Inhibitors): In patients who are elderly, volume-depleted (including those on diuretic therapy), or with compromised renal function, coadministration of NSAIDs, including selective COX-2 inhibitors, with angiotensin II receptor antagonists, including valsartan, may result in deterioration of renal function, including possible acute renal failure. These effects are usually reversible. Monitor renal function periodically in patients receiving valsartan and NSAID therapy.

The antihypertensive effect of angiotensin II receptor antagonists, including valsartan may be attenuated by NSAIDs including selective COX-2 inhibitors.

Potassium: Concomitant use of valsartan with other agents that block the renin-angiotensin system, potassium sparing diuretics (e.g., spironolactone, triamterene, amiloride), potassium supplements, or salt substitutes containing potassium may lead to increases in serum potassium and in heart failure patients to increases in serum creatinine. If comedication is considered necessary, monitoring of serum potassium is advisable.

Dual Blockade of the Renin-Angiotensin System (RAS): Dual blockade of the RAS with angiotensin receptor blockers, ACE inhibitors, or aliskiren is associated with increased risks of hypotension, hyperkalemia, and changes in renal function (including acute renal failure) compared to monotherapy. Closely monitor blood pressure, renal function, and electrolytes in patients on Diovan HCT and other agents that affect the RAS.

Do not coadminister aliskiren with Diovan HCT in patients with diabetes. Avoid use of aliskiren with Diovan HCT in patients with renal impairment (GFR <60 mL/min).

Hydrochlorothiazide: When administered concurrently, the following drugs may interact with thiazide diuretics:

Antidiabetic Drugs (oral agents and insulin) - Dosage adjustment of the antidiabetic drug may be required.

Nonsteroidal Anti-inflammatory Drugs (NSAIDs and COX-2 selective inhibitors) - When Diovan HCT and nonsteroidal anti-inflammatory agents are used concomitantly, the patient should be observed closely to determine if the desired effect of the diuretic is obtained.

Carbamazepine – May lead to symptomatic hyponatremia.

Ion exchange resins: Staggering the dosage of hydrochlorothiazide and ion exchange resins (e.g., cholestyramine, colestipol) such that hydrochlorothiazide is administered at least 4 hours before or 4 to 6 hours after the administration of resins would potentially minimize the interaction [see Clinical Pharmacology (12.3)].

Cyclosporine: Concomitant treatment with cyclosporine may increase the risk of hyperuricemia and gout-type complications.

8 USE IN SPECIFIC POPULATIONS

8.1 Pregnancy

Pregnancy Category D

Use of drugs that act on the renin-angiotensin system during the second and third trimesters of pregnancy reduces fetal renal function and increases fetal and neonatal morbidity and death. Resulting oligohydramnios can be associated with fetal lung hypoplasia and skeletal deformations. Potential neonatal adverse effects include skull hypoplasia, anuria, hypotension, renal failure, and death. When pregnancy is detected, discontinue Diovan HCT as soon as possible. These adverse outcomes are usually associated with use of these drugs in the second and third trimester of pregnancy. Most epidemiologic studies examining fetal abnormalities after exposure to antihypertensive use in the first trimester have not distinguished drugs affecting the renin-angiotensin system from other antihypertensive agents. Appropriate management of maternal hypertension during pregnancy is important to optimize outcomes for both mother and fetus.

In the unusual case that there is no appropriate alternative to therapy with drugs affecting the renin-angiotensin system for a particular patient, apprise the mother of the potential risk to the fetus. Perform serial ultrasound examinations to assess the intra-amniotic environment. If oligohydramnios is observed, discontinue Diovan HCT, unless it is considered lifesaving for the mother. Fetal testing may be appropriate, based on the week of pregnancy. Patients and physicians should be aware, however, that oligohydramnios may not appear until after the fetus has sustained irreversible injury. Closely observe infants with histories of in utero exposure to Diovan HCT for hypotension, oliguria, and hyperkalemia *[see Use in Specific Populations (8.4)]*.

Hydrochlorothiazide
Thiazides can cross the placenta, and concentrations reached in the umbilical vein approach those in the maternal plasma. Hydrochlorothiazide, like other diuretics, can cause placental hypoperfusion. It accumulates in the amniotic fluid, with reported concentrations up to 19 times higher than in umbilical vein plasma. Use of thiazides during pregnancy is associated with a risk of fetal or neonatal jaundice or thrombocytopenia. Since they do not prevent or alter the course of EPH (Edema, Proteinuria, Hypertension) gestosis (pre-eclampsia), these drugs should not be used to treat hypertension in pregnant women. The use of hydrochlorothiazide for other indications (e.g., heart disease) in pregnancy should be avoided.

8.3 Nursing Mothers
It is not known whether valsartan is excreted in human milk. Valsartan was excreted into the milk of lactating rats; however, animal breast milk drug levels may not accurately reflect human breast milk levels. Hydrochlorothiazide is excreted in human breast milk. Because many drugs are excreted into human milk and because of the potential for adverse reactions in nursing infants from Diovan HCT, a decision should be made whether to discontinue nursing or discontinue the drug, taking into account the importance of the drug to the mother.

8.4 Pediatric Use
Safety and effectiveness of Diovan HCT in pediatric patients have not been established.
Neonates with a history of in utero exposure to Diovan HCT:
If oliguria or hypotension occurs, direct attention toward support of blood pressure and renal perfusion. Exchange transfusions or dialysis may be required as a means of reversing hypotension and/or substituting for disordered renal function.

8.5 Geriatric Use
In the controlled clinical trials of Diovan HCT, 764 (17.5%) patients treated with valsartan-hydrochlorothiazide were ≥65 years and 118 (2.7%) were ≥75 years. No overall difference in the efficacy or safety of valsartan-hydrochlorothiazide was observed between these patients and younger patients, but greater sensitivity of some older individuals cannot be ruled out.

8.6 Renal Impairment
Safety and effectiveness of Diovan HCT in patients with severe renal impairment (CrCl ≤30 mL/min) have not been established. No dose adjustment is required in patients with mild (CrCl 60 to 90 mL/min) or moderate (CrCl 30 to 60 mL/min) renal impairment.

8.7 Hepatic Impairment
Valsartan
No dose adjustment is necessary for patients with mild-to-moderate liver disease. No dosing recommendations can be provided for patients with severe liver disease.
Hydrochlorothiazide
Minor alterations of fluid and electrolyte balance may precipitate hepatic coma in patients with impaired hepatic function or progressive liver disease.

10 OVERDOSAGE
Valsartan – Hydrochlorothiazide: Limited data are available related to overdosage in humans. The most likely manifestations of overdosage would be hypotension and tachycardia; bradycardia could occur from parasympathetic (vagal) stimulation. Depressed level of consciousness, circulatory collapse and shock have been reported. If symptomatic hypotension should occur, supportive treatment should be instituted.
Valsartan is not removed from the plasma by dialysis.
The degree to which hydrochlorothiazide is removed by hemodialysis has not been established. The most common signs and symptoms observed in patients are those caused by electrolyte depletion (hypokalemia, hypochloremia, hyponatremia) and dehydration resulting from excessive diuresis. If digitalis has also been administered, hypokalemia may accentuate cardiac arrhythmias.

In rats and marmosets, single oral doses of valsartan up to 1524 and 762 mg/kg in combination with hydrochlorothiazide at doses up to 476 and 238 mg/kg, respectively, were very well tolerated without any treatment-related effects. These no adverse effect doses in rats and marmosets, respectively, represent 46.5 and 23 times the maximum recommended human dose (MRHD) of valsartan and 188 and 113 times the MRHD of hydrochlorothiazide on a mg/m^2 basis. (Calculations assume an oral dose of 320 mg/day valsartan in combination with 25 mg/day hydrochlorothiazide and a 60-kg patient.)

Valsartan: Valsartan was without grossly observable adverse effects at single oral doses up to 2000 mg/kg in rats and up to 1000 mg/kg in marmosets, except for salivation and diarrhea in the rat and vomiting in the marmoset at the highest dose (60 and 31 times, respectively, the MRHD on a mg/m^2 basis). (Calculations assume an oral dose of 320 mg/day and a 60-kg patient.)

Hydrochlorothiazide: The oral LD$_{50}$ of hydrochlorothiazide is greater than 10 g/kg in both mice and rats, which represents 2027 and 4054 times, respectively, the MRHD on a mg/m^2 basis. (Calculations assume an oral dose of 25 mg/day and a 60-kg patient.)

11 DESCRIPTION
Diovan HCT (valsartan and hydrochlorothiazide, USP) is a combination of valsartan, an orally active, specific angiotensin II receptor blocker (ARB) acting on the AT$_1$ receptor subtype, and hydrochlorothiazide, a diuretic.
Valsartan, a nonpeptide molecule, is chemically described as *N*-(1-oxopentyl)-*N*-[[2′-(1*H*-tetrazol-5-yl)[1,1′-biphenyl]-4-yl]methyl]-L-Valine. Its empirical formula is C$_{24}$H$_{29}$N$_5$O$_3$, its molecular weight is 435.5, and its structural formula is:

Valsartan is a white to practically white fine powder. It is soluble in ethanol and methanol and slightly soluble in water.
Hydrochlorothiazide USP is a white, or practically white, practically odorless, crystalline powder. It is slightly soluble in water; freely soluble in sodium hydroxide solution, in *n*-butylamine, and in dimethylformamide; sparingly soluble in methanol; and insoluble in ether, in chloroform, and in dilute mineral acids. Hydrochlorothiazide is chemically described as 6-chloro-3,4-dihydro-2*H*-1,2,4-benzothiadiazine-7-sulfonamide 1,1-dioxide.
Hydrochlorothiazide is a thiazide diuretic. Its empirical formula is C$_7$H$_8$ClN$_3$O$_4$S$_2$, its molecular weight is 297.73, and its structural formula is:

Diovan HCT tablets are formulated for oral administration to contain valsartan and hydrochlorothiazide, USP 80/12.5 mg, 160/12.5 mg, 160/25 mg, 320/12.5 mg, and 320/25 mg. The inactive ingredients of the tablets are colloidal silicon dioxide, crospovidone, hydroxypropyl methylcellulose, iron oxides, magnesium stearate, microcrystalline cellulose, polyethylene glycol, talc, and titanium dioxide.

12 CLINICAL PHARMACOLOGY
12.1 Mechanism of Action
Angiotensin II is formed from angiotensin I in a reaction catalyzed by angiotensin-converting enzyme (ACE, kininase II). Angiotensin II is the principal pressor agent of the renin-angiotensin system, with effects that include vasoconstriction, stimulation of synthesis and release of aldosterone, cardiac stimulation, and renal reabsorption of sodium. Valsartan blocks the vasoconstrictor and aldosterone-secreting effects of angiotensin II by selectively blocking the binding of angiotensin II to the AT$_1$ receptor in many tissues, such as vascular smooth muscle and the adrenal gland. Its action is therefore independent of the pathways for angiotensin II synthesis.
There is also an AT$_2$ receptor found in many tissues, but AT$_2$ is not known to be associated with cardiovascular homeostasis. Valsartan has much greater affinity (about 20000-fold) for the AT$_1$ receptor than for the AT$_2$ receptor. The pri-

mary metabolite of valsartan is essentially inactive with an affinity for the AT$_1$ receptor about one 200th that of valsartan itself.
Blockade of the renin-angiotensin system with ACE inhibitors, which inhibit the biosynthesis of angiotensin II from angiotensin I, is widely used in the treatment of hypertension. ACE inhibitors also inhibit the degradation of bradykinin, a reaction also catalyzed by ACE. Because valsartan does not inhibit ACE (kininase II) it does not affect the response to bradykinin. Whether this difference has clinical relevance is not yet known. Valsartan does not bind to or block other hormone receptors or ion channels known to be important in cardiovascular regulation.
Blockade of the angiotensin II receptor inhibits the negative regulatory feedback of angiotensin II on renin secretion, but the resulting increased plasma renin activity and angiotensin II circulating levels do not overcome the effect of valsartan on blood pressure.
Hydrochlorothiazide is a thiazide diuretic. Thiazides affect the renal tubular mechanisms of electrolyte reabsorption, directly increasing excretion of sodium and chloride in approximately equivalent amounts. Indirectly, the diuretic action of hydrochlorothiazide reduces plasma volume, with consequent increases in plasma renin activity, increases in aldosterone secretion, increases in urinary potassium loss, and decreases in serum potassium. The renin-aldosterone link is mediated by angiotensin II, so coadministration of an angiotensin II receptor antagonist tends to reverse the potassium loss associated with these diuretics.
The mechanism of the antihypertensive effect of thiazides is unknown.

12.2 Pharmacodynamics
Valsartan: Valsartan inhibits the pressor effect of angiotensin II infusions. An oral dose of 80 mg inhibits the pressor effect by about 80% at peak with approximately 30% inhibition persisting for 24 hours. No information on the effect of larger doses is available.
Removal of the negative feedback of angiotensin II causes a 2- to 3-fold rise in plasma renin and consequent rise in angiotensin II plasma concentration in hypertensive patients. Minimal decreases in plasma aldosterone were observed after administration of valsartan; very little effect on serum potassium was observed.
Hydrochlorothiazide: After oral administration of hydrochlorothiazide, diuresis begins within 2 hours, peaks in about 4 hours and lasts about 6 to 12 hours.
Drug Interactions
Hydrochlorothiazide:
Alcohol, barbiturates, or narcotics. Potentiation of orthostatic hypotension may occur.
Skeletal muscle relaxants: Possible increased responsiveness to muscle relaxants such as curare derivatives.
Digitalis glycosides. Thiazide-induced hypokalemia or hypomagnesemia may predispose the patient to digoxin toxicity.

12.3 Pharmacokinetics
Valsartan: Valsartan peak plasma concentration is reached 2 to 4 hours after dosing. Valsartan shows biexponential decay kinetics following intravenous administration, with an average elimination half-life of about 6 hours. Absolute bioavailability for the capsule formulation is about 25% (range 10% to 35%). Food decreases the exposure (as measured by AUC) to valsartan by about 40% and peak plasma concentration (C$_{max}$) by about 50%. AUC and C$_{max}$ values of valsartan increase approximately linearly with increasing dose over the clinical dosing range. Valsartan does not accumulate appreciably in plasma following repeated administration.
Hydrochlorothiazide: The estimated absolute bioavailability of hydrochlorothiazide after oral administration is about 70%. Peak plasma hydrochlorothiazide concentrations (C$_{max}$) are reached within 2 to 5 hours after oral administration. There is no clinically significant effect of food on the bioavailability of hydrochlorothiazide.
Hydrochlorothiazide binds to albumin (40% to 70%) and distributes into erythrocytes. Following oral administration, plasma hydrochlorothiazide concentrations decline biexponentially, with a mean distribution half-life of about 2 hours and an elimination half-life of about 10 hours.
Diovan HCT: Diovan HCT may be administered with or without food.
Distribution
Valsartan: The steady state volume of distribution of valsartan after intravenous administration is small (17 L), indicating that valsartan does not distribute into tissues extensively. Valsartan is highly bound to serum proteins (95%), mainly serum albumin.
Metabolism
Valsartan: The primary metabolite, accounting for about 9% of dose, is valeryl 4-hydroxy valsartan. *In vitro* metabolism studies involving recombinant CYP 450 enzymes indicated that CYP 2C9 isoenzyme is responsible for the formation of valeryl-4-hydroxy valsartan. Valsartan does not inhibit CYP 450 isozymes at clinically relevant concentra-

tions. CYP 450 mediated drug interaction between valsartan and coadministered drugs are unlikely because of the low extent of metabolism.

Hydrochlorothiazide: Is not metabolized.

Excretion

Valsartan: Valsartan, when administered as an oral solution, is primarily recovered in feces (about 83% of dose) and urine (about 13% of dose). The recovery is mainly as unchanged drug, with only about 20% of dose recovered as metabolites.

Following intravenous administration, plasma clearance of valsartan is about 2 L/h and its renal clearance is 0.62 L/h (about 30% of total clearance).

Hydrochlorothiazide: About 70% of an orally administered dose of hydrochlorothiazide is eliminated in the urine as unchanged drug.

Special Populations

Geriatric: Exposure (measured by AUC) to valsartan is higher by 70% and the half-life is longer by 35% in the elderly than in the young. A limited amount of data suggest that the systemic clearance of hydrochlorothiazide is reduced in both healthy and hypertensive elderly subjects compared to young healthy volunteers.

Gender: Pharmacokinetics of valsartan do not differ significantly between males and females.

Race: Pharmacokinetic differences due to race have not been studied.

Renal Insufficiency: There is no apparent correlation between renal function (measured by creatinine clearance) and exposure (measured by AUC) to valsartan in patients with different degrees of renal impairment. Valsartan has not been studied in patients with severe impairment of renal function (creatinine clearance <10 mL/min). Valsartan is not removed from the plasma by hemodialysis.

In a study in individuals with impaired renal function, the mean elimination half-life of hydrochlorothiazide was doubled in individuals with mild/moderate renal impairment (30< CrCl <90 mL/min) and tripled in severe renal impairment (CrCl ≤30 mL/min), compared to individuals with normal renal function (CrCl >90 mL/min) [see Use in Specific Populations (8.6)].

Hepatic Insufficiency: On average, patients with mild-to-moderate chronic liver disease have twice the exposure (measured by AUC values) to valsartan of healthy volunteers (matched by age, sex, and weight) [see Use in Specific Populations (8.7)].

Drug Interactions

Hydrochlorothiazide:

Drugs that alter gastrointestinal motility: The bioavailability of thiazide-type diuretics may be increased by anticholinergic agents (e.g., atropine, biperiden), apparently due to a decrease in gastrointestinal motility and the stomach emptying rate. Conversely, pro-kinetic drugs may decrease the bioavailability of thiazide diuretics.

Cholestyramine: In a dedicated drug interaction study, administration of cholestyramine 2 hours before hydrochlorothiazide resulted in a 70% reduction in exposure to hydrochlorothiazide. Further, administration of hydrochlorothiazide 2 hours before cholestyramine resulted in 35% reduction in exposure to hydrochlorothiazide.

Antineoplastic agents (e.g., cyclophosphamide, methotrexate): Concomitant use of thiazide diuretics may reduce renal excretion of cytotoxic agents and enhance their myelosuppressive effects.

13 NONCLINICAL TOXICOLOGY

13.1 Carcinogenesis, Mutagenesis, Impairment of Fertility

Valsartan-Hydrochlorothiazide: No carcinogenicity, mutagenicity, or fertility studies have been conducted with the combination of valsartan and hydrochlorothiazide. However, these studies have been conducted for valsartan as well as hydrochlorothiazide alone. Based on the preclinical safety and human pharmacokinetic studies, there is no indication of any adverse interaction between valsartan and hydrochlorothiazide.

Valsartan: There was no evidence of carcinogenicity when valsartan was administered in the diet to mice and rats for up to 2 years at doses up to 160 and 200 mg/kg/day, respectively. These doses in mice and rats are about 2.6 and 6 times, respectively, the MRHD on a mg/m² basis. (Calculations assume an oral dose of 320 mg/day and a 60-kg patient.)

Mutagenicity assays did not reveal any valsartan-related effects at either the gene or chromosome level. These assays included bacterial mutagenicity tests with *Salmonella* (Ames) and *E. coli*; a gene mutation test with Chinese hamster V79 cells; a cytogenetic test with Chinese hamster ovary cells; and a rat micronucleus test.

Valsartan had no adverse effects on the reproductive performance of male or female rats at oral doses up to 200 mg/kg/day. This dose is about 6 times the MRHD on a mg/m² basis. (Calculations assume an oral dose of 320 mg/day and a 60-kg patient.)

Hydrochlorothiazide: Two-year feeding studies in mice and rats conducted under the auspices of the National Toxicology Program (NTP) uncovered no evidence of a carcinogenic potential of hydrochlorothiazide in female mice (at doses of up to approximately 600 mg/kg/day) or in male and female rats (at doses of up to approximately 100 mg/kg/day). The NTP, however, found equivocal evidence for hepatocarcinogenicity in male mice.

Hydrochlorothiazide was not genotoxic *in vitro* in the Ames mutagenicity assay of *Salmonella Typhimurium* strains TA 98, TA 100, TA 1535, TA 1537, and TA 1538 and in the Chinese Hamster Ovary (CHO) test for chromosomal aberrations, or *in vivo* in assays using mouse germinal cell chromosomes, Chinese hamster bone marrow chromosomes, and the Drosophila sex-linked recessive lethal trait gene. Positive test results were obtained only in the *in vitro* CHO Sister Chromatid Exchange (clastogenicity) and in the Mouse Lymphoma Cell (mutagenicity) assays, using concentrations of hydrochlorothiazide from 43 to 1300 mcgm/mL, and in the Aspergillus Nidulans non-disjunction assay at an unspecified concentration.

Hydrochlorothiazide had no adverse effects on the fertility of mice and rats of either sex in studies wherein these species were exposed, via their diet, to doses of up to 100 and 4 mg/kg, respectively, prior to mating and throughout gestation. These doses of hydrochlorothiazide in mice and rats represent 19 and 1.5 times, respectively, the MRHD on a mg/m² basis. (Calculations assume an oral dose of 25 mg/day and a 60-kg patient.)

13.3 Developmental Toxicity Studies

Valsartan-Hydrochlorothiazide: There was no evidence of teratogenicity in mice, rats, or rabbits treated orally with valsartan at doses up to 600, 100, and 10 mg/kg/day, respectively, in combination with hydrochlorothiazide at doses up to 188, 31, and 3 mg/kg/day. These non-teratogenic doses in mice, rats and rabbits, respectively, represent 9, 3.5, and 0.5 times the MRHD of valsartan and 38, 13, and 2 times the MRHD of hydrochlorothiazide on a mg/m² basis. (Calculations assume an oral dose of 320 mg/day valsartan in combination with 25 mg/day hydrochlorothiazide and a 60-kg patient.)

Fetotoxicity was observed in association with maternal toxicity in rats and rabbits at valsartan doses of ≥200 and 10 mg/kg/day, respectively, in combination with hydrochlorothiazide doses of ≥63 and 3 mg/kg/day. Fetotoxicity in rats was considered to be related to decreased fetal weights and included fetal variations of sternebrae, vertebrae, ribs and/or renal papillae. Fetotoxicity in rabbits included increased numbers of late resorptions with resultant increases in total resorptions, postimplantation losses, and decreased number of live fetuses. The no observed adverse effect doses in mice, rats and rabbits for valsartan were 600, 100, and 3 mg/kg/day, respectively, in combination with hydrochlorothiazide doses of 188, 31, and 1 mg/kg/day. These no adverse effect doses in mice, rats, and rabbits, respectively, represent 9, 3, and 0.18 times the MRHD of valsartan and 38, 13, and 0.5 times the MRHD of hydrochlorothiazide on a mg/m² basis. (Calculations assume an oral dose of 320 mg/day valsartan in combination with 25 mg/day hydrochlorothiazide and a 60-kg patient.)

Valsartan: No teratogenic effects were observed when valsartan was administered to pregnant mice and rats at oral doses up to 600 mg/kg/day and to pregnant rabbits at oral doses up to 10 mg/kg/day. However, significant decreases in fetal weight, pup birth weight, pup survival rate, and slight delays in developmental milestones were observed in studies in which parental rats were treated with valsartan at oral, maternally toxic (reduction in body weight gain and food consumption) doses of 600 mg/kg/day during organogenesis or late gestation and lactation. In rabbits, fetotoxicity (i.e., resorptions, litter loss, abortions, and low body weight) associated with maternal toxicity (mortality) was observed at doses of 5 and 10 mg/kg/day. The no observed adverse effect doses of 600, 200, and 2 mg/kg/day in mice, rats, and rabbits represent 9, 6, and 0.1 times, respectively, the MRHD on a mg/m² basis. (Calculations assume an oral dose of 320 mg/day and a 60-kg patient.)

Hydrochlorothiazide: Under the auspices of the National Toxicology Program, pregnant mice and rats that received hydrochlorothiazide via gavage at doses up to 3000 and 1000 mg/kg/day, respectively, on gestation days 6 through 15 showed no evidence of teratogenicity. These doses of hydrochlorothiazide in mice and rats represent 608 and 405 times, respectively, the MRHD on a mg/m² basis. (Calculations assume an oral dose of 25 mg/day and a 60-kg patient.)

14 CLINICAL STUDIES

14.1 Hypertension

Valsartan-Hydrochlorothiazide: In controlled clinical trials including over 7600 patients, 4372 patients were exposed to valsartan (80, 160, and 320 mg) and concomitant hydrochlorothiazide (12.5 and 25 mg). Two factorial trials compared various combinations of 80/12.5 mg, 80/25 mg, 160/12.5 mg, 160/25 mg, 320/12.5 mg, and 320/25 mg with

their respective components and placebo. The combination of valsartan and hydrochlorothiazide resulted in additive placebo-adjusted decreases in systolic and diastolic blood pressure at trough of 14-21/8-11 mmHg at 80/12.5 mg to 320/25 mg, compared to 7-10/4-5 mmHg for valsartan 80 mg to 320 mg, and 5-11/2-5 mmHg for hydrochlorothiazide 12.5 mg to 25 mg alone.

Three other controlled trials investigated the addition of hydrochlorothiazide to patients who did not respond adequately to valsartan 80 mg to valsartan 320 mg, resulted in the additional lowering of systolic and diastolic blood pressure by approximately 4-12/2-5 mmHg.

The maximal antihypertensive effect was attained 4 weeks after the initiation of therapy, the first time point at which blood pressure was measured in these trials.

In long-term follow-up studies (without placebo control) the effect of the combination of valsartan and hydrochlorothiazide appeared to be maintained for up to 2 years. The antihypertensive effect is independent of age or gender. The overall response to the combination was similar for black and non-black patients.

There was essentially no change in heart rate in patients treated with the combination of valsartan and hydrochlorothiazide in controlled trials.

There are no trials of the Diovan HCT combination tablet demonstrating reductions in cardiovascular risk in patients with hypertension, but the hydrochlorothiazide component and several ARBs, which are the same pharmacological class as the valsartan component, have demonstrated such benefits.

Valsartan: The antihypertensive effects of valsartan were demonstrated principally in 7 placebo-controlled, 4- to 12-week trials (1 in patients over 65 years) of dosages from 10 to 320 mg/day in patients with baseline diastolic blood pressures of 95-115 mmHg. The studies allowed comparison of once-daily and twice-daily regimens of 160 mg/day; comparison of peak and trough effects; comparison (in pooled data) of response by gender, age, and race; and evaluation of incremental effects of hydrochlorothiazide.

Administration of valsartan to patients with essential hypertension results in a significant reduction of sitting, supine, and standing systolic and diastolic blood pressure, usually with little or no orthostatic change.

In most patients, after administration of a single oral dose, onset of antihypertensive activity occurs at approximately 2 hours, and maximum reduction of blood pressure is achieved within 6 hours. The antihypertensive effect persists for 24 hours after dosing, but there is a decrease from peak effect at lower doses (40 mg) presumably reflecting loss of inhibition of angiotensin II. At higher doses, however (160 mg), there is little difference in peak and trough effect. During repeated dosing, the reduction in blood pressure with any dose is substantially present within 2 weeks, and maximal reduction is generally attained after 4 weeks. In long-term follow-up studies (without placebo control) the effect of valsartan appeared to be maintained for up to 2 years. The antihypertensive effect is independent of age, gender or race. The latter finding regarding race is based on pooled data and should be viewed with caution, because antihypertensive drugs that affect the renin-angiotensin system (that is, ACE inhibitors and angiotensin II blockers) have generally been found to be less effective in low-renin hypertensives (frequently blacks) than in high-renin hypertensives (frequently whites). In pooled, randomized, controlled trials of Diovan that included a total of 140 blacks and 830 whites, valsartan and an ACE-inhibitor control were generally at least as effective in blacks as whites. The explanation for this difference from previous findings is unclear.

Abrupt withdrawal of valsartan has not been associated with a rapid increase in blood pressure.

The 7 studies of valsartan monotherapy included over 2000 patients randomized to various doses of valsartan and about 800 patients randomized to placebo. Doses below 80 mg were not consistently distinguished from those of placebo at trough, but doses of 80, 160 and 320 mg produced dose-related decreases in systolic and diastolic blood pressure, with the difference from placebo of approximately 6-9/3-5 mmHg at 80 to 160 mg and 9/6 mmHg at 320 mg.

Patients with an inadequate response to 80 mg once daily were titrated to either 160 mg once daily or 80 mg twice daily, which resulted in a comparable response in both groups.

In another 4-week study, 1876 patients randomized to valsartan 320 mg once daily had an incremental blood pressure reduction 3/1 mmHg lower than did 1900 patients randomized to valsartan 160 mg once daily.

In controlled trials, the antihypertensive effect of once daily valsartan 80 mg was similar to that of once daily enalapril 20 mg or once daily lisinopril 10 mg.

There was essentially no change in heart rate in valsartan-treated patients in controlled trials.

14.2 Initial Therapy - Hypertension

The safety and efficacy of Diovan HCT as initial therapy for patients with severe hypertension (defined as a sitting diastolic blood pressure ≥110 mmHg and systolic blood pressure ≥140 mmHg off all antihypertensive therapy) was studied in a 6-week multicenter, randomized, double-blind study. Patients were randomized to either Diovan HCT (valsartan and hydrochlorothiazide 160/12.5 mg once daily) or to valsartan (160 mg once daily) and followed for blood pressure response. Patients were force-titrated at 2-week intervals. Patients on combination therapy were subsequently titrated to 160/25 mg followed by 320/25 mg valsartan/hydrochlorothiazide. Patients on monotherapy were subsequently titrated to 320 mg valsartan followed by a titration to 320 mg valsartan to maintain the blind.

The study randomized 608 patients, including 261 (43%) females, 147 (24%) blacks, and 75 (12%) ≥65 years of age. The mean blood pressure at baseline for the total population was 168/112 mmHg. The mean age was 52 years. After 4 weeks of therapy, reductions in systolic and diastolic blood pressure were 9/5 mmHg greater in the group treated with Diovan HCT compared to valsartan. Similar trends were seen when the patients were grouped according to gender, race, or age.

16 HOW SUPPLIED/STORAGE AND HANDLING

Diovan HCT (valsartan and hydrochlorothiazide, USP) is available as non-scored tablets containing valsartan/hydrochlorothiazide 80/12.5 mg, 160/12.5 mg, 160/25 mg, 320/12.5 mg, and 320/25 mg. Strengths are available as follows.

80/12.5 mg Tablet - Light orange, ovaloid, with slightly convex faces debossed CG on 1 side and HGH on the other side.

Bottles of 90	NDC 0078-0314-34
Bottles of 14,000	NDC 0078-0314-33
Unit Dose (blister pack) Box of 100 (strips of 10)	NDC 0078-0314-06

160/12.5 mg Tablet - Dark red, ovaloid, with slightly convex faces debossed CG on 1 side and HHH on the other side.

Bottles of 90	NDC 0078-0315-34
Bottles of 7,000	NDC 0078-0315-17
Unit Dose (blister pack) Box of 100 (strips of 10)	NDC 0078-0315-06
Unit Dose (blister pack of 30)	NDC 0078-0315-15

160/25 mg Tablet - Brown orange, ovaloid, with slightly convex faces debossed NVR on 1 side and HXH on the other side.

Bottles of 90	NDC 0078-0383-34
Bottles of 7,000	NDC 0078-0383-17
Unit Dose (blister pack) Box of 100 (strips of 10)	NDC 0078-0383-06
Unit Dose (blister pack of 30)	NDC 0078-0383-15

320/12.5 mg Tablet - Pink, ovaloid, with beveled edge, debossed NVR on 1 side and HIL on the other side.

Bottles of 90	NDC 0078-0471-34
Bottles of 3,500	NDC 0078-0471-11
Unit Dose (blister pack) Box of 100 (strips of 10)	NDC 0078-0471-06
Unit Dose (blister pack of 30)	NDC 0078-0471-15

320/25 mg Tablet - Yellow, ovaloid, with beveled edge, debossed NVR on 1 side and CTI on the other side.

Bottles of 90	NDC 0078-0472-34
Bottles of 3,500	NDC 0078-0472-11
Unit Dose (blister pack) Box of 100 (strips of 10)	NDC 0078-0472-06
Unit Dose (blister pack of 30)	NDC 0078-0472-15

Store at 25°C (77°F); excursions permitted to 15-30°C (59-86°F) [see USP Controlled Room Temperature].
Protect from moisture.
Dispense in tight container (USP).

17 PATIENT COUNSELING INFORMATION

Information for Patients

Pregnancy: Female patients of childbearing age should be told about the consequences of exposure to Diovan HCT during pregnancy. Discuss treatment options with women planning to become pregnant. Patients should be asked to report pregnancies to their physicians as soon as possible.

Symptomatic Hypotension: A patient receiving Diovan HCT should be cautioned that lightheadedness can occur, especially during the first days of therapy, and that it should be reported to the prescribing physician. The patients should be told that if syncope occurs, Diovan HCT should be discontinued until the physician has been consulted.

All patients should be cautioned that inadequate fluid intake, excessive perspiration, diarrhea, or vomiting can lead to an excessive fall in blood pressure, with the same consequences of lightheadedness and possible syncope.

Potassium Supplements: A patient receiving Diovan HCT should be told not to use potassium supplements or salt substitutes containing potassium without consulting the prescribing physician.

T2014-30
March 2014

FDA-Approved Patient Labeling
PATIENT INFORMATION
DIOVAN HCT (DYE'-o-van HCT)
(valsartan and hydrochlorothiazide)
Tablets

Read the Patient Information that comes with DIOVAN HCT before you start taking it and each time you get a refill. There may be new information. This leaflet does not take the place of talking with your doctor about your condition and treatment. If you have any questions about DIOVAN HCT, ask your doctor or pharmacist.

> **What is the most important information I should know about DIOVAN HCT?**
>
> Diovan HCT can cause harm or death to an unborn baby. Talk to your doctor about other ways to lower your blood pressure if you plan to become pregnant. If you get pregnant while taking Diovan HCT, tell your doctor right away.

What is DIOVAN HCT?
DIOVAN HCT contains 2 prescription medicines:
1. valsartan, an angiotensin receptor blocker (ARB)
2. hydrochlorothiazide (HCTZ), a water pill (diuretic)
DIOVAN HCT may be used to lower high blood pressure (hypertension) in adults-
* when 1 medicine to lower your high blood pressure is not enough.
* as the first medicine to lower high blood pressure if your doctor decides you are likely to need more than 1 medicine.
DIOVAN HCT has not been studied in children under 18 years of age.

Who should not take DIOVAN HCT?
Do not take DIOVAN HCT if you:
* are allergic to any of the ingredients in DIOVAN HCT. See the end of this leaflet for a complete list of ingredients in DIOVAN HCT.
* make less urine due to kidney problems.
* are allergic to medicines that contain sulfonamides.

What should I tell my doctor before taking DIOVAN HCT?
Tell your doctor about all your medical conditions including if you:
* are pregnant or plan to become pregnant. See "What is the most important information I should know about DIOVAN HCT?"
* are breastfeeding. DIOVAN HCT passes into breast milk. You should choose either to take DIOVAN HCT or breast-feed, but not both.
* have liver problems
* have kidney problems
* have or had gallstones
* have Lupus
* have low levels of potassium (with or without symptoms such as muscle weakness, muscle spasms, abnormal heart rhythm) or magnesium in your blood
* have high levels of calcium in your blood (with or without symptoms such as nausea, vomiting, constipation, stomach pain, frequent urination, thirst, muscle weakness and twitching).
* have high levels of uric acid in the blood.
* have ever had a reaction called angioedema, to another blood pressure medication. Angioedema causes swelling of the face, lips, tongue, throat and may cause difficulty breathing.
Tell your doctor about all the medicines you take including prescription and nonprescription medicines, vitamins and herbal supplements. Some of your other medicines and DIOVAN HCT could affect each other, causing serious side effects. Especially, tell your doctor if you take:
* other medicines for high blood pressure or a heart problem
* water pills (diuretics)
* potassium supplements. Your doctor may check the amount of potassium in your blood periodically.
* a salt substitute. Your doctor may check the amount of potassium in your blood periodically.
* antidiabetic medicines including insulin
* narcotic pain medicines
* sleeping pills
* lithium, a medicine used in some types of depression (Eskalith®, Lithobid®, Lithium Carbonate, Lithium Citrate)
* aspirin or other medicines called Non-Steroidal Anti-Inflammatory Drugs (NSAIDs), like ibuprofen or naproxen
* digoxin or other digitalis glycosides (a heart medicine)
* muscle relaxants (medicines used during operations)
* certain cancer medicines, like cyclophosphamide or methotrexate

---

* certain antibiotics (rifamycin group), a drug used to protect against transplant rejection (cyclosporin) or an anti-retroviral drug used to treat HIV/AIDS infection (ritonavir). These drugs may increase the effect of valsartan.
Ask your doctor if you are not sure if you are taking 1 of these medicines.
Know the medicines you take. Keep a list of your medicines with you to show to your doctor and pharmacist when a new medicine is prescribed. Talk to your doctor or pharmacist before you start taking any new medicine. Your doctor or pharmacist will know what medicines are safe to take together.

How should I take DIOVAN HCT?
* Take DIOVAN HCT exactly as prescribed by your doctor. Your doctor may change your dose if needed.
* Take DIOVAN HCT once each day.
* DIOVAN HCT can be taken with or without food.
* If you miss a dose, take it as soon as you remember. If it is close to your next dose, do not take the missed dose. Just take the next dose at your regular time.
* If you take too much DIOVAN HCT, call your doctor or Poison Control Center, or go to the nearest hospital emergency room.

What should I avoid while taking DIOVAN HCT?
You should not take DIOVAN HCT during pregnancy. See "What is the most important information I should know about DIOVAN HCT?"

What are the possible side effects of DIOVAN HCT?
DIOVAN HCT may cause serious side effects including:
* **Harm to an unborn baby** causing injury and even death. See "What is the most important information I should know about DIOVAN HCT?"
* **Low blood pressure (hypotension).** Low blood pressure is most likely to happen if you:
  ○ take water pills
  ○ are on a low salt diet
  ○ get dialysis treatments
  ○ have heart problems
  ○ get sick with vomiting or diarrhea
  ○ drink alcohol
Lie down if you feel faint or dizzy. Call your doctor right away.
* **Allergic reactions.** People with and without allergy problems or asthma who take DIOVAN HCT may get allergic reactions.
* **Worsening of Lupus.** Hydrochlorothiazide, 1 of the medicines in DIOVAN HCT may cause Lupus to become active or worse.
* **Fluid and electrolyte (salt) problems.** Tell your doctor about any of the following signs and symptoms of fluid and electrolyte problems:

• dry mouth	• drowsiness	• muscle fatigue
• thirst	• restlessness	• very low urine
• lack of energy	• confusion	output
(lethargic)	• seizures	• fast heartbeat
• weakness	• muscle pain or	• nausea and
	cramps	vomiting

* **Kidney problems.** Kidney problems may become worse in people that already have kidney disease. Some people will have changes on blood tests for kidney function and may need a lower dose of DIOVAN HCT. Call your doctor if you get swelling in your feet, ankles, or hands, or unexplained weight gain. If you have heart failure, your doctor should check your kidney function before prescribing DIOVAN HCT.
* **Skin rash.** Call your doctor right away if you have an unusual skin rash.
* **Eye Problems.** One of the medicines in DIOVAN HCT can cause eye problems that may lead to vision loss. Symptoms of eye problems can happen within hours to weeks of starting DIOVAN HCT. Tell your doctor right away if you have:
  • decrease in vision
  • eye pain
Other side effects were generally mild and brief. They generally have not caused patients to stop taking DIOVAN HCT.
Tell your doctor if you have any side effect that bothers you or that does not go away.
These are not all the possible side effects of DIOVAN HCT. For a complete list, ask your doctor or pharmacist.
Call your doctor for medical advice about side effects. You may report side effects to FDA at 1-800-FDA-1088.

How do I store DIOVAN HCT?
* Store DIOVAN HCT tablets at room temperature between 59°F to 86°F (15°C to 30°C).
* Keep DIOVAN HCT in a closed container in a dry place.
Keep DIOVAN HCT and all medicines out of the reach of children.

General information about DIOVAN HCT

Medicines are sometimes prescribed for conditions that are not mentioned in patient information leaflets. Do not use DIOVAN HCT for a condition for which it was not prescribed. Do not give DIOVAN HCT to other people, even if they have the same symptoms you have. It may harm them. This leaflet summarizes the most important information about DIOVAN HCT. If you would like more information, talk with your doctor. You can ask your doctor or pharmacist for information about DIOVAN HCT that is written for health professionals. For more information about DIOVAN HCT, go to www.DIOVAN.com or call 1-866-404-6359.

What are the ingredients in DIOVAN HCT?

Active ingredients: Valsartan and hydrochlorothiazide
Inactive ingredients: colloidal silicon dioxide, crospovidone, hydroxypropyl methylcellulose, iron oxides, magnesium stearate, microcrystalline cellulose, polyethylene glycol, talc, and titanium dioxide.

What is high blood pressure (hypertension)?

Blood pressure is the force in your blood vessels when your heart beats and when your heart rests. You have high blood pressure when the force is too much. DIOVAN HCT can help your blood vessels relax and reduce the amount of water in your body so your blood pressure is lower. Medicines that lower blood pressure lower your risk of having a stroke or heart attack.

High blood pressure makes the heart work harder to pump blood throughout the body and causes damage to the blood vessels. If high blood pressure is not treated, it can lead to stroke, heart attack, heart failure, kidney failure, and vision problems.

Eskalith® and Lithobid® are registered trademarks of Noven Pharmaceuticals, Inc.
Distributed by:
Novartis Pharmaceuticals Corporation
East Hanover, New Jersey 07936
© Novartis
T2014-31
March 2014
Shown in Product Identification Guide, page 310

EXELON® PATCH
[ĕx´ə-lŏn]
(rivastigmine transdermal system)

℞

The following prescribing information is based on official labeling in effect July 2013.

HIGHLIGHTS OF PRESCRIBING INFORMATION

These highlights do not include all the information needed to use EXELON PATCH safely and effectively. See full prescribing information for EXELON PATCH.
EXELON® PATCH (rivastigmine transdermal system)
Initial U.S. Approval: 2000

———RECENT MAJOR CHANGES———
Indications and Usage (1.1)   06/2013
Dosage and Administration (2.1, 2.2)   06/2013
Contraindications (4)   06/2013
Warnings and Precautions (5.3)   06/2013

———INDICATIONS AND USAGE———
Exelon Patch is an acetylcholinesterase inhibitor indicated for treatment of:
• Mild, moderate, and severe dementia of the Alzheimer's type (1.1)
• Mild to moderate dementia associated with Parkinson's disease (1.2)

———DOSAGE AND ADMINISTRATION———
• Apply patch on intact skin for a 24-hour period; replace with a new patch every 24 hours (2.1, 2.4)
• **Initiate treatment with 4.6 mg/24 hours Exelon Patch (2.1)**
• **After a minimum of 4 weeks, if tolerated, increase dose to 9.5 mg/24 hours, which is the minimum effective dose (2.1)**
• **Following a minimum additional 4 weeks, may increase dosage to maximum dosage of 13.3 mg/24 hours (2.1)**
• **Mild to Moderate Alzheimer's Disease and Parkinson's Disease Dementia:** Exelon Patch 9.5 mg/24 hours or 13.3 mg/24 hours once daily (2.1)
• **Severe Alzheimer's Disease:** Exelon Patch 13.3 mg/24 hours once daily (2.1)
• For treatment interruption longer than 3 days, retitrate dosage starting at 4.6 mg/24 hours (2.1)
• Consider dose adjustments in patients with (2.2):
  ◦ Mild to moderate hepatic impairment (8.7)
  ◦ Low (<50 kg) body weight (8.8)

———DOSAGE FORMS AND STRENGTHS———
Exelon Patch: 4.6 mg/24 hours or 9.5 mg/24 hours or 13.3 mg/24 hours (3)

———CONTRAINDICATIONS———
Patients with known hypersensitivity to rivastigmine, other carbamate derivatives, or other components of the formulation or previous history of application site reactions with rivastigmine transdermal patch suggestive of allergic contact dermatitis (4, 6.2)

———WARNINGS AND PRECAUTIONS———
• *Overdose from medication errors:* Hospitalization and, rarely, death have been reported due to application of multiple patches at same time. Ensure patients or caregivers receive instruction on proper dosing and administration. (5.1)
• *Gastrointestinal adverse reactions:* May include significant nausea, vomiting, diarrhea, anorexia/decreased appetite, and weight loss, and may necessitate treatment interruption. Dehydration may result from prolonged vomiting or diarrhea and can be associated with serious outcomes. (5.2)
• *Skin reactions:* Application site reactions may occur with the patch form of rivastigmine. Discontinue treatment if application site reactions spread beyond the patch size, if there is evidence of a more intense local reaction (e.g., increasing erythema, edema, papules, vesicles), and if symptoms do not significantly improve within 48 hours after patch removal. (5.3)

———ADVERSE REACTIONS———
Most commonly observed adverse reactions (>5% and higher than with placebo): Nausea, vomiting, and diarrhea (6.1)

To report SUSPECTED ADVERSE REACTIONS, contact Novartis Pharmaceuticals Corporation at 1-888-669-6682 or FDA at 1-800-FDA-1088 or www.fda.gov/medwatch.

———DRUG INTERACTIONS———
Cholinomimetic and anticholinergic drugs: Avoid concomitant use unless clinically necessary (7.1)

———USE IN SPECIFIC POPULATIONS———
See 17 for PATIENT COUNSELING INFORMATION and FDA-approved patient labeling

Revised: 7/2013

FULL PRESCRIBING INFORMATION: CONTENTS*
* Sections or subsections omitted from the full prescribing information are not listed

FULL PRESCRIBING INFORMATION

1   INDICATIONS AND USAGE
1.1   Alzheimer's Disease
Exelon Patch is indicated for the treatment of dementia of the Alzheimer's type (AD). Efficacy has been demonstrated in patients with mild, moderate, and severe Alzheimer's disease.

1.2   Parkinson's Disease Dementia
Exelon Patch is indicated for the treatment of mild to moderate dementia associated with Parkinson's disease (PDD).

2   DOSAGE AND ADMINISTRATION
2.1   Recommended Dosing
Initial Dose
Initiate treatment with one 4.6 mg/24 hours Exelon Patch applied to the skin once daily [see Dosage and Administration (2.4)].

Dose Titration
Increase the dose only after a minimum of 4 weeks at the previous dose, and only if the previous dose has been well tolerated. For mild to moderate AD and PDD patients continue the recommended effective dose of 9.5 mg/24 hours for as long as therapeutic benefit persists. Patients can then be increased to the maximum effective dose of 13.3 mg/24 hours dose. For patients with severe AD, 13.3 mg/24 hours is the recommended effective dose. Doses higher than 13.3 mg/24 hours confer no appreciable additional benefit, and are associated with an increase in the incidence of adverse reactions [see Warnings and Precautions (5.2), Adverse Reactions (6.1)].

Mild to Moderate Alzheimer's Disease and Mild to Moderate Parkinson's Disease Dementia
The effective dosage of Exelon Patch is 9.5 mg/24 hours or 13.3 mg/24 hours administered once per day; replace with a new patch every 24 hours.

Severe Alzheimer's Disease
The effective dosage of Exelon Patch in patients with severe Alzheimer's disease is 13.3 mg/24 hours administered once per day; replace with a new patch every 24 hours.

Interruption of Treatment
If dosing is interrupted for 3 days or fewer, restart treatment with the same or lower strength Exelon Patch. If dosing is interrupted for more than 3 days, restart treatment with the 4.6 mg/24 hours Exelon Patch and titrate as described above.

2.2   Dosing in Specific Populations
Dosing Modifications in Patients with Hepatic Impairment
Consider using the 4.6 mg/24 hours Exelon Patch as both the initial and maintenance dose in patients with mild (Child-Pugh score 5 to 6) to moderate (Child-Pugh score 7 to 9) hepatic impairment [see Use in Specific Populations (8.7), Clinical Pharmacology (12.3)].
Dosing Modifications in Patients with Low Body Weight
Because rivastigmine blood levels vary with weight [see Use in Specific Populations (8.8), Clinical Pharmacology (12.3)], carefully titrate and monitor patients with low body weight (<50kg) for toxicities (e.g., excessive nausea, vomiting) and consider reducing the maintenance dose to the 4.6 mg/24 hours Exelon Patch if such toxicities develop.

2.3   Switching to Exelon Patch from Exelon Capsules or Exelon Oral Solution
Patients treated with Exelon Capsules or Oral Solution may be switched to Exelon Patch as follows:
• A patient who is on a total daily dose of <6 mg of oral rivastigmine can be switched to the 4.6 mg/24 hours Exelon Patch.
• A patient who is on a total daily dose of 6 mg to 12 mg of oral rivastigmine can be switched to the 9.5 mg/24 hours Exelon Patch.
Instruct patients or caregivers to apply the first patch on the day following the last oral dose.

2.4   Important Administration Instructions
Exelon Patch is for transdermal use on intact skin.
(a) Do not use the patch if the pouch seal is broken or the patch is cut, damaged, or changed in any way.
(b) Apply the Exelon Patch once a day
• Press down firmly for 30 seconds until the edges stick well when applying to clean, dry, hairless, intact healthy skin in a place that will not be rubbed against by tight clothing.
• Use the upper or lower back as the site of application because the patch is less likely to be removed by the patient. If sites on the back are not accessible, apply the patch to the upper arm or chest.
• Do not apply to a skin area where cream, lotion, or powder has recently been applied.
(c) Do not apply to skin that is red, irritated, or cut.
(d) Replace the Exelon Patch with a new patch every 24 hours. Instruct patients to only wear 1 patch at a time (remove the previous day's patch before applying a new patch) [see Warnings and Precautions (5.1) and Overdosage (10)]. If a patch falls off or if a dose is missed, apply a new patch immediately and then replace this patch the following day at the usual application time.
(e) Change the site of patch application daily to minimize potential irritation, although a new patch can be applied to the same general anatomic site (e.g., another spot on the upper back) on consecutive days. Do not apply a new patch to the same location for at least 14 days.
(f) May wear the patch during bathing and in hot weather. But avoid long exposure to external heat sources (excessive sunlight, saunas, solariums).
(g) Place used patches in the previously saved pouch and discard in the trash, away from pets or children.

3 DOSAGE FORMS AND STRENGTHS

Exelon Patch is available in 3 strengths. Each patch has a beige backing layer labeled as either:
- EXELON® PATCH 4.6 mg/24 hours, AMCX
- EXELON® PATCH 9.5 mg/24 hours, BHDI
- EXELON® PATCH 13.3 mg/24 hours, CNFU

4 CONTRAINDICATIONS

Exelon Patch (rivastigmine transdermal system) is contraindicated in patients with:
- known hypersensitivity to rivastigmine, other carbamate derivatives, or other components of the formulation [see Description (11)].
- previous history of application site reactions with rivastigmine transdermal patch suggestive of allergic contact dermatitis [see Warnings and Precautions (5.3)].

Isolated cases of generalized skin reactions have been described in postmarketing experience [see Adverse Reactions (6.2)].

5 WARNINGS AND PRECAUTIONS

5.1 Medication Errors Resulting in Overdose

Medication errors with Exelon Patch have resulted in serious adverse reactions; some cases have required hospitalization, and rarely, led to death. The majority of medication errors have involved not removing the old patch when putting on a new one and the use of multiple patches at one time. Instruct patients and their caregivers on important administration instructions for Exelon Patch. [see Dosage and Administration (2.4)].

5.2 Gastrointestinal Adverse Reactions

Exelon Patch can cause gastrointestinal adverse reactions, including significant nausea, vomiting, diarrhea, anorexia/decreased appetite, and weight loss. Dehydration may result from prolonged vomiting or diarrhea and can be associated with serious outcomes. The incidence and severity of these reactions are dose-related [see Adverse Reactions (6.1)]. For this reason, initiate treatment with Exelon Patch at a dose of 4.6 mg/24 hours and titrate to a dose of 9.5 mg/24 hours and then to a dose of 13.3 mg/24 hours, if appropriate [see Dosage and Administration (2.1)].

If treatment is interrupted for more than 3 days because of intolerance, reinitiate Exelon Patch with the 4.6 mg/24 hours dose to reduce the possibility of severe vomiting and its potentially serious sequelae. A postmarketing report described a case of severe vomiting with esophageal rupture following inappropriate reinitiation of treatment of an oral formulation of rivastigmine without retitration after 8 weeks of treatment interruption.

Inform caregivers to monitor for gastrointestinal adverse reactions and to inform the physician if they occur. It is critical to inform caregivers that if therapy has been interrupted for more than 3 days because of intolerance, the next dose should not be administered without contacting the physician regarding proper retitration.

5.3 Skin Reactions

Skin reactions (application site reactions) may occur with Exelon Patch and are usually mild or moderate in intensity. These reactions are not in themselves an indication of sensitization. However, use of rivastigmine patch may lead to allergic contact dermatitis.

Allergic contact dermatitis should be suspected if application site reactions spread beyond the patch size, if there is evidence of a more intense local reaction (e.g. increasing erythema, edema, papules, vesicles) and if symptoms do not significantly improve within 48 hours after patch removal. In these cases, treatment should be discontinued [see Contraindications (4)].

In patients who develop application site reactions to Exelon Patch suggestive of allergic contact dermatitis and who still require rivastigmine, treatment should be switched to oral rivastigmine only after negative allergy testing and under close medical supervision. It is possible that some patients sensitized to rivastigmine by exposure to rivastigmine patch may not be able to take rivastigmine in any form.

There have been isolated postmarketing reports of patients experiencing disseminated hypersensitivity reactions of the skin when administered rivastigmine irrespective of the route of administration (oral or transdermal). In these cases, treatment should be discontinued [see Contraindications (4)]. Patients and caregivers should be instructed accordingly.

5.4 Other Adverse Reactions from Increased Cholinergic Activity

Neurologic Effects

Extrapyramidal Symptoms: Cholinomimetics, including rivastigmine may exacerbate or induce extrapyramidal symptoms. Worsening of parkinsonism symptoms, particularly tremor, has been observed in patients with dementia associated with Parkinson's disease who were treated with Exelon Capsules.

Seizures: Drugs that increase cholinergic activity are believed to have some potential for causing seizures. However, seizure activity also may be a manifestation of Alzheimer's disease.

Table 1: Proportion of Adverse Reactions Observed with a Frequency of ≥2% and Occurring at a Rate Greater Than Placebo in Study 1

	Exelon Patch 9.5 mg/24 hours	Exelon Patch 17.4 mg/24 hours	Exelon Capsule 6 mg twice daily	Placebo
Total Patients Studied	291	303	294	302
Total Percentage of Patients with ARs (%)	51	66	63	46
Nausea	7	21	23	5
Vomiting*	6	19	17	3
Diarrhea	6	10	5	3
Depression	4	4	4	1
Headache	3	4	6	2
Anxiety	3	3	2	1
Anorexia/Decreased Appetite	3	9	9	2
Weight Decreased**	3	8	5	1
Dizziness	2	7	7	2
Abdominal Pain	2	4	2	1
Urinary Tract Infection	2	2	1	1
Asthenia	2	3	6	1
Fatigue	2	2	1	1
Insomnia	1	4	2	2
Abdominal Pain Upper	1	3	2	2
Vertigo	0	2	1	1

*Vomiting was severe in 0% of patients who received Exelon Patch 9.5 mg/24 hours, 1% of patients who received Exelon Patch 17.4 mg/24 hours, 1% of patients who received the Exelon Capsule at doses up to 6 mg BID, and 0% of those who received placebo.

**Weight Decreased as presented in Table 1 is based upon clinical observations and/or adverse events reported by patients or caregivers. Body weight was also monitored at prespecified time points throughout the course of the clinical study. The proportion of patients who had weight loss equal to or greater than 7% of their baseline weight was 8% of those treated with Exelon Patch 9.5 mg/24 hours, 12% of those treated with Exelon Patch 17.4 mg/24 hours, 11% of patients who received the Exelon Capsule at doses up to 6 mg BID and 6% of those who received placebo. It is not clear how much of the weight loss was associated with anorexia, nausea, vomiting, and the diarrhea associated with the drug.

Peptic Ulcers/Gastrointestinal Bleeding

Cholinesterase inhibitors, including rivastigmine, may increase gastric acid secretion due to increased cholinergic activity. Monitor patients using Exelon Patch for symptoms of active or occult gastrointestinal bleeding, especially those at increased risk for developing ulcers, e.g., those with a history of ulcer disease or those receiving concurrent nonsteroidal anti-inflammatory drugs (NSAIDs). Clinical studies of rivastigmine have shown no significant increase, relative to placebo, in the incidence of either peptic ulcer disease or gastrointestinal bleeding.

Use with Anesthesia

Rivastigmine, as a cholinesterase inhibitor, is likely to exaggerate succinylcholine-type muscle relaxation during anesthesia.

Cardiac Conduction Effects

Because rivastigmine increases cholinergic activity, use of the Exelon Patch may have vagotonic effects on heart rate (e.g., bradycardia). The potential for this action may be particularly important in patients with sick sinus syndrome or other supraventricular cardiac conduction conditions. In clinical trials, rivastigmine was not associated with any increased incidence of cardiovascular adverse events, heart rate or blood pressure changes, or ECG abnormalities.

Genitourinary Effects

Although not observed in clinical trials of rivastigmine, drugs that increase cholinergic activity may cause urinary obstruction.

Pulmonary Effects

Drugs that increase cholinergic activity, including Exelon Patch should be used with care in patients with a history of asthma or obstructive pulmonary disease.

5.5 Impairment in Driving or Use of Machinery

Dementia may cause gradual impairment of driving performance or compromise the ability to use machinery. The administration of rivastigmine may also result in adverse reactions that are detrimental to these functions. During treatment with the Exelon Patch, routinely evaluate the patient's ability to continue driving or operating machinery.

6 ADVERSE REACTIONS

Significant gastrointestinal adverse reactions including nausea, vomiting, anorexia, and weight loss are described below and elsewhere in the labeling [see Warnings and Precautions (5.2)].

6.1 Clinical Trials Experience

Because clinical trials are conducted under widely varying conditions, adverse reaction rates observed in the clinical trials of a drug cannot be directly compared to rates in the clinical trials of another drug and may not reflect the rates observed in practice.

Exelon Patch has been administered to 2348 patients with Alzheimer's disease during clinical trials worldwide. Of these, 1954 patients have been treated for at least 12 weeks, 1643 patients have been treated for at least 24 weeks, and 847 patients have been treated for at least 48 weeks.

Mild to Moderate Alzheimer's Disease

24-Week International Placebo-Controlled Trial (Study 1)

Most Commonly Observed Adverse Reactions

The most commonly observed adverse reactions in patients administered Exelon Patch in Study 1 [see Clinical Studies (14)], defined as those occurring at a frequency of at least 5% in the 9.5 mg/24 hours Exelon Patch arm and at a frequency at higher than in the placebo group, were nausea, vomiting, and diarrhea. These reactions were dose-related, with each being more common in patients using the 17.4 mg/24 hours Exelon Patch than in those using the 9.5 mg/24 hours Exelon Patch.

Discontinuation Rates

In Study 1, which randomized a total of 1195 patients, the proportions of patients in the Exelon Patch 9.5 mg/24 hours, Exelon Capsules 6 mg twice daily, and placebo groups who discontinued treatment due to adverse events were 9.6%, 8.1%, and 5.0%, respectively.

The most common adverse reactions in the Exelon Patch-treated groups that led to treatment discontinuation in this study were nausea and vomiting. The proportions of patients who discontinued treatment due to nausea were 0.7%, 1.7%, and 1.3% in the Exelon Patch 9.5 mg/24 hours, Exelon Capsules 6 mg twice daily, and placebo groups, respectively. The proportions of patients who discontinued treatment due to vomiting were 0%, 2.0%, and 0.3% in the Exelon Patch 9.5 mg/24 hours, Exelon Capsules 6 mg twice daily, and placebo groups, respectively.

Adverse Reactions Observed at an Incidence of ≥2%

Table 1 lists adverse reactions seen at an incidence of ≥2% in either Exelon Patch-treated group in Study 1 and for which the rate of occurrence was greater than for those treated with that dose of Exelon Patch than for those treated with placebo. The unapproved 17.4 mg/24 hours Exelon Patch arm is included to demonstrate the increased rates of gastrointestinal adverse reactions over those seen with the 9.5 mg/24 hours Exelon Patch.

[See table 1 above]

48-Week International Active Comparator-Controlled Trial (Study 2)

Most Commonly Observed Adverse Reactions

In Study 2 [see Clinical Studies (14)] of the commonly observed adverse reactions (≥3% in any treatment group) the most frequent event in the Exelon Patch 13.3 mg/24 hours group was nausea, followed by vomiting, fall, weight decreased, application site erythema, decreased appetite, diarrhea and urinary tract infection (Table 3). The percentage of patients with these events was higher in the Exelon Patch 13.3 mg/24 hours group than in the Exelon Patch 9.5 mg/24 hours group. Patients with nausea, vomiting, diarrhea and decreased appetite experienced these reactions more often during the first 4 weeks of the double-blind treatment phase. These reactions decreased over time in each treatment group. Weight decreased was reported to have increased over time in each treatment group.

Discontinuation Rates

Table 2 displays the most common adverse reactions leading to discontinuation during the 48-week, double-blind treatment phase in Study 2.

Table 2: Proportion of Most Common Adverse Reactions (>1% at Any Dose) Leading to Discontinuation During 48-week Double-Blind Treatment Phase in Study 2

	Exelon Patch 13.3 mg/ 24 hours	Exelon Patch 9.5 mg/ 24 hours	Total
Total Patients Studied	280	283	563
Total Percentage of Patients with ARs Leading to Discontinuation (%)	9.6	12.7	11.2
Vomiting	1.4	0.4	0.9
Application site pruritus	1.1	1.1	1.1
Aggression	0.4	1.1	0.7

Most Commonly Observed Adverse Reactions ≥3%

Other adverse reactions of interest which occurred less frequently, but which were observed in a markedly higher percentage of patients in the Exelon Patch 13.3 mg/24 hours group than in the Exelon Patch 9.5 mg/24 hours group in Study 2, included dizziness and upper abdominal pain. The percentage of patients with these reactions decreased over time in each treatment group (Table 3). The majority of patients reported adverse events of mild to moderate severity. The adverse event severity profile was generally similar for both the Exelon Patch 13.3 mg/24 hours and 9.5 mg/24 hours groups.

[See table 3 below]

Severe Alzheimer's Disease

24-Week US Controlled Trial (Study 3)

Most Commonly Observed Adverse Reactions

The most commonly observed adverse reactions in patients administered Exelon Patch in the controlled clinical trial, defined as those occurring at a frequency of at least 5% in the 13.3 mg/24 hours Exelon Patch arm and at a frequency higher than in the 4.6 mg/24 hours Exelon Patch were: application site erythema, fall, insomnia, vomiting, diarrhea, weight decreased, and nausea (Table 4). Patients in the lower dose group reported more events of agitation, urinary tract infection, and hallucinations than patients in the higher dose group.

Discontinuation Rates

In Study 3 *[see Clinical Studies (14)]*, the proportions of patients in the Exelon Patch 13.3 mg/24 hours (n=355) and

Exelon Patch 4.6 mg/24 hours (n=359), who discontinued treatment due to adverse reactions were 20.5% and 14.2%, respectively.

The most frequent adverse reaction leading to discontinuation in the 13.3 mg/24 hours treatment group versus the 4.6 mg/24 hours treatment group was agitation (2.8% versus 2.2%), followed by vomiting (2.5% and 1.1%), nausea (1.7% and 1.1%), decreased appetite (1.7% and 0%), aggression (1.1% and 0.3%), fall (1.1% and 0.3%) and syncope (1.1% and 0.3%). Otherwise, all AEs leading to discontinuation were reported in <1% of patients.

Most Commonly Observed Adverse Reactions ≥5%

Other adverse reactions of interest which were observed in a higher percentage of patients in the Exelon Patch 13.3 mg/24 hours group than in the Exelon Patch 4.6 mg/24 hours group, included application site erythema, fall, insomnia, vomiting, diarrhea, weight decreased, and nausea (Table 4). Overall, the majority of patients in this study experienced adverse reactions that were mild (30.7%) or moderate (32.1%) in severity. Slightly more patients in the 4.6 mg/24 hours patch group reported mild events than in the 13.3 mg/24 hours patch group, while the numbers of patients reporting moderate events were comparable between groups. Severe adverse reactions were reported at a slightly higher percentage at the higher dose (12.4%) than at the lower dose (10%) treatment groups. With the exception of severe adverse reactions of agitation (13.3 mg: 1.1%; 4.6 mg: 1.4%), fall (13.3 mg: 1.1%) and urinary tract infection (4.6 mg: 1.1%), all adverse reactions reported as severe occurred in less than 1% of patients in either treatment group.

Table 4: Proportion of Adverse Reactions in the 24-week Double-Blind (DB) Treatment Phase (at Least 5% in Any Treatment Group) in Study 3

Preferred term	Exelon Patch 13.3 mg/ 24 hours	Exelon Patch 4.6 mg/ 24 hours
Total number of patients studied	355	359
Total percentage of patients with ARs (%)	75	73
Application site erythema	13	12
Agitation	12	14
Urinary tract infection	8	10
Fall	8	6
Insomnia	7	4

Vomiting	7	3
Diarrhea	7	5
Weight decreased*	7	3
Nausea	6	3
Depression	5	4
Decreased appetite	5	1
Anxiety	5	5
Hallucination	2	5

*Weight Decreased as presented in Table 4 is based upon clinical observations and/or adverse events reported by patients or caregivers. Body weight was monitored as a vital sign at prespecified time points throughout the course of the clinical study. The proportion of patients who had weight loss equal to or greater than 7% of their baseline weight was 11% of those treated with Exelon Patch 4.6 mg/24 hours and 14.1% of those treated with Exelon Patch 13.3 mg/24 hours during the 24-week double-blind treatment.

Application Site Reactions in Studies 1, 2, and 3

A direct comparison of the rates of application site reactions reported in the placebo-controlled and active comparator controlled clinical trials cannot be made due to differences in the method of data collection employed in each of the trials.

In Study 1, cases of skin irritation were captured separately on an investigator-rated skin irritation scale and not as adverse events unless they fulfilled the criteria for a serious adverse event. Among the skin reactions reported were the following: application site reactions, application site dermatitis, and application site irritation.

In Study 2, cases of application site reactions were captured as patient or caregiver reported adverse events. The most commonly reported skin irritation events for both treatment groups were application site erythema and application site pruritus. These events occurred more frequently during the first 24 weeks of the double-blind period and decreased over time in each treatment group after 24 weeks (Table 3). The most common reason for discontinuation due to application site reactions was application site pruritus which occurred in 1.1% of the patients in each treatment group (Table 2).

In Study 3, cases of application site reactions were captured as patient or caregiver reported adverse events. The most commonly reported skin irritation events during the 24 weeks of the study were application site erythema and application site pruritus (Table 4). The most common reason for discontinuation due to application site reactions were application site erythema and application site pruritus which occurred in less than 1% of patients in each treatment group.

Other Adverse Events Observed During Clinical Trials

The frequencies represent the proportion of 2348 patients from 3 controlled and 4 open-label trials in North America, Europe, Latin America, Asia, and Japan who experienced that event while receiving Exelon Patch. All patch doses are pooled.

All adverse events occurring in approximately 0.1% of patients are included, except for those already listed elsewhere in labeling, too general to be informative, or relatively minor events.

Events are classified by system organ class and listed using the following definitions: *Frequent*–those occurring in at least 1/100 patients; *Infrequent*–those occurring in 1/100 to 1/1000 patients. These adverse events are not necessarily related to Exelon Patch treatment and in most cases were observed at a similar frequency in placebo-treated patients in the controlled studies.

Cardiac Disorders: *Infrequent:* Bradycardia, atrial fibrillation, atrioventricular block, arrhythmia, supraventricular extrasystole.

Ear and Labyrinth Disorders: *Infrequent:* Tinnitus.

Eye Disorders: *Infrequent:* Vision blurred.

Gastrointestinal System: *Frequent:* Constipation, gastritis. *Infrequent:* Gastroesophageal reflux disease, hematochezia, hematemesis, pancreatitis, salivary hypersecretion.

General Disorders and Administration Site Conditions: *Infrequent:* Chest pain.

Injury, Poisoning and Procedural Complications: *Infrequent:* Hip fracture.

Investigations: *Infrequent:* Blood creatine phosphokinase increased, lipase increased, blood amylase increased, electrocardiogram QT prolonged.

Metabolic and Nutritional Disorders: *Frequent:* Dehydration. *Infrequent:* Hypokalemia, hyponatremia.

Nervous System Disorders: *Infrequent:* Migraine.

Psychiatric Disorders: *Infrequent:* Delirium.

Respiratory, Thoracic, and Mediastinal Disorders: *Infrequent:* Dyspnea, bronchospasm.

Skin and Subcutaneous Tissue Disorders: *Frequent:* Pruritus. *Infrequent:* Erythema, eczema, dermatitis, rash erythematous, skin ulcer.

Table 3: Proportion of Adverse Reactions Over Time in the 48-week Double-Blind (DB) Treatment Phase (at Least 3% in any Treatment Group) in Study 2

	Cumulative Week 0 to 48 (DB Phase)		Week 0 to 24 (DB Phase)		Week >24 to 48 (DB Phase)	
Preferred Term	Exelon Patch 13.3 mg/ 24 hours	Exelon Patch 9.5 mg/ 24 hours	Exelon Patch 13.3 mg/ 24 hours	Exelon Patch 9.5 mg/ 24 hours	Exelon Patch 13.3 mg/ 24 hours	Exelon Patch 9.5 mg/ 24 hours
Total Patients Studied	280	283	280	283	241	246
Total Percentage of Patients with ARs (%)	75	68	65	55	42	40
Nausea	12	5	10	4	4	2
Vomiting	10	5	9	3	3	2
Fall	8	6	4	4	4	3
Weight decreased*	7	3	3	1	5	2
Application site erythema	6	6	6	5	1	2
Decreased appetite	6	3	5	2	2	<1
Diarrhea	6	5	5	4	2	<1
Urinary tract infection	5	4	3	3	3	2
Agitation	5	5	4	3	1	2
Depression	5	5	3	3	3	2
Dizziness	4	1	3	<1	2	<1
Application site pruritus	4	4	4	3	<1	1
Headache	4	4	4	4	<1	<1
Insomnia	4	3	2	1	3	2
Abdominal pain upper	4	1	3	1	1	<1
Anxiety	4	3	2	2	2	1
Hypertension	3	3	3	2	1	1
Urinary incontinence	3	2	2	2	1	<1
Psychomotor hyperactivity	3	3	2	3	2	1
Aggression	2	3	1	3	1	1

*Decreased Weight as presented in Table 3 is based upon clinical observations and/or adverse events reported by patients or caregivers. Body weight was monitored as a vital sign at pre-specified time points throughout the course of the clinical study. The proportion of patients who had weight loss equal to or greater than 7% of their baseline weight was 15.2% of those treated with Exelon Patch 9.5 mg/24 hours and 18.6% of those treated with Exelon Patch 13.3 mg/24 hours during the 48-week double-blind treatment period.

Vascular Disorders: *Infrequent*: Hypotension, cerebrovascular accident.

Other Adverse Reactions Observed with Exelon Capsules or Oral Solution
The following additional adverse reactions have been observed with Exelon Capsules/Oral Solution:
Confusion, duodenal ulcers, angina pectoris, myocardial infarction, tremor

Parkinson's Disease Dementia
76-week International Open-Label Trial (Study 4)
Exelon Patch has been administered to 288 patients with mild to moderate Parkinson's Disease Dementia in a single, 76-week, open-label, active-comparator safety study. Of these, 256 have been treated for at least 12 weeks, 232 for at least 24 weeks, and 196 for at least 52 weeks.
Treatment with Exelon Patch was initiated at 4.6 mg/24 hours and if well tolerated the dose was increased after 4 weeks to 9.5 mg/24 hours. Exelon Capsule (target maintenance dose of 12 mg/day) served as the active comparator and was administered to 294 patients. Treatment emergent adverse reactions are presented in Table 5.

Table 5: Proportion of Adverse Reactions Reported at a Rate ≥2% During the Initial 24-Week Period in Study 4

Adverse drug reactions	Exelon Patch
Total patients studied	288
	Percentage (%)
Psychiatric disorders	
Insomnia	6
Depression	6
Anxiety	5
Agitation	3
Nervous system disorders	
Tremor	7
Dizziness	6
Somnolence	4
Hypokinesia	4
Bradykinesia	4
Cogwheel rigidity	3
Dyskinesia	3
Gastrointestinal disorders	
Abdominal pain	2
Vascular disorders	
Hypertension	3
General disorders and administration site conditions	
Fall	12
Application site erythema	11
Application site irritation, pruritus, rash	3; 5; 2
Fatigue	4
Asthenia	2
Gait disturbance	4

Additional adverse reactions observed during the 76-week prospective, open-label study in patients with dementia associated with Parkinson's disease treated with Exelon transdermal patches: Frequent (those occurring in at least 1/100 patients): dehydration, weight decreased, aggression, hallucination visual.
In patients with dementia associated with Parkinson's disease the following adverse drug reactions have only been observed in clinical trials with Exelon Capsules: Frequent: nausea, vomiting, decreased appetite, restlessness, worsening of Parkinson's disease, bradycardia, diarrhea, dyspepsia, salivary hypersecretion, sweating increased; Infrequent (those occurring between 1/100 to 1/1000 patients): dystonia, atrial fibrillation, atrioventricular block.

6.2 Postmarketing Experience
The following additional adverse reactions have been identified based on postmarketing spontaneous reports and are not listed above. Because these reactions are reported voluntarily from a population of uncertain size, it is not always possible to reliably estimate their frequency or establish a causal relationship to drug exposure.
Hypertension, application site hypersensitivity, urticaria, blister, allergic dermatitis, seizure, worsening of Parkinson's disease in patients with Parkinson's disease who were treated with Exelon Patch, tachycardia, abnormal liver function tests, disseminated cutaneous hypersensitivity reactions.

7 DRUG INTERACTIONS
7.1 Cholinomimetic and Anticholinergic Drugs
Rivastigmine may increase the cholinergic effects of other cholinomimetic drugs. Rivastigmine may also interfere with the activity of anticholinergic medications. Avoid concomitant use of rivastigmine with drugs having these pharmacologic effects unless deemed clinically necessary.

8 USE IN SPECIFIC POPULATIONS
8.1 Pregnancy
Pregnancy Category B
There are no adequate and well-controlled studies in pregnant women. No dermal reproduction studies in animals have been conducted. Oral reproduction studies conducted in pregnant rats and rabbits revealed no evidence of teratogenicity. Studies in rats showed slightly decreased fetal/pup weight, usually at doses causing some maternal toxicity. Because animal reproduction studies are not always predictive of human response, this drug should be used during pregnancy only if clearly needed.

8.3 Nursing Mothers
Rivastigmine and its metabolites are excreted in rat milk following oral administration of rivastigmine; levels of rivastigmine plus metabolites in rat milk are approximately 2 times that in maternal plasma. It is not known whether rivastigmine is excreted in human milk. Because many drugs are excreted in human milk and because of the potential for serious adverse reactions in nursing infants from Exelon Patch, a decision should be made whether to discontinue nursing or to discontinue the drug, taking into account the importance of the drug to the mother.

8.4 Pediatric Use
Safety and effectiveness in pediatric patients have not been established. Use of Exelon Patch in children and adolescents (below 18 years of age) is not recommended.

8.5 Geriatric Use
Of the total number of subjects in clinical studies of Exelon Patch, 88% were 65 years and over, while 55% were 75 years and over. No overall differences in safety or effectiveness were observed between these subjects and younger subjects, and other reported clinical experience has not identified differences in responses between the elderly and younger patients, but greater sensitivity of some older individuals cannot be ruled out.

8.6 Renal Impairment
No dose adjustment is necessary for patients with renal impairment *[see Clinical Pharmacology (12.3)]*.

8.7 Hepatic Impairment
In patients with mild or moderate hepatic impairment (Child-Pugh score 5 to 9), clearance of oral rivastigmine was reduced *[see Clinical Pharmacology (12.3)]*. In these patients, consider using the lowest dose Exelon Patch (4.6 mg/24 hours) for both initial and maintenance therapy. No data are available on the use of rivastigmine in patients with severe hepatic impairment.

8.8 Low or High Body Weight
Because rivastigmine blood levels vary with weight [see Clinical Pharmacology (12.3)], careful titration and monitoring should be performed in patients with low or high body weights. In patients with low body weight (<50 kg), monitor closely for toxicities (e.g., excessive nausea, vomiting), and consider reducing the maintenance dose to the 4.6 mg/24 hour Exelon Patch if such toxicities develop. In patients with body weight >100 kg, consider the use of doses higher than 9.5 mg/24 hours.

10 OVERDOSAGE
Overdose with Exelon Patch has been reported in the postmarketing setting *[see Warnings and Precautions (5.1)]*. Overdoses have occurred from application of more than one patch at one time and not removing the previous day's patch before applying a new patch. The symptoms reported in these overdose cases are similar to those seen in cases of overdose associated with rivastigmine oral formulations.
Because strategies for the management of overdose are continually evolving, it is advisable to contact a Poison Control Center to determine the latest recommendations for the management of an overdose of any drug. As rivastigmine has a plasma half-life of about 3.4 hours after patch administration and a duration of acetylcholinesterase inhibition of about 9 hours, it is recommended that in cases of asymptomatic overdose the patch should be immediately removed and no further patch should be applied for the next 24 hours.
As in any case of overdose, general supportive measures should be utilized. Overdosage with cholinesterase inhibitors can result in cholinergic crisis characterized by severe nausea, vomiting, salivation, sweating, bradycardia, hypotension, respiratory depression, and convulsions. Increasing muscle weakness is a possibility and may result in death if respiratory muscles are involved in the event of an overdose. Atypical responses in blood pressure and heart rate have been reported with other drugs that increase cholinergic activity when coadministered with quaternary anticholinergics such as glycopyrrolate. Due to the short plasma elimination half-life of rivastigmine after patch administration, dialysis (hemodialysis, peritoneal dialysis, or hemofiltration) would not be clinically indicated in the event of an overdose.
In overdose accompanied by severe nausea and vomiting, the use of antiemetics should be considered.

11 DESCRIPTION
Exelon Patch (rivastigmine transdermal system) contains rivastigmine, a reversible cholinesterase inhibitor known chemically as (S)-3-[1-(dimethylamino) ethyl]phenyl ethylmethylcarbamate. It has an empirical formula of $C_{14}H_{22}N_2O_2$ as the base and a molecular weight of 250.34 (as the base). Rivastigmine is a viscous, clear, and colorless to yellow to very slightly brown liquid that is sparingly soluble in water and very soluble in ethanol, acetonitrile, n-octanol and ethyl acetate.
The distribution coefficient at 37°C in n-octanol/phosphate buffer solution pH 7 is 4.27.

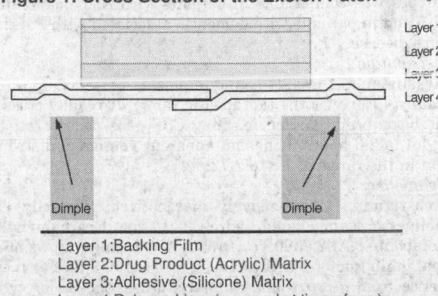

Exelon Patch is for transdermal administration. The patch is a 4-layer laminate containing the backing layer, drug matrix, adhesive matrix and overlapping release liner (see Figure 1). The release liner is removed and discarded prior to use.

Figure 1: Cross Section of the Exelon Patch

Layer 1
Layer 2
Layer 3
Layer 4

Dimple   Dimple

Layer 1: Backing Film
Layer 2: Drug Product (Acrylic) Matrix
Layer 3: Adhesive (Silicone) Matrix
Layer 4: Release Liner (removed at time of use)

Excipients within the formulation include acrylic copolymer, poly(butylmethacrylate, methylmethacrylate), silicone adhesive applied to a flexible polymer backing film, silicone oil, and vitamin E.

12 CLINICAL PHARMACOLOGY
12.1 Mechanism of Action
Although the precise mechanism of action of rivastigmine is unknown, it is thought to exert its therapeutic effect by enhancing cholinergic function. This is accomplished by increasing the concentration of acetylcholine through reversible inhibition of its hydrolysis by cholinesterase. The effect of rivastigmine may lessen as the disease process advances and fewer cholinergic neurons remain functionally intact. There is no evidence that rivastigmine alters the course of the underlying dementing process.

12.2 Pharmacodynamics
After a 6-mg oral dose of rivastigmine in humans, anticholinesterase activity is present in cerebrospinal fluid for about 10 hours, with a maximum inhibition of about 60% 5 hours after dosing.
In vitro and *in vivo* studies demonstrate that the inhibition of cholinesterase by rivastigmine is not affected by the concomitant administration of memantine, an N-methyl-D-aspartate receptor antagonist.

12.3 Pharmacokinetics
Absorption
After the initial application of Exelon Patch, there is a lag time of 0.5 to 1 hour in the absorption of rivastigmine. Concentrations then rise slowly typically reaching a maximum after 8 hours, although maximum values (C_{max}) can also occur later (at 10 to 16 hours). After the peak, plasma concentrations slowly decrease over the remainder of the 24-hour period of application. At steady state, trough levels are approximately 60 to 80% of peak levels.
Exelon Patch 9.5 mg/24 hours gave exposure approximately the same as that provided by an oral dose of 6 mg twice daily (i.e., 12 mg/day). Inter-subject variability in exposure was lower (43% to 49%) for the Exelon Patch formulation as compared with the oral formulations (73% to 103%). Fluctuation (between C_{max} and C_{min}) is less for Exelon Patch than for the oral formulation of rivastigmine.
Figure 2 displays rivastigmine plasma concentrations over 24 hours for the 3 available patch strengths.
[See figure 2 at top of next column]
Over a 24-hour dermal application, approximately 50% of the drug content of the patch is released from the system. Exposure (AUC_∞) to rivastigmine (and metabolite NAP266-90) was highest when the patch was applied to the upper back, chest, or upper arm. Two other sites (abdomen and thigh) could be used if none of the 3 other sites is available, but the practitioner should be aware that the rivastigmine plasma exposure associated with these sites was approximately 20% to 30% lower.
There was no relevant accumulation of rivastigmine or the metabolite NAP226-90 in plasma in patients with Alzheimer's disease with daily dosing.

Figure 2: Rivastigmine Plasma Concentrations Following Dermal 24-Hour Patch Application

The pharmacokinetic profile of rivastigmine transdermal patches was comparable in patients with Alzheimer's disease and in patients with dementia associated with Parkinson's disease.

Distribution
Rivastigmine is weakly bound to plasma proteins (approximately 40%) over the therapeutic range. It readily crosses the blood-brain barrier, reaching CSF peak concentrations in 1.4 to 2.6 hours. It has an apparent volume of distribution in the range of 1.8 to 2.7 L/kg.

Metabolism
Rivastigmine is extensively metabolized primarily via cholinesterase-mediated hydrolysis to the decarbamylated metabolite NAP226-90. *In vitro*, this metabolite shows minimal inhibition of acetylcholinesterase (<10%). Based on evidence from *in vitro* and animal studies, the major cytochrome P450 isoenzymes are minimally involved in rivastigmine metabolism.

The metabolite-to-parent AUC_∞ ratio was about 0.7 after Exelon Patch application versus 3.5 after oral administration, indicating that much less metabolism occurred after dermal treatment. Less NAP226-90 is formed following patch application, presumably because of the lack of presystemic (hepatic first pass) metabolism. Based on *in vitro* studies, no unique metabolic routes were detected in human skin.

Elimination
Renal excretion of the metabolites is the major route of elimination. Unchanged rivastigmine is found in trace amounts in the urine. Following administration of ^{14}C-rivastigmine, renal elimination was rapid and essentially complete (>90%) within 24 hours. Less than 1% of the administered dose is excreted in the feces. The apparent elimination half-life in plasma is approximately 3 hours after patch removal. Renal clearance was approximately 2.1 to 2.8 L/hr.

Renal Impairment
No study was conducted with Exelon Patch in subjects with renal impairment. Based on population analysis creatinine clearance did not show any clear effect on steady state concentrations of rivastigmine or its metabolite. No dosage adjustment is necessary in patients with renal impairment.

Hepatic Impairment
No pharmacokinetic study was conducted with Exelon Patch in subjects with hepatic impairment. After multiple 6-mg twice daily oral dosing, the mean clearance of rivastigmine was 65% lower in mild (n=7, Child-Pugh score 5 to 6) and moderate (n=3, Child-Pugh score 7 to 9) hepatically impaired patients (biopsy proven, liver cirrhosis) than in healthy subjects (n=10) *[see Dosage and Administration (2.2), Specific Population (8.7)]*.

Body Weight
A relationship between drug exposure at steady state (rivastigmine and metabolite NAP226-90) and body weight was observed in Alzheimer's dementia patients. Rivastigmine exposure is higher in subjects with low body weight. Compared to a patient with a body weight of 65 kg, the rivastigmine steady-state concentrations in a patient with a body weight of 35 kg would be approximately doubled, while for a patient with a body weight of 100 kg the concentrations would be approximately halved *[see Dosage and Administration (2.2)]*.

Age
Age had no impact on the exposure to rivastigmine in Alzheimer's disease patients treated with Exelon Patch.

Gender or Race
No specific pharmacokinetic study was conducted to investigate the effect of gender and race on the disposition of Exelon Patch. A population pharmacokinetic analysis of oral rivastigmine indicated that neither gender (n=277 males and 348 females) nor race (n=575 Caucasian, 34 Black, 4 Asian, and 12 Other) affected clearance of the drug. Similar results were seen with analyses of pharmacokinetic data obtained after the administration of Exelon Patch.

Smoking
Population pharmacokinetic analysis showed that nicotine use increased the oral clearance of rivastigmine by 23% (n=75 smokers and 549 nonsmokers).

Drug Interaction Studies
No specific interaction studies have been conducted with Exelon Patch. Information presented below is from studies with oral rivastigmine.

Effect of Rivastigmine on the Metabolism of Other Drugs
Rivastigmine is primarily metabolized through hydrolysis by esterases. Minimal metabolism occurs via the major cytochrome P450 isoenzymes. Based on *in vitro* studies, no pharmacokinetic drug interactions with drugs metabolized by the following isoenzyme systems are expected: CYP1A2, CYP2D6, CYP3A4/5, CYP2E1, CYP2C9, CYP2C8, CYP2C19, or CYP2B6.

No pharmacokinetic interaction was observed between rivastigmine taken orally and digoxin, warfarin, diazepam or fluoxetine in studies in healthy volunteers. The increase in prothrombin time induced by warfarin is not affected by administration of rivastigmine.

Effect of Other Drugs on the Metabolism of Rivastigmine
Drugs that induce or inhibit CYP450 metabolism are not expected to alter the metabolism of rivastigmine.
Population pharmacokinetic analysis with a database of 625 patients showed that the pharmacokinetics of rivastigmine taken orally were not influenced by commonly prescribed medications such as antacids (n=77), antihypertensives (n=72), ß-blockers (n=42), calcium channel blockers (n=75), antidiabetics (n=21), nonsteroidal anti-inflammatory drugs (n=79), estrogens (n=70), salicylate analgesics (n=177), antianginals (n=35), and antihistamines (n=15).

13 NONCLINICAL TOXICOLOGY

13.1 Carcinogenesis, Mutagenesis, Impairment of Fertility

Carcinogenesis
In oral carcinogenicity studies conducted at doses up to 1.1 mg base/kg/day in rats and 1.6 mg base/kg/day in mice, rivastigmine was not carcinogenic.
In a dermal carcinogenicity study conducted at doses up to 0.75 mg base/kg/day in mice, rivastigmine was not carcinogenic. The mean rivastigmine plasma exposure (AUC) at this dose was less than that in humans at the maximum recommended human dose (13.3 mg/24 hours).

Mutagenesis
Rivastigmine was clastogenic in *in vitro* chromosomal aberration assays in mammalian cells in the presence, but not the absence, of metabolic activation. Rivastigmine was negative in an *in vitro* bacterial reverse mutation (Ames) assay, an *in vitro* HGPRT assay, and in an *in vivo* mouse micronucleus test.

Impairment of Fertility
No fertility or reproduction studies of dermal rivastigmine have been conducted in animals. Rivastigmine had no effect on fertility or reproductive performance in rats at oral doses up to 1.1 mg base/kg/day.

14 CLINICAL STUDIES

The effectiveness of the Exelon Patch in dementia of the Alzheimer's type and dementia associated with Parkinson's disease was based on the results of 3 controlled trials of Exelon Patch in patients with Alzheimer's disease (Studies 1, 2, and 3) (see below); 3 controlled trials of oral rivastigmine in patients with dementia of the Alzheimer's type; and 1 controlled trial of oral rivastigmine in patients with dementia associated with Parkinson's disease. See the prescribing information for oral rivastigmine for details of the four studies of oral rivastigmine.

Mild to Moderate Alzheimer's Disease
International 24-Week Study of Exelon Patch in Dementia of the Alzheimer's Type (Study 1)
This study was a randomized double-blind, double dummy clinical investigation in patients with Alzheimer's disease [diagnosed by NINCDS-ADRDA and DSM-IV criteria, Mini-Mental Status Examination (MMSE) score ≥10 and ≤20] (Study 1). The mean age of patients participating in this trial was 74 years with a range of 50 to 90 years. Approximately 67% of patients were women, and 33% were men. The racial distribution was Caucasian 75%, Black 1%, Asian 9%, and other races 15%.
The effectiveness of the Exelon Patch was evaluated in Study 1 using a dual outcome assessment strategy, evaluating for changes in both cognitive performance and overall clinical effect.
The ability of the Exelon Patch to improve cognitive performance was assessed with the cognitive subscale of the Alzheimer's Disease Assessment Scale (ADAS-Cog), a multi-item instrument that has been extensively validated in longitudinal cohorts of Alzheimer's disease patients. The ADAS-Cog examines selected aspects of cognitive performance including elements of memory, orientation, attention, reasoning, language, and praxis. The ADAS-Cog scoring range is from 0 to 70, with higher scores indicating

greater cognitive impairment. Elderly normal adults may score as low as 0 or 1, but it is not unusual for nondemented adults to score slightly higher.
The ability of the Exelon Patch to produce an overall clinical effect was assessed using the Alzheimer's Disease Cooperative Study-Clinical Global Impression of Change (ADCS-CGIC). The ADCS-CGIC is a more standardized form of the Clinician's Interview-Based Impression Of Change-Plus (CIBIC-Plus) and is also scored as a 7-point categorical rating; scores range from 1, indicating "markedly improved," to 4, indicating "no change," to 7, indicating "marked worsening."
In Study 1, 1195 patients were randomized to 1 of the following 4 treatments: Exelon Patch 9.5 mg/24 hours, Exelon Patch 17.4 mg/24 hours, Exelon Capsules in a dose of 6 mg twice daily, or placebo. This 24-week study was divided into a 16-week titration phase followed by an 8-week maintenance phase. In the active treatment arms of this study, doses below the target dose were permitted during the maintenance phase in the event of poor tolerability.
Figure 3 illustrates the time course for the change from baseline in ADAS-Cog scores for all 4 treatment groups over the 24-week study. At 24 weeks, the mean differences in the ADAS-Cog change scores for the Exelon-treated patients compared to the patients on placebo, were 1.8, 2.9, and 1.8 units for the Exelon Patch 9.5 mg/24 hours, Exelon Patch 17.4 mg/24 hours, and Exelon Capsule 6 mg twice daily groups, respectively. The difference between each of these groups and placebo was statistically significant. Although a slight improvement was observed with the 17.4 mg/24 hours patch compared to the 9.5 mg/24 hours patch on this outcome measure, no meaningful difference between the two was seen on the global evaluation (see Figure 4).

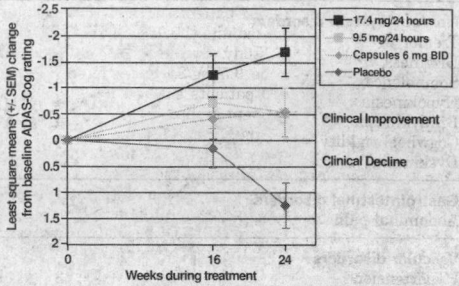

Figure 3: Time Course of the Change from Baseline in ADAS-Cog Score for Patients Observed at Each Time Point in Study 1

Figure 4 presents the distribution of patients' scores on the ADCS-CGIC for all 4 treatment groups. At 24 weeks, the mean difference in the ADCS-CGIC scores for the comparison of patients in each of the Exelon-treated groups with the patients on placebo was 0.2 units. The difference between each of these groups and placebo was statistically significant.

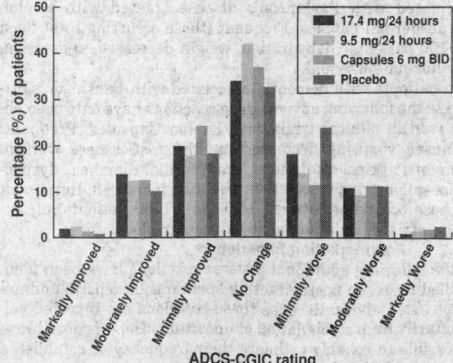

Figure 4: Distribution of ADCS-CGIC Scores for Patients Completing Study 1

International 48-Week Study of Exelon Patch in Dementia of the Alzheimer's Type (Study 2)
This study was a randomized double-blind clinical investigation in patients with Alzheimer's disease [diagnosed by NINCDS-ADRDA and DSM-IV criteria, Mini-Mental State Examination (MMSE) score ≥10 and ≤24] (Study 2). The mean age of patients participating in this trial was 76 years with a range of 50 to 85 years. Approximately 65% of patients were women and 35% were men. The racial distribution was approximately Caucasian 97%, Black 2%, Asian

0.5%, and other races 1%. Approximately 27% of the patients were taking memantine throughout the entire duration of the study.

Alzheimer's disease patients who received 24 to 48 weeks open-label treatment with Exelon Patch 9.5mg/24 hours and who demonstrated functional and cognitive decline were randomized into treatment with either Exelon Patch 9.5 mg/24 hours or Exelon Patch 13.3 mg/24 hours in a 48-week, double-blind treatment phase. Functional decline was assessed by the investigator and cognitive decline was defined as a decrease in the MMSE score of ≥2 points from the previous visit or a decrease of ≥3 points from baseline.

Study 2 was designed to compare the efficacy of Exelon Patch 13.3 mg/24 hours versus that of Exelon Patch 9.5 mg/24 hours during the 48-week, double-blind treatment phase.

The ability of the Exelon Patch 13.3 mg/24 hours to improve cognitive performance over that provided by the Exelon Patch 9.5 mg/24 hours was assessed by the cognitive subscale of the Alzheimer's Disease Assessment Scale (ADAS-Cog) [see Clinical Studies, International 24-Week Study (14)].

The ability of the Exelon Patch 13.3 mg/24 hours to improve overall function versus that provided by Exelon Patch 9.5 mg/24 hours was assessed by the instrumental subscale of the Alzheimer's Disease Cooperative Study Activities of Daily Living (ADCS-IADL). The ADCS-IADL subscale is composed of items 7 to 23 of the caregiver-based ADCS-ADL scale. The ADCS-IADL assesses activities such as those necessary for communicating and interacting with other people, maintaining a household, and conducting hobbies and interests. A sum score is calculated by adding the scores of the individual items and can range from 0 to 56, with higher scores indicating less impairment.

Out of a total of 1584 patients enrolled in the initial open-label phase of the study, 567 patients were classified as decliners and were randomized into the 48-week double-blind treatment phase of the study. Two hundred eighty-seven (287) patients entered the 9.5 mg/24 hours Exelon Patch treatment group and 280 patients entered the 13.3 mg/24 hours Exelon Patch treatment group.

Figure 5 illustrates the time course for the mean change from double-blind baseline in ADCS-IADL scores for each treatment group over the course of the 48-week treatment phase of the study. Decline in the mean ADCS-IADL score from the double-blind baseline for the Intent to Treat–Last Observation Carried Forward (ITT-LOCF) analysis was less at each timepoint in the 13.3 mg/24 hour Exelon Patch treatment group than in the 9.5 mg/24 hours Exelon Patch treatment group. The 13.3 mg/24 hours dose was statistically significantly superior to the 9.5mg/24 hours dose at weeks 16, 24, 32, and 48 (primary endpoint).

Figure 6 illustrates the time course for the mean change from double-blind baseline in ADAS-Cog scores for both treatment groups over the 48-week treatment phase. The between-treatment group difference for Exelon Patch 13.3 mg/24 hours versus Exelon Patch 9.5 mg/24 hours was nominally statistically significant at week 24 (p=0.027), but not at week 48 (p=0.227), which was the primary endpoint.

X: p<0.05 for Exelon Patch 13.3 mg/24hr vs. 9.5 mg/24hr

Figure 5: Time Course of the Change from Double-Blind Baseline in ADCS-IADL Score for Patients Observed at Each Time Point in Study 2

[See figure 6 at top of next column]

Severe Alzheimer's Disease
24-Week United States Study with Exelon Patch in Severe Alzheimer's Disease (Study 3)
This was a 24-week randomized double-blind, clinical investigation in patients with severe Alzheimer's disease [diagnosed by NINCDS-ADRDA and DSM-IV criteria, Mini-Mental State Examination (MMSE) score ≥3 and ≤12]. The mean age of patients participating in this trial was 78 years with a range of 51 to 96 years with 62% aged >75 years. Approximately 65% of patients were women and 35% were men. The racial distribution was approximately Caucasian 87%, Black 7%, Asian 1%, and other races 5%. Patients on a stable dose of memantine were permitted to enter the study.

X: p<0.05 for Exelon Patch 13.3 mg/24hr vs. 9.5 mg/24hr

Figure 6: Time Course of the Change from Double-Blind Baseline in ADAS-Cog Score for Patients Observed at Each Time Point in Study 2

Approximately 61% of the patients in each treatment group were taking memantine throughout the entire duration of the study.

The study was designed to compare the efficacy of Exelon Patch 13.3 mg/24 hours versus that of Exelon Patch 4.6 mg/24 hours during the 24-week double-blind treatment phase.

The ability of the 13.3 mg/24 hours Exelon Patch to improve cognitive performance versus that provided by the 4.6 mg/24 hours Exelon Patch was assessed with the Severe Impairment Battery (SIB) which uses a validated 40-item scale developed for the evaluation of the severity of cognitive dysfunction in more advanced AD patients. The domains assessed included social interaction, memory, language, attention, orientation, praxis, visuospatial ability, construction, and orienting to name. The SIB was scored from 0 to 100, with higher scores reflecting higher levels of cognitive ability.

The ability of the 13.3 mg/24 hours Exelon Patch to improve overall function versus that provided by the 4.6 mg/24 hours Exelon Patch was assessed with the Alzheimer's Disease Cooperative Study-Activities of Daily Living-Severe Impairment Version (ADCS-ADL-SIV) which is a caregiver-based ADL scale composed of 19 items developed for use in clinical studies of dementia. It is designed to assess the patient's performance of both basic and instrumental activities of daily living such as those necessary for personal care, communicating and interacting with other people, maintaining a household, conducting hobbies and interests, and making judgments and decisions. A sum score is calculated by adding the scores of the individual items and can range from 0 to 54, with higher scores indicating less functional impairment.

In this study, 716 patients were randomized into one of the following treatments: Exelon Patch 13.3 mg/24 hours or Exelon Patch 4.6 mg/24 hours in a 1:1 ratio. This 24-week study was divided into an 8-week titration phase followed by a 16-week maintenance phase. In the active treatment arms of this study, temporary dose adjustments below the target dose were permitted during the titration and maintenance phase in the event of poor tolerability.

Figure 7 illustrates the time course for the mean change from baseline SIB scores for each treatment group over the course of the 24-week treatment phase of the study. Decline in the mean SIB score from the baseline for the Modified Full Analysis Set (MFAS)-Last Observation Carried Forward (LOCF) analysis was less at each timepoint in the 13.3 mg/24 hour Exelon Patch treatment group than in the 4.6 mg/24 hours Exelon Patch treatment group. The 13.3 mg/24 hours dose was statistically significantly superior to the 4.6 mg/24 hours dose at weeks 16 and 24 (primary endpoint).

Figure 8 illustrates the time course for the mean change from baseline in ADCS-ADL-SIV scores for each treatment group over the course of the 24-week treatment phase of the study. Decline in the mean ADCS-ADL-SIV score from baseline for the MFAS-LOCF analysis was less at each timepoint in the 13.3 mg/24 hour Exelon Patch treatment group than in the 4.6 mg/24 hours Exelon Patch treatment group. The 13.3 mg/24 hours dose was statistically significantly superior to the 4.6 mg/24 hours dose at weeks 16 and 24 (primary endpoint).

[See figure 7 at top of next column]
[See figure 8 at top of next column]

16   HOW SUPPLIED/STORAGE AND HANDLING
Exelon Patch: 4.6 mg/24 hours
Each patch of 5 cm² contains 9 mg rivastigmine base with *in vivo* release rate of 4.6 mg/24 hours.
   Carton of 30 ....NDC 0078-0501-15
Exelon Patch: 9.5 mg/24 hours
Each patch of 10 cm² contains 18 mg rivastigmine base with *in vivo* release rate of 9.5 mg/24 hours.
   Carton of 30 ....NDC 0078-0502-15

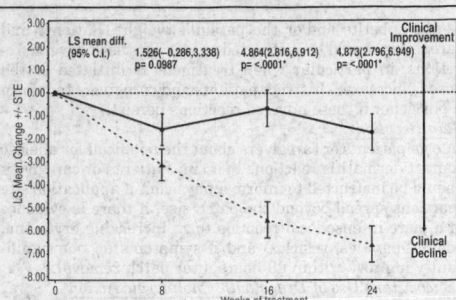

Least squares means (LS means) and the standard errors of the LS means (STE) are based on an analysis of covariance model adjusted for pooled center and baseline.
* indicating statistical significance at a level of 0.05

Figure 7: Time Course of the Change from Baseline in SIB Score for Patients Observed at Each Time Point (Modified Full Analysis Set-LOCF)

Least squares means (LS means) and the standard errors of the LS means (STE) are based on an analysis of covariance model adjusted for pooled center and baseline.
* indicating statistical significance at a level of 0.05

Figure 8: Time Course of the Change from Baseline in ADCS-ADL-SIV Score for Patients Observed at Each Time Point (Modified Full Analysis Set-LOCF)

Exelon Patch: 13.3 mg/24 hours
Each patch of 15 cm² contains 27 mg rivastigmine base with *in vivo* release rate of 13.3 mg/24 hours.
   Carton of 30 ....NDC 0078-0503-15
Store at 25°C (77°F); excursions permitted to 15°C to 30°C (59°F to 86°F) [see USP Controlled Room Temperature]. Keep Exelon Patch in the individual sealed pouch until use. Each pouch contains 1 patch. Used systems should be folded, with the adhesive surfaces pressed together, and discarded safely.

17   PATIENT COUNSELING INFORMATION
See FDA-approved patient labeling (Patient Information).
Importance of Correct Usage
Inform patients or caregivers of the importance of applying the correct dose on the correct part of the body. They should be instructed to rotate the application site in order to minimize skin irritation. The same site should not be used within 14 days. The previous day's patch must be removed before applying a new patch to a different skin location. Exelon Patch should be replaced every 24 hours and the time of day should be consistent. It may be helpful for this to be part of a daily routine, such as the daily bath or shower. Only 1 patch should be worn at a time.
Instruct patients or caregivers to avoid exposure of the patch to external heat sources (excessive sunlight, saunas, solariums) for long periods of time.
Instruct patients who have missed a dose to apply a new patch immediately. They may apply the next patch at the usual time the next day. Instruct patients to not apply 2 patches to make up for 1 missed.
Inform the patient or caregiver to contact the physician for retitration instructions if treatment has been interrupted.
Discarding Used Patches
Instruct patients or caregivers to fold the patch in half after use, return the used patch to its original pouch, and discard it out of the reach and sight of children and pets. They should also be informed that drug still remains in the patch after 24-hour usage. They should be instructed to avoid eye contact and to wash their hands after handling the patch. In case of accidental contact with the eyes, or if their eyes become red after handling the patch, they should be instructed to rinse immediately with plenty of water and to seek medical advice if symptoms do not resolve.
Gastrointestinal Adverse Reactions
Inform patients or caregivers of the potential gastrointestinal adverse reactions such as nausea, vomiting, and diarrhea, including the possibility of dehydration due to these symptoms. Explain that Exelon Patch may affect the pa-

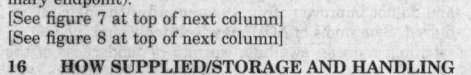

tient's appetite and/or the patient's weight. Patients and caregivers should be instructed to look for these adverse reactions, in particular when treatment is initiated or the dose is increased. Instruct patients and caregivers to inform a physician if these adverse reactions persist.

Skin Reactions
Inform patients or caregivers about the potential for allergic contact dermatitis reactions to occur. Patients or caregivers should be instructed to inform a physician if application site reactions spread beyond the patch size, if there is evidence of a more intense local reaction (e.g., increasing erythema, edema, papules, vesicles) and if symptoms do not significantly improve within 48 hours after patch removal.

Concomitant Use of Drugs with Cholinergic Action
Inform patients or caregivers that while wearing Exelon Patch, patients should not be taking Exelon Capsules or Exelon Oral Solution or other drugs with cholinergic effects.
T2013-66
July 2013

Patient Information
Exelon (ECS-'el-on) Patch
(rivastigmine transdermal system)
Exelon Patch is for skin use only.

What is Exelon Patch?
Exelon Patch is a prescription medicine used to treat:
• Mild, moderate, and severe memory problems (dementia) associated with Alzheimer's disease.
• Mild to moderate memory problems (dementia) associated with Parkinson's disease.
Based on clinical trials conducted over 6 to 12 months Exelon Patch was shown to help with cognition which includes (memory, understanding communication, reasoning) and with doing daily tasks. Exelon Patch does not work the same in all people. Some people treated with Exelon Patch may:
• Seem much better
• Get better in small ways or stay the same
• Get worse but slower than expected
• Not change and then get worse as expected
Some patients will not benefit from treatment with Exelon Patch. Exelon Patch does not cure Alzheimer's disease. All patients with Alzheimer's disease get worse over time.
Exelon Patch comes as a transdermal system that delivers rivastigmine (the medicine in Exelon Patch) through the skin.
It is not known if Exelon Patch is safe or effective in children under 18 years of age.

Who should not use Exelon Patch?
Do not use Exelon Patch if you:
• are allergic to rivastigmine, carbamate derivatives, or any of the ingredients in Exelon Patch. See the end of this leaflet for a complete list of ingredients in Exelon Patch.
• have had a skin reaction that:
  ○ spread beyond the Exelon Patch size
  ○ had blisters, increased skin redness, or swelling
  ○ did not get better within 48 hours after you removed the Exelon Patch
Ask your healthcare provider if you are not sure if you should use Exelon Patch.

What should I tell my healthcare provider before using Exelon Patch?
Before you use Exelon Patch, tell your healthcare provider if you:
• have or have had a stomach ulcer
• are planning to have surgery
• have or have had problems with your heart
• have problems passing urine
• have or have had seizures
• have problems with movement (tremors)
• have asthma or breathing problems
• have a loss of appetite or are losing weight
• have had a skin reaction to rivastigmine (the medicine in Exelon Patch) in the past.
• have any other medical conditions
• are pregnant or plan to become pregnant. It is not known if the medicine in Exelon Patch will harm your unborn baby. Talk to your healthcare provider if you are pregnant or plan to become pregnant.
• are breastfeeding or plan to breastfeed. It is not known if the medicine in Exelon Patch passes into your breast milk. You and your healthcare provider should decide if you will use Exelon Patch or breastfeed. You should not do both.
Tell your healthcare provider about all the medicines you take, including prescription and over-the counter medicines, vitamins, and herbal supplements.
Especially tell your healthcare provider if you take:
• a medicine used to treat inflammation [nonsteroidal anti-inflammatory drugs (NSAIDs)]
• other medicines used to treat Alzheimer's or Parkinson's disease
• an anticholinergic medicine, such as an allergy or cold medicine, a medicine to treat bladder or bowel spasms, or certain asthma medicines, or certain medicines to prevent motion or travel sickness

Ask your healthcare provider if you are not sure if your medicine is one listed above.
Know the medicines you take. Keep a list of them to show to your healthcare provider and pharmacist when you get a new medicine.

How should I use Exelon Patch?
• Use Exelon Patch exactly as your healthcare provider tells you to use it.
• Exelon Patches come in 3 different dosage strengths.
• Your healthcare provider may change your dose as needed.
• Wear only 1 Exelon Patch at a time.
• Exelon Patch is for skin use only.
• Only apply Exelon Patch to healthy skin that is clean, dry, hairless, and free of redness, irritation, burns or cuts.
• Avoid applying Exelon Patch to areas on your body that will be rubbed against tight clothing.
• Do not apply Exelon Patch to skin that has cream, lotion, or powder on it.
• Change your Exelon Patch every 24 hours at the same time of day. You may write the date and time you put on the Exelon Patch with a ballpoint pen before applying the patch to help you remember when to remove it.
• Change your application site every day to avoid skin irritation. You can use the same area, but do not use the exact same spot for at least 14 days after your last application.
• Check to see if the Exelon Patch has become loose when you are bathing, swimming, or showering.
• Exelon Patch is designed to deliver medication during the time it is worn. If your Exelon Patch falls off before its usual replacement time, put on a new Exelon Patch right away. Replace the new patch the next day at the same time as usual. Do not use overlays, bandages, or tape to secure an Exelon Patch that has become loose or try to reapply an Exelon Patch that has fallen off.
• If you miss a dose or forget to change your Exelon Patch apply your next Exelon Patch as soon as you remember. Do not apply 2 Exelon Patches to make up for the missed dose.
• If you miss more than 3 doses of applying Exelon Patch, call your healthcare provider before putting on a new Exelon Patch. You may need to restart Exelon Patch at a lower dose.
• Always remove the old Exelon Patch from the previous day before you apply a new one.
• **Having more than 1 Exelon Patch on your body at the same time can cause you to get too much medicine.** If you accidentally use more than 1 Exelon Patch at a time, call your healthcare provider right away. If you are unable to reach your healthcare provider, call your local Poison Control Center at 1-800-222-1222 or go to the nearest hospital emergency room right away.

What should I avoid while using Exelon Patch?
• Do not touch your eyes after you touch the Exelon Patch. In case of accidental contact with your eyes or if your eyes become red after handling the patch, rinse immediately with plenty of water and seek medical advice if symptoms do not resolve.
• Exelon Patch can cause drowsiness, dizziness, weakness, or fainting. Do not drive, operate heavy machinery, or do other dangerous activities until you know how Exelon Patch affects you.
• Avoid exposure to heat sources such as excessive sunlight, saunas, or sun-rooms for long periods of time.

What are the possible side effects of Exelon Patch?
Exelon Patch may cause serious side effects, including:
• **Medication overdose.** Hospitalization and rarely death may happen when people accidentally wear more than 1 patch at the same time. It is important that the old Exelon Patch be removed before you apply a new one. Do not wear more than 1 Exelon Patch at a time.
• **Stomach or bowel (intestinal) problems, including:**
  ○ nausea
  ○ vomiting
  ○ diarrhea
  ○ dehydration
  ○ loss of appetite
  ○ weight loss
  ○ bleeding in your stomach (ulcers)
• **Skin reactions.** Some people have had a serious skin reaction called allergic contact dermatitis (ACD) when using Exelon Patch. Stop using Exelon Patch and call your healthcare provider right away if you experience reactions that spread beyond the patch size, are intense in nature and do not improve within 48 hours after the patch is removed. Symptoms of ACD may be intense and include:
  ○ itching, redness, swelling, warmth or tenderness of the skin
  ○ peeling or blistering of the skin that may ooze, drain or crust over
• **heart problems**
• **seizures**
• **problems with movement (tremors)**
The most common side effects of Exelon Patch include:
• depression
• headache

• anxiety
• dizziness
• stomach pain
• urinary tract infections
• muscle weakness
• tiredness
• trouble sleeping
Tell your healthcare provider if you have any side effect that bothers you or that does not go away.
These are not all the possible side effects of Exelon Patch. For more information, ask your healthcare provider or pharmacist.
Call your doctor for medical advice about side effects. You may report side effects to the FDA at 1-800-FDA-1088.

How should I store Exelon Patch?
• Store Exelon Patch between 68°F to 77°F (20°C to 25°C).
• Keep Exelon Patch in the sealed pouch until ready to use.
Keep Exelon Patch and all medicines out of the reach of children.

General information about the safe and effective use of Exelon Patch.
Medicines are sometimes prescribed for purposes other than those listed in the Patient Information leaflet. Do not use Exelon Patch for a condition for which it was not prescribed. Do not give Exelon Patch to other people, even if they have the same symptoms you have. It may harm them.
This Patient Information leaflet summarizes the most important information about Exelon Patch. If you would like more information, talk with your healthcare provider. You can ask your pharmacist or healthcare provider for information about Exelon Patch that is written for health professionals.
For more information, go to www.EXELONPATCH.com or call 1-888-669-6682.

What are the ingredients of Exelon Patch?
Active ingredient: rivastigmine
Excipients include: acrylic copolymer, poly (butylmethacrylate, methylmethacrylate), silicone adhesive applied to a flexible polymer backing film, silicone oil, and vitamin E
T2013-67
July 2013

Instructions for Use
Exelon (ECS-'el-on) Patch
(rivastigmine transdermal system)
You will need the following supplies (See Figure A):
Exelon Patch is supplied in cartons containing 30 patches (see Figure A)

Figure A

• Exelon Patch is a thin, beige, plastic patch that sticks to the skin. Each Exelon Patch is sealed in a pouch that protects it until you are ready to put it on (See Figure A).
• **Only 1 Exelon Patch should be worn at a time. Do not apply more than 1 Exelon Patch at a time to the body.**
• Do not open the pouch or remove the Exelon Patch until you are ready to apply it.

Using Exelon Patch:
Step 1. Choose an area to apply the Exelon Patch (See Figure B).
• **Instructions for Caregivers:** Apply Exelon Patch to the upper or lower back if it is likely that the patient will remove it. If this is not a concern, the Exelon Patch can be applied **instead** to the upper arm **or** chest. Do not apply the Exelon Patch to areas where it can be rubbed off by tight clothing or belts.
• Only apply the Exelon Patch to healthy skin that is clean, dry, hairless, and free of redness, irritation, burns or cuts.

Figure B

The diagram represents areas on the body where Exelon Patch may be applied. Only 1 patch should be worn at a time. Do not apply multiple patches to the body.
Step 2. Remove the Exelon Patch from the pouch (See Figure C).
Carefully cut the pouch along the dotted line to open and remove the Exelon Patch. Save the pouch for later use.

Figure C

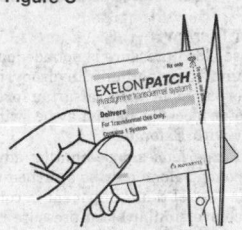

- Do not cut or fold the Exelon Patch itself.
Step 3. Remove 1 side of the adhesive liner (See Figure D).
- A protective liner covers the sticky (adhesive) side of the Exelon Patch. Peel off 1 side of the protective cover. Do not touch the sticky part of the Exelon Patch with your fingers.

Figure D
Protective Liners

Sticky surface of patch

Step 4. Apply the Exelon Patch to your skin (See Figure E).
- Apply the sticky (adhesive) side of the Exelon Patch to your chosen area of skin **and** then peel off the other side of the protective cover.

Figure E

- Press down on the Exelon Patch firmly for 30 seconds to make sure that the edges stick to your skin (See Figure F).

Figure F

Step 5: Wash your hands with soap and water right away.
Note:
- If your Exelon Patch falls off, select a new area, and repeat Steps 2 to 5 to apply a new Exelon Patch.
- Be sure to replace the new Exelon Patch the next day at the same time as usual.

Removing your Exelon Patch:
Step 6. Remove the Exelon Patch from the skin (See Figure G).
- Gently pull on 1 edge of the Exelon Patch to remove it from your skin.

Figure G

Throwing away the used Exelon Patch:
Step 7. Throw away the used Exelon Patch (See Figure H).
- Fold the used Exelon Patch in half (with the sticky sides together) and put it back into the pouch that you saved.

Figure H

Fold sticky sides together	Slide folded patch into empty pouch you saved	Place in trash Keep from Children and Pets

- Throw away the used Exelon Patch safely and out of the reach of children and pets.
- Some medicine stays in the patch for 24 hours after you use it and should be folded together (sticky side together) and safely thrown away. Do not try to re-use Exelon Patches.
Step 8: Wash your hands with soap and water right away.
- After you remove the Exelon Patch, if any adhesive remains on your skin, you can use soap and water or an oil-based substance (such as baby oil) to remove the adhesive. Alcohol or other dissolving liquids (such as nail polish) should not be used.
This Patient Information and Instructions for Use have been approved by the U.S. Food and Drug Administration.
Distributed by:
Novartis Pharmaceuticals Corporation
East Hanover, New Jersey 07936
©Novartis
T2013-68
July 2013
Shown in Product Identification Guide, page 310

EXFORGE ℞
[X-phorj]
(amlodipine and valsartan)
Tablets

The following prescribing information is based on official labeling in effect July 2014.
HIGHLIGHTS OF PRESCRIBING INFORMATION
These highlights do not include all the information needed to use Exforge safely and effectively. See full prescribing information for Exforge.
Exforge (amlodipine and valsartan) Tablets
Initial U.S. Approval: 2007

> **WARNING: FETAL TOXICITY**
> *See full prescribing information for complete boxed warning.*
> - **When pregnancy is detected, discontinue Exforge as soon as possible. (5.1)**
> - **Drugs that act directly on the renin-angiotensin system can cause injury and death to the developing fetus. (5.1)**

————INDICATIONS AND USAGE————
Exforge is the combination tablet of amlodipine, a dihydropyridine calcium channel blocker (DHP CCB), and valsartan, an angiotensin II receptor blocker (ARB). Exforge is indicated for the treatment of hypertension, to lower blood pressure:
- In patients not adequately controlled on monotherapy (1)
- As initial therapy in patients likely to need multiple drugs to achieve their blood pressure goals (1)
Lowering blood pressure reduces the risk of fatal and non-fatal cardiovascular events, primarily strokes and myocardial infarctions.

————DOSAGE AND ADMINISTRATION————
General Considerations:
- Majority of effect attained within 2 weeks (2.1)
- May be administered with other antihypertensive agents (2.1)
Hypertension:
- May be used as add-on therapy for patients not controlled on monotherapy (2.2)

- Patients who experience dose-limiting adverse reactions on monotherapy may be switched to Exforge containing a lower dose of that component (2.2)
- May be substituted for titrated components (2.3)
- When used as initial therapy: Initiate with 5/160 mg, then titrate upwards as necessary to a maximum of 10/320 mg once daily (2.4)

————DOSAGE FORMS AND STRENGTHS————
Tablets (amlodipine/valsartan mg): 5/160, 10/160, 5/320, 10/320 (3)

————CONTRAINDICATIONS————
Known hypersensitivity to any component;
Do not coadminister aliskiren with Exforge in patients with diabetes (4)

————WARNINGS AND PRECAUTIONS————
- Hypotension: Correct volume depletion prior to initiation (5.2)
- Increased angina and/or myocardial infarction (5.3)
- Monitor renal function and potassium in susceptible patients (5.4, 5.5)

————ADVERSE REACTIONS————
In placebo-controlled clinical trials, discontinuation due to side effects occurred in 1.8% of patients in the Exforge-treated patients and 2.1% in the placebo-treated group. The most common reasons for discontinuation of therapy with Exforge were peripheral edema and vertigo. The adverse experiences that occurred in clinical trials (≥2% of patients) at a higher incidence than placebo included peripheral edema, nasopharyngitis, upper respiratory tract infection, and dizziness. (6.1)
To report SUSPECTED ADVERSE REACTIONS, contact Novartis Pharmaceuticals Corporation at 1-888-669-6682 or FDA at 1-800-FDA-1088 or www.fda.gov/medwatch.

————DRUG INTERACTIONS————
- If simvastatin is coadministered with amlodipine, do not exceed doses greater than 20 mg daily of simvastatin (7)
- NSAID use may lead to increased risk of renal impairment and loss of anti-hypertensive effect (7)
- Dual inhibition of the renin-angiotensin system: Increased risk of renal impairment, hypotension, and hyperkalemia (7)
- Lithium: Increases in serum lithium concentrations and lithium toxicity (7)

————USE IN SPECIFIC POPULATIONS————
Start amlodipine or add amlodipine at 2.5 mg in patients ≥75 years old or in patients with hepatic impairment. (8.5, 8.7)
Nursing Mothers: Avoid use while nursing – discontinue either nursing or drug (8.3)
See 17 for PATIENT COUNSELING INFORMATION and FDA-approved patient labeling
Revised: 6/2014

FULL PRESCRIBING INFORMATION

> **WARNING: FETAL TOXICITY**
> • **When pregnancy is detected, discontinue Exforge as soon as possible. (5.1)**
> • **Drugs that act directly on the renin-angiotensin system can cause injury and death to the developing fetus. (5.1)**

1 INDICATIONS AND USAGE

1.1 Hypertension

Exforge (amlodipine and valsartan) is indicated for the treatment of hypertension, to lower blood pressure. Lowering blood pressure reduces the risk of fatal and nonfatal cardiovascular events, primarily strokes and myocardial infarctions. These benefits have been seen in controlled trials of antihypertensive drugs from a wide variety of pharmacologic classes, including amlodipine and the ARB class to which valsartan principally belongs. There are no controlled trials demonstrating risk reduction with Exforge.

Control of high blood pressure should be part of comprehensive cardiovascular risk management, including, as appropriate, lipid control, diabetes management, antithrombotic therapy, smoking cessation, exercise, and limited sodium intake. Many patients will require more than 1 drug to achieve blood pressure goals. For specific advice on goals and management, see published guidelines, such as those of the National High Blood Pressure Education Program's Joint National Committee on Prevention, Detection, Evaluation, and Treatment of High Blood Pressure (JNC).

Numerous antihypertensive drugs, from a variety of pharmacologic classes and with different mechanisms of action, have been shown in randomized controlled trials to reduce cardiovascular morbidity and mortality, and it can be concluded that it is blood pressure reduction, and not some other pharmacologic property of the drugs, that is largely responsible for those benefits. The largest and most consistent cardiovascular outcome benefit has been a reduction in the risk of stroke, but reductions in myocardial infarction and cardiovascular mortality also have been seen regularly. Elevated systolic or diastolic pressure causes increased cardiovascular risk, and the absolute risk increase per mmHg is greater at higher blood pressures, so that even modest reductions of severe hypertension can provide substantial benefit. Relative risk reduction from blood pressure reduction is similar across populations with varying absolute risk, so the absolute benefit is greater in patients who are at higher risk independent of their hypertension (for example, patients with diabetes or hyperlipidemia), and such patients would be expected to benefit from more aggressive treatment to a lower blood pressure goal.

Some antihypertensive drugs have smaller blood pressure effects (as monotherapy) in black patients, and many antihypertensive drugs have additional approved indications and effects (e.g., on angina, heart failure, or diabetic kidney disease). These considerations may guide selection of therapy. Exforge (amlodipine and valsartan) is indicated for the treatment of hypertension.

Exforge may be used in patients whose blood pressure is not adequately controlled on either monotherapy.

Exforge may also be used as initial therapy in patients who are likely to need multiple drugs to achieve their blood pressure goals.

The choice of Exforge as initial therapy for hypertension should be based on an assessment of potential benefits and risks including whether the patient is likely to tolerate the lowest dose of Exforge.

Patients with stage 2 hypertension (moderate or severe) are at a relatively higher risk for cardiovascular events (such as strokes, heart attacks, and heart failure), kidney failure and vision problems, so prompt treatment is clinically relevant. The decision to use a combination as initial therapy should be individualized and should be shaped by considerations such as baseline blood pressure, the target goal and the incremental likelihood of achieving goal with a combination compared to monotherapy. Individual blood pressure goals may vary based upon the patient's risk.

Data from the high-dose multifactorial study *[see Clinical Studies (14)]* provide estimates of the probability of reaching a blood pressure goal with Exforge compared to amlodipine or valsartan monotherapy. The figures below provide estimates of the likelihood of achieving systolic or diastolic blood pressure control with Exforge 10/320 mg, based upon baseline systolic or diastolic blood pressure. The curve of each treatment group was estimated by logistic regression modeling. The estimated likelihood at the right tail of each curve is less reliable due to small numbers of subjects with high baseline blood pressures.

[See figures 1-4 below]

For example, a patient with a baseline blood pressure of 160/100 mmHg has about a 67% likelihood of achieving a goal of <140 mmHg (systolic) and 80% likelihood of achieving <90 mmHg (diastolic) on amlodipine alone, and the likelihood of achieving these goals on valsartan alone is about 47% (systolic) or 62% (diastolic). The likelihood of achieving these goals on Exforge rises to about 80% (systolic) or 85% (diastolic). The likelihood of achieving these goals on placebo is about 28% (systolic) or 37% (diastolic).

2 DOSAGE AND ADMINISTRATION

2.1 General Considerations

Dose once daily. The dosage can be increased after 1 to 2 weeks of therapy to a maximum of one 10/320mg tablet once daily as needed to control blood pressure. The majority of the antihypertensive effect is attained within 2 weeks after initiation of therapy or a change in dose.

Exforge may be administered with or without food.

Exforge may be administered with other antihypertensive agents.

2.2 Add-on Therapy

A patient whose blood pressure is not adequately controlled with amlodipine (or another dihydropyridine calcium-channel blocker) alone or with valsartan (or another angiotensin II receptor blocker) alone may be switched to combination therapy with Exforge.

A patient who experiences dose-limiting adverse reactions on either component alone may be switched to Exforge containing a lower dose of that component in combination with the other to achieve similar blood pressure reductions. The clinical response to Exforge should be subsequently evaluated and if blood pressure remains uncontrolled after 3 to 4 weeks of therapy, the dose may be titrated up to a maximum of 10/320 mg.

2.3 Replacement Therapy

For convenience, patients receiving amlodipine and valsartan from separate tablets may instead wish to receive tablets of Exforge containing the same component doses.

2.4 Initial Therapy

A patient may be initiated on Exforge if it is unlikely that control of blood pressure would be achieved with a single agent. The usual starting dose is Exforge 5/160 mg once daily in patients who are not volume-depleted.

3 DOSAGE FORMS AND STRENGTHS

5/160 mg tablets, debossed with NVR/ECE (side 1/side 2)
10/160 mg tablets, debossed with NVR/UIC
5/320 mg tablets, debossed with NVR/CSF
10/320 mg tablets, debossed with NVR/LUF

4 CONTRAINDICATIONS

Do not use in patients with known hypersensitivity to any component.

Do not coadminister aliskiren with Exforge in patients with diabetes *[see Drug Interactions (7)]*.

5 WARNINGS AND PRECAUTIONS

5.1 Fetal Toxicity

Pregnancy Category D

Use of drugs that act on the renin-angiotensin system during the second and third trimesters of pregnancy reduces fetal renal function and increases fetal and neonatal morbidity and death. Resulting oligohydramnios can be associated with fetal lung hypoplasia and skeletal deformations. Potential neonatal adverse effects include skull hypoplasia, anuria, hypotension, renal failure, and death. When pregnancy is detected, discontinue Exforge as soon as possible *[see Use in Specific Populations (8.1)]*.

5.2 Hypotension

Excessive hypotension was seen in 0.4% of patients with uncomplicated hypertension treated with Exforge in placebo-controlled studies. In patients with an activated renin-angiotensin system, such as volume- and/or salt-depleted patients receiving high doses of diuretics, symptomatic hypotension may occur in patients receiving angiotensin receptor blockers. Volume depletion should be corrected prior to administration of Exforge. Treatment with Exforge should start under close medical supervision.

Initiate therapy cautiously in patients with heart failure or recent myocardial infarction and in patients undergoing surgery or dialysis. Patients with heart failure or post-myocardial infarction patients given valsartan commonly have some reduction in blood pressure, but discontinuation of therapy because of continuing symptomatic hypotension usually is not necessary when dosing instructions are followed. In controlled trials in heart failure patients, the incidence of hypotension in valsartan-treated patients was 5.5% compared to 1.8% in placebo-treated patients. In the Valsartan in Acute Myocardial Infarction Trial (VALIANT), hypotension in post-myocardial infarction patients led to permanent discontinuation of therapy in 1.4% of valsartan-treated patients and 0.8% of captopril-treated patients.

Since the vasodilation induced by amlodipine is gradual in onset, acute hypotension has rarely been reported after oral administration. Nonetheless, caution, as with any other peripheral vasodilator, should be exercised when administering amlodipine, particularly in patients with severe aortic stenosis.

If excessive hypotension occurs with Exforge, the patient should be placed in a supine position and, if necessary, given an intravenous infusion of normal saline. A transient hypotensive response is not a contraindication to further treatment, which usually can be continued without difficulty once the blood pressure has stabilized.

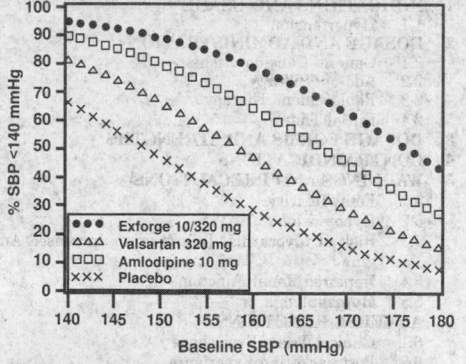

Figure 1: Probability of Achieving Systolic Blood Pressure <140 mmHg at Week 8

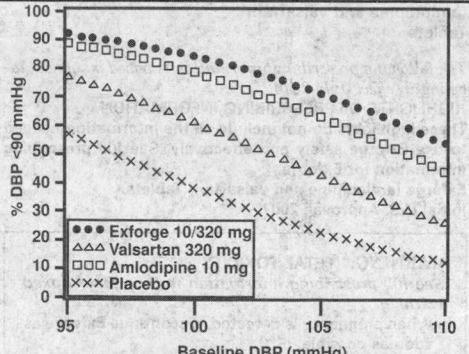

Figure 2: Probability of Achieving Diastolic Blood Pressure <90 mmHg at Week 8

Figure 3: Probability of Achieving Systolic Blood Pressure <130 mmHg at Week 8

Figure 4: Probability of Achieving Diastolic Blood Pressure <80 mmHg at Week 8

5.3 Risk of Myocardial Infarction or Increased Angina

Worsening angina and acute myocardial infarction can develop after starting or increasing the dose of amlodipine, particularly in patients with severe obstructive coronary artery disease.

5.4 Impaired Renal Function

Changes in renal function including acute renal failure can be caused by drugs that inhibit the renin-angiotensin system and by diuretics. Patients whose renal function may depend in part on the activity of the renin-angiotensin system (e.g., patients with renal artery stenosis, chronic kidney disease, severe congestive heart failure, or volume depletion) may be at particular risk of developing acute renal failure on Exforge. Monitor renal function periodically in these patients. Consider withholding or discontinuing therapy in patients who develop a clinically significant decrease in renal function on Exforge *[see Drug Interactions (7)]*.

5.5 Hyperkalemia

Drugs that inhibit the renin-angiotensin system can cause hyperkalemia. Monitor serum electrolytes periodically. Some patients with heart failure have developed increases in potassium with valsartan therapy. These effects are usually minor and transient, and they are more likely to occur in patients with pre-existing renal impairment. Dosage reduction and/or discontinuation of Exforge may be required *[see Adverse Reactions (6.1)]*.

6 ADVERSE REACTIONS

6.1 Clinical Trials Experience

Because clinical trials are conducted under widely varying conditions, adverse reaction rates observed in the clinical trials of a drug cannot be directly compared to rates in the clinical trials of another drug and may not reflect the rates observed in practice. The adverse reaction information from clinical trials does, however, provide a basis for identifying the adverse events that appear to be related to drug use and for approximating rates.

Studies with Exforge:

Exforge has been evaluated for safety in over 2600 patients with hypertension; over 1440 of these patients were treated for at least 6 months and over 540 of these patients were treated for at least 1 year. Adverse reactions have generally been mild and transient in nature and have only infrequently required discontinuation of therapy.

The hazards *[see Warnings and Precautions (5)]* of valsartan are generally independent of dose; those of amlodipine are a mixture of dose-dependent phenomena (primarily peripheral edema) and dose-independent phenomena, the former much more common than the latter.

The overall frequency of adverse reactions was neither dose-related nor related to gender, age, or race. In placebo-controlled clinical trials, discontinuation due to side effects occurred in 1.8% of patients in the Exforge-treated patients and 2.1% in the placebo-treated group. The most common reasons for discontinuation of therapy with Exforge were peripheral edema (0.4%), and vertigo (0.2%).

The adverse reactions that occurred in placebo-controlled clinical trials in at least 2% of patients treated with Exforge but at a higher incidence in amlodipine/valsartan patients (n=1437) than placebo (n=337) included peripheral edema (5.4% vs 3.0%), nasopharyngitis (4.3% vs 1.8%), upper respiratory tract infection (2.9% vs 2.1%) and dizziness (2.1% vs 0.9%).

Orthostatic events (orthostatic hypotension and postural dizziness) were seen in less than 1% of patients.

Other adverse reactions that occurred in placebo-controlled clinical trials with Exforge (≥0.2%) are listed below. It cannot be determined whether these events were causally related to Exforge.

Blood and Lymphatic System Disorders: Lymphadenopathy

Cardiac Disorders: Palpitations, tachycardia

Ear and Labyrinth Disorders: Ear pain

Gastrointestinal Disorders: Diarrhea, nausea, constipation, dyspepsia, abdominal pain, abdominal pain upper, gastritis, vomiting, abdominal discomfort, abdominal distention, dry mouth, colitis

General Disorders and Administration Site Conditions: Fatigue, chest pain, asthenia, pitting edema, pyrexia, edema

Immune System Disorders: Seasonal allergies

Infections and Infestations: Nasopharyngitis, sinusitis, bronchitis, pharyngitis, gastroenteritis, pharyngotonsillitis, bronchitis acute, tonsillitis

Injury and Poisoning: Epicondylitis, joint sprain, limb injury

Metabolism and Nutrition Disorders: Gout, non-insulin-dependent diabetes mellitus, hypercholesterolemia

Musculoskeletal and Connective Tissue Disorders: Arthralgia, back pain, muscle spasms, pain in extremity, myalgia, osteoarthritis, joint swelling, musculoskeletal chest pain

Nervous System Disorders: Headache, sciatica, paresthesia, cervicobrachial syndrome, carpal tunnel syndrome, hypoesthesia, sinus headache, somnolence

Psychiatric Disorders: Insomnia, anxiety, depression

Renal and Urinary Disorders: Hematuria, nephrolithiasis, pollakiuria

Reproductive System and Breast Disorders: Erectile dysfunction

Respiratory, Thoracic and Mediastinal Disorders: Cough, pharyngolaryngeal pain, sinus congestion, dyspnea, epistaxis, productive cough, dysphonia, nasal congestion

Skin and Subcutaneous Tissue Disorders: Pruritus, rash, hyperhidrosis, eczema, erythema

Vascular Disorders: Flushing, hot flush

Isolated cases of the following clinically notable adverse reactions were also observed in clinical trials: exanthema, syncope, visual disturbance, hypersensitivity, tinnitus, and hypotension.

Studies with Amlodipine:

Norvasc®* has been evaluated for safety in more than 11000 patients in U.S. and foreign clinical trials. Other adverse events that have been reported <1% but >0.1% of patients in controlled clinical trials or under conditions of open trials or marketing experience where a causal relationship is uncertain were:

Cardiovascular: arrhythmia (including ventricular tachycardia and atrial fibrillation), bradycardia, chest pain, peripheral ischemia, syncope, postural hypotension, vasculitis

Central and Peripheral Nervous System: neuropathy peripheral, tremor

Gastrointestinal: anorexia, dysphagia, pancreatitis, gingival hyperplasia

General: allergic reaction, hot flushes, malaise, rigors, weight gain, weight loss

Musculoskeletal System: arthrosis, muscle cramps

Psychiatric: sexual dysfunction (male and female), nervousness, abnormal dreams, depersonalization

Respiratory System: dyspnea

Skin and Appendages: angioedema, erythema multiforme, rash erythematous, rash maculopapular

Special Senses: abnormal vision, conjunctivitis, diplopia, eye pain, tinnitus

Urinary System: micturition frequency, micturition disorder, nocturia

Autonomic Nervous System: sweating increased

Metabolic and Nutritional: hyperglycemia, thirst

Hemopoietic: leukopenia, purpura, thrombocytopenia

Other events reported with amlodipine at a frequency of ≤0.1% of patients include: cardiac failure, pulse irregularity, extrasystoles, skin discoloration, urticaria, skin dryness, alopecia, dermatitis, muscle weakness, twitching, ataxia, hypertonia, migraine, cold and clammy skin, apathy, agitation, amnesia, gastritis, increased appetite, loose stools, rhinitis, dysuria, polyuria, parosmia, taste perversion, abnormal visual accommodation, and xerophthalmia. Other reactions occurred sporadically and cannot be distinguished from medications or concurrent disease states such as myocardial infarction and angina.

Adverse reactions reported for amlodipine for indications other than hypertension may be found in the prescribing information for Norvasc.

Studies with Valsartan:

Diovan® has been evaluated for safety in more than 4000 hypertensive patients in clinical trials. In trials in which valsartan was compared to an ACE inhibitor with or without placebo, the incidence of dry cough was significantly greater in the ACE inhibitor group (7.9%) than in the groups who received valsartan (2.6%) or placebo (1.5%). In a 129-patient trial limited to patients who had had dry cough when they had previously received ACE inhibitors, the incidences of cough in patients who received valsartan, HCTZ, or lisinopril were 20%, 19%, and 69% respectively (p<0.001). Other adverse reactions, not listed above, occurring in >0.2% of patients in controlled clinical trials with valsartan are:

Body as a Whole: allergic reaction, asthenia

Musculoskeletal: muscle cramps

Neurologic and Psychiatric: paresthesia

Respiratory: sinusitis, pharyngitis

Urogenital: impotence

Other reported events seen less frequently in clinical trials were: angioedema.

Adverse reactions reported for valsartan for indications other than hypertension may be found in the prescribing information for Diovan.

Clinical Lab Test Findings:

Creatinine: In hypertensive patients, greater than 50% increases in creatinine occurred in 0.4% of patients receiving Exforge and 0.6% receiving placebo. In heart failure patients, greater than 50% increases in creatinine were observed in 3.9% of valsartan-treated patients compared to 0.9% of placebo-treated patients. In post-myocardial infarction patients, doubling of serum creatinine was observed in 4.2% of valsartan-treated patients and 3.4% of captopril-treated patients.

Liver Function Tests: Occasional elevations (greater than 150%) of liver chemistries occurred in Exforge-treated patients.

Serum Potassium: In hypertensive patients, greater than 20% increases in serum potassium were observed in 2.8% of Exforge-treated patients compared to 3.4% of placebo-treated patients. In heart failure patients, greater than 20% increases in serum potassium were observed in 10% of valsartan-treated patients compared to 5.1% of placebo-treated patients.

Blood Urea Nitrogen (BUN): In hypertensive patients, greater than 50% increases in BUN were observed in 5.5% of Exforge-treated patients compared to 4.7% of placebo-treated patients. In heart failure patients, greater than 50% increases in BUN were observed in 16.6% of valsartan-treated patients compared to 6.3% of placebo-treated patients.

Neutropenia: Neutropenia was observed in 1.9% of patients treated with Diovan and 0.8% of patients treated with placebo.

6.2 Postmarketing Experience

Amlodipine: Gynecomastia has been reported infrequently and a causal relationship is uncertain. Jaundice and hepatic enzyme elevations (mostly consistent with cholestasis or hepatitis), in some cases severe enough to require hospitalization, have been reported in association with use of amlodipine.

Valsartan: The following additional adverse reactions have been reported in postmarketing experience with valsartan:

Blood and Lymphatic: Decrease in hemoglobin, decrease in hematocrit, neutropenia

Hypersensitivity: There are rare reports of angioedema. Some of these patients previously experienced angioedema with other drugs including ACE inhibitors. Exforge should not be re-administered to patients who have had angioedema.

Digestive: Elevated liver enzymes and very rare reports of hepatitis

Renal: Impaired renal function, renal failure

Clinical Laboratory Tests: Hyperkalemia

Dermatologic: Alopecia, bullous dermatitis

Vascular: Vasculitis

Rare cases of rhabdomyolysis have been reported in patients receiving angiotensin II receptor blockers.

7 DRUG INTERACTIONS

No drug interaction studies have been conducted with Exforge and other drugs, although studies have been conducted with the individual amlodipine and valsartan components.

Studies with Amlodipine

Simvastatin: Coadministration of simvastatin with amlodipine increases the systemic exposure of simvastatin. Limit the dose of simvastatin in patients on amlodipine to 20 mg daily.

CYP3A4 Inhibitors: Coadministration with CYP3A4 inhibitors (moderate and strong) result in increased systemic exposure to amlodipine warranting dose reduction. Monitor for symptoms of hypotension and edema when amlodipine is coadministered with CYP3A4 inhibitors to determine the need for dose adjustment.

CYP3A4 Inducers: No information is available on the quantitative effects of CYP3A4 inducers on amlodipine. Blood pressure should be monitored when amlodipine is coadministered with CYP3A4 inducers.

Studies with Valsartan

No clinically significant pharmacokinetic interactions were observed when valsartan was coadministered with amlodipine, atenolol, cimetidine, digoxin, furosemide, glyburide, hydrochlorothiazide, or indomethacin. The valsartan-atenolol combination was more antihypertensive than either component, but it did not lower the heart rate more than atenolol alone.

Warfarin: Coadministration of valsartan and warfarin did not change the pharmacokinetics of valsartan or the time-course of the anticoagulant properties of warfarin.

Non-Steroidal Anti-Inflammatory Agents including Selective Cyclooxygenase-2 Inhibitors (COX-2 Inhibitors): In patients who are elderly, volume-depleted (including those on diuretic therapy), or with compromised renal function, coadministration of NSAIDs, including selective COX-2 inhibitors, with angiotensin II receptor antagonists, including valsartan, may result in deterioration of renal function, including possible acute renal failure. These effects are usually reversible. Monitor renal function periodically in patients receiving valsartan and NSAID therapy.

The antihypertensive effect of angiotensin II receptor antagonists, including valsartan may be attenuated by NSAIDs including selective COX-2 inhibitors.

Potassium: Concomitant use of valsartan with other agents that block the renin-angiotensin system, potassium sparing diuretics (e.g., spironolactone, triamterene, amiloride), potassium supplements, or salt substitutes containing potassium may lead to increases in serum potassium and in heart failure patients to increases in serum creatinine. If co-medication is considered necessary, monitoring of serum potassium is advisable.

CYP 450 Interactions: In vitro metabolism studies indicate that CYP 450 mediated drug interactions between valsartan and coadministered drugs are unlikely because of low extent of metabolism *[see Pharmacokinetics, Valsartan (12.3)].*

Transporters: The results from an *in vitro* study with human liver tissue indicate that valsartan is a substrate of the hepatic uptake transporter OATP1B1 and the hepatic efflux transporter MRP2. Coadministration of inhibitors of the uptake transporter (rifampin, cyclosporine) or efflux transporter (ritonavir) may increase the systemic exposure to valsartan.

Dual Blockade of the Renin-Angiotensin System (RAS): Dual blockade of the RAS with angiotensin receptor blockers, ACE inhibitors, or aliskiren is associated with increased risks of hypotension, hyperkalemia, and changes in renal function (including acute renal failure) compared to monotherapy. Closely monitor blood pressure, renal function, and electrolytes in patients on Exforge and other agents that affect the RAS.

Do not coadminister aliskiren with Exforge in patients with diabetes. Avoid use of aliskiren with Exforge in patients with renal impairment (GFR <60 mL/min).

Lithium: Increases in serum lithium concentrations and lithium toxicity have been reported during concomitant administration of lithium with angiotensin II receptor antagonists, including valsartan. Monitor serum lithium levels during concomitant use.

8 USE IN SPECIFIC POPULATIONS

8.1 Pregnancy

Pregnancy Category D

Use of drugs that act on the renin-angiotensin system during the second and third trimesters of pregnancy reduces fetal renal function and increases fetal and neonatal morbidity and death. Resulting oligohydramnios can be associated with fetal lung hypoplasia and skeletal deformations. Potential neonatal adverse effects include skull hypoplasia, anuria, hypotension, renal failure, and death. When pregnancy is detected, discontinue Exforge as soon as possible. These adverse outcomes are usually associated with use of these drugs in the second and third trimesters of pregnancy. Most epidemiologic studies examining fetal abnormalities after exposure to antihypertensive use in the first trimester have not distinguished drugs affecting the renin-angiotensin system from other antihypertensive agents. Appropriate management of maternal hypertension during pregnancy is important to optimize outcomes for both mother and fetus.

In the unusual case that there is no appropriate alternative to therapy with drugs affecting the renin-angiotensin system for a particular patient, apprise the mother of the potential risk to the fetus. Perform serial ultrasound examinations to assess the intra-amniotic environment. If oligohydramnios is observed, discontinue Exforge, unless it is considered lifesaving for the mother. Fetal testing·may be appropriate, based on the week of pregnancy. Patients and physicians should be aware, however, that oligohydramnios may not appear until after the fetus has sustained irreversible injury.

Closely observe infants with histories of *in utero* exposure to Exforge for hypotension, oliguria, and hyperkalemia *[see Use in Specific Populations (8.4)].*

8.2 Labor and Delivery

The effect of Exforge on labor and delivery has not been studied.

8.3 Nursing Mothers

It is not known whether amlodipine is excreted in human milk. In the absence of this information, it is recommended that nursing be discontinued while amlodipine is administered.

It is not known whether valsartan is excreted in human milk. Valsartan was excreted into the milk of lactating rats; however, animal breast milk drug levels may not accurately reflect human breast milk levels. Because many drugs are excreted into human milk and because of the potential for adverse reactions in nursing infants from Exforge, a decision should be made whether to discontinue nursing or discontinue the drug, taking into account the importance of the drug to the mother.

8.4 Pediatric Use

Safety and effectiveness of Exforge in pediatric patients have not been established.

Neonates with a history of *in utero* exposure to Exforge: If oliguria or hypotension occurs, direct attention toward support of blood pressure and renal perfusion. Exchange

transfusions or dialysis may be required as a means of reversing hypotension and/or substituting for disordered renal function.

8.5 Geriatric Use

In controlled clinical trials, 323 (22.5%) hypertensive patients treated with Exforge were ≥65 years and 79 (5.5%) were ≥75 years. No overall differences in the efficacy or safety of Exforge was observed in this patient population, but greater sensitivity of some older individuals cannot be ruled out.

Amlodipine: Clinical studies of amlodipine besylate tablets did not include sufficient numbers of subjects aged 65 and over to determine whether they respond differently from younger subjects. Other reported clinical experience has not identified differences in responses between the elderly and younger patients. In general, dose selection for an elderly patient should be cautious, usually starting at the low end of the dosing range, reflecting the greater frequency of decreased hepatic, renal or cardiac function, and of concomitant disease or other drug therapy. Elderly patients have decreased clearance of amlodipine with a resulting increase of AUC of approximately 40% to 60%, and a lower initial dose may be required.

Valsartan: In the controlled clinical trials of valsartan, 1214 (36.2%) of hypertensive patients treated with valsartan were ≥65 years and 265 (7.9%) were ≥75 years. No overall difference in the efficacy or safety of valsartan was observed in this patient population, but greater sensitivity of some older individuals cannot be ruled out.

8.6 Renal Impairment

Safety and effectiveness of Exforge in patients with severe renal impairment (CrCl<30 mL/min) have not been established. No dose adjustment is required in patients with mild (CrCl 60 to 90 mL/min) or moderate (CrCl 30 to 60 mL/min) renal impairment.

8.7 Hepatic Impairment

Amlodipine

Exposure to amlodipine is increased in patients with hepatic insufficiency, thus consider using lower doses of Exforge *[see Clinical Pharmacology (12.3)].*

Valsartan

No dose adjustment is necessary for patients with mild-to-moderate disease. No dosing recommendations can be provided for patients with severe liver disease.

10 OVERDOSAGE

Information on Amlodipine

Single oral doses of amlodipine maleate equivalent to 40 mg/kg and 100 mg/kg amlodipine in mice and rats, respectively, caused deaths. Single oral doses equivalent to 4 or more mg/kg amlodipine in dogs (11 or more times the maximum recommended human dose on a mg/m^2 basis) caused a marked peripheral vasodilation and hypotension. Overdosage might be expected to cause excessive peripheral vasodilation with marked hypotension. In humans, experience with intentional overdosage of amlodipine is limited. Marked and potentially prolonged systemic hypotension up to and including shock with fatal outcome have been reported.

If massive overdose should occur, initiate active cardiac and respiratory monitoring. Frequent blood pressure measurements are essential. Should hypotension occur, cardiovascular support including elevation of the extremities and the judicious administration of fluids should be initiated. If hypotension remains unresponsive to these conservative measures, consider administration of vasopressors (such as phenylephrine) with attention to circulating volume and urine output. As amlodipine is highly protein bound, hemodialysis is not likely to be of benefit. Administration of activated charcoal to healthy volunteers immediately or up to two hours after ingestion of amlodipine has been shown to significantly decrease amlodipine absorption.

Information on Valsartan

Limited data are available related to overdosage in humans. The most likely effect of overdose with valsartan would be peripheral vasodilation, hypotension, and tachycardia; bradycardia could occur from parasympathetic (vagal) stimulation. Depressed level of consciousness, circulatory collapse, and shock have been reported. If symptomatic hypotension should occur, supportive treatment should be instituted.

Valsartan is not removed from the plasma by hemodialysis. Valsartan was without grossly observable adverse effects at single oral doses up to 2000 mg/kg in rats and up to 1000 mg/kg in marmosets, except for the salivation and diarrhea in the rat and vomiting in the marmoset at the highest dose (60 and 37 times, respectively, the maximum recommended human dose (MRHD) on a mg/m^2 basis). (Calculations assume an oral dose of 320 mg/day and a 60 kg patient.)

11 DESCRIPTION

Exforge is a fixed combination of amlodipine and valsartan. Exforge contains the besylate salt of amlodipine, a dihydropyridine calcium-channel blocker (CCB). Amlodipine besylate is a white to pale yellow crystalline powder, slightly soluble in water and sparingly soluble in ethanol. Amlodipine besylate's chemical name is 3-Ethyl-5-methyl(4RS)-2-[(2-aminoethoxy)methyl]-4-(2-chlorophenyl)-6-methyl-1,4-dihydropyridine-3,5-dicarboxylate benzenesulphonate; its structural formula is:

Its empirical formula is $C_{20}H_{25}ClN_2O_5 \cdot C_6H_6O_3S$ and its molecular weight is 567.1.

Valsartan is a nonpeptide, orally active, and specific angiotensin II antagonist acting on the AT_1 receptor subtype. Valsartan is a white to practically white fine powder, soluble in ethanol and methanol and slightly soluble in water. Valsartan's chemical name is N-(1-oxopentyl)-N-[[2'-(1H-tetrazol-5-yl) [1,1'-biphenyl]-4-yl]methyl]-L-valine; its structural formula is:

Its empirical formula is $C_{24}H_{29}N_5O_3$ and its molecular weight is 435.5.

Exforge tablets are formulated in 4 strengths for oral administration with a combination of amlodipine besylate, equivalent to 5 mg or 10 mg of amlodipine free-base, with 160 mg, or 320 mg of valsartan providing for the following available combinations: 5/160 mg, 10/160 mg, 5/320 mg, and 10/320 mg.

The inactive ingredients for all strengths of the tablets are colloidal silicon dioxide, crospovidone, magnesium stearate, and microcrystalline cellulose. Additionally the 5/320 mg and 10/320 mg strengths contain iron oxide yellow and sodium starch glycolate. The film coating contains hypromellose, iron oxides, polyethylene glycol, talc, and titanium dioxide.

12 CLINICAL PHARMACOLOGY

12.1 Mechanism of Action

Amlodipine

Amlodipine is a dihydropyridine calcium channel blocker that inhibits the transmembrane influx of calcium ions into vascular smooth muscle and cardiac muscle. Experimental data suggest that amlodipine binds to both dihydropyridine and nondihydropyridine binding sites. The contractile processes of cardiac muscle and vascular smooth muscle are dependent upon the movement of extracellular calcium ions into these cells through specific ion channels. Amlodipine inhibits calcium ion influx across cell membranes selectively, with a greater effect on vascular smooth muscle cells than on cardiac muscle cells. Negative inotropic effects can be detected *in vitro* but such effects have not been seen in intact animals at therapeutic doses. Serum calcium concentration is not affected by amlodipine. Within the physiologic pH range, amlodipine is an ionized compound (pKa=8.6); and its kinetic interaction with the calcium channel receptor is characterized by a gradual rate of association and dissociation with the receptor binding site, resulting in a gradual onset of effect.

Amlodipine is a peripheral arterial vasodilator that acts directly on vascular smooth muscle to cause a reduction in peripheral vascular resistance and reduction in blood pressure.

Valsartan

Angiotensin II is formed from angiotensin I in a reaction catalyzed by angiotensin-converting enzyme (ACE, kininase II). Angiotensin II is the principal pressor agent of the renin-angiotensin system, with effects that include vasoconstriction, stimulation of synthesis and release of aldosterone, cardiac stimulation, and renal reabsorption of sodium. Valsartan blocks the vasoconstrictor and aldosterone-secreting effects of angiotensin II by selectively blocking the binding of angiotensin II to the AT_1 receptor in many tissues, such as vascular smooth muscle and the adrenal gland. Its action is therefore independent of the pathways for angiotensin II synthesis.

There is also an AT_2 receptor found in many tissues, but AT_2 is not known to be associated with cardiovascular homeostasis. Valsartan has much greater affinity (about 20,000-fold) for the AT_1 receptor than for the AT_2 receptor. The increased plasma levels of angiotensin following AT_1 receptor blockade with valsartan may stimulate the unblocked AT_2 receptor. The primary metabolite of valsartan is essentially inactive with an affinity for the AT_1 receptor about one-200th that of valsartan itself.

Blockade of the renin-angiotensin system with ACE inhibitors, which inhibit the biosynthesis of angiotensin II from angiotensin I, is widely used in the treatment of hypertension. ACE inhibitors also inhibit the degradation of bradykinin, a reaction also catalyzed by ACE. Because valsartan does not inhibit ACE (kininase II), it does not affect the response to bradykinin. Whether this difference has clinical relevance is not yet known. Valsartan does not bind to or block other hormone receptors or ion channels known to be important in cardiovascular regulation.

Blockade of the angiotensin II receptor inhibits the negative regulatory feedback of angiotensin II on renin secretion, but the resulting increased plasma renin activity and angiotensin II circulating levels do not overcome the effect of valsartan on blood pressure.

12.2 Pharmacodynamics

Amlodipine

Following administration of therapeutic doses to patients with hypertension, amlodipine produces vasodilation resulting in a reduction of supine and standing blood pressures. These decreases in blood pressure are not accompanied by a significant change in heart rate or plasma catecholamine levels with chronic dosing. Although the acute intravenous administration of amlodipine decreases arterial blood pressure and increases heart rate in hemodynamic studies of patients with chronic stable angina, chronic oral administration of amlodipine in clinical trials did not lead to clinically significant changes in heart rate or blood pressures in normotensive patients with angina.

With chronic, once-daily administration, antihypertensive effectiveness is maintained for at least 24 hours. Plasma concentrations correlate with effect in both young and elderly patients. The magnitude of reduction in blood pressure with amlodipine is also correlated with the height of pretreatment elevation; thus, individuals with moderate hypertension (diastolic pressure 105-114 mmHg) had about a 50% greater response than patients with mild hypertension (diastolic pressure 90-104 mmHg). Normotensive subjects experienced no clinically significant change in blood pressure (+1/-2 mmHg).

In hypertensive patients with normal renal function, therapeutic doses of amlodipine resulted in a decrease in renal vascular resistance and an increase in glomerular filtration rate and effective renal plasma flow without change in filtration fraction or proteinuria.

As with other calcium channel blockers, hemodynamic measurements of cardiac function at rest and during exercise (or pacing) in patients with normal ventricular function treated with amlodipine have generally demonstrated a small increase in cardiac index without significant influence on dP/dt or on left ventricular end diastolic pressure or volume. In hemodynamic studies, amlodipine has not been associated with a negative inotropic effect when administered in the therapeutic dose range to intact animals and man, even when coadministered with beta-blockers to man. Similar findings, however, have been observed in normal or well-compensated patients with either heart failure with agents possessing significant negative inotropic effects.

Amlodipine does not change sinoatrial nodal function or atrioventricular (AV) conduction in intact animals or man. In patients with chronic stable angina, intravenous administration of 10 mg did not significantly alter A-H and H-V conduction and sinus node recovery time after pacing. Similar results were obtained in patients receiving amlodipine and concomitant beta-blockers. In clinical studies in which amlodipine was administered in combination with beta-blockers to patients with either hypertension or angina, no adverse effects of electrocardiographic (ECG) parameters were observed. In clinical trials with angina patients alone, amlodipine therapy did not alter electrocardiographic intervals or produce higher degrees of AV blocks.

Amlodipine has indications other than hypertension which can be found in the Norvasc* package insert.

Valsartan

Valsartan inhibits the pressor effect of angiotensin II infusions. An oral dose of 80 mg inhibits the pressor effect by about 80% at peak with approximately 30% inhibition persisting for 24 hours. No information on the effect of larger doses is available.

Removal of the negative feedback of angiotensin II causes a 2- to 3-fold rise in plasma renin and consequent rise in angiotensin II plasma concentration in hypertensive patients. Minimal decreases in plasma aldosterone were observed after administration of valsartan; very little effect on serum potassium was observed.

In multiple dose studies in hypertensive patients with stable renal insufficiency and patients with renovascular hypertension, valsartan had no clinically significant effects on glomerular filtration rate, filtration fraction, creatinine clearance, or renal plasma flow.

Administration of valsartan to patients with essential hypertension results in a significant reduction of sitting, supine, and standing systolic blood pressure, usually with little or no orthostatic change. Valsartan has indications other than hypertension which can be found in the Diovan package insert.

Exforge

Exforge has been shown to be effective in lowering blood pressure. Both amlodipine and valsartan lower blood pressure by reducing peripheral resistance, but calcium influx blockade and reduction of angiotensin II vasoconstriction are complementary mechanisms.

12.3 Pharmacokinetics

Amlodipine

Peak plasma concentrations of amlodipine are reached 6 to 12 hours after administration of amlodipine alone. Absolute bioavailability has been estimated to be between 64% and 90%. The bioavailability of amlodipine is not altered by the presence of food.

The apparent volume of distribution of amlodipine is 21 L/kg. Approximately 93% of circulating amlodipine is bound to plasma proteins in hypertensive patients.

Amlodipine is extensively (about 90%) converted to inactive metabolites via hepatic metabolism with 10% of the parent compound and 60% of the metabolites excreted in the urine. Elimination of amlodipine from the plasma is biphasic with a terminal elimination half-life of about 30 to 50 hours. Steady state plasma levels of amlodipine are reached after 7 to 8 days of consecutive daily dosing.

Valsartan

Following oral administration of valsartan alone peak plasma concentrations of valsartan are reached in 2 to 4 hours. Absolute bioavailability is about 25% (range 10% to 35%). Food decreases the exposure (as measured by AUC) to valsartan by about 40% and peak plasma concentration (C_{max}) by about 50%.

The steady state volume of distribution of valsartan after intravenous administration is 17 L indicating that valsartan does not distribute into tissues extensively. Valsartan is highly bound to serum proteins (95%), mainly serum albumin.

Valsartan shows biexponential decay kinetics following intravenous administration with an average elimination half-life of about 6 hours. The recovery is mainly as unchanged drug, with only about 20% of dose recovered as metabolites. The primary metabolite, accounting for about 9% of dose, is valeryl 4-hydroxy valsartan. In vitro metabolism studies involving recombinant CYP 450 enzymes indicated that the CYP 2C9 isoenzyme is responsible for the formation of valeryl-4-hydroxy valsartan. Valsartan does not inhibit CYP 450 isozymes at clinically relevant concentrations. CYP 450 mediated drug interaction between valsartan and coadministered drugs are unlikely because of the low extent of metabolism.

Valsartan, when administered as an oral solution, is primarily recovered in feces (about 83% of dose) and urine (about 13% of dose). Following intravenous administration, plasma clearance of valsartan is about 2 L/h and its renal clearance is 0.62 L/h (about 30% of total clearance).

Exforge

Following oral administration of Exforge in normal healthy adults, peak plasma concentrations of valsartan and amlodipine are reached in 3 and 6 to 8 hours, respectively. The rate and extent of absorption of valsartan and amlodipine from Exforge are the same as when administered as individual tablets. The bioavailabilities of amlodipine and valsartan are not altered by the coadministration of food.

Special Populations

Geriatric

Studies with Amlodipine: Elderly patients have decreased clearance of amlodipine with a resulting increase in peak plasma levels, elimination half-life and AUC.

Studies with Valsartan: Exposure (measured by AUC) to valsartan is higher by 70% and the half-life is longer by 35% in the elderly than in the young. No dosage adjustment is necessary.

Gender

Studies with Valsartan: Pharmacokinetics of valsartan does not differ significantly between males and females.

Renal Insufficiency

Studies with Amlodipine: The pharmacokinetics of amlodipine is not significantly influenced by renal impairment.

Studies with Valsartan: There is no apparent correlation between renal function (measured by creatinine clearance) and exposure (measured by AUC) to valsartan in patients with different degrees of renal impairment. Consequently, dose adjustment is not required in patients with mild-to-moderate renal dysfunction. No studies have been performed in patients with severe impairment of renal function (creatinine clearance <10 mL/min). Valsartan is not removed from the plasma by hemodialysis. In the case of severe renal disease, exercise care with dosing of valsartan.

Hepatic Insufficiency

Studies with Amlodipine: Patients with hepatic insufficiency have decreased clearance of amlodipine with resulting increase in AUC of approximately 40% to 60%.

Studies with Valsartan: On average, patients with mild-to-moderate chronic liver disease have twice the exposure (measured by AUC values) to valsartan of healthy volunteers (matched by age, sex and weight). In general, no dosage adjustment is needed in patients with mild-to-moderate liver disease. Care should be exercised in patients with liver disease.

Drug Interactions

In vitro data in human plasma indicate that amlodipine has no effect on the protein binding of digoxin, phenytoin, warfarin and indomethacin.

Cimetidine: Coadministration of amlodipine with cimetidine did not alter the pharmacokinetics of amlodipine.

Grapefruit juice: Coadministration of 240 mL of grapefruit juice with a single oral dose of amlodipine 10 mg in 20 healthy volunteers had no significant effect on the pharmacokinetics of amlodipine.

Maalox® (antacid): Coadministration of the antacid Maalox with a single dose of amlodipine had no significant effect on the pharmacokinetics of amlodipine.

Sildenafil: A single 100 mg dose of sildenafil (Viagra®**) in subjects with essential hypertension had no effect on the pharmacokinetic parameters of amlodipine. When amlodipine and sildenafil were used in combination, each agent independently exerted its own blood pressure lowering effect.

Atorvastatin: Coadministration of multiple 10 mg doses of amlodipine with 80 mg of atorvastatin resulted in no significant change in the steady state pharmacokinetic parameters of atorvastatin.

Digoxin: Coadministration of amlodipine with digoxin did not change serum digoxin levels or digoxin renal clearance in normal volunteers.

Warfarin: Coadministration of amlodipine with warfarin did not change the warfarin prothrombin response time.

Simvastatin: Coadministration of multiple doses of 10 mg of amlodipine with 80 mg simvastatin resulted in a 77% increase in exposure to simvastatin compared to simvastatin alone. Limit the dose of simvastatin in patients on amlodipine to 20 mg daily.

CYP3A4 Inhibitors: Coadministration of a 180 mg daily dose of diltiazem with 5 mg amlodipine in elderly hypertensive patients resulted in a 60% increase in amlodipine systemic exposure. Erythromycin coadministration in healthy volunteers did not significantly change amlodipine systemic exposure. However, strong inhibitors of CYP3A4 (i.e., ketoconazole, itraconazole, ritonavir) may increase the plasma concentrations of amlodipine to a greater extent.

13 NONCLINICAL TOXICOLOGY

13.1 Carcinogenesis, Mutagenesis, Impairment of Fertility

Studies with Amlodipine

Rats and mice treated with amlodipine maleate in the diet for up to 2 years, at concentrations calculated to provide daily dosage levels of 0.5, 1.25, and 2.5 mg amlodipine/kg/day, showed no evidence of a carcinogenic effect of the drug. For the mouse, the highest dose was, on mg/m^2 basis, similar to the MRHD of 10 mg amlodipine/day. For the rat, the highest dose was, on a mg/m^2 basis, about 2.5 the MRHD. (Calculations based on a 60 kg patient.)

Mutagenicity studies conducted with amlodipine maleate revealed no drug-related effects at either the gene or chromosome level.

There was no effect on the fertility of rats treated orally with amlodipine maleate (males for 64 days and females for 14 days prior to mating) at doses of up to 10 mg amlodipine/kg/day (about 10 times the MRHD of 10 mg/day on a mg/m^2 basis).

Studies with Valsartan

There was no evidence of carcinogenicity when valsartan was administered in the diet to mice and rats for up to 2 years at concentrations calculated to provide doses of up to 160 and 200 mg/kg/day, respectively. These doses in mice and rats are about 2.4 and 6 times, respectively, the MRHD of 320 mg/day on a mg/m^2 basis. (Calculations based on a 60 kg patient.)

Mutagenicity assays did not reveal any valsartan-related effects at either the gene or chromosome level. These assays included bacterial mutagenicity tests with Salmonella and E. coli, a gene mutation test with Chinese hamster V79 cells, a cytogenetic test with Chinese hamster ovary cells, and a rat micronucleus test.

Table 1: Effect of Exforge on Sitting Diastolic Blood Pressure

Amlodipine dosage	Valsartan dosage							
	0 mg		80 mg		160 mg		320 mg	
	Mean Change*	Placebo-subtracted	Mean Change*	Placebo-subtracted	Mean Change*	Placebo-subtracted	Mean Change*	Placebo-subtracted
0 mg	-6.4	---	-9.5	-3.1	-10.9	-4.5	-13.2	-6.7
5 mg	-11.1	-4.7	-14.2	-7.8	-14.0	-7.6	-15.7	-9.3

*Mean Change and Placebo-Subtracted Mean Change from Baseline (mmHg) at Week 8 in Sitting Diastolic Blood Pressure. Mean baseline diastolic BP was 99.3 mmHg.

Table 2: Effect of Exforge on Sitting Systolic Blood Pressure

Amlodipine dosage	Valsartan dosage							
	0 mg		80 mg		160 mg		320 mg	
	Mean Change*	Placebo-subtracted	Mean Change*	Placebo-subtracted	Mean Change*	Placebo-subtracted	Mean Change*	Placebo-subtracted
0 mg	-6.2	---	-12.9	-6.8	-14.3	-8.2	-16.3	-10.1
5 mg	-14.8	-8.6	-20.7	-14.5	-19.4	-13.2	-22.4	-16.2

*Mean Change and Placebo-Subtracted Mean Change from Baseline (mmHg) at Week 8 in Sitting Systolic Blood Pressure. Mean baseline systolic BP was 152.8 mmHg.

Table 3: Effect of Exforge on Sitting Diastolic Blood Pressure

Amlodipine dosage	Valsartan dosage					
	0 mg		160 mg		320 mg	
	Mean Change*	Placebo-subtracted	Mean Change*	Placebo-subtracted	Mean Change*	Placebo-subtracted
0 mg	-8.2	---	-12.8	-4.5	-12.8	-4.5
10 mg	-15.0	-6.7	-17.2	-9.0	-18.1	-9.9

*Mean Change and Placebo-Subtracted Mean Change from Baseline (mmHg) at Week 8 in Sitting Diastolic Blood Pressure. Mean baseline diastolic BP was 99.1 mmHg.

Table 4: Effect of Exforge on Sitting Systolic Blood Pressure

Amlodipine dosage	Valsartan dosage					
	0 mg		160 mg		320 mg	
	Mean Change*	Placebo-subtracted	Mean Change*	Placebo-subtracted	Mean Change*	Placebo-subtracted
0 mg	-11.0	---	-18.1	-7.0	-18.5	-7.5
10 mg	-22.2	-11.2	-26.6	-15.5	-26.9	-15.9

*Mean Change and Placebo-Subtracted Mean Change from Baseline (mmHg) at Week 8 in Sitting Systolic Blood Pressure. Mean baseline systolic BP was 156.7 mmHg.

Valsartan had no adverse effects on the reproductive performance of male or female rats at oral doses of up to 200 mg/kg/day. This dose is about 6 times the MRHD on a mg/m² basis.

13.3 Developmental Toxicity Studies

Studies with Amlodipine

No evidence of teratogenicity or other embryo/fetal toxicity was found when pregnant rats and rabbits were treated orally with amlodipine maleate at doses of up to 10 mg amlodipine/kg/day (respectively, about 10 and 20 times the MRHD of 10 mg amlodipine on a mg/m² basis) during their respective periods of major organogenesis. (Calculations based on a patient weight of 60 kg.) However, litter size was significantly decreased (by about 50%) and the number of intrauterine deaths was significantly increased (about 5-fold) for rats receiving amlodipine maleate at a dose equivalent to 10 mg amlodipine/kg/day for 14 days before mating and throughout gestation. Amlodipine maleate has been shown to prolong both the gestation period and the duration of labor in rats at this dose. There are no adequate and well-controlled studies in pregnant women. Amlodipine should be used during pregnancy only if the potential benefit justifies the potential risk to the fetus.

Studies with Valsartan

No teratogenic effects were observed when valsartan was administered to pregnant mice and rats at oral doses of up to 600 mg/kg/day and to pregnant rabbits at oral doses of up to 10 mg/kg/day. However, significant decreases in fetal weight, pup birth weight, pup survival rate, and slight delays in developmental milestones were observed in studies in which parental rats were treated with valsartan at oral, maternally toxic (reduction in body weight gain and food consumption) doses of 600 mg/kg/day during organogenesis or late gestation and lactation. In rabbits, fetotoxicity (i.e., resorptions, litter loss, abortions, and low body weight) associated with maternal toxicity (mortality) was observed at doses of 5 and 10 mg/kg/day. The no observed adverse effect doses of 600, 200, and 2 mg/kg/day in mice, rats and rabbits, respectively, are about 9, 6, and 0.1 times the MRHD of 320 mg/day on a mg/m² basis. (Calculations based on a patient weight of 60 kg.)

Studies with Amlodipine Besylate and Valsartan

In the oral embryofetal development study in rats using amlodipine besylate plus valsartan at doses equivalent to 5 mg/kg/day amlodipine plus 80 mg/kg/day valsartan, 10 mg/kg/day amlodipine plus 160 mg/kg/day valsartan, and 20 mg/kg/day amlodipine plus 320 mg/kg/day valsartan, treatment-related maternal and fetal effects (developmental delays and alterations noted in the presence of significant maternal toxicity) were noted with the high dose combination. The no-observed-adverse-effect level (NOAEL) for embryofetal effects was 10 mg/kg/day amlodipine plus 160 mg/kg/day valsartan. On a systemic exposure [AUC$_{(0-\infty)}$] basis, these doses are, respectively, 4.3, and 2.7 times the systemic exposure [AUC$_{(0-\infty)}$] in humans receiving the MRHD (10/320 mg/60 kg).

14 CLINICAL STUDIES

Exforge was studied in 2 placebo-controlled and 4 active-controlled trials in hypertensive patients. In a double-blind, placebo-controlled study, a total of 1012 patients with mild-to-moderate hypertension received treatments of 3 combinations of amlodipine and valsartan (5/80, 5/160, 5/320 mg) or amlodipine alone (5 mg), valsartan alone (80, 160, or 320 mg) or placebo. All doses with the exception of the 5/320 mg dose were initiated at the randomized dose. The high dose was titrated to that dose after a week at a dose of 5/160 mg. At week 8, the combination treatments were statistically significantly superior to their monotherapy components in reduction of diastolic and systolic blood pressures.

[See table 1 above]

[See table 2 above]

In a double-blind, placebo-controlled study, a total of 1246 patients with mild to moderate hypertension received treatments of 2 combinations of amlodipine and valsartan (10/160, 10/320 mg), valsartan alone (10 mg), valsartan alone (160 or 320 mg) or placebo. With the exception of the 10/320 mg dose, treatment was initiated at the randomized dose. The high dose was initiated at a dose of 5/160 mg and titrated to the randomized dose after 1 week. At week 8, the combination treatments were statistically significantly superior to their monotherapy components in reduction of diastolic and systolic blood pressures.

[See table 3 above]

[See table 4 above]

In a double-blind, active-controlled study, a total of 947 patients with mild to moderate hypertension who were not adequately controlled on valsartan 160 mg received treatments of 2 combinations of amlodipine and valsartan (10/160, 5/160 mg) or valsartan alone (160 mg). At week 8, the combination treatments were statistically significantly superior to the monotherapy component in reduction of diastolic and systolic blood pressures.

[See table 5 at top of next page]

In a double-blind, active-controlled study, a total of 944 patients with mild to moderate hypertension who were not adequately controlled on amlodipine 10 mg received a combination of amlodipine and valsartan (10/160 mg) or amlodipine alone (10 mg). At week 8, the combination treatment was statistically significantly superior to the monotherapy component in reduction of diastolic and systolic blood pressures.

[See table 6 at top of next page]

Exforge was also evaluated for safety in a 6-week, double-blind, active-controlled trial of 130 hypertensive patients with severe hypertension (mean baseline BP of 171/113 mmHg). Adverse events were similar in patients with severe hypertension and mild/moderate hypertension treated with Exforge.

A wide age range of the adult population, including the elderly was studied (range 19 to 92 years, mean 54.7 years). Women comprised almost half of the studied population (47.3%). Of the patients in the studied Exforge group, 87.6% were Caucasian. Black and Asian patients each represented approximately 4% of the population in the studied Exforge group.

Two additional double-blind, active-controlled studies were conducted in which Exforge was administered as initial therapy. In 1 study, a total of 572 black patients with moderate to severe hypertension were randomized to receive either combination amlodipine/valsartan or amlodipine monotherapy for 12 weeks. The initial dose of amlodipine/valsartan was 5/160 mg for 2 weeks with forced titration to 10/160 mg for 2 weeks, followed by optional titration to 10/320 mg for 4 weeks and optional addition of HCTZ 12.5 mg for 4 weeks. The initial dose of amlodipine was 5 mg for 2 weeks with forced titration to 10 mg for 2 weeks, followed by optional titration to 10 mg for 4 weeks and optional addition of HCTZ 12.5 mg for 4 weeks. At the primary endpoint of 8 weeks, the treatment difference between amlodipine/valsartan and amlodipine was 6.7/2.8 mmHg.

In the other study of similar design, a total of 646 patients with moderate to severe hypertension (MSSBP of ≥160 mmHg and <200 mmHg) were randomized to receive either combination amlodipine/valsartan or amlodipine monotherapy for 8 weeks. The initial dose of amlodipine/valsartan was 5/160 mg for 2 weeks with forced titration to 10/160 mg for 2 weeks, followed by the optional addition of HCTZ 12.5 mg for 4 weeks. The initial dose of amlodipine was 5 mg for 2 weeks with forced titration to 10 mg for 2 weeks, followed by the optional addition of HCTZ 12.5 mg for 4 weeks. At the primary endpoint of 4 weeks, the treatment difference between amlodipine/valsartan and amlodipine was 6.6/3.9 mmHg.

There are no trials of the Exforge combination tablet demonstrating reductions in cardiovascular risk in patients with hypertension, but the amlodipine component and several ARBs, which are the same pharmacological class as the valsartan component, have demonstrated such benefits.

16   HOW SUPPLIED/STORAGE AND HANDLING

Exforge is available as non-scored tablets containing amlodipine besylate equivalent to 5 mg, or 10 mg of amlodipine free-base with valsartan 160 mg or 320 mg, providing for the following available combinations: 5/160 mg, 10/160 mg, 5/320 mg, and 10/320 mg.

All strengths are packaged in bottles and blisters of 30 tablets.

5/160 mg Tablets - dark yellow, ovaloid shaped, film-coated tablet with beveled edge, debossed with "NVR" on one side and "ECE" on the other side.

Bottles of 30	NDC 0078-0488-15
Unit Dose (blister pack of 30)	NDC 0078-0488-30

10/160 mg Tablets - light yellow, ovaloid shaped, film-coated tablet with beveled edge, debossed with "NVR" on one side and "UIC" on the other side.

Bottles of 30	NDC 0078-0489-15
Unit Dose (blister pack of 30)	NDC 0078-0489-30

5/320 mg Tablets - very dark yellow, ovaloid shaped, film-coated tablet with beveled edge, debossed with "NVR" on one side and "CSF" on the other side.

Bottles of 30	NDC 0078-0490-15
Unit Dose (blister pack of 30)	NDC 0078-0490-30

10/320 mg Tablets - dark yellow, ovaloid shaped, film-coated tablet with beveled edge, debossed with "NVR" on one side and "LUF" on the other side.

Bottles of 30	NDC 0078-0491-15
Unit Dose (blister pack of 30)	NDC 0078-0491-30

Store at 25°C (77°F); excursions permitted to 15-30°C (59-86°F). [See USP Controlled Room Temperature.] Protect from moisture.

17   PATIENT COUNSELING INFORMATION

Information for Patients

Pregnancy: Female patients of childbearing age should be told about the consequences of exposure to Exforge during pregnancy. Discuss treatment options with women planning to become pregnant. Patients should be asked to report pregnancies to their physicians as soon as possible.

T2014-62
June 2014

FDA-APPROVED PATIENT LABELING
PATIENT INFORMATION
EXFORGE (X-phorj)
(amlodipine and valsartan)
Tablets

Read the Patient Information that comes with EXFORGE before you start taking it and each time you get a refill. There may be new information. This leaflet does not take the place of talking with your doctor about your medical condition or treatment. If you have any questions about EXFORGE, ask your doctor or pharmacist.

What is the most important information I should know about EXFORGE?
- EXFORGE can cause harm or death to an unborn baby.
- Talk to your doctor about other ways to lower your blood pressure if you plan to become pregnant.
- If you get pregnant while taking EXFORGE, tell your doctor right away.

What is EXFORGE?
EXFORGE contains 2 prescription medicines:
1. amlodipine, a calcium channel blocker
2. valsartan, an angiotensin receptor blocker (ARB).
EXFORGE may be used to lower high blood pressure (hypertension) in adults
- when 1 medicine to lower your high blood pressure is not enough
- as the first medicine to lower high blood pressure if your doctor decides you are likely to need more than 1 medicine.
EXFORGE has not been studied in children under 18 years of age.

What should I tell my doctor before taking EXFORGE?
Tell your doctor about all of your medical conditions, including if you:

Table 5: Effect of Exforge on Sitting Diastolic/Systolic Blood Pressure

Treatment Group	Diastolic BP		Systolic BP	
	Mean change*	Treatment Difference**	Mean change*	Treatment Difference**
Exforge 10/160 mg	-11.4	-4.8	-13.9	-5.7
Exforge 5/160 mg	-9.6	-3.1	-12.0	-3.9
Valsartan 160 mg	-6.6	---	-8.2	---

*Mean Change from Baseline at Week 8 in Sitting Diastolic/Systolic Blood Pressure. Mean baseline BP was 149.5/96.5 (systolic/diastolic) mmHg
**Treatment Difference = difference in mean BP reduction between Exforge and the control group (Valsartan 160 mg)

Table 6: Effect of Exforge on Sitting Diastolic/Systolic Blood Pressure

Treatment Group	Diastolic BP		Systolic BP	
	Mean change*	Treatment Difference**	Mean change*	Treatment Difference**
Exforge 10/160 mg	-11.8	-1.8	-12.7	-1.9
Amlodipine 10 mg	-10.0	---	-10.8	---

*Mean Change from Baseline at Week 8 in Sitting Diastolic/Systolic Blood Pressure. Mean baseline BP was 147.0/95.1 (systolic/diastolic) mmHg
**Treatment Difference = difference in mean BP reduction between Exforge and the control group (Amlodipine 10 mg)

- are pregnant or plan to become pregnant. See "What is the most important information I should know about EXFORGE?"
- are breastfeeding or plan to breastfeed. EXFORGE may pass into your milk. Do not breastfeed while you are taking EXFORGE.
- have heart problems
- have liver problems
- have kidney problems
- are vomiting or having a lot of diarrhea
- have ever had a reaction called angioedema, to another blood pressure medicine. Angioedema causes swelling of the face, lips, tongue, throat, and may cause difficulty breathing.

Tell your doctor about all the medicines you take, including prescription and nonprescription medicines, vitamins, and herbal supplements. Some of your other medicines and EXFORGE could affect each other, causing serious side effects.
Especially tell your doctor if you take:
- simvastatin or other cholesterol lowering medicine
- other medicines for high blood pressure or a heart problem
- water pills (diuretics)
- potassium supplements. Your doctor may check the amount of potassium in your blood periodically.
- a salt substitute. Your doctor may check the amount of potassium in your blood periodically.
- nonsteroidal anti-inflammatory drugs (like ibuprofen or naproxen)
- medicines used to prevent and treat fungal skin infections (such as Ketoconazole, itraconazole)
- medicines used to treat bacterial infections (such as clarithromycin, telithromycin)
- certain antibiotics (rifamycin group), a drug used to protect against transplant rejection (cyclosporin) or an antiretroviral drug used to treat HIV/AIDS infection (ritonavir). These drugs may increase the effect of valsartan.
- lithium, a medicine used in some types of depression
Know the medicines you take. Keep a list of your medicines and show it to your doctor or pharmacist when you get a new medicine. Talk to your doctor or pharmacist before you start taking any new medicine. Your doctor or pharmacist will know what medicines are safe to take together.

How should I take EXFORGE?
- Take EXFORGE exactly as your doctor tells you.
- Take EXFORGE once each day.
- EXFORGE can be taken with or without food.
- If you miss a dose, take it as soon as you remember. If it is close to your next dose, do not take the missed dose. Just take the next dose at your regular time.
- If you take too much EXFORGE, call your doctor or Poison Control Center, or go to the emergency room.
- Tell all your doctors or dentist you are taking EXFORGE if you:
  ○ are going to have surgery
  ○ go for kidney dialysis

What should I avoid while taking EXFORGE?
You should not take EXFORGE during pregnancy. See "What is the most important information I should know about EXFORGE?"

What are the possible side effects of EXFORGE?
EXFORGE may cause serious side effects including:
- harm to an unborn baby causing injury and even death. See "What is the most important information I should know about EXFORGE?"
- low blood pressure (hypotension). Low blood pressure is most likely to happen if you:
  ○ take water pills
  ○ are on a low-salt diet
  ○ get dialysis treatments
  ○ have heart problems
  ○ get sick with vomiting or diarrhea
  ○ drink alcohol
Lie down if you feel faint or dizzy. Call your doctor right away.
- more heart attacks and chest pain (angina) in people that already have severe heart problems. This may happen when you start EXFORGE or when there is an increase in your dose of EXFORGE. Get emergency help if you get worse chest pain or chest pain that does not go away.
- kidney problems. Kidney problems may become worse in people that already have kidney disease. Some people will have changes in blood tests for kidney function and may need a lower dose of EXFORGE. Call your doctor if you have swelling in your feet, ankles, or hands or unexplained weight gain. If you have heart failure, your doctor should check your kidney function before prescribing EXFORGE.
- laboratory blood test changes in people with heart failure. Some people with heart failure who take valsartan, 1 of the medicines in EXFORGE, have changes in blood tests including increased potassium and decreased kidney function.
The most common side effects of EXFORGE include:
- swelling (edema) of the hands, ankles, or feet
- nasal congestion, sore throat, and discomfort when swallowing
- upper respiratory tract infection (head or chest cold)
- dizziness
Tell your doctor if you have any side effect that bothers you or that does not go away.
These are not all the possible side effects of EXFORGE. For more information, ask your doctor or pharmacist.
Call your doctor for medical advice about side effects. You may report side effects to FDA at 1-800-FDA-1088.

How should I store EXFORGE?
- Store EXFORGE at room temperature between 59°F to 86°F (15°C to 30°C).
- Keep EXFORGE dry (protect it from moisture).
Keep EXFORGE and all medicines out of the reach of children.

General Information about EXFORGE
Medicines are sometimes prescribed for conditions that are not mentioned in the patient information leaflet. Do not use EXFORGE for a condition for which it was not prescribed. Do not give EXFORGE to other people, even if they have the same symptoms that you have. It may harm them.
This patient information leaflet summarizes the most important information about EXFORGE. If you would like more information about EXFORGE, talk with your doctor. You can ask your doctor or pharmacist for information about

EXFORGE that is written for health professionals. For more information go to www.EXFORGE.com or call 1-888-839-3674.

What are the ingredients in EXFORGE?
Active ingredients: Amlodipine besylate and valsartan
The inactive ingredients of all strengths of the tablets are colloidal silicon dioxide, crospovidone, magnesium stearate, and microcrystalline cellulose. Additionally, the 5/320 mg and 10/320 mg strengths contain iron oxide yellow and sodium starch glycolate. The film coating contains hypromellose, iron oxides, polyethylene glycol, talc, and titanium dioxide.

What is high blood pressure (hypertension)?
Blood pressure is the force of blood in your blood vessels when your heart beats and when your heart rests. You have high blood pressure when the force is too much. EXFORGE can help your blood vessels relax so your blood pressure is lower. Medicines that lower blood pressure lower your chance of having a stroke or heart attack.
High blood pressure makes the heart work harder to pump blood throughout the body and causes damage to blood vessels. If high blood pressure is not treated, it can lead to stroke, heart attack, heart failure, kidney failure, and vision problems.

*Norvasc® is a registered trademark of Pfizer, Inc.
**Viagra® is a registered trademark of Pfizer, Inc.
Distributed by:
Novartis Pharmaceuticals Corporation
East Hanover, New Jersey 07936
©Novartis
T2014-33
March 2014
Shown in Product Identification Guide, page 310

EXFORGE HCT®   ℞
[X-phorj HCT]
(amlodipine, valsartan, hydrochlorothiazide)
Tablets

The following prescribing information is based on official labeling in effect July 2014.
HIGHLIGHTS OF PRESCRIBING INFORMATION
These highlights do not include all the information needed to use Exforge HCT safely and effectively. See full prescribing information for Exforge HCT.
Exforge HCT® (amlodipine, valsartan, hydrochlorothiazide) Tablets
Initial U.S. Approval: 2009

> **WARNING: FETAL TOXICITY**
> *See full prescribing information for complete boxed warning.*
> - **When pregnancy is detected, discontinue Exforge HCT as soon as possible. (5.1)**
> - **Drugs that act directly on the renin-angiotensin system can cause injury and death to the developing fetus. (5.1)**

──────── INDICATIONS AND USAGE ────────
- Exforge HCT is a combination tablet of amlodipine, a dihydropyridine calcium channel blocker (DHP CCB), valsartan, an angiotensin II receptor blocker (ARB), and hydrochlorothiazide, a thiazide diuretic. Exforge HCT is indicated for the treatment of hypertension to lower blood pressure. Lowering blood pressure reduces the risk of fatal and nonfatal cardiovascular events, primarily strokes, and myocardial infarctions. (1)
- Not indicated for initial therapy

──────── DOSAGE AND ADMINISTRATION ────────
- Dose once-daily. Titrate up to a maximum dose of 10/320/25 mg
- Exforge HCT may be used as add-on/switch therapy for patients not adequately controlled on any two of the following antihypertensive classes: calcium channel blockers, angiotensin receptor blockers, and diuretics.
- Exforge HCT may be substituted for its individually titrated components (2).

──── DOSAGE FORMS AND STRENGTHS ────
Tablets: (amlodipine/valsartan/hydrochlorothiazide mg) 5/160/12.5, 10/160/12.5, 5/160/25, 10/160/25, 10/320/25 (3)

──────── CONTRAINDICATIONS ────────
- Anuria (4)
- Hypersensitivity to sulfonamide-derived drugs (4)
- Known hypersensitivity to any component (4)
- Do not coadminister aliskiren with Exforge HCT in patients with diabetes (4)

──── WARNINGS AND PRECAUTIONS ────
- Hypotension: Correct volume depletion prior to initiation (5.2)
- Increased angina and/or myocardial infarction (5.3)
- Monitor renal function and potassium in susceptible patients (5.4, 5.5)

- Exacerbation or activation of systemic lupus erythematosus (5.7)
- Observe for signs of fluid or electrolyte imbalance (5.9)
- Acute angle-closure glaucoma (5.10)

──────── ADVERSE REACTIONS ────────
Most common adverse events (≥2% incidence) are dizziness, peripheral edema, headache, dyspepsia, fatigue, muscle spasms, back pain, nausea and nasopharyngitis. (6.1)
To report SUSPECTED ADVERSE REACTIONS, contact Novartis Pharmaceuticals Corporation at 1-888-669-6682 or FDA at 1-800-FDA-1088 or www.fda.gov/medwatch.

──────── DRUG INTERACTIONS ────────
- If simvastatin is coadministered with amlodipine, do not exceed doses greater than 20 mg daily of simvastatin (7)
- Antidiabetic drugs: Dosage adjustment of antidiabetic may be required (7)
- Cholestyramine and colestipol: Reduced absorption of thiazides (12.3)
- Lithium: Increased risk of lithium toxicity. Monitor serum lithium concentrations during concurrent use. (7)
- NSAID use may lead to increased risk of renal impairment and loss of anti-hypertensive effect (7)
- Dual inhibition of the renin-angiotensin system: Increased risk of renal impairment, hypotension, and hyperkalemia (7)

──── USE IN SPECIFIC POPULATIONS ────
Nursing Mothers: Avoid use while nursing – discontinue either nursing or drug (8.3)
See 17 for PATIENT COUNSELING INFORMATION and FDA-approved patient labeling
                                        Revised: 6/2014

FULL PRESCRIBING INFORMATION: CONTENTS*
WARNING: FETAL TOXICITY

FULL PRESCRIBING INFORMATION

> **WARNING: FETAL TOXICITY**
> - **When pregnancy is detected, discontinue Exforge HCT as soon as possible. (5.1)**
> - **Drugs that act directly on the renin-angiotensin system can cause injury and death to the developing fetus. (5.1)**

1 INDICATIONS AND USAGE
Exforge HCT (amlodipine, valsartan, hydrochlorothiazide) is indicated for the treatment of hypertension, to lower blood pressure. Lowering blood pressure reduces the risk of fatal and nonfatal cardiovascular events, primarily strokes and myocardial infarctions. These benefits have been seen in controlled trials of antihypertensive drugs from a wide variety of pharmacologic classes, including amlodipine, hydrochlorothiazide, and the ARB class to which valsartan principally belongs. There are no controlled trials demonstrating risk reduction with Exforge HCT.

Control of high blood pressure should be part of comprehensive cardiovascular risk management, including, as appropriate, lipid control, diabetes management, antithrombotic therapy, smoking cessation, exercise, and limited sodium intake. Many patients will require more than 1 drug to achieve blood pressure goals. For specific advice on goals and management, see published guidelines, such as those of the National High Blood Pressure Education Program's Joint National Committee on Prevention, Detection, Evaluation, and Treatment of High Blood Pressure (JNC).

Numerous antihypertensive drugs, from a variety of pharmacologic classes and with different mechanisms of action, have been shown in randomized controlled trials to reduce cardiovascular morbidity and mortality, and it can be concluded that it is blood pressure reduction, and not some other pharmacologic property of the drugs, that is largely responsible for those benefits. The largest and most consistent cardiovascular outcome benefit has been a reduction in the risk of stroke, but reductions in myocardial infarction and cardiovascular mortality also have been seen regularly. Elevated systolic or diastolic pressure causes increased cardiovascular risk, and the absolute risk increase per mmHg is greater at higher blood pressures, so that even modest reductions of severe hypertension can provide substantial benefit. Relative risk reduction from blood pressure reduction is similar across populations with varying absolute risk, so the absolute benefit is greater in patients who are at higher risk independent of their hypertension (e.g., patients with diabetes or hyperlipidemia), and such patients would be expected to benefit from more aggressive treatment to a lower blood pressure goal.

Some antihypertensive drugs have smaller blood pressure effects (as monotherapy) in black patients, and many antihypertensive drugs have additional approved indications and effects (e.g., on angina, heart failure, or diabetic kidney disease). These considerations may guide selection of therapy.

This fixed combination drug is not indicated for the initial therapy of hypertension *[see Dosage and Administration (2)]*.

2 DOSAGE AND ADMINISTRATION
2.1 General Considerations
Dose once-daily. The dosage may be increased after 2 weeks of therapy. The full blood pressure lowering effect was achieved 2 weeks after being on the maximal dose of Exforge HCT. The maximum recommended dose of Exforge HCT is 10/320/25 mg.
2.2 Add-on / Switch Therapy
Exforge HCT may be used for patients not adequately controlled on any 2 of the following antihypertensive classes: calcium channel blockers, angiotensin receptor blockers, and diuretics.
A patient who experiences dose-limiting adverse reactions to an individual component while on any dual combination of the components of Exforge HCT may be switched to Exforge HCT containing a lower dose of that component to achieve similar blood pressure reductions.
2.3 Replacement Therapy
Exforge HCT may be substituted for the individually titrated components.
2.4 Use with Other Antihypertensive Drugs
Exforge HCT may be administered with other antihypertensive agents.

3 DOSAGE FORMS AND STRENGTHS
- 5 mg amlodipine /160 mg valsartan /12.5 mg hydrochlorothiazide Tablets – White, non-scored, film-coated tablet, ovaloid, biconvex with beveled edge with debossing "NVR" on one side and "VCL" on the other side.
- 10 mg amlodipine /160 mg valsartan /12.5 mg hydrochlorothiazide Tablets – Pale yellow, non-scored, film-coated tablet, ovaloid, biconvex with beveled edge with debossing "NVR" on one side and "VDL" on the other side.
- 5 mg amlodipine /160 mg valsartan /25 mg hydrochlorothiazide Tablets – Yellow, non-scored, film-coated tablet, ovaloid, biconvex with beveled edge with debossing "NVR" on one side and "VEL" on the other side.
- 10 mg amlodipine /160 mg valsartan /25 mg hydrochlorothiazide Tablets – Brown-yellow, non-scored, film-coated tablet, ovaloid, biconvex with beveled edge with debossing "NVR" on one side and "VHL" on the other side.

- 10 mg amlodipine /320 mg valsartan /25 mg hydrochlorothiazide Tablets – Brown-yellow, non-scored, film-coated tablet, ovaloid, biconvex with beveled edge with debossing "NVR" on one side and "VFL" on the other side.

4 CONTRAINDICATIONS

Do not use in patients with anuria, hypersensitivity to other sulfonamide-derived drugs, or hypersensitivity to any component of this product.

Do not coadminister aliskiren with Exforge HCT in patients with diabetes [see Drug Interactions (7)].

5 WARNINGS AND PRECAUTIONS

5.1 Fetal Toxicity

Pregnancy Category D

Use of drugs that act on the renin-angiotensin system during the second and third trimesters of pregnancy reduces fetal renal function and increases fetal and neonatal morbidity and death. Resulting oligohydramnios can be associated with fetal lung hypoplasia and skeletal deformations. Potential neonatal adverse effects include skull hypoplasia, anuria, hypotension, renal failure, and death. When pregnancy is detected, discontinue Exforge HCT as soon as possible [see Use in Specific Populations (8.1)].

5.2 Hypotension in Volume- or Salt-Depleted Patients

Excessive hypotension, including orthostatic hypotension, was seen in 1.7% of patients treated with the maximum dose of Exforge HCT (10/320/25 mg) compared to 1.8% of valsartan/HCTZ (320/25 mg) patients, 0.4% of amlodipine/valsartan (10/320 mg) patients, and 0.2% of HCTZ/amlodipine (25/10 mg) patients in a controlled trial in patients with moderate to severe uncomplicated hypertension. In patients with an activated renin-angiotensin system, such as volume- or salt-depleted patients receiving high doses of diuretics, symptomatic hypotension may occur in patients receiving angiotensin receptor blockers. Correct this condition prior to administration of Exforge HCT.

Exforge HCT has not been studied in patients with heart failure, recent myocardial infarction, or in patients undergoing surgery or dialysis. Patients with heart failure or post-myocardial infarction patients given valsartan commonly have some reduction in blood pressure, but discontinuation of therapy because of continuing symptomatic hypotension usually is not necessary when dosing instructions are followed. In controlled trials in heart failure patients, the incidence of hypotension in valsartan-treated patients was 5.5% compared to 1.8% in placebo-treated patients. In the Valsartan in Acute Myocardial Infarction Trial (VALIANT), hypotension in post-myocardial infarction patients led to permanent discontinuation of therapy in 1.4% of valsartan-treated patients and 0.8% of captopril-treated patients.

Since the vasodilation induced by amlodipine is gradual in onset, acute hypotension has rarely been reported after oral administration. Do not initiate treatment with Exforge HCT in patients with aortic or mitral stenosis or obstructive hypertrophic cardiomyopathy.

If excessive hypotension occurs with Exforge HCT, the patient should be placed in a supine position and, if necessary, given an intravenous infusion of normal saline. A transient hypotensive response is not a contraindication to further treatment, which usually can be continued without difficulty once the blood pressure has stabilized.

5.3 Increased Angina and/or Myocardial Infarction

Worsening angina and acute myocardial infarction can develop after starting or increasing the dose of amlodipine, particularly in patients with severe obstructive coronary artery disease.

5.4 Impaired Renal Function

Changes in renal function including acute renal failure can be caused by drugs that inhibit the renin-angiotensin system and by diuretics. Patients whose renal function may depend in part on the activity of the renin-angiotensin system (e.g., patients with renal artery stenosis, chronic kidney disease, severe congestive heart failure, or volume depletion) may be at particular risk of developing acute renal failure on Exforge HCT. Monitor renal function periodically in these patients. Consider withholding or discontinuing therapy in patients who develop a clinically significant decrease in renal function on Exforge HCT [see Drug Interactions (7)].

5.5 Potassium Abnormalities

In the controlled trial of Exforge HCT in moderate to severe hypertensive patients, the incidence of hypokalemia (serum potassium <3.5 mEq/L) at any time post-baseline with the maximum dose of Exforge HCT (10/320/25 mg) was 10% compared to 25% with HCTZ/amlodipine (25/10 mg), 7% with valsartan/HCTZ (320/25 mg), and 3% with amlodipine/valsartan (10/320 mg). One patient (0.2%) discontinued therapy due to an adverse event of hypokalemia in each of the Exforge HCT and HCTZ/amlodipine groups. The incidence of hyperkalemia (serum potassium >5.7 mEq/L) was 0.4% with Exforge HCT compared to 0.2% to 0.7% with the dual therapies.

Some patients with heart failure have developed increases in potassium on valsartan. These effects are usually minor and transient, and they are more likely to occur in patients with pre-existing renal impairment. Dosage reduction and/or discontinuation of the diuretic and/or valsartan may be required.

Hydrochlorothiazide can cause hypokalemia and hyponatremia. Hypomagnesemia can result in hypokalemia which appears difficult to treat despite potassium repletion. Drugs that inhibit the renin-angiotensin system can cause hyperkalemia. Monitor serum electrolytes periodically.

If hypokalemia is accompanied by clinical signs (e.g., muscular weakness, paresis, or ECG alterations), Exforge HCT should be discontinued. Correction of hypokalemia and any coexisting hypomagnesemia is recommended prior to the initiation of thiazides.

5.6 Hypersensitivity Reaction

Hypersensitivity reactions to hydrochlorothiazide may occur in patients with or without a history of allergy or bronchial asthma, but are more likely in patients with such a history.

5.7 Systemic Lupus Erythematosus

Thiazide diuretics have been reported to cause exacerbation or activation of systemic lupus erythematosus.

5.8 Lithium Interaction

Increases in serum lithium concentrations and lithium toxicity have been reported with concomitant use of valsartan or thiazide diuretics. Monitor lithium levels in patients receiving Exforge HCT and lithium [see Drug Interactions (7)].

5.9 Metabolic Imbalances

Hydrochlorothiazide may alter glucose tolerance and raise serum levels of cholesterol and triglycerides.

Hydrochlorothiazide may raise the serum uric acid level due to reduced clearance of uric acid and may cause or exacerbate hyperuricemia and precipitate gout in susceptible patients.

Hydrochlorothiazide decreases urinary calcium excretion and may cause elevations of serum calcium. Monitor calcium levels in patients with hypercalcemia receiving Exforge HCT.

5.10 Acute Myopia and Secondary Angle-Closure Glaucoma

Hydrochlorothiazide, a sulfonamide, can cause an idiosyncratic reaction, resulting in acute transient myopia and acute angle-closure glaucoma. Symptoms include acute onset of decreased visual acuity or ocular pain and typically occur within hours to weeks of drug initiation. Untreated acute angle-closure glaucoma can lead to permanent vision loss. The primary treatment is to discontinue hydrochlorothiazide as rapidly as possible. Prompt medical or surgical treatments may need to be considered if the intraocular pressure remains uncontrolled. Risk factors for developing acute angle-closure glaucoma may include a history of sulfonamide or penicillin allergy.

6 ADVERSE REACTIONS

6.1 Clinical Trials Experience

Because clinical studies are conducted under widely varying conditions, adverse reaction rates observed in the clinical studies of a drug cannot be directly compared to rates in the clinical studies of another drug and may not reflect the rates observed in clinical practice.

In the controlled trial of Exforge HCT, where only the maximum dose (10/320/25 mg) was evaluated, safety data were obtained in 582 patients with hypertension. Adverse reactions have generally been mild and transient in nature and have only infrequently required discontinuation of therapy. The overall frequency of adverse reactions was similar between men and women, younger (<65 years) and older (≥65 years) patients, and black and white patients. In the active controlled clinical trial, discontinuation because of adverse events occurred in 4.0% of patients treated with Exforge HCT 10/320/25 mg compared to 2.9% of patients treated with valsartan/HCTZ 320/25 mg, 1.6% of patients treated with amlodipine/valsartan 10/320 mg, and 3.4% of patients treated with HCTZ/amlodipine 25/10 mg. The most common reasons for discontinuation of therapy with Exforge HCT were dizziness (1.0%) and hypotension (0.7%).

Preferred Term	Aml/Val/HCTZ 10/320/25 mg N=582 n (%)	Val/HCTZ 320/25 mg N=559 n (%)	Aml/Val 10/320 mg N=566 n (%)	HCTZ/Aml 25/10 mg N=561 n (%)
Dizziness	48 (8.2)	40 (7.2)	14 (2.5)	23 (4.1)
Edema	38 (6.5)	8 (1.4)	65 (11.5)	63 (11.2)
Headache	30 (5.2)	31 (5.5)	30 (5.3)	40 (7.1)
Dyspepsia	13 (2.2)	5 (0.9)	6 (1.1)	2 (0.4)
Fatigue	13 (2.2)	15 (2.7)	12 (2.1)	8 (1.4)
Muscle spasms	13 (2.2)	7 (1.3)	7 (1.2)	5 (0.9)
Back pain	12 (2.1)	13 (2.3)	5 (0.9)	12 (2.1)
Nausea	12 (2.1)	7 (1.3)	10 (1.8)	12 (2.1)
Nasopharyngitis	12 (2.1)	13 (2.3)	13 (2.3)	12 (2.1)

The most frequent adverse events that occurred in the active controlled clinical trial in at least 2% of patients treated with Exforge HCT are presented in the following table. [See table above]

Orthostatic events (orthostatic hypotension and postural dizziness) were seen in 0.5% of patients. Other adverse reactions that occurred in clinical trials with Exforge HCT (>0.2%) are listed below. It cannot be determined whether these events were causally related to Exforge HCT.

Cardiac Disorders: tachycardia

Ear and Labyrinth Disorders: vertigo, tinnitus

Eye Disorders: vision blurred

Gastrointestinal Disorders: diarrhea, abdominal pain upper, vomiting, abdominal pain, toothache, dry mouth, gastritis, hemorrhoids

General Disorders and Administration Site Conditions: asthenia, noncardiac chest pain, chills, malaise

Infections and Infestations: upper respiratory tract infection, bronchitis, influenza, pharyngitis, tooth abscess, gastroenteritis viral, respiratory tract infection, rhinitis, urinary tract infection

Injury, Poisoning and Procedural Complications: back injury, contusion, joint sprain, procedural pain

Investigations: blood uric acid increased, blood creatine phosphokinase increased, weight decreased

Metabolism and Nutrition Disorders: hypokalemia, diabetes mellitus, hyperlipidemia, hyponatremia

Musculoskeletal and Connective Tissue Disorders: pain in extremity, arthralgia, musculoskeletal pain, muscular weakness, musculoskeletal weakness, musculoskeletal stiffness, joint swelling, neck pain, osteoarthritis, tendonitis

Nervous System Disorders: paresthesia, somnolence, syncope, carpal tunnel syndrome, disturbance in attention, dizziness postural, dysgeusia, head discomfort, lethargy, sinus headache, tremor

Psychiatric Disorders: anxiety, depression, insomnia

Renal and Urinary Disorders: pollakiuria

Reproductive System and Breast Disorders: erectile dysfunction

Respiratory, Thoracic and Mediastinal Disorders: dyspnea, nasal congestion, cough, pharyngolaryngeal pain

Skin and Subcutaneous Tissue Disorders: pruritus, hyperhidrosis, night sweats, rash

Vascular Disorders: hypotension

Isolated cases of the following clinically notable adverse reactions were also observed in clinical trials: anorexia, constipation, dehydration, dysuria, increased appetite, viral infection.

Amlodipine

Amlodipine has been evaluated for safety in more than 11000 patients in US and foreign clinical trials. Other adverse reactions not listed above that have been reported in <1% but >0.1% of patients in controlled clinical trials or under conditions of open trials or marketing experience where a causal relationship is uncertain were:

Cardiovascular: arrhythmia (including ventricular tachycardia and atrial fibrillation), bradycardia, chest pain, peripheral ischemia, syncope, postural hypotension, vasculitis

Central and Peripheral Nervous System: neuropathy peripheral, tremor

Gastrointestinal: anorexia, dysphagia, pancreatitis, gingival hyperplasia

General: allergic reaction, hot flushes, malaise, rigors, weight gain

Musculoskeletal System: arthrosis, muscle cramps

Psychiatric: sexual dysfunction (male and female), nervousness, abnormal dreams, depersonalization

Skin and Appendages: angioedema, erythema multiforme, rash erythematous, rash maculopapular

Special Senses: abnormal vision, conjunctivitis, diplopia, eye pain, tinnitus

Urinary System: micturition frequency, micturition disorder, nocturia

Autonomic Nervous System: sweating increased

Metabolic and Nutritional: hyperglycemia, thirst

Hemopoietic: leukopenia, purpura, thrombocytopenia

Other adverse reactions reported with amlodipine at a frequency of ≤0.1% of patients include: cardiac failure, pulse irregularity, extrasystoles, skin discoloration, urticaria, skin dryness, alopecia, dermatitis, muscle weakness, twitching, ataxia, hypertonia, migraine, cold and clammy skin, apathy, agitation, amnesia, gastritis, increased appetite, loose stools, rhinitis, dysuria, polyuria, parosmia, taste perversion, abnormal visual accommodation, and xerophthalmia. Other reactions occurred sporadically and cannot be distinguished from medications or concurrent disease states such as myocardial infarction and angina.

Adverse reactions reported for amlodipine for indications other than hypertension may be found in its full prescribing information.

Valsartan

Valsartan has been evaluated for safety in more than 4000 hypertensive patients in clinical trials. In trials in which valsartan was compared to an ACE inhibitor with or without placebo, the incidence of dry cough was significantly greater in the ACE inhibitor group (7.9%) than in the groups who received valsartan (2.6%) or placebo (1.5%). In a 129-patient trial limited to patients who had dry cough when they had previously received ACE inhibitors, the incidences of cough in patients who received valsartan, HCTZ, or lisinopril were 20%, 19%, and 69% respectively (p <0.001).

Other adverse reactions, not listed above, occurring in >0.2% of patients in controlled clinical trials with valsartan are:

Digestive: flatulence
Respiratory: sinusitis, pharyngitis
Urogenital: impotence

Adverse reactions reported for valsartan for indications other than hypertension may be found in the prescribing information for Diovan.

Hydrochlorothiazide

Other adverse reactions not listed above that have been reported with hydrochlorothiazide, without regard to causality, are listed below:

Body as a Whole: weakness
Digestive: pancreatitis, jaundice (intrahepatic cholestatic jaundice), sialadenitis, cramping, gastric irritation
Hematologic: aplastic anemia, agranulocytosis, hemolytic anemia
Hypersensitivity: photosensitivity, urticaria, necrotizing angiitis (vasculitis and cutaneous vasculitis), fever, respiratory distress including pneumonitis and pulmonary edema, anaphylactic reactions
Metabolic: glycosuria, hyperuricemia
Nervous System/Psychiatric: restlessness
Renal: renal failure, renal dysfunction, interstitial nephritis
Skin: erythema multiforme including Stevens-Johnson syndrome, exfoliative dermatitis including toxic epidermal necrolysis
Special Senses: transient blurred vision, xanthopsia.

Clinical Laboratory Test Findings

Clinical laboratory test findings for Exforge HCT were obtained in a controlled trial of Exforge HCT administered at the maximal dose of 10/320/25 mg compared to maximal doses of dual therapies, i.e., valsartan/HCTZ 320/25 mg, amlodipine/valsartan 10/320 mg, and HCTZ/amlodipine 25/10 mg. Findings for the components of Exforge HCT were obtained from other trials.

Creatinine: In hypertensive patients, greater than 50% increases in creatinine occurred in 2.1% of Exforge HCT patients compared to 2.4% of valsartan/HCTZ patients, 0.7% of amlodipine/valsartan patients, and 1.8% of HCTZ/amlodipine patients.

In heart failure patients, greater than 50% increases in creatinine were observed in 3.9% of valsartan-treated patients compared to 0.9% of placebo-treated patients. In postmyocardial infarction patients, doubling of serum creatinine was observed in 4.2% of valsartan-treated patients and 3.4% of captopril-treated patients.

Liver Function Tests: Occasional elevations (greater than 150%) of liver chemistries occurred in Exforge HCT-treated patients.

Blood Urea Nitrogen (BUN): In hypertensive patients, greater than 50% increases in BUN were observed in 30% of Exforge HCT-treated patients compared to 29% of valsartan/HCTZ patients, 15.8% of amlodipine/valsartan patients, and 18.5% of HCTZ/amlodipine patients. The majority of BUN values remained within normal limits.

In heart failure patients, greater than 50% increases in BUN were observed in 17% of valsartan-treated patients compared to 6% of placebo-treated patients.

Serum Electrolytes (Potassium): In hypertensive patients, greater than 20% decreases in serum potassium were observed in 6.5% of Exforge HCT-treated patients compared to 3.3% of valsartan/HCTZ patients, 0.4% of amlodipine/valsartan patients, and 19.3% of HCTZ/amlodipine patients. Greater than 20% increases in potassium were observed in 3.5% of Exforge HCT-treated patients compared to 2.4% of valsartan/HCTZ patients, 6.2% of amlodipine/valsartan patients, and 2.2% of HCTZ/amlodipine patients.

In heart failure patients, greater than 20% increases in serum potassium were observed in 10% of valsartan-treated patients compared to 5.1% of placebo-treated patients [see Warnings and Precautions (5.5)].

Neutropenia: Neutropenia (<1500/L) was observed in 1.9% of patients treated with valsartan and 0.8% of patients treated with placebo.

6.2 Postmarketing Experience

The following additional adverse reactions have been reported in postmarketing experience. Because these reactions are reported voluntarily from a population of uncertain size, it is not always possible to reliably estimate their frequency or establish a causal relationship to drug exposure.

Amlodipine

With amlodipine, gynecomastia has been reported infrequently and a causal relationship is uncertain. Jaundice and hepatic enzyme elevations (mostly consistent with cholestasis or hepatitis), in some cases severe enough to require hospitalization, have been reported in association with use of amlodipine.

Valsartan

The following additional adverse reactions have been reported in postmarketing experience with valsartan or valsartan/hydrochlorothiazide:

Blood and Lymphatic: Decrease in hemoglobin, decrease in hematocrit, neutropenia

Hypersensitivity: There are rare reports of angioedema. Some of these patients previously experienced angioedema with other drugs including ACE inhibitors. Exforge HCT should not be re-administered to patients who have had angioedema.

Digestive: Elevated liver enzymes and very rare reports of hepatitis

Renal: Impaired renal function, renal failure

Clinical Laboratory Tests: Hyperkalemia

Dermatologic: Alopecia, bullous dermatitis

Vascular: Vasculitis

Nervous System: Syncope

Rare cases of rhabdomyolysis have been reported in patients receiving angiotensin II receptor blockers.

Hydrochlorothiazide

The following additional adverse reactions have been reported in post-marketing experience with hydrochlorothiazide:

Acute renal failure, renal disorder, aplastic anemia, erythema multiforme, pyrexia, muscle spasm, asthenia, acute angle-closure glaucoma, bone marrow failure, worsening of diabetes control, hypokalemia, blood lipids increased, hyponatremia, hypomagnesemia, hypercalcemia, hypochloremic alkalosis, impotence, visual impairment.

Pathological changes in the parathyroid gland of patients with hypercalcemia and hypophosphatemia have been observed in a few patients on prolonged thiazide therapy. If hypercalcemia occurs, further diagnostic evaluation is necessary.

7 DRUG INTERACTIONS

No drug interaction studies have been conducted with Exforge HCT and other drugs, although studies have been conducted with the individual components. A pharmacokinetic drug-drug interaction study has been conducted to address the potential for pharmacokinetic interaction between the triple combination, Exforge HCT, and the corresponding 3 double combinations. No clinically relevant interaction was observed.

Amlodipine

Simvastatin: Coadministration of simvastatin with amlodipine increases the systemic exposure of simvastatin. Limit the dose of simvastatin in patients on amlodipine to 20 mg daily.

CYP3A4 Inhibitors: Coadministration with CYP3A inhibitors (moderate and strong) result in increased systemic exposure to amlodipine warranting dose reduction. Monitor for symptoms of hypotension and edema when amlodipine is coadministered with CYP3A4 inhibitors to determine the need for dose adjustment.

CYP3A4 Inducers: No information is available on the quantitative effects of CYP3A4 inducers on amlodipine. Blood pressure should be monitored when amlodipine is coadministered with CYP3A4 inducers.

Valsartan

No clinically significant pharmacokinetic interactions were observed when valsartan was coadministered with amlodipine, atenolol, cimetidine, digoxin, furosemide, glyburide, hydrochlorothiazide, or indomethacin. The valsartan-atenolol combination was more antihypertensive than either component/HCT, but it did not lower the heart rate more than atenolol alone.

In vitro metabolism studies have indicated that CYP450 mediated drug interaction between valsartan and coadministered drugs are unlikely because of the low extent of metabolism [see Pharmacokinetics – Valsartan, (12.3)].

Coadministration of valsartan and warfarin did not change the pharmacokinetics of valsartan or the time-course of the anticoagulant properties of warfarin.

Potassium: Concomitant use of valsartan with other agents that block the renin-angiotensin system, potassium-sparing diuretics (e.g., spironolactone, triamterene, amiloride), potassium supplements, or salt substitutes containing potassium may lead to increases in serum potassium and in heart failure patients to increases in serum creatinine. If co-medication is considered necessary, monitoring of serum potassium is advisable.

Non-Steroidal Anti-Inflammatory Agents including Selective Cyclooxygenase-2 Inhibitors (COX-2 Inhibitors): In patients who are elderly, volume-depleted (including those on diuretic therapy), or with compromised renal function, coadministration of NSAIDs, including selective COX-2 inhibitors, with angiotensin II receptor antagonists, including valsartan, may result in deterioration of renal function, including possible acute renal failure. These effects are usually reversible. Monitor renal function periodically in patients receiving valsartan and NSAID therapy.

The antihypertensive effect of angiotensin II receptor antagonists, including valsartan may be attenuated by NSAIDs including selective COX-2 inhibitors.

Dual Blockade of the Renin-Angiotensin System (RAS): Dual blockade of the RAS with angiotensin receptor blockers, ACE inhibitors, or aliskiren is associated with increased risks of hypotension, hyperkalemia, and changes in renal function (including acute renal failure) compared to monotherapy. Closely monitor blood pressure, renal function, and electrolytes in patients on Exforge HCT and other agents that affect the RAS.

Do not coadminister aliskiren with Exforge HCT in patients with diabetes. Avoid use of aliskiren with Exforge HCT in patients with renal impairment (GFR <60 mL/min).

Valsartan – Hydrochlorothiazide

Lithium: Increases in serum lithium concentrations and lithium toxicity have been reported during concomitant administration of lithium with angiotensin II receptor antagonists or thiazides. Monitor lithium levels in patients taking Exforge HCT.

Hydrochlorothiazide

When administered concurrently the following drugs may interact with thiazide diuretics:

Antidiabetic drugs (oral agents and insulin): Dosage adjustment of the antidiabetic drug may be required.

Non-steroidal anti-inflammatory drugs (NSAIDs and COX-2 selective inhibitors): When Exforge HCT and nonsteroidal anti-inflammatory agents are used concomitantly, the patient should be observed closely to determine if the desired effect of diuretic is obtained.

Carbamazepine: May lead to symptomatic hyponatremia.

Ion exchange resins: Staggering the dosage of hydrochlorothiazide and ion exchange resins (e.g., cholestyramine, colestipol) such that hydrochlorothiazide is administered at least 4 hours before or 4 to 6 hours after the administration of resins would potentially minimize the interaction [see Clinical Pharmacology (12.3)].

Cyclosporine: Concomitant treatment with cyclosporine may increase the risk of hyperuricemia and gout-type complications.

8 USE IN SPECIFIC POPULATIONS
8.1 Pregnancy

Pregnancy Category D

Use of drugs that act on the renin-angiotensin system during the second and third trimesters of pregnancy reduces fetal renal function and increases fetal and neonatal morbidity and death. Resulting oligohydramnios can be associated with fetal lung hypoplasia and skeletal deformations. Potential neonatal adverse effects include skull hypoplasia, anuria, hypotension, renal failure, and death. When pregnancy is detected, discontinue Exforge HCT as soon as possible. These adverse outcomes are usually associated with use of these drugs in the second and third trimesters of pregnancy. Most epidemiologic studies examining fetal abnormalities after exposure to antihypertensive use in the first trimester have not distinguished drugs affecting the renin-angiotensin system from other antihypertensive agents. Appropriate management of maternal hypertension during pregnancy is important to optimize outcomes for both mother and fetus.

In the unusual case that there is no appropriate alternative to therapy with drugs affecting the renin-angiotensin system for a particular patient, apprise the mother of the potential risk to the fetus. Perform serial ultrasound examinations to assess the intra-amniotic environment. If oligohydramnios is observed, discontinue Exforge HCT, unless it is considered lifesaving for the mother. Fetal testing may be appropriate, based on the week of pregnancy. Patients and physicians should be aware, however, that oligohydramnios may not appear until after the fetus has sustained irreversible injury. Closely observe infants with histories of in utero exposure to Exforge HCT for hypotension, oliguria, and hyperkalemia *[see Use in Specific Populations (8.4)]*.

Hydrochlorothiazide
Thiazides can cross the placenta, and concentrations reached in the umbilical vein approach those in the maternal plasma. Hydrochlorothiazide, like other diuretics, can cause placental hypoperfusion. It accumulates in the amniotic fluid, with required concentrations up to 19 times higher than in umbilical vein plasma. Use of thiazides during pregnancy is associated with a risk of fetal or neonatal jaundice of thrombocytopenia. Since they do not prevent or alter the course of EPH (Edema, Proteinuria, Hypertension) gestosis (pre-eclampsia), these drugs should not be used to treat hypertension in pregnant women. The use of hydrochlorothiazide for other indications (e.g., heart disease) in pregnancy should be avoided.

8.3 Nursing Mothers
It is not known whether amlodipine and valsartan are excreted in human milk, but thiazides are excreted in human milk and valsartan is excreted in rat milk. Because of the potential for adverse effects on the nursing infant, a decision should be made whether to discontinue nursing or discontinue the drug, taking into account the importance of the drug to the mother.

8.4 Pediatric Use
The safety and effectiveness of Exforge HCT in pediatric patients have not been established.
Neonates with a history of in utero exposure to Exforge HCT: If oliguria or hypotension occurs, direct attention toward support of blood pressure and renal perfusion. Exchange transfusions or dialysis may be required as a means of reversing hypotension and/or substituting for disordered renal function.

8.5 Geriatric Use
Exposure to amlodipine is increased in elderly patients, thus consider lower initial doses of Exforge HCT *[see Clinical Pharmacology (12.3)]*.
In controlled clinical trials, 82 hypertensive patients treated with Exforge HCT were ≥65 years and 13 were ≥75 years. No overall differences in the efficacy or safety of Exforge HCT were observed in this patient population, but greater sensitivity of some older individuals cannot be ruled out.

8.6 Renal Impairment
Safety and effectiveness of Exforge HCT in patients with severe renal impairment (CrCl <30 mL/min) have not been established. No dose adjustment is required in patients with mild (CrCl 60 to 90 mL/min) or moderate (CrCl 30 to 60 mL/min) renal impairment.

8.7 Hepatic Impairment
Amlodipine
Exposure to amlodipine is increased in patients with hepatic insufficiency, thus consider using lower doses of Exforge HCT *[see Clinical Pharmacology (12.3)]*.
Valsartan
No dose adjustment is necessary for patients with mild-to-moderate disease. No dosing recommendations can be provided for patients with severe liver disease.
Hydrochlorothiazide
Minor alterations of fluid and electrolyte balance may precipitate hepatic coma in patients with impaired hepatic function or progressive liver disease.

10 OVERDOSAGE

Limited data are available related to overdosage in humans. The most likely manifestations of overdosage would be hypotension and tachycardia; bradycardia could occur from parasympathetic (vagal) stimulation. If symptomatic hypotension should occur, supportive treatment should be instituted.

Amlodipine
Single oral doses of amlodipine maleate equivalent to 40 mg/kg and 100 mg/kg amlodipine in mice and rats, respectively, caused deaths. Single oral doses equivalent to 4 or more mg/kg amlodipine in dogs (11 or more times the maximum recommended human dose on a mg/m² basis) caused a marked peripheral vasodilation and hypotension. Overdosage might be expected to cause excessive peripheral vasodilation with marked hypotension. In humans, experience with intentional overdosage of amlodipine is limited. Marked and potentially prolonged systemic hypotension up to and including shock with fatal outcome have been reported.
If massive overdose should occur, initiate active cardiac and respiratory monitoring. Frequent blood pressure measurements are essential. Should hypotension occur, initiate cardiovascular support including elevation of the extremities and the judicious administration of fluids. If hypotension remains unresponsive to these conservative measures, consider administration of vasopressors (such as phenylephrine) with attention to circulating volume and urine output.

As amlodipine is highly protein bound, hemodialysis is not likely to be of benefit. Administration of activated charcoal to healthy volunteers immediately or up to two hours after ingestion of amlodipine has been shown to significantly decrease amlodipine absorption.

Valsartan
Depressed level of consciousness, circulatory collapse, and shock have been reported.
Valsartan is not removed from the plasma by hemodialysis. Valsartan was without grossly observable adverse effects at single oral doses up to 2000 mg/kg in rats and up to 1000 mg/kg in marmosets, except for salivation and diarrhea in the rat and vomiting in the marmoset at the highest dose (60 and 31 times, respectively, the maximum recommended human dose (MRHD) on a mg/m² basis). (Calculations assume an oral dose of 320 mg/day and a 60 kg patient.)

Hydrochlorothiazide
The degree to which hydrochlorothiazide is removed by hemodialysis has not been established. The most common signs and symptoms observed in patients are those caused by electrolyte depletion (hypokalemia, hypochloremia, hyponatremia) and dehydration resulting from excessive diuresis. If digitalis has also been administered, hypokalemia may accentuate cardiac arrhythmias.
The oral LD$_{50}$ of hydrochlorothiazide is greater than 10 g/kg in both mice and rats, 2000 and 4000 times, respectively, the MRHD on a mg/m² basis. (Calculations assume an oral dose of 25 mg/day and a 60-kg patient.)

Valsartan and Hydrochlorothiazide
In rats and marmosets, single oral doses of valsartan up to 1524 and 762 mg/kg in combination with hydrochlorothiazide at doses up to 476 and 238 mg/kg, respectively, were very well tolerated without any treatment-related effects. These no adverse effect doses in rats and marmosets, respectively, represent 46.5 and 23 times the MRHD of valsartan and 188 and 113 times the MRHD of hydrochlorothiazide on a mg/m² basis. (Calculations assume an oral dose of 320 mg/day valsartan in combination with 25 mg/day hydrochlorothiazide and a 60 kg patient.)

11 DESCRIPTION

Exforge HCT is a fixed combination of amlodipine, valsartan, and hydrochlorothiazide.
Exforge HCT contains the besylate salt of amlodipine, a dihydropyridine calcium channel blocker (CCB). Amlodipine besylate, USP is a white to pale yellow crystalline powder, slightly soluble in water and sparingly soluble in ethanol. Amlodipine besylate's chemical name is 3-Ethyl 5-methyl (±)-2-[(2-aminoethoxy)methyl]-4-(o-chlorophenyl)-1,4-dihydro-6-methyl-3,5-pyridinedicarboxylate, monobenzenesulfonate ; its structural formula is:

Its empirical formula is $C_{20}H_{25}ClN_2O_5 \cdot C_6H_6O_3S$ and its molecular weight is 567.1.
Valsartan, USP is a nonpeptide, orally active, and specific angiotensin II antagonist acting on the AT$_1$ receptor subtype. Valsartan is a white to practically white fine powder, soluble in ethanol and methanol and slightly soluble in water. Valsartan's chemical name is N-(1-oxopentyl)-N-[[2'-(1H-tetrazol-5-yl) [1,1'-biphenyl]-4-yl]methyl]-L-valine; its structural formula is:

Its empirical formula is $C_{24}H_{29}N_5O_3$ and its molecular weight is 435.5.
Hydrochlorothiazide, USP is a white, or practically white, practically odorless, crystalline powder. It is slightly soluble in water; freely soluble in sodium hydroxide solution, in n-butylamine, and in dimethylformamide; sparingly soluble in methanol; and insoluble in ether, in chloroform, and in dilute mineral acids. Hydrochlorothiazide is chemically described as 6-chloro-3,4-dihydro-2H-1,2,4-benzothiadiazine-7-sulfonamide 1,1-dioxide.

Hydrochlorothiazide is a thiazide diuretic. Its empirical formula is $C_7H_8ClN_3O_4S_2$, its molecular weight is 297.73, and its structural formula is:

Exforge HCT film-coated tablets are formulated in 5 strengths for oral administration with a combination of amlodipine besylate, valsartan, and hydrochlorothiazide, providing for the following available combinations: 5/160/12.5 mg, 10/160/12.5 mg, 5/160/25 mg, 10/160/25 mg, and 10/320/25 mg amlodipine besylate/valsartan/hydrochlorothiazide. The inactive ingredients for all strengths of the tablets include microcrystalline cellulose; crospovidone; colloidal anhydrous silica; magnesium stearate; hypromellose, macrogol 4000, and talc. Additionally, the 5/160/12.5 mg strength contains titanium dioxide; the 10/160/12.5 mg strength contains titanium dioxide and yellow and red iron oxides; the 5/160/25 mg strength contains titanium dioxide and yellow iron oxide, and the 10/160/25 mg and 10/320/25 mg strengths both contain yellow iron oxide.

12 CLINICAL PHARMACOLOGY

12.1 Mechanism of Action
The active ingredients of Exforge HCT target 3 separate mechanisms involved in blood pressure regulation. Specifically, amlodipine blocks the contractile effects of calcium on cardiac and vascular smooth muscle cells; valsartan blocks the vasoconstriction and sodium retaining effects of angiotensin II on cardiac, vascular smooth muscle, adrenal and renal cells; and hydrochlorothiazide directly promotes the excretion of sodium and chloride in the kidney leading to reductions in intravascular volume. A more detailed description of the mechanism of action of each individual component follows.

Amlodipine
Amlodipine is a dihydropyridine calcium channel blocker that inhibits the transmembrane influx of calcium ions into vascular smooth muscle and cardiac muscle. Experimental data suggest that amlodipine binds to both dihydropyridine and nondihydropyridine binding sites. The contractile processes of cardiac muscle and vascular smooth muscle are dependent upon the movement of extracellular calcium ions into these cells through specific ion channels. Amlodipine inhibits calcium ion influx across cell membranes selectively, with a greater effect on vascular smooth muscle cells than on cardiac muscle cells. Negative inotropic effects can be detected in vitro but such effects have not been seen in intact animals at therapeutic doses. Serum calcium concentration is not affected by amlodipine. Within the physiologic pH range, amlodipine is an ionized compound (pKa=8.6), and its kinetic interaction with the calcium channel receptor is characterized by a gradual rate of association and dissociation with the receptor binding site, resulting in a gradual onset of effect.
Amlodipine is a peripheral arterial vasodilator that acts directly on vascular smooth muscle to cause a reduction in peripheral vascular resistance and reduction in blood pressure.

Valsartan
Angiotensin II is formed from angiotensin I in a reaction catalyzed by angiotensin-converting enzyme (ACE, kininase II). Angiotensin II is the principal pressor agent of the renin-angiotensin system, with effects that include vasoconstriction, stimulation of synthesis and release of aldosterone, cardiac stimulation, and renal reabsorption of sodium. Valsartan blocks the vasoconstrictor and aldosterone-secreting effects of angiotensin II by selectively blocking the binding of angiotensin II to the AT$_1$ receptor in many tissues, such as vascular smooth muscle and the adrenal gland. Its action is therefore independent of the pathways for angiotensin II synthesis.
There is also an AT$_2$ receptor found in many tissues, but AT$_2$ is not known to be associated with cardiovascular homeostasis. Valsartan has much greater affinity (about 20000-fold) for the AT$_1$ receptor than for the AT$_2$ receptor. The increased plasma levels of angiotensin following AT$_1$ receptor blockade with valsartan may stimulate the unblocked AT$_2$ receptor. The primary metabolite of valsartan is essentially inactive with an affinity for the AT$_1$ receptor about one-200th that of valsartan itself.
Blockade of the renin-angiotensin system with ACE inhibitors, which inhibit the biosynthesis of angiotensin II from angiotensin I, is widely used in the treatment of hypertension. ACE inhibitors also inhibit the degradation of bradykinin, a reaction also catalyzed by ACE. Because valsartan does not inhibit ACE (kininase II), it does not affect the response to bradykinin. Whether this difference has clinical

relevance is not yet known. Valsartan does not bind to or block other hormone receptors or ion channels known to be important in cardiovascular regulation.

Blockade of the angiotensin II receptor inhibits the negative regulatory feedback of angiotensin II on renin secretion, but the resulting increased plasma renin activity and angiotensin II circulating levels do not overcome the effect of valsartan on blood pressure.

Hydrochlorothiazide

Hydrochlorothiazide is a thiazide diuretic. Thiazides affect the renal tubular mechanisms of electrolyte reabsorption, directly increasing excretion of sodium and chloride in approximately equivalent amounts. Indirectly, the diuretic action of hydrochlorothiazide reduces plasma volume, with consequent increases in plasma renin activity, increases in aldosterone secretion, increases in urinary potassium loss, and decreases in serum potassium. The renin-aldosterone link is mediated by angiotensin II, so coadministration of an angiotensin II receptor antagonist tends to reverse the potassium loss associated with these diuretics.

The mechanism of the antihypertensive effect of thiazides is unknown.

12.2   Pharmacodynamics

Exforge HCT has been shown to be effective in lowering blood pressure. The 3 components of Exforge HCT (amlodipine, valsartan, hydrochlorothiazide) lower the blood pressure through complementary mechanisms, each working at a separate site and blocking different effector pathways. The pharmacodynamics of each individual component are described below.

Exforge HCT has not been studied in indications other than hypertension.

Amlodipine

Following administration of therapeutic doses to patients with hypertension, amlodipine produces vasodilation resulting in a reduction of supine and standing blood pressures. These decreases in blood pressure are not accompanied by a significant change in heart rate or plasma catecholamine levels with chronic dosing. Although the acute intravenous administration of amlodipine decreases arterial blood pressure and increases heart rate in hemodynamic studies of patients with chronic stable angina, chronic oral administration of amlodipine in clinical trials did not lead to clinically significant changes in heart rate or blood pressures in normotensive patients with angina.

With chronic, once-daily administration, antihypertensive effectiveness is maintained for at least 24 hours. Plasma concentrations correlate with effect in both young and elderly patients. The magnitude of reduction in blood pressure with amlodipine is also correlated with the height of pretreatment elevation; thus, individuals with moderate hypertension (diastolic pressure 105-114 mmHg) had about a 50% greater response than patients with mild hypertension (diastolic pressure 90-104 mmHg). Normotensive subjects experienced no clinically significant change in blood pressure (+1/-2 mmHg).

In hypertensive patients with normal renal function, therapeutic doses of amlodipine resulted in a decrease in renal vascular resistance and an increase in glomerular filtration rate and effective renal plasma flow without change in filtration fraction or proteinuria.

As with other calcium channel blockers, hemodynamic measurements of cardiac function at rest and during exercise (or pacing) in patients with normal ventricular function treated with amlodipine have generally demonstrated a small increase in cardiac index without significant influence on dP/dt or on left ventricular end diastolic pressure or volume. In hemodynamic studies, amlodipine has not been associated with a negative inotropic effect when administered in the therapeutic dose range to intact animals and man, even when coadministered with beta-blockers to man. Similar findings, however, have been observed in normal or well-compensated patients with heart failure with agents possessing significant negative inotropic effects.

Amlodipine does not change sinoatrial nodal function or atrioventricular conduction in intact animals or man. In patients with chronic stable angina, intravenous administration of 10 mg did not significantly alter A-H and H-V conduction and sinus node recovery time after pacing. Similar results were obtained in patients receiving amlodipine and concomitant beta-blockers. In clinical studies in which amlodipine was administered in combination with beta-blockers to patients with either hypertension or angina, no adverse effects of electrocardiographic (ECG) parameters were observed. In clinical trials with angina patients alone, amlodipine therapy did not alter ECG intervals or produce higher degrees of AV blocks.

Amlodipine has indications other than hypertension which are described in its full prescribing information.

Valsartan

Valsartan inhibits the pressor effect of angiotensin II infusions. An oral dose of 80 mg inhibits the pressor effect by about 80% at peak with approximately 30% inhibition persisting for 24 hours. No information on the effect of larger doses is available.

Removal of the negative feedback of angiotensin II causes a 2- to 3-fold rise in plasma renin and consequent rise in angiotensin II plasma concentration in hypertensive patients. Minimal decreases in plasma aldosterone were observed after administration of valsartan; very little effect on serum potassium was observed.

Administration of valsartan to patients with essential hypertension results in a significant reduction of sitting, supine, and standing systolic blood pressure, usually with little or no orthostatic change.

Valsartan has indications other than hypertension which are described in its full prescribing information.

Hydrochlorothiazide

After oral administration of hydrochlorothiazide, diuresis begins within 2 hours, peaks in about 4 hours and lasts about 6 to 12 hours.

12.3   Pharmacokinetics

Exforge HCT

Following oral administration of Exforge HCT in normal healthy adults, peak plasma concentrations of amlodipine, valsartan and HCTZ are reached in about 6 hours, 3 hours, and 2 hours, respectively. The rate and extent of absorption of amlodipine, valsartan and HCTZ from Exforge HCT are the same as when administered as individual dosage forms. The bioavailability of amlodipine, valsartan, and HCTZ were not altered when Exforge HCT was administered with food. Exforge HCT may be administered with or without food.

Amlodipine

Peak plasma concentrations of amlodipine are reached 6 to 12 hours after administration of amlodipine alone. Absolute bioavailability has been estimated to be between 64% and 90%. The apparent volume of distribution of amlodipine is 21 L/kg. Approximately 93% of circulating amlodipine is bound to plasma proteins in hypertensive patients.

Amlodipine is extensively (about 90%) converted to inactive metabolites via hepatic metabolism with 10% of the parent compound and 60% of the metabolites excreted in the urine. Elimination of amlodipine from the plasma is biphasic with a terminal elimination half-life of about 30 to 50 hours. Steady state plasma levels of amlodipine are reached after 7 to 8 days of consecutive daily dosing.

Valsartan

Following oral administration of valsartan alone peak plasma concentrations of valsartan are reached in 2 to 4 hours. Absolute bioavailability is about 25% (range 10% to 35%).

The steady state volume of distribution of valsartan after intravenous administration is 17 L indicating that valsartan does not distribute into tissues extensively. Valsartan is highly bound to serum proteins (95%), mainly serum albumin.

Valsartan shows biexponential decay kinetics following intravenous administration with an average elimination half-life of about 6 hours. The recovery is mainly as unchanged drug, with only about 20% of dose recovered as metabolites. The primary metabolite, accounting for about 9% of dose, is valeryl 4-hydroxy valsartan. In vitro metabolism studies involving recombinant CYP450 enzymes indicated that the CYP2C9 isoenzyme is responsible for the formation of valeryl-4-hydroxy valsartan. Valsartan does not inhibit CYP450 isozymes at clinically relevant concentrations. CYP450 mediated drug interaction between valsartan and coadministered drugs are unlikely because of the low extent of metabolism.

Valsartan, when administered as an oral solution, is primarily recovered in feces (about 83% of dose) and urine (about 13% of dose). Following intravenous administration, plasma clearance of valsartan is about 2 L/h and its renal clearance is 0.62 L/h (about 30% of total clearance).

Hydrochlorothiazide

The estimated absolute bioavailability of hydrochlorothiazide after oral administration is about 70%. Peak plasma hydrochlorothiazide concentrations (C_{max}) are reached within 2 to 5 hours after oral administration. There is no clinically significant effect of food on the bioavailability of hydrochlorothiazide.

Hydrochlorothiazide binds to albumin (40% to 70%) and distributes into erythrocytes. Following oral administration, plasma hydrochlorothiazide concentrations decline biexponentially, with a mean distribution half-life of about 2 hours and an elimination half-life of about 10 hours.

About 70% of an orally administered dose of hydrochlorothiazide is eliminated in the urine as unchanged drug.

Special Populations

Geriatric: Elderly patients have decreased clearance of amlodipine with a resulting increase in peak plasma levels, elimination half-life, and AUC. Exposure (measured by AUC) to valsartan is higher by 70% and the half-life is longer by 35% in the elderly than in the young. Limited amount of data suggest that the systemic clearance of hydrochlorothiazide is reduced in both healthy and hypertensive elderly subjects compared to young healthy volunteers.

Gender: Pharmacokinetics of valsartan do not differ significantly between males and females.

Race: Pharmacokinetic differences due to race have not been studied.

Renal Insufficiency: The pharmacokinetics of amlodipine are not significantly influenced by renal impairment. There is no apparent correlation between renal function (measured by creatinine clearance) and exposure (measured by AUC) to valsartan in patients with different degrees of renal impairment. Valsartan has not been studied in patients with severe impairment of renal function (creatinine clearance <10 mL/min). Valsartan is not removed from the plasma by hemodialysis.

In a study in individuals with impaired renal function, the mean elimination half-life of hydrochlorothiazide was doubled in individuals with mild/moderate renal impairment (30< CrCl ≤90 mL/min) and tripled in severe renal impairment (CrCl ≤30 mL/min), compared to individuals with normal renal function (CrCl >90 mL/min) *[see Use in Specific Populations (8.6)].*

Hepatic Insufficiency: Patients with hepatic insufficiency have decreased clearance of amlodipine with resulting increase in AUC of approximately 40% to 60%. On average, patients with mild-to-moderate chronic liver disease have twice the exposure (measured by AUC values) to valsartan of healthy volunteers (matched by age, sex, and weight) *[see Use in Specific Populations (8.7)].*

Drug Interactions

Amlodipine:

In vitro data in human plasma indicate that amlodipine has no effect on the protein binding of digoxin, phenytoin, warfarin, and indomethacin.

Cimetidine: Coadministration of amlodipine with cimetidine did not alter the pharmacokinetics of amlodipine.

Grapefruit juice: Coadministration of 240 mL of grapefruit juice with a single oral dose of amlodipine 10 mg in 20 healthy volunteers had no significant effect on the pharmacokinetics of amlodipine.

Maalox® (antacid): Coadministration of the antacid Maalox with a single dose of amlodipine had no significant effect on the pharmacokinetics of amlodipine.

Sildenafil: A single 100 mg dose of sildenafil in subjects with essential hypertension had no effect on the pharmacokinetic parameters of amlodipine. When amlodipine and sildenafil were used in combination, each agent independently exerted its own blood pressure lowering effect.

Atorvastatin: Coadministration of multiple 10 mg doses of amlodipine with 80 mg of atorvastatin resulted in no significant change in the steady state pharmacokinetic parameters of atorvastatin.

Digoxin: Coadministration of amlodipine with digoxin did not change serum digoxin levels or digoxin renal clearance in normal volunteers.

Ethanol (alcohol): Single and multiple 10 mg doses of amlodipine had no significant effect on the pharmacokinetics of ethanol.

Warfarin: Coadministration of amlodipine with warfarin did not change the warfarin prothrombin response time.

Simvastatin: Coadministration of multiple doses of 10 mg of amlodipine with 80 mg simvastatin resulted in a 77% increase in exposure to simvastatin compared to simvastatin alone. Limit the dose of simvastatin in patients on amlodipine to 20 mg daily.

CYP3A4 Inhibitors: Coadministration of a 180 mg daily dose of diltiazem with 5 mg amlodipine in elderly hypertensive patients resulted in a 60% increase in amlodipine systemic exposure. Erythromycin coadministration in healthy volunteers did not significantly change amlodipine systemic exposure. However, strong inhibitors of CYP3A4 (e.g., ketoconazole, itraconazole, ritonavir) may increase the plasma concentrations of amlodipine to a greater extent.

Hydrochlorothiazide

Drugs that alter gastrointestinal motility: The bioavailability of thiazide-type diuretics may be increased by anticholinergic agents (e.g., atropine, biperiden), apparently due to a decrease in gastrointestinal motility and the stomach emptying rate. Conversely, pro-kinetic drugs may decrease the bioavailability of thiazide diuretics.

Cholestyramine: In a dedicated drug interaction study, administration of cholestyramine 2 hours before hydrochlorothiazide resulted in a 70% reduction in exposure to hydrochlorothiazide. Further, administration of hydrochlorothiazide 2 hours before cholestyramine resulted in 35% reduction in exposure to hydrochlorothiazide.

Antineoplastic agents (e.g., cyclophosphamide, methotrexate): Concomitant use of thiazide diuretics may reduce renal excretion of cytotoxic agents and enhance their myelosuppressive effects.

Alcohol, barbiturates, or narcotics: Potentiation of orthostatic hypotension may occur.

Skeletal muscle relaxants: Possible increased responsiveness to muscle relaxants such as curare derivatives.
Digitalis glycosides: Thiazide-induced hypokalemia or hypomagnesemia may predispose the patient to digoxin toxicity.

13 NONCLINICAL TOXICOLOGY

13.1 Carcinogenesis, Mutagenesis, Impairment of Fertility

Studies with amlodipine/valsartan/hydrochlorothiazide: No carcinogenicity, mutagenicity, or fertility studies have been conducted with this combination. However, these studies have been conducted for amlodipine, valsartan and hydrochlorothiazide alone. Based on the preclinical safety and human pharmacokinetic studies, there is no indication of any toxicologically significant adverse interaction between these components.

Studies with amlodipine: Rats and mice treated with amlodipine maleate in the diet for up to two years, at concentrations calculated to provide daily dosage levels of 0.5, 1.25, and 2.5 mg amlodipine/kg/day, showed no evidence of a carcinogenic effect of the drug. For the mouse, the highest dose was, on mg/m² basis, similar to the MRHD of 10 mg amlodipine/day. For the rat, the highest dose was, on a mg/m² basis, about 2.5 times the MRHD. (Calculations based on a 60 kg patient.)

Mutagenicity studies conducted with amlodipine maleate revealed no drug-related effects at either the gene or chromosome level.

There was no effect on the fertility of rats treated orally with amlodipine maleate (males for 64 days and females for 14 days prior to mating) at doses of up to 10 mg amlodipine/kg/day (about 10 times the MRHD of 10 mg/day on a mg/m² basis).

Studies with valsartan: There was no evidence of carcinogenicity when valsartan was administered in the diet to mice and rats for up to 2 years at concentrations calculated to provide doses of up to 160 and 200 mg/kg/day, respectively. These doses in mice and rats are about 2.4 and 6 times, respectively, the MRHD of 320 mg/day on a mg/m² basis. (Calculations based on a 60 kg patient.)

Mutagenicity assays did not reveal any valsartan-related effects at either the gene or chromosome level. These assays included bacterial mutagenicity tests with Salmonella and E. coli, a gene mutation test with Chinese hamster V79 cells, a cytogenetic test with Chinese hamster ovary cells, and a rat micronucleus test.

Valsartan had no adverse effects on the reproductive performance of male or female rats at oral doses of up to 200 mg/day. This dose is about 6 times the MRHD on a mg/m² basis.

Studies with hydrochlorothiazide: Two-year feeding studies in mice and rats conducted under the auspices of the National Toxicology Program (NTP) uncovered no evidence of a carcinogenic potential of hydrochlorothiazide in female mice (at doses of up to approximately 600 mg/kg/day) or in male and female rats (at doses of up to approximately 100 mg/kg/day). The NTP, however, found equivocal evidence for hepatocarcinogenicity in male mice.

Hydrochlorothiazide was not genotoxic *in vitro* in the Ames mutagenicity assay of Salmonella Typhimurium strains TA 98, TA 100, TA 1535, TA 1537, and TA 1538 and in the Chinese Hamster Ovary (CHO) test for chromosomal aberrations, or *in vivo* in assays using mouse germinal cell chromosomes, Chinese hamster bone marrow chromosomes, and the Drosophila sex-linked recessive lethal trait gene. Positive test results were obtained in the *in vitro* CHO Sister Chromatid Exchange (clastogenicity) and Mouse Lymphoma Cell (mutagenicity) assays and in the Aspergillus Nidulans non-disjunction assay.

Hydrochlorothiazide had no adverse effects on the fertility of mice and rats of either sex in studies wherein these species were exposed via diet at doses of up to 100 and 4 mg/kg, respectively, prior to mating and throughout gestation. These doses of hydrochlorothiazide in mice and rats are 19 and 1.5 times, respectively, the MRHD on a mg/m² basis. (Calculations assume an oral dose of 25 mg/day and a 60-kg patient.)

13.3 Developmental Toxicity

Studies with amlodipine: No evidence of teratogenicity or other embryo/fetal toxicity was found when pregnant rats and rabbits were treated orally with amlodipine maleate at doses of up to 10 mg amlodipine/kg/day (respectively, about 10 and 20 times the MRHD of 10 mg amlodipine on a mg/m² basis) during their respective periods of major organogenesis. (Calculations based on a patient weight of 60 kg.) However, litter size was significantly decreased (by about 50%) and the number of intrauterine deaths was significantly increased (about 5-fold) for rats receiving amlodipine maleate at a dose equivalent to 10 mg amlodipine/kg/day for 14 days before mating and throughout mating and gestation. Amlodipine maleate has been shown to prolong both the gestation period and the duration of labor in rats at this dose. There are no adequate and well controlled studies in pregnant women.

Studies with valsartan: No teratogenic effects were observed when valsartan was administered to pregnant mice and rats at oral doses of up to 600 mg/kg/day and to pregnant rabbits at oral doses of up to 10 mg/kg/day. However, significant decreases in fetal weight, pup birth weight, pup survival rate, and slight delays in developmental milestones were observed in studies in which parental rats were treated with valsartan at oral, maternally toxic (reduction in body weight gain and food consumption) doses of 600 mg/kg/day during organogenesis or late gestation and lactation. In rabbits, fetotoxicity (i.e., resorptions, litter loss, abortions, and low body weight) associated with maternal toxicity (mortality) was observed at doses of 5 and 10 mg/kg/day. The no observed adverse effect doses of 600, 200 and 2 mg/kg/day in mice, rats and rabbits, respectively, are about 9, 6 and 0.1 times the MRHD of 320 mg/day on a mg/m² basis. (Calculations based on a patient weight of 60 kg.)

Studies with hydrochlorothiazide: Under the auspices of the National Toxicology Program, pregnant mice and rats that received hydrochlorothiazide via gavage at doses up to 3000 and 1000 mg/kg/day, respectively, on gestation days 6 through 15 showed no evidence of teratogenicity. These doses of hydrochlorothiazide in mice and rats are 608 and 405 times, respectively, the MRHD on a mg/m² basis. (Calculations assume an oral dose of 25 mg/day and a 60-kg patient.)

Studies with amlodipine and valsartan: In the oral embryofetal development study in rats using amlodipine besylate plus valsartan at doses equivalent to 5 mg/kg/day amlodipine plus 80 mg/kg/day valsartan, 10 mg/kg/day amlodipine plus 160 mg/kg/day valsartan, and 20 mg/kg/day amlodipine plus 320 mg/kg/day valsartan, treatment-related maternal and fetal effects (developmental delays and alterations noted in the presence of significant maternal toxicity) were noted with the high dose combination. The no-observed-adverse-effect level (NOAEL) for embryofetal effects was 10 mg/kg/day amlodipine plus 160 mg/kg/day valsartan. On a systemic exposure [AUC$_{(0-\infty)}$] basis, these doses are, respectively, 4.3 and 2.7 times the systemic exposure [AUC$_{(0-\infty)}$] in humans receiving the MRHD (10/320 mg/60 kg).

Studies with valsartan and hydrochlorothiazide: There was no evidence of teratogenicity in mice, rats, or rabbits treated orally with valsartan at doses up to 600, 100, and 10 mg/kg/day, respectively, in combination with hydrochlorothiazide at doses up to 188, 31, and 3 mg/kg/day. These non-teratogenic doses in mice, rats and rabbits are, respectively, 9, 3.5, and 0.5 times the MRHD of valsartan and 38, 13 and 2 times the MRHD of hydrochlorothiazide on a mg/m² basis. (Calculations assume an oral dose of 320 mg/day valsartan in combination with 25 mg/day hydrochlorothiazide in a 60-kg patient.)

Fetotoxicity was observed in association with maternal toxicity in rats at valsartan/hydrochlorothiazide doses ≥200/63 mg/kg/day and in rabbits at valsartan/hydrochlorothiazide doses of 10/3 mg/kg/day. Evidence of fetotoxicity in rats consisted of decreased fetal weight and fetal variations of sternebrae, vertebrae, ribs, and/or renal papillae. Evidence of fetotoxicity in rabbits included increased numbers of late resorptions with resultant increases in total resorptions, postimplantation losses, and decreased number of live fetuses. The no observed adverse effect doses of the valsartan/hydrochlorothiazide combination in mice, rats and rabbits were 600/188, 100/31 and 3/1 mg/kg/day, respectively. These doses in mice, rats and rabbits are, respectively, 9, 3 and 0.18 times the MRHD of valsartan and 38, 13, and 0.5 times the MRHD of hydrochlorothiazide on a mg/m² basis. (Calculations assume an oral dose of 320 mg/day valsartan in combination with 25 mg/day hydrochlorothiazide in a 60-kg patient.)

14 CLINICAL STUDIES

Exforge HCT was studied in a double-blind, active controlled study in hypertensive patients. A total of 2271 patients with moderate to severe hypertension (mean baseline systolic/diastolic blood pressure was 170/107 mmHg) received treatments of amlodipine/valsartan/HCTZ 10/320/25 mg, valsartan/HCTZ 320/25 mg, amlodipine/valsartan 10/320 mg, or HCTZ/amlodipine 25/10 mg. At study initiation patients assigned to the 2-component arms received lower doses of their treatment combination while patients assigned to the Exforge HCT arm received 160/12.5 mg valsartan/hydrochlorothiazide. After 1 week, Exforge HCT patients were titrated to 5/160/12.5 mg amlodipine/valsartan/hydrochlorothiazide, while all other patients continued receiving their initial doses. After 2 weeks, all patients were titrated to their full treatment dose. A total of 55% of patients were male, 14% were 65 years or older, 72% were Caucasian, and 17% were black.

At week 8, the triple combination therapy produced greater reductions in blood pressure than each of the 3 dual combination treatments (p<0.0001 for both diastolic and systolic blood pressures reductions). The reductions in systolic/

diastolic blood pressure with Exforge HCT were 7.6/5.0 mmHg greater than with valsartan/HCTZ, 6.2/3.3 mmHg greater than with amlodipine/valsartan, and 8.2/5.3 mmHg greater than with amlodipine/HCTZ (see Figure 1). The full blood pressure lowering effect was achieved 2 weeks after being on the maximal dose of Exforge HCT (see Figure 2 and Figure 3). As the pivotal study was an active-controlled trial, the treatment effects shown in Figures 1, 2, and 3 include a placebo effect of unknown size.

Figure 1: Reduction in Mean Blood Pressure at Endpoint

Figure 2: Mean Sitting Diastolic Blood Pressure by Treatment and Week

Figure 3: Mean Sitting Systolic Blood Pressure by Treatment and Week

A subgroup of 283 patients was studied with ambulatory blood pressure monitoring. The blood pressure lowering effect in the triple therapy group was maintained throughout the 24-hour period (see Figure 4 and Figure 5).

Figure 4: Mean Ambulatory Diastolic Blood Pressure at Endpoint by Treatment and Hour

[See figure 5 at top of next column]

There are no trials of the Exforge HCT combination tablet demonstrating reductions in cardiovascular risk in patients with hypertension, but both the amlodipine and hydrochlorothiazide components and several ARBs, which are the same pharmacological class as the valsartan component, have demonstrated such benefits.

Figure 5: Mean Ambulatory Systolic Blood Pressure at Endpoint by Treatment and Hour

16 HOW SUPPLIED/STORAGE AND HANDLING

Exforge HCT (amlodipine, valsartan, hydrochlorothiazide) is available as film-coated tablets containing amlodipine besylate equivalent to 5 mg or 10 mg of amlodipine free-base with valsartan 160 mg or 320 mg, and hydrochlorothiazide 12.5 mg or 25 mg, providing for the following available combinations: 5/160/12.5 mg, 10/160/12.5 mg, 5/160/25 mg, 10/160/25 mg, and 10/320/25 mg. All strengths are packaged in bottles and blisters of 30 tablets.

5 mg amlodipine /160 mg valsartan /12.5 mg hydrochlorothiazide Tablets – White, non-scored, film-coated tablet, ovaloid, biconvex with beveled edge with debossing "NVR" on one side and "VCL" on the other side.

Bottles of 30	NDC 0078-0559-15
Unit Dose (blister pack of 30)	NDC 0078-0559-30

10 mg amlodipine /160 mg valsartan /12.5 mg hydrochlorothiazide Tablets – Pale yellow, non-scored, film-coated tablet, ovaloid, biconvex with beveled edge with debossing "NVR" on one side and "VDL" on the other side.

Bottles of 30	NDC 0078-0561-15
Unit Dose (blister pack of 30)	NDC 0078-0561-30

5 mg amlodipine /160 mg valsartan /25 mg hydrochlorothiazide Tablets – Yellow, non-scored, film-coated tablet, ovaloid, biconvex with beveled edge with debossing "NVR" on one side and "VEL" on the other side.

Bottles of 30	NDC 0078-0560-15
Unit Dose (blister pack of 30)	NDC 0078-0560-30

10 mg amlodipine /160 mg valsartan /25 mg hydrochlorothiazide Tablets – Brown-yellow, non-scored, film-coated tablet, ovaloid, biconvex with beveled edge with debossing "NVR" on one side and "VHL" on the other side.

Bottles of 30	NDC 0078-0562-15
Unit Dose (blister pack of 30)	NDC 0078-0562-30

10 mg amlodipine /320 mg valsartan /25 mg hydrochlorothiazide Tablets – Brown-yellow, non-scored, film-coated tablet, ovaloid, biconvex with beveled edge with debossing "NVR" on one side and "VFL" on the other side.

Bottles of 30	NDC 0078-0563-15
Unit Dose (blister pack of 30)	NDC 0078-0563-30

Store at 25°C (77°F); excursions permitted to 15-30°C (59-86°F), [see USP controlled room temperature.]
Protect from moisture.
Dispense in tight container (USP).

17 PATIENT COUNSELING INFORMATION

Pregnancy: Female patients of childbearing age should be told about the consequences of exposure to Exforge HCT during pregnancy. Discuss treatment options with women planning to become pregnant. Patients should be asked to report pregnancies to their physicians as soon as possible.

Symptomatic Hypotension: A patient receiving Exforge HCT should be cautioned that lightheadedness can occur, especially during the first days of therapy, and that it should be reported to the prescribing physician. The patients should be told that if syncope occurs, Exforge HCT should be discontinued until the physician has been consulted.

All patients should be cautioned that inadequate fluid intake, excessive perspiration diarrhea, or vomiting can lead to an excessive fall in blood pressure, with the same consequences of lightheadedness and possible syncope.

Potassium Supplements: A patient receiving Exforge HCT should be told not to use potassium supplements or salt substitutes containing potassium without consulting the prescribing physician.

T2014-64
June 2014
Information for Patients
Patient Information
Exforge HCT (X-phorj HCT)
(amlodipine and valsartan and hydrochlorothiazide) Tablets
Read the Patient Information that comes with EXFORGE HCT before you start taking it and each time you get a refill. There may be new information. This leaflet does not take the place of talking with your doctor about your medical condition or treatment.

What is the most important information I should know about EXFORGE HCT?
• EXFORGE HCT can cause harm or death to an unborn baby.
• Talk to your doctor about other ways to lower your blood pressure if you plan to become pregnant.
• If you get pregnant while taking EXFORGE HCT, tell your doctor right away.

What is EXFORGE HCT?
EXFORGE HCT contains 3 prescription medicines:
1. amlodipine, a calcium channel blocker
2. valsartan, an angiotensin receptor blocker, and
3. hydrochlorothiazide, a diuretic (water pill)
EXFORGE HCT may be used to lower blood pressure in adults when 2 medicines to lower your high blood pressure are not enough.
EXFORGE HCT has not been studied in children under 18 years of age.

Who should not take EXFORGE HCT?
Do not take EXFORGE HCT if you have low or no urine output (anuria).

What should I tell my doctor before taking EXFORGE HCT?
Tell your doctor about all of your medical conditions, including if you:
• **are pregnant or plan to become pregnant.** See "What is the most important information I should know about EXFORGE HCT?"
• **are breastfeeding or plan to breastfeed.** EXFORGE HCT may pass into your milk. Do not breastfeed while you are taking EXFORGE HCT.
• are allergic to any of the ingredients in EXFORGE HCT. See the end of this leaflet for a list of the ingredients in EXFORGE HCT.
• have heart problems
• have liver problems
• have kidney problems
• are vomiting or having a lot of diarrhea
• have or had gallstones
• have Lupus
• have low levels of potassium (with or without symptoms such as muscle weakness, muscle spasms, abnormal heart rhythm) or magnesium in your blood
• have high levels of calcium in your blood (with or without symptoms such as nausea, vomiting, constipation, stomach pain, frequent urination, thirst, muscle weakness, and twitching).
• have high levels of uric acid in the blood.
• have ever had a reaction called angioedema, to another blood pressure medicine. Angioedema causes swelling of the face, lips, tongue, and may cause difficulty breathing.
Tell your doctor about all the medicines you take, including prescription and nonprescription medicines, vitamins, and herbal supplements. Some of your other medicines and EXFORGE HCT could affect each other, causing serious side effects.
Especially tell your doctor if you take:
• simvastatin or other cholesterol lowering medicine
• other medicines for high blood pressure or a heart problem
• water pills ("diuretics")
• potassium supplements. Your doctor may check the amount of potassium in your blood periodically.
• salt substitute containing potassium. Your doctor may check the amount of potassium in your blood periodically.
• diabetes medicine including insulin
• narcotic pain medicines
• sleeping pills and antiseizure medicines called barbiturates
• lithium, a medicine used to treat some types of depression
• aspirin or other medicines called nonsteroidal anti-inflammatory drugs (NSAIDs), like ibuprofen or naproxen
• steroids
• alcohol
• digoxin or other digitalis glycosides (a heart medicine)
• muscle relaxants (medicines used during operations)
• certain cancer medicines, like cyclophosphamide or methotrexate
• medicines used to prevent and treat fungal infections (such as ketoconazole, itraconazole)
• medicines used to treat bacterial infections (such as clarithromycin, telithromycin)
• certain antibiotics (rifamycin group), a drug used to protect against transplant rejection (cyclosporin) or an anti-retroviral drug used to treat HIV/AIDS infection (ritonavir). These drugs may increase the effect of valsartan.
Know the medicines you take. Keep a list of your medicines and show it to your doctor or pharmacist when you get a new medicine.

How should I take EXFORGE HCT?
• Take EXFORGE HCT exactly as your doctor tells you.
• Take EXFORGE HCT one time each day.
• EXFORGE HCT can be taken with or without food.
• If you miss a dose, take it as soon as you remember. If it is close to your next dose, do not take the missed dose. Just take the next dose at the regular time.

• If you take too much EXFORGE HCT, call your doctor or Poison Control Center, or go to the emergency room.
• Tell all your doctors and dentist you are taking EXFORGE HCT. This is especially important if you:
  ◦ are going to have surgery
  ◦ go for kidney dialysis
What are the possible side effects of EXFORGE HCT?
EXFORGE HCT may cause **serious side effects** including:
• **harm to an unborn baby causing injury or death.** See "What is the most important information I should know about EXFORGE HCT?"
• **low blood pressure** (hypotension). Low blood pressure is most likely to happen if you:
  ◦ take water pills
  ◦ are on a low salt diet
  ◦ have heart problems
  ◦ get dialysis treatments
  ◦ get sick with vomiting or diarrhea
  ◦ drink alcohol.
Lie down if you feel faint or dizzy. If you faint (lose consciousness), stop taking EXFORGE HCT. Call your doctor right away.
• Get emergency help if you get worse chest pain or chest pain that does not go away.
• **kidney problems.** Kidney problems may become worse in people that already have kidney disease. Some people will have changes in blood tests for kidney function and may need a lower dose of EXFORGE HCT. Call your doctor if you have swelling in your feet, ankles, or hands, or unexplained weight gain. If you have heart failure, your doctor should check your kidney function before prescribing EXFORGE HCT.
• **laboratory blood test changes in people with heart failure.** Some people with heart failure who take valsartan, one of the medicines in EXFORGE HCT, have changes in blood tests including increased potassium and decreased kidney function.
• **allergic reactions**
• **skin rash.** Call your doctor right away if you get an unusual skin rash.
• **eye problems.** One of the medicines in EXFORGE HCT can cause eye problems that may lead to vision loss. Symptoms of eye problems can happen within hours to weeks of starting EXFORGE HCT. Tell your doctor right away if you have:
  • decrease in vision
  • eye pain
The **most common** side effects of EXFORGE HCT include:
• dizziness
• swelling (edema) of the hands, ankles, or feet
• headache
• indigestion
• tiredness
• muscle spasms
• back pain
• nausea
Tell your doctor if you have any side effect that bothers you or that does not go away.
These are not all the possible side effects of EXFORGE HCT. For more information, ask your doctor or pharmacist. Call your doctor for medical advice about side effects. You may report side effects to FDA at 1-800-FDA-1088.
How should I store EXFORGE HCT?
• Store EXFORGE HCT at room temperature between 59°F to 86°F (15°C to 30°C).
• Keep EXFORGE HCT dry (protect it from moisture).
Keep EXFORGE HCT and all medicines out of the reach of children.
General Information about EXFORGE HCT
Medicines are sometimes prescribed for conditions that are not mentioned in the patient information leaflet. Do not use EXFORGE HCT for a condition for which it was not prescribed. Do not give EXFORGE HCT to other people, even if they have the same symptoms that you have. It may harm them.
This patient information leaflet summarizes the most important information about EXFORGE HCT. If you would like more information about EXFORGE HCT, talk with your doctor. You can ask your doctor or pharmacist for information about EXFORGE HCT that is written for health professionals. For more information go to www.EXFORGE.com or call 1-888-839-3674.
What are the ingredients in EXFORGE HCT?
Active ingredients: amlodipine besylate, valsartan, and hydrochlorothiazide
The inactive ingredients of all strengths of the tablets are crospovidone, magnesium stearate, microcrystalline cellulose, and colloidal anhydrous silica. The film coating contains hypromellose, talc, macrogol 4000, and may contain titanium dioxide or yellow and red iron oxides.
What is high blood pressure (hypertension)?
Blood pressure is the force of blood in your blood vessels when your heart beats and when your heart rests. You have high blood pressure when the force is too much. EXFORGE

HCT can help your blood vessels relax so your blood pressure is lower. Medicines that lower blood pressure lower your chance of having a stroke or heart attack.

High blood pressure makes the heart work harder to pump blood throughout the body and causes damage to blood vessels. If high blood pressure is not treated, it can lead to stroke, heart attack, heart failure, kidney failure, and vision problems.

Distributed by:
Novartis Pharmaceuticals Corporation
East Hanover, New Jersey 07936
© Novartis
T2014-65
June 2014

Shown in Product Identification Guide, page 310

EXJADE®

[x-jāde]
(deferasirox)
tablets, for oral suspension

℞

The following prescribing information is based on official labeling in effect July 2014.

HIGHLIGHTS OF PRESCRIBING INFORMATION
These highlights do not include all the information needed to use EXJADE safely and effectively. See full prescribing information for EXJADE.
EXJADE® (deferasirox) tablets, for oral suspension
Initial U.S. Approval: 2005

WARNING: RENAL FAILURE, HEPATIC FAILURE, AND GASTROINTESTINAL HEMORRHAGE
See full prescribing information for complete boxed warning
Exjade may cause:
• renal toxicity, including failure (5.1)
• hepatic toxicity, including failure (5.2)
• gastrointestinal hemorrhage (5.3)
Exjade therapy requires close patient monitoring, including laboratory tests of renal and hepatic function. (5)

RECENT MAJOR CHANGES

Indications and Usage (1)	5/2013
Dosage and Administration (2)	5/2013
Warnings and Precautions (5)	10/2013

INDICATIONS AND USAGE

Exjade is an iron chelator indicated for the treatment of chronic iron overload due to blood transfusions in patients 2 years of age and older. This indication is based on reduction in serum ferritin and liver iron concentration (LIC). An improvement in survival or disease-related symptoms has not been established. (1.1)

Exjade is indicated for the treatment of chronic iron overload in patients 10 years of age and older with non-transfusion-dependent thalassemia (NTDT) syndromes and with a liver iron (Fe) concentration (LIC) of at least 5 mg Fe per gram of dry weight and a serum ferritin greater than 300 mcg/L. This indication is based on achievement of an LIC less than 5 mg Fe/g dw. An improvement in survival or disease-related symptoms has not been established. (1.2)

Limitation of Use
Controlled clinical trials of Exjade in patients with myelodysplastic syndromes (MDS) and chronic iron overload due to blood transfusion have not been performed. (1.3)
The safety and efficacy of Exjade when administered with other iron chelation therapy have not been established. (1.3)

DOSAGE AND ADMINISTRATION

• In patients with transfusional iron overload, the recommended initial daily dose is 20 mg per kg body weight once daily, as oral suspension. Calculate dose to the nearest whole tablet. (2.1)
• In patients with NTDT syndromes, the recommended initial daily dose is 10 mg per kg body weight once daily, as oral suspension. Calculate dose to the nearest whole tablet. (2.2)
• Monitor serum ferritin monthly and adjust dose accordingly. (2.1, 2.2)
• Monitor LIC every 6 months and adjust dose accordingly. (2.2)
• Do not chew or swallow tablets whole. (2.3)
• Take on an empty stomach at least 30 minutes before food. Disperse tablets by stirring in an appropriate amount of water, orange juice, or apple juice. (2.3)
• Reduce the starting dose in patients with moderate (Child-Pugh B) hepatic impairment by 50%. Avoid the use of Exjade in patients with severe (Child-Pugh C) hepatic impairment. (2.4)
• Reduce the starting dose by 50% in patients with renal impairment (ClCr 40-60 mL/min). (2.4)

DOSAGE FORMS AND STRENGTHS

Tablets for oral suspension: 125 mg, 250 mg, 500 mg. (3)

CONTRAINDICATIONS

• Serum creatinine greater than 2 times the age-appropriate upper limit of normal or creatinine clearance less than 40 mL/min. (4)
• Patients with poor performance status. (4)
• Patients with high-risk myelodysplastic syndromes (MDS). (4)
• Patients with advanced malignancies. (4)
• Patients with platelet counts <50 × 10⁹/L. (4)
• Known hypersensitivity to deferasirox or any component of Exjade. (4)

WARNINGS AND PRECAUTIONS

• Renal toxicity: Measure serum creatinine and creatinine clearance in duplicate before starting therapy. Monitor renal function during Exjade therapy and reduce dose or interrupt therapy for toxicity. (2.4, 5.1)
• Hepatic toxicity: Monitor hepatic function. Reduce dose or interrupt therapy for toxicity. (5.2)
• Fatal and nonfatal gastrointestinal bleeding, ulceration, and irritation: Risk may be greater in patients who are taking Exjade in combination with drugs that have known ulcerogenic or hemorrhagic potential. (5.3)
• Bone marrow suppression: Neutropenia, agranulocytosis, worsening anemia, and thrombocytopenia, including fatal events; monitor blood counts during Exjade therapy. Interrupt therapy for toxicity. (5.4)
• Elderly: Monitor closely for toxicity due to the greater frequency of decreased hepatic, renal, and/or cardiac function. (5.5)
• Serious and severe hypersensitivity reactions: Discontinue Exjade and institute medical intervention. (5.6)
• Severe skin reactions including Stevens Johnson Syndrome: Discontinue Exjade and evaluate. (5.7)

ADVERSE REACTIONS

In patients with transfusional iron overload, the most frequently occurring (>5%) adverse reactions are diarrhea, vomiting, nausea, abdominal pain, skin rashes, and increases in serum creatinine. In Exjade-treated patients with NTDT syndromes, the most frequently occurring (>5%) adverse reactions are diarrhea, rash and nausea. (6.1)

To report SUSPECTED ADVERSE REACTIONS, contact Novartis Pharmaceuticals Corporation at 1-888-669-6682 or FDA at 1-800-FDA-1088 or www.fda.gov/medwatch.

DRUG INTERACTIONS

• Avoid the use of Exjade with aluminum-containing antacid preparations. (7.1)
• Exjade increases the exposure of the CYP2C8 substrate repaglinide. Consider repaglinide dose reduction and monitor blood glucose levels. (7.3)
• Avoid the use of Exjade with CYP1A2 substrate theophylline. (7.4)

USE IN SPECIFIC POPULATIONS

• Pregnancy: Based on animal studies, may cause fetal harm. (8.1)
• Nursing Mothers: Discontinue drug or nursing, taking into consideration importance of drug to mother. (8.3)

See 17 for PATIENT COUNSELING INFORMATION
Revised: 10/2013

FULL PRESCRIBING INFORMATION

WARNING: RENAL FAILURE, HEPATIC FAILURE, AND GASTROINTESTINAL HEMORRHAGE

Renal Failure
• Exjade can cause acute renal failure and death, particularly in patients with comorbidities and those who are in the advanced stages of their hematologic disorders.
• Measure serum creatinine and determine creatinine clearance in duplicate prior to initiation of therapy and monitor renal function at least monthly thereafter. For patients with baseline renal impairment or increased risk of acute renal failure, monitor creatinine weekly for the first month, then at least monthly. Consider dose reduction, interruption, or discontinuation based on increases in serum creatinine *[see Dosage and Administration (2.4, 2.5), Warnings and Precautions (5.1)]*.

Hepatic Failure
• Exjade can cause hepatic injury including hepatic failure and death.
• Measure serum transaminases and bilirubin in all patients prior to initiating treatment, every 2 weeks during the first month, and at least monthly thereafter.
• Avoid use of Exjade in patients with severe (Child-Pugh C) hepatic impairment and reduce the dose in patients with moderate (Child Pugh B) hepatic impairment *[see Dosage and Administration (2.4), Warnings and Precautions (5.2)]*.

Gastrointestinal Hemorrhage
• Exjade can cause gastrointestinal (GI) hemorrhages, which may be fatal, especially in elderly patients who have advanced hematologic malignancies and/or low platelet counts.
• Monitor patients and discontinue Exjade for suspected GI ulceration or hemorrhage *[see Warnings and Precautions (5.3)]*.

---

1   INDICATIONS AND USAGE

1.1   Treatment of Chronic Iron Overload Due to Blood Transfusions (Transfusional Iron Overload)
Exjade is indicated for the treatment of chronic iron overload due to blood transfusions (transfusional hemosiderosis) in patients 2 years of age and older. This indication is based on a reduction of liver iron concentration and serum ferritin levels *[see Clinical Studies (14)]*. An improvement in survival or disease-related symptoms has not been established *[see Indications and Usage (1.3)]*.

1.2 Treatment of Chronic Iron Overload in Non-Transfusion-Dependent Thalassemia Syndromes

Exjade is indicated for the treatment of chronic iron overload in patients 10 years of age and older with non-transfusion-dependent thalassemia (NTDT) syndromes and with a liver iron concentration (LIC) of at least 5 milligrams of iron per gram of liver dry weight (mg Fe/g dw) and a serum ferritin greater than 300 mcg/L. This indication is based on achievement of an LIC less than 5 mg Fe/g dw [see *Clinical Studies (14)*]. An improvement in survival or disease-related symptoms has not been established.

1.3 Limitation of Use

Controlled clinical trials of Exjade with myelodysplastic syndromes (MDS) and chronic iron overload due to blood transfusions have not been performed [see *Clinical Studies (14)*].

The safety and efficacy of Exjade when administered with other iron chelation therapy have not been established.

2 DOSAGE AND ADMINISTRATION

2.1 Transfusional Iron Overload

Exjade therapy should only be considered when a patient has evidence of chronic transfusional iron overload. The evidence should include the transfusion of at least 100 mL/kg of packed red blood cells (e.g., at least 20 units of packed red blood cells for a 40 kg person or more in individuals weighing more than 40 kg), and a serum ferritin consistently greater than 1000 mcg/L.

Prior to starting therapy, obtain:
* serum ferritin level
* baseline serum creatinine in duplicate (due to variations in measurements) and determine the creatinine clearance (Cockcroft-Gault method) [see *Dosage and Administration (2.4), Warnings and Precautions (5.1)*]
* serum transaminases and bilirubin [see *Dosage and Administration (2.4), Warnings and Precautions (5.2)*]
* baseline auditory and ophthalmic examinations [see *Warnings and Precautions (5.9)*]

The recommended initial dose of Exjade for patients 2 years of age and older is 20 mg per kg body weight orally, once daily. Calculate doses (mg per kg per day) to the nearest whole tablet.

After commencing therapy, monitor serum ferritin monthly and adjust the dose of Exjade, if necessary, every 3-6 months based on serum ferritin trends. Make dose adjustments in steps of 5 or 10 mg per kg and tailor adjustments to the individual patient's response and therapeutic goals. In patients not adequately controlled with doses of 30 mg per kg (e.g., serum ferritin levels persistently above 2500 mcg/L and not showing a decreasing trend over time), doses of up to 40 mg per kg may be considered. Doses above 40 mg per kg are not recommended.

If the serum ferritin falls consistently below 500 mcg/L, consider temporarily interrupting therapy with Exjade [see *Warnings and Precautions (5.10)*].

2.2 Iron Overload in Non-Transfusion-Dependent Thalassemia Syndromes

Exjade therapy should only be considered when a patient with NTDT syndrome has an LIC of at least 5 mg Fe/g dw and a serum ferritin greater than 300 mcg/L.

Prior to starting therapy, obtain:
* LIC by liver biopsy or by an FDA-cleared or approved method for identifying patients for treatment with deferasirox therapy
* Serum ferritin level on at least 2 measurements 1 month apart [see *Clinical Studies (14)*]
* Baseline serum creatinine in duplicate (due to variations in measurements) and determine the creatinine clearance (Cockcroft-Gault method) [see *Dosage and Administration (2.4), Warnings and Precautions (5.1)*]
* Serum transaminases and bilirubin [see *Dosage and Administration (2.4), Warnings and Precautions (5.2)*]
* Baseline auditory and ophthalmic examinations [see *Warnings and Precautions (5.9)*]

Initiating therapy:
* The recommended initial dose of Exjade is 10 mg per kg body weight orally once daily. Calculate doses (mg per kg per day) to the nearest whole tablet.
* If the baseline LIC is greater than 15 mg Fe/g dw, consider increasing the dose to 20 mg/kg/day after 4 weeks.

During therapy:
* Monitor serum ferritin monthly. Interrupt treatment when serum ferritin is less than 300 mcg/L and obtain an LIC to determine whether the LIC has fallen to less than 3 mg Fe/g dw.
* Monitor LIC every 6 months.
* After 6 months of therapy, if the LIC remains greater than 7 mg Fe/g dw, increase the dose of deferasirox to a maximum of 20 mg/kg/day. Do not exceed a maximum of 20 mg/kg/day.
* If after 6 months of therapy, the LIC is 3-7 mg Fe/g dw, continue treatment with deferasirox at no more than 10 mg/kg/day.

* When the LIC is less than 3 mg Fe/g dw, interrupt treatment with deferasirox and continue to monitor the LIC.
* Monitor blood counts, hepatic function, and renal function [see *Warnings and Precautions (5.1, 5.2, 5.4)*].

Restart treatment when the LIC rises again to more than 5 mg Fe/g dw.

2.3 Administration

Do not chew tablets or swallow them whole.

Take Exjade once daily on an empty stomach at least 30 minutes before food, preferably at the same time each day. Completely disperse tablets by stirring in water, orange juice, or apple juice until a fine suspension is obtained. Disperse doses of less than 1 g in 3.5 ounces of liquid and doses of 1 g or greater in 7 ounces of liquid. After swallowing the suspension, resuspend any residue in a small volume of liquid and swallow. Do not take Exjade with aluminum-containing antacid products [see *Drug Interactions (7.1)*].

2.4 Use in Patients with Baseline Hepatic or Renal Impairment

Patients with Baseline Hepatic Impairment

Mild (Child-Pugh A) hepatic impairment: No dose adjustment is necessary.

Moderate (Child-Pugh B) hepatic impairment: Reduce the starting dose by 50%.

Severe (Child-Pugh C) hepatic impairment: Avoid Exjade [see *Warnings and Precautions (5.2), Use in Specific Populations (8.7)*].

Patients with Baseline Renal Impairment

For patients with renal impairment (ClCr 40–60 mL/min), reduce the starting dose by 50% [see *Use in Specific Populations (8.6)*]. Do not use Exjade in patients with serum creatinine greater than 2 times the upper limit of normal or creatinine clearance less than 40 mL/min [see *Contraindications (4)*].

2.5 Dose Modifications for Increases in Serum Creatinine on Exjade

For serum creatinine increases while receiving Exjade [see *Warnings and Precautions (5.1)*] modify the dose as follows:

Transfusional Iron Overload

Adults and Adolescents (ages 16 years and older):
◦ If the serum creatinine increases by 33% or more above the average baseline measurement, repeat the serum creatinine within 1 week, and if still elevated by 33% or more, reduce the dose by 10 mg per kg.

Pediatric Patients (ages 2-15 years):
◦ Reduce the dose by 10 mg per kg if serum creatinine increases to greater than 33% above the average baseline measurement and greater than the age appropriate upper limit of normal.

All Patients (regardless of age):
◦ Discontinue therapy for serum creatinine greater than 2 times the age-appropriate upper limit of normal or for creatinine clearance <40 mL/min. [see *Contraindications (4)*]

Non-Transfusion-Dependent Thalassemia Syndromes

Adults and Adolescents (ages 16 years and older):
◦ If the serum creatinine increases by 33% or more above the average baseline measurement, repeat the serum creatinine within 1 week, and if still elevated by 33% or more, interrupt therapy if the dose is 5 mg per kg, or reduce by 50% if the dose is 10 or 20 mg per kg.

Pediatric Patients (ages 10-15 years):
◦ Reduce the dose by 5 mg per kg if serum creatinine increases to greater than 33% above the average baseline measurement and greater than the age appropriate upper limit of normal.

All Patients (regardless of age):
◦ Discontinue therapy for serum creatinine greater than 2 times the age-appropriate upper limit of normal or for creatinine clearance <40 mL/min [see *Contraindications (4)*].

2.6 Dose Modifications Based on Concomitant Medications

UDP-glucuronosyltransferases (UGT) Inducers

Concomitant use of UGT inducers decreases Exjade systemic exposure. Avoid the concomitant use of potent UGT inducers (e.g., rifampicin, phenytoin, phenobarbital, ritonavir) with Exjade. If you must administer Exjade with 1 of these agents, consider increasing the initial dose of Exjade by 50%, and monitor serum ferritin levels and clinical responses for further dose modification [see *Dosage and Administration (2.1, 2.2), Drug Interactions (7.5)*].

Bile Acid Sequestrants

Concomitant use of bile acid sequestrants decreases Exjade systemic exposure. Avoid the concomitant use of bile acid sequestrants (e.g., cholestyramine, colesevelam, colestipol) with Exjade. If you must administer Exjade with 1 of these agents, consider increasing the initial dose of Exjade by 50%, and monitor serum ferritin levels and clinical responses for further dose modification [see *Dosage and Administration (2.1, 2.2), Drug Interactions (7.6)*].

3 DOSAGE FORMS AND STRENGTHS

* 125 mg tablets
  Off-white, round, flat tablet with beveled edge and imprinted with "J" and "125" on one side and "NVR" on the other.

* 250 mg tablets
  Off-white, round, flat tablet with beveled edge and imprinted with "J" and "250" on one side and "NVR" on the other.

* 500 mg tablets
  Off-white, round, flat tablet with beveled edge and imprinted with "J" and "500" on one side and "NVR" on the other.

4 CONTRAINDICATIONS

Exjade is contraindicated in patients with:
* Serum creatinine greater than 2 times the age-appropriate upper limit of normal or creatinine clearance less than 40 mL/min [see *Warning and Precautions (5.1)*];
* Poor performance status;
* High-risk myelodysplastic syndromes;
* Advanced malignancies;
* Platelet counts <50 × 10^9/L;
* Known hypersensitivity to deferasirox or any component of Exjade [see *Warnings and Precautions (5.6), Adverse Reactions (6.2)*].

5 WARNINGS AND PRECAUTIONS

5.1 Renal Toxicity, Renal Failure, and Proteinuria

Exjade can cause acute renal failure, fatal in some patients and requiring dialysis in others. Postmarketing experience showed that most fatalities occurred in patients with multiple comorbidities and who were in advanced stages of their hematological disorders. In the clinical trials, Exjade-treated patients experienced dose-dependent increases in serum creatinine. In patients with transfusional iron overload, these increases in creatinine occurred at a greater frequency compared to deferoxamine-treated patients (38% versus 14%, respectively, in Study 1 and 36% versus 22%, respectively, in Study 3) [see *Adverse Reactions (6.1, 6.2)*].

Measure serum creatinine in duplicate (due to variations in measurements) and determine the creatinine clearance (estimated by the Cockcroft-Gault method) before initiating therapy in all patients in order to establish a reliable pretreatment baseline. Monitor serum creatinine weekly during the first month after initiation or modification of therapy and at least monthly thereafter. Monitor serum creatinine and/or creatinine clearance more frequently if creatinine levels are increasing. Dose reduction, interruption, or discontinuation based on increases in serum creatinine may be necessary [see *Dosage and Administration (2.5)*].

Exjade is contraindicated in patients with creatinine clearance less than 40 mL/minute or serum creatinine greater than 2 times the age appropriate upper limit of normal.

Renal tubular damage, including Fanconi's Syndrome, has been reported in patients treated with Exjade, most commonly in children and adolescents with beta-thalassemia and serum ferritin levels <1500 mcg/L.

Intermittent proteinuria (urine protein/creatinine ratio >0.6 mg/mg) occurred in 18.6% of Exjade-treated patients compared to 7.2% of deferoxamine-treated patients in Study 1. In clinical trials in patients with transfusional iron overload, Exjade was temporarily withheld until the urine protein/creatinine ratio fell below 0.6 mg/mg. Monthly monitoring for proteinuria is recommended. The mechanism and clinical significance of the proteinuria are uncertain [see *Adverse Reactions (6.1)*].

5.2 Hepatic Toxicity and Failure

Exjade can cause hepatic injury, fatal in some patients. In Study 1, 4 patients (1.3%) discontinued Exjade because of hepatic toxicity (drug-induced hepatitis in 2 patients and increased serum transaminases in 2 additional patients). Hepatic toxicity appears to be more common in patients greater than 55 years of age. Hepatic failure was more common in patients with significant comorbidities, including liver cirrhosis and multiorgan failure [see *Adverse Reactions (6.1)*].

Measure transaminases (AST and ALT) and bilirubin in all patients before the initiation of treatment and every 2 weeks during the first month and at least monthly thereafter. Consider dose modifications or interruption of treatment for severe or persistent elevations.

Avoid the use of Exjade in patients with severe (Child-Pugh C) hepatic impairment. Reduce the starting dose in patients with moderate (Child-Pugh B) hepatic impairment [see *Dosage and Administration (2.4), Use in Specific Populations (8.7)*]. Patients with mild (Child-Pugh A) or moderate (Child-Pugh B) hepatic impairment may be at higher risk for hepatic toxicity.

5.3 Gastrointestinal (GI) Hemorrhage

GI hemorrhage, including deaths, has been reported, especially in elderly patients who had advanced hematologic malignancies and/or low platelet counts. Nonfatal upper GI irritation, ulceration and hemorrhage have been reported in patients, including children and adolescents, receiving Exjade [see *Adverse Reactions (6.1)*]. Monitor for signs and symptoms of GI ulceration and hemorrhage during Exjade therapy and promptly initiate additional evaluation and treatment if a serious GI adverse event is suspected. The risk of gastrointestinal hemorrhage may be increased when administering Exjade in combination with drugs that have ulcerogenic or hemorrhagic potential, such as nonsteroidal anti-inflammatory drugs (NSAIDs), corticosteroids, oral bisphosphonates, or anticoagulants.

5.4 Bone Marrow Suppression

Neutropenia, agranulocytosis, worsening anemia, and thrombocytopenia, including fatal events, have been reported in patients treated with Exjade. Preexisting hematologic disorders may increase this risk. Monitor blood counts in all patients. Interrupt treatment with Exjade in patients who develop cytopenias until the cause of the cytopenia has been determined. Exjade is contraindicated in patients with platelet counts below 50×10^9/L.

5.5 Increased Risk of Toxicity in the Elderly

Exjade has been associated with serious and fatal adverse reactions in the postmarketing setting, predominantly in elderly patients. Monitor elderly patients treated with Exjade more frequently for toxicity [see Use in Specific Populations (8.5)].

5.6 Hypersensitivity

Exjade may cause serious hypersensitivity reactions (such as anaphylaxis and angioedema), with the onset of the reaction usually occurring within the first month of treatment [see Adverse Reactions (6.2)]. If reactions are severe, discontinue Exjade and institute appropriate medical intervention. Exjade is contraindicated in patients with known hypersensitivity to Exjade.

5.7 Severe Skin Reactions

Severe skin reactions, including Stevens-Johnson syndrome (SJS) and erythema multiforme, have been reported during Exjade therapy [see Adverse Reactions (6.2)]. If SJS or erythema multiforme is suspected, discontinue Exjade and evaluate.

5.8 Skin Rash

Rashes may occur during Exjade treatment [see Adverse Reactions (6.1)]. For rashes of mild to moderate severity, Exjade may be continued without dose adjustment, since the rash often resolves spontaneously. In severe cases, interrupt treatment with Exjade. Reintroduction at a lower dose with escalation may be considered in combination with a short period of oral steroid administration.

5.9 Auditory and Ocular Abnormalities

Auditory disturbances (high frequency hearing loss, decreased hearing), and ocular disturbances (lens opacities, cataracts, elevations in intraocular pressure, and retinal disorders) were reported at a frequency of <1% with Exjade therapy in the clinical studies. Perform auditory and ophthalmic testing (including slit lamp examinations and dilated fundoscopy) before starting Exjade treatment and thereafter at regular intervals (every 12 months). If disturbances are noted, monitor more frequently. Consider dose reduction or interruption.

5.10 Overchelation

For patients with transfusional iron overload, measure serum ferritin monthly to assess for possible overchelation of iron. If the serum ferritin falls below 500 mcg/L, consider interrupting therapy with Exjade, since overchelation may increase Exjade toxicity [see Dosage and Administration (2.1)].

For patients with NTDT, measure LIC by liver biopsy or by using an FDA-cleared or approved method for monitoring patients receiving deferasirox therapy every 6 months on treatment. Interrupt Exjade administration when the LIC is less than 3 mg Fe/g dw. Measure serum ferritin monthly, and if the serum ferritin falls below 300 mcg/L, interrupt Exjade and obtain a confirmatory LIC [see Clinical Studies (14)].

6 ADVERSE REACTIONS

6.1 Clinical Trials Experience

The following adverse reactions are also discussed in other sections of the labeling:
- Renal Toxicity, Renal Failure, and Proteinuria [see Warnings and Precautions (5.1)]
- Hepatic Toxicity and Failure [see Warnings and Precautions (5.2)]
- Gastrointestinal (GI) Hemorrhage [see Warnings and Precautions (5.3)]
- Bone Marrow Suppression [see Warnings and Precautions (5.4)]
- Hypersensitivity [see Warnings and Precautions (5.6)]
- Severe Skin Reactions [see Warnings and Precautions (5.7)]
- Skin Rash [see Warnings and Precautions (5.8)]
- Auditory and Ocular Abnormalities [see Warnings and Precautions (5.9)]

Because clinical trials are conducted under widely varying conditions, adverse reaction rates observed in the clinical trials of a drug cannot be directly compared to rates in the clinical trials of another drug and may not reflect the rates observed in practice.

Table 1. Adverse Reactions* Occurring in >5% of Exjade-treated Patients in Study 1, Study 3, and MDS Pool

| Preferred Term | Study 1 (Beta-thalassemia) | | Study 3 (Sickle Cell Disease) | | MDS Pool |
	EXJADE N=296 n (%)	Deferoxamine N=290 n (%)	EXJADE N=132 n (%)	Deferoxamine N=63 n (%)	EXJADE N=627 n (%)
Abdominal Pain**	63 (21)	41 (14)	37 (28)	9 (14)	145 (23)
Diarrhea	35 (12)	21 (7)	26 (20)	3 (5)	297 (47)
Creatinine Increased***	33 (11)	0 (0)	9 (7)	0	89 (14)
Nausea	31 (11)	14 (5)	30 (23)	7 (11)	161 (26)
Vomiting	30 (10)	28 (10)	28 (21)	10 (16)	83 (13)
Rash	25 (8)	9 (3)	14 (11)	3 (5)	83 (13)

*Adverse reaction frequencies are based on adverse events reported regardless of relationship to study drug.
**Includes 'abdominal pain', 'abdominal pain lower', and 'abdominal pain upper' which were reported as adverse events.
***Includes 'blood creatinine increased' and 'blood creatinine abnormal' which were reported as adverse events. Also see Table 2.

Table 2. Number (%) of Patients with Increases in Serum Creatinine or SGPT/ALT in Study 1, Study 3, and MDS Pool

| Laboratory Parameter | Study 1 (Beta-thalassemia) | | Study 3 (Sickle Cell Disease) | | MDS Pool |
	EXJADE N=296 n (%)	Deferoxamine N=290 n (%)	EXJADE N=132 n (%)	Deferoxamine N=63 n (%)	EXJADE N=627 n (%)
Serum Creatinine					
Creatinine increase >33% at 2 consecutive postbaseline visits	113 (38)	41 (14)	48 (36)	14 (22)	229 (37)
Creatinine increase >33% and >ULN at 2 consecutive postbaseline visits	7 (2)	1 (0)	3 (2)	2 (3)	126 (20)
SGPT/ALT					
SGPT/ALT >5 × ULN at 2 postbaseline visits	25 (8)	7 (2)	2 (2)	0	9 (1)
SGPT/ALT >5 × ULN at 2 consecutive postbaseline visits	17 (6)	5 (2)	5 (4)	0	5 (1)

Transfusional Iron Overload

A total of 700 adult and pediatric patients were treated with Exjade (deferasirox) for 48 weeks in premarketing studies. These included 469 patients with beta-thalassemia, 99 with rare anemias, and 132 with sickle cell disease. Of these patients, 45% were male, 70% were Caucasian and 292 patients were <16 years of age. In the sickle cell disease population, 89% of patients were black. Median treatment duration among the sickle cell patients was 51 weeks. Of the 700 patients treated, 469 (403 beta-thalassemia and 66 rare anemias) were entered into extensions of the original clinical protocols. In ongoing extension studies, median durations of treatment were 88-205 weeks.

Six hundred twenty-seven patients with MDS were enrolled across 5 uncontrolled trials. These studies varied in duration from 1 to 5 years. The discontinuation rate across studies in the first year was 46% (AEs 20%, withdrawal of consent 10%, death 8%, other 4%, lab abnormalities 3%, and lack of efficacy 1%). Among 47 patients enrolled in the study of 5-year duration, 10 remained on Exjade at the completion of the study.

Table 1 displays adverse reactions occurring in >5% of Exjade-treated beta-thalassemia patients (Study 1), sickle cell disease patients (Study 3), and patients with MDS (MDS pool). Abdominal pain, nausea, vomiting, diarrhea, skin rashes, and increases in serum creatinine were the most frequent adverse reactions reported with a suspected relationship to Exjade. Gastrointestinal symptoms, increases in serum creatinine, and skin rash were dose related.

[See table 1 above]

In Study 1, a total of 113 (38%) patients treated with Exjade had increases in serum creatinine >33% above baseline on 2 separate occasions (Table 2) and 25 (8%) patients required dose reductions. Increases in serum creatinine appeared to be dose related [see Warnings and Precautions (5.1)]. In this study, 17 (6%) patients treated with Exjade developed elevations in SGPT/ALT levels >5 times the upper limit of normal at 2 consecutive visits. Of these, 2 patients had liver biopsy proven drug-induced hepatitis and both discontinued Exjade therapy [see Warnings and Precautions (5.2)]. An additional 2 patients, who did not have elevations in SGPT/ALT >5 times the upper limit of normal, discontinued Exjade because of increased SGPT/ALT. Increases in transaminases did not appear to be dose related. Adverse reactions that led to discontinuations included abnormal liver function tests (2 patients) and drug-induced hepatitis (2 patients), skin rash, glycosuria/proteinuria, Henoch Schönlein purpura, hyperactivity/insomnia, drug fever, and cataract (1 patient each).

In Study 3, a total of 48 (36%) patients treated with Exjade had increases in serum creatinine >33% above baseline on 2 separate occasions (Table 2) [see Warnings and Precautions (5.1)]. Of the patients who experienced creatinine increases in Study 3, 8 Exjade-treated patients required dose reductions. In this study, 5 patients in the Exjade group developed elevations in SGPT/ALT levels >5 times the upper limit of normal at 2 consecutive visits and 1 patient subsequently had Exjade permanently discontinued. Four additional patients discontinued Exjade due to adverse reactions with a suspected relationship to study drug, including diarrhea, pancreatitis associated with gallstones, atypical tuberculosis, and skin rash.

In the MDS pool, in the first year, a total of 229 (37%) patients treated with Exjade had increases in serum creatinine >33% above baseline on 2 consecutive occasions (Table 2) and 8 (3.5%) patients permanently discontinued [see Warnings and Precautions (5.1)]. A total of 5 (0.8%) patients developed SGPT/ALT levels >5 times the upper limit of normal at 2 consecutive visits. The most frequent adverse reactions that led to discontinuation included increases in serum creatinine, diarrhea, nausea, rash, and vomiting. Death was reported in the first year in 52 (8%) of patients [see Clinical Studies (14)].

[See table 2 above]

Non-Transfusion-Dependent Thalassemia Syndromes

In Study 4, 110 patients with NTDT received 1 year of treatment with Exjade 5 or 10 mg/kg/day and 56 patients received placebo in a double-blind, randomized trial. In Study 5, 130 of the patients who completed Study 4 were treated with open-label Exjade at 5, 10, or 20 mg/kg/day (depending on the baseline LIC) for 1 year [see Clinical Studies (14)]. Table 3 displays adverse reactions occurring in >5% in any group. The most frequent adverse reactions with a suspected relationship to study drug were nausea, rash, and diarrhea.

Table 3. Adverse Reactions Occurring in >5% in NTDT Patients

| | Study 4 | | Study 5 |
	EXJADE N=110 n (%)	Placebo N=56 n (%)	EXJADE N=130 n (%)
Any adverse reaction	31 (28)	9 (16)	27 (21)
Nausea	7 (6)	4 (7)	2 (2)
Rash	7 (6)	1 (2)	2 (2)
Diarrhea	5 (5)	1 (2)	7 (5)

In Study 4, 1 patient in the placebo 10 mg/kg/day group experienced an ALT increase to >5 times ULN and >2 times baseline (Table 4). Three Exjade-treated patients (all in the 10 mg/kg/day group) had 2 consecutive serum creatinine level increases >33% from baseline and >ULN. Serum creatinine returned to normal in all 3 patients (in 1 spontaneously and in the other 2 after drug interruption). Two additional cases of ALT increase and 2 additional cases of serum creatinine increase were observed in the 1-year extension of Study 4.

Table 4. Number (%) of NTDT Patients with Increases in Serum Creatinine or SGPT/ALT

Laboratory Parameter	Study 4		Study 5
	EXJADE N=110 n (%)	Placebo N=56 n (%)	EXJADE N=130 n (%)
Serum creatinine (>33% increase from baseline and >ULN at ≥2 consecutive postbaseline values)	3 (3%)	0	2 (2%)
SGPT/ALT (>5 × ULN and >2 × baseline)	1 (1%)	1 (2%)	2 (2%)

Proteinuria
In clinical studies, urine protein was measured monthly. Intermittent proteinuria (urine protein/creatinine ratio >0.6 mg/mg) occurred in 18.6% of Exjade-treated patients compared to 7.2% of deferoxamine-treated patients in Study 1 *[see Warnings and Precautions (5.1)]*.

Other Adverse Reactions
In the population of more than 5,000 patients with transfusional iron overload who have been treated with Exjade during clinical trials, adverse reactions occurring in 0.1% to 1% of patients included gastritis, edema, sleep disorder, pigmentation disorder, dizziness, anxiety, maculopathy, cholelithiasis, pyrexia, fatigue, pharyngolaryngeal pain, early cataract, hearing loss, gastrointestinal hemorrhage, gastric ulcer (including multiple ulcers), duodenal ulcer, and renal tubulopathy (Fanconi's Syndrome). Adverse reactions occurring in 0.01% to 0.1% of patients included optic neuritis, esophagitis, and erythema multiforme. Adverse reactions which most frequently led to dose interruption or dose adjustment during clinical trials were rash, gastrointestinal disorders, infections, increased serum creatinine, and increased serum transaminases.

6.2   Postmarketing Experience
The following adverse reactions have been spontaneously reported during post-approval use of Exjade in the transfusional iron overload setting. Because these reactions are reported voluntarily from a population of uncertain size, in which patients may have received concomitant medication, it is not always possible to reliably estimate frequency or establish a causal relationship to drug exposure.
Skin and subcutaneous tissue disorders: Stevens-Johnson syndrome (SJS), leukocytoclastic vasculitis, urticaria, alopecia
Immune system disorders: hypersensitivity reactions (including anaphylaxis and angioedema)
Renal and urinary disorders: acute renal failure, tubulointerstitial nephritis
Hepatobiliary disorders: hepatic failure
Gastrointestinal disorders: gastrointestinal hemorrhage
Blood and lymphatic system disorders: worsening anemia

7   DRUG INTERACTIONS
7.1   Aluminum Containing Antacid Preparations
The concomitant administration of Exjade and aluminum-containing antacid preparations has not been formally studied. Although deferasirox has a lower affinity for aluminum than for iron, avoid use of Exjade with aluminum-containing antacid preparations due to the mechanism of action of Exjade.
7.2   Agents Metabolized by CYP3A4
Deferasirox may induce CYP3A4 resulting in a decrease in CYP3A4 substrate concentration when these drugs are co-administered. Closely monitor patients for signs of reduced effectiveness when deferasirox is administered with drugs metabolized by CYP3A4 (e.g., alfentanil, aprepitant, budesonide, buspirone, conivaptan, cyclosporine, darifenacin, darunavir, dasatinib, dihydroergotamine, dronedarone, eletriptan, eplerenone, ergotamine, everolimus, felodipine, fentanyl, hormonal contraceptive agents, indinavir, fluticasone, lopinavir, lovastatin, lurasidone, maraviroc, midazolam, nisoldipine, pimozide, quetiapine, quinidine, saquinavir, sildenafil, simvastatin, sirolimus, tacrolimus, tolvaptan, tipranavir, triazolam, ticagrelor, and vardenafil) *[see Clinical Pharmacology (12.3)]*.
7.3   Agents Metabolized by CYP2C8
Deferasirox inhibits CYP2C8 resulting in an increase in CYP2C8 substrate (e.g., repaglinide and paclitaxel) concentration when these drugs are coadministered. If Exjade and

repaglinide are used concomitantly, consider decreasing the dose of repaglinide and perform careful monitoring of blood glucose levels. Closely monitor patients for signs of exposure related toxicity when Exjade is coadministered with other CYP2C8 substrates *[see Clinical Pharmacology (12.3)]*.
7.4   Agents Metabolized by CYP1A2
Deferasirox inhibits CYP1A2 resulting in an increase in CYP1A2 substrate (e.g., alosetron, caffeine, duloxetine, melatonin, ramelteon, tacrine, theophylline, tizanidine) concentration when these drugs are coadministered. An increase in theophylline plasma concentrations could lead to clinically significant theophylline induced CNS or other adverse reactions. Avoid the concomitant use of theophylline or other CYP1A2 substrates with a narrow therapeutic index (e.g., tizanidine) with Exjade. Monitor theophylline concentrations and consider theophylline dose modification if you must coadminister theophylline with Exjade. Closely monitor patients for signs of exposure related toxicity when Exjade is coadministered with other drugs metabolized by CYP1A2 [see Clinical Pharmacology (12.3)].
7.5   Agents Inducing UDP-glucuronosyltransferase (UGT) Metabolism
Deferasirox is a substrate of UGT1A1 and to a lesser extent UGT1A3. The concomitant use of Exjade with potent UGT inducers (e.g., rifampicin, phenytoin, phenobarbital, ritonavir) may result in a decrease in Exjade efficacy due to a possible decrease in deferasirox concentration. Avoid the concomitant use of potent UGT inducers with Exjade. Consider increasing the initial dose of Exjade if you must coadminister these agents together *[see Dosage and Administration (2.5), Clinical Pharmacology (12.3)]*.
7.6   Bile Acid Sequestrants
Avoid the concomitant use of bile acid sequestrants (e.g., cholestyramine, colesevelam, colestipol) with Exjade due to a possible decrease in deferasirox concentration. If you must coadminister these agents together, consider increasing the initial dose of Exjade *[see Dosage and Administration (2.5), Clinical Pharmacology (12.3)]*.

8   USE IN SPECIFIC POPULATIONS
8.1   Pregnancy
Pregnancy Category C
There are no adequate and well-controlled studies with Exjade in pregnant women. Administration of deferasirox to animals during pregnancy and lactation resulted in decreased offspring viability and an increase in renal anomalies in male offspring at exposures that were less than the recommended human exposure. Exjade should be used during pregnancy only if the potential benefit justifies the potential risk to the fetus.
In embryofetal developmental studies, pregnant rats and rabbits received oral deferasirox during the period of organogenesis at doses up to (100 mg per kg/day in rats and 50 mg per kg/day in rabbits) 0.8 times the maximum recommended human dose (MRHD) on a mg/m^2 basis. These doses resulted in maternal toxicity but no fetal harm was observed.
In a prenatal and postnatal developmental study, pregnant rats received oral deferasirox daily from organogenesis through lactation day 20 at doses (10, 30, and 90 mg per kg/day) 0.08, 0.2, and 0.7 times the MRHD on a mg/m^2 basis. Maternal toxicity, loss of litters, and decreased offspring viability occurred at 0.7 times the MRHD on a mg/m^2 basis, and increases in renal anomalies in male offspring occurred at 0.2 times the MRHD on a mg/m^2 basis.
8.3   Nursing Mothers
It is not known whether Exjade is excreted in human milk. Deferasirox and its metabolites were excreted in rat milk. Because many drugs are excreted in human milk and because of the potential for serious adverse reactions in nursing infants from deferasirox and its metabolites, a decision should be made whether to discontinue nursing or to discontinue the drug, taking into account the importance of the drug to the mother.
8.4   Pediatric Use
Of the 700 patients with transfusional iron overload who received Exjade during clinical studies, 292 were pediatric patients 2-<16 years of age with various congenital and acquired anemias, including 52 patients age 2-<6 years, 121 patients age 6-<12 years and 119 patients age 12-<16 years. Seventy percent of these patients had beta-thalassemia. Children between the ages of 2-<6 years have a systemic exposure to Exjade approximately 50% of that of adults *[see Clinical Pharmacology (12.3)]*. However, the safety and efficacy of Exjade in pediatric patients was similar to that of adult patients, and younger pediatric patients responded similarly to older pediatric patients. The recommended starting dose and dosing modification are the same for children and adults *[see Clinical Studies (14), Indications and Usage (1), Dosage and Administration (2.1)]*.
Growth and development in patients with chronic iron overload due to blood transfusions were within normal limits in children followed for up to 5 years in clinical trials.

Sixteen pediatric patients (10 to <16 years of age) with chronic iron overload and NTDT were treated with Exjade in clinical studies. The safety and efficacy of Exjade in these children was similar to that seen in the adults. The recommended starting dose and dosing modification are the same for children and adults with chronic iron overload in NTDT *[see Clinical Studies (14), Indications and Usage (1.2), Dosage and Administration (2.2)]*.
Safety and effectiveness have not been established in pediatric patients with chronic iron overload due to blood transfusions who are less than 2 years of age or pediatric patients with chronic iron overload and NTDT who are less than 10 years of age.
8.5   Geriatric Use
Four hundred thirty-one (431) patients ≥65 years of age were studied in clinical trials of Exjade in the transfusional iron overload setting. The majority of these patients had myelodysplastic syndrome (MDS) (n=393). In these trials, elderly patients experienced a higher frequency of adverse reactions than younger patients. Monitor elderly patients for early signs or symptoms of adverse reactions that may require a dose adjustment. Elderly patients are at increased risk for toxicity due to the greater frequency of decreased hepatic, renal, or cardiac function, and of concomitant disease or other drug therapy. Dose selection for an elderly patient should be cautious, usually starting at the low end of the dosing range.
8.6   Renal Impairment
For patients with renal impairment (ClCr 40-60 mL/min), reduce the starting dose by 50% *[see Dosage and Administration (2.4), Clinical Pharmacology (12.3)]*. Exjade is contraindicated in patients with a creatinine clearance <40 mL/min or serum creatinine >2 times the age-appropriate upper limit of normal *[see Contraindications (4)]*.
Exjade can cause renal failure. Monitor serum creatinine and calculate creatinine clearance (using Cockcroft-Gault method) during treatment in all patients. Reduce, interrupt or discontinue Exjade dosing based on increases in serum creatinine *[see Dosage and Administration (2.4, 2.5), Warnings and Precautions (5.1)]*.
8.7   Hepatic Impairment
In a single dose (20 mg/kg) study in patients with varying degrees of hepatic impairment, deferasirox exposure was increased compared to patients with normal hepatic function. The average total (free and bound) AUC of deferasirox increased 16% in 6 patients with mild (Child-Pugh A) hepatic impairment, and 76% in 6 patients with moderate (Child-Pugh B) hepatic impairment compared to 6 patients with normal hepatic function. The impact of severe (Child-Pugh C) hepatic impairment was assessed in only 1 patient. Avoid the use of Exjade in patients with severe (Child-Pugh C) hepatic impairment. For patients with moderate (Child-Pugh B) hepatic impairment, the starting dose should be reduced by 50%. Closely monitor patients with mild (Child-Pugh A) or moderate (Child-Pugh B) hepatic impairment for efficacy and adverse reactions that may require dose titration *[see Dosage and Administration (2.4), Warnings and Precautions (5.2)]*.

10   OVERDOSAGE
Cases of overdose (2-3 times the prescribed dose for several weeks) have been reported. In 1 case, this resulted in hepatitis which resolved without long-term consequences after a dose interruption. Single doses up to 80 mg per kg per day in iron overloaded beta-thalassemic patients have been tolerated with nausea and diarrhea noted. In healthy volunteers, single doses of up to 40 mg per kg per day were tolerated. There is no specific antidote for Exjade. In case of overdose, induce vomiting and employ gastric lavage.

11   DESCRIPTION
Exjade (deferasirox) is an iron chelating agent. Exjade tablets for oral suspension contain 125 mg, 250 mg, or 500 mg deferasirox. Deferasirox is designated chemically as 4-[3,5-Bis (2-hydroxyphenyl)-1H-1,2,4-triazol-1-yl]-benzoic acid and its structural formula is:

Deferasirox is a white to slightly yellow powder. Its molecular formula is $C_{21}H_{15}N_3O_4$ and its molecular weight is 373.4.
Inactive Ingredients: Lactose monohydrate (NF), crospovidone (NF), povidone (K30) (NF), sodium lauryl sulphate (NF), microcrystalline cellulose (NF), silicon dioxide (NF), and magnesium stearate (NF).

12 CLINICAL PHARMACOLOGY

12.1 Mechanism of Action

Exjade (deferasirox) is an orally active chelator that is selective for iron (as Fe^{3+}). It is a tridentate ligand that binds iron with high affinity in a 2:1 ratio. Although deferasirox has very low affinity for zinc and copper there are variable decreases in the serum concentration of these trace metals after the administration of deferasirox. The clinical significance of these decreases is uncertain.

12.2 Pharmacodynamics

Pharmacodynamic effects tested in an iron balance metabolic study showed that deferasirox (10, 20, and 40 mg per kg per day) was able to induce a mean net iron excretion (0.119, 0.329, and 0.445 mg Fe/kg body weight per day, respectively) within the clinically relevant range (0.1-0.5 mg per kg per day). Iron excretion was predominantly fecal.

12.3 Pharmacokinetics

Absorption

Exjade is absorbed following oral administration with median times to maximum plasma concentration (t_{max}) of about 1.5-4 hours. The C_{max} and AUC of deferasirox increase approximately linearly with dose after both single administration and under steady-state conditions. Exposure to deferasirox increased by an accumulation factor of 1.3-2.3 after multiple doses. The absolute bioavailability (AUC) of deferasirox tablets for oral suspension is 70% compared to an intravenous dose. The bioavailability (AUC) of deferasirox was variably increased when taken with a meal.

Distribution

Deferasirox is highly (~99%) protein bound almost exclusively to serum albumin. The percentage of deferasirox confined to the blood cells was 5% in humans. The volume of distribution at steady state (V_{ss}) of deferasirox is 14.37 ± 2.69 L in adults.

Metabolism

Glucuronidation is the main metabolic pathway for deferasirox, with subsequent biliary excretion. Deconjugation of glucuronidates in the intestine and subsequent reabsorption (enterohepatic recycling) is likely to occur. Deferasirox is mainly glucuronidated by UGT1A1 and to a lesser extent UGT1A3. CYP450-catalyzed (oxidative) metabolism of deferasirox appears to be minor in humans (about 8%). Deconjugation of glucuronide metabolites in the intestine and subsequent reabsorption (enterohepatic recycling) was confirmed in a healthy volunteer study in which the administration of cholestyramine 12 g twice daily (strongly binds to deferasirox and its conjugates) 4 and 10 hours after a single dose of deferasirox resulted in a 45% decrease in deferasirox exposure (AUC) by interfering with the enterohepatic recycling of deferasirox.

Excretion

Deferasirox and metabolites are primarily (84% of the dose) excreted in the feces. Renal excretion of deferasirox and metabolites is minimal (8% of the administered dose). The mean elimination half-life ($t_{1/2}$) ranged from 8-16 hours following oral administration.

Drug Interactions

Midazolam: In healthy volunteers, the concomitant administration of Exjade and midazolam (a CYP3A4 probe substrate) resulted in a decrease of midazolam peak concentration by 23% and exposure by 17%. In the clinical setting, this effect may be more pronounced. The study was not adequately designed to conclusively assess the potential induction of CYP3A4 by deferasirox [see Drug Interactions (7.2)].

Repaglinide: In a healthy volunteer study, the concomitant administration of Exjade (30 mg per kg/day for 4 days) and the CYP2C8 probe substrate repaglinide (single dose of 0.5 mg) resulted in an increase in repaglinide systemic exposure (AUC) to 2.3-fold of control and an increase in C_{max} of 62% [see Drug Interactions (7.3)].

Theophylline: In a healthy volunteer study, the concomitant administration of Exjade (repeated dose of 30 mg per kg/day) and the CYP1A2 substrate theophylline (single dose of 120 mg) resulted in an approximate doubling of the theophylline AUC and elimination half-life. The single dose C_{max} was not affected, but an increase in theophylline C_{max} is expected to occur with chronic dosing [see Drug Interactions (7.4)].

Rifampicin: In a healthy volunteer study, the concomitant administration of Exjade (single dose of 30 mg per kg) and the potent UDP-glucuronosyltransferase (UGT) inducer rifampicin (600 mg/day for 9 days) resulted in a decrease of deferasirox systemic exposure (AUC) by 44% [see Drug Interactions (7.5)].

Cholestyramine: The concomitant use of Exjade with bile acid sequestrants may result in a decrease in Exjade efficacy. In healthy volunteers, the administration of cholestyramine after a single dose of deferasirox resulted in a 45% decrease in deferasirox exposure (AUC) [see Drug Interactions (7.6)].

In vitro studies:

• Cytochrome P450 Enzymes: Deferasirox inhibits human CYP3A4, CYP2C8, CYP1A2, CYP2A6, CYP2D6, and CYP2C19 in vitro.

• Transporter Systems: The addition of cyclosporin A (PgP/MRP1/MRP2 inhibitor) or verapamil (PgP/MRP1 inhibitor) did not influence ICL670 permeability in vitro.

Pharmacokinetics in Specific Populations

Pediatric: Following oral administration of single or multiple doses, systemic exposure of adolescents and children to deferasirox was less than in adult patients. In children <6 years of age, systemic exposure was about 50% lower than in adults.

Geriatric: The pharmacokinetics of deferasirox have not been studied in elderly patients (65 years of age or older).

Gender: Females have a moderately lower apparent clearance (by 17.5%) for deferasirox compared to males.

Renal Impairment: Compared to patients with MDS and ClCr >60 mL/min, patients with MDS and ClCr 40 to 60 mL/min (n=34) had approximately 50% higher mean deferasirox trough plasma concentrations.

12.6 QT Prolongation

The effect of 20 and 40 mg per kg per day of deferasirox on the QT interval was evaluated in a single-dose, double-blind, randomized, placebo- and active-controlled (moxifloxacin 400 mg), parallel group study in 182 healthy male and female volunteers age 18-65 years. No evidence of prolongation of the QTc interval was observed in this study.

13 NONCLINICAL TOXICOLOGY

13.1 Carcinogenesis, Mutagenesis, Impairment of Fertility

A 104-week oral carcinogenicity study in Wistar rats showed no evidence of carcinogenicity from deferasirox at doses up to 60 mg per kg per day (0.48 times the MRHD on a mg/m² basis). A 26-week oral carcinogenicity study in p53 (+/-) transgenic mice has shown no evidence of carcinogenicity from deferasirox at doses up to 200 mg per kg per day (0.81 times the MRHD on a mg/m² basis) in males and 300 mg per kg per day (1.21 times the MRHD on a mg/m² basis) in females.

Deferasirox was negative in the Ames test and chromosome aberration test with human peripheral blood lymphocytes. It was positive in 1 of 3 in vivo oral rat micronucleus tests. Deferasirox at oral doses up to 75 mg per kg per day (0.6 times the MRHD on a mg/m² basis) was found to have no adverse effect on fertility and reproductive performance of male and female rats.

14 CLINICAL STUDIES

Transfusional Iron Overload

The primary efficacy study, Study 1, was a multicenter, open-label, randomized, active-comparator control study to compare Exjade (deferasirox) and deferoxamine in patients with beta-thalassemia and transfusional hemosiderosis. Patients ≥2 years of age were randomized in a 1:1 ratio to receive either oral Exjade at starting doses of 5, 10, 20, or 30 mg per kg once daily or subcutaneous Desferal (deferoxamine) at starting doses of 20 to 60 mg per kg for at least 5 days per week based on LIC at baseline (2-3, >3-7, >7-14, and >14 mg Fe/g dry weight). Patients randomized to deferoxamine who had LIC values <7 mg Fe/g dry weight were permitted to continue on their prior deferoxamine dose, even though the dose may have been higher than specified in the protocol.

Patients were to have a liver biopsy at baseline and end of study (after 12 months) for LIC. The primary efficacy endpoint was defined as a reduction in LIC of ≥3 mg Fe/g dry weight for baseline values ≥10 mg Fe/g dry weight, reduction of baseline values between 7 and <10 to <7 mg Fe/g dry weight, or maintenance or reduction for baseline values <7 mg Fe/g dry weight.

A total of 586 patients were randomized and treated, 296 with Exjade and 290 with deferoxamine. The mean age was 17.1 years (range, 2-53 years); 52% were females and 88% were Caucasian. The primary efficacy population consisted of 553 patients (Exjade n=276; deferoxamine n=277) who had LIC evaluated at baseline and 12 months or discontinued due to an adverse event. The percentage of patients achieving the primary endpoint was 52.9% for Exjade and 66.4% for deferoxamine. The relative efficacy of Exjade to deferoxamine cannot be determined from this study.

In patients who had an LIC at baseline and at end of study, the mean change in LIC was -2.4 mg Fe/g dry weight in patients treated with Exjade and -2.9 mg Fe/g dry weight in patients treated with deferoxamine.

Reduction of LIC and serum ferritin was observed with Exjade doses of 20 to 30 mg per kg per day. Exjade doses below 20 mg per kg per day failed to provide consistent lowering of LIC and serum ferritin levels (Figure 1). Therefore, a starting dose of 20 mg per kg per day is recommended [see Dosage and Administration (2.1)].

Figure 1. Changes in Liver Iron Concentration and Serum Ferritin Following EXJADE (5-30 mg/kg per day) in Study 1

Study 2 was an open-label, noncomparative trial of efficacy and safety of Exjade given for 1 year to patients with chronic anemias and transfusional hemosiderosis. Similar to Study 1, patients received 5, 10, 20, or 30 mg per kg per day of Exjade based on baseline LIC.

A total of 184 patients were treated in this study: 85 patients with beta-thalassemia and 99 patients with other congenital or acquired anemias (myelodysplastic syndromes, n=47; Diamond-Blackfan syndrome, n=30; other, n=22). 19% of patients were <16 years of age and 16% were ≥65 years of age. There was a reduction in the absolute LIC from baseline to end of study (-4.2 mg Fe/g dry weight).

Study 3 was a multicenter, open-label, randomized trial of the safety and efficacy of Exjade relative to deferoxamine given for 1 year in patients with sickle cell disease and transfusional hemosiderosis. Patients were randomized to Exjade at doses of 5, 10, 20, or 30 mg per kg per day or subcutaneous deferoxamine at doses of 20-60 mg per kg per day for 5 days per week according to baseline LIC.

A total of 195 patients were treated in this study: 132 with Exjade and 63 with deferoxamine. 44% of patients were <16 years of age and 91% were black. At end of study, the mean change in LIC (as measured by magnetic susceptometry by a superconducting quantum interference device) in the per protocol-1 (PP-1) population, which consisted of patients who had at least 1 post-baseline LIC assessment, was -1.3 mg Fe/g dry weight for patients receiving Exjade (n=113) and -0.7 mg Fe/g dry weight for patients receiving deferoxamine (n=54).

One-hundred five (105) patients with thalassemia major and cardiac iron overload were enrolled in a study assessing the change in cardiac MRI T2* value (measured in milliseconds, ms) before and after treatment with Exjade. Cardiac T2* values at baseline ranged from 5 to <20 ms. The geometric mean of cardiac T2* in the 68 patients who completed 3 years of Exjade therapy increased from 11.98 ms at baseline to 17.12 ms at 3 years. Cardiac T2* values improved in patients with severe cardiac iron overload (<10 ms) and in those with mild to moderate cardiac iron overload (≥10 to <20 ms). The clinical significance of these observations is unknown.

Six hundred twenty-seven patients with MDS were enrolled across 5 uncontrolled trials. Two hundred thirty-nine of the 627 patients were enrolled in trials that limited enrollment to patients with IPSS Low or Intermediate 1 risk MDS and the remaining 388 patients were enrolled in trials that did not specify MDS risk stratification but required a life expectancy of greater than 1 year. Planned duration of treatment in these trials ranged from 1 year (365 patients) to 5 years (47 patients). These trials evaluated the effects of Exjade therapy on parameters of iron overload, including LIC (125 patients) and serum ferritin (627 patients). Percent of patients completing planned duration of treatment was 51% in the largest 1 year study, 52% in the 3-year study and 22% in the 5 year study. The major causes for treatment discontinuation were withdrawal of consent, adverse reaction, and death. Over 1 year of follow-up across these pooled studies, mean change in serum ferritin was -332.8 (±2615.59) mcg/L (n=593) and mean change in LIC was -5.9 (±8.32) mg Fe/g dw (n=68). Results of these pooled studies in 627 patients with MDS suggest a progressive decrease in serum ferritin and LIC beyond 1 year in those patients who are able to continue Exjade. No controlled trials have been performed to demonstrate that these reductions improve morbidity or mortality in patients with MDS. Adverse reactions with Exjade therapy occur more frequently in older patients [see Use in Specific Populations (8.5)]. In elderly patients, including those with MDS, individualize the decision to remove accumulated iron based on clinical circumstances and the anticipated clinical benefit and risks of Exjade therapy.

Non-Transfusion Dependent Thalassemia

Study 4 was a randomized, double-blind, placebo-controlled trial of treatment with Exjade for patients 10 years of age or older with NTDT syndromes and iron overload. Eligible patients had an LIC of at least 5 mg Fe/g dw measured by R2 MRI and a serum ferritin exceeding 300 mcg/L at screening (2 consecutive values at least 14 days apart from each other). A total of 166 patients were randomized, 55 to the Exjade 5 mg/kg/day dose group, 55 to the Exjade 10 mg/kg/

Table 5. Absolute Change in LIC at Week 52 in NTDT Patients

	Placebo	EXJADE 5 mg/kg/day	EXJADE 10 mg/kg/day	EXJADE 20 mg/kg/day
		Starting Dose[1]		
Study 4[2]				
Number of Patients	n=54	n=51	n=54	-
Mean LIC at Baseline (mg Fe/g dw)	16.1	13.4	14.4	-
Mean Change (mg Fe/g dw)	+0.4	-2.0	-3.8	-
(95% Confidence Interval)	(-0.6, +1.3)	(-2.9, -1.0)	(-4.8, -2.9)	-
Study 5				
Number of Patients	-	n=8	n=77	n=43
Mean LIC at Baseline (mg Fe/g dw)	-	5.6	8.8	23.5
Mean Change (mg Fe/g dw)	-	-1.5	-2.8	-9.1
(95% Confidence Interval)	-	(-3.7, +0.7)	(-3.4, -2.2)	(-11.0, -7.3)

[1]Randomized dose in Study 4 or assigned starting dose in Study 5
[2]Least square mean change for Study 4

day dose group, and 56 to placebo (28 to each matching placebo group). Doses could be increased after 6 months if the LIC exceeded 7 mg Fe/g dw and the LIC reduction from baseline was less than 15%. The patients enrolled included 89 males and 77 females. The underlying disease was beta-thalassemia intermedia in 95 (57%) patients, HbE beta-thalassemia in 49 (30%) patients, and alpha-thalassemia in 22 (13%) patients. There were 17 pediatric patients in the study. Caucasians comprised 57% of the study population and Asians comprised 42%. The median baseline LIC (range) for all patients was 12.1 (2.6-49.1) mg Fe/g dw. Follow-up was for 1 year. The primary efficacy endpoint of change in LIC from baseline to Week 52 was statistically significant in favor of both Exjade dose groups compared with placebo (p ≤0.001) (Table 5). Furthermore, a statistically significant dose effect of Exjade was observed in favor of the 10 mg/kg/day dose group (10 versus 5 mg/kg/day, p=0.009). In a descriptive analysis, the target LIC (less than 5 mg Fe/g dw) was reached by 15 (27%) of 55 patients in the 10 mg/kg/day arm, 8 (15%) of 55 patients in the 5 mg/kg/day arm and 2 (4%) of 56 patients in the combined placebo groups.

[See table 5 above]

Study 5 was an open-label trial of Exjade for the treatment of patients previously enrolled on Study 4, including crossover to active treatment for those previously treated with placebo. The starting dose of Exjade in Study 5 was assigned based on the patient's LIC at completion of Study 4, being 20 mg/kg/day for an LIC exceeding 15 mg Fe/g dw, 10 mg/kg/day for LIC 3-15 mg Fe/g dw, and observation if the LIC was less than 3 mg Fe/g dw. Patients could continue on 5 mg/kg/day if they had previously exhibited at least a 30% reduction in LIC. Doses could be increased to a maximum of 20 mg/kg/day after 6 months if the LIC was more than 7 mg Fe/g dw and the LIC reduction from baseline was less than 15%. The primary efficacy endpoint in Study 5 was the proportion of patients achieving an LIC less than 5 mg Fe/g dw. A total of 133 patients were enrolled. Twenty patients began Study 5 with an LIC less than 5 mg Fe/g dw. Of the 113 patients with a baseline LIC of at least 5 mg Fe/g dw in Study 5, the target LIC (less than 5 mg Fe/g dw) was reached by 39 (35%). The responders included 4 (10%) of 39 patients treated at 20 mg/kg/day for a baseline LIC exceeding 15 mg Fe/g dw, and 31 (51%) of 61 patients treated at 10 mg/kg/day for a baseline LIC between 5 and 15 mg Fe/g dw. The absolute change in LIC at Week 52 by starting dose is shown in Table 5 above.

16   HOW SUPPLIED/STORAGE AND HANDLING

Exjade is provided as 125 mg, 250 mg, and 500 mg tablets for oral suspension.

125 mg
Off-white, round, flat tablet with beveled edge and imprinted with "J" and "125" on one side and "NVR" on the other.

Bottles of 30 tablets...............................(NDC 0078-0468-15)

250 mg
Off-white, round, flat tablet with beveled edge and imprinted with "J" and "250" on one side and "NVR" on the other.

Bottles of 30 tablets...............................(NDC 0078-0469-15)

500 mg
Off-white, round, flat tablet with beveled edge and imprinted with "J" and "500" on one side and "NVR" on the other.

Bottles of 30 tablets...............................(NDC 0078-0470-15)

Store Exjade tablets at 25°C (77°F); excursions are permitted to 15°C-30°C (59°F-86°F) [see USP Controlled Room Temperature]. Protect from moisture.

17   PATIENT COUNSELING INFORMATION

- Advise patients to take Exjade once daily on an empty stomach at least 30 minutes prior to food, preferably at the same time every day. Instruct patients to completely disperse the tablets in water, orange juice, or apple juice, and drink the resulting suspension immediately. After the suspension has been swallowed, resuspend any residue in a small volume of the liquid and swallow [see Dosage and Administration (2.3)].
- Advise patients not to chew tablets or swallow them whole [see Dosage and Administration (2.3)].
- Caution patients not to take aluminum-containing antacids and Exjade simultaneously [see Drug Interactions (7.1)].
- Because auditory and ocular disturbances have been reported with Exjade, conduct auditory testing and ophthalmic testing before starting Exjade treatment and thereafter at regular intervals [see Warnings and Precautions (5.9)].
- Caution patients experiencing dizziness to avoid driving or operating machinery [see Adverse Reactions (6.1)].
- Caution patients about the potential for the development of GI ulcers or bleeding when taking Exjade in combination with drugs that have ulcerogenic or hemorrhagic potential, such as NSAIDs, corticosteroids, oral bisphosphonates, or anticoagulants [see Warnings and Precautions (5.3)].
- Caution patients about potential loss of effectiveness of drugs metabolized by CYP3A4 (e.g., cyclosporine, simvastatin, hormonal contraceptive agents) when Exjade is administered with these drugs [see Drug Interactions (7.2)].
- Caution patients about potential loss of effectiveness of Exjade when administered with drugs that are potent UGT inducers (e.g., rifampicin, phenytoin, phenobarbital, ritonavir). Based on serum ferritin levels and clinical response, consider increases in the dose of Exjade when concomitantly used with potent UGT inducers [see Drug Interactions (7.5)].
- Caution patients about potential loss of effectiveness of Exjade when administered with drugs that are bile acid sequestrants (e.g., cholestyramine, colesevelam, colestipol). Based on serum ferritin levels and clinical response, consider increases in the dose of Exjade when concomitantly used with bile acid sequestrants [see Drug Interactions (7.6)].
- Perform careful monitoring of glucose levels when repaglinide is used concomitantly with Exjade. An interaction between Exjade and other CYP2C8 substrates like paclitaxel cannot be excluded [see Drug Interactions (7.3)].
- Advise patients that blood tests will be performed because Exjade may affect your kidneys, liver, or blood cells. The blood tests will be performed every month or more frequently if you are at increased risk of complications (e.g., preexisting kidney condition, are elderly, have multiple medical conditions, or are taking medicine that affects your organs). There have been reports of severe kidney and liver problems, blood disorders, stomach hemorrhage and death in patients taking Exjade [see Warnings and Precautions (5.1, 5.2, 5.3, 5.4, 5.5)].
- Skin rashes may occur during Exjade treatment and if severe, interrupt treatment. Serious allergic reactions (which include swelling of the throat) have been reported in patients taking Exjade, usually within the first month of treatment. If reactions are severe, advise patients to stop taking Exjade and contact their doctor immediately [see Warnings and Precautions (5.6, 5.7, 5.8)].

Manufactured by:
Novartis Pharma Stein AG
Stein, Switzerland

Distributed by:
Novartis Pharmaceuticals Corporation
East Hanover, New Jersey 07936
© Novartis
T2013-93
October 2013

Shown in Product Identification Guide, page 310

FANAPT®   Rx
[fan-apt]
(iloperidone)
tablets

The following prescribing information is based on official labeling in effect July 2014.

HIGHLIGHTS OF PRESCRIBING INFORMATION
These highlights do not include all the information needed to use FANAPT safely and effectively. See full prescribing information for FANAPT.
FANAPT® (iloperidone) tablets
Initial U.S. Approval: 2009

> **WARNING: INCREASED MORTALITY IN ELDERLY PATIENTS WITH DEMENTIA-RELATED PSYCHOSIS**
> *See full prescribing information for complete boxed warning.*
> Elderly patients with dementia-related psychosis treated with antipsychotic drugs are at an increased risk of death. FANAPT is not approved for use in patients with dementia-related psychosis. (5.1)

—————RECENT MAJOR CHANGES—————
Dosage and Administration (2.2)   4/2014

—————INDICATIONS AND USAGE—————
FANAPT is an atypical antipsychotic agent indicated for the treatment of schizophrenia in adults. (1) Efficacy was established in two short-term (4- and 6-week) placebo- and active-controlled studies of adult patients with schizophrenia. (14) In choosing among treatments, prescribers should consider the ability of FANAPT to prolong the QT interval and the use of other drugs first. Prescribers should also consider the need to titrate FANAPT slowly to avoid orthostatic hypotension, which may lead to delayed effectiveness compared to some other drugs that do not require similar titration.

—————DOSAGE AND ADMINISTRATION—————
The recommended target dosage of FANAPT tablets is 12 to 24 mg/day administered twice daily. This target dosage range is achieved by daily dosage adjustments, alerting patients to symptoms of orthostatic hypotension, starting at a dose of 1 mg twice daily, then moving to 2 mg, 4 mg, 6 mg, 8 mg, 10 mg, and 12 mg twice daily on Days 2, 3, 4, 5, 6, and 7 respectively, to reach the 12 mg/day to 24 mg/day dose range. FANAPT can be administered without regard to meals. (2.1)

—————DOSAGE FORMS AND STRENGTHS—————
1 mg, 2 mg, 4 mg, 6 mg, 8 mg, 10 mg and 12 mg tablets. (3)

—————CONTRAINDICATIONS—————
Known hypersensitivity to FANAPT or to any components in the formulation. (4)

—————WARNINGS AND PRECAUTIONS—————
- *Elderly patients with dementia-related psychosis* who are treated with atypical antipsychotic drugs are at an increased risk of death and cerebrovascular-related adverse events, including stroke. (5.1)
- *QT prolongation:* Prolongs QT interval and may be associated with arrhythmia and sudden death-consider using other antipsychotics first. Avoid use of FANAPT in combination with other drugs that are known to prolong QTc; use caution and consider dose modification when prescribing FANAPT with other drugs that inhibit FANAPT metabolism. Monitor serum potassium and magnesium in patients at risk for electrolyte disturbances. (1, 5.2, 7.1, 7.3, 12.3)
- *Neuroleptic Malignant Syndrome:* Manage with immediate discontinuation of drug and close monitoring. (5.3)
- *Tardive dyskinesia:* Discontinue if clinically appropriate. (5.4)
- *Metabolic Changes:* Atypical antipsychotic drugs have been associated with metabolic changes that may increase cardiovascular/cerebrovascular risk. These metabolic changes include hyperglycemia, dyslipidemia, and weight gain. (5.5)
  - *Hyperglycemia and diabetes mellitus:* Monitor patients for symptoms of hyperglycemia including polydipsia, polyuria, polyphagia, and weakness. Monitor glucose regularly in patients at risk for diabetes. (5.5)
  - *Dyslipidemia:* Undesirable alterations have been observed in patients treated with atypical antipsychotics. (5.5)
  - *Weight Gain:* Weight gain has been reported. Monitor weight. (5.5)

- *Seizures:* Use cautiously in patients with a history of seizures or with conditions that lower seizure threshold. (5.6)
- *Orthostatic hypotension:* Dizziness, tachycardia, and syncope can occur with standing. (5.7)
- *Leukopenia, Neutropenia, and Agranulocytosis* have been reported with antipsychotics. Patients with a pre-existing low white blood cell count (WBC) or a history of leukopenia/neutropenia should have their complete blood count (CBC) monitored frequently during the first few months of therapy and should discontinue FANAPT at the first sign of a decline in WBC in the absence of other causative factors. (5.8)
- *Suicide:* Close supervision of high risk patients. (5.12)
- *Priapism:* Cases have been reported in association with FANAPT treatment. (5.13)
- *Potential for cognitive and motor impairment:* Use caution when operating machinery. (5.14)
- See Full Prescribing Information for additional *WARNINGS and PRECAUTIONS.*

---------------------ADVERSE REACTIONS---------------------

Commonly observed adverse reactions (incidence ≥5% and 2-fold greater than placebo) were: dizziness, dry mouth, fatigue, nasal congestion, orthostatic hypotension, somnolence, tachycardia, and weight increased. (6.1)

To report SUSPECTED ADVERSE REACTIONS, contact Novartis Pharmaceuticals Corporation at 1-888-669-6682 or FDA at 1-800-FDA-1088 or www.fda.gov/medwatch.

---------------------DRUG INTERACTIONS---------------------

- The dose of FANAPT should be reduced in patients co-administered a strong CYP2D6 or CYP3A4 inhibitor. (2.2, 7.1)

---------------USE IN SPECIFIC POPULATIONS---------------

- Pregnancy: No human or animal data. Use only if clearly needed. (8.1)
- Nursing Mothers: Should not breastfeed. (8.3)
- Pediatric Use: Safety and effectiveness not established in children and adolescents. (8.4)
- Hepatic Impairment: FANAPT is not recommended for patients with severe hepatic impairment. (2.2, 8.7)
- The dose of FANAPT should be reduced in patients who are poor metabolizers of CYP2D6. (2.2, 12.3)

See 17 for PATIENT COUNSELING INFORMATION

Revised: 4/2014

FULL PRESCRIBING INFORMATION: CONTENTS*
WARNING: INCREASED MORTALITY IN ELDERLY PATIENTS WITH DEMENTIA-RELATED PSYCHOSIS

FULL PRESCRIBING INFORMATION

> **WARNING: INCREASED MORTALITY IN ELDERLY PATIENTS WITH DEMENTIA-RELATED PSYCHOSIS**
>
> Elderly patients with dementia-related psychosis treated with antipsychotic drugs are at an increased risk of death. Analysis of seventeen placebo-controlled trials (modal duration 10 weeks), largely in patients taking atypical antipsychotic drugs, revealed a risk of death in the drug-treated patients of between 1.6 to 1.7 times the risk of death in placebo-treated patients. Over the course of a typical 10-week controlled trial, the rate of death in drug-treated patients was about 4.5%, compared to a rate of about 2.6% in the placebo group. Although the causes of death were varied, most of the deaths appeared to be either cardiovascular (e.g., heart failure, sudden death) or infectious (e.g., pneumonia) in nature. Observational studies suggest that, similar to atypical antipsychotic drugs, treatment with conventional antipsychotic drugs may increase mortality. The extent to which the findings of increased mortality in observational studies may be attributed to the antipsychotic drug as opposed to some characteristic(s) of the patients is not clear. FANAPT is not approved for the treatment of patients with Dementia-Related Psychosis. *[See Warnings and Precautions (5.1)]*

1 INDICATIONS AND USAGE

FANAPT® tablets are indicated for the treatment of adults with schizophrenia. Efficacy was established in two short-term (4- and 6-week) placebo and active-controlled studies of adult patients with schizophrenia *[see Clinical Studies (14)]*.

When deciding among the alternative treatments available for this condition, the prescriber should consider the finding that FANAPT is associated with prolongation of the QTc interval *[see Warnings and Precautions (5.2)]*. Prolongation of the QTc interval is associated in some other drugs with the ability to cause torsade de pointes-type arrhythmia, a potentially fatal polymorphic ventricular tachycardia which can result in sudden death. In many cases this would lead to the conclusion that other drugs should be tried first. Whether FANAPT will cause torsade de pointes or increase the rate of sudden death is not yet known.

Patients must be titrated to an effective dose of FANAPT. Thus, control of symptoms may be delayed during the first 1 to 2 weeks of treatment compared to some other antipsychotic drugs that do not require a similar titration. Prescribers should be mindful of this delay when selecting an antipsychotic drug for the treatment of schizophrenia *[see Dosage and Administration (2.1) and Clinical Studies (14)]*. The effectiveness of FANAPT in long-term use, that is, for more than 6 weeks, has not been systematically evaluated in controlled trials. Therefore, the physician who elects to use FANAPT for extended periods should periodically re-evaluate the long-term usefulness of the drug for the individual patient *[see Dosage and Administration (2.3)]*.

2 DOSAGE AND ADMINISTRATION

2.1 Usual Dose

FANAPT must be titrated slowly from a low starting dose to avoid orthostatic hypotension due to its alpha-adrenergic blocking properties. The recommended starting dose for FANAPT tablets is 1 mg twice daily. Dose increases to reach the target range of 6 to 12 mg twice daily (12 to 24 mg/day) may be made with daily dosage adjustments not to exceed 2 mg twice daily (4 mg/day). The maximum recommended dose is 12 mg twice daily (24 mg/day). FANAPT doses above 24 mg/day have not been systematically evaluated in the clinical trials. Efficacy was demonstrated with FANAPT in a dose range of 6 to 12 mg twice daily. Prescribers should be mindful of the fact that patients need to be titrated to an effective dose of FANAPT. Thus, control of symptoms may be delayed during the first 1 to 2 weeks of treatment compared to some other antipsychotic drugs that do not require similar titration. Prescribers should also be aware that some adverse effects associated with FANAPT use are dose related.

FANAPT can be administered without regard to meals.

2.2 Dosage in Special Populations

Dosage adjustments are not routinely indicated on the basis of age, gender, race, or renal impairment status *[see Use in Specific Populations (8.6, 8.7)]*.

Dosage adjustment for patients taking FANAPT concomitantly with potential CYP2D6 inhibitors: FANAPT dose should be reduced by one-half when administered concomitantly with strong CYP2D6 inhibitors such as fluoxetine or paroxetine. When the CYP2D6 inhibitor is withdrawn from the combination therapy, FANAPT dose should then be increased to where it was before *[see Drug Interactions (7.1)]*.

Dosage adjustment for patients taking FANAPT concomitantly with potential CYP3A4 inhibitors: FANAPT dose should be reduced by one-half when administered concomitantly with strong CYP3A4 inhibitors such as ketoconazole or clarithromycin. When the CYP3A4 inhibitor is withdrawn from the combination therapy, FANAPT dose should be increased to where it was before *[see Drug Interactions (7.1)]*.

Dosage adjustment for patients taking FANAPT who are poor metabolizers of CYP2D6: FANAPT dose should be reduced by one-half for poor metabolizers of CYP2D6 *[see Clinical Pharmacology (12.3)]*.

Hepatic Impairment: No dose adjustment to FANAPT is needed in patients with mild hepatic impairment. Exercise caution when administering it to patients with moderate hepatic impairment. FANAPT is not recommended for patients with severe hepatic impairment *[see Use in Specific Populations (8.7)]*.

2.3 Maintenance Treatment

Although there is no body of evidence available to answer the question of how long the patient treated with FANAPT should be maintained, it is generally recommended that responding patients be continued beyond the acute response. Patients should be periodically reassessed to determine the need for maintenance treatment.

2.4 Reinitiation of Treatment in Patients Previously Discontinued

Although there are no data to specifically address reinitiation of treatment, it is recommended that the initiation titration schedule be followed whenever patients have had an interval off FANAPT of more than 3 days.

2.5 Switching from Other Antipsychotics

There are no specific data to address how patients with schizophrenia can be switched from other antipsychotics to FANAPT or how FANAPT can be used concomitantly with other antipsychotics. Although immediate discontinuation of the previous antipsychotic treatment may be acceptable for some patients with schizophrenia, more gradual discontinuation may be most appropriate for others. In all cases, the period of overlapping antipsychotic administration should be minimized.

3 DOSAGE FORMS AND STRENGTHS

FANAPT tablets are available in the following strengths: 1 mg, 2 mg, 4 mg, 6 mg, 8 mg, 10 mg, and 12 mg. The tablets are white, round, flat, beveled-edged and identified with a logo debossed on one side and tablet strength "1", "2", "4", "6", "8", "10", or "12" debossed on the other side.

4 CONTRAINDICATIONS

FANAPT is contraindicated in individuals with a known hypersensitivity reaction to the product. Reactions have included pruritus and urticaria.

5 WARNINGS AND PRECAUTIONS

5.1 Increased Risks in Elderly Patients with Dementia-Related Psychosis

Increased Mortality

Elderly patients with dementia-related psychosis treated with atypical antipsychotic drugs are at an increased risk of death compared to placebo. FANAPT is not approved for the treatment of patients with dementia-related psychosis *[see Boxed Warning]*.

Cerebrovascular Adverse Events, Including Stroke

In placebo-controlled trials with risperidone, aripiprazole, and olanzapine in elderly patients with dementia, there was a higher incidence of cerebrovascular adverse events (cerebrovascular accidents and transient ischemic attacks) including fatalities compared to placebo-treated patients. FANAPT is not approved for the treatment of patients with dementia-related psychosis *[see Boxed Warning]*.

5.2 QT Prolongation

In an open-label QTc study in patients with schizophrenia or schizoaffective disorder (n=160), FANAPT was associated with QTc prolongation of 9 msec at an iloperidone dose of 12 mg twice daily. The effect of FANAPT on the QT interval was augmented by the presence of CYP450 2D6 or 3A4 metabolic inhibition (paroxetine 20 mg once daily and ketoconazole 200 mg twice daily, respectively). Under conditions of metabolic inhibition for both 2D6 and 3A4, FANAPT 12 mg twice daily was associated with a mean QTcF increase from baseline of about 19 msec.

No cases of torsade de pointes or other severe cardiac arrhythmias were observed during the pre-marketing clinical program.

The use of FANAPT should be avoided in combination with other drugs that are known to prolong QTc including Class 1A (e.g., quinidine, procainamide) or Class III (e.g., amiodarone, sotalol) antiarrhythmic medications, antipsychotic medications (e.g., chlorpromazine, thioridazine), antibiotics (e.g., gatifloxacin, moxifloxacin), or any other class of medications known to prolong the QTc interval (e.g., pentamidine, levomethadyl acetate, methadone). FANAPT should also be avoided in patients with congenital long QT syndrome and in patients with a history of cardiac arrhythmias.

Certain circumstances may increase the risk of torsade de pointes and/or sudden death in association with the use of drugs that prolong the QTc interval, including (1) bradycardia; (2) hypokalemia or hypomagnesemia; (3) concomitant use of other drugs that prolong the QTc interval; and (4) presence of congenital prolongation of the QT interval; (5) recent acute myocardial infarction; and/or (6) uncompensated heart failure.

Caution is warranted when prescribing FANAPT with drugs that inhibit FANAPT metabolism [see Drug Interactions (7.1)], and in patients with reduced activity of CYP2D6 [see Clinical Pharmacology (12.3)].

It is recommended that patients being considered for FANAPT treatment who are at risk for significant electrolyte disturbances have baseline serum potassium and magnesium measurements with periodic monitoring. Hypokalemia (and/or hypomagnesemia) may increase the risk of QT prolongation and arrhythmia. FANAPT should be avoided in patients with histories of significant cardiovascular illness, e.g., QT prolongation, recent acute myocardial infarction, uncompensated heart failure, or cardiac arrhythmia. FANAPT should be discontinued in patients who are found to have persistent QTc measurements >500 msec.

If patients taking FANAPT experience symptoms that could indicate the occurrence of cardiac arrhythmias, e.g., dizziness, palpitations, or syncope, the prescriber should initiate further evaluation, including cardiac monitoring.

5.3 Neuroleptic Malignant Syndrome (NMS)

A potentially fatal symptom complex sometimes referred to as Neuroleptic Malignant Syndrome (NMS) has been reported in association with administration of antipsychotic drugs, including FANAPT. Clinical manifestations include hyperpyrexia, muscle rigidity, altered mental status (including catatonic signs) and evidence of autonomic instability (irregular pulse or blood pressure, tachycardia, diaphoresis, and cardiac dysrhythmia). Additional signs may include elevated creatine phosphokinase, myoglobinuria (rhabdomyolysis), and acute renal failure.

The diagnostic evaluation of patients with this syndrome is complicated. In arriving at a diagnosis, it is important to identify cases in which the clinical presentation includes both serious medical illness (e.g., pneumonia, systemic infection, etc.) and untreated or inadequately treated extrapyramidal signs and symptoms (EPS). Other important considerations in the differential diagnosis include central anticholinergic toxicity, heat stroke, drug fever, and primary central nervous system (CNS) pathology.

The management of this syndrome should include: (1) immediate discontinuation of the antipsychotic drugs and other drugs not essential to concurrent therapy, (2) intensive symptomatic treatment and medical monitoring, and (3) treatment of any concomitant serious medical problems for which specific treatments are available. There is no general agreement about specific pharmacological treatment regimens for NMS.

If a patient requires antipsychotic drug treatment after recovery from NMS, the potential reintroduction of drug therapy should be carefully considered. The patient should be carefully monitored, since recurrences of NMS have been reported.

5.4 Tardive Dyskinesia

Tardive dyskinesia is a syndrome consisting of potentially irreversible, involuntary, dyskinetic movements, which may develop in patients treated with antipsychotic drugs. Although the prevalence of the syndrome appears to be highest among the elderly, especially elderly women, it is impossible to rely on prevalence estimates to predict, at the inception of antipsychotic treatment, which patients are likely to develop the syndrome. Whether antipsychotic drug products differ in their potential to cause tardive dyskinesia is unknown.

The risk of developing tardive dyskinesia and the likelihood that it will become irreversible are believed to increase as the duration of treatment and the total cumulative dose of antipsychotic administered increases. However, the syndrome can develop, although much less commonly, after relatively brief treatment periods at low doses.

There is no known treatment for established cases of tardive dyskinesia, although the syndrome may remit, partially or completely, if antipsychotic treatment is withdrawn. Antipsychotic treatment itself, however, may suppress (or partially suppress) the signs and symptoms of the syndrome and thereby may possibly mask the underlying process. The effect that symptomatic suppression has upon the long-term course of the syndrome is unknown.

Given these considerations, FANAPT should be prescribed in a manner that is most likely to minimize the occurrence of tardive dyskinesia. Chronic antipsychotic treatment should generally be reserved for patients who suffer from a chronic illness that (1) is known to respond to antipsychotic drugs, and (2) for whom alternative, equally effective, but potentially less harmful treatments are not available or appropriate. In patients who do require chronic treatment, the smallest dose and the shortest duration of treatment producing a satisfactory clinical response should be sought. The need for continued treatment should be reassessed periodically.

If signs and symptoms of tardive dyskinesia appear in a patient on FANAPT, drug discontinuation should be considered. However, some patients may require treatment with FANAPT despite the presence of the syndrome.

5.5 Metabolic Changes

Atypical antipsychotic drugs have been associated with metabolic changes that may increase cardiovascular/cerebrovascular risk. These metabolic changes include hyperglycemia, dyslipidemia, and body weight gain [see Patient Counseling Information (17.3)]. While all atypical antipsychotic drugs have been shown to produce some metabolic changes, each drug in the class has its own specific risk profile.

Hyperglycemia and Diabetes Mellitus

Hyperglycemia, in some cases extreme and associated with ketoacidosis or hyperosmolar coma or death, has been reported in patients treated with atypical antipsychotics including FANAPT. Assessment of the relationship between atypical antipsychotic use and glucose abnormalities is complicated by the possibility of an increased background risk of diabetes mellitus in patients with schizophrenia and the increasing incidence of diabetes mellitus in the general population. Given these confounders, the relationship between atypical antipsychotic use and hyperglycemia-related adverse events is not completely understood. However, epidemiological studies suggest an increased risk of treatment-emergent hyperglycemia-related adverse events in patients treated with the atypical antipsychotics included in these studies. Because FANAPT was not marketed at the time these studies were performed, it is not known if FANAPT is associated with this increased risk.

Patients with an established diagnosis of diabetes mellitus who are started on atypical antipsychotics should be monitored regularly for worsening of glucose control. Patients with risk factors for diabetes mellitus (e.g., obesity, family history of diabetes) who are starting treatment with atypical antipsychotics should undergo fasting blood glucose testing at the beginning of treatment and periodically during treatment. Any patient treated with atypical antipsychotics should be monitored for symptoms of hyperglycemia including polydipsia, polyuria, polyphagia, and weakness. Patients who develop symptoms of hyperglycemia during treatment with atypical antipsychotics should undergo fasting blood glucose testing. In some cases, hyperglycemia has resolved when the atypical antipsychotic was discontinued; however, some patients required continuation of antidiabetic treatment despite discontinuation of the suspect drug. Data from a 4-week, fixed-dose study in adult subjects with schizophrenia, in which fasting blood samples were drawn, are presented in Table 1.

Table 1: Change in Fasting Glucose

	Placebo	FANAPT 24 mg/day
	Mean Change from Baseline(mg/dL)	
	n=114	n=228
Serum Glucose Change from Baseline	-0.5	6.6
	Proportion of Patients with Shifts	
Serum Glucose Normal to High	2.5 %	10.7 %
(<100 mg/dL to ≥126 mg/dL)	(2/80)	(18/169)

Pooled analyses of glucose data from clinical studies including longer term trials are shown in Table 2.

Table 2: Change in Glucose

Mean Change from Baseline (mg/dL)			
	3-6 months	6-12 months	>12 months
FANAPT 10-16 mg/day	1.8 (N=773)	5.4 (N=723)	5.4 (N=425)
FANAPT 20-24 mg/day	-3.6 (N=34)	-9.0 (N=31)	-18.0 (N=20)

Dyslipidemia

Undesirable alterations in lipids have been observed in patients treated with atypical antipsychotics.

Data from a placebo-controlled, 4-week, fixed-dose study, in which fasting blood samples were drawn, in adult subjects with schizophrenia are presented in Table 3.

Table 3: Change in Fasting Lipids

	Placebo	FANAPT 24 mg/day
	Mean Change from Baseline (mg/dL)	
Cholesterol	n=114	n=228
Change from baseline	-2.17	8.18
LDL	n=109	n=217
Change from baseline	-1.41	9.03
HDL	n=114	n=228
Change from baseline	-3.35	0.55
Triglycerides	n=114	n=228
Change from baseline	16.47	-0.83
	Proportion of Patients with Shifts	
Cholesterol		
Normal to High	1.4%	3.6%
(<200 mg/dL to ≥240 mg/dL)	(1/72)	(5/141)
LDL		
Normal to High	2.4%	1.1%
(<100 mg/dL to ≥160 mg/dL)	(1/42)	(1/90)
HDL		
Normal to Low	23.8%	12.1%
(≥40 mg/dL to <40 mg/dL)	(19/80)	(20/166)
Triglycerides		
Normal to High	8.3%	10.1%
(<150 mg/dL to ≥200 mg/dL)	(6/72)	(15/148)

Pooled analyses of cholesterol and triglyceride data from clinical studies including longer term trials are shown in Tables 4 and 5.

Table 4: Change in Cholesterol

Mean Change from Baseline (mg/dL)			
	3-6 months	6-12 months	>12 months
FANAPT 10-16 mg/day	-3.9 (N=783)	-3.9 (N=726)	-7.7 (N=428)
FANAPT 20-24 mg/day	-19.4 (N=34)	-23.2 (N=31)	-19.4 (N=20)

Table 5: Change in Triglycerides

Mean Change from Baseline (mg/dL)			
	3-6 months	6-12 months	>12 months
FANAPT 10-16 mg/day	-8.9 (N=783)	-8.9 (N=726)	-17.7 (N=428)
FANAPT 20-24 mg/day	-26.6 (N=34)	-35.4 (N=31)	-17.7 (N=20)

Weight Gain

Weight gain has been observed with atypical antipsychotic use. Clinical monitoring of weight is recommended.

Across all short- and long-term studies, the overall mean change from baseline at endpoint was 2.1 kg.

Changes in body weight (kg) and the proportion of subjects with ≥7% gain in body weight from 4 placebo-controlled, 4- or 6-week, fixed- or flexible-dose studies in adult subjects are presented in Table 6.

Table 6: Change in Body Weight

	Placebo n=576	FANAPT 10-16 mg/ day n=481	FANAPT 20-24 mg/ day n=391
Weight (kg) Change from Baseline	-0.1	2.0	2.7
Weight Gain ≥7% increase from Baseline	4%	12%	18%

5.6 Seizures

In short-term placebo-controlled trials (4- to 6-weeks), seizures occurred in 0.1% (1/1344) of patients treated with FANAPT compared to 0.3% (2/587) on placebo. As with other antipsychotics, FANAPT should be used cautiously in patients with a history of seizures or with conditions that potentially lower the seizure threshold, e.g., Alzheimer's dementia. Conditions that lower the seizure threshold may be more prevalent in a population of 65 years or older.

5.7 Orthostatic Hypotension and Syncope

FANAPT can induce orthostatic hypotension associated with dizziness, tachycardia, and syncope. This reflects its alpha1-adrenergic antagonist properties. In double-blind placebo-controlled short-term studies, where the dose was increased slowly, as recommended above, syncope was reported in 0.4% (5/1344) of patients treated with FANAPT, compared with 0.2% (1/587) on placebo. Orthostatic hypotension was reported in 5% of patients given 20 to 24 mg/day, 3% of patients given 10 to 16 mg/day, and 1% of patients given placebo. More rapid titration would be expected to increase the rate of orthostatic hypotension and syncope.

FANAPT should be used with caution in patients with known cardiovascular disease (e.g., heart failure, history of myocardial infarction, ischemia, or conduction abnormalities), cerebrovascular disease, or conditions that predispose the patient to hypotension (dehydration, hypovolemia, and treatment with antihypertensive medications). Monitoring of orthostatic vital signs should be considered in patients who are vulnerable to hypotension.

5.8 Leukopenia, Neutropenia and Agranulocytosis

In clinical trial and postmarketing experience, events of leukopenia/neutropenia have been reported temporally related to antipsychotic agents. Agranulocytosis (including fatal cases) has also been reported.

Possible risk factors for leukopenia/neutropenia include preexisting low white blood cell count (WBC) and history of drug induced leukopenia/neutropenia. Patients with a pre-existing low WBC or a history of drug induced leukopenia/neutropenia should have their complete blood count (CBC) monitored frequently during the first few months of therapy and should discontinue FANAPT at the first sign of a decline in WBC in the absence of other causative factors. Patients with neutropenia should be carefully monitored for fever or other symptoms or signs of infection and treated promptly if such symptoms or signs occur. Patients with severe neutropenia (absolute neutrophil count <1000/mm³) should discontinue FANAPT and have their WBC followed until recovery.

5.9 Hyperprolactinemia

As with other drugs that antagonize dopamine D2 receptors, FANAPT elevates prolactin levels.

Hyperprolactinemia may suppress hypothalamic GnRH, resulting in reduced pituitary gonadotropin secretion. This, in turn, may inhibit reproductive function by impairing gonadalsteroidogenesis in both female and male patients. Galactorrhea, amenorrhea, gynecomastia, and impotence have been reported with prolactin-elevating compounds. Longstanding hyperprolactinemia when associated with hypogonadism may lead to decreased bone density in both female and male patients.

Tissue culture experiments indicate that approximately one-third of human breast cancers are prolactin-dependent *in vitro*, a factor of potential importance if the prescription of these drugs is contemplated in a patient with previously detected breast cancer. Mammary gland proliferative changes and increases in serum prolactin were seen in mice and rats treated with FANAPT *[see Nonclinical Toxicology (13.1)]*. Neither clinical studies nor epidemiologic studies conducted to date have shown an association between chronic administration of this class of drugs and tumorigenesis in humans; the available evidence is considered too limited to be conclusive at this time.

In a short-term placebo-controlled trial (4-weeks), the mean change from baseline to endpoint in plasma prolactin levels for the FANAPT 24 mg/day-treated group was an increase of 2.6 ng/mL compared to a decrease of 6.3 ng/mL in the placebo-group. In this trial, elevated plasma prolactin levels were observed in 26% of adults treated with FANAPT compared to 12% in the placebo-group. In the short-term trials, FANAPT was associated with modest levels of prolactin elevation compared to greater prolactin elevations observed with some other antipsychotic agents. In pooled analysis from clinical studies including longer term trials, in 3210 adults treated with iloperidone, gynecomastia was reported in 2 male subjects (0.1%) compared to 0% in placebo-treated patients, and galactorrhea was reported in 8 female subjects (0.2%) compared to 3 female subjects (0.5%) in placebo-treated patients.

5.10 Body Temperature Regulation

Disruption of the body's ability to reduce core body temperature has been attributed to antipsychotic agents. Appropriate care is advised when prescribing FANAPT for patients who will be experiencing conditions which may contribute to an elevation in core body temperature, e.g., exercising strenuously, exposure to extreme heat, receiving concomitant medication with anticholinergic activity, or being subject to dehydration.

5.11 Dysphagia

Esophageal dysmotility and aspiration have been associated with antipsychotic drug use. Aspiration pneumonia is a common cause of morbidity and mortality in elderly patients, in particular those with advanced Alzheimer's dementia. FANAPT and other antipsychotic drugs should be used cautiously in patients at risk for aspiration pneumonia *[see Boxed Warning]*.

5.12 Suicide

The possibility of a suicide attempt is inherent in psychotic illness, and close supervision of high-risk patients should accompany drug therapy. Prescriptions for FANAPT should be written for the smallest quantity of tablets consistent with good patient management in order to reduce the risk of overdose.

5.13 Priapism

Three cases of priapism were reported in the premarketing FANAPT program. Drugs with alpha-adrenergic blocking effects have been reported to induce priapism. FANAPT shares this pharmacologic activity. Severe priapism may require surgical intervention.

5.14 Potential for Cognitive and Motor Impairment

FANAPT, like other antipsychotics, has the potential to impair judgment, thinking or motor skills. In short-term, placebo-controlled trials, somnolence (including sedation) was reported in 11.9% (104/874) of adult patients treated with FANAPT at doses of 10 mg/day or greater versus 5.3% (31/587) treated with placebo. Patients should be cautioned about operating hazardous machinery, including automobiles, until they are reasonably certain that therapy with FANAPT does not affect them adversely.

Table 7: Percentage of Treatment-Emergent Adverse Reactions in Short-Term, Fixed- or Flexible-Dose, Placebo-Controlled Trials in Adult Patients*

Body System or Organ Class Dictionary-derived Term	Placebo (%) (N=587)	FANAPT 10-16 mg/day (%) (N=483)	FANAPT 20-24 mg/day (%) (N=391)
Body as a Whole			
Arthralgia	2	3	3
Fatigue	3	4	6
Musculoskeletal Stiffness	1	1	3
Weight Increased	1	1	9
Cardiac Disorders			
Tachycardia	1	3	12
Eye Disorders			
Vision Blurred	2	3	1
Gastrointestinal Disorders			
Nausea	8	7	10
Dry Mouth	1	8	10
Diarrhea	4	5	7
Abdominal Discomfort	1	1	3
Infections			
Nasopharyngitis	3	4	3
Upper Respiratory Tract Infection	1	2	3
Nervous System Disorders			
Dizziness	7	10	20
Somnolence	5	9	15
Extrapyramidal Disorder	4	5	4
Tremor	2	3	3
Lethargy	1	3	1
Reproductive System			
Ejaculation Failure	<1	2	2
Respiratory			
Nasal Congestion	2	5	8
Dyspnea	<1	2	2
Skin			
Rash	2	3	2
Vascular Disorders			
Orthostatic Hypotension	1	3	5
Hypotension	<1	<1	3

* Table includes adverse reactions that were reported in 2% or more of patients in any of the FANAPT dose groups and which occurred at greater incidence than in the placebo-group. Figures rounded to the nearest integer.

6 ADVERSE REACTIONS

6.1 Clinical Studies Experience

Because clinical trials are conducted under widely varying conditions, adverse reaction rates observed in the clinical trial of a drug cannot be directly compared to rates in the clinical trials of another drug and may not reflect the rates observed in clinical practice. The information below is derived from a clinical trial database for FANAPT consisting of 2070 patients exposed to FANAPT at doses of 10 mg/day or greater, for the treatment of schizophrenia. Of these, 806 received FANAPT for at least 6 months, with 463 exposed to FANAPT for at least 12 months. All of these patients who received FANAPT were participating in multiple-dose clinical trials. The conditions and duration of treatment with FANAPT varied greatly and included (in overlapping categories), open-label and double-blind phases of studies, inpatients and outpatients, fixed-dose and flexible-dose studies, and short-term and longer-term exposure.

Adverse reactions during exposure were obtained by general inquiry and recorded by clinical investigators using their own terminology. Consequently, to provide a meaningful estimate of the proportion of individuals experiencing adverse reactions, reactions were grouped in standardized categories using MedDRA terminology.

The stated frequencies of adverse reactions represent the proportions of individuals who experienced a treatment-emergent adverse reaction of the type listed. A reaction was considered treatment-emergent if it occurred for the first time or worsened while receiving therapy following baseline evaluation.

The information presented in these sections was derived from pooled data from 4 placebo-controlled, 4- or 6-week, fixed- or flexible-dose studies in patients who received FANAPT at daily doses within a range of 10 to 24 mg (n=874).

Adverse Reactions Occurring at an Incidence of 2% or More among FANAPT-Treated Patients and More Frequent than Placebo

Table 7 enumerates the pooled incidences of treatment-emergent adverse reactions that were spontaneously reported in four placebo-controlled, 4- or 6-week, fixed- or flexible-dose studies, listing those reactions that occurred in 2% or more of patients treated with FANAPT in any of the dose groups, and for which the incidence in FANAPT-treated patients in any dose group was greater than the incidence in patients treated with placebo.

[See table 7 above]

Help Patients Save on Rx Drugs: PDR.net/PharmacyDiscountCard

Dose-Related Adverse Reactions in Clinical Trials

Based on the pooled data from 4 placebo-controlled, 4- or 6-week, fixed-dose studies, adverse reactions that occurred with a greater than 2% incidence in the patients treated with FANAPT, and for which the incidence in patients treated with FANAPT 20 to 24 mg/day were twice than the incidence in patients treated with FANAPT 10 to 16 mg/day were: abdominal discomfort, dizziness, hypotension, musculoskeletal stiffness, tachycardia, and weight increased.

Common and Drug-Related Adverse Reactions in Clinical Trials

Based on the pooled data from 4 placebo-controlled, 4- or 6-week, fixed- or flexible-dose studies, the following adverse reactions occurred in ≥5% incidence in the patients treated with FANAPT and at least twice the placebo rate for at least 1 dose: dizziness, dry mouth, fatigue, nasal congestion, somnolence, tachycardia, orthostatic hypotension, and weight increased. Dizziness, tachycardia, and weight increased were at least twice as common on 20 to 24 mg/day as on 10 to 16 mg/day.

Extrapyramidal Symptoms (EPS) in Clinical Trials

Pooled data from the 4 placebo-controlled, 4- or 6-week, fixed- or flexible-dose studies provided information regarding treatment-emergent EPS. Adverse event data collected from those trials showed the following rates of EPS-related adverse events as shown in Table 8.

Table 8: Percentage of EPS Compared to Placebo

Adverse Event Term	Placebo (%) (N=587)	FANAPT 10-16 mg/ day (%) (N=483)	FANAPT 20-24 mg/ day (%) (N=391)
All EPS events	**11.6**	**13.5**	**15.1**
Akathisia	2.7	1.7	2.3
Bradykinesia	0	0.6	0.5
Dyskinesia	1.5	1.7	1.0
Dystonia	0.7	1.0	0.8
Parkinsonism	0	0.2	0.3
Tremor	1.9	2.5	3.1

Adverse Reactions Associated with Discontinuation of Treatment in Clinical Trials

Based on the pooled data from 4 placebo-controlled, 4- or 6-week, fixed- or flexible-dose studies, there was no difference in the incidence of discontinuation due to adverse events between FANAPT-treated (5%) and placebo-treated (5%) patients. The types of adverse events that led to discontinuation were similar for the FANAPT- and placebo-treated patients.

Demographic Differences in Adverse Reactions in Clinical Trials

An examination of population subgroups in the 4 placebo-controlled, 4- or 6-week, fixed- or flexible-dose studies did not reveal any evidence of differences in safety on the basis of age, gender or race *[see Warnings and Precautions (5.1)]*.

Laboratory Test Abnormalities in Clinical Trials

There were no differences between FANAPT and placebo in the incidence of discontinuation due to changes in hematology, urinalysis, or serum chemistry.

In short-term placebo-controlled trials (4- to 6-weeks), there were 1.0% (13/1342) iloperidone-treated patients with hematocrit at least one time below the extended normal range during post-randomization treatment, compared to 0.3% (2/585) on placebo. The extended normal range for lowered hematocrit was defined in each of these trials as the value 15% below the normal range for the centralized laboratory that was used in the trial.

Other Reactions During the Premarketing Evaluation of FANAPT

The following is a list of MedDRA terms that reflect treatment-emergent adverse reactions in patients treated with FANAPT at multiple doses ≥4 mg/day during any phase of a trial with the database of 3210 FANAPT-treated patients. All reported reactions are included except those already listed in Table 7, or other parts of the *Adverse Reactions (6)* section, those considered in the *Warnings and Precautions (5)*, those reaction terms which were so general as to be uninformative, reactions reported in fewer than 3 patients and which were neither serious nor life-threatening, reactions that are otherwise common as background reactions, and reactions considered unlikely to be drug related. It is important to emphasize that, although the reactions reported occurred during treatment with FANAPT, they were not necessarily caused by it.

Reactions are further categorized by MedDRA system organ class and listed in order of decreasing frequency according to the following definitions: frequent adverse events are those occurring in at least 1/100 patients (only those not listed in Table 7 appear in this listing); infrequent adverse reactions are those occurring in 1/100 to 1/1000 patients; rare events are those occurring in fewer than 1/1000 patients.

Blood and Lymphatic Disorders: Infrequent – anemia, iron deficiency anemia; *Rare* – leukopenia

Cardiac Disorders: Frequent – palpitations; *Rare* – arrhythmia, atrioventricular block first degree, cardiac failure (including congestive and acute)

Ear and Labyrinth Disorders: Infrequent – vertigo, tinnitus

Endocrine Disorders: Infrequent – hypothyroidism

Eye Disorders: Frequent – conjunctivitis (including allergic); *Infrequent* – dry eye, blepharitis, eyelid edema, eye swelling, lenticular opacities, cataract, hyperemia (including conjunctival)

Gastrointestinal Disorders: Infrequent – gastritis, salivary hypersecretion, fecal incontinence, mouth ulceration; *Rare* - aphthous stomatitis, duodenal ulcer, hiatus hernia, hyperchlorhydria, lip ulceration, reflux esophagitis, stomatitis

General Disorders and Administrative Site Conditions: Infrequent – edema (general, pitting, due to cardiac disease), difficulty in walking, thirst; *Rare* - hyperthermia

Hepatobiliary Disorders: Infrequent – cholelithiasis

Investigations: Frequent - weight decreased; *Infrequent* – hemoglobin decreased, neutrophil count increased, hematocrit decreased

Metabolism and Nutrition Disorders: Infrequent – increased appetite, dehydration, hypokalemia, fluid retention

Musculoskeletal and Connective Tissue Disorders: Frequent – myalgia, muscle spasms; *Rare* – torticollis

Nervous System Disorders: Infrequent – paresthesia, psychomotor hyperactivity, restlessness, amnesia, nystagmus; *Rare* – restless legs syndrome

Psychiatric Disorders: Frequent – restlessness, aggression, delusion; *Infrequent* – hostility, libido decreased, paranoia, anorgasmia, confusional state, mania, catatonia, mood swings, panic attack, obsessive-compulsive disorder, bulimia nervosa, delirium, polydipsia psychogenic, impulse-control disorder, major depression

Renal and Urinary Disorders: Frequent – urinary incontinence; *Infrequent* – dysuria, pollakiuria, enuresis, nephrolithiasis; *Rare* – urinary retention, renal failure acute

Reproductive System and Breast Disorders: Frequent – erectile dysfunction; *Infrequent* – testicular pain, amenorrhea, breast pain; *Rare* – menstruation irregular, gynecomastia, menorrhagia, metrorrhagia, postmenopausal hemorrhage, prostatitis.

Respiratory, Thoracic and Mediastinal Disorders: Infrequent – epistaxis, asthma, rhinorrhea, sinus congestion, nasal dryness; *Rare* – dry throat, sleep apnea syndrome, dyspnea exertional

6.2   Postmarketing Experience

The following adverse reactions have been identified during post-approval use of FANAPT: retrograde ejaculation. Because these reactions were reported voluntarily from a population of uncertain size, it is not possible to reliably estimate their frequency or establish a causal relationship to drug exposure.

7   DRUG INTERACTIONS

Given the primary CNS effects of FANAPT, caution should be used when it is taken in combination with other centrally acting drugs and alcohol. Due to its alpha1-adrenergic receptor antagonism, FANAPT has the potential to enhance the effect of certain antihypertensive agents.

7.1   Potential for Other Drugs to Affect FANAPT

Iloperidone is not a substrate for CYP1A1, CYP1A2, CYP2A6, CYP2B6, CYP2C8, CYP2C9, CYP2C19, or CYP2E1 enzymes. This suggests that an interaction of iloperidone with inhibitors or inducers of these enzymes, or other factors, like smoking, is unlikely.

Both CYP3A4 and CYP2D6 are responsible for iloperidone metabolism. Inhibitors of CYP3A4 (e.g., ketoconazole) or CYP2D6 (e.g., fluoxetine, paroxetine) can inhibit iloperidone elimination and cause increased blood levels.

Ketoconazole: Co-administration of ketoconazole (200 mg twice daily for 4 days), a potent inhibitor of CYP3A4, with a 3 mg single dose of iloperidone to 19 healthy volunteers, ages 18 to 45 years, increased the area under the curve (AUC) of iloperidone and its metabolites P88 and P95 by 57%, 55% and 35%, respectively. Iloperidone doses should be reduced by about one-half when administered with ketoconazole or other strong inhibitors of CYP3A4 (e.g., itraconazole). Weaker inhibitors (e.g., erythromycin, grapefruit juice) have not been studied. When the CYP3A4 inhibitor is withdrawn from the combination therapy, the iloperidone dose should be returned to the previous level.

Fluoxetine: Co-administration of fluoxetine (20 mg twice daily for 21 days), a potent inhibitor of CYP2D6, with a single 3 mg dose of iloperidone to 23 healthy volunteers, ages 29 to 44 years, who were classified as CYP2D6 extensive metabolizers, increased the AUC of iloperidone and its metabolite P88, by about 2- to 3-fold, and decreased the AUC of its metabolite P95 by one-half. Iloperidone doses should be reduced by one-half when administered with fluoxetine. When fluoxetine is withdrawn from the combination therapy, the iloperidone dose should be returned to the previous level. Other strong inhibitors of CYP2D6 would be expected to have similar effects and would need appropriate dose reductions. When the CYP2D6 inhibitor is withdrawn from the combination therapy, iloperidone dose could then be increased to the previous level.

Paroxetine: Co-administration of paroxetine (20 mg/day for 5 to 8 days), a potent inhibitor of CYP2D6, with multiple doses of iloperidone (8 or 12 mg twice daily) to patients with schizophrenia ages 18 to 65 years resulted in increased mean steady-state peak concentrations of iloperidone and its metabolite P88, by about 1.6-fold, and decreased mean steady-state peak concentrations of its metabolite P95 by one-half. Iloperidone doses should be reduced by one-half when administered with paroxetine. When paroxetine is withdrawn from the combination therapy, the iloperidone dose should be returned to the previous level. Other strong inhibitors of CYP2D6 would be expected to have similar effects and would need appropriate dose reductions. When the CYP2D6 inhibitor is withdrawn from the combination therapy, iloperidone dose could then be increased to previous levels.

Paroxetine and Ketoconazole: Co-administration of paroxetine (20 mg once daily for 10 days), a CYP2D6 inhibitor, and ketoconazole (200 mg twice daily) with multiple doses of iloperidone (8 or 12 mg twice daily) to patients with schizophrenia ages 18 to 65 years resulted in a 1.4-fold increase in steady-state concentrations of iloperidone and its metabolite P88 and a 1.4-fold decrease in the P95 in the presence of paroxetine. So giving iloperidone with inhibitors of both of its metabolic pathways did not add to the effect of either inhibitor given alone. Iloperidone doses should therefore be reduced by about one-half if administered concomitantly with both a CYP2D6 and CYP3A4 inhibitor.

7.2   Potential for FANAPT to Affect Other Drugs

In vitro studies in human liver microsomes showed that iloperidone does not substantially inhibit the metabolism of drugs metabolized by the following cytochrome P450 isozymes: CYP1A1, CYP1A2, CYP2A6, CYP2B6, CYP2C8, CYP2C9, or CYP2E1. Furthermore, *in vitro* studies in human liver microsomes showed that iloperidone does not have enzyme inducing properties, specifically for the following cytochrome P450 isozymes: CYP1A2, CYP2C8, CYP2C9, CYP2C19, CYP3A4 and CYP3A5.

Dextromethorphan: A study in healthy volunteers showed that changes in the pharmacokinetics of dextromethorphan (80 mg dose) when a 3 mg dose of iloperidone was co-administered resulted in a 17% increase in total exposure and a 26% increase in the maximum plasma concentrations (C_{max}) of dextromethorphan. Thus, an interaction between iloperidone and other CYP2D6 substrates is unlikely.

Fluoxetine: A single 3 mg dose of iloperidone had no effect on the pharmacokinetics of fluoxetine (20 mg twice daily).

Midazolam (a sensitive CYP 3A4 substrate): A study in patients with schizophrenia showed a less than 50% increase in midazolam total exposure at iloperidone steady state (14 days of oral dosing at up to 10 mg iloperidone twice daily) and no effect on midazolam C_{max}. Thus, an interaction between iloperidone and other CYP3A4 substrates is unlikely.

7.3   Drugs that Prolong the QT Interval

FANAPT should not be used with any other drugs that prolong the QT interval *[see Warnings and Precautions (5.2)]*.

8   USE IN SPECIFIC POPULATIONS

8.1   Pregnancy

Pregnancy Category C

FANAPT caused developmental toxicity, but was not teratogenic, in rats and rabbits.

In an embryo-fetal development study, pregnant rats were given 4, 16, or 64 mg/kg/day (1.6, 6.5, and 26 times the maximum recommended human dose (MRHD) of 24 mg/day on a mg/m² basis) of iloperidone orally during the period of organogenesis. The highest dose caused increased early intrauterine deaths, decreased fetal weight and length, decreased fetal skeletal ossification, and an increased incidence of minor fetal skeletal anomalies and variations; this dose also caused decreased maternal food consumption and weight gain.

In an embryo-fetal development study, pregnant rabbits were given 4, 10, or 25 mg/kg/day (3, 8, and 20 times the MRHD on a mg/m² basis) of iloperidone during the period of organogenesis. The highest dose caused increased early intrauterine deaths and decreased fetal viability at term; this dose also caused maternal toxicity.

In additional studies in which rats were given iloperidone at doses similar to the above beginning from either pre-conception or from day 17 of gestation and continuing through weaning, adverse reproductive effects included prolonged pregnancy and parturition, increased stillbirth rates, increased incidence of fetal visceral variations, decreased fetal and pup weights, and decreased post-partum pup survival. There were no drug effects on the neurobehavioral or reproductive development of the surviving pups. No-effect doses ranged from 4 to 12 mg/kg except for the increase in stillbirth rates which occurred at the lowest dose tested of 4 mg/kg, which is 1.6 times the MRHD on a mg/m² basis. Maternal toxicity was seen at the higher doses in these studies.

The iloperidone metabolite P95, which is a major circulating metabolite of iloperidone in humans but is not present in significant amounts in rats, was given to pregnant rats during the period of organogenesis at oral doses of 20, 80, or 200 mg/kg/day. No teratogenic effects were seen. Delayed skeletal ossification occurred at all doses. No significant maternal toxicity was produced. Plasma levels of P95 (AUC) at the highest dose tested were 2 times those in humans receiving the MRHD of iloperidone.

There are no adequate and well-controlled studies in pregnant women.

Non-teratogenic Effects

Neonates exposed to antipsychotic drugs, during the third trimester of pregnancy are at risk for extrapyramidal and/or withdrawal symptoms following delivery. There have been reports of agitation, hypertonia, hypotonia, tremor, somnolence, respiratory distress and feeding disorder in these neonates. These complications have varied in severity; while in some cases symptoms have been self-limited, in other cases neonates have required intensive care unit support and prolonged hospitalization.

FANAPT should be used during pregnancy only if the potential benefit justifies the potential risk to the fetus.

8.2 Labor and Delivery
The effect of FANAPT on labor and delivery in humans is unknown.

8.3 Nursing Mothers
FANAPT was excreted in milk of rats during lactation. It is not known whether FANAPT or its metabolites are excreted in human milk. It is recommended that women receiving FANAPT should not breastfeed.

8.4 Pediatric Use
Safety and effectiveness in pediatric and adolescent patients have not been established.

8.5 Geriatric Use
Clinical Studies of FANAPT in the treatment of schizophrenia did not include sufficient numbers of patients aged 65 years and over to determine whether or not they respond differently than younger adult patients. Of the 3210 patients treated with FANAPT in premarketing trials, 25 (0.5%) were ≥65 years old and there were no patients ≥75 years old.

Studies of elderly patients with psychosis associated with Alzheimer's disease have suggested that there may be a different tolerability profile (i.e., increased risk in mortality and cerebrovascular events including stroke) in this population compared to younger patients with schizophrenia [see Boxed Warning and Warnings and Precautions (5.1)]. The safety and efficacy of FANAPT in the treatment of patients with psychosis associated with Alzheimer's disease has not been established. If the prescriber elects to treat such patients with FANAPT, vigilance should be exercised.

8.6 Renal Impairment
Because FANAPT is highly metabolized, with less than 1% of the drug excreted unchanged, renal impairment alone is unlikely to have a significant impact on the pharmacokinetics of FANAPT. Renal impairment (creatinine clearance <30 mL/min) had minimal effect on C_{max} of iloperidone (given in a single dose of 3 mg) and its metabolites P88 and P95 in any of the 3 analytes measured. $AUC_{0-\infty}$ was increased by 24%, decreased by 6%, and increased by 52% for iloperidone, P88 and P95, respectively, in subjects with renal impairment.

8.7 Hepatic Impairment
No dose adjustment to FANAPT is needed in patients with mild hepatic impairment. Exercise caution when administering it to patients with moderate hepatic impairment. FANAPT is not recommended for patients with severe hepatic impairment [see Dosage in Special Populations (2.2)]. In adult subjects with mild hepatic impairment no relevant difference in pharmacokinetics of iloperidone, P88 or P95 (total or unbound) was observed compared to healthy adult controls. In subjects with moderate hepatic impairment a higher (2-fold) and more variable free exposure to the active metabolites P88 was observed compared to healthy controls, whereas exposure to iloperidone and P95 was generally similar (less than 50% change compared to control). Since a study in severe liver impaired subjects has not been conducted, FANAPT is not recommended for patients with severe hepatic impairment.

8.8 Smoking Status
Based on in vitro studies utilizing human liver enzymes, FANAPT is not a substrate for CYP1A2; smoking should therefore not have an effect on the pharmacokinetics of FANAPT.

9 DRUG ABUSE AND DEPENDENCE
9.1 Controlled Substance
FANAPT is not a controlled substance.

9.2 Abuse
FANAPT has not been systematically studied in animals or humans for its potential for abuse, tolerance, or physical dependence. While the clinical trials did not reveal any tendency for drug-seeking behavior, these observations were not systematic and it is not possible to predict on the basis of this experience the extent to which a CNS active drug, FANAPT, will be misused, diverted, and/or abused once marketed. Consequently, patients should be evaluated carefully for a history of drug abuse, and such patients should be observed closely for signs of FANAPT misuse or abuse (e.g., development of tolerance, increases in dose, drug-seeking behavior).

10 OVERDOSAGE
10.1 Human Experience
In premarketing trials involving over 3210 patients, accidental or intentional overdose of FANAPT was documented in 8 patients ranging from 48 mg to 576 mg taken at once and 292 mg taken over a 3-day period. No fatalities were reported from these cases. The largest confirmed single ingestion of FANAPT was 576 mg; no adverse physical effects were noted for this patient. The next largest confirmed ingestion of FANAPT was 438 mg over a 4-day period; extrapyramidal symptoms and a QTc interval of 507 msec were reported for this patient with no cardiac sequelae. This patient resumed FANAPT treatment for an additional 11 months. In general, reported signs and symptoms were those resulting from an exaggeration of the known pharmacological effects (e.g., drowsiness and sedation, tachycardia and hypotension) of FANAPT.

10.2 Management of Overdose
There is no specific antidote for FANAPT. Therefore appropriate supportive measures should be instituted. In case of acute overdose, the physician should establish and maintain an airway and ensure adequate oxygenation and ventilation. Gastric lavage (after intubation, if patient is unconscious) and administration of activated charcoal together with a laxative should be considered. The possibility of obtundation, seizures or dystonic reaction of the head and neck following overdose may create a risk of aspiration with induced emesis. Cardiovascular monitoring should commence immediately and should include continuous ECG monitoring to detect possible arrhythmias. If antiarrhythmic therapy is administered, disopyramide, procainamide and quinidine should not be used, as they have the potential for QT-prolonging effects that might be additive to those of FANAPT. Similarly, it is reasonable to expect that the alpha-blocking properties of bretylium might be additive to those of FANAPT, resulting in problematic hypotension. Hypotension and circulatory collapse should be treated with appropriate measures such as intravenous fluids or sympathomimetic agents (epinephrine and dopamine should not be used, since beta stimulation may worsen hypotension in the setting of FANAPT-induced alpha blockade). In cases of severe extrapyramidal symptoms, anticholinergic medication should be administered. Close medical supervision should continue until the patient recovers.

11 DESCRIPTION
FANAPT is a psychotropic agent belonging to the chemical class of piperidinyl-benzisoxazole derivatives. Its chemical name is 4'-[3-[4-(6-Fluoro-1,2-benzisoxazol-3-yl)piperidino] propoxy]-3'-methoxyacetophenone. Its molecular formula is $C_{24}H_{27}FN_2O_4$ and its molecular weight is 426.48. The structural formula is:

Iloperidone is a white to off-white finely crystalline powder. It is practically insoluble in water, very slightly soluble in 0.1 N HCl and freely soluble in chloroform, ethanol, methanol, and acetonitrile.

FANAPT tablets are intended for oral administration only. Each round, uncoated tablet contains 1 mg, 2 mg, 4 mg, 6 mg, 8 mg, 10 mg, or 12 mg of iloperidone. Inactive ingredients are: lactose monohydrate, microcrystalline cellulose, hydroxypropylmethylcellulose, crospovidone, magnesium stearate, colloidal silicon dioxide, and purified water (removed during processing). The tablets are white, round, flat, beveled-edged and identified with a logo ☞ debossed on one side and tablet strength "1", "2", "4", "6", "8", "10", or "12" debossed on the other side.

12 CLINICAL PHARMACOLOGY
12.1 Mechanism of Action
The mechanism of action of FANAPT, as with other drugs having efficacy in schizophrenia, is unknown. However it is proposed that the efficacy of FANAPT is mediated through a combination of dopamine type 2 (D_2) and serotonin type 2 ($5-HT_2$) antagonisms.

12.2 Pharmacodynamics
FANAPT exhibits high (nM) affinity binding to serotonin $5-HT_{2A}$ dopamine D_2 and D_3 receptors, and norepinephrine $NE\alpha1$ receptors (K_i values of 5.6, 6.3, 7.1, and 0.36 nM, respectively). FANAPT has moderate affinity for dopamine D_4, and serotonin $5-HT_6$ and $5-HT_7$ receptors (K_i values of 25, 43, and 22, nM respectively), and low affinity for the serotonin $5-HT_{1A}$, dopamine D_1, and histamine H_1 receptors (K_i values of 168, 216 and 437 nM, respectively). FANAPT has no appreciable affinity ($K_i >1000$ nM) for cholinergic muscarinic receptors. FANAPT functions as an antagonist at the dopamine D_2, D_3, serotonin $5-HT_{1A}$ and norepinephrine α_1/α_{2C} receptors. The affinity of the FANAPT metabolite P88 is generally equal or less than that of the parent compound. In contrast, the metabolite P95 only shows affinity for $5-HT_{2A}$ (K_i value of 3.91) and the $NE_{\alpha1A}$, $NE_{\alpha1B}$, $NE_{\alpha1D}$, and $NE_{\alpha2C}$ receptors (K_i values of 4.7, 2.7, 8.8, and 4.7 nM respectively).

12.3 Pharmacokinetics
The observed mean elimination half-lives for iloperidone, P88 and P95 in CYP2D6 extensive metabolizers (EM) are 18, 26, and 23 hours, respectively, and in poor metabolizers (PM) are 33, 37, and 31 hours, respectively. Steady-state concentrations are attained within 3 to 4 days of dosing. Iloperidone accumulation is predictable from single-dose pharmacokinetics. The pharmacokinetics of iloperidone is more than dose proportional. Elimination of iloperidone is mainly through hepatic metabolism involving 2 P450 isozymes, CYP2D6 and CYP3A4.

Absorption: Iloperidone is well absorbed after administration of the tablet with peak plasma concentrations occurring within 2 to 4 hours; while the relative bioavailability of the tablet formulation compared to oral solution is 96%. Administration of iloperidone with a standard high-fat meal did not significantly affect the C_{max} or AUC of iloperidone, P88, or P95, but delayed T_{max} by 1 hour for iloperidone, 2 hours for P88 and 6 hours for P95. FANAPT can be administered without regard to meals.

Distribution: Iloperidone has an apparent clearance (clearance/bioavailability) of 47 to 102 L/h, with an apparent volume of distribution of 1340 to 2800 L. At therapeutic concentrations, the unbound fraction of iloperidone in plasma is ~3% and of each metabolite (P88 and P95) it is ~8%.

Metabolism and Elimination: Iloperidone is metabolized primarily by 3 biotransformation pathways: carbonyl reduction, hydroxylation (mediated by CYP2D6) and O-demethylation (mediated by CYP3A4). There are 2 predominant iloperidone metabolites, P95 and P88. The iloperidone metabolite P95 represents 47.9% of the AUC of iloperidone and its metabolites in plasma at steady-state for extensive metabolizers (EM) and 25% for poor metabolizers (PM). The active metabolite P88 accounts for 19.5% and 34.0% of total plasma exposure in EM and PM, respectively. Approximately 7% to 10% of Caucasians and 3% to 8% of black/African Americans lack the capacity to metabolize CYP2D6 substrates and are classified as poor metabolizers (PM), whereas the rest are intermediate, extensive or ultrarapid metabolizers. Co-administration of FANAPT with known strong inhibitors of CYP2D6 like fluoxetine results in a 2.3-fold increase in iloperidone plasma exposure, and therefore one-half of the FANAPT dose should be administered.

Similarly, PMs of CYP2D6 have higher exposure to iloperidone compared with EMs and PMs should have their dose reduced by one-half. Laboratory tests are available to identify CYP2D6 PMs.

The bulk of the radioactive materials were recovered in the urine (mean 58.2% and 45.1% in EM and PM, respectively), with feces accounting for 19.9% (EM) to 22.1% (PM) of the dosed radioactivity.

Transporter Interaction: Iloperidone and P88 are not substrates of P-gp and iloperidone is a weak P-gp inhibitor.

13 NONCLINICAL TOXICOLOGY
13.1 Carcinogenesis, Mutagenesis, Impairment of Fertility
Carcinogenesis: Lifetime carcinogenicity studies were conducted in CD-1 mice and Sprague Dawley rats. Iloperidone was administered orally at doses of 2.5, 5.0, and 10 mg/kg/day to CD-1 mice and 4, 8, and 16 mg/kg/day to Sprague Dawley rats (0.5, 1.0, and 2.0 times and 1.6, 3.2, and 6.5 times, respectively, the MRHD of 24 mg/day on a mg/m² basis). There was an increased incidence of malignant mammary gland tumors in female mice treated with the lowest dose (2.5 mg/kg/day) only. There were no treatment-related increases in neoplasia in rats.

The carcinogenic potential of the iloperidone metabolite P95, which is a major circulating metabolite of iloperidone in humans but is not present at significant amounts in mice or rats, was assessed in a lifetime carcinogenicity study in Wistar rats at oral doses of 25, 75, and 200 mg/kg/day in males and 50, 150, and 250 (reduced from 400) mg/kg/day in females.

Drug-related neoplastic changes occurred in males, in the pituitary gland (pars distalis adenoma) at all doses and in the pancreas (islet cell adenoma) at the high dose. Plasma levels of P95 (AUC) in males at the tested doses (25, 75, and 200 mg/kg/day) were approximately 0.4, 3, and 23 times, respectively, the human exposure to P95 at the MRHD of iloperidone.

An increase in mammary, pituitary and endocrine pancreas neoplasms has been found in rodents after chronic administration of other antipsychotic drugs and is considered to be mediated by prolonged dopamine D2 antagonism and hyperprolactinemia. Increases in serum prolactin were seen in mice and rats treated with iloperidone. The relevance of these tumor findings in rodents in terms of human risk is unknown.

Mutagenesis: Iloperidone was negative in the Ames test and in the *in vivo* mouse bone marrow and rat liver micronucleus tests. Iloperidone induced chromosomal aberrations in Chinese Hamster Ovary (CHO) cells *in vitro* at concentrations which also caused some cytotoxicity.

The iloperidone metabolite P95 was negative in the Ames test, the V79 chromosome aberration test, and an *in vivo* mouse bone marrow micronucleus test.

Impairment of Fertility: Iloperidone decreased fertility at 12 and 36 mg/kg in a study in which both male and female rats were treated. The no-effect dose was 4 mg/kg, which is 1.6 times the MRHD of 24 mg/day on a mg/m^2 basis.

14 CLINICAL STUDIES

The efficacy of FANAPT in the treatment of schizophrenia was supported by 2 placebo- and active-controlled short-term (4- and 6-week) trials. Both trials enrolled patients who met the DSM-III/IV criteria for schizophrenia.

Two instruments were used for assessing psychiatric signs and symptoms in these studies. The Positive and Negative Syndrome Scale (PANSS) and Brief Psychiatric Rating Scale (BPRS) are both multi-item inventories of general psychopathology usually used to evaluate the effects of drug treatment in schizophrenia.

A 6-week, placebo-controlled trial (n=706) involved 2 flexible dose ranges of FANAPT (12 to 16 mg/day or 20 to 24 mg/day) compared to placebo and an active-control (risperidone). For the 12 to 16 mg/day group, the titration schedule of FANAPT was 1 mg twice daily on Days 1 and 2, 2 mg twice daily on Days 3 and 4, 4 mg twice daily on Days 5 and 6, and 6 mg twice daily on Day 7. For the 20 to 24 mg/day group, the titration schedule of FANAPT was 1 mg twice daily on Day 1, 2 mg twice daily on Day 2, 4 mg twice daily on Day 3, 6 mg twice daily on Days 4 and 5, 8 mg twice daily on Day 6, and 10 mg twice daily on Day 7. The primary endpoint was change from baseline on the BPRS total score at the end of treatment (Day 42). Both the 12 to 16 mg/day and the 20 to 24 mg/day dose ranges of FANAPT were superior to placebo on the BPRS total score. The active-control antipsychotic drug appeared to be superior to FANAPT in this trial within the first 2 weeks, a finding that may in part be explained by the more rapid titration that was possible for that drug. In patients in this study who remained on treatment for at least 2 weeks, iloperidone appeared to have had comparable efficacy to the active-control.

A 4-week, placebo-controlled trial (n=604) involved one fixed dose of FANAPT (24 mg/day) compared to placebo- and an active-control (ziprasidone). The titration schedule for this study was similar to that for the 6-week study. This study involved titration of FANAPT starting at 1 mg twice daily on Day 1 and increasing to 2, 4, 6, 8, 10, and 12 mg twice daily on Days 2, 3, 4, 5, 6, and 7. The primary endpoint was change from baseline on the PANSS total score at the end of treatment (Day 28). The 24 mg/day FANAPT dose was superior to placebo in the PANSS total score. FANAPT appeared to have similar efficacy to the active-control drug which also needed a slow titration to the target dose.

16 HOW SUPPLIED/STORAGE AND HANDLING

FANAPT tablets are white, round and identified with a logo "⌖" debossed on one side and tablet strength "1", "2", "4", "6", "8", "10", or "12" debossed on the other side. Tablets are supplied in the following strengths and package configurations:

Package Configuration	Tablet Strength (mg)	NDC Code
Bottles of 60	1 mg	0078-0595-20
Bottles of 60	2 mg	0078-0596-20
Bottles of 60	4 mg	0078-0597-20
Bottles of 60	6 mg	0078-0598-20
Bottles of 60	8 mg	0078-0599-20
Bottles of 60	10 mg	0078-0600-20
Bottles of 60	12 mg	0078-0601-20
Titration Pack	2×1 mg, 2×2 mg, 2×4 mg, 2×6 mg (Total of 8 tablets)	0078-0602-08

Storage

Store FANAPT tablets at controlled room temperature, 25°C (77°F); excursions permitted to 15° to 30 °C (59° to 86°F) [See USP Controlled Room Temperature]. Protect FANAPT tablets from exposure to light and moisture.

17 PATIENT COUNSELING INFORMATION

Physicians are advised to discuss the following issues with patients for whom they prescribe FANAPT:

17.1 QT Interval Prolongation

Patients should be advised to consult their physician immediately if they feel faint, lose consciousness or have heart palpitations. Patients should be counseled not to take FANAPT with other drugs that cause QT interval prolongation [see Warnings and Precautions (5.2)]. Patients should be told to inform physicians that they are taking FANAPT before any new drug is taken.

17.2 Neuroleptic Malignant Syndrome

Patients and caregivers should be counseled that a potentially fatal symptom complex sometimes referred to as NMS has been reported in association with administration of antipsychotic drugs, including FANAPT. Signs and symptoms of NMS include hyperpyrexia, muscle rigidity, altered mental status, and evidence of autonomic instability (irregular pulse or blood pressure, tachycardia, diaphoresis, and cardiac dysrhythmia) [see Warnings and Precautions (5.3)].

17.3 Metabolic Changes

Patients should be aware of the symptoms of hyperglycemia (high blood sugar) and diabetes mellitus. Patients who are diagnosed with diabetes, those with risk factors for diabetes, or those who develop these symptoms during treatment should have their blood glucose monitored at the beginning of and periodically during treatment. Patients should be counseled that weight gain has occurred during treatment with FANAPT. Clinical monitoring of weight is recommended [see Warnings and Precautions (5.5)].

17.4 Orthostatic Hypotension

Patients should be advised of the risk of orthostatic hypotension, particularly at the time of initiating treatment, re-initiating treatment, or increasing the dose [see Warnings and Precautions (5.7)].

17.5 Interference with Cognitive and Motor Performance

Because FANAPT may have the potential to impair judgment, thinking, or motor skills, patients should be cautioned about operating hazardous machinery, including automobiles, until they are reasonably certain that FANAPT therapy does not affect them adversely [see Warnings and Precautions (5.14)].

17.6 Pregnancy

Patients should be advised to notify their physician if they become pregnant or intend to become pregnant during therapy with FANAPT [see Use in Specific Populations (8.1)].

17.7 Nursing

Patients should be advised not to breastfeed an infant if they are taking FANAPT [see Use in Specific Populations (8.3)].

17.8 Concomitant Medication

Patients should be advised to inform their physicians if they are taking, or plan to take, any prescription or over-the-counter drugs, since there is a potential for interactions [see Drug Interactions (7)].

17.9 Alcohol

Patients should be advised to avoid alcohol while taking FANAPT.

17.10 Heat Exposure and Dehydration

Patients should be advised regarding appropriate care in avoiding overheating and dehydration.

Fanapt® is a registered trademark of Vanda Pharmaceuticals Inc. and is used by Novartis Pharmaceuticals Corporation under license.

Distributed by:
Novartis Pharmaceuticals Corporation
East Hanover, NJ 07936
T2014-48
April 2014

Shown in Product Identification Guide, page 310

FEMARA ℞
[fĕm-ara]
(letrozole)
tablets

The following prescribing information is based on official labeling in effect July 2014.

HIGHLIGHTS OF PRESCRIBING INFORMATION
These highlights do not include all the information needed to use FEMARA safely and effectively. See full prescribing information for FEMARA.
Femara (letrozole) tablets
Initial U.S. Approval: 1997

──────────INDICATIONS AND USAGE──────────
Femara is an aromatase inhibitor indicated for:
• Adjuvant treatment of postmenopausal women with hormone receptor positive early breast cancer (1.1)
• Extended adjuvant treatment of postmenopausal women with early breast cancer who have received prior standard adjuvant tamoxifen therapy (1.2)
• First and second-line treatment of postmenopausal women with hormone receptor positive or unknown advanced breast cancer (1.3)

──────DOSAGE AND ADMINISTRATION──────
Femara tablets are taken orally without regard to meals (2):
• Recommended dose: 2.5 mg once daily (2.1)
• Patients with cirrhosis or severe hepatic impairment: 2.5 mg every other day (2.5, 5.3)

──────DOSAGE FORMS AND STRENGTHS──────
2.5 milligram tablets (3)

──────────CONTRAINDICATIONS──────────
Women of premenopausal endocrine status, including pregnant women (4)

──────WARNINGS AND PRECAUTIONS──────
• Decreases in bone mineral density may occur. Consider bone mineral density monitoring (5.1)
• Increases in total cholesterol may occur. Consider cholesterol monitoring. (5.2)
• Fatigue, dizziness and somnolence may occur. Exercise caution when operating machinery (5.4)

──────────ADVERSE REACTIONS──────────
The most common adverse reactions (>20%) were hot flashes, arthralgia (6.1); flushing, asthenia, edema, arthralgia, headache, dizziness, hypercholesterolemia, sweating increased, bone pain (6.2, 6.3); and musculoskeletal (6.4).

To report SUSPECTED ADVERSE REACTIONS, contact Novartis Pharmaceuticals Corporation at 1-888-669-6682 or FDA at 1-800-FDA-1088 or www.fda.gov/medwatch.

See 17 for PATIENT COUNSELING INFORMATION
Revised: 1/2014

FULL PRESCRIBING INFORMATION

1   INDICATIONS AND USAGE

1.1   Adjuvant Treatment of Early Breast Cancer

Femara (letrozole) is indicated for the adjuvant treatment of postmenopausal women with hormone receptor positive early breast cancer.

1.2   Extended Adjuvant Treatment of Early Breast Cancer

Femara is indicated for the extended adjuvant treatment of early breast cancer in postmenopausal women, who have received 5 years of adjuvant tamoxifen therapy. The effectiveness of Femara in extended adjuvant treatment of early breast cancer is based on an analysis of disease-free survival in patients treated with Femara for a median of 60 months [see Clinical Studies (14.2, 14.3)].

1.3   First and Second-Line Treatment of Advanced Breast Cancer

Femara is indicated for first-line treatment of postmenopausal women with hormone receptor positive or unknown, locally advanced or metastatic breast cancer. Femara is also indicated for the treatment of advanced breast cancer in postmenopausal women with disease progression following antiestrogen therapy [see Clinical Studies (14.4, 14.5)].

2   DOSAGE AND ADMINISTRATION

2.1   Recommended Dose

The recommended dose of Femara is one 2.5 mg tablet administered once a day, without regard to meals.

2.2   Use in Adjuvant Treatment of Early Breast Cancer

In the adjuvant setting, the optimal duration of treatment with letrozole is unknown. The planned duration of treatment in the study was 5 years with 73% of the patients having completed adjuvant therapy. Treatment should be discontinued at relapse [see Clinical Studies (14.1)].

2.3   Use in Extended Adjuvant Treatment of Early Breast Cancer

In the extended adjuvant setting, the optimal treatment duration with Femara is not known. The planned duration of treatment in the study was 5 years. In the final updated analysis, conducted at a median follow-up of 62 months, the median treatment duration was 60 months. Seventy-one percent of patients were treated for at least 3 years and 58% of patients completed at least 4.5 years of extended adjuvant treatment. The treatment should be discontinued at tumor relapse [see Clinical Studies (14.2)].

2.4   Use in First and Second-Line Treatment of Advanced Breast Cancer

In patients with advanced disease, treatment with Femara should continue until tumor progression is evident [see Clinical Studies (14.4, 14.5)].

2.5   Use in Hepatic Impairment

No dosage adjustment is recommended for patients with mild to moderate hepatic impairment, although Femara blood concentrations were modestly increased in subjects with moderate hepatic impairment due to cirrhosis. The dose of Femara in patients with cirrhosis and severe hepatic dysfunction should be reduced by 50% [see Warnings and Precautions (5.3)]. The recommended dose of Femara for such patients is 2.5 mg administered every other day. The effect of hepatic impairment on Femara exposure in noncirrhotic cancer patients with elevated bilirubin levels has not been determined.

2.6   Use in Renal Impairment

No dosage adjustment is required for patients with renal impairment if creatinine clearance is ≥10 mL/min [see Clinical Pharmacology (12.3)].

3   DOSAGE FORMS AND STRENGTHS

2.5 mg tablets: dark yellow, film-coated, round, slightly biconvex, with beveled edges (imprinted with the letters FV on one side and CG on the other side).

4   CONTRAINDICATIONS

Femara may cause fetal harm when administered to a pregnant woman and the clinical benefit to premenopausal women with breast cancer has not been demonstrated. Femara is contraindicated in women who are or may become pregnant. If Femara is used during pregnancy, or if the patient becomes pregnant while taking this drug, the patient should be apprised of the potential hazard to a fetus [see Use in Specific Populations (8.1)].

5   WARNINGS AND PRECAUTIONS

5.1   Bone Effects

Use of Femara may cause decreases in bone mineral density (BMD). Consideration should be given to monitoring BMD. Results of a substudy to evaluate safety in the adjuvant setting comparing the effect on lumbar spine (L2-L4) bone mineral density (BMD) of adjuvant treatment with letrozole to that with tamoxifen showed at 24 months a median decrease in lumbar spine BMD of 4.1% in the letrozole arm compared to a median increase of 0.3% in the tamoxifen arm (difference = 4.4%) (P<0.0001) [see Adverse reactions (6.1)]. Updated results from the BMD substudy in the extended adjuvant setting demonstrated that at 2 years patients receiving letrozole had a median decrease from baseline of 3.8% in hip BMD compared to a median decrease of 2.0% in the placebo group. The changes from baseline in lumbar spine BMD in letrozole and placebo treated groups were not significantly different [see Adverse Reactions (6.2)]. In the adjuvant trial the incidence of bone fractures at any time after randomization was 13.8% for letrozole and 10.5% for tamoxifen. The incidence of osteoporosis was 5.1% for letrozole and 2.7% for tamoxifen [see Adverse Reactions (6.1)]. In the extended adjuvant trial the incidence of bone fractures at any time after randomization was 13.3% for letrozole and 7.8% for placebo. The incidence of new osteoporosis was 14.5% for letrozole and 7.8% for placebo [see Adverse Reactions (6.3)].

5.2   Cholesterol

Consideration should be given to monitoring serum cholesterol. In the adjuvant trial hypercholesterolemia was reported in 52.3% of letrozole patients and 28.6% of tamoxifen patients. CTC grade 3-4 hypercholesterolemia was reported in 0.4% of letrozole patients and 0.1% of tamoxifen patients. Also in the adjuvant setting, an increase of ≥1.5 × ULN in total cholesterol (generally non-fasting) was observed in patients on monotherapy who had baseline total serum cholesterol within the normal range (i.e., <=1.5 × ULN) in 151/1843 (8.2%) on letrozole vs 57/1840 (3.2%). Lipid lowering medications were required for 25% of patients on letrozole and 16% on tamoxifen [see Adverse Reactions (6.1)].

Table 1: Patients with Adverse Reactions (CTC Grades 1-4, Irrespective of Relationship to Study Drug) in the Adjuvant Study – Monotherapy Arms Analysis (Median Follow-up 73 Months; Median Treatment 60 Months)

Adverse Reaction	Grades 1-4		Grades 3-4	
	Femara N=2448 n (%)	tamoxifen N=2447 n (%)	Femara N=2448 n (%)	tamoxifen N=2447 n (%)
Pts with any adverse event	2310 (94.4)	2214 (90.5)	635 (25.9)	604 (24.7)
Hypercholesterolemia	1280 (52.3)	700 (28.6)	11 (0.4)	6 (0.2)
Hot Flashes/Flushes	821 (33.5)	929 (38.0)	0 -	0 -
Arthralgia/Arthritis	618 (25.2)	501 (20.4)	85 (3.5)	50 (2.0)
Night Sweats	357 (14.6)	426 (17.4)	0 -	0 -
Bone Fractures[2]	338 (13.8)	257 (10.5)	- -	- -
Weight Increase	317 (12.9)	378 (15.4)	27 (1.1)	39 (1.6)
Nausea	283 (11.6)	277 (11.3)	6 (0.2)	9 (0.4)
Bone Fractures[1]	247 (10.1)	174 (7.1)	- -	- -
Fatigue (Lethargy, Malaise, Asthenia)	235 (9.6)	250 (10.2)	6 (0.2)	7 (0.3)
Myalgia	217 (8.9)	212 (8.7)	18 (0.7)	14 (0.6)
Edema	164 (6.7)	160 (6.5)	3 (0.1)	1 (<0.1)
Weight Decrease	140 (5.7)	129 (5.3)	8 (0.3)	5 (0.2)
Vaginal Bleeding	128 (5.2)	320 (13.1)	1 (<0.1)	8 (0.3)
Back Pain	125 (5.1)	136 (5.6)	7 (0.3)	11 (0.4)
Osteoporosis NOS	124 (5.1)	66 (2.7)	10 (0.4)	5 (0.2)
Bone pain	123 (5.0)	109 (4.5)	6 (0.2)	4 (0.2)
Depression	119 (4.9)	114 (4.7)	16 (0.7)	14 (0.6)
Vaginal Irritation	111 (4.5)	77 (3.1)	2 (<0.1)	2 (<0.1)
Headache	105 (4.3)	94 (3.8)	9 (0.4)	5 (0.2)
Pain in extremity	103 (4.2)	79 (3.2)	6 (0.2)	4 (0.2)
Osteopenia	87 (3.6)	74 (3.0)	0 -	2 (<0.1)
Dizziness/Light-Headedness	84 (3.4)	84 (3.4)	1 (<0.1)	6 (0.2)
Alopecia	83 (3.4)	84 (3.4)	0 -	0 -
Vomiting	80 (3.3)	80 (3.3)	3 (0.1)	5 (0.2)
Cataract	49 (2.0)	54 (2.2)	16 (0.7)	17 (0.7)
Constipation	49 (2.0)	71 (2.9)	3 (0.1)	1 (<0.1)
Breast pain	37 (1.5)	43 (1.8)	1 (<0.1)	0 -
Anorexia	20 (0.8)	20 (0.8)	1 (<0.1)	1 (<0.1)
Endometrial Hyperplasia/Cancer[2, 3]	11/1909 (0.6)	70/1943 (3.6)	- -	- -
Endometrial Proliferation Disorders	10 (0.3)	71 (1.8)	0 -	0 -
Endometrial Hyperplasia/Cancer[1, 3]	6/1909 (0.3)	57/1943 (2.9)	- -	14 (0.6)
Other Endometrial Disorders	2 (<0.1)	3 (0.1)	0 -	0 -
Myocardial Infarction[1]	24 (1.0)	12 (0.5)	- -	- -
Myocardial Infarction[2]	37 (1.5)	25 (1.0)	- -	- -
Myocardial Ischemia	6 (0.2)	9 (0.4)	- -	- -
Cerebrovascular Accident[1]	52 (2.1)	46 (1.9)	- -	- -
Cerebrovascular Accident[2]	70 (2.9)	63 (2.6)	- -	- -
Angina[1]	26 (1.1)	24 (1.0)	- -	- -
Angina[2]	32 (1.3)	31 (1.3)	- -	- -
Thromboembolic Event[1]	51 (2.1)	89 (3.6)	- -	- -
Thromboembolic Event[2]	71 (2.9)	111 (4.5)	- -	- -
Other Cardiovascular[1]	260 (10.6)	256 (10.5)	- -	- -
Other Cardiovascular[2]	312 (12.7)	337 (13.8)	- -	- -
Second Malignancies[1]	53 (2.2)	78 (3.2)	- -	- -
Second Malignancies[2]	102 (4.2)	119 (4.9)	- -	- -

[1] During study treatment, based on Safety Monotherapy population
[2] Any time after randomization, including post treatment follow-up
[3] Excluding women who had undergone hysterectomy before study entry
Note: Cardiovascular (including cerebrovascular and thromboembolic), skeletal and urogenital/endometrial events and second malignancies were collected life-long. All of these events were assumed to be of CTC Grade 3 to 5 and were not individually graded.

Table 2: Percentage of Patients with Adverse Reactions

	Number (%) of Patients with Grade 1-4 Adverse Reaction		Number (%) of Patients with Grade 3-4 Adverse Reaction	
	Femara N=2563	Placebo N=2573	Femara N=2563	Placebo N=2573
Any Adverse Reaction	2232 (87.1)	2174 (84.5)	419 (16.3)	389 (15.1)
Vascular Disorders	1375 (53.6)	1230 (47.8)	59 (2.3)	74 (2.9)
Flushing	1273 (49.7)	1114 (43.3)	3 (0.1)	0
General Disorders	1154 (45)	1090 (42.4)	30 (1.2)	28 (1.1)
Asthenia	862 (33.6)	826 (32.1)	16 (0.6)	7 (0.3)
Edema NOS	471 (18.4)	416 (16.2)	4 (0.2)	3 (0.1)
Musculoskeletal Disorders	978 (38.2)	836 (32.5)	71 (2.8)	50 (1.9)
Arthralgia	565 (22)	465 (18.1)	25 (1)	20 (0.8)
Arthritis NOS	173 (6.7)	124 (4.8)	10 (0.4)	5 (0.2)
Myalgia	171 (6.7)	122 (4.7)	8 (0.3)	6 (0.2)
Back Pain	129 (5)	112 (4.4)	8 (0.3)	7 (0.3)
Nervous System Disorders	863 (33.7)	819 (31.8)	65 (2.5)	58 (2.3)
Headache	516 (20.1)	508 (19.7)	18 (0.7)	17 (0.7)
Dizziness	363 (14.2)	342 (13.3)	9 (0.4)	6 (0.2)
Skin Disorders	830 (32.4)	787 (30.6)	17 (0.7)	16 (0.6)
Sweating Increased	619 (24.2)	577 (22.4)	1 (<0.1)	0
Gastrointestinal Disorders	725 (28.3)	731 (28.4)	43 (1.7)	42 (1.6)
Constipation	290 (11.3)	304 (11.8)	6 (0.2)	2 (<0.1)
Nausea	221 (8.6)	212 (8.2)	3 (0.1)	10 (0.4)
Diarrhea NOS	128 (5)	143 (5.6)	12 (0.5)	8 (0.3)
Metabolic Disorders	551 (21.5)	537 (20.9)	24 (0.9)	32 (1.2)
Hypercholesterolemia	401 (15.6)	398 (15.5)	2 (<0.1)	5 (0.2)
Reproductive Disorders	303 (11.8)	357 (13.9)	9 (0.4)	8 (0.3)
Vaginal Hemorrhage	123 (4.8)	171 (6.6)	2 (<0.1)	5 (0.2)
Vulvovaginal Dryness	137 (5.3)	127 (4.9)	0	0
Psychiatric Disorders	320 (12.5)	276 (10.7)	21 (0.8)	16 (0.6)
Insomnia	149 (5.8)	120 (4.7)	2 (<0.1)	2 (<0.1)
Respiratory Disorders	279 (10.9)	260 (10.1)	30 (1.2)	28 (1.1)
Dyspnea	140 (5.5)	137 (5.3)	21 (0.8)	18 (0.7)
Investigations	184 (7.2)	147 (5.7)	13 (0.5)	13 (0.5)
Infections and Infestations	166 (6.5)	163 (6.3)	40 (1.6)	33 (1.3)
Renal Disorders	130 (5.1)	100 (3.9)	12 (0.5)	6 (0.2)

5.3 Hepatic Impairment

Subjects with cirrhosis and severe hepatic impairment who were dosed with 2.5 mg of Femara experienced approximately twice the exposure to Femara as healthy volunteers with normal liver function. Therefore, a dose reduction is recommended for this patient population. The effect of hepatic impairment on Femara exposure in cancer patients with elevated bilirubin levels has not been determined [see Dosage and Administration (2.5)].

5.4 Fatigue and Dizziness

Because fatigue, dizziness, and somnolence have been reported with the use of Femara, caution is advised when driving or using machinery until it is known how the patient reacts to Femara use.

5.5 Laboratory Test Abnormalities

No dose-related effect of Femara on any hematologic or clinical chemistry parameter was evident. Moderate decreases in lymphocyte counts, of uncertain clinical significance, were observed in some patients receiving Femara 2.5 mg. This depression was transient in about half of those affected. Two patients on Femara developed thrombocytopenia; relationship to the study drug was unclear. Patient withdrawal due to laboratory abnormalities, whether related to study treatment or not, was infrequent.

6 ADVERSE REACTIONS

The most serious adverse reactions from the use of Femara are:
- Bone effects [see Warnings and Precautions (5.1)]
- Increases in cholesterol [see Warnings and Precautions (5.2)]

Because clinical trials are conducted under widely varying conditions, adverse reactions rates observed in the clinical trials of a drug cannot be directly compared to rates in the clinical trials of another drug and may not reflect the rates observed in practice.

6.1 Adjuvant Treatment of Early Breast Cancer

The median treatment duration of adjuvant treatment was 60 months and the median duration of follow-up for safety was 73 months for patients receiving Femara and tamoxifen.

Certain adverse reactions were prospectively specified for analysis, based on the known pharmacologic properties and side effect profiles of the two drugs.

Adverse reactions were analyzed irrespective of whether a symptom was present or absent at baseline. Most adverse reactions reported (approximately 75% of patients reporting 1 or more AE) were Grade 1 or Grade 2 applying the Common Toxicity Criteria Version 2.0/ Common Terminology Criteria for Adverse Events, version 3.0. Table 1 describes adverse reactions (Grades 1-4) irrespective of relationship to study treatment in the adjuvant trial for the monotherapy arms analysis (safety population).

[See table 1 at top of previous page]

When considering all grades during study treatment, a higher incidence of events was seen for Femara regarding fractures (10.1% vs 7.1%), myocardial infarctions (1.0% vs 0.5%), and arthralgia (25.2% vs 20.4%) (Femara vs tamoxifen respectively). A higher incidence was seen for tamoxifen regarding thromboembolic events (2.1% vs 3.6%), endometrial hyperplasia/cancer (0.3% vs 2.9%), and endometrial proliferation disorders (0.3% vs 1.8%) (Femara vs tamoxifen respectively).

At a median follow up of 73 months, a higher incidence of events was seen for Femara (13.8%) than for tamoxifen (10.5%) regarding fractures. A higher incidence was seen for tamoxifen compared to Femara regarding thromboembolic events (4.5% vs 2.9%), and endometrial hyperplasia or cancer (2.9% vs 0.4%) (tamoxifen vs Femara, respectively).

Bone Study: Results of a phase 3 safety trial in 262 postmenopausal women with resected receptor positive early breast cancer in the adjuvant setting comparing the effect on lumbar spine (L2-L4) bone mineral density (BMD) of adjuvant treatment with letrozole to that with tamoxifen showed at 24 months a median decrease in lumbar spine BMD of 4.1% in the letrozole arm compared to a median increase of 0.3% in the tamoxifen arm (difference = 4.4%) (P<0.0001). No patients with a normal BMD at baseline became osteoporotic over the 2 years and only 1 patient with osteopenia at baseline (T score of -1.9) developed osteoporosis during the treatment period (assessment by central review). The results for total hip BMD were similar, although the differences between the two treatments were less pronounced. During the 2 year period, fractures were reported by 4 of 103 patients (4%) in the letrozole arm, and 6 of 97 patients (6%) in the tamoxifen arm.

Lipid Study: In a phase 3 safety trial in 262 postmenopausal women with resected receptor positive early breast cancer at 24 months comparing the effects on lipid profiles of adjuvant letrozole to tamoxifen, 12% of patients on letrozole had at least one total cholesterol value of a higher CTCAE grade than at baseline compared with 4% of patients on tamoxifen.

6.2 Extended Adjuvant Treatment of Early Breast Cancer, Median Treatment Duration of 24 Months

The median duration of extended adjuvant treatment was 24 months and the median duration of follow-up for safety was 28 months for patients receiving Femara and placebo.

Table 2 describes the adverse reactions occurring at a frequency of at least 5% in any treatment group during treatment. Most adverse reactions reported were Grade 1 and Grade 2 based on the Common Toxicity Criteria Version 2.0. In the extended adjuvant setting, the reported drug-related adverse reactions that were significantly different from placebo were hot flashes, arthralgia/arthritis, and myalgia. [See table 2 above]

Based on a median follow-up of patients for 28 months, the incidence of clinical fractures from the core randomized study in patients who received Femara was 5.9% (152) and placebo was 5.5% (142). The incidence of self-reported osteoporosis was higher in patients who received Femara 6.9% (176) than in patients who received placebo 5.5% (141). Bisphosphonates were administered to 21.1% of the patients who received Femara and 18.7% of the patients who received placebo.

The incidence of cardiovascular ischemic events from the core randomized study was comparable between patients who received Femara 6.8% (175) and placebo 6.5% (167).

A patient-reported measure that captures treatment impact on important symptoms associated with estrogen deficiency demonstrated a difference in favor of placebo for vasomotor and sexual symptom domains.

Bone Sub-study: [see Warnings and Precautions (5.1)].

Lipid Sub-study: In the extended adjuvant setting, based on a median duration of follow-up of 62 months, there was no significant difference between Femara and placebo in total cholesterol or in any lipid fraction at any time over 5 years. Use of lipid lowering drugs or dietary management of elevated lipids was allowed [see Warnings and Precautions (5.2)].

6.3 Updated Analysis, Extended Adjuvant Treatment of Early Breast Cancer, Median Treatment Duration of 60 Months

The extended adjuvant treatment trial was unblinded early [see Adverse Reactions (6.2)]. At the updated (final analysis), overall the side effects seen were consistent to those seen at a median treatment duration of 24 months.

During treatment or within 30 days of stopping treatment (median duration of treatment 60 months) a higher rate of fractures was observed for Femara (10.4%) compared to placebo (5.8%), as also a higher rate of osteoporosis (Femara 12.2% vs placebo 6.4%).

Based on 62 months median duration of follow-up in the randomized letrozole arm in the safety population the incidence of new fractures at any time after randomization was 13.3% for letrozole and 7.8% for placebo. The incidence of new osteoporosis was 14.5% for letrozole and 7.8% for placebo.

During treatment or within 30 days of stopping treatment (median duration of treatment 60 months) the incidence of cardiovascular events was 9.8% for Femara and 7.0% for placebo.

Based on 62 months median duration of follow-up in the randomized letrozole arm in the safety population the incidence of cardiovascular disease at any time after randomization was 14.4% for letrozole and 9.8% for placebo.

Lipid sub-study: In the extended adjuvant setting, based on a median duration of follow-up of 62 months, there was no significant difference between Femara and placebo in total cholesterol or in any lipid fraction over 5 years. Use of lipid lowering drugs or dietary management of elevated lipids was allowed [see Warnings and Precautions (5.2)].

6.4 First-Line Treatment of Advanced Breast Cancer

A total of 455 patients were treated for a median time of exposure of 11 months. The incidence of adverse reactions was similar for Femara and tamoxifen. The most frequently reported adverse reactions were bone pain, hot flushes, back pain, nausea, arthralgia and dyspnea. Discontinuations for adverse reactions other than progression of tumor occurred in 10/455 (2%) of patients on Femara and in 15/455 (3%) of patients on tamoxifen.

Adverse reactions, regardless of relationship to study drug, that were reported in at least 5% of the patients treated with Femara 2.5 mg or tamoxifen 20 mg in the first-line treatment study are shown in Table 3.

Table 3: Percentage (%) of Patients with Adverse Reactions

Adverse Reaction	Femara 2.5 mg (N=455) %	tamoxifen 20 mg (N=455) %
General Disorders		
Fatigue	13	13
Chest Pain	8	9
Edema Peripheral	5	6
Pain NOS	5	7
Weakness	6	4
Investigations		
Weight Decreased	7	5
Vascular Disorders		
Hot Flushes	19	16
Hypertension	8	4
Gastrointestinal Disorders		
Nausea	17	17
Constipation	10	11

Diarrhea	8	4
Vomiting	7	8
Infections/Infestations		
Influenza	6	4
Urinary Tract Infection NOS	6	3
Injury, Poisoning and Procedural Complications		
Post-Mastectomy Lymphedema	7	7
Metabolism and Nutrition Disorders		
Anorexia	4	6
Musculoskeletal and Connective Tissue Disorders		
Bone Pain	22	21
Back Pain	18	19
Arthralgia	16	15
Pain in Limb	10	8
Nervous System Disorders		
Headache NOS	8	7
Psychiatric Disorders		
Insomnia	7	4
Reproductive System and Breast Disorders		
Breast Pain	7	7
Respiratory, Thoracic and Mediastinal Disorders		
Dyspnea	18	17
Cough	13	13
Chest Wall Pain	6	6

Other less frequent (≤2%) adverse reactions considered consequential for both treatment groups, included peripheral thromboembolic events, cardiovascular events, and cerebrovascular events. Peripheral thromboembolic events included venous thrombosis, thrombophlebitis, portal vein thrombosis and pulmonary embolism. Cardiovascular events included angina, myocardial infarction, myocardial ischemia, and coronary heart disease. Cerebrovascular events included transient ischemic attacks, thrombotic or hemorrhagic strokes and development of hemiparesis.

6.5 Second-Line Treatment of Advanced Breast Cancer
Study discontinuations in the megestrol acetate comparison study for adverse reactions other than progression of tumor were 5/188 (2.7%) on Femara 0.5 mg, in 4/174 (2.3%) on Femara 2.5 mg, and in 15/190 (7.9%) on megestrol acetate. There were fewer thromboembolic events at both Femara doses than on the megestrol acetate arm (0.6% vs 4.7%). There was also less vaginal bleeding (0.3% vs 3.2%) on Femara than on megestrol acetate. In the aminoglutethimide comparison study, discontinuations for reasons other than progression occurred in 6/193 (3.1%) on 0.5 mg Femara, 7/185 (3.8%) on 2.5 mg Femara, and 7/178 (3.9%) of patients on aminoglutethimide.

Comparisons of the incidence of adverse reactions revealed no significant differences between the high and low dose Femara groups in either study. Most of the adverse reactions observed in all treatment groups were mild to moderate in severity and it was generally not possible to distinguish adverse reactions due to treatment from the consequences of the patient's metastatic breast cancer, the effects of estrogen deprivation, or intercurrent illness.

Adverse reactions, regardless of relationship to study drug, that were reported in at least 5% of the patients treated with Femara 0.5 mg, Femara 2.5 mg, megestrol acetate, or aminoglutethimide in the two controlled trials are shown in Table 4.

[See table 4 above]

Other less frequent (<5%) adverse reactions considered consequential and reported in at least 3 patients treated with Femara, included hypercalcemia, fracture, depression, anxiety, pleural effusion, alopecia, increased sweating and vertigo.

6.6 First and Second-Line Treatment of Advanced Breast Cancer
In the combined analysis of the first- and second-line metastatic trials and post-marketing experiences other adverse reactions that were reported were cataract, eye irritation, palpitations, cardiac failure, tachycardia, dysesthesia (including hypesthesia/paresthesia), arterial thrombosis, memory impairment, irritability, nervousness, urticaria, increased urinary frequency, leukopenia, stomatitis cancer pain, pyrexia, vaginal discharge, appetite increase, dryness of skin and mucosa (including dry mouth), and disturbances of taste and thirst.

6.7 Postmarketing Experience
Cases of blurred vision, increased hepatic enzymes, angioedema, anaphylactic reactions, toxic epidermal necrolysis, erythema multiforme, and hepatitis have been reported. Cases of carpal tunnel syndrome and trigger finger have been identified during post approval use of Femara.

Table 4: Percentage (%) of Patients with Adverse Reactions

Adverse Reaction	Pooled Femara 2.5 mg (N=359) %	Pooled Femara 0.5 mg (N=380) %	megestrol acetate 160 mg (N=189) %	aminoglutethimide 500 mg (N=178) %
Body as a Whole				
Fatigue	8	6	11	3
Chest Pain	6	3	7	3
Peripheral Edema[1]	5	5	8	3
Asthenia	4	5	4	5
Weight Increase	2	2	9	3
Cardiovascular				
Hypertension	5	7	5	6
Digestive System				
Nausea	13	15	9	14
Vomiting	7	7	5	9
Constipation	6	7	9	7
Diarrhea	6	5	3	4
Pain-Abdominal	6	5	9	8
Anorexia	5	3	5	5
Dyspepsia	3	4	6	5
Infections/Infestations				
Viral Infection	6	5	6	3
Lab Abnormality				
Hypercholesterolemia	3	3	0	6
Musculoskeletal System				
Musculoskeletal[2]	21	22	30	14
Arthralgia	8	8	8	3
Nervous System				
Headache	9	12	9	7
Somnolence	3	2	2	9
Dizziness	3	5	7	3
Respiratory System				
Dyspnea	7	9	16	5
Coughing	6	6	7	5
Skin and Appendages				
Hot Flushes	6	5	4	3
Rash[3]	5	4	3	12
Pruritus	1	2	5	3

[1] Includes peripheral edema, leg edema, dependent edema, edema
[2] Includes musculoskeletal pain, skeletal pain, back pain, arm pain, leg pain
[3] Includes rash, erythematous rash, maculopapular rash, psoriasiform rash, vesicular rash

7 DRUG INTERACTIONS

Tamoxifen
Coadministration of Femara and tamoxifen 20 mg daily resulted in a reduction of letrozole plasma levels of 38% on average. Clinical experience in the second-line breast cancer trials indicates that the therapeutic effect of Femara therapy is not impaired if Femara is administered immediately after tamoxifen.

Cimetidine
A pharmacokinetic interaction study with cimetidine showed no clinically significant effect on letrozole pharmacokinetics.

Warfarin
An interaction study with warfarin showed no clinically significant effect of letrozole on warfarin pharmacokinetics.

Other anticancer agents
There is no clinical experience to date on the use of Femara in combination with other anticancer agents.

8 USE IN SPECIFIC POPULATIONS

8.1 Pregnancy
Pregnancy Category X *[see Contraindications (4)]*. Femara may cause fetal harm when administered to a pregnant woman and the clinical benefit to premenopausal women with breast cancer has not been demonstrated. Femara is contraindicated in women who are or may become pregnant. If this drug is used during pregnancy, or if the patient becomes pregnant while taking this drug, the patient should be apprised of the potential hazard to a fetus.

Femara caused adverse pregnancy outcomes, including congenital malformations, in rats and rabbits at doses much smaller than the daily maximum recommended human dose (MRHD) on a mg/m² basis. Effects included increased postimplantation pregnancy loss and resorptions, fewer live fetuses, and fetal malformations affecting the renal and skeletal systems. Animal data and letrozole's mechanism of action raise concerns that letrozole could be a human teratogen as well.

Reproduction studies in rats showed embryo and fetal toxicity at letrozole doses during organogenesis equal to or greater than 1/100 the daily maximum recommended human dose (MRHD) (mg/m² basis). Adverse effects included: intrauterine mortality; increased resorptions and postimplantation loss; decreased numbers of live fetuses; and fetal anomalies including absence and shortening of renal papilla, dilation of ureter, edema and incomplete ossi-

cation of frontal skull and metatarsals. Letrozole doses 1/10 the daily MHRD (mg/m² basis) caused fetal domed head and cervical/centrum vertebral fusion. In rabbits, letrozole caused embryo and fetal toxicity at doses about 1/100,000 and 1/10,000 the daily MHRD respectively (mg/m² basis). Fetal anomalies included incomplete ossification of the skull, sternebrae, and fore- and hind legs *[see Nonclinical Toxicology (13.2)]*.

Physicians should discuss the need for adequate contraception with women who are recently menopausal. Contraception should be used until postmenopausal status is clinically well established.

8.3 Nursing Mothers
It is not known if letrozole is excreted in human milk. Because many drugs are excreted in human milk and because of the potential for serious adverse reactions in nursing infants from letrozole, a decision should be made whether to discontinue nursing or to discontinue the drug, taking into account the importance of the drug to the mother.

8.4 Pediatric Use
The safety and effectiveness in pediatric patients have not been established.

8.5 Geriatric Use
The median age of patients in all studies of first-line and second-line treatment of metastatic breast cancer was 64-65 years. About 1/3 of the patients were ≥70 years old. In the first-line study, patients ≥70 years of age experienced longer time to tumor progression and higher response rates than patients <70.

For the extended adjuvant setting, more than 5,100 postmenopausal women were enrolled in the clinical study. In total, 41% of patients were aged 65 years or older at enrollment, while 12% were 75 or older. In the extended adjuvant setting, no overall differences in safety or efficacy were observed between these older patients and younger patients, and other reported clinical experience has not identified differences in responses between the elderly and younger patients, but greater sensitivity of some older individuals cannot be ruled out.

In the adjuvant setting, more than 8,000 postmenopausal women were enrolled in the clinical study. In total, 36% of patients were aged 65 years or older at enrollment, while 12% were 75 or older. More adverse reactions were generally reported in elderly patients irrespective of study treatment allocation. However, in comparison to tamoxifen, no overall differences with regards to the safety and efficacy profiles were observed between elderly patients and younger patients.

10 OVERDOSAGE

Isolated cases of Femara overdose have been reported. In these instances, the highest single dose ingested was 62.5 mg or 25 tablets. While no serious adverse reactions were reported in these cases, because of the limited data available, no firm recommendations for treatment can be made. However, emesis could be induced if the patient is alert. In general, supportive care and frequent monitoring of vital signs are also appropriate. In single-dose studies, the highest dose used was 30 mg, which was well tolerated; in multiple-dose trials, the largest dose of 10 mg was well tolerated.

Lethality was observed in mice and rats following single oral doses that were equal to or greater than 2,000 mg/kg (about 4,000 to 8,000 times the daily maximum recommended human dose on a mg/m^2 basis); death was associated with reduced motor activity, ataxia and dyspnea. Lethality was observed in cats following single IV doses that were equal to or greater than 10 mg/kg (about 50 times the daily maximum recommended human dose on a mg/m^2 basis); death was preceded by depressed blood pressure and arrhythmias.

11 DESCRIPTION

Femara tablets for oral administration contains 2.5 mg of letrozole, a nonsteroidal aromatase inhibitor (inhibitor of estrogen synthesis). It is chemically described as 4,4'-(1H-1,2,4-Triazol-1-ylmethylene)dibenzonitrile, and its structural formula is

Letrozole is a white to yellowish crystalline powder, practically odorless, freely soluble in dichloromethane, slightly soluble in ethanol, and practically insoluble in water. It has a molecular weight of 285.31, empirical formula $C_{17}H_{11}N_5$, and a melting range of 184°C to 185°C.

Femara is available as 2.5 mg tablets for oral administration.

Inactive Ingredients: Colloidal silicon dioxide, ferric oxide, hydroxypropyl methylcellulose, lactose monohydrate, magnesium stearate, maize starch, microcrystalline cellulose, polyethylene glycol, sodium starch glycolate, talc, and titanium dioxide.

12 CLINICAL PHARMACOLOGY

12.1 Mechanism of Action

The growth of some cancers of the breast is stimulated or maintained by estrogens. Treatment of breast cancer thought to be hormonally responsive (i.e., estrogen and/or progesterone receptor positive or receptor unknown) has included a variety of efforts to decrease estrogen levels (ovariectomy, adrenalectomy, hypophysectomy) or inhibit estrogen effects (antiestrogens and progestational agents). These interventions lead to decreased tumor mass or delayed progression of tumor growth in some women.

In postmenopausal women, estrogens are mainly derived from the action of the aromatase enzyme, which converts adrenal androgens (primarily androstenedione and testosterone) to estrone and estradiol. The suppression of estrogen biosynthesis in peripheral tissues and in the cancer tissue itself can therefore be achieved by specifically inhibiting the aromatase enzyme.

Letrozole is a nonsteroidal competitive inhibitor of the aromatase enzyme system; it inhibits the conversion of androgens to estrogens. In adult nontumor- and tumor-bearing female animals, letrozole is as effective as ovariectomy in reducing uterine weight, elevating serum LH, and causing the regression of estrogen-dependent tumors. In contrast to ovariectomy, treatment with letrozole does not lead to an increase in serum FSH. Letrozole selectively inhibits gonadal steroidogenesis but has no significant effect on adrenal mineralocorticoid or glucocorticoid synthesis.

Letrozole inhibits the aromatase enzyme by competitively binding to the heme of the cytochrome P450 subunit of the enzyme, resulting in a reduction of estrogen biosynthesis in all tissues. Treatment of women with letrozole significantly lowers serum estrone, estradiol and estrone sulfate and has not been shown to significantly affect adrenal corticosteroid synthesis, aldosterone synthesis, or synthesis of thyroid hormones.

12.2 Pharmacodynamics

In postmenopausal patients with advanced breast cancer, daily doses of 0.1 mg to 5 mg Femara (letrozole) suppress plasma concentrations of estradiol, estrone, and estrone sulfate by 75% to 95% from baseline with maximal suppression achieved within two-three days. Suppression is dose-related, with doses of 0.5 mg and higher giving many values of estrone and estrone sulfate that were below the limit of detection in the assays. Estrogen suppression was maintained throughout treatment in all patients treated at 0.5 mg or higher.

Letrozole is highly specific in inhibiting aromatase activity. There is no impairment of adrenal steroidogenesis. No clinically-relevant changes were found in the plasma concentrations of cortisol, aldosterone, 11-deoxycortisol, 17-hydroxy-progesterone, ACTH or in plasma renin activity among postmenopausal patients treated with a daily dose of Femara 0.1 mg to 5 mg. The ACTH stimulation test performed after 6 and 12 weeks of treatment with daily doses of 0.1, 0.25, 0.5, 1, 2.5, and 5 mg did not indicate any attenuation of aldosterone or cortisol production. Glucocorticoid or mineralocorticoid supplementation is, therefore, not necessary.

No changes were noted in plasma concentrations of androgens (androstenedione and testosterone) among healthy postmenopausal women after 0.1, 0.5, and 2.5 mg single doses of Femara or in plasma concentrations of androstenedione among postmenopausal patients treated with daily doses of 0.1 mg to 5 mg. This indicates that the blockade of estrogen biosynthesis does not lead to accumulation of androgenic precursors. Plasma levels of LH and FSH were not affected by letrozole in patients, nor was thyroid function as evaluated by TSH levels, T3 uptake, and T4 levels.

12.3 Pharmacokinetics

Absorption and Distribution: Letrozole is rapidly and completely absorbed from the gastrointestinal tract and absorption is not affected by food. It is metabolized slowly to an inactive metabolite whose glucuronide conjugate is excreted renally, representing the major clearance pathway. About 90% of radiolabeled letrozole is recovered in urine. Letrozole's terminal elimination half-life is about 2 days and steady-state plasma concentration after daily 2.5 mg dosing is reached in 2-6 weeks. Plasma concentrations at steady state are 1.5 to 2 times higher than predicted from the concentrations measured after a single dose, indicating a slight non-linearity in the pharmacokinetics of letrozole upon daily administration of 2.5 mg. These steady-state levels are maintained over extended periods, however, and continuous accumulation of letrozole does not occur. Letrozole is weakly protein bound and has a large volume of distribution (approximately 1.9 L/kg).

Metabolism and Excretion: Metabolism to a pharmacologically-inactive carbinol metabolite (4,4'-methanol-bisbenzonitrile) and renal excretion of the glucuronide conjugate of this metabolite is the major pathway of letrozole clearance. Of the radiolabel recovered in urine, at least 75% was the glucuronide of the carbinol metabolite, about 9% was two unidentified metabolites, and 6% was unchanged letrozole.

In human microsomes with specific CYP isozyme activity, CYP3A4 metabolized letrozole to the carbinol metabolite while CYP2A6 formed both this metabolite and its ketone analog. In human liver microsomes, letrozole strongly inhibited CYP2A6 and moderately inhibited CYP2C19.

Pediatric, Geriatric and Race: In the study populations (adults ranging in age from 35 to >80 years), no change in pharmacokinetic parameters was observed with increasing age. Differences in letrozole pharmacokinetics between adult and pediatric populations have not been studied. Differences in letrozole pharmacokinetics due to race have not been studied.

Renal Impairment: In a study of volunteers with varying renal function (24-hour creatinine clearance: 9 to 116 mL/min), no effect of renal function on the pharmacokinetics of single doses of 2.5 mg of Femara was found. In addition, in a study of 347 patients with advanced breast cancer, about half of whom received 2.5 mg Femara and half 0.5 mg Femara, renal impairment (calculated creatinine clearance: 20 to 50 mL/min) did not affect steady-state plasma letrozole concentrations.

Hepatic Impairment: In a study of subjects with mild to moderate non-metastatic hepatic dysfunction (e.g., cirrhosis, Child-Pugh classification A and B), the mean AUC values of the volunteers with moderate hepatic impairment were 37% higher than in normal subjects, but still within the range seen in subjects without impaired function. In a pharmacokinetic study, subjects with liver cirrhosis and severe hepatic impairment (Child-Pugh classification C, which included bilirubins about 2-11 times ULN with minimal to severe ascites) had two-fold increase in exposure (AUC) and 47% reduction in systemic clearance. Breast cancer patients with severe hepatic impairment are thus expected to be exposed to higher levels of letrozole than patients with normal liver function receiving similar doses of this drug [see Dosage and Administration (2.5)].

13 NONCLINICAL TOXICOLOGY

13.1 Carcinogenesis, Mutagenesis, Impairment of Fertility

A conventional carcinogenesis study in mice at doses of 0.6 to 60 mg/kg/day (about 1 to 100 times the daily maximum recommended human dose on a mg/m^2 basis) administered by oral gavage for up to 2 years revealed a dose-related increase in the incidence of benign ovarian stromal tumors. The incidence of combined hepatocellular adenoma and carcinoma showed a significant trend in females when the high dose group was excluded due to low survival. In a separate study, plasma AUC$_{0-12hr}$ levels in mice at 60 mg/kg/day were 55 times higher than the AUC$_{0-24hr}$ level in breast cancer patients at the recommended dose. The carcinogenicity study in rats at oral doses of 0.1 to 10 mg/kg/day (about 0.4 to 40 times the daily maximum recommended human dose on a mg/m^2 basis) for up to 2 years also produced an increase in the incidence of benign ovarian stromal tumors at 10 mg/kg/day. Ovarian hyperplasia was observed in females at doses equal to or greater than 0.1 mg/kg/day. At 10 mg/kg/day, plasma AUC$_{0-24hr}$ levels in rats were 80 times higher than the level in breast cancer patients at the recommended dose. The benign ovarian stromal tumors observed in mice and rats were considered to be related to the pharmacological inhibition of estrogen synthesis and may be due to increased luteinizing hormone resulting from the decrease in circulating estrogen.

Femara (letrozole) was not mutagenic in *in vitro* tests (Ames and E.coli bacterial tests) but was observed to be a potential clastogen in *in vitro* assays (CHO K1 and CCL 61 Chinese hamster ovary cells). Letrozole was not clastogenic *in vivo* (micronucleus test in rats).

Studies to investigate the effect of letrozole on fertility have not been conducted; however, repeated dosing caused sexual inactivity in females and atrophy of the reproductive tract in males and females at doses of 0.6, 0.1 and 0.03 mg/kg in mice, rats and dogs, respectively (about one, 0.4 and 0.4 the daily maximum recommended human dose on a mg/m^2 basis, respectively). Oral administration of letrozole to female rats starting 2 weeks before mating until pregnancy day 6 resulted in decreases in the incidence of successful mating and pregnancy at equal to or greater than 0.03 mg/kg/day (approximately 0.1 times the recommended human dose on a mg/m^2 basis). An increase in pre-implantation loss was observed at doses equal to or greater than 0.003 mg/kg/day (approximately 0.01 times the recommended human dose on a mg/m^2 basis).

Letrozole administered to young (postnatal day 7) rats for 12 weeks duration at 0.003, 0.03, 0.3 mg/kg/day by oral gavage, resulted in adverse skeletal/growth effects (bone maturation, bone mineral density) and neuroendocrine and reproductive developmental perturbations of the hypothalamic-pituitary axis at exposures less than exposure anticipated at the clinical dose of 2.5 mg/day. Decreased fertility was accompanied by hypertrophy of the hypophysis and testicular changes that included degeneration of the seminiferous tubular epithelium and atrophy of the female reproductive tract. Young rats in this study were allowed to recover following discontinuation of letrozole treatment for 42 days. Histopathological changes were not reversible at clinically relevant exposures.

13.2 Animal Toxicology and/or Pharmacology

Reproductive Toxicology: Reproduction studies in rats at letrozole doses equal to or greater than 0.003 mg/kg (about 1/100 the daily maximum recommended human dose on a mg/m^2 basis) administered during the period of organogenesis, have shown that letrozole is embryotoxic and fetotoxic, as indicated by intrauterine mortality, increased resorption, increased postimplantation loss, decreased numbers of live fetuses and fetal anomalies including absence and shortening of renal papilla, dilation of ureter, edema and incomplete ossification of frontal skull and metatarsals. Letrozole was teratogenic in rats. A 0.03 mg/kg dose (about 1/10 the daily maximum recommended human dose on a mg/m^2 basis) caused fetal domed head and cervical/centrum vertebral fusion.

Letrozole is embryotoxic at doses equal to or greater than 0.002 mg/kg and fetotoxic when administered to rabbits at 0.02 mg/kg (about 1/100,000 and 1/10,000 the daily maximum recommended human dose on a mg/m^2 basis, respectively). Fetal anomalies included incomplete ossification of the skull, sternebrae, and fore- and hind legs.

14 CLINICAL STUDIES

14.1 Updated Adjuvant Treatment of Early Breast Cancer

In a multicenter study enrolling over 8,000 postmenopausal women with resected, receptor-positive early breast cancer, one of the following treatments was randomized in a double-blind manner:

Option 1:
A. tamoxifen for 5 years
B. Femara for 5 years
C. tamoxifen for 2 years followed by Femara for 3 years
D. Femara for 2 years followed by tamoxifen for 3 years
Option 2:
A. tamoxifen for 5 years
B. Femara for 5 years

The study in the adjuvant setting, BIG 1-98 was designed to answer two primary questions: whether Femara for 5 years was superior to tamoxifen for 5 years (Primary Core Analysis) and whether switching endocrine treatments at 2 years was superior to continuing the same agent for a total of 5 years (Sequential Treatments Analysis). Selected baseline characteristics for the study population are shown in Table 5.

The primary endpoint of this trial was disease-free survival (DFS) (i.e., interval between randomization and earliest occurrence of a local, regional, or distant recurrence, or invasive contralateral breast cancer, or death from any cause). The secondary endpoints were overall survival (OS), systemic disease-free survival (SDFS), invasive contralateral breast cancer, time to breast cancer recurrence (TBR) and time to distant metastasis (TDM).

The Primary Core Analysis (PCA) included all patients and all follow-up in the monotherapy arms in both randomization options, but follow-up in the two sequential treatments arms was truncated 30 days after switching treatments. The PCA was conducted at a median treatment duration of 24 months and a median follow-up of 26 months. Femara was superior to tamoxifen in all endpoints except overall survival and contralateral breast cancer [e.g., DFS: hazard ratio, HR 0.79; 95% CI (0.68, 0.92); P=0.002; SDFS: HR 0.83; 95% CI (0.70, 0.97); TDM: HR 0.73; 95% CI (0.60, 0.88); OS: HR 0.86; 95% CI (0.70, 1.06).

In 2005, based on recommendations by the independent Data Monitoring Committee, the tamoxifen arms were unblinded and patients were allowed to complete initial adjuvant therapy with Femara (if they had received tamoxifen for at least 2 years) or to start extended adjuvant treatment with Femara (if they had received tamoxifen for at least 4.5 years) if they remained alive and disease-free. In total, 632 patients crossed to Femara or another aromatase inhibitor. Approximately 70% (448) of these 632 patients crossed to Femara to complete initial adjuvant therapy and most of these crossed in years 3 to 4. All of these patients were in Option 1. A total of 184 patients started extended adjuvant therapy with Femara (172 patients) or with another aromatase inhibitor (12 patients). To explore the impact of this selective crossover, results from analyses censoring follow-up at the date of the selective crossover (in the tamoxifen arm) are presented for the Monotherapy Arms Analysis (MAA).

The PCA allowed the results of Femara for 5 years compared with tamoxifen for 5 years to be reported in 2005 after a median follow-up of only 26 months. The design of the PCA is not optimal to evaluate the effect of Femara after a longer time (because follow-up was truncated in two arms at around 25 months). The Monotherapy Arms Analysis (ignoring the two sequential treatment arms) provided follow-up equally as long in each treatment and did not over-emphasize early recurrences as the PCA did. The MAA thus provides the clinically appropriate updated efficacy results in answer to the first primary question, despite the confounding of the tamoxifen reference arm by the selective crossover to Femara. The updated results for the MAA are summarized in Table 6. Median follow-up for this analysis is 73 months.

The Sequential Treatments Analysis (STA) addresses the second primary question of the study. The primary analysis for the Sequential Treatments Analysis (STA) was from switch (or equivalent time-point in monotherapy arms) + 30 days (STA-S) with a two-sided test applied to each pair-wise comparison at the 2.5% level. Additional analyses were conducted from randomization (STA-R) but these comparisons (added in light of changing medical practice) were underpowered for efficacy.

[See table 5 above]

[See table 6 above]

Figure 1 shows the Kaplan-Meier curves for Disease-Free Survival Monotherapy Analysis

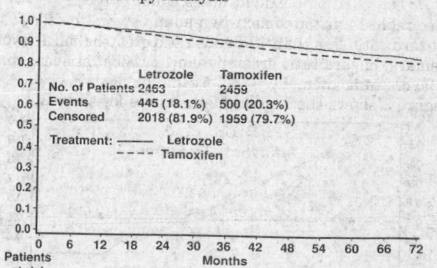

Figure 1 Disease-Free Survival (Median follow-up 73 months, ITT Approach)

DFS events defined as loco-regional recurrence, distant metastasis, invasive contralateral breast cancer, or death from any cause (i.e., definition excludes second non-breast primary cancers).

Table 5: Adjuvant Study - Patient and Disease Characteristics (ITT Population)

Characteristic	Primary Core Analysis (PCA) Femara N=4003 n (%)	Primary Core Analysis (PCA) tamoxifen N=4007 n (%)	Monotherapy Arms Analysis (MAA) Femara N=2463 n (%)	Monotherapy Arms Analysis (MAA) tamoxifen N=2459 n (%)
Age (median, years)	61	61	61	61
Age range (years)	38-89	39-90	38-88	39-90
Hormone receptor status (%)				
ER+ and/or PgR+	99.7	99.7	99.7	99.7
Both unknown	0.3	0.3	0.3	0.3
Nodal status (%)				
Node negative	52	52	50	52
Node positive	41	41	43	41
Nodal status unknown	7	7	7	7
Prior adjuvant chemotherapy (%)	24	24	24	24

Table 6: Updated Adjuvant Study Results - Monotherapy Arms Analysis (Median Follow-up 73 Months)

		Femara N=2463 Events (%)	Femara N=2463 5-year rate	tamoxifen N=2459 Events (%)	tamoxifen N=2459 5-year rate	Hazard ratio (95% CI)	P
Disease-free survival[1]	ITT	445 (18.1)	87.4	500 (20.3)	84.7	0.87 (0.76, 0.99)	0.03
	Censor	445	87.4	483	84.2	0.84 (0.73, 0.95)	
0 positive nodes	ITT	165	92.2	189	90.3	0.88 (0.72, 1.09)	
1-3 positive nodes	ITT	151	85.6	163	83.0	0.85 (0.68, 1.06)	
>=4 positive nodes	ITT	123	71.2	142	62.6	0.81 (0.64, 1.03)	
Adjuvant chemotherapy	ITT	119	86.4	150	80.6	0.77 (0.60, 0.98)	
No chemotherapy	ITT	326	87.8	350	86.1	0.91 (0.78, 1.06)	
Systemic DFS[2]	ITT	401	88.5	446	86.6	0.88 (0.77,1.01)	
Time to distant metastasis[3]	ITT	257	92.4	298	90.1	0.85 (0.72, 1.00)	
Adjuvant chemotherapy	ITT	84	-	109	-	0.75 (0.56-1.00)	
No chemotherapy	ITT	173	-	189	-	0.90 (0.73,1.11)	
Distant DFS[4]	ITT	385	89.0	432	87.1	0.87 (0.76,1.00)	
Contralateral breast cancer	ITT	34	99.2	44	98.6	0.76 (0.49, 1.19)	
Overall survival	ITT	303	91.8	343	90.9	0.87 (0.75, 1.02)	
	Censor	303	91.8	338	90.1	0.82 (0.70, 0.96)	
0 positive nodes	ITT	107	95.2	121	94.8	0.90 (0.69,1.16)	
1-3 positive nodes	ITT	99	90.8	114	90.6	0.81 (0.62,1.06)	
>=4 positive nodes	ITT	92	80.2	104	73.6	0.86 (0.65, 1.14)	
Adjuvant chemotherapy	ITT	76	91.5	96	88.4	0.79 (0.58, 1.06)	
No chemotherapy	ITT	227	91.9	247	91.8	0.91 (0.76, 1.08)	

Definition of:
[1] Disease-free survival: Interval from randomization to earliest event of invasive loco-regional recurrence, distant metastasis, invasive contralateral breast cancer, or death without a prior event
[2] Systemic disease-free survival: Interval from randomization to invasive regional recurrence, distant metastasis, or death without a prior cancer event
[3] Time to distant metastasis: Interval from randomization to distant metastasis
[4] Distant disease-free survival: Interval from randomization to earlier event of relapse in a distant site or death from any cause
ITT analysis ignores selective crossover in tamoxifen arms
Censored analysis censors follow-up at the date of selective crossover in 632 patients who crossed to Femara or another aromatase inhibitor after the tamoxifen arms were unblinded in 2005

The medians of overall survival for both arms were not reached for the Monotherapy Arms Analysis (MAA). There was no statistically significant difference in overall survival. The hazard ratio for survival in the Femara arm compared to the tamoxifen arm was 0.87, with 95% CI (0.75, 1.02) (see Table 6).

There were no significant differences in DFS, OS, SDFS, and Distant DFS from switch in the Sequential Treatments Analysis with respect to either monotherapy (e.g., [Tamoxifen 2 years followed by] Femara 3 years versus tamoxifen beyond 2 years, DFS HR 0.89; 97.5% CI 0.68, 1.15 and [Femara 2 years followed by] tamoxifen 3 years versus Femara beyond 2 years, DFS HR 0.93; 97.5% CI 0.71, 1.22). There were no significant differences in DFS, OS, SDFS, and Distant DFS from randomization in the Sequential Treatments Analyses.

14.2 Extended Adjuvant Treatment of Early Breast Cancer, Median Treatment Duration of 24 Months

A double-blind, randomized, placebo-controlled trial of Femara was performed in over 5,100 postmenopausal women with receptor-positive or unknown primary breast cancer who were disease free after 5 years of adjuvant treatment with tamoxifen.

The planned duration of treatment for patients in the study was 5 years, but the trial was terminated early because of an interim analysis showing a favorable Femara effect on time without recurrence or contralateral breast cancer. At the time of unblinding, women had been followed for a median of 28 months, 30% of patients had completed 3 or more years of follow-up and less than 1% of patients had completed 5 years of follow-up.

Selected baseline characteristics for the study population are shown in Table 7.

Table 7: Selected Study Population Demographics (Modified ITT Population)

Baseline Status	Femara N=2582	Placebo N=2586
Hormone Receptor Status (%)		
ER+ and/or PgR+	98	98
Both Unknown	2	2
Nodal Status (%)		
Node Negative	50	50
Node Positive	46	46
Nodal Status Unknown	4	4
Chemotherapy	46	46

Table 8 shows the study results. Disease-free survival was measured as the time from randomization to the earliest event of loco-regional or distant recurrence of the primary disease or development of contralateral breast cancer or death. DFS by hormone receptor status, nodal status and adjuvant chemotherapy were similar to the overall results. Data were premature for an analysis of survival.

[See table 8 at top of next page]

14.3 Updated Analyses of Extended Adjuvant Treatment of Early Breast Cancer, Median Treatment Duration of 60 Months

[See table 9 at top of next page]

Updated analyses were conducted at a median follow-up of 62 months. In the Femara arm, 71% of the patients were treated for at least 3 years and 58% of patients completed at least 4.5 years of extended adjuvant treatment. After the

Table 8: Extended Adjuvant Study Results

	Femara N = 2582	Placebo N = 2586	Hazard Ratio (95% CI)	P-Value
Disease Free Survival (DFS)[1] Events	122 (4.7%)	193 (7.5%)	0.62 (0.49, 0.78)[2]	0.00003
Local Breast Recurrence	9	22		
Local Chest Wall Recurrence	2	8		
Regional Recurrence	7	4		
Distant Recurrence	55	92	0.61 (0.44 - 0.84)	0.003
Contralateral Breast Cancer	19	29		
Deaths Without Recurrence or Contralateral Breast Cancer	30	38		

CI = confidence interval for hazard ratio. Hazard ratio of less than 1.0 indicates difference in favor of Femara (lesser risk of recurrence); hazard ratio greater than 1.0 indicates difference in favor of placebo (higher risk of recurrence with Femara).
[1] First event of loco-regional recurrence, distant relapse, contralateral breast cancer or death from any cause
[2] Analysis stratified by receptor status, nodal status and prior adjuvant chemotherapy (stratification factors as at randomization). P-value based on stratified logrank test.

Table 9: Update of Extended Adjuvant Study Results

	Femara N = 2582 (%)	Placebo N = 2586 (%)	Hazard Ratio[1] (95% CI)	P-Value[2]
Disease Free Survival (DFS) events[3]	344 (13.3)	402 (15.5)	0.89 (0.77, 1.03)	0.12
Breast cancer recurrence	209	286	0.75 (0.63, 0.89)	0.001
(Protocol definition of DFS events[4])				
Local Breast Recurrence	15	44		
Local Chest Wall Recurrence	6	14		
Regional Recurrence	10	8		
Distant Recurrence	140	167		
Distant Recurrence (first or subsequent events)	142	169	0.88 (0.70,1.10)	0.246
Contralateral Breast Cancer	37	53		
Deaths Without Recurrence or Contralateral Breast Cancer	135	116		

[1] Adjusted by receptor status, nodal status and prior chemotherapy
[2] Stratified logrank test, stratified by receptor status, nodal status and prior chemotherapy
[3] DFS events defined as earliest of loco-regional recurrence, distant metastasis, contralateral breast cancer or death from any cause, and ignoring switches to Femara in 60% of the placebo arm.
[4] Protocol definition does not include deaths from any cause

Table 11: Results of First-Line Treatment of Advanced Breast Cancer

	Femara 2.5 mg N=453	tamoxifen 20 mg N=454	Hazard or Odds Ratio (95% CI) P-Value (2-Sided)
Median Time to Progression	9.4 months	6.0 months	0.72 (0.62, 0.83)[1] P<0.0001
Objective Response Rate (CR + PR)	145 (32%)	95 (21%)	1.77 (1.31, 2.39)[2] P=0.0002
(CR)	42 (9%)	15 (3%)	2.99 (1.63, 5.47)[2] P=0.0004
Duration of Objective Response Median	18 months (N=145)	16 months (N=95)	
Overall Survival	35 months (N=458)	32 months (N=458)	P=0.5136[3]

[1] Hazard ratio
[2] Odds ratio
[3] Overall logrank test

unblinding of the study at a median follow-up of 28 months, approximately 60% of the selected patients in the placebo arm opted to switch to Femara.

In this updated analysis shown in Table 9, Femara significantly reduced the risk of breast cancer recurrence or contralateral breast cancer compared with placebo (HR 0.75; 95% CI 0.63, 0.89; P=0.001). However, in the updated DFS analysis (interval between randomization and earliest event of loco-regional recurrence, distant metastasis, contralateral breast cancer, or death from any cause) the treatment difference was heavily diluted by 60% of the patients in the placebo arm switching to Femara and accounting for 64% of the total placebo patient-years of follow-up. Ignoring these switches, the risk of DFS event was reduced by a non-significant 11% (HR 0.89; 95% CI 0.77, 1.03). There was no significant difference in distant disease-free survival or overall survival.

14.4   First-Line Treatment of Advanced Breast Cancer
A randomized, double-blind, multinational trial compared Femara 2.5 mg with tamoxifen 20 mg in 916 postmenopausal patients with locally advanced (Stage IIIB or loco-regional recurrence not amenable to treatment with surgery or radiation) or metastatic breast cancer. Time to progression (TTP) was the primary endpoint of the trial. Selected baseline characteristics for this study are shown in Table 10.

Table 10: Selected Study Population Demographics

Baseline Status	Femara N=458	tamoxifen N=458
Stage of Disease		
IIIB	6%	7%
IV	93%	92%
Receptor Status		
ER and PgR Positive	38%	41%
ER or PgR Positive	26%	26%
Both Unknown	34%	33%
ER⁻ or PgR⁻/Other Unknown	<1%	0
Previous Antiestrogen Therapy		
Adjuvant	19%	18%
None	81%	82%
Dominant Site of Disease		
Soft Tissue	25%	25%
Bone	32%	29%
Viscera	43%	46%

Femara was superior to tamoxifen in TTP and rate of objective tumor response (see Table 11).
Table 11 summarizes the results of the trial, with a total median follow-up of approximately 32 months. (All analyses are unadjusted and use 2-sided P-values.)
[See table 11 above]
Figure 2 shows the Kaplan-Meier curves for TTP.

Figure 2 Kaplan-Meier Estimates of Time to Progression (Tamoxifen Study)

Table 12 shows results in the subgroup of women who had received prior antiestrogen adjuvant therapy, Table 13, results by disease site and Table 14, the results by receptor status.

Table 12: Efficacy in Patients Who Received Prior Antiestrogen Therapy

Variable	Femara 2.5 mg N=84	tamoxifen 20 mg N=83
Median Time to Progression (95% CI)	8.9 months (6.2, 12.5)	5.9 months (3.2, 6.2)
Hazard Ratio for TTP (95% CI)	0.60 (0.43, 0.84)	
Objective Response Rate (CR + PR)	22 (26%)	7 (8%)
Odds Ratio for Response (95% CI)	3.85 (1.50, 9.60)	

Hazard ratio less than 1 or odds ratio greater than 1 favors Femara; hazard ratio greater than 1 or odds ratio less than 1 favors tamoxifen.

Table 13: Efficacy by Disease Site

	Femara 2.5 mg	tamoxifen 20 mg
Dominant Disease Site		
Soft Tissue:	N=113	N=115
Median TTP	12.1 months	6.4 months
Objective Response Rate	50%	34%
Bone:	N=145	N=131
Median TTP	9.5 months	6.3 months
Objective Response Rate	23%	15%
Viscera:	N=195	N=208
Median TTP	8.3 months	4.6 months
Objective Response Rate	28%	17%

[See table 14 at top of next page]
Hazard ratio less than 1 or odds ratio greater than 1 favors Femara; hazard ratio greater than 1 or odds ratio less than 1 favors tamoxifen.
Figure 3 shows the Kaplan-Meier curves for survival.

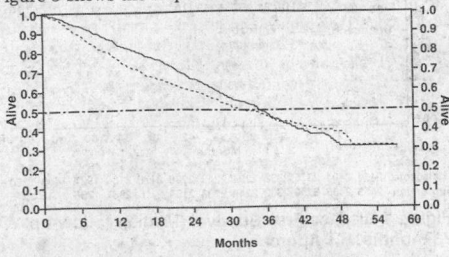

Figure 3 Survival by Randomized Treatment Arm

Legend: Randomized Femara: n=458, events 57%, median overall survival 35 months (95% CI 32 to 38 months)

Table 14: Efficacy by Receptor Status

Variable	Femara 2.5 mg	tamoxifen 20 mg
Receptor Positive	N=294	N=305
Median Time to Progression (95% CI)	9.4 months (8.9, 11.8)	6.0 months (5.1, 8.5)
Hazard Ratio for TTP (95% CI)	0.69 (0.58, 0.83)	
Objective Response Rate (CR+PR)	97 (33%)	66 (22%)
Odds Ratio for Response 95% CI	1.78 (1.20, 2.60)	
Receptor Unknown	N=159	N=149
Median Time to Progression (95% CI)	9.2 months (6.1, 12.3)	6.0 months (4.1, 6.4)
Hazard Ratio for TTP (95% CI)	0.77 (0.60, 0.99)	
Objective Response Rate (CR+PR)	48 (30%)	29 (20%)
Odds Ratio for Response (95% CI)	1.79 (1.10, 3.00)	

Table 16: Megestrol Acetate Study Results

	Femara 0.5 mg N=188	Femara 2.5 mg N=174	megestrol acetate N=190
Objective Response (CR + PR)	22 (11.7%)	41 (23.6%)	31 (16.3%)
Median Duration of Response	552 days	(Not reached)	561 days
Median Time to Progression	154 days	170 days	168 days
Median Survival	633 days	730 days	659 days
Odds Ratio for Response	Femara 2.5: Femara 0.5=2.33 (95% CI: 1.32, 4.17); P=0.004*		Femara 2.5: megestrol=1.58 (95% CI: 0.94, 2.66); P=0.08*
Relative Risk of Progression	Femara 2.5: Femara 0.5=0.81 (95% CI: 0.63, 1.03); P=0.09*		Femara 2.5: megestrol=0.77 (95% CI: 0.60, 0.98); P=0.03*

* two-sided *P*-value

Table 17: Aminoglutethimide Study Results

	Femara 0.5 mg N=193	Femara 2.5 mg N=185	aminoglutethimide N=179
Objective Response (CR + PR)	34 (17.6%)	34 (18.4%)	22 (12.3%)
Median Duration of Response	619 days	706 days	450 days
Median Time to Progression	103 days	123 days	112 days
Median Survival	636 days	792 days	592 days
Odds Ratio for Response	Femara 2.5: Femara 0.5=1.05 (95% CI: 0.62, 1.79); P=0.85*		Femara 2.5: aminoglutethimide=1.61 (95% CI: 0.90, 2.87); P=0.11*
Relative Risk of Progression	Femara 2.5: Femara 0.5=0.86 (95% CI: 0.68, 1.11); P=0.25*		Femara 2.5: aminoglutethimide=0.74 (95% CI: 0.57, 0.94); P=0.02*

* 2-sided *P*-value

Randomized tamoxifen: n=458, events 57%, median overall survival 32 months (95% CI 28 to 37 months)

Overall logrank P=0.5136 (i.e., there was no significant difference between treatment arms in overall survival).

The median overall survival was 35 months for the Femara group and 32 months for the tamoxifen group, with a P-value 0.5136. Study design allowed patients to cross over upon progression to the other therapy. Approximately 50% of patients crossed over to the opposite treatment arm and almost all patients who crossed over had done so by 36 months. The median time to crossover was 17 months (Femara to tamoxifen) and 13 months (tamoxifen to Femara). In patients who did not cross over to the opposite treatment arm, median survival was 35 months with Femara (n=219, 95% CI 29 to 43 months) vs 20 months with tamoxifen (n=229, 95% CI 16 to 26 months).

14.5 Second-Line Treatment of Advanced Breast Cancer

Femara was initially studied at doses of 0.1 mg to 5.0 mg daily in six non-comparative Phase I/II trials in 181 postmenopausal estrogen/progesterone receptor positive or unknown advanced breast cancer patients previously treated with at least antiestrogen therapy. Patients had received other hormonal therapies and also may have received cytotoxic therapy. Eight (20%) of forty patients treated with Femara 2.5 mg daily in Phase I/II trials achieved an objective tumor response (complete or partial response).

Two large randomized, controlled, multinational (predominantly European) trials were conducted in patients with advanced breast cancer who had progressed despite antiestrogen therapy. Patients were randomized to Femara 0.5 mg daily, Femara 2.5 mg daily, or a comparator (megestrol acetate 160 mg daily in one study; and aminoglutethimide 250 mg b.i.d. with corticosteroid supplementation in the other study). In each study over 60% of the patients had received therapeutic antiestrogens, and about one-fifth of these patients had an objective response. The megestrol acetate controlled study was double-blind; the other study was open label. Selected baseline characteristics for each study are shown in Table 15.

Table 15: Selected Study Population Demographics

Parameter	megestrol acetate study	aminoglutethimide study
No. of Participants	552	557
Receptor Status		
ER/PR Positive	57%	56%
ER/PR Unknown	43%	44%
Previous Therapy		
Adjuvant Only	33%	38%
Therapeutic +/- Adj.	66%	62%
Sites of Disease		
Soft Tissue	56%	50%
Bone	50%	55%
Viscera	40%	44%

Confirmed objective tumor response (complete response plus partial response) was the primary endpoint of the trials. Responses were measured according to the Union Internationale Contre le Cancer (UICC) criteria and verified by independent, blinded review. All responses were confirmed by a second evaluation 4 to 12 weeks after the documentation of the initial response.

Table 16 shows the results for the first trial, with a minimum follow-up of 15 months, that compared Femara 0.5 mg, Femara 2.5 mg, and megestrol acetate 160 mg daily. (All analyses are unadjusted.)

[See table 16 above]

The Kaplan-Meier curves for progression for the megestrol acetate study are shown in Figure 4.

[See figure 4 at top of next column]

The results for the study comparing Femara to aminoglutethimide, with a minimum follow-up of 9 months, are shown in Table 17. (Unadjusted analyses are used.)

[See table 17 above]

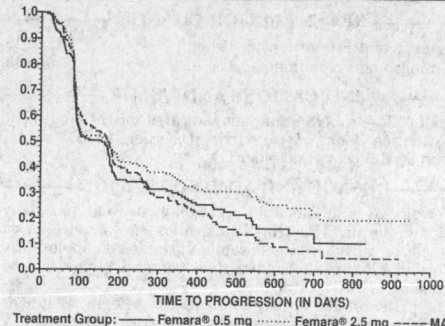

Figure 4 Kaplan-Meier Estimates of Time to Progression (Megestrol Acetate Study)

The Kaplan-Meier curves for progression for the aminoglutethimide study is shown in Figure 5.

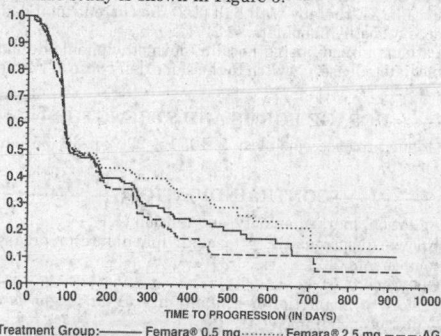

Figure 5 Kaplan-Meier Estimates of Time to Progression (Aminoglutethimide Study)

16 HOW SUPPLIED/STORAGE AND HANDLING

Packaged in HDPE bottles with a safety screw cap.

2.5 milligram tablets

Bottles of 30 tablets ....NDC 0078-0249-15

Store at 25°C (77°F); excursions permitted to 15 to 30°C (59 to 86°F) [see USP Controlled Room Temperature].

17 PATIENT COUNSELING INFORMATION

Information for Patients

Pregnancy: Femara is contraindicated in women of premenopausal endocrine status. The physician needs to discuss the necessity of adequate contraception with women who have the potential to become pregnant including women who are perimenopausal or who recently became postmenopausal, until their postmenopausal status is fully established.

Fatigue and Dizziness: Since fatigue and dizziness have been observed with the use of Femara and somnolence was uncommonly reported, caution is advised when driving or using machinery.

Bone Effects: Consideration should be given to monitoring bone mineral density.

Novartis Pharmaceuticals Corporation

East Hanover, New Jersey, 07936

© Novartis

T2014-01

January 2014

Shown in Product Identification Guide, page 310

FOCALIN XR

[fōk'ä-lǐn X-R]

(dexmethylphenidate hydrochloride)

Extended-Release Capsules CII for oral use

The following prescribing information is based on official labeling in effect July 2014.

HIGHLIGHTS OF PRESCRIBING INFORMATION

These highlights do not include all the information needed to use FOCALIN XR safely and effectively. See full prescribing information for FOCALIN XR.

FOCALIN XR (dexmethylphenidate hydrochloride) Extended-Release Capsules CII for oral use

Initial U.S. Approval: 2005

> **WARNING: DRUG DEPENDENCE**
>
> *See full prescribing information for complete boxed warning*
>
> **Focalin XR should be given cautiously to patients with a history of drug dependence or alcoholism. Chronic abusive use can lead to marked tolerance and psychological dependence, with varying degrees of abnormal behavior.**

RECENT MAJOR CHANGES

Warnings and Precautions (5.10)	12/2013
Warnings and Precautions (5.11)	6/2013

INDICATIONS AND USAGE

Focalin XR is a CNS stimulant indicated for the treatment of Attention Deficit Hyperactivity Disorder (ADHD) in patients aged 6 years and older (1)

DOSAGE AND ADMINISTRATION

- Focalin XR is intended for oral administration once daily in the morning. Focalin XR capsules may be swallowed whole, or capsule contents can be sprinkled on applesauce. Focalin XR capsules and/or their contents should not be crushed, chewed, or divided. (2)
- For patients new to methylphenidate: Begin treatment with Focalin XR at 5 mg/day for pediatrics and 10 mg/day for adults, titrating the dose weekly in 5 mg increments for pediatrics and in 10 mg increments for adults. Doses above 30 mg/day in children and 40 mg/day in adults have not been studied. (2.1)
- For patients already using methylphenidate: Initiate Focalin XR therapy with half (1/2) the current total daily dose of methylphenidate. (2.2)
- Patients already using Focalin (dexmethylphenidate) immediate release: switch to the same daily dose of Focalin XR. (2.2)

DOSAGE FORMS AND STRENGTHS

Extended-release capsules: 5, 10, 15, 20, 25, 30, 35, and 40 mg (3)

CONTRAINDICATIONS

- Agitation, marked anxiety, and tension (4.1)
- Known hypersensitivity to methylphenidate or product components (4.2)
- Glaucoma (4.3)
- History of motor tics or a family history or diagnosis of Tourette's syndrome (4.4)
- During, or within a minimum of 14 days following discontinuation of treatment with a monoamine oxidase inhibitor (MAOI) (4.5)

WARNINGS AND PRECAUTIONS

- Serious Cardiovascular Events: Sudden death has been reported in association with CNS stimulant treatment at usual doses in children and adolescents with structural cardiac abnormalities or other serious heart problems. Sudden death, stroke, and myocardial infarction have been reported in adults taking stimulant drugs at usual doses for ADHD. Stimulant products generally should not be used in patients with known structural cardiac abnormalities, cardiomyopathy, serious heart rhythm abnormalities, coronary artery disease, or other serious heart problems. (5.1)
- Increased Blood Pressure and Heart Rate: have been reported. Monitor patients for changes in blood pressure and heart rate. Caution should be exercised in treating patients whose underlying medical conditions might be compromised by increases in blood pressure or heart rate. (5.2)
- Assess Cardiovascular Status: prior to stimulant treatment, assess for cardiac disease with history and exam and, if suggested by findings, conduct further cardiac evaluation. Patients with emerging symptoms suggestive of cardiac disease should undergo a prompt cardiac evaluation. (5.3)
- Psychotic Symptoms: may be exacerbated in patients with psychotic disorders. (5.4)
- Bipolar Disorder: Use with particular care in ADHD patients with comorbid Bipolar Disorder. Before initiating stimulant therapy, obtain a detailed psychiatric history for patients with comorbid depressive symptoms, in order to determine risk for Bipolar Disorder. (5.5)
- Emergence of New Psychotic or Manic Symptoms: Treatment-emergent psychotic or manic symptoms without a prior history can be caused by stimulants at usual doses. Discontinuation of stimulant therapy may be indicated. (5.6)
- Aggression: Monitor for appearance of or worsening of aggressive behavior or hostility. (5.7)
- Long-Term Suppression of Growth: monitor height and weight in pediatric patients at appropriate intervals. Patients who are not growing or gaining weight as expected may need to have their treatment interrupted. (5.8)
- Seizures: The threshold for seizures may be lowered. In the presence of seizure, discontinue treatment. (5.9)
- Priapism: Cases of painful and prolonged penile erections and priapism have been reported with methylphenidate products. Immediate medical attention should be sought if signs or symptoms of prolonged penile erections or priapism are observed. (5.10)
- Peripheral Vasculopathy, including Raynaud's phenomenon: Stimulants used to treat ADHD are associated with peripheral vasculopathy, including Raynaud's phenomenon. Careful observation for digital changes is necessary during treatment with ADHD stimulants. (5.11)

- Visual Disturbance: difficulties with accommodation and blurring of vision have been reported with stimulant treatment. (5.12)
- Hematologic Monitoring: periodic monitoring of CBC with differential is advised during prolonged therapy. (5.14)

ADVERSE REACTIONS

Most common adverse reactions (at least 5% and twice the incidence among placebo-treated patients) are dyspepsia, decreased appetite, headache, and anxiety for pediatric patients and dry mouth, dyspepsia, headache, and anxiety for adult patients (6).

To report SUSPECTED ADVERSE REACTIONS, contact Novartis Pharmaceuticals Corporation at 1-888-669-6682 or FDA at 1-800-FDA-1088 or www.fda.gov/medwatch.

DRUG INTERACTIONS

- Focalin XR should not be used in patients being treated (currently or within the preceding two weeks) with MAO Inhibitors (4.5)
- Focalin XR should be used cautiously with pressor agents (7)
- Antacids or acid suppressants could alter the release of Focalin XR (7)
- Racemic methylphenidate may inhibit the metabolism of coumarin anticoagulants, anticonvulsants, and tricyclic drugs (7)

USE IN SPECIFIC POPULATIONS

- Focalin XR should not be used in children under 6 years of age. (5.13)
- Pregnancy: Limited human data. Based on animal data, may cause fetal harm. (8.1)
- Nursing Mothers: Caution should be exercised when administered to a nursing woman. (8.3)

See 17 for PATIENT COUNSELING INFORMATION and Medication Guide

Revised: 12/2013

FULL PRESCRIBING INFORMATION

> **WARNING: DRUG DEPENDENCE**
>
> Focalin XR should be given cautiously to patients with a history of drug dependence or alcoholism. Chronic abusive use can lead to marked tolerance and psychological dependence with varying degrees of abnormal behavior. Frank psychotic episodes can occur, especially with parenteral abuse. Careful supervision is required during withdrawal from abusive use, since severe depression may occur. Withdrawal following chronic therapeutic use may unmask symptoms of the underlying disorder that may require follow-up.

1   INDICATIONS AND USAGE

Focalin XR is indicated for the treatment of Attention Deficit Hyperactivity Disorder (ADHD) in patients aged 6 years and older.

The effectiveness of Focalin XR in the treatment of ADHD in patients aged 6 years and older was established in 2 placebo-controlled studies in patients meeting DSM-IV criteria for ADHD [see *Clinical Studies (14)*].

A diagnosis of Attention Deficit Hyperactivity Disorder (ADHD; DSM-IV) implies the presence of hyperactive-impulsive or inattentive symptoms that caused impairment and were present before age 7 years. The symptoms must cause clinically significant impairment, e.g., in social, academic, or occupational functioning, and be present in 2 or more settings, e.g., school (or work) and at home. The symptoms must not be better accounted for by another mental disorder. For the Inattentive Type, at least 6 of the following symptoms must have persisted for at least 6 months: lack of attention to details/careless mistakes; lack of sustained attention; poor listener; failure to follow through on tasks; poor organization; avoids tasks requiring sustained mental effort; loses things; easily distracted; forgetful. For the Hyperactive-Impulsive Type, at least 6 of the following symptoms must have persisted for at least 6 months: fidgeting/squirming; leaving seat; inappropriate running/climbing; difficulty with quiet activities; "on the go"; excessive talking; blurting answers; can't wait turn; intrusive. The Combined Types requires both inattentive and hyperactive-impulsive criteria to be met.

Special Diagnostic Considerations

Specific etiology of this syndrome is unknown, and there is no single diagnostic test. Adequate diagnosis requires the use not only of medical but of special psychological, educational, and social resources. Learning may or may not be impaired. The diagnosis must be based upon a complete history and evaluation of the child and not solely on the presence of the required number of DSM-IV characteristics.

Need for Comprehensive Treatment Program

Focalin XR is indicated as an integral part of a total treatment program for ADHD that may include other measures (psychological, educational, social) for patients with this syndrome. Drug treatment may not be indicated for all children with this syndrome. Stimulants are not intended for use in the child who exhibits symptoms secondary to environmental factors and/or other primary psychiatric disorders, including psychosis. Appropriate educational placement is essential and psychosocial intervention is often helpful. When remedial measures alone are insufficient, the decision to prescribe stimulant medication will depend upon the physician's assessment of the chronicity and severity of the child's symptoms.

Long-Term Use

The effectiveness of Focalin XR for long-term use, i.e., for more than 7 weeks, has not been systematically evaluated in controlled trials. Therefore, the physician who elects to use Focalin XR for extended periods should periodically re-evaluate the long-term usefulness of the drug for the individual patient [see Dosage and Administration (2.3)].

2 DOSAGE AND ADMINISTRATION

Focalin XR is for oral administration once daily in the morning.

Focalin XR may be swallowed as whole capsules or alternatively may be administered by sprinkling the capsule contents on a small amount of applesauce (see specific instructions below). Focalin XR capsules and/or their contents should not be crushed, chewed, or divided.

The capsules may be carefully opened and the beads sprinkled over a spoonful of applesauce. The mixture of drug and applesauce should be consumed immediately in its entirety. The drug and applesauce mixture should not be stored for future use.

Dosage should be individualized according to the needs and responses of the patient.

2.1 Patients New to Methylphenidate

The recommended starting dose of Focalin XR for patients who are not currently taking dexmethylphenidate or racemic methylphenidate, or for patients who are on stimulants other than methylphenidate, is 5 mg/day for pediatric patients and 10 mg/day for adult patients.

Dosage may be adjusted in 5 mg increments for pediatric patients and in 10 mg increments for adult patients. In general, dosage adjustments may proceed at approximately weekly intervals. The patient should be observed for a sufficient duration at a given dose to ensure that a maximal benefit has been achieved before a dose increase is considered. In dose-response (fixed-dose) studies (pediatric from 10 to 30 mg/day and adult from 20 to 40 mg/day), all doses were effective vs. placebo. There was no clear finding, however, of greater average benefits for the higher doses compared to the lower doses. Adverse events and discontinuations, however, were dose-related. Doses above 30 mg/day in pediatrics and 40 mg/day in adults have not been studied and are not recommended.

2.2 Patients Currently Using Methylphenidate

For patients currently using methylphenidate, the recommended starting dose of Focalin XR is half the total daily dose of racemic methylphenidate. Patients currently using Focalin (dexmethylphenidate) may be switched to the same daily dose of Focalin XR.

2.3 Maintenance/Extended Treatment

There is no body of evidence available from controlled trials to indicate how long the patient with ADHD should be treated with Focalin XR. It is generally agreed, however, that pharmacological treatment of ADHD may be needed for extended periods. Nevertheless, the physician who elects to use Focalin XR for extended periods in patients with ADHD should periodically reevaluate the long-term usefulness of the drug for the individual patient with periods off medication to assess the patient's functioning without pharmacotherapy. Improvement may be sustained when the drug is either temporarily or permanently discontinued.

2.4 Dose Reduction and Discontinuation

If paradoxical aggravation of symptoms or other adverse events occur, the dosage should be reduced, or, if necessary, the drug should be discontinued.

If improvement is not observed after appropriate dosage adjustment over a 1-month period, the drug should be discontinued.

3 DOSAGE FORMS AND STRENGTHS

5 mg extended-release capsules
10 mg extended-release capsules
15 mg extended-release capsules
20 mg extended-release capsules
25 mg extended-release capsules
30 mg extended-release capsules
35 mg extended-release capsules
40 mg extended-release capsules

4 CONTRAINDICATIONS

4.1 Agitation

Focalin XR is contraindicated in patients with marked anxiety, tension, and agitation, since the drug may aggravate these symptoms.

4.2 Hypersensitivity to Methylphenidate

Focalin XR is contraindicated in patients known to be hypersensitive to methylphenidate, or other components of the product. Hypersensitivity reactions, including angioedema and anaphylactic reactions, have been observed in patients treated with methylphenidate [see Adverse Reactions (6.5, 6.6)].

4.3 Glaucoma

Focalin XR is contraindicated in patients with glaucoma.

4.4 Tics

Focalin XR is contraindicated in patients with motor tics or with a family history or diagnosis of Tourette's syndrome [see Adverse Reactions (6.1)].

4.5 Monoamine Oxidase Inhibitors

Focalin XR is contraindicated during treatment with monoamine oxidase inhibitors, and also within a minimum of 14 days following discontinuation of treatment with a monoamine oxidase inhibitor (hypertensive crises may result).

5 WARNINGS AND PRECAUTIONS

5.1 Sudden Death and Preexisting Structural Cardiac Abnormalities or Other Serious Heart Problems

Children and Adolescents

Sudden death has been reported in association with CNS stimulant treatment at usual doses in children and adolescents with structural cardiac abnormalities or other serious heart problems. Although some serious heart problems alone carry an increased risk of sudden death, stimulant products generally should not be used in children or adolescents with known serious structural cardiac abnormalities, cardiomyopathy, serious heart rhythm abnormalities, or other serious cardiac problems that may place them at increased vulnerability to the sympathomimetic effects of a stimulant drug.

Adults

Sudden death, stroke, and myocardial infarction have been reported in adults taking stimulant drugs at usual doses for ADHD. Although the role of stimulants in these adult cases is also unknown, adults have a greater likelihood than children of having serious structural cardiac abnormalities, cardiomyopathy, serious heart rhythm abnormalities, coronary artery disease, or other serious cardiac problems. Adults with such abnormalities should also generally not be treated with stimulant drugs.

5.2 Hypertension and Other Cardiovascular Conditions

Stimulant medications cause a modest increase in average blood pressure (about 2-4 mmHg) and average heart rate (about 3-6 bpm), and individuals may have larger increases. While the mean changes alone would not be expected to have short-term consequences, all patients should be monitored for larger changes in heart rate and blood pressure. Caution is indicated in treating patients whose underlying medical conditions might be compromised by increases in blood pressure or heart rate, e.g., those with preexisting hypertension, heart failure, recent myocardial infarction, or ventricular arrhythmia.

5.3 Assessing Cardiovascular Status in Patients being Treated with Stimulant Medications

Children, adolescents, or adults who are being considered for treatment with stimulant medications should have a careful history (including assessment for a family history of sudden death or ventricular arrhythmia) and physical exam to assess for the presence of cardiac disease, and should receive further cardiac evaluation if findings suggest such disease (e.g., electrocardiogram and echocardiogram). Patients who develop symptoms such as exertional chest pain, unexplained syncope, or other symptoms suggestive of cardiac disease during stimulant treatment should undergo a prompt cardiac evaluation.

5.4 Preexisting Psychosis

Administration of stimulants may exacerbate symptoms of behavior disturbance and thought disorder in patients with a preexisting psychotic disorder.

5.5 Bipolar Illness

Particular care should be taken in using stimulants to treat ADHD in patients with comorbid bipolar disorder because of concern for possible induction of a mixed/manic episode in such patients. Prior to initiating treatment with a stimulant, patients with comorbid depressive symptoms should be adequately screened to determine if they are at risk for bipolar disorder; such screening should include a detailed psychiatric history, including a family history of suicide, bipolar disorder, and depression.

5.6 Emergence of New Psychotic or Manic Symptoms

Treatment emergent psychotic or manic symptoms, e.g., hallucinations, delusional thinking, or mania in children and adolescents without a prior history of psychotic illness or mania can be caused by stimulants at usual doses. If such symptoms occur, consideration should be given to a possible causal role of the stimulant, and discontinuation of treatment may be appropriate. In a pooled analysis of multiple short-term, placebo-controlled studies, such symptoms occurred in about 0.1% (4 patients with events out of 3,482 exposed to methylphenidate or amphetamine for several weeks at usual doses) of stimulant-treated patients compared to 0 in placebo-treated patients.

5.7 Aggression

Aggressive behavior or hostility is often observed in children and adolescents with ADHD, and has been reported in clinical trials and the post marketing experience of some medications indicated for the treatment of ADHD. Although there is no systematic evidence that stimulants cause aggressive behavior or hostility, patients beginning treatment for ADHD should be monitored for the appearance of or worsening of aggressive behavior or hostility.

Long-Term Suppression of Growth

[partially obscured] nonmeasure-up of weight and height in children ages 7 to in nature randomized to either methylphenidate or and nonmedication treatment groups over 14 months, as well as ages of 10 to 13 groups of newly methylphenidate-treated children (i.e., treated children over 36 months (to the year) have a temporary or 7 days per week throughout the a total of about 2 cm growing in growth rate (on average, growth in weight over 3 growth in height and 2.7 kg less rebound during this period without evidence of growth double-blind, placebo-controlled week study of Focalin XR, the mean weight gain was greater (+0.4 kg) than for patients receiving receiving placebo Focalin XR (-0.5 kg). Published data are inadequate chronic use of amphetamines may cause whether sion of growth, however, it is anticipated similar suppression have this effect as well. Therefore, growth at they likely tored during treatment with stimulants, and should be monitored are not growing or gaining height or weight patients who may need to have their treatment interrupted. expected

5.9 Seizures

There is some clinical evidence that stimulants may lower the convulsive threshold in patients with prior history of seizures, in patients with prior EEG abnormalities in absence of seizures, and, very rarely, in patients without a history of seizures and no prior EEG evidence of seizures. In the presence of seizures, the drug should be discontinued.

5.10 Priapism

Prolonged and painful erections, sometimes requiring surgical intervention, have been reported with methylphenidate products in both pediatric and adult patients. Priapism was not reported with drug initiation but developed after some time on the drug, often subsequent to an increase in dose. Priapism has also appeared during a period of drug withdrawal (drug holidays or during discontinuation). Patients who develop abnormally sustained or frequent and painful erections should seek immediate medical attention.

5.11 Peripheral Vasculopathy, Including Raynaud's Phenomenon

Stimulants, including Focalin XR, used to treat ADHD are associated with peripheral vasculopathy, including Raynaud's phenomenon. Signs and symptoms are usually intermittent and mild; however, very rare sequelae include digital ulceration and/or soft tissue breakdown. Effects of peripheral vasculopathy, including Raynaud's phenomenon, were observed in postmarketing reports at different times and at therapeutic doses in all age groups throughout the course of treatment. Signs and symptoms generally improve after reduction in dose or discontinuation of drug. Careful observation for digital changes is necessary during treatment with ADHD stimulants. Further clinical evaluation (e.g., rheumatology referral) may be appropriate for certain patients.

5.12 Visual Disturbance

Difficulties with accommodation and blurring of vision have been reported with stimulant treatment.

5.13 Use in Children Under Six Years of Age

Focalin XR should not be used in children under 6 years of age, since safety and efficacy in this age group have not been established.

5.14 Hematologic Monitoring

Periodic CBC, differential, and platelet counts are advised during prolonged therapy.

6 ADVERSE REACTIONS

Focalin XR was administered to 46 children and 7 adolescents with ADHD for up to 7 weeks and 206 adults with ADHD in clinical studies. During the clinical studies, 101 adult patients were treated for at least 6 months.

Adverse events during exposure were obtained primarily by general inquiry and recorded by clinical investigators using terminology of their own choosing. Consequently, it is not possible to provide a meaningful estimate of the proportion of individuals experiencing adverse events without first grouping similar types of events into a smaller number of standardized event categories. In the tables and listings that follow, MedDRA terminology has been used to classify reported adverse events. The stated frequencies of adverse events represent the proportion of individuals who experienced, at least once, a treatment-emergent adverse event of the type listed. An event was considered treatment emergent if it occurred for the first time or worsened while receiving therapy following baseline evaluation.

6.1 Adverse Events Associated with Discontinuation of Treatment in Acute Clinical Studies with Focalin XR- Children

Overall, 50 of 684 children treated with Focalin immediate-release formulation (7.3%) experienced an adverse event that resulted in discontinuation. The most common reasons

Help Patients Save on Rx Drugs: PDR.net/PharmacyDiscountCard

for discontinuation were twitching (described anatximately 1% each). None of the 53 Focalin XR-vocal tics), anorexia, insomnia, and tachycarents in ric patients discontinued treatment due to ... of 5% or the 7-week, placebo-controlled study.

6.2   Adverse Events Occurring at an ... dren
More Among Focalin XR-Treated Pat;... ...rse events for
Table 1 enumerates treatment-emer... ly in children and the placebo-controlled, parallel-gr... ocalin XR doses of adolescents with ADHD at fle... ly those events that 5-30 mg/day. The table incl...treated with Focalin XR occurred in 5% or more of p...ients treated with Focalin and for which the inciden...ience in placebo-treated pa-XR was at least twice th... be aware that these figures tients. The prescriber ...e incidence of adverse events in cannot be used to pr...cal practice where patient charac-the course of usua...lors differ from those which prevailed teristics and oth... Similarly, the cited frequencies cannot in the clinical ...figures obtained from other clinical inves-be compared,...ing different treatments, uses, and investigations in...ted figures, however, do provide the prescrib-gators. Th...ian with some basis for estimating the relative ing ph...tion of drug and nondrug factors to the adverse contr...incidence rate in the population studied.
even...

able 1.Treatment-Emergent Adverse Events[1] Occurring During Double-Blind Treatment–Pediatric Patients

	Focalin XR N=53	Placebo N=47
No. of Patients with AEs		
Total	76%	57%
Primary System Organ Class/ Adverse Event Preferred Term		
Gastrointestinal Disorders	38%	19%
Dyspepsia	8%	4%
Metabolism and Nutrition Disorders	34%	11%
Decreased Appetite	30%	9%
Nervous System Disorders	30%	13%
Headache	25%	11%
Psychiatric Disorders	26%	15%
Anxiety	6%	0%

[1]Events, regardless of causality, for which the incidence for patients treated with Focalin XR was at least 5% and twice the incidence among placebo-treated patients. Incidence has been rounded to the nearest whole number.

Table 2 below enumerates the incidence of dose-related adverse events that occurred during a fixed-dose, double-blind, placebo-controlled trial of Focalin XR up to 30mg/day versus placebo in children and adolescents with ADHD.
[See table 2 above]

6.3   Adverse Events Associated with Discontinuation of Treatment in Clinical Studies with Focalin XR-Adults
In the adult placebo-controlled study, 10.7% of the Focalin XR-treated patients and 7.5% of the placebo-treated patients discontinued for adverse events. Among Focalin XR-treated patients, insomnia (1.8%, n=3), feeling jittery (1.8%, n=3), anorexia (1.2%, n=2), and anxiety (1.2%, n=2) were the reasons for discontinuation reported by more than 1 patient.

6.4   Adverse Events Occurring at an Incidence of 5% or More Among Focalin XR-Treated Patients-Adults
Table 3 enumerates treatment-emergent adverse events for the placebo-controlled, parallel-group study in adults with ADHD at fixed Focalin XR doses of 20, 30, and 40 mg/day. The table includes only those events that occurred in 5% or more of patients in a Focalin XR dose group and for which the incidences in patients treated with Focalin XR appeared to increase with dose. The prescriber should be aware that these figures cannot be used to predict the incidence of adverse events in the course of usual medical practice where patient characteristics and other factors differ from those which prevailed in the clinical trials. Similarly, the cited frequencies cannot be compared with figures obtained from other clinical investigations involving different treatments, uses, and investigators. The cited figures, however, do provide the prescribing physician with some basis for estimating the relative contribution of drug and non-drug factors to the adverse event incidence rate in the population studied.
[See table 3 above]
Two other adverse reactions occurring in clinical trials with Focalin XR at a frequency greater than placebo, but which were not dose related were: feeling jittery (12% and 2%, respectively) and dizziness (6% and 2%, respectively).
Table 4 summarizes changes in vital signs and weight that were recorded in the adult study (N=218) of Focalin XR in the treatment of ADHD.
[See table 4 above]

Table 2. Dose-related Adverse Events from a Fixed-dose Study of Double-Blind Treatment in Pediatric Patients by Organ-System and Preferred Term

ADVERSE EVENT	Focalin XR 10 mg/d N=64	Focalin XR 20 mg/d N=60	Focalin XR 30 mg/d N=58	Placebo N=63
Gastrointestinal Disorders	22%	23%	29%	24%
Vomiting	2%	8%	9%	0
Metabolism and Nutritional Disorders	16%	17%	22%	5%
Anorexia	5%	5%	7%	0
Psychiatric Disorders	19%	20%	38%	8%
Insomnia	5%	8%	17%	3%
Depression	0	0	3%	0
Mood Swings	0	0	3%	2%
Other Adverse Events				
Irritability	0	2%	5%	0
Nasal Congestion	0	0	5%	0
Pruritus	0	0	3%	0

Table 3. Treatment-Emergent Adverse Events[1] Occurring During Double-Blind Treatment–Adults

	Focalin XR 20 mg N=57	Focalin XR 30 mg N=54	Focalin XR 40 mg N=54	Placebo N=53
No. of Patients with AEs				
Total	84%	94%	85%	68%
Primary System Organ Class/ Adverse Event Preferred Term				
Gastrointestinal Disorders	28%	32%	44%	19%
Dry Mouth	7%	20%	20%	4%
Dyspepsia	5%	9%	9%	2%
Nervous System Disorders	37%	39%	50%	28%
Headache	26%	30%	39%	19%
Psychiatric Disorders	40%	43%	46%	30%
Anxiety	5%	11%	11%	2%
Respiratory, Thoracic and Mediastinal Disorders	16%	9%	15%	8%
Pharyngolaryngeal Pain	4%	4%	7%	2%

[1]Events, regardless of causality, for which the incidence was at least 5% in a Focalin XR group and which appeared to increase with randomized dose. Incidence has been rounded to the nearest whole number.

Table 4. Changes (Mean ± SD) in Vital Signs and Weight by Randomized Dose During Double-Blind Treatment-Adults

	Focalin XR 20 mg (N=57)	Focalin XR 30 mg (N=54)	Focalin XR 40 mg (N=54)	Placebo (N=53)
Pulse (bpm)	3.1 ± 11.1	4.3 ± 11.7	6.0 ± 10.1	-1.4 ± 9.3
Diastolic BP (mmHg)	-0.2 ± 8.2	1.2 ± 8.9	2.1 ± 8.0	0.3 ± 7.8
Weight (kg)	-1.4 ± 2.0	-1.2 ± 1.9	-1.7 ± 2.3	-0.1 ± 3.9

6.5   Postmarketing Experience
The following additional adverse reactions have been identified during postapproval use of Focalin XR. Because these reactions are reported voluntarily from a population of uncertain size, it is not always possible to reliably estimate their frequency:
Immune System Disorders: hypersensitivity reactions, including angioedema and anaphylaxis

6.6   Adverse Events with Other Methylphenidate HCl Dosage Forms
Nervousness and insomnia are the most common adverse reactions reported with other methylphenidate products. In children, loss of appetite, abdominal pain, weight loss during prolonged therapy, insomnia, and tachycardia may occur more frequently; however, any of the other adverse reactions listed below may also occur.
Other reactions include:
Cardiac: angina, arrhythmia, palpitations, pulse increased or decreased, tachycardia
Gastrointestinal: abdominal pain, nausea
Immune: hypersensitivity reactions including skin rash, urticaria, fever, arthralgia, exfoliative dermatitis, erythema multiforme with histopathological findings of necrotizing vasculitis, and thrombocytopenic purpura
Metabolism/Nutrition: anorexia, weight loss during prolonged therapy
Nervous System: dizziness, drowsiness, dyskinesia, headache, rare reports of Tourette's syndrome, toxic psychosis
Vascular: blood pressure increased or decreased, cerebral arteritis and/or occlusion
Although a definite causal relationship has not been established, the following have been reported in patients taking methylphenidate:
Blood/Lymphatic: leukopenia and/or anemia
Hepatobiliary: abnormal liver function, ranging from transaminase elevation to hepatic coma

Psychiatric: transient depressed mood, aggressive behavior, libido changes
Skin/Subcutaneous: scalp hair loss
Urogenital: priapism
Very rare reports of neuroleptic malignant syndrome (NMS) have been received, and, in most of these, patients were concurrently receiving therapies associated with NMS. In a single report, a 10-year-old boy who had been taking methylphenidate for approximately 18 months experienced an NMS-like event within 45 minutes of ingesting his first dose of venlafaxine. It is uncertain whether this case represented a drug-drug interaction, a response to either drug alone, or some other cause.

7   DRUG INTERACTIONS
Focalin XR should not be used in patients being treated (currently or within the preceding 2 weeks) with MAO Inhibitors [see Contraindications (4.5)].
Because of possible effects on blood pressure, Focalin XR should be used cautiously with pressor agents.
Methylphenidate may decrease the effectiveness of drugs used to treat hypertension.
Dexmethylphenidate is metabolized primarily to *d*-ritalinic acid by de-esterification and not through oxidative pathways.
The effects of gastrointestinal pH alterations on the absorption of dexmethylphenidate from Focalin XR have not been studied. Since the modified release characteristics of Focalin XR are pH dependent, the coadministration of antacids or acid suppressants could alter the release of dexmethylphenidate.
Human pharmacologic studies have shown that racemic methylphenidate may inhibit the metabolism of coumarin anticoagulants, anticonvulsants (e.g., phenobarbital, phenytoin, primidone), and tricyclic drugs (e.g., imipramine, clomipramine, desipramine). Downward dose adjustments of

these drugs may be required when given concomitantly with methylphenidate. It may be necessary to adjust the dosage and monitor plasma drug concentration (or, in the case of coumarin, coagulation times), when initiating or discontinuing methylphenidate.

8 USE IN SPECIFIC POPULATIONS

8.1 Pregnancy
Pregnancy Category C:
There are no adequate and well controlled studies of Focalin in pregnant women. Dexmethylphenidate did not cause major malformations in rats or rabbits; however, it did cause delayed skeletal ossification and decreased postweaning weight gain in rats. Focalin XR should be used during pregnancy only if the potential benefit justifies the potential risk to the fetus.

In studies conducted in rats and rabbits, dexmethylphenidate was administered orally at doses of up to 20 and 100 mg/kg/day, respectively, during the period of organogenesis. No evidence of teratogenic activity was found in either the rat or rabbit study; however, delayed fetal skeletal ossification was observed at the highest dose level in rats. When dexmethylphenidate was administered to rats throughout pregnancy and lactation at doses of up to 20 mg/kg/day, postweaning body weight gain was decreased in male offspring at the highest dose, but no other effects on postnatal development were observed. At the highest doses tested, plasma levels (AUCs) of dexmethylphenidate in pregnant rats and rabbits were approximately 5 and 1 times, respectively, those in adults dosed with 20 mg/day. Racemic methylphenidate has been shown to have teratogenic effects in rabbits when given in doses of 200 mg/kg/day throughout organogenesis.

8.2 Labor and Delivery
Focalin XR has not been studied in labor and delivery.

8.3 Nursing Mothers
It is not known whether dexmethylphenidate is excreted in human milk. Because many drugs are excreted in human milk, caution should be exercised if Focalin XR is administered to a nursing woman. Information from 4 published case reports on the use of racemic methylphenidate during breastfeeding suggest that at maternal doses of 35-80 mg/day, milk concentrations of methylphenidate range from undetectable to 15.4 ng/mL. Based on these limited data, the calculated infant daily dose for an exclusively breastfed infant would be about 0.4-2.9 µg/kg/day or about 0.2-0.7% of the maternal weight adjusted dose.

8.4 Pediatric Use
The safety and efficacy of Focalin XR in children under 6 years old have not been established. Long-term effects of Focalin in children have not been well established [see *Warnings and Precautions (5.13)*].

In a study conducted in young rats, racemic methylphenidate was administered orally at doses of up to 100 mg/kg/day for 9 weeks, starting early in the postnatal period (Postnatal Day 7) and continuing through sexual maturity (Postnatal Week 10). When these animals were tested as adults (Postnatal Weeks 13-14), decreased spontaneous locomotor activity was observed in males and females previously treated with 50 mg/kg/day (approximately 6 times the maximum recommended human dose [MRHD] of racemic methylphenidate on a mg/m^2 basis) or greater, and a deficit in the acquisition of a specific learning task was seen in females exposed to the highest dose (12 times the racemic MRHD on a mg/m^2 basis). The no effect dose for juvenile neurobehavioral development in rats was 5 mg/kg/day (half the racemic MRHD on a mg/m^2 basis). The clinical significance of the long-term behavioral effects observed in rats is unknown.

8.5 Geriatric Use
Focalin XR has not been studied in the geriatric population.

9 DRUG ABUSE AND DEPENDENCE

9.1 Controlled Substance Class
Focalin XR, like other methylphenidate products, is classified as a Schedule II controlled substance by Federal regulation.

9.2 Abuse, Dependence, Tolerance
See the complete boxed warning for drug abuse and dependence information at the beginning of *Full Prescribing Information*.

10 OVERDOSAGE

10.1 Signs and Symptoms
Signs and symptoms of acute methylphenidate overdosage, resulting principally from overstimulation of the CNS and from excessive sympathomimetic effects, may include the following: vomiting, agitation, tremors, hyperreflexia, muscle twitching, convulsions (may be followed by coma), euphoria, confusion, hallucinations, delirium, sweating, flushing, headache, hyperpyrexia, tachycardia, palpitations, cardiac arrhythmias, hypertension, mydriasis, and dryness of mucous membranes.

10.2 Poison Control Center
The physician may wish to consider contacting a poison control center for up-to-date information on the management of overdosage with methylphenidate.

10.3 Recommended Treatment
As with the management of all overdosage, the possibility of multiple drug ingestion should be considered.

When treating overdose, practitioners should bear in mind that there is a prolonged release of dexmethylphenidate from Focalin XR.

Treatment consists of appropriate supportive measures. The patient must be protected against self-injury and against external stimuli that would aggravate overstimulation already present. Gastric contents may be evacuated by gastric lavage as indicated. Before performing gastric lavage, control agitation and seizures if present and protect the airway. Other measures to detoxify the gut include administration of activated charcoal and a cathartic. Intensive care must be provided to maintain adequate circulation and respiratory exchange; external cooling procedures may be required for hyperpyrexia.

Efficacy of peritoneal dialysis for Focalin overdosage has not been established.

11 DESCRIPTION

Focalin XR is an extended-release formulation of dexmethylphenidate with a bi-modal release profile. Focalin XR uses the proprietary SODAS® (Spheroidal Oral Drug Absorption System) technology. Each bead-filled Focalin XR capsule contains half the dose as immediate-release beads and half as enteric-coated, delayed-release beads, thus providing an immediate release of dexmethylphenidate and a second delayed release of dexmethylphenidate. Focalin XR is available as 5, 10, 15, 20, 25, 30, 35, and 40 mg extended-release capsules. Focalin XR 5, 10, 15, 20, 25, 30, 35, and 40 mg extended-release capsules provide in a single dose the same amount of dexmethylphenidate as dosages of 2.5, 5, 7.5, 10, 12.5, 15, 17.5, or 20 mg of Focalin given b.i.d. as tablets.

Dexmethylphenidate hydrochloride, the *d-threo* enantiomer of racemic methylphenidate hydrochloride, is a central nervous system (CNS) stimulant.

Dexmethylphenidate hydrochloride is methyl α-phenyl-2-piperidineacetate hydrochloride, (R,R')-(+)-. Its empirical formula is $C_{14}H_{19}NO_2 \cdot HCl$. Its molecular weight is 269.77 and its structural formula is:

Note* = asymmetric carbon center

Dexmethylphenidate hydrochloride is a white to off white powder. Its solutions are acid to litmus. It is freely soluble in water and in methanol, soluble in alcohol, and slightly soluble in chloroform and in acetone.

Inactive ingredients: ammonio methacrylate copolymer, FD&C Blue #2 (5 mg, 15 mg, 25 mg, 35 mg, and 40 mg strengths), FDA/E172 yellow iron oxide (10 mg, 15 mg, 30 mg, 35 mg, and 40 mg strengths), gelatin, ink Tan SW-8010, methacrylic acid copolymer, polyethylene glycol, sugar spheres, talc, titanium dioxide, and triethyl citrate.

12 CLINICAL PHARMACOLOGY

12.1 Mechanism of Action
Dexmethylphenidate hydrochloride, the active ingredient in Focalin XR, is a central nervous system stimulant. Dexmethylphenidate, the more pharmacologically active *d*-enantiomer of racemic methylphenidate, is thought to block the reuptake of norepinephrine and dopamine into the presynaptic neuron and increase the release of these monoamines into the extraneuronal space. The mode of therapeutic action in Attention Deficit Hyperactivity Disorder (ADHD) is not known.

12.2 Pharmacodynamics
Effects on QT Interval
The effect of Focalin XR on the QT interval was evaluated in a double-blind, placebo- and open-label active (moxifloxacin)-controlled study following single doses of Focalin XR 40mg in 75 healthy volunteers. ECGs were collected up to 12 hours postdose. Frederica's method for heart rate correction was employed to derive the corrected QT interval (QTcF). The maximum mean prolongation of QTcF intervals was <5 ms, and the upper limit of the 90% confidence interval was below 10 ms for all time matched comparisons versus placebo. This was below the threshold of clinical concern and there was no evident-exposure response relationship.

12.3 Pharmacokinetics
Absorption
Focalin XR produces a bi-modal plasma concentration-time profile (i.e., 2 distinct peaks approximately 4 hours apart) when orally administered to healthy adults. The initial rate of absorption for Focalin XR is similar to that of Focalin tablets as shown by the similar rate parameters between the 2 formulations, i.e., first peak concentration (C_{max1}), and time to the first peak (t_{max1}), which is reached in 1.5 hours (typ-

ical range 1-4 hours). The mean time to the interpeak minimum (t_{minip}) is slightly shorter, and time to the second peak (t_{max2}) is slightly longer for Focalin XR given once daily (about 6.5 hours, range 4.5-7 hours) compared to Focalin tablets given in 2 doses 4 hours apart (see Figure 1), although the ranges observed are greater for Focalin XR. Focalin XR given once daily exhibits a lower second peak concentration (C_{max2}), higher interpeak minimum concentrations (C_{minip}), and fewer peak and trough fluctuations than Focalin tablets given in 2 doses given 4 hours apart. This is due to an earlier onset and more prolonged absorption from the delayed-release beads (see Figure 1).

The AUC (exposure) after administration of Focalin XR given once daily is equivalent to the same total dose of Focalin tablets given in 2 doses 4 hours apart. The variability in C_{max}, C_{min}, and AUC is similar between Focalin XR and Focalin IR with approximately a 3-fold range in each. Radiolabeled racemic methylphenidate is well absorbed after oral administration with approximately 90% of the radioactivity recovered in urine. However, due to first pass metabolism the mean absolute bioavailability of dexmethylphenidate when administered in various formulations was 22%-25%.

Figure 1. Mean Dexmethylphenidate Plasma Concentration-Time Profiles After Administration of 1 x 20 mg Focalin XR (n=24) Capsules and 2 x 10 mg Focalin Immediate-Release Tablets (n=25)

Dose Proportionality
Dose proportionality of Focalin XR was evaluated in a randomized, single-dose, 5-period, cross-over study with administration of single doses of 5, 10, 20, 30, and 40 mg to healthy adults. Results confirmed dose proportionality within this dose range.

Food Effects
Administration times relative to meals and meal composition may need to be individually titrated.

No food effect study was performed with Focalin XR. However, the effect of food has been studied in adults with racemic methylphenidate in the same type of extended-release formulation. The findings of that study are considered applicable to Focalin XR. After a high fat breakfast, there was a longer lag time until absorption began and variable delays in the time until the first peak concentration, the time until the interpeak minimum, and the time until the second peak. The first peak concentration and the extent of absorption were unchanged after food relative to the fasting state, although the second peak was approximately 25% lower. The effect of a high fat lunch was not examined. There is no evidence of dose dumping in the presence or absence of food. There were no differences in the plasma concentration-time profile, when administered with applesauce, compared to administration in the fasting condition. The results are expected not to differ for Focalin XR.

For patients unable to swallow the capsule, the contents may be sprinkled on applesauce and administered [see *Dosage and Administration (2)*].

Distribution
The plasma protein binding of dexmethylphenidate is not known; racemic methylphenidate is bound to plasma proteins by 12%-15%, independent of concentration. Dexmethylphenidate shows a volume of distribution of 2.65±1.11 L/kg. Plasma dexmethylphenidate concentrations decline monophasically following oral administration of Focalin XR.

Metabolism and Excretion
In humans, dexmethylphenidate is metabolized primarily to *d*-α-phenyl-piperidine acetic acid (also known as *d*-ritalinic acid) by de-esterification. This metabolite has little or no pharmacological activity. There is no *in vivo* interconversion to the *l-threo*-enantiomer, based on a finding of no levels of *l-threo*-methylphenidate being detectable after administration of up to 40 mg dexmethylphenidate in adults. After oral dosing of radiolabeled racemic methylphenidate in humans, about 90% of the radioactivity was recovered in urine. The main urinary metabolite of racemic (*d,l-*) methylphenidate was *d,l*-ritalinic acid, accountable for approximately 80% of the dose. Urinary excretion of parent compound accounted for 0.5% of an intravenous dose.

In vitro studies showed that dexmethylphenidate did not inhibit cytochrome P450 isoenzymes at concentrations observed after therapeutic doses.

Intravenous dexmethylphenidate was eliminated with a mean clearance of 0.40 ± 0.12 L/kg.h^{-1} corresponding to 0.56 ± 0.18 L/min. The mean terminal elimination half-life of dexmethylphenidate was just over 3 hours in healthy adults and typically varied between 2 and 4.5 hours with an occasional subject exhibiting a terminal half-life between 5 and 7 hours. Children tend to have slightly shorter half-lives with means of 2–3 hours.

Special Populations
Gender
After administration of Focalin XR the first peak, (C_{max1}), was on average 45% higher in women. The interpeak minimum and the second peak also tended to be slightly higher in women although the difference was not statistically significant, and these patterns remained even after weight normalization. Pharmacokinetic parameters for dexmethylphenidate after Focalin immediate-release tablets were similar for boys and girls.

Race
There is insufficient experience with the use of Focalin XR to detect ethnic variations in pharmacokinetics.

Age
The pharmacokinetics of dexmethylphenidate after Focalin XR administration have not been studied in children less than 18 years of age. When a similar formulation of racemic methylphenidate was examined in 15 children between 10 and 12 years of age and 3 children with ADHD between 7 and 9 years of age, the time to the first peak was similar, although the time until the between peak minimum, and the time until the second peak were delayed and more variable in children compared to adults. After administration of the same dose to children and adults, concentrations in children were approximately twice the concentrations observed in adults. This higher exposure is almost completely due to smaller body size as no relevant age-related differences in dexmethylphenidate pharmacokinetic parameters (i.e., clearance and volume of distribution) are observed after normalization to dose and weight.

Renal Insufficiency
There is no experience with the use of Focalin XR in patients with renal insufficiency. After oral administration of radiolabeled racemic methylphenidate in humans, methylphenidate was extensively metabolized and approximately 80% of the radioactivity was excreted in the urine in the form of racemic ritalinic acid which is pharmacologically inactive. Very little unchanged drug is excreted in the urine, thus renal insufficiency is expected to have little effect on the pharmacokinetics of Focalin XR.

Hepatic Insufficiency
There is no experience with the use of Focalin XR in patients with hepatic insufficiency *[see Drug Interactions (7)].*

13   NONCLINICAL TOXICOLOGY
13.1 Carcinogenesis, Mutagenesis, and Impairment of Fertility
Carcinogenesis
Lifetime carcinogenicity studies have not been carried out with dexmethylphenidate. In a lifetime carcinogenicity study carried out in B6C3F1 mice, racemic methylphenidate caused an increase in hepatocellular adenomas, and in males only, an increase in hepatoblastomas at a daily dose of approximately 60 mg/kg/day. Hepatoblastoma is a relatively rare rodent malignant tumor type. There was no increase in total malignant hepatic tumors. The mouse strain used is sensitive to the development of hepatic tumors, and the significance of these results to humans is unknown.

Racemic methylphenidate did not cause any increase in tumors in a lifetime carcinogenicity study carried out in F344 rats; the highest dose used was approximately 45 mg/kg/day.

In a 24-week study of racemic methylphenidate in the transgenic mouse strain p53+/-, which is sensitive to genotoxic carcinogens, there was no evidence of carcinogenicity. Mice were fed diets containing the same concentrations as in the lifetime carcinogenicity study; the high-dose group was exposed to 60-74 mg/kg/day of racemic methylphenidate.

Mutagenesis
Dexmethylphenidate was not mutagenic in the *in vitro* Ames reverse mutation assay, the *in vitro* mouse lymphoma cell forward mutation assay, or the *in vivo* mouse bone marrow micronucleus test.

Racemic methylphenidate was not mutagenic in the *in vitro* Ames reverse mutation assay or the *in vitro* mouse lymphoma cell forward mutation assay, and was negative *in vivo* in the mouse bone marrow micronucleus assay. However, sister chromatid exchanges and chromosome aberrations were increased, indicative of a weak clastogenic response, in an *in vitro* assay of racemic methylphenidate in cultured Chinese Hamster Ovary (CHO) cells.

Impairment of Fertility
Racemic methylphenidate did not impair fertility in male or female mice that were fed diets containing the drug in an 18-week Continuous Breeding study. The study was conducted at doses of up to 160 mg/kg/day.

14   CLINICAL STUDIES
The effectiveness of Focalin XR in the treatment of ADHD was established in randomized, double-blind, placebo-controlled studies in children and adolescents and in adults who met Diagnostic and Statistical Manual 4th edition (DSM-IV) criteria for ADHD *[see Indications and Usage (1)].*

14.1 Children and Adolescents
The effectiveness of Focalin XR was established in a randomized, double-blind, placebo-controlled, parallel-group study in 103 pediatric patients (ages 6 to 12, n=86; ages 13 to 17, n=17) who met DSM-IV criteria for ADHD. Patients were randomized to receive either a flexible dose of Focalin XR (5 to 30 mg/day) or placebo once daily for 7 weeks. During the first 5 weeks of treatment patients were titrated to their optimal dose and in the last 2 weeks of the study patients remained on their optimal dose without dose changes or interruption.

Signs and symptoms of ADHD were evaluated by comparing the mean change from baseline to endpoint for Focalin XR– and placebo-treated patients using an intent-to-treat analysis of the primary efficacy outcome measure, the DSM-IV total subscale score of the Conners ADHD/DSM-IV Scales for teachers (CADS-T).

There was a statistically significant treatment effect in favor of Focalin XR. There were insufficient adolescents enrolled in this study to assess the efficacy for Focalin XR in the adolescent population. However, pharmacokinetic considerations and evidence of effectiveness of immediate-release Focalin in adolescents support the effectiveness of Focalin XR in this population.

In 2 additional studies in pediatric patients aged 6-12 years who received 20 mg Focalin XR or placebo in a cross-over design, Focalin XR was found to have a statistically significant treatment effect versus placebo on the Swanson, Kotkin, Agler, M-Flynn & Pelham (SKAMP) rating scale combined score at all time points after dosing in each study (0.5, 1, 3, 4, 5, 7, 9, 10, 11, and 12 hours in one study and 1, 2, 4, 6, 8, 9, 10, 11, and 12 hours in the other study). A treatment effect was also observed 0.5 hours after administration of Focalin XR 20 mg in an additional study of ADHD patients aged 6-12 years. The SKAMP is a reliable and validated scale that assesses specific classroom behaviors related to attention (e.g., getting started, sticking with activities, completing work, and stopping for transition) and deportment or behavior (e.g., remaining quiet, remaining seated, interacting with other students, and interacting with the teacher.) Each item is rated on a 7-point impairment scale, and an average rating per item is calculated for the subscales of Attention and Deportment.

14.2 Adults
The effectiveness of Focalin XR was established in a randomized, double-blind, placebo-controlled, parallel-group study in 221 adult patients (ages 18 to 60) who met DSM-IV criteria for ADHD. Patients were randomized to receive either a fixed dose of Focalin XR (20, 30, or 40 mg/day) or placebo once daily for 5 weeks. Patients randomized to Focalin XR were initiated on a 10 mg/day starting dose and titrated in increments of 10 mg/week to the randomly assigned fixed dose. Patients were maintained on their fixed dose (20, 30, or 40 mg/day) for a minimum of 2 weeks.

Signs and symptoms of ADHD were evaluated by comparing the mean change from baseline to endpoint for Focalin XR– and placebo-treated patients using an intent-to-treat analysis of the primary efficacy outcome measure, the investigator-administered DSM-IV Attention-Deficit/Hyperactivity Disorder Rating Scale (DSM-IV ADHD RS).

All three Focalin XR doses were statistically significantly superior to placebo. There was no obvious increase in effectiveness with increasing dose.

15   REFERENCES
American Psychiatric Association. Diagnosis and Statistical Manual of Mental Disorders. 4th ed. Washington DC: American Psychiatric Association 1994.

16   HOW SUPPLIED/STORAGE AND HANDLING
5 mg Extended-Release Capsules (NDC 0078-0430-05) light-blue, (imprinted NVR D5) supplied in bottles of 100

10 mg Extended-Release Capsules (NDC 0078-0431-05) light caramel (imprinted NVR D10) supplied in bottles of 100

15 mg Extended-Release Capsules (NDC 0078-0493-05) green (imprinted NVR D15) supplied in bottles of 100

20 mg Extended-Release Capsules (NDC 0078-0432-05) white (imprinted NVR D20) supplied in bottles of 100

25 mg Extended-Release Capsules (NDC 0078-0608-05) light-blue and white (imprinted NVR D25) supplied in bottles of 100

30 mg Extended-Release Capsules (NDC 0078-0433-05) light caramel and white (imprinted NVR D30) supplied in bottles of 100

35 mg Extended-Release Capsules (NDC 0078-0609-05) light-blue and light caramel (imprinted NVR D35) supplied in bottles of 100

40 mg Extended-Release Capsules (NDC 0078-0434-05) green and white (imprinted NVR D40) supplied in bottles of 100

Store FOCALIN XR at 25°C (77°F), excursions permitted 15°-30°C (59°-86°F). [See USP Controlled Room Temperature.]

Dispense in tight container (USP).

17   PATIENT COUNSELING INFORMATION
17.1 Information for Patients
Prescribers or other health professionals should inform patients, their families, and their caregivers about the benefits and risks associated with treatment with dexmethylphenidate and should counsel them in its appropriate use. A patient Medication Guide is available for Focalin XR. The prescriber or health professional should instruct patients, their families, and their caregivers to read the Medication Guide and should assist them in understanding its contents. Patients should be given the opportunity to discuss the contents of the Medication Guide and to obtain answers to any questions they may have. The complete text of the Medication Guide is reprinted at the end of this document.

Priapism
Advise patients, caregivers, and family members of the possibility of painful or prolonged penile erections (priapism). Instruct the patient to seek immediate medical attention in the event of priapism *[see Warnings and Precautions (5.10)].*

Circulation problems in fingers and toes [Peripheral vasculopathy, including Raynaud's phenomenon]
- Instruct patients beginning treatment with Focalin XR about the risk of peripheral vasculopathy, including Raynaud's Phenomenon, and associated signs and symptoms: fingers or toes may feel numb, cool, painful, and/or may change color from pale, to blue, to red.
- Instruct patients to report to their physician any new numbness, pain, skin color change, or sensitivity to temperature in fingers or toes.
- **Instruct patients to call their physician immediately with any signs of unexplained wounds appearing on fingers or toes while taking Focalin XR.**
- Further clinical evaluation (e.g., rheumatology referral) may be appropriate for certain patients.

T2013-121
December 2013

MEDICATION GUIDE
FOCALIN XR
(dexmethylphenidate hydrochloride)
extended-release capsules CII
Read the Medication Guide that comes with FOCALIN XR before you or your child starts taking it and each time you get a refill. There may be new information. This Medication Guide does not take the place of talking to your doctor about your or your child's treatment with FOCALIN XR.

What is the most important information I should know about FOCALIN XR?
The following have been reported with use of dexmethylphenidate hydrochloride and other stimulant medicines.
1. Heart-related problems:
- **sudden death in patients who have heart problems or heart defects**
- **stroke and heart attack in adults**
- **increased blood pressure and heart rate**

Tell your doctor if you or your child have any heart problems, heart defects, high blood pressure, or a family history of these problems.
Your doctor should check you or your child carefully for heart problems before starting FOCALIN XR.
Your doctor should check your or your child's blood pressure and heart rate regularly during treatment with FOCALIN XR.
Call your doctor right away if you or your child has any signs of heart problems such as chest pain, shortness of breath, or fainting while taking FOCALIN XR.
2. Mental (Psychiatric) problems:
All Patients
- **new or worse behavior and thought problems**
- **new or worse bipolar illness**
- **new or worse aggressive behavior or hostility**

Children and Teenagers
- **new psychotic symptoms (such as hearing voices, believing things that are not true, are suspicious) or new manic symptoms**

Tell your doctor about any mental problems you or your child have, or about a family history of suicide, bipolar illness, or depression.

Call your doctor right away if you or your child have any new or worsening mental symptoms or problems while taking FOCALIN XR, especially seeing or hearing things that are not real, believing things that are not real, or are suspicious.

3. **Circulation problems in fingers and toes** [Peripheral vasculopathy, including Raynaud's phenomenon]: fingers or toes may feel numb, cool, painful, and/or may change color from pale, to blue, to red.

- Tell your doctor if you have or your child has numbness, pain, skin color change, or sensitivity to temperature in the fingers or toes.
- **Call your doctor right away if you have or your child has any signs of unexplained wounds appearing on fingers or toes while taking FOCALIN XR.**

What Is FOCALIN XR?

FOCALIN XR is a central nervous system stimulant prescription medicine. **It is used for the treatment of attention deficit and hyperactivity disorder (ADHD).** FOCALIN XR may help increase attention and decrease impulsiveness and hyperactivity in patients with ADHD.

FOCALIN XR should be used as a part of a total treatment program for ADHD that may include counseling or other therapies.

> **FOCALIN XR is a federally controlled substance (CII) because it can be abused or lead to dependence. Keep FOCALIN XR in a safe place to prevent misuse and abuse. Selling or giving away FOCALIN XR may harm others, and is against the law.**
>
> Tell your doctor if you or your child have (or have a family history of) ever abused or been dependent on alcohol, prescription medicines or street drugs.

Who should not take FOCALIN XR?
FOCALIN XR should not be taken if you or your child:

- are very anxious, tense, or agitated.
- have an eye problem called glaucoma.
- have tics or Tourette's syndrome, or a family history of Tourette's syndrome. Tics are hard-to-control repeated movements or sounds.
- are taking or have taken within the past 14 days an anti-depression medicine called a monoamine oxidase inhibitor or MAOI.
- are allergic to anything in FOCALIN XR. See the end of this Medication Guide for a complete list of ingredients.

FOCALIN XR should not be used in children less than 6 years old because it has not been studied in this age group.

FOCALIN XR may not be right for you or your child. Before starting FOCALIN XR tell your or your child's doctor about all health conditions (or a family history of) including:

- heart problems, heart defects, high blood pressure
- mental problems including psychosis, mania, bipolar illness, or depression
- tics or Tourette's syndrome
- seizures or have had an abnormal brain wave test (EEG)
- circulation problems in fingers or toes

Tell your doctor if you or your child is pregnant, planning to become pregnant, or breastfeeding.

Can FOCALIN XR be taken with other medicines?
Tell your doctor about all of the medicines that you or your child takes including prescription and nonprescription medicines, vitamins, and herbal supplements. FOCALIN XR and some medicines may interact with each other and cause serious side effects. Sometimes the doses of other medicines will need to be adjusted while taking FOCALIN XR.

Your doctor will decide whether FOCALIN XR can be taken with other medicines.

Especially tell your doctor if you or your child takes:

- anti-depression medicines including MAOIs
- seizure medicines
- blood thinner medicines
- blood pressure medicines
- antacids
- cold or allergy medicines that contain decongestants

Know the medicines that you or your child takes. Keep a list of your medicines with you to show your doctor and pharmacist.

Do not start any new medicine while taking FOCALIN XR without talking to your doctor first.

How should FOCALIN XR be taken?

- **Take FOCALIN XR exactly as prescribed.** Your doctor may adjust the dose until it is right for you or your child.
- Take FOCALIN XR once each day in the morning. FOCALIN XR is an extended-release capsule. It releases medicine into your body throughout the day.
- FOCALIN XR can be taken with or without food. Taking FOCALIN XR with food may slow the time it takes for the medicine to start working.

- Swallow FOCALIN XR capsules whole with water or other liquids. **Do not chew, crush, or divide the capsules or the beads in the capsule.** If you or your child cannot swallow the capsule, open it and sprinkle the small beads of medicine over a spoonful of applesauce and swallow it right away without chewing.
- From time to time, your doctor may stop FOCALIN XR treatment for a while to check ADHD symptoms.
- Your doctor may do regular checks of the blood, heart, and blood pressure while taking FOCALIN XR. Children should have their height and weight checked often while taking FOCALIN XR. FOCALIN XR treatment may be stopped if a problem is found during these check-ups.
- **If you or your child takes too much FOCALIN XR or overdoses, call your doctor or poison control center right away, or get emergency treatment.**

What are possible side effects of FOCALIN XR?
See "What is the most important information I should know about FOCALIN XR?" for information on reported heart and mental problems.

Other serious side effects include:

- serious allergic reactions (symptoms can be difficulty breathing, swelling of the face, neck and throat, rashes and hives, fever)
- slowing of growth (height and weight) in children
- seizures, mainly in patients with a history of seizures
- painful and prolonged erections (priapism) have occurred with methylphenidate. If you or your child develop priapism seek medical help right away. Because of the potential for lasting damage, priapism should be evaluated by a doctor immediately.
- eyesight changes or blurred vision

Common side effects include:

• headache	• decreased appetite
• upset stomach	• dry mouth
• trouble sleeping	• dizziness
• anxiety	• nervousness

Talk to your doctor if you or your child has side effects that are bothersome or do not go away.

This is not a complete list of possible side effects. Ask your doctor or pharmacist for more information.

How should I store FOCALIN XR?

- Store FOCALIN XR in a safe place at room temperature, 59 to 86°F (15 to 30°C).
- **Keep FOCALIN XR and all medicines out of the reach of children.**

General information about FOCALIN XR.
Medicines are sometimes prescribed for purposes other than those listed in a Medication Guide. Do not use FOCALIN XR for a condition for which it was not prescribed. Do not give FOCALIN XR to other people, even if they have the same condition. It may harm them and it is against the law.

This Medication Guide summarizes the most important information about FOCALIN XR. If you would like more information, talk with your doctor. You can ask your doctor or pharmacist for information about FOCALIN XR that was written for healthcare professionals. For more information about FOCALIN XR call 1-888-669-6682.

What are the ingredients in FOCALIN XR?
Active Ingredient: dexmethylphenidate hydrochloride
Inactive Ingredients: ammonio methacrylate copolymer, FD&C Blue #2 (5 mg, 15 mg, 25 mg, 35 mg, and 40 mg strengths), FDA/E172 yellow iron oxide (10 mg, 15 mg, 30 mg, 35 mg, and 40 mg strengths), gelatin, ink Tan SW-8010, methacrylic acid copolymer, polyethylene glycol, sugar spheres, talc, titanium dioxide, and triethyl citrate.

This Medication Guide has been approved by the U.S. Food and Drug Administration.

Focalin XR is a trademark of Novartis AG
SODAS® is a registered trademark of Alkermes Pharma Ireland Limited
This product is covered by US patents including 5,837,284, 5,908,850, 6,228,398, 6,355,656, and 6,635,284.
Manufactured for
Novartis Pharmaceuticals Corporation
East Hanover, New Jersey 07936
By Alkermes Gainesville LLC
Gainesville, GA 30504
© Novartis
T2013-122
December 2013

Shown in Product Identification Guide, page 310

GILENYA
[je-LEN-yah]
(fingolimod)
capsules

℞

The following prescribing information is based on official labeling in effect July 2014.
HIGHLIGHTS OF PRESCRIBING INFORMATION
These highlights do not include all the information needed to use GILENYA® safely and effectively. See full prescribing information for GILENYA.

GILENYA (fingolimod) capsules
Initial U.S. Approval: 2010

──────RECENT MAJOR CHANGES──────

Dosage and Administration (2)	4/2014
Warnings and Precautions: (5.2, 5.4, 5.8)	4/2014

──────INDICATIONS AND USAGE──────
GILENYA is a sphingosine 1-phosphate receptor modulator indicated for the treatment of patients with relapsing forms of multiple sclerosis (MS) to reduce the frequency of clinical exacerbations and to delay the accumulation of physical disability. (1)

──────DOSAGE AND ADMINISTRATION──────

- Recommended dose: 0.5 mg orally once daily, with or without food (2)
- First Dose Monitoring:
  - Observe all patients for bradycardia for at least 6 hours after first dose with hourly pulse and blood pressure measurement. Obtain electrocardiogram (ECG) prior to dosing and at end of observation period.
  - Patients who develop heart rate <45 bpm, 2nd degree or higher atrioventricular (AV) block, or in whom lowest postdose heart rate is at the end of the observation period should be monitored until resolution.
  - If symptomatic bradycardia occurs, begin continuous ECG monitoring until resolved. If pharmacological intervention is required, continue this monitoring overnight, and repeat first-dose monitoring for the second dose.
  - Patients at higher risk of symptomatic bradycardia or heart block (2, 7), or prolonged QTc interval, or taking drugs with known risk of torsades de pointes should be observed overnight (2, 7).

──────DOSAGE FORMS AND STRENGTHS──────
0.5 mg hard capsules (3)

──────CONTRAINDICATIONS──────

- Recent (within the last 6 months) myocardial infarction, unstable angina, stroke, transient ischemic attack, decompensated heart failure requiring hospitalization, or Class III/IV heart failure (4)
- History of Mobitz Type II 2nd degree or 3rd degree AV block or sick sinus syndrome, unless patient has a pacemaker (4)
- Baseline QTc interval ≥500 msec (4)
- Treatment with Class Ia or Class III anti-arrhythmic drugs (4)

──────WARNINGS AND PRECAUTIONS──────

- Bradycardia and/or atrioventricular conduction after first dose: Monitor patients. (2, 5.1)
- Infections: GILENYA may increase the risk of infections. A recent CBC should be available before initiating treatment. Monitor for infection during treatment and for 2 months after discontinuation. Do not start in patients with active infections. (5.2)
- Macular edema: Perform an ophthalmologic evaluation before and 3-4 months after treatment initiation. Patients with diabetes mellitus or a history of uveitis are at increased risk. (5.3)
- Posterior reversible encephalopathy syndrome (PRES): If suspected, discontinue GILENYA (5.4)
- Decrease in pulmonary function tests (PFT): Obtain PFT when clinically indicated. (5.5)
- Liver injury: liver enzyme results should be available before initiation. Discontinue if significant liver injury occurs (5.6)
- Women of childbearing potential should use effective contraception during and for 2 months after stopping GILENYA (5.7)
- Blood pressure (BP): Monitor BP during treatment (5.8)

──────ADVERSE REACTIONS──────
Most common adverse reactions (incidence ≥10% and > placebo): Headache, influenza, diarrhea, back pain, liver transaminase elevations, and cough. (6.1)

To report SUSPECTED ADVERSE REACTIONS, contact Novartis Pharmaceuticals Corporation at 1-888-669-6682 or FDA at 1-800-FDA-1088 or www.fda.gov/medwatch.

──────DRUG INTERACTIONS──────

- Ketoconazole: Closely monitor during concomitant use with systemic ketoconazole (7, 12.3)
- Vaccines: Avoid live attenuated vaccines during, and for 2 months after stopping GILENYA treatment. (5.2, 7)

──────USE IN SPECIFIC POPULATIONS──────

- Pregnancy: Based on animal data, may cause fetal harm. (8.1)
- Hepatic impairment: Closely monitor patients with severe hepatic impairment. (5.6, 8.6, 12.3)

See 17 for PATIENT COUNSELING INFORMATION and Medication Guide

Revised: 4/2014

──────────────────────

FULL PRESCRIBING INFORMATION: CONTENTS*

1   **INDICATIONS AND USAGE**
2   **DOSAGE AND ADMINISTRATION**
3   **DOSAGE FORMS AND STRENGTHS**
4   **CONTRAINDICATIONS**

FULL PRESCRIBING INFORMATION

1   INDICATIONS AND USAGE

GILENYA is indicated for the treatment of patients with relapsing forms of multiple sclerosis (MS) to reduce the frequency of clinical exacerbations and to delay the accumulation of physical disability.

2   DOSAGE AND ADMINISTRATION

Recommended Dose

The recommended dose of GILENYA is 0.5 mg orally once daily. Fingolimod doses higher than 0.5 mg are associated with a greater incidence of adverse reactions without additional benefit. GILENYA can be taken with or without food.

First Dose Monitoring

Initiation of GILENYA treatment results in a decrease in heart rate [see Warnings and Precautions (5.1) and Clinical Pharmacology (12.2)]. After the first dose of GILENYA, the heart rate decrease starts within an hour and the Day 1 nadir generally occurs within approximately 6 hours, although the nadir can be observed up to 24 hours after the first dose in some patients.

The first dose of GILENYA should be administered in a setting in which resources to appropriately manage symptomatic bradycardia are available. In order to assess patient response to the first dose of fingolimod, observe all patients for 6 hours for signs and symptoms of bradycardia with hourly pulse and blood pressure measurement. Obtain in all patients an electrocardiogram (ECG) prior to dosing, and at the end of the observation period.

Additional observation should be instituted until the finding has resolved in the following situations:

• The heart rate 6 hours postdose is <45 bpm
• The heart rate 6 hours postdose is at the lowest value postdose (suggesting that the maximum pharmacodynamic effect on the heart may not have occurred)
• The ECG 6-hours postdose shows new onset second degree or higher atrioventricular (AV) block

Should postdose symptomatic bradycardia occur, initiate appropriate management, begin continuous ECG monitoring, and continue observation until the symptoms have resolved.

Should a patient require pharmacologic intervention for symptomatic bradycardia, continuous overnight ECG monitoring in a medical facility should be instituted, and the first dose monitoring strategy should be repeated after the second dose of GILENYA.

Patients with some preexisting conditions (e.g., ischemic heart disease, history of myocardial infarction, congestive heart failure, history of cardiac arrest, cerebrovascular disease, uncontrolled hypertension, history of symptomatic bradycardia, history of recurrent syncope, severe untreated sleep apnea, AV block, sinoatrial heart block) may poorly tolerate the GILENYA-induced bradycardia, or experience serious rhythm disturbances after the first dose of GILENYA. Prior to treatment with GILENYA, these pa-

tients should have a cardiac evaluation by a physician appropriately trained to conduct such evaluation, and, if treated with GILENYA, should be monitored overnight with continuous ECG in a medical facility after the first dose. GILENYA is contraindicated in patients who in the last 6 months experienced myocardial infarction, unstable angina, stroke, transient ischemic attack (TIA), decompensated heart failure requiring hospitalization or Class III/IV heart failure) [see Contraindications (4)].

Since initiation of GILENYA treatment results in decreased heart rate and may prolong the QT interval, patients with a prolonged QTc interval (>450 msec males, >470 msec females) before dosing or during 6 hour observation, or at additional risk for QT prolongation (e.g., hypokalemia, hypomagnesemia, congenital long-QT syndrome), or on concurrent therapy with QT prolonging drugs with a known risk of torsades de pointes (e.g., citalopram, chlorpromazine, haloperidol, methadone, erythromycin) should be monitored overnight with continuous ECG in a medical facility [see Drug Interactions (7)].

Experience with GILENYA is limited in patients receiving concurrent therapy with drugs that slow heart rate or atrioventricular conduction (e.g., beta blockers, heart-rate lowering calcium channel blockers such as diltiazem or verapamil, or digoxin). Because the initiation of GILENYA treatment is also associated with slowing of the heart rate, concomitant use of these drugs during GILENYA initiation may be associated with severe bradycardia or heart block. The possibility to switch to drugs that do not slow the heart rate or atrioventricular conduction should be evaluated by the physician prescribing these drugs before initiating GILENYA. Patients who cannot switch should have overnight continuous ECG monitoring after the first dose [see Drug Interactions (7)].

Clinical data indicate effects of GILENYA on heart rate are maximal after the first dose although milder effects on heart rate may persist for, on average, 2 to 4 weeks after initiation of therapy at which time heart rate generally returns to baseline. Physicians should continue to be alert to patient reports of cardiac symptoms.

Reinitiation of Therapy Following Discontinuation

If GILENYA treatment is discontinued for more than 14 days, after the first month of treatment, the effects on heart rate and AV conduction may recur on reintroduction of GILENYA treatment and the same precautions (first dose monitoring) as for initial dosing should apply. Within the first 2 weeks of treatment, first dose procedures are recommended after interruption of 1 day or more; during weeks 3 and 4 of treatment first dose procedures are recommended after treatment interruption of more than 7 days.

3   DOSAGE FORMS AND STRENGTHS

GILENYA is available as 0.5 mg hard capsules with a white opaque body and bright yellow cap imprinted with "FTY 0.5 mg" on the cap and 2 radial bands imprinted on the capsule body with yellow ink.

4   CONTRAINDICATIONS

Patients who in the last 6 months experienced myocardial infarction, unstable angina, stroke, TIA, decompensated heart failure requiring hospitalization or Class III/IV heart failure

History or presence of Mobitz Type II second-degree or third-degree atrioventricular (AV) block or sick sinus syndrome, unless patient has a functioning pacemaker

Baseline QTc interval ≥500 msec

Treatment with Class Ia or Class III anti-arrhythmic drugs

5   WARNINGS AND PRECAUTIONS

5.1   Bradyarrhythmia and Atrioventricular Blocks

Because of a risk for bradyarrhythmia and atrioventricular (AV) blocks, patients should be monitored during GILENYA treatment initiation [see Dosage and Administration (2)].

Reduction in Heart Rate

After the first dose of GILENYA, the heart rate decrease starts within an hour. On Day 1, the maximal decline in heart rate generally occurs within 6 hours and recovers, although not to baseline levels, by 8- 10 hours postdose. Because of physiological diurnal variation, there is a second period of heart rate decrease within 24 hours after the first dose. In some patients, heart rate decrease during the second period is more pronounced than the decrease observed in the first 6 hours. Heart rates below 40 beats per minute were rarely observed. Adverse reactions of symptomatic bradycardia following the first dose were reported in 0.5% of patients receiving GILENYA 0.5 mg, but in no patient on placebo. Patients who experienced bradycardia were generally asymptomatic, but some patients experienced hypotension, dizziness, fatigue, palpitations, and chest pain that usually resolved within the first 24 hours on treatment. Following the second dose, a further decrease in heart rate may occur when compared to the heart rate prior to the second dose, but this change is of a smaller magnitude than that observed following the first dose. With continued dosing, the heart rate returns to baseline within 1 month of chronic treatment.

Atrioventricular Blocks

Initiation of GILENYA treatment has resulted in transient AV conduction delays. In controlled clinical trials, adverse reactions of first-degree AV block (prolonged PR interval on ECG) following the first dose were reported in 0.1% of patients receiving GILENYA 0.5 mg, but in no patient on placebo. Second-degree AV blocks following the first dose were also identified in 0.1% of patients receiving GILENYA 0.5 mg, but in no patient on placebo. In a study of 698 patients with available 24-hour Holter monitoring data after their first dose (N=351 on GILENYA 0.5 mg and N=347 on placebo), second-degree AV blocks, Mobitz types I (Wenckebach) and/or II, were reported in 3.7% (N=13) of patients receiving GILENYA 0.5 mg and 2% (N=7) of patients on placebo. The conduction abnormalities were usually transient and asymptomatic, and resolved within the first 24 hours on treatment, but they occasionally required treatment with atropine or isoproterenol.

Postmarketing Experience

In the postmarketing setting, third-degree AV block and AV block with junctional escape have been observed during the first-dose 6-hour observation period with GILENYA. Isolated delayed onset events, including transient asystole and unexplained death, have occurred within 24 hours of the first dose. These events were confounded by concomitant medications and/or preexisting disease, and the relationship to GILENYA is uncertain. Cases of syncope were also reported after the first dose of GILENYA.

5.2   Infections

Risk of Infections

GILENYA causes a dose-dependent reduction in peripheral lymphocyte count to 20%–30% of baseline values because of reversible sequestration of lymphocytes in lymphoid tissues. GILENYA may therefore increase the risk of infections, some serious in nature [see Clinical Pharmacology (12.2)].

Before initiating treatment with GILENYA, a recent CBC (i.e., within 6 months) should be available. Consider suspending treatment with GILENYA if a patient develops a serious infection, and reassess the benefits and risks prior to reinitiation of therapy. Because the elimination of fingolimod after discontinuation may take up to 2 months, continue monitoring for infections throughout this period. Instruct patients receiving GILENYA to report symptoms of infections to a physician. Patients with active acute or chronic infections should not start treatment until the infection(s) is resolved.

Two patients died of herpetic infections during GILENYA controlled studies in the premarketing database (1 disseminated primary herpes zoster and 1 herpes simplex encephalitis). In both cases, the patients were receiving a fingolimod dose (1.25 mg) higher than recommended for the treatment of MS (0.5 mg), and had received high-dose corticosteroid therapy for suspected MS relapse. No deaths due to viral infections occurred in patients treated with GILENYA 0.5 mg in the premarketing database.

In MS controlled studies, the overall rate of infections (72%) and serious infections (2%) with GILENYA 0.5 mg was similar to placebo. However, bronchitis and, to a lesser extent, pneumonia were more common in GILENYA-treated patients.

Prior and Concomitant Treatment with Antineoplastic, Immunosuppressive, or Immune-Modulating Therapies

GILENYA has not been administered concomitantly with antineoplastic, immunosuppressive, or immune-modulating therapies used for treatment of MS. Concomitant use of GILENYA with any of these therapies would be expected to increase the risk of immunosuppression [see Drug Interactions (7)].

When switching from other immunosuppressive medications, the duration and mode of action of such substances must be considered when initiating Gilenya to avoid additive immunosuppressive effects.

Varicella Zoster Virus Antibody Testing/Vaccination

As for any immune-modulating drug, before initiating GILENYA therapy, patients without a history of chickenpox or without vaccination against varicella zoster virus (VZV) should be tested for antibodies to VZV. VZV vaccination of antibody-negative patients should be considered prior to commencing treatment with GILENYA, following which initiation of treatment with GILENYA should be postponed for 1 month to allow the full effect of vaccination to occur.

5.3   Macular Edema

In patients receiving GILENYA 0.5 mg, macular edema occurred in 0.4% of patients. An adequate ophthalmologic evaluation should be performed at baseline and 3-4 months after treatment initiation. If patients report visual disturbances at any time while on GILENYA therapy, additional ophthalmologic evaluation should be undertaken.

In MS controlled studies involving 1204 patients treated with GILENYA 0.5 mg and 861 patients treated with placebo, macular edema with or without visual symptoms was reported in 0.4% of patients treated with GILENYA 0.5 mg and 0.1% of patients treated with placebo; it occurred predominantly in the first 3-4 months of therapy. Some patients presented with blurred vision or decreased visual acuity, but others were asymptomatic and diagnosed on routine ophthalmologic examination. Macular edema generally improved or resolved with or without treatment after drug discontinuation, but some patients had residual visual acuity loss even after resolution of macular edema.

Continuation of GILENYA in patients who develop macular edema has not been evaluated. A decision on whether or not to discontinue GILENYA therapy should include an assessment of the potential benefits and risks for the individual patient. The risk of recurrence after rechallenge has not been evaluated.

Macular Edema in Patients with History of Uveitis or Diabetes Mellitus

Patients with a history of uveitis and patients with diabetes mellitus are at increased risk of macular edema during GILENYA therapy. The incidence of macular edema is also increased in MS patients with a history of uveitis. The rate was approximately 20% in patients with a history of uveitis versus 0.6% in those without a history of uveitis, in the combined experience with all doses of fingolimod. MS patients with diabetes mellitus or a history of uveitis should undergo an ophthalmologic evaluation prior to initiating GILENYA therapy and have regular follow-up ophthalmologic evaluations while receiving GILENYA therapy. GILENYA has not been tested in MS patients with diabetes mellitus.

5.4 Posterior Reversible Encephalopathy Syndrome

There have been rare cases of posterior reversible encephalopathy syndrome (PRES) reported in patients receiving Gilenya. Symptoms reported included sudden onset of severe headache, altered mental status, visual disturbances, and seizure. Symptoms of PRES are usually reversible but may evolve into ischemic stroke or cerebral hemorrhage. Delay in diagnosis and treatment may lead to permanent neurological sequelae. If PRES is suspected, GILENYA should be discontinued.

5.5 Respiratory Effects

Dose-dependent reductions in forced expiratory volume over 1 second (FEV1) and diffusion lung capacity for carbon monoxide (DLCO) were observed in patients treated with GILENYA as early as 1 month after treatment initiation. At Month 24, the reduction from baseline in the percent of predicted values for FEV1 was 3.1% for GILENYA 0.5 mg and 2% for placebo. For DLCO, the reductions from baseline in percent of predicted values at Month 24 were 3.8% for GILENYA 0.5 mg and 2.7% for placebo. The changes in FEV1 appear to be reversible after treatment discontinuation. There is insufficient information to determine the reversibility of the decrease of DLCO after drug discontinuation. In MS controlled trials, dyspnea was reported in 5% of patients receiving GILENYA 0.5 mg and 4% of patients receiving placebo. Several patients discontinued GILENYA because of unexplained dyspnea during the extension (uncontrolled) studies. GILENYA has not been tested in MS patients with compromised respiratory function.

Spirometric evaluation of respiratory function and evaluation of DLCO should be performed during therapy with GILENYA if clinically indicated.

5.6 Liver Injury

Elevations of liver enzymes may occur in patients receiving GILENYA. Recent (i.e., within last 6 months) transaminase and bilirubin levels should be available before initiation of GILENYA therapy.

During clinical trials, 3-fold the upper limit of normal (ULN) or greater elevation in liver transaminases occurred in 8% of patients treated with GILENYA 0.5 mg, as compared to 2% of patients on placebo. Elevations 5-fold the ULN occurred in 2% of patients on GILENYA and 1% of patients on placebo. In clinical trials, GILENYA was discontinued if the elevation exceeded 5 times the ULN. Recurrence of liver transaminase elevations occurred with rechallenge in some patients, supporting a relationship to drug. The majority of elevations occurred within 6-9 months. Serum transaminase levels returned to normal within approximately 2 months after discontinuation of GILENYA.

Liver enzymes should be monitored in patients who develop symptoms suggestive of hepatic dysfunction, such as unexplained nausea, vomiting, abdominal pain, fatigue, anorexia, or jaundice and/or dark urine. GILENYA should be discontinued if significant liver injury is confirmed. Patients with preexisting liver disease may be at increased risk of developing elevated liver enzymes when taking GILENYA.

Because GILENYA exposure is doubled in patients with severe hepatic impairment, these patients should be closely monitored, as the risk of adverse reactions is greater [see Use in Specific Populations (8.6), Clinical Pharmacology (12.3)].

5.7 Fetal Risk

Based on animal studies, GILENYA may cause fetal harm. Because it takes approximately 2 months to eliminate GILENYA from the body, women of childbearing potential should use effective contraception to avoid pregnancy during and for 2 months after stopping GILENYA treatment.

5.8 Blood Pressure Effects

In MS clinical trials, patients treated with GILENYA 0.5 mg had an average increase over placebo of approximately 3 mmHg in systolic pressure, and approximately 2 mmHg in diastolic pressure, first detected after approximately 1 month of treatment initiation, and persisting with continued treatment. Hypertension was reported as an adverse reaction in 8% of patients on GILENYA 0.5 mg and in 4% of patients on placebo. Blood pressure should be monitored during treatment with GILENYA.

5.9 Immune System Effects Following GILENYA Discontinuation

Fingolimod remains in the blood and has pharmacodynamic effects, including decreased lymphocyte counts, for up to 2 months following the last dose of GILENYA. Lymphocyte counts generally return to the normal range within 1-2 months of stopping therapy [see Clinical Pharmacology (12.2)]. Because of the continuing pharmacodynamic effects of fingolimod, initiating other drugs during this period warrants the same considerations needed for concomitant administration (e.g., risk of additive immunosuppressant effects) [see Drug Interactions (7)].

6 ADVERSE REACTIONS

The following serious adverse reactions are described elsewhere in labeling:

- Bradyarrhythmia and Atrioventricular Blocks [see Warnings and Precautions (5.1)]
- Infections [see Warnings and Precautions (5.2)]
- Macular Edema [see Warnings and Precautions (5.3)]
- Posterior Reversible Encephalopathy Syndrome [see Warnings and Precautions (5.4)]
- Respiratory Effects [see Warnings and Precautions (5.5)]
- Liver Injury [see Warnings and Precautions (5.6)]

The most frequent adverse reactions (incidence ≥10% and >placebo) for GILENYA 0.5 mg were headache, influenza, diarrhea, back pain, liver enzyme elevations, and cough. The only adverse event leading to treatment interruption reported at an incidence >1% for GILENYA 0.5 mg was serum transaminase elevations (3.8%).

6.1 Clinical Trials Experience

A total of 1703 patients on GILENYA (0.5 or 1.25 mg once daily) constituted the safety population in the 2 controlled studies in patients with relapsing-remitting MS (RRMS) [see Clinical Studies (14)].

Study 1 was a 2-year placebo-controlled clinical study in 1272 MS patients treated with GILENYA 0.5 mg (N=425), GILENYA 1.25 mg (N=429), or placebo (N=418).

Table 1 Adverse Reactions in Study 1 (Occurring in ≥1% of Patients and Reported for GILENYA 0.5 mg at ≥1% Higher Rate than for Placebo)

Primary System Organ Class Preferred Term	GILENYA 0.5 mg N=425 %	Placebo N=418 %
Infections		
Influenza viral infections	13	10
Herpes viral infections	9	8
Bronchitis	8	4
Sinusitis	7	5
Gastroenteritis	5	3
Tinea infections	4	1
Cardiac Disorders		
Bradycardia	4	1
Nervous system disorders		
Headache	25	23
Dizziness	7	6
Paresthesia	5	4
Migraine	5	1
Gastrointestinal disorders		
Diarrhea	12	7
General disorders and administration site conditions		
Asthenia	3	1
Musculoskeletal and connective tissue disorders		
Back pain	12	7
Skin and subcutaneous tissue disorders		
Alopecia	4	2
Eczema	3	2
Pruritus	3	1
Investigations		
ALT/AST increased	14	5
GGT increased	5	1
Weight decreased	5	3
Blood triglycerides increased	3	1
Respiratory, thoracic, and mediastinal disorders		
Cough	10	8
Dyspnea	8	5
Psychiatric disorders		
Depression	8	7
Eye disorders		
Vision blurred	4	1
Eye pain	3	1
Vascular disorders		
Hypertension	6	4
Blood and lymphatic system disorders		
Lymphopenia	4	1
Leukopenia	3	<1

Adverse reactions in Study 2, a 1-year active-controlled (versus interferon beta-1a, n=431) study including 849 patients with MS treated with fingolimod, were generally similar to those in Study 1.

Vascular Events

Vascular events, including ischemic and hemorrhagic strokes, and peripheral arterial occlusive disease were reported in premarketing clinical trials in patients who received GILENYA doses (1.25-5 mg) higher than recommended for use in MS. Similar events have been reported with GILENYA 0.5 mg in the postmarketing setting although a causal relationship has not been established.

Lymphomas

Cases of lymphoma (cutaneous T-cell lymphoproliferative disorders or diffuse B-cell lymphoma) were reported in premarketing clinical trials in MS patients receiving GILENYA at, or above, the recommended dose of 0.5 mg. Based on the small number of cases and short duration of exposure, the relationship to GILENYA remains uncertain.

7 DRUG INTERACTIONS

QT Prolonging Drugs

GILENYA has not been studied in patients treated with drugs that prolong the QT interval. Drugs that prolong the QT interval have been associated with cases of torsades de pointes in patients with bradycardia. Since initiation of GILENYA treatment results in decreased heart rate and may prolong the QT interval, patients on QT prolonging drugs with a known risk of torsades de pointes (e.g., citalopram, chlorpromazine, haloperidol, methadone, erythromycin) should be monitored overnight with continuous ECG in a medical facility [see Dosage and Administration (2) and Warnings and Precautions (5.1)].

Ketoconazole

The blood levels of fingolimod and fingolimod-phosphate are increased by 1.7-fold when used concomitantly with ketoconazole. Patients who use GILENYA and systemic ketoconazole concomitantly should be closely monitored, as the risk of adverse reactions is greater.

Vaccines

GILENYA reduces the immune response to vaccination. Vaccination may be less effective during and for up to 2 months after discontinuation of treatment with GILENYA [see Clinical Pharmacology (12.2)]. The use of live attenuated vaccines should be avoided during and for 2 months after treatment with GILENYA because of the risk of infection.

Antineoplastic, Immunosuppressive, or Immunomodulating Therapies

Antineoplastic, immunosuppressive, or immune-modulating therapies are expected to increase the risk of immunosuppression. Use caution when switching patients from long-acting therapies with immune effects such as natalizumab or mitoxantrone [see Warnings and Precautions (5.2)].

Drugs That Slow Heart Rate or Atrioventricular Conduction (e.g., beta blockers or diltiazem)

Experience with GILENYA in patients receiving concurrent therapy with drugs that slow the heart rate or atrioventricular conduction (e.g., beta blockers, digoxin, or heart rate-slowing calcium channel blockers such as diltiazem or verapamil) is limited. Because initiation of GILENYA treatment may result in an additional decrease in heart rate, concomitant use of these drugs during GILENYA initiation may be associated with severe bradycardia or heart block. Seek advice from the prescribing physician regarding the possibility to switch to drugs that do not slow the heart rate or atrioventricular conduction before initiating GILENYA. Patients who cannot switch, should have overnight continuous ECG monitoring after the first dose [see Dosage and Administration (2) and Warnings and Precautions (5.1)].

Laboratory Test Interaction

Because GILENYA reduces blood lymphocyte counts via redistribution in secondary lymphoid organs, peripheral blood lymphocyte counts cannot be utilized to evaluate the lymphocyte subset status of a patient treated with GILENYA. A recent CBC should be available before initiating treatment with GILENYA.

8 USE IN SPECIFIC POPULATIONS

8.1 Pregnancy

Pregnancy Category C

There are no adequate and well-controlled studies in pregnant women. In oral studies conducted in rats and rabbits, fingolimod demonstrated developmental toxicity, including teratogenicity (rats) and embryolethality, when given to pregnant animals. In rats, the highest no-effect dose was less than the recommended human dose (RHD) of 0.5 mg/day on a body surface area (mg/m2) basis. The most common fetal visceral malformations in rats included persistent truncus arteriosus and ventricular septal defect. The receptor affected by fingolimod (sphingosine 1-phosphate receptor) is known to be involved in vascular formation during embryogenesis. Because it takes approximately 2 months to eliminate fingolimod from the body, potential risks to the fetus may persist after treatment ends [see Warnings and Precautions (5.7, 5.9)]. GILENYA should be used during pregnancy only if the potential benefit justifies the potential risk to the fetus.

Pregnancy Registry

A pregnancy registry has been established to collect information about the effect of GILENYA use during pregnancy. Physicians are encouraged to enroll pregnant patients, or pregnant women may register themselves in the GILENYA pregnancy registry by calling Outcome at 1-877-598-7237, sending an email to gpr@outcome.com or visiting www.gilenyapregnancyregistry.com.

Animal Data

When fingolimod was orally administered to pregnant rats during the period of organogenesis (0, 0.03, 0.1, and 0.3 mg/kg/day or 0, 1, 3, and 10 mg/kg/day), increased incidences of fetal malformations and embryo-fetal deaths were observed at all but the lowest dose tested (0.03 mg/kg/day), which is less than the RHD on a mg/m^2 basis. Oral administration to pregnant rabbits during organogenesis (0, 0.5, 1.5, and 5 mg/kg/day) resulted in increased incidences of embryo-fetal mortality and fetal growth retardation at the mid and high doses. The no-effect dose for these effects in rabbits (0.5 mg/kg/day) is approximately 20 times the RHD on a mg/m^2 basis.

When fingolimod was orally administered to female rats during pregnancy and lactation (0, 0.05, 0.15, and 0.5 mg/kg/day), pup survival was decreased at all doses and a neurobehavioral (learning) deficit was seen in offspring at the high dose. The low-effect dose of 0.05 mg/kg/day is similar to the RHD on a mg/m^2 basis.

8.2 Labor and Delivery

The effects of GILENYA on labor and delivery are unknown.

8.3 Nursing Mothers

Fingolimod is excreted in the milk of treated rats. It is not known whether this drug is excreted in human milk. Because many drugs are excreted in human milk and because of the potential for serious adverse reactions in nursing infants from GILENYA, a decision should be made whether to discontinue nursing or to discontinue the drug, taking into account the importance of the drug to the mother.

8.4 Pediatric Use

The safety and effectiveness of GILENYA in pediatric patients with MS below the age of 18 years have not been established.

In a study in which fingolimod (0.3, 1.5, or 7.5 mg/kg/day) was orally administered to young rats from weaning through sexual maturity, changes in bone mineral density and persistent neurobehavioral impairment (altered auditory startle) were observed at all doses. Delayed sexual maturation was noted in females at the highest dose tested and in males at all doses. The bone changes observed in fingolimod-treated juvenile rats are consistent with a reported role of S1P in the regulation of bone mineral homeostasis.

When fingolimod (0.5 or 5 mg/kg/day) was orally administered to rats from the neonatal period through sexual maturity, a marked decrease in T-cell dependent antibody response was observed at both doses. This effect had not fully recovered by 6-8 weeks after the end of treatment.

8.5 Geriatric Use

Clinical MS studies of GILENYA did not include sufficient numbers of patients aged 65 years and over to determine whether they respond differently than younger patients. GILENYA should be used with caution in patients aged 65 years and over, reflecting the greater frequency of decreased hepatic, or renal, function and of concomitant disease or other drug therapy.

8.6 Hepatic Impairment

Because fingolimod, but not fingolimod-phosphate, exposure is doubled in patients with severe hepatic impairment, patients with severe hepatic impairment should be closely monitored, as the risk of adverse reactions may be greater [see Warnings and Precautions (5.6) and Clinical Pharmacology (12.3)].

No dose adjustment is needed in patients with mild or moderate hepatic impairment.

8.7 Renal Impairment

The blood level of some GILENYA metabolites is increased (up to 13-fold) in patients with severe renal impairment [see Clinical Pharmacology (12.3)]. The toxicity of these metabolites has not been fully explored. The blood level of these metabolites has not been assessed in patients with mild or moderate renal impairment.

10 OVERDOSAGE

GILENYA can induce bradycardia as well as AV conduction blocks (including complete AV block). The decline in heart rate usually starts within 1 hour of the first dose and is maximal within 6 hours in most patients [see Warnings and Precautions (5.1)]. In case of GILENYA overdosage, observe patients overnight with continuous ECG monitoring in a medical facility, and obtain regular measurements of blood pressure [see Dosage and Administration (2)].

Neither dialysis nor plasma exchange results in removal of fingolimod from the body.

11 DESCRIPTION

Fingolimod is a sphingosine 1-phosphate receptor modulator.

Chemically, fingolimod is 2-amino-2-[2-(4-octylphenyl)ethyl]propan-1,3-diol hydrochloride. Its structure is shown below:

Fingolimod hydrochloride is a white to practically white powder that is freely soluble in water and alcohol and soluble in propylene glycol. It has a molecular weight of 343.93. GILENYA is provided as 0.5 mg hard gelatin capsules for oral use. Each capsule contains 0.56 mg of fingolimod hydrochloride, equivalent to 0.5 mg of fingolimod.

Each GILENYA 0.5 mg capsule contains the following inactive ingredients: gelatin, magnesium stearate, mannitol, titanium dioxide, yellow iron oxide.

12 CLINICAL PHARMACOLOGY

12.1 Mechanism of Action

Fingolimod is metabolized by sphingosine kinase to the active metabolite, fingolimod-phosphate. Fingolimod-phosphate is a sphingosine 1-phosphate receptor modulator, and binds with high affinity to sphingosine 1-phosphate receptors 1, 3, 4, and 5. Fingolimod-phosphate blocks the capacity of lymphocytes to egress from lymph nodes, reducing the number of lymphocytes in peripheral blood. The mechanism by which fingolimod exerts therapeutic effects in multiple sclerosis is unknown, but may involve reduction of lymphocyte migration into the central nervous system.

12.2 Pharmacodynamics

Heart Rate and Rhythm

Fingolimod causes a transient reduction in heart rate and AV conduction at treatment initiation [see Warnings and Precautions (5.1)].

Heart rate progressively increases after the first day, returning to baseline values within 1 month of the start of chronic treatment.

Autonomic responses of the heart, including diurnal variation of heart rate and response to exercise, are not affected by fingolimod treatment.

Fingolimod treatment is not associated with a decrease in cardiac output.

Potential to Prolong the QT Interval

In a thorough QT interval study of doses of 1.25 or 2.5 mg fingolimod at steady-state, when a negative chronotropic effect of fingolimod was still present, fingolimod treatment resulted in a prolongation of QTc, with the upper bound of the 90% confidence interval (CI) of 14.0 msec. There is no consistent signal of increased incidence of QTc outliers, either absolute or change from baseline, associated with fingolimod treatment. In MS studies, there was no clinically relevant prolongation of QT interval, but patients at risk for QT prolongation were not included in clinical studies.

Immune System

Effects on Immune Cell Numbers in the Blood

In a study in which 12 subjects received GILENYA 0.5 mg daily, the lymphocyte count decreased to approximately 60% of baseline within 4-6 hours after the first dose. With continued daily dosing, the lymphocyte count continued to decrease over a 2-week period, reaching a nadir count of approximately 500 cells/µL or approximately 30% of baseline. In a placebo-controlled study in 1272 MS patients (of whom 425 received fingolimod 0.5 mg daily and 418 received placebo), 18% (N=78) of patients on fingolimod 0.5 mg reached a nadir of <200 cells/µL on at least 1 occasion. No patient on placebo reached a nadir of <200 cells/µL. Low lymphocyte counts are maintained with chronic daily dosing of GILENYA 0.5 mg daily.

Chronic fingolimod dosing leads to a mild decrease in the neutrophil count to approximately 80% of baseline. Monocytes are unaffected by fingolimod.

Peripheral lymphocyte count increases are evident within days of stopping fingolimod treatment and typically normal counts are reached within 1 to 2 months.

Effect on Antibody Response

GILENYA reduces the immune response to vaccination, as evaluated in 2 studies.

In the first study, the immunogenicity of keyhole limpet hemocyanin (KLH) and pneumococcal polysaccharide vaccine (PPV-23) immunization were assessed by IgM and IgG titers in a steady-state, randomized, placebo-controlled study in healthy volunteers. Compared to placebo, antigen-specific IgM titers were decreased by 91% and 25% in response to KLH and PPV-23, respectively, in subjects on GILENYA 0.5 mg. Similarly, IgG titers were decreased by 45% and 50%, in response to KLH and PPV-23, respectively, in subjects on GILENYA 0.5 mg daily compared to placebo. The responder rate for GILENYA 0.5 mg as measured by the number of subjects with a >4-fold increase in KLH IgG was comparable to placebo and 25% lower for PPV-23 IgG, while the number of subjects with a >4 fold increase in KLH and PPV-23 IgM was 75% and 40% lower, respectively, compared to placebo. The capacity to mount a skin delayed-type hypersensitivity reaction to Candida and tetanus toxoid was decreased by approximately 30% in subjects on GILENYA 0.5 mg daily, compared to placebo. Immunologic responses were further decreased with fingolimod 1.25 mg (a dose higher than recommended in MS) [see Warnings and Precautions (5.2)].

In the second study, the immunogenicity of Northern hemisphere seasonal influenza and tetanus toxoid vaccination was assessed in a 12-week steady-state, randomized, placebo-controlled study of GILENYA 0.5 mg in multiple sclerosis patients (n=136). The responder rate 3 weeks after vaccination, defined as seroconversion or a ≥4-fold increase in antibody directed against at least 1 of the 3 influenza strains, was 54% for GILENYA 0.5 mg and 85% in the placebo group. The responder rate 3 weeks after vaccination, defined as seroconversion or a ≥4-fold increase in antibody directed against tetanus toxoid was 40% for GILENYA 0.5 mg and 61% in the placebo group.

Pulmonary Function

Single fingolimod doses ≥5 mg (10-fold the recommended dose) are associated with a dose-dependent increase in airway resistance. In a 14-day study of 0.5, 1.25, or 5 mg/day, fingolimod was not associated with impaired oxygenation or oxygen desaturation with exercise or an increase in airway responsiveness to methacholine. Subjects on fingolimod treatment had a normal bronchodilator response to inhaled beta-agonists.

In a 14-day placebo-controlled study of patients with moderate asthma, no effect was seen for GILENYA 0.5 mg (recommended dose in MS). A 10% reduction in mean FEV1 at 6 hours after dosing was observed in patients receiving fingolimod 1.25 mg (a dose higher than recommended for use in MS) on Day 10 of treatment. Fingolimod 1.25 mg was associated with a 5-fold increase in the use of rescue short acting beta-agonists.

12.3 Pharmacokinetics

Absorption

The T_{max} of fingolimod is 12-16 hours. The apparent absolute oral bioavailability is 93%.

Food intake does not alter C_{max} or exposure (AUC) of fingolimod or fingolimod-phosphate. Therefore GILENYA may be taken without regard to meals.

Steady-state blood concentrations are reached within 1 to 2 months following once-daily administration and steady-state levels are approximately 10-fold greater than with the initial dose.

Distribution

Fingolimod highly (86%) distributes in red blood cells. Fingolimod-phosphate has a smaller uptake in blood cells of <17%. Fingolimod and fingolimod-phosphate are >99.7% protein bound. Fingolimod and fingolimod-phosphate protein binding is not altered by renal or hepatic impairment. Fingolimod is extensively distributed to body tissues with a volume of distribution of about 1200±260 L.

Metabolism

The biotransformation of fingolimod in humans occurs by 3 main pathways: by reversible stereoselective phosphorylation to the pharmacologically active (S)-enantiomer of fingolimod-phosphate, by oxidative biotransformation mainly via the cytochrome P450 4F2 isoenzyme and subsequent fatty acid-like degradation to inactive metabolites, and by formation of pharmacologically inactive non-polar ceramide analogs of fingolimod.

Fingolimod is primarily metabolized via human CYP4F2 with a minor contribution of CYP2D6, 2E1, 3A4, and 4F12. Inhibitors or inducers of these isozymes might alter the exposure of fingolimod or fingolimod-phosphate. The involvement of multiple CYP isoenzymes in the oxidation of fingolimod suggests that the metabolism of fingolimod will not be subject to substantial inhibition in the presence of an inhibitor of a single specific CYP isozyme.

Following single oral administration of [^{14}C] fingolimod, the major fingolimod-related components in blood, as judged from their contribution to the AUC up to 816 hours postdose of total radiolabeled components, are fingolimod itself (23.3%), fingolimod-phosphate (10.3%), and inactive metabolites [M3 carboxylic acid metabolite (8.3%), M29 ceramide metabolite (8.9%), and M30 ceramide metabolite (7.3%)].

Elimination

Fingolimod blood clearance is 6.3±2.3 L/h, and the average apparent terminal half-life ($t_{1/2}$) is 6 to 9 days. Blood levels of fingolimod-phosphate decline in parallel with those of fingolimod in the terminal phase, yielding similar half-lives for both.

After oral administration, about 81% of the dose is slowly excreted in the urine as inactive metabolites. Fingolimod and fingolimod-phosphate are not excreted intact in urine but are the major components in the feces with amounts of each representing less than 2.5% of the dose.

Special Populations

Renal Impairment

In patients with severe renal impairment, fingolimod C_{max} and AUC are increased by 32% and 43%, respectively, and fingolimod-phosphate C_{max} and AUC are increased by 25% and 14%, respectively, with no change in apparent elimination half-life. Based on these findings, the GILENYA 0.5 mg dose is appropriate for use in patients with renal impairment. The systemic exposure of 2 metabolites (M2 and M3) is increased by 3- and 13-fold, respectively. The toxicity of these metabolites has not been fully characterized.

A study in patients with mild or moderate renal impairment has not been conducted.

Hepatic Impairment

In subjects with mild, moderate, or severe hepatic impairment, no change in fingolimod C_{max} was observed, but fingolimod AUC was increased respectively by 12%, 44%, and 103%. In patients with severe hepatic impairment, fingolimod-phosphate C_{max} was decreased by 22% and AUC was not substantially changed. The pharmacokinetics of fingolimod-phosphate was not evaluated in patients with mild or moderate hepatic impairment. The apparent elimination half-life of fingolimod is unchanged in subjects with mild hepatic impairment, but is prolonged by about 50% in patients with moderate or severe hepatic impairment. Patients with severe hepatic impairment should be closely monitored, as the risk of adverse reactions is greater [see Warnings and Precautions (5.6)].

No dose adjustment is needed in patients with mild or moderate hepatic impairment.

Race

The effects of race on fingolimod and fingolimod-phosphate pharmacokinetics cannot be adequately assessed due to a low number of non-white patients in the clinical program.

Gender

Gender has no clinically significant influence on fingolimod and fingolimod-phosphate pharmacokinetics.

Geriatric Patients

The mechanism for elimination and results from population pharmacokinetics suggest that dose adjustment would not be necessary in elderly patients. However, clinical experience in patients aged above 65 years is limited.

Pharmacokinetic Interactions

Ketoconazole

The coadministration of ketoconazole (a potent inhibitor of CYP3A and CYP4F) 200 mg twice daily at steady-state and a single dose of fingolimod 5 mg led to a 70% increase in AUC of fingolimod and fingolimod-phosphate. Patients who use GILENYA and systemic ketoconazole concomitantly should be closely monitored, as the risk of adverse reactions is greater [see Drug Interactions (7)].

Carbamazepine

The coadministration of carbamazepine (a potent CYP450 enzyme inducer) 600 mg twice daily at steady-state and a single dose of fingolimod 2 mg decreased blood concentrations (AUC) of fingolimod and fingolimod-phosphate by approximately 40%. The clinical impact of this decrease is unknown.

Other strong CYP450 enzyme inducers, e.g., rifampicin, phenytoin, phenobarbital, and St. John's wort, may also reduce AUC of fingolimod and fingolimod-phosphate. The clinical impact of this potential decrease is unknown.

Potential of Fingolimod and Fingolimod-phosphate to Inhibit the Metabolism of Comedications

In vitro inhibition studies in pooled human liver microsomes and specific metabolic probe substrates demonstrate that fingolimod has little or no capacity to inhibit the activity of the following CYP450 enzymes: CYP1A2, CYP2A6, CYP2B6, CYP2C8, CYP2C9, CYP2C19, CYP2D6, CYP2E1, CYP3A4/5, or CYP4A9/11, and similarly fingolimod-phosphate has little or no capacity to inhibit the activity of CYP1A2, CYP2A6, CYP2B6, CYP2C8, CYP2C9, CYP2C19, CYP2D6, CYP2E1, or CYP3A4 at concentrations

up to 3 orders of magnitude of therapeutic concentrations. Therefore, fingolimod and fingolimod-phosphate are unlikely to reduce the clearance of drugs that are mainly cleared through metabolism by the major cytochrome P450 isoenzymes described above.

Potential of Fingolimod and Fingolimod-phosphate to Induce its Own and/or the Metabolism of Comedications

Fingolimod was examined for its potential to induce human CYP3A4, CYP1A2, CYP4F2, and MDR1 (P-glycoprotein) mRNA and CYP3A, CYP1A2, CYP2B6, CYP2C8, CYP2C9, CYP2C19, and CYP4F2 activity in primary human hepatocytes. Fingolimod did not induce mRNA or activity of the different CYP450 enzymes and MDR1 with respect to the vehicle control; therefore, no clinically relevant induction of the tested CYP450 enzymes or MDR1 by fingolimod are expected at therapeutic concentrations. Fingolimod-phosphate was also examined for its potential to induce mRNA and/or activity of human CYP1A2, CYP2B6, CYP2C8, CYP2C9, CYP2C19, CYP3A, CYP4F2, CYP4F3B, and CYP4F12. Fingolimod-phosphate is not expected to have clinically significant induction effects on these enzymes at therapeutic dose of fingolimod.

Transporters

Fingolimod as well as fingolimod-phosphate are not expected to inhibit the uptake of comedications and/or biologics transported by OATP1B1, OATP1B3, or NTCP. Similarly, they are not expected to inhibit the efflux of comedications and/or biologics transported by the breast cancer resistant protein (MXR), the bile salt export pump (BSEP), the multidrug resistance-associated protein 2 (MRP2), and MDR1-mediated transport at therapeutic concentrations.

Oral Contraceptives

The coadministration of fingolimod 0.5 mg daily with oral contraceptives (ethinylestradiol and levonorgestrel) did not elicit any clinically significant change in oral contraceptives exposure. Fingolimod and fingolimod-phosphate exposure were consistent with those from previous studies. No interaction studies have been performed with oral contraceptives containing other progestagens; however, an effect of fingolimod on their exposure is not expected.

Cyclosporine

The pharmacokinetics of single-dose fingolimod was not altered during coadministration with cyclosporine at steady-state, nor was cyclosporine steady-state pharmacokinetics altered by fingolimod. These data indicate that GILENYA is unlikely to reduce the clearance of drugs mainly cleared by CYP3A4 and show that the potent inhibition of transporters MDR1, MRP2, and OATP-C does not influence fingolimod disposition.

Isoproterenol, Atropine, Atenolol, and Diltiazem

Single-dose fingolimod and fingolimod-phosphate exposure was not altered by coadministered isoproterenol or atropine. Likewise, the single-dose pharmacokinetics of fingolimod and fingolimod-phosphate and the steady-state pharmacokinetics of both atenolol and diltiazem were unchanged during the coadministration of the latter 2 drugs individually with fingolimod.

Population Pharmacokinetics Analysis

A population pharmacokinetics evaluation performed in MS patients did not provide evidence for a significant effect of fluoxetine and paroxetine (strong CYP2D6 inhibitors) on fingolimod or fingolimod-phosphate predose concentrations. In addition, the following commonly coprescribed substances had no clinically relevant effect (<20%) on fingolimod or fingolimod-phosphate predose concentrations: baclofen, gabapentin, oxybutynin, amantadine, modafinil, amitriptyline, pregabalin, and corticosteroids.

13   NONCLINICAL TOXICOLOGY

13.1   Carcinogenesis, Mutagenesis, Impairment of Fertility

Oral carcinogenicity studies of fingolimod were conducted in mice and rats. In mice, fingolimod was administered at oral doses of 0, 0.025, 0.25, and 2.5 mg/kg/day for up to 2 years. The incidence of malignant lymphoma was increased in males and females at the mid and high dose. The lowest dose tested (0.025 mg/kg/day) is less than the recommended human dose (RHD) of 0.5 mg/day on a body surface area (mg/m^2) basis. In rats, fingolimod was administered at oral doses of 0, 0.05, 0.15, 0.5, and 2.5 mg/kg/day. No increase in tumors was observed. The highest dose tested (2.5 mg/kg/day) is approximately 50 times the RHD on a mg/m^2 basis.

Fingolimod was negative in a battery of in vitro (Ames, mouse lymphoma thymidine kinase, chromosomal aberration in mammalian cells) and in vivo (micronucleus in mouse and rat) assays.

When fingolimod was administered orally (0, 1, 3, and 10 mg/kg/day) to male and female rats prior to and during mating, and continuing to Day 7 of gestation in females, no effect on fertility was observed up to the highest dose tested (10 mg/kg), which is approximately 200 times the RHD on a mg/m^2 basis.

13.2   Animal Toxicology and/or Pharmacology

Lung toxicity was observed in 2 different strains of rats and in dogs and monkeys. The primary findings included increase in lung weight, associated with smooth muscle hypertrophy, hyperdistension of the alveoli, and/or increased collagen. Insufficient or lack of pulmonary collapse at necropsy, generally correlated with microscopic changes, was observed in all species. In rats and monkeys, lung toxicity was observed at all oral doses tested in chronic studies. The lowest doses tested in rats (0.05 mg/kg/day in the 2-year carcinogenicity study) and monkeys (0.5 mg/kg/day in the 39-week toxicity study) are similar to and approximately 20 times the RHD on a mg/m^2 basis, respectively.

In the 52-week oral study in monkeys, respiratory distress associated with ketamine administration was observed at doses of 3 and 10 mg/kg/day; the most affected animal became hypoxic and required oxygenation. As ketamine is not generally associated with respiratory depression, this effect was attributed to fingolimod. In a subsequent study in rats, ketamine was shown to potentiate the bronchoconstrictive effects of fingolimod. The relevance of these findings to humans is unknown.

14   CLINICAL STUDIES

The efficacy of GILENYA was demonstrated in 2 studies that evaluated once-daily doses of GILENYA 0.5 mg and 1.25 mg in patients with relapsing-remitting MS (RRMS). Both studies included patients who had experienced at least 2 clinical relapses during the 2 years prior to randomization or at least 1 clinical relapse during the 1 year prior to randomization, and had an Expanded Disability Status Scale (EDSS) score from 0 to 5.5. Study 1 was a 2-year randomized, double-blind, placebo-controlled study in patients with RRMS who had not received any interferon-beta or glatiramer acetate for at least the previous 3 months and had not received any natalizumab for at least the previous 6 months. Neurological evaluations were performed at screening, every 3 months and at time of suspected relapse. MRI evaluations were performed at screening, Month 6, Month 12, and Month 24. The primary endpoint was the annualized relapse rate.

Median age was 37 years, median disease duration was 6.7 years and median EDSS score at baseline was 2.0. Patients were randomized to receive GILENYA 0.5 mg (N=425), 1.25 mg (N=429), or placebo (N=418) for up to 24 months. Median time on study drug was 717 days on 0.5 mg, 715 days on 1.25 mg and 719 days on placebo.

The annualized relapse rate was significantly lower in patients treated with GILENYA than in patients who received placebo. The secondary endpoint was the time to 3-month confirmed disability progression as measured by at least a 1-point increase from baseline in EDSS (0.5 point increase for patients with baseline EDSS of 5.5) sustained for 3 months. Time to onset of 3-month confirmed disability progression was significantly delayed with GILENYA treatment compared to placebo. The 1.25 mg dose resulted in no additional benefit over the GILENYA 0.5 mg dose. The results for this study are shown in Table 2 and Figure 1.

[See table 2 at top of next page]

Figure 1 Time to 3-month Confirmed Disability Progression – Study 1 (ITT population)

Study 2 was a 1-year randomized, double-blind, doubledummy, active-controlled study in patients with RRMS who had not received any natalizumab in the previous 6 months. Prior therapy with interferon-beta or glatiramer acetate up to the time of randomization was permitted.

Neurological evaluations were performed at screening, every 3 months, and at the time of suspected relapses. MRI evaluations were performed at screening and at month 12. The primary endpoint was the annualized relapse rate.

Median age was 36 years, median disease duration was 5.9 years, and median EDSS score at baseline was 2.0. Patients were randomized to receive GILENYA 0.5 mg (N=431), 1.25 mg (N=426), or interferon beta-1a, 30 micrograms via the intramuscular route (IM) once weekly (N=435) for up to

Table 2 Clinical and MRI Results of Study 1

	GILENYA 0.5 mg N=425	Placebo N=418	p-value
Clinical Endpoints			
Annualized relapse rate (primary endpoint)	0.18	0.40	<0.001
Percentage of patients without relapse	70%	46%	<0.001
Hazard ratio‡ of disability progression	0.70		0.02
(95% CI)	(0.52, 0.96)		
MRI Endpoint			
Mean (median) number of new or newly enlarging T2 lesions over 24 months	2.5 (0)	9.8 (5.0)	<0.001
Mean (median) number of T1 Gd-enhancing lesions at Month 24	0.2 (0)	1.1 (0)	<0.001

All analyses of clinical endpoints were intent-to-treat. MRI analysis used evaluable dataset.
‡ Hazard ratio is an estimate of the relative risk of having the event of disability progression on GILENYA as compared to placebo.

Table 3 Clinical and MRI Results of Study 2

	GILENYA 0.5 mg N=429	Interferon beta-1a IM 30 µg N=431	p-value
Clinical Endpoints			
Annualized relapse rate (primary endpoint)	0.16	0.33	<0.001
Percentage of patients without relapse	83%	70%	<0.001
Hazard ratio‡ of disability progression	0.71		0.21
(95% CI)	(0.42, 1.21)		
MRI Endpoint			
Mean (median) number of new or newly enlarging T2 lesions over 12 months	1.6 (0)	2.6 (1.0)	0.002
Mean (median) number of T1 Gd-enhancing lesions at Month 12	0.2 (0)	0.5 (0)	<0.001

All analyses of clinical endpoints were intent-to-treat. MRI analysis used evaluable dataset.
‡ Hazard ratio is an estimate of the relative risk of having the event of disability progression on GILENYA as compared to control.

12 months. Median time on study drug was 365 days on GILENYA 0.5 mg, 354 days on 1.25 mg, and 361 days on interferon beta-1a IM.

The annualized relapse rate was significantly lower in patients treated with GILENYA 0.5 mg than in patients who received interferon beta-1a IM. The key secondary endpoints were number of new and newly enlarging T2 lesions and time to onset of 3-month confirmed disability progression as measured by at least a 1-point increase from baseline in EDSS (0.5 point increase for those with baseline EDSS of 5.5) sustained for 3 months. The number of new and newly enlarging T2 lesions was significantly lower in patients treated with GILENYA than in patients who received interferon beta-1a IM. There was no significant difference in the time to 3-month confirmed disability progression between GILENYA and interferon beta-1a-treated patients at 1 year. The 1.25 mg dose resulted in no additional benefit over the GILENYA 0.5 mg dose. The results for this study are shown in Table 3.
[See Table 3 above]

Pooled results of study 1 and study 2 showed a consistent and statistically significant reduction of annualized relapse rate compared to comparator in subgroups defined by gender, age, prior MS therapy, and disease activity.

16 HOW SUPPLIED/STORAGE AND HANDLING

0.5 mg GILENYA capsules are hard gelatin capsules with a white opaque body and bright yellow cap imprinted with "FTY 0.5 mg" on the cap and 2 radial bands imprinted on the capsule body with yellow ink.
GILENYA capsules are supplied in blister packs.
Carton of 28 capsules containing 2 folded blister cards of 14 capsules per blister card   NDC 0078-0607-51
Carton of 7 capsules containing 1 blister card of 7 capsules per blister card   NDC 0078-0607-89
GILENYA capsules should be stored at 25°C (77°F); excursions permitted to 15°C–30°C (59°F–86°F). Protect from moisture.

17 PATIENT COUNSELING INFORMATION

See Medication Guide.
A Medication Guide is required for distribution with GILENYA. Encourage patients to read the GILENYA Medication Guide. The complete text of the Medication Guide is reprinted at the end of this document.

Benefits and Risks
Summarize for patients the benefits and potential risks of treatment with GILENYA. Tell patients to take GILENYA once daily as prescribed. Tell patients not to discontinue GILENYA without first discussing this with the prescribing physician. Advise patients to contact their physician if they accidently take more Gilenya than prescribed.

Cardiac Effects
Advise patients that initiation of GILENYA treatment results in a transient decrease in heart rate. Inform patients that they will need to be observed in the doctor's office or other facility for at least 6 hours after the first dose. Advise patients that if GILENYA is discontinued for more than 14 days, effects similar to those observed on treatment initiation may be seen and observation for at least 6 hours will be needed on treatment reinitiation, and that the same precautions will be taken if treatment is interrupted for more than 1 day within the first 2 weeks of treatment, or for more than 7 days during week 3 and 4 of treatment.

Risk of Infections
Inform patients that they may be more likely to get infections when taking GILENYA, and that they should contact their physician if they develop symptoms of infection. Advise patients that the use of some vaccines should be avoided during treatment with GILENYA and for 2 months after discontinuation. Advise patients who have not had chickenpox or vaccination to consider VZV vaccination prior to commencing treatment with GILENYA. Inform patients that prior or concomitant use of drugs that suppress the immune system may increase the risk of infection.

Macular Edema
Advise patients that GILENYA may cause macular edema, and that they should contact their physician if they experience any changes in their vision. Inform patients with diabetes mellitus or a history of uveitis that their risk of macular edema is increased.

Respiratory Effects
Advise patients that they should contact their physician if they experience new onset or worsening of dyspnea.

Hepatic Effects
Inform patients that GILENYA may increase liver enzymes. Advise patients that they should contact their physician if they have any unexplained nausea, vomiting, abdominal pain, fatigue, anorexia, or jaundice and/or dark urine.

Fetal Risk
Inform patients that, based on animal studies, GILENYA may cause fetal harm. Discuss with women of childbearing age whether they are pregnant, might be pregnant or are trying to become pregnant. Advise women of childbearing age of the need for effective contraception during GILENYA treatment and for 2 months after stopping GILENYA. Advise the patient that if she should nevertheless become pregnant, she should immediately inform her physician.

Persistence of GILENYA Effects After Drug Discontinuation
Advise patients that GILENYA remains in the blood and continues to have effects, including decreased blood lymphocyte counts, for up to 2 months following the last dose.
T2014-53
April 2014

MEDICATION GUIDE
GILENYA® (je-LEN-yah)
(fingolimod)
capsules

Read this Medication Guide before you start using Gilenya and each time you get a refill. There may be new information. This information does not take the place of talking with your doctor about your health problem or treatment.

What is the most important information I should know about GILENYA?
GILENYA may cause serious side effects, including:
1. Slow heart rate (bradycardia or bradyarrhythmia) when you start taking GILENYA. GILENYA can cause your heart rate to slow down, especially after you take your first dose. You will have a test to check the electrical activity of your heart (ECG) before you take your first dose of GILENYA. **You will be observed by a healthcare professional for at least 6 hours after you take your first dose of GILENYA.**
After you take your first dose of GILENYA:
• Your pulse and blood pressure should be checked every hour.
• You should be observed by a healthcare professional to see if you have any serious side effects. If your heart rate slows down too much, you may have symptoms such as:
  ○ dizziness
  ○ tiredness
  ○ feeling like your heart is beating slowly or skipping beats
• If you have any of the symptoms of slow heart rate, they will usually happen during the first 6 hours after your first dose of GILENYA. Symptoms can happen up to 24 hours after you take your first GILENYA dose.
• 6 hours after you take your first dose of GILENYA you will have another ECG. If your ECG shows any heart problems or if your heart rate is still too low or continues to decrease, you will continue to be observed.
• If you have any serious side effects after your first dose of GILENYA, especially those that require treatment with other medicines, you will stay in the medical facility to be observed overnight. You will also be observed for any serious side effects for at least 6 hours after you take your second dose of GILENYA the next day.
• If you have certain types of heart problems, or if you are taking certain types of medicines that can affect your heart, you will be observed overnight after you take your first dose of GILENYA.
Your slow heart rate will usually return to normal within 1 month after you start taking GILENYA. Call your doctor or go to the nearest hospital emergency room right away if you have any symptoms of a slow heart rate.
If you miss 1 or more doses of GILENYA you may need to be observed by a healthcare professional when you take your next dose. Call your doctor if you miss a dose of GILENYA. See "How should I take GILENYA?"
2. Infections. GILENYA can increase your risk of serious infections and decrease the way vaccines work in your body to prevent certain diseases, especially the chicken pox vaccine. GILENYA lowers the number of white blood cells (lymphocytes) in your blood. This will usually go back to normal within 2 months of stopping treatment. Your doctor may do a blood test before you start taking GILENYA. Call your doctor right away if you have any of these symptoms of an infection:
• fever
• tiredness
• body aches
• chills
• nausea
• vomiting
3. A problem with your vision called macular edema. Macular edema can cause some of the same vision symptoms as an MS attack (optic neuritis). You may not notice any symptoms with macular edema. If macular edema happens, it usually starts in the first 3 to 4 months after you start taking GILENYA. Your doctor should test your vision before you start taking GILENYA and 3 to 4 months after you start taking GILENYA, or any time you notice vision changes during treatment with GILENYA. Your risk of macular edema may be higher if you have diabetes or have had an inflammation of your eye called uveitis.
Call your doctor right away if you have any of the following:
• blurriness or shadows in the center of your vision
• a blind spot in the center of your vision
• sensitivity to light
• unusually colored (tinted) vision
What is GILENYA?
GILENYA is a prescription medicine used to treat relapsing forms of multiple sclerosis (MS) in adults. GILENYA can decrease the number of MS flare-ups (relapses). GILENYA does not cure MS, but it can help slow down the physical problems that MS causes.
It is not known if GILENYA is safe and effective in children under 18 years of age.

Who should not take GILENYA?

Do not take GILENYA if you:

- have had a heart attack, unstable angina, stroke or warning stroke or certain types of heart failure in the last 6 months
- have certain types of irregular or abnormal heartbeat (arrhythmia), including patients in whom a heart finding called prolonged QT is seen on ECG before starting GILENYA
- are taking certain medicines that change your heart rhythm

If any of the above situations apply to you, tell your doctor.

What should I tell my doctor before taking GILENYA?

Before you take GILENYA, tell your doctor about all your medical conditions, including if you had or now have:

- an irregular or abnormal heartbeat (arrhythmia)
- a history of stroke or warning stroke
- heart problems, including heart attack or angina
- a history of repeated fainting (syncope)
- a fever or infection, or you are unable to fight infections due to a disease or taking medicines that lower your immune system. Tell your doctor if you have had chicken pox or have received the vaccine for chicken pox. Your doctor may do a blood test for chicken pox virus. You may need to get the vaccine for chicken pox and then wait 1 month before you start taking GILENYA.
- eye problems, especially an inflammation of the eye called uveitis.
- diabetes
- breathing problems, including during your sleep
- liver problems
- high blood pressure
- Are pregnant or plan to become pregnant. GILENYA may harm your unborn baby. Talk to your doctor if you are pregnant or are planning to become pregnant.
  - Tell your doctor right away if you become pregnant while taking GILENYA or if you become pregnant within 2 months after you stop taking GILENYA.
  - If you are a female who can become pregnant, you should use effective birth control during your treatment with GILENYA and for at least 2 months after you stop taking GILENYA.

  Pregnancy Registry: There is a registry for women who become pregnant during treatment with GILENYA. If you become pregnant while taking GILENYA, talk to your doctor about registering with the GILENYA Pregnancy Registry. The purpose of this registry is to collect information about your health and your baby's health. For more information, contact the GILENYA Pregnancy Registry by calling Outcome at 1-877-598-7237, by sending an email to gpr@outcome.com, or go to www.gilenyapregnancyregistry.com.
- Are breastfeeding or plan to breastfeed. It is not known if GILENYA passes into your breast milk. You and your doctor should decide if you will take GILENYA or breastfeed. You should not do both.

Tell your doctor about all the medicines you take or have recently taken, including prescription and over-the-counter medicines, vitamins, and herbal supplements. Especially tell your doctor if you take medicines that affect your immune system, or have taken them in the past.

Know the medicines you take. Keep a list of your medicines with you to show your doctor and pharmacist when you get a new medicine.

Using GILENYA and other medicines together may affect each other causing serious side effects.

Especially tell your doctor if you take vaccines. Tell your doctor if you have been vaccinated within 1 month before you start taking GILENYA. You should not get certain vaccines while you take GILENYA and for at least 2 months after you stop taking GILENYA. If you take certain vaccines, you may get the infection the vaccine should have prevented. Vaccines may not work as well as when given during GILENYA treatment.

How should I take GILENYA?

- You will be observed by a healthcare professional for at least 6 hours after your first dose of GILENYA. See "What is the most important information I should know about GILENYA?"
- Take GILENYA exactly as your doctor tells you to take it.
- Take GILENYA 1 time each day.
- If you take too much GILENYA, call your doctor or go to the nearest hospital emergency room right away.
- Take GILENYA with or without food.
- Do not stop taking GILENYA without talking with your doctor first.
- Call your doctor right away if you miss a dose of GILENYA. You may need to be observed by a healthcare professional for at least 6 hours when you take your next dose. If you need to be observed by a healthcare professional when you take your next dose of GILENYA you will have:
  - an ECG before you take your dose

  - hourly pulse and blood pressure measurements after you take the dose
  - an ECG 6 hours after your dose
- If you have certain types of heart problems, or if you are taking certain types of medicines that can affect your heart, you will be observed overnight by a healthcare professional in a medical facility after you take your dose of GILENYA.
- If you have serious side effects after taking a dose of GILENYA, especially those that require treatment with other medicines, you will stay in the medical facility to be observed overnight. If you were observed overnight, you will also be observed for any serious side effects for at least 6 hours after you take your second dose of GILENYA. See "What is the most important information I should know about GILENYA?"

What are possible side effects of GILENYA?

GILENYA can cause serious side effects.

See "What is the most important information I should know about GILENYA?"

Serious side effects include:

- **swelling and narrowing of the blood vessels in your brain that may lead to a stroke or bleeding.** This problem usually gets better when you stop taking GILENYA. Call your doctor right away if you have any of the following symptoms of a stroke or bleeding in your brain, including:
  - sudden headache
  - confusion
  - seizures
  - loss of vision
  - weakness
- **breathing problems.** Some people who take GILENYA have shortness of breath. Call your doctor right away if you have trouble breathing.
- **liver problems.** GILENYA may cause liver problems. Your doctor should do blood tests to check your liver before you start taking GILENYA. Call your doctor right away if you have any of the following symptoms of liver problems:
  - nausea
  - vomiting
  - stomach pain
  - loss of appetite
  - tiredness
  - your skin or the whites of your eyes turn yellow
  - dark urine

The most common side effects of GILENYA include:

- headache
- flu
- diarrhea
- back pain
- abnormal liver tests
- cough

Tell your doctor if you have any side effect that bothers you or that does not go away.

These are not all of the possible side effects of GILENYA. For more information, ask your doctor or pharmacist. Call your doctor for medical advice about side effects. You may report side effects to FDA at 1-800-FDA-1088.

How do I store GILENYA?

- Store GILENYA in the original blister pack in a dry place.
- Store GILENYA at room temperature between 59°F to 86°F (15°C to 30°C).
- Keep GILENYA and all medicines out of the reach of children.

General information about GILENYA

Medicines are sometimes prescribed for purposes other than those listed in a Medication Guide. Do not use GILENYA for a condition for which it was not prescribed. Do not give GILENYA to other people, even if they have the same symptoms you have. It may harm them.

This Medication Guide summarizes the most important information about GILENYA. If you would like more information, talk with your doctor. You can ask your doctor or pharmacist for information about GILENYA that is written for healthcare professionals.

For more information, go to www.pharma.US.Novartis.com or call 1-888-669-6682.

What are the ingredients in GILENYA?

Active ingredient: fingolimod

Inactive ingredients: gelatin, magnesium stearate, mannitol, titanium dioxide, yellow iron oxide.

This Medication Guide has been approved by the U.S. Food and Drug Administration.

GILENYA is a registered trademark of Novartis AG.

Manufactured by:
Novartis Pharma Stein AG
Stein, Switzerland

Distributed by:
Novartis Pharmaceuticals Corporation
East Hanover, New Jersey 07936

© Novartis

T2014-54

Revised: April 2014

Shown in Product Identification Guide, page 310

GLEEVEC

[glē-věk]
(imatinib mesylate)
tablets for oral use

℞

The following prescribing information is based on official labeling in effect July 2014.

HIGHLIGHTS OF PRESCRIBING INFORMATION
These highlights do not include all the information needed to use Gleevec safely and effectively. See full prescribing information for Gleevec.
GLEEVEC (imatinib mesylate) tablets for oral use
Initial U.S. Approval: 2001

——————INDICATIONS AND USAGE——————

Gleevec is a kinase inhibitor indicated for the treatment of:

- Newly diagnosed adult and pediatric patients with Philadelphia chromosome positive chronic myeloid leukemia (Ph+ CML) in chronic phase (1.1)
- Patients with Philadelphia chromosome positive chronic myeloid leukemia (Ph+ CML) in blast crisis (BC), accelerated phase (AP), or in chronic phase (CP) after failure of interferon-alpha therapy (1.2)
- Adult patients with relapsed or refractory Philadelphia chromosome positive acute lymphoblastic leukemia (Ph+ ALL) (1.3)
- Pediatric patients with newly diagnosed Philadelphia chromosome positive acute lymphoblastic leukemia (Ph+ ALL) in combination with chemotherapy (1.4)
- Adult patients with myelodysplastic/ myeloproliferative diseases (MDS/MPD) associated with PDGFR (platelet-derived growth factor receptor) gene re-arrangements (1.5)
- Adult patients with aggressive systemic mastocytosis (ASM) without the D816V c-Kit mutation or with c-Kit mutational status unknown (1.6)
- Adult patients with hypereosinophilic syndrome (HES) and/or chronic eosinophilic leukemia (CEL) who have the FIP1L1-PDGFRα fusion kinase (mutational analysis or FISH demonstration of CHIC2 allele deletion) and for patients with HES and/or CEL who are FIP1L1-PDGFRα fusion kinase negative or unknown (1.7)
- Adult patients with unresectable, recurrent and/or metastatic dermatofibrosarcoma protuberans (DFSP) (1.8)
- Patients with Kit (CD117) positive unresectable and/or metastatic malignant gastrointestinal stromal tumors (GIST) (1.9)
- Adjuvant treatment of adult patients following resection of Kit (CD117) positive GIST (1.10)

——————DOSAGE AND ADMINISTRATION——————

- Adults with Ph+ CML CP (2.1): 400 mg/day
- Adults with Ph+ CML AP or BC (2.1): 600 mg/day
- Pediatrics with Ph+ CML CP (2.2): 340 mg/m²/day
- Adults with Ph+ ALL (2.3): 600 mg/day
- Pediatrics with Ph+ ALL (2.4): 340 mg/m²/day
- Adults with MDS/MPD (2.5): 400 mg/day
- Adults with ASM (2.6): 100 mg/day or 400 mg/day
- Adults with HES/CEL (2.7): 100 mg/day or 400 mg/day
- Adults with DFSP (2.8): 800 mg/day
- Adults with metastatic and/or unresectable GIST (2.9): 400 mg/day
- Adjuvant treatment of adults with GIST (2.10): 400 mg/day
- Patients with mild to moderate hepatic impairment (2.11): 400 mg/day
- Patients with severe hepatic impairment (2.11): 300 mg/day

All doses of Gleevec should be taken with a meal and a large glass of water. Doses of 400 mg or 600 mg should be administered once daily, whereas a dose of 800 mg should be administered as 400 mg twice a day. Gleevec can be dissolved in water or apple juice for patients having difficulty swallowing. Daily dosing of 800 mg and above should be accomplished using the 400 mg tablet to reduce exposure to iron.

——————DOSAGE FORMS AND STRENGTHS——————

Tablets (scored): 100 mg and 400 mg (3)

——————CONTRAINDICATIONS——————

None (4)

——————WARNINGS AND PRECAUTIONS——————

- Edema and severe fluid retention have occurred. Weigh patients regularly and manage unexpected rapid weight gain by drug interruption and diuretics (5.1, 6.1, 6.11)
- Cytopenias, particularly anemia, neutropenia, and thrombocytopenia, have occurred. Manage with dose reduction or dose interruption and in rare cases discontinuation of treatment. Perform complete blood counts weekly for the first month, biweekly for the second month, and periodically thereafter (5.2)
- Severe congestive heart failure and left ventricular dysfunction have been reported, particularly in patients with comorbidities and risk factors. Patients with cardiac disease or risk factors for cardiac failure should be monitored and treated (5.3)
- Severe hepatotoxicity including fatalities may occur. Assess liver function before initiation of treatment and

monthly thereafter or as clinically indicated. Monitor liver function when combined with chemotherapy known to be associated with liver dysfunction (5.4)

- Grade 3/4 hemorrhage has been reported in clinical studies in patients with newly diagnosed CML and with GIST. GI tumor sites may be the source of GI bleeds in GIST (5.5)
- Gastrointestinal perforations, some fatal, have been reported (5.6)
- Cardiogenic shock/left ventricular dysfunction has been associated with the initiation of Gleevec in patients with conditions associated with high eosinophil levels (e.g., HES, MDS/MPD and ASM) (5.7)
- Bullous dermatologic reactions (e.g., erythema multiforme and Stevens-Johnson syndrome) have been reported with the use of Gleevec (5.8)
- Hypothyroidism has been reported in thyroidectomy patients undergoing levothyroxine replacement. Closely monitor TSH levels in such patients (5.9)
- Consider potential toxicities, specifically, liver, kidney, and cardiac toxicity, and immunosuppression from long-term use (5.10)
- Fetal harm can occur when administered to a pregnant woman. Women should be apprised of the potential harm to the fetus (5.11, 8.1)
- Growth retardation occurring in children and pre-adolescents receiving Gleevec has been reported. Close monitoring of growth in children under Gleevec treatment is recommended (5.12, 6.13)
- Tumor lysis syndrome. Close monitoring is recommended (5.13)
- Reports of motor vehicle accidents have been received in patients receiving Gleevec. Caution patients about driving a car or operating machinery (5.14)

------ADVERSE REACTIONS------

The most frequently reported adverse reactions (>30%) were edema, nausea, vomiting, muscle cramps, musculoskeletal pain, diarrhea, rash, fatigue and abdominal pain (6.1, 6.11)

To report SUSPECTED ADVERSE REACTIONS, contact Novartis Pharmaceuticals Corporation at 1-888-669-6682 or FDA at 1-800-FDA-1088 or www.fda.gov/medwatch.

------DRUG INTERACTIONS------

- CYP3A4 inducers may decrease Gleevec C_{max} and AUC (2.11, 7.1)
- CYP3A4 inhibitors may increase Gleevec C_{max} and AUC (7.2)
- Gleevec is an inhibitor of CYP3A4 and CYP2D6 which may increase the C_{max} and AUC of other drugs (7.3, 7.4)
- Patients who require anticoagulation should receive low-molecular weight or standard heparin and not warfarin (7.3)

------USE IN SPECIFIC POPULATIONS------

- There is no experience in children less than 1 year of age (8.4)
- Pregnancy: Sexually active female patients should use highly effective contraception during treatment (5.11)

See 17 for PATIENT COUNSELING INFORMATION and FDA-approved patient labeling

Revised: 5/2014

Table 1 Dose Adjustments for Neutropenia and Thrombocytopenia

Condition (starting dose)	ANC / platelets	Action
ASM associated with eosinophilia (starting dose 100 mg)	ANC <1.0×10^9/L and/or platelets <50×10^9/L	1. Stop Gleevec until ANC ≥1.5×10^9/L and platelets ≥75×10^9/L 2. Resume treatment with Gleevec at previous dose (i.e., dose before severe adverse reaction)
HES/CEL with FIP1L1-PDGFRα fusion kinase (starting dose 100 mg)	ANC <1.0×10^9/L and/or platelets <50×10^9/L	1. Stop Gleevec until ANC ≥1.5×10^9/L and platelets ≥75×10^9/L 2. Resume treatment with Gleevec at previous dose (i.e., dose before severe adverse reaction)
Chronic Phase CML (starting dose 400 mg) MDS/MPD, ASM and HES/CEL (starting dose 400 mg) GIST (starting dose 400 mg)	ANC <1.0×10^9/L and/or platelets <50×10^9/L	1. Stop Gleevec until ANC ≥1.5×10^9/L and platelets ≥75×10^9/L 2. Resume treatment with Gleevec at the original starting dose of 400 mg 3. If recurrence of ANC <1.0×10^9/L and/or platelets <50×10^9/L, repeat step 1 and resume Gleevec at a reduced dose of 300 mg
Ph+ CML : Accelerated Phase and Blast Crisis (starting dose 600 mg) Ph+ ALL (starting dose 600 mg)	ANC <0.5×10^9/L and/or platelets <10×10^9/L	1. Check if cytopenia is related to leukemia (marrow aspirate or biopsy) 2. If cytopenia is unrelated to leukemia, reduce dose of Gleevec to 400 mg 3. If cytopenia persists 2 weeks, reduce further to 300 mg 4. If cytopenia persists 4 weeks and is still unrelated to leukemia, stop Gleevec until ANC ≥1×10^9/L and platelets ≥20×10^9/L and then resume treatment at 300 mg
DFSP (starting dose 800 mg)	ANC <1.0×10^9/L and/or platelets <50×10^9/L	1. Stop Gleevec until ANC ≥1.5×10^9/L and platelets ≥75×10^9/L 2. Resume treatment with Gleevec at 600 mg 3. In the event of recurrence of ANC <1.0×10^9/L and/or platelets <50×10^9/L, repeat step 1 and resume Gleevec at reduced dose of 400 mg
Pediatric newly diagnosed chronic phase CML (starting dose 340 mg/m²)	ANC <1.0×10^9/L and/or platelets <50×10^9/L	1. Stop Gleevec until ANC ≥1.5×10^9/L and platelets ≥75×10^9/L 2. Resume treatment with Gleevec at previous dose (i.e., dose before severe adverse reaction) 3. In the event of recurrence of ANC <1.0×10^9/L and/or platelets <50×10^9/L, repeat step 1 and resume Gleevec at reduced dose of 260 mg/m²

FULL PRESCRIBING INFORMATION

1 INDICATIONS AND USAGE
1.1 Newly Diagnosed Philadelphia Positive Chronic Myeloid Leukemia (Ph+ CML)
Newly diagnosed adult and pediatric patients with Philadelphia chromosome positive chronic myeloid leukemia in chronic phase.
1.2 Ph+ CML in Blast Crisis (BC), Accelerated Phase (AP) or Chronic Phase (CP) After Interferon-alpha (IFN) Therapy
Patients with Philadelphia chromosome positive chronic myeloid leukemia in blast crisis, accelerated phase, or in chronic phase after failure of interferon-alpha therapy.

1.3 Adult patients with Ph+ Acute Lymphoblastic Leukemia (ALL)

Adult patients with relapsed or refractory Philadelphia chromosome positive acute lymphoblastic leukemia.

1.4 Pediatric patients with Ph+ Acute Lymphoblastic Leukemia (ALL)

Pediatric patients with newly diagnosed Philadelphia chromosome positive acute lymphoblastic leukemia (Ph+ ALL) in combination with chemotherapy.

1.5 Myelodysplastic/Myeloproliferative Diseases (MDS/MPD)

Adult patients with myelodysplastic/ myeloproliferative diseases associated with PDGFR (platelet-derived growth factor receptor) gene re-arrangements.

1.6 Aggressive Systemic Mastocytosis (ASM)

Adult patients with aggressive systemic mastocytosis without the D816V c-Kit mutation or with c-Kit mutational status unknown.

1.7 Hypereosinophilic Syndrome (HES) and/or Chronic Eosinophilic Leukemia (CEL)

Adult patients with hypereosinophilic syndrome and/or chronic eosinophilic leukemia who have the FIP1L1-PDGFRα fusion kinase (mutational analysis or FISH demonstration of CHIC2 allele deletion) and for patients with HES and/or CEL who are FIP1L1-PDGFRα fusion kinase negative or unknown.

1.8 Dermatofibrosarcoma Protuberans (DFSP)

Adult patients with unresectable, recurrent and/or metastatic dermatofibrosarcoma protuberans.

1.9 Kit+ Gastrointestinal Stromal Tumors (GIST)

Patients with Kit (CD117) positive unresectable and/or metastatic malignant gastrointestinal stromal tumors.

1.10 Adjuvant Treatment of GIST

Adjuvant treatment of adult patients following complete gross resection of Kit (CD117) positive GIST.

2 DOSAGE AND ADMINISTRATION

Therapy should be initiated by a physician experienced in the treatment of patients with hematological malignancies or malignant sarcomas, as appropriate. The prescribed dose should be administered orally, with a meal and a large glass of water. Doses of 400 mg or 600 mg should be administered once daily, whereas a dose of 800 mg should be administered as 400 mg twice a day.

In children, Gleevec treatment can be given as a once-daily dose in CML and Ph+ ALL. Alternatively, in children with CML the daily dose may be split into two - one portion dosed in the morning and one portion in the evening. There is no experience with Gleevec treatment in children under 1 year of age.

For patients unable to swallow the film-coated tablets, the tablets may be dispersed in a glass of water or apple juice. The required number of tablets should be placed in the appropriate volume of beverage (approximately 50 mL for a 100 mg tablet, and 200 mL for a 400 mg tablet) and stirred with a spoon. The suspension should be administered immediately after complete disintegration of the tablet(s).

For daily dosing of 800 mg and above, dosing should be accomplished using the 400 mg tablet to reduce exposure to iron.

Treatment may be continued as long as there is no evidence of progressive disease or unacceptable toxicity.

2.1 Adult Patients with Ph+ CML CP, AP, and BC

The recommended dose of Gleevec is 400 mg/day for adult patients in chronic phase CML and 600 mg/day for adult patients in accelerated phase or blast crisis.

In CML, a dose increase from 400 mg to 600 mg in adult patients with chronic phase disease, or from 600 mg to 800 mg (given as 400 mg twice daily) in adult patients in accelerated phase or blast crisis may be considered in the absence of severe adverse drug reaction and severe non-leukemia related neutropenia or thrombocytopenia in the following circumstances: disease progression (at any time), failure to achieve a satisfactory hematologic response after at least 3 months of treatment, failure to achieve a cytogenetic response after 6-12 months of treatment, or loss of a previously achieved hematologic or cytogenetic response.

2.2 Pediatric Patients with Ph+ CML CP

The recommended dose of Gleevec for children with newly diagnosed Ph+ CML is 340 mg/m²/day (not to exceed 600 mg).

2.3 Adults Patients with Ph+ ALL

The recommended dose of Gleevec is 600 mg/day for adult patients with relapsed/refractory Ph+ ALL.

2.4 Pediatric Patients with Ph+ ALL

The recommended dose of Gleevec to be given in combination with chemotherapy to children with newly diagnosed Ph+ ALL is 340mg/m²/day (not to exceed 600mg).

2.5 MDS/MPD

The recommended dose of Gleevec is 400 mg/day for adult patients with MDS/MPD.

2.6 ASM

The recommended dose of Gleevec is 400 mg/day for adult patients with ASM without the D816V c-Kit mutation. If

c-Kit mutational status is not known or unavailable, treatment with Gleevec 400 mg/day may be considered for patients with ASM not responding satisfactorily to other therapies. For patients with ASM associated with eosinophilia, a clonal hematological disease related to the fusion kinase FIP1L1-PDGFRα, a starting dose of 100 mg/day is recommended. Dose increase from 100 mg to 400 mg for these patients may be considered in the absence of adverse drug reactions if assessments demonstrate an insufficient response to therapy.

2.7 HES/CEL

The recommended dose of Gleevec is 400 mg/day for adult patients with HES/CEL. For HES/CEL patients with demonstrated FIP1L1-PDGFRα fusion kinase, a starting dose of 100 mg/day is recommended. Dose increase from 100 mg to 400 mg for these patients may be considered in the absence of adverse drug reactions if assessments demonstrate an insufficient response to therapy.

2.8 DFSP

The recommended dose of Gleevec is 800 mg/day for adult patients with DFSP.

2.9 Metastatic or Unresectable GIST

The recommended dose of Gleevec is 400 mg/day for adult patients with unresectable and/or metastatic, malignant GIST. A dose increase up to 800 mg daily (given as 400 mg twice daily) may be considered, as clinically indicated, in patients showing clear signs or symptoms of disease progression at a lower dose and in the absence of severe adverse drug reactions.

2.10 Adjuvant GIST

The recommended dose of Gleevec is 400 mg/day for the adjuvant treatment of adult patients following complete gross resection of GIST. In clinical trials one year of Gleevec and three years of Gleevec were studied. In the patient population defined in Study 2, three years of Gleevec is recommended [see Clinical Studies (14.8)]. The optimal treatment duration with Gleevec is not known.

2.11 Dose Modification Guidelines

Concomitant Strong CYP3A4 inducers: The use of concomitant strong CYP3A4 inducers should be avoided (e.g., dexamethasone, phenytoin, carbamazepine, rifampin, rifabutin, rifampacin, phenobarbital). If patients must be co-administered a strong CYP3A4 inducer, based on pharmacokinetic studies, the dosage of Gleevec should be increased by at least 50%, and clinical response should be carefully monitored [see Drug Interactions (7.1)].

Hepatic Impairment: Patients with mild and moderate hepatic impairment do not require a dose adjustment and should be treated per the recommended dose. A 25% decrease in the recommended dose should be used for patients with severe hepatic impairment [see Use in Specific Populations (8.6)].

Renal Impairment: Patients with moderate renal impairment (CrCL=20-39 mL/min) should receive a 50% decrease in the recommended starting dose and future doses can be increased as tolerated. Doses greater than 600 mg are not recommended in patients with mild renal impairment (CrCL=40-59 mL/min). For patients with moderate renal impairment doses greater than 400 mg are not recommended.

Imatinib should be used with caution in patients with severe renal impairment. A dose of 100 mg/day was tolerated in two patients with severe renal impairment [See Warnings and Precautions (5.3), Use in Specific Populations (8.7)].

2.12 Dose Adjustment for Hepatotoxicity and Non-Hematologic Adverse Reactions

If elevations in bilirubin >3 × institutional upper limit of normal (IULN) or in liver transaminases >5 × IULN occur, Gleevec should be withheld until bilirubin levels have returned to a <1.5 × IULN and transaminase levels to <2.5 × IULN. In adults, treatment with Gleevec may then be continued at a reduced daily dose (i.e., 400 mg to 300 mg, 600 mg to 400 mg or 800 mg to 600 mg). In children, daily doses can be reduced under the same circumstances from 340 mg/m²/day to 260 mg/m²/day.

If a severe non-hematologic adverse reaction develops (such as severe hepatotoxicity or severe fluid retention), Gleevec should be withheld until the event has resolved. Thereafter, treatment can be resumed as appropriate depending on the initial severity of the event.

2.13 Dose Adjustment for Hematologic Adverse Reactions

Dose reduction or treatment interruptions for severe neutropenia and thrombocytopenia are recommended as indicated in Table 1.

[See table 1 at top of previous page]

3 DOSAGE FORMS AND STRENGTHS

100 mg film coated tablets
Very dark yellow to brownish orange, film-coated tablets, round, biconvex with bevelled edges, debossed with "NVR" on one side, and "SA" with score on the other side
400 mg film coated tablets
Very dark yellow to brownish orange, film-coated tablets, ovaloid, biconvex with bevelled edges, debossed with "400" on one side with score on the other side, and "SL" on each side of the score

Table 2 Adverse Reactions Regardless of Relationship to Study Drug Reported in Newly Diagnosed CML Clinical Trial (≥10% of Gleevec Treated Patients)[1]

Preferred Term	All Grades		CTC Grades 3/4	
	Gleevec N=551 (%)	IFN+Ara–C N=533 (%)	Gleevec N=551 (%)	IFN+Ara–C N=533 (%)
Fluid Retention	61.7	11.1	2.5	0.9
– Superficial Edema	59.9	9.6	1.5	0.4
– Other Fluid Retention Reactions[2]	6.9	1.9	1.3	0.6
Nausea	49.5	61.5	1.3	5.1
Muscle Cramps	49.2	11.8	2.2	0.2
Musculoskeletal Pain	47.0	44.8	5.4	8.6
Diarrhea	45.4	43.3	3.3	3.2
Rash and Related Terms	40.1	26.1	2.9	2.4
Fatigue	38.8	67.0	1.8	25.1
Headache	37.0	43.3	0.5	3.8
Joint Pain	31.4	38.1	2.5	7.7
Abdominal Pain	36.5	25.9	4.2	3.9
Nasopharyngitis	30.5	8.8	0	0.4
Hemorrhage	28.9	21.2	1.8	1.7
- GI Hemorrhage	1.6	1.1	0.5	0.2
- CNS Hemorrhage	0.2	0.4	0	0.4
Myalgia	24.1	38.8	1.5	8.3
Vomiting	22.5	27.8	2.0	3.4
Dyspepsia	18.9	8.3	0	0.8
Cough	20.0	23.1	0.2	0.6
Pharyngolaryngeal Pain	18.1	11.4	0.2	0
Upper Respiratory Tract Infection	21.2	8.4	0.2	0.4
Dizziness	19.4	24.4	0.9	3.8
Pyrexia	17.8	42.6	0.9	3.0
Weight Increased	15.6	2.6	2.0	0.4
Insomnia	14.7	18.6	0	2.3
Depression	14.9	35.8	0.5	13.1
Influenza	13.8	6.2	0.2	0.2
Bone Pain	11.3	15.6	1.6	3.4
Constipation	11.4	14.4	0.7	0.2
Sinusitis	11.4	6.0	0.2	0.2

[1]All adverse reactions occurring in ≥10% of Gleevec treated patients are listed regardless of suspected relationship to treatment.
[2]Other fluid retention reactions include pleural effusion, ascites, pulmonary edema, pericardial effusion, anasarca, edema aggravated, and fluid retention not otherwise specified.

Help Patients Save on Rx Drugs: PDR.net/PharmacyDiscountCard

Table 3 Adverse Reactions Regardless of Relationship to Study Drug Reported in Other CML Clinical Trials (≥10% of All Patients in any Trial)[1]

Preferred Term	Myeloid Blast Crisis (n=260) % All Grades	Myeloid Blast Crisis (n=260) % Grade 3/4	Accelerated Phase (n=235) % All Grades	Accelerated Phase (n=235) % Grade 3/4	Chronic Phase, IFN Failure (n=532) % All Grades	Chronic Phase, IFN Failure (n=532) % Grade 3/4
Fluid Retention	72	11	76	6	69	4
-Superficial Edema	66	6	74	3	67	2
-Other Fluid Retention Reactions [2]	22	6	15	4	7	2
Nausea	71	5	73	5	63	3
Muscle Cramps	28	1	47	0.4	62	2
Vomiting	54	4	58	3	36	2
Diarrhea	43	4	57	5	48	3
Hemorrhage	53	19	49	11	30	2
- CNS Hemorrhage	9	7	3	3	2	1
- GI Hemorrhage	8	4	6	5	2	0.4
Musculoskeletal Pain	42	9	49	9	38	2
Fatigue	30	4	46	4	48	1
Skin Rash	36	5	47	5	47	3
Pyrexia	41	7	41	8	21	2
Arthralgia	25	5	34	6	40	1
Headache	27	5	32	2	36	0.6
Abdominal Pain	30	6	33	4	32	1
Weight Increased	5	1	17	5	32	7
Cough	14	0.8	27	0.9	20	0
Dyspepsia	12	0	22	0	27	0
Myalgia	9	0	24	2	27	0.2
Nasopharyngitis	10	0	17	0	22	0
Asthenia	18	5	21	5	15	0.2
Dyspnea	15	4	21	7	12	0.9
Upper Respiratory Tract Infection	3	0	12	0.4	19	0
Anorexia	14	2	17	2	7	0
Night Sweats	13	0.8	17	1	14	0.2
Constipation	16	2	16	0.9	9	0.4
Dizziness	12	0.4	13	0	16	0.2
Pharyngitis	10	0	12	0	15	0
Insomnia	10	0	14	0	14	0.2
Pruritus	8	1	14	0.9	14	0.8
Hypokalemia	13	4	9	2	6	0.8
Pneumonia	13	7	10	7	4	1
Anxiety	8	0.8	12	0	8	0.4
Liver Toxicity	10	5	12	6	6	3
Rigors	10	0	12	0.4	10	0
Chest Pain	7	2	10	0.4	11	0.8
Influenza	0.8	0.4	6	0	11	0.2
Sinusitis	4	0.4	11	0.4	9	0.4

[1] All adverse reactions occurring in ≥10% of patients are listed regardless of suspected relationship to treatment.
[2] Other fluid retention reactions include pleural effusion, ascites, pulmonary edema, pericardial effusion, anasarca, edema aggravated, and fluid retention not otherwise specified.

Table 4 Lab Abnormalities in Newly Diagnosed CML Clinical Trial

CTC Grades	Gleevec N=551 % Grade 3	Gleevec N=551 % Grade 4	IFN+Ara–C N=533 % Grade 3	IFN+Ara–C N=533 % Grade 4
Hematology Parameters*				
– Neutropenia*	13.1	3.6	20.8	4.5
– Thrombocytopenia*	8.5	0.4	15.9	0.6
– Anemia	3.3	1.1	4.1	0.2
Biochemistry Parameters				
– Elevated Creatinine	0	0	0.4	0
– Elevated Bilirubin	0.9	0.2	0.2	0
– Elevated Alkaline Phosphatase	0.2	0	0.8	0
– Elevated SGOT /SGPT	4.7	0.5	7.1	0.4

*p<0.001 (difference in Grade 3 plus 4 abnormalities between the two treatment groups)

4 CONTRAINDICATIONS

None

5 WARNINGS AND PRECAUTIONS

5.1 Fluid Retention and Edema

Gleevec is often associated with edema and occasionally serious fluid retention [see Adverse Reactions (6.1)]. Patients should be weighed and monitored regularly for signs and symptoms of fluid retention. An unexpected rapid weight gain should be carefully investigated and appropriate treatment provided. The probability of edema was increased with higher Gleevec dose and age >65 years in the CML studies. Severe superficial edema was reported in 1.5% of newly diagnosed CML patients taking Gleevec, and in 2%-6% of other adult CML patients taking Gleevec. In addition, other severe fluid retention (e.g., pleural effusion, pericardial effusion, pulmonary edema, and ascites) reactions were reported in 1.3% of newly diagnosed CML patients taking Gleevec, and in 2%-6% of other adult CML patients taking Gleevec. Severe fluid retention was reported in 9% to 13.1% of patients taking Gleevec for GIST [see Adverse Reactions (6.11)].

5.2 Hematologic Toxicity

Treatment with Gleevec is associated with anemia, neutropenia, and thrombocytopenia. Complete blood counts should be performed weekly for the first month, biweekly for the second month, and periodically thereafter as clinically indicated (for example, every 2-3 months). In CML, the occurrence of these cytopenias is dependent on the stage of disease and is more frequent in patients with accelerated phase CML or blast crisis than in patients with chronic phase CML. In pediatric CML patients the most frequent toxicities observed were Grade 3 or 4 cytopenias including neutropenia, thrombocytopenia and anemia. These generally occur within the first several months of therapy [see Dosage and Administration (2.12)].

5.3 Severe Congestive Heart Failure and Left Ventricular Dysfunction

Severe congestive heart failure and left ventricular dysfunction have been reported in patients taking Gleevec. Most of the patients with reported cardiac reactions have had other co-morbidities and risk factors, including advanced age and previous medical history of cardiac disease. In an international randomized phase 3 study in 1,106 patients with newly diagnosed Ph+ CML in chronic phase, severe cardiac failure and left ventricular dysfunction were observed in 0.7% of patients taking Gleevec compared to 0.9% of patients taking IFN + Ara-C. Patients with cardiac disease or risk factors for cardiac or history of renal failure should be monitored carefully and any patient with signs or symptoms consistent with cardiac or renal failure should be evaluated and treated.

5.4 Hepatotoxicity

Hepatotoxicity, occasionally severe, may occur with Gleevec [see Adverse Reactions (6.3)]. Cases of fatal liver failure and severe liver injury requiring liver transplants have been reported with both short-term and long-term use of Gleevec. Liver function (transaminases, bilirubin, and alkaline phosphatase) should be monitored before initiation of treatment and monthly, or as clinically indicated. Laboratory abnormalities should be managed with Gleevec interruption and/or dose reduction [see Dosage and Administration (2.12)].

When Gleevec is combined with chemotherapy, liver toxicity in the form of transaminase elevation and hyperbilirubinemia has been observed. Additionally, there have been reports of acute liver failure. Monitoring of hepatic function is recommended.

5.5 Hemorrhage

In the newly diagnosed CML trial, 1.8% of patients had Grade 3/4 hemorrhage. In the Phase 3 unresectable or metastatic GIST studies 211 patients (12.9%) reported Grade 3/4 hemorrhage at any site. In the Phase 2 unresectable or metastatic GIST study 7 patients (5%) had a total of 8 CTC Grade 3/4 hemorrhages; gastrointestinal (GI) (3 patients), intra-tumoral (3 patients) or both (1 patient). Gastrointestinal tumor sites may have been the source of GI hemorrhages. Patients should therefore be monitored for gastrointestinal symptoms at the start of therapy.

5.6 Gastrointestinal Disorders

Gleevec is sometimes associated with GI irritation. Gleevec should be taken with food and a large glass of water to minimize this problem. There have been rare reports, including fatalities, of gastrointestinal perforation.

5.7 Hypereosinophilic Cardiac Toxicity

In patients with hypereosinophilic syndrome with occult infiltration of HES cells within the myocardium, cases of cardiogenic shock/left ventricular dysfunction have been associated with HES cell degranulation upon the initiation of Gleevec therapy. The condition was reported to be reversible with the administration of systemic steroids, circulatory support measures and temporarily withholding Gleevec. Myelodysplastic/ myeloproliferative disease and systemic mastocytosis may be associated with high eosinophil levels. Performance of an echocardiogram and determination of serum troponin should therefore be considered in patients with HES/CEL, and in patients with MDS/MPD or ASM associated with high eosinophil levels. If either is abnormal, the prophylactic use of systemic steroids (1-2 mg/kg) for one to two weeks concomitantly with Gleevec should be considered at the initiation of therapy.

5.8 Dermatologic Toxicities

Bullous dermatologic reactions, including erythema multiforme and Stevens-Johnson syndrome, have been reported with use of Gleevec. In some cases of bullous dermatologic reactions, including erythema multiforme and Stevens-Johnson syndrome reported during postmarketing surveillance, a recurrent dermatologic reaction was observed upon re-challenge. Several foreign post-marketing reports have described cases in which patients tolerated the reintroduction of Gleevec therapy after resolution or improvement of the bullous reaction. In these instances, Gleevec was resumed at a dose lower than that at which the reaction occurred and some patients also received concomitant treatment with corticosteroids or antihistamines.

5.9 Hypothyroidism

Clinical cases of hypothyroidism have been reported in thyroidectomy patients undergoing levothyroxine replacement during treatment with Gleevec. TSH levels should be closely monitored in such patients.

5.10 Toxicities from Long-Term Use

It is important to consider potential toxicities suggested by animal studies, specifically, liver, kidney, and cardiac toxicity and immunosuppression. Severe liver toxicity was observed in dogs treated for 2 weeks, with elevated liver enzymes, hepatocellular necrosis, bile duct necrosis, and bile duct hyperplasia. Renal toxicity was observed in monkeys treated for 2 weeks, with focal mineralization and dilation of the renal tubules and tubular nephrosis. Increased BUN and creatinine were observed in several of these animals. An increased rate of opportunistic infections was observed with chronic imatinib treatment in laboratory animal studies. In a 39-week monkey study, treatment with imatinib resulted in worsening of normally suppressed malarial infections in these animals. Lymphopenia was observed in animals (as in humans). Additional long-term toxicities were identified in a 2-year rat study. Histopathological examination of the treated rats that died on study revealed cardiomyopathy (both sexes), chronic progressive nephropathy (females) and preputial gland papilloma as principal causes of death or reasons for sacrifice. Non-neoplastic lesions seen in this 2-year study which were not identified in earlier preclinical studies were the cardiovascular system, pancreas, endocrine organs and teeth. The most important changes included cardiac hypertrophy and dilatation, leading to signs of cardiac insufficiency in some animals.

5.11 Embryo-fetal Toxicity

Gleevec can cause fetal harm when administered to a pregnant woman. Imatinib mesylate was teratogenic in rats when administered during organogenesis at doses approximately equal to the maximum human dose of 800 mg/day based on body surface area. Significant post-implantation loss was seen in female rats administered imatinib mesylate at doses approximately one-half the maximum human dose of 800 mg/day based on body surface area. Sexually active female patients of reproductive potential taking Gleevec should use highly effective contraception. If this drug is used during pregnancy or if the patient becomes pregnant while taking this drug, the patient should be apprised of the potential hazard to a fetus [see Use in Specific Populations (8.1)].

5.12 Children and Adolescents

Growth retardation has been reported in children and pre-adolescents receiving Gleevec. The long term effects of prolonged treatment with Gleevec on growth in children are unknown. Therefore, close monitoring of growth in children under Gleevec treatment is recommended [see Adverse Reactions (6.13)].

5.13 Tumor Lysis Syndrome

Cases of Tumor Lysis Syndrome (TLS), including fatal cases, have been reported in patients with CML, GIST, ALL and eosinophilic leukemia receiving Gleevec. The patients at risk of TLS are those with tumors having a high proliferative rate or high tumor burden prior to treatment. These patients should be monitored closely and appropriate precautions taken. Due to possible occurrence of TLS, correction of clinically significant dehydration and treatment of high uric acid levels are recommended prior to initiation of Gleevec.

5.14 Driving and Using Machinery

Reports of motor vehicle accidents have been received in patients receiving Gleevec. While most of these reports are not suspected to be caused by Gleevec, patients should be advised that they may experience undesirable effects such as dizziness, blurred vision or somnolence during treatment with Gleevec. Therefore, caution should be recommended when driving a car or operating machinery.

6 ADVERSE REACTIONS

Because clinical trials are conducted under widely varying conditions, the adverse reaction rates observed cannot be directly compared to rates on other clinical trials and may not reflect the rates observed in clinical practice.

6.1 Chronic Myeloid Leukemia

The majority of Gleevec-treated patients experienced adverse reactions at some time. Most reactions were of mild-to-moderate grade, but drug was discontinued for drug-related adverse reactions in 2.4% of newly diagnosed patients, 4% of patients in chronic phase after failure of interferon-alpha therapy, 4% in accelerated phase and 5% in blast crisis.

The most frequently reported drug-related adverse reactions were edema, nausea and vomiting, muscle cramps, musculoskeletal pain, diarrhea and rash (Table 2 for newly diagnosed CML, Table 3 for other CML patients). Edema was most frequently periorbital or in lower limbs and was managed with diuretics, other supportive measures, or by reducing the dose of Gleevec [see Dosage and Administration (2.12)]. The frequency of severe superficial edema was 1.5%-6%.

A variety of adverse reactions represent local or general fluid retention including pleural effusion, ascites, pulmonary edema and rapid weight gain with or without superficial edema. These reactions appear to be dose related, were more common in the blast crisis and accelerated phase studies (where the dose was 600 mg/day), and are more common in the elderly. These reactions were usually managed by interrupting Gleevec treatment and using diuretics or other appropriate supportive care measures. A few of these reactions may be serious or life threatening, and one patient with blast crisis died with pleural effusion, congestive heart failure, and renal failure.

Adverse reactions, regardless of relationship to study drug, that were reported in at least 10% of the Gleevec treated patients are shown in Tables 2 and 3.

Table 5 Lab Abnormalities in Other CML Clinical Trials

CTC Grades[1]	Myeloid Blast Crisis (n=260) 600 mg n=223 400 mg n=37 %		Accelerated Phase (n=235) 600 mg n=158 400 mg n=77 %		Chronic Phase, IFN Failure (n=532) 400 mg %	
	Grade 3	Grade 4	Grade 3	Grade 4	Grade 3	Grade 4
Hematology Parameters						
– Neutropenia	16	48	23	36	27	9
– Thrombocytopenia	30	33	31	13	21	<1
– Anemia	42	11	34	7	6	1
Biochemistry Parameters						
– Elevated Creatinine	1.5	0	1.3	0	0.2	0
– Elevated Bilirubin	3.8	0	2.1	0	0.6	0
– Elevated Alkaline Phosphatase	4.6	0	5.5	0.4	0.2	0
– Elevated SGOT (AST)	1.9	0	3.0	0	2.3	0
– Elevated SGPT (ALT)	2.3	0.4	4.3	0	2.1	0

[1]CTC Grades: neutropenia (Grade 3 $\geq$0.5-1.0 $\times$ 10^9/L, Grade 4 <0.5 $\times$ 10^9/L), thrombocytopenia (Grade 3 $\geq$10-50 $\times$ 10^9/L, Grade 4 <10 $\times$ 10^9/L), anemia (hemoglobin $\geq$65-80 g/L, Grade 4 <65 g/L), elevated creatinine (Grade 3 >3-6 $\times$ upper limit normal range [ULN], Grade 4 >6 $\times$ ULN), elevated bilirubin (Grade 3 >3-10 $\times$ ULN, Grade 4 >10 $\times$ ULN), elevated alkaline phosphatase (Grade 3 >5-20 $\times$ ULN, Grade 4 >20 $\times$ ULN), elevated SGOT or SGPT (Grade 3 >5-20 $\times$ ULN, Grade 4 >20 $\times$ ULN)

Table 6 Adverse Reactions Reported More Frequently in Patients Treated with Study Drug (>5%) or in Cycles with Study Drug (>1%)

Adverse Event	Per Patient Incidence Ph+ALL With Gleevec N = 92	Per Patient Incidence Ph- ALL No Gleevec N = 65	Per Patient Per Cycle Incidence With Gleevec* N = 778	Per Patient Per Cycle Incidence No Gleevec** N = 647
Grade 3 and 4 Adverse Events				
Nausea and/or Vomiting	15 (16%)	6 (9%)	28 (4%)	8 (1%)
Hypokalemia	31 (34%)	16 (25%)	72 (9%)	32(5%)
Pneumonitis	7 (8%)	1 (1%)	7(1%)	1(<1%)
Pleural effusion	6 (7%)	0	6 (1%)	0
Abdominal Pain	8 (9%)	2 (3%)	9 (1%)	3(<1%)
Anorexia	10 (11%)	3 (5%)	19 (2%)	4 (1%)
Hemorrhage	11 (12%)	4 (6%)	17 (2%)	8 (1%)
Hypoxia	8 (9%)	2 (3%)	12 (2%)	2 (<1%)
Myalgia	5 (5%)	0	4 (1%)	1 (<1%)
Stomatitis	15 (16%)	8 (12%)	22 (3%)	14 (2%)
Diarrhea	8 (9%)	3 (5%)	12 (2%)	3 (<1%)
Rash / Skin Disorder	4 (4%)	0	5 (1%)	0
Infection	49 (53%)	32 (49%)	131 (17%)	92 (14%)
Hepatic (transaminase and/or bilirubin)	52 (57%)	38 (58%)	172 (22%)	113 (17%)
Hypotension	10 (11%)	5 (8%)	16 (2%)	6 (1%)
Myelosuppression				
Neutropenia (<750/µL)	92 (100%)	63 (97%)	556 (71%)	218 (34%)
Thrombocytopenia (<75,000/µL)	90 (92%)	63 (97%)	431 (55%)	329 (51%)

* Defined as the frequency of AEs per patient per treatment cycles that included Gleevec (includes patients with Ph+ ALL that received cycles with Gleevec
** Defined as the frequency of AEs per patient per treatment cycles that did not include Gleevec (includes patients with Ph+ALL that received cycles without Gleevec as well as all patients with Ph- ALL who did not receive Gleevec in any treatment cycle)

[See table 2 at top of page 1909]
[See table 3 at top of previous page]

6.2 Hematologic Toxicity

Cytopenias, and particularly neutropenia and thrombocytopenia, were a consistent finding in all studies, with a higher frequency at doses $\geq$750 mg (Phase 1 study). The occurrence of cytopenias in CML patients was also dependent on the stage of the disease.

In patients with newly diagnosed CML, cytopenias were less frequent than in the other CML patients (see Tables 4 and 5). The frequency of Grade 3 or 4 neutropenia and thrombocytopenia was between 2- and 3-fold higher in blast crisis and accelerated phase compared to chronic phase (see Tables 4 and 5). The median duration of the neutropenic and thrombocytopenic episodes varied from 2 to 3 weeks, and from 2 to 4 weeks, respectively.

These reactions can usually be managed with either a reduction of the dose or an interruption of treatment with Gleevec, but in rare cases require permanent discontinuation of treatment.

[See table 4 at top of previous page]
[See table 5 above]

6.3 Hepatotoxicity

Severe elevation of transaminases or bilirubin occurred in approximately 5% of CML patients (see Tables 4 and 5) and were usually managed with dose reduction or interruption (the median duration of these episodes was approximately 1 week). Treatment was discontinued permanently because of liver laboratory abnormalities in less than 1.0% of CML pa-

tients. One patient, who was taking acetaminophen regularly for fever, died of acute liver failure. In the Phase 2 GIST trial, Grade 3 or 4 SGPT (ALT) elevations were observed in 6.8% of patients and Grade 3 or 4 SGOT (AST) elevations were observed in 4.8% of patients. Bilirubin elevation was observed in 2.7% of patients.

6.4 Adverse Reactions in Pediatric Population

Single agent therapy

The overall safety profile of pediatric patients treated with Gleevec in 93 children studied was similar to that found in studies with adult patients, except that musculoskeletal pain was less frequent (20.5%) and peripheral edema was not reported. Nausea and vomiting were the most commonly reported individual adverse reactions with an incidence similar to that seen in adult patients. Although most patients experienced adverse reactions at some time during the study, the incidence of Grade 3/4 adverse reactions was low.

In combination with multi-agent chemotherapy

Pediatric and young adult patients with very high risk ALL, defined as those with an expected 5 year event-free survival (EFS) less than 45%, were enrolled after induction therapy on a multicenter, non-randomized cooperative group pilot protocol. The study population included patients with a median age of 10 years (1 to 21 years), 61% of whom were male, 75% were white, 7% were black and 6% were Asian/Pacific Islander. Patients with Ph+ ALL (n=92) were assigned to receive Gleevec and treated in 5 successive cohorts. Gleevec exposure was systematically increased in successive cohorts by earlier introduction and more prolonged duration.

The safety of Gleevec given in combination with intensive chemotherapy was evaluated by comparing the incidence of grade 3 and 4 adverse events, neutropenia (<750/µL) and thrombocytopenia (<75,000/ µL) in the 92 patients with Ph+ ALL compared to 65 patients with Ph- ALL enrolled on the trial who did not receive Gleevec. The safety was also evaluated comparing the incidence of adverse events in cycles of therapy administered with or without Gleevec. The protocol included up to 18 cycles of therapy. Patients were exposed to a cumulative total of 1425 cycles of therapy, 778 with Gleevec and 647 without Gleevec. The adverse events that were reported with a 5% or greater incidence in patients with Ph+ ALL compared to Ph- ALL or with a 1% or greater incidence in cycles of therapy that included Gleevec are presented in Table 6.

[See table 6 at top of previous page]

6.5 Adverse Reactions in Other Subpopulations

In older patients (≥65 years old), with the exception of edema, where it was more frequent, there was no evidence of an increase in the incidence or severity of adverse reactions. In women there was an increase in the frequency of neutropenia, as well as Grade 1/2 superficial edema, headache, nausea, rigors, vomiting, rash, and fatigue. No differences were seen that were related to race but the subsets were too small for proper evaluation.

6.6 Acute Lymphoblastic Leukemia

The adverse reactions were similar for Ph+ ALL as for Ph+ CML. The most frequently reported drug-related adverse reactions reported in the Ph+ ALL studies were mild nausea and vomiting, diarrhea, myalgia, muscle cramps and rash, which were easily manageable. Superficial edema was a common finding in all studies and were described primarily as periorbital or lower limb edemas. These edemas were rarely severe and may be managed with diuretics, other supportive measures, or in some patients by reducing the dose of Gleevec.

6.7 Myelodysplastic/Myeloproliferative Diseases

Adverse reactions, regardless of relationship to study drug, that were reported in at least 10% of the patients treated with Gleevec for MDS/MPD in the phase 2 study, are shown in Table 7.

Table 7 Adverse Reactions Regardless of Relationship to Study Drug Reported (More than One Patient) in MPD Patients in the Phase 2 Study (≥10% All Patients) All Grades

Preferred Term	N=7 n (%)
Nausea	4 (57.1)
Diarrhea	3 (42.9)
Anemia	2 (28.6)
Fatigue	2 (28.6)
Muscle Cramp	3 (42.9)
Arthralgia	2 (28.6)
Periorbital Edema	2 (28.6)

6.8 Aggressive Systemic Mastocytosis

All ASM patients experienced at least one adverse reaction at some time. The most frequently reported adverse reactions were diarrhea, nausea, ascites, muscle cramps, dyspnea, fatigue, peripheral edema, anemia, pruritus, rash and lower respiratory tract infection. None of the 5 patients in the phase 2 study with ASM discontinued Gleevec due to drug-related adverse reactions or abnormal laboratory values.

6.9 Hypereosinophilic Syndrome and Chronic Eosinophilic Leukemia

The safety profile in the HES/CEL patient population does not appear to be different from the safety profile of Gleevec observed in other hematologic malignancy populations, such as Ph+ CML. All patients experienced at least one adverse reaction, the most common being gastrointestinal, cutaneous and musculoskeletal disorders. Hematological abnormalities were also frequent, with instances of CTC Grade 3 leukopenia, neutropenia, lymphopenia, and anemia.

6.10 Dermatofibrosarcoma Protuberans

Adverse reactions, regardless of relationship to study drug, that were reported in at least 10% of the 12 patients treated with Gleevec for DFSP in the phase 2 study are shown in Table 8.

Table 8 Adverse Reactions Regardless of Relationship to Study Drug Reported in DFSP Patients in the Phase 2 Study (≥10% All Patients) All Grades

Preferred term	N=12 n (%)
Nausea	5 (41.7)
Diarrhea	3 (25.0)
Vomiting	3 (25.0)
Periorbital Edema	4 (33.3)
Face Edema	2 (16.7)
Rash	3 (25.0)
Fatigue	5 (41.7)
Edema Peripheral	4 (33.3)
Pyrexia	2 (16.7)
Eye Edema	4 (33.3)
Lacrimation Increased	3 (25.0)
Dyspnea Exertional	2 (16.7)
Anemia	3 (25.0)
Rhinitis	2 (16.7)
Anorexia	2 (16.7)

Clinically relevant or severe laboratory abnormalities in the 12 patients treated with Gleevec for DFSP in the phase 2 study are presented in Table 9.

Table 9 Laboratory Abnormalities Reported in DFSP Patients in the Phase 2 Study

CTC Grades[1]	N=12	
	Grade 3	Grade 4
Hematology Parameters		
- Anemia	17 %	0 %
- Thrombocytopenia	17 %	0 %
- Neutropenia	0 %	8 %
Biochemistry Parameters		
- Elevated Creatinine	0 %	8 %

[1]CTC Grades: neutropenia (Grade 3 ≥0.5-1.0 × 10⁹/L, Grade 4 <0.5 × 10⁹/L), thrombocytopenia (Grade 3 ≥10 - 50 × 10⁹/L, Grade 4 <10 × 10⁹/L), anemia (Grade 3 ≥65-80 g/L, Grade 4 <65 g/L), elevated creatinine (Grade 3 >3-6 × upper limit normal range [ULN], Grade 4 >6 × ULN),

6.11 Gastrointestinal Stromal Tumors
Unresectable and/or Malignant Metastatic GIST

In the Phase 3 trials the majority of Gleevec-treated patients experienced adverse reactions at some time. The most frequently reported adverse reactions were edema, fatigue, nausea, abdominal pain, diarrhea, rash, vomiting, myalgia, anemia, and anorexia. Drug was discontinued for adverse reactions in a total of 89 patients (5.4%). Superficial edema, most frequently periorbital or lower extremity edema was managed with diuretics, other supportive measures, or by

Table 10 Number (%) of Patients with Adverse Reactions Regardless of Relationship to Study Drug where Frequency is ≥10% in any One Group (Full Analysis Set) in the Phase 3 Unresectable and/or Malignant Metastatic GIST Clinical Trials

Reported or Specified Term	Imatinib 400 mg N=818		Imatinib 800 mg N=822	
	All Grades %	Grades 3/4/5 %	All Grades %	Grades 3/4/5 %
Edema	76.7	9.0	86.1	13.1
Fatigue/lethargy, malaise, asthenia	69.3	11.7	74.9	12.2
Nausea	58.1	9.0	64.5	7.8
Abdominal pain/cramping	57.2	13.8	55.2	11.8
Diarrhea	56.2	8.1	58.2	8.6
Rash/desquamation	38.1	7.6	49.8	8.9
Vomiting	37.4	9.2	40.6	7.5
Myalgia	32.2	5.6	30.2	3.8
Anemia	32.0	4.9	34.8	6.4
Anorexia	31.1	6.6	35.8	4.7
Other GI toxicity	25.2	8.1	28.1	6.6
Headache	22.0	5.7	19.7	3.6
Other pain (excluding tumor related pain)	20.4	5.9	20.8	5.0
Other dermatology /skin toxicity	17.6	5.9	20.1	5.7
Leukopenia	17.0	0.7	19.6	1.6
Other constitutional symptoms	16.7	6.4	15.2	4.4
Cough	16.1	4.5	14.5	3.2
Infection (without neutropenia)	15.5	6.6	16.5	5.6
Pruritus	15.4	5.4	18.9	4.3
Other neurological toxicity	15.0	6.4	15.2	4.9
Constipation	14.8	5.1	14.4	4.1
Other renal/genitourinary toxicity	14.2	6.5	13.6	5.2
Arthralgia (joint pain)	13.6	4.8	12.3	3.0
Dyspnea (shortness of breath)	13.6	6.8	14.2	5.6
Fever in absence of neutropenia (ANC<1.0 × 10⁹/L)	13.2	4.9	12.9	3.4
Sweating	12.7	4.6	8.5	2.3
Other hemorrhage	12.3	6.7	13.3	6.1
Weight gain	12.0	1.0	10.6	0.6
Alopecia	11.9	4.3	14.8	3.2
Dyspepsia/heartburn	11.5	0.6	10.9	0.5
Neutropenia/ granulocytopenia	11.5	3.1	16.1	4.1
Rigors/chills	11.0	4.6	10.2	3.0
Dizziness/ lightheadedness	11.0	4.8	10.0	2.8
Creatinine increase	10.8	0.4	10.1	0.6
Flatulence	10.0	0.2	10.1	0.1
Stomatitis/pharyngitis (oral/pharyngeal mucositis)	9.2	5.4	10.0	4.3
Lymphopenia	6.0	0.7	10.1	1.9

reducing the dose of Gleevec [see Dosage and Administration (2.12)]. Severe (CTC Grade 3/4) edema was observed in 182 patients (11.1%).

Adverse reactions, regardless of relationship to study drug, that were reported in at least 10% of the patients treated with Gleevec are shown in Table 10.

Overall the incidence of all grades of adverse reactions and the incidence of severe adverse reactions (CTC Grade 3 and above) were similar between the two treatment arms except for edema, which was reported more frequently in the 800 mg group.

[See table 10 above]

Clinically relevant or severe abnormalities of routine hematologic or biochemistry laboratory values were not reported or evaluated in the Phase 3 GIST trials. Severe abnormal laboratory values reported in the Phase 2 GIST trial are presented in Table 11.

[See table 11 at top of next page]

Adjuvant Treatment of GIST

In Study 1, the majority of both Gleevec and placebo treated patients experienced at least one adverse reaction at some time. The most frequently reported adverse reactions were similar to those reported in other clinical studies in other patient populations and include diarrhea, fatigue, nausea, edema, decreased hemoglobin, rash, vomiting, and abdominal pain. No new adverse reactions were reported in the adjuvant GIST treatment setting that had not been previously reported in other patient populations including patients with unresectable and/or malignant metastatic GIST. Drug was discontinued for adverse reactions in 57 patients (17%) and 11 patients (3%) of the Gleevec and placebo treated patients respectively. Edema, gastrointestinal disturbances (nausea, vomiting, abdominal distention and diarrhea), fatigue, low hemoglobin, and rash were the most frequently reported adverse reactions at the time of discontinuation.

In Study 2, discontinuation of therapy due to adverse reactions occurred in 15 patients (8%) and 27 patients (14%) of the Gleevec 12-month and 36-month treatment arms, respectively. As in previous trials the most common adverse reactions were diarrhea, fatigue, nausea, edema, decreased hemoglobin, rash, vomiting, and abdominal pain.

Adverse reactions, regardless of relationship to study drug, that were reported in at least 5% of the patients treated with Gleevec are shown in Table 12 (Study 1) and Table 13 (Study 2). There were no deaths attributable to Gleevec treatment in either trial.

[See table 12 at top of next page]
[See table 13 at top of page 1914]

Table 11 Laboratory Abnormalities in the Phase 2 Unresectable and/or Malignant Metastatic GIST Trial

CTC Grades[1]	400 mg (n=73) %		600 mg (n=74) %	
	Grade 3	Grade 4	Grade 3	Grade 4
Hematology Parameters				
– Anemia	3	0	8	1
– Thrombocytopenia	0	0	1	0
– Neutropenia	7	3	8	3
Biochemistry Parameters				
– Elevated Creatinine	0	0	3	0
– Reduced Albumin	3	0	4	0
– Elevated Bilirubin	1	0	1	3
– Elevated Alkaline Phosphatase	0	0	3	0
– Elevated SGOT (AST)	4	0	3	3
– Elevated SGPT (ALT)	6	0	7	1

[1]CTC Grades: neutropenia (Grade 3 ≥0.5-1.0 × 10⁹/L, Grade 4 <0.5 × 10⁹/L), thrombocytopenia (Grade 3 ≥10 - 50 × 10⁹/L, Grade 4 <10 × 10⁹/L), anemia (Grade 3 ≥65-80 g/L, Grade 4 <65 g/L), elevated creatinine (Grade 3 >3-6 × upper limit normal range [ULN], Grade 4 >6 × ULN), elevated bilirubin (Grade 3 >3-10 × ULN, Grade 4 >10 × ULN), elevated alkaline phosphatase, SGOT or SGPT (Grade 3 >5-20 × ULN, Grade 4 >20 × ULN), albumin (Grade 3 <20 g/L)

Table 12: Adverse Reactions Regardless of Relationship to Study Drug Reported in Study 1 (≥5% of Gleevec Treated Patients)[1]

Preferred Term	All CTC Grades		CTC Grade 3 and above	
	Gleevec (n=337) %	Placebo (n=345) %	Gleevec (n=337) %	Placebo (n=345) %
Diarrhea	59.3	29.3	3.0	1.4
Fatigue	57.0	40.9	2.1	1.2
Nausea	53.1	27.8	2.4	1.2
Periorbital Edema	47.2	14.5	1.2	0
Hemoglobin Decreased	46.9	27.0	0.6	0
Peripheral Edema	26.7	14.8	0.3	0
Rash (Exfoliative)	26.1	12.8	2.7	0
Vomiting	25.5	13.9	2.4	0.6
Abdominal Pain	21.1	22.3	3.0	1.4
Headache	19.3	20.3	0.6	0
Dyspepsia	17.2	13.0	0.9	0
Anorexia	16.9	8.7	0.3	0
Weight Increased	16.9	11.6	0.3	0
Liver enzymes (ALT) Increased	16.6	13.0	2.7	0
Muscle spasms	16.3	3.3	0	0
Neutrophil Count Decreased	16.0	6.1	3.3	0.9
Arthralgia	15.1	14.5	0	0.3
White Blood Cell Count Decreased	14.5	4.3	0.6	0.3
Constipation	12.8	17.7	0	0.3
Dizziness	12.5	10.7	0	0.3
Liver Enzymes (AST) Increased	12.2	7.5	2.1	0
Myalgia	12.2	11.6	0	0.3
Blood Creatinine Increased	11.6	5.8	0	0.3
Cough	11.0	11.3	0	0
Pruritus	11.0	7.8	0.9	0
Weight Decreased	10.1	5.2	0	0
Hyperglycemia	9.8	11.3	0.6	1.7
Insomnia	9.8	7.2	0.9	0
Lacrimation Increased	9.8	3.8	0	0
Alopecia	9.5	6.7	0	0
Flatulence	8.9	9.6	0	0
Rash	8.9	5.2	0.9	0
Abdominal Distension	7.4	6.4	0.3	0.3
Back Pain	7.4	8.1	0.6	0
Pain in Extremity	7.4	7.2	0.3	0
Hypokalemia	7.1	2.0	0.9	0.6
Depression	6.8	6.4	0.9	0.6
Facial Edema	6.8	1.2	0.3	0
Blood Alkaline Phosphatase Increased	6.5	7.5	0	0
Dry skin	6.5	5.2	0	0
Dysgeusia	6.5	2.9	0	0
Abdominal Pain Upper	6.2	6.4	0.3	0
Neuropathy Peripheral	5.9	6.4	0	0
Hypocalcemia	5.6	1.7	0.3	0
Leukopenia	5.0	2.6	0.3	0
Platelet Count Decreased	5.0	3.5	0	0
Stomatitis	5.0	1.7	0.6	0
Upper Respiratory Tract Infection	5.0	3.5	0	0
Vision Blurred	5.0	2.3	0	0

[1]All adverse reactions occurring in ≥5% of patients are listed regardless of suspected relationship to treatment. A patient with multiple occurrences of an adverse reaction is counted only once in the adverse reaction category.

6.12   Additional Data from Multiple Clinical Trials

The following adverse reactions have been reported during clinical trials of Gleevec.

Cardiac Disorders:
Estimated 0.1%-1%: congestive cardiac failure, tachycardia, palpitations, pulmonary edema
Estimated 0.01%-0.1%: arrhythmia, atrial fibrillation, cardiac arrest, myocardial infarction, angina pectoris, pericardial effusion

Vascular Disorders:
Estimated 1%-10%: flushing, hemorrhage
Estimated 0.1%-1%: hypertension, hypotension, peripheral coldness, Raynauds phenomenon, hematoma, subdural hematoma

Clinical Laboratory Tests:
Estimated 0.1%-1%: blood CPK increased, blood LDH increased
Estimated 0.01%-0.1%: blood amylase increased

Dermatologic:
Estimated 1%-10%: dry skin, alopecia, face edema, erythema, photosensitivity reaction
Estimated 0.1%-1%: exfoliative dermatitis, bullous eruption, nail disorder, purpura, psoriasis, rash pustular, contusion, sweating increased, urticaria, ecchymosis, increased tendency to bruise, hypotrichosis, skin hypopigmentation, skin hyperpigmentation, onychoclasis, folliculitis, petechiae
Estimated 0.01%-0.1%: vesicular rash, Stevens-Johnson syndrome, acute generalized exanthematous pustulosis, acute febrile neutrophilic dermatosis (Sweet's syndrome), nail discoloration, angioneurotic edema, erythema multiforme, leucocytoclastic vasculitis

Digestive:
Estimated 1%-10%: abdominal distention, gastroesophageal reflux, dry mouth, gastritis
Estimated 0.1%-1%: gastric ulcer, stomatitis, mouth ulceration, eructation, melena, esophagitis, ascites, hematemesis, chelitis, dysphagia, pancreatitis
Estimated 0.01%-0.1%: colitis, ileus, inflammatory bowel disease

General Disorders and Administration Site Conditions:
Estimated 1%-10%: weakness, anasarca, chills
Estimated 0.1%-1%: malaise

Hematologic:
Estimated 1%-10%: pancytopenia, febrile neutropenia
Estimated 0.1%-1%: thrombocythemia, lymphopenia, bone marrow depression, eosinophilia, lymphadenopathy
Estimated 0.01%-0.1%: hemolytic anemia, aplastic anemia

Hepatobiliary:
Estimated 0.1%-1%: hepatitis, jaundice
Estimated 0.01%-0.1%: hepatic failure and hepatic necrosis[1]

Hypersensitivity:
Estimated 0.01%-0.1%: angioedema

Infections:
Estimated 0.1%-1%: sepsis, herpes simplex, herpes zoster, cellulitis, urinary tract infection, gastroenteritis
Estimated 0.01%-0.1%: fungal infection

Metabolic and Nutritional:
Estimated 1%-10%: weight decreased
Estimated 0.1%-1%: hypophosphatemia, dehydration, gout, increased appetite, decreased appetite, hyperuricemia, hypercalcemia, hyperglycemia, hyponatremia
Estimated 0.01%-0.1%: hyperkalemia, hypomagnesemia

Musculoskeletal:
Estimated 1%-10%: joint swelling
Estimated 0.1%-1%: joint and muscle stiffness
Estimated 0.01%-0.1%: muscular weakness, arthritis

Nervous System/Psychiatric:
Estimated 1%-10%: paresthesia, hypesthesia
Estimated 0.1%-1%: syncope, peripheral neuropathy, somnolence, migraine, memory impairment, libido decreased, sciatica, restless leg syndrome, tremor
Estimated 0.01%-0.1%: increased intracranial pressure[1], confusional state, convulsions, optic neuritis

Renal:
Estimated 0.1%-1%: renal failure acute, urinary frequency increased, hematuria, renal pain

Reproductive:
Estimated 0.1%-1%: breast enlargement, menorrhagia, sexual dysfunction, gynecomastia, erectile dysfunction, menstruation irregular, nipple pain, scrotal edema

Respiratory:
Estimated 1%-10%: epistaxis
Estimated 0.1%-1%: pleural effusion
Estimated 0.01%-0.1%: interstitial pneumonitis, pulmonary fibrosis, pleuritic pain, pulmonary hypertension, pulmonary hemorrhage

Special Senses:
Estimated 1%-10%: conjunctivitis, vision blurred, eyelid edema, conjunctival hemorrhage, dry eye
Estimated 0.1%-1%: vertigo, tinnitus, eye irritation, eye pain, orbital edema, scleral hemorrhage, retinal hemorrhage, blepharitis, macular edema, hearing loss
Estimated 0.01%-0.1%: papilledema[1], glaucoma, cataract

[1]Including some fatalities

6.13   Postmarketing Experience

The following additional adverse reactions have been identified during post approval use of Gleevec. Because these re-

Table 13: Adverse Reactions Regardless of Relationship to Study Drug by Preferred Term All Grades and 3/4 Grades (≥5% of Gleevec Treated Patients) Study 2[1]

Preferred Term	All CTC Grades		CTC Grades 3 and above	
	Gleevec 12 Months (N=194) %	Gleevec 36 Months (N=198) %	Gleevec 12 Months (N=194) %	Gleevec 36 Months (N=198) %
Patients with at least one AE	99.0	100.0	20.1	32.8
Hemoglobin decreased	72.2	80.3	0.5	0.5
Periorbital edema	59.3	74.2	0.5	1.0
Blood lactate dehydrogenase increased	43.3	60.1	0	0
Diarrhea	43.8	54.0	0.5	2.0
Nausea	44.8	51.0	1.5	0.5
Muscle spasms	30.9	49.0	0.5	1.0
Fatigue	48.5	48.5	1.0	0.5
White blood cell count decreased	34.5	47.0	2.1	3.0
Pain	25.8	45.5	1.0	3.0
Blood creatinine increased	30.4	44.4	0	0
Edema peripheral	33.0	40.9	0.5	1.0
Dermatitis	29.4	38.9	2.1	1.5
Aspartate aminotransferase increased	30.9	37.9	1.5	3.0
Alanine aminotransferase increased	28.9	34.3	2.1	3.0
Neutrophil count decreased	24.2	33.3	4.6	5.1
Hypoproteinemia	23.7	31.8	0	0
Infection	13.9	27.8	1.5	2.5
Weight increased	13.4	26.8	0	0.5
Pruritus	12.9	25.8	0	0
Flatulence	19.1	24.7	1.0	0.5
Vomiting	10.8	22.2	0.5	1.0
Dyspepsia	17.5	21.7	0.5	1.0
Hypoalbuminemia	11.9	21.2	0	0
Edema	10.8	19.7	0	0.5
Abdominal distension	11.9	19.2	0.5	0
Headache	8.2	18.2	0	0
Lacrimation increased	18.0	17.7	0	0
Arthralgia	8.8	17.2	0	1.0
Blood alkaline phosphatase increased	10.8	16.7	0	0.5
Dyspnea	6.2	16.2	0.5	1.5
Myalgia	9.3	15.2	0	1.0
Platelet count decreased	11.3	14.1	0	0
Blood bilirubin increased	11.3	13.1	0	0
Dysgeusia	9.3	12.6	0	0
Paresthesia	5.2	12.1	0	0.5
Vision blurred	10.8	11.1	1.0	0.5
Alopecia	11.3	10.6	0	0
Decreased appetite	9.8	10.1	0	0
Constipation	8.8	9.6	0	0
Pyrexia	6.2	9.6	0	0
Depression	3.1	8.1	0	0
Abdominal pain	2.6	7.6	0	0
Conjunctivitis	5.2	7.6	0	0
Photosensitivity reaction	3.6	7.1	0	0
Dizziness	4.6	6.6	0.5	0
Hemorrhage	3.1	6.6	0	0
Dry skin	6.7	6.1	0.5	0
Nasopharyngitis	1.0	6.1	0	0.5
Palpitations	5.2	5.1	0	0

[1]All adverse reactions occurring in ≥5% of patients are listed regardless of suspected relationship to treatment. A patient with multiple occurrences of an adverse reaction is counted only once in the adverse reaction category.

actions are reported voluntarily from a population of uncertain size, it is not always possible to reliably estimate their frequency or establish a causal relationship to drug exposure.

Nervous system disorders: cerebral edema[1]
Eye disorders: vitreous hemorrhage
Cardiac disorders: pericarditis, cardiac tamponade[1]
Vascular disorders: thrombosis/embolism, anaphylactic shock
Respiratory, thoracic and mediastinal disorders: acute respiratory failure[1], interstitial lung disease
Gastrointestinal disorders: ileus/intestinal obstruction, tumor hemorrhage/tumor necrosis, gastrointestinal perforation[1] [see Warnings and Precautions (5.6)], diverticulitis
Skin and subcutaneous tissue disorders: lichenoid keratosis, lichen planus, toxic epidermal necrolysis, palmarplantar erythrodysesthesia syndrome, drug rash with eosinophilia and systemic symptoms (DRESS)
Musculoskeletal and connective tissue disorders: avascular necrosis/hip osteonecrosis, rhabdomyolysis/myopathy, growth retardation in children
Reproduction disorders: hemorrhagic corpus luteum/hemorrhagic ovarian cyst
[1]Including some fatalities

7   DRUG INTERACTIONS
7.1   Agents Inducing CYP3A Metabolism
Pretreatment of healthy volunteers with multiple doses of rifampin followed by a single dose of Gleevec, increased Gleevec oral-dose clearance by 3.8-fold, which significantly (p<0.05) decreased mean C_{max} and AUC.

Similar findings were observed in patients receiving 400-1200 mg/day Gleevec concomitantly with enzyme-inducing anti-epileptic drugs (EIAED) (e.g., carbamazepine, oxcarbamazepine, phenytoin, fosphenytoin, phenobarbital, and primidone). The mean dose normalized AUC for imatinib in the patients receiving EIAED's decreased by 73% compared to patients not receiving EIAED.

Concomitant administration of Gleevec and St. John's Wort led to a 30% reduction in the AUC of imatinib.

Consider alternative therapeutic agents with less enzyme induction potential in patients when rifampin or other CYP3A4 inducers are indicated. Gleevec doses up to 1200 mg/day (600 mg BID) have been given to patients receiving concomitant strong CYP3A4 inducers [see Dosage and Administration (2.11)].

7.2   Agents Inhibiting CYP3A Metabolism
There was a significant increase in exposure to imatinib (mean C_{max} and AUC increased by 26% and 40%, respectively) in healthy subjects when Gleevec was co-administered with a single dose of ketoconazole (a CYP3A4 inhibitor). Caution is recommended when administering Gleevec with strong CYP3A4 inhibitors (e.g., ketoconazole, itraconazole, clarithromycin, atazanavir, indinavir, nefazodone, nelfinavir, ritonavir, saquinavir, telithromycin, and voriconazole). Grapefruit juice may also increase plasma concentrations of imatinib and should be avoided. Substances that inhibit the cytochrome P450 isoenzyme (CYP3A4) activity may decrease metabolism and increase imatinib concentrations.

7.3   Interactions with Drugs Metabolized by CYP3A4
Gleevec increases the mean C_{max} and AUC of simvastatin (CYP3A4 substrate) 2- and 3.5-fold, respectively, suggesting

an inhibition of the CYP3A4 by Gleevec. Particular caution is recommended when administering Gleevec with CYP3A4 substrates that have a narrow therapeutic window (e.g., alfentanil, cyclosporine, diergotamine, ergotamine, fentanyl, pimozide, quinidine, sirolimus or tacrolimus).

Gleevec will increase plasma concentration of other CYP3A4 metabolized drugs (e.g., triazolo-benzodiazepines, dihydropyridine calcium channel blockers, certain HMG-CoA reductase inhibitors, etc.).

Because warfarin is metabolized by CYP2C9 and CYP3A4, patients who require anticoagulation should receive low-molecular weight or standard heparin instead of warfarin.

7.4   Interactions with Drugs Metabolized by CYP2D6
Gleevec increased the mean C_{max} and AUC of metoprolol by approximately 23% suggesting that Gleevec has a weak inhibitory effect on CYP2D6-mediated metabolism. No dose adjustment is necessary, however, caution is recommended when administering Gleevec with CYP2D6 substrates that have a narrow therapeutic window.

7.5   Interaction with Acetaminophen
In vitro, Gleevec inhibits the acetaminophen O-glucuronidate pathway (K_i 58.5 µM). Co-administration of Gleevec (400 mg/day for eight days) with acetaminophen (1000 mg single dose on day eight) in patients with CML did not result in any changes in the pharmacokinetics of acetaminophen. Gleevec pharmacokinetics were not altered in the presence of single-dose acetaminophen. There is no pharmacokinetic or safety data on the concomitant use of Gleevec at doses >400 mg/day or the chronic use of concomitant acetaminophen and Gleevec.

8   USE IN SPECIFIC POPULATIONS
8.1   Pregnancy
Pregnancy Category D [see Warnings and Precautions (5.11)].

Risk Summary
Gleevec can cause fetal harm when administered to a pregnant woman. There have been post-market reports of spontaneous abortions and infant congenital anomalies from women who have taken Gleevec. Imatinib was teratogenic in animals. Women should be advised not to become pregnant when taking Gleevec. If this drug is used during pregnancy, or if the patient becomes pregnant while taking this drug, the patient should be apprised of the potential hazard to the fetus.

Animal Data
Imatinib mesylate was teratogenic in rats when administered orally during organogenesis at doses ≥100 mg/kg (approximately equal to the maximum human dose of 800 mg/day based on body surface area). Teratogenic effects included exencephaly or encephalocele, absent/reduced frontal and absent parietal bones. Female rats administered doses ≥45 mg/kg (approximately one-half the maximum human dose of 800 mg/day based on body surface area) also experienced significant post-implantation loss as evidenced by early fetal resorption or stillbirths, nonviable pups and early pup mortality between postpartum Days 0 and 4. At doses higher than 100 mg/kg, total fetal loss was noted in all animals. Fetal loss was not seen at doses ≤30 mg/kg (one-third the maximum human dose of 800 mg).

8.3   Nursing Mothers
Imatinib and its active metabolite are excreted into human milk. Based on data from three breastfeeding women taking Gleevec, the milk:plasma ratio is about 0.5 for imatinib and about 0.9 for the active metabolite. Considering the combined concentration of imatinib and active metabolite, a breastfed infant could receive up to 10% of the maternal therapeutic dose based on body weight. Because of the potential for serious adverse reactions in nursing infants from Gleevec, a decision should be made whether to discontinue nursing or to discontinue the drug, taking into account the importance of the drug to the mother.

8.4   Pediatric Use
Gleevec safety and efficacy have been demonstrated in children with newly diagnosed Ph+ chronic phase CML and Ph+ ALL. There are no data in children under 1 year of age. As in adult patients, imatinib was rapidly absorbed after oral administration in pediatric patients, with a C_{max} of 2-4 hours. Apparent oral clearance was similar to adult values (11.0 L/hr/m^2 in children vs. 10.0 L/hr/m^2 in adults), as was the half-life (14.8 hours in children vs. 17.1 hours in adults). Dosing in children at both 260 mg/m^2 and 340 mg/m^2 achieved an AUC similar to the 400 mg dose in adults. The comparison of AUC on Day 8 vs. Day 1 at 260 mg/m^2 and 340 mg/m^2 dose levels revealed a 1.5- and 2.2-fold drug accumulation, respectively, after repeated once-daily dosing. Mean imatinib AUC did not increase proportionally with increasing dose.

Based on pooled population pharmacokinetic analysis in pediatric patients with hematological disorders (CML, Ph+

ALL, or other hematological disorders treated with imatinib), clearance of imatinib increases with increasing body surface area (BSA). After correcting for the BSA effect, other demographics such as age, body weight and body mass index did not have clinically significant effects on the exposure of imatinib. The analysis confirmed that exposure of imatinib in pediatric patients receiving 260 mg/m² once daily (not exceeding 400 mg once daily) or 340 mg/m² once daily (not exceeding 600 mg once daily) were similar to those in adult patients who received imatinib 400 mg or 600 mg once daily.

8.5 Geriatric Use
In the CML clinical studies, approximately 20% of patients were older than 65 years. In the study of patients with newly diagnosed CML, 6% of patients were older than 65 years. No difference was observed in the safety profile in patients older than 65 years as compared to younger patients, with the exception of a higher frequency of edema [see Warnings and Precautions (5.1)]. The efficacy of Gleevec was similar in older and younger patients.

In the unresectable or metastatic GIST study, 16% of patients were older than 65 years. No obvious differences in the safety or efficacy profile were noted in patients older than 65 years as compared to younger patients, but the small number of patients does not allow a formal analysis. In the adjuvant GIST study, 221 patients (31%) were older than 65 years. No difference was observed in the safety profile in patients older than 65 years as compared to younger patients, with the exception of a higher frequency of edema. The efficacy of Gleevec was similar in patients older than 65 years and younger patients.

8.6 Hepatic Impairment
The effect of hepatic impairment on the pharmacokinetics of both imatinib and its major metabolite, CGP74588, was assessed in 84 cancer patients with varying degrees of hepatic impairment (Table 14) at imatinib doses ranging from 100-800 mg. Exposure to both imatinib and CGP74588 was comparable between each of the mildly and moderately hepatically-impaired groups and the normal group. Patients with severe hepatic impairment tend to have higher exposure to both imatinib and its metabolite than patients with normal hepatic function. At steady state, the mean C_{max}/dose and AUC/dose for imatinib increased by about 63% and 45%, respectively, in patients with severe hepatic impairment compared to patients with normal hepatic function. The mean C_{max}/dose and AUC/dose for CGP74588 increased by about 56% and 55%, respectively, in patients with severe hepatic impairment compared to patients with normal hepatic function [see Dosage and Administration (2.11)].
[See table 14 above]

8.7 Renal Impairment
The effect of renal impairment on the pharmacokinetics of imatinib was assessed in 59 cancer patients with varying degrees of renal impairment (Table 15) at single and steady state imatinib doses ranging from 100 to 800 mg/day. The mean exposure to imatinib (dose normalized AUC) in patients with mild and moderate renal impairment increased 1.5- to 2-fold compared to patients with normal renal function. The AUCs did not increase for doses greater than 600 mg in patients with mild renal impairment. The AUCs did not increase for doses greater than 400 mg in patients with moderate renal impairment. Two patients with severe renal impairment were dosed with 100 mg/day and their exposures were similar to those seen in patients with normal renal function receiving 400 mg/day. Dose reductions are necessary for patients with moderate and severe renal impairment [See Dosage and Administration (2.11)].

Table 15 Renal Function Classification

Renal Dysfunction	Renal Function Tests
Mild	CrCL = 40-59 mL/min
Moderate	CrCL = 20-39 mL/min
Severe	CrCL = <20 mL/min

CrCL = Creatinine Clearance

10 OVERDOSAGE
Experience with doses greater than 800 mg is limited. Isolated cases of Gleevec overdose have been reported. In the event of overdosage, the patient should be observed and appropriate supportive treatment given.

Adult Overdose
1,200 to 1,600 mg (duration varying between 1 to 10 days): Nausea, vomiting, diarrhea, rash erythema, edema, swelling, fatigue, muscle spasms, thrombocytopenia, pancytopenia, abdominal pain, headache, decreased appetite.
1,800 to 3,200 mg (as high as 3,200 mg daily for 6 days): Weakness, myalgia, increased CPK, increased bilirubin, gastrointestinal pain.
6,400 mg (single dose): One case in the literature reported one patient who experienced nausea, vomiting, abdominal pain, pyrexia, facial swelling, neutrophil count decreased, increase transaminases.

Table 14 Liver Function Classification

Liver Function Test	Normal (n=14)	Mild (n=30)	Moderate (n=20)	Severe (n=20)
Total Bilirubin	≤ULN	>1.0-1.5× ULN	>1.5-3× ULN	>3-10× ULN
SGOT	≤ULN	>ULN (can be normal if Total Bilirubin is >ULN)	Any	Any

ULN=upper limit of normal for the institution

8 to 10 g (single dose): Vomiting and gastrointestinal pain have been reported.
A patient with myeloid blast crisis experienced Grade 1 elevations of serum creatinine, Grade 2 ascites and elevated liver transaminase levels, and Grade 3 elevations of bilirubin after inadvertently taking 1,200 mg of Gleevec daily for 6 days. Therapy was temporarily interrupted and complete reversal of all abnormalities occurred within 1 week. Treatment was resumed at a dose of 400 mg daily without recurrence of adverse reactions. Another patient developed severe muscle cramps after taking 1,600 mg of Gleevec daily for 6 days. Complete resolution of muscle cramps occurred following interruption of therapy and treatment was subsequently resumed. Another patient that was prescribed 400 mg daily, took 800 mg of Gleevec on Day 1 and 1,200 mg on Day 2. Therapy was interrupted, no adverse reactions occurred and the patient resumed therapy.

Pediatric Overdose
One 3 year-old male exposed to a single dose of 400 mg experienced vomiting, diarrhea and anorexia and another 3 year-old male exposed to a single dose of 980 mg experienced decreased white blood cell count and diarrhea.

11 DESCRIPTION
Imatinib is a small molecule kinase inhibitor. Gleevec film-coated tablets contain imatinib mesylate equivalent to 100 mg or 400 mg of imatinib free base. Imatinib mesylate is designated chemically as 4-[(4-Methyl-1-piperazinyl)methyl]-N-[4-methyl-3-[[4-(3-pyridinyl)-2-pyrimidinyl]amino]-phenyl]benzamide methanesulfonate and its structural formula is

Imatinib mesylate is a white to off-white to brownish or yellowish tinged crystalline powder. Its molecular formula is $C_{29}H_{31}N_7O \cdot CH_4SO_3$ and its molecular weight is 589.7. Imatinib mesylate is soluble in aqueous buffers ≤pH 5.5 but is very slightly soluble to insoluble in neutral/alkaline aqueous buffers. In non-aqueous solvents, the drug substance is freely soluble to very slightly soluble in dimethyl sulfoxide, methanol, and ethanol, but is insoluble in n-octanol, acetone, and acetonitrile.
Inactive Ingredients: colloidal silicon dioxide (NF); crospovidone (NF); hydroxypropyl methylcellulose (USP); magnesium stearate (NF); and microcrystalline cellulose (NF). Tablet coating: ferric oxide, red (NF); ferric oxide, yellow (NF); hydroxypropyl methylcellulose (USP); polyethylene glycol (NF) and talc (USP).

12 CLINICAL PHARMACOLOGY
12.1 Mechanism of Action
Imatinib mesylate is a protein-tyrosine kinase inhibitor that inhibits the bcr-abl tyrosine kinase, the constitutive abnormal tyrosine kinase created by the Philadelphia chromosome abnormality in CML. Imatinib inhibits proliferation and induces apoptosis in bcr-abl positive cell lines as well as fresh leukemic cells from Philadelphia chromosome positive chronic myeloid leukemia. Imatinib inhibits colony formation in assays using ex vivo peripheral blood and bone marrow samples from CML patients.
In vivo, imatinib inhibits tumor growth of bcr-abl transfected murine myeloid cells as well as bcr-abl positive leukemia lines derived from CML patients in blast crisis.
Imatinib is also an inhibitor of the receptor tyrosine kinases for platelet-derived growth factor (PDGF) and stem cell factor (SCF), c-kit, and inhibits PDGF- and SCF-mediated cellular events. In vitro, imatinib inhibits proliferation and induces apoptosis in GIST cells, which express an activating c-kit mutation.

12.3 Pharmacokinetics
The pharmacokinetics of Gleevec have been evaluated in studies in healthy subjects and in population pharmacokinetic studies in over 900 patients. The pharmacokinetics of Gleevec are similar in CML and GIST patients. Imatinib is well absorbed after oral administration with C_{max} achieved within 2-4 hours post-dose. Mean absolute bioavailability is 98%. Following oral administration in healthy volunteers, the elimination half-lives of imatinib and its major active metabolite, the N-demethyl derivative (CGP74588), are approximately 18 and 40 hours, respectively. Mean imatinib AUC increases proportionally with increasing doses ranging from 25 mg-1,000 mg. There is no significant change in the pharmacokinetics of imatinib on repeated dosing, and accumulation is 1.5- to 2.5-fold at steady state when Gleevec is dosed once daily. At clinically relevant concentrations of imatinib, binding to plasma proteins in in vitro experiments is approximately 95%, mostly to albumin and α1-acid glycoprotein.
CYP3A4 is the major enzyme responsible for metabolism of imatinib. Other cytochrome P450 enzymes, such as CYP1A2, CYP2D6, CYP2C9, and CYP2C19, play a minor role in its metabolism. The main circulating active metabolite in humans is the N-demethylated piperazine derivative, formed predominantly by CYP3A4. It shows in vitro potency similar to the parent imatinib. The plasma AUC for this metabolite is about 15% of the AUC for imatinib. The plasma protein binding of N-demethylated metabolite CGP74588 is similar to that of the parent compound. Human liver microsome studies demonstrated that Gleevec is a potent competitive inhibitor of CYP2C9, CYP2D6, and CYP3A4/5 with Ki values of 27, 7.5, and 8 μM, respectively.
Imatinib elimination is predominately in the feces, mostly as metabolites. Based on the recovery of compound(s) after an oral ¹⁴C-labeled dose of imatinib, approximately 81% of the dose was eliminated within 7 days, in feces (68% of dose) and urine (13% of dose). Unchanged imatinib accounted for 25% of the dose (5% urine, 20% feces), the remainder being metabolites.
Typically, clearance of imatinib in a 50-year-old patient weighing 50 kg is expected to be 8 L/h, while for a 50-year-old patient weighing 100 kg the clearance will increase to 14 L/h. The inter-patient variability of 40% in clearance does not warrant initial dose adjustment based on body weight and/or age but indicates the need for close monitoring for treatment-related toxicity.

13 NONCLINICAL TOXICOLOGY
13.1 Carcinogenesis, Mutagenesis, Impairment of Fertility
In the 2-year rat carcinogenicity study administration of imatinib at 15, 30, and 60 mg/kg/day resulted in a statistically significant reduction in the longevity of males at 60 mg/kg/day and females at ≥30 mg/kg/day. Target organs for neoplastic changes were the kidneys (renal tubule and renal pelvis), urinary bladder, urethra, preputial and clitoral gland, small intestine, parathyroid glands, adrenal glands and non-glandular stomach. Neoplastic lesions were not seen at: 30 mg/kg/day for the kidneys, urinary bladder, urethra, small intestine, parathyroid glands, adrenal glands and non-glandular stomach, and 15 mg/kg/day for the preputial and clitoral gland. The papilloma/carcinoma of the preputial/clitoral gland were noted at 30 and 60 mg/kg/day, representing approximately 0.5 to 4 or 0.3 to 2.4 times the human daily exposure (based on AUC) at 400 mg/day or 800 mg/day, respectively, and 0.4 to 3.0 times the daily exposure in children (based on AUC) at 340 mg/m². The renal tubule adenoma/carcinoma, renal pelvis transitional cell neoplasms, the urinary bladder and urethra transitional cell papillomas, the small intestine adenocarcinomas, the parathyroid glands adenomas, the benign and malignant medullary tumors of the adrenal glands and the non-glandular stomach papillomas/carcinomas were noted at 60 mg/kg/day. The relevance of these findings in the rat carcinogenicity study for humans is not known.
Positive genotoxic effects were obtained for imatinib in an in vitro mammalian cell assay (Chinese hamster ovary) for clastogenicity (chromosome aberrations) in the presence of metabolic activation. Two intermediates of the manufacturing process, which are also present in the final product, are positive for mutagenesis in the Ames assay. One of these intermediates was also positive in the mouse lymphoma assay. Imatinib was not genotoxic when tested in an in vitro

bacterial cell assay (Ames test), an *in vitro* mammalian cell assay (mouse lymphoma) and an *in vivo* rat micronucleus assay.

In a study of fertility, male rats were dosed for 70 days prior to mating and female rats were dosed 14 days prior to mating and through to gestational Day 6. Testicular and epididymal weights and percent motile sperm were decreased at 60 mg/kg, approximately three-fourths the maximum clinical dose of 800 mg/day based on body surface area. This was not seen at doses ≤20 mg/kg (one-fourth the maximum human dose of 800 mg). The fertility of male and female rats was not affected.

In a pre- and post-natal development study in female rats dosed with imatinib mesylate at 45 mg/kg (approximately one-half the maximum human dose of 800 mg/day, based on body surface area) from gestational Day 6 until the end of lactation, red vaginal discharge was noted on either gestational Day 14 or 15. In the first generation offspring at this same dose level, mean body weights were reduced from birth until terminal sacrifice. First generation offspring fertility was not affected but reproductive effects were noted at 45 mg/kg/day including an increased number of resorptions and a decreased number of viable fetuses.

Fertility was not affected in the preclinical fertility and early embryonic development study although lower testes and epididymal weights as well as a reduced number of motile sperm were observed in the high dose males rats. In the preclinical pre- and postnatal study in rats, fertility in the first generation offspring was also not affected by Gleevec. Human studies on male patients receiving Gleevec and its affect on male fertility and spermatogenesis have not been performed. Male patients concerned about their fertility on Gleevec treatment should consult with their physician.

14 CLINICAL STUDIES

14.1 Chronic Myeloid Leukemia

Chronic Phase, Newly Diagnosed: An open-label, multicenter, international randomized Phase 3 study has been conducted in patients with newly diagnosed Philadelphia chromosome positive (Ph+) chronic myeloid leukemia (CML) in chronic phase. This study compared treatment with either single-agent Gleevec or a combination of interferon-alpha (IFN) plus cytarabine (Ara-C). Patients were allowed to cross over to the alternative treatment arm if they failed to show a complete hematologic response (CHR) at 6 months, a major cytogenetic response (MCyR) at 12 months, or if they lost a CHR or MCyR. Patients with increasing WBC or severe intolerance to treatment were also allowed to cross over to the alternative treatment arm with the permission of the study monitoring committee (SMC). In the Gleevec arm, patients were treated initially with 400 mg daily. Dose escalations were allowed from 400 mg daily to 600 mg daily, then from 600 mg daily to 800 mg daily. In the IFN arm, patients were treated with a target dose of IFN of 5 MIU/m²/day subcutaneously in combination with subcutaneous Ara-C 20 mg/m²/day for 10 days/month.

A total of 1,106 patients were randomized from 177 centers in 16 countries, 553 to each arm. Baseline characteristics were well balanced between the two arms. Median age was 51 years (range 18-70 years), with 21.9% of patients ≥60 years of age. There were 59% males and 41% females; 89.9% Caucasian and 4.7% Black patients. At the cut-off for this analysis (7 years after last patient had been recruited), the median duration of first-line treatment was 82 and 8 months in the Gleevec and IFN arm, respectively. The median duration of second-line treatment with Gleevec was 64 months. Sixty percent of patients randomized to Gleevec are still receiving first-line treatment. In these patients, the average dose of Gleevec was 403 mg ± 57 mg. Overall, in patients receiving first line Gleevec, the average daily dose delivered was 406 mg ± 76 mg. Due to discontinuations and cross-overs, only 2% of patients randomized to IFN were still on first-line treatment. In the IFN arm, withdrawal of consent (14%) was the most frequent reason for discontinuation of first-line therapy, and the most frequent reason for cross over to the Gleevec arm was severe intolerance to treatment (26%) and progression (14%).

The primary efficacy endpoint of the study was progression-free survival (PFS). Progression was defined as any of the following events: progression to accelerated phase or blast crisis (AP/BC), death, loss of CHR or MCyR, or in patients not achieving a CHR an increasing WBC despite appropriate therapeutic management. The protocol specified that the progression analysis would compare the intent to treat (ITT) population: patients randomized to receive Gleevec were compared with patients randomized to receive IFN. Patients that crossed over prior to progression were not censored at the time of cross-over, and events that occurred in these patients following cross-over were attributed to the original randomized treatment. The estimated rate of progression-free survival at 84 months in the ITT population was 81.2 % [95% CI: 78, 85] in the Gleevec arm and 60.6 % [56, 65] in the IFN arm (p<0.0001, log-rank test), (Figure 1). With 7 years follow up there were 93 (16.8%) pro-

gression events in the Gleevec arm: 37(6.7%) progression to AP/BC, 31(5.6%) loss of MCyR, 15 (2.7%) loss of CHR or increase in WBC and 10 (1.8%) CML unrelated deaths. In contrast, there were 165 (29.8%) events in the IFN+Ara-C arm of which 130 occurred during first-line treatment with IFN-Ara-C. The estimated rate of patients free of progression to accelerated phase (AP) or blast crisis (BC) at 84 months was 92.5%[90, 95] in the Gleevec arm compared to the 85.1%, [82, 89] (p≤0.001) in the IFN arm, (Figure 2). The annual rates of any progression events have decreased with time on therapy. The probability of remaining progression free at 60 months was 95% for patients who were in complete cytogenetic response (CCyR) with molecular response (≥3 log reduction in Bcr-Abl transcripts as measured by quantitative reverse transcriptase polymerase chain reaction) at 12 months, compared to 89% for patients in complete cytogenetic response but without a major molecular response and 70% in patients who were not in complete cytogenetic response at this time point (p<0.001).

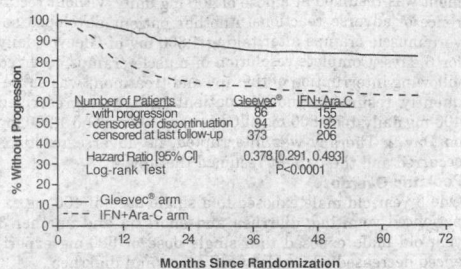

Figure 1 Progression Free Survival (ITT Principle)

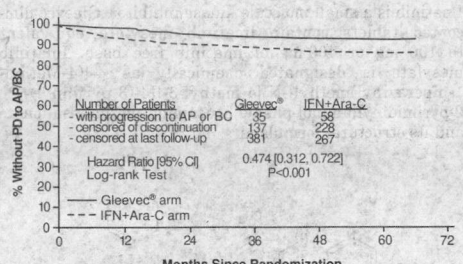

**Figure 2 Time to Progression to AP or BC
(ITT Principle)**

A total of 71 (12.8%) and 85 (15.4%) patients died in the Gleevec and IFN+Ara-C group, respectively. At 84 months the estimated overall survival was 86.4% (83, 90) vs. 83.3% (80, 87) in the randomized Gleevec and the IFN+Ara-C group, respectively (p=0.073 log-rank test). The hazard ratio is 0.750 with 95% CI 0.547-1.028. This time-to-event endpoint may be affected by the high crossover rate from IFN+Ara-C to Gleevec. Major cytogenetic response, hematologic response, evaluation of minimal residual disease (molecular response), time to accelerated phase or blast crisis and survival were main secondary endpoints. Response data are shown in Table 16. Complete hematologic response, major cytogenetic response and complete cytogenetic response were also statistically significantly higher in the Gleevec arm compared to the IFN + Ara-C arm (no cross-over data considered for evaluation of responses). Median time to CCyR in the 454 responders was 6 months (range 2-64 months, 25th to 75th percentiles=3 to 11 months) with 10% of responses seen only after 22 months of therapy).

**Table 16 Response in Newly Diagnosed CML Study
(84-Month Data)**

(Best Response Rate)	Gleevec n=553	IFN+Ara-C n=553
Hematologic Response[1]		
CHR Rate n (%)	534 (96.6%)*	313 (56.6%)*
[95% CI]	[94.7%, 97.9%]	[52.4%, 60.8%]
Cytogenetic Response[2]		
Major Cytogenetic Response n (%)	472 (85.4 %)*	93 (16.8%)*
[95% CI]	[82.1%, 88.2%]	[13.8%, 20.2%]
Unconfirmed[3]	88.6%*	23.3%*
Complete Cytogenetic Response n (%)	413 (74.7%)*	36 (6.5%)*
[95% CI]	[70.8, 78.3]	[4.6, 8.9]

Unconfirmed[3]	82.5%*	11.6%*

*p<0.001, Fischer's exact test

[1]**Hematologic response criteria** (all responses to be confirmed after ≥4 weeks):
WBC<10 × 10⁹/L, platelet <450 × 10⁹/L, myelocyte + metamyelocyte <5% in blood, no blasts and promyelocytes in blood, no extramedullary involvement.

[2]**Cytogenetic response criteria** (confirmed after ≥4 weeks): complete (0% Ph+ metaphases) or partial (1%-35%). A major response (0%-35%) combines both complete and partial responses.

[3]**Unconfirmed cytogenetic response** is based on a single bone marrow cytogenetic evaluation, therefore unconfirmed complete or partial cytogenetic responses might have had a lesser cytogenetic response on a subsequent bone marrow evaluation.

Molecular response was defined as follows: in the peripheral blood, after 12 months of therapy, reduction of ≥3 logarithms in the amount of bcr-abl transcripts (measured by real-time quantitative reverse transcriptase PCR assay) over a standardized baseline. Molecular response was only evaluated in a subset of patients who had a complete cytogenetic response by 12 months or later (N=333). The molecular response rate in patients who had a complete cytogenetic response in the Gleevec arm was 59% at 12 months and 72% at 24 months.

Physical, functional, and treatment-specific biologic response modifier scales from the FACT-BRM (Functional Assessment of Cancer Therapy - Biologic Response Modifier) instrument were used to assess patient-reported general effects of interferon toxicity in 1,067 patients with CML in chronic phase. After one month of therapy to six months of therapy, there was a 13%-21% decrease in median index from baseline in patients treated with IFN, consistent with increased symptoms of IFN toxicity. There was no apparent change from baseline in median index for patients treated with Gleevec.

Late Chronic Phase CML and Advanced Stage CML: Three international, open-label, single-arm phase 2 studies were conducted to determine the safety and efficacy of Gleevec in patients with Ph+ CML: 1) in the chronic phase after failure of IFN therapy, 2) in accelerated phase disease, or 3) in myeloid blast crisis. About 45% of patients were women and 6% were Black. In clinical studies 38%-40% of patients were ≥60 years of age and 10%-12% of patients were ≥70 years of age.

Chronic Phase, Prior Interferon-Alpha Treatment: 532 patients were treated at a starting dose of 400 mg; dose escalation to 600 mg was allowed. The patients were distributed in three main categories according to their response to prior interferon: failure to achieve (within 6 months), or loss of a complete hematologic response (29%), failure to achieve (within 1 year) or loss of a major cytogenetic response (35%), or intolerance to interferon (36%). Patients had received a median of 14 months of prior IFN therapy at doses ≥25 × 10⁶ IU/week and were all in late chronic phase, with a median time from diagnosis of 32 months. Effectiveness was evaluated on the basis of the rate of hematologic response and by bone marrow exams to assess the rate of major cytogenetic response (up to 35% Ph+ metaphases) or complete cytogenetic response (0% Ph+ metaphases). Median duration of treatment was 29 months with 81% of patients treated for ≥24 months (maximum = 31.5 months). Efficacy results are reported in Table 16. Confirmed major cytogenetic response rates were higher in patients with IFN intolerance (66%) and cytogenetic failure (64%), than in patients with hematologic failure (47%). Hematologic response was achieved in 98% of patients with cytogenetic failure, 94% of patients with hematologic failure, and 92% of IFN-intolerant patients.

Accelerated Phase: 235 patients with accelerated phase disease were enrolled. These patients met one or more of the following criteria: ≥15%-<30% blasts in PB or BM; ≥30% blasts + promyelocytes in PB or BM; ≥20% basophils in PB; and <100 × 10⁹/L platelets. The first 77 patients were started at 400 mg, with the remaining 158 patients starting at 600 mg.

Effectiveness was evaluated primarily on the basis of the rate of hematologic response, reported as either complete hematologic response, no evidence of leukemia (i.e., clearance of blasts from the marrow and the blood, but without a full peripheral blood recovery as for complete responses), or return to chronic phase CML. Cytogenetic responses were also evaluated. Median duration of treatment was 18 months with 45% of patients treated for ≥24 months (maximum=35 months). Efficacy results are reported in Table 17. Response rates in accelerated phase CML were higher for the 600 mg dose group than for the 400 mg group: hematologic response (75% vs. 64%), confirmed and unconfirmed major cytogenetic response (31% vs. 19%).

Myeloid Blast Crisis: 260 patients with myeloid blast crisis were enrolled. These patients had ≥30% blasts in PB or BM and/or extramedullary involvement other than spleen or liver; 95 (37%) had received prior chemotherapy for treatment of either accelerated phase or blast crisis ("pretreated patients") whereas 165 (63%) had not ("untreated patients"). The first 37 patients were started at 400 mg; the remaining 223 patients were started at 600 mg.

Effectiveness was evaluated primarily on the basis of rate of hematologic response, reported as either complete hematologic response, no evidence of leukemia, or return to chronic phase CML using the same criteria as for the study in accelerated phase. Cytogenetic responses were also assessed. Median duration of treatment was 4 months with 21% of patients treated for ≥12 months and 10% for ≥24 months (maximum=35 months). Efficacy results are reported in Table 17. The hematologic response rate was higher in untreated patients than in treated patients (36% vs. 22%, respectively) and in the group receiving an initial dose of 600 mg rather than 400 mg (33% vs. 16%). The confirmed and unconfirmed major cytogenetic response rate was also higher for the 600 mg dose group than for the 400 mg dose group (17% vs. 8%).

[See table 17 above]

The median time to hematologic response was 1 month. In late chronic phase CML, with a median time from diagnosis of 32 months, an estimated 87.8% of patients who achieved MCyR maintained their response 2 years after achieving their initial response. After 2 years of treatment, an estimated 85.4% of patients were free of progression to AP or BC, and estimated overall survival was 90.8% [88.3, 93.2]. In accelerated phase, median duration of hematologic response was 28.8 months for patients with an initial dose of 600 mg (16.5 months for 400 mg). An estimated 63.8% of patients who achieved MCyR were still in response 2 years after achieving initial response. The median survival was 20.9 [13.1, 34.4] months for the 400 mg group and was not yet reached for the 600 mg group (p=0.0097). An estimated 46.2% [34.7, 57.7] vs. 65.8% [58.4, 73.3] of patients were still alive after 2 years of treatment in the 400 mg vs. 600 mg dose groups, respectively. In blast crisis, the estimated median duration of hematologic response is 10 months. An estimated 27.2% [16.8, 37.7] of hematologic responders maintained their response 2 years after achieving their initial response. Median survival was 6.9 [5.8, 8.6] months, and an estimated 18.3% [13.4, 23.3] of all patients with blast crisis were alive 2 years after start of study.

Efficacy results were similar in men and women and in patients younger and older than age 65. Responses were seen in Black patients, but there were too few Black patients to allow a quantitative comparison.

14.2   Pediatric CML

A total of 51 pediatric patients with newly diagnosed and untreated CML in chronic phase were enrolled in an open-label, multicenter, single arm phase 2 trial. Patients were treated with Gleevec 340 mg/m²/day, with no interruptions in the absence of dose limiting toxicity. Complete hematologic response (CHR) was observed in 78% of patients after 8 weeks of therapy. The complete cytogenetic response rate (CCyR) was 65%, comparable to the results observed in adults. Additionally, partial cytogenetic response (PCyR) was observed in 16%. The majority of patients who achieved a CCyR developed the CCyR between months 3 and 10 with a median time to response based on the Kaplan-Meier estimate of 6.74 months. Patients were allowed to be removed from protocol therapy to undergo alternative therapy including hematopoietic stem cell transplantation. Thirty one children received stem cell transplantation. Of the 31 children, 5 were transplanted after disease progression on study and 1 withdrew from study during first week treatment and received transplant approximately 4 months after withdrawal. Twenty five children withdrew from protocol therapy to undergo stem cell transplant after receiving a median of 9 twenty-eight day courses (range 4 to 24). Of the 25 patients 13 (52%) had CCyR and 5 (20%) had PCyR at the end of protocol therapy.

One open-label, single-arm study enrolled 14 pediatric patients with Ph+ chronic phase CML recurrent after stem cell transplant or resistant to interferon-alpha therapy. These patients had not previously received Gleevec and ranged in age from 3-20 years old; 3 were 3-11 years old, 9 were 12-18 years old, and 2 were >18 years old. Patients were treated at doses of 260 mg/m²/day (n=3), 340 mg/m²/day (n=4), 440 mg/m²/day (n=5) and 570 mg/m²/day (n=2). In the 13 patients for whom cytogenetic data are available, 4 achieved a major cytogenetic response, 7 achieved a complete cytogenetic response, and 2 had a minimal cytogenetic response.

In a second study, 2 of 3 patients with Ph+ chronic phase CML resistant to interferon-alpha therapy achieved a complete cytogenetic response at doses of 242 and 257 mg/m²/day.

14.3   Acute Lymphoblastic Leukemia

A total of 48 Philadelphia chromosome positive acute lymphoblastic leukemia (Ph+ ALL) patients with relapsed/refractory disease were studied, 43 of whom received the rec-

Table 17 Response in CML Studies

	Chronic Phase IFN Failure (n=532) 400 mg	Accelerated Phase (n=235) 600 mg n=158 400 mg n=77	Myeloid Blast Crisis (n=260) 600 mg n=223 400 mg n=37
	% of patients [CI ₉₅%]		
Hematologic Response[1]	95% [92.3–96.3]	71% [64.8-76.8]	31% [25.2–36.8]
Complete Hematologic Response (CHR)	95%	38%	7%
No Evidence of Leukemia (NEL)	Not applicable	13%	5%
Return to Chronic Phase (RTC)	Not applicable	20%	18%
Major Cytogenetic Response[2]	60% [55.3–63.8]	21% [16.2–27.1]	7% [4.5–11.2]
(Unconfirmed[3])	(65%)	(27%)	(15%)
Complete[4] (Unconfirmed[3])	39% (47%)	16% (20%)	2% (7%)

[1] **Hematologic response criteria** (all responses to be confirmed after ≥4 weeks):
CHR:Chronic phase study [WBC <10 × 10⁹/L, platelet <450 × 10⁹/L, myelocytes + metamyelocytes <5% in blood, no blasts and promyelocytes in blood, basophils <20%, no extramedullary involvement] and in the accelerated and blast crisis studies [ANC ≥1.5 × 10⁹/L, platelets ≥100 × 10⁹/L, no blood blasts, BM blasts <5% and no extramedullary disease]
NEL: Same criteria as for CHR but ANC ≥1 × 10⁹/L and platelets ≥20 × 10⁹/L (accelerated and blast crisis studies)
RTC: <15% blasts BM and PB, <30% blasts + promyelocytes in BM and PB, <20% basophils in PB, no extramedullary disease other than spleen and liver (accelerated and blast crisis studies).
BM=bone marrow, PB=peripheral blood
[2] **Cytogenetic response criteria** (confirmed after ≥4 weeks): complete (0% Ph+ metaphases) or partial (1%-35%). A major response (0%-35%) combines both complete and partial responses.
[3] **Unconfirmed cytogenetic response** is based on a single bone marrow cytogenetic evaluation, therefore unconfirmed complete or partial cytogenetic responses might have had a lesser cytogenetic response on a subsequent bone marrow evaluation.
[4] **Complete cytogenetic response** confirmed by a second bone marrow cytogenetic evaluation performed at least 1 month after the initial bone marrow study.

ommended Gleevec dose of 600 mg/day. In addition 2 patients with relapsed/refractory Ph+ ALL received Gleevec 600 mg/day in a phase 1 study.

Confirmed and unconfirmed hematologic and cytogenetic response rates for the 43 relapsed/refractory Ph+ALL phase 2 study patients and for the 2 phase 1 patients are shown in Table 18. The median duration of hematologic response was 3.4 months and the median duration of MCyR was 2.3 months.

Table 18 Effect of Gleevec on Relapsed/Refractory Ph+ ALL.

	Phase 2 Study (N=43)	Phase 1 Study (N=2)
CHR	8 (19%)	2 (100%)
NEL	5 (12%)	
RTC/PHR	11 (26%)	
MCyR	15 (35%)	
CCyR	9 (21%)	
PCyR	6 (14%)	

14.4   Pediatric ALL

Pediatric and young adult patients with very high risk ALL, defined as those with an expected 5 year event-free survival (EFS) less than 45%, were enrolled after induction therapy on a multicenter, non-randomized cooperative group pilot protocol.

The safety and effectiveness of Gleevec (340 mg/m²/day) in combination with intensive chemotherapy was evaluated in a subgroup of patients with Ph+ ALL. The protocol included intensive chemotherapy and hematopoietic stem cell transplant after 2 courses of chemotherapy for patients with an appropriate HLA-matched family donor. There were 92 eligible patients with Ph+ ALL enrolled. The median age was 9.5 years (1 to 21 years), 64% were male, 75% were white, 9% were Asian/Pacific Islander, and 5% were black. In 5 successive cohorts of patients, Gleevec exposure was systematically increased by earlier introduction and prolonged duration. Cohort 1 received the lowest intensity and cohort 5 received the highest intensity of Gleevec exposure.

There were 50 patients with Ph+ ALL assigned to cohort 5 all of whom received Gleevec plus chemotherapy; 30 were treated exclusively with chemotherapy and Gleevec and 20 received chemotherapy plus Gleevec and then underwent hematopoietic stem cell transplant, followed by further Gleevec treatment. Patients in cohort 5 treated with chemotherapy received continuous daily exposure to Gleevec beginning in the first course of post induction chemotherapy continuing through maintenance cycles 1 through 4 chemotherapy. During maintenance cycles 5 through 12 Gleevec was administered 28 days out of the 56 day cycle. Patients who underwent hematopoietic stem cell transplant received 42 days of Gleevec prior to HSCT, and 28 weeks (196 days) of Gleevec after the immediate post transplant period. The estimated 4-year EFS of patients in cohort 5 was 70% (95% CI: 54, 81). The median follow-up time for EFS at data cutoff in cohort 5 was 40.5 months.

14.5   Myelodysplastic/Myeloproliferative Diseases

An open label, multicenter, phase 2 clinical trial was conducted testing Gleevec in diverse populations of patients suffering from life-threatening diseases associated with Abl, Kit or PDGFR protein tyrosine kinases. This study included 7 patients with MDS/MPD. These patients were treated with Gleevec 400 mg daily. The ages of the enrolled patients ranged from 20 to 86 years. A further 24 patients with MDS/MPD aged 2 to 79 years were reported in 12 published case reports and a clinical study. These patients also received Gleevec at a dose of 400 mg daily with the exception of three patients who received lower doses. Of the total population of 31 patients treated for MDS/MPD, 14 (45%) achieved a complete hematological response and 12 (39%) a major cytogenetic response (including 10 with a complete cytogenetic response). Sixteen patients had a translocation, involving chromosome 5q33 or 4q12, resulting in a PDGFR gene rearrangement. All of these patients responded hematologically (13 completely). Cytogenetic response was evaluated in 12 out of 14 patients, all of whom responded (10 patients completely). Only 1(7%) out of the 14 patients without a translocation associated with PDGFR gene re-arrangement achieved a complete hematological response and none achieved a major cytogenetic response. A further patient with a PDGFR gene re-arrangement in molecular relapse after bone marrow transplant responded molecularly. Median duration of therapy was 12.9 months (0.8-26.7) in the 7 patients treated within the phase 2 study and ranged between 1 week and more than 18 months in responding patients in the published literature. Results are provided in Table 19. Response durations of phase 2 study patients ranged from 141+ days to 457+ days.

Table 19 Response in MDS/MPD

	N	Complete Hematologic Response N (%)	Major Cytogenetic Response N (%)
Overall Population	31	14 (45)	12 (39)
Chromosome 5 Translocation	14	11 (79)	11 (79)
Chromosome 4 Translocation	2	2 (100)	1 (50)
Others / no Translocation	14	1 (7)	0 (0)
Molecular Relapse	1	NE[1]	NE[1]

[1] NE: Not Evaluable

14.6   Aggressive Systemic Mastocytosis

One open-label, multicenter, phase 2 study was conducted testing Gleevec in diverse populations of patients with life-threatening diseases associated with Abl, Kit or PDGFR protein tyrosine kinases. This study included 5 patients with aggressive systemic mastocytosis (ASM) treated with 100 mg to 400 mg of Gleevec daily. These 5 patients ranged from 49 to 74 years of age. In addition to these 5 patients, 10 published case reports and case series describe the use of

Table 20 Response in ASM

Cytogenetic Abnormality	Number of Patients	Complete Hematologic Response N (%)	Partial Hematologic Response N (%)
FIP1L1-PDGFRα Fusion Kinase (or CHIC2 Deletion)	7	7(100%)	0%
Juxtamembrane Mutation	2	0 (0%)	2 (100%)
Unknown or No Cytogenetic Abnormality Detected	15	0(0%)	7 (44%)
D816V Mutation	4	1* (25%)	0%
Total	28	8 (29%)	9 (32%)

* Patient had concomitant CML and ASM

Table 21 Response in HES/CEL

Cytogenetic Abnormality	Number of Patients	Complete Hematological Response N (%)	Partial Hematological Response N (%)
Positive FIP1L1-PDGFRα Fusion Kinase	61	61 (100%)	0%
Negative FIP1L1-PDGFRα Fusion Kinase	56	12 (21%)	9 (16%)
Unknown Cytogenetic Abnormality	59	34 (58%)	7 (12%)
Total	176	107 (61%)	23 (13%)

Gleevec in 23 additional patients with ASM aged 26 to 85 years who also received 100 mg to 400 mg of Gleevec daily.

Cytogenetic abnormalities were evaluated in 20 of the 28 ASM patients treated with Gleevec from the published reports and in the phase 2 study. Seven of these 20 patients had the FIP1L1-PDGFRα fusion kinase (or CHIC2 deletion). Patients with this cytogenetic abnormality were predominantly males and had eosinophilia associated with their systemic mast cell disease. Two patients had a Kit mutation in the juxtamembrane region (one Phe522Cys and one K509I) and four patients had a D816V c-Kit mutation (not considered sensitive to Gleevec), one with concomitant CML.

Of the 28 patients treated for ASM, 8 (29%) achieved a complete hematologic response and 9 (32%) a partial hematologic response (61% overall response rate). Median duration of Gleevec therapy for the 5 ASM patients in the phase 2 study was 13 months (range 1.4-22.3 months) and between 1 month and more than 30 months in the responding patients described in the published medical literature. A summary of the response rates to Gleevec in ASM is provided in Table 20. Response durations of literature patients ranged from 1+ to 30+ months.

[See table 20 above]

Gleevec has not been shown to be effective in patients with less aggressive forms of systemic mastocytosis (SM). Gleevec is therefore not recommended for use in patients with cutaneous mastocytosis, indolent systemic mastocytosis (smoldering SM or isolated bone marrow mastocytosis), SM with an associated clonal hematological non-mast cell lineage disease, mast cell leukemia, mast cell sarcoma or extracutaneous mastocytoma. Patients that harbor the D816V mutation of c-Kit are not sensitive to Gleevec and should not receive Gleevec.

14.7 Hypereosinophilic Syndrome/Chronic Eosinophilic Leukemia

One open-label, multicenter, phase 2 study was conducted testing Gleevec in diverse populations of patients with life-threatening diseases associated with Abl, Kit or PDGFR protein tyrosine kinases. This study included 14 patients with Hypereosinophilic Syndrome/Chronic Eosinophilic Leukemia (HES/CEL). HES patients were treated with 100 mg to 1000 mg of Gleevec daily. The ages of these patients ranged from 16 to 64 years. A further 162 patients with HES/CEL aged 11 to 78 years were reported in 35 published case reports and case series. These patients received Gleevec at doses of 75 mg to 800 mg daily. Hematologic response rates are summarized in Table 21. Response durations for literature patients ranged from 6+ weeks to 44 months.

[See table 21 above]

14.8 Dermatofibrosarcoma Protuberans

Dermatofibrosarcoma Protuberans (DFSP) is a cutaneous soft tissue sarcoma. It is characterized by a translocation of chromosomes 17 and 22 that results in the fusion of the collagen type 1 alpha 1 gene and the PDGF B gene.

An open-label, multicenter, phase 2 study was conducted testing Gleevec in a diverse population of patients with life-threatening diseases associated with Abl, Kit or PDGFR protein tyrosine kinases. This study included 12 patients with DFSP who were treated with Gleevec 800 mg daily (age range 23 to 75 years). DFSP was metastatic, locally recurrent following initial surgical resection and not consid-

ered amenable to further surgery at the time of study entry. A further 6 DFSP patients treated with Gleevec are reported in 5 published case reports, their ages ranging from 18 months to 49 years. The total population treated for DFSP therefore comprises 18 patients, 8 of them with metastatic disease. The adult patients reported in the published literature were treated with either 400 mg (4 cases) or 800 mg (1 case) Gleevec daily. A single pediatric patient received 400 mg/m²/daily, subsequently increased to 520 mg/m²/daily. Ten patients had the PDGF B gene rearrangement, 5 had no available cytogenetics and 3 had complex cytogenetic abnormalities. Responses to treatment are described in Table 22.

Table 22 Response in DFSP

	Number of Patients (n=18)	%
Complete Response	7	39
Partial Response *	8	44
Total Responders	15	83

* 5 patients made disease free by surgery

Twelve of these 18 patients either achieved a complete response (7 patients) or were made disease free by surgery after a partial response (5 patients, including one child) for a total complete response rate of 67%. A further 3 patients achieved a partial response, for an overall response rate of 83%. Of the 8 patients with metastatic disease, five responded (62%), three of them completely (37%). For the 10 study patients with the PDGF B gene rearrangement there were 4 complete and 6 partial responses. The median duration of response in the phase 2 study was 6.2 months, with a maximum duration of 24.3 months, while in the published literature it ranged between 4 weeks and more than 20 months.

14.9 Gastrointestinal Stromal Tumors
Unresectable and/or Malignant Metastatic GIST

Two open-label, randomized, multinational Phase 3 studies were conducted in patients with unresectable or metastatic malignant gastrointestinal stromal tumors (GIST). The two study designs were similar allowing a predefined combined analysis of safety and efficacy. A total of 1640 patients were enrolled into the two studies and randomized 1:1 to receive either 400 mg or 800 mg orally daily continuously until disease progression or unacceptable toxicity. Patients in the 400 mg daily treatment group who experienced disease progression were permitted to crossover to receive treatment with 800 mg daily. The studies were designed to compare response rates, progression-free survival and overall survival between the dose groups. Median age at patient entry was 60 years. Males comprised 58% of the patients enrolled. All patients had a pathologic diagnosis of CD117 positive unresectable and/or metastatic malignant GIST.

The primary objective of the two studies was to evaluate either progression-free survival (PFS) with a secondary objective of overall survival (OS) in one study or overall survival with a secondary objective of PFS in the other study. A planned analysis of both OS and PFS from the combined datasets from these two studies was conducted. Results from this combined analysis are shown in Table 23.

Table 23 Overall Survival, Progression-Free Survival and Tumor Response Rates in the Phase 3 GIST Trials

	Gleevec 400 mg N=818	Gleevec 800 mg N=822
Progression-Free Survival (months)		
Median	18.9	23.2
95% CI	17.4-21.2	20.8-24.9
Overall Survival (months)	49.0	48.7
95% CI	45.3-60.0	45.3-51.6
Best Overall Tumor Response		
Complete Response (CR)	43 (5.3%)	41 (5.0%)
Partial Response (PR)	377 (46.1%)	402 (48.9%)

Median follow up for the combined studies was 37.5 months. There were no observed differences in overall survival between the treatment groups (p=0.98). Patients who crossed over following disease progression from the 400 mg/day treatment group to the 800 mg/day treatment group (n=347) had a 3.4 month median and a 7.7 month mean exposure to Gleevec following crossover.

One open-label, multinational Phase 2 study was conducted in patients with Kit (CD117) positive unresectable or metastatic malignant GIST. In this study, 147 patients were enrolled and randomized to receive either 400 mg or 600 mg orally q.d. for up to 36 months. The primary outcome of the study was objective response rate. Tumors were required to be measurable at entry in at least one site of disease, and response characterization was based on Southwestern Oncology Group (SWOG) criteria. There were no differences in response rates between the 2 dose groups. The response rate was 68.5% for the 400 mg group and 67.6% for the 600 mg group. The median time to response was 12 weeks (range was 3-98 weeks) and the estimated median duration of response is 118 weeks (95% CI: 86, not reached).

Adjuvant Treatment of GIST

In the adjuvant setting, Gleevec was investigated in a multicenter, double-blind, placebo-controlled, randomized trial involving 713 patients (Study 1). Patients were randomized one to one to Gleevec at 400 mg/day or matching placebo for 12 months. The ages of these patients ranged from 18 to 91 years. Patients were included who had a histologic diagnosis of primary GIST, expressing KIT protein by immunochemistry and a tumor size ≥3 cm in maximum dimension with complete gross resection of primary GIST within 14 to 70 days prior to registration.

Recurrence-free survival (RFS) was defined as the time from date of randomization to the date of recurrence or death from any cause. In a planned interim analysis, the median follow up was 15 months in patients without a RFS event; there were 30 RFS events in the 12-month Gleevec arm compared to 70 RFS events in the placebo arm with a hazard ratio of 0.398 (95% CI: 0.259, 0.610), p<0.0001. After the interim analysis of RFS, 79 of the 354 patients initially randomized to the placebo arm were eligible to cross over to the 12-month Gleevec arm. Seventy-two of these 79 patients subsequently crossed over to Gleevec therapy. In an updated analysis, the median follow-up for patients without a RFS event was 50 months. There were 74 (21%) RFS events in the 12-month Gleevec arm compared to 98 (28%) events in the placebo arm with a hazard ratio of 0.718 (95% CI: 0.531-0.971) (Figure 3). The median follow-up for OS in patients still living was 61 months. There were 26 (7%) and 33 (9%) deaths in the 12-month Gleevec and placebo arms, respectively with a hazard ratio of 0.816 (95% CI: 0.488-1.365).

Figure 3 Study 1 Recurrence-Free Survival (ITT Population)

A second randomized, multicenter, open label, phase 3 trial in the adjuvant setting (Study 2) compared 12 months of Gleevec treatment to 36 months of Gleevec treatment at 400 mg/day in adult patients with KIT (CD117) positive GIST after surgical resection with one of the following: tumor diameter >5 cm and mitotic count >5/50 high power fields (HPF), or tumor diameter >10 cm and any mitotic

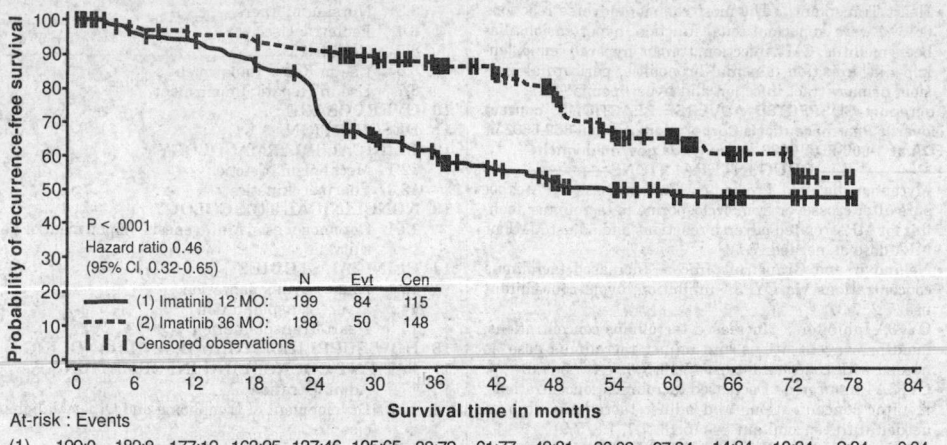

Figure 4 Study 2 Recurrence-Free Survival (ITT Population)

Figure 5 Study 2 Overall Survival (ITT Population)

count, or tumor of any size with mitotic count >10/50 HPF, or tumors ruptured into the peritoneal cavity. There were a total of 397 patients randomized in the trial with 199 patients on the 12-month treatment arm and 198 patients on the 36-month treatment arm. The median age was 61 years (range 22 to 84 years).

RFS was defined as the time from date of randomization to the date of recurrence or death from any cause. The median follow-up for patients without a RFS event was 42 months. There were 84 (42%) RFS events in the 12-month treatment arm and 50 (25%) RFS events in the 36-month treatment arm. Thirty-six months of Gleevec treatment significantly prolonged RFS compared to 12 months of Gleevec treatment with a hazard ratio of 0.46 (95% CI: 0.32, 0.65), p<0.0001 (Figure 4).

The median follow-up for overall survival (OS) in patients still living was 48 months. There were 25 (13%) deaths in the 12-month treatment arm and 12 (6%) deaths in the 36-month treatment arm. Thirty-six months of Gleevec treatment significantly prolonged OS compared to 12 months of Gleevec treatment with a hazard ratio of 0.45 (95% CI: 0.22, 0.89), p=0.0187 (Figure 5).

[See figure 4 above]
[See figure 5 above]

15   REFERENCES

1. OSHA Hazardous Drugs. OSHA. [Accessed on 20-September- 2013, from http://www.osha.gov/SLTC/hazardousdrugs/index.html]

16   HOW SUPPLIED/STORAGE AND HANDLING

Each film-coated tablet contains 100 mg or 400 mg of imatinib free base.
100 mg Tablets
Very dark yellow to brownish orange, film-coated tablets, round, biconvex with bevelled edges, debossed with "NVR" on one side, and "SA" with score on the other side.

Bottles of 90 tablets ....NDC 0078-0401-34
400 mg Tablets
Very dark yellow to brownish orange, film-coated tablets, ovaloid, biconvex with bevelled edges, debossed with "400" on one side with score on the other side, and "SL" on each side of the score.
Bottles of 30 tablets ....NDC 0078-0438-15
Storage and Handling
Store at 25°C (77°F); excursions permitted to 15°C-30°C (59°F-86°F) [see USP Controlled Room Temperature]. Protect from moisture.
Dispense in a tight container, USP.
Gleevec is an antineoplastic product. Follow special handling and disposal procedures¹
Gleevec tablets should not be crushed. Direct contact of crushed tablets with the skin or mucous membranes should be avoided. If such contact occurs, wash thoroughly as outlined in the references. Personnel should avoid exposure to crushed tablets.

17   PATIENT COUNSELING INFORMATION
17.1   Dosing and Administration
Patients should be informed to take Gleevec exactly as prescribed, not to change their dose or to stop taking Gleevec unless they are told to do so by their doctor. If patients miss a dose they should be advised to take their dose as soon as possible unless it is almost time for their next dose in which case the missed dose should not be taken. A double dose should not be taken to make up for any missed dose. Patients should be advised to take Gleevec with a meal and a large glass of water.
17.2   Pregnancy and Breast-Feeding
Patients should be advised to inform their doctor if they are or think they may be pregnant. Women of reproductive potential should be advised to avoid becoming pregnant while taking Gleevec. Sexually active female patients taking Gleevec should use highly effective contraception. Patients should also be advised not to breast feed while taking Gleevec.

17.3   Adverse Reactions
Patients should be advised to tell their doctor if they experience side effects during Gleevec therapy including fever, shortness of breath, blood in their stools, jaundice, sudden weight gain, symptoms of cardiac failure, or if they have a history of cardiac disease or risk factors for cardiac failure.
17.4   Drug Interactions
Patients should be advised not to take any other medications, including over-the-counter medications such as herbal products without talking to their doctor or pharmacist first. Examples of other medications that should not be taken with Gleevec are warfarin, erythromycin, and phenytoin. Patients should also be advised to tell their doctor if they are taking or plan to take iron supplements. Patients should also avoid grapefruit juice and other foods known to inhibit CYP3A4 while taking Gleevec.
17.5   Pediatric
Patients should be advised that growth retardation has been reported in children and pre-adolescents receiving Gleevec. The long term effects of prolonged treatment with Gleevec on growth in children are unknown. Therefore, close monitoring of growth in children under Gleevec treatment is recommended.
17.6   Driving and Using Machines
Patients should be advised that they may experience undesirable effects such as dizziness, blurred vision or somnolence during treatment with Gleevec. Therefore, caution patients about driving a car or operating machinery.

Distributed by:
Novartis Pharmaceuticals Corporation
East Hanover, New Jersey 07936
© Novartis
T2014-59
May 2014

Shown in Product Identification Guide, page 310

HECORIA™   ℞
(tacrolimus capsules, USP)

The following prescribing information is based on official labeling in effect July 2014.
HIGHLIGHTS OF PRESCRIBING INFORMATION
These highlights do not include all the information needed to use Hecoria safely and effectively. See full prescribing information for Hecoria.
Hecoria™ (tacrolimus capsules, USP)
Initial U.S. Approval: 1994

> **WARNING: MALIGNANCIES AND SERIOUS INFECTIONS**
> *See full prescribing information for complete boxed warning*
> - **Increased risk of development of lymphoma and other malignancies, particularly of the skin, due to immunosuppression (5.2)**
> - **Increased susceptibility to bacterial, viral, fungal, and protozoal infections, including opportunistic infections (5.3, 5.4, 5.5)**
> - **Only physicians experienced in immunosuppressive therapy and management of organ transplant patients should prescribe Hecoria (tacrolimus) capsules (5.1)**

——RECENT MAJOR CHANGES——

Warnings and Precautions, Use with CYP3A4 Inhibitors and Inducers (5.13)	8/2013
Warnings and Precautions, QT Prolongation (5.14)	8/2013
Warnings and Precautions, Gastrointestinal Perforation (5.18)	8/2013

——INDICATIONS AND USAGE——

Hecoria (tacrolimus capsules, USP) is a calcineurin-inhibitor immunosuppressant indicated for (1)
- Prophylaxis of organ rejection in patients receiving allogeneic liver, kidney, or heart transplants (1.1, 1.2, 1.3)
- Use concomitantly with adrenal corticosteroids; in kidney and heart transplant, use in conjunction with azathioprine or mycophenolate mofetil (MMF) (1.1, 1.2, 1.3)
- Limitations of Use (1.4):
  ○ Do not use simultaneously with cyclosporine
  ○ Intravenous use reserved for patients who cannot tolerate capsules orally
  ○ Use with sirolimus is not recommended in liver and heart transplant; use with sirolimus in kidney transplant has not been established

——DOSAGE AND ADMINISTRATION——

Summary of Initial Oral Dosage Recommendation and Observed Whole Blood Trough Concentrations (2.1, 2.2).

Patient Population	Recommended Initial Oral Dosage (two divided doses every 12 hours)	Observed Whole Blood Trough Concentrations
Adult Kidney transplant In combination with azathioprine	0.2 mg/kg/day	month 1 to 3: 7 to 20 ng/mL month 4 to 12: 5 to 15 ng/mL
In combination with MMF/IL-2 receptor antagonist	0.1 mg/kg/day	month 1 to 12: 4 to 11 ng/mL
Adult Liver transplant	0.10 to 0.15 mg/kg/day	month 1 to 12: 5 to 20 ng/mL
Pediatric Liver transplant	0.15 to 0.20 mg/kg/day	month 1 to 12: 5 to 20 ng/mL
Adult Heart transplant	0.075 mg/kg/day	month 1 to 3: 10 to 20 ng/mL month ≥4: 5 to 15 ng/mL

- Careful and frequent monitoring of tacrolimus trough concentrations is recommended; Black patients may require higher doses in order to achieve comparable trough concentrations (2.1)
- Hepatic/Renal impaired patients should receive doses at the lowest value of the recommended initial oral dosing range (2.3, 2.4)
- Administer capsules consistently with or without food; do not drink grapefruit juice (2.5, 7.2)

————DOSAGE FORMS AND STRENGTHS————
- Capsules: 0.5 mg, 1 mg and 5 mg (3)

————————CONTRAINDICATIONS————————
- Hypersensitivity to tacrolimus (4)

————WARNINGS AND PRECAUTIONS————
- Lymphoma and Other Malignancies: Risk of lymphomas, including post transplant lymphoproliferative disorder (PTLD); appears related to intensity and duration of use. Avoid prolonged exposure to UV light and sunlight (5.2)
- Serious infections: Increased risk of bacterial, viral, fungal and protozoal infections, including opportunistic infections: combination immunosuppression should be used with caution (5.3)
- Polyoma Virus Infections: Serious, sometimes fatal outcomes, including polyoma virus-associated nephropathy (PVAN), mostly due to BK virus, and JC virus-associated progressive multifocal leukoencephalopathy (PML); consider reducing immunosuppression (5.4)
- Cytomegalovirus (CMV) Infections: Increased risk of CMV viremia and disease; consider reducing immunosuppression (5.5)
- New Onset Diabetes After Transplant: Monitor blood glucose (5.6)
- Nephrotoxicity: Acute and/or chronic; reduce the dose; use caution with other nephrotoxic drugs (5.7)
- Neurotoxicity: Risk of Posterior Reversible Encephalopathy Syndrome, monitor for neurologic abnormalities; reduce or discontinue tacrolimus and other immunosuppressants (5.8)
- Hyperkalemia: Monitor serum potassium levels. Careful consideration should be given prior to use of other agents also associated with hyperkalemia (5.9)
- Hypertension: May require antihypertensive therapy. Monitor relevant drug-drug interactions (5.10)
- Anaphylactic Reactions with IV formulation: Observe patients receiving tacrolimus injection for signs and symptoms of anaphylaxis (5.11)
- Use with Sirolimus: Not recommended in liver and heart transplant due to increased risk of serious adverse reactions (5.12)
- Myocardial Hypertrophy: Consider dosage reduction or discontinuation (5.15)
- Immunizations: Use of live vaccines should be avoided (5.16)
- Pure Red Cell Aplasia: Discontinuation should be considered (5.17)

————————ADVERSE REACTIONS————————
- Kidney Transplant: The most common adverse reactions (≥30%) were infection, tremor, hypertension, abnormal renal function, constipation, diarrhea, headache, abdominal pain, insomnia, nausea, hypomagnesemia, urinary tract infection, hypophosphatemia, peripheral edema, asthenia, pain, hyperlipidemia, hyperkalemia, and anemia (6.1)
- Liver Transplant: The most common adverse reactions (≥40%) were tremor, headache, diarrhea, hypertension, nausea, abnormal renal function, abdominal pain, insomnia, paresthesia, anemia, pain, fever, asthenia, hyperkalemia, hypomagnesemia, and hyperglycemia (6.1)

- Heart Transplant: The most common adverse reactions (≥15%) were abnormal renal function, hypertension, diabetes mellitus, CMV infection, tremor, hyperglycemia, leukopenia, infection, anemia, bronchitis, pericardial effusion, urinary tract infection and hyperlipemia (6.1)

To report SUSPECTED ADVERSE REACTIONS, contact Novartis Pharmaceuticals Corporation at 1-888-669-6682 or FDA at 1-800-FDA-1088 or www.fda.gov/medwatch

————————DRUG INTERACTIONS————————
- Mycophenolic Acid Products: Can increase MPA exposure after crossover from cyclosporine to tacrolimus; monitor for MPA-related adverse reactions and adjust MMF or MPA-dose as needed (7.1)
- Nelfinavir and Grapefruit Juice: Increased tacrolimus concentrations via CYP3A inhibition; avoid concomitant use (7.2, 7.3)
- CYP3A Inhibitors: Increased tacrolimus concentrations; monitor concentrations and adjust tacrolimus dose as needed with concomitant use (5.13, 7.3, 7.4, 7.5, 7.6)
- CYP3A4 Inducers: Decreased tacrolimus concentrations; monitor concentrations and adjust tacrolimus dose as needed with concomitant use (5.13, 7.7, 7.8, 7.9)

————USE IN SPECIFIC POPULATIONS————
- Pregnancy: Based on animal data may cause fetal harm. Use only if the potential benefit justifies the risk (8.1)
- Nursing Mothers: Discontinue nursing taking into consideration importance of drug to mother (8.3)
- Hepatic/Renal impaired patients: Administer at the lower end of the recommended starting dose. Monitor renal function in patients with impaired renal function (2.3, 2.4, 8.6, 8.7)

See 17 for PATIENT COUNSELING INFORMATION and FDA-approved patient labeling

Revised: 9/2013

———————————————————————————————————
FULL PRESCRIBING INFORMATION: CONTENTS*
BOXED WARNING - MALIGNANCIES AND SERIOUS INFECTIONS

FULL PRESCRIBING INFORMATION

BOXED WARNING - MALIGNANCIES AND SERIOUS INFECTIONS
- Increased risk of development of lymphoma and other malignancies, particularly of the skin, due to immunosuppression [see WARNINGS AND PRECAUTIONS (5.2)].
- Increased susceptibility to bacterial, viral, fungal, and protozoal infections, including opportunistic infections [see WARNINGS AND PRECAUTIONS (5.3, 5.4, 5.5)].
- Only physicians experienced in immunosuppressive therapy and management of organ transplant patients should prescribe Hecoria (tacrolimus) capsules. Patients receiving the drug should be managed in facilities equipped and staffed with adequate laboratory and supportive medical resources. The physician responsible for maintenance therapy should have complete information requisite for the follow-up of the patient [see WARNINGS AND PRECAUTIONS (5.1)].

1 INDICATIONS AND USAGE
1.1 Prophylaxis of Organ Rejection in Kidney Transplant
Hecoria (tacrolimus capsules, USP) is indicated for the prophylaxis of organ rejection in patients receiving allogeneic kidney transplants. It is recommended that Hecoria be used concomitantly with azathioprine or mycophenolate mofetil (MMF) and adrenal corticosteroids [see CLINICAL STUDIES (14.1)]. Therapeutic drug monitoring is recommended for all patients receiving Hecoria [see DOSAGE AND ADMINISTRATION (2.6)].
1.2 Prophylaxis of Organ Rejection in Liver Transplant
Hecoria (tacrolimus capsules, USP) is indicated for the prophylaxis of organ rejection in patients receiving allogeneic liver transplants. It is recommended that Hecoria be used concomitantly with adrenal corticosteroids [see CLINICAL STUDIES (14.2)]. Therapeutic drug monitoring is recommended for all patients receiving Hecoria [see DOSAGE AND ADMINISTRATION (2.6)].
1.3 Prophylaxis of Organ Rejection in Heart Transplant
Hecoria (tacrolimus capsules, USP) is indicated for the prophylaxis of organ rejection in patients receiving allogeneic heart transplants. It is recommended that Hecoria be used concomitantly with azathioprine or mycophenolate mofetil (MMF) and adrenal corticosteroids [see CLINICAL STUDIES (14.3)]. Therapeutic drug monitoring is recommended for all patients receiving Hecoria [see DOSAGE AND ADMINISTRATION (2.6)].
1.4 Limitations of Use
Hecoria (tacrolimus capsules, USP) should not be used simultaneously with cyclosporine [see DOSAGE AND ADMINISTRATION (2.5)].

Tacrolimus injection should be reserved for patients unable to take Hecoria capsules orally [see DOSAGE AND ADMINISTRATION (2.1) and WARNINGS AND PRECAUTIONS (5.11)].

Use with sirolimus is not recommended in liver and heart transplant. The safety and efficacy of Hecoria with sirolimus has not been established in kidney transplant [see **WARNINGS AND PRECAUTIONS (5.12)**].

2 DOSAGE AND ADMINISTRATION

2.1 Dosage in Adult Kidney, Liver, or Heart Transplant Patients

The initial oral dosage recommendations for adult patients with kidney, liver, or heart transplants along with recommendations for whole blood trough concentrations are shown in **Table 1**. The initial dose of Hecoria (tacrolimus capsules, USP) should be administered no sooner than 6 hours after transplantation in the liver and heart transplant patients. In kidney transplant patients, the initial dose of Hecoria may be administered within 24 hours of transplantation, but should be delayed until renal function has recovered. For blood concentration monitoring details see **DOSAGE AND ADMINISTRATION (2.6)**.

Table 1. Summary of Initial Oral Dosage Recommendations and Observed Whole Blood Trough Concentrations in Adults

Patient Population	Recommended Hecoria Initial Oral Dosage Note: daily doses should be administered as two divided doses, every 12 hours	Observed Tacrolimus Whole Blood Trough Concentrations
Adult kidney transplant patients In combination with azathioprine	0.2 mg/kg/day	month 1 to 3: 7 to 20 ng/mL month 4 to 12: 5 to 15 ng/mL
In combination with MMF/IL-2 receptor antagonist[a]	0.1 mg/kg/day	month 1 to 12: 4 to 11 ng/mL
Adult liver transplant patients	0.10 to 0.15 mg/kg/day	month 1 to 12: 5 to 20 ng/mL
Adult heart transplant patients	0.075 mg/kg/day	month 1 to 3: 10 to 20 ng/mL month ≥4: 5 to 15 ng/mL

[a]In a second smaller trial, the initial dose of tacrolimus was 0.15 to 0.2 mg/kg/day and observed tacrolimus concentrations were 6 to 16 ng/mL during months 1 to 3 and 5 to 12 ng/mL during months 4 to 12 [see **CLINICAL STUDIES (14.1)**].

Dosing should be titrated based on clinical assessments of rejection and tolerability. Lower Hecoria dosages than the recommended initial dosage may be sufficient as maintenance therapy. Adjunct therapy with adrenal corticosteroids is recommended early post-transplant.

The data in kidney transplant patients indicate that the Black patients required a higher dose to attain comparable trough concentrations compared to Caucasian patients (**Table 2**).

[See table 2 above]

Initial Dose – Injection

Tacrolimus injection should be used only as a continuous IV infusion and when the patient cannot tolerate oral administration of Hecoria (tacrolimus capsules, USP). Tacrolimus injection should be discontinued as soon as the patient can tolerate oral administration of Hecoria capsules, usually within 2 to 3 days. In a patient receiving an IV infusion, the first dose of oral therapy should be given 8 to 12 hours after discontinuing the IV infusion.

The observed trough concentrations described above pertain to oral administration of Hecoria only; while monitoring Hecoria concentrations in patients receiving tacrolimus injection as a continuous IV infusion may have some utility, the observed concentrations will not represent comparable exposures to those estimated by the trough concentrations observed in patients on oral therapy.

The recommended starting dose of tacrolimus injection is 0.03 to 0.05 mg/kg/day in kidney and liver transplant and 0.01 mg/kg/day in heart transplant given as a continuous IV infusion. Adult patients should receive doses at the lower end of the dosing range. Concomitant adrenal corticosteroid therapy is recommended early post-transplantation.

Anaphylactic reactions have occurred with injectables containing castor oil derivatives, such as tacrolimus injection [see **WARNINGS AND PRECAUTIONS (5.11)**].

2.2 Dosage in Pediatric Liver Transplant Patients
The initial oral dosage recommendations for pediatric patients with liver transplants along with recommendations

Table 2. Comparative Dose and Trough Concentrations Based on Race

Time After Transplant	Caucasian n=114		Black n=56	
	Dose (mg/kg)	Trough Concentrations (ng/mL)	Dose (mg/kg)	Trough Concentrations (ng/mL)
Day 7	0.18	12	0.23	10.9
Month 1	0.17	12.8	0.26	12.9
Month 6	0.14	11.8	0.24	11.5
Month 12	0.13	10.1	0.19	11

for whole blood trough concentrations are shown in **Table 3**. For blood concentration monitoring details see **DOSAGE AND ADMINISTRATION (2.6)**. If necessary, pediatric patients may start on an IV dose of 0.03 to 0.05 mg/kg/day.

Table 3. Summary of Initial Oral Dosage Recommendations and Observed Whole Blood Trough Concentrations in Children

Patient Population	Recommended Hecoria Initial Oral Dosage Note: daily doses should be administered as two divided doses, every 12 hours	Observed Tacrolimus Whole Blood Trough Concentrations
Pediatric liver transplant patients	0.15 to 0.20 mg/kg/day	Month 1 to 12: 5 to 20 ng/mL

Pediatric liver transplantation patients without pre-existing renal or hepatic dysfunction have required and tolerated higher doses than adults to achieve similar blood concentrations.

Experience in pediatric kidney and heart transplantation patients is limited.

2.3 Dosage Adjustment in Patients with Renal Impairment
Due to its potential for nephrotoxicity, consideration should be given to dosing Hecoria (tacrolimus capsules, USP) at the lower end of the therapeutic dosing range in patients who have received a liver or heart transplant and have pre-existing renal impairment. Further reductions in dose below the targeted range may be required.

In kidney transplant patients with post-operative oliguria, the initial dose of Hecoria should be administered no sooner than 6 hours and within 24 hours of transplantation, but may be delayed until renal function shows evidence of recovery.

2.4 Dosage Adjustments in Patients with Hepatic Impairment
Due to the reduced clearance and prolonged half-life, patients with severe hepatic impairment (Child Pugh ≥ 10) may require lower doses of Hecoria (tacrolimus capsules, USP). Close monitoring of blood concentrations is warranted.

The use of Hecoria in liver transplant recipients experiencing post-transplant hepatic impairment may be associated with increased risk of developing renal insufficiency related to high whole-blood concentrations of tacrolimus. These patients should be monitored closely and dosage adjustments should be considered. Some evidence suggests that lower doses should be used in these patients [see **DOSAGE AND ADMINISTRATION (2.1)**, **USE IN SPECIFIC POPULATIONS (8.7)** and **CLINICAL PHARMACOLOGY (12.3)**].

2.5 Administration Instructions
It is recommended that patients initiate oral therapy with Hecoria (tacrolimus capsules, USP) if possible.

Initial dosage and observed tacrolimus whole blood trough concentrations for adults are shown in **Table 1** and for pediatrics in **Table 3** [see **DOSAGE AND ADMINISTRATION (2.1, 2.2)**]; for blood concentration monitoring details in kidney transplant patients [see **DOSAGE AND ADMINISTRATION (2.1)**].

It is important to take Hecoria capsules consistently every day either with or without food because the presence and composition of food decreases the bioavailability of Hecoria [see **CLINICAL PHARMACOLOGY (12.3)**].

Patients should not eat grapefruit or drink grapefruit juice in combination with Hecoria [see **DRUG INTERACTIONS (7.2)**].

Hecoria should not be used simultaneously with cyclosporine. Hecoria or cyclosporine should be discontinued at least 24 hours before initiating the other. In the presence of elevated Hecoria or cyclosporine concentrations, dosing with the other drug usually should be further delayed.

In patients unable to take oral Hecoria (tacrolimus capsules, USP), therapy may be initiated with tacrolimus injection as a continuous IV infusion. If IV therapy is necessary, conversion from IV to oral tacrolimus is recommended as soon as oral therapy can be tolerated. This usually occurs within 2 to 3 days. In patients receiving an IV infusion, the first dose of oral therapy should be given 8 to 12 hours after discontinuing the IV infusion.

2.6 Therapeutic Drug Monitoring
Monitoring of tacrolimus blood concentrations in conjunction with other laboratory and clinical parameters is considered an essential aid to patient management for the evaluation of rejection, toxicity, dose adjustments and compliance. Observed whole blood trough concentrations can be found in **Table 1**. Factors influencing frequency of monitoring include but are not limited to hepatic or renal dysfunction, the addition or discontinuation of potentially interacting drugs and the post-transplant time. Blood concentration monitoring is not a replacement for renal and liver function monitoring and tissue biopsies. Data from clinical trials show that tacrolimus whole blood concentrations were most variable during the first week post-transplantation.

The relative risks of toxicity and efficacy failure are related to tacrolimus whole blood trough concentrations. Therefore, monitoring of whole blood trough concentrations is recommended to assist in the clinical evaluation of toxicity and efficacy failure.

Methods commonly used for the assay of tacrolimus include high performance liquid chromatography with tandem mass spectrometric detection (HPLC/MS/MS) and immunoassays. Immunoassays may react with metabolites as well as parent compound. Therefore assay results obtained with immunoassays may have a positive bias relative to results of HPLC/MS. The bias may depend upon the specific assay and laboratory. Comparison of the concentrations in published literature to patient concentrations using the current assays must be made with detailed knowledge of the assay methods and biological matrices employed. Whole blood is the matrix of choice and specimens should be collected into tubes containing ethylene diamine tetraacetic acid (EDTA) anti-coagulant. Heparin anti-coagulation is not recommended because of the tendency to form clots on storage. Samples which are not analyzed immediately should be stored at room temperature or in a refrigerator and assayed within 7 days; see assay instructions for specifics. If samples are to be kept longer they should be deep frozen at -20°C. One study showed drug recovery >90% for samples stored at -20°C for 6 months, with reduced recovery observed after 6 months.

3 DOSAGE FORMS AND STRENGTHS

Hecoria (tacrolimus capsules, USP) is available in 0.5 mg, 1 mg, and 5 mg strengths.

Hecoria (tacrolimus capsules, USP) containing white to off white powder equivalent to 0.5 mg of anhydrous tacrolimus, are hard gelatin capsules with white opaque body and ivory cap. The body is imprinted "0.5 mg" and cap is imprinted "HECORIA" in black ink.

Hecoria (tacrolimus capsules, USP) containing white to off white powder equivalent to 1 mg of anhydrous tacrolimus, are hard gelatin capsules with white opaque body and brown cap. The body is imprinted "1 mg" and cap is imprinted "HECORIA" in black ink.

Hecoria (tacrolimus capsules, USP) containing white to off white powder equivalent to 5 mg of anhydrous tacrolimus, are hard gelatin capsules with white opaque body and orange cap. The body is imprinted "5 mg" and cap is imprinted "HECORIA" in black ink.

4 CONTRAINDICATIONS

Hecoria (tacrolimus) capsules are contraindicated in patients with a hypersensitivity to tacrolimus. Hypersensitivity symptoms reported include dyspnea, rash, pruritus, and acute respiratory distress syndrome [see **ADVERSE REACTIONS (6)**].

5 WARNINGS AND PRECAUTIONS
5.1 Management of Immunosuppression
Only physicians experienced in immunosuppressive therapy and management of organ transplant patients should

use Hecoria (tacrolimus) capsules. Patients receiving the drug should be managed in facilities equipped and staffed with adequate laboratory and supportive medical resources. The physicians responsible for maintenance therapy should have complete information requisite for the follow-up of the patient [see **BOXED WARNING**].

5.2 Lymphoma and Other Malignancies

Patients receiving immunosuppressants, including Hecoria (tacrolimus) capsules, are at increased risk of developing lymphomas and other malignancies, particularly of the skin [see **BOXED WARNING**]. The risk appears to be related to the intensity and duration of immunosuppression rather than to the use of any specific agent.

As usual for patients with increased risk for skin cancer, exposure to sunlight and UV light should be limited by wearing protective clothing and using a sunscreen with a high protection factor.

Post transplant lymphoproliferative disorder (PTLD) has been reported in immunosuppressed organ transplant recipients. The majority of PTLD events appear related to Epstein Barr Virus (EBV) infection. The risk of PTLD appears greatest in those individuals who are EBV seronegative, a population which includes many young children.

5.3 Serious Infections

Patients receiving immunosuppressants, including Hecoria (tacrolimus) capsules, are at increased risk of developing bacterial, viral, fungal, and protozoal infections, including opportunistic infections [see **BOXED WARNING** and **WARNINGS AND PRECAUTIONS (5.4, 5.5)**]. These infections may lead to serious, including fatal, outcomes. Because of the danger of oversuppression of the immune system which can increase susceptibility to infection, combination immunosuppressant therapy should be used with caution.

5.4 Polyoma Virus Infections

Patients receiving immunosuppressants, including Hecoria (tacrolimus) capsules, are at increased risk for opportunistic infections, including polyoma virus infections. Polyoma virus infections in transplant patients may have serious, and sometimes fatal, outcomes. These include polyoma virus-associated nephropathy (PVAN), mostly due to BK virus infection, and JC virus-associated progressive multifocal leukoencephalopathy (PML) which have been observed in patients receiving tacrolimus [see **ADVERSE REACTIONS (6.2)**].

PVAN is associated with serious outcomes, including deteriorating renal function and kidney graft loss [see **ADVERSE REACTIONS (6.2)**]. Patient monitoring may help detect patients at risk for PVAN.

Cases of PML have been reported in patients treated with Hecoria. PML, which is sometimes fatal, commonly presents with hemiparesis, apathy, confusion, cognitive deficiencies and ataxia. Risk factors for PML include treatment with immunosuppressant therapies and impairment of immune function. In immunosuppressed patients, physicians should consider PML in the differential diagnosis in patients reporting neurological symptoms and consultation with a neurologist should be considered as clinically indicated.

Reductions in immunosuppression should be considered for patients who develop evidence of PVAN or PML. Physicians should also consider the risk that reduced immunosuppression represents to the functioning allograft.

5.5 Cytomegalovirus (CMV) Infections

Patients receiving immunosuppressants, including Hecoria (tacrolimus) capsules, are at increased risk of developing CMV viremia and CMV disease. The risk of CMV disease is highest among transplant recipients seronegative for CMV at time of transplant who receive a graft from a CMV seropositive donor. Therapeutic approaches to limiting CMV disease exist and should be routinely provided. Patient monitoring may help detect patients at risk for CMV disease. Consideration should be given to reducing the amount of immunosuppression in patients who develop CMV viremia and/or CMV disease.

5.6 New Onset Diabetes After Transplant

Tacrolimus was shown to cause new onset diabetes mellitus in clinical trials of kidney, liver, and heart transplantation. New onset diabetes after transplantation may be reversible in some patients. Black and Hispanic kidney transplant patients are at an increased risk. Blood glucose concentrations should be monitored closely in patients using Hecoria (tacrolimus) capsules [see **ADVERSE REACTIONS (6.1)**].

5.7 Nephrotoxicity

Hecoria (tacrolimus) capsules, like other calcineurin-inhibitors, can cause acute or chronic nephrotoxicity, particularly when used in high doses. Acute nephrotoxicity is most often related to vasoconstriction of the afferent renal arteriole, is characterized by increasing serum creatinine, hyperkalemia, and/or a decrease in urine output, and is typically reversible. Chronic calcineurin-inhibitor nephrotoxicity is associated with increased serum creatinine, decreased kidney graft life, and characteristic histologic changes observed on renal biopsy; the changes associated with chronic calcineurin-inhibitor nephrotoxicity are typically progressive. Patients with impaired renal function should be monitored closely as the dosage of tacrolimus may need to be reduced. In patients with persistent elevations of serum creatinine who are unresponsive to dosage adjustments, consideration should be given to changing to another immunosuppressive therapy.

Based on reported adverse reactions terms related to decreased renal function, nephrotoxicity was reported in approximately 52% of kidney transplantation patients and in 40% and 36% of liver transplantation patients receiving tacrolimus in the U.S. and European randomized trials, respectively, and in 59% of heart transplantation patients in a European randomized trial [see **ADVERSE REACTIONS (6.1)**].

Due to the potential for additive or synergistic impairment of renal function, care should be taken when administering Hecoria with drugs that may be associated with renal dysfunction. These include, but are not limited to, aminoglycosides, ganciclovir, amphotericin B, cisplatin, nucleotide reverse transcriptase inhibitors (e.g., tenofovir) and protease inhibitors (e.g., ritonavir, indinavir). Similarly, care should be exercised when administering with CYP3A4 inhibitors such as antifungal drugs (e.g., ketoconazole), calcium channel blockers (e.g., diltiazem, verapamil), and macrolide antibiotics (e.g., clarithromycin, erythromycin, troleandomycin) which will result in increased tacrolimus whole blood concentrations due to inhibition of tacrolimus metabolism [see **DRUG INTERACTIONS (7.3, 7.4, 7.5, 7.6)**].

5.8 Neurotoxicity

Hecoria (tacrolimus) capsules may cause a spectrum of neurotoxicities, particularly when used in high doses. The most severe neurotoxicities include posterior reversible encephalopathy syndrome (PRES), delirium, and coma. Patients treated with tacrolimus have been reported to develop PRES. Symptoms indicating PRES include headache, altered mental status, seizures, visual disturbances and hypertension. Diagnosis may be confirmed by radiological procedure. If PRES is suspected or diagnosed, blood pressure control should be maintained and immediate reduction of immunosuppression is advised. This syndrome is characterized by reversal of symptoms upon reduction or discontinuation of immunosuppression.

Coma and delirium, in the absence of PRES, have also been associated with high plasma concentrations of tacrolimus. Seizures have occurred in adult and pediatric patients receiving Hecoria [see **ADVERSE REACTIONS (6.1)**].

Less severe neurotoxicities, include tremors, parathesias, headache, and other changes in motor function, mental status, and sensory function [see **ADVERSE REACTIONS (6.1)**]. Tremor and headache have been associated with high whole-blood concentrations of tacrolimus and may respond to dosage adjustment.

5.9 Hyperkalemia

Hyperkalemia has been reported with Hecoria (tacrolimus) capsule use. Serum potassium levels should be monitored. Careful consideration should be given prior to use of other agents also associated with hyperkalemia (e.g., potassium-sparing diuretics, ACE inhibitors, angiotensin receptor blockers) during Hecoria therapy [see **ADVERSE REACTIONS (6.1)**].

5.10 Hypertension

Hypertension is a common adverse effect of Hecoria (tacrolimus) capsules therapy and may require antihypertensive therapy [see **ADVERSE REACTIONS (6.1)**]. The control of blood pressure can be accomplished with any of the common antihypertensive agents, though careful consideration should be given prior to use of antihypertensive agents associated with hyperkalemia (e.g., potassium-sparing diuretics, ACE inhibitors, angiotensin receptor blockers) [see **WARNINGS AND PRECAUTIONS (5.9)**]. Calcium-channel blocking agents may increase tacrolimus blood concentrations and therefore require dosage reduction of Hecoria [see **DRUG INTERACTIONS (7.5)**].

5.11 Anaphylactic Reactions with Tacrolimus Injection

Anaphylactic reactions have occurred with injectables containing castor oil derivatives, including tacrolimus, in a small percentage of patients (0.6%). The exact cause of these reactions is not known. Tacrolimus injection should be reserved for patients who are unable to take tacrolimus capsules [see **INDICATIONS AND USAGE (1.4)**].

Patients receiving tacrolimus injection should be under continuous observation for at least the first 30 minutes following the start of the infusion and at frequent intervals thereafter. If signs or symptoms of anaphylaxis occur, the infusion should be stopped. An aqueous solution of epinephrine should be available at the bedside as well as a source of oxygen.

5.12 Use with Sirolimus

The safety and efficacy of Hecoria (tacrolimus) capsules with sirolimus has not been established in kidney transplant patients.

Use of sirolimus with tacrolimus in studies of de novo liver transplant patients was associated with an excess mortality, graft loss, and hepatic artery thrombosis (HAT) and is not recommended [see **INDICATIONS AND USAGE (1.4)**]. Use of sirolimus (2 mg per day) with tacrolimus in heart transplant patients in a U.S. trial was associated with increased risk of renal function impairment, wound healing complications, and insulin-dependent post–transplant diabetes mellitus, and is not recommended [see **CLINICAL STUDIES (14.3)**].

5.13 Use with CYP3A4 Inhibitors and Inducers

When coadministering Hecoria (tacrolimus) with strong CYP3A4-inhibitors (e.g., telaprevir, boceprevir, ritonavir, ketoconazole, itraconazole, voriconazole, clarithromycin) and strong inducers (e.g., rifampin, rifabutin) adjustments in the dosing regimen of Hecoria (tacrolimus) and subsequent frequent monitoring of tacrolimus whole blood trough concentrations and tacrolimus-associated adverse reactions are recommended [see **DRUG INTERACTIONS (7)**].

5.14 QT Prolongation

Hecoria (tacrolimus) may prolong the QT/QTc interval and may cause Torsade de Pointes. Avoid Hecoria (tacrolimus) in patients with congenital long QT syndrome. In patients with congestive heart failure, bradyarrhythmias, those taking certain antiarrhythmic medications or other medicinal products that lead to QT prolongation and those with electrolyte disturbances such as hypokalemia, hypocalcemia, or hypomagnesemia, consider obtaining electrocardiograms and monitoring electrolytes (magnesium, potassium, calcium) periodically during treatment.

When coadministering tacrolimus with other substrates and/or inhibitors of CYP3A4 that also have the potential to prolong the QT interval, a reduction in tacrolimus dose, frequent monitoring of tacrolimus whole blood concentrations, and monitoring for QT prolongation is recommended. Use of tacrolimus with amiodarone has been reported to result in increased tacrolimus whole blood concentrations with or without concurrent QT prolongation [see **DRUG INTERACTIONS (7)**].

5.15 Myocardial Hypertrophy

Myocardial hypertrophy has been reported in infants, children, and adults, particularly those with high tacrolimus trough concentrations, and is generally manifested by echocardiographically demonstrated concentric increases in left ventricular posterior wall and interventricular septum thickness. This condition appears reversible in most cases following dose reduction or discontinuance of therapy. In patients who develop renal failure or clinical manifestations of ventricular dysfunction while receiving tacrolimus therapy, echocardiographic evaluation should be considered. If myocardial hypertrophy is diagnosed, dosage reduction or discontinuation of Hecoria (tacrolimus) capsules should be considered [see **ADVERSE REACTIONS (6.2)**].

5.16 Immunizations

The use of live vaccines should be avoided during treatment with tacrolimus; examples include (not limited to) the following: intranasal influenza, measles, mumps, rubella, oral polio, BCG, yellow fever, varicella, and TY21a typhoid vaccines.

5.17 Pure Red Cell Aplasia

Cases of pure red cell aplasia (PRCA) have been reported in patients treated with tacrolimus. A mechanism for tacrolimus-induced PRCA has not been elucidated. All patients reported risk factors for PRCA such as parvovirus B19 infection, underlying disease, or concomitant medications associated with PRCA. If PRCA is diagnosed, discontinuation of Hecoria (tacrolimus) capsules should be considered [see **ADVERSE REACTIONS (6.2)**].

5.18 Gastrointestinal Perforation

Gastrointestinal perforation has been reported in patients treated with Hecoria (tacrolimus); all reported cases were considered to be a complication of transplant surgery or accompanied by infection, diverticulum, or malignant neoplasm. As gastrointestinal perforation may be serious or life-threatening, appropriate medical/surgical management should be instituted promptly [see **ADVERSE REACTIONS (6.1)**].

6 ADVERSE REACTIONS

The following serious and otherwise important adverse drug reactions are discussed in greater detail in other sections of labeling:

- Lymphoma and Other Malignancies [see **BOXED WARNING, WARNINGS AND PRECAUTIONS (5.2)**]
- Serious Infections [see **BOXED WARNING, WARNINGS AND PRECAUTIONS (5.3)**]
- Polyoma Virus Infections [see **BOXED WARNING, WARNINGS AND PRECAUTIONS (5.4)**]
- CMV Infections [see **BOXED WARNING, WARNINGS AND PRECAUTIONS (5.5)**]
- New Onset Diabetes After Transplant [see **WARNINGS AND PRECAUTIONS (5.6)**]
- Nephrotoxicity [see **WARNINGS AND PRECAUTIONS (5.7)**]
- Neurotoxicity [see **WARNINGS AND PRECAUTIONS (5.8)**]

- Hyperkalemia [see **WARNINGS AND PRECAUTIONS** (5.9)]
- Hypertension [see **WARNINGS AND PRECAUTIONS** (5.10)]
- Anaphylaxis with Tacrolimus Injection [see **WARNINGS AND PRECAUTIONS** (5.11)]
- Myocardial Hypertrophy [see **WARNINGS AND PRECAUTIONS** (5.15)]
- Pure Red Cell Aplasia [see **WARNINGS AND PRECAUTIONS** (5.17)]
- Gastrointestinal Perforation [see **WARNINGS AND PRECAUTIONS** (5.18)]

6.1 Clinical Studies Experience

Because clinical trials are conducted under widely varying conditions, adverse reaction rates observed in the clinical trials of a drug cannot be directly compared to rates in the clinical trials of another drug and may not reflect the rates observed in practice. In addition, the clinical trials were not designed to establish comparative differences across study arms with regards to the adverse reactions discussed below.

Kidney Transplant

The incidence of adverse reactions was determined in three randomized kidney transplant trials. One of the trials used azathioprine (AZA) and corticosteroids and two of the trials used mycophenolate mofetil (MMF) and corticosteroids concomitantly for maintenance immunosuppression.

Tacrolimus-based immunosuppression in conjunction with azathioprine and corticosteroids following kidney transplantation was assessed in trial where 205 patients received tacrolimus based immunosuppression and 207 patients received cyclosporine based immunosuppression. The trial population had a mean age of 43 years (mean±sd was 43±13 years on tacrolimus and 44±12 years on cyclosporine arm), the distribution was 61% male, and the composition was White (58%), Black (25%), Hispanic (12%) and Other (5%). The 12 month post-transplant information from this trial is presented below.

The most common adverse reactions (≥ 30%) observed in tacrolimus-treated kidney transplant patients are: infection, tremor, hypertension, abnormal renal function, constipation, diarrhea, headache, abdominal pain, insomnia, nausea, hypomagnesemia, urinary tract infection, hypophosphatemia, peripheral edema, asthenia, pain, hyperlipidemia, hyperkalemia and anemia.

Adverse reactions that occurred in ≥ 15% of kidney transplant patients treated with tacrolimus in conjunction with azathioprine are presented below:

Table 4. Kidney Transplantation: Adverse Reactions Occurring in ≥ 15% of Patients Treated with Tacrolimus in Conjunction with Azathioprine (AZA)

	Tacrolimus/ AZA (N=205)	Cyclosporine/ AZA (N=207)
Nervous System		
Tremor	54%	34%
Headache	44%	38%
Insomnia	32%	30%
Paresthesia	23%	16%
Dizziness	19%	16%
Gastrointestinal		
Diarrhea	44%	41%
Nausea	38%	36%
Constipation	35%	43%
Vomiting	29%	23%
Dyspepsia	28%	20%
Cardiovascular		
Hypertension	50%	52%
Chest Pain	19%	13%
Urogenital		
Creatinine Increased	45%	42%
Urinary Tract Infection	34%	35%
Metabolic and Nutritional		
Hypophosphatemia	49%	53%
Hypomagnesemia	34%	17%
Hyperlipemia	31%	38%
Hyperkalemia	31%	32%
Diabetes Mellitus	24%	9%
Hypokalemia	22%	25%
Hyperglycemia	22%	16%
Edema	18%	19%
Hemic and Lymphatic		
Anemia	30%	24%
Leukopenia	15%	17%
Miscellaneous		
Infection	45%	49%
Peripheral Edema	36%	48%
Asthenia	34%	30%
Abdominal Pain	33%	31%
Pain	32%	30%
Fever	29%	29%
Back Pain	24%	20%
Respiratory System		
Dyspnea	22%	18%
Cough Increased	18%	15%
Musculoskeletal		
Arthralgia	25%	24%
Skin		
Rash	17%	12%
Pruritus	15%	7%

Two trials were conducted for tacrolimus-based immunosuppression in conjunction with MMF and corticosteroids. In the non-US trial (Study 1), the incidence of adverse reactions was based on 1195 kidney transplant patients that received tacrolimus (Group C, n=403), or one of two cyclosporine (CsA) regimens (Group A, n=384 and Group B, n=408) in combination with MMF and corticosteroids; all patients, except those in one of the two cyclosporine groups, also received induction with daclizumab. The trial population had a mean age of 46 years (range 17 to 76), the distribution was 65% male, and the composition was 93% Caucasian. The 12 month post-transplant information from this trial is presented below.

Adverse reactions that occurred in ≥ 10% of kidney transplant patients treated with tacrolimus in conjunction with MMF in Study 1 [Note: This trial was conducted entirely outside of the United States. Such trials often report a lower incidence of adverse reactions in comparison to U.S. trials] are presented below:

Table 5. Kidney Transplantation: Adverse Reactions Occurring in ≥ 10% of Patients Treated with Tacrolimus in Conjunction with MMF (Study 1)

	Tacrolimus (Group C) (N=403)	Cyclosporine (Group A) (N=384)	Cyclosporine (Group B) (N=408)
Diarrhea	25%	16%	13%
Urinary Tract Infection	24%	28%	24%
Anemia	17%	19%	17%
Hypertension	13%	14%	12%
Leukopenia	13%	10%	10%
Edema Peripheral	11%	12%	13%
Hyperlipidemia	10%	15%	13%

Key: Group A = CsA/MMF/CS, B = CsA/MMF/CS/Daclizumab, C = Tac/MMF/CS/Daclizumab
CsA = Cyclosporine, CS = Corticosteroids, Tac = Tacrolimus, MMF = mycophenolate mofetil

[See table above]

In the U.S. trial (Study 2) with tacrolimus-based immunosuppression in conjunction with MMF and corticosteroids, 424 kidney transplant patients received tacrolimus (n=212) or cyclosporine (n=212) in combination with MMF 1 gram twice daily, basiliximab induction, and corticosteroids. The trial population had a mean age of 48 years (range 17 to 77), the distribution was 63% male, and the composition was White (74%), Black (20%), Asian (3%) and other (3%). The 12 month post-transplant information from this trial is presented below.

Adverse reactions that occurred in ≥15% of kidney transplant patients treated with tacrolimus in conjunction with MMF in Study 2 are presented below:

Table 6. Kidney Transplantation: Adverse Reactions Occurring in ≥ 15% of Patients Treated with Tacrolimus in Conjunction with MMF (Study 2)

	Tacrolimus/ MMF (N=212)	Cyclosporine/ MMF (N=212)
Gastrointestinal Disorders		
Diarrhea	44%	26%
Nausea	39%	47%
Constipation	36%	41%
Vomiting	26%	25%
Dyspepsia	18%	15%
Injury, Poisoning, and Procedural Complications		
Post-Procedural Pain	29%	27%
Incision Site Complication	28%	23%
Graft Dysfunction	24%	18%
Metabolism and Nutrition Disorders		
Hypomagnesemia	28%	22%
Hypophosphatemia	28%	21%
Hyperkalemia	26%	19%
Hyperglycemia	21%	15%
Hyperlipidemia	18%	25%
Hypokalemia	16%	18%
Nervous System Disorders		
Tremor	34%	20%
Headache	24%	25%
Blood and Lymphatic System Disorders		
Anemia	30%	28%

Leukopenia	16%	12%
Miscellaneous		
Edema Peripheral	35%	46%
Hypertension	32%	35%
Insomnia	30%	21%
Urinary Tract Infection	26%	22%
Blood Creatinine Increased	23%	23%

Less frequently observed adverse reactions in both liver transplantation and kidney transplantation patients are described under the subsection *Less Frequently Reported Adverse Reactions*.

Liver Transplantation

There were two randomized comparative liver transplant trials. In the U.S. trial, 263 adult and pediatric patients received tacrolimus and steroids and 266 patients received cyclosporine-based immunosuppressive regimen (CsA/AZA). The trial population had a mean age of 44 years (range 0.4 to 70), the distribution was 52% male, and the composition was White (78%), Black (5%), Asian (2%), Hispanic (13%) and Other (2%). In the European trial, 270 patients received tacrolimus and steroids and 275 patients received CsA/AZA. The trial population had a mean age of 46 years (range 15 to 68), the distribution was 59% male, and the composition was White (95.4%), Black (1%), Asian (2%) and Other (2%). The proportion of patients reporting more than one adverse event was > 99% in both the tacrolimus group and the CsA/AZA group. Precautions must be taken when comparing the incidence of adverse reactions in the U.S. trial to that in the European trial. The 12-month post-transplant information from the U.S. trial and from the European trial is presented below. The two trials also included different patient populations and patients were treated with immunosuppressive regimens of differing intensities. Adverse reactions reported in ≥15% in tacrolimus patients (combined trial results) are presented below for the two controlled trials in liver transplantation.

The most common adverse reactions (≥ 40%) observed in tacrolimus-treated liver transplant patients are: tremor, headache, diarrhea, hypertension, nausea, abnormal renal function, abdominal pain, insomnia, paresthesia, anemia, pain, fever, asthenia, hyperkalemia, hypomagnesemia, and hyperglycemia. These all occur with oral administration of tacrolimus and some may respond to a reduction in dosing (e.g., tremor, headache, paresthesia, hypertension). Diarrhea was sometimes associated with other gastrointestinal complaints such as nausea and vomiting.

[See table 7 above]

Less frequently observed adverse reactions in both liver transplantation and kidney transplantation patients are described under the subsection *Less Frequently Reported Adverse Reactions*.

Heart Transplantation

The incidence of adverse reactions was determined based on two trials in primary orthotopic heart transplantation. In a trial conducted in Europe, 314 patients received a regimen of antibody induction, corticosteroids and azathioprine (AZA) in combination with tacrolimus (n=157) or cyclosporine (n=157) for 18 months. The trial population had a mean age of 51 years (range 18 to 65), the distribution was 82% male, and the composition was White (96%), Black (3%) and other (1%).

The most common adverse reactions (≥15%) observed in tacrolimus-treated heart transplant patients are: abnormal renal function, hypertension, diabetes mellitus, CMV infection, tremor, hyperglycemia, leukopenia, infection, anemia, bronchitis, pericardial effusion, urinary tract infection and hyperlipemia.

Adverse reactions in heart transplant patients in the European trial are presented below:

Table 8. Heart Transplantation: Adverse Reactions Occurring in ≥15% of Patients Treated with Tacrolimus in Conjunction with Azathioprine (AZA)

	Tacrolimus/ AZA	Cyclosporine/ AZA
	(n=157)	(n=157)
Cardiovascular System		
Hypertension	62%	69%
Pericardial Effusion	15%	14%

Table 7. Liver Transplantation: Adverse Reactions Occurring in ≥ 15% of Patients Treated with Tacrolimus

	U.S. TRIAL		EUROPEAN TRIAL	
	Tacrolimus (N=250)	Cyclosporine/AZA (N=250)	Tacrolimus (N=264)	Cyclosporine/AZA (N=265)
Nervous System				
Headache	64%	60%	37%	26%
Insomnia	64%	68%	32%	23%
Tremor	56%	46%	48%	32%
Paresthesia	40%	30%	17%	17%
Gastrointestinal				
Diarrhea	72%	47%	37%	27%
Nausea	46%	37%	32%	27%
LFT Abnormal	36%	30%	6%	5%
Anorexia	34%	24%	7%	5%
Vomiting	27%	15%	14%	11%
Constipation	24%	27%	23%	21%
Cardiovascular				
Hypertension	47%	56%	38%	43%
Urogenital				
Kidney Function Abnormal	40%	27%	36%	23%
Creatinine Increased	39%	25%	24%	19%
BUN Increased	30%	22%	12%	9%
Oliguria	18%	15%	19%	12%
Urinary Tract Infection	16%	18%	21%	19%
Metabolic and Nutritional				
Hypomagnesemia	48%	45%	16%	9%
Hyperglycemia	47%	38%	33%	22%
Hyperkalemia	45%	26%	13%	9%
Hypokalemia	29%	34%	13%	16%
Hemic and Lymphatic				
Anemia	47%	38%	5%	1%
Leukocytosis	32%	26%	8%	8%
Thrombocytopenia	24%	20%	14%	19%
Miscellaneous				
Pain	63%	57%	24%	22%
Abdominal Pain	59%	54%	29%	22%
Asthenia	52%	48%	11%	7%
Fever	48%	56%	19%	22%
Back Pain	30%	29%	17%	17%
Ascites	27%	22%	7%	8%
Peripheral Edema	26%	26%	12%	14%
Respiratory System				
Pleural Effusion	30%	32%	36%	35%
Dyspnea	29%	23%	5%	4%
Atelectasis	28%	30%	5%	4%
Skin and Appendages				
Pruritus	36%	20%	15%	7%
Rash	24%	19%	10%	4%

Body as a Whole		
CMV Infection	32%	30%
Infection	24%	21%
Metabolism and Nutrition Disorders		
Diabetes Mellitus	26%	16%
Hyperglycemia	23%	17%
Hyperlipemia	18%	27%
Hemic and Lymphatic System		
Anemia	50%	36%
Leukopenia	48%	39%
Urogenital System		
Kidney Function Abnormal	56%	57%
Urinary Tract Infection	16%	12%
Respiratory System		
Bronchitis	17%	18%
Nervous System		
Tremor	15%	6%

In the European trial, the cyclosporine trough concentrations were above the pre-defined target range (i.e., 100 to 200 ng/mL) at Day 122 and beyond in 32 to 68% of the patients in the cyclosporine treatment arm, whereas the tacrolimus trough concentrations were within the pre-defined target range (i.e., 5 to 15 ng/mL) in 74 to 86% of the patients in the tacrolimus treatment arm.

In the U.S. trial, the incidence of adverse reactions was based on 331 heart transplant patients that received corticosteroids and tacrolimus in combination with sirolimus (n=109), tacrolimus in combination with MMF (n=107) or cyclosporine modified in combination with MMF (n=115) for 1 year. The trial population had a mean age of 53 years (range 18 to 75), the distribution was 78% male, and the composition was White (83%), Black (13%) and other (4%). Only selected targeted treatment-emergent adverse reactions were collected in the U.S. heart transplantation trial. Those reactions that were reported at a rate of 15% or greater in patients treated with tacrolimus and MMF include the following: any target adverse reactions (99%), hypertension (89%), hyperglycemia requiring antihyperglycemic therapy (70%), hypertriglyceridemia (65%), anemia (hemoglobin <10 g/dL) (65%), fasting blood glucose >140 mg/dL (on two separate occasions) (61%), hypercholesterolemia (57%), hyperlipidemia (34%), WBCs <3000 cells/mcL (34%), serious bacterial infections (30%), magnesium <1.2 mEq/L (24%), platelet count <75,000 cells/mcL (19%), and other opportunistic infections (15%).

Other targeted treatment-emergent adverse reactions in tacrolimus-treated patients occurred at a rate of less than 15%, and include the following: Cushingoid features, impaired wound healing, hyperkalemia, *Candida* infection, and CMV infection/syndrome.

New Onset Diabetes After Transplant
Kidney Transplant
New Onset Diabetes After Transplant (NODAT) is defined as a composite of fasting plasma glucose ≥126 mg/dL, HbA$_{1C}$ ≥ 6%, insulin use ≥ 30 days or oral hypoglycemic use. In a trial in kidney transplant patients (Study 2), NODAT was observed in 75% in the tacrolimus-treated and 61% in the Neoral-treated patients without pre-transplant history of diabetes mellitus (Table 9) [see **CLINICAL STUDIES (14.1)**].

Table 9. Incidence of New Onset Diabetes After Transplant at 1 Year in Kidney Transplant Recipients in a Phase 3 Trial (Study 2)

Parameter	Treatment Group	
	Tacrolimus/MMF (n = 212)	Neoral/MMF (n = 212)
NODAT	112/150 (75%)	93/152 (61%)
Fasting Plasma Glucose ≥ 126 mg/dL	96/150 (64%)	80/152 (53%)
HbA$_{1C}$ ≥ 6%	59/150 (39%)	28/152 (18%)

Table 12. Incidence of Post-Transplant Diabetes Mellitus and Insulin Use at 1 Year in Liver Transplant Recipients

Status of PTDM[a]	US Trial		European Trial	
	Tacrolimus	Cyclosporine	Tacrolimus	Cyclosporine
Patients at risk[b]	239	236	239	249
New Onset PTDM[a]	42 (18%)	30 (13%)	26 (11%)	12 (5%)
Patients still on insulin at 1 year	23 (10%)	19 (8%)	18 (8%)	6 (2%)

[a] Use of insulin for 30 or more consecutive days, with < 5 day gap, without a prior history of insulin-dependent diabetes mellitus or non-insulin dependent diabetes mellitus.
[b] Patients without pre-transplant history of diabetes mellitus.

Insulin Use ≥ 30 days	9/150 (6%)	4/152 (3%)
Oral Hypoglycemic Use	15/150 (10%)	5/152 (3%)

In early trials of tacrolimus, Post-Transplant Diabetes Mellitus (PTDM) was evaluated with a more limited criteria of "use of insulin for 30 or more consecutive days with < 5 day gap" in patients without a prior history of insulin-dependent diabetes mellitus or non-insulin dependent diabetes mellitus. Data are presented in **Tables 10 to 13**. PTDM was reported in 20% of tacrolimus/Azathioprine (AZA)-treated kidney transplant patients without pre-transplant history of diabetes mellitus in a Phase 3 trial (**Table 10**). The median time to onset of PTDM was 68 days. Insulin dependence was reversible in 15% of these PTDM patients at one year and in 50% at 2 years post-transplant. Black and Hispanic kidney transplant patients were at an increased risk of development of PTDM (**Table 11**).

Table 10. Incidence of Post-Transplant Diabetes Mellitus and Insulin Use at 2 Years in Kidney Transplant Recipients in a Phase 3 Trial using Azathioprine (AZA)

Status of PTDM[a]	Tacrolimus/AZA	CsA/AZA
Patients without pre-transplant history of diabetes mellitus	151	151
New onset PTDM[a], 1st Year	30/151 (20%)	6/151 (4%)
Still insulin-dependent at one year in those without prior history of diabetes	25/151 (17%)	5/151 (3%)
New onset PTDM[a] post 1 year	1	0
Patients with PTDM[a] at 2 years	16/151 (11%)	5/151 (3%)

[a] Use of insulin for 30 or more consecutive days, with < 5 day gap, without a prior history of insulin-dependent diabetes mellitus or non-insulin dependent diabetes mellitus.

Table 11. Development of Post-Transplant Diabetes Mellitus by Race or Ethnicity and by Treatment Group During First Year Post Kidney Transplantation in a Phase 3 Trial

Patient Race	Patients Who Developed PTDM[a]	
	Tacrolimus	Cyclosporine
Black	15/41 (37%)	3 (8%)
Hispanic	5/17 (29%)	1 (6%)
Caucasian	10/82 (12%)	1 (1%)
Other	0/11 (0%)	1 (10%)
Total	30/151 (20%)	6 (4%)

[a] Use of insulin for 30 or more consecutive days, with < 5 day gap, without a prior history of insulin-dependent diabetes mellitus or non-insulin dependent diabetes mellitus.

Liver Transplant
Insulin-dependent PTDM was reported in 18% and 11% of tacrolimus-treated liver transplant patients and was reversible in 45% and 31% of these patients at 1 year post-transplant, in the U.S. and European randomized trials, respectively (**Table 12**). Hyperglycemia was associated with

the use of tacrolimus in 47% and 33% of liver transplant recipients in the U.S. and European randomized trials, respectively, and may require treatment [see **ADVERSE REACTIONS (6.1)**].
[See table 12 above]
Heart Transplant
Insulin-dependent PTDM was reported in 13% and 22% of tacrolimus-treated heart transplant patients receiving mycophenolate mofetil (MMF) or azathioprine (AZA) and was reversible in 30% and 17% of these patients at one year post-transplant, in the U.S. and European randomized trials, respectively (Table 13). Hyperglycemia defined as two fasting plasma glucose levels ≥126 mg/dL was reported with the use of tacrolimus plus MMF or AZA in 32% and 35% of heart transplant recipients in the U.S. and European randomized trials, respectively, and may require treatment [see **ADVERSE REACTIONS (6.1)**].
[See table 13 at top of next page]
Less Frequently Reported Adverse Reactions (>3% and <15%)
The following adverse reactions were reported in either liver, kidney, and/or heart transplant recipients who were treated with tacrolimus in clinical trials.
Nervous System [see **WARNINGS AND PRECAUTIONS (5.8)**]
Abnormal dreams, agitation, amnesia, anxiety, confusion, convulsion, crying, depression, elevated mood, emotional lability, encephalopathy, hemorrhagic stroke, hallucinations, hypertonia, incoordination, monoparesis, myoclonus, nerve compression, nervousness, neuralgia, neuropathy, paralysis flaccid, psychomotor skills impaired, psychosis, quadriparesis, somnolence, thinking abnormal, vertigo, writing impaired
Special Senses
Abnormal vision, amblyopia, ear pain, otitis media, tinnitus
Gastrointestinal
Cholangitis, cholestatic jaundice, duodenitis, dysphagia, esophagitis, flatulence, gastritis, gastroesophagitis, gastrointestinal hemorrhage, GGT increase, GI disorder, GI perforation, hepatitis, hepatitis granulomatous, ileus, increased appetite, jaundice, liver damage, esophagitis ulcerative, oral moniliasis, pancreatic pseudocyst, rectal disorder, stomatitis
Cardiovascular
Abnormal ECG, angina pectoris, arrhythmia, atrial fibrillation, atrial flutter, bradycardia, cardiac fibrillation, cardiopulmonary failure, cardiovascular disorder, congestive heart failure, deep thrombophlebitis, echocardiogram abnormal, electrocardiogram QRS complex abnormal, electrocardiogram ST segment abnormal, heart failure, heart rate decreased, hemorrhage, hypotension, peripheral vascular disorder, phlebitis, postural hypotension, syncope, tachycardia, thrombosis, vasodilatation
Urogenital
Acute kidney failure [see **WARNINGS AND PRECAUTIONS (5.7)**], albuminuria, BK nephropathy, bladder spasm, cystitis, dysuria, hematuria, hydronephrosis, kidney failure, kidney tubular necrosis, nocturia, pyuria, toxic nephropathy, urge incontinence, urinary frequency, urinary incontinence, urinary retention, vaginitis
Metabolic/Nutritional
Acidosis, alkaline phosphatase increased, alkalosis, ALT (SGPT) increased, AST (SGOT) increased, bicarbonate decreased, bilirubinemia, dehydration, GGT increased, gout, healing abnormal, hypercalcemia, hypercholesterolemia, hyperphosphatemia, hyperuricemia, hypervolemia, hypocalcemia, hypoglycemia, hyponatremia, hypoproteinemia, lactic dehydrogenase increase, weight gain
Endocrine
Cushing's syndrome
Hemic/Lymphatic
Coagulation disorder, ecchymosis, hematocrit increased, hemoglobin abnormal, hypochromic anemia, leukocytosis, polycythemia, prothrombin decreased, serum iron decreased
Miscellaneous
Abdomen enlarged, abscess, accidental injury, allergic reaction, cellulitis, chills, fall, feeling abnormal, flu syndrome,

Table 13. Incidence of Post-Transplant Diabetes Mellitus and Insulin Use at 1 Year in Heart Transplant Recipients

Status of PTDM[a]	US Trial		European Trial	
	Tacrolimus/MMF	Cyclosporine/MMF	Tacrolimus/AZA	Cyclosporine/AZA
Patients at risk[b]	75	83	132	138
New Onset PTDM[a]	10 (13%)	6 (7%)	29 (22%)	5 (4%)
Patients still on insulin at 1 year[c]	7 (9%)	1 (1%)	24 (18%)	4 (3%)

[a] Use of insulin for 30 or more consecutive days without a prior history of insulin-dependent diabetes mellitus or non-insulin dependent diabetes mellitus.
[b] Patients without pre-transplant history of diabetes mellitus.
[c] 7 to 12 months for the U.S. trial.

generalized edema, hernia, mobility decreased, peritonitis, photosensitivity reaction, sepsis, temperature intolerance, ulcer

Musculoskeletal
Arthralgia, cramps, generalized spasm, joint disorder, leg cramps, myalgia, myasthenia, osteoporosis

Respiratory
Asthma, emphysema, hiccups, lung disorder, lung function decreased, pharyngitis, pneumonia, pneumothorax, pulmonary edema, respiratory disorder, rhinitis, sinusitis, voice alteration

Skin
Acne, alopecia, exfoliative dermatitis, fungal dermatitis, herpes simplex, herpes zoster, hirsutism, neoplasm skin benign, skin discoloration, skin disorder, skin ulcer, sweating

6.2 Postmarketing Adverse Reactions
The following adverse reactions have been reported from worldwide marketing experience with tacrolimus. Because these reactions are reported voluntarily from a population of uncertain size it is not always possible to reliably estimate their frequency or establish a causal relationship to drug exposure. Decisions to include these reactions in labeling are typically based on one or more of the following factors: (1) seriousness of the reaction, (2) frequency of the reporting, or (3) strength of causal connection to the drug. Other reactions include:

Cardiovascular
Atrial fibrillation, atrial flutter, cardiac arrhythmia, cardiac arrest, electrocardiogram T wave abnormal, flushing, myocardial infarction, myocardial ischaemia, pericardial effusion, QT prolongation, Torsade de Pointes, venous thrombosis deep limb, ventricular extrasystoles, ventricular fibrillation, myocardial hypertrophy [see **WARNINGS AND PRECAUTIONS (5.15)**].

Gastrointestinal
Bile duct stenosis, colitis, enterocolitis, gastroenteritis, gastroesophageal reflux disease, hepatic cytolysis, hepatic necrosis, hepatotoxicity, impaired gastric emptying, liver fatty, mouth ulceration, pancreatitis haemorrhagic, pancreatitis necrotizing, stomach ulcer, venoocclusive liver disease

Hemic/Lymphatic
Agranulocytosis, disseminated intravascular coagulation, hemolytic anemia, neutropenia, pancytopenia, thrombocytopenic purpura, thrombotic thrombocytopenic purpura, pure red cell aplasia [see **WARNINGS AND PRECAUTIONS (5.17)**]

Infections
Cases of progressive multifocal leukoencephalopathy (PML), sometimes fatal; polyoma virus-associated nephropathy, (PVAN) including graft loss [see **WARNINGS AND PRECAUTIONS (5.4)**]

Metabolic/Nutritional
Glycosuria, increased amylase including pancreatitis, weight decreased

Miscellaneous
Feeling hot and cold, feeling jittery, hot flushes, multi-organ failure, primary graft dysfunction

Nervous System
Carpal tunnel syndrome, cerebral infarction, hemiparesis, leukoencephalopathy, mental disorder, mutism, posterior reversible encephalopathy syndrome (PRES) [see **WARNINGS AND PRECAUTIONS (5.8)**], progressive multifocal leukoencephalopathy (PML) [see **WARNINGS AND PRECAUTIONS (5.4)**], quadriplegia, speech disorder, syncope

Respiratory
Acute respiratory distress syndrome, interstitial lung disease, lung infiltration, respiratory distress, respiratory failure

Skin
Stevens-Johnson syndrome, toxic epidermal necrolysis

Special Senses
Blindness, blindness cortical, hearing loss including deafness, photophobia

Urogenital
Acute renal failure, cystitis haemorrhagic, hemolytic-uremic syndrome, micturition disorder

7 DRUG INTERACTIONS
Since tacrolimus is metabolized mainly by CYP3A enzymes, drugs or substances known to inhibit these enzymes may increase tacrolimus whole blood concentrations. Drugs known to induce CYP3A enzymes may decrease tacrolimus whole blood concentrations [see **WARNINGS AND PRECAUTIONS (5.13)** and **CLINICAL PHARMACOLOGY (12.3)**]. Dose adjustments may be needed along with frequent monitoring of tacrolimus whole blood trough concentrations when Hecoria is administered with CYP3A inhibitors or inducers. In addition, patients should be monitored for adverse reactions including changes in renal function and QT prolongation [see **WARNINGS AND PRECAUTIONS (5.7)** and **(5.14)**].

7.1 Mycophenolic Acid Products
With a given dose of mycophenolic acid (MPA) products, exposure to MPA is higher with tacrolimus co-administration than with cyclosporine co-administration because cyclosporine interrupts the enterohepatic recirculation of MPA while tacrolimus does not. Clinicians should be aware that there is also a potential for increased MPA exposure after crossover from cyclosporine to Hecoria (tacrolimus) capsules in patients concomitantly receiving MPA-containing products.

7.2 Grapefruit Juice
Grapefruit juice inhibits CYP3A-enzymes resulting in increased tacrolimus whole blood trough concentrations, and patients should avoid eating grapefruit or drinking grapefruit juice with tacrolimus [see **DOSAGE AND ADMINISTRATION (2.5)**].

7.3 Protease Inhibitors
Most protease inhibitors inhibit CYP3A enzymes and may increase tacrolimus whole blood concentrations. It is recommended to avoid concomitant use of tacrolimus with nelfinavir unless the benefits outweigh the risks [see **CLINICAL PHARMACOLOGY (12.3)**]. Whole blood concentrations of tacrolimus are markedly increased when coadministered with telaprevir or with boceprevir [see **CLINICAL PHARMACOLOGY (12.3)**]. Monitoring of tacrolimus whole blood concentrations and tacrolimus-associated adverse reactions, and appropriate adjustments in the dosing regimen of tacrolimus are recommended when tacrolimus and protease inhibitors (e.g., ritonavir, telaprevir, boceprevir) are used concomitantly.

7.4 Antifungal Agents
Frequent monitoring of whole blood concentrations and appropriate dosage adjustments of tacrolimus are recommended when concomitant use of the following antifungal drugs with tacrolimus is initiated or discontinued [see **CLINICAL PHARMACOLOGY (12.3)**].
Azoles: Voriconazole, posaconazole, itraconazole, ketoconazole, fluconazole and clotrimazole inhibit CYP3A metabolism of tacrolimus and increase tacrolimus whole blood concentrations. When initiating therapy with voriconazole or posaconazole in patients already receiving tacrolimus, it is recommended that the tacrolimus dose be initially reduced to one-third of the original dose and the subsequent tacrolimus doses be adjusted based on the tacrolimus whole blood concentrations.
Caspofungin is an inducer of CYP3A and decreases whole blood concentrations of tacrolimus.

7.5 Calcium Channel Blockers
Verapamil, diltiazem, nifedipine, and nicardipine inhibit CYP3A metabolism of tacrolimus and may increase tacrolimus whole blood concentrations. Monitoring of whole blood concentrations and appropriate dosage adjustments of tacrolimus are recommended when these calcium channel blocking drugs and tacrolimus are used concomitantly.

7.6 Antibacterials
Erythromycin, clarithromycin, troleandomycin and chloramphenicol inhibit CYP3A metabolism of tacrolimus and

may increase tacrolimus whole blood concentrations. Monitoring of blood concentrations and appropriate dosage adjustments of tacrolimus are recommended when these drugs and tacrolimus are used concomitantly.

7.7 Antimycobacterials
Rifampin [see **CLINICAL PHARMACOLOGY (12.3)**] and rifabutin are inducers of CYP3A enzymes and may decrease tacrolimus whole blood concentrations. Monitoring of whole blood concentrations and appropriate dosage adjustments of tacrolimus are recommended when these antimycobacterial drugs and tacrolimus are used concomitantly.

7.8 Anticonvulsants
Phenytoin, carbamazepine and phenobarbital induce CYP3A enzymes and may decrease tacrolimus whole blood concentrations. Monitoring of whole blood concentrations and appropriate dosage adjustments of tacrolimus are recommended when these drugs and tacrolimus are used concomitantly.
Concomitant administration of phenytoin with tacrolimus may also increase phenytoin plasma concentrations. Thus, frequent monitoring of phenytoin plasma concentrations and adjusting the phenytoin dose as needed are recommended when tacrolimus and phenytoin are administered concomitantly.

7.9 St. John's Wort (*Hypericum perforatum*)
St. John's Wort induces CYP3A enzymes and may decrease tacrolimus whole blood concentrations. Monitoring of whole blood concentrations and appropriate dosage adjustments of tacrolimus are recommended when St. John's Wort and tacrolimus are coadministered.

7.10 Gastric Acid Suppressors/Neutralizers
Lansoprazole and omeprazole, as CYP2C19 and CYP3A4 substrates, may potentially inhibit the CYP3A4 metabolism of tacrolimus and thereby substantially increase tacrolimus whole blood concentrations, especially in transplant patients who are intermediate or poor CYP2C19 metabolizers, as compared to those patients who are efficient CYP2C19 metabolizers.
Cimetidine may also inhibit the CYP3A4 metabolism of tacrolimus and thereby substantially increase tacrolimus whole blood concentrations.
Coadministration with magnesium and aluminum hydroxide antacids increase tacrolimus whole blood concentrations [see **CLINICAL PHARMACOLOGY (12.3)**]. Monitoring of whole blood concentrations and appropriate dosage adjustments of tacrolimus are recommended when these drugs and tacrolimus are used concomitantly.

7.11 Others
Bromocriptine, nefazodone, metoclopramide, danazol, ethinyl estradiol, amiodarone and methylprednisolone may inhibit CYP3A metabolism of tacrolimus and increase tacrolimus whole blood concentrations. Monitoring of blood concentrations and appropriate dosage adjustments of tacrolimus are recommended when these drugs and tacrolimus are coadministered.

8 USE IN SPECIFIC POPULATIONS

8.1 Pregnancy
Pregnancy Category C - There are no adequate and well-controlled studies in pregnant women. Tacrolimus is transferred across the placenta. The use of tacrolimus during pregnancy in humans has been associated with neonatal hyperkalemia and renal dysfunction. Tacrolimus given orally to pregnant rabbits at 0.5 to 4.3 times the clinical dose and pregnant rats at 0.8 to 6.9 times the clinical dose was associated with an increased incidence of fetal death *in utero*, fetal malformations (cardiovascular, skeletal, omphalocele, and gallbladder agenesis) and maternal toxicity. Hecoria (tacrolimus) capsules should be used during pregnancy only if the potential benefit to the mother justifies the potential risk to the fetus.
In pregnant rabbits, tacrolimus at oral doses of 0.32 and 1 mg/kg, 0.5 to 4.3 times the clinical dose range (0.075 to 0.2 mg/kg) based on body surface area, was associated with maternal toxicity as well as an increased incidence of abortions. At the 1 mg/kg dose, fetal rabbits showed an increased incidence of malformations (ventricular hypoplasia, interventricular septal defect, bulbous aortic arch, stenosis of ductus arteriosis, interrupted ossification of vertebral arch, vertebral and rib malformations, omphalocele, and gallbladder agenesis) and developmental variations. In pregnant rats, tacrolimus at oral doses of 3.2 mg/kg, 2.6 to 6.9 times the clinical dose range was associated with maternal toxicity, an increase in late resorptions, decreased numbers of live births, and decreased pup weight and viability. Tacrolimus, given orally to pregnant rats after organogenesis and during lactation at 1 and 3.2 mg/kg, 0.8 to 6.9 times the recommended clinical dose range was associated with reduced pup weights and pup viability (3.2 mg/kg only); among the high dose pups that died early, an increased incidence of kidney hydronephrosis was observed.

8.3 Nursing Mothers
Tacrolimus is excreted in human milk. As the effect of chronic exposure to tacrolimus in healthy infants is not established, patients maintained on Hecoria (tacrolimus) capsules should discontinue nursing taking into consideration importance of drug to the mother.

8.4 Pediatric Use

The safety and efficacy of Hecoria (tacrolimus) capsules in pediatric kidney and heart transplant patients have not been established. Successful liver transplants have been performed in pediatric patients (ages up to 16 years) using tacrolimus. Two randomized active-controlled trials of tacrolimus in primary liver transplantation included 56 pediatric patients. Thirty-one patients were randomized to tacrolimus-based and 25 to cyclosporine-based therapies. Additionally, a minimum of 122 pediatric patients were studied in an uncontrolled trial of tacrolimus in living related donor liver transplantation. Pediatric patients generally required higher doses of tacrolimus to maintain blood trough concentrations of tacrolimus similar to adult patients [see **DOSAGE AND ADMINISTRATION (2.2)**].

8.5 Geriatric Use

Clinical trials of tacrolimus did not include sufficient numbers of subjects aged 65 and over to determine whether they respond differently from younger subjects. Other reported clinical experience has not identified differences in responses between the elderly and younger patients. In general, dose selection for an elderly patient should be cautious, usually starting at the low end of the dosing range, reflecting the greater frequency of decreased hepatic, renal, or cardiac function, and of concomitant disease or other drug therapy.

8.6 Use in Renal Impairment

The pharmacokinetics of tacrolimus in patients with renal impairment was similar to that in healthy volunteers with normal renal function. However, consideration should be given to dosing Hecoria (tacrolimus) capsules at the lower end of the therapeutic dosing range in patients who have received a liver or heart transplant and have pre-existing renal impairment. Further reductions in dose below the targeted range may be required [see **DOSAGE AND ADMINISTRATION (2.3)** and **CLINICAL PHARMACOLOGY (12.3)**].

8.7 Use in Hepatic Impairment

The mean clearance of tacrolimus was substantially lower in patients with severe hepatic impairment (mean Child-Pugh score: >10) compared to healthy volunteers with normal hepatic function. Close monitoring of tacrolimus trough concentrations is warranted in patients with hepatic impairment [see **CLINICAL PHARMACOLOGY (12.3)**].

The use of Hecoria (tacrolimus) capsules in liver transplant recipients experiencing post-transplant hepatic impairment may be associated with increased risk of developing renal insufficiency related to high whole-blood trough concentrations of tacrolimus. These patients should be monitored closely and dosage adjustments should be considered. Some evidence suggests that lower doses should be used in these patients [see **DOSAGE AND ADMINISTRATION (2.3)** and **CLINICAL PHARMACOLOGY (12.3)**].

10 OVERDOSAGE

Limited overdosage experience is available. Acute overdosages of up to 30 times the intended dose have been reported. Almost all cases have been asymptomatic and all patients recovered with no sequelae. Acute overdosage was sometimes followed by adverse reactions consistent with those listed in **ADVERSE REACTIONS (6)** (including tremors, abnormal renal function, hypertension, and peripheral edema); in one case of acute overdosage, transient urticaria and lethargy were observed. Based on the poor aqueous solubility and extensive erythrocyte and plasma protein binding, it is anticipated that tacrolimus is not dialyzable to any significant extent; there is no experience with charcoal hemoperfusion. The oral use of activated charcoal has been reported in treating acute overdoses, but experience has not been sufficient to warrant recommending its use. General supportive measures and treatment of specific symptoms should be followed in all cases of overdosage.

In acute oral and IV toxicity studies, mortalities were seen at or above the following doses: in adult rats, 52 times the recommended human oral dose; in immature rats, 16 times the recommended oral dose; and in adult rats, 16 times the recommended human IV dose (all based on body surface area corrections).

11 DESCRIPTION

Hecoria is available for oral administration as capsules (tacrolimus capsules) containing the equivalent of 0.5 mg, 1 mg or 5 mg of anhydrous tacrolimus. In addition, each capsule contains the following inactive ingredients: croscarmellose sodium, hypromellose, lactose monohydrate, and magnesium stearate.

The Hecoria (tacrolimus) capsule shell for 0.5 mg strength consists of gelatin, titanium dioxide and yellow iron oxide. The Hecoria (tacrolimus) capsule shell for 1 mg strength consists of black iron oxide, gelatin, red iron oxide, titanium dioxide, and yellow iron oxide. The Hecoria (tacrolimus) capsule shell for 5 mg strength consists of red iron oxide, gelatin, and titanium dioxide. Hecoria (tacrolimus capsules, USP) 0.5 mg, 1 mg and 5 mg are printed with edible black ink. The black ink is comprised of ammonia, black iron oxide, butyl alcohol, potassium hydroxide, propylene glycol, and shellac.

Table 14. Pharmacokinetics Parameters (mean±S.D.) of Tacrolimus in Healthy Volunteers and Patients

Population	N	Route (Dose)	C_{max} (ng/mL)	T_{max} (hr)	AUC (ng·hr/mL)	$t_{1/2}$ (hr)	Cl (L/hr/kg)	V (L/kg)
Healthy Volunteers	8	IV (0.025 mg/kg/4hr)	a	a	598[b] ± 125	34.2 ± 7.7	0.040 ± 0.009	1.91 ± 0.31
	16	PO (5 mg)	29.7 ± 7.2	1.6 ± 0.7	243[c] ± 73	34.8 ± 11.4	0.041[d] ± 0.008	1.94[d] ± 0.53
Kidney Transplant Patients	26	IV (0.02 mg/kg/12 hr)	a	a	294[e] ± 262	18.8 ± 16.7	0.083 ± 0.050	1.41 ± 0.66
		PO (0.2 mg/kg/day)	19.2 ± 10.3	3	203[e] ± 42	f	f	f
		PO (0.3 mg/kg/day)	24.2 ± 15.8	1.5	288[e] ± 93	f	f	f
Liver Transplant Patients	17	IV (0.05 mg/kg/12 hr)	a	a	3300[e] ± 2130	11.7 ± 3.9	0.053 ± 0.017	0.85 ± 0.30
		PO (0.3 mg/kg/day)	68.5 ± 30	2.3 ± 1.5	519[e] ± 179	f	f	f
Heart Transplant Patients	11	IV (0.01 mg/kg/day as a continuous infusion)	a	a	954[g] ± 334	23.6 ± 9.22	0.051 ± 0.015	f
	11	PO (0.075 mg/kg/day)[h]	14.7 ± 7.79	2.1 [0.5-6][i]	82.7[j] ± 63.2	a	f	f
	14	PO (0.15 mg/kg/day)[h]	24.5 ± 13.7	1.5 [0.4-4][i]	142[j] ± 116	a	f	f

[a] not applicable
[b] AUC_{0-120}
[c] AUC_{0-72}
[d] Corrected for individual bioavailability
[e] AUC_{0-inf}
[f] not available
[g] AUC_{0-t}
[h] Determined after the first dose
[i] Median [range]
[j] AUC_{0-12}

Tacrolimus, previously known as FK506, is the active ingredient in Hecoria (tacrolimus capsules, USP). Tacrolimus is a macrolide immunosuppressant produced by *Streptomyces tsukubaensis*. Chemically, tacrolimus is designated as [3S-[3R*[E(1S*,3S*,4S*)],4S*,5R*,8S*,9E,12R*,14R*, 15S*, 16R*,18S*,19S*,26aR*]] 5,6,8,11,12,13,14,15,16,17, 18,19, 24,25,26,26a-hexadecahydro-5,19-dihydroxy-3-[2-(4-hydroxy-3-methoxycyclohexyl)-1-methylethenyl]-14,16-dimethoxy-4,10,12,18-tetramethyl-8-(2-propenyl)-15,19-epoxy-3H-pyrido[2,1-c][1,4] oxaazacyclotricosine-1,7,20, 21(4H,23H)-tetrone, monohydrate.

The chemical structure of tacrolimus is:

Tacrolimus has a molecular formula of $C_{44}H_{69}NO_{12} \cdot H_2O$ and a formula weight of 822.03. Tacrolimus appears as white crystals or crystalline powder. It is practically insoluble in water, freely soluble in ethanol, and very soluble in methanol and chloroform.

USP Dissolution test 2 and Organic Impurities procedure 2 used.

12 CLINICAL PHARMACOLOGY

12.1 Mechanism of Action

Tacrolimus inhibits T-lymphocyte activation, although the exact mechanism of action is not known. Experimental evidence suggests that tacrolimus binds to an intracellular protein, FKBP-12. A complex of tacrolimus-FKBP-12, calcium, calmodulin, and calcineurin is then formed and the phosphatase activity of calcineurin inhibited. This effect may prevent the dephosphorylation and translocation of nuclear factor of activated T-cells (NF-AT), a nuclear component thought to initiate gene transcription for the formation of lymphokines (such as interleukin-2, gamma interferon). The net result is the inhibition of T-lymphocyte activation (i.e., immunosuppression).

Tacrolimus prolongs the survival of the host and transplanted graft in animal transplant models of liver, kidney, heart, bone marrow, small bowel and pancreas, lung and trachea, skin, cornea, and limb.

In animals, tacrolimus has been demonstrated to suppress some humoral immunity and, to a greater extent, cell-mediated reactions such as allograft rejection, delayed type hypersensitivity, collagen-induced arthritis, experimental allergic encephalomyelitis, and graft versus host disease.

12.3 Pharmacokinetics

Tacrolimus activity is primarily due to the parent drug. The pharmacokinetic parameters (mean±S.D.) of tacrolimus have been determined following intravenous (IV) and/or oral (PO) administration in healthy volunteers, and in kidney transplant, liver transplant, and heart transplant patients (**Table 14**).

[See table 14 above]

Due to intersubject variability in tacrolimus pharmacokinetics, individualization of dosing regimen is necessary for optimal therapy [see **DOSAGE AND ADMINISTRATION (2.6)**]. Pharmacokinetic data indicate that whole blood concentrations rather than plasma concentrations serve as the more appropriate sampling compartment to describe tacrolimus pharmacokinetics.

Absorption

Absorption of tacrolimus from the gastrointestinal tract after oral administration is incomplete and variable. The absolute bioavailability of tacrolimus was 17±10% in adult kidney transplant patients (N=26), 22±6% in adult liver transplant patients (N=17), 23±9% in adult heart transplant patients (N=11) and 18±5% in healthy volunteers (N=16).

A single dose trial conducted in 32 healthy volunteers established the bioequivalence of the 1 mg and 5 mg capsules. Another single dose trial in 32 healthy volunteers established the bioequivalence of the 0.5 mg and 1 mg capsules. Tacrolimus maximum blood concentrations (C_{max}) and area

Table 15. Pharmacokinetic In Renal and Hepatic Impaired Patients

Population (No. of Patients)	Dose	AUC_{0-t} (ng·hr/mL)	$t_{1/2}$ (hr)	V (L/kg)	CI (L/hr/kg)
Renal Impairment (n=12)	0.02 mg/kg/4hr IV	393±123 (t=60 hr)	26.3±9.2	1.07 ±0.20	0.038 ±0.014
Mild Hepatic Impairment (n=6)	0.02 mg/kg/4hr IV	367±107 (t=72 hr)	60.6±43.8 Range: 27.8 to 141	3.1±1.6	0.042 ±0.02
	7.7 mg PO	488±320 (t=72 hr)	66.1±44.8 Range: 29.5 to 138	3.7±4.7[a]	0.034 ±0.019[a]
Severe Hepatic Impairment (n=6, IV)	0.02 mg/kg/4hr IV (n=2) 0.01 mg/kg/8hr IV (n=4)	762±204 (t=120 hr) 289±117 (t=144 hr)	198±158 Range: 81 to 436	3.9±1	0.017 ±0.013
(n=5, PO)[b]	8 mg PO (n=1) 5 mg PO (n=4) 4 mg PO (n=1)	658 (t=120 hr) 533±156 (t=144 hr)	119±35 Range: 85 to 178	3.1±3.4[a]	0.016 ±0.011[a]

[a] corrected for bioavailability
[b] 1 patient did not receive the PO dose

under the curve (AUC) appeared to increase in a dose-proportional fashion in 18 fasted healthy volunteers receiving a single oral dose of 3, 7, and 10 mg.

In 18 kidney transplant patients, tacrolimus trough concentrations from 3 to 30 ng/mL measured at 10 to 12 hours post-dose (C_{min}) correlated well with the AUC (correlation coefficient 0.93). In 24 liver transplant patients over a concentration range of 10 to 60 ng/mL, the correlation coefficient was 0.94. In 25 heart transplant patients over a concentration range of 2 to 24 ng/mL, the correlation coefficient was 0.89 after an oral dose of 0.075 or 0.15 mg/kg/day at steady-state.

Food Effects
The rate and extent of tacrolimus absorption were greatest under fasted conditions. The presence and composition of food decreased both the rate and extent of tacrolimus absorption when administered to 15 healthy volunteers.

The effect was most pronounced with a high-fat meal (848 kcal, 46% fat): mean AUC and C_{max} were decreased 37% and 77%, respectively; T_{max} was lengthened 5-fold. A high-carbohydrate meal (668 kcal, 85% carbohydrate) decreased mean AUC and mean C_{max} by 28% and 65%, respectively.

In healthy volunteers (N=16), the time of the meal also affected tacrolimus bioavailability. When given immediately following the meal, mean C_{max} was reduced 71%, and mean AUC was reduced 39%, relative to the fasted condition. When administered 1.5 hours following the meal, mean C_{max} was reduced 63%, and mean AUC was reduced 39%, relative to the fasted condition.

In 11 liver transplant patients, tacrolimus administered 15 minutes after a high fat (400 kcal, 34% fat) breakfast, resulted in decreased AUC (27±18%) and C_{max} (50±19%), as compared to a fasted state.

Hecoria (tacrolimus) capsules should be taken consistently every day either with or without food because the presence and composition of food decreases the bioavailability of Hecoria [see **DOSAGE AND ADMINISTRATION (2.5)**].

Distribution
The plasma protein binding of tacrolimus is approximately 99% and is independent of concentration over a range of 5 to 50 ng/mL. Tacrolimus is bound mainly to albumin and alpha-1-acid glycoprotein, and has a high level of association with erythrocytes. The distribution of tacrolimus between whole blood and plasma depends on several factors, such as hematocrit, temperature at the time of plasma separation, drug concentration, and plasma protein concentration. In a U.S. trial, the ratio of whole blood concentration to plasma concentration averaged 35 (range 12 to 67).

Metabolism
Tacrolimus is extensively metabolized by the mixed-function oxidase system, primarily the cytochrome P-450 system (CYP3A). A metabolic pathway leading to the formation of 8 possible metabolites has been proposed. Demethylation and hydroxylation were identified as the primary mechanisms of biotransformation *in vitro*. The major metabolite identified in incubations with human liver microsomes is 13-demethyl tacrolimus. In *in vitro* studies, a 31-demethyl metabolite has been reported to have the same activity as tacrolimus.

Excretion
The mean clearance following IV administration of tacrolimus is 0.040, 0.083, 0.053, and 0.051 L/hr/kg in healthy volunteers, adult kidney transplant patients, adult liver transplant patients, and adult heart transplant patients, respectively. In man, less than 1% of the dose administered is excreted unchanged in urine.

In a mass balance study of IV administered radiolabeled tacrolimus to 6 healthy volunteers, the mean recovery of radiolabel was 77.8±12.7%. Fecal elimination accounted for 92.4±1% and the elimination half-life based on radioactivity was 48.1±15.9 hours whereas it was 43.5±11.6 hours based on tacrolimus concentrations. The mean clearance of radiolabel was 0.029±0.015 L/hr/kg and clearance of tacrolimus was 0.029±0.009 L/hr/kg. When administered PO, the mean recovery of the radiolabel was 94.9±30.7%. Fecal elimination accounted for 92.6±30.7%, urinary elimination accounted for 2.3±1.1% and the elimination half-life based on radioactivity was 31.9±10.5 hours whereas it was 48.4±12.3 hours based on tacrolimus concentrations. The mean clearance of radiolabel was 0.226±0.116 L/hr/kg and clearance of tacrolimus 0.172±0.088 L/hr/kg.

Specific Populations
Pediatric
Pharmacokinetics of tacrolimus have been studied in liver transplantation patients, 0.7 to 13.2 years of age. Following oral administration to 9 patients, mean AUC and C_{max} were 337±167 ng·hr/mL and 48.4±27.9 ng/mL, respectively. The absolute bioavailability was 31±24%.

Whole blood trough concentrations from 31 patients less than 12 years old showed that pediatric patients needed higher doses than adults to achieve similar tacrolimus trough concentrations [see **DOSAGE AND ADMINISTRATION (2.2)**].

Pharmacokinetics of tacrolimus have also been studied in kidney transplantation patients, 8.2±2.4 years of age. Following oral administration, mean AUC and C_{max} were 181±65 (range 81 to 300) ng·hr/mL and 30±11 (range 14 to 49) ng/mL, respectively. The absolute bioavailability was 19±14 (range 5.2 to 56) %.

Renal and Hepatic Impairment
The mean pharmacokinetic parameters for tacrolimus following single administrations to patients with renal and hepatic impairment are given in **Table 15**.
[See table 15 above]

Renal Impairment: Tacrolimus pharmacokinetics following a single IV administration were determined in 12 patients (7 not on dialysis and 5 on dialysis, serum creatinine of 3.9±1.6 and 12±2.4 mg/dL, respectively) prior to their kidney transplant. The pharmacokinetic parameters obtained were similar for both groups. The mean clearance of tacrolimus in patients with renal dysfunction was similar to that in normal volunteers (**Table 15**) [see **DOSAGE AND ADMINISTRATION (2.3)** and **USE IN SPECIFIC POPULATIONS (8.6)**].

Hepatic Impairment: Tacrolimus pharmacokinetics have been determined in six patients with mild hepatic dysfunction (mean Pugh score: 6.2) following oral administrations. The mean clearance of tacrolimus in patients with mild hepatic dysfunction was not substantially different from that in normal volunteers (see previous table). Tacrolimus pharmacokinetics were studied in 6 patients with severe hepatic dysfunction (mean Pugh score: >10). The mean clearance was substantially lower in patients with severe hepatic dysfunction, irrespective of the route of administration [see **DOSAGE AND ADMINISTRATION (2.4)** and **USE IN SPECIFIC POPULATIONS (8.7)**].

Race
The pharmacokinetics of tacrolimus have been studied following single IV and oral administration of tacrolimus to 10 African-American, 12 Latino-American, and 12 Caucasian healthy volunteers. There were no significant pharmacokinetic differences among the three ethnic groups following a 4-hour IV infusion of 0.015 mg/kg. However, after single oral administration of 5 mg, mean (±SD) tacrolimus C_{max} in African-Americans (23.6±12.1 ng/mL) was significantly lower than in Caucasians (40.2±12.6 ng/mL) and the Latino-Americans (36.2±15.8 ng/mL) (p<0.01). Mean AUC_{0-inf} tended to be lower in African-Americans (203±115 ng·hr/mL) than Caucasians (344±186 ng·hr/mL) and Latino-Americans (274±150 ng·hr/mL). The mean (±SD) absolute oral bioavailability (F) in African-Americans (12±4.5%) and Latino-Americans (14±7.4%) was significantly lower than in Caucasians (19±5.8%, p=0.011). There was no significant difference in mean terminal $T_{1/2}$ among the three ethnic groups (range from approximately 25 to 30 hours). A retrospective comparison of African-American and Caucasian kidney transplant patients indicated that African-American patients required higher tacrolimus doses to attain similar trough concentrations [see **DOSAGE AND ADMINISTRATION (2.1)**].

Gender
A formal trial to evaluate the effect of gender on tacrolimus pharmacokinetics has not been conducted, however, there was no difference in dosing by gender in the kidney transplant trial. A retrospective comparison of pharmacokinetics in healthy volunteers, and in kidney, liver, and heart transplant patients indicated no gender-based differences.

Drug Interactions
Frequent monitoring of whole blood concentrations and appropriate dosage adjustments of tacrolimus are recommended when concomitant use of the following drugs with tacrolimus is initiated or discontinued [see **DRUG INTERACTIONS (7)**].

Telaprevir: In a single dose study in 9 healthy volunteers, coadministration of tacrolimus (0.5 mg single dose) with telaprevir (750 mg three times daily for 13 days) increased the tacrolimus dose-normalized Cmax by 9.3-fold and AUC by 70-fold compared to tacrolimus alone [see **DRUG INTERACTIONS (7.3)**].

Boceprevir: In a single dose study in 12 subjects, coadministration of tacrolimus (0.5 mg single dose) with boceprevir (800 mg three times daily for 11 days) increased tacrolimus C_{max} by 9.9-fold and AUC by 17-fold compared to tacrolimus alone [see **DRUG INTERACTIONS (7.3)**].

Nelfinavir: Based on a clinical study of 5 liver transplant recipients, coadministration of tacrolimus with nelfinavir increased blood concentrations of tacrolimus significantly and, as a result, a reduction in the tacrolimus dose by an average of 16-fold was needed to maintain mean trough tacrolimus blood concentrations of 9.7 ng/mL. It is recommended to avoid concomitant use of Hecoria (tacrolimus) capsules and nelfinavir unless the benefits outweigh the risks [see **DRUG INTERACTIONS (7.3)**].

Rifampin: In a study of 6 normal volunteers, a significant decrease in tacrolimus oral bioavailability (14±6% vs. 7±3%) was observed with concomitant rifampin administration (600 mg). In addition, there was a significant increase in tacrolimus clearance (0.036±0.008 L/hr/kg vs. 0.053±0.010 L/hr/kg) with concomitant rifampin administration [see **DRUG INTERACTIONS (7.7)**].

Magnesium-aluminum-hydroxide: In a single-dose crossover study in healthy volunteers, coadministration of tacrolimus and magnesium-aluminum-hydroxide resulted in a 21% increase in the mean tacrolimus AUC and a 10% decrease in the mean tacrolimus C_{max} relative to tacrolimus administration alone [see **DRUG INTERACTIONS (7.10)**].

Ketoconazole: In a study of 6 normal volunteers, a significant increase in tacrolimus oral bioavailability (14±5% vs. 30±8%) was observed with concomitant ketoconazole administration (200 mg). The apparent oral clearance of tacrolimus during ketoconazole administration was significantly decreased compared to tacrolimus alone (0.430±0.129 L/hr/kg vs. 0.148±0.043 L/hr/kg). Overall, IV clearance of tacrolimus was not significantly changed by ketoconazole coadministration, although it was highly variable between patients [see **DRUG INTERACTIONS (7.4)**].

Voriconazole (see complete prescribing information for Voriconazole): Repeat oral dose administration of voriconazole (400 mg every 12 hours for one day, then 200 mg every 12 hours for 6 days) increased tacrolimus (0.1 mg/kg single dose) C_{max} and $AUC\tau$ in healthy subjects by an average of 2-fold (90% CI: 1.9, 2.5) and 3-fold (90% CI: 2.7, 3.8), respectively [see **DRUG INTERACTIONS (7.4)**].

Posaconazole (see complete prescribing information for Noxafil®): Repeat oral administration of posaconazole (400 mg twice daily for 7 days) increased tacrolimus (0.05 mg/kg single dose) C_{max} and AUC in healthy volunteers by an average of 2-fold (90% CI: 2.01, 2.42) and 4.5-fold (90% CI: 4.03, 5.19), respectively [see **DRUG INTERACTIONS (7.4)**].

Caspofungin (see complete prescribing information for CANCIDAS®): Caspofungin reduced the blood AUC_{0-12} of tacrolimus by approximately 20%, peak blood concentration (C_{max}) by 16%, and 12-hour blood concentration (C_{12hr}) by 26% in healthy adult subjects when tacrolimus (2 doses of 0.1 mg/kg 12 hours apart) was administered on the 10th day of CANCIDAS® 70 mg daily, as compared to results from a control period in which tacrolimus was administered alone [see **DRUG INTERACTIONS (7.4)**].

13 NONCLINICAL TOXICOLOGY

13.1 Carcinogenesis, Mutagenesis, Impairment of Fertility

Carcinogenicity studies were conducted in male and female rats and mice. In the 80-week mouse oral study and in the 104-week rat oral study, no relationship of tumor incidence to tacrolimus dosage was found. The highest dose used in the mouse was 3 mg/kg/day (0.9 to 2.2 times the AUC at clinical doses of 0.075 to 0.2 mg/kg/day) and in the rat was 5 mg/kg/day (0.265 to 0.65 times the AUC at clinical doses of 0.075 to 0.2 mg/kg/day) [see **BOXED WARNING** and **WARNINGS AND PRECAUTIONS (5.2)**].

A 104-week dermal carcinogenicity study was performed in mice with tacrolimus ointment (0.03% - 3%), equivalent to tacrolimus doses of 1.1-118 mg/kg/day or 3.3-354 mg/m²/day. In the study, the incidence of skin tumors was minimal and the topical application of tacrolimus was not associated with skin tumor formation under ambient room lighting. However, a statistically significant elevation in the incidence of pleomorphic lymphoma in high dose male (25/50) and female animals (27/50) and in the incidence of undifferentiated lymphoma in high dose female animals (13/50) was noted in the mouse dermal carcinogenicity study. Lymphomas were noted in the mouse dermal carcinogenicity study at a daily dose of 3.5 mg/kg (0.1% tacrolimus ointment). No drug-related tumors were noted in the mouse dermal carcinogenicity study at a daily dose of 1.1 mg/kg (0.03% tacrolimus ointment). The relevance of topical administration of tacrolimus in the setting of systemic tacrolimus use is unknown.

The implications of these carcinogenicity studies to the human condition are limited; doses of tacrolimus were administered that likely induced immunosuppression in these animals impairing their immune system's ability to inhibit unrelated carcinogenesis.

No evidence of genotoxicity was seen in bacterial (*Salmonella* and *E. coli*) or mammalian (Chinese hamster lung-derived cells) *in vitro* assays of mutagenicity, the *in vitro* CHO/HGPRT assay of mutagenicity, or *in vivo* clastogenicity assays performed in mice; tacrolimus did not cause unscheduled DNA synthesis in rodent hepatocytes.

Tacrolimus given orally at 1 mg/kg (0.8 to 2.2 times the clinical dose range of 0.075 to 0.2 mg/kg/day based on body surface area) to male and female rats, prior to and during mating, as well as to dams during gestation and lactation, was associated with embryolethality and adverse effects on female reproduction. Effects on female reproductive function (parturition) and embryolethal effects were indicated by a higher rate of pre-implantation loss and increased numbers of undelivered and nonviable pups. When given at 3.2 mg/kg (2.6 to 6.9 times the clinical dose range based on body surface area), tacrolimus was associated with maternal and paternal toxicity as well as reproductive toxicity including marked adverse effects on estrus cycles, parturition, pup viability, and pup malformations.

14 CLINICAL STUDIES

14.1 Kidney Transplantation

Tacrolimus/azathioprine (AZA)

Tacrolimus-based immunosuppression in conjunction with azathioprine and corticosteroids following kidney transplantation was assessed in a randomized, multicenter, non-blinded, prospective trial. There were 412 kidney transplant patients enrolled at 19 clinical sites in the United States. Study therapy was initiated when renal function was stable as indicated by a serum creatinine ≤4 mg/dL (median of 4 days after transplantation, range 1 to 14 days). Patients less than 6 years of age were excluded.

There were 205 patients randomized to tacrolimus-based immunosuppression and 207 patients were randomized to cyclosporine-based immunosuppression. All patients received prophylactic induction therapy consisting of an anti-lymphocyte antibody preparation, corticosteroids and azathioprine. Overall 1-year patient and graft survival was 96.1% and 89.6%, respectively.

Data from this trial of tacrolimus in conjunction with azathioprine indicate that during the first three months of that trial, 80% of the patients maintained trough concentrations between 7 to 20 ng/mL, and then between 5 to 15 ng/mL, through 1 year.

Tacrolimus/mycophenolate mofetil (MMF)

Tacrolimus-based immunosuppression in conjunction with MMF, corticosteroids, and induction has been studied. In a randomized, open-label, multi-center trial (Study 1), 1,589 kidney transplant patients received tacrolimus (Group C, n=401), sirolimus (Group D, n=399), or one of two cyclosporine (CsA) regimens (Group A, n=390 and Group B, n=399) in combination with MMF and corticosteroids; all patients, except those in one of the two cyclosporine groups, also received induction with daclizumab. The trial was conducted outside the United States; the trial population was 93% Caucasian. In this trial, mortality at 12 months in patients receiving tacrolimus/MMF was similar (3%) compared to patients receiving cyclosporine/MMF (3% and 2%) or sirolimus/MMF (3%). Patients in the tacrolimus group exhibited higher estimated creatinine clearance rates (eCL_{cr}) using the Cockcroft-Gault formula (**Table 16**) and experienced fewer efficacy failures, defined as biopsy proven acute rejection (BPAR), graft loss, death, and/or lost to follow-up (**Table 17**) in comparison to each of the other three groups. Patients randomized to tacrolimus/MMF were more likely to develop diarrhea and diabetes after the transplantation and experienced similar rates of infections compared to patients randomized to either cyclosporine/MMF regimen [see **ADVERSE REACTIONS (6.1)**].

[See table 16 above]
[See table 17 above]

The protocol-specified target tacrolimus trough concentrations ($C_{trough,Tac}$) were 3 to 7 ng/mL; however, the observed median $C_{troughs,Tac}$ approximated 7 ng/mL throughout the 12-month trial (**Table 18**). Approximately 80% of patients maintained tacrolimus whole blood concentrations between 4 to 11 ng/mL through 1 year post-transplant.

The protocol-specified target cyclosporine trough concentrations ($C_{trough,CsA}$) for Group B were 50 to 100 ng/mL; however, the observed median $C_{trough,CsA}$ approximated 100 ng/mL throughout the 12-month trial. The protocol-specified target $C_{troughs,CsA}$ for Group A were 150 to 300 ng/mL for the first 3 months and 100 to 200 ng/mL from month 4 to month 12; the observed median $C_{troughs,CsA}$ approximated 225 ng/mL for the first 3 months and 140 ng/mL from month 4 to month 12.

While patients in all groups started MMF at 1gram twice daily, the MMF dose was reduced to less than 2 g per day in 63% of patients in the tacrolimus treatment arm by month 12 (**Table 19**); approximately 50% of these MMF dose reductions were due to adverse reactions. By comparison, the MMF dose was reduced to less than 2 g per day in 49% and 45% of patients in the two cyclosporine arms (Group A and Group B, respectively), by month 12 and approximately 40% of MMF dose reductions were due to adverse reactions.

Table 16. Estimated Creatinine Clearance at 12 Months (Study 1)

Group	eCL$_{cr}$ [mL/min] at Month 12[a]				
	N	MEAN	SD	MEDIAN	Treatment Difference with Group C (99.2% CI[b])
(A) CsA/MMF/CS	390	56.5	25.8	56.9	-8.6 (-13.7, -3.7)
(B) CsA/MMF/CS/Daclizumab	399	58.9	25.6	60.9	-6.2 (-11.2, -1.2)
(C) Tac/MMF/CS/Daclizumab	401	65.1	27.4	66.2	-
(D) Siro/MMF/CS/Daclizumab	399	56.2	27.4	57.3	-8.9 (-14.1, -3.9)
Total	1,589	59.2	26.8	60.5	

Key: CsA =Cyclosporine, CS=Corticosteroids, Tac=Tacrolimus, Siro=Sirolimus

[a] All death/graft loss (n=41, 27, 23 and 42 in Groups A, B, C and D) and patients whose last recorded creatinine values were prior to month 3 visit (n=10, 9, 7 and 9 in Groups A, B, C and D, respectively) were imputed with Glomerular Filtration Rate (GFR) of 10 mL/min; a subject's last observed creatinine value from month 3 on was used for the remainder of subjects with missing creatinine at month 12 (n=11, 12, 15 and 19 for Groups A, B, C and D, respectively). Weight was also imputed in the calculation of estimated GFR, if missing.
[b] Adjusted for multiple (6) pairwise comparisons using Bonferroni corrections.

Table 17. Incidence of BPAR, Graft Loss, Death or Loss to Follow-up at 12 Months (Study 1)

	Group A N=390	Group B N=399	Group C N=401	Group D N=399
Overall Failure	141 (36.2%)	126 (31.6%)	82 (20.4%)	185 (46.4%)
Components of efficacy failure				
BPAR	113 (29%)	106 (26.6%)	60 (15%)	152 (38.1%)
Graft loss excluding death	28 (7.2%)	20 (5%)	12 (3%)	30 (7.5%)
Mortality	13 (3.3%)	7 (1.8%)	11 (2.7%)	12 (3%)
Lost to follow-up	5 (1.3%)	7 (1.8%)	5 (1.3%)	6 (1.5%)
Treatment Difference of efficacy failure compared to Group C (99.2% CI[a])	15.8% (7.1%, 24.3%)	11.2% (2.7%, 19.5%)	-	26% (17.2%, 34.7%)

Key: Group A=CsA/MMF/CS, B=CsA/MMF/CS/Daclizumab, C=Tac/MMF/CS/Daclizumab, and D=Siro/MMF/CS/Daclizumab

[a] Adjusted for multiple (6) pairwise comparisons using Bonferroni corrections.

Table 18. Tacrolimus Whole Blood Trough Concentrations (Study 1)

Time	Median (P10-P90[a]) tacrolimus whole blood trough concentrations (ng/mL)
Day 30 (N=366)	6.9 (4.4 to 11.3)
Day 90 (N=351)	6.8 (4.1 to 10.7)
Day 180 (N=355)	6.5 (4 to 9.6)
Day 365 (N=346)	6.5 (3.8 to 10)

[a] 10 to the 90th Percentile: range of $C_{trough,Tac}$ that excludes lowest 10% and highest 10% of $C_{trough,Tac}$

Table 19. MMF Dose Over Time in Tacrolimus/MMF (Group C) (Study 1)

Time period (Days)	Time-averaged MMF dose (grams per day)[a]		
	Less than 2	2	Greater than 2
0 to 30 (N=364)	37%	60%	2%
0 to 90 (N=373)	47%	51%	2%
0 to 180 (N=377)	56%	42%	2%

0 to 365 (N=380)	63%	36%	1%

Key: Time-averaged MMF dose = (total MMF dose)/(duration of treatment)

[a] Percentage of patients for each time-averaged MMF dose range during various treatment periods. Administration of 2 g per day of time-averaged MMF dose means that MMF dose was not reduced in those patients during the treatment periods.

In a second randomized, open-label, multi-center trial (Study 2), 424 kidney transplant patients received tacrolimus (N=212) or cyclosporine (N=212) in combination with MMF 1 gram twice daily, basiliximab induction, and corticosteroids. In this trial, the rate for the combined endpoint of BPAR, graft failure, death, and/or lost to follow-up at 12 months in the tacrolimus/MMF group was similar to the rate in the cyclosporine/MMF group. There was, however, an imbalance in mortality at 12 months in those patients receiving tacrolimus/MMF (4%) compared to those receiving cyclosporine/MMF (2%), including cases attributed to overimmunosuppression (Table 20).

Table 20. Incidence of BPAR, Graft Loss, Death or Loss to Follow-up at 12 Months (Study 2)

	Tacrolimus/MMF	Cyclosporine/MMF
	(N=212)	(N=212)
Overall Failure	32 (15.1%)	36 (17%)
Components of efficacy failure		
BPAR	16 (7.5%)	29 (13.7%)
Graft loss excluding death	6 (2.8%)	4 (1.9%)
Mortality	9 (4.2%)	5 (2.4%)
Lost to follow-up	4 (1.9%)	1 (0.5%)
Treatment Difference of efficacy failure compared to tacrolimus/MMF group (95% CI[a])		1.9% (-5.2%, 9%)

[a] 95% confidence interval calculated using Fisher's Exact Test

The protocol-specified target tacrolimus whole blood trough concentrations ($C_{trough,Tac}$) in Study 2 were 7 to 16 ng/mL for the first three months and 5 to 15 ng/mL thereafter. The observed median $C_{troughs,Tac}$ approximated 10 ng/mL during the first three months and 8 ng/mL from month 4 to month 12 (Table 21). Approximately 80% of patients maintained tacrolimus whole trough blood concentrations between 6 to 16 ng/mL during months 1 through 3 and, then, between 5 to 12 ng/mL from month 4 through 1 year.

Table 21. Tacrolimus Whole Blood Trough Concentrations (Study 2)

Time	Median (P10-P90[a]) tacrolimus whole blood trough concentrations (ng/mL)
Day 30 (N=174)	10.5 (6.3 to 16.8)
Day 60 (N=179)	9.2 (5.9 to 15.3)
Day 120 (N=176)	8.3 (4.6 to 13.3)
Day 180 (N=171)	7.8 (5.5 to 13.2)
Day 365 (N=178)	7.1 (4.2 to 12.4)

[a] 10 to 90th Percentile: range of $C_{trough,Tac}$ that excludes lowest 10% and highest 10% of $C_{trough, Tac}$

The protocol-specified target cyclosporine whole blood concentrations ($C_{trough,CsA}$) were 125 to 400 ng/mL for the first three months, and 100 to 300 ng/mL thereafter. The observed median $C_{troughs, CsA}$ approximated 280 ng/mL during the first three months and 190 ng/mL from month 4 to month 12.
Patients in both groups started MMF at 1gram twice daily. The MMF dose was reduced to less than 2 grams per day by month 12 in 62% of patients in the tacrolimus/MMF group (Table 22) and in 47% of patients in the cyclosporine/MMF

group. Approximately 63% and 55% of these MMF dose reductions were because of adverse reactions in the tacrolimus/MMF group and the cyclosporine/MMF group, respectively [see **ADVERSE REACTIONS (6.1)**].

Table 22. MMF Dose Over Time in the Tacrolimus/MMF Group (Study 2)

Time period (Days)	Time-averaged MMF dose (grams per day)[a]		
	Less than 2	2	Greater than 2
0 to 30 (N=212)	25%	69%	6%
0 to 90 (N=212)	41%	53%	6%
0 to 180 (N=212)	52%	41%	7%
0 to 365 (N=212)	62%	34%	4%

Key: Time-averaged MMF dose=(total MMF dose)/(duration of treatment)

[a] Percentage of patients for each time-averaged MMF dose range during various treatment periods. Two grams per day of time-averaged MMF dose means that MMF dose was not reduced in those patients during the treatment periods.

14.2 Liver Transplantation

The safety and efficacy of tacrolimus-based immunosuppression following orthotopic liver transplantation were assessed in two prospective, randomized, non-blinded multicenter trials. The active control groups were treated with a cyclosporine-based immunosuppressive regimen (CsA/AZA). Both trials used concomitant adrenal corticosteroids as part of the immunosuppressive regimens. These trials compared patient and graft survival rates at 12 months following transplantation.

In one trial, 529 patients were enrolled at 12 clinical sites in the United States; prior to surgery, 263 were randomized to the tacrolimus-based immunosuppressive regimen and 266 to the CsA/AZA. In 10 of the 12 sites, the same CsA/AZA protocol was used, while 2 sites used different control protocols. This trial excluded patients with renal dysfunction, fulminant hepatic failure with Stage IV encephalopathy, and cancers; pediatric patients (≤ 12 years old) were allowed.

In the second trial, 545 patients were enrolled at 8 clinical sites in Europe; prior to surgery, 270 were randomized to the tacrolimus-based immunosuppressive regimen and 275 to CsA/AZA. In this trial, each center used its local standard CsA/AZA protocol in the active-control arm. This trial excluded pediatric patients, but did allow enrollment of subjects with renal dysfunction, fulminant hepatic failure in Stage IV encephalopathy, and cancers other than primary hepatic with metastases.

One-year patient survival and graft survival in the tacrolimus-based treatment groups were similar to those in the CsA/AZA treatment groups in both trials. The overall 1-year patient survival (CsA/AZA and tacrolimus-based treatment groups combined) was 88% in the U.S. trial and 78% in the European trial. The overall 1-year graft survival (CsA/AZA and tacrolimus-based treatment groups combined) was 81% in the U.S. trial and 73% in the European trial. In both trials, the median time to convert from IV to oral tacrolimus dosing was 2 days.

Although there is a lack of direct correlation between tacrolimus concentrations and drug efficacy, data from clinical trials of liver transplant patients have shown an increasing incidence of adverse reactions with increasing trough blood concentrations. Most patients are stable when trough whole blood concentrations are maintained between 5 to 20 ng/mL. Long-term post-transplant patients often are maintained at the low end of this target range.

Data from the U.S. clinical trial show that the median trough blood concentrations, measured at intervals from the second week to one year post-transplantation ranged from 9.8 ng/mL to 19.4 ng/mL.

14.3 Heart Transplantation

Two open-label, randomized, comparative trials evaluated the safety and efficacy of tacrolimus-based and cyclosporine-based immunosuppression in primary orthotopic heart transplantation. In a trial conducted in Europe, 314 patients received a regimen of antibody induction, corticosteroids and azathioprine in combination with tacrolimus or cyclosporine modified for 18 months. In a 3-arm trial conducted in the US, 331 patients received corticosteroids and tacrolimus plus sirolimus, tacrolimus plus mycophenolate mofetil (MMF) or cyclosporine modified plus MMF for 1 year.

In the European trial, patient/graft survival at 18 months post-transplant was similar between treatment arms, 92%

in the tacrolimus group and 90% in the cyclosporine group. In the U.S. trial, patient and graft survival at 12 months was similar with 93% survival in the tacrolimus plus MMF group and 86% survival in the cyclosporine modified plus MMF group. In the European trial, the cyclosporine trough concentrations were above the pre-defined target range (i.e., 100 to 200 ng/mL) at Day 122 and beyond in 32 to 68% of the patients in the cyclosporine treatment arm, whereas the tacrolimus trough concentrations were within the pre-defined target range (i.e., 5 to 15 ng/mL) in 74 to 86% of the patients in the tacrolimus treatment arm. Data from this European trial indicate that from 1 week to 3 months post-transplant, approximately 80% of patients maintained trough concentrations between 8 to 20 ng/mL and, from 3 months through 18 months post-transplant, approximately 80% of patients maintained trough concentrations between 6 to 18 ng/mL. The U.S. trial contained a third arm of a combination regimen of sirolimus, 2 mg per day, and full-dose tacrolimus; however, this regimen was associated with increased risk of wound healing complications, renal function impairment, and insulin-dependent post-transplant diabetes mellitus, and is not recommended [see **WARNINGS AND PRECAUTIONS (5.12)**].

16   HOW SUPPLIED/STORAGE AND HANDLING

Hecoria (tacrolimus capsules, USP) containing white to off-white powder equivalent to 0.5 mg of anhydrous tacrolimus, are hard gelatin capsules with white opaque body and ivory cap. The body is imprinted "0.5 mg" and cap is imprinted "HECORIA" in black ink.
They are supplied as follows:
NDC 0078-0616-05, bottle of 100 capsules with child-resistant closure

Hecoria (tacrolimus capsules, USP) containing white to off-white powder equivalent to 1 mg of anhydrous tacrolimus, are hard gelatin capsules with white opaque body and brown cap. The body is imprinted "1 mg" and cap is imprinted "HECORIA" in black ink.
They are supplied as follows:
NDC 0078-0617-05, bottle of 100 capsules with child-resistant closure

Hecoria (tacrolimus capsules, USP) containing white to off-white powder equivalent to 5 mg of anhydrous tacrolimus, are hard gelatin capsules with white opaque body and orange cap. The body is imprinted "5 mg" and cap is imprinted "HECORIA" in black ink.
They are supplied as follows:
NDC 0078-0618-05, bottle of 100 capsules with child-resistant closure.

Hecoria capsules should be stored at 20° to 25°C (68° to 77°F) [see USP Controlled Room Temperature].

17   PATIENT COUNSELING INFORMATION

17.1   Administration

Advise patients to:
- Take Hecoria (tacrolimus) capsules at the same 12-hour intervals every day to achieve consistent blood concentrations.
- Take Hecoria consistently either with or without food because the presence and composition of food decreases the bioavailability of Hecoria.
- Not to eat grapefruit or drink grapefruit juice in combination with Hecoria [see **DRUG INTERACTIONS (7.2)**].

17.2   Development of Lymphoma and Other Malignancies

Inform patients they are at increased risk of developing lymphomas and other malignancies, particularly of the skin, due to immunosuppression. Advise patients to limit exposure to sunlight and ultraviolet (UV) light by wearing protective clothing and use a sunscreen with a high protection factor [see **WARNINGS AND PRECAUTIONS (5.2)**].

17.3   Increased Risk of Infection

Inform patients they are at increased risk of developing a variety of infections, including opportunistic infections, due to immunosuppression and to contact their physician if they develop any symptoms of infection [see **WARNINGS AND PRECAUTIONS (5.3, 5.4, 5.5)**].

17.4   New Onset Diabetes After Transplant

Inform patients that Hecoria (tacrolimus) capsules can cause diabetes mellitus and should be advised to contact their physician if they develop frequent urination, increased thirst or hunger [see **WARNINGS AND PRECAUTIONS (5.6)**].

17.5   Nephrotoxicity

Inform patients that Hecoria (tacrolimus) capsules can have toxic effects on the kidney that should be monitored. Advise patients to attend all visits and complete all blood tests ordered by their medical team [see **WARNINGS AND PRECAUTIONS (5.7)**].

17.6   Neurotoxicity

Inform patients that they are at risk of developing adverse neurologic effects including seizure, altered mental status, and tremor. Advise patients to contact their physician should they develop vision changes, deliriums, or tremors [see **WARNINGS AND PRECAUTIONS (5.8)**].

17.7 Hyperkalemia

Inform patients that Hecoria (tacrolimus) capsules can cause hyperkalemia. Monitoring of potassium levels may be necessary, especially with concomitant use of other drugs known to cause hyperkalemia [see **WARNINGS AND PRECAUTIONS (5.9)**].

17.8 Hypertension

Inform patients that Hecoria (tacrolimus) capsules can cause high blood pressure which may require treatment with anti-hypertensive therapy [see **WARNINGS AND PRECAUTIONS (5.10)**].

17.9 Drug Interactions

Instruct patients to tell their health care providers when they start or stop taking all the medicines, including prescription medicines and non-prescription medicines, natural or herbal remedies, nutritional supplements and vitamins [see **DRUG INTERACTIONS (7)**].

17.10 Pregnant Women and Nursing Mothers

Instruct patients to tell their healthcare providers if they plan to become pregnant or breast-feed their infant [see **USE IN SPECIFIC POPULATIONS (8.1, 8.3)**]

17.11 Immunizations

Inform patients that Hecoria (tacrolimus) capsules can interfere with the usual response to immunizations and that they should avoid live vaccines [see **WARNINGS AND PRECAUTIONS (5.16)**].

T2013-83
September 2013

PATIENT INFORMATION
Hecoria™ (tacrolimus capsules, USP)

Read this Patient Information before you start taking Hecoria (tacrolimus) capsules and each time you get a refill. There may be new information. This information does not take the place of talking with your doctor about your medical condition or your treatment.

What is the most important information I should know about Hecoria (tacrolimus) capsules?

Hecoria (tacrolimus) capsules can cause serious side effects, including:

1. Increased risk of cancer. People who take Hecoria have an increased risk of getting some kinds of cancer, including skin and lymph gland cancer (lymphoma).

2. Increased risk of infection. Hecoria is a medicine that affects your immune system. Hecoria can lower the ability of your immune system to fight infections. Serious infections can happen in people receiving Hecoria that can cause death. **Call your doctor right away if you have symptoms of an infection such as:**
• fever
• sweats or chills
• cough or flu-like symptoms
• muscle aches
• warm, red, or painful areas on your skin

What are Hecoria (tacrolimus) capsules?

Hecoria is a prescription medicine used with other medicines to help prevent organ rejection in people who have had a kidney, liver, or heart transplant and Hecoria is not for use with medicines called cyclosporines (Gengraf®, Neoral®, and Sandimmune®).

Hecoria is not for use with a medicine called sirolimus (Rapamune®) in people who have had a liver or heart transplant.

It is not known if Hecoria is safe and effective when used with sirolimus in people who have had kidney transplants.

It is not known if Hecoria is safe and effective in children who have had a kidney or heart transplant.

Who should not take Hecoria (tacrolimus) capsules?

Do not take Hecoria if you are allergic to tacrolimus or any of the ingredients in Hecoria. See the end of this leaflet for a complete list of ingredients in Hecoria.

What should I tell my doctor before taking Hecoria (tacrolimus) capsules?

Before you take Hecoria, tell your doctor if you:
• plan to receive any live vaccines
• have or have had liver, kidney or heart problems
• are pregnant or plan to become pregnant. Hecoria may harm your unborn baby. Talk to your doctor if you are pregnant or plan to become pregnant.
• Are breastfeeding or plan to breastfeed. Hecoria can pass into your breast milk. You and your doctor should decide if you will take Hecoria or breastfeed. You should not do both.

Tell your doctor about all the medicines you take, including prescription and non-prescription medicines, vitamins, and herbal supplements.

Especially tell your doctor if you take:
• cyclosporine (Gengraf®, Neoral®, and Sandimmune®)
• sirolimus (Rapamune®)
• nelfinavir (Viracept®)
• telaprevir (Incivek™)
• boceprevir (Victrelis™)

• amiodarone (Cordarone™, Nexterone™, Pacerone™)

Ask your doctor or pharmacist if you are not sure if you take any of the medicines listed above.

Hecoria may affect the way other medicines work, and other medicines may affect how Hecoria works.

Know the medicines you take. Keep a list of your medicines and show it to your doctor and pharmacist when you get a new medicine.

How should I take Hecoria (tacrolimus) capsules?
• Take Hecoria exactly as your doctor tells you to take it.
• Your doctor will tell you how many Hecoria capsules to take and when to take them.
• Your doctor may change your Hecoria dose if needed. Do not stop taking or change your dose of Hecoria without talking to your doctor.
• Take Hecoria with or without food.
• Take Hecoria the same way every day. For example, if you choose to take Hecoria with food, you should always take Hecoria with food.
• Take Hecoria at the same time each day, 12 hours apart. For example, if you take your first dose at 7:00 a.m. you should take your second dose at 7:00 p.m.
   ○ Taking Hecoria at the same time each day helps to keep enough medicine in your body to give your transplanted organ the around-the-clock medicine it needs.
• **Do not** eat grapefruit or drink grapefruit juice while taking Hecoria.
• If you take too much Hecoria, call your doctor or go to the nearest hospital emergency room right away.

What should I avoid while taking Hecoria (tacrolimus) capsules?
• While you take Hecoria you should not receive any live vaccines such as:
   ○ flu vaccine through your nose
   ○ measles
   ○ mumps
   ○ rubella
   ○ polio by mouth
   ○ BCG (TB vaccine)
   ○ yellow fever
   ○ chicken pox (varicella)
   ○ typhoid
• Avoid exposure to sunlight and UV light such as tanning machines. Wear protective clothing and use a sunscreen.

What are the possible side effects of Hecoria (tacrolimus) capsules?

Hecoria may cause serious side effects, including:
• See "What is the most important information I should know about Hecoria?"
• **high blood sugar (diabetes).** Your doctor may do certain tests to check for diabetes while you take Hecoria. Call your doctor right away if you have:
   ○ frequent urination
   ○ increased thirst or hunger
   ○ blurred vision
   ○ confusion
   ○ drowsiness
   ○ loss of appetite
   ○ fruity smell on your breath
   ○ nausea, vomiting, or stomach pain
• **kidney problems.** Your doctor may do certain tests to check your kidney function while you take Hecoria.
• **nervous system problems.** Call your doctor right away if you get any of these symptoms while taking Hecoria. These could be signs of a serious nervous system problem:
   ○ confusion
   ○ coma
   ○ muscle tremors
   ○ numbness and tingling
   ○ headache
   ○ seizures
   ○ vision changes
• **high levels of potassium in your blood.** Your doctor may do certain tests to check your potassium level while you take Hecoria.
• **high blood pressure.** Your doctor will monitor your blood pressure while you take Hecoria.
• **heart problems (myocardial hypertrophy).** Tell your doctor right away if you get any of these symptoms of heart problems while taking Hecoria:
   ○ shortness of breath
   ○ chest pain
   ○ feel lightheaded
   ○ feel faint

The most common side effects of Hecoria (tacrolimus) capsules in people receiving kidney transplant are:
• infection
• tremors (shaking of the body)
• high blood pressure
• kidney problems
• constipation
• diarrhea
• headache
• stomach pain

• trouble sleeping
• nausea
• low levels of phosphate in your blood
• swelling of the hands, ankles, or legs
• weakness
• pain
• high levels of fat in your blood
• high levels of potassium in your blood
• low red blood cell count (anemia)

The most common side effects of Hecoria (tacrolimus) capsules in people receiving liver transplants are:
• shaking of the body tremors
• headache
• diarrhea
• high blood pressure
• nausea
• kidney problems
• stomach pain
• trouble sleeping
• numbness or tingling in your hands or feet
• anemia
• pain
• fever
• weakness
• high levels of potassium in the blood
• low levels of magnesium in the blood

The most common side effects of Hecoria (tacrolimus) capsules for heart transplant patients are:
• kidney problems
• high blood pressure

Tell your doctor if you have any side effect that bothers you or that does not go away.

These are not all the possible side effects of Hecoria. For more information, ask your doctor or pharmacist.

Call your doctor for medical advice about side effects. You may report side effects to FDA at 1-800-FDA-1088.

How should I store Hecoria (tacrolimus) capsules?
• Store Hecoria at 20° to 25°C (68° to 77°F).
• Safely throw away medicine that is out of date or no longer needed.

Keep Hecoria and all medicines out of reach of children.

General information about the safe and effective use of Hecoria (tacrolimus) capsules

Medicines are sometimes prescribed for purposes other than those listed in a Patient Information leaflet. Do not use Hecoria for a condition for which it was not prescribed. Do not give Hecoria to other people, even if they have the same symptoms that you have. It may harm them.

How do Hecoria (tacrolimus) capsules protect my new organ?

The body's immune system protects the body against anything that it does not recognize as part of the body. For example, when the immune system detects a virus or bacteria it tries to get rid of it to prevent infection. When a person has a liver, kidney, or heart transplant, the immune system does not recognize the new organ as a part of the body and tries to get rid of it, too. This is called "rejection." Hecoria protects your new organ by slowing down the body's immune system.

This Patient Information leaflet summarizes the most important information about Hecoria. If you would like more information, talk with your doctor. You can ask your pharmacist or doctor for information about Hecoria that is written for health professionals.

For more information contact Novartis Pharmaceuticals Corporation at 1-888-669-6682.

What are the ingredients in Hecoria (tacrolimus) capsules?

Active ingredient: tacrolimus

Inactive ingredients: croscarmellose sodium, hypromellose, lactose monohydrate, and magnesium stearate.

The Hecoria capsule shell for 0.5 mg strength consists of gelatin, titanium dioxide and yellow iron oxide.

The Hecoria capsule shell for 1 mg strength consists of black iron oxide, gelatin, red iron oxide, titanium dioxide, and yellow iron oxide.

The Hecoria capsule shell for 5 mg strength consists of red iron oxide, gelatin, and titanium dioxide.

Hecoria capsules 0.5 mg, 1 mg and 5 mg are printed with edible black ink. The black ink is comprised of ammonia, black iron oxide, butyl alcohol, potassium hydroxide, propylene glycol, and shellac.

This Patient Information has been approved by the U.S. Food and Drug Administration.

Manufactured in India by Sandoz Private Limited
Distributed by: Novartis Pharmaceuticals Corporation
East Hanover, NJ 07936
© Novartis
T2013-84
September 2013

ILARIS
(canakinumab)
injection for subcutaneous use   ℞

The following prescribing information is based on official labeling in effect July 2013.

HIGHLIGHTS OF PRESCRIBING INFORMATION
These highlights do not include all the information needed to use ILARIS safely and effectively. See full prescribing information for ILARIS
ILARIS (canakinumab) injection for subcutaneous use
Initial U.S. Approval: 2009

RECENT MAJOR CHANGES

Indications and Usage, Systemic Juvenile Idiopathic Arthritis (SJIA) (1.2)	05/2013
Dosage and Administration, Systemic Juvenile Idiopathic Arthritis (SJIA) (2.3)	05/2013
Warnings and Precautions, Macrophage Activation Syndrome (SJIA) (5.5)	05/2013

INDICATIONS AND USAGE
ILARIS is an interleukin-1β blocker indicated for the treatment of:
Cryopyrin-Associated Periodic Syndromes (CAPS), in adults and children 4 years of age and older including:
• Familial Cold Autoinflammatory Syndrome (FCAS) (1.1)
• Muckle-Wells Syndrome (MWS) (1.1)
Active Systemic Juvenile Idiopathic Arthritis (SJIA) in patients aged 2 years and older (1.2)

DOSAGE AND ADMINISTRATION
Cryopyrin-Associated Periodic Syndromes
150 mg for CAPS patients with body weight greater than 40 kg and 2 mg/kg for CAPS patients with body weight greater than or equal to 15 kg and less than or equal to 40 kg. For children 15 to 40 kg with an inadequate response, the dose can be increased to 3 mg/kg. Administer subcutaneously every 8 weeks. (2.2)
Systemic Juvenile Idiopathic Arthritis (SJIA)
4 mg/kg (with a maximum of 300mg) for patients with a body weight greater than or equal to 7.5kg. Administer subcutaneously every 4 weeks. (2.3)

DOSAGE FORMS AND STRENGTHS
Sterile, single-use, glass vial containing 180 mg of ILARIS as a lyophilized powder for reconstitution. (3)

CONTRAINDICATIONS
Confirmed hypersensitivity to the active substance or to any of the excipients. (4)

WARNINGS AND PRECAUTIONS
• Interleukin-1 blockade may interfere with immune response to infections. Treatment with medications that work through inhibition of IL-1 has been associated with an increased risk of serious infections. ILARIS has been associated with an increased incidence of serious infections. Physicians should exercise caution when administering ILARIS to patients with infections, a history of recurring infections or underlying conditions which may predispose them to infections. Discontinue treatment with ILARIS if a patient develops a serious infection. Do not administer ILARIS to patients during an active infection requiring medical intervention. (5.1)
• Live vaccines should not be given concurrently with ILARIS. Prior to initiation of therapy with ILARIS, patients should receive all recommended vaccinations. (5.4)

ADVERSE REACTIONS
CAPS: The most common adverse reactions greater than 10% reported by patients with CAPS treated with ILARIS are nasopharyngitis, diarrhea, influenza, headache and nausea. (6)
SJIA: The most common adverse drug reactions greater than 10% reported by patients with SJIA treated with ILARIS are infections (nasopharyngitis and upper respiratory tract infections), abdominal pain and injection site reactions. (6)
To report SUSPECTED ADVERSE REACTIONS, contact Novartis Pharmaceuticals Corporation at 1-888-669-6682 or FDA at 1-800-FDA-1088 or www.fda.gov/medwatch

DRUG INTERACTIONS
No formal drug interaction studies have been conducted with ILARIS. (7)

USE IN SPECIFIC POPULATIONS
• Pregnancy: No Human data. Because animal reproduction studies are not always predictive of human response, this drug should be used during pregnancy only if clearly needed. (8.1)
• Nursing Mothers: Caution should be exercised when administered to a nursing woman. (8.3)
See 17 for PATIENT COUNSELING INFORMATION and Medication Guide

Revised: 5/2013

FULL PRESCRIBING INFORMATION: CONTENTS*

FULL PRESCRIBING INFORMATION

1 INDICATIONS AND USAGE
1.1 Cryopyrin-Associated Periodic Syndromes (CAPS)
ILARIS (canakinumab) is an interleukin-1β blocker indicated for the treatment of Cryopyrin-Associated Periodic Syndromes (CAPS), in adults and children 4 years of age and older including:
• Familial Cold Autoinflammatory Syndrome (FCAS)
• Muckle-Wells Syndrome (MWS)
1.2 Systemic Juvenile Idiopathic Arthritis (SJIA)
ILARIS is indicated for the treatment of active Systemic Juvenile Idiopathic Arthritis (SJIA) in patients aged 2 years and older.

2 DOSAGE AND ADMINISTRATION
2.1 General Dosing Information
INJECTION FOR SUBCUTANEOUS USE ONLY.
2.2 Cryopyrin-Associated Periodic Syndromes (CAPS)
The recommended dose of ILARIS is 150 mg for CAPS patients with body weight greater than 40 kg. For CAPS patients with body weight greater than or equal to 15 kg and less than or equal to 40 kg, the recommended dose is 2 mg/kg. For children 15 to 40 kg with an inadequate response, the dose can be increased to 3 mg/kg.
ILARIS is administered every eight weeks as a single dose via subcutaneous injection.
2.3 Systemic Juvenile Idiopathic Arthritis (SJIA)
The recommended dose of ILARIS for SJIA patients with a body weight greater than or equal to 7.5kg is 4mg/kg (with a maximum of 300mg) administered every four weeks via subcutaneous injection.
2.4 Four Steps for Preparation and Administration
STEP 1: Using aseptic technique, reconstitute each vial of ILARIS by slowly injecting 1 mL of preservative-free Sterile Water for Injection with a 1 mL syringe and an 18 gauge × 2" needle.
STEP 2: Swirl the vial slowly at an angle of about 45° for approximately 1 minute and allow to stand for 5 minutes. Do not shake. Then gently turn the vial upside down and back again ten times. Avoid touching the rubber stopper with your fingers.
STEP 3: Allow to stand for about 15 minutes at room temperature to obtain a clear solution. The reconstituted solution has a final concentration of 150mg/mL. Do not shake. Do not use if particulate matter is present in the solution. Tap the side of the vial to remove any residual liquid from the stopper. The reconstituted solution should be essentially free from particulates, and clear to opalescent. The solution should be colorless or may have a slight brownish-yellow tint. If the solution has a distinctly brown discoloration it should not be used. If not used within 60 minutes of reconstitution, the solution should be stored in the refrigerator at 2 to 8° C (36 to 46° F) and used within 4 hours. Slight foaming of the product upon reconstitution is not unusual.
STEP 4: Using a sterile syringe and needle carefully withdraw the required volume depending on the dose to be administered (0.2 mL to 1 mL) and subcutaneously inject using a 27 gauge × 0.5" needle.
Injection into scar tissue should be avoided as this may result in insufficient exposure to ILARIS.
ILARIS 180-mg powder for solution for injection is supplied in a single-use vial. Any unused product or waste material should be disposed of in accordance with local requirements.

3 DOSAGE FORMS AND STRENGTHS
ILARIS is supplied as a 180 mg white lyophilized powder for solution for subcutaneous injection. Reconstitution with 1 mL of preservative-free Sterile Water for Injection is required prior to subcutaneous administration of the drug, resulting in a total volume of 1.2 mL reconstituted solution. The reconstituted ILARIS is a clear to slightly opalescent, colorless to a slight brownish yellow tint, essentially free from particulates, 150 mg/mL solution.

4 CONTRAINDICATIONS
Confirmed hypersensitivity to the active substance or to any of the excipients [see Warnings and Precautions (5.3) and Adverse Reactions (6.2)].

5 WARNINGS AND PRECAUTIONS
5.1 Serious Infections
ILARIS has been associated with an increased risk of serious infections. Physicians should exercise caution when administering ILARIS to patients with infections, a history of recurring infections or underlying conditions which may predispose them to infections. ILARIS should not be administered to patients during an active infection requiring medical intervention. Administration of ILARIS should be discontinued if a patient develops a serious infection.
Infections, predominantly of the upper respiratory tract, in some instances serious, have been reported with ILARIS. Generally, the observed infections responded to standard therapy. Isolated cases of unusual or opportunistic infections were reported during ILARIS treatment. In clinical trials, ILARIS has not been administered concomitantly with tumor necrosis factor (TNF) inhibitors. An increased incidence of serious infections has been associated with administration of another IL-1 blocker in combination with TNF inhibitors. Co-administration of ILARIS with TNF inhibitors is not recommended because this may increase the risk of serious infections [see Drug Interactions (7.1)].
Drugs that affect the immune system by blocking TNF have been associated with an increased risk of new tuberculosis and reactivation of latent tuberculosis (TB). It is possible that use of IL-1 inhibitors such as ILARIS increases the risk of reactivation of tuberculosis or of opportunistic infections. Prior to initiating immunomodulatory therapies, including ILARIS, patients should be evaluated for active and latent tuberculosis infection. Appropriate screening tests should be performed in all patients. ILARIS has not been studied in patients with a positive tuberculosis screen, and the safety of ILARIS in individuals with latent tuberculosis infection is unknown. Patients testing positive in tuberculosis screening should be treated according to standard medical practice prior to therapy with ILARIS. All patients should be instructed to seek medical advice if signs, symptoms, or high risk exposure suggestive of tuberculosis (e.g. persistent cough, weight loss, subfebrile temperature) appear during or after ILARIS therapy.
Healthcare providers should follow current CDC guidelines both to evaluate for and to treat possible latent tuberculosis infections before initiating therapy with ILARIS.
5.2 Immunosuppression
The impact of treatment with anti-interleukin-1 (IL-1) therapy on the development of malignancies is not known. However, treatment with immunosuppressants, including ILARIS, may result in an increase in the risk of malignancies.
5.3 Hypersensitivity
Hypersensitivity reactions have been reported with ILARIS therapy. During clinical trials, no anaphylactic reactions have been reported. It should be recognized that symptoms of the underlying disease being treated may be similar to symptoms of hypersensitivity. ILARIS should not be administered to any patients with known clinical hypersensitivity to ILARIS [see Contraindications (4) and Adverse Reactions (6.2)].
5.4 Immunizations
Live vaccines should not be given concurrently with ILARIS [see Drug Interactions (7.2)]. Since no data are available on either the efficacy or on the risks of secondary transmission of infection by live vaccines in patients receiving ILARIS,

live vaccines should not be given concurrently with ILARIS. In addition, because ILARIS may interfere with normal immune response to new antigens, vaccinations may not be effective in patients receiving ILARIS. No data are available on the effectiveness of vaccinations with inactivated (killed) antigens in patients receiving ILARIS. [see Drug Interactions (7.2)].

Because IL-1 blockade may interfere with immune response to infections, it is recommended that prior to initiation of therapy with ILARIS, adult and pediatric patients receive all recommended vaccinations, as appropriate, including pneumococcal vaccine and inactivated influenza vaccine. (See current recommended immunization schedules at the website of the Centers for Disease Control, http://www.cdc.gov/vaccines/recs/schedules/).

5.5 Macrophage Activation Syndrome

Macrophage activation syndrome (MAS) is a known, life-threatening disorder that may develop in patients with rheumatic conditions, in particular SJIA, and should be aggressively treated. Physicians should be attentive to symptoms of infection or worsening of SJIA, as these are known triggers for MAS. Eleven cases of MAS were observed in 201 SJIA patients treated with canakinumab in clinical trials. Based on the clinical trial experience, ILARIS does not appear to increase the incidence of MAS in SJIA patients, but no definitive conclusion can be made.

6 ADVERSE REACTIONS

395 patients, including approximately 250 children (aged 2 to 17 years) have been treated with ILARIS in interventional trials in CAPS or SJIA. The most frequently reported adverse drug reactions were infections predominantly of the upper respiratory tract. The majority of the events were mild to moderate although serious infections were observed. The type and frequency of adverse drug reactions appeared to be consistent over time.

6.1 Clinical Trial Experience

Because clinical trials are conducted under widely varying conditions, adverse reaction rates observed in the clinical trials of a drug cannot be directly compared to rates in the clinical trials of another drug and may not reflect the rates observed in practice.

Treatment of CAPS

The data described herein reflect exposure to ILARIS in 104 adult and pediatric CAPS patients, (including 20 FCAS, 72 MWS, 10 MWS/NOMID (Neonatal Onset Multisystem Inflammatory Disorder) overlap, 1 non-FCAS non-MWS, and 1 mis-diagnosed in placebo-controlled (35 patients) and uncontrolled trials. Sixty-two patients were exposed to ILARIS for at least 6 months, 56 for at least 1 year and 4 for at least 3 years. A total of 9 serious adverse reactions were reported for CAPS patients. Among these were vertigo (2 patients), infections (3 patients), including intra-abdominal abscess following appendectomy (1 patient). The most commonly reported adverse reactions associated with ILARIS treatment in the CAPS patients were nasopharyngitis, diarrhea, influenza, headache, and nausea. One patient discontinued treatment due to potential infection.

CAPS Study 1 investigated the safety of ILARIS in an 8-week, open-label period (Part 1), followed by a 24-week, randomized withdrawal period (Part 2), followed by a 16-week, open-label period (Part 3). All patients were treated with ILARIS 150 mg subcutaneously or 2 mg/kg if body weight was greater than or equal to 15 kg and less than or equal to 40 kg (see Table 1).

Since all CAPS patients received ILARIS in Part 1, there are no controlled data on adverse events (AEs). Data in Table 1 are for all AEs for all CAPS patients receiving canakinumab. In CAPS Study 1, no pattern was observed for any type or frequency of adverse events throughout the three study periods.

Table 1 Number (%) of Patients with AEs by Preferred Terms, in > 10% of Patients in Parts 1 to 3 of the Phase 3 Trial for CAPS Patients

Preferred Term	ILARIS N=35 n (%)
n % of Patients with Adverse Events	35 (100)
Nasopharyngitis	12 (34)
Diarrhea	7 (20)
Influenza	6 (17)
Rhinitis	6 (17)
Nausea	5 (14)
Headache	5 (14)
Bronchitis	4 (11)
Gastroenteritis	4 (11)
Pharyngitis	4 (11)
Weight increased	4 (11)
Musculoskeletal pain	4 (11)
Vertigo	4 (11)

Table 2 Tabulated summary of adverse drug reactions from pivotal SJIA clinical trials

	SJIA Study 2			SJIA Study 1	
	Part I	Part II			
	ILARIS N=177 n (%) (IR)^	ILARIS N=50 n (%) (IR)	Placebo N=50 n (%) (IR)	ILARIS N=43 n (%) (IR)	Placebo N=41 n (%) (IR)
Infections and infestations					
Infection (e.g. nasopharyngitis, (viral) upper respiratory tract infection, pneumonia, rhinitis, pharyngitis, tonsillitis, sinusitis, urinary tract infection, gastroenteritis, viral infection)	97 (54.8%) (0.91)	27 (54%) (0.59)	19 (38%) (0.63)	13 (30.2%) (1.26)	5 (12.2%) (1.37)
Gastrointestinal disorders					
Abdominal pain (upper)	25 (14.1%) (0.16)	8 (16%) (0.15)	6 (12%) (0.08)	3 (7%) (0.25)	1 (2.4%) (0.23)
Skin and subcutaneous tissue disorders					
Injection site reaction*					
mild	19 (10.7%)	6 (12.0%)	2 (4.0%)	0	3 (7.3%)
moderate	2 (1.1%)	1 (2.0%)	0	0	0

n= number of patients
^ IR=Exposure adjusted incidence rate per 100 patient-days
* No injection site reaction led to study discontinuation

Vertigo

Vertigo has been reported in 9 to 14% of patients in CAPS studies, exclusively in MWS patients, and reported as a serious adverse event in two cases. All events resolved with continued treatment with ILARIS.

Injection Site Reactions

In CAPS Study 1, subcutaneous injection site reactions were observed in 9% of patients in Part 1 with mild tolerability reactions; in Part 2, one patient each (7%) had a mild or a moderate tolerability reaction and, in Part 3, one patient had a mild local tolerability reaction. No severe injection-site reactions were reported and none led to discontinuation of treatment.

Treatment of SJIA

A total of 201 SJIA patients aged 2 to less than 20 years have received ILARIS in clinical trials. The safety of ILARIS compared to placebo was investigated in two phase 3 studies [see Clinical Studies (14.2)]. Patients in SJIA Study 1 received a single dose of ILARIS 4mg/kg (n=43) or placebo (n=41) via subcutaneous injection and were assessed at Day 15 for the efficacy endpoints and had a safety analysis up to Day 29. SJIA Study 2 was a two-part study with an open-label, single-arm active treatment period (Part I) followed by a randomized, double-blind, placebo-controlled, event-driven withdrawal design (Part II). Overall, 177 patients were enrolled into the study and received ILARIS 4 mg/kg (up to 300 mg maximum) in Part I, and 100 patients received ILARIS 4mg/kg (up to 300mg maximum) every 4 weeks or placebo in Part II. Adverse drug reactions listed in Table 2 showed higher rates than placebo from both trials. The adverse drug reactions associated with ILARIS treatment in SJIA patients were infections, abdominal pain, and injection site reactions.

Adverse reactions are listed according to MedDRA version 15.0 system organ class.

[See table 2 above]

6.2 Hypersensitivity

During clinical trials, no anaphylactic reactions have been reported. In CAPS trials one patient discontinued and in SJIA trials no patients discontinued due to hypersensitivity reactions. ILARIS should not be administered to any patients with known clinical hypersensitivity to ILARIS [see Contraindications (4) and Warnings and Precautions (5.3)].

6.3 Immunogenicity

A biosensor binding assay or a bridging immunoassay was used to detect antibodies directed against canakinumab in patients who received ILARIS. Antibodies against ILARIS were observed in approximately 1.5% and 3.1% of the patients treated with ILARIS for CAPS and SJIA, respectively. No neutralizing antibodies were detected. No apparent correlation of antibody development to clinical response or adverse events was observed. The CAPS clinical studies employed the biosensor binding assay, and most of the SJIA clinical studies employed the bridging assay. The data obtained in an assay are highly dependent on several factors including assay sensitivity and specificity, assay methodology, sample handling, timing of sample collection, concomitant medications, underlying disease, and the number of patients tested. For these reasons, comparison of the incidence of antibodies to canakinumab between the CAPS and SJIA clinical studies or with the incidence of antibodies to other products may be misleading.

6.4 Laboratory Findings

Hematology

During clinical trials with ILARIS, mean values decreased for white blood cells, neutrophils and platelets.

In the randomized, placebo-controlled portion of SJIA Study 2 decreased white blood cell counts (WBC) less than or equal to 0.8× lower limit of normal (LLN) were reported in 5 patients (10.4%)in the ILARIS group compared to 2 (4.0%) in the placebo group. Transient decreases in absolute neutrophil counts (ANC) to less than 1×10^9/L were reported in 3 patients (6.0%) in the ILARIS group compared to1 patient (2.0%) in the placebo group. One case of ANC counts less than 0.5×10^9/L was observed in the ILARIS group and none in the placebo group.

Mild (less than LLN and greater than 75×10^9/L) and transient decreases in platelet counts were observed in 3 (6.3%) ILARIS treated patients versus 1 (2.0%) placebo-treated patient.

Hepatic transaminases

Elevations of transaminases have been observed in patients treated with ILARIS.

In the randomized, placebo-controlled portion of SJIA Study 2, high ALT and/or AST greater than or equal to 3× upper limit of normal (ULN) were reported in 2 (4.1%) ILARIS-treated patients and 1 (2.0%) placebo patient. All patients had normal values at the next visit.

Bilirubin

Asymptomatic and mild elevations of serum bilirubin have been observed in patients treated with ILARIS without concomitant elevations of transaminases.

7 DRUG INTERACTIONS

Interactions between ILARIS and other medicinal products have not been investigated in formal studies.

7.1 TNF-Blocker and IL-1 Blocking Agent

An increased incidence of serious infections and an increased risk of neutropenia have been associated with administration of another IL-1 blocker in combination with TNF inhibitors in another patient population. Use of ILARIS with TNF inhibitors may also result in similar toxicities and is not recommended because this may increase the risk of serious infections [see Warnings and Precautions (5.1)].

The concomitant administration of ILARIS with other drugs that block IL-1 has not been studied. Based upon the potential for pharmacological interactions between ILARIS and a recombinant IL-1ra, concomitant administration of ILARIS and other agents that block IL-1 or its receptors is not recommended.

7.2 Immunization

No data are available on either the effects of live vaccination or the secondary transmission of infection by live vaccines

Table 3 Physician's Global Assessment of Auto-Inflammatory Disease Activity and Assessment of Skin Disease: Frequency Table and Treatment Comparison in Part 2 (Using LOCF, ITT Population)

	ILARIS N= 15			Placebo N= 16	
	Baseline	Start of Part 2 (Week 8)	End of Part 2	Start of Part 2 (Week 8)	End of Part 2
Physician's Global Assessment of Auto-Inflammatory Disease Activity - n (%)					
Absent	0/31 (0)	9/15 (60)	8/15 (53)	8/16 (50)	0/16 (0)
Minimal	1/31 (3)	4/15 (27)	7/15 (47)	8/16 (50)	4/16 (25)
Mild	7/31 (23)	2/15 (13)	0/15 (0)	0/16 (0)	8/16 (50)
Moderate	19/31 (61)	0/15 (0)	0/15 (0)	0/16 (0)	4/16 (25)
Severe	4/31 (13)	0/15 (0)	0/15 (0)	0/16 (0)	0/16 (0)
Assessment of Skin Disease – n (%)					
Absent	3/31 (10)	13/15 (87)	14/15 (93)	13/16 (81)	5/16 (31)
Minimal	6/31 (19)	2/15 (13)	1/15 (7)	3/16 (19)	3/16 (19)
Mild	9/31 (29)	0/15 (0)	0/15 (0)	0/16 (0)	5/16 (31)
Moderate	12/31 (39)	0/15 (0)	0/15 (0)	0/16 (0)	3/16 (19)
Severe	1/32 (3)	0/15 (0)	0/15 (0)	0/16 (0)	0/16 (0)

in patients receiving ILARIS. Therefore, live vaccines should not be given concurrently with ILARIS. It is recommended that, if possible, pediatric and adult patients should complete all immunizations in accordance with current immunization guidelines prior to initiating ILARIS therapy [see Warnings and Precautions (5.4)].

7.3 Cytochrome P450 Substrates
The formation of CYP450 enzymes is suppressed by increased levels of cytokines (e.g., IL-1) during chronic inflammation. Thus it is expected that for a molecule that binds to IL-1, such as canakinumab, the formation of CYP450 enzymes could be normalized. This is clinically relevant for CYP450 substrates with a narrow therapeutic index, where the dose is individually adjusted (e.g., warfarin). Upon initiation of canakinumab, in patients being treated with these types of medicinal products, therapeutic monitoring of the effect or drug concentration should be performed and the individual dose of the medicinal product may need to be adjusted as needed.

8 USE IN SPECIFIC POPULATIONS
8.1 Pregnancy
Pregnancy Category C
Canakinumab has been shown to produce delays in fetal skeletal development when evaluated in marmoset monkeys using doses 11-fold the maximum recommended human dose (MRHD) and greater (based on a plasma area under the time-concentration curve [AUC] comparison). Doses producing exposures within the clinical exposure range at the MRHD were not evaluated. Similar delays in fetal skeletal development were observed in mice administered a murine analog of canakinumab. There are no adequate and well-controlled studies of ILARIS in pregnant women. Because animal reproduction studies are not always predictive of human response, this drug should be used during pregnancy only if clearly needed.

Embryofetal developmental toxicity studies were performed in marmoset monkeys and mice. Pregnant marmoset monkeys were administered canakinumab subcutaneously twice weekly at doses of 15, 50 or 150 mg/kg (representing 11 to 110-fold the human dose based on a plasma AUC comparison at the MRHD) from gestation days 25 to 109 which revealed no evidence of embryotoxicity or fetal malformations. There were increases in the incidence of incomplete ossification of the terminal caudal vertebra and misaligned and/or bipartite vertebra in fetuses at all dose levels when compared to concurrent controls suggestive of delay in skeletal development in the marmoset. Since canakinumab does not cross-react with mouse or rat IL-1, pregnant mice were subcutaneously administered a murine analog of canakinumab at doses of 15, 50, or 150 mg/kg on gestation days 6, 11 and 17. The incidence of incomplete ossification of the parietal and frontal skull bones of fetuses was increased in a dose-dependent manner at all dose levels tested.

8.3 Nursing Mothers
It is not known whether canakinumab is excreted in human milk. Because many drugs are excreted in human milk, caution should be exercised when ILARIS is administered to a nursing woman.

8.4 Pediatric Use
The CAPS trials with ILARIS included a total of 23 pediatric patients with an age range from 4 years to 17 years (11 adolescents were treated subcutaneously with 150 mg , and 12 children were treated with 2 mg/kg based on body weight greater than or equal to 15 kg and less than or equal to 40 kg). The majority of patients achieved improvement in clinical symptoms and objective markers of inflammation (e.g., Serum Amyloid A and C-Reactive Protein). Overall, the efficacy and safety of ILARIS in pediatric and adult patients were comparable. Infections of the upper respiratory tract were the most frequently reported infection. The

safety and effectiveness of ILARIS in CAPS patients under 4 years of age has not been established [see Pharmacokinetics (12.3)].
The safety and efficacy of ILARIS in SJIA patients under 2 years of age have not been established [see Pharmacokinetics (12.3)].

8.5 Geriatric Use
Clinical studies of ILARIS did not include sufficient numbers of subjects aged 65 and over to determine whether they respond differently from younger subjects.

8.6 Patients with Renal Impairment
No formal studies have been conducted to examine the pharmacokinetics of ILARIS administered subcutaneously in patients with renal impairment.

8.7 Patients with Hepatic Impairment
No formal studies have been conducted to examine the pharmacokinetics of ILARIS administered subcutaneously in patients with hepatic impairment.

10 OVERDOSAGE
No confirmed case of overdose has been reported. In the case of overdose, it is recommended that the subject be monitored for any signs and symptoms of adverse reactions or effects, and appropriate symptomatic treatment be instituted immediately.

11 DESCRIPTION
Canakinumab is a recombinant, human anti-human-IL-1β monoclonal antibody that belongs to the IgG1/κ isotype subclass. It is expressed in a murine Sp2/0-Ag14 cell line and comprised of two 447- (or 448-) residue heavy chains and two 214-residue light chains, with a molecular mass of 145157 Daltons when deglycosylated. Both heavy chains of canakinumab contain oligosaccharide chains linked to the protein backbone at asparagine 298 (Asn 298).
The biological activity of canakinumab is measured by comparing its inhibition of IL-1β-dependent expression of the reporter gene luciferase to that of a canakinumab internal reference standard, using a stably transfected cell line.
ILARIS is supplied in a sterile, single-use, colorless, 6 mL glass vial with coated stopper and aluminum flip-off cap. Each vial contains 180 mg of canakinumab as a white, preservative-free, lyophilized powder. Reconstitution with 1 mL of preservative-free Sterile Water for Injection is required prior to subcutaneous administration of the drug. The reconstituted canakinumab is a 150 mg/mL solution essentially free of particulates, clear to slightly opalescent, and is colorless or may have a slightly brownish-yellow tint. A volume of up to 1 mL can be withdrawn for delivery of 150 mg/mL canakinumab for subcutaneous administration. Each reconstituted vial contains 180 mg canakinumab, sucrose, L-histidine, L-histidine HCl monohydrate, polysorbate 80 and Sterile Water for Injection. No preservatives are present.

12 CLINICAL PHARMACOLOGY
12.1 Mechanism of Action
Canakinumab is a human monoclonal anti-human IL-1β antibody of the IgG1/κ isotype. Canakinumab binds to human IL-1β and neutralizes its activity by blocking its interaction with IL-1 receptors, but it does not bind IL-1α or IL-1 receptor antagonist (IL-1ra).
CAPS refer to rare genetic syndromes generally caused by mutations in the NLRP-3 [nucleotide-binding domain, leucine rich family (NLR), pyrin domain containing 3] gene (also known as Cold-Induced Auto-inflammatory Syndrome-1 [CIAS1]). CAPS disorders are inherited in an autosomal dominant pattern with male and female offspring equally affected. Features common to all disorders include fever, urticaria-like rash, arthralgia, myalgia, fatigue, and conjunctivitis.

The NLRP-3 gene encodes the protein cryopyrin, an important component of the inflammasome. Cryopyrin regulates the protease caspase-1 and controls the activation of interleukin-1 beta (IL-1β). Mutations in NLRP-3 result in an overactive inflammasome resulting in excessive release of activated IL-1β that drives inflammation. Systemic juvenile idiopathic arthritis (SJIA) is a severe autoinflammatory disease, driven by innate immunity by means of proinflammatory cytokines such as interleukin 1β (IL-1β).

12.2 Pharmacodynamics
C-reactive protein and Serum Amyloid A (SAA) are indicators of inflammatory disease activity that are elevated in patients with CAPS. Elevated SAA has been associated with the development of systemic amyloidosis in patients with CAPS. Following ILARIS treatment, CRP and SAA levels normalize within 8 days. In SJIA the median percent reduction in CRP from baseline to Day 15 was 91%. Improvement in pharmacodynamic markers may not be representative of clinical response.

12.3 Pharmacokinetics
Absorption
The peak serum canakinumab concentration (Cmax) of 16 ± 3.5 µg/mL occurred approximately 7 days after subcutaneous administration of a single, 150-mg dose subcutaneously to adult CAPS patients. The mean terminal half-life was 26 days. The absolute bioavailability of subcutaneous canakinumab was estimated to be 66%. Exposure parameters (such as AUC and Cmax) increased in proportion to dose over the dose range of 0.30 to 10 mg/kg given as intravenous infusion or from 150 to 300 mg as subcutaneous injection.

Distribution
Canakinumab binds to serum IL-1β. Canakinumab volume of distribution (Vss) varied according to body weight and was estimated to be 6.01 liters in a typical CAPS patient weighing 70 kg, and 3.2 liters in a SJIA patient weighing 33 kg. The expected accumulation ratio was 1.3-fold for CAPS patients and 1.6-fold for SJIA patients following 6 months of subcutaneous dosing of 150 mg ILARIS every 8 weeks and 4mg/kg every 4 weeks, respectively.

Elimination
Clearance (CL) of canakinumab varied according to body weight and was estimated to be 0.174 L/day in a typical CAPS patient weighing 70 kg and 0.11 L/day in a SJIA patient weighing 33 kg. There was no indication of accelerated clearance or time-dependent change in the pharmacokinetic properties of canakinumab following repeated administration. No gender- or age-related pharmacokinetic differences were observed after correction for body weight.

Pediatrics
Pharmacokinetic properties are similar in CAPS and SJIA pediatric populations.
In CAPS patients, peak concentrations of canakinumab occurred between 2 to 7 days following single subcutaneous administration of ILARIS 150 mg or 2 mg/kg in pediatric patients. The terminal half-life ranged from 22.9 to 25.7 days, similar to the pharmacokinetic properties observed in adults.
In SJIA, exposure parameters (such as AUC and Cmax) were comparable across age groups from 2 years of age and above following subcutaneous administration of canakinumab 4 mg/kg every 4 weeks.

13 NONCLINICAL TOXICOLOGY
13.1 Carcinogenesis, Mutagenesis, Impairment of Fertility
Long-term animal studies have not been performed to evaluate the carcinogenic potential of canakinumab.
The mutagenic potential of canakinumab was not evaluated.
As canakinumab does not cross-react with rodent IL-1β, male and female fertility was evaluated in a mouse model using a murine analog of canakinumab. Male mice were treated weekly beginning 4 weeks prior to mating and continuing through 3 weeks after mating. Female mice were treated weekly for 2 weeks prior to mating through gestation day 3 or 4. The murine analog of canakinumab did not alter either male or female fertility parameters at subcutaneous doses up to 150 mg/kg.

14 CLINICAL STUDIES
14.1 Treatment of CAPS
The efficacy and safety of ILARIS for the treatment of CAPS was demonstrated in CAPS Study 1, a 3-part trial in patients 9 to 74 years of age with the MWS phenotype of CAPS. Throughout the trial, patients weighing more than 40 kg received ILARIS 150 mg and patients weighing 15 to 40 kg received 2 mg/kg. Part 1 was an 8-week open-label, single-dose period where all patients received ILARIS. Patients who achieved a complete clinical response and did not relapse by Week 8 were randomized into Part 2, a 24-week randomized, double-blind, placebo-controlled withdrawal period. Patients who completed Part 2 or experienced a disease flare entered Part 3, a 16-week open-label active treatment phase. A complete response was defined as ratings of minimal or better for physician's assessment of disease activity (PHY) and assessment of skin disease (SKD) and had

serum levels of C-Reactive Protein (CRP) and Serum Amyloid A (SAA) less than 10 mg/L. A disease flare was defined as a CRP and/or SAA values greater than 30 mg/L and either a score of mild or worse for PHY or a score of minimal or worse for PHY and SKD.

In Part 1, a complete clinical response was observed in 71% of patients one week following initiation of treatment and in 97% of patients by Week 8 (see Figure 1 and Table 2). In the randomized withdrawal period, a total of 81% of the patients randomized to placebo flared as compared to none (0%) of the patients randomized to ILARIS. The 95% confidence interval for treatment difference in the proportion of flares was 53% to 96%. At the end of Part 2, all 15 patients treated with ILARIS had absent or minimal disease activity and skin disease (see Table 3).

In a second trial, patients 4 to 74 years of age with both MWS and FCAS phenotypes of CAPS were treated in an open-label manner. Treatment with ILARIS resulted in clinically significant improvement of signs and symptoms and in normalization of high CRP and SAA in a majority of patients within 1 week.

[See table 3 at top of previous page]

Markers of inflammation CRP and SAA normalized within 8 days of treatment in the majority of patients. Normal mean CRP (Figure 1) and SAA values were sustained throughout CAPS Study 1 in patients continuously treated with canakinumab. After withdrawal of canakinumab in Part 2 CRP (figure 1) and SAA values again returned to abnormal values and subsequently normalized after reintroduction of canakinumab in Part 3. The pattern of normalization of CRP and SAA was similar.

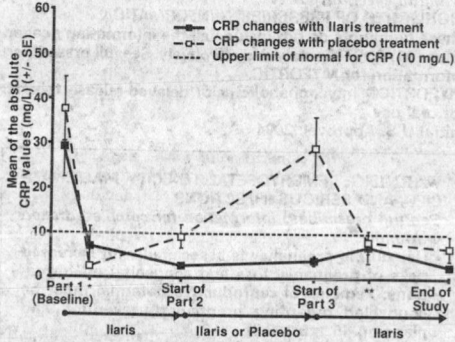

Figure 1. Mean C-Reactive Protein Levels at the End of Parts 1, 2 and 3 of CAPS Study 1

14.2 Treatment of SJIA

The efficacy of ILARIS for the treatment of active SJIA was assessed in two phase 3 studies (SJIA Study 1 and SJIA Study 2). Patients enrolled were aged 2 to less than 20 years (mean age at baseline: 8.5 years) with a confirmed diagnosis of SJIA at least 2 months before enrollment (mean disease duration at baseline: 3.5 years). Patients had active disease defined as greater than or equal to 2 joints with active arthritis (mean number of active joints at baseline: 15.4), documented spiking, intermittent fever (body temperature greater than 38°C) for at least 1 day within 1 week before study drug administration, and CRP greater than 30 mg/L (normal range less than 10 mg/L)(mean CRP at baseline: 200.5 mg/L). Patients were allowed to continue their stable dose of methotrexate, corticosteroids, and/or NSAIDs without change, except for tapering of the corticosteroid dose as per study design in SJIA Study 2 (see below).

SJIA Study 1 was a randomized, double-blind, placebo-controlled, single-dose 4-week study assessing the short term efficacy of ILARIS in 84 patients randomized to receive a single subcutaneous dose of 4 mg/kg ILARIS or placebo (43 patients received ILARIS and 41 patients received placebo). The primary objective of this study was to demonstrate the superiority of ILARIS versus placebo in the proportion of patients who achieved at least 30% improvement in an adapted pediatric American College of Rheumatology (ACR) response criterion which included both the pediatric ACR core set (ACR30 response) and absence of fever (temperature less than or equal to 38°C in the preceding 7 days) at Day 15.

Pediatric ACR responses are defined by achieving levels of percentage improvement (30%, 50%, and 70%) from baseline in at least 3 of the 6 core outcome variables, with worsening of greater than or equal to 30% in no more than one of the remaining variables. Core outcome variables included a physician global assessment of disease activity, parent or patient global assessment of wellbeing, number of joints with active arthritis, number of joints with limited range of motion, CRP, and functional ability (Childhood Health Assessment Questionnaire - CHAQ).

Table 4 Pediatric ACR response at Days 15 and 29

	Day 15			Day 29		
	ILARIS N=43	Placebo N=41	Weighted Difference[1] (95% CI)[2]	ILARIS N=43	Placebo N=41	Weighted Difference[1] (95% CI)[2]
ACR30	84%	10%	70% (56%, 84%)	81%	10%	70% (56%, 84%)
ACR50	67%	5%	65% (50%, 80%)	79%	5%	76% (63%, 88%)
ACR70	60%	2%	64% (49%, 79%)	67%	2%	67% (52%, 81%)

[1]Weighted difference is the difference between the ILARIS and placebo response rates, adjusted for the stratification factors (number of active joints, previous response to anakinra, and level of oral corticosteroid use)
[2]CI: confidence interval for the weighted difference

Figure 2. Kaplan Meier Estimates of the Probability to Stay Flare-Free in Part II of SJIA Study 2 by Treatment
*Very few patients were followed for more than 48 weeks

Percentages of patients by pediatric ACR response are presented in Table 4.

[See table 4 above]

Results for the components of the pediatric ACR core set were consistent with the overall ACR response results, for systemic and arthritic components including the reduction in the total number of active joints and joints with limited range of motion. Among the patients who returned for a Day 15 visit, the mean change in patient pain score (0-100 mm visual analogue scale) was -50.0 mm on ILARIS (N=43), as compared to +4.5 mm on placebo (N=25). The mean change in pain score among ILARIS treated patients was consistent through Day 29. All patients treated with ILARIS had no fever at Day 3 compared to 87% of patients treated with placebo.

SJIA Study 2 was a randomized, double-blind, placebo-controlled, withdrawal study of flare prevention by ILARIS in patients with active SJIA. Flare was defined by worsening of greater than or equal to 30% in at least 3 of the 6 core Pediatric ACR response variables combined with improvement of greater than or equal to 30% in no more than 1 of the 6 variables, or reappearance of fever not due to infection for at least 2 consecutive days. The study consisted of two major parts. 177 patients were enrolled in the study and received 4mg/kg ILARIS subcutaneously every 4 weeks in Part I and 100 of these patients continued into Part II to receive either ILARIS 4mg/kg or placebo subcutaneously every 4 weeks.

Corticosteroid dose tapering

Of the total 128 patients who entered the open-label portion of Study 2 taking corticosteroids, 92 attempted corticosteroid tapering. Fifty-seven (62%) of the 92 patients who attempted to taper were able to successfully taper their corticosteroid dose and 42 (46%) discontinued corticosteroids

Time to Flare

Part II was a randomized withdrawal design to demonstrate that the time to flare was longer with ILARIS than with placebo. Follow-up stopped when 37 events had been observed resulting in patients being followed for different lengths of time. The probability of experiencing a flare over time in Part II was statistically lower for the ILARIS treatment group than for the placebo group (Figure 2). This corresponded to a 64% relative reduction in the risk of flare for patients in the ILARIS group as compared to those in the placebo group (hazard ratio of 0.36; 95% CI: 0.17 to 0.75).

[See figure 2 above]

16 HOW SUPPLIED/STORAGE AND HANDLING

Carton of 1 vial   NDC 0078-0582-61

Each single-use vial of ILARIS contains a sterile, preservative free, white lyophilized powder containing 180 mg of canakinumab. Each vial is to be reconstituted with 1 mL of preservative-free Sterile Water for Injection resulting in a final concentration of 150 mg/mL.

Special Precautions for Storage

The unopened vial must be stored refrigerated at 2 to 8° C (36 to 46° F). Do not freeze. Store in the original carton to protect from light. Do not use beyond the date stamped on the label. After reconstitution, ILARIS should be kept from light, and can be kept at room temperature if used within 60 minutes of reconstitution. Otherwise, it should be refrigerated at 2 to 8° C (36 to 46° F) and used within 4 hours of reconstitution. ILARIS does not contain preservatives. Unused portions of ILARIS should be discarded.

Keep this and all drugs out of the reach of children.

17 PATIENT COUNSELING INFORMATION

See FDA-approved patient labeling (Medication Guide)
Patients should be advised of the potential benefits and risks of ILARIS. Physicians should instruct their patients to read the Medication Guide before starting ILARIS therapy.

Drug Administration

Patients should be advised that healthcare providers should perform administration of ILARIS, by the subcutaneous injection route.

Infections

Patients should be cautioned that ILARIS use has been associated with serious infections. Patients should be counseled to contact their healthcare professional immediately if they develop an infection after starting ILARIS. Treatment with ILARIS should be discontinued if a patient develops a serious infection. Patients should be counseled not to take any IL-1 blocking drug, including ILARIS, if they are also taking a drug that blocks TNF such as etanercept, infliximab, or adalimumab. Use of ILARIS with other IL-1 blocking agents, such as rilonacept and anakinra is not recommended. Patients should be cautioned not to receive ILARIS if they have a chronic or active infection, including HIV, Hepatitis B or Hepatitis C.

Vaccinations

Prior to initiation of therapy with ILARIS, physicians should review with adult and pediatric patients their vaccination history relative to current medical guidelines for vaccine use, including taking into account the potential of increased risk of infection during treatment with ILARIS.

Injection-site Reactions

Physicians should explain to patients that a very small number of patients in the clinical trials experienced a reaction at the subcutaneous injection site. Injection-site reactions may include pain, erythema, swelling, pruritus, bruising, mass, inflammation, dermatitis, edema, urticaria, vesicles, warmth, and hemorrhage. Healthcare providers should be cautioned to avoid injecting into an area that is already swollen or red. Any persistent reaction should be brought to the attention of the prescribing physician.

Hypersensitivity

Patients should be counseled to contact their healthcare provider immediately if they develop signs of allergic reaction such as difficulty breathing or swallowing, nausea, dizziness, skin rash, itching, hives, palpitations or low blood pressure.

Manufactured by:
Novartis Pharma Stein AG
Stein, Switzerland
Distributed by:
Novartis Pharmaceuticals Corporation
East Hanover, New Jersey 07936
© Novartis
T2013-33
May 2013

Medication Guide
ILARIS® (i-LAHR-us)
(canakinumab)
injection for subcutaneous use

What is the most important information I should know about ILARIS?
ILARIS can cause serious side effects, including:
• **Increased risk of serious infections.** ILARIS can lower the ability of your immune system to fight infections. Your healthcare provider should:
• test you for tuberculosis (TB) before you receive ILARIS
• monitor you closely for symptoms of TB during treatment with ILARIS
• check you for symptoms of any type of infection before, during, and after your treatment with ILARIS
Tell your healthcare provider right away if you have any symptoms of an infection such as fever, sweats or chills, cough, flu-like symptoms, weight loss, shortness of breath, blood in your phlegm, sores on your body, warm or painful areas on your body, diarrhea or stomach pain, or feeling very tired.

What is ILARIS?
ILARIS is a prescription medicine injected by your healthcare provider just below the skin (subcutaneous) used to treat:
• Adults and children 4 years of age and older who have auto-inflammatory diseases called Cryopyrin-Associated Syndromes (CAPS), including:
  ○ Familial Cold Auto-inflammatory Syndrome (FCAS)
  ○ Muckle-Wells Syndrome (MWS)
• Systemic Juvenile Idiopathic Arthritis (SJIA) in children 2 years of age and older.
It is not known if ILARIS is safe and effective when used to treat SJIA in children under 2 years of age or when used to treat CAPS in children under 4 years of age.

Who should not receive ILARIS?
• Do not receive ILARIS if you are allergic to canakinumab or any of the ingredients in ILARIS. See the end of this Medication Guide for a complete list of ingredients in ILARIS.

What should I tell my healthcare provider before receiving ILARIS?
Before you receive ILARIS, tell your healthcare provider about all your medical conditions, including if you:
• think you have or are being treated for an active infection
• have symptoms of an infection
• have a history of infections that keep coming back
• have a history of low white blood cells
• have or have had HIV, Hepatitis B, or Hepatitis C
• are scheduled to receive any immunizations (vaccines). You should not get 'live vaccines' if you are receiving ILARIS.
• are pregnant or planning to become pregnant. It is not known if ILARIS will harm your unborn baby. Tell your healthcare provider right away if you become pregnant while receiving ILARIS.
• are breastfeeding or planning to breastfeed. It is not known if ILARIS passes into your breast milk. You and your healthcare provider should decide if you will receive ILARIS or breastfeed. You should not do both.

Tell your healthcare provider about all the medicines you take, including prescription and nonprescription medicines, vitamins, and herbal supplements. Especially tell your healthcare provider if you take:

• Medicines that affect your immune system
• Medicines called IL-1 blocking agents such as Kineret® (anakinra), Arcalyst® (rilonacept)
• Medicines called Tumor Necrosis Factor (TNF) inhibitors such as Enbrel® (etanercept), Humira® (adalimumab), Remicade® (infliximab), Simponi® (golimumab), or Cimzia® (certolizumab pegol)
• Medicines that effect enzyme metabolism
Ask your healthcare provider if you are not sure.

How will I receive ILARIS?
• ILARIS is given by your healthcare provider every 8 weeks for CAPS and every 4 weeks for SJIA.

What are the possible side effects of ILARIS?
ILARIS can cause serious side effects, including:
• See "What is the most important information I should know about ILARIS?"
• **decreased ability of your body to fight infections (immunosuppression).** For people treated with medicines that cause immunosuppression like ILARIS, the chances of getting cancer may increase.
• **allergic reactions.** Allergic reactions can happen while you are receiving ILARIS. Call your healthcare provider right away if you have any of these symptoms of an allergic reaction:
  ○ rash
  ○ itching and hives
  ○ difficulty breathing or swallowing
  ○ dizziness or feeling faint
• **risk of infection with live vaccines.** You should not get live vaccines if you are receiving ILARIS. Tell your healthcare provider if you are scheduled to receive any vaccines.

The most common side effects of ILARIS include:
When ILARIS is used for the treatment of CAPS:
• cold symptoms
• diarrhea
• flu (influenza)
• runny nose
• nausea
• headache
• cough
• weight gain
• body aches
• feeling like you are spinning (vertigo)
• injection site reactions (such as redness, swelling, warmth, or itching)

When ILARIS is used for treatment of the SJIA:
• cold symptoms
• upper respiratory tract infection
• pneumonia
• runny nose
• sore throat
• urinary tract infection
• nausea, vomiting, and diarrhea (gastroenteritis)
• stomach pain
• injection site reactions
Tell your healthcare provider about any side effect that bothers you or does not go away. These are not all the possible side effects of ILARIS. For more information, ask your healthcare provider or pharmacist.
Call your doctor for medical advice about side effects. You may report side effects to FDA at 1-800-FDA-1088.

General information about the safe and effective use of ILARIS.
Medicines are sometimes prescribed for purposes other than those listed in Medication Guide. Do not use ILARIS for a condition for which it was not prescribed. Do not give ILARIS to other people, even if they have the same condition as you. It may harm them.
This Medication Guide summarizes the most important information about ILARIS. If you would like more information, talk with your healthcare provider. You can ask your healthcare provider or pharmacist for information about ILARIS that was written for health professionals. For more information about ILARIS, call 1-877-452-7471 or visit www.ILARIS.com.

What are the ingredients in ILARIS?
Active ingredient: canakinumab
Inactive ingredients: sucrose, L-histidine, L-histidine HCl monohydrate, polysorbate 80, preservative-free sterile water for injection

What are CAPS?
CAPS are a group of illnesses that run in families where patients make too much IL-1β. The IL-1β triggers inflammation. This leads to symptoms such as rash, fever/chills, joint pain, fatigue, and eye pain and redness.

What is SJIA?
SJIA is an autoinflammatory disorder which can be caused by having too much or being too sensitive to certain proteins, including interleukin-1β (IL-1β), and can lead to symptoms such as fever, rash, headache, fatigue, or painful joints and muscles.

What is Macrophage Activation Syndrome (MAS)?
MAS is a syndrome associated with SJIA that can lead to death. Tell your healthcare provider right away if your SJIA symptoms get worse or if you have any of these symptoms of an infection:
○ a fever lasting longer than 3 days
○ a cough that does not go away
○ redness in one part of your body
○ warm feeling or swelling of your skin
This Medication Guide has been approved by the U.S. Food and Drug Administration.
Manufactured by:
Novartis Pharma Stein AG
Stein, Switzerland
Distributed by:
Novartis Pharmaceuticals Corporation
East Hanover, New Jersey 07936
© Novartis
Kineret®, Arcalyst®, Enbrel®, Humira®, Remicade®, Simponi®, and Cimzia® are trademarks of Amgen, Regeneron, Immunex Corporation, Abbott Laboratories, Centocor Ortho Biotech Inc., Janssen Biotech Inc., and the UCB Group of companies, respectively.
T2013-34
Revised: May 2013
Shown in Product Identification Guide, page 310

MYFORTIC® ℞
[mi-for-tic]
(mycophenolic acid)
delayed-release tablets, for oral use

The following prescribing information is based on official labeling in effect July 2014.
HIGHLIGHTS OF PRESCRIBING INFORMATION
These highlights do not include all the information needed to use MYFORTIC safely and effectively. See full prescribing information for MYFORTIC.
MYFORTIC® (mycophenolic acid) delayed-release tablets, for oral use
Initial U.S. Approval: 2004

WARNING: EMBRYOFETAL TOXICITY, MALIGNANCIES, AND SERIOUS INFECTIONS
See full prescribing information for complete boxed warning
• **Use during pregnancy is associated with increased risks of pregnancy loss and congenital malformations. Females of reproductive potential must be counseled regarding pregnancy prevention and planning. (5.1, 8.1, 8.6)**
• **Increased risk of development of lymphoma and other malignancies, particularly of the skin, due to immunosuppression. (5.4)**
• **Increased susceptibility to bacterial, viral, fungal, and protozoal infections, including opportunistic infections. (5.5, 5.6)**
• **Only physicians experienced in immunosuppressive therapy and management of organ transplant patients should prescribe Myfortic. (5.3)**

——RECENT MAJOR CHANGES——
Warnings and Precautions, New or Reactivated
Viral Infections (5.6)   9/2013
——INDICATIONS AND USAGE——
• Myfortic is an antimetabolite immunosuppressant indicated for prophylaxis of organ rejection in adult patients receiving kidney transplants and in pediatric patients at least 5 years of age and older who are at least 6 months post kidney transplant. (1.1)
• Use in combination with cyclosporine and corticosteroids. (1.1)
Limitations of Use:
• Myfortic delayed release tablets and mycophenolate mofetil tablets and capsules should not be used interchangeably. (1.2)
——DOSAGE AND ADMINISTRATION——
• In adults: 720 mg by mouth, twice daily (1440 mg total daily dose) on an empty stomach, 1 hour before or 2 hours after food intake. (2.1)
• In children: 5 years of age and older (who are at least 6 months post kidney transplant), 400 mg/m² by mouth, twice daily (up to a maximum of 720 mg twice daily). (2.2)
• Do not crush, chew, or cut tablet prior to ingestion. (2.3)
——DOSAGE FORMS AND STRENGTHS——
Myfortic is available as 180 mg and 360 mg tablets. (3)
——CONTRAINDICATIONS——
Known hypersensitivity to mycophenolate sodium, mycophenolic acid, mycophenolate mofetil, or to any of its excipients. (4.1)
——WARNINGS AND PRECAUTIONS——
• New or Reactivated Viral Infections: Consider reducing immunosuppression. (5.6)
• Blood Dyscrasias including Pure Red Cell Aplasia (PRCA): Monitor for neutropenia or anemia; consider treatment interruption or dose reduction. (5.7)

- Serious GI Tract Complications (gastrointestinal bleeding, perforations and ulcers): Administer with caution to patients with active digestive system disease. (5.8)
- Immunizations: Avoid live vaccines. (5.9)
- Patients with Hereditary Deficiency of Hypoxanthine-guanine Phosphoribosyl-transferase (HGPRT): May cause exacerbation of disease symptoms; avoid use. (5.10)

-------ADVERSE REACTIONS-------

Most common adverse reactions (≥20%): anemia, leukopenia, constipation, nausea, diarrhea, vomiting, dyspepsia, urinary tract infection, CMV infection, insomnia, and postoperative pain. (6.2)

To report SUSPECTED ADVERSE REACTIONS, contact Novartis Pharmaceuticals Corporation at 1-888-669-6682 or FDA at 1-800-FDA-1088 or www.fda.gov/medwatch.

-------DRUG INTERACTIONS-------

- Antacids with Magnesium and Aluminum Hydroxides: Decreases concentrations of mycophenolic acid (MPA); concomitant use is not recommended. (7.1)
- Azathioprine: Competition for purine metabolism; concomitant administration is not recommended. (7.2)
- Cholestyramine, Bile Acid Sequestrates, Oral Activated Charcoal, and Other Drugs that Interfere with Enterohepatic Recirculation: May decrease MPA concentrations; concomitant use is not recommended. (7.3)
- Sevelamer: May decrease MPA concentrations; concomitant use is not recommended. (7.4)
- Cyclosporine: May decrease MPA concentrations; exercise caution when switching from cyclosporine to other drugs or from other drugs to cyclosporine. (7.5)
- Norfloxacin and Metronidazole: May decrease MPA concentrations; concomitant use with both drugs is not recommended. (7.6)
- Rifampin: May decrease MPA concentrations; concomitant use is not recommended unless the benefit outweighs the risk. (7.7)
- Hormonal Contraceptives: Additional barrier contraceptive methods must be used. (5.2, 7.8)
- Acyclovir, Valacyclovir, Ganciclovir, Valganciclovir, and Other Drugs that Undergo Renal Tubular Secretion: May increase concentrations of mycophenolic acid glucuronide (MPAG) and coadministered drug; monitor blood cell counts. (7.9)

-------USE IN SPECIFIC POPULATIONS-------

- Pregnancy: Can cause fetal harm. (5.1, 8.1)
- Nursing Mothers: Discontinue drug or discontinue nursing while on treatment or within 6 weeks after stopping therapy, taking into consideration the importance of the drug to the mother. (8.3)
- Females of reproductive potential must be counseled regarding pregnancy prevention and planning. (5.2, 8.6)

See 17 for PATIENT COUNSELING INFORMATION and Medication Guide

Revised: 9/2013

FULL PRESCRIBING INFORMATION: CONTENTS*

FULL PRESCRIBING INFORMATION

> **WARNING: EMBRYOFETAL TOXICITY, MALIGNANCIES, AND SERIOUS INFECTIONS**
> - Use during pregnancy is associated with increased risks of pregnancy loss and congenital malformations. Females of reproductive potential must be counseled regarding pregnancy prevention and planning [see *Warnings and Precautions (5.1), Use in Specific Populations (8.1, 8.6)*].
> - Increased risk of development of lymphoma and other malignancies, particularly of the skin, due to immunosuppression [see *Warnings and Precautions (5.4)*].
> - Increased susceptibility to bacterial, viral, fungal, and protozoal infections, including opportunistic infections [see *Warnings and Precautions (5.5, 5.6)*].
> - Only physicians experienced in immunosuppressive therapy and management of organ transplant patients should prescribe Myfortic. Patients receiving Myfortic should be managed in facilities equipped and staffed with adequate laboratory and supportive medical resources. The physician responsible for maintenance therapy should have complete information requisite for the follow-up of the patient [see *Warnings and Precautions (5.3)*].

1 INDICATIONS AND USAGE

1.1 Prophylaxis of Organ Rejection in Kidney Transplant

Myfortic® (mycophenolic acid) is indicated for the prophylaxis of organ rejection in adult patients receiving a kidney transplant.

Myfortic is indicated for the prophylaxis of organ rejection in pediatric patients 5 years of age and older who are at least 6 months post kidney transplant.

Myfortic is to be used in combination with cyclosporine and corticosteroids.

1.2 Limitations of Use

Myfortic delayed-release tablets and mycophenolate mofetil (MMF) tablets and capsules should not be used interchangeably without physician supervision because the rate of absorption following the administration of these two products is not equivalent.

2 DOSAGE AND ADMINISTRATION

2.1 Dosage in Adult Kidney Transplant Patients

The recommended dose of Myfortic is 720 mg administered twice daily (1440 mg total daily dose).

2.2 Dosage in Pediatric Kidney Transplant Patients

The recommended dose of Myfortic in conversion (at least 6 months post-transplant) pediatric patients age 5 years and older is 400 mg/m² body surface area (BSA) administered twice daily (up to a maximum dose of 720 mg administered twice daily).

2.3 Administration

Myfortic tablets should be taken on an empty stomach, 1 hour before or 2 hours after food intake [see *Clinical Pharmacology (12.3)*].

Myfortic tablets should not be crushed, chewed, or cut prior to ingesting. The tablets should be swallowed whole in order to maintain the integrity of the enteric coating.

Pediatric patients with a BSA of 1.19 to 1.58 m² may be dosed either with three Myfortic 180 mg tablets, or one 180 mg tablet plus one 360 mg tablet twice daily (1080 mg daily dose). Patients with a BSA of >1.58 m² may be dosed either with four Myfortic 180 mg tablets, or two Myfortic 360 mg tablets twice daily (1440 mg daily dose). Pediatric doses for patients with BSA <1.19 m² cannot be accurately administered using currently available formulations of Myfortic tablets.

3 DOSAGE FORMS AND STRENGTHS

Myfortic is available as 360 mg and 180 mg tablets.

Table 1: Description of Myfortic (mycophenolic acid) Delayed-Release Tablets

Dosage Strength	360 mg tablet	180 mg tablet
Active ingredient	mycophenolic acid as mycophenolate sodium	mycophenolic acid as mycophenolate sodium
Appearance	Pale orange-red film-coated ovaloid tablet	Lime green film-coated round tablet with bevelled edges
Imprint	"CT" on one side	"C" on one side

4 CONTRAINDICATIONS

4.1 Hypersensitivity Reactions

Myfortic is contraindicated in patients with a hypersensitivity to mycophenolate sodium, mycophenolic acid, mycophenolate mofetil, or to any of its excipients. Reactions like rash, pruritus, hypotension, and chest pain have been observed in clinical trials and post marketing reports [see *Adverse Reactions (6)*].

5 WARNINGS AND PRECAUTIONS

5.1 Embryofetal Toxicity

Use of Myfortic during pregnancy is associated with an increased risk of first trimester pregnancy loss and an increased risk of congenital malformations, especially external ear and other facial abnormalities including cleft lip and palate, and anomalies of the distal limbs, heart, esophagus, and kidney [see *Use in Specific Populations (8.1)*].

5.2 Pregnancy Exposure Prevention and Planning

Females of reproductive potential must be aware of the increased risk of first trimester pregnancy loss and congenital malformations and must be counseled regarding pregnancy prevention and planning. For recommended pregnancy testing and contraception methods see *Use in Specific Populations (8.6)*.

5.3 Management of Immunosuppression

Only physicians experienced in immunosuppressive therapy and management of organ transplant patients should prescribe Myfortic. Patients receiving the drug should be managed in facilities equipped and staffed with adequate laboratory and supportive medical resources. The physicians responsible for maintenance therapy should have complete information requisite for the follow-up of the patient [see *Boxed Warning*].

5.4 Lymphoma and Other Malignancies

Patients receiving immunosuppressants, including Myfortic, are at increased risk of developing lymphomas and other malignancies, particularly of the skin [see *Adverse Reactions (6)*]. The risk appears to be related to the intensity and duration of immunosuppression rather than to the use of any specific agent.

As usual for patients with increased risk for skin cancer, exposure to sunlight and UV light should be limited by wearing protective clothing and using a sunscreen with a high protection factor.

Post-transplant lymphoproliferative disorder (PTLD) has been reported in immunosuppressed organ transplant recipients. The majority of PTLD events appear related to Epstein Barr Virus (EBV) infection. The risk of PTLD appears greatest in those individuals who are EBV seronegative, a population which includes many young children.

5.5 Serious Infections

Patients receiving immunosuppressants, including Myfortic, are at increased risk of developing bacterial, viral, fungal, and protozoal infections, and new or reactivated viral infections including opportunistic infections [see *Warnings and Precautions (5.6)*]. These infections may lead to serious, including fatal outcomes. Because of the danger of oversuppression of the immune system which can increase susceptibility to infection, combination immunosuppressant therapy should be used with caution.

5.6 New or Reactivated Viral Infections

Polyomavirus associated nephropathy (PVAN), JC virus associated progressive multifocal leukoencephalopathy (PML), cytomegalovirus (CMV) infections, reactivation of hepatitis B (HBV) or hepatitis C (HCV) have been reported in patients treated with immunosuppressants, including the mycophenolic acid (MPA) derivatives Myfortic and

Table 2: Adverse Reactions (%) Reported in ≥10% of de novo Kidney Transplant Patients in Either Treatment Group

System organ class Adverse drug reactions	de novo Renal Trial	
	Myfortic 1.44 grams per day (n=213) (%)	mycophenolate mofetil (MMF) 2 grams per day (n=210) (%)
Blood and Lymphatic System Disorders		
Anemia	22	22
Leukopenia	19	21
Gastrointestinal System Disorders		
Constipation	38	40
Nausea	29	27
Diarrhea	24	25
Vomiting	23	20
Dyspepsia	23	19
Abdominal pain upper	14	14
Flatulence	10	13
General and Administrative Site Disorders		
Edema	17	18
Edema lower limb	16	17
Pyrexia	13	19
Investigations		
Increased blood creatinine	15	10
Infections and Infestations		
Urinary Tract Infection	29	33
CMV Infection	20	18
Metabolism and Nutrition Disorders		
Hypocalcemia	11	15
Hyperuricemia	13	13
Hyperlipidemia	12	10
Hypokalemia	13	9
Hypophosphatemia	11	9
Musculoskeletal, Connective Tissue and Bone Disorders		
Back pain	12	6
Arthralgia	7	11
Nervous System Disorder		
Insomnia	24	24
Tremor	12	14
Headache	13	11
Vascular Disorders		
Hypertension	18	18

**The trial was not designed to support comparative claims for Myfortic for the adverse reactions reported in this table.

MMF. Reduction in immunosuppression should be considered for patients who develop evidence of new or reactivated viral infections. Physicians should also consider the risk that reduced immunosuppression represents to the functioning allograft.

PVAN, especially due to BK virus infection, is associated with serious outcomes, including deteriorating renal function and renal graft loss. Patient monitoring may help detect patients at risk for PVAN.

PML, which is sometimes fatal, commonly presents with hemiparesis, apathy, confusion, cognitive deficiencies, and ataxia. Risk factors for PML include treatment with immunosuppressant therapies and impairment of immune function. In immunosuppressed patients, physicians should consider PML in the differential diagnosis in patients reporting neurological symptoms and consultation with a neurologist should be considered as clinically indicated.

The risk of CMV viremia and CMV disease is highest among transplant recipients seronegative for CMV at time of transplant who receive a graft from a CMV seropositive donor. Therapeutic approaches to limiting CMV disease exist and should be routinely provided. Patient monitoring may help detect patients at risk for CMV disease. [see Adverse Reactions (6.1)].

Viral reactivation has been reported in patients infected with HBV or HCV. Monitoring infected patients for clinical and laboratory signs of active HBV or HCV infection is recommended.

5.7   Blood Dyscrasias Including Pure Red Cell Aplasia
Cases of pure red cell aplasia (PRCA) have been reported in patients treated with MPA derivatives in combination with other immunosuppressive agents. The mechanism for MPA derivatives induced PRCA is unknown; the relative contribution of other immunosuppressants and their combinations in an immunosuppressive regimen is also unknown. In some cases PRCA was found to be reversible with dose reduction or cessation of therapy with MPA derivatives. In transplant patients, however, reduced immunosuppression may place the graft at risk. Changes to Myfortic therapy should only be undertaken under appropriate supervision in transplant recipients in order to minimize the risk of graft rejection.

Patients receiving Myfortic should be monitored for blood dyscrasias (e.g., neutropenia or anemia). The development of neutropenia may be related to Myfortic itself, concomitant medications, viral infections, or some combination of these reactions. Complete blood count should be performed weekly during the first month, twice monthly for the second and the third month of treatment, then monthly through the first year. If blood dyscrasias occur [neutropenia develops (ANC <1.3 × 10³/mcL) or anemia], dosing with Myfortic should be interrupted or the dose reduced, appropriate tests performed, and the patient managed accordingly.

5.8   Serious GI Tract Complications
Gastrointestinal bleeding (requiring hospitalization), intestinal perforations, gastric ulcers, and duodenal ulcers have been reported in patients treated with Myfortic. Myfortic should be administered with caution in patients with active serious digestive system disease.

5.9   Immunizations
The use of live attenuated vaccines should be avoided during treatment with Myfortic; examples include (but not limited to) the following: intranasal influenza, measles, mumps, rubella, oral polio, BCG, yellow fever, varicella, and TY21a typhoid vaccines.

5.10   Rare Hereditary Deficiencies
Myfortic is an inosine monophosphate dehydrogenase inhibitor (IMPDH Inhibitor). Myfortic should be avoided in patients with rare hereditary deficiency of hypoxanthine-guanine phosphoribosyl-transferase (HGPRT) such as Lesch-Nyhan and Kelley-Seegmiller syndromes because it may cause an exacerbation of disease symptoms characterized by the overproduction and accumulation of uric acid leading to symptoms associated with gout such as acute arthritis, tophi, nephrolithiasis or urolithiasis and renal disease including renal failure.

6   ADVERSE REACTIONS
The following adverse reactions are discussed in greater detail in other sections of the label.
- Embryofetal Toxicity [see Boxed Warning, Warnings and Precautions (5.1)]
- Lymphomas and Other Malignancies [see Boxed Warning, Warnings and Precautions (5.4)]
- Serious Infections [see Boxed Warning, Warnings and Precautions (5.5)]
- New or Reactivated Viral Infections [see Warnings and Precautions (5.6)]
- Blood Dyscrasias Including Pure Red Cell Aplasia [see Warnings and Precautions (5.7)]
- Serious GI Tract Complications [see Warnings and Precautions (5.8)]
- Rare Hereditary Deficiencies [see Warnings and Precautions (5.10)]

6.1   Clinical Studies Experience
Because clinical trials are conducted under widely varying conditions, adverse reaction rates observed in the clinical trials of a drug cannot be directly compared to rates in the clinical trials of another drug and may not reflect the rates observed in practice.

The data described below derive from two randomized, comparative, active-controlled, double-blind, double-dummy trials in prevention of acute rejection in de novo and converted stable kidney transplant patients.

In the de novo trial, patients were administered either Myfortic 1.44 grams per day (N=213) or MMF 2 grams per day (N=210) within 48 hours post-transplant for 12 months in combination with cyclosporine, USP MODIFIED and corticosteroids. Forty-one percent of patients also received antibody therapy as induction treatment. In the conversion trial, renal transplant patients who were at least 6 months post-transplant and receiving 2 grams per day MMF in combination with cyclosporine USP MODIFIED, with or without corticosteroids for at least two weeks prior to entry in the trial were randomized to Myfortic 1.44 grams per day (N=159) or MMF 2 grams per day (N=163) for 12 months.

The average age of patients in both studies was 47 years and 48 years (de novo study and conversion study, respectively), ranging from 22 to 75 years. Approximately 66% of patients were male; 82% were white, 12% were black, and 6% other races. About 40% of patients were from the United States and 60% from other countries.

In the de novo trial, the overall incidence of discontinuation due to adverse reactions was 18% (39/213) and 17% (35/210) in the Myfortic and MMF arms, respectively. The most common adverse reactions leading to discontinuation in the Myfortic arm were graft loss (2%), diarrhea (2%), vomiting (1%), renal impairment (1%), CMV infection (1%), and leukopenia (1%). The overall incidence of patients reporting dose reduction at least once during the 0 to 12 month study period was 59% and 60% in the Myfortic and MMF arms, respectively. The most frequent reasons for dose reduction in the Myfortic arm were adverse reactions (44%), dose reductions according to protocol guidelines (17%), dosing errors (11%) and missing data (2%).

The most common adverse reactions (≥20%) associated with the administration of Myfortic were anemia, leukopenia, constipation, nausea, diarrhea, vomiting, dyspepsia, urinary tract infection, CMV infection, insomnia, and postoperative pain.

The adverse reactions reported in ≥10% of patients in the de novo trial are presented in Table 2 below.
[See table 2 above]

Table 3 summarizes the incidence of opportunistic infections in de novo transplant patients.

Table 3: Viral and Fungal Infections (%) Reported Over 0 to 12 Months

	de novo Renal Trial	
	Myfortic 1.44 grams per day (n=213) (%)	mycophenolate mofetil (MMF) 2 grams per day (n=210) (%)
Any Cytomegalovirus	22	21
- Cytomegalovirus Disease	5	4
Herpes Simplex	8	6
Herpes Zoster	5	4
Any Fungal Infection	11	12
- Candida NOS	6	6
- Candida albicans	2	4

Lymphoma developed in 2 de novo patients (1%), (1 diagnosed 9 days after treatment initiation) and in 2 conversion patients (1%) receiving Myfortic with other immunosuppressive agents in the 12-month controlled clinical trials. Nonmelanoma skin carcinoma occurred in 1% de novo and 12% conversion patients. Other types of malignancy occurred in 1% de novo and 1% conversion patients [see Warnings and Precautions (5.4)].

The adverse reactions reported in <10% of de novo or conversion patients treated with Myfortic in combination with cyclosporine and corticosteroids are listed in Table 4.

Table 4: Adverse Reactions Reported in <10% of Patients Treated with Myfortic in Combination with Cyclosporine* and Corticosteroids

Blood and Lymphatic Disorders	Lymphocele, thrombocytopenia
Cardiac Disorder	Tachycardia
Eye Disorder	Vision blurred
Gastrointestinal Disorders	Abdominal pain, abdominal distension, gastroesophageal reflux disease, gingival hyperplasia
General Disorders and Administration Site Conditions	Fatigue, peripheral edema
Infections and Infestations	Nasopharyngitis, herpes simplex, upper respiratory infection, oral candidiasis, herpes zoster, sinusitis, influenza, wound infection, implant infection, pneumonia, sepsis
Investigations	Hemoglobin decrease, liver function tests abnormal
Metabolism and Nutrition Disorders	Hypercholesterolemia, hyperkalemia, hypomagnesemia, diabetes mellitus, hyperglycemia
Musculoskeletal and Connective Tissue Disorders	Arthralgia, pain in limb, peripheral swelling, muscle cramps, myalgia
Nervous System Disorders	Dizziness (excluding vertigo)
Psychiatric Disorders	Anxiety
Renal and Urinary Disorders	Renal tubular necrosis, renal impairment, hematuria, urinary retention
Respiratory, Thoracic and Mediastinal Disorders	Cough, dyspnea, dyspnea exertional
Skin and Subcutaneous Tissue Disorders	Acne, pruritus, rash
Vascular Disorders	Hypertension aggravated, hypotension

* USP MODIFIED

The following additional adverse reactions have been associated with the exposure to mycophenolic acid (MPA) when administered as a sodium salt or as mofetil ester:

Gastrointestinal: Intestinal perforation, gastrointestinal hemorrhage, gastric ulcers, duodenal ulcers [see *Warnings and Precautions (5.8)*], colitis (including CMV colitis), pancreatitis, esophagitis, and ileus.

Infections: Serious life-threatening infections such as meningitis and infectious endocarditis, tuberculosis, and atypical mycobacterial infection [see *Warnings and Precautions (5.5)*].

Respiratory: Interstitial lung disorders, including fatal pulmonary fibrosis.

6.2 Postmarketing Experience

The following adverse reactions have been identified during post-approval use of Myfortic or other MPA derivatives. Because these reactions are reported voluntarily from a population of uncertain size, it is not always possible to reliably estimate their frequency or establish a causal relationship to drug exposure.

- Congenital malformations and an increased incidence of first trimester pregnancy loss have been reported following exposure to MMF during pregnancy [see *Boxed Warning, Warnings and Precautions (5.1)*].
- Infections [see *Warnings and Precautions (5.5, 5.6)*]
  ○ Cases of progressive multifocal leukoencephalopathy (PML), sometimes fatal.
  ○ Polyomavirus associated nephropathy (PVAN), especially due to BK virus infection, associated with serious outcomes, including deteriorating renal function and renal graft loss.
  ○ Viral reactivation in patients infected with HBV or HCV.

- Cases of pure red cell aplasia (PRCA) have been reported in patients treated with MPA derivatives in combination with other immunosuppressive agents [see *Warnings and Precautions (5.7)*].

The following additional adverse reactions have been identified during postapproval use of Myfortic: agranulocytosis, asthenia, osteomyelitis, lymphadenopathy, lymphopenia, wheezing, dry mouth, gastritis, peritonitis, anorexia, alopecia, pulmonary edema, Kaposi's sarcoma.

7 DRUG INTERACTIONS

7.1 Antacids with Magnesium and Aluminum Hydroxides

Concomitant use of Myfortic and antacids decreased plasma concentrations of mycophenolic acid (MPA). It is recommended that Myfortic and antacids not be administered simultaneously [see *Clinical Pharmacology (12.3)*].

7.2 Azathioprine

Given that azathioprine and MMF inhibit purine metabolism, it is recommended that Myfortic not be administered concomitantly with azathioprine or MMF.

7.3 Cholestyramine, Bile Acid Sequestrates, Oral Activated Charcoal and Other Drugs that Interfere with Enterohepatic Recirculation

Drugs that interrupt enterohepatic recirculation may decrease MPA plasma concentrations when coadministered with MMF. Therefore, do not administer Myfortic with cholestyramine or other agents that may interfere with enterohepatic recirculation or drugs that may bind bile acids, e.g., bile acid sequestrates or oral activated charcoal, because of the potential to reduce the efficacy of Myfortic [see *Clinical Pharmacology (12.3)*].

7.4 Sevelamer

Concomitant administration of sevelamer and MMF may decrease MPA plasma concentrations. Sevelamer and other calcium free phosphate binders should not be administered simultaneously with Myfortic [see *Clinical Pharmacology (12.3)*].

7.5 Cyclosporine

Cyclosporine inhibits the enterohepatic recirculation of MPA, and therefore, MPA plasma concentrations may be decreased when Myfortic is coadministered with cyclosporine. Clinicians should be aware that there is also a potential change of MPA plasma concentrations after switching from cyclosporine to other immunosuppressive drugs or from other immunosuppressive drugs to cyclosporine in patients concomitantly receiving Myfortic [see *Clinical Pharmacology (12.3)*].

7.6 Norfloxacin and Metronidazole

MPA plasma concentrations may be decreased when MMF is administrated with norfloxacin and metronidazole. Therefore, Myfortic is not recommended to be given with the combination of norfloxacin and metronidazole. Although there will be no effect on MPA plasma concentrations when Myfortic is concomitantly administered with norfloxacin or metronidazole when given separately [see *Clinical Pharmacology (12.3)*].

7.7 Rifampin

The concomitant administration of MMF and rifampin may decrease MPA plasma concentrations. Therefore, Myfortic is not recommended to be given with rifampin concomitantly unless the benefit outweighs the risk [see *Clinical Pharmacology (12.3)*].

7.8 Hormonal Contraceptives

In a drug interaction study, mean levonorgestrel AUC was decreased by 15% when coadministered with MMF. Although Myfortic may not have any influence on the ovulation-suppressing action of oral contraceptives, it is recommended to coadminister Myfortic with hormonal contraceptives (e.g., birth control pill, transdermal patch, vaginal ring, injection, and implant) with caution, and additional barrier contraceptive methods must be used [see *Warnings and Precautions (5.2), Use in Specific Populations (8.6), and Clinical Pharmacology (12.3)*].

7.9 Acyclovir (Valacyclovir), Ganciclovir (Valganciclovir), and Other Drugs that Undergo Renal Tubular Secretion

The coadministration of MMF and acyclovir or ganciclovir may increase plasma concentrations of mycophenolic acid glucuronide (MPAG) and acyclovir/valacyclovir/ganciclovir/ valganciclovir as their coexistence competes for tubular secretion. Both acyclovir/valacyclovir/ganciclovir/valganciclovir and MPAG concentrations will be also increased in the presence of renal impairment.

Acyclovir/valacyclovir/ganciclovir/ valganciclovir may be taken with Myfortic; however, during the period of treatment, physicians should monitor blood cell counts [see *Clinical Pharmacology (12.3)*].

7.10 Ciprofloxacin, Amoxicillin plus Clavulanic Acid and Other Drugs that Alter the Gastrointestinal Flora

Drugs that alter the gastrointestinal flora such as ciprofloxacin or amoxicillin plus clavulanic acid may interact with MMF by disrupting enterohepatic recirculation. Interference of MPAG hydrolysis may lead to less MPA available for absorption when Myfortic is concomitantly administered

with ciprofloxacin or amoxicillin plus clavulanic acid. The clinical relevance of this interaction is unclear; however, no dose adjustment of Myfortic is needed when coadministered with these drugs [see *Clinical Pharmacology (12.3)*].

7.11 Pantoprazole

Administration of a pantoprazole at a dose of 40 mg twice daily for 4 days to healthy volunteers did not alter the pharmacokinetics of a single dose of Myfortic [see *Clinical Pharmacology (12.3)*].

8 USE IN SPECIFIC POPULATIONS

8.1 Pregnancy

Pregnancy Category D [*See Warnings and Precautions (5.1)*]

For those females using Myfortic at any time during pregnancy and those becoming pregnant within 6 weeks of discontinuing therapy, the healthcare practitioner should report the pregnancy to the Mycophenolate Pregnancy Registry (1-800-617-8191). The healthcare practitioner should strongly encourage the patient to enroll in the pregnancy registry. The information provided to the registry will help the Health Care Community to better understand the effects of mycophenolate in pregnancy.

Risk Summary

Following oral or intravenous (IV) administration, MMF is metabolized to mycophenolic acid (MPA), the active ingredient in Myfortic and the active form of the drug. Use of MMF during pregnancy is associated with an increased risk of first trimester pregnancy loss and an increased risk of congenital malformations, especially external ear and other facial abnormalities including cleft lip and palate, and anomalies of the distal limbs, heart, esophagus, and kidney. In animal studies, congenital malformations and pregnancy loss occurred when pregnant rats and rabbits received mycophenolic acid at dose multiples similar to and less than clinical doses.

Risks and benefits of Myfortic should be discussed with the patient. When appropriate, consider alternative immunosuppressants with less potential for embryofetal toxicity. In certain situations, the patient and her healthcare practitioner may decide that the maternal benefits outweigh the risks to the fetus. If this drug is used during pregnancy, or if the patient becomes pregnant while taking this drug, the patient should be apprised of the potential hazard to the fetus.

Data

Human Data

In the National Transplantation Pregnancy Registry (NTPR), there were data on 33 MMF-exposed pregnancies in 24 transplant patients; there were 15 spontaneous abortions (45%) and 18 live-born infants. Four of these 18 infants had structural malformations (22%). In postmarketing data (collected from 1995 to 2007) on 77 women exposed to systemic MMF during pregnancy, 25 had spontaneous abortions and 14 had a malformed infant or fetus. Six of 14 malformed offspring had ear abnormalities. Because these postmarketing data are reported voluntarily, it is not always possible to reliably estimate the frequency of particular adverse outcomes. These malformations are similar to findings in animal reproductive toxicology studies. For comparison, the background rate for congenital anomalies in the United States is about 3%, and NTPR data show a rate of 4%–5% among babies born to organ transplant patients using other immunosuppressive drugs. There are no relevant qualitative or quantitative differences in the teratogenic potential of mycophenolate sodium and MMF.

Animal Data

In a teratology study performed with mycophenolate sodium in rats, at a dose as low as 1 mg per kg, malformations in the offspring were observed, including anophthalmia, exencephaly, and umbilical hernia. The systemic exposure at this dose represents 0.05 times the clinical exposure at the dose of 1440 mg per day Myfortic. In teratology studies in rabbits, fetal resorptions and malformations occurred at doses equal to or greater than 80 mg per kg per day, in the absence of maternal toxicity (which corresponds to about 1.1 times the recommended clinical dose, based on body surface area).

8.3 Nursing Mothers

It is not known whether MPA is excreted in human milk. Because many drugs are excreted in human milk and because of the potential for serious adverse reactions in nursing infants from Myfortic, a decision should be made whether to discontinue nursing or discontinue the drug, taking into account the importance of the drug to the mother.

8.4 Pediatric Use

The safety and effectiveness of Myfortic have been established in pediatric kidney transplant patients 5 to 16 years of age who were initiated on Myfortic at least 6 months post-transplant. Use of Myfortic in this age group is supported by evidence from adequate and well-controlled studies of Myfortic in a similar population of adult kidney transplant patients with additional pharmacokinetic data in pediatric kidney transplant patients [see Dosage and Administration (2.2, 2.3), Clinical Pharmacology (12.3)]. Pediatric doses for patients with BSA <1.19 m² cannot be accurately administered using currently available formulations of Myfortic tablets.

The safety and effectiveness of Myfortic in de novo pediatric kidney transplant patients and in pediatric kidney transplant patients below the age of 5 years have not been established.

8.5 Geriatric Use

Clinical studies of Myfortic did not include sufficient numbers of subjects aged 65 and over to determine whether they respond differently from younger subjects. Of the 372 patients treated with Myfortic in the clinical trials, 6% (N=21) were 65 years of age and older and 0.3% (N=1) were 75 years of age and older. Other reported clinical experience has not identified differences in responses between the elderly and younger patients. In general, dose selection for an elderly patient should be cautious, reflecting the greater frequency of decreased hepatic, renal, or cardiac function, and of concomitant disease or other drug therapy.

8.6 Females of Reproductive Potential

Pregnancy Exposure Prevention and Planning

Females of reproductive potential must be made aware of the increased risk of first trimester pregnancy loss and congenital malformations and must be counseled regarding pregnancy prevention and planning.

Females of reproductive potential include girls who have entered puberty and all women who have a uterus and have not passed through menopause. Menopause is the permanent end of menstruation and fertility. Menopause should be clinically confirmed by a patient's healthcare practitioner. Some commonly used diagnostic criteria include 1) 12 months of spontaneous amenorrhea (not amenorrhea induced by a medical condition or medical therapy), or 2) postsurgical from a bilateral oophorectomy.

Pregnancy Testing

To prevent unplanned exposure during pregnancy, females of reproductive potential should have a serum or urine pregnancy test with a sensitivity of at least 25 mIU/mL immediately before starting Myfortic. Another pregnancy test with the same sensitivity should be done 8 to 10 days later. Repeat pregnancy tests should be performed during routine follow-up visits. Results of all pregnancy tests should be discussed with the patient.

In the event of a positive pregnancy test, females should be counseled with regard to whether the maternal benefits of mycophenolate treatment may outweigh the risks to the fetus in certain situations.

Contraception

Females of reproductive potential taking Myfortic must receive contraceptive counseling and use acceptable contraception (see Table 5 for Acceptable Contraception Methods). Patients must use acceptable birth control during entire Myfortic therapy, and for 6 weeks after stopping Myfortic, unless the patient chooses abstinence (she chooses to avoid heterosexual intercourse completely).

Patients should be aware that Myfortic reduces blood levels of the hormones in the oral contraceptive pill and could theoretically reduce its effectiveness [see Patient Counseling Information (17), Drug Interactions (7.8)].

Table 5: Acceptable Contraception Methods for Females of Reproductive Potential

Pick from the following birth control options:

Option 1		
Methods to Use Alone	Intrauterine devices (IUDs) Tubal sterilization Patient's partner had a vasectomy	

OR

Option 2	Hormone Methods choose 1	Barrier Methods choose 1
Choose One Hormone Method AND One Barrier Method	**Estrogen and Progesterone** Oral Contraceptive Pill Transdermal patch Vaginal ring **Progesterone-only** Injection	*AND* Diaphragm with spermicide Cervical cap with spermicide Contraceptive sponge Male condom Female condom

OR

Option 3	Barrier Methods choose 1		Barrier Methods choose 1
Choose One Barrier Method from each column (must choose two methods)	Diaphragm with spermicide Cervical cap with spermicide Contraceptive sponge	*AND*	Male condom Female condom

Pregnancy Planning

For patients who are considering pregnancy, consider alternative immunosuppressants with less potential for embryofetal toxicity. Risks and benefits of Myfortic should be discussed with the patient.

10 OVERDOSAGE

Signs and Symptoms

There have been anecdotal reports of deliberate or accidental overdoses with Myfortic, whereas not all patients experienced related adverse reactions.

In those overdose cases in which adverse reactions were reported, the reactions fall within the known safety profile of the class. Accordingly an overdose of Myfortic could possibly result in oversuppression of the immune system and may increase the susceptibility to infection including opportunistic infections, fatal infections and sepsis. If blood dyscrasias occur (e.g., neutropenia with absolute neutrophil count <1.5 × 10³/mcL or anemia), it may be appropriate to interrupt or discontinue Myfortic.

Possible signs and symptoms of acute overdose could include the following: hematological abnormalities such as leukopenia and neutropenia, and gastrointestinal symptoms such as abdominal pain, diarrhea, nausea and vomiting, and dyspepsia.

Treatment and Management

General supportive measures and symptomatic treatment should be followed in all cases of overdosage. Although dialysis may be used to remove the inactive metabolite mycophenolic acid glucuronide (MPAG), it would not be expected to remove clinically significant amounts of the active moiety, mycophenolic acid, due to the 98% plasma protein binding of mycophenolic acid. By interfering with enterohepatic circulation of mycophenolic acid, activated charcoal or bile sequestrates, such as cholestyramine, may reduce the systemic mycophenolic acid exposure.

11 DESCRIPTION

Myfortic® (mycophenolic acid) delayed-release tablets are an enteric formulation of mycophenolate sodium that delivers the active moiety mycophenolic acid (MPA). Myfortic is an immunosuppressive agent. As the sodium salt, MPA is chemically designated as (E)-6-(4-hydroxy-6-methoxy-7-methyl-3-oxo-1,3-dihydroisobenzofuran-5-yl)-4-methylhex-4-enoic acid sodium salt.

Its empirical formula is $C_{17}H_{19}O_6Na$. The molecular weight is 342.32 and the structural formula is:

Myfortic, as the sodium salt, is a white to off-white, crystalline powder and is highly soluble in aqueous media at physiological pH and practically insoluble in 0.1N hydrochloric acid.

Myfortic is available for oral use as delayed-release tablets containing either 180 mg or 360 mg of mycophenolic acid. Inactive ingredients include colloidal silicon dioxide, crospovidone, lactose anhydrous, magnesium stearate, povidone (K-30), and starch. The enteric coating of the tablet consists of hypromellose phthalate, titanium dioxide, iron oxide yellow, and indigotine (180 mg) or iron oxide red (360 mg).

12 CLINICAL PHARMACOLOGY

12.1 Mechanism of Action

Mycophenolic acid (MPA), an immunosuppressant, is an uncompetitive and reversible inhibitor of inosine monophosphate dehydrogenase (IMPDH), and therefore inhibits the de novo pathway of guanosine nucleotide synthesis without incorporation to DNA. T- and B-lymphocytes are critically dependent for their proliferation on de novo synthesis of purines, whereas other cell types can utilize salvage pathways. MPA has cytostatic effects on lymphocytes.

Mycophenolate sodium has been shown to prevent the occurrence of acute rejection in rat models of kidney and heart allotransplantation. Mycophenolate sodium also decreases antibody production in mice.

12.3 Pharmacokinetics

Myfortic exhibits linear and dose-proportional pharmacokinetics over the dose-range (360 to 2160 mg) evaluated. The absolute bioavailability of Myfortic in stable renal transplant patients on cyclosporine was 72%. MPA is highly protein bound (>98% bound to albumin). The predominant metabolite of MPA is the phenolic glucuronide (MPAG) which is pharmacologically inactive. A minor metabolite AcMPAG which is an acyl glucuronide of MPA is also formed and has pharmacological activity comparable to MPA. MPAG undergoes renal elimination. A fraction of MPAG also undergoes biliary excretion, followed by deconjugation by gut flora and subsequent reabsorption as MPA. The mean elimination half-lives of MPA and MPAG ranged between 8 and 16 hours, and 13 and 17 hours, respectively.

Absorption

In vitro studies demonstrated that the enteric-coated Myfortic tablet does not release MPA under acidic conditions (pH <5) as in the stomach but is highly soluble in neutral pH conditions as in the intestine. Following Myfortic oral administration without food in several pharmacokinetic studies conducted in renal transplant patients, consistent with its enteric-coated formulation, the median delay (T_{lag}) in the rise of MPA concentration ranged between 0.25 and 1.25 hours and the median time to maximum concentration (T_{max}) of MPA ranged between 1.5 and 2.75 hours. In comparison, following the administration of MMF, the median T_{max} ranged between 0.5 and 1.0 hours. In stable renal transplant patients on cyclosporine, USP MODIFIED based immunosuppression, gastrointestinal absorption and absolute bioavailability of MPA following the administration of Myfortic delayed-release tablet was 93% and 72%, respectively. Myfortic pharmacokinetics is dose proportional over the dose range of 360 to 2160 mg.

Distribution

The mean (± SD) volume of distribution at steady state and elimination phase for MPA is 54 (± 25) L and 112 (± 48) L, respectively. MPA is highly protein bound to albumin, >98%. The protein binding of mycophenolic acid glucuronide (MPAG) is 82%. The free MPA concentration may increase under conditions of decreased protein binding (uremia, hepatic failure, and hypoalbuminemia).

Metabolism

MPA is metabolized principally by glucuronyl transferase to glucuronidated metabolites. The phenolic glucuronide of MPA, mycophenolic acid glucuronide (MPAG), is the predominant metabolite of MPA and does not manifest pharmacological activity. The acyl glucuronide is a minor metabolite and has comparable pharmacological activity to MPA. In stable renal transplant patients on cyclosporine, USP MODIFIED based immunosuppression, approximately 28% of the oral Myfortic dose was converted to MPAG by presystemic metabolism. The AUC ratio of MPA:MPAG:acyl glucuronide is approximately 1:24:0.28 at steady state. The mean clearance of MPA was 140 (± 30) mL/min.

Elimination

The majority of MPA dose administered is eliminated in the urine primarily as MPAG (>60%) and approximately 3% as unchanged MPA following Myfortic administration to stable renal transplant patients. The mean renal clearance of MPAG was 15.5 (± 5.9) mL/min. MPAG is also secreted in the bile and available for deconjugation by gut flora. MPA resulting from the deconjugation may then be reabsorbed and produce a second peak of MPA approximately 6 to 8 hours after Myfortic dosing. The mean elimination half-life of MPA and MPAG ranged between 8 and 16 hours, and 13 and 17 hours, respectively.

Food Effect

Compared to the fasting state, administration of Myfortic 720 mg with a high-fat meal (55 g fat, 1000 calories) had no effect on the systemic exposure (AUC) of MPA. However, there was a 33% decrease in the maximal concentration (C_{max}), a 3.5-hour delay in the T_{lag} (range, -6 to 18 hours), and 5.0-hour delay in the T_{max} (range, -9 to 20 hours) of MPA. To avoid the variability in MPA absorption between doses, Myfortic should be taken on an empty stomach [see Dosage and Administration (2.3)].

Pharmacokinetics in Renal Transplant Patients

The mean pharmacokinetic parameters for MPA following the administration of Myfortic in renal transplant patients on cyclosporine, USP MODIFIED based immunosuppression are shown in Table 6. Single-dose Myfortic pharmacokinetics predicts multiple-dose pharmacokinetics. However, in the early post-transplant period, mean MPA AUC and C_{max} were approximately one-half of those measured 6 months post-transplant.

After near equimolar dosing of Myfortic 720 mg twice daily and MMF 1000 mg twice daily (739 mg as MPA) in both the single- and multiple-dose cross-over trials, mean systemic MPA exposure (AUC) was similar.

[See table 6 above]

Specific Populations

Renal Insufficiency: No specific pharmacokinetic studies in individuals with renal impairment were conducted with Myfortic. However, based on studies of renal impairment with MMF, MPA exposure is not expected to be appreciably increased over the range of normal to severely impaired renal function following Myfortic administration. In contrast, MPAG exposure would be increased markedly with decreased renal function; MPAG exposure being approximately 8-fold higher in the setting of anuria. Although dialysis may be used to remove the inactive metabolite MPAG, it would not be expected to remove clinically significant amounts of the active moiety MPA. This is in large part due to the high plasma protein binding of MPA.

Hepatic Insufficiency: No specific pharmacokinetic studies in individuals with hepatic impairment were conducted with Myfortic. In a single dose (MMF 1000 mg) trial of 18 volunteers with alcoholic cirrhosis and 6 healthy volunteers, hepatic MPA glucuronidation processes appeared to be relatively unaffected by hepatic parenchymal disease when the pharmacokinetic parameters of healthy volunteers and alcoholic cirrhosis patients within this trial were compared. However, it should be noted that for unexplained reasons, the healthy volunteers in this trial had about a 50% lower AUC compared to healthy volunteers in other studies, thus making comparison between volunteers with alcoholic cirrhosis and healthy volunteers difficult. Effects of hepatic disease on this process probably depend on the particular disease. Hepatic disease, such as primary biliary cirrhosis, with other etiologies may show a different effect.

Pediatrics: Limited data are available on the use of Myfortic at a dose of 450 mg/m² body surface area in children. The mean MPA pharmacokinetic parameters for stable pediatric renal transplant patients, 5 to 16 years, on cyclosporine, USP MODIFIED are shown in Table 6. At the same dose administered based on body surface area, the respective mean C_{max} and AUC of MPA determined in children were higher by 33% and 18% than those determined for adults. The clinical impact of the increase in MPA exposure is not known [see *Dosage and Administration (2.2, 2.3)*].

Gender: There are no significant gender differences in Myfortic pharmacokinetics.

Elderly: Pharmacokinetics in the elderly have not been formally studied.

Ethnicity: Following a single dose administration of 720 mg of Myfortic to 18 Japanese and 18 Caucasian healthy subjects, the exposure (AUC_{inf}) for MPA and MPAG were 15% and 22% lower in Japanese subjects compared to Caucasians. The peak concentrations (C_{max}) for MPAG were similar between the two populations, however, Japanese subjects had 9.6% higher C_{max} for MPA. These results do not suggest any clinically relevant differences.

Drug Interactions:

Antacids with Magnesium and Aluminum Hydroxides: Absorption of a single dose of Myfortic was decreased when administered to 12 stable kidney transplant patients also taking magnesium-aluminum-containing antacids (30 mL): the mean C_{max} and $AUC_{(0-t)}$ values for MPA were 25% and 37% lower, respectively, than when Myfortic was administered alone under fasting conditions [see *Drug Interactions (7.1)*].

Pantoprazole: In a trial conducted in 12 healthy volunteers, the pharmacokinetics of MPA were observed to be similar when a single dose of 720 mg of Myfortic was administered alone and following concomitant administration of Myfortic and pantoprazole, which was administered at a dose of 40 mg twice daily for 4 days [see *Drug Interactions (7.11)*].

The following drug interaction studies were conducted following the administration of MMF:

Cholestyramine: Following single-dose oral administration of 1.5 grams MMF to 12 healthy volunteers pretreated with 4 grams three times daily of cholestyramine for 4 days, MPA AUC decreased approximately 40%. This decrease is consistent with interruption of enterohepatic recirculation which may be due to binding of recirculating MPAG with cholestyramine in the intestine [see *Drug Interactions (7.3)*].

Sevelamer: Concomitant administration of sevelamer and MMF in stable adult and pediatric kidney transplant patients decreased the mean MPA C_{max} and $AUC_{(0-12h)}$ by 36% and 26% respectively [see *Drug Interactions (7.4)*].

Cyclosporine: Cyclosporine (Sandimmune®) pharmacokinetics (at doses of 275 to 415 mg/day) was unaffected by single and multiple doses of 1.5 grams twice daily of MMF in 10 stable kidney transplant patients. The mean (±SD) $AUC_{(0-12h)}$ and C_{max} of cyclosporine after 14 days of multiple doses of MMF were 3290 (±822) ng•h/mL and 753 (±161) ng/mL, respectively, compared to 3245 (±1088) ng•h/mL and 700 (±246) ng/mL, respectively, 1 week before administration of MMF.

A total of 73 *de novo* kidney allograft recipients on MMF therapy received either low dose cyclosporine withdrawal by 6 months post-transplant (50 to 100 ng/mL for up to 3 months post-transplant followed by complete withdrawal at month 6 post-transplant) or standard dose cyclosporine (150 to 300 ng/mL from baseline through to month 4 post-transplant and 100 to 200 ng/mL thereafter). At month 12 post-transplant, the mean MPA ($AUC_{(0-12h)}$) in the cyclosporine withdrawal group was approximately 40% higher, than that of the standard dose cyclosporine group.

Cyclosporine inhibits multidrug-resistance-associated protein 2 (MRP-2) transporter in the biliary tract, thereby preventing the excretion of MPAG into the bile that would lead to enterohepatic recirculation of MPA [see *Drug Interactions (7.5)*].

Norfloxacin and Metronidazole: Following single-dose administration of MMF (1 g) to 11 healthy volunteers on day 4 of a 5-day course of a combination of norfloxacin and metronidazole, the mean MPA $AUC_{(0-48h)}$ was reduced by 33% compared to the administration of MMF alone (p<0.05). There was no significant effect on mean MPA $AUC_{(0-48h)}$ when MMF was concomitantly administered with norfloxacin or metronidazole separately. The mean (±SD) MPA $AUC_{(0-48h)}$ after coadministration of MMF with norfloxacin or metronidazole separately was 48.3 (±24) mcg•h/mL and 42.7 (±23) mcg•h/mL, respectively, compared with 56.2 (±24) mcg•h/mL after administration of MMF alone [see *Drug Interactions (7.6)*].

Rifampin: In a single heart-lung transplant patient on MMF therapy (1 gram twice daily), a 67% decrease in MPA exposure ($AUC_{(0-12h)}$) was observed with concomitant administration of MMF and 600 mg rifampin daily.

In 8 kidney transplant patients on stable MMF therapy (1 gram twice daily), administration of 300 mg rifampin twice daily resulted in a 17.5% decrease in MPA $AUC_{(0-12h)}$ due to inhibition of enterohepatic recirculation of MPAG by rifampin. Rifampin coadministration also resulted in a 22.4% increase in MPAG $AUC_{(0-12h)}$ [see *Drug Interactions (7.7)*].

Oral Contraceptives: In a drug-drug interaction trial, mean AUCs were similar for ethinyl estradiol and norethindrone, when coadministered with MMF as compared to administration of the oral contraceptives alone [see *Drug Interactions (7.8)*].

Acyclovir: Coadministration of MMF (1 gram) and acyclovir (800 mg) to 12 healthy volunteers resulted in no significant change in MPA AUC and C_{max}. However, MPAG and acyclovir plasma mean $AUC_{(0-24h)}$ were increased 10% and 18%, respectively. Because MPAG plasma concentrations are increased in the presence of kidney impairment, as are acyclovir concentrations, the potential exists for mycophenolate and acyclovir or its prodrug (e.g., valacyclovir) to compete for tubular secretion, further increasing the concentrations of both drugs [see *Drug Interactions (7.9)*].

Ganciclovir: Following single-dose administration to 12 stable kidney transplant patients, no pharmacokinetic interaction was observed between MMF (1.5 grams) and intravenous ganciclovir (5 mg per kg). Mean (±SD) ganciclovir AUC and C_{max} (n=10) were 54.3 (±19.0) mcg•h/mL and 11.5 (±1.8) mcg/mL, respectively, after coadministration of the two drugs, compared to 51.0 (±17.0) mcg•h/mL and 10.6 (±2.0) mcg/mL, respectively, after administration of intravenous ganciclovir alone. The mean (±SD) AUC and C_{max} of MPA (n=12) after coadministration were 80.9 (±21.6) mcg•h/mL and 27.8 (±13.9) mcg/mL, respectively, compared to values of 80.3 (±16.4) mcg•h/mL and 30.9 (±11.2) mcg/mL, respectively, after administration of MMF alone.

Because MPAG plasma concentrations are increased in the presence of renal impairment, as are ganciclovir concentrations, the two drugs will compete for tubular secretion and thus further increases in concentrations of both drugs may occur. In patients with renal impairment in which MMF and ganciclovir or its prodrug (e.g., valganciclovir) are coadministered, patients should be monitored carefully [see *Drug Interactions (7.9)*].

Ciprofloxacin and Amoxicillin plus Clavulanic Acid: A total of 64 MMF treated kidney transplant recipients received either oral ciprofloxacin 500 mg twice daily or amoxicillin plus clavulanic acid 375 mg three times daily for 7 or at least 14 days. Approximately 50% reductions in median trough MPA concentrations (predose) from baseline (MMF alone) were observed in 3 days following commencement of oral ciprofloxacin or amoxicillin plus clavulanic acid. These reductions in trough MPA concentrations tended to diminish within 14 days of antibiotic therapy and ceased within 3 days after discontinuation of antibiotics. The postulated mechanism for this interaction is an antibiotic-induced reduction in glucuronidase-possessing enteric organisms leading to a decrease in enterohepatic recirculation of MPA. The change in trough level may not accurately represent changes in overall MPA exposure; therefore, clinical relevance of these observations is unclear [see *Drug Interactions (7.10)*].

13 NONCLINICAL TOXICOLOGY

13.1 Carcinogenesis, Mutagenesis, Impairment of Fertility

In a 104-week oral carcinogenicity study in rats, mycophenolate sodium was not tumorigenic at daily doses up to 9 mg per kg, the highest dose tested. This dose resulted in approximately 0.6 to 1.2 times the systemic exposure (based on plasma AUC) observed in renal transplant patients at the recommended dose of 1440 mg per day. Similar results were observed in a parallel study in rats performed with MMF. In a 104-week oral carcinogenicity study in mice, MMF was not tumorigenic at a daily dose level as high as 180 mg per kg (which corresponds to 0.6 times the recommended mycophenolate sodium therapeutic dose, based on body surface area).

The genotoxic potential of mycophenolate sodium was determined in five assays. Mycophenolate sodium was genotoxic in the mouse lymphoma/thymidine kinase assay, the micronucleus test in V79 Chinese hamster cells, and the in vivo mouse micronucleus assay. Mycophenolate sodium was not genotoxic in the bacterial mutation assay (*Salmonella typhimurium* TA 1535, 97a, 98, 100, and 102) or the chromosomal aberration assay in human lymphocytes.

Mycophenolate mofetil generated similar genotoxic activity. The genotoxic activity of mycophenolic acid (MPA) is probably due to the depletion of the nucleotide pool required for DNA synthesis as a result of the pharmacodynamic mode of action of MPA (inhibition of nucleotide synthesis).

Mycophenolate sodium had no effect on male rat fertility at daily oral doses as high as 18 mg per kg and exhibited no testicular or spermatogenic effects at daily oral doses of 20 mg per kg for 13 weeks (approximately 2 times the systemic exposure of MPA at the recommended therapeutic dose). No effects on female fertility were seen up to a daily dose of 20 mg per kg (approximately 3 times the systemic exposure of MPA at the recommended therapeutic dose).

14 CLINICAL STUDIES

14.1 Prophylaxis of Organ Rejection in Patients Receiving Allogeneic Renal Transplants

The safety and efficacy of Myfortic in combination with cyclosporine, USP MODIFIED and corticosteroids for the prevention of organ rejection was assessed in two multicenter, randomized, double-blind, active-controlled trials in *de novo* and conversion renal transplant patients compared to MMF. The *de novo* trial was conducted in 423 renal transplant patients (ages 18–75 years) in Austria, Canada, Germany, Hungary, Italy, Norway, Spain, UK, and USA. Eighty-four percent of randomized patients received kidneys from deceased donors. Patients were excluded if they had second or multiorgan (e.g., kidney and pancreas) transplants, or pre-

Table 6: Mean ± SD Pharmacokinetic Parameters for MPA Following the Oral Administration of Myfortic to Renal Transplant Patients on Cyclosporine, USP MODIFIED Based Immunosuppression

Patient	Myfortic Dosing	N	Dose (mg)	T_{max}*(h)	C_{max} (mcg/mL)	$AUC_{(0-12h)}$ (mcg*h/mL)
Adult	Single	24	720	2 (0.8-8)	26.1 ± 12.0	66.5 ± 22.6**
Pediatric***	Single	10	450/m²	2.5 (1.5-24)	36.3 ± 20.9	74.3 ± 22.5**
Adult	Multiple x6 days, twice daily	10	720	2 (1.5-3.0)	37.0 ± 13.3	67.9 ± 20.3
Adult	Multiple x28 days, twice daily	36	720	2.5 (1.5-8)	31.2 ± 18.1	71.2 ± 26.3
Adult	Chronic, multiple dose, twice daily					
	2 weeks post-transplant	12	720	1.8 (1.0-5.3)	15.0 ± 10.7	28.6 ± 11.5
	3 months post-transplant	12	720	2 (0.5-2.5)	26.2 ± 12.7	52.3 ± 17.4
	6 months post-transplant	12	720	2 (0-3)	24.1 ± 9.6	57.2 ± 15.3
Adult	Chronic, multiple dose, twice daily	18	720	1.5 (0-6)	18.9 ± 7.9	57.4 ± 15.0

*median (range), **AUC_{inf}, ***age range of 5–16 years

Table 7: Treatment Failure in de novo Renal Transplant Patients (Percent of Patients) at 6 and 12 Months of Treatment when Administered in Combination with Cyclosporine* and Corticosteroids

	Myfortic 1.44 grams per day (n=213)	mycophenolate mofetil (MMF) 2 grams per day (n=210)
6 Months	n (%)	n (%)
Treatment failure#	55 (25.8)	55 (26.2)
Biopsy-proven acute rejection	46 (21.6)	48 (22.9)
Graft loss	7 (3.3)	9 (4.3)
Death	1 (0.5)	2 (1.0)
Lost to follow-up**	3 (1.4)	0
12 Months	n (%)	n (%)
Graft loss or death or lost to follow-up***	20 (9.4)	18 (8.6)
Treatment failure##	61 (28.6)	59 (28.1)
Biopsy-proven acute rejection	48 (22.5)	51 (24.3)
Graft loss	9 (4.2)	9 (4.3)
Death	2 (0.9)	5 (2.4)
Lost to follow-up**	5 (2.3)	0

*USP MODIFIED
**Lost to follow-up indicates patients who were lost to follow-up without prior biopsy-proven acute rejection, graft loss or death
***Lost to follow-up indicates patients who were lost to follow-up without prior graft loss or death (9 Myfortic patients and 4 MMF patients)
#95% confidence interval of the difference in treatment failure at 6 months (Myfortic–MMF) is (-8.7%, 8.0%).
##95% confidence interval of the difference in treatment failure at 12 months (Myfortic–MMF) is (-8.0%, 9.1%).

Table 8: Treatment Failure in Conversion Transplant Patients (Percent of Patients) at 6 and 12 Months of Treatment when Administered in Combination with Cyclosporine* and with or without Corticosteroids

	Myfortic 1.44 grams per day (n=159)	mycophenolate mofetil (MMF) 2 grams per day (n=163)
6 Months	n (%)	n (%)
Treatment failure#	7 (4.4)	11 (6.7)
Biopsy-proven acute rejection	2 (1.3)	2 (1.2)
Graft loss	0	1 (0.6)
Death	0	1 (0.6)
Lost to follow-up**	5 (3.1)	7 (4.3)
12 Months	n (%)	n (%)
Graft loss or death or lost to follow-up***	10 (6.3)	17 (10.4)
Treatment failure##	12 (7.5)	20 (12.3)
Biopsy-proven acute rejection	2 (1.3)	5 (3.1)
Graft loss	0	1 (0.6)
Death	2 (1.3)	4 (2.5)
Lost to follow-up**	8 (5.0)	10 (6.1)

*USP MODIFIED
**Lost to follow-up indicates patients who were lost to follow-up without prior biopsy-proven acute rejection, graft loss, or death
***Lost to follow-up indicates patients who were lost to follow-up without prior graft loss or death (8 Myfortic patients and 12 MMF patients)
#95% confidence interval of the difference in treatment failure at 6 months (Myfortic–MMF) is (-7.3%, 2.7%).
##95% confidence interval of the difference in treatment failure at 12 months (Myfortic–MMF) is (-11.2%, 1.8%).

vious transplant with any other organs; kidneys from non-heart beating donors; panel reactive antibodies (PRA) of >50% at last assessment prior to transplantation, and presence of severe diarrhea, active peptic ulcer disease, or uncontrolled diabetes mellitus. Patients were administered either Myfortic 1.44 grams per day or MMF 2 grams per day within 48 hours post-transplant for 12 months in combination with cyclosporine, USP MODIFIED and corticosteroids. Forty-one percent of patients received antibody therapy as induction treatment. Treatment failure was defined as the first occurrence of biopsy proven acute rejection, graft loss, death or lost to follow-up at 6 months.
The incidence of treatment failure was similar in Myfortic- and MMF-treated patients at 6 and 12 months (Table 7). The cumulative incidence of graft loss, death and lost to follow-up at 12 months is also shown in Table 7.
[See table 7 above]
The conversion trial was conducted in 322 renal transplant patients (ages 18–75 years), who were at least 6 months post-transplant and had undergone primary or secondary, deceased donor, living related, or unrelated donor kidney transplant, stable graft function (serum creatinine <2.3 mg/mL), no change in immunosuppressive regimen due to graft malfunction, and no known clinically significant physical and/or laboratory changes for at least 2 months prior to enrollment. Patients were excluded if they had 3 or more kidney transplants, multiorgan transplants (e.g., kidney and pancreas), previous organ transplants, evidence of graft rejection or who had been treated for acute rejection within 2 months prior to screening, clinically significant infections requiring continued therapy, presence of severe diarrhea, active peptic ulcer disease, or uncontrolled diabetes mellitus.

Patients received 2 grams per day MMF in combination with cyclosporine USP MODIFIED, with or without corticosteroids for at least two weeks prior to entry in the trial. Patients were randomized to Myfortic 1.44 grams per day or MMF 2 grams per day for 12 months. The trial was conducted in Austria, Belgium, Canada, Germany, Italy, Spain, and USA. Treatment failure was defined as the first occurrence of biopsy-proven acute rejection, graft loss, death, or lost to follow-up at 6 and 12 months.
The incidences of treatment failure at 6 and 12 months were similar between Myfortic- and MMF-treated patients (Table 8). The cumulative incidence of graft loss, death and lost to follow-up at 12 months is also shown in Table 8.
[See table 8 above]

16 HOW SUPPLIED/STORAGE AND HANDLING

360 mg tablet: Pale orange-red film-coated ovaloid tablet with imprint (debossing) "CT" on one side, containing 360 mg mycophenolic acid (MPA) as mycophenolate sodium.

Bottles of 120.. NDC 0078-0386-66

180 mg tablet: Lime green film-coated round tablet with bevelled edges and the imprint (debossing) "C" on one side, containing 180 mg mycophenolic acid (MPA) as mycophenolate sodium.

Bottles of 120.. NDC 0078-0385-66

Storage
Store at 25°C (77°F); excursions permitted to 15-30°C (59-86°F) [see USP Controlled Room Temperature]. Protect from moisture. **Dispense in a tight container (USP).**

Handling
Keep out of reach and sight of children. Myfortic tablets should not be crushed or cut in order to maintain the integrity of the enteric coating [see Dosage and Administration (2.3)].
Teratogenic effects have been observed with mycophenolate sodium [see Warnings and Precautions (5.1)]. If for any reason, the Myfortic tablets must be crushed, avoid inhalation of the powder, or direct contact of the powder, with skin or mucous membranes.

17 PATIENT COUNSELING INFORMATION
See FDA-approved patient labeling (Medication Guide)
Embryofetal Toxicity
• Inform pregnant women and females of reproductive potential that use of Myfortic in pregnancy is associated with an increased risk of first trimester pregnancy loss and an increased risk of congenital malformations [see Use in Specific Populations (8.1)].
• In the event of a positive pregnancy test, discuss the risks and benefits of Myfortic with the patient. Encourage her to enroll in the pregnancy registry. (1-800-617-8191). [see Use in Specific Populations (8.1)].
Pregnancy Exposure Prevention and Planning
• Discuss pregnancy testing, pregnancy prevention and planning with females of reproductive potential [see Females of Reproductive Potential (8.6)].
• Inform females of reproductive potential must use acceptable birth control during entire Myfortic therapy and for 6 weeks after stopping Myfortic, unless the patient chooses to avoid heterosexual sexual intercourse completely (abstinence) [see Warnings and Precautions (5.2) and Females of Reproductive Potential (8.6)].
• For patients who are considering pregnancy, discuss appropriate alternative immunosuppressants with less potential for embryofetal toxicity. Risks and benefits of Myfortic should be discussed with the patient [see Females of Reproductive Potential (8.6)].
Nursing Mothers
Advise patients that they should not breastfeed during Myfortic therapy [see Nursing Mothers (8.3)].
Development of Lymphoma and Other Malignancies
• Inform patients they are at increased risk of developing lymphomas and other malignancies, particularly of the skin, due to immunosuppression.
• Advise patients to limit exposure to sunlight and ultraviolet (UV) light by wearing protective clothing and use a sunscreen with a high protection factor.
Increased Risk of Infection
Inform patients they are at increased risk of developing a variety of infections, including opportunistic infections, due to immunosuppression and to contact their physician if they develop any symptoms of infection [see Warnings and Precautions (5.5, 5.6)].
Blood Dyscrasias
Inform patients they are at increased risk for developing blood dyscrasias (e.g., neutropenia or anemia) and to immediately contact their healthcare provider if they experience any evidence of infection, unexpected bruising, bleeding, or any other manifestation of bone marrow suppression [see Warnings and Precautions (5.7)].
Gastrointestinal Tract Complications
Inform patients that Myfortic can cause gastrointestinal tract complications including bleeding, intestinal perforations, and gastric or duodenal ulcers. Advise the patient to contact their healthcare provider if they have symptoms of gastrointestinal bleeding or sudden onset or persistent abdominal pain [see Warnings and Precautions (5.8)].
Immunizations
Inform patients that Myfortic can interfere with the usual response to immunizations and that they should avoid live vaccines [see Warnings and Precautions (5.9)].
Administration Instructions
Advise patients to swallow Myfortic tablets whole, and not crush, chew, or cut the tablets. Inform patients to take Myfortic on an empty stomach, 1 hour before or 2 hours after food intake.
Drug Interactions
Patients should be advised to report to their doctor the use of any other medications while taking Myfortic. The simultaneous administration of any of the following drugs with Myfortic may result in clinically significant adverse reactions:
Antacids with magnesium and aluminum hydroxides
Azathioprine
Cholestyramine
Hormonal Contraceptives (e.g., birth control pill, transdermal patch, vaginal ring, injection, and implant)
Manufactured by:
Novartis Pharma Stein AG
Stein, Switzerland
Distributed by:
Novartis Pharmaceuticals Corporation
East Hanover, New Jersey 07936
T2013-78
September 2013

MEDICATION GUIDE

MYFORTIC® (my-for-tic)
(mycophenolic acid)
delayed-release tablets

Read the Medication Guide that comes with Myfortic before you start taking it and each time you get a refill. There may be new information. This Medication Guide does not take the place of talking with your healthcare provider about your medical condition or treatment. If you have any questions about Myfortic, ask your doctor.

What is the most important information I should know about Myfortic?

Myfortic can cause serious side effects including:

- **Increased risk of loss of pregnancy (miscarriage) and higher risk of birth defects.** Females who take Myfortic during pregnancy, have a higher risk of miscarriage during the first 3 months (first trimester), and a higher risk that their baby will be born with birth defects.
If you are a female who can become pregnant:
- your doctor must talk with you about acceptable birth control methods (contraceptive counseling) while taking Myfortic.
- you should have a pregnancy test immediately before starting Myfortic and another pregnancy test 8 to 10 days later. Pregnancy tests should be repeated during routine follow-up visits with your doctor. Talk to your doctor about the results of all of your pregnancy tests.
- you must use acceptable birth control during your entire Myfortic therapy and for 6 weeks after stopping Myfortic, unless at any time you choose to avoid sexual intercourse (abstinence) with a man completely. Myfortic decreases blood levels of the hormones in birth control pills that you take by mouth. Birth control pills may not work as well while you take Myfortic and you could become pregnant. If you decide to take birth control pills while using Myfortic, you must also use another form of birth control. Talk to your doctor about other birth control methods that can be used while taking Myfortic.

If you plan to become pregnant, talk with your doctor. Your doctor will decide if other medicines to prevent rejection may be right for you.

- **If you become pregnant while taking Myfortic, do not stop taking Myfortic. Call your doctor right away.** In certain situations, you and your doctor may decide that taking Myfortic is more important to your health than the possible risks to your unborn baby.
- You and your doctor should report your pregnancy to
- Mycophenolate Pregnancy Registry (1-800-617-8191)
The purpose of this registry is to gather information about the health of your baby.
- **Increased risk of getting serious infections.** Myfortic weakens the body's immune system and affects your ability to fight infections. Serious infections can happen with Myfortic and can lead to death. These serious infections can include:
  - **Viral infections.** Certain viruses can live in your body and cause active infections when your immune system is weak. Viral infections that can happen with Myfortic include:
    - Shingles, other herpes infections, and cytomegalovirus (CMV). CMV can cause serious tissue and blood infections.
    - BK virus. BK virus can affect how your kidney works and cause your transplanted kidney to fail.
    - Hepatitis B and C viruses. Hepatitis viruses can affect how your liver works. Talk to your doctor about how hepatitis viruses may affect you.
- **A brain infection called Progressive Multifocal Leukoencephalopathy (PML).** In some patients Myfortic may cause an infection of the brain that may cause death. You are at risk for this brain infection because you have a weakened immune system. You should tell your healthcare provider right away if you have any of the following symptoms:
  - Weakness on one side of the body
  - You do not care about things that you usually care about (apathy)
  - You are confused or have problems thinking
  - You cannot control your muscles
- **Fungal infections.** Yeast and other types of fungal infections can happen with Myfortic and cause serious tissue and blood infections. See "What are the possible side effects of Myfortic?"

Call your doctor right away if you have any of these signs and symptoms of infection:
- Temperature of 100.5°F or greater
- Cold symptoms, such as a runny nose or sore throat
- Flu symptoms, such as an upset stomach, stomach pain, vomiting, or diarrhea
- Earache or headache
- Pain during urination or you need to urinate often
- White patches in the mouth or throat
- Unexpected bruising or bleeding
- Cuts, scrapes, or incisions that are red, warm, and oozing pus

- **Increased risk of getting certain cancers.** People who take Myfortic have a higher risk of getting lymphoma, and other cancers, especially skin cancer. Tell your doctor if you have:
  - unexplained fever, tiredness that does not go away, weight loss, or lymph node swelling
  - a brown or black skin lesion with uneven borders, or one part of the lesion does not look like other parts
  - a change in the size or color of a mole
  - a new skin lesion or bump
  - any other changes to your health

See the section "What are the possible side effects of Myfortic?" for other serious side effects.

What is Myfortic?

Myfortic is a prescription medicine given to prevent rejection (antirejection medicine) in people who have received a kidney transplant. Rejection is when the body's immune system senses the new organ as "foreign" and attacks it. Myfortic is used with other medicines containing cyclosporine (Sandimmune®, Gengraf®, and Neoral®) and corticosteroids.

Myfortic can be used to prevent rejection in children who are 5 years or older and are stable after having a kidney transplant. It is not known if Myfortic is safe and works in children younger than 5 years. It is not known how Myfortic works in children who have just received a new kidney transplant.

Who should not take Myfortic?

Do not take Myfortic if you are allergic to mycophenolic acid, mycophenolate sodium, mycophenolate mofetil, or any of the ingredients in Myfortic. See the end of this Medication Guide for a complete list of ingredients in Myfortic.

What should I tell my doctor before I start taking Myfortic?

Tell your healthcare provider about all of your medical conditions, including if you:

- **have any digestive problems, such as ulcers**
- **plan to receive any vaccines.** You should not receive live vaccines while you take Myfortic. Some vaccines may not work as well during treatment with Myfortic.
- **have Lesch-Nyhan or Kelley-Seegmiller syndrome or another rare inherited deficiency of hypoxanthine-guanine phosphoribosyl-transferase (HGPRT).** You should not take Myfortic if you have one of these disorders.
- **are pregnant or planning to become pregnant. See "What is the most important information I should know about Myfortic?"**
- **are breastfeeding or plan to breastfeed.** It is not known if Myfortic passes into breast milk. You and your doctor will decide if you will take Myfortic or breastfeed.

Tell your doctor about all the medicines you take, including prescription and nonprescription medicines, vitamins, and herbal supplements.

Some medicines may affect the way Myfortic works and Myfortic may affect how some medicines work. Especially tell your doctor if you take:

- birth control pills (oral contraceptives). **See "What is the most important information I should know about Myfortic?"**
- antacids that contain aluminum or magnesium. Myfortic and antacids should not be taken at the same time.
- acyclovir (Zovirax®), Ganciclovir (Cytovene® IV, Valcyte®)
- azathioprine (Azasan®, Imuran®)
- cholestyramine (Questran® Light, Questran®, Locholest Light, Prevalite®)

Know the medicines you take. Keep a list of your medicines with you to show your healthcare provider and pharmacist when you get a new medicine. Do not take any new medicine without talking to your doctor.

How should I take Myfortic?

- Take Myfortic exactly as prescribed. Your healthcare provider will tell you how much Myfortic to take.
- Do not stop taking or change your dose of Myfortic without talking to your healthcare provider.
- Take Myfortic on an empty stomach, either 1 hour before or 2 hours after a meal.
- Swallow Myfortic whole. Do not crush, chew, or cut Myfortic. The Myfortic tablets have a coating so that the medicine will pass through your stomach and dissolve in your intestine.
- **If you forget to take Myfortic,** take it as soon as you remember and then take your next dose at its regular time. If it is almost time for your next dose, skip the missed dose. Do not take two doses at the same time. Call your doctor or pharmacist if you are not sure what to do.
- **If you take more than the prescribed dose of Myfortic,** call your doctor right away.
- **Do not change (substitute) between using Myfortic delayed-release tablets and mycophenolate mofetil tablets, capsules, or oral suspension for one another unless your healthcare provider tells you to.** These medicines are absorbed differently. This may affect the amount of medicine in your blood.
- Be sure to keep all appointments at your transplant clinic. During these visits, your doctor may perform regular blood tests.

What should I avoid while taking Myfortic?

Avoid pregnancy. See "What is the most important information I should know about Myfortic?"

- Limit the amount of time you spend in sunlight. Avoid using tanning beds and sunlamps. People who take Myfortic have a higher risk of getting skin cancer. See "What is the most important information I should know about Myfortic?" Wear protective clothing when you are in the sun and use a sunscreen with a high sun protection factor (SPF 30 and above). This is especially important if your skin is fair (light colored) or you have a family history of skin cancer.
- Elderly patients 65 years of age or older may have more side effects with Myfortic because of a weaker immune system.

What are the possible side effects of Myfortic?

Myfortic can cause serious side effects.

See "What is the most important information I should know about Myfortic?"

Stomach and intestinal bleeding can happen in people who take Myfortic. Bleeding can be severe and you may have to be hospitalized for treatment.

The most common side effects of taking Myfortic include:
In people with a new transplant:
- low blood cell counts
  - red blood cells
  - white blood cells
  - platelets
- constipation
- nausea
- diarrhea
- vomiting
- urinary tract infections
- stomach upset

In people who take Myfortic for a long time (long-term) after transplant:
- low blood cell counts
  - red blood cells
  - white blood cells
- nausea
- diarrhea
- sore throat

Your healthcare provider will do blood tests before you start taking Myfortic and during treatment with Myfortic to check your blood cell counts. Tell your healthcare provider right away if you have any signs of infection (see "What is the most important information I should know about Myfortic?"), or any unexpected bruising or bleeding. Also, tell your healthcare provider if you have unusual tiredness, dizziness, or fainting.

These are not all the possible side effects of Myfortic. Your healthcare provider may be able to help you manage these side effects.

Call your doctor for medical advice about side effects. You may report side effects to
- FDA MedWatch at 1-800-FDA-1088 or
- Novartis Drug Safety at 888-NOW-NOVA (1-888-669-6682).

How should I store Myfortic?

- Store Myfortic tablets at room temperature, 59° to 86°F (15° to 30°C). Myfortic does not need to be refrigerated.
- Keep the container tightly closed. Store Myfortic in a dry place.
- **Keep Myfortic and all medicines out of the reach of children.**

General information about Myfortic

Medicines are sometimes prescribed for purposes other than those listed in a Medication Guide. Do not use Myfortic for a condition for which it was not prescribed. Do not give Myfortic to other people, even if they have the same symptoms you have. It may harm them.

This Medication Guide summarizes the most important information about Myfortic. If you would like more information, talk with your doctor. You can ask your doctor or pharmacist for information about Myfortic that is written for healthcare professionals. You can also call 1-888-669-6682 or visit the Myfortic website at www.myfortic.com.

What are the ingredients in Myfortic?

Active ingredient: mycophenolic acid (as mycophenolate sodium)

Inactive ingredients: colloidal silicon dioxide, crospovidone, lactose anhydrous, magnesium stearate, povidone (K-30), and starch. The enteric coating of the tablet consists of hypromellose phthalate, titanium dioxide, iron oxide yellow, and indigotine (for the 180-mg tablet) or iron oxide red (for the 360-mg tablet)

This Medication Guide has been approved by the U.S. Food and Drug Administration.

Sandimmune and Neoral are registered trademarks of Novartis Pharmaceuticals Corporation.

Any other trademarks in this document are the property of their respective owners.

Manufactured by:
Novartis Pharma Stein AG Stein, Switzerland

Distributed by:
Novartis Pharmaceuticals Corporation
East Hanover, New Jersey 07936
© Novartis
T2013-79
September 2013
Shown in Product Identification Guide, page 310

NEORAL® SOFT GELATIN CAPSULES   ℞

[nĕŏ′ral]
(cyclosporine capsules, USP)
MODIFIED
NEORAL® ORAL SOLUTION
(cyclosporine oral solution, USP)
MODIFIED
Rx only
Prescribing Information

The following prescribing information is based on official labeling in effect July 2013.

Patient Population	Dose/day[1] (mg/d)	Dose/weight (mg/kg/d)	AUC[2] (ng·hr/mL)	Cmax (ng/mL)	Trough[3] (ng/mL)	CL/F (mL/min)	CL/F (mL/min/kg)
			Pharmacokinetic Parameters (mean±SD)				
De novo renal transplant[4] Week 4 (N=37)	597±174	7.95±2.81	8772±2089	1802±428	361±129	593±204	7.8±2.9
Stable renal transplant[4] (N=55)	344±122	4.10±1.58	6035±2194	1333±469	251±116	492±140	5.9±2.1
De novo liver transplant[5] Week 4 (N=18)	458±190	6.89±3.68	7187±2816	1555±740	268±101	577±309	8.6±5.7
De novo rheumatoid arthritis[6] (N=23)	182±55.6	2.37±0.36	2641±877	728±263	96.4±37.7	613±196	8.3±2.8
De novo psoriasis[6] Week 4 (N=18)	189±69.8	2.48±0.65	2324±1048	655±186	74.9±46.7	723±186	10.2±3.9

[1]Total daily dose was divided into two doses administered every 12 hours
[2]AUC was measured over one dosing interval
[3]Trough concentration was measured just prior to the morning Neoral® dose, approximately 12 hours after the previous dose
[4]Assay: TDx specific monoclonal fluorescence polarization immunoassay
[5]Assay: Cyclo-trac specific monoclonal radioimmunoassay
[6]Assay: INCSTAR specific monoclonal radioimmunoassay

WARNING

Only physicians experienced in management of systemic immunosuppressive therapy for the indicated disease should prescribe Neoral®. At doses used in solid organ transplantation, only physicians experienced in immunosuppressive therapy and management of organ transplant recipients should prescribe Neoral®. Patients receiving the drug should be managed in facilities equipped and staffed with adequate laboratory and supportive medical resources. The physician responsible for maintenance therapy should have complete information requisite for the follow-up of the patient.

Neoral®, a systemic immunosuppressant, may increase the susceptibility to infection and the development of neoplasia. In kidney, liver, and heart transplant patients Neoral® may be administered with other immunosuppressive agents. Increased susceptibility to infection and the possible development of lymphoma and other neoplasms may result from the increase in the degree of immunosuppression in transplant patients.

Neoral® Soft Gelatin Capsules (cyclosporine capsules, USP) MODIFIED and Neoral® Oral Solution (cyclosporine oral solution, USP) MODIFIED have increased bioavailability in comparison to Sandimmune® Soft Gelatin Capsules (cyclosporine capsules, USP) and Sandimmune® Oral Solution (cyclosporine oral solution, USP). Neoral® and Sandimmune® are not bioequivalent and cannot be used interchangeably without physician supervision. For a given trough concentration, cyclosporine exposure will be greater with Neoral® than with Sandimmune®. If a patient who is receiving exceptionally high doses of Sandimmune® is converted to Neoral®, particular caution should be exercised. Cyclosporine blood concentrations should be monitored in transplant and rheumatoid arthritis patients taking Neoral® to avoid toxicity due to high concentrations. Dose adjustments should be made in transplant patients to minimize possible organ rejection due to low concentrations. Comparison of blood concentrations in the published literature with blood concentrations obtained using current assays must be done with detailed knowledge of the assay methods employed.

For Psoriasis Patients (See also BOXED WARNING above)

Psoriasis patients previously treated with PUVA and to a lesser extent, methotrexate or other immunosuppressive agents, UVB, coal tar, or radiation therapy, are at an increased risk of developing skin malignancies when taking Neoral®.

Cyclosporine, the active ingredient in Neoral®, in recommended dosages, can cause systemic hypertension and nephrotoxicity. The risk increases with increasing dose and duration of cyclosporine therapy. Renal dysfunction, including structural kidney damage, is a potential consequence of cyclosporine, and therefore, renal function must be monitored during therapy.

DESCRIPTION

Neoral® is an oral formulation of cyclosporine that immediately forms a microemulsion in an aqueous environment. Cyclosporine, the active principle in Neoral®, is a cyclic polypeptide immunosuppressant agent consisting of 11 amino acids. It is produced as a metabolite by the fungus species *Beauveria nivea*.

Chemically, cyclosporine is designated as [R-[R*,R*-(E)]]-cyclic-(L-alanyl-D-alanyl-N-methyl-L-leucyl-N-methyl-L-leucyl-N-methyl-L-valyl-3-hydroxy-N,4-dimethyl-L-2-amino-6-octenoyl-L-α-amino-butyryl-N-methylglycyl-N-methyl-L-leucyl-L-valyl-N-methyl-L-leucyl).

Neoral® Soft Gelatin Capsules

(cyclosporine capsules, USP) MODIFIED are available in 25 mg and 100 mg strengths.
Each 25 mg capsule contains:

cyclosporine..25 mg
alcohol, USP dehydrated   11.9% v/v (9.5% wt/vol.)
Each 100 mg capsule contains:

cyclosporine..100 mg
alcohol, USP dehydrated..................11.9% v/v (9.5% wt/vol.)
Inactive Ingredients: Corn oil-mono-di-triglycerides, polyoxyl 40 hydrogenated castor oil NF, DL-α-tocopherol USP, gelatin NF, glycerol, iron oxide black, propylene glycol USP, titanium dioxide USP, carmine, and other ingredients.

Neoral® Oral Solution

(cyclosporine oral solution, USP) MODIFIED is available in 50 mL bottles.
Each mL contains:

cyclosporine..100 mg/mL
alcohol, USP dehydrated...............11.9% v/v (9.5% wt/vol.)
Inactive Ingredients: Corn oil-mono-di-triglycerides, polyoxyl 40 hydrogenated castor oil NF, DL-α -tocopherol USP, propylene glycol USP.
The chemical structure of cyclosporine (also known as cyclosporin A) is:

$C_{62}H_{111}N_{11}O_{12}$ Mol. Wt. 1202.63

CLINICAL PHARMACOLOGY

Cyclosporine is a potent immunosuppressive agent that in animals prolongs survival of allogeneic transplants involving skin, kidney, liver, heart, pancreas, bone marrow, small intestine, and lung. Cyclosporine has been demonstrated to suppress some humoral immunity and to a greater extent, cell-mediated immune reactions such as allograft rejection, delayed hypersensitivity, experimental allergic encephalomyelitis, Freund's adjuvant arthritis, and graft vs. host disease in many animal species for a variety of organs.

The effectiveness of cyclosporine results from specific and reversible inhibition of immunocompetent lymphocytes in the G_0- and G_1-phase of the cell cycle. T-lymphocytes are preferentially inhibited. The T-helper cell is the main target, although the T-suppressor cell may also be suppressed. Cyclosporine also inhibits lymphokine production and release including interleukin-2.

No effects on phagocytic function (changes in enzyme secretions, chemotactic migration of granulocytes, macrophage migration, carbon clearance *in vivo*) have been detected in animals. Cyclosporine does not cause bone marrow suppression in animal models or man.

Pharmacokinetics

The immunosuppressive activity of cyclosporine is primarily due to parent drug. Following oral administration, absorption of cyclosporine is incomplete. The extent of absorption of cyclosporine is dependent on the individual patient, the patient population, and the formulation. Elimination of cyclosporine is primarily biliary with only 6% of the dose (parent drug and metabolites) excreted in urine. The disposition of cyclosporine from blood is generally biphasic, with a terminal half-life of approximately 8.4 hours (range 5-18 hours). Following intravenous administration, the blood clearance of cyclosporine (assay: HPLC) is approximately 5-7 mL/min/kg in adult recipients of renal or liver allografts. Blood cyclosporine clearance appears to be slightly slower in cardiac transplant patients.

The Neoral® Soft Gelatin Capsules (cyclosporine capsules, USP) MODIFIED and Neoral® Oral Solution (cyclosporine oral solution, USP) MODIFIED are bioequivalent. Neoral® Oral Solution diluted with orange juice or apple juice is bioequivalent to Neoral® Oral Solution diluted with water. The effect of milk on the bioavailability of cyclosporine when administered as Neoral® Oral Solution has not been evaluated. The relationship between administered dose and exposure (area under the concentration versus time curve, AUC) is linear within the therapeutic dose range. The intersubject variability (total, %CV) of cyclosporine exposure (AUC) when Neoral® or Sandimmune® is administered ranges from approximately 20% to 50% in renal transplant patients. This intersubject variability contributes to the need for individualization of the dosing regimen for optimal therapy (See DOSAGE AND ADMINISTRATION). Intrasubject variability of AUC in renal transplant recipients (%CV) was 9%-21% for Neoral® and 19%-26% for Sandimmune®. In the same studies, intrasubject variability of trough concentrations (%CV) was 17%-30% for Neoral® and 16%-38% for Sandimmune®.

Absorption

Neoral® has increased bioavailability compared to Sandimmune®. The absolute bioavailability of cyclosporine administered as Sandimmune® is dependent on the patient population, estimated to be less than 10% in liver transplant patients and as great as 89% in some renal transplant patients. The absolute bioavailability of cyclosporine administered as Neoral® has not been determined in adults. In studies of renal transplant, rheumatoid arthritis and psoriasis patients, the mean cyclosporine AUC was approximately 20% to 50% greater and the peak blood cyclosporine concentration (Cmax) was approximately 40% to 106% greater following administration of Neoral® compared to following administration of Sandimmune®. The dose normalized AUC in *de novo* liver transplant patients administered Neoral® 28 days after transplantation was 50% greater and Cmax was 90% greater than in those patients administered Sandimmune®. AUC and Cmax are also increased (Neoral® relative to Sandimmune®) in heart transplant patients, but data are very limited. Although the AUC and Cmax values are higher on Neoral® relative to Sandimmune®, the predose trough concentrations (dose-normalized) are similar for the two formulations.

Following oral administration of Neoral®, the time to peak blood cyclosporine concentrations (Tmax) ranged from 1.5-2.0 hours. The administration of food with Neoral® decreases the cyclosporine AUC and Cmax. A high fat meal (669 kcal, 45 grams fat) consumed within one-half hour before Neoral® administration decreased the AUC by 13% and Cmax by 33%. The effects of a low fat meal (667 kcal, 15 grams fat) were similar.

The effect of T-tube diversion of bile on the absorption of cyclosporine from Neoral® was investigated in eleven *de novo* liver transplant patients. When the patients were administered Neoral® with and without T-tube diversion of bile, very little difference in absorption was observed, as measured by the change in maximal cyclosporine blood concentrations from pre-dose values with the T-tube closed relative to when it was open: 6.9±41% (range -55% to 68%). [See table at top of previous page]

Distribution

Cyclosporine is distributed largely outside the blood volume. The steady state volume of distribution during intravenous dosing has been reported as 3-5 L/kg in solid organ transplant recipients. In blood, the distribution is concentration dependent. Approximately 33%-47% is in plasma, 4%-9% in lymphocytes, 5%-12% in granulocytes, and 41%-58% in erythrocytes. At high concentrations, the binding capacity of leukocytes and erythrocytes becomes saturated. In plasma, approximately 90% is bound to proteins, primarily lipoproteins. Cyclosporine is excreted in human milk. (*See PRECAUTIONS, Nursing Mothers*)

Metabolism

Cyclosporine is extensively metabolized by the cytochrome P-450 3A enzyme system in the liver, and to a lesser degree in the gastrointestinal tract, and the kidney. The metabolism of cyclosporine can be altered by the coadministration of a variety of agents. (*See PRECAUTIONS, Drug Interactions*) At least 25 metabolites have been identified from human bile, feces, blood, and urine. The biological activity of the metabolites and their contributions to toxicity are considerably less than those of the parent compound. The major metabolites (M1, M9, and M4N) result from oxidation at the 1-beta, 9-gamma, and 4-N-demethylated positions, respectively. At steady state following the oral administration of Sandimmune®, the mean AUCs for blood concentrations of M1, M9, and M4N are about 70%, 21%, and 7.5% of the AUC for blood cyclosporine concentrations, respectively. Based on blood concentration data from stable renal transplant patients (13 patients administered Neoral® and Sandimmune® in a crossover study), and bile concentration data from *de novo* liver transplant patients (4 administered Neoral®, 3 administered Sandimmune®), the percentage of dose present as M1, M9, and M4N metabolites is similar when either Neoral® or Sandimmune® is administered.

Excretion

Only 0.1% of a cyclosporine dose is excreted unchanged in the urine. Elimination is primarily biliary with only 6% of the dose (parent drug and metabolites) excreted in the urine. Neither dialysis nor renal failure alters cyclosporine clearance significantly.

Drug Interactions

(*See PRECAUTIONS, Drug Interactions*) When diclofenac or methotrexate was coadministered with cyclosporine in rheumatoid arthritis patients, the AUC of diclofenac and methotrexate, each was significantly increased. (*See PRECAUTIONS, Drug Interactions*) No clinically significant pharmacokinetic interactions occurred between cyclosporine and aspirin, ketoprofen, piroxicam, or indomethacin.

Specific Populations

Renal Impairment

In a study performed in 4 subjects with end-stage renal disease (creatinine clearance <5 mL/min), an intravenous infusion of 3.5 mg/kg of cyclosporine over 4 hours administered at the end of a hemodialysis session resulted in a mean volume of distribution (Vdss) of 3.49 L/kg and systemic clearance (CL) of 0.369 L/hr/kg. This systemic CL (0.369 L/hr/kg) was approximately two thirds of the mean systemic CL (0.56 L/hr/kg) of cyclosporine in historical control subjects with normal renal function. In 5 liver transplant patients, the mean clearance of cyclosporine on and off hemodialysis was 463 mL/min and 398 mL/min, respectively. Less than 1% of the dose of cyclosporine was recovered in the dialysate.

Hepatic Impairment

Cyclosporine is extensively metabolized by the liver. Since severe hepatic impairment may result in significantly increased cyclosporine exposures, the dosage of cyclosporine may need to be reduced in these patients.

Pediatric Population

Pharmacokinetic data from pediatric patients administered Neoral® or Sandimmune® are very limited. In 15 renal transplant patients aged 3-16 years, cyclosporine whole blood clearance after IV administration of Sandimmune® was 10.6±3.7 mL/min/kg (assay: Cyclo-trac specific RIA). In a study of 7 renal transplant patients aged 2-16, the cyclosporine clearance ranged from 9.8-15.5 mL/min/kg. In 9 liver transplant patients aged 0.6-5.6 years, clearance was 9.3±5.4 mL/min/kg (assay: HPLC).

In the pediatric population, Neoral® also demonstrates an increased bioavailability as compared to Sandimmune®. In 7 liver *de novo* transplant patients aged 1.4-10 years, the absolute bioavailability of Neoral® was 43% (range 30%-68%) and for Sandimmune® in the same individuals absolute bioavailability was 28% (range 17%-42%).

Pediatric Pharmacokinetic Parameters (mean±SD)						
Patient Population	Dose/day (mg/d)	Dose/weight (mg/kg/d)	AUC[1] (ng·hr/mL)	C_{max} (ng/mL)	CL/F (mL/min)	CL/F (mL/min/kg)
Stable liver transplant[2]						
Age 2-8, Dosed TID (N=9)	101±25	5.95±1.32	2163±801	629±219	285±94	16.6±4.3
Age 8-15, Dosed BID (N=8)	188±55	4.96±2.09	4272±1462	975±281	378±80	10.2±4.0
Stable liver transplant[3]						
Age 3, Dosed BID (N=1)	120	8.33	5832	1050	171	11.9
Age 8-15, Dosed BID (N=5)	158±55	5.51±1.91	4452±2475	1013±635	328±121	11.0±1.9
Stable renal transplant[3]						
Age 7-15, Dosed BID (N=5)	328±83	7.37±4.11	6922±1988	1827±487	418±143	8.7±2.9

[1]AUC was measured over one dosing interval
[2]Assay: Cyclo-trac specific monoclonal radioimmunoassay
[3]Assay: TDx specific monoclonal fluorescence polarization immunoassay

numbers on columns are p-values vs. placebo, unless indicated otherwise
ACR Responders
Randomized

[See table above]

Geriatric Population

Comparison of single dose data from both normal elderly volunteers (N=18, mean age 69 years) and elderly rheumatoid arthritis patients (N=16, mean age 68 years) to single dose data in young adult volunteers (N=16, mean age 26 years) showed no significant difference in the pharmacokinetic parameters.

CLINICAL TRIALS

Rheumatoid Arthritis

The effectiveness of Sandimmune® and Neoral® in the treatment of severe rheumatoid arthritis was evaluated in 5 clinical studies involving a total of 728 cyclosporine treated patients and 273 placebo treated patients.

A summary of the results is presented for the "responder" rates per treatment group, with a responder being defined as a patient having *completed* the trial with a 20% improvement in the tender and the swollen joint count and a 20% improvement in 2 of 4 of investigator global, patient global, disability, and erythrocyte sedimentation rates (ESR) for the Studies 651 and 652 and 3 of 5 of investigator global, patient global, disability, visual analog pain, and ESR for Studies 2008, 654 and 302.

Study 651 enrolled 264 patients with active rheumatoid arthritis with at least 20 involved joints, who had failed at least one major RA drug, using a 3:3:2 randomization to one of the following three groups: (1) cyclosporine dosed at 2.5-5 mg/kg/day, (2) methotrexate at 7.5-15 mg/week, or (3) placebo. Treatment duration was 24 weeks. The mean cyclosporine dose at the last visit was 3.1 mg/kg/day. See Graph below.

Study 652 enrolled 250 patients with active RA with >6 active painful or tender joints who had failed at least one major RA drug. Patients were randomized using a 3:3:2 randomization to 1 of 3 treatment arms: (1) 1.5-5 mg/kg/day of cyclosporine, (2) 2.5-5 mg/kg/day of cyclosporine, and (3) placebo. Treatment duration was 16 weeks. The mean cyclosporine dose for group 2 at the last visit was 2.92 mg/kg/day. See Graph below.

Study 2008 enrolled 144 patients with active RA and >6 active joints who had unsuccessful treatment courses of aspirin and gold or Penicillamine. Patients were randomized to 1 of 2 treatment groups (1) cyclosporine 2.5-5 mg/kg/day with adjustments after the first month to achieve a target trough level and (2) placebo. Treatment duration was 24 weeks. The mean cyclosporine dose at the last visit was 3.63 mg/kg/day. See Graph below.

Study 654 enrolled 148 patients who remained with active joint counts of 6 or more despite treatment with maximally tolerated methotrexate doses for at least three months. Patients continued to take their current dose of methotrexate and were randomized to receive, in addition, one of the following medications: (1) cyclosporine 2.5 mg/kg/day with dose increases of 0.5 mg/kg/day at weeks 2 and 4 if there was no evidence of toxicity and further increases of 0.5 mg/kg/day at weeks 8 and 16 if a <30% decrease in active joint count occurred without any significant toxicity; dose decreases could be made at any time for toxicity or (2) placebo. Treatment duration was 24 weeks. The mean cyclosporine dose at the last visit was 2.8 mg/kg/day (range: 1.3-4.1). See Graph below.

Study 302 enrolled 299 patients with severe active RA, 99% of whom were unresponsive or intolerant to at least one prior major RA drug. Patients were randomized to 1 of 2 treatment groups (1) Neoral® and (2) cyclosporine, both of which were started at 2.5 mg/kg/day and increased after 4 weeks for inefficacy in increments of 0.5 mg/kg/day to a maximum of 5 mg/kg/day and decreased at any time for toxicity. Treatment duration was 24 weeks. The mean cyclosporine dose at the last visit was 2.91 mg/kg/day (range: 0.72-5.17) for Neoral® and 3.27 mg/kg/day (range: 0.73-5.68) for cyclosporine. See Graph below. [See figure above]

INDICATIONS AND USAGE

Kidney, Liver, and Heart Transplantation

Neoral® is indicated for the prophylaxis of organ rejection in kidney, liver, and heart allogeneic transplants. Neoral® has been used in combination with azathioprine and corticosteroids.

Rheumatoid Arthritis

Neoral® is indicated for the treatment of patients with severe active, rheumatoid arthritis where the disease has not adequately responded to methotrexate. Neoral® can be used in combination with methotrexate in rheumatoid arthritis patients who do not respond adequately to methotrexate alone.

Psoriasis

Neoral® is indicated for the treatment of *adult, nonimmunocompromised* patients with severe (i.e., extensive and/or

Nephrotoxicity vs. Rejection

Parameter	Nephrotoxicity	Rejection
History	Donor >50 years old or hypotensive Prolonged kidney preservation Prolonged anastomosis time Concomitant nephrotoxic drugs	Anti-donor immune response Retransplant patient
Clinical	Often >6 weeks postop[b] Prolonged initial nonfunction (acute tubular necrosis)	Often < 4 weeks postop[b] Fever > 37.5°C Weight gain > 0.5 kg Graft swelling and tenderness Decrease in daily urine volume > 500 mL (or 50%)
Laboratory	CyA serum trough level > 200 ng/mL Gradual rise in Cr (< 0.15 mg/dl/day)[a] Cr plateau < 25% above baseline BUN/Cr ≥ 20	CyA serum trough level < 150 ng/mL Rapid rise in Cr (> 0.3 mg/dl/day)[a] Cr > 25% above baseline BUN/Cr < 20
Biopsy	Arteriolopathy (medial hypertrophy [a], hyalinosis, nodular deposits, intimal thickening, endothelial vacuolization, progressive scarring) Tubular atrophy, isometric vacuolization, isolated calcifications Minimal edema Mild focal infiltrates[c] Diffuse interstitial fibrosis, often striped form	Endovasculitis[c] (proliferation[a], intimal arteritis[b], necrosis, sclerosis) Tubulitis with RBC[b] and WBC[b] casts, some irregular vacuolization Interstitial edema[c] and hemorrhage[b] Diffuse moderate to severe mononuclear infiltrates[d] Glomerulitis (mononuclear cells)[c]
Aspiration Cytology	CyA deposits in tubular and endothelial cells Fine isometric vacuolization of tubular cells	Inflammatory infiltrate with mononuclear phagocytes, macrophages, lymphoblastoid cells, and activated T-cells These strongly express HLA-DR antigens
Urine Cytology	Tubular cells with vacuolization and granularization	Degenerative tubular cells, plasma cells, and lymphocyturia > 20% of sediment
Manometry	Intracapsular pressure < 40 mm Hg[b]	Intracapsular pressure > 40 mm Hg[b]
Ultrasonography	Unchanged graft cross sectional area	Increase in graft cross sectional area AP diameter ≥ Transverse diameter
Magnetic Resonance Imagery	Normal appearance	Loss of distinct corticomedullary junction, swelling image intensity of parachyma approaching that of psoas, loss of hilar fat Patchy arterial flow
Radionuclide Scan	Normal or generally decreased perfusion Decrease in tubular function ([131] I-hippuran) > decrease in perfusion ([99m] Tc DTPA)	Decrease in perfusion > decrease in tubular function Increased uptake of Indium 111 labeled platelets or Tc-99m in colloid
Therapy	Responds to decreased cyclosporine	Responds to increased steroids or antilymphocyte globulin

[a] p < 0.05, [b] p < 0.01, [c] p < 0.001, [d] p < 0.0001

disabling), recalcitrant, plaque psoriasis who have failed to respond to at least one systemic therapy (e.g., PUVA, retinoids, or methotrexate) or in patients for whom other systemic therapies are contraindicated, or cannot be tolerated. While rebound rarely occurs, most patients will experience relapse with Neoral® as with other therapies upon cessation of treatment.

CONTRAINDICATIONS
General
Neoral® is contraindicated in patients with a hypersensitivity to cyclosporine or to any of the ingredients of the formulation.

Rheumatoid Arthritis
Rheumatoid arthritis patients with abnormal renal function, uncontrolled hypertension, or malignancies should not receive Neoral®.

Psoriasis
Psoriasis patients who are treated with Neoral® should not receive concomitant PUVA or UVB therapy, methotrexate or other immunosuppressive agents, coal tar or radiation therapy. Psoriasis patients with abnormal renal function, uncontrolled hypertension, or malignancies should not receive Neoral®.

WARNINGS
(See also BOXED WARNING)
All Patients
Cyclosporine, the active ingredient of Neoral®, can cause nephrotoxicity and hepatotoxicity. The risk increases with increasing doses of cyclosporine. Renal dysfunction including structural kidney damage is a potential consequence of Neoral® and therefore renal function must be monitored during therapy. **Care should be taken in using cyclosporine with nephrotoxic drugs. (See PRECAUTIONS.)**
Patients receiving Neoral® require frequent monitoring of serum creatinine. *(See Special Monitoring under DOSAGE AND ADMINISTRATION)* Elderly patients should be monitored with particular care, since decreases in renal function also occur with age. If patients are not properly monitored and doses are not properly adjusted, cyclosporine therapy can be associated with the occurrence of structural kidney damage and persistent renal dysfunction.
An increase in serum creatinine and BUN may occur during Neoral® therapy and reflect a reduction in the glomerular

filtration rate. Impaired renal function at any time requires close monitoring, and frequent dosage adjustment may be indicated. The frequency and severity of serum creatinine elevations increase with dose and duration of cyclosporine therapy. These elevations are likely to become more pronounced without dose reduction or discontinuation.
Because Neoral® is not bioequivalent to Sandimmune®, conversion from Neoral® to Sandimmune® using a 1:1 ratio (mg/kg/day) may result in lower cyclosporine blood concentrations. Conversion from Neoral® to Sandimmune® should be made with increased monitoring to avoid the potential of underdosing.
Kidney, Liver, and Heart Transplant
Nephrotoxicity
Cyclosporine, the active ingredient of Neoral®, can cause nephrotoxicity and hepatotoxicity when used in high doses. It is not unusual for serum creatinine and BUN levels to be elevated during cyclosporine therapy. These elevations in renal transplant patients do not necessarily indicate rejection, and each patient must be fully evaluated before dosage adjustment is initiated.
Based on the historical Sandimmune® experience with oral solution, nephrotoxicity associated with cyclosporine had been noted in 25% of cases of renal transplantation, 38% of cases of cardiac transplantation, and 37% of cases of liver transplantation. Mild nephrotoxicity was generally noted 2-3 months after renal transplant and consisted of an arrest in the fall of the pre-operative elevations of BUN and creatinine at a range of 35-45 mg/dl and 2.0-2.5 mg/dl respectively. These elevations were often responsive to cyclosporine dosage reduction.
More overt nephrotoxicity was seen early after transplantation and was characterized by a rapidly rising BUN and creatinine. Since these events are similar to renal rejection episodes, care must be taken to differentiate between them. This form of nephrotoxicity is usually responsive to cyclosporine dosage reduction.
Although specific diagnostic criteria which reliably differentiate renal graft rejection from drug toxicity have not been found, a number of parameters have been significantly associated with one or the other. It should be noted however, that up to 20% of patients may have simultaneous nephrotoxicity and rejection.
[See table above]

A form of a cyclosporine-associated nephropathy is characterized by serial deterioration in renal function and morphologic changes in the kidneys. From 5%-15% of transplant recipients who have received cyclosporine will fail to show a reduction in rising serum creatinine despite a decrease or discontinuation of cyclosporine therapy. Renal biopsies from these patients will demonstrate one or several of the following alterations: tubular vacuolization, tubular microcalcifications, peritubular capillary congestion, arteriolopathy, and a striped form of interstitial fibrosis with tubular atrophy. Though none of these morphologic changes is entirely specific, a diagnosis of cyclosporine-associated structural nephrotoxicity requires evidence of these findings.
When considering the development of cyclosporine-associated nephropathy, it is noteworthy that several authors have reported an association between the appearance of interstitial fibrosis and higher cumulative doses or persistently high circulating trough concentrations of cyclosporine. This is particularly true during the first 6 post-transplant months when the dosage tends to be highest and when, in kidney recipients, the organ appears to be most vulnerable to the toxic effects of cyclosporine. Among other contributing factors to the development of interstitial fibrosis in these patients are prolonged perfusion time, warm ischemia time, as well as episodes of acute toxicity, and acute and chronic rejection. The reversibility of interstitial fibrosis and its correlation to renal function have not yet been determined. Reversibility of arteriolopathy has been reported after stopping cyclosporine or lowering the dosage.
Impaired renal function at any time requires close monitoring, and frequent dosage adjustment may be indicated.
In the event of severe and unremitting rejection, when rescue therapy with pulse steroids and monoclonal antibodies fail to reverse the rejection episode, it may be preferable to switch to alternative immunosuppressive therapy rather than increase the Neoral® dose to excessive blood concentrations.
Due to the potential for additive or synergistic impairment of renal function, caution should be exercised when coadministering Neoral® with other drugs that may impair renal function. *(See PRECAUTIONS, Drug Interactions)*
Thrombotic Microangiopathy
Occasionally patients have developed a syndrome of thrombocytopenia and microangiopathic hemolytic anemia which may result in graft failure. The vasculopathy can occur in the absence of rejection and is accompanied by avid platelet consumption within the graft as demonstrated by Indium 111 labeled platelet studies. Neither the pathogenesis nor the management of this syndrome is clear. Though resolution has occurred after reduction or discontinuation of cyclosporine and 1) administration of streptokinase and heparin or 2) plasmapheresis, this appears to depend upon early detection with Indium 111 labeled platelet scans. *(See ADVERSE REACTIONS)*
Hyperkalemia
Significant hyperkalemia (sometimes associated with hyperchloremic metabolic acidosis) and hyperuricemia have been seen occasionally in individual patients.
Hepatotoxicity
Cases of hepatotoxicity and liver injury including cholestasis, jaundice, hepatitis, and liver failure have been reported in patients treated with cyclosporine. Most reports included patients with significant co-morbidities, underlying conditions and other confounding factors including infectious complications and comedications with hepatotoxic potential. In some cases, mainly in transplant patients, fatal outcomes have been reported. *(See ADVERSE REACTIONS, Postmarketing Experience, Kidney, Liver and Heart Transplantation)*
Hepatotoxicity, usually manifested by elevations in hepatic enzymes and bilirubin, was reported in patients treated with cyclosporine in clinical trials: 4% in renal transplantation, 7% in cardiac transplantation, and 4% in liver transplantation. This was usually noted during the first month of therapy when high doses of cyclosporine were used. The chemistry elevations usually decreased with a reduction in dosage.
Malignancies
As in patients receiving other immunosuppressants, those patients receiving cyclosporine are at increased risk for development of lymphomas and other malignancies, particularly those of the skin. Patients taking cyclosporine should be warned to avoid excess ultraviolet light exposure. The increased risk appears related to the intensity and duration of immunosuppression rather than to the use of specific agents. Because of the danger of oversuppression of the immune system resulting in increased risk of infection or malignancy, a treatment regimen containing multiple immunosuppressants should be used with caution. Some malignancies may be fatal. Transplant patients receiving cyclosporine are at increased risk for serious infection with fatal outcome.

Serious Infections

Patients receiving immunosuppressants, including Neoral, are at increased risk of developing bacterial, viral, fungal, and protozoal infections, including opportunistic infections. These infections may lead to serious, including fatal, outcomes. (See BOXED WARNING, and ADVERSE REACTIONS)

Polyoma Virus Infections

Patients receiving immunosuppressants, including Neoral, are at increased risk for opportunistic infections, including polyoma virus infections. Polyoma virus infections in transplant patients may have serious, and sometimes fatal outcomes. These include cases of JC virus-associated progressive multifocal leukoencephalopathy (PML), and polyoma virus-associated nephropathy (PVAN), especially due to BK virus infection, which have been observed in patients receiving cyclosporine. PVAN is associated with serious outcomes, including deteriorating renal function and renal graft loss, (See ADVERSE REACTIONS, Postmarketing Experience, Kidney, Liver and Heart Transplantation). Patient monitoring may help detect patients at risk for PVAN.

Cases of PML have been reported in patients treated with Neoral. PML, which is sometimes fatal, commonly presents with hemiparesis, apathy, confusion, cognitive deficiencies and ataxia. Risk factors for PML include treatment with immunosuppressant therapies and impairment of immune function. In immunosuppressed patients, physicians should consider PML in the differential diagnosis in patients reporting neurological symptoms and consultation with a neurologist should be considered as clinically indicated.

Consideration should be given to reducing the total immunosuppression in transplant patients who develop PML or PVAN. However, reduced immunosuppression may place the graft at risk.

Neurotoxicity

There have been reports of convulsions in adult and pediatric patients receiving cyclosporine, particularly in combination with high dose methylprednisolone.

Encephalopathy, including Posterior Reversible Encephalopathy Syndrome (PRES), has been described both in postmarketing reports and in the literature. Manifestations include impaired consciousness, convulsions, visual disturbances (including blindness), loss of motor function, movement disorders and psychiatric disturbances. In many cases, changes in the white matter have been detected using imaging techniques and pathologic specimens. Predisposing factors such as hypertension, hypomagnesemia, hypocholesterolemia, high-dose corticosteroids, high cyclosporine blood concentrations, and graft-versus-host disease have been noted in many but not all of the reported cases. The changes in most cases have been reversible upon discontinuation of cyclosporine, and in some cases improvement was noted after reduction of dose. It appears that patients receiving liver transplant are more susceptible to encephalopathy than those receiving kidney transplant. Another rare manifestation of cyclosporine-induced neurotoxicity, occurring in transplant patients more frequently than in other indications, is optic disc edema including papilloedema, with possible visual impairment, secondary to benign intracranial hypertension.

Care should be taken in using cyclosporine with nephrotoxic drugs. (See PRECAUTIONS)

Rheumatoid Arthritis

Cyclosporine nephropathy was detected in renal biopsies of 6 out of 60 (10%) rheumatoid arthritis patients after the average treatment duration of 19 months. Only one patient, out of these 6 patients, was treated with a dose ≤4 mg/kg/day. Serum creatinine improved in all but one patient after discontinuation of cyclosporine. The "maximal creatinine increase" appears to be a factor in predicting cyclosporine nephropathy.

There is a potential, as with other immunosuppressive agents, for an increase in the occurrence of malignant lymphomas with cyclosporine. It is not clear whether the risk with cyclosporine is greater than that in rheumatoid arthritis patients or in rheumatoid arthritis patients on cytotoxic treatment for this indication. Five cases of lymphoma were detected: four in a survey of approximately 2,300 patients treated with cyclosporine for rheumatoid arthritis, and another case of lymphoma was reported in a clinical trial. Although other tumors (12 skin cancers, 24 solid tumors of diverse types, and 1 multiple myeloma) were also reported in this survey, epidemiologic analyses did not support a relationship to cyclosporine other than for malignant lymphomas.

Patients should be thoroughly evaluated before and during Neoral® treatment for the development of malignancies. Moreover, use of Neoral® therapy with other immunosuppressive agents may induce an excessive immunosuppression which is known to increase the risk of malignancy.

Psoriasis

(See also BOXED WARNING for Psoriasis)

Since cyclosporine is a potent immunosuppressive agent with a number of potentially serious side effects, the risks and benefits of using Neoral® should be considered before treatment of patients with psoriasis. Cyclosporine, the active ingredient in Neoral®, can cause nephrotoxicity and hypertension (See PRECAUTIONS) and the risk increases with increasing dose and duration of therapy. Patients who may be at increased risk such as those with abnormal renal function, uncontrolled hypertension or malignancies, should not receive Neoral®.

Renal dysfunction is a potential consequence of Neoral® therefore renal function must be monitored during therapy. Patients receiving Neoral® require frequent monitoring of serum creatinine. (See Special Monitoring under DOSAGE AND ADMINISTRATION) Elderly patients should be monitored with particular care, since decreases in renal function also occur with age. If patients are not properly monitored and doses are not properly adjusted, cyclosporine therapy can cause structural kidney damage and persistent renal dysfunction.

An increase in serum creatinine and BUN may occur during Neoral® therapy and reflects a reduction in the glomerular filtration rate.

Kidney biopsies from 86 psoriasis patients treated for a mean duration of 23 months with 1.2-7.6 mg/kg/day of cyclosporine showed evidence of cyclosporine nephropathy in 18/86 (21%) of the patients. The pathology consisted of renal tubular atrophy and interstitial fibrosis. On repeat biopsy of 13 of these patients maintained on various dosages of cyclosporine for a mean of 2 additional years, the number with cyclosporine induced nephropathy rose to 26/86 (30%). The majority of patients (19/26) were on a dose of ≥5.0 mg/kg/day (the highest recommended dose is 4 mg/kg/day). The patients were also on cyclosporine for greater than 15 months (18/26) and/or had a clinically significant increase in serum creatinine for greater than 1 month (21/26). Creatinine levels returned to normal range in 7 of 11 patients in whom cyclosporine therapy was discontinued.

There is an increased risk for the development of skin and lymphoproliferative malignancies in cyclosporine-treated psoriasis patients. The relative risk of malignancies is comparable to that observed in psoriasis patients treated with other immunosuppressive agents.

Tumors were reported in 32 (2.2%) of 1439 psoriasis patients treated with cyclosporine worldwide from clinical trials. Additional tumors have been reported in 7 patients in cyclosporine postmarketing experience. Skin malignancies were reported in 16 (1.1%) of these patients; all but 2 of them had previously received PUVA therapy. Methotrexate was received by 7 patients. UVB and coal tar had been used by 2 and 3 patients, respectively. Seven patients had either a history of previous skin cancer or a potentially predisposing lesion was present prior to cyclosporine exposure. Of the 16 patients with skin cancer, 11 patients had 18 squamous cell carcinomas and 7 patients had 10 basal cell carcinomas. There were two lymphoproliferative malignancies; one case of non-Hodgkin's lymphoma which required chemotherapy, and one case of mycosis fungoides which regressed spontaneously upon discontinuation of cyclosporine. There were four cases of benign lymphocytic infiltration: 3 regressed spontaneously upon discontinuation of cyclosporine, while the fourth regressed despite continuation of the drug. The remainder of the malignancies, 13 cases (0.9%), involved various organs.

Patients should not be treated concurrently with cyclosporine and PUVA or UVB, other radiation therapy, or other immunosuppressive agents, because of the possibility of excessive immunosuppression and the subsequent risk of malignancies. (See CONTRAINDICATIONS) Patients should also be warned to protect themselves appropriately when in the sun, and to avoid excessive sun exposure. Patients should be thoroughly evaluated before and during treatment for the presence of malignancies remembering that malignant lesions may be hidden by psoriatic plaques. Skin lesions not typical of psoriasis should be biopsied before starting treatment. Patients should be treated with Neoral® only after complete resolution of suspicious lesions, and only if there are no other treatment options. (See Special Monitoring for Psoriasis Patients)

Special Excipients

Alcohol (ethanol)

The alcohol content (See DESCRIPTION) of Neoral should be taken into account when given to patients in whom alcohol intake should be avoided or minimized, e.g., pregnant or breastfeeding women, in patients presenting with liver disease or epilepsy, in alcoholic patients, or pediatric patients. For an adult weighing 70 kg, the maximum daily oral dose would deliver about 1 gram of alcohol which is approximately 6% of the amount of alcohol contained in a standard drink.

PRECAUTIONS

General

Hypertension

Cyclosporine is the active ingredient of Neoral®. Hypertension is a common side effect of cyclosporine therapy which may persist. (See ADVERSE REACTIONS and DOSAGE AND ADMINISTRATION for monitoring recommendations) Mild or moderate hypertension is encountered more frequently than severe hypertension and the incidence decreases over time. In recipients of kidney, liver, and heart allografts treated with cyclosporine, antihypertensive therapy may be required. (See Special Monitoring of Rheumatoid Arthritis and Psoriasis Patients) However, since cyclosporine may cause hyperkalemia, potassium-sparing diuretics should not be used. While calcium antagonists can be effective agents in treating cyclosporine-associated hypertension, they can interfere with cyclosporine metabolism. (See Drug Interactions)

Vaccination

During treatment with cyclosporine, vaccination may be less effective; and the use of live attenuated vaccines should be avoided.

Special Monitoring of Rheumatoid Arthritis Patients

Before initiating treatment, a careful physical examination, including blood pressure measurements (on at least two occasions) and two creatinine levels to estimate baseline should be performed. Blood pressure and serum creatinine should be evaluated every 2 weeks during the initial 3 months and then monthly if the patient is stable. It is advisable to monitor serum creatinine and blood pressure always after an increase of the dose of nonsteroidal anti-inflammatory drugs and after initiation of new nonsteroidal anti-inflammatory drug therapy during Neoral® treatment. If coadministered with methotrexate, CBC and liver function tests are recommended to be monitored monthly. (See also PRECAUTIONS, General, Hypertension)

In patients who are receiving cyclosporine, the dose of Neoral® should be decreased by 25%-50% if hypertension occurs. If hypertension persists, the dose of Neoral® should be further reduced or blood pressure should be controlled with antihypertensive agents. In most cases, blood pressure has returned to baseline when cyclosporine was discontinued.

In placebo-controlled trials of rheumatoid arthritis patients, systolic hypertension (defined as an occurrence of two systolic blood pressure readings >140 mmHg) and diastolic hypertension (defined as two diastolic blood pressure readings >90 mmHg) occurred in 33% and 19% of patients treated with cyclosporine, respectively. The corresponding placebo rates were 22% and 8%.

Special Monitoring for Psoriasis Patients

Before initiating treatment, a careful dermatological and physical examination, including blood pressure measurements (on at least two occasions) should be performed. Since Neoral® is an immunosuppressive agent, patients should be evaluated for the presence of occult infection on their first physical examination and for the presence of tumors initially, and throughout treatment with Neoral®. Skin lesions not typical for psoriasis should be biopsied before starting Neoral®. Patients with malignant or premalignant changes of the skin should be treated with Neoral® only after appropriate treatment of such lesions and if no other treatment option exists.

Baseline laboratories should include serum creatinine (on two occasions), BUN, CBC, serum magnesium, potassium, uric acid, and lipids.

The risk of cyclosporine nephropathy is reduced when the starting dose is low (2.5 mg/kg/day), the maximum dose does not exceed 4.0 mg/kg/day, serum creatinine is monitored regularly while cyclosporine is administered, and the dose of Neoral® is decreased when the rise in creatinine is greater than or equal to 25% above the patient's pretreatment level. The increase in creatinine is generally reversible upon timely decrease of the dose of Neoral® or its discontinuation.

Serum creatinine and BUN should be evaluated every 2 weeks during the initial 3 months of therapy and then monthly if the patient is stable. If the serum creatinine is greater than or equal to 25% above the patient's pretreatment level, serum creatinine should be repeated within two weeks. If the change in serum creatinine remains greater than or equal to 25% above baseline, Neoral® should be reduced by 25%-50%. If at any time the serum creatinine increases by greater than or equal to 50% above pretreatment level, Neoral® should be reduced by 25%-50%. Neoral® should be discontinued if reversibility (within 25% of baseline) of serum creatinine is not achievable after two dosage modifications. It is advisable to monitor serum creatinine after an increase of the dose of nonsteroidal anti-inflammatory drug and after initiation of new nonsteroidal anti-inflammatory therapy during Neoral® treatment.

Blood pressure should be evaluated every 2 weeks during the initial 3 months of therapy and then monthly if the patient is stable, or more frequently when dosage adjustments are made. Patients without a history of previous hypertension before initiation of treatment with Neoral®, should have the drug reduced by 25%-50% if found to have sustained hypertension. If the patient continues to be hypertensive despite multiple reductions of Neoral®, then Neoral® should be discontinued. For patients with treated hyperten-

Help Patients Save on Rx Drugs: PDR.net/PharmacyDiscountCard

Antibiotics	Antineoplastics	Antifungals	Anti-inflammatory Drugs	Gastrointestinal Agents	Immunosuppressives	Other Drugs
ciprofloxacin	melphalan	amphotericin B	azapropazon	cimetidine	tacrolimus	fibric acid derivatives
gentamicin		ketoconazole	colchicine	ranitidine		(e.g., bezafibrate,
tobramycin			diclofenac			fenofibrate)
vancomycin			naproxen			methotrexate
trimethoprim with			sulindac			
sulfamethoxazole						

sion, before the initiation of Neoral® therapy, their medication should be adjusted to control hypertension while on Neoral®. Neoral® should be discontinued if a change in hypertension management is not effective or tolerable.

CBC, uric acid, potassium, lipids, and magnesium should also be monitored every 2 weeks for the first 3 months of therapy, and then monthly if the patient is stable or more frequently when dosage adjustments are made. Neoral® dosage should be reduced by 25%-50% for any abnormality of clinical concern.

In controlled trials of cyclosporine in psoriasis patients, cyclosporine blood concentrations did not correlate with either improvement or with side effects such as renal dysfunction.

Information for Patients: Patients should be advised that any change of cyclosporine formulation should be made cautiously and only under physician supervision because it may result in the need for a change in dosage.

Patients should be informed of the necessity of repeated laboratory tests while they are receiving cyclosporine. Patients should be advised of the potential risks during pregnancy and informed of the increased risk of neoplasia. Patients should also be informed of the risk of hypertension and renal dysfunction.

Patients should be advised that during treatment with cyclosporine, vaccination may be less effective and the use of live attenuated vaccines should be avoided.

Patients should be given careful dosage instructions. Neoral® Oral Solution (cyclosporine oral solution, USP) MODIFIED should be diluted, preferably with orange or apple juice that is at room temperature. The combination of Neoral® Oral Solution (cyclosporine oral solution, USP) MODIFIED with milk can be unpalatable.

Patients should be advised to take Neoral® on a consistent schedule with regard to time of day and relation to meals. Grapefruit and grapefruit juice affect metabolism, increasing blood concentration of cyclosporine, thus should be avoided.

Laboratory Tests

In all patients treated with cyclosporine, renal and liver functions should be assessed repeatedly by measurement of serum creatinine, BUN, serum bilirubin, and liver enzymes. Serum lipids, magnesium, and potassium should also be monitored. Cyclosporine blood concentrations should be routinely monitored in transplant patients (See DOSAGE AND ADMINISTRATION, Blood Concentration Monitoring in Transplant Patients), and periodically monitored in rheumatoid arthritis patients.

Drug Interactions

A. Effect of Drugs and Other Agents on Cyclosporine Pharmacokinetics and/or Safety

All of the individual drugs cited below are well substantiated to interact with cyclosporine. In addition, concomitant use of non-steroidal anti-inflammatory drugs with cyclosporine, particularly in the setting of dehydration, may potentiate renal dysfunction. Caution should be exercised when using other drugs which are known to impair renal function. (See WARNINGS, Nephrotoxicity)

Drugs That May Potentiate Renal Dysfunction

[See table above]

During the concomitant use of a drug that may exhibit additive or synergistic renal impairment with cyclosporine, close monitoring of renal function (in particular serum creatinine) should be performed. If a significant impairment of renal function occurs, the dosage of the coadministered drug should be reduced or an alternative treatment considered. Cyclosporine is extensively metabolized by CYP 3A isoenzymes, in particular CYP3A4, and is a substrate of the multidrug efflux transporter P-glycoprotein. Various agents are known to either increase or decrease plasma or whole blood concentrations of cyclosporine usually by inhibition or induction of CYP3A4 or P-glycoprotein transporter or both. Compounds that decrease cyclosporine absorption such as orlistat should be avoided. Appropriate Neoral® dosage adjustment to achieve the desired cyclosporine concentration is essential when drugs that significantly alter cyclosporine concentrations are used concomitantly. (See Blood Concentration Monitoring)

1. Drugs That Increase Cyclosporine Concentrations

[See first table below]

HIV Protease inhibitors

The HIV protease inhibitors (e.g., indinavir, nelfinavir, ritonavir, and saquinavir) are known to inhibit cytochrome P-450 3A and thus could potentially increase the concentra-

tions of cyclosporine, however no formal studies of the interaction are available. Care should be exercised when these drugs are administered concomitantly.

Grapefruit juice

Grapefruit and grapefruit juice affect metabolism, increasing blood concentrations of cyclosporine, thus should be avoided.

2. Drugs/Dietary Supplements That Decrease Cyclosporine Concentrations

[See second table below]

Bosentan

Coadministration of bosentan (250–1000 mg every 12 hours based on tolerability) and cyclosporine (300 mg every 12 hours for 2 days then dosing to achieve a C_{min} of 200–250 ng/mL) for 7 days in healthy subjects resulted in decreases in the cyclosporine mean dose-normalized AUC, C_{max}, and trough concentration of approximately 50%, 30%, and 60%, respectively, compared to when cyclosporine was given alone (See also Effect of Cyclosporine on the Pharmacokinetics and/or Safety of Other Drugs or Agents).

Boceprevir

Coadministration of boceprevir (800 mg three times daily for 7 days) and cyclosporine (100 mg single dose) in healthy subjects resulted in increases in the mean AUC and C_{max} of cyclosporine approximately 2.7-fold and 2-fold, respectively, compared to when cyclosporine was given alone.

Telaprevir

Coadministration of telaprevir (750 mg every 8 hours for 11 days) with cyclosporine (10 mg on day 8) in healthy subjects resulted in increases in the mean dose-normalized AUC and C_{max} of cyclosporine approximately 4.5-fold and 1.3-fold, respectively, compared to when cyclosporine (100 mg single dose) was given alone.

St. John's Wort

There have been reports of a serious drug interaction between cyclosporine and the herbal dietary supplement St. John's Wort. This interaction has been reported to produce a marked reduction in the blood concentrations of cyclosporine, resulting in subtherapeutic levels, rejection of transplanted organs, and graft loss.

Rifabutin

Rifabutin is known to increase the metabolism of other drugs metabolized by the cytochrome P-450 system. The interaction between rifabutin and cyclosporine has not been studied. Care should be exercised when these two drugs are administered concomitantly.

B. Effect of Cyclosporine on the Pharmacokinetics and/or Safety of Other Drugs or Agents

Cyclosporine is an inhibitor of CYP3A4 and of the multidrug efflux transporter P-glycoprotein and may increase plasma concentrations of comedications that are substrates of CYP3A4 or P-glycoprotein or both.

Cyclosporine may reduce the clearance of digoxin, colchicine, prednisolone, HMG-CoA reductase inhibitors (statins), and, aliskiren, repaglinide, NSAIDs, sirolimus, etoposide, and other drugs. See the full prescribing information of the other drug for further information and specific recommendations. The decision on coadministration of cyclosporine with other drugs or agents should be made by the physician following the careful assessment of benefits and risks.

Digoxin

Severe digitalis toxicity has been seen within days of starting cyclosporine in several patients taking digoxin. If digoxin is used concurrently with cyclosporine, serum digoxin concentrations should be monitored.

Colchicine

There are reports on the potential of cyclosporine to enhance the toxic effects of colchicine such as myopathy and neuropathy, especially in patients with renal dysfunction. Concomitant administration of cyclosporine and colchicine results in significant increases in colchicine plasma concentrations. If colchicine is used concurrently with cyclosporine, a reduction in the dosage of colchicine is recommended.

HMG-CoA reductase inhibitors (statins)

Literature and postmarketing cases of myotoxicity, including muscle pain and weakness, myositis, and rhabdomyolysis, have been reported with concomitant administration of cyclosporine with lovastatin, simvastatin, atorvastatin, pravastatin, and, rarely fluvastatin. When concurrently administered with cyclosporine, the dosage of these statins should be reduced according to label recommendations. Statin therapy needs to be temporarily withheld or discontinued in patients with signs and symptoms of myopathy or those with risk factors predisposing to severe renal injury, including renal failure, secondary to rhabdomyolysis.

Repaglinide

Cyclosporine may increase the plasma concentrations of repaglinide and thereby increase the risk of hypoglycemia. In 12 healthy male subjects who received two doses of 100mg cyclosporine capsule orally 12 hours apart with a single dose of 0.25mg repaglinide tablet (one half of a 0.5mg tablet) orally 13 hours after the cyclosporine initial dose, the repaglinide mean Cmax and AUC were increased 1.8 fold (range: 0.6-3.7 fold) and 2.4 fold (range 1.2-5.3 fold), respectively. Close monitoring of blood glucose level is advisable for a patient taking cyclosporine and repaglinide concomitantly.

Ambrisentan

Coadministration of ambrisentan (5 mg daily) and cyclosporine (100–150 mg twice daily initially, then dosing to achieve C_{min} 150–200 ng/mL) for 8 days in healthy subjects resulted in mean increases in ambrisentan AUC and C_{max} of approximately 2-fold and 1.5–fold, respectively, compared to ambrisentan alone.

Anthracycline antibiotics

High doses of cyclosporine (e.g., at starting intravenous dose of 16 mg/kg/day) may increase the exposure to anthracycline antibiotics (e.g., doxorubicin, mitoxantrone, daunorubicin) in cancer patients.

Aliskiren

Cyclosporine alters the pharmacokinetics of aliskiren, a substrate of P-glycoprotein and CYP3A4. In 14 healthy subjects who received concomitantly single doses of cyclosporine (200 mg) and reduced dose aliskiren (75 mg), the mean Cmax of aliskiren was increased by approximately 2.5 fold (90% CI: 1.96-3.17) and the mean AUC by approximately 4.3 fold (90% CI: 3.52-5.21), compared to when these subjects received aliskiren alone. The concomitant administration of aliskiren with cyclosporine prolonged the median aliskiren elimination half-life (26 hours versus 43 to 45 hours) and the T_{max} (0.5 hours versus 1.5 to 2.0 hours). The mean AUC and C_{max} of cyclosporine were com-

Calcium Channel Blockers	Antifungals	Antibiotics	Glucocorticoids	Other Drugs
diltiazem	fluconazole	azithromycin	methylprednisolone	Allopurinol
nicardipine	itraconazole	clarithromycin		Amiodarone
verapamil	ketoconazole	erythromycin		Bromocriptine
	voriconazole	quinupristin/ dalfopristin		colchicine
				danazol
				imatinib
				metoclopramide
				nefazodone
				oral contraceptives

Antibiotics	Anticonvulsants	Other Drugs/Dietary Supplements	
nafcillin	carbamazepine	bosentan	St. John's Wort
rifampin	oxcarbazepine	octreotide	
	phenobarbital	orlistat	
	phenytoin	sulfinpyrazone	
		terbinafine	
		ticlopidine	

parable to reported literature values. Coadministration of cyclosporine and aliskiren in these subjects also resulted in an increase in the number and/or intensity of adverse events, mainly headache, hot flush, nausea, vomiting, and somnolence. The coadministration of cyclosporine with aliskiren is not recommended.

Bosentan

In healthy subjects, coadministration of bosentan and cyclosporine resulted in mean increases in dose-normalized bosentan trough concentrations on day 1 and day 8 of approximately 21-fold and 2-fold, respectively, compared to when bosentan was given alone as a single dose on day 1. *(See also Effect of Drugs and Other Agents on Cyclosporine Pharmacokinetics and/or Safety)*

Potassium-Sparing Diuretics

Cyclosporine should not be used with potassium-sparing diuretics because hyperkalemia can occur. Caution is also required when cyclosporine is coadministered with potassium sparing drugs (e.g., angiotensin converting enzyme inhibitors, angiotensin II receptor antagonists), potassium containing drugs as well as in patients on a potassium rich diet. Control of potassium levels in these situations is advisable.

Nonsteroidal Anti-inflammatory Drug (NSAID) Interactions

Clinical status and serum creatinine should be closely monitored when cyclosporine is used with nonsteroidal anti-inflammatory agents in rheumatoid arthritis patients. *(See WARNINGS)*

Pharmacodynamic interactions have been reported to occur between cyclosporine and both naproxen and sulindac, in that concomitant use is associated with additive decreases in renal function, as determined by ^{99m}Tc-diethylenetriaminepentaacetic acid (DTPA) and (p-aminohippuric acid) PAH clearances. Although concomitant administration of diclofenac does not affect blood concentrations of cyclosporine, it has been associated with approximate doubling of diclofenac blood concentrations and occasional reports of reversible decreases in renal function. Consequently, the dose of diclofenac should be in the lower end of the therapeutic range.

Methotrexate Interaction

Preliminary data indicate that when methotrexate and cyclosporine were coadministered to rheumatoid arthritis patients (N=20), methotrexate concentrations (AUCs) were increased approximately 30% and the concentrations (AUCs) of its metabolite, 7-hydroxy methotrexate, were decreased by approximately 80%. The clinical significance of this interaction is not known. Cyclosporine concentrations do not appear to have been altered (N=6).

Sirolimus

Elevations in serum creatinine were observed in studies using sirolimus in combination with full-dose cyclosporine. This effect is often reversible with cyclosporine dose reduction. Simultaneous coadministration of cyclosporine significantly increases blood levels of sirolimus. To minimize increases in sirolimus concentrations, it is recommended that sirolimus be given 4 hours after cyclosporine administration.

Nifedipine

Frequent gingival hyperplasia when nifedipine is given concurrently with cyclosporine has been reported. The concomitant use of nifedipine should be avoided in patients in whom gingival hyperplasia develops as a side effect of cyclosporine.

Methylprednisolone

Convulsions when high dose methylprednisolone is given concurrently with cyclosporine have been reported.

Other Immunosuppressive Drugs and Agents

Psoriasis patients receiving other immunosuppressive agents or radiation therapy (including PUVA and UVB) should not receive concurrent cyclosporine because of the possibility of excessive immunosuppression.

C. Effect of Cyclosporine on the Efficacy of Live Vaccines

During treatment with cyclosporine, vaccination may be less effective. The use of live vaccines should be avoided.

For additional information on Cyclosporine Drug Interactions please contact Novartis Medical Affairs Department at 888-NOW-NOVA [888-669-6682].

Carcinogenesis, Mutagenesis, and Impairment of Fertility

Carcinogenicity studies were carried out in male and female rats and mice. In the 78-week mouse study, evidence of a statistically significant trend was found for lymphocytic lymphomas in females, and the incidence of hepatocellular carcinomas in mid-dose males significantly exceeded the control value. In the 24-month rat study, pancreatic islet cell adenomas significantly exceeded the control rate in the low dose level. Doses used in the mouse and rat studies were 0.01 to 0.16 times the clinical maintenance dose (6 mg/kg). The hepatocellular carcinomas and pancreatic islet cell adenomas were not dose related. Published reports indicate that co-treatment of hairless mice with UV irradiation and cyclosporine or other immunosuppressive agents shorten the time to skin tumor formation compared to UV irradiation alone.

Cyclosporine was not mutagenic in appropriate test systems. Cyclosporine has not been found to be mutagenic/genotoxic in the Ames Test, the V79-HGPRT Test, the micronucleus test in mice and Chinese hamsters, the chromosome-aberration tests in Chinese hamster bone-marrow, the mouse dominant lethal assay, and the DNA-repair test in sperm from treated mice. A recent study analyzing sister chromatid exchange (SCE) induction by cyclosporine using human lymphocytes *in vitro* gave indication of a positive effect (i.e., induction of SCE), at high concentrations in this system. In two published research studies, rabbits exposed to cyclosporine *in utero* (10 mg/kg/day subcutaneously) demonstrated reduced numbers of nephrons, renal hypertrophy, systemic hypertension and progressive renal insufficiency up to 35 weeks of age. Pregnant rats which received 12 mg/kg/day of cyclosporine intravenously (twice the recommended human intravenous dose) had fetuses with an increased incidence of ventricular septal defect. These findings have not been demonstrated in other species and their relevance for humans is unknown. No impairment in fertility was demonstrated in studies in male and female rats.

Widely distributed papillomatosis of the skin was observed after chronic treatment of dogs with cyclosporine at 9 times the human initial psoriasis treatment dose of 2.5 mg/kg, where doses are expressed on a body surface area basis. This papillomatosis showed a spontaneous regression upon discontinuation of cyclosporine.

An increased incidence of malignancy is a recognized complication of immunosuppression in recipients of organ transplants and patients with rheumatoid arthritis and psoriasis. The most common forms of neoplasms are non-Hodgkin's lymphoma and carcinomas of the skin. The risk of malignancies in cyclosporine recipients is higher than in the normal, healthy population but similar to that in patients receiving other immunosuppressive therapies. Reduction or discontinuance of immunosuppression may cause the lesions to regress.

In psoriasis patients on cyclosporine, development of malignancies, especially those of the skin has been reported. *(See WARNINGS)* Skin lesions not typical for psoriasis should be biopsied before starting cyclosporine treatment. Patients with malignant or premalignant changes of the skin should be treated with cyclosporine only after appropriate treatment of such lesions and if no other treatment option exists.

Pregnancy

Pregnancy Category C

Animal studies have shown reproductive toxicity in rats and rabbits. Cyclosporine gave no evidence of mutagenic or teratogenic effects in the standard test systems with oral application (rats up to 17 mg/kg and rabbits up to 30 mg/kg per day orally.) Only at dose levels toxic to dams, were adverse effects seen in reproduction studies in rats. Cyclosporine has been shown to be embryo- and fetotoxic in rats and rabbits following oral administration at maternally toxic doses. Fetal toxicity was noted in rats at 0.8 and rabbits at 5.4 times the transplant doses in humans of 6.0 mg/kg, where dose corrections are based on body surface area. Cyclosporine was embryo- and fetotoxic as indicated by increased pre- and postnatal mortality and reduced fetal weight together with related skeletal retardation.

There are no adequate and well-controlled studies in pregnant women therefore, Neoral® should not be used during pregnancy unless the potential benefit to the mother justifies the potential risk to the fetus.

In pregnant transplant recipients who are being treated with immunosuppressants the risk of premature birth is increased. The following data represent the reported outcomes of 116 pregnancies in women receiving cyclosporine during pregnancy, 90% of whom were transplant patients, and most of whom received cyclosporine throughout the entire gestational period. The only consistent patterns of abnormality were premature birth (gestational period of 28 to 36 weeks) and low birth weight for gestational age. Sixteen fetal losses occurred. Most of the pregnancies (85 of 100) were complicated by disorders; including, preeclampsia, eclampsia, premature labor, abruptio placentae, oligohydramnios, Rh incompatibility, and fetoplacental dysfunction. Pre-term delivery occurred in 47%. Seven malformations were reported in 5 viable infants and in 2 cases of fetal loss. Twenty-eight percent of the infants were small for gestational age. Neonatal complications occurred in 27%. Therefore, the risks and benefits of using Neoral® during pregnancy should be carefully weighed.

A limited number of observations in children exposed to cyclosporine *in utero* are available, up to an age of approximately 7 years. Renal function and blood pressure in these children were normal.

Because of the possible disruption of maternal-fetal interaction, the risk/benefit ratio of using Neoral® in psoriasis patients during pregnancy should carefully be weighed with serious consideration for discontinuation of Neoral®.

The alcohol content of the Neoral formulations should also be taken into account in pregnant women. (See WARNINGS, Special Excipients)

Nursing Mothers

Cyclosporine is present in breast milk. Because of the potential for serious adverse drug reactions in nursing infants from Neoral, a decision should be made whether to discontinue nursing or to discontinue the drug, taking into account the importance of the drug to the mother. Neoral contains ethanol. Ethanol will be present in human milk at levels similar to that found in maternal serum and if present in breast milk will be orally absorbed by a nursing infant (See WARNINGS).

Pediatric Use

Although no adequate and well-controlled studies have been completed in children, transplant recipients as young as one year of age have received Neoral® with no unusual adverse effects. The safety and efficacy of Neoral® treatment in children with juvenile rheumatoid arthritis or psoriasis below the age of 18 have not been established.

Geriatric Use

In rheumatoid arthritis clinical trials with cyclosporine, 17.5% of patients were age 65 or older. These patients were more likely to develop systolic hypertension on therapy, and more likely to show serum creatinine rises ≥50% above the baseline after 3-4 months of therapy.

Clinical studies of Neoral® in transplant and psoriasis patients did not include a sufficient number of subjects aged 65 and over to determine whether they respond differently from younger subjects. Other reported clinical experiences have not identified differences in response between the elderly and younger patients. In general, dose selection for an elderly patient should be cautious, usually starting at the low end of the dosing range, reflecting the greater frequency of decreased hepatic, renal, or cardiac function, and of concomitant disease or other drug therapy.

ADVERSE REACTIONS

Kidney, Liver, and Heart Transplantation

The principal adverse reactions of cyclosporine therapy are renal dysfunction, tremor, hirsutism, hypertension, and gum hyperplasia.

Hypertension

Hypertension, which is usually mild to moderate, may occur in approximately 50% of patients following renal transplantation and in most cardiac transplant patients.

Glomerular Capillary Thrombosis

Glomerular capillary thrombosis has been found in patients treated with cyclosporine and may progress to graft failure. The pathologic changes resembled those seen in the hemolytic-uremic syndrome and included thrombosis of the renal microvasculature, with platelet-fibrin thrombi occluding glomerular capillaries and afferent arterioles, microangiopathic hemolytic anemia, thrombocytopenia, and decreased renal function. Similar findings have been observed when other immunosuppressives have been employed post-transplantation.

Hypomagnesemia

Hypomagnesemia has been reported in some, but not all, patients exhibiting convulsions while on cyclosporine therapy. Although magnesium-depletion studies in normal subjects suggest that hypomagnesemia is associated with neurologic disorders, multiple factors, including hypertension, high dose methylprednisolone, hypocholesterolemia, and nephrotoxicity associated with high plasma concentrations of cyclosporine appear to be related to the neurological manifestations of cyclosporine toxicity.

Clinical Studies

In controlled studies, the nature, severity, and incidence of the adverse events that were observed in 493 transplanted patients treated with Neoral® were comparable with those observed in 208 transplanted patients who received Sandimmune® in these same studies when the dosage of the two drugs was adjusted to achieve the same cyclosporine blood trough concentrations.

Based on the historical experience with Sandimmune®, the following reactions occurred in 3% or greater of 892 patients involved in clinical trials of kidney, heart, and liver transplants.

[See first table at top of next page]

Among 705 kidney transplant patients treated with cyclosporine oral solution (Sandimmune®) in clinical trials, the reason for treatment discontinuation was renal toxicity in 5.4%, infection in 0.9%, lack of efficacy in 1.4%, acute tubular necrosis in 1.0%, lymphoproliferative disorders in 0.3%, hypertension in 0.3%, and other reasons in 0.7% of the patients.

The following reactions occurred in 2% or less of cyclosporine-treated patients: allergic reactions, anemia, anorexia, confusion, conjunctivitis, edema, fever, brittle fingernails, gastritis, hearing loss, hiccups, hyperglycemia, migraine (Neoral®), muscle pain, peptic ulcer, thrombocytopenia, tinnitus.

The following reactions occurred rarely: anxiety, chest pain, constipation, depression, hair breaking, hematuria, joint pain, lethargy, mouth sores, myocardial infarction,

Body System	Adverse Reactions	Randomized Kidney Patients		Cyclosporine Patients (Sandimmune®)		
		Sandimmune® (N=227)%	Azathioprine (N=228)%	Kidney (N=705)%	Heart (N=112)%	Liver (N=75)%
Genitourinary	Renal Dysfunction	32	6	25	38	37
Cardiovascular	Hypertension	26	18	13	53	27
	Cramps	4	<1	2	<1	0
Skin	Hirsutism	21	<1	21	28	45
	Acne	6	8	2	2	1
Central Nervous System	Tremor	12	0	21	31	55
	Convulsions	3	1	1	4	5
	Headache	2	<1	2	15	4
Gastrointestinal	Gum Hyperplasia	4	0	9	5	16
	Diarrhea	3	<1	3	4	8
	Nausea/Vomiting	2	<1	4	10	4
	Hepatotoxicity	<1	<1	4	7	4
	Abdominal Discomfort	<1	0	<1	7	0
Autonomic Nervous System	Paresthesia	3	0	1	2	1
	Flushing	<1	0	4	0	4
Hematopoietic	Leukopenia	2	19	<1	6	0
	Lymphoma	<1	0	1	6	1
Respiratory	Sinusitis	<1	0	4	3	7
Miscellaneous	Gynecomastia	<1	0	<1	4	3

Infectious Complications in Historical Randomized Studies in Renal Transplant Patients Using Sandimmune®

Complication	Cyclosporine Treatment (N=227) % of Complications	Azathioprine with Steroids* (N=228) % of Complications
Septicemia	5.3	4.8
Abscesses	4.4	5.3
Systemic Fungal Infection	2.2	3.9
Local Fungal Infection	7.5	9.6
Cytomegalovirus	4.8	12.3
Other Viral Infections	15.9	18.4
Urinary Tract Infections	21.1	20.2
Wound and Skin Infections	7.0	10.1
Pneumonia	6.2	9.2

*Some patients also received ALG.

night sweats, pancreatitis, pruritus, swallowing difficulty, tingling, upper GI bleeding, visual disturbance, weakness, weight loss.

Patients receiving immunosuppressive therapies, including cyclosporine and cyclosporine -containing regimens, are at increased risk of infections (viral, bacterial, fungal, parasitic). Both generalized and localized infections can occur. Pre-existing infections may also be aggravated. Fatal outcomes have been reported. (See WARNINGS)

[See second table above]

Postmarketing Experience, Kidney, Liver and Heart Transplantation

Hepatotoxicity

Cases of hepatotoxicity and liver injury including cholestasis, jaundice, hepatitis and liver failure; serious and/or fatal outcomes have been reported. (See WARNINGS, Hepatotoxicity)

Increased Risk of Infections

Cases of JC virus-associated progressive multifocal leukoencephalopathy (PML), sometimes fatal; and polyoma virus-associated nephropathy (PVAN), especially BK virus resulting in graft loss have been reported. (See WARNINGS, Polyoma Virus Infection)

Headache, including Migraine

Cases of migraine have been reported. In some cases, patients have been unable to continue cyclosporine, however, the final decision on treatment discontinuation should be made by the treating physician following the careful assessment of benefits versus risks.

Rheumatoid Arthritis

The principal adverse reactions associated with the use of cyclosporine in rheumatoid arthritis are renal dysfunction (See WARNINGS), hypertension (See PRECAUTIONS), headache, gastrointestinal disturbances, and hirsutism/hypertrichosis.

In rheumatoid arthritis patients treated in clinical trials within the recommended dose range, cyclosporine therapy was discontinued in 5.3% of the patients because of hypertension and in 7% of the patients because of increased creatinine. These changes are usually reversible with timely dose decrease or drug discontinuation. The frequency and severity of serum creatinine elevations increase with dose and duration of cyclosporine therapy. These elevations are likely to become more pronounced without dose reduction or discontinuation.

The following adverse events occurred in controlled clinical trials:

[See table on pages 1951 and 1952]

In addition, the following adverse events have been reported in 1% to <3% of the rheumatoid arthritis patients in the cyclosporine treatment group in controlled clinical trials.

Autonomic Nervous System: dry mouth, increased sweating

Body as a Whole: allergy, asthenia, hot flushes, malaise, overdose, procedure NOS*, tumor NOS*, weight decrease, weight increase

Cardiovascular: abnormal heart sounds, cardiac failure, myocardial infarction, peripheral ischemia

Central and Peripheral Nervous System: hypoesthesia, neuropathy, vertigo

Endocrine: goiter

Gastrointestinal: constipation, dysphagia, enanthema, eructation, esophagitis, gastric ulcer, gastritis, gastroenteritis, gingival bleeding, glossitis, peptic ulcer, salivary gland enlargement, tongue disorder, tooth disorder

Infection: abscess, bacterial infection, cellulitis, folliculitis, fungal infection, herpes simplex, herpes zoster, renal abscess, moniliasis, tonsillitis, viral infection

Hematologic: anemia, epistaxis, leukopenia, lymphadenopathy

Liver and Biliary System: bilirubinemia

Metabolic and Nutritional: diabetes mellitus, hyperkalemia, hyperuricemia, hypoglycemia

Musculoskeletal System: arthralgia, bone fracture, bursitis, joint dislocation, myalgia, stiffness, synovial cyst, tendon disorder

Neoplasms: breast fibroadenosis, carcinoma

Psychiatric: anxiety, confusion, decreased libido, emotional lability, impaired concentration, increased libido, nervousness, paroniria, somnolence

Reproductive (Female): breast pain, uterine hemorrhage

Respiratory System: abnormal chest sounds, bronchospasm

Skin and Appendages: abnormal pigmentation, angioedema, dermatitis, dry skin, eczema, nail disorder, pruritus, skin disorder, urticaria

Special Senses: abnormal vision, cataract, conjunctivitis, deafness, eye pain, taste perversion, tinnitus, vestibular disorder

Urinary System: abnormal urine, hematuria, increased BUN, micturition urgency, nocturia, polyuria, pyelonephritis, urinary incontinence

*NOS=Not Otherwise Specified

Psoriasis

The principal adverse reactions associated with the use of cyclosporine in patients with psoriasis are renal dysfunction, headache, hypertension, hypertriglyceridemia, hirsutism/hypertrichosis, paresthesia or hyperesthesia, influenza-like symptoms, nausea/vomiting, diarrhea, abdominal discomfort, lethargy, and musculoskeletal or joint pain.

In psoriasis patients treated in US controlled clinical studies within the recommended dose range, cyclosporine therapy was discontinued in 1.0% of the patients because of hypertension and in 5.4% of the patients because of increased creatinine. In the majority of cases, these changes were reversible after dose reduction or discontinuation of cyclosporine.

There has been one reported death associated with the use of cyclosporine in psoriasis. A 27-year-old male developed renal deterioration and was continued on cyclosporine. He had progressive renal failure leading to death.

Frequency and severity of serum creatinine increases with dose and duration of cyclosporine therapy. These elevations are likely to become more pronounced and may result in irreversible renal damage without dose reduction or discontinuation.

[See second table at top of page 1952]

The following events occurred in 1% to less than 3% of psoriasis patients treated with cyclosporine:

Body as a Whole: fever, flushes, hot flushes

Cardiovascular: chest pain

Central and Peripheral Nervous System: appetite increased, insomnia, dizziness, nervousness, vertigo

Gastrointestinal: abdominal distention, constipation, gingival bleeding

Liver and Biliary System: hyperbilirubinemia

Neoplasms: skin malignancies [squamous cell (0.9%) and basal cell (0.4%) carcinomas]

Reticuloendothelial: platelet, bleeding, and clotting disorders, red blood cell disorder

Respiratory: infection, viral and other infection

Skin and Appendages: acne, folliculitis, keratosis, pruritus, rash, dry skin

Urinary System: micturition frequency

Vision: abnormal vision

Mild hypomagnesemia and hyperkalemia may occur but are asymptomatic. Increases in uric acid may occur and attacks of gout have been rarely reported. A minor and dose related hyperbilirubinemia has been observed in the absence of hepatocellular damage. Cyclosporine therapy may be associated with a modest increase of serum triglycerides or cholesterol. Elevations of triglycerides (>750 mg/dL) occur in about 15% of psoriasis patients; elevations of cholesterol (>300 mg/dL) are observed in less than 3% of psoriasis patients. Generally these laboratory abnormalities are reversible upon dose reduction or discontinuation of cyclosporine.

Postmarketing Experience, Psoriasis

Cases of transformation to erythrodermic psoriasis or generalized pustular psoriasis upon either withdrawal or reduction of cyclosporine in patients with chronic plaque psoriasis have been reported.

OVERDOSAGE

There is a minimal experience with cyclosporine overdosage. Forced emesis and gastric lavage can be of value up to 2 hours after administration of Neoral®. Transient hepatotoxicity and nephrotoxicity may occur which should resolve following drug withdrawal. Oral doses of cyclosporine up to 10 g (about 150 mg/kg) have been tolerated with relatively minor clinical consequences, such as vomiting, drowsiness, headache, tachycardia and, in a few patients, moderately severe, reversible impairment of renal function. However, serious symptoms of intoxication have been reported following accidental parenteral overdosage with cyclosporine in premature neonates. General supportive measures and symptomatic treatment should be followed in all cases of overdosage. Cyclosporine is not dialyzable to any great extent, nor is it cleared well by charcoal hemoperfusion. The oral dosage at which half of experimental animals are estimated to die is 31 times, 39 times, and >54 times the human maintenance dose for transplant patients (6mg/kg; corrections based on body surface area) in mice, rats, and rabbits.

DOSAGE AND ADMINISTRATION

Neoral® Soft Gelatin Capsules (cyclosporine capsules, USP) MODIFIED and Neoral® Oral Solution (cyclosporine oral solution, USP) MODIFIED

Neoral® has increased bioavailability in comparison to Sandimmune®. Neoral® and Sandimmune® are not bioequivalent and cannot be used interchangeably without physician supervision.

The daily dose of Neoral® should always be given in two divided doses (BID). It is recommended that Neoral® be administered on a consistent schedule with regard to time of day and relation to meals. Grapefruit and grapefruit juice affect metabolism, increasing blood concentration of cyclosporine, thus should be avoided.

Specific Populations

Renal Impairment in Kidney, Liver, and Heart Transplantation

Cyclosporine undergoes minimal renal elimination and its pharmacokinetics do not appear to be significantly altered in patients with end-stage renal disease who receive routine hemodialysis treatments (See CLINICAL PHARMACOLOGY). However, due to its nephrotoxic potential (See WARNINGS), careful monitoring of renal function is recommended; cyclosporine dosage should be reduced if indicated. (See WARNINGS and PRECAUTIONS)

Renal Impairment in Rheumatoid Arthritis and Psoriasis Patients with impaired renal function should not receive cyclosporine. (See CONTRAINDICATIONS, WARNINGS and PRECAUTIONS)

Hepatic Impairment

The clearance of cyclosporine may be significantly reduced in severe liver disease patients (See CLINICAL PHARMACOLOGY). Dose reduction may be necessary in patients with severe liver impairment to maintain blood concentrations within the recommended target range (See WARNINGS and PRECAUTIONS).

Newly Transplanted Patients

The initial oral dose of Neoral® can be given 4-12 hours prior to transplantation or be given postoperatively. The initial dose of Neoral® varies depending on the transplanted organ and the other immunosuppressive agents included in the immunosuppressive protocol. In newly transplanted patients, the initial oral dose of Neoral® is the same as the initial oral dose of Sandimmune®. Suggested initial doses are available from the results of a 1994 survey of the use of Sandimmune® in US transplant centers. The mean ± SD initial doses were 9±3 mg/kg/day for renal transplant patients (75 centers), 8±4 mg/kg/day for liver transplant patients (30 centers), and 7±3 mg/kg/day for heart transplant patients (24 centers). Total daily doses were divided into two equal daily doses. The Neoral® dose is subsequently adjusted to achieve a pre-defined cyclosporine blood concentration. (See Blood Concentration Monitoring in Transplant Patients, below) If cyclosporine trough blood concentrations are used, the target range is the same for Neoral® as for Sandimmune®. Using the same trough concentration target range for Neoral® as for Sandimmune® results in greater cyclosporine exposure when Neoral® is administered. (See Pharmacokinetics, Absorption) Dosing should be titrated based on clinical assessments of rejection and tolerability. Lower Neoral® doses may be sufficient as maintenance therapy.

Adjunct therapy with adrenal corticosteroids is recommended initially. Different tapering dosage schedules of prednisone appear to achieve similar results. A representative dosage schedule based on the patient's weight started with 2.0 mg/kg/day for the first 4 days tapered to 1.0 mg/kg/day by 1 week, 0.6 mg/kg/day by 2 weeks, 0.3 mg/kg/day by 1 month, and 0.15 mg/kg/day by 2 months and thereafter as a maintenance dose. Steroid doses may be further tapered on an individualized basis depending on status of patient and function of graft. Adjustments in dosage of prednisone must be made according to the clinical situation.

Conversion from Sandimmune® to Neoral® in Transplant Patients

In transplanted patients who are considered for conversion to Neoral® from Sandimmune®, Neoral® should be started with the same daily dose as was previously used with Sandimmune® (1:1 dose conversion). The Neoral® dose should subsequently be adjusted to attain the pre-conversion cyclosporine blood trough concentration. Using the same trough concentration target range for Neoral® as for Sandimmune® results in greater cyclosporine exposure when Neoral® is administered. (See Pharmacokinetics, Absorption) Patients with suspected poor absorption of Sandimmune® require different dosing strategies. (See Transplant Patients with Poor Absorption of Sandimmune®, below) In some patients, the increase in blood trough concentration is more pronounced and may be of clinical significance.

Until the blood trough concentration attains the pre-conversion value, it is strongly recommended that the cyclosporine blood trough concentration be monitored every 4 to 7 days after conversion to Neoral®. In addition, clinical safety parameters such as serum creatinine and blood pressure should be monitored every two weeks during the first two months after conversion. If the blood trough concentrations are outside the desired range and/or if the clinical safety parameters worsen, the dosage of Neoral® must be adjusted accordingly.

Transplant Patients with Poor Absorption of Sandimmune®

Patients with lower than expected cyclosporine blood trough concentrations in relation to the oral dose of Sandimmune® may have poor or inconsistent absorption of cyclosporine from Sandimmune®. After conversion to Neoral®, patients tend to have higher cyclosporine concentrations. **Due to the increase in bioavailability of cyclosporine following conversion to Neoral®, the cyclosporine blood trough concentration may exceed the target range. Particular caution should be exercised when converting patients to Neoral® at doses greater than 10 mg/kg/day.** The dose of Neoral® should be titrated individually based on cyclosporine trough concentrations, tolerability, and clinical response. In this population the cyclosporine blood trough concentration should be measured more frequently, at least twice a week (daily, if initial dose exceeds 10 mg/kg/day) until the concentration stabilizes within the desired range.

Rheumatoid Arthritis

The initial dose of Neoral® is 2.5 mg/kg/day, taken twice daily as a divided (BID) oral dose. Salicylates, nonsteroidal anti-inflammatory agents, and oral corticosteroids may be continued. (See WARNINGS and PRECAUTIONS, Drug Interactions) Onset of action generally occurs between 4 and 8 weeks. If insufficient clinical benefit is seen and tolerability is good (including serum creatinine less than 30% above

Neoral®/Sandimmune® Rheumatoid Arthritis
Percentage of Patients with Adverse Events ≥3% in any Cyclosporine Treated Group

Body System	Preferred Term	Studies 651+652+2008 Sandimmune®† (N=269)	Study 302 Sandimmune® (N=155)	Study 654 Methotrexate & Sandimmune® (N=74)	Study 654 Methotrexate & Placebo (N=73)	Study 302 Neoral® (N=143)	Studies 651+652+2008 Placebo (N=201)
Autonomic Nervous System Disorders							
	Flushing	2%	2%	3%	0%	5%	2%
Body As A Whole–General Disorders							
	Accidental Trauma	0%	1%	10%	4%	4%	0%
	Edema NOS*	5%	14%	12%	4%	10%	<1%
	Fatigue	6%	3%	8%	12%	3%	7%
	Fever	2%	3%	0%	0%	2%	4%
	Influenza-like symptoms	<1%	6%	1%	0%	3%	2%
	Pain	6%	9%	10%	15%	13%	4%
	Rigors	1%	1%	4%	0%	3%	1%
Cardiovascular Disorders							
	Arrhythmia	2%	5%	5%	6%	2%	1%
	Chest Pain	4%	5%	1%	1%	6%	1%
	Hypertension	8%	26%	16%	12%	25%	2%
Central and Peripheral Nervous System Disorders							
	Dizziness	8%	6%	7%	3%	8%	3%
	Headache	17%	23%	22%	11%	25%	9%
	Migraine	2%	3%	0%	0%	3%	1%
	Paresthesia	8%	7%	8%	4%	11%	1%
	Tremor	8%	7%	7%	3%	13%	4%
Gastrointestinal System Disorders							
	Abdominal Pain	15%	15%	15%	7%	15%	10%
	Anorexia	3%	3%	1%	0%	3%	3%
	Diarrhea	12%	12%	18%	15%	13%	8%
	Dyspepsia	12%	12%	10%	8%	8%	4%
	Flatulence	5%	5%	5%	4%	4%	1%
	Gastrointestinal Disorder NOS*	0%	2%	1%	4%	4%	0%
	Gingivitis	4%	3%	0%	0%	0%	1%
	Gum Hyperplasia	2%	4%	1%	3%	4%	1%
	Nausea	23%	14%	24%	15%	18%	14%
	Rectal Hemorrhage	0%	3%	0%	0%	1%	1%
	Stomatitis	7%	5%	16%	12%	6%	8%
	Vomiting	9%	8%	14%	7%	6%	5%
Hearing and Vestibular Disorders							
	Ear Disorder NOS*	0%	5%	0%	0%	1%	0%
Metabolic and Nutritional Disorders							
	Hypomagnesemia	0%	4%	0%	0%	6%	0%
Musculoskeletal System Disorders							
	Arthropathy	0%	5%	0%	1%	4%	0%
	Leg Cramps/ Involuntary Muscle Contractions	2%	11%	11%	3%	12%	1%
Psychiatric Disorders							
	Depression	3%	6%	3%	1%	1%	2%
	Insomnia	4%	1%	1%	0%	3%	2%
Renal							
	Creatinine elevations ≥30%	43%	39%	55%	19%	48%	13%
	Creatinine elevations ≥50%	24%	18%	26%	8%	18%	3%
Reproductive Disorders, Female							
	Leukorrhea	1%	0%	4%	0%	1%	0%
	Menstrual Disorder	3%	2%	1%	0%	1%	1%
Respiratory System Disorders							
	Bronchitis	1%	3%	1%	0%	1%	3%
	Coughing	5%	3%	5%	7%	4%	4%
	Dyspnea	5%	1%	3%	3%	1%	2%
	Infection NOS*	9%	5%	0%	7%	3%	10%
	Pharyngitis	3%	5%	5%	6%	4%	4%
	Pneumonia	1%	0%	4%	0%	1%	1%
	Rhinitis	0%	3%	11%	10%	1%	0%
	Sinusitis	4%	4%	8%	4%	3%	3%
	Upper Respiratory Tract	0%	14%	23%	15%	13%	0%

(Table continued on next page)

Neoral®/Sandimmune® Rheumatoid Arthritis
Percentage of Patients with Adverse Events ≥3% in any Cyclosporine Treated Group (cont.)

	Studies 651+652+2008	Study 302	Study 654	Study 654	Study 302	Studies 651+652+2008
			Methotrexate & Sandimmune®	Methotrexate & Placebo	Neoral®	Placebo
Body System	Preferred Term	Sandimmune®† (N=269)	Sandimmune® (N=155)	(N=74)	(N=73)	(N=143)	(N=201)
Skin and Appendages Disorders							
	Alopecia	3%	0%	1%	1%	4%	4%
	Bullous Eruption	1%	0%	4%	1%	1%	1%
	Hypertrichosis	19%	17%	12%	0%	15%	3%
	Rash	7%	12%	10%	7%	8%	10%
	Skin Ulceration	1%	1%	3%	4%	0%	2%
Urinary System Disorders							
	Dysuria	0%	0%	11%	3%	1%	2%
	Micturition Frequency	2%	4%	3%	1%	2%	2%
	NPN, Increased	0%	19%	12%	0%	18%	0%
	Urinary Tract Infection	0%	3%	5%	4%	3%	0%
Vascular (Extracardiac) Disorders							
	Purpura	3%	4%	1%	1%	2%	0%

† Includes patients in 2.5 mg/kg/day dose group only. *NOS=Not Otherwise Specified.

Adverse Events Occurring in 3% or More of Psoriasis Patients in Controlled Clinical Trials

Body System*	Preferred Term	Neoral® (N=182)	Sandimmune® (N=185)
Infection or Potential Infection		24.7%	24.3%
	Influenza-Like Symptoms	9.9%	8.1%
	Upper Respiratory Tract Infections	7.7%	11.3%
Cardiovascular System		28.0%	25.4%
	Hypertension**	27.5%	25.4%
Urinary System		24.2%	16.2%
	Increased Creatinine	19.8%	15.7%
Central and Peripheral Nervous System		26.4%	20.5%
	Headache	15.9%	14.0%
	Paresthesia	7.1%	4.8%
Musculoskeletal System		13.2%	8.7%
	Arthralgia	6.0%	1.1%
Body As a Whole– General		29.1%	22.2%
	Pain	4.4%	3.2%
Metabolic and Nutritional		9.3%	9.7%
Reproductive, Female		8.5% (4 of 47 females)	11.5% (6 of 52 females)
Resistance Mechanism		18.7%	21.1%
Skin and Appendages		17.6%	15.1%
	Hypertrichosis	6.6%	5.4%
Respiratory System		5.0%	6.5%
	Bronchospasm, Coughing, Dyspnea, Rhinitis	5.0%	4.9%
Psychiatric		5.0%	3.8%
Gastrointestinal System		19.8%	28.7%
	Abdominal Pain	2.7%	6.0%
	Diarrhea	5.0%	5.9%
	Dyspepsia	2.2%	3.2%
	Gum Hyperplasia	3.8%	6.0%
	Nausea	5.5%	5.9%
White cell and RES		4.4%	2.7%

*Total percentage of events within the system
**Newly occurring hypertension = SBP≥160 mm Hg and/or DBP≥90 mm Hg

baseline), the dose may be increased by 0.5-0.75 mg/kg/day after 8 weeks and again after 12 weeks to a maximum of 4 mg/kg/day. If no benefit is seen by 16 weeks of therapy, Neoral® therapy should be discontinued.

Dose decreases by 25%-50% should be made at any time to control adverse events, e.g., hypertension elevations in serum creatinine (30% above patient's pretreatment level) or clinically significant laboratory abnormalities. (See WARNINGS and PRECAUTIONS)

If dose reduction is not effective in controlling abnormalities or if the adverse event or abnormality is severe, Neoral® should be discontinued. The same initial dose and dosage range should be used if Neoral® is combined with the recommended dose of methotrexate. Most patients can be treated with Neoral® doses of 3 mg/kg/day or below when combined with methotrexate doses of up to 15 mg/week. (See CLINICAL PHARMACOLOGY, Clinical Trials)

There is limited long-term treatment data. Recurrence of rheumatoid arthritis disease activity is generally apparent within 4 weeks after stopping cyclosporine.

Psoriasis
The initial dose of Neoral® should be 2.5 mg/kg/day. Neoral® should be taken twice daily, as a divided (1.25 mg/kg BID) oral dose. Patients should be kept at that dose for at least 4 weeks, barring adverse events. If significant clinical improvement has not occurred in patients by that time, the patient's dosage should be increased at 2-week intervals. Based on patient response, dose increases of approximately 0.5 mg/kg/day should be made to a maximum of 4.0 mg/kg/day.

Dose decreases by 25%-50% should be made at any time to control adverse events, e.g., hypertension, elevations in serum creatinine (≥25% above the patient's pretreatment level), or clinically significant laboratory abnormalities. If dose reduction is not effective in controlling abnormalities, or if the adverse event or abnormality is severe, Neoral® should be discontinued. (See Special Monitoring of Psoriasis Patients)

Patients generally show some improvement in the clinical manifestations of psoriasis in 2 weeks. Satisfactory control and stabilization of the disease may take 12-16 weeks to achieve. Results of a dose-titration clinical trial with Neoral® indicate that an improvement of psoriasis by 75% or more (based on PASI) was achieved in 51% of the patients after 8 weeks and in 79% of the patients after 16 weeks. Treatment should be discontinued if satisfactory response cannot be achieved after 6 weeks at 4 mg/kg/day or the patient's maximum tolerated dose. Once a patient is adequately controlled and appears stable the dose of Neoral® should be lowered, and the patient treated with the lowest dose that maintains an adequate response (this should not necessarily be total clearing of the patient). In clinical trials, cyclosporine doses at the lower end of the recommended dosage range were effective in maintaining a satisfactory response in 60% of the patients. Doses below 2.5 mg/kg/day may also be equally effective.

Upon stopping treatment with cyclosporine, relapse will occur in approximately 6 weeks (50% of the patients) to 16 weeks (75% of the patients). In the majority of patients rebound does not occur after cessation of treatment with cyclosporine. Thirteen cases of transformation of chronic plaque psoriasis to more severe forms of psoriasis have been reported. There were 9 cases of pustular and 4 cases of erythrodermic psoriasis. Long term experience with Neoral® in psoriasis patients is limited and continuous treatment for extended periods greater than one year is not recommended. Alternation with other forms of treatment should be considered in the long term management of patients with this life long disease.

Neoral® Oral Solution (cyclosporine oral solution, USP) MODIFIED–Recommendations for Administration
To make Neoral® Oral Solution (cyclosporine oral solution, USP) MODIFIED more palatable, it should be diluted with orange or apple juice that is at room temperature. Patients should avoid switching diluents frequently. Grapefruit juice affects metabolism of cyclosporine and should be avoided. The combination of Neoral® solution with milk can be unpalatable. The effect of milk on the bioavailability of cyclosporine when administered as Neoral Oral Solution has not been evaluated.

Take the prescribed amount of Neoral® Oral Solution (cyclosporine oral solution, USP) MODIFIED from the container using the dosing syringe supplied, after removal of the protective cover, and transfer the solution to a glass of orange or apple juice. Stir well and drink at once. Do not allow diluted oral solution to stand before drinking. Use a glass container (not plastic). Rinse the glass with more diluent to ensure that the total dose is consumed. After use, dry the outside of the dosing syringe with a clean towel and replace the protective cover. Do not rinse the dosing syringe with water or other cleaning agents. If the syringe requires cleaning, it must be completely dry before resuming use.

Blood Concentration Monitoring in Transplant Patients
Transplant centers have found blood concentration monitoring of cyclosporine to be an essential component of patient management. Of importance to blood concentration analysis are the type of assay used, the transplanted organ, and other immunosuppressant agents being administered. While no fixed relationship has been established, blood concentration monitoring may assist in the clinical evaluation of rejection and toxicity, dose adjustments, and the assessment of compliance.

Various assays have been used to measure blood concentrations of cyclosporine. Older studies using a nonspecific assay often cited concentrations that were roughly twice those of the specific assays. Therefore, comparison between concentrations in the published literature and an individual patient concentration using current assays must be made with detailed knowledge of the assay methods employed. Current assay results are not interchangeable and their use should be guided by their approved labeling. A discussion of the different assay methods is contained in Annals of Clinical Biochemistry 1994;31:420-446. While several assays and assay matrices are available, there is a consensus that parent-compound-specific assays correlate best with clinical events. Of these, HPLC is the standard reference, but the monoclonal antibody RIAs and the monoclonal antibody FPIA offer sensitivity, reproducibility, and convenience. Most clinicians base their monitoring on trough cyclosporine concentrations. Applied Pharmacokinetics, Principles of Therapeutic Drug Monitoring (1992) contains a broad discussion of cyclosporine pharmacokinetics and drug monitoring techniques. Blood concentration monitoring is not a replacement for renal function monitoring or tissue biopsies.

HOW SUPPLIED

Neoral® Soft Gelatin Capsules (cyclosporine capsules, USP) MODIFIED

25 mg

Oval, blue-gray imprinted in red, "Neoral" over "25 mg."
Packages of 30 unit-dose blisters (NDC 0078-0246-15).

100 mg

Oblong, blue-gray imprinted in red, "NEORAL" over "100 mg."

Packages of 30 unit-dose blisters (NDC 0078-0248-15).

Store and Dispense

In the original unit-dose container at controlled room temperature 68°-77°F (20°-25°C).

Neoral® Oral Solution (cyclosporine oral solution, USP) MODIFIED

A clear, yellow liquid supplied in 50 mL bottles containing 100 mg/mL (NDC 0078-0274-22).

Store and Dispense

In the original container at controlled room temperature 68°-77°F (20°-25°C). Do not store in the refrigerator. Once opened, the contents must be used within two months. At temperatures below 68°F (20°C) the solution may gel; light flocculation or the formation of a light sediment may also occur. There is no impact on product performance or dosing using the syringe provided. Allow to warm to room temperature 77°F (25°C) to reverse these changes.

Neoral® Soft Gelatin Capsules (cyclosporine capsules, USP) MODIFIED

Neoral® Oral Solution (cyclosporine oral solution, USP) MODIFIED

Distributed by:

Novartis Pharmaceuticals Corporation, East Hanover, New Jersey 07936

© Novartis

T2013-38

May 2013

Shown in Product Identification Guide, page 310

RECLAST®

[RE-klast]

(zoledronic acid)

Injection

℞

The following prescribing information is based on official labeling in effect July 2014.

HIGHLIGHTS OF PRESCRIBING INFORMATION

These highlights do not include all the information needed to use RECLAST safely and effectively. See full prescribing information for RECLAST.

Reclast® (zoledronic acid) Injection

Initial U.S. Approval: 2001

———————RECENT MAJOR CHANGES———————

Indications and Usage (1.6)   04/2013

———————INDICATIONS AND USAGE———————

Reclast is a bisphosphonate indicated for:

• Treatment and prevention of postmenopausal osteoporosis (1.1, 1.2)

• Treatment to increase bone mass in men with osteoporosis (1.3)

• Treatment and prevention of glucocorticoid-induced osteoporosis (1.4)

• Treatment of Paget's disease of bone in men and women (1.5)

Limitations of Use

Optimal duration of use has not been determined. For patients at low-risk for fracture, consider drug discontinuation after 3 to 5 years of use (1.6)

———————DOSAGE AND ADMINISTRATION———————

Infusion given intravenously over no less than 15 minutes:

• Treatment of postmenopausal osteoporosis (2.2); treatment to increase bone mass in men with osteoporosis (2.4); treatment and prevention of glucocorticoid-induced osteoporosis (2.5): 5 mg once a year

• Prevention of postmenopausal osteoporosis: 5 mg once every 2 years (2.3)

• Treatment of Paget's disease of bone: a single 5 mg infusion. Patients should receive 1500 mg elemental calcium and 800 international units vitamin D daily (2.6)

———————DOSAGE FORMS AND STRENGTHS———————

5 mg in a 100 mL ready-to-infuse solution (3)

———————CONTRAINDICATIONS———————

• Hypocalcemia (4)

• Patients with creatinine clearance less than 35 mL/min and in those with evidence of acute renal impairment (4, 5.3)

• Hypersensitivity to any component of Reclast (4, 6.2)

———————WARNINGS AND PRECAUTIONS———————

• *Products Containing Same Active Ingredient:* Patients receiving Zometa should not receive Reclast (5.1)

• *Hypocalcemia may worsen during treatment.* Patients must be adequately supplemented with calcium and vitamin D (5.2)

• *Renal Impairment:* A single dose should not exceed 5 mg and the duration of infusion should be no less than 15 minutes. Renal toxicity may be greater in patients with underlying renal impairment or with other risk factors, including advanced age or dehydration. Monitor creatinine clearance before each dose (2.7, 5.3)

• *Osteonecrosis of the Jaw (ONJ)* has been reported. All patients should have a routine oral exam by the prescriber prior to treatment (5.4)

• *Atypical Femur Fractures* have been reported. Patients with thigh or groin pain should be evaluated to rule out a femoral fracture (5.5)

• *Pregnancy:* Reclast can cause fetal harm. Women of childbearing potential should be advised (5.6, 8.1)

• *Severe Bone, Joint, and Muscle Pain* may occur. Withhold future doses of Reclast if severe symptoms occur (5.7)

———————ADVERSE REACTIONS———————

The most common adverse reactions (greater than 10%) were pyrexia, myalgia, headache, arthralgia, pain in extremity (6.1). Other important adverse reactions were flu-like illness, nausea, vomiting, diarrhea (6.2), and eye inflammation (6.1).

To report SUSPECTED ADVERSE REACTIONS, contact Novartis Pharmaceuticals Corporation at 1-888-669-6682 or FDA at 1-800-FDA-1088 or www.fda.gov/medwatch.

———————DRUG INTERACTIONS———————

• Aminoglycosides: May lower serum calcium for prolonged periods (7.1)

• Loop diuretics: May increase risk of hypocalcemia (7.2)

• Nephrotoxic drugs: Use with caution (7.3)

• Drugs primarily excreted by the kidney: Exposure may be increased with renal impairment. Monitor serum creatinine in patients at risk (7.4)

———————USE IN SPECIFIC POPULATIONS———————

Nursing Mothers: Reclast should not be given to nursing women (8.3)

Pediatric Use: Not indicated for use in pediatric patients (8.4)

Geriatric Use: Special care to monitor renal function (8.5)

See 17 for PATIENT COUNSELING INFORMATION and Medication Guide

Revised: 4/2013

FULL PRESCRIBING INFORMATION

1 INDICATIONS AND USAGE

1.1 Treatment of Osteoporosis in Postmenopausal Women

Reclast is indicated for treatment of osteoporosis in postmenopausal women. In postmenopausal women with osteoporosis, diagnosed by bone mineral density (BMD) or prevalent vertebral fracture, Reclast reduces the incidence of fractures (hip, vertebral and non-vertebral osteoporosis-related fractures). In patients at high risk of fracture, defined as a recent low-trauma hip fracture, Reclast reduces the incidence of new clinical fractures [see Clinical Studies (14.1)].

1.2 Prevention of Osteoporosis in Postmenopausal Women

Reclast is indicated for prevention of osteoporosis in postmenopausal women [see Clinical Studies (14.2)].

1.3 Osteoporosis in Men

Reclast is indicated for treatment to increase bone mass in men with osteoporosis [see Clinical Studies (14.3)].

1.4 Glucocorticoid-Induced Osteoporosis

Reclast is indicated for the treatment and prevention of glucocorticoid-induced osteoporosis in men and women who are either initiating or continuing systemic glucocorticoids in a daily dosage equivalent to 7.5 mg or greater of prednisone and who are expected to remain on glucocorticoids for at least 12 months [see Clinical Studies (14.4)].

1.5 Paget's Disease of Bone

Reclast is indicated for treatment of Paget's disease of bone in men and women. Treatment is indicated in patients with Paget's disease of bone with elevations in serum alkaline phosphatase of two times or higher than the upper limit of the age-specific normal reference range, or those who are symptomatic, or those at risk for complications from their disease [see Clinical Studies (14.5)].

1.6 Important Limitations of Use

The safety and effectiveness of Reclast for the treatment of osteoporosis is based on clinical data of three years duration. The optimal duration of use has not been determined. All patients on bisphosphonate therapy should have the need for continued therapy re-evaluated on a periodic basis. Patients at low-risk for fracture should be considered for drug discontinuation after 3 to 5 years of use. Patients who discontinue therapy should have their risk for fracture re-evaluated periodically.

2 DOSAGE AND ADMINISTRATION

2.1 Important Administration Instructions

Reclast injection must be administered as an intravenous infusion over no less than 15 minutes.

• Patients must be appropriately hydrated prior to administration of Reclast [see Warnings and Precautions (5.3)].

• Parenteral drug products should be inspected visually for particulate matter and discoloration prior to administration, whenever solution and container permit.

• Intravenous infusion should be followed by a 10 mL normal saline flush of the intravenous line.

• Administration of acetaminophen following Reclast administration may reduce the incidence of acute-phase reaction symptoms.

2.2 Treatment of Osteoporosis in Postmenopausal Women

The recommended regimen is a 5 mg infusion once a year given intravenously over no less than 15 minutes.

2.3 Prevention of Osteoporosis in Postmenopausal Women

The recommended regimen is a 5 mg infusion given once every 2 years intravenously over no less than 15 minutes.

2.4 Osteoporosis in Men

The recommended regimen is a 5 mg infusion once a year given intravenously over no less than 15 minutes.

2.5 Treatment and Prevention of Glucocorticoid-Induced Osteoporosis

The recommended regimen is a 5 mg infusion once a year given intravenously over no less than 15 minutes.

2.6 Treatment of Paget's Disease of Bone

The recommended dose is a 5 mg infusion. The infusion time must be not less than 15 minutes given over a constant infusion rate.

Help Patients Save on Rx Drugs: PDR.net/PharmacyDiscountCard

Table 1. Adverse Reactions Occurring in greater than or equal to 2.0% of Patients with Osteoporosis and More Frequently than in Placebo-Treated Patients

System Organ Class	Study 1		Study 2	
	5 mg IV Reclast once per year % (N=3862)	Placebo once per year % (N=3852)	5 mg IV Reclast once per year % (N=1054)	Placebo once per year % (N=1057)
Blood and the Lymphatic System Disorders				
Anemia	4.4	3.6	5.3	5.2
Metabolism and Nutrition Disorders				
Dehydration	0.6	0.6	2.5	2.3
Anorexia	2.0	1.1	1.0	1.0
Nervous System Disorders				
Headache	12.4	8.1	3.9	2.5
Dizziness	7.6	6.7	2.0	4.0
Ear and Labyrinth Disorders				
Vertigo	4.3	4.0	1.3	1.7
Cardiac Disorders				
Atrial Fibrillation	2.4	1.9	2.8	2.6
Vascular Disorders				
Hypertension	12.7	12.4	6.8	5.4
Gastrointestinal Disorders				
Nausea	8.5	5.2	4.5	4.5
Diarrhea	6.0	5.6	5.2	4.7
Vomiting	4.6	3.2	3.4	3.4
Abdominal Pain Upper	4.6	3.1	0.9	1.5
Dyspepsia	4.3	4.0	1.7	1.6
Musculoskeletal, Connective Tissue and Bone Disorders				
Arthralgia	23.8	20.4	17.9	18.3
Myalgia	11.7	3.7	4.9	2.7
Pain in Extremity	11.3	9.9	5.9	4.8
Shoulder Pain	6.9	5.6	0.0	0.0
Bone Pain	5.8	2.3	3.2	1.0
Neck Pain	4.4	3.8	1.4	1.1
Muscle Spasms	3.7	3.4	1.5	1.7
Osteoarthritis	9.1	9.7	5.7	4.5
Musculoskeletal Pain	0.4	0.3	3.1	1.2
General Disorders and Administrative Site Conditions				
Pyrexia	17.9	4.6	8.7	3.1
Influenza-like Illness	8.8	2.7	0.8	0.4
Fatigue	5.4	3.5	2.1	1.2
Chills	5.4	1.0	1.5	0.5
Asthenia	5.3	2.9	3.2	3.0
Peripheral Edema	4.6	4.2	5.5	5.3
Pain	3.3	1.3	1.5	0.5
Malaise	2.0	1.0	1.1	0.5
Hyperthermia	0.3	<0.1	2.3	0.3
Chest Pain	1.3	1.1	2.4	1.8
Investigations				
Creatinine Renal Clearance Decreased	2.0	2.4	2.1	1.7

Re-treatment of Paget's Disease

After a single treatment with Reclast in Paget's disease an extended remission period is observed. Specific re-treatment data are not available. However, re-treatment with Reclast may be considered in patients who have relapsed, based on increases in serum alkaline phosphatase, or in those patients who failed to achieve normalization of their serum alkaline phosphatase, or in those patients with symptoms, as dictated by medical practice.

2.7 Laboratory Testing and Oral Examination Prior to Administration

• Prior to administration of each dose of Reclast, obtain a serum creatinine and creatinine clearance should be calculated based on actual body weight using Cockcroft-Gault formula before each Reclast dose. Reclast is contraindicated in patients with creatinine clearance less than 35 mL/min and in those with evidence of acute renal impairment. A 5 mg dose of Reclast administered intravenously is recommended for patients with creatinine clearance greater than or equal to 35 mL/min. There are no safety or efficacy data to support the adjustment of the Reclast dose based on baseline renal function. Therefore, no dose adjustment is required in patients with CrCl greater than or equal to 35 mL/min [*see Contraindications (4), Warnings and Precautions (5.3)*].

• A routine oral examination should be performed by the prescriber prior to initiation of Reclast treatment [*see Warnings and Precautions (5.4)*].

2.8 Calcium and Vitamin D Supplementation

• Instruct patients being treated for Paget's disease of bone on the importance of calcium and vitamin D supplementation in maintaining serum calcium levels, and on the symptoms of hypocalcemia. All patients should take 1500 mg elemental calcium daily in divided doses (750 mg two times a day, or 500 mg three times a day) and 800 in-ternational units vitamin D daily, particularly in the 2 weeks following Reclast administration [*see Warnings and Precautions (5.2)*].

• Instruct patients being treated for osteoporosis to take supplemental calcium and vitamin D if their dietary intake is inadequate. An average of at least 1200 mg calcium and 800-1000 international units vitamin D daily is recommended.

2.9 Method of Administration

The Reclast infusion time must not be less than 15 minutes given over a constant infusion rate.

The i.v. infusion should be followed by a 10 mL normal saline flush of the intravenous line.

Reclast solution for infusion must not be allowed to come in contact with any calcium or other divalent cation-containing solutions, and should be administered as a single intravenous solution through a separate vented infusion line.

If refrigerated, allow the refrigerated solution to reach room temperature before administration. After opening, the solution is stable for 24 hours at 2°C–8°C (36°F - 46°F) [*see How Supplied/Storage and Handling (16)*].

3 DOSAGE FORMS AND STRENGTHS

5 mg in a 100 mL ready to infuse solution.

4 CONTRAINDICATIONS

Reclast is contraindicated in patients with the following conditions:

• Hypocalcemia [*see Warnings and Precautions (5.2)*]

• Creatinine clearance less than 35 mL/min and in those with evidence of acute renal impairment due to an increased risk of renal failure [*see Warnings and Precautions (5.3)*].

• Known hypersensitivity to zoledronic acid or any components of Reclast. Hypersensitivity reactions including urticaria, angioedema, and anaphylactic reaction/shock have been reported [*see Post-Marketing Experience (6.2)*].

5 WARNINGS AND PRECAUTIONS

5.1 Drug Products with Same Active Ingredient

Reclast contains the same active ingredient found in Zometa, used for oncology indications, and a patient being treated with Zometa should not be treated with Reclast.

5.2 Hypocalcemia and Mineral Metabolism

Pre-existing hypocalcemia and disturbances of mineral metabolism (e.g., hypoparathyroidism, thyroid surgery, parathyroid surgery; malabsorption syndromes, excision of small intestine) must be effectively treated before initiating therapy with Reclast. Clinical monitoring of calcium and mineral levels (phosphorus and magnesium) is highly recommended for these patients [*see Contraindications (4)*].

Hypocalcemia following Reclast administration is a significant risk in Paget's disease. All patients should be instructed about the symptoms of hypocalcemia and the importance of calcium and vitamin D supplementation in maintaining serum calcium levels [*see Dosage and Administration (2.8), Adverse Reactions (6.1), Information for Patients (17)*].

All osteoporosis patients should be instructed on the importance of calcium and vitamin D supplementation in maintaining serum calcium levels [*see Dosage and Administration (2.8), Adverse Reactions (6.1), Information for Patients (17)*].

5.3 Renal Impairment

A single dose of Reclast should not exceed 5 mg and the duration of infusion should be no less than 15 minutes [*see Dosage and Administration (2)*].

Reclast is contraindicated in patients with creatinine clearance less than 35 mL/min and in those with evidence of acute renal impairment [*see Contraindications (4)*]. If history or physical signs suggest dehydration, Reclast therapy should be withheld until normovolemic status has been achieved [*see Post-Marketing Experience (6.2)*].

Reclast should be used with caution in patients with chronic renal impairment. Acute renal impairment, including renal failure, has been observed following the administration of zoledronic acid, especially in patients with pre-existing renal compromise, advanced age, concomitant nephrotoxic medications, concomitant diuretic therapy, or severe dehydration occurring before or after Reclast administration. Acute renal failure (ARF) has been observed in patients after a single administration. Rare reports of hospitalization and/or dialysis or fatal outcome occurred in patients with underlying moderate to severe renal impairment or with any of the risk factors described in this section [*see Post-Marketing Experience (6.2)*]. Renal impairment may lead to increased exposure of concomitant medications and/or their metabolites that are primarily renally excreted [*see Drug Interactions (7.4)*].

Creatinine clearance should be calculated based on actual body weight using Cockcroft-Gault formula before each Reclast dose. Transient increase in serum creatinine may be greater in patients with impaired renal function; interim monitoring of creatinine clearance should be performed in at-risk patients. Elderly patients and those receiving diuretic therapy are at increased risk of acute renal failure. These patients should have their fluid status assessed and be appropriately hydrated prior to administration of Reclast. Reclast should be used with caution with other nephrotoxic drugs [*see Drug Interactions (7.3)*]. Consider monitoring creatinine clearance in patients at-risk for ARF who are taking concomitant medications that are primarily excreted by the kidney [*see Drug Interactions (7.4)*].

5.4 Osteonecrosis of the Jaw

Osteonecrosis of the jaw (ONJ) has been reported in patients treated with bisphosphonates, including zoledronic acid. Most cases have been in cancer patients treated with intravenous bisphosphonates undergoing dental procedures. Some cases have occurred in patients with postmenopausal osteoporosis treated with either oral or intravenous bisphosphonates. A routine oral examination should be performed by the prescriber prior to initiation of bisphosphonate treatment. A dental examination with appropriate preventive dentistry should be considered prior to treatment with bisphosphonates in patients with a history of concomitant risk factors (e.g., cancer, chemotherapy, radiotherapy, corticosteroids, poor oral hygiene, pre-existing dental disease or infection, anemia, coagulopathy).

While on treatment, patients with concomitant risk factors should avoid invasive dental procedures if possible. For patients who develop ONJ while on bisphosphonate therapy, dental surgery may exacerbate the condition. For patients requiring dental procedures, there are no data available to suggest whether discontinuation of bisphosphonate treatment reduces the risk of ONJ. The clinical judgment of the treating physician should guide the management plan of each patient based on individual benefit/risk assessment [*see Adverse Reactions (6.1)*].

5.5 Atypical Subtrochanteric and Diaphyseal Femoral Fractures

Atypical, low-energy, or low trauma fractures of the femoral shaft have been reported in bisphosphonate-treated patients. These fractures can occur anywhere in the femoral shaft from just below the lesser trochanter to above the supracondylar flare and are transverse or short oblique in orientation without evidence of comminution. Causality has not been established as these fractures also occur in osteoporotic patients who have not been treated with bisphosphonates.

Atypical femur fractures most commonly occur with minimal or no trauma to the affected area. They may be bilateral and many patients report prodromal pain in the affected area, usually presenting as dull, aching thigh pain, weeks to months before a complete fracture occurs. A number of reports note that patients were also receiving treatment with glucocorticoids (e.g., prednisone) at the time of fracture.

Any patient with a history of bisphosphonate exposure who presents with thigh or groin pain should be suspected of having an atypical fracture and should be evaluated to rule out an incomplete femur fracture. Patients presenting with an atypical femur fracture should also be assessed for symptoms and signs of fracture in the contralateral limb. Interruption of bisphosphonate therapy should be considered, pending a risk/benefit assessment, on an individual basis.

5.6 Pregnancy

RECLAST SHOULD NOT BE USED DURING PREGNANCY. Reclast may cause fetal harm when administered to a pregnant woman. If the patient becomes pregnant while taking this drug, the patient should be apprised of the potential harm to the fetus. Women of childbearing potential should be advised to avoid becoming pregnant while on Reclast therapy [see Use in Specific Populations (8.1)].

5.7 Musculoskeletal Pain

In post-marketing experience, severe and occasionally incapacitating bone, joint, and/or muscle pain have been infrequently reported in patients taking bisphosphonates, including Reclast. The time to onset of symptoms varied from one day to several months after starting the drug. Consider withholding future Reclast treatment if severe symptoms develop. Most patients had relief of symptoms after stopping. A subset had recurrence of symptoms when rechallenged with the same drug or another bisphosphonate [see Adverse Reactions (6.2)].

5.8 Patients with Asthma

While not observed in clinical trials with Reclast, there have been reports of bronchoconstriction in aspirin-sensitive patients receiving bisphosphonates. Use Reclast with caution in aspirin-sensitive patients.

6 ADVERSE REACTIONS

6.1 Clinical Studies Experience

Because clinical trials are conducted under widely varying conditions, adverse reaction rates observed in the clinical trials of a drug cannot be directly compared to rates in the clinical trials of another drug and may not reflect the rates observed in practice.

Treatment of Osteoporosis in Postmenopausal Women

The safety of Reclast in the treatment of postmenopausal osteoporosis was assessed in Study 1, a large, randomized, double-blind, placebo-controlled, multinational study of 7736 postmenopausal women aged 65-89 years with osteoporosis, diagnosed by bone mineral density or the presence of a prevalent vertebral fracture. The duration of the trial was three years with 3862 patients exposed to Reclast and 3852 patients exposed to placebo administered once annually as a single 5 mg dose in 100 mL solution infused over at least 15 minutes, for a total of three doses. All women received 1000 to 1500 mg of elemental calcium plus 400 to 1200 international units of vitamin D supplementation per day.

The incidence of all-cause mortality was similar between groups: 3.4% in the Reclast group and 2.9% in the placebo group. The incidence of serious adverse events was 29.2% in the Reclast group and 30.1% in the placebo group. The percentage of patients who withdrew from the study due to adverse events was 5.4% and 4.8% for the Reclast and placebo groups, respectively.

The safety of Reclast in the treatment of osteoporosis patients with a recent (within 90 days) low-trauma hip fracture was assessed in Study 2, a randomized, double-blind, placebo-controlled, multinational endpoint-driven study of 2127 men and women aged 50-95 years; 1065 patients were randomized to Reclast and 1062 patients were randomized to placebo. Reclast was administered once annually as a single 5 mg dose in 100 mL solution infused over at least 15 minutes. The study continued until at least 211 patients had a confirmed clinical fracture in the study population who were followed for an average of approximately 2 years on study drug. Vitamin D levels were not routinely measured but a loading dose of vitamin D (50,000 to 125,000 international units orally or IM) was given to patients and they were started on 1000 to 1500 mg of elemental calcium

plus 800 to 1200 international units of vitamin D supplementation per day for at least 14 days prior to the study drug infusions.

The incidence of all-cause mortality was 9.6% in the Reclast group and 13.3% in the placebo group. The incidence of serious adverse events was 38.3% in the Reclast group and 41.3% in the placebo group. The percentage of patients who withdrew from the study due to adverse events was 5.3% and 4.7% for the Reclast and placebo groups, respectively. Adverse reactions reported in at least 2% of patients with osteoporosis and more frequently in the Reclast-treated patients than placebo-treated patients in either osteoporosis trial are shown below in Table 1.

[See table 1 at top of previous page]

Renal Impairment

Treatment with intravenous bisphosphonates, including zoledronic acid, has been associated with renal impairment manifested as deterioration in renal function (i.e., increased serum creatinine) and in rare cases, acute renal failure. In the clinical trial for postmenopausal osteoporosis, patients with baseline creatinine clearance less than 30 mL/min (based on actual body weight), urine dipstick greater than or equal to 2+ protein or increase in serum creatinine of greater than 0.5 mg/dL during the screening visits were excluded. The change in creatinine clearance (measured annually prior to dosing) and the incidence of renal failure and impairment was comparable for both the Reclast and placebo treatment groups over 3 years, including patients with creatinine clearance between 30-60 mL/min at baseline. Overall, there was a transient increase in serum creatinine observed within 10 days of dosing in 1.8% of Reclast-treated patients versus 0.8% of placebo-treated patients which resolved without specific therapy [see Warnings and Precautions (5.3)].

Acute Phase Reaction

The signs and symptoms of acute phase reaction occurred in Study 1 following Reclast infusion including fever (18%), myalgia (9%), flu-like symptoms (8%), headache (7%), and arthralgia (7%). The majority of these symptoms occurred within the first 3 days following the dose of Reclast and usually resolved within 3 days of onset but resolution could take up to 7-14 days. In Study 2, patients without a contraindication to acetaminophen were provided with a standard oral dose at the time of the IV infusion and instructed to use additional acetaminophen at home for the next 72 hours as needed. Reclast was associated with fewer signs and symptoms of a transient acute phase reaction in this trial: fever (7%) and arthralgia (3%). The incidence of these symptoms decreased with subsequent doses of Reclast.

Laboratory Findings

In Study 1, in women with postmenopausal osteoporosis, approximately 0.2% of patients had notable declines of serum calcium levels (less than 7.5 mg/dL) following Reclast administration. No symptomatic cases of hypocalcemia were observed. In Study 2, following pre-treatment with vitamin D, no patients had treatment emergent serum calcium levels below 7.5 mg/dL.

Injection Site Reactions

In the osteoporosis trials, local reactions at the infusion site such as itching, redness and/or pain have been reported in 0% to 0.7% of patients following the administration of Reclast and 0% to 0.5% of patients following administration of placebo.

Osteonecrosis of the Jaw

In the postmenopausal osteoporosis trial, Study 1, in 7736 patients, after initiation of therapy, symptoms consistent with ONJ occurred in one patient treated with placebo and one patient treated with Reclast. Both cases resolved after

Table 2. Adverse Reactions Occurring in greater than or equal to 2% of Patients with Osteopenia and More Frequently than in Placebo-Treated Patients

System Organ Class	5 mg IV Reclast Once Per Year % (n=198)	5 mg IV Reclast Once % (n=181)	Placebo once per year % (n=202)
Metabolism and nutrition disorders			
Anorexia	2.0	0.6	0.0
Nervous system disorders			
Headache	14.6	20.4	11.4
Dizziness	7.6	6.1	3.5
Hypoesthesia	5.6	2.2	2.0
Ear and labyrinth disorders			
Vertigo	2.0	1.7	1.0
Vascular disorders			
Hypertension	5.1	8.3	6.9
Gastrointestinal disorders			
Nausea	17.7	11.6	7.9
Diarrhea	8.1	6.6	7.9
Vomiting	7.6	5.0	7.9
Dyspepsia	7.1	6.6	4.5
Abdominal pain*	8.6	6.6	5.0
Constipation	6.6	7.2	7.9
Abdominal discomfort	2.0	1.1	0.5
Abdominal distension	2.0	0.6	0.0
Skin and subcutaneous tissue disorders			
Rash	3.0	2.2	2.5
Musculoskeletal and connective tissue disorders			
Arthralgia	27.3	18.8	19.3
Myalgia	19.2	22.7	6.9
Back pain	18.2	16.6	11.9
Pain in extremity	11.1	16.0	9.9
Muscle spasms	5.6	2.8	5.0
Musculoskeletal pain**	8.1	7.2	7.9
Bone pain	5.1	3.3	1.0
Neck pain	5.1	6.6	5.0
Arthritis	4.0	2.2	1.5
Joint stiffness	3.5	1.1	2.0
Joint swelling	3.0	0.6	2.0
Flank pain	2.0	0.6	0.0
Pain in jaw	2.0	3.9	2.5
General disorders and administration site conditions			
Pain	24.2	14.9	3.5
Pyrexia	21.7	21.0	4.5
Chills	18.2	18.2	3.0
Fatigue	14.6	9.9	4.0
Asthenia	6.1	2.8	1.0
Peripheral edema	5.6	3.9	3.5
Non-cardiac chest pain	3.5	7.7	3.0
Influenza-like illness	1.5	3.3	2.0
Malaise	1.0	2.2	0.5

* Combined abdominal pain, abdominal pain upper, and abdominal pain lower as one ADR
** Combined musculoskeletal pain and musculoskeletal chest pain as one ADR

appropriate treatment [see *Warnings and Precautions (5.4)*]. No reports of osteonecrosis of the jaw were reported in either treatment group in Study 2.

Atrial Fibrillation

In the postmenopausal osteoporosis trial, Study 1, adjudicated serious adverse events of atrial fibrillation in the zoledronic acid treatment group occurred in 1.3% of patients (50 out of 3862) compared to 0.4% (17 out of 3852) in the placebo group. The overall incidence of all atrial fibrillation adverse events in the zoledronic acid treatment group was reported in 2.5% of patients (96 out of 3862) in the Reclast group vs. 1.9% of patients (75 out of 3852) in the placebo group. Over 90% of these events in both treatment groups occurred more than a month after the infusion. In an ECG sub-study, ECG measurements were performed on a subset of 559 patients before and 9 to 11 days after treatment. There was no difference in the incidence of atrial fibrillation between treatment groups suggesting these events were not related to the acute infusions. In Study 2, adjudicated serious adverse events of atrial fibrillation in the zoledronic acid treatment group occurred in 1.0% of patients (11 out of 1054) compared to 1.2% (13 out of 1057) in the placebo group demonstrating no difference between treatment groups.

Ocular Adverse Events

Cases of iritis/uveitis/episcleritis/conjunctivitis have been reported in patients treated with bisphosphonates, including zoledronic acid. In the osteoporosis trials, 1 (less than 0.1%) to 9 (0.2%) patients treated with Reclast and 0 (0%) to 1 (less than 0.1%) patient treated with placebo developed iritis/uveitis/episcleritis.

Prevention of Osteoporosis in Postmenopausal Women

The safety of Reclast in postmenopausal women with osteopenia (low bone mass) was assessed in a 2-year randomized, multi-center, double-blind, placebo-controlled study of 581 postmenopausal women aged greater than or equal to 45 years. Patients were randomized to one of three treatment groups: (1) Reclast given at randomization and Month 12 (n=198); (2) Reclast given at randomization and placebo at Month 12 (n=181); and (3) placebo given at randomization and Month 12 (n=202). Reclast was administered as a single 5 mg dose in 100 mL solution infused over at least 15 minutes. All women received 500 to 1200 mg elemental calcium plus 400 to 800 international units vitamin D supplementation per day.

The incidence of serious adverse events was similar for subjects given (1) Reclast at randomization and at Month 12 (10.6%), (2) Reclast at randomization and placebo given at Month 12 (9.4%), and (3) placebo at randomization and at Month 12 (11.4%). The percentages of patients who withdrew from the study due to adverse events were 7.1%, 7.2%, and 3.0% in the two Reclast groups and placebo group, respectively. Adverse reactions reported in at least 2% of patients with osteopenia and more frequently in the Reclast-treated patients than placebo-treated patients are shown in Table 2.

[See table 2 at top of previous page]

Ocular Adverse Events

Cases of iritis/uveitis/episcleritis/conjunctivitis have been reported in patients treated with bisphosphonates, including zoledronic acid. In the osteoporosis prevention trial, 4 (1.1%) patients treated with Reclast and 0 (0%) patients treated with placebo developed iritis/uveitis.

Acute Phase Reaction

In patients given Reclast at randomization and placebo at Month 12, Reclast was associated with signs and symptoms of an acute phase reaction: myalgia (20.4%), fever (19.3%), chills (18.2%), pain (13.8%), headache (13.3%), fatigue (8.3%), arthralgia (6.1%), pain in extremity (3.9%), influenza-like illness (3.3%), and back pain (1.7%), which occurred within the first 3 days following the dose of Reclast. The majority of these symptoms were mild to moderate and resolved within 3 days of the event onset but resolution could take up to 7-14 days.

Osteoporosis in Men

The safety of Reclast in men with osteoporosis or osteoporosis secondary to hypogonadism was assessed in a two year randomized, multicenter, double-blind, active controlled group study of 302 men aged 25-86 years. One hundred fifty three (153) patients were exposed to Reclast administered once annually with a 5 mg dose in 100 mL infused over 15 minutes for up to a total of two doses, and 148 patients were exposed to a commercially-available oral weekly bisphosphonate (active control) for up to two years. All participants received 1000 mg of elemental calcium plus 800 to 1000 international units of vitamin D supplementation per day.

The incidence of all-cause mortality (one in each group) and serious adverse events were similar between the Reclast and active control treatment groups. The percentage of patients experiencing at least one adverse event was comparable between the Reclast and active control groups, with the exception of a higher incidence of post-dose symptoms in

the Reclast group that occurred within 3 days after infusion. The overall safety and tolerability of Reclast was similar to the active control.

Adverse reactions reported in at least 2% of men with osteoporosis and more frequently in the Reclast-treated patients than the active control-treated patients and either (1) not reported in the postmenopausal osteoporosis treatment trial or (2) reported more frequently in the trial of osteoporosis in men are presented in Table 3. Therefore, Table 3 should be viewed in conjunction with Table 1.

Table 3: Adverse Reactions Occurring in greater than or equal to 2% of Men with Osteoporosis and More Frequently in the Reclast-Treated Patients than the Active Control-Treated Patients and either (1) Not Reported in the Postmenopausal Osteoporosis Treatment Trial or (2) Reported More Frequently in this Trial

System Organ Class	5 mg IV Reclast once per year % (N=153)	Active Control once weekly % (N=148)
Nervous System Disorders		
Headache	15.0	6.1
Lethargy	3.3	1.4
Eye Disorders		
Eye pain	2.0	0.0
Cardiac Disorders		
Atrial fibrillation	3.3	2.0
Palpitations	2.6	0.0
Respiratory, Thoracic and Mediastinal Disorders		
Dyspnea	6.5	4.7
Abdominal pain*	7.9	4.1
Skin and Subcutaneous Tissue Disorders		
Hyperhidrosis	2.6	2.0
Musculoskeletal, Connective Tissue and Bone Disorders		
Myalgia	19.6	6.8
Musculoskeletal pain**	12.4	10.8
Musculoskeletal stiffness	4.6	0.0
Renal and Urinary Disorders		
Blood creatinine increased	2.0	0.7
General Disorders and Administrative Site Conditions		
Fatigue	17.6	6.1
Pain	11.8	4.1
Chills	9.8	2.7
Influenza-like illness	9.2	2.0
Malaise	7.2	0.7
Acute phase reaction	3.9	0.0
Investigations		
C-reactive protein increased	4.6	1.4

* Combined abdominal pain, abdominal pain upper, and abdominal pain lower as one ADR
** Combined musculoskeletal pain and musculoskeletal chest pain as one ADR

Renal Impairment

Creatinine clearance was measured annually prior to dosing and changes in long-term renal function over 24 months were comparable in the Reclast and active control groups [see *Warnings and Precautions (5.3)*].

Acute Phase Reaction

Reclast was associated with signs and symptoms of an acute phase reaction: myalgia (17.1%), fever (15.7%), fatigue (12.4%), arthralgia (11.1%), pain (10.5%), chills (9.8%), headache (9.8%), influenza-like illness (8.5%), malaise (5.2%), and back pain (3.3%), which occurred within the first 3 days following the dose of Reclast. The majority of these symptoms were mild to moderate and resolved within 3 days of the event onset but resolution could take up to 7-14 days. The incidence of these symptoms decreased with subsequent doses of Reclast.

Atrial Fibrillation

The incidence of all atrial fibrillation adverse events in the Reclast treatment group was 3.3% (5 out of 153) compared to 2.0% (3 out of 148) in the active control group. However, there were no patients with adjudicated serious adverse events of atrial fibrillation in the Reclast treatment group.

Laboratory Findings

There were no patients who had treatment emergent serum calcium levels below 7.5 mg/dL.

Injection Site Reactions

There were 4 patients (2.6%) on Reclast vs. 2 patients (1.4%) on active control with local site reactions.

Osteonecrosis of the Jaw

In this trial there were no cases of osteonecrosis of the jaw [see *Warnings and Precautions (5.4)*].

Glucocorticoid-Induced Osteoporosis

The safety of Reclast in men and women in the treatment and prevention of glucocorticoid-induced osteoporosis was assessed in a randomized, multicenter, double-blind, active controlled, stratified study of 833 men and women aged 18-85 years treated with greater than or equal to 7.5 mg/day oral prednisone (or equivalent). Patients were stratified according to the duration of their pre-study corticosteroid therapy: less than or equal to 3 months prior to randomization (prevention subpopulation), and greater than 3 months prior to randomization (treatment subpopulation).

The duration of the trial was one year with 416 patients exposed to Reclast administered once as a single 5 mg dose in 100 mL infused over 15 minutes, and 417 patients exposed to a commercially-available oral daily bisphosphonate (active control) for one year. All participants received 1000 mg of elemental calcium plus 400 to 1000 international units of vitamin D supplementation per day.

The incidence of all-cause mortality was similar between treatment groups: 0.9% in the Reclast group and 0.7% in the active control group. The incidence of serious adverse events was similar between the Reclast treatment and prevention groups, 18.4% and 18.1%, respectively, and the active control treatment and prevention groups, 19.8% and 16.0%, respectively. The percentage of subjects who withdrew from the study due to adverse events was 2.2% in the Reclast group vs. 1.4% in the active control group. The overall safety and tolerability were similar between Reclast and active control groups with the exception of a higher incidence of post-dose symptoms in the Reclast group that occurred within 3 days after infusion. The overall safety and tolerability profile of Reclast in glucocorticoid-induced osteoporosis was similar to the adverse events reported in the Reclast postmenopausal osteoporosis clinical trial.

Adverse reactions reported in at least 2% of patients that were either not reported in the postmenopausal osteoporosis treatment trial or reported more frequently in the treatment and prevention of glucocorticoid-induced osteoporosis trial included the following: abdominal pain (Reclast 7.5%; active control 5.0%), and musculoskeletal pain (Reclast 3.1%; active control 1.7%). Other musculoskeletal events included back pain (Reclast 4.3%, active control 6.2%), bone pain (Reclast 3.1%, active control 2.2%), and pain in the extremity (Reclast 3.1%, active control 1.2%). In addition, the following adverse events occurred more frequently than in the postmenopausal osteoporosis trial: nausea (Reclast 9.6%; active control 8.4%), and dyspepsia (Reclast 5.5%; active control 4.3%).

Renal Impairment

Renal function measured prior to dosing and at the end of the 12 month study was comparable in the Reclast and active control groups [see *Warnings and Precautions (5.3)*].

Acute Phase Reaction

Reclast was associated with signs and symptoms of a transient acute phase reaction that was similar to that seen in the Reclast postmenopausal osteoporosis clinical trial.

Atrial Fibrillation

The incidence of atrial fibrillation adverse events was 0.7% (3 of 416) in the Reclast group compared to no adverse events in the active control group. All subjects had a prior history of atrial fibrillation and no cases were adjudicated as serious adverse events. One patient had atrial flutter in the active control group.

Laboratory Findings

There were no patients who had treatment emergent serum calcium levels below 7.5 mg/dL.

Injection Site Reactions

There were no local reactions at the infusion site.

Osteonecrosis of the Jaw

In this trial there were no cases of osteonecrosis of the jaw [see *Warnings and Precautions (5.4)*].

Paget's Disease of Bone

In the Paget's disease trials, two 6-month, double-blind, comparative, multinational studies of 349 men and women aged greater than 30 years with moderate to severe disease and with confirmed Paget's disease of bone, 177 patients were exposed to Reclast and 172 patients exposed to risedronate. Reclast was administered once as a single 5 mg dose in 100 mL solution infused over at least 15 minutes. Risedronate was given as an oral daily dose of 30 mg for 2 months.

The incidence of serious adverse events was 5.1% in the Reclast group and 6.4% in the risedronate group. The percentage of patients who withdrew from the study due to adverse events was 1.7% and 1.2% for the Reclast and risedronate groups, respectively.

Adverse reactions occurring in at least 2% of the Paget's patients receiving Reclast (single 5 mg intravenous infusion) or risedronate (30 mg oral daily dose for 2 months) over a 6-month study period are listed by system organ class in Table 4.

Table 4. Adverse Reactions Reported in at Least 2% of Paget's Patients Receiving Reclast (Single 5 mg intravenous Infusion) or Risedronate (Oral 30 mg Daily for 2 Months) Over a 6-Month Follow-Up Period

System Organ Class	5 mg IV Reclast % (N = 177)	30 mg/day × 2 Months risedronate % (N = 172)
Infections and Infestations		
Influenza	7	5
Metabolism and Nutrition Disorders		
Hypocalcemia	3	1
Anorexia	2	2
Nervous System Disorders		
Headache	11	10
Dizziness	9	4
Lethargy	5	1
Paresthesia	2	0
Respiratory, Thoracic and Mediastinal Disorders		
Dyspnea	5	1
Gastrointestinal Disorders		
Nausea	9	6
Diarrhea	6	6
Constipation	6	5
Dyspepsia	5	4
Abdominal Distension	2	1
Abdominal Pain	2	2
Vomiting	2	2
Abdominal Pain Upper	1	2
Skin and Subcutaneous Tissue Disorders		
Rash	3	2
Musculoskeletal, Connective Tissue and Bone Disorders		
Arthralgia	9	11
Bone Pain	9	5
Myalgia	7	4
Back Pain	4	7
Musculoskeletal Stiffness	2	1
General Disorders and Administrative Site Conditions		
Influenza-like Illness	11	6
Pyrexia	9	2
Fatigue	8	4
Rigors	8	1
Pain	5	4
Peripheral Edema	3	1
Asthenia	2	1

Laboratory Findings
In the Paget's disease trials, early, transient decreases in serum calcium and phosphate levels were observed. Approximately 21% of patients had serum calcium levels less than 8.4 mg/dL 9-11 days following Reclast administration.

Renal Impairment
In clinical trials in Paget's disease there were no cases of renal deterioration following a single 5 mg 15-minute infusion [see Warnings and Precautions (5.3)].

Acute Phase Reaction
The signs and symptoms of acute phase reaction (influenza-like illness, pyrexia, myalgia, arthralgia, and bone pain) were reported in 25% of patients in the Reclast-treated group compared to 8% in the risedronate-treated group. Symptoms usually occur within the first 3 days following Reclast administration. The majority of these symptoms resolved within 4 days of onset.

Osteonecrosis of the Jaw
Osteonecrosis of the jaw has been reported with zoledronic acid [see Warnings and Precautions (5.4)].

6.2   Post-Marketing Experience
Because these reactions are reported voluntarily from a population of uncertain size, it is not always possible to reliably estimate their frequency or establish a causal relationship to drug exposure.
The following adverse reactions have been identified during post approval use of Reclast:

Acute Phase Reactions
Fever, headache, flu-like symptoms, nausea, vomiting, diarrhea, arthralgia, and myalgia. Symptoms may be significant and lead to dehydration.

Acute Renal Failure
Acute renal failure requiring hospitalization and/or dialysis or with a fatal outcome have been rarely reported. Increased serum creatinine was reported in patients with 1) underlying renal disease, 2) dehydration secondary to fever, sepsis, gastrointestinal losses, or diuretic therapy, or 3) other risk factors such as advanced age, or concomitant nephrotoxic drugs in the post-infusion period. Transient rise in serum creatinine can be correctable with intravenous fluids.

Allergic Reactions
Allergic reaction with intravenous zoledronic acid including anaphylactic reaction/shock, urticaria, angioedema, and bronchoconstriction have been reported.

Asthma Exacerbations
Asthma exacerbations have been reported.

Hypocalcemia
Hypocalcemia has been reported.

Osteonecrosis of the Jaw
Osteonecrosis of the jaw has been reported.

Ocular Adverse Events
Cases of the following events have been reported: conjunctivitis, iritis, iridocyclitis, uveitis, episcleritis, scleritis and orbital inflammation/edema.

Other
Hypotension in patients with underlying risk factors has been reported.

7   DRUG INTERACTIONS
No in vivo drug interaction studies have been performed for Reclast. In vitro and ex vivo studies showed low affinity of zoledronic acid for the cellular components of human blood. In vitro mean zoledronic acid protein binding in human plasma ranged from 28% at 200 ng/mL to 53% at 50 ng/mL. In vivo studies showed that zoledronic acid is not metabolized, and is excreted into the urine as the intact drug.

7.1   Aminoglycosides
Caution is advised when bisphosphonates, including zoledronic acid, are administered with aminoglycosides, since these agents may have an additive effect to lower serum calcium level for prolonged periods. This effect has not been reported in zoledronic acid clinical trials.

7.2   Loop Diuretics
Caution should also be exercised when Reclast is used in combination with loop diuretics due to an increased risk of hypocalcemia.

7.3   Nephrotoxic Drugs
Caution is indicated when Reclast is used with other potentially nephrotoxic drugs such as nonsteroidal anti-inflammatory drugs.

7.4   Drugs Primarily Excreted by the Kidney
Renal impairment has been observed following the administration of zoledronic acid in patients with pre-existing renal compromise or other risk factors [see Warnings and Precautions (5.3)]. In patients with renal impairment, the exposure to concomitant medications that are primarily renally excreted (e.g., digoxin) may increase. Consider monitoring serum creatinine in patients at risk for renal impairment who are taking concomitant medications that are primarily excreted by the kidney.

8   USE IN SPECIFIC POPULATIONS
8.1   Pregnancy
Pregnancy Category D [see Warnings and Precautions (5.6)]. RECLAST SHOULD NOT BE USED DURING PREGNANCY. If the patient becomes pregnant while taking this drug, the patient should be apprised of the potential harm to the fetus. Women of childbearing potential should be advised to avoid becoming pregnant while receiving Reclast.
Bisphosphonates are incorporated into the bone matrix, from where they are gradually released over periods of weeks to years. The extent of bisphosphonate incorporation into adult bone, and hence, the amount available for release back into the systemic circulation, is directly related to the total dose and duration of bisphosphonate use. Although there are no data on fetal risk in humans, bisphosphonates do cause fetal harm in animals, and animal data suggest that uptake of bisphosphonates into fetal bone is greater than into maternal bone. Therefore, there is a theoretical risk of fetal harm (e.g., skeletal and other abnormalities) if a woman becomes pregnant after completing a course of bisphosphonate therapy. The impact of variables such as time between cessation of bisphosphonate therapy to conception space, the particular bisphosphonate used, and the route of administration (intravenous versus oral) on this risk has not been established.
In female rats given daily subcutaneous doses of zoledronic acid beginning 15 days before mating and continuing through gestation, the number of stillbirths was increased and survival of neonates was decreased at approximately greater than or equal to 0.3 times the anticipated human systemic exposure following a 5 mg intravenous dose (based on an AUC comparison). Adverse maternal effects were observed in all dose groups at greater than or equal to 0.1 times the human systemic exposure following a 5 mg intravenous dose (based on an AUC comparison) and included dystocia and periparturient mortality in pregnant rats allowed to deliver. Maternal mortality was considered related to drug-induced inhibition of skeletal calcium mobilization, resulting in periparturient hypocalcemia. This appears to be a bisphosphonate class effect.

In pregnant rats given daily subcutaneous dose of zoledronic acid during gestation, adverse fetal effects were observed at about 2 and 4 times human systemic exposure following a 5 mg intravenous dose (based on an AUC comparison). These adverse effects included increases in pre- and post-implantation losses, decreases in viable fetuses, and fetal skeletal, visceral, and external malformations.
In pregnant rabbits given daily subcutaneous doses of zoledronic acid during gestation at doses less than or equal to 0.4 times the anticipated human systemic exposure following a 5 mg intravenous dose (based on a mg/m^2 comparison) no adverse fetal effects were observed. Maternal mortality and abortion occurred in all treatment groups (at doses greater than or equal to 0.04 times the human 5 mg intravenous dose, based on a mg/m^2 comparison). Adverse maternal effects were associated with, and may have been caused by, drug-induced hypocalcemia [see Nonclinical Toxicology (13.3)].

8.3   Nursing Mothers
It is not known whether Reclast is excreted in human milk. Because many drugs are excreted in human milk, and because Reclast binds to bone long-term, Reclast should not be administered to a nursing woman.

8.4   Pediatric Use
Reclast is not indicated for use in children.
The safety and effectiveness of zoledronic acid was studied in a one-year active controlled trial of 152 pediatric subjects (74 receiving zoledronic acid). The enrolled population was subjects with severe osteogenesis imperfecta, aged 1-17 years, 55% male, 84% Caucasian, with a mean lumbar spine BMD of 0.431 gm/cm^2, which is 2.7 standard deviations below the mean for age-matched controls (BMD Z-score of -2.7). At one year, increases in BMD were observed in the zoledronic acid treatment group. However, changes in BMD in individual patients with severe osteogenesis imperfecta did not necessarily correlate with the risk for fracture or the incidence or severity of chronic bone pain. The adverse events observed with zoledronic acid use in children did not raise any new safety findings beyond those previously seen in adults treated for Paget's disease of bone and treatment of osteoporosis including osteonecrosis of the jaw (ONJ) and renal impairment. However, adverse reactions seen more commonly in pediatric patients included pyrexia (61%), arthralgia (26%), hypocalcemia (22%) and headache (22%). These reactions, excluding arthralgia, occurred most frequently within three days after the first infusion and became less common with repeat dosing. No cases of ONJ or renal impairment were observed in this study. Because of long-term retention in bone, Reclast should only be used in children if the potential benefit outweighs the potential risk.
Plasma zoledronic acid concentration data was obtained from 10 patients with severe osteogenesis imperfecta (4 in the age group of 3-8 years and 6 in the age group of 9-17 years) infused with 0.05 mg/kg dose over 30 minutes. Mean C_{max} and $AUC_{(0-last)}$ was 167 ng/mL and 220 ng.h/mL respectively. The plasma concentration time profile of zoledronic acid in pediatric patients represent a multi-exponential decline, as observed in adult cancer patients at an approximately equivalent mg/kg dose.

8.5   Geriatric Use
The combined osteoporosis trials included 4863 Reclast-treated patients who were at least 65 years of age, while 2101 patients were at least 75 years old. No overall differences in efficacy or safety were observed between patients under 75 years of age with those at least 75 years of age, except that the acute phase reactions occurred less frequently in the older patients.
Of the patients receiving Reclast in the osteoporosis study in men, glucocorticoid-induced osteoporosis, and Paget's disease studies, 83, 116, and 132 patients, respectively were 65 years of age or over, while 24, 29, and 68 patients, respectively were at least 75 years of age.
However, because decreased renal function occurs more commonly in the elderly, special care should be taken to monitor renal function.

8.6   Renal Impairment
Reclast is contraindicated in patients with creatinine clearance less than 35 mL/min and in those with evidence of acute renal impairment. There are no safety or efficacy data to support the adjustment of the Reclast dose based on baseline renal function. Therefore, no dosage adjustment is required in patients with a creatinine clearance of greater than or equal to 35 mL/min [see Warnings and Precautions (5.3), Clinical Pharmacology (12.3)]. Risk of acute renal failure may increase with underlying renal disease and dehydration secondary to fever, sepsis, gastrointestinal losses, diuretic therapy, advanced age, etc. [see Post-Marketing Experience (6.2)].

8.7   Hepatic Impairment
Reclast is not metabolized in the liver. No clinical data are available for use of Reclast in patients with hepatic impairment.

10 OVERDOSAGE

Clinical experience with acute overdosage of zoledronic acid (Reclast) solution for intravenous infusion is limited. Patients who have received doses higher than those recommended should be carefully monitored. Overdosage may cause clinically significant renal impairment, hypocalcemia, hypophosphatemia, and hypomagnesemia. Clinically relevant reductions in serum levels of calcium, phosphorus, and magnesium should be corrected by intravenous administration of calcium gluconate, potassium or sodium phosphate, and magnesium sulfate, respectively.

Single doses of Reclast should not exceed 5 mg and the duration of the intravenous infusion should be no less than 15 minutes [see Dosage and Administration (2)].

11 DESCRIPTION

Reclast contains zoledronic acid, a bisphosphonic acid which is an inhibitor of osteoclastic bone resorption. Zoledronic acid is designated chemically as (1-Hydroxy-2-imidazol-1-yl-phosphonoethyl) phosphonic acid monohydrate and its structural formula is:

Zoledronic acid monohydrate is a white crystalline powder. Its molecular formula is $C_5H_{10}N_2O_7P_2 \cdot H_2O$ and a molar mass of 290.1 g/Mol. Zoledronic acid monohydrate is highly soluble in 0.1N sodium hydroxide solution, sparingly soluble in water and 0.1N hydrochloric acid, and practically insoluble in organic solvents. The pH of the Reclast solution for infusion is approximately 6.0 – 7.0.

Reclast Injection is available as a sterile solution in bottles for intravenous infusion. One bottle with 100 mL solution contains 5.330 mg of zoledronic acid monohydrate, equivalent to 5 mg zoledronic acid on an anhydrous basis.

Inactive Ingredients: 4950 mg of mannitol, USP; and 30 mg of sodium citrate, USP.

12 CLINICAL PHARMACOLOGY

12.1 Mechanism of Action

Reclast is a bisphosphonate and acts primarily on bone. It is an inhibitor of osteoclast-mediated bone resorption.

The selective action of bisphosphonates on bone is based on their high affinity for mineralized bone. Intravenously administered zoledronic acid rapidly partitions to bone and localizes preferentially at sites of high bone turnover. The main molecular target of zoledronic acid in the osteoclast is the enzyme farnesyl pyrophosphate synthase. The relatively long duration of action of zoledronic acid is attributable to its high binding affinity for bone mineral.

12.2 Pharmacodynamics

In the osteoporosis treatment trial, the effect of Reclast treatment on markers of bone resorption (serum beta-C-telopeptides [b-CTx]) and bone formation (bone specific alkaline phosphatase [BSAP], serum N-terminal propeptide of type I collagen [P1NP]) was evaluated in patients (subsets ranging from 517 to 1246 patients) at periodic intervals. Treatment with a 5 mg annual dose of Reclast reduces bone turnover markers to the pre-menopausal range with an approximate 55% reduction in b-CTx, a 29% reduction in BSAP and a 52% reduction in P1NP over 36 months. There was no progressive reduction of bone turnover markers with repeated annual dosing.

12.3 Pharmacokinetics

Pharmacokinetic data in patients with osteoporosis and Paget's disease of bone are not available.

Distribution: Single or multiple (x 28 days) 5-minute or 15-minute infusions of 2, 4, 8 or 16 mg zoledronic acid were given to 64 patients with cancer and bone metastases. The post-infusion decline of zoledronic acid concentrations in plasma was consistent with a triphasic process showing a rapid decrease from peak concentrations at end-of-infusion to less than 1% of C_{max} 24 hours post infusion with population half-lives of $t_{1/2\alpha}$ 0.24 hour and $t_{1/2\beta}$ 1.87 hours for the early disposition phases of the drug. The terminal elimination phase of zoledronic acid was prolonged, with very low concentrations in plasma between Days 2 and 28 post infusion, and a terminal elimination half-life $t_{1/2\gamma}$ of 146 hours. The area under the plasma concentration versus time curve (AUC_{0-24h}) of zoledronic acid was dose proportional from 2 to 16 mg. The accumulation of zoledronic acid measured over three cycles was low, with mean AUC_{0-24h} ratios for cycles 2 and 3 versus 1 of 1.13 ± 0.30 and 1.16 ± 0.36, respectively. *In vitro* and *ex vivo* studies showed low affinity of zoledronic acid for the cellular components of human blood. *In vitro* mean zoledronic acid protein binding in human plasma ranged from 28% at 200 ng/mL to 53% at 50 ng/mL.

Metabolism: Zoledronic acid does not inhibit human P450 enzymes *in vitro*. Zoledronic acid does not undergo biotransformation *in vivo*. In animal studies, less than 3% of the administered intravenous dose was found in the feces, with the balance either recovered in the urine or taken up by bone, indicating that the drug is eliminated intact via the kidney. Following an intravenous dose of 20 nCi ^{14}C-zoledronic acid in a patient with cancer and bone metastases, only a single radioactive species with chromatographic properties identical to those of parent drug was recovered in urine, which suggests that zoledronic acid is not metabolized.

Excretion: In 64 patients with cancer and bone metastases on average (± SD) 39 ± 16% of the administered zoledronic acid dose was recovered in the urine within 24 hours, with only trace amounts of drug found in urine post Day 2. The cumulative percent of drug excreted in the urine over 0-24 hours was independent of dose. The balance of drug not recovered in urine over 0-24 hours, representing drug presumably bound to bone, is slowly released back into the systemic circulation, giving rise to the observed prolonged low plasma concentrations. The 0-24 hour renal clearance of zoledronic acid was 3.7 ± 2.0 L/h.

Zoledronic acid clearance was independent of dose but dependent upon the patient's creatinine clearance. In a study in patients with cancer and bone metastases, increasing the infusion time of a 4 mg dose of zoledronic acid from 5 minutes (n=5) to 15 minutes (n=7) resulted in a 34% decrease in the zoledronic acid concentration at the end of the infusion ([mean ± SD] 403 ± 118 ng/mL vs. 264 ± 86 ng/mL) and a 10% increase in the total AUC (378 ± 116 ng × h/mL vs. 420 ± 218 ng × h/mL). The difference between the AUC means was not statistically significant.

Specific Populations

Pediatrics: Reclast is not indicated for use in children [see Pediatric Use (8.4)].

Geriatrics: The pharmacokinetics of zoledronic acid was not affected by age in patients with cancer and bone metastases whose age ranged from 38 years to 84 years.

Race: The pharmacokinetics of zoledronic acid was not affected by race in patients with cancer and bone metastases.

Hepatic Impairment: No clinical studies were conducted to evaluate the effect of hepatic impairment on the pharmacokinetics of zoledronic acid.

Renal Impairment: The pharmacokinetic studies conducted in 64 cancer patients represented typical clinical populations with normal to moderately-impaired renal function. Compared to patients with creatinine clearance greater than 80 mL/min (N=37), patients with creatinine clearance = 50-80 mL/min (N=15) showed an average increase in plasma AUC of 15%, whereas patients with creatinine clearance = 30-50 mL/min (N=11) showed an average increase in plasma AUC of 43%. No dosage adjustment is required in patients with a creatinine clearance of greater than or equal to 35 mL/min. Reclast is contraindicated in patients with creatinine clearance less than 35 mL/min and in those with evidence of acute renal impairment due to an increased risk of renal failure [see Contraindications (4), Warnings and Precautions (5.3), Use in Specific Populations (8.6)].

13 NONCLINICAL TOXICOLOGY

13.1 Carcinogenesis, Mutagenesis, Impairment of Fertility

Carcinogenesis: Standard lifetime carcinogenicity bioassays were conducted in mice and rats. Mice were given daily oral doses of zoledronic acid of 0.1, 0.5, or 2.0 mg/kg/day. There was an increased incidence of Harderian gland adenomas in males and females in all treatment groups (at doses greater than or equal to 0.002 times the human intravenous dose of 5 mg, based on a mg/m² comparison). Rats were given daily oral doses of zoledronic acid of 0.1, 0.5, or 2.0 mg/kg/day. No increased incidence of tumors was observed (at doses less than or equal to 0.1 times the human intravenous dose of 5 mg, based on a mg/m² comparison).

Mutagenesis: Zoledronic acid was not genotoxic in the Ames bacterial mutagenicity assay, in the Chinese hamster ovary cell assay, or in the Chinese hamster gene mutation assay, with or without metabolic activation. Zoledronic acid was not genotoxic in the *in vivo* rat micronucleus assay.

Impairment of Fertility: Female rats were given daily subcutaneous doses of zoledronic acid of 0.01, 0.03, or 0.1 mg/kg beginning 15 days before mating and continuing through gestation. Effects observed in the high-dose group (equivalent to human systemic exposure following a 5 mg intravenous dose, based on an AUC comparison) included inhibition of ovulation and a decrease in the number of pregnant rats. Effects observed in both the mid-dose group and high-dose group (0.3 to 1 times human systemic exposure following a 5 mg intravenous dose, based on an AUC comparison) included an increase in pre-implantation losses and a decrease in the number of implantations and live fetuses.

13.2 Animal Pharmacology

Bone Safety Studies: Zoledronic acid is a potent inhibitor of osteoclastic bone resorption. In the ovariectomized rat, single IV doses of zoledronic acid of 4-500 µg/kg (less than 0.1 to 3.5 times human exposure at the 5 mg intravenous dose, based on a mg/m² comparison) suppressed bone turnover and protected against trabecular bone loss, cortical thinning and the reduction in vertebral and femoral bone strength in a dose-dependent manner. At a dose equivalent to human exposure at the 5 mg intravenous dose, the effect persisted for 8 months, which corresponds to approximately 8 remodeling cycles or 3 years in humans.

In ovariectomized rats and monkeys, weekly treatment with zoledronic acid dose-dependently suppressed bone turnover and prevented the decrease in cancellous and cortical BMD and bone strength, at yearly cumulative doses up to 3.5 times the intravenous human dose of 5 mg, based on a mg/m² comparison. Bone tissue was normal and there was no evidence of a mineralization defect, no accumulation of osteoid, and no woven bone.

13.3 Reproductive and Developmental Toxicology

In female rats given subcutaneous doses of zoledronic acid of 0.01, 0.03, or 0.1 mg/kg/day beginning 15 days before mating and continuing through gestation, the number of stillbirths was increased and survival of neonates was decreased in the mid- and high-dose groups (greater than or equal to 0.3 times the anticipated human systemic exposure following a 5 mg intravenous dose, based on an AUC comparison). Adverse maternal effects were observed in all dose groups (greater than or equal to 0.1 times the human systemic exposure following a 5 mg intravenous dose, based on an AUC comparison) and included dystocia and periparturient mortality in pregnant rats allowed to deliver. Maternal mortality was considered related to drug-induced inhibition of skeletal calcium mobilization, resulting in periparturient hypocalcemia. This appears to be a bisphosphonate class effect.

In pregnant rats given daily subcutaneous dose of zoledronic acid of 0.1, 0.2, or 0.4 mg/kg during gestation, adverse fetal effects were observed in the mid- and high-dose groups (about 2 and 4 times human systemic exposure following a 5 mg intravenous dose, based on an AUC comparison). These adverse effects included increases in pre- and post-implantation losses, decreases in viable fetuses, and fetal skeletal, visceral, and external malformations. Fetal skeletal effects observed in the high-dose group included unossified or incompletely ossified bones, thickened, curved or shortened bones, wavy ribs, and shortened jaw. Other adverse fetal effects observed in the high-dose group included reduced lens, rudimentary cerebellum, reduction or absence of liver lobes, reduction of lung lobes, vessel dilation, cleft palate, and edema. Skeletal variations were also observed in the low-dose group (about 1.2 times the anticipated human systemic exposure, based on an AUC comparison). Signs of maternal toxicity were observed in the high-dose group and included reduced body weights and food consumption, indicating that maximal exposure levels were achieved in this study.

In pregnant rabbits given subcutaneous doses of zoledronic acid of 0.01, 0.03, or 0.1 mg/kg/day during gestation (at doses less than or equal to 0.4 times the anticipated human systemic exposure following a 5 mg intravenous dose, based on a mg/m² comparison) no adverse fetal effects were observed. Maternal mortality and abortion occurred in all treatment groups (at doses greater than or equal to 0.04 times the human 5 mg intravenous dose, based on a mg/m² comparison). Adverse maternal effects were associated with, and may have been caused by, drug-induced hypocalcemia.

14 CLINICAL STUDIES

14.1 Treatment of Postmenopausal Osteoporosis

Study 1: The efficacy and safety of Reclast in the treatment of postmenopausal osteoporosis was demonstrated in Study 1, a randomized, double-blind, placebo-controlled, multinational study of 7736 women aged 65-89 years (mean age of 73) with either: a femoral neck BMD T-score less than or equal to -1.5 and at least two mild or one moderate existing vertebral fracture(s); or a femoral neck BMD T-score less than or equal to -2.5 with or without evidence of an existing vertebral fracture(s). Women were stratified into two groups: Stratum I: no concomitant use of osteoporosis therapy or Stratum II: baseline concomitant use of osteoporosis therapies which included calcitonin, raloxifene, tamoxifen, and hormone replacement therapy, but excluded other bisphosphonates.

Women enrolled in Stratum I (n=5661) were evaluated annually for incidence of vertebral fractures. All women (Strata I and II) were evaluated for the incidence of hip and other clinical fractures. Reclast was administered once a year for three consecutive years, as a single 5 mg dose in 100 mL solution infused over at least 15 minutes, for a total of three doses. All women received 1000 to 1500 mg of elemental calcium plus 400 to 1200 international units of vitamin D supplementation per day.

The two primary efficacy variables were the incidence of morphometric vertebral fractures at 3 years and the incidence of hip fractures over a median duration of 3 years. The diagnosis of an incident vertebral fracture was based on both qualitative diagnosis by the radiologist and quantitative morphometric criterion. The morphometric criterion required the dual occurrence of 2 events: a relative height ratio or relative height reduction in a vertebral body of at least 20%, together with at least a 4 mm absolute decrease in height.

Effect on Vertebral Fractures

Reclast significantly decreased the incidence of new vertebral fractures at one, two, and three years as shown in Table 5.

[See table 5 above]

The reductions in vertebral fractures over three years were consistent (including new/worsening and multiple vertebral fractures) and significantly greater than placebo regardless of age, geographical region, baseline body mass index, number of baseline vertebral fractures, femoral neck BMD T-score, or prior bisphosphonate usage.

Effect on Hip Fracture over 3 years

Reclast demonstrated a 1.1% absolute reduction and 41% relative reduction in the risk of hip fractures over a median duration of follow-up of 3 years. The hip fracture event rate was 1.4% for Reclast-treated patients compared to 2.5% for placebo-treated patients.

Figure 1. Cumulative Incidence of Hip Fracture Over 3 Years

The reductions in hip fractures over three years were greater for Reclast than placebo regardless of femoral neck BMD T-score.

Effect on All Clinical Fractures

Reclast demonstrated superiority to placebo in reducing the incidence of all clinical fractures, clinical (symptomatic) vertebral and non-vertebral fractures (excluding finger, toe, facial, and clinical thoracic and lumbar vertebral fractures). All clinical fractures were verified based on the radiographic and/or clinical evidence. A summary of results is presented in Table 6.

[See table 6 above]

Effect on Bone Mineral Density (BMD)

Reclast significantly increased BMD at the lumbar spine, total hip and femoral neck, relative to treatment with placebo at time points 12, 24, and 36 months. Treatment with Reclast resulted in a 6.7% increase in BMD at the lumbar spine, 6.0% at the total hip, and 5.1% at the femoral neck, over 3 years as compared to placebo.

Bone Histology

Bone biopsy specimens were obtained between Months 33 and 36 from 82 postmenopausal patients with osteoporosis treated with 3 annual doses of Reclast. Of the biopsies obtained, 81 were adequate for qualitative histomorphometry assessment, 59 were adequate for partial quantitative histomorphometry assessment, and 38 were adequate for full quantitative histomorphometry assessment. Micro CT analysis was performed on 76 specimens. Qualitative, quantitative and micro CT assessments showed bone of normal architecture and quality without mineralization defects.

Effect on Height

In the 3-year osteoporosis study, standing height was measured annually using a stadiometer. The Reclast group revealed less height loss compared to placebo (4.2 mm vs. 7.0 mm, respectively [p<0.001]).

Study 2: The efficacy and safety of Reclast in the treatment of patients with osteoporosis who suffered a recent low-trauma hip fracture was demonstrated in Study 2, a randomized, double-blind, placebo-controlled, multinational endpoint study of 2127 men and women aged 50-95 years (mean age of 74.5). Concomitant osteoporosis therapies excluding other bisphosphonates and parathyroid hormone were allowed. Reclast was administered once a year as a single 5 mg dose in 100 mL solution, infused over at least 15 minutes. The study continued until at least 211 patients had confirmed clinical fractures in the study population. Vitamin D levels were not routinely measured but a loading dose of vitamin D (50,000 to 125,000 international units orally or IM) was given to patients and they were started on 1000 to 1500 mg of elemental calcium plus 800 to 1200 international units of vitamin D supplementation per day for at least 14 days prior to the study drug infusions. The primary efficacy variable was the incidence of clinical fractures over the duration of the study.

Reclast significantly reduced the incidence of any clinical fracture by 35%. There was also a 46% reduction in the risk of a clinical vertebral fracture (Table 7).

Table 5. Proportion of Patients with New Morphometric Vertebral Fractures

Outcome	Reclast (%)	Placebo (%)	Absolute Reduction in Fracture Incidence % (95% CI)	Relative Reduction in Fracture Incidence % (95% CI)
At least one new vertebral fracture (0–1 year)	1.5	3.7	2.2 (1.4, 3.1)	60 (43, 72)*
At least one new vertebral fracture (0–2 years)	2.2	7.7	5.5 (4.4, 6.6)	71 (62, 78)*
At least one new vertebral fracture (0–3 years)	3.3	10.9	7.6 (6.3, 9.0)	70 (62, 76)*

* p <0.0001

Table 6. Between–Treatment Comparisons of the Incidence of Clinical Fracture Variables Over 3 Years

Outcome	Reclast (N= 3875) Event Rate n (%)+	Placebo (N= 3861) Event Rate n (%)+	Absolute Reduction in Fracture Incidence % (95% CI)+	Relative Risk Reduction in Fracture Incidence % (95% CI)
Any clinical fracture [1]	308 (8.4)	456 (12.8)	4.4 (3.0, 5.8)	33 (23, 42)**
Clinical vertebral fracture [2]	19 (0.5)	84 (2.6)	2.1 (1.5, 2.7)	77 (63, 86)**
Non-vertebral fracture [3]	292 (8.0)	388 (10.7)	2.7 (1.4, 4.0)	25 (13, 36)*

*p-value < 0.001, **p-value <0.0001
+ Event rates based on Kaplan-Meier estimates at 36 months
[1] Excluding finger, toe, and facial fractures
[2] Includes clinical thoracic and clinical lumbar vertebral fractures
[3] Excluding finger, toe, facial, and clinical thoracic and lumbar vertebral fractures

Table 7. Between-Treatment Comparisons of the Incidence of Key Clinical Fracture Variables

Outcome	Reclast (N=1065) Event Rate n (%)+	Placebo (N=1062) Event Rate n (%)+	Absolute Reduction in Fracture Incidence % (95% CI)+	Relative Risk Reduction in Fracture Incidence % (95% CI)
Any clinical fracture [1]	92 (8.6)	139 (13.9)	5.3 (2.3, 8.3)	35 (16, 50)**
Clinical vertebral fracture [2]	21 (1.7)	39 (3.8)	2.1 (0.5, 3.7)	46 (8, 68)*

*p-value <0.05, **p-value <0.005
+ Event rates based on Kaplan-Meier estimates at 24 months
[1] Excluding finger, toe and facial fractures
[2] Including clinical thoracic and clinical lumbar vertebral fractures

[See table 7 above]

Effect on Bone Mineral Density (BMD)

Reclast significantly increased BMD relative to placebo at the hip and femoral neck at all timepoints (12, 24, and 36 months). Treatment with Reclast resulted in a 6.4% increase in BMD at the total hip and a 4.3% increase at the femoral neck over 36 months as compared to placebo.

14.2   Prevention of Postmenopausal Osteoporosis

The efficacy and safety of Reclast in postmenopausal women with osteopenia (low bone mass) was assessed in a 2-year randomized, multi-center, double-blind, placebo-controlled study of 581 postmenopausal women aged greater than or equal to 45 years, who were stratified by years since menopause: Stratum I women less than 5 years from menopause (n=224); Stratum II women greater than or equal to 5 years from menopause (n=357). Patients within Stratum I and II were randomized to one of three treatment groups: (1) Reclast given at randomization and at Month 12 (n=77) in Stratum I and (n=121) in Stratum II; (2) Reclast given at randomization and placebo at Month 12 (n=70) in Stratum I and (n=111) in Stratum II; and (3) Placebo given at randomization and Month 12 (n=202). Reclast was administered as a single 5 mg dose in 100 mL solution infused over at least 15 minutes. All women received 500 to 1200 mg elemental calcium plus 400 to 800 international units vitamin D supplementation per day. The primary efficacy variable was the percent change of BMD at 24 Months relative to baseline.

Effect on Bone Mineral Density (BMD)

Reclast significantly increased lumbar spine BMD relative to placebo at Month 24 across both strata. Reclast given once at randomization (and placebo given at Month 12) resulted in 4.0% increase in BMD in Stratum I patients and 4.8% increase in Stratum II patients over 24 months. Placebo given at randomization and at Month 12 resulted in 2.2% decrease in BMD in Stratum I patients and 0.7% decrease in BMD in Stratum II patients over 24 months. Therefore, Reclast given once at randomization (and pla-

cebo given at Month 12) resulted in a 6.3% increase in BMD in Stratum I patients and 5.4% increase in Stratum II patients over 24 months as compared to placebo (both p<0.0001).

Reclast also significantly increased total hip BMD relative to placebo at Month 24 across both strata. Reclast given once at randomization (and placebo given at Month 12) resulted in 2.6% increase in BMD in Stratum I patients and 2.1% in Stratum II patients over 24 months. Placebo given at randomization and at Month 12 resulted in 2.1% decrease in BMD in Stratum I patients and 1.0% decrease in BMD in Stratum II patients over 24 months. Therefore, Reclast given once at randomization (and placebo given at Month 12) resulted in a 4.7% increase in BMD in Stratum I patients and 3.2% increase in Stratum II patients over 24 months as compared to placebo (both p<0.0001).

14.3   Osteoporosis in Men

The efficacy and safety of Reclast in men with osteoporosis or significant osteoporosis secondary to hypogonadism, was assessed in a randomized, multicenter, double-blind, active controlled, study of 302 men aged 25-86 years (mean age of 64). The duration of the trial was two years. Patients were randomized to either Reclast which was administered once annually as a 5 mg dose in 100 mL infused over 15 minutes for a total of up to two doses, or to an oral weekly bisphosphonate (active control) for up to two years. All participants received 1000 mg of elemental calcium plus 800 to 1000 international units of vitamin D supplementation per day.

Effect on Bone Mineral Density (BMD)

An annual infusion of Reclast was non-inferior to the oral weekly bisphosphonate active control based on the percentage change in lumbar spine BMD at Month 24 relative to baseline (Reclast: 6.1% increase; active control: 6.2% increase).

14.4   Treatment and Prevention of Glucocorticoid-Induced Osteoporosis

The efficacy and safety of Reclast to prevent and treat glucocorticoid-induced osteoporosis (GIO) was assessed in a

Figure 2. Therapeutic Response/Serum Alkaline Phosphatase (SAP) Normalization Over Time

randomized, multicenter, double-blind, stratified, active controlled study of 833 men and women aged 18-85 years (mean age of 54.4 years) treated with greater than or equal to 7.5 mg/day oral prednisone (or equivalent). Patients were stratified according to the duration of their pre-study corticosteroid therapy: less than or equal to 3 months prior to randomization (prevention subpopulation), and greater than 3 months prior to randomization (treatment subpopulation). The duration of the trial was one year. Patients were randomized to either Reclast which was administered once as a 5 mg dose in 100 mL infused over 15 minutes, or to an oral daily bisphosphonate (active control) for one year. All participants received 1000 mg of elemental calcium plus 400 to 1000 international units of vitamin D supplementation per day.

Effect on Bone Mineral Density (BMD)
In the GIO treatment subpopulation, Reclast demonstrated a significant mean increase in lumbar spine BMD compared to the active control at one year (Reclast 4.1%, active control 2.7%) with a treatment difference of 1.4% (p<0.001). In the GIO prevention subpopulation, Reclast demonstrated a significant mean increase in lumbar spine BMD compared to active control at one year (Reclast 2.6%, active control 0.6%) with a treatment difference of 2.0% (p<0.001).

Bone Histology
Bone biopsy specimens were obtained from 23 patients (12 in the Reclast treatment group and 11 in the active control treatment group) at Month 12 treated with an annual dose of Reclast or daily oral active control. Qualitative assessments showed bone of normal architecture and quality without mineralization defects. Apparent reductions in activation frequency and remodeling rates were seen when compared with the histomorphometry results seen with Reclast in the postmenopausal osteoporosis population. The long-term consequences of this degree of suppression of bone remodeling in glucocorticoid-treated patients is unknown.

14.5   Treatment of Paget's Disease of Bone
Reclast was studied in male and female patients with moderate to severe Paget's disease of bone, defined as serum alkaline phosphatase level at least twice the upper limit of the age-specific normal reference range at the time of study entry. Diagnosis was confirmed by radiographic evidence.
The efficacy of one infusion of 5 mg Reclast vs. oral daily doses of 30 mg risedronate for 2 months was demonstrated in two identically designed 6-month randomized, double blind trials. The mean age of patients in the two trials was 70. Ninety-three percent (93%) of patients were Caucasian. Therapeutic response was defined as either normalization of serum alkaline phosphatase (SAP) or a reduction of at least 75% from baseline in total SAP excess at the end of 6 months. SAP excess was defined as the difference between the measured level and midpoint of normal range.
In both trials Reclast demonstrated a superior and more rapid therapeutic response compared with risedronate and returned more patients to normal levels of bone turnover, as evidenced by biochemical markers of formation (SAP, serum N-terminal propeptide of type I collagen [P1NP] and resorption (serum CTx 1 [cross-linked C-telopeptides of type I collagen] and urine α-CTx).
The 6-month combined data from both trials showed that 96% (169/176) of Reclast-treated patients achieved a therapeutic response as compared with 74% (127/171) of patients treated with risedronate. Most Reclast patients achieved a therapeutic response by the Day 63 visit. In addition, at 6 months, 89% (156/176) of Reclast-treated patients achieved normalization of SAP levels, compared to 58% (99/171) of patients treated with risedronate (p<0.0001) (see Figure 2). [See figure 2 above]
The therapeutic response to Reclast was similar across demographic and disease-severity groups defined by gender, age, previous bisphosphonate use, and disease severity. At 6 months, the percentage of Reclast-treated patients who achieved therapeutic response was 97% and 95%, respectively, in each of the baseline disease severity subgroups (baseline SAP less than 3xULN, greater than or equal to

3xULN) compared to 75% and 74%, respectively, for the same disease severity subgroups of risedronate-treated patients.
In patients who had previously received treatment with oral bisphosphonates, therapeutic response rates were 96% and 55% for Reclast and risedronate, respectively. The comparatively low risedronate response was due to the low response rate (7/23, 30%) in patients previously treated with risedronate. In patients naïve to previous treatment, a greater therapeutic response was also observed with Reclast (98%) relative to risedronate (86%). In patients with symptomatic pain at screening, therapeutic response rates were 94% and 70% for Reclast and risedronate respectively. For patients without pain at screening, therapeutic response rates were 100% and 82% for Reclast and risedronate respectively.
Bone histology was evaluated in 7 patients with Paget's disease 6 months after being treated with Reclast 5 mg. Bone biopsy results showed bone of normal quality with no evidence of impaired bone remodeling and no evidence of mineralization defect.

16   HOW SUPPLIED/STORAGE AND HANDLING
Each bottle contains 5 mg/100 mL. NDC 0078-0435-61
Handling
After opening the solution, it is stable for 24 hours at 2°C–8°C (36°F-46°F).
If refrigerated, allow the refrigerated solution to reach room temperature before administration.
Storage
Store at 25°C (77°F); excursions permitted to 15°C-30°C (59°F-86°F) [see USP Controlled Room Temperature].

17   PATIENT COUNSELING INFORMATION
See FDA-Approved Medication Guide
Information for Patients
Patients should be made aware that Reclast contains the same active ingredient (zoledronic acid) found in Zometa®, and that patients being treated with Zometa should not be treated with Reclast.
Reclast is contraindicated in patients with creatinine clearance less than 35 mL/min [*see Contraindications (4)*].
Before being given Reclast, patients should tell their doctor if they have kidney problems and what medications they are taking.
Reclast should not be given if the patient is pregnant or plans to become pregnant, or if she is breast-feeding [*see Warnings and Precautions (5.6)*].
There have been reports of bronchoconstriction in aspirin-sensitive patients receiving bisphosphonates, including Reclast. Before being given Reclast, patients should tell their doctor if they are aspirin-sensitive.
If the patient had surgery to remove some or all of the parathyroid glands in their neck, or had sections of their intestine removed, or are unable to take calcium supplements they should tell their doctor.
Reclast is given as an infusion into a vein by a nurse or a doctor, and the infusion time must not be less than 15 minutes.
On the day of treatment the patient should eat and drink normally, which includes drinking at least 2 glasses of fluid such as water within a few hours prior to the infusion, as directed by their doctor, before receiving Reclast.
After getting Reclast it is strongly recommended patients with Paget's disease take calcium in divided doses (for example, 2 to 4 times a day) for a total of 1500 mg calcium a day to prevent low blood calcium levels. This is especially important for the two weeks after getting Reclast [*see Warnings and Precautions (5.2)*].
Adequate calcium and vitamin D intake is important in patients with osteoporosis and the current recommended daily intake of calcium is 1200 mg and vitamin D is 800 international units – 1000 international units daily. All patients should be instructed on the importance of calcium and vitamin D supplementation in maintaining serum calcium levels.

Patients should be aware of the most commonly associated side effects of therapy. Patients may experience one or more side effects that could include: fever, flu-like symptoms, myalgia, arthralgia, and headache. Most of these side effects occur within the first 3 days following the dose of Reclast. They usually resolve within 3 days of onset but may last for up to 7 to 14 days. Patients should consult their physician if they have questions or if these symptoms persist. The incidence of these symptoms decreased markedly with subsequent doses of Reclast.
Administration of acetaminophen following Reclast administration may reduce the incidence of these symptoms.
Physicians should inform their patients that there have been reports of persistent pain and/or a non-healing sore of the mouth or jaw, primarily in patients treated with bisphosphonates for other illnesses. If they experience these symptoms, they should inform their physician or dentist.
Severe and occasionally incapacitating bone, joint, and/or muscle pain have been infrequently reported in patients taking bisphosphonates, including Reclast. Consider withholding future Reclast treatment if severe symptoms develop.
Atypical femur fractures in patients on bisphosphonate therapy have been reported; patients with thigh or groin pain should be evaluated to rule out a femoral fracture.
T2013-39
April 2013
MEDICATION GUIDE
Reclast® (RE-clast)
(zoledronic acid)
Injection
Read the Medication Guide that comes with Reclast before you start taking it and each time you get a refill. There may be new information. This Medication Guide does not take the place of talking with your doctor about your medical condition or treatment. Talk to your doctor if you have any questions about Reclast.
What is the most important information I should know about Reclast?
You should not receive Reclast if you are already receiving Zometa. Both Reclast and Zometa contain zoledronic acid.
Reclast can cause serious side effects including:
1. Low calcium levels in your blood (hypocalcemia)
2. Severe kidney problems
3. Severe jaw bone problems (osteonecrosis)
4. Bone, joint or muscle pain
5. Unusual thigh bone fractures
1. Low calcium levels in your blood (hypocalcemia).
Reclast may lower the calcium levels in your blood. If you have low blood calcium before you start taking Reclast, it may get worse during treatment. Your low blood calcium must be treated before you take Reclast. Most people with low blood calcium levels do not have symptoms, but some people may have symptoms. Call your doctor right away if you have symptoms of low blood calcium such as:
• Spasms, twitches, or cramps in your muscles
• Numbness or tingling in your fingers, toes, or around your mouth
Your doctor may prescribe calcium and vitamin D to help prevent low calcium levels in your blood, while you take Reclast. Take calcium and vitamin D as your doctor tells you to.
2. Severe kidney problems.
Severe kidney problems may happen when you take Reclast. Severe kidney problems may lead to hospitalization or kidney dialysis and can be life-threatening. Your risk of kidney problems is higher if you:
• already have kidney problems
• take a diuretic or "water pill"
• do not have enough water in your body (dehydrated) before or after you receive Reclast
• are of advanced age since the risk increases as you get older
• take any medicines known to harm your kidneys
You should drink at least 2 glasses of fluid within a few hours before receiving Reclast to reduce the risk of kidney problems.
3. Severe jaw bone problems (osteonecrosis).
Severe jaw bone problems may happen when you take Reclast. Your doctor should examine your mouth before you start Reclast. Your doctor may tell you to see your dentist before you start Reclast. It is important for you to practice good mouth care during treatment with Reclast.
4. Unusual thigh bone fractures.
Some people have developed unusual fractures in their thigh bone. Symptoms of a fracture may include new or unusual pain in your hip, groin, or thigh.
5. Possible harm to your unborn baby.
Reclast should not be used if you are pregnant. Tell your doctor right away if you are pregnant or plan to become pregnant. Reclast may harm your unborn baby.
6. Bone, joint, or muscle pain.
Some people who take bisphosphonates develop severe bone, joint, or muscle pain.
Call your doctor right away if you have any of these side effects.

What is Reclast?

Reclast is a prescription medicine used to:

- Treat or prevent osteoporosis in women after menopause. Reclast helps reduce the chance of having a hip or spinal fracture (break).
- Increase bone mass in men with osteoporosis.
- Treat or prevent osteoporosis in either men or women who will be taking corticosteroid medicines for at least one year.
- Treat certain men and women who have Paget's disease of the bone.

It is not known how long Reclast works for the treatment and prevention of osteoporosis. You should see your doctor regularly to determine if Reclast is still right for you.
Reclast is not for use in children.

Who should not take Reclast?

Do not take Reclast if you:

- Have low levels of calcium in your blood
- Have kidney problems
- Are allergic to zoledronic acid or any of its ingredients. A list of ingredients is at the end of this leaflet.

What should I tell my doctor before taking Reclast?

Before you start Reclast, be sure to talk to your doctor if you:

- Have low blood calcium.
- Have kidney problems.
- Had parathyroid or thyroid surgery (glands in your neck).
- Have been told you have trouble absorbing minerals in your stomach or intestines (malabsorption syndrome) or have had parts of your intestine removed.
- Have asthma (wheezing) from taking aspirin.
- Plan to have dental surgery or teeth removed.
- Are pregnant, or plan to become pregnant. Reclast may harm your unborn baby. **Reclast should not be used if you are pregnant.**
- Are breastfeeding or plan to breastfeed. It is not known if Reclast passes into your milk and may harm your baby.

Tell your doctor about all the medicines you take, including prescription and non-prescription medicines, vitamins, and herbal supplements. Certain medicines may affect how Reclast works.

Especially tell your doctor if you are taking:

- An antibiotic. Certain antibiotic medicines called aminoglycosides may increase the effect of Reclast in lowering your blood calcium for a long period of time.
- A diuretic or "water pill".
- Non-steroidal anti-inflammatory medicines (NSAIDS).

Ask your doctor or pharmacist for a list of these medicines, if you are not sure.

Know the medicines you take. Keep a list of them and show it to your doctor and pharmacist each time you get a new medicine.

How will I receive Reclast?

- Your doctor will tell you how often you will receive Reclast.
- Reclast is given by infusion into your vein (intravenously). Your infusion should last at least 15 minutes.
- Before you receive Reclast, drink at least 2 glasses of fluid (such as water) within a few hours as directed by your doctor.
- You may eat before your treatment with Reclast.
- If you miss a dose of Reclast, call your doctor or healthcare provider to schedule your next dose.

What are the possible side effects of Reclast?

Reclast may cause serious side effects.

- See **"What is the most important information I should know about Reclast?"**

The most common side effects of Reclast included:

- Fever
- Pain in your bones, joints or muscles
- Pain in your arms and legs
- Headache
- Flu-like illness (fever, chills, bone, joint, or muscle pain, fatigue)
- Nausea
- Vomiting
- Diarrhea

Talk to your doctor about things you can do to help decrease some of these side effects that might happen with a Reclast infusion.

You may get allergic reactions, such as hives, swelling of your face, lips, tongue, or throat.

Tell your doctor if you have any side effect that bothers you or that does not go away.

These are not all the possible side effects of Reclast. For more information, ask your doctor or pharmacist.

Call your doctor for medical advice about side effects. You may report side effects to FDA at 1-800-FDA-1088.

General information about safe and effective use of Reclast.

Medicines are sometimes prescribed for purposes other than those listed in a Medication Guide.

This Medication Guide summarizes the most important information about Reclast. If you would like more information, talk with your doctor. You can ask your doctor or pharmacist for information about Reclast that is written for health professionals.

For more information, go to: www.RECLAST.com or call 1-866-732-5278.

What are the ingredients in Reclast?

Active ingredient: zoledronic acid monohydrate.
Inactive ingredients: mannitol and sodium citrate.
Distributed by:
Novartis Pharmaceuticals Corporation
East Hanover, New Jersey 07936
This Medication Guide has been approved by the U.S. Food and Drug Administration.
© Novartis
T2013-40
April 2013

Shown in Product Identification Guide, page 310

SANDIMMUNE®
(cyclosporine capsules, USP)
Soft Gelatin Capsules
SANDIMMUNE®
(cyclosporine oral solution, USP)
Oral Solution
SANDIMMUNE®
(cyclosporine injection, USP)
Injection
FOR INFUSION ONLY
Rx only
Prescribing Information

℞

The following prescribing information is based on official labeling in effect July 2013.

WARNING

Only physicians experienced in immunosuppressive therapy and management of organ transplant patients should prescribe Sandimmune® (cyclosporine). Patients receiving the drug should be managed in facilities equipped and staffed with adequate laboratory and supportive medical resources. The physician responsible for maintenance therapy should have complete information requisite for the follow-up of the patient.

Sandimmune® (cyclosporine) should be administered with adrenal corticosteroids but not with other immunosuppressive agents. Increased susceptibility to infection and the possible development of lymphoma may result from immunosuppression.

Sandimmune® Soft Gelatin Capsules (cyclosporine capsules, USP) and Sandimmune® Oral Solution (cyclosporine oral solution, USP) have decreased bioavailability in comparison to Neoral® Soft Gelatin Capsules (cyclosporine capsules, USP) MODIFIED and Neoral® Oral Solution (cyclosporine oral solution, USP) MODIFIED.

Sandimmune® and Neoral® are not bioequivalent and cannot be used interchangeably without physician supervision.

The absorption of cyclosporine during chronic administration of Sandimmune® Soft Gelatin Capsules and Oral Solution was found to be erratic. It is recommended that patients taking the soft gelatin capsules or oral solution over a period of time be monitored at repeated intervals for cyclosporine blood concentrations and subsequent dose adjustments be made in order to avoid toxicity due to high concentrations and possible organ rejection due to low absorption of cyclosporine. This is of special importance in liver transplants. Numerous assays are being developed to measure blood concentrations of cyclosporine. Comparison of concentrations in published literature to patient concentrations using current assays must be done with detailed knowledge of the assay methods employed. (See Blood Concentration Monitoring under DOSAGE AND ADMINISTRATION)

DESCRIPTION

Cyclosporine, the active principle in Sandimmune® (cyclosporine) is a cyclic polypeptide immunosuppressant agent consisting of 11 amino acids. It is produced as a metabolite by the fungus species *Beauveria nivea*.

Chemically, cyclosporine is designated as $[R-[R^*,R^*-(E)]]$-cyclic(L-alanyl-D-alanyl-*N*-methyl-L-leucyl-*N*-methyl-L-leucyl-*N*-methyl-L-valyl-3-hydroxy-*N*,4-dimethyl-L-2-amino-6-octenoyl-L-α-amino-butyryl-*N*-methylglycyl-*N*-methyl-L-leucyl-L-valyl-*N*-methyl-L-leucyl).

Sandimmune® Soft Gelatin Capsules (cyclosporine capsules, USP) are available in 25 mg and 100 mg strengths.

Each 25 mg capsule contains:

cyclosporine, USP	25 mg
alcohol, USP dehydrated	max 12.7% by volume

Each 100 mg capsule contains:

cyclosporine, USP	100 mg
alcohol, USP dehydrated	max 12.7% by volume

Inactive Ingredients: corn oil, gelatin, iron oxide red, linoleoyl macrogolglycerides, sorbitol, and titanium dioxide. May also contain glycerol. 100 mg capsules may contain iron oxide yellow.

Sandimmune® Oral Solution (cyclosporine oral solution, USP) is available in 50 mL bottles.

Each mL contains:

cyclosporine, USP	100 mg
alcohol, Ph. Helv.	12.5% by volume

dissolved in an olive oil, Ph. Helv./Labrafil M 1944 CS (polyoxyethylated oleic glycerides) vehicle which must be further diluted with milk, chocolate milk, or orange juice before oral administration.

Sandimmune® Injection (cyclosporine injection, USP) is available in a 5 mL sterile ampul for I.V. administration.

Each mL contains:

cyclosporine, USP	50 mg
*Cremophor® EL (polyoxyethylated castor oil)	650 mg
alcohol, Ph. Helv.	32.9% by volume
nitrogen	qs

which must be diluted further with 0.9% Sodium Chloride Injection or 5% Dextrose Injection before use.

The chemical structure of cyclosporine (also known as cyclosporin A) is

$C_{62}H_{111}N_{11}O_{12}$ Mol. Wt. 1202.63

CLINICAL PHARMACOLOGY

Sandimmune® (cyclosporine) is a potent immunosuppressive agent which in animals prolongs survival of allogeneic transplants involving skin, heart, kidney, pancreas, bone marrow, small intestine, and lung. Sandimmune® (cyclosporine) has been demonstrated to suppress some humoral immunity and to a greater extent, cell-mediated reactions such as allograft rejection, delayed hypersensitivity, experimental allergic encephalomyelitis, Freund's adjuvant arthritis, and graft vs. host disease in many animal species for a variety of organs.

Successful kidney, liver, and heart allogeneic transplants have been performed in man using Sandimmune® (cyclosporine).

The exact mechanism of action of Sandimmune® (cyclosporine) is not known. Experimental evidence suggests that the effectiveness of cyclosporine is due to specific and reversible inhibition of immunocompetent lymphocytes in the G_0- or G_1-phase of the cell cycle. T-lymphocytes are preferentially inhibited. The T-helper cell is the main target, although the T-suppressor cell may also be suppressed. Sandimmune® (cyclosporine) also inhibits lymphokine production and release including interleukin-2 or T-cell growth factor (TCGF).

No functional effects on phagocytic (changes in enzyme secretions not altered, chemotactic migration of granulocytes, macrophage migration, bacteria clearance *in vivo*) or tumor cells (growth rate, metastasis) can be detected in animals. Sandimmune® (cyclosporine) does not cause bone marrow suppression in animal models or man.

The absorption of cyclosporine from the gastrointestinal tract is incomplete and variable. Peak concentrations (C_{max}) in blood and plasma are achieved at about 3.5 hours. C_{max} and area under the plasma or blood concentration/time curve (AUC) increase with the administered dose; for blood, the relationship is curvilinear (parabolic) between 0 and 1400 mg. As determined by a specific assay, C_{max} is approximately 1.0 ng/mL/mg of dose for plasma and 2.7-1.4 ng/mL/mg of dose for blood (for low to high doses). Compared to an intravenous infusion, the absolute bioavailability of the oral solution is approximately 30% based upon the results in 2 patients. The bioavailability of Sandimmune® Soft Gelatin Capsules (cyclosporine capsules, USP) is equivalent to Sandimmune® Oral Solution, (cyclosporine oral solution, USP).

Cyclosporine is distributed largely outside the blood volume. In blood, the distribution is concentration dependent. Approximately 33%-47% is in plasma, 4%-9% in lymphocytes, 5%-12% in granulocytes, and 41%-58% in erythrocytes. At high concentrations, the uptake by leukocytes and erythrocytes becomes saturated. In plasma, approximately 90% is bound to proteins, primarily lipoproteins.

Nephrotoxicity vs. Rejection

Parameter	Nephrotoxicity	Rejection
History	Donor > 50 years old or hypotensive Prolonged kidney preservation Prolonged anastomosis time Concomitant nephrotoxic drugs	Antidonor immune response Retransplant patient
Clinical	Often > 6 weeks postop[b] Prolonged initial nonfunction (acute tubular necrosis)	Often < 4 weeks postop[b] Fever > 37.5°C Weight gain > 0.5 kg Graft swelling and tenderness Decrease in daily urine volume > 500 mL (or 50%)
Laboratory	CyA serum trough level > 200 ng/mL Gradual rise in Cr (< 0.15 mg/dl/day)[a] Cr plateau < 25% above baseline BUN/Cr ≥ 20 Arteriolopathy (medial hypertrophy[a], hyalinosis, nodular deposits, intimal thickening, endothelial vacuolization, progressive scarring)	CyA serum trough level < 150 ng/mL Rapid rise in Cr (> 0.3 mg/dl/day)[a] Cr > 25% above baseline BUN/Cr < 20 Endovasculitis[c] (proliferation[a], intimal arteritis[b], necrosis, sclerosis)
Biopsy	Tubular atrophy, isometric vacuolization, isolated calcifications Minimal edema Mild focal infiltrates[c] Diffuse interstitial fibrosis, often striped form CyA deposits in tubular and endothelial cells	Tubulitis with RBC[b] and WBC[b] casts, some irregular vacuolization Interstitial edema[c] and hemorrhage[b] Diffuse moderate to severe mononuclear infiltrates[d] Glomerulitis (mononuclear cells)[c]
Aspiration Cytology	Fine isometric vacuolization of tubular cells	Inflammatory infiltrate with mononuclear phagocytes, macrophages, lymphoblastoid cells, and activated T-cells These strongly express HLA-DR antigens
Urine Cytology	Tubular cells with vacuolization and granularization	Degenerative tubular cells, plasma cells, and lymphocyturia > 20% of sediment
Manometry	Intracapsular pressure < 40 mm Hg[b]	Intracapsular pressure > 40 mm Hg[b]
Ultrasonography	Unchanged graft cross-sectional area	Increase in graft cross-sectional area AP diameter ≥ Transverse diameter
Magnetic Resonance Imagery	Normal appearance	Loss of distinct corticomedullary junction, swelling, image intensity of parachyma approaching that of psoas, loss of hilar fat
Radionuclide Scan	Normal or generally decreased perfusion Decrease in tubular function (^{131}I-hippuran) > decrease in perfusion (^{99m}Tc DTPA)	Patchy arterial flow Decrease in perfusion > decrease in tubular function Increased uptake of Indium 111 labeled platelets or Tc-99m in colloid
Therapy	Responds to decreased Sandimmune® (cyclosporine)	Responds to increased steroids or antilymphocyte globulin

[a] p <0.05, [b] p <0.01, [c] p <0.001, [d] p <0.0001

The disposition of cyclosporine from blood is biphasic with a terminal half-life of approximately 19 hours (range: 10-27 hours). Elimination is primarily biliary with only 6% of the dose excreted in the urine.

Cyclosporine is extensively metabolized but there is no major metabolic pathway. Only 0.1% of the dose is excreted in the urine as unchanged drug. Of 15 metabolites characterized in human urine, 9 have been assigned structures. The major pathways consist of hydroxylation of the Cγ-carbon of 2 of the leucine residues, Cη-carbon hydroxylation, and cyclic ether formation (with oxidation of the double bond) in the side chain of the amino acid 3-hydroxyl-N,4-dimethyl-L-2-amino-6-octenoic acid and N-demethylation of N-methyl leucine residues. Hydrolysis of the cyclic peptide chain or conjugation of the aforementioned metabolites do not appear to be important biotransformation pathways.

Specific Populations
Renal Impairment
In a study performed in 4 subjects with end-stage renal disease (creatinine clearance <5mL/min), an intravenous infusion of 3.5 mg/kg of cyclosporine over 4 hours administered at the end of a hemodialysis session resulted in a mean volume of distribution (Vdss) of 3.49 L/kg and systemic clearance (CL) of 0.369 L/hr/kg. This systemic CL (0.369 L/hr/kg) was approximately two thirds of the mean systemic CL (0.56 L/hr/kg) of cyclosporine in historical control subjects with normal renal function. In 5 liver transplant patients, the mean clearance of cyclosporine on and off hemodialysis was 463 mL/min and 398 mL/min, respectively. Less than 1% of the dose of cyclosporine was recovered in the dialysate.

Hepatic Impairment
Cyclosporine is extensively metabolized by the liver. Since severe hepatic impairment may result in significantly increased cyclosporine exposures, the dosage of cyclosporine may need to be reduced in these patients.

INDICATIONS AND USAGE
Sandimmune® (cyclosporine) is indicated for the prophylaxis of organ rejection in kidney, liver, and heart allogeneic transplants. It is always to be used with adrenal corticoster-

oids. The drug may also be used in the treatment of chronic rejection in patients previously treated with other immunosuppressive agents.

Because of the risk of anaphylaxis, Sandimmune® Injection (cyclosporine injection, USP) should be reserved for patients who are unable to take the soft gelatin capsules or oral solution.

CONTRAINDICATIONS
Sandimmune® Injection (cyclosporine injection, USP) is contraindicated in patients with a hypersensitivity to Sandimmune® (cyclosporine) and/or Cremophor® EL (polyoxyethylated castor oil).

WARNINGS
Kidney, Liver and Heart Transplant
(See BOXED WARNING): Sandimmune® (cyclosporine), when used in high doses, can cause hepatotoxicity and nephrotoxicity.

Nephrotoxicity
It is not unusual for serum creatinine and BUN levels to be elevated during Sandimmune® (cyclosporine) therapy. These elevations in renal transplant patients do not necessarily indicate rejection, and each patient must be fully evaluated before dosage adjustment is initiated.

Nephrotoxicity has been noted in 25% of cases of renal transplantation, 38% of cases of cardiac transplantation, and 37% of cases of liver transplantation. Mild nephrotoxicity was generally noted 2-3 months after transplant and consisted of an arrest in the fall of the preoperative elevations of BUN and creatinine at a range of 35-45 mg/dl and 2.0-2.5 mg/dl, respectively. These elevations were often responsive to dosage reduction.

More overt nephrotoxicity was seen early after transplantation and was characterized by a rapidly rising BUN and creatinine. Since these events are similar to rejection episodes, care must be taken to differentiate between them. This form of nephrotoxicity is usually responsive to Sandimmune® (cyclosporine) dosage reduction.

Although specific diagnostic criteria which reliably differentiate renal graft rejection from drug toxicity have not been

found, a number of parameters have been significantly associated to one or the other. It should be noted however, that up to 20% of patients may have simultaneous nephrotoxicity and rejection.
[See table above]
A form of chronic progressive cyclosporine-associated nephrotoxicity is characterized by serial deterioration in renal function and morphologic changes in the kidneys. From 5%-15% of transplant recipients will fail to show a reduction in a rising serum creatinine despite a decrease or discontinuation of cyclosporine therapy. Renal biopsies from these patients will demonstrate an interstitial fibrosis with tubular atrophy. In addition, toxic tubulopathy, peritubular capillary congestion, arteriolopathy, and a striped form of interstitial fibrosis with tubular atrophy may be present. Though none of these morphologic changes is entirely specific, a histologic diagnosis of chronic progressive cyclosporine-associated nephrotoxicity requires evidence of these.

When considering the development of chronic nephrotoxicity it is noteworthy that several authors have reported an association between the appearance of interstitial fibrosis and higher cumulative doses or persistently high circulating trough concentrations of cyclosporine. This is particularly true during the first 6 posttransplant months when the dosage tends to be highest and when, in kidney recipients, the organ appears to be most vulnerable to the toxic effects of cyclosporine. Among other contributing factors to the development of interstitial fibrosis in these patients must be included, prolonged perfusion time, warm ischemia time, as well as episodes of acute toxicity, and acute and chronic rejection. The reversibility of interstitial fibrosis and its correlation to renal function have not yet been determined.

Impaired renal function at any time requires close monitoring, and frequent dosage adjustment may be indicated. In patients with persistent high elevations of BUN and creatinine who are unresponsive to dosage adjustments, consideration should be given to switching to other immunosuppressive therapy. In the event of severe and unremitting rejection, it is preferable to allow the kidney transplant to be rejected and removed rather than increase the Sandimmune® (cyclosporine) dosage to a very high level in an attempt to reverse the rejection.

Due to the potential for additive or synergistic impairment of renal function, caution should be exercised when co-administering Sandimmune with other drugs that may impair renal function. (See PRECAUTIONS, Drug Interactions)

Thrombotic Microangiopathy
Occasionally patients have developed a syndrome of thrombocytopenia and microangiopathic hemolytic anemia which may result in graft failure. The vasculopathy can occur in the absence of rejection and is accompanied by avid platelet consumption within the graft as demonstrated by Indium 111 labeled platelet studies. Neither the pathogenesis nor the management of this syndrome is clear. Though resolution has occurred after reduction or discontinuation of Sandimmune® (cyclosporine) and 1) administration of streptokinase and heparin or 2) plasmapheresis, this appears to depend upon early detection with Indium 111 labeled platelet scans. (See ADVERSE REACTIONS)

Hyperkalemia
Significant hyperkalemia (sometimes associated with hyperchloremic metabolic acidosis) and hyperuricemia have been seen occasionally in individual patients.

Hepatotoxicity
Cases of hepatotoxicity and liver injury including cholestasis, jaundice, hepatitis, and liver failure have been reported in patients treated with cyclosporine. Most reports included patients with significant co-morbidities, underlying conditions and other confounding factors including infectious complications and comedications with hepatotoxic potential. In some cases, mainly in transplant patients, fatal outcomes have been reported (See ADVERSE REACTIONS, Postmarketing Experience)

Hepatotoxicity, usually manifested by elevations in hepatic enzymes and bilirubin, was reported in patients treated with cyclosporine in clinical trials: 4% in renal transplantation, 7% in cardiac transplantation, and 4% in liver transplantation. This was usually noted during the first month of therapy when high doses of Sandimmune® (cyclosporine) were used. The chemistry elevations usually decreased with a reduction in dosage.

Malignancies
As in patients receiving other immunosuppressants, those patients receiving Sandimmune® (cyclosporine) are at increased risk for development of lymphomas and other malignancies, particularly those of the skin. The increased risk appears related to the intensity and duration of immunosuppression rather than to the use of specific agents. Because of the danger of oversuppression of the immune system, which can also increase susceptibility to infection, Sandimmune® (cyclosporine) should not be administered with other immunosuppressive agents except adrenal corticosteroids. The efficacy and safety of cyclosporine in combi-

Drugs That May Potentiate Renal Dysfunction

Antibiotics	*Antineoplastic*	*Antifungals*	*Anti-Inflammatory Drugs*	*Gastrointestinal Agents*	*Immunosuppressives*	*Other Drugs*
ciprofloxacin	melphalan	amphotericin B	azapropazon	cimetidine	tacrolimus	fibric acid derivatives (e.g., bezafibrate, fenofibrate)
gentamicin		ketoconazole	colchicine	ranitidine		methotrexate
tobramycin			diclofenac			
trimethoprim with sulfamethoxazole			naproxen			
vancomycin			sulindac			

nation with other immunosuppressive agents have not been determined. Some malignancies may be fatal. Transplant patients receiving cyclosporine are at increased risk for serious infection with fatal outcome.

Serious Infections

Patients receiving immunosuppressants, including Sandimmune, are at increased risk of developing bacterial, viral, fungal, and protozoal infections, including opportunistic infections. These infections may lead to serious, including fatal, outcomes (See BOXED WARNING, and ADVERSE REACTIONS).

Polyoma Virus Infections

Patients receiving immunosuppressants, including Sandimmune, are at increased risk for opportunistic infections, including polyoma virus infections. Polyoma virus infections in transplant patients may have serious, and sometimes, fatal outcomes. These include cases of JC virus-associated progressive multifocal leukoencephalopathy (PML), and polyoma virus-associated nephropathy (PVAN), especially due to BK virus infection, which have been observed in patients receiving cyclosporine.

PVAN is associated with serious outcomes, including deteriorating renal function and renal graft loss, (See ADVERSE REACTIONS/Postmarketing Experience). Patient monitoring may help detect patients at risk for PVAN.

Cases of PML have been reported in patients treated with Sandimmune. PML, which is sometimes fatal, commonly presents with hemiparesis, apathy, confusion, cognitive deficiencies and ataxia. Risk factors for PML include treatment with immunosuppressant therapies and impairment of immune function. In immunosuppressed patients, physicians should consider PML in the differential diagnosis in patients reporting neurological symptoms and consultation with a neurologist should be considered as clinically indicated.

Consideration should be given to reducing the total immunosuppression in transplant patients who develop PML or PVAN. However, reduced immunosuppression may place the graft at risk.

Neurotoxicity

There have been reports of convulsions in adult and pediatric patients receiving cyclosporine, particularly in combination with high-dose methylprednisolone.

Encephalopathy, including Posterior Reversible Encephalopathy Syndrome (PRES), has been described both in post-marketing reports and in the literature. Manifestations include impaired consciousness, convulsions, visual disturbances (including blindness), loss of motor function, movement disorders and psychiatric disturbances. In many cases, changes in the white matter have been detected using imaging techniques and pathologic specimens. Predisposing factors such as hypertension, hypomagnesemia, hypocholesterolemia, high-dose corticosteroids, high cyclosporine blood concentrations, and graft-versus-host disease have been noted in many but not all of the reported cases. The changes in most cases have been reversible upon discontinuation of cyclosporine, and in some cases, improvement was noted after reduction of dose. It appears that patients receiving liver transplant are more susceptible to encephalopathy than those receiving kidney transplant. Another rare manifestation of cyclosporine-induced neurotoxicity is optic disc edema including papilloedema, with possible visual impairment, secondary to benign intracranial hypertension.

Specific Excipients

Anaphylactic Reactions

Rarely (approximately 1 in 1000), patients receiving Sandimmune® Injection (cyclosporine injection, USP) have experienced anaphylactic reactions. Although the exact cause of these reactions is unknown, it is believed to be due to the Cremophor® EL (polyoxyethylated castor oil) used as the vehicle for the I.V. formulation. These reactions can consist of flushing of the face and upper thorax, and noncardiogenic pulmonary edema, with acute respiratory distress, dyspnea, wheezing, blood pressure changes, and tachycardia. One patient died after respiratory arrest and aspiration pneumonia. In some cases, the reaction subsided after the infusion was stopped.

Patients receiving Sandimmune® Injection (cyclosporine injection, USP) should be under continuous observation for at least the first 30 minutes following the start of the infusion and at frequent intervals thereafter. If anaphylaxis occurs, the infusion should be stopped. An aqueous solution of epinephrine 1:1000 should be available at the bedside as well as a source of oxygen.

Anaphylactic reactions have not been reported with the soft gelatin capsules or oral solution which lack Cremophor® EL (polyoxyethylated castor oil). In fact, patients experiencing anaphylactic reactions have been treated subsequently with the soft gelatin capsules or oral solution without incident.

Alcohol (ethanol)

The alcohol content (See DESCRIPTION) of Sandimmune should be taken into account when given to patients in whom alcohol intake should be avoided or minimized, e.g. pregnant or breastfeeding women, in patients presenting with liver disease or epilepsy, in alcoholic patients, or pediatric patients. For an adult weighing 70 kg, the maximum daily oral dose would deliver about 1 gram of alcohol which is approximately 6% of the amount of alcohol contained in a standard drink. The daily intravenous dose would deliver approximately 15% of the amount of alcohol contained in a standard drink.

Care should be taken in using Sandimmune® (cyclosporine) with nephrotoxic drugs. (See PRECAUTIONS)

Conversion from Neoral to Sandimmune

Because Sandimmune® (cyclosporine) is not bioequivalent to Neoral®, conversion from Neoral® to Sandimmune® (cyclosporine) using a 1:1 ratio (mg/kg/day) may result in a lower cyclosporine blood concentration. Conversion from Neoral® to Sandimmune® (cyclosporine) should be made with increased blood concentration monitoring to avoid the potential of underdosing.

PRECAUTIONS

General

Patients with malabsorption may have difficulty in achieving therapeutic concentrations with Sandimmune® Soft Gelatin Capsules or Oral Solution.

Hypertension

Hypertension is a common side effect of Sandimmune® (cyclosporine) therapy. (See ADVERSE REACTIONS) Mild or moderate hypertension is more frequently encountered than severe hypertension and the incidence decreases over time. Antihypertensive therapy may be required. Control of blood pressure can be accomplished with any of the common antihypertensive agents. However, since cyclosporine may cause hyperkalemia, potassium-sparing diuretics should not be used. While calcium antagonists can be effective agents in treating cyclosporine-associated hypertension, care should be taken since interference with cyclosporine metabolism may require a dosage adjustment. (See Drug Interactions)

Vaccination

During treatment with Sandimmune® (cyclosporine), vaccination may be less effective and the use of live attenuated vaccines should be avoided.

Information for Patients

Patients should be advised that any change of cyclosporine formulation should be made cautiously and only under physician supervision because it may result in the need for a change in dosage.

Patients should be informed of the necessity of repeated laboratory tests while they are receiving the drug. They should be given careful dosage instructions, advised of the potential risks during pregnancy, and informed of the increased risk of neoplasia.

Patients using cyclosporine oral solution with its accompanying syringe for dosage measurement should be cautioned not to rinse the syringe either before or after use. Introduction of water into the product by any means will cause variation in dose.

Laboratory Tests

Renal and liver functions should be assessed repeatedly by measurement of BUN, serum creatinine, serum bilirubin, and liver enzymes.

Drug Interactions

A. Effect of Drugs and Other Agents on Cyclosporine Pharmacokinetics and/or Safety

All of the individual drugs cited below are well substantiated to interact with cyclosporine. In addition, concomitant use of nonsteroidal anti-inflammatory drugs with cyclosporine, particularly in the setting of dehydration, may potentiate renal dysfunction. Caution should be exercised when using other drugs which are known to impair renal function. (See WARNINGS, Nephrotoxicity)

[See table above]

During the concomitant use of a drug that may exhibit additive or synergistic renal impairment potential with cyclosporine, close monitoring of renal function (in particular serum creatinine) should be performed. If a significant impairment of renal function occurs, reduction in the dosage of cyclosporine and/or co-administered drug or an alternative treatment should be considered.

Cyclosporine is extensively metabolized by CYP 3A isoenzymes, in particular CYP3A4, and is a substrate of the multidrug efflux transporter P-glycoprotein. Various agents are known to either increase or decrease plasma or whole blood concentrations of cyclosporine usually by inhibition or induction of CYP3A4 or P-glycoprotein transporter or both. Compounds that decrease cyclosporine absorption such as orlistat should be avoided. Appropriate Sandimmune® (cyclosporine) dosage adjustment to achieve the desired cyclosporine concentrations is essential when drugs that significantly alter cyclosporine concentrations are used concomitantly. (See Blood Concentration Monitoring)

[See first table at top of next page]

HIV Protease inhibitors

The HIV protease inhibitors (e.g., indinavir, nelfinavir, ritonavir, and saquinavir) are known to inhibit cytochrome P-450 3A and thus could potentially increase the concentrations of cyclosporine, however no formal studies of the interaction are available. Care should be exercised when these drugs are administered concomitantly.

Grapefruit juice

Grapefruit and grapefruit juice affect metabolism, increasing blood concentrations of cyclosporine, thus should be avoided.

[See second table at top of next page]

Bosentan

Co-administration of bosentan (250-1000 mg every 12 hours based on tolerability) and cyclosporine (300 mg every 12 hours for 2 days then dosing to achieve a C_{min} of 200-250 ng/mL) for 7 days in healthy subjects resulted in decreases in the cyclosporine mean dose-normalized AUC, C_{max}, and trough concentration of approximately 50%, 30% and 60%, respectively, compared to when cyclosporine was given alone. (See also Effect of Cyclosporine on the Pharmacokinetics and/or Safety of Other Drugs or Agents)

Boceprevir

Co-administration of boceprevir (800 mg three times daily for 7 days) and cyclosporine (100 mg single dose) in healthy subjects resulted in increases in the mean AUC and C_{max} of cyclosporine approximately 2.7-fold and 2-fold, respectively, compared to when cyclosporine was given alone.

Telaprevir

Co-administration of telaprevir (750 mg every 8 hours for 11 days) with cyclosporine (10 mg on day 8) in healthy subjects resulted in increases in the mean dose-normalized AUC and C_{max} of cyclosporine approximately 4.5-fold and 1.3-fold, respectively, compared to when cyclosporine (100 mg single dose) was given alone.

St. John's Wort

There have been reports of a serious drug interaction between cyclosporine and the herbal dietary supplement, St. John's Wort. This interaction has been reported to produce a marked reduction in the blood concentrations of cyclosporine, resulting in subtherapeutic levels, rejection of transplanted organs, and graft loss.

Rifabutin

Rifabutin is known to increase the metabolism of other drugs metabolized by the cytochrome P-450 system. The in-

1. Drugs That Increase Cyclosporine Concentrations

Calcium Channel Blockers	Antifungals	Antibiotics	Glucocorticoids	Other Drugs
diltiazem	fluconazole	azithromycin	methylprednisolone	allopurinol
nicardipine	itraconazole	clarithromycin		amiodarone
verapamil	ketoconazole	erythromycin		bromocriptine
	voriconazole	quinupristin/		colchicine
		dalfopristin		
				danazol
				imatinib
				metoclopramide
				nefazodone
				oral contraceptives

2. Drugs/Dietary Supplements That Decrease Cyclosporine Concentrations

Antibiotics	Anticonvulsants	Other Drugs / Dietary Supplements	
nafcillin	carbamazepine	bosentan	St. John's Wort
rifampin	oxcarbazepine	octreotide	
	phenobarbital	orlistat	
	phenytoin	sulfinpyrazone	
		terbinafine	
		ticlopidine	

teraction between rifabutin and cyclosporine has not been studied. Care should be exercised when these two drugs are administered concomitantly.

B. Effect of Cyclosporine on the Pharmacokinetics and/or Safety of Other Drugs or Agents
Cyclosporine is an inhibitor of CYP3A4 and of the multidrug efflux transporter P-glycoprotein and may increase plasma concentrations of comedications that are substrates of CYP3A4 or P-glycoprotein or both.
Cyclosporine may reduce the clearance of digoxin, colchicine, prednisolone, HMG-CoA reductase inhibitors (statins) and aliskiren, repaglinide, NSAIDs, sirolimus, etoposide, and other drugs. See the full prescribing information of the other drug for further information and specific recommendations. The decision on co-administration of cyclosporine with other drugs or agents should be made by the physician following the careful assessment of benefits and risks.
Digoxin
Severe digitalis toxicity has been seen within days of starting cyclosporine in several patients taking digoxin. If digoxin is used concurrently with cyclosporine, serum digoxin concentrations should be monitored.
Colchicine
There are reports on the potential of cyclosporine to enhance the toxic effects of colchicine such as myopathy and neuropathy, especially in patients with renal dysfunction. Concomitant administration of cyclosporine and colchicine results in significant increases in colchicine plasma concentrations. If colchicine is used concurrently with cyclosporine, a reduction in the dosage of colchicine is recommended.
HMG Co-A reductase inhibitors (statins)
Literature and postmarketing cases of myotoxicity, including muscle pain and weakness, myositis, and rhabdomyolysis, have been reported with concomitant administration of cyclosporine with lovastatin, simvastatin, atorvastatin, pravastatin, and rarely, fluvastatin. When concurrently administered with cyclosporine, the dosage of these statins should be reduced according to label recommendations. Statin therapy needs to be temporarily withheld or discontinued in patients with signs and symptoms of myopathy or those with risk factors predisposing to severe renal injury, including renal failure, secondary to rhabdomyolysis.
Repaglinide
Cyclosporine may increase the plasma concentrations of repaglinide and thereby increase the risk of hypoglycemia. In 12 healthy male subjects who received two doses of 100 mg cyclosporine capsule orally 12 hours apart with a single dose of 0.25 mg repaglinide tablet (one half of a 0.5 mg tablet) orally 13 hours after the cyclosporine initial dose, the repaglinide mean C_{max} and AUC were increased 1.8 fold (range: 0.6-3.7 fold) and 2.4 fold (range 1.2-5.3 fold), respectively. Close monitoring of blood glucose level is advisable for a patient taking cyclosporine and repaglinide concomitantly.
Ambrisentan
Co-administration of ambrisentan (5 mg daily) and cyclosporine (100-150 mg twice daily initially, then dosing to achieve C_{min} 150-200 ng/mL) for 8 days in healthy subjects resulted mean increases in ambrisentan AUC and C_{max} of approximately 2-fold and 1.5-fold, respectively, compared to ambrisentan alone.
Anthracycline antibiotics
High doses of cyclosporine (e.g., at starting intravenous dose of 16 mg/kg/day) may increase the exposure to anthracycline antibiotics (e.g., doxorubicin, mitoxantrone, daunorubicin) in cancer patients.

Aliskiren
Cyclosporine alters the pharmacokinetics of aliskiren, a substrate of P-glycoprotein and CYP3A4. In 14 healthy subjects who received concomitantly single doses of cyclosporine (200 mg) and reduced dose aliskiren (75 mg), the mean C_{max} of aliskiren was increased by approximately 2.5 fold (90% CI: 1.96-3.17) and the mean AUC by approximately 4.3 fold (90% CI: 3.52-5.21), compared to when these subjects received aliskiren alone. The concomitant administration of aliskiren with cyclosporine prolonged the median aliskiren elimination half-life (26 hours versus 43 to 45 hours) and the T_{max} (0.5 hours versus 1.5 to 2.0 hours). The mean AUC and C_{max} of cyclosporine were comparable to reported literature values. Coadministration of cyclosporine and aliskiren in these subjects also resulted in an increase in the number and/or intensity of adverse events, mainly headache, hot flush, nausea, vomiting, and somnolence. The coadministration of cyclosporine with aliskiren is not recommended.
Bosentan
In healthy subjects, co-administration of bosentan and cyclosporine resulted in mean increases in dose-normalized bosentan trough concentrations on day 1 and day 8 of approximately 21-fold and 2-fold , respectively, compared to when bosentan was given alone as a single dose on day 1. (See also Effect of Drugs and Other Agents on Cyclosporine Pharmacokinetics and/or Safety)
Potassium sparing diuretics
Cyclosporine should not be used with potassium-sparing diuretics because hyperkalemia can occur. Caution is also required when cyclosporine is coadministered with potassium-sparing drugs (e.g., angiotensin-converting enzyme inhibitors, angiotensin II receptor antagonists), potassium-containing drugs as well as in patients on a potassium-rich diet. Control of potassium levels in these situations is advisable.
Nonsteroidal Anti-inflammatory Drug (NSAID) Interactions
Clinical status and serum creatinine should be closely monitored when cyclosporine is used with nonsteroidal anti-inflammatory agents in rheumatoid arthritis patients. (See WARNINGS)
Pharmacodynamic interactions have been reported to occur between cyclosporine and both naproxen and sulindac, in that concomitant use is associated with additive decreases in renal function, as determined by 99mTc-diethylenetriaminepentaacetic acid (DTPA) and (p-aminohippuric acid) PAH clearances. Although concomitant administration of diclofenac does not affect blood concentrations of cyclosporine, it has been associated with approximate doubling of diclofenac blood levels and occasional reports of reversible decreases in renal function. Consequently, the dose of diclofenac should be in the lower end of the therapeutic range.
Methotrexate Interaction
Preliminary data indicate that when methotrexate and cyclosporine were coadministered to rheumatoid arthritis patients (N=20), methotrexate concentrations (AUCs) were increased approximately 30% and the concentrations (AUCs) of its metabolite, 7-hydroxy methotrexate, were decreased by approximately 80%. The clinical significance of this interaction is not known. Cyclosporine concentrations do not appear to have been altered (N=6).
Sirolimus
Elevations in serum creatinine were observed in studies using sirolimus in combination with full-dose cyclosporine. This effect is often reversible with cyclosporine dose reduction. Simultaneous coadministration of cyclosporine signifi-

cantly increases blood levels of sirolimus. To minimize increases in sirolimus blood concentrations, it is recommended that sirolimus be given 4 hours after cyclosporine administration.
Nifedipine
Frequent gingival hyperplasia when nifedipine is given concurrently with cyclosporine has been reported. The concomitant use of nifedipine should be avoided in patients in whom gingival hyperplasia develops as a side effect of cyclosporine.
Methylprednisolone
Convulsions when high dose methylprednisolone is given concomitantly with cyclosporine have been reported.
Other Immunosuppressive Drugs and Agents
Psoriasis patients receiving other immunosuppressive agents or radiation therapy (including PUVA and UVB) should not receive concurrent cyclosporine because of the possibility of excessive immunosuppression.
C. Effect of Cyclosporine on the Efficacy of Live Vaccines
During treatment with cyclosporine, vaccination may be less effective. The use of live vaccines should be avoided.
For additional information on Cyclosporine Drug Interactions please contact Novartis Medical Affairs Department at 888-NOW-NOVA (888-669-6682).
Carcinogenesis, Mutagenesis, and Impairment of Fertility
Cyclosporine gave no evidence of mutagenic or teratogenic effects in appropriate test systems. Only at dose levels toxic to dams, were adverse effects seen in reproduction studies in rats. (See Pregnancy)
Carcinogenicity studies were carried out in male and female rats and mice. In the 78-week mouse study, at doses of 1, 4, and 16 mg/kg/day, evidence of a statistically significant trend was found for lymphocytic lymphomas in females, and the incidence of hepatocellular carcinomas in mid-dose males significantly exceeded the control value. In the 24-month rat study, conducted at 0.5, 2, and 8 mg/kg/day, pancreatic islet cell adenomas significantly exceeded the control rate in the low-dose level. The hepatocellular carcinomas and pancreatic islet cell adenomas were not dose related. No impairment in fertility was demonstrated in studies in male and female rats.
Cyclosporine has not been found mutagenic/genotoxic in the Ames Test, the V79-HGPRT Test, the micronucleus test in mice and Chinese hamsters, the chromosome-aberration tests in Chinese hamster bone marrow, the mouse dominant lethal assay, and the DNA-repair test in sperm from treated mice. A recent study analyzing sister chromatid exchange (SCE) induction by cyclosporine using human lymphocytes in vitro gave indication of a positive effect (i.e., induction of SCE), at high concentrations in this system. In two published research studies, rabbits exposed to cyclosporine in utero (10 mg/kg/day subcutaneously) demonstrated reduced numbers of nephrons, renal hypertrophy, systemic hypertension and progressive renal insufficiency up to 35 weeks of age. Pregnant rats which received 12 mg/kg/day of cyclosporine intravenously (twice the recommended human intravenous dose) had fetuses with an increased incidence of ventricular septal defect. These findings have not been demonstrated in other species and their relevance for humans is unknown.
An increased incidence of malignancy is a recognized complication of immunosuppression in recipients of organ transplants. The most common forms of neoplasms are non-Hodgkin's lymphoma and carcinomas of the skin. The risk of malignancies in cyclosporine recipients is higher than in the normal, healthy population, but similar to that in patients receiving other immunosuppressive therapies. It has been reported that reduction or discontinuance of immunosuppression may cause the lesions to regress.
Pregnancy
Pregnancy Category C
Animal studies have shown reproductive toxicity in rats and rabbits. Cyclosporine gave no evidence of mutagenic or teratogenic effects in the standard test systems with oral application (rats up to 17 mg/kg and rabbits up to 30 mg/kg per day orally). Sandimmune® Oral Solution (cyclosporine oral solution, USP) has been shown to be embryo-and fetotoxic in rats and rabbits when given in doses 2-5 times the human dose. At toxic doses (rats at 30 mg/kg/day and rabbits at 100 mg/kg/day), Sandimmune® Oral Solution (cyclosporine oral solution, USP) was embryo- and fetotoxic as indicated by increased pre- and postnatal mortality and reduced fetal weight together with related skeletal retardations. In the well-tolerated dose range (rats at up to 17 mg/kg/day and rabbits at up to 30 mg/kg/day), Sandimmune® Oral Solution (cyclosporine oral solution, USP) proved to be without any embryolethal or teratogenic effects.
There are no adequate and well-controlled studies in pregnant women and therefore, Sandimmune® (cyclosporine) should not be used during pregnancy unless the potential benefit to the mother justifies the potential risk to the fetus.

In pregnant transplant recipients who are being treated with immunosuppressants, the risk of premature birth is increased. The following data represent the reported outcomes of 116 pregnancies in women receiving Sandimmune® (cyclosporine) during pregnancy, 90% of whom were transplant patients, and most of whom received Sandimmune® (cyclosporine) throughout the entire gestational period. Since most of the patients were not prospectively identified, the results are likely to be biased toward negative outcomes. The only consistent patterns of abnormality were premature birth (gestational period of 28 to 36 weeks) and low birth weight for gestational age. It is not possible to separate the effects of Sandimmune® (cyclosporine) on these pregnancies from the effects of the other immunosuppressants, the underlying maternal disorders, or other aspects of the transplantation milieu. Sixteen fetal losses occurred. Most of the pregnancies (85 of 100) were complicated by disorders; including, preeclampsia, eclampsia, premature labor, abruptio placentae, oligohydramnios, Rh incompatibility and fetoplacental dysfunction. Preterm delivery occurred in 47%. Seven malformations were reported in 5 viable infants and in 2 cases of fetal loss. Twenty-eight percent of the infants were small for gestational age. Neonatal complications occurred in 27%. In a report of 23 children followed up to 4 years, postnatal development was said to be normal. More information on cyclosporine use in pregnancy is available from Novartis Pharmaceuticals Corporation.

A limited number of observations in children exposed to cyclosporine in utero are available, up to an age of approximately 7 years. Renal function and blood pressure in these children were normal.

The alcohol content of the Sandimmune formulations should also be taken into account in pregnant women. (See WARNINGS, Special Excipients)

Nursing Mothers

Cyclosporine is present in breast milk. Because of the potential for serious adverse drug reactions in nursing infants from Sandimmune, a decision should be made whether to discontinue nursing or to discontinue the drug, taking into account the importance of the drug to the mother. Sandimmune contains ethanol. Ethanol will be present in human milk at levels similar to that found in maternal serum and if present in breast milk will be orally absorbed by a nursing infant. (See WARNINGS)

Pediatric Use

Although no adequate and well-controlled studies have been conducted in children, patients as young as 6 months of age have received the drug with no unusual adverse effects.

Geriatric Use

Clinical studies of Sandimmune® (cyclosporine) did not include sufficient numbers of subjects aged 65 and over to determine whether they respond differently from younger patients. Other reported clinical experience has not identified differences in responses between the elderly and younger patients. In general, dose selection for an elderly patient should be cautious, usually starting at the low end of the dosing range, reflecting the greater frequency of decreased hepatic, renal, or cardiac function, and of concomitant disease or other drug therapy.

ADVERSE REACTIONS

The principal adverse reactions of Sandimmune® (cyclosporine) therapy are renal dysfunction, tremor, hirsutism, hypertension, and gum hyperplasia.

Hypertension

Hypertension, which is usually mild to moderate, may occur in approximately 50% of patients following renal transplantation and in most cardiac transplant patients.

Glomerular Capillary Thrombosis

Glomerular capillary thrombosis has been found in patients treated with cyclosporine and may progress to graft failure. The pathologic changes resemble those seen in the hemolytic-uremic syndrome and include thrombosis of the renal microvasculature, with platelet-fibrin thrombi occluding glomerular capillaries and afferent arterioles, microangiopathic hemolytic anemia, thrombocytopenia, and decreased renal function. Similar findings have been observed when other immunosuppressives have been employed post-transplantation.

Hypomagnesemia

Hypomagnesemia has been reported in some, but not all, patients exhibiting convulsions while on cyclosporine therapy. Although magnesium-depletion studies in normal subjects suggest that hypomagnesemia is associated with neurologic disorders, multiple factors, including hypertension, high-dose methylprednisolone, hypocholesterolemia, and nephrotoxicity associated with high plasma concentrations of cyclosporine appear to be related to the neurological manifestations of cyclosporine toxicity.

Clinical Studies

The following reactions occurred in 3% or greater of 892 patients involved in clinical trials of kidney, heart, and liver transplants:
[See first table above]

Body System/ Adverse Reactions	Randomized Kidney Patients Sandimmune® (N=227) %	Azathioprine (N=228) %	All Sandimmune® (cyclosporine) Patients Kidney (N=705) %	Heart (N=112) %	Liver (N=75) %
Genitourinary					
Renal Dysfunction	32	6	25	38	37
Cardiovascular					
Hypertension	26	18	13	53	27
Cramps	4	< 1	2	< 1	0
Skin					
Hirsutism	21	< 1	21	28	45
Acne	6	8	2	2	1
Central Nervous System					
Tremor	12	0	21	31	55
Convulsions	3	1	1	4	5
Headache	2	< 1	2	15	4
Gastrointestinal					
Gum Hyperplasia	4	0	9	5	16
Diarrhea	3	< 1	3	4	8
Nausea/Vomiting	2	< 1	4	10	4
Hepatotoxicity	< 1	< 1	4	7	4
Abdominal Discomfort	< 1	0	< 1	7	0
Autonomic Nervous System					
Paresthesia	3	0	1	2	1
Flushing	< 1	0	4	0	4
Hematopoietic					
Leukopenia	2	19	< 1	6	0
Lymphoma	< 1	0	1	6	1
Respiratory					
Sinusitis	< 1	0	4	3	7
Miscellaneous					
Gynecomastia	< 1	0	< 1	4	3

Reason for Discontinuation	Renal Transplant Patients in Whom Therapy Was Discontinued Randomized Patients Sandimmune® (N=227) %	Azathioprine (N=228) %	All Sandimmune® Patients (N=705) %
Renal Toxicity	5.7	0	5.4
Infection	0	0.4	0.9
Lack of Efficacy	2.6	0.9	1.4
Acute Tubular Necrosis	2.6	0	1.0
Lymphoma/Lymphoproliferative Disease	0.4	0	0.3
Hypertension	0	0	0.3
Hematological Abnormalities	0	0.4	0
Other	0	0	0.7

Sandimmune® (cyclosporine) was discontinued on a temporary basis and then restarted in 18 additional patients.

The following reactions occurred in 2% or less of patients: allergic reactions, anemia, anorexia, confusion, conjunctivitis, edema, fever, brittle fingernails, gastritis, hearing loss, hiccups, hyperglycemia, muscle pain, peptic ulcer, thrombocytopenia, tinnitus.

The following reactions occurred rarely: anxiety, chest pain, constipation, depression, hair breaking, hematuria, joint pain, lethargy, mouth sores, myocardial infarction, night sweats, pancreatitis, pruritus, swallowing difficulty, tingling, upper GI bleeding, visual disturbance, weakness, weight loss.

[See second table above]

Patients receiving immunosuppressive therapies, including cyclosporine and cyclosporine -containing regimens, are at increased risk of infections (viral, bacterial, fungal, parasitic). Both generalized and localized infections can occur. Pre-existing infections may also be aggravated. Fatal outcomes have been reported. (see WARNINGS)

Complication	Infectious Complications in the Randomized Renal Transplant Patients Sandimmune® Treatment (N=227) % of Complications	Standard Treatment* (N=228) % of Complications
Septicemia	5.3	4.8
Abscesses	4.4	5.3
Systemic Fungal Infection	2.2	3.9
Local Fungal Infection	7.5	9.6
Cytomegalovirus	4.8	12.3
Other Viral Infections	15.9	18.4
Urinary Tract Infections	21.1	20.2
Wound and Skin Infections	7.0	10.1
Pneumonia	6.2	9.2

*Some patients also received ALG.

Cremophor® EL (polyoxyethylated castor oil) is known to cause hyperlipemia and electrophoretic abnormalities of lipoproteins. These effects are reversible upon discontinuation of treatment but are usually not a reason to stop treatment.

Postmarketing Experience

Hepatotoxicity

Cases of hepatotoxicity and liver injury including cholestasis, jaundice, hepatitis and liver failure; serious and/or fatal outcomes have been reported. (See WARNINGS, Hepatotoxicity)

Increased Risk of Infections

Cases of JC virus-associated progressive multifocal leukoencephalopathy (PML), sometimes fatal; and polyoma virus-associated nephropathy (PVAN), especially BK virus resulting in graft loss have been reported. (See WARNINGS, Polyoma Virus Infection)

Headache, including Migraine

Cases of migraine have been reported. In some cases, patients have been unable to continue cyclosporine, however, the final decision on treatment discontinuation should be made by the treating physician following the careful assessment of benefits versus risks.

OVERDOSAGE

There is a minimal experience with overdosage. Because of the slow absorption of Sandimmune® Soft Gelatin Capsules or Oral Solution, forced emesis and gastric lavage would be of value up to 2 hours after administration. Transient hepatotoxicity and nephrotoxicity may occur which should resolve following drug withdrawal. Oral doses of cyclosporine up to 10 g (about 150 mg/kg) have been tolerated with relatively minor clinical consequences, such as vomiting, drowsiness, headache, tachycardia and, in a few patients, moderately severe, reversible impairment of renal function. However, serious symptoms of intoxication have been reported following accidental parenteral overdosage with cyclosporine in premature neonates. General supportive measures and symptomatic treatment should be followed in all cases of overdosage. Sandimmune® (cyclosporine) is not dialyzable to any great extent, nor is it cleared well by charcoal hemoperfusion. The oral LD_{50} is 2329 mg/kg in mice, 1480 mg/kg in rats, and >1000 mg/kg in rabbits. The I.V. LD_{50} is 148 mg/kg in mice, 104 mg/kg in rats, and 46 mg/kg in rabbits.

DOSAGE AND ADMINISTRATION

Sandimmune® Soft Gelatin Capsules (cyclosporine capsules, USP) and Sandimmune® Oral Solution (cyclosporine oral solution, USP)

Sandimmune® Soft Gelatin Capsules (cyclosporine capsules, USP) and Sandimmune® Oral Solution (cyclosporine oral solution, USP) have decreased bioavailability in comparison to Neoral® Soft Gelatin Capsules (cyclosporine capsules, USP) MODIFIED and Neoral® Oral Solution (cyclosporine oral solution, USP) MODIFIED. Sandimmune® and Neoral® are not bioequivalent and cannot be used interchangeably without physician supervision. The initial oral dose of Sandimmune® (cyclosporine) should be given 4-12 hours prior to transplantation as a single dose of 15 mg/kg. Although a daily single dose of 14-18 mg/kg was used in most clinical trials, few centers continue to use the highest dose, most favoring the lower end of the scale. There is a trend towards use of even lower initial doses for renal transplantation in the ranges of 10-14 mg/kg/day. The initial single daily dose is continued postoperatively for 1-2 weeks and then tapered by 5% per week to a maintenance dose of 5-10 mg/kg/day. Some centers have successfully tapered the maintenance dose to as low as 3 mg/kg/day in selected *renal* transplant patients without an apparent rise in rejection rate.

(See Blood Concentration Monitoring, below.)

Specific Populations

Renal Impairment

Cyclosporine undergoes minimal renal elimination and its pharmacokinetics do not appear to be significantly altered in patients with end-stage renal disease who receive routine hemodialysis treatments (See CLINICAL PHARMACOLOGY). However, due to its nephrotoxic potential (see WARNINGS), careful monitoring of renal function is recommended; cyclosporine dosage should be reduced if indicated. (See WARNINGS and PRECAUTIONS)

Hepatic Impairment

The clearance of cyclosporine may be significantly reduced in severe liver disease patients (See CLINICAL PHARMACOLOGY). Dose reduction may be necessary in patients with severe liver impairment to maintain blood concentrations within the recommended target range. (See WARNINGS and PRECAUTIONS)

Pediatrics

In pediatric usage, the same dose and dosing regimen may be used as in adults although in several studies, children have required and tolerated higher doses than those used in adults.

Adjunct therapy with adrenal corticosteroids is recommended. Different tapering dosage schedules of prednisone appear to achieve similar results. A dosage schedule based on the patient's weight started with 2.0 mg/kg/day for the first 4 days tapered to 1.0 mg/kg/day by 1 week, 0.6 mg/kg/day by 2 weeks, 0.3 mg/kg/day by 1 month, and 0.15 mg/kg/day by 2 months and thereafter as a maintenance dose. Another center started with an initial dose of 200 mg tapered by 40 mg/day until reaching 20 mg/day. After 2 months at this dose, a further reduction to 10 mg/day was made. Adjustments in dosage of prednisone must be made according to the clinical situation.

To make Sandimmune® Oral Solution (cyclosporine oral solution, USP) more palatable, the oral solution may be diluted with milk, chocolate milk, or orange juice preferably at room temperature. Patients should avoid switching diluents frequently. Sandimmune® Soft Gelatin Capsules and Oral Solution should be administered on a consistent schedule with regard to time of day and relation to meals.

Take the prescribed amount of Sandimmune® (cyclosporine) from the container using the dosage syringe supplied after removal of the protective cover, and transfer the solution to a glass of milk, chocolate milk, or orange juice. Stir well and drink at once. Do not allow to stand before drinking. It is best to use a glass container and rinse it with more diluent to ensure that the total dose is taken. After use, replace the dosage syringe in the protective cover. Do not rinse the dosage syringe with water or other cleaning agents either before or after use. If the dosage syringe requires cleaning, it must be completely dry before resuming use. Introduction of water into the product by any means will cause variation in dose.

Sandimmune® Injection (cyclosporine injection, USP)
FOR INFUSION ONLY
Note: Anaphylactic reactions have occurred with Sandimmune® Injection (cyclosporine injection, USP). (See WARNINGS)

Patients unable to take Sandimmune® Soft Gelatin Capsules or Oral Solution pre- or postoperatively may be treated with the I.V. concentrate. **Sandimmune® Injection (cyclosporine injection, USP) is administered at 1/3 the oral dose.** The initial dose of Sandimmune® Injection (cyclosporine injection, USP) should be given 4-12 hours prior to transplantation as a single I.V. dose of 5-6 mg/kg/day. This daily single dose is continued postoperatively until the patient can tolerate the soft gelatin capsules or oral solution. Patients should be switched to Sandimmune® Soft Gelatin Capsules or Oral Solution as soon as possible after surgery. In pediatric usage, the same dose and dosing regimen may be used, although higher doses may be required. Adjunct steroid therapy is to be used. (See aforementioned.)

Immediately before use, the I.V. concentrate should be diluted 1 mL Sandimmune® Injection (cyclosporine injection, USP) in 20 mL-100 mL 0.9% Sodium Chloride Injection or 5% Dextrose Injection and given in a slow intravenous infusion over approximately 2-6 hours.

Diluted infusion solutions should be discarded after 24 hours.

The Cremophor® EL (polyoxyethylated castor oil) contained in the concentrate for intravenous infusion can cause phthalate stripping from PVC.

Parenteral drug products should be inspected visually for particulate matter and discoloration prior to administration, whenever solution and container permit.

Blood Concentration Monitoring

Several study centers have found blood concentration monitoring of cyclosporine useful in patient management. While no fixed relationships have yet been established, in one series of 375 consecutive cadaveric renal transplant recipients, dosage was adjusted to achieve specific whole blood 24-hour trough concentrations of 100-200 ng/mL as determined by high-pressure liquid chromatography (HPLC).

Of major importance to blood concentration analysis is the type of assay used. The above concentrations are specific to the parent cyclosporine molecule and correlate directly to the new monoclonal specific radioimmunoassays (mRIA-sp). Nonspecific assays are also available which detect the parent compound molecule and various of its metabolites. Older studies often cited concentrations using a nonspecific assay which were roughly twice those of specific assays. Assay results are not interchangeable and their use should be guided by their approved labeling. If plasma specimens are employed, concentrations will vary with the temperature at the time of separation from whole blood. Plasma concentrations may range from 1/2-1/5 of whole blood concentrations. Refer to individual assay labeling for complete instructions. In addition, *Transplantation Proceedings* (June 1990) contains position papers and a broad consensus generated at the Cyclosporine-Therapeutic Drug Monitoring conference that year. Blood concentration monitoring is not a replacement for renal function monitoring or tissue biopsies.

HOW SUPPLIED

Sandimmune® Soft Gelatin Capsules (cyclosporine capsules, USP)
25 mg: Oblong, pink, branded "△ 78/240". Unit dose packages of 30 capsules,

3 blister cards of 10 capsules ....NDC 0078-0240-15
100 mg: Oblong, dusty rose, branded "△ 78/241". Unit dose packages of 30 capsules,

3 blister cards of 10 capsules ....NDC 0078-0241-15
Store and Dispense: Store at 25°C (77°F); excursions permitted to 15-30°C (59-86°F) [see USP Controlled Room Temperature].

An odor may be detected upon opening the unit dose container, which will dissipate shortly thereafter. This odor does not affect the quality of the product.

Sandimmune® Oral Solution (cyclosporine oral solution, USP)
Supplied in 50 mL bottles containing 100 mg of cyclosporine per mL   NDC 0078-0110-22
A dosage syringe is provided for dispensing.
Store and Dispense: In the original container at temperatures below 30°C (86°F). Do not store in the refrigerator. Protect from freezing. Once opened, the contents must be used within 2 months.

Sandimmune® Injection (cyclosporine injection, USP)
FOR INTRAVENOUS INFUSION
Supplied as a 5 mL sterile ampul containing 50 mg of cyclosporine per mL,

in boxes of 10 ampuls ....NDC 0078-0109-01
Store and Dispense: At temperatures below 30°C (86°F). Protect from light.

FOR INFUSION ONLY
*Cremophor® is the registered trademark of BASF Aktiengesellschaft.

Distributed by:
Novartis Pharmaceuticals Corporation
East Hanover, New Jersey 07936
© Novartis
T2013-37
May 2013

SANDOSTATIN®   ℞
[săn-dō-stă-tĭn]
octreotide acetate
Injection

The following prescribing information is based on official labeling in effect July 2012.

DESCRIPTION

Sandostatin® (octreotide acetate) Injection, a cyclic octapeptide prepared as a clear sterile solution of octreotide, acetate salt, in a buffered lactic acid solution for administration by deep subcutaneous (intrafat) or intravenous injection. Octreotide acetate, known chemically as L-Cysteinamide, D-phenylalanyl-L-cysteinyl-L-phenylalanyl-D-tryptophyl-L-lysyl-L-threonyl-N-[2-hydroxy-1-(hydroxymethyl)propyl]-, cyclic (2→7)-disulfide; [R-(R*, R*)] acetate salt, is a long-acting octapeptide with pharmacologic actions mimicking those of the natural hormone somatostatin.

Sandostatin Injection is available as: sterile 1-mL ampuls in 3 strengths, containing 50, 100, or 500 mcg octreotide (as acetate), and sterile 5-mL multi-dose vials in 2 strengths, containing 200 and 1000 mcg/mL of octreotide (as acetate). Each ampul also contains:
lactic acid, USP   3.4 mg
mannitol, USP   45 mg
sodium bicarbonate, USP   qs to pH 4.2 ± 0.3
water for injection, USP   qs to 1 mL
Each mL of the multi-dose vials also contains:
lactic acid, USP   3.4 mg
mannitol, USP   45 mg
phenol, USP   5.0 mg
sodium bicarbonate, USP   qs to pH 4.2 ± 0.3
water for injection, USP   qs to 1 mL
Lactic acid and sodium bicarbonate are added to provide a buffered solution, pH to 4.2 ± 0.3.

The molecular weight of octreotide acetate is 1019.3 (free peptide, $C_{49}H_{66}N_{10}O_{10}S_2$) and its amino acid sequence is:

H-D-Phe-Cys-Phe-D-Trp-Lys-Thr-Cys-Thr-ol,
xCH₃COOH   where x = 1.4 to 2.5

CLINICAL PHARMACOLOGY

Sandostatin® (octreotide acetate) exerts pharmacologic actions similar to the natural hormone, somatostatin. It is an even more potent inhibitor of growth hormone, glucagon, and insulin than somatostatin. Like somatostatin, it also suppresses LH response to GnRH, decreases splanchnic blood flow, and inhibits release of serotonin, gastrin, vasoactive intestinal peptide, secretin, motilin, and pancreatic polypeptide.

By virtue of these pharmacological actions, Sandostatin has been used to treat the symptoms associated with metastatic carcinoid tumors (flushing and diarrhea), and Vasoactive Intestinal Peptide (VIP) secreting adenomas (watery diarrhea).

Sandostatin substantially reduces growth hormone and/or IGF-I (somatomedin C) levels in patients with acromegaly. Single doses of Sandostatin have been shown to inhibit gallbladder contractility and to decrease bile secretion in normal volunteers. In controlled clinical trials the incidence of gallstone or biliary sludge formation was markedly increased (*see* WARNINGS).

Sandostatin suppresses secretion of thyroid stimulating hormone (TSH).

Pharmacokinetics

After subcutaneous injection, octreotide is absorbed rapidly and completely from the injection site. Peak concentrations of 5.2 ng/mL (100-mcg dose) were reached 0.4 hours after dosing. Using a specific radioimmunoassay, intravenous and subcutaneous doses were found to be bioequivalent. Peak concentrations and area under the curve values were dose proportional after intravenous single doses up to 200 mcg and subcutaneous single doses up to 500 mcg and after subcutaneous multiple doses up to 500 mcg t.i.d. (1500 mcg/day).

In healthy volunteers the distribution of octreotide from plasma was rapid (tα1/2 = 0.2 h), the volume of distribution (Vdss) was estimated to be 13.6 L, and the total body clearance ranged from 7 L/hr to 10 L/hr. In blood, the distribution into the erythrocytes was found to be negligible and about 65% was bound in the plasma in a concentration-independent manner. Binding was mainly to lipoprotein and, to a lesser extent, to albumin.

The elimination of octreotide from plasma had an apparent half-life of 1.7 to 1.9 hours compared with 1-3 minutes with the natural hormone. The duration of action of Sandostatin is variable but extends up to 12 hours depending upon the type of tumor. About 32% of the dose is excreted unchanged into the urine. In an elderly population, dose adjustments may be necessary due to a significant increase in the half-life (46%) and a significant decrease in the clearance (26%) of the drug.

In patients with acromegaly, the pharmacokinetics differ somewhat from those in healthy volunteers. A mean peak concentration of 2.8 ng/mL (100-mcg dose) was reached in 0.7 hours after subcutaneous dosing. The volume of distribution (Vdss) was estimated to be 21.6 ± 8.5 L and the total body clearance was increased to 18 L/h. The mean percent of the drug bound was 41.2%. The disposition and elimination half-lives were similar to normals.

In patients with renal impairment the elimination of octreotide from plasma was prolonged and total body clearance reduced. In mild renal impairment (Cl_{CR} 40-60 mL/min) octreotide $t_{1/2}$ was 2.4 hours and total body clearance was 8.8 L/hr, in moderate impairment (Cl_{CR} 10-39 mL/min) $t_{1/2}$ was 3.0 hours and total body clearance 7.3 L/hr, and in severely renally impaired patients not requiring dialysis (Cl_{CR} <10 mL/min) $t_{1/2}$ was 3.1 hours and total body clearance was 7.6 L/hr. In patients with severe renal failure requiring dialysis, total body clearance was reduced to about half that found in healthy subjects (from approximately 10 L/hr to 4.5 L/hr).

Patients with liver cirrhosis showed prolonged elimination of drug, with octreotide $t_{1/2}$ increasing to 3.7 hr and total body clearance decreasing to 5.9 L/hr, whereas patients with fatty liver disease showed $t_{1/2}$ increased to 3.4 hr and total body clearance of 8.2 L/hr.

INDICATIONS AND USAGE
Acromegaly
Sandostatin® (octreotide acetate) is indicated to reduce blood levels of growth hormone and IGF-I (somatomedin C) in acromegaly patients who have had inadequate response to or cannot be treated with surgical resection, pituitary irradiation, and bromocriptine mesylate at maximally tolerated doses. The goal is to achieve normalization of growth hormone and IGF-I (somatomedin C) levels (see DOSAGE AND ADMINISTRATION). In patients with acromegaly, Sandostatin reduces growth hormone to within normal ranges in 50% of patients and reduces IGF-I (somatomedin C) to within normal ranges in 50%-60% of patients. Since the effects of pituitary irradiation may not become maximal for several years, adjunctive therapy with Sandostatin to reduce blood levels of growth hormone and IGF-I (somatomedin C) offers potential benefit before the effects of irradiation are manifested.

Improvement in clinical signs and symptoms or reduction in tumor size or rate of growth were not shown in clinical trials performed with Sandostatin; these trials were not optimally designed to detect such effects.

Carcinoid Tumors
Sandostatin is indicated for the symptomatic treatment of patients with metastatic carcinoid tumors where it suppresses or inhibits the severe diarrhea and flushing episodes associated with the disease.

Sandostatin studies were not designed to show an effect on the size, rate of growth or development of metastases.

Vasoactive Intestinal Peptide Tumors (VIPomas)
Sandostatin is indicated for the treatment of the profuse watery diarrhea associated with VIP-secreting tumors.

Sandostatin studies were not designed to show an effect on the size, rate of growth or development of metastases.

CONTRAINDICATIONS
Sensitivity to this drug or any of its components.

WARNINGS
Single doses of Sandostatin® (octreotide acetate) have been shown to inhibit gallbladder contractility and decrease bile secretion in normal volunteers. In clinical trials (primarily patients with acromegaly or psoriasis), the incidence of biliary tract abnormalities was 63% (27% gallstones, 24% sludge without stones, 12% biliary duct dilatation). The incidence of stones or sludge in patients who received Sandostatin for 12 months or longer was 52%. Less than 2% of patients treated with Sandostatin for 1 month or less developed gallstones. The incidence of gallstones did not appear related to age, sex or dose. Like patients without gallbladder abnormalities, the majority of patients developing gallbladder abnormalities on ultrasound had gastrointestinal symptoms. The symptoms were not specific for gallbladder disease. A few patients developed acute cholecystitis, ascending cholangitis, biliary obstruction, cholestatic hepatitis, or pancreatitis during Sandostatin therapy or following its withdrawal. One patient developed ascending cholangitis during Sandostatin therapy and died.

PRECAUTIONS
General
Sandostatin® (octreotide acetate) alters the balance between the counter-regulatory hormones, insulin, glucagon

and growth hormone, which may result in hypoglycemia or hyperglycemia. Sandostatin also suppresses secretion of thyroid stimulating hormone, which may result in hypothyroidism. Cardiac conduction abnormalities have also occurred during treatment with Sandostatin. However, the incidence of these adverse events during long-term therapy was determined vigorously only in acromegaly patients who, due to their underlying disease and/or the subsequent treatment they receive, are at an increased risk for the development of diabetes mellitus, hypothyroidism, and cardiovascular disease. Although the degree to which these abnormalities are related to Sandostatin therapy is not clear, new abnormalities of glycemic control, thyroid function and ECG developed during Sandostatin therapy as described below.

Risk of Pregnancy with Normalization of IGF-1 and GH
Although acromegaly may lead to infertility, there are reports of pregnancy in acromegalic women. In women with active acromegaly who have been unable to become pregnant, normalization of GH and IGF-1 may restore fertility. Female patients of childbearing potential should be advised to use adequate contraception during treatment with octreotide.

The hypoglycemia or hyperglycemia which occurs during Sandostatin therapy is usually mild, but may result in overt diabetes mellitus or necessitate dose changes in insulin or other hypoglycemic agents. Hypoglycemia and hyperglycemia occurred on Sandostatin in 3% and 16% of acromegalic patients, respectively. Severe hyperglycemia, subsequent pneumonia, and death following initiation of Sandostatin therapy was reported in one patient with no history of hyperglycemia.

In patients with concomitant Type I diabetes mellitus, Sandostatin Injection and Sandostatin LAR® Depot (octreotide acetate for injectable suspension) are likely to affect glucose regulation, and insulin requirements may be reduced. Symptomatic hypoglycemia, which may be severe, has been reported in these patients. In non-diabetics and Type II diabetics with partially intact insulin reserves, Sandostatin Injection or Sandostatin LAR Depot administration may result in decreases in plasma insulin levels and hyperglycemia. It is therefore recommended that glucose tolerance and antidiabetic treatment be periodically monitored during therapy with these drugs.

In acromegalic patients, 12% developed biochemical hypothyroidism only, 8% developed goiter, and 4% required initiation of thyroid replacement therapy while receiving Sandostatin. Baseline and periodic assessment of thyroid function (TSH, total and/or free T_4) is recommended during chronic therapy.

In acromegalics, bradycardia (<50 bpm) developed in 25%; conduction abnormalities occurred in 10% and arrhythmias occurred in 9% of patients during Sandostatin therapy. Other EKG changes observed included QT prolongation, axis shifts, early repolarization, low voltage, R/S transition, and early R wave progression. These ECG changes are not uncommon in acromegalic patients. Dose adjustments in drugs such as beta-blockers that have bradycardia effects may be necessary. In one acromegalic patient with severe congestive heart failure, initiation of Sandostatin therapy resulted in worsening of CHF with improvement when drug was discontinued. Confirmation of a drug effect was obtained with a positive rechallenge.

Several cases of pancreatitis have been reported in patients receiving Sandostatin therapy.

Sandostatin may alter absorption of dietary fats in some patients.

In patients with severe renal failure requiring dialysis, the half-life of Sandostatin may be increased, necessitating adjustment of the maintenance dosage.

Depressed vitamin B_{12} levels and abnormal Schilling's tests have been observed in some patients receiving Sandostatin therapy, and monitoring of vitamin B_{12} levels is recommended during chronic Sandostatin therapy.

Information for Patients
Careful instruction in sterile subcutaneous injection technique should be given to the patients and to other persons who may administer Sandostatin Injection.

Laboratory Tests
Laboratory tests that may be helpful as biochemical markers in determining and following patient response depend on the specific tumor. Based on diagnosis, measurement of the following substances may be useful in monitoring the progress of therapy:

Acromegaly: Growth Hormone, IGF-I (somatomedin C) Responsiveness to Sandostatin may be evaluated by determining growth hormone levels at 1-4 hour intervals for 8-12 hours post dose. Alternatively, a single measurement of IGF-I (somatomedin C) level may be made two weeks after drug initiation or dosage change.

Carcinoid: 5-HIAA (urinary 5-hydroxyindole acetic acid), plasma serotonin, plasma Substance P

VIPoma: VIP (plasma vasoactive intestinal peptide)

Baseline and periodic total and/or free T_4 measurements should be performed during chronic therapy (see PRECAUTIONS – General).

Drug Interactions
Sandostatin has been associated with alterations in nutrient absorption, so it may have an effect on absorption of orally administered drugs. Concomitant administration of Sandostatin with cyclosporine may decrease blood levels of cyclosporine and result in transplant rejection.

Patients receiving insulin, oral hypoglycemic agents, beta blockers, calcium channel blockers, or agents to control fluid and electrolyte balance, may require dose adjustments of these therapeutic agents.

Concomitant administration of octreotide and bromocriptine increases the availability of bromocriptine. Limited published data indicate that somatostatin analogs might decrease the metabolic clearance of compounds known to be metabolized by cytochrome P450 enzymes, which may be due to the suppression of growth hormones. Since it cannot be excluded that octreotide may have this effect, other drugs mainly metabolized by CYP3A4 and which have a low therapeutic index (e.g., quinidine, terfenadine) should therefore be used with caution.

Drug Laboratory Test Interactions
No known interference exists with clinical laboratory tests, including amine or peptide determinations.

Carcinogenesis/Mutagenesis/Impairment of Fertility
Studies in laboratory animals have demonstrated no mutagenic potential of Sandostatin.

No carcinogenic potential was demonstrated in mice treated subcutaneously for 85-99 weeks at doses up to 2000 mcg/kg/day (8× the human exposure based on body surface area). In a 116-week subcutaneous study in rats, a 27% and 12% incidence of injection site sarcomas or squamous cell carcinomas was observed in males and females, respectively, at the highest dose level of 1250 mcg/kg/day (10× the human exposure based on body surface area) compared to an incidence of 8%-10% in the vehicle-control groups. The increased incidence of injection site tumors was most probably caused by irritation and the high sensitivity of the rat to repeated subcutaneous injections at the same site. Rotating injection sites would prevent chronic irritation in humans. There have been no reports of injection site tumors in patients treated with Sandostatin for up to 5 years. There was also a 15% incidence of uterine adenocarcinomas in the 1250 mcg/kg/day females compared to 7% in the saline-control females and 0% in the vehicle-control females. The presence of endometritis coupled with the absence of corpora lutea, the reduction in mammary fibroadenomas, and the presence of uterine dilatation suggest that the uterine tumors were associated with estrogen dominance in the aged female rats which does not occur in humans.

Sandostatin did not impair fertility in rats at doses up to 1000 mcg/kg/day, which represents 7× the human exposure based on body surface area.

Pregnancy Category B
There are no adequate and well-controlled studies of octreotide use in pregnant women. Reproduction studies have been performed in rats and rabbits at doses up to 16 times the highest recommended human dose based on body surface area and revealed no evidence of harm to the fetus due to octreotide. However, because animal reproduction studies are not always predictive of human response, this drug should be used during pregnancy only if clearly needed.

In postmarketing data, a limited number of exposed pregnancies have been reported in patients with acromegaly. Most women were exposed to octreotide during the first trimester of pregnancy at doses ranging from 100-300 mcg/day of Sandostatin s.c. or 20-30 mg/month of Sandostatin LAR, however some women elected to continue octreotide therapy throughout pregnancy. In cases with a known outcome, no congenital malformations were reported.

Nursing Mothers
It is not known whether octreotide is excreted into human milk. Because many drugs are excreted in human milk, caution should be exercised when octreotide is administered to a nursing woman.

Pediatric Use
Safety and efficacy of Sandostatin Injection in the pediatric population have not been demonstrated.

No formal controlled clinical trials have been performed to evaluate the safety and effectiveness of Sandostatin in pediatric patients under age 6 years. In post-marketing reports, serious adverse events, including hypoxia, necrotizing enterocolitis, and death, have been reported with Sandostatin use in children, most notably in children under 2 years of age. The relationship of these events to octreotide has not been established as the majority of these pediatric patients had serious underlying co-morbid conditions.

The efficacy and safety of Sandostatin using the Sandostatin LAR Depot formulation was examined in a single randomized, double-blind, placebo-controlled, six-month pharmacokinetics study in 60 pediatric patients age 6-17 years with hypothalamic obesity resulting from cranial insult. The mean octreotide concentration after 6 doses of 40 mg Sandostatin LAR Depot administered by IM injection every four weeks was approximately 3 ng/ml. Steady-state concentrations was achieved after 3 injections of a 40 mg dose. Mean BMI increased 0.1 kg/m² in Sandostatin LAR Depot-treated subjects compared to 0.0 kg/m² in saline control-treated subjects. Efficacy was not demonstrated. Diarrhea occurred in 11 of 30 (37%) patients treated with Sandostatin LAR Depot. No unexpected adverse events were observed. However, with Sandostatin LAR Depot 40 mg once a month, the incidence of new cholelithiasis in this pediatric population (33%) was higher than that seen in other adults indications such as acromegaly (22%) or malignant carcinoid syndrome (24%), where Sandostatin LAR Depot was 10 to 30 mg once a month.

Geriatric Use
Clinical studies of Sandostatin did not include sufficient numbers of subjects aged 65 and over to determine whether they respond differently from younger subjects. Other reported clinical experience has not identified differences in responses between the elderly and younger patients. In general, dose selection for an elderly patient should be cautious, usually starting at the low end of the dosing range, reflecting the greater frequency of decreased hepatic, renal, or cardiac function, and of concomitant disease or other drug therapy.

ADVERSE REACTIONS
Gallbladder Abnormalities
Gallbladder abnormalities, especially stones and/or biliary sludge, frequently develop in patients on chronic Sandostatin® (octreotide acetate) therapy (see WARNINGS).
Cardiac
In acromegalics, sinus bradycardia (<50 bpm) developed in 25%; conduction abnormalities occurred in 10% and arrhythmias developed in 9% of patients during Sandostatin therapy (see PRECAUTIONS – General).
Gastrointestinal
Diarrhea, loose stools, nausea and abdominal discomfort were each seen in 34%-61% of acromegalic patients in U.S. studies although only 2.6% of the patients discontinued therapy due to these symptoms. These symptoms were seen in 5%-10% of patients with other disorders.

The frequency of these symptoms was not dose-related, but diarrhea and abdominal discomfort generally resolved more quickly in patients treated with 300 mcg/day than in those treated with 750 mcg/day. Vomiting, flatulence, abnormal stools, abdominal distention, and constipation were each seen in less than 10% of patients.

In rare instances, gastrointestinal side effects may resemble acute intestinal obstruction, with progressive abdominal distension, severe epigastric pain, abdominal tenderness and guarding.
Hypo/Hyperglycemia
Hypoglycemia and hyperglycemia occurred in 3% and 16% of acromegalic patients, respectively, but only in about 1.5% of other patients. Symptoms of hypoglycemia were noted in approximately 2% of patients.
Hypothyroidism
In acromegalics, biochemical hypothyroidism alone occurred in 12% while goiter occurred in 6% during Sandostatin therapy (see PRECAUTIONS – General). In patients without acromegaly, hypothyroidism has only been reported in several isolated patients and goiter has not been reported.
Other Adverse Events
Pain on injection was reported in 7.7%, headache in 6% and dizziness in 5%. Pancreatitis was also observed (see WARNINGS and PRECAUTIONS).
Other Adverse Events 1%-4%
Other events (relationship to drug not established), each observed in 1%-4% of patients, included fatigue, weakness, pruritus, joint pain, backache, urinary tract infection, cold symptoms, flu symptoms, injection site hematoma, bruise, edema, flushing, blurred vision, pollakiuria, fat malabsorption, hair loss, visual disturbance and depression.
Other Adverse Events <1%
Events reported in less than 1% of patients and for which relationship to drug is not established are listed: Gastrointestinal: hepatitis, jaundice, increase in liver enzymes, GI bleeding, hemorrhoids, appendicitis, gastric/peptic ulcer, gallbladder polyp; Integumentary: rash, cellulitis, petechiae, urticaria, basal cell carcinoma; Musculoskeletal: arthritis, joint effusion, muscle pain, Raynaud's phenomenon; Cardiovascular: chest pain, shortness of breath, thrombophlebitis, ischemia, congestive heart failure, hypertension, hypertensive reaction, palpitations, orthostatic BP decrease, tachycardia; CNS: anxiety, libido decrease, syncope, tremor, seizure, vertigo, Bell's Palsy, paranoia, pituitary apoplexy, increased intraocular pressure, amnesia, hearing loss, neuritis; Respiratory: pneumonia, pulmonary nodule, status asthmaticus; Endocrine: galactorrhea, hypoadrenalism, diabetes insipidus, gynecomastia, amenorrhea, polymenorrhea, oligomenorrhea, vaginitis; Urogenital: nephrolithia-

sis, hematuria; Hematologic: anemia, iron deficiency, epistaxis; Miscellaneous: otitis, allergic reaction, increased CK, weight loss.

Evaluation of 20 patients treated for at least 6 months has failed to demonstrate titers of antibodies exceeding background levels. However, antibody titers to Sandostatin were subsequently reported in three patients and resulted in prolonged duration of drug action in two patients. Anaphylactoid reactions, including anaphylactic shock, have been reported in several patients receiving Sandostatin.
Postmarketing Experience
The following adverse reactions have been identified during the postapproval use of Sandostatin. Because these reactions are reported voluntarily from a population of uncertain size, it is not always possible to reliably estimate their frequency or establish a causal relationship to drug exposure.

Gastrointestinal: intestinal obstruction
Hematologic: thrombocytopenia

OVERDOSAGE
A limited number of accidental overdoses of Sandostatin® in adults have been reported. In adults, the doses ranged from 2,400–6,000 micrograms/day administered by continuous infusion (100-250 micrograms/hour) or subcutaneously (1,500 micrograms t.i.d.). Adverse events in some patients included arrhythmia, hypotension, cardiac arrest, brain hypoxia, pancreatitis, hepatitis steatosis, hepatomegaly, lactic acidosis, flushing, diarrhea, lethargy, weakness, and weight loss.

Sandostatin Injection given in intravenous boluses of 1 mg (1000 mcg) to healthy volunteers did not result in serious ill effects, nor did doses of 30 mg (30,000 mcg) given intravenously over 20 minutes and of 120 mg (120,000 mcg) given intravenously over 8 hours to research patients.

If overdose occurs, symptomatic management is indicated. Up-to-date information about the treatment of overdose can often be obtained from the National Poison Control Center at 1-800-222-1222.
Drug Abuse and Dependence
There is no indication that Sandostatin has potential for drug abuse or dependence. Sandostatin levels in the central nervous system are negligible, even after doses up to 30,000 mcg.

DOSAGE AND ADMINISTRATION
Sandostatin® (octreotide acetate) may be administered subcutaneously or intravenously. Subcutaneous injection is the usual route of administration of Sandostatin for control of symptoms. Pain with subcutaneous administration may be reduced by using the smallest volume that will deliver the desired dose. Multiple subcutaneous injections at the same site within short periods of time should be avoided. Sites should be rotated in a systematic manner.

Parenteral drug products should be inspected visually for particulate matter and discoloration prior to administration. **Do not use if particulates and/or discoloration are observed.** Proper sterile technique should be used in the preparation of parenteral admixtures to minimize the possibility of microbial contamination. **Sandostatin is not compatible in Total Parenteral Nutrition (TPN) solutions because of the formation of a glycosyl octreotide conjugate which may decrease the efficacy of the product.**

Sandostatin is stable in sterile isotonic saline solutions or sterile solutions of dextrose 5% in water for 24 hours. It may be diluted in volumes of 50-200 mL and infused intravenously over 15-30 minutes or administered by IV push over 3 minutes. In emergency situations (e.g., carcinoid crisis) it may be given by rapid bolus.

The initial dosage is usually 50 mcg administered twice or three times daily. Upward dose titration is frequently required. Dosage information for patients with specific tumors follows.
Acromegaly
Dosage may be initiated at 50 mcg t.i.d. Beginning with this low dose may permit adaptation to adverse gastrointestinal effects for patients who will require higher doses. IGF-I (somatomedin C) levels every 2 weeks can be used to guide titration. Alternatively, multiple growth hormone levels at 0-8 hours after Sandostatin® (octreotide acetate) administration permit more rapid titration of dose. The goal is to achieve growth hormone levels less than 5 ng/mL or IGF-I (somatomedin C) levels less than 1.9 U/mL in males and less than 2.2 U/mL in females. The dose most commonly found to be effective is 100 mcg t.i.d., but some patients require up to 500 mcg t.i.d. for maximum effectiveness. Doses greater than 300 mcg/day seldom result in additional biochemical benefit, and if an increase in dose fails to provide additional benefit, the dose should be reduced. IGF-I (somatomedin C) or growth hormone levels should be re-evaluated at 6-month intervals.

Sandostatin should be withdrawn yearly for approximately 4 weeks from patients who have received irradiation to as-

sess disease activity. If growth hormone or IGF-I (somatomedin C) levels increase and signs and symptoms recur, Sandostatin therapy may be resumed.
Carcinoid Tumors
The suggested daily dosage of Sandostatin during the first 2 weeks of therapy ranges from 100-600 mcg/day in 2-4 divided doses (mean daily dosage is 300 mcg). In the clinical studies, the **median** daily maintenance dosage was approximately 450 mcg, but clinical and biochemical benefits were obtained in some patients with as little as 50 mcg, while others required doses up to 1500 mcg/day. However, experience with doses above 750 mcg/day is limited.
VIPomas
Daily dosages of 200-300 mcg in 2-4 divided doses are recommended during the initial 2 weeks of therapy (range 150-750 mcg) to control symptoms of the disease. On an individual basis, dosage may be adjusted to achieve a therapeutic response, but usually doses above 450 mcg/day are not required.

HOW SUPPLIED
Sandostatin® (octreotide acetate) Injection is available in 1-mL ampuls and 5-mL multi-dose vials as follows:
Ampuls
50 mcg/mL octreotide (as acetate)
Package of 10 ampuls   NDC 0078-0180-01
100 mcg/mL octreotide (as acetate)
Package of 10 ampuls   NDC 0078-0181-01
500 mcg/mL octreotide (as acetate)
Package of 10 ampuls   NDC 0078-0182-01
Multi-Dose Vials
200 mcg/mL octreotide (as acetate)
Box of one   NDC 0078-0183-25
1000 mcg/mL octreotide (as acetate)
Box of one   NDC 0078-0184-25
Storage
For prolonged storage, Sandostatin ampuls and multi-dose vials should be stored at refrigerated temperatures 2°C-8°C (36°F-46°F) and store in outer carton in order to protect from light. At room temperature, (20°C-30°C or 70°F-86°F), Sandostatin is stable for 14 days if protected from light. The solution can be allowed to come to room temperature prior to administration. Do not warm artificially. After initial use, multiple-dose vials should be discarded within 14 days. Ampuls should be opened just prior to administration and the unused portion discarded. Dispose unused product or waste properly.

Manufactured by:
Novartis Pharma Stein AG
Stein, Switzerland
Distributed by:
Novartis Pharmaceuticals Corporation
East Hanover, NJ 07936
© Novartis
T2012-71
March 2012

Shown in Product Identification Guide, page 311

SANDOSTATIN® LAR DEPOT   ℞
[săn-dō-stă-tĭn]
(octreotide acetate for injectable suspension)

The following prescribing information is based on official labeling in effect July 2014.

HIGHLIGHTS OF PRESCRIBING INFORMATION
These highlights do not include all the information needed to use Sandostatin LAR safely and effectively. See full prescribing information for Sandostatin LAR.
Sandostatin® LAR Depot (octreotide acetate for injectable suspension)
Initial U.S. Approval: 1988

--------INDICATIONS AND USAGE--------
Sandostatin LAR is a somatostatin analogue indicated for: Treatment in patients who have responded to and tolerated Sandostatin Injection subcutaneous injection for:
• Acromegaly (1.1)
• Severe diarrhea/flushing episodes associated with metastatic carcinoid tumors (1.2)
• Profuse watery diarrhea associated with VIP-secreting tumors (1.3)

--------DOSAGE AND ADMINISTRATION--------
Patients not currently receiving Sandostatin Injection subcutaneously:
• Acromegaly: 50 mcg three times daily Sandostatin Injection subcutaneously for 2 weeks followed by Sandostatin LAR 20 mg intragluteally every 4 weeks for 3 months (2.1)
• Carcinoid Tumors and VIPomas: Sandostatin Injection subcutaneously 100-600 mcg/day in 2-4 divided doses for 2 weeks followed by Sandostatin LAR 20 mg every 4 weeks for 2 months (2.2)
Patients currently receiving Sandostatin Injection subcutaneously:
• Acromegaly: 20 mg every 4 weeks for 3 months (2.1)

- Carcinoid Tumors and VIPomas: 20 mg every 4 weeks for 2 months (2.2)

Renal Impairment, patients on dialysis: 10 mg every 4 weeks (2.3)

Hepatic Impairment, patients with cirrhosis: 10 mg every 4 weeks (2.4)

---------------------DOSAGE FORMS AND STRENGTHS--------------------

For Injectable Suspension; Strengths 10 mg per 6 mL, 20 mg per 6 mL, or 30 mg per 6 mL vials (3)

-----------------------------CONTRAINDICATIONS-----------------------------

None (4)

--------------------WARNINGS AND PRECAUTIONS--------------------

- Gallbladder abnormalities may occur. Monitor periodically. (5.1)
- Glucose Metabolism: Hypoglycemia or hyperglycemia may occur. Glucose monitoring is recommended and antidiabetic treatment may need adjustment. (5.2)
- Thyroid Function: Hypothyroidism may occur. Monitor thyroid levels periodically. (5.3)
- Cardiac Function: Bradycardia, arrhythmia, or conduction abnormalities may occur. Use with caution in at-risk patients. (5.4)

-----------------------------ADVERSE REACTIONS-----------------------------

The most common adverse reactions, occurring in ≥20% of patients are:

- Acromegaly: diarrhea, cholelithiasis, abdominal pain, flatulence (6.1)
- Carcinoid Syndrome: back pain, fatigue, headache, abdominal pain, nausea, dizziness (6.1)

To report SUSPECTED ADVERSE REACTIONS, contact Novartis Pharmaceuticals Corporation at 1-888-669-6682 or FDA at 1-800-FDA-1088 or www.fda.gov/medwatch.

-----------------------------DRUG INTERACTIONS-----------------------------

The following drugs require monitoring and possible dose adjustment when used with Sandostatin LAR: cyclosporine, insulin, oral hypoglycemic agents, beta-blockers, bromocriptine (7)

See 17 for PATIENT COUNSELING INFORMATION

Revised: 7/2014

FULL PRESCRIBING INFORMATION: CONTENTS*

FULL PRESCRIBING INFORMATION

1 INDICATIONS AND USAGE

Sandostatin LAR Depot 10 mg, 20 mg, and 30 mg is indicated in patients in whom initial treatment with Sandostatin Injection has been shown to be effective and tolerated.

1.1 Acromegaly

Long-term maintenance therapy in acromegalic patients who have had an inadequate response to surgery and/or radiotherapy, or for whom surgery and/or radiotherapy is not an option. The goal of treatment in acromegaly is to reduce GH and IGF-1 levels to normal *[see Clinical Studies (14) and Dosage and Administration (2)]*.

1.2 Carcinoid Tumors

Long-term treatment of the severe diarrhea and flushing episodes associated with metastatic carcinoid tumors.

1.3 Vasoactive Intestinal Peptide Tumors (VIPomas)

Long-term treatment of the profuse watery diarrhea associated with VIP-secreting tumors.

1.4 Important Limitations of Use

In patients with carcinoid syndrome and VIPomas, the effect of Sandostatin Injection and Sandostatin LAR Depot on tumor size, rate of growth and development of metastases, has not been determined.

2 DOSAGE AND ADMINISTRATION

- Sandostatin LAR Depot should be administered by a trained healthcare provider. It is important to closely follow the mixing instructions included in the packaging. Sandostatin LAR Depot must be administered immediately after mixing.
- **Do not directly inject diluent without preparing suspension.**
- The recommended needle size for administration of Sandostatin LAR Depot is the 1½" 20 gauge safety injection needle (supplied in the drug product kit). For patients with a greater skin to muscle depth, a size 2" 20 gauge needle (not supplied) may be used.
- Sandostatin LAR Depot should be administered intramuscularly in the gluteal region at 4-week intervals. Administration of Sandostatin LAR Depot at intervals greater than 4 weeks is not recommended.
- Injection sites should be rotated in a systematic manner to avoid irritation. Deltoid injections should be avoided due to significant discomfort at the injection site when given in that area.
- **Sandostatin LAR Depot should never be administered intravenously or subcutaneously.**

The following dosage regimens are recommended.

2.1 Acromegaly

Patients Not Currently Receiving Octreotide Acetate

Patients not currently receiving octreotide acetate should begin therapy with Sandostatin Injection given subcutaneously in an initial dose of 50 mcg three times daily which may be titrated. Most patients require doses of 100 mcg to 200 mcg three times daily for maximum effect but some patients require up to 500 mcg three times daily.

Patients should be maintained on Sandostatin Injection subcutaneous for at least 2 weeks to determine tolerance to octreotide. Patients who are considered to be "responders" to the drug, based on GH and IGF-1 levels and who tolerate the drug can then be switched to Sandostatin LAR Depot in the dosage scheme described below (Patients Currently Receiving Sandostatin Injection).

Patients Currently Receiving Sandostatin Injection

Patients currently receiving Sandostatin Injection can be switched directly to Sandostatin LAR Depot in a dose of 20 mg given IM intragluteally at 4-week intervals for 3 months. After 3 months, dosage may be adjusted as follows:

- GH ≤2.5 ng/mL, IGF-1 normal, and clinical symptoms controlled: maintain Sandostatin LAR Depot dosage at 20 mg every 4 weeks.
- GH >2.5 ng/mL, IGF-1 elevated, and/or clinical symptoms uncontrolled, increase Sandostatin LAR Depot dosage to 30 mg every 4 weeks.
- GH ≤1 ng/mL, IGF-1 normal, and clinical symptoms controlled, reduce Sandostatin LAR Depot dosage to 10 mg every 4 weeks.
- If GH, IGF-1, or symptoms are not adequately controlled at a dose of 30 mg, the dose may be increased to 40 mg every 4 weeks. Doses higher than 40 mg are not recommended.

In patients who have received pituitary irradiation, Sandostatin LAR Depot should be withdrawn yearly for approximately 8 weeks to assess disease activity. If GH or IGF-1 levels increase and signs and symptoms recur, Sandostatin LAR Depot therapy may be resumed.

2.2 Carcinoid Tumors and VIPomas

Patients Not Currently Receiving Octreotide Acetate

Patients not currently receiving octreotide acetate should begin therapy with Sandostatin Injection given subcutaneously. The suggested daily dosage for carcinoid tumors during the first 2 weeks of therapy ranges from 100-600 mcg/day in 2-4 divided doses (mean daily dosage is 300 mcg). Some patients may require doses up to 1500 mcg/day. The suggested daily dosage for VIPomas is 200-300 mcg in 2-4 divided doses (range 150-750 mcg); dosage may be adjusted on an individual basis to control symptoms but usually doses above 450 mcg/day are not required. Sandostatin Injection should be continued for at least 2 weeks. Thereafter, patients who are considered "responders" to octreotide acetate and who tolerate the drug may be switched to Sandostatin LAR Depot in the dosage regimen as described below (Patients Currently Receiving Sandostatin Injection).

Patients Currently Receiving Sandostatin Injection

Patients currently receiving Sandostatin Injection can be switched to Sandostatin LAR Depot in a dosage of 20 mg given IM intragluteally at 4-week intervals for 2 months. Because of the need for serum octreotide to reach therapeutically effective levels following initial injection of Sandostatin LAR Depot, carcinoid tumor and VIPoma patients should continue to receive Sandostatin Injection subcutaneously for at least 2 weeks in the same dosage they were taking before the switch. Failure to continue subcutaneous injections for this period may result in exacerbation of symptoms. (Some patients may require 3 or 4 weeks of such therapy.)

After 2 months, dosage may be adjusted as follows:

- If symptoms are adequately controlled, consider a dose reduction to 10 mg for a trial period. If symptoms recur, dosage should then be increased to 20 mg every 4 weeks. Many patients can, however, be satisfactorily maintained at a 10-mg dose every 4 weeks.
- If symptoms are not adequately controlled, increase Sandostatin LAR Depot to 30 mg every 4 weeks. Patients who achieve good control on a 20-mg dose may have their dose lowered to 10 mg for a trial period. If symptoms recur, dosage should then be increased to 20 mg every 4 weeks.
- Dosages higher than 30 mg are not recommended.

Despite good overall control of symptoms, patients with carcinoid tumors and VIPomas often experience periodic exacerbation of symptoms (regardless of whether they are being maintained on Sandostatin Injection or Sandostatin LAR Depot). During these periods they may be given Sandostatin Injection subcutaneously for a few days at the dosage they were receiving prior to switching to Sandostatin LAR Depot. When symptoms are again controlled, the Sandostatin Injection subcutaneous can be discontinued.

2.3 Special Populations: Renal Impairment

In patients with renal failure requiring dialysis, the starting dose should be 10 mg every 4 weeks. In other patients with renal impairment, the starting dose should be similar to a nonrenal patient (i.e., 20 mg every 4 weeks) *[see Clinical Pharmacology (12)]*.

2.4 Special Populations: Hepatic Impairment – Cirrhotic Patients

In patients with established cirrhosis of the liver, the starting dose should be 10 mg every 4 weeks *[see Clinical Pharmacology (12.3)]*.

3 DOSAGE FORMS AND STRENGTHS

Sandostatin LAR Depot is available in single-use kits for injectable suspension containing a 6-mL vial of 10 mg, 20 mg, or 30 mg strength, a syringe containing 2 mL of diluent, one vial adapter, and one sterile 1½" 20 gauge safety injection needle. An instruction booklet for the preparation of drug suspension for injection is also included with each kit.

4 CONTRAINDICATIONS

None

5 WARNINGS AND PRECAUTIONS

5.1 Cholelithiasis and Gallbladder Sludge

Sandostatin may inhibit gallbladder contractility and decrease bile secretion, which may lead to gallbladder abnormalities or sludge. Patients should be monitored periodically *[see Adverse Reactions (6)]*.

5.2 Hyperglycemia and Hypoglycemia

Octreotide alters the balance between the counter-regulatory hormones, insulin, glucagon, and growth hormone, which may result in hypoglycemia or hyperglycemia. Blood glucose levels should be monitored when Sandostatin LAR treatment is initiated, or when the dose is altered. Antidiabetic treatment should be adjusted accordingly *[see Adverse Reactions (6)]*.

5.3 Thyroid Function Abnormalities

Octreotide suppresses the secretion of thyroid-stimulating hormone (TSH), which may result in hypothyroidism. Baseline and periodic assessment of thyroid function (TSH, total and/or free T_4) is recommended during chronic octreotide therapy *[see Adverse Reactions (6)]*.

5.4 Cardiac Function Abnormalities

In both acromegalic and carcinoid syndrome patients, bradycardia, arrhythmias and conduction abnormalities have been reported during octreotide therapy. Other ECG changes were observed such as QT prolongation, axis shifts, early repolarization, low voltage, R/S transition, early R wave progression, and nonspecific ST-T wave changes. The relationship of these events to octreotide acetate is not established because many of these patients have underlying cardiac disease. Dose adjustments in drugs such as beta-blockers that have bradycardic effects may be necessary. In one acromegalic patient with severe congestive heart failure (CHF), initiation of Sandostatin Injection therapy resulted in worsening of CHF with improvement when drug was discontinued. Confirmation of a drug effect was obtained with a positive rechallenge *[see Adverse Reactions (6)]*.

5.5 Nutrition

Octreotide may alter absorption of dietary fats.

Depressed vitamin B_{12} levels and abnormal Schilling tests have been observed in some patients receiving octreotide therapy, and monitoring of vitamin B_{12} levels is recommended during therapy with Sandostatin LAR Depot.

Octreotide has been investigated for the reduction of excessive fluid loss from the GI tract in patients with conditions producing such a loss. If such patients are receiving total parenteral nutrition (TPN), serum zinc may rise excessively when the fluid loss is reversed. Patients on TPN and octreotide should have periodic monitoring of zinc levels.

5.6 Monitoring: Laboratory Tests

Laboratory tests that may be helpful as biochemical markers in determining and following patient response depend on the specific tumor. Based on diagnosis, measurement of the following substances may be useful in monitoring the progress of therapy *[see Dosage and Administration (2.1, 2.2)]*.

Acromegaly: Growth Hormone, IGF-1 (somatomedin C)
Carcinoid: 5-HIAA (urinary 5-hydroxyindole acetic acid), plasma serotonin, plasma Substance P
VIPoma: VIP (plasma vasoactive intestinal peptide) baseline and periodic total and/or free T_4 measurements should be performed during chronic therapy

5.7 Drug Interactions

Octreotide has been associated with alterations in nutrient absorption, so it may have an effect on absorption of orally administered drugs. Concomitant administration of octreotide injection with cyclosporine may decrease blood levels of cyclosporine *[see Drug Interactions (7.1)]*.

6 ADVERSE REACTIONS

6.1 Clinical Studies Experience

Because clinical trials are conducted under widely varying conditions, adverse reaction rates observed in the clinical trials of a drug cannot be directly compared to rates in the clinical trial of another drug and may not reflect the rates observed in practice.

Acromegaly

The safety of Sandostatin LAR in the treatment of acromegaly has been evaluated in three phase 3 studies in 261 patients, including 209 exposed for 48 weeks and 96 exposed for greater than 108 weeks. Sandostatin LAR was studied primarily in a double-blind, cross-over manner. Patients on subcutaneous Sandostatin Injection were switched to the LAR formulation followed by an open-label extension. The population age range was 14-81 years old and 53% were female. Approximately 35% of these acromegaly patients had not been treated with surgery and/or radiation. Most patients received a starting dose of 20 mg every 4 weeks intramuscularly. Dose was up or down titrated based on efficacy and tolerability to a final dose between 10-60 mg every 4 weeks. Table 1 below reflects adverse events from these studies regardless of presumed causality to study drug.

Table 1. Adverse Events Occurring in ≥10% of Acromegalic Patients in the Phase 3 Studies

WHO Preferred Term	Phase 3 Studies (Pooled) Number (%) of Subjects with AE's 10 mg/20 mg/30 mg (n=261) n (%)
Diarrhea	93 (35.6)
Abdominal Pain	75 (28.7)
Flatulence	66 (25.3)
Influenza-Like Symptoms	52 (19.9)
Constipation	46 (17.6)
Headache	40 (15.3)
Anemia	40 (15.3)
Injection Site Pain	36 (13.8)
Cholelithiasis	35 (13.4)
Hypertension	33 (12.6)
Dizziness	30 (11.5)
Fatigue	29 (11.1)

The safety of Sandostatin LAR in the treatment of acromegaly was also evaluated in a postmarketing randomized phase 4 study. One-hundred four (104) patients were randomized to either pituitary surgery or 20 mg of Sandostatin LAR. All the patients were treatment naïve ('de novo'). Crossover was allowed according to treatment response and a total of 76 patients were exposed to Sandostatin LAR. Approximately half of the patients initially randomized to Sandostatin LAR were exposed to Sandostatin LAR up to 1 year. The population age range was between 20-76 years old, 45% were female, 93% were Caucasian, and 1% black. The majority of these patients were exposed to 30 mg every 4 weeks. Table 2 below reflects the adverse events occurring in this study regardless of presumed causality to study drug.

Table 2. Adverse Events Occurring in ≥10% of Acromegalic Patients in Phase 4 Study

WHO Preferred Term	Phase 4 Study SAS LAR N=76 n (%)	Phase 4 Study Surgery N=64 n (%)
Diarrhea	36 (47.4)	2 (3.1)
Cholelithiasis	29 (38.2)	3 (4.7)
Abdominal Pain	19 (25.0)	2 (3.1)
Nausea	12 (15.8)	5 (7.8)
Alopecia	10 (13.2)	5 (7.8)
Injection Site Pain	9 (11.8)	0
Abdominal Pain Upper	8 (10.5)	0
Headache	8 (10.5)	6 (9.4)
Epistaxis	0	7 (10.9)

Gallbladder Abnormalities

Single doses of Sandostatin Injection have been shown to inhibit gallbladder contractility and decrease bile secretion in normal volunteers. In clinical trials with Sandostatin Injection (primarily patients with acromegaly or psoriasis) in patients who had not previously received octreotide, the incidence of biliary tract abnormalities was 63% (27% gallstones, 24% sludge without stones, 12% biliary duct dilatation). The incidence of stones or sludge in patients who received Sandostatin Injection for 12 months or longer was 52%. The incidence of gallbladder abnormalities did not appear to be related to age, sex, or dose but was related to duration of exposure.

In clinical trials 52% of acromegalic patients, most of whom received Sandostatin LAR Depot for 12 months or longer, developed new biliary abnormalities including gallstones, microlithiasis, sediment, sludge, and dilatation. The incidence of new cholelithiasis was 22%, of which 7% were microstones.

Across all trials, a few patients developed acute cholecystitis, ascending cholangitis, biliary obstruction, cholestatic hepatitis, or pancreatitis during octreotide therapy or following its withdrawal. One patient developed ascending cholangitis during Sandostatin Injection therapy and died. Despite the high incidence of new gallstones in patients receiving octreotide, 1% of patients developed acute symptoms requiring cholecystectomy.

Glucose Metabolism - Hypoglycemia/Hyperglycemia

In acromegaly patients treated with either Sandostatin Injection or Sandostatin LAR Depot, hypoglycemia occurred in approximately 2% and hyperglycemia in approximately 15% of patients *[see Warnings and Precautions (5.2)]*.

Hypothyroidism

In acromegaly patients receiving Sandostatin Injection, 12% developed biochemical hypothyroidism, 8% developed goiter, and 4% required initiation of thyroid replacement therapy while receiving Sandostatin Injection. In acromegalic patients treated with Sandostatin LAR Depot, hypothyroidism was reported as an adverse event in 2% and goiter in 2%. Two patients receiving Sandostatin LAR Depot required initiation of thyroid hormone replacement therapy *[see Warnings and Precautions (5.3)]*.

Table 3. Number (%) of Acromegalic Patients with Common GI Adverse Events

Adverse Event	Sandostatin Injection S.C. Three Times Daily n=114 n	Sandostatin Injection S.C. Three Times Daily n=114 %	Sandostatin LAR Depot Every 28 Days n=261 n	Sandostatin LAR Depot Every 28 Days n=261 %
Diarrhea	66	(57.9)	95	(36.4)
Abdominal Pain or Discomfort	50	(43.9)	76	(29.1)
Nausea	34	(29.8)	27	(10.3)
Flatulence	15	(13.2)	67	(25.7)
Constipation	10	(8.8)	49	(18.8)
Vomiting	5	(4.4)	17	(6.5)

Cardiac

In acromegalic patients, sinus bradycardia (<50 bpm) developed in 25%; conduction abnormalities occurred in 10% and arrhythmias developed in 9% of patients during Sandostatin Injection therapy. The relationship of these events to octreotide acetate is not established because many of these patients have underlying cardiac disease *[see Warnings and Precautions (5.4)]*.

Gastrointestinal

The most common symptoms are gastrointestinal. The overall incidence of the most frequent of these symptoms in clinical trials of acromegalic patients treated for approximately 1 to 4 years is shown in Table 3.

[See table 3 above]

Only 2.6% of the patients on Sandostatin Injection in US clinical trials discontinued therapy due to these symptoms. No acromegalic patient receiving Sandostatin LAR Depot discontinued therapy for a GI event.

In patients receiving Sandostatin LAR Depot, the incidence of diarrhea was dose related. Diarrhea, abdominal pain, and nausea developed primarily during the first month of treatment with Sandostatin LAR Depot. Thereafter, new cases of these events were uncommon. The vast majority of these events were mild-to-moderate in severity.

In rare instances, gastrointestinal adverse effects may resemble acute intestinal obstruction, with progressive abdominal distention, severe epigastric pain, abdominal tenderness, and guarding.

Dyspepsia, steatorrhea, discoloration of feces, and tenesmus were reported in 4%-6% of patients.

In a clinical trial of carcinoid syndrome, nausea, abdominal pain, and flatulence were reported in 27%-38% and constipation or vomiting in 15%-21% of patients treated with Sandostatin LAR Depot. Diarrhea was reported as an adverse event in 14% of patients but since most of the patients had diarrhea as a symptom of carcinoid syndrome, it is difficult to assess the actual incidence of drug-related diarrhea.

Pain at the Injection Site

Pain on injection, which is generally mild-to-moderate, and short lived (usually about 1 hour) is dose related, being reported by 2%, 9%, and 11% of acromegalic patients receiving doses of 10 mg, 20 mg, and 30 mg, respectively, of Sandostatin LAR Depot. In carcinoid patients, where a diary was kept, pain at the injection site was reported by about 20%-25% at a 10-mg dose and about 30%-50% at the 20-mg and 30-mg dose.

Antibodies to Octreotide

Studies to date have shown that antibodies to octreotide develop in up to 25% of patients treated with octreotide acetate. These antibodies do not influence the degree of efficacy response to octreotide; however, in two acromegalic patients who received Sandostatin Injection, the duration of GH suppression following each injection was about twice as long as in patients without antibodies. It has not been determined whether octreotide antibodies will also prolong the duration of GH suppression in patients being treated with Sandostatin LAR Depot.

Carcinoid and VIPomas

The safety of Sandostatin LAR in the treatment of carcinoid tumors and VIPomas has been evaluated in one phase 3 study. Study 1 randomized 93 patients with carcinoid syndrome to Sandostatin LAR 10 mg, 20 mg, or 30 mg in a blind fashion or to open-label Sandostatin Injection subcutaneously. The population age range was between 25-78 years old and 44% were female, 95% were Caucasian and 3% black. All the patients had symptom control on their previous Sandostatin subcutaneous treatment. 80 patients finished the initial 24 weeks of Sandostatin exposure in Study 1. In Study 1, comparable numbers of patients were randomized to each dose. Table 4 below reflects the adverse events occurring in ≥15% of patients regardless of presumed causality to study drug.

[See table 4 at top of next page]

Gallbladder Abnormalities

In clinical trials, 62% of malignant carcinoid patients who received Sandostatin LAR Depot for up to 18 months developed new biliary abnormalities including jaundice, gallstones, sludge, and dilatation. New gallstones occurred in a total of 24% of patients.

Glucose Metabolism - Hypoglycemia/Hyperglycemia
In carcinoid patients, hypoglycemia occurred in 4% and hyperglycemia in 27% of patients treated with Sandostatin LAR Depot [see Warnings and Precautions (5.2)].

Hypothyroidism
In carcinoid patients, hypothyroidism has only been reported in isolated patients and goiter has not been reported [see Warnings and Precautions (5.3)].

Cardiac
Electrocardiograms were performed only in carcinoid patients receiving Sandostatin LAR Depot. In carcinoid syndrome patients, sinus bradycardia developed in 19%, conduction abnormalities occurred in 9%, and arrhythmias developed in 3%. The relationship of these events to octreotide acetate is not established because many of these patients have underlying cardiac disease [see Warnings and Precautions (5.4)].

Other Clinical Studies Adverse Events
Other clinically significant adverse events (relationship to drug not established) in acromegalic and/or carcinoid syndrome patients receiving Sandostatin LAR Depot were malignant hyperpyrexia, cerebral vascular disorder, rectal bleeding, ascites, pulmonary embolism, pneumonia, and pleural effusion.

Table 4. Adverse Events Occurring in ≥15% of Carcinoid Tumor and VIPoma Patients in Study 1

WHO Preferred Term	Number (%) of Subjects with AE's (n=93)			
	Sc N=26	10 mg N=22	20 mg N=20	30 mg N=25
Abdominal Pain	8 (30.8)	8 (35.4)	2 (10.0)	5 (20.0)
Arthropathy	5 (19.2)	2 (9.1)	3 (15.0)	2 (8.0)
Back Pain	7 (26.9)	6 (27.3)	2 (10.0)	2 (8.0)
Dizziness	4 (15.4)	4 (18.2)	4 (20.0)	5 (20.0)
Fatigue	3 (11.5)	7 (31.8)	2 (10.0)	2 (8.0)
Flatulence	3 (11.5)	2 (9.1)	2 (10.0)	4 (16.0)
Generalized Pain	4 (15.4)	2 (9.1)	3 (15.0)	1 (4.0)
Headache	5 (19.2)	4 (18.2)	6 (30.0)	4 (16.0)
Musculoskeletal Pain	4 (15.4)	0	1 (5.0)	0
Myalgia	0	4 (18.2)	1 (5.0)	1 (4.0)
Nausea	8 (30.8)	9 (40.9)	6 (30.0)	6 (24.0)
Pruritus	0	4 (18.2)	0	0
Rash	1 (3.8)	0	3 (15.0)	0
Sinusitis	4 (15.4)	0	1 (5.0)	3 (12.0)
URTI	6 (23.1)	4 (18.2)	2 (10.0)	3 (12.0)
Vomiting	3 (11.5)	0	0	4 (16.0)

6.2 Postmarketing Experience
The following adverse reactions have been identified during the postapproval use of Sandostatin. Because these reactions are reported voluntarily from a population of uncertain size, it is not always possible to reliably estimate their frequency or establish a causal relationship to drug exposure.

Myocardial infarction has been observed in the postmarketing setting, mainly in patients with cardiovascular risk factors. Hypoadrenalism has been reported in some reports in patients 18 months of age and under.

Additional events reported in the postmarketing setting include anaphylactoid reactions, including anaphylactic shock, cardiac arrest, renal failure, renal insufficiency, convulsions, atrial fibrillation, aneurysm, hepatitis, increased liver enzymes, gastrointestinal hemorrhage, pancreatitis, pancytopenia, thrombocytopenia, arterial thrombosis of the arm, retinal vein thrombosis, intracranial hemorrhage, hemiparesis, paresis, deafness, visual field defect, aphasia, scotoma, status asthmaticus, pulmonary hypertension, diabetes mellitus, intestinal obstruction, peptic/gastric ulcer, appendicitis, creatinine increased, CK increased, arthritis, joint effusion, pituitary apoplexy, breast carcinoma, suicide attempt, paranoia, migraines, urticaria, facial edema, generalized edema, hematuria, orthostatic hypotension, Raynaud's syndrome, glaucoma, pulmonary nodule, pneumothorax aggravated, cellulitis, Bell's palsy, diabetes insipidus, gynecomastia, galactorrhea, gallbladder polyp, fatty liver, abdomen enlarged, libido decrease, and petechiae.

7 DRUG INTERACTIONS

7.1 Cyclosporine
Concomitant administration of octreotide injection with cyclosporine may decrease blood levels of cyclosporine and result in transplant rejection.

7.2 Insulin and Oral Hypoglycemic Drugs
Octreotide inhibits the secretion of insulin and glucagon. Therefore, blood glucose levels should be monitored when Sandostatin LAR treatment is initiated or when the dose is altered and antidiabetic treatment should be adjusted accordingly.

7.3 Bromocriptine
Concomitant administration of octreotide and bromocriptine increases the availability of bromocriptine.

7.4 Other Concomitant Drug Therapy
Concomitant administration of bradycardia-inducing drugs (e.g., beta-blockers) may have an additive effect on the reduction of heart rate associated with octreotide. Dose adjustments of concomitant medication may be necessary.
Octreotide has been associated with alterations in nutrient absorption, so it may have an effect on absorption of orally administered drugs.

7.5 Drug Metabolism Interactions
Limited published data indicate that somatostatin analogs may decrease the metabolic clearance of compounds known to be metabolized by cytochrome P450 enzymes, which may be due to the suppression of growth hormone. Since it cannot be excluded that octreotide may have this effect, other drugs mainly metabolized by CYP3A4 and which have a low therapeutic index (e.g., quinidine, terfenadine) should therefore be used with caution.

8 USE IN SPECIFIC POPULATIONS

8.1 Pregnancy
Pregnancy Category B
There are no adequate and well-controlled studies in pregnant women. Reproduction studies have been performed in rats and rabbits at doses up to 16× the highest recommended human dose and have revealed no evidence of harm to the fetus due to octreotide. However, because animal reproduction studies are not always predictive of human response, this drug should be used during pregnancy only if clearly needed [see Nonclinical Toxicology (13.2)].

8.3 Nursing Mothers
It is not known whether octreotide is excreted into human milk. Because many drugs are excreted in human milk, caution should be exercised when Sandostatin LAR Depot is administered to a nursing woman.

8.4 Pediatric Use
Safety and efficacy of Sandostatin LAR Depot in the pediatric population have not been demonstrated.
No formal controlled clinical trials have been performed to evaluate the safety and effectiveness of Sandostatin LAR Depot in pediatric patients under 6 years of age. In postmarketing reports, serious adverse events, including hypoxia, necrotizing enterocolitis, and death, have been reported with Sandostatin use in children, most notably in children under 2 years of age. The relationship of these events to octreotide has not been established as the majority of these pediatric patients had serious underlying comorbid conditions.
The efficacy and safety of Sandostatin LAR Depot was examined in a single randomized, double-blind, placebo-controlled, 6-month pharmacokinetics study in 60 pediatric patients age 6-17 years with hypothalamic obesity resulting from cranial insult. The mean octreotide concentration after 6 doses of 40 mg Sandostatin LAR Depot administered by IM injection every four weeks was approximately 3 ng/mL. Steady-state concentrations were achieved after 3 injections of a 40 mg dose. Mean BMI increased 0.1 kg/m² in Sandostatin LAR Depot-treated subjects compared to 0.0 kg/m² in saline control-treated subjects. Efficacy was not demonstrated. Diarrhea occurred in 11 of 30 (37%) patients treated with Sandostatin LAR Depot. No unexpected adverse events were observed. However, with Sandostatin LAR Depot 40 mg once a month, the incidence of new cholelithiasis in this pediatric population (33%) was higher than that seen in other adult indications such as acromegaly (22%) or malignant carcinoid syndrome (24%), where Sandostatin LAR Depot was dosed at 10 to 30 mg once a month.

8.5 Geriatric Use
Clinical studies of Sandostatin did not include sufficient numbers of subjects age 65 years and over to determine whether they respond differently from younger subjects. Other reported clinical experience has not identified differences in responses between the elderly and younger patients. In general, dose selection for an elderly patient should be cautious, usually starting at the low end of the dosing range, reflecting the greater frequency of decreased hepatic, renal, or cardiac function, and of concomitant disease or other drug therapy.

8.6 Renal Impairment
In patients with renal failure requiring dialysis, the starting dose should be 10 mg. This dose should be up titrated based on clinical response and speed of response as deemed necessary by the physician. In patients with mild, moderate, or severe renal impairment there is no need to adjust the starting dose of Sandostatin. The maintenance dose should be adjusted thereafter based on clinical response and tolerability as in nonrenal patients [see Clinical Pharmacology (12)].

8.7 Hepatic Impairment-Cirrhotic Patients
In patients with established liver cirrhosis, the starting dose should be 10 mg. This dose should be up titrated based on clinical response and speed of response as deemed necessary by the physician. Once at a higher dose, patient should be maintained or dose adjusted based on response and tolerability as in any noncirrhotic patients [see Clinical Pharmacology (12)].

10 OVERDOSAGE
No frank overdose has occurred in any patient to date. Sandostatin Injection given in intravenous bolus doses of 1 mg (1000 mcg) to healthy volunteers did not result in serious ill effects, nor did doses of 30 mg (30,000 mcg) given intravenously over 20 minutes and of 120 mg (120,000 mcg) given intravenously over 8 hours to research patients. Doses of 2.5 mg (2500 mcg) of Sandostatin Injection subcutaneously have, however, caused hypoglycemia, flushing, dizziness, and nausea.
Up-to-date information about the treatment of overdose can often be obtained from a certified Regional Poison Control Center. Telephone numbers of certified Regional Poison Control Centers are listed in the Physicians' Desk Reference®**.
Mortality occurred in mice and rats given 72 mg/kg and 18 mg/kg intravenously, respectively, of octreotide.

11 DESCRIPTION
Octreotide is the acetate salt of a cyclic octapeptide. It is a long-acting octapeptide with pharmacologic properties mimicking those of the natural hormone somatostatin. Octreotide is known chemically as L-Cysteinamide, D-phenylalanyl-L-cysteinyl-L-phenylalanyl-D-tryptophyl-L-lysyl-L-threonyl-N-[2-hydroxy-1- (hydroxy-methyl) propyl]-, cyclic (2→7)-disulfide; [R-(R*,R*)].
The molecular weight of octreotide is 1019.3 (free peptide, $C_{49}H_{66}N_{10}O_{10}S_2$) and its amino acid sequence is:

H-D-Phe-Cys-Phe-D-Trp-Lys-Thr-Cys-Thr-ol•xCH₃COOH
where x = 1.4 to 2.5

Sandostatin LAR Depot is available in a vial containing the sterile drug product, which when mixed with diluent, becomes a suspension that is given as a monthly intragluteal injection. The octreotide is uniformly distributed within the microspheres which are made of a biodegradable glucose star polymer, D,L-lactic and glycolic acids copolymer. Sterile mannitol is added to the microspheres to improve suspendability.
Sandostatin LAR Depot is available as: sterile 6-mL vials in 3 strengths delivering 10 mg, 20 mg, or 30 mg octreotide-free peptide. Each vial of Sandostatin LAR Depot delivers:

Name of Ingredient	10 mg	20 mg	30 mg
octreotide acetate	11.2 mg*	22.4 mg*	33.6 mg*
D,L-lactic and glycolic acids copolymer	188.8 mg	377.6 mg	566.4 mg
mannitol	41.0 mg	81.9 mg	122.9 mg

*Equivalent to 10/20/30 mg octreotide base.

Each syringe of diluent contains:

carboxymethylcellulose sodium	14.0 mg
mannitol	12.0 mg
poloxamer 188	4.0 mg
water for injection	2.0 mL

Table 5. Hormonal Response in Acromegalic Patients Receiving 27 to 28 Injections During[1] Treatment with Sandostatin LAR Depot

Mean Hormone Level	Sandostatin Injection S.C.		Sandostatin LAR Depot	
	n	%	n	%
GH <5.0 ng/mL	69/88	78	73/88	83
<2.5 ng/mL	44/88	50	41/88	47
<1.0 ng/mL	6/88	7	10/88	11
IGF-1 normalized	36/88	41	45/88	51
GH <5.0 ng/mL + IGF-1 normalized	36/88	41	45/88	51
<2.5 ng/mL + IGF-1 normalized	30/88	34	37/88	42
<1.0 ng/mL + IGF-1 normalized	5/88	6	10/88	11

[1]Average of monthly levels of GH and IGF-1 over the course of the trials.

12 CLINICAL PHARMACOLOGY

Sandostatin LAR Depot is a long-acting dosage form consisting of microspheres of the biodegradable glucose star polymer, D,L-lactic and glycolic acids copolymer, containing octreotide. It maintains all of the clinical and pharmacological characteristics of the immediate-release dosage form Sandostatin Injection with the added feature of slow release of octreotide from the site of injection, reducing the need for frequent administration. This slow release occurs as the polymer biodegrades, primarily through hydrolysis. Sandostatin LAR Depot is designed to be injected intramuscularly (intragluteally) once every 4 weeks.

12.1 Mechanism of Action

Octreotide exerts pharmacologic actions similar to the natural hormone, somatostatin. It is an even more potent inhibitor of growth hormone, glucagon, and insulin than somatostatin. Like somatostatin, it also suppresses LH response to GnRH, decreases splanchnic blood flow, and inhibits release of serotonin, gastrin, vasoactive intestinal peptide, secretin, motilin, and pancreatic polypeptide.

By virtue of these pharmacological actions, octreotide has been used to treat the symptoms associated with metastatic carcinoid tumors (flushing and diarrhea), and Vasoactive Intestinal Peptide (VIP) secreting adenomas (watery diarrhea).

12.2 Pharmacodynamics

Octreotide substantially reduces and in many cases can normalize growth hormone and/or IGF-1 (somatomedin C) levels in patients with acromegaly.

Single doses of Sandostatin Injection given subcutaneously have been shown to inhibit gallbladder contractility and to decrease bile secretion in normal volunteers. In controlled clinical trials, the incidence of gallstone or biliary sludge formation was markedly increased [see Warnings and Precautions (5.1)].

Octreotide may cause clinically significant suppression of thyroid-stimulating hormone (TSH).

12.3 Pharmacokinetics

Sandostatin Injection

According to data obtained with the immediate-release formulation, Sandostatin Injection solution, after subcutaneous injection, octreotide is absorbed rapidly and completely from the injection site. Peak concentrations of 5.2 ng/mL (100-mcg dose) were reached 0.4 hours after dosing. Using a specific radioimmunoassay, intravenous and subcutaneous doses were found to be bioequivalent. Peak concentrations and area-under-the-curve (AUC) values were dose proportional both after subcutaneous or intravenous single doses up to 400 mcg and with multiple doses of 200 mcg 3 times daily (600 mcg/day). Clearance was reduced by about 66% suggesting nonlinear kinetics of the drug at daily doses of 600 mcg/day compared to 150 mcg/day. The relative decrease in clearance with doses above 600 mcg/day is not defined.

In healthy volunteers, the distribution of octreotide from plasma was rapid ($t\alpha_{1/2}$=0.2 h), the volume of distribution (Vdss) was estimated to be 13.6 L and the total body clearance was 10 L/h.

In blood, the distribution of octreotide into the erythrocytes was found to be negligible and about 65% was bound in the plasma in a concentration-independent manner. Binding was mainly to lipoprotein and, to a lesser extent, to albumin.

The elimination of octreotide from plasma had an apparent half-life of 1.7 hours, compared with the 1-3 minutes with the natural hormone, somatostatin. The duration of action of subcutaneously administered Sandostatin Injection solution is variable but extends up to 12 hours depending upon the type of tumor, necessitating multiple daily dosing with this immediate-release dosage form. About 32% of the dose is excreted unchanged into the urine. In an elderly population, dose adjustments may be necessary due to a significant increase in the half-life (46%) and a significant decrease in the clearance (26%) of the drug.

In patients with acromegaly, the pharmacokinetics differ somewhat from those in healthy volunteers. A mean peak concentration of 2.8 ng/mL (100-mcg dose) was reached in 0.7 hours after subcutaneous dosing. The Vdss was estimated to be 21.6 ± 8.5 L and the total body clearance was increased to 18 L/h. The mean percent of the drug bound was 41.2%. The disposition and elimination half-lives were similar to normals.

The half-life in renal-impaired patients was slightly longer than normal subjects (2.4-3.1 h versus 1.9 h). The clearance in renal-impaired patients was 7.3-8.8 L/h as compared to 8.3 L/h in healthy subjects. In patients with severe renal failure requiring dialysis, clearance was reduced to about half that found in healthy subjects (from approximately 10 L/h to 4.5 L/h).

Patients with liver cirrhosis showed prolonged elimination of drug, with octreotide half-life increasing to 3.7 h and total body clearance decreasing to 5.9 L/h, whereas patients with fatty liver disease showed half-life increasing to 3.4 h and total body clearance of 8.4 L/h. In normal subjects, octreotide half-life is 1.9 h and the clearance is 8.3 L/h which is comparable with the clearance in fatty-liver patients.

Sandostatin LAR Depot

The magnitude and duration of octreotide serum concentrations after an intramuscular injection of the long-acting depot formulation Sandostatin LAR Depot reflect the release of drug from the microsphere polymer matrix. Drug release is governed by the slow biodegration of the microspheres in the muscle, but once present in the systemic circulation, octreotide distributes and is eliminated according to its known pharmacokinetic properties which are as follows.

After a single IM injection of the long-acting depot dosage form Sandostatin LAR Depot in healthy volunteer subjects, the serum octreotide concentration reached a transient initial peak of about 0.03 ng/mL/mg within 1 hour after administration progressively declining over the following 3-5 days to a nadir of <0.01 ng/mL/mg, then slowly increasing and reaching a plateau about 2-3 weeks postinjection. Plateau concentrations were maintained over a period of nearly 2-3 weeks, showing dose proportional peak concentrations of about 0.07 ng/mL/mg. After about 6 weeks postinjection, octreotide concentration slowly decreased, to <0.01 ng/mL/mg by Weeks 12 to 13, concomitant with the terminal degradation phase of the polymer matrix of the dosage form. The relative bioavailability of the long-acting release Sandostatin LAR Depot compared to immediate-release Sandostatin Injection solution given subcutaneously was 60%-63%.

In patients with acromegaly, the octreotide concentrations after single doses of 10 mg, 20 mg, and 30 mg Sandostatin LAR Depot were dose proportional. The transient Day 1 peak, amounting to 0.3 ng/mL, 0.8 ng/mL, and 1.3 ng/mL, respectively, was followed by plateau concentrations of 0.5 ng/mL, 1.3 ng/mL, and 2.0 ng/mL, respectively, achieved about 3 weeks postinjection. These plateau concentrations were maintained for nearly 2 weeks.

Following multiple doses of Sandostatin LAR Depot given every 4 weeks, steady-state octreotide serum concentrations were achieved after the third injection. Concentrations were dose proportional and higher by a factor of approximately 1.6 to 2.0 compared to the concentrations after a single dose. The steady-state octreotide concentrations were 1.2 ng/mL and 2.1 ng/mL, respectively, at trough and 1.6 ng/mL and 2.6 ng/mL, respectively, at peak with 20 mg and 30 mg Sandostatin LAR Depot given every 4 weeks. No accumulation of octreotide beyond that expected from the overlapping release profiles occurred over a duration of up to 28 monthly injections of Sandostatin LAR Depot. With the long-acting depot formulation Sandostatin LAR Depot administered IM every 4 weeks the peak-to-trough variation in octreotide concentrations ranged from 44%-68%, compared to the 163%-209% variation encountered with the daily subcutaneous three times daily regimen of Sandostatin Injection solution.

In patients with carcinoid tumors, the mean octreotide concentrations after 6 doses of 10 mg, 20 mg, and 30 mg Sandostatin LAR Depot administered by IM injection every 4 weeks were 1.2 ng/mL, 2.5 ng/mL, and 4.2 ng/mL, respectively. Concentrations were dose proportional and steady-state concentrations were reached after 2 injections of 20 mg and 30 mg and after 3 injections of 10 mg.

Sandostatin LAR Depot has not been studied in patients with renal impairment.

Sandostatin LAR Depot has not been studied in patients with hepatic impairment.

13 NONCLINICAL TOXICOLOGY

13.1 Carcinogenesis, Mutagenesis, Impairment of Fertility

Studies in laboratory animals have demonstrated no mutagenic potential of Sandostatin. No mutagenic potential of the polymeric carrier in Sandostatin LAR Depot, D,L-lactic and glycolic acids copolymer, was observed in the Ames mutagenicity test.

No carcinogenic potential was demonstrated in mice treated subcutaneously with octreotide for 85-99 weeks at doses up to 2000 mcg/kg/day (8× the human exposure based on body surface area). In a 116-week subcutaneous study in rats administered octreotide, a 27% and 12% incidence of injection site sarcomas or squamous cell carcinomas was observed in males and females, respectively, at the highest dose level of 1250 mcg/kg/day (10× the human exposure based on body surface area) compared to an incidence of 8%-10% in the vehicle-control groups. The increased incidence of injection site tumors was most probably caused by irritation and the high sensitivity of the rat to repeated subcutaneous injections at the same site. Rotating injection sites would prevent chronic irritation in humans. There have been no reports of injection site tumors in patients treated with Sandostatin Injection for at least 5 years. There was also a 15% incidence of uterine adenocarcinomas in the 1250 mcg/kg/day females compared to 7% in the saline-control females and 0% in the vehicle-control females. The presence of endometritis coupled with the absence of corpora lutea, the reduction in mammary fibroadenomas, and the presence of uterine dilatation suggest that the uterine tumors were associated with estrogen dominance in the aged female rats which does not occur in humans.

Octreotide did not impair fertility in rats at doses up to 1000 mcg/kg/day, which represents 7x the human exposure based on body surface area.

13.2 Reproductive Toxicology Studies

Reproduction studies have been performed in rats and rabbits at doses up to 16x the highest recommended human dose based on body surface area and have revealed no evidence of harm to the fetus due to octreotide.

14 CLINICAL STUDIES

14.1 Acromegaly

The clinical trials of Sandostatin LAR Depot were performed in patients who had been receiving Sandostatin Injection for a period of weeks to as long as 10 years. The acromegaly studies with Sandostatin LAR Depot described below were performed in patients who achieved GH levels of <10 ng/mL (and, in most cases <5 ng/mL) while on subcutaneous Sandostatin Injection. However, some patients enrolled were partial responders to subcutaneous Sandostatin Injection, i.e., GH levels were reduced by >50% on subcutaneous Sandostatin Injection compared to the untreated state, although not suppressed to <5 ng/mL.

Sandostatin LAR Depot was evaluated in three clinical trials in acromegalic patients.

In two of the clinical trials, a total of 101 patients were entered who had, in most cases, achieved a GH level <5 ng/mL on Sandostatin Injection given in doses of 100 mcg or 200 mcg three times daily. Most patients were switched to 20 mg or 30 mg doses of Sandostatin LAR Depot given once every 4 weeks for up to 27 to 28 injections. A few patients received doses of 10 mg and a few required doses of 40 mg. Growth hormone and IGF-1 levels were at least as well controlled with Sandostatin LAR Depot as they had been on Sandostatin Injection and this level of control remained for the entire duration of the trials.

A third trial was a 12-month study that enrolled 151 patients who had a GH level <10 ng/mL after treatment with Sandostatin Injection (most had levels <5 ng/mL). The starting dose of Sandostatin LAR Depot was 20 mg every 4 weeks for 3 doses. Thereafter, patients received 10 mg, 20 mg, or 30 mg every 4 weeks, depending upon the degree of GH suppression [see Dosage and Administration (2)]. Growth hormone and IGF-1 were at least as well controlled on Sandostatin LAR Depot as they had been on Sandostatin Injection.

Table 5 summarizes the data on hormonal control (GH and IGF-1) for those patients in the first two clinical trials who received all 27 to 28 injections of Sandostatin LAR Depot.

[See table 5 above]

For the 88 patients in Table 5, a mean GH level of <2.5 ng/mL was observed in 47% receiving Sandostatin LAR Depot. Over the course of the trials, 42% of patients maintained mean growth hormone levels of <2.5 ng/mL and mean normal IGF-1 levels.

Table 6. Hormonal Response in Acromegalic Patients Receiving 12 Injections During[1] Treatment with Sandostatin LAR Depot

Mean Hormone Level	Sandostatin Injection S.C.		Sandostatin LAR Depot	
	n	%	n	%
GH <5.0 ng/mL	116/122	95	118/122	97
<2.5 ng/mL	84/122	69	80/122	66
<1.0 ng/mL	25/122	21	28/122	23
IGF-1 normalized	82/122	67	82/122	67
GH <5.0 ng/mL + IGF-1 normalized	80/122	66	82/122	67
<2.5 ng/mL + IGF-1 normalized	65/122	53	70/122	57
<1.0 ng/mL + IGF-1 normalized	23/122	19	27/122	22

[1]Average of monthly levels of GH and IGF-1 over the course of the trial

Table 7. Average Number of Daily Stools and Flushing Episodes in Patients with Malignant Carcinoid Syndrome

Treatment	n	Daily Stools (Average Number)		Daily Flushing Episodes (Average Number)	
		Baseline	Last Visit	Baseline	Last Visit
Sandostatin Injection S.C.	26	3.7	2.6	3.0	0.5
Sandostatin LAR Depot					
10 mg	22	4.6	2.8	3.0	0.9
20 mg	20	4.0	2.1	5.9	0.6
30 mg	24	4.9	2.8	6.1	1.0

Table 6 summarizes the data on hormonal control (GH and IGF-1) for those patients in the third clinical trial who received all 12 injections of Sandostatin LAR Depot.
[See table 6 above]
For the 122 patients in Table 6, who received all 12 injections in the third trial, a mean GH level of <2.5 ng/mL was observed in 66% receiving Sandostatin LAR Depot. Over the course of the trial, 57% of patients maintained mean growth hormone levels of <2.5 ng/mL and mean normal IGF-1 levels. In comparing the hormonal responses in these trials, note that a higher percentage of patients in the third trial suppressed their mean GH to <5 ng/mL on subcutaneous Sandostatin Injection, 95%, compared to 78% across the two previous trials.
In all three trials, GH, IGF-1, and clinical symptoms were similarly controlled on Sandostatin LAR Depot as they had been on Sandostatin Injection.
Of the 25 patients who completed the trials and were partial responders to Sandostatin Injection (GH >5.0 ng/mL but reduced by >50% relative to untreated levels), 1 patient (4%) responded to Sandostatin LAR Depot with a reduction of GH to <2.5 ng/mL and 8 patients (32%) responded with a reduction of GH to <5.0 ng/mL.
Two open-label clinical studies investigated a 48-week treatment with Sandostatin LAR Depot in 143 untreated (de novo) acromegalic patients. The median reduction in tumor volume was 20.6% in Study 1 (49 patients) at 24 weeks and 24.5% in Study 2 (94 patients) at 24 weeks and 36.2% at 48 weeks.

14.2 Carcinoid Syndrome
A 6-month clinical trial of malignant carcinoid syndrome was performed in 93 patients who had previously been shown to be responsive to Sandostatin Injection. Sixty-seven (67) patients were randomized at baseline to receive double-blind doses of 10 mg, 20 mg, or 30 mg Sandostatin LAR Depot every 28 days and 26 patients continued, unblinded, on their previous Sandostatin Injection regimen (100-300 mcg three times daily).
In any given month after steady-state levels of octreotide were reached, approximately 35%-40% of the patients who received Sandostatin LAR Depot required supplemental subcutaneous Sandostatin Injection therapy usually for a few days, to control exacerbation of carcinoid symptoms. In any given month, the percentage of patients randomized to subcutaneous Sandostatin Injection who required supplemental treatment with an increased dose of Sandostatin Injection was similar to the percentage of patients randomized to Sandostatin LAR Depot. Over the 6-month treatment period, approximately 50%-70% of patients who completed the trial on Sandostatin LAR Depot required subcutaneous Sandostatin Injection supplemental therapy to control exacerbation of carcinoid symptoms although steady-state serum Sandostatin LAR Depot levels had been reached.
Table 7 presents the average number of daily stools and flushing episodes in malignant carcinoid patients.
[See table 7 above]
Overall, mean daily stool frequency was as well controlled on Sandostatin LAR Depot as on Sandostatin Injection (approximately 2-2.5 stools/day).
Mean daily flushing episodes were similar at all doses of Sandostatin LAR Depot and on Sandostatin Injection (approximately 0.5-1 episode/day).

In a subset of patients with variable severity of disease, median 24 hour urinary 5-HIAA (5-hydroxyindole acetic acid) levels were reduced by 38%-50% in the groups randomized to Sandostatin LAR Depot.
The reductions are within the range reported in the published literature for patients treated with octreotide (about 10%-50%).
Seventy-eight (78) patients with malignant carcinoid syndrome who had participated in this 6-month trial, subsequently participated in a 12-month extension study in which they received 12 injections of Sandostatin LAR Depot at 4-week intervals. For those who remained in the extension trial, diarrhea and flushing were as well controlled as during the 6-month trial. Because malignant carcinoid disease is progressive, as expected, a number of deaths (8 patients: 10%) occurred due to disease progression or complications from the underlying disease. An additional 22% of patients prematurely discontinued Sandostatin LAR Depot due to disease progression or worsening of carcinoid symptoms.

16 HOW SUPPLIED/STORAGE AND HANDLING
Sandostatin LAR Depot is available in single-use kits containing a 6-mL vial of 10 mg, 20 mg or 30 mg strength, a syringe containing 2 mL of diluent, one vial adapter, and one sterile 1½" 20 gauge safety injection needle. An instruction booklet for the preparation of drug suspension for injection is also included with each kit.
Drug Product Kits

10 mg kit	NDC 0078-0646-81
20 mg kit	NDC 0078-0647-81
30 mg kit	NDC 0078-0648-81

Demonstration kit NDC 0078-9648-81
For prolonged storage, Sandostatin LAR Depot should be stored at refrigerated temperatures between 2°C to 8°C (36°F to 46°F) and protected from light until the time of use. Sandostatin LAR Depot drug product kit should remain at room temperature for 30-60 minutes prior to preparation of the drug suspension. However, after preparation the drug suspension must be administered immediately.

17 PATIENT COUNSELING INFORMATION
Patients with carcinoid tumors and VIPomas should be advised to adhere closely to their scheduled return visits for reinjection in order to minimize exacerbation of symptoms. Patients with acromegaly should also be urged to adhere to their return visit schedule to help assure steady control of GH and IGF-1 levels.
**Trademark of PDR Network.
Sandostatin® LAR Depot vials are manufactured by:
Sandoz GmbH, Schaftenau, Austria
(Subsidiary of Novartis Pharma AG, Basle, Switzerland)
The diluent syringes are manufactured by:
Abbott Biologicals B.V.
Olst, The Netherlands
Distributed by:
Novartis Pharmaceuticals Corporation
East Hanover, New Jersey 07936
© Novartis
T2014-74
Shown in Product Identification Guide, page 311

SIMULECT®
[sĭm ew lĕkt]
(basiliximab)
For Injection
Rx only

Rx

Prescribing Information
The following prescribing information is based on official labeling in effect July 2014.

WARNING

Only physicians experienced in immunosuppression therapy and management of organ transplantation patients should prescribe Simulect® (basiliximab). The physician responsible for Simulect administration should have complete information requisite for the follow-up of the patient. Patients receiving the drug should be managed in facilities equipped and staffed with adequate laboratory and supportive medical resources.

DESCRIPTION
Simulect® (basiliximab) is a chimeric (murine/human) monoclonal antibody (IgG$_{1\kappa}$), produced by recombinant DNA technology, that functions as an immunosuppressive agent, specifically binding to and blocking the interleukin-2 receptor α-chain (IL-2Rα, also known as CD25 antigen) on the surface of activated T-lymphocytes. Based on the amino acid sequence, the calculated molecular weight of the protein is 144 kilodaltons. It is a glycoprotein obtained from fermentation of an established mouse myeloma cell line genetically engineered to express plasmids containing the human heavy and light chain constant region genes and mouse heavy and light chain variable region genes encoding the RFT5 antibody that binds selectively to the IL-2Rα.
The active ingredient, basiliximab, is water soluble. The drug product, Simulect, is a sterile lyophilisate which is available in 6 mL colorless glass vials and is available in 10 mg and 20 mg strengths.
Each 10-mg vial contains 10 mg basiliximab, 3.61 mg monobasic potassium phosphate, 0.50 mg disodium hydrogen phosphate (anhydrous), 0.80 mg sodium chloride, 10 mg sucrose, 40 mg mannitol and 20 mg glycine, to be reconstituted in 2.5 mL of Sterile Water for Injection, USP. No preservatives are added.
Each 20-mg vial contains 20 mg basiliximab, 7.21 mg monobasic potassium phosphate, 0.99 mg disodium hydrogen phosphate (anhydrous), 1.61 mg sodium chloride, 20 mg sucrose, 80 mg mannitol and 40 mg glycine, to be reconstituted in 5 mL of Sterile Water for Injection, USP. No preservatives are added.

CLINICAL PHARMACOLOGY
General
Mechanism of Action: Basiliximab functions as an IL-2 receptor antagonist by binding with high affinity ($K_a = 1 \times 10^{10}$ M^{-1}) to the alpha chain of the high affinity IL-2 receptor complex and inhibiting IL-2 binding. Basiliximab is specifically targeted against IL-2Rα, which is selectively expressed on the surface of activated T-lymphocytes. This specific high affinity binding of Simulect® (basiliximab) to IL-2Rα competitively inhibits IL-2-mediated activation of lymphocytes, a critical pathway in the cellular immune response involved in allograft rejection.
While in the circulation, Simulect impairs the response of the immune system to antigenic challenges. Whether the ability to respond to repeated or ongoing challenges with those antigens returns to normal after Simulect is cleared is unknown (see PRECAUTIONS).
Pharmacokinetics
Adults: Single-dose and multiple-dose pharmacokinetic studies have been conducted in patients undergoing first kidney transplantation. Cumulative doses ranged from 15 mg up to 150 mg. Peak mean ± SD serum concentration following intravenous infusion of 20 mg over 30 minutes is 7.1 ± 5.1 mg/L. There is a dose-proportional increase in C_{max} and AUC up to the highest tested single dose of 60 mg. The volume of distribution at steady state is 8.6 ± 4.1 L. The extent and degree of distribution to various body compartments have not been fully studied. The terminal half-life is 7.2 ± 3.2 days. Total body clearance is 41 ± 19 mL/h. No clinically relevant influence of body weight or gender on distribution volume or clearance has been observed in adult patients. Elimination half-life was not influenced by age (20-69 years), gender or race (see DOSAGE AND ADMINISTRATION).
Pediatric: The pharmacokinetics of Simulect have been assessed in 39 pediatric patients undergoing renal transplantation. In infants and children (1-11 years of age, n=25), the distribution volume and clearance were reduced by about

Table 1. Efficacy Parameters (Percentage of Patients)

| | Dual-therapy Regimen (cyclosporine* and corticosteroids) | | | | | |
	Placebo (N=185)	Study 1 Simulect® (N=190)	p-value	Placebo (N=173)	Study 2 Simulect® (N=173)	p-value
Primary endpoint						
Death, graft loss or acute rejection episode (0-6 months)	57%	42%	0.003	55%	38%	0.002
Secondary endpoints						
Death, graft loss or acute rejection episode (0-12 months)	60%	46%	0.007	58%	41%	0.001
Biopsy-confirmed rejection episode (0-6 months)	44%	30%	0.007	46%	33%	0.015
Biopsy-confirmed rejection episode (0-12 months)	46%	32%	0.005	49%	35%	0.009
Patient survival (12 months)	97%	95%	0.29	96%	97%	0.56
Patients with functioning graft (12 months)	87%	88%	0.70	93%	95%	0.50

* USP (MODIFIED)

Table 2. Efficacy Parameters (Percentage of Patients)

| | Study 3: Triple-therapy Regimen (cyclosporine*, corticosteroids, and azathioprine) | | |
	Placebo (N=172)	Simulect® (N=168)	p-value
Primary endpoint			
Acute rejection episode (0-6 months)	35%	21%	0.005
Secondary endpoints			
Death, graft loss or acute rejection episode (0-6 months)	40%	26%	0.008
Biopsy-confirmed rejection episode (0-6 months)	29%	18%	0.023
Patient survival (12 months)	97%	98%	1.000
Patients with functioning graft (12 months)	88%	90%	0.599

*USP (MODIFIED)

50% compared to adult renal transplantation patients. The volume of distribution at steady state was 4.8 ± 2.1 L, half-life was 9.5 ± 4.5 days and clearance was 17 ± 6 mL/h. Disposition parameters were not influenced to a clinically relevant extent by age (1-11 years of age), body weight (9-37 kg) or body surface area (0.44-1.20 m^2) in this age group. In adolescents (12-16 years of age, n=14), disposition was similar to that in adult renal transplantation patients. The volume of distribution at steady state was 7.8 ± 5.1 L, half-life was 9.1 ± 3.9 days and clearance was 31 ± 19 mL/h (see DOSAGE AND ADMINISTRATION).

Pharmacodynamics

Complete and consistent binding to IL-2Rα in adults is maintained as long as serum Simulect levels exceed 0.2 µg/mL. As concentrations fall below this threshold, the IL-2Rα sites are no longer fully bound and the number of T-cells expressing unbound IL-2Rα returns to pretherapy values within 1-2 weeks. The relationship between serum concentration and receptor saturation was assessed in 13 pediatric patients and was similar to that characterized in adult renal transplantation patients. In vitro studies using human tissues indicate that Simulect binds only to lymphocytes.

The duration of clinically relevant IL-2 receptor blockade after the recommended course of Simulect is not known. When basiliximab was added to a regimen of cyclosporine, USP (MODIFIED) and corticosteroids in adult patients, the duration of IL-2Rα saturation was 36 ± 14 days (mean ± SD), similar to that observed in pediatric patients (36 ± 14 days) (see DOSAGE AND ADMINISTRATION). When basiliximab was added to a triple therapy regimen consisting of cyclosporine, USP (MODIFIED), corticosteroids, and azathioprine in adults, the duration was 50 ± 20 days and when added to cyclosporine, USP (MODIFIED), corticosteroids, and mycophenolate mofetil in adults, the duration was 59 ± 17 days (see PRECAUTIONS, Drug Interactions). No significant changes to circulating lymphocyte numbers or cell phenotypes were observed by flow cytometry.

CLINICAL STUDIES

The safety and efficacy of Simulect® (basiliximab) for the prophylaxis of acute organ rejection in adults following cadaveric- or living-donor renal transplantation were assessed in four randomized, double-blind, placebo-controlled clinical studies (1,184 patients). Of these four, two studies (Study 1 [EU/CAN] and Study 2 [US Study]) compared two 20-mg doses of Simulect with placebo, each administered intravenously as an infusion, as part of a standard immunosuppressive regimen comprised of cyclosporine, USP (MODIFIED) and corticosteroids. The other two controlled studies compared two 20-mg doses of Simulect with placebo, each administered intravenously as a bolus injection, as part of a standard triple-immunosuppressive regimen comprised of cyclosporine, USP (MODIFIED), corticosteroids and either azathioprine or mycophenolate mofetil (Study 3 and Study 4, respectively). The first dose of Simulect or placebo was administered within 2 hours prior to transplantation surgery (Day 0) and the second dose administered on Day 4 post-transplantation. The regimen of Simulect was chosen to provide 30-45 days of IL-2Rα saturation.

729 patients were enrolled in the two studies using a dual maintenance immunosuppressive regimen comprised of cyclosporine, USP (MODIFIED) and corticosteroids, of which 363 patients were treated with Simulect and 358 patients were placebo-treated. Study 1 was conducted at 21 sites in Europe and Canada (EU/CAN Study); Study 2 was conducted at 21 sites in the USA (US Study). Patients 18-75 years of age undergoing first cadaveric- (Study 1 and Study 2) or living-donor (Study 2 only) renal transplantation, with ≥1 HLA mismatch, were enrolled.[1,2]

The primary efficacy endpoint in both studies was the incidence of death, graft loss or an episode of acute rejection during the first 6 months post-transplantation. Secondary efficacy endpoints included the primary efficacy variable measured during the first 12 months post-transplantation, the incidence of biopsy-confirmed acute rejection during the first 6 and 12 months post-transplantation, and patient survival and graft survival, each measured at 12 months post-transplantation. Table 1 summarizes the results of these studies. Figure 1 displays the Kaplan-Meier estimates of the percentage of patients by treatment group experiencing the primary efficacy endpoint during the first 12 months post-transplantation for Study 2. Patients in both studies receiving Simulect experienced a significantly lower incidence of biopsy-confirmed rejection episodes at both 6 and 12 months post-transplantation. There was no difference in the rate of delayed graft function, patient survival, or graft survival between Simulect-treated patients and placebo-treated patients in either study.

There was no evidence that the clinical benefit of Simulect was limited to specific subpopulations based on age, gender, race, donor type (cadaveric or living donor allograft) or history of diabetes mellitus.

[See table 1 above]

Figure 1
Kaplan-Meier Estimate of the Percentage of Subjects with Death, Graft Loss or First Rejection Episode (Dual Therapy)
Month: 0 – 12

Two double-blind, randomized, placebo-controlled studies (Study 3 and Study 4) assessed the safety and efficacy of Simulect for the prophylaxis of acute renal transplant rejection in adults when used in combination with a triple immunosuppressive regimen. In Study 3, 340 patients were concomitantly treated with cyclosporine, USP (MODIFIED), corticosteroids and azathioprine (AZA), of which 168 patients were treated with Simulect and 172 patients were treated with placebo. In Study 4, 123 patients were concomitantly treated with cyclosporine, USP (MODIFIED), corticosteroids and mycophenolate mofetil (MMF), of which 59 patients were treated with Simulect and 64 patients were treated with placebo. Patients 18-70 years of age undergoing first or second cadaveric or living donor (related or unrelated) renal transplantation were enrolled in both studies. The results of Study 3 are shown in Table 2. These results are consistent with the findings from Study 1 and Study 2.

In Study 4, the percentage of patients experiencing biopsy-proven acute rejection by 6 months was 15% (9 of 59 patients) in the Simulect group and 27% (17 of 64 patients) in the placebo group. Although numerically lower, the difference in acute rejection was not significant.

In a multicenter, randomized, double-blind, placebo-controlled trial of Simulect for the prevention of allograft rejection in liver transplant recipients (n=381) receiving concomitant cyclosporine, USP (MODIFIED) and steroids, the incidence of the combined endpoint of death, graft loss, or first biopsy-confirmed rejection episode at either 6 or 12 months was similar between patients randomized to receive Simulect and those randomized to receive placebo.

The efficacy of Simulect for the prophylaxis of acute rejection in recipients of a second renal allograft has not been demonstrated.

Long Term Follow-up

Five-year patient survival and graft survival data were provided by 71% and 58% of the original subjects of Study 1 and Study 2, respectively. Subjects in both studies continued to receive a dual-therapy regimen with cyclosporine, USP (MODIFIED) and corticosteroid. No difference was observed between groups in the 5-year graft survival in either Study 1 (91% Simulect group, 92% placebo group) or Study 2 (85% Simulect group, 86% placebo group). In Study 1, patient survival was lower in the Simulect-treated patients compared to the placebo-treated patients (142/163 [87%] vs. 156/164 [95%], respectively). The cause of this difference in survival is unknown. The data do not indicate an increase in malignancy- or infection-related mortality. In Study 2, patient survival in the placebo group (90%) was the same compared to Simulect group (90%).

INDICATIONS AND USAGE

Simulect® (basiliximab) is indicated for the prophylaxis of acute organ rejection in patients receiving renal transplantation when used as part of an immunosuppressive regimen that includes cyclosporine, USP (MODIFIED) and corticosteroids.

The efficacy of Simulect for the prophylaxis of acute rejection in recipients of other solid organ allografts has not been demonstrated.

CONTRAINDICATIONS

Simulect® (basiliximab) is contraindicated in patients with known hypersensitivity to basiliximab or any other component of the formulation. See composition of Simulect under DESCRIPTION.

WARNINGS. See Boxed WARNING.
General

Simulect® (basiliximab) should be administered under qualified medical supervision. Patients should be informed of the potential benefits of therapy and the risks associated with administration of immunosuppressive therapy.

While neither the incidence of lymphoproliferative disorders nor opportunistic infections was higher in Simulect-treated patients than in placebo-treated patients, patients on immunosuppressive therapy are at increased risk for developing these complications and should be monitored accordingly.

Hypersensitivity

Severe acute (onset within 24 hours) hypersensitivity reactions including anaphylaxis have been observed both on initial exposure to Simulect and/or following re-exposure after several months. These reactions may include hypotension, tachycardia, cardiac failure, dyspnea, wheezing, bronchospasm, pulmonary edema, respiratory failure, urticaria, rash, pruritus, and/or sneezing. Extreme caution should be exercised in all patients previously given Simulect when being administered a subsequent course of Simulect. A subgroup of patients may be particularly at risk of developing severe hypersensitivity reactions on re-administration. These are patients in whom concomitant immunosuppression was discontinued prematurely (e.g., due to abandoned transplantation or early loss of the graft) following the initial administration of Simulect. If a severe hypersensitivity reaction occurs, therapy with Simulect should be permanently discontinued. Medications for the treatment of severe hypersensitivity reactions including anaphylaxis should be available for immediate use.

PRECAUTIONS

General

It is not known whether Simulect® (basiliximab) use will have a long-term effect on the ability of the immune system to respond to antigens first encountered during Simulect-induced immunosuppression.

Immunogenicity

Of renal transplantation patients treated with Simulect and tested for anti-idiotype antibodies, 4/339 developed an anti-idiotype antibody response, with no deleterious clinical effect upon the patient. In none of these cases was there evidence that the presence of anti-idiotype antibody accelerated Simulect clearance or decreased the period of receptor saturation. In Study 2, the incidence of human anti-murine antibody (HAMA) in renal transplantation patients treated with Simulect was 2/138 in patients not exposed to muromonab-CD3 and 4/34 in patients who subsequently received muromonab-CD3. The available clinical data on the use of muromonab-CD3 in patients previously treated with Simulect suggest that subsequent use of muromonab-CD3 or other murine anti-lymphocytic antibody preparations is not precluded.

These data reflect the percentage of patients whose test results were considered positive for antibodies to Simulect in an ELISA assay, and are highly dependent on the sensitivity and specificity of the assay. Additionally the observed incidence of antibody positivity in an assay may be influenced by several factors including sample handling, concomitant medications, and underlying disease. For these reasons, comparison of the incidence of antibodies to Simulect with the incidence of antibodies to other products may be misleading.

Drug Interactions

No dose adjustment is necessary when Simulect is added to triple-immunosuppression regimens including cyclosporine, corticosteroids, and either azathioprine or mycophenolate mofetil. Three clinical trials have investigated Simulect use in combination with triple-therapy regimens. Pharmacokinetics were assessed in two of these trials. Total body clearance of Simulect was reduced by an average 22% and 51% when azathioprine and mycophenolate mofetil, respectively, were added to a regimen consisting of cyclosporine, USP (MODIFIED) and corticosteroids. Nonetheless, the range of individual Simulect clearance values in the presence of azathioprine (12-57 mL/h) or mycophenolate mofetil (7-54 mL/h) did not extend outside the range observed with dual therapy (10-78 mL/h). The following medications have been administered in clinical trials with Simulect with no increase in adverse reactions: ATG/ALG, azathioprine, corticosteroids, cyclosporine, mycophenolate mofetil, and muromonab-CD3.

Carcinogenesis/Mutagenesis/Impairment of Fertility

No mutagenic potential of Simulect was observed in the in vitro assays with Salmonella (Ames) and V79 Chinese hamster cells. No long-term or fertility studies in laboratory animals have been performed to evaluate the potential of Simulect to produce carcinogenicity or fertility impairment, respectively.

Pregnancy Category B

There are no adequate and well-controlled studies in pregnant women. No maternal toxicity, embryotoxicity, or teratogenicity was observed in cynomolgus monkeys 100 days post coitum following dosing with basiliximab during the organogenesis period; blood levels in pregnant monkeys were 13-fold higher than those seen in human patients. Immunotoxicology studies have not been performed in the offspring. Because IgG molecules are known to cross the placental barrier, because the IL-2 receptor may play an important role in development of the immune system, and because animal reproduction studies are not always predictive of human response, Simulect should only be used in pregnant women when the potential benefit justifies the potential risk to the fetus. Women of childbearing potential should use effective contraception before beginning Simulect therapy, during therapy, and for 4 months after completion of Simulect therapy.

Nursing Mothers

It is not known whether Simulect is excreted in human milk. Because many drugs including human antibodies are excreted in human milk, and because of the potential for adverse reactions, a decision should be made to discontinue nursing or to discontinue the drug, taking into account the importance of the drug to the mother.

Pediatric Use

No randomized, placebo-controlled studies have been completed in pediatric patients. In a safety and pharmacokinetic study, 41 pediatric patients (1-11 years of age [n=27], 12-16 years of age [n=14], median age 8.1 years) were treated with Simulect via intravenous bolus injection in addition to standard immunosuppressive agents including cy-

closporine, USP (MODIFIED), corticosteroids, azathioprine, and mycophenolate mofetil. The acute rejection rate at 6 months was comparable to that in adults in the triple-therapy trials. The most frequently reported adverse events were hypertension, hypertrichosis, and rhinitis (49% each), urinary tract infections (46%), and fever (39%). Overall, the adverse event profile was consistent with general clinical experience in the pediatric renal transplantation population and with the profile in the controlled adult renal transplantation studies. The available pharmacokinetic data in children and adolescents are described in CLINICAL PHARMACOLOGY and DOSAGE AND ADMINISTRATION.

It is not known whether the immune response to vaccines, infection, and other antigenic stimuli administered or encountered during Simulect therapy is impaired or whether such response will remain impaired after Simulect therapy.

Geriatric Use

Controlled clinical studies of Simulect have included a small number of patients 65 years and older (Simulect 28; placebo 32). From the available data comparing Simulect and placebo-treated patients, the adverse event profile in patients ≥65 years of age is not different from patients <65 years of age and no age-related dosing adjustment is required. Caution must be used in giving immunosuppressive drugs to elderly patients.

ADVERSE REACTIONS

Because clinical trials are conducted under widely varying conditions, adverse reaction rates observed in the clinical trials of a drug cannot be directly compared to rates in the clinical trials of another drug and may not reflect the rates observed in practice. The adverse reaction information from clinical trials does, however, provide a basis for identifying the adverse events that appear to be related to drug use and for approximating rates.

The incidence of adverse events for Simulect® (basiliximab) was determined in four randomized, double-blind, placebo-controlled clinical trials for the prevention of renal allograft rejection. Two of the studies (Study 1 and Study 2), used a dual maintenance immunosuppressive regimen comprised of cyclosporine, USP (MODIFIED) and corticosteroids, whereas the other two studies (Study 3 and Study 4) used a triple-immunosuppressive regimen comprised of cyclosporine, USP (MODIFIED), corticosteroids, and either azathioprine or mycophenolate mofetil.

Simulect did not appear to add to the background of adverse events seen in organ transplantation patients as a consequence of their underlying disease and the concurrent administration of immunosuppressants and other medications. Adverse events were reported by 96% of the patients in the placebo-treated group and 96% of the patients in the Simulect-treated group. In the four placebo-controlled studies, the pattern of adverse events in 590 patients treated with the recommended dose of Simulect was similar to that in 594 patients treated with placebo. Simulect did not increase the incidence of serious adverse events observed compared with placebo.

The most frequently reported adverse events were gastrointestinal disorders, reported in 69% of Simulect-treated patients and 67% of placebo-treated patients.

The incidence and types of adverse events were similar in Simulect-treated and placebo-treated patients. The following adverse events occurred in ≥10% of Simulect-treated patients: *Gastrointestinal System:* constipation, nausea, abdominal pain, vomiting, diarrhea, dyspepsia; *Body as a Whole-General:* pain, peripheral edema, fever, viral infection; *Metabolic and Nutritional:* hyperkalemia, hypokalemia, hyperglycemia, hypercholesterolemia, hypophosphatemia, hyperuricemia; *Urinary System:* urinary tract infection; *Respiratory System:* dyspnea, upper respiratory tract infection; *Skin and Appendages:* surgical wound complications, acne; *Cardiovascular Disorders-General:* hypertension; *Central and Peripheral Nervous System:* headache, tremor; *Psychiatric:* insomnia; *Red Blood Cell:* anemia.

The following adverse events, not mentioned above, were reported with an incidence of ≥3% and <10% in pooled analysis of patients treated with Simulect in the four controlled clinical trials, or in an analysis of the two dual-therapy trials: *Body as a Whole-General:* accidental trauma, asthenia, chest pain, increased drug level, infection, face edema, fatigue, dependent edema, generalized edema, leg edema, malaise, rigors, sepsis; *Cardiovascular:* abnormal heart sounds, aggravated hypertension, angina pectoris, cardiac failure, chest pain, hypotension; *Endocrine:* increased glucocorticoids; *Gastrointestinal:* enlarged abdomen, esophagitis, flatulence, gastrointestinal disorder, gastroenteritis, GI hemorrhage, gum hyperplasia, melena, moniliasis, ulcerative stomatitis; *Heart Rate and Rhythm:* arrhythmia, atrial fibrillation, tachycardia; *Metabolic and Nutritional:* acidosis, dehydration, diabetes mellitus, fluid overload, hypercalcemia, hyperlipemia, hypertriglyceridemia, hypocalcemia, hypoglycemia, hypomagnesemia, hypoproteinemia, weight increase; *Musculoskeletal:* arthralgia, ar-

thropathy, back pain, bone fracture, cramps, hernia, myalgia, leg pain; *Nervous System:* dizziness, neuropathy, paraesthesia, hypoesthesia; *Platelet and Bleeding:* hematoma, hemorrhage, purpura, thrombocytopenia, thrombosis; *Psychiatric:* agitation, anxiety, depression; *Red Blood Cell:* polycythemia; *Reproductive Disorders, Male:* genital edema, impotence; *Respiratory:* bronchitis, bronchospasm, abnormal chest sounds, coughing, pharyngitis, pneumonia, pulmonary disorder, pulmonary edema, rhinitis, sinusitis; *Skin and Appendages:* cyst, herpes simplex, herpes zoster, hypertrichosis, pruritus, rash, skin disorder, skin ulceration; *Urinary:* albuminuria, bladder disorder, dysuria, frequent micturition, hematuria, increased nonprotein nitrogen, oliguria, abnormal renal function, renal tubular necrosis, surgery, ureteral disorder, urinary retention; *Vascular Disorders:* vascular disorder; *Vision Disorders:* cataract, conjunctivitis, abnormal vision; *White Blood Cell:* leucopenia. Among these events, leucopenia and hypertriglyceridemia occurred more frequently in the two triple-therapy studies using azathioprine and mycophenolate mofetil than in the dual-therapy studies.

Malignancies

The incidence of malignancies in the controlled clinical trials of renal transplant was not significantly different between groups at 1 year (9/590 Simulect-treated patients vs. 12/594 placebo-treated patients) or among patients with 5-year follow-up from Studies 1 and 2 (21/295 Simulect-treated patients vs. 21/291 placebo-treated patients). The incidence of lymphoproliferative disease was not significantly different between groups, and less than 1% in the Simulect-treated patients.

Infections

The overall incidence of cytomegalovirus infection was similar in Simulect- and placebo-treated patients (15% vs. 17%) receiving a dual- or triple-immunosuppression regimen. However, in patients receiving a triple-immunosuppression regimen, the incidence of serious cytomegalovirus infection was higher in Simulect-treated patients compared to placebo-treated patients (11% vs. 5%). The rates of infections, serious infections, and infectious organisms were similar in the Simulect- and placebo-treatment groups among dual- and triple-therapy treated patients.

Post-Marketing Experience

Severe acute hypersensitivity reactions including anaphylaxis characterized by hypotension, tachycardia, cardiac failure, dyspnea, wheezing, bronchospasm, pulmonary edema, respiratory failure, urticaria, rash, pruritus, and/or sneezing, as well as capillary leak syndrome and cytokine release syndrome, have been reported during post-marketing experience with Simulect.

OVERDOSAGE

A maximum tolerated dose of Simulect® (basiliximab) has not been determined in patients. During the course of clinical studies, Simulect has been administered to adult renal transplantation patients in single doses of up to 60 mg, or in divided doses over 3-5 days of up to 120 mg, without any associated serious adverse events. There has been one spontaneous report of a pediatric renal transplantation patient who received a single 20-mg dose (2.3 mg/kg) without adverse events.

DOSAGE AND ADMINISTRATION

Simulect® (basiliximab) is used as part of an immunosuppressive regimen that includes cyclosporine, USP (MODIFIED) and corticosteroids. Simulect is for central or peripheral intravenous administration only. Reconstituted Simulect should be given either as a bolus injection or diluted to a volume of 25 mL (10-mg vial) or 50 mL (20-mg vial) with normal saline or dextrose 5% and administered as an intravenous infusion over 20 to 30 minutes. Bolus administration may be associated with nausea, vomiting and local reactions, including pain.

Simulect should only be administered once it has been determined that the patient will receive the graft and concomitant immunosuppression. Patients previously administered Simulect should only be re-exposed to a subsequent course of therapy with extreme caution due to the potential risk of hypersensitivity (see WARNINGS).

Parenteral drug products should be inspected visually for particulate matter and discoloration before administration. After reconstitution, Simulect should be a clear-to-opalescent, colorless solution. If particulate matter is present or the solution is colored, do not use.

Care must be taken to assure sterility of the prepared solution because the drug product does not contain any antimicrobial preservatives or bacteriostatic agents.

It is recommended that after reconstitution, the solution should be used immediately. If not used immediately, it can be stored at 2°C to 8°C for 24 hours or at room temperature for 4 hours. Discard the reconstituted solution if not used within 24 hours.

No incompatibility between Simulect and polyvinyl chloride bags or infusion sets has been observed. No data are avail-

Help Patients Save on Rx Drugs: PDR.net/PharmacyDiscountCard

able on the compatibility of Simulect with other intravenous substances. Other drug substances should not be added or infused simultaneously through the same intravenous line.

Adults

In adult patients, the recommended regimen is two doses of 20 mg each. The first 20-mg dose should be given within 2 hours prior to transplantation surgery. The recommended second 20-mg dose should be given 4 days after transplantation. The second dose should be withheld if complications such as severe hypersensitivity reactions to Simulect or graft loss occur.

Pediatric

In pediatric patients weighing less than 35 kg, the recommended regimen is two doses of 10 mg each. In pediatric patients weighing 35 kg or more, the recommended regimen is two doses of 20 mg each. The first dose should be given within 2 hours prior to transplantation surgery. The recommended second dose should be given 4 days after transplantation. The second dose should be withheld if complications such as severe hypersensitivity reactions to Simulect or graft loss occur.

Reconstitution of 10 mg Simulect® Vial

To prepare the reconstituted solution, add 2.5 mL of Sterile Water for Injection, USP, using aseptic technique, to the vial containing the Simulect powder. Shake the vial gently to dissolve the powder.

The reconstituted solution is isotonic and may be given either as a bolus injection or diluted to a volume of 25 mL with normal saline or dextrose 5% for infusion. When mixing the solution, gently invert the bag in order to avoid foaming; DO NOT SHAKE.

Reconstitution of 20 mg Simulect® Vial

To prepare the reconstituted solution, add 5 mL of Sterile Water for Injection, USP, using aseptic technique, to the vial containing the Simulect powder. Shake the vial gently to dissolve the powder.

The reconstituted solution is isotonic and may be given either as a bolus injection or diluted to a volume of 50 mL with normal saline or dextrose 5% for infusion. When mixing the solution, gently invert the bag in order to avoid foaming; DO NOT SHAKE.

HOW SUPPLIED

Simulect® (basiliximab) is supplied in a single-use glass vial.

Each carton contains one of the following
1 Simulect 10 mg vial ....NDC 0078-0393-61
1 Simulect 20 mg vial ....NDC 0078-0331-84
Store lyophilized Simulect under refrigerated conditions (2°C to 8°C; 36°F to 46°F).
Do not use beyond the expiration date stamped on the vial.

REFERENCES

1. Kahan, B.D., Rajagopalan P.R. and Hall M., Transplantation, 67, 276-284 (1999).
2. Nashan, B., Moore R., Amlot P., Schmidt A.-G., Abeywickrama K. and Soulillou J.-P., Lancet 350, 1193-1198 (1997).
T2005-28
2027722
US License No. 1244
REV: September 2005
Novartis Pharmaceuticals Corporation
East Hanover, New Jersey 07936
©Novartis

Shown in Product Identification Guide, page 311

TASIGNA®

[ta-sig-na]
(nilotinib)
Capsules for oral use   ℞

The following prescribing information is based on official labeling in effect July 2014.

HIGHLIGHTS OF PRESCRIBING INFORMATION
These highlights do not include all the information needed to use TASIGNA safely and effectively. See full prescribing information for TASIGNA.
TASIGNA®(nilotinib) Capsules for oral use
Initial U.S. Approval: 2007

WARNING: QT PROLONGATION AND SUDDEN DEATHS
See full prescribing information for complete boxed warning.

- Tasigna prolongs the QT interval. Prior to Tasigna administration and periodically, monitor for hypokalemia or hypomagnesemia and correct deficiencies (5.2). Obtain ECGs to monitor the QTc at baseline, seven days after initiation, and periodically thereafter, and following any dose adjustments (5.2, 5.3, 5.7, 5.14).
- Sudden deaths have been reported in patients receiving nilotinib (5.3). Do not administer Tasigna to patients with hypokalemia, hypomagnesemia, or long QT syndrome (4, 5.2).

- Avoid use of concomitant drugs known to prolong the QT interval and strong CYP3A4 inhibitors (5.8).
- Avoid food 2 hours before and 1 hour after taking the dose (5.9).

RECENT MAJOR CHANGES
Dosage and Administration (2.1, 2.2) 9/2013
Warnings and Precautions (5) 1/2014

INDICATIONS AND USAGE
Tasigna is a kinase inhibitor indicated for:
The treatment of newly diagnosed adult patients with Philadelphia chromosome positive chronic myeloid leukemia (Ph+ CML) in chronic phase. The study is ongoing and further data will be required to determine long-term outcome. (1.1)
The treatment of chronic phase (CP) and accelerated phase (AP) Ph+ CML in adult patients resistant to or intolerant to prior therapy that included imatinib. (1.2)

DOSAGE AND ADMINISTRATION
- Recommended Dose: Newly diagnosed Ph+ CML-CP: 300 mg orally twice daily. Resistant or intolerant Ph+ CML-CP and CML-AP: 400 mg orally twice daily. (2.1)
- Take each Tasigna dose approximately 12 hours apart. Tasigna must be taken on an empty stomach. Avoid food for at least 2 hours before the dose is taken and avoid food for at least 1 hour after the dose is taken. (2.1)
- Swallow the capsules whole with water. (2.1)
- Dose adjustment may be required for hematologic and non-hematologic toxicities, and drug interactions. (2.2)
- A lower starting dose is recommended in patients with hepatic impairment (at baseline). (2.2)

DOSAGE FORMS AND STRENGTHS
150 mg and 200 mg hard capsules (3)

CONTRAINDICATIONS
Do not use in patients with hypokalemia, hypomagnesemia, or long QT syndrome. (4)

WARNINGS AND PRECAUTIONS
- Myelosuppression: Associated with neutropenia, thrombocytopenia and anemia. CBC should be done every 2 weeks for the first 2 months, then monthly. Reversible by withholding dose. Dose reduction may be required. (5.1)
- QT Prolongation: Tasigna prolongs the QT interval. Correct hypokalemia or hypomagnesemia prior to administration and monitor periodically. (5.2) Avoid drugs known to prolong the QT interval and strong CYP3A4 inhibitors. (5.8) Use with caution in patients with hepatic impairment (5.10). Obtain ECGs at baseline, seven days after initiation, and periodically thereafter, as well as following any dose adjustments. (5.2, 5.3, 5.7, 5.14)
- Sudden deaths: Sudden deaths have been reported in patients with resistant or intolerant Ph+ CML receiving nilotinib. Ventricular repolarization abnormalities may have contributed to their occurrence. (5.3)
- Cardiac and Vascular Events: Cardiovascular events including ischemic heart disease, peripheral arterial occlusive disease and ischemic cerebrovascular events have been reported in patients with newly diagnosed Ph+CML receiving nilotinib. Cardiovascular status should be evaluated and cardiovascular risk factors monitored and managed during Tasigna therapy. (5.4)
- Pancreatitis and elevated serum lipase: Monitor serum lipase monthly or as clinically indicated. In case lipase elevations are accompanied by abdominal symptoms, interrupt doses and consider appropriate diagnostics to exclude pancreatitis. (5.5)
- Hepatotoxicity: Tasigna may result in elevations in bilirubin, AST/ALT, and alkaline phosphatase. Monitor hepatic function tests monthly or as clinically indicated. (5.6)
- Electrolyte abnormalities: Tasigna can cause hypophosphatemia, hypokalemia, hyperkalemia, hypocalcemia, and hyponatremia. Correct electrolyte abnormalities prior to initiating Tasigna and monitor periodically during therapy. (5.7, 5.14)
- Hepatic impairment: Nilotinib exposure is increased in patients with impaired hepatic function (at baseline). A dose reduction is recommended in these patients and QT interval should be monitored closely. (5.10)
- Tumor lysis syndrome: Tumor lysis syndrome cases have been reported in Tasigna treated patients with resistant or intolerant CML. Due to potential for tumor lysis syndrome, maintain adequate hydration and correct uric acid levels prior to initiating therapy with Tasigna. (5.11)
- Drug interactions: Avoid concomitant use of strong inhibitors or inducers of CYP3A4. If patients must be coadministered a strong CYP3A4 inhibitor, dose reduction should be considered and the QT interval should be monitored closely. (5.8)
- Food effects: Food increases blood levels of Tasigna. Avoid food 2 hours before and 1 hour after a dose. (5.9)
- Total gastrectomy: More frequent follow-up of these patients should be considered. If necessary, dose increase may be considered. (5.12)

- Embryo-fetal toxicity: Fetal harm can occur when administered to a pregnant woman. Women should be advised not to become pregnant when taking Tasigna. (5.15)

ADVERSE REACTIONS
The most commonly reported non-hematologic adverse reactions (≥20% in patients with newly diagnosed Ph+ CML-CP, resistant or intolerant Ph+ CML-CP, or resistant or intolerant Ph+ CML-AP) were nausea, rash, headache, fatigue, pruritus, vomiting, diarrhea, cough, constipation, arthralgia, nasopharyngitis, pyrexia, and night sweats. Hematologic adverse drug reactions include myelosuppression: thrombocytopenia, neutropenia and anemia. (6.1)

To report SUSPECTED ADVERSE REACTIONS, contact NOVARTIS Pharmaceuticals Corporation at 1-888-669-6682 or FDA at 1-800-FDA-1088 or www.fda.gov/medwatch.

DRUG INTERACTIONS
- Tasigna is an inhibitor of CYP3A4, CYP2C8, CYP2C9, CYP2D6. It may also induce CYP2B6, CYP2C8 and CYP2C9. Therefore, Tasigna may alter serum concentration of other drugs (7.1)
- CYP3A4 inhibitors may affect serum concentration (7.2)
- CYP3A4 inducers may affect serum concentration (7.2)

USE IN SPECIFIC POPULATIONS
- Should not breastfeed (8.3)
- No data to support use in pediatrics (8.4)
- A lower starting dose is recommended in patients with hepatic impairment (at baseline). (2.2, 8.7)

See 17 for PATIENT COUNSELING INFORMATION and Medication Guide

Revised: 1/2014

FULL PRESCRIBING INFORMATION: CONTENTS*
WARNING: QT PROLONGATION AND SUDDEN DEATHS

* Sections or subsections omitted from the full prescribing information are not listed

FULL PRESCRIBING INFORMATION

> **WARNING: QT PROLONGATION AND SUDDEN DEATHS**
> - Tasigna prolongs the QT interval. Prior to Tasigna administration and periodically, monitor for hypokalemia or hypomagnesemia and correct deficiencies (5.2). Obtain ECGs to monitor the QTc at baseline, seven days after initiation, and periodically thereafter, and following any dose adjustments (5.2, 5.3, 5.7, 5.14).
> - Sudden deaths have been reported in patients receiving nilotinib (5.3). Do not administer Tasigna to patients with hypokalemia, hypomagnesemia, or long QT syndrome (4, 5.2).
> - Avoid use of concomitant drugs known to prolong the QT interval and strong CYP3A4 inhibitors (5.8).
> - Avoid food 2 hours before and 1 hour after taking the dose (5.9).

1 INDICATIONS AND USAGE

1.1 Newly Diagnosed Ph+ CML-CP

Tasigna (nilotinib) is indicated for the treatment of adult patients with newly diagnosed Philadelphia chromosome positive chronic myeloid leukemia (Ph+ CML) in chronic phase. The effectiveness of Tasigna is based on major molecular response and cytogenetic response rates [see Clinical Studies (14.1)]. The study is ongoing and further data will be required to determine long-term outcome.

1.2 Resistant or Intolerant Ph+ CML-CP and CML-AP

Tasigna is indicated for the treatment of chronic phase and accelerated phase Philadelphia chromosome positive chronic myelogenous leukemia (Ph+ CML) in adult patients resistant or intolerant to prior therapy that included imatinib. The effectiveness of Tasigna is based on hematologic and cytogenetic response rates [see Clinical Studies (14.2)].

2 DOSAGE AND ADMINISTRATION

2.1 Recommended Dosing

Tasigna should be taken twice daily at approximately 12-hour intervals and must be taken on an empty stomach. No food should be consumed for at least 2 hours before the dose is taken and for at least 1 hour after the dose is taken. Advise patients to swallow the capsules whole with water [see Boxed Warning, Warnings and Precautions (5.9), Clinical Pharmacology (12.3)].

For patients who are unable to swallow capsules, the contents of each capsule may be dispersed in 1 teaspoon of applesauce (puréed apple). The mixture should be taken immediately (within 15 minutes) and should not be stored for future use [see Clinical Pharmacology (12.3)].

Tasigna may be given in combination with hematopoietic growth factors such as erythropoietin or G-CSF if clinically indicated. Tasigna may be given with hydroxyurea or anagrelide if clinically indicated.

Newly Diagnosed Ph+ CML-CP

The recommended dose of Tasigna is 300 mg orally twice daily [see Clinical Pharmacology (12.3)].

Resistant or Intolerant Ph+ CML-CP and CML-AP

The recommended dose of Tasigna (nilotinib) is 400 mg orally twice daily [see Clinical Pharmacology (12.3)].

2.2 Dose Adjustments or Modifications

QT Interval Prolongation:

Table 1: Dose Adjustments for QT Prolongation

ECGs with a QTc >480 msec	1. Withhold Tasigna, and perform an analysis of serum potassium and magnesium, and if below lower limit of normal, correct with supplements to within normal limits. Concomitant medication usage must be reviewed. 2. Resume within 2 weeks at prior dose if QTcF returns to <450 msec and to within 20 msec of baseline. 3. If QTcF is between 450 msec and 480 msec after 2 weeks, reduce the dose to 400 mg once daily. 4. If, following dose-reduction to 400 mg once daily, QTcF returns to >480 msec, Tasigna should be discontinued. 5. An ECG should be repeated approximately 7 days after any dose adjustment.

Myelosuppression

Withhold or dose reduce Tasigna for hematological toxicities (neutropenia, thrombocytopenia) that are not related to underlying leukemia (Table 2).

[See table 2 above]

Table 2: Dose Adjustments for Neutropenia and Thrombocytopenia

Newly diagnosed Ph+ CML in chronic phase at 300 mg twice daily	ANC* <1.0 × 10⁹/L and/or platelet counts <50 × 10⁹/L	1. Stop Tasigna, and monitor blood counts 2. Resume within 2 weeks at prior dose if ANC >1.0 × 10⁹/L and platelets >50 × 10⁹/L 3. If blood counts remain low for >2 weeks, reduce the dose to 400 mg once daily
Resistant or intolerant Ph+ CML in chronic phase or accelerated phase at 400 mg twice daily		

*ANC = absolute neutrophil count

Table 4: Dose Adjustments for Hepatic Impairment (At Baseline)

Newly diagnosed Ph+ CML in chronic phase at 300 mg twice daily	Mild, Moderate, or Severe*	An initial dosing regimen of 200 mg twice daily followed by dose escalation to 300 mg twice daily based on tolerability
Resistant or intolerant Ph+ CML in chronic phase or accelerated phase at 400 mg twice daily	Mild or Moderate*	An initial dosing regimen of 300 mg twice daily followed by dose escalation to 400 mg twice daily based on tolerability
	Severe*	A starting dose of 200 mg twice daily followed by a sequential dose escalation to 300 mg twice daily and then to 400 mg twice daily based on tolerability

*Mild = mild hepatic impairment (Child-Pugh Class A); Moderate = moderate hepatic impairment (Child-Pugh Class B); Severe = severe hepatic impairment (Child-Pugh Class C) [see Warnings and Precautions (5.10), Use in Specific Populations (8.7)].

See Table 3 for dose adjustments for elevations of lipase, amylase, bilirubin, and/or hepatic transaminases [see Adverse Reactions (6.1)].

Table 3: Dose Adjustments for Selected Non-hematologic Laboratory Abnormalities

Elevated serum lipase or amylase ≥Grade 3	1. Withhold Tasigna, and monitor serum lipase or amylase 2. Resume treatment at 400 mg once daily if serum lipase or amylase returns to ≤Grade 1
Elevated bilirubin ≥Grade 3	1. Withhold Tasigna, and monitor bilirubin 2. Resume treatment at 400 mg once daily if bilirubin returns to ≤Grade 1
Elevated hepatic transaminases ≥Grade 3	1. Withhold Tasigna, and monitor hepatic transaminases 2. Resume treatment at 400 mg once daily if hepatic transaminases returns to ≤Grade 1

Other Non-hematologic Toxicities

If other clinically significant moderate or severe non-hematologic toxicity develops, withhold dosing, and resume at 400 mg once daily when the toxicity has resolved. If clinically appropriate, escalation of the dose back to 300 mg (newly diagnosed Ph+ CML-CP) or 400 mg (resistant or intolerant Ph+ CML-CP and CML-AP) twice daily should be considered. For Grade 3 to 4 lipase elevations, dosing should be withheld, and may be resumed at 400 mg once daily. Test serum lipase levels monthly or as clinically indicated. For Grade 3 to 4 bilirubin or hepatic transaminase elevations, dosing should be withheld, and may be resumed at 400 mg once daily. Test bilirubin and hepatic transaminases levels monthly or as clinically indicated [see Warnings and Precautions (5.5, 5.6), Use in Specific Populations (8.7)].

Hepatic Impairment

If possible, consider alternative therapies. If Tasigna must be administered to patients with hepatic impairment, consider the following dose reduction:

[See table 4 above]

Concomitant Strong CYP3A4 Inhibitors

Avoid the concomitant use of strong CYP3A4 inhibitors (e.g., ketoconazole, itraconazole, clarithromycin, atazanavir, indinavir, nefazodone, nelfinavir, ritonavir, saquinavir, telithromycin, voriconazole). Avoid grapefruit products since they may also increase serum concentrations of nilotinib. Should treatment with any of these agents be required, therapy with Tasigna should be interrupted. If patients must be coadministered a strong CYP3A4 inhibitor, based on pharmacokinetic studies, consider a dose reduction to 300 mg once daily in patients with resistant or intolerant Ph+ CML or to 200 mg once daily in patients with newly diagnosed Ph+ CML-CP. However, there are no clinical data with this dose adjustment in patients receiving strong CYP3A4 inhibitors. If the strong inhibitor is discontinued, a washout period should be allowed before the Tasigna dose is adjusted upward to the indicated dose. For patients who cannot avoid use of strong CYP3A4 inhibitors, monitor closely for prolongation of the QT interval [see Boxed Warning, Warnings and Precautions (5.2, 5.8), Drug Interactions (7.2)].

Concomitant Strong CYP3A4 Inducers

Avoid the concomitant use of strong CYP3A4 inducers (e.g., dexamethasone, phenytoin, carbamazepine, rifampin, rifabutin, rifapentine, phenobarbital). Also inform patients not to take St. John's Wort since these agents may reduce the concentration of Tasigna. Based on the nonlinear pharmacokinetic profile of nilotinib, increasing the dose of Tasigna when coadministered with such agents is unlikely to compensate for the loss of exposure [see Drug Interactions (7.2)].

3 DOSAGE FORMS AND STRENGTHS

150 mg red opaque hard gelatin capsules with black axial imprint "NVR/BCR".

200 mg light yellow opaque hard gelatin capsules with a red axial imprint "NVR/TKI".

4 CONTRAINDICATIONS

Do not use in patients with hypokalemia, hypomagnesemia, or long QT syndrome [see Boxed Warning].

5 WARNINGS AND PRECAUTIONS

5.1 Myelosuppression

Treatment with Tasigna can cause Grade 3/4 thrombocytopenia, neutropenia and anemia. Perform complete blood counts every 2 weeks for the first 2 months and then monthly thereafter, or as clinically indicated. Myelosuppression was generally reversible and usually managed by withholding Tasigna temporarily or dose reduction [see Dosage and Administration (2.2)].

5.2 QT Prolongation

Tasigna has been shown to prolong cardiac ventricular repolarization as measured by the QT interval on the surface ECG in a concentration-dependent manner [see Adverse Reactions (6.1), Clinical Pharmacology (12.6)]. Prolongation of the QT interval can result in a type of ventricular tachycardia called torsade de pointes, which may result in syncope, seizure, and/or death. ECGs should be performed at baseline, 7 days after initiation of Tasigna, and periodically as clinically indicated and following dose adjustments [see Warnings and Precautions (5.14)].

Tasigna should not be used in patients who have hypokalemia, hypomagnesemia or long QT syndrome. Before initiating Tasigna and periodically, test electrolyte, calcium and magnesium blood levels. Hypokalemia or hypomagnesemia must be corrected prior to initiating Tasigna and these electrolytes should be monitored periodically during therapy [see Warnings and Precautions (5.14)].

Significant prolongation of the QT interval may occur when Tasigna is inappropriately taken with food and/or strong CYP3A4 inhibitors and/or medicinal products with a known potential to prolong QT. Therefore, coadministration with food must be avoided and concomitant use with strong CYP3A4 inhibitors and/or medicinal products with a known

Table 5: Most Frequently Reported Non-hematologic Adverse Reactions (Regardless of Relationship to Study Drug) in Patients with Newly Diagnosed Ph+ CML-CP (≥10% in Tasigna 300 mg Twice Daily or Imatinib 400 mg Once Daily Groups) 48-Month Analysis[a]

Body System and Preferred Term		Patients with Newly Diagnosed Ph+ CML-CP			
		TASIGNA 300 mg twice daily	Imatinib 400 mg once daily	TASIGNA 300 mg twice daily	Imatinib 400 mg once daily
		N=279	N=280	N=279	N=280
		All Grades (%)		CTC Grades[b] 3/4 (%)	
Skin and subcutaneous tissue disorders	Rash	38	18	<1	2
	Pruritus	21	7	<1	0
	Alopecia	13	7	0	0
	Dry skin	12	6	0	0
Gastrointestinal disorders	Nausea	22	41	2	1
	Constipation	19	8	<1	0
	Diarrhea	18	45	<1	3
	Vomiting	15	26	<1	<1
	Abdominal pain upper	17	13	1	<1
	Abdominal pain	15	12	2	0
	Dyspepsia	9	12	0	0
Nervous system disorders	Headache	32	23	3	<1
	Dizziness	11	10	<1	<1
General disorders and administration site conditions	Fatigue	23	19	1	1
	Pyrexia	13	13	<1	0
	Asthenia	14	12	<1	0
	Peripheral edema	10	21	<1	0
	Face edema	<1	14	0	<1
Musculoskeletal and connective tissue disorders	Myalgia	19	19	<1	<1
	Arthralgia	20	16	<1	<1
	Muscle spasms	12	34	0	1
	Pain in extremity	13	15	<1	<1
	Back pain	17	16	1	1
Respiratory, thoracic and mediastinal disorders	Cough	17	13	0	0
	Oropharyngeal pain	11	6	0	0
	Dyspnea	10	6	2	<1
Infections and infestations	Nasopharyngitis	25	21	0	0
	Upper respiratory tract infection	16	14	<1	0
	Influenza	12	9	0	0
Eye disorders	Eyelid edema	1	18	0	<1
	Periorbital edema	<1	15	0	0
Psychiatric disorders	Insomnia	11	9	0	0

[a]Excluding laboratory abnormalities
[b]NCI Common Terminology Criteria for Adverse Events, Version 3.0

potential to prolong QT should be avoided *[see Warnings and Precautions (5.8, 5.9)]*. The presence of hypokalemia and hypomagnesemia may further prolong the QT interval *[see Warnings and Precautions (5.7, 5.14)]*.

5.3   Sudden Deaths
Sudden deaths have been reported in 0.3% of patients with CML treated with nilotinib in clinical studies of 5,661 patients. The relative early occurrence of some of these deaths

relative to the initiation of nilotinib suggests the possibility that ventricular repolarization abnormalities may have contributed to their occurrence.

5.4   Cardiac and Vascular Events
Cardiovascular events, including arterial vascular occlusive events, were reported in a randomized, clinical trial in newly diagnosed CML patients and observed in the postmarketing reports of patients receiving nilotinib therapy.

With a median time on therapy of 48 months in the clinical trial, cases of cardiovascular events included ischemic heart disease-related events (5.0% and 5.8% in the nilotinib 300 mg and 400 mg bid arms respectively, and 1.8% in the imatinib arm), peripheral arterial occlusive disease (1.8% and 2.2% in the nilotinib 300 mg and 400 mg bid arms respectively, and 0% in the imatinib arm), and ischemic cerebrovascular events (1.1% and 1.8% in the nilotinib 300 mg and 400 mg bid arms respectively, and 0.7% in the imatinib arm). If acute signs or symptoms of cardiovascular events occur, advise patients to seek immediate medical attention. The cardiovascular status of patients should be evaluated and cardiovascular risk factors should be monitored and actively managed during Tasigna therapy according to standard guidelines *[see Dosage and Administration (2.2)]*.

5.5   Pancreatitis and Elevated Serum Lipase
Tasigna can cause increases in serum lipase. Patients with a previous history of pancreatitis may be at greater risk of elevated serum lipase. If lipase elevations are accompanied by abdominal symptoms, interrupt dosing and consider appropriate diagnostics to exclude pancreatitis. Test serum lipase levels monthly or as clinically indicated.

5.6   Hepatotoxicity
Tasigna may result in hepatotoxicity as measured by elevations in bilirubin, AST/ALT, and alkaline phosphatase. Monitor hepatic function tests monthly or as clinically indicated *[see Warnings and Precautions (5.14)]*.

5.7   Electrolyte Abnormalities
The use of Tasigna can cause hypophosphatemia, hypokalemia, hyperkalemia, hypocalcemia, and hyponatremia. Electrolyte abnormalities must be corrected prior to initiating Tasigna and these electrolytes should be monitored periodically during therapy *[see Warnings and Precautions (5.14)]*.

5.8   Drug Interactions
Avoid administration of Tasigna with agents that may increase nilotinib exposure (e.g., strong CYP3A4 inhibitors) or anti-arrhythmic drugs (including, but not limited to amiodarone, disopyramide, procainamide, quinidine and sotalol) and other drugs that may prolong QT interval (including, but not limited to chloroquine, clarithromycin, haloperidol, methadone, moxifloxacin and pimozide). Should treatment with any of these agents be required, interrupt therapy with Tasigna. If interruption of treatment with Tasigna is not possible, patients who require treatment with a drug that prolongs QT or strongly inhibits CYP3A4 should be closely monitored for prolongation of the QT interval *[see Boxed Warning, Dosage and Administration (2.2), Drug Interactions (7.2)]*.

5.9   Food Effects
The bioavailability of nilotinib is increased with food, thus Tasigna must not be taken with food. No food should be consumed for at least 2 hours before and for at least 1 hour after the dose is taken. Also avoid grapefruit products and other foods that are known to inhibit CYP3A4 *[see Boxed Warning, Drug Interactions (7.2) and Clinical Pharmacology (12.3)]*.

5.10   Hepatic Impairment
Nilotinib exposure is increased in patients with impaired hepatic function. Use a lower starting dose for patients with mild to severe hepatic impairment (at baseline) and monitor the QT interval frequently *[see Dosage and Administration (2.2) and Use in Specific Populations (8.7)]*.

5.11   Tumor Lysis Syndrome
Tumor lysis syndrome cases have been reported in Tasigna treated patients with resistant or intolerant CML. Malignant disease progression, high WBC counts and/or dehydration were present in the majority of these cases. Due to potential for tumor lysis syndrome, maintain adequate hydration and correct uric acid levels prior to initiating therapy with Tasigna.

5.12   Total Gastrectomy
Since the exposure of nilotinib is reduced in patients with total gastrectomy, perform more frequent monitoring of these patients. Consider dose increase or alternative therapy in patients with total gastrectomy *[see Clinical Pharmacology 12.3)]*.

5.13   Lactose
Since the capsules contain lactose, Tasigna is not recommended for patients with rare hereditary problems of galactose intolerance, severe lactase deficiency with a severe degree of intolerance to lactose-containing products, or of glucose-galactose malabsorption.

5.14   Monitoring Laboratory Tests
Complete blood counts should be performed every 2 weeks for the first 2 months and then monthly thereafter. Chemistry panels, including electrolytes, calcium, magnesium, lipid profile, and glucose should be checked prior to therapy and periodically. ECGs should be obtained at baseline, 7 days after initiation and periodically thereafter, as well as following dose adjustments *[see Warnings and Precautions (5.2)]*. Laboratory monitoring for patients receiving Tasigna may need to be performed more or less frequently at the physician's discretion.

5.15 Embryo-Fetal Toxicity

There are no adequate and well controlled studies of Tasigna in pregnant women. However, Tasigna may cause fetal harm when administered to a pregnant woman. Nilotinib caused embryo-fetal toxicities in animals at maternal exposures that were lower than the expected human exposure at the recommended doses of nilotinib. If this drug is used during pregnancy, or if the patient becomes pregnant while taking this drug, the patient should be apprised of the potential hazard to the fetus. Women of child-bearing potential should avoid becoming pregnant while taking Tasigna *[see Use in Specific Populations (8.1)]*.

6   ADVERSE REACTIONS

The following serious adverse reactions can occur with Tasigna and are discussed in greater detail in other sections of the package insert *[see Boxed Warning, Warnings and Precautions (5)]*.

- Myelosuppression *[see Warnings and Precautions (5.1)]*
- QT Prolongation *[see Boxed Warning, Warnings and Precautions (5.2)]*
- Sudden Deaths *[see Boxed Warning, Warnings and Precautions (5.3)]*
- Pancreatitis and Elevated Serum Lipase *[see Warnings and Precautions (5.5)]*
- Hepatotoxicity *[see Warnings and Precautions (5.6)]*
- Electrolyte Abnormalities *[see Boxed Warning, Warnings and Precautions (5.7)]*

6.1   Clinical Trials Experience

Because clinical trials are conducted under widely varying conditions, adverse reaction rates observed in the clinical trials of a drug cannot be directly compared to rates in the clinical trials of another drug and may not reflect the rates observed in practice.

In Patients with Newly Diagnosed Ph+ CML-CP

The data below reflect exposure to Tasigna from a randomized trial in patients with newly diagnosed Ph+ CML in chronic phase treated at the recommended dose of 300 mg twice daily (n=279). The median time on treatment in the nilotinib 300 mg twice daily group was 48 months (range 0.1 to 59 months). The median actual dose intensity was 594 mg/day in the nilotinib 300 mg twice daily group.

The most common (>10%) non-hematologic adverse drug reactions were rash, pruritus, headache, nausea, fatigue, alopecia and myalgia. Upper abdominal pain, constipation, diarrhea, dry skin, muscle spasms, arthralgia, abdominal pain, peripheral edema, vomiting, and asthenia were observed less commonly (≤10% and >5%) and have been of mild to moderate severity, manageable and generally did not require dose reduction. Pleural and pericardial effusions, occurred in 1% and <1% of patients, respectively. Gastrointestinal hemorrhage was reported in 3% of patients.

Increase in QTcF >60 msec from baseline was observed in 1 patient (0.4%) in the 300 mg twice daily treatment group. No patient had an absolute QTcF of >500 msec while on study drug.

The most common hematologic adverse drug reactions (all grades) were myelosuppression including: thrombocytopenia (18%), neutropenia (15%) and anemia (7%). See Table 7 for Grade 3/4 laboratory abnormalities.

Discontinuation due to adverse reactions, regardless of relationship to study drug, was observed in 10% of patients.

In Patients with Resistant or Intolerant Ph+ CML-CP and CML-AP

In the single open-label multicenter clinical trial, a total of 458 patients with Ph+ CML-CP and CML-AP resistant to or intolerant to at least one prior therapy including imatinib were treated (CML-CP=321; CML-AP=137) at the recommended dose of 400 mg twice daily.

The median duration of exposure in days for CML-CP and CML-AP patients is 561 (range 1 to 1096) and 264 (range 2 to 1160), respectively. The median dose intensity for patients with CML-CP and CML-AP is 789 mg/day (range 151 to 1110) and 780 mg/day (range 150 to 1149), respectively and corresponded to the planned 400 mg twice daily dosing. The median cumulative duration in days of dose interruptions for the CML-CP patients was 20 (range 1 to 345), and the median duration in days of dose interruptions for the CML-AP patients was 23 (range 1 to 234).

In patients with CML-CP, the most commonly reported non-hematologic adverse drug reactions (≥10%) were rash, pruritus, nausea, fatigue, headache, constipation, diarrhea, vomiting and myalgia. The common serious drug-related adverse reactions (≥1% and <10%) were thrombocytopenia, neutropenia and anemia.

In patients with CML-AP, the most commonly reported non-hematologic adverse drug reactions (≥10%) were rash, pruritus and fatigue. The common serious adverse drug reactions (≥1% and <10%) were thrombocytopenia, neutropenia, febrile neutropenia, pneumonia, leukopenia, intracranial hemorrhage, elevated lipase and pyrexia.

Sudden deaths and QT prolongation were reported. The maximum mean QTcF change from baseline at steady-state was 10 msec. Increase in QTcF >60 msec from baseline was observed in 4.1% of the patients and QTcF of >500 msec was observed in 4 patients (<1%) *[see Boxed Warning, Warnings and Precautions (5.2, 5.3), Clinical Pharmacology (12.6)]*. Discontinuation due to adverse drug reactions was observed in 16% of CML-CP and 10% of CML-AP patients.

Most Frequently Reported Adverse Reactions

Tables 5 and 6 show the percentage of patients experiencing non-hematologic adverse reactions (excluding laboratory abnormalities) regardless of relationship to study drug. Adverse reactions reported in greater than 10% of patients who received at least 1 dose of Tasigna are listed.

[See table 5 at top of previous page]

[See table 6 above]

Laboratory Abnormalities

Table 7 shows the percentage of patients experiencing treatment-emergent Grade 3/4 laboratory abnormalities in patients who received at least one dose of Tasigna.

[See table 7 at top of next page]

6.2   Additional Data from Clinical Trials

The following adverse drug reactions were reported in patients in the Tasigna clinical studies at the recommended doses. These adverse drug reactions are ranked under a heading of frequency, the most frequent first using the following convention: common (≥1% and <10%), uncommon

Table 6: Most Frequently Reported Non-hematologic Adverse Reactions in Patients with Resistant or Intolerant Ph+ CML Receiving Tasigna 400 mg Twice Daily (Regardless of Relationship to Study Drug) (≥10% in any Group) 24-Month Analysis[a]

Body System and Preferred Term		CML-CP N=321		CML-AP N=137	
		All Grades (%)	CTC Grades[b] 3/4 (%)	All Grades (%)	CTC Grades[b] 3/4 (%)
Skin and subcutaneous tissue disorders	Rash	36	2	29	0
	Pruritus	32	<1	20	0
	Night sweat	12	<1	27	0
	Alopecia	11	0	12	0
Gastrointestinal disorders	Nausea	37	1	22	<1
	Constipation	26	<1	19	0
	Diarrhea	28	3	24	2
	Vomiting	29	<1	13	0
	Abdominal pain	15	2	16	3
	Abdominal pain upper	14	<1	12	<1
	Dyspepsia	10	<1	4	0
Nervous system disorders	Headache	35	2	20	1
General disorders and administration site conditions	Fatigue	32	3	23	<1
	Pyrexia	22	<1	28	2
	Asthenia	16	0	14	1
	Peripheral edema	15	<1	12	0
Musculoskeletal and connective tissue disorders	Myalgia	19	2	16	<1
	Arthralgia	26	2	16	0
	Muscle spasms	13	<1	15	0
	Bone pain	14	<1	15	2
	Pain in extremity	20	2	18	1
	Back pain	17	2	15	<1
	Musculoskeletal pain	11	<1	12	1
Respiratory, thoracic and mediastinal disorders	Cough	27	<1	18	0
	Dyspnea	15	2	9	2
	Oropharyngeal pain	11	0	7	0
Infections and infestations	Nasopharyngitis	24	<1	15	0
	Upper respiratory tract infection	12	0	10	0
Metabolism and nutrition disorders	Decreased appetite[c]	15	<1	17	<1
Psychiatric disorders	Insomnia	12	1	7	0
Vascular disorders	Hypertension	10	2	11	<1

[a]Excluding laboratory abnormalities
[b]NCI Common Terminology Criteria for Adverse Events, Version 3.0
[c]Also includes preferred term anorexia

Table 7: Percent Incidence of Clinically Relevant Grade 3/4* Laboratory Abnormalities

	Patient Population			
	Newly Diagnosed Ph+ CML-CP		Resistant or Intolerant Ph+	
			CML-CP	CML-AP
	TASIGNA 300 mg twice daily N=279 (%)	Imatinib 400 mg once daily N=280 (%)	TASIGNA 400 mg twice daily N=321 (%)	TASIGNA 400 mg twice daily N=137 (%)
Hematologic Parameters				
Thrombocytopenia	10	9	30[1]	42[3]
Neutropenia	12	21	31[2]	42[4]
Anemia	4	6	11	27
Biochemistry Parameters				
Elevated lipase	9	4	18	18
Hyperglycemia	6	<1	12	6
Hypophosphatemia	6	10	17	15
Elevated bilirubin (total)	4	<1	7	9
Elevated SGPT (ALT)	4	3	4	4
Hyperkalemia	2	1	6	4
Hyponatremia	1	<1	7	7
Hypokalemia	<1	2	2	9
Elevated SGOT (AST)	1	1	3	2
Decreased albumin	0	<1	4	3
Hypocalcemia	<1	<1	2	5
Elevated alkaline phosphatase	0	<1	<1	1
Elevated creatinine	0	<1	<1	<1

*NCI Common Terminology Criteria for Adverse Events, version 3.0
[1] CML-CP: Thrombocytopenia: 12% were Grade 3, 18% were Grade 4
[2] CML-CP: Neutropenia: 16% were Grade 3, 15% were Grade 4
[3] CML-AP: Thrombocytopenia: 11% were Grade 3, 32% were Grade 4
[4] CML-AP: Neutropenia: 16% were Grade 3, 26% were Grade 4

(≥0.1% and <1%), and unknown frequency (single events). For laboratory abnormalities, very common events (≥10%), which were not included in Tables 5 and 6, are also reported. These adverse reactions are included based on clinical relevance and ranked in order of decreasing seriousness within each category, obtained from 2 clinical studies:
1. Newly diagnosed Ph+CML-CP 48 month analysis and,
2. Resistant or intolerant Ph+CML-CP and CMP-AP 24 months' analysis.

Infections and Infestations: Common: folliculitis, upper respiratory tract infection (including pharyngitis, nasopharyngitis, rhinitis). Uncommon: pneumonia, bronchitis, urinary tract infection, candidiasis (including oral candidiasis), gastroenteritis. Unknown frequency: sepsis, subcutaneous abscess, anal abscess, furuncle, tinea pedis.
Neoplasms Benign, Malignant, and Unspecified: Common: skin papilloma. Unknown frequency: oral papilloma, paraproteinemia.
Blood and Lymphatic System Disorders: Common: eosinophilia, febrile neutropenia, pancytopenia, lymphopenia. Unknown frequency: thrombocythemia, leukocytosis.
Immune System Disorders: Unknown frequency: hypersensitivity.
Endocrine Disorders: Uncommon: hyperthyroidism, hypothyroidism. Unknown frequency: hyperparathyroidism secondary, thyroiditis.
Metabolism and Nutrition Disorders: Very Common: hypophosphatemia. Common: electrolyte imbalance (including hypomagnesemia, hyperkalemia, hypokalemia, hyponatremia, hypocalcemia, hypercalcemia, hyperphosphatemia), diabetes mellitus, hyperglycemia, hypercholesterolemia, hyperlipidemia, hypertriglyceridemia. Uncommon: gout, dehydration, increased appetite. Unknown frequency: hyperuricemia, hypoglycemia.
Psychiatric Disorders: Common: depression, insomnia, anxiety. Unknown frequency: disorientation, confusional state, amnesia, dysphoria.
Nervous System Disorders: Common: dizziness, peripheral neuropathy, hypoesthesia, paresthesia. Uncommon: intra-cranial hemorrhage, migraine, loss of consciousness (including syncope), tremor, disturbance in attention, hyperesthesia. Unknown frequency: transient ischemic attack, brain edema, optic neuritis, lethargy, dysesthesia, restless legs syndrome.
Eye Disorders: Common: eye hemorrhage, periorbital edema, eye pruritus, conjunctivitis, dry eye (including xerophthalmia). Uncommon: vision impairment, vision blurred, visual acuity reduced, photopsia, hyperemia (scleral, conjunctival, ocular), eye irritation, conjunctival hemorrhage. Unknown frequency: papilloedema, diplopia, photophobia, eye swelling, blepharitis, eye pain, chorioretinopathy, conjunctivitis allergic, ocular surface disease.
Ear and Labyrinth Disorders: Common: vertigo. Unknown frequency: hearing impaired, ear pain, tinnitus.
Cardiac Disorders: Common: angina pectoris, arrhythmia (including atrioventricular block, cardiac flutter, extrasystoles, atrial fibrillation, tachycardia, bradycardia), palpitations, electrocardiogram QT prolonged. Uncommon: cardiac failure, pericardial effusion, coronary artery disease, cyanosis, cardiac murmur. Unknown frequency: myocardial infarction, ventricular dysfunction, pericarditis, ejection fraction decrease.
Vascular Disorders: Common: hypertension, flushing. Uncommon: hypertensive crisis, peripheral arterial occlusive disease, intermittent claudication, arterial stenosis limb, hematoma, arteriosclerosis. Unknown frequency: shock hemorrhagic, hypotension, thrombosis.
Respiratory, Thoracic and Mediastinal Disorders: Common: dyspnea, dyspnea exertional, epistaxis, cough, dysphonia. Uncommon: pulmonary edema, pleural effusion, interstitial lung disease, pleuritic pain, pleurisy, pharyngolaryngeal pain, throat irritation. Unknown frequency: pulmonary hypertension, wheezing, oropharyngeal pain.
Gastrointestinal Disorders: Common: pancreatitis, abdominal discomfort, abdominal distension, dyspepsia, dysgeusia, flatulence. Uncommon: gastrointestinal hemorrhage, melena, mouth ulceration, gastroesophageal reflux, stomatitis, esophageal pain, dry mouth, gastritis, sensitiv-ity of teeth. Unknown frequency: gastrointestinal ulcer perforation, retroperitoneal hemorrhage, hematemesis, gastric ulcer, esophagitis ulcerative, subileus, enterocolitis, hemorrhoids, hiatus hernia, rectal hemorrhage, gingivitis.
Hepatobiliary Disorders: Very Common: hyperbilirubinemia. Common: hepatic function abnormal. Uncommon: hepatotoxicity, toxic hepatitis, jaundice. Unknown frequency: cholestasis, hepatomegaly.
Skin and Subcutaneous Tissue Disorders: Common: night sweats, eczema, urticaria, erythema, hyperhidrosis, contusion, acne, dermatitis (including allergic, exfoliative and acneiform), dry skin. Uncommon: exfoliative rash, drug eruption, pain of skin, ecchymosis, swelling of face. Unknown frequency: psoriasis, erythema multiforme, erythema nodosum, skin ulcer, palmar-plantar erythrodysesthesia syndrome, petechiae, photosensitivity, blister, dermal cyst, sebaceous hyperplasia, skin atrophy, skin discoloration, skin exfoliation, skin hyperpigmentation, skin hypertrophy, hyperkeratosis.
Musculoskeletal and Connective Tissue Disorders: Common: bone pain, musculoskeletal chest pain, musculoskeletal pain, back pain, neck pain, flank pain. Uncommon: musculoskeletal stiffness, muscular weakness, joint swelling. Unknown frequency: arthritis.
Renal and Urinary Disorders: Common: pollakiuria. Uncommon: dysuria, micturition urgency, nocturia. Unknown frequency: renal failure, hematuria, urinary incontinence, chromaturia.
Reproductive System and Breast Disorders: Uncommon: breast pain, gynecomastia, erectile dysfunction. Unknown frequency: breast induration, menorrhagia, nipple swelling.
General Disorders and Administration Site Conditions: Common: pyrexia, chest pain (including non-cardiac chest pain), pain, chest discomfort, malaise. Uncommon: face edema, gravitational edema, influenza-like illness, chills, feeling body temperature change (including feeling hot, feeling cold). Unknown frequency: localized edema.
Investigations: Very Common: alanine aminotransferase increased, aspartate aminotransferase increased, lipase increased. Common: hemoglobin decreased, blood amylase increased, gamma-glutamyltransferase increased, blood creatinine phosphokinase increased, blood alkaline phosphatase increased, weight decreased, weight increased, lipoprotein increased (including very low density and high density). Uncommon: blood lactate dehydrogenase increased, blood urea increased, globulins decreased. Unknown frequency: troponin increased, blood bilirubin unconjugated increased, insulin C-peptide decreased, blood parathyroid hormone increased.

7 DRUG INTERACTIONS

7.1 Effects of Nilotinib on Drug Metabolizing Enzymes and Drug Transport Systems

Nilotinib is a competitive inhibitor of CYP3A4, CYP2C8, CYP2C9, CYP2D6 and UGT1A1 *in vitro*, potentially increasing the concentrations of drugs eliminated by these enzymes. *In vitro* studies also suggest that nilotinib may induce CYP2B6, CYP2C8 and CYP2C9, and decrease the concentrations of drugs which are eliminated by these enzymes.

Single-dose administration of Tasigna with midazolam (a CYP3A4 substrate) to healthy subjects increased midazolam exposure by 30%. Single-dose administration of Tasigna to healthy subjects did not change the pharmacokinetics and pharmacodynamics of warfarin (a CYP2C9 substrate). The ability of Tasigna to induce metabolism has not been determined *in vivo*. Exercise caution when coadministering Tasigna with substrates for these enzymes that have a narrow therapeutic index.

Nilotinib inhibits human P-glycoprotein (P-gp). If Tasigna is administered with drugs that are substrates of P-gp, increased concentrations of the substrate drug are likely, and caution should be exercised.

7.2 Drugs that Inhibit or Induce Cytochrome P450 3A4 Enzymes

Nilotinib undergoes metabolism by CYP3A4, and concomitant administration of strong inhibitors or inducers of CYP3A4 can increase or decrease nilotinib concentrations significantly. The administration of Tasigna with agents that are strong CYP3A4 inhibitors should be avoided *[see Boxed Warning, Dosage and Administration (2.2), Warnings and Precautions (5.2, 5.8)]*. Concomitant use of Tasigna with medicinal products and herbal preparations that are potent inducers of CYP3A4 is likely to reduce exposure to nilotinib to a clinically relevant extent. Therefore, in patients receiving Tasigna, concomitant use of alternative therapeutic agents with less potential for CYP3A4 induction should be selected.

Ketoconazole: In healthy subjects receiving ketoconazole, a CYP3A4 inhibitor, at 400 mg once daily for 6 days, systemic exposure (AUC) to nilotinib was increased approximately 3-fold.

Rifampicin: In healthy subjects receiving the CYP3A4 inducer, rifampicin, at 600 mg daily for 12 days, systemic exposure (AUC) to nilotinib was decreased approximately 80%.

7.3 Drugs that Affect Gastric pH

Nilotinib has pH-dependent solubility, with decreased solubility at higher pH. Drugs such as proton pump inhibitors that inhibit gastric acid secretion to elevate the gastric pH may decrease the solubility of nilotinib and reduce its bioavailability. In healthy subjects, coadministration of a single 400 mg dose of Tasigna with multiple doses of esomeprazole (a proton pump inhibitor) at 40 mg daily decreased the nilotinib AUC by 34%. Increasing the dose of Tasigna when coadministered with such agents is not likely to compensate for the loss of exposure. Since proton pump inhibitors affect pH of the upper GI tract for an extended period, separation of doses may not eliminate the interaction. The concomitant use of proton pump inhibitors with Tasigna is not recommended.

In healthy subjects, no significant change in nilotinib pharmacokinetics was observed when a single 400 mg dose of Tasigna was administered 10 hours after and 2 hours before famotidine (an H2 blocker). Therefore, when the concurrent use of a H2 blocker is necessary, it may be administered approximately 10 hours before and approximately 2 hours after the dose of Tasigna.

Administration of an antacid (aluminum hydroxide/magnesium hydroxide/simethicone) to healthy subjects, 2 hours before or 2 hours after a single 400 mg dose of Tasigna did not alter nilotinib pharmacokinetics. Therefore, if necessary, an antacid may be administered approximately 2 hours before or approximately 2 hours after the dose of Tasigna.

7.4 Drugs that Inhibit Drug Transport Systems

Nilotinib is a substrate of the efflux transporter P-glycoprotein (P-gp, ABCB1). If Tasigna is administered with drugs that inhibit P-gp, increased concentrations of nilotinib are likely, and caution should be exercised.

7.5 Drugs that May Prolong the QT Interval

The administration of Tasigna with agents that may prolong the QT interval such as anti-arrhythmic medicines should be avoided [see Boxed Warning, Dosage and Administration (2.2), Warnings and Precautions (5.2, 5.8)].

8 USE IN SPECIFIC POPULATIONS

8.1 Pregnancy

Pregnancy Category D [see Warnings and Precautions (5.15)].

Risk Summary

Based on its mechanism of action and findings in animals, Tasigna may cause fetal harm when administered to a pregnant woman. Women should be advised to avoid becoming pregnant while on Tasigna. If this drug is used during pregnancy, or if the patient becomes pregnant while taking this drug, the patient should be apprised of the potential hazard to the fetus.

Animal Data

Nilotinib was studied for effects on embryo-fetal development in pregnant rats and rabbits given oral doses of 10, 30, 100 mg/kg/day, and 30, 100, 300 mg/kg/day, respectively, during organogenesis. In rats, nilotinib at doses of 100 mg/kg/day (approximately 5.7 times the AUC in patients at the dose of 400 mg twice daily) was associated with maternal toxicity (decreased gestation weight, gravid uterine weight, net weight gain, and food consumption). Nilotinib at doses ≥30 mg/kg/day (approximately 2 times the AUC in patients at the dose of 400 mg twice daily) resulted in embryo-fetal toxicity as shown by increased resorption and post-implantation loss, and at 100 mg/kg/day, a decrease in viable fetuses. In rabbits, maternal toxicity at 300 mg/kg/day (approximately one-half the human exposure based on AUC) was associated with mortality, abortion, decreased gestation weights and decreased food consumption. Embryonic toxicity (increased resorption) and minor skeletal anomalies were observed at a dose of 300 mg/kg/day. Nilotinib is not considered teratogenic.

When pregnant rats were dosed with nilotinib during organogenesis and through lactation, the adverse effects included a longer gestational period, lower pup body weights until weaning and decreased fertility indices in the pups when they reached maturity, all at a maternal dose of 360 mg/m^2 (approximately 0.7 times the clinical dose of 400 mg twice daily based on body surface area). At doses up to 120 mg/m^2 (approximately 0.25 times the clinical dose of 400 mg twice daily based on body surface area) no adverse effects were seen in the maternal animals or the pups.

8.3 Nursing Mothers

It is not known whether nilotinib is excreted in human milk. One study in lactating rats demonstrates that nilotinib is excreted into milk. Because many drugs are excreted in human milk and because of the potential for serious adverse reactions in nursing infants from Tasigna, a decision should be made whether to discontinue nursing or to discontinue the drug, taking into account the importance of the drug to the mother.

8.4 Pediatric Use

The safety and effectiveness of Tasigna in pediatric patients have not been established.

8.5 Geriatric Use

In the clinical trials of Tasigna (patients with newly diagnosed Ph+ CML-CP and resistant or intolerant Ph+ CML-CP and CML-AP), approximately 12% and 30% of patients were 65 years or over respectively.

• Patients with newly diagnosed Ph+ CML-CP: There was no difference in major molecular response between patients aged <65 years and those ≥65 years.

• Patients with resistant or intolerant CML-CP: There was no difference in major cytogenetic response rate between patients aged <65 years and those ≥65 years.

• Patients with resistant or intolerant CML-AP: The hematologic response rate was 44% in patients <65 years of age and 29% in patients ≥65 years.

No major differences for safety were observed in patients ≥65 years of age as compared to patients <65 years.

8.6 Cardiac Disorders

In the clinical trials, patients with a history of uncontrolled or significant cardiovascular disease, including recent myocardial infarction, congestive heart failure, unstable angina or clinically significant bradycardia, were excluded. Caution should be exercised in patients with relevant cardiac disorders [see Boxed Warning, Warnings and Precautions (5.2)].

8.7 Hepatic Impairment

Nilotinib exposure is increased in patients with impaired hepatic function. In a study of subjects with mild to severe hepatic impairment following a single dose administration of 200 mg of Tasigna, the mean AUC values were increased on average of 35%, 35%, and 56% in subjects with mild (Child-Pugh class A, score 5 to 6), moderate (Child-Pugh class B, score 7 to 9) and severe hepatic impairment (Child-Pugh class C, score 10 to 15), respectively, compared to a control group of subjects with normal hepatic function. Table 8 summarizes the Child-Pugh Liver Function Classification applied in this study. A lower starting dose is recommended in patients with hepatic impairment and the QT interval should be monitored closely in these patients [see Dosage and Administration (2.2), Warnings and Precautions (5.10)].

Table 8: Child-Pugh Liver Function Classification

Assessment	Degree of Abnormality	Score
Encephalopathy Grade	None	1
	1 or 2	2
	3 or 4	3
Ascites	Absent	1
	Slight	2
	Moderate	3
Total Bilirubin (mg/dL)	<2	1
	2-3	2
	>3	3
Serum Albumin (g/dL)	>3.5	1
	2.8-3.5	2
	<2.8	3
Prothrombin Time (seconds prolonged)	<4	1
	4-6	2
	>6	3

8.8 Renal Impairment

Clinical studies have not been performed in patients with impaired renal function. Clinical studies have excluded patients with serum creatinine concentration >1.5 times the upper limit of the normal range.

Since nilotinib and its metabolites are not renally excreted, a decrease in total body clearance is not anticipated in patients with renal impairment.

10 OVERDOSAGE

Overdose with nilotinib has been reported, where an unspecified number of Tasigna capsules were ingested in combination with alcohol and other drugs. Events included neutropenia, vomiting, and drowsiness. In the event of overdose, the patient should be observed and appropriate supportive treatment given.

11 DESCRIPTION

Tasigna (nilotinib) belongs to a pharmacologic class of drugs known as kinase inhibitors.

Nilotinib drug substance, a monohydrate monohydrochloride, is a white to slightly yellowish to slightly greenish yellow powder with the anhydrous molecular formula and weight, respectively, of $C_{28}H_{22}F_3N_7O$•HCl • H_2O and 584. The solubility of nilotinib in aqueous solutions decreases with increasing pH. Nilotinib is not optically active. The pK$_a$1 was determined to be 2.1; pK$_a$2 was estimated to be 5.4.

The chemical name of nilotinib is 4-methyl-N-[3-(4-methyl-1H-imidazol-1-yl)-5-(trifluoromethyl)phenyl]-3-[[4-(3-pyridinyl)-2-pyrimidinyl]amino]-benzamide, monohydrochloride, monohydrate. Its structure is shown below:

Tasigna (nilotinib) capsules, for oral use, contain 150 mg or 200 mg nilotinib base, anhydrous (as hydrochloride, monohydrate) with the following inactive ingredients: colloidal silicon dioxide, crospovidone, lactose monohydrate, magnesium stearate and poloxamer 188. The capsules contain gelatin, iron oxide (red), iron oxide (yellow), iron oxide (black), and titanium dioxide.

12 CLINICAL PHARMACOLOGY

12.1 Mechanism of Action

Nilotinib is an inhibitor of the BCR-ABL kinase. Nilotinib binds to and stabilizes the inactive conformation of the kinase domain of ABL protein. *In vitro*, nilotinib inhibited BCR-ABL mediated proliferation of murine leukemic cell lines and human cell lines derived from patients with Ph+ CML. Under the conditions of the assays, nilotinib was able to overcome imatinib resistance resulting from BCR-ABL kinase mutations, in 32 out of 33 mutations tested. *In vivo*, nilotinib reduced the tumor size in a murine BCR-ABL xenograft model. Nilotinib inhibited the autophosphorylation of the following kinases at IC50 values as indicated: BCR-ABL (20 to 60 nM), PDGFR (69 nM), c-KIT (210 nM), CSF-1R (125 to 250 nM), and DDR1 (3.7 nM).

12.3 Pharmacokinetics

Absorption and Distribution

The absolute bioavailability of nilotinib has not been determined. As compared to an oral drink solution (pH of 1.2 to 1.3), relative bioavailability of nilotinib capsule is approximately 50%. Peak concentrations of nilotinib are reached 3 hours after oral administration.

Steady-state nilotinib exposure was dose-dependent with less than dose-proportional increases in systemic exposure at dose levels higher than 400 mg given as once daily dosing. Daily serum exposure to nilotinib following 400 mg twice daily dosing at steady state was 35% higher than with 800 mg once daily dosing. Steady state exposure (AUC) of nilotinib with 400 mg twice daily dosing was 13% higher than with 300 mg twice daily dosing. The average steady state nilotinib trough and peak concentrations did not change over 12 months. There was no relevant increase in exposure to nilotinib when the dose was increased from 400 mg twice daily to 600 mg twice daily.

The bioavailability of nilotinib was increased when given with a meal. Compared to the fasted state, the systemic exposure (AUC) increased by 82% when the dose was given 30 minutes after a high fat meal.

Single dose administration of two 200 mg nilotinib capsules each dispersed in 1 teaspoon of applesauce and administered within 15 minutes was shown to be bioequivalent to a single dose administration of two 200 mg intact capsules. The blood-to-serum ratio of nilotinib is 0.68. Serum protein binding is approximately 98% on the basis of *in vitro* experiments.

Median steady-state trough concentration of nilotinib was decreased by 53% in patients with total gastrectomy compared to patients who had not undergone surgeries [see Warnings and Precautions (5.12)].

Pharmacokinetics, Metabolism and Excretion

The apparent elimination half-life estimated from the multiple dose pharmacokinetic studies with daily dosing was approximately 17 hours. Inter-patient variability in nilotinib AUC was 32% to 64%. Steady state conditions were achieved by Day 8. An increase in serum exposure to nilotinib between the first dose and steady state was approximately 2-fold for daily dosing and 3.8-fold for twice-daily dosing.

Main metabolic pathways identified in healthy subjects are oxidation and hydroxylation. Nilotinib is the main circulating component in the serum. None of the metabolites contribute significantly to the pharmacological activity of nilotinib.

After a single dose of radiolabeled nilotinib in healthy subjects, more than 90% of the administered dose was eliminated within 7 days: mainly in feces (93% of the dose). Parent drug accounted for 69% of the dose.

Age, body weight, gender, or ethnic origin did not significantly affect the pharmacokinetics of nilotinib.

Drug-Drug Interactions

In a Phase 1 trial of nilotinib 400 mg twice daily in combination with imatinib 400 mg daily or 400 mg twice daily, the AUC increased 30% to 50% for nilotinib and approximately 20% for imatinib.

12.5 Pharmacogenomics

Tasigna can increase bilirubin levels. A pharmacogenetic analysis of 97 patients evaluated the polymorphisms of UGT1A1 and its potential association with hyperbilirubinemia during Tasigna treatment. In this study, the (TA)7/(TA)7 genotype was associated with a statistically significant increase in the risk of hyperbilirubinemia relative to the (TA)6/(TA)6 and (TA)6/(TA)7 genotypes. However, the largest increases in bilirubin were observed in the (TA)7/(TA)7 genotype (UGT1A1*28) patients [see *Warnings and Precautions (5.6)*].

12.6 QT/QTc Prolongation

In a placebo-controlled study in healthy volunteers designed to assess the effects of Tasigna on the QT interval, administration of Tasigna was associated with concentration-dependent QT prolongation; the maximum mean placebo-adjusted QTcF change from baseline was 18 msec (1-sided 95% Upper CI: 26 msec). A positive control was not included in the QT study of healthy volunteers. Peak plasma concentrations in the QT study were 26% lower than those observed in patients enrolled in the single-arm study [see *Boxed Warning, Warnings and Precautions (5.2), and Adverse Reactions (6.1)*].

13 NONCLINICAL TOXICOLOGY

13.1 Carcinogenesis, Mutagenesis, Impairment of Fertility

A 2-year carcinogenicity study was conducted orally in rats at nilotinib doses of 5, 15, and 40 mg/kg/day. Exposures in animals at the highest dose tested were approximately 2 to 3 fold the human exposure (based on AUC) at the nilotinib dose of 400 mg twice daily. The study was negative for carcinogenic findings.

Nilotinib was not mutagenic in a bacterial mutagenesis (Ames) assay, was not clastogenic in a chromosome aberration assay in human lymphocytes, did not induce DNA damage (comet assay) in L5178Y mouse lymphoma cells, nor was it clastogenic in an *in vivo* rat bone marrow micronucleus assay with two oral treatments at doses up to 2000 mg/kg/dose.

There were no effects on male or female rat and female rabbit mating or fertility at doses up to 180 mg/kg in rats (approximately 4 to 7 fold for males and females, respectively, the AUC in patients at the dose of 400 mg twice daily) or 300 mg/kg in rabbits (approximately one-half the AUC in patients at the dose of 400 mg twice daily). The effect of Tasigna on human fertility is unknown. In a study where male and female rats were treated with nilotinib at oral doses of 20 to 180 mg/kg/day (approximately 1 to 6.6 fold the AUC in patients at the dose of 400 mg twice daily) during the pre-mating and mating periods and then mated, and dosing of pregnant rats continued through gestation Day 6, nilotinib increased post-implantation loss and early resorption, and decreased the number of viable fetuses and litter size at all doses tested.

14 CLINICAL STUDIES

14.1 Newly Diagnosed Ph+ CML-CP

An open-label, multicenter, randomized trial was conducted to determine the efficacy of Tasigna versus imatinib tablets in adult patients with cytogenetically confirmed newly diagnosed Ph+ CML-CP. Patients were within 6 months of diagnosis and were previously untreated for CML-CP, except for hydroxyurea and/or anagrelide. Efficacy was based on a total of 846 patients: 283 patients in the imatinib 400 mg once daily group, 282 patients in the nilotinib 300 mg twice daily group, 281 patients in the nilotinib 400 mg twice daily group.

Median age was 46 years in the imatinib group and 47 years in both nilotinib groups, with 12%, 13%, and 10% of patients ≥65 years of age in imatinib 400 mg once daily, nilotinib 300 mg twice daily and nilotinib 400 mg twice daily treatment groups, respectively. There were slightly more male than female patients in all groups (56%, 56%, and 62% in imatinib 400 mg once daily, nilotinib 300 mg twice daily and nilotinib 400 mg twice daily treatment groups, respectively). More than 60% of all patients were Caucasian, and 25% were Asian.

The primary data analysis was performed when all 846 patients completed 12 months of treatment (or discontinued earlier). Subsequent analyses were done when patients completed 24, 36, and 48 months of treatment (or discontinued earlier). The median time on treatment was approxi-

mately 48 months in all three treatment groups. This study is on-going and further data will be required to determine long-term outcome.

The primary efficacy endpoint was major molecular response (MMR) at 12 months after the start of study medication. MMR was defined as ≤0.1% BCR-ABL/ABL % by international scale measured by RQ-PCR, which corresponds to a ≥3 log reduction of BCR-ABL transcript from standardized baseline. Efficacy endpoints are summarized in Table 9 below.

Three patients in the nilotinib arm progressed to either accelerated phase (including clonal evolution) or blast crisis (2 within the first 6 months of treatment and 1 within 36 to 48 months while 17 patients on the imatinib arm progressed to either accelerated phase (including clonal evolution) or blast crisis (8 patients within first 6 months, 4 within 6 to 12 months, 4 within 12 to 18 months and 1 within 18 to 24 months).

Table 9: Efficacy (MMR and CCyR) of TASIGNA Compared to Imatinib in Newly Diagnosed Ph+ CML-CP

	TASIGNA 300 mg twice daily	Imatinib 400 mg once daily
	N = 282	N = 283
MMR at 12 months (95% CI)	44% (38.4, 50.3)	22% (17.6, 27.6)
P-Value[a]	<0.0001	
CCyR[b] by 12 months (95% CI)	80% (75.0, 84.6)	65% (59.2, 70.6)
MMR at 24 months (95% CI)	62% (55.8, 67.4)	38% (31.8, 43.4)
CCyR[b] by 24 months (95% CI)	87% (82.4, 90.6)	77% (71.7, 81.8)

[a]CMH test stratified by Sokal risk group
[b]CCyR: 0% Ph+ metaphases. Cytogenetic responses were based on the percentage of Ph-positive metaphases among ≥20 metaphase cells in each bone marrow sample.

14.2 Patients with Resistant or Intolerant Ph+ CML-CP and CML-AP

A single-arm, open-label, multicenter study was conducted to evaluate the efficacy and safety of Tasigna (400 mg twice daily) in patients with imatinib-resistant or -intolerant CML with separate cohorts for chronic and accelerated phase disease. The definition of imatinib resistance included failure to achieve a complete hematologic response (by 3 months), cytogenetic response (by 6 months) or major cytogenetic response (by 12 months) or progression of disease after a previous cytogenetic or hematologic response. Imatinib intolerance was defined as discontinuation of treatment due to toxicity and lack of a major cytogenetic response at time of study entry. At the time of data cut-off, 321 patients with CML-CP and 137 patients with CML-AP with a minimum follow-up of 24 months were enrolled. In this study, about 50% of CML-CP and CML-AP patients were males, over 90% (CML-CP) and 80% (CML-AP) were Caucasian, and approximately 30% were age 65 years or older.

Overall, 73% of patients were imatinib resistant while 27% were imatinib intolerant. The median time of prior imatinib treatment was approximately 32 (CML-CP) and 28 (CML-AP) months. Prior therapy included hydroxyurea in 85% of patients, interferon in 56% and stem cell or bone marrow transplant in 8%. The median highest prior imatinib dose was 600 mg/day for patients with CML-CP and CML-AP, and the highest prior imatinib dose was ≥600 mg/day in 74% of all patients with 40% of patients receiving imatinib doses ≥800 mg/day.

Median duration of nilotinib treatment was 18.4 months in patients with CML-CP and 8.7 months in patients with CML-AP.

The efficacy endpoint in CML-CP was unconfirmed major cytogenetic response (MCyR) which included complete and partial cytogenetic responses.

The efficacy endpoint in CML-AP was confirmed hematologic response (HR), defined as either a complete hematologic response (CHR) or no evidence of leukemia (NEL). The rates of response for CML-CP and CML-AP patients are reported in Table 10.

Median durations of response had not been reached at the time of data analysis.

Table 10: Efficacy of Tasigna in Resistant or Intolerant Ph+ CML-CP and CML-AP

Cytogenetic Response Rate (Unconfirmed) (%)[a]	Chronic Phase (n = 321)
Major (95% CI)	51% (46% - 57%)
Complete (95% CI)	37% (32% - 42%)
Partial (95% CI)	15% (11% – 19%)
	Accelerated Phase (n = 137)
Hematologic Response Rate (Confirmed) (95% CI)[b]	39% (31% - 48%)
Complete Hematologic Response Rate (95% CI)	30% (22% - 38%)
No Evidence of Leukemia (95% CI)	9% (5% -16%)

[a]Cytogenetic response criteria: Complete (0% Ph + metaphases) or partial (1% to 35%). Cytogenetic responses were based on the percentage of Ph-positive metaphases among ≥20 metaphase cells in each bone marrow sample.
[b]Hematologic response=CHR + NEL (all responses confirmed after 4 weeks).
CHR (CML-CP): WBC <10 × 10⁹/L, platelets <450,000/mm³, no blasts or promyelocytes in peripheral blood, <5% myelocytes + metamyelocytes in bone marrow, <20% basophils in peripheral blood, and no extramedullary involvement.
CHR (CML-AP): neutrophils ≥1.5 x 10⁹/L, platelets ≥100 × 10⁹/L, no myeloblasts in peripheral blood, myeloblasts <5% in bone marrow, and no extramedullary involvement.
NEL: same criteria as for CHR but neutrophils ≥1.0 × 10⁹/L and platelets >20 × 10⁹/L without transfusions or bleeding.

Patients with Chronic Phase

The MCyR rate in 321 CML-CP patients was 51%. The median time to MCyR among responders was 2.8 months (range 1 to 28 months). The median duration of MCyR cannot be estimated. The median duration of exposure on this single arm-trial was 18.4 months. Among the CML-CP patients who achieved MCyR, 62% of them had MCyR lasting more than 18 months. The CCyR rate was 37%.

Patients with Accelerated Phase

The overall confirmed hematologic response rate in 137 patients with CML-AP was 39%. The median time to first hematologic response among responders was 1 month (range 1 to 14 months). Among the CML-AP patients who achieved HR, 44% of them had a response lasting for more than 18 months.

After imatinib failure, 24 different BCR-ABL mutations were noted in 42% of chronic phase and 54% of accelerated phase CML patients who were evaluated for mutations.

16 HOW SUPPLIED/STORAGE AND HANDLING

Tasigna (nilotinib) 150 mg capsules are red opaque hard gelatin capsules, size 1 with black axial imprint "NVR/BCR". Tasigna (nilotinib) 200 mg capsules are light yellow opaque hard gelatin capsules, size 0 with the red axial imprint "NVR/TKI." Tasigna capsules are supplied in blister packs.

150 mg

Carton of 4 blister packs of (4x28).....	NDC 0078-0592-87
Blisters of 28 capsules	NDC 0078-0592-51

200 mg

Carton of 4 blister packs of (4x28).....	NDC 0078-0526-87
Blisters of 28 capsules	NDC 0078-0526-51

Tasigna (nilotinib) capsules should be stored at 25°C (77°F); excursions permitted between 15° to 30°C (59° to 86°F) [see USP Controlled Room Temperature].

17 PATIENT COUNSELING INFORMATION

See FDA-Approved Patient Labeling (Medication Guide). A Medication Guide is required for distribution with Tasigna. Encourage patients to read the Tasigna Medication Guide. The complete text of the Medication Guide is reprinted at the end of this document.

Cardiac and Vascular Events

Advise patients that cardiovascular events (including ischemic heart disease, peripheral arterial occlusive disease, and ischemic cerebrovascular events) have been reported. Advise patients to seek immediate medical attention with any symptoms suggestive of a cardiovascular event. Cardiovascular status of patients should be evaluated and cardiovascular risk factors should be monitored and managed during Tasigna therapy according to standard guidelines [see *Warnings and Precautions (5.4)*].

Taking Tasigna

Advise patients to take Tasigna doses twice daily approximately 12 hours apart. The capsules should be swallowed whole with water.

Advise patients to take Tasigna on an empty stomach. No food should be consumed for at least 2 hours before the dose is taken and for at least 1 hour after the dose is taken. Patients should not consume grapefruit products and other foods that are known to inhibit CYP3A4 at any time during Tasigna treatment *[see Dosage and Administration (2.1), Warnings and Precautions (5.8, 5.9) and Medication Guide]*. If the patient missed a dose of Tasigna, the patient should take the next scheduled dose at its regular time. The patient should not take two doses at the same time.

Should patients be unable to swallow capsules, the contents of each capsule can be dispersed in one teaspoon of applesauce and the mixture swallowed immediately (within 15 minutes).

Drug Interactions

Tasigna and certain other medicines, including over the counter medications or herbal supplements (such as St. John's Wort), can interact with each other *[see Warnings and Precautions (5.8) and Drug Interactions (7)]*.

Pregnancy

Advise patients that the use of Tasigna during pregnancy may cause harm to the fetus and that Tasigna should not be taken during pregnancy unless necessary. Women of childbearing potential should use highly effective contraceptives while taking Tasigna. Sexually active female patients taking Tasigna should use adequate contraception *[see Warnings and Precautions (5.15) and Use in Specific Populations (8.1)]*.

Compliance

Advise patients of the following:
- Continue taking Tasigna every day for as long as their doctor tells them.
- This is a long-term treatment.
- Do not change dose or stop taking Tasigna without first consulting their doctor.
- If a dose is missed, take the next dose as scheduled. Do not take a double dose to make up for the missed capsules.

T2014-02
January 2014

Medication Guide
TASIGNA® (ta-sig-na)
(nilotinib)
Capsules

Read this Medication Guide before you start taking TASIGNA and each time you get a refill. There may be new information. This information does not take the place of talking to your doctor about your medical condition or treatment.

What is the most important information I should know about Tasigna?

Tasigna can cause a possible life-threatening heart problem called QTc prolongation. QTc prolongation causes an irregular heartbeat, which may lead to sudden death.

Your doctor should check the electrical activity of your heart with a test called an electrocardiogram (ECG):
- before starting Tasigna
- 7 days after starting Tasigna
- with any dose changes
- regularly during Tasigna treatment

You may lower your chances for having QTc prolongation with Tasigna if you:
- **Take Tasigna on an empty stomach:**
  - Avoid eating food for at least 2 hours before the dose is taken, and
  - Avoid eating food for at least 1 hour after the dose is taken.
- Avoid grapefruit, grapefruit juice, and any supplement containing grapefruit extract while taking Tasigna. Food and grapefruit products increase the amount of Tasigna in your body.
- Avoid taking other medicines or supplements with Tasigna that can also cause QTc prolongation.
- Tasigna can interact with many medicines and supplements and increase your chance for serious and life-threatening side effects.
- Do not take any other medicine while taking Tasigna unless your doctor tells you it is okay to do so.
- If you cannot swallow Tasigna capsules whole, you may open the Tasigna capsule and sprinkle the contents of each capsule in 1 teaspoon of applesauce (puréed apple). Swallow the mixture right away (within 15 minutes). For more information, see "How should I take Tasigna?"

Call your doctor right away if you feel lightheaded, faint, or have an irregular heartbeat while taking Tasigna. These can be symptoms of QTc prolongation.

What is Tasigna?

Tasigna is a prescription medicine used to treat a type of leukemia called Philadelphia chromosome positive chronic myeloid leukemia (Ph+ CML) in adults who:

- are newly diagnosed, **or**
- are no longer benefiting from previous other treatments, including treatment with imatinib (Gleevec®), **or**
- have taken other treatments, including imatinib (Gleevec), and cannot tolerate them

It is not known if Tasigna is safe and effective in children.

Who should not take Tasigna?

Do not take if you have:
- low levels of potassium or magnesium in your blood
- long QTc syndrome

What should I tell my doctor before starting Tasigna?

Before taking Tasigna, tell your doctor about all of your medical conditions, including if you have:
- heart problems
- had a stroke or other problems due to decreased blood flow to the brain
- problems with decreased blood flow to your legs
- irregular heartbeat
- QTc prolongation or a family history of it
- liver problems
- had pancreatitis
- low blood levels of potassium or magnesium in your blood
- a severe problem with lactose (milk sugar) or other sugars. Tasigna capsules contain lactose. Most patients who have mild or moderate lactose intolerance can take Tasigna.
- had a surgical procedure involving the removal of the entire stomach (total gastrectomy)
- are pregnant or plan to become pregnant. Tasigna may harm your unborn baby. If you are able to become pregnant, you should use effective birth control during treatment with Tasigna. Talk to your doctor about the best birth control methods to prevent pregnancy while you are taking Tasigna.
- are breastfeeding or plan to breastfeed. It is not known if Tasigna passes into your breast milk. You and your doctor should decide if you will take Tasigna or breastfeed. You should not do both.

Tell your doctor about all the medicines you take, including prescription and nonprescription medicines, vitamins and herbal supplements.

If you need to take antacids (medicines to treat heartburn) do not take them at the same time that you take Tasigna. If you take:
- **a medicine to block the amount of acid produced in the stomach (H₂ blocker):** Take these medicines **about 10 hours before** you take Tasigna, **or about 2 hours after** you take Tasigna.
- **an antacid that contains aluminum hydroxide, magnesium hydroxide, and simethicone to reduce the amount of acid in the stomach:** Take these medicines **about 2 hours before or about 2 hours after** you take Tasigna.

Tasigna can interact with many medicines and supplements and increase your chance for serious and life-threatening side effects. **See "What is the most important information I should know about Tasigna?"**

Know the medicines you take. Keep a list of them and show it to your doctor and pharmacist when you get a new medicine.

How should I take Tasigna?
- Take Tasigna exactly as your doctor tells you to take it. Do not change your dose or stop taking Tasigna unless your doctor tells you.
- Tasigna is a long-term treatment.
- Your doctor will tell you how many Tasigna capsules to take and when to take them.
- **Tasigna must be taken on an empty stomach.**
  - **Avoid eating food for at least 2 hours before the dose is taken, and**
  - **Avoid eating food for at least 1 hour after the dose is taken.**
- Swallow Tasigna capsules whole with water. If you cannot swallow Tasigna capsules whole, tell your doctor.
- **If you cannot swallow Tasigna capsules whole:**
  - Open the Tasigna capsules and sprinkle the contents in 1 teaspoon of applesauce (puréed apple).
    - Do not use more than 1 teaspoon of applesauce.
    - Only use applesauce. Do not sprinkle Tasigna onto other foods.
  - Swallow the mixture right away (within 15 minutes).
- Do not drink grapefruit juice, eat grapefruit, or take supplements containing grapefruit extract at any time during treatment. **See "What is the most important information I should know about Tasigna?"**
- If you miss a dose, just take your next dose at your regular time. Do not take 2 doses at the same time to make up for a missed dose.
- If you take too much Tasigna, call your doctor or poison control center right away. Symptoms may include vomiting and drowsiness. During treatment with Tasigna your doctor will do tests to check for side effects and to see how well Tasigna is working for you. The tests will check your:
  - heart
  - blood cells (white blood cells, red blood cells, and platelets). Your blood cells should be checked every 2 weeks for the first 2 months and then monthly.
  - electrolytes (potassium, magnesium)
  - pancreas and liver function
  - bone marrow samples
- Your doctor may change your dose. Your doctor may have you stop Tasigna for some time or lower your dose if you have side effects with it.

What are the possible side effects of Tasigna?

Tasigna may cause serious side effects including:
- See "What is the most important information I should know about Tasigna?"
- **Decreased blood flow to the leg, heart, or brain.** People who have recently been diagnosed with Ph+ CML and take Tasigna may develop decreased blood flow to the leg, the heart, or brain.

  Get medical help right away if you suddenly develop any of the following symptoms:
  - chest pain or discomfort
  - numbness or weakness
  - problems walking or speaking
  - leg pain
  - your leg feels cold
  - change in the skin color of your leg
- **Low blood counts.** Low blood counts are common with Tasigna. Your doctor will check your blood counts regularly during treatment with Tasigna. Symptoms of low blood counts include:
  - unexplained bleeding or bruising
  - blood in urine or stool
  - unexplained weakness
- **Liver problems.** Symptoms include yellow skin and eyes.
- **Pancreas inflammation (pancreatitis).** Symptoms include sudden stomach area pain with nausea and vomiting.
- **Bleeding in the brain.** Symptoms include sudden headache, changes in your eyesight, not being aware of what is going on around you and becoming unconscious.
- **Tumor Lysis Syndrome (TLS).** TLS is caused by a fast breakdown of cancer cells. TLS can cause you to have:
  - kidney failure and the need for dialysis treatment
  - an abnormal heart beat

Your doctor may do blood tests to check you for TLS.

The most common side effects of Tasigna include:
- low blood count
- nausea
- rash
- headache
- tiredness
- itching
- vomiting
- diarrhea
- cough
- constipation
- muscle and joint pain
- runny or stuffy nose, sneezing, sore throat
- fever
- night sweats

Tell your doctor if you have any side effect that bothers you or does not go away.

These are not all of the possible side effects of Tasigna. For more information, ask your doctor or pharmacist.

Call your doctor for medical advice about side effects. You may report side effects to FDA at 1-800-FDA-1088.

How should I store Tasigna?
- Store Tasigna at room temperature between 68°F to 77°F (20°C to 25°C).
- Safely throw away medicine that is out of date or no longer needed.
- **Keep Tasigna and all medicines out of the reach of children.**

General information about Tasigna

Medicines are sometimes prescribed for purposes other than those listed in a Medication Guide. Do not use Tasigna for a condition for which it was not prescribed. Do not give Tasigna to other people, even if they have the same problem you have. It may harm them.

This Medication Guide summarizes the most important information about Tasigna. If you would like more information, talk with your doctor. You can ask your doctor or pharmacist for information about Tasigna that is written for health professionals.

For more information, go to www.us.tasigna.com or call 1-866-411-8274.

What are the ingredients in Tasigna?

Active ingredient: nilotinib

Inactive ingredients: colloidal silicon dioxide, crospovidone, lactose monohydrate, magnesium stearate and poloxamer 188.

The capsule shell contains gelatin, iron oxide (red), iron oxide (yellow), iron oxide (black), and titanium dioxide.

This Medication Guide has been approved by the U.S. Food and Drug Administration.

Manufactured by:
Novartis Pharma Stein AG
Stein, Switzerland
Distributed by:
Novartis Pharmaceuticals Corporation
East Hanover, New Jersey 07936
Revised: January 2014
© Novartis
T2014-03
January 2014

Shown in Product Identification Guide, page 311

TEKAMLO
[tĕk'-ăm-lō]
(aliskiren and amlodipine)
tablets, for oral use

The following prescribing information is based on official labeling in effect July 2014.

HIGHLIGHTS OF PRESCRIBING INFORMATION
These highlights do not include all the information needed to use TEKAMLO safely and effectively. See full prescribing information for TEKAMLO.

Tekamlo (aliskiren and amlodipine) tablets, for oral use
Initial U.S. Approval: 2010

> **WARNING: FETAL TOXICITY**
> *See full prescribing information for complete boxed warning.*
> • When pregnancy is detected, discontinue Tekamlo as soon as possible. (5.1)
> • Drugs that act directly on the renin-angiotensin system can cause injury and death to the developing fetus. (5.1)

RECENT MAJOR CHANGES
Warnings and Precautions (5.4)   11/2013

INDICATIONS AND USAGE
Tekamlo is a combination of aliskiren, a renin inhibitor, and amlodipine, a dihydropyridine calcium channel blocker, indicated for the treatment of hypertension, to lower blood pressure:
• As initial therapy in patients likely to need multiple drugs to achieve their blood pressure goals. (1)
• In patients not adequately controlled with monotherapy. (1)
• As a substitute for its titrated components. (1)

Lowering blood pressure reduces the risk of fatal and nonfatal cardiovascular events, primarily strokes and myocardial infarctions.

DOSAGE AND ADMINISTRATION
• Add-on therapy or initial therapy: Initiate with 150 mg/5 mg. Titrate as needed up to a maximum of 300 mg/10 mg. (2.1, 2.2)
• The blood pressure lowering effect is largely attained within 1-2 weeks. (2.1)
• Replacement therapy: may substitute for titrated components. (2.3)
• Administer one tablet daily with a routine pattern with regard to meals. (2.5)

DOSAGE FORMS AND STRENGTHS
Tablets (aliskiren/amlodipine): 150 mg/5 mg, 150 mg/10 mg, 300 mg/5 mg, 300 mg/10 mg. (3)

CONTRAINDICATIONS
Do not use with angiotensin receptor blockers (ARBs) or ACE inhibitors (ACEIs) in patients with diabetes (4)
Known hypersensitivity to any component (4)

WARNINGS AND PRECAUTIONS
• Avoid concomitant use with ARBs or ACEI in patients with renal impairment (GFR<60 mL/min) (5.2)
• Anaphylactic Reactions and Head and Neck Angioedema: Discontinue Tekamlo and monitor until signs and symptoms resolve. (5.3)
• Hypotension in volume- and/or salt-depleted patients or with combined use of other agents acting on RAAS: Correct imbalances before initiating therapy with Tekamlo. (5.4)
• Increased angina or myocardial infarction with calcium channel blockers may occur upon dosage initiation or increase. (5.5)
• Impaired renal function: Monitor serum creatinine periodically. (5.6)
• Hyperkalemia: Monitor potassium levels periodically. (5.8)

ADVERSE REACTIONS
The most common adverse event (incidence ≥2 % and more common than with placebo) is peripheral edema. (6.1)

To report SUSPECTED ADVERSE REACTIONS, contact Novartis Pharmaceuticals Corporation at 1-888-669-6682 or FDA at 1-800-FDA-1088 or www.fda.gov/medwatch.

DRUG INTERACTIONS
• Cyclosporine: Avoid concomitant use (7, 12.3)
• Itraconazole: Avoid concomitant use (7, 12.3)
• NSAIDs use may lead to increased risk of renal impairment and loss of antihypertensive effect (7)
• If simvastatin is co-administered with amlodipine, do not exceed doses greater than 20 mg daily of simvastatin (7)

USE IN SPECIFIC POPULATIONS
Nursing Mothers: Discontinue drug or nursing. (8.3)

See 17 for PATIENT COUNSELING INFORMATION and FDA-approved patient labeling

Revised: 3/2014

FULL PRESCRIBING INFORMATION: CONTENTS*
WARNING: FETAL TOXICITY
1 INDICATIONS AND USAGE
2 DOSAGE AND ADMINISTRATION
  2.1 General Considerations
  2.2 Add-on Therapy
  2.3 Replacement Therapy
  2.4 Use with Other Antihypertensive Drugs
  2.5 Relationship to Meals
3 DOSAGE FORMS AND STRENGTHS
4 CONTRAINDICATIONS
5 WARNINGS AND PRECAUTIONS
  5.1 Fetal Toxicity
  5.2 Renal Impairment/Hyperkalemia/Hypotension when Tekamlo is given in combination with ARBs or ACEIs
  5.3 Anaphylactic Reactions and Head and Neck Angioedema
  5.4 Hypotension
  5.5 Risk of Myocardial Infarction or Increased Angina
  5.6 Impaired Renal Function
  5.7 Cyclosporine or Itraconazole
  5.8 Hyperkalemia
6 ADVERSE REACTIONS
  6.1 Clinical Studies Experience
  6.2 Post-marketing Experience
7 DRUG INTERACTIONS
8 USE IN SPECIFIC POPULATIONS
  8.1 Pregnancy
  8.3 Nursing Mothers
  8.4 Pediatric Use
  8.5 Geriatric Use
  8.6 Hepatic Impairment
  8.7 Renal Impairment
10 OVERDOSAGE
11 DESCRIPTION
12 CLINICAL PHARMACOLOGY
  12.1 Mechanism of Action
  12.2 Pharmacodynamics
  12.3 Pharmacokinetics
13 NONCLINICAL TOXICOLOGY
  13.1 Carcinogenesis, Mutagenesis, Impairment of Fertility
  13.2 Animal Toxicology and/or Pharmacology
14 CLINICAL STUDIES
  14.1 Tekamlo
  14.2 Aliskiren in Patients with Diabetes treated with ARB or ACEI (ALTITUDE study)
16 HOW SUPPLIED/STORAGE AND HANDLING
17 PATIENT COUNSELING INFORMATION
* Sections or subsections omitted from the full prescribing information are not listed

FULL PRESCRIBING INFORMATION

> **WARNING: FETAL TOXICITY**
> • When pregnancy is detected, discontinue Tekamlo as soon as possible. (5.1)
> • Drugs that act directly on the renin-angiotensin system can cause injury and death to the developing fetus. (5.1)

1 INDICATIONS AND USAGE
Tekamlo is indicated for the treatment of hypertension, alone or with other antihypertensive agents, to lower blood pressure. Lowering blood pressure reduces the risk of fatal and nonfatal cardiovascular events, primarily strokes and myocardial infarctions. These benefits have been seen in controlled trials of antihypertensive drugs from a wide variety of pharmacologic classes including amlodipine. There are no controlled trials demonstrating risk reduction with Tekamlo.

Control of high blood pressure should be part of comprehensive cardiovascular risk management, including, as appropriate, lipid control, diabetes management, antithrombotic therapy, smoking cessation, exercise, and limited sodium intake. Many patients will require more than one drug to achieve blood pressure goals. For specific advice on goals and management, see published guidelines, such as those of the National High Blood Pressure Education Program's Joint National Committee on Prevention, Detection, Evaluation, and Treatment of High Blood Pressure (JNC).

Numerous antihypertensive drugs, from a variety of pharmacologic classes and with different mechanisms of action, have been shown in randomized controlled trials to reduce cardiovascular morbidity and mortality, and it can be concluded that it is blood pressure reduction, and not some other pharmacologic property of the drugs, that is largely responsible for those benefits. The largest and most consistent cardiovascular outcome benefit has been a reduction in

---

the risk of stroke, but reductions in myocardial infarction and cardiovascular mortality also have been seen regularly. Elevated systolic or diastolic pressure causes increased cardiovascular risk, and the absolute risk increase per mmHg is greater at higher blood pressures, so that even modest reductions of severe hypertension can provide substantial benefit. Relative risk reduction from blood pressure reduction is similar across populations with varying absolute risk, so the absolute benefit is greater in patients who are at higher risk independent of their hypertension (for example, patients with diabetes or hyperlipidemia), and such patients would be expected to benefit from more aggressive treatment to a lower blood pressure goal.

Some antihypertensive drugs have smaller blood pressure effects (as monotherapy) in black patients, and many antihypertensive drugs have additional approved indications and effects (e.g., on angina, heart failure, or diabetic kidney disease). These considerations may guide selection of therapy.

Data from the high-dose multifactorial study *[see Clinical Studies (14)]* provide estimates of the probability of reaching a target blood pressure with Tekamlo compared to aliskiren or amlodipine monotherapy. The figures below provide estimates of the likelihood of achieving systolic or diastolic blood pressure control with Tekamlo 300 mg/10 mg, based upon baseline systolic or diastolic blood pressure. The curve of each treatment group was estimated by logistic regression modeling. The estimated likelihood at the right tail of each curve is less reliable because of a small number of subjects with high baseline blood pressures.

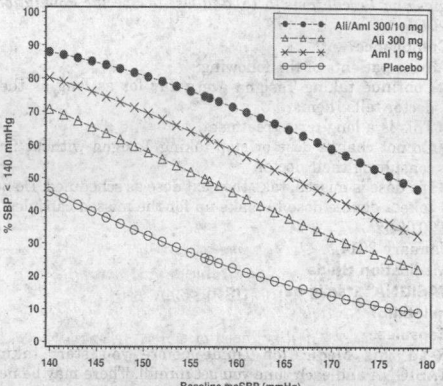

Figure 1: Probability of Achieving Systolic Blood Pressure (SBP) <140 mmHg

Figure 2: Probability of Achieving Diastolic Blood Pressure (DBP) <90 mmHg

[See figure 3 at top of next column]
[See figure 4 at top of next column]
The figures above provide an approximation of the likelihood of reaching a targeted blood pressure goal (e.g. SBP<140 mmHg or <130 mmHg) for the high dose groups evaluated in the study. At all levels of baseline blood pressure, the probability of achieving any given diastolic or systolic goal is greater with the combination than for either monotherapy. For example, the mean baseline SBP/DBP for patients participating in this multifactorial study was 157/100 mmHg. A patient with a baseline blood pressure of 157/100 mmHg has about a 49% likelihood of achieving a goal of <140 mmHg (systolic) and 50% likelihood of achieving <90 mmHg (diastolic) on aliskiren alone, and the likelihood of achieving these goals on amlodipine alone is about 62% (systolic) and 69% (diastolic). The likelihood of achieving these goals on Tekamlo rises to about 74% (systolic) and

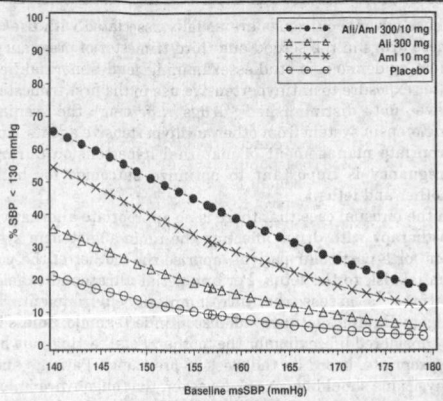

Figure 3: Probability of Achieving Systolic Blood Pressure (SBP) <130 mmHg

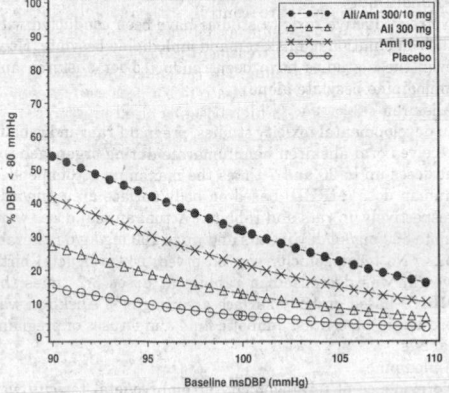

Figure 4: Probability of Achieving Diastolic Blood Pressure (DBP) <80 mmHg

83% (diastolic). The likelihood of achieving these goals on placebo is about 25% (systolic) and 27% (diastolic) [see Dosage and Administration (2) and Clinical Studies (14)].

2   DOSAGE AND ADMINISTRATION
2.1   General Considerations
The recommended initial once-daily dose of Tekamlo is 150 mg/5 mg. Titrate as needed to a maximum of 300 mg/10 mg.

The blood pressure lowering effects are largely attained within 1-2 weeks. If blood pressure remains uncontrolled after 2 to 4 weeks of therapy, titrate the dose to a maximum of Tekamlo 300 mg/10 mg once daily.

2.2   Add-on Therapy
Use Tekamlo for patients not adequately controlled with aliskiren alone or amlodipine besylate (or another dihydropyridine calcium channel blocker) alone.

Switch a patient who experiences dose-limiting adverse reactions on either component alone to Tekamlo containing a lower dose of that component in combination with the other to achieve similar blood pressure reductions.

2.3   Replacement Therapy
Switch patients receiving aliskiren and amlodipine besylate from separate tablets to a single tablet of Tekamlo containing the same component doses. When substituting for individual components, increase the dose of one or both of the components if blood pressure control has not been satisfactory.

2.4   Use with Other Antihypertensive Drugs
Tekamlo may be administered with some other antihypertensive agents. In diabetics, do not use in combination with angiotensin receptor blockers (ARBs) or angiotensin converting enzyme inhibitors (ACEIs) [see Contraindications (4)]. Concomitant use of aliskiren with an ARB or ACEI is not recommended in patients with GFR <60 ml/min [see Warnings and Precautions (5.2)]. It is not known whether Tekamlo decreases blood pressure further when added to maximum dosages of ACE inhibitors and beta blockers [see Clinical Studies (14)].

2.5   Relationship to Meals
Advise patients to establish a routine pattern for taking Tekamlo with regard to meals. High-fat meals decrease absorption substantially [see Clinical Pharmacology (12.3)].

3   DOSAGE FORMS AND STRENGTHS
- 150 mg aliskiren/5 mg amlodipine tablets: Non-scored light yellow, ovaloid convex shaped film-coated tablet with a beveled edge with debossing "T2" on one side and "NVR" on the reverse side of the tablet.

- 150 mg aliskiren/10 mg amlodipine tablets: Non-scored yellow, ovaloid convex shaped film-coated tablet with a beveled edge with debossing "T7" on one side and "NVR" on the reverse side of the tablet.
- 300 mg aliskiren/5 mg amlodipine tablets: Non-scored dark yellow, ovaloid convex shaped film-coated tablet with a beveled edge with debossing "T11" on one side and "NVR" on the reverse side of the tablet.
- 300 mg aliskiren/10 mg amlodipine tablets: Non-scored brown yellow, ovaloid convex shaped film-coated tablet with a beveled edge with debossing "T12" on one side and "NVR" on the reverse side of the tablet.

4   CONTRAINDICATIONS
Do not use aliskiren with ARBs or ACEIs in patients with diabetes [see Warnings and Precautions (5.2), Clinical Studies (14.2)].

Tekamlo is contraindicated in patients with known hypersensitivity to any of the components.

5   WARNINGS AND PRECAUTIONS
5.1   Fetal Toxicity
Pregnancy Category D

Use of drugs that act on the renin-angiotensin system during the second and third trimesters of pregnancy reduces fetal renal function and increases fetal and neonatal morbidity and death. Resulting oligohydramnios can be associated with fetal lung hypoplasia and skeletal deformations. Potential neonatal adverse effects include skull hypoplasia, anuria, hypotension, renal failure, and death. When pregnancy is detected, discontinue Tekamlo as soon as possible [see Use in Specific Populations (8.1)].

5.2   Renal   Impairment/Hyperkalemia/Hypotension when Tekamlo is given in combination with ARBs or ACEIs
Tekamlo is contraindicated in patients with diabetes who are receiving ARBs or ACEIs because of the increased risk of renal impairment, hyperkalemia, and hypotension [see Contraindications (4) and Clinical Studies (14.2)].

Avoid use of Tekamlo with ARBs or ACEIs in patients with moderate renal impairment (GFR <60 ml/min).

5.3   Anaphylactic Reactions and Head and Neck Angioedema
Aliskiren

Hypersensitivity reactions such as anaphylactic reactions and angioedema of the face, extremities, lips, tongue, glottis and/or larynx have been reported in patients treated with aliskiren and has necessitated hospitalization and intubation. This may occur at any time during treatment and has occurred in patients with and without a history of angioedema with ACE inhibitors or angiotensin receptor antagonists. Anaphylactic reactions have been reported from postmarketing experience with unknown frequency. If angioedema involves the throat, tongue, glottis or larynx, or if the patient has a history of upper respiratory surgery, airway obstruction may occur and be fatal. Patients who experience these effects, even without respiratory distress, require prolonged observation and appropriate monitoring measures since treatment with antihistamines and corticosteroids may not be sufficient to prevent respiratory involvement. Prompt administration of subcutaneous epinephrine solution 1:1000 (0.3 to 0.5 ml) and measures to ensure a patent airway may be necessary.

Discontinue Tekamlo immediately in patients who develop anaphylactic reactions or angioedema and do not readminister.

5.4   Hypotension
Symptomatic hypotension may occur after initiation of treatment with Tekamlo in patients with marked volume depletion, patients with salt depletion, or with combined use of aliskiren and other agents acting on the renin-angiotensin-aldosterone system. The volume or salt depletion should be corrected prior to administration of Tekamlo, or the treatment should start under close medical supervision.

A transient hypotensive response is not a contraindication to further treatment, which usually can be continued without difficulty once the blood pressure has stabilized.

Amlodipine besylate

Symptomatic hypotension is possible, particularly in patients with severe aortic stenosis. Because of the gradual onset of action, acute hypotension is unlikely.

5.5   Risk of Myocardial Infarction or Increased Angina
Worsening angina and acute myocardial infarction can develop after starting or increasing the dose of amlodipine, particularly with severe obstructive coronary artery disease.

5.6   Impaired Renal Function
Monitor renal function periodically in patients treated with Tekamlo. Changes in renal function, including acute renal failure, can be caused by drugs that affect the renin-angiotensin-aldosterone system. Patients whose renal function may depend in part on the activity of the renin-angiotensin-aldosterone system (e.g., patients with renal artery stenosis, severe heart failure, post-myocardial infarc-

tion or volume depletion) or patients receiving ARB, ACEI or non-steroidal anti-inflammatory (NSAID) therapy may be at particular risk for developing acute renal failure on Tekamlo [see Contraindications (4), Warnings and Precautions (5.2), Clinical Studies (14.2)]. Consider withholding or discontinuing therapy in patients who develop a clinically significant decrease in renal function.

5.7   Cyclosporine or Itraconazole
Aliskiren

When aliskiren was given with cyclosporine or itraconazole, the blood concentrations of aliskiren were significantly increased. Avoid concomitant use of aliskiren with cyclosporine or intraconazole [see Drug Interactions (7)].

5.8   Hyperkalemia
Aliskiren

Monitor serum potassium periodically in patients receiving aliskiren. Drugs that affect the renin-angiotensin-aldosterone system can cause hyperkalemia. Risk factors for the development of hyperkalemia include renal insufficiency, diabetes, combination use with ARBs or ACEI [see Contraindications (4), Warnings and Precautions (5.2), and Clinical Studies (14.2)], NSAIDs, or potassium supplements or potassium sparing diuretics.

6   ADVERSE REACTIONS
6.1   Clinical Studies Experience
The following serious adverse reactions are discussed in greater detail in other sections of the label:
- Risk of fetal/neonatal morbidity and mortality [see Warnings and Precautions (5.1)]
- Head and neck angioedema [see Warnings and Precautions (5.3)]
- Hypotension [see Warnings and Precautions (5.4)]

Because clinical trials are conducted under widely varying conditions, adverse reaction rates observed in the clinical trials of a drug cannot be directly compared to rates in clinical trials of another drug and may not reflect the rates observed in practice.

Tekamlo

Tekamlo has been evaluated for safety in more than 2800 patients, including 372 patients for 1 year or longer.

In a placebo-controlled study, there were 51% males, 62% Caucasians, 20% Blacks, 18% Hispanics, and 17% who were over 65 years of age. In this study, the overall incidence of adverse events on therapy with Tekamlo was similar to the individual components. Discontinuation of therapy due to a clinical adverse event in this study occurred in 1.7% of patients treated with Tekamlo (2.2% in the highest dose group) versus 1.5% of patients given placebo.

Peripheral edema is a known, dose-dependent adverse effect of amlodipine. The incidence of peripheral edema for Tekamlo in short-term double-blind placebo-controlled studies was lower than or equal to that of the corresponding amlodipine doses.

The adverse event in a placebo-controlled trial that occurred in at least 2% of patients treated with Tekamlo and at a higher incidence than placebo was peripheral edema (6.2% versus 1.0%). The incidence rate of peripheral edema at high dose was 8.9%.

In a long-term safety trial, the safety profile of adverse events was similar to that seen in the short-term controlled trials.

Aliskiren

Aliskiren has been evaluated for safety in 6460 patients, including 1740 treated for longer than 6 months, and 1250 for longer than 1 year. In placebo-controlled clinical trials, discontinuation of therapy because of a clinical adverse event, including uncontrolled hypertension, occurred in 2.2% of patients treated with aliskiren versus 3.5% of patients given placebo. These data do not include information from the ALTITUDE study which evaluated the use of aliskiren in combination with ARBs or ACEI [see Contraindications (4), Warnings and Precautions (5.2), and Clinical Studies (14.2)].

Two cases of angioedema with respiratory symptoms were reported with aliskiren use in the clinical studies. Two other cases of periorbital edema without respiratory symptoms were reported as possible angioedema and resulted in discontinuation. The rate of these angioedema cases in the completed studies was 0.06%.

In addition, 26 other cases of edema involving the face, hands, or whole body were reported with aliskiren use, including 4 leading to discontinuation.

In the placebo-controlled studies, however, the incidence of edema involving the face, hands, or whole body was 0.4% with aliskiren compared with 0.5% with placebo. In a long-term active-controlled study with aliskiren and HCTZ arms, the incidence of edema involving the face, hands, or whole body was 0.4% in both treatment arms.

Aliskiren produces dose-related gastrointestinal (GI) adverse reactions. Diarrhea was reported by 2.3% of patients at 300 mg, compared to 1.2% in placebo patients. In women and the elderly (age ≥65) increases in diarrhea rates were evident starting at a dose of 150 mg daily, with rates for these subgroups at 150 mg similar to those seen at 300 mg for men or younger patients (all rates about 2%). Other GI symptoms included abdominal pain, dyspepsia, and gastroesophageal reflux, although increased rates for abdominal pain and dyspepsia were distinguished from placebo only at 600 mg daily. Diarrhea and other GI symptoms were typically mild and rarely led to discontinuation.

Aliskiren was associated with a slight increase in cough in the placebo-controlled studies (1.1% for any aliskiren use versus 0.6% for placebo). In active-controlled trials with ACE inhibitor (ramipril, lisinopril) arms, the rates of cough for the aliskiren arms were about one-third to one-half the rates in the ACE inhibitor arms.

Other adverse reactions with increased rates for aliskiren compared to placebo included rash (1% versus 0.3%), elevated uric acid (0.4% versus 0.1%), gout (0.2% versus 0.1%), and renal stones (0.2% versus 0%).

Single episodes of tonic-clonic seizures with loss of consciousness were reported in two patients treated with aliskiren in the clinical trials. One patient had predisposing causes for seizures and had a negative electroencephalogram (EEG) and cerebral imaging following the seizures; for the other patient, EEG and imaging results were not reported. Aliskiren was discontinued and there was no rechallenge in either case.

No clinically meaningful changes in vital signs or in ECG (including QTc interval) were observed in patients treated with aliskiren.

Amlodipine besylate
Amlodipine (Norvasc®) has been evaluated for safety in more than 11,000 patients in U.S. and foreign clinical trials. Other adverse events that have been reported <1% but >0.1% of patients in controlled clinical trials or under conditions of open trials or marketing experience where a causal relationship is uncertain were:

Cardiovascular: arrhythmia (including ventricular tachycardia and atrial fibrillation), bradycardia, chest pain, peripheral ischemia, syncope, postural hypotension, vasculitis
Central and Peripheral Nervous System: neuropathy peripheral, paresthesia, tremor, vertigo
Gastrointestinal: anorexia, constipation, dyspepsia,** dysphagia, diarrhea, flatulence, pancreatitis, vomiting, gingival hyperplasia
General: allergic reaction, asthenia,** back pain, hot flushes, malaise, pain, rigors, weight gain, weight decrease
Musculoskeletal System: arthralgia, arthrosis, muscle cramps,** myalgia
Psychiatric: sexual dysfunction (male** and female), insomnia, nervousness, depression, abnormal dreams, anxiety, depersonalization
Respiratory System: dyspnea, epistaxis
Skin and Appendages: angioedema, erythema multiforme, pruritus,** rash,** rash erythematous, rash maculopapular
**These events occurred in less than 1% in placebo-controlled trials, but the incidence of these side effects was between 1% and 2% in all multiple dose studies.
Special Senses: abnormal vision, conjunctivitis, diplopia, eye pain, tinnitus
Urinary System: micturition frequency, micturition disorder, nocturia
Autonomic Nervous System: dry mouth, sweating increased
Metabolic and Nutritional: hyperglycemia, thirst
Hemopoietic: leukopenia, purpura, thrombocytopenia
Other events reported with amlodipine at a frequency of ≤0.1% of patients include: cardiac failure, pulse irregularity, extrasystoles, skin discoloration, urticaria, skin dryness, alopecia, dermatitis, muscle weakness, twitching, ataxia, hypertonia, migraine, cold and clammy skin, apathy, agitation, amnesia, gastritis, increased appetite, loose stools, rhinitis, dysuria, polyuria, parosmia, taste perversion, abnormal visual accommodation, and xerophthalmia. Other reactions occurred sporadically and cannot be distinguished from medications or concurrent disease states such as myocardial infarction and angina.

Clinical Laboratory Test Abnormalities
RBC count, hemoglobin and hematocrit: Small mean changes from baseline were seen in RBC count, hemoglobin and hematocrit in patients treated with both Tekamlo and aliskiren monotherapy. This effect is also seen with other agents acting on the renin angiotensin system. In aliskiren monotherapy trials these decreases led to slight increases in rates of anemia compared to placebo (0.1% for any aliskiren use, 0.3% for aliskiren 600 mg daily, vs. 0% for placebo). No patients discontinued due to anemia.
Blood Urea Nitrogen (BUN)/Creatinine: In patients with hypertension not concomitantly treated with an ARB or ACEI, elevations in BUN (> 40 mg/dL) and creatinine (>2.0 mg/dL) in patients treated with Tekamlo were <1.0%.
Serum Potassium: In patients with hypertension not concomitantly treated with an ARB or ACEI, increases in

serum potassium >5.5 mEq/L were infrequent (0.9% compared to 0.6% with placebo) *[see Contraindications (4) and Warnings and Precautions (5.10)]*.

6.2 Post-marketing Experience
The following adverse reactions have been identified during postapproval use of either aliskiren or amlodipine. Because these reactions are reported voluntarily from a population of uncertain size, it is not always possible to estimate their frequency or establish a causal relationship to drug exposure:
Hypersensitivity: angioedema requiring airway management and hospitalization
Aliskiren: Peripheral edema, severe cutaneous adverse reactions, including Stevens-Johnson syndrome and toxic epidermal necrolysis, urticaria, hepatic enzyme increase with clinical symptoms of hepatic dysfunction, pruritus, erythema
Hypersensitivity: anaphylactic reactions and angioedema requiring airway management and hospitalization
Amlodipine: The following postmarketing event has been reported infrequently where a causal relationship is uncertain: gynecomastia. In postmarketing experience, jaundice and hepatic enzyme elevations (mostly consistent with cholestasis or hepatitis), in some cases severe enough to require hospitalization, have been reported in association with use of amlodipine.

7 DRUG INTERACTIONS
No drug interaction studies have been conducted with Tekamlo and other drugs, although studies with the individual aliskiren and amlodipine besylate components are described below.
Aliskiren
Cyclosporine: Avoid co-administration of cyclosporine with aliskiren.
Itraconazole: Avoid co-administration of itraconazole with aliskiren *[see Clinical Pharmacology (12.3)]*.
Non-Steroidal Anti-Inflammatory Agents(NSAIDs) including selective Cyclooxygenase-2 inhibitors (COX-2 inhibitors): In patients who are elderly, volume-depleted (including those on diuretic therapy), or with compromised renal function, co-administration of NSAIDs, including selective COX-2 inhibitors with agents that affect the renin-angiotensin-aldosterone system, including aliskiren, may result in deterioration of renal function, including possible acute renal failure. These effects are usually reversible. Monitor renal function periodically in patients receiving aliskiren and NSAID therapy.
The antihypertensive effect of aliskiren may be attenuated by NSAIDs.
Dual Blockade of the renin-angiotensin-aldosterone system: The concomitant use of aliskiren with other agents acting on the renin-angiotensin-aldosterone system such as ACEIs or ARBs is associated with an increased risk of hypotension, hyperkalemia, and changes in renal function (including acute renal failure) compared to monotherapy. Monitor blood pressure, renal function, and electrolytes in patients on aliskiren and other agents that affect the renin-angiotensin-aldosterone system *[see Warnings and Precautions (5.4, 5.6, 5.8)]*.
The concomitant use of aliskiren with an ARB or an ACEI in diabetic patients is contraindicated and should be avoided in patients with moderate renal impairment *[see Contraindications (4) and Warnings and Precautions (5.2)]*.
Furosemide: Oral co-administration of aliskiren and furosemide reduced exposure to furosemide. Monitor diuretic effects when furosemide is co-administered with aliskiren.
Amlodipine besylate
Simvastatin: Co-administration of simvastatin with amlodipine increases the systemic exposure of simvastatin. Limit the dose of simvastatin in patients on amlodipine to 20 mg daily.
CYP3A4 Inhibitors: Co-administration with CYP3A inhibitors (moderate and strong) result in increased systemic exposure to amlodipine warranting dose reduction. Monitor for symptoms of hypotension and edema when amlodipine is co-administered with CYP3A4 inhibitors to determine the need for dose adjustment.
CYP3A4 Inducers: No information is available on the quantitative effects of CYP3A4 inducers on amlodipine. Blood pressure should be monitored when amlodipine is co-administered with CYP3A4 inducers.

8 USE IN SPECIFIC POPULATIONS
8.1 Pregnancy
Pregnancy Category D
Use of drugs that act on the renin-angiotensin system during the second and third trimesters of pregnancy reduces fetal renal function and increases fetal and neonatal morbidity and death. Resulting oligohydramnios can be associated with fetal lung hypoplasia and skeletal deformations. Potential neonatal adverse effects include skull hypoplasia, anuria, hypotension, renal failure, and death. When pregnancy is detected, discontinue Tekamlo as soon as possible.

These adverse outcomes are usually associated with use of these drugs in the second and third trimester of pregnancy. Most epidemiologic studies examining fetal abnormalities after exposure to antihypertensive use in the first trimester have not distinguished drugs affecting the renin-angiotensin system from other antihypertensive agents. Appropriate management of maternal hypertension during pregnancy is important to optimize outcomes for both mother and fetus.

In the unusual case that there is no appropriate alternative to therapy with drugs affecting the renin-angiotensin system for a particular patient, apprise the mother of the potential risk to the fetus. Perform serial ultrasound examinations to assess the intra-amniotic environment. If oligohydramnios is observed, discontinue Tekamlo, unless it is considered lifesaving for the mother. Fetal testing may be appropriate, based on the week of pregnancy. Patients and physicians should be aware, however, that oligohydramnios may not appear until after the fetus has sustained irreversible injury. Closely observe infants with histories of in utero exposure to Tekamlo for hypotension, oliguria, and hyperkalemia. *[see Use in Specific Populations (8.4)]*

Animal Data
No reproductive toxicity studies have been conducted with the combination of aliskiren and amlodipine besylate. However, these studies have been conducted for aliskiren and amlodipine besylate alone.

Aliskiren
In developmental toxicity studies, pregnant rats and rabbits received oral aliskiren hemifumarate during organogenesis at doses up to 20 and 7 times the maximum recommended human dose (MRHD) based on body surface area (mg/m²), respectively, in rats and rabbits. (Actual animal doses were up to 600 mg/kg/day in rats and up to 100 mg/kg/day in rabbits.) No teratogenicity was observed; however, fetal birth weight was decreased in rabbits at doses 3.2 times the MRHD based on body surface area (mg/m²). Aliskiren was present in placentas, amniotic fluid and fetuses of pregnant rabbits.

Amlodipine
No evidence of teratogenicity or embryo/fetal toxicity was found when pregnant rats and rabbits were treated orally with amlodipine maleate at doses up to 10 mg amlodipine/kg/day during their respective periods of major organogenesis. However, litter size was significantly decreased (by about 50%) and the number of intrauterine deaths was significantly increased (about 5-fold). Amlodipine has been shown to prolong both the gestation period and the duration of labor in rats at this dose.

8.3 Nursing Mothers
It is not known whether aliskiren or amlodipine is excreted in human milk. Both aliskiren and amlodipine are secreted in the milk of lactating rats. Because of the potential for serious adverse reactions in human milk-fed infants from Tekamlo, a decision should be made whether to discontinue nursing or discontinue Tekamlo, taking into account the importance of the drug to the mother.

8.4 Pediatric Use
Safety and effectiveness of Tekamlo in pediatric patients have not been established.
Neonates with a history of in utero exposure to Tekamlo:
If oliguria or hypotension occurs, direct attention toward support of blood pressure and renal perfusion. Exchange transfusions or dialysis may be required as a means of reversing hypotension and/or substituting for disordered renal function.

8.5 Geriatric Use
Exposure to aliskiren and amlodipine is increased in elderly patients, thus consider lower initial doses of Tekamlo *[see Clinical Pharmacology (12.3)]*.
In the short-term controlled clinical trials of Tekamlo, 17% of patients treated with Tekamlo were ≥ 65 years. No overall differences in safety or effectiveness were observed between these subjects and younger subjects. Other reported clinical experience has not identified differences in responses between the elderly and younger patients, but greater sensitivity of some older individuals cannot be ruled out.

8.6 Hepatic Impairment
Exposure to amlodipine is increased in patients with hepatic insufficiency, thus consider using lower doses of Tekamlo *[see Clinical Pharmacology (12.3)]*.

8.7 Renal Impairment
There is no impact of renal function on the pharmacokinetics of aliskiren and amlodipine. However, safety and effectiveness of Tekamlo in patients with severe renal impairment (creatinine clearance <30 mL/min) have not been established as these patients were excluded in clinical trials *[see Warnings and Precautions (5.6), Clinical Pharmacology (12.3) and Clinical Studies (14)]*.

10 OVERDOSAGE

Aliskiren

Limited data are available related to overdosage in humans. The most likely manifestation of overdosage would be hypotension. If symptomatic hypotension should occur, provide supportive treatment.

Aliskiren is poorly dialyzed. Therefore, hemodialysis is not adequate to treat aliskiren overexposure *[see Clinical Pharmacology (12.3)]*.

Amlodipine besylate

Overdosage might be expected to cause excessive peripheral vasodilation with marked hypotension and possibly a reflex tachycardia. Marked and potentially prolonged systemic hypotension up to and including shock with fatal outcome have been reported. In humans, experience with intentional overdosage of amlodipine is limited. Single oral doses of amlodipine maleate equivalent to 40 mg amlodipine/kg and 100 mg amlodipine/kg in mice and rats, respectively, caused deaths. Single oral amlodipine maleate doses equivalent to 4 or more mg amlodipine/kg or higher in dogs (11 or more times the maximum recommended human dose on a mg/m2 basis) caused a marked peripheral vasodilation and hypotension.

If massive overdose should occur, initiate active cardiac and respiratory monitoring. Frequent blood pressure measurements are essential. Should hypotension occur, provide cardiovascular support including elevation of the extremities and the judicious administration of fluids. If hypotension remains unresponsive to these conservative measures, consider administration of vasopressors (such as phenylephrine) with attention to circulating volume and urine output. As amlodipine is highly protein bound, hemodialysis is not likely to be of benefit. Administration of activated charcoal to healthy volunteers immediately or up to two hours after ingestion of amlodipine has been shown to significantly decrease amlodipine absorption.

11 DESCRIPTION

Tekamlo is a single tablet for oral administration of aliskiren hemifumarate (an orally active, nonpeptide, potent direct renin inhibitor) and amlodipine besylate (a dihydropyridine calcium channel blocker).

Aliskiren hemifumarate

Aliskiren hemifumarate is chemically described as (2S,4S,5S,7S)-N-(2-carbamoyl-2-methylpropyl)-5-amino-4-hydroxy-2,7-diisopropyl-8-[4-methoxy-3-(3-methoxypropoxy)phenyl]-octanamide hemifumarate and its structural formula is:

Molecular formula: $C_{30}H_{53}N_3O_6 \cdot 0.5\ C_4H_4O_4$

Aliskiren hemifumarate is a white to slightly yellowish powder with a molecular weight of 609.8 (free base- 551.8). It is highly soluble in water, and freely soluble in methanol, ethanol and isopropanol.

Amlodipine besylate

Amlodipine besylate, USP is chemically described as 3-Ethyl 5-methyl (±)-2-[(2-aminoethoxy)methyl]-4-(o-chlorophenyl)-1,4-dihydro-6-methyl-3,5-pyridinedicarboxylate, monobenzenesulfonate, and its structural formula is:

Molecular formula: $C_{20}H_{25}ClN_2O_5 \cdot C_6H_6O_3S$

Amlodipine besylate is a white to pale yellow crystalline powder with a molecular weight of 567.1. It is slightly soluble in water and sparingly soluble in ethanol.

Tekamlo tablets are formulated for oral administration to contain aliskiren hemifumarate and amlodipine besylate providing for the following available combinations: 150 mg/5 mg, 150 mg/10 mg, 300 mg/5 mg and 300 mg/10 mg aliskiren/amlodipine. The inactive ingredients for all strengths of the tablets may contain colloidal silicon dioxide, crospovidone, hypromellose, iron oxide red, iron oxide yellow, magnesium stearate, microcrystalline cellulose, polyethylene glycol, povidone, talc, and titanium dioxide.

12 CLINICAL PHARMACOLOGY

12.1 Mechanism of Action

Aliskiren

Renin is secreted by the kidney in response to decreases in blood volume and renal perfusion. Renin cleaves angiotensinogen to form the inactive decapeptide angiotensin I (Ang I). Ang I is converted to the active octapeptide angiotensin II (Ang II) by angiotensin-converting enzyme (ACE) and non-ACE pathways. Ang II is a powerful vasoconstrictor and leads to the release of catecholamines from the adrenal medulla and prejunctional nerve endings. It also promotes aldosterone secretion and sodium reabsorption. Together, these effects increase blood pressure. Ang II also inhibits renin release, thus providing a negative feedback to the system. This cycle, from renin through angiotensin to aldosterone and its associated negative feedback loop, is known as the renin-angiotensin-aldosterone system (RAAS). Aliskiren is a direct renin inhibitor, decreasing plasma renin activity (PRA) and inhibiting the conversion of angiotensinogen to Ang I. Whether aliskiren affects other RAAS components, e.g., ACE or non-ACE pathways, is not known. All agents that inhibit the RAAS, including renin inhibitors, suppress the negative feedback loop, leading to a compensatory rise in plasma renin concentration. When this rise occurs during treatment with ACE inhibitors and ARBs, the result is increased levels of PRA. During treatment with aliskiren, however, the effect of increased renin levels is blocked, so that PRA, Ang I and Ang II are all reduced, whether aliskiren is used as monotherapy or in combination with other antihypertensive agents.

Amlodipine besylate

Amlodipine is a dihydropyridine calcium channel blocker that inhibits the transmembrane influx of calcium ions into vascular smooth muscle and cardiac muscle. Experimental data suggest that amlodipine binds to both dihydropyridine and nondihydropyridine binding sites. The contractile processes of cardiac muscle and vascular smooth muscle are dependent upon the movement of extracellular calcium ions into these cells through specific ion channels. Amlodipine inhibits calcium ion influx across cell membranes selectively, with a greater effect on vascular smooth muscle cells than on cardiac muscle cells. Negative inotropic effects can be detected *in vitro* but such effects have not been seen in intact animals at therapeutic doses. Serum calcium concentration is not affected by amlodipine. Within the physiologic pH range, amlodipine is an ionized compound (pKa=8.6), and its kinetic interaction with the calcium channel receptor is characterized by a gradual rate of association and dissociation with the receptor binding site, resulting in a gradual onset of effect.

Amlodipine is a peripheral arterial vasodilator that acts directly on vascular smooth muscle to cause a reduction in peripheral vascular resistance and reduction in blood pressure.

Tekamlo

The effects of combined treatment of aliskiren and amlodipine arise from the actions of these two agents on different, but complementary mechanisms that regulate blood pressure, calcium channel-mediated vasoconstriction and RAAS-mediated effects on vascular tone and sodium excretion.

12.2 Pharmacodynamics

Aliskiren

PRA reductions in clinical trials ranged from approximately 50% to 80%, were not dose-related and did not correlate with blood pressure reductions. The clinical implications of the differences in effect on PRA are not known.

Amlodipine besylate

Following administration of therapeutic doses to patients with hypertension, amlodipine produces vasodilation resulting in a reduction of supine and standing blood pressures. These decreases in blood pressure are not accompanied by a significant change in heart rate or plasma catecholamine levels with chronic dosing. Although the acute intravenous administration of amlodipine decreases arterial blood pressure and increase heart rate in hemodynamic studies of patients with chronic stable angina, chronic oral administration of amlodipine in clinical trials did not lead to clinically significant changes in heart rate or blood pressures in normotensive patients with angina.

With chronic once daily administration, antihypertensive effectiveness is maintained for at least 24 hours. Plasma concentrations correlate with effect in both young and elderly patients. The magnitude of reduction in blood pressure with amlodipine is also correlated with the height of pretreatment elevation; thus, individuals with moderate hypertension (diastolic pressure 105-114 mmHg) had about 50% greater response than patients with mild hypertension (diastolic pressure 90-104 mmHg). Normotensive subjects experienced no clinically significant change in blood pressure (+1/-2 mmHg).

In hypertensive patients with normal renal function, therapeutic doses of amlodipine resulted in a decrease in renal vascular resistance and an increase in glomerular filtration rate and effective renal plasma flow without change in filtration fraction or proteinuria.

As with other calcium channel blockers, hemodynamic measurements of cardiac function at rest and during exercise (or pacing) in patients with normal ventricular function treated with amlodipine have generally demonstrated a small increase in cardiac index without significant influence on dP/dt or on left ventricular end diastolic pressure or volume. In hemodynamic studies, amlodipine has not been associated with a negative inotropic effect when administered in therapeutic dose range to intact animals and man, even when co-administered with beta-blockers to man. Similar findings, however, have been observed in normal or well-compensated patients with heart failure with agents possessing significant negative inotropic effects.

Amlodipine does not change sinoatrial nodal function or atrioventricular conduction in intact animals or man. In patients with chronic stable angina, intravenous administration of 10 mg did not significantly alter A-H and H-V conduction and sinus node recovery time after pacing. Similar results were obtained in patients receiving amlodipine and concomitant beta-blockers. In clinical studies in which amlodipine was administered in combination with beta-blockers to patients with either hypertension or angina, no adverse effects of electrocardiographic parameters were observed. In clinical trials with angina patients alone, amlodipine therapy did not alter electrocardiographic intervals or produce higher degrees of AV blocks.

Amlodipine has indications other than hypertension which can be found in the Norvasc® package insert.

Tekamlo

In a placebo-controlled study in hypertensive patients, amlodipine was associated with an increase in PRA (59-73% increase) whereas aliskiren monotherapy was associated with a 61-68% reduction in PRA. Aliskiren in combination with amlodipine reduced PRA (55-68% reduction).

12.3 Pharmacokinetics

Absorption and Distribution

Tekamlo

Following oral administration of the aliskiren/amlodipine combination tablets, the median peak plasma concentration times are within 3.0 hours for aliskiren and 8.0 hours for amlodipine. The rate and extent of absorption of aliskiren and amlodipine from Tekamlo are the same as when administered as individual tablets. When taken with food, mean AUC and C_{max} of aliskiren are decreased by 79% and 90%, respectively, while there is no impact of food on the AUC and C_{max} of amlodipine.

Aliskiren

Aliskiren is poorly absorbed (bioavailability about 2.5%) with an accumulation half life of about 24 hours. Steady state blood levels are reached in about 7-8 days. Following oral administration, peak plasma concentrations of aliskiren are reached within 1-3 hours. When taken with a high fat meal, mean AUC and Cmax of aliskiren are decreased by 71% and 85% respectively. In the clinical trials, aliskiren was administered without a fixed relation to meals.

Amlodipine besylate

Peak plasma concentrations of amlodipine are reached 6-12 hours after an oral administration of amlodipine. Absolute bioavailability has been estimated to be between 64% and 90%. The bioavailability of amlodipine is not altered by the presence of food.

The apparent volume of distribution of amlodipine is about 21 L/kg. Approximately 93% of circulating amlodipine is bound to plasma proteins in hypertensive patients.

Metabolism and Elimination

Aliskiren

About one-fourth of the absorbed dose appears in the urine as parent drug. How much of the absorbed dose is metabolized is unknown. Based on the in vitro studies, the major enzyme responsible for aliskiren metabolism appears to be CYP 3A4. Aliskiren does not inhibit the CYP450 isoenzymes (CYP 1A2, 2C8, 2C9, 2C19, 2D6, 2E1, and 3A) or induce CYP 3A4.

Transporters: Pgp (MDR1/Mdr1a/1b) was found to be the major efflux system involved in absorption and disposition of aliskiren in preclinical studies. The potential for drug interactions at the Pgp site will likely depend on the degree of inhibition of this transporter.

Drug interactions: The effect of co-administered drugs on the pharmacokinetics of aliskiren and vice versa, were studied in several single and multiple dose studies. Pharmacokinetic measures indicating the magnitude of these interactions are presented in Figure 5 (impact of co-administered drugs on aliskiren) and Figure 6 (impact on co-administered drugs).

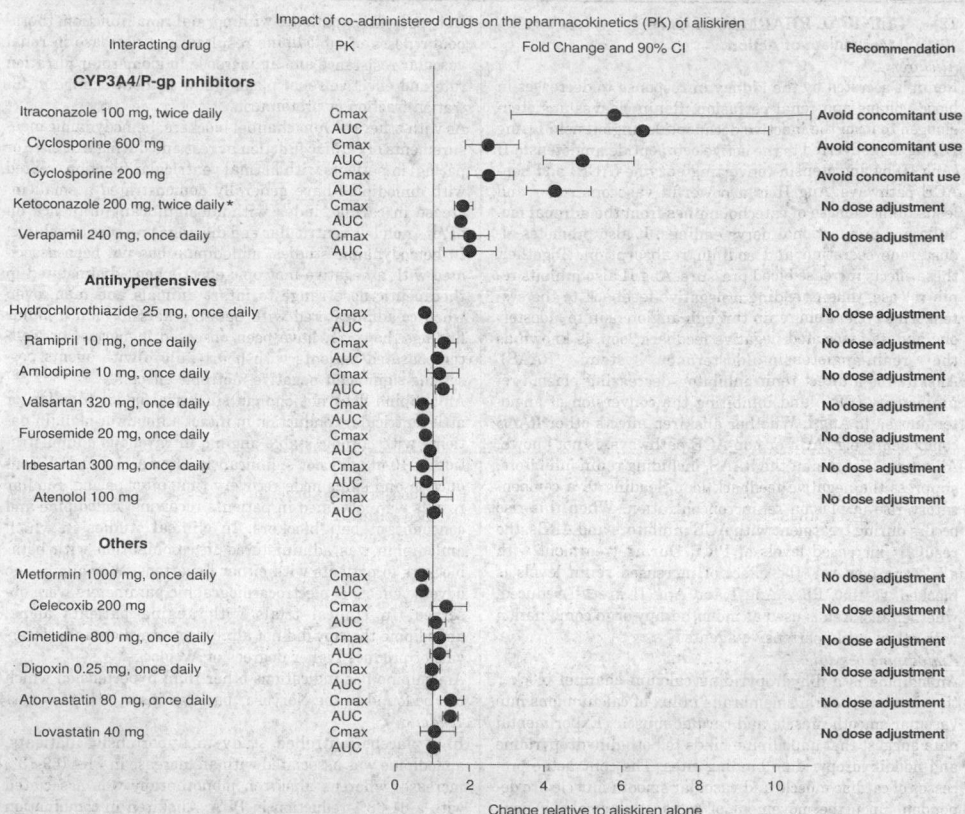

Figure 5: The impact of co-administered drugs on the pharmacokinetics of aliskiren.

*A 400 mg once daily dose was not studied, but would be expected to increase aliskiren blood levels further.

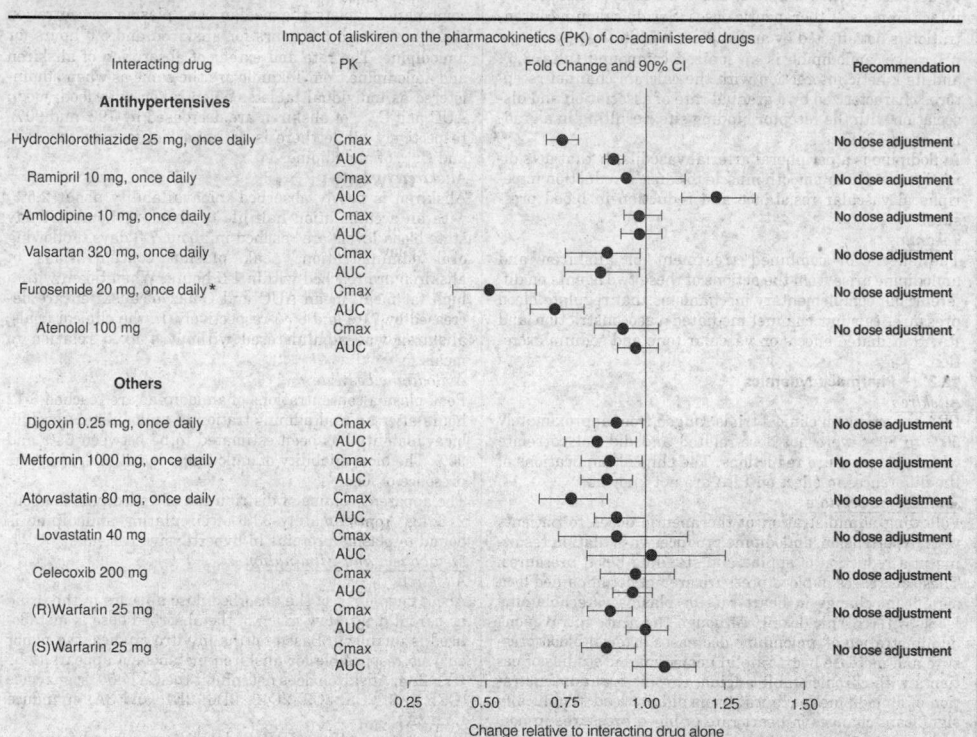

*Patients receiving furosemide could find its effect diminished after starting aliskiren.

Figure 6: The impact of aliskiren on the pharmacokinetics of co-administered drugs.

[See figure 5 above]
Warfarin: There was no clinically significant effect of a single dose of warfarin 25 mg on the pharmacokinetics of aliskiren.
[See figure 6 above]

Furosemide: In patients with heart failure, co-administration of aliskiren (300 mg/day) reduced plasma AUC and Cmax of oral furosemide (60 mg/day) by 17% and 27%, respectively, and reduced 24 hour urinary furosemide excretion by 29%. This change in exposure did not result in statistically significant difference in total urine volume and urinary sodium excretion over 24 hours. However, a transient decrease in urinary sodium excretion and urine volume effects up to 12 hours were observed when furosemide was co-administered with aliskiren 300 mg/day.

Amlodipine besylate
Amlodipine is extensively (about 90%) converted to inactive metabolites via hepatic metabolism with 10% of the parent compound and 60% of the metabolites excreted in the urine. Elimination of amlodipine from the plasma is biphasic with a terminal elimination half-life of about 30-50 hours Steady state plasma levels are reached after once-daily dosing for 7-8 days.

Drug interactions:
Aliskiren exposure is increased slightly (AUC increased 29%) when aliskiren is co-administered with amlodipine, while amlodipine exposure remains unchanged when co-administered with aliskiren. The slight exposure increase of aliskiren in the presence of amlodipine is not clinically relevant.
In vitro data in human plasma indicate that amlodipine has no effect on the protein binding of digoxin, phenytoin, warfarin, and indomethacin.
Cimetidine: Co-administration of amlodipine with cimetidine did not alter the pharmacokinetics of amlodipine.
Grapefruit juice: Co-administration of 240 mL of grapefruit juice with a single oral dose of amlodipine 10 mg in 20 healthy volunteers had no significant effect on the pharmacokinetics of amlodipine.
Maalox® (antacid): Co-administration of the antacid Maalox with a single dose of amlodipine had no significant effect on the pharmacokinetics of amlodipine.
Sildenafil: A single 100 mg dose of sildenafil in subjects with essential hypertension had no effect on the pharmacokinetic parameters of amlodipine. When amlodipine and sildenafil were used in combination, each agent independently exerted its own blood pressure lowering effect.
Atorvastatin: Co-administration of multiple 10 mg doses of amlodipine with 80 mg of atorvastatin resulted in no significant change in the steady-state pharmacokinetic parameters of atorvastatin.
Digoxin: Co-administration of amlodipine with digoxin did not change serum digoxin levels or digoxin renal clearance in normal volunteers.
Ethanol (alcohol): Single and multiple 10 mg doses of amlodipine had no significant effect on the pharmacokinetics of ethanol.
Warfarin: Co-administration of amlodipine with warfarin did not change the warfarin prothrombin response time.
Simvastatin: Co-administration of multiple doses of 10 mg of amlodipine with 80 mg simvastatin resulted in a 77% increase in exposure to simvastatin compared to simvastatin alone.
CYP3A inhibitors: Co-administration of a 180 mg daily dose of diltiazem with 5 mg amlodipine in elderly hypertensive patients resulted in a 60% increase in amlodipine systemic exposure. Erythromycin co-administration in healthy volunteers did not significantly change amlodipine systemic exposure. However, strong inhibitors of CYP3A4 (e.g. ketoconazole, itraconazole, ritonavir) may increase the plasma concentrations of amlodipine to a greater extent.

Special Populations
Pediatric Patients
The pharmacokinetics of Tekamlo have not been investigated in patients <18 years of age.
Geriatric Patients
Impact of aging on aliskiren pharmacokinetics has been assessed. When compared to young adults (18-40 years), aliskiren mean AUC and Cmax in elderly subjects (> 65 years) are increased by 57% and 28%, respectively. In the elderly, clearance of amlodipine is decreased with resulting increases in peak plasma levels, elimination half-life and area-under-the-plasma-concentration curve [see Use in Specific Populations (8.5)].
Race
With Tekamlo, pharmacokinetic differences due to race have not been studied. The pharmacokinetic differences among Blacks, Caucasians, and Japanese are minimal with aliskiren therapy.
Hepatic Impairment
The pharmacokinetics of aliskiren is not significantly affected in patients with mild-to-severe liver disease. Patients with hepatic insufficiency have decreased clearance of amlodipine with resulting increase in AUC of approximately 40%-60% [see Use in Specific Populations (8.6)].
Renal Impairment
The pharmacokinetics of aliskiren was evaluated in patients with varying degrees of renal impairment. Rate and extent of exposure (AUC and Cmax) of aliskiren in subjects with renal impairment did not show a consistent correlation with the severity of renal impairment.
The pharmacokinetics of aliskiren following administration of a single oral dose of 300 mg was evaluated in patients with End Stage Renal Disease (ESRD) undergoing hemodi-

alysis. When compared to healthy subjects, changes in the rate and extent of aliskiren exposure (Cmax and AUC) in ESRD patients undergoing hemodialysis was not clinically significant. Timing of hemodialysis did not significantly alter the pharmacokinetics of aliskiren in ESRD patients. The pharmacokinetics of amlodipine is not significantly influenced by renal impairment [see Warnings and Precautions (5.6) and Use in Specific Populations (8.7)].

13 NONCLINICAL TOXICOLOGY

13.1 Carcinogenesis, Mutagenesis, Impairment of Fertility

Studies with Aliskiren hemifumarate and Amlodipine besylate

No carcinogenicity, mutagenicity or fertility studies have been conducted with the combination of aliskiren hemifumarate and amlodipine besylate alone. However, these studies have been conducted for aliskiren hemifumarate and amlodipine besylate alone.

Studies with Aliskiren hemifumarate

Carcinogenic potential was assessed in a 2-year rat study and a 6-month transgenic (rasH2) mouse study with aliskiren hemifumarate at oral doses of up to 1500 mg aliskiren/kg/day. Although there were no statistically significant increases in tumor incidence associated with exposure to aliskiren, mucosal epithelial hyperplasia (with or without erosion/ulceration) was observed in the lower gastrointestinal tract at doses of 750 or more mg/kg/day in both species, with a colonic adenoma identified in one rat and a cecal adenocarcinoma identified in another, rare tumors in the strain of rat studied. On a systemic exposure (AUC$_{0-24hr}$) basis, 1500 mg/kg/day in the rat is about 4 times and in the mouse about 1.5 times the maximum recommended human dose (300 mg aliskiren/day). Mucosal hyperplasia in the cecum or colon of rats was also observed at doses of 250 mg/kg/day (the lowest tested dose) as well as at higher doses in 4- and 13-week studies.

Aliskiren hemifumarate was devoid of genotoxic potential in the Ames reverse mutation assay with *S. typhimurium* and *E. coli*, the in vitro Chinese hamster ovary cell chromosomal aberration assay, the in vitro Chinese hamster V79 cell gene mutation test and the in vivo rat bone marrow micronucleus assay.

Fertility of male and female rats was unaffected at doses of up to aliskiren 250 mg/kg/day (8 times the maximum recommended human dose of aliskiren 300 mg/60 kg on a mg/m^2 basis).

Studies with Amlodipine besylate

Rats and mice treated with amlodipine maleate in the diet for up to two years, at concentrations calculated to provide daily dosage levels of 0.5, 1.25, and 2.5 mg amlodipine/kg/day, showed no evidence of a carcinogenic effect of the drug. For the mouse, the highest dose was, on mg/m^2 basis, similar to the maximum recommended human dose (MRHD) of 10 mg amlodipine/day. For the rat, the highest dose was, on a mg/m^2 basis, about twice the MRHD.

Mutagenicity studies conducted with amlodipine maleate revealed no drug-related effects at either the gene or chromosome level.

There was no effect on the fertility of rats treated orally with amlodipine maleate (males for 64 days and females for 14 days prior to mating) at doses of up to 10 mg amlodipine/kg/day (about 8 times the MRHD of 10 mg/day on a mg/m^2 basis).

13.2 Animal Toxicology and/or Pharmacology

Preclinical safety studies have demonstrated that the combination of aliskiren hemifumarate and amlodipine besylate was well tolerated in rats. The findings from the 2- and 13-week oral toxicity studies in rats were consistent with those of aliskiren hemifumarate and amlodipine besylate when both drugs were administered alone. There were no new toxicities or increased severity of the toxicities which were associated with either component.

Animal reproductive and developmental toxicology findings are described elsewhere [see Use in Specific Populations (8.1)].

14 CLINICAL STUDIES

14.1 Tekamlo

Tekamlo was studied in a total of 5549 patients with mild to moderate hypertension (diastolic blood pressure between 90 mmHg and 109 mmHg).

Aliskiren 150 mg and 300 mg and amlodipine besylate 5 mg and 10 mg were studied alone and in combination in an 8-week, randomized, double-blind, placebo-controlled, multifactorial study comparing the combinations 150 mg/5 mg, 150 mg/10 mg, 300 mg/5 mg and 300 mg/10 mg of aliskiren and amlodipine with their components and placebo. The combination of aliskiren and amlodipine resulted in placebo-adjusted decreases in systolic/diastolic blood pressure at trough of 14-17/9-11 mmHg compared to 4-9/3-5 mmHg for aliskiren alone and 9-14/6-8 mmHg for amlodipine alone.

Treatment with Tekamlo resulted overall in significantly greater reductions in diastolic and systolic blood pressure compared to the respective monotherapy components.

Table 1: Incidence of Selected Adverse Events During the Treatment Phase in ALTITUDE

	Aliskiren N=4272		Placebo N=4285	
	Serious Adverse Events* (%)	Adverse Events (%)	Serious Adverse Events* (%)	Adverse Events (%)
Renal impairment †	5.7	14.5	4.3	12.4
Hypotension ††	2.3	19.9	1.9	16.3
Hyperkalemia †††	1.0	38.9	0.5	28.8

†renal failure, renal failure acute, renal failure chronic, renal impairment
††dizziness, dizziness postural, hypotension, orthostatic hypotension, presyncope, syncope
††† Given the variable baseline potassium levels of patients with renal insufficiency on dual RAAS therapy, the reporting of adverse event of hyperkalemia was at the discretion of the investigator.
* A Serious Adverse Event (SAE) is defined as: an event which is fatal or life-threatening, results in persistent or significant disability/incapacity, constitutes a congenital anomaly/birth defect, requires inpatient hospitalization or prolongation of existing hospitalization, or is medically significant (i.e. defined as an event that jeopardizes the patient or may require medical or surgical intervention to prevent one of the outcomes previously listed).

The antihypertensive effect of Tekamlo was similar in patients with and without diabetes, obese and non-obese patients, in patients ≥65 years of age and <65 years of age, and in women and men.

A subgroup of 819 patients was studied with ambulatory blood pressure monitoring. The blood pressure lowering effect in the aliskiren/amlodipine group was maintained throughout the 24-hour period (see Figure 7 and Figure 8).

Figure 7: Mean Ambulatory Diastolic Blood Pressure at Endpoint by Treatment and Hour

Figure 8: Mean Ambulatory Systolic Blood Pressure at Endpoint by Treatment and Hour

Two additional double-blind, active-controlled studies of similar design were conducted in which Tekamlo was administered as initial therapy in patients with moderate to severe hypertension (SBP 160-200 mmHg). Patients were randomized to receive either combination aliskiren/amlodipine or amlodipine monotherapy. The initial dose of aliskiren/amlodipine was 150 mg/5 mg for 1 week with forced titration to 300 mg/10 mg for 7 weeks. The initial dose of amlodipine was 5 mg for 1 week with forced titration to 10 mg for 7 weeks. In one study of 443 Black patients, at the primary endpoint of 8 weeks, the treatment difference between aliskiren/amlodipine and amlodipine was 5.2/3.8 mmHg. In the other study of 484 patients, at the primary endpoint of 8 weeks, the treatment difference between aliskiren/amlodipine and amlodipine was 7.1/3.8 mmHg.

The blood pressure lowering effects of Tekamlo are largely attained within 1-2 weeks.

There are no trials of the Tekamlo combination tablet demonstrating reductions in cardiovascular risk in patients with hypertension, but the amlodipine component has demonstrated such benefits.

14.2 Aliskiren in Patients with Diabetes treated with ARB or ACEI (ALTITUDE study)

Patients with diabetes with renal disease (defined either by the presence of albuminuria or reduced GFR) were randomized to aliskiren 300 mg daily (n=4296) or placebo (n=4310). All patients were receiving background therapy with an ARB or ACEI. The primary efficacy outcome was the time to the first event of the primary composite endpoint consisting of cardiovascular death, resuscitated sudden death, nonfatal myocardial infarction, non-fatal stroke, unplanned hospitalization for heart failure, onset of end stage renal disease, renal death, and doubling of serum creatinine concentration from baseline sustained for at least one month. After a median follow up of about 32 months, the trial was terminated early for lack of efficacy. Higher risk of renal impairment, hypotension and hyperkalemia was observed in aliskiren compared to placebo treated patients, as shown in the table below.

[See table 1 above]

The risk of stroke (3.4% aliskiren vs 2.7% placebo) and death (8.4% aliskiren vs. 8.0% placebo) were also numerically higher in aliskiren treated patients.

16 HOW SUPPLIED/STORAGE AND HANDLING

Tekamlo (aliskiren and amlodipine) is supplied as follows:
150 mg aliskiren/5 mg amlodipine Tablets - Non-scored light yellow, ovaloid convex-shaped, film-coated tablet with a beveled edge with debossing "T2" on one side and "NVR" on the reverse side of the tablet. The tablet dimensions are approximately 16 × 6.3 mm.
150 mg aliskiren/10 mg amlodipine Tablets - Non-scored yellow, ovaloid convex shaped, film-coated tablet with a beveled edge with debossing "T7" on one side and "NVR" on the reverse side of the tablet. The tablet dimensions are approximately 16 × 6.3 mm.
300 mg aliskiren/5 mg amlodipine Tablets - Non-scored dark yellow, ovaloid convex-shaped, film-coated tablet with a beveled edge with debossing "T11" on one side and "NVR" on the reverse side of the tablet. The tablet dimensions are approximately 21 × 8.3 mm.
300 mg aliskiren/10 mg amlodipine Tablets - Non-scored brown yellow, ovaloid convex shaped, film-coated tablet with a beveled edge with debossing "T12" on one side and "NVR" on the reverse side of the tablet. The tablet dimensions are approximately 21 × 8.3 mm.
All strengths are packaged in bottles and unit-dose blister packages (10 strips of 10 tablets) as described below.
[See table 2 at top of next page]

Storage
Store at 25°C (77°F); excursions permitted to 15-30°C (59-86°F) in original container.
Protect from heat and moisture.
Dispense in original container.

17 PATIENT COUNSELING INFORMATION

See FDA-Approved Patient Labeling (Patient Information)
Healthcare professionals should instruct their patients to read the Patient Package Insert before starting Tekamlo and to reread each time the prescription is renewed. Patients should be instructed to inform their doctor or pharmacist if they develop any unusual symptom, or if any known symptom persists or worsens.

Table 2: Tekamlo Tablets Supply

Tablet	Color	Debossed	Debossed	NDC 0078- XXXX-XX		
Aliskiren hemifumarate/ amlodipine besylate		Side 1	Side 2	Bottle of 30	Bottle of 90	Blister Packages of 100
150 mg/5 mg	Light yellow	T2	NVR	0603-15	0603-34	0603-35
150 mg/10 mg	Yellow	T7	NVR	0604-15	0604-34	0604-35
300 mg/5 mg	Dark yellow	T11	NVR	0605-15	0605-34	0605-35
300 mg/10 mg	Brown yellow	T12	NVR	0606-15	0606-34	0606-35

Pregnancy

Female patients of childbearing age should be told about the consequences of exposure to Tekamlo during pregnancy. Discuss treatment options with women planning to become pregnant. Patients should be asked to report pregnancies to their physician as soon as possible.

Symptomatic Hypotension

Caution patients receiving Tekamlo that lightheadedness can occur, especially during the first days of therapy, and that it should be reported to the prescribing physician. Tell patients that if syncope occurs, discontinue Tekamlo until the physician has been consulted.

Caution all patients that inadequate fluid intake, excessive perspiration, diarrhea, or vomiting can lead to an excessive fall in blood pressure, with the same consequences of lightheadedness and possible syncope.

Anaphylactic Reactions and Angioedema

Patients should be advised and told to report immediately any signs or symptoms suggesting a severe allergic reaction (difficulty breathing or swallowing, tightness of the chest, hives, general rash, swelling, itching, dizziness, vomiting, or abdominal pain) or angioedema (swelling of face, extremities, eyes, lips, tongue, difficulty in swallowing or breathing) and to take no more drug until they have consulted with the prescribing physician. Angioedema, including laryngeal edema, may occur at any time during treatment with Tekamlo.

Potassium Supplements

Tell patients receiving Tekamlo not to use potassium supplements or salt substitutes containing potassium without consulting the prescribing physician.

Relationship to Meals

Patients should establish a routine pattern for taking Tekamlo with regard to meals. High-fat meals decrease absorption substantially.

T2014-22
March 2014
FDA-Approved Patient Labeling
Patient Information
Tekamlo™ *(tĕk'-ăm-lō)*
Tekamlo
(aliskiren and amlodipine)
Tablets

Read the Patient Information that comes with Tekamlo before you start taking it and each time you get a refill. There may be new information. This information does not take the place of talking with your doctor about your condition and treatment. If you have any questions about Tekamlo, ask your doctor or pharmacist.

What is the most important information I should know about Tekamlo?

Tekamlo can cause harm or death to an unborn baby. Talk to your doctor about other ways to lower your blood pressure if you plan to become pregnant. If you get pregnant while taking Tekamlo, tell your doctor right away.

What is Tekamlo?

Tekamlo is a prescription medicine that may be used:

- as the first medicine to lower your high blood pressure if your doctor decides that you are likely to need more than one medicine.
- to treat your high blood pressure when one medicine to lower your high blood pressure has not worked well enough.
- if you are already taking the medicines aliskiren and amlodipine to treat your high blood pressure.

Tekamlo contains:

- aliskiren, a direct renin inhibitor (DRI)
- amlodipine, a calcium channel blocker (CCB)

Your doctor may prescribe other medicines for you to take along with Tekamlo to treat your high blood pressure.

It is not known if Tekamlo is safe and works in children under 18 years of age.

Who should not take Tekamlo?

- If you get pregnant, stop taking Tekamlo and call your doctor right away. If you plan to become pregnant, talk to your doctor about other treatment options for your high blood pressure.
- If you have diabetes and are taking a kind of medicine called an angiotensin-receptor-blocker or angiotensin-converting-enzyme-inhibitor.

- **If you are allergic** (hypersensitive) to aliskiren, amlodipine or other dihydropyridines (calcium-channel blockers, a group of medicines to lower blood pressure to which amlodipine belongs) or any of the other ingredients of Tekamlo listed at the end of this leaflet.

What should I tell my doctor before taking Tekamlo?

Before taking Tekamlo, tell your doctor if you:

- have kidney problems
- have liver problems
- have ever had an allergic reaction to another blood pressure medicine. Symptoms may include: swelling of the face, lips, tongue, throat, arms and legs, and trouble breathing.
- suffer from heart disorders or if you experienced a heart attack
- have any other medical problems
- are pregnant or planning to become pregnant. See "What is the most important information I should know about Tekamlo?"
- are breastfeeding. It is not known if Tekamlo passes into your breast milk and if it can harm your baby. You and your doctor should decide if you will take Tekamlo or breastfeed. You should not do both.

Tell your doctor about all the medicines you take including prescription and nonprescription medicines, vitamins and herbal supplements. Tekamlo and certain other medicines may affect each other and cause side effects.

Especially tell your doctor if you take:

- a kind of medicine called angiotensin receptor blocker or angiotensin converting enzyme inhibitor
- water pills (also called "diuretics")
- medicines for treating fungus or fungal infections
- cyclosporine (Gengraf®, Neoral, Sandimmune), a medicine used to suppress the immune system
- potassium-containing medicines, potassium supplements, or salt substitutes containing potassium
- simvastatin (Zocor®) or atorvastatin (Lipitor®)
- non-steroidal anti-inflammatory drugs (like ibuprofen or naproxen)
- medicines used to treat AIDS or HIV infections (such as ritonavir, indinavir)

Know your medicines. Keep a list of all your medicines. Show this list to your doctor or pharmacist when you get a new medicine. Your doctor or pharmacist will know what medicines are safe to take together.

How should I take Tekamlo?

- Take Tekamlo exactly as prescribed by your doctor. It is important to take Tekamlo every day to control your blood pressure.
- Take Tekamlo one time a day, about the same time each day.
- Take Tekamlo the same way every day, either with or without a meal.
- Your doctor may change your dose of Tekamlo if needed. Do not change the amount of Tekamlo you take without talking to your doctor.
- If you miss a dose of Tekamlo, take it as soon as you remember. If it is close to your next dose, do not take the missed dose. Just take the next dose at your regular time.
- If you take too much Tekamlo, call your doctor or a Poison Control Center, or go to the nearest hospital emergency room.

What are the possible side effects of Tekamlo?

Tekamlo may cause serious side effects:

- **Harm to an unborn baby, causing injury or death. See "What is the most important information I should know about Tekamlo?"**
- **Severe Allergic Reactions and Angioedema.** Aliskiren, one of the medicines in Tekamlo, can cause difficulty breathing or swallowing, tightness of the chest, hives, general rash, swelling, itching, dizziness, vomiting, or abdominal pain (signs of a severe allergic reaction). Aliskiren can also cause swelling of your face, lips, tongue, throat, arms and legs, or the whole body (signs of angioedema). Get medical help right away and tell your doctor if you get any one or more of these symptoms. Angioedema can happen at any time while you are taking Tekamlo.
- **Low blood pressure (hypotension).** Your blood pressure may get too low if you also take water pills, are on a low-

salt diet, get dialysis treatments, have heart problems, or get sick with vomiting or diarrhea. Lie down if you feel faint or get dizzy. Call your doctor right away.

- **Possible increased chest pain or risk of heart attack.** It is rare, but when you first start taking Tekamlo or increase your dose, you may have a heart attack or your angina may get worse. If that happens, call your doctor right away or go directly to a hospital emergency room.
- **Renal impairment or failure.** Aliskiren, one of the medicines in Tekamlo, may cause renal disorder with symptoms such as severely decreased urine output or decreased urine output (signs of renal impairment or failure).

The most common side effects of Tekamlo include:

- Swelling of your lower legs

Common side effects of Tekamlo include:

- diarrhea
- cough
- dizziness
- flu-like symptoms
- tiredness
- high levels of potassium in the blood (hyperkalemia)

Less common side effects include rash, severe skin reactions (signs may include severe blistering of the lips, eyes or mouth, rash with fever and skin peeling) and liver disorder (signs may include nausea, loss of appetite, dark colored urine or yellowing of skin and eyes).

Tell your doctor if you have any side effect that bothers you or that does not go away.

These are not all of the possible side effects of Tekamlo. For more information, ask your doctor or pharmacist.

Call your doctor for medical advice about side effects. You may report side effects to FDA at 1-800-FDA-1088.

How do I store Tekamlo?

- Store Tekamlo tablets at room temperature between 59°F to 86°F (15°C to 30°C).
- Keep the original prescription bottle and store in a dry place.
- Protect Tekamlo from heat and moisture.

Keep Tekamlo and all medicines out of the reach of children.

General information about Tekamlo

Medicines are sometimes prescribed for conditions not listed in the patient information leaflet. Do not take Tekamlo for a condition for which it was not prescribed. Do not give Tekamlo to other people, even if they have the same condition or symptoms you have. It may harm them.

This leaflet summarizes the most important information about Tekamlo. If you have questions about Tekamlo talk with your doctor. You can ask your doctor or pharmacist for information that is written for healthcare professionals.

For more information about Tekamlo, visit www.Tekamlo.com, or call 1-888-NOW-NOVA (1-888-669-6682).

What are the ingredients in Tekamlo?

Active Ingredients: Aliskiren hemifumarate and amlodipine

Inactive ingredients: Colloidal silicon dioxide, crospovidone, hypromellose, iron oxide red, iron oxide yellow, magnesium stearate, microcrystalline cellulose, polyethylene glycol, povidone, talc, and titanium dioxide.

What is high blood pressure (hypertension)?

Blood pressure is the force of blood in your blood vessels when your heart beats and when your heart rests. You have high blood pressure when the force is too much.

High blood pressure makes the heart work harder to pump blood through the body and causes damage to blood vessels. Tekamlo can help your blood vessels relax so your blood pressure is lower. Medicines that lower your blood pressure may lower your chance of having a stroke or heart attack.

Distributed by:
Novartis Pharmaceuticals Corporation
East Hanover, New Jersey 07936
© Novartis
T2013-109
November 2013
Shown in Product Identification Guide, page 311

TEKTURNA® ℞
[tek-turn-a]
(aliskiren)
tablets, for oral use

The following prescribing information is based on official labeling in effect July 2014.
HIGHLIGHTS OF PRESCRIBING INFORMATION
These highlights do not include all the information needed to use TEKTURNA® safely and effectively. See full prescribing information for TEKTURNA®.
Tekturna® (aliskiren) tablets, for oral use
Initial U.S. Approval: 2007

WARNING: FETAL TOXICITY
See full prescribing information for complete boxed warning
• When pregnancy is detected, discontinue Tekturna as soon as possible. (5.1)

• Drugs that act directly on the renin-angiotensin system can cause injury and death to the developing fetus. (5.1)

——————RECENT MAJOR CHANGES——————
Warnings and Precautions (5.4)   11/2013
——————INDICATIONS AND USAGE——————
Tekturna is a renin inhibitor (RI) indicated for:
• The treatment of hypertension, to lower blood pressure (1.1)
Lowering blood pressure reduces the risk of fatal and nonfatal cardiovascular events, primarily strokes and myocardial infarctions.
——————DOSAGE AND ADMINISTRATION——————
• Starting dose: 150 mg once daily with a routine pattern with regard to meals. If blood pressure remains uncontrolled titrate up to 300 mg daily (2.1, 2.3)
• Majority of effect of given dose attained in 2 weeks (2.1)
——————DOSAGE FORMS AND STRENGTHS——————
Tablets: 150 mg, 300 mg (3)
——————CONTRAINDICATIONS——————
Do not use with angiotensin receptor blockers (ARBs) or ACE inhibitors (ACEIs) in patients with diabetes (4)
——————WARNINGS AND PRECAUTIONS——————
• Avoid concomitant use with ARBs or ACEIs in patients with renal impairment (GFR<60 mL/min) (5.2)
• Anaphylactic Reactions and Head and Neck Angioedema: Discontinue use of Tekturna and monitor until signs and symptoms resolve (5.3)
• Hypotension in volume and/or salt depleted patients or with combined use of other agents acting on RAAS: Correct imbalances before initiating therapy with Tekturna (5.4)
• Impaired renal function: Monitor serum creatinine periodically. (5.5)
• Hyperkalemia: Monitor potassium levels periodically. (5.6)
——————ADVERSE REACTIONS——————
Most common adverse reaction: diarrhea (incidence 2.3%) (6.1)

To report SUSPECTED ADVERSE REACTIONS, contact Novartis Pharmaceuticals Corporation at 1-888-669-6682 or FDA at 1-800-FDA-1088 or www.fda.gov/medwatch.
——————DRUG INTERACTIONS——————
• Cyclosporine: Avoid concomitant use (7, 12.3)
• Itraconazole: Avoid concomitant use (7, 12.3)
• NSAIDs use may lead to increased risk of renal impairment and loss of antihypertensive effect (7)
——————USE IN SPECIFIC POPULATIONS——————
Nursing Mothers: Adverse reactions may occur in nursing infants (8.3)

See 17 for PATIENT COUNSELING INFORMATION and FDA-approved patient labeling
                                    Revised: 3/2014

FULL PRESCRIBING INFORMATION: CONTENTS*
WARNING: FETAL TOXICITY

FULL PRESCRIBING INFORMATION

WARNING: FETAL TOXICITY
• When pregnancy is detected, discontinue Tekturna as soon as possible. (5.1)
• Drugs that act directly on the renin-angiotensin system can cause injury and death to the developing fetus. (5.1)

1 INDICATIONS AND USAGE
1.1 Hypertension
Tekturna is indicated for the treatment of hypertension, to lower blood pressure. Lowering blood pressure reduces the risk of fatal and nonfatal cardiovascular events, primarily strokes and myocardial infarctions. These benefits have been seen in controlled trials of antihypertensive drugs from a wide variety of pharmacologic classes. There are no controlled trials demonstrating risk reduction with Tekturna.

Control of high blood pressure should be part of comprehensive cardiovascular risk management, including, as appropriate, lipid control, diabetes management, antithrombotic therapy, smoking cessation, exercise, and limited sodium intake. Many patients will require more than one drug to achieve blood pressure goals. For specific advice on goals and management, see published guidelines, such as those of the National High Blood Pressure Education Program's Joint National Committee on Prevention, Detection, Evaluation, and Treatment of High Blood Pressure (JNC).

Numerous antihypertensive drugs, from a variety of pharmacologic classes and with different mechanisms of action, have been shown in randomized controlled trials to reduce cardiovascular morbidity and mortality, and it can be concluded that it is blood pressure reduction, and not some other pharmacologic property of the drugs, that is largely responsible for those benefits. The largest and most consistent cardiovascular outcome benefit has been a reduction in the risk of stroke, but reductions in myocardial infarction and cardiovascular mortality also have been seen regularly. Elevated systolic or diastolic pressure causes increased cardiovascular risk, and the absolute risk increase per mmHg is greater at higher blood pressures, so that even modest reductions of severe hypertension can provide substantial benefit. Relative risk reduction from blood pressure reduction is similar across populations with varying absolute risk, so the absolute benefit is greater in patients who are at higher risk independent of their hypertension (for example, patients with diabetes or hyperlipidemia), and such patients would be expected to benefit from more aggressive treatment to a lower blood pressure goal.

Some antihypertensive drugs have smaller blood pressure effects (as monotherapy) in black patients, and many antihypertensive drugs have additional approved indications and effects (e.g., on angina, heart failure, or diabetic kidney disease). These considerations may guide selection of therapy.

2 DOSAGE AND ADMINISTRATION
2.1 Hypertension
The usual recommended starting dose of Tekturna is 150 mg once daily. In patients whose blood pressure is not adequately controlled, the daily dose may be increased to 300 mg. Doses above 300 mg did not give an increased blood pressure response but resulted in an increased rate of diarrhea. The antihypertensive effect of a given dose is substantially attained (85-90%) by 2 weeks.
2.2 Use with Other Antihypertensives
Tekturna may be administered with some other antihypertensive agents. In diabetics, do not use in combination with angiotensin receptor blockers (ARBs) or angiotensin converting enzyme inhibitors (ACEIs) [see Contraindications (4)]. Concomitant use of aliskiren with an ARB or ACEI is not recommended in patients with GFR <60 ml/min [see Warnings and Precautions (5.2)]. Most exposure to date is with diuretics, an angiotensin receptor blocker (valsartan) or a calcium channel blocker (amlodipine). Aliskiren used together with these drugs has a greater effect at their maximum recommended doses than either drug alone. It is not

known whether additive effects are present when Tekturna is used with angiotensin-converting enzyme inhibitors (ACEIs) or beta blockers (BB).
2.3 Relationship to Meals
Patients should establish a routine pattern for taking Tekturna with regard to meals. High fat meals decrease absorption substantially [see Clinical Pharmacology (12.3)].

3 DOSAGE FORMS AND STRENGTHS
150 mg light pink biconvex round tablet, imprinted NVR/IL (Side 1/Side 2)
300 mg light red biconvex ovaloid round tablet, imprinted NVR/IU (Side 1/Side 2)

4 CONTRAINDICATIONS
Do not use aliskiren with ARBs or ACEIs in patients with diabetes [see Warnings and Precautions (5.2), Clinical Studies (14.3)].

5 WARNINGS AND PRECAUTIONS
5.1 Fetal Toxicity
Pregnancy Category D
Use of drugs that act on the renin-angiotensin system during the second and third trimesters of pregnancy reduces fetal renal function and increases fetal and neonatal morbidity and death. Resulting oligohydramnios can be associated with fetal lung hypoplasia and skeletal deformations. Potential neonatal adverse effects include skull hypoplasia, anuria, hypotension, renal failure, and death. When pregnancy is detected, discontinue Tekturna as soon as possible [see Use in Specific Populations (8.1)].
5.2 Renal Impairment/Hyperkalemia/Hypotension when Tekturna is given in combination with ARBs or ACEIs
Tekturna is contraindicated in patients who are receiving ARBs or ACEIs because of the increased risk of renal impairment, hyperkalemia, and hypotension [see Contraindications (4) and Clinical Studies (14.3)].
Avoid use of Tekturna with ARBs or ACEIs in patients with moderate renal impairment (GFR <60 ml/min).
5.3 Anaphylactic Reactions and Head and Neck Angioedema
Hypersensitivity reactions such as anaphylactic reactions and angioedema of the face, extremities, lips, tongue, glottis and/or larynx have been reported in patients treated with Tekturna and has necessitated hospitalization and intubation. This may occur at any time during treatment and has occurred in patients with and without a history of angioedema with ACE inhibitors or angiotensin receptor antagonists. Anaphylactic reactions have been reported from postmarketing experience with unknown frequency. If angioedema involves the throat, tongue, glottis or larynx, or if the patient has a history of upper respiratory surgery, airway obstruction may occur and be fatal. Patients who experience these effects, even without respiratory distress, require prolonged observation and appropriate monitoring measures since treatment with antihistamines and corticosteroids may not be sufficient to prevent respiratory involvement. Prompt administration of subcutaneous epinephrine solution 1:1000 (0.3 to 0.5 ml) and measures to ensure a patent airway may be necessary.
Discontinue Tekturna immediately in patients who develop anaphylactic reactions or angioedema, and do not readminister.
5.4 Hypotension
Symptomatic hypotension may occur after initiation of treatment with Tekturna in patients with marked volume depletion, patients with salt depletion, or with combined use of aliskiren and other agents acting on the renin-angiotensin-aldosterone system. The volume or salt depletion should be corrected prior to administration of Tekturna, or the treatment should start under close medical supervision.
A transient hypotensive response is not a contraindication to further treatment, which usually can be continued without difficulty once the blood pressure has stabilized.
5.5 Impaired Renal Function
Monitor renal function periodically in patients treated with Tekturna. Changes in renal function, including acute renal failure, can be caused by drugs that affect the renin-angiotensin-aldosterone system. Patients whose renal function may depend in part on the activity of the renin-angiotensin-aldosterone system (e.g., patients with renal artery stenosis, severe heart failure, post-myocardial infarction or volume depletion) or patients receiving ARB, ACEI or non-steroidal anti-inflammatory (NSAID) therapy may be at particular risk for developing acute renal failure on Tekturna [see Contraindications (4), Warnings and Precautions (5.2), Clinical Studies (14.3)]. Consider withholding or discontinuing therapy in patients who develop a clinically significant decrease in renal function.
5.6 Hyperkalemia
Monitor serum potassium periodically in patients receiving Tekturna. Drugs that affect the renin-angiotensin-aldosterone system can cause hyperkalemia. Risk factors for the development of hyperkalemia include renal insuffi-

ciency, diabetes, combination use with ARBs or ACEIs [see Contraindications (4), Warnings and Precautions (5.2), and Clinical Studies (14.3)], NSAIDs, or potassium supplements or potassium sparing diuretics.

5.7 Cyclosporine or Itraconazole
When aliskiren was given with cyclosporine or itraconazole, the blood concentrations of aliskiren were significantly increased. Avoid concomitant use of aliskiren with cyclosporine or itraconazole [see Drug Interactions (7)].

6 ADVERSE REACTIONS
6.1 Clinical Trials Experience
Because clinical trials are conducted under widely varying conditions, adverse reaction rates observed in the clinical trials of a drug cannot be directly compared to rates in clinical trials of another drug and may not reflect the rates observed in practice.

Data described below reflect the evaluation of the safety of Tekturna in more than 6,460 patients, including over 1,740 treated for longer than 6 months, and more than 1,250 patients for longer than 1 year. In placebo controlled clinical trials, discontinuation of therapy due to a clinical adverse event, including uncontrolled hypertension occurred in 2.2% of patients treated with Tekturna vs. 3.5% of patients given placebo. These data do not include information from the ALTITUDE study which evaluated the use of aliskiren in combination with ARBs or ACEIs [see Contraindications (4), Warnings and Precautions (5.2), and Clinical Studies (14.3)].

Angioedema: Two cases of angioedema with respiratory symptoms were reported with Tekturna use in the clinical studies. Two other cases of periorbital edema without respiratory symptoms were reported as possible angioedema and resulted in discontinuation. The rate of these angioedema cases in the completed studies was 0.06%. In addition, 26 other cases of edema involving the face, hands, or whole body were reported with Tekturna use including 4 leading to discontinuation. In the placebo controlled studies, however, the incidence of edema involving the face, hands or whole body was 0.4% with Tekturna compared with 0.5% with placebo. In a long term active control study with Tekturna and HCTZ arms, the incidence of edema involving the face, hand or whole body was 0.4% in both treatment arms [see Warnings and Precautions (5.2)].

Gastrointestinal: Tekturna produces dose-related gastrointestinal (GI) adverse reactions. Diarrhea was reported by 2.3% of patients at 300 mg, compared to 1.2% in placebo patients. In women and the elderly (age ≥ 65) increases in diarrhea rates were evident starting at a dose of 150 mg daily, with rates for these subgroups at 150 mg comparable to those seen at 300 mg for men or younger patients (all rates about 2.0-2.3%). Other GI symptoms included abdominal pain, dyspepsia, and gastroesophageal reflux, although increased rates for abdominal pain and dyspepsia were distinguished from placebo only at 600 mg daily. Diarrhea and other GI symptoms were typically mild and rarely led to discontinuation.

Cough: Tekturna was associated with a slight increase in cough in the placebo-controlled studies (1.1% for any Tekturna use vs. 0.6% for placebo). In active-controlled trials with ACE inhibitor (ramipril, lisinopril) arms, the rates of cough for the Tekturna arms were about one-third to one-half the rates in the ACE inhibitor arms.

Seizures: Single episodes of tonic-clonic seizures with loss of consciousness were reported in two patients treated with Tekturna in the clinical trials. One of these patients did have predisposing causes for seizures and had a negative electroencephalogram (EEG) and cerebral imaging following the seizures (for the other patient EEG and imaging results were not reported). Tekturna was discontinued and there was no re-challenge.

Other adverse effects with increased rates for Tekturna compared to placebo included rash (1% vs. 0.3%), elevated uric acid (0.4% vs. 0.1%), gout (0.2% vs. 0.1%) and renal stones (0.2% vs. 0%).

Aliskiren's effect on ECG intervals was studied in a randomized, double-blind, placebo and active-controlled (moxifloxacin), 7-day repeat dosing study with Holter-monitoring and 12 lead ECGs throughout the interdosing interval. No effect of aliskiren on QT interval was seen.

Clinical Laboratory Findings
In controlled clinical trials, clinically relevant changes in standard laboratory parameters were rarely associated with the administration of Tekturna in patients with hypertension not concomitantly treated with an ARB or ACEI. In multiple-dose studies in hypertensive patients, Tekturna had no clinically important effects on total cholesterol, HDL, fasting triglycerides, or fasting glucose.

Blood Urea Nitrogen, Creatinine: In patients with hypertension not concomitantly treated with an ARB or ACEI, minor increases in blood urea nitrogen (BUN) or serum creatinine were observed in less than 7% of patients treated with Tekturna alone vs. 6% on placebo [see Warnings and Precautions (5.2)].

Hemoglobin and Hematocrit: Small decreases in hemoglobin and hematocrit (mean decreases of approximately 0.08 g/dL and 0.16 volume percent, respectively, for all aliskiren monotherapy) were observed. The decreases were dose-related and were 0.24 g/dL and 0.79 volume percent for 600 mg daily. This effect is also seen with other agents acting on the renin angiotensin system, such as angiotensin inhibitors and angiotensin receptor blockers and may be mediated by reduction of angiotensin II which stimulates erythropoietin production via the AT1 receptor. These decreases led to slight increases in rates of anemia with aliskiren compared to placebo were observed (0.1% for any aliskiren use, 0.3% for aliskiren 600 mg daily, vs 0% for placebo). No patients discontinued therapy due to anemia.

Serum Potassium: In patients with hypertension not concomitantly treated with an ARB or ACEI, increases in serum potassium >5.5 mEq/L were infrequent (0.9% compared to 0.6% with placebo) [See Contraindications (4) and Warnings and Precautions (5.6)].

Serum Uric Acid: Aliskiren monotherapy produced small median increases in serum uric acid levels (about 6 µmol/L) while HCTZ produced larger increases (about 30 µmol/L). The combination of aliskiren with HCTZ appears to be additive (about 40 µmol/L increase). The increases in uric acid appear to lead to slight increases in uric acid-related AEs: elevated uric acid (0.4% vs 0.1%), gout (0.2% vs. 0.1%), and renal stones (0.2% vs 0%).

Creatine Kinase: Increases in creatine kinase of >300% were recorded in about 1% of aliskiren monotherapy patients vs. 0.5% of placebo patients. Five cases of creatine kinase rises, three leading to discontinuation and one diagnosed as subclinical rhabdomyolysis, and another as myositis, were reported as adverse events with aliskiren use in the clinical trials. No cases were associated with renal dysfunction.

6.2 Postmarketing Experience
The following adverse reactions have been reported in aliskiren post-marketing experience. Because these reactions are reported voluntarily from a population of uncertain size, it is not always possible to estimate their frequency or establish a causal relationship to drug exposure.

Hypersensitivity: anaphylactic reactions and angioedema requiring airway management and hospitalization

Urticaria

Peripheral edema

Hepatic enzyme increase with clinical symptoms of hepatic dysfunction

Severe cutaneous adverse reactions, including Stevens-Johnson syndrome and toxic epidermal necrolysis

Pruritus

Erythema

7 DRUG INTERACTIONS
Cyclosporine: Avoid co-administration of cyclosporine with aliskiren.

Itraconazole: Avoid co-administration of itraconazole with aliskiren [See Clinical Pharmacology (12.3)].

Non-Steroidal Anti-Inflammatory Agents (NSAIDs) including selective Cyclooxygenase-2 inhibitors (COX-2 inhibitors): In patients who are elderly, volume-depleted (including those on diuretic therapy), or with compromised renal function, co-administration of NSAIDs, including selective COX-2 inhibitors with agents that affect the renin-angiotensin-aldosterone system, including aliskiren, may result in deterioration of renal function, including possible acute renal failure. These effects are usually reversible. Monitor renal function periodically in patients receiving aliskiren and NSAID therapy.

The antihypertensive effect of aliskiren may be attenuated by NSAIDs.

Dual Blockade of the renin-angiotensin-aldosterone system: The concomitant use of aliskiren with other agents acting on the renin-angiotensin-aldosterone system such as ACEIs or ARBs is associated with an increased risk of hypotension, hyperkalemia, and changes in renal function (including acute renal failure) compared to monotherapy. Monitor blood pressure, renal function, and electrolytes in patients on aliskiren and other agents that affect the renin-angiotensin-aldosterone system [see Warnings and Precautions (5.4, 5.5, 5.6)].

The concomitant use of aliskiren with an ARB or an ACEI in diabetic patients is contraindicated and should be avoided in patients with moderate renal impairment [see Contraindications (4) and Warnings and Precautions (5.2)].

Furosemide: Oral co-administration of aliskiren and furosemide reduced exposure to furosemide. Monitor diuretic effects when furosemide is co-administered with aliskiren.

8 USE IN SPECIFIC POPULATIONS
8.1 Pregnancy
Pregnancy Category D

Use of drugs that act on the renin-angiotensin system during the second and third trimesters of pregnancy reduces fetal renal function and increases fetal and neonatal mor-

bidity and death. Resulting oligohydramnios can be associated with fetal lung hypoplasia and skeletal deformations. Potential neonatal adverse effects include skull hypoplasia, anuria, hypotension, renal failure, and death. When pregnancy is detected, discontinue Tekturna as soon as possible. These adverse outcomes are usually associated with use of these drugs in the second and third trimester of pregnancy. Most epidemiologic studies examining fetal abnormalities after exposure to antihypertensive use in the first trimester have not distinguished drugs affecting the renin-angiotensin system from other antihypertensive agents. Appropriate management of maternal hypertension during pregnancy is important to optimize outcomes for both mother and fetus.

In the unusual case that there is no appropriate alternative to therapy with drugs affecting the renin-angiotensin system for a particular patient, apprise the mother of the potential risk to the fetus. Perform serial ultrasound examinations to assess the intra-amniotic environment. If oligohydramnios is observed, discontinue Tekturna, unless it is considered lifesaving for the mother. Fetal testing may be appropriate, based on the week of pregnancy. Patients and physicians should be aware, however, that oligohydramnios may not appear until after the fetus has sustained irreversible injury. Closely observe infants with histories of in utero exposure to Tekturna for hypotension, oliguria, and hyperkalemia. [see Use in Specific Populations (8.4)]

8.3 Nursing Mothers
It is not known whether aliskiren is excreted in human breast milk. Aliskiren was secreted in the milk of lactating rats. Because of the potential for adverse effects on the nursing infant, a decision should be made whether to discontinue nursing or discontinue the drug, taking into account the importance of the drug to the mother.

8.4 Pediatric Use
Safety and effectiveness of aliskiren in pediatric patients <18 years have not been established.

Neonates with a history of in utero exposure to Tekturna: If oliguria or hypotension occurs, direct attention toward support of blood pressure and renal perfusion. Exchange transfusions or dialysis may be required as a means of reversing hypotension and/or substituting for disordered renal function.

8.5 Geriatric Use
Of the total number of patients receiving aliskiren in clinical studies, 1,275 (19%) were 65 years or older and 231 (3.4%) were 75 years or older. No overall differences in safety or effectiveness were observed between these subjects and younger subjects. Other reported clinical experience has not identified differences in responses between the elderly and younger patients, but greater sensitivity of some older individuals cannot be ruled out.

8.6 Renal Impairment
Safety and effectiveness of Tekturna in patients with severe renal impairment (CrCL <30 ml/min) have not been established as patients with eGFR <30ml/min were excluded in clinical trials [see Clinical Studies (14)].

10 OVERDOSAGE
Limited data are available related to overdosage in humans. The most likely manifestation of overdosage would be hypotension. If symptomatic hypotension occurs, supportive treatment should be initiated.

Aliskiren is poorly dialyzed. Therefore, hemodialysis is not adequate to treat aliskiren overexposure [see Clinical Pharmacology (12.3)].

11 DESCRIPTION
Tekturna contains aliskiren hemifumarate, a renin inhibitor, that is provided as tablets for oral administration. Aliskiren hemifumarate is chemically described as (2S, 4S,5S,7S)-N-(2-carbamoyl-2-methylpropyl)-5-amino-4-hydroxy-2,7-diisopropyl-8-[4-methoxy-3-(3-methoxypropoxy) phenyl]-octanamide hemifumarate and its structural formula is

Molecular formula: $C_{30}H_{53}N_3O_6 \cdot 0.5\ C_4H_4O_4$

Aliskiren hemifumarate is a white to slightly yellowish crystalline powder with a molecular weight of 609.8 (free base- 551.8). It is soluble in phosphate buffer, n-octanol, and highly soluble in water.

12 CLINICAL PHARMACOLOGY
12.1 Mechanism of Action
Renin is secreted by the kidney in response to decreases in blood volume and renal perfusion. Renin cleaves angiotensin-

ogen to form the inactive decapeptide angiotensin I (Ang I). Ang I is converted to the active octapeptide angiotensin II (Ang II) by angiotensin-converting enzyme (ACE) and non-ACE pathways. Ang II is a powerful vasoconstrictor and leads to the release of catecholamines from the adrenal medulla and prejunctional nerve endings. It also promotes aldosterone secretion and sodium reabsorption. Together, these effects increase blood pressure. Ang II also inhibits renin release, thus providing a negative feedback to the system. This cycle, from renin through angiotensin to aldosterone and its associated negative feedback loop, is known as the renin-angiotensin-aldosterone system (RAAS). Aliskiren is a direct renin inhibitor, decreasing plasma renin activity (PRA) and inhibiting the conversion of angiotensinogen to Ang I. Whether aliskiren affects other RAAS components, e.g., ACE or non-ACE pathways, is not known.

All agents that inhibit the RAAS, including renin inhibitors, suppress the negative feedback loop, leading to a compensatory rise in plasma renin concentration. When this rise occurs during treatment with ACE inhibitors and ARBs, the result is increased levels of PRA. During treatment with aliskiren, however, the effect of increased renin levels is blocked so that PRA, Ang I and Ang II are all reduced, whether aliskiren is used as monotherapy or in combination with other antihypertensive agents.

12.2 Pharmacodynamics

In placebo controlled clinical trials, plasma renin activity (PRA) was decreased in a range of 50-80%. This reduction in PRA was not dose-related and did not correlate with blood pressure reductions. The clinical implications of the differences in effect on PRA are not known.

12.3 Pharmacokinetics

Aliskiren is poorly absorbed (bioavailability about 2.5%) with an approximate accumulation half life of 24 hours. Steady state blood levels are reached in about 7-8 days.

Absorption and Distribution

Following oral administration, peak plasma concentrations of aliskiren are reached within 1 – 3 hours. When taken with a high fat meal, mean AUC and C_{max} of aliskiren are decreased by 71% and 85% respectively. In the clinical trials of aliskiren, it was administered without requiring a fixed relation of administration to meals.

Metabolism and Elimination

About one fourth of the absorbed dose appears in the urine as parent drug. How much of the absorbed dose is metabolized is unknown. Based on the in vitro studies, the major enzyme responsible for aliskiren metabolism appears to be CYP 3A4. Aliskiren does not inhibit the CYP450 isoenzymes (CYP 1A2, 2C8, 2C9, 2C19, 2D6, 2E1, and 3A) or induce CYP 3A4.

Transporters: Pgp (MDR1/Mdr1a/1b) was found to be the major efflux system involved in absorption and disposition of aliskiren in preclinical studies. The potential for drug interactions at the Pgp site will likely depend on the degree of inhibition of this transporter.

Drug interactions

The effect of co-administered drugs on the pharmacokinetics of aliskiren and vice versa, were studied in several single and multiple dose studies. Pharmacokinetic measures indicating the magnitude of these interactions are presented in Figure 1 (impact of co-administered drugs on aliskiren) and Figure 2 (impact of aliskiren on co-administered drugs).

[See figure 1 above]

Warfarin: There was no clinically significant effect of a single dose of warfarin 25 mg on the pharmacokinetics of aliskiren.

[See figure 2 above]

Furosemide: In patients with heart failure, co-administration of aliskiren (300 mg/day) reduced plasma AUC and Cmax of oral furosemide (60 mg/day) by 17% and 27%, respectively, and reduced 24 hour urinary furosemide excretion by 29%. This change in exposure did not result in statistically significant difference in total urine volume and urinary sodium excretion over 24 hours. However, a transient decrease in urinary sodium excretion and urine volume effects up to 12 hours were observed when furosemide was co-administered with aliskiren 300 mg/day.

Special Populations

Renally Impaired Patients: Aliskiren was evaluated in patients with varying degrees of renal insufficiency. The rate and extent of exposure (AUC and C_{max}) of aliskiren in subjects with renal impairment did not show a consistent correlation with the severity of renal impairment. Adjustment of the starting dose is not required in these patients [see Warnings and Precautions (5.2)].

The pharmacokinetics of aliskiren following administration of a single oral dose of 300 mg was evaluated in patients with End Stage Renal Disease (ESRD) undergoing hemodialysis. When compared to matched healthy subjects, changes in the rate and extent of aliskiren exposure (C_{max} and AUC) in ESRD patients undergoing hemodialysis was not clinically significant.

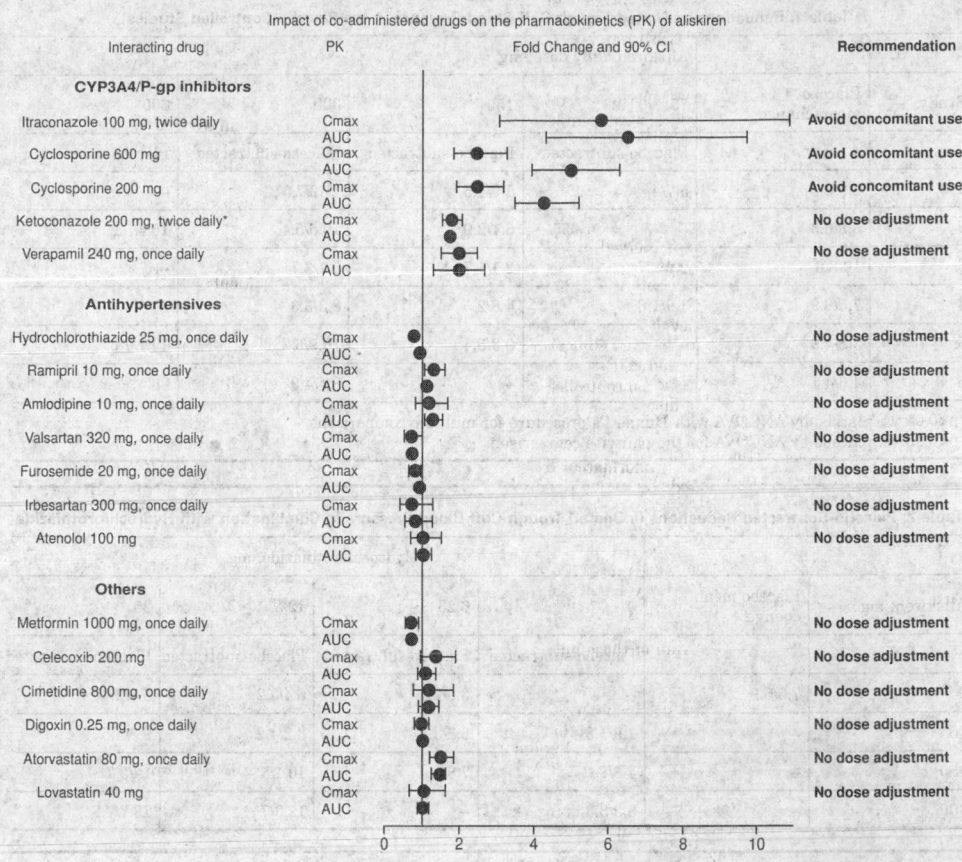

Figure 1: The impact of co-administered drugs on the pharmacokinetics of aliskiren.

Figure 2: The impact of aliskiren on the pharmacokinetics of co-administered drugs.

Timing of hemodialysis did not significantly alter the pharmacokinetics of aliskiren in ESRD patients. Therefore, no dose adjustment is warranted in ESRD patients receiving hemodialysis.

Hepatically Impaired Patients: The pharmacokinetics of aliskiren were not significantly affected in patients with mild to severe liver disease. Consequently, adjustment of the starting dose is not required in these patients.

Table 1: Reductions in Seated Trough Cuff Blood Pressure in the Placebo-Controlled Studies

Study	Placebo mean change	Aliskiren daily dose, mg			
		75	150	300	600
		Placebo-subtracted	Placebo-subtracted	Placebo-subtracted	Placebo-subtracted
1	2.9/3.3	5.7/4*	5.9/4.5*	11.2/7.5*	--
2	5.3/6.3	--	6.1/2.9*	10.5/5.4*	10.4/5.2*
3	10/8.6	2.2/1.7	2.1/1.7	5.1/3.7*	--
4	7.5/6.9	1.9/1.8	4.8/2*	8.3/3.3*	--
5	3.8/4.9	--	9.3/5.4*	10.9/6.2*	12.1/7.6*
6	4.6/4.1	--	--	8.4/4.9†	

*$p<0.05$ vs. placebo by ANCOVA with Dunnett's procedure for multiple comparisons
†$p<0.05$ vs. placebo by ANCOVA for the pairwise comparison.

Table 2: Placebo-Subtracted Reductions in Seated Trough Cuff Blood Pressure in Combination with Hydrochlorothiazide

Aliskiren, mg	Placebo mean change	Hydrochlorothiazide, mg			
		0	6.25	12.5	25
		Placebo-subtracted	Placebo-subtracted	Placebo-subtracted	Placebo-subtracted
0	7.5/6.9	--	3.5/2.1	6.4/3.2	6.8/2.4
75	--	1.9/1.8	6.8/3.8	8.2/4.2	9.8/4.5
150	--	4.8/2	7.8/3.4	10.1/5	12/5.7
300	--	8.3/3.3	--	12.3/7	13.7/7.3

Table 3: Placebo-Subtracted Reductions in Seated Trough Cuff Blood Pressure in Combination with Valsartan

Aliskiren, mg	Placebo mean change	Valsartan, mg		
		0	160	320
0	4.6/4.1*	--	5.6/3.9	8.2/5.6
150	--	5.4/2.7	10.0/5.7	--
300	--	8.4/4.9	--	12.6/8.1

* The placebo change is 5.2/4.8 for week 4 endpoint which was used for the dose groups containing Aliskiren 150 mg or Valsartan 160 mg.

Table 4: Placebo-Subtracted Reductions in Seated Trough Cuff Blood Pressure in Combination with Amlodipine

Aliskiren, mg	Placebo mean change	Amlodipine, mg		
		0	5	10
0	5.4/6.8	--	5.6/9.0	8.5/14.3
150	--	2.6/3.9	8.6/13.9	10.8/17.1
300	--	4.9/8.6	9.6/15.0	11.1/16.4

Pediatric Patients: The pharmacokinetics of aliskiren have not been investigated in patients <18 years of age.
Geriatric Patients: Exposure (measured by AUC) is increased in elderly patients ≥65 years. Adjustment of the starting dose is not required in these patients.
Race: The pharmacokinetic differences between Blacks, Caucasians, and the Japanese are minimal.

13   NONCLINICAL TOXICOLOGY
13.1   Carcinogenesis, Mutagenesis, Impairment of Fertility
Carcinogenic potential was assessed in a 2-year rat study and a 6-month transgenic (rasH2) mouse study with aliskiren hemifumarate at oral doses of up to 1500 mg aliskiren/kg/day. Although there were no statistically significant increases in tumor incidence associated with exposure to aliskiren, mucosal epithelial hyperplasia (with or without erosion/ulceration) was observed in the lower gastrointestinal tract at doses of ≥750 mg/kg/day in both species, with a colonic adenoma identified in one rat and a cecal adenocarcinoma identified in another, rare tumors in the strain of rat studied. On a systemic exposure (AUC_{0-24hr}) basis, 1500 mg/kg/day in the rat is about 4 times and in the mouse about 1.5 times the maximum recommended human dose (300 mg aliskiren/day). Mucosal hyperplasia in the cecum or colon of rats was also observed at doses of 250 mg/kg/day (the lowest tested dose) as well as at higher doses in 4- and 13-week studies.
Aliskiren hemifumarate was devoid of genotoxic potential in the Ames reverse mutation assay with *S. typhimurium* and *E. coli*, the in vitro Chinese hamster ovary cell chromosomal aberration assay, the in vitro Chinese hamster V79 cell gene mutation test and the in vivo mouse bone marrow micronucleus assay.
Fertility of male and female rats was unaffected at doses of up to 250 mg aliskiren/kg/day (8 times the maximum recommended human dose of 300 mg Tekturna/60 kg on a mg/m² basis.)

13.2   Animal Toxicology and/or Pharmacology
Reproductive Toxicology Studies: Reproductive toxicity studies of aliskiren hemifumarate did not reveal any evidence of teratogenicity at oral doses up to 600 mg aliskiren/kg/day (20 times the maximum recommended human dose (MRHD) of 300 mg/day on a mg/m² basis) in pregnant rats or up to 100 mg aliskiren/kg/day (7 times the MRHD on a mg/m² basis) in pregnant rabbits. Fetal birth weight was adversely affected in rabbits at 50 mg/kg/day (3.2 times the MRHD on a mg/m² basis). Aliskiren was present in placenta, amniotic fluid and fetuses of pregnant rabbits.

14   CLINICAL STUDIES
14.1   Aliskiren Monotherapy
The antihypertensive effects of Tekturna have been demonstrated in six randomized, double-blind, placebo-controlled 8-week clinical trials in patients with mild-to-moderate hypertension. The placebo response and placebo-subtracted changes from baseline in seated trough cuff blood pressure are shown in Table 1.
[See table 1 above]
The studies included approximately 2,730 patients given doses of 75-600 mg of aliskiren and 1,231 patients given placebo. As shown in Table 1, there is some increase in response with administered dose in all studies, with reasonable effects seen at 150-300 mg, and no clear further increases at 600 mg. A substantial proportion (85%-90%) of the blood pressure lowering effect was observed within 2 weeks of treatment studies with ambulatory blood pressure monitoring showed reasonable control throughout the inter-dosing interval; the ratios of mean daytime to mean nighttime ambulatory BP range from 0.6 to 0.9.
Patients in the placebo-controlled trials continued open-label aliskiren for up to one year. A persistent blood pressure lowering effect was demonstrated by a randomized withdrawal study (patients randomized to continue drug or placebo), which showed a statistically significant difference between patients kept on aliskiren and those randomized to placebo. With cessation of treatment, blood pressure gradually returned toward baseline levels over a period of several weeks. There was no evidence of rebound hypertension after abrupt cessation of therapy.
Aliskiren lowered blood pressure in all demographic subgroups, although Black patients tended to have smaller reduction than Caucasians and Asians, as has been seen with ACE inhibitors and ARBs.
There are no studies of Tekturna or members of the direct renin inhibitors demonstrating reductions in cardiovascular risk in patients with hypertension.

14.2   Aliskiren in Combination with Other Antihypertensives
Hydrochlorothiazide
Aliskiren 75, 150, and 300 mg and hydrochlorothiazide 6.25, 12.5, and 25 mg were studied alone and in combination in an 8-week, 2,776-patient, randomized, double-blind, placebo-controlled, parallel-group, 15-arm factorial study. Blood pressure reductions with the combinations were greater than the reductions with the monotherapies as shown in Table 2.
[See table 2 above]

Valsartan
Aliskiren 150 and 300 mg and valsartan 160 and 320 mg were studied alone and in combination in an 8-week, 1,797-patient, randomized, double-blind, placebo-controlled, parallel-group, 4-arm, dose-escalation study. The dosages of aliskiren and valsartan were started at 150 and 160 mg, respectively, and increased at four weeks to 300 mg and 320 mg, respectively. Seated trough cuff blood pressure was measured at baseline, 4, and 8 weeks. Blood pressure reductions with the combinations were greater than the reductions with the monotherapies as shown in Table 3.
[See table 3 above]

Amlodipine
Aliskiren 150 mg and 300 mg and amlodipine besylate 5 mg and 10 mg were studied alone and in combination in an 8-week, 1,685-patient, randomized, double-blind, placebo-controlled, multifactorial study. Treatment with aliskiren and amlodipine resulted overall in significantly greater reductions in diastolic and systolic blood pressure compared to the respective monotherapy components as shown in Table 4.
[See table 4 above]

ACE inhibitors
Aliskiren has not been studied when added to maximal doses of ACE inhibitors to determine whether aliskiren produces additional blood pressure reduction.

14.3   Aliskiren in Patients with Diabetes treated with ARB or ACEI (ALTITUDE study)
Patients with diabetes with renal disease (defined either by the presence of albuminuria or reduced GFR) were randomized to aliskiren 300 mg daily (n=4296) or placebo (n=4310). All patients were receiving background therapy with an ARB or ACEI. The primary efficacy outcome was the time to the first event of the primary composite endpoint consisting of cardiovascular death, resuscitated sudden death, non-fatal myocardial infarction, non-fatal stroke, unplanned hospitalization for heart failure, onset of end stage renal disease, renal death, and doubling of serum creatinine concentration from baseline sustained for at least one month. After a median follow up of about 32 months, the trial was terminated early for lack of efficacy. Higher risk of renal im-

pairment, hypotension and hyperkalemia was observed in aliskiren compared to placebo treated patients, as shown in the table below.
[See table 5 above]
The risk of stroke (3.4% aliskiren vs 2.7% placebo) and death (8.4% aliskiren vs. 8.0% placebo) were also numerically higher in aliskiren treated patients.

16   HOW SUPPLIED/STORAGE AND HANDLING

Tekturna is supplied as a light-pink, biconvex round tablet containing 150 mg of aliskiren, and as a light-red biconvex ovaloid tablet containing 300 mg of aliskiren. Tablets are imprinted with NVR on one side and IL, IU, on the other side of the 150, and 300 mg tablets, respectively.
All strengths are packaged in bottles and unit-dose blister packages (10 strips or 10 tablets) as described below in Table 6.
[See table 6 above]
Store at 25°C (77°F); excursions permitted to 15-30°C (59-86°F) [See USP Controlled Room Temperature]. Protect from moisture.
Dispense in original container.

17   PATIENT COUNSELING INFORMATION

See FDA-approved patient labeling (Patient Information)
Information for Patients
Pregnancy: Female patients of child bearing age should be told about the consequences of exposure to Tekturna during pregnancy. Discuss treatment options with women planning to become pregnant. Patients should be asked to report pregnancies to their physicians as soon as possible.
Anaphylactic Reactions and Angioedema: Patients should be advised and told to report immediately any signs or symptoms suggesting a severe allergic reaction (difficulty breathing or swallowing, tightness of the chest, hives, general rash, swelling, itching, dizziness, vomiting, or abdominal pain) or angioedema (swelling of face, extremities, eyes, lips, tongue, difficulty in swallowing or breathing) and to take no more drug until they have consulted with the prescribing physicians. Angioedema, including laryngeal edema, may occur at any time during treatment with Tekturna.
Symptomatic Hypotension: A patient receiving Tekturna should be cautioned that lightheadedness can occur, especially during the first days of therapy, and that it should be reported to the prescribing physician. The patients should be told that if syncope occurs, Tekturna should be discontinued until the physician has been consulted.
All patients should be cautioned that inadequate fluid intake, excessive perspiration, diarrhea, or vomiting can lead to an excessive fall in blood pressure, with the same consequences of lightheadedness and possible syncope.
Potassium Supplements: A patient receiving Tekturna should be told not to use potassium supplements or salt substitutes containing potassium without consulting the prescribing physician.
Relationship to Meals: Patients should establish a routine pattern for taking Tekturna with regard to meals. High-fat meals decrease absorption substantially.
T2014-23
March 2014
FDA approved patient labeling
PATIENT INFORMATION
Tekturna (pronounced tek-turn-a)
(aliskiren)
Tablets
Dosing Strengths:
150 mg tablets
300 mg tablets
Available by Prescription Only
Read the patient information that comes with Tekturna before you start taking it and each time you get a refill. There may be new information. This leaflet does not replace talking to your doctor about your condition or treatment. If you have any questions about Tekturna, ask your doctor or pharmacist.
What is the most important information I should know about Tekturna?
Tekturna can cause harm or death to an unborn baby. Talk to your doctor about other ways to lower your blood pressure if you plan to become pregnant. If you get pregnant while taking Tekturna, tell your doctor right away.
What Is Tekturna?
Tekturna can help your blood vessels relax and widen so blood pressure is lower. Tekturna is a type of prescription medicine called a direct renin inhibitor. By reducing renin, it helps to reduce blood pressure.
What Is High Blood Pressure (Hypertension)?
Blood pressure is the force that pushes the blood through your blood vessels to all the organs of your body. You have high blood pressure when the force of your blood moving through your blood vessels is too great. Renin (pronounced REE-nin) is a chemical in the body that starts a process that

Table 5: Incidence of Selected Adverse Events During the Treatment Phase in ALTITUDE

	Aliskiren N=4272		Placebo N=4285	
	Serious Adverse Events* (%)	Adverse Events (%)	Serious Adverse Events* (%)	Adverse Events (%)
Renal impairment †	5.7	14.5	4.3	12.4
Hypotension ††	2.3	19.9	1.9	16.3
Hyperkalemia †††	1.0	38.9	0.5	28.8

†renal failure, renal failure acute, renal failure chronic, renal impairment
††dizziness, dizziness postural, hypotension, orthostatic hypotension, presyncope, syncope
††† Given the variable baseline potassium levels of patients with renal insufficiency on dual RAAS therapy, the reporting of adverse event of hyperkalemia was at the discretion of the investigator.
* A Serious Adverse Event (SAE) is defined as: an event which is fatal or life-threatening, results in persistent or significant disability/incapacity, constitutes a congenital anomaly/birth defect, requires inpatient hospitalization or prolongation of existing hospitalization, or is medically significant (i.e. defined as an event that jeopardizes the patient or may require medical or surgical intervention to prevent one of the outcomes previously listed).

Table 6: Tekturna Tablets Supply

Tablet	Color	Imprint	Imprint	NDC 0078-XXXX-XX		
		Side 1	Side 2	Bottle of 30	Bottle of 90	Blister Packages of 100
150 mg	Light-Pink	NVR	IL	0485-15	0485-34	0485-35
300 mg	Light-Red	NVR	IU	0486-15	0486-34	0486-35

makes blood vessels narrow, leading to high blood pressure. Drugs that lower blood pressure lower your risk of having a stroke or heart attack.
High blood pressure makes the heart work harder to pump blood throughout the body and causes damage to the blood vessels. If high blood pressure is not treated, it can lead to stroke, heart attack, heart failure, kidney failure, and vision problems.
Who Should Not Take Tekturna?
• **If you get pregnant, stop taking Tekturna and call your doctor right away. If you plan to become pregnant, talk to your doctor about other treatment options for your high blood pressure.**
• **If you have diabetes and are taking a kind of medicine called an angiotensin-receptor-blocker or angiotensin-converting-enzyme-inhibitor.**
• **Do not take Tekturna if you are allergic to any of its ingredients. See the end of this leaflet for a complete list of the ingredients in Tekturna.**
• **Tekturna has not been studied in children under 18 years of age.**
What Should I Tell My Doctor Before Taking Tekturna?
Tell your doctor about all your medical conditions, including whether you:
• have kidney problems.
• are pregnant or planning to become pregnant, see "What is the most important information I should know about Tekturna?"
• are breast-feeding. It is not known if Tekturna passes into your breast milk. You should choose either to take Tekturna or breast-feed, but not both.
• are allergic to any of the ingredients in Tekturna, see "What are the ingredients in Tekturna?"
• have ever had a reaction called angioedema, to an ACE inhibitor medicine. Angioedema causes swelling of the face, lips, tongue, throat, arms, and legs, and may cause difficulty breathing.
Tell your doctor about all the medicines you take including prescription and nonprescription medicines, vitamins and herbal supplements. Especially tell your doctor if you are taking:
• a kind of medicine called angiotensin receptor blocker or angiotensin converting enzyme inhibitor
• Atorvastatin (medicine to lower cholesterol in your blood).
• water pills (also called "diuretics").
• medicines for treating fungus or fungal infections.
• cyclosporine (a medicine used to suppress the immune system).
• potassium-containing medicines, potassium supplements, or salt substitutes containing potassium.
• nonsteroidal anti-inflammatory drugs (like ibuprofen or naproxen).
Your doctor or pharmacist will know what medicines are safe to take together.
How Should I Take Tekturna?
• Take Tekturna once a day, at the same time each day. As with any blood pressure medication, it is important to take Tekturna on a regular daily basis exactly as prescribed by your doctor.

• Tekturna can be taken by itself or safely in combination with other medicines to lower high blood pressure. Your doctor may change your dose if needed.
• Tekturna can be taken with or without food.
• If you miss a dose, take it as soon as you remember. If it is close to your next dose, do not take the missed dose. Just take the next dose at your regular time.
• If you take too much Tekturna, call your doctor or Poison Control Center, or go to the nearest hospital emergency room.
What Are Possible Side Effects Of Tekturna?
Tekturna may cause serious side effects:
• **Injury or death to an unborn baby.** See "What is the most important information I should know about Tekturna?"
• **Low blood pressure (hypotension).** Your blood pressure may get too low if you also take water pills, are on a low-salt diet, get dialysis treatments, have heart problems, or get sick with vomiting or diarrhea. Lie down if you feel faint or dizzy. Call your doctor right away.
• **Severe Allergic Reactions and Angioedema.** Aliskiren may cause difficulty breathing or swallowing, tightness of the chest, hives, general rash, swelling, itching, dizziness, vomiting, or abdominal pain (signs of a severe allergic reaction). Aliskiren can also cause swelling of the face, lips, tongue, throat, arms and legs or the whole body (signs of angioedema). Get medical help right away and tell your doctor if you get any one or more of these symptoms. Angioedema can happen at any time while you are taking Tekturna.
• **Renal impairment or failure.** Aliskiren may cause renal disorder with symptoms such as severely decreased urine output or decreased urine output (signs of renal impairment or failure).
Common side effects of Tekturna include:
   diarrhea
   cough
   dizziness
   headache
   flu-like symptoms
   back pain
   tiredness
   high levels of potassium in the blood (hyperkalemia)
Less common side effects include rash, severe skin reactions (signs may include severe blistering of the lips, eyes or mouth, rash with fever and skin peeling) and liver disorder (signs may include nausea, loss of appetite, dark colored urine or yellowing of skin and eyes).
Tell your doctor if you have any side effect that bothers you or that does not go away. These are not all of the possible side effects of Tekturna. For a complete list of side effects, ask your doctor or pharmacist.
How Do I Store Tekturna?
• Store Tekturna tablets at room temperature between 59° to 86°F (15°-30°C).
• Keep Tekturna in the original prescription bottle in a dry place. Do not remove the desiccant (drying agent) from the bottle.
• Keep Tekturna and all medicines out of the reach of children.

General Information About Tekturna

Medicines are sometimes prescribed for conditions not listed in the patient information leaflet. Do not take Tekturna for a condition for which it was not prescribed. Do not give Tekturna to other people, even if they have the same condition or symptoms you have. It may harm them. This leaflet summarizes the most important information about Tekturna. If you have more questions about Tekturna talk with your doctor. You can ask your doctor or pharmacist for information that is written for healthcare professionals. For more information about Tekturna, ask your doctor or pharmacist, visit www.Tekturna.com, or call 1-888-Tekturna (1-888-835-8876).

What are the ingredients in Tekturna?
Active Ingredients: Aliskiren (Tekturna)
Inactive Ingredients: colloidal silicone dioxide, crospovidone, hypromellose, iron oxide colorants, magnesium stearate, microcrystalline cellulose, polyethylene glycol, talc, and titanium dioxide.
Manufactured by:
Novartis Pharma AG, Stein, Switzerland
Novartis Pharma Produktions GmbH, Wehr, Germany
Distributed by:
Novartis Pharmaceuticals Corporation
East Hanover, NJ 07936
© Novartis
T2013-111
November 2013
Shown in Product Identification Guide, page 311

TEKTURNA HCT

[tek-turn-a HCT]
(aliskiren and hydrochlorothiazide)
tablets, for oral use

℞

The following prescribing information is based on official labeling in effect July 2014.

HIGHLIGHTS OF PRESCRIBING INFORMATION

These highlights do not include all the information needed to use TEKTURNA HCT safely and effectively. See full prescribing information for TEKTURNA HCT.

Tekturna HCT (aliskiren and hydrochlorothiazide) tablets, for oral use

Initial U.S. Approval: 2008

> **WARNING: FETAL TOXICITY**
> *See full prescribing information for complete boxed warning*
> - When pregnancy is detected, discontinue Tekturna HCT as soon as possible. (5.1)
> - Drugs that act directly on the renin-angiotensin system can cause injury and death to the developing fetus. (5.1)

——————RECENT MAJOR CHANGES——————

Warnings and Precautions (5.4)   11/2013

——————INDICATIONS AND USAGE——————

Tekturna HCT is a combination of aliskiren, a renin inhibitor, and hydrochlorothiazide (HCTZ), a thiazide diuretic, indicated for the treatment of hypertension, to lower blood pressure:
- In patients not adequately controlled with monotherapy
- As initial therapy in patients likely to need multiple drugs to achieve their blood pressure goals (1)

Lowering blood pressure reduces the risk of fatal and nonfatal cardiovascular events, primarily strokes and myocardial infarction.

——————DOSAGE AND ADMINISTRATION——————

- The antihypertensive effect is largely manifested within 1 week, with maximal effects seen at around 4 weeks. If blood pressure remains uncontrolled after 2 to 4 weeks of therapy, titrate up to a maximum of 300/25 mg. (2.2)
- Order of increasing mean effect: 150/12.5 mg, 150/25 mg or 300/12.5 mg, and 300/25 mg (2.1)
- One tablet daily, with a routine pattern with regard to meals. (2.7)
- Add-on or Initial therapy: Initiate with 150/12.5mg. Titrate as needed up to a maximum of 300/25 mg. (2.3, 2.5)
- Replacement therapy: May be substituted for titrated components (2.4)

——————DOSAGE FORMS AND STRENGTHS——————

Tablets (mg aliskiren/mg HCTZ): 150/12.5, 150/25, 300/12.5, 300/25 (3)

——————CONTRAINDICATIONS——————

Do not use with angiotensin receptor blockers (ARBs) or ACE inhibitors (ACEIs) in patients with diabetes (4)
Anuria (4)
Hypersensitivity to sulfonamide-derived drugs (4)

——————WARNINGS AND PRECAUTIONS——————

- Avoid concomitant use with ARBs or ACEIs in patients with renal impairment (GFR<60 mL/min) (5.2)

- Anaphylactic Reactions and Head and Neck Angioedema: Discontinue Tekturna HCT and monitor until signs and symptoms resolve. (5.3)
- Hypotension in volume and/or salt depleted patients or with combined use of other agents acting on RAAS: Correct imbalances prior to initiating therapy with Tekturna HCT. (5.4)
- Impaired renal function: Monitor serum creatinine periodically. (5.5)
- Hypersensitivity Reactions: May occur from HCTZ component (5.6)
- Hyperkalemia: Monitor potassium levels periodically. (5.9)
- Hydrochlorothiazide has been associated with acute angle-closure glaucoma (5.11)

——————ADVERSE REACTIONS——————

The most common adverse reactions (incidence ≥1.5% and more common than with placebo) are: dizziness and diarrhea. (6.1)

To report SUSPECTED ADVERSE REACTIONS, contact Novartis Pharmaceuticals Corporation at 1-888-669-6682 or FDA at 1-800-FDA-1088 or www.fda.gov/medwatch.

——————DRUG INTERACTIONS——————

- Cyclosporine: Avoid concomitant use (7, 12.3)
- Itraconazole: Avoid concomitant use (7, 12.3)
- NSAIDs use may lead to increased risk of renal impairment and loss of antihypertensive effect (7)
- Antidiabetic Drugs: Dosage adjustment of antidiabetic may be required (7)
- Cholestyramine and Colestipol: Reduced absorption of thiazides (7)
- Lithium: Increased risk of lithium toxicity when used with diuretics. Monitor serum lithium concentrations during concurrent use. (7)

——————USE IN SPECIFIC POPULATIONS——————

Nursing Mothers: Nursing or drug should be discontinued. (8.3)

See 17 for PATIENT COUNSELING INFORMATION and FDA-approved patient labeling

Revised: 3/2014

FULL PRESCRIBING INFORMATION

> **WARNING: FETAL TOXICITY**
> - When pregnancy is detected, discontinue Tekturna HCT as soon as possible. (5.1)
> - Drugs that act directly on the renin-angiotensin system can cause injury and death to the developing fetus. (5.1)

1   INDICATIONS AND USAGE

Tekturna HCT is indicated for the treatment of hypertension, to lower blood pressure. Lowering blood pressure reduces the risk of fatal and nonfatal cardiovascular events, primarily strokes and myocardial infarctions. These benefits have been seen in controlled trials of antihypertensive drugs from a wide variety of pharmacologic classes including hydrochlorothiazide. There are no controlled trials demonstrating risk reduction with Tekturna HCT.

Control of high blood pressure should be part of comprehensive cardiovascular risk management, including, as appropriate, lipid control, diabetes management, antithrombotic therapy, smoking cessation, exercise, and limited sodium intake. Many patients will require more than one drug to achieve blood pressure goals. For specific advice on goals and management, see published guidelines, such as those of the National High Blood Pressure Education Program's Joint National Committee on Prevention, Detection, Evaluation, and Treatment of High Blood Pressure (JNC).

Numerous antihypertensive drugs, from a variety of pharmacologic classes and with different mechanisms of action, have been shown in randomized controlled trials to reduce cardiovascular morbidity and mortality, and it can be concluded that it is blood pressure reduction, and not some other pharmacologic property of the drugs, that is largely responsible for those benefits. The largest and most consistent cardiovascular outcome benefit has been a reduction in the risk of stroke, but reductions in myocardial infarction and cardiovascular mortality also have been seen regularly. Elevated systolic or diastolic pressure causes increased cardiovascular risk, and the absolute risk increase per mmHg is greater at higher blood pressures, so that even modest reductions of severe hypertension can provide substantial benefit. Relative risk reduction from blood pressure reduction is similar across populations with varying absolute risk, so the absolute benefit is greater in patients who are at higher risk independent of their hypertension (for example, patients with diabetes or hyperlipidemia), and such patients would be expected to benefit from more aggressive treatment to a lower blood pressure goal.

Some antihypertensive drugs have smaller blood pressure effects (as monotherapy) in black patients, and many antihypertensive drugs have additional approved indications and effects (e.g., on angina, heart failure, or diabetic kidney disease). These considerations may guide selection of therapy.

Add-On Therapy

A patient whose blood pressure is not adequately controlled with aliskiren alone or hydrochlorothiazide alone may be switched to combination therapy with Tekturna HCT.

A patient whose blood pressure is controlled with hydrochlorothiazide alone but who experiences hypokalemia may be switched to combination therapy with Tekturna HCT.

A patient who experiences dose-limiting adverse reactions on either component alone may be switched to Tekturna HCT containing a lower dose of that component in combination with the other to achieve similar blood pressure reductions.

Replacement Therapy

Tekturna HCT may be substituted for the titrated components.

Initial Therapy

Tekturna HCT may be used as initial therapy in patients who are likely to need multiple drugs to achieve their blood pressure goals.

The choice of Tekturna HCT as initial therapy should be based on an assessment of potential benefits and risks.

Patients with Stage 2 hypertension are at a relatively high risk for cardiovascular events (such as strokes, heart attacks, and heart failure), kidney failure, and vision problems, so prompt treatment is clinically relevant. The decision to use a combination as initial therapy should be individualized and should be shaped by considerations such as baseline blood pressure, the target goal, and the incremental likelihood of achieving goal with a combination compared to monotherapy. Individual blood pressure goals may vary based upon the patient's risk.

Data from the high-dose multifactorial study [see Clinical Studies (14)] provide estimates of the probability of reaching a target blood pressure with Tekturna HCT compared to aliskiren or hydrochlorothiazide monotherapy. The figures below provide estimates of the likelihood of achieving systolic or diastolic blood pressure control with Tekturna HCT 300/25 mg, based upon baseline systolic or diastolic blood pressure. The curve of each treatment group was estimated by logistic regression modeling. The estimated likelihood at the right tail of each curve is less reliable because of small numbers of subjects with high baseline blood pressures.

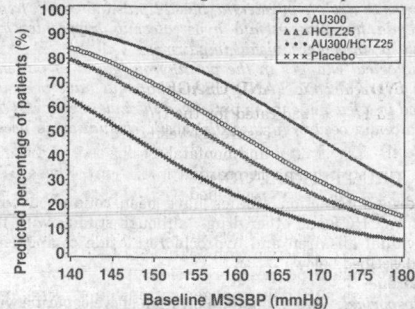

Figure 1: Probability of Achieving Systolic Blood Pressure (SBP) <140 mmHg

Figure 2: Probability of Achieving Systolic Blood Pressure (SBP) <130 mmHg

Figure 3: Probability of Achieving Diastolic Blood Pressure (DBP) <90 mmHg

[See figure 4 at top of next column]

At all levels of baseline blood pressure, the probability of achieving any given diastolic or systolic goal is greater with the combination than for either monotherapy. For example, the mean baseline msSBP/msDBP for patients participating in this multifactorial study was 154/99 mmHg. A patient with a baseline blood pressure of 154/99 mmHg has about a 62% chance of achieving a goal of <140 mmHg (systolic) and 61% chance of achieving <90 mmHg (diastolic) on aliskiren alone, and the chance of achieving these goals on hydrochlorothiazide alone is about 54% (systolic) and 49% (diastolic). The chance of achieving these goals on Tekturna HCT rises to about 77% (systolic) and 74% (diastolic). The chance of achieving these goals on placebo is about 34% (systolic) and 37% (diastolic) [see Dosage and Administration (2) and Clinical Studies (14)].

2   DOSAGE AND ADMINISTRATION
2.1   Dose Selection
The recommended once-daily doses of Tekturna HCT in order of increasing mean effect are 150/12.5 mg, 150/25 mg or 300/12.5 mg, and 300/25 mg.

Figure 4: Probability of Achieving Diastolic Blood Pressure (DBP) <80 mmHg

2.2   Dose Titration
The antihypertensive effect of Tekturna HCT is largely manifested within 1 week, with maximal effects generally seen at around 4 weeks. If blood pressure remains uncontrolled after 2 to 4 weeks of therapy, the dose may be titrated up to a maximum of aliskiren 300 mg/hydrochlorothiazide 25 mg.
2.3   Add-On Therapy
A patient whose blood pressure is not adequately controlled with aliskiren alone or hydrochlorothiazide alone may be switched to combination therapy with Tekturna HCT. The usual recommended starting dose is 150/12.5 mg once daily as needed to control blood pressure. The dose may be titrated up to a maximum of aliskiren 300 mg/hydrochlorothiazide 25 mg once daily.
2.4   Replacement Therapy
Tekturna HCT may be substituted for the individually titrated components.
2.5   Initial Therapy
The usual recommended starting dose is 150/12.5 mg once daily as needed to control blood pressure. The dose may be titrated up to a maximum of aliskiren 300 mg/hydrochlorothiazide 25 mg once daily.
Tekturna HCT is not recommended for use as initial therapy in patients with intravascular volume depletion [see Warnings and Precautions (5.4)].
2.6   Use with Other Antihypertensive Drugs
Tekturna HCT may be administered with some other antihypertensive agents. In diabetics, do not use in combination with angiotensin receptor blockers (ARBs) or angiotensin converting enzyme inhibitors (ACEIs) [see Contraindications (4)]. Concomitant use of aliskiren with an ARB or ACEI is not recommended in patients with GFR <60 ml/min [see Warnings and Precautions (5.2)]. There are no data available with use of Tekturna HCT with angiotensin-converting enzyme inhibitors or beta blockers [see Clinical Studies (14)].
2.7   Relationship to Meals
Patients should establish a routine pattern for taking Tekturna HCT with regard to meals. High-fat meals decrease absorption substantially [see Clinical Pharmacology (12.3)].

3   DOSAGE FORMS AND STRENGTHS
- 150 mg/12.5 mg tablets: white, biconvex ovaloid, film-coated tablets imprinted with NVR/LCI
- 150 mg/25 mg tablets: pale yellow, biconvex ovaloid, film-coated tablets imprinted with NVR/CLL
- 300 mg/12.5 mg tablets: violet white, biconvex ovaloid, film-coated tablets imprinted with NVR/CVI
- 300 mg/25 mg tablets: light yellow, biconvex ovaloid, film-coated tablets imprinted with NVR/CVV

4   CONTRAINDICATIONS
Do not use aliskiren with ARBs or ACEIs in patients with diabetes [see Warnings and Precautions (5.2), Clinical Studies (14.4)].
Because of the hydrochlorothiazide component, Tekturna HCT is contraindicated in patients with anuria or hypersensitivity to sulfonamide-derived drugs [see Warnings and Precautions (5.6) and Adverse Reactions (6.1)]. Hypersensitivity reactions may range from urticaria to anaphylaxis [see Adverse Reactions (6.1)].

5   WARNINGS AND PRECAUTIONS
5.1   Fetal Toxicity
Pregnancy Category D
Use of drugs that act on the renin-angiotensin system during the second and third trimesters of pregnancy reduces fetal renal function and increases fetal and neonatal morbidity and death. Resulting oligohydramnios can be associated with fetal lung hypoplasia and skeletal deformations. Potential neonatal adverse effects include skull hypoplasia, anuria, hypotension, renal failure, and death. When pregnancy is detected, discontinue Tekturna HCT as soon as possible [see Use in Specific Populations (8.1)].

Thiazides cross the placenta, and use of thiazides during pregnancy is associated with a risk of fetal or neonatal jaundice, thrombocytopenia, and possible other adverse reactions that have occurred in Tekturna HCT.
5.2   Renal   Impairment/Hyperkalemia/Hypotension when Tekturna HCT is given in combination with ARBs or ACEIs
Tekturna HCT is contraindicated in patients with diabetes who are receiving ARBs or ACEIs because of the increased risk of renal impairment, hyperkalemia, and hypotension [see Contraindications (4) and Clinical Studies (14.4)].
Avoid use of Tekturna HCT with ARBs or ACEIs in patients with moderate renal impairment (GFR <60 ml/min).
5.3   Anaphylactic   Reactions   and   Head   and   Neck Angioedema
Aliskiren
Hypersensitivity reactions such as anaphylactic reactions and angioedema of the face, extremities, lips, tongue, glottis and/or larynx have been reported in patients treated with Tekturna and has necessitated hospitalization and intubation. This may occur at any time during treatment and has occurred in patients with and without a history of angioedema with ACE inhibitors or angiotensin receptor antagonists. Anaphylactic reactions have been reported from post-marketing experience with unknown frequency. If angioedema involves the throat, tongue, glottis or larynx, or if the patient has a history of upper respiratory surgery, airway obstruction may occur and be fatal. Patients who experience these effects, even without respiratory distress, require prolonged observation and appropriate monitoring measures since treatment with antihistamines and corticosteroids may not be sufficient to prevent respiratory involvement. Prompt administration of subcutaneous epinephrine solution 1:1000 (0.3 to 0.5 ml) and measures to ensure a patent airway may be necessary.
Discontinue Tekturna HCT immediately in patients who develop anaphylactic reactions or angioedema, and do not readminister.
5.4   Hypotension
Symptomatic hypotension may occur after initiation of treatment with Tekturna HCT in patients with marked volume depletion, patients with salt depletion, or with combined use of aliskiren and other agents acting on the renin-angiotensin-aldosterone system. The volume or salt depletion should be corrected prior to administration of Tekturna HCT, or the treatment should start under close medical supervision.
A transient hypotensive response is not a contraindication to further treatment, which usually can be continued without difficulty once the blood pressure has stabilized.
5.5   Impaired Renal Function
Monitor renal function periodically in patients treated with Tekturna HCT. Changes in renal function, including acute renal failure, can be caused by drugs that affect the renin-angiotensin-aldosterone system and by diuretics. Patients whose renal function may depend in part on the activity of the renin-angiotensin-aldosterone system (e.g., patients with renal artery stenosis, severe heart failure, post-myocardial infarction or volume depletion) or patients receiving ARB, ACEI or non-steroidal anti-inflammatory (NSAID) therapy may be at particular risk of developing acute renal failure on Tekturna HCT [see Contraindications (4), Warnings and Precautions (5.2), Clinical Studies (14.4)]. Consider withholding or discontinuing therapy in patients who develop a clinically significant decrease in renal function on Tekturna HCT.
5.6   Hypersensitivity Reactions
Hydrochlorothiazide
Hypersensitivity reactions to hydrochlorothiazide may occur in patients with or without a history of allergy or bronchial asthma, but are more likely in patients with such a history.
5.7   Systemic Lupus Erythematosus
Hydrochlorothiazide
Thiazide diuretics have been reported to cause exacerbation or activation of systemic lupus erythematosus.
5.8   Lithium Interaction
Hydrochlorothiazide
Lithium generally should not be given with thiazides [see Drug Interactions (7)].
5.9   Serum Electrolyte Abnormalities
Tekturna HCT
In the short-term controlled trials of various doses of Tekturna HCT, in patients with hypertension not concomitantly treated with an ARB or ACEI, the incidence of hypertensive patients who developed hypokalemia (serum potassium <3.5 mEq/L) was 2.2%; the incidence of hyperkalemia (serum potassium >5.5 mEq/L) was 0.8%. No patients discontinued due to increase or decrease of serum potassium.
Aliskiren
Monitor serum potassium periodically in patients receiving aliskiren. Drugs that affect the renin-angiotensin-aldosterone system can cause hyperkalemia. Risk factors for the development of hyperkalemia include renal insuffi-

ciency, diabetes, combination use with ARBs or ACEI *[see Contraindications (4), Warnings and Precautions (5.2), and Clinical Studies (14.4)]*, NSAIDs, or potassium supplements or potassium sparing diuretics.

Hydrochlorothiazide

Hydrochlorothiazide can cause hypokalemia and hyponatremia. Hypomagnesemia can result in hypokalemia which appears difficult to treat despite potassium repletion.

If hypokalemia is accompanied by clinical signs (e.g., muscular weakness, paresis, or ECG alterations), Tekturna HCT should be discontinued. Correction of hypokalemia and any coexisting hypomagnesemia is recommended prior to the initiation of thiazides.

5.10 Cyclosporine or Itraconazole

Aliskiren

When aliskiren was given with cyclosporine or itraconazole, the blood concentrations of aliskiren were significantly increased. Avoid concomitant use of aliskiren with cyclosporine or itraconazole *[see Drug Interactions (7)]*.

5.11 Acute Myopia and Secondary Angle-Closure Glaucoma

Hydrochlorothiazide, a sulfonamide, can cause an idiosyncratic reaction, resulting in acute transient myopia and acute angle-closure glaucoma. Symptoms include acute onset of decreased visual acuity or ocular pain and typically occur within hours to weeks of drug initiation. Untreated acute angle-closure glaucoma can lead to permanent vision loss. The primary treatment is to discontinue hydrochlorothiazide as rapidly as possible. Prompt medical or surgical treatments may need to be considered if the intraocular pressure remains uncontrolled. Risk factors for developing acute angle-closure glaucoma may include a history of sulfonamide or penicillin allergy.

5.12 Metabolic Disturbances

Hydrochlorothiazide

Hydrochlorothiazide may alter glucose tolerance and raise serum levels of cholesterol and triglycerides.

Hydrochlorothiazide may raise the serum uric acid level due to reduced clearance of uric acid and may cause or exacerbate hyperuricemia and precipitate gout in susceptible patients.

Hydrochlorothiazide decreases urinary calcium excretion and may cause elevations of serum calcium. Monitor calcium levels in patients with hypercalcemia receiving Tekturna HCT.

6 ADVERSE REACTIONS

6.1 Clinical Studies Experience

The following serious adverse reactions are discussed in greater detail in other sections of the label:

- Risk of fetal/neonatal morbidity and mortality *[see Warnings and Precautions (5.1)]*.
- Head and neck angioedema *[see Warnings and Precautions (5.3)]*.
- Hypotension in volume- and/or salt-depleted patients *[see Warnings and Precautions (5.4)]*.

Because clinical trials are conducted under widely varying conditions, adverse reaction rates observed in the clinical trials of a drug cannot be directly compared to rates in clinical trials of another drug and may not reflect the rates observed in practice.

Tekturna HCT

Tekturna HCT has been evaluated for safety in more than 2,700 patients, including over 700 treated for 6 months and 190 for over 1 year. In placebo-controlled clinical trials, discontinuation of therapy due to a clinical adverse event (including uncontrolled hypertension) occurred in 2.7% of patients treated with Tekturna HCT versus 3.6% of patients given placebo.

Adverse events in placebo-controlled trials that occurred in at least 1% of patients treated with Tekturna HCT and at a higher incidence than placebo included dizziness (2.3% vs. 1%), influenza (2.3% vs. 1.6%), diarrhea (1.6% vs. 0.5%), cough (1.3% vs. 0.5%), vertigo (1.2% vs. 0.5%), asthenia (1.2% vs. 0%), and arthralgia (1% vs. 0.5%).

Aliskiren

Aliskiren has been evaluated for safety in 6,460 patients, including 1,740 treated for longer than 6 months, and 1,250 for longer than 1 year. In placebo-controlled clinical trials, discontinuation of therapy due to a clinical adverse event, including uncontrolled hypertension occurred in 2.2% of patients treated with aliskiren, versus 3.5% of patients given placebo. These data do not include information from the ALTITUDE study which evaluated the use of aliskiren in combination with ARBs or ACEIs *[see Contraindications (4), Warnings and Precautions (5.2), and Clinical Studies (14.4)]*.

Two cases of angioedema with respiratory symptoms were reported with aliskiren use in the clinical studies. Two other cases of periorbital edema without respiratory symptoms were reported as possible angioedema and resulted in discontinuation. The rate of these angioedema cases in the completed studies was 0.06%.

In addition, 26 other cases of edema involving the face, hands, or whole body were reported with aliskiren use, including 4 leading to discontinuation.

In the placebo-controlled studies, however, the incidence of edema involving the face, hands, or whole body was 0.4% with aliskiren compared with 0.5% with placebo. In a long-term active-controlled study with aliskiren and HCTZ arms, the incidence of edema involving the face, hands, or whole body was 0.4% in both treatment arms.

Aliskiren produces dose-related gastrointestinal (GI) adverse reactions. Diarrhea was reported by 2.3% of patients at 300 mg, compared to 1.2% in placebo patients. In women and the elderly (age ≥65) increases in diarrhea rates were evident starting at a dose of 150 mg daily, with rates for these subgroups at 150 mg comparable to those seen at 300 mg for men or younger patients (all rates about 2% to 2.3%). Other GI symptoms included abdominal pain, dyspepsia, and gastroesophageal reflux, although increased rates for abdominal pain and dyspepsia were distinguished from placebo only at 600 mg daily. Diarrhea and other GI symptoms were typically mild and rarely led to discontinuation.

Aliskiren was associated with a slight increase in cough in the placebo-controlled studies (1.1% for any aliskiren use vs. 0.6% for placebo). In active-controlled trials with ACE inhibitor (ramipril, lisinopril) arms, the rates of cough for the aliskiren arms were about one-third to one-half the rates in the ACE inhibitor arms.

Other adverse reactions with increased rates for aliskiren compared to placebo included rash (1% vs. 0.3%) and renal stones (0.2% vs. 0%).

Single episodes of tonic-clonic seizures with loss of consciousness were reported in two patients treated with aliskiren in the clinical trials. One patient had predisposing causes for seizures and had a negative electroencephalogram (EEG) and cerebral imaging following the seizures; for the other patient, EEG and imaging results were not reported. Aliskiren was discontinued and there was no rechallenge in either case.

No clinically meaningful changes in vital signs or in ECG (including QTc interval) were observed in patients treated with aliskiren.

Hydrochlorothiazide

Other adverse reactions that have been reported with hydrochlorothiazide, without regard to causality, are listed below:

Body As A Whole: weakness

Digestive: pancreatitis, jaundice (intrahepatic cholestatic jaundice), sialadenitis, cramping, gastric irritation

Hematologic: aplastic anemia, agranulocytosis, leukopenia, hemolytic anemia, thrombocytopenia;

Hypersensitivity: purpura, photosensitivity, urticaria, necrotizing angiitis (vasculitis and cutaneous vasculitis), fever, respiratory distress including pneumonitis and pulmonary edema, anaphylactic reactions

Metabolic: hyperglycemia, glycosuria, hyperuricemia

Musculoskeletal: muscle spasm

Nervous System/Psychiatric: restlessness

Renal: renal failure, renal dysfunction, interstitial nephritis

Skin: erythema multiforme including Stevens-Johnson syndrome, exfoliative dermatitis including toxic epidermal necrolysis

Special Senses: transient blurred vision, xanthopsia

Clinical Laboratory Test Abnormalities

In controlled clinical trials, clinically important changes in standard laboratory parameters were rarely associated with administration of Tekturna HCT in patients with hypertension not concomitantly treated with an ARB or ACEI.

Blood Urea Nitrogen (BUN)/Creatinine: In patients with hypertension not concomitantly treated with an ARB or ACEI, elevations (greater than 50% increase) in BUN and creatinine occurred in 11.8% and 0.9%, respectively, of patients taking Tekturna HCT, and 7% and 1.1%, respectively, of patients given placebo in short-term controlled clinical trials. No patients were discontinued due to an increase in either BUN or creatinine.

Hemoglobin and Hematocrit: A greater than 20% decrease in hemoglobin and hematocrit were observed in <0.1% and 0.1%, respectively, of patients treated with Tekturna HCT, compared with 0% in placebo-treated patients. No patients were discontinued due to anemia.

Liver Function Tests: Occasional elevations (greater than 150%) in ALT (SGPT) were observed in 1.2% of patients treated with Tekturna HCT, compared with 0% in placebo-treated patients. No patients were discontinued due to abnormal liver function tests.

6.2 Post-Marketing Experience

The following adverse reactions have been reported in aliskiren or hydrochlorothiazide post-marketing experience. Because these reactions are reported voluntarily from a population of uncertain size, it is not always possible to estimate their frequency or establish a causal relationship to drug exposure.

Aliskiren

Hypersensitivity: anaphylactic reactions and angioedema requiring airway management and hospitalization

Urticaria

Peripheral edema

Hepatic enzyme increase with clinical symptoms of hepatic dysfunction

Severe cutaneous adverse reactions, including Stevens-Johnson syndrome and toxic epidermal necrolysis

Pruritus

Erythema

Hydrochlorothiazide

Acute renal failure, renal disorder, aplastic anemia, erythema mutliforme, pyrexia, muscle spasm, asthenia, acute angle-closure glaucoma, bone marrow failure, worsening of diabetes control, hypokalemia, blood lipids increased, hyponatremia, hypomagnesemia, hypercalcemia, hyperchloremic alkalosis, impotence, visual impairment

Pathological changes in the parathyroid gland of patients with hypercalcemia and hypophosphatemia have been observed in a few patients on prolonged thiazide therapy. If hypercalcemia occurs, further diagnostic evaluation is necessary.

7 DRUG INTERACTIONS

No drug interaction studies have been conducted with Tekturna HCT and other drugs, although studies with the individual aliskiren and hydrochlorothiazide components are described below.

Aliskiren

Cyclosporine: Avoid co-administration of cyclosporine with aliskiren.

Itraconazole: Avoid co-administration of itraconazole with aliskiren *[See Clinical Pharmacology (12.3)]*.

Non-Steroidal Anti-Inflammatory Agents (NSAIDs) including selective Cyclooxygenase-2 inhibitors (COX-2 inhibitors): In patients who are elderly, volume-depleted (including those on diuretic therapy), or with compromised renal function, co-administration of NSAIDs, including selective COX-2 inhibitors with agents that affect the renin-angiotensin-aldosterone system, including aliskiren, may result in deterioration of renal function, including possible acute renal failure. These effects are usually reversible. Monitor renal function periodically in patients receiving aliskiren and NSAID therapy.

The antihypertensive effect of aliskiren may be attenuated by NSAIDs.

Dual Blockade of the renin-angiotensin-aldosterone system: The concomitant use of aliskiren with other agents acting on the renin-angiotensin-aldosterone system such as ACEIs or ARBs is associated with an increased risk of hypotension, hyperkalemia, and changes in renal function (including acute renal failure) compared to monotherapy. Monitor blood pressure, renal function, and electrolytes in patients on aliskiren and other agents that affect the renin-angiotensin-aldosterone system *[see Warnings and Precautions (5.4, 5.5, 5.9)]*.

The concomitant use of aliskiren with an ARB or an ACEI in diabetic patients is contraindicated and should be avoided in patients with moderate renal impairment *[see Contraindications (4) and Warnings and Precautions (5.2)]*.

Furosemide: Oral co-administration of aliskiren and furosemide reduced exposure to furosemide. Monitor diuretic effects when furosemide is co-administered with aliskiren.

Hydrochlorothiazide

When administered concurrently, the following drugs may interact with thiazide diuretics.

Antidiabetic drugs (oral agents and insulin): Dosage adjustment of the antidiabetic drug may be required.

Lithium: Diuretic agents increase the risk of lithium toxicity. Refer to the package insert for lithium before use of such preparation with Tekturna HCT. Monitoring of serum lithium concentrations is recommended during concurrent use.

Nonsteroidal anti-inflammatory drugs: When Tekturna HCT and nonsteroidal anti-inflammatory agents are used concomitantly, the patient should be observed closely to determine if the desired effect of the diuretic is obtained.

Ion exchange resins: Staggering the dosage of hydrochlorothiazide and ion exchange resins (e.g., cholestyramine, colestipol) such that hydrochlorothiazide is administered at least 4 hours before or 4-6 hours after the administration of resins would potentially minimize the interaction *[see Clinical Pharmacology (12.3)]*.

8 USE IN SPECIFIC POPULATIONS

8.1 Pregnancy

Pregnancy Category D

Use of drugs that act on the renin-angiotensin system during the second and third trimesters of pregnancy reduces fetal renal function and increases fetal and neonatal morbidity and death. Resulting oligohydramnios can be associated with fetal lung hypoplasia and skeletal deformations. Potential neonatal adverse effects include skull hypoplasia, anuria, hypotension, renal failure, and death. When pregnancy is detected, discontinue Tekturna HCT as soon as possible. These adverse outcomes are usually associated with use of these drugs in the second and third trimester of pregnancy. Most epidemiologic studies examining fetal abnormalities after exposure to antihypertensive use in the first trimester have not distinguished drugs affecting the renin-angiotensin system from other antihypertensive agents. Appropriate management of maternal hypertension during pregnancy is important to optimize outcomes for both mother and fetus.

In the unusual case that there is no appropriate alternative to therapy with drugs affecting the renin-angiotensin system for a particular patient, apprise the mother of the potential risk to the fetus. Perform serial ultrasound examinations to assess the intra-amniotic environment. If oligohydramnios is observed, discontinue Tekturna HCT, unless it is considered lifesaving for the mother. Fetal testing may be appropriate, based on the week of pregnancy. Patients and physicians should be aware, however, that oligohydramnios may not appear until after the fetus has sustained irreversible injury. Closely observe infants with histories of in utero exposure to Tekturna HCT for hypotension, oliguria, and hyperkalemia. *[see Use in Specific Populations (8.4)]*

Thiazides cross the placenta, and use of thiazides during pregnancy is associated with a risk of fetal or neonatal jaundice, thrombocytopenia, and possible other adverse reactions that have occurred in adults.

Reproductive toxicity studies of aliskiren hemifumarate did not reveal any evidence of teratogenicity at oral doses up to 600 mg aliskiren/kg/day (20 times the maximum recommended human dose [MRHD] of 300 mg/day on a mg/m^2 basis) in pregnant rats or up to 100 mg aliskiren/kg/day (seven times the MRHD on a mg/m^2 basis) in pregnant rabbits. Fetal birth weight was adversely affected in rabbits at 50 mg/kg/day (3.2 times the MRHD on a mg/m^2 basis). Aliskiren was present in placenta, amniotic fluid and fetuses of pregnant rabbits.

When pregnant mice and rats were given hydrochlorothiazide at doses up to 3000 and 1000 mg/kg/day, respectively (about 600 and 400 times the MRHD) during their respective periods of major organogenesis, there was no evidence of fetal harm.

Hydrochlorothiazide
Thiazides can cross the placenta, and concentrations reached in the umbilical vein approach those in the maternal plasma. Hydrochlorothiazide, like other diuretics, can cause placental hypoperfusion. It accumulates in the amniotic fluid, with reported concentrations up to 19 times higher than in umbilical vein plasma. Use of thiazides during pregnancy is associated with a risk of fetal or neonatal jaundice or thrombocytopenia. Since they do not prevent or alter the course of EPH (Edema, Proteinuria, Hypertension) gestosis (pre eclampsia), these drugs should not be used to treat hypertension in pregnant women. The use of hydrochlorothiazide for other indications (e.g. heart disease) in pregnancy should be avoided.

8.3 Nursing Mothers
It is not known whether aliskiren is excreted in human milk, but aliskiren was secreted in the milk of lactating rats. Thiazides appear in human milk. Because of the potential for adverse effects on the nursing infant, a decision should be made whether to discontinue nursing or discontinue the drug, taking into account the importance of the drug to the mother.

8.4 Pediatric Use
Safety and effectiveness in pediatric patients have not been established.

Neonates with a history of in utero exposure to Tekturna HCT:
If oliguria or hypotension occurs, direct attention toward support of blood pressure and renal perfusion. Exchange transfusions or dialysis may be required as a means of reversing hypotension and/or substituting for disordered renal function.

8.5 Geriatric Use
In the short-term controlled clinical trials of Tekturna HCT, 325 (19.6%) patients treated with Tekturna HCT were ≥65 years and 53 (3.2%) were ≥75 years.

No overall differences in safety or effectiveness were observed between these subjects and younger subjects, and other reported clinical experience has not identified differences in responses between the elderly and younger patients, but greater sensitivity of some older individuals cannot be ruled out.

8.6 Renal Impairment
Safety and effectiveness of Tekturna HCT in patients with severe renal impairment (CrCl ≤ 30 mL/min) have not been established. No dose adjustment is required in patients with mild (CrCl 60-90 mL/min) or moderate (CrCl 30-60) renal impairment.

8.7 Hepatic Impairment
Aliskiren
No dose adjustment is necessary for patients with mild-to-severe liver disease.

Hydrochlorothiazide
Minor alterations of fluid and electrolyte balance may precipitate hepatic coma in patients with impaired hepatic function or progressive liver disease.

10 OVERDOSAGE
Aliskiren
Limited data are available related to overdosage in humans. The most likely manifestation of overdosage would be hypotension. If symptomatic hypotension should occur, supportive treatment should be initiated.

Aliskiren is poorly dialyzed. Therefore, hemodialysis is not adequate to treat aliskiren overexposure *[see Clinical Pharmacology (12.3)]*.

Hydrochlorothiazide
The most common signs and symptoms of overdose observed in humans are those caused by electrolyte depletion (hypokalemia, hypochloremia, hyponatremia) and dehydration resulting from excessive diuresis. If digitalis has also been administered, hypokalemia may accentuate cardiac arrhythmias. The degree to which hydrochlorothiazide is removed by hemodialysis has not been established. The oral LD_{50} of hydrochlorothiazide is greater than 10 g/kg in both mice and rats.

11 DESCRIPTION
Tekturna HCT is a fixed combination of aliskiren, an orally active, nonpeptide, direct renin inhibitor, and hydrochlorothiazide, a thiazide diuretic that is provided as tablets for oral administration.

Aliskiren
Aliskiren hemifumarate is chemically described as (2S, 4S,5S,7S)-N-(2-carbamoyl-2-methylpropyl)-5-amino-4-hydroxy-2,7-diisopropyl-8-[4-methoxy-3-(3-methoxypropoxy)-phenyl]-octanamide hemifumarate and its structural formula is

Molecular formula: $C_{30}H_{53}N_3O_6 \cdot 0.5\ C_4H_4O_4$

Aliskiren hemifumarate is a white to slightly yellowish crystalline powder with a molecular weight of 609.8 (free base- 551.8). It is soluble in phosphate buffer, n-octanol, and highly soluble in water.

Hydrochlorothiazide
Hydrochlorothiazide USP is a white, or practically white, practically odorless, crystalline powder. It is slightly soluble in water; freely soluble in sodium hydroxide solution, in n-butylamine, and in dimethylformamide; sparingly soluble in methanol; and insoluble in ether, in chloroform, and in dilute mineral acids. Hydrochlorothiazide is chemically described as 6-chloro-3,4-dihydro-2H-1,2,4-benzothiadiazine-7-sulfonamide 1,1-dioxide.

Hydrochlorothiazide is a thiazide diuretic. Its empirical formula is $C_7H_8ClN_3O_4S_2$, its molecular weight is 297.73, and its structural formula is

Tekturna HCT tablets are formulated for oral administration to contain aliskiren and hydrochlorothiazide, USP 150/12.5 mg, 150/25 mg, 300/12.5 mg and 300/25 mg. The inactive ingredients for all strengths of the tablets are colloidal silicon dioxide, crospovidone, hydroxypropyl methylcellulose, iron oxide colorants, lactose, magnesium stearate, microcrystalline cellulose, polyethylene glycol, povidone, talc, titanium dioxide, and wheat starch.

12 CLINICAL PHARMACOLOGY
12.1 Mechanism of Action
Aliskiren
Renin is secreted by the kidney in response to decreases in blood volume and renal perfusion. Renin cleaves angiotensinogen to form the inactive decapeptide angiotensin I (Ang I). Ang I is converted to the active octapeptide angiotensin II (Ang II) by angiotensin-converting enzyme (ACE) and non-ACE pathways. Ang II is a powerful vasoconstrictor and leads to the release of catecholamines from the adrenal medulla and prejunctional nerve endings. It also promotes aldosterone secretion and sodium reabsorption. Together, these effects increase blood pressure. Ang II also

inhibits renin release, thus providing a negative feedback to the system. This cycle, from renin through angiotensin to aldosterone and its associated negative feedback loop, is known as the renin-angiotensin-aldosterone system (RAAS). Aliskiren is a direct renin inhibitor, decreasing plasma renin activity (PRA) and inhibiting the conversion of angiotensinogen to Ang I. Whether aliskiren affects other RAAS components, e.g., ACE or non-ACE pathways, is not known.

All agents that inhibit the RAAS, including renin inhibitors, suppress the negative feedback loop, leading to a compensatory rise in plasma renin concentration. When this rise occurs during treatment with ACE inhibitors and ARBs, the result is increased levels of PRA. During treatment with aliskiren, however, the effect of increased renin levels is blocked, so that PRA, Ang I and Ang II are all reduced, whether aliskiren is used as monotherapy or in combination with other antihypertensive agents.

Hydrochlorothiazide
Hydrochlorothiazide is a thiazide diuretic. Thiazides affect the renal tubular mechanisms of electrolyte reabsorption, directly increasing excretion of sodium and chloride in approximately equivalent amounts. Indirectly, the diuretic action of hydrochlorothiazide reduces plasma volume, with consequent increases in plasma renin activity, increases in aldosterone secretion, increases in urinary potassium loss, and decreases in serum potassium. The renin-aldosterone link is mediated by angiotensin II, so coadministration of agents that block the production or function of angiotensin II tends to reverse the potassium loss associated with these diuretics.

The mechanism of action of the antihypertensive effect of thiazides is unknown.

12.2 Pharmacodynamics
Tekturna HCT
In placebo-controlled clinical trials, PRA was decreased with aliskiren monotherapy (ranging from 54% to 65%) and increased with hydrochlorothiazide monotherapy (ranging from 4% to 72%). Treatment with Tekturna HCT resulted in PRA reductions ranging from approximately 46% to 63% in various doses despite the increase in PRA with hydrochlorothiazide treatment. The clinical implications of the differences in effect on PRA are not known.

Aliskiren
PRA reductions in clinical trials ranged from approximately 50% to 80%, were not dose-related and did not correlate with blood pressure reductions. The clinical implications of the differences in effect on PRA are not known.

Hydrochlorothiazide
After oral administration of hydrochlorothiazide, diuresis begins within 2 hours, peaks in about 4 hours, and lasts about 6 to 12 hours.

Drug Interactions
Hydrochlorothiazide
Alcohol, barbiturates, or narcotics: Potentiation of orthostatic hypotension may occur.

Skeletal muscle relaxants: Possible increased responsiveness to muscle relaxants such as curare derivatives.

Digitalis glycosides: Thiazide-induced hypokalemia or hypomagnesemia may predispose the patient to digoxin toxicity.

12.3 Pharmacokinetics
Absorption and Distribution
Tekturna HCT
Following oral administration of Tekturna HCT combination tablets, the median peak plasma concentration time is within 1 hour for aliskiren and 2.5 hours for hydrochlorothiazide. When taken with food, mean AUC and C_{max} of aliskiren are decreased by 60% and 82%, respectively; mean AUC and C_{max} of hydrochlorothiazide increased by 13% and 10%, respectively. As a result, patients should establish a routine pattern for taking Tekturna HCT with regard to meals.

Aliskiren
Aliskiren is poorly absorbed (bioavailability about 2.5%). Following oral administration, peak plasma concentrations of aliskiren are reached within 1 to 3 hours. When taken with a high fat meal, mean AUC and C_{max} of aliskiren are decreased by 71% and 85% respectively. In the clinical trials of aliskiren, it was administered without requiring a fixed relation of administration to meals.

Hydrochlorothiazide
The estimated absolute bioavailability of hydrochlorothiazide after oral administration is about 70%. Peak plasma hydrochlorothiazide concentrations (C_{max}) are reached within 2 to 5 hours after oral administration. There is no clinically significant effect of food on the bioavailability of hydrochlorothiazide.

Hydrochlorothiazide binds to albumin (40 to 70%) and distributes into erythrocytes. Following oral administration, plasma hydrochlorothiazide concentrations decline biexponentially, with a mean distribution half-life of about 2 hours and an elimination half-life of about 10 hours.

Figure 5: The impact of co-administered drugs on the pharmacokinetics of aliskiren

*A 400 mg once daily dose was not studied, but would be expected to increase aliskiren blood levels further.

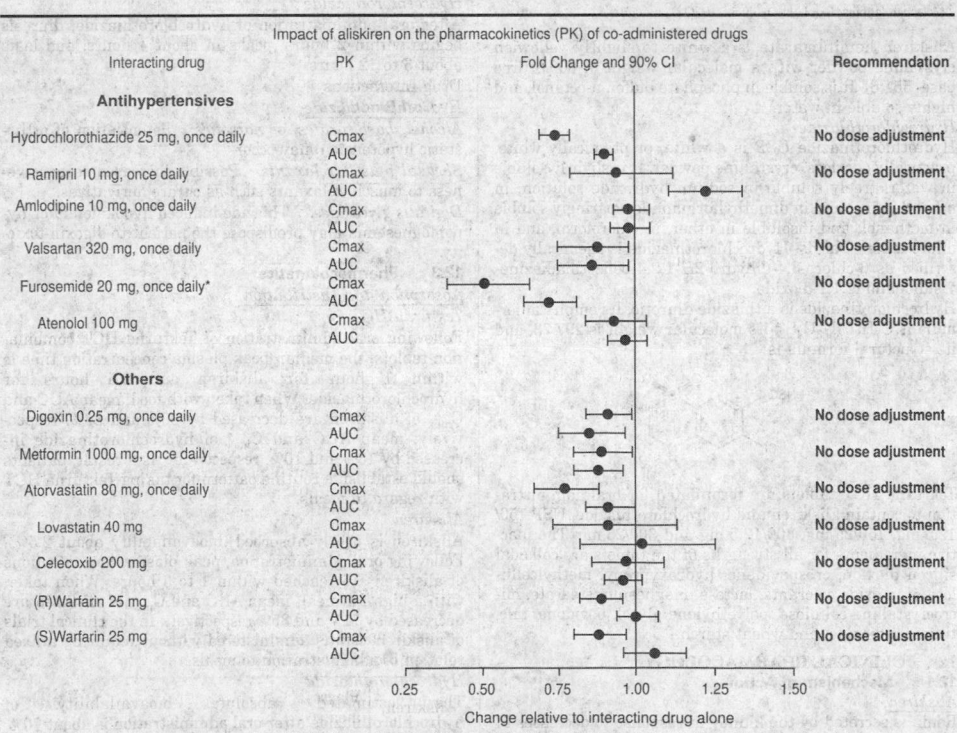

*Patients receiving furosemide could find its effect diminished after starting aliskiren.

Figure 6: The impact of aliskiren on the pharmacokinetics of co-administered drugs

Aliskiren does not inhibit the CYP450 isoenzymes (CYP 1A2, 2C8, 2C9, 2C19, 2D6, 2E1, and 3A) or induce CYP 3A4.

Transporters: Pgp (MDR1/Mdr1a/1b) was found to be the major efflux system involved in absorption and disposition of aliskiren in preclinical studies. The potential for drug interactions at the Pgp site will likely depend on the degree of inhibition of this transporter.

Hydrochlorothiazide
About 70% of an orally administered dose of hydrochlorothiazide is eliminated in the urine as unchanged drug.

Drug interactions:
Aliskiren
The effect of co-administered drugs on the pharmacokinetics of aliskiren and vice versa, were studied in several single and multiple dose studies. Pharmacokinetic measures indicating the magnitude of these interactions are presented in Figure 5 (impact of co-administered drugs on aliskiren) and Figure 6 (impact on co-administered drugs).
[See figure 5 above]
Warfarin: There was no clinically significant effect of a single dose of warfarin 25 mg on the pharmacokinetics of aliskiren.
[See figure 6 above]
Furosemide: In patients with heart failure, co-administration of aliskiren (300 mg/day) reduced plasma AUC and Cmax of oral furosemide (60 mg/day) by 17% and 27%, respectively, and reduced 24 hour urinary furosemide excretion by 29%. This change in exposure did not result in statistically significant difference in total urine volume and urinary sodium excretion over 24 hours. However, a transient decrease in urinary sodium excretion and urine volume effects up to 12 hours were observed when furosemide was co-administered with aliskiren 300 mg/day.

Hydrochlorothiazide
Drugs that alter gastrointestinal motility: The bioavailability of thiazide-type diuretics may be increased by anticholinergic agents (e.g. atropine, biperiden), apparently due to a decrease in gastrointestinal motility and the stomach emptying rate. Conversely, pro-kinetic drugs may decrease the bioavailability of thiazide diuretics.
Cholestyramine: In a dedicated drug interaction study, administration of cholestyramine 2 hours before hydrochlorothiazide resulted in a 70% reduction in exposure to hydrochlorothiazide. Further, administration of hydrochlorothiazide 2 hours before cholestyramine, resulted in 35% reduction in exposure to hydrochlorothiazide.
Antineoplastic agents (e.g. cyclophosphamide, methotrexate): Concomitant use of thiazide diuretics may reduce renal excretion of cytotoxic agents and enhance their myelosuppressive effects.

Special Populations
Pediatric Patients
The pharmacokinetics of aliskiren have not been investigated in patients <18 years of age.
Geriatric Patients
Aliskiren
The pharmacokinetics of aliskiren were studied in the elderly (≥65 years). Exposure (measured by AUC) is increased in elderly patients.
Hydrochlorothiazide
A limited amount of data suggest that the systemic clearance of hydrochlorothiazide is reduced in both healthy and hypertensive elderly subjects compared to young healthy volunteers.
Race
Too few non-Caucasians have been studied with Tekturna HCT to assess pharmacokinetic differences among races. The pharmacokinetic differences among Blacks, Caucasians, and Japanese are minimal with aliskiren therapy.
Renal Impairment
Aliskiren
The pharmacokinetics of aliskiren were evaluated in patients with varying degrees of renal impairment. Rate and extent of exposure (AUC and C_{max}) of aliskiren in subjects with renal impairment did not show a consistent correlation with the severity of renal impairment [see Use in Specific Populations (8.6)].
The pharmacokinetics of aliskiren following administration of a single oral dose of 300 mg was evaluated in patients with End Stage Renal Disease (ESRD) undergoing hemodialysis. When compared to matched healthy subjects, changes in the rate and extent of aliskiren exposure (Cmax and AUC) in ESRD patients undergoing hemodialysis were not clinically significant.
Timing of hemodialysis did not significantly alter the pharmacokinetics of aliskiren in ESRD patients. Therefore, no dose adjustment is warranted in ESRD patients receiving hemodialysis.
Hydrochlorothiazide
In a study in individuals with impaired renal function, the mean elimination half-life of hydrochlorothiazide was doubled in individuals with mild/moderate renal impairment (30 < CLcr < 90 mL/min) and tripled in severe renal impairment (≤ 30 mL/min), compared to individuals with normal renal function (CLcr > 90 mL/min) [see Use in Specific Populations (8.6)].

Metabolism and Elimination
Aliskiren
The effective half-life for aliskiren is 24 hours. Steady state blood levels are reached in about 7 – 8 days. About one-

fourth of the absorbed dose appears in the urine as parent drug. How much of the absorbed dose is metabolized is unknown. Based on the *in vitro* studies, the major enzyme responsible for aliskiren metabolism appears to be CYP 3A4.

Hepatic Impairment
Aliskiren
The pharmacokinetics of aliskiren were not significantly affected in patients with mild-to-severe liver disease *[see Use in Specific Populations (8.7)]*.

13 NONCLINICAL TOXICOLOGY

13.1 Carcinogenesis, Mutagenesis, Impairment of Fertility

Tekturna HCT
No carcinogenicity, mutagenicity or fertility studies have been conducted with Tekturna HCT. However, these studies have been conducted for aliskiren as well as hydrochlorothiazide alone.

Aliskiren
Carcinogenic potential was assessed in a 2-year rat study and a 6-month transgenic (rasH2) mouse study with aliskiren hemifumarate at oral doses of up to 1500 mg aliskiren/kg/day. Although there were no statistically significant increases in tumor incidence associated with exposure to aliskiren, mucosal epithelial hyperplasia (with or without erosion/ulceration) was observed in the lower gastrointestinal tract at doses of 750 or more mg/kg/day in both species, with a colonic adenoma identified in one rat and a cecal adenocarcinoma identified in another, rare tumors in the strain of rat studied. On a systemic exposure (AUC_{0-24hr}) basis, 1500 mg/kg/day in the rat is about 4 times and in the mouse about 1.5 times the maximum recommended human dose (300 mg aliskiren/day). Mucosal hyperplasia in the cecum or colon of rats was also observed at doses of 250 mg/kg/day (the lowest tested dose) as well as at higher doses in 4- and 13-week studies.

Aliskiren hemifumarate was devoid of genotoxic potential in the Ames reverse mutation assay with *S. typhimurium* and *E. coli*, the in vitro Chinese hamster ovary cell chromosomal aberration assay, the in vitro Chinese hamster V79 cell gene mutation test and the in vivo mouse bone marrow micronucleus assay.

Fertility of male and female rats was unaffected at doses of up to 250 mg aliskiren/kg/day (8 times the maximum recommended human dose of 300 mg Tekturna/60 kg on a mg/m² basis).

Hydrochlorothiazide
Two-year feeding studies in mice and rats conducted under the auspices of the National Toxicology Program (NTP) uncovered no evidence of a carcinogenic potential of hydrochlorothiazide in female mice (at doses of up to approximately 600 mg/kg/day) or in male and female rats (at doses of up to approximately 100 mg/kg/day). The NTP, however, found equivocal evidence for hepatocarcinogenicity in male mice.

Hydrochlorothiazide was not genotoxic in vitro in the Ames mutagenicity assay of *S. typhimurium* strains TA 98, TA 100, TA 1535, TA 1537, and TA 1538 and in the Chinese Hamster Ovary (CHO) test for chromosomal aberrations, or in vivo in assays using mouse germinal cell chromosomes, Chinese hamster bone marrow chromosomes, and the Drosophila sex-linked recessive lethal trait gene. Positive test results were obtained only in the in vitro CHO Sister Chromatid Exchange (clastogenicity) and in the Mouse Lymphoma Cell (mutagenicity) assays, using concentrations of hydrochlorothiazide from 43 to 1300 mcgm/mL, and in the Aspergillums Nidulans nondisjunction assay at an unspecified concentration.

Hydrochlorothiazide was not teratogenic and had no adverse effects on the fertility of mice and rats of either sex in studies wherein these species were exposed, via their diet, to doses of up to 100 and 4 mg/kg, respectively, prior to mating and throughout gestation. These doses of hydrochlorothiazide in mice and rats represent 19 and 1.5 times, respectively, the maximum recommended human dose on a mg/m² basis. (Calculations assume an oral dose of 25 mg/day and a 60-kg patient.)

14 CLINICAL STUDIES

14.1 Tekturna HCT

In all clinical trials including over 6,200 patients, more than 2,700 patients were exposed to combinations of aliskiren and hydrochlorothiazide. The safety and efficacy of Tekturna HCT were evaluated in patients with mild-to-moderate hypertension in an 8-week, randomized, double-blind, placebo-controlled, parallel-group, 15-arm factorial trial (n=2762). Patients were randomized to receive various combinations of aliskiren (75 mg to 300 mg) plus hydrochlorothiazide (6.25 mg to 25 mg) once daily (without titrating up from monotherapy) and followed for blood pressure response. The combination of aliskiren and hydrochlorothiazide resulted in additive placebo-adjusted decreases in systolic and diastolic blood pressure at trough of 10-14/5-7 mmHg at doses of 150-300 mg/12.5-25 mg, compared to 5-8/2-3 mmHg for aliskiren 150 mg to 300 mg and 6-7/2-3 mmHg for hydrochlorothiazide 12.5 mg to 25 mg, alone. Blood pressure reductions with the combinations were greater than the reductions with the monotherapies as shown in Table 1.

[See table 1 above]
The safety and efficacy of Tekturna HCT as initial therapy was evaluated in this trial. All patients randomized to the combination groups received the combination treatment of Tekturna HCT at assigned doses as initial therapy without titration from monotherapy. The figures *[see Indications and Usage (1)]* display the probability that a patient will achieve systolic or diastolic blood pressure goal with Tekturna HCT 300/25 mg, based upon their baseline systolic or diastolic blood pressure. At all levels of baseline blood pressure, the probability of achieving any given diastolic or systolic goal is greater with the combination than for either monotherapy.

The antihypertensive effect of Tekturna HCT was largely manifested within 1 week. The maximum antihypertensive effect was generally attained after about 4 weeks of therapy. One active-controlled trial investigated the addition of 300 mg aliskiren in obese hypertensive patients who did not respond adequately to hydrochlorothiazide 25 mg, and showed incremental decreases of systolic and diastolic blood pressure of approximately 7/4 mmHg.

In long-term follow-up studies (without placebo control) the effect of the combination of aliskiren and hydrochlorothiazide was maintained for over 1 year.

The antihypertensive effect was independent of age and gender. There were too few non-Caucasians to assess differences in blood pressure effects by race.

14.2 Aliskiren Monotherapy

The antihypertensive effects of aliskiren have been demonstrated in six randomized, double-blind, placebo-controlled, 8-week clinical trials in patients with mild-to-moderate hypertension. The placebo response and placebo-subtracted changes from baseline in seated trough cuff blood pressure are shown in Table 2.

[See table 2 above]
The studies included approximately 2,730 patients given doses of 75 mg to 600 mg of aliskiren and 1,231 patients given placebo. As shown in Table 2, there is some increase in response with administered dose in all studies, with reasonable effects seen at 150 mg to 300 mg, and no clear further increase at 600 mg. A substantial proportion (85% to 90%) of the blood pressure lowering effect was observed within 2 weeks of treatment. Studies with ambulatory blood pressure monitoring showed reasonable control throughout the interdosing interval, e.g., the ratios of mean daytime to mean nighttime ambulatory BP ranged from 0.6 to 0.9.

Patients in the placebo-controlled trials continued open-label aliskiren for up to one year. A persistent blood pressure lowering effect was demonstrated by a randomized withdrawal study (patients randomized to continued drug or placebo), which showed a statistically significant difference between patients kept on aliskiren and those randomized to placebo. With cessation of treatment, blood pressure gradually returned toward baseline levels over a period of several weeks. There was no evidence of rebound hypertension after abrupt cessation of therapy.

The effectiveness of aliskiren was demonstrated across all demographic subgroups, although Black patients tended to have smaller reductions in blood pressure than Caucasians and Asians, as has been seen with ACE inhibitors and ARBs.

14.3 Aliskiren in Combination with Other Antihypertensives

Valsartan
Aliskiren 150 mg and 300 mg and valsartan 160 mg and 320 mg were studied alone and in combination in an 8-week, 1,797-patient, randomized, double-blind, placebo-controlled, parallel-group, 4-arm, dose-escalation study. The dosages of aliskiren and valsartan were started at 150 mg and 160 mg, respectively, and increased at four weeks to 300 mg and 320 mg, respectively. Seated trough cuff blood pressure was measured at baseline, 4, and 8 weeks. Blood pressure reductions with the combinations were greater than the reductions with the monotherapies as shown in Table 3.

Amlodipine
Aliskiren 150 mg and 300 mg and amlodipine besylate 5 mg and 10 mg were studied alone and in combination in an 8-week, 1,685-patient, randomized, double-blind, placebo-controlled, multifactorial study. Treatment with aliskiren and amlodipine resulted overall in significantly greater reductions in diastolic and systolic blood pressure compared to the respective monotherapy components as shown in Table 4.

Table 1: Placebo-Subtracted Reductions in Seated Trough Cuff Blood Pressure in Combination with Hydrochlorothiazide

| | Hydrochlorothiazide, mg | | | | |
| | 0 | | 6.25 | 12.5 | 25 |
Aliskiren, mg	Placebo Mean Change	Placebo-subtracted	Placebo-subtracted	Placebo-subtracted	Placebo-subtracted
0	7.5/6.9	--	3.5/2.1	6.4/3.2	6.8/2.4
75	--	1.9/1.8	6.8/3.8	8.2/4.2	9.8/4.5
150	--	4.8/2	7.8/3.4	10.1/5	12/5.7
300	--	8.3/3.3	--	12.3/7	13.7/7.3

Table 2: Reductions in Seated Trough Cuff Blood Pressure in the Placebo-Controlled Studies of Aliskiren Monotherapy

| | | Aliskiren Daily Dose, mg | | | |
| | | 75 | 150 | 300 | 600 |
Study	Placebo Mean Change	Placebo-subtracted	Placebo-subtracted	Placebo-subtracted	Placebo-subtracted
1	2.9/3.3	5.7/4*	5.9/4.5*	11.2/7.5*	--
2	5.3/6.3	--	6.1/2.9*	10.5/5.4*	10.4/5.2*
3	10/8.6	2.2/1.7	2.1/1.7	5.1/3.7*	--
4	7.5/6.9	1.9/1.8	4.8/2*	8.3/3.3*	--
5	3.8/4.9	--	9.3/5.4*	10.9/6.2*	12.1/7.6*
6	4.6/4.1	--	--	8.4/4.9†	--

*p<0.05 vs. placebo by ANCOVA with Dunnett's procedure for multiple comparisons.
†p<0.05 vs. placebo by ANCOVA for the pairwise comparison.

Table 3: Placebo-Subtracted Reductions in Seated Trough Cuff Blood Pressure of Aliskiren in Combination with Valsartan

| | | Valsartan, mg | | |
Aliskiren, mg	Placebo Mean Change	0	160	320
0	4.6/4.1*	--	5.6/3.9	8.2/5.6
150	--	5.4/2.7	10.0/5.7	--
300	--	8.4/4.9	--	12.6/8.1

* The placebo change is 5.2/4.8 for Week 4 endpoint which was used for the dose groups containing aliskiren 150 mg or valsartan 160 mg.

Table 4: Placebo-Subtracted Reductions in Seated Trough Cuff Blood Pressure in Combination with Amlodipine

| Aliskiren, mg | Placebo mean change | Amlodipine, mg | | |
		0	5	10
0	5.4/6.8	--	5.6/9.0	8.5/14.3
150	--	2.6/3.9	8.6/13.9	10.8/17.1
300	--	4.9/8.6	9.6/15.0	11.1/16.4

Table 5: Incidence of Selected Adverse Events During the Treatment Phase in ALTITUDE

	Aliskiren N=4272		Placebo N=4285	
	Serious Adverse Events* (%)	Adverse Events (%)	Serious Adverse Events* (%)	Adverse Events (%)
Renal impairment †	5.7	14.5	4.3	12.4
Hypotension ††	2.3	19.9	1.9	16.3
Hyperkalemia †††	1.0	38.9	0.5	28.8

†renal failure, renal failure acute, renal failure chronic, renal impairment
††dizziness, dizziness postural, hypotension, orthostatic hypotension, presyncope, syncope
††† Given the variable baseline serum potassium levels of patients with renal insufficiency on dual RAAS therapy, the reporting of adverse event of hyperkalemia was at the discretion of the investigator.
* A Serious Adverse Event (SAE) is defined as: an event which is fatal or life-threatening, results in persistent or significant disability/incapacity, constitutes a congenital anomaly/birth defect, requires inpatient hospitalization or prolongation of existing hospitalization, or is medically significant (i.e. defined as an event that jeopardizes the patient or may require medical or surgical intervention to prevent one of the outcomes previously listed).

Table 6: Tekturna HCT Tablets Supply

Tablet	Color	Imprint Side 1	Imprint Side 2	NDC 0078- XXXX-XX Bottle of 30	Bottle of 90	Blister Packages of 100
Aliskiren/HCTZ						
150 mg/12.5 mg	White	NVR	LCI	0521-15	0521-34	0521-35
150 mg/25 mg	Pale Yellow	NVR	CLL	0522-15	0522-34	0522-35
300 mg/12.5 mg	Violet White	NVR	CVI	0523-15	0523-34	0523-35
300 mg/25 mg	Light Yellow	NVR	CVV	0524-15	0524-34	0524-35

ACE Inhibitors
Aliskiren has not been studied when added to maximal doses of ACE inhibitors to determine whether aliskiren produces additional blood pressure reduction.
There are no trials of the Tekturna HCT combination tablet demonstrating reductions in cardiovascular risk in patients with hypertension, but the hydrochlorothiazide component has demonstrated such benefits.

14.4   Aliskiren in Patients with Diabetes treated with ARB or ACEI (ALTITUDE study)
Patients with diabetes with renal disease (defined either by the presence of albuminuria or reduced GFR) were randomized to aliskiren 300 mg daily (n=4296) or placebo (n=4310). All patients were receiving background therapy with an ARB or ACEI. The primary efficacy outcome was the time to the first event of the primary composite endpoint consisting of cardiovascular death, resuscitated sudden death, non-fatal myocardial infarction, non-fatal stroke, unplanned hospitalization for heart failure, onset of end stage renal disease, renal death, and doubling of serum creatinine concentration from baseline sustained for at least one month. After a median follow up of about 32 months, the trial was terminated early for lack of efficacy. Higher risk of renal impairment, hypotension and hyperkalemia was observed in aliskiren compared to placebo treated patients, as shown in the table below.
[See table 5 above]
The risk of stroke (3.4% aliskiren vs 2.7% placebo) and death (8.4% aliskiren vs. 8.0% placebo) were also numerically higher in aliskiren treated patients.

16   HOW SUPPLIED/STORAGE AND HANDLING
Tekturna HCT is supplied as biconvex, ovaloid film-coated tablets.
All strengths are packaged in bottles and unit-dose blister packages (10 strips of 10 tablets) as described below.
[See table 6 above]
Storage
Store at 25°C (77°F); excursions permitted to 15-30°C (59-86°F) *[See USP Controlled Room Temperature]*.
Protect from moisture.
Dispense in original container.

17   PATIENT COUNSELING INFORMATION
See FDA-approved patient labeling (Patient Information)
Healthcare professionals should instruct their patients to read the Patient Package Insert before starting Tekturna HCT and to reread each time the prescription is renewed. Patients should be instructed to inform their doctor or pharmacist if they develop any unusual symptom, or if any known symptom persists or worsens.
Pregnancy
Female patients of childbearing age should be told about the consequences of exposure to Tekturna HCT during pregnancy. Discuss treatment options with women planning to become pregnant. Patients should be asked to report pregnancies to their physicians as soon as possible.

Symptomatic Hypotension
A patient receiving Tekturna HCT should be cautioned that lightheadedness can occur, especially during the first days of therapy, and that it should be reported to the prescribing physician. The patients should be told that if syncope occurs, Tekturna HCT should be discontinued until the physician has been consulted.
All patients should be cautioned that inadequate fluid intake, excessive perspiration, diarrhea, or vomiting can lead to an excessive fall in blood pressure, with the same consequences of lightheadedness and possible syncope.
Anaphylactic Reactions and Angioedema
Patients should be advised and told to report immediately any signs or symptoms suggesting a severe allergic reaction (difficulty breathing or swallowing, tightness of the chest, hives, general rash, swelling, itching, dizziness, vomiting, or abdominal pain) or angioedema (swelling of face, extremities, eyes, lips, tongue, difficulty in swallowing or breathing) and to take no more drug until they have consulted with the prescribing physician. Angioedema, including laryngeal edema, may occur at any time during treatment with Tekturna HCT.
Potassium Supplements
A patient receiving Tekturna HCT should be told not to use potassium supplements or salt substitutes containing potassium without consulting the prescribing physician.
Relationship to Meals
Patients should establish a routine pattern for taking Tekturna HCT with regard to meals. High-fat meals decrease absorption substantially.

T2014-24
March 2014
FDA-Approved Patient Labeling
Patient Information
Tekturna HCT® (tek-turn-a HCT)
(aliskiren and hydrochlorothiazide, USP)
Combination Tablets
Read the Patient Information that comes with Tekturna HCT before you start taking it and each time you get a refill. There may be new information. This leaflet does not take the place of talking with your doctor about your condition and treatment.
What is the most important information I should know about Tekturna HCT?
Tekturna HCT can cause harm or death to an unborn baby. Talk to your doctor about other ways to lower your blood pressure if you plan to become pregnant. If you get pregnant while taking Tekturna HCT, tell your doctor right away.
What is Tekturna HCT?
Tekturna HCT contains two prescription medicines in one tablet that work together to lower blood pressure. It contains:
• aliskiren (Tekturna), a direct renin inhibitor (DRI)
• hydrochlorothiazide, a diuretic (water pill)

Aliskiren (Tekturna) reduces the effect of renin, and the harmful process that narrows blood vessels. Aliskiren also helps blood vessels relax and widen so blood pressure is lower. Hydrochlorothiazide reduces the amount of salt and water in your body so your blood pressure is lower.
Tekturna HCT may be used to lower high blood pressure in adults
• when one medicine to lower high blood pressure is not enough
• as the first medicine to lower high blood pressure if your doctor decides that you are likely to need more than one medicine
Tekturna HCT has not been studied in children under 18 years of age.
Your doctor may prescribe other medicines for you to take along with Tekturna HCT to treat your high blood pressure.
What is high blood pressure (hypertension)?
Blood pressure is the force that pushes the blood through your blood vessels to all the organs of your body. You have high blood pressure when the force of your blood moving through your blood vessels is too great. One cause of high blood pressure is renin, a chemical in the body that starts a process that makes blood vessels narrow, leading to high blood pressure.
Tekturna HCT reduces high blood pressure. Medicines that lower your blood pressure lower your chance of having a stroke or heart attack. High blood pressure makes the heart work harder to pump blood throughout the body and causes damage to the blood vessels. If high blood pressure is not treated, it can lead to stroke, heart attack, heart failure, kidney failure, and vision problems.
Who should not take Tekturna HCT?
• **If you get pregnant, stop taking Tekturna HCT and call your doctor right away. If you plan to become pregnant, talk to your doctor about other treatment options for your high blood pressure.**
• **If you have diabetes and are taking a kind of medicine called an angiotensin-receptor-blocker or angiotensin-converting-enzyme-inhibitor**
• **Do not take Tekturna HCT if you make very little or no urine due to kidney problems.**
• **Do not take Tekturna HCT if you are allergic to any of its ingredients. See the end of this leaflet for a complete list of the ingredients in Tekturna HCT.**
What should I tell my doctor before taking Tekturna HCT?
Tell your doctor about all your medical conditions, including whether you:
• have kidney problems
• are pregnant or planning to become pregnant. See "What is the most important information I should know about Tekturna HCT?"
• have any allergies or asthma
• have liver problems
• have systemic lupus erythematosus (SLE). Tekturna HCT can make your SLE active or worse.
• have ever had a reaction called angioedema, to an ACE inhibitor medicine. Angioedema causes swelling of the face, lips, tongue, throat, arms and legs, and may cause difficulty breathing.
• are breast-feeding. It is not known if Tekturna HCT passes into your breast milk.
Tell your doctor about all the medicines you take including prescription and nonprescription medicines, vitamins and herbal supplements. Especially tell your doctor if you are taking:
• a kind of medicine called angiotensin receptor blocker or angiotensin converting enzyme inhibitor
• atorvastatin (medicine to lower cholesterol in your blood)
• water pills (also called "diuretics")
• medicines for treating fungus or fungal infections
• cyclosporine (a medicine used to suppress the immune system)
• potassium-containing medicines, potassium supplements, or salt substitutes containing potassium
• cholestyramine (for example; Questran, Questran Light, Cholestyramine Light, Locholest Light, Locholest, Prevalite) (medicines to lower the cholesterol in your blood)
• colestipol (for example; Colestipol hydrochloride, Colestid, Flavored Colestid) (medicines to lower the cholesterol in your blood)
• medicines to treat diabetes, including insulin
• lithium, a medicine used in some types of depression. Do not take Tekturna HCT if you are taking lithium.
• Nonsteroidal anti-inflammatory (NSAIDs) medicines. Ask your doctor if you are not sure if you are taking one of these medicines.
• blood thinners
• barbiturate or narcotic medicines. Ask your doctor if you are not sure if you are taking one of these medicines.
Your doctor or pharmacist will know what medicines are safe to take together. Know your medicines. Keep a list of your medicines and show it to your doctor or pharmacist when you get a new medicine.

How should I take Tekturna HCT?

- Take Tekturna HCT exactly as prescribed by your doctor. It is important to take Tekturna HCT every day to control your blood pressure.
- Take Tekturna HCT once each day, about the same time each day.
- Take Tekturna HCT the same way every day, either with or without a meal.
- Your doctor may change your dose of Tekturna HCT if needed.
- If you miss a dose of Tekturna HCT, take it as soon as you remember. If it is close to your next dose, do not take the missed dose. Just take the next dose at your regular time.
- If you take too much Tekturna HCT, call your doctor or a Poison Control Center, or go to the nearest hospital emergency room.

What are the possible side effects of Tekturna HCT?

Tekturna HCT may cause serious side effects:

- **Injury or death to an unborn baby.** See "What is the most important information I should know about Tekturna HCT?"
- **Low blood pressure (hypotension).** Your blood pressure may get too low if you also take water pills, are on a low-salt diet, get dialysis treatments, have heart problems, or get sick with vomiting or diarrhea. Drinking alcohol and taking certain medicines (barbiturates or narcotics) can cause low blood pressure to get worse. Lie down if you feel faint or dizzy, and call your doctor right away.
- **Severe Allergic Reactions and Angioedema.** Aliskiren, one of the medicines in Tekturna HCT, can cause difficulty breathing or swallowing, tightness of the chest, hives, general rash, swelling, itching, dizziness, vomiting, or abdominal pain (signs of a severe allergic reaction). Aliskiren can also cause swelling of the face, lips, tongue, throat, arms and legs, or the whole body (signs of angioedema). Get medical help right away and tell your doctor if you get any one or more of these symptoms. Angioedema can happen at any time while you are taking Tekturna HCT.
- **Renal impairment or failure.** Aliskiren, one of the medicines in Tekturna HCT, may cause renal disorder with symptoms such as severely decreased urine output or decreased urine output (signs of renal impairment or failure).
- **Active or worsened Systemic Lupus Erythematosus (SLE).** If you have SLE, tell your doctor right away if you get any new or worse symptoms.
- **Eye problems.** One of the medicines in Tekturna HCT can cause eye problems that may lead to vision loss. Symptoms of eye problems can happen within hours to weeks of starting Tekturna HCT. Tell your doctor right away if you have:
  - Decrease in vision
  - Eye pain

Common side effects of Tekturna HCT include:

- dizziness
- flu-like symptoms
- diarrhea
- cough
- tiredness
- high levels of potassium in the blood (hyperkalemia)

Less common side effects include skin rash, severe skin reactions (signs may include severe blistering of the lips, eyes or mouth, rash with fever and skin peeling) and liver disorder (signs may include nausea, loss of appetite, dark colored urine or yellowing of skin and eyes).

Tell your doctor if you have any side effect that bothers you or that does not go away. These are not all of the possible side effects of Tekturna HCT. For a complete list of side effects, ask your doctor or pharmacist.

How do I store Tekturna HCT?

- Store Tekturna HCT tablets at room temperature between 59°F-86°F (15°C-30°C).
- Keep Tekturna HCT in the original prescription bottle in a dry place. Do not remove the desiccant (drying agent) from the bottle.

Keep Tekturna HCT and all medicines out of the reach of children.

General information about Tekturna HCT

Medicines are sometimes prescribed for conditions not listed in the patient information leaflet. Do not take Tekturna HCT for a condition for which it was not prescribed. Do not give Tekturna HCT to other people, even if they have the same condition or symptoms you have. It may harm them.

This leaflet summarizes the most important information about Tekturna HCT. If you have questions about Tekturna HCT talk with your doctor. You can ask your doctor or pharmacist for information that is written for healthcare professionals.

For more information about Tekturna HCT, visit www.TekturnaHCT.com, or call 1-888-669-6682.

What are the ingredients in Tekturna HCT?

Active ingredients: Aliskiren and hydrochlorothiazide
Inactive ingredients: Colloidal silicon dioxide, crospovidone, hydroxypropyl methylcellulose, iron oxide colorants, lactose, magnesium stearate, microcrystalline cellulose, polyethylene glycol, povidone, talc, titanium dioxide, and wheat starch.

Call your doctor for medical advice about side effects. You may report side effects to FDA at 1-800-FDA-1088.

Manufactured by:
Novartis Pharma Produktions GmbH
Wehr, Germany
Distributed by:
Novartis Pharmaceuticals Corporation
East Hanover, New Jersey 07936
© Novartis
T2014-25
March 2014

Shown in Product Identification Guide, page 311

TOBI® ℞

[toe-bye]
(tobramycin inhalation solution, USP)
Nebulizer Solution – For Inhalation Use Only
Rx only
Prescribing Information

The following prescribing information is based on official labeling in effect July 2014.

DESCRIPTION

TOBI® is a tobramycin solution for inhalation. It is a sterile, clear, slightly yellow, non-pyrogenic, aqueous solution with the pH and salinity adjusted specifically for administration by a compressed air driven reusable nebulizer. The chemical formula for tobramycin is $C_{18}H_{37}N_5O_9$ and the molecular weight is 467.52. Tobramycin is O-3-amino-3-deoxy-α-D-glucopyranosyl-(1→4)-O-[2,6-diamino-2,3,6-trideoxy-α-D-ribo-hexopyranosyl-(1→6)]-2-deoxy-L-streptamine. The structural formula for tobramycin is:

Each single-use 5 mL ampule contains 300 mg tobramycin and 11.25 mg sodium chloride in sterile water for injection. Sulfuric acid and sodium hydroxide are added to adjust the pH to 6.0. Nitrogen is used for sparging. All ingredients meet USP requirements. The formulation contains no preservatives.

CLINICAL PHARMACOLOGY

TOBI® is specifically formulated for administration by inhalation. When inhaled, tobramycin is concentrated in the airways.

Pharmacokinetics

TOBI® contains tobramycin, a cationic polar molecule that does not readily cross epithelial membranes.[1] The bioavailability of TOBI® may vary because of individual differences in nebulizer performance and airway pathology.[2] Following administration of TOBI®, tobramycin remains concentrated primarily in the airways.

Sputum Concentrations: Ten minutes after inhalation of the first 300-mg dose of TOBI®, the average concentration of tobramycin was 1237 µg/g (ranging from 35 to 7417 µg/g) in sputum. Tobramycin does not accumulate in sputum; after 20 weeks of therapy with the TOBI® regimen, the average concentration of tobramycin at ten minutes after inhalation was 1154 µg/g (ranging from 39 to 8085 µg/g) in sputum. High variability of tobramycin concentration in sputum was observed. Two hours after inhalation, sputum concentrations declined to approximately 14% of tobramycin levels at ten minutes after inhalation.

Serum Concentrations: The average serum concentration of tobramycin one hour after inhalation of a single 300-mg dose of TOBI® by cystic fibrosis patients was 0.95 µg/mL. After 20 weeks of therapy on the TOBI® regimen, the average serum tobramycin concentration one hour after dosing was 1.05 µg/mL.

Elimination: The elimination half-life of tobramycin from serum is approximately 2 hours after intravenous (IV) administration. Assuming tobramycin absorbed following inhalation behaves similarly to tobramycin following IV administration, systemically absorbed tobramycin is elimi-

nated principally by glomerular filtration. Unabsorbed tobramycin, following TOBI® administration, is probably eliminated primarily in expectorated sputum.

Microbiology

Tobramycin is an aminoglycoside antibiotic produced by *Streptomyces tenebrarius*.[1] It acts primarily by disrupting protein synthesis, leading to altered cell membrane permeability, progressive disruption of the cell envelope, and eventual cell death.[3]

Tobramycin has *in-vitro* activity against a wide range of gram-negative organisms including *Pseudomonas aeruginosa*. It is bactericidal at concentrations equal to or slightly greater than inhibitory concentrations.

Susceptibility Testing

A single sputum sample from a cystic fibrosis patient may contain multiple morphotypes of *Pseudomonas aeruginosa* and each morphotype may have a different level of *in-vitro* susceptibility to tobramycin. Treatment for 6 months with TOBI® in two clinical studies did not affect the susceptibility of the majority of *P. aeruginosa* isolates tested; however, increased minimum inhibitory concentrations (MICs) were noted in some patients. The clinical significance of this information has not been clearly established in the treatment of *P. aeruginosa* in cystic fibrosis patients. For additional information regarding the effects of TOBI® on *P. aeruginosa* MIC values and bacterial sputum density, please refer to the CLINICAL STUDIES section.

The *in-vitro* antimicrobial susceptibility test methods used for parenteral tobramycin therapy can be used to monitor the susceptibility of *P. aeruginosa* isolated from cystic fibrosis patients. If decreased susceptibility is noted, the results should be reported to the clinician.

Susceptibility breakpoints established for parenteral administration of tobramycin do not apply to aerosolized administration of TOBI®. The relationship between *in-vitro* susceptibility test results and clinical outcome with TOBI® therapy is not clear.

INDICATIONS AND USAGE

TOBI® is indicated for the management of cystic fibrosis patients with *P. aeruginosa*.

Safety and efficacy have not been demonstrated in patients under the age of 6 years, patients with forced expiratory volume in 1 second (FEV_1) <25% or >75% predicted, or patients colonized with *Burkholderia cepacia* (see CLINICAL STUDIES).

CONTRAINDICATIONS

TOBI® is contraindicated in patients with a known hypersensitivity to any aminoglycoside.

WARNINGS

Caution should be exercised when prescribing TOBI® to patients with known or suspected renal, auditory, vestibular, or neuromuscular dysfunction. Patients receiving concomitant parenteral aminoglycoside therapy should be monitored as clinically appropriate.

Aminoglycosides can cause fetal harm when administered to a pregnant woman. Aminoglycosides cross the placenta, and streptomycin has been associated with several reports of total, irreversible, bilateral congenital deafness in pediatric patients exposed *in utero*. Patients who use TOBI® during pregnancy, or become pregnant while taking TOBI® should be apprised of the potential hazard to the fetus.

Ototoxicity

Ototoxicity, as measured by complaints of hearing loss or by audiometric evaluations, did not occur with TOBI® therapy during clinical studies. However, transient tinnitus occurred in eight TOBI®-treated patients versus no placebo patients in the clinical studies. Tinnitus may be a sentinel symptom of ototoxicity, and therefore the onset of this symptom warrants caution (see ADVERSE REACTIONS). Ototoxicity, manifested as both auditory and vestibular toxicity, has been reported with parenteral aminoglycosides. Vestibular toxicity may be manifested by vertigo, ataxia or dizziness.

In postmarketing experience, patients receiving TOBI® have reported hearing loss. Some of these reports occurred in patients with previous or concomitant treatment with systemic aminoglycosides. Patients with hearing loss frequently reported tinnitus.

Nephrotoxicity

Nephrotoxicity was not seen during TOBI® clinical studies but has been associated with aminoglycosides as a class. If nephrotoxicity occurs in a patient receiving TOBI®, tobramycin therapy should be discontinued until serum concentrations fall below 2 µg/mL.

Muscular Disorders

TOBI® should be used cautiously in patients with neuromuscular disorders, such as myasthenia gravis or Parkinson's disease, since aminoglycosides may aggravate muscle weakness because of a potential curare-like effect on neuromuscular function.

Bronchospasm

Bronchospasm can occur with inhalation of TOBI®. In clinical studies of TOBI®, changes in FEV_1 measured after the inhaled dose were similar in the TOBI® and placebo groups. Bronchospasm should be treated as medically appropriate.

PRECAUTIONS

Information for Patients

NOTE: In addition to information provided below, a Patient Medication Guide providing instructions for proper use of TOBI® is contained inside the package.

Safety Information

TOBI® is in a class of antibiotics that have caused hearing loss, dizziness, kidney damage, and harm to a fetus. Ringing in the ears and hoarseness were two symptoms that were seen in more patients taking TOBI® than placebo in research studies. Patients with cystic fibrosis can have many symptoms. Some of these symptoms may be related to your medications. If you have new or worsening symptoms, you should tell your doctor.

Hearing: You should tell your doctor if you have ringing in the ears, dizziness, or any changes in hearing.

Kidney Damage: Inform your doctor if you have any history of kidney problems.

Pregnancy: If you want to become pregnant or are pregnant while on TOBI®, you should talk with your doctor about the possibility of TOBI® causing any harm.

Nursing Mothers: If you are nursing a baby, you should talk with your doctor before using TOBI®.

TOBI® Packaging

TOBI® comes in a single dose, ready-to-use ampule containing 300 mg tobramycin. Each foil pouch contains 4 ampules, for 2 days of TOBI® therapy.

Dosage

The 300 mg dose of TOBI® is the same for patients regardless of age or weight. TOBI® has not been studied in patients less than 6 years old. Doses should be inhaled as close to 12 hours apart as possible and not less than 6 hours apart.

You should not mix TOBI® with dornase alfa (PULMOZYME®, Genentech) in the nebulizer.

If you are taking several medications the recommended order is as follows: bronchodilator first, followed by chest physiotherapy, then other inhaled medications and, finally, TOBI®.

Treatment Schedule

You should take TOBI® in repeated cycles of 28 days on drug followed by 28 days off drug. You should take TOBI® twice a day during the 28-day period on drug.

How To Administer TOBI®

THIS INFORMATION IS NOT INTENDED TO REPLACE CONSULTATION WITH YOUR PHYSICIAN AND CF CARE TEAM ABOUT PROPERLY TAKING MEDICATION OR USING INHALATION EQUIPMENT.

TOBI® is specifically formulated for inhalation using a PARI LC PLUS™ Reusable Nebulizer and a DeVilbiss® Pulmo-Aide® air compressor. TOBI® can be taken at home, school, or at work. The following are instructions on how to use the DeVilbiss® Pulmo-Aide® air compressor and PARI LC PLUS™ Reusable Nebulizer to administer TOBI®.

You will need the following supplies:
- TOBI® plastic ampule (vial)
- DeVilbiss® Pulmo-Aide® air compressor
- PARI LC PLUS™ Reusable Nebulizer
- Tubing to connect the nebulizer and compressor
- Clean paper or cloth towels
- Nose clips (optional)

It is important that your nebulizer and compressor function properly before starting your TOBI® therapy.

Note: Please refer to the manufacturers' care and use instructions for important information.

Preparing Your TOBI® for Inhalation

1. Wash your hands thoroughly with soap and water.

2a. TOBI® is packaged with 4 ampules per foil pouch.

2b. Separate one ampule by gently pulling apart at the bottom tabs. Store all remaining ampules in the refrigerator as directed.

3. Lay out the contents of a PARI LC PLUS™ Reusable Nebulizer package on a clean, dry paper or cloth towel. You should have the following parts:
- Nebulizer Top and Bottom (Nebulizer Cup) Assembly
- Inspiratory Valve Cap
- Mouthpiece with Valve
- Tubing

4. Remove the Nebulizer Top from the Nebulizer Cup by twisting the Nebulizer Top counter-clockwise, and then lifting off. Place the Nebulizer Top on the clean paper or cloth towel. Stand the Nebulizer Cup upright on the towel.

5. Connect one end of the tubing to the compressor air outlet. The tubing should fit snugly. Plug in your compressor to an electrical outlet.

6. Open the TOBI® ampule by holding the bottom tab with one hand and twisting off the top of the ampule with the other hand. Be careful not to squeeze the ampule until you are ready to empty its contents into the Nebulizer Cup.

7. Squeeze **all** the contents of the ampule into the Nebulizer Cup.

8. Replace the Nebulizer Top. Note: In order to insert the Nebulizer Top into the Nebulizer Cup, the semi-circle halfway down the stem of the Nebulizer Top should face the Nebulizer Outlet.

9. Attach the Mouthpiece to the Nebulizer Outlet. Then firmly push the Inspiratory Valve Cap in place on the Nebulizer Top. Note: the Inspiratory Valve Cap will fit snugly.

10. Connect the free end of the tubing from the compressor to the Air Intake on the bottom of the nebulizer, making sure to keep the nebulizer upright. Press the tubing on the Air Intake firmly.

TOBI® Treatment

1. Turn on the compressor.

2. Check for a steady mist from the Mouthpiece. If there is no mist, check all tubing connections and confirm that the compressor is working properly.

3. Sit or stand in an upright position that will allow you to breathe normally.

4. Place Mouthpiece between your teeth and on top of your tongue and breathe normally only through your mouth. Nose clips may help you breathe through your mouth and not through your nose. Do not block airflow with your tongue.

5. Continue treatment until all your TOBI® is gone, and there is no longer any mist being produced. You may hear a sputtering sound when the Nebulizer Cup is empty. The entire TOBI® treatment should take approximately 15 minutes to complete. Note: if you are interrupted, need to cough or rest during your TOBI® treatment, turn off the compressor to save your medication. Turn the compressor back on when you are ready to resume your therapy.

6. Follow the nebulizer cleaning and disinfecting instructions after completing therapy.

Cleaning Your Nebulizer

To reduce the risk of infection, illness or injury from contamination, you must thoroughly clean all parts of the nebulizer as instructed after each treatment. Never use a nebulizer with a clogged nozzle. If the nozzle is clogged, no aerosol mist is produced, which will alter the effectiveness of the treatment. Replace the nebulizer if clogging occurs.

1. Remove tubing from nebulizer and disassemble nebulizer parts.

2. Wash all parts (except tubing) with warm water and liquid dish soap.

3. Rinse thoroughly with warm water and shake out water.

4. Air dry or hand dry nebulizer parts on a clean, lint-free cloth. Reassemble nebulizer when dry, and store.

5. You can also wash all parts of the nebulizer in a dishwasher (except tubing). Place the nebulizer parts in a dishwasher basket, then place on the top rack of the dishwasher. Remove and dry the parts when the cycle is complete.

Disinfecting Your Nebulizer

Your nebulizer is for your use only - Do not share your nebulizer with other people. You must regularly disinfect the nebulizer. Failure to do so could lead to serious or fatal illness.

Clean the nebulizer as described above. Every other treatment day, disinfect the nebulizer parts (except tubing) by boiling them in water for a full 10 minutes. Dry parts on a clean, lint-free cloth.

Care and Use of Your Pulmo-Aide® Compressor

Follow the manufacturer's instructions for care and use of your compressor.

Filter Change:

1. DeVilbiss® Compressor filters should be changed every six months or sooner if filter turns completely gray in color.

Compressor Cleaning:

1. With power switch in the "Off" position, unplug power cord from wall outlet.

2. Wipe outside of the compressor cabinet with a clean, damp cloth every few days to keep dust free.

Caution: Do not submerge in water; doing so will result in compressor damage.

Storage Instructions

You should store TOBI® ampules in a refrigerator (2-8°C or 36-46°F). However, when you don't have a refrigerator available (e.g., transporting your TOBI®), you may store the foil pouches (opened or unopened) at room temperature (up to 25°C/77°F) for up to 28 days.

Avoid exposing TOBI® ampules to intense light.

Unrefrigerated TOBI®, which is normally slightly yellow, may darken with age; however, the color change does not indicate any change in the quality of the product.

You should not use TOBI® if it is cloudy, if there are particles in the solution, or if it has been stored at room temperature for more than 28 days. You should not use TOBI® beyond the expiration date stamped on the ampule.

Additional Information

Nebulizer: 1-800-327-8632

Compressor: 1-800-338-1988

TOBI®: 1-888-NOW-NOVA (1-888-669-6682)

Laboratory Tests

Audiograms

Clinical studies of TOBI® did not identify hearing loss using audiometric tests which evaluated hearing up to 8000 Hz. **Physicians should consider an audiogram for patients who show any evidence of auditory dysfunction, or who are at increased risk for auditory dysfunction.** Tinnitus may be a sentinel symptom of ototoxicity, and therefore the onset of this symptom warrants caution.

Serum Concentrations

In patients with normal renal function treated with TOBI®, serum tobramycin concentrations are approximately 1 µg/mL 1 hour after dose administration and do not require routine monitoring. Serum concentrations of tobramycin in patients with renal dysfunction or patients treated with concomitant parenteral tobramycin should be monitored at the discretion of the treating physician.

The serum concentration of tobramycin should only be monitored through venipuncture and not finger prick blood sampling. Contamination of the skin of the fingers with tobramycin may lead to falsely increased measurements of serum levels of the drug. This contamination cannot be completely avoided by hand washing before testing.

Renal Function

The clinical studies of TOBI® did not reveal any imbalance in the percentage of patients in the TOBI® and placebo groups who experienced at least a 50% rise in serum creatinine from baseline (see ADVERSE REACTIONS). Laboratory tests of urine and renal function should be conducted at the discretion of the treating physician.

Drug Interactions

In clinical studies of TOBI®, patients taking TOBI® concomitantly with dornase alfa (PULMOZYME®, Genentech), ß-agonists, inhaled corticosteroids, other anti-pseudomonal antibiotics, or parenteral aminoglycosides demonstrated adverse experience profiles similar to the study population as a whole.

Concurrent and/or sequential use of TOBI® with other drugs with neurotoxic, nephrotoxic, or ototoxic potential should be avoided. Some diuretics can enhance aminoglycoside toxicity by altering antibiotic concentrations in serum and tissue. TOBI® should not be administered concomitantly with ethacrynic acid, furosemide, urea, or intravenous mannitol. The interaction between inhaled mannitol and TOBI® has not been evaluated.

Carcinogenesis, Mutagenesis, Impairment of Fertility

A two-year rat inhalation toxicology study to assess carcinogenic potential of TOBI® has been completed. Rats were exposed to TOBI® for up to 1.5 hours per day for 95 weeks. The clinical formulation of the drug was used for this carcinogenicity study. Serum levels of tobramycin of up to 35 mcg/mL were measured in rats, in contrast to the average 1 mcg/mL levels observed in cystic fibrosis patients in clinical trials. There was no drug-related increase in the incidence of any variety of tumor.

Additionally, TOBI® has been evaluated for genotoxicity in a battery of *in-vitro* and *in-vivo* tests. The Ames bacterial reversion test, conducted with 5 tester strains, failed to show a significant increase in revertants with or without metabolic activation in all strains. Tobramycin was negative in the mouse lymphoma forward mutation assay, did not induce chromosomal aberrations in Chinese hamster ovary cells, and was negative in the mouse micronucleus test.

Subcutaneous administration of up to 100 mg/kg of tobramycin did not affect mating behavior or cause impairment of fertility in male or female rats.

Pregnancy

Teratogenic Effects – Pregnancy Category D

(See WARNINGS.)

No reproduction toxicology studies have been conducted with TOBI®. However, subcutaneous administration of tobramycin at doses of 100 or 20 mg/kg/day during organogenesis was not teratogenic in rats or rabbits, respectively. Doses of tobramycin ≥40 mg/kg/day were severely maternally toxic to rabbits and precluded the evaluation of teratogenicity. Aminoglycosides can cause fetal harm (e.g., congenital deafness) when administered to a pregnant woman. Ototoxicity was not evaluated in offspring during nonclinical reproduction toxicity studies with tobramycin. If TOBI® is used during pregnancy, or if the patient becomes pregnant while taking TOBI®, the patient should be apprised of the potential hazard to the fetus.

Nursing Mothers

It is not known if TOBI® will reach sufficient concentrations after administration by inhalation to be excreted in human breast milk. Because of the potential for ototoxicity and nephrotoxicity in infants, a decision should be made whether to terminate nursing or discontinue TOBI®.

Pediatric Use

The safety and efficacy of TOBI® have not been studied in pediatric patients under 6 years of age.

Geriatric Use

Clinical studies of TOBI® did not include patients aged 65 years and over. Tobramycin is known to be substantially excreted by the kidney, and the risk of adverse reactions to this drug may be greater in patients with impaired renal function. Because elderly patients are more likely to have decreased renal function, it may be useful to monitor renal function (see WARNINGS – Nephrotoxicity; PRECAUTIONS – Serum Concentrations).

ADVERSE REACTIONS

TOBI® was generally well tolerated during two clinical studies in 258 cystic fibrosis patients ranging in age from 6 to 48 years. Patients received TOBI® in alternating periods of 28 days on and 28 days off drug in addition to their standard cystic fibrosis therapy for a total of 24 weeks.

Voice alteration and tinnitus were the only adverse experiences reported by significantly more TOBI®-treated patients. Thirty-three patients (13%) treated with TOBI® complained of voice alteration compared to 17 (7%) placebo patients. Voice alteration was more common in the on-drug periods.

Eight patients from the TOBI® group (3%) reported tinnitus compared to no placebo patients. All episodes were transient, resolved without discontinuation of the TOBI® treatment regimen, and were not associated with loss of hearing in audiograms. Tinnitus is one of the sentinel symptoms of cochlear toxicity, and patients with this symptom should be carefully monitored for high frequency hearing loss. The numbers of patients reporting vestibular adverse experiences such as dizziness were similar in the TOBI® and placebo groups.

Nine (3%) patients in the TOBI® group and nine (3%) patients in the placebo group had increases in serum creatinine of at least 50% over baseline. In all nine patients in the TOBI® group, creatinine decreased at the next visit.

Table 1 lists the percent of patients with treatment-emergent adverse experiences (spontaneously reported and solicited) that occurred in >5% of TOBI® patients during the two Phase III studies.

Table 1: Percent of Patients With Treatment Emergent Adverse Experiences Occurring in >5% of TOBI® Patients

Adverse Event	TOBI® (n=258) %	Placebo (n=262) %
Cough Increased	46.1	47.3
Pharyngitis	38.0	39.3
Sputum Increased	37.6	39.7
Asthenia	35.7	39.3
Rhinitis	34.5	33.6
Dyspnea	33.7	38.5
Fever[1]	32.9	43.5
Lung Disorder	31.4	31.3
Headache	26.7	32.1
Chest Pain	26.0	29.8
Sputum Discoloration	21.3	19.8
Hemoptysis	19.4	23.7
Anorexia	18.6	27.9
Lung Function Decreased[2]	16.3	15.3
Asthma	15.9	20.2
Vomiting	14.0	22.1
Abdominal Pain	12.8	23.7
Voice Alteration	12.8	6.5
Nausea	11.2	16.0
Weight Loss	10.1	15.3
Pain	8.1	12.6
Sinusitis	8.1	9.2
Ear Pain	7.4	8.8
Back Pain	7.0	8.0
Epistaxis	7.0	6.5
Taste Perversion	6.6	6.9
Diarrhea	6.2	10.3
Malaise	6.2	5.3
Lower Respiratory Tract Infection	5.8	8.0
Dizziness	5.8	7.6
Hyperventilation	5.4	9.9
Rash	5.4	6.1

[1]Includes subjective complaints of fever.
[2]Includes reported decreases in pulmonary function tests or decreased lung volume on chest radiograph associated with intercurrent illness or study drug administration.

Adverse drug reactions (<5%) occurring more frequently with TOBI in the placebo-controlled studies and assessed as drug-related in ≥1% of patients:

Ear and labyrinth disorders
Tinnitus (3.1%, vs 0% for placebo)

Musculoskeletal and connective tissue disorders
Myalgia (4.7%, vs 2.7% for placebo)

Infections and infestations
Laryngitis (4.3%, vs 3.1% for placebo)

Adverse drug reactions derived from spontaneous reports
The following adverse reactions have been identified during postapproval use of TOBI. Because these reactions are re-

ported voluntarily from a population of uncertain size, it is not always possible to reliably estimate their frequency or establish a causal relationship to drug exposure.

Ear and labyrinth disorders
Hearing loss (see WARNINGS – Ototoxicity)

Skin and subcutaneous tissue disorders
Hypersensitivity, pruritus, urticaria, rash

Nervous system disorders
Aphonia, dysgeusia

Respiratory, thoracic, and mediastinal disorders
Bronchospasm (see WARNINGS – Bronchospasm), oropharyngeal pain

OVERDOSAGE

Signs and symptoms of acute toxicity from overdosage of IV tobramycin might include dizziness, tinnitus, vertigo, loss of high-tone hearing acuity, respiratory failure, neuromuscular blockade, and renal impairment. Administration by inhalation results in low systemic bioavailability of tobramycin. Tobramycin is not significantly absorbed following oral administration. Tobramycin serum concentrations may be helpful in monitoring overdosage.

In all cases of suspected overdosage, physicians should contact the Regional Poison Control Center for information about effective treatment. In the case of any overdosage, the possibility of drug interactions with alterations in drug disposition should be considered.

DOSAGE AND ADMINISTRATION

The recommended dosage for both adults and pediatric patients 6 years of age and older is 1 single-use ampule (300 mg) administered BID for 28 days. Dosage is not adjusted by weight. All patients should be administered 300 mg BID. The doses should be taken as close to 12 hours apart as possible; they should not be taken less than 6 hours apart.

TOBI® is inhaled while the patient is sitting or standing upright and breathing normally through the mouthpiece of the nebulizer. Nose clips may help the patient breathe through the mouth.

TOBI® is administered BID in alternating periods of 28 days. After 28 days of therapy, patients should stop TOBI® therapy for the next 28 days, and then resume therapy for the next 28 day on/28 day off cycle.

TOBI® is supplied as a single-use ampule and is administered by inhalation, using a hand-held PARI LC PLUS™ Reusable Nebulizer with a DeVilbiss® Pulmo-Aide® compressor. TOBI® is not for subcutaneous, intravenous or intrathecal administration.

Usage

TOBI® is administered by inhalation over an approximately 15-minute period, using a hand-held PARI LC PLUS™ Reusable Nebulizer with a DeVilbiss® Pulmo-Aide® compressor. TOBI® should not be diluted or mixed with dornase alfa (PULMOZYME®, Genentech) or other medications in the nebulizer.

During clinical studies, patients on multiple therapies were instructed to take them first, followed by TOBI®.

HOW SUPPLIED

TOBI® 300 mg is available as follows:
NDC 0078-0494-71
5 mL single-dose ampule (carton of 56)

Storage

TOBI® should be stored under refrigeration at 2-8°C/36-46°F. Upon removal from the refrigerator, or if refrigeration is unavailable, TOBI® pouches (opened or unopened) may be stored at room temperature (up to 25°C/77°F) for up to 28 days. TOBI® should not be used beyond the expiration date stamped on the ampule when stored under refrigeration (2-8°C/36-46°F) or beyond 28 days when stored at room temperature (25°C/77°F).

TOBI® ampules should not be exposed to intense light. The solution in the ampule is slightly yellow, but may darken with age if not stored in the refrigerator; however, the color change does not indicate any change in the quality of the product as long as it is stored within the recommended storage conditions.

Clinical Studies

Two identically designed, double-blind, randomized, placebo-controlled, parallel group, 24-week clinical studies

Table 2: Dosing Regimens in Clinical Studies

	Cycle 1		Cycle 2		Cycle 3	
	28 days	28 days	28 days	28 days	28 days	28 days
TOBI® regimen n=258	TOBI® 300 mg BID	No drug	TOBI® 300 mg BID	No drug	TOBI® 300 mg BID	No drug
Placebo regimen n=262	placebo BID	No drug	placebo BID	No drug	placebo BID	No drug

(Study 1 and Study 2) at a total of 69 cystic fibrosis centers in the United States were conducted in cystic fibrosis patients with *P. aeruginosa*. Subjects who were less than 6 years of age, had a baseline creatinine of >2 mg/dL, or had *Burkholderia cepacia* isolated from sputum were excluded. All subjects had baseline FEV₁ % predicted between 25% and 75%. In these clinical studies, 258 patients received TOBI® therapy on an outpatient basis (see Table 2) using a hand-held PARI LC PLUS™ Reusable Nebulizer with a DeVilbiss® Pulmo-Aide® compressor.
[See table 2 above]

All patients received either TOBI® or placebo (saline with 1.25 mg quinine for flavoring) in addition to standard treatment recommended for cystic fibrosis patients, which included oral and parenteral anti-pseudomonal therapy, β₂-agonists, cromolyn, inhaled steroids, and airway clearance techniques. In addition, approximately 77% of patients were concurrently treated with dornase alfa (PULMOZYME®, Genentech).

In each study, TOBI®-treated patients experienced significant improvement in pulmonary function. Improvement was demonstrated in the TOBI® group in Study 1 by an average increase in FEV₁ % predicted of about 11% relative to baseline (Week 0) during 24 weeks compared to no average change in placebo patients. In Study 2, TOBI®-treated patients had an average increase of about 7% compared to an average decrease of about 1% in placebo patients. Figure 1 shows the average relative change in FEV₁% predicted over 24 weeks for both studies.

Figure 1: Relative Change From Baseline in FEV₁% Predicted

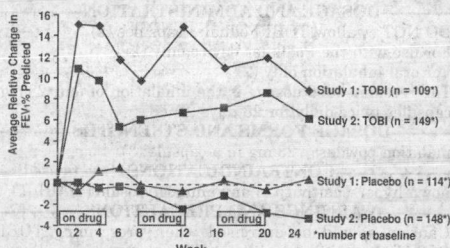

In each study, TOBI® therapy resulted in a significant reduction in the number of *P. aeruginosa* colony forming units (CFUs) in sputum during the on-drug periods. Sputum bacterial density returned to baseline during the off-drug periods. Reductions in sputum bacterial density were smaller in each successive cycle. (see Figure 2).

Figure 2: Absolute Change From Baseline in Log₁₀ CFUs

Patients treated with TOBI® were hospitalized for an average of 5.1 days compared to 8.1 days for placebo patients. Patients treated with TOBI® required an average of 9.6 days of parenteral anti-pseudomonal antibiotic treatment compared to 14.1 days for placebo patients. During the 6 months of treatment, 40% of TOBI® patients and 53% of placebo patients were treated with parenteral anti-pseudomonal antibiotics.

The relationship between *in-vitro* susceptibility test results and clinical outcome with TOBI® therapy is not clear. However, 4 TOBI® patients who began the clinical trial with *P. aeruginosa* isolates having MIC values ≥128 µg/mL did not experience an improvement in FEV₁ or a decrease in sputum bacterial density.

Treatment with TOBI® did not affect the susceptibility of the majority of *P. aeruginosa* isolates during the 6-month studies. However, some *P. aeruginosa* isolates did exhibit increased tobramycin MICs. The percentage of patients with *P. aeruginosa* isolates with tobramycin MICs ≥16 µg/mL was 13% at the beginning, and 23% at the end of 6 months of the TOBI® regimen.

REFERENCES

1. Neu HC. Tobramycin: an overview. [Review]. J Infect Dis 1976; Suppl 134:S3-19.
2. Weber A, Smith A, Williams-Warren J et al. Nebulizer delivery of tobramycin to the lower respiratory tract. Pediatr Pulmonol 1994; 17 (5):331-9.
3. Bryan LE. Aminoglycoside resistance. Bryan LE, Ed. Antimicrobial drug resistance. Orlando, FL: Academic Press, 1984: 241-77.

U.S. Patent 5,508,269; other patents pending.
Distributed by:
Novartis Pharmaceuticals Corporation
East Hanover, New Jersey 07936
© Novartis
T2014-52
April 2014
Shown in Product Identification Guide, page 311

TOBI® PODHALER™   ℞
(tobramycin inhalation powder)
for oral inhalation use

The following prescribing information is based on official labeling in effect July 2014.

HIGHLIGHTS OF PRESCRIBING INFORMATION
These highlights do not include all the information needed to use TOBI Podhaler safely and effectively. See full prescribing information for TOBI Podhaler.
TOBI® PODHALER™ (tobramycin inhalation powder), for oral inhalation use
Initial U.S. Approval: 1975
────────INDICATIONS AND USAGE────────
TOBI Podhaler is an antibacterial aminoglycoside indicated for the management of cystic fibrosis patients with *Pseudomonas aeruginosa*.
Safety and efficacy have not been demonstrated in patients under the age of 6 years, patients with forced expiratory volume in 1 second (FEV$_1$) <25% or >80%, or patients colonized with *Burkholderia cepacia* (1).
────────DOSAGE AND ADMINISTRATION────────
• DO NOT swallow TOBI Podhaler capsules (2)
• For use with the Podhaler device only (2)
• For oral inhalation only (2)
• The recommended dosage is the inhalation of four 28 mg capsules twice-daily for 28 days (2)
────────DOSAGE FORMS AND STRENGTHS────────
Inhalation powder: 28 mg in a capsule (3)
────────CONTRAINDICATIONS────────
Known hypersensitivity to any aminoglycoside (4)
────────WARNINGS AND PRECAUTIONS────────
• Caution should be exercised when prescribing TOBI Podhaler to patients with known or suspected auditory, vestibular, renal, or neuromuscular dysfunction (5.1, 5.2, 5.3)
• Ototoxicity, as measured by complaints of hearing loss or tinnitus, was reported in clinical trials (5.1)
• Aminoglycosides may aggravate muscle weakness because of a potential curare-like effect on neuromuscular function (5.3)
• Bronchospasm can occur with inhalation of TOBI Podhaler (5.4)
• Audiograms, serum concentrations, and renal function should be monitored as appropriate (5.5)
• Fetal harm can occur when aminoglycosides are administered to a pregnant woman. Apprise women of the potential hazard to the fetus (5.6)
────────ADVERSE REACTIONS────────
The most common adverse reactions (≥10 % of TOBI Podhaler and TOBI patients in primary safety population) are cough, lung disorder, productive cough, dyspnea, pyrexia, oropharyngeal pain, dysphonia, hemoptysis, and headache (6.1)
To report SUSPECTED ADVERSE REACTIONS, contact Novartis Pharmaceuticals Corporation at 1-888-669-6682 or FDA at 1-800-FDA-1088 or www.fda.gov/medwatch.
────────DRUG INTERACTIONS────────
Concurrent and/or sequential use of TOBI Podhaler with other drugs with neurotoxic, nephrotoxic, or ototoxic potential should be avoided (7)
────────USE IN SPECIFIC POPULATIONS────────
• Aminoglycosides can cause fetal harm when administered to a pregnant woman (8.1)
• Nursing mother: discontinue drug or nursing, taking into consideration the importance of the drug to the mother (8.3)
See 17 for PATIENT COUNSELING INFORMATION and FDA-approved patient labeling
                                                       Revised: 4/2014

FULL PRESCRIBING INFORMATION

1   INDICATIONS AND USAGE

TOBI Podhaler is indicated for the management of cystic fibrosis patients with *Pseudomonas aeruginosa*.
Safety and efficacy have not been demonstrated in patients under the age of 6 years, patients with forced expiratory volume in 1 second (FEV$_1$) <25% or >80% predicted, or patients colonized with *Burkholderia cepacia* [see *Clinical Studies (14)*].

2   DOSAGE AND ADMINISTRATION

DO NOT SWALLOW TOBI PODHALER CAPSULES
FOR USE WITH THE PODHALER DEVICE ONLY
FOR ORAL INHALATION ONLY
TOBI Podhaler capsules must not be swallowed as the intended effects in the lungs will not be obtained. The contents of TOBI Podhaler capsules are only for oral inhalation and should only be used with the Podhaler device.
The recommended dosage of TOBI Podhaler for both adults and pediatric patients 6 years of age and older is the inhalation of the contents of four 28 mg TOBI Podhaler capsules twice-daily for 28 days using the Podhaler device.
Refer to the Instructions For Use (IFU) for full administration information.
Dosage is not adjusted by weight. Each dose of four capsules should be taken as close to 12 hours apart as possible; each dose should not be taken less than 6 hours apart.
TOBI Podhaler is administered twice-daily in alternating periods of 28 days. After 28 days of therapy, patients should stop TOBI Podhaler therapy for the next 28 days, and then resume therapy for the next 28 day on and 28 day off cycle. TOBI Podhaler capsules should always be stored in the blister and each capsule should only be removed IMMEDIATELY BEFORE USE.
For patients taking several different inhaled medications and/or performing chest physiotherapy, the order of therapies should follow the physician's recommendation. It is recommended that TOBI Podhaler is taken last.

3   DOSAGE FORMS AND STRENGTHS

Inhalation powder:
28 mg: clear, colorless hypromellose capsule with "NVR AVCI" in blue radial imprint on one part of the capsule and the Novartis logo "ɕ" in blue radial imprint on the other part of the capsule.

---

4   CONTRAINDICATIONS

TOBI Podhaler is contraindicated in patients with a known hypersensitivity to any aminoglycoside.

5   WARNINGS AND PRECAUTIONS

5.1   Ototoxicity
Caution should be exercised when prescribing TOBI Podhaler to patients with known or suspected auditory or vestibular dysfunction.
Ototoxicity, as measured by complaints of hearing loss or tinnitus, was reported by patients in the TOBI Podhaler clinical studies [see *Adverse Reactions (6.1)*]. Tinnitus may be a sentinel symptom of ototoxicity, and therefore the onset of this symptom warrants caution. Ototoxicity, manifested as both auditory (hearing loss) and vestibular toxicity, has been reported with parenteral aminoglycosides. Vestibular toxicity may be manifested by vertigo, ataxia or dizziness.

5.2   Nephrotoxicity
Caution should be exercised when prescribing TOBI Podhaler to patients with known or suspected renal dysfunction.
Nephrotoxicity was not observed during TOBI Podhaler clinical studies but has been associated with aminoglycosides as a class.

5.3   Neuromuscular Disorders
Caution should be exercised when prescribing TOBI Podhaler to patients with known or suspected neuromuscular dysfunction.
TOBI Podhaler should be used cautiously in patients with neuromuscular disorders, such as myasthenia gravis or Parkinson's disease, since aminoglycosides may aggravate muscle weakness because of a potential curare-like effect on neuromuscular function.

5.4   Bronchospasm
Bronchospasm can occur with inhalation of TOBI Podhaler [see *Adverse Reactions (6.1)*]. Bronchospasm should be treated as medically appropriate.

5.5   Laboratory Tests
Audiograms
Physicians should consider an audiogram at baseline, particularly for patients at increased risk of auditory dysfunction.
If a patient reports tinnitus or hearing loss during TOBI Podhaler therapy, the physician should refer that patient for audiological assessment.
Serum Concentrations
In patients treated with TOBI Podhaler, serum tobramycin concentrations are approximately 1 to 2 µg/mL one hour after dose administration and do not require routine monitoring. Serum concentrations of tobramycin in patients with known or suspected auditory or renal dysfunction or patients treated with a concomitant parenteral aminoglycoside (or other nephrotoxic or ototoxic medications) should be monitored at the discretion of the treating physician. If ototoxicity or nephrotoxicity occurs in a patient receiving TOBI Podhaler, tobramycin therapy should be discontinued until serum concentrations fall below 2 µg/mL.
The serum concentration of tobramycin should only be monitored through venipuncture and not finger prick blood sampling. Contamination of the skin of the fingers with tobramycin may lead to falsely increased measurements of serum levels of the drug. This contamination cannot be completely avoided by hand washing before testing.
Renal Function
Laboratory tests of urine and renal function should be conducted at the discretion of the treating physician.

5.6   Use in Pregnancy
Aminoglycosides can cause fetal harm when administered to a pregnant woman. Aminoglycosides cross the placenta, and streptomycin has been associated with several reports of total, irreversible, bilateral congenital deafness in pediatric patients exposed *in utero*. Patients who use TOBI Podhaler during pregnancy, or become pregnant while taking TOBI Podhaler should be apprised of the potential hazard to the fetus [see *Use in Specific Populations (8.1)*].

6   ADVERSE REACTIONS

6.1   Clinical Trials Experience
Because clinical trials are conducted under widely varying conditions, adverse reaction rates observed in the clinical trials of a drug cannot be directly compared to rates in the clinical trials of another drug and may not reflect the rates observed in practice.
TOBI Podhaler has been evaluated for safety in 425 cystic fibrosis patients exposed to at least one dose of TOBI Podhaler, including 273 patients who were exposed across three cycles (6 months) of treatment. Each cycle consisted of 28 days on-treatment (with 112 mg administered twice daily) and 28 days off-treatment. Patients with serum creatinine and blood urea nitrogen (BUN) ≥ 40 mg/dL were excluded from clinical studies. There were 218 males and 207 females in this population, and reflecting the cystic fibrosis population in the U.S., the vast majority of patients were Caucasian. There were 221 patients ≥ 20

years old, 121 patients ≥ 13 to < 20 years old, and 83 patients ≥ 6 to < 13 years old. There were 239 patients with screening FEV_1 % predicted ≥ 50%, 156 patients with screening FEV_1 % predicted < 50%, and 30 patients with missing FEV_1 % predicted.

The primary safety population reflects patients from Study 1, an open-label study comparing TOBI Podhaler with TOBI (tobramycin inhalation solution, USP) over three cycles of 4 weeks on treatment followed by 4 weeks off treatment. Randomization, in a planned 3:2 ratio, resulted in 308 patients treated with TOBI Podhaler and 209 patients treated with TOBI. For both the TOBI Podhaler and TOBI groups, mean exposure to medication for each cycle was 28-29 days. The mean age for both arms was between 25 and 26 years old. The mean baseline FEV_1 % predicted for both arms was 53%.

Table 1 displays adverse drug reactions reported by at least 2% of TOBI Podhaler patients in Study 1, inclusive of all cycles (on and off treatment). Adverse drug reactions are listed according to MedDRA system organ class and sorted within system organ class group in descending order of frequency.

Table 1: Adverse reactions reported in Study 1 (occurring in ≥2% of TOBI Podhaler patients)

Primary System Organ Class Preferred Term	TOBI Podhaler N=308 %	TOBI N=209 %
Respiratory, thoracic, and mediastinal disorders		
Cough	48.4	31.1
Lung disorder[1]	33.8	30.1
Productive cough	18.2	19.6
Dyspnea	15.6	12.4
Oropharyngeal pain	14.0	10.5
Dysphonia	13.6	3.8
Hemoptysis	13.0	12.4
Nasal congestion	8.1	7.2
Rales	7.1	6.2
Wheezing	6.8	6.2
Chest discomfort	6.5	2.9
Throat irritation	4.5	1.9
Gastrointestinal disorders		
Nausea	7.5	9.6
Vomiting	6.2	5.7
Diarrhea	4.2	1.9
Dysgeusia	3.9	0.5
Infections and infestations		
Upper respiratory tract infection	6.8	8.6
Investigations		
Pulmonary function test decreased	6.8	8.1
Forced expiratory volume decreased	3.9	1.0
Blood glucose increased	2.9	0.5
Vascular disorders		
Epistaxis	2.6	1.9
Nervous system disorders		
Headache	11.4	12.0
General disorders and administration site conditions		
Pyrexia	15.6	12.4
Musculoskeletal and connective tissue disorders		
Musculoskeletal chest pain	4.5	4.8
Skin and subcutaneous tissue disorders		
Rash	2.3	2.4

[1]This includes adverse events of pulmonary or cystic fibrosis exacerbations

Adverse drug reactions that occurred in <2% of patients treated with TOBI Podhaler in Study 1 were: bronchospasm (TOBI Podhaler 1.6%, TOBI 0.5%); deafness including deafness unilateral (reported as mild to moderate hearing loss or increased hearing loss) (TOBI Podhaler 1.0%, TOBI 0.5%); and tinnitus (TOBI Podhaler 1.9%, TOBI 2.4%).

Discontinuations in Study 1 were higher in the TOBI Podhaler arm compared to TOBI (27% TOBI Podhaler vs 18% TOBI). This was driven primarily by discontinuations due to adverse events (14% TOBI Podhaler vs 8% TOBI). Higher rates of discontinuation were seen in subjects ≥ 20 years old and those with baseline FEV_1 % predicted < 50%. Respiratory related hospitalizations occurred in 24% of the patients in the TOBI Podhaler arm and 22% of the patients in the TOBI arm. There was an increased new usage of antipseudomonal medication in the TOBI Podhaler arm (65% TOBI Podhaler vs 55% TOBI). This included oral antibiotics in 55% of TOBI Podhaler patients and 40% of TOBI patients and intravenous antibiotics in 35% of TOBI Podhaler pa-

tients and 33% of TOBI patients. Median time to first antipseudomonal usage was 89 days in the TOBI Podhaler arm and 112 days in the TOBI arm.

The supportive safety population reflects patients from two studies: Study 2, a double-blind, placebo-controlled design for the first treatment cycle, followed by all patients receiving TOBI Podhaler (replaced placebo) for two additional cycles, and Study 3, a double-blind, placebo-controlled trial for one treatment cycle only. Placebo in these studies was inhaled powder without the active ingredient, tobramycin. The patient population for these studies was much younger than in Study 1 (mean age 13 years old).

Adverse drug reactions reported more frequently by TOBI Podhaler patients in the placebo-controlled cycle (Cycle 1) of Study 2, which included 46 TOBI Podhaler and 49 placebo patients, were:

Respiratory, thoracic, and mediastinal disorders
Pharyngolaryngeal pain (TOBI Podhaler 10.9%, placebo 0%); dysphonia (TOBI Podhaler 4.3%, placebo 0%)

Gastrointestinal disorders
Dysgeusia (TOBI Podhaler 6.5%, placebo 2.0%)

Adverse drug reactions reported more frequently by TOBI Podhaler patients in Study 3, which included 30 TOBI Podhaler and 32 placebo patients, were:

Respiratory, thoracic, and mediastinal disorders
Cough (TOBI Podhaler 10%, placebo 0%)

Ear and labyrinth disorders
Hypoacusis (TOBI Podhaler 10%, placebo 6.3%)

Audiometric assessment
In Study 1, audiology testing was performed in a subset of approximately 25% of TOBI Podhaler (n=78) and TOBI (n=45) patients. Using the criteria for either ear of ≥ 10 dB loss at two consecutive frequencies, ≥ 20 dB loss at any frequency, or loss of response at three consecutive frequencies where responses were previously obtained, five TOBI Podhaler patients and three TOBI patients were judged to have ototoxicity, a ratio similar to the planned 3:2 randomization for this study.

Audiology testing was also performed in a subset of patients in both Study 2 (n=13 from the TOBI Podhaler group and n=9 from the placebo group) and Study 3 (n=14 from the TOBI Podhaler group and n=11 from the placebo group). In Study 2, no patients reported hearing complaints but two TOBI Podhaler patients met the criteria for ototoxicity. In Study 3, three TOBI Podhaler and two placebo patients had reports of 'hypoacusis'. One TOBI Podhaler and two placebo patients met the criteria for ototoxicity. In some patients, ototoxicity was transient or may have been related to a conductive defect.

Cough
Cough is a common symptom in cystic fibrosis, reported in 42% of the patients in Study 1 at baseline. Cough was the most frequently reported adverse event in Study 1 and was more common in the TOBI Podhaler arm (48% TOBI Podhaler vs 31% TOBI). There was a higher rate of cough adverse event reporting during the first week of active treatment with TOBI Podhaler (i.e., the first week of Cycle 1). The time to first cough event in the TOBI Podhaler and TOBI groups were similar thereafter. In some patients, cough resulted in discontinuation of TOBI Podhaler treatment. Sixteen patients (5%) receiving treatment with TOBI Podhaler discontinued study treatment due to cough events compared with 2 (1%) in the TOBI treatment group. Children and adolescents coughed more than adults when treated with TOBI Podhaler, yet the adults were more likely to discontinue: of the 16 patients on TOBI Podhaler in Study 1 who discontinued treatment due to cough events, 14 were ≥20 years of age, one patient was between the ages of 13 and <20, and one was between the ages of 6 and <13. The rates of bronchospasm (as measured by ≥20% decrease in FEV_1 % predicted post-dose) were approximately 5% in both treatment groups, and none of these patients experienced concomitant cough.

In Study 2, cough was the most commonly reported adverse event during the first cycle of treatment (the double blind period of treatment) and occurred more frequently in placebo-treated patients (26.5%) than patients treated with TOBI Podhaler (13%). Similar percentages of patients in both treatment groups reported cough as a baseline symptom. In Study 3, cough events were reported by three patients in the TOBI Podhaler group (10%) and none in the placebo group (0%).

6.2   Post-Marketing Experience
The following adverse reaction has been identified during postapproval use of TOBI Podhaler. Because these reactions are reported voluntarily from a population of uncertain size, it is not always possible to reliably estimate their frequency or establish a causal relationship to drug exposure.

Nervous system disorders
Aphonia

7   DRUG INTERACTIONS

No clinical drug interaction studies have been performed with TOBI Podhaler. In clinical studies, patients receiving

TOBI Podhaler continued to take dornase alfa, bronchodilators, inhaled corticosteroids, and macrolides. No clinical signs of drug interactions with these medicines were identified.

Concurrent and/or sequential use of TOBI Podhaler with other drugs with neurotoxic, nephrotoxic, or ototoxic potential should be avoided.

Some diuretics can enhance aminoglycoside toxicity by altering antibiotic concentrations in serum and tissue. TOBI Podhaler should not be administered concomitantly with ethacrynic acid, furosemide, urea, or intravenous mannitol. The interaction between inhaled mannitol and TOBI Podhaler has not been evaluated.

8   USE IN SPECIFIC POPULATIONS

8.1   Pregnancy
Teratogenic Effects – Pregnancy Category D [see *Warnings and Precautions (5.6)*]

No reproduction toxicology studies have been conducted with TOBI Podhaler. However, subcutaneous administration of tobramycin at doses of 100 or 20 mg/kg/day during organogenesis was not teratogenic in rats or rabbits, respectively. Doses of tobramycin ≥ 40 mg/kg/day were severely maternally toxic to rabbits and precluded the evaluation of teratogenicity. Ototoxicity was not evaluated in offspring during nonclinical reproduction toxicity studies with tobramycin.

Aminoglycosides can cause fetal harm (e.g., congenital deafness) when administered to a pregnant woman. No adequate and well-controlled studies of TOBI Podhaler in pregnant women have been conducted. If TOBI Podhaler is used during pregnancy, or if the patient becomes pregnant while taking TOBI Podhaler, the patient should be apprised of the potential hazard to the fetus.

8.3   Nursing Mothers
The amount of tobramycin excreted in human breast milk after administration by inhalation is not known. Because of the potential for ototoxicity and nephrotoxicity in infants, a decision should be made whether to terminate nursing or discontinue the drug, taking into account the importance of the drug to the mother.

8.4   Pediatric Use
Patients 6 years and older were included in the Phase 3 studies with TOBI Podhaler; 206 patients below 20 years of age received TOBI Podhaler. No dosage adjustments are needed based on age. The overall pattern of adverse events in pediatric patients was similar to the adults. Dysgeusia (taste disturbance) was more commonly reported in younger patients six to 19 years of age than in patients 20 years and older, 7.4% vs 2.7%, respectively. Safety and effectiveness in pediatric patients below the age of 6 years have not been established.

8.5   Geriatric Use
Clinical studies of TOBI Podhaler did not include sufficient numbers of subjects aged 65 years and over to determine whether they respond differently from younger subjects. Tobramycin is known to be substantially excreted by the kidney, and the risk of adverse reactions to this drug may be greater in patients with impaired renal function. Because elderly patients are more likely to have decreased renal function, it may be useful to monitor renal function [see *Warnings and Precautions (5.2, 5.5)*].

8.6   Renal Impairment
Tobramycin is primarily excreted unchanged in the urine and renal function is expected to affect the exposure to tobramycin. The risk of adverse reactions to this drug may be greater in patients with impaired renal function. Patients with serum creatinine > 2 mg/dL and blood urea nitrogen (BUN) > 40 mg/dL have not been included in clinical studies and there are no data in this population to support a recommendation regarding dose adjustment with TOBI Podhaler [see *Warnings and Precautions (5.2, 5.5)*].

8.7   Hepatic Impairment
No studies have been performed in patients with hepatic impairment. As tobramycin is not metabolized, an effect of hepatic impairment on the exposure to tobramycin is not expected.

8.8   Organ Transplantation
Adequate data do not exist for the use of TOBI Podhaler in patients after organ transplantation.

10   OVERDOSAGE

The maximum tolerated daily dose of TOBI Podhaler has not been established.

In the event of accidental oral ingestion of TOBI Podhaler capsules, systemic toxicity is unlikely as tobramycin is poorly absorbed. Tobramycin serum concentrations may be helpful in monitoring overdosage.

Acute toxicity should be treated with immediate withdrawal of TOBI Podhaler, and baseline tests of renal function should be undertaken.

Hemodialysis may be helpful in removing tobramycin from the body.

In all cases of suspected overdosage, physicians should contact the Regional Poison Control Center for information about effective treatment. In the case of any overdosage, the possibility of drug interactions with alterations in drug disposition should be considered.

11 DESCRIPTION

TOBI Podhaler consists of a dry powder formulation of tobramycin for oral inhalation only with the Podhaler device. The inhalation powder is filled into clear, colorless hypromellose capsules.

Each clear, colorless hypromellose capsule contains a spray dried powder of 28 mg of tobramycin active ingredient with 1,2-distearoyl-sn-glycero-3-phosphocholine (DSPC), calcium chloride, and sulfuric acid (for pH adjustment).

The active component of TOBI Podhaler is tobramycin. Tobramycin is an aminoglycoside antibiotic. Its chemical name is O-3-amino-3-deoxy-α-D-glucopyranosyl-(1→4)-O-[2,6-diamino-2,3,6-trideoxy-α-D-ribo-hexopyranosyl-(1→6)]-2-deoxy-L-streptamine; its structural formula is:

Tobramycin has a molecular weight of 467.52, and its empirical formula is $C_{18}H_{37}N_5O_9$. Tobramycin is a white to almost white powder; visually free from any foreign contaminants. Tobramycin is freely soluble in water, very slightly soluble in ethanol, and practically insoluble in chloroform and ether.

The Podhaler device is a plastic device used to inhale the dry powder contained in the TOBI Podhaler capsule. Under standardized *in vitro* testing at a fixed flow rate of 60 L/min and volume of 2 L for 2 seconds, the Podhaler device has a target delivered dose of 102 mg of tobramycin from the mouthpiece (4 capsules per dose). Peak inspiratory flow rate and inhaled volumes were explored in 96 cystic fibrosis patients aged 6 years and older. Older patients with significant disease progression and associated decreases in forced expiratory volume (FEV_1) and younger patients with inhaled volumes < 1 L were able to generate inspiratory flow rates and volumes required to receive their medication when following the instructions for use. However, no pediatric patients aged 6 to 10 years with FEV_1 less than 40% predicted were evaluated.

12 CLINICAL PHARMACOLOGY

12.1 Mechanism of Action

Tobramycin is an aminoglycoside antibiotic [see *Clinical Pharmacology (12.4)*].

12.3 Pharmacokinetics

Absorption

TOBI Podhaler contains tobramycin, a cationic polar molecule that does not readily cross epithelial membranes. TOBI Podhaler is specifically formulated for administration by oral inhalation. The systemic exposure to tobramycin after inhalation of TOBI Podhaler is expected to result from pulmonary absorption of the dose fraction delivered to the lungs as tobramycin and is not absorbed to any appreciable extent when administered via the oral route.

Serum concentrations

After inhalation of a 112 mg single dose (4 × 28 mg capsules) of TOBI Podhaler in cystic fibrosis patients, the maximum serum concentration (C_{max}) of tobramycin was 1.02 ± 0.53 µg/mL (mean ± SD) and the median time to reach the peak concentration (T_{max}) was 1 hour. In comparison, after inhalation of a single 300 mg dose of TOBI, C_{max} was 1.04 ± 0.58 µg/mL and median T_{max} was 1 hour. The extent of systemic exposure (AUC_{0-12}) was also similar: 4.6 ± 2.0 µg·h/mL following the 112 mg TOBI Podhaler dose and 4.8 ± 2.5 µg·h/mL following the 300 mg TOBI dose. At the end of a 4-week dosing cycle of TOBI Podhaler (112 mg twice daily), the maximum serum concentration of tobramycin 1 hour after dosing ranged from 1.48 ± 0.69 µg/mL to 1.99 ± 0.59 µg/mL (mean ± SD).

Sputum concentrations

After inhalation of a 112 mg single dose (4 × 28 mg capsules) of TOBI Podhaler in cystic fibrosis patients, sputum C_{max} of tobramycin was 1048 ± 1080 µg/g (mean ± SD). In compar-

ison, after inhalation of a single 300 mg dose of TOBI, sputum C_{max} was 737 ± 1028 µg/g. The variability in pharmacokinetic parameters was higher in sputum as compared to serum.

Distribution

A population pharmacokinetic analysis for TOBI Podhaler in cystic fibrosis patients estimated the apparent volume of distribution of tobramycin in the central compartment to be 85.1 L for a typical CF patient.

Binding of tobramycin to serum proteins is negligible.

Metabolism

Tobramycin is not metabolized and is primarily excreted unchanged in the urine.

Elimination

Tobramycin is eliminated from the systemic circulation primarily by glomerular filtration of the unchanged compound. Systemically absorbed tobramycin following TOBI Podhaler administration is also expected to be eliminated principally by glomerular filtration.

The apparent terminal half-life of tobramycin in serum after inhalation of a 112 mg single dose of TOBI Podhaler was approximately 3 hours in cystic fibrosis patients and consistent with the half-life of tobramycin after TOBI inhalation. A population pharmacokinetic analysis for TOBI Podhaler in cystic fibrosis patients aged 6 to 58 years estimated the apparent serum clearance of tobramycin to be 14.5 L/h. No clinically relevant covariates that were predictive of tobramycin clearance were identified from this analysis.

12.4 Microbiology

Mechanism of Action

Tobramycin is an aminoglycoside antimicrobial produced by *Streptomyces tenebrarius*. It acts primarily by disrupting protein synthesis leading to altered cell membrane permeability, progressive disruption of the cell envelope, and eventual cell death.

Tobramycin has *in vitro* activity against Gram-negative bacteria including *P. aeruginosa*. It is bactericidal *in vitro* at peak concentrations equal to or slightly greater than the minimum inhibitory concentration.

Susceptibility Testing

Interpretive criteria for inhaled antibacterial products are not defined. The *in vitro* antimicrobial susceptibility test methods used to determine the susceptibility for parenteral tobramycin therapy can be used to monitor the susceptibility of *P. aeruginosa* isolated from cystic fibrosis patients [1, 2, 3]. The relationship between *in vitro* susceptibility test results and clinical outcome with TOBI Podhaler therapy is not clear. A single sputum sample from a cystic fibrosis patient may contain multiple morphotypes of *P. aeruginosa* and each morphotype may require a different concentration of tobramycin to inhibit its growth *in vitro*. Patients should be monitored for changes in tobramycin susceptibility.

Development of Resistance

In clinical studies, some increases from baseline to the end of the treatment period were observed in the tobramycin MIC for *P. aeruginosa* morphotypes. In general, a higher percentage of patients treated with TOBI Podhaler had increases in tobramycin MIC compared with placebo or patients treated with TOBI inhalation solution.

The clinical significance of changes in MICs for *P. aeruginosa* has not been clearly established in the treatment of cystic fibrosis patients.

Cross-Resistance

Some emerging resistance to aztreonam, ceftazidime, ciprofloxacin, imipenem, or meropenem were observed in the TOBI Podhaler clinical trials. As other anti-pseudomonal antibiotics were concomitantly utilized in many patients in the clinical trials, the association with TOBI Podhaler is not clear.

Other

No trends were observed in the isolation of treatment-emergent bacterial respiratory pathogens (*Burkholderia cepacia*, *Stenotrophomonas maltophilia*, *Staphylococcus aureus* and *Achromobacter xylosoxidans*).

13 NONCLINICAL TOXICOLOGY

13.1 Carcinogenesis, Mutagenesis, Impairment of Fertility

Carcinogenicity studies were not conducted with TOBI Podhaler. A two-year rat inhalation toxicology study to assess carcinogenic potential of TOBI (tobramycin inhalation solution, USP) has been completed. Rats were exposed to TOBI for up to 1.5 hours per day for 95 weeks. Serum levels of tobramycin of up to 35 µg/mL were measured in rats, in contrast to the maximum 1.99 ± 0.59 µg/mL level observed in cystic fibrosis patients in TOBI Podhaler clinical trials. There was no drug-related increase in the incidence of any variety of tumor.

Additionally, tobramycin has been evaluated for genotoxicity in a battery of *in vitro* and *in vivo* tests. The Ames bacterial reversion test, conducted with 5 tester strains, failed to show a significant increase in revertants with or without metabolic activation in all strains. Tobramycin was negative in the mouse lymphoma forward mutation assay, did not induce chromosomal aberrations in Chinese hamster ovary cells, and was negative in the mouse micronucleus test. Subcutaneous administration of up to 100 mg/kg of tobramycin did not affect mating behavior or cause impairment of fertility in male or female rats.

14 CLINICAL STUDIES

The Phase 3 clinical development program included two placebo-controlled studies (Studies 2 and 3) and one open-label study (Study 1), which randomized and dosed 157 and 517 patients, respectively, with a clinical diagnosis of cystic fibrosis, confirmed by quantitative pilocarpine iontophoresis sweat chloride test, well-characterized disease causing mutations in each CFTR gene, or abnormal nasal transepithelial potential difference characteristic of cystic fibrosis.

In the placebo-controlled studies, all patients were aged between 6 and 21 years old and had an FEV_1 at screening within the range of 25% to 80% (inclusive) of predicted normal values for their age, sex, and height based upon Knudson criteria. In addition, all patients were infected with *P. aeruginosa* as demonstrated by a positive sputum or throat culture (or bronchoalveolar lavage) within 6 months prior to screening, and also in a sputum culture taken at the screening visit. Among the 76 patients treated with TOBI Podhaler, 37% were males and 63% were females. Thirty-six patients were between 6 and 12 years of age, and 40 patients were between 13 and 21 years of age. Patients had a mean baseline FEV_1 of 56% of predicted normal value.

In both studies, >90% of patients received concomitant therapies for cystic fibrosis related indications. The most frequently used other antibacterial drugs (any route of administration) were azithromycin, ciprofloxacin, and ceftazidime. Consistent with the population of cystic fibrosis patients, the most frequently used concomitant medications included oral pancreatic enzyme preparations, mucolytics (especially dornase alfa), and selective β_2-adrenoreceptor agonists.

Study 2

Study 2 was a randomized, three-cycle, two-arm trial. Each cycle comprised of 28 days on treatment followed by 28 days off treatment. The first cycle was double-blind, placebo-controlled with eligible patients randomized 1:1 to TOBI Podhaler (4 × 28 mg capsules twice daily) or placebo. Upon completion of the first cycle, patients who were randomized to the placebo treatment group received TOBI Podhaler for Cycles 2 and 3. The total treatment period was 24 weeks.

A total of 95 patients were randomized into Study 2 and received TOBI Podhaler (n=46) or placebo (n=49) in Cycle 1. All patients were less than 22 years of age (mean age 13.3 years) and had not received inhaled antipseudomonal antibiotics within four months prior to screening; 56% were female and 84% were Caucasian. This study was stopped early for demonstrated benefit and the primary analysis used the set of patients included in the interim analysis (n=79); 16 patients did not have data on the primary endpoint at that time. Of the 79 patients included in the interim analysis, 18 patients were excluded due to a failure to meet spirometry quality review criteria as determined by an external review panel. This resulted in a total of 61 patients, 29 in the TOBI Podhaler arm and 32 in the placebo arm, who were included in the primary analysis.

In the primary analysis, TOBI Podhaler significantly improved lung function compared with placebo as measured by the relative change in FEV_1 % predicted from baseline to the end of Cycle 1 dosing. This analysis adjusted for the covariates of baseline FEV_1 % predicted, age, and region, and imputed for missing data. Treatment with TOBI Podhaler and placebo resulted in relative increases in FEV_1 % predicted of 12.54% and 0.09%, respectively (LS mean difference = 12.44%; 95% CI: 4.89, 20.00; p=0.002). Analysis of absolute changes in FEV_1 % predicted showed LS means of 6.38% for TOBI Podhaler and -0.52% for placebo with a difference of 6.90% (95% CI: 2.40, 11.40). Improvements in lung function were achieved during the subsequent cycles of treatment with TOBI Podhaler, although the magnitude was reduced (Figure 1).

The percentage of patients using new antipseudomonal antibiotics in Cycle 1 was greater in the placebo treatment group (18.4%) compared with the TOBI Podhaler treatment group (13.1%). During the first cycle, 8.7% of TOBI Podhaler patients and 10.2% of placebo patients were treated with parenteral antipseudomonal antibiotics. In Cycle 1, two patients (4.4%) in the TOBI Podhaler treatment group required respiratory-related hospitalizations, compared with six patients (12.2%) in the placebo treatment group.

Figure 1 – Study 2: Mean relative change in FEV_1 % predicted from baseline in Cycles 1-3 by treatment group

Error bars represent the mean relative change (95% CI)

Study 3

Study 3 was a randomized, double-blind, placebo-controlled trial, similar in design to Study 2. Eligible patients were randomized 1:1 to receive TOBI Podhaler (4×28 mg capsules twice daily) or placebo for one cycle (28 days on-treatment and 28 days off-treatment).

A total of 62 patients were randomized into Study 3 and allocated to TOBI Podhaler (n=32) or placebo (n=30). All patients were less than 22 years of age (mean age 12.9 years) and had not received inhaled antipseudomonal antibiotics within 4 months prior to screening; 64.5% were female and 98.4% were Caucasian.

In this study, the results were not statistically significant for the primary lung function endpoint when adjusting for the covariates of age (<13 years, ≥13 years) and FEV_1 % predicted at screening (< 50%, ≥ 50%) and imputing for missing data. Improvement in lung function for TOBI Podhaler compared with placebo was evaluated using the relative change in FEV_1 % predicted from baseline to the end of Cycle 1 dosing. Treatment with TOBI Podhaler (8.19%) compared to placebo (2.27%) failed to achieve statistical significance in relative change in FEV_1 % predicted (LS mean difference = 5.91%; 95% CI: -2.54, 14.37; p=0.167). Analyses of absolute changes in FEV_1 % predicted showed LS means of 4.86% for TOBI Podhaler and 0.48% for placebo with a difference of 4.38% (95% CI:-0.17, 8.94).

Study 1

Study 1 was a randomized, open-label, active-controlled parallel arm trial. Eligible patients were randomized 3:2 to TOBI Podhaler (4×28 mg capsules twice daily) or TOBI (300 mg/5 mL twice daily). Treatment was administered for 28 days, followed by 28 days off therapy (one cycle) for three cycles. The total treatment period was 24 weeks. The time to administer a dose of TOBI Podhaler (10th to 90th percentiles) ranged from 2-7 minutes at the end of the dosing period for Cycle 1, and 2-6 minutes at the end of the dosing period for Cycle 2.

A total of 517 patients were randomized in Study 1 and received TOBI Podhaler (n=308) or TOBI (n=209). Patients were predominantly 20 years of age or older (mean age 25.6 years) with no inhaled antipseudomonal antibiotic use within 28 days prior to study drug administration; 45% were female and 91% were Caucasian.

The primary purpose of Study 1 was to evaluate safety. Interpretation of efficacy results in Study 1 is limited by several factors including open-label design, testing of multiple secondary endpoints, and missing values for the outcome of FEV_1 % predicted. The number (%) of patients with missing values for FEV_1 % predicted at Weeks 5 and 25 in the TOBI Podhaler treated group were 40 (13.0%) and 86 (27.9%) compared to 15 (7.2%) and 40 (19.1%) in the TOBI treated group. Using imputation of the missing data, the mean differences (TOBI Podhaler minus TOBI) in the percent relative change from baseline in FEV_1 % predicted at Weeks 5 and 25 were -0.87 (95% CI: -3.80, 2.07) and 1.62 (95% CI: -0.90, 4.14), respectively.

15 REFERENCES

1. Clinical and Laboratory Standards Institute (CLSI). Methods for Dilution Antimicrobial Susceptibility Tests for Bacteria that Grow Aerobically – Ninth Edition; Approved Standard. CLSI Document M7-A9. CLSI, 950 West Valley Rd., Suite 2500, Wayne, PA 19087, 2012.
2. CLSI. Performance Standards for Antimicrobial Disk Susceptibility Tests; Approved Standard – 11th ed. CLSI document M02-A11. CLSI, 2012.
3. CLSI. Performance Standards for Antimicrobial Susceptibility Testing; 22nd Informational Supplement. CLSI document M100-S22. CLSI, 2012

16 HOW SUPPLIED/STORAGE AND HANDLING

16.1 How Supplied

TOBI Podhaler contains aluminum blister-packaged 28 mg TOBI Podhaler (tobramycin inhalation powder) clear, colorless hypromellose capsules with "NVR AVCI" in blue radial imprint on one part of the capsule and the Novartis logo "⬙" in blue radial imprint on the other part of the capsule, and Podhaler devices.

Each Podhaler device consists of the inhaler body, mouthpiece, capsule chamber and blue push button. The Podhaler device is provided in a case that protects the device during shipment, storage and its one week in-use period.

Unit Dose (blister pack), Box of 224 capsules contains: NDC 0078-0630-35
4 weekly packs, each containing:
56 capsules (7 blister cards of 8 capsules)
1 Podhaler device
1 reserve Podhaler device

16.2 Information for Patients

Store at 25°C (77°F); excursions permitted to 15-30°C (59-86°F)

Protect TOBI Podhaler from moisture.

• TOBI Podhaler capsules should be used with the Podhaler device only. The Podhaler device should not be used with any other capsules.

• Capsules should always be stored in the blister and each capsule should only be removed immediately before use.

• Always use the new Podhaler device provided with each weekly pack.

Keep this and all drugs out of the reach of children.

17 PATIENT COUNSELING INFORMATION

See *FDA-Approved Patient Labeling*

Information for Patients

Information on the long term efficacy and safety of TOBI Podhaler is limited. There is no information in patients with limited pulmonary reserve (FEV_1 <25% predicted). Decreased susceptibility of Pseudomonas aeruginosa to tobramycin has been seen with use of TOBI Podhaler. The relationship between in vitro susceptibility test results and clinical outcome with TOBI Podhaler therapy is not clear. Occurrence of decreased susceptibility on treatment should be monitored, and treatment with an alternative therapy should be considered if clinical worsening is observed.

TOBI Podhaler may not be tolerated by all patients. Patients should be instructed to consider alternative therapy if they are unable to tolerate TOBI Podhaler. Patients should be advised to complete a full 28-day course of TOBI Podhaler, even if they are feeling better. After 28 days of therapy, patients should stop TOBI Podhaler therapy for the next 28 days, and then resume therapy for the next 28 day on and 28 day off cycle.

It is important for patients to understand how to correctly administer TOBI Podhaler capsules using the Podhaler device. It is recommended that caregivers and patients be adequately trained in the proper use of the TOBI Podhaler prior to use. [See Instructions for Use at the end of the Patient Information leaflet.] Caregivers should provide assistance to children using TOBI Podhaler (including preparing the dose for inhalation) particularly for those aged 10 years or younger, and should continue to supervise them until they are able to use the Podhaler device properly without help.

For patients taking several different inhaled medications and/or performing chest physiotherapy, advise the patient regarding the order they should take the therapies. It is recommended that TOBI Podhaler be taken last.

17.1 Ototoxicity

Inform patients that ototoxicity, as measured by complaints of hearing loss or tinnitus, was reported by patients in the TOBI Podhaler clinical studies. Physicians should consider an audiogram at baseline, particularly for patients at increased risk of auditory dysfunction. If a patient reports tinnitus or hearing loss during TOBI Podhaler therapy, the physician should refer that patient for audiological assessment.

Patients should be reminded that vestibular toxicity may manifest as vertigo, ataxia, or dizziness.

17.2 Bronchospasm

Inform patients that bronchospasm can occur with inhalation of TOBI Podhaler.

17.3 Risks Associated with Aminoglycosides

Inform patients of adverse reactions associated with aminoglycosides such as nephrotoxicity and neuromuscular disorders.

17.4 Laboratory Tests

Inform patients of the need to monitor hearing, serum concentrations of tobramycin, or renal function as necessary during treatment with TOBI Podhaler.

17.5 Pregnancy

Inform patients that aminoglycosides can cause fetal harm when administered to a pregnant woman. Advise them to inform their doctor if they are pregnant, become pregnant, or plan to become pregnant.

17.6 Cough

Inform patients that cough was reported with the use of TOBI Podhaler in clinical trials. If coughing that may be experienced with TOBI Podhaler becomes bothersome or cannot be tolerated, advise patients that tobramycin inhalation solution or alternative therapeutic options may be considered.

T2014-51
April 2014
Patient Information
TOBI (TOH-bee) Podhaler (POD-hay-ler)
(tobramycin inhalation powder)
For Oral Inhalation

Important information: Do not swallow TOBI Podhaler capsules. TOBI Podhaler capsules are used only with the Podhaler device and inhaled through your mouth (oral inhalation). Never place a capsule in the mouthpiece of the Podhaler device.

Read this Patient Information before you start using TOBI Podhaler and each time you get a refill. There may be new information. This information does not take the place of talking to your healthcare provider about your medical condition or treatment.

What is TOBI Podhaler?

TOBI Podhaler is a prescription medicine used to treat people with cystic fibrosis who have a bacterial infection called Pseudomonas aeruginosa. TOBI Podhaler contains an antibacterial medicine called tobramycin (an aminoglycoside).

It is not known if TOBI Podhaler is safe and effective:
• in children under 6 years of age
• in people who have an FEV1 less than 25% predicted
• in people who are colonized with a bacterium called *Burkholderia cepacia*
• when used for more than 3 cycles

Who should not use TOBI Podhaler?

Do not use TOBI Podhaler if you are allergic to tobramycin, any of the ingredients in TOBI Podhaler, or to any other aminoglycoside antibacterial.

What should I tell my healthcare provider before using TOBI Podhaler?

Before you use TOBI Podhaler, tell your healthcare provider if you:
• have or have had hearing problems (including noises in your ears such as ringing or hissing)
• have dizziness
• have or have had kidney problems
• have or have had problems with muscle weakness such as myasthenia gravis or Parkinson's disease
• have or have had breathing problems such as wheezing, coughing, or chest tightness
• have had an organ transplant
• are pregnant or plan to become pregnant
• are breastfeeding or plan to breastfeed. It is not known if TOBI Podhaler passes into your breast milk.

Tell your healthcare provider about all the medicines you take, including prescription and non-prescription medicines, vitamins, and herbal supplements.

Using TOBI Podhaler with certain other medicines can cause serious side effects.

If you are using TOBI Podhaler, you should discuss with your healthcare provider if you should take:
• other medicines that may harm your nervous system, kidneys, or hearing
• "water pills" (diuretics) such as Edecrin (ethacrynic acid), Lasix (furosemide), or intravenous mannitol
• urea

Ask your healthcare provider or pharmacist for a list of these medicines, if you are not sure.

Know the medicines you take. Keep a list of them and show it to your healthcare provider and pharmacist when you get a new medicine.

How should I use TOBI Podhaler?

• See the step-by-step Instructions for Use at the end of this Patient Information leaflet about the right way to use TOBI Podhaler. Do not use TOBI Podhaler unless your healthcare provider has taught you how to use it the right way. Ask your healthcare provider or pharmacist if you are not sure.

• Always use TOBI Podhaler exactly as your healthcare provider tells you to use it. Ask your healthcare provider or pharmacist if you are not sure.

• The usual dose for adults and children over 6 years of age is:
  ○ The content of 4 TOBI Podhaler capsules inhaled by mouth in the morning using your Podhaler device and the content of 4 TOBI Podhaler capsules inhaled by mouth in the evening using your Podhaler device.
  ○ Check to see that each capsule is empty after inhaling. If powder remains in the capsule, repeat inhalation until the capsule is empty.

• Each dose of 4 TOBI Podhaler capsules should be taken as close to 12 hours as possible.

• You should not take your dose of 4 TOBI Podhaler capsules less than 6 hours apart.

• If you forget to take TOBI Podhaler and there are at least 6 hours to your next dose, take your dose as soon as you can. Otherwise, wait for your next dose. Do not double the dose to make up for the missed dose.

- After using TOBI Podhaler for 28 days, you should stop using it and wait 28 days. After you have stopped using TOBI Podhaler for 28 days, you should start using TOBI Podhaler again for 28 days. Complete the full 28 day course even if you are feeling better. It is important that you keep to the 28-day on, 28-day off cycle (See Figure A).

ON TOBI Podhaler	OFF TOBI Podhaler
Take TOBI Podhaler twice a day, every day for 28 days	Do not take any TOBI Podhaler for the next 28 days

Repeat cycle
(Figure A)

- If you are taking several different medicines inhaled through your mouth, your healthcare provider will tell you how to take your medicines the right way.
- If you are doing therapies for cystic fibrosis (chest physiotherapy), you should take TOBI Podhaler after your therapies are done.
- If you inhale too much TOBI Podhaler, tell your healthcare provider right away.
- If you accidentally swallow TOBI Podhaler capsules, tell your healthcare provider right away.
- Use a new Podhaler device every 7 days.
- Caregivers should help children who are 10 years of age and younger use TOBI Podhaler, and should keep watching them use their TOBI Podhaler until they are able to use it the right way without help.

What are the possible side effects of TOBI Podhaler?
TOBI Podhaler can cause serious side effects, including:

- hearing loss or ringing in the ears (ototoxicity). Tell your healthcare provider right away if you have hearing loss or you hear noises in your ears such as ringing or hissing. Tell your healthcare provider if you develop vertigo, difficulty with balance or dizziness.
- worsening kidney problems (nephrotoxicity). TOBI Podhaler is in a class of drugs which may cause worsening kidney problems, especially in people with known or suspected kidney problems. Your healthcare provider may do a blood test to check how your kidneys are working while you are using TOBI Podhaler.
- worsening muscle weakness. TOBI Podhaler is in a class of drugs which can cause muscle weakness to get worse in people who already have problems with muscle weakness (myasthenia gravis or Parkinson's disease).
- severe breathing problems (bronchospasm). Tell your healthcare provider right away if you get any of these symptoms of bronchospasm with using TOBI Podhaler:
  ○ shortness of breath with wheezing
  ○ coughing and chest tightness
- TOBI Podhaler is in a class of drugs which may cause harm to an unborn baby.

The most common side effects of TOBI Podhaler include:
- cough
- worsening of lung problems or cystic fibrosis
- productive cough
- shortness of breath
- fever
- sore throat
- changes in your voice (hoarseness)
- coughing up blood
- headache
- altered taste

Laboratory tests show reduced tobramycin activity against *Pseudomonas aeruginosa* bacteria in some patients with the use of TOBI Podhaler. The relationship between these lab results and how well TOBI Podhaler works is not clear. Let your healthcare provider know if your symptoms worsen. Some patients may be unable to continue TOBI Podhaler and need to consider alternative therapies. Tell your healthcare provider about any side effect that bothers you enough to stop treatment or that does not go away.

These are not all of the possible side effects of TOBI Podhaler. For more information, ask your healthcare provider or pharmacist.

Call your doctor for medical advice about side effects. You may report side effects to FDA at 1-800-FDA-1088.

General information about the safe and effective use of TOBI Podhaler

Medicines are sometimes prescribed for purposes other than those listed in a patient information leaflet. Do not use TOBI Podhaler for a condition for which it was not prescribed. Do not give TOBI Podhaler to other people, even if they have the same problem you have. It may harm them. This leaflet summarizes the most important information about TOBI Podhaler. If you would like more information, talk with your healthcare provider. You can ask your healthcare provider or pharmacist for information about TOBI Podhaler that was written for healthcare professionals.

For more information, go to www.TOBIPodhaler.com or call 1-877-999-TOBI (8624).

What are the ingredients in TOBI Podhaler?
Active ingredient: tobramycin
Inactive ingredients: 1,2-distearoyl-sn-glycero-3-phosphocholine (DSPC), calcium chloride, and sulfuric acid (for pH adjustment)

What is *Pseudomonas aeruginosa*?
It is a very common bacterium that infects the lungs of nearly everyone with cystic fibrosis at some time during their lives. Some people do not get this infection until later in their lives, while others get it very young. It is one of the most damaging bacteria for people with cystic fibrosis. If the infection is not properly managed, it will continue to damage your lungs causing further problems to your breathing.
T2013-91
November 2013

Instructions for Use
TOBI Podhaler
Follow the instructions below for using your TOBI Podhaler. You will breathe in (inhale) the medicine in the TOBI Podhaler capsules using the Podhaler device. If you have any questions, ask your healthcare provider or pharmacist. Each TOBI Podhaler package contains (See Figure A):
- 4 weekly packs (28-day supply), each containing:
  ○ 56 capsules (7 blister cards of 8 capsules). Each blister card contains 8 TOBI Podhaler capsules (4 capsules for inhalation in the morning and 4 capsules for inhalation in the evening).
  ○ 1 Podhaler device and its storage case
- 1 reserve Podhaler device (to be used if needed) and its storage case

(Figure A)

Please note the following:
- **Do not** swallow TOBI Podhaler capsules. The powder in the capsule is for you to inhale using the Podhaler device.
- Only use the Podhaler device contained in this pack. **Do not** use TOBI Podhaler capsules with any other device, and **do not** use the Podhaler device to take any other medicine.
- When you start a new weekly (7 day) pack of capsules, use the new Podhaler device that is supplied in the pack and discard the used device and its case. Each Podhaler device is only used for one week (7 days).
- Always keep the TOBI Podhaler capsules in the blister card. Only remove 1 capsule at a time just before you are going to use it.
- Doses should be inhaled as close to 12 hours apart as possible and not less than 6 hours apart.
- Once in a while, very small pieces of the capsules can get into your mouth and you may be able to feel these pieces on your tongue. These small pieces will not hurt you if you swallow or inhale them.
- The reserve Podhaler device provided in the package may be used if the Podhaler device:
  ○ is wet, dirty, or broken
  ○ has been dropped
  ○ does not seem to be piercing the capsule properly (see Step 17)

Getting ready:
- **Wash and dry your hands completely** (See Figure B).

Figure B

Preparing your TOBI Podhaler dose
Step 1: Just before use, hold the base of the Podhaler device and unscrew the lid in a counter-clockwise direction (See Figure C). Set the lid aside.

Figure C

Step 2: Stand the Podhaler device upright in the base of the case (See Figure D).

Figure D

Step 3: Hold the body of the Podhaler device and unscrew the mouthpiece in a counter-clockwise direction (See Figure E). Set the mouthpiece aside on a clean, dry surface.

Figure E

Step 4: Take 1 blister card and tear the pre-cut lines along the length (See Figure F) then tear at the pre-cut lines along the width (See Figure G).

Figure F   **Figure G**

Step 5: Peel (by rolling back) the foil that covers 1 TOBI Podhaler capsule on the blister card (See Figure H). Always hold the foil close to where you are peeling.

Figure I

Figure H

Step 6: Take out 1 TOBI Podhaler capsule from the blister card (See Figure I). Only remove one capsule at a time just before you are going to use it in the device.
[See figure I at top of previous page]

Step 7: Immediately, place the TOBI Podhaler capsule in the capsule chamber at the top of the Podhaler device (See Figure J). **Do not** put the capsule directly into the top of the mouthpiece.

Figure J

Step 8: Put the mouthpiece back on your Podhaler device and screw the mouthpiece in a clockwise direction until it is tight (See Figure K). **Do not** overtighten.

Figure K

Step 9: Hold the Podhaler device with the mouthpiece pointing down. Put your thumb on the blue button and press the blue button all the way down (See Figure L). Let go of the blue button. **Do not** press the blue button more than 1 time. The chances of the capsule breaking into pieces will be increased if the capsule is accidentally pierced more than once.

Figure L

Taking your TOBI Podhaler dose:
You will need to inhale at least twice from each capsule in order to get the full dose.

Step 10: Breathe out (exhale) all the way (See Figure M). **Do not** blow or exhale into the mouthpiece.

Figure M

Step 11: Place your mouth over the mouthpiece and close your lips tightly around it (See Figure N).

Figure N

Step 12: Inhale deeply with a single breath (See Figure O).

Figure O

Step 13: Remove the Podhaler device from your mouth, and hold your breath for about 5 seconds, then exhale normally away from the Podhaler device.

Step 14: Take a few normal breaths away from the Podhaler device. **Do not** blow or exhale into the mouthpiece.

Step 15: For your second inhalation, repeat steps 10 through 13 using the same capsule.

Step 16: Unscrew the mouthpiece and remove the TOBI Podhaler capsule from the capsule chamber (See Figure P).

Figure P

Step 17: Look at the used capsule. It should be pierced and empty. There will be a fine coating of powder remaining on the inside of the capsule (See Figure Q). If it is pierced and empty, throw it away and go to Step 18.

piercing marks

Figure Q

• If the capsule is pierced but still contains more than just a fine coating of powder (See Figure R for an example):

piercing marks   powder level

Figure R

○ Put the capsule back into the Podhaler device capsule-chamber (See Figure J) with the pierced side of the capsule pointing down (See Figure R). Put the mouthpiece back on and repeat Steps 10 to 13.

• If the capsule does not look pierced (See Figure S):

no piercing marks   powder level

Figure S

○ Put the capsule back into the Podhaler device capsule-chamber (See Figure J). Put the mouthpiece back on and repeat Steps 9 to 17.

■ If the capsule still does not look pierced and still has some powder in it, use the reserve Podhaler device provided in the TOBI Podhaler package and repeat Steps 1 to 3, then 7 to 17.

Step 18: Repeat Steps 6 to 17 for 3 more times until your whole dose (4 capsules) has been taken (See Figure T).

1 dose =

Figure T

After your TOBI Podhaler dose:

Step 19: Throw away all the empty TOBI Podhaler capsules. **Do not** store the TOBI Podhaler capsules in the Podhaler device.

Step 20: Put the mouthpiece back on to your Podhaler device and twist the mouthpiece in a clockwise direction until it is tight (See Figure K). **Do not** overtighten.

Step 21: Wipe the mouthpiece with a clean, dry cloth (See Figure U).

Figure U

• **Do not** wash the Podhaler device with water. Your Podhaler device needs to stay dry at all times to work the right way.

Step 22: Place your Podhaler device back in the storage case base.

Step 23: Place the lid back on the storage case base and screw the cover in a clockwise direction until it is tight (See Figure V).

Figure V

How should I store TOBI Podhaler?
• Store your Podhaler device and blister-packaged capsules at room temperature between 68°F to 77°F (20°C to 25°C).
• Keep the TOBI Podhaler capsules and Podhaler device in a dry place.
• Store the Podhaler device tightly closed in its case when you are not using it.
• Keep TOBI Podhaler capsules, Podhaler device, and all medicines out of the reach of children.

This Patient Information and Instructions for Use have been approved by the U.S. Food and Drug Administration.

Distributed by:
Novartis Pharmaceuticals Corporation
East Hanover, NJ 07936
© Novartis
T2013-22
March 2013

Shown in Product Identification Guide, page 311

ZOMETA®   ℞
[zō-mĕ-ta]
(zoledronic acid)
Injection
Ready-to-Use Solution for Intravenous Infusion
(For Single Use)
Concentrate for Intravenous Infusion

The following prescribing information is based on official labeling in effect July 2014.

HIGHLIGHTS OF PRESCRIBING INFORMATION
These highlights do not include all the information needed to use ZOMETA safely and effectively. See full prescribing information for ZOMETA.
ZOMETA® (zoledronic acid) Injection
Ready-to-Use Solution for Intravenous Infusion
(For Single Use)
Concentrate for Intravenous Infusion
Initial U.S. Approval: 2001

————————RECENT MAJOR CHANGES————————
Warnings and Precautions, Hypocalcemia (5.10)   9/2013

————————INDICATIONS AND USAGE————————
Zometa is a bisphosphonate indicated for the treatment of:
• Hypercalcemia of malignancy. (1.1)
• Patients with multiple myeloma and patients with documented bone metastases from solid tumors, in conjunction with standard antineoplastic therapy. Prostate cancer should have progressed after treatment with at least one hormonal therapy. (1.2)

Important limitation of use: The safety and efficacy of Zometa has not been established for use in hyperparathyroidism or nontumor-related hypercalcemia. (1.3)

————————DOSAGE AND ADMINISTRATION————————
Hypercalcemia of malignancy (2.1)
• 4 mg as a single-use intravenous infusion over no less than 15 minutes.
• 4 mg as retreatment after a minimum of 7 days.
Multiple myeloma and bone metastasis from solid tumors. (2.2)
• 4 mg as a single-use intravenous infusion over no less than 15 minutes every 3-4 weeks for patients with creatinine clearance of greater than 60 mL/min.
• Reduce the dose for patients with renal impairment.
• Coadminister oral calcium supplements of 500 mg and a multiple vitamin containing 400 international units of Vitamin D daily.

Administer through a separate vented infusion line and do not allow to come in contact with any calcium or divalent cation-containing solutions. (2.3)

----------DOSAGE FORMS AND STRENGTHS----------

4 mg/100 mL single-use ready-to-use bottle (3)
4 mg/5 mL single-use vial of concentrate (3)

----------CONTRAINDICATIONS----------

Hypersensitivity to any component of Zometa (4)

----------WARNINGS AND PRECAUTIONS----------

- Patients being treated with Zometa should not be treated with Reclast®. (5.1)
- Adequately rehydrate patients with hypercalcemia of malignancy prior to administration of Zometa and monitor electrolytes during treatment. (5.2)
- Renal toxicity may be greater in patients with renal impairment. Do not use doses greater than 4 mg. Treatment in patients with severe renal impairment is not recommended. Monitor serum creatinine before each dose. (5.3)
- Osteonecrosis of the jaw has been reported. Preventive dental exams should be performed before starting Zometa. Avoid invasive dental procedures. (5.4)
- Severe incapacitating bone, joint, and/or muscle pain may occur. Discontinue Zometa if severe symptoms occur. (5.5)
- Zometa can cause fetal harm. Women of childbearing potential should be advised of the potential hazard to the fetus and to avoid becoming pregnant. (5.9, 8.1)
- Atypical subtrochanteric and diaphyseal femoral fractures have been reported in patients receiving bisphosphonate therapy. These fractures may occur after minimal or no trauma. Evaluate patients with thigh or groin pain to rule out a femoral fracture. Consider drug discontinuation in patients suspected to have an atypical femur fracture. (5.6)
- Hypocalcemia: Correct before initiating Zometa. Adequately supplement patients with calcium and vitamin D (5.10)

----------ADVERSE REACTIONS----------

The most common adverse events (greater than 25%) were nausea, fatigue, anemia, bone pain, constipation, fever, vomiting, and dyspnea (6.1)

To report SUSPECTED ADVERSE REACTIONS, contact Novartis Pharmaceuticals Corporation at 1-888-669-6682 or FDA at 1-800-FDA-1088 or www.fda.gov/medwatch.

----------DRUG INTERACTIONS----------

- Aminoglycosides: May have an additive effect to lower serum calcium for prolonged periods. (7.1)
- Loop diuretics: Concomitant use with Zometa may increase risk of hypocalcemia. (7.2)
- Nephrotoxic drugs: Use with caution. (7.3)

----------USE IN SPECIFIC POPULATIONS----------

- Nursing Mothers: It is not known whether Zometa is excreted in human milk. (8.3)
- Pediatric Use: Not indicated for use in pediatric patients. (8.4)
- Geriatric Use: Special care to monitor renal function. (8.5)

See 17 for PATIENT COUNSELING INFORMATION
Revised: 4/2014

FULL PRESCRIBING INFORMATION: CONTENTS*
WARNING:

* Sections or subsections omitted from the full prescribing information are not listed

FULL PRESCRIBING INFORMATION

1   INDICATIONS AND USAGE

1.1   Hypercalcemia of Malignancy

Zometa is indicated for the treatment of hypercalcemia of malignancy defined as an albumin-corrected calcium (cCa) of greater than or equal to 12 mg/dL [3.0 mmol/L] using the formula: cCa in mg/dL=Ca in mg/dL + 0.8 (4.0 g/dL - patient albumin [g/dL]).

1.2   Multiple Myeloma and Bone Metastases of Solid Tumors

Zometa is indicated for the treatment of patients with multiple myeloma and patients with documented bone metastases from solid tumors, in conjunction with standard antineoplastic therapy. Prostate cancer should have progressed after treatment with at least one hormonal therapy.

1.3   Important Limitation of Use

The safety and efficacy of Zometa in the treatment of hypercalcemia associated with hyperparathyroidism or with other nontumor-related conditions have not been established.

2   DOSAGE AND ADMINISTRATION

Parenteral drug products should be inspected visually for particulate matter and discoloration prior to administration, whenever solution and container permit.

2.1   Hypercalcemia of Malignancy

The maximum recommended dose of Zometa in hypercalcemia of malignancy (albumin-corrected serum calcium greater than or equal to 12 mg/dL [3.0 mmol/L]) is 4 mg. The 4-mg dose must be given as a single-dose intravenous infusion over **no less than 15 minutes**. Patients who receive Zometa should have serum creatinine assessed prior to each treatment.

Dose adjustments of Zometa are not necessary in treating patients for hypercalcemia of malignancy presenting with mild-to-moderate renal impairment prior to initiation of therapy (serum creatinine less than 400 μmol/L or less than 4.5 mg/dL).

Patients should be adequately rehydrated prior to administration of Zometa [see Warnings and Precautions (5.2)].

Consideration should be given to the severity of, as well as the symptoms of, tumor-induced hypercalcemia when considering use of Zometa. Vigorous saline hydration, an integral part of hypercalcemia therapy, should be initiated promptly and an attempt should be made to restore the urine output to about 2 L/day throughout treatment. Mild or asymptomatic hypercalcemia may be treated with conservative measures (i.e., saline hydration, with or without loop diuretics). Patients should be hydrated adequately throughout the treatment, but overhydration, especially in those patients who have cardiac failure, must be avoided. Diuretic therapy should not be employed prior to correction of hypovolemia.

Retreatment with Zometa 4 mg may be considered if serum calcium does not return to normal or remain normal after initial treatment. It is recommended that a minimum of 7 days elapse before retreatment, to allow for full response to the initial dose. Renal function must be carefully monitored in all patients receiving Zometa and serum creatinine must be assessed prior to retreatment with Zometa [see Warnings and Precautions (5.2)].

2.2   Multiple Myeloma and Metastatic Bone Lesions of Solid Tumors

The recommended dose of Zometa in patients with multiple myeloma and metastatic bone lesions from solid tumors for patients with creatinine clearance (CrCl) greater than 60 mL/min is 4 mg infused over **no less than 15 minutes** every 3 to 4 weeks. The optimal duration of therapy is not known.

Upon treatment initiation, the recommended Zometa doses for patients with reduced renal function (mild and moderate renal impairment) are listed in Table 1. These doses are calculated to achieve the same area under the curve (AUC) as that achieved in patients with creatinine clearance of 75 mL/min. CrCl is calculated using the Cockcroft-Gault formula [see Warnings and Precautions (5.2)].

Table 1: Reduced Doses for Patients with Baseline CrCl Less than or Equal to 60 mL/min

Baseline Creatinine Clearance (mL/min)	Zometa Recommended Dose*
greater than 60	4 mg
50-60	3.5 mg
40-49	3.3 mg
30-39	3 mg

*Doses calculated assuming target AUC of 0.66(mg•hr/L) (CrCl=75 mL/min)

During treatment, serum creatinine should be measured before each Zometa dose and treatment should be withheld for renal deterioration. In the clinical studies, renal deterioration was defined as follows:
For patients with normal baseline creatinine, increase of 0.5 mg/dL
For patients with abnormal baseline creatinine, increase of 1.0 mg/dL
In the clinical studies, Zometa treatment was resumed only when the creatinine returned to within 10% of the baseline value. Zometa should be reinitiated at the same dose as that prior to treatment interruption.

Patients should also be administered an oral calcium supplement of 500 mg and a multiple vitamin containing 400 international units of Vitamin D daily.

2.3   Preparation of Solution

Zometa must not be mixed with calcium or other divalent cation-containing infusion solutions, such as Lactated Ringer's solution, and should be administered as a single intravenous solution in a line separate from all other drugs.

4 mg/100 mL Single-Use Ready-to-Use Bottle

Bottles of Zometa ready-to-use solution for infusion contain overfill allowing for the administration of 100 mL of solution (equivalent to 4 mg zoledronic acid). This solution is ready-to-use and may be administered directly to the patient without further preparation. For single use only.

To prepare reduced doses for patients with baseline CrCl less than or equal to 60 mL/min, withdraw the specified volume of the Zometa solution from the bottle (see Table 2) and replace with an equal volume of sterile 0.9% Sodium Chloride, USP, or 5% Dextrose Injection, USP. Administer the newly-prepared dose-adjusted solution to the patient by infusion. Follow proper aseptic technique. Properly discard previously withdrawn volume of ready-to-use solution - do not store or reuse.

Table 2: Preparation of Reduced Doses–Zometa Ready-to-Use Bottle

Remove and discard the following Zometa ready-to-use solution (mL)	Replace with the following volume of sterile 0.9% Sodium Chloride, USP or 5% Dextrose Injection, USP (mL)	Dose (mg)
12.0	12.0	3.5
18.0	18.0	3.3
25.0	25.0	3.0

If not used immediately after dilution with infusion media, for microbiological integrity, the solution should be refrigerated at 2°C–8°C (36°F–46°F). The refrigerated solution should then be equilibrated to room temperature prior to administration. The total time between dilution, storage in the refrigerator, and end of administration must not exceed 24 hours.

4 mg/5 mL Single-Use Vial

Vials of Zometa concentrate for infusion contain overfill allowing for the withdrawal of 5 mL of concentrate (equivalent to 4 mg zoledronic acid). This concentrate should immediately be diluted in 100 mL of sterile 0.9% Sodium Chloride, USP, or 5% Dextrose Injection, USP, following proper aseptic technique, and administered to the patient by infusion. Do not store undiluted concentrate in a syringe, to avoid inadvertent injection.

To prepare reduced doses for patients with baseline CrCl less than or equal to 60 mL/min, withdraw the specified volume of the Zometa concentrate from the vial for the dose required (see Table 3).

Table 3: Preparation of Reduced Doses – Zometa Concentrate

Remove and Use Zometa Volume (mL)	Dose (mg)
4.4	3.5
4.1	3.3
3.8	3.0

The withdrawn concentrate must be diluted in 100 mL of sterile 0.9% Sodium Chloride, USP, or 5% Dextrose Injection, USP.

If not used immediately after dilution with infusion media, for microbiological integrity, the solution should be refrigerated at 2°C-8°C (36°F-46°F). The refrigerated solution should then be equilibrated to room temperature prior to administration. The total time between dilution, storage in the refrigerator, and end of administration must not exceed 24 hours.

2.4 Method of Administration

Due to the risk of clinically significant deterioration in renal function, which may progress to renal failure, single doses of Zometa should not exceed 4 mg and the duration of infusion should be no less than 15 minutes [see Warnings and Precautions (5.3)]. In the trials and in postmarketing experience, renal deterioration, progression to renal failure and dialysis, have occurred in patients, including those treated with the approved dose of 4 mg infused over 15 minutes. There have been instances of this occurring after the initial Zometa dose.

3 DOSAGE FORMS AND STRENGTHS

4 mg/100 mL single-use ready-to-use bottle
4 mg/5 mL single-use vial of concentrate

4 CONTRAINDICATIONS

4.1 Hypersensitivity to Zoledronic Acid or Any Components of Zometa

Hypersensitivity reactions including rare cases of urticaria and angioedema, and very rare cases of anaphylactic reaction/shock have been reported [see Adverse Reactions (6.2)].

5 WARNINGS AND PRECAUTIONS

5.1 Drugs with Same Active Ingredient or in the Same Drug Class

Zometa contains the same active ingredient as found in Reclast® (zoledronic acid). Patients being treated with Zometa should not be treated with Reclast or other bisphosphonates.

5.2 Hydration and Electrolyte Monitoring

Patients with hypercalcemia of malignancy must be adequately rehydrated prior to administration of Zometa. Loop diuretics should not be used until the patient is adequately rehydrated and should be used with caution in combination with Zometa in order to avoid hypocalcemia. Zometa should be used with caution with other nephrotoxic drugs.

Standard hypercalcemia-related metabolic parameters, such as serum levels of calcium, phosphate, and magnesium, as well as serum creatinine, should be carefully monitored following initiation of therapy with Zometa. If hypocalcemia, hypophosphatemia, or hypomagnesemia occur, short-term supplemental therapy may be necessary.

5.3 Renal Impairment

Zometa is excreted intact primarily via the kidney, and the risk of adverse reactions, in particular renal adverse reactions, may be greater in patients with impaired renal function. Safety and pharmacokinetic data are limited in patients with severe renal impairment and the risk of renal deterioration is increased [see Adverse Reactions (6.1)]. Pre-existing renal insufficiency and multiple cycles of Zometa and other bisphosphonates are risk factors for subsequent renal deterioration with Zometa. Factors predisposing to renal deterioration, such as dehydration or the use of other nephrotoxic drugs, should be identified and managed, if possible.

Zometa treatment in patients with hypercalcemia of malignancy with severe renal impairment should be considered only after evaluating the risks and benefits of treatment. In the clinical studies, patients with serum creatinine greater than 400 μmol/L or greater than 4.5 mg/dL were excluded. Zometa treatment is not recommended in patients with bone metastases with severe renal impairment. In the clinical studies, patients with serum creatinine greater than 265 μmol/L or greater than 3.0 mg/dL were excluded and there were only 8 of 564 patients treated with Zometa 4 mg by 15-minute infusion with a baseline creatinine greater than 2 mg/dL. Limited pharmacokinetic data exists in patients with creatinine clearance less than 30 mL/min [see Clinical Pharmacology (12.3)].

5.4 Osteonecrosis of the Jaw

Osteonecrosis of the jaw (ONJ) has been reported predominantly in cancer patients treated with intravenous bisphosphonates, including Zometa. Many of these patients were

Table 4: Percentage of Patients with Adverse Events ≥10% Reported in Hypercalcemia of Malignancy Clinical Trials by Body System

	Zometa 4 mg n (%)		Pamidronate 90 mg n (%)	
Patients Studied				
Total No. of Patients Studied	86	(100)	103	(100)
Total No. of Patients with any AE	81	(94)	95	(92)
Body as a Whole				
Fever	38	(44)	34	(33)
Progression of Cancer	14	(16)	21	(20)
Cardiovascular				
Hypotension	9	(11)	2	(2)
Digestive				
Nausea	25	(29)	28	(27)
Constipation	23	(27)	13	(13)
Diarrhea	15	(17)	17	(17)
Abdominal Pain	14	(16)	13	(13)
Vomiting	12	(14)	17	(17)
Anorexia	8	(9)	14	(14)
Hemic and Lymphatic System				
Anemia	19	(22)	18	(18)
Infections				
Moniliasis	10	(12)	4	(4)
Laboratory Abnormalities				
Hypophosphatemia	11	(13)	2	(2)
Hypokalemia	10	(12)	16	(16)
Hypomagnesemia	9	(11)	5	(5)
Musculoskeletal				
Skeletal Pain	10	(12)	10	(10)
Nervous				
Insomnia	13	(15)	10	(10)
Anxiety	12	(14)	8	(8)
Confusion	11	(13)	13	(13)
Agitation	11	(13)	8	(8)
Respiratory				
Dyspnea	19	(22)	20	(19)
Coughing	10	(12)	12	(12)
Urogenital				
Urinary Tract Infection	12	(14)	15	(15)

also receiving chemotherapy and corticosteroids which may be risk factors for ONJ. Postmarketing experience and the literature suggest a greater frequency of reports of ONJ based on tumor type (advanced breast cancer, multiple myeloma), and dental status (dental extraction, periodontal disease, local trauma including poorly fitting dentures). Many reports of ONJ involved patients with signs of local infection including osteomyelitis.

Cancer patients should maintain good oral hygiene and should have a dental examination with preventive dentistry prior to treatment with bisphosphonates.

While on treatment, these patients should avoid invasive dental procedures if possible. For patients who develop ONJ while on bisphosphonate therapy, dental surgery may exacerbate the condition. For patients requiring dental procedures, there are no data available to suggest whether discontinuation of bisphosphonate treatment reduces the risk of ONJ. Clinical judgment of the treating physician should guide the management plan of each patient based on individual benefit/risk assessment [see Adverse Reactions (6.2)].

5.5 Musculoskeletal Pain

In postmarketing experience, severe and occasionally incapacitating bone, joint, and/or muscle pain has been reported in patients taking bisphosphonates, including Zometa. The time to onset of symptoms varied from one day to several months after starting the drug. Discontinue use if severe symptoms develop. Most patients had relief of symptoms after stopping. A subset had recurrence of symptoms when rechallenged with the same drug or another bisphosphonate [see Adverse Reactions (6.2)].

5.6 Atypical Subtrochanteric and Diaphyseal Femoral Fractures

Atypical subtrochanteric and diaphyseal femoral fractures have been reported in patients receiving bisphosphonate therapy, including Zometa. These fractures can occur anywhere in the femoral shaft from just below the lesser trochanter to just above the supracondylar flare and are transverse or short oblique in orientation without evidence of comminution. These fractures occur after minimal or no trauma. Patients may experience thigh or groin pain weeks to months before presenting with a completed femoral fracture. Fractures are often bilateral; therefore the contralateral femur should be examined in bisphosphonate-treated patients who have sustained a femoral shaft fracture. Poor healing of these fractures has also been reported. A number of case reports noted that patients were also receiving treatment with glucocorticoids (such as prednisone or dexamethasone) at the time of fracture. Causality with bisphosphonate therapy has not been established.

Any patient with a history of bisphosphonate exposure who presents with thigh or groin pain in the absence of trauma should be suspected of having an atypical fracture and should be evaluated. Discontinuation of Zometa therapy in patients suspected to have an atypical femur fracture should be considered pending evaluation of the patient, based on an individual benefit risk assessment. It is unknown whether the risk of atypical femur fracture continues after stopping therapy.

5.7 Patients with Asthma

While not observed in clinical trials with Zometa, there have been reports of bronchoconstriction in aspirin-sensitive patients receiving bisphosphonates.

5.8 Hepatic Impairment

Only limited clinical data are available for use of Zometa to treat hypercalcemia of malignancy in patients with hepatic insufficiency, and these data are not adequate to provide guidance on dosage selection or how to safely use Zometa in these patients.

5.9 Use in Pregnancy

Bisphosphonates, such as Zometa, are incorporated into the bone matrix, from where they are gradually released over periods of weeks to years. There may be a risk of fetal harm (e.g., skeletal and other abnormalities) if a woman becomes pregnant after completing a course of bisphosphonate therapy.

Zometa may cause fetal harm when administered to a pregnant woman. In reproductive studies in pregnant rats, subcutaneous doses equivalent to 2.4 or 4.8 times the human systemic exposure resulted in pre- and postimplantation losses, decreases in viable fetuses and fetal skeletal, visceral, and external malformations. There are no adequate and well controlled studies in pregnant women. If this drug is used during pregnancy, or if the patient becomes pregnant while taking this drug, the patient should be apprised of the potential hazard to a fetus [see Use in Specific Populations (8.1)].

5.10 Hypocalcemia

Hypocalcemia has been reported in patients treated with Zometa. Cardiac arrhythmias and neurologic adverse events (seizures, tetany, and numbness) have been reported secondary to cases of severe hypocalcemia. In some instances, hypocalcemia may be life-threatening. Hypocalcemia must be corrected before initiating Zometa. Adequately supplement patients with calcium and vitamin D.

6 ADVERSE REACTIONS

6.1 Clinical Studies Experience

Because clinical trials are conducted under widely varying conditions, adverse reaction rates observed in the clinical

Table 5: Grade 3 Laboratory Abnormalities for Serum Creatinine, Serum Calcium, Serum Phosphorus, and Serum Magnesium in Two Clinical Trials in Patients with HCM

| Laboratory Parameter | Grade 3 | | | |
| | Zometa 4 mg | | Pamidronate 90 mg | |
	n/N	(%)	n/N	(%)
Serum Creatinine[1]	2/86	(2%)	3/100	(3%)
Hypocalcemia[2]	1/86	(1%)	2/100	(2%)
Hypophosphatemia[3]	36/70	(51%)	27/81	(33%)
Hypomagnesemia[4]	0/71	—	0/84	—

Table 6: Grade 4 Laboratory Abnormalities for Serum Creatinine, Serum Calcium, Serum Phosphorus, and Serum Magnesium in Two Clinical Trials in Patients with HCM

| Laboratory Parameter | Grade 4 | | | |
| | Zometa 4 mg | | Pamidronate 90 mg | |
	n/N	(%)	n/N	(%)
Serum Creatinine[1]	0/86	—	1/100	(1%)
Hypocalcemia[2]	0/86	—	0/100	—
Hypophosphatemia[3]	1/70	(1%)	4/81	(5%)
Hypomagnesemia[4]	0/71	—	1/84	(1%)

[1] Grade 3 (greater than 3× Upper Limit of Normal); Grade 4 (greater than 6× Upper Limit of Normal)
[2] Grade 3 (less than 7 mg/dL); Grade 4 (less than 6 mg/dL)
[3] Grade 3 (less than 2 mg/dL); Grade 4 (less than 1 mg/dL)
[4] Grade 3 (less than 0.8 mEq/L); Grade 4 (less than 0.5 mEq/L)

trials of a drug cannot be directly compared to rates in the clinical trials of another drug and may not reflect the rates observed in practice.

Hypercalcemia of Malignancy
The safety of Zometa was studied in 185 patients with hypercalcemia of malignancy (HCM) who received either Zometa 4 mg given as a 5-minute intravenous infusion (n=86) or pamidronate 90 mg given as a 2-hour intravenous infusion (n=103). The population was aged 33-84 years, 60% male and 81% Caucasian, with breast, lung, head and neck, and renal cancer as the most common forms of malignancy. NOTE: pamidronate 90 mg was given as a 2-hour intravenous infusion. The relative safety of pamidronate 90 mg given as a 2-hour intravenous infusion compared to the same dose given as a 24-hour intravenous infusion has not been adequately studied in controlled clinical trials.

Renal Toxicity
Administration of Zometa 4 mg given as a 5-minute intravenous infusion has been shown to result in an increased risk of renal toxicity, as measured by increases in serum creatinine, which can progress to renal failure. The incidence of renal toxicity and renal failure has been shown to be reduced when Zometa 4 mg is given as a 15-minute intravenous infusion. Zometa should be administered by intravenous infusion over no less than 15 minutes [see Warnings and Precautions (5.3), Dosage and Administration (2.4)].

The most frequently observed adverse events were fever, nausea, constipation, anemia, and dyspnea (see Table 4).

Table 4 provides adverse events that were reported by 10% or more of the 189 patients treated with Zometa 4 mg or pamidronate 90 mg from the two HCM trials. Adverse events are listed regardless of presumed causality to study drug.

[See table 4 at top of previous page]

The following adverse events from the two controlled multicenter HCM trials (n=189) were reported by a greater percentage of patients treated with Zometa 4 mg than with pamidronate 90 mg and occurred with a frequency of greater than or equal to 5% but less than 10%. Adverse events are listed regardless of presumed causality to study drug: asthenia, chest pain, leg edema, mucositis, dysphagia, granulocytopenia, thrombocytopenia, pancytopenia, nonspecific infection, hypocalcemia, dehydration, arthralgias, headache and somnolence.

Rare cases of rash, pruritus, and chest pain have been reported following treatment with Zometa.

Acute Phase Reaction
Within three days after Zometa administration, an acute phase reaction has been reported in patients with symptoms including pyrexia, fatigue, bone pain and/or arthralgias, myalgias, chills, and influenza-like illness. These symptoms usually resolve within a few days. Pyrexia has been the most commonly associated symptom, occurring in 44% of patients.

Mineral and Electrolyte Abnormalities
Electrolyte abnormalities, most commonly hypocalcemia, hypophosphatemia, and hypomagnesemia, can occur with bisphosphonate use.

Grade 3 and Grade 4 laboratory abnormalities for serum creatinine, serum calcium, serum phosphorus, and serum magnesium observed in two clinical trials of Zometa in patients with HCM are shown in Table 5 and 6.
[See table 5 above]
[See table 6 above]

Injection Site Reactions
Local reactions at the infusion site, such as redness or swelling, were observed infrequently. In most cases, no specific treatment is required and the symptoms subside after 24-48 hours.

Ocular Adverse Events
Ocular inflammation such as uveitis and scleritis can occur with bisphosphonate use, including Zometa. No cases of iritis, scleritis, or uveitis were reported during these clinical trials. However, cases have been seen in postmarketing use [see Adverse Reactions (6.2)].

Multiple Myeloma and Bone Metastases of Solid Tumors
The safety analysis includes patients treated in the core and extension phases of the trials. The analysis includes the 2042 patients treated with Zometa 4 mg, pamidronate 90 mg, or placebo in the three controlled multicenter bone metastases trials, including 969 patients completing the efficacy phase of the trial, and 619 patients that continued in the safety extension phase. Only 347 patients completed the extension phases and were followed for 2 years (or 21 months for the other solid tumor patients). The median duration of exposure for safety analysis for Zometa 4 mg (core plus extension phases) was 12.8 months for breast cancer and multiple myeloma, 10.8 months for prostate cancer, and 4.0 months for other solid tumors.

Table 7 describes adverse events that were reported by 10% or more of patients. Adverse events are listed regardless of presumed causality to study drug.
[See table 7 at top of next page]
Grade 3 and Grade 4 laboratory abnormalities for serum creatinine, serum calcium, serum phosphorus, and serum magnesium observed in three clinical trials of Zometa in patients with bone metastases are shown in Tables 8 and 9.
[See table 8 at top of next page]
[See table 9 at top of page 2016]

Among the less frequently occurring adverse events (less than 15% of patients), rigors, hypokalemia, influenza-like illness, and hypocalcemia showed a trend for more events with bisphosphonate administration (Zometa 4 mg and pamidronate groups) compared to the placebo group.

Less common adverse events reported more often with Zometa 4 mg than pamidronate included decreased weight, which was reported in 16% of patients in the Zometa 4 mg group compared with 9% in the pamidronate group. Decreased appetite was reported in slightly more patients in the Zometa 4 mg group (13%) compared with the pamidronate (9%) and placebo (10%) groups, but the clinical significance of these small differences is not clear.

Renal Toxicity
In the bone metastases trials, renal deterioration was defined as an increase of 0.5 mg/dL for patients with normal baseline creatinine (less than 1.4 mg/dL) or an increase of

1.0 mg/dL for patients with an abnormal baseline creatinine (greater than or equal to 1.4 mg/dL). The following are data on the incidence of renal deterioration in patients receiving Zometa 4 mg over 15 minutes in these trials (see Table 10).
[See table 10 at top of page 2016]
The risk of deterioration in renal function appeared to be related to time on study, whether patients were receiving Zometa (4 mg over 15 minutes), placebo, or pamidronate.
In the trials and in postmarketing experience, renal deterioration, progression to renal failure, and dialysis have occurred in patients with normal and abnormal baseline renal function, including patients treated with 4 mg infused over a 15-minute period. There have been instances of this occurring after the initial Zometa dose.

6.2 Postmarketing Experience
The following adverse reactions have been reported during postapproval use of Zometa. Because these reports are from a population of uncertain size and are subject to confounding factors, it is not possible to reliably estimate their frequency or establish a causal relationship to drug exposure.

Osteonecrosis of the Jaw
Cases of osteonecrosis (primarily involving the jaws) have been reported predominantly in cancer patients treated with intravenous bisphosphonates including Zometa. Many of these patients were also receiving chemotherapy and corticosteroids which may be a risk factor for ONJ. Data suggests a greater frequency of reports of ONJ in certain cancers, such as advanced breast cancer and multiple myeloma. The majority of the reported cases are in cancer patients following invasive dental procedures, such as tooth extraction. It is therefore prudent to avoid invasive dental procedures as recovery may be prolonged [see Warnings and Precautions (5.4)].

Acute Phase Reaction
Within three days after Zometa administration, an acute phase reaction has been reported, with symptoms including pyrexia, fatigue, bone pain and/or arthralgias, myalgias, chills, influenza-like illness and arthritis with subsequent joint swelling; these symptoms usually resolve within three days of onset, but resolution could take up to 7 to 14 days. However, some of these symptoms have been reported to persist for a longer duration.

Musculoskeletal Pain
Severe and occasionally incapacitating bone, joint, and/or muscle pain has been reported with bisphosphonate use [see Warnings and Precautions (5.5)].

Atypical Subtrochanteric and Diaphyseal Femoral Fractures
Atypical subtrochanteric and diaphyseal femoral fractures have been reported with bisphosphonate therapy, including Zometa [see Warnings and Precautions (5.6)].

Ocular Adverse Events
Cases of uveitis, scleritis, episcleritis, conjunctivitis, iritis, and orbital inflammation including orbital edema have been reported during postmarketing use. In some cases, symptoms resolved with topical steroids.

Hypersensitivity Reactions
There have been rare reports of allergic reaction with intravenous zoledronic acid including angioedema and bronchoconstriction. Very rare cases of anaphylactic reaction/shock have also been reported.
Additional adverse reactions reported in postmarketing use include:
CNS: taste disturbance, hyperesthesia, tremor; *Special Senses*: blurred vision; *Gastrointestinal*: dry mouth; *Skin*: Increased sweating; *Musculoskeletal*: muscle cramps; *Cardiovascular*: hypertension, bradycardia, hypotension (associated with syncope or circulatory collapse primarily in patients with underlying risk factors); *Respiratory*: bronchospasms, interstitial lung disease (ILD) with positive rechallenge; *Renal*: hematuria, proteinuria; *General Disorders and Administration Site*: weight increase, influenza-like illness (pyrexia, asthenia, fatigue or malaise) persisting for greater than 30 days; *Laboratory Abnormalities*: hyperkalemia, hypernatremia.

7 DRUG INTERACTIONS
In vitro studies indicate that the plasma protein binding of zoledronic acid is low, with the unbound fraction ranging from 60%-77%. *In vitro* studies also indicate that zoledronic acid does not inhibit microsomal CYP450 enzymes. *In vivo* studies showed that zoledronic acid is not metabolized, and is excreted into the urine as the intact drug.

7.1 Aminoglycosides
Caution is advised when bisphosphonates are administered with aminoglycosides, since these agents may have an additive effect to lower serum calcium level for prolonged periods. This effect has not been reported in Zometa clinical trials.

7.2 Loop Diuretics
Caution should also be exercised when Zometa is used in combination with loop diuretics due to an increased risk of hypocalcemia.

7.3 Nephrotoxic Drugs

Caution is indicated when Zometa is used with other potentially nephrotoxic drugs.

7.4 Thalidomide

No dose adjustment for Zometa 4 mg is needed when coadministered with thalidomide. In a pharmacokinetic study of 24 patients with multiple myeloma, Zometa 4 mg given as a 15-minute infusion was administered either alone or with thalidomide (100 mg once daily on days 1-14 and 200 mg once daily on days 15-28). Coadministration of thalidomide with Zometa did not significantly change the pharmacokinetics of zoledronic acid or creatinine clearance.

8 USE IN SPECIFIC POPULATIONS

8.1 Pregnancy

Pregnancy Category D *[see Warnings and Precautions (5.9)]*
There are no adequate and well-controlled studies of Zometa in pregnant women. Zometa may cause fetal harm when administered to a pregnant woman. Bisphosphonates, such as Zometa, are incorporated into the bone matrix and are gradually released over periods of weeks to years. The extent of bisphosphonate incorporation into adult bone, and hence, the amount available for release back into the systemic circulation, is directly related to the total dose and duration of bisphosphonate use. Although there are no data on fetal risk in humans, bisphosphonates do cause fetal harm in animals, and animal data suggest that uptake of bisphosphonates into fetal bone is greater than into maternal bone. Therefore, there is a theoretical risk of fetal harm (e.g., skeletal and other abnormalities) if a woman becomes pregnant after completing a course of bisphosphonate therapy. The impact of variables such as time between cessation of bisphosphonate therapy to conception, the particular bisphosphonate used, and the route of administration (intravenous versus oral) on this risk has not been established. If this drug is used during pregnancy or if the patient becomes pregnant while taking or after taking this drug, the patient should be apprised of the potential hazard to the fetus.

In female rats given subcutaneous doses of zoledronic acid of 0.01, 0.03, or 0.1 mg/kg/day beginning 15 days before mating and continuing through gestation, the number of stillbirths was increased and survival of neonates was decreased in the mid- and high-dose groups ($\geq$0.2 times the human systemic exposure following an intravenous dose of 4 mg, based on an AUC comparison). Adverse maternal effects were observed in all dose groups (with a systemic exposure of $\geq$0.07 times the human systemic exposure following an intravenous dose of 4 mg, based on an AUC comparison) and included dystocia and periparturient mortality in pregnant rats allowed to deliver. Maternal mortality may have been related to drug-induced inhibition of skeletal calcium mobilization, resulting in periparturient hypocalcemia. This appears to be a bisphosphonate-class effect.

In pregnant rats given a subcutaneous dose of zoledronic acid of 0.1, 0.2, or 0.4 mg/kg/day during gestation, adverse fetal effects were observed in the mid- and high-dose groups (with systemic exposures of 2.4 and 4.8 times, respectively, the human systemic exposure following an intravenous dose of 4 mg, based on an AUC comparison). These adverse effects included increases in pre- and postimplantation losses, decreases in viable fetuses, and fetal skeletal, visceral, and external malformations. Fetal skeletal effects observed in the high-dose group included unossified or incompletely ossified bones, thickened, curved, or shortened bones, wavy ribs, and shortened jaw. Other adverse fetal effects observed in the high-dose group included reduced lens, rudimentary cerebellum, reduction or absence of liver lobes, reduction of lung lobes, vessel dilation, cleft palate, and edema. Skeletal variations were also observed in the low-dose group (with systemic exposure of 1.2 times the human systemic exposure following an intravenous dose of 4 mg, based on an AUC comparison). Signs of maternal toxicity were observed in the high-dose group and included reduced body weights and food consumption, indicating that maximal exposure levels were achieved in this study.

In pregnant rabbits given subcutaneous doses of zoledronic acid of 0.01, 0.03, or 0.1 mg/kg/day during gestation ($\leq$0.5 times the human intravenous dose of 4 mg, based on a comparison of relative body surface areas), no adverse fetal effects were observed. Maternal mortality and abortion occurred in all treatment groups (at doses $\geq$0.05 times the human intravenous dose of 4 mg, based on a comparison of relative body surface areas). Adverse maternal effects were associated with, and may have been caused by, drug-induced hypocalcemia.

8.3 Nursing Mothers

It is not known whether zoledronic acid is excreted in human milk. Because many drugs are excreted in human milk, and because of the potential for serious adverse reactions in nursing infants from Zometa, a decision should be made to discontinue nursing or to discontinue the drug, taking into account the importance of the drug to the mother. Zoledronic acid binds to bone long term and may be released over weeks to years.

Table 7: Percentage of Patients with Adverse Events ≥10% Reported in Three Bone Metastases Clinical Trials by Body System

	Zometa 4 mg n (%)		Pamidronate 90 mg n (%)		Placebo n (%)	
Patients Studied						
Total No. of Patients	1031	(100)	556	(100)	455	(100)
Total No. of Patients with any AE	1015	(98)	548	(99)	445	(98)
Blood and Lymphatic						
Anemia	344	(33)	175	(32)	128	(28)
Neutropenia	124	(12)	83	(15)	35	(8)
Thrombocytopenia	102	(10)	53	(10)	20	(4)
Gastrointestinal						
Nausea	476	(46)	266	(48)	171	(38)
Vomiting	333	(32)	183	(33)	122	(27)
Constipation	320	(31)	162	(29)	174	(38)
Diarrhea	249	(24)	162	(29)	83	(18)
Abdominal Pain	143	(14)	81	(15)	48	(11)
Dyspepsia	105	(10)	74	(13)	31	(7)
Stomatitis	86	(8)	65	(12)	14	(3)
Sore Throat	82	(8)	61	(11)	17	(4)
General Disorders and Administration Site						
Fatigue	398	(39)	240	(43)	130	(29)
Pyrexia	328	(32)	172	(31)	89	(20)
Weakness	252	(24)	108	(19)	114	(25)
Edema Lower Limb	215	(21)	126	(23)	84	(19)
Rigors	112	(11)	62	(11)	28	(6)
Infections						
Urinary Tract Infection	124	(12)	50	(9)	41	(9)
Upper Respiratory Tract Infection	101	(10)	82	(15)	30	(7)
Metabolism						
Anorexia	231	(22)	81	(15)	105	(23)
Weight Decreased	164	(16)	50	(9)	61	(13)
Dehydration	145	(14)	60	(11)	59	(13)
Appetite Decreased	130	(13)	48	(9)	45	(10)
Musculoskeletal						
Bone Pain	569	(55)	316	(57)	284	(62)
Myalgia	239	(23)	143	(26)	74	(16)
Arthralgia	216	(21)	131	(24)	73	(16)
Back Pain	156	(15)	106	(19)	40	(9)
Pain in Limb	143	(14)	84	(15)	52	(11)
Neoplasms						
Malignant Neoplasm Aggravated	205	(20)	97	(17)	89	(20)
Nervous						
Headache	191	(19)	149	(27)	50	(11)
Dizziness (excluding vertigo)	180	(18)	91	(16)	58	(13)
Insomnia	166	(16)	111	(20)	73	(16)
Paresthesia	149	(15)	85	(15)	35	(8)
Hypoesthesia	127	(12)	65	(12)	43	(10)
Psychiatric						
Depression	146	(14)	95	(17)	49	(11)
Anxiety	112	(11)	73	(13)	37	(8)
Confusion	74	(7)	39	(7)	47	(10)
Respiratory						
Dyspnea	282	(27)	155	(28)	107	(24)
Cough	224	(22)	129	(23)	65	(14)
Skin						
Alopecia	125	(12)	80	(14)	36	(8)
Dermatitis	114	(11)	74	(13)	38	(8)

Table 8: Grade 3 Laboratory Abnormalities for Serum Creatinine, Serum Calcium, Serum Phosphorus, and Serum Magnesium in Three Clinical Trials in Patients with Bone Metastases

			Grade 3			
Laboratory Parameter	Zometa 4 mg		Pamidronate 90 mg		Placebo	
	n/N	(%)	n/N	(%)	n/N	(%)
Serum Creatinine[1]*	7/529	(1%)	4/268	(2%)	4/241	(2%)
Hypocalcemia[2]	6/973	(<1%)	4/536	(<1%)	0/415	—
Hypophosphatemia[3]	115/973	(12%)	38/537	(7%)	14/415	(3%)
Hypermagnesemia[4]	19/971	(2%)	2/535	(<1%)	8/415	(2%)
Hypomagnesemia[5]	1/971	(<1%)	0/535	—	1/415	(<1%)

[1] Grade 3 (greater than 3× Upper Limit of Normal); Grade 4 (greater than 6× Upper Limit of Normal)
* Serum creatinine data for all patients randomized after the 15-minute infusion amendment
[2] Grade 3 (less than 7 mg/dL); Grade 4 (less than 6 mg/dL)
[3] Grade 3 (less than 2 mg/dL); Grade 4 (less than 1 mg/dL)
[4] Grade 3 (greater than 3 mEq/L); Grade 4 (greater than 8 mEq/L)
[5] Grade 3 (less than 0.9 mEq/L); Grade 4 (less than 0.7 mEq/L)

8.4 Pediatric Use

Zometa is not indicated for use in children.
The safety and effectiveness of zoledronic acid was studied in a one-year, active-controlled trial of 152 pediatric subjects (74 receiving zoledronic acid). The enrolled population was subjects with severe osteogenesis imperfecta, aged 1-17 years, 55% male, 84% Caucasian, with a mean lumbar spine bone mineral density (BMD) of 0.431 gm/cm^2, which is 2.7 standard deviations below the mean for age-matched controls (BMD Z-score of -2.7). At one year, increases in BMD were observed in the zoledronic acid treatment group. However, changes in BMD in individual patients with severe osteogenesis imperfecta did not necessarily correlate with the risk for fracture or the incidence or severity of chronic bone pain. The adverse events observed with Zometa use in children did not raise any new safety findings beyond those previously seen in adults treated for hypercalcemia of malignancy or bone metastases. However, adverse reactions seen

Table 9: Grade 4 Laboratory Abnormalities for Serum Creatinine, Serum Calcium, Serum Phosphorus, and Serum Magnesium in Three Clinical Trials in Patients with Bone Metastases

| Laboratory Parameter | Grade 4 | | | | | |
| | Zometa 4 mg | | Pamidronate 90 mg | | Placebo | |
	n/N	(%)	n/N	(%)	n/N	(%)
Serum Creatinine[1]*	2/529	(<1%)	1/268	(<1%)	0/241	—
Hypocalcemia[2]	7/973	(<1%)	3/536	(<1%)	2/415	(<1%)
Hypophosphatemia[3]	5/973	(<1%)	0/537	—	1/415	(<1%)
Hypermagnesemia[4]	0/971	—	0/535	—	2/415	(<1%)
Hypomagnesemia[5]	2/971	(<1%)	1/535	(<1%)	0/415	—

[1] Grade 3 (greater than 3× Upper Limit of Normal); Grade 4 (greater than 6× Upper Limit of Normal)
* Serum creatinine data for all patients randomized after the 15-minute infusion amendment
[2] Grade 3 (less than 7 mg/dL); Grade 4 (less than 6 mg/dL)
[3] Grade 3 (less than 2 mg/dL); Grade 4 (less than 1 mg/dL)
[4] Grade 3 (greater than 3 mEq/L); Grade 4 (greater than 8 mEq/L)
[5] Grade 3 (less than 0.9 mEq/L); Grade 4 (less than 0.7 mEq/L)

Table 10: Percentage of Patients with Treatment-Emergent Renal Function Deterioration by Baseline Serum Creatinine*

Patient Population/Baseline Creatinine				
Multiple Myeloma and Breast Cancer	Zometa 4 mg		Pamidronate 90 mg	
	n/N	(%)	n/N	(%)
Normal	27/246	(11%)	23/246	(9%)
Abnormal	2/26	(8%)	2/22	(9%)
Total	29/272	(11%)	25/268	(9%)
Solid Tumors	Zometa 4 mg		Placebo	
	n/N	(%)	n/N	(%)
Normal	17/154	(11%)	10/143	(7%)
Abnormal	1/11	(9%)	1/20	(5%)
Total	18/165	(11%)	11/163	(7%)
Prostate Cancer	Zometa 4 mg		Placebo	
	n/N	(%)	n/N	(%)
Normal	12/82	(15%)	8/68	(12%)
Abnormal	4/10	(40%)	2/10	(20%)
Total	16/92	(17%)	10/78	(13%)

*Table includes only patients who were randomized to the trial after a protocol amendment that lengthened the infusion duration of Zometa to 15 minutes.

more commonly in pediatric patients included pyrexia (61%), arthralgia (26%), hypocalcemia (22%) and headache (22%). These reactions, excluding arthralgia, occurred most frequently within 3 days after the first infusion and became less common with repeat dosing. Because of long-term retention in bone, Zometa should only be used in children if the potential benefit outweighs the potential risk.

Plasma zoledronic acid concentration data was obtained from 10 patients with severe osteogenesis imperfecta (4 in the age group of 3-8 years and 6 in the age group of 9-17 years) infused with 0.05 mg/kg dose over 30 min. Mean C_{max} and $AUC_{(0-last)}$ was 167 ng/mL and 220 ng•h/mL, respectively. The plasma concentration time profile of zoledronic acid in pediatric patients represent a multi-exponential decline, as observed in adult cancer patients at an approximately equivalent mg/kg dose.

8.5   Geriatric Use

Clinical studies of Zometa in hypercalcemia of malignancy included 34 patients who were 65 years of age or older. No significant differences in response rate or adverse reactions were seen in geriatric patients receiving Zometa as compared to younger patients. Controlled clinical studies of Zometa in the treatment of multiple myeloma and bone metastases of solid tumors in patients over age 65 revealed similar efficacy and safety in older and younger patients. Because decreased renal function occurs more commonly in the elderly, special care should be taken to monitor renal function.

10   OVERDOSAGE

Clinical experience with acute overdosage of Zometa is limited. Two patients received Zometa 32 mg over 5 minutes in clinical trials. Neither patient experienced any clinical or laboratory toxicity. Overdosage may cause clinically significant hypocalcemia, hypophosphatemia, and hypomagnesemia. Clinically relevant reductions in serum levels of calcium, phosphorus, and magnesium should be corrected by intravenous administration of calcium gluconate, potassium or sodium phosphate, and magnesium sulfate, respectively. In an open-label study of zoledronic acid 4 mg in breast cancer patients, a female patient received a single 48-mg dose of zoledronic acid in error. Two days after the overdose, the patient experienced a single episode of hyperthermia (38°C), which resolved after treatment. All other evaluations were normal, and the patient was discharged seven days after the overdose.

A patient with non-Hodgkin's lymphoma received zoledronic acid 4 mg daily on four successive days for a total dose of 16 mg. The patient developed paresthesia and abnormal liver function tests with increased GGT (nearly 100 U/L, each value unknown). The outcome of this case is not known.

In controlled clinical trials, administration of Zometa 4 mg as an intravenous infusion over 5 minutes has been shown to increase the risk of renal toxicity compared to the same dose administered as a 15-minute intravenous infusion. In controlled clinical trials, Zometa 8 mg has been shown to be associated with an increased risk of renal toxicity compared to Zometa 4 mg, even when given as a 15-minute intravenous infusion, and was not associated with added benefit in patients with hypercalcemia of malignancy [see Dosage and Administration (2.4)].

11   DESCRIPTION

Zometa contains zoledronic acid, a bisphosphonic acid which is an inhibitor of osteoclastic bone resorption. Zoledronic acid is designated chemically as (1-Hydroxy-2-imidazol-1-yl-phosphonoethyl) phosphonic acid monohydrate and its structural formula is:

Zoledronic acid is a white crystalline powder. Its molecular formula is $C_5H_{10}N_2O_7P_2•H_2O$ and its molar mass is 290.1g/mol. Zoledronic acid is highly soluble in 0.1N sodium hydroxide solution, sparingly soluble in water and 0.1N hydrochloric acid, and practically insoluble in organic solvents. The pH of a 0.7% solution of zoledronic acid in water is approximately 2.0.

Zometa is available in 100 mL bottles as a sterile liquid ready-to-use solution for intravenous infusion and in 5 mL vials as a sterile liquid concentrate solution for intravenous infusion.

• Each 100 mL ready-to-use bottle contains 4.264 mg zoledronic acid monohydrate, corresponding to 4 mg zoledronic acid on an anhydrous basis, 5100 mg of mannitol, USP, water for injection, and 24 mg of sodium citrate, USP.

• Each 5 mL concentrate vial contains 4.264 mg zoledronic acid monohydrate, corresponding to 4 mg zoledronic acid on an anhydrous basis, 220 mg of mannitol, USP, water for injection, and 24 mg of sodium citrate, USP.

Inactive Ingredients: mannitol, USP, as bulking agent, water for injection, and sodium citrate, USP, as buffering agent.

12   CLINICAL PHARMACOLOGY

12.1   Mechanism of Action

The principal pharmacologic action of zoledronic acid is inhibition of bone resorption. Although the antiresorptive mechanism is not completely understood, several factors are thought to contribute to this action. In vitro, zoledronic acid inhibits osteoclastic activity and induces osteoclast apoptosis. Zoledronic acid also blocks the osteoclastic resorption of mineralized bone and cartilage through its binding to bone. Zoledronic acid inhibits the increased osteoclastic activity and skeletal calcium release induced by various stimulatory factors released by tumors.

12.2   Pharmacodynamics

Clinical studies in patients with hypercalcemia of malignancy (HCM) showed that single-dose infusions of Zometa are associated with decreases in serum calcium and phosphorus and increases in urinary calcium and phosphorus excretion.

Osteoclastic hyperactivity resulting in excessive bone resorption is the underlying pathophysiologic derangement in hypercalcemia of malignancy (HCM, tumor-induced hypercalcemia) and metastatic bone disease. Excessive release of calcium into the blood as bone is resorbed results in polyuria and gastrointestinal disturbances, with progressive dehydration and decreasing glomerular filtration rate. This, in turn, results in increased renal resorption of calcium, setting up a cycle of worsening systemic hypercalcemia. Reducing excessive bone resorption and maintaining adequate fluid administration are, therefore, essential to the management of hypercalcemia of malignancy.

Patients who have hypercalcemia of malignancy can generally be divided into two groups according to the pathophysiologic mechanism involved: humoral hypercalcemia and hypercalcemia due to tumor invasion of bone. In humoral hypercalcemia, osteoclasts are activated and bone resorption is stimulated by factors such as parathyroid hormone-related protein, which are elaborated by the tumor and circulate systemically. Humoral hypercalcemia usually occurs in squamous cell malignancies of the lung or head and neck or in genitourinary tumors such as renal cell carcinoma or ovarian cancer. Skeletal metastases may be absent or minimal in these patients.

Extensive invasion of bone by tumor cells can also result in hypercalcemia due to local tumor products that stimulate bone resorption by osteoclasts. Tumors commonly associated with locally mediated hypercalcemia include breast cancer and multiple myeloma.

Total serum calcium levels in patients who have hypercalcemia of malignancy may not reflect the severity of hypercalcemia, since concomitant hypoalbuminemia is commonly present. Ideally, ionized calcium levels should be used to diagnose and follow hypercalcemic conditions; however, these are not commonly or rapidly available in many clinical situations. Therefore, adjustment of the total serum calcium value for differences in albumin levels (corrected serum calcium, CSC) is often used in place of measurement of ionized calcium; several nomograms are in use for this type of calculation [see Dosage and Administration (2.1)].

12.3   Pharmacokinetics

Pharmacokinetic data in patients with hypercalcemia are not available.

Distribution

Single or multiple (q 28 days) 5-minute or 15-minute infusions of 2, 4, 8, or 16 mg Zometa were given to 64 patients with cancer and bone metastases. The postinfusion decline of zoledronic acid concentrations in plasma was consistent with a triphasic process showing a rapid decrease from peak concentrations at end of infusion to less than 1% of C_{max} 24 hours postinfusion with population half-lives of $t_{1/2\alpha}$ 0.24 hours and $t_{1/2\beta}$ 1.87 hours for the early disposition phases of the drug. The terminal elimination phase of zoledronic acid was prolonged, with very low concentrations in plasma between Days 2 and 28 postinfusion, and a terminal elimination half-life $t_{1/2\gamma}$ of 146 hours. The area under the plasma concentration versus time curve (AUC_{0-24h}) of zoledronic acid was dose proportional from 2-16 mg. The accumulation of zoledronic acid measured over three cycles was low, with mean AUC_{0-24h} ratios for cycles 2 and 3 versus 1 of 1.13 ± 0.30 and 1.16 ± 0.36, respectively.

In vitro and ex vivo studies showed low affinity of zoledronic acid for the cellular components of human blood, with a mean blood to plasma concentration ratio of 0.59 in a concentration range of 30 ng/mL to 5000 ng/mL. In vitro, the plasma protein binding is low, with the unbound fraction ranging from 60% at 2 ng/mL to 77% at 2000 ng/mL of zoledronic acid.

Metabolism

Zoledronic acid does not inhibit human P450 enzymes *in vitro*. Zoledronic acid does not undergo biotransformation *in vivo*. In animal studies, less than 3% of the administered intravenous dose was found in the feces, with the balance either recovered in the urine or taken up by bone, indicating that the drug is eliminated intact via the kidney. Following an intravenous dose of 20 nCi ^{14}C-zoledronic acid in a patient with cancer and bone metastases, only a single radioactive species with chromatographic properties identical to those of parent drug was recovered in urine, which suggests that zoledronic acid is not metabolized.

Excretion

In 64 patients with cancer and bone metastases, on average (± SD) 39 ± 16% of the administered zoledronic acid dose was recovered in the urine within 24 hours, with only trace amounts of drug found in urine post-Day 2. The cumulative percent of drug excreted in the urine over 0-24 hours was independent of dose. The balance of drug not recovered in urine over 0-24 hours, representing drug presumably bound to bone, is slowly released back into the systemic circulation, giving rise to the observed prolonged low plasma concentrations. The 0-24 hour renal clearance of zoledronic acid was 3.7 ± 2.0 L/h.

Zoledronic acid clearance was independent of dose but dependent upon the patient's creatinine clearance. In a study in patients with cancer and bone metastases, increasing the infusion time of a 4-mg dose of zoledronic acid from 5 minutes (n=5) to 15 minutes (n=7) resulted in a 34% decrease in the zoledronic acid concentration at the end of the infusion ([mean ± SD] 403 ± 118 ng/mL versus 264 ± 86 ng/mL) and a 10% increase in the total AUC (378 ± 116 ng × h/mL versus 420 ± 218 ng × h/mL). The difference between the AUC means was not statistically significant.

Special Populations

Pediatrics

Zometa is not indicated for use in children *[see Use in Specific Populations (8.4)]*.

Geriatrics

The pharmacokinetics of zoledronic acid were not affected by age in patients with cancer and bone metastases who ranged in age from 38 years to 84 years.

Race

Population pharmacokinetic analyses did not indicate any differences in pharmacokinetics among Japanese and North American (Caucasian and African American) patients with cancer and bone metastases.

Hepatic Insufficiency

No clinical studies were conducted to evaluate the effect of hepatic impairment on the pharmacokinetics of zoledronic acid.

Renal Insufficiency

The pharmacokinetic studies conducted in 64 cancer patients represented typical clinical populations with normal to moderately impaired renal function. Compared to patients with normal renal function (N=37), patients with mild renal impairment (N=15) showed an average increase in plasma AUC of 15%, whereas patients with moderate renal impairment (N=11) showed an average increase in plasma AUC of 43%. Limited pharmacokinetic data are available for Zometa in patients with severe renal impairment (creatinine clearance less than 30 mL/min). Based on population PK/PD modeling, the risk of renal deterioration appears to increase with AUC, which is doubled at a creatinine clearance of 10 mL/min. Creatinine clearance is calculated by the Cockcroft-Gault formula:

[See first table above]

Zometa systemic clearance in individual patients can be calculated from the population clearance of Zometa, CL $(L/h)=6.5(CrCl/90)^{0.4}$. These formulae can be used to predict the Zometa AUC in patients, where $CL=Dose/AUC_{0-\infty}$. The average AUC_{0-24} in patients with normal renal function was 0.42 mg•h/L and the calculated $AUC_{0-\infty}$ for a patient with creatinine clearance of 75 mL/min was 0.66 mg•h/L following a 4-mg dose of Zometa. However, efficacy and safety of adjusted dosing based on these formulae have not been prospectively assessed *[see Warnings and Precautions (5.3)]*.

13 NONCLINICAL TOXICOLOGY

13.1 Carcinogenesis, Mutagenesis, Impairment of Fertility

Standard lifetime carcinogenicity bioassays were conducted in mice and rats. Mice were given oral doses of zoledronic acid of 0.1, 0.5, or 2.0 mg/kg/day. There was an increased incidence of Harderian gland adenomas in males and females in all treatment groups (at doses ≥0.002 times a human intravenous dose of 4 mg, based on a comparison of relative body surface areas). Rats were given oral doses of zoledronic acid of 0.1, 0.5, or 2.0 mg/kg/day. No increased incidence of tumors was observed (at doses ≤0.2 times the human intravenous dose of 4 mg, based on a comparison of relative body surface areas).

Zoledronic acid was not genotoxic in the Ames bacterial mutagenicity assay, in the Chinese hamster ovary cell assay, or in the Chinese hamster gene mutation assay, with or without metabolic activation. Zoledronic acid was not genotoxic in the *in vivo* rat micronucleus assay.

Female rats were given subcutaneous doses of zoledronic acid of 0.01, 0.03, or 0.1 mg/kg/day beginning 15 days before mating and continuing through gestation. Effects observed in the high-dose group (with systemic exposure of 1.2 times the human systemic exposure following an intravenous dose of 4 mg, based on AUC comparison) included inhibition of ovulation and a decrease in the number of pregnant rats. Effects observed in both the mid-dose group (with systemic exposure of 0.2 times the human systemic exposure following an intravenous dose of 4 mg, based on an AUC comparison) and high-dose group included an increase in preimplantation losses and a decrease in the number of implantations and live fetuses.

14 CLINICAL STUDIES

14.1 Hypercalcemia of Malignancy

Two identical multicenter, randomized, double-blind, double-dummy studies of Zometa 4 mg given as a 5-minute intravenous infusion or pamidronate 90 mg given as a 2-hour intravenous infusion were conducted in 185 patients with hypercalcemia of malignancy (HCM). NOTE: Administration of Zometa 4 mg given as a 5-minute intravenous infusion has been shown to result in an increased risk of renal toxicity, as measured by increases in serum creatinine, which can progress to renal failure. The incidence of renal toxicity and renal failure has been shown to be reduced when Zometa 4 mg is given as a 15-minute intravenous infusion. Zometa should be administered by intravenous infusion over no less than 15 minutes *[see Warnings and Precautions (5.1 and 5.2) and Dosage and Administration (2.4)]*. The treatment groups in the clinical studies were generally well balanced with regards to age, sex, race, and tumor types. The mean age of the study population was 59 years; 81% were Caucasian, 15% were Black, and 4% were of other races. 60% of the patients were male. The most common tumor types were lung, breast, head and neck, and renal.

In these studies, HCM was defined as a corrected serum calcium (CSC) concentration of greater than or equal to 12.0 mg/dL (3.00 mmol/L). The primary efficacy variable was the proportion of patients having a complete response, defined as the lowering of the CSC to less than or equal to 10.8 mg/dL (2.70 mmol/L) within 10 days after drug infusion.

To assess the effects of Zometa versus those of pamidronate, the two multicenter HCM studies were combined in a pre-planned analysis. The results of the primary analysis revealed that the proportion of patients that had normalization of corrected serum calcium by Day 10 were 88% and 70% for Zometa 4 mg and pamidronate 90 mg, respectively (P=0.002) (see Figure 1). In these studies, no additional benefit was seen for Zometa 8 mg over Zometa 4 mg; however, the risk of renal toxicity of Zometa 8 mg was significantly greater than that seen with Zometa 4 mg.

$$CrCl= \frac{[140\text{-age (years)}] \times \text{weight (kg)}}{[72 \times \text{serum creatinine (mg/dL)}]} \quad [\times\ 0.85\ \text{for female patients}]$$

Table 11: Secondary Efficacy Variables in Pooled HCM Studies

	Zometa 4 mg		Pamidronate 90 mg	
Complete Response	N	Response Rate	N	Response Rate
By Day 4	86	45.3%	99	33.3%
By Day 7	86	82.6%*	99	63.6%
Duration of Response	N	Median Duration (Days)	N	Median Duration (Days)
Time to Relapse	86	30*	99	17
Duration of Complete Response	76	32	69	18

* P less than 0.05 versus pamidronate 90 mg.

Table 12: Overview of Efficacy Population for Phase III Studies

Patient Population	No. of Patients	Zometa Dose	Control	Median Duration (Planned Duration) Zometa 4 mg
Multiple myeloma or metastatic breast cancer	1,648	4 and 8* mg Q3-4 weeks	Pamidronate 90 mg Q3-4 weeks	12.0 months (13 months)
Metastatic prostate cancer	643	4 and 8* mg Q3 weeks	Placebo	10.5 months (15 months)
Metastatic solid tumor other than breast or prostate cancer	773	4 and 8* mg Q3 weeks	Placebo	3.8 months (9 months)

* Patients who were randomized to the 8 mg Zometa group are not included in any of the analyses in this package insert.

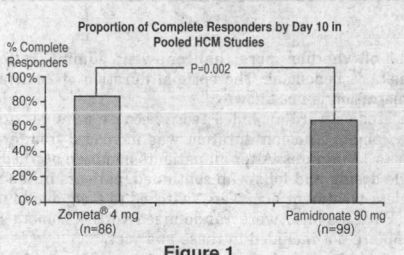

Figure 1

Proportion of Complete Responders by Day 10 in Pooled HCM Studies — P=0.002 — Zometa® 4 mg (n=86); Pamidronate 90 mg (n=99); % Complete Responders

Secondary efficacy variables from the pooled HCM studies included the proportion of patients who had normalization of corrected serum calcium (CSC) by Day 4; the proportion of patients who had normalization of CSC by Day 7; time to relapse of HCM; and duration of complete response. Time to relapse of HCM was defined as the duration (in days) of normalization of serum calcium from study drug infusion until the last CSC value less than 11.6 mg/dL (less than 2.90 mmol/L). Patients who did not have a complete response were assigned a time to relapse of 0 days. Duration of complete response was defined as the duration (in days) from the occurrence of a complete response until the last CSC ≤10.8 mg/dL (2.70 mmol/L). The results of these secondary analyses for Zometa 4 mg and pamidronate 90 mg are shown in Table 11.

[See table 11 above]

14.2 Clinical Trials in Multiple Myeloma and Bone Metastases of Solid Tumors

Table 12 describes an overview of the efficacy population in three randomized Zometa trials in patients with multiple myeloma and bone metastases of solid tumors. These trials included a pamidronate-controlled study in breast cancer and multiple myeloma, a placebo-controlled study in prostate cancer, and a placebo-controlled study in other solid tumors. The prostate cancer study required documentation of previous bone metastases and 3 consecutive rising PSAs while on hormonal therapy. The other placebo-controlled solid tumor study included patients with bone metastases from malignancies other than breast cancer and prostate cancer, including NSCLC, renal cell cancer, small cell lung cancer, colorectal cancer, bladder cancer, GI/genitourinary cancer, head and neck cancer, and others. These trials were comprised of a core phase and an extension phase. In the solid tumor, breast cancer and multiple myeloma trials, only the core phase was evaluated for efficacy as a high percentage of patients did not choose to participate in the extension phase. In the prostate cancer trials, both the core and extension phases were evaluated for efficacy showing the Zometa effect during the first 15 months was maintained without decrement or improvement for another 9 months. The design of these clinical trials does not permit assess-

Table 13: Zometa Compared to Placebo in Patients with Bone Metastases from Prostate Cancer or Other Solid Tumors

Study	Study Arm & Patient Number	I. Analysis of Proportion of Patients with a SRE[1]			II. Analysis of Time to the First SRE		
		Proportion	Difference[2] & 95% CI	P-value	Median (Days)	Hazard Ratio[3] & 95% CI	P-value
Prostate Cancer	Zometa 4 mg (n=214)	33%	-11% (-20%, -1%)	0.02	Not Reached	0.67 (0.49, 0.91)	0.011
	Placebo (n=208)	44%			321		
Solid Tumors	Zometa 4 mg (n=257)	38%	-7% (-15%, 2%)	0.13	230	0.73 (0.55, 0.96)	0.023
	Placebo (n=250)	44%			163		

[1]SRE=Skeletal-Related Event
[2]Difference for the proportion of patients with a SRE of Zometa 4 mg versus placebo.
[3]Hazard ratio for the first occurrence of a SRE of Zometa 4 mg versus placebo.

Table 14: Zometa Compared to Pamidronate in Patients with Multiple Myeloma or Bone Metastases from Breast Cancer

Study	Study Arm & Patient Number	I. Analysis of Proportion of Patients with a SRE[1]			II. Analysis of Time to the First SRE		
		Proportion	Difference[2] & 95% CI	P-value	Median (Days)	Hazard Ratio[3] & 95% CI	P-value
Multiple Myeloma & Breast Cancer	Zometa 4 mg (n=561)	44%	-2% (-7.9%, 3.7%)	0.46	373	0.92 (0.77, 1.09)	0.32
	Pamidronate (n=555)	46%			363		

[1]SRE=Skeletal-Related Event
[2]Difference for the proportion of patients with a SRE of Zometa 4 mg versus pamidronate 90 mg.
[3]Hazard ratio for the first occurrence of a SRE of Zometa 4 mg versus pamidronate 90 mg.

ment of whether more than one-year administration of Zometa is beneficial. The optimal duration of Zometa administration is not known.

The studies were amended twice because of renal toxicity. The Zometa infusion duration was increased from 5 minutes to 15 minutes. After all patients had been accrued, but while dosing and follow-up continued, patients in the 8 mg Zometa treatment arm were switched to 4 mg due to toxicity. Patients who were randomized to the Zometa 8 mg group are not included in these analyses.
[See table 12 at top of previous page]
Each study evaluated skeletal-related events (SREs), defined as any of the following: pathologic fracture, radiation therapy to bone, surgery to bone, or spinal cord compression. Change in antineoplastic therapy due to increased pain was a SRE in the prostate cancer study only. Planned analyses included the proportion of patients with a SRE during the study and time to the first SRE. Results for the two Zometa placebo-controlled studies are given in Table 13. [See table 13 above]
In the breast cancer and myeloma trial, efficacy was determined by a noninferiority analysis comparing Zometa to pamidronate 90 mg for the proportion of patients with a SRE. This analysis required an estimation of pamidronate efficacy. Historical data from 1,128 patients in three pamidronate placebo-controlled trials demonstrated that pamidronate decreased the proportion of patients with a SRE by 13.1% (95% CI=7.3%, 18.9%). Results of the comparison of treatment with Zometa compared to pamidronate are given in Table 14.
[See table 14 above]

16　HOW SUPPLIED/STORAGE AND HANDLING

4 mg/100 mL single-use ready-to-use bottle
Carton of 1 bottle ....NDC 0078-0590-61
Store at 25°C (77°F); excursions permitted to 15-30°C (59-86°F) [see USP Controlled Room Temperature].

4 mg/5 mL single-use vial of concentrate
Carton of 1 vial...NDC 0078-0387-25
Store at 25°C (77°F); excursions permitted to 15-30°C (59-86°F) [see USP Controlled Room Temperature].

17　PATIENT COUNSELING INFORMATION

- Patients should be instructed to tell their doctor if they have kidney problems before being given Zometa.
- Patients should be informed of the importance of getting their blood tests (serum creatinine) during the course of their Zometa therapy.
- Zometa should not be given if the patient is pregnant or plans to become pregnant, or if she is breastfeeding.
- Patients should be advised to have a dental examination prior to treatment with Zometa and should avoid invasive dental procedures during treatment.
- Patients should be informed of the importance of good dental hygiene and routine dental care.

- Patients with multiple myeloma and bone metastasis of solid tumors should be advised to take an oral calcium supplement of 500 mg and a multiple vitamin containing 400 international units of Vitamin D daily.
- Patients should be advised to report any thigh, hip, or groin pain. It is unknown whether the risk of atypical femur fracture continues after stopping therapy.
- Patients should be aware of the most common side effects including: anemia, nausea, vomiting, constipation, diarrhea, fatigue, fever, weakness, lower limb edema, anorexia, decreased weight, bone pain, myalgia, arthralgia, back pain, malignant neoplasm aggravated, headache, dizziness, insomnia, paresthesia, dyspnea, cough, and abdominal pain.
- There have been reports of bronchoconstriction in aspirin-sensitive patients receiving bisphosphonates, including zoledronic acid. Before being given zoledronic acid, patients should tell their doctor if they are aspirin-sensitive.

Manufactured by
Novartis Pharma Stein AG
Stein, Switzerland for
Novartis Pharmaceuticals Corporation
East Hanover, New Jersey 07936
© Novartis
T2014-40
April 2014
Shown in Product Identification Guide, page 311

ZORTRESS®　　　　　　　　　　　　　　　　　　℞
[ZOR-tres]
(everolimus)
Tablets for oral use

The following prescribing information is based on official labeling in effect July 2013.
HIGHLIGHTS OF PRESCRIBING INFORMATION
These highlights do not include all the information needed to use ZORTRESS® (everolimus) safely and effectively. See full prescribing information for ZORTRESS.
ZORTRESS (everolimus) tablets for oral use.
Initial U.S. Approval: 2010

WARNING: MALIGNANCIES AND SERIOUS INFECTIONS, KIDNEY GRAFT THROMBOSIS; NEPHROTOXICITY; AND MORTALITY IN HEART TRANSPLANTATION
See Full Prescribing Information for Complete Boxed Warning

- Only physicians experienced in immunosuppressive therapy and management of transplant patients should use Zortress. (5.1)
- Increased susceptibility to infection and the possible development of malignancies may result from immunosuppression. (5.2, 5.3)

- Increased incidence of kidney graft thrombosis. (5.4)
- Reduced doses of cyclosporine are required for use in combination with Zortress in order to reduce nephrotoxicity. (2.1, 2.3, 5.6, 12.7, 12.8)
- Increased mortality in a heart transplant clinical trial. Use in heart transplantation is not recommended. (5.7)

RECENT MAJOR CHANGES

Boxed Warning:　Mortality in Heart Transplantation	04/2012
Indications and Usage:　Prophylaxis of Organ Rejection in Liver Transplantation (1.2)	02/2013
Warnings and Precautions (5.5)	02/2013
Warnings and Precautions (5.7, 5.13)	04/2012

INDICATIONS AND USAGE

- Zortress is indicated for the prophylaxis of organ rejection in adult patients:
- Kidney transplant:　at low-moderate immunologic risk. (1.1) Use in combination with basiliximab, cyclosporine (reduced doses) and corticosteroids.
- Liver transplant:　Administer no earlier than 30 days post-transplant. Use in combination with tacrolimus (reduced doses) and corticosteroids. (1.2, 5.5)
Limitations of Use (1.3)
Safety and efficacy has not been established in the following:
- Kidney transplant patients at high immunologic risk.
- Recipients of transplanted organs other than kidney or liver
- Pediatric patients (<18 years)

DOSAGE AND ADMINISTRATION

- Kidney transplantation:　starting oral dose of 0.75 mg twice daily as soon as possible after transplantation. (2.1)
- Liver transplantation:　starting oral dose of 1.0 mg twice daily starting 30 days after transplantation. (2.2)
- Monitor everolimus concentrations:　Adjust maintenance dose to achieve trough concentrations within the 3-8 ng/mL target range (using LC/MS/MS assay method (2.1, 2.2, 2.3)
- Administer consistently with or without food at the same time as cyclosporine or tacrolimus. (2.6, 12.5)
- Mild hepatic impairment:　Reduce initial daily dose by one-third. (2.7)
- Moderate or Severe hepatic impairment:　Reduce initial daily dose by one-half. (2.7)

DOSAGE FORMS AND STRENGTHS

Zortress is available as 0.25 mg, 0.5 mg, and 0.75 mg tablets. (3)

CONTRAINDICATIONS

- Hypersensitivity to everolimus, sirolimus, or to components of the drug product. (4)

WARNINGS AND PRECAUTIONS

- Angioedema (increased risk with concomitant ACE inhibitors):　Monitor for symptoms and treat promptly. (5.8)
- Delayed Wound Healing/Fluid Accumulation:　Monitor symptoms; treat promptly to minimize complications. (5.9)
- Interstitial Lung Disease/Non-Infectious Pneumonitis:　Monitor for symptoms or radiologic changes; manage by dose reduction or discontinuation until symptoms resolve; consider use of corticosteroids. (5.10)
- Hyperlipidemia (elevations of serum cholesterol and triglycerides):　Monitor and consider anti-lipid therapy. (5.11)
- Proteinuria (increased risk with higher trough concentrations):　Monitor urine protein. (5.12)
- Polyoma Virus Infections (activation of latent viral infections; BK-virus associated nephropathy):　Consider reducing immunosuppression. (5.13)
- TMA/TTP/HUS (concomitant use with cyclosporine may increase risk):　Monitor for hematological changes or symptoms. (5.15)
- New Onset Diabetes After Transplantation:　Monitor serum glucose. (5.16)
- Male Infertility:　Azospermia or oligospermia may occur. (5.17, 13.1)
- Immunizations:　Avoid live vaccines. (5.18)

ADVERSE REACTIONS

Most common adverse reactions were as follows:
Kidney transplantation (incidence ≥20%):　peripheral edema, constipation, hypertension, nausea, anemia, UTI, and hyperlipidemia. (6.1);
Liver transplantation (incidence>10%):　diarrhea, headache, peripheral edema, hypertension, nausea, pyrexia, abdominal pain, and leukopenia (6.1)

To report SUSPECTED ADVERSE REACTIONS, contact Novartis Pharmaceuticals Corporation at 1-888-669-6682 or FDA at 1-800-FDA-1088 or www.fda.gov/medwatch.

DRUG INTERACTIONS

Strong-moderate CYP3A4 inhibitors (e.g., cyclosporine, ketoconazole, erythromycin, verapamil) and CYP3A4 inducers (e.g., rifampin) may affect everolimus concentrations. Consider Zortress dose adjustment (5.14)

USE IN SPECIFIC POPULATIONS

- Pregnancy: Based on animal data may cause fetal harm. (8.1)
- Nursing Mothers: Discontinue drug or nursing. (8.3)

See 17 for PATIENT COUNSELING INFORMATION and Medication Guide

Revised: 02/2013

FULL PRESCRIBING INFORMATION: CONTENTS*
WARNING: MALIGNANCIES AND SERIOUS INFECTIONS, KIDNEY GRAFT THROMBOSIS; NEPHROTOXICITY; AND MORTALITY IN HEART TRANSPLANTATION

* Sections or subsections omitted from the full prescribing information are not listed

---

FULL PRESCRIBING INFORMATION

> **WARNING: MALIGNANCIES AND SERIOUS INFECTIONS, KIDNEY GRAFT THROMBOSIS; NEPHROTOXICITY; AND MORTALITY IN HEART TRANSPLANTATION**
>
> **Malignancies and Serious Infections**
> - Only physicians experienced in immunosuppressive therapy and management of transplant patients should prescribe Zortress. Patients receiving the drug should be managed in facilities equipped and staffed with adequate laboratory and supportive medical resources. The physician responsible for maintenance therapy should have complete information requisite for the follow-up of the patient. [*See Warnings and Precautions (5.1)*]
> - Increased susceptibility to infection and the possible development of malignancies such as lymphoma and skin cancer may result from immunosuppression. [*See Warnings and Precautions (5.2 and 5.3)*]
>
> **Kidney Graft Thrombosis**
> - An increased risk of kidney arterial and venous thrombosis, resulting in graft loss, was reported, mostly within the first 30 days post-transplantation. [*See Warnings and Precautions (5.4)*]
>
> **Nephrotoxicity**
> - Increased nephrotoxicity can occur with use of standard doses of cyclosporine in combination with Zortress. Therefore reduced doses of cyclosporine should be used in combination with Zortress in order to reduce renal dysfunction. It is important to monitor the cyclosporine and everolimus whole blood trough concentrations. [*See Dosage and Administration (2.2 and 2.3) and Warnings and Precautions (5.5) and Clinical Pharmacology (12.7 and 12.8)*]
>
> **Mortality in Heart Transplantation**
> - Increased mortality, often associated with serious infections, within the first three months post-transplantation was observed in a clinical trial of *de novo* heart transplant patients receiving immunosuppressive regimens with or without induction therapy. Use in heart transplantation is not recommended. [*See Warnings and Precautions (5.7)*]

1   INDICATIONS AND USAGE

1.1   Prophylaxis of Organ Rejection in Kidney Transplantation

Zortress is indicated for the prophylaxis of organ rejection in adult patients at low-moderate immunologic risk receiving a kidney transplant. [*See Clinical Studies (14.1)*] Zortress is to be administered in combination with basiliximab induction and concurrently with reduced doses of cyclosporine and with corticosteroids. Therapeutic drug monitoring of everolimus and cyclosporine is recommended for all patients receiving these products. [*See Dosage and Administration (2.2 and 2.3)*]

1.2   Prophylaxis of Organ Rejection in Liver Transplantation

Zortress is indicated for the prophylaxis of allograft rejection in adult patients receiving a liver transplant. Zortress is to be administered no earlier than 30 days post-transplant concurrently in combination with reduced doses of tacrolimus and with corticosteroids [*See Warnings and Precautions (5.5) and Clinical Studies (14.2)*]. Therapeutic drug monitoring of everolimus and tacrolimus is recommended for all patients receiving these products. [*See Dosage and Administration (2.3 and 2.5)*]

1.3   Limitations of Use

The safety and efficacy of Zortress has not been established in the following populations:

  Kidney transplant patients at high immunologic risk
  Recipients of transplanted organs other than kidney and liver [*See Warnings and Precautions (5.7)*]
  Pediatric patients (<18 years).

2   DOSAGE AND ADMINISTRATION

Patients receiving Zortress may require dose adjustments based on everolimus blood concentrations achieved, tolerability, individual response, change in concomitant medications and the clinical situation. Optimally, dose adjustments of Zortress should be based on trough concentrations obtained 4 or 5 days after a previous dosing change. [*See Therapeutic Drug Monitoring (2.3)*]

2.1   Dosage in Adult Kidney Transplant Patients

An initial Zortress dose of 0.75 mg orally twice daily (1.5 mg per day) is recommended for adult kidney transplant patients in combination with reduced dose cyclosporine, administered as soon as possible after transplantation. [*See Therapeutic Drug Monitoring (2.3 and 2.4), Clinical Studies (14.1)*]

Oral prednisone should be initiated once oral medication is tolerated. Steroid doses may be further tapered on an individualized basis depending on the clinical status of patient and function of graft.

2.2   Dosage in Adult Liver Transplant Patients

Start Zortress at least 30 days post-transplant. An initial dose of 1.0 mg orally twice daily (2.0 mg per day) is recommended for adult liver transplant patients in combination with reduced dose tacrolimus. [*See Therapeutic Drug Monitoring (2.3 and 2.5), Clinical Studies (14.2)*]

Steroid doses may be further tapered on an individualized basis depending on the clinical status of patient and function of graft.

2.3   Therapeutic Drug Monitoring - Everolimus

Routine everolimus whole blood therapeutic drug concentration monitoring is recommended for all patients. The recommended everolimus therapeutic range is 3 to 8 ng/mL. [*See Clinical Pharmacology (12.7)*] Careful attention should be made to clinical signs and symptoms, tissue biopsies, and laboratory parameters. It is important to monitor everolimus blood concentrations, in patients with hepatic impairment, during concomitant administration of CYP3A4 inducers or inhibitors, when switching cyclosporine formulations and/or when cyclosporine dosing is reduced according to recommended target concentrations. [*See Clinical Pharmacology (12.7 and 12.8)*]

There is an interaction of cyclosporine on everolimus, and consequently, everolimus concentrations may decrease if cyclosporine exposure is reduced. There is little to no pharmacokinetic interaction of tacrolimus on everolimus, and thus, everolimus concentrations do not decrease if the tacrolimus exposure is reduced. [*See Drug Interactions (7.2)*]

The everolimus recommended therapeutic range of 3 to 8 ng/mL is based on an LC/MS/MS assay method. Currently in clinical practice, everolimus whole blood trough concentrations may be measured by chromatographic or immunoassay methodologies. Because the measured everolimus whole blood trough concentrations depend on the assay used, individual patient sample concentration values from different assays may not be interchangeable. Consideration of assay results must be made with knowledge of the specific assay used. Therefore, communication should be maintained with the laboratory performing the assay.

2.4   Therapeutic Drug Monitoring- Cyclosporine in Kidney Transplant Patients

Both cyclosporine doses and the target range for whole blood trough concentrations should be reduced, when given in a regimen with Zortress, in order to minimize the risk of nephrotoxicity. [*See Warnings and Precautions (5.6) and Drug Interactions (7.2), Clinical Pharmacology (12.8)*]

The recommended cyclosporine therapeutic ranges when administered and with Zortress are 100 to 200 ng/mL through

Month 1 post-transplant, 75 to 150 ng/mL at Months 2 and 3 post-transplant, 50 to 100 ng/mL at Month 4 post-transplant, and 25 to 50 ng/mL from Month 6 through Month 12 post-transplant. The median trough concentrations observed in the clinical trial ranged between 161 to 185 ng/mL through Month 1 post-transplant and between 111 to 140 ng/mL at Months 2 and 3 post-transplant. The median trough concentration was 99 ng/mL at Month 4 post-transplant and ranged between 46 to 75 ng/mL from Months 6 through Month 12 post-transplant. [See Clinical Pharmacology (12.8) and Clinical Studies (14.1)]

Cyclosporine, USP Modified is to be administered as oral capsules twice daily unless cyclosporine oral solution or intravenous administration of cyclosporine cannot be avoided. Cyclosporine, USP Modified should be initiated as soon as possible - and no later than 48 hours - after reperfusion of the graft and dose adjusted to target concentrations from Day 5 onwards.

If impairment of renal function is progressive the treatment regimen should be adjusted. In renal transplant patients, the cyclosporine dose should be based on cyclosporine whole blood trough concentrations. [See Clinical Pharmacology (12.8)]

In renal transplantation, there are limited data regarding dosing Zortress with reduced cyclosporine trough concentrations of 25 to 50 ng/mL after 12 months. Zortress has not been evaluated in clinical trials with other formulations of cyclosporine. Prior to dose reduction of cyclosporine it should be ascertained that steady-state everolimus whole blood trough concentration is at least 3 ng/mL. There is an interaction of cyclosporine on everolimus, and consequently, everolimus concentrations may decrease if cyclosporine exposure is reduced. [See Drug Interactions (7.2)]

2.5 Therapeutic Drug Monitoring- Tacrolimus in Liver Transplant Patients

Both tacrolimus doses and the target range for whole blood trough concentrations should be reduced, when given in a regimen with Zortress, in order to minimize the potential risk of nephrotoxicity. [See Warnings and Precautions (5.6) and Clinical Pharmacology (12.9)]

The recommended tacrolimus therapeutic range when administered with Zortress are whole blood trough (C-0h) concentrations of 3 to 5 ng/mL by three weeks after the first dose of Zortress (approximately Month 2) and through Month 12 post transplant.

The median tacrolimus trough concentrations observed in the clinical trial ranged between 8.6 to 9.5 ng/mL at Weeks 2 and 4 post-transplant (prior to initiation of everolimus). The median tacrolimus trough concentrations ranged between 7 to 8.1 ng/mL at Weeks 5 and 6 post-transplant, between 5.2 to 5.6 ng/mL at Months 2 and 3 post-transplant, and between 4.3 to 4.9 ng/mL between Months 4 and 12 post-transplant. [See Clinical Pharmacology (12.9) and Clinical Studies (14.2)]

Tacrolimus is to be administered as oral capsules twice daily unless intravenous administration of tacrolimus cannot be avoided.

In liver transplant patients, the tacrolimus dose should be based on tacrolimus whole blood trough concentrations. [See Clinical Pharmacology (12.9)]

In liver transplantation, there are limited data regarding dosing Zortress with reduced tacrolimus trough concentrations of 3 to 5 ng/mL after 12 months. Prior to dose reduction of tacrolimus it should be ascertained that the steady-state everolimus whole blood trough concentration is at least 3 ng/mL. Unlike the interaction between cyclosporine and everolimus, tacrolimus does not affect everolimus trough concentrations, and consequently, everolimus concentrations do not decrease if the tacrolimus exposure is reduced.

2.6 Administration

Zortress tablets should be swallowed whole with a glass of water and not crushed before use.

Administer Zortress consistently approximately 12 hours apart with or without food to minimize variability in absorption and at the same time as cyclosporine or tacrolimus. [See Clinical Pharmacology (12.5)]

2.7 Hepatic Impairment

Whole blood trough concentrations of everolimus should be closely monitored in patients with impaired hepatic function. For patients with mild hepatic impairment (Child-Pugh Class A), the initial daily dose should be reduced by approximately one-third of the normally recommended daily dose. For patients with moderate or severe hepatic impairment (Child-Pugh B or C), the initial daily dose should be reduced to approximately one-half of the normally recommended daily dose. Further dose adjustment and/or dose titration should be made if a patient's whole blood trough concentration of everolimus, as measured by an LC/MS/MS assay, is not within the target trough concentration range of 3 to 8 ng/mL. [See Clinical Pharmacology (12.5)]

3 DOSAGE FORMS AND STRENGTHS

Zortress is available as 0.25 mg, 0.5 mg, and 0.75 mg tablets.

Table 1. Description of Zortress (everolimus) Tablets

Dosage Strength	0.25 mg	0.5 mg	0.75 mg
Appearance	White to yellowish, marbled, round, flat tablets with bevelled edge		
Imprint	"C" on one side and "NVR" on the other	"CH" on one side and "NVR" on the other	"CL" on one side and "NVR" on the other

4 CONTRAINDICATIONS

4.1 Hypersensitivity Reactions

Zortress is contraindicated in patients with known hypersensitivity to everolimus, sirolimus, or to components of the drug product.

5 WARNINGS AND PRECAUTIONS

5.1 Management of Immunosuppression

Only physicians experienced in management of systemic immunosuppressant therapy in transplantation should prescribe Zortress. Patients receiving the drug should be managed in facilities equipped and staffed with adequate laboratory and supportive medical resources. The physician responsible for the maintenance therapy should have complete information requisite for the follow-up of the patient.

5.2 Lymphomas and Other Malignancies

Patients receiving immunosuppressants, including Zortress, are at increased risk of developing lymphomas and other malignancies, particularly of the skin. The risk appears to be related to the intensity and duration of immunosuppression rather than to the use of any specific agent. As usual for patients with increased risk for skin cancer, exposure to sunlight and ultraviolet light should be limited by wearing protective clothing and using a sunscreen with a high protection factor.

5.3 Serious Infections

Patients receiving immunosuppressants, including Zortress, are at increased risk of developing bacterial, viral, fungal, and protozoal infections, including opportunistic infections. [See Warnings and Precautions (5.13) and Adverse Reactions (6.1, 6.2)] These infections may lead to serious, including fatal, outcomes. Because of the danger of over immunosuppression, which can cause increased susceptibility to infection, combination immunosuppressant therapy should be used with caution.

Antimicrobial prophylaxis for Pneumocystis jiroveci (carinii) pneumonia and prophylaxis for cytomegalovirus (CMV) is recommended in transplant recipients.

5.4 Kidney Graft Thrombosis

An increased risk of kidney arterial and venous thrombosis, resulting in graft loss, has been reported, usually within the first 30 days post-transplantation. [See Boxed Warning]

5.5 Hepatic Artery Thrombosis

Mammalian target of rapamycin (mTOR) inhibitors are associated with an increase in hepatic artery thrombosis (HAT). Reported cases mostly have occurred within the first 30 days post-transplant and most also lead to graft loss or death. Therefore, Zortress should not be administered earlier than 30 days after liver transplant.

5.6 Zortress and Calcineurin Inhibitor-Induced Nephrotoxicity

In kidney transplant recipients, Zortress with standard dose cyclosporine increases the risk of nephrotoxicity resulting in a lower glomerular filtration rate. Reduced doses of cyclosporine are required for use in combination with Zortress in order to reduce renal dysfunction. [See Boxed Warning, Indications and Usage (1.1), Clinical Pharmacology (12.8)]

In liver transplant recipients, Zortress has not been studied with standard dose tacrolimus. Reduced doses of tacrolimus should be used in combination with Zortress in order to minimize the potential risk of nephrotoxicity. [See Indications and Usage (1.2), Clinical Pharmacology (12.9)]

Renal function should be monitored during the administration of Zortress. Consider switching to other immunosuppressive therapies if renal function does not improve after dose adjustments or if the dysfunction is thought to be drug related. Caution should be exercised when using other drugs which are known to impair renal function.

5.7 Heart Transplantation

In a clinical trial of de novo heart transplant patients, Zortress in an immunosuppressive regimen with or without induction therapy, resulted in an increased mortality often associated with serious infections within the first three months post-transplantation compared to the control regimen. Use of Zortress in heart transplantation is not recommended.

5.8 Angioedema

Zortress has been associated with the development of angioedema. The concomitant use of Zortress with other drugs known to cause angioedema, such as angiotensin converting enzyme (ACE) inhibitors may increase the risk of developing angioedema.

5.9 Wound Healing and Fluid Accumulation

Zortress increases the risk of delayed wound healing and increases the occurrence of wound-related complications like wound dehiscence, wound infection, incisional hernia, lymphocele and seroma. These wound-related complications may require more surgical intervention. Generalized fluid accumulation, including peripheral edema (e.g., lymphoedema) and other types of localized fluid collection, such as pericardial and pleural effusions and ascites have also been reported.

5.10 Interstitial Lung Disease/Non-Infectious Pneumonitis

A diagnosis of interstitial lung disease (ILD) should be considered in patients presenting with symptoms consistent with infectious pneumonia but not responding to antibiotic therapy and in whom infectious, neoplastic and other non-drug causes have been ruled-out through appropriate investigations. Cases of ILD have been reported with Zortress, which generally resolve on drug interruption with or without glucocorticoid therapy. However, fatal cases have also occurred.

5.11 Hyperlipidemia

Increased serum cholesterol and triglycerides, requiring the need for anti-lipid therapy, have been reported to occur following initiation of Zortress and the risk of hyperlipidemia is increased with higher everolimus whole blood trough concentrations. [See Adverse Reactions (6.2)] Use of anti-lipid therapy may not normalize lipid levels in patients receiving Zortress.

Any patient who is administered Zortress should be monitored for hyperlipidemia. If detected, interventions, such as diet, exercise, and lipid-lowering agents should be initiated as outlined by the National Cholesterol Education Program guidelines. The risk/benefit should be considered in patients with established hyperlipidemia before initiating an immunosuppressive regimen containing Zortress. Similarly, the risk/benefit of continued Zortress therapy should be re-evaluated in patients with severe refractory hyperlipidemia. Zortress has not been studied in patients with baseline cholesterol levels >350 mg/dL.

Due to an interaction with cyclosporine, clinical trials of Zortress and cyclosporine in kidney transplant patients strongly discouraged patients from receiving the HMG-CoA reductase inhibitors simvastatin and lovastatin. During Zortress therapy with cyclosporine, patients administered an HMG-CoA reductase inhibitor and/or fibrate should be monitored for the possible development of rhabdomyolysis and other adverse effects, as described in the respective labeling for these agents. [See Drug Interactions (7.7)]

5.12 Proteinuria

The use of Zortress in transplant patients has been associated with increased proteinuria. The risk of proteinuria increased with higher everolimus whole blood trough concentrations. Patients receiving Zortress should be monitored for proteinuria. [See Adverse Reactions (6.2)]

5.13 Polyoma Virus Infections

Patients receiving immunosuppressants, including Zortress, are at increased risk for opportunistic infections; including polyoma virus infections. Polyoma virus infections in transplant patients may have serious, and sometimes fatal, outcomes. These include polyoma virus-associated nephropathy (PVAN), mostly due to BK virus infection, and JC virus associated progressive multiple leukoencephalopathy (PML). PVAN has been observed in patients receiving immunosuppressants, including Zortress. PVAN is associated with serious outcomes; including deteriorating renal function and kidney graft loss. [See Adverse Reactions (6.2)] Patient monitoring may help detect patients at risk for PVAN. Reductions in immunosuppression should be considered for patients who develop evidence of PVAN or PML. Physicians should also consider the risk that reduced immunosuppression represents to the functioning allograft.

5.14 Interaction with Strong Inhibitors and Inducers of CYP3A4

Co-administration of Zortress with strong CYP3A4-inhibitors (e.g., ketoconazole, itraconazole, voriconazole, clarithromycin, telithromycin, ritonavir, boceprevir, telaprevir) and strong CYP3A4 inducers (e.g., rifampin, rifabutin) is not recommended without close monitoring of everolimus whole blood trough concentrations. [See Drug Interactions (7)]

5.15 Thrombotic Microangiopathy/Thrombotic Thrombocytopenic Purpura/Hemolytic Uremic Syndrome (TMA/TTP/HUS)

The concomitant use of Zortress with cyclosporine may increase the risk of thrombotic microangiopathy/thrombotic thrombocytopenic purpura/hemolytic uremic syndrome. Monitor hematologic parameters. [See Adverse Reactions (6.2)]

5.16 New Onset Diabetes After Transplant

Zortress has been shown to increase the risk of new onset diabetes mellitus after transplant. Blood glucose concentrations should be monitored closely in patients using Zortress.

5.17 Male Infertility

Azospermia or oligospermia may be observed. [See Adverse Reactions (6.2) and Carcinogenesis, Mutagenesis, Impairment of Fertility (13.1)] Zortress is an anti-proliferative drug and affects rapidly dividing cells like the germ cells.

5.18 Immunizations

The use of live vaccines should be avoided during treatment with Zortress; examples include (not limited to) the following: intranasal influenza, measles, mumps, rubella, oral polio, BCG, yellow fever, varicella, and TY21a typhoid vaccines.

5.19 Interaction with Grapefruit Juice

Grapefruit and grapefruit juice inhibit cytochrome P450 3A4 and P-gp activity and should therefore be avoided with concomitant use of Zortress and cyclosporine or tacrolimus.

5.20 Patients with Hereditary Disorders/Other

Patients with rare hereditary problems of galactose intolerance, the Lapp lactase deficiency or glucose-galactose malabsorption should not take Zortress as this may result in diarrhea and malabsorption.

6 ADVERSE REACTIONS

6.1 Serious and Otherwise Important Adverse Reactions

The following adverse reactions are discussed in greater detail in other sections of the label.

- Hypersensitivity reactions [See Contraindications (4.1)]
- Lymphomas and Other Malignancies [See Boxed Warning, Warnings and Precautions (5.2)]
- Serious Infections [See Warnings and Precautions (5.3)]
- Kidney Graft Thrombosis [See Warnings and Precautions (5.4)]
- Hepatic Artery Thrombosis [See Warnings and Precautions (5.5)]
- Zortress and Calcineurin Inhibitor-Induced Nephrotoxicity [See Warnings and Precautions (5.6)]
- Heart Transplantation [See Warnings and Precautions (5.7)]
- Angioedema [See Warnings and Precautions (5.8)]
- Wound Healing and Fluid Accumulation [See Warnings and Precautions (5.9)]
- Interstitial Lung Disease/Non-Infectious Pneumonitis [See Warnings and Precautions (5.10)]
- Hyperlipidemia [See Warnings and Precautions (5.11)]
- Proteinuria [See Warnings and Precautions (5.12)]
- Polyoma Virus Infections [See Warnings and Precautions (5.13)]
- Thrombotic Microangiopathy/Thrombotic Thrombocytopenic Purpura/Hemolytic Uremic Syndrome (TMA/TTP/HUS) [See Warnings and Precautions (5.15)]
- New Onset Diabetes After Transplant [See Warnings and Precautions (5.16)]
- Male Infertility [See Warnings and Precautions (5.17)]

6.2 Clinical Studies Experience

Because clinical trials are conducted under widely varying conditions, the adverse reaction rates observed cannot be directly compared to rates in other trials and may not reflect the rates observed in clinical practice.

Kidney transplantation

The data described below reflect exposure to Zortress in an open-label, randomized trial of de novo kidney transplant patients of concentration-controlled everolimus at an initial Zortress starting dose of 1.5 mg per day [target trough concentrations 3 to 8 ng/mL with reduced exposure cyclosporine (N=274) compared to mycophenolic acid (N=273) with standard exposure cyclosporine]. All patients received basiliximab induction therapy and corticosteroids. The population was between 18 and 70 years, more than 43% were 50 years of age or older (mean age was 46 years in the Zortress group, 47 years control group); a majority of recipients were male (64% in the Zortress group, 69% control group); and a majority of patients were Caucasian (70% in the Zortress group, 69% control group). Demographic characteristics were comparable between treatment groups. The most frequent diseases leading to transplantation were balanced between groups and included hypertension/nephrosclerosis, glomerulonephritis/glomerular disease and diabetes mellitus. Significantly more patients discontinued Zortress 1.5 mg per day treatment (83/277, 30%) than discontinued the control regimen (60/277, 22%). Of those patients who prematurely discontinued treatment, most discontinuations were due to adverse reactions: 18% in the Zortress group compared to 9% in the control group (p-value = 0.004). This difference was more prominent between treatment groups among female patients. In those patients discontinuing study medication, adverse reactions were collected up to 7 days after study medication discontinuation and serious adverse reactions up to 30 days after study medication discontinuation.

Discontinuation of Zortress at a higher dose (3 mg per day) was 95/279, 34%, including 20% due to adverse reactions, and this regimen is not recommended (see below).

The overall incidences of serious adverse reactions were 57% (159/278) in the Zortress group and 52% (141/273) in

the mycophenolic acid group. Infections and infestations reported as serious adverse reactions had the highest incidence in both groups [20% (54/274) in the Zortress group and 25% (69/273) in the control group]. The difference was mainly due to the higher incidence of viral infections in the mycophenolic acid group, mainly CMV and BK virus infections. Injury, poisoning and procedural complications reported as serious adverse reactions had the second highest incidence in both groups [14% (39/274) in the Zortress group and 12% (32/273) in the control group] followed by renal and urinary disorders [10% (28/274) in the Zortress group and 13% (36/273) in the control group] and vascular disorders [10% (26/274) in the Zortress group and 7% (20/273) in the control group].

A total of 13 patients died during the first 12 months of study; 7 (3%) in the Zortress group and 6 (2%) in the control group. The most common causes of death across the study groups were related to cardiac conditions and infections. There were 12 (4%) graft losses in the Zortress group and 8 (3%) in the control group over the 12 month study period. Of the graft losses, 4 were due to renal artery and two due to renal vein thrombosis in the Zortress group (2%) compared to two renal artery thromboses in the control group (1%). [See Boxed Warning and Warnings and Precautions (5.4)]

The most common (≥20%) adverse reactions observed in the Zortress group were: peripheral edema, constipation, hypertension, nausea, anemia, urinary tract infection, and hyperlipidemia.

Infections

The overall incidence of bacterial, fungal and viral infections reported as adverse reactions was higher in the control group (68%) compared to the Zortress group (64%) and

Table 2. Incidence Rates of Frequent (≥10% in Any Treatment Group) Adverse Reactions by Primary System Organ Class and Preferred Term

Primary System Organ Class Preferred Term	Zortress (everolimus) 1.5 mg With reduced exposure cyclosporine N=274 n (%)	Mycophenolic acid 1.44 g With standard exposure cyclosporine N=273 n (%)
Any Adverse Reactions*	271 (99)	270 (99)
Blood lymphatic system disorders	93 (34)	111 (41)
Anemia	70 (26)	68 (25)
Leukopenia	8 (3)	33 (12)
Gastrointestinal disorders	196 (72)	207 (76)
Constipation	105 (38)	117 (43)
Nausea	79 (29)	85 (31)
Diarrhea	51 (19)	54 (20)
Vomiting	40 (15)	60 (22)
Abdominal pain	36 (13)	42 (15)
Dyspepsia	12 (4)	31 (11)
Abdominal pain upper	9 (3)	30 (11)
General disorders and administrative site conditions	181 (66)	160 (59)
Edema peripheral	123 (45)	108 (40)
Pyrexia	51 (19)	40 (15)
Fatigue	25 (9)	28 (10)
Infections and infestations	169 (62)	185 (68)
Urinary tract infection	60 (22)	63 (23)
Upper respiratory tract infection	44 (16)	49 (18)
Injury, poisoning and procedural complications	163 (60)	163 (60)
Incision site pain	45 (16)	47 (17)
Procedural pain	40 (15)	37 (14)
Investigations	137 (50)	133 (49)
Blood creatinine increased	48 (18)	59 (22)
Metabolism and nutrition disorders	222 (81)	199 (73)
Hyperlipidemia	57 (21)	43 (16)
Hyperkalemia	49 (18)	48 (18)
Hypercholesterolemia	47 (17)	34 (13)
Dyslipidemia	41 (15)	24 (9)
Hypomagnesemia	37 (14)	40 (15)
Hypophosphatemia	35 (13)	35 (13)
Hyperglycemia	34 (12)	38 (14)
Hypokalemia	32 (12)	32 (12)

(Table continued on next page)

Table 2 (cont.). Incidence Rates of Frequent (≥10% in Any Treatment Group) Adverse Reactions by Primary System Organ Class and Preferred Term

Primary System Organ Class Preferred Term	Zortress (everolimus) 1.5 mg With reduced exposure cyclosporine N=274 n (%)	Mycophenolic acid 1.44 g With standard exposure cyclosporine N=273 n (%)
Musculoskeletal and connective tissue disorders	112 (41)	105 (39)
Pain in extremity	32 (12)	29 (11)
Back pain	30 (11)	28 (10)
Nervous system disorders	92 (34)	109 (40)
Headache	49 (18)	40 (15)
Tremor	23 (8)	38 (14)
Psychiatric disorders	90 (33)	72 (26)
Insomnia	47 (17)	43 (16)
Renal and urinary disorders	112 (41)	124 (45)
Hematuria	33 (12)	33 (12)
Dysuria	29 (11)	28 (10)
Respiratory, thoracic and mediastinal disorders	86 (31)	93 (34)
Cough	20 (7)	30 (11)
Vascular disorders	122 (45)	124 (45)
Hypertension	81 (30)	82 (30)

* As reported in the safety analysis population defined as all randomized patients who received at least one dose of treatment and had at least one post-baseline safety assessment.

was primarily due to an increased number of viral infections (21% in the control group and 10% in the Zortress group). The incidence of cytomegalovirus (CMV) infections reported as adverse reactions was 8% in the control group compared to 1% in the Zortress group; and 3% of the serious CMV infections in the control group versus 0% in the Zortress group were considered serious. [See Warnings and Precautions (5.3)]

BK Virus

BK virus infections were lower in incidence in the Zortress group (2 patients, 1%) compared to the control group (11 patients, 4%). One of the two BK virus infections in the Zortress group and two of the 11 BK virus infections in the control group were also reported as serious adverse reactions. BK virus infections did not result in graft loss in any of the groups in the clinical trial.

Wound Healing and Fluid Collections

Wound healing-related reactions were identified through a retrospective search and request for additional data. The overall incidence of wound-related reactions, including lymphocele, seroma, hematoma, dehiscence, incisional hernia, and infections was 35% in the Zortress group compared to 26% in the control group. More patients required intraoperative repair debridement or drainage of incisional wound complications and more required drainage of lymphoceles and seromas in the Zortress group compared to control. Adverse reactions due to major fluid collections such as edema and other types of fluid collections was 45% in the Zortress group and 40% in the control group. [See Warnings and Precautions (5.9)]

Neoplasms

Adverse reactions due to malignant and benign neoplasms were reported in 3% of patients in the Zortress group and 6% in the control group. The most frequently reported neoplasms in the control group were basal cell carcinoma, squamous cell carcinoma, skin papilloma and seborrheic keratosis. One patient in the Zortress group who underwent a melanoma excision prior to transplantation died due to metastatic melanoma. [See Boxed Warning and Warnings and Precautions (5.2)]

New Onset Diabetes Mellitus (NODM)

NODM reported based on adverse reactions and random serum glucose values, was 9% in the Zortress group compared to 7% in the control group.

Endocrine Effects in Males

In the Zortress group, serum testosterone levels significantly decreased while the FSH levels significantly increased without significant changes being observed in the control group. In both the Zortress and the control groups mean testosterone and FSH levels remained within the nor-mal range with the mean FSH level in the Zortress group being at the upper limit of the normal range (11.1 U/L). More patients were reported with erectile dysfunction in the Zortress treatment group compared to the control group (5% compared to 2%, respectively).

Table 2 compares the incidence of treatment-emergent adverse reactions reported with an incidence of ≥10% for patients receiving Zortress with reduced dose cyclosporine or mycophenolic acid with standard dose cyclosporine. Within each MedDRA system organ class, the adverse reactions are presented in order of decreasing frequency.

[See table 2 on previous page and above]

Adverse reaction that occurred with at least a 5% higher frequency in the Zortress 1.5 mg group compared to the control group were: peripheral edema (45% compared to 40%), hyperlipidemia (21% compared to 16%), dyslipidemia (15% compared to 9%), and stomatitis/mouth ulceration (8% compared to 3%).

A third treatment group of Zortress 3.0 mg per day (1.5 mg twice daily; target trough concentrations 6 to 12 ng/mL) with reduced exposure cyclosporine was included in the study described above. Although as effective as the lower dose Zortress group, the overall safety was worse and consequently higher doses of Zortress cannot be recommended. Out of 279 patients, 95 (34%) discontinued the study medication with 57 (20%) doing so because of adverse reactions. The most frequent adverse reactions leading to discontinuation of Zortress when used at this higher dose were injury, poisoning and procedural complications (Zortress 1.5 mg: 5%, Zortress 3.0 mg: 7%, and control: 2%), infections (2%, 6%, and 3%, respectively), renal and urinary disorders (4%, 7%, and 4%, respectively) and gastrointestinal disorders (1%, 3%, and 2%).

The combination of fixed dose Zortress and standard doses cyclosporine in previous kidney clinical trials resulted in frequent elevations of serum creatinine with higher mean and median serum creatinine values was observed than in the current study with reduced exposure cyclosporine. These results indicate that Zortress increases the cyclosporine-induced nephrotoxicity; and therefore should only be used in a concentration-controlled regimen with reduced exposure cyclosporine. [See Boxed Warnings, Indications and Usage (1.1) and Warnings and Precautions (5.6)]

Liver transplantation

The data described below reflect exposure to Zortress starting 30 days after transplantation in an open-label, randomized trial of liver transplant patients. Seven hundred and nineteen (719) patients who fulfilled the inclusion/exclusion criteria [see Clinical Trials section (14.2)] were randomized into one of the three treatment groups of the study. During the first 30 days prior to randomization patients received tacrolimus and corticosteroids, with or without mycophenolate mofetil (about 70 to 80% received MMF). No induction antibody was administered. At randomization, MMF was discontinued and patients were randomized to Zortress initial dose of 1.0 mg twice per day (2.0 mg daily) and adjusted to protocol specified target trough concentrations of 3 to 8 ng/mL with reduced exposure tacrolimus [protocol specified target troughs 3 to 5 ng/mL] (N=245) or to a control group of standard exposure tacrolimus [protocol specified target troughs 8 to 12 ng/mL up to Month 4 post-transplant, then 6 to 10 ng/mL Month 4 through Month 12 post-transplant] (N=241). A third randomized group was discontinued prematurely [See Clinical Studies (14.2)] and is not described in this section.

The population was between 18 and 70 years, more than 50% were 50 years of age (mean age was 54 years in the Zortress group, 55 years in the tacrolimus control group); 74% were male in both Zortress and control groups, respectively, and a majority were Caucasian (86% Zortress group, 80% control group). Demographic characteristics were comparable between treatment groups. The most frequent diseases leading to transplantation were balanced between groups. The most frequent causes of end-stage liver disease (ESLD) were alcoholic cirrhosis, hepatitis C, and hepatocellular carcinoma and were balanced between groups.

Twenty-seven percent discontinued study drug in the Zortress group compared with 22% for the tacrolimus control group. The most common reason for discontinuation of study medication was due to adverse reactions (19% and 11%, respectively), including proteinuria, recurrent hepatitis C, and pancytopenia in the Zortress group.

The overall incidences of serious adverse reactions were 50% (122/245) in the Zortress group and 43% (104/241) in the control group. Infections and infestations were reported as serious adverse reactions with the highest incidence followed by Gastrointestinal disorders and Hepatobiliary disorders.

During the first 12 months of study, 13 deaths were reported in the Zortress group (one patient never took Zortress). In the same 12 month period, 7 deaths were reported in the tacrolimus control group. Deaths occurred in both groups for a variety of reasons and were mostly associated with liver-related issues, infections and sepsis.

The most common adverse reactions (reported for ≥10% patients in any group) in the Zortress group were: diarrhea, headache, peripheral edema, hypertension, nausea, pyrexia, abdominal pain, and leukopenia (see Table 3).

Infections

The overall incidence of infections reported as adverse reactions was 50% for Zortress and 44% in the control group. The types of infections were reported as follows: bacterial 16% vs 12%, viral 17% vs 13%; and fungal infections 2% vs 5% for Zortress and control, respectively. [See Warnings and Precautions (5.3)]

Wound Healing and Fluid Collections

Wound healing complications were reported as adverse reactions for 11% of patients in the Zortress group compared to 8% of patients in the control group. Pleural effusions were reported in 5% in both groups, and ascites in 4% of patients in the Zortress group and 3% in the control arm.

Neoplasms

Malignant and benign neoplasms were reported as adverse reactions in 4% of patients in the Zortress group and 7% in the control group. In the Zortress group 3 malignant tumors were reported compared to 9 cases in the control group. For the Zortress group this included lymphoma, lymphoproliferative disorder and a hepatocellular carcinoma, and for the control group included Kaposi's sarcoma (2), metastatic colorectal cancer, glioblastoma, malignant hepatic neoplasm, pancreatic neuroendocrine tumor, hemophagocytic histiocytosis, and squamous cell carcinomas. [See Boxed Warning and Warnings and Precautions (5.2)]

Lipid abnormalities

Hyperlipidemia adverse reactions (including the preferred terms: hyperlipidemia, hypercholesterolemia, blood cholesterol increased, blood triglycerides increased, hypertriglyceridemia lipids increased, total cholesterol/HDL ratio increased, and dyslipidemia) were reported for 24% Zortress patients, and 10% control patients.

New Onset of Diabetes After Transplant (NODAT)

Of the patients without diabetes mellitus at randomization, NODAT was reported in 32% in the Zortress group compared to 29% in the control group.

Table 3 compares the incidence of treatment-emergent adverse reactions reported with an incidence of ≥10% for patients receiving Zortress with reduced exposure tacrolimus or standard dose tacrolimus. Within each MedDRA system organ class, the adverse reactions are presented in order of decreasing frequency.

[See table 3 at top of next page]

Primary system organ classes are presented alphabetically.
* No *de novo* hepatitis C cases were reported

Less common adverse reactions, occurring overall in ≥1% to <10% of kidney and liver transplant patients treated with Zortress include:

Blood and Lymphatic System Disorders: leukocytosis, lymphadenopathy, neutropenia, pancytopenia, thrombocythemia, thrombocytopenia

Cardiac and Vascular Disorders: angina pectoris, atrial fibrillation, cardiac failure congestive, palpitations, tachycardia, hypertension including hypertensive crisis, hypotension, deep vein thrombosis

Endocrine Disorders: Cushingoid, hyperparathyroidism

Eye Disorders: cataract, conjunctivitis, vision blurred

Gastrointestinal Disorders: abdominal distention, dyspepsia, dysphagia, epigastric discomfort, flatulence, gastroesophageal reflux disease, gingival hypertrophy, hematemesis, hemorrhoids, ileus, mouth ulceration, peritonitis, stomatitis

General Disorders and Administrative Site Conditions: chest discomfort, chest pain, chills, fatigue, incisional hernia, malaise, edema including generalized edema, pain

Hepatobiliary Disorders: hepatic enzyme increased, bilirubin increased

Infections and Infestations: BK virus infection [*See Warnings and Precautions (5.13)*], bacteremia, bronchitis, candidiasis, cellulitis, folliculitis, gastroenteritis, herpes infections, influenza, lower respiratory tract, nasopharyngitis, onychomycosis, oral candidiasis, oral herpes, osteomyelitis, pneumonia, pyelonephritis, sepsis, sinusitis, tinea pedis, urethritis, wound infection [*See Boxed Warning and Warnings and Precautions (5.3)*]

Injury Poisoning and Procedural Complications: incision site complications including infections, perinephric collection, seroma, wound dehiscence, incisional hernia, perinephric hematoma, localized intraabdominal fluid collection, impaired healing, lymphocele, lymphorrhea

Investigations: blood alkaline phosphatase increased, white blood cell count decreased, transaminases increased

Metabolism and Nutrition Disorders: blood urea increased, acidosis, anorexia, dehydration, diabetes mellitus [*See Warnings and Precautions (5.16)*], decreased appetite, fluid retention, gout, hypercalcemia, hypertriglyceridemia, hyperuricemia, hypocalcemia, hypoglycemia, hyponatremia, iron deficiency, new onset diabetes mellitus, vitamin B12 deficiency

Musculoskeletal and Connective Tissues Disorders: arthralgia, joint swelling, muscle spasms, muscular weakness, musculoskeletal pain, myalgia, osteonecrosis, osteopenia, osteoporosis, spondylitis

Nervous System Disorders: dizziness, hemiparesis, hypoaesthesia, lethargy, migraine, neuralgia, paresthesia, somnolence, syncope, tremor

Psychiatric Disorders: agitation, anxiety, depression, hallucination

Renal and Urinary Disorders: bladder spasm, hydronephrosis, micturition urgency, nephritis interstitial, pollakiuria, polyuria, proteinuria [*See Warnings and Precautions (5.12)*], pyuria, renal artery thrombosis [*See Boxed Warning and Warnings and Precautions (5.4)*], acute renal failure, renal impairment [*See Warnings and Precautions (5.6)*], urinary retention

Reproductive System and Breast Disorders: erectile dysfunction, ovarian cyst, scrotal edema

Respiratory, Thoracic, Mediastinal Disorders: atelectasis, dyspnea, epistaxis, nasal congestion, oropharyngeal pain, pleural effusions, pulmonary edema, rhinorrhea, sinus congestion, wheezing

Skin and Subcutaneous Tissue Disorders: acne, alopecia, dermatitis acneiform, hirsutism, hyperhydrosis, hypertrichosis, night sweats, pruritus, rash

Vascular Disorders: venous thromboembolism (including deep vein thrombosis), pulmonary embolism

Less common, serious adverse reactions include:

- Interstitial Lung Disease/Non-infectious Pneumonitis [*See Warnings and Precautions (5.10) and Adverse Reactions (6.1)*]
- Thrombotic Microangiopathy (TMA), Thrombotic Thrombocytopenic Purpura (TTP), and Hemolytic Uremic Syndrome (HUS) [*See Warnings and Precautions (5.15)*]

6.3   Post Marketing Experience

Adverse reactions identified from the post-marketing use of the combination regimen of Zortress and cyclosporine that are not specific to any one transplant indication include angioedema [*See Warnings and Precautions (5.8)*], pancreatitis and pulmonary embolism. There have also been reports of male infertility with mTOR inhibitors including Zortress. [*See Warnings and Precautions (5.17)*]

7   DRUG INTERACTIONS

7.1   Interactions with Strong Inhibitors or Inducers of CYP3A4 and P-glycoprotein

Everolimus is mainly metabolized by CYP3A4 in the liver and to some extent in the intestinal wall and is a substrate

Table 3. Incidence Rates of most Frequent (≥ 10% in Any Treatment Group) Adverse Reactions by Primary System Organ Class and Preferred Term and treatment (Safety population – 12 month analysis)

Primary System Organ Class Preferred Term	Zortress (everolimus) with reduced exposure Tacrolimus N=245 n (%)	Tacrolimus (standard exposure) N=241 n (%)
Any Adverse Reaction/Infection	232 (95)	229 (95)
Blood & lymphatic system disorders	66 (27)	47 (20)
Leukopenia	29 (12)	12 (5)
Gastrointestinal disorders	136 (56)	121 (50)
Diarrhea	47 (19)	50 (21)
Nausea	33 (14)	28 (12)
Abdominal pain	32 (13)	22 (9)
General disorders and administration site conditions	94 (38)	85 (35)
Peripheral edema	43 (18)	26 (11)
Pyrexia	32 (13)	25 (10)
Fatigue	22 (9)	26 (11)
Infections and infestations	123 (50)	105 (44)
Hepatitis C*	28 (11)	19 (8)
Investigations	81 (33)	78 (32)
Liver function test abnormal	16 (7)	24 (10)
Nervous system disorders	89 (36)	85 (35)
Headache	47 (19)	46 (19)
Tremor	23 (9)	29 (12)
Vascular disorders	56 (23)	57 (24)
Hypertension	42 (17)	38 (16)

for the multidrug efflux pump, P-glycoprotein (P-gp). Therefore, absorption and subsequent elimination of systemically absorbed everolimus may be influenced by medicinal products that affect CYP3A4 and/or P-gp. Concurrent treatment with strong inhibitors (e.g., ketoconazole, itraconazole, voriconazole, clarithromycin, telithromycin, ritonavir, boceprevir, telaprevir) and inducers (e.g., rifampin, rifabutin) of CYP3A4 is not recommended. Inhibitors of P-gp (e.g., digoxin, cyclosporine) may decrease the efflux of everolimus from intestinal cells and increase everolimus blood concentrations. *In vitro,* everolimus was a competitive inhibitor of CYP3A4 and of CYP2D6, potentially increasing the concentrations of medicinal products eliminated by these enzymes. Thus, caution should be exercised when co-administering Zortress with CYP3A4 and CYP2D6 substrates with a narrow therapeutic index. [*See Therapeutic Drug Monitoring (2.3)*]

All *in vivo* interaction studies were conducted without concomitant cyclosporine. Pharmacokinetic interactions between Zortress and concomitantly administered drugs are discussed below. Drug interaction studies have not been conducted with drugs other than those described below.

7.2   Cyclosporine (CYP3A4/P-gp inhibitor and CYP3A4 substrate)

The steady-state C_{max} and AUC estimates of everolimus were significantly increased by co-administration of single dose cyclosporine. [*See Clinical Pharmacology (12.5)*] Dose adjustment of Zortress might be needed if the cyclosporine dose is altered. [*See Dosage and Administration (2.3)*] Zortress had a clinically minor influence on cyclosporine pharmacokinetics in transplant patients receiving cyclosporine (Neoral).

7.3   Ketoconazole and Other Strong CYP3A4 Inhibitors

Multiple-dose ketoconazole administration to healthy volunteers significantly increased single dose estimates of everolimus C_{max}, AUC, and half-life. It is recommended that strong inhibitors of CYP3A4 (e.g., ketoconazole, itraconazole, voriconazole, clarithromycin, telithromycin, ritonavir, boceprevir, telaprevir) should not be co-administered with Zortress. [*See Warnings and Precautions (5.14), and Clinical Pharmacology (12.5)*]

7.4   Erythromycin (Moderate CYP3A4 Inhibitor)

Multiple-dose erythromycin administration to healthy volunteers significantly increased single dose estimates of

everolimus C_{max}, AUC, and half-life. If erythromycin is co-administered, everolimus blood concentrations should be monitored and a dose adjustment made as necessary. [*See Clinical Pharmacology (12.5)*]

7.5   Verapamil (CYP3A4 and P-gp Substrate)

Multiple-dose verapamil administration to healthy volunteers significantly increased single dose estimates of everolimus C_{max} and AUC. Everolimus half-life was not changed. If verapamil is co-administered, everolimus blood concentrations should be monitored and a dose adjustment made as necessary. [*See Clinical Pharmacology (12.5)*]

7.6   Atorvastatin (CYP3A4 substrate) and Pravastatin (P-gp substrate)

Single-dose administration of Zortress with either atorvastatin or pravastatin to healthy subjects did not influence the pharmacokinetics of atorvastatin, pravastatin and everolimus, as well as total HMG-CoA reductase bioreactivity in plasma to a clinically relevant extent. However, these results cannot be extrapolated to other HMG-CoA reductase inhibitors. Patients should be monitored for the development of rhabdomyolysis and other adverse reactions as described in the respective labeling for these products.

7.7   Simvastatin and Lovastatin

Due to an interaction with cyclosporine, clinical studies of Zortress with cyclosporine conducted in kidney transplant patients strongly discouraged patients with receiving HMG-CoA reductase inhibitors such as simvastatin and lovastatin. [*See Warnings and Precautions (5.11)*]

7.8   Rifampin (Strong CYP3A4/P-gp Inducers)

Pretreatment of healthy subjects with multiple-dose rifampin followed by a single dose of Zortress increased everolimus clearance and decreased the everolimus C_{max} and AUC estimates. Combination with rifampin is not recommended. [*See Warnings and Precautions (5.14) and Clinical Pharmacology (12.5)*]

7.9   Midazolam (CYP3A4/5 substrate)

Single-dose administration of midazolam to healthy volunteers following administration of multiple-dose Zortress indicated that everolimus is a weak inhibitor of CYP3A4/5. Dose adjustment of midazolam or other CYP3A4/5 substrates is not necessary when Zortress is coadministered with midazolam or other CYP3A4/5 substrates. [*See Clinical Pharmacology (12.5)*]

7.10   Other Possible Interactions

Moderate inhibitors of CYP3A4 and P-gp may increase everolimus blood concentrations (e.g., fluconazole; macro-

Table 4. Steady-State Pharmacokinetic Parameters (mean +/- SD) Following the Administration of 0.75 mg Twice Daily

C_{max}	T_{max}	AUC	CL/F[1]	Vc/F[1]	Half-life ($T_{1/2}$)
11.1 ± 4.6 ng/mL	1-2 h	75 + 31 ng•h/mL	8.8 L/h	110 L	30 ± 11h

[1] population pharmacokinetic analysis

lide antibiotics; nicardipine, diltiazem; nelfinavir, indinavir, amprenavir). Inducers of CYP3A4 may increase the metabolism of everolimus and decrease everolimus blood concentrations (e.g., St. John's Wort [*Hypericum perforatum*]; anticonvulsants: carbamazepine, phenobarbital, phenytoin; efavirenz, nevirapine).

7.11   Tacrolimus

There is little to no pharmacokinetic interaction of tacrolimus on everolimus, and consequently, dose adjustment of Zortress is not necessary when Zortress is co-administered with tacrolimus.

8   USE IN SPECIFIC POPULATIONS

8.1   Pregnancy

Pregnancy Category C

There are no adequate and well-controlled studies of Zortress in pregnant women. In rats and rabbits, everolimus crossed the placenta and was toxic to the conceptus. The potential risk for humans is unknown. Zortress should be given to pregnant women only if the potential benefit to the mother justifies the potential risk to the fetus. Women of childbearing potential should be advised to use effective contraception methods while they are receiving Zortress and up to 8 weeks after treatment has been stopped.

Everolimus administered daily to pregnant rats by oral gavage at 0.1 mg/kg from before mating through organogenesis resulted in increased preimplantation loss and early resorptions of fetal implants. AUCs in rats at this dose were approximately one-third those in humans administered the starting dose (0.75 mg twice daily). Everolimus administered daily by oral gavage at 0.8 mg/kg to pregnant rabbits during organogenesis resulted in increased late resorptions of fetal implants. At this dose, AUCs in rabbits were slightly less than the AUCs in humans administered the starting clinical dose.

8.3   Nursing Mothers

It is not known whether everolimus is excreted in human milk. Everolimus and/or its metabolites readily transferred into milk of lactating rats at a concentration 3.5 times higher than in maternal serum. Because many drugs are excreted in human milk and because of the potential for serious adverse reactions in nursing infants from everolimus, women should avoid breast-feeding during treatment with Zortress.

8.4   Pediatric Use

The safe and effective use of Zortress in kidney or liver transplant patients younger than 18 years of age has not been established. [*See Clinical Pharmacology (12.5)*]

8.5   Geriatric Use

There is limited clinical experience on the use of Zortress in patients of age 65 or older. There is no evidence to suggest that elderly patients will require a different dosage recommendation from younger adult patients. [*See Clinical Pharmacology (12.5)*]

8.6   Hepatic Impairment

Everolimus whole blood trough concentrations should be closely monitored in patients with impaired hepatic function. For patients with mild hepatic impairment (Child-Pugh Class A), the dose should be reduced by approximately one-third of the normally recommended daily dose. For patients with moderate or severe hepatic impairment (Child-Pugh B or C), the initial daily dose should be reduced to approximately half of the normally recommended daily dose. Further dose adjustment and/or dose titration should be made if a patient's whole blood trough concentration of everolimus, as measured by an LC/MS/MS assay, is not within the target trough concentration range of 3 to 8 ng/mL. [*See Clinical Pharmacology (12.5)*]

8.7   Renal Impairment

No dose adjustment is needed in patients with renal impairment. [*See Clinical Pharmacology (12.5)*]

10   OVERDOSAGE

Reported experience with overdose in humans is very limited. There is a single case of an accidental ingestion of 1.5 mg everolimus in a 2-year-old child where no adverse reactions were observed. Single doses up to 25 mg have been administered to transplant patients with acceptable acute tolerability. Single doses up to 70 mg (without cyclosporine) have been given with acceptable acute tolerability. General supportive measures should be followed in all cases of overdose. Everolimus is not considered dialyzable to any relevant degree (<10% of everolimus removed within 6 hours of hemodialysis). In animal studies, everolimus

showed a low acute toxic potential. No lethality or severe toxicity was observed after single oral doses of 2000 mg/kg (limit test) in either mice or rats.

11   DESCRIPTION

Zortress (everolimus) is a macrolide immunosuppressant. The chemical name of everolimus is (1R, 9S, 12S, 15R, 16E, 18R, 19R, 21R, 23S, 24E, 26E, 28E, 30S, 32S, 35R)-1, 18-dihydroxy-12 -[(1R)-2-[(1S,3R,4R)-4-(2-hydroxyethoxy)-3-methoxycyclohexyl]-1-methylethyl]-19,30-dimethoxy-15, 17, 21, 23, 29, 35-hexamethyl-11, 36-dioxa-4-aza-tricyclo[30.3.1.0^{4,9}] hexatriaconta-16,24,26,28-tetraene-2, 3,10,14,20-pentaone.

The molecular formula is $C_{53}H_{83}NO_{14}$ and the molecular weight is 958.25. The structural formula is:

Zortress is supplied as tablets for oral administration containing 0.25 mg, 0.5 mg, and 0.75 mg of everolimus together with butylated hydroxytoluene, magnesium stearate, lactose monohydrate, hypromellose, crospovidone and lactose anhydrous as inactive ingredients.

12   CLINICAL PHARMACOLOGY

12.1   Mechanism of Action

Everolimus inhibits antigenic and interleukin (IL-2 and IL-15) stimulated activation and proliferation of T and B lymphocytes.

In cells, everolimus binds to a cytoplasmic protein, the FK506 Binding Protein-12 (FKBP-12), to form an immunosuppressive complex (everolimus: FKBP-12) that binds to and inhibits the mammalian Target Of Rapamycin (mTOR), a key regulatory kinase. In the presence of everolimus phosphorylation of p70 S6 ribosomal protein kinase (p70S6K), a substrate of mTOR, is inhibited. Consequently, phosphorylation of the ribosomal S6 protein and subsequent protein synthesis and cell proliferation are inhibited. The everolimus: FKBP-12 complex has no effect on calcineurin activity.

In rats and nonhuman primate models, everolimus effectively reduces kidney allograft rejection resulting in prolonged graft survival.

12.3   Pharmacokinetics

Everolimus pharmacokinetics have been characterized after oral administration of single and multiple doses to adult kidney transplant patients, hepatically-impaired patients, and healthy subjects.

Absorption

After oral dosing, peak everolimus concentrations occur 1 to 2 h post dose. Over the dose range of 0.5 mg to 2 mg twice daily, everolimus C_{max} and AUC are dose proportional in transplant patients at steady-state.

Food Effect

In 24 healthy subjects, a high-fat breakfast (44.5 g fat) reduced everolimus C_{max} by 60%, delayed t_{max} by a median 1.3 hours, and reduced AUC by 16% compared with a fasting administration. To minimize variability, everolimus should be taken consistently with or without food. [*See Dosage and Administration (2.6)*]

Distribution

The blood-to-plasma ratio of everolimus is concentration dependent ranging from 17% to 73% over the range of 5 ng/mL to 5000 ng/mL. Plasma protein binding is approximately 74% in healthy subjects and in patients with moderate hepatic impairment. The apparent distribution volume associated with the terminal phase (Vz/F) from a single-dose pharmacokinetic study in maintenance kidney transplant patients is 342 to 107 L (range 128 to 589 L).

Metabolism

Everolimus is a substrate of CYP3A4 and P-gp. The main metabolic pathways identified in man were monohydroxylations and O-dealkylations. Two main metabolites were formed by hydrolysis of the cyclic lactone. Everolimus was the main circulating component in blood. None of the main metabolites contribute significantly to the immunosuppressive activity of everolimus.

Excretion

After a single dose of radiolabeled everolimus was given to transplant patients receiving cyclosporine, the majority (80%) of radioactivity was recovered from the feces and only a minor amount (5%) was excreted in urine. Parent drug was not detected in urine and feces.

Pharmacokinetics in Kidney Transplant Patients

Steady-state is reached by Day 4 with an accumulation in blood levels of 2- to 3-fold compared with the exposure after the first dose. Table 4 below provides a summary of the steady-state pharmacokinetic parameters.

[See table above]

The half-life estimates from 12 maintenance renal transplant patients who received single doses of everolimus capsules at 0.75 mg or 2.5 mg with their maintenance cyclosporine regimen indicate that the pharmacokinetics of everolimus are linear over the clinically-relevant dose range. Results indicate the half-life of everolimus in maintenance renal transplant patients receiving single doses of 0.75 mg or 2.5 mg Zortress during steady-state cyclosporine treatment was 30 ± 11 hours (range 19 to 53 hours).

12.5   Drug-Drug Interactions

Everolimus is known to be a substrate for both cytochrome CYP3A4 and P-gp. The pharmacokinetic interaction between everolimus and concomitantly administered drugs is discussed below. Drug interaction studies have not been conducted with drugs other than those described below. [*See Warnings and Precautions (5.14), and Drug Interactions (7)*]

Cyclosporine (CYP3A4/P-gp inhibitor and CYP3A4 substrate): Zortress should be taken concomitantly with cyclosporine in kidney transplant patients. Everolimus concentrations may decrease when doses of cyclosporine are reduced, unless the Zortress dose is increased. [*See Dosage and Administration (2.1), Drug Interactions (7.2)*]

In a single-dose study in healthy subjects, cyclosporine (Neoral) administered at a dose of 175 mg increased everolimus AUC by 168% (range, 46% to 365%) and C_{max} by 82% (range, 25% to 158%) when administered with 2 mg Zortress compared with administration of Zortress alone. [*See Drug Interactions (7.2)*]

Ketoconazole and Other Strong CYP3A4 Inhibitors: Multiple-dose administration of 200 mg ketoconazole twice daily for 5 days to 12 healthy volunteers significantly increased everolimus C_{max}, AUC, and half-life by 3.9-fold, 15-fold, and 89%, respectively, when co-administered with 2 mg Zortress. It is recommended that strong inhibitors of CYP3A4 (e.g., ketoconazole, itraconazole, voriconazole, clarithromycin, telithromycin, ritonavir, boceprevir, telaprevir) should not be co-administered with Zortress. [*See Warnings and Precautions (5.14) and Drug Interactions (7.3)*]

Erythromycin (Moderate CYP3A4 Inhibitor): Multiple-dose administration of 500 mg erythromycin three times daily for 5 days to 16 healthy volunteers significantly increased everolimus C_{max}, AUC, and half-life by 2.0-fold, 4.4-fold, and 39%, respectively, when co-administered with 2 mg Zortress. If erythromycin is co-administered, everolimus blood concentrations should be monitored and a dose adjustment made as necessary. [*See Drug Interactions (7.4)*]

Verapamil (CYP3A4 Inhibitor and P-gp Substrate): Multiple-dose administration of 80 mg verapamil three times daily for 5 days to 16 healthy volunteers significantly increased everolimus C_{max} and AUC by 2.3-fold and 3.5-fold, respectively, when co-administered with 2 mg Zortress. Everolimus half-life was not changed. If verapamil is co-administered, everolimus blood concentrations should be monitored and a dose adjustment made as necessary. [*See Drug Interactions (7.5)*]

Atorvastatin (CYP3A4 Substrate) and Pravastatin (P-gp Substrate): Following administration of a single dose of 2 mg Zortress to 12 healthy subjects, the concomitant administration of a single oral dose administration of atorvastatin 20 mg or pravastatin 20 mg only slightly decreased everolimus C_{max} and AUC by 9% and 10%, respectively. There was no apparent change in the mean $T_{1/2}$ or median T_{max}. In the same study, the concomitant Zortress dose slightly increased the mean C_{max} of atorvastatin by 11% and slightly decreased the AUC by 7%. The concomitant Zortress dose decreased the mean C_{max} and AUC of pravastatin by 10% and 5%, respectively. No dosage adjustments are needed for concomitant administration of Zortress and atorvastatin and pravastatin. [*See Drug Interactions (7.6)*]

Midazolam (CYP3A4/5 Substrate): In 25 healthy male subjects, co-administration of a single dose of midazolam 4 mg oral solution with steady-state everolimus (10 mg daily dose for 5 days) resulted in a 25% increase in midazolam C_{max} and a 30% increase in midazolam AUC; whereas, the terminal half-life of midazolam and the metabolic AUC-ratio (1-hydroxymidazolam/midazolam) were not affected. [*See Drug Interactions (7.9)*]

Rifampin (*Strong CYP3A4 and P-gp Inducer*): Pretreatment of 12 healthy subjects with multiple-dose rifampin (600 mg once-daily for 8 days) followed by a single dose of 4 mg Zortress increased everolimus clearance nearly 3-fold, and decreased C_{max} by 58% and AUC by 63%. Combination with rifampin is not recommended. [*See Drug Interactions (7.8)*]

12.6 Specific Populations

Hepatic Impairment
Relative to the AUC of everolimus in subjects with normal hepatic function, the average AUC in 6 patients with mild hepatic impairment (Child-Pugh Class A) was 1.6-fold higher following administration of a 10 mg single-dose. In two independently studied groups of 8 and 9 patients with moderate hepatic impairment (Child-Pugh Class B) the average AUC was 2.1-fold and 3.3-fold higher following administration of a 2 mg or a 10 mg single-dose, respectively; and in 6 patients with severe hepatic impairment (Child-Pugh Class C) the average AUC was 3.6-fold higher following administration of a 10 mg single-dose. For patients with mild hepatic impairment (Child-Pugh Class A), the dose should be reduced by approximately one-third of the normally recommended daily dose. For patients with moderate or severe hepatic impairment (Child-Pugh B or C), the initial daily dose should be reduced to approximately one-half of the normally recommended daily dose. Further dose adjustment and/or dose titration should be made if a patient's whole blood trough concentration of everolimus, as measured by an LC/MS/MS assay, is not within the target trough concentration range of 3 to 8 ng/mL. [*See Dosage and Administration (2.7)*]

Renal Impairment
No pharmacokinetic studies in patients with renal impairment were conducted. Post-transplant renal function (creatinine clearance range 11 to 107 mL/min) did not affect the pharmacokinetics of everolimus, therefore, no dosage adjustments are needed in patients with renal impairment.

Pediatrics
The safety and efficacy of Zortress has not been established in pediatric patients.

Geriatrics
A limited reduction in everolimus oral CL of 0.33% per year was estimated in adults (age range studied was 16 to 70 years). There is no evidence to suggest that elderly patients will require a different dosage recommendation from younger adult patients.

Race
Based on analysis of population pharmacokinetics, oral clearance (CL/F) is, on average, 20% higher in black transplant patients.

12.7 Everolimus Whole Blood Concentrations Observed in Kidney and in Liver Transplant Patients

Everolimus in Kidney Transplantation
Based on exposure-efficacy and exposure-safety analyses of clinical trials and using an LC/MS/MS assay method, kidney transplant patients achieving everolimus whole blood trough concentrations ≥3.0 ng/mL have been found to have a lower incidence of treated biopsy-proven acute rejection compared with patients whose trough concentrations were below 3.0 ng/mL. Patients who attained everolimus trough concentrations within the range of 6 to 12 ng/mL had similar efficacy and more adverse reactions than patients who attained lower trough concentrations between 3 to 8 ng/mL. [*See Dosage and Administration (2.3)*]
In the kidney clinical trial [*See Clinical Studies (14.1)*], everolimus whole blood trough concentrations were measured at Days 3, 7, and 14 and Months 1, 2, 3, 4, 6, 7, 9, and 12. The proportion of patients receiving 0.75 mg twice daily Zortress treatment regimen who had everolimus whole blood trough concentrations within the protocol specified target range of 3 to 8 ng/mL at Days 3, 7, and 14 were 55%, 71% and 69%, respectively. Approximately 80% of patients had everolimus whole blood trough concentrations within the 3 to 8 ng/mL target range by Month 1 and remained stable within range through Month 12. The median everolimus trough concentration for the 0.75 mg twice daily treatment group was between 3 and 8 ng/mL throughout the study duration.

Everolimus in Liver Transplantation
In the liver clinical trial [*See Clinical Studies (14.2)*] Zortress dosing was initiated after 30 days following transplantation. Whole blood trough everolimus concentrations were measured within 5 days after first dose, followed by weekly intervals for 3 to 4 weeks, and then monthly thereafter. Approximately 49%, 37%, and 18% of patients, respectively, were below 3 ng/mL at 1, 2, and 4 weeks after initiation of Zortress dosing. The majority of patients (approximately 70 to 80%) had everolimus trough blood concentrations within the target range of 3-8 ng/mL after Month 2 through Month 12.

Table 5. Cyclosporine Trough Concentrations Over 12 Months - Kidney Study Median Values (ng/mL) with 10th and 90th Percentiles

Treatment group	Visit	N	Target (ng/mL)	Median	10th Percentile	90th Percentile
Zortress 0.75 mg twice daily	Day 3	242	100-200	172	46	388
	Day 7	265	100-200	185	75	337
	Day 14	243	100-200	182	97	309
	Month 1	245	100-200	161	85	274
	Month 2	232	75-150	140	84	213
	Month 3	220	75-150	111	68	187
	Month 4	208	50-100	99	56	156
	Month 6	200	25-50	75	43	142
	Month 7	199	25-50	59	36	117
	Month 9	194	25-50	49	28	91
	Month 12	186	25-50	46	25	100

Table 6. Tacrolimus Trough Concentrations Over 12 Months – Liver Study Median Values (ng/mL) with 10th and 90th Percentiles

Treatment group	Visit	N	Target (ng/mL)	Median	10th Percentile	90th Percentile
Predose group	Week 4	234	3-5	9.5	5.8	14.6
Zortress 1.0 mg twice daily (initiated at month 1)	Week 5	219	3-5	8.1	4.5	13.8
	Week 6	233	3-5	7.0	4.1	12.0
	Month 2	219	3-5	5.6	3.4	10.3
	Month 3	218	3-5	5.2	3.1	9.7
	Month 4	196	3-5	4.9	2.9	7.7
	Month 5	195	3-5	4.8	2.7	7.3
	Month 6	200	3-5	4.6	3.0	7.5
	Month 9	186	3-5	4.4	2.9	8.0
	Month 12	175	3-5	4.3	2.6	7.3

12.8 Cyclosporine Concentrations Observed in Kidney Transplant Patients

In the kidney transplant clinical trial [*See Clinical Studies (14.1)*], the target cyclosporine whole blood trough concentration for the Zortress treatment arm of 0.75 mg twice daily were 100 to 200 ng/mL through Month 1 post-transplant, 75 to 150 ng/mL at Months 2 and 3 post-transplant, 50 to 100 ng/mL at Month 4 post-transplant, and 25 to 50 ng/mL from Month 6 through Month 12 post-transplant. Table 5 below provides a summary of the observed cyclosporine whole blood trough concentrations during the study.
[See table 5 above]

12.9 Tacrolimus Concentrations in Liver Transplant

In the liver transplant clinical trial [*See Clinical Studies (14.2)*], the target tacrolimus whole blood trough concentrations were greater than or equal to 8 ng/mL in the first 30 days post-transplant. The protocol required that patients had a tacrolimus trough concentration of at least 8 ng/mL in the week prior to initiation of Zortress. Zortress was initiated after 30 days post-transplant. At that time, the target tacrolimus trough concentrations were reduced to 3 to 5 ng/mL. Table 6 below provides a summary of the tacrolimus whole blood trough concentrations observed during the study.
[See table 6 above]

13 NONCLINICAL TOXICOLOGY

13.1 Carcinogenesis, Mutagenesis, Impairment of Fertility

Everolimus was not carcinogenic in mice or rats when administered daily by oral gavage for 2 years at doses of 0.9 mg/kg. In these studies, AUCs in mice were much higher (at least 20 times) than those in humans receiving 0.75 mg twice daily, and AUCs in rats were in the same range as those in humans receiving 0.75 mg twice daily.
Everolimus was not mutagenic in the bacterial reverse mutation, the mouse lymphoma thymidine kinase assay, or the

chromosome aberration assay using V79 Chinese hamster cells, or *in vivo* following two daily doses of 500 mg/kg in the mouse micronucleus assay.
In a 13-week male fertility oral gavage study in rats, testicular morphology was affected at 0.5 mg/kg and above, and sperm motility, sperm head count and plasma testosterone concentrations were diminished at 5 mg/kg which caused a decrease in male fertility. There was evidence of reversibility of these findings in animals examined after 13 weeks post-dosing. The 0.5 mg/kg dose in male rats resulted in AUCs in the range of clinical exposures, and the 5 mg/kg dose resulted in AUCs approximately 5 times the AUCs in humans receiving 0.75 mg twice daily. Everolimus did not affect female fertility in nonclinical studies, but everolimus crossed the placenta and was toxic to the conceptus. [*See Pregnancy (8.1)*]

14 CLINICAL STUDIES

14.1 Prevention of Organ Rejection after Renal Transplantation

A 24-month, multi-national, open-label, randomized (1:1:1) trial was conducted comparing two concentration-controlled Zortress regimens of 1.5 mg per day starting dose (targeting 3 to 8 ng/mL using an LC/MS/MS assay method and 3.0 mg per day starting dose (targeting 6 to 12 ng/mL using an LC/MS/MS assay method) with reduced exposure cyclosporine and corticosteroids, to 1.44 g per day of mycophenolic acid with standard exposure cyclosporine and corticosteroids. The mean cyclosporine starting dose was 5.2, 5.0 and 5.7 mg/kg body weight/day in the Zortress 1.5 mg, 3.0 mg and in mycophenolic acid groups, respectively. The cyclosporine dose in the Zortress group was then adjusted to the blood trough concentration ranges indicated in Table 5, whereas in the mycophenolic acid group the target ranges were 200-300 ng/mL starting Day 5: 200-300 ng/mL, and 100-250 ng/mL from Month 2 to Month 12.
All patients received basiliximab induction therapy. The study population consisted of 18 to 70 year old male and

Table 7. Efficacy Failure by Treatment Group (ITT Population) at 12 Months

	Zortress (everolimus) 1.5 mg per day With reduced exposure CsA N=277 n (%)	Mycophenolic Acid 1.44 g per day With standard exposure CsA N=277 n (%)
Efficacy Endpoints[1]		
Efficacy Failure Endpoint[2]	70 (25.3)	67 (24.2)
Treated Biopsy Proven Acute Rejection	45 (16.2)	47 (17.0)
Death	7 (2.5)	6 (2.2)
Graft Loss	12 (4.3)	9 (3.2)
Loss to Follow-up	12 (4.3)	9 (3.2)
Graft Loss or Death or Loss to Follow-up[3]	32 (11.6)	26 (9.4)
Graft Loss or Death	18 (6.5)	15 (5.4)
Loss to Follow-up[3]	14 (5.1)	11 (4.0)

* Treated biopsy-proven acute rejection (tBPAR) was defined as a histologically confirmed acute rejection with a biopsy graded as IA, IB, IIA, IIB, or III according to 1997 Banff criteria that was treated with anti-rejection medication.
[1] The difference in rates (Zortress–mycophenolic acid) with 95% CI for primary efficacy failure endpoint is 1.1% (-6.1%, 8.3%); and for the graft loss, death or loss to follow-up endpoint is 2.2% (-2.9%, 7.3%).
[2] Includes treated BPAR, graft loss, death or loss to follow-up by Month 12 where loss to follow-up represents patient who did not experience treated BPAR, graft loss or death and whose last contact date is prior to 12 month visit
[3] Loss to follow-up (for Graft Loss, Death, or Loss to Follow-up) represents patient who did not experience death or graft loss and whose last contact date is prior to 12 month visit

Table 8. Estimated Glomerular Filtration Rates (mL/min/1.73m^2) by MDRD at 12 Months Post-Transplant*

Month 12 GFR (MDRD)	Zortress (everolimus) 1.5 mg per day with reduced exposure CsA N=276	Mycophenolic Acid 1.44 g per day with standard exposure CsA N=277
Mean (SD)**	54.6 (21.7)	52.3 (26.5)
Median (Range)	55.0 (0-140.9)	50.1 (0.0-366.4)

* Analysis based on using a subject's last observation carried forward for missing data at 12 months due to death or lost to follow-up data, a value of zero is used for subjects who experienced a graft loss.
** SD=standard deviation

Table 9. Efficacy Failure by Treatment Group (ITT Population) at 12 Months

	Zortress (everolimus) With reduced Exposure Tacrolimus N=245 n (%)	Tacrolimus (standard exposure) N=243 n (%)
Efficacy Endpoints[1]		
Efficacy Failure Endpoint[2]	22 (9.0)	33 (13.6)
Treated Biopsy Proven Acute Rejection*	7 (2.9)	17 (7.0)
Death	13 (5.3)	7 (2.9)
Graft Loss	6 (2.4)	3 (1.2)
Loss to Follow-up	4 (1.6)	9 (3.7)
Graft Loss or Death or Loss to Follow-up[3]	18 (7.3)	18 (7.4)
Graft Loss or Death	14 (5.7)	8 (3.3)
Loss to Follow-up[3]	4 (1.6)	10 (4.1)

* Treated biopsy-proven acute rejection (tBPAR) was defined as histologically confirmed acute rejection with a rejection activity index (RAI) ≥ RAI score 3 that received anti-rejection treatment.
[1] The difference in rates (Zortress – control) with 97.5% CI for efficacy failure endpoint is -4.6% (-11.4%, 2.2%); and for the graft loss, death or loss to follow-up endpoint is -0.1% (-5.4%, 5.3%).
[2] Includes treated BPAR, graft loss, death or loss to follow-up by Month 12 where loss to follow-up represents patients who did not experience treated BPAR, graft loss or death and whose last contact date is prior to 12 month visit
[3] Loss to follow-up (for Graft Loss, Death, or Loss to Follow-up) represents patients who did not experience death or graft loss and whose last contact date is prior to 12 month visit

female low to moderate risk renal transplant recipients undergoing their first transplant. Low to moderate immunologic risk was defined in the study as an ABO blood type compatible first organ or tissue transplant recipient with anti-HLA Class I PRA <20% by a complement dependent cytotoxicity-based assay, or <50% by a flow cytometry or ELISA-based assay, and with a negative T-cell cross match. Eight hundred thirty-three (833) patients were randomized after transplantation; 277 randomized to the Zortress 1.5 mg per day group, 279 to the Zortress 3.0 mg per day group and 277 to the mycophenolic acid 1.44 g per day group. The study was conducted at 79 renal transplant centers across Europe, South Africa, North and South America, and Asia-Pacific. There were no major baseline differences between treatment groups with regard to recipient or donor disease characteristics. The majority of transplant recipients in all groups (70% to 76%) had three or more HLA mismatches; mean percentage of panel reactive antibodies ranged from 1% to 2%. The rate of premature treatment discontinuation at 12 months was 30% and 22% in the Zortress 1.5 mg and control groups, respectively, (p=0.03, Fisher's exact test) and was more prominent between groups among female patients. Results at 12 months indicated that Zortress 1.5 mg per day is comparable to control with respect to efficacy failure, defined as treated biopsy-proven acute rejection*, graft loss, death or loss to follow-up. The percentage of patients experiencing this endpoint and each individual variable in the Zortress and control groups is shown in Table 7.
[See table 7 above]
The estimated mean glomerular filtration rate (using the MDRD equation) for Zortress 1.5 mg (target trough concentrations 3 to 8 ng/mL) and mycophenolic acid groups were comparable at Month 12 in the ITT population (Table 8).
[See table 8 above]
Two earlier studies compared fixed doses of Zortress 1.5 mg per day and 3 mg per day, without therapeutic drug monitoring, combined with standard exposure cyclosporine and corticosteroids to mycophenolate mofetil 2.0 g per day and corticosteroids. Antilymphocyte antibody induction was prohibited in both studies. Both were multicenter, double-blind (for first 12 months), randomized trials (1:1:1) of 588 and 583 de novo renal transplant patients, respectively. The 12 month analysis of GFR showed increased rates of renal impairment in both the Zortress groups compared to the mycophenolate mofetil group in both studies. Therefore, reduced exposure cyclosporine should be used in combination with Zortress in order to avoid renal dysfunction and everolimus trough concentrations should be adjusted using therapeutic drug monitoring to maintain trough concentrations between 3 to 8 ng/mL. [See Boxed Warning, Dosage and Administration (2.4) and Warnings and Precautions (5.6)]

14.2 Prevention of Organ Rejection after Liver Transplantation

A 24-month, multinational, open-label, randomized (1:1:1) trial was conducted in liver transplant patients starting 30 days post-transplant. During the first 30 days, after transplant and prior to randomization, patients received tacrolimus and corticosteroids, with or without mycophenolate mofetil. No induction antibody was administered. Approximately 70 to 80% of patients received at least one dose of mycophenolate mofetil at a median total daily dose of 1.5 g during the first 30 days. For eligibility, patients had to have a tacrolimus trough concentration of at least 8 ng/mL in the week prior to randomization.
At randomization, mycophenolate mofetil was discontinued and patients were randomized to one of two Zortress treatment groups [initial dose of 1 mg twice per day (2 mg daily) and adjusted to target trough concentrations using an LC/MS/MS assay of 3 to 8 ng/mL] either with reduced exposure of tacrolimus (target trough whole blood concentrations of 3 to 5 ng/mL) or tacrolimus elimination. In the tacrolimus elimination group, at Month 4 post-transplant, once the everolimus trough concentrations were within the target range of 6 to 10 ng/mL, reduced exposure tacrolimus was eliminated. The Zortress with tacrolimus elimination group was discontinued early due to higher incidence of acute rejection. In the control group, patients received standard exposure tacrolimus (target trough whole blood concentrations of 8 to 12 ng/mL tapered to 6 to 10 ng/mL by month 4 post-transplant). All patients received corticosteroids during the trial.
The study population consisted of 18 to 70 year old male and female liver transplant recipients undergoing their first transplant, mean age was approximately 54 years, more than 70% of patients were male, and the majority of patients were Caucasian, with approximately 89% of patients per treatment group completing the study. Key stratification parameters of HCV status (31-32% HCV positive across groups) and renal function (mean baseline eGFR range 79-83 mL/min/1.73m^2) were also balanced between groups.
A total of 1147 patients were enrolled into the run-in period of this trial. At 30 days post-transplant a total 719 patients, who were eligible according to study inclusion/exclusion criteria, were randomized into one of three treatment groups: Zortress with reduced exposure tacrolimus; N=245, Zortress with tacrolimus elimination (tacrolimus elimination group); N=231, or standard dose/exposure tacrolimus (tacrolimus control); N=243. The study was conducted at 89 liver transplant centers across Europe, including the United Kingdom and Ireland, North and South America, and Australia.
Key inclusion criteria were recipients 18-70 years of age, eGFR ≥30 mL/min/1.73m^2, tacrolimus trough level of ≥8 ng/mL in the week prior to randomization, and the ability to take oral medication.

Key exclusion criteria were recipients of multiple solid organ transplants, history of malignancy (except hepatocellular carcinoma within Milan criteria), human immunodeficiency virus, and any surgical or medical condition which significantly alter the absorption, distribution, metabolism and excretion of study drug.

There were no major baseline differences between treatment groups with regard to recipient or donor disease characteristics. Mean MELD scores at time of transplantation, cold ischemia times (CIT), and ABO matching were similar across groups. Overall the treatment groups were comparable with respect to the key determinants of liver transplantation.

The tacrolimus elimination group was stopped prematurely due to a higher incidence of acute rejection and adverse reactions leading to treatment discontinuation reported during the elimination phase of tacrolimus. Therefore, a treatment regimen of Zortress with tacrolimus elimination is not recommended.

Results at 12 months indicated that Zortress with reduced exposure tacrolimus is comparable to standard exposure tacrolimus with respect to efficacy failure, defined as treated biopsy-proven acute rejection, graft loss, death or loss to follow-up. The percentage of patients experiencing this endpoint and each individual variable in the Zortress and control group is shown in Table 9.

[See table 9 at top of previous page]

The estimated mean glomerular filtration rate (using the MDRD equation) for the Zortress group was 80.9 mL/min/1.73m^2 and the tacrolimus control was 70.3 mL/min/1.73m^2 at Month 12 for patients with estimated GFR (eGFR) in the ITT population (Table 10).

Table 10. Estimated Glomerular Filtration Rates (mL/min/1.73m^2) by MDRD at 12 Months Post-Transplant

Month 12 GFR (MDRD)	Zortress (everolimus) with reduced exposure Tacrolimus N=215	Tacrolimus (standard exposure) N=209
Mean (SD)	80.9 (27.3)	70.3 (23.1)
Median* (Range)	78.3 (28.4-153.1)	66.4 (27.9-155.8)

Figure 1. Mean and 95% CI of eGFR (MDRD 4) [mL/min/1.73m^2] by Visit Window and Treatment (ITT population – 12 Month Analysis)*

* Zortress dosing was initiated 30 days after transplantation

16   HOW SUPPLIED/STORAGE AND HANDLING

Zortress (everolimus) Tablets are packed in child-resistant blisters.

Table 11. Description of Zortress (everolimus) Tablets

Dosage Strength	0.25 mg	0.5 mg	0.75 mg
Appearance	White to yellowish, marbled, round, flat tablets with beveled edge		
Imprint	"C" on one side and "NVR" on the other	"CH" on one side and "NVR" on the other	"CL" on one side and "NVR" on the other
NDC Number	0078-0417-20	0078-0414-20	0078-0415-20

Each strength is available in boxes of 60 tablets (6 blister strips of 10 tablets each).

Storage

Store at 25°C (77°F); excursions permitted to 15-30°C (59-86°F). [see USP Controlled Room Temperature]
Protect from light and moisture.

17   PATIENT COUNSELING INFORMATION

17.1   Administration

Inform patients that Zortress should be taken orally twice a day approximately 12 hours apart consistently either with or without food.

Inform patients to avoid grapefruit and grapefruit juice which increase blood drug concentrations of Zortress. [See Warnings and Precautions (5.19)]

Advise patients that Zortress should be used concurrently with reduced doses of cyclosporine and that any change in doses of these medications should be made under physician supervision. A change in the cyclosporine dose may also require a change in the dosage of Zortress.

Inform patients of the necessity of repeated laboratory tests according to physician recommendations while they are taking Zortress.

17.2   Development of Lymphomas and Other Malignancies

Inform patients they are at risk of developing lymphomas and other malignancies, particularly of the skin, due to immunosuppression. Advise patients to limit exposure to sunlight and ultraviolet (UV) light by wearing protective clothing and using a sunscreen with a high protection factor. [See Warnings and Precautions (5.2)]

17.3   Increased Risk of Infection

Inform patients they are at increased risk of developing a variety of infections, including opportunistic infections, due to immunosuppression. Advise patients to contact their physician if they develop any symptoms of infection. [See Warnings and Precautions (5.3, 5.13)]

17.4   Kidney Graft Thrombosis

Inform patients that Zortress has been associated with an increased risk of kidney arterial and venous thrombosis, resulting in graft loss, usually within the first 30 days post-transplantation. [See Warnings and Precautions (5.4)]

17.5   Zortress and Calcineurin Inhibitor-Induced Nephrotoxicity

Advise patients of the risks of impaired kidney function with the combination of Zortress and cyclosporine as well as the need for routine blood concentration monitoring for both drugs. Advise patients of the importance of serum creatinine monitoring. [See Warnings and Precautions (5.6)]

17.6   Angioedema

Inform patients of the risk of angioedema and that concomitant use of angiotensin converting enzyme (ACE) inhibitors may increase this risk. Advise patients to seek prompt medical attention if symptoms occur. [See Warnings and Precautions (5.8)]

17.7   Wound Healing Complications and Fluid Accumulation

Inform patients the use of Zortress has been associated with impaired or delayed wound healing, fluid accumulation and the need for careful observation of their incision site. [See Warnings and Precautions (5.9)]

17.8   Interstitial lung disease/Non-Infectious Pneumonitis

Inform patients the use of Zortress may increase the risk of non-infectious pneumonitis. Advise patients to seek medical attention if they develop clinical symptoms consistent with pneumonia. [See Warnings and Precautions (5.10)]

17.9   Hyperlipidemia

Inform patients the use of Zortress has been associated with increased serum cholesterol and triglycerides that may require treatment and the need for monitoring of blood lipid concentrations. [See Warnings and Precautions (5.11)]

17.10   Proteinuria

Inform patients the use of Zortress has been associated with an increased risk of proteinuria. [See Warnings and Precautions (5.12)]

17.11   Pregnancy

Advise women of childbearing age to avoid becoming pregnant throughout treatment and for 8 weeks after Zortress therapy has stopped.

17.12   Medications that Interfere with Zortress

Some medications can increase or decrease blood concentrations of Zortress. Advise patients to inform their physician if they are taking any of the following: antifungals, antibiotics, antivirals, anti-epileptic medicines including carbamazepine, phenytoin and barbiturates, herbal/dietary supplements (St. John's Wort), and/or rifampin. [See Warnings and Precautions (5.14)]

17.13   New Onset Diabetes

Inform patients the use of Zortress may increase the risk of diabetes mellitus and to contact their physician if they develop symptoms. [See Warnings and Precautions (5.16)]

17.14   Immunizations

Inform patients that vaccinations may be less effective while they are being treated with Zortress. Advise patients live vaccines should be avoided. [See Warnings and Precautions (5.18)]

17.15   Patient with Hereditary Disorders

Advise patients to inform their physicians that if they have hereditary disorders of galactose intolerance (Lapp-lactase deficiency or glucose-galactose malabsorption) not to take Zortress. [See Warnings and Precautions (5.20)]

Manufactured by:
Novartis Pharma Stein AG
Stein, Switzerland
Distributed by:
Novartis Pharmaceuticals Corporation
East Hanover, New Jersey 07936
© Novartis
T2013-09
February 2013

MEDICATION GUIDE
ZORTRESS (ZOR-tres)
(everolimus)
Tablets

Read this Medication Guide before you start using ZORTRESS and each time you get a refill. There may be new information. This information does not take the place of talking with your doctor about your medical condition or treatment.

What is the most important information i should know about ZORTRESS?

ZORTRESS can cause serious side effects, including:

• **Increased risk of getting certain cancers.** People who take ZORTRESS have a higher chance of getting lymphoma and other cancers, especially skin cancer. Talk to your doctor about your risk for cancer.

• **Increased risk of serious infections.** ZORTRESS weakens the body's immune system and affects your ability to fight infections. Serious infections can happen with ZORTRESS that may lead to death. People taking ZORTRESS have a higher chance of getting infections caused by viruses, bacteria, and fungi (yeast).
  ○ Call your doctor if you have symptoms of infection including fever or chills.

• **Blood clot in the blood vessels of your transplanted kidney.** If this happens, it usually occurs within the first 30 days after your kidney transplant. Tell your doctor right away if you:
  ○ have pain in your groin, lower back, side or stomach (abdomen)
  ○ make less urine or you do not pass any urine
  ○ have blood in your urine or dark colored urine (tea-colored)
  ○ have fever, nausea, or vomiting

• **Serious problems with your transplanted kidney (nephrotoxicity).** You will need to start with a lower dose of cyclosporine when you take it with ZORTRESS. Your Doctor should do regular blood tests to check your levels of both ZORTRESS and cyclosporine.

• **Increased risk of death that can be related to infection, in people who have had a heart transplant.** You should not take Zortress if you have had a heart transplant without talking to your doctor.

See the section "What are the possible side effects of ZORTRESS?" for information about other serious side effects.

What is ZORTRESS?

ZORTRESS is a prescription medicine used to prevent transplant rejection (antirejection medicine) in people who have received a kidney transplant or liver transplant. Transplant rejection happens when the body's immune system perceives the new transplanted kidney as "foreign" and attacks it.

ZORTRESS is used with other medicines called cyclosporine, corticosteroids and certain other transplant medicines to prevent rejection of your transplanted kidney. Zortress is used with other medicines called tacrolimus and corticosteroids to prevent rejection of your transplanted liver.

It is not known if ZORTRESS is safe and effective in transplanted organs other than the kidney and liver.

It is not known if ZORTRESS is safe and effective in children under 18 years of age.

Who should not take ZORTRESS?

Do not take ZORTRESS if you are allergic to:

• everolimus (ZORTRESS/AFINITOR®) or any of the ingredients in ZORTRESS. See the end of this Medication Guide for a complete list of ingredients in ZORTRESS.
• sirolimus (Rapamune®)

What should I tell my doctor before taking ZORTRESS?
Before taking ZORTRESS, tell your doctor if you:

• have liver problems
• have skin cancer or it runs in your family
• have high cholesterol or triglycerides (fat in your blood)
• have Lapp lactase deficiency or glucose-galactose malabsorption. You should not take ZORTRESS if you have this disorder.
• have any other medical conditions

- are pregnant or plan to become pregnant. It is not known if ZORTRESS will harm your unborn baby. Talk with your doctor if you are pregnant or plan to become pregnant.
  - Women who may become pregnant should use effective birth control (contraception) while taking ZORTRESS and for 8 weeks after stopping ZORTRESS.
- are breastfeeding or plan to breastfeed. It is not known if ZORTRESS passes into your breast milk. You and your doctor should decide if you will take ZORTRESS or breast-feed. You should not do both.

Tell your doctor about all the medicines you take, including prescription and non-prescription medicines, vitamins, and herbal supplements. ZORTRESS may affect the way other medicines work, and other medicines may affect how ZORTRESS works.

Especially tell your doctor if you take:
- antifungal medicine
- antibiotic medicine
- heart medicine
- high blood pressure medicine
- a medicine to lower cholesterol or triglycerides
- cyclosporine (Sandimmune, Gengraf, Neoral)
- tuberculosis (TB) medicine
- HIV medicine
- St. John's Wort
- seizure (anticonvulsant) medicine

Know the medicines you take. Keep a list of them to show your doctor and pharmacist when you get a new medicine. Do not take any new medicine without talking with your doctor first.

How should I take ZORTRESS?
- Take ZORTRESS exactly as your doctor tells you.
- **Do not** stop taking ZORTRESS or change your dose unless your doctor tells you to.
- Take ZORTRESS at the same time as your dose of cyclosporine medicine.
- **Do not** stop taking or change your dose of cyclosporine or tacrolimus medicine unless your doctor tells you to.
- If your doctor changes your dose of cyclosporine your dose of ZORTRESS may change.
- Take ZORTRESS 2 times a day about 12 hours apart.
- Swallow ZORTRESS tablets whole with a glass of water. Do not crush or chew ZORTRESS tablets.
- Take ZORTRESS tablets with or without food. If you take ZORTRESS tablets **with food,** always take ZORTRESS tablets **with food.** If you take ZORTRESS tablets **without food,** always take ZORTRESS tablets **without food.**
- **Your doctor will do regular blood tests to check your kidney function while you take ZORTRESS. It is important that you get these tests done when your doctor tells you to. Blood tests will monitor how your kidneys are working and make sure you are getting the right dose of ZORTRESS and other transplant medications they may be on (cyclosporine and tacrolimus).**
- If you take too much ZORTRESS, call your doctor or go to the nearest hospital emergency room right away.

What should I avoid while taking ZORTRESS?
- Avoid receiving any live vaccines while taking ZORTRESS. Some vaccines may not work as well while you are taking ZORTRESS.
- Do not eat grapefruit or drink grapefruit juice while you are taking ZORTRESS. Grapefruit may increase your blood level of ZORTRESS.
- Limit the amount of time you spend in the sunlight. Avoid using tanning beds or sunlamps. People who take ZORTRESS have a higher risk of getting skin cancer. See the section "What is the most important information I should know about ZORTRESS?" Wear protective clothing when you are in the sun and use a sunscreen with a high protection factor (SPF 30 and above). This is especially important if you have fair skin or if you have a family history of skin cancer.
- Avoid becoming pregnant. See the section "What should I tell my doctor before taking ZORTRESS?"

What are possible side effects of ZORTRESS?
ZORTRESS can cause serious side effects, including:
- See **"What is the most important information I should know about ZORTRESS?"**
- **swelling under your skin especially around your mouth, eyes and in your throat (angioedema).** Your chance of having swelling under your skin is higher if you take ZORTRESS along with certain other medicines. Tell your doctor right away or go to the nearest emergency room if you have any of these symptoms of angioedema:
  - sudden swelling of your face, mouth, throat, tongue or hands
  - hives or welts
  - itchy or painful swollen skin
  - trouble breathing
- **delayed wound healing.** ZORTRESS can cause your incision to heal slowly or not heal well. Call your doctor right away if you have any of the following symptoms:
  - your incision is red, warm or painful
  - blood, fluid, or pus in your incision

- your incision opens up
- swelling of your incision
- **lung or breathing problems.** Tell your doctor right away if you have new or worsening cough, shortness of breath, difficulty breathing or wheezing. In some patients lung or breathing problems have been severe, and can even lead to death. Your doctor may need to stop ZORTRESS or lower your dose.
- **increased cholesterol and triglycerides (fat in your blood).** If your cholesterol and triglyceride levels are high your doctor may want to lower them with diet, exercise and certain medicines.
- **protein in your urine (proteinuria).**
- **change in kidney function.** ZORTRESS may cause kidney problems when taken along with a standard dose of cyclosporine medicine instead of a lower dose.

Your doctor should do blood and urine tests to monitor your cholesterol, triglycerides and kidney function.
- **viral infections.** Certain viruses can live in your body and cause active infections when your immune system is weak. Viral infections that can happen with ZORTRESS include BK virus-associated nephropathy. BK virus can affect how your kidney works and cause your transplanted kidney to fail.
- **blood clotting problems.**
- **diabetes.** Tell your doctor if you have frequent urination, increased thirst or hunger.
- **male infertility (low or no sperm count).**

The most common side effects of ZORTRESS in people who have had a kidney or liver transplant include:
These common side effects have been reported in both kidney and liver transplant patients:
- nausea
- swelling of the lower legs, ankles and feet
- high blood pressure

The most common side effects of ZORTRESS in people who have had a kidney transplant include:
- constipation
- low red blood cell count (anemia)
- urinary tract infection
- increased fat in the blood (cholesterol and triglycerides)

The most common side effects of ZORTRESS in people who have had a liver transplant include:
- diarrhea
- headache
- fever
- abdominal pain
- low white blood cells

These are not all of the possible side effects of ZORTRESS. Tell your doctor about any side effect that bothers you or that does not go away.

Call your doctor for medical advice about side effects. You may report side effects to the FDA at 1-800-FDA-1088.

How do I store ZORTRESS?
- Store ZORTRESS tablets between 59°F to 86°F (15°C to 30°C).
- Keep ZORTRESS out of the light.
- Keep ZORTRESS tablets dry.

Keep ZORTRESS and all medicines out of the reach of children.

General information about the safe and effective use of ZORTRESS.

Medicines are sometimes prescribed for purposes other than those listed in a Medication Guide. Do not use ZORTRESS for a condition for which it was not prescribed. Do not give ZORTRESS to other people, even if they have the same symptoms you have. It may harm them.

This Medication Guide summarizes the most important information about ZORTRESS. For more information, talk with your doctor. You can ask your doctor or pharmacist for information about ZORTRESS that is written for healthcare professionals. For more information, call 1-888-669-6682 or visit www.zortress.com.

What are the ingredients in ZORTRESS?
Active ingredient: everolimus
Inactive ingredients: butylated hydroxytoluene, magnesium stearate, lactose monohydrate, hypromellose, crospovidone and lactose anhydrous.

This Medication Guide has been approved by the U.S. Food and Drug Administration.

Any other trademarks in this document are the property of their respective owners.

Manufactured by:
Novartis Pharma Stein AG
Stein, Switzerland
Distributed by:
Novartis Pharmaceuticals Corporation
East Hanover, New Jersey 07936
© Novartis
Rapamune® is a registered trademark of Pfizer Inc
Gengraf® is a registered trademark of Abbott Laboratories
T2013-10
February 2013
Shown in Product Identification Guide, page 311

ZYKADIA™
(ceritinib)
capsules, for oral use

Ŗ

The following prescribing information is based on official labeling in effect July 2014.

HIGHLIGHTS OF PRESCRIBING INFORMATION
These highlights do not include all the information needed to use ZYKADIA safely and effectively. See full prescribing information for ZYKADIA.
ZYKADIA™ (ceritinib) capsules, for oral use
Initial U.S. Approval: 2014

————————**INDICATIONS AND USAGE**————————
ZYKADIA is a kinase inhibitor indicated for the treatment of patients with anaplastic lymphoma kinase (ALK)-positive metastatic non-small cell lung cancer (NSCLC) who have progressed on or are intolerant to crizotinib. This indication is approved under accelerated approval based on tumor response rate and duration of response. An improvement in survival or disease-related symptoms has not been established. Continued approval for this indication may be contingent upon verification and description of clinical benefit in confirmatory trials. (1)

————————**DOSAGE AND ADMINISTRATION**————————
- 750 mg orally once daily. Administer ZYKADIA on an empty stomach (i.e., do not administer within 2 hours of a meal). (2.1)

————————**DOSAGE FORMS AND STRENGTHS**————————
Capsules: 150 mg (3)

————————**CONTRAINDICATIONS**————————
None (4)

————————**WARNINGS AND PRECAUTIONS**————————
- Severe or Persistent Gastrointestinal Toxicity: Dose modification due to diarrhea, nausea, vomiting or abdominal pain occurred in 38% of patients. Withhold if not responsive to anti-emetics or anti-diarrheals, then dose reduce ZYKADIA. (2.2, 5.1)
- Hepatotoxicity: ZYKADIA can cause hepatotoxicity. Monitor liver laboratory tests at least monthly. Withhold then dose reduce, or permanently discontinue ZYKADIA. (2.2, 5.2)
- Interstitial Lung Disease (ILD)/Pneumonitis: Occurred in 4% of patients. Permanently discontinue ZYKADIA in patients diagnosed with treatment-related ILD/pneumonitis. (2.2, 5.3)
- QT Interval Prolongation: ZYKADIA can cause QTc interval prolongation. Monitor electrocardiograms and electrolytes in patients with congestive heart failure, bradyarrhythmias, electrolyte abnormalities, or those who are taking medications that are known to prolong the QTc interval. Withhold then dose reduce, or permanently discontinue ZYKADIA. (2.2, 5.4)
- Hyperglycemia: ZYKADIA can cause hyperglycemia. Monitor glucose and initiate or optimize antihyperglycemic medications as indicated. Withhold then dose reduce, or permanently discontinue ZYKADIA. (2.2, 5.5)
- Bradycardia: ZYKADIA can cause bradycardia. Monitor heart rate and blood pressure regularly. Withhold then dose reduce, or permanently discontinue ZYKADIA. (2.2, 5.6)
- Embryofetal Toxicity: ZYKADIA may cause fetal harm. Advise females of reproductive potential of the potential risk to a fetus. (5.7, 8.1, 8.7)

————————**ADVERSE REACTIONS**————————
The most common adverse reactions (incidence of at least 25%) are diarrhea, nausea, elevated transaminases, vomiting, abdominal pain, fatigue, decreased appetite, and constipation. (6)
To report SUSPECTED ADVERSE REACTIONS, contact Novartis Pharmaceuticals Corporation at 1-888-669-6682 or FDA at 1-800-FDA-1088 or www.fda.gov/medwatch.

————————**DRUG INTERACTIONS**————————
- CYP3A Inhibitors and Inducers: Avoid concurrent use of ZYKADIA with strong CYP3A inhibitors or inducers. If concurrent use of a strong CYP3A inhibitor is unavoidable, reduce the dose of ZYKADIA. (2.3, 7.1)
- CYP3A and CYP2C9 Substrates: Avoid concurrent use of ZYKADIA with CYP3A or CYP2C9 substrates with narrow therapeutic indices. (7.2)

See 17 for PATIENT COUNSELING INFORMATION and FDA-approved patient labeling.

Revised: 4/2014

FULL PRESCRIBING INFORMATION: CONTENTS*
1   **INDICATIONS AND USAGE**
2   **DOSAGE AND ADMINISTRATION**
     2.1   Dosing and Administration
     2.2   Dose Modifications for Adverse Reactions
     2.3   Dose Modification for Strong CYP3A4 Inhibitors
3   **DOSAGE FORMS AND STRENGTHS**

4 CONTRAINDICATIONS
5 WARNINGS AND PRECAUTIONS
5.1 Severe or Persistent Gastrointestinal Toxicity
5.2 Hepatotoxicity
5.3 Interstitial Lung Disease (ILD)/Pneumonitis
5.4 QT Interval Prolongation
5.5 Hyperglycemia
5.6 Bradycardia
5.7 Embryofetal Toxicity
6 ADVERSE REACTIONS
6.1 Clinical Trials Experience
7 DRUG INTERACTIONS
7.1 Effect of Other Drugs on Ceritinib
7.2 Effect of Ceritinib on Other Drugs
8 USE IN SPECIFIC POPULATIONS
8.1 Pregnancy
8.3 Nursing Mothers
8.4 Pediatric Use
8.5 Geriatric Use
8.6 Hepatic Impairment
8.7 Females and Males of Reproductive Potential
11 DESCRIPTION
12 CLINICAL PHARMACOLOGY
12.1 Mechanism of Action
12.2 Pharmacodynamics
12.3 Pharmacokinetics
13 NONCLINICAL TOXICOLOGY
13.1 Carcinogenesis, Mutagenesis, Impairment of Fertility
13.2 Animal Toxicology and/or Pharmacology
14 CLINICAL STUDIES
16 HOW SUPPLIED/STORAGE AND HANDLING
17 PATIENT COUNSELING INFORMATION
* Sections or subsections omitted from the full prescribing information are not listed.

FULL PRESCRIBING INFORMATION

1 INDICATIONS AND USAGE

ZYKADIA is indicated for the treatment of patients with anaplastic lymphoma kinase (ALK)-positive metastatic non-small cell lung cancer (NSCLC) who have progressed on or are intolerant to crizotinib.

This indication is approved under accelerated approval based on tumor response rate and duration of response [see Clinical Studies (14)]. An improvement in survival or disease-related symptoms has not been established. Continued approval for this indication may be contingent upon verification and description of clinical benefit in confirmatory trials.

2 DOSAGE AND ADMINISTRATION
2.1 Dosing and Administration

The recommended dose of ZYKADIA is 750 mg orally once daily until disease progression or unacceptable toxicity. Administer ZYKADIA on an empty stomach (i.e., do not administer within 2 hours of a meal) [see Clinical Pharmacology (12.3)].

A recommended dose has not been determined for patients with moderate to severe hepatic impairment [see Use in Specific Populations (8.6)].

If a dose of ZYKADIA is missed, make up that dose unless the next dose is due within 12 hours.

2.2 Dose Modifications for Adverse Reactions

Recommendations for dose modifications of ZYKADIA for adverse reactions are provided in Table 1.

Approximately 60% of patients initiating treatment at the recommended dose required at least one dose reduction and the median time to first dose reduction was 7 weeks.

Discontinue ZYKADIA for patients unable to tolerate 300 mg daily.

Table 1: ZYKADIA Dose Interruption, Reduction, or Discontinuation Recommendations

Criteria	ZYKADIA Dosing
• ALT or AST elevation greater than 5 times ULN with • total bilirubin elevation less than or equal to 2 times ULN	Withhold until recovery to baseline or less than or equal to 3 times ULN, then resume ZYKADIA with a 150 mg dose reduction.
• ALT or AST elevation greater than 3 times ULN with • total bilirubin elevation greater than 2 times ULN in the absence of cholestasis or hemolysis	Permanently discontinue ZYKADIA.
Any Grade treatment-related ILD/pneumonitis	Permanently discontinue ZYKADIA.
QTc interval greater than 500 msec on at least 2 separate ECGs	Withhold until QTc interval is less than 481 msec or recovery to baseline if baseline QTc is greater than or equal to 481 msec, then resume ZYKADIA with a 150 mg dose reduction.
QTc interval prolongation in combination with Torsade de pointes or polymorphic ventricular tachycardia or signs/symptoms of serious arrhythmia	Permanently discontinue ZYKADIA.
Severe or intolerable nausea, vomiting or diarrhea despite optimal anti-emetic or anti-diarrheal therapy	Withhold until improved, then resume ZYKADIA with a 150 mg dose reduction.
Persistent hyperglycemia greater than 250 mg/dL despite optimal anti-hyperglycemic therapy	Withhold until hyperglycemia is adequately controlled, then resume ZYKADIA with a 150 mg dose reduction. If adequate hyperglycemic control cannot be achieved with optimal medical management, discontinue ZYKADIA.
Symptomatic bradycardia that is not life-threatening	Withhold until recovery to asymptomatic bradycardia or to a heart rate of 60 bpm or above, evaluate concomitant medications known to cause bradycardia, and adjust the dose of ZYKADIA.
Clinically significant bradycardia requiring intervention or life-threatening bradycardia in patients taking a concomitant medication also known to cause bradycardia or a medication known to cause hypotension	Withhold until recovery to asymptomatic bradycardia or to a heart rate of 60 bpm or above. If the concomitant medication can be adjusted or discontinued, resume ZYKADIA with a 150 mg dose reduction, with frequent monitoring.
Life-threatening bradycardia in patients who are not taking a concomitant medication also known to cause bradycardia or known to cause hypotension	Permanently discontinue ZYKADIA.

CTCAE, Common Terminology Criteria for Adverse Events v4.03
ALT, alanine aminotransferase; AST, aspartate aminotransferase; ULN, upper limit of normal; ILD, interstitial lung disease; ECG, electrocardiogram

2.3 Dose Modification for Strong CYP3A4 Inhibitors

Avoid concurrent use of strong CYP3A inhibitors during treatment with ZYKADIA [see Drug Interactions (7.1) and Clinical Pharmacology (12.3)].

If concomitant use of a strong CYP3A inhibitor is unavoidable, reduce the ZYKADIA dose by approximately one-third, rounded to the nearest 150 mg dosage strength. After discontinuation of a strong CYP3A inhibitor, resume the ZYKADIA dose that was taken prior to initiating the strong CYP3A4 inhibitor.

3 DOSAGE FORMS AND STRENGTHS

150 mg hard gelatin capsule with opaque blue cap and opaque white body containing a white to off-white powder. The opaque blue cap is marked in black ink with "LDK 150MG" and the opaque white body is marked in black ink with "NVR".

4 CONTRAINDICATIONS

None

5 WARNINGS AND PRECAUTIONS
5.1 Severe or Persistent Gastrointestinal Toxicity

Diarrhea, nausea, vomiting, or abdominal pain occurred in 96% of 255 patients including severe cases in 14% of patients treated with ZYKADIA in Study 1. Dose modification due to diarrhea, nausea, vomiting, or abdominal pain occurred in 38% of patients.

Monitor and manage patients using standards of care, including anti-diarrheals, anti-emetics, or fluid replacement, as indicated. Based on the severity of the adverse drug reaction, withhold ZYKADIA with resumption at a reduced dose as described in Table 1 [see Dosage and Administration (2.2) and Adverse Reactions (6)].

5.2 Hepatotoxicity

Drug-induced hepatotoxicity occurred in patients treated with ZYKADIA. Elevations in alanine aminotransferase (ALT) greater than 5 times the upper limit of normal (ULN) occurred in 27% of 255 patients in Study 1. One patient (0.4%) required permanent discontinuation due to elevated transaminases and jaundice.

Monitor with liver laboratory tests including ALT, aspartate aminotransferase (AST), and total bilirubin once a month and as clinically indicated, with more frequent testing in patients who develop transaminase elevations. Based on the severity of the adverse drug reaction, withhold ZYKADIA with resumption at a reduced dose, or permanently discontinue ZYKADIA as described in Table 1 [see Dosage and Administration (2.2) and Adverse Reactions (6)].

5.3 Interstitial Lung Disease (ILD)/Pneumonitis

Severe, life-threatening, or fatal ILD/pneumonitis can occur in patients treated with ZYKADIA. In Study 1, pneumonitis was reported in 4% of 255 patients treated with ZYKADIA. CTCAE Grade 3 or 4 ILD/pneumonitis was reported in 3% of patients, and fatal ILD/pneumonitis was reported in 1 patient (0.4%) in Study 1. One percent (1%) of patients discontinued ZYKADIA in Study 1 due to ILD/pneumonitis.

Monitor patients for pulmonary symptoms indicative of ILD/pneumonitis. Exclude other potential causes of ILD/pneumonitis, and permanently discontinue ZYKADIA in patients diagnosed with treatment-related ILD/pneumonitis [see Dosage and Administration (2.2) and Adverse Reactions (6)].

5.4 QT Interval Prolongation

QTc interval prolongation occurs in patients treated with ZYKADIA. Three percent (3%) of 255 patients experienced a QTc interval increase over baseline greater than 60 msec in Study 1. Across the development program of ZYKADIA, one of 304 patients (less than 1%) treated with ZYKADIA doses ranging from 50 to 750 mg was found to have a QTc greater than 500 msec and 3% of patients had an increase from baseline QTc greater than 60 msec. A pharmacokinetic analysis suggested that ZYKADIA causes concentration-dependent increases in the QTc interval.

When possible, avoid use of ZYKADIA in patients with congenital long QT syndrome. Conduct periodic monitoring with electrocardiograms (ECGs) and electrolytes in patients with congestive heart failure, bradyarrhythmias, electrolyte abnormalities, or those who are taking medications that are known to prolong the QTc interval. Withhold ZYKADIA in patients who develop a QTc interval greater than 500 msec on at least 2 separate ECGs until the QTc interval is less than 481 msec or recovery to baseline if the QTc interval is greater than or equal to 481 msec, then resume ZYKADIA at a reduced dose as described in Table 1. Permanently discontinue ZYKADIA in patients who develop QTc interval prolongation in combination with Torsade de pointes or polymorphic ventricular tachycardia or signs/symptoms of serious arrhythmia [see Dosage and Administration (2.2) and Clinical Pharmacology (12.2)].

5.5 Hyperglycemia

Hyperglycemia can occur in patients receiving ZYKADIA. In Study 1, CTCAE Grade 3–4 hyperglycemia, based on laboratory values, occurred in 13% of 255 patients. There was a 6-fold increase in the risk of CTCAE Grade 3–4 hyperglycemia in patients with diabetes or glucose intolerance and a 2-fold increase in patients taking corticosteroids.

Monitor serum glucose levels as clinically indicated. Initiate or optimize anti-hyperglycemic medications as indicated. Based on the severity of the adverse drug reaction, withhold ZYKADIA until hyperglycemia is adequately controlled, then resume ZYKADIA at a reduced dose as described in Table 1. If adequate hyperglycemic control cannot be achieved with optimal medical management, permanently discontinue ZYKADIA [see Dosage and Administration (2.2) and Adverse Reactions (6)].

5.6 Bradycardia

Bradycardia can occur in patients receiving ZYKADIA. In Study 1, sinus bradycardia, defined as a heart rate of less than 50 beats per minute, was noted as a new finding in 1% of 255 patients. Bradycardia was reported as an adverse drug reaction in 3% of patients in Study 1.

Avoid using ZYKADIA in combination with other agents known to cause bradycardia (e.g., beta-blockers, non-dihydropyridine calcium channel blockers, clonidine, and digoxin) to the extent possible. Monitor heart rate and blood pressure regularly. In cases of symptomatic bradycardia that is not life-threatening, withhold ZYKADIA until recovery to asymptomatic bradycardia or to a heart rate of 60 bpm or above, evaluate the use of concomitant medications, and adjust the dose of ZYKADIA. Permanently discontinue ZYKADIA for life-threatening bradycardia if no contributing concomitant medication is identified; however, if associated with a concomitant medication known to cause bradycardia or hypotension, withhold ZYKADIA until recovery to asymptomatic bradycardia or to a heart rate of 60 bpm or above, and if the concomitant medication can be adjusted or discontinued, resume ZYKADIA at a reduced dose as described in Table 1 upon recovery to asymptomatic bradycardia or to a heart rate of 60 bpm or above, with frequent monitoring [see Dosage and Administration (2.2) and Adverse Reactions (6)].

5.7 Embryofetal Toxicity

Based on its mechanism of action, ZYKADIA may cause fetal harm when administered to a pregnant woman. In animal studies, administration of ceritinib to rats and rabbits during organogenesis at maternal plasma exposures below the recommended human dose of 750 mg daily caused increases in skeletal anomalies in rats and rabbits. Apprise women of reproductive potential of the potential hazard to a fetus [see Use in Specific Populations (8.1)]. Advise females of reproductive potential to use effective contraception during treatment with ZYKADIA and for at least 2 weeks following completion of therapy [see Use in Specific Populations (8.7)].

6 ADVERSE REACTIONS

The following adverse reactions are discussed in greater detail in other sections of the labeling:

• Severe or Persistent Gastrointestinal Toxicity [see Warnings and Precautions (5.1)]
• Hepatotoxicity [see Warnings and Precautions (5.2)]
• Interstitial Lung Disease/Pneumonitis [see Warnings and Precautions (5.3)]
• QT Interval Prolongation [see Warnings and Precautions (5.4) and Clinical Pharmacology (12.2)]
• Hyperglycemia [see Warnings and Precautions (5.5)]
• Bradycardia [see Warnings and Precautions (5.6) and Clinical Pharmacology (12.2)]

6.1 Clinical Trials Experience

Because clinical trials are conducted under widely varying conditions, adverse reaction rates observed in the clinical trials of a drug cannot be directly compared to rates in the clinical trials of another drug and may not reflect the rates observed in practice.

The safety evaluation of ZYKADIA is based on 255 ALK-positive patients in Study 1 (246 patients with NSCLC and 9 patients with other cancers who received ZYKADIA at a dose of 750 mg daily. The median duration of exposure to ZYKADIA was 6 months. The study population characteristics were: median age 53 years, age less than 65 (84%), female (53%), Caucasian (63%), Asian (34%), NSCLC adenocarcinoma histology (90%), never or former smoker (97%), ECOG PS 0 or 1 (89%), brain metastasis (49%), and number of prior therapies 2 or more (67%).

Dose reductions due to adverse reactions occurred in 59% of patients treated with ZYKADIA. The most frequent adverse reactions, reported in at least 10% of patients, that led to dose reductions or interruptions were: increased ALT (29%), nausea (20%), increased AST (16%), diarrhea (16%), and vomiting (16%). Serious adverse drug reactions reported in 2% or more of patients in Study 1 were convulsion, pneumonia, ILD/pneumonitis, dyspnea, dehydration, hyperglycemia, and nausea. Fatal adverse reactions in patients treated with ZYKADIA occurred in 5% of patients, consisting of: pneumonia (4 patients), respiratory failure, ILD/pneumonitis, pneumothorax, gastric hemorrhage, general physical health deterioration, pulmonary tuberculosis, cardiac tamponade, and sepsis (1 patient each). Discontinuation of therapy due to adverse reactions occurred in 10% of patients treated with ZYKADIA. The most frequent adverse drug reactions that led to discontinuation in 1% or more of patients in Study 1 were pneumonia, ILD/pneumonitis, and decreased appetite.

Tables 2 and 3 summarize the common adverse reactions and laboratory abnormalities observed in ZYKADIA-treated patients.

Table 2: Adverse Reactions (>10% for All NCI CTCAE* Grades or ≥2% for Grades 3-4) in ALK-Positive Patients Treated with ZYKADIA in Study 1

	ZYKADIA N=255	
	All Grades	Grade 3–4
	%	%
Gastrointestinal disorders		
Diarrhea	86	6
Nausea	80	4
Vomiting	60	4
Abdominal pain[a]	54	2
Constipation	29	0
Esophageal disorder[b]	16	1
General disorders and administration site conditions		
Fatigue[c]	52	5
Metabolism and nutrition disorders		
Decreased appetite	34	1
Skin and subcutaneous tissue disorders		
Rash[d]	16	0
Respiratory, thoracic and mediastinal disorders		
Interstitial lung disease/ pneumonitis	4	3

*National Cancer Institute Common Terminology Criteria for Adverse Events (version 4.03)

[a] Abdominal pain (abdominal pain, upper abdominal pain, abdominal discomfort, epigastric discomfort)
[b] Esophageal disorder (dyspepsia, gastroesophageal reflux disease, dysphagia)
[c] Fatigue (fatigue, asthenia)
[d] Rash (rash, maculopapular rash, acneiform dermatitis)

Additional clinically significant adverse reactions occurring in 2% or more of patients treated with ZYKADIA included neuropathy (17%; comprised of paresthesia, muscular weakness, gait disturbance, peripheral neuropathy, hypoesthesia, peripheral sensory neuropathy, dysesthesia, neuralgia, peripheral motor neuropathy, hypotonia, or polyneuropathy), vision disorder (9%; comprised of vision impairment, blurred vision, photopsia, accommodation disorder, presbyopia, or reduced visual acuity), prolonged QT interval (4%), and bradycardia (3%).

Table 3: Key Laboratory Abnormalities Occurring in >10% (All NCI CTCAE Grades) of ALK-Positive Patients Treated with ZYKADIA in Study 1

	ZYKADIA N=255	
	All Grades	Grade 3–4
	%	%
Hemoglobin decreased	84	5
Alanine transaminase (ALT) increased	80	27
Aspartate transaminase (AST) increased	75	13
Creatinine increased	58	2
Glucose increased	49	13
Phosphate decreased	36	7
Lipase increased	28	10
Bilirubin (total) increased	15	1

7 DRUG INTERACTIONS

7.1 Effect of Other Drugs on Ceritinib

Ceritinib is primarily metabolized by CYP3A4 and is a substrate of the efflux transporter P-glycoprotein (P-gp).

Strong CYP3A Inhibitors
Ketoconazole (a strong CYP3A4/P-gp inhibitor) increased the systemic exposure of ceritinib [see Clinical Pharmacology (12.3)]. Avoid concurrent use of strong CYP3A inhibitors during treatment with ZYKADIA. If concomitant use of strong CYP3A inhibitors including certain antivirals (e.g., ritonavir), macrolide antibiotics (e.g., telithromycin), antifungals (e.g., ketoconazole), and nefazodone is unavoidable, reduce the ZYKADIA dose by approximately one-third, rounded to the nearest 150 mg dosage strength. After discontinuation of a strong CYP3A inhibitor, resume the ZYKADIA dose that was taken prior to initiating the strong CYP3A4 inhibitor.

Do not consume grapefruit and grapefruit juice as they may inhibit CYP3A.

Strong CYP3A Inducers
Rifampin (a strong CYP3A4/P-gp inducer) decreased the systemic exposure of ceritinib [see Clinical Pharmacology (12.3)]. Avoid concurrent use of strong CYP3A inducers (e.g., carbamazepine, phenytoin, rifampin, and St. John's Wort) during treatment with ZYKADIA.

7.2 Effect of Ceritinib on Other Drugs

Ceritinib may inhibit CYP3A and CYP2C9 at clinical concentrations [see Clinical Pharmacology (12.3)]. Avoid concurrent use of CYP3A and CYP2C9 substrates known to have narrow therapeutic indices or substrates primarily metabolized by CYP3A and CYP2C9 during treatment with ZYKADIA. If use of these medications is unavoidable, consider dose reduction of CYP3A substrates with narrow therapeutic indices (e.g., alfentanil, cyclosporine, dihydroergotamine, ergotamine, fentanyl, pimozide, quinidine, sirolimus, tacrolimus) and CYP2C9 substrates with narrow therapeutic indices (e.g., phenytoin, warfarin).

8 USE IN SPECIFIC POPULATIONS

8.1 Pregnancy

Pregnancy Category D

Risk Summary
Based on its mechanism of action, ZYKADIA may cause fetal harm when administered to a pregnant woman. In animal studies, administration of ceritinib to rats and rabbits during organogenesis at maternal plasma exposures below the recommended human dose caused increases in skeletal anomalies in rats and rabbits. If this drug is used during pregnancy, or if the patient becomes pregnant while taking this drug, apprise the patient of the potential hazard to a fetus.

Animal Data
In an embryo-fetal development study in which pregnant rats were administered daily doses of ceritinib during organogenesis, dose-related skeletal anomalies were observed at doses as low as 50 mg/kg (less than 0.5-fold the human exposure by AUC at the recommended dose). Findings included delayed ossifications and skeletal variations.

In pregnant rabbits administered ceritinib daily during organogenesis, dose-related skeletal anomalies, including incomplete ossification, were observed at doses equal to or greater than 2 mg/kg/day (approximately 0.015-fold the human exposure by AUC at the recommended dose). A low incidence of visceral anomalies, including absent or malpositioned gallbladder and retroesophageal subclavian cardiac artery, was observed at doses equal to or greater than 10 mg/kg/day (approximately 0.13-fold the human exposure by AUC at the recommended dose). Maternal toxicity and abortion occurred in rabbits at doses of 35 mg/kg or greater. In addition, embryolethality was observed in rabbits at a dose of 50 mg/kg.

8.3 Nursing Mothers

It is not known whether ceritinib or its metabolites are present in human milk. Because many drugs are present in human milk and because of the potential for serious adverse reactions in nursing infants from ceritinib, advise mothers to discontinue nursing.

8.4 Pediatric Use

The safety and effectiveness of ZYKADIA in pediatric patients have not been established.

8.5 Geriatric Use

Clinical studies of ZYKADIA did not include sufficient numbers of subjects aged 65 years and older to determine whether they respond differently from younger subjects. Of the 255 patients in Study 1 who received ZYKADIA at the recommended dose, 40 (16%) were 65 years or older.

8.6 Hepatic Impairment

As ceritinib is eliminated primarily via the liver, patients with hepatic impairment may have increased exposure. Dose adjustment is not recommended for patients with mild hepatic impairment (total bilirubin less than or equal to ULN and AST greater than ULN or total bilirubin greater than 1.0 to 1.5 times ULN and any AST) based on results of the population pharmacokinetic analysis [see Clinical Pharmacology (12.3)]. A recommended dose has not been determined for patients with moderate to severe hepatic impairment.

8.7 Females and Males of Reproductive Potential
Contraception
Based on its mechanism of action, ZYKADIA may cause fetal harm when administered to a pregnant woman [see Use in Specific Populations (8.1)]. Advise females of reproductive potential to use effective contraception during treatment with ZYKADIA and for at least 2 weeks following completion of therapy.

11 DESCRIPTION

ZYKADIA (ceritinib) is a tyrosine kinase inhibitor for oral administration. The molecular formula for ceritinib is $C_{28}H_{36}N_5O_3ClS$. The molecular weight is 558.14 g/mole. Ceritinib is described chemically as 5-Chloro-N4-[2-[(1-methylethyl)sulfonyl]phenyl]-N2-[5-methyl-2-(1-methylethoxy)-4-(4-piperidinyl)phenyl]-2,4-pyrimidinediamine. The chemical structure of ceritinib is shown below:

Ceritinib is a white to almost white or light yellow or light brown powder with a pKa of 9.7 and 4.1.
ZYKADIA is supplied as printed hard-gelatin capsules containing 150 mg of ceritinib and the following inactive ingredients: colloidal anhydrous silica, L-hydroxypropylcellulose, magnesium stearate, microcrystalline cellulose, sodium starch glycolate, and hard gelatin capsule shells. The capsule shell is composed of gelatin, indigotine, and titanium dioxide.

12 CLINICAL PHARMACOLOGY
12.1 Mechanism of Action
Ceritinib is a kinase inhibitor. Targets of ceritinib inhibition identified in either biochemical or cellular assays at clinically relevant concentrations include ALK, insulin-like growth factor 1 receptor (IGF-1R), insulin receptor (InsR), and ROS1. Among these, ceritinib is most active against ALK. Ceritinib inhibited autophosphorylation of ALK, ALK-mediated phosphorylation of the downstream signaling protein STAT3, and proliferation of ALK-dependent cancer cells in in vitro and in vivo assays.
Ceritinib inhibited the in vitro proliferation of cell lines expressing EML4-ALK and NPM-ALK fusion proteins and demonstrated dose-dependent inhibition of EML4-ALK-positive NSCLC xenograft growth in mice and rats. Ceritinib exhibited dose-dependent anti-tumor activity in mice bearing EML4-ALK-positive NSCLC xenografts with demonstrated resistance to crizotinib, at concentrations within a clinically relevant range.

12.2 Pharmacodynamics
Cardiac Electrophysiology
Serial ECGs were collected following a single dose and at steady-state to evaluate the effect of ceritinib on the QT interval in an open-label, dose-escalation, and expansion study. A total of 304 patients were treated with ZYKADIA doses ranging from 50 to 750 mg with 255 patients treated with ZYKADIA 750 mg. One of 304 patients (less than 1%) was found to have a QTc greater than 500 msec and 10 patients (3%) had an increase from baseline QTc greater than 60 msec. A central tendency analysis of the QTc data at average steady-state concentrations demonstrated that the upper bound of the 2-sided 90% CI for QTc was 16 msec at ZYKADIA 750 mg. A pharmacokinetic/pharmacodynamic analysis suggested concentration-dependent QTc interval prolongation [see Warnings and Precautions (5.4)].
Based on central review of ECG data, 2 of 304 patients (0.7%) had bradycardia defined as less than 50 beats per minute. Bradycardia was reported as an adverse drug reaction in 3% of patients in Study 1.

12.3 Pharmacokinetics
Absorption
After single oral administration of ZYKADIA in patients, peak plasma levels (C_{max}) of ceritinib were achieved at approximately 4 to 6 hours, and area under the curve (AUC) and C_{max} increased dose proportionally over 50 to 750 mg. The absolute bioavailability of ZYKADIA has not been determined.
Following ZYKADIA 750 mg once daily dosing, steady-state was reached by approximately 15 days with a geometric

mean accumulation ratio of 6.2 after 3 weeks. Systemic exposure increased in a greater than dose proportional manner after repeat doses of 50 to 750 mg once daily.
Systemic exposure of ceritinib was increased when administered with a meal. A food effect study conducted in healthy subjects with a single 500 mg ceritinib dose showed that a high–fat meal (containing approximately 1000 calories and 58 grams of fat) increased ceritinib AUC by 73% and C_{max} by 41% and a low-fat meal (containing approximately 330 calories and 9 grams of fat) increased ceritinib AUC by 58% and C_{max} by 43% as compared with the fasted state. A 600 mg or higher ZYKADIA dose taken with a meal is expected to result in systemic exposure exceeding that of a 750 mg ZYKADIA dose taken in the fasted state, and may increase adverse drug reactions.
Distribution
Ceritinib is 97% bound to human plasma proteins, independent of drug concentration. The apparent volume of distribution (V_d/F) is 4230 L following a single 750 mg ZYKADIA dose in patients. Ceritinib also has a slight preferential distribution to red blood cells, relative to plasma, with a mean in vitro blood-to-plasma ratio of 1.35.
Elimination
Following a single 750 mg ZYKADIA dose, the geometric mean apparent plasma terminal half-life ($t_{1/2}$) of ceritinib was 41 hours in patients. Ceritinib demonstrates nonlinear PK over time. The geometric mean apparent clearance (CL/F) of ceritinib was lower at steady-state (33.2 L/h) after 750 mg daily dosing than after a single 750 mg dose (88.5 L/h).
Metabolism: In vitro studies demonstrated that CYP3A was the major enzyme involved in the metabolic clearance of ceritinib. Following oral administration of a single 750 mg radiolabeled ceritinib dose, ceritinib as the parent compound was the main circulating component (82%) in human plasma.
Excretion: Following oral administration of a single 750 mg radiolabeled ceritinib dose, 92.3% of the administered dose was recovered in the feces (with 68% as unchanged parent compound) while 1.3% of the administered dose was recovered in the urine.
Specific Populations
Age, Gender, Race, and Body Weight: Age, gender, race, and body weight had no clinically important effect on the systemic exposure of ceritinib based on population pharmacokinetic analyses.
Hepatic Impairment: As ceritinib is eliminated primarily via the liver, patients with hepatic impairment may have increased exposure. A pharmacokinetic trial in patients with hepatic impairment has not been conducted. Based on a population pharmacokinetic analysis of 48 patients with mild hepatic impairment (total bilirubin less than or equal to ULN and AST greater than ULN or total bilirubin greater than 1.0 to 1.5 times ULN and any AST) and 254 patients with normal hepatic function (total bilirubin less than or equal to ULN and AST less than or equal to ULN), ceritinib exposures were similar in patients with mild hepatic impairment and normal hepatic function. The pharmacokinetics of ceritinib has not been studied in patients with moderate to severe hepatic impairment [see Use in Specific Populations (8.6)].
Renal Impairment: A pharmacokinetic trial in patients with renal impairment has not been conducted as ceritinib elimination via the kidney is low (1.3% of a single oral administered dose). Based on a population pharmacokinetic analysis of 97 patients with mild renal impairment (CLcr 60 to less than 90 mL/min), 22 patients with moderate renal impairment (CLcr 30 to less than 60 mL/min) and 183 patients with normal renal function (greater than or equal to 90 mL/min), ceritinib exposures were similar in patients with mild and moderate renal impairment and normal renal function. Patients with severe renal impairment (CLcr less than 30 mL/min) were not included in the clinical trial.
Pediatrics: No trials have been conducted to evaluate the pharmacokinetics of ceritinib in pediatric patients.
Drug Interactions
Effect of Strong CYP3A Inhibitors on Ceritinib: In vitro studies show that ceritinib is a substrate of CYP3A. Coadministration of a single 450 mg ZYKADIA dose with ketoconazole (a strong CYP3A inhibitor) 200 mg twice daily for 14 days increased ceritinib AUC (90% CI) by 2.9-fold (2.5, 3.3) and C_{max} (90% CI) by 22% (7%, 39%) in 19 healthy subjects [see Drug Interactions (7.1)]. The steady-state AUC of ceritinib at reduced doses after coadministration with ketoconazole 200 mg twice daily for 14 days was predicted by simulations to be similar to the steady-state AUC of ceritinib alone [see Dosage and Administration (2.3)].
Effect of Strong CYP3A Inducers on Ceritinib: Coadministration of a single 750 mg ZYKADIA dose with rifampin (a strong CYP3A inducer) 600 mg daily for 14 days decreased ceritinib AUC (90% CI) by 70% (61%, 77%) and C_{max} (90% CI) by 44% (24%, 59%) in 19 healthy subjects [see Drug Interactions (7.1)].

Effect of Ceritinib on CYP Substrates: Based on in vitro data, ceritinib may inhibit CYP3A and CYP2C9 at clinical concentrations [see Drug Interactions (7.2)]. Time-dependent inhibition of CYP3A was also observed.
Effect of Transporters on Ceritinib Disposition: Ceritinib is a substrate of efflux transporter P-gp, but is not a substrate of Breast Cancer Resistance Protein (BCRP), Multidrug Resistance Protein (MRP2), Organic Cation Transporter (OCT1), Organic Anion Transporter (OAT2), or Organic Anion Transporting Polypeptide (OATP1B1) in vitro. Drugs that inhibit P-gp may increase ceritinib concentrations.
Effect of Ceritinib on Transporters: Based on in vitro data, ceritinib does not inhibit apical efflux transporters, P-gp, BCRP, or MRP2, hepatic uptake transporters OATP1B1 and OATP1B3, renal organic anion uptake transporters OAT1 and OAT3, or organic cation uptake transporters OCT1 and OCT2 at clinical concentrations.
Effect of Gastric Acid Reducing Agents on Ceritinib: Gastric acid reducing agents (e.g., proton pump inhibitors, H_2-receptor antagonists, antacids) may alter the solubility of ceritinib and reduce its bioavailability as ceritinib demonstrates pH-dependent solubility and becomes poorly soluble as pH increases in vitro. A dedicated study has not been conducted to evaluate the effect of gastric acid reducing agents on the bioavailability of ceritinib.

13 NONCLINICAL TOXICOLOGY
13.1 Carcinogenesis, Mutagenesis, Impairment of Fertility
Carcinogenicity studies have not been performed with ceritinib.
Ceritinib was not mutagenic in vitro in the bacterial reverse mutation (Ames) assay but induced numerical aberrations (aneugenic) in the in vitro cytogenetic assay using human lymphocytes, and micronuclei in the in vitro micronucleus test using TK6 cells. Ceritinib was not clastogenic in the in vivo rat micronucleus assay.
There are no data on the effect of ceritinib on human fertility. Fertility/early embryonic development studies were not conducted with ceritinib. There were no adverse effects on male or female reproductive organs in general toxicology studies conducted in monkeys and rats at exposures equal to or greater than 0.5- and 1.5-fold, respectively, of the human exposure by AUC at the recommended dose of 750 mg.

13.2 Animal Toxicology and/or Pharmacology
Target organs in nonclinical animal models included, but were not limited to, the pancreas, biliopancreatic/bile ducts, gastrointestinal tract, and liver. Pancreatic focal acinar cell atrophy was observed in rats at 1.5-fold the human exposure by AUC at the recommended dose. Biliopancreatic duct and bile duct necrosis was observed in rats at exposures equal to or greater than 5% of the human exposure by AUC at the recommended dose. Bile duct inflammation and vacuolation were also noted in monkeys at exposures equal to or greater than 0.5-fold the human exposure by AUC at the recommended dose. Frequent minimal necrosis and hemorrhage of the duodenum was exhibited in monkeys at 0.5-fold the human exposure by AUC, and in rats at an exposure similar to that observed clinically.
Ceritinib crossed the blood brain barrier in rats with a brain-to-blood exposure (AUC_{inf}) ratio of approximately 15%.

14 CLINICAL STUDIES
The efficacy of ZYKADIA was established in a multicenter, single-arm, open-label clinical trial (Study 1). A total of 163 patients with metastatic ALK-positive NSCLC who progressed while receiving or were intolerant to crizotinib were enrolled. All patients received ZYKADIA at a dose of 750 mg once daily. The major efficacy outcome measure was objective response rate (ORR) according to RECIST v1.0 as evaluated by both investigators and a Blinded Independent Central Review Committee (BIRC). Duration of response (DOR) was an additional outcome measure.
The study population characteristics were: median age 52 years, age less than 65 (87%), female (54%), Caucasian (66%), Asian (29%), never or former smoker (97%), ECOG PS 0 or 1 (87%), progression on previous crizotinib (91%), number of prior therapies 2 or more (84%), and adenocarcinoma histology (93%). Sites of extra-thoracic metastasis included brain (60%), liver (42%), and bone (42%). ALK-positivity was verified retrospectively by review of local test results for 99% of patients.
Efficacy results from Study 1 are summarized in Table 4.

Table 4: Overall Response Rate and Duration of Response[1] in Patients with ALK-Positive NSCLC who Received Prior Crizotinib in Study 1

Efficacy Parameter	Investigator Assessment (N=163)	BIRC Assessment (N=163)
Overall Response Rate (95% CI)	54.6% (47, 62)	43.6% (36, 52)

CR	1.2%	2.5%
PR	53.4%	41.1%
Duration of Response, median (months) (95% CI)	7.4 (5.4, 10.1)	7.1 (5.6, NE)

[1]Overall Response Rate and Duration of Response determined by RECIST v1.0
BIRC, blinded independent review committee; CR, complete response; NE, not estimable; PR, partial response.

The analysis by the BIRC assessment was similar to the analysis by the investigator assessment.

16 HOW SUPPLIED/STORAGE AND HANDLING

ZYKADIA 150 mg capsules
Hard gelatin capsule with opaque blue cap and opaque white body; opaque blue cap marked in black ink with "LDK 150MG", opaque white body marked in black ink with "NVR". Available in:
Bottles of 70 capsules ....NDC 0078-0640-70
Store at 25°C (77°F); excursions permitted between 15°C to 30°C (59°F to 86°F) [see USP Controlled Room Temperature].

17 PATIENT COUNSELING INFORMATION

Advise the patient to read the FDA-approved patient labeling (Patient Information).
• Inform patients that diarrhea, nausea, vomiting, and abdominal pain are the most commonly reported adverse reactions in patients treated with ZYKADIA. Inform patients of supportive care options such as anti-emetic and anti-diarrheal medications. Advise patients to contact their healthcare provider for severe or persistent gastrointestinal symptoms [see Warnings and Precautions (5.1)].
• Inform patients of the signs and symptoms of hepatotoxicity. Advise patients to contact their healthcare provider immediately for signs or symptoms of hepatotoxicity [see Warnings and Precautions (5.2)].
• Inform patients of the risks of severe or fatal ILD/pneumonitis. Advise patients to contact their healthcare provider immediately to report new or worsening respiratory symptoms [see Warnings and Precautions (5.3)].
• Inform patients of the risks of QTc interval prolongation and bradycardia. Advise patients to contact their healthcare provider immediately to report new chest pain or discomfort, changes in heartbeat, palpitations, dizziness, lightheadedness, fainting, and changes in or new use of heart or blood pressure medications [see Warnings and Precautions (5.4, 5.6)].
• Inform patients of the signs and symptoms of hyperglycemia. Advise patients to contact their healthcare provider immediately for signs or symptoms of hyperglycemia [see Warnings and Precautions (5.5)].
• Advise females to inform their healthcare provider if they are pregnant. Inform females of reproductive potential of the risk to a fetus. Advise females of reproductive potential to use effective contraception during treatment with ZYKADIA and for at least 2 weeks following completion of therapy [see Warnings and Precautions (5.7) and Use in Specific Populations (8.1, 8.7)].
• Advise females not to breastfeed during treatment with ZYKADIA [see Use in Specific Populations (8.3)].
• Inform patients not to consume grapefruit and grapefruit juice during treatment with ZYKADIA [see Drug Interactions (7.1)].
• Take ZYKADIA on an empty stomach (i.e., do not take within 2 hours of a meal) [see Dosage and Administration (2.1)].
• Advise patients to make up a missed dose of ZYKADIA unless the next dose is due within 12 hours [see Dosage and Administration (2.1)].
T2014-41

PATIENT INFORMATION
ZYKADIA™ (zye kaye' dee ah)
(ceritinib) capsules

What is the most important information I should know about ZYKADIA?
ZYKADIA may cause serious side effects, including:
Stomach and intestinal (gastrointestinal) problems. ZYKADIA causes stomach and intestinal problems in most people, including diarrhea, nausea, vomiting, and stomach-area pain. These problems can sometimes be severe. Follow your healthcare provider's instructions about taking medicines to help these symptoms. Call your healthcare provider for advice if your symptoms are severe or do not go away.

Liver problems. ZYKADIA may cause liver injury. Your healthcare provider should do blood tests at least every month to check your liver while you are taking ZYKADIA. Tell your healthcare provider right away if you get any of the following:

• you feel tired
• your skin or the whites of your eyes turn yellow
• you have a decreased appetite
• your urine turns dark or brown (tea color)
• you have itchy skin
• you have nausea or vomiting
• you have pain on the right side of your stomach-area
• you bleed or bruise more easily than normal

Lung problems (pneumonitis). ZYKADIA may cause severe or life-threatening swelling (inflammation) of the lungs during treatment that can lead to death. Symptoms may be similar to those symptoms from lung cancer. Tell your healthcare provider right away if you have any new or worsening symptoms, including:

• trouble breathing or shortness of breath
• fever
• cough with or without mucous
• chest pain

Heart problems. ZYKADIA may cause very slow, very fast, or abnormal heartbeats. Your healthcare provider may check your heart during treatment with ZYKADIA. Tell your healthcare provider right away if you feel new chest pain or discomfort, dizziness or lightheadedness, if you faint, or have abnormal heartbeats. Tell your healthcare provider if you start to take or have any changes in heart or blood pressure medicines.
See "What are possible side effects of ZYKADIA?" for more information about side effects.

What is ZYKADIA?
ZYKADIA is a prescription medicine that is used to treat people with non-small cell lung cancer (NSCLC) that:
• is caused by a defect in a gene called anaplastic lymphoma kinase (ALK), and
• has spread to other parts of the body, and
• who have taken the medicine crizotinib, but their NSCLC worsened or they cannot tolerate taking crizotinib.
It is not known if ZYKADIA is safe and effective in children.

What should I tell my healthcare provider before taking ZYKADIA?
Before you take ZYKADIA, tell your healthcare provider about all of your medical conditions, including if you:
• have liver problems
• have diabetes or high blood sugar
• have heart problems, including a condition called long QT syndrome
• are pregnant or plan to become pregnant. ZYKADIA may harm your unborn baby. Women who are able to become pregnant should use an effective method of birth control during treatment with ZYKADIA and for at least 2 weeks after stopping ZYKADIA. Talk to your healthcare provider about birth control methods that may be right for you.
• are breastfeeding or plan to breastfeed. It is not known if ZYKADIA passes into your breast milk. You should not breastfeed if you take ZYKADIA.
Tell your healthcare provider about all the medicines you take, including prescription medicines, over-the-counter medicines, vitamins, and herbal supplements.

How should I take ZYKADIA?
• Take ZYKADIA exactly as your healthcare provider tells you. Do not change your dose or stop taking unless your healthcare provider tells you to.
• Take ZYKADIA 1 time each day.
• Take ZYKADIA on an empty stomach, do not eat for 2 hours before and do not eat for 2 hours after taking ZYKADIA.
• If you miss a dose of ZYKADIA, take it as soon as you remember. If your next dose is due within 12 hours, then skip the missed dose. Just take the next dose at your regular time.

What should I avoid while taking ZYKADIA?
• You should not drink grapefruit juice or eat grapefruit during treatment with ZYKADIA. It may make

the amount of ZYKADIA in your blood increase to a harmful level.

What are the possible side effects of ZYKADIA?
ZYKADIA may cause serious side effects, including:
• See "What is the most important information I should know about ZYKADIA?"
• **High blood sugar (hyperglycemia).** People who have diabetes or glucose intolerance or who take a corticosteroid medicine have an increased risk of high blood sugar with ZYKADIA. Follow your healthcare provider's instructions about monitoring your blood sugar. Call your healthcare provider right away if you have any symptoms of high blood sugar, including:
• increased thirst
• increased hunger
• headaches
• trouble thinking or concentrating
• urinating often
• blurred vision
• tiredness
• your breath smells like fruit
The most common side effects of ZYKADIA include:
• stomach and intestinal (gastrointestinal) problems.
See "What is the most important information I should know about ZYKADIA?"
• tiredness, decreased appetite, and constipation
These are not all of the possible side effects of ZYKADIA. For more information, ask your healthcare provider or pharmacist. Call your doctor for medical advice about side effects. You may report side effects to FDA at 1-800-FDA-1088.

How should I store ZYKADIA?
• Store ZYKADIA at room temperature between 68°F to 77°F (20°C to 25°C).
Keep ZYKADIA and all medicines out of the reach of children.

General information about the safe and effective use of ZYKADIA
Medicines are sometimes prescribed for purposes other than those listed in a Patient Information leaflet. Do not use ZYKADIA for a condition for which it was not prescribed. Do not give it to other people, even if they have the same symptoms you have. It may harm them. You can ask your healthcare provider or pharmacist for more information about ZYKADIA.

What are the ingredients in ZYKADIA?
Active ingredient: ceritinib
Inactive ingredients: colloidal anhydrous silica, L-hydroxypropylcellulose, magnesium stearate, microcrystalline cellulose, and sodium starch glycolate
Capsule shell contains: gelatin, indiogotine, and titanium dioxide

Distributed by: Novartis Pharmaceuticals Corporation East Hanover, New Jersey 07936
For more information, go to www.US.ZYKADIA.com or call 888-669-6682.

This Patient Information has been approved by the U.S. Food and Drug Administration.
T2014-42
Issued: April 2014
Shown in Product Identification Guide, page 311

For the first time, the trusted *Physicians' Desk Reference®* is now available as a convenient eBook. Visit PDR.net to download your free copy today.

Novo Nordisk Inc.
800 SCUDDERS MILL ROAD
PLAINSBORO, NJ 08536

Direct Inquiries to:
Novo Nordisk Inc.
(800) 727-6500
8:30 AM - 6 PM EST M–F

LEVEMIR® ℞
[lev'e-mīr]
(insulin detemir [rDNA origin] injection)
solution for subcutaneous injection

HIGHLIGHTS OF PRESCRIBING INFORMATION
These highlights do not include all the information needed to use LEVEMIR® safely and effectively.
See full prescribing information for LEVEMIR.
LEVEMIR® (insulin detemir [rDNA origin] injection) solution for subcutaneous injection
Initial U.S. Approval: 2005

────────RECENT MAJOR CHANGES────────
Warnings and Precautions (5.8) 3/2013

────────INDICATIONS AND USAGE────────
LEVEMIR is a long-acting human insulin analog indicated to improve glycemic control in adults and children with diabetes mellitus. (1)
Important Limitations of Use:
• Not recommended for treating diabetic ketoacidosis. Use intravenous, rapid-acting or short-acting insulin instead.

────────DOSAGE AND ADMINISTRATION────────
• The starting dose should be individualized based on the type of diabetes and whether the patient is insulin-naïve (2.1, 2.2, 2.3)
• Administer subcutaneously once daily or in divided doses twice daily. Once daily administration should be given with the evening meal or at bedtime (2.1)
• Rotate injection sites within an injection area (abdomen, thigh, or deltoid) to reduce the risk of lipodystrophy (2.1)
• Converting from other insulin therapies may require adjustment of timing and dose of LEVEMIR. Closely monitor glucoses especially upon converting to LEVEMIR and during the initial weeks thereafter (2.3)

────────DOSAGE FORMS AND STRENGTHS────────
Solution for injection 100 Units/mL (U-100) in
• 3 mL LEVEMIR FlexPen®
• 3 mL LEVEMIR FlexTouch®
• 10 mL vial (3)

────────CONTRAINDICATIONS────────
• Do not use in patients with hypersensitivity to LEVEMIR or any of its excipients (4)

────────WARNINGS AND PRECAUTIONS────────
• Dose adjustment and monitoring: Monitor blood glucose in all patients treated with insulin. Insulin regimens should be modified cautiously and only under medical supervision (5.1)
• Administration: Do not dilute or mix with any other insulin or solution. Do not administer subcutaneously via an insulin pump, intramuscularly, or intravenously because severe hypoglycemia can occur (5.2)
• Hypoglycemia is the most common adverse reaction of insulin therapy and may be life-threatening (5.3, 6.1)
• Allergic reactions: Severe, life-threatening, generalized allergy, including anaphylaxis, can occur (5.4)
• Renal or hepatic impairment: May require adjustment of the LEVEMIR dose (5.5, 5.6)
• Fluid retention and heart failure can occur with concomitant use of thiazolidinediones (TZDs), which are PPAR-gamma agonists, and insulin, including LEVEMIR (5.8)

────────ADVERSE REACTIONS────────
Adverse reactions associated with LEVEMIR include hypoglycemia, allergic reactions, injection site reactions, lipodystrophy, rash and pruritus (6)
To report SUSPECTED ADVERSE REACTIONS, contact Novo Nordisk Inc. at 1-800-727-6500 or FDA at 1-800-FDA-1088 or www.fda.gov/medwatch

────────DRUG INTERACTIONS────────
• Certain drugs may affect glucose metabolism requiring insulin dose adjustment and close monitoring of blood glucose (7)
• The signs of hypoglycemia may be reduced or absent in patients taking anti-adrenergic drugs (e.g., beta-blockers, clonidine, guanethidine, and reserpine) (7)

────────USE IN SPECIFIC POPULATIONS────────
Pediatric: Has not been studied in children with type 2 diabetes. Has not been studied in children with type 1 diabetes < 2 years of age (8.4)
See 17 for PATIENT COUNSELING INFORMATION and FDA-approved patient labeling
Revised: 10/2013

FULL PRESCRIBING INFORMATION

1   INDICATIONS AND USAGE
LEVEMIR is indicated to improve glycemic control in adults and children with diabetes mellitus.
Important Limitations of Use:
• LEVEMIR is not recommended for the treatment of diabetic ketoacidosis. Intravenous rapid-acting or short-acting insulin is the preferred treatment for this condition.

2   DOSAGE AND ADMINISTRATION
2.1   Dosing
LEVEMIR is a recombinant human insulin analog for once- or twice-daily subcutaneous administration.
Patients treated with LEVEMIR once-daily should administer the dose with the evening meal or at bedtime.
Patients who require twice-daily dosing can administer the evening dose with the evening meal, at bedtime, or 12 hours after the morning dose.
The dose of LEVEMIR must be individualized based on clinical response. Blood glucose monitoring is essential in all patients receiving insulin therapy.
Patients adjusting the amount or timing of dosing with LEVEMIR should only do so under medical supervision with appropriate glucose monitoring [see Warnings and Precautions (5.1)].
In patients with type 1 diabetes, LEVEMIR must be used in a regimen with rapid-acting or short-acting insulin.
As with all insulins, injection sites should be rotated within the same region (abdomen, thigh, or deltoid) from one injection to the next to reduce the risk of lipodystrophy [see Adverse Reactions (6.1)].
LEVEMIR can be injected subcutaneously in the thigh, abdominal wall, or upper arm. As with all insulins, the rate of absorption, and consequently the onset and duration of action, may be affected by exercise and other variables, such as stress, intercurrent illness, or changes in co-administered medications or meal patterns.

When using LEVEMIR with a glucagon-like peptide (GLP)-1 receptor agonist, administer as separate injections. Never mix. It is acceptable to inject LEVEMIR and a GLP-1 receptor agonist in the same body region but the injections should not be adjacent to each other.
2.2   Initiation of LEVEMIR Therapy
The recommended starting dose of LEVEMIR in patients with type 1 diabetes should be approximately one-third of the total daily insulin requirements. Rapid-acting or short-acting, pre-meal insulin should be used to satisfy the remainder of the daily insulin requirements.
The recommended starting dose of LEVEMIR in patients with type 2 diabetes inadequately controlled on oral antidiabetic medications is 10 Units (or 0.1-0.2 Units/kg) given once daily in the evening or divided into a twice daily regimen.
The recommended starting dose of LEVEMIR in patients with type 2 diabetes inadequately controlled on a GLP-1 receptor agonist is 10 Units given once daily in the evening. LEVEMIR doses should subsequently be adjusted based on blood glucose measurements. The dosages of LEVEMIR should be individualized under the supervision of a healthcare provider.
2.3   Converting to LEVEMIR from other insulin therapies
If converting from insulin glargine to LEVEMIR, the change can be done on a unit-to-unit basis.
If converting from NPH insulin, the change can be done on a unit-to-unit basis. However, some patients with type 2 diabetes may require more LEVEMIR than NPH insulin, as observed in one trial [see Clinical Studies (14)].
As with all insulins, close glucose monitoring is recommended during the transition and in the initial weeks thereafter. Doses and timing of concurrent rapid-acting or short-acting insulins or other concomitant antidiabetic treatment may need to be adjusted.

3   DOSAGE FORMS AND STRENGTHS
LEVEMIR solution for injection 100 Unit per mL is available as:
• 3 mL LEVEMIR FlexPen®
• 3 mL LEVEMIR FlexTouch®
• 10 mL vial

4   CONTRAINDICATIONS
LEVEMIR is contraindicated in patients with hypersensitivity to LEVEMIR or any of its excipients. Reactions have included anaphylaxis [see Warnings and Precautions (5.4) and Adverse Reactions (6.1)].

5   WARNINGS AND PRECAUTIONS
5.1   Dosage adjustment and monitoring
Glucose monitoring is essential for all patients receiving insulin therapy. Changes to an insulin regimen should be made cautiously and only under medical supervision.
Changes in insulin strength, manufacturer, type, or method of administration may result in the need for a change in the insulin dose or an adjustment of concomitant anti-diabetic treatment.
As with all insulin preparations, the time course of action for LEVEMIR may vary in different individuals or at different times in the same individual and is dependent on many conditions, including the local blood supply, local temperature, and physical activity.
5.2   Administration
LEVEMIR should only be administered subcutaneously.
Do not administer LEVEMIR intravenously or intramuscularly. The intended duration of activity of LEVEMIR is dependent on injection into subcutaneous tissue. Intravenous or intramuscular administration of the usual subcutaneous dose could result in severe hypoglycemia [see Warnings and Precautions (5.3)].
Do not use LEVEMIR in insulin infusion pumps.
Do not dilute or mix LEVEMIR with any other insulin or solution. If LEVEMIR is diluted or mixed, the pharmacokinetic or pharmacodynamic profile (e.g., onset of action, time to peak effect) of LEVEMIR and the mixed insulin may be altered in an unpredictable manner.
5.3   Hypoglycemia
Hypoglycemia is the most common adverse reaction of insulin therapy, including LEVEMIR. The risk of hypoglycemia increases with intensive glycemic control.
When a GLP-1 receptor agonist is used in combination with LEVEMIR, the LEVEMIR dose may need to be lowered or more conservatively titrated to minimize the risk of hypoglycemia [see Adverse Reactions (6.1)].
All patients must be educated to recognize and manage hypoglycemia. Severe hypoglycemia can lead to unconsciousness or convulsions and may result in temporary or permanent impairment of brain function or death. Severe hypoglycemia requiring the assistance of another person or parenteral glucose infusion, or glucagon administration has been observed in clinical trials with insulin, including trials with LEVEMIR.
The timing of hypoglycemia usually reflects the time-action profile of the administered insulin formulations. Other fac-

tors such as changes in food intake (e.g., amount of food or timing of meals), exercise, and concomitant medications may also alter the risk of hypoglycemia [see Drug Interactions (7)].

The prolonged effect of subcutaneous LEVEMIR may delay recovery from hypoglycemia.

As with all insulins, use caution in patients with hypoglycemia unawareness and in patients who may be predisposed to hypoglycemia (e.g., the pediatric population and patients who fast or have erratic food intake). The patient's ability to concentrate and react may be impaired as a result of hypoglycemia. This may present a risk in situations where these abilities are especially important, such as driving or operating other machinery.

Early warning symptoms of hypoglycemia may be different or less pronounced under certain conditions, such as long-standing diabetes, diabetic neuropathy, use of medications such as beta-blockers, or intensified glycemic control [see Drug Interactions (7)]. These situations may result in severe hypoglycemia (and, possibly, loss of consciousness) prior to the patient's awareness of hypoglycemia.

5.4 Hypersensitivity and allergic reactions

Severe, life-threatening, generalized allergy, including anaphylaxis, can occur with insulin products, including LEVEMIR.

5.5 Renal Impairment

No difference was observed in the pharmacokinetics of insulin detemir between non-diabetic individuals with renal impairment and healthy volunteers. However, some studies with human insulin have shown increased circulating insulin concentrations in patients with renal impairment. Careful glucose monitoring and dose adjustments of insulin, including LEVEMIR, may be necessary in patients with renal impairment [see Clinical Pharmacology (12.3)].

5.6 Hepatic Impairment

Non-diabetic individuals with severe hepatic impairment had lower systemic exposures to insulin detemir compared to healthy volunteers. However, some studies with human insulin have shown increased circulating insulin concentrations in patients with liver impairment. Careful glucose monitoring and dose adjustments of insulin, including LEVEMIR, may be necessary in patients with hepatic impairment [see Clinical Pharmacology (12.3)].

5.7 Drug interactions

Some medications may alter insulin requirements and subsequently increase the risk for hypoglycemia or hyperglycemia [see Drug Interactions (7)].

5.8 Fluid retention and heart failure with concomitant use of PPAR-gamma agonists

Thiazolidinediones (TZDs), which are peroxisome proliferator-activated receptor (PPAR)-gamma agonists, can cause dose-related fluid retention, particularly when used in combination with insulin. Fluid retention may lead to or exacerbate heart failure. Patients treated with insulin, including LEVEMIR, and a PPAR-gamma agonist should be observed for signs and symptoms of heart failure. If heart failure develops, it should be managed according to current standards of care, and discontinuation or dose reduction of the PPAR-gamma agonist must be considered.

6 ADVERSE REACTIONS

The following adverse reactions are discussed elsewhere:
• Hypoglycemia [see Warnings and Precautions (5.3)]
• Hypersensitivity and allergic reactions [see Warnings and Precautions (5.4)]

6.1 Clinical trial experience

Because clinical trials are conducted under widely varying designs, the adverse reaction rates reported in one clinical trial may not be easily compared to those rates reported in another clinical trial, and may not reflect the rates actually observed in clinical practice.

The frequencies of adverse reactions (excluding hypoglycemia) reported during LEVEMIR clinical trials in patients with type 1 diabetes mellitus and type 2 diabetes mellitus are listed in Tables 1-4 below. See Tables 5 and 6 for the hypoglycemia findings.

In the LEVEMIR add-on to liraglutide+metformin trial, all patients received liraglutide 1.8 mg + metformin during a 12-week run-in period. During the run-in period, 167 patients (17% of enrolled total) withdrew from the trial: 76 (46% of withdrawals) of these patients doing so because of gastrointestinal adverse reactions and 15 (9% of withdrawals) doing so due to other adverse events. Only those patients who completed the run-in period with inadequate glycemic control were randomized to 26 weeks of add-on therapy with LEVEMIR or continued, unchanged treatment with liraglutide 1.8 mg + metformin. During this randomized 26-week period, diarrhea was the only adverse reaction reported in ≥5% of patients treated with liraglutide 1.8 mg + metformin (11.7%) and greater than in patients treated with liraglutide 1.8 mg and metformin alone (6.9%).

In two pooled trials, a total of 1155 adults with type 1 diabetes were exposed to individualized doses of LEVEMIR (n=767) or NPH (n=388). The mean duration of exposure to

LEVEMIR was 153 days, and the total exposure to LEVEMIR was 321 patient-years. The most common adverse reactions are summarized in Table 1.

Table 1: Adverse reactions (excluding hypoglycemia) in two pooled clinical trials of 16 weeks and 24 weeks duration in adults with type 1 diabetes (adverse reactions with incidence ≥ 5%)

	LEVEMIR, % (n = 767)	NPH, % (n = 388)
Upper respiratory tract infection	26.1	21.4
Headache	22.6	22.7
Pharyngitis	9.5	8.0
Influenza-like illness	7.8	7.0
Abdominal Pain	6.0	2.6

A total of 320 adults with type 1 diabetes were exposed to individualized doses of LEVEMIR (n=161) or insulin glargine (n=159). The mean duration of exposure to LEVEMIR was 176 days, and the total exposure to LEVEMIR was 78 patient-years. The most common adverse reactions are summarized in Table 2.

Table 2: Adverse reactions (excluding hypoglycemia) in a 26-week trial comparing insulin aspart + LEVEMIR to insulin aspart + insulin glargine in adults with type 1 diabetes (adverse reactions with incidence ≥ 5%)

	LEVEMIR, % (n = 161)	Glargine, % (n = 159)
Upper respiratory tract infection	26.7	32.1
Headache	14.3	19.5
Back pain	8.1	6.3
Influenza-like illness	6.2	8.2
Gastroenteritis	5.6	4.4
Bronchitis	5.0	1.9

In two pooled trials, a total of 869 adults with type 2 diabetes were exposed to individualized doses of Levemir (n=432) or NPH (n=437). The mean duration of exposure to LEVEMIR was 157 days, and the total exposure to LEVEMIR was 186 patient-years. The most common adverse reactions are summarized in Table 3.

Table 3: Adverse reactions (excluding hypoglycemia) in two pooled clinical trials of 22 weeks and 24 weeks duration in adults with type 2 diabetes (adverse reactions with incidence ≥ 5%)

	LEVEMIR, % (n = 432)	NPH, % (n = 437)
Upper respiratory tract infection	12.5	11.2
Headache	6.5	5.3

A total of 347 children and adolescents (6-17 years) with type 1 diabetes were exposed to individualized doses of LEVEMIR (n=232) or NPH (n=115). The mean duration of exposure to LEVEMIR was 180 days, and the total exposure to LEVEMIR was 114 patient-years. The most common adverse reactions are summarized in Table 4.

Table 4: Adverse reactions (excluding hypoglycemia) in one 26-week clinical trial of children and adolescents with type 1 diabetes (adverse reactions with incidence ≥ 5%)

	LEVEMIR, % (n = 232)	NPH, % (n = 115)
Upper respiratory tract infection	35.8	42.6
Headache	31.0	32.2
Pharyngitis	17.2	20.9
Gastroenteritis	16.8	11.3
Influenza-like illness	13.8	20.9
Abdominal pain	13.4	13.0
Pyrexia	10.3	6.1
Cough	8.2	4.3
Viral infection	7.3	7.8
Nausea	6.5	7.0
Rhinitis	6.5	3.5
Vomiting	6.5	10.4

Pregnancy

A randomized, open-label, controlled clinical trial has been conducted in pregnant women with type 1 diabetes. [see Use in Specific Populations (8.1)]

• Hypoglycemia

Hypoglycemia is the most commonly observed adverse reaction in patients using insulin, including LEVEMIR [see Warnings and Precautions (5.3)].

Tables 5 and 6 summarize the incidence of severe and non-severe hypoglycemia in the LEVEMIR clinical trials.

For the adult trials and one of the pediatric trials (Study D), severe hypoglycemia was defined as an event with symptoms consistent with hypoglycemia requiring assistance of another person and associated with either a plasma glucose value below 56 mg/dL (blood glucose below 50 mg/dL) or prompt recovery after oral carbohydrate, intravenous glucose or glucagon administration. For the other pediatric trial (Study I), severe hypoglycemia was defined as an event with semi-consciousness, unconsciousness, coma and/or convulsions in a patient who could not assist in the treatment and who may have required glucagon or intravenous glucose.

For the adult trials and pediatric Study D, non-severe hypoglycemia was defined as an asymptomatic or symptomatic plasma glucose < 56 mg/dL (or equivalently blood glucose <50 mg/dL as used in Study A and C) that was self-treated by the patient. For pediatric Study I, non-severe hypoglycemia included asymptomatic events with plasma glucose <65 mg/dL as well as symptomatic events that the patient could self-treat or treat by taking oral therapy provided by the caregiver.

The rates of hypoglycemia in the LEVEMIR clinical trials (see Section 14 for a description of the study designs) were comparable between LEVEMIR-treated patients and non-LEVEMIR-treated patients (see Tables 5 and 6).

[See table 5 at top of next page]
[See table 6 at top of next page]

• Insulin Initiation and Intensification of Glucose Control

Intensification or rapid improvement in glucose control has been associated with a transitory, reversible ophthalmologic refraction disorder, worsening of diabetic retinopathy, and acute painful peripheral neuropathy. However, long-term glycemic control decreases the risk of diabetic retinopathy and neuropathy.

• Lipodystrophy

Long-term use of insulin, including LEVEMIR, can cause lipodystrophy at the site of repeated insulin injections. Lipodystrophy includes lipohypertrophy (thickening of adipose tissue) and lipoatrophy (thinning of adipose tissue), and may affect insulin absorption. Rotate insulin injection sites within the same region to reduce the risk of lipodystrophy [see Dosage and Administration (2.1)].

• Weight Gain

Weight gain can occur with insulin therapy, including LEVEMIR, and has been attributed to the anabolic effects of insulin and the decrease in glucosuria [see Clinical Studies (14)].

• Peripheral Edema

Insulin, including LEVEMIR, may cause sodium retention and edema, particularly if previously poor metabolic control is improved by intensified insulin therapy.

• Allergic Reactions

Local Allergy

As with any insulin therapy, patients taking LEVEMIR may experience injection site reactions, including localized erythema, pain, pruritus, urticaria, edema, and inflammation. In clinical studies in adults, three patients treated with LEVEMIR reported injection site pain (0.25%) compared to one patient treated with NPH insulin (0.12%). The reports of pain at the injection site did not result in discontinuation of therapy.

Rotation of the injection site within a given area from one injection to the next may help to reduce or prevent these reactions. In some instances, these reactions may be related to factors other than insulin, such as irritants in a skin cleansing agent or poor injection technique. Most minor reactions to insulin usually resolve in a few days to a few weeks.

Systemic Allergy

Severe, life-threatening, generalized allergy, including anaphylaxis, generalized skin reactions, angioedema, bronchospasm, hypotension, and shock may occur with any insulin, including LEVEMIR, and may be life-threatening *[see Warnings and Precautions (5.4)].*

• *Antibody Production*

All insulin products can elicit the formation of insulin antibodies. These insulin antibodies may increase or decrease the efficacy of insulin and may require adjustment of the insulin dose. In phase 3 clinical trials of LEVEMIR, antibody development has been observed with no apparent impact on glycemic control.

6.2   Postmarketing experience

The following adverse reactions have been identified during post approval use of LEVEMIR. Because these reactions are reported voluntarily from a population of uncertain size, it is not always possible to reliably estimate their frequency or establish a causal relationship to drug exposure.

Medication errors have been reported during post-approval use of LEVEMIR in which other insulins, particularly rapid-acting or short-acting insulins, have been accidentally administered instead of LEVEMIR *[see Patient Counseling Information (17)].* To avoid medication errors between LEVEMIR and other insulins, patients should be instructed always to verify the insulin label before each injection.

7   DRUG INTERACTIONS

A number of medications affect glucose metabolism and may require insulin dose adjustment and particularly close monitoring.

The following are examples of medications that may increase the blood-glucose-lowering effect of insulins including LEVEMIR and, therefore, increase the susceptibility to hypoglycemia: oral antidiabetic medications, pramlintide acetate, angiotensin converting enzyme (ACE) inhibitors, disopyramide, fibrates, fluoxetine, monoamine oxidase (MAO) inhibitors, propoxyphene, pentoxifylline, salicylates, somatostatin analogs, and sulfonamide antibiotics.

The following are examples of medications that may reduce the blood-glucose-lowering effect of insulins including LEVEMIR: corticosteroids, niacin, danazol, diuretics, sympathomimetic agents (e.g., epinephrine, albuterol, terbutaline), glucagon, isoniazid, phenothiazine derivatives, somatropin, thyroid hormones, estrogens, progestogens (e.g., in oral contraceptives), protease inhibitors and atypical antipsychotic medications (e.g. olanzapine and clozapine).

Beta-blockers, clonidine, lithium salts, and alcohol may either increase or decrease the blood-glucose-lowering effect of insulin. Pentamidine may cause hypoglycemia, which may sometimes be followed by hyperglycemia.

The signs of hypoglycemia may be reduced or absent in patients taking anti-adrenergic drugs such as beta-blockers, clonidine, guanethidine, and reserpine.

8   USE IN SPECIFIC POPULATIONS

8.1   Pregnancy

Pregnancy Category B

Risk Summary

The background risk of birth defects, pregnancy loss, or other adverse events that exists for all pregnancies is increased in pregnancies complicated by hyperglycemia. Female patients should be advised to tell their physician if they intend to become, or if they become pregnant while taking LEVEMIR. A randomized controlled clinical trial of pregnant women with type I diabetes using LEVEMIR during pregnancy did not show an increase in the risk of fetal abnormalities. Reproductive toxicology studies in nondiabetic rats and rabbits that included concurrent human insulin control groups indicated that insulin detemir and human insulin had similar effects regarding embryotoxicity and teratogenicity that were attributed to maternal hypoglycemia.

Clinical Considerations

The increased risk of adverse events in pregnancies complicated by hyperglycemia may be decreased with good glucose control before conception and throughout pregnancy. Because insulin requirements vary throughout pregnancy and in the post-partum period, careful monitoring of glucose control is essential in pregnant women.

Human Data

In an open-label, clinical study, women with type 1 diabetes who were (between weeks 8 and 12 of gestation) or intended to become pregnant were randomized 1:1 to LEVEMIR (once or twice daily) or NPH insulin (once, twice or thrice daily). Insulin aspart was administered before each meal. A total of 152 women in the LEVEMIR arm and 158 women in the NPH arm were or became pregnant during the study (Total pregnant women = 310). Approximately one half of the study participants in each arm were randomized as pregnant and were exposed to NPH or to other insulins prior to conception and in the first 8 weeks of gestation. In the 310 pregnant women, the mean glycosylated hemoglobin (HbA$_{1c}$) was < 7% at 10, 12, and 24 weeks of gestation in

Table 5: Hypoglycemia in Patients with Type 1 Diabetes

		Severe Hypoglycemia		Non-Severe Hypoglycemia	
		Percent of patients with at least 1 event (n/total N)	Event/patient/year	Percent of patients (n/total N)	Event/patient/year
Study A Type 1 Diabetes Adults 16 weeks In combination with insulin aspart	Twice-Daily LEVEMIR	8.7 (24/276)	0.52	88.0 (243/276)	26.4
	Twice-Daily NPH	10.6 (14/132)	0.43	89.4 (118/132)	37.5
Study B Type 1 Diabetes Adults 26 weeks In combination with insulin aspart	Twice-Daily LEVEMIR	5.0 (8/161)	0.13	82.0 (132/161)	20.2
	Once-Daily Glargine	10.1 (16/159)	0.31	77.4 (123/159)	21.8
Study C Type 1 Diabetes Adults 24 weeks In combination with regular insulin	Once-Daily LEVEMIR	7.5 (37/491)	0.35	88.4 (434/491)	31.1
	Once-Daily NPH	10.2 (26/256)	0.32	87.9 (225/256)	33.4
Study D Type 1 Diabetes Pediatrics 26 weeks In combination with insulin aspart	Once- or Twice Daily LEVEMIR	15.9 (37/232)	0.91	93.1 (216/232)	31.6
	Once- or Twice Daily NPH	20.0 (23/115)	0.99	95.7 (110/115)	37.0
Study I Type 1 Diabetes Pediatrics 52 weeks In combination with insulin aspart	Once- or Twice Daily LEVEMIR	1.7 (3/177)	0.02	94.9 (168/177)	56.1
	Once- or Twice Daily NPH	7.1 (12/170)	0.09	97.6 (166/170)	70.7

Table 6: Hypoglycemia in Patients with Type 2 Diabetes

		Study E Type 2 Diabetes Adults 24 weeks In combination with oral agents		Study F Type 2 Diabetes Adults 22 weeks In combination with insulin aspart		Study H Type 2 Diabetes Adults 26 weeks in combination with Liraglutide and Metformin	
		Twice-Daily LEVEMIR	Twice-Daily NPH	Once- or Twice Daily LEVEMIR	Once- or Twice Daily NPH	Once Daily LEVEMIR + Liraglutide + Metformin	Liraglutide + Metformin
Severe hypoglycemia	Percent of patients with at least 1 event (n/total N)	0.4 (1/237)	2.5 (6/238)	1.5 (3/195)	4.0 (8/199)	0	0
	Event/patient/year	0.01	0.08	0.04	0.13	0	0
Non-severe hypoglycemia	Percent of patients (n/total N)	40.5 (96/237)	64.3 (153/238)	32.3 (63/195)	32.2 (64/199)	9.2 (15/163)	1.3 (2/158*)
	Event/patient/year	3.5	6.9	1.6	2.0	0.29	0.03

* One subject is an outlier and was excluded due to 25 hypoglycemic episodes that the patient was able to self-treat. This patient had a history of frequent hypoglycemia prior to the study

both arms. In the intent-to-treat population, the adjusted mean HbA$_{1c}$ (standard error) at gestational week 36 was 6.27% (0.053) in LEVEMIR-treated patient (n=138) and 6.33% (0.052) in NPH-treated patients (n=145); the difference was not clinically significant.

Adverse reactions in pregnant patients occurring at an incidence of ≥5% are shown in Table 7. The two most common adverse reactions were nasopharyngitis and headache. These are consistent with findings from other type 1 diabetes trials (see Table 1, Section 6.1.), and are not repeated in Table 7.

The incidence of adverse reactions of pre-eclampsia was 10.5% (16 cases) and 7.0% (11 cases) in the LEVEMIR and NPH insulin groups respectively. Out of the total number of cases of pre-eclampsia, eight (8) cases in the LEVEMIR group and 1 case in the NPH insulin group required hospi-

talization. The rates of pre-eclampsia observed in the study are within expected rates for pregnancy complicated by diabetes. Pre-eclampsia is a syndrome defined by symptoms, hypertension and proteinuria; the definition of pre-eclampsia was not standardized in the trial making it difficult to establish a link between a given treatment and an increased risk of pre-eclampsia. All events were considered unlikely related to trial treatment. In all nine (9) cases requiring hospitalization the women had healthy infants. Events of hypertension, proteinuria and edema were reported less frequently in the LEVEMIR group than in the NPH insulin group as a whole. There was no difference between the treatment groups in mean blood pressure during pregnancy and there was no indication of a general increase in blood pressure.

In the NPH insulin group there were 6 serious adverse reactions in four mothers of the following placental disorders,

Table 8: Hypoglycemia in Pregnant Women with Type 1 Diabetes

		Study G Type 1 Diabetes Pregnancy In combination with insulin aspart	
		LEVEMIR	NPH
Severe hypoglycemia*	Percent of patients with at least 1 event (n/total N)	16.4 (25/152)	20.9 (33/158)
	Events/patient/year	1.1	1.2
Non-severe hypoglycemia*	Percent of patients with at least 1 event (n/total N)	94.7 (144/152)	92.4 (146/158)
	Events/patient/year	114.2	108.4

* For definition regarding severe and non-severe hypoglycemia see section 6, Hypoglycemia.

Figure 1: Structural Formula of insulin detemir

'Placenta previa', 'Placenta previa hemorrhage', and 'Premature separation of placenta' and 1 serious adverse reaction of 'Antepartum haemorrhage'. There were none reported in the LEVEMIR group.
The incidence of early fetal death (abortions) was similar in LEVEMIR and NPH treated patients; 6.6% and 5.1%, respectively. The abortions were reported under the following terms: 'Abortion spontaneous', 'Abortion missed', 'Blighted ovum', 'Cervical incompetence' and 'Abortion incomplete'.

Table 7: Adverse reactions during pregnancy in a trial comparing insulin aspart + LEVEMIR to insulin aspart + NPH insulin in pregnant women with type 1 diabetes (adverse reactions with incidence ≥ 5%)*

	LEVEMIR, % (n = 152)	NPH, % (n = 158)
Anemia	13.2	10.8
Diarrhea	11.8	5.1
Pre-eclampsia	10.5	7.0
Urinary tract infection	9.9	5.7
Gastroenteritis	8.6	5.1
Abdominal pain upper	5.9	3.8
Vomiting	5.3	4.4
Abortion spontaneous	5.3	2.5
Abdominal pain	5.3	6.3
Oropharyngeal pain	5.3	6.3

* Because clinical trials are conducted under widely varying designs, the adverse reaction rates reported in one clinical trial may not be easily compared to those rates reported in another clinical trial, and may not reflect the rates actually observed in clinical practice.
The proportion of subjects experiencing severe hypoglycemia was 16.4% and 20.9% in LEVEMIR and NPH treated patients respectively. The rate of severe hypoglycemia was 1.1 and 1.2 events per patient-year in LEVEMIR and NPH treated patients respectively. Proportion and incidence rates for non-severe episodes of hypoglycemia were similar in both treatment groups (Table 8).

[See table 8 above]

In about a quarter of infants, LEVEMIR was detected in the infant cord blood at levels above the lower level of quantification (<25 pmol/L).
No differences in pregnancy outcomes or the health of the fetus and newborn were seen with LEVEMIR use.
Animal Data
In a fertility and embryonic development study, insulin detemir was administered to female rats before mating, during mating, and throughout pregnancy at doses up to 300 nmol/kg/day (3 times a human dose of 0.5 Units/kg/day, based on plasma area under the curve (AUC) ratio). Doses of 150 and 300 nmol/kg/day produced numbers of litters with visceral anomalies. Doses up to 900 nmol/kg/day (approximately 135 times a human dose of 0.5 Units/kg/day based on AUC ratio) were given to rabbits during organogenesis. Drug and dose related increases in the incidence of fetuses with gallbladder abnormalities such as small, bilobed, bifurcated, and missing gallbladders were observed at a dose of 900 nmol/kg/day. The rat and rabbit embryofetal development studies that included concurrent human insulin control groups indicated that insulin detemir and human insulin had similar effects regarding embryotoxicity and teratogenicity suggesting that the effects seen were the result of hypoglycemia resulting from insulin exposure in normal animals.
8.3 Nursing Mothers
It is unknown whether LEVEMIR is excreted in human milk. Because many drugs, including human insulin, are excreted in human milk, use caution when administering LEVEMIR to a nursing woman. Women with diabetes who are lactating may require adjustments of their insulin doses.
8.4 Pediatric Use
The pharmacokinetics, safety and effectiveness of subcutaneous injections of LEVEMIR have been established in pediatric patients (age 2 to 17 years) with type 1 diabetes [see Clinical Pharmacology (12.3) and Clinical Studies (14)]. LEVEMIR has not been studied in pediatric patients younger than 2 years of age with type 1 diabetes. LEVEMIR has not been studied in pediatric patients with type 2 diabetes.
The dose recommendation when converting to LEVEMIR is the same as that described for adults [see Dosage and Administration (2) and Clinical Studies (14)]. As in adults, the dosage of LEVEMIR must be individualized in pediatric patients based on metabolic needs and frequent monitoring of blood glucose.
8.5 Geriatric Use
In controlled clinical trials comparing LEVEMIR to NPH insulin or insulin glargine, 64 of 1624 patients (3.9%) in the type 1 diabetes trials and 309 of 1082 patients (28.6%) in the type 2 diabetes trials were ≥65 years of age. A total of 52

(7 type 1 and 45 type 2) patients (1.9%) were ≥75 years of age. No overall differences in safety or effectiveness were observed between these patients and younger patients, but small sample sizes, particularly for patients ≥65 years of age in the type 1 diabetes trials and for patients ≥75 years of age in all trials limits conclusions. Greater sensitivity of some older individuals cannot be ruled out. In elderly patients with diabetes, the initial dosing, dose increments, and maintenance dosage should be conservative to avoid hypoglycemia. Hypoglycemia may be difficult to recognize in the elderly.
10 OVERDOSAGE
An excess of insulin relative to food intake, energy expenditure, or both may lead to severe and sometimes prolonged and life-threatening hypoglycemia. Mild episodes of hypoglycemia usually can be treated with oral glucose. Adjustments in drug dosage, meal patterns, or exercise may be needed.
More severe episodes with coma, seizure, or neurologic impairment may be treated with intramuscular/subcutaneous glucagon or concentrated intravenous glucose. After apparent clinical recovery from hypoglycemia, continued observation and additional carbohydrate intake may be necessary to avoid recurrence of hypoglycemia [see Warnings and Precautions (5.3)].
11 DESCRIPTION
LEVEMIR (insulin detemir [rDNA origin] injection) is a sterile solution of insulin detemir for use as a subcutaneous injection. Insulin detemir is a long-acting (up to 24-hour duration of action) recombinant human insulin analog. LEVEMIR is produced by a process that includes expression of recombinant DNA in *Saccharomyces cerevisiae* followed by chemical modification.
Insulin detemir differs from human insulin in that the amino acid threonine in position B30 has been omitted, and a C14 fatty acid chain has been attached to the amino acid B29. Insulin detemir has a molecular formula of $C_{267}H_{402}O_{76}N_{64}S_6$ and a molecular weight of 5916.9. It has the following structure:
[See figure 1 above]
LEVEMIR is a clear, colorless, aqueous, neutral sterile solution. Each milliliter of LEVEMIR contains 100 units (14.2 mg/mL) insulin detemir, 65.4 mcg zinc, 2.06 mg m-cresol, 16.0 mg glycerol, 1.80 mg phenol, 0.89 mg disodium phosphate dihydrate, 1.17 mg sodium chloride, and water for injection. Hydrochloric acid and/or sodium hydroxide may be added to adjust pH. LEVEMIR has a pH of approximately 7.4.
12 CLINICAL PHARMACOLOGY
12.1 Mechanism of Action
The primary activity of insulin detemir is the regulation of glucose metabolism. Insulins, including insulin detemir, exert their specific action through binding to insulin receptors. Receptor-bound insulin lowers blood glucose by facilitating cellular uptake of glucose into skeletal muscle and adipose tissue and by inhibiting the output of glucose from the liver. Insulin inhibits lipolysis in the adipocyte, inhibits proteolysis, and enhances protein synthesis.
12.2 Pharmacodynamics
Insulin detemir is a soluble, long-acting basal human insulin analog with up to a 24-hour duration of action. The pharmacodynamic profile of LEVEMIR is relatively constant with no pronounced peak.
The duration of action of LEVEMIR is mediated by slowed systemic absorption of insulin detemir molecules from the injection site due to self-association of the drug molecules. In addition, the distribution of insulin detemir to peripheral target tissues is slowed because of binding to albumin.
Figure 2 shows results from a study in patients with type 1 diabetes conducted for a maximum of 24 hours after the subcutaneous injection of LEVEMIR or NPH insulin. The mean time between injection and the end of pharmacological effect for insulin detemir ranged from 7.6 hours to > 24 hours (24 hours was the end of the observation period).
[See figure 2 at top of next column]
For doses in the interval of 0.2 to 0.4 Units/kg, insulin detemir exerts more than 50% of its maximum effect from 3 to 4 hours up to approximately 14 hours after dose administration.
Figure 3 shows glucose infusion rate results from a 16-hour glucose clamp study in patients with type 2 diabetes. The clamp study was terminated at 16 hours according to protocol.
[See figure 3 at top of next column]
12.3 Pharmacokinetics
Absorption and Bioavailability
After subcutaneous injection of LEVEMIR in healthy subjects and in patients with diabetes, insulin detemir serum concentrations had a relatively constant concentration/time profile over 24 hours with the maximum serum concentration (Cmax) reached between 6-8 hours post-dose. Insulin detemir was more slowly absorbed after subcutaneous administration to the thigh where AUC_{0-5h} was 30-40% lower

Pharmacodynamic Parameters for LEVEMIR and NPH			
	LEVEMIR		NPH
	0.2 U/kg	0.4 U/kg	0.3 IU/kg
AUC$_{GIR}$ (mg/kg)	419	1184	743
GIR$_{max}$ (mg/kg/min)	1.1	1.7	1.6

LEVEMIR 0.2 Units/kg — LEVEMIR 0.4 Units/kg
NPH 0.3 International Units/kg

AUC$_{GIR}$: Area Under Curve for Glucose Infusion Rate
GIR$_{max}$: Maximum Glucose Infusion Rate

Figure 2: Activity Profiles in Patients with Type 1 Diabetes in a 24-hour Glucose Clamp Study

Pharmacodynamic Parameters for LEVEMIR and NPH			
	LEVEMIR		NPH
	0.6 U/kg	1.2 U/kg	0.6 IU/kg	1.2 IU/kg
AUC$_{GIR}$ (mg/kg)	1359	2333	1900	3220
GIR$_{max}$ (mg/kg/min)	2.3	3.7	3.2	4.8

LEVEMIR 0.6 Units/kg — LEVEMIR 1.2 Units/kg
NPH 0.6 International Units/kg — NPH 1.2 International Units/kg

AUC$_{GIR}$: Area Under Curve for Glucose Infusion Rate
GIR$_{max}$: Maximum Glucose Infusion Rate

Figure 3: Activity Profiles in Patients with Type 2 Diabetes in a 16-hour Glucose Clamp Study

and AUC$_{0-inf}$ was 10% lower than the corresponding AUCs with subcutaneous injections to the deltoid and abdominal regions.

The absolute bioavailability of insulin detemir is approximately 60%.

Distribution and Elimination

More than 98% of insulin detemir in the bloodstream is bound to albumin. The results of *in vitro* and *in vivo* protein binding studies demonstrate that there is no clinically relevant interaction between insulin detemir and fatty acids or other protein-bound drugs.

Insulin detemir has an apparent volume of distribution of approximately 0.1 L/kg. After subcutaneous administration in patients with type 1 diabetes, insulin detemir has a terminal half-life of 5 to 7 hours depending on dose.

Specific Populations

Children and Adolescents- The pharmacokinetic properties of LEVEMIR were investigated in children (6-12 years), adolescents (13-17 years), and adults with type 1 diabetes. In children, the insulin detemir plasma area under the curve (AUC) and C$_{max}$ were increased by 10% and 24%, respectively, as compared to adults. There was no difference in pharmacokinetics between adolescents and adults.

Geriatrics- In a clinical trial investigating differences in pharmacokinetics of a single subcutaneous dose of LEVEMIR in young (20 to 35 years) versus elderly (≥68 years) healthy subjects, the insulin detemir AUC was up to 35% higher among the elderly subjects due to reduced clearance. As with other insulin preparations, LEVEMIR should always be titrated according to individual requirements.

Gender- No clinically relevant differences in pharmacokinetic parameters of LEVEMIR are observed between males and females.

Race- In two clinical pharmacology studies conducted in healthy Japanese and Caucasian subjects, there were no clinically relevant differences seen in pharmacokinetic parameters. The pharmacokinetics and pharmacodynamics of LEVEMIR were investigated in a clamp study comparing patients with type 2 diabetes of Caucasian, African-American, and Latino origin. Dose-response relationships for LEVEMIR were comparable in these three populations.

Renal impairment- A single subcutaneous dose of 0.2 Units/kg (1.2 nmol/kg) of LEVEMIR was administered to healthy subjects and those with varying degrees of renal impairment (mild, moderate, severe, and hemodialysis-dependent). In this study, there were no differences in the pharmacokinetics of LEVEMIR between healthy subjects and those with renal impairment. However, some studies with human insulin have shown increased circulating levels of insulin in patients with renal impairment. Careful glucose monitoring and dose adjustments of insulin, including LEVEMIR, may be necessary in patients with renal impairment *[see Warnings and Precautions (5.5)]*.

Hepatic impairment- A single subcutaneous dose of 0.2 Units/kg (1.2 nmol/kg) of LEVEMIR was administered to healthy subjects and those with varying degrees of hepatic impairment (mild, moderate and severe). LEVEMIR exposure as estimated by AUC decreased with increasing degrees of hepatic impairment with a corresponding increase in apparent clearance. However, some studies with human insulin have shown increased circulating levels of insulin in patients with liver impairment. Careful glucose monitoring and dose adjustments of insulin, including LEVEMIR, may be necessary in patients with hepatic impairment *[see Warnings and Precautions (5.6)]*.

Pregnancy- The effect of pregnancy on the pharmacokinetics and pharmacodynamics of LEVEMIR has not been studied *[see Use in Specific Populations (8.1)]*.

Smoking- The effect of smoking on the pharmacokinetics and pharmacodynamics of LEVEMIR has not been studied.

Liraglutide -No pharmacokinetic interaction was observed between liraglutide and LEVEMIR when separate subcutaneous injections of LEVEMIR 0.5 Unit/kg (single-dose) and liraglutide 1.8 mg (steady state) were administered in patients with type 2 diabetes.

13   NONCLINICAL TOXICOLOGY

13.1   Carcinogenesis, Mutagenesis, Impairment of Fertility

Standard 2-year carcinogenicity studies in animals have not been performed. Insulin detemir tested negative for genotoxic potential in the *in vitro* reverse mutation study in bacteria, human peripheral blood lymphocyte chromosome aberration test, and the *in vivo* mouse micronucleus test.

In a fertility and embryonic development study, insulin detemir was administered to female rats before mating, during mating, and throughout pregnancy at doses up to 300 nmol/kg/day (3 times a human dose of 0.5 Units/kg/day, based on plasma AUC ratio). There were no effects on fertility in the rat.

14   CLINICAL STUDIES

The efficacy and safety of LEVEMIR given once-daily at bedtime or twice-daily (before breakfast and at bedtime, before breakfast and with the evening meal, or at 12-hour intervals) was compared to that of once-daily or twice-daily NPH insulin in open-label, randomized, parallel studies of 1155 adults with type 1 diabetes mellitus, 347 pediatric patients with type 1 diabetes mellitus, and 869 adults with type 2 diabetes mellitus. The efficacy and safety of LEVEMIR given twice-daily was compared to once-daily insulin glargine in an open-label, randomized, parallel study of 320 patients with type 1 diabetes. The evening LEVEMIR dose was titrated in all trials according to predefined targets for fasting blood glucose. The pre-dinner blood glucose was used to titrate the morning LEVEMIR dose in those trials that also administered LEVEMIR in the morning. In general, the reduction in glycosylated hemoglobin (HbA$_{1c}$) with LEVEMIR was similar to that with NPH insulin or insulin glargine.

Type 1 Diabetes – Adult

In a 16-week open-label clinical study (Study A, n=409), adults with type 1 diabetes were randomized to treatment

Table 9: Type 1 Diabetes Mellitus – Adult

	Study A 16 weeks NovoLog® (insulin aspart)		Study B 26 weeks NovoLog® (insulin aspart)		Study C 24 weeks Human Soluble Insulin (regular insulin)	
Treatment duration / Treatment in combination with	Twice-daily LEVEMIR	Twice-daily NPH	Twice-daily LEVEMIR	Once-daily insulin glargine	Once-daily LEVEMIR	Once-daily NPH
Number of patients treated	276	133	161	159	492	257
HbA1c (%)						
Baseline HbA1c	8.6	8.5	8.9	8.8	8.4	8.3
Adj. mean change from baseline	-0.8*	-0.7*	-0.6†	-0.5†	-0.1*	0.0*
LEVEMIR – NPH	-0.2		-0.0		-0.1	
95% CI for Treatment difference	(-0.3, -0.0)		(-0.2, 0.2)		(-0.3, 0.0)	
Basal insulin dose (units/day)						
Baseline mean	21	24	27	23	12	24
Mean change from baseline	16	10	10	4	9	2
Total insulin dose (units/day)						
Baseline mean	48	54	56	51	46	57
Mean change from baseline	17	10	9	6	11	3
Fasting blood glucose (mg/dL)						
Baseline mean	209	220	153	150	213	206
Adj. mean change from baseline	-44*	-9*	-38†	-41†	-30*	-9*
Body weight (kg)						
Baseline mean	74.6	75.5	77.5	75.1	76.5	76.9
Adj.Mean change from baseline	0.2*	0.8*	0.5†	1.0†	-0.3*	0.3*

* From an ANCOVA model adjusted for baseline value and country.
† From an ANCOVA model adjusted for baseline value and study site.

Table 10: Type 1 Diabetes Mellitus – Pediatric

	Study D 26 weeks NovoLog® (insulin aspart)		Study I 52 weeks NovoLog® (insulin aspart)	
Treatment duration / Treatment in combination with	Once- or Twice Daily LEVEMIR	Once- or Twice Daily NPH	Once- or Twice Daily LEVEMIR	Once- or Twice Daily NPH
Number of subjects treated	232	115	177	170
HbA1c (%)				
Baseline HbA1c	8.8	8.8	8.4	8.4
Adj. mean change from baseline	-0.7*	-0.8*	0.3†	0.2†
LEVEMIR – NPH	0.1		0.1	
95% CI for Treatment difference	-0.1; 0.3		-0.1; 0.4	
Basal insulin dose (units/day)				
Baseline mean	24	26	17	17
Mean change from baseline	8	6	8	7
Total insulin dose (units/day)				
Baseline mean	48	50	35	34
Mean change from baseline	9	7	10	8
Fasting blood glucose (mg/dL)				
Baseline mean	181	181	135	141
Adj. mean change from baseline	-39	-21	-10†	0†
Body weight (kg)				
Baseline mean	46.3	46.2	37.4	36.5
Adj.Mean change from baseline	1.6*	2.7*	2.7†	3.6†

* From an ANCOVA model adjusted for baseline value, geographical region, gender and age (covariate)
† From an ANCOVA model adjusted for baseline value, country, pubertal status at baseline and age (stratification factor).

Table 11: Type 2 Diabetes Mellitus – Adult

	Study E 24 weeks oral agents		Study F 22 weeks insulin aspart	
Treatment duration Treatment in combination with	Twice-daily LEVEMIR	Twice-daily NPH	Once- or Twice Daily LEVEMIR	Once- or Twice Daily NPH
Number of subjects treated	237	239	195	200
HbA1c (%)				
Baseline HbA1c	8.6	8.5	8.2	8.1
Adj. mean change from baseline	-2.0*	-2.1*	-0.6†	-0.6†
LEVEMIR – NPH	0.1		-0.1	
95% CI for Treatment difference	(-0.0, 0.3)		(-0.2, 0.1)	
Basal insulin dose (units/day)				
Baseline mean	18	17	22	22
Mean change from baseline	48	28	26	15
Total insulin dose‡ (units/day)				
Baseline mean	-	-	22	22
Mean change from baseline	-	-	57	42
Fasting blood glucose§ (mg/dL)				
Baseline mean	179	173	-	-
Adj. mean change from baseline	-69*	-74*	-	-
Body weight (kg)				
Baseline mean	82.5	82.3	82.0	79.6
Adj.Mean change from baseline	1.2*	2.8*	0.5†	1.2†

* From an ANCOVA model adjusted for baseline value, country and oral antidiabetic treatment category.
† From an ANCOVA model adjusted for baseline value and country.
‡ Study E – Conducted in insulin-naïve patients
§ Study F - Fasting blood glucose data not collected

Table 12: Results of a 26-week open-label trial of LEVEMIR as add on to liraglutide + metformin compared to continued treatment with liraglutide + metformin alone in patients not achieving HbA1c < 7% after 12 weeks of Metformin and Liraglutide

	Study H	
	LEVEMIR + Liraglutide +Metformin	Liraglutide+ Metformin
Intent-to-Treat Population (N)*	162	157
HbA$_{1c}$ (%) (Mean)		
Baseline (week 0)	7.6	7.6
Adjusted mean change from baseline	-0.5†	0†
Difference from liraglutide + metformin arm (LS mean)‡	-0.5§	
95% Confidence Interval	(-0.7, -0.4)	
Percentage of patients achieving A$_{1c}$ <7%	43¶	17¶
Fasting Plasma Glucose (mg/dL) (Mean)		
Baseline (week 0)	166	159
Adjusted mean change from baseline	-38†	-7†
Difference from liraglutide + metformin arm (LS mean)‡	-31§	
95% Confidence Interval	(-39 , -23)	

* Intent-to-treat population using last observation on study
† From an ANCOVA model adjusted for baseline value, country and previous oral antidiabetic treatment category
‡ Least squares mean adjusted for baseline value
§ p-value <0.0001
¶ From a logistic regression model adjusted for baseline HbA1c.

with either LEVEMIR at 12-hour intervals, LEVEMIR administered in the morning and bedtime or NPH insulin administered in the morning and bedtime. Insulin aspart was also administered before each meal. At 16 weeks of treatment, the combined LEVEMIR-treated patients had similar HbA$_{1c}$ and fasting plasma glucose (FPG) reductions compared to the NPH-treated patients (Table 9). Differences in timing of LEVEMIR administration had no effect on HbA$_{1c}$, fasting plasma glucose (FPG), or body weight.

In a 26-week, open-label clinical study (Study B, n=320), adults with type 1 diabetes were randomized to twice-daily LEVEMIR (administered in the morning and bedtime) or once-daily insulin glargine (administered at bedtime). Insulin aspart was administered before each meal. LEVEMIR-treated patients had a decrease in HbA$_{1c}$ similar to that of insulin glargine-treated patients.

In a 24-week, open-label clinical study (Study C, n=749), adults with type 1 diabetes were randomized to once-daily LEVEMIR or once-daily NPH insulin, both administered at bedtime and in combination with regular human insulin before each meal. LEVEMIR and NPH insulin had a similar effect on HbA$_{1c}$.
[See table 9 at top of previous page]

Type 1 Diabetes – Pediatric
Two open-label, randomized, controlled clinical studies have been conducted in pediatric patients with type 1 diabetes. One study was 26 weeks in duration and enrolled patients 6-17 years of age. The other study was 52 weeks in duration and enrolled patients 2-16 years of age. In both studies, LEVEMIR and NPH insulin were administered once- or twice-daily. Bolus insulin aspart was administered before each meal. In the 26-week study, LEVEMIR-treated patients had a mean decrease in HbA$_{1c}$ similar to that of NPH insulin (Table 10). In the 52-week study, the randomization was stratified by age (2-5 years, n=82, and 6-16 years, n=265) and the mean HbA$_{1c}$ increased in both treatment arms, with similar findings in the 2-5 year-old age group (n=80) and the 6-16 year-old age group (n=258) (Table 10).
[See table 10 at top of previous page]

Type 2 Diabetes – Adult
In a 24-week, open-label, randomized, clinical study (Study E, n=476), LEVEMIR administered twice-daily (before breakfast and evening) was compared to NPH insulin administered twice-daily (before breakfast and evening) as part of a regimen of stable combination therapy with one or two of the following oral antidiabetic medications: metformin, an insulin secretagogue, or an alpha–glucosidase inhibitor. All patients were insulin-naïve at the time of randomization. LEVEMIR and NPH insulin similarly lowered HbA$_{1c}$ from baseline (Table 11).

In a 22-week, open-label, randomized, clinical study (Study F, n=395) in adults with type 2 diabetes, LEVEMIR and NPH insulin were given once- or twice-daily as part of a basal-bolus regimen with insulin aspart. As measured by HbA$_{1c}$ or FPG, LEVEMIR had efficacy similar to that of NPH insulin.
[See table 11 above]

Combination Therapy with Metformin and Liraglutide
This 26-week open-label trial enrolled 988 patients with inadequate glycemic control (HbA1c 7-10%) on metformin (≥1500 mg/day) alone or inadequate glycemic control (HbA1c 7-8.5%) on metformin (≥1500 mg/day) and a sulfonylurea. Patients who were on metformin and a sulfonylurea discontinued the sulfonylurea then all patients entered a 12-week run-in period during which they received add-on therapy with liraglutide titrated to 1.8 mg once-daily. At the end of the run-in period, 498 patients (50%) achieved HbA1c <7% with liraglutide 1.8 mg and metformin and continued treatment in a non-randomized, observational arm. Another 167 patients (17%) withdrew from the trial during the run-in period with approximately one-half of these patients doing so because of gastrointestinal adverse reactions [see Adverse Reactions (6.1)]. The remaining 323 patients with HbA1c ≥7% (33% of those who entered the run-in period) were randomized to 26 weeks of once-daily LEVEMIR administered in the evening as add-on therapy (N=162) or to continued, unchanged treatment with liraglutide 1.8 mg and metformin (N=161). The starting dose of LEVEMIR was 10 units/day and the mean dose at the end of the 26-week randomized period was 39 units/day. During the 26-week randomized treatment period, the percentage of patients who discontinued due to ineffective therapy was 11.2% in the group randomized to continued treatment with liraglutide 1.8 mg and metformin and 1.2% in the group randomized to add-on therapy with LEVEMIR.

Treatment with LEVEMIR as add-on to liraglutide 1.8 mg + metformin resulted in statistically significant reductions in HbA1c and FPG compared to continued, unchanged treatment with liraglutide 1.8 mg + metformin alone (Table 12). From a mean baseline body weight of 96 kg after randomization, there was a mean reduction of 0.3 kg in the patients who received LEVEMIR add-on therapy compared to a mean reduction of 1.1 kg in the patients who continued on unchanged treatment with liraglutide 1.8 mg + metformin alone.
[See table 12 above]

Pregnancy
A randomized, open-label, controlled clinical trial has been conducted in pregnant women with type 1 diabetes. [see Use in Specific Populations (8.1)]

16 HOW SUPPLIED/STORAGE AND HANDLING
16.1 How Supplied
LEVEMIR is available in the following package sizes: each presentation containing 100 Units of insulin detemir per mL (U-100).
3 mL LEVEMIR FlexPen® NDC 0169-6439-10
3 mL LEVEMIR FlexTouch® NDC 0169-6438-10
10 mL vial NDC 0169-3687-12
FlexPen and FlexTouch can be used with NovoFine® or NovoTwist® disposable needles. Each FlexPen or FlexTouch is for use by a single patient. LEVEMIR FlexPen and LEVEMIR FlexTouch should never be shared between patients, even if the needle is changed.

16.2 Storage
Unused (unopened) LEVEMIR should be stored in the refrigerator between 2° and 8°C (36° to 46°F). Do not store in the freezer or directly adjacent to the refrigerator cooling element. **Do not freeze. Do not use LEVEMIR if it has been frozen.**

Unused (unopened) LEVEMIR can be kept until the expiration date printed on the label if it is stored in a refrigerator. Keep unused LEVEMIR in the carton so that it stays clean and protected from light.

If refrigeration is not possible, unused (unopened) LEVEMIR can be kept unrefrigerated at room temperature, below 30°C (86°F) as long as it is kept as cool as possible and away from direct heat and light. Unrefrigerated LEVEMIR should be discarded 42 days after it is first kept out of the refrigerator, even if the FlexPen, FlexTouch or vial still contains insulin.

Vials:
After initial use, vials should be stored in a refrigerator, never in a freezer. If refrigeration is not possible, the in-use vial can be kept unrefrigerated at room temperature, below 30°C (86°F) as long as it is kept as cool as possible and away from direct heat and light. Refrigerated LEVEMIR vials should be discarded 42 days after initial use. Unrefrigerated LEVEMIR vials should be discarded 42 days after they are first kept out of the refrigerator.

LEVEMIR FlexPen or LEVEMIR FlexTouch
After initial use, the LEVEMIR FlexPen or LEVEMIR FlexTouch must NOT be stored in a refrigerator and must

NOT be stored with the needle in place. Keep the opened (in use) LEVEMIR FlexPen or LEVEMIR FlexTouch away from direct heat and light at room temperature, below 30°C (86°F). Unrefrigerated LEVEMIR FlexPen or LEVEMIR FlexTouch should be discarded 42 days after they are first kept out of the refrigerator.

The storage conditions are summarized in Table 13:

Table 13: Storage Conditions for LEVEMIR FlexPen, LEVEMIR FlexTouch, and vial

	Not in-use (unopened) Refrigerated	Not in-use (unopened) Room Temperature (below 30°C)	In-use (opened)
3 mL LEVEMIR FlexPen	Until expiration date	42 days*	42 days* Room Temperature (below 30°C) (Do not refrigerate)
3 mL LEVEMIR FlexTouch	Until expiration date	42 days*	42 days* Room Temperature (below 30°C) (Do not refrigerate)
10 mL vial	Until expiration date	42 days*	42 days* Refrigerated or Room Temperature (below 30°C)

* The total time allowed at room temperature (below 30°C) is 42 days regardless of whether the product is in-use or not in-use.

16.3   Preparation and handling
Parenteral drug products should be inspected visually for particulate matter and discoloration prior to administration, whenever solution and container permit. LEVEMIR should be inspected visually prior to administration and should only be used if the solution appears clear and colorless.

Mixing and diluting: LEVEMIR must NOT be mixed or diluted with any other insulin or solution [See Warnings and Precautions (5.2)].

17   PATIENT COUNSELING INFORMATION
See FDA-Approved Patient Labeling (Patient Information and Instructions for Use)

17.1   Instructions for Patients
Patients should be informed that changes to insulin regimens must be made cautiously and only under medical supervision. Patients should be informed about the potential side effects of insulin therapy, including hypoglycemia, weight gain, lipodystrophy (and the need to rotate injection sites within the same body region), and allergic reactions. Patients should be informed that the ability to concentrate and react may be impaired as a result of hypoglycemia. This may present a risk in situations where these abilities are especially important, such as driving or operating other machinery. Patients who have frequent hypoglycemia or reduced or absent warning signs of hypoglycemia should be advised to use caution when driving or operating machinery.

Accidental mix-ups between LEVEMIR and other insulins, particularly short-acting insulins, have been reported. To avoid medication errors between LEVEMIR and other insulins, patients should be instructed to always check the insulin label before each injection.

LEVEMIR must only be used if the solution is clear and colorless with no particles visible. Patients must be advised that LEVEMIR must NOT be diluted or mixed with any other insulin or solution.

Patients should be instructed on self-management procedures including glucose monitoring, proper injection technique, and management of hypoglycemia and hyperglycemia. Patients should be instructed on handling of special situations such as intercurrent conditions (illness, stress, or emotional disturbances), an inadequate or skipped insulin dose, inadvertent administration of an increased insulin dose, inadequate food intake, and skipped meals.

Patients should receive proper training on how to use Levemir. Instruct patients that when injecting Levemir, they must press and hold down the dose button until the dose counter shows 0 and then keep the needle in the skin and count slowly to 6. When the dose counter returns to 0, the prescribed dose is not completely delivered until 6 seconds later. If the needle is removed earlier, they may see a stream of insulin coming from the needle tip. If so, the full dose will not be delivered (a possible under-dose may occur by as much as 20%), and they should increase the frequency of checking their blood glucose levels and possible additional insulin administration may be necessary.

• If 0 does not appear in the dose counter after continuously pressing the dose button, the patient may have used a blocked needle. In this case they would **not** have received **any** insulin – even though the dose counter has moved from the original dose that was set.

• If the patient did have a blocked needle, instruct them to change the needle as described in Section 5 of the Instructions for Use and repeat all steps in the IFU starting with Section 1: Prepare your pen with a new needle. **Make sure the patient selects the full dose needed.**

Patients with diabetes should be advised to inform their healthcare professional if they are pregnant or are contemplating pregnancy. Refer patients to the LEVEMIR "Patient Information" for additional information.

17.2   Never Share a LEVEMIR FlexPen or LEVEMIR FlexTouch Between Patients
Counsel patients that they should never share a LEVEMIR FlexPen or LEVEMIR FlexTouch with another person, even if the needle is changed. Sharing of the FlexPen or FlexTouch between patients may pose a risk of transmission of infection.

Novo Nordisk®, Levemir®, NovoLog®, FlexPen®, FlexTouch®, NovoFine®, and NovoTwist® are registered trademarks of Novo Nordisk A/S.

LEVEMIR® is covered by US Patent Nos. 5,750,497, 5,866,538, 6,011,007, 6,869,930 and other patents pending.
FlexPen® is covered by US Patent Nos. RE 41,956, 6,004,297, RE 43,834 and other patents pending.
FlexTouch® is covered by US patent Nos. 7,686,786, 6,899,699, and other patents pending.
© 2005-2013 Novo Nordisk
Manufactured by:
Novo Nordisk A/S
DK-2880 Bagsvaerd, Denmark
For information about LEVEMIR contact:
Novo Nordisk Inc.
800 Scudders Mill Road
Plainsboro, New Jersey 08536
1-800-727-6500
www.novonordisk-us.com

Patient Information

Patient Information
LEVEMIR® (LEV–uh-mere)
(insulin detemir [rDNA origin] injection)

What is Levemir?
• Levemir is a man-made insulin that is used to control high blood sugar in adults and children with diabetes mellitus.
• Levemir is not meant for use to treat diabetic ketoacidosis.

Who should not take Levemir?
Do not take Levemir if you:
• have an allergy to Levemir or any of the ingredients in Levemir.

Before taking Levemir, tell your healthcare provider about all your medical conditions including, if you are:
• pregnant, planning to become pregnant, or are breastfeeding.
• taking new prescription or over-the-counter medicines, vitamins, or herbal supplements.
Before you start taking Levemir, talk to your healthcare provider about low blood sugar and how to manage it.

How should I take Levemir?
• **Read the Instructions for Use** that come with your Levemir.
• Take Levemir exactly as your healthcare provider tells you to.
• Know the type and strength of insulin you take. **Do not** change the type of insulin you take unless your healthcare provider tells you to. The amount of insulin and the best time for you to take your insulin may need to change if you take different types of insulin.
• **Check your blood sugar levels.** Ask your healthcare provider what your blood sugars should be and when you should check your blood sugar levels.
• **Do not share your Levemir FlexPen, FlexTouch or needles with another person.** You may give another person an infection or get an infection from them.
• **Never** inject Levemir into a vein or muscle.

What should I avoid while taking Levemir?
While taking Levemir do not:
• Drive or operate heavy machinery, until you know how Levemir affects you.
• Drink alcohol or use prescription or over-the-counter medicines that contain alcohol.

What are the possible side effects of Levemir?
Levemir may cause serious side effects that can lead to death, including:
Low blood sugar (hypoglycemia). Signs and symptoms that may indicate low blood sugar include:
• dizziness or light-headedness
• sweating
• confusion
• headache
• blurred vision
• slurred speech
• shakiness
• fast heart beat
• anxiety, irritability, or mood changes
• hunger
Your insulin dose may need to change because of:
• change in level of physical activity or exercise
• weight gain or loss
• increased stress
• illness
• change in diet
Other common side effects of Levemir may include:
• Reactions at the injection site, itching, rash, serious allergic reactions (whole body reactions), skin thickening or pits at the injection site (lipodystrophy), weight gain, and swelling of your hands and feet.
Get emergency medical help if you have:
• trouble breathing, shortness of breath, fast heartbeat, swelling of your face, tongue, or throat, sweating, extreme drowsiness, dizziness, confusion.
These are not all the possible side effects of Levemir. Call your doctor for medical advice about side effects. You may report side effects to FDA at 1-800-FDA-1088.

General information about the safe and effective use of Levemir.
Medicines are sometimes prescribed for purposes other than those listed in a Patient Information leaflet. You can ask your pharmacist or healthcare provider for information about Levemir that is written for health professionals. Do not use Levemir for a condition for which it was not prescribed. Do not give Levemir to other people, even if they have the same symptoms that you have. It may harm them.

What are the ingredients in Levemir?
Active Ingredient: insulin detemir (rDNA origin)
Inactive Ingredients: zinc, m-cresol, glycerol, phenol, disodium phosphate dihydrate, sodium chloride and water for injection. Hydrochloric acid or sodium hydroxide may be added.
Manufactured by:
Novo Nordisk A/S
DK-2880 Bagsvaerd, Denmark
For more information, go to **www.novonordisk-us.com** or call 1-800-727-6500.

This Patient Information has been approved by the U.S. Food and Drug Administration
Revised: 10/2013
For more information go to
www.levemirflextouch.com
© 2005-2013 Novo Nordisk

Patient Instructions For Use
LEVEMIR® 10 mL vial
Please read the following Instructions for use carefully before using your LEVEMIR® 10 mL vial and each time you get a refill. You should read the instructions in this manual even if you have used an insulin 10 mL vial before.
How should I use the LEVEMIR 10 mL vial?
Using the 10 mL vial:

---

1. Check to make sure that you have the correct type of insulin. This is especially important if you use different types of insulin.
2. Look at the vial and the insulin. The LEVEMIR insulin should be clear and colorless. The tamper-resistant cap should be in place before the first use. If the cap has been removed before your first use of the vial, or if the insulin is cloudy or colored, **Do not** use the insulin and return it to your pharmacy.
3. Wash your hands with soap and water.

Levemir® FlexPen®: Pen cap, Rubber stopper, Cartridge, Cartridge scale, Pointer, Dose selector, Push-button

NovoFine® Needle: Big outer needle cap, Inner needle cap, Needle, Protective tab

4. If you are using a new vial, pull off the tamper-resistant cap.
Before each use, wipe the rubber stopper with an alcohol wipe.

5. Do not roll or shake the vial. Shaking the vial right before the dose is drawn into the syringe may cause bubbles or foam. This can cause you to draw up the wrong dose of insulin. The insulin should be used only if it is clear and colorless.

6. Pull back the plunger on your syringe until the black tip reaches the marking for the number of units you will inject.

7. Push the needle through the rubber stopper into the vial.

8. Push the plunger all the way in. This inserts air into the vial.

9. Turn the vial and syringe upside down and slowly pull the plunger back to a few units beyond the correct dose that you need.

10. If there are air bubbles, tap the syringe gently with your finger to raise the air bubbles to the top of the needle. Then slowly push the plunger to the correct unit marking for your dose.

11. Check to make sure you have the right dose of LEVEMIR in the syringe.
12. Pull the syringe out of the vial.
13. Inject your LEVEMIR right away as instructed by your healthcare provider.

How should I inject LEVEMIR with a syringe?

If you clean your injection site with an alcohol swab, let the injection site dry before you inject. Talk with your healthcare provider about how to rotate injection sites and how to give an injection.

1. Pinch your skin between two fingers, push the needle into the skinfold, using a dart-like motion and push the plunger to inject the insulin under your skin. The needle will be straight in.

2. Keep the needle under your skin for at least 6 seconds to make sure you have injected all the insulin. After you pull the needle from your skin you may see a drop of Levemir at the needle tip. This is normal and has no effect on the dose you just received.
3. If blood appears after you pull the needle from your skin, press the injection site lightly with an alcohol swab. Do not rub the area.
4. After each injection, **remove the needle without recapping** and dispose of it in a puncture-resistant container. Used syringes, needles, and lancets should be placed in sharps containers (such as red biohazard containers), hard plastic containers (such as detergent bottles), or metal containers (such as an empty coffee can). Such containers should be sealed and disposed of properly.

Revised: March 2013
Novo Nordisk® and LEVEMIR® are registered trademarks of Novo Nordisk A/S.
LEVEMIR® is covered by US Patent Nos. 5,750,497, 5,866,538, 6,011,007, 6,869,930, and other patents pending.
© 2005-2013 Novo Nordisk
Manufactured by:
Novo Nordisk A/S
DK-2880 Bagsvaerd, Denmark
For information about LEVEMIR® contact:
Novo Nordisk Inc.
800 Scudders Mill Road
Plainsboro, New Jersey 08536

Instructions For Use
LEVEMIR® FlexPen®

Please carefully read the following Instructions for use before using your LEVEMIR® FlexPen® and each time you get a refill. You should read the instructions in this manual even if you have used a LEVEMIR FlexPen before.
LEVEMIR FlexPen is a disposable dial-a-dose insulin pen. You can select doses from 1 to 60 units in increments of 1 unit. LEVEMIR FlexPen is designed to be used with NovoFine® needles.
Δ LEVEMIR FlexPen should not be used by people who are blind or have severe eyesight problems without the help of a person who has good eyesight and who is trained to use the LEVEMIR FlexPen the right way.

Getting ready
Make sure you have the following items:
• LEVEMIR FlexPen
• NovoFine disposable needles
• Alcohol swab
[See figure above]

PREPARING YOUR LEVEMIR FLEXPEN
Wash your hands with soap and water. Before you start to prepare your injection, check the label to make sure that you are taking the right type of insulin. This is especially important if you take more than 1 type of insulin. LEVEMIR should look clear and colorless.

A. Pull off the pen cap (see diagram A).
Wipe the rubber stopper with an alcohol swab.

B. Attaching the needle
Remove the protective tab from a new disposable needle.

Attach the needle tightly onto your FlexPen. It is important that the needle is put on straight (see diagram B). Never place a disposable needle on your LEVEMIR FlexPen until you are ready to give your injection.

C. Pull off the big outer needle cap (see diagram C).

D. Pull off the inner needle cap and throw it away (see diagram D).

Δ Always use a new needle for each injection to cut down the chance of infection and to prevent blocked needles.
Δ Be careful not to bend or damage the needle before use.
Δ To reduce the risk of needle sticks, never put the inner needle cap back on the needle.

Giving the airshot before each injection
Before each injection, small amounts of air may collect in the cartridge during normal use. To avoid injecting air and to ensure you take the right dose of insulin:

E. Turn the dose selector to select 2 units (see diagram E).

2 units selected

F. Hold your LEVEMIR FlexPen with the needle pointing up. Tap the cartridge gently with your finger a few times to make any air bubbles collect at the top of the cartridge (see diagram F).

G. While you keep the needle pointing upwards, press the push-button all the way in (see diagram G). The dose selector returns to 0.
A drop of insulin should appear at the needle tip. If not, change the needle and repeat the procedure no more than 6 times.
If you do not see a drop of insulin after 6 times, do not use the LEVEMIR FlexPen and contact Novo Nordisk at 1-800-727-6500.

A small air bubble may remain at the needle tip, but it will not be injected.

NovoFine®
Outer needle cap · Inner needle cap · Needle · Paper tab

NovoTwist®
Outer needle cap · Inner needle cap · Needle · Paper tab

Pen cap

Insulin scale · Insulin window · Dose counter · Dose selector

Levemir FlexTouch

Dose pointer · Dose button

(Figure A)

SELECTING YOUR DOSE

Check and make sure that the dose selector is set at 0.

H. Turn the dose selector to the number of units you need to inject. The pointer should line up with your dose. The dose can be corrected either up or down by turning the dose selector in either direction until the correct dose lines up with the pointer (see diagram H). When turning the dose selector, be careful not to press the push-button as insulin will come out.
You cannot select a dose larger than the number of units left in the cartridge.

5 units selected

24 units selected

You will hear a click for every single unit dialed. Do not set the dose by counting the number of clicks you hear.
Δ Do not use the cartridge scale printed on the cartridge to measure your dose of insulin.

GIVING THE INJECTION

Do the injection exactly as shown to you by your healthcare provider. Your healthcare provider should tell you if you need to pinch the skin before injecting. Wipe the skin with an alcohol swab and let the area dry.

I. Insert the needle into your skin.
Inject the dose by pressing the push-button all the way in until the 0 lines up with the pointer (see diagram I). Be careful only to push the button after the needle is in the skin. Turning the dose selector will not inject insulin.

J. Keep the needle in the skin for at least 6 seconds, and keep the push-button pressed all the way in until the needle has been pulled out from the skin (see diagram J). This will make sure that the full dose has been given.
You may see a drop of LEVEMIR at the needle tip.

This is normal and has no effect on the dose you just received. If blood appears after you take the needle out of your skin, press the injection site lightly with an alcohol swab. **Do not rub the area.**

After the injection

Carefully remove the needle from the pen after each injection. This helps to prevent infection and leakage of insulin. You can carefully recap the needle with the bigger outer cap to help make it easier to remove the needle.
Δ **Do not recap the needle with the small inner cap.** Recapping with this small part can increase your chances of having a needle stick injury.
Δ Put the needle in a sharps container or some type of hard plastic or metal container with a screw top such as a detergent bottle or empty coffee can. These containers should be sealed and thrown away the right way. Check with your

healthcare provider about the right way to throw away used syringes and needles. There may be local or state laws about how to throw away used needles and syringes. Do not throw away used needles and syringes in household trash or recycling bins.

K. Put the pen cap on the LEVEMIR FlexPen and store the LEVEMIR FlexPen without the needle attached (see diagram K).
The LEVEMIR FlexPen prevents the cartridge from being completely emptied.
It can deliver 300 units then you should throw it away in a sharps container or some type of hard plastic or metal container with a screw top, such as a detergent bottle or empty coffee can.

FUNCTION CHECK

L. If your LEVEMIR FlexPen is not working the right way, follow the steps below:
• Attach a new NovoFine needle.
• Remove the big outer needle cap and the inner needle cap.
• Do an airshot as described in "Giving the airshot before each injection" (see diagram E through G).
• Put the big outer needle cap onto the needle. Do not put on the inner needle cap.
• Turn the dose selector so the dose indicator window shows 20 units.
• Hold the LEVEMIR FlexPen so the needle is pointing down.
• Press the push-button all the way in.

The insulin should fill the lower part of the big outer needle cap to the marker (see diagram L). If LEVEMIR FlexPen has released too much or too little insulin, do the function check again. If the same problem happens again, do not use your LEVEMIR FlexPen and contact Novo Nordisk at 1-800-727-6500.

Maintenance

Your FlexPen is designed to work accurately and safely. It must be handled with care. If you drop your FlexPen it could get damaged. If you are concerned that your FlexPen is damaged, use a new one. You can clean the outside of your FlexPen by wiping it with a damp cloth. Do not soak or wash your FlexPen. Soaking or washing the FlexPen could damage it. Do not refill your FlexPen.
Δ Remove the needle from the LEVEMIR FlexPen after each injection. This helps to cut down your chance of infection, prevent leakage of insulin. Be careful when handling used needles to avoid needle sticks and transfer of infections.
Δ Keep your LEVEMIR FlexPen and needles out of the reach of children.
Δ Use LEVEMIR FlexPen as directed to treat your diabetes. Needles and LEVEMIR FlexPen must not be shared.
Δ Always use a new needle for each injection.
Δ Novo Nordisk is not responsible for harm due to using this insulin pen with products not recommended by Novo Nordisk.
Δ As a safety measure, always carry a spare insulin delivery device in case your LEVEMIR FlexPen is lost or damaged.
Δ Remember to keep the disposable LEVEMIR FlexPen with you. Do not leave it in a car or other location where it can get too hot or too cold.

Revised: May 2013
Novo Nordisk®, LEVEMIR®, FlexPen®, and NovoFine® are registered trademarks of Novo Nordisk A/S.
LEVEMIR® is covered by US Patent Nos. 5,750,497, 5,866,538, 6,011,007, 6,869,930, and other patents pending.

FlexPen® is covered by US Patent Nos. 6,004,297, RE 43,834, RE 41,956 and other patents pending.
© 2005-2013 Novo Nordisk
Manufactured by:
Novo Nordisk A/S
DK-2880 Bagsvaerd, Denmark
For information about LEVEMIR® contact:
Novo Nordisk Inc.
800 Scudders Mill Road
Plainsboro, New Jersey 08536

Instructions for Use
Levemir® (LEV–uh-mere) FlexTouch® Pen
(insulin detemir [rDNA origin] injection)

• **Levemir FlexTouch Pen ("Pen") is a prefilled disposable pen** containing 300 units of U-100 Levemir (insulin detemir [rDNA origin] injection) insulin. You can inject from 1 to 80 units in a single injection.
• **Do not share your Levemir FlexTouch Pen with another person. You may give an infection to them or get an infection from them.**
• **This Pen is not recommended for use by the blind or visually impaired without the assistance of a person trained in the proper use of the product.**
Supplies you will need to give your Levemir injection:
• Levemir FlexTouch Pen
• a new NovoFine or NovoTwist needle
• alcohol swab
• 1 sharps container for throwing away used Pens and needles. See "Disposing of used Levemir FlexTouch Pens and needles" at the end of these instructions.
Preparing your Levemir FlexTouch Pen:
• Wash your hands with soap and water.
• **Before you start to prepare your injection, check the Levemir FlexTouch Pen label to make sure you are taking the right type of insulin. This is especially important if you take more than 1 type of insulin.**
• **Levemir should look clear and colorless. Do not use Levemir if it is thick, cloudy, or is colored.**
• **Do not use Levemir past the expiration date printed on the label or 42 days after you start using the Pen.**
• **Always use a new needle for each injection to help ensure sterility and prevent blocked needles.**
[See figure above]

Step 1:
• Pull Pen cap straight off (See Figure B).

(Figure B)

Step 2:
• **Check the liquid in the Pen** (See Figure C). Levemir should look clear and colorless. **Do not** use it if it looks cloudy or colored.

(Figure C)

Step 3:
• **Select a new needle.**
• Pull off the paper tab from the outer needle cap (See Figure D).

NovoFine® NovoTwist®

(Figure D)

Step 4:
• Push the capped needle straight onto the Pen and twist the needle on until it is tight (See Figure E).

NovoFine® NovoTwist®

(Figure E)

Step 5:
Pull off the outer needle cap. **Do not** throw it away (See Figure F).

(Figure F)

Step 6:
Pull off the inner needle cap and throw it away (See Figure G).

(Figure G)

Priming your Levemir FlexTouch Pen:

Step 7:
Turn the dose selector to **select 2 units** (See Figure H).

2 units selected

(Figure H)

Step 8:
• Hold the Pen with the needle pointing up. Tap the top of the Pen gently a few times to let any air bubbles rise to the top (See Figure I).

(Figure I)

Step 9:
• Hold the Pen with the needle pointing up. Press and hold in the dose button until the dose counter shows "0". The "0" must line up with the dose pointer.
• A drop of insulin should be seen at the needle tip (See Figure J).
  ○ If you **do not** see a drop of insulin, repeat steps 7 to 9, no more than 6 times.
  ○ If you **still do not** see a drop of insulin, change the needle and repeat steps 7 to 9.

(Figure J)

Selecting your dose:

Step 10:
• **Turn the dose selector to select the number of units you need to inject.** The dose pointer should line up with your dose (See Figure K).
  ○ If you select the wrong dose, you can turn the dose selector forwards or backwards to the correct dose.
  ○ The **even** numbers are printed on the dial.
  ○ The **odd** numbers are shown as lines.

Examples

5 units selected

24 units selected

(Figure K)

• The Levemir FlexTouch Pen insulin scale will show you how much insulin is left in your Pen (See Figure L).
• **To see how much insulin is left in your Levemir FlexTouch Pen:**
  ○ Turn the dose selector until it stops. The dose counter will line up with the number of units of insulin that is left in your Pen. If the dose counter shows 80, there are **at least 80** units left in your Pen.
  ○ If the dose counter shows **less than 80**, the number shown in the dose counter is the number of units left in your Pen.

Example| Approx. 200 units left

(Figure L)

Giving your injection:
• Inject your Levemir exactly as your healthcare provider has shown you. Your healthcare provider should tell you if you need to pinch the skin before injecting.
• Levemir can be injected under the skin (subcutaneously) of your stomach area (abdomen), buttocks, upper legs (thighs) or upper arms.
• Change (rotate) your injection sites within the area you choose for each dose. **Do not** use the same injection site for each injection.

Step 11:
• Choose your injection site and wipe the skin with an alcohol swab. Let the injection site dry before you inject your dose (See Figure M).

(Figure M)

Step 12:
• **Insert the needle into your skin** (See Figure N).
  ○ **Make sure you can see the dose counter. Do not** cover it with your fingers, this can stop your injection.

(Figure N)

Step 13:
• **Press and hold down the dose button until the dose counter shows "0"** (See Figure O).
  ○ The "0" must line up with the dose pointer. You may then hear or feel a click.

(Figure O)

• **Keep the needle in your skin after** the dose counter has returned to "0" and **slowly count to 6** (See Figure P).
  ○ When the dose counter returns to "0", you will not get your full dose until 6 seconds later.
  ○ If the needle is removed before you count to 6, you may see a stream of insulin coming from the needle tip.
  ○ If you see a stream of insulin coming from the needle tip you will not get your full dose. If this happens you should check your blood sugar levels more often because you may need more insulin.

Count slowly:

1-2-3-4-5-6

(Figure P)

Step 14:
• **Pull the needle out of your skin** (See Figure Q).
  ○ If you see blood after you take the needle out of your skin, press the injection site lightly with a piece of gauze or an alcohol swab. **Do not** rub the area.

(Figure Q)

Step 15:
• **Carefully remove the needle from the Pen and throw it away** (See Figure R).
  ○ **Do not** recap the needle. Recapping the needle can lead to needle stick injury.
• If you **do not** have a sharps container, carefully slip the needle into the outer needle cap (See Figure S). Safely remove the needle and throw it away as soon as you can.
  ○ **Do not** store the Pen with the needle attached. Storing without the needle attached helps prevent leaking, blocking of the needle, and air from entering the Pen.

(Figure R)

(Figure S)

Step 16:
• Replace the Pen cap by pushing it straight on (See Figure T).

(Figure T)

After your injection:
• Put your used Levemir FlexTouch Pen and needles in a FDA-cleared sharps disposal container right away after use. Do not throw away (dispose of) loose needles and Pens in your household trash.
• If you do not have a FDA-cleared sharps disposal container, you may use a household container that is:
  ○ made of a heavy-duty plastic
  ○ can be closed with a tight-fitting, puncture-resistant lid, without sharps being able to come out
  ○ upright and stable during use
  ○ leak-resistant
  ○ properly labeled to warn of hazardous waste inside the container
• When your sharps disposal container is almost full, you will need to follow your community guidelines for the right way to dispose of your sharps disposal container. There may be state or local laws about how you should throw away used needles and syringes. For more information about the safe sharps disposal, and for specific information about sharps disposal in the state that you live in, go to the FDA's website at: http://www.fda.gov/safesharpsdisposal.

- Do not dispose of your used sharps disposal container in your household trash unless your community guidelines permit this. Do not recycle your used sharps disposal container.

How should I store my Levemir FlexTouch Pen?
- Store unused Levemir FlexTouch Pens in the refrigerator at 36°F to 46°F (2°C to 8°C).
- Store the Pen you are currently using out of the refrigerator below 86°F.
- **Do not** freeze Levemir. **Do not** use Levemir if it has been frozen.
- Keep Levemir away from heat or light.
- Unused Pens may be used until the expiration date printed on the label, if kept in the refrigerator.
- The Levemir FlexTouch Pen you are using should be thrown away after 42 days, even if it still has insulin left in it.

General Information about the safe and effective use of Levemir.
- **Keep Levemir FlexTouch Pens and needles out of the reach of children.**
- **Always** use a new needle for each injection.
- **Do not** share Pens or needles.

This Instructions for Use has been approved by the U.S. Food and Drug Administration.

Manufactured By:
Novo Nordisk A/S
DK-2880 Bagsvaerd, Denmark
Revised: 10/2013

Shown in Product Identification Guide, page 311

NOVOLOG®   ℞

[NO-vō-log]
(insulin aspart [rDNA origin] injection)
solution for subcutaneous use

HIGHLIGHTS OF PRESCRIBING INFORMATION
These highlights do not include all the information needed to use NovoLog safely and effectively.
See full prescribing information for NovoLog.
NovoLog® (insulin aspart [rDNA origin] injection) solution for subcutaneous use
Initial U.S. Approval: 2000

────INDICATIONS AND USAGE────
- NovoLog is an insulin analog indicated to improve glycemic control in adults and children with diabetes mellitus (1.1).

────DOSAGE AND ADMINISTRATION────
- The dosage of NovoLog must be individualized.
- *Subcutaneous injection:* NovoLog should generally be given immediately (within 5-10 minutes) prior to the start of a meal (2.2).
- *Use in pumps:* Change the NovoLog in the reservoir at least every 6 days, change the infusion set, and the infusion set insertion site at least every 3 days. NovoLog should not be mixed with other insulins or with a diluent when it is used in the pump (2.3).
- *Intravenous use:* NovoLog should be used at concentrations from 0.05 U/mL to 1.0 U/mL insulin aspart in infusion systems using polypropylene infusion bags. NovoLog has been shown to be stable in infusion fluids such as 0.9% sodium chloride (2.4).

────DOSAGE FORMS AND STRENGTHS────
Each presentation contains 100 Units of insulin aspart per mL (U-100)
- 10 mL vials (3)
- 3 mL PenFill® cartridges for the 3 mL PenFill cartridge device (3)
- 3 mL NovoLog FlexPen® (3)
- 3 mL NovoLog FlexTouch® (3)

────CONTRAINDICATIONS────
- Do not use during episodes of hypoglycemia (4).
- Do not use in patients with hypersensitivity to NovoLog or one of its excipients.

────WARNINGS AND PRECAUTIONS────
- Hypoglycemia is the most common adverse effect of insulin therapy. Glucose monitoring is recommended for all patients with diabetes. Any change of insulin dose should be made cautiously and only under medical supervision (5.1, 5.2).
- Insulin, particularly when given intravenously or in settings of poor glycemic control, can cause hypokalemia. Use caution in patients predisposed to hypokalemia (5.3).
- Like all insulins, NovoLog requirements may be reduced in patients with renal impairment or hepatic impairment (5.4, 5.5).
- Severe, life-threatening, generalized allergy, including anaphylaxis, may occur with insulin products, including NovoLog (5.6).

- Fluid retention and heart failure can occur with concomitant use of thiazolidinediones (TZDs), which are PPAR-gamma agonists, and insulin, including NovoLog (5.10).

────ADVERSE REACTIONS────
Adverse reactions observed with NovoLog include hypoglycemia, allergic reactions, local injection site reactions, lipodystrophy, rash and pruritus (6).

To report SUSPECTED ADVERSE REACTIONS, contact Novo Nordisk Inc. at 1-800-727-6500 or FDA at 1-800-FDA-1088 or www.fda.gov/medwatch.

────DRUG INTERACTIONS────
- The following may increase the blood-glucose-lowering effect and susceptibility to hypoglycemia: oral antidiabetic products, pramlintide, ACE inhibitors, disopyramide, fibrates, fluoxetine, monoamine oxidase inhibitors, propoxyphene, salicylates, somatostatin analogs, sulfonamide antibiotics (7).
- The following may reduce the blood-glucose-lowering effect: corticosteroids, niacin, danazol, diuretics, sympathomimetic agents (e.g., epinephrine, salbutamol, terbutaline), isoniazid, phenothiazine derivatives, somatropin, thyroid hormones, estrogens, progestogens (e.g., in oral contraceptives), atypical antipsychotics (7).
- Beta-blockers, clonidine, lithium salts, and alcohol may either potentiate or weaken the blood-glucose-lowering effect of insulin (7).
- Pentamidine may cause hypoglycemia, which may sometimes be followed by hyperglycemia (7).
- The signs of hypoglycemia may be reduced or absent in patients taking sympatholytic products such as beta-blockers, clonidine, guanethidine, and reserpine (7).

────USE IN SPECIFIC POPULATIONS────
- Pediatric: Has not been studied in children with type 2 diabetes. Has not been studied in children with type 1 diabetes <2 years of age (8.4).

See 17 for PATIENT COUNSELING INFORMATION and FDA-approved patient labeling

Revised: 04/2014

FULL PRESCRIBING INFORMATION: CONTENTS*
* Sections or subsections omitted from the full prescribing information are not listed

---

FULL PRESCRIBING INFORMATION

1   INDICATIONS AND USAGE
1.1   Treatment of Diabetes Mellitus
NovoLog is an insulin analog indicated to improve glycemic control in adults and children with diabetes mellitus.

2   DOSAGE AND ADMINISTRATION
2.1   Dosing
NovoLog is an insulin analog with an earlier onset of action than regular human insulin. The dosage of NovoLog must be individualized. NovoLog given by subcutaneous injection should generally be used in regimens with an intermediate or long-acting insulin [*see Warnings and Precautions (5), How Supplied/Storage and Handling (16.2)*]. The total daily insulin requirement may vary and is usually between 0.5 to 1.0 units/kg/day. When used in a meal-related subcutaneous injection treatment regimen, 50 to 70% of total insulin requirements may be provided by NovoLog and the remainder provided by an intermediate-acting or long-acting insulin. Because of NovoLog's comparatively rapid onset and short duration of glucose lowering activity, some patients may require more basal insulin and more total insulin to prevent pre-meal hyperglycemia when using NovoLog than when using human regular insulin.
Do not use NovoLog that is viscous (thickened) or cloudy; use only if it is clear and colorless. NovoLog should not be used after the printed expiration date.
2.2   Subcutaneous Injection
NovoLog should be administered by subcutaneous injection in the abdominal region, buttocks, thigh, or upper arm. Because NovoLog has a more rapid onset and a shorter duration of activity than human regular insulin, it should be injected immediately (within 5-10 minutes) before a meal. Injection sites should be rotated within the same region to reduce the risk of lipodystrophy. As with all insulins, the duration of action of NovoLog will vary according to the dose, injection site, blood flow, temperature, and level of physical activity.
NovoLog may be diluted with Insulin Diluting Medium for NovoLog for subcutaneous injection. Diluting one part NovoLog to nine parts diluent will yield a concentration one-tenth that of NovoLog (equivalent to U-10). Diluting one part NovoLog to one part diluent will yield a concentration one-half that of NovoLog (equivalent to U-50).
2.3   Continuous Subcutaneous Insulin Infusion (CSII) by External Pump
NovoLog can also be infused subcutaneously by an external insulin pump [*see Warnings and Precautions (5.8, 5.9), How Supplied/Storage and Handling (16.2)*]. Diluted insulin should not be used in external insulin pumps. Because NovoLog has a more rapid onset and a shorter duration of activity than human regular insulin, pre-meal boluses of NovoLog should be infused immediately (within 5-10 minutes) before a meal. Infusion sites should be rotated within the same region to reduce the risk of lipodystrophy. The initial programming of the external insulin infusion pump should be based on the total daily insulin dose of the previous regimen. Although there is significant interpatient variability, approximately 50% of the total dose is usually given as meal-related boluses of NovoLog and the remainder is given as a basal infusion. **Change the NovoLog in the reservoir at least every 6 days, change the infusion sets and the infusion set insertion site at least every 3 days.**
The following insulin pumps† have been used in NovoLog clinical or in vitro studies conducted by Novo Nordisk, the manufacturer of NovoLog:
- Medtronic Paradigm® 512 and 712
- MiniMed 508
- Disetronic® D-TRON® and H-TRON®
Before using a different insulin pump with NovoLog, read the pump label to make sure the pump has been evaluated with NovoLog.
2.4   Intravenous Use
NovoLog can be administered intravenously under medical supervision for glycemic control with close monitoring of blood glucose and potassium levels to avoid hypoglycemia and hypokalemia [*see Warnings and Precautions (5), How Supplied/Storage and Handling (16.2)*]. For intravenous use, NovoLog should be used at concentrations from 0.05 U/mL to 1.0 U/mL insulin aspart in infusion systems using polypropylene infusion bags. NovoLog has been shown to be stable in infusion fluids such as 0.9% sodium chloride.
Inspect NovoLog for particulate matter and discoloration prior to parenteral administration.

3   DOSAGE FORMS AND STRENGTHS
NovoLog is available in the following package sizes: each presentation contains 100 units of insulin aspart per mL (U-100).

Table 1: Treatment-Emergent Adverse Events in Patients with Type 1 Diabetes Mellitus (Adverse events with frequency ≥ 5% and occurring more frequently with NovoLog compared to human regular insulin are listed)

Preferred Term	NovoLog + NPH N= 596		Human Regular Insulin + NPH N= 286	
	N	(%)	N	(%)
Hypoglycemia*	448	75%	205	72%
Headache	70	12%	28	10%
Injury accidental	65	11%	29	10%
Nausea	43	7%	13	5%
Diarrhea	28	5%	9	3%

* Hypoglycemia is defined as an episode of blood glucose concentration <45 mg/dL, with or without symptoms. See Section 14 for the incidence of serious hypoglycemia in the individual clinical trials.

- 10 mL vials
- 3 mL PenFill cartridges for the 3 mL PenFill cartridge delivery device (with or without the addition of a NovoPen® 3 PenMate®) with NovoFine® disposable needles
- 3 mL NovoLog FlexPen
- 3 mL NovoLog FlexTouch

4   CONTRAINDICATIONS
NovoLog is contraindicated
- during episodes of hypoglycemia
- in patients with hypersensitivity to NovoLog or one of its excipients.

5   WARNINGS AND PRECAUTIONS
5.1   Administration
NovoLog has a more rapid onset of action and a shorter duration of activity than regular human insulin. An injection of NovoLog should immediately be followed by a meal within 5-10 minutes. Because of NovoLog's short duration of action, a longer acting insulin should also be used in patients with type 1 diabetes and may also be needed in patients with type 2 diabetes. Glucose monitoring is recommended for all patients with diabetes and is particularly important for patients using external pump infusion therapy.

Any change of insulin dose should be made cautiously and only under medical supervision. Changing from one insulin product to another or changing the insulin strength may result in the need for a change in dosage. As with all insulin preparations, the time course of NovoLog action may vary in different individuals or at different times in the same individual and is dependent on many conditions, including the site of injection, local blood supply, temperature, and physical activity. Patients who change their level of physical activity or meal plan may require adjustment of insulin dosages. Insulin requirements may be altered during illness, emotional disturbances, or other stresses.

Patients using continuous subcutaneous insulin infusion pump therapy must be trained to administer insulin by injection and have alternate insulin therapy available in case of pump failure.

Needles, NovoLog FlexPen and NovoLog FlexTouch must not be shared.

5.2   Hypoglycemia
Hypoglycemia is the most common adverse effect of all insulin therapies, including NovoLog. Severe hypoglycemia may lead to unconsciousness and/or convulsions and may result in temporary or permanent impairment of brain function or death. Severe hypoglycemia requiring the assistance of another person and/or parenteral glucose infusion or glucagon administration has been observed in clinical trials with insulin, including trials with NovoLog.

The timing of hypoglycemia usually reflects the time-action profile of the administered insulin formulations [see Clinical Pharmacology (12)]. Other factors such as changes in food intake (e.g., amount of food or timing of meals), injection site, exercise, and concomitant medications may also alter the risk of hypoglycemia [see Drug Interactions (7)]. As with all insulins, use caution in patients with hypoglycemia unawareness and in patients who may be predisposed to hypoglycemia (e.g., patients who are fasting or have erratic food intake). The patient's ability to concentrate and react may be impaired as a result of hypoglycemia. This may present a risk in situations where these abilities are especially important, such as driving or operating other machinery.

Rapid changes in serum glucose levels may induce symptoms of hypoglycemia in persons with diabetes, regardless of the glucose value. Early warning symptoms of hypoglycemia may be different or less pronounced under certain conditions, such as longstanding diabetes, diabetic nerve disease, use of medications such as beta-blockers, or intensified diabetes control [see Drug Interactions (7)]. These situations may result in severe hypoglycemia (and, possibly, loss of consciousness) prior to the patient's awareness of hypoglycemia. Intravenously administered insulin has a more rapid onset of action than subcutaneously administered insulin, requiring more close monitoring for hypoglycemia.

5.3   Hypokalemia
All insulin products, including NovoLog, cause a shift in potassium from the extracellular to intracellular space, possibly leading to hypokalemia that, if left untreated, may cause respiratory paralysis, ventricular arrhythmia, and death. Use caution in patients who may be at risk for hypokalemia (e.g., patients using potassium-lowering medications, patients taking medications sensitive to serum potassium concentrations, and patients receiving intravenously administered insulin).

5.4   Renal Impairment
As with other insulins, the dose requirements for NovoLog may be reduced in patients with renal impairment [see Clinical Pharmacology (12.3)].

5.5   Hepatic Impairment
As with other insulins, the dose requirements for NovoLog may be reduced in patients with hepatic impairment [see Clinical Pharmacology (12.3)].

5.6   Hypersensitivity and Allergic Reactions
Local Reactions - As with other insulin therapy, patients may experience redness, swelling, or itching at the site of NovoLog injection. These reactions usually resolve in a few days to a few weeks, but in some occasions, may require discontinuation of NovoLog. In some instances, these reactions may be related to factors other than insulin, such as irritants in a skin cleansing agent or poor injection technique. Localized reactions and generalized myalgias have been reported with injected metacresol, which is an excipient in NovoLog.

Systemic Reactions - Severe, life-threatening, generalized allergy, including anaphylaxis, may occur with any insulin product, including NovoLog. Anaphylactic reactions with NovoLog have been reported post-approval. Generalized allergy to insulin may also cause whole body rash (including pruritus), dyspnea, wheezing, hypotension, tachycardia, or diaphoresis. In controlled clinical trials, allergic reactions were reported in 3 of 735 patients (0.4%) treated with regular human insulin and 10 of 1394 patients (0.7%) treated with NovoLog. In controlled and uncontrolled clinical trials, 3 of 2341 (0.1%) NovoLog-treated patients discontinued due to allergic reactions.

5.7   Antibody Production
Increases in anti-insulin antibody titers that react with both human insulin and insulin aspart have been observed in patients treated with NovoLog. Increases in anti-insulin antibodies are observed more frequently with NovoLog than with regular human insulin. Data from a 12-month controlled trial in patients with type 1 diabetes suggest that the increase in these antibodies is transient, and the differences in antibody levels between the regular human insulin and insulin aspart treatment groups observed at 3 and 6 months were no longer evident at 12 months. In this study these antibodies did not appear to cause deterioration in glycemic control or necessitate increases in insulin dose.

In rare cases, the presence of such insulin antibodies may necessitate adjustment of the insulin dose in order to correct a tendency towards hyperglycemia or hypoglycemia.

5.8   Mixing of Insulins
- Mixing NovoLog with NPH human insulin immediately before injection attenuates the peak concentration of NovoLog, without significantly affecting the time to peak concentration or total bioavailability of NovoLog. If NovoLog is mixed with NPH human insulin, NovoLog should be drawn into the syringe first, and the mixture should be injected immediately after mixing.
- The efficacy and safety of mixing NovoLog with insulin preparations produced by other manufacturers have not been studied.
- Insulin mixtures should not be administered intravenously.

5.9   Continuous Subcutaneous Insulin Infusion by External Pump
When used in an external subcutaneous insulin infusion pump, NovoLog should not be mixed with any other insulin or diluent. When using NovoLog in an external insulin pump, the NovoLog-specific information should be followed (e.g., in-use time, frequency of changing infusion sets) because NovoLog-specific information may differ from general pump manual instructions.

Pump or infusion set malfunctions or insulin degradation can lead to a rapid onset of hyperglycemia and ketosis because of the small subcutaneous depot of insulin. This is especially pertinent for rapid-acting insulin analogs that are more rapidly absorbed through skin and have a shorter duration of action. Prompt identification and correction of the cause of hyperglycemia or ketosis is necessary. Interim therapy with subcutaneous injection may be required [see Dosage and Administration (2.3), Warnings and Precautions (5.8, 5.9), How Supplied/Storage and Handling (16.2), and Patient Counseling Information (17.2)].

NovoLog should not be exposed to temperatures greater than 37°C (98.6°F). **NovoLog that will be used in a pump should not be mixed with other insulin or with a diluent** [see Dosage and Administration (2.3), Warnings and Precautions (5.8, 5.9), How Supplied/Storage and Handling (16.2), and Patient Counseling Information (17.2)].

5.10   Fluid retention and heart failure with concomitant use of PPAR-gamma agonists
Thiazolidinediones (TZDs), which are peroxisome proliferator-activated receptor (PPAR)-gamma agonists, can cause dose-related fluid retention, particularly when used in combination with insulin. Fluid retention may lead to or exacerbate heart failure. Patients treated with insulin, including NovoLog, and a PPAR-gamma agonist should be observed for signs and symptoms of heart failure. If heart failure develops, it should be managed according to current standards of care, and discontinuation or dose reduction of the PPAR-gamma agonist must be considered.

6   ADVERSE REACTIONS
Clinical Trial Experience
Because clinical trials are conducted under widely varying designs, the adverse reaction rates reported in one clinical trial may not be easily compared to those rates reported in another clinical trial, and may not reflect the rates actually observed in clinical practice.

- *Hypoglycemia*
Hypoglycemia is the most commonly observed adverse reaction in patients using insulin, including NovoLog [see Warnings and Precautions (5)].
- *Insulin initiation and glucose control intensification*
Intensification or rapid improvement in glucose control has been associated with a transitory, reversible ophthalmologic refraction disorder, worsening of diabetic retinopathy, and acute painful peripheral neuropathy. However, long-term glycemic control decreases the risk of diabetic retinopathy and neuropathy.
- *Lipodystrophy*
Long-term use of insulin, including NovoLog, can cause lipodystrophy at the site of repeated insulin injections or infusion. Lipodystrophy includes lipohypertrophy (thickening of adipose tissue) and lipoatrophy (thinning of adipose tissue), and may affect insulin absorption. Rotate insulin injection or infusion sites within the same region to reduce the risk of lipodystrophy.
- *Weight gain*
Weight gain can occur with some insulin therapies, including NovoLog, and has been attributed to the anabolic effects of insulin and the decrease in glucosuria.
- *Peripheral Edema*
Insulin may cause sodium retention and edema, particularly if previously poor metabolic control is improved by intensified insulin therapy.
- *Frequencies of adverse drug reactions*
The frequencies of adverse drug reactions during NovoLog clinical trials in patients with type 1 diabetes mellitus and type 2 diabetes mellitus are listed in the tables below.
[See table 1 above]
[See table 2 at top of next page]

Postmarketing Data
The following additional adverse reactions have been identified during postapproval use of NovoLog. Because these adverse reactions are reported voluntarily from a population of uncertain size, it is generally not possible to reliably estimate their frequency. Medication errors in which other insulins have been accidentally substituted for NovoLog have been identified during postapproval use [see Patient Counseling Information (17)].

7   DRUG INTERACTIONS
A number of substances affect glucose metabolism and may require insulin dose adjustment and particularly close monitoring.

- The following are examples of substances that may increase the blood-glucose-lowering effect and susceptibility to hypoglycemia: oral antidiabetic products, pramlintide, ACE inhibitors, disopyramide, fibrates, fluoxetine, monoamine oxidase (MAO) inhibitors, propoxyphene, salicylates, somatostatin analog (e.g., octreotide), sulfonamide antibiotics.
- The following are examples of substances that may reduce the blood-glucose-lowering effect: corticosteroids, niacin, danazol, diuretics, sympathomimetic agents (e.g., epinephrine, salbutamol, terbutaline), isoniazid, phenothiazine derivatives, somatropin, thyroid hormones, estrogens, progestogens (e.g., in oral contraceptives), atypical antipsychotics.
- Beta-blockers, clonidine, lithium salts, and alcohol may either potentiate or weaken the blood-glucose-lowering effect of insulin.
- Pentamidine may cause hypoglycemia, which may sometimes be followed by hyperglycemia.
- The signs of hypoglycemia may be reduced or absent in patients taking sympatholytic products such as beta-blockers, clonidine, guanethidine, and reserpine.

8 USE IN SPECIFIC POPULATIONS

8.1 Pregnancy

Pregnancy Category B. All pregnancies have a background risk of birth defects, loss, or other adverse outcome regardless of drug exposure. This background risk is increased in pregnancies complicated by hyperglycemia and may be decreased with good metabolic control. It is essential for patients with diabetes or history of gestational diabetes to maintain good metabolic control before conception and throughout pregnancy. Insulin requirements may decrease during the first trimester, generally increase during the second and third trimesters, and rapidly decline after delivery. Careful monitoring of glucose control is essential in these patients. Therefore, female patients should be advised to tell their physician if they intend to become, or if they become pregnant while taking NovoLog.

An open-label, randomized study compared the safety and efficacy of NovoLog (n=157) versus regular human insulin (n=165) in 322 pregnant women with type 1 diabetes. Two-thirds of the enrolled patients were already pregnant when they entered the study. Because only one-third of the patients enrolled before conception, the study was not large enough to evaluate the risk of congenital malformations. Both groups achieved a mean HbA1c of ~ 6% during pregnancy, and there was no significant difference in the incidence of maternal hypoglycemia.

Subcutaneous reproduction and teratology studies have been performed with NovoLog and regular human insulin in rats and rabbits. In these studies, NovoLog was given to female rats before mating, during mating, and throughout pregnancy, and to rabbits during organogenesis. The effects of NovoLog did not differ from those observed with subcutaneous regular human insulin. NovoLog, like human insulin, caused pre- and post-implantation losses and visceral/skeletal abnormalities in rats at a dose of 200 U/kg/day (approximately 32 times the human subcutaneous dose of 1.0 U/kg/day, based on U/body surface area) and in rabbits at a dose of 10 U/kg/day (approximately three times the human subcutaneous dose of 1.0 U/kg/day, based on U/body surface area). The effects are probably secondary to maternal hypoglycemia at high doses. No significant effects were observed in rats at a dose of 50 U/kg/day and in rabbits at a dose of 3 U/kg/day. These doses are approximately 8 times the human subcutaneous dose of 1.0 U/kg/day for rats and equal to the human subcutaneous dose of 1.0 U/kg/day for rabbits, based on U/body surface area.

8.3 Nursing Mothers

It is unknown whether insulin aspart is excreted in human milk. Use of NovoLog is compatible with breastfeeding, but women with diabetes who are lactating may require adjustments of their insulin doses.

8.4 Pediatric Use

NovoLog is approved for use in children for subcutaneous daily injections and for subcutaneous continuous infusion by external insulin pump. NovoLog has not been studied in pediatric patients younger than 2 years of age. NovoLog has not been studied in pediatric patients with type 2 diabetes. Please see *Section 14 CLINICAL STUDIES* for summaries of clinical studies.

8.5 Geriatric Use

Of the total number of patients (n= 1,375) treated with NovoLog in 3 controlled clinical studies, 2.6% (n=36) were 65 years of age or over. One-half of these patients had type 1 diabetes (18/1285) and the other half had type 2 diabetes (18/90). The HbA1c response to NovoLog, as compared to human insulin, did not differ by age, particularly in patients with type 2 diabetes. Additional studies in larger populations of patients 65 years of age or over are needed to permit conclusions regarding the safety of NovoLog in elderly compared to younger patients. Pharmacokinetic/pharmacodynamic studies to assess the effect of age on the onset of NovoLog action have not been performed.

Table 2: Treatment-Emergent Adverse Events in Patients with Type 2 Diabetes Mellitus (except for hypoglycemia, adverse events with frequency ≥ 5% and occurring more frequently with NovoLog compared to human regular insulin are listed)

	NovoLog + NPH N= 91		Human Regular Insulin + NPH N= 91	
	N	(%)	N	(%)
Hypoglycemia*	25	27%	33	36%
Hyporeflexia	10	11%	6	7%
Onychomycosis	9	10%	5	5%
Sensory disturbance	8	9%	6	7%
Urinary tract infection	7	8%	6	7%
Chest pain	5	5%	3	3%
Headache	5	5%	3	3%
Skin disorder	5	5%	2	2%
Abdominal pain	5	5%	1	1%
Sinusitis	5	5%	1	1%

* Hypoglycemia is defined as an episode of blood glucose concentration <45 mg/dL, with or without symptoms. See Section 14 for the incidence of serious hypoglycemia in the individual clinical trials.

10 OVERDOSAGE

Excess insulin administration may cause hypoglycemia and, particularly when given intravenously, hypokalemia. Mild episodes of hypoglycemia usually can be treated with oral glucose. Adjustments in drug dosage, meal patterns, or exercise, may be needed. More severe episodes with coma, seizure, or neurologic impairment may be treated with intramuscular/subcutaneous glucagon or concentrated intravenous glucose. Sustained carbohydrate intake and observation may be necessary because hypoglycemia may recur after apparent clinical recovery. Hypokalemia must be corrected appropriately.

11 DESCRIPTION

NovoLog (insulin aspart [rDNA origin] injection) is a rapid-acting human insulin analog used to lower blood glucose. NovoLog is homologous with regular human insulin with the exception of a single substitution of the amino acid proline by aspartic acid in position B28, and is produced by recombinant DNA technology utilizing *Saccharomyces cerevisiae* (baker's yeast). Insulin aspart has the empirical formula $C_{256}H_{381}N_{65}O_{79}S_6$ and a molecular weight of 5825.8.

Figure 1. Structural formula of insulin aspart.

NovoLog is a sterile, aqueous, clear, and colorless solution, that contains insulin aspart 100 Units/mL, glycerin 16 mg/mL, phenol 1.50 mg/mL, metacresol 1.72 mg/mL, zinc 19.6 mcg/mL, disodium hydrogen phosphate dihydrate 1.25 mg/mL, sodium chloride 0.58 mg/mL and water for injection. NovoLog has a pH of 7.2-7.6. Hydrochloric acid 10% and/or sodium hydroxide 10% may be added to adjust pH.

12 CLINICAL PHARMACOLOGY

12.1 Mechanism of Action

The primary activity of NovoLog is the regulation of glucose metabolism. Insulins, including NovoLog, bind to the insulin receptors on muscle and fat cells and lower blood glucose by facilitating the cellular uptake of glucose and simultaneously inhibiting the output of glucose from the liver.

12.2 Pharmacodynamics

Studies in normal volunteers and patients with diabetes demonstrated that subcutaneous administration of NovoLog has a more rapid onset of action than regular human insulin.

In a study in patients with type 1 diabetes (n=22), the maximum glucose-lowering effect of NovoLog occurred between 1 and 3 hours after subcutaneous injection (see Figure 2). The duration of action for NovoLog is 3 to 5 hours. The time course of action of insulin and insulin analogs such as NovoLog may vary considerably in different individuals or within the same individual. The parameters of NovoLog activity (time of onset, peak time and duration) as designated

in Figure 2 should be considered only as general guidelines. The rate of insulin absorption and onset of activity is affected by the site of injection, exercise, and other variables [see *Warnings and Precautions (5.1)*].

Figure 2. Serial mean serum glucose collected up to 6 hours following a single pre-meal dose of NovoLog (solid curve) or regular human insulin (hatched curve) injected immediately before a meal in 22 patients with type 1 diabetes.

A double-blind, randomized, two-way cross-over study in 16 patients with type 1 diabetes demonstrated that intravenous infusion of NovoLog resulted in a blood glucose profile that was similar to that after intravenous infusion with regular human insulin. NovoLog or human insulin was infused until the patient's blood glucose decreased to 36 mg/dL, or until the patient demonstrated signs of hypoglycemia (rise in heart rate and onset of sweating), defined as the time of autonomic reaction (R) (see Figure 3).

Note: The slashes on the mean profile indicate a jump on the time axis

Figure 3. Mean blood glucose profiles following intravenous infusion of NovoLog (hatched curve) and regular human insulin (solid curve) in 16 patients with type 1 diabetes. R represents the time of autonomic reaction.

12.3 Pharmacokinetics

The single substitution of the amino acid proline with aspartic acid at position B28 in NovoLog reduces the molecule's tendency to form hexamers as observed with regular human insulin. NovoLog is, therefore, more rapidly absorbed after subcutaneous injection compared to regular human insulin.

In a randomized, double-blind, crossover study 17 healthy Caucasian male subjects between 18 and 40 years of age received an intravenous infusion of either NovoLog or regular human insulin at 1.5 mU/kg/min for 120 minutes. The mean insulin clearance was similar for the two groups with mean values of 1.2 l/h/kg for the NovoLog group and 1.2 l/h/kg for the regular human insulin group.

Bioavailability and Absorption - NovoLog has a faster absorption, a faster onset of action, and a shorter duration of action than regular human insulin after subcutaneous injection (see Figure 2 and Figure 4). The relative bioavailability of NovoLog compared to regular human insulin indicates that the two insulins are absorbed to a similar extent.

Figure 4. Serial mean serum free insulin concentration collected up to 6 hours following a single pre-meal dose of NovoLog (solid curve) or regular human insulin (hatched curve) injected immediately before a meal in 22 patients with type 1 diabetes.

In studies in healthy volunteers (total n=107) and patients with type 1 diabetes (total n=40), NovoLog consistently reached peak serum concentrations approximately twice as fast as regular human insulin. The median time to maximum concentration in these trials was 40 to 50 minutes for NovoLog versus 80 to 120 minutes for regular human insulin. In a clinical trial in patients with type 1 diabetes, NovoLog and regular human insulin, both administered subcutaneously at a dose of 0.15 U/kg body weight, reached mean maximum concentrations of 82 and 36 mU/L, respectively. Pharmacokinetic/pharmacodynamic characteristics of insulin aspart have not been established in patients with type 2 diabetes.

The intra-individual variability in time to maximum serum insulin concentration for healthy male volunteers was significantly less for NovoLog than for regular human insulin. The clinical significance of this observation has not been established.

In a clinical study in healthy non-obese subjects, the pharmacokinetic differences between NovoLog and regular human insulin described above, were observed independent of the site of injection (abdomen, thigh, or upper arm).

Distribution and Elimination - NovoLog has low binding to plasma proteins (<10%), similar to that seen with regular human insulin. After subcutaneous administration in normal male volunteers (n=24), NovoLog was more rapidly eliminated than regular human insulin with an average apparent half-life of 81 minutes compared to 141 minutes for regular human insulin.

Specific Populations

Children and Adolescents - The pharmacokinetic and pharmacodynamic properties of NovoLog and regular human insulin were evaluated in a single dose study in 18 children (6-12 years, n=9) and adolescents (13-17 years [Tanner grade > 2], n=9) with type 1 diabetes. The relative differences in pharmacokinetics and pharmacodynamics in children and adolescents with type 1 diabetes between NovoLog and regular human insulin were similar to those in healthy adult subjects and adults with type 1 diabetes.

Gender - In healthy volunteers, no difference in insulin aspart levels was seen between men and women when body weight differences were taken into account. There was no significant difference in efficacy noted (as assessed by HbA1c) between genders in a trial in patients with type 1 diabetes.

Obesity - A single subcutaneous dose of 0.1 U/kg NovoLog was administered in a study of 23 patients with type 1 diabetes and a wide range of body mass index (BMI, 22-39 kg/m²). The pharmacokinetic parameters, AUC and C_{max}, of NovoLog were generally unaffected by BMI in the different groups – BMI 19-23 kg/m² (N=4); BMI 23-27 kg/m² (N=7); BMI 27-32 kg/m² (N=6) and BMI >32 kg/m² (N=6). Clearance of NovoLog was reduced by 28% in patients with BMI >32 kg/m² compared to patients with BMI <23 kg/m².

Renal Impairment - Some studies with human insulin have shown increased circulating levels of insulin in patients with renal failure. A single subcutaneous dose of 0.08 U/kg NovoLog was administered in a study to subjects with either normal (N=6) creatinine clearance (CLcr) (> 80 ml/min) or mild (N=7; CLcr = 50-80 ml/min), moderate (N=3; CLcr = 30-50 ml/min) or severe (but not requiring hemodialysis) (N=2; CLcr = <30 ml/min) renal impairment. In this small study, there was no apparent effect of creatinine clearance values on AUC and C_{max} of NovoLog. Careful glucose

monitoring and dose adjustments of insulin, including NovoLog, may be necessary in patients with renal dysfunction [*see Warnings and Precautions (5.4)*].

Hepatic Impairment - Some studies with human insulin have shown increased circulating levels of insulin in patients with liver failure. A single subcutaneous dose of 0.06 U/kg NovoLog was administered in an open-label, single-dose study of 24 subjects (N=6/group) with different degree of hepatic impairment (mild, moderate and severe) having Child-Pugh Scores ranging from 0 (healthy volunteers) to 12 (severe hepatic impairment). In this small study, there was no correlation between the degree of hepatic failure and any NovoLog pharmacokinetic parameter. Careful glucose monitoring and dose adjustments of insulin, including NovoLog, may be necessary in patients with hepatic dysfunction [*see Warnings and Precautions (5.5)*].

The effect of age, ethnic origin, pregnancy and smoking on the pharmacokinetics and pharmacodynamics of NovoLog has not been studied.

13 NONCLINICAL TOXICOLOGY

13.1 Carcinogenesis, Mutagenesis, Impairment of Fertility

Standard 2-year carcinogenicity studies in animals have not been performed to evaluate the carcinogenic potential of NovoLog. In 52-week studies, Sprague-Dawley rats were dosed subcutaneously with NovoLog at 10, 50, and 200 U/kg/day (approximately 2, 8, and 32 times the human subcutaneous dose of 1.0 U/kg/day, based on U/body surface area, respectively). At a dose of 200 U/kg/day, NovoLog increased the incidence of mammary gland tumors in females when compared to untreated controls. The incidence of mammary tumors for NovoLog was not significantly different than for regular human insulin. The relevance of these findings to humans is not known. NovoLog was not genotoxic in the following tests: Ames test, mouse lymphoma cell forward gene mutation test, human peripheral blood lymphocyte chromosome aberration test, *in vivo* micronucleus test in mice, and in *ex vivo* UDS test in rat liver hepatocytes. In fertility studies in male and female rats, at subcutaneous doses up to 200 U/kg/day (approximately 32 times the human subcutaneous dose, based on U/body surface area), no direct adverse effects on male and female fertility, or general reproductive performance of animals was observed.

13.2 Animal Toxicology and/or Pharmacology

In standard biological assays in mice and rabbits, one unit of NovoLog has the same glucose-lowering effect as one unit of regular human insulin. In humans, the effect of NovoLog is more rapid in onset and of shorter duration, compared to regular human insulin, due to its faster absorption after subcutaneous injection (see *Section 12 CLINICAL PHARMACOLOGY* Figure 2 and Figure 4).

14 CLINICAL STUDIES

14.1 Subcutaneous Daily Injections

Two six-month, open-label, active-controlled studies were conducted to compare the safety and efficacy of NovoLog to Novolin R in adult patients with type 1 diabetes. Because the two study designs and results were similar, data are shown for only one study (see Table 3). NovoLog was administered by subcutaneous injection immediately prior to meals and regular human insulin was administered by subcutaneous injection 30 minutes before meals. NPH insulin was administered as the basal insulin in either single or divided daily doses. Changes in HbA1c and the incidence rates of severe hypoglycemia (as determined from the number of events requiring intervention from a third party) were comparable for the two treatment regimens in this study (Table 3) as well as in the other clinical studies that are cited in this section. Diabetic ketoacidosis was not reported in any of the adult studies in either treatment group.

Table 3. Subcutaneous NovoLog Administration in Type 1 Diabetes (24 weeks; n=882)

	NovoLog + NPH	Novolin R + NPH
N	596	286
Baseline HbA1c (%)*	7.9 ±1.1	8.0 ± 1.2
Change from Baseline HbA1c (%)	-0.1 ± 0.8	0.0 ± 0.8
Treatment Difference in HbA1c, Mean (95% confidence interval)	-0.2 (-0.3, -0.1)	
Baseline insulin dose (IU/kg/ 24 hours)*	0.7 ± 0.2	0.7 ± 0.2
End-of-Study insulin dose (IU/kg/24 hours)*	0.7 ± 0.2	0.7 ± 0.2
Patients with severe hypoglycemia (n, %)†	104 (17%)	54 (19%)

	NovoLog + NPH	Novolin R + NPH
Baseline body weight (kg)*	75.3 ± 14.5	75.9 ± 13.1
Weight Change from baseline (kg)*	0.5 ± 3.3	0.9 ± 2.9

* Values are Mean ± SD
† Severe hypoglycemia refers to hypoglycemia associated with central nervous system symptoms and requiring the intervention of another person or hospitalization.

A 24-week, parallel-group study of children and adolescents with type 1 diabetes (n = 283) aged 6 to 18 years compared two subcutaneous multiple-dose treatment regimens: NovoLog (n = 187) or Novolin R (n = 96). NPH insulin was administered as the basal insulin. NovoLog achieved glycemic control comparable to Novolin R, as measured by change in HbA1c (Table 4) and both treatment groups had a comparable incidence of hypoglycemia. Subcutaneous administration of NovoLog and regular human insulin have also been compared in children with type 1 diabetes (n=26) aged 2 to 6 years with similar effects on HbA1c and hypoglycemia.

Table 4. Pediatric Subcutaneous Administration of NovoLog in Type 1 Diabetes (24 weeks; n=283)

	NovoLog + NPH	Novolin R + NPH
N	187	96
Baseline HbA1c (%)*	8.3 ± 1.2	8.3 ± 1.3
Change from Baseline HbA1c (%)	0.1± 1.0	0.1± 1.1
Treatment Difference in HbA1c, Mean (95% confidence interval)	0.1 (-0.5, 0.1)	
Baseline insulin dose (IU/kg/ 24 hours)*	0.4 ± 0.2	0.6 ± 0.2
End-of-Study insulin dose (IU/kg/24 hours)*	0.4 ± 0.2	0.7 ± 0.2
Patients with severe hypoglycemia (n, %)†	11 (6%)	9 (9%)
Diabetic ketoacidosis (n, %)	10 (5%)	2 (2%)
Baseline body weight (kg)* Weight Change from baseline (kg)*	50.6 ± 19.6 2.7 ± 3.5	48.7 ± 15.8 2.4 ± 2.6

* Values are Mean ± SD
† Severe hypoglycemia refers to hypoglycemia associated with central nervous system symptoms and requiring the intervention of another person or hospitalization.

One six-month, open-label, active-controlled study was conducted to compare the safety and efficacy of NovoLog to Novolin R in patients with type 2 diabetes (Table 5). NovoLog was administered by subcutaneous injection immediately prior to meals and regular human insulin was administered by subcutaneous injection 30 minutes before meals. NPH insulin was administered as the basal insulin in either single or divided daily doses. Changes in HbA1c and the rates of severe hypoglycemia (as determined from the number of events requiring intervention from a third party) were comparable for the two treatment regimens.

Table 5. Subcutaneous NovoLog Administration in Type 2 Diabetes (6 months; n=176)

	NovoLog + NPH	Novolin R + NPH
N	90	86
Baseline HbA1c (%)*	8.1 ± 1.2	7.8 ± 1.1
Change from Baseline HbA1c (%)	-0.3 ± 1.0	-0.1 ± 0.8
Treatment Difference in HbA1c, Mean (95% confidence interval)	- 0.1 (-0.4, -0.1)	
Baseline insulin dose (IU/kg/24 hours)*	0.6 ± 0.3	0.6 ± 0.3
End-of-Study insulin dose (IU/kg/24 hours)*	0.7 ± 0.3	0.7 ± 0.3
Patients with severe hypoglycemia (n, %)†	9 (10%)	5 (8%)

Baseline body weight (kg)*	88.4 ± 13.3	85.8 ± 14.8
Weight Change from baseline (kg)*	1.2 ± 3.0	0.4 ± 3.1

* Values are Mean ± SD

† Severe hypoglycemia refers to hypoglycemia associated with central nervous system symptoms and requiring the intervention of another person or hospitalization.

14.2 Continuous Subcutaneous Insulin Infusion (CSII) by External Pump

Two open-label, parallel design studies (6 weeks [n=29] and 16 weeks [n=118]) compared NovoLog to buffered regular human insulin (Velosulin) in adults with type 1 diabetes receiving a subcutaneous infusion with an external insulin pump. The two treatment regimens had comparable changes in HbA$_{1c}$ and rates of severe hypoglycemia.

Table 6. Adult Insulin Pump Study in Type 1 Diabetes (16 weeks; n=118)

	NovoLog	Buffered human insulin
N	59	59
Baseline HbA$_{1c}$ (%)*	7.3 ± 0.7	7.5 ± 0.8
Change from Baseline HbA$_{1c}$ (%)	0.0 ± 0.5	0.2 ± 0.6
Treatment Difference in HbA$_{1c}$, Mean (95% confidence interval)	0.3 (-0.1, 0.4)	
Baseline insulin dose (IU/kg/24 hours)*	0.7 ± 0.8	0.6 ± 0.2
End-of-Study insulin dose (IU/kg/24 hours)*	0.7 ± 0.7	0.6 ± 0.2
Patients with severe hypoglycemia (n, %)†	1 (2%)	2 (3%)
Baseline body weight (kg)* Weight Change from baseline (kg)*	77.4 ± 16.1 0.1 ± 3.5	74.8 ± 13.8 -0.0 ± 1.7

* Values are Mean ± SD

† Severe hypoglycemia refers to hypoglycemia associated with central nervous system symptoms and requiring the intervention of another person or hospitalization.

A randomized, 16-week, open-label, parallel design study of children and adolescents with type 1 diabetes (n=298) aged 4-18 years compared two subcutaneous infusion regimens administered via an external insulin pump: NovoLog (n=198) or insulin lispro (n=100). These two treatments resulted in comparable changes from baseline in HbA$_{1c}$ and comparable rates of hypoglycemia after 16 weeks of treatment (see Table 7).

Table 7. Pediatric Insulin Pump Study in Type 1 Diabetes (16 weeks; n=298)

	NovoLog	Lispro
N	198	100
Baseline HbA$_{1c}$ (%)*	8.0 ± 0.9	8.2 ± 0.8
Change from Baseline HbA$_{1c}$ (%)	-0.1 ± 0.8	-0.1 ± 0.7
Treatment Difference in HbA$_{1c}$, Mean (95% confidence interval)	-0.1 (-0.3, 0.1)	
Baseline insulin dose (IU/kg/24 hours)*	0.9 ± 0.3	0.9 ± 0.3
End-of-Study insulin dose (IU/kg/24 hours)*	0.9 ± 0.2	0.9 ± 0.2
Patients with severe hypoglycemia (n, %)†	19 (10%)	8 (8%)
Diabetic ketoacidosis (n, %)	1 (0.5%)	0 (0)
Baseline body weight (kg)* Weight Change from baseline (kg)*	54.1 ± 19.7 1.8 ± 2.1	55.5 ± 19.0 1.6 ± 2.1

* Values are Mean ± SD

Table 9. Storage conditions for vial, PenFill cartridges, NovoLog FlexPen, and NovoLog FlexTouch

NovoLog presentation	Not in-use (unopened) Room Temperature (below 30°C)	Not in-use (unopened) Refrigerated	In-use (opened) Room Temperature (below 30°C)
10 mL vial	28 days	Until expiration date	28 days (refrigerated/room temperature)
3 mL PenFill cartridges	28 days	Until expiration date	28 days (Do not refrigerate)
3 mL NovoLog FlexPen	28 days	Until expiration date	28 days (Do not refrigerate)
3 mL NovoLog FlexTouch	28 days	Until expiration date	28 days (Do not refrigerate)

† Severe hypoglycemia refers to hypoglycemia associated with central nervous system symptoms and requiring the intervention of another person or hospitalization.

An open-label, 16-week parallel design trial compared preprandial NovoLog injection in conjunction with NPH injections to NovoLog administered by continuous subcutaneous infusion in 127 adults with type 2 diabetes. The two treatment groups had similar reductions in HbA$_{1c}$ and rates of severe hypoglycemia (Table 8) [*see Indications and Usage (1), Dosage and Administration (2), Warnings and Precautions (5) and How Supplied/Storage and Handling (16.2)*].

Table 8. Pump Therapy in Type 2 Diabetes (16 weeks; n=127)

	NovoLog pump	NovoLog + NPH
N	66	61
Baseline HbA$_{1c}$ (%)*	8.2 ± 1.4	8.0 ± 1.1
Change from Baseline HbA$_{1c}$ (%)	-0.6 ± 1.1	-0.5 ± 0.9
Treatment Difference in HbA$_{1c}$, Mean (95% confidence interval)	0.1 (0.4, 0.3)	
Baseline insulin dose (IU/kg/24 hours)*	0.7 ± 0.3	0.8 ± 0.5
End-of-Study insulin dose (IU/kg/24 hours)*	0.9 ± 0.4	0.9 ± 0.5
Baseline body weight (kg)* Weight Change from baseline (kg)*	96.4 ± 17.0 1.7 ± 3.7	96.9 ± 17.9 0.7 ± 4.1

* Values are Mean ± SD

14.3 Intravenous Administration of NovoLog
See *Section 12.2 CLINICAL PHARMACOLOGY/Pharmacodynamics*.

16 HOW SUPPLIED/STORAGE AND HANDLING
16.1 How Supplied
NovoLog is available in the following package sizes: each presentation containing 100 Units of insulin aspart per mL (U-100).

10 mL vials	NDC 0169-7501-11
3 mL PenFill cartridges*	NDC 0169-3303-12
3 mL NovoLog FlexPen	NDC 0169-6339-10
3 mL NovoLog FlexTouch	NDC 0169-6338-10

* NovoLog PenFill cartridges are designed for use with Novo Nordisk 3 mL PenFill cartridge compatible insulin delivery devices (with or without the addition of a NovoPen 3 PenMate) with NovoFine disposable needles. FlexPen and FlexTouch can be used with NovoFine or NovoTwist disposable needles.

16.2 Recommended Storage
Unused NovoLog should be stored in a refrigerator between 2° and 8°C (36° to 46°F). Do not store in the freezer or directly adjacent to the refrigerator cooling element. **Do not freeze NovoLog and do not use NovoLog if it has been frozen.** NovoLog should not be drawn into a syringe and stored for later use.
Vials: After initial use a vial may be kept at temperatures below 30°C (86°F) for up to 28 days, but should not be exposed to excessive heat or light. Opened vials may be refrigerated.

Unpunctured vials can be used until the expiration date printed on the label if they are stored in a refrigerator. Keep unused vials in the carton so they will stay clean and protected from light.
PenFill cartridges or NovoLog FlexPen and NovoLog FlexTouch:
Once a cartridge or NovoLog FlexPen or NovoLog FlexTouch is punctured, it should be kept at temperatures below 30°C (86°F) for up to 28 days, but should not be exposed to excessive heat or sunlight. A NovoLog FlexPen or NovoLog FlexTouch or cartridge in use must NOT be stored in the refrigerator. Keep the NovoLog FlexPen or NovoLog FlexTouch and all PenFill cartridges away from direct heat and sunlight. Unpunctured NovoLog FlexPen or NovoLog FlexTouch and PenFill cartridges can be used until the expiration date printed on the label if they are stored in a refrigerator. Keep unused NovoLog FlexPen or NovoLog FlexTouch and PenFill cartridges in the carton so they will stay clean and protected from light.
Always remove the needle after each injection and store the 3 mL PenFill cartridge delivery device or NovoLog FlexPen or NovoLog FlexTouch without a needle attached. This prevents contamination and/or infection, or leakage of insulin, and will ensure accurate dosing. Always use a new needle for each injection to prevent contamination.
Pump:
NovoLog in the pump reservoir should be discarded after at least every 6 days of use or after exposure to temperatures that exceed 37°C (98.6°F). The infusion set and the infusion set insertion site should be changed at least every 3 days.
Summary of Storage Conditions:
The storage conditions are summarized in the following table:
[See table 9 above]
Storage of Diluted NovoLog
NovoLog diluted with Insulin Diluting Medium for NovoLog to a concentration equivalent to U-10 or equivalent to U-50 may remain in patient use at temperatures below 30°C (86°F) for 28 days.
Storage of NovoLog in Infusion Fluids
Infusion bags prepared as indicated under *Dosage and Administration (2)* are stable at room temperature for 24 hours. Some insulin will be initially adsorbed to the material of the infusion bag.

17 PATIENT COUNSELING INFORMATION
[See *FDA Approved Patient Labeling (17.3)*]
17.1 Physician Instructions
Maintenance of normal or near-normal glucose control is a treatment goal in diabetes mellitus and has been associated with a reduction in diabetic complications. Patients should be informed about potential risks and benefits of NovoLog therapy including the possible adverse reactions. Patients should also be offered continued education and advice on insulin therapies, injection technique, life-style management, regular glucose monitoring, periodic glycosylated hemoglobin testing, recognition and management of hypo- and hyperglycemia, adherence to meal planning, complications of insulin therapy, timing of dose, instruction in the use of injection or subcutaneous infusion devices, and proper storage of insulin. Patients should be informed that frequent, patient-performed blood glucose measurements are needed to achieve optimal glycemic control and avoid both hyper- and hypoglycemia.
Patients should receive proper training on how to use NovoLog. Instruct patients that when injecting NovoLog, they must press and hold down the dose button until the dose counter shows 0 and then keep the needle in the skin and count slowly to 6. When the dose counter returns to 0, the prescribed dose is not completely delivered until 6 seconds later. If the needle is removed earlier, they may see a stream of insulin coming from the needle tip. If so, the full dose will not be delivered (a possible under-dose may occur by as much as 20%), and they should increase the frequency of checking their blood glucose levels and possible additional insulin administration may be necessary.

- If 0 does not appear in the dose counter after continuously pressing the dose button, the patient may have used a blocked needle. In this case they would **not** have received **any** insulin – even though the dose counter has moved from the original dose that was set.
- If the patient did have a blocked needle, instruct them to change the needle as described in Section 5 of the Instructions for Use and repeat all steps in the IFU starting with Section 1: Prepare your pen with a new needle. **Make sure the patient selects the full dose needed.**

The patient's ability to concentrate and react may be impaired as a result of hypoglycemia. This may present a risk in situations where these abilities are especially important, such as driving or operating other machinery. Patients who have frequent hypoglycemia or reduced or absent warning signs of hypoglycemia should be advised to use caution when driving or operating machinery.

Accidental substitutions between NovoLog and other insulin products have been reported. Patients should be instructed to always carefully check that they are administering the appropriate insulin to avoid medication errors between NovoLog and any other insulin. **The written prescription for NovoLog should be written clearly, to avoid confusion with other insulin products, for example, NovoLog Mix 70/30.**

17.2 Patients Using Pumps

Patients using external pump infusion therapy should be trained in intensive insulin therapy with multiple injections and in the function of their pump and pump accessories.

The following insulin pumps† have been used in NovoLog clinical or *in vitro* studies conducted by Novo Nordisk, the manufacturer of NovoLog:

- Medtronic Paradigm® 512 and 712
- MiniMed 508
- Disetronic® D-TRON® and H-TRON®

Before using another insulin pump with NovoLog, read the pump label to make sure the pump has been evaluated with NovoLog.

NovoLog is recommended for use in any reservoir and infusion sets that are compatible with insulin and the specific pump. Please see recommended reservoir and infusion sets in the pump manual.

To avoid insulin degradation, infusion set occlusion, and loss of the preservative (metacresol), insulin in the reservoir should be replaced at least every 6 days; infusion sets and infusion set insertion sites should be changed at least every 3 days.

Insulin exposed to temperatures higher than 37°C (98.6°F) should be discarded. The temperature of the insulin may exceed ambient temperature when the pump housing, cover, tubing, or sport case is exposed to sunlight or radiant heat. Infusion sites that are erythematous, pruritic, or thickened should be reported to medical personnel, and a new site selected because continued infusion may increase the skin reaction and/or alter the absorption of NovoLog. Pump or infusion set malfunctions or insulin degradation can lead to hyperglycemia and ketosis in a short time because of the small subcutaneous depot of insulin. This is especially pertinent for rapid-acting insulin analogs that are more rapidly absorbed through skin and have shorter duration of action. These differences are particularly relevant when patients are switched from multiple injection therapy. Prompt identification and correction of the cause of hyperglycemia or ketosis is necessary. Problems include pump malfunction, infusion set occlusion, leakage, disconnection or kinking, and degraded insulin. Less commonly, hypoglycemia from pump malfunction may occur. If these problems cannot be promptly corrected, patients should resume therapy with subcutaneous insulin injection and contact their physician [*see Dosage and Administration (2), Warnings and Precautions (5) and How Supplied/Storage and Handling (16.2)*].

17.3 FDA Approved Patient Labeling

See separate leaflet.

Rx only

Date of Issue: April 25, 2014
Version: 22

Novo Nordisk®, NovoLog®, NovoPen® 3, PenFill®, Novolin®, FlexPen®, FlexTouch®, PenMate®, NovoFine® and NovoTwist® are registered trademarks of Novo Nordisk A/S. NovoLog® is covered by US Patent Nos. 5,618,913, 5,866,538, and other patents pending.

FlexPen® is covered by US Patent Nos. RE 41,956, 6,004,297, RE 43,834, and other patents pending.

FlexTouch® pen is covered by US Patent Nos. 7,686,786, 6,899,699, and other patents pending.

PenFill® is covered by US Patent No. 5,693,027.

†The brands listed are the registered trademarks of their respective owners and are not trademarks of Novo Nordisk A/S.

© 2002-2014 Novo Nordisk
Manufactured by:
Novo Nordisk A/S
DK-2880 Bagsvaerd, Denmark

For information about NovoLog contact:
Novo Nordisk Inc.
800 Scudders Mill Road
Plainsboro, New Jersey 08536
1-800-727-6500
www.novonordisk-us.com

PATIENT INFORMATION

NovoLog® (NŌ-vō-log)
(insulin aspart [rDNA origin] injection)

What is NovoLog?
- NovoLog is a man-made insulin that is used to control high blood sugar in adults and children with diabetes mellitus.

Who should not take NovoLog?
Do not take NovoLog if you:
- are having an episode of low blood sugar (hypoglycemia).
- have an allergy to NovoLog or any of the ingredients in NovoLog.

Before taking NovoLog, tell your healthcare provider about all your medical conditions including, if you are:
- pregnant, planning to become pregnant, or are breastfeeding.
- taking new prescription or over-the-counter medicines, vitamins, or herbal supplements.

Before you start taking NovoLog, talk to your healthcare provider about low blood sugar and how to manage it.

How should I take NovoLog?
- **Read the Instructions for Use** that come with your NovoLog.
- Take NovoLog exactly as your healthcare provider tells you to.
- **NovoLog starts acting fast.** You should eat a meal within 5 to 10 minutes after you take your dose of NovoLog.
- Know the type and strength of insulin you take. **Do not** change the type of insulin you take unless your healthcare provider tells you to. The amount of insulin and the best time for you to take your insulin may need to change if you take different types of insulin.
- **Check your blood sugar levels.** Ask your healthcare provider what your blood sugars should be and when you should check your blood sugar levels.
- **Do not share your NovoLog FlexPen, FlexTouch or needles with another person.** You may give another person an infection or get an infection from them.

What should I avoid while taking NovoLog?
While taking NovoLog do not:
- Drive or operate heavy machinery, until you know how NovoLog affects you.
- Drink alcohol or use prescription or over-the-counter medicines that contain alcohol.

What are the possible side effects of NovoLog?
NovoLog may cause serious side effects that can lead to death, including:
Low blood sugar (hypoglycemia). Signs and symptoms that may indicate low blood sugar include:
- dizziness or light-headedness
- blurred vision
- anxiety, irritability, or mood changes
- sweating
- slurred speech
- hunger
- confusion
- shakiness
- headache
- fast heart beat

Your insulin dose may need to change because of:
- change in level of physical activity or exercise
- increased stress
- change in diet
- weight gain or loss
- illness

Other common side effects of NovoLog may include:
- low potassium in your blood (hypokalemia), reactions at the injection site, itching, rash, serious allergic reactions (whole body reactions), skin thickening or pits at the injection site (lipodystrophy), weight gain, and swelling of your hands and feet.

Get emergency medical help if you have:
- trouble breathing, shortness of breath, fast heartbeat, swelling of your face, tongue, or throat, sweating, extreme drowsiness, dizziness, confusion.

These are not all the possible side effects of NovoLog. Call your doctor for medical advice about side effects. You may report side effects to FDA at 1-800-FDA-1088.

General information about the safe and effective use of NovoLog.
Medicines are sometimes prescribed for purposes other than those listed in a Patient Information leaflet. You can ask your pharmacist or healthcare provider for information about NovoLog that is written for health professionals. Do not use NovoLog for a condition for which it was not prescribed. Do not give NovoLog to other people, even if they have the same symptoms that you have. It may harm them.

What are the ingredients in NovoLog?
Active Ingredient: insulin aspart (rDNA origin)
Inactive Ingredients: glycerin, phenol, metacresol, zinc, disodium hydrogen phosphate dihydrate, sodium chloride and water for injection
Manufactured by:
Novo Nordisk A/S
DK-2880 Bagsvaerd, Denmark
For more information, go to www.novonordisk-us.com or call 1-800-727-6500.
This Patient Information has been approved by the U.S. Food and Drug Administration
Revised: 10/2013
For more information go to
www.novologflextouch.com
© 2002-2013 Novo Nordisk

PATIENT INSTRUCTIONS FOR USE

NovoLog® (NŌ-vō-log)
(insulin aspart [rDNA origin] injection)
10 mL vial (100 Units/mL, U-100)
Read this Instructions for Use before you start taking NovoLog® and each time you get a refill. There may be new information. This information does not take the place of talking to your healthcare provider about your medical condition or your treatment.

Supplies you will need to give your NovoLog® injection:
- 10 mL NovoLog® vial
- insulin syringe and needle
- alcohol swab

Preparing your NovoLog® dose:
- Wash your hands with soap and water.
- Before you start to prepare your injection, check the NovoLog® label to make sure that you are taking the right type of insulin. This is especially important if you use more than 1 type of insulin.
- NovoLog® should look clear and colorless. **Do not** use NovoLog® if it is thick, cloudy, or is colored.
- **Do not** use NovoLog® past the expiration date printed on the label.

Step 1: Pull off the tamper resistant cap (See Figure A).
Step 2: Wipe the rubber stopper with an alcohol swab (See Figure B).

(Figure A Figure B)

Step 3: Hold the syringe with the needle pointing up. Pull down on the plunger until the black tip reaches the line for the number of units for your prescribed dose (See Figure C).

(Figure C)

Step 4: Push the needle through the rubber stopper of the NovoLog® vial (See Figure D).

(Figure D)

Step 5: Push the plunger all the way in. This puts air into the NovoLog® vial (See Figure E).

(Figure E)

Step 6: Turn the NovoLog® vial and syringe upside down and slowly pull the plunger down until the black tip is a few units past the line for your dose (See Figure F).

(Figure F)

• If there are air bubbles, tap the syringe gently a few times to let any air bubbles rise to the top (See Figure G).

(Figure G)

Step 7: Slowly push the plunger up until the black tip reaches the line for your NovoLog® dose (See Figure H).

(Figure H)

Step 8: Check the syringe to make sure you have the right dose of NovoLog®.

Step 9: Pull the syringe out of the vial's rubber stopper (See Figure I).

(Figure I)

Giving your Injection:
• Inject your NovoLog® exactly as your healthcare provider has shown you. Your healthcare provider should tell you if you need to pinch the skin before injecting.
• NovoLog® can be injected under the skin (subcutaneously) of your stomach area, buttocks, upper legs or upper arms, infused in an insulin pump, or given through a needle in your arm (intravenously) by your healthcare provider.

• If you inject NovoLog®, change (rotate) your injection sites within the area you choose for each dose. **Do not** use the same injection site for each injection.
• If you use NovoLog® in an insulin pump, you should change your insertion site every 3 days. The insulin in the reservoir should be changed at least every 6 days even if you have not used all of the insulin.
• If you use NovoLog® in an insulin pump, see your insulin pump manual for instructions or talk to your healthcare provider.
• NPH insulin is the only type of insulin that can be mixed with NovoLog®. **Do not** mix NovoLog® with any other type of insulin.
• NovoLog® should **only** be mixed with NPH insulin if it is going to be injected right away under your skin (subcutaneously).
• NovoLog® should be drawn up into the syringe **before** you draw up your NPH insulin.
• Talk to your healthcare provider if you are not sure about the right way to mix NovoLog® and NPH insulin.

Step 10: Choose your injection site and wipe the skin with an alcohol swab. Let the injection site dry before you inject your dose (See Figure J).

Front

Back

(Figure J)

Step 11: Insert the needle into your skin. Push down on the plunger to inject your dose (See Figure K). **Needle should remain in the skin for at least 6 seconds to make sure you have injected all the insulin.**

(Figure K)

Step 12: Pull the needle out of your skin. After that, you may see a drop of NovoLog® at the needle tip. This is normal and does not affect the dose you just received (See Figure L).
• If you see blood after you take the needle out of your skin, press the injection site lightly with a piece of gauze or an alcohol swab. **Do not** rub the area.

(Figure L)

After your injection:
• **Do not** recap the needle. Recapping the needle can lead to a needle stick injury.
• Throw away empty insulin vials, used syringes, and needles in a sharps container or some type of hard plastic or metal container with a screw on cap such as a detergent bottle or empty coffee can. Check with your healthcare provider about the right way to throw away the container. There may be local or state laws about how to throw away used syringes and needles. Do not throw away used syringes and needles in household trash or recycling bins.

How should I store NovoLog®?
Do not freeze NovoLog®. **Do not** use NovoLog® if it has been frozen.
• Keep NovoLog® away from heat or light.
• Store opened and unopened NovoLog® vials in the refrigerator at 36°F to 46°F (2°C to 8°C). Opened NovoLog® vials can also be stored out of the refrigerator below 86°F (30°C).
• Unopened vials may be used until the expiration date printed on the label, if they are kept in the refrigerator.
• Opened NovoLog® vials should be thrown away after 28 days, even if they still have insulin left in them.

General information about the safe and effective use of NovoLog®
• Always use a new syringe and needle for each injection.
• Do not share syringes or needles.
• Keep NovoLog® vials, syringes, and needles out of the reach of children.
This Instructions for Use has been approved by the U.S. Food and Drug Administration.
Manufactured by:
Novo Nordisk A/S
DK-2880 Bagsvaerd, Denmark
NovoLog® is a registered trademark of Novo Nordisk A/S.
NovoLog® is covered by US Patent Nos. 5,618,913, 5,866,538, and other patents pending.
© 2002-2013 Novo Nordisk
For information about NovoLog® contact:
Novo Nordisk Inc.
800 Scudders Mill Road
Plainsboro, New Jersey 08536
1-800-727-6500
www.novonordisk-us.com
Revised: March 2013

PATIENT INSTRUCTIONS FOR USE
NovoLog® 3 mL PenFill® cartridge (100 Units/mL, U-100)
Before using the NovoLog® cartridge
1. Talk with your healthcare provider for information about where to inject NovoLog® (injection sites) and how to give an injection with your insulin delivery device.
2. Read the instruction manual that comes with your insulin delivery device for complete instructions on how to use the PenFill® cartridge with the device.

How to use the NovoLog® cartridge
1. **Check your insulin.** Just before using your NovoLog® cartridge, check to make sure that you have the right type of insulin. This is especially important if you use different types of insulin.
2. **Carefully look at the cartridge and the insulin inside it.** The insulin should be clear and colorless. The tamper-resistant foil should be in place before the first use. If the foil has been broken or removed before your first use of the cartridge, or if the insulin is cloudy or colored, do not use it. Call Novo Nordisk at 1-800-727-6500.
3. **Wash your hands** well with soap and water. If you clean your injection site with an alcohol swab, let the injection site dry before you inject. Talk with your healthcare provider for guidance on injection sites and how to give an injection with your insulin delivery device.
4. Gather your supplies for injecting NovoLog®.
5. Insert a 3 mL cartridge into your Novo Nordisk 3 mL PenFill® cartridge compatible insulin delivery device. Wipe the front rubber stopper of the 3 mL PenFill® cartridge with an alcohol swab, then attach a new needle. For NovoFine® needles, remove the big outer needle cap and the inner needle cap. Always use a new needle for each injection to prevent infection.

Giving the airshot before each injection:
To prevent the injection of air and to make sure insulin is delivered, you must do an airshot before each injection. Hold the device with the needle pointing up and gently tap the PenFill® cartridge holder with your finger a few times to raise any air bubbles to the top of the cartridge. Do the airshot as described in the device instruction manual.

Giving the injection
6. Dial the number of units on the insulin delivery device that you need to inject. Inject the right way as shown to you by your healthcare provider.
7. Insert the needle into the skin. Inject the dose by pressing the push button all the way in. Keep the needle in the skin for at least 6 seconds, and keep the push button pressed all the way in until the needle has been pulled out from the skin. This will make sure that the full dose has been given. You may see a drop of NovoLog® at the needle tip. This is normal and has no effect on the dose you just received. If blood appears after you take the needle out of your skin, press the injection site lightly with a finger. **Do not** rub the area.

After the injection
8. **Do not recap the needle.** Recapping can lead to a needle stick injury.
9. Remove the needle from the PenFill® cartridge after each injection. Keep the 3 mL PenFill® cartridge in the insulin delivery device. The needle should not be attached to the 3 mL PenFill® cartridge during storage. This will prevent infection or leakage of insulin and will help ensure that you receive the right dose of NovoLog®.
10. Put the used needle and cartridge in a sharps container, or some type of hard plastic or metal container with a screw on top such as a detergent bottle or coffee can. Check with your healthcare provider about the right way to throw away used needles and cartridges. There may be local or state laws about how to throw away used needles and syringes. Do not throw used needles and cartridges in household trash or recycling bins.
11. Put the pen cap back on the Novo Nordisk 3 mL PenFill® cartridge compatible insulin delivery device.

Date of Issue: March 2013
Version: 9

NovoFine®
Outer needle cap | Inner needle cap | Needle | Paper tab

NovoTwist®
Outer needle cap | Inner needle cap | Needle | Paper tab

Pen cap | Insulin scale | Insulin window | Dose counter | Dose selector | Dose pointer | Dose button

(Figure A)

Novo Nordisk®, NovoLog®, PenFill®, and NovoFine® are registered trademarks of Novo Nordisk A/S.
NovoLog® is covered by US Patent Nos. 5,618,913, 5,866,538, and other patents pending.
PenFill® is covered by US Patent No. 5,693,027.
© 2002-2013 Novo Nordisk
Manufactured by:
Novo Nordisk A/S
DK-2880 Bagsvaerd, Denmark
For information about NovoLog® contact:
Novo Nordisk Inc.
800 Scudders Mill Road
Plainsboro, New Jersey 08536

PATIENT INSTRUCTIONS FOR USE
NovoLog® (NŌ-vō-log)FlexTouch® Pen
(insulin aspart [rDNA origin] injection)
- **NovoLog FlexTouch Pen ("Pen") is a prefilled disposable pen** containing 300 units of U-100 NovoLog (insulin aspart [rDNA origin] injection) insulin. You can inject from 1 to 80 units in a single injection.
- **Do not share your NovoLog FlexTouch Pen with another person. You may give an infection to them or get an infection from them.**
- **This Pen is not recommended for use by the blind or visually impaired without the assistance of a person trained in the proper use of the product.**
Supplies you will need to give your NovoLog injection:
- NovoLog FlexTouch Pen
- a new NovoFine or NovoTwist needle
- alcohol swab
- 1 sharps container for throwing away used Pens and needles. See "Disposing of used NovoLog FlexTouch Pens and needles" at the end of these instructions.
Preparing your NovoLog FlexTouch Pen:
- Wash your hands with soap and water.
- **Before you start to prepare your injection, check the NovoLog FlexTouch Pen label to make sure you are taking the right type of insulin. This is especially important if you take more than 1 type of insulin.**
- NovoLog should look clear and colorless. **Do not** use NovoLog if it is thick, cloudy, or is colored.
- **Do not** use NovoLog past the expiration date printed on the label or 28 days after you start using the Pen.
- **Always use a new needle for each injection to help ensure sterility and prevent blocked needles.**
[See figure above]
Step 1:
- Pull Pen cap straight off (See Figure B).

(Figure B)

Step 2:
- **Check the liquid in the Pen** (See Figure C). NovoLog should look clear and colorless. **Do not** use it if it looks cloudy or colored.

(Figure C)

Step 3:
- **Select a new needle.**
- Pull off the paper tab from the outer needle cap (See Figure D).

NovoFine® | NovoTwist®

(Figure D)

Step 4:
- Push the capped needle straight onto the Pen and twist the needle on until it is tight (See Figure E).

NovoFine® | NovoTwist®

(Figure E)

Step 5:
- Pull off the outer needle cap. **Do not** throw it away (See Figure F).

NovoFine® | NovoTwist®

(Figure F)

Step 6:
- Pull off the inner needle cap and throw it away (See Figure G).

NovoFine® | NovoTwist®

(Figure G)

Priming your NovoLog FlexTouch Pen:
Step 7:
- Turn the dose selector to **select 2 units** (See Figure H).

2 units selected

(Figure H)

Step 8:
- Hold the Pen with the needle pointing up. Tap the top of the Pen gently a few times to let any air bubbles rise to the top (See Figure I).

(Figure I)

Step 9:
- **Hold the Pen with the needle pointing up.** Press and hold in the dose button until the dose counter shows "0". The "0" must line up with the dose pointer.
- A drop of insulin should be seen at the needle tip (See Figure J).
- If you **do not** see a drop of insulin, repeat steps 7 to 9, no more than 6 times.
- If you **still do not** see a drop of insulin, change the needle and repeat steps 7 to 9.

(Figure J)

Selecting your dose:
Step 10:
- **Turn the dose selector to select the number of units you need to inject.** The dose pointer should line up with your dose (See Figure K).
  - If you select the wrong dose, you can turn the dose selector forwards or backwards to the correct dose.
  - The **even** numbers are printed on the dial.
  - The **odd** numbers are shown as lines.

Examples

5 units selected

24 units selected

(Figure K)

- The NovoLog FlexTouch Pen insulin scale will show you how much insulin is left in your Pen (See Figure L).

Example Approx. 200 units left

(Figure L)

- **To see how much insulin is left in your NovoLog FlexTouch Pen:**
  - Turn the dose selector until it stops. The dose counter will line up with the number of units of insulin that is left in your Pen. If the dose counter shows 80, there are **at least 80** units left in your Pen.

- If the dose counter shows **less than 80,** the number shown in the dose counter is the number of units left in your Pen.

Giving your injection:

- Inject your NovoLog exactly as your healthcare provider has shown you. Your healthcare provider should tell you if you need to pinch the skin before injecting.
- NovoLog can be injected under the skin (subcutaneously) of your stomach area (abdomen), buttocks, upper legs (thighs) or upper arms.
- Change (rotate) your injection sites within the area you choose for each dose. **Do not** use the same injection site for each injection.

Step 11:

- Choose your injection site and wipe the skin with an alcohol swab. Let the injection site dry before you inject your dose (See Figure M).

(Figure M)

Step 12:

- Insert the needle into your skin (See Figure N).
  - **Make sure you can see the dose counter. Do not** cover it with your fingers, this can stop your injection.

(Figure N)

Step 13:

- **Press and hold down the dose button until the dose counter shows "0"** (See Figure O).
  - The "0" must line up with the dose pointer. You may then hear or feel a click.

(Figure O)

- **Keep the needle in your skin after** the dose counter has returned to "0" and **slowly count to 6** (See Figure P).

Count slowly:

1-2-3-4-5-6

(Figure P)

- **When the dose counter returns to "0", you will not get your full dose until 6 seconds later.**
- **If the needle is removed before you count to 6, you may see a stream of insulin coming from the needle tip.**
- **If you see a stream of insulin coming from the needle tip you will not get your full dose. If this happens you should check your blood sugar levels more often because you may need more insulin.**

Step 14:

- **Pull the needle out of your skin** (See Figure Q).
  - If you see blood after you take the needle out of your skin, press the injection site lightly with a piece of gauze or an alcohol swab. **Do not** rub the area.

[See figure Q at top of next column]

Step 15:

- **Carefully remove the needle from the Pen and throw it away** (See Figure R).

NovoLog® FlexPen®

Pen cap   Rubber stopper   Cartridge   Cartridge scale   Pointer   Dose selector   Push-button

(Figure Q)

- **Do not** recap the needle. Recapping the needle can lead to needle stick injury.

NovoFine®   NovoTwist®

(Figure R)

- If you **do not** have a sharps container, carefully slip the needle into the outer needle cap (See Figure S). Safely remove the needle and throw it away as soon as you can.

(Figure S)

- **Do not** store the Pen with the needle attached. Storing without the needle attached helps prevent leaking, blocking of the needle, and air from entering the Pen.

Step 16:

- Replace the Pen cap by pushing it straight on (See Figure T).

(Figure T)

After your injection:

- Put your used NovoLog FlexTouch Pen and needles in a FDA-cleared sharps disposal container right away after use. Do not throw away (dispose of) loose needles and Pens in your household trash.
- If you do not have a FDA-cleared sharps disposal container, you may use a household container that is:
  - made of a heavy-duty plastic
  - can be closed with a tight-fitting, puncture-resistant lid, without sharps being able to come out
  - upright and stable during use
  - leak-resistant
  - properly labeled to warn of hazardous waste inside the container
- When your sharps disposal container is almost full, you will need to follow your community guidelines for the right way to dispose of your sharps disposal container. There may be state or local laws about how you should throw away used needles and syringes. For more information about the safe sharps disposal, and for specific information about sharps disposal in the state that you live in, go to the FDA's website at: http://www.fda.gov/safesharpsdisposal.

- Do not dispose of your used sharps disposal container in your household trash unless your community guidelines permit this. Do not recycle your used sharps disposal container.

How should I store my NovoLog FlexTouch Pen?

- Store unused NovoLog FlexTouch Pens in the refrigerator at 36°F to 46°F (2°C to 8°C).
- Store the Pen you are currently using out of the refrigerator below 86°F.
- **Do not** freeze NovoLog. **Do not** use NovoLog if it has been frozen.
- Keep NovoLog away from heat or light.
- Unused Pens may be used until the expiration date printed on the label, if kept in the refrigerator.
- The NovoLog FlexTouch Pen you are using should be thrown away after 28 days, even if it still has insulin left in it.

General Information about the safe and effective use of NovoLog.

- **Keep NovoLog FlexTouch Pens and needles out of the reach of children.**
- **Always** use a new needle for each injection.
- **Do not** share Pens or needles.

This Instructions for Use has been approved by the U.S. Food and Drug Administration.

Manufactured By:
Novo Nordisk A/S
DK-2880 Bagsvaerd, Denmark
Revised: 10/2013

PATIENT INSTRUCTIONS FOR USE
NovoLog® FlexPen®
Introduction
Please read the following instructions carefully before using your NovoLog® FlexPen®.
NovoLog FlexPen is a disposable dial-a-dose insulin pen. You can select doses from 1 to 60 units in increments of 1 unit. NovoLog FlexPen is designed to be used with NovoFine® needles.

△ NovoLog FlexPen should not be used by people who are blind or have severe visual problems without the help of a person who has good eyesight and who is trained to use the NovoLog FlexPen the right way.

Getting ready
Make sure you have the following items:
- NovoLog FlexPen
- New NovoFine needle
- Alcohol swab

[See figure above]

NovoFine® needle

Big outer needle cap   Inner needle cap   Needle   Protective tab

Preparing Your NovoLog FlexPen
Wash your hands with soap and water. Before you start to prepare your injection, check the label to make sure that you are taking the right type of insulin. This is especially important if you take more than 1 type of insulin. NovoLog should look clear.
A. Pull off the pen cap (see diagram A).

A

Wipe the rubber stopper with an alcohol swab.

B. Attaching the needle
Remove the protective tab from a disposable needle. Screw the needle tightly onto your FlexPen. It is important that the needle is put on straight (see diagram B).

Never place a disposable needle on your NovoLog FlexPen until you are ready to take your injection.
C. Pull off the big outer needle cap (see diagram C).

D. Pull off the inner needle cap and dispose of it (see diagram D).

Δ Always use a new needle for each injection to help ensure sterility and prevent blocked needles.
Δ Be careful not to bend or damage the needle before use.
Δ To reduce the risk of unexpected needle sticks, never put the inner needle cap back on the needle.
Giving the airshot before each injection
Before each injection small amounts of air may collect in the cartridge during normal use. To avoid injecting air and to ensure proper dosing:
E. Turn the dose selector to select 2 units (see diagram E).

2 units selected

F. Hold your NovoLog FlexPen with the needle pointing up. Tap the cartridge gently with your finger a few times to make any air bubbles collect at the top of the cartridge (see diagram F).

G. Keep the needle pointing upwards, press the push-button all the way in (see diagram G). The dose selector returns to 0.

A drop of insulin should appear at the needle tip. If not, change the needle and repeat the procedure no more than 6 times.
If you do not see a drop of insulin after 6 times, do not use the NovoLog FlexPen and contact Novo Nordisk at 1-800-727-6500.
A small air bubble may remain at the needle tip, but it will not be injected.

Selecting your dose
Check and make sure that the dose selector is set at 0.
H. Turn the dose selector to the number of units you need to inject. The pointer should line up with your dose.
The dose can be corrected either up or down by turning the dose selector in either direction until the correct dose lines up with the pointer (see diagram H). When turning the dose selector, be careful not to press the push-button as insulin will come out.

5 units selected

24 units selected

You cannot select a dose larger than the number of units left in the cartridge.
You will hear a click for every single unit dialed. Do not set the dose by counting the number of clicks you hear.
Δ Do not use the cartridge scale printed on the cartridge to measure your dose of insulin.
Giving the injection
Do the injection exactly as shown to you by your healthcare provider. Your healthcare provider should tell you if you need to pinch the skin before injecting.
I. Insert the needle into your skin.
Inject the dose by pressing the push-button all the way in until the 0 lines up with the pointer (see diagram I). Be careful only to push the button when injecting.

Turning the dose selector will not inject insulin.
J. Keep the needle in the skin for at least 6 seconds, and keep the push-button pressed all the way in until the needle has been pulled out from the skin (see diagram J). This will make sure that the full dose has been given.
You may see a drop of NovoLog at the needle tip. This is normal and has no effect on the dose you just received. If blood appears after you take the needle out of your skin, press the injection site lightly with a finger. **Do not rub the area.**

After the injection
Do not recap the needle. Recapping can lead to a needle stick injury. Remove the needle from the NovoLog FlexPen after each injection. This helps to prevent infection, leakage of insulin, and will help to make sure you inject the right dose of insulin.
Δ Put the needle and any empty NovoLog FlexPen or any used NovoLog FlexPen still containing insulin in a sharps container or some type of hard plastic or metal container with a screw top such as a detergent bottle or empty coffee can. These containers should be sealed and thrown away the right way. Check with your healthcare provider about the right way to throw away used syringes and needles. There may be local or state laws about how to throw away used needles and syringes. Do not throw away used needles and syringes in household trash or recycling bins. The NovoLog FlexPen prevents the cartridge from being completely emptied. It is designed to deliver 300 units.
K. Put the pen cap on the NovoLog FlexPen and store the NovoLog FlexPen without the needle attached (see diagram K).

L Function Check
If your NovoLog FlexPen is not working the right way, follow the steps below:
• Screw on a new NovoFine needle.
• Remove the big outer needle cap and the inner needle cap.
• Do an airshot as described in "Giving the airshot before each injection".
• Put the big outer needle cap onto the needle. Do not put on the inner needle cap.
• Turn the dose selector so the dose indicator window shows 20 units.
• Hold the NovoLog FlexPen so the needle is pointing down.
• Press the push-button all the way in.
The insulin should fill the lower part of the big outer needle cap (see diagram L). If the NovoLog FlexPen has released too much or too little insulin, do the function check again. If the same problem happens again, do not use your NovoLog FlexPen and contact Novo Nordisk at 1-800-727-6500.

20

Maintenance
Your FlexPen is designed to work accurately and safely. It must be handled with care. Avoid dropping your FlexPen as it may damage it. If you are concerned that your FlexPen is damaged, use a new one. You can clean the outside of your FlexPen by wiping it with a damp cloth. Do not soak or wash your FlexPen as it may damage it. Do not refill your FlexPen.
Δ Remove the needle from the NovoLog FlexPen after each injection. This helps to ensure sterility, prevent leakage of insulin, and will help to make sure you inject the right dose of insulin for future injections.
Δ Be careful when handling used needles to avoid needle sticks and transfer of infectious diseases.
Δ Keep your NovoLog FlexPen and needles out of the reach of children.
Δ Use NovoLog FlexPen as directed to treat your diabetes. Needles and NovoLog FlexPen must not be shared.
Δ Always use a new needle for each injection.
Δ Novo Nordisk is not responsible for harm due to using this insulin pen with products not recommended by Novo Nordisk.
Δ As a precautionary measure, always carry a spare insulin delivery device in case your NovoLog FlexPen is lost or damaged.
Δ Remember to keep the disposable NovoLog FlexPen with you. Do not leave it in a car or other location where it can get too hot or too cold.

NOVOLOG® MIX 70/30 ℞
[NŌ-vō-log-MIX-SEV-en-tee-THIR-tee]
(70% insulin aspart protamine suspension and 30% insulin aspart injection, [rDNA origin])
Suspension for subcutaneous injection

HIGHLIGHTS OF PRESCRIBING INFORMATION
These highlights do not include all the information needed to use NovoLog Mix 70/30 safely and effectively. See full prescribing information for NovoLog Mix 70/30.
NovoLog® Mix 70/30 (70% insulin aspart protamine suspension and 30% insulin aspart injection, [rDNA origin])
Suspension for subcutaneous injection
Initial U.S. Approval: 2001

————INDICATIONS AND USAGE————
NovoLog Mix 70/30 is an insulin analog indicated to improve glycemic control in patients with diabetes mellitus. Important Limitations of Use: In premix insulins, such as NovoLog Mix 70/30, the proportions of rapid acting and long acting insulins are fixed and do not allow for basal versus prandial dose adjustments (1).

————DOSAGE AND ADMINISTRATION————
• Only for subcutaneous injection (2.1).
  Type 1 DM: dose within 15 minutes before meal initiation.
  Type 2 DM: dose within 15 minutes before or after starting a meal.
• Do not administer intravenously (2.1).

- Do not use in insulin infusion pumps (2.1).
- Must be resuspended immediately before use (2.2).

DOSAGE FORMS AND STRENGTHS

Each presentation contains 100 Units of insulin aspart per mL (U-100) (3)
- 10 mL vials
- 3 mL NovoLog Mix 70/30 FlexPen

CONTRAINDICATIONS

- Do not use during episodes of hypoglycemia (4).
- Do not use in patients with hypersensitivity to NovoLog Mix 70/30 or one of its excipients (4).

WARNINGS AND PRECAUTIONS

- NovoLog Mix 70/30 should not be mixed with any other insulin product (5.1).
- Hypoglycemia is the most common adverse effect of insulin therapy. Glucose monitoring is recommended for all patients with diabetes. Any change of insulin dose should be made cautiously and only under medical supervision (5.1, 5.2).
- Insulin, particularly when given in settings of poor glycemic control, can cause hypokalemia. Use caution in patients predisposed to hypokalemia (5.3).
- Like all insulins, NovoLog Mix 70/30 requirements may be reduced in patients with renal impairment or hepatic impairment (5.4, 5.5).
- Severe, life-threatening, generalized allergy, including anaphylaxis, may occur with insulin products, including NovoLog Mix 70/30 (5.6).
- Fluid retention and heart failure can occur with concomitant use of thiazolidinediones (TZDs), which are PPAR-gamma agonists, and insulin, including NovoLog Mix 70/30 (5.8).

ADVERSE REACTIONS

Adverse reactions observed with insulin therapy include hypoglycemia, allergic reactions, local injection site reactions, lipodystrophy, rash and pruritus (6).

To report SUSPECTED ADVERSE REACTIONS, contact Novo Nordisk Inc. at 1-800-727-6500 or FDA at 1-800-FDA-1088 or www.fda.gov/medwatch.

DRUG INTERACTIONS

- The following may increase the blood-glucose-lowering effect and susceptibility to hypoglycemia: oral antidiabetic products, pramlintide, ACE inhibitors, disopyramide, fibrates, fluoxetine, monoamine oxidase (MAO) inhibitors, propoxyphene, salicylates, somatostatin analog (e.g. octreotide), sulfonamide antibiotics (7).
- The following may reduce the blood-glucose-lowering effect: corticosteroids, niacin, danazol, diuretics, sympathomimetic agents (e.g., epinephrine, salbutamol, terbutaline), isoniazid, phenothiazine derivatives, somatropin, thyroid hormones, estrogens, progestogens (e.g., in oral contraceptives), atypical antipsychotics (7).
- Beta-blockers, clonidine, lithium salts, and alcohol may either potentiate or weaken the blood-glucose-lowering effect of insulin (7).
- Pentamidine may cause hypoglycemia, which may be followed by hyperglycemia (7).
- The signs of hypoglycemia may be reduced or absent in patients taking sympatholytic products such as beta-blockers, clonidine, guanethidine, and reserpine (7).

See 17 for PATIENT COUNSELING INFORMATION and FDA-approved patient labeling

Revised: 06/2014

FULL PRESCRIBING INFORMATION: CONTENTS*

General advice about NovoLog® Mix 70/30

* Sections or subsections omitted from the full prescribing information are not listed

---

FULL PRESCRIBING INFORMATION

1   INDICATIONS AND USAGE

NovoLog Mix 70/30 is an insulin analog indicated to improve glycemic control in patients with diabetes mellitus.
Important Limitations of Use:
In premix insulins, such as NovoLog Mix 70/30, the proportions of rapid acting and long acting insulins are fixed and do not allow for basal versus prandial dose adjustments.

2   DOSAGE AND ADMINISTRATION

2.1   Dosing

NovoLog Mix 70/30 is an insulin analog with an earlier onset and intermediate duration of action in comparison to the basal human insulin premix. The addition of protamine to the rapid-acting aspart insulin analog (NovoLog) results in insulin activity that is 30% short-acting and 70% long-acting. NovoLog Mix 70/30 is typically dosed on a twice-daily basis (with each dose intended to cover 2 meals or a meal and a snack). The dosage of NovoLog Mix 70/30 must be individualized. The written prescription for NovoLog Mix 70/30 should include the full name, to avoid confusion with NovoLog (insulin aspart) and Novolin 70/30 (human premix).

NovoLog Mix 70/30 should appear uniformly white and cloudy. Do not use it if it looks clear or if it contains solid particles. NovoLog Mix 70/30 should not be used after the printed expiration date.

NovoLog Mix 70/30 should be administered by subcutaneous injection in the abdominal region, buttocks, thigh, or upper arm. NovoLog Mix 70/30 has a faster onset of action than human insulin premix 70/30 and should be dosed within 15 minutes before meal initiation for patients with type 1 diabetes. For patients with type 2 diabetes, dosing should occur within 15 minutes before or after meal initiation. Injection sites should be rotated within the same region to reduce the risk of lipodystrophy. As with all insulins, the duration of action may vary according to the dose, injection site, blood flow, temperature, and level of physical activity.

NovoLog Mix 70/30 should not be administered intravenously or used in insulin infusion pumps. Dose regimens of NovoLog Mix 70/30 will vary among patients and should be determined by the health care professional familiar with the patient's recommended glucose treatment goals, metabolic needs, eating habits, and other lifestyle variables.

2.2   Resuspension

NovoLog Mix 70/30 is a suspension that must be visually inspected and resuspended immediately before use.

The NovoLog Mix 70/30 vial should be rolled gently in your hands in a horizontal position 10 times to mix it. The rolling procedure must be repeated until the suspension appears uniformly white and cloudy. Inject immediately. Resuspension is easier when the insulin has reached room temperature.

The NovoLog Mix 70/30 FlexPen should be rolled 10 times gently between your hands in a horizontal position. Thereafter, turn the NovoLog Mix 70/30 FlexPen upside down so that the glass ball moves from one end of the reservoir to the other. Do this at least 10 times. The rolling and turning procedure must be repeated until the suspension appears uniformly white and cloudy. Inject immediately. Before each subsequent injection, turn the disposable NovoLog Mix 70/30 FlexPen upside down so that the glass ball moves from one end of the reservoir to the other at least 10 times and until the suspension appears uniformly white and cloudy. Inject immediately.

3   DOSAGE FORMS AND STRENGTHS

NovoLog Mix 70/30 is available in the following package sizes: each presentation contains 100 units of insulin aspart per mL (U-100).

- 10 mL vials
- 3 mL NovoLog Mix 70/30 FlexPen

4   CONTRAINDICATIONS

NovoLog Mix 70/30 is contraindicated
- during episodes of hypoglycemia
- in patients with hypersensitivity to NovoLog Mix 70/30 or one of its excipients.

5   WARNINGS AND PRECAUTIONS

5.1   Administration

The short and long-acting components of insulin mixes, including NovoLog Mix 70/30, cannot be titrated independently. Because NovoLog Mix 70/30 has peak pharmacodynamic activity between 1-4 hours after injection, it should be administered within 15 minutes of meal initiation [see Clinical Pharmacology (12)]. The dose of insulin required to provide adequate glycemic control for one of the meals may result in hyper- or hypoglycemia for the other meal. The pharmacodynamic profile may also be inadequate for patients who require more frequent meals.

NovoLog Mix 70/30 should not be mixed with any other insulin product.

NovoLog Mix 70/30 should not be used intravenously.

NovoLog Mix 70/30 should not be used in insulin infusion pumps.

Glucose monitoring is recommended for all patients with diabetes. Any change of insulin dose should be made cautiously and only under medical supervision. Changing from one insulin product to another or changing the insulin strength may result in the need for a change in dosage. Changes may also be necessary during illness, emotional stress, and other physiologic stress in addition to changes in meals and exercise.

The pharmacokinetic and pharmacodynamic profiles of all insulins may be altered by the site used for injection and the degree of vascularization of the site. Smoking, temperature, and exercise contribute to variations in blood flow and insulin absorption. These and other factors contribute to inter- and intra-patient variability.

Needles and NovoLog Mix 70/30 FlexPen must not be shared.

5.2   Hypoglycemia

Hypoglycemia is the most common adverse effect of insulin therapy, including NovoLog Mix 70/30. Severe hypoglycemia may lead to unconsciousness and/or convulsions and may result in temporary or permanent impairment of brain function or even death. Severe hypoglycemia requiring the assistance of another person and/or parenteral glucose infusion or glucagon administration has been observed in clinical trials with insulin, including trials with NovoLog Mix 70/30.

The timing of hypoglycemia may reflect the time-action profile of the insulin formulation [see Clinical Pharmacology (12)]. Other factors, such as changes in dietary intake (e.g., amount of food or timing of meals), injection site, exercise, and concomitant medications may also alter the risk of hypoglycemia [see Drug Interactions (7)]. As with all insulins, use caution in patients with hypoglycemia unawareness and in patients who may be predisposed to hypoglycemia (e.g. patients who are fasting or have erratic food intake). The patient's ability to concentrate and react may be impaired as a result of hypoglycemia. This may present a risk in situations where these abilities are especially important, such as driving or operating machinery.

Rapid changes in serum glucose levels may induce symptoms of hypoglycemia in persons with diabetes, regardless of the glucose value. Early warning symptoms of hypoglycemia may be different or less pronounced under certain conditions, such as long duration of diabetes, diabetic nerve disease, use of medications such as beta-blockers, or intensified diabetes control [see Drug Interactions (7)].

5.3   Hypokalemia

All insulin products, including NovoLog Mix 70/30, cause a shift in potassium from the extracellular to intracellular space, possibly leading to hypokalemia that, if left untreated, may cause respiratory paralysis, ventricular arrhythmia, and death. Use caution in patients who may be at risk for hypokalemia (e.g. patients using potassium-lowering medications or patients taking medications sensitive to potassium concentrations).

5.4   Renal Impairment

Clinical or pharmacology studies with NovoLog Mix 70/30 in diabetic patients with various degrees of renal impairment have not been conducted. As with other insulins, the requirements for NovoLog Mix 70/30 may be reduced in patients with renal impairment [see Clinical Pharmacology (12.3)].

5.5   Hepatic Impairment

Clinical or pharmacology studies with NovoLog Mix 70/30 in diabetic patients with various degrees of hepatic impairment have not been conducted. As with other insulins, the requirements for NovoLog Mix 70/30 may be reduced in patients with hepatic impairment [see Clinical Pharmacology (12.3)].

Help Patients Save on Rx Drugs: PDR.net/PharmacyDiscountCard

Table 1: Treatment-Emergent Adverse Events in Patients with Type 1 diabetes mellitus (Adverse events with frequency ≥ 5% are included.)

Preferred Term	NovoLog Mix 70/30 (N=55)		Novolin 70/30 (N=49)	
	N	%	N	%
Hypoglycemia	38	69	37	76
Headache	19	35	6	12
Influenza-like symptoms	7	13	1	2
Dyspepsia	5	9	3	6
Back pain	4	7	2	4
Diarrhea	4	7	3	6
Pharyngitis	4	7	1	2
Rhinitis	3	5	6	12
Skeletal pain	3	5	2	4
Upper respiratory tract infection	3	5	1	2

Table 2: Treatment-Emergent Adverse Events in Patients with Type 2 diabetes mellitus (Adverse events with frequency ≥ 5% are included.)

Preferred Term	NovoLog Mix 70/30 (N=85)		Novolin 70/30 (N=102)	
	N	%	N	%
Hypoglycemia	40	47	51	50
Upper respiratory tract infection	10	12	6	6
Headache	8	9	8	8
Diarrhea	7	8	2	2
Neuropathy	7	8	2	2
Pharyngitis	5	6	4	4
Abdominal pain	4	5	0	0
Rhinitis	4	5	2	2

5.6 Hypersensitivity and Allergic Reactions

Local Reactions- As with other insulin therapy, patients may experience reactions such as erythema, edema or pruritus at the site of NovoLog Mix 70/30 injection. These reactions usually resolve in a few days to a few weeks, but in some occasions, may require discontinuation of NovoLog Mix 70/30. In some instances, these reactions may be related to the insulin molecule, other components in the insulin preparation including protamine and cresol, components in skin cleansing agents, or injection techniques. Localized reactions and generalized myalgias have been reported with the use of cresol as an injectable excipient.

Systemic Reactions- Less common, but potentially more serious, is generalized allergy to insulin, which may cause rash (including pruritus) over the whole body, shortness of breath, wheezing, reduction in blood pressure, rapid pulse, or sweating. Severe cases of generalized allergy, including anaphylactic reaction, may be life threatening.

5.7 Antibody Production

Specific anti-insulin antibodies as well as cross-reacting anti-insulin antibodies were monitored in a 3-month, open-label comparator trial as well as in a long-term extension trial. Changes in cross-reactive antibodies were more common after NovoLog Mix 70/30 than with Novolin 70/30 but these changes did not correlate with change in HbA_{1c} or increase in insulin dose. In this study, antibodies did not increase further after long-term exposure (>6 months) to NovoLog Mix 70/30. The presence of such insulin antibodies may necessitate adjustment of the insulin dose in order to correct a tendency towards hyperglycemia or hypoglycemia.

5.8 Fluid retention and heart failure can occur with concomitant use of PPAR-gamma agonists

Thiazolidinediones (TZDs), which are peroxisome proliferator-activated receptor (PPAR)-gamma agonists, can cause dose-related fluid retention, particularly when used in combination with insulin. Fluid retention may lead to or exacerbate heart failure. Patients treated with insulin, including NovoLog Mix 70/30, and a PPAR-gamma agonist should be observed for signs and symptoms of heart failure. If heart failure develops, it should be managed according to current standards of care; and discontinuation or dose reduction of the PPAR-gamma agonist must be considered.

6 ADVERSE REACTIONS

Clinical Trial Experience

Clinical trials are conducted under widely varying designs, therefore, the adverse reaction rates reported in one clinical trial may not be easily compared to those rates reported in another clinical trial, and may not reflect the rates actually observed in clinical practice.

• *Hypoglycemia*

Hypoglycemia is the most commonly observed adverse reaction in patients using insulin, including NovoLog Mix 70/30 *[see Warnings and Precautions (5.2)]*. NovoLog Mix 70/30 should not be used during episodes of hypoglycemia *[see Contraindications (4) and Warnings and Precautions (5)]*.

• *Insulin initiation and glucose control intensification*

Intensification or rapid improvement in glucose control has been associated with transitory, reversible ophthalmologic refraction disorder, worsening of diabetic retinopathy, and acute painful peripheral neuropathy. However, long-term glycemic control decreases the risk of diabetic retinopathy and neuropathy.

• *Lipodystrophy*

Long-term use of insulin, including NovoLog Mix 70/30, can cause lipodystrophy at the site of repeated insulin injections. Lipodystrophy includes lipohypertrophy (thickening of adipose tissue) and lipoatrophy (thinning of adipose tissue), and may affect insulin absorption. Rotate insulin injection sites within the same region to reduce the risk of lipodystrophy.

• *Weight gain*

Weight gain can occur with some insulin therapies, including NovoLog Mix 70/30, and has been attributed to the anabolic effects of insulin and the decrease in glycosuria.

• *Peripheral Edema*

Insulin may cause sodium retention and edema, particularly if previously poor metabolic control is improved by intensified insulin therapy.

• *Frequencies of adverse drug reactions*

The frequencies of adverse drug reactions during a clinical trial with NovoLog Mix 70/30 in patients with type 1 diabetes mellitus and type 2 diabetes mellitus are listed in the tables below. The trial was a three-month, open-label trial in patients with type 1 or type 2 diabetes who were treated twice daily (before breakfast and before supper) with NovoLog Mix 70/30.
[See table 1 above]
[See table 2 above]

Postmarketing Data

Additional adverse reactions have been identified during post-approval use of NovoLog Mix 70/30. Because these adverse reactions are reported voluntarily from a population of uncertain size, it is generally not possible to reliably estimate their frequency. They include medication errors in which other insulins have been accidentally substituted for NovoLog Mix 70/30 *[see Patient Counseling Information (17)]*.

7 DRUG INTERACTIONS

A number of substances affect glucose metabolism and may require insulin dose adjustment and particularly close monitoring.

• The following are examples of substances that may increase the blood-glucose-lowering effect and susceptibility to hypoglycemia: oral antidiabetic products, pramlintide, ACE inhibitors, disopyramide, fibrates, fluoxetine, monoamine oxidase (MAO) inhibitors, propoxyphene, salicylates, somatostatin analog (e.g. octreotide), sulfonamide antibiotics.

• The following are examples of substances that may reduce the blood-glucose-lowering effect: corticosteroids, niacin, danazol, diuretics, sympathomimetic agents (e.g., epinephrine, salbutamol, terbutaline), isoniazid, phenothiazine derivatives, somatropin, thyroid hormones, estrogens, progestogens (e.g., in oral contraceptives), atypical antipsychotics.

• Beta-blockers, clonidine, lithium salts, and alcohol may either potentiate or weaken the blood-glucose-lowering effect of insulin.

• Pentamidine may cause hypoglycemia, which may sometimes be followed by hyperglycemia.

• The signs of hypoglycemia may be reduced or absent in patients taking sympatholytic products such as beta-blockers, clonidine, guanethidine, and reserpine.

8 USE IN SPECIFIC POPULATIONS

8.1 Pregnancy

Pregnancy Category B.

All pregnancies have a background risk of birth defects, loss, or other adverse outcome regardless of drug exposure. This background risk is increased in pregnancies complicated by hyperglycemia and may be decreased with good metabolic control. It is essential for patients with diabetes or history of gestational diabetes to maintain good metabolic control before conception and throughout pregnancy. Insulin requirements may decrease during the first trimester, generally increase during the second and third trimesters, and rapidly decline after delivery. Careful monitoring of glucose control is essential in such patients.

An open-label, randomized study compared the safety and efficacy of NovoLog (the rapid-acting component of NovoLog Mix 70/30) versus human insulin in the treatment of pregnant women with type 1 diabetes (322 exposed pregnancies (NovoLog: 157, human insulin: 165)). Two-thirds of the enrolled patients were already pregnant when they entered the study. Since only one-third of the patients enrolled before conception, the study was not large enough to evaluate the risk of congenital malformations. Mean HbA_{1c} of ~ 6% was observed in both groups during pregnancy, and there was no significant difference in the incidence of maternal hypoglycemia.

Animal reproduction studies have not been conducted with NovoLog Mix 70/30. However, subcutaneous reproduction and teratology studies have been performed with NovoLog (the rapid-acting component of NovoLog Mix 70/30) and regular human insulin in rats and rabbits. In these studies, NovoLog was given to female rats before mating, during mating, and throughout pregnancy, and to rabbits during organogenesis. The effects of NovoLog did not differ from those observed with subcutaneous regular human insulin. NovoLog, like human insulin, caused pre- and post-implantation losses and visceral/skeletal abnormalities in rats at a dose of 200 U/kg/day (approximately 32-times the human subcutaneous dose of 1.0 U/kg/day, based on U/body surface area), and in rabbits at a dose of 10 U/kg/day (approximately three times the human subcutaneous dose of 1.0 U/kg/day, based on U/body surface area). The effects are probably secondary to maternal hypoglycemia at high doses. No significant effects were observed in rats at a dose of 50 U/kg/day and rabbits at a dose of 3 U/kg/day. These doses are approximately 8 times the human subcutaneous dose of 1.0 U/kg/day for rats and equal to the human subcutaneous dose of 1.0 U/kg/day for rabbits based on U/body surface area.

Female patients should be advised to discuss with their physician if they intend to, or if they become pregnant. There are no adequate and well-controlled studies of the use of NovoLog Mix 70/30 in pregnant women.

8.3 Nursing Mothers

It is unknown whether insulin aspart is excreted in human milk as occurs with human insulin. There are no adequate and well-controlled studies of the use of NovoLog Mix 70/30 or NovoLog in lactating women. Women with diabetes who are lactating may require adjustments of their insulin doses.

8.4 Pediatric Use

Safety and effectiveness of NovoLog Mix 70/30 have not been established in pediatric patients.

8.5 Geriatric Use

Clinical studies of NovoLog Mix 70/30 did not include sufficient numbers of patients aged 65 and over to determine whether they respond differently than younger patients. In general, dose selection for an elderly patient should be cautious, usually starting at the low end of the dosing range reflecting the greater frequency of decreased hepatic, renal, or cardiac function, and of concomitant disease or other drug therapy in this population.

10 OVERDOSAGE

Hypoglycemia may occur as a result of an excess of insulin relative to food intake, energy expenditure, or both. Mild episodes of hypoglycemia usually can be treated with oral glucose. Adjustments in drug dosage, meal patterns, or exercise, may be needed. More severe episodes with coma, seizure, or neurologic impairment may be treated with intramuscular/subcutaneous glucagon or concentrated intravenous glucose. Sustained carbohydrate intake and observation may be necessary because hypoglycemia may recur after apparent clinical recovery.

11 DESCRIPTION

NovoLog Mix 70/30 (70% insulin aspart protamine suspension and 30% insulin aspart injection, [rDNA origin]) is a human insulin analog suspension containing 70% insulin aspart protamine crystals and 30% soluble insulin aspart. NovoLog Mix 70/30 is a blood-glucose-lowering agent with an earlier onset and an intermediate duration of action. Insulin aspart is homologous with regular human insulin with the exception of a single substitution of the amino acid proline by aspartic acid in position B28, and is produced by recombinant DNA technology utilizing *Saccharomyces cerevisiae* (baker's yeast). Insulin aspart (NovoLog) has the empirical formula $C_{256}H_{381}N_{65}O_{79}S_6$ and a molecular weight of 5825.8 Da.

Figure 1. Structural formula of insulin aspart

NovoLog Mix 70/30 is a uniform, white, sterile suspension that contains insulin aspart 100 Units/mL.
Inactive ingredients are glycerol 16.0 mg/mL, phenol 1.50 mg/mL, metacresol 1.72 mg/mL, zinc 19.6 µg/mL, disodium hydrogen phosphate dihydrate 1.25 mg/mL, sodium chloride 0.877 mg/mL, and protamine sulfate 0.32 mg/mL. NovoLog Mix 70/30 has a pH of 7.20 - 7.44. Hydrochloric acid or sodium hydroxide may be added to adjust pH.

12 CLINICAL PHARMACOLOGY

12.1 Mechanism of Action

The primary activity of NovoLog Mix 70/30 is the regulation of glucose metabolism. Insulins, including NovoLog Mix 70/30, bind to the insulin receptors on muscle, liver and fat cells and lower blood glucose by facilitating the cellular uptake of glucose and simultaneously inhibiting the output of glucose from the liver.

12.2 Pharmacodynamics

The two euglycemic clamp studies described below *[see Clinical Pharmacology (12.3)]* assessed glucose utilization after dosing of healthy volunteers. NovoLog Mix 70/30 has an earlier onset of action than human premix 70/30 in studies of normal volunteers and patients with diabetes. The onset of action is between 10-20 minutes for NovoLog Mix 70/30 compared to 30 minutes for Novolin 70/30. The mean ± SD time to peak activity for NovoLog Mix 70/30 is 2.4 hr ± 0.8 hr compared to 4.2 hr ± 0.4 hr for Novolin 70/30. The duration of action may be as long as 24 hours (see Figure 2).
[See figure 2 at top of next column]

12.3 Pharmacokinetics

The single substitution of the amino acid proline with aspartic acid at position B28 in insulin aspart (NovoLog) reduces the molecule's tendency to form hexamers as observed with regular human insulin. The rapid absorption characteristics of NovoLog are maintained by NovoLog Mix 70/30. The insulin aspart in the soluble component of NovoLog Mix 70/30 is absorbed more rapidly from the subcutaneous layer

Figure 2. Pharmacodynamic Activity Profile of NovoLog Mix 70/30 and Novolin 70/30 in healthy subjects.

than regular human insulin. The remaining 70% is in crystalline form as insulin aspart protamine which has a prolonged absorption profile after subcutaneous injection.
Bioavailability and Absorption- The relative bioavailability of NovoLog Mix 70/30 compared to NovoLog and Novolin 70/30 indicates that the insulins are absorbed to similar extent. In euglycemic clamp studies in healthy volunteers (n=23) after dosing with NovoLog Mix 70/30 (0.2 U/kg), a mean maximum serum concentration (C_{max}) of 23.4 ± 5.3 mU/L was reached after 60 minutes. The mean half-life ($t_{1/2}$) of NovoLog Mix 70/30 was about 8 to 9 hours. Serum insulin levels returned to baseline 15 to 18 hours after a subcutaneous dose of NovoLog Mix 70/30. Similar data were seen in a separate euglycemic clamp study in healthy volunteers (n=24) after dosing with NovoLog Mix 70/30 (0.3 U/kg). A C_{max} of 61.3 ± 20.1 mU/L was reached after 85 minutes. Serum insulin levels returned to baseline 12 hours after a subcutaneous dose.
The C_{max} and the area under the insulin concentration-time curve (AUC) after administration of NovoLog Mix 70/30 was approximately 20% greater than those after administration of Novolin 70/30, (see Fig. 3 for pharmacokinetic profiles).

Points represent mean ± 2 SEM

Figure 3. Pharmacokinetic Profiles of NovoLog Mix 70/30 and Novolin 70/30

Distribution and Elimination- NovoLog has a low binding to plasma proteins, 0 to 9%, similar to regular human insulin. After subcutaneous administration in normal male volunteers (n=24), NovoLog was more rapidly eliminated than regular human insulin with an average apparent half-life of 81 minutes compared to 141 minutes for regular human insulin.
The effect of sex, age, obesity, ethnic origin, renal and hepatic impairment, pregnancy, or smoking, on the pharmacodynamics and pharmacokinetics of NovoLog Mix 70/30 has not been studied.

13 NONCLINICAL TOXICOLOGY

13.1 Carcinogenesis, Mutagenesis, Impairment of Fertility

Standard 2-year carcinogenicity studies in animals have not been performed to evaluate the carcinogenic potential of NovoLog Mix 70/30. In 52-week studies, Sprague-Dawley rats were dosed subcutaneously with NovoLog, the rapid-acting component of NovoLog Mix 70/30, at 10, 50, and 200 U/kg/day (approximately 2, 8, and 32 times the human subcutaneous dose of 1.0 U/kg/day, based on U/body surface area, respectively). At a dose of 200 U/kg/day, NovoLog increased the incidence of mammary gland tumors in females when compared to untreated controls. The incidence of mammary tumors found with NovoLog was not significantly different from that found with regular human insulin. The relevance of these findings to humans is not known.
NovoLog was not genotoxic in the following tests: Ames test, mouse lymphoma cell forward gene mutation test, human peripheral blood lymphocyte chromosome aberration test, *in vivo* micronucleus test in mice, and in *ex vivo* UDS test in rat liver hepatocytes.
In fertility studies in male and female rats, NovoLog at subcutaneous doses up to 200 U/kg/day (approximately 32

times the human subcutaneous dose, based on U/body surface area) had no direct adverse effects on male and female fertility, or on general reproductive performance of animals.

13.2 Animal Toxicology and/or Pharmacology

In standard biological assays in mice and rabbits, one unit of NovoLog has the same glucose-lowering effect as one unit of regular human insulin. However, the effect of NovoLog Mix 70/30 is more rapid in onset compared to Novolin (human insulin) 70/30 due to its faster absorption after subcutaneous injection.

14 CLINICAL STUDIES

14.1 NovoLog Mix 70/30 versus Novolin 70/30

In a three-month, open-label trial, patients with type 1 (n=104) or type 2 (n=187) diabetes were treated twice daily (before breakfast and before supper) with NovoLog Mix 70/30 or Novolin 70/30. Patients had received insulin for at least 24 months before the study. Oral hypoglycemic agents were not allowed within 1 month prior to the study or during the study. The small changes in HbA1c were comparable across the treatment groups (see Table 3).

Table 3: Glycemic Parameters at the End of Treatment [Mean ± SD (N subjects)]

	NovoLog Mix 70/30	Novolin 70/30
Type 1, N=104		
Fasting Blood Glucose (mg/dL)	174 ± 64 (48)	142 ± 59 (44)
1.5 Hour Post Breakfast (mg/dL)	187 ± 82 (48)	200 ± 82 (42)
1.5 Hour Post Dinner (mg/dL)	162 ± 77 (47)	171 ± 66 (41)
HbA1c (%) Baseline	8.4 ± 1.2 (51)	8.5 ± 1.1 (46)
HbA1c (%) Week 12	8.4 ± 1.1 (51)	8.3 ± 1.0 (47)
Type 2, N=187		
Fasting Blood Glucose (mg/dL)	153 ± 40 (76)	152 ± 69 (93)
1.5 Hour Post Breakfast (mg/dL)	182 ± 65 (75)	200 ± 80 (92)
1.5 Hour Post Dinner (mg/dL)	168 ± 51 (75)	191 ± 65 (93)
HbA1c (%) Baseline	8.1 ± 1.2 (82)	8.2 ± 1.3 (98)
HbA1c (%) Week 12	7.9 ± 1.0 (81)	8.1 ± 1.1 (96)

The significance, with respect to the long-term clinical sequelae of diabetes, of the differences in postprandial hyperglycemia between treatment groups has not been established.
Specific anti-insulin antibodies as well as cross-reacting anti-insulin antibodies were monitored in the 3-month, open-label comparator trial as well as in a long-term extension trial.

14.2 Combination Therapy: Insulin and Oral Agents in Patients with Type 2 Diabetes

Trial 1:
In a 34-week, open-label trial, insulin-naïve patients with type 2 diabetes currently treated with 2 oral antidiabetic agents were switched to treatment with metformin and pioglitazone. During an 8-week optimization period metformin and pioglitazone were increased to 2500 mg per day and 30 or 45 mg per day, respectively. After the optimization period, subjects were randomized to receive either NovoLog Mix 70/30 twice daily added on to the metformin and pioglitazone regimen or continue the current optimized metformin and pioglitazone therapy. NovoLog Mix 70/30 was started at a dose of 6 IU twice daily (before breakfast and before supper). Insulin doses were titrated to a pre-meal glucose goal of 80-110 mg/dL. The total daily insulin dose at the end of the study was 56.9 ± 30.5 IU.
[See table 4 at top of next page]

Trial 2:
In a 28-week, open-label trial, insulin-naïve patients with type 2 diabetes with fasting plasma glucose above 140 mg/dL currently treated with metformin ± thiazolidinedione therapy were randomized to receive either NovoLog Mix 70/30 twice daily [before breakfast and before supper] or insulin glargine once daily[1] (see Table 5). NovoLog Mix 70/30 was started at an average dose of 5-6 IU (0.07 ± 0.03 IU/kg) twice daily (before breakfast and before supper), and bedtime insulin glargine was started at 10-12 IU (0.13 ± 0.03 IU/kg). Insulin doses were titrated

Table 4: Combination Therapy with Oral Agents and Insulin in Patients with Type 2 Diabetes Mellitus [Mean (SD)]

Treatment duration 24-weeks	NovoLog Mix 70/30 + Metformin + Pioglitazone	Metformin + Pioglitazone
HbA$_{1c}$		
Baseline mean ± SD (n)	8.1 ± 1.0 (102)	8.1 ± 1.0 (98)
End-of-study mean ± SD (n) - LOCF	6.6 ± 1.0 (93)	7.8 ± 1.2 (87)
Adjusted Mean change from baseline ± SE (n)*	-1.6 ± 0.1 (93)	-0.3 ± 0.1 (87)
Treatment difference mean ± SE* 95% CI*	-1.3 ± 0.1 (-1.6, -1.0)	
Percentage of subjects reaching HbA$_{1c}$ <7.0%	76%	24%
Percentage of subjects reaching HbA$_{1c}$ ≤6.5%	59%	12%
Fasting Blood Glucose (mg/dL)		
Baseline Mean ± SD (n)	173 ± 39.8 (93)	163 ± 35.4 (88)
End of Study Mean ± SD (n) - LOCF	130 ± 50.0 (90)	162 ± 40.8 (84)
Adjusted Mean change from baseline ± SE (n)*	-43.0 ± 5.3 (90)	-3.9 ± 5.3 (84)
End-of-Study Blood Glucose (Plasma) (mg/dL)		
2 Hour Post Breakfast	138 ± 42.8 (86)	188 ± 57.7 (74)
2 Hour Post Lunch	150 ± 41.5 (86)	176 ± 56.5 (74)
2 Hour Post Dinner	141 ± 57.8 (86)	195 ± 60.1 (74)
% of patients with severe hypoglycemia**	3	0
% of patients with minor hypoglycemia**	52	3
Weight gain at end of study (kg)**	4.6 ± 4.3 (92)	0.8 ± 3.2 (86)

*Adjusted mean per group, treatment difference, and 95% CI were obtained based on an ANCOVA model with treatment, FPG stratum, and secretagogue stratum as fixed factors and baseline HbA$_{1c}$ as the covariate.
**If metabolic control is improved by intensified insulin therapy, an increased risk of hypoglycemia and weight gain may occur.

	Not in-use (unopened) Room Temperature (below 30°C [86°F])	Not in-use (unopened) Refrigerated (2°C - 8°C [36°F - 46°F])	In-use (opened) Room Temperature (below 30°C [86°F])
10 mL vial	28 days	Until expiration date	28 days (refrigerated/room temperature)
3 mL NovoLog Mix 70/30 FlexPen	14 days	Until expiration date	14 days (Do not refrigerate)

weekly by decrements or increments of -2 to +6 units per injection to a pre-meal glucose goal of 80-110 mg/dL. The metformin dose was adjusted to 2550 mg/day. Approximately one-third of the patients in each group were also treated with pioglitazone (30 mg/day). Insulin secretagogues were discontinued in order to reduce the risk of hypoglycemia. Most patients were Caucasian (53%), and the mean initial weight was 90 kg.

Table 5: Combination Therapy with Oral Agents and Two Types of Insulin in Patients with Type 2 Diabetes Mellitus [Mean (SD)]

Treatment duration 28-weeks	NovoLog Mix 70/30 + Metformin ± Pioglitazone	Insulin Glargine + Metformin ± Pioglitazone
Number of patients	117	116
HbA$_{1c}$		
Baseline mean (%)	9.7 ± 1.5 (117)	9.8 ± 1.4 (114)
End-of-study mean (± SD)	6.9 ± 1.2 (108)	7.4 ± 1.2 (114)
Mean change from baseline	-2.7 ± 1.6 (108)	-2.4 ± 1.5 (114)
Percentage of subjects reaching HbA$_{1c}$ <7.0%	66%	40%

Total Daily Insulin Dose at end of study (U)	78 ± 40 (117)	51 ± 27 (116)
% of patients with severe hypoglycemia	0	0
% of minor hypoglycemia	43	16
Weight gain at end of study	5.4 ± 4.8 (117)	3.5 ± 4.5 (116)

15 REFERENCES

1. Raskin R, Allen E, Hollander P, et al. Initiating insulin therapy in type 2 diabetes: a comparison of biphasic and basal insulin analogs. *Diabetes Care.* 2005; 28:260-265.

16 HOW SUPPLIED/STORAGE AND HANDLING
16.1 How Supplied
NovoLog Mix 70/30 is available in the following package sizes: each presentation contains 100 Units of insulin aspart per mL (U-100).

10 mL vials	NDC 0169-3685-12
3 mL NovoLog Mix 70/30 FlexPen	NDC 0169-3696-19

NovoLog Mix 70/30 vials and NovoLog Mix 70/30 FlexPen are latex free.
16.2 Recommended Storage
Unused NovoLog Mix 70/30 should be stored in a refrigerator between 2°C and 8°C (36°F to 46°F). Do not store in the freezer or directly adjacent to the refrigerator cooling element. **Do not freeze NovoLog Mix 70/30 or use NovoLog Mix 70/30 if it has been frozen.**
Vials: After initial use, a vial may be kept at temperatures below 30°C (86°F) for up to 28 days, but should not be exposed to excessive heat or sunlight. Open vials may be refrigerated.
Unpunctured vials can be used until the expiration date printed on the label if they are stored in a refrigerator. Keep unused vials in the carton so they will stay clean and protected from light.
NovoLog Mix 70/30 FlexPen: Once a NovoLog Mix 70/30 FlexPen is punctured, it should be kept at temperatures below 30°C (86°F) for up to 14 days, but should not be exposed to excessive heat or sunlight. A NovoLog Mix 70/30 FlexPen in use must NOT be stored in the refrigerator. Keep the disposable NovoLog Mix 70/30 FlexPen away from direct heat and sunlight. An unpunctured NovoLog Mix 70/30 FlexPen can be used until the expiration date printed on the label if they are stored in a refrigerator. Keep any unused NovoLog Mix 70/30 FlexPen in the carton so it will stay clean and protected from light.
These storage conditions are summarized in the following table:
[See table above]

17 PATIENT COUNSELING INFORMATION
[see FDA-Approved Patient Labeling]
17.1 Physician Instructions
Maintenance of normal or near-normal glucose control is a treatment goal in diabetes mellitus and has been associated with a reduction in diabetic complications. Patients should be informed about potential risks and advantages of NovoLog Mix 70/30 therapy including the possible adverse reactions. Patients should also be offered continued education and advice on insulin therapies, injection technique, life-style management, regular glucose monitoring, periodic glycosylated hemoglobin testing, recognition and management of hypo- and hyperglycemia, adherence to meal planning, complications of insulin therapy, timing of dose, instruction for use of injection devices, and proper storage of insulin. See Patient Information supplied with the product. Patients should be informed that frequent, patient-performed blood glucose measurements are needed to achieve optimal glycemic control and avoid both hyper- and hypoglycemia, and diabetic ketoacidosis.
The patient's ability to concentrate and react may be impaired as a result of hypoglycemia. This may present a risk in situations where these abilities are especially important, such as driving or operating other machinery. Patients who have frequent hypoglycemia or reduced or absent warning signs of hypoglycemia should be advised to use caution when driving or operating machinery.
Accidental substitutions between NovoLog Mix 70/30 and other insulin products have been reported. Patients should be instructed to always carefully check that they are administering the appropriate insulin to avoid medication errors between NovoLog Mix 70/30 and any other insulin. **The prescription for NovoLog Mix 70/30 should be written clearly in order to avoid confusion with other insulin products, for example, NovoLog or Novolin 70/30. In addition, the written prescription should clearly indicate the presentation, for example FlexPen or vial.**

Rx only
Date of Issue: June 13, 2014
Version: 12
Novo Nordisk®, NovoLog®, FlexPen®, and Novolin® are registered trademarks of Novo Nordisk® A/S.
NovoLog® Mix 70/30 is covered by US Patent Nos. 5,547,930, 5,618,913, 5,834,422, 5,840,680, 5,866,538 and other patents pending.
FlexPen® is covered by US Patent Nos. 6,004,297, RE 43,834, RE 41,956 and other patents pending.
© 2002 – 2014 Novo Nordisk
Manufactured by:
Novo Nordisk A/S
DK-2880 Bagsvaerd, Denmark
For information about NovoLog Mix 70/30 contact:
Novo Nordisk Inc.
800 Scudders Mill Road
Plainsboro, New Jersey 08536
1-800-727-6500
www.novonordisk-us.com
PATIENT INFORMATION
NovoLog® Mix 70/30
(NŌ-vō-log-MIX-SEV-en-tee-THIR-tee)
(70% insulin aspart protamine suspension and 30% insulin aspart injection, [rDNA origin])
Read the Patient Information leaflet that comes with NovoLog® Mix 70/30 before you start taking it and each time you get a refill. There may be new information. This leaflet does not take the place of talking with your healthcare provider about your diabetes or your treatment. Make sure you know how to manage your diabetes. Ask your healthcare provider if you have any questions about managing your diabetes.

What is NovoLog® Mix 70/30?

NovoLog® Mix 70/30 is a man-made insulin that is used to control high blood sugar in adults with diabetes mellitus. It is not known if NovoLog® Mix 70/30 is safe or effective in children.

Who should not use NovoLog® Mix 70/30?

Do not take NovoLog® Mix 70/30 if:

• Your blood sugar is too low (hypoglycemia)
• You are allergic to any of the ingredients in NovoLog® Mix 70/30. See the end of this leaflet for a complete list of ingredients in NovoLog® Mix 70/30. Check with your healthcare provider if you are not sure.

What should I tell my healthcare provider before taking NovoLog® Mix 70/30?

Before you use NovoLog® Mix 70/30, tell your healthcare provider if you:

• have kidney or liver problems
• take any other medicines, especially ones commonly called TZDs (thiazolidinediones).
• **have heart failure or other heart problems.** If you have heart failure, it may get worse while you take TZDs with NovoLog® Mix 70/30.
• **have any other medical conditions.** Medical conditions can affect your insulin needs and your dose of NovoLog® Mix 70/30.
• **are pregnant or plan to become pregnant.** It is not known if NovoLog® Mix 70/30 will harm your unborn baby. Talk to your healthcare provider if you are pregnant or plan to become pregnant. You and your healthcare provider should decide about the best way to manage your diabetes while you are pregnant.
• **are breastfeeding or plan to breastfeed.** It is not known if NovoLog® Mix 70/30 passes into your breast milk. You and your healthcare provider should decide if you will take NovoLog® Mix 70/30 while you breastfeed.

Tell your healthcare provider about all medicines you take, including prescriptions and non-prescription medicines, vitamins and herbal supplements.

NovoLog® Mix 70/30 may affect the way other medicines work, and other medicines may affect how NovoLog® Mix 70/30 works. Your NovoLog® Mix 70/30 dose may change if you take other medicines.

Know the medicines you take. Keep a list of your medicines with you to show your healthcare providers and pharmacist when you get a new medicine.

How should I take NovoLog® Mix 70/30?

• Take NovoLog® Mix 70/30 exactly as your healthcare provider tells you to take it.
• Your healthcare provider will tell you how much NovoLog® Mix 70/30 to take and when to take it.
• Do not make any changes to your dose or type of insulin unless your healthcare provider tells you to.
• **NovoLog® Mix 70/30 starts acting fast. If you have Type 1 diabetes, inject it up to 15 minutes before you eat a meal.** Do not inject NovoLog® Mix 70/30 if you are not planning to eat within 15 minutes.
• **If you have Type 2 diabetes, you may inject NovoLog® Mix 70/30 up to 15 minutes before or after starting your meal.**
• **Do Not mix** NovoLog® Mix 70/30 with other insulin products.
• **Do Not** use NovoLog® Mix 70/30 in an insulin pump.
• **Inject NovoLog® Mix 70/30 under the skin (subcutaneously) of your stomach area, upper arms, buttocks or upper legs.** NovoLog® Mix 70/30 may affect your blood sugar levels faster if you inject it under the skin of your stomach area. Never inject NovoLog® Mix 70/30 into a vein or into a muscle.
• **Change (rotate) injection sites** within the area you choose with each dose. **Do not** inject into the exact same spot for each injection.
• **Read the instructions for use that come with your NovoLog® Mix 70/30.** Talk to your healthcare provider if you have any questions. Your healthcare provider should show you how to inject NovoLog® Mix 70/30 before you start using it.
• NovoLog® Mix 70/30 comes in:
  • 10 mL vials for use with a syringe
  • 3 mL NovoLog® Mix 70/30 FlexPen®
• **If you take too much NovoLog® Mix 70/30, your blood sugar may fall too low (hypoglycemia).** You can treat mild low blood sugar (hypoglycemia) by drinking or eating something sugary right away (fruit juice, sugar candies, or glucose tablets). It is important to treat low blood sugar (hypoglycemia) right away because it could get worse and you could pass out (loss of consciousness).
• **If you forget to take your dose of NovoLog® Mix 70/30, your blood sugar may go too high (hyperglycemia).** If high blood sugar (hyperglycemia) is not treated it can lead to serious problems, like passing out (loss of consciousness), coma or even death. Follow your healthcare provider's instructions for treating high blood sugar. Know your symptoms of high blood sugar which may include:

• increased thirst
• frequent urination
• drowsiness
• loss of appetite
• a hard time breathing
• fruity smell on the breath
• high amounts of sugar and ketones in your urine
• nausea, vomiting (throwing up) or stomach pain

Do not share needles, insulin pens or syringes with others.

Check your blood sugar levels. Ask your healthcare provider what your blood sugars should be and when you should check your blood sugar levels.

Your insulin dosage may need to change because of:

• illness
• stress
• other medicines you take
• change in diet
• change in physical activity or exercise

See the end of this patient information for instructions about preparing and giving your injection.

What should I consider while using NovoLog® Mix 70/30?

• **Alcohol.** Drinking alcohol may affect your blood sugar when you take NovoLog® Mix 70/30.
• **Driving and operating machinery.** You may have trouble paying attention or reacting if you have low blood sugar (hypoglycemia). Be careful when you drive a car or operate machinery. Ask your healthcare provider if it is alright for you to drive if you often have:
  • low blood sugar
  • decreased or no warning signs of low blood sugar

What are the possible side effects of NovoLog® Mix 70/30?

NovoLog® Mix 70/30 may cause serious side effects, including:

• **low blood sugar (hypoglycemia).** Symptoms of low blood sugar may include:

• sweating
• dizziness or lightheadedness
• shakiness
• hunger
• fast heart beat
• tingling of lips and tongue
• trouble concentrating or confusion
• blurred vision
• slurred speech
• anxiety, irritability or mood changes
• headache

Very low blood sugar can cause you to pass out (loss of consciousness), seizures, and death. Talk to your healthcare provider about how to tell if you have low blood sugar and what to do if this happens while taking NovoLog® Mix 70/30. Know your symptoms of low blood sugar. Follow your healthcare provider's instructions for treating low blood sugar.

Talk to your healthcare provider if low blood sugar is a problem for you. Your dose of NovoLog® Mix 70/30 may need to be changed.

• **Low potassium in your blood (hypokalemia)**
• **Reactions at the injection site (local allergic reaction).** You may get redness, swelling, and itching at the injection site. If you keep having skin reactions or they are serious talk to your healthcare provider.
• **Serious allergic reaction (whole body reaction). Get medical help right away,** if you have any of these symptoms of an allergic reaction:
  • a rash over your whole body
  • have trouble breathing
  • a fast heartbeat
  • sweating
  • feel faint
• **Swelling of your hands and feet**
• **Heart Failure.** Taking certain diabetes pills called thiazolidinediones or "TZDs" with NovoLog® Mix 70/30 may cause heart failure in some people. This can happen even if you have never had heart failure or heart problems before. If you already have heart failure it may get worse while you take TZDs with NovoLog® Mix 70/30. Your healthcare provider should monitor you closely while you are taking TZDs with NovoLog® Mix 70/30. Tell your healthcare provider if you have any new or worse symptoms of heart failure including:
  • shortness of breath
  • swelling of your ankles or feet
  • sudden weight gain
  Treatment with TZDs and NovoLog® Mix 70/30 may need to be adjusted or stopped by your healthcare provider if you have new or worse heart failure.

The most common side effects of NovoLog® Mix 70/30 include:

• **Skin thickening or pits at the injection site (lipodystrophy).** Change (rotate) where you inject your insulin to help to prevent these skin changes from happening. Do not inject insulin into this type of skin.
• **Weight gain**
• **Swelling of your hands and feet**
• **Vision changes**

These are not all of the possible side effects from NovoLog® Mix 70/30. Ask your healthcare provider or pharmacist for more information.

Call your doctor for medical advice about side effects. You may report side effects to FDA at 1-800-FDA-1088.

How should I store NovoLog® Mix 70/30?

All Unopened NovoLog® Mix 70/30:

• Keep all unopened NovoLog® Mix 70/30 in the refrigerator between 36°F to 46°F (2°C to 8°C).
• **Do not freeze or store next to the refrigerator cooling element.** Do not use NovoLog® Mix 70/30 if it has been frozen.
• Keep unopened NovoLog® Mix 70/30 in the carton to protect from light.
• Unopened vials can be used until the expiration date on the NovoLog® Mix 70/30 label, if the medicine has been stored in a refrigerator.
• Unused NovoLog® Mix 70/30 FlexPen® can be used until the expiration date on the NovoLog® Mix 70/30 FlexPen® label, if the medicine has been stored in a refrigerator.

After NovoLog® Mix 70/30 has been opened:

• **Vials**
  • Keep in the refrigerator or at room temperature below 86°F (30°C) for up to 28 days.
  • Keep vials away from direct heat or light.
  • Throw away an opened vial after 28 days of use, even if there is insulin left in the vial.
• **NovoLog® Mix 70/30 FlexPen®**
  • Keep at room temperature below 86°F (30°C) for up to 14 days.
  • **Do not** store a NovoLog® Mix 70/30 FlexPen® that you are using in the refrigerator.
  • Keep NovoLog® Mix 70/30 FlexPen® away from direct heat or light.
  • Throw away a used NovoLog® Mix 70/30 FlexPen® after 14 days, even if there is insulin left in the syringe.

Never use insulin after the expiration date that is printed on the label and carton.

Keep NovoLog® Mix 70/30 and all medicines out of the reach of children.

General advice about NovoLog® Mix 70/30

Medicines are sometimes prescribed for conditions that are not mentioned in the patient leaflet. Do not use NovoLog® Mix 70/30 for a condition for which it was not prescribed. Do not give NovoLog® Mix 70/30 to other people, even if they have the same symptoms you have. It may harm them.

This leaflet summarizes the most important information about NovoLog® Mix 70/30. If you would like more information about NovoLog® Mix 70/30 or diabetes, talk with your healthcare provider. You can ask your healthcare provider or pharmacist for information about NovoLog® Mix 70/30 that is written for healthcare professionals. For more information call 1-800-727-6500 or go to www.novonordisk-us.com.

What are the ingredients in NovoLog® Mix 70/30?

• **Active Ingredients in NovoLog® Mix 70/30:** 70% insulin aspart protamine suspension and 30% insulin aspart injection (rDNA origin).
• **Inactive Ingredients in NovoLog® Mix 70/30:** glycerol, phenol, metacresol, zinc, disodium hydrogen phosphate dihydrate, sodium chloride, protamine sulfate, water for injection, hydrochloric acid or sodium hydroxide.

All NovoLog® Mix 70/30 vials and NovoLog® Mix 70/30 FlexPen® are latex free.

Helpful information for people with diabetes is published by the American Diabetes Association, 1701 N Beauregard Street, Alexandria, VA 22311 and is available at www.diabetes.org.

Date of Issue: March 9, 2013
Version: 9

Novo Nordisk®, NovoLog®, and FlexPen® are registered trademarks of Novo Nordisk A/S.

NovoLog® Mix 70/30 is covered by US Patent Nos. 5,547,930, 5,618,913, 5,834,422, 5,840,680, 5,866,538 and other patents pending.

FlexPen® is covered by US Patent Nos. 6,582,404, 6,004,297, 6,235,004 and other patents pending.

© 2002-2013 Novo Nordisk

Manufactured by:
Novo Nordisk A/S
DK-2880 Bagsvaerd, Denmark
For information about NovoLog® Mix 70/30 contact:
Novo Nordisk Inc.
800 Scudders Mill Road
Plainsboro, New Jersey 08536
1-800-727-6500
www.novonordisk-us.com

PATIENT INSTRUCTIONS FOR USE

NovoLog® Mix 70/30 (NOvōLog-MIX-SEV-en-tee-THIR-tee)
(70% insulin aspart protamine suspension and 30% insulin aspart (rDNA origin) injection)
10 mL vial (100 Units/mL, U-100)

Read this Instructions for Use before you start taking NovoLog® Mix 70/30 and each time you get a refill. There may be new information. This information does not take the place of talking to your healthcare provider about your medical condition or your treatment.

Supplies you will need to give your NovoLog® Mix 70/30 injection:

• 10 mL NovoLog® Mix 70/30 vial
• insulin syringe and needle
• alcohol swab

Preparing your NovoLog® Mix 70/30 dose:

• Wash your hands with soap and water.
• Before you start to prepare your injection, check the NovoLog® Mix 70/30 label to make sure that you are taking the right type of insulin. This is especially important if you use more than 1 type of insulin.
• NovoLog® Mix 70/30 should look white and cloudy after mixing. **Do not** use NovoLog Mix 70/30 if it looks clear or contains any lumps or particles.
• NovoLog® Mix 70/30 is easier to mix when it is at room temperature.
• After mixing NovoLog® Mix 70/30, inject your dose right away. If you wait to inject your dose, the insulin will need to be mixed again.
• **Do not** use NovoLog® Mix 70/30 past the expiration date printed on the label.

Step 1: If you are using a new vial, pull off the tamper-resistant cap (See Figure A).
Step 2: Wipe the rubber stopper with an alcohol swab (See Figure B).

(Figure A Figure B)

Step 3: Roll the NovoLog Mix 70/30 vial between your hands 10 times. Keep the vial in a horizontal (flat) position (See Figure C). Roll the vial between your hands until the NovoLog® Mix 70/30 looks white and cloudy. Do not shake the vial.

(Figure C)

Step 4: Hold the syringe with the needle pointing up. Pull down on the plunger until the black tip reaches the line for the number of units for your prescribed dose (See Figure D). [See figure D at top of next column]
Step 5: Push the needle through the rubber stopper of the NovoLog® Mix 70/30 vial (See Figure E). [See figure E at top of next column]
Step 6: Push the plunger all the way in. This puts air into the NovoLog® Mix 70/30 vial (See Figure F). [See figure F at top of next column]

(Figure D)

(Figure E)

(Figure F)

Step 7: Turn the NovoLog® Mix 70/30 vial and syringe upside down and slowly pull the plunger down until the black tip is a few units past the line for your dose (See Figure G).

(Figure G)

• If there are air bubbles, tap the syringe gently a few times to let any air bubbles rise to the top (See Figure H).

(Figure H)

Step 8: Slowly push the plunger up until the black tip reaches the line for your NovoLog® Mix 70/30 dose (See Figure I).

(Figure I)

Step 9: Check the syringe to make sure you have the right dose of NovoLog® Mix 70/30.
Step 10: Pull the syringe out of the vial's rubber stopper (See Figure J).

(Figure J)

Giving your injection:

• Inject your NovoLog® Mix 70/30 exactly as your healthcare provider has shown you. Your healthcare provider should tell you if you need to pinch the skin before injecting.
• NovoLog® Mix 70/30 is injected under the skin (subcutaneously) of your stomach area, buttocks, upper legs, or upper arms.
• Change (rotate) your injection sites within the area you choose for each dose. **Do not** use the same injection site for each injection.

Step 11: Choose your injection site and wipe the skin with an alcohol swab. Let the injection site dry before you inject your dose (See Figure K).

(Figure K)

Step 12: Insert the needle into your skin. Push down on the plunger to inject your dose (See Figure L). Needle should remain in the skin for at least 6 seconds to make sure you have injected all the insulin.

(Figure L)

Step 13: Pull the needle out of your skin. After that, you may see a drop of NovoLog® Mix 70/30 at the needle tip. This is normal and does not affect the dose you just received (See Figure M).

• If you see blood after you take the needle out of your skin, press the injection site lightly with a piece of gauze or an alcohol swab. **Do not** rub the area.

(Figure M)

After your injection:

• **Do not** recap the needle. Recapping the needle can lead to a needle stick injury.
• Throw away empty insulin vials, used syringes and needles in a sharps container or some type of hard plastic or metal container with a screw on cap such as a detergent bottle or coffee can. Check with your healthcare provider about the right way to throw away the container. There may be local or state laws about how to throw away used syringes and needles. **Do not** throw away used syringes and needles in household trash or recycling bins.

How should I store NovoLog® Mix 70/30?

• **Do not** freeze NovoLog® Mix 70/30. **Do not** use NovoLog® Mix 70/30 if it has been frozen.
• Keep NovoLog® Mix 70/30 away from heat or light.
• Store opened and unopened NovoLog® Mix 70/30 vials in the refrigerator at 36°F to 46°F (2°C to 8°C). Opened NovoLog® Mix 70/30 vials can also be stored out of the refrigerator below 86°F (30°C).
• Unopened vials may be used until the expiration date printed on the label, if they are kept in the refrigerator.
• Opened NovoLog® Mix 70/30 vials should be thrown away after 28 days, even if they still have insulin left in them.

General information about the safe and effective use of NovoLog® Mix 70/30

• Always use a new syringe and needle for each injection.
• Do not share syringes or needles.
• Keep NovoLog® Mix 70/30 vials, syringes, and needles out of the reach of children.

This Instructions for Use has been approved by the U.S. Food and Drug Administration.

NovoLog® Mix 70/30 FlexPen®: Pen cap, Rubber stopper, 12 Units, Glass ball, Cartridge, Cartridge scale, Pointer, Dose selector button, Push-button. NovoFine® needle: Big outer needle cap, Inner needle cap, Needle, Protective tab

Manufactured by:
Novo Nordisk A/S
DK-2880 Bagsvaerd, Denmark
Revised: March 2013
NovoLog is a registered trademark of Novo Nordisk A/S.
NovoLog® Mix 70/30 is covered by US Patent Nos. 5,547,930, 5,618,913, 5,834,422, 5,840,680, 5,866,538 and other patents pending.
© 2002-2013 Novo Nordisk
For information about NovoLog® Mix 70/30 contact:
Novo Nordisk Inc.
800 Scudders Mill Road
Plainsboro, New Jersey 08536
1-800-727-6500
www.novonordisk-us.com

PATIENT INSTRUCTIONS FOR USE
NovoLog® Mix 70/30 FlexPen®
Read the following instructions carefully before you start using your NovoLog® Mix 70/30 FlexPen® and each time you get a refill. There may be new information. You should read the instructions even if you have used NovoLog® Mix 70/30 FlexPen® before.
NovoLog® Mix 70/30 FlexPen® is a disposable dial-a-dose insulin pen. You can select doses from 1 to 60 units in increments of 1 unit. NovoLog® Mix 70/30 FlexPen® is designed to be used with NovoFine® needles.
NovoLog® Mix 70/30 FlexPen® should not be used by people who are blind or have severe visual problems without the help of a person who has good eyesight and who is trained to use the NovoLog® Mix 70/30 FlexPen® the right way.

Getting ready
Make sure you have the following items:
• NovoLog® Mix 70/30 FlexPen®
• New NovoFine® needle
• Alcohol swab
[See figure above]

PREPARING YOUR NOVOLOG® MIX 70/30 FLEXPEN®
• Wash your hands with soap and water.
• Before you start to prepare your injection, check the label to make sure that you are taking the right type of insulin. This is especially important if you take more than 1 type of insulin. NovoLog® Mix 70/30 should look cloudy after mixing.
Before your first injection with a new NovoLog® Mix 70/30 FlexPen® you must mix the insulin:
A. Let the insulin reach room temperature before you use it. This makes it easier to mix.
Pull off the pen cap (see diagram A).

B. Roll the pen between your palms 10 times - it is important that the pen is kept horizontal (see diagram B).

C. Then gently move the pen up and down ten times between position **1** and **2** as shown, so the glass ball moves from one end of the cartridge to the other (see diagram C).

Repeat rolling and moving the pen until the liquid appears white and cloudy.
For every following injection move the pen up and down between positions 1 and 2 at least ten times until the liquid appears white and cloudy.
After mixing, complete all the following steps of the injection right away. If there is a delay, the insulin will need to be mixed again.
Wipe the rubber stopper with an alcohol swab.
△ Before you inject, there must be at least 12 units of insulin left in the cartridge to make sure the remaining insulin is evenly mixed. If there are less than 12 units left, use a new NovoLog® Mix 70/30 FlexPen®.

Attaching the needle
D. Remove the protective tab from a disposable needle. Screw the needle tightly onto your NovoLog® Mix 70/30 FlexPen®. It is important that the needle is put on straight (see diagram D).

Never place a disposable needle on your NovoLog® Mix 70/30 FlexPen® until you are ready to take your injection.
E. Pull off the big outer needle cap (see diagram E).

F. Pull off the inner needle cap and dispose of it (see diagram F).

△ Always use a new needle for each injection to help ensure sterility and prevent blocked needles.
△ Be careful not to bend or damage the needle before use.
△ To reduce the risk of a needle stick, **never put the inner needle cap back on the needle.**
Giving the airshot before each injection
Before each injection small amounts of air may collect in the cartridge during normal use. **To avoid injecting air and to make sure you take the right dose of insulin:**
G. Turn the dose selector to select 2 units (see diagram G).

2 units selected

H. Hold your NovoLog® Mix 70/30 FlexPen® with the needle pointing up. Tap the cartridge gently with your finger a few times to make any air bubbles collect at the top of the cartridge (see diagram H).

I. Keep the needle pointing upwards, press the push-button all the way in (see diagram I). The dose selector returns to 0.

A drop of insulin should appear at the needle tip. If not, change the needle and repeat the procedure no more than 6 times.
If you do not see a drop of insulin after 6 times, do not use the NovoLog® Mix 70/30 FlexPen® and contact Novo Nordisk at 1-800-727-6500.

A small air bubble may remain at the needle tip, but it will not be injected.
SELECTING YOUR DOSE
Check and make sure that the dose selector is set at 0.
J. Turn the dose selector to the number of units you need to inject. The pointer should line up with your dose.
The dose can be corrected either up or down by turning the dose selector in either direction until the correct dose lines up with the pointer (see diagram J). When turning the dose selector, be careful not to press the push-button as insulin will come out.
You cannot select a dose larger than the number of units left in the cartridge.
You will hear a click for every single unit dialed. Do not set the dose by counting the number of clicks you hear.

5 units selected

24 units selected

△ Do not use the cartridge scale printed on the cartridge to measure your dose of insulin.
GIVING THE INJECTION
Do the injection exactly as shown to you by your healthcare provider. Your healthcare provider should tell you if you need to pinch the skin before injecting. Wipe the skin with an alcohol swab and let the area dry.
K. Insert the needle into your skin.
Inject the dose by pressing the push-button all the way in until the 0 lines up with the pointer (see diagram K). Be careful only to push the button when injecting.
Turning the dose selector will not inject insulin.

L. Keep the needle in the skin for at least 6 seconds, and keep the push-button pressed all the way in until the needle has been pulled out from the skin (see diagram L). This will make sure that the full dose has been given.

You may see a drop of NovoLog® Mix 70/30 at the needle tip. This is normal and has no effect on the dose you just received. If blood appears after you take the needle out of your skin, press the injection site lightly with an alcohol swab. **Do not rub the area.**
After the injection
Do not recap the needle. Recapping can lead to a needle stick injury. Remove the needle from the NovoLog® Mix 70/30 FlexPen® after each injection. This helps to prevent infection, leakage of insulin, and will help to make sure you inject the right dose of insulin.
△ Put the needle and any empty NovoLog® Mix 70/30 FlexPen® or any used NovoLog® Mix 70/30 FlexPen® still containing insulin in a sharps container or some type of hard plastic or metal container with a screw top such as a detergent bottle or empty coffee can. These containers should be sealed and thrown away the right way. Check with your

healthcare provider about the right way to throw away used syringes and needles. There may be local or state laws about how to throw away used needles and syringes. Do not throw away used needles and syringes in household trash or recycling bins.

The NovoLog® Mix 70/30 FlexPen® prevents the cartridge from being completely emptied. It is designed to deliver 300 units.

M. Put the pen cap on the NovoLog® Mix 70/30 FlexPen® and store the NovoLog® Mix 70/30 FlexPen® without the needle attached (see diagram M).

FUNCTION CHECK

N. If your NovoLog® Mix 70/30 FlexPen® is not working the right way, follow the steps below:

- Screw on a new NovoFine® needle.
- Remove the big outer needle cap and the inner needle cap.
- Do an airshot as described in "Giving the airshot before each injection".
- Put the big outer needle cap onto the needle. Do not put on the inner needle cap.
- Turn the dose selector so the dose indicator window shows 20 units.
- Hold the NovoLog® Mix 70/30 FlexPen® so the needle is pointing down.
- Press the push-button all the way in.

The insulin should fill the lower part of the big outer needle cap (see diagram N). If NovoLog® Mix 70/30 FlexPen® has released too much or too little insulin, do the function check again. If the same problem happens again, do not use your NovoLog® Mix 70/30 FlexPen® and contact Novo Nordisk at 1-800-727-6500.

Maintenance

Your NovoLog® Mix 70/30 FlexPen® is designed to work accurately and safely. It must be handled with care. Avoid dropping your NovoLog® Mix 70/30 FlexPen® as it may damage it. If you are concerned that your NovoLog® Mix 70/30 FlexPen® is damaged, use a new one. You can clean the outside of your NovoLog® Mix 70/30 FlexPen® by wiping it with a damp cloth. Do not soak or wash your NovoLog® Mix 70/30 FlexPen® as it may damage it. Do not refill your NovoLog® Mix 70/30 FlexPen®.

Δ Remove the needle from the NovoLog® Mix 70/30 FlexPen® after each injection. This helps to ensure sterility, prevent leakage of insulin, and will help to make sure you inject the right dose of insulin for future injections.

Δ Be careful when handling used needles to avoid needle sticks and transfer of infectious diseases.

Δ Keep your NovoLog® Mix 70/30 FlexPen® and needles out of the reach of children.

Δ Use NovoLog® Mix 70/30 FlexPen® as directed to treat your diabetes. Needles and NovoLog® Mix 70/30 FlexPen® must not be shared.

Δ Always use a new needle for each injection.

Δ Novo Nordisk is not responsible for harm due to using this insulin pen with products not recommended by Novo Nordisk.

Δ As a precautionary measure, always carry a spare insulin delivery device in case your NovoLog® Mix 70/30 FlexPen® is lost or damaged.

Remember to keep the disposable NovoLog® Mix 70/30 FlexPen® with you. Do not leave it in a car or other location where it can get too hot or too cold.

Date of Issue: March 2013

Version: 9

Novo Nordisk®, NovoLog®, FlexPen®, and NovoFine® are registered trademarks of Novo Nordisk A/S.

NovoLog® Mix 70/30 is covered by US Patent Nos. 5,547,930, 5,618,913, 5,834,422, 5,840,680, 5,866,538 and other patents pending.

FlexPen® is covered by US Patent Nos. 6,582,404, 6,004,297, 6,235,004 and other patents pending.

© 2002-2013 Novo Nordisk

Manufactured by:
Novo Nordisk A/S
DK-2880 Bagsvaerd, Denmark
For information about NovoLog® Mix 70/30 contact:
Novo Nordisk Inc.
800 Scudders Mill Road
Plainsboro, New Jersey 08536
1-800-727-6500
www.novonordisk-us.com

VICTOZA®   ℞

[VIC-tow-za]
(liraglutide (rDNA origin) injection)
solution for subcutaneous use

HIGHLIGHTS OF PRESCRIBING INFORMATION

These highlights do not include all the information needed to use Victoza safely and effectively. See full prescribing information for Victoza.

Victoza® (liraglutide [rDNA origin] injection), solution for subcutaneous use

Initial U.S. Approval: 2010

> **WARNING: RISK OF THYROID C-CELL TUMORS**
> *See full prescribing information for complete boxed warning.*
> - **Liraglutide causes thyroid C-cell tumors at clinically relevant exposures in rodents. It is unknown whether Victoza causes thyroid C-cell tumors, including medullary thyroid carcinoma (MTC), in humans, as human relevance could not be determined by clinical or nonclinical studies (5.1).**
> - **Victoza is contraindicated in patients with a personal or family history of MTC or in patients with Multiple Endocrine Neoplasia syndrome type 2 (MEN 2) (5.1).**

——————RECENT MAJOR CHANGES——————

Indications and Usage:	
Important Limitations of Use (1.1)	04/2013
Warnings and Precautions:	
Pancreatitis (5.2)	04/2013

——————INDICATIONS AND USAGE——————

Victoza is a glucagon-like peptide-1 (GLP-1) receptor agonist indicated as an adjunct to diet and exercise to improve glycemic control in adults with type 2 diabetes mellitus (1).

Important Limitations of Use (1.1):

- Not recommended as first-line therapy for patients inadequately controlled on diet and exercise (5.1).
- Has not been studied in patients with a history of pancreatitis. Consider other antidiabetic therapies in patients with a history of pancreatitis (5.2).
- Not for treatment of type 1 diabetes mellitus or diabetic ketoacidosis.
- Has not been studied in combination with prandial insulin.

——————DOSAGE AND ADMINISTRATION——————

- Administer once daily at any time of day, independently of meals (2).
- Inject subcutaneously in the abdomen, thigh or upper arm (2).
- The injection site and timing can be changed without dose adjustment (2).
- Initiate at 0.6 mg per day for one week. This dose is intended to reduce gastrointestinal symptoms during initial titration, and is not effective for glycemic control. After one week, increase the dose to 1.2 mg. If the 1.2 mg dose does not result in acceptable glycemic control, the dose can be increased to 1.8 mg (2).

——————DOSAGE FORMS AND STRENGTHS——————

- Solution for subcutaneous injection, pre-filled, multi-dose pen that delivers doses of 0.6 mg, 1.2 mg, or 1.8 mg (6 mg/mL, 3 mL) (3).

——————CONTRAINDICATIONS——————

Do not use in patients with a personal or family history of medullary thyroid carcinoma or in patients with Multiple Endocrine Neoplasia syndrome type 2 (4).

Do not use if history of serious hypersensitivity to Victoza or any product components (4).

——————WARNINGS AND PRECAUTIONS——————

- Thyroid C-cell tumors in animals: Counsel patients regarding the risk of medullary thyroid carcinoma and the symptoms of thyroid tumors (5.1).
- Pancreatitis: Postmarketing reports, including fatal and non-fatal hemorrhagic or necrotizing pancreatitis. Discon-

---

tinue promptly if pancreatitis is suspected. Do not restart if pancreatitis is confirmed. Consider other antidiabetic therapies in patients with a history of pancreatitis (5.2).

- Serious hypoglycemia: Can occur when Victoza is used with an insulin secretagogue (e.g. a sulfonylurea) or insulin. Consider lowering the dose of the insulin secretagogue or insulin to reduce the risk of hypoglycemia (5.3).
- Renal Impairment: Has been reported postmarketing, usually in association with nausea, vomiting, diarrhea, or dehydration which may sometimes require hemodialysis. Use caution when initiating or escalating doses of Victoza in patients with renal impairment (5.4).
- Hypersensitivity: Postmarketing reports of serious hypersensitivity reactions (e.g., anaphylactic reactions and angioedema). The patient should discontinue Victoza and other suspect medications and promptly seek medical advice (5.5).
- Macrovascular outcomes: There have been no studies establishing conclusive evidence of macrovascular risk reduction with Victoza or any other antidiabetic drug (5.6).

——————ADVERSE REACTIONS——————

- The most common adverse reactions, reported in ≥5% of patients treated with Victoza and more commonly than in patients treated with placebo, are: headache, nausea, diarrhea and anti-liraglutide antibody formation (6).
- Immunogenicity-related events, including urticaria, were more common among Victoza-treated patients (0.8%) than among comparator-treated patients (0.4%) in clinical trials (6).

To report SUSPECTED ADVERSE REACTIONS, contact Novo Nordisk Inc. at 1-877-484-2869 or FDA at 1-800-FDA-1088 or www.fda.gov/medwatch.

——————DRUG INTERACTIONS——————

- Victoza delays gastric emptying. May impact absorption of concomitantly administered oral medications. Use caution (7).

——————USE IN SPECIFIC POPULATIONS——————

- Limited data in patients with renal or hepatic impairment. (8.6, 8.7).

See 17 for PATIENT COUNSELING INFORMATION and Medication Guide

Revised: 04/2013

FULL PRESCRIBING INFORMATION: CONTENTS*

WARNING: RISK OF THYROID C-CELL TUMORS

17.6   Never Share a Victoza Pen Between Patients
17.7   Instructions
17.8   Laboratory Tests
* Sections or subsections omitted from the full prescribing information are not listed

FULL PRESCRIBING INFORMATION

WARNING: RISK OF THYROID C-CELL TUMORS

Liraglutide causes dose-dependent and treatment-duration-dependent thyroid C-cell tumors at clinically relevant exposures in both genders of rats and mice. It is unknown whether Victoza causes thyroid C-cell tumors, including medullary thyroid carcinoma (MTC), in humans, as human relevance could not be ruled out by clinical or nonclinical studies. Victoza is contraindicated in patients with a personal or family history of MTC and in patients with Multiple Endocrine Neoplasia syndrome type 2 (MEN 2). Based on the findings in rodents, monitoring with serum calcitonin or thyroid ultrasound was performed during clinical trials, but this may have increased the number of unnecessary thyroid surgeries. It is unknown whether monitoring with serum calcitonin or thyroid ultrasound will mitigate human risk of thyroid C-cell tumors. Patients should be counseled regarding the risk and symptoms of thyroid tumors [see Contraindications (4), Warnings and Precautions (5.1) and Nonclinical Toxicology (13.1)].

1   INDICATIONS AND USAGE

Victoza is indicated as an adjunct to diet and exercise to improve glycemic control in adults with type 2 diabetes mellitus.

1.1   Important Limitations of Use

• Because of the uncertain relevance of the rodent thyroid C-cell tumor findings to humans, prescribe Victoza only to patients for whom the potential benefits are considered to outweigh the potential risk. Victoza is not recommended as first-line therapy for patients who have inadequate glycemic control on diet and exercise.
• Based on spontaneous postmarketing reports, acute pancreatitis, including fatal and non-fatal hemorrhagic or necrotizing pancreatitis has been observed in patients treated with Victoza. Victoza has not been studied in patients with a history of pancreatitis. It is unknown whether patients with a history of pancreatitis are at increased risk for pancreatitis while using Victoza. Other antidiabetic therapies should be considered in patients with a history of pancreatitis.
• Victoza is not a substitute for insulin. Victoza should not be used in patients with type 1 diabetes mellitus or for the treatment of diabetic ketoacidosis, as it would not be effective in these settings.
• The concurrent use of Victoza and prandial insulin has not been studied.

2   DOSAGE AND ADMINISTRATION

Victoza can be administered once daily at any time of day, independently of meals, and can be injected subcutaneously in the abdomen, thigh or upper arm. The injection site and timing can be changed without dose adjustment.
For all patients, Victoza should be initiated with a dose of 0.6 mg per day for one week. The 0.6 mg dose is a starting dose intended to reduce gastrointestinal symptoms during initial titration, and is not effective for glycemic control. After one week at 0.6 mg per day, the dose should be increased to 1.2 mg. If the 1.2 mg dose does not result in acceptable glycemic control, the dose can be increased to 1.8 mg.
When initiating Victoza, consider reducing the dose of concomitantly administered insulin secretagogues (such as sulfonylureas) to reduce the risk of hypoglycemia [see Warnings and Precautions (5.3) and Adverse Reactions (6)].
When using Victoza with insulin, administer as separate injections. Never mix. It is acceptable to inject Victoza and insulin in the same body region but the injections should not be adjacent to each other.
Victoza solution should be inspected prior to each injection, and the solution should be used only if it is clear, colorless, and contains no particles.
If a dose is missed, the once-daily regimen should be resumed as prescribed with the next scheduled dose. An extra dose or increase in dose should not be taken to make-up for the missed dose.
Based on the elimination half-life, patients should be advised to reinitiate Victoza at 0.6 mg if more than 3 days have elapsed since the last Victoza dose. This approach will mitigate any gastrointestinal symptoms associated with reinitiation of treatment. Upon reinitiation, Victoza should be titrated at the discretion of the prescribing healthcare provider.

3   DOSAGE FORMS AND STRENGTHS

Solution for subcutaneous injection, pre-filled, multi-dose pen that delivers doses of 0.6 mg, 1.2 mg, or 1.8 mg (6 mg/mL, 3 mL).

4   CONTRAINDICATIONS

Do not use in patients with a personal or family history of medullary thyroid carcinoma (MTC) or in patients with Multiple Endocrine Neoplasia syndrome type 2 (MEN 2).
Do not use in patients with a prior serious hypersensitivity reaction to Victoza or to any of the product components.

5   WARNINGS AND PRECAUTIONS

5.1   Risk of Thyroid C-cell Tumors

Liraglutide causes dose-dependent and treatment-duration-dependent thyroid C-cell tumors (adenomas and/or carcinomas) at clinically relevant exposures in both genders of rats and mice [see Nonclinical Toxicology (13.1)]. Malignant thyroid C-cell carcinomas were detected in rats and mice. A statistically significant increase in cancer was observed in rats receiving liraglutide at 8-times clinical exposure compared to controls. It is unknown whether Victoza will cause thyroid C-cell tumors, including medullary thyroid carcinoma (MTC), in humans, as the human relevance of liraglutide-induced rodent thyroid C-cell tumors could not be determined by clinical or nonclinical studies [see Boxed Warning, Contraindications (4)].
In the clinical trials, there have been 6 reported cases of thyroid C-cell hyperplasia among Victoza-treated patients and 2 cases in comparator-treated patients (1.3 vs. 1.0 cases per 1000 patient-years). One comparator-treated patient with MTC had pre-treatment serum calcitonin concentrations >1000 ng/L suggesting pre-existing disease. All of these cases were diagnosed after thyroidectomy, which was prompted by abnormal results on routine, protocol-specified measurements of serum calcitonin. Five of the six Victoza-treated patients had elevated calcitonin concentrations at baseline and throughout the trial. One Victoza and one non-Victoza-treated patient developed elevated calcitonin concentrations while on treatment.
Calcitonin, a biological marker of MTC, was measured throughout the clinical development program. The serum calcitonin assay used in the Victoza clinical trials had a lower limit of quantification (LLOQ) of 0.7 ng/L and the upper limit of the reference range was 5.0 ng/L for women and 8.4 ng/L for men. At Weeks 26 and 52 in the clinical trials, adjusted mean serum calcitonin concentrations were higher in Victoza-treated patients compared to placebo-treated patients but not compared to patients receiving active comparator. At these timepoints, the adjusted mean serum calcitonin values (~ 1.0 ng/L) were just above the LLOQ with between-group differences in adjusted mean serum calcitonin values of approximately 0.1 ng/L or less. Among patients with pre-treatment serum calcitonin below the upper limit of the reference range, shifts to above the upper limit of the reference range which persisted in subsequent measurements occurred most frequently among patients treated with Victoza 1.8 mg/day. In trials with on-treatment serum calcitonin measurements out to 5-6 months, 1.9% of patients treated with Victoza 1.8 mg/day developed new and persistent calcitonin elevations above the upper limit of the reference range compared to 0.8-1.1% of patients treated with control medication or the 0.6 and 1.2 mg doses of Victoza. In trials with on-treatment serum calcitonin measurements out to 12 months, 1.3% of patients treated with Victoza 1.8 mg/day had new and persistent elevations of calcitonin from below or within the reference range to above the upper limit of the reference range, compared to 0.6%, 0% and 1.0% of patients treated with Victoza 1.2 mg, placebo and active control, respectively. Otherwise, Victoza did not produce consistent dose-dependent or time-dependent increases in serum calcitonin.
Patients with MTC usually have calcitonin values >50 ng/L. In Victoza clinical trials, among patients with pre-treatment serum calcitonin <50 ng/L, one Victoza-treated patient and no comparator-treated patients developed serum calcitonin >50 ng/L. The Victoza-treated patient who developed serum calcitonin >50 ng/L had an elevated pre-treatment serum calcitonin of 10.7 ng/L that increased to 30.7 ng/L at Week 12 and 53.5 ng/L at the end of the 6-month trial. Follow-up serum calcitonin was 22.3 ng/L more than 2.5 years after the last dose of Victoza. The largest increase in serum calcitonin in a comparator-treated patient was seen with glimepiride in a patient whose serum calcitonin increased from 19.3 ng/L at baseline to 44.8 ng/L at Week 65 and 38.1 ng/L at Week 104. Among patients who began with serum calcitonin <20 ng/L, calcitonin elevations to >20 ng/L occurred in 0.7% of Victoza-treated patients, 0.3% of placebo-treated patients, and 0.5% of active-comparator-treated patients, with an incidence of 1.1% among patients treated with 1.8 mg/day of Victoza. The clinical significance of these findings is unknown.
Counsel patients regarding the risk for MTC and the symptoms of thyroid tumors (e.g. a mass in the neck, dysphagia,

dyspnea or persistent hoarseness). It is unknown whether monitoring with serum calcitonin or thyroid ultrasound will mitigate the potential risk of MTC, and such monitoring may increase the risk of unnecessary procedures, due to low test specificity for serum calcitonin and a high background incidence of thyroid disease. Patients with thyroid nodules noted on physical examination or neck imaging obtained for other reasons should be referred to an endocrinologist for further evaluation. Although routine monitoring of serum calcitonin is of uncertain value in patients treated with Victoza, if serum calcitonin is measured and found to be elevated, the patient should be referred to an endocrinologist for further evaluation.

5.2   Pancreatitis

Based on spontaneous postmarketing reports, acute pancreatitis, including fatal and non-fatal hemorrhagic or necrotizing pancreatitis, has been observed in patients treated with Victoza. After initiation of Victoza, observe patients carefully for signs and symptoms of pancreatitis (including persistent severe abdominal pain, sometimes radiating to the back and which may or may not be accompanied by vomiting). If pancreatitis is suspected, Victoza should promptly be discontinued and appropriate management should be initiated. If pancreatitis is confirmed, Victoza should not be restarted. Consider antidiabetic therapies other than Victoza in patients with a history of pancreatitis.

In clinical trials of Victoza, there have been 13 cases of pancreatitis among Victoza-treated patients and 1 case in a comparator (glimepiride) treated patient (2.7 vs. 0.5 cases per 1000 patient-years). Nine of the 13 cases with Victoza were reported as acute pancreatitis and four were reported as chronic pancreatitis. In one case in a Victoza-treated patient, pancreatitis, with necrosis, was observed and led to death; however clinical causality could not be established. Some patients had other risk factors for pancreatitis, such as a history of cholelithiasis or alcohol abuse.

5.3   Use with Medications Known to Cause Hypoglycemia

Patients receiving Victoza in combination with an insulin secretagogue (e.g., sulfonylurea) or insulin may have an increased risk of hypoglycemia. The risk of hypoglycemia may be lowered by a reduction in the dose of sulfonylurea (or other concomitantly administered insulin secretagogues) or insulin [see Adverse Reactions (6.1)].

5.4   Renal Impairment

Victoza has not been found to be directly nephrotoxic in animal studies or clinical trials. There have been postmarketing reports of acute renal failure and worsening of chronic renal failure, which may sometimes require hemodialysis in Victoza-treated patients [see Adverse Reactions (6.2)]. Some of these events were reported in patients without known underlying renal disease. A majority of the reported events occurred in patients who had experienced nausea, vomiting, diarrhea, or dehydration [see Adverse Reactions (6.1)]. Some of the reported events occurred in patients receiving one or more medications known to affect renal function or hydration status. Altered renal function has been reversed in many of the reported cases with supportive treatment and discontinuation of potentially causative agents, including Victoza. Use caution when initiating or escalating doses of Victoza in patients with renal impairment [see Use in Specific Populations (8.6)].

5.5   Hypersensitivity Reactions

There have been postmarketing reports of serious hypersensitivity reactions (e.g., anaphylactic reactions and angioedema) in patients treated with Victoza. If a hypersensitivity reaction occurs, the patient should discontinue Victoza and other suspect medications and promptly seek medical advice.
Angioedema has also been reported with other GLP-1 receptor agonists. Use caution in a patient with a history of angioedema with another GLP-1 receptor agonist because it is unknown whether such patients will be predisposed to angioedema with Victoza.

5.6   Macrovascular Outcomes

There have been no clinical studies establishing conclusive evidence of macrovascular risk reduction with Victoza or any other antidiabetic drug.

6   ADVERSE REACTIONS

6.1   Clinical Trials Experience

Because clinical trials are conducted under widely varying conditions, adverse reaction rates observed in the clinical trials of a drug cannot be directly compared to rates in the clinical trials of another drug and may not reflect the rates observed in practice.
The safety of Victoza has been evaluated in 8 clinical trials [see Clinical Studies (14)]:
• A double-blind 52-week monotherapy trial compared Victoza 1.2 mg daily, Victoza 1.8 mg daily, and glimepiride 8 mg daily.
• A double-blind 26 week add-on to metformin trial compared Victoza 0.6 mg once-daily, Victoza 1.2 mg once-daily, Victoza 1.8 mg once-daily, placebo, and glimepiride 4 mg once-daily.

Table 2 Adverse reactions reported in ≥5% of Victoza-treated patients and occurring more frequently with Victoza compared to placebo: 26-week combination therapy trials

Add-on to Metformin Trial

	All Victoza + Metformin N = 724	Placebo + Metformin N = 121	Glimepiride + Metformin N = 242
Adverse Reaction	(%)	(%)	(%)
Nausea	15.2	4.1	3.3
Diarrhea	10.9	4.1	3.7
Headache	9.0	6.6	9.5
Vomiting	6.5	0.8	0.4

Add-on to Glimepiride Trial

	All Victoza + Glimepiride N = 695	Placebo + Glimepiride N = 114	Rosiglitazone + Glimepiride N = 231
Adverse Reaction	(%)	(%)	(%)
Nausea	7.5	1.8	2.6
Diarrhea	7.2	1.8	2.2
Constipation	5.3	0.9	1.7
Dyspepsia	5.2	0.9	2.6

Add-on to Metformin + Glimepiride

	Victoza 1.8 + Metformin + Glimepiride N = 230	Placebo + Metformin + Glimepiride N = 114	Glargine + Metformin + Glimepiride N = 232
Adverse Reaction	(%)	(%)	(%)
Nausea	13.9	3.5	1.3
Diarrhea	10.0	5.3	1.3
Headache	9.6	7.9	5.6
Dyspepsia	6.5	0.9	1.7
Vomiting	6.5	3.5	0.4

Add-on to Metformin + Rosiglitazone

	All Victoza + Metformin + Rosiglitazone N = 355	Placebo + Metformin + Rosiglitazone N = 175
Adverse Reaction	(%)	(%)
Nausea	34.6	8.6
Diarrhea	14.1	6.3
Vomiting	12.4	2.9
Headache	8.2	4.6
Constipation	5.1	1.1

• A double-blind 26 week add-on to glimepiride trial compared Victoza 0.6 mg daily, Victoza 1.2 mg once-daily, Victoza 1.8 mg once-daily, placebo, and rosiglitazone 4 mg once-daily.
• A 26 week add-on to metformin + glimepiride trial, compared double-blind Victoza 1.8 mg once-daily, double-blind placebo, and open-label insulin glargine once-daily.
• A double-blind 26-week add-on to metformin + rosiglitazone trial compared Victoza 1.2 mg once-daily, Victoza 1.8 mg once-daily and placebo.
• An open-label 26-week add-on to metformin and/or sulfonylurea trial compared Victoza 1.8 mg once-daily and exenatide 10 mcg twice-daily.
• An open-label 26-week add-on to metformin trial compared Victoza 1.2 mg once-daily, Victoza 1.8 mg once-daily, and sitagliptin 100 mg once-daily.
• An open-label 26-week trial compared insulin detemir as add-on to Victoza 1.8 mg + metformin to continued treatment with Victoza + metformin alone.

Withdrawals
The incidence of withdrawal due to adverse events was 7.8% for Victoza-treated patients and 3.4% for comparator-treated patients in the five double-blind controlled trials of 26 weeks duration or longer. This difference was driven by withdrawals due to gastrointestinal adverse reactions, which occurred in 5.0% of Victoza-treated patients and 0.5% of comparator-treated patients. In these five trials, the most common adverse reactions leading to withdrawal for Victoza-treated patients were nausea (2.8% versus 0% for comparator) and vomiting (1.5% versus 0.1% for comparator). Withdrawal due to gastrointestinal adverse events mainly occurred during the first 2-3 months of the trials.
Common adverse reactions
Tables 1, 2, 3 and 4 summarize common adverse reactions (hypoglycemia is discussed separately) reported in seven of the eight controlled trials of 26 weeks duration or longer. Most of these adverse reactions were gastrointestinal in nature.
In the five double-blind clinical trials of 26 weeks duration or longer, gastrointestinal adverse reactions were reported in 41% of Victoza-treated patients and were dose-related. Gastrointestinal adverse reactions occurred in 17% of comparator-treated patients. Common adverse reactions that occurred at a higher incidence among Victoza-treated patients included nausea, vomiting, diarrhea, dyspepsia and constipation.

In the five double-blind and three open-label clinical trials of 26 weeks duration or longer, the percentage of patients who reported nausea declined over time. In the five double-blind trials approximately 13% of Victoza-treated patients and 2% of comparator-treated patients reported nausea during the first 2 weeks of treatment.
In the 26-week open-label trial comparing Victoza to exenatide, both in combination with metformin and/or sulfonylurea, gastrointestinal adverse reactions were reported at a similar incidence in the Victoza and exenatide treatment groups (Table 3).
In the 26-week open-label trial comparing Victoza 1.2 mg, Victoza 1.8 mg and sitagliptin 100 mg, all in combination with metformin, gastrointestinal adverse reactions were reported at a higher incidence with Victoza than sitagliptin (Table 4).
In the remaining 26-week trial, all patients received Victoza 1.8 mg + metformin during a 12-week run-in period. During the run-in period, 167 patients (17% of enrolled total) withdrew from the trial: 76 (46% of withdrawals) of these patients doing so because of gastrointestinal adverse reactions and 15 (9% of withdrawals) doing so due to other adverse events. Only those patients who completed the run-in period with inadequate glycemic control were randomized to 26 weeks of add-on therapy with insulin detemir or continued, unchanged treatment with Victoza 1.8 mg + metformin. During this randomized 26-week period, diarrhea was the only adverse reaction reported in ≥5% of patients treated with Victoza 1.8 mg + metformin + insulin detemir (11.7%) and greater than in patients treated with Victoza 1.8 mg and metformin alone (6.9%).

Table 1 Adverse reactions reported in ≥5% of Victoza-treated patients in a 52-week monotherapy trial

	All Victoza N = 497	Glimepiride N = 248
Adverse Reaction	(%)	(%)
Nausea	28.4	8.5
Diarrhea	17.1	8.9
Vomiting	10.9	3.6
Constipation	9.9	4.8
Headache	9.1	9.3

[See table 2 above]

Table 3 Adverse Reactions reported in ≥5% of Victoza-treated patients in a 26-Week Open-Label Trial versus Exenatide

	Victoza 1.8 mg once daily + metformin and/or sulfonylurea N = 235	Exenatide 10 mcg twice daily + metformin and/or sulfonylurea N = 232
Adverse Reaction	(%)	(%)
Nausea	25.5	28.0
Diarrhea	12.3	12.1
Headache	8.9	10.3
Dyspepsia	8.9	4.7
Vomiting	6.0	9.9
Constipation	5.1	2.6

Table 4 Adverse Reactions in ≥5% of Victoza-treated patients in a 26-Week Open-Label Trial versus Sitagliptin

	All Victoza + metformin N = 439	Sitagliptin 100 mg/day + metformin N = 219
Adverse Reaction	(%)	(%)
Nausea	23.9	4.6
Headache	10.3	10.0
Diarrhea	9.3	4.6
Vomiting	8.7	4.1

Immunogenicity

Consistent with the potentially immunogenic properties of protein and peptide pharmaceuticals, patients treated with Victoza may develop anti-liraglutide antibodies. Approximately 50-70% of Victoza-treated patients in the five double-blind clinical trials of 26 weeks duration or longer were tested for the presence of anti-liraglutide antibodies at the end of treatment. Low titers (concentrations not requiring dilution of serum) of anti-liraglutide antibodies were detected in 8.6% of these Victoza-treated patients. Sampling was not performed uniformly across all patients in the clinical trials, and this may have resulted in an underestimate of the actual percentage of patients who developed antibodies. Cross-reacting anti-liraglutide antibodies to native glucagon-like peptide-1 (GLP-1) occurred in 6.9% of the Victoza-treated patients in the double-blind 52-week monotherapy trial and in 4.8% of the Victoza-treated patients in the double-blind 26-week add-on combination therapy trials. These cross-reacting antibodies were not tested for neutralizing effect against native GLP-1, and thus the potential for clinically significant neutralization of native GLP-1 was not assessed. Antibodies that had a neutralizing effect on liraglutide in an *in vitro* assay occurred in 2.3% of the Victoza-treated patients in the double-blind 52-week monotherapy trial and in 1.0% of the Victoza-treated patients in the double-blind 26-week add-on combination therapy trials.

Among Victoza-treated patients who developed anti-liraglutide antibodies, the most common category of adverse events was that of infections, which occurred among 40% of these patients compared to 36%, 34% and 35% of antibody-negative Victoza-treated, placebo-treated and active-control-treated patients, respectively. The specific infections which occurred with greater frequency among Victoza-treated antibody-positive patients were primarily nonserious upper respiratory tract infections, which occurred among 11% of Victoza-treated antibody-positive patients; and among 7%, 7% and 5% of antibody-negative Victoza-treated, placebo-treated and active-control-treated patients, respectively. Among Victoza-treated antibody-negative patients, the most common category of adverse events was that of gastrointestinal events, which occurred in 43%, 18% and 19% of antibody-negative Victoza-treated, placebo-treated and active-control-treated patients, respectively. Antibody formation was not associated with reduced efficacy of Victoza when comparing mean HbA$_{1c}$ of all antibody-positive and all antibody-negative patients. However, the 3 patients with the highest titers of anti-liraglutide antibodies had no reduction in HbA$_{1c}$ with Victoza treatment.

In the five double-blind clinical trials of Victoza, events from a composite of adverse events potentially related to immunogenicity (e.g. urticaria, angioedema) occurred among 0.8% of Victoza-treated patients and among 0.4% of comparator-treated patients. Urticaria accounted for approximately one-half of the events in this composite for Victoza-treated patients. Patients who developed anti-liraglutide antibodies were not more likely to develop events from the immunogenicity events composite than were patients who did not develop anti-liraglutide antibodies.

Injection site reactions

Injection site reactions (e.g., injection site rash, erythema) were reported in approximately 2% of Victoza-treated patients in the five double-blind clinical trials of at least 26 weeks duration. Less than 0.2% of Victoza-treated patients discontinued due to injection site reactions.

Papillary thyroid carcinoma

In clinical trials of Victoza, there were 7 reported cases of papillary thyroid carcinoma in patients treated with Victoza and 1 case in a comparator-treated patient (1.5 vs. 0.5 cases per 1000 patient-years). Most of these papillary thyroid carcinomas were <1 cm in greatest diameter and were diagnosed in surgical pathology specimens after thyroidectomy prompted by findings on protocol-specified screening with serum calcitonin or thyroid ultrasound.

Hypoglycemia

In the eight clinical trials of at least 26 weeks duration, hypoglycemia requiring the assistance of another person for treatment occurred in 11 Victoza-treated patients (2.3 cases per 1000 patient-years) and in two exenatide-treated patients. Of these 11 Victoza-treated patients, six patients were concomitantly using metformin and a sulfonylurea, one was concomitantly using a sulfonylurea, two were concomitantly using metformin (blood glucose values were 65 and 94 mg/dL) and two were using Victoza as monotherapy (one of these patients was undergoing an intravenous glucose tolerance test and the other was receiving insulin as treatment during a hospital stay). For these two patients on Victoza monotherapy, the insulin treatment was the likely explanation for the hypoglycemia.

In the 26-week open-label trial comparing Victoza to sitagliptin, the incidence of hypoglycemic events defined as symptoms accompanied by a fingerstick glucose <56 mg/dL was comparable among the treatment groups (approximately 5%).

Table 5 Incidence (%) and Rate (episodes/patient year) of Hypoglycemia in the 52-Week Monotherapy Trial and in the 26-Week Combination Therapy Trials

	Victoza Treatment	Active Comparator	Placebo Comparator
Monotherapy	**Victoza (N = 497)**	**Glimepiride (N = 248)**	**None**
Patient not able to self-treat	0	0	-
Patient able to self-treat	9.7 (0.24)	25.0 (1.66)	-
Not classified	1.2 (0.03)	2.4 (0.04)	-
Add-on to Metformin	**Victoza + Metformin (N = 724)**	**Glimepiride + Metformin (N = 242)**	**Placebo + Metformin (N = 121)**
Patient not able to self-treat	0.1 (0.001)	0	0
Patient able to self-treat	3.6 (0.05)	22.3 (0.87)	2.5 (0.06)
Add-on to Victoza + Metformin	**Insulin detemir + Victoza + Metformin (N = 163)**	**Continued Victoza + Metformin alone (N = 158*)**	**None**
Patient not able to self-treat	0	0	-
Patient able to self-treat	9.2 (0.29)	1.3 (0.03)	-
Add-on to Glimepiride	**Victoza + Glimepiride (N = 695)**	**Rosiglitazone + Glimepiride (N = 231)**	**Placebo + Glimepiride (N = 114)**
Patient not able to self-treat	0.1 (0.003)	0	0
Patient able to self-treat	7.5 (0.38)	4.3 (0.12)	2.6 (0.17)
Not classified	0.9 (0.05)	0.9 (0.02)	0
Add-on to Metformin + Rosiglitazone	**Victoza + Metformin + Rosiglitazone (N = 355)**	**None**	**Placebo + Metformin + Rosiglitazone (N = 175)**
Patient not able to self-treat	0	-	0
Patient able to self-treat	7.9 (0.49)	-	4.6 (0.15)
Not classified	0.6 (0.01)	-	1.1 (0.03)
Add-on to Metformin + Glimepiride	**Victoza + Metformin + Glimepiride (N = 230)**	**Insulin glargine + Metformin + Glimepiride (N = 232)**	**Placebo + Metformin + Glimepiride (N = 114)**
Patient not able to self-treat	2.2 (0.06)	0	0
Patient able to self-treat	27.4 (1.16)	28.9 (1.29)	16.7 (0.95)
Not classified	0	1.7 (0.04)	0

* One patient is an outlier and was excluded due to 25 hypoglycemic episodes that the patient was able to self-treat. This patient had a history of frequent hypoglycemia prior to the study.

[See table 5 above]

In a pooled analysis of clinical trials, the incidence rate (per 1,000 patient-years) for malignant neoplasms (based on investigator-reported events, medical history, pathology reports, and surgical reports from both blinded and open-label study periods) was 10.9 for Victoza, 6.3 for placebo, and 7.2 for active comparator. After excluding papillary thyroid carcinoma events *[see Adverse Reactions (6.1)]*, no particular cancer cell type predominated. Seven malignant neoplasm events were reported beyond 1 year of exposure to study medication, six events among Victoza-treated patients (4 colon, 1 prostate and 1 nasopharyngeal), no events with placebo and one event with active comparator (colon). Causality has not been established.

Laboratory Tests

In the five clinical trials of at least 26 weeks duration, mildly elevated serum bilirubin concentrations (elevations to no more than twice the upper limit of the reference range) occurred in 4.0% of Victoza-treated patients, 2.1% of placebo-treated patients and 3.5% of active-comparator-treated patients. This finding was not accompanied by abnormalities in other liver tests. The significance of this isolated finding is unknown.

Vital signs

Victoza did not have adverse effects on blood pressure. Mean increases from baseline in heart rate of 2 to 3 beats per minute have been observed with Victoza compared to placebo. The long-term clinical effects of the increase in pulse rate have not been established *[see Warnings and Precautions (5.6)]*.

6.2   Post-Marketing Experience

The following additional adverse reactions have been reported during post-approval use of Victoza. Because these events are reported voluntarily from a population of uncertain size, it is generally not possible to reliably estimate their frequency or establish a causal relationship to drug exposure.

- Dehydration resulting from nausea, vomiting and diarrhea. *[see Warnings and Precautions (5.4) and Patient Counseling Information (17.3)]*
- Increased serum creatinine, acute renal failure or worsening of chronic renal failure, sometimes requiring hemodialysis. *[see Warnings and Precautions (5.4) and Patient Counseling Information (17.3)]*
- Angioedema and anaphylactic reactions. *[see Contraindications (4), Warnings and Precautions (5.5), Patient counseling Information (17.5)]*
- Allergic reactions: rash and pruritus
- Acute pancreatitis, hemorrhagic and necrotizing pancreatitis sometimes resulting in death *[see Warnings and Precautions (5.2)]*

7   DRUG INTERACTIONS

7.1   Oral Medications

Victoza causes a delay of gastric emptying, and thereby has the potential to impact the absorption of concomitantly administered oral medications. In clinical pharmacology trials, Victoza did not affect the absorption of the tested orally administered medications to any clinically relevant degree. Nonetheless, caution should be exercised when oral medications are concomitantly administered with Victoza.

8 USE IN SPECIFIC POPULATIONS

8.1 Pregnancy
Pregnancy Category C.
There are no adequate and well-controlled studies of Victoza in pregnant women. Victoza should be used during pregnancy only if the potential benefit justifies the potential risk to the fetus. Liraglutide has been shown to be teratogenic in rats at or above 0.8 times the human systemic exposures resulting from the maximum recommended human dose (MRHD) of 1.8 mg/day based on plasma area under the time-concentration curve (AUC). Liraglutide has been shown to cause reduced growth and increased total major abnormalities in rabbits at systemic exposures below human exposure at the MRHD based on plasma AUC.
Female rats given subcutaneous doses of 0.1, 0.25 and 1.0 mg/kg/day liraglutide beginning 2 weeks before mating through gestation day 17 had estimated systemic exposures 0.8-, 3-, and 11-times the human exposure at the MRHD based on plasma AUC comparison. The number of early embryonic deaths in the 1 mg/kg/day group increased slightly. Fetal abnormalities and variations in kidneys and blood vessels, irregular ossification of the skull, and a more complete state of ossification occurred at all doses. Mottled liver and minimally kinked ribs occurred at the highest dose. The incidence of fetal malformations in liraglutide-treated groups exceeding concurrent and historical controls were misshapen oropharynx and/or narrowed opening into larynx at 0.1 mg/kg/day and umbilical hernia at 0.1 and 0.25 mg/kg/day.
Pregnant rabbits given subcutaneous doses of 0.01, 0.025 and 0.05 mg/kg/day liraglutide from gestation day 6 through day 18 inclusive, had estimated systemic exposures less than the human exposure at the MRHD of 1.8 mg/day at all doses, based on plasma AUC. Liraglutide decreased fetal weight and dose-dependently increased the incidence of total major fetal abnormalities at all doses. The incidence of malformations exceeded concurrent and historical controls at 0.01 mg/kg/day (kidneys, scapula), ≥ 0.01 mg/kg/day (eyes, forelimb), 0.025 mg/kg/day (brain, tail and sacral vertebrae, major blood vessels and heart, umbilicus), ≥ 0.025 mg/kg/day (sternum) and at 0.05 mg/kg/day (parietal bones, major blood vessels). Irregular ossification and/or skeletal abnormalities occurred in the skull and jaw, vertebrae and ribs, sternum, pelvis, tail, and scapula; and dose-dependent minor skeletal variations were observed. Visceral abnormalities occurred in blood vessels, lung, liver, and esophagus. Bilobed or bifurcated gallbladder was seen in all treatment groups, but not in the control group.
In pregnant female rats given subcutaneous doses of 0.1, 0.25 and 1.0 mg/kg/day liraglutide from gestation day 6 through weaning or termination of nursing on lactation day 24, estimated systemic exposures were 0.8-, 3-, and 11-times human exposure at the MRHD of 1.8 mg/day, based on plasma AUC. A slight delay in parturition was observed in the majority of treated rats. Group mean body weight of neonatal rats from liraglutide-treated dams was lower than neonatal rats from control group dams. Bloody scabs and agitated behavior occurred in male rats descended from dams treated with 1 mg/kg/day liraglutide. Group mean body weight from birth to postpartum day 14 trended lower in F_2 generation rats descended from liraglutide-treated rats compared to F_2 generation rats descended from controls, but differences did not reach statistical significance for any group.

8.3 Nursing Mothers
It is not known whether Victoza is excreted in human milk. Because many drugs are excreted in human milk and because of the potential for tumorigenicity shown for liraglutide in animal studies, a decision should be made whether to discontinue nursing or to discontinue Victoza, taking into account the importance of the drug to the mother. In lactating rats, liraglutide was excreted unchanged in milk at concentrations approximately 50% of maternal plasma concentrations.

8.4 Pediatric Use
Safety and effectiveness of Victoza have not been established in pediatric patients. Victoza is not recommended for use in pediatric patients.

8.5 Geriatric Use
In the Victoza clinical trials, a total of 797 (20%) of the patients were 65 years of age and over and 113 (2.8%) were 75 years of age and over. No overall differences in safety or effectiveness were observed between these patients and younger patients, but greater sensitivity of some older individuals cannot be ruled out.

8.6 Renal Impairment
There is limited experience with Victoza in patients with mild, moderate, and severe renal impairment, including

end-stage renal disease. However, there have been post-marketing reports of acute renal failure and worsening of chronic renal failure, which may sometimes require hemodialysis [see Warnings and Precautions (5.4) and Adverse Reactions (6.2)]. Victoza should be used with caution in this patient population. No dose adjustment of Victoza is recommended for patients with renal impairment [see Clinical Pharmacology (12.3)].

8.7 Hepatic Impairment
There is limited experience in patients with mild, moderate or severe hepatic impairment. Therefore, Victoza should be used with caution in this patient population. No dose adjustment of Victoza is recommended for patients with hepatic impairment [see Clinical Pharmacology (12.3)].

8.8 Gastroparesis
Victoza slows gastric emptying. Victoza has not been studied in patients with pre-existing gastroparesis.

10 OVERDOSAGE
Overdoses have been reported in clinical trials and post-marketing use of Victoza. Effects have included severe nausea and severe vomiting. In the event of overdosage, appropriate supportive treatment should be initiated according to the patient's clinical signs and symptoms.

11 DESCRIPTION
Victoza contains liraglutide, an analog of human GLP-1 and acts as a GLP-1 receptor agonist. The peptide precursor of liraglutide, produced by a process that includes expression of recombinant DNA in Saccharomyces cerevisiae, has been engineered to be 97% homologous to native human GLP-1 by substituting arginine for lysine at position 34. Liraglutide is made by attaching a C-16 fatty acid (palmitic acid) with a glutamic acid spacer on the remaining lysine residue at position 26 of the peptide precursor. The molecular formula of liraglutide is $C_{172}H_{265}N_{43}O_{51}$ and the molecular weight is 3751.2 Daltons. The structural formula (Figure 1) is:

Figure 1 Structural Formula of liraglutide

Victoza is a clear, colorless solution. Each 1 mL of Victoza solution contains 6 mg of liraglutide. Each pre-filled pen contains a 3 mL solution of Victoza equivalent to 18 mg liraglutide (free-base, anhydrous) and the following inactive ingredients: disodium phosphate dihydrate, 1.42 mg; propylene glycol, 14 mg; phenol, 5.5 mg; and water for injection.

12 CLINICAL PHARMACOLOGY

12.1 Mechanism of Action
Liraglutide is an acylated human Glucagon-Like Peptide-1 (GLP-1) receptor agonist with 97% amino acid sequence homology to endogenous human GLP-1(7-37). GLP-1(7-37) represents <20% of total circulating endogenous GLP-1. Like GLP-1(7-37), liraglutide activates the GLP-1 receptor, a membrane-bound cell-surface receptor coupled to adenylyl cyclase by the stimulatory G-protein, Gs, in pancreatic beta cells. Liraglutide increases intracellular cyclic AMP (cAMP) leading to insulin release in the presence of elevated glucose concentrations. This insulin secretion subsides as blood glucose concentrations decrease and approach euglycemia. Liraglutide also decreases glucagon secretion in a glucose-dependent manner. The mechanism of blood glucose lowering also involves a delay in gastric emptying.
GLP-1(7-37) has a half-life of 1.5-2 minutes due to degradation by the ubiquitous endogenous enzymes, dipeptidyl peptidase IV (DPP-IV) and neutral endopeptidases (NEP). Unlike native GLP-1, liraglutide is stable against metabolic degradation by both peptidases and has a plasma half-life of 13 hours after subcutaneous administration. The pharmacokinetic profile of liraglutide, which makes it suitable for once daily administration, is a result of self-association that delays absorption, plasma protein binding and stability against metabolic degradation by DPP-IV and NEP.

12.2 Pharmacodynamics
Victoza's pharmacodynamic profile is consistent with its pharmacokinetic profile observed after single subcutaneous administration as Victoza lowered fasting, premeal and postprandial glucose throughout the day [see Clinical Pharmacology (12.3)].
Fasting and postprandial glucose was measured before and up to 5 hours after a standardized meal after treatment to steady state with 0.6, 1.2 and 1.8 mg Victoza or placebo.

Compared to placebo, the postprandial plasma glucose $AUC_{0-300min}$ was 35% lower after Victoza 1.2 mg and 38% lower after Victoza 1.8 mg.

Glucose-dependent insulin secretion
The effect of a single dose of 7.5 mcg/kg (~ 0.7 mg) Victoza on insulin secretion rates (ISR) was investigated in 10 patients with type 2 diabetes during graded glucose infusion. In these patients, on average, the ISR response was increased in a glucose-dependent manner (Figure 2).

Figure 2 Mean Insulin Secretion Rate (ISR) versus Glucose Concentration Following Single-Dose Victoza 7.5 mcg/kg (~ 0.7 mg) or Placebo in Patients with Type 2 Diabetes (N=10) During Graded Glucose Infusion

Glucagon secretion
Victoza lowered blood glucose by stimulating insulin secretion and lowering glucagon secretion. A single dose of Victoza 7.5 mcg/kg (~ 0.7 mg) did not impair glucagon response to low glucose concentrations.

Gastric emptying
Victoza causes a delay of gastric emptying, thereby reducing the rate at which postprandial glucose appears in the circulation.

Cardiac Electrophysiology (QTc)
The effect of Victoza on cardiac repolarization was tested in a QTc study. Victoza at steady state concentrations with daily doses up to 1.8 mg did not produce QTc prolongation.

12.3 Pharmacokinetics
Absorption - Following subcutaneous administration, maximum concentrations of liraglutide are achieved at 8-12 hours post dosing. The mean peak (C_{max}) and total (AUC) exposures of liraglutide were 35 ng/mL and 960 ng•h/mL, respectively, for a subcutaneous single dose of 0.6 mg. After subcutaneous single dose administrations, C_{max} and AUC of liraglutide increased proportionally over the therapeutic dose range of 0.6 mg to 1.8 mg. At 1.8 mg Victoza, the average steady state concentration of liraglutide over 24 hours was approximately 128 ng/mL. $AUC_{0-\infty}$ was equivalent between upper arm and abdomen, and between upper arm and thigh. $AUC_{0-\infty}$ from thigh was 22% lower than that from abdomen. However, liraglutide exposures were considered comparable among these three subcutaneous injection sites. Absolute bioavailability of liraglutide following subcutaneous administration is approximately 55%.
Distribution - The mean apparent volume of distribution after subcutaneous administration of Victoza 0.6 mg is approximately 13 L. The mean volume of distribution after intravenous administration of Victoza is 0.07 L/kg. Liraglutide is extensively bound to plasma protein (>98%).
Metabolism - During the initial 24 hours following administration of a single [³H]-liraglutide dose to healthy subjects, the major component in plasma was intact liraglutide. Liraglutide is endogenously metabolized in a similar manner to large proteins without a specific organ as a major route of elimination.
Elimination - Following a [³H]-liraglutide dose, intact liraglutide was not detected in urine or feces. Only a minor part of the administered radioactivity was excreted as liraglutide-related metabolites in urine or feces (6% and 5%, respectively). The majority of urine and feces radioactivity was excreted during the first 6-8 days. The mean apparent clearance following subcutaneous administration of a single dose of liraglutide is approximately 1.2 L/h with an elimination half-life of approximately 13 hours, making Victoza suitable for once daily administration.

Specific Populations
Elderly - Age had no effect on the pharmacokinetics of Victoza based on a pharmacokinetic study in healthy elderly subjects (65 to 83 years) and population pharmacokinetic analyses of patients 18 to 80 years of age [see Use in Specific Populations (8.5)].
Gender - Based on the results of population pharmacokinetic analyses, females have 34% lower weight-adjusted clearance of Victoza compared to males. Based on the exposure response data, no dose adjustment is necessary based on gender.
Race and Ethnicity - Race and ethnicity had no effect on the pharmacokinetics of Victoza based on the results of population pharmacokinetic analyses that included Caucasian, Black, Asian and Hispanic/Non-Hispanic subjects.
Body Weight - Body weight significantly affects the pharmacokinetics of Victoza based on results of population pharma-

cokinetic analyses. The exposure of liraglutide decreases with an increase in baseline body weight. However, the 1.2 mg and 1.8 mg daily doses of Victoza provided adequate systemic exposures over the body weight range of 40 – 160 kg evaluated in the clinical trials. Liraglutide was not studied in patients with body weight >160 kg.

Pediatric - Victoza has not been studied in pediatric patients [see Use in Specific Populations (8.4)].

Renal Impairment - The single-dose pharmacokinetics of Victoza were evaluated in subjects with varying degrees of renal impairment. Subjects with mild (estimated creatinine clearance 50-80 mL/min) to severe (estimated creatinine clearance <30 mL/min) renal impairment and subjects with end-stage renal disease requiring dialysis were included in the trial. Compared to healthy subjects, liraglutide AUC in mild, moderate, and severe renal impairment and in end-stage renal disease was on average 35%, 19%, 29% and 30% lower, respectively [see Use in Specific Populations (8.6)].

Hepatic Impairment - The single-dose pharmacokinetics of Victoza were evaluated in subjects with varying degrees of hepatic impairment. Subjects with mild (Child Pugh score 5-6) to severe (Child Pugh score > 9) hepatic impairment were included in the trial. Compared to healthy subjects, liraglutide AUC in subjects with mild, moderate and severe hepatic impairment was on average 11%, 14% and 42% lower, respectively [see Use in Specific Populations (8.7)].

Drug Interactions

In vitro assessment of drug-drug interactions

Victoza has low potential for pharmacokinetic drug-drug interactions related to cytochrome P450 (CYP) and plasma protein binding.

In vivo assessment of drug-drug interactions

The drug-drug interaction studies were performed at steady state with Victoza 1.8 mg/day. Before administration of concomitant treatment, subjects underwent a 0.6 mg weekly dose increase to reach the maximum dose of 1.8 mg/day. Administration of the interacting drugs was timed so that C_{max} of Victoza (8-12 h) would coincide with the absorption peak of the co-administered drugs.

Digoxin

A single dose of digoxin 1 mg was administered 7 hours after the dose of Victoza at steady state. The concomitant administration with Victoza resulted in a reduction of digoxin AUC by 16%; C_{max} decreased by 31%. Digoxin median time to maximal concentration (T_{max}) was delayed from 1 h to 1.5 h.

Lisinopril

A single dose of lisinopril 20 mg was administered 5 minutes after the dose of Victoza at steady state. The co-administration with Victoza resulted in a reduction of lisinopril AUC by 15%; C_{max} decreased by 27%. Lisinopril median T_{max} was delayed from 6 h to 8 h with Victoza.

Atorvastatin

Victoza did not change the overall exposure (AUC) of atorvastatin following a single dose of atorvastatin 40 mg, administered 5 hours after the dose of Victoza at steady state. Atorvastatin C_{max} was decreased by 38% and median T_{max} was delayed from 1 h to 3 h with Victoza.

Acetaminophen

Victoza did not change the overall exposure (AUC) of acetaminophen following a single dose of acetaminophen 1000 mg, administered 8 hours after the dose of Victoza at steady state. Acetaminophen C_{max} was decreased by 31% and median T_{max} was delayed up to 15 minutes.

Griseofulvin

Victoza did not change the overall exposure (AUC) of griseofulvin following co-administration of a single dose of griseofulvin 500 mg with Victoza at steady state. Griseofulvin C_{max} increased by 37% while median T_{max} did not change.

Oral Contraceptives

A single dose of an oral contraceptive combination product containing 0.03 mg ethinylestradiol and 0.15 mg levonorgestrel was administered under fed conditions and 7 hours after the dose of Victoza at steady state. Victoza lowered ethinylestradiol and levonorgestrel C_{max} by 12% and 13%, respectively. There was no effect of Victoza on the overall exposure (AUC) of ethinylestradiol. Victoza increased the levonorgestrel $AUC_{0-\infty}$ by 18%. Victoza delayed T_{max} for both ethinylestradiol and levonorgestrel by 1.5 h.

Insulin Detemir

No pharmacokinetic interaction was observed between Victoza and insulin detemir when separate subcutaneous injections of insulin detemir 0.5 Unit/kg (single-dose) and Victoza 1.8 mg (steady state) were administered in patients with type 2 diabetes.

13   NONCLINICAL TOXICOLOGY

13.1   Carcinogenesis, Mutagenesis, Impairment of Fertility

A 104-week carcinogenicity study was conducted in male and female CD-1 mice at doses of 0.03, 0.2, 1.0, and 3.0 mg/kg/day liraglutide administered by bolus subcutaneous injection yielding systemic exposures 0.2-, 2-, 10- and 45-times the human exposure, respectively, at the MRHD of

1.8 mg/day based on plasma AUC comparison. A dose-related increase in benign thyroid C-cell adenomas was seen in the 1.0 and the 3.0 mg/kg/day groups with incidences of 13% and 19% in males and 6% and 20% in females, respectively. C-cell adenomas did not occur in control groups or 0.03 and 0.2 mg/kg/day groups. Treatment-related malignant C-cell carcinomas occurred in 3% of females in the 3.0 mg/kg/day group. Thyroid C-cell tumors are rare findings during carcinogenicity testing in mice. A treatment-related increase in fibrosarcomas was seen on the dorsal skin and subcutis, the body surface used for drug injection, in males in the 3 mg/kg/day group. These fibrosarcomas were attributed to the high local concentration of drug near the injection site. The liraglutide concentration in the clinical formulation (6 mg/mL) is 10-times higher than the concentration in the formulation used to administer 3 mg/kg/day liraglutide to mice in the carcinogenicity study (0.6 mg/mL).

A 104-week carcinogenicity study was conducted in male and female Sprague Dawley rats at doses of 0.075, 0.25 and 0.75 mg/kg/day liraglutide administered by bolus subcutaneous injection with exposures 0.5-, 2- and 8-times the human exposure, respectively, resulting from the MRHD based on plasma AUC comparison. A treatment-related increase in benign thyroid C-cell adenomas was seen in males in 0.25 and 0.75 mg/kg/day liraglutide groups with incidences of 12%, 16%, 42%, and 46% and in all female liraglutide-treated groups with incidences of 10%, 27%, 33%, and 56% in 0 (control), 0.075, 0.25, and 0.75 mg/kg/day groups, respectively. A treatment-related increase in malignant thyroid C-cell carcinomas was observed in all male liraglutide-treated groups with incidences of 2%, 8%, 6%, and 14% and in females at 0.25 and 0.75 mg/kg/day with incidences of 0%, 0%, 4%, and 6% in 0 (control), 0.075, 0.25, and 0.75 mg/kg/day groups, respectively. Thyroid C-cell carcinomas are rare findings during carcinogenicity testing in rats. Human relevance of thyroid C-cell tumors in mice and rats is unknown and could not be determined by clinical studies or nonclinical studies [see Boxed Warning and Warnings and Precautions (5.1)].

Liraglutide was negative with and without metabolic activation in the Ames test for mutagenicity and in a human peripheral blood lymphocyte chromosome aberration test for clastogenicity. Liraglutide was negative in repeat-dose *in vivo* micronucleus tests in rats.

In rat fertility studies using subcutaneous doses of 0.1, 0.25 and 1.0 mg/kg/day liraglutide, males were treated for 4 weeks prior to and throughout mating and females were treated 2 weeks prior to and throughout mating until gestation day 17. No direct adverse effects on male fertility was observed at doses up to 1.0 mg/kg/day, a high dose yielding

an estimated systemic exposure 11- times the human exposure at the MRHD, based on plasma AUC. In female rats, an increase in early embryonic deaths occurred at 1.0 mg/kg/day. Reduced body weight gain and food consumption were observed in females at the 1.0 mg/kg/day dose.

14   CLINICAL STUDIES

A total of 6090 patients with type 2 diabetes participated in 8 phase 3 trials. There were 5 double-blind (one of these trials had an open-label active control insulin glargine arm), randomized, controlled clinical trials, one of 52 weeks duration and four of 26 weeks duration. There were also three 26 week open-label trials; one comparing Victoza to twice-daily exenatide, one comparing Victoza to sitagliptin and one comparing Victoza+metformin+insulin detemir to Victoza+metformin alone. These multinational trials were conducted to evaluate the glycemic efficacy and safety of Victoza in type 2 diabetes as monotherapy and in combination with one or two oral anti-diabetic medications or insulin detemir. The 7 add-on combination therapy trials enrolled patients who were previously treated with anti-diabetic therapy, and approximately two-thirds of patients in the monotherapy trial also were previously treated with anti-diabetic therapy. In total, 272 (4%) of the 6090 patients in these 8 trials were new to anti-diabetic therapy. In these 8 clinical trials, patients ranged in age from 18-80 years old and 54% were men. Approximately 82% of patients were Caucasian, and 6% were Black. In the 5 trials where ethnicity was captured, 10% of patients were Hispanic/Latino (n=630).

In each of the placebo controlled trials, treatment with Victoza produced clinically and statistically significant improvements in hemoglobin A_{1c} and fasting plasma glucose (FPG) compared to placebo.

All Victoza-treated patients started at 0.6 mg/day. The dose was increased in weekly intervals by 0.6 mg to reach 1.2 mg or 1.8 mg for patients randomized to these higher doses. Victoza 0.6 mg is not effective for glycemic control and is intended only as a starting dose to reduce gastrointestinal intolerance [see Dosage and Administration (2)].

14.1   Monotherapy

In this 52-week trial, 746 patients were randomized to Victoza 1.2 mg, Victoza 1.8 mg, or glimepiride 8 mg. Patients who were randomized to glimepiride were initially treated with 2 mg daily for two weeks, increasing to 4 mg daily for another two weeks, and finally increasing to 8 mg daily. Treatment with Victoza 1.8 mg and 1.2 mg resulted in a statistically significant reduction in HbA_{1c} compared to glimepiride (Table 6). The percentage of patients who discontinued due to ineffective therapy was 3.6% in the Victoza

Table 6 Results of a 52-week monotherapy trial*

	Victoza 1.8 mg	Victoza 1.2 mg	Glimepiride 8 mg
Intent-to-Treat Population (N)	246	251	248
HbA_{1c} (%) (Mean)			
Baseline	8.2	8.2	8.2
Change from baseline (adjusted mean)[†]	-1.1	-0.8	-0.5
Difference from glimepiride arm (adjusted mean)[†]	-0.6[‡]	-0.3[§]	
95% Confidence Interval	(-0.8, -0.4)	(-0.5, -0.1)	
Percentage of patients achieving A_{1c} <7%	51	43	28
Fasting Plasma Glucose (mg/dL) (Mean)			
Baseline	172	168	172
Change from baseline (adjusted mean)[†]	-26	-15	-5
Difference from glimepiride arm (adjusted mean)[†]	-20[‡]	-10[§]	
95% Confidence Interval	(-29, -12)	(-19, -1)	
Body Weight (kg) (Mean)			
Baseline	92.6	92.1	93.3
Change from baseline (adjusted mean)[†]	-2.5	-2.1	+1.1
Difference from glimepiride arm (adjusted mean)[†]	-3.6[‡]	-3.2[‡]	
95% Confidence Interval	(-4.3, -2.9)	(-3.9, -2.5)	

* Intent-to-treat population using last observation on study
† Least squares mean adjusted for baseline value
‡ p-value <0.0001
§ p-value <0.05

Table 7 Results of a 26-week trial of Victoza as add-on to metformin*

	Victoza 1.8 mg + Metformin	Victoza 1.2 mg + Metformin	Placebo + Metformin	Glimepiride 4 mg[†] + Metformin
Intent-to-Treat Population (N)	242	240	121	242
HbA$_{1c}$ (%) (Mean)				
Baseline	8.4	8.3	8.4	8.4
Change from baseline (adjusted mean)[‡]	-1.0	-1.0	+0.1	-1.0
Difference from placebo + metformin arm (adjusted mean)[‡]	-1.1[§]	-1.1[§]		
95% Confidence Interval	(-1.3, -0.9)	(-1.3, -0.9)		
Difference from glimepiride + metformin arm (adjusted mean)[‡]	0.0	0.0		
95% Confidence Interval	(-0.2, 0.2)	(-0.2, 0.2)		
Percentage of patients achieving A$_{1c}$ <7%	42	35	11	36
Fasting Plasma Glucose (mg/dL) (Mean)				
Baseline	181	179	182	180
Change from baseline (adjusted mean)[‡]	-30	-30	+7	-24
Difference from placebo + metformin arm (adjusted mean)[‡]	-38[§]	-37[§]		
95% Confidence Interval	(-48, -27)	(-47, -26)		
Difference from glimepiride + metformin arm (adjusted mean)[‡]	-7	-6		
95% Confidence Interval	(-16, 2)	(-15, 3)		
Body Weight (kg) (Mean)				
Baseline	88.0	88.5	91.0	89.0
Change from baseline (adjusted mean)[‡]	-2.8	-2.6	-1.5	+1.0
Difference from placebo + metformin arm (adjusted mean)[‡]	-1.3[¶]	-1.1[¶]		
95% Confidence Interval	(-2.2, -0.4)	(-2.0, -0.2)		
Difference from glimepiride + metformin arm (adjusted mean)[‡]	-3.8[§]	-3.5[§]		
95% Confidence Interval	(-4.5, -3.0)	(-4.3, -2.8)		

* Intent-to-treat population using last observation on study
† For glimepiride, one-half of the maximal approved United States dose.
‡ Least squares mean adjusted for baseline value
§ p-value <0.0001
¶ p-value <0.05

1.8 mg treatment group, 6.0% in the Victoza 1.2 mg treatment group, and 10.1% in the glimepiride-treatment group.
[See table 6 at top of previous page]

*p-value = 0.0014 for VICTOZA 1.2 mg compared to glimepiride.
†p-value < 0.0001 for VICTOZA 1.8 mg compared to glimepiride.
P values derived from change from baseline ANCOVA model.

Figure 3 Mean HbA$_{1c}$ for patients who completed the 52-week trial and for the Last Observation Carried Forward (LOCF, intent-to-treat) data at Week 52 (Monotherapy)

14.2   Combination Therapy
Add-on to Metformin
In this 26-week trial, 1091 patients were randomized to Victoza 0.6 mg, Victoza 1.2 mg, Victoza 1.8 mg, placebo, or glimepiride 4 mg (one-half of the maximal approved dose in the United States), all as add-on to metformin. Randomiza-

tion occurred after a 6-week run-in period consisting of a 3-week initial forced metformin titration period followed by a maintenance period of another 3 weeks. During the titration period, doses of metformin were increased up to 2000 mg/day.
Treatment with Victoza 1.2 mg and 1.8 mg as add-on to metformin resulted in a significant mean HbA$_{1c}$ reduction relative to placebo add-on to metformin and resulted in a similar mean HbA$_{1c}$ reduction relative to glimepiride 4 mg add-on to metformin (Table 7). The percentage of patients who discontinued due to ineffective therapy was 5.4% in the Victoza 1.8 mg + metformin treatment group, 3.3% in the Victoza 1.2 mg + metformin treatment group, 23.8% in the placebo + metformin treatment group, and 3.7% in the glimepiride + metformin treated group.
[See table 7 above]

Victoza Compared to Sitagliptin, Both as Add-on to Metformin

In this 26–week, open-label trial, 665 patients on a background of metformin ≥1500 mg per day were randomized to Victoza 1.2 mg once-daily, Victoza 1.8 mg once-daily or sitagliptin 100 mg once-daily, all dosed according to approved labeling. Patients were to continue their current treatment on metformin at a stable, pre-trial dose level and dosing frequency.
The primary endpoint was the change in HbA1c from baseline to Week 26. Treatment with Victoza 1.2 mg and Victoza 1.8 mg resulted in statistically significant reductions in HbA1c relative to sitagliptin 100 mg (Table 8). The percentage of patients who discontinued due to ineffective therapy

was 3.1% in the Victoza 1.2 mg group, 0.5% in the Victoza 1.8 mg treatment group, and 4.1% in the sitagliptin 100 mg treatment group. From a mean baseline body weight of 94 kg, there was a mean reduction of 2.7 kg for Victoza 1.2 mg, 3.3 kg for Victoza 1.8 mg, and 0.8 kg for sitagliptin 100 mg.
[See table 8 at top of next page]

*p-value <0.0001 for Victoza compared with sitagliptin
P values derived from change from baseline ANCOVA model

Figure 4 Mean HbA$_{1c}$ for patients who completed the 26-week trial and for the Last Observation Carried Forward (LOCF, intent-to-treat) data at Week 26

Combination Therapy with Metformin and Insulin
This 26-week open-label trial enrolled 988 patients with inadequate glycemic control (HbA1c 7-10%) on metformin (≥1500 mg/day) alone or inadequate glycemic control (HbA1c 7-8.5%) on metformin (≥1500 mg/day) and a sulfonylurea. Patients who were on metformin and a sulfonylurea discontinued the sulfonylurea then all patients entered a 12-week run-in period during which they received add-on therapy with Victoza titrated to 1.8 mg once-daily. At the end of the run-in period, 498 patients (50%) achieved HbA1c <7% with Victoza 1.8 mg and metformin and continued treatment in a non-randomized, observational arm. Another 167 patients (17%) withdrew from the trial during the run-in period with approximately one-half of these patients doing so because of gastrointestinal adverse reactions *[see Adverse Reactions (6.1)]*. The remaining 323 patients with HbA1c ≥7% (33% of those who entered the run-in period) were randomized to 26 weeks of once-daily insulin detemir administered in the evening as add-on therapy (N=162) or to continued, unchanged treatment with Victoza 1.8 mg and metformin (N=161). The starting dose of insulin detemir was 10 units/day and the mean dose at the end of the 26-week randomized period was 39 units/day. During the 26 week randomized treatment period, the percentage of patients who discontinued due to ineffective therapy was 11.2% in the group randomized to continued treatment with Victoza 1.8 mg and metformin and 1.2% in the group randomized to add-on therapy with insulin detemir.
Treatment with insulin detemir as add-on to Victoza 1.8 mg + metformin resulted in statistically significant reductions in HbA$_{1c}$ and FPG compared to continued, unchanged treatment with Victoza 1.8 mg + metformin alone (Table 9). From a mean baseline body weight of 96 kg after randomization, there was a mean reduction of 0.3 kg in the patients who received insulin detemir add-on therapy compared to a mean reduction of 1.1 kg in the patients who continued on unchanged treatment with Victoza 1.8 mg + metformin alone.
[See table 9 at top of next page]
Add-on to Sulfonylurea
In this 26-week trial, 1041 patients were randomized to Victoza 0.6 mg, Victoza 1.2 mg, Victoza 1.8 mg, placebo, or rosiglitazone 4 mg (one-half of the maximal approved dose in the United States), all as add-on to glimepiride. Randomization occurred after a 4-week run-in period consisting of an initial, 2-week, forced-glimepiride titration period followed by a maintenance period of another 2 weeks. During the titration period, doses of glimepiride were increased to 4 mg/day. The doses of glimepiride could be reduced (at the discretion of the investigator) from 4 mg/day to 3 mg/day or 2 mg/day (minimum) after randomization, in the event of unacceptable hypoglycemia or other adverse events.
Treatment with Victoza 1.2 mg and 1.8 mg as add-on to glimepiride resulted in a statistically significant reduction in mean HbA$_{1c}$ compared to placebo add-on to glimepiride (Table 10). The percentage of patients who discontinued due to ineffective therapy was 3.0% in the Victoza 1.8 mg + glimepiride treatment group, 3.5% in the Victoza 1.2 mg + glimepiride treatment group, 17.5% in the placebo + glimepiride treatment group, and 6.9% in the rosiglitazone + glimepiride treatment group.
[See table 10 at top of page 2068]
Add-on to Metformin and Sulfonylurea
In this 26-week trial, 581 patients were randomized to Victoza 1.8 mg, placebo, or insulin glargine, all as add-on to metformin and glimepiride. Randomization took place after a 6-week run-in period consisting of a 3-week forced metformin and glimepiride titration period followed by a main-

tenance period of another 3 weeks. During the titration period, doses of metformin and glimepiride were to be increased up to 2000 mg/day and 4 mg/day, respectively. After randomization, patients randomized to Victoza 1.8 mg underwent a 2 week period of titration with Victoza. During the trial, the Victoza and metformin doses were fixed, although glimepiride and insulin glargine doses could be adjusted. Patients titrated glargine twice-weekly during the first 8 weeks of treatment based on self-measured fasting plasma glucose on the day of titration. After Week 8, the frequency of insulin glargine titration was left to the discretion of the investigator, but, at a minimum, the glargine dose was to be revised, if necessary, at Weeks 12 and 18. Only 20% of glargine-treated patients achieved the prespecified target fasting plasma glucose of ≤100 mg/dL. Therefore, optimal titration of the insulin glargine dose was not achieved in most patients.

Treatment with Victoza as add-on to glimepiride and metformin resulted in a statistically significant mean reduction in HbA1c compared to placebo add-on to glimepiride and metformin (Table 11). The percentage of patients who discontinued due to ineffective therapy was 0.9% in the Victoza 1.8 mg + metformin + glimepiride treatment group, 0.4% in the insulin glargine + metformin + glimepiride treatment group, and 11.3% in the placebo + metformin + glimepiride treatment group.

[See table 11 at top of page 2069]

Victoza Compared to Exenatide, Both as Add-on to Metformin and/or Sulfonylurea Therapy

In this 26–week, open-label trial, 464 patients on a background of metformin monotherapy, sulfonylurea monotherapy or a combination of metformin and sulfonylurea were randomized to once daily Victoza 1.8 mg or exenatide 10 mcg twice daily. Maximally tolerated doses of background therapy were to remain unchanged for the duration of the trial. Patients randomized to exenatide started on a dose of 5 mcg twice-daily for 4 weeks and then were escalated to 10 mcg twice daily.

Treatment with Victoza 1.8 mg resulted in statistically significant reductions in HbA1c and FPG relative to exenatide (Table 12). The percentage of patients who discontinued for ineffective therapy was 0.4% in the Victoza treatment group and 0% in the exenatide treatment group. Both treatment groups had a mean decrease from baseline in body weight of approximately 3 kg.

[See table 12 at top of page 2069]

Add-on to Metformin and Thiazolidinedione

In this 26-week trial, 533 patients were randomized to Victoza 1.2 mg, Victoza 1.8 mg or placebo, all as add-on to rosiglitazone (8 mg) plus metformin (2000 mg). Patients underwent a 9 week run-in period (3-week forced dose escalation followed by a 6-week dose maintenance phase) with rosiglitazone (starting at 4 mg and increasing to 8 mg/day within 2 weeks) and metformin (starting at 500 mg with increasing weekly increments of 500 mg to a final dose of 2000 mg/day). Only patients who tolerated the final dose of rosiglitazone (8 mg/day) and metformin (2000 mg/day) and completed the 6-week dose maintenance phase were eligible for randomization into the trial.

Treatment with Victoza as add-on to metformin and rosiglitazone produced a statistically significant reduction in mean HbA1c compared to placebo add-on to metformin and rosiglitazone (Table 13). The percentage of patients who discontinued to ineffective therapy was 1.7% in the Victoza 1.8 mg + metformin + rosiglitazone treatment group, 1.7% in the Victoza 1.2 mg + metformin + rosiglitazone treatment group, and 16.4% in the placebo + metformin + rosiglitazone treatment group.

[See table 13 at top of page 2070]

16 HOW SUPPLIED/STORAGE AND HANDLING

16.1 How Supplied

Victoza is available in the following package sizes containing disposable, pre-filled, multi-dose pens. Each individual pen delivers doses of 0.6 mg, 1.2 mg, or 1.8 mg (6 mg/mL, 3 mL).

2 × Victoza pen NDC 0169-4060-12

3 × Victoza pen NDC 0169-4060-13

Each Victoza pen is for use by a single patient. A Victoza pen should never be shared between patients, even if the needle is changed.

16.2 Recommended Storage

Prior to first use, Victoza should be stored in a refrigerator between 36°F to 46°F (2°C to 8°C) (Table 14). Do not store in the freezer or directly adjacent to the refrigerator cooling element. Do not freeze Victoza and do not use Victoza if it has been frozen.

After initial use of the Victoza pen, the pen can be stored for 30 days at controlled room temperature (59°F to 86°F; 15°C to 30°C) or in a refrigerator (36°F to 46°F; 2°C to 8°C). Keep the pen cap on when not in use. Victoza should be protected from excessive heat and sunlight. Always remove and safely discard the needle after each injection and store the Victoza

Table 8 Results of a 26-week open-label trial of Victoza Compared to Sitagliptin (both in combination with metformin)*

	Victoza 1.8 mg + Metformin	Victoza 1.2 mg + Metformin	Sitagliptin 100 mg + Metformin
Intent-to-Treat Population (N)	218	221	219
HbA1c (%) (Mean)			
Baseline	8.4	8.4	8.5
Change from baseline (adjusted mean)	-1.5	-1.2	-0.9
Difference from sitagliptin arm (adjusted mean)†	-0.6‡	-0.3‡	
95% Confidence Interval	(-0.8, -0.4)	(-0.5, -0.2)	
Percentage of patients achieving A1c <7%	56	44	22
Fasting Plasma Glucose (mg/dL) (Mean)			
Baseline	179	182	180
Change from baseline (adjusted mean)	-39	-34	-15
Difference from sitagliptin arm (adjusted mean)†	-24‡	-19‡	
95% Confidence Interval	(-31, -16)	(-26, -12)	

* Intent-to-treat population using last observation on study
† Least squares mean adjusted for baseline value
‡ p-value <0.0001

Table 9 Results of a 26-week open label trial of Insulin detemir as add on to Victoza + metformin compared to continued treatment with Victoza + metformin alone in patients not achieving HbA1c < 7% after 12 weeks of Metformin and Victoza*

	Insulin detemir + Victoza + Metformin	Victoza + Metformin
Intent-to-Treat Population (N)	162	157
HbA1c (%) (Mean)		
Baseline (week 0)	7.6	7.6
Change from baseline (adjusted mean)	-0.5	0
Difference from Victoza + metformin arm (LS mean)†	-0.5‡	
95% Confidence Interval	(-0.7, -0.4)	
Percentage of patients achieving A1c <7%	43	17
Fasting Plasma Glucose (mg/dL) (Mean)		
Baseline (week 0)	166	159
Change from baseline (adjusted mean)	-39	-7
Difference from Victoza + metformin arm (LS mean)†	-31‡	
95% Confidence Interval	(-39 , -23)	

* Intent-to-treat population using last observation on study
† Least squares mean adjusted for baseline value
‡ p-value <0.0001

pen without an injection needle attached. This will reduce the potential for contamination, infection, and leakage while also ensuring dosing accuracy.

Table 14 Recommended Storage Conditions for the Victoza Pen

Prior to first use	After first use	
Refrigerated 36°F to 46°F (2°C to 8°C)	Room Temperature 59°F to 86°F (15°C to 30°C)	Refrigerated 36°F to 46°F (2°C to 8°C)
Until expiration date	30 days	

17 PATIENT COUNSELING INFORMATION

17.1 FDA-Approved Medication Guide

See separate leaflet.

17.2 Risk of Thyroid C-cell Tumors

Patients should be informed that liraglutide causes benign and malignant thyroid C-cell tumors in mice and rats and that the human relevance of this finding is unknown. Patients should be counseled to report symptoms of thyroid tumors (e.g., a lump in the neck, hoarseness, dysphagia or dyspnea) to their physician.

17.3 Dehydration and Renal Failure

Patients treated with Victoza should be advised of the potential risk of dehydration due to gastrointestinal adverse reactions and take precautions to avoid fluid depletion. Patients should be informed of the potential risk for worsening renal function, which in some cases may require dialysis.

17.4 Pancreatitis

Patients should be informed of the potential risk for pancreatitis. Explain that persistent severe abdominal pain that may radiate to the back and which may or may not be accompanied by vomiting, is the hallmark symptom of acute pancreatitis. Instruct patients to discontinue Victoza

promptly and contact their physician if persistent severe abdominal pain occurs *[see Warnings and Precautions (5.2)]*.

17.5 Hypersensitivity Reactions

Patients should be informed that serious hypersensitivity reactions have been reported during postmarketing use of Victoza. If symptoms of hypersensitivity reactions occur, patients must stop taking Victoza and seek medical advice promptly *[see Warnings and Precautions (5.5)]*.

17.6 Never Share a Victoza Pen Between Patients

Counsel patients that they should never share a Victoza pen with another person, even if the needle is changed. Sharing of the pen between patients may pose a risk of transmission of infection.

17.7 Instructions

Patients should be informed of the potential risks and benefits of Victoza and of alternative modes of therapy. Patients should also be informed about the importance of adherence to dietary instructions, regular physical activity, periodic blood glucose monitoring and A1c testing, recognition and management of hypoglycemia and hyperglycemia, and assessment for diabetes complications. During periods of stress such as fever, trauma, infection, or surgery, medication requirements may change and patients should be advised to seek medical advice promptly.

Patients should be advised that the most common side effects of Victoza are headache, nausea and diarrhea. Nausea is most common when first starting Victoza, but decreases over time in the majority of patients and does not typically require discontinuation of Victoza.

Physicians should instruct their patients to read the Patient Medication Guide before starting Victoza therapy and to reread each time the prescription is renewed. Patients should be instructed to inform their doctor or pharmacist if they develop any unusual symptom, or if any known symptom persists or worsens.

Inform patients not to take an extra dose of Victoza to make up for a missed dose. If a dose is missed, the once-daily regimen should be resumed as prescribed with the next scheduled dose.

Table 10 Results of a 26-week trial of Victoza as add-on to sulfonylurea*

	Victoza 1.8 mg + Glimepiride	Victoza 1.2 mg + Glimepiride	Placebo + Glimepiride	Rosiglitazone 4 mg[†] + Glimepiride
Intent-to-Treat Population (N)	234	228	114	231
HbA$_{1c}$ (%) (Mean)				
Baseline	8.5	8.5	8.4	8.4
Change from baseline (adjusted mean)[‡]	-1.1	-1.1	+0.2	-0.4
Difference from placebo + glimepiride arm (adjusted mean)[‡]	-1.4[§]	-1.3[§]		
95% Confidence Interval	(-1.6, -1.1)	(-1.5, -1.1)		
Percentage of patients achieving A$_{1c}$ <7%	42	35	7	22
Fasting Plasma Glucose (mg/dL) (Mean)				
Baseline	174	177	171	179
Change from baseline (adjusted mean)[‡]	-29	-28	+18	-16
Difference from placebo + glimepiride arm (adjusted mean)[‡]	-47[§]	-46[§]		
95% Confidence Interval	(-58, -35)	(-58, -35)		
Body Weight (kg) (Mean)				
Baseline	83.0	80.0	81.9	80.6
Change from baseline (adjusted mean)[‡]	-0.2	+0.3	-0.1	+2.1
Difference from placebo + glimepiride arm (adjusted mean)[‡]	-0.1	0.4		
95% Confidence Interval	(-0.9, 0.6)	(-0.4, 1.2)		

* Intent-to-treat population using last observation on study
† For rosiglitazone, one-half of the maximal approved United States dose.
‡ Least squares mean adjusted for baseline value
§ p-value <0.0001

If more than 3 days have elapsed since the last dose, the patient should be advised to reinitiate Victoza at 0.6 mg to mitigate any gastrointestinal symptoms associated with re-initiation of treatment. Victoza should be titrated at the discretion of the prescribing physician [see Dosage and Administration (2)].

17.8   Laboratory Tests
Patients should be informed that response to all diabetic therapies should be monitored by periodic measurements of blood glucose and A$_{1c}$ levels, with a goal of decreasing these levels towards the normal range. A$_{1c}$ is especially useful for evaluating long-term glycemic control.
Date of Issue: April 16, 2013
Version: 6
Victoza® is a registered trademark of Novo Nordisk A/S.
Victoza® is covered by US Patent Nos. 6,268,343, 6,458,924, 7,235,627, 8,114,833 and other patents pending.
Victoza® Pen is covered by US Patent Nos. 6,004,297, RE 43,834, RE 41,956 and other patents pending.
© 2010-13 Novo Nordisk
Manufactured by:
Novo Nordisk A/S
DK-2880 Bagsvaerd, Denmark
For information about Victoza contact:
Novo Nordisk Inc.
800 Scudders Mill Road
Plainsboro, NJ 08536
1-877-484-2869
Medication Guide
Victoza® (VIC-tow-za)
(liraglutide [rDNA origin]) Injection
Read this Medication Guide and Patient Instructions for Use that come with Victoza before you start using Victoza and each time you get a refill. There may be new information. This Medication Guide does not take the place of talking with your healthcare provider about your medical condition or your treatment. If you have questions about Victoza after reading this information, ask your healthcare provider or pharmacist.
What is the most important information I should know about Victoza?
Serious side effects may happen in people who take Victoza, including:
1. Possible thyroid tumors, including cancer. During the drug testing process, the medicine in Victoza caused rats and mice to develop tumors of the thyroid gland. Some of

these tumors were cancers. It is not known if Victoza will cause thyroid tumors or a type of thyroid cancer called medullary thyroid cancer in people. If medullary thyroid cancer occurs, it may lead to death if not detected and treated early. If you develop tumors or cancer of the thyroid, your thyroid may have to be surgically removed.
• Before you start taking Victoza, tell your healthcare provider if you or any of your family members have had thyroid cancer, especially medullary thyroid cancer, or Multiple Endocrine Neoplasia syndrome type 2. Do not take Victoza if you or any of your family members have medullary thyroid cancer, or if you have Multiple Endocrine Neoplasia syndrome type 2. People with these conditions already have a higher chance of developing medullary thyroid cancer in general and should not take Victoza.
• While taking Victoza, tell your healthcare provider if you get a lump or swelling in your neck, hoarseness, trouble swallowing, or shortness of breath. These may be symptoms of thyroid cancer.
2. Inflammation of the pancreas (pancreatitis), which may be severe and lead to death.
Before taking Victoza, tell your healthcare provider if you have had:
• pancreatitis
• stones in your gallbladder (gallstones)
• a history of alcoholism
• high blood triglyceride levels
These medical conditions can make you more likely to get pancreatitis in general. It is not known if having these conditions will lead to a higher chance of getting pancreatitis while taking Victoza.
While taking Victoza:
Stop taking Victoza and call your healthcare provider right away if you have pain in your stomach area (abdomen) that is severe and will not go away. The pain may happen with or without vomiting. The pain may be felt going from your abdomen through to your back. This type of pain may be a symptom of pancreatitis.
What is Victoza?
• Victoza is an injectable prescription medicine that may improve blood sugar (glucose) in adults with type 2 diabetes mellitus, and should be used along with diet and exercise.
• Victoza is not recommended as the first choice of medication for treating diabetes.
• Victoza is not a substitute for insulin.

• Victoza is not for use in people with type 1 diabetes or people with diabetic ketoacidosis.
• It is not known if Victoza is safe and effective in children. Victoza is not recommended for use in children.
Who should not use Victoza?
Do not use Victoza if:
• you or any of your family members have a history of medullary thyroid cancer.
• you have Multiple Endocrine Neoplasia syndrome type 2 (MEN 2). This is a disease where people have tumors in more than one gland in their body.
• you are allergic to liraglutide or any of the ingredients in Victoza. See the end of this Medication Guide for a complete list of ingredients in Victoza. Symptoms of a serious allergic reaction may include:
  ◦ swelling of your face, lips, tongue, or throat
  ◦ fainting or feeling dizzy
  ◦ very rapid heartbeat
  ◦ problems breathing or swallowing
  ◦ severe rash or itching
Talk with your healthcare provider if you are not sure if you have any of these conditions.
What should I tell my healthcare provider before using Victoza?
Before taking Victoza, tell your healthcare provider if you:
• have any of the conditions listed in the section "What is the most important information I should know about Victoza?"
• are allergic to liraglutide or any of the other ingredients in Victoza. See the end of this Medication Guide for a list of ingredients in Victoza.
• have severe problems with your stomach, such as slowed emptying of your stomach (gastroparesis) or problems with digesting food.
• have or have had kidney or liver problems.
• have any other medical conditions.
• are pregnant or plan to become pregnant. It is not known if Victoza will harm your unborn baby. Tell your healthcare provider if you become pregnant while taking Victoza.
• are breastfeeding or plan to breastfeed. It is not known if Victoza passes into your breast milk. You and your healthcare provider should decide if you will take Victoza or breastfeed. You should not do both without talking with your healthcare provider first.
Tell your healthcare provider about all the medicines you take including prescription and non-prescription medicines, vitamins, and herbal supplements. Victoza slows stomach emptying and can affect medicines that need to pass through the stomach quickly. Victoza may affect the way some medicines work and some other medicines may affect the way Victoza works. Tell your healthcare provider if you take other diabetes medicines, especially sulfonylurea medicines or insulin.
Know the medicines you take. Keep a list of them with you to show your healthcare provider and pharmacist each time you get a new medicine.
How should I use Victoza?
• Use Victoza exactly as prescribed by your healthcare provider. Your dose should be increased after using Victoza for one week. After that, do not change your dose unless your healthcare provider tells you to.
• Victoza is injected 1 time each day, at any time during the day.
• You can take Victoza with or without food.
• Victoza comes in a prefilled pen.
• Your healthcare provider must teach you how to inject Victoza before you use it for the first time. If you have questions or do not understand the instructions, talk to your healthcare provider or pharmacist. See the Patient Instructions for Use that come with this Medication Guide for detailed information about the right way to use your Victoza pen.
• Pen needles are not included. Use the Victoza pen with Novo Nordisk disposable needles. You may need a prescription to get pen needles from your pharmacist. Ask your healthcare provider which needle size is best for you.
• When starting a new prefilled Victoza pen, you must follow the "First Time Use for Each New Pen" (see the detailed Patient Instructions for Use that comes with this Medication Guide). You only need to do this 1 time with each new pen. You should also do this if you drop your pen. If you do the "First Time Use for Each New Pen" before each injection, you will run out of medicine too soon.
• Inject your dose of Victoza under the skin (subcutaneous injection) in your stomach area (abdomen), upper leg (thigh), or upper arm, as instructed by your healthcare provider. **Do not inject into a vein or muscle.**
• If you also give yourself insulin injections in addition to Victoza, **never mix insulin and Victoza together.** Give yourself 2 separate injections. You may give both injections in the same body area (for example, your stomach area), but you should not give the injections right next to each other.
• If you take too much Victoza, call your healthcare provider right away. Too much Victoza may cause severe nausea and vomiting.

- If you miss your daily dose of Victoza, use Victoza as soon as you remember. Then take your next daily dose as usual on the following day. Do not take an extra dose of Victoza or increase your dose on the following day to make up for your missed dose. If you miss your dose of Victoza for **3 days or more**, call your healthcare provider to talk about how to restart your treatment.
- Follow your healthcare provider's instructions for diet, exercise, how often to test your blood sugar, and when to get your HbA$_{1c}$ checked. If you stop using Victoza your blood sugar levels may increase. First talk to your healthcare provider if you want to stop taking Victoza.
- Your dose of diabetes medicines may need to be changed if your body is under certain types of stress. Tell your healthcare provider if you:
  - have fever
  - have trauma
  - have an infection
  - plan to have or have had surgery
- Never share your Victoza pen or needles with another person. You may give an infection to them, or get an infection from them.

What are the possible side effects of Victoza?
Victoza may cause serious side effects, including:
- See "What is the most important information I should know about Victoza?"
- **Low blood sugar (hypoglycemia).** Your risk for getting low blood sugar is higher if you take Victoza with another medicine that can cause low blood sugar, such as a sulfonylurea or insulin. In some people, the blood sugar may get so low that they need another person to help them. The dose of your sulfonylurea medicine or insulin may need to be lowered while you use Victoza. Signs and symptoms of low blood sugar may include:
- shakiness
- sweating
- headache
- drowsiness
- weakness
- dizziness
- confusion
- irritability
- hunger
- fast heartbeat
- feeling jittery

Talk to your healthcare provider about how to recognize and treat low blood sugar. Make sure that your family and other people who are around you a lot know how to recognize and treat low blood sugar.
- **Kidney problems (kidney failure).** Victoza may cause nausea, vomiting or diarrhea leading to loss of fluids (dehydration). Dehydration may cause kidney failure which can lead to the need for dialysis. This can happen in people who have never had kidney problems before. Drinking plenty of fluids may reduce your chance of dehydration.
Call your healthcare provider right away if you have nausea, vomiting, or diarrhea that does not go away, or if you cannot drink liquids by mouth.
- **Serious allergic reactions.** Serious allergic reactions can happen with Victoza. Stop using Victoza, and get medical help right away if you have any symptom of a serious allergic reaction **See "Who should not use Victoza?"**
Common side effects of Victoza include:
- headache
- nausea
- diarrhea

Nausea is most common when first starting Victoza, but decreases over time in most people as their body gets used to the medicine.
Tell your healthcare provider if you have any side effect that bothers you or that does not go away.
These are not all the side effects with Victoza. For more information, ask your healthcare provider or pharmacist.
Call your doctor for medical advice about side effects. You may report side effects to FDA at 1-800-FDA-1088.

How should I store Victoza?
Before use:
- Store your new, unused Victoza pen in the refrigerator at 36°F to 46°F (2°C to 8°C).
- Do not freeze Victoza or use Victoza if it has been frozen. Do not store Victoza near the refrigerator cooling element.
Pen in use:
- Store your Victoza pen for 30 days either at 59°F to 86°F (15°C to 30°C), or in a refrigerator at 36°F to 46°F (2°C to 8°C).
- When carrying the pen away from home, store the pen at a temperature between 59°F to 86°F (15°C to 30°C) and keep it dry.
- If Victoza has been exposed to temperatures above 86°F (30°C), it should be thrown away.
- Protect your Victoza pen from heat and sunlight.
- Keep the pen cap on when your Victoza pen is not in use.
- Use your Victoza pen within 30 days after the first day it is stored outside the refrigerator. After these 30 days, throw away your Victoza pen even if some medicine is left in the pen.
- Do not use Victoza after the expiration date printed on the carton.

Do not store the Victoza pen with the needle attached. Always safely remove and safely throw away the needle after each injection. This may help prevent contamination, infection and leakage. It also helps to make sure that you get the correct dose of Victoza. See the Patient Instructions for Use for information about how to dispose of used pen needles and used Victoza pens.
Keep your Victoza pen, pen needles, and all medicines out of the reach of children.
General information about Victoza
Medicines are sometimes prescribed for purposes other than those listed in a Medication Guide. Do not use Victoza for a condition for which it was not prescribed. Do not give Victoza to other people, even if they have the same symptoms you have. It may harm them.

This Medication Guide summarizes the most important information you should know about using Victoza. If you would like more information, talk with your healthcare provider. You can ask your pharmacist or healthcare provider for information about Victoza that is written for health professionals.
For more information, go to victoza.com or call 1-877-484-2869.
What are the ingredients in Victoza?
Active Ingredient: liraglutide
Inactive Ingredients: disodium phosphate dihydrate, propylene glycol, phenol and water for injection
Manufactured by:
Novo Nordisk A/S
DK-2880 Bagsvaerd, Denmark

Table 11 Results of a 26-week trial of Victoza as add-on to metformin and sulfonylurea*

	Victoza 1.8 mg + Metformin + Glimepiride	Placebo + Metformin + Glimepiride	Insulin glargine[†] + Metformin + Glimepiride
Intent-to-Treat Population (N)	230	114	232
HbA$_{1c}$ (%) (Mean)			
Baseline	8.3	8.3	8.1
Change from baseline (adjusted mean)[‡]	-1.3	-0.2	-1.1
Difference from placebo + metformin + glimepiride arm (adjusted mean)[‡]	-1.1[§]		
95% Confidence Interval	(-1.3, -0.9)		
Percentage of patients achieving A$_{1c}$ <7%	53	15	46
Fasting Plasma Glucose (mg/dL) (Mean)			
Baseline	165	170	164
Change from baseline (adjusted mean)[‡]	-28	+10	-32
Difference from placebo + metformin + glimepiride arm (adjusted mean)[‡]	-38[§]		
95% Confidence Interval	(-46, -30)		
Body Weight (kg) (Mean)			
Baseline	85.8	85.4	85.2
Change from baseline (adjusted mean)[‡]	-1.8	-0.4	1.6
Difference from placebo + metformin + glimepiride arm (adjusted mean)[‡]	-1.4[¶]		
95% Confidence Interval	(-2.1, -0.7)		

* Intent-to-treat population using last observation on study
† For insulin glargine, optimal titration regimen was not achieved for 80% of patients.
‡ Least squares mean adjusted for baseline value
§ p-value <0.0001
¶ p-value <0.05

Table 12 Results of a 26-week open-label trial of Victoza versus Exenatide (both in combination with metformin and/or sulfonylurea)*

	Victoza 1.8 mg once daily + metformin and/or sulfonylurea	Exenatide 10 mcg twice daily + metformin and/or sulfonylurea
Intent-to-Treat Population (N)	233	231
HbA$_{1c}$ (%) (Mean)		
Baseline	8.2	8.1
Change from baseline (adjusted mean)[†]	-1.1	-0.8
Difference from exenatide arm (adjusted mean)[†]	-0.3[‡]	
95% Confidence Interval	(-0.5, -0.2)	
Percentage of patients achieving A$_{1c}$ <7%	54	43
Fasting Plasma Glucose (mg/dL) (Mean)		
Baseline	176	171
Change from baseline (adjusted mean)[†]	-29	-11
Difference from exenatide arm (adjusted mean)[†]	-18[‡]	
95% Confidence Interval	(-25, -12)	

* Intent-to-treat population using last observation carried forward
† Least squares mean adjusted for baseline value
‡ p-value <0.0001

Table 13 Results of a 26-week trial of Victoza as add-on to metformin and thiazolidinedione*

	Victoza 1.8 mg + Metformin + Rosiglitazone	Victoza 1.2 mg + Metformin + Rosiglitazone	Placebo + Metformin + Rosiglitazone
Intent-to-Treat Population (N)	178	177	175
HbA$_{1c}$ (%) (Mean)			
Baseline	8.6	8.5	8.4
Change from baseline (adjusted mean)†	-1.5	-1.5	-0.5
Difference from placebo + metformin + rosiglitazone arm (adjusted mean)†	-0.9‡	-0.9‡	
95% Confidence Interval	(-1.1, -0.8)	(-1.1, -0.8)	
Percentage of patients achieving A$_{1c}$ <7%	54	57	28
Fasting Plasma Glucose (mg/dL) (Mean)			
Baseline	185	181	179
Change from baseline (adjusted mean)†	-44	-40	-8
Difference from placebo + metformin + rosiglitazone arm (adjusted mean)†	-36‡	-32‡	
95% Confidence Interval	(-44, -27)	(-41, -23)	
Body Weight (kg) (Mean)			
Baseline	94.9	95.3	98.5
Change from baseline (adjusted mean)†	-2.0	-1.0	+0.6
Difference from placebo + metformin + rosiglitazone arm (adjusted mean)†	-2.6‡	-1.6‡	
95% Confidence Interval	(-3.4, -1.8)	(-2.4, -1.0)	

* Intent-to-treat population using last observation on study
† Least squares mean adjusted for baseline value
‡ p-value <0.0001

For information about Victoza contact:
Novo Nordisk Inc.
800 Scudders Mill Road
Plainsboro, NJ 08536
1-877-484-2869
Issued: April 2013
Version: 4
This Medication Guide has been approved by the U.S. Food and Drug Administration.
Victoza® is a registered trademark of Novo Nordisk A/S.
Victoza® is covered by US Patent Nos. 6,268,343, 6,458,924, 7,235,627, 8,114,833 and other patents pending.
Victoza® pen is covered by US Patent Nos. 6,004,297, RE 43,834, RE 41,956 and other patents pending.
© 2010-2013 Novo Nordisk

PATIENT INSTRUCTIONS FOR USE
Victoza (liraglutide [rDNA origin]) injection

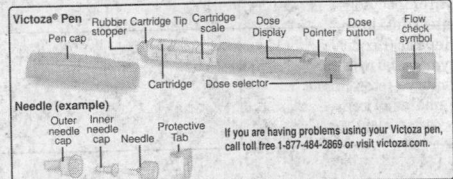

First read the Medication Guide that comes with your Victoza pen and then read these Patient Instructions for Use for information about how to use your Victoza pen the right way.
These instructions do not take the place of talking with your healthcare provider about your medical condition or your treatment.
Your Victoza pen contains 3 mL of Victoza and will deliver doses of 0.6 mg, 1.2 mg or 1.8 mg. The number of doses that you can take with a Victoza pen depends on the dose of medicine that is prescribed for you. Your healthcare provider will tell you how much Victoza to take.
Victoza pen should be used with Novo Nordisk disposable needles. Talk to your healthcare provider or pharmacist for more information about needles for your Victoza pen.
Important Information
- Do not share your Victoza pen or needles with anyone else. You may give an infection to them or get an infection from them.

- Always use a new needle for each injection.
- Keep your Victoza pen and all medicines out of the reach of children.
- If you drop your Victoza pen, repeat "First Time Use For Each New Pen" (steps A through D).
- Be careful not to bend or damage the needle.
- Do not use the cartridge scale to measure how much Victoza to inject.
- Be careful when handling used needles to avoid needle stick injuries.
- You can use your Victoza pen for up to 30 days after you use it the first time.
Caring for your Victoza pen
- After removing the needle, put the pen cap on your Victoza pen and store your Victoza pen without the needle attached.

- Do not try to refill your Victoza pen - it is prefilled and is disposable.
- Do not try to repair your pen or pull it apart.
- Keep your Victoza pen away from dust, dirt and liquids.
- If cleaning is needed, wipe the outside of the pen with a clean, damp cloth.
How should I store Victoza?
Before use:
- Store your new, unused Victoza pen in the refrigerator at 36°F to 46°F (2°C to 8°C).
- If Victoza is stored outside of refrigeration (by mistake) prior to first use, it should be used or thrown away within 30 days.
- Do not freeze Victoza or use Victoza if it has been frozen. Do not store Victoza near the refrigerator cooling element.
Pen in use:
- Store your Victoza pen for 30 days at 59°F to 86°F (15°C to 30°C), or in a refrigerator at 36°F to 46°F (2°C to 8°C).
- When carrying the pen away from home, store the pen at a temperature between 59°F to 86°F (15°C to 30°C).

- If Victoza has been exposed to temperatures above 86°F (30°C), it should be thrown away.
- Protect your Victoza pen from heat and sunlight.
- Keep the pen cap on when your Victoza pen is not in use.
- Use a Victoza pen for only 30 days. Throw away a used Victoza pen after 30 days, even if some medicine is left in the pen.
First Time Use for Each New Pen
Step A. Check the Pen
- Take your new Victoza pen out of the refrigerator.
- Wash hands with soap and water before use.
- Check pen label before each use to make sure it is your Victoza pen.
- Pull off pen cap.

- Check Victoza in the cartridge. The liquid should be clear, colorless and free of particles. If not, do not use.
- Wipe the rubber stopper with an alcohol swab.
Step B. Attach the Needle
- Remove protective tab from outer needle cap.
- Push outer needle cap containing the needle straight onto the pen, then screw needle on until secure.

- Pull off outer needle cap. Do not throw away.

- Pull off inner needle cap and throw away. A small drop of liquid may appear. This is normal.

Step C. Dial to the Flow Check Symbol
This step is done only ONCE for each new pen and is ONLY required the first time you use a new pen.
- Turn dose selector until flow check symbol (- --) lines up with pointer. The flow check symbol does not administer the dose as prescribed by your healthcare provider.
- To select the dose prescribed by your healthcare provider, continue to Step G under "Routine Use".

Flow check symbol selected

Step D. Prepare the Pen
- Hold pen with needle pointing up.
- Tap cartridge gently with your finger a few times to bring any air bubbles to the top of the cartridge.

- Keep needle pointing up and press dose button until 0 mg lines up with pointer. Repeat steps C and D, up to 6 times, until a drop of Victoza appears at the needle tip. If you still see no drop of Victoza, use a new pen and contact Novo Nordisk at 1-877-484-2869.
  Continue to Step G under "Routine Use" →

Routine Use
Step E. Check the Pen
- Take your Victoza pen from where it is stored.
- Wash hands with soap and water before use.
- Check pen label before each use to make sure it is your Victoza pen.
- Pull off pen cap.

- Check Victoza in the cartridge. The liquid should be clear, colorless and free of particles. If not, do not use.
- Wipe the rubber stopper with an alcohol swab.

Step F. Attach the Needle
- Remove protective tab from outer needle cap.
- Push outer needle cap containing the needle straight onto the pen, then screw needle on until secure.

- Pull off outer needle cap. Do not throw away.

- Pull off inner needle cap and throw away. A small drop of liquid may appear. This is normal.

Step G. Dial the Dose
- Victoza pen can give a dose of 0.6 mg (starting dose), 1.2 mg or 1.8 mg. Be sure that you know the dose of Victoza that is prescribed for you.

- Turn the dose selector until your needed dose lines up with the pointer (0.6 mg, 1.2 mg or 1.8 mg).
  [See figure at top of next column]
- You will hear a "click" every time you turn the dose selector. **Do not set the dose by counting the number of clicks you hear.**
- If you select a wrong dose, change it by turning the dose selector backwards or forwards until the correct dose lines

	0.6 mg selected
	1.2 mg selected
	1.8 mg selected

up with the pointer. Be careful not to press the dose button when turning the dose selector. This may cause Victoza to come out.

Step H. Injecting the Dose
- Insert needle into your skin in the stomach, thigh or upper arm. Use the injection technique shown to you by your healthcare provider. **Do not inject Victoza into a vein or muscle.**

- Press down on the center of the dose button to inject until 0 mg lines up with the pointer.
- Be careful not to touch the dose display with your other fingers. This may block the injection.
- Keep the dose button pressed down and make sure that you keep the needle under the skin for a full count of 6 seconds to make sure the full dose is injected. Keep your thumb on the injection button until you remove the needle from your skin.

- Change (rotate) your injection sites within the area you choose for each dose. **Do not** use the same injection site for each injection.

Step I. Withdraw Needle
- You may see a drop of Victoza at the needle tip. This is normal and it does not affect the dose you just received. If blood appears after you take the needle out of your skin, apply light pressure, but **do not rub the area.**

Step J. Remove and Dispose of the Needle
- Carefully put the outer needle cap over the needle. Unscrew the needle.

- Safely remove the needle from your Victoza pen after each use.
- Place used needles in a closeable, puncture-resistant container. If your Victoza pen is empty or if you have been using it for 30 days (even if it is not empty), throw away the used pen. You may use a sharps container (such as a red biohazard container), a hard plastic container (such as an empty detergent bottle), or metal container with a screw top (such as an empty coffee can).
- Ask your healthcare provider for instructions on the right way to dispose of your used needles, pens, and the container. Do not throw the disposal container in the household trash. Do not recycle.

Shown in Product Identification Guide, page 311

Onyx Pharmaceuticals, Inc.
249 E. GRAND AVENUE
SOUTH SAN FRANCISCO, CA 94080

Direct Inquires to:
Phone: 877-ONYX-121(669-9121)
Fax: 877-ONX-PHRM(669-7476)
medinfo@onyx.com

KYPROLIS ℞

HIGHLIGHTS OF PRESCRIBING INFORMATION
These highlights do not include all the information needed to use KYPROLIS safely and effectively. See full prescribing information for KYPROLIS.
Initial U.S. Approval: [2012]

———————INDICATIONS AND USAGE———————
KYPROLIS is a proteasome inhibitor indicated for the treatment of patients with multiple myeloma who have received at least two prior therapies including bortezomib and an immunomodulatory agent and have demonstrated disease progression on or within 60 days of completion of the last therapy. Approval is based on response rate. Clinical benefit, such as improvement in survival or symptoms, has not been verified. (1, 14)

———————DOSAGE AND ADMINISTRATION———————
- Administer intravenously over 2 to 10 minutes, on two consecutive days each week for three weeks (Days 1, 2, 8, 9, 15, and 16), followed by a 12-day rest period (Days 17 to 28). (2.1)
- Recommended Cycle 1 dose is 20 mg/m²/day and if tolerated increase Cycle 2 dose and subsequent cycles doses to 27 mg/m²/day. (2.1)
- Hydrate patients prior to and following administration. (2.2)
- Pre-medicate with dexamethasone prior to all Cycle 1 doses, during the first cycle of dose escalation, and if infusion reaction symptoms develop or reappear. (2.3)
- Modify dosing based on toxicity. (2.4)

———————DOSAGE FORMS AND STRENGTHS———————
Single-use vial: 60 mg sterile lyophilized powder (3)

———————CONTRAINDICATIONS———————
None (4)

———————WARNINGS AND PRECAUTIONS———————
- Cardiac Adverse Reactions including heart failure and ischemia: Monitor for cardiac complications. Treat promptly and withhold KYPROLIS. (2.4, 5.1)
- Pulmonary Hypertension: Withhold dosing if suspected. (2.4, 5.2)
- Pulmonary Complications: Monitor for and manage dyspnea immediately; interrupt KYPROLIS until symptoms have resolved or returned to baseline. (2.4, 5.3)
- Infusion Reactions: Pre-medicate with dexamethasone to prevent. (2.3) Advise patients to seek immediate medical attention if symptoms develop. (5.4)
- Tumor Lysis Syndrome (TLS): Hydrate patients to prevent. (2.2) Monitor for TLS and treat promptly. (5.5)
- Thrombocytopenia: Monitor platelet counts; reduce or interrupt dosing as clinically indicated. (2.4, 5.6)
- Hepatic Toxicity and Hepatic Failure: Monitor liver enzymes and withhold dosing if suspected. (2.4, 5.7)
- Embryo-fetal Toxicity: KYPROLIS can cause fetal harm. Females of reproductive potential should avoid becoming pregnant while being treated. (5.8, 8.1)

———————ADVERSE REACTIONS———————
Most commonly reported adverse reactions (incidence ≥ 30%) are fatigue, anemia, nausea, thrombocytopenia, dyspnea, diarrhea, and pyrexia. (6)
To report SUSPECTED ADVERSE REACTIONS, contact Onyx Pharmaceuticals, Inc. at 1-877-669-9121 or FDA at 1-800-FDA-1088 or *www.fda.gov/medwatch.*

———————USE IN SPECIFIC POPULATIONS———————
- Patients on dialysis: Administer KYPROLIS after the dialysis procedure. (8.6)
See 17 for PATIENT COUNSELING INFORMATION
Revised: 07/2012

———————————————————————————————————————
FULL PRESCRIBING INFORMATION: CONTENTS*

FULL PRESCRIBING INFORMATION

1   INDICATIONS AND USAGE

KYPROLIS is indicated for the treatment of patients with
multiple myeloma who have received at least two prior therapies including bortezomib and an immunomodulatory
agent and have demonstrated disease progression on or
within 60 days of completion of the last therapy. Approval is
based on response rate [see *Clinical Studies (14.1)*]. Clinical
benefit, such as improvement in survival or symptoms, has
not been verified.

2   DOSAGE AND ADMINISTRATION

2.1   Dosing Guidelines

KYPROLIS is administered intravenously over 2 to 10 minutes, on two consecutive days, each week for three weeks
(Days 1, 2, 8, 9, 15, and 16), followed by a 12-day rest period
(Days 17 to 28). Each 28-day period is considered one treatment cycle (Table 1).
In Cycle 1, KYPROLIS is administered at a dose of 20 mg/
m^2. If tolerated in Cycle 1, the dose should be escalated to
27 mg/m^2 beginning in Cycle 2 and continued at 27 mg/m^2
in subsequent cycles. Treatment may be continued until disease progression or until unacceptable toxicity occurs [see
Dosage and Administration (2.4)].

The dose is calculated using the patient's actual body surface area at baseline. Patients with a body surface area
greater than 2.2 m^2 should receive a dose based upon a body
surface are of 2.2 m^2. Dose adjustments do not need to be
made for weight changes of less than or equal to 20%.
[See table 1 below]

2.2   Hydration and Fluid Monitoring

Hydrate patients to reduce the risk of renal toxicity and of
tumor lysis syndrome (TLS) with KYPROLIS treatment
[see *Warnings and Precautions (5.5)*]. Maintain adequate
fluid volume status throughout treatment and monitor
blood chemistries closely. Prior to each dose in Cycle 1, give
250 mL to 500 mL of intravenous normal saline or other appropriate intravenous fluid. Give an additional 250 mL to
500 mL of intravenous fluids as needed following
KYPROLIS administration. Continue intravenous hydration, as needed, in subsequent cycles. Also monitor patients
during this period for fluid overload [see *Warnings and Precautions (5.1)*].

2.3   Dexamethasone Premedication

Pre-medicate with dexamethasone 4 mg orally or intravenously prior to all doses of KYPROLIS during Cycle 1 and
prior to all KYPROLIS doses during the first cycle of dose
escalation to 27 mg/m^2 to reduce the incidence and severity
of infusion reactions [see *Warnings and Precautions (5.4)*].
Reinstate dexamethasone premedication (4 mg orally or intravenously) if these symptoms develop or reappear during
subsequent cycles.

2.4   Dose Modifications Based on Toxicities

Recommended actions and dose modifications are presented
in Table 2.

**Table 2: Dose Modifications for Toxicity* during
KYPROLIS Treatment**

Hematologic Toxicity	Recommended Action
● Grade 3[a] or 4 Neutropenia ● Grade 4 Thrombocytopenia [see *Warnings and Precautions (5.6)*]	● Withhold dose. ● If fully recovered before next scheduled dose, continue at same dose level. ● If recovered to Grade 2 neutropenia or Grade 3 thrombocytopenia, reduce dose by one dose level (from 27 mg/m^2 to 20 mg/m^2, OR from 20 mg/m^2 to 15 mg/m^2). ● If tolerated, the reduced dose may be escalated to the previous dose at the discretion of the physician.

Non-Hematologic Toxicity	Recommended Action
Cardiac Toxicity Grade 3 or 4, new onset or worsening of: ● congestive heart failure; ● decreased left ventricular function; ● or myocardial ischemia [see *Warnings and Precautions (5.1)*]	● Withhold until resolved or returned to baseline. ● After resolution, consider if restarting KYPROLIS at a reduced dose is appropriate (from 27 mg/m^2 to 20 mg/m^2, OR from 20 mg/m^2 to 15 mg/m^2). ● If tolerated, the reduced dose may be escalated to the previous dose at the discretion of the physician.
Pulmonary Hypertension [see *Warnings and Precautions (5.2)*]	● Withhold until resolved or returned to baseline. ● Restart at the dose used prior to the event or reduced dose (from 27 mg/m^2 to 20 mg/m^2, OR from 20 mg/m^2 to 15 mg/m^2), at the discretion of the physician. ● If tolerated, the reduced dose may be escalated to the previous dose at the discretion of the physician.
Pulmonary Complications ● Grade 3 or 4 [see *Warnings and Precautions (5.3)*]	● Withhold until resolved or returned to baseline. ● Consider restarting at the next scheduled treatment with one dose level reduction (from 27 mg/m^2 to 20 mg/m^2, OR from 20 mg/m^2 to 15 mg/m^2). ● If tolerated, the reduced dose may be escalated to the previous dose at the discretion of the physician.
Hepatic Toxicity ● Grade 3 or 4 elevation of transaminases, bilirubin or other liver abnormalities [see *Warnings and Precautions (5.7)*]	● Withhold until resolved or returned to baseline. ● After resolution, consider if restarting KYPROLIS is appropriate; may be reinitiated at a reduced dose (from 27 mg/m^2 to 20 mg/m^2, OR from 20 mg/m^2 to 15 mg/m^2) with frequent monitoring of liver function. ● If tolerated, the reduced dose may be escalated to the previous dose at the discretion of the physician.
Renal Toxicity ● Serum creatinine equal to or greater than 2 × baseline [see *Adverse Reactions (6.1)*]	● Withhold until renal function has recovered to Grade 1 or to baseline and monitor renal function. ● If attributable to KYPROLIS, restart at the next scheduled treatment at a reduced dose (from 27 mg/m^2 to 20 mg/m^2, OR from 20 mg/m^2 to 15 mg/m^2). ● If not attributable to KYPROLIS, restart at the dose used prior to the event. ● If tolerated, the reduced dose may be escalated to the previous dose at the discretion of the physician.
Peripheral Neuropathy ● Grade 3 or 4 [see *Adverse Reactions (6.1)*]	● Withhold until resolved or returned to baseline. ● Restart at the dose used prior to the event or reduced dose (from 27 mg/m^2 to 20 mg/m^2, OR from 20 mg/m^2 to 15 mg/m^2), at the discretion of the physician. ● If tolerated, the reduced dose may be escalated to the previous dose at the discretion of the physician.
Other ● Grade 3 or 4 non-hematological toxicities	● Withhold until resolved or returned to baseline. ● Consider restarting at the next scheduled treatment with one dose level reduction (from 27 mg/m^2 to 20 mg/m^2, OR from 20 mg/m^2 to 15 mg/m^2). ● If tolerated, the reduced dose may be escalated to the previous dose at the discretion of the physician.

* National Cancer Institute Common Terminology
Criteria for Adverse Events (NCI CTCAE) Version 3.0

2.5   Administration Precautions

The quantity of KYPROLIS contained in one single-use vial
(60 mg carfilzomib) may exceed the required dose. Caution
should be used in calculating the quantity delivered to prevent overdosing.

Table 1: KYPROLIS Dosage Regimen for Patients with Multiple Myeloma

	Cycle 1									
	Week 1			Week 2			Week 3			Week 4
KYPROLIS (20 mg/m^2):	Day 1	Day 2	Days 3-7	Day 8	Day 9	Days 10-14	Day 15	Day 16	Days 17-21	Days 22-28
	20	20	No Dosing	20	20	No Dosing	20	20	No Dosing	No Dosing

	Cycles 2 and Beyond*									
	Week 1			Week 2			Week 3			Week 4
KYPROLIS (27 mg/m^2):	Day 1	Day 2	Days 3-7	Day 8	Day 9	Days 10-14	Day 15	Day 16	Days 17-21	Days 22-28
	27	27	No Dosing	27	27	No Dosing	27	27	No Dosing	No Dosing

* If previous cycle dosage is tolerated.

Do not mix KYPROLIS with or administer as an infusion with other medicinal products.

The intravenous administration line should be flushed with normal saline or 5% Dextrose Injection, USP immediately before and after KYPROLIS administration. KYPROLIS should not be administered as a bolus. KYPROLIS should be administered over 2 to 10 minutes.

2.6 Reconstitution and Preparation for Intravenous Administration

KYPROLIS vials contain no antimicrobial preservatives and are intended only for single use. Unopened vials of KYPROLIS are stable until the date indicated on the package when stored in the original package at 2°C to 8°C (36°F to 46°F). The reconstituted solution contains carfilzomib at a concentration of 2 mg/mL. Read the complete preparation instructions prior to reconstitution.

Reconstitution/Preparation Steps:

1. Remove vial from refrigerator just prior to use.
2. Aseptically reconstitute each vial by slowly injecting **29 mL** Sterile Water for Injection, USP, directing the solution onto the INSIDE WALL OF THE VIAL to minimize foaming.

3. Gently swirl and/or invert the vial slowly for about 1 minute, or until complete dissolution of any cake or powder occurs. DO NOT SHAKE to avoid foam generation. If foaming occurs, allow solution to rest in vial for about 2 to 5 minutes, until foaming subsides.
4. After reconstitution, KYPROLIS is ready for intravenous administration. The reconstituted product should be a clear, colorless solution. If any discoloration or particulate matter is observed, do not use the reconstituted product.
5. When administering in an intravenous bag, withdraw the calculated dose [see *Dosage and Administration (2.1)*] from the vial and dilute into **50 mL** 5% Dextrose Injection, USP intravenous bag.
6. Immediately discard the vial containing the unused portion.

The stabilities of reconstituted KYPROLIS under various temperature and container conditions are shown in Table 3. [See table 3 above]

3 DOSAGE FORMS AND STRENGTHS

KYPROLIS single-use vial contains 60 mg of carfilzomib as a sterile, white to off-white lyophilized cake or powder.

4 CONTRAINDICATIONS

None.

5 WARNINGS AND PRECAUTIONS

5.1 Cardiac Arrest, Congestive Heart Failure, Myocardial Ischemia

Death due to cardiac arrest has occurred within a day of KYPROLIS administration. New onset or worsening of pre-existing congestive heart failure with decreased left ventricular function or myocardial ischemia have occurred following administration of KYPROLIS. Cardiac failure events (e.g., cardiac failure congestive, pulmonary edema, ejection fraction decreased) were reported in 7% of patients. Monitor for cardiac complications and manage promptly. Withhold KYPROLIS for Grade 3 or 4 cardiac events until recovery and consider whether to restart KYPROLIS based on a benefit/risk assessment [see *Dosage and Administration (2.4)*]. Patients with New York Heart Association Class III and IV heart failure, myocardial infarction in the preceding 6 months, and conduction abnormalities uncontrolled by medications were not eligible for the clinical trials. These patients may be at greater risk for cardiac complications.

5.2 Pulmonary Hypertension

Pulmonary arterial hypertension (PAH) was reported in 2% of patients treated with KYPROLIS and was Grade 3 or greater in less than 1% of patients. Evaluate with cardiac imaging and/or other tests as indicated. Withhold KYPROLIS for pulmonary hypertension until resolved or returned to baseline and consider whether to restart KYPROLIS based on a benefit/risk assessment [see *Dosage and Administration (2.4)*].

5.3 Pulmonary Complications

Dyspnea was reported in 35% of patients enrolled in clinical trials. Grade 3 dyspnea occurred in 5%; no Grade 4 events, and 1 death (Grade 5) was reported. Monitor and manage

Table 3: Stability of Reconstituted KYPROLIS

Storage Conditions of Reconstituted KYPROLIS	Stability*per Container		
	Vial	Syringe	IV Bag (D5W†)
Refrigerated (2°C to 8°C; 36°F to 46°F)	24 hours	24 hours	24 hours
Room Temperature (15°C to 30°C; 59°F to 86°F)	4 hours	4 hours	4 hours

* Total time from reconstitution to administration should not exceed 24 hours.
† 5% Dextrose Injection, USP.

dyspnea immediately; interrupt KYPROLIS until symptoms have resolved or returned to baseline [see *Dosage and Administration (2.4)* and *Adverse Reactions (6.1)*].

5.4 Infusion Reactions

Infusion reactions were characterized by a spectrum of systemic symptoms including fever, chills, arthralgia, myalgia, facial flushing, facial edema, vomiting, weakness, shortness of breath, hypotension, syncope, chest tightness, or angina. These reactions can occur immediately following or up to 24 hours after administration of KYPROLIS. Administer dexamethasone prior to KYPROLIS to reduce the incidence and severity of reactions [see *Dosage and Administration (2.3)*]. Inform patients of the risk and symptoms and to contact physician if symptoms of an infusion reaction occur [see *Patient Counseling Information (17)*].

5.5 Tumor Lysis Syndrome

Tumor lysis syndrome (TLS) occurred following KYPROLIS administration in < 1% of patients. Patients with multiple myeloma and a high tumor burden should be considered to be at greater risk for TLS. Prior to receiving KYPROLIS, ensure that patients are well hydrated [see *Dosage and Administration (2.2)*]. Monitor for evidence of TLS during treatment, and manage promptly. Interrupt KYPROLIS until TLS is resolved [see *Dosage and Administration (2.4)*].

5.6 Thrombocytopenia

KYPROLIS causes thrombocytopenia with platelet nadirs occurring around Day 8 of each 28-day cycle and recovery to baseline by the start of the next 28-day cycle. In patients with multiple myeloma, 36% of patients experienced thrombocytopenia, including Grade 4 in 10%. Thrombocytopenia following KYPROLIS administration resulted in a dose reduction in 1% of patients and discontinuation of treatment with KYPROLIS in < 1% of patients. Monitor platelet counts frequently during treatment with KYPROLIS. Reduce or interrupt dose as clinically indicated [see *Dosage and Administration (2.4)*].

5.7 Hepatic Toxicity and Hepatic Failure

Cases of hepatic failure, including fatal cases, have been reported (< 1%). KYPROLIS can cause elevations of serum transaminases and bilirubin. Withhold KYPROLIS in patients experiencing Grade 3 or greater elevations of transaminases, bilirubin, or other liver abnormalities until resolved or returned to baseline. After resolution, consider if restarting KYPROLIS is appropriate. Monitor liver enzymes frequently [see *Dosage and Administration (2.4)* and *Adverse Reactions (6.1)*].

5.8 Embryo-fetal Toxicity

KYPROLIS can cause fetal harm when administered to a pregnant woman based on its mechanism of action and findings in animals. There are no adequate and well-controlled studies in pregnant women using KYPROLIS. Carfilzomib caused embryo-fetal toxicity in pregnant rabbits at doses that were lower than in patients receiving the recommended dose.

Females of reproductive potential should be advised to avoid becoming pregnant while being treated with KYPROLIS. If this drug is used during pregnancy, or if the patient becomes pregnant while taking this drug, the patient should be apprised of the potential hazard to the fetus [see *Use in Specific Populations (8.1)*].

6 ADVERSE REACTIONS

The following adverse reactions are discussed in greater detail in other sections of the labeling:
- Cardiac Arrest, Congestive Heart Failure, Myocardial Ischemia [see *Warnings and Precautions (5.1)*]
- Pulmonary Hypertension [see *Warnings and Precautions (5.2)*]
- Pulmonary Complications [see *Warnings and Precautions (5.3)*]
- Infusion Reactions [see *Warnings and Precautions (5.4)*]
- Tumor Lysis Syndrome [see *Warnings and Precautions (5.5)*]
- Thrombocytopenia [see *Warnings and Precautions (5.6)*]
- Hepatic Toxicity and Hepatic Failure [see *Warnings and Precautions (5.7)*]

The most common adverse reactions (incidence of 30% or greater) to KYPROLIS observed in clinical trials of patients with multiple myeloma were fatigue, anemia, nausea, thrombocytopenia, dyspnea, diarrhea, and pyrexia.

6.1 Clinical Trials Safety Experience

Because clinical trials are conducted under widely varying conditions, adverse reaction rates observed in the clinical trials of a drug cannot be directly compared with rates in the clinical trials of another drug, and may not reflect the rates observed in medical practice.

A total of 526 patients with relapsed and/or refractory multiple myeloma received KYPROLIS as monotherapy or with pre-dose dexamethasone. Patients received a median of four treatment cycles with a median cumulative KYPROLIS dose of 993.4 mg.

Deaths due to all causes within 30 days of the last dose of KYPROLIS occurred in 37/526 (7%) of patients. Deaths not attributed to disease progression were cardiac in 5 patients (acute coronary syndrome, cardiac arrest, cardiac disorder), end-organ failure in 4 patients (multi-organ failure, hepatic failure, renal failure), infection in 4 patients (sepsis, pneumonia, respiratory tract bacterial infection), dyspnea and intracranial hemorrhage in 1 patient each, and 1 patient found dead of unknown causes.

Serious adverse reactions were reported in 45% patients. The most common serious adverse reactions were pneumonia (10%), acute renal failure (4%), pyrexia (3%), and congestive heart failure (3%). Adverse reactions leading to discontinuation of KYPROLIS occurred in 15% of patients and included congestive heart failure (2%), cardiac arrest, dyspnea, increased blood creatinine, and acute renal failure (1% each).

Adverse reactions occurring at a rate of 10% or greater are presented in Table 4.

Table 4: Incidence of Adverse Reactions Occurring in ≥ 10% of Multiple Myeloma Patients Treated with KYPROLIS

Event	Patients (N = 526) [n (%)]		
	All Grades*	Grade 3 Events	Grade 4 Events
Fatigue	292 (55.5)	38 (7.2)	2 (0.4)
Anemia	246 (46.8)	111 (21.1)	7 (1.3)
Nausea	236 (44.9)	7 (1.3)	0
Thrombocytopenia	191 (36.3)	69 (13.1)	54 (10.3)
Dyspnea	182 (34.6)	25 (4.8)	1 (0.2)†
Diarrhea	172 (32.7)	4 (0.8)	1 (0.2)
Pyrexia	160 (30.4)	7 (1.3)	2 (0.4)
Upper respiratory tract infection	149 (28.3)	17 (3.2)	0
Headache	145 (27.6)	7 (1.3)	0
Cough	137 (26.0)	1 (0.2)	0
Blood creatinine increased	127 (24.1)	13 (2.5)	1 (0.2)
Lymphopenia	126 (24.0)	84 (16.0)	11 (2.1)
Edema peripheral	126 (24.0)	3 (0.6)	0
Vomiting	117 (22.2)	5 (1.0)	0
Constipation	110 (20.9)	1 (0.2)	0
Neutropenia	109 (20.7)	50 (9.5)	4 (0.8)
Back pain	106 (20.2)	15 (2.9)	0
Insomnia	94 (17.9)	0	0
Chills	84 (16.0)	1 (0.2)	0
Arthralgia	83 (15.8)	7 (1.3)	0
Muscle spasms	76 (14.4)	2 (0.4)	0
Hypertension	75 (14.3)	15 (2.9)	2 (0.4)
Asthenia	73 (13.9)	12 (2.3)	1 (0.2)
Hypokalemia	72 (13.7)	14 (2.7)	3 (0.6)
Hypomagnesemia	71 (13.5)	2 (0.4)	0
Leukopenia	71 (13.5)	27 (5.1)	1 (0.2)
Pain in extremity	70 (13.3)	7 (1.3)	0
Pneumonia	67 (12.7)	52 (9.9)	3 (0.6)†
Aspartate aminotransferase increased	66 (12.5)	15 (2.9)	1 (0.2)
Dizziness	66 (12.5)	5 (1.0)	1 (0.2)
Hypoesthesia	64 (12.2)	3 (0.6)	0
Anorexia	63 (12.0)	1 (0.2)	0
Pain	63 (12.0)	12 (2.3)	1 (0.2)
Hyperglycemia	62 (11.8)	16 (3.0)	3 (0.6)
Chest wall pain	60 (11.4)	3 (0.6)	0

Hypercalcemia	58 (11.0)	13 (2.5)	8 (1.5)
Hypophosphatemia	55 (10.5)	24 (4.6)	3 (0.6)
Hyponatremia	54 (10.3)	31 (5.9)	3 (0.6)

* National Cancer Institute Common Terminology Criteria for Adverse Events (NCI CTCAE) Version 3.0
† One event was Grade 5 severity.

Description of Selected Adverse Drug Reactions
Renal Events
The most common renal adverse reactions were increase in blood creatinine (24%) and renal failure (9%), which were mostly Grade 1 or Grade 2 in severity. Grade 3 renal adverse reactions occurred in 6% of patients and Grade 4 events occurred in 1%. Discontinuations due to increased blood creatinine and acute renal failure were 1% each. In one patient, death occurred with concurrent sepsis and worsening renal function [see *Dosage and Administration (2.4)*].
Peripheral Neuropathy
Peripheral neuropathy (including all events of peripheral sensory neuropathy and peripheral motor neuropathy) occurred in 14% of patients enrolled in clinical trials. Grade 3 peripheral neuropathy occurred in 1% of patients. Serious peripheral neuropathy events occurred in < 1% of patients, which resulted in dose reduction in < 1% and treatment discontinuation in < 1%. Withhold or discontinue treatment as recommended [see *Dosage and Administration (2.4)*].
Herpes Virus Infection
Herpes zoster reactivation was reported in 2% of patients. Consider antiviral prophylaxis for patients who have a history of herpes zoster infection.

7 DRUG INTERACTIONS
Carfilzomib is primarily metabolized via peptidase and epoxide hydrolase activities, and as a result, the pharmacokinetic profile of carfilzomib is unlikely to be affected by concomitant administration of cytochrome P450 inhibitors and inducers. Carfilzomib is not expected to influence exposure of other drugs [see *Clinical Pharmacology (12.3)*].

8 USE IN SPECIFIC POPULATIONS
8.1 Pregnancy
Pregnancy Category D [*see Warnings and Precautions (5.8)*]. Females of reproductive potential should be advised to avoid becoming pregnant while being treated with KYPROLIS. Based on its mechanism of action and findings in animals, KYPROLIS can cause fetal harm when administered to a pregnant woman. Carfilzomib caused embryofetal toxicity in pregnant rabbits at doses that were lower than in patients receiving the recommended dose. If KYPROLIS is used during pregnancy, or if the patient becomes pregnant while taking this drug, the patient should be apprised of the potential hazard to the fetus.
Carfilzomib was administered intravenously to pregnant rats and rabbits during the period of organogenesis at doses of 0.5, 1, and 2 mg/kg/day in rats and 0.2, 0.4, and 0.8 mg/kg/day in rabbits. Carfilzomib was not teratogenic at any dose tested. In rabbits, there was an increase in preimplantation loss at ≥ 0.4 mg/kg/day and an increase in early resorptions and post-implantation loss and a decrease in fetal weight at the maternally toxic dose of 0.8 mg/kg/day. The doses of 0.4 and 0.8 mg/kg/day in rabbits are approximately 20% and 40%, respectively, of the recommended dose in humans of 27 mg/m^2 based on body surface area.
8.3 Nursing Mothers
It is not known whether KYPROLIS is excreted in human milk. Since many drugs are excreted in human milk and because of the potential for serious adverse reactions in nursing infants from KYPROLIS, a decision should be made whether to discontinue nursing or to discontinue the drug, taking into account the importance of the drug to the mother.
8.4 Pediatric Use
The safety and effectiveness of KYPROLIS in pediatric patients have not been established.
8.5 Geriatric Use
In studies of KYPROLIS there were no clinically significant differences observed in safety and efficacy between patients less than 65 years of age and patients 65 years of age and older.
8.6 Renal Impairment
The pharmacokinetics and safety of KYPROLIS were evaluated in a Phase 2 trial in patients with normal renal function and those with mild, moderate, and severe renal impairment and patients on chronic dialysis. On average, patients were treated for 5.5 cycles using KYPROLIS doses of 15 mg/m^2 on Cycle 1, 20 mg/m^2 on Cycle 2, and 27 mg/m^2 on Cycles 3 and beyond. The pharmacokinetics and safety of KYPROLIS were not influenced by the degree of baseline renal impairment, including the patients on dialysis. Since dialysis clearance of KYPROLIS concentrations has not been studied, the drug should be administered after the dialysis procedure [see *Clinical Pharmacology (12.3)*].
8.7 Hepatic Impairment
The safety, efficacy and pharmacokinetics of KYPROLIS have not been evaluated in patients with baseline hepatic impairment. Patients with the following laboratory values were excluded from the KYPROLIS clinical trials: ALT/AST ≥ 3 × upper limit of normal (ULN) and bilirubin ≥ 2 × ULN [see *Clinical Pharmacology (12.3)*].
8.8 Cardiac Impairment
Patients with New York Heart Association Class III and IV heart failure were not eligible for the clinical trials. Safety in this population has not been evaluated.

10 OVERDOSAGE
There is no known specific antidote for KYPROLIS overdosage. In the event of an overdosage, monitor the patient and provide appropriate supportive care.

11 DESCRIPTION
KYPROLIS (carfilzomib) for Injection is an antineoplastic agent available for intravenous use only. KYPROLIS is a sterile, white to off-white lyophilized powder and is available as a single-use vial. Each vial of KYPROLIS contains 60 mg of carfilzomib, 3000 mg sulfobutylether beta-cyclodextrin, 57.7 mg citric acid, and sodium hydroxide for pH adjustment (target pH 3.5).
Carfilzomib is a modified tetrapeptidyl epoxide, isolated as the crystalline free base. The chemical name for carfilzomib is (2S)-N-((S)-1-((S)-4-methyl-1-((R)-2-methyloxiran-2-yl)-1-oxopentan-2-ylcarbamoyl)-2-phenylethyl)-2-((S)-2-(2-morpholinoacetamido)-4-phenylbutanamido)-4-methylpentanamide. Carfilzomib has the following structure:

Carfilzomib is a crystalline substance with a molecular weight of 719.9. The molecular formula is $C_{40}H_{57}N_5O_7$. Carfilzomib is practically insoluble in water, and very slightly soluble in acidic conditions.

12 CLINICAL PHARMACOLOGY
12.1 Mechanism of Action
Carfilzomib is a tetrapeptide epoxyketone proteasome inhibitor that irreversibly binds to the N-terminal threonine-containing active sites of the 20S proteasome, the proteolytic core particle within the 26S proteasome. Carfilzomib had antiproliferative and proapoptotic activities *in vitro* in solid and hematologic tumor cells. In animals, carfilzomib inhibited proteasome activity in blood and tissue and delayed tumor growth in models of multiple myeloma, hematologic, and solid tumors.
12.2 Pharmacodynamics
Intravenous carfilzomib administration resulted in suppression of proteasome chymotrypsin-like activity when measured in blood 1 hour after the first dose. On Day 1 of Cycle 1, proteasome inhibition in peripheral blood mononuclear cells (PBMCs) ranged from 79% to 89% at 15 mg/m^2, and from 82% to 83% at 20 mg/m^2. In addition, carfilzomib administration resulted in inhibition of the LMP2 and MECL1 subunits of the immunoproteasome ranging from 26% to 32% and 41% to 49%, respectively, at 20 mg/m^2. Proteasome inhibition was maintained for ≥ 48 hours following the first dose of carfilzomib for each week of dosing.
12.3 Pharmacokinetics
Absorption: The C_{max} and AUC following a single intravenous dose of 27 mg/m^2 was 4232 ng/mL and 379 ng•hr/mL, respectively. Following repeated doses of carfilzomib at 15 and 20 mg/m^2, systemic exposure (AUC) and half-life were similar on Days 1 and 15 or 16 of Cycle 1, suggesting there was no systemic carfilzomib accumulation. At doses between 20 and 36 mg/m^2, there was a dose-dependent increase in exposure.
Distribution: The mean steady-state volume of distribution of a 20 mg/m^2 dose of carfilzomib was 28 L. When tested *in vitro*, the binding of carfilzomib to human plasma proteins averaged 97% over the concentration range of 0.4 to 4 micromolar.
Metabolism: Carfilzomib was rapidly and extensively metabolized. The predominant metabolites measured in human plasma and urine, and generated *in vitro* by human hepatocytes, were peptide fragments and the diol of carfilzomib, suggesting that peptidase cleavage and epoxide hydrolysis were the principal pathways of metabolism. Cytochrome P450-mediated mechanisms played a minor role in overall carfilzomib metabolism. The metabolites have no known biologic activity.
Elimination: Following intravenous administration of doses ≥ 15 mg/m^2, carfilzomib was rapidly cleared from the systemic circulation with a half-life of ≤ 1 hour on Day 1 of Cycle 1. The systemic clearance ranged from 151 to 263 L/hour, and exceeded hepatic blood flow, suggesting that carfilzomib was largely cleared extrahepatically. The pathways of carfilzomib elimination have not been characterized in humans.

Age: Analysis of population pharmacokinetics data after the first dose of Cycle 1 (Day 1) in 154 patients who had received an IV dose of 20 mg/m^2 showed no clinically significant difference in exposure between patients < 65 years and ≥ 65 years of age.
Gender: Mean dose-normalized AUC and C_{max} values were comparable between male and female patients in the population pharmacokinetics study.
Hepatic Impairment: No pharmacokinetic studies were performed with KYPROLIS in patients with hepatic impairment [see *Warnings and Precautions (5.7)*].
Renal Impairment: A pharmacokinetic study was conducted in which 43 multiple myeloma patients who had various degrees of renal impairment and who were classified according to their creatinine clearances (CLcr) into the following groups: normal function (CLcr > 80 mL/min, n = 8), mild impairment (CLcr 50–80 mL/min, n = 12), moderate impairment (CLcr 30–49 mL/min, n = 8), severe impairment (CLcr < 30 mL/min, n = 7), and chronic dialysis (n = 8). KYPROLIS was administered intravenously over 2 to 10 minutes, on two consecutive days, weekly for three weeks (Days 1, 2, 8, 9, 15, and 16), followed by a 12-day rest period every 28 days. Patients received an initial dose of 15 mg/m^2, which could be escalated to 20 mg/m^2 starting in Cycle 2 if 15 mg/m^2 was well tolerated in Cycle 1. In this study, renal function status had no effect on the clearance or exposure of carfilzomib following a single or repeat-dose administration [see *Use in Specific Populations (8.6)*].
Cytochrome P450: In an *in vitro* study using human liver microsomes, carfilzomib showed modest direct and time-dependent inhibitory effect on human cytochrome CYP3A4/5. *In vitro* studies indicated that carfilzomib did not induce human CYP1A2 and CYP3A4 in cultured fresh human hepatocytes. Cytochrome P450-mediated mechanisms play a minor role in the overall metabolism of carfilzomib. A clinical trial of 17 patients using oral midazolam as a CYP3A probe demonstrated that the pharmacokinetics of midazolam were unaffected by concomitant carfilzomib administration. KYPROLIS is not expected to inhibit CYP3A4/5 activities and/or affect the exposure to CYP3A4/5 substrates.
P-gp: Carfilzomib is a P-glycoprotein (P-gp) substrate and showed marginal inhibitory effects on P-gp in a Caco-2 monolayer system. Given that KYPROLIS is administrated intravenously and is extensively metabolized, the pharmacokinetic profile of KYPROLIS is unlikely to be affected by P-gp inhibitors or inducers.

13 NONCLINICAL TOXICOLOGY
13.1 Carcinogenesis, Mutagenesis, Impairment of Fertility
Carcinogenicity studies have not been conducted with carfilzomib.
Carfilzomib was clastogenic in the *in vitro* chromosomal aberration test in peripheral blood lymphocytes. Carfilzomib was not mutagenic in the *in vitro* bacterial reverse mutation (Ames) test and was not clastogenic in the *in vivo* mouse bone marrow micronucleus assay.
Fertility studies with carfilzomib have not been conducted. No effects on reproductive tissues were noted during 28-day repeat-dose rat and monkey toxicity studies or in 6-month rat and 9-month monkey chronic toxicity studies.
13.2 Animal Toxicology and/or Pharmacology
Monkeys administered a single bolus intravenous dose of carfilzomib at 3 mg/kg (approximately 1.3 times recommended dose in humans of 27 mg/m^2 based on body surface area) experienced hypotension, increased heart rate, and increased serum levels of troponin-T. The repeated bolus intravenous administration of carfilzomib at ≥ 2 mg/kg/dose in rats and 2 mg/kg/dose in monkeys using dosing schedules similar to those used clinically resulted in mortalities that were due to toxicities occurring in the cardiovascular (cardiac failure, cardiac fibrosis, pericardial fluid accumulation, cardiac hemorrhage/degeneration), gastrointestinal (necrosis/hemorrhage), renal (glomerulonephropathy, tubular necrosis, dysfunction), and pulmonary (hemorrhage/inflammation) systems. The dose of 2 mg/kg/dose in rats is approximately half the recommended dose in humans of 27 mg/m^2 based on body surface area. The dose of 2 mg/kg/dose in monkeys is approximately equivalent to the recommended dose in humans based on body surface area.

14 CLINICAL STUDIES
14.1 Relapsed Multiple Myeloma
The safety and efficacy of KYPROLIS were evaluated in a single-arm, multicenter clinical trial. Two hundred and sixty-six patients with relapsed multiple myeloma who had received at least two prior therapies (including bortezomib and thalidomide and/or lenalidomide) were enrolled. Patients were enrolled in the trial whose disease had a less than or equal to 25% response to the most recent therapy or had disease progression during or within 60 days of the most recent therapy. Patients were excluded from the trial with total bilirubin levels ≥ 2 × upper limit of normal (ULN); creatinine clearance rates < 30 mL/min; New York Heart Association Class III to IV congestive heart failure; symptomatic cardiac ischemia; myocardial infarction within the last 6 months; peripheral neuropathy Grade 3 or 4, or

Table 5: Demographics and Baseline Disease Characteristics

Characteristic	Number of Patients (%)
Patient Characteristics	
Enrolled patients	266 (100)
Median age, years (range)	63.0 (37, 87)
Age group, < 65 / ≥ 65 (years)	146 (54.9) / 120 (45.1)
Gender (male / female)	155 (58.3) / 111 (41.7)
Race (White / Black / Asian / Other)	190 (71.4) / 53 (19.9) / 6 (2.3) / 17 (6.4)
Disease Characteristics	
Number of Prior Regimens (median)	5*
Prior Transplant	198 (74.4)
Refractory Status to Most Recent Therapy[†]	
Refractory: Progression during most recent therapy	198 (74.4)
Refractory: Progression within 60 days after completion of most recent therapy	
Refractory: ≤ 25% response to treatment	38 (14.3)
Relapsed: Progression after 60 days post treatment	16 (6.0)
	14 (5.3)
Years since diagnosis, median (range)	5.35 (0.5, 22.3)
Plasma cell involvement	
(< 50% / ≥ 50% / unknown or missing)	143 (53.8) / 106 (39.8) / 17 (6.4)
Cytogenetics or FISH analyses	
Normal/Favorable	159 (59.8)
Poor Prognosis	75 (28.2)
Unknown/Not tested	32 (12.0)
Serum Beta-2 Microglobulin	
median (range)	4.3 (0.4, 20.5)
Creatinine clearance < 30 (mL/min)	6 (2.3)

* Range: 1, 20.
† Categories for refractory status are derived by programmatic assessment using available laboratory data.

peripheral neuropathy Grade 2 with pain; active infections requiring treatment; and pleural effusion.
KYPROLIS was administered intravenously over 2 to 10 minutes on two consecutive days each week for three weeks, followed by a 12-day rest period (28-day treatment cycle), until disease progression, unacceptable toxicity, or for a maximum of 12 cycles. Patients received 20 mg/m² at each dose in Cycle 1, and 27 mg/m² in subsequent cycles. To reduce the incidence and severity of fever, rigors, chills, dyspnea, myalgia, and arthralgia, dexamethasone 4 mg by mouth or by intravenous infusion was administered prior to all KYPROLIS doses during the first cycle and prior to all KYPROLIS doses during the first dose-escalation (27 mg/m²) cycle. Dexamethasone premedication (4 mg orally or intravenously) was reinstated if these symptoms reappeared during subsequent cycles.
Baseline patient and disease characteristics are summarized in Table 5.
[See table 5 above]
The median number of cycles started was four.
The primary endpoint was the overall response rate (ORR) as determined by Independent Review Committee assessment using International Myeloma Working Group criteria. The ORR (stringent complete response [sCR] + complete response [CR] + very good partial response [VGPR] + partial response [PR]) was 22.9% (95% CI: 18.0, 28.5) (N = 266) (see Table 6). The median duration of response (DOR) was 7.8 months (95% CI: 5.6, 9.2).

Table 6: Response Categories

Characteristic	Study Patients n (%)
Number of patients (%)	266 (100)
Response category*	
Complete response	1 (0.4)
Very good partial response	13 (4.9)
Partial response	47 (17.7)
Overall response	61 (22.9)
95% CI[†]	(18.0, 28.5)

* As assessed by the Independent Review Committee.
† Exact confidence interval.

16 HOW SUPPLIED/STORAGE AND HANDLING
16.1 How Supplied
KYPROLIS (carfilzomib) for Injection is supplied as an individually cartoned single-use vial containing a dose of 60 mg of carfilzomib as a white to off-white lyophilized cake or powder.
• NDC 76075-101-01, 60 mg carfilzomib per vial
16.2 Storage and Handling
Unopened vials should be stored refrigerated (2°C to 8°C; 36°F to 46°F). Retain in original package to protect from light.

17 PATIENT COUNSELING INFORMATION
Discuss the following with patients prior to treatment with KYPROLIS:
Instruct patients to contact their physician if they develop any of the following symptoms: fever, chills, rigors, chest pain, cough, or swelling of the feet or legs.
Advise patients that KYPROLIS may cause fatigue, dizziness, fainting, and/or drop in blood pressure. Advise patients not to drive or operate machinery if they experience any of these symptoms.
Advise patients that they may experience shortness of breath (dyspnea) during treatment with KYPROLIS. This most commonly occurs within a day of dosing. Advise patients to contact their physicians if they experience shortness of breath.
Counsel patients to avoid dehydration, since patients receiving KYPROLIS therapy may experience vomiting and/or diarrhea. Instruct patients to seek medical advice if they experience symptoms of dizziness, lightheadedness, or fainting spells.
Counsel females of reproductive potential to use effective contraceptive measures to prevent pregnancy during treatment with KYPROLIS. Advise the patient that if she becomes pregnant during treatment, to contact her physician immediately. Advise patients not to take KYPROLIS treatment while pregnant or breastfeeding. If a patient wishes to restart breastfeeding after treatment, advise her to discuss the appropriate timing with her physician.
Advise patients to discuss with their physician any medication they are currently taking prior to starting treatment with KYPROLIS, or prior to starting any new medication(s) during treatment with KYPROLIS.
Manufactured for:
Onyx Pharmaceuticals, Inc.
249 East Grand Avenue
South San Francisco, CA 94080
U.S. Patent Numbers: 7,232,818; 7,417,042; 7,491,704; 7,737,112
05-1088-00
Shown in Product Identification Guide, page 311

Register at PDR.net to receive free PDR® Drug Alerts, monthly Drug Updates, and FDA-required Drug Safety Alerts via email from PDR Network.

Otsuka America Pharmaceutical, Inc.
2440 RESEARCH BOULEVARD
ROCKVILLE, MD 20850

Direct Inquiries to:
Medical Affairs
Otsuka America Pharmaceutical, Inc.
(800) 441-6763
FAX: 301-212-8634
To Request Routine or Emergency Medical Information, or to Report an Adverse Experience:
(800) 438-9927

ABILIFY MAINTENA™   ℞
(aripiprazole)
for extended-release injectable suspension, for intramuscular use

HIGHLIGHTS OF PRESCRIBING INFORMATION
These highlights do not include all the information needed to use ABILIFY MAINTENA safely and effectively. See full prescribing information for ABILIFY MAINTENA.
ABILIFY MAINTENA™ (aripiprazole) for extended-release injectable suspension, for intramuscular use
Initial U.S. Approval: 2002

> **WARNING: INCREASED MORTALITY IN ELDERLY PATIENTS WITH DEMENTIA-RELATED PSYCHOSIS**
> *See full prescribing information for complete boxed warning.*
> • Elderly patients with dementia-related psychosis treated with antipsychotic drugs are at an increased risk of death (5.1)
> • ABILIFY MAINTENA is not approved for the treatment of patients with dementia-related psychosis (5.1)

——————INDICATIONS AND USAGE——————
ABILIFY MAINTENA is an atypical antipsychotic indicated for the treatment of schizophrenia (1)

——————DOSAGE AND ADMINISTRATION——————
• Only to be administered by intramuscular injection in the gluteal muscle by a healthcare professional (2.1)
• For patients naïve to aripiprazole, establish tolerability with oral aripiprazole prior to initiating ABILIFY MAINTENA (2.1)
• Recommended starting and maintenance dose is 400 mg administered monthly as a single injection (2.1)
• In conjunction with first dose, take 14 consecutive days of concurrent oral aripiprazole (10 mg to 20 mg) or current oral antipsychotic (2.1)
• Some patients may benefit from a reduction to a 300 mg dose (2.1)
• Dosage adjustments are required for missed doses (2.2)
• See instructions for use for reconstitution procedures (2.4, 2.5, 2.6, 2.7, 2.8)
• Dosage adjustments for patients who are CYP2D6 poor metabolizers and for patients taking CYP2D6 inhibitors, CYP3A4 inhibitors, or CYP3A4 inducers for greater than 14 days (2.3):

	Adjusted Dose
CYP2D6 Poor Metabolizers	
CYP2D6 Poor Metabolizers	300 mg
CYP2D6 Poor Metabolizers taking concomitant CYP3A4 inhibitors	200 mg
Patients Taking 400 mg of ABILIFY MAINTENA	
Strong CYP2D6 **or** CYP3A4 inhibitors	300 mg
CYP2D6 **and** CYP3A4 inhibitors	200 mg
CYP3A4 inducers	Avoid use
Patients Taking 300 mg of ABILIFY MAINTENA	
Strong CYP2D6 **or** CYP3A4 inhibitors	200 mg
CYP2D6 **and** CYP3A4 inhibitors	160 mg
CYP3A4 inducers	Avoid use

DOSAGE FORMS AND STRENGTHS

For extended-release injectable suspension: 400 mg/vial and 300 mg/vial of lyophilized powder for reconstitution (3)

CONTRAINDICATIONS

Known hypersensitivity to aripiprazole (4)

WARNINGS AND PRECAUTIONS

- *Cerebrovascular Adverse Reactions in Elderly Patients with Dementia-Related Psychosis:* Increased incidence of cerebrovascular adverse reactions (e.g., stroke, transient ischemic attack, including fatalities) (5.2)
- *Neuroleptic Malignant Syndrome:* Manage with immediate discontinuation and close monitoring (5.3)
- *Tardive Dyskinesia:* Discontinue if clinically appropriate (5.4)
- *Metabolic Changes:* Atypical antipsychotic drugs have been associated with metabolic changes that may increase cardiovascular/cerebrovascular risk. These metabolic changes include hyperglycemia, dyslipidemia, and weight gain (5.5)
  - *Hyperglycemia and Diabetes Mellitus:* Monitor patients for symptoms of hyperglycemia including polydipsia, polyuria, polyphagia, and weakness. Monitor glucose regularly in patients with and at risk for diabetes (5.5)
  - *Dyslipidemia:* Undesirable alterations have been observed in patients treated with atypical antipsychotics (5.5)
  - *Weight Gain:* Gain in body weight has been observed; clinical monitoring of weight is recommended (5.5)
- *Orthostatic Hypotension:* Use with caution in patients with known cardiovascular or cerebrovascular disease (5.6)
- *Leukopenia, Neutropenia, and Agranulocytosis:* Perform complete blood counts in patients with a history of a clinically significant low white blood cell count (WBC). Consider discontinuation if clinically significant decline in WBC in the absence of other causative factors (5.7)
- *Seizures:* Use cautiously in patients with a history of seizures or with conditions that lower the seizure threshold (5.8)
- *Potential for Cognitive and Motor Impairment:* Use caution when operating machinery (5.9)

ADVERSE REACTIONS

Most commonly observed adverse reaction with oral aripiprazole (incidence ≥5% and at least twice that for placebo) was akathisia (6.1)

To report SUSPECTED ADVERSE REACTIONS, contact Otsuka America Pharmaceutical, Inc. at 1-800-438-9927 or FDA at 1-800-FDA-1088 (*www.fda.gov/medwatch*).

USE IN SPECIFIC POPULATIONS

- *Pregnancy:* Based on animal data, may cause fetal harm (8.1)
- *Nursing Mothers:* Discontinue drug or nursing, taking into consideration importance of drug to the mother (8.3)

See 17 for PATIENT COUNSELING INFORMATION and Medication Guide

Revised: 02/2013

FULL PRESCRIBING INFORMATION: CONTENTS*

FULL PRESCRIBING INFORMATION

> **WARNING: INCREASED MORTALITY IN ELDERLY PATIENTS WITH DEMENTIA-RELATED PSYCHOSIS**
>
> **Elderly patients with dementia-related psychosis treated with antipsychotic drugs are at an increased risk of death. ABILIFY MAINTENA is not approved for the treatment of patients with dementia-related psychosis [see Warnings and Precautions (5.1)].**

1   INDICATIONS AND USAGE

ABILIFY MAINTENA (aripiprazole) is indicated for the treatment of schizophrenia.

Efficacy was demonstrated in a placebo-controlled, randomized-withdrawal maintenance trial in patients with schizophrenia and additional support for efficacy was derived from oral aripiprazole trials [see Clinical Studies (14)].

2   DOSAGE AND ADMINISTRATION

2.1   Dosing Information

ABILIFY MAINTENA is only to be administered by intramuscular injection by a healthcare professional. For patients who have never taken aripiprazole, establish tolerability with oral aripiprazole prior to initiating treatment with ABILIFY MAINTENA. The recommended starting and maintenance dose of ABILIFY MAINTENA is 400 mg monthly (no sooner than 26 days after the previous injection).

After the first ABILIFY MAINTENA injection, continue treatment with oral aripiprazole (10 mg to 20 mg) or other oral antipsychotic for 14 consecutive days to maintain therapeutic antipsychotic concentrations during initiation of therapy.

If there are adverse reactions with the 400 mg dosage, consider reducing the dosage to 300 mg once monthly.

2.2   Dosage Adjustments for Missed Doses

If the second or third doses are missed:
- **If more than 4 weeks and less than 5 weeks have elapsed since the last injection,** administer the injection as soon as possible.
- **If more than 5 weeks have elapsed since the last injection,** restart concomitant oral aripiprazole for 14 days with the next administered injection.

If the fourth or subsequent doses are missed:
- **If more than 4 weeks and less than 6 weeks have elapsed since the last injection,** administer the injection as soon as possible.
- **If more than 6 weeks have elapsed since the last injection,** restart concomitant oral aripiprazole for 14 days with the next administered injection.

2.3   CYP2D6 Poor Metabolizers and with Concomitant Use of CYP3A4 Inhibitors, CYP2D6 Inhibitors, or CYP3A4 Inducers

Dosage adjustments are recommended in patients who are CYP2D6 poor metabolizers and in patients taking concomitant CYP3A4 inhibitors or CYP2D6 inhibitors for greater than 14 days (see Table 1). If the CYP3A4 inhibitor, or CYP2D6 inhibitor is withdrawn, the ABILIFY MAINTENA dosage may need to be increased [see Dosage and Administration (2.1)].

Avoid the concomitant use of CYP3A4 inducers with ABILIFY MAINTENA for greater than 14 days because the blood levels of aripiprazole are decreased and may be below the effective levels.

Dosage adjustments are not recommended for patients with concomitant use of CYP3A4 inhibitors, CYP2D6 inhibitors or CYP3A4 inducers for less than 14 days.

Table 1: Dose Adjustments of ABILIFY MAINTENA in Patients who are CYP2D6 Poor Metabolizers and Patients Taking Concomitant CYP2D6 Inhibitors, 3A4 Inhibitors, and/or CYP3A4 Inducers for Greater than 14 days

	Adjusted Dose
CYP2D6 Poor Metabolizers	
CYP2D6 Poor Metabolizers	300 mg
CYP2D6 Poor Metabolizers taking concomitant CYP3A4 inhibitors	200 mg
Patients Taking 400 mg of ABILIFY MAINTENA	
Strong CYP2D6 **or** CYP3A4 inhibitors	300 mg
CYP2D6 **and** CYP3A4 inhibitors	200 mg
CYP3A4 inducers	Avoid use
Patients Taking 300 mg of ABILIFY MAINTENA	
Strong CYP2D6 **or** CYP3A4 inhibitors	200 mg
CYP2D6 **and** CYP3A4 inhibitors	160 mg
CYP3A4 inducers	Avoid use

2.4   Preparation Prior to Reconstitution of the Lyophilized ABILIFY MAINTENA Powder

For deep intramuscular gluteal injection by healthcare professionals only. Do not administer by any other route. Inject immediately after reconstitution. Administer once monthly.

(a) Lay out and confirm that components listed below are provided in the kit:
- Vial of ABILIFY MAINTENA™ (aripiprazole) for extended-release injectable suspension lyophilized powder
- 5 mL vial of Sterile Water for Injection, USP
- One 3 mL Luer Lock syringe with pre-attached 21 gauge, 1.5 inch (38 mm) Hypodermic Needle-Pro® safety needle with needle protection device
- One 3 mL BD Luer-Lok™ disposable syringe with BD Luer-Lok tip
- One vial adapter
- One 21 gauge, 1.5 inch (38 mm) Hypodermic Needle-Pro® safety needle with needle protection device
- One 21 gauge, 2 inch (50 mm) Hypodermic Needle-Pro® safety needle for obese patients with needle protection device

(b) ABILIFY MAINTENA should be suspended using the Sterile Water for Injection as supplied in the kit.

(c) The Sterile Water for Injection and ABILIFY MAINTENA vials are for single-use only.

(d) Use appropriate aseptic techniques throughout reconstitution and reconstitute at room temperature.

(e) Select the amount of Sterile Water for Injection needed for reconstitution (see Table 2).

Table 2: Amount of Sterile Water for Injection Needed for Reconstitution

400 mg Vial		300 mg Vial	
Dose	Sterile Water for Injection	Dose	Sterile Water for Injection
400 mg	1.9 mL	300 mg	1.5 mL

Important: There is more Sterile Water for Injection in the vial than is needed to reconstitute ABILIFY MAINTENA (aripiprazole) for extended-release injectable suspension. The vial will have excess Sterile Water for Injection; discard any unused portion.

2.5 Reconstitution of the Lyophilized Powder

(a) Remove the cap of the vial of Sterile Water for Injection and remove the cap of the vial containing ABILIFY MAINTENA lyophilized powder and wipe the tops with a sterile alcohol swab.

(b) Using the syringe with pre-attached Hypodermic Needle-Pro needle, withdraw the pre-determined Sterile Water for Injection volume from the vial of Sterile Water for Injection into the syringe (see Figure 1). Residual Sterile Water for Injection will remain in the vial following withdrawal; discard any unused portion.

Figure 1

(c) Slowly inject the Sterile Water for Injection into the vial containing the ABILIFY MAINTENA lyophilized powder (see Figure 2).

Figure 2

(d) Withdraw air to equalize the pressure in the vial by pulling back slightly on the plunger. Subsequently, remove the needle from the vial. Engage the needle safety device by using the one-handed technique (see Figure 3). Gently press the sheath against a flat surface until the needle is firmly engaged in the needle protection sheath. Visually confirm that the needle is fully engaged into the needle protection sheath, and discard.

Figure 3

(e) Shake the vial vigorously for 30 seconds until the reconstituted suspension appears uniform (see Figure 4). [See figure 4 at top of next column]

(f) Visually inspect the reconstituted suspension for particulate matter and discoloration prior to administration. The reconstituted ABILIFY MAINTENA is a uniform, homogeneous suspension that is opaque and milky-white in color.

Figure 4

(g) If the injection is not performed immediately after reconstitution keep the vial at room temperature and shake the vial vigorously for at least 60 seconds to re-suspend prior to injection.

(h) Do not store the reconstituted suspension in a syringe.

2.6 Preparation Prior to Injection

(a) Use appropriate aseptic techniques throughout injection of the reconstituted ABILIFY MAINTENA suspension.

(b) Remove the cover from the vial adapter package (see Figure 5). Do not remove the vial adapter from the package.

Figure 5

(c) Using the vial adapter package to handle the vial adapter, attach the prepackaged BD Luer-Lok syringe to the vial adapter (see Figure 6).

Figure 6

(d) Use the BD Luer-Lok syringe to remove the vial adapter from the package and discard the vial adapter package (see Figure 7). Do not touch the spike tip of the adapter at any time.

Figure 7

(e) Determine the recommended volume for injection (Table 3).

Table 3: ABILIFY MAINTENA Reconstituted Suspension Volume to Inject

400 mg Vial		300 mg Vial	
Dose	Volume to Inject	Dose	Volume to Inject
400 mg	2 mL	---	---
300 mg	1.5 mL	300 mg	1.5 mL
200 mg	1 mL	200 mg	1 mL
160 mg	0.8 mL	160 mg	0.8 mL

(f) Wipe the top of the vial of the reconstituted ABILIFY MAINTENA suspension with a sterile alcohol swab.

(g) Place and hold the vial of the reconstituted ABILIFY MAINTENA suspension on a hard surface. Attach the adapter-syringe assembly to the vial by holding the outside

of the adapter and pushing the adapter's spike firmly through the rubber stopper, until the adapter snaps in place (see Figure 8).

Figure 8

(h) Slowly withdraw the recommended volume from the vial into the BD Luer-Lok syringe to allow for injection (see Figure 9). A small amount of excess product will remain in the vial.

Figure 9

2.7 Injection Procedure

(a) Detach the BD Luer-Lok syringe containing the recommended volume of reconstituted ABILIFY MAINTENA suspension from the vial.

(b) Select one of the following Hypodermic Needle-Pro needles and attach the needle to the BD Luer-Lok syringe containing the suspension for injection. Ensure the needle is firmly seated on the Needle-Pro safety device with a push and clockwise twist and then pull the needle cap straight away from the needle (see Figure 10).

• 21 gauge, 1.5 inch (38 mm) Hypodermic Needle-Pro needle with needle protection device for non-obese patients.

• 21 gauge, 2 inch (50 mm) Hypodermic Needle-Pro safety needle for obese patients.

Figure 10

(c) Slowly inject the recommended volume as a single intramuscular injection into the gluteal muscle. Do not massage the injection site. Do not administer intravenously or subcutaneously.

2.8 Procedures After Injection

(a) Engage the needle safety device as described in Section 2.5, Step (d). Dispose of the vials, adapter, needles, and syringe appropriately after injection. **The Sterile Water for Injection and ABILIFY MAINTENA vials are for single-use only.**

(b) Rotate sites of injections between the two gluteal muscles.

2.9 Different Aripiprazole Formulations

There are two aripiprazole formulations for intramuscular use with different dosages, dosing frequencies, and indications. ABILIFY MAINTENA is a long-acting aripiprazole formulation with 4 week dosing intervals indicated for the treatment of schizophrenia. In contrast, aripiprazole injection (9.75 mg per vial) is a short-acting formulation indicated for agitation in patients with schizophrenia or mania. Do not substitute these products. Refer to the prescribing information for aripiprazole injection for more information about aripiprazole injection.

3   DOSAGE FORMS AND STRENGTHS

For extended-release injectable suspension: 300 mg and 400 mg, lyophilized powder in a single-use vial for reconsti-

Table 4: Changes in Fasting Glucose From Placebo-Controlled Monotherapy Trials in Adult Patients

Category Change (at least once) from Baseline		Treatment Arm	n/N	%
Fasting Glucose	Normal to High (<100 mg/dL to ≥126 mg/dL)	Aripiprazole	31/822	3.8
		Placebo	22/605	3.6
	Borderline to High (≥100 mg/dL and <126 mg/dL to ≥126 mg/dL)	Aripiprazole	31/176	17.6
		Placebo	13/142	9.2

tution. The reconstituted extended-release injectable suspension is a uniform, homogeneous suspension that is opaque and milky-white in color.

4 CONTRAINDICATIONS

ABILIFY MAINTENA is contraindicated in patients with a known hypersensitivity to aripiprazole. Hypersensitivity reactions ranging from pruritus/urticaria to anaphylaxis have been reported in patients receiving aripiprazole [see Adverse Reactions (6.2)].

5 WARNINGS AND PRECAUTIONS

5.1 Increased Mortality in Elderly Patients with Dementia- Related Psychosis

Elderly patients with dementia-related psychosis treated with antipsychotic drugs are at an increased risk of death. Analyses of 17 placebo-controlled trials (modal duration of 10 weeks), largely in patients taking atypical antipsychotic drugs, revealed a risk of death in drug-treated patients of between 1.6 to 1.7 times the risk of death in placebo-treated patients. Over the course of a typical 10–week controlled trial, the rate of death in drug-treated patients was about 4.5%, compared to a rate of about 2.6% in the placebo group. Although the causes of death were varied, most of the deaths appeared to be either cardiovascular (e.g., heart failure, sudden death) or infectious (e.g., pneumonia) in nature. Observational studies suggest that, similar to atypical antipsychotic drugs, treatment with conventional antipsychotic drugs may increase mortality. The extent to which the findings of increased mortality in observational studies may be attributed to the antipsychotic drug as opposed to some characteristic(s) of the patients is not clear. ABILIFY MAINTENA is not approved for the treatment of patients with dementia-related psychosis.

5.2 Cerebrovascular Adverse Reactions, Including Stroke in Elderly Patients with Dementia-Related Psychosis

In placebo-controlled clinical studies (two flexible dose and one fixed dose study) of dementia-related psychosis, there was an increased incidence of cerebrovascular adverse reactions (e.g., stroke, transient ischemic attack), including fatalities, in oral aripiprazole-treated patients (mean age: 84 years; range: 78–88 years). In the fixed-dose study, there was a statistically significant dose response relationship for cerebrovascular adverse reactions in patients treated with oral aripiprazole. ABILIFY MAINTENA is not approved for the treatment of patients with dementia-related psychosis.

5.3 Neuroleptic Malignant Syndrome

A potentially fatal symptom complex sometimes referred to as Neuroleptic Malignant Syndrome (NMS) may occur with administration of antipsychotic drugs, including ABILIFY MAINTENA. Rare cases of NMS occurred during aripiprazole treatment in the worldwide clinical database. Clinical manifestations of NMS are hyperpyrexia, muscle rigidity, altered mental status, and evidence of autonomic instability (irregular pulse or blood pressure, tachycardia, diaphoresis, and cardiac dysrhythmia). Additional signs may include elevated creatine phosphokinase, myoglobinuria (rhabdomyolysis), and acute renal failure.

The diagnostic evaluation of patients with this syndrome is complicated. In arriving at a diagnosis, it is important to exclude cases where the clinical presentation includes both serious medical illness (e.g., pneumonia, systemic infection) and untreated or inadequately treated extrapyramidal signs and symptoms (EPS). Other important considerations in the differential diagnosis include central anticholinergic toxicity, heat stroke, drug fever, and primary central nervous system pathology.

The management of NMS should include: 1) immediate discontinuation of antipsychotic drugs and other drugs not essential to concurrent therapy; 2) intensive symptomatic treatment and medical monitoring; and 3) treatment of any concomitant serious medical problems for which specific treatments are available. There is no general agreement about specific pharmacological treatment regimens for uncomplicated NMS.

If a patient requires antipsychotic drug treatment after recovery from NMS, the potential reintroduction of drug therapy should be carefully considered. The patient should be carefully monitored, since recurrences of NMS have been reported.

5.4 Tardive Dyskinesia

A syndrome of potentially irreversible, involuntary, dyskinetic movements, may develop in patients treated with antipsychotic drugs. Although the prevalence of the syndrome appears to be highest among the elderly, especially elderly women, it is impossible to rely upon prevalence estimates to predict, at the inception of antipsychotic treatment, which patients are likely to develop the syndrome. Whether antipsychotic drug products differ in their potential to cause tardive dyskinesia is unknown.

The risk of developing tardive dyskinesia and the likelihood that it will become irreversible are believed to increase as the duration of treatment and the total cumulative dose of antipsychotic drugs administered to the patient increase. However, the syndrome can develop, although much less commonly, after relatively brief treatment periods at low doses.

There is no known treatment for established tardive dyskinesia, although the syndrome may remit, partially or completely, if antipsychotic treatment is withdrawn. Antipsychotic treatment, itself, however, may suppress (or partially suppress) the signs and symptoms of the syndrome and, thereby, may possibly mask the underlying process. The effect of symptomatic suppression on the long-term course of the syndrome is unknown.

Given these considerations, ABILIFY MAINTENA should be prescribed in a manner that is most likely to minimize the occurrence of tardive dyskinesia. Chronic antipsychotic treatment should generally be reserved for patients who suffer from a chronic illness that 1) is known to respond to antipsychotic drugs and 2) for whom alternative, equally effective, but potentially less harmful treatments are not available or appropriate. In patients who do require chronic treatment, the smallest dose and the shortest duration of treatment producing a satisfactory clinical response should be sought. The need for continued treatment should be reassessed periodically.

If signs and symptoms of tardive dyskinesia appear in a patient treated with ABILIFY MAINTENA drug discontinuation should be considered. However, some patients may require treatment with ABILIFY MAINTENA despite the presence of the syndrome.

5.5 Metabolic Changes

Atypical antipsychotic drugs have been associated with metabolic changes that include hyperglycemia/diabetes mellitus, dyslipidemia, and weight gain. While all drugs in the class have been shown to produce some metabolic changes, each drug has its own specific risk profile. Although the following metabolic data were collected in patients treated with oral formulations of aripiprazole, the findings pertain to patients receiving ABILIFY MAINTENA as well.

Hyperglycemia/Diabetes Mellitus

Hyperglycemia, in some cases extreme and associated with diabetic ketoacidosis, hyperosmolar coma, or death, has been reported in patients treated with atypical antipsychotics. There have been reports of hyperglycemia in patients treated with aripiprazole [see Adverse Reactions (6.1)]. Assessment of the relationship between atypical antipsychotic use and glucose abnormalities is complicated by the possibility of an increased background risk of diabetes mellitus in patients with schizophrenia and the increasing incidence of diabetes mellitus in the general population. Given these confounders, the relationship between atypical antipsychotic use and hyperglycemia-related adverse reactions is not completely understood. However, epidemiological studies suggest an increased risk of hyperglycemia-related adverse reactions in patients treated with the atypical antipsychotics. Because aripiprazole was not marketed at the time these studies were performed, it is not known if aripiprazole is associated with this increased risk. Precise risk estimates for hyperglycemia-related adverse reactions in patients treated with atypical antipsychotics are not available. Patients with an established diagnosis of diabetes mellitus who are started on atypical antipsychotics should be monitored regularly for worsening of glucose control. Patients with risk factors for diabetes mellitus (e.g., obesity, family history of diabetes), who are starting treatment with atypical antipsychotics should undergo fasting blood glucose

testing at the beginning of treatment and periodically during treatment. Any patient treated with atypical antipsychotics should be monitored for symptoms of hyperglycemia including polydipsia, polyuria, polyphagia, and weakness. Patients who develop symptoms of hyperglycemia during treatment with atypical antipsychotics should undergo fasting blood glucose testing. In some cases, hyperglycemia has resolved when the atypical antipsychotic was discontinued; however, some patients required continuation of anti-diabetic treatment despite discontinuation of the atypical antipsychotic drug.

In an analysis of 13 placebo-controlled monotherapy trials in adults, primarily with schizophrenia or bipolar disorder, the mean change in fasting glucose in aripiprazole-treated patients (+4.4 mg/dL; median exposure 25 days; N=1057) was not significantly different than in placebo-treated patients (+2.5 mg/dL; median exposure 22 days; N=799). Table 4 shows the proportion of aripiprazole-treated patients with normal and borderline fasting glucose at baseline (median exposure 25 days) that had high fasting glucose measurements compared to placebo-treated patients (median exposure 22 days).

[See table 4 above]

At 24 weeks, the mean change in fasting glucose in aripiprazole-treated patients was not significantly different than in placebo-treated patients [+2.2 mg/dL (n=42) and +9.6 mg/dL (n=28), respectively].

Dyslipidemia

Undesirable alterations in lipids have been observed in patients treated with atypical antipsychotics.

There were no significant differences between aripiprazole- and placebo-treated patients in the proportion with changes from normal to clinically significant levels for fasting/non-fasting total cholesterol, fasting triglycerides, fasting LDLs, and fasting/nonfasting HDLs. Analyses of patients with at least 12 or 24 weeks of exposure were limited by small numbers of patients.

Table 5 shows the proportion of adult patients, primarily from pooled schizophrenia and bipolar disorder monotherapy placebo-controlled trials, with changes in total cholesterol (pooled from 17 trials; median exposure 21 to 25 days), fasting triglycerides (pooled from eight trials; median exposure 42 days), fasting LDL cholesterol (pooled from eight trials; median exposure 39 to 45 days, except for placebo-treated patients with baseline normal fasting LDL measurements, who had median treatment exposure of 24 days) and HDL cholesterol (pooled from nine trials; median exposure 40 to 42 days).

Table 5: Changes in Blood Lipid Parameters From Placebo-Controlled Monotherapy Trials in Adults

	Treatment Arm	n/N	%
Total Cholesterol Normal to High (<200 mg/dL to ≥240 mg/dL)	Aripiprazole	34/1357	2.5
	Placebo	27/973	2.8
Fasting Triglycerides Normal to High (<150 mg/dL to ≥200 mg/dL)	Aripiprazole	40/539	7.4
	Placebo	30/431	7.0
Fasting LDL Cholesterol Normal to High (<100 mg/dL to ≥160 mg/dL)	Aripiprazole	2/332	0.6
	Placebo	2/268	0.7
HDL Cholesterol Normal to Low (≥40 mg/dL to <40 mg/dL)	Aripiprazole	121/1066	11.4
	Placebo	99/794	12.5

In monotherapy trials in adults, the proportion of patients at 12 weeks and 24 weeks with changes from Normal to High in total cholesterol (fasting/nonfasting), fasting triglycerides, and fasting LDL cholesterol were similar between aripiprazole- and placebo-treated patients: at 12 weeks, Total Cholesterol (fasting/nonfasting), 1/71 (1.4%) vs. 3/74 (4.1%); Fasting Triglycerides, 8/62 (12.9%) vs. 5/37 (13.5%); Fasting LDL Cholesterol, 0/34 (0%) vs. 1/25 (4.0%), respectively; and at 24 weeks, Total Cholesterol (fasting/nonfasting), 1/42 (2.4%) vs. 3/37 (8.1%); Fasting Triglycerides, 5/34 (14.7%) vs. 5/20 (25%); Fasting LDL Cholesterol, 0/22 (0%) vs. 1/18 (5.6%), respectively.

Weight Gain

Weight gain has been observed with atypical antipsychotic use. Clinical monitoring of weight is recommended.

In an analysis of 13 placebo-controlled monotherapy trials, primarily from pooled schizophrenia and bipolar disorder, with a median exposure of 21 to 25 days, the mean change in body weight in aripiprazole-treated patients was +0.3 kg (N=1673) compared to -0.1 kg (N=1100) in placebo-controlled patients. At 24 weeks, the mean change from baseline in body weight in aripiprazole-treated patients was -1.5 kg (n=73) compared to -0.2 kg (n=46) in placebo-treated patients.

Table 6 shows the percentage of adult patients with weight gain ≥7% of body weight in the 13 pooled placebo-controlled monotherapy trials.
[See table 6 above]

5.6 Orthostatic Hypotension

Aripiprazole may cause orthostatic hypotension, perhaps due to its α_1-adrenergic receptor antagonism. Orthostasis occurred in 4/576 (0.7%) patients treated with ABILIFY MAINTENA during the stabilization phase, including abnormal orthostatic blood pressure (1/576, 0.2%), postural dizziness (1/576, 0.2%), presyncope (1/576, 0.2%) and orthostatic hypotension (1/576, 0.2%).

In the stabilization phase, the incidence of significant orthostatic change in blood pressure (defined as a decrease in systolic blood pressure ≥20 mmHg accompanied by an increase in heart rate ≥25 when comparing standing to supine values) was 0.2% (1/575).

5.7 Leukopenia, Neutropenia, and Agranulocytosis

Class Effect: In clinical trials and post-marketing experience, leukopenia and neutropenia have been reported temporally related to antipsychotic agents, including oral aripiprazole. Agranulocytosis has also been reported.

Possible risk factors for leukopenia/neutropenia include pre-existing low white blood cell count (WBC) and history of drug-induced leukopenia/neutropenia. In patients with a history of a clinically significant low WBC or drug-induced leukopenia/neutropenia perform a complete blood count (CBC) frequently during the first few months of therapy. In such patients, consider discontinuation of ABILIFY MAINTENA at the first sign of a clinically significant decline in WBC in the absence of other causative factors. Monitor patients with clinically significant neutropenia for fever or other symptoms or signs of infection and treat promptly if such symptoms or signs occur. Discontinue ABILIFY MAINTENA in patients with severe neutropenia (absolute neutrophil count <1000/mm³) and follow their WBC counts until recovery.

5.8 Seizures

As with other antipsychotic drugs, use ABILIFY MAINTENA cautiously in patients with a history of seizures or with conditions that lower the seizure threshold. Conditions that lower the seizure threshold may be more prevalent in a population of 65 years or older.

5.9 Potential for Cognitive and Motor Impairment

ABILIFY MAINTENA, like other antipsychotics, may impair judgment, thinking, or motor skills. Instruct patients to avoid operating hazardous machinery, including automobiles, until they are reasonably certain that therapy with ABILIFY MAINTENA does not affect them adversely.

5.10 Body Temperature Regulation

Disruption of the body's ability to reduce core body temperature has been attributed to antipsychotic agents. Appropriate care is advised when prescribing ABILIFY MAINTENA for patients who will be experiencing conditions which may contribute to an elevation in core body temperature, (e.g., exercising strenuously, exposure to extreme heat, receiving concomitant medication with anticholinergic activity, or being subject to dehydration).

5.11 Dysphagia

Esophageal dysmotility and aspiration have been associated with antipsychotic drug use, including ABILIFY MAINTENA. ABILIFY MAINTENA and other antipsychotic drugs should be used cautiously in patients at risk for aspiration pneumonia *[see Warnings and Precautions (5.1)]*.

6 ADVERSE REACTIONS

The following adverse reactions are discussed in more detail in other sections of the labeling:

- Increased Mortality in Elderly Patients with Dementia-Related Psychosis Use *[see Boxed Warning and Warnings and Precautions (5.1)]*
- Cerebrovascular Adverse Reactions, Including Stroke in Elderly Patients with Dementia-Related Psychosis *[see Boxed Warning and Warnings and Precautions 5.2]*
- Neuroleptic Malignant Syndrome *[see Warnings and Precautions (5.3)]*
- Tardive Dyskinesia *[see Warnings and Precautions (5.4)]*
- Metabolic Changes *[see Warnings and Precautions (5.5)]*
- Orthostatic Hypotension *[see Warnings and Precautions (5.6)]*
- Leukopenia, Neutropenia, and Agranulocytosis *[see Warnings and Precautions (5.7)]*
- Seizures *[see Warnings and Precautions (5.8)]*
- Potential for Cognitive and Motor Impairment *[see Warnings and Precautions (5.9)]*
- Body Temperature Regulation *[see Warnings and Precautions (5.10)]*
- Dysphagia *[see Warnings and Precautions (5.11)]*

6.1 Clinical Trials Experience

Because clinical trials are conducted under widely varying conditions, adverse reaction rates observed in the clinical trials of a drug cannot be directly compared to rates in the clinical trials of another drug and may not reflect the rates observed in practice.

Table 6: Percentage of Patients From Placebo-Controlled Trials in Adult Patients with Weight Gain ≥7% of Body Weight

	Indication	Treatment Arm	N	Patients n (%)
Weight gain ≥7% of body weight	Schizophrenia*	Aripiprazole	852	69 (8.1)
		Placebo	379	12 (3.2)
	Bipolar Mania†	Aripiprazole	719	16 (2.2)
		Placebo	598	16 (2.7)

* 4–6 weeks duration.
† 3 weeks duration.

Safety Database of ABILIFY MAINTENA and Oral Aripiprazole

Aripiprazole has been evaluated for safety in 16,114 adult patients who participated in multiple-dose, clinical trials in schizophrenia and other indications, and who had approximately 8,578 patient–years of exposure to oral aripiprazole. A total of 3,901 patients were treated with oral aripiprazole for at least 180 days, 2,259 patients were treated with oral aripiprazole for at least 360 days, and 933 patients continuing aripiprazole treatment for at least 720 days.

ABILIFY MAINTENA 300–400 mg every 4 weeks has been evaluated for safety in 1,287 adult patients in clinical trials in schizophrenia, with approximately 1,281 patient–years of exposure to ABILIFY MAINTENA. A total of 832 patients were treated with ABILIFY MAINTENA for at least 180 days (at least 7 consecutive injections) and 630 patients treated with ABILIFY MAINTENA had at least 1 year of exposure (at least 13 consecutive injections).

The conditions and duration of treatment with ABILIFY MAINTENA included double-blind and open-label studies. The safety profile of ABILIFY MAINTENA is expected to be similar to that of oral aripiprazole. Therefore, most of the safety data presented below are derived from trials with the oral formulation. In patients who tolerated and responded to treatment with oral aripiprazole and single-blind ABILIFY MAINTENA and were then randomized to receive ABILIFY MAINTENA or placebo injections under double-blind conditions, the incidence of adverse reactions was similar between the two treatment groups.

Adverse Reactions of ABILIFY MAINTENA and Oral Aripiprazole

Adverse Reactions Associated with Discontinuation of Oral Aripiprazole

Based on a pool of five placebo-controlled trials (four 4–week and one 6–week) in which oral aripiprazole was administered to adults with schizophrenia in doses ranging from 2 mg/day to 30 mg/day, the incidence of discontinuation due to adverse reactions was 7% in oral aripiprazole-treated and 9% in placebo-treated patients. The types of adverse reactions that led to discontinuation were similar for the aripiprazole-treated and placebo-treated patients.

Commonly Observed Adverse Reactions of Oral Aripiprazole

Based on a pool of five placebo-controlled trials (four 4–week and one 6–week) in which oral aripiprazole was administered to adults with schizophrenia in doses ranging from 2 mg/day to 30 mg/day, the only commonly observed adverse reaction associated with the use of oral aripiprazole in patients with schizophrenia (incidence of 5% or greater and aripiprazole incidence at least twice that for placebo) was akathisia (aripiprazole 8%; placebo 4%).

Less Common Adverse Reactions in Adults Treated with Oral Aripiprazole

Table 7 enumerates the pooled incidence, rounded to the nearest percent, of adverse reactions that occurred during acute therapy (up to 6 weeks in schizophrenia and up to 3 weeks in bipolar mania), including only those reactions that occurred in 2% or more of patients treated with oral aripiprazole (doses ≥2 mg/day) and for which the incidence in patients treated with aripiprazole was greater than the incidence in patients treated with placebo in the combined dataset.

Table 7: Adverse Reactions in Short-Term, Placebo-Controlled Trials in Adult Patients Treated with Oral Aripiprazole

System Organ Class Preferred Term	Percentage of Patients Reporting Reaction*	
	Oral Aripiprazole (n=1843)	Placebo (n=1166)
Eye Disorders		
Blurred Vision	3	1
Gastrointestinal Disorders		
Nausea	15	11
Constipation	11	7
Vomiting	11	6
Dyspepsia	9	7
Dry Mouth	5	4
Toothache	4	3
Abdominal Discomfort	3	2
Stomach Discomfort	3	2
General Disorders and Administration Site Conditions		
Fatigue	6	4
Pain	3	2
Musculoskeletal and Connective Tissue Disorders		
Musculoskeletal Stiffness	4	3
Pain in Extremity	4	2
Myalgia	2	1
Muscle Spasms	2	1
Nervous System Disorders		
Headache	27	23
Dizziness	10	7
Akathisia	10	4
Sedation	7	4
Extrapyramidal Disorder	5	3
Tremor	5	3
Somnolence	5	3
Psychiatric Disorders		
Agitation	19	17
Insomnia	18	13
Anxiety	17	13
Restlessness	5	3
Respiratory, Thoracic, and Mediastinal Disorders		
Pharyngolaryngeal Pain	3	2
Cough	3	2

* Adverse reactions reported by at least 2% of patients treated with oral aripiprazole, except adverse reactions which had an incidence equal to or less than placebo.

An examination of population subgroups did not reveal any clear evidence of differential adverse reaction incidence on the basis of age, gender, or race.

Dose-Related Adverse Reactions of Oral Aripiprazole

Dose response relationships for the incidence of treatment-emergent adverse events were evaluated from four trials in adult patients with schizophrenia comparing various fixed oral doses of aripiprazole (2 mg/day, 5 mg/day, 10 mg/day, 15 mg/day, 20 mg/day, and 30 mg/day) to placebo. This analysis, stratified by study, indicated that the only adverse reaction to have a possible dose response relationship, and then most prominent only with 30 mg, was somnolence [including sedation]; (incidences were placebo, 7.1%; 10 mg, 8.5%; 15 mg, 8.7%; 20 mg, 7.5%; 30 mg, 12.6%).

Injection Site Reactions of ABILIFY MAINTENA

In the open-label, stabilization phase of a study with ABILIFY MAINTENA in patients with schizophrenia, the percent of patients reporting any injection site-related adverse reaction was 6.3% for ABILIFY MAINTENA-treated patients. The mean intensity of injection pain reported by subjects using a visual analog scale (0=no pain to 100=unbearably painful) was minimal and improved in subjects receiving ABILIFY MAINTENA from the first to the last injection in the open-label, stabilization phase (6.1 to 4.9). Investigator evaluation of the injection site for pain, swelling, redness and induration following injections of ABILIFY MAINTENA in the open-label, stabilization phase were rated as absent for 74%-96% of subjects following the first injection and 77%-96% of subjects following the last injection.

Extrapyramidal Symptoms of Oral Aripiprazole

In short-term, placebo-controlled trials in schizophrenia, the incidence of reported EPS-related events, excluding events related to akathisia, for oral aripiprazole-treated patients was 13% vs. 12% for placebo; and the incidence of akathisia-related events for aripiprazole-treated patients was 8% vs. 4% for placebo.

Objectively collected data from those trials was collected on the Simpson Angus Rating Scale (for EPS), the Barnes Akathisia Scale (for akathisia), and the Abnormal Involuntary Movement Scale (for dyskinesias). In the schizophrenia trials, the objectively collected data did not show a difference between aripiprazole and placebo, with the exception of the Barnes Akathisia Scale (aripiprazole, 0.08; placebo, -0.05). Similarly, in a long-term (26-week), placebo-controlled trial of schizophrenia in adults, objectively collected data on the Simpson Angus Rating Scale (for EPS), the Barnes Akathisia Scale (for akathisia), and the Abnormal Involuntary Movement Scale (for dyskinesias) did not show a difference between aripiprazole and placebo.

Dystonia
Class Effect: Symptoms of dystonia, prolonged abnormal contractions of muscle groups, may occur in susceptible individuals during the first few days of treatment. Dystonic symptoms include: spasm of the neck muscles, sometimes progressing to tightness of the throat, swallowing difficulty, difficulty breathing, and/or protrusion of the tongue. While these symptoms can occur at low doses, they occur more frequently and with greater severity with high potency and at higher doses of first generation antipsychotic drugs. An elevated risk of acute dystonia is observed in males and younger age groups.

Adverse Reactions in Long-Term, Double-Blind, Placebo-Controlled Trials of Oral Aripiprazole
The adverse reactions reported in a 26-week, double-blind trial comparing oral aripiprazole and placebo in patients with schizophrenia were generally consistent with those reported in the short-term, placebo-controlled trials, except for a higher incidence of tremor [8% (12/153) for oral aripiprazole vs. 2% (3/153) for placebo]. In this study, the majority of the cases of tremor were of mild intensity (8/12 mild and 4/12 moderate), occurred early in therapy (9/12 ≤49 days), and were of limited duration (7/12 ≤10 days). Tremor infrequently led to discontinuation (<1%) of oral aripiprazole. In addition, in a long-term, active-controlled study, the incidence of tremor was 5% (40/859) for oral aripiprazole.

Other Adverse Reactions Observed During the Premarketing Evaluation of Oral Aripiprazole
Following is a list of MedDRA terms that reflect adverse reactions reported by patients treated with oral aripiprazole at multiple doses ≥2 mg/day during any phase of a trial within the database of 13,543 adult patients. All events assessed as possible adverse drug reactions have been included with the exception of more commonly occurring events. In addition, medically/clinically meaningful adverse reactions, particularly those that are likely to be useful to the prescriber or that have pharmacologic plausibility, have been included. Events already listed in other parts of *Adverse Reactions (6)*, or those considered in *Warnings and Precautions (5)* or *Overdosage (10)* have been excluded. Although the reactions reported occurred during treatment with aripiprazole, they were not necessarily caused by it. Events are further categorized by MedDRA system organ class and listed in order of decreasing frequency according to the following definitions: those occurring in at least 1/100 patients (only those not already listed in the tabulated results from placebo-controlled trials appear in this listing); those occurring in 1/100 to 1/1000 patients; and those occurring in fewer than 1/1000 patients.

Blood and Lymphatic System Disorders:
≥1/1000 patients and <1/100 patients - thrombocytopenia
Cardiac Disorders:
≥1/1000 patients and <1/100 patients - palpitations, cardiopulmonary failure, myocardial infarction, cardiorespiratory arrest, atrioventricular block, extrasystoles, angina pectoris, myocardial ischemia; <1/1000 patients - atrial flutter, supraventricular tachycardia, ventricular tachycardia
Eye Disorders:
≥1/1000 patients and <1/100 patients - photophobia, diplopia, eyelid edema, photopsia
Gastrointestinal Disorders:
≥1/1000 patients and <1/100 patients - gastroesophageal reflux disease, swollen tongue, esophagitis; <1/1000 patients - pancreatitis
General Disorders and Administration Site Conditions:
≥1/100 patients - asthenia, peripheral edema, chest pain; ≥1/1000 patients and <1/100 patients - face edema, angioedema; <1/1000 patients - hypothermia
Hepatobiliary Disorders:
<1/1000 patients - hepatitis, jaundice
Immune System Disorders:
≥1/1000 patients and <1/100 patients - hypersensitivity
Injury, Poisoning, and Procedural Complications:
≥1/100 patients - fall; <1/1000 patients - heat stroke
Investigations:
≥1/1000 patients and <1/100 patients - blood prolactin increased, blood urea increased, blood creatinine increased, blood bilirubin increased; <1/1000 patients - blood lactate dehydrogenase increased, glycosylated hemoglobin increased
Metabolism and Nutrition Disorders:
≥1/1000 patients and <1/100 patients - anorexia, hyponatremia, hypoglycemia, polydipsia; <1/1000 patients - diabetic ketoacidosis

Musculoskeletal and Connective Tissue Disorders:
≥1/1000 patients and <1/100 patients - muscle rigidity, muscular weakness, muscle tightness, mobility decreased; <1/1000 patients - rhabdomyolysis
Nervous System Disorders:
≥1/100 patients - coordination abnormal; ≥1/1000 patients and <1/100 patients - speech disorder, hypokinesia, hypotonia, myoclonus, akinesia, bradykinesia; <1/1000 patients - choreoathetosis
Psychiatric Disorders:
≥1/100 patients - suicidal ideation; ≥1/1000 patients and <1/100 patients - loss of libido, suicide attempt, hostility, libido increased, anger, anorgasmia, delirium, intentional self injury, completed suicide, tic, homicidal ideation; <1/1000 patients - catatonia, sleep walking
Renal and Urinary Disorders:
≥1/1000 patients and <1/100 patients - urinary retention, polyuria, nocturia
Reproductive System and Breast Disorders:
≥1/1000 patients and <1/100 patients - menstruation irregular, erectile dysfunction, amenorrhea, breast pain; <1/1000 patients - gynecomastia, priapism
Respiratory, Thoracic, and Mediastinal Disorders:
≥1/100 patients - nasal congestion, dyspnea
Skin and Subcutaneous Tissue Disorders:
≥1/100 patients - rash (including erythematous, exfoliative, generalized, macular, maculopapular, papular rash; acneiform, allergic, contact, exfoliative, seborrheic dermatitis, neurodermatitis, and drug eruption); hyperhydrosis; ≥1/1000 patients and <1/100 patients - pruritus, photosensitivity reaction, alopecia, urticaria

6.2   Postmarketing Experience
The following adverse reactions have been identified during post-approval use of oral aripiprazole. Because these reactions are reported voluntarily from a population of uncertain size, it is not always possible to reliably estimate their frequency or establish a causal relationship to drug exposure: rare occurrences of allergic reaction (anaphylactic reaction, angioedema, laryngospasm, pruritus/urticaria, or oropharyngeal spasm).

7   DRUG INTERACTIONS
7.1   Carbamazepine or Other CYP3A4 Inducers
Concomitant use of ABILIFY MAINTENA with carbamazepine or other CYP3A4 inducers decreases the concentrations of aripiprazole. Avoid use of ABILIFY MAINTENA in combination with carbamazepine and other inducers of CYP3A4 for greater than 14 days *[see Dosage and Administration (2.3) and Clinical Pharmacology (12.3)]*.
7.2   Ketoconazole or Other Strong CYP3A4 Inhibitors
Concomitant use of ABILIFY MAINTENA with ketoconazole or other CYP3A4 inhibitors for more than 14 days increases the concentrations of aripiprazole and reduction of the ABILIFY MAINTENA dose is recommended *[see Dosage and Administration (2.3) and Clinical Pharmacology (12.3)]*. Due to prolonged-release characteristics of ABILIFY MAINTENA, short-term co-administration of ketoconazole or other inhibitors of CYP3A4 with ABILIFY MAINTENA does not require a dose adjustment.
7.3   Quinidine or Other Strong CYP2D6 Inhibitors
Concomitant use of ABILIFY MAINTENA with quinidine or other CYP2D6 inhibitors increases the concentrations of aripiprazole after longer-term use (i.e., over 14 days) and reduction of the ABILIFY MAINTENA is recommended *[see Dosage and Administration (2.3) and Clinical Pharmacology (12.3)]*. Due to prolonged-release characteristics of ABILIFY MAINTENA, short-term co-administration of quinidine or other CYP2D6 inhibitors with ABILIFY MAINTENA does not require a dose adjustment.
7.4   CNS Depressants
Given the CNS depressant effects of aripiprazole, use caution when ABILIFY MAINTENA is taken in combination with other centrally-acting drugs or alcohol.
7.5   Anti-Hypertensive Agents
Due to its alpha adrenergic antagonism, aripiprazole has the potential to enhance the effect of certain antihypertensive agents.

8   USE IN SPECIFIC POPULATIONS
8.1   Pregnancy
Pregnancy Category C:
Risk Summary
Adequate and well controlled studies with aripiprazole have not been conducted in pregnant women. Neonates exposed to antipsychotic drugs (including ABILIFY MAINTENA) during the third trimester of pregnancy are at risk for extrapyramidal and/or withdrawal symptoms following delivery. In animal studies, aripiprazole demonstrated developmental toxicity, including possible teratogenic effects in rats and rabbits at doses 1 – 10 times the oral maximum recommended human dose [MRHD] of 30 mg/day based on a mg/m² body surface area. ABILIFY MAINTENA should be used during pregnancy only if the potential benefit justifies the potential risk to the fetus.
Clinical Considerations
Fetal/Neonatal Adverse Reactions
Monitor neonates exhibiting extrapyramidal or withdrawal symptoms. Some neonates recover within hours or days

without specific treatment; others may require prolonged hospitalization.
Animal Data
Pregnant rats were treated with oral doses of 3 mg/kg/day, 10 mg/kg/day, and 30 mg/kg/day (1 times, 3 times, and 10 times the oral maximum recommended human dose [MRHD] of 30 mg/day on a mg/m² body surface area) of aripiprazole during the period of organogenesis. Gestation was slightly prolonged at 30 mg/kg. Treatment caused a slight delay in fetal development, as evidenced by decreased fetal weight (30 mg/kg), undescended testes (30 mg/kg), and delayed skeletal ossification (10 mg/kg and 30 mg/kg). There were no adverse effects on embryofetal or pup survival. Delivered offspring had decreased body weights (10 mg/kg and 30 mg/kg), and increased incidences of hepatodiaphragmatic nodules and diaphragmatic hernia at 30 mg/kg (the other dose groups were not examined for these findings). A low incidence of diaphragmatic hernia was also seen in the fetuses exposed to 30 mg/kg. Postnatally, delayed vaginal opening was seen at 10 mg/kg and 30 mg/kg and impaired reproductive performance (decreased fertility rate, corpora lutea, implants, live fetuses, and increased post-implantation loss, likely mediated through effects on female offspring) was seen at 30 mg/kg. Some maternal toxicity was seen at 30 mg/kg; however, there was no evidence to suggest that these developmental effects were secondary to maternal toxicity.
In pregnant rats receiving aripiprazole injection intravenously (3 mg/kg/day, 9 mg/kg/day, and 27 mg/kg/day) during the period of organogenesis, decreased fetal weight and delayed skeletal ossification were seen at the highest dose, which also caused some maternal toxicity.
Pregnant rabbits were treated with oral doses of 10 mg/kg/day, 30 mg/kg/day, and 100 mg/kg/day (2 times, 3 times, and 11 times human exposure at the oral MRHD of 30 mg/day based on AUC and 6 times, 19 times, and 65 times the oral MRHD of 30 mg/day based on mg/m² body surface area) of aripiprazole during the period of organogenesis. Decreased maternal food consumption and increased abortions were seen at 100 mg/kg. Treatment caused increased fetal mortality (100 mg/kg), decreased fetal weight (30 mg/kg and 100 mg/kg), increased incidence of a skeletal abnormality (fused sternebrae at 30 mg/kg and 100 mg/kg), and minor skeletal variations (100 mg/kg).
In pregnant rabbits receiving aripiprazole injection intravenously (3 mg/kg/day, 10 mg/kg/day, and 30 mg/kg/day) during the period of organogenesis, the highest dose, which caused pronounced maternal toxicity, resulted in decreased fetal weight, increased fetal abnormalities (primarily skeletal), and decreased fetal skeletal ossification. The fetal noeffect dose was 10 mg/kg, which produced 5 times the human exposure at the oral MRHD based on AUC and is 6 times the oral MRHD of 30 mg/day based on mg/m² body surface area.
In a study in which rats were treated with oral doses of 3 mg/kg/day, 10 mg/kg/day, and 30 mg/kg/day (1 times, 3 times, and 10 times the oral MRHD of 30 mg/day on a mg/m² body surface area) of aripiprazole perinatally and postnatally (from day 17 of gestation through day 21 postpartum), slight maternal toxicity and slightly prolonged gestation were seen at 30 mg/kg. An increase in stillbirths and decreases in pup weight (persisting into adulthood) and survival were seen at this dose.
In rats receiving aripiprazole injection intravenously (3 mg/kg/day, 8 mg/kg/day, and 20 mg/kg/day) from day 6 of gestation through day 20 postpartum, an increase in stillbirths was seen at 8 mg/kg and 20 mg/kg, and decreases in early postnatal pup weights and survival were seen at 20 mg/kg. These doses produced some maternal toxicity. There were no effects on postnatal behavioral and reproductive development.
8.3   Nursing Mothers
Aripiprazole is excreted in human breast milk. A decision should be made whether to discontinue nursing or to discontinue the drug, taking into account the importance of the drug to the mother.
8.4   Pediatric Use
Safety and effectiveness of ABILIFY MAINTENA in patients <18 years of age have not been evaluated.
8.5   Geriatric Use
Safety and effectiveness of ABILIFY MAINTENA in patients >60 years of age have not been evaluated.
In oral single-dose pharmacokinetic studies (with aripiprazole given in a single oral dose of 15 mg), aripiprazole clearance was 20% lower in elderly (≥65 years) subjects compared to younger adult subjects (18 to 64 years). There was no detectable age effect, however, in the population pharmacokinetic analysis of oral aripiprazole in schizophrenia patients. Also, the pharmacokinetics of oral aripiprazole after multiple doses in elderly patients appeared similar to that observed in young, healthy subjects. No dosage adjustment of ABILIFY MAINTENA is recommended for elderly patients *[see Boxed Warning and Warnings and Precautions (5.1)]*.
8.6   CYP2D6 Poor Metabolizers
Approximately 8% of Caucasians and 3–8% of Black/African Americans cannot metabolize CYP2D6 substrates and are

classified as poor metabolizers (PM). Dosage adjustment is recommended in CYP2D6 poor metabolizers due to high aripiprazole concentrations [see Dosage and Administration (2.3) and Clinical Pharmacology (12.3)].

10 OVERDOSAGE

10.1 Human Experience

The largest known case of acute ingestion with a known outcome involved 1260 mg of oral aripiprazole (42 times the maximum recommended daily dose) in a patient who fully recovered.

Common adverse reactions (reported in at least 5% of all overdose cases) reported with oral aripiprazole overdosage (alone or in combination with other substances) include vomiting, somnolence, and tremor. Other clinically important signs and symptoms observed in one or more patients with aripiprazole overdoses (alone or with other substances) include acidosis, aggression, aspartate aminotransferase increased, atrial fibrillation, bradycardia, coma, confusional state, convulsion, blood creatinine phosphokinase increased, depressed level of consciousness, hypertension, hypokalemia, hypotension, lethargy, loss of consciousness, QRS complex prolonged, QT prolonged, pneumonia aspiration, respiratory arrest, status epilepticus, and tachycardia.

10.2 Management of Overdosage

In case of overdosage, call the Poison Control Center immediately at 1-800-222-1222.

11 DESCRIPTION

Aripiprazole is an atypical antipsychotic which is present in ABILIFY MAINTENA as its monohydrate polymorphic form. Aripiprazole monohydrate is 7-[4-[4-(2,3-dichlorophenyl)-1-piperazinyl] butoxy]-3,4 dihydrocarbostyril monohydrate. The empirical formula is $C_{23}H_{27}Cl_2N_3O_2 \cdot H_2O$ and its molecular weight is 466.40. The chemical structure is:

ABILIFY MAINTENA (aripiprazole) is an extended-release injectable suspension available in 400 mg or 300 mg strength vials. The labeled strengths are calculated based on the anhydrous form (aripiprazole). Inactive ingredients include carboxymethyl cellulose sodium, mannitol, sodium phosphate monobasic monohydrate and sodium hydroxide.

12 CLINICAL PHARMACOLOGY

12.1 Mechanism of Action

The mechanism of action of aripiprazole in the treatment of schizophrenia is unknown.

However, the efficacy of aripiprazole may be mediated through a combination of partial agonist activity at D_2 and 5-HT_{1A} receptors and antagonist activity at 5-HT_{2A} receptors. Actions at receptors other than D_2, 5-HT_{1A}, and 5-HT_{2A} may explain some of the other adverse reactions of aripiprazole (e.g., the orthostatic hypotension observed with aripiprazole may be explained by its antagonist activity at adrenergic alpha$_1$ receptors).

12.2 Pharmacodynamics

Aripiprazole exhibits high affinity for dopamine D_2 and D_3, serotonin 5-HT_{1A} and 5-HT_{2A} receptors (K_i values of 0.34 nM, 0.8 nM, 1.7 nM, and 3.4 nM, respectively), moderate affinity for dopamine D_4, serotonin 5-HT_{2C} and 5-HT_7, alpha$_1$-adrenergic and histamine H_1 receptors (K_i values of 44 nM, 15 nM, 39 nM, 57 nM, and 61 nM, respectively), and moderate affinity for the serotonin reuptake site (K_i=98 nM). Aripiprazole has no appreciable affinity for cholinergic muscarinic receptors (IC_{50}>1000 nM). Aripiprazole functions as a partial agonist at the dopamine D_2 and the serotonin 5-HT_{1A} receptors, and as an antagonist at serotonin 5-HT_{2A} receptor.

Alcohol

There was no significant difference between oral aripiprazole co-administered with ethanol and placebo co-administered with ethanol on performance of gross motor skills or stimulus response in healthy subjects. As with most psychoactive medications, patients should be advised to avoid alcohol while taking ABILIFY MAINTENA.

12.3 Pharmacokinetics

ABILIFY MAINTENA activity is presumably primarily due to the parent drug, aripiprazole, and to a lesser extent, to its major metabolite, dehydro-aripiprazole, which has been shown to have affinities for D_2 receptors similar to the parent drug and represents about 29% of the parent drug exposure in plasma.

Aripiprazole absorption into the systemic circulation is slow and prolonged following intramuscular injection due to low solubility of aripiprazole particles. Following a single intramuscular dose, the plasma concentrations of aripiprazole gradually rise to reach maximum plasma concentrations at a median T_{max} of 5–7 days. The mean aripiprazole terminal elimination half–life was 29.9 days and 46.5 days after every 4–week injection of ABILIFY MAINTENA 300 mg and 400 mg, respectively, and steady state concentrations were attained by the fourth dose. Approximate dose-proportional increases in aripiprazole and dehydro-aripiprazole concen-

trations and AUC parameters were observed after every four week ABILIFY MAINTENA injections of 300 mg and 400 mg.

Elimination of aripiprazole is mainly through hepatic metabolism involving two P450 isozymes, CYP2D6 and CYP3A4. Aripiprazole is not a substrate of CYP1A1, CYP1A2, CYP2A6, CYP2B6, CYP2C8, CYP2C9, CYP2C19, or CYP2E1 enzymes. Aripiprazole also does not undergo direct glucuronidation.

Drug Interaction Studies

No specific drug interaction studies have been performed with ABILIFY MAINTENA. The information below is obtained from studies with oral aripiprazole.

Potential for Other Drugs to Affect ABILIFY MAINTENA

Ketoconazole and Other Strong CYP3A4 Inhibitors

Co-administration of ketoconazole (200 mg/day for 14 days) with a 15 mg single oral dose of aripiprazole increased the AUC of aripiprazole and its active metabolite by 63% and 77%, respectively. The effect of a higher ketoconazole dose (400 mg/day) has not been studied.

Other strong inhibitors of CYP3A4 (itraconazole) would be expected to have similar effects and need similar dose reductions; moderate inhibitors (erythromycin, grapefruit juice) have not been studied [see Dosage and Administration (2.3) and Drug Interactions (7.2)].

Quinidine and Other Strong CYP2D6 Inhibitors

Co-administration of a 10 mg single oral dose of aripiprazole with quinidine (166 mg/day for 13 days), a potent inhibitor of CYP2D6, increased the AUC of aripiprazole by 112% but decreased the AUC of its active metabolite, dehydro-aripiprazole, by 35%. Other significant inhibitors of CYP2D6, such as fluoxetine or paroxetine, would be expected to have similar effects [see Dosage and Administration (2.3) and Drug Interactions (7.3)].

Carbamazepine and Other CYP3A4 Inducers

Co-administration of carbamazepine (200 mg twice daily), a potent CYP3A4 inducer, with oral aripiprazole (30 mg/day) resulted in an approximate 70% decrease in C_{max} and AUC values of both aripiprazole and its active metabolite, dehydro-aripiprazole [see Dosage and Administration (2.3) and Drug Interactions (7.1)].

Valproate

When valproate (500 mg/day–1500 mg/day) and oral aripiprazole (30 mg/day) were co-administered, at steady-state the C_{max} and AUC of aripiprazole were decreased by 25%. No dosage adjustment of ABILIFY MAINTENA is required when administered concomitantly with valproate.

Lithium

A pharmacokinetic interaction of ABILIFY MAINTENA with lithium is unlikely because lithium is not bound to plasma proteins, is not metabolized, and is almost entirely excreted unchanged in urine. Co-administration of therapeutic doses of lithium (1200 mg/day–1800 mg/day) for 21 days with oral aripiprazole (30 mg/day) did not result in clinically significant changes in the pharmacokinetics of aripiprazole or its active metabolite, dehydro-aripiprazole (C_{max} and AUC increased by less than 20%). No dosage adjustment of ABILIFY MAINTENA is required when administered concomitantly with lithium.

Potential for ABILIFY MAINTENA to Affect Other Drugs

Aripiprazole is unlikely to cause clinically important pharmacokinetic interactions with drugs metabolized by cytochrome P450 enzymes. In vivo studies, 10 mg/day to 30 mg/day doses of oral aripiprazole had no significant effect on metabolism by CYP2D6 (dextromethorphan), CYP2C9 (warfarin), CYP2C19 (omeprazole, warfarin), and CYP3A4 (dextromethorphan) substrates. Additionally, aripiprazole and dehydro-aripiprazole did not show potential for altering CYP1A2-mediated metabolism in vitro.

No effect of oral aripiprazole was seen on the pharmacokinetics of lithium or valproate.

Valproate

When oral aripiprazole (30 mg/day) and valproate (1000 mg/day) were co-administered, at steady state there were no clinically significant changes in the C_{max} or AUC of valproate. No dosage adjustment of valproate is required when administered concomitantly with ABILIFY MAINTENA.

Lithium

Co-administration of oral aripiprazole (30 mg/day) with lithium (900 mg/day) did not result in clinically significant changes in the pharmacokinetics of lithium. No dosage adjustment of lithium is required when administered concomitantly with ABILIFY MAINTENA.

Dextromethorphan

Oral aripiprazole at doses of 10 mg/day to 30 mg/day for 14 days had no effect on dextromethorphan's O-dealkylation to its major metabolite, dextrorphan, a pathway dependent on CYP2D6 activity. Oral aripiprazole also had no effect on dextromethorphan's N-demethylation to its metabolite 3-methoxymorphinan, a pathway dependent on CYP3A4 activity. No dosage adjustment of dextromethorphan is required when administered concomitantly with ABILIFY MAINTENA.

Warfarin

Oral aripiprazole 10 mg/day for 14 days had no effect on the pharmacokinetics of R-warfarin and S-warfarin or on the

pharmacodynamic end-point of International Normalized Ratio, indicating the lack of a clinically relevant effect of aripiprazole on CYP2C9 and CYP2C19 metabolism or the binding of highly protein-bound warfarin. No dosage adjustment of warfarin is required when administered concomitantly with ABILIFY MAINTENA.

Omeprazole

Oral aripiprazole 10 mg/day for 15 days had no effect on the pharmacokinetics of a single 20 mg dose of omeprazole, a CYP2C19 substrate, in healthy subjects. No dosage adjustment of omeprazole is required when administered concomitantly with ABILIFY MAINTENA.

Escitalopram

Co-administration of 10 mg/day doses of oral aripiprazole for 14 days to healthy subjects had no effect on the steady-state pharmacokinetics of 10 mg/day escitalopram, a substrate of CYP2C19 and CYP3A4. No dosage adjustment of escitalopram is required when ABILIFY MAINTENA is added to escitalopram.

Venlafaxine

Co-administration of 10 mg/day to 20 mg/day doses of oral aripiprazole for 14 days to healthy subjects had no effect on the steady-state pharmacokinetics of venlafaxine and O-desmethylvenlafaxine following 75 mg/day venlafaxine XR, a CYP2D6 substrate. No dosage adjustment of venlafaxine is required when ABILIFY MAINTENA is added to venlafaxine.

Specific Population Studies

No specific pharmacokinetic studies have been performed with ABILIFY MAINTENA in specific populations. All the information is obtained from studies with oral aripiprazole.

CYP2D6 Poor Metabolizers

Approximately 8% of Caucasians and 3–8% of Black/African Americans cannot metabolize CYP2D6 substrates and are classified as poor metabolizers (PMs). People who are not PMs are classified as extensive metabolizers (EMs). Laboratory tests are available to identify CYP2D6 PMs. PMs have about an 80% increase in aripiprazole exposure and about a 30% decrease in exposure to the active metabolite compared to EMs, resulting in about a 60% higher exposure to the total active moieties from a given dose of aripiprazole compared to EMs. The mean elimination half-lives for aripiprazole are about 75 and 146 hours in EMs and PMs, respectively. Hence, the recommended dosage of ABILIFY MAINTENA is lower [see Dosage and Administration (2.3) and Use in Specific Populations (8.6)].

Aripiprazole does not inhibit or induce the CYP2D6 pathway.

Gender

C_{max} and AUC of aripiprazole and its active metabolite, dehydro-aripiprazole, are 30% to 40% higher in women than in men, and correspondingly, the apparent oral clearance of aripiprazole is lower in women. These differences, however, are largely explained by differences in body weight (25%) between men and women. No dosage adjustment of ABILIFY MAINTENA is recommended based on gender.

Race

Although no specific pharmacokinetic study was conducted to investigate the effects of race on the disposition of aripiprazole, population pharmacokinetic evaluation revealed no evidence of clinically significant race-related differences in the pharmacokinetics of aripiprazole. No dosage adjustment of ABILIFY MAINTENA is recommended based on race.

Smoking

Based on studies utilizing human liver enzymes in vitro, aripiprazole is not a substrate for CYP1A2 and also does not undergo direct glucuronidation. Smoking should, therefore, not have an effect on the pharmacokinetics of aripiprazole. Consistent with these in vitro results, population pharmacokinetic evaluation did not reveal any significant pharmacokinetic differences between smokers and nonsmokers. No dosage adjustment of ABILIFY MAINTENA is recommended based on smoking status.

Renal Impairment

In patients with severe renal impairment (creatinine clearance <30 mL/min), C_{max} of oral aripiprazole (given in a single dose of oral 15 mg) and dehydro-aripiprazole increased by 36% and 53%, respectively, but AUC was 15% lower for aripiprazole and 7% higher for dehydro-aripiprazole. Renal excretion of both unchanged aripiprazole and dehydro-aripiprazole is less than 1% of the dose. No dosage adjustment of ABILIFY MAINTENA is required for doses in subjects with renal impairment.

Hepatic Impairment

In a single-dose trial (15 mg of oral aripiprazole) in subjects with varying degrees of liver cirrhosis (Child-Pugh Classes A, B, and C), the AUC of aripiprazole, compared to healthy subjects, increased 31% in mild hepatic impairment, increased 8% in moderate hepatic impairment, and decreased 20% in severe hepatic impairment. None of these differences would require dose adjustment of ABILIFY MAINTENA.

13 NONCLINICAL TOXICOLOGY

13.1 Carcinogenesis, Mutagenesis, Impairment of Fertility

Carcinogenesis

Lifetime carcinogenicity studies were conducted in ICR mice and in Sprague-Dawley (SD) and F344 rats.

Aripiprazole was administered for 2 years in the diet at doses of 1 mg/kg/day, 3 mg/kg/day, 10 mg/kg/day, and 30 mg/kg/day to ICR mice and 1 mg/kg/day, 3 mg/kg/day, and 10 mg/kg/day to F344 rats (0.2 times to 5 times and 0.3 times to 3 times the oral maximum recommended human dose [MRHD] of 30 mg/day based on mg/m² body surface area, respectively). In addition, SD rats were dosed orally for 2 years at 10 mg/kg/day, 20 mg/kg/day, 40 mg/kg/day, and 60 mg/kg/day (3 times to 19 times the oral MRHD of 30 mg/day based on mg/m² body surface area). Aripiprazole did not induce tumors in male mice or rats. In female mice, the incidences of pituitary gland adenomas and mammary gland adenocarcinomas and adenoacanthomas were increased at dietary doses of 3 mg/kg/day to 30 mg/kg/day (0.1 times to approximately 1 times human exposure at the oral MRHD of 30 mg/day based on AUC and 0.5 times to 5 times the oral MRHD of 30 mg/day based on mg/m² body surface area). In female rats, the incidence of mammary gland fibroadenomas was increased at a dietary dose of 10 mg/kg/day (0.1 times human exposure at the oral MRHD of 30 mg/day based on AUC and 3 times the oral MRHD of 30 mg/day based on mg/m² body surface area); and the incidences of adrenocortical carcinomas and combined adrenocortical adenomas/carcinomas were increased at an oral dose of 60 mg/kg/day (14 times human exposure at the oral MRHD of 30 mg/day based on AUC and 19 times the oral MRHD of 30 mg/day based on mg/m² body surface area).

Proliferative changes in the pituitary and mammary gland of rodents have been observed following chronic administration of other antipsychotic agents and are considered prolactin-mediated. Serum prolactin was not measured in the aripiprazole carcinogenicity studies. However, increases in serum prolactin levels were observed in female mice in a 13–week dietary study at the doses associated with mammary gland and pituitary tumors. Serum prolactin was not increased in female rats in 4–week and 13–week dietary studies at the dose associated with mammary gland tumors. The relevance for human risk of the findings of prolactin-mediated endocrine tumors in rodents is unknown.

Mutagenesis
Aripiprazole was not mutagenic when tested in the *in vitro* bacterial mutation assay, the *in vitro* bacterial DNA repair assay, and the *in vitro* mouse lymphoma gene mutation assay. The clastogenic potential of aripiprazole was tested in the *in vitro* chromosomal aberration assay in Chinese hamster lung (CHL) cells, the *in vivo* micronucleus assay in mice, and the unscheduled DNA synthesis assay in rats. Aripiprazole and its metabolite (2,3-DCPP) were clastogenic in the *in vitro* chromosomal aberration assay in CHL cells both in the presence and absence of metabolic activation. The metabolite, 2,3-DCPP, produced increases in numerical aberrations in the *in vitro* assay in CHL cells in the absence of metabolic activation. A positive response was obtained in the oral *in vivo* micronucleus assay in mice; however, the response was due to a mechanism not considered relevant to humans.

Impairment of Fertility
Female rats were treated with oral doses of 2 mg/kg/day, 6 mg/kg/day, and 20 mg/kg/day (0.6 times, 2 times, and 6 times the oral maximum recommended human dose [MRHD] of 30 mg/day on a mg/m² body surface area) of aripiprazole from 2 weeks prior to mating through day 7 of gestation. Estrus cycle irregularities and increased corpora lutea were seen at all doses, but no impairment of fertility was seen. Increased pre-implantation loss was seen at 6 mg/kg and 20 mg/kg and decreased fetal weight was seen at 20 mg/kg.

Male rats were treated with oral doses of 20 mg/kg/day, 40 mg/kg/day, and 60 mg/kg/day (6 times, 13 times, and 19 times the oral MRHD of 30 mg/day on a mg/m² body surface area) of aripiprazole from 9 weeks prior to mating through mating. Disturbances in spermatogenesis were seen at 60 mg/kg and prostate atrophy was seen at 40 mg/kg and 60 mg/kg, but no impairment of fertility was seen.

13.2   Animal Toxicity and/or Pharmacology
Oral Aripiprazole
Aripiprazole produced retinal degeneration in albino rats in a 26–week chronic toxicity study at a dose of 60 mg/kg and in a 2–year carcinogenicity study at doses of 40 mg/kg and 60 mg/kg. The 40 mg/kg and 60 mg/kg doses are 13 times and 19 times the oral maximum recommended human dose (MRHD) of 30 mg/day based on mg/m² body surface area based on AUC. Evaluation of the retinas of albino mice and of monkeys did not reveal evidence of retinal degeneration. Additional studies to further evaluate the mechanism have not been performed. The relevance of this finding to human risk is unknown.

Intramuscular Aripiprazole
The toxicological profile for aripiprazole administered to experimental animals by intramuscular injection is generally similar to that seen following oral administration at comparable plasma levels of the drug. With intramuscular injection, however, injection-site tissue reactions are observed that consist of localized inflammation, swelling, scabbing and foreign-body reactions to deposited drug. These effects gradually resolved with discontinuation of dosing.

After 26 weeks of treatment in rats, the no-observed-adverse-effect level (NOAEL) was 50 mg/kg in male rats and 100 mg/kg in female rats, which are approximately 1 and 2 times, respectively, the maximum recommended human 400 mg dose of aripiprazole extended-release injectable suspension on a mg/m² body surface area. At the NOAEL in rats, the AUC_{7d} values were 14.4 µg•h/mL in males and 104.1 µg•h/mL in females. In dogs at 52 weeks of treatment at the NOAEL of 40 mg/kg, which is approximately 3 times the MRHD (400 mg) on a mg/m² body surface area, the AUC_{7d} values were approximately 59 µg•h/mL in males and 44 µg•h/mL in females. In patients at the MRHD of 400 mg, the $AUC\tau$ (0-28 days) was 163 µg•h/mL. For comparison to this human AUC, extrapolating the animal AUC_{7d} values to an AUC_{28d} results in AUC_{28d} values of approximately 58 and 416 µg•h/mL for male and female rats, respectively, and 236 and 175 µg•h/mL for male and female dogs, respectively.

14   CLINICAL STUDIES
The efficacy of ABILIFY MAINTENA in the treatment of patients with schizophrenia was established, in part, on the basis of efficacy data from trials with the oral formulation of aripiprazole. In addition, the efficacy of ABILIFY MAINTENA in maintaining symptomatic control in schizophrenia was established in a randomized-withdrawal, double-blind, placebo-controlled, trial in adult patients who met DSM-IV-TR criteria for schizophrenia and who were being treated with at least one antipsychotic medication. Patients had at least a 3 year history of illness and a history of relapse or symptom exacerbation when not receiving antipsychotic treatment.
Clinical ratings during this trial included:
• The Positive and Negative Syndrome Scale (PANSS). The PANSS is a 30 item scale that measures positive symptoms of schizophrenia (7 items), negative symptoms of schizophrenia (7 items), and general psychopathology (16 items), each rated on a scale of 1 (absent) to 7 (extreme). Total PANSS scores range from 30 to 210.
• The Clinical Global Impression-Severity (CGI-S) scale. The CGI-S rates the severity of mental illness on a scale of 1 (normal) to 7 (among the most extremely ill) based on the total clinical experience of the rater in treating patients with schizophrenia.
• The Clinical Global Impression-Improvement (CGI-I) scale. The CGI-I rates improvement in mental illness on a scale of 1 (very much improved) to 7 (very much worse) based on the change from baseline in clinical condition.
• The Clinical Global Impression- Severity of Suicide (CGI-SS) scale, which is comprised of 2 parts: Part 1 rates the severity of suicidal thoughts and behavior on a scale of 1 (not at all suicidal) to 5 (attempted suicide) based on the most severe level in the last 7 days from all information available to the rater and Part 2 rates the change from baseline in suicidal thoughts and behavior on a scale of 1 (very much improved) to 7 (very much worse).
This trial included:
• A 4–6 week open-label, oral conversion phase for patients on antipsychotic medications other than aripiprazole. A total of 633 patients entered this phase.
• An open-label, oral aripiprazole stabilization phase (target dose of 10 mg to 30 mg once daily). A total of 710 patients entered this phase. Patients were 18 to 60 years old (mean 40 years) and 60% were male. The mean PANSS total score was 66 (range 33 to 124). The mean CGI-S score was 3.5 (mildly to moderately ill). Prior to the next phase, stabilization was required. Stabilization was defined as having all of the following for four consecutive weeks: an outpatient status, PANSS total score ≤80, CGI-S ≤4 (moderately ill), and CGI-SS score ≤2 (mildly suicidal) on Part 1 and ≤5 (minimally worsened) on Part 2; and a score of ≤4 on each of the following PANSS items: conceptual disorganization, suspiciousness, hallucinatory behavior, and unusual thought content.
• A minimum 12–week uncontrolled, single-blind ABILIFY MAINTENA stabilization phase (treatment with 400 mg of ABILIFY MAINTENA given every 4 weeks in conjunction with oral aripiprazole [10 mg to 20 mg/day] for the first 2 weeks). The dose of ABILIFY MAINTENA may have been decreased to 300 mg due to adverse reactions. A total of 576 patients entered this phase. The mean PANSS total score was 59 (range 30 to 80) and the mean CGI-S score was 3.2 (mildly ill). Prior to the next phase, stabilization was required (see above for the definition of stabilization) for 12 consecutive weeks.
• A double-blind, placebo-controlled randomized-withdrawal phase to observe for relapse (defined below). A total of 403 patients were randomized 2:1 to the same dose of ABILIFY MAINTENA they were receiving at the end of the stabilization phase, (400 mg or 300 mg administered once every 4 weeks) or placebo. Patients had a mean PANSS total score of 55 (range 31 to 80) and a CGI-S score of 2.9 (mildly ill) at entry. The dose could be adjusted up and down or down and up within the range of 300 to 400 mg on a one time basis.

The primary efficacy endpoint was time from randomization to relapse. Relapse was defined as the first occurrence of one or more of the following criteria:
1) CGI-I of ≥5 (minimally worse) and
a) an increase on any of the following individual PANSS items (conceptual disorganization, hallucinatory behavior, suspiciousness, unusual thought content) to a score >4 with an absolute increase of ≥2 on that specific item since randomization or
b) an increase on any of the following individual PANSS items (conceptual disorganization, hallucinatory behavior, suspiciousness, unusual thought content) to a score >4 and an absolute increase ≥4 on the combined four PANSS items (conceptual disorganization, hallucinatory behavior, suspiciousness, unusual thought content) since randomization
2) Hospitalization due to worsening of psychotic symptoms (including partial hospitalization), but excluding hospitalization for psychosocial reasons
3) CGI-SS of 4 (severely suicidal) or 5 (attempted suicide) on Part 1 and/or 6 (much worse) or 7 (very much worse) on Part 2, or
4) Violent behavior resulting in clinically significant self-injury, injury to another person, or property damage.

A pre-planned interim analysis demonstrated a statistically significantly longer time to relapse in patients randomized to the ABILIFY MAINTENA group compared to placebo-treated patients and the trial was subsequently terminated early because maintenance of efficacy was demonstrated. The final analysis demonstrated a statistically significantly longer time to relapse in patients randomized to the ABILIFY MAINTENA group than compared to placebo-treated patients (log-rank test p<0.0001). The Kaplan-Meier curves of the time from randomization to relapse during the double-blind treatment phase for ABILIFY MAINTENA and placebo groups are shown in Figure 11.

Figure 11: Time to Relapse *

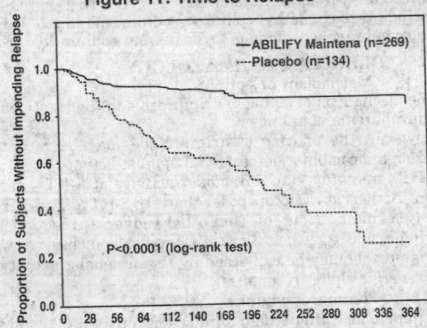

ABILIFY
Maintena (n) 269 244 201 186 153 130 104 76 63 44 36 30 23
Placebo (n) 134 118 85 68 53 45 37 27 22 14 12 9   5   3

* This figure is based on a total of 80 relapse events

The key secondary efficacy endpoint, percentage of subjects meeting the exacerbation of psychotic symptoms/ relapse criteria, was statistically significantly lower in patients randomized to the ABILIFY MAINTENA group (10%) than in the placebo group (40%).

16   HOW SUPPLIED/STORAGE AND HANDLING
16.1   How Supplied
ABILIFY MAINTENA™ (aripiprazole) extended-release injectable suspension is available in 300 mg or 400 mg strength vials.
The 300 mg kit includes (NDC 59148-018-71):
• 300 mg vial of ABILIFY MAINTENA (aripiprazole) extended-release injectable suspension lyophilized powder
• 5 mL vial of Sterile Water for Injection, USP
• One 3 mL Luer Lock syringe with pre-attached 21 gauge, 1.5 inch Hypodermic Needle-Pro® safety needle with needle protection device
• One 3 mL BD Luer-Lok™ disposable syringe with BD Luer-Lok tip
• One vial adapter
• One 21 gauge, 1.5 inch (38 mm) Hypodermic Needle-Pro® safety needle with needle protection device
• One 21 gauge, 2 inch (50 mm) Hypodermic Needle-Pro® safety needle with needle protection device
The 400 mg kit includes (NDC 59148-019-71):
• 400 mg vial of ABILIFY MAINTENA (aripiprazole) extended-release injectable suspension lyophilized powder
• 5 mL vial of Sterile Water for Injection, USP
• One 3 mL Luer Lock syringe with pre-attached 21 gauge, 1.5 inch Hypodermic Needle-Pro® safety needle with needle protection device

- One 3 mL BD Luer-Lok™ disposable syringe with BD Luer-Lok tip
- One vial adapter
- One 21 gauge, 1.5 inch (38 mm) Hypodermic Needle-Pro® safety needle with needle protection device
- One 21 gauge, 2 inch (50 mm) Hypodermic Needle-Pro® safety needle with needle protection device

16.2 Storage

Store at 25 °C (77 °F), excursions permitted between 15 °C and 30 °C (59 °F to 86 °F) [see USP Controlled Room Temperature].

Keep out of reach of children.

17 PATIENT COUNSELING INFORMATION

See FDA-approved patient labeling (Medication Guide)

Physicians are advised to discuss the following issues with patients for whom they prescribe ABILIFY MAINTENA.

17.1 Increased Mortality in Elderly Patients with Dementia-Related Psychosis

Patients and caregivers should be advised that elderly patients with dementia-related psychoses treated with antipsychotic drugs are at increased risk of death. Aripiprazole is not approved for elderly patients with dementia-related psychosis [see Warning and Precautions (5.1)].

17.2 Neuroleptic Malignant Syndrome

Counsel patients and caregivers that a potentially fatal symptom complex sometimes referred to as NMS has been reported in association with administration of antipsychotic drugs. Signs and symptoms of NMS include hyperpyrexia, muscle rigidity, altered mental status, and evidence of autonomic instability (irregular pulse or blood pressure, tachycardia, diaphoresis, and cardiac dysrhythmia) [see Warnings and Precautions (5.3)].

17.3 Tardive Dyskinesia

Advise patients that abnormal involuntary movements have been associated with the administration of antipsychotic drugs. Counsel patients to notify their physician if they notice any movements which they cannot control in their face, tongue, or other body part [see Warnings and Precautions (5.4)].

17.4 Hyperglycemia and Diabetes mellitus

Advise patients of the symptoms of hyperglycemia and diabetes mellitus. Patients who are diagnosed with diabetes, those with risk factors for diabetes, or those that develop these symptoms during treatment should have their blood glucose monitored at the beginning of and periodically during treatment [see Warnings and Precautions (5.5)].

17.5 Orthostatic Hypotension

Advise patients of the risk of orthostatic hypotension, particularly at the time of initiating treatment, re-initiating treatment, or increasing the dose [see Warnings and Precautions (5.6)].

17.6 Leukopenia/Neutropenia

Advise patients with a pre-existing low WBC count or a history of drug-induced leukopenia/neutropenia that they should have their CBC monitored while receiving ABILIFY MAINTENA [see Warnings and Precautions (5.7)].

17.7 Interference with Cognitive and Motor Performance

Because ABILIFY MAINTENA may have the potential to impair judgment, thinking, or motor skills, instruct patients to be cautious about operating hazardous machinery, including automobiles, until they are reasonably certain that ABILIFY MAINTENA therapy does not affect them adversely [see Warnings and Precautions (5.9)].

17.8 Heat Exposure and Dehydration

Advise patients regarding appropriate care in avoiding overheating and dehydration [see Warnings and Precautions (5.10)].

17.9 Concomitant Medication

Advise patients to inform their physicians if they are taking, or plan to take, any prescription or over-the-counter drugs, since there is a potential for interactions [see Drug Interactions (7)].

17.10 Pregnancy

Advise patients to notify their physician if they become pregnant or intend to become pregnant during therapy with ABILIFY MAINTENA [see Use in Specific Populations (8.1)].

17.11 Nursing

Aripiprazole is excreted in human breast milk. A decision should be made whether to discontinue nursing or to discontinue ABILIFY MAINTENA, taking into account the importance of the drug to the mother [see Use in Specific Populations (8.3)].

17.12 Alcohol

Advise patients to avoid alcohol while taking ABILIFY MAINTENA [see Clinical Pharmacology (12.2)].

Distributed and marketed by Otsuka America Pharmaceutical, Inc., Rockville, MD 20850 USA

Marketed by Lundbeck, Deerfield, IL 60015 USA

ABILIFY MAINTENA is a trademark of Otsuka Pharmaceutical Company.

Luer-Lok is a trademark of Becton, Dickinson and Company, NJ.

Needle-Pro is a registered trademark of Smiths Medical ASD, Inc., DE.

09US12L-1001

February 2013

© 2013, Otsuka Pharmaceutical Co., Ltd., Tokyo, 101-8535 Japan

MEDICATION GUIDE

ABILIFY MAINTENA™ (a-BIL-i-fy main-TEN-a)

(aripiprazole)

extended-release injectable suspension, for intramuscular use

Read this Medication Guide before you receive your first injection of ABILIFY MAINTENA and before each injection. There may be new information. This information does not take the place of talking to your healthcare provider about your medical condition or your treatment.

What is the most important information I should know about ABILIFY MAINTENA?

ABILIFY MAINTENA may cause serious side effects, including:

- **Increased risk of death in elderly people with dementia-related psychosis.** ABILIFY MAINTENA is not for the treatment of people who have lost touch with reality (psychosis) due to confusion and memory loss (dementia).
- **Neuroleptic malignant syndrome (NMS) a serious condition that can lead to death.** Tell your healthcare provider right away if you have some or all of the following symptoms of NMS:
  ◦ high fever
  ◦ stiff muscles
  ◦ confusion
  ◦ sweating
  ◦ changes in pulse, heart rate, and blood pressure

Call your healthcare provider right away if you have any of these symptoms.

What is ABILIFY MAINTENA?

ABILIFY MAINTENA is a prescription medicine used to treat schizophrenia.

It is not known if ABILIFY MAINTENA is safe and effective in children under 18 years of age.

Who should not receive ABILIFY MAINTENA?

Do not receive ABILIFY MAINTENA if you are allergic to aripiprazole or any of the ingredients in ABILIFY MAINTENA. See the end of this leaflet for a complete list of ingredients in ABILIFY MAINTENA.

What should I tell my healthcare provider before receiving ABILIFY MAINTENA?

Before you receive ABILIFY MAINTENA, tell your healthcare provider if you:

- have never taken ABILIFY (aripiprazole) before
- have diabetes or high blood sugar or a family history of diabetes or high blood sugar. Your healthcare provider should check your blood sugar before you start receiving ABILIFY MAINTENA and during your treatment.
- have or had seizures (convulsions)
- have or had low or high blood pressure
- have or had heart problems or a stroke
- have or had a low white blood cell count
- have any other medical problems including problems that may affect you receiving an injection in your buttocks
- are pregnant or plan to become pregnant. It is not known if ABILIFY MAINTENA will harm your unborn baby.
- are breastfeeding or plan to breastfeed. ABILIFY MAINTENA can pass into your milk and may harm your baby. Talk to your healthcare provider about the best way to feed your baby if you receive ABILIFY MAINTENA.

Tell your healthcare provider about all the medicines you take, including prescription medicines, non-prescription medicines, vitamins, and herbal supplements.

ABILIFY MAINTENA and other medicines may affect each other causing possible serious side effects. ABILIFY MAINTENA may affect the way other medicines work, and other medicines may affect how ABILIFY MAINTENA works.

Your healthcare provider can tell you if it is safe to take ABILIFY MAINTENA with your other medicines. Do not start or stop any medicines while taking ABILIFY MAINTENA without talking to your healthcare provider first.

Know the medicines you take. Keep a list of them to show your healthcare provider and pharmacist when you get a new medicine.

How should I receive ABILIFY MAINTENA?

- ABILIFY MAINTENA is an injection given in your buttock by your healthcare provider 1 time a month. You may feel a little pain in your buttock during your injection.
- After your first injection of ABILIFY MAINTENA you should continue your current antipsychotic medicine for 2 weeks.
- You should not miss a dose of ABILIFY MAINTENA. If you miss a dose for some reason, call your healthcare provider right away to discuss what you should do next.

What should I avoid while receiving ABILIFY MAINTENA?

- Do not drive, operate machinery, or do other dangerous activities until you know how ABILIFY MAINTENA affects you. ABILIFY MAINTENA may make you feel drowsy.
- Do not drink alcohol while you receive ABILIFY MAINTENA.
- Do not become too hot or dehydrated while you receive ABILIFY MAINTENA.
  ◦ Do not exercise too much.
  ◦ In hot weather, stay inside in a cool place if possible.
  ◦ Stay out of the sun.
  ◦ Do not wear too much clothing or heavy clothing.
  ◦ Drink plenty of water.

What are the possible side effects of ABILIFY MAINTENA?

ABILIFY MAINTENA may cause serious side effects, including:

- See "What is the most important information I should know about ABILIFY MAINTENA?"
- **Uncontrolled body movements (tardive dyskinesia).** ABILIFY MAINTENA may cause movements that you cannot control in your face, tongue, or other body parts. Tardive dyskinesia may not go away, even if you stop receiving ABILIFY MAINTENA. Tardive dyskinesia may also start after you stop receiving ABILIFY MAINTENA.
- **Problems with your metabolism such as:**
  ◦ **High blood sugar (hyperglycemia):** Increases in blood sugar can happen in some people who take ABILIFY MAINTENA. Extremely high blood sugar can lead to coma or death. If you have diabetes or risk factors for diabetes (such as being overweight or a family history of diabetes), your healthcare provider should check your blood sugar before you start receiving ABILIFY MAINTENA and during your treatment.

Call your healthcare provider if you have any of these symptoms of high blood sugar while receiving ABILIFY MAINTENA:

- feel very thirsty
- need to urinate more than usual
- feel very hungry
- feel weak or tired
- feel sick to your stomach
- feel confused, or your breath smells fruity
  ◦ **Increased fat levels (cholesterol and triglycerides) in your blood.**
  ◦ **Weight gain.** You and your healthcare provider should check your weight regularly.
- **Decreased blood pressure (orthostatic hypotension).** You may feel lightheaded or faint when you rise too quickly from a sitting or lying position.
- **Low white blood cell count**
- **Seizures (convulsions)**
- **Problems controlling your body temperature so that you feel too warm. See "What should I avoid while receiving ABILIFY MAINTENA?"**
- **Difficulty swallowing**

The most common side effect of ABILIFY MAINTENA includes feeling like you need to move to stop unpleasant feelings in your legs (restless leg syndrome or akathisia).

Tell your healthcare provider if you have any side effect that bothers you or does not go away.

These are not all the possible side effects of ABILIFY MAINTENA. For more information, ask your healthcare provider or pharmacist.

Call your doctor for medical advice about side effects. You may report side effects to FDA at 1-800-FDA-1088.

General information about the safe and effective use of ABILIFY MAINTENA

This Medication Guide summarizes the most important information about ABILIFY MAINTENA. If you would like more information, talk with your healthcare provider.

You can ask your healthcare provider or pharmacist for information about ABILIFY MAINTENA. If you would like more information, talk with your healthcare provider. You can ask your pharmacist or healthcare provider for information about ABILIFY MAINTENA that is written for healthcare professionals.

For more information about ABILIFY MAINTENA, go to www.ABILIFYMAINTENA.com or call 1-800-441-6763.

What are the ingredients in ABILIFY MAINTENA?

Active ingredient: aripiprazole monohydrate

Inactive ingredients: carboxymethyl cellulose sodium, mannitol, sodium phosphate monobasic monohydrate and sodium hydroxide

This Medication Guide has been approved by the U.S. Food and Drug Administration.

ABILIFY MAINTENA is a trademark of Otsuka Pharmaceutical Company.

Luer-Lok is a trademark of Becton, Dickinson and Company, NJ

Needle-Pro is a registered trademark of Smiths Medical ASD, Inc., DE

09US12L-1001C

February 2013

© 2013, Otsuka Pharmaceutical Co., Ltd., Tokyo, 101-8535 Japan

Shown in Product Identification Guide, page 311

Pfizer Inc.
235 EAST 42ND STREET
NEW YORK, NY 10017–5755

For updates to the product information listed below, please check the Pfizer Web site, http://www.pfizerpro.com, or call (800) 438-1985. For complete product listing, please see the Manufacturers' Index.

For Medical Information, Contact:
(800) 438-1985
24 hours a day, 7 days a week

Distribution:
1855 Shelby Oaks Drive North
Memphis, TN 38134
(901) 387-5200

Customer Service:
(800) 533-4535

Pfizer Companies Include:
Agouron Pharmaceuticals
King Pharmaceuticals Inc.
Pharmaceuticals Inc.
Parke-Davis
Pharmacia & Upjohn
G.D. Searle & Co.
Wyeth Pharmaceuticals – see Wyeth Pharmaceuticals

VIAGRA®   ℞
[vI-AG-ra]
(sildenafil citrate)
tablets, for oral use

HIGHLIGHTS OF PRESCRIBING INFORMATION
These highlights do not include all the information needed to use VIAGRA safely and effectively. See full prescribing information for VIAGRA.
VIAGRA® (sildenafil citrate) tablets, for oral use
Initial U.S. Approval: 1998

———————INDICATIONS AND USAGE———————
VIAGRA is a phosphodiesterase-5 (PDE5) inhibitor indicated for the treatment of erectile dysfunction (ED) (1)

—————DOSAGE AND ADMINISTRATION—————
• For most patients, the recommended dose is 50 mg taken, as needed, approximately 1 hour before sexual activity. However, VIAGRA may be taken anywhere from 30 minutes to 4 hours before sexual activity (2.1)
• Based on effectiveness and toleration, may increase to a maximum of 100 mg or decrease to 25 mg (2.1)
• Maximum recommended dosing frequency is once per day (2.1)

—————DOSAGE FORMS AND STRENGTHS—————
Tablets: 25 mg, 50 mg, 100 mg (3)

———————CONTRAINDICATIONS———————
• Administration of VIAGRA to patients using nitric oxide donors, such as organic nitrates or organic nitrites in any form. VIAGRA was shown to potentiate the hypotensive effect of nitrates (4.1, 7.1, 12.2)
• Known hypersensitivity to sildenafil or any component of tablet (4.2)

—————WARNINGS AND PRECAUTIONS—————
• Patients should not use VIAGRA if sexual activity is inadvisable due to cardiovascular status (5.1)
• Patients should seek emergency treatment if an erection lasts >4 hours. Use VIAGRA with caution in patients predisposed to priapism (5.2)
• Patients should stop VIAGRA and seek medical care if a sudden loss of vision occurs in one or both eyes, which could be a sign of non arteritic anterior ischemic optic neuropathy (NAION). VIAGRA should be used with caution, and only when the anticipated benefits outweigh the risks, in patients with a history of NAION. Patients with a "crowded" optic disc may also be at an increased risk of NAION. (5.3)
• Patients should stop VIAGRA and seek prompt medical attention in the event of sudden decrease or loss of hearing (5.4)
• Caution is advised when VIAGRA is co-administered with alpha-blockers or anti-hypertensives. Concomitant use may lead to hypotension (5.5)
• Decreased blood pressure, syncope, and prolonged erection may occur at higher sildenafil exposures. In patients taking strong CYP inhibitors, such as ritonavir, sildenafil exposure is increased. Decrease in VIAGRA dosage is recommended (2.4, 5.6)

———————ADVERSE REACTIONS———————
Most common adverse reactions (≥ 2%) include headache, flushing, dyspepsia, abnormal vision, nasal congestion, back pain, myalgia, nausea, dizziness and rash (6.1)
To report SUSPECTED ADVERSE REACTIONS, contact Pfizer at 1-800-438-1985 or FDA at 1-800-FDA-1088 or www.fda.gov/medwatch.

———————DRUG INTERACTIONS———————
• VIAGRA can potentiate the hypotensive effects of nitrates, alpha blockers, and anti-hypertensives (4.1, 5.5, 7.1, 7.2, 7.3, 12.2)
• With concomitant use of alpha blockers, initiate VIAGRA at 25 mg dose (2.3)
• CYP3A4 inhibitors (e.g., ritonavir, ketoconazole, itraconazole, erythromycin): Increase VIAGRA exposure (2.4, 7.4, 12.3)
 ▪ Ritonavir: Do not exceed a maximum single dose of 25 mg in a 48 hour period (2.4, 5.6)
 ▪ Erythromycin or strong CYP3A4 inhibitors (e.g., ketoconazole, itraconazole, saquinavir): Consider a starting dose of 25 mg (2.4, 7.4)

—————USE IN SPECIFIC POPULATIONS—————
• Geriatric use: Consider a starting dose of 25 mg (2.5, 8.5)
• Severe renal impairment: Consider a starting dose of 25 mg (2.5, 8.6)
• Hepatic impairment: Consider a starting dose of 25 mg (2.5, 8.7)

See 17 for PATIENT COUNSELING INFORMATION and FDA-approved patient labeling
                                    Revised: 03/2014

FULL PRESCRIBING INFORMATION: CONTENTS*

FULL PRESCRIBING INFORMATION

1   INDICATIONS AND USAGE
VIAGRA is indicated for the treatment of erectile dysfunction.

2   DOSAGE AND ADMINISTRATION
2.1   Dosage Information
For most patients, the recommended dose is 50 mg taken, as needed, approximately 1 hour before sexual activity. However, VIAGRA may be taken anywhere from 30 minutes to 4 hours before sexual activity.
The maximum recommended dosing frequency is once per day.
Based on effectiveness and toleration, the dose may be increased to a maximum recommended dose of 100 mg or decreased to 25 mg.
2.2   Use with Food
VIAGRA may be taken with or without food.
2.3   Dosage Adjustments in Specific Situations
VIAGRA was shown to potentiate the hypotensive effects of nitrates and its administration in patients who use nitric oxide donors such as organic nitrates or organic nitrites in any form is therefore contraindicated [see Contraindications (4.1), Drug Interactions (7.1), and Clinical Pharmacology (12.2)].
When VIAGRA is co-administered with an alpha-blocker, patients should be stable on alpha-blocker therapy prior to initiating VIAGRA treatment and VIAGRA should be initiated at 25 mg [see Warnings and Precautions (5.5), Drug Interactions (7.2), and Clinical Pharmacology (12.2)].
2.4   Dosage Adjustments Due to Drug Interactions
Ritonavir
The recommended dose for ritonavir-treated patients is 25 mg prior to sexual activity and the recommended maximum dose is 25 mg within a 48 hour period because concomitant administration increased the blood levels of sildenafil by 11-fold [see Warnings and Precautions (5.6), Drug Interactions (7.4), and Clinical Pharmacology (12.3)].
CYP3A4 Inhibitors
Consider a starting dose of 25 mg in patients treated with strong CYP3A4 inhibitors (e.g., ketoconazole, itraconazole, or saquinavir) or erythromycin. Clinical data have shown that co-administration with saquinavir or erythromycin increased plasma levels of sildenafil by about 3 fold [see Drug Interactions (7.4) and Clinical Pharmacology (12.3)].
2.5   Dosage Adjustments in Special Populations
Consider a starting dose of 25 mg in patients > 65 years, patients with hepatic impairment (e.g., cirrhosis), and patients with severe renal impairment (creatinine clearance <30 mL/minute) because administration of VIAGRA in these patients resulted in higher plasma levels of sildenafil [see Use in Specific Populations (8.5, 8.6, 8.7) and Clinical Pharmacology (12.3)].

3   DOSAGE FORMS AND STRENGTHS
VIAGRA is supplied as blue, film-coated, rounded-diamond-shaped tablets containing sildenafil citrate equivalent to 25 mg, 50 mg, or 100 mg of sildenafil. Tablets are debossed with PFIZER on one side and VGR25, VGR50 or VGR100 on the other to indicate the dosage strengths.

4   CONTRAINDICATIONS
4.1   Nitrates
Consistent with its known effects on the nitric oxide/cGMP pathway [see Clinical Pharmacology (12.1, 12.2)], VIAGRA was shown to potentiate the hypotensive effects of nitrates, and its administration to patients who are using nitric oxide donors such as organic nitrates or organic nitrites in any form either regularly and/or intermittently is therefore contraindicated.
After patients have taken VIAGRA, it is unknown when nitrates, if necessary, can be safely administered. Although plasma levels of sildenafil at 24 hours post dose are much lower than at peak concentration, it is unknown whether nitrates can be safely co-administered at this time point [see Dosage and Administration (2.3), Drug Interactions (7.1), and Clinical Pharmacology (12.2)].
4.2   Hypersensitivity Reactions
VIAGRA is contraindicated in patients with a known hypersensitivity to sildenafil, as contained in VIAGRA and REVATIO, or any component of the tablet. Hypersensitivity reactions have been reported, including rash and urticaria [see Adverse Reactions (6.1)].

5   WARNINGS AND PRECAUTIONS
5.1   Cardiovascular
There is a potential for cardiac risk of sexual activity in patients with preexisting cardiovascular disease. Therefore, treatments for erectile dysfunction, including VIAGRA, should not be generally used in men for whom sexual activity is inadvisable because of their underlying cardiovascular status. The evaluation of erectile dysfunction should include a determination of potential underlying causes and the

identification of appropriate treatment following a complete medical assessment.

VIAGRA has systemic vasodilatory properties that resulted in transient decreases in supine blood pressure in healthy volunteers (mean maximum decrease of 8.4/5.5 mmHg), [see *Clinical Pharmacology (12.2)*]. While this normally would be expected to be of little consequence in most patients, prior to prescribing VIAGRA, physicians should carefully consider whether their patients with underlying cardiovascular disease could be affected adversely by such vasodilatory effects, especially in combination with sexual activity. Use with caution in patients with the following underlying conditions which can be particularly sensitive to the actions of vasodilators including VIAGRA – those with left ventricular outflow obstruction (e.g., aortic stenosis, idiopathic hypertrophic subaortic stenosis) and those with severely impaired autonomic control of blood pressure.

There are no controlled clinical data on the safety or efficacy of VIAGRA in the following groups; if prescribed, this should be done with caution.

- Patients who have suffered a myocardial infarction, stroke, or life-threatening arrhythmia within the last 6 months;
- Patients with resting hypotension (BP <90/50 mmHg) or hypertension (BP >170/110 mmHg);
- Patients with cardiac failure or coronary artery disease causing unstable angina.

5.2 Prolonged Erection and Priapism

Prolonged erection greater than 4 hours and priapism (painful erections greater than 6 hours in duration) have been reported infrequently since market approval of VIAGRA. In the event of an erection that persists longer than 4 hours, the patient should seek immediate medical assistance. If priapism is not treated immediately, penile tissue damage and permanent loss of potency could result.

VIAGRA should be used with caution in patients with anatomical deformation of the penis (such as angulation, cavernosal fibrosis or Peyronie's disease), or in patients who have conditions which may predispose them to priapism (such as sickle cell anemia, multiple myeloma, or leukemia). However, there are no controlled clinical data on the safety or efficacy of VIAGRA in patients with sickle cell or related anemias.

5.3 Effects on the Eye

Physicians should advise patients to stop use of all phosphodiesterase type 5 (PDE5) inhibitors, including VIAGRA, and seek medical attention in the event of a sudden loss of vision in one or both eyes. Such an event may be a sign of nonarteritic anterior ischemic optic neuropathy (NAION), a rare condition and a cause of decreased vision including permanent loss of vision, that has been reported rarely postmarketing in temporal association with the use of all PDE5 inhibitors. Based on published literature, the annual incidence of NAION is 2.5–11.8 cases per 100,000 in males aged ≥ 50. An observational study evaluated whether recent use of PDE5 inhibitors, as a class, was associated with acute onset of NAION. The results suggest an approximate 2 fold increase in the risk of NAION within 5 half-lives of PDE5 inhibitor use. From this information, it is not possible to determine whether these events are related directly to the use of PDE5 inhibitors or to other factors [see *Adverse Reactions (6.2)*].

Physicians should consider whether their patients with underlying NAION risk factors could be adversely affected by use of PDE5 inhibitors. Individuals who have already experienced NAION are at increased risk of NAION recurrence. Therefore, PDE5 inhibitors, including VIAGRA, should be used with caution in these patients and only when the anticipated benefits outweigh the risks. Individuals with "crowded" optic disc are also considered at greater risk for NAION compared to the general population, however, evidence is insufficient to support screening of prospective users of PDE5 inhibitors, including VIAGRA, for this uncommon condition.

There are no controlled clinical data on the safety or efficacy of VIAGRA in patients with retinitis pigmentosa (a minority of these patients have genetic disorders of retinal phosphodiesterases).

5.4 Hearing Loss

Physicians should advise patients to stop taking PDE5 inhibitors, including VIAGRA, and seek prompt medical attention in the event of sudden decrease or loss of hearing. These events, which may be accompanied by tinnitus and dizziness, have been reported in temporal association to the intake of PDE5 inhibitors, including VIAGRA. It is not possible to determine whether these events are related directly to the use of PDE5 inhibitors or to other factors [see *Adverse Reactions (6.1, 6.2)*].

5.5 Hypotension when Co-administered with Alpha-blockers or Anti-hypertensives

Alpha-blockers

Caution is advised when PDE5 inhibitors are co-administered with alpha-blockers. PDE5 inhibitors, including VIAGRA, and alpha-adrenergic blocking agents are both

Table 1: Adverse Reactions Reported by ≥2% of Patients Treated with VIAGRA and More Frequent than Placebo in Fixed-Dose Phase II/III Studies

Adverse Reaction	25 mg (n=312)	50 mg (n=511)	100 mg (n=506)	Placebo (n=607)
Headache	16%	21%	28%	7%
Flushing	10%	19%	18%	2%
Dyspepsia	3%	9%	17%	2%
Abnormal vision*	1%	2%	11%	1%
Nasal congestion	4%	4%	9%	2%
Back pain	3%	4%	4%	2%
Myalgia	2%	2%	4%	1%
Nausea	2%	3%	3%	1%
Dizziness	3%	4%	3%	2%
Rash	1%	2%	3%	1%

* Abnormal Vision: Mild to moderate in severity and transient, predominantly color tinge to vision, but also increased sensitivity to light, or blurred vision.

vasodilators with blood pressure lowering effects. When vasodilators are used in combination, an additive effect on blood pressure may occur. In some patients, concomitant use of these two drug classes can lower blood pressure significantly [see *Drug Interactions (7.2)* and *Clinical Pharmacology (12.2)*] leading to symptomatic hypotension (e.g., dizziness, lightheadedness, fainting).

Consideration should be given to the following:

- Patients who demonstrate hemodynamic instability on alpha-blocker therapy alone are at increased risk of symptomatic hypotension with concomitant use of PDE5 inhibitors. Patients should be stable on alpha-blocker therapy prior to initiating a PDE5 inhibitor.
- In those patients who are stable on alpha-blocker therapy, PDE5 inhibitors should be initiated at the lowest dose [see *Dosage and Administration (2.3)*].
- In those patients already taking an optimized dose of a PDE5 inhibitor, alpha-blocker therapy should be initiated at the lowest dose. Stepwise increase in alpha-blocker dose may be associated with further lowering of blood pressure when taking a PDE5 inhibitor.
- Safety of combined use of PDE5 inhibitors and alpha-blockers may be affected by other variables, including intravascular volume depletion and other anti-hypertensive drugs.

Anti-hypertensives

VIAGRA has systemic vasodilatory properties and may further lower blood pressure in patients taking anti-hypertensive medications.

In a separate drug interaction study, when amlodipine, 5 mg or 10 mg, and VIAGRA, 100 mg were orally administered concomitantly to hypertensive patients mean additional blood pressure reduction of 8 mmHg systolic and 7 mmHg diastolic were noted [see *Drug Interactions (7.3)* and *Clinical Pharmacology (12.2)*].

5.6 Adverse Reactions with the Concomitant Use of Ritonavir

The concomitant administration of the protease inhibitor ritonavir substantially increases serum concentrations of sildenafil (11-fold increase in AUC). If VIAGRA is prescribed to patients taking ritonavir, caution should be used. Data from subjects exposed to high systemic levels of sildenafil are limited. Decreased blood pressure, syncope, and prolonged erection were reported in some healthy volunteers exposed to high doses of sildenafil (200–800 mg). To decrease the chance of adverse reactions in patients taking ritonavir, a decrease in sildenafil dosage is recommended [see *Dosage and Administration (2.4)*, *Drug Interactions (7.4)*, and *Clinical Pharmacology (12.3)*].

5.7 Combination with other PDE5 Inhibitors or Other Erectile Dysfunction Therapies

The safety and efficacy of combinations of VIAGRA with other PDE5 Inhibitors, including REVATIO or other pulmonary arterial hypertension (PAH) treatments containing sildenafil, or other treatments for erectile dysfunction have not been studied. Such combinations may further lower blood pressure. Therefore, the use of such combinations is not recommended.

5.8 Effects on Bleeding

There have been postmarketing reports of bleeding events in patients who have taken VIAGRA. A causal relationship between VIAGRA and these events has not been established. In humans, VIAGRA has no effect on bleeding time when taken alone or with aspirin. However, *in vitro* studies with human platelets indicate that sildenafil potentiates the antiaggregatory effect of sodium nitroprusside (a nitric oxide donor). In addition, the combination of heparin and VIAGRA had an additive effect on bleeding time in the anesthetized rabbit, but this interaction has not been studied in humans.

The safety of VIAGRA is unknown in patients with bleeding disorders and patients with active peptic ulceration.

5.9 Counseling Patients About Sexually Transmitted Diseases

The use of VIAGRA offers no protection against sexually transmitted diseases. Counseling of patients about the protective measures necessary to guard against sexually transmitted diseases, including the Human Immunodeficiency Virus (HIV), may be considered.

6 ADVERSE REACTIONS

The following are discussed in more detail in other sections of the labeling:

- Cardiovascular [see *Warnings and Precautions (5.1)*]
- Prolonged Erection and Priapism [see *Warnings and Precautions (5.2)*]
- Effects on the Eye [see *Warnings and Precautions (5.3)*]
- Hearing Loss [see *Warnings and Precautions (5.4)*]
- Hypotension when Co-administered with Alpha-blockers or Anti-hypertensives [see *Warnings and Precautions (5.5)*]
- Adverse Reactions with the Concomitant Use of Ritonavir [see *Warnings and Precautions (5.6)*]
- Combination with other PDE5 Inhibitors or Other Erectile Dysfunction Therapies [see *Warnings and Precautions (5.7)*]
- Effects on Bleeding [see *Warnings and Precautions (5.8)*]
- Counseling Patients About Sexually Transmitted Diseases [see *Warnings and Precautions (5.9)*]

The most common adverse reactions reported in clinical trials (≥ 2%) are headache, flushing, dyspepsia, abnormal vision, nasal congestion, back pain, myalgia, nausea, dizziness, and rash.

6.1 Clinical Trials Experience

Because clinical trials are conducted under widely varying conditions, adverse reaction rates observed in the clinical trials of a drug cannot be directly compared to rates in the clinical trials of another drug and may not reflect the rates observed in clinical practice.

VIAGRA was administered to over 3700 patients (aged 19–87 years) during pre-marketing clinical trials worldwide. Over 550 patients were treated for longer than one year.

In placebo-controlled clinical studies, the discontinuation rate due to adverse reactions for VIAGRA (2.5%) was not significantly different from placebo (2.3%).

In fixed-dose studies, the incidence of some adverse reactions increased with dose. The type of adverse reactions in flexible-dose studies, which reflect the recommended dosage regimen, was similar to that for fixed-dose studies. At doses above the recommended dose range, adverse reactions were similar to those detailed in Table 1 below but generally were reported more frequently.

[See table 1 above]

When VIAGRA was taken as recommended (on an as-needed basis) in flexible-dose, placebo-controlled clinical trials of two to twenty-six weeks duration, patients took VIAGRA at least once weekly, and the following adverse reactions were reported:

Table 2. Adverse Reactions Reported by ≥2% of Patients Treated with VIAGRA and More Frequent than Placebo in Flexible-Dose Phase II/III Studies

Adverse Reaction	VIAGRA	PLACEBO
	N=734	N=725
Headache	16%	4%
Flushing	10%	1%
Dyspepsia	7%	2%
Nasal Congestion	4%	2%
Abnormal Vision*	3%	0%
Back pain	2%	2%
Dizziness	2%	1%
Rash	2%	1%

* Abnormal Vision: Mild and transient, predominantly color tinge to vision, but also increased sensitivity to light or blurred vision. In these studies, only one patient discontinued due to abnormal vision.

The following events occurred in <2% of patients in controlled clinical trials; a causal relationship to VIAGRA is uncertain. Reported events include those with a plausible relation to drug use; omitted are minor events and reports too imprecise to be meaningful:

Body as a Whole: face edema, photosensitivity reaction, shock, asthenia, pain, chills, accidental fall, abdominal pain, allergic reaction, chest pain, accidental injury.

Cardiovascular: angina pectoris, AV block, migraine, syncope, tachycardia, palpitation, hypotension, postural hypotension, myocardial ischemia, cerebral thrombosis, cardiac arrest, heart failure, abnormal electrocardiogram, cardiomyopathy.

Digestive: vomiting, glossitis, colitis, dysphagia, gastritis, gastroenteritis, esophagitis, stomatitis, dry mouth, liver function tests abnormal, rectal hemorrhage, gingivitis.

Hemic and Lymphatic: anemia and leukopenia.

Metabolic and Nutritional: thirst, edema, gout, unstable diabetes, hyperglycemia, peripheral edema, hyperuricemia, hypoglycemic reaction, hypernatremia.

Musculoskeletal: arthritis, arthrosis, myalgia, tendon rupture, tenosynovitis, bone pain, myasthenia, synovitis.

Nervous: ataxia, hypertonia, neuralgia, neuropathy, paresthesia, tremor, vertigo, depression, insomnia, somnolence, abnormal dreams, reflexes decreased, hypesthesia.

Respiratory: asthma, dyspnea, laryngitis, pharyngitis, sinusitis, bronchitis, sputum increased, cough increased.

Skin and Appendages: urticaria, herpes simplex, pruritus, sweating, skin ulcer, contact dermatitis, exfoliative dermatitis.

Special Senses: sudden decrease or loss of hearing, mydriasis, conjunctivitis, photophobia, tinnitus, eye pain, ear pain, eye hemorrhage, cataract, dry eyes.

Urogenital: cystitis, nocturia, urinary frequency, breast enlargement, urinary incontinence, abnormal ejaculation, genital edema and anorgasmia.

Analysis of the safety database from controlled clinical trials showed no apparent difference in adverse reactions in patients taking VIAGRA with and without antihypertensive medication. This analysis was performed retrospectively, and was not powered to detect any prespecified difference in adverse reactions.

6.2   Postmarketing Experience

The following adverse reactions have been identified during post approval use of VIAGRA. Because these reactions are reported voluntarily from a population of uncertain size, it is not always possible to reliably estimate their frequency or establish a causal relationship to drug exposure. These events have been chosen for inclusion either due to their seriousness, reporting frequency, lack of clear alternative causation, or a combination of these factors.

Cardiovascular and cerebrovascular

Serious cardiovascular, cerebrovascular, and vascular events, including myocardial infarction, sudden cardiac death, ventricular arrhythmia, cerebrovascular hemorrhage, transient ischemic attack, hypertension, subarachnoid and intracerebral hemorrhages, and pulmonary hemorrhage have been reported post-marketing in temporal association with the use of VIAGRA. Most, but not all, of these patients had preexisting cardiovascular risk factors. Many of these events were reported to occur during or shortly after sexual activity, and a few were reported to occur shortly after the use of VIAGRA without sexual activity. Others were reported to have occurred hours to days after

the use of VIAGRA and sexual activity. It is not possible to determine whether these events are related directly to VIAGRA, to sexual activity, to the patient's underlying cardiovascular disease, to a combination of these factors, or to other factors [see Warnings and Precautions (5.1) and Patient Counseling Information (17.3)].

Hemic and Lymphatic: vaso-occlusive crisis: In a small, prematurely terminated study of REVATIO (sildenafil) in patients with pulmonary arterial hypertension (PAH) secondary to sickle cell disease, vaso-occlusive crises requiring hospitalization were more commonly reported in patients who received sildenafil than in those randomized to placebo. The clinical relevance of this finding to men treated with VIAGRA for ED is not known.

Nervous: seizure, seizure recurrence, anxiety, and transient global amnesia.

Respiratory: epistaxis

Special senses:

Hearing: Cases of sudden decrease or loss of hearing have been reported postmarketing in temporal association with the use of PDE5 inhibitors, including VIAGRA. In some of the cases, medical conditions and other factors were reported that may have also played a role in the otologic adverse events. In many cases, medical follow-up information was limited. It is not possible to determine whether these reported events are related directly to the use of VIAGRA, to the patient's underlying risk factors for hearing loss, to a combination of these factors, or to other factors [see Warnings and Precautions (5.4) and Patient Counseling Information (17.5)].

Ocular: diplopia, temporary vision loss/decreased vision, ocular redness or bloodshot appearance, ocular burning, ocular swelling/pressure, increased intraocular pressure, retinal edema, retinal vascular disease or bleeding, and vitreous traction/detachment.

Non-arteritic anterior ischemic optic neuropathy (NAION), a cause of decreased vision including permanent loss of vision, has been reported rarely post-marketing in temporal association with the use of phosphodiesterase type 5 (PDE5) inhibitors, including VIAGRA. Most, but not all, of these patients had underlying anatomic or vascular risk factors for developing NAION, including but not necessarily limited to: low cup to disc ratio ("crowded disc"), age over 50, diabetes, hypertension, coronary artery disease, hyperlipidemia and smoking. It is not possible to determine whether these events are related directly to the use of PDE5 inhibitors, to the patient's underlying vascular risk factors or anatomical defects, to a combination of these factors, or to other factors [see Warnings and Precautions (5.3) and Patient Counseling Information (17.4)].

Urogenital: prolonged erection, priapism [see Warnings and Precautions (5.2) and Patient Counseling Information (17.6)], and hematuria.

7   DRUG INTERACTIONS

7.1   Nitrates

Administration of VIAGRA with nitric oxide donors such as organic nitrates or organic nitrites in any form is contraindicated. Consistent with its known effects on the nitric oxide/cGMP pathway, VIAGRA was shown to potentiate the hypotensive effects of nitrates [see Dosage and Administration (2.3), Contraindications (4.1), Clinical Pharmacology (12.2)].

7.2   Alpha-blockers

Use caution when co-administering alpha-blockers with VIAGRA because of potential additive blood pressure-lowering effects. When VIAGRA is co-administered with an alpha-blocker, patients should be stable on alpha-blocker therapy prior to initiating VIAGRA treatment and VIAGRA should be initiated at the lowest dose [see Dosage and Administration (2.3), Warnings and Precautions (5.5), Clinical Pharmacology (12.2)].

7.3   Amlodipine

When VIAGRA 100 mg was co-administered with amlodipine (5 mg or 10 mg) to hypertensive patients, the mean additional reduction on supine blood pressure was 8 mmHg systolic and 7 mmHg diastolic [see Warnings and Precautions (5.5), Clinical Pharmacology (12.2)].

7.4   Ritonavir and other CYP3A4 inhibitors

Co-administration of ritonavir, a strong CYP3A4 inhibitor, greatly increased the systemic exposure of sildenafil (11-fold increase in AUC). It is therefore recommended not to exceed a maximum single dose of 25 mg of VIAGRA in a 48 hour period [see Dosage and Administration (2.4), Warnings and Precautions (5.6), Clinical Pharmacology (12.3)].

Co-administration of erythromycin, a moderate CYP3A4 inhibitor, resulted in a 160% and 182% increases in sildenafil C_{max} and AUC, respectively. Co-administration of saquinavir, a strong CYP3A4 inhibitor, resulted in 140% and 210% increases in sildenafil C_{max} and AUC, respectively. Stronger CYP3A4 inhibitors such as ketoconazole or itraconazole could be expected to have greater effects than seen with saquinavir. A starting dose of 25 mg of VIAGRA should be considered in patients taking erythromycin or strong CYP3A4

inhibitors (such as saquinavir, ketoconazole, itracanozole) [see Dosage and Administration (2.4), Clinical Pharmacology (12.3)].

7.5   Alcohol

In a drug-drug interaction study sildenafil 50 mg given with alcohol 0.5 g/kg in which mean maximum blood alcohol levels of 0.08% was achieved, sildenafil did not potentiate the hypotensive effect of alcohol in healthy volunteers [see Clinical Pharmacology (12.2)].

8   USE IN SPECIFIC POPULATIONS

8.1   Pregnancy

Pregnancy Category B.

VIAGRA is not indicated for use in women. There are no adequate and well-controlled studies of sildenafil in pregnant women.

Risk Summary

Based on animal data, VIAGRA is not predicted to increase the risk of adverse developmental outcomes in humans.

Animal Data

No evidence of teratogenicity, embryotoxicity or fetotoxicity was observed in rats and rabbits which received up to 200 mg/kg/day during organogenesis. These doses represent, respectively, about 20 and 40 times the Maximum Recommended Human Dose (MRHD) on a mg/m^2 basis in a 50 kg subject. In the rat pre- and postnatal development study, the no observed adverse effect dose was 30 mg/kg/day given for 36 days. In the nonpregnant rat the AUC at this dose was about 20 times human AUC.

8.4   Pediatric Use

VIAGRA is not indicated for use in pediatric patients. Safety and effectiveness have not been established in pediatric patients.

8.5   Geriatric Use

Healthy elderly volunteers (65 years or over) had a reduced clearance of sildenafil resulting in approximately 84% and 107% higher plasma AUC values of sildenafil and its active N-desmethyl metabolite, respectively, compared to those seen in healthy young volunteers (18–45 years) [see Clinical Pharmacology (12.3)]. Due to age-differences in plasma protein binding, the corresponding increase in the AUC of free (unbound) sildenafil and its active N-desmethyl metabolite were 45% and 57%, respectively [see Clinical Pharmacology (12.3)].

Of the total number of subjects in clinical studies of Viagra, 18% were 65 years and older, while 2% were 75 years and older. No overall differences in safety or efficacy were observed between older (≥ 65 years of age) and younger (< 65 years of age) subjects.

However, since higher plasma levels may increase the incidence of adverse reactions, a starting dose of 25 mg should be considered in older subjects due to the higher systemic exposure [see Dosage and Administration (2.5)].

8.6   Renal Impairment

No dose adjustment is required for mild (CLcr=50–80 mL/min) and moderate (CLcr=30–49 mL/min) renal impairment. In volunteers with severe renal impairment (Clcr<30 mL/min), sildenafil clearance was reduced, resulting in higher plasma exposure of sildenafil (~2 fold), approximately doubling of C_{max} and AUC. A starting dose of 25 mg should be considered in patients with severe renal impairment [see Dosage and Administration (2.5) and Clinical Pharmacology (12.3)].

8.7   Hepatic Impairment

In volunteers with hepatic impairment (Child-Pugh Class A and B), sildenafil clearance was reduced, resulting in higher plasma exposure of sildenafil (47% for C_{max} and 85% for AUC). The pharmacokinetics of sildenafil in patients with severely impaired hepatic function (Child-Pugh Class C) have not been studied. A starting dose of 25 mg should be considered in patients with any degree of hepatic impairment [see Dosage and Administration (2.5) and Clinical Pharmacology (12.3)].

10   OVERDOSAGE

In studies with healthy volunteers of single doses up to 800 mg, adverse reactions were similar to those seen at lower doses but incidence rates and severities were increased.

In cases of overdose, standard supportive measures should be adopted as required. Renal dialysis is not expected to accelerate clearance as sildenafil is highly bound to plasma proteins and it is not eliminated in the urine.

11   DESCRIPTION

VIAGRA (sildenafil citrate), an oral therapy for erectile dysfunction, is the citrate salt of sildenafil, a selective inhibitor of cyclic guanosine monophosphate (cGMP)-specific phosphodiesterase type 5 (PDE5).

Sildenafil citrate is designated chemically as 1-[[3-(6,7-dihydro-1-methyl-7-oxo-3-propyl-1H-pyrazolo[4,3-d]pyrimidin-5-yl)-4-ethoxyphenyl]sulfonyl]-4-methylpiperazine citrate and has the following structural formula:

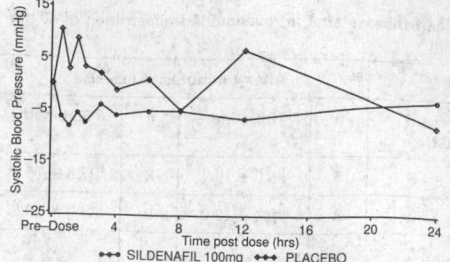

Sildenafil citrate is a white to off-white crystalline powder with a solubility of 3.5 mg/mL in water and a molecular weight of 666.7.

VIAGRA is formulated as blue, film-coated rounded-diamond-shaped tablets equivalent to 25 mg, 50 mg and 100 mg of sildenafil for oral administration. In addition to the active ingredient, sildenafil citrate, each tablet contains the following inactive ingredients: microcrystalline cellulose, anhydrous dibasic calcium phosphate, croscarmellose sodium, magnesium stearate, hypromellose, titanium dioxide, lactose, triacetin, and FD & C Blue #2 aluminum lake.

12   CLINICAL PHARMACOLOGY

12.1   Mechanism of Action

The physiologic mechanism of erection of the penis involves release of nitric oxide (NO) in the corpus cavernosum during sexual stimulation. NO then activates the enzyme guanylate cyclase, which results in increased levels of cyclic guanosine monophosphate (cGMP), producing smooth muscle relaxation in the corpus cavernosum and allowing inflow of blood.

Sildenafil enhances the effect of NO by inhibiting phosphodiesterase type 5 (PDE5), which is responsible for degradation of cGMP in the corpus cavernosum. Sildenafil has no direct relaxant effect on isolated human corpus cavernosum. When sexual stimulation causes local release of NO, inhibition of PDE5 by sildenafil causes increased levels of cGMP in the corpus cavernosum, resulting in smooth muscle relaxation and inflow of blood to the corpus cavernosum. Sildenafil at recommended doses has no effect in the absence of sexual stimulation.

Binding Characteristics

Studies in vitro have shown that sildenafil is selective for PDE5. Its effect is more potent on PDE5 than on other known phosphodiesterases (10-fold for PDE6, >80-fold for PDE1, >700-fold for PDE2, PDE3, PDE4, PDE7, PDE8, PDE9, PDE10, and PDE11). Sildenafil is approximately 4,000-fold more selective for PDE5 compared to PDE3. PDE3 is involved in control of cardiac contractility. Sildenafil is only about 10-fold as potent for PDE5 compared to PDE6, an enzyme found in the retina which is involved in the phototransduction pathway of the retina. This lower selectivity is thought to be the basis for abnormalities related to color vision [see Clinical Pharmacology (12.2)].

In addition to human corpus cavernosum smooth muscle, PDE5 is also found in other tissues including platelets, vascular and visceral smooth muscle, and skeletal muscle, brain, heart, liver, kidney, lung, pancreas, prostate, bladder, testis, and seminal vesicle. The inhibition of PDE5 in some of these tissues by sildenafil may be the basis for the enhanced platelet antiaggregatory activity of NO observed in vitro, an inhibition of platelet thrombus formation in vivo and peripheral arterial-venous dilatation in vivo.

12.2   Pharmacodynamics

Effects of VIAGRA on Erectile Response: In eight double-blind, placebo-controlled crossover studies of patients with either organic or psychogenic erectile dysfunction, sexual stimulation resulted in improved erections, as assessed by an objective measurement of hardness and duration of erections (RigiScan®), after VIAGRA administration compared with placebo. Most studies assessed the efficacy of VIAGRA approximately 60 minutes post dose. The erectile response, as assessed by RigiScan®, generally increased with increasing sildenafil dose and plasma concentration. The time course of effect was examined in one study, showing an effect for up to 4 hours but the response was diminished compared to 2 hours.

Effects of VIAGRA on Blood Pressure: Single oral doses of sildenafil (100 mg) administered to healthy volunteers produced decreases in sitting blood pressure (mean maximum decrease in systolic/diastolic blood pressure of 8.3/5.3 mmHg). The decrease in sitting blood pressure was most notable approximately 1–2 hours after dosing, and was not different than placebo at 8 hours. Similar effects on blood pressure were noted with 25 mg, 50 mg and 100 mg of VIAGRA, therefore the effects are not related to dose or plasma levels within this dosage range. Larger effects were recorded among patients receiving concomitant nitrates [see Contraindications (4.1)].

Figure 1: Mean Change from Baseline in Sitting Systolic Blood Pressure, Healthy Volunteers.

Effects of VIAGRA on Blood Pressure When Nitroglycerin is Subsequently Administered: Based on the pharmacokinetic profile of a single 100 mg oral dose given to healthy normal volunteers, the plasma levels of sildenafil at 24 hours post dose are approximately 2 ng/mL (compared to peak plasma levels of approximately 440 ng/mL). In the following patients: age >65 years, hepatic impairment (e.g., cirrhosis), severe renal impairment (e.g., creatinine clearance <30 mL/min), and concomitant use of erythromycin or strong CYP3A4 inhibitors, plasma levels of sildenafil at 24 hours post dose have been found to be 3 to 8 times higher than those seen in healthy volunteers. Although plasma levels of sildenafil at 24 hours post dose are much lower than at peak concentration, it is unknown whether nitrates can be safely co-administered at this time point [see Contraindications (4.1)].

Effects of VIAGRA on Blood Pressure When Co-administered with Alpha-Blockers: Three double-blind, placebo-controlled, randomized, two-way crossover studies were conducted to assess the interaction of VIAGRA with doxazosin, an alpha-adrenergic blocking agent.

Study 1:   VIAGRA with Doxazosin

In the first study, a single oral dose of VIAGRA 100 mg or matching placebo was administered in a 2-period crossover design to 4 generally healthy males with benign prostatic hyperplasia (BPH). Following at least 14 consecutive daily doses of doxazosin, VIAGRA 100 mg or matching placebo was administered simultaneously with doxazosin. Following a review of the data from these first 4 subjects (details provided below), the VIAGRA dose was reduced to 25 mg. Thereafter, 17 subjects were treated with VIAGRA 25 mg or matching placebo in combination with doxazosin 4 mg (15 subjects) or doxazosin 8 mg (2 subjects). The mean subject age was 66.5 years.

For the 17 subjects who received VIAGRA 25 mg and matching placebo, the placebo-subtracted mean maximum decreases from baseline (95% CI) in systolic blood pressure were as follows:

Placebo-subtracted mean maximum decrease in systolic blood pressure (mm Hg)	VIAGRA 25 mg
Supine	7.4 (-0.9, 15.7)
Standing	6.0 (-0.8, 12.8)

The mean profiles of the change from baseline in standing systolic blood pressure in subjects treated with doxazosin in combination with 25 mg VIAGRA or matching placebo are shown in Figure 2.

Figure 2: Mean Standing Systolic Blood Pressure Change from Baseline

Blood pressure was measured immediately pre-dose and at 15, 30, 45 minutes, and 1, 1.5, 2, 2.5, 3, 4, 6 and 8 hours after VIAGRA or matching placebo. Outliers were defined as subjects with a standing systolic blood pressure of <85 mmHg or a decrease from baseline in standing systolic blood pressure of >30 mmHg at one or more timepoints. There were no subjects treated with VIAGRA 25 mg who had a standing SBP < 85mmHg. There were three subjects

with a decrease from baseline in standing systolic BP >30mmHg following VIAGRA 25 mg, one subject with a decrease from baseline in standing systolic BP > 30 mmHg following placebo and two subjects with a decrease from baseline in standing systolic BP > 30 mmHg following both VIAGRA and placebo. No severe adverse events potentially related to blood pressure effects were reported in this group. Of the four subjects who received VIAGRA 100 mg in the first part of this study, a severe adverse event related to blood pressure effect was reported in one patient (postural hypotension that began 35 minutes after dosing with VIAGRA with symptoms lasting for 8 hours), and mild adverse events potentially related to blood pressure effects were reported in two others (dizziness, headache and fatigue at 1 hour after dosing; and dizziness, lightheadedness and nausea at 4 hours after dosing). There were no reports of syncope among these patients. For these four subjects, the placebo-subtracted mean maximum decreases from baseline in supine and standing systolic blood pressures were 14.8 mmHg and 21.5 mmHg, respectively. Two of these subjects had a standing SBP < 85mmHg. Both of these subjects were protocol violators, one due to a low baseline standing SBP, and the other due to baseline orthostatic hypotension.

Study 2:   VIAGRA with Doxazosin

In the second study, a single oral dose of VIAGRA 50 mg or matching placebo was administered in a 2-period crossover design to 20 generally healthy males with BPH. Following at least 14 consecutive days of doxazosin, VIAGRA 50 mg or matching placebo was administered simultaneously with doxazosin 4 mg (17 subjects) or with doxazosin 8 mg (3 subjects). The mean subject age in this study was 63.9 years. Twenty subjects received VIAGRA 50 mg, but only 19 subjects received matching placebo. One patient discontinued the study prematurely due to an adverse event of hypotension following dosing with VIAGRA 50 mg. This patient had been taking minoxidil, a potent vasodilator, during the study.

For the 19 subjects who received both VIAGRA and matching placebo, the placebo-subtracted mean maximum decreases from baseline (95% CI) in systolic blood pressure were as follows:

Placebo-subtracted mean maximum decrease in systolic blood pressure (mm Hg)	VIAGRA 50 mg (95% CI)
Supine	9.08 (5.48, 12.68)
Standing	11.62 (7.34, 15.90)

The mean profiles of the change from baseline in standing systolic blood pressure in subjects treated with doxazosin in combination with 50 mg VIAGRA or matching placebo are shown in Figure 3.

Figure 3: Mean Standing Systolic Blood Pressure Change from Baseline

Blood pressure was measured after administration of VIAGRA at the same times as those specified for the first doxazosin study. There were two subjects who had a standing SBP of < 85 mmHg. In these two subjects, hypotension was reported as a moderately severe adverse event, beginning at approximately 1 hour after administration of VIAGRA 50 mg and resolving after approximately 7.5 hours. There was one subject with a decrease from baseline in standing systolic BP >30mmHg following VIAGRA 50 mg and one subject with a decrease from baseline in standing systolic BP > 30 mmHg following both VIAGRA 50 mg and placebo. There were no severe adverse events potentially related to blood pressure and no episodes of syncope reported in this study.

Study 3:   VIAGRA with Doxazosin

In the third study, a single oral dose of VIAGRA 100 mg or matching placebo was administered in a 3-period crossover design to 20 generally healthy males with BPH. In dose period 1, subjects were administered open-label doxazosin and a single dose of VIAGRA 50 mg simultaneously, after at least 14 consecutive days of doxazosin. If a subject did not successfully complete this first dosing period, he was discontinued from the study. Subjects who had successfully completed the previous doxazosin interaction study (using VIAGRA 50 mg), including no significant hemodynamic ad-

Table 3. Hemodynamic Data in Patients with Stable Ischemic Heart Disease after Intravenous Administration of 40 mg of Sildenafil

Means ± SD	At rest				After 4 minutes of exercise			
	N	Baseline (B2)	n	Sildenafil (D1)	n	Baseline	n	Sildenafil
PAOP (mmHg)	8	8.1 ± 5.1	8	6.5 ± 4.3	8	36.0 ± 13.7	8	27.8 ± 15.3
Mean PAP (mmHg)	8	16.7 ± 4	8	12.1 ± 3.9	8	39.4 ± 12.9	8	31.7 ± 13.2
Mean RAP (mmHg)	7	5.7 ± 3.7	8	4.1 ± 3.7	-	-	-	-
Systolic SAP (mmHg)	8	150.4 ± 12.4	8	140.6 ± 16.5	8	199.5 ± 37.4	8	187.8 ± 30.0
Diastolic SAP (mmHg)	8	73.6 ± 7.8	8	65.9 ± 10	8	84.6 ± 9.7	8	79.5 ± 9.4
Cardiac output (L/min)	8	5.6 ± 0.9	8	5.2 ± 1.1	8	11.5 ± 2.4	8	10.2 ± 3.5
Heart rate (bpm)	8	67 ± 11.1	8	66.9 ± 12	8	101.9 ± 11.6	8	99.0 ± 20.4

verse events, were allowed to skip dose period 1. Treatment with doxazosin continued for at least 7 days after dose period 1. Thereafter, VIAGRA 100 mg or matching placebo was administered simultaneously with doxazosin 4 mg (14 subjects) or doxazosin 8 mg (6 subjects) in standard crossover fashion. The mean subject age in this study was 66.4 years.

Twenty-five subjects were screened. Two were discontinued after study period 1: one failed to meet pre-dose screening qualifications and the other experienced symptomatic hypotension as a moderately severe adverse event 30 minutes after dosing with open-label VIAGRA 50 mg. Of the twenty subjects who were ultimately assigned to treatment, a total of 13 subjects successfully completed dose period 1, and seven had successfully completed the previous doxazosin study (using VIAGRA 50 mg).

For the 20 subjects who received VIAGRA 100 mg and matching placebo, the placebo-subtracted mean maximum decreases from baseline (95% CI) in systolic blood pressure were as follows:

Placebo-subtracted mean maximum decrease in systolic blood pressure (mm Hg)	VIAGRA 100 mg
Supine	7.9 (4.6, 11.1)
Standing	4.3 (-1.8, 10.3)

The mean profiles of the change from baseline in standing systolic blood pressure in subjects treated with doxazosin in combination with 100 mg VIAGRA or matching placebo are shown in Figure 4.

Figure 4: Mean Standing Systolic Blood Pressure Change from Baseline

Blood pressure was measured after administration of VIAGRA at the same times as those specified for the previous doxazosin studies. There were three subjects who had a standing SBP of < 85 mmHg. All three were taking VIAGRA 100 mg, and all three reported mild adverse events at the time of reductions in standing SBP, including vasodilation and lightheadedness. There were four subjects with a decrease from baseline in standing systolic BP > 30 mmHg following VIAGRA 100 mg, one subject with a decrease from baseline in standing systolic BP > 30 mmHg following placebo and one subject with a decrease from baseline in standing systolic BP > 30 mmHg following both VIAGRA and placebo. While there were no severe adverse events potentially related to blood pressure reported in this study, one subject reported moderate vasodilatation after both VIAGRA 50 mg and 100 mg. There were no episodes of syncope reported in this study.

Effect of VIAGRA on Blood Pressure When Co-administered with Anti-hypertensives: When VIAGRA 100 mg oral was

co-administered with amlodipine, 5 mg or 10 mg oral, to hypertensive patients, the mean additional reduction on supine blood pressure was 8 mmHg systolic and 7 mmHg diastolic.

Effect of VIAGRA on Blood Pressure When Co-administered with Alcohol: VIAGRA (50 mg) did not potentiate the hypotensive effect of alcohol (0.5 g/kg) in healthy volunteers with mean maximum blood alcohol levels of 0.08%. The maximum observed decrease in systolic blood pressure was -18.5 mmHg when sildenafil was co-administered with alcohol versus -17.4 mmHg when alcohol was administered alone. The maximum observed decrease in diastolic blood pressure was -17.2 mmHg when sildenafil was co-administered with alcohol versus -11.1 mmHg when alcohol was administered alone. There were no reports of postural dizziness or orthostatic hypotension. The maximum recommended dose of 100 mg sildenafil was not evaluated in this study [*see Drug Interactions (7.5)*].

Effects of VIAGRA on Cardiac Parameters: Single oral doses of sildenafil up to 100 mg produced no clinically relevant changes in the ECGs of normal male volunteers.

Studies have produced relevant data on the effects of VIAGRA on cardiac output. In one small, open-label, uncontrolled, pilot study, eight patients with stable ischemic heart disease underwent Swan-Ganz catheterization. A total dose of 40 mg sildenafil was administered by four intravenous infusions.

The results from this pilot study are shown in Table 3; the mean resting systolic and diastolic blood pressures decreased by 7% and 10% compared to baseline in these patients. Mean resting values for right atrial pressure, pulmonary artery pressure, pulmonary artery occluded pressure and cardiac output decreased by 28%, 28%, 20% and 7% respectively. Even though this total dosage produced plasma sildenafil concentrations which were approximately 2 to 5 times higher than the mean maximum plasma concentrations following a single oral dose of 100 mg in healthy male volunteers, the hemodynamic response to exercise was preserved in these patients.

[See table 3 above]

In a double-blind study, 144 patients with erectile dysfunction and chronic stable angina limited by exercise, not receiving chronic oral nitrates, were randomized to a single dose of placebo or VIAGRA 100 mg 1 hour prior to exercise testing. The primary endpoint was time to limiting angina in the evaluable cohort. The mean times (adjusted for baseline) to onset of limiting angina were 423.6 and 403.7 seconds for sildenafil (N=70) and placebo, respectively. These results demonstrated that the effect of VIAGRA on the primary endpoint was statistically non-inferior to placebo.

Effects of VIAGRA on Vision: At single oral doses of 100 mg and 200 mg, transient dose-related impairment of color discrimination was detected using the Farnsworth-Munsell 100-hue test, with peak effects near the time of peak plasma levels. This finding is consistent with the inhibition of PDE6, which is involved in phototransduction in the retina. Subjects in the study reported this finding as difficulties in discriminating blue/green. An evaluation of visual function at doses up to twice the maximum recommended dose revealed no effects of VIAGRA on visual acuity, intraocular pressure, or pupillometry.

Effects of VIAGRA on Sperm: There was no effect on sperm motility or morphology after single 100 mg oral doses of VIAGRA in healthy volunteers.

12.3   Pharmacokinetics

VIAGRA is rapidly absorbed after oral administration, with a mean absolute bioavailability of 41% (range 25–63%). The pharmacokinetics of sildenafil are dose-proportional over

the recommended dose range. It is eliminated predominantly by hepatic metabolism (mainly CYP3A4) and is converted to an active metabolite with properties similar to the parent, sildenafil. Both sildenafil and the metabolite have terminal half lives of about 4 hours.

Mean sildenafil plasma concentrations measured after the administration of a single oral dose of 100 mg to healthy male volunteers is depicted below:

Figure 5: Mean Sildenafil Plasma Concentrations in Healthy Male Volunteers.

Absorption and Distribution: VIAGRA is rapidly absorbed. Maximum observed plasma concentrations are reached within 30 to 120 minutes (median 60 minutes) of oral dosing in the fasted state. When VIAGRA is taken with a high fat meal, the rate of absorption is reduced, with a mean delay in T_{max} of 60 minutes and a mean reduction in C_{max} of 29%. The mean steady state volume of distribution (Vss) for sildenafil is 105 L, indicating distribution into the tissues. Sildenafil and its major circulating N-desmethyl metabolite are both approximately 96% bound to plasma proteins. Protein binding is independent of total drug concentrations.

Based upon measurements of sildenafil in semen of healthy volunteers 90 minutes after dosing, less than 0.001% of the administered dose may appear in the semen of patients.

Metabolism and Excretion: Sildenafil is cleared predominantly by the CYP3A4 (major route) and CYP2C9 (minor route) hepatic microsomal isoenzymes. The major circulating metabolite results from N-desmethylation of sildenafil, and is itself further metabolized. This metabolite has a PDE selectivity profile similar to sildenafil and an *in vitro* potency for PDE5 approximately 50% of the parent drug. Plasma concentrations of this metabolite are approximately 40% of those seen for sildenafil, so that the metabolite accounts for about 20% of sildenafil's pharmacologic effects.

After either oral or intravenous administration, sildenafil is excreted as metabolites predominantly in the feces (approximately 80% of administered oral dose) and to a lesser extent in the urine (approximately 13% of the administered oral dose). Similar values for pharmacokinetic parameters were seen in normal volunteers and in the patient population, using a population pharmacokinetic approach.

Pharmacokinetics in Special Populations

Geriatrics: Healthy elderly volunteers (65 years or over) had a reduced clearance of sildenafil, resulting in approximately 84% and 107% higher plasma AUC values of sildenafil and its active N-desmethyl metabolite, respectively, compared to those seen in healthy younger volunteers (18–45 years). Due to age-differences in plasma protein binding, the corresponding increase in the AUC of free (unbound) sildenafil and its active N-desmethyl metabolite were 45% and 57%, respectively [*see Dosage and Administration (2.5), and Use in Specific Populations (8.5)*]

Renal Impairment: In volunteers with mild (CLcr= 50–80 mL/min) and moderate (CLcr=30–49 mL/min) renal impairment, the pharmacokinetics of a single oral dose of VIAGRA (50 mg) were not altered. In volunteers with severe (CLcr <30 mL/min) renal impairment, sildenafil clearance was reduced, resulting in approximately doubling of AUC and C_{max} compared to age-matched volunteers with no renal impairment [*see Dosage and Administration (2.5), and Use in Specific Populations (8.6)*].

In addition, N-desmethyl metabolite AUC and C_{max} values significantly increased by 200% and 79%, respectively in subjects with severe renal impairment compared to subjects with normal renal function.

Hepatic Impairment: In volunteers with hepatic impairment (Child-Pugh Class A and B), sildenafil clearance was reduced, resulting in increases in AUC (85%) and C_{max} (47%) compared to age-matched volunteers with no hepatic impairment. The pharmacokinetics of sildenafil in patients with severely impaired hepatic function (Child-Pugh Class C) have not been studied [*see Dosage and Administration (2.5), and Use in Specific Populations (8.7)*].

Therefore, age >65, hepatic impairment and severe renal impairment are associated with increased plasma levels of sildenafil. A starting oral dose of 25 mg should be considered in those patients [*see Dosage and Administration (2.5)*].

Drug Interaction Studies
Effects of Other Drugs on VIAGRA
Sildenafil metabolism is principally mediated by CYP3A4 (major route) and CYP2C9 (minor route). Therefore, inhibitors of these isoenzymes may reduce sildenafil clearance and inducers of these isoenzymes may increase sildenafil clearance. The concomitant use of erythromycin or strong CYP3A4 inhibitors (e.g., saquinavir, ketoconazole, itraconazole) as well as the nonspecific CYP inhibitor, cimetidine, is associated with increased plasma levels of sildenafil [*see Dosage and Administration (2.4)*].
In vivo studies:
Cimetidine (800 mg), a nonspecific CYP inhibitor, caused a 56% increase in plasma sildenafil concentrations when co-administered with VIAGRA (50 mg) to healthy volunteers. When a single 100 mg dose of VIAGRA was administered with erythromycin, a moderate CYP3A4 inhibitor, at steady state (500 mg bid for 5 days), there was a 160% increase in sildenafil C_{max} and a 182% increase in sildenafil AUC. In addition, in a study performed in healthy male volunteers, co-administration of the HIV protease inhibitor saquinavir, also a CYP3A4 inhibitor, at steady state (1200 mg tid) with Viagra (100 mg single dose) resulted in a 140% increase in sildenafil C_{max} and a 210% increase in sildenafil AUC. Viagra had no effect on saquinavir pharmacokinetics. A stronger CYP3A4 inhibitor such as ketoconazole or itraconazole could be expected to have greater effect than that seen with saquinavir. Population pharmacokinetic data from patients in clinical trials also indicated a reduction in sildenafil clearance when it was co-administered with CYP3A4 inhibitors (such as ketoconazole, erythromycin, or cimetidine) [*see Dosage and Administration (2.4) and Drug Interactions (7.4)*].
In another study in healthy male volunteers, co-administration with the HIV protease inhibitor ritonavir, which is a highly potent P450 inhibitor, at steady state (500 mg bid) with VIAGRA (100 mg single dose) resulted in a 300% (4-fold) increase in sildenafil C_{max} and a 1000% (11-fold) increase in sildenafil plasma AUC. At 24 hours the plasma levels of sildenafil were still approximately 200 ng/mL, compared to approximately 5 ng/mL when sildenafil was dosed alone. This is consistent with ritonavir's marked effects on a broad range of P450 substrates. VIAGRA had no effect on ritonavir pharmacokinetics [*see Dosage and Administration (2.4) and Drug Interactions (7.4)*].
Although the interaction between other protease inhibitors and sildenafil has not been studied, their concomitant use is expected to increase sildenafil levels.
In a study of healthy male volunteers, co-administration of sildenafil at steady state (80 mg t.i.d.) with endothelin receptor antagonist bosentan (a moderate inducer of CYP3A4, CYP2C9 and possibly of CYP2C19) at steady state (125 mg b.i.d.) resulted in a 63% decrease of sildenafil AUC and a 55% decrease in sildenafil C_{max}. Concomitant administration of strong CYP3A4 inducers, such as rifampin, is expected to cause greater decreases in plasma levels of sildenafil.
Single doses of antacid (magnesium hydroxide/aluminum hydroxide) did not affect the bioavailability of VIAGRA.
In healthy male volunteers, there was no evidence of a clinically significant effect of azithromycin (500 mg daily for 3 days) on the systemic exposure of sildenafil or its major circulating metabolite.
Pharmacokinetic data from patients in clinical trials showed no effect on sildenafil pharmacokinetics of CYP2C9 inhibitors (such as tolbutamide, warfarin), CYP2D6 inhibitors (such as selective serotonin reuptake inhibitors, tricyclic antidepressants), thiazide and related diuretics, ACE inhibitors, and calcium channel blockers. The AUC of the active metabolite, N-desmethyl sildenafil, was increased 62% by loop and potassium-sparing diuretics and 102% by nonspecific beta-blockers. These effects on the metabolite are not expected to be of clinical consequence.
Effects of VIAGRA on Other Drugs
In vitro studies:
Sildenafil is a weak inhibitor of the CYP isoforms 1A2, 2C9, 2C19, 2D6, 2E1 and 3A4 (IC50 >150 μM). Given sildenafil peak plasma concentrations of approximately 1 μM after recommended doses, it is unlikely that VIAGRA will alter the clearance of substrates of these isoenzymes.
In vivo studies:
No significant interactions were shown with tolbutamide (250 mg) or warfarin (40 mg), both of which are metabolized by CYP2C9.
In a study of healthy male volunteers, sildenafil (100 mg) did not affect the steady state pharmacokinetics of the HIV protease inhibitors, saquinavir and ritonavir, both of which are CYP3A4 substrates.
VIAGRA (50 mg) did not potentiate the increase in bleeding time caused by aspirin (150 mg).
Sildenafil at steady state, at a dose not approved for the treatment of erectile dysfunction (80 mg t.i.d.) resulted in a 50% increase in AUC and a 42% increase in C_{max} of bosentan (125 mg b.i.d.).

13 NONCLINICAL TOXICOLOGY
13.1 Carcinogenesis, Mutagenesis, Impairment of Fertility
Carcinogenesis
Sildenafil was not carcinogenic when administered to rats for 24 months at a dose resulting in total systemic drug exposure (AUCs) for unbound sildenafil and its major metabolite of 29- and 42- times, for male and female rats, respectively, the exposures observed in human males given the Maximum Recommended Human Dose (MRHD) of 100 mg. Sildenafil was not carcinogenic when administered to mice for 18–21 months at dosages up to the Maximum Tolerated Dose (MTD) of 10 mg/kg/day, approximately 0.6 times the MRHD on a mg/m^2 basis.
Mutagenesis
Sildenafil was negative in *in vitro* bacterial and Chinese hamster ovary cell assays to detect mutagenicity, and *in vitro* human lymphocytes and *in vivo* mouse micronucleus assays to detect clastogenicity.
Impairment of Fertility
There was no impairment of fertility in rats given sildenafil up to 60 mg/kg/day for 36 days to females and 102 days to males, a dose producing an AUC value of more than 25 times the human male AUC.

14 CLINICAL STUDIES
In clinical studies, VIAGRA was assessed for its effect on the ability of men with erectile dysfunction (ED) to engage in sexual activity and in many cases specifically on the ability to achieve and maintain an erection sufficient for satisfactory sexual activity. VIAGRA was evaluated primarily at doses of 25 mg, 50 mg and 100 mg in 21 randomized, double-blind, placebo-controlled trials of up to 6 months in duration, using a variety of study designs (fixed dose, titration, parallel, crossover). VIAGRA was administered to more than 3,000 patients aged 19 to 87 years, with ED of various etiologies (organic, psychogenic, mixed) with a mean duration of 5 years. VIAGRA demonstrated statistically significant improvement compared to placebo in all 21 studies. The studies that established benefit demonstrated improvements in success rates for sexual intercourse compared with placebo.
Efficacy Endpoints in Controlled Clinical Studies
The effectiveness of VIAGRA was evaluated in most studies using several assessment instruments. The primary measure in the principal studies was a sexual function questionnaire (the International Index of Erectile Function - IIEF) administered during a 4-week treatment-free run-in period, at baseline, at follow-up visits, and at the end of double-blind, placebo-controlled, at-home treatment. Two of the questions from the IIEF served as primary study endpoints; categorical responses were elicited to questions about (1) the ability to achieve erections sufficient for sexual intercourse and (2) the maintenance of erections after penetration. The patient addressed both questions at the final visit for the last 4 weeks of the study. The possible categorical responses to these questions were (0) no attempted intercourse, (1) never or almost never, (2) a few times, (3) sometimes, (4) most times, and (5) almost always or always. Also collected as part of the IIEF was information about other aspects of sexual function, including information on erectile function, orgasm, desire, satisfaction with intercourse, and overall sexual satisfaction. Sexual function data were also recorded by patients in a daily diary. In addition, patients were asked a global efficacy question and an optional partner questionnaire was administered.
Efficacy Results from Controlled Clinical Studies
The effect on one of the major end points, maintenance of erections after penetration, is shown in Figure 6, for the pooled results of 5 fixed-dose, dose-response studies of greater than one month duration, showing response according to baseline function. Results with all doses have been pooled, but scores showed greater improvement at the 50 and 100 mg doses than at 25 mg. The pattern of responses was similar for the other principal question, the ability to achieve an erection sufficient for intercourse. The titration studies, in which most patients received 100 mg, showed similar results. Figure 6 shows that regardless of the baseline levels of function, subsequent function in patients treated with VIAGRA was better than that seen in patients treated with placebo. At the same time, on-treatment function was better in treated patients who were less impaired at baseline.
[See Figure 6 at top of next column]
The frequency of patients reporting improvement of erections in response to a global question in four of the randomized, double-blind, parallel, placebo-controlled fixed dose studies (1797 patients) of 12 to 24 weeks duration is shown in Figure 7. These patients had erectile dysfunction at baseline that was characterized by median categorical scores of 2 (a few times) on principal IIEF questions. Erectile dysfunction was attributed to organic (58%; generally not characterized, but including diabetes and excluding spinal cord injury), psychogenic (17%), or mixed (24%) etiologies. Sixty-

Effect of VIAGRA on Maintenance of Erection by Baseline Score

Effect of Placebo on Maintenance of Erection by Baseline Score

Figure 6. Effect of VIAGRA and Placebo on Maintenance of Erection by Baseline Score.

three percent, 74%, and 82% of the patients on 25 mg, 50 mg and 100 mg of VIAGRA, respectively, reported an improvement in their erections, compared to 24% on placebo. In the titration studies (n=644) (with most patients eventually receiving 100 mg), results were similar.

Overall treatment p<0.0001

Figure 7. Percentage of Patients Reporting an Improvement in Erections.

The patients in studies had varying degrees of ED. One-third to one-half of the subjects in these studies reported successful intercourse at least once during a 4-week, treatment-free run-in period.
In many of the studies, of both fixed dose and titration designs, daily diaries were kept by patients. In these studies, involving about 1600 patients, analyses of patient diaries showed no effect of VIAGRA on attempted intercourse (about 2 per week), but there was clear treatment-related improvement in sexual function: per patient weekly success rates averaged 1.3 on 50–100 mg of VIAGRA vs 0.4 on placebo; similarly, group mean success rates (total successes divided by total attempts) were about 66% on VIAGRA vs about 20% on placebo.
During 3 to 6 months of double-blind treatment or longer-term (1 year), open-label studies, few patients withdrew from active treatment for any reason, including lack of effectiveness. At the end of the long-term study, 88% of patients reported that VIAGRA improved their erections.
Men with untreated ED had relatively low baseline scores for all aspects of sexual function measured (again using a 5-point scale) in the IIEF. VIAGRA improved these aspects of sexual function: frequency, firmness and maintenance of erections; frequency of orgasm; frequency and level of desire; frequency, satisfaction and enjoyment of intercourse; and overall relationship satisfaction.
One randomized, double-blind, flexible-dose, placebo-controlled study included only patients with erectile dysfunction attributed to complications of diabetes mellitus (n=268). As in the other titration studies, patients were started on 50 mg and allowed to adjust the dose up to 100 mg or down to 25 mg of VIAGRA; all patients, however, were receiving 50 mg or 100 mg at the end of the study. There were highly statistically significant improvements on the two principal IIEF questions (frequency of successful penetration during sexual activity and maintenance of erections after penetration) on VIAGRA compared to placebo. On a global improvement question, 57% of VIAGRA pa-

Help Patients Save on Rx Drugs: PDR.net/PharmacyDiscountCard

	25 mg	50 mg	100 mg
Obverse	VGR25	VGR50	VGR100
Reverse	PFIZER	PFIZER	PFIZER
Bottle of 30	NDC-0069-4200-30	NDC-0069-4210-30	NDC-0069-4220-30
Bottle of 100	N/A	NDC-0069-4210-66	NDC-0069-4220-66

tients reported improved erections versus 10% on placebo. Diary data indicated that on VIAGRA, 48% of intercourse attempts were successful versus 10% on placebo.

One randomized, double-blind, placebo-controlled, cross-over, flexible-dose (up to 100 mg) study of patients with erectile dysfunction resulting from spinal cord injury (n=178) was conducted. The changes from baseline in scoring on the two end point questions (frequency of successful penetration during sexual activity and maintenance of erections after penetration) were highly statistically significantly in favor of VIAGRA. On a global improvement question, 83% of patients reported improved erections on VIAGRA versus 12% on placebo. Diary data indicated that on VIAGRA, 59% of attempts at sexual intercourse were successful compared to 13% on placebo.

Across all trials, VIAGRA improved the erections of 43% of radical prostatectomy patients compared to 15% on placebo. Subgroup analyses of responses to a global improvement question in patients with psychogenic etiology in two fixed-dose studies (total n=179) and two titration studies (total n=149) showed 84% of VIAGRA patients reported improvement in erections compared with 26% of placebo. The changes from baseline in scoring on the two end point questions (frequency of successful penetration during sexual activity and maintenance of erections after penetration) were highly statistically significantly in favor of VIAGRA. Diary data in two of the studies (n=178) showed rates of successful intercourse per attempt of 70% for VIAGRA and 29% for placebo.

Efficacy Results in Subpopulations in Controlled Clinical Studies

A review of population subgroups demonstrated efficacy regardless of baseline severity, etiology, race and age. VIAGRA was effective in a broad range of ED patients, including those with a history of coronary artery disease, hypertension, other cardiac disease, peripheral vascular disease, diabetes mellitus, depression, coronary artery bypass graft (CABG), radical prostatectomy, transurethral resection of the prostate (TURP) and spinal cord injury, and in patients taking antidepressants/antipsychotics and anti-hypertensives/diuretics.

16   HOW SUPPLIED/STORAGE AND HANDLING

VIAGRA (sildenafil citrate) is supplied as blue, film-coated, rounded-diamond-shaped tablets containing sildenafil citrate equivalent to the nominally indicated amount of sildenafil and debossed on the obverse and reverse sides as follows:

[See table above]

Recommended Storage: Store at 25°C (77°F); excursions permitted to 15–30°C (59–86°F) [see USP Controlled Room Temperature].

17   PATIENT COUNSELING INFORMATION

See FDA-approved patient labeling (Patient Information)

Nitrates

Physicians should discuss with patients the contraindication of VIAGRA with regular and/or intermittent use of nitric oxide donors, such as organic nitrates or organic nitrites in any form [see *Contraindications (4.1)*].

Concomitant Use with Drugs Which Lower Blood Pressure

Physicians should advise patients of the potential for VIAGRA to augment the blood pressure lowering effect of alpha-blockers and anti-hypertensive medications. Concomitant administration of VIAGRA and an alpha-blocker may lead to symptomatic hypotension in some patients. Therefore, when VIAGRA is co-administered with alpha-blockers, patients should be stable on alpha-blocker therapy prior to initiating VIAGRA treatment and VIAGRA should be initiated at the lowest dose [see *Warnings and Precautions (5.5)*].

Cardiovascular Considerations

Physicians should discuss with patients the potential cardiac risk of sexual activity in patients with preexisting cardiovascular risk factors. Patients who experience symptoms (e.g., angina pectoris, dizziness, nausea) upon initiation of sexual activity should be advised to refrain from further activity and should discuss the episode with their physician [see *Warnings and Precautions (5.1)*].

Sudden Loss of Vision

Physicians should advise patients to stop use of all PDE5 inhibitors, including VIAGRA, and seek medical attention in the event of a sudden loss of vision in one or both eyes. Such an event may be a sign of non-arteritic anterior ischemic optic neuropathy (NAION), a cause of decreased vi-

sion including possible permanent loss of vision, that has been reported rarely post-marketing in temporal association with the use of all PDE5 inhibitors. It is not possible to determine whether these events are related directly to the use of PDE5 inhibitors or to other factors. Physicians should discuss with patients the increased risk of NAION in individuals who have already experienced NAION in one eye. Physicians should also discuss with patients the increased risk of NAION among the general population in patients with a "crowded" optic disc, although evidence is insufficient to support screening of prospective users of PDE5 inhibitor, including VIAGRA, for this uncommon condition [see *Warnings and Precautions (5.3) and Adverse Reactions (6.2)*].

Sudden Hearing Loss

Physicians should advise patients to stop taking PDE5 inhibitors, including VIAGRA, and seek prompt medical attention in the event of sudden decrease or loss of hearing. These events, which may be accompanied by tinnitus and dizziness, have been reported in temporal association to the intake of PDE5 inhibitors, including VIAGRA. It is not possible to determine whether these events are related directly to the use of PDE5 inhibitors or to other factors [see *Warnings and Precautions (5.4) and Adverse Reactions (6.2)*].

Priapism

Physicians should warn patients that prolonged erections greater than 4 hours and priapism (painful erections greater than 6 hours in duration) have been reported infrequently since market approval of VIAGRA. In the event of an erection that persists longer than 4 hours, the patient should seek immediate medical assistance. If priapism is not treated immediately, penile tissue damage and permanent loss of potency may result [see *Warnings and Precautions (5.2)*].

Avoid Use with other PDE5 Inhibitors

Physicians should inform patients not to take VIAGRA with other PDE5 inhibitors including REVATIO or other pulmonary arterial hypertension (PAH) treatments containing sildenafil. Sildenafil is also marketed as REVATIO for the treatment of PAH. The safety and efficacy of VIAGRA with other PDE5 inhibitors, including REVATIO, have not been studied [see *Warnings and Precautions (5.7)*].

Sexually Transmitted Disease

The use of VIAGRA offers no protection against sexually transmitted diseases. Counseling of patients about the protective measures necessary to guard against sexually transmitted diseases, including the Human Immunodeficiency Virus (HIV), may be considered [see *Warnings and Precautions (5.9)*].

Distributed by

Pfizer Labs

Division of Pfizer Inc, NY, NY 10017

LAB-0221-13.0

Patient Information

VIAGRA® (vi-AG-rah)

(sildenafil citrate)

Tablets

What is the most important information I should know about VIAGRA?

VIAGRA can cause your blood pressure to drop suddenly to an unsafe level if it is taken with certain other medicines. Do not take VIAGRA if you take any other medicines called "nitrates." Nitrates are used to treat chest pain (angina). A sudden drop in blood pressure can cause you to feel dizzy, faint, or have a heart attack or stroke.

Tell all your healthcare providers that you take VIAGRA. If you need emergency medical care for a heart problem, it will be important for your healthcare provider to know when you last took VIAGRA.

Stop sexual activity and get medical help right away if you get symptoms such as chest pain, dizziness, or nausea during sex.

Sexual activity can put an extra strain on your heart, especially if your heart is already weak from a heart attack or heart disease. Ask your doctor if your heart is healthy enough to handle the extra strain of having sex.

VIAGRA does not protect you or your partner from getting sexually transmitted diseases, including HIV—the virus that causes AIDS.

What is VIAGRA?

VIAGRA is a prescription medicine used to treat erectile dysfunction (ED). You will not get an erection just by taking

this medicine. VIAGRA helps a man with erectile dysfunction get and keep an erection only when he is sexually excited (stimulated).

VIAGRA is not for use in women or children.

It is not known if VIAGRA is safe and effective in women or children under 18 years of age.

Who should not take VIAGRA?

Do not take VIAGRA if you:

- take medicines called "nitrates" (such as nitroglycerin)
- use street drugs called "poppers" such as amyl nitrate or amyl nitrite, and butyl nitrate
- are allergic to sildenafil, as contained in VIAGRA and REVATIO, or any of the ingredients in VIAGRA. See the end of this leaflet for a complete list of ingredients in VIAGRA.

What should I tell my healthcare provider before taking VIAGRA?

Before you take VIAGRA, tell your healthcare provider if you:

- have or have had heart problems such as a heart attack, irregular heartbeat, angina, chest pain, narrowing of the aortic valve or heart failure
- have had heart surgery within the last 6 months
- have had a stroke
- have low blood pressure, or high blood pressure that is not controlled
- have a deformed penis shape
- have had an erection that lasted for more than 4 hours
- have problems with your blood cells such as sickle cell anemia, multiple myeloma, or leukemia
- have retinitis pigmentosa, a rare genetic (runs in families) eye disease
- have ever had severe vision loss, including an eye problem called non-arteritic anterior ischemic optic neuropathy (NAION)
- have bleeding problems
- have or have had stomach ulcers
- have liver problems
- have kidney problems or are having kidney dialysis
- have any other medical conditions

Tell your healthcare provider about all the medicines you take[1], including prescription and over-the-counter medicines, vitamins, and herbal supplements.

VIAGRA may affect the way other medicines work, and other medicines may affect the way VIAGRA works causing side effects. Especially tell your healthcare provider if you take any of the following:

- medicines called nitrates (see **"What is the most important information I should know about VIAGRA?"**)
- medicines called alpha blockers such as Hytrin (terazosin HCl), Flomax (tamsulosin HCl), Cardura (doxazosin mesylate), Minipress (prazosin HCl), Uroxatral (alfuzosin HCl), Jalyn (dutasteride and tamsulosin HCl), or Rapaflo (silodosin). Alpha-blockers are sometimes prescribed for prostate problems or high blood pressure. In some patients, the use of VIAGRA with alpha-blockers can lead to a drop in blood pressure or to fainting.
- medicines called HIV protease inhibitors, such as ritonavir (Norvir), indinavir sulfate (Crixivan), saquinavir (Fortovase or Invirase) or atazanavir sulfate (Reyataz)
- some types of oral antifungal medicines, such as ketoconazole (Nizoral), and itraconazole (Sporanox)
- some types of antibiotics, such as clarithromycin (Biaxin), telithromycin (Ketek), or erythromycin
- other medicines that treat high blood pressure
- other medicines or treatments for ED
- VIAGRA contains sildenafil, which is the same medicine found in another drug called REVATIO. REVATIO is used to treat a rare disease called pulmonary arterial hypertension (PAH). VIAGRA should not be used with REVATIO or with other PAH treatments containing sildenafil or any other PDE5 inhibitors (such as Adcirca [tadalafil]).

Ask your healthcare provider or pharmacist for a list of these medicines, if you are not sure.

Know the medicines you take. Keep a list of them to show to your healthcare provider and pharmacist when you get a new medicine.

How should I take VIAGRA?

- Take VIAGRA exactly as your healthcare provider tells you to take it.
- Your healthcare provider will tell you how much VIAGRA to take and when to take it.
- Your healthcare provider may change your dose if needed.
- Take VIAGRA about 1 hour before sexual activity. You may take VIAGRA between 30 minutes to 4 hours before sexual activity if needed.
- VIAGRA can be taken with or without food. If you take VIAGRA after a high fat meal (such as a cheeseburger and french fries), VIAGRA may take a little longer to start working
- **Do** not take VIAGRA more than 1 time a day.
- If you accidentally take too much VIAGRA, call your doctor or go to the nearest hospital emergency room right away.

Register at PDR.net to Receive Email Drug Alerts

What are the possible side effects of VIAGRA?

VIAGRA can cause serious side effects. Rarely reported side effects include:

- **an erection that will not go away (priapism).** If you have an erection that lasts more than 4 hours, get medical help right away. If it is not treated right away, priapism can permanently damage your penis.
- **sudden vision loss in one or both eyes.** Sudden vision loss in one or both eyes can be a sign of a serious eye problem called non-arteritic anterior ischemic optic neuropathy (NAION). Stop taking VIAGRA and call your healthcare provider right away if you have sudden vision loss in one or both eyes.
- **sudden hearing decrease or hearing loss.** Some people may also have ringing in their ears (tinnitus) or dizziness. If you have these symptoms, stop taking VIAGRA and contact a doctor right away.

The most common side effects of VIAGRA are:

- headache
- flushing
- upset stomach
- abnormal vision, such as changes in color vision (such as having a blue color tinge) and blurred vision
- stuffy or runny nose
- back pain
- muscle pain
- nausea
- dizziness
- rash

In addition, heart attack, stroke, irregular heartbeats and death have happened rarely in men taking VIAGRA. Most, but not all, of these men had heart problems before taking VIAGRA. It is not known if VIAGRA caused these problems. Tell your healthcare provider if you have any side effect that bothers you or does not go away.

These are not all the possible side effects of VIAGRA. For more information, ask your healthcare provider or pharmacist.

Call your doctor for medical advice about side effects. You may report side effects to FDA at 1-800-FDA-1088.

How should I store VIAGRA?

- Store VIAGRA at room temperature between 68°F to 77°F (20°C to 25°C).

Keep VIAGRA and all medicines out of the reach of children.

General information about the safe and effective use of VIAGRA.

Medicines are sometimes prescribed for purposes other than those listed in a Patient Information leaflet. Do not use VIAGRA for a condition for which it was not prescribed. Do not give VIAGRA to other people, even if they have the same symptoms that you have. It may harm them.

This Patient Information leaflet summarizes the most important information about VIAGRA. If you would like more information, talk with your healthcare provider. You can ask your healthcare provider or pharmacist for information about VIAGRA that is written for health professionals.

For more information, go to www.viagra.com, or call 1-888-4VIAGRA

What are the ingredients in VIAGRA?

Active ingredient: sildenafil citrate

Inactive ingredients: microcrystalline cellulose, anhydrous dibasic calcium phosphate, croscarmellose sodium, magnesium stearate, hypromellose, titanium dioxide, lactose, triacetin, and FD & C Blue #2 aluminum lake

This Patient Information has been approved by the U.S. Food and Drug Administration.

Distributed by

Pfizer Labs

Division of Pfizer Inc, NY, NY 10017

LAB-0220-8.0

03/2014

This product's label may have been updated. For current full prescribing information, please visit www.pfizer.com.

Viagra (sildenafil citrate), Revatio (sildenafil), Cardura (doxazosin mesylate), and Minipress (prazosin HCl) are registered trademarks of Pfizer Inc.

[1]The other brands listed are trademarks of their respective owners and are not trademarks of Pfizer Inc. The makers of these brands are not affiliated with and do not endorse Pfizer Inc or its products.

XELJANZ®

(tofacitinib)
tablets for oral administration

℞

HIGHLIGHTS OF PRESCRIBING INFORMATION

These highlights do not include all the information needed to use XELJANZ safely and effectively. See full prescribing information for XELJANZ.

XELJANZ ® (tofacitinib) tablets, for oral use
Initial U.S. Approval: 2012

WARNING: SERIOUS INFECTIONS AND MALIGNANCY

See full prescribing information for complete boxed warning.

- Serious infections leading to hospitalization or death, including tuberculosis and bacterial, invasive fungal, viral, and other opportunistic infections, have occurred in patients receiving XELJANZ. (5.1)
- If a serious infection develops, interrupt XELJANZ until the infection is controlled. (5.1)
- Prior to starting XELJANZ, perform a test for latent tuberculosis; if it is positive, start treatment for tuberculosis prior to starting XELJANZ. (5.1)
- Monitor all patients for active tuberculosis during treatment, even if the initial latent tuberculosis test is negative. (5.1)
- Lymphoma and other malignancies have been observed in patients treated with XELJANZ. Epstein Barr Virus-associated post-transplant lymphoproliferative disorder has been observed at an increased rate in renal transplant patients treated with XELJANZ and concomitant immunosuppressive medications. (5.2)

RECENT MAJOR CHANGES

INDICATIONS AND USAGE

- XELJANZ is an inhibitor of Janus kinases (JAKs) indicated for the treatment of adult patients with moderately to severely active rheumatoid arthritis who have had an inadequate response or intolerance to methotrexate. It may be used as monotherapy or in combination with methotrexate or other nonbiologic disease-modifying antirheumatic drugs (DMARDs). (1.1)
- Limitations of Use: Use of XELJANZ in combination with biologic DMARDs or potent immunosuppressants such as azathioprine and cyclosporine is not recommended. (1.1)

DOSAGE AND ADMINISTRATION

Rheumatoid Arthritis

- Recommended dose of XELJANZ is 5 mg twice daily. (2.1)
- Moderate and severe renal impairment and moderate hepatic impairment: Reduce dose to 5 mg once daily. (2.4, 8.6, 8.7)

DOSAGE FORMS AND STRENGTHS

Tablets: 5 mg (3)

CONTRAINDICATIONS

None (4)

WARNINGS AND PRECAUTIONS

- Avoid use of XELJANZ during an active serious infection, including localized infections. (5.1)
- Gastrointestinal Perforations – Use with caution in patients that may be at increased risk. (5.3)
- Laboratory Monitoring –Recommended due to potential changes in lymphocytes, neutrophils, hemoglobin, liver enzymes and lipids. (5.4)
- Immunizations – Live vaccines: Avoid use with XELJANZ. (5.5)

ADVERSE REACTIONS

The most commonly reported adverse reactions during the first 3 months in controlled clinical trials (occurring in greater than or equal to 2% of patients treated with XELJANZ monotherapy or in combination with DMARDs) were upper respiratory tract infections, headache, diarrhea and nasopharyngitis. (6.1)

To report SUSPECTED ADVERSE REACTIONS, contact Pfizer, Inc at 1-800-438-1985 or FDA at 1-800-FDA-1088 or www.fda.gov/medwatch.

DRUG INTERACTIONS

- Potent inhibitors of Cytochrome P450 3A4 (CYP3A4) (e.g., ketoconazole): Reduce dose to 5 mg once daily. (2.3, 7.1)
- One or more concomitant medications that result in both moderate inhibition of CYP3A4 and potent inhibition of CYP2C19 (e.g., fluconazole): Reduce dose to 5 mg once daily. (2.3, 7.2)

- Potent CYP inducers (e.g., rifampin): May result in loss of or reduced clinical response. (2.3, 7.3)

See 17 for PATIENT COUNSELING INFORMATION and Medication Guide

Revised: 05/2014

FULL PRESCRIBING INFORMATION: CONTENTS*

FULL PRESCRIBING INFORMATION

WARNING: SERIOUS INFECTIONS AND MALIGNANCY

SERIOUS INFECTIONS

Patients treated with XELJANZ are at increased risk for developing serious infections that may lead to hospitalization or death *[see Warnings and Precautions (5.1) and Adverse Reactions (6.1)]*. Most patients who developed these infections were taking concomitant immunosuppressants such as methotrexate or corticosteroids.

If a serious infection develops, interrupt XELJANZ until the infection is controlled.

Reported infections include:

- Active tuberculosis, which may present with pulmonary or extrapulmonary disease. Patients should be tested for latent tuberculosis before XELJANZ use and during therapy. Treatment for latent infection should be initiated prior to XELJANZ use.
- Invasive fungal infections, including cryptococcosis and pneumocystosis. Patients with invasive fungal infections may present with disseminated, rather than localized, disease.
- Bacterial, viral, and other infections due to opportunistic pathogens.

The risks and benefits of treatment with XELJANZ should be carefully considered prior to initiating therapy in patients with chronic or recurrent infection.

Patients should be closely monitored for the development of signs and symptoms of infection during and after treatment with XELJANZ, including the possible development of tuberculosis in patients who tested negative for latent tuberculosis infection prior to initiating therapy *[see Warnings and Precautions (5.1)]*.

MALIGNANCIES

Lymphoma and other malignancies have been observed in patients treated with XELJANZ. Epstein Barr Virus-associated post-transplant lymphoproliferative disorder has been observed in renal transplant patients treated with XELJANZ and concomitant immunosuppressive medications *[see Warnings and Precautions (5.2)]*.

1 INDICATIONS AND USAGE
1.1 Rheumatoid Arthritis
- XELJANZ (tofacitinib) is indicated for the treatment of adult patients with moderately to severely active rheumatoid arthritis who have had an inadequate response or intolerance to methotrexate. It may be used as monotherapy or in combination with methotrexate or other nonbiologic disease-modifying antirheumatic drugs (DMARDs).
- Limitations of Use: Use of XELJANZ in combination with biologic DMARDs or with potent immunosuppressants such as azathioprine and cyclosporine is not recommended.

2 DOSAGE AND ADMINISTRATION
2.1 Dosage in Rheumatoid Arthritis
- XELJANZ may be used as monotherapy or in combination with methotrexate or other nonbiologic disease-modifying antirheumatic drugs (DMARDs). The recommended dose of XELJANZ is 5 mg twice daily.
- XELJANZ is given orally with or without food.
2.2 Dosage Modifications due to Serious Infections and Cytopenias
(See Tables 1, 2, and 3 below.)
- It is recommended that XELJANZ not be initiated in patients with an absolute lymphocyte count less than 500 cells/mm³, an absolute neutrophil count (ANC) less than 1000 cells/mm³ or who have hemoglobin levels less than 9 g/dL.
- Dose interruption is recommended for management of lymphopenia, neutropenia and anemia *[see Warnings and Precautions (5.4) and Adverse Reactions (6.1)]*.
- Avoid use of XELJANZ if a patient develops a serious infection until the infection is controlled.
2.3 Dosage Modifications due to Drug Interactions
- XELJANZ dosage should be reduced to 5 mg once daily in patients:
  - receiving potent inhibitors of Cytochrome P450 3A4 (CYP3A4) (e.g., ketoconazole).
  - receiving one or more concomitant medications that result in both moderate inhibition of CYP3A4 and potent inhibition of CYP2C19 (e.g., fluconazole).
- Coadministration of potent inducers of CYP3A4 (e.g., rifampin) with XELJANZ may result in loss of or reduced clinical response to XELJANZ. Coadministration of potent inducers of CYP3A4 with XELJANZ is not recommended.
2.4 Dosage Modifications in Patients with Renal or Hepatic Impairment
- XELJANZ dosage should be reduced to 5 mg once daily in patients:
  - with moderate or severe renal insufficiency.
  - with moderate hepatic impairment.
- Use of XELJANZ in patients with severe hepatic impairment is not recommended.

Table 1: Dose Adjustments for Lymphopenia

Low Lymphocyte Count *[see Warnings and Precautions (5.4)]*

Lab Value (cells/mm³)	Recommendation
Lymphocyte count greater than or equal to 500	Maintain dose
Lymphocyte count less than 500 (Confirmed by repeat testing)	Discontinue XELJANZ

Table 2: Dose Adjustments for Neutropenia

Low ANC *[see Warnings and Precautions (5.4)]*

Lab Value (cells/mm³)	Recommendation
ANC greater than 1000	Maintain dose
ANC 500–1000	For persistent decreases in this range, interrupt dosing until ANC is greater than 1000
	When ANC is greater than 1000, resume XELJANZ 5 mg twice daily
ANC less than 500 (Confirmed by repeat testing)	Discontinue XELJANZ

Table 3: Dose Adjustments for Anemia

Low Hemoglobin Value *[see Warnings and Precautions (5.4)]*

Lab Value (g/dL)	Recommendation
Less than or equal to 2 g/dL decrease and greater than or equal to 9.0 g/dL	Maintain dose
Greater than 2 g/dL decrease or less than 8.0 g/dL (Confirmed by repeat testing)	Interrupt the administration of XELJANZ until hemoglobin values have normalized

3 DOSAGE FORMS AND STRENGTHS
XELJANZ is provided as 5 mg tofacitinib (equivalent to 8 mg tofacitinib citrate) tablets: White, round, immediate-release film-coated tablets, debossed with "Pfizer" on one side, and "JKI 5" on the other side.

4 CONTRAINDICATIONS
None

5 WARNINGS AND PRECAUTIONS
5.1 Serious Infections
Serious and sometimes fatal infections due to bacterial, mycobacterial, invasive fungal, viral, or other opportunistic pathogens have been reported in rheumatoid arthritis patients receiving XELJANZ. The most common serious infections reported with XELJANZ included pneumonia, cellulitis, herpes zoster and urinary tract infection *[see Adverse Reactions (6.1)]*. Among opportunistic infections, tuberculosis and other mycobacterial infections, cryptococcosis, esophageal candidiasis, pneumocystosis, multidermatomal herpes zoster, cytomegalovirus, and BK virus were reported with XELJANZ. Some patients have presented with disseminated rather than localized disease, and were often taking concomitant immunomodulating agents such as methotrexate or corticosteroids.

Other serious infections that were not reported in clinical studies may also occur (e.g., histoplasmosis, coccidioidomycosis, and listeriosis).

Avoid use of XELJANZ in patients with an active, serious infection, including localized infections. The risks and benefits of treatment should be considered prior to initiating XELJANZ in patients:
- with chronic or recurrent infection
- who have been exposed to tuberculosis
- with a history of a serious or an opportunistic infection
- who have resided or traveled in areas of endemic tuberculosis or endemic mycoses; or
- with underlying conditions that may predispose them to infection.

Patients should be closely monitored for the development of signs and symptoms of infection during and after treatment with XELJANZ. XELJANZ should be interrupted if a patient develops a serious infection, an opportunistic infection, or sepsis. A patient who develops a new infection during treatment with XELJANZ should undergo prompt and complete diagnostic testing appropriate for an immunocompromised patient; appropriate antimicrobial therapy should be initiated, and the patient should be closely monitored.

Tuberculosis
Patients should be evaluated and tested for latent or active infection prior to administration of XELJANZ.

Anti-tuberculosis therapy should also be considered prior to administration of XELJANZ in patients with a past history of latent or active tuberculosis in whom an adequate course of treatment cannot be confirmed, and for patients with a negative test for latent tuberculosis but who have risk factors for tuberculosis infection. Consultation with a physician with expertise in the treatment of tuberculosis is recommended to aid in the decision about whether initiating anti-tuberculosis therapy is appropriate for an individual patient.

Patients should be closely monitored for the development of signs and symptoms of tuberculosis, including patients who tested negative for latent tuberculosis infection prior to initiating therapy.

Patients with latent tuberculosis should be treated with standard antimycobacterial therapy before administering XELJANZ.

Viral Reactivation
Viral reactivation, including cases of herpes virus reactivation (e.g., herpes zoster), were observed in clinical studies with XELJANZ. The impact of XELJANZ on chronic viral hepatitis reactivation is unknown. Patients who screened positive for hepatitis B or C were excluded from clinical trials. Screening for viral hepatitis should be performed in accordance with clinical guidelines before starting therapy with XELJANZ.

5.2 Malignancy and Lymphoproliferative Disorders
Consider the risks and benefits of XELJANZ treatment prior to initiating therapy in patients with a known malignancy other than a successfully treated non-melanoma skin cancer (NMSC) or when considering continuing XELJANZ in patients who develop a malignancy. Malignancies were observed in clinical studies of XELJANZ *[see Adverse Reactions (6.1)]*.

In the seven controlled rheumatoid arthritis clinical studies, 11 solid cancers and one lymphoma were diagnosed in 3328 patients receiving XELJANZ with or without DMARD, compared to 0 solid cancers and 0 lymphomas in 809 patients in the placebo with or without DMARD group during the first 12 months of exposure. Lymphomas and solid cancers have also been observed in the long-term extension studies in rheumatoid arthritis patients treated with XELJANZ.

In Phase 2B, controlled dose-ranging trials in *de-novo* renal transplant patients, all of whom received induction therapy with basiliximab, high-dose corticosteroids, and mycophenolic acid products, Epstein Barr Virus-associated post-transplant lymphoproliferative disorder was observed in 5 out of 218 patients treated with XELJANZ (2.3%) compared to 0 out of 111 patients treated with cyclosporine.

Non-Melanoma Skin Cancer
Non-melanoma skin cancers (NMSCs) have been reported in patients treated with XELJANZ. Periodic skin examination is recommended for patients who are at increased risk for skin cancer.

5.3 Gastrointestinal Perforations
Events of gastrointestinal perforation have been reported in clinical studies with XELJANZ in rheumatoid arthritis patients, although the role of JAK inhibition in these events is not known.

XELJANZ should be used with caution in patients who may be at increased risk for gastrointestinal perforation (e.g., patients with a history of diverticulitis). Patients presenting with new onset abdominal symptoms should be evaluated promptly for early identification of gastrointestinal perforation *[see Adverse Reactions (6.1)]*.

5.4 Laboratory Abnormalities
Lymphocyte Abnormalities
Treatment with XELJANZ was associated with initial lymphocytosis at one month of exposure followed by a gradual decrease in mean absolute lymphocyte counts below the baseline of approximately 10% during 12 months of therapy. Lymphocyte counts less than 500 cells/mm³ were associated with an increased incidence of treated and serious infections.

Avoid initiation of XELJANZ treatment in patients with a low lymphocyte count (i.e., less than 500 cells/mm³). In patients who develop a confirmed absolute lymphocyte count less than 500 cells/mm³ treatment with XELJANZ is not recommended.

Monitor lymphocyte counts at baseline and every 3 months thereafter. For recommended modifications based on lymphocyte counts *see Dosage and Administration (2.2)*.

Neutropenia
Treatment with XELJANZ was associated with an increased incidence of neutropenia (less than 2000 cells/mm³) compared to placebo.

Avoid initiation of XELJANZ treatment in patients with a low neutrophil count (i.e., ANC less than 1000 cells/mm³). For patients who develop a persistent ANC of 500–1000 cells/mm³, interrupt XELJANZ dosing until ANC is greater than or equal to 1000 cells/mm³. In patients who develop an ANC less than 500 cells/mm³, treatment with XELJANZ is not recommended.

Monitor neutrophil counts at baseline and after 4–8 weeks of treatment and every 3 months thereafter. For recommended modifications based on ANC results *see Dosage and Administration (2.2)*.

Anemia
Avoid initiation of XELJANZ treatment in patients with a low hemoglobin level (i.e. less than 9 g/dL). Treatment with XELJANZ should be interrupted in patients who develop hemoglobin levels less than 8 g/dL or whose hemoglobin level drops greater than 2 g/dL on treatment.

Monitor hemoglobin at baseline and after 4–8 weeks of treatment and every 3 months thereafter. For recommended modifications based on hemoglobin results *see Dosage and Administration (2.2)*.

Liver Enzyme Elevations

Treatment with XELJANZ was associated with an increased incidence of liver enzyme elevation compared to placebo. Most of these abnormalities occurred in studies with background DMARD (primarily methotrexate) therapy.

Routine monitoring of liver tests and prompt investigation of the causes of liver enzyme elevations is recommended to identify potential cases of drug-induced liver injury. If drug-induced liver injury is suspected, the administration of XELJANZ should be interrupted until this diagnosis has been excluded.

Lipid Elevations

Treatment with XELJANZ was associated with increases in lipid parameters including total cholesterol, low-density lipoprotein (LDL) cholesterol, and high-density lipoprotein (HDL) cholesterol. Maximum effects were generally observed within 6 weeks. The effect of these lipid parameter elevations on cardiovascular morbidity and mortality has not been determined.

Assessment of lipid parameters should be performed approximately 4–8 weeks following initiation of XELJANZ therapy.

Manage patients according to clinical guidelines [e.g., National Cholesterol Educational Program (NCEP)] for the management of hyperlipidemia.

5.5 Vaccinations

No data are available on the response to vaccination or on the secondary transmission of infection by live vaccines to patients receiving XELJANZ. Avoid use of live vaccines concurrently with XELJANZ.

Update immunizations in agreement with current immunization guidelines prior to initiating XELJANZ therapy.

6 ADVERSE REACTIONS

6.1 Clinical Trial Experience

Because clinical studies are conducted under widely varying conditions, adverse reaction rates observed in the clinical studies of a drug cannot be directly compared to rates in the clinical studies of another drug and may not predict the rates observed in a broader patient population in clinical practice.

Although other doses have been studied, the recommended dose of XELJANZ is 5 mg twice daily.

The following data includes two Phase 2 and five Phase 3 double-blind, controlled, multicenter trials. In these trials, patients were randomized to doses of XELJANZ 5 mg twice daily (292 patients) and 10 mg twice daily (306 patients) monotherapy, XELJANZ 5 mg twice daily (1044 patients) and 10 mg twice daily (1043 patients) in combination with DMARDs (including methotrexate) and placebo (809 patients). All seven protocols included provisions for patients taking placebo to receive treatment with XELJANZ at Month 3 or Month 6 either by patient response (based on uncontrolled disease activity) or by design, so that adverse events cannot always be unambiguously attributed to a given treatment. Therefore some analyses that follow include patients who changed treatment by design or by patient response from placebo to XELJANZ in both the placebo and XELJANZ group of a given interval. Comparisons between placebo and XELJANZ were based on the first 3 months of exposure, and comparisons between XELJANZ 5 mg twice daily and XELJANZ 10 mg twice daily were based on the first 12 months of exposure.

The long-term safety population includes all patients who participated in a double-blind, controlled trial (including earlier development phase studies) and then participated in one of two long-term safety studies. The design of the long-term safety studies allowed for modification of XELJANZ doses according to clinical judgment. This limits the interpretation of the long-term safety data with respect to dose. The most common serious adverse reactions were serious infections [see Warnings and Precautions (5.1)].

The proportion of patients who discontinued treatment due to any adverse reaction during the 0 to 3 months exposure in the double-blind, placebo-controlled trials was 4% for patients taking XELJANZ and 3% for placebo-treated patients.

Overall Infections

In the seven controlled trials, during the 0 to 3 months exposure, the overall frequency of infections was 20% and 22% in the 5 mg twice daily and 10 mg twice daily groups, respectively, and 18% in the placebo group.

The most commonly reported infections with XELJANZ were upper respiratory tract infections, nasopharyngitis, and urinary tract infections (4%, 3%, and 2% of patients, respectively).

Serious Infections

In the seven controlled trials, during the 0 to 3 months exposure, serious infections were reported in 1 patient (0.5 events per 100 patient-years) who received placebo and 11 patients (1.7 events per 100 patient-years) who received XELJANZ 5 mg or 10 mg twice daily. The rate difference between treatment groups (and the corresponding 95% confi-

dence interval) was 1.1 (-0.4, 2.5) events per 100 patient-years for the combined 5 mg twice daily and 10 mg twice daily XELJANZ group minus placebo.

In the seven controlled trials, during the 0 to 12 months exposure, serious infections were reported in 34 patients (2.7 events per 100 patient-years) who received 5 mg twice daily of XELJANZ and 33 patients (2.7 events per 100 patient-years) who received 10 mg twice daily of XELJANZ. The rate difference between XELJANZ doses (and the corresponding 95% confidence interval) was -0.1 (-1.3, 1.2) events per 100 patient-years for 10 mg twice daily XELJANZ minus 5 mg twice daily XELJANZ.

The most common serious infections included pneumonia, cellulitis, herpes zoster, and urinary tract infection [see Warnings and Precautions (5.1)].

Tuberculosis

In the seven controlled trials, during the 0 to 3 months exposure, tuberculosis was not reported in patients who received placebo, 5 mg twice daily of XELJANZ, or 10 mg twice daily of XELJANZ.

In the seven controlled trials, during the 0 to 12 months exposure, tuberculosis was reported in 0 patients who received 5 mg twice daily of XELJANZ and 6 patients (0.5 events per 100 patient-years) who received 10 mg twice daily of XELJANZ. The rate difference between XELJANZ doses (and the corresponding 95% confidence interval) was 0.5 (0.1, 0.9) events per 100 patient-years for 10 mg twice daily XELJANZ minus 5 mg twice daily XELJANZ.

Cases of disseminated tuberculosis were also reported. The median XELJANZ exposure prior to diagnosis of tuberculosis was 10 months (range from 152 to 960 days) [see Warnings and Precautions (5.1)].

Opportunistic Infections (excluding tuberculosis)

In the seven controlled trials, during the 0 to 3 months exposure, opportunistic infections were not reported in patients who received placebo, 5 mg twice daily of XELJANZ, or 10 mg twice daily of XELJANZ.

In the seven controlled trials, during the 0 to 12 months exposure, opportunistic infections were reported in 4 patients (0.3 events per 100 patient-years) who received 5 mg twice daily of XELJANZ and 4 patients (0.3 events per 100 patient-years) who received 10 mg twice daily of XELJANZ. The rate difference between XELJANZ doses (and the corresponding 95% confidence interval) was 0 (-0.5, 0.5) events per 100 patient-years for 10 mg twice daily XELJANZ minus 5 mg twice daily XELJANZ.

The median XELJANZ exposure prior to diagnosis of an opportunistic infection was 8 months (range from 41 to 698 days) [see Warnings and Precautions (5.1)].

Malignancy

In the seven controlled trials, during the 0 to 3 months exposure, malignancies excluding NMSC were reported in 0 patients who received placebo and 2 patients (0.3 events per 100 patient-years) who received either XELJANZ 5 mg or 10 mg twice daily. The rate difference between treatment groups (and the corresponding 95% confidence interval) was 0.3 (-0.1, 0.7) events per 100 patient-years for the combined 5 mg and 10 mg twice daily XELJANZ group minus placebo.

In the seven controlled trials, during the 0 to 12 months exposure, malignancies excluding NMSC were reported in 5 patients (0.4 events per 100 patient-years) who received 5 mg twice daily of XELJANZ and 7 patients (0.6 events per 100 patient-years) who received 10 mg twice daily of XELJANZ. The rate difference between XELJANZ doses (and the corresponding 95% confidence interval) was 0.2 (-0.4, 0.7) events per 100 patient-years for 10 mg twice daily XELJANZ minus 5 mg twice daily XELJANZ. One of these malignancies was a case of lymphoma that occurred during the 0 to 12 month period in a patient treated with XELJANZ 10 mg twice daily.

The most common types of malignancy, including malignancies observed during the long-term extension, were lung and breast cancer, followed by gastric, colorectal, renal cell, prostate cancer, lymphoma, and malignant melanoma [see Warnings and Precautions (5.2)].

Laboratory Abnormalities

Lymphopenia

In the controlled clinical trials, confirmed decreases in absolute lymphocyte counts below 500 cells/mm³ occurred in 0.04% of patients for the 5 mg twice daily and 10 mg twice daily XELJANZ groups combined during the first 3 months of exposure.

Confirmed lymphocyte counts less than 500 cells/mm³ were associated with an increased incidence of treated and serious infections [see Warnings and Precautions (5.4)].

Neutropenia

In the controlled clinical trials, confirmed decreases in ANC below 1000 cells/mm³ occurred in 0.07% of patients for the 5 mg twice daily and 10 mg twice daily XELJANZ groups combined during the first 3 months of exposure.

There were no confirmed decreases in ANC below 500 cells/mm³ observed in any treatment group.

There was no clear relationship between neutropenia and the occurrence of serious infections.

In the long-term safety population, the pattern and incidence of confirmed decreases in ANC remained consistent with what was seen in the controlled clinical trials [see Warnings and Precautions (5.4)].

Liver Enzyme Elevations

Confirmed increases in liver enzymes greater than 3 times the upper limit of normal (3× ULN) were observed in patients treated with XELJANZ. In patients experiencing liver enzyme elevation, modification of treatment regimen, such as reduction in the dose of concomitant DMARD, interruption of XELJANZ, or reduction in XELJANZ dose, resulted in decrease or normalization of liver enzymes.

In the controlled monotherapy trials (0–3 months), no differences in the incidence of ALT or AST elevations were observed between the placebo, and XELJANZ 5 mg, and 10 mg twice daily groups.

In the controlled background DMARD trials (0–3 months), ALT elevations greater than 3× ULN were observed in 1.0%, 1.3% and 1.2% of patients receiving placebo, 5 mg, and 10 mg twice daily, respectively. In these trials, AST elevations greater than 3× ULN were observed in 0.6%, 0.5% and 0.4% of patients receiving placebo, 5 mg, and 10 mg twice daily, respectively.

One case of drug-induced liver injury was reported in a patient treated with XELJANZ 10 mg twice daily for approximately 2.5 months. The patient developed symptomatic elevations of AST and ALT greater than 3× ULN and bilirubin elevations greater than 2× ULN, which required hospitalizations and a liver biopsy.

Lipid Elevations

In the controlled clinical trials, dose-related elevations in lipid parameters (total cholesterol, LDL cholesterol, HDL cholesterol, triglycerides) were observed at one month of exposure and remained stable thereafter. Changes in lipid parameters during the first 3 months of exposure in the controlled clinical trials are summarized below:

- Mean LDL cholesterol increased by 15% in the XELJANZ 5 mg twice daily arm and 19% in the XELJANZ 10 mg twice daily arm.
- Mean HDL cholesterol increased by 10% in the XELJANZ 5 mg twice daily arm and 12% in the XELJANZ 10 mg twice daily arm.
- Mean LDL/HDL ratios were essentially unchanged in XELJANZ-treated patients.

In a controlled clinical trial, elevations in LDL cholesterol and ApoB decreased to pretreatment levels in response to statin therapy.

In the long-term safety population, elevations in lipid parameters remained consistent with what was seen in the controlled clinical trials.

Serum Creatinine Elevations

In the controlled clinical trials, dose-related elevations in serum creatinine were observed with XELJANZ treatment. The mean increase in serum creatinine was <0.1 mg/dL in the 12-month pooled safety analysis; however with increasing duration of exposure in the long-term extensions, up to 2% of patients were discontinued from XELJANZ treatment due to the protocol-specified discontinuation criterion of an increase in creatinine by more than 50% of baseline. The clinical significance of the observed serum creatinine elevations is unknown.

Other Adverse Reactions

Adverse reactions occurring in 2% or more of patients on 5 mg twice daily or 10 mg twice daily XELJANZ and at least 1% greater than that observed in patients on placebo with or without DMARD are summarized in Table 4.

Table 4: Adverse Reactions Occurring in at Least 2% or More of Patients on 5 or 10 mg Twice Daily XELJANZ With or Without DMARD (0–3 months) and at Least 1% Greater Than That Observed in Patients on Placebo

Preferred Term	XELJANZ 5 mg Twice Daily	XELJANZ 10 mg Twice Daily*	Placebo
	N = 1336 (%)	N = 1349 (%)	N = 809 (%)
Diarrhea	4.0	2.9	2.3
Nasopharyngitis	3.8	2.8	2.8
Upper respiratory tract infection	4.5	3.8	3.3
Headache	4.3	3.4	2.1
Hypertension	1.6	2.3	1.1

N reflects randomized and treated patients from the seven clinical trials

* The recommended dose of XELJANZ is 5 mg twice daily.

Other adverse reactions occurring in controlled and open-label extension studies included:

Blood and lymphatic system disorders: Anemia
Metabolism and nutrition disorders: Dehydration
Psychiatric disorders: Insomnia
Nervous system disorders: Paresthesia
Respiratory, thoracic and mediastinal disorders: Dyspnea, cough, sinus congestion
Gastrointestinal disorders: Abdominal pain, dyspepsia, vomiting, gastritis, nausea
Hepatobiliary disorders: Hepatic steatosis
Skin and subcutaneous tissue disorders: Rash, erythema, pruritus
Musculoskeletal, connective tissue and bone disorders: Musculoskeletal pain, arthralgia, tendonitis, joint swelling
Neoplasms benign, malignant and unspecified (including cysts and polyps): Non-melanoma skin cancers
General disorders and administration site conditions: Pyrexia, fatigue, peripheral edema

Clinical Experience in Methotrexate-Naïve Patients
Study VI was an active-controlled clinical trial in methotrexate-naïve patients *[see Clinical Studies (14)]*. The safety experience in these patients was consistent with Studies I–V.

7 DRUG INTERACTIONS
7.1 Potent CYP3A4 Inhibitors
Tofacitinib exposure is increased when XELJANZ is coadministered with potent inhibitors of cytochrome P450 (CYP) 3A4 (e.g., ketoconazole) *[see Dosage and Administration (2.3) and Figure 3]*.
7.2 Moderate CYP3A4 and Potent CYP2C19 Inhibitors
Tofacitinib exposure is increased when XELJANZ is coadministered with medications that result in both moderate inhibition of CYP3A4 and potent inhibition of CYP2C19 (e.g., fluconazole) *[see Dosage and Administration (2.3) and Figure 3]*.
7.3 Potent CYP3A4 Inducers
Tofacitinib exposure is decreased when XELJANZ is coadministered with potent CYP3A4 inducers (e.g., rifampin) *[see Dosage and Administration (2.3) and Figure 3]*.
7.4 Immunosuppressive Drugs
There is a risk of added immunosuppression when XELJANZ is coadministered with potent immunosuppressive drugs (e.g., azathioprine, tacrolimus, cyclosporine). Combined use of multiple-dose XELJANZ with potent immunosuppressants has not been studied in rheumatoid arthritis. Use of XELJANZ in combination with biologic DMARDs or potent immunosuppressants such as azathioprine and cyclosporine is not recommended.

8 USE IN SPECIFIC POPULATIONS
8.1 Pregnancy
Teratogenic effects:
Pregnancy Category C. There are no adequate and well-controlled studies in pregnant women. XELJANZ should be used during pregnancy only if the potential benefit justifies the potential risk to the fetus. Tofacitinib has been shown to be fetocidal and teratogenic in rats and rabbits when given at exposures 146 times and 13 times, respectively, the maximum recommended human dose (MRHD).

In a rat embryofetal developmental study, tofacitinib was teratogenic at exposure levels approximately 146 times the MRHD (on an AUC basis at oral doses of 100 mg/kg/day). Teratogenic effects consisted of external and soft tissue malformations of anasarca and membranous ventricular septal defects, respectively, and skeletal malformations or variations (absent cervical arch; bent femur, fibula, humerus, radius, scapula, tibia, and ulna; sternoschisis; absent rib; misshapen femur; branched rib; fused rib; fused sternebra; and hemicentric thoracic centrum). In addition, there was an increase in post-implantation loss, consisting of early and late resorptions, resulting in a reduced number of viable fetuses. Mean fetal body weight was reduced. No developmental toxicity was observed in rats at exposure levels approximately 58 times the MRHD (on an AUC basis at oral doses of 30 mg/kg/day). In the rabbit embryofetal developmental study, tofacitinib was teratogenic at exposure levels approximately 13 times the MRHD (on an AUC basis at oral doses of 30 mg/kg/day) in the absence of signs of maternal toxicity. Teratogenic effects included thoracogastroschisis, omphalocele, membranous ventricular septal defects, and cranial/skeletal malformations (microstomia, microphthalmia), mid-line and tail defects. In addition, there was an increase in post-implantation loss associated with late resorptions. No developmental toxicity was observed in rabbits at exposure levels approximately 3 times the MRHD (on an AUC basis at oral doses of 10 mg/kg/day).

Nonteratogenic effects:
In a peri- and postnatal rat study, there were reductions in live litter size, postnatal survival, and pup body weights at exposure levels approximately 73 times the MRHD (on an AUC basis at oral doses of 50 mg/kg/day). There was no effect on behavioral and learning assessments, sexual maturation or the ability of the F1 generation rats to mate and produce viable F2 generation fetuses in rats at exposure levels approximately 17 times the MRHD (on an AUC basis at oral doses of 10 mg/kg/day).

Pregnancy Registry: To monitor the outcomes of pregnant women exposed to XELJANZ, a pregnancy registry has been established. Physicians are encouraged to register patients and pregnant women are encouraged to register themselves by calling 1-877-311-8972.

8.3 Nursing Mothers
Tofacitinib was secreted in milk of lactating rats. It is not known whether tofacitinib is excreted in human milk. Because many drugs are excreted in human milk and because of the potential for serious adverse reactions in nursing infants from tofacitinib, a decision should be made whether to discontinue nursing or to discontinue the drug, taking into account the importance of the drug for the mother.
8.4 Pediatric Use
The safety and effectiveness of XELJANZ in pediatric patients have not been established.
8.5 Geriatric Use
Of the 3315 patients who enrolled in Studies I to V, a total of 505 rheumatoid arthritis patients were 65 years of age and older, including 71 patients 75 years and older. The frequency of serious infection among XELJANZ-treated subjects 65 years of age and older was higher than among those under the age of 65. As there is a higher incidence of infections in the elderly population in general, caution should be used when treating the elderly.
8.6 Hepatic Impairment
XELJANZ-treated patients with moderate hepatic impairment had greater tofacitinib levels than XELJANZ-treated patients with normal hepatic function *[see Clinical Pharmacology (12.3)]*. Higher blood levels may increase the risk of some adverse reactions, therefore, XELJANZ dose should be reduced to 5 mg once daily in patients with moderate hepatic impairment *[see Dosage and Administration (2.4)]*. XELJANZ has not been studied in patients with severe hepatic impairment; therefore, use of XELJANZ in patients with severe hepatic impairment is not recommended. No dose adjustment is required in patients with mild hepatic impairment. The safety and efficacy of XELJANZ have not been studied in patients with positive hepatitis B virus or hepatitis C virus serology.
8.7 Renal Impairment
XELJANZ-treated patients with moderate and severe renal impairment had greater tofacitinib blood levels than XELJANZ-treated patients with normal renal function; therefore, XELJANZ dose should be reduced to 5 mg once daily in patients with moderate and severe renal impairment *[see Dosage and Administration (2.4)]*. In clinical trials, XELJANZ was not evaluated in rheumatoid arthritis patients with baseline creatinine clearance values (estimated by the Cockroft-Gault equation) less than 40 mL/min. No dose adjustment is required in patients with mild renal impairment.

10 OVERDOSAGE
Signs, Symptoms, and Laboratory Findings of Acute Overdosage in Humans
There is no experience with overdose of XELJANZ.
Treatment or Management of Overdose
Pharmacokinetic data up to and including a single dose of 100 mg in healthy volunteers indicate that more than 95% of the administered dose is expected to be eliminated within 24 hours.
There is no specific antidote for overdose with XELJANZ. In case of an overdose, it is recommended that the patient be monitored for signs and symptoms of adverse reactions. Patients who develop adverse reactions should receive appropriate treatment.

11 DESCRIPTION
XELJANZ is the citrate salt of tofacitinib, a JAK inhibitor. Tofacitinib citrate is a white to off-white powder with the following chemical name: (3R,4R)-4-methyl-3-(methyl-7H-pyrrolo [2,3-d]pyrimidin-4-ylamino)-ß-oxo-1-piperidinepropanenitrile, 2-hydroxy-1,2,3-propanetricarboxylate (1:1). The solubility of tofacitinib citrate in water is 2.9 mg/mL. Tofacitinib citrate has a molecular weight of 504.5 Daltons (or 312.4 Daltons as the tofacitinib free base) and a molecular formula of $C_{16}H_{20}N_6O \cdot C_6H_8O_7$. The chemical structure of tofacitinib citrate is:

XELJANZ is supplied for oral administration as 5 mg tofacitinib (equivalent to 8 mg tofacitinib citrate) white round, immediate-release film-coated tablet. Each tablet of XELJANZ contains the appropriate amount of XELJANZ as a citrate salt and the following inactive ingredients: microcrystalline cellulose, lactose monohydrate, croscarmellose sodium, magnesium stearate, HPMC 2910/Hypromellose 6cP, titanium dioxide, macrogol/PEG3350, and triacetin.

12 CLINICAL PHARMACOLOGY
12.1 Mechanism of Action
Tofacitinib is a Janus kinase (JAK) inhibitor. JAKs are intracellular enzymes which transmit signals arising from cytokine or growth factor-receptor interactions on the cellular membrane to influence cellular processes of hematopoiesis and immune cell function. Within the signaling pathway, JAKs phosphorylate and activate Signal Transducers and Activators of Transcription (STATs) which modulate intracellular activity including gene expression. Tofacitinib modulates the signaling pathway at the point of JAKs, preventing the phosphorylation and activation of STATs. JAK enzymes transmit cytokine signaling through pairing of JAKs (e.g., JAK1/JAK3, JAK1/JAK2, JAK1/TyK2, JAK2/JAK2). Tofacitinib inhibited the *in vitro* activities of JAK1/JAK2, JAK1/JAK3, and JAK2/JAK2 combinations with IC_{50} of 406, 56, and 1377 nM, respectively. However, the relevance of specific JAK combinations to therapeutic effectiveness is not known.
12.2 Pharmacodynamics
Treatment with XELJANZ was associated with dose-dependent reductions of circulating CD16/56+ natural killer cells, with estimated maximum reductions occurring at approximately 8–10 weeks after initiation of therapy. These changes generally resolved within 2–6 weeks after discontinuation of treatment. Treatment with XELJANZ was associated with dose-dependent increases in B cell counts. Changes in circulating T-lymphocyte counts and T-lymphocyte subsets (CD3+, CD4+ and CD8+) were small and inconsistent. The clinical significance of these changes is unknown.
Total serum IgG, IgM, and IgA levels after 6-month dosing in patients with rheumatoid arthritis were lower than placebo; however, changes were small and not dose-dependent. After treatment with XELJANZ in patients with rheumatoid arthritis, rapid decreases in serum C-reactive protein (CRP) were observed and maintained throughout dosing. Changes in CRP observed with XELJANZ treatment do not reverse fully within 2 weeks after discontinuation, indicating a longer duration of pharmacodynamic activity compared to the pharmacokinetic half-life.
12.3 Pharmacokinetics
Following oral administration of XELJANZ, peak plasma concentrations are reached within 0.5–1 hour, elimination half-life is ~3 hours and a dose-proportional increase in systemic exposure was observed in the therapeutic dose range. Steady state concentrations are achieved in 24–48 hours with negligible accumulation after twice daily administration.
Absorption
The absolute oral bioavailability of tofacitinib is 74%. Coadministration of XELJANZ with a high-fat meal resulted in no changes in AUC while C_{max} was reduced by 32%. In clinical trials, XELJANZ was administered without regard to meals.
Distribution
After intravenous administration, the volume of distribution is 87 L. The protein binding of tofacitinib is ~40%. Tofacitinib binds predominantly to albumin and does not appear to bind to α1-acid glycoprotein. Tofacitinib distributes equally between red blood cells and plasma.
Metabolism and Elimination
Clearance mechanisms for tofacitinib are approximately 70% hepatic metabolism and 30% renal excretion of the parent drug. The metabolism of tofacitinib is primarily mediated by CYP3A4 with minor contribution from CYP2C19. In a human radiolabeled study, more than 65% of the total circulating radioactivity was accounted for by unchanged tofacitinib, with the remaining 35% attributed to 8 metabolites, each accounting for less than 8% of total radioactivity. The pharmacologic activity of tofacitinib is attributed to the parent molecule.
Pharmacokinetics in Rheumatoid Arthritis Patients
Population PK analysis in rheumatoid arthritis patients indicated no clinically relevant change in tofacitinib exposure, after accounting for differences in renal function (i.e., creatinine clearance) between patients, based on age, weight, gender and race (Figure 1). An approximately linear relationship between body weight and volume of distribution was observed, resulting in higher peak (C_{max}) and lower trough (C_{min}) concentrations in lighter patients. However, this difference is not considered to be clinically relevant. The between-subject variability (% coefficient of variation) in AUC of tofacitinib is estimated to be approximately 27%.

Figure 1: Impact of Intrinsic Factors on Tofacitinib Pharmacokinetics

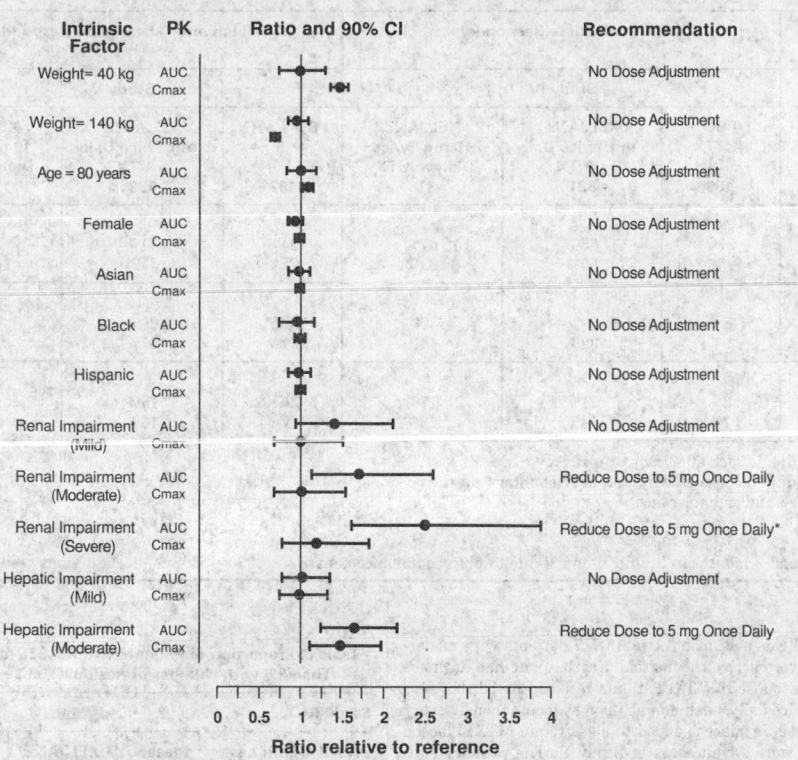

*Supplemental doses are not necessary in patients after dialysis

Figure 3. Impact of Other Drugs on PK of XELJANZ

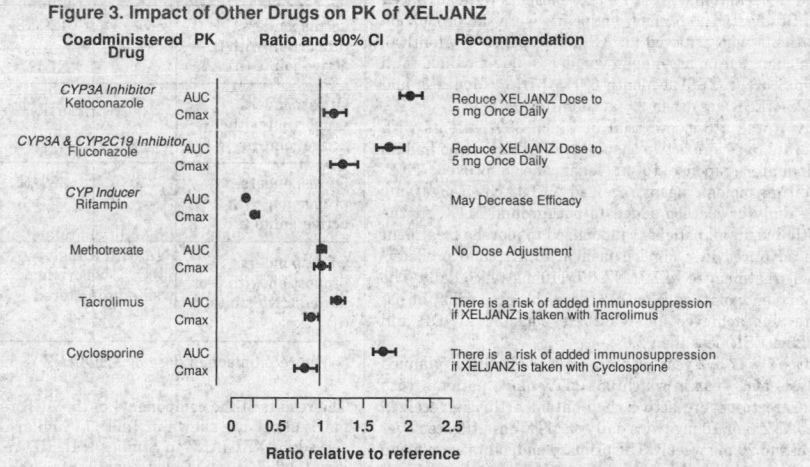

Figure 2. Impact of XELJANZ on PK of Other Drugs

stantially alter the PK of tofacitinib. Dosing recommendations for XELJANZ for administration with CYP inhibitors or inducers are shown in Figure 3.

[See figure 3 above]

Note: Reference group is administration of tofacitinib alone

13 NONCLINICAL TOXICOLOGY

13.1 Carcinogenesis, Mutagenesis, Impairment of Fertility

In a 39-week toxicology study in monkeys, tofacitinib at exposure levels approximately 6 times the MRHD (on an AUC basis at oral doses of 5 mg/kg twice daily) produced lymphomas. No lymphomas were observed in this study at exposure levels 1 times the MRHD (on an AUC basis at oral doses of 1 mg/kg twice daily).

The carcinogenic potential of tofacitinib was assessed in 6-month rasH2 transgenic mouse carcinogenicity and 2-year rat carcinogenicity studies. Tofacitinib, at exposure levels approximately 34 times the MRHD (on an AUC basis at oral doses of 200 mg/kg/day) was not carcinogenic in mice.

In the 24-month oral carcinogenicity study in Sprague-Dawley rats, tofacitinib caused benign Leydig cell tumors, hibernomas (malignancy of brown adipose tissue), and benign thymomas at doses greater than or equal to 30 mg/kg/day (approximately 42 times the exposure levels at the MRHD on an AUC basis). The relevance of benign Leydig cell tumors to human risk is not known.

Tofacitinib was not mutagenic in the bacterial reverse mutation assay. It was positive for clastogenicity in the *in vitro* chromosome aberration assay with human lymphocytes in the presence of metabolic enzymes, but negative in the absence of metabolic enzymes. Tofacitinib was negative in the *in vivo* rat micronucleus assay and in the *in vitro* CHO-HGPRT assay and the *in vivo* rat hepatocyte unscheduled DNA synthesis assay.

In rats, tofacitinib at exposure levels approximately 17 times the MRHD (on an AUC basis at oral doses of 10 mg/kg/day) reduced female fertility due to increased post-implantation loss. There was no impairment of female rat fertility at exposure levels of tofacitinib equal to the MRHD (on an AUC basis at oral doses of 1 mg/kg/day). Tofacitinib exposure levels at approximately 133 times the MRHD (on an AUC basis at oral doses of 100 mg/kg/day) had no effect on male fertility, sperm motility, or sperm concentration.

14 CLINICAL STUDIES

The XELJANZ clinical development program included two dose-ranging trials and five confirmatory trials. Although other doses have been studied, the recommended dose of XELJANZ is 5 mg twice daily.

DOSE-RANGING TRIALS

Dose selection for XELJANZ was based on two pivotal dose-ranging trials.

Dose-Ranging Study 1 was a 6-month monotherapy trial in 384 patients with active rheumatoid arthritis who had an inadequate response to a DMARD. Patients who previously received adalimumab therapy were excluded. Patients were randomized to 1 of 7 monotherapy treatments: XELJANZ 1, 3, 5, 10 or 15 mg twice daily, adalimumab 40 mg subcutaneously every other week for 10 weeks followed by XELJANZ 5 mg twice daily for 3 months, or placebo.

Dose-Ranging Study 2 was a 6-month trial in which 507 patients with active rheumatoid arthritis who had an inadequate response to MTX alone received one of 6 dose regimens of XELJANZ (20 mg once daily; 1, 3, 5, 10 or 15 mg twice daily), or placebo added to background MTX.

The results of XELJANZ-treated patients achieving ACR20 responses in Studies 1 and 2 are shown in Figure 4. Although a dose-response relationship was observed in Study 1, the proportion of patients with an ACR20 response did

Specific Populations

The effect of renal and hepatic impairment and other intrinsic factors on the pharmacokinetics of tofacitinib is shown in Figure 1.

[See figure 1 above]

Reference values for weight, age, gender, and race comparisons are 70 kg, 55 years, male, and White, respectively; reference groups for renal and hepatic impairment data are subjects with normal renal and hepatic function.

Drug Interactions

Potential for XELJANZ to Influence the PK of Other Drugs

In vitro studies indicate that tofacitinib does not significantly inhibit or induce the activity of the major human drug-metabolizing CYPs (CYP1A2, CYP2B6, CYP2C8, CYP2C9, CYP2C19, CYP2D6, and CYP3A4) at concentrations exceeding 185 times the steady state C_{max} of a 5 mg twice daily dose. These *in vitro* results were confirmed by a human drug interaction study showing no changes in the PK of midazolam, a highly sensitive CYP3A4 substrate, when coadministered with XELJANZ.

In rheumatoid arthritis patients, the oral clearance of tofacitinib does not vary with time, indicating that tofacitinib does not normalize CYP enzyme activity in rheumatoid arthritis patients. Therefore, coadministration with XELJANZ is not expected to result in clinically relevant increases in the metabolism of CYP substrates in rheumatoid arthritis patients.

In vitro data indicate that the potential for tofacitinib to inhibit transporters such as P-glycoprotein, organic anionic or cationic transporters at therapeutic concentrations is low. Dosing recommendations for coadministered drugs following administration with XELJANZ are shown in Figure 2.

[See figure 2 at top of next column]

Note: Reference group is administration of concomitant medication alone; OCT = Organic Cationic Transporter; MATE = Multidrug and Toxic Compound Extrusion

Potential for Other Drugs to Influence the PK of Tofacitinib

Since tofacitinib is metabolized by CYP3A4, interaction with drugs that inhibit or induce CYP3A4 is likely. Inhibitors of CYP2C19 alone or P-glycoprotein are unlikely to sub-

Table 5: Proportion of Patients with an ACR Response

N§	Percent of Patients								
	Monotherapy in Nonbiologic or Biologic DMARD Inadequate Responders*			MTX Inadequate Responders†			TNF Inhibitor Inadequate Responders‡		
	Study I			Study IV			Study V		
	PBO	XELJANZ 5 mg Twice Daily	XELJANZ 10 mg Twice Daily¶	PBO + MTX	XELJANZ 5 mg Twice Daily + MTX	XELJANZ 10 mg Twice Daily + MTX¶	PBO + MTX	XELJANZ 5 mg Twice Daily + MTX	XELJANZ 10 mg Twice Daily + MTX¶
	122	243	245	160	321	316	132	133	134
ACR20									
Month 3	26%	59%	65%	27%	55%	67%	24%	41%	48%
Month 6	NA#	69%	70%	25%	50%	62%	NA	51%	54%
ACR50									
Month 3	12%	31%	36%	8%	29%	37%	8%	26%	28%
Month 6	NA	42%	46%	9%	32%	44%	NA	37%	30%
ACR70									
Month 3	6%	15%	20%	3%	11%	17%	2%	14%	10%
Month 6	NA	22%	29%	1%	14%	23%	NA	16%	16%

* Inadequate response to at least one DMARD (biologic or nonbiologic) due to lack of efficacy or toxicity.
† Inadequate response to MTX defined as the presence of sufficient residual disease activity to meet the entry criteria.
‡ Inadequate response to a least one TNF inhibitor due to lack of efficacy and/or intolerance.
§ N is number of randomized and treated patients.
¶ The recommended dose of XELJANZ is 5 mg twice daily.
# NA Not applicable, as data for placebo treatment is not available beyond 3 months in Studies I and V due to placebo advancement.

not clearly differ between the 10 mg and 15 mg doses. In Study 2, a smaller proportion of patients achieved an ACR20 response in the placebo and XELJANZ 1 mg groups compared to patients treated with the other XELJANZ doses. However, there was no difference in the proportion of responders among patients treated with XELJANZ 3, 5, 10, 15 mg twice daily or 20 mg once daily doses.

Figure 4: Proportion of Patients with ACR20 Response at Month 3 in Dose-Ranging Studies 1 and 2

* XELJANZ twice daily dosing in mg, except for 20 mg which is once daily dosing in mg.
PBO is placebo; ADA is adalimumab 40 mg subcutaneous injection every other week.

Study 1 was a dose-ranging monotherapy trial not designed to provide comparative effectiveness data and should not be interpreted as evidence of superiority to adalimumab.

CONFIRMATORY TRIALS

Study I was a 6-month monotherapy trial in which 610 patients with moderate to severe active rheumatoid arthritis who had an inadequate response to a DMARD (nonbiologic or biologic) received XELJANZ 5 or 10 mg twice daily or placebo. At the Month 3 visit, all patients randomized to placebo treatment were advanced in a blinded fashion to a second predetermined treatment of XELJANZ 5 or 10 mg twice daily. The primary endpoints at Month 3 were the proportion of patients who achieved an ACR20 response, changes in Health Assessment Questionnaire – Disability Index (HAQ-DI), and rates of Disease Activity Score DAS28-4(ESR) less than 2.6.

Study II was a 12-month trial in which 792 patients with moderate to severe active rheumatoid arthritis who had an inadequate response to a nonbiologic DMARD received XELJANZ 5 or 10 mg twice daily or placebo added to background DMARD treatment (excluding potent immunosuppressive treatments such as azathioprine or cyclosporine). At the Month 3 visit, nonresponding patients were advanced in a blinded fashion to a second predetermined treatment of XELJANZ 5 or 10 mg twice daily. At the end of Month 6, all placebo patients were advanced to their second predetermined treatment in a blinded fashion. The primary endpoints were the proportion of patients who achieved an ACR20 response at Month 6, changes in HAQ-DI at Month 3, and rates of DAS28-4(ESR) less than 2.6.

Study III was a 12-month trial in 717 patients with moderate to severe active rheumatoid arthritis who had an inadequate response to MTX. Patients received XELJANZ 5 or 10 mg twice daily, adalimumab 40 mg subcutaneously every other week, or placebo added to background MTX. Placebo patients were advanced as in Study II. The primary endpoints were the proportion of patients who achieved an ACR20 response at Month 6, HAQ-DI at Month 3, and DAS28-4(ESR) less than 2.6 at Month 6.

Study IV was a 2-year trial with a planned analysis at 1 year in which 797 patients with moderate to severe active rheumatoid arthritis who had an inadequate response to MTX received XELJANZ 5 or 10 mg twice daily or placebo added to background MTX. Placebo patients were advanced as in Study II. The primary endpoints were the proportion of patients who achieved an ACR20 response at Month 6, mean change from baseline in van der Heijde-modified total Sharp Score (mTSS) at Month 6, HAQ-DI at Month 3, and DAS28-4(ESR) less than 2.6 at Month 6.

Study V was a 6-month trial in which 399 patients with moderate to severe active rheumatoid arthritis who had an inadequate response to at least one approved TNF-inhibiting biologic agent received XELJANZ 5 or 10 mg twice daily or placebo added to background MTX. At the Month 3 visit, all patients randomized to placebo treatment were advanced in a blinded fashion to a second predetermined treatment of XELJANZ 5 or 10 mg twice daily. The primary endpoints at Month 3 were the proportion of patients who achieved an ACR20 response, HAQ-DI, and DAS28-4(ESR) less than 2.6.

Study VI was a 2-year monotherapy trial with a planned analysis at 1 year in which 952 MTX-naïve patients with moderate to severe active rheumatoid arthritis received XELJANZ 5 or 10 mg twice daily or MTX dose-titrated over 8 weeks to 20 mg weekly. The primary endpoints were mean change from baseline in van der Heijde-modified Total Sharp Score (mTSS) at Month 6 and the proportion of patients who achieved an ACR70 response at Month 6.

Clinical Response

The percentages of XELJANZ-treated patients achieving ACR20, ACR50, and ACR70 responses in Studies I, IV, and V are shown in Table 5. Similar results were observed with Studies II and III. In trials I–V, patients treated with either 5 or 10 mg twice daily XELJANZ had higher ACR20, ACR50, and ACR70 response rates versus placebo, with or without background DMARD treatment, at Month 3 and Month 6. Higher ACR20 response rates were observed within 2 weeks compared to placebo. In the 12-month trials, ACR response rates in XELJANZ-treated patients were consistent at 6 and 12 months.
[See table 5 above]

In Study IV, a greater proportion of patients treated with XELJANZ 5 mg or 10 mg twice daily plus MTX achieved a low level of disease activity as measured by a DAS28-4(ESR) less than 2.6 at 6 months compared to those treated with MTX alone (Table 6).

Table 6: Proportion of Patients with DAS28-4(ESR) Less Than 2.6 with Number of Residual Active Joints

Study IV

DAS28-4(ESR) Less Than 2.6	Placebo + MTX 160	XELJANZ 5 mg Twice Daily + MTX 321	XELJANZ 10 mg Twice Daily + MTX* 316
Proportion of responders at Month 6 (n)	1% (2)	6% (19)	13% (42)
Of responders, proportion with 0 active joints (n)	50% (1)	42% (8)	36% (15)
Of responders, proportion with 1 active joint (n)	0	5% (1)	17% (7)
Of responders, proportion with 2 active joints (n)	0	32% (6)	7% (3)
Of responders, proportion with 3 or more active joints (n)	50% (1)	21% (4)	40% (17)

* The recommended dose of XELJANZ is 5 mg twice daily.

The results of the components of the ACR response criteria for Study IV are shown in Table 7. Similar results were observed for XELJANZ in Studies I, II, III, V, and VI.
[See table 7 at top of next page]

The percent of ACR20 responders by visit for Study IV is shown in Figure 5. Similar responses were observed for XELJANZ in Studies I, II, III, V, and VI.
[See figure 5 at top of next column]

Radiographic Response

Two studies were conducted to evaluate the effect of XELJANZ on structural joint damage. In Study IV and Study VI, progression of structural joint damage was assessed radiographically and expressed as change from baseline in mTSS and its components, the erosion score and joint space narrowing score, at Months 6 and 12. The proportion of patients with no radiographic progression (mTSS change less than or equal to 0) was also assessed.

In Study IV, XELJANZ 10 mg twice daily plus background MTX reduced the progression of structural damage compared to placebo plus MTX at Month 6. When given at a dose of 5 mg twice daily, XELJANZ exhibited similar effects on mean progression of structural damage (not statistically significant). These results are shown in Table 8. Analyses of erosion and joint space narrowing scores were consistent with the overall results.

Figure 5: Percentage of ACR20 Responders by Visit for Study IV

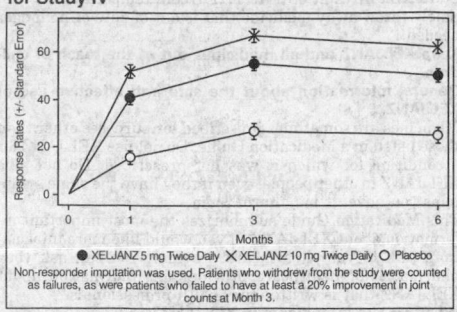

Non-responder imputation was used. Patients who withdrew from the study were counted as failures, as were patients who failed to have at least a 20% improvement in joint counts at Month 3.

● XELJANZ 5 mg Twice Daily X XELJANZ 10 mg Twice Daily ○ Placebo

In the placebo plus MTX group, 74% of patients experienced no radiographic progression at Month 6 compared to 84% and 79% of patients treated with XELJANZ plus MTX 5 or 10 mg twice daily.

In Study VI, XELJANZ monotherapy inhibited the progression of structural damage compared to MTX at Months 6 and 12 as shown in Table 8. Analyses of erosion and joint space narrowing scores were consistent with the overall results.

In the MTX group, 55% of patients experienced no radiographic progression at Month 6 compared to 73% and 77% of patients treated with XELJANZ 5 or 10 mg twice daily. [See table 8 above]

Physical Function Response

Improvement in physical functioning was measured by the HAQ-DI. Patients receiving XELJANZ 5 and 10 mg twice daily demonstrated greater improvement from baseline in physical functioning compared to placebo at Month 3.

The mean (95% CI) difference from placebo in HAQ-DI improvement from baseline at Month 3 in Study III was -0.22 (-0.35, -0.10) in patients receiving 5 mg XELJANZ twice daily and -0.32 (-0.44, -0.19) in patients receiving 10 mg XELJANZ twice daily. Similar results were obtained in Studies I, II, IV and V. In the 12-month trials, HAQ-DI results in XELJANZ-treated patients were consistent at 6 and 12 months.

Other Health-Related Outcomes

General health status was assessed by the Short Form health survey (SF-36). In studies I, IV, and V, patients receiving XELJANZ 5 mg twice daily or XELJANZ 10 mg twice daily demonstrated greater improvement from baseline compared to placebo in physical component summary (PCS), mental component summary (MCS) scores and in all 8 domains of the SF-36 at Month 3.

16 HOW SUPPLIED/STORAGE AND HANDLING

XELJANZ is provided as 5 mg tofacitinib (equivalent to 8 mg tofacitinib citrate) tablets: White, round, immediate-release film-coated tablets, debossed with "Pfizer" on one side, and "JKI 5" on the other side, and available in:

Bottles of 28:	NDC 0069-1001-03
Bottles of 60:	NDC 0069-1001-01
Bottles of 180:	NDC 0069-1001-02

Storage and Handling

Store at 20°C to 25°C (68°F to 77°F). [See USP Controlled Room Temperature].

Do not repackage.

17 PATIENT COUNSELING INFORMATION

See FDA-approved patient labeling (Medication Guide). Advise the patient to read the FDA-approved patient labeling (Medication Guide).

Patient Counseling

Advise patients of the potential benefits and risks of XELJANZ.

Serious Infection

Inform patients that XELJANZ may lower the ability of their immune system to fight infections. Advise patients not to start taking XELJANZ if they have an active infection. Instruct patients to contact their healthcare provider immediately during treatment if symptoms suggesting infection appear in order to ensure rapid evaluation and appropriate treatment [see Warnings and Precautions (5.1)].

Malignancies and Lymphoproliferative Disorders

Inform patients that XELJANZ may increase their risk of certain cancers, and that lymphoma and other cancers have been observed in patients taking XELJANZ. Instruct patients to inform their healthcare provider if they have ever had any type of cancer [see Warnings and Precautions (5.2)].

Important Information on Laboratory Abnormalities

Inform patients that XELJANZ may affect certain lab test results, and that blood tests are required before and during XELJANZ treatment [see Warnings and Precautions (5.4)].

Pregnancy

Inform patients that XELJANZ should not be used during pregnancy unless clearly necessary, and advise patients to inform their doctors right away if they become pregnant while taking XELJANZ. Inform patients that Pfizer has a registry for pregnant women who have taken XELJANZ during pregnancy. Advise patients to contact the registry at 1-877-311-8972 to enroll [see Pregnancy (8.1)].

This product's label may have been updated. For current full prescribing information, please visit www.pfizer.com.

LAB-0445-7.0

MEDICATION GUIDE

XELJANZ (ZEL' JANS')

(tofacitinib)

Read this Medication Guide before you start taking XELJANZ and each time you get a refill. There may be new information. This Medication Guide does not take the place of talking to your healthcare provider about your medical condition or treatment.

What is the most important information I should know about XELJANZ?

XELJANZ may cause serious side effects including:

1. Serious infections.

XELJANZ is a medicine that affects your immune system. XELJANZ can lower the ability of your immune system to fight infections. Some people have serious infections while taking XELJANZ, including tuberculosis (TB), and infections caused by bacteria, fungi, or viruses that can spread throughout the body. Some people have died from these infections.

- Your healthcare provider should test you for TB before starting XELJANZ.
- Your healthcare provider should monitor you closely for signs and symptoms of TB infection during treatment with XELJANZ.

You should not start taking XELJANZ if you have any kind of infection unless your healthcare provider tells you it is okay.

Table 7: Components of ACR Response at Month 3

Component (mean) [†]	Study IV					
	XELJANZ 5 mg Twice Daily + MTX N=321		XELJANZ 10 mg* Twice Daily + MTX N=316		Placebo + MTX N=160	
	Baseline	Month 3[†]	Baseline	Month 3[†]	Baseline	Month 3[†]
Number of tender joints (0–68)	24 (14)	13 (14)	23 (15)	10 (12)	23 (13)	18 (14)
Number of swollen joints (0–66)	14 (8)	6 (8)	14 (8)	6 (7)	14 (9)	10 (9)
Pain[‡]	58 (23)	34 (23)	58 (24)	29 (22)	55 (24)	47 (24)
Patient global assessment[‡]	58 (24)	35 (23)	57 (23)	29 (20)	54 (23)	47 (24)
Disability index (HAQ-DI)[§]	1.41 (0.68)	0.99 (0.65)	1.40 (0.66)	0.84 (0.64)	1.32 (0.67)	1.19 (0.68)
Physician global assessment[‡]	59 (16)	30 (19)	58 (17)	24 (17)	56 (18)	43 (22)
CRP (mg/L)	15.3 (19.0)	7.1 (19.1)	17.1 (26.9)	4.4 (8.6)	13.7 (14.9)	14.6 (18.7)

* The recommended dose of XELJANZ is 5 mg twice daily.
† Data shown is mean (Standard Deviation) at Month 3.
‡ Visual analog scale: 0 = best, 100 = worst.
§ Health Assessment Questionnaire Disability Index: 0 = best, 3 = worst; 20 questions; categories: dressing and grooming, arising, eating, walking, hygiene, reach, grip, and activities.

Table 8: Radiographic Changes at Months 6 and 12

	Study IV				
	Placebo N=139 Mean (SD)[†]	XELJANZ 5 mg Twice Daily N=277 Mean (SD)[†]	XELJANZ 5 mg Twice Daily Mean Difference from Placebo[‡] (CI)	XELJANZ 10 mg Twice Daily* N=290 Mean (SD)[†]	XELJANZ 10 mg Twice Daily Mean Difference from Placebo[‡] (CI)
mTSS[§]					
Baseline	33 (42)	31 (48)	-	37 (54)	-
Month 6	0.5 (2.0)	0.1 (1.7)	-0.3 (-0.7, 0.0)	0.1 (2.0)	-0.4 (-0.8, 0.0)
	Study VI				
	MTX N=166 Mean (SD)[†]	XELJANZ 5 mg Twice Daily N=346 Mean (SD)[†]	XELJANZ 5 mg Twice Daily Mean Difference from MTX[‡] (CI)	XELJANZ 10 mg Twice Daily* N=369 Mean (SD)[†]	XELJANZ 10 mg Twice Daily Mean Difference from MTX[‡] (CI)
mTSS[§]					
Baseline	17 (29)	20 (40)	-	19 (39)	-
Month 6	0.8 (2.7)	0.2 (2.3)	-0.7 (-1.0, -0.3)	0.0 (1.2)	-0.8 (-1.2, -0.4)
Month 12	1.3 (3.7)	0.4 (3.0)	-0.9 (-1.4, -0.4)	0.0 (1.5)	-1.3 (-1.8, -0.8)

* The recommended dose of XELJANZ is 5 mg twice daily.
† SD = Standard Deviation
‡ Difference between least squares means XELJANZ minus placebo or MTX (95% CI = 95% confidence interval)
§ Month 6 and Month 12 data are mean change from baseline.

Before starting XELJANZ, tell your healthcare provider if you:

- think you have an infection or have symptoms of an infection such as:

  - fever, sweating, or chills
  - muscle aches
  - cough
  - shortness of breath
  - blood in phlegm
  - weight loss

  - warm, red, or painful skin or sores on your body
  - diarrhea or stomach pain
  - burning when you urinate or urinating more often than normal
  - feeling very tired

- are being treated for an infection
- get a lot of infections or have infections that keep coming back
- have diabetes, HIV, or a weak immune system. People with these conditions have a higher chance for infections.
- have TB, or have been in close contact with someone with TB
- live or have lived, or have traveled to certain parts of the country (such as the Ohio and Mississippi River valleys and the Southwest) where there is an increased chance for getting certain kinds of fungal infections (histoplasmosis, coccidioidomycosis, or blastomycosis). These infections may happen or become more severe if you use XELJANZ. Ask your healthcare provider if you do not know whether you have lived in an area where these infections are common.
- have or have had hepatitis B or C

After starting XELJANZ, call your healthcare provider right away if you have any symptoms of an infection. XELJANZ can make you more likely to get infections or make worse any infection that you have.

2. Cancer and immune system problems.
XELJANZ may increase your risk of certain cancers by changing the way your immune system works.

- Lymphoma and other cancers including skin cancers can happen in patients taking XELJANZ. Tell your healthcare provider if you have ever had any type of cancer.
- Some people who have taken XELJANZ with certain other medicines to prevent kidney transplant rejection have had a problem with certain white blood cells growing out of control (Epstein Barr Virus-associated post transplant lymphoproliferative disorder).

3. Tears (perforation) in the stomach or intestines.

- Tell your healthcare provider if you have had diverticulitis (inflammation in parts of the large intestine) or ulcers in your stomach or intestines. Some people taking XELJANZ get tears in their stomach or intestine. This happens most often in people who also take nonsteroidal anti-inflammatory drugs (NSAIDs), corticosteroids, or methotrexate.
- Tell your healthcare provider right away if you have fever and stomach-area pain that does not go away, and a change in your bowel habits.

4. Changes in certain laboratory test results. Your healthcare provider should do blood tests before you start receiving XELJANZ and while you take XELJANZ to check for the following side effects:

- **changes in lymphocyte counts.** Lymphocytes are white blood cells that help the body fight off infections.
- **low neutrophil counts.** Neutrophils are white blood cells that help the body fight off infections.
- **low red blood cell count.** This may mean that you have anemia, which may make you feel weak and tired.

Your healthcare provider should routinely check certain liver tests.

You should not receive XELJANZ if your lymphocyte count, neutrophil count, or red blood cell count is too low or your liver tests are too high.

Your healthcare provider may stop your XELJANZ treatment for a period of time if needed because of changes in these blood test results.

You may also have changes in other laboratory tests, such as your blood cholesterol levels. Your healthcare provider should do blood tests to check your cholesterol levels 4 to 8 weeks after you start receiving XELJANZ, and as needed after that. Normal cholesterol levels are important to good heart health.

See "What are the possible side effects of XELJANZ?" for more information about side effects.

What is XELJANZ?
XELJANZ is a prescription medicine called a Janus kinase (JAK) inhibitor. XELJANZ is used to treat adults with moderately to severely active rheumatoid arthritis in which methotrexate did not work well.

It is not known if XELJANZ is safe and effective in people with Hepatitis B or C.

XELJANZ is not for people with severe liver problems.

It is not known if XELJANZ is safe and effective in children.

What should I tell my healthcare provider before taking XELJANZ?
XELJANZ may not be right for you. Before taking XELJANZ, tell your healthcare provider if you:

- have an infection. See "What is the most important information I should know about XELJANZ?"
- have liver problems
- have kidney problems
- have any stomach area (abdominal) pain or been diagnosed with diverticulitis or ulcers in your stomach or intestines
- have had a reaction to tofacitinib or any of the ingredients in XELJANZ
- have recently received or are scheduled to receive a vaccine. People who take XELJANZ should not receive live vaccines. People taking XELJANZ can receive non-live vaccines.
- have any other medical conditions
- plan to become pregnant or are pregnant. It is not known if XELJANZ will harm an unborn baby.
  Pregnancy Registry: Pfizer has a registry for pregnant women who take XELJANZ. The purpose of this registry is to check the health of the pregnant mother and her baby. If you are pregnant or become pregnant while taking XELJANZ, talk to your healthcare provider about how you can join this pregnancy registry or you may contact the registry at 1-877-311-8972 to enroll.
- plan to breastfeed or are breastfeeding. You and your healthcare provider should decide if you will take XELJANZ or breastfeed. You should not do both.

Tell your healthcare provider about all the medicines you take, including prescription and non-prescription medicines, vitamins, and herbal supplements. XELJANZ and other medicines may affect each other causing side effects. Especially tell your healthcare provider if you take:

- any other medicines to treat your rheumatoid arthritis. You should not take tocilizumab (Actemra®), etanercept (Enbrel®), adalimumab (Humira®), infliximab (Remicade®), rituximab (Rituxan®), abatacept (Orencia®), anakinra (Kineret®), certolizumab (Cimzia®), golimumab (Simponi®), azathioprine, cyclosporine, or other immunosuppressive drugs while you are taking XELJANZ. Taking XELJANZ with these medicines may increase your risk of infection.
- medicines that affect the way certain liver enzymes work. Ask your healthcare provider if you are not sure if your medicine is one of these.

Know the medicines you take. Keep a list of them to show your healthcare provider and pharmacist when you get a new medicine.

How should I take XELJANZ?

- Take XELJANZ as your healthcare provider tells you to take it.
- Take XELJANZ 2 times a day with or without food.
- If you take too much XELJANZ, call your healthcare provider or go to the nearest hospital emergency room right away.

What are possible side effects of XELJANZ?
XELJANZ may cause serious side effects, including:

- See "What is the most important information I should know about XELJANZ?"
- **Hepatitis B or C activation infection** in people who carry the virus in their blood. If you are a carrier of the hepatitis B or C virus (viruses that affect the liver), the virus may become active while you use XELJANZ. Your healthcare provider may do blood tests before you start treatment with XELJANZ and while you are using XELJANZ. Tell your healthcare provider if you have any of the following symptoms of a possible hepatitis B or C infection:

  - feel very tired
  - skin or eyes look yellow
  - little or no appetite
  - vomiting
  - clay-colored bowel movements

  - fevers
  - chills
  - stomach discomfort
  - muscle aches
  - dark urine
  - skin rash

Common side effects of XELJANZ include:

- upper respiratory tract infections (common cold, sinus infections)
- headache
- diarrhea
- nasal congestion, sore throat, and runny nose (nasopharyngitis)

Tell your healthcare provider if you have any side effect that bothers you or that does not go away.

These are not all the possible side effects of XELJANZ. For more information, ask your healthcare provider or pharmacist.

Call your doctor for medical advice about side effects. You may report side effects to FDA at 1-800-FDA-1088.
You may also report side effects to Pfizer at 1-800-438-1985.

How should I store XELJANZ?
Store XELJANZ at 68°F to 77°F (room temperature).
Safely throw away medicine that is out of date or no longer needed.
Keep XELJANZ and all medicines out of the reach of children.
General information about the safe and effective use of XELJANZ.
Medicines are sometimes prescribed for purposes other than those listed in a Medication Guide. Do not use XELJANZ for a condition for which it was not prescribed. Do not give XELJANZ to other people, even if they have the same symptoms you have. It may harm them.
This Medication Guide summarizes the most important information about XELJANZ. If you would like more information, talk to your healthcare provider. You can ask your pharmacist or healthcare provider for information about XELJANZ that is written for health professionals.
What are the ingredients in XELJANZ?
Active ingredient: tofacitinib citrate
Inactive ingredients: microcrystalline cellulose, lactose monohydrate, croscarmellose sodium, magnesium stearate, HPMC 2910/Hypromellose 6cP, titanium dioxide, macrogol/PEG3350, and triacetin.
This Medication Guide has been approved by the U.S. Food and Drug Administration.
LAB-0535-2.0
March 2014

Pivotal Therapeutics Inc.
81 ZENWAY BOULEVARD
UNIT #10
WOODBRIDGE, ONTARIO L4H 0S5
CANADA
Telephone: 1-905-856-9797

Pivotal Therapeutics (US), Inc.
3651 FAU Blvd., Suite 400
Boca Raton, FL 33431
United States
Telephone: 1-888-358-2080
Telephone: 1-561-288-5231
Email: info@pivotaltherapeutics.us
Website: www.pivotaltherapeutics.us

VASCAZEN®   ℞

RECOMMENDED USE

VASCAZEN® (omega-3-acid ethyl esters) is a prescription only Medical Food intended for the dietary management of Omega-3 Deficiency in patients with Cardiovascular Disease (CVD).
Must be administered under physician supervision. Dispensed by prescription only.
VASCAZEN® softgel capsules to be administered orally, and is dispensed by prescription only for the dietary management of Omega-3 Deficiency in patients with CVD. The adult dose is four (4) capsules daily, supplying 3g/day of eicosapentaenoic acid (EPA) and docosahexaenoic acid (DHA). VASCAZEN® should only be taken under the supervision of a physician, and is only dispensed by prescription. Do not take VASCAZEN® if you have a known allergy to fish or soy. If you are pregnant, nursing, or under the age of 18 years, consult your physician prior to taking VASCAZEN®.

PRODUCT DESCRIPTION
Primary Ingredients
VASCAZEN® consists of a proprietary formulation of Omega-3 fatty acid ethyl esters, containing a minimum of 900mg of Omega-3 fatty acid ethyl esters, including 680mg of EPA and 110mg of DHA in a ratio of 6:1, per 1g capsule.
Other Ingredients
VASCAZEN® contains the following inactive carriers or excipients: mixed natural tocopherols, gelatin, glycerol, purified water, and trace amounts of soy.

MEDICAL FOODS

Medical Food products are often used in hospitals and outside of a hospital setting under a physician's care for the dietary management of diseases in patients with particular, unique or distinctive medical or metabolic needs due to their disease or condition. Congress defined "Medical Food" in the Orphan Drug Act and Amendments of 1988 as "a food which is formulated to be consumed or administered enterally [or orally] under the supervision of a physician and which is intended for the specific dietary management of a disease or condition for which distinctive nutritional requirements, based on recognized scientific principles, are established by medical evaluation." Medical Foods are complex formulated products, requiring sophisticated and exacting technology, and that are used only for a patient receiving active and ongoing medical supervision wherein the patient requires medical care on a recurring basis for, among other things, instructions on the use of the Medical Food. **VASCAZEN®** has been developed, manufactured and labeled in accordance with the statutory definition of a Medical Food. **VASCAZEN®** must be used while the patient is under the ongoing care of a physician.

BACKGROUND
Omega-3 Deficiency
A critical component of the definition of a Medical Food is that the product must address the distinct nutritional requirements of a particular disease or condition. **VASCAZEN®** meets the definition of distinctive nutritional requirements as follows: "the dietary management" of patients with specific diseases requires, in some instances, the ability to meet nutritional requirements that differ substantially from the needs of healthy persons. For example, in establishing the recommended dietary allowances for the general, healthy population, the Food and Nutrition Board of the Institute of Medicine National Academy of Sciences recognized that different or distinctive physiologic requirements may exist for certain persons with special nutritional needs arising from metabolic disorders, chronic diseases, or other medical conditions. Thus, the distinctive nutritional needs associated with a disease reflects the total amount needed by a healthy person to support life or maintain homeostasis, adjusted for the distinctive changes in the nutritional needs of the patient as a result of the effects of the disease process on absorption, metabolism, and excretion. It was also proposed that in patients with certain disease states who respond to nutritional therapies, a physiologic deficiency of the nutrient is assumed to exist. For example, more than 80% of patients with CVD are Omega-3 Deficient, i.e. residing in the highest risk quartiles as defined[1,2] by measuring either the Omega-Score™ or Omega-3 Index. The Omega-Score™ is a measure of Omega-3 fatty acid (EPA, DHA and docosapentaenoic acid (DPA)) levels in blood and the Omega-3 Index is a measure of EPA and DHA in red blood cells. Epidemiological and subsequent human studies have established that Omega-3 fatty acids are essential nutrients and have pleiotropic effects in cell function and regulate multiple metabolic pathways controlling blood lipids, inflammatory factors, cellular and molecular events in heart cells, and vascular endothelial cells. Metabolic deficiency of Omega-3 fatty acids can lead to high blood pressure, a change in the blood lipid profile, with elevations in low density lipoprotein cholesterol (LDL-C; "bad cholesterol"), decrease in high density lipoprotein cholesterol (HDL-C; "good cholesterol"), triglyceride (TG) increase, with increased inflammation (excess of 2-series eicosanoids). Correction of Omega-3 Deficiency is thought to have a positive effect on the above and can promote a shift from 2-series (pro-inflammatory), to 3-series (less inflammatory) eicosanoids as the ratio of arachidonic acid (AA)/EPA decreases[3]. **VASCAZEN®** is a prescription Medical Food for the dietary management of Omega-3 Deficiency in patients with CVD, providing EPA and DHA to levels not attainable through normal dietary modifications alone. This deficiency can be corrected by providing prescription **VASCAZEN®**, reducing a key risk factor in patients with CVD.

A review of the scientific and medical literature identifies there are medically determined Omega-3 nutrient requirements in patients with CVD[1,2,4,5], supporting the recommendation of consuming 3g of EPA and DHA per day[6]. It would be difficult to achieve and sustain this high level of EPA and DHA through mere modification of the "normal" diet. Consumption of fatty fish every day may approach the level of 3g of EPA and DHA per day. However, the typical American diet consists of approximately 1/15th of these levels[7] and increasing fish consumption 15-fold, to reach the clinically beneficial EPA and DHA levels through diet alone, would not be considered "normal" as required under the Medical Food definition. **VASCAZEN®** delivers 3g/day of EPA and DHA, levels not reasonably achievable through diet modifications alone.

Omega-3 Fatty Acids
Omega-3 fatty acids are polyunsaturated fatty acids with a double bond at the third carbon atom from the end of the carbon chain (methyl terminal). The main Omega-3 fatty acids are EPA and DHA. Dietary sources of EPA and DHA are largely from cold water, oily fish including anchovies, sardines, mackerel and salmon and have demonstrated therapeutic benefits for overall cardiovascular health[3,8]. However, to attain the sustained and stable levels of Omega-3 required for cardio-protective effects, a diet consisting predominantly of fish can be difficult to maintain on a daily basis. There is also a growing public concern for toxin accumulation in fish (e.g. mercury, other heavy metals, PCBs etc.), contributing to lower desire to include fish as a regular dietary staple.

Structural formulas for EPA and DHA ethyl esters are:
Eicosapentaenoic Acid (EPA) Ethyl Ester

Docosahexaenoic Acid (DHA) Ethyl Ester

The molecular weight of EPA ethyl ester is 330.5 and has an empirical formula of $C_{22}H_{34}O_2$, and DHA ethyl ester has a molecular weight of 356.6 and an empirical formula of $C_{24}H_{36}O_2$.

Physical Description
VASCAZEN® is distributed as an ultra-purified, light yellow, fish oil-filled, transparent softgel capsule in 15-count blister cards. Capsules are intended for oral administration and contain a minimum of 900mg Omega-3 fatty acids by weight comprised of a combination of at least 680mg EPA and 110mg DHA in a weight ratio of 6:1 in each 1g capsule. **VASCAZEN®** undergoes multiple independent third party testing for safety and purity.

CLINICAL PHARMACOLOGY OF OMEGA-3's
VASCAZEN® is intended to restore and sustain healthy levels of EPA and DHA in Omega-3 Deficient patients with CVD. Increasing dietary levels of EPA and DHA have been shown to have a host of cardio-protective benefits[9,10]. Scientific literature suggests a correlation between high circulating blood levels of EPA and DHA with a reduction in the risk of cardiovascular events[2,5]. Beneficial effects of EPA and DHA have been documented in a number of clinical studies[9,10]. These include positive effects on lipid metabolism, blood pressure, heart rate, platelet aggregation, inflammation and helping to reduce the risk of cardiovascular disease[2,3,8].

CLINICAL EXPERIENCE
Clinical dietary management of Omega-3 Deficiency in patients with CVD can be achieved with **VASCAZEN®** at a dose of four (4) capsules per day.

VASCAZEN® Open Label Safety and Efficacy Study
The safety and efficacy of **VASCAZEN®** was evaluated in an open label clinical study that assessed Omega-3 Deficiency and efficacy of **VASCAZEN®** treatment for two to six weeks. The study involved a treatment regime consisting of four capsules daily of **VASCAZEN®** and monitoring of blood Omega-3 levels over a six week period. The Open label study consisted of 143 study subjects enrolled for baseline Omega-3 Deficiency assessment, of which 63 subjects were scheduled to receive **VASCAZEN®** (3g EPA and DHA at a ratio of 6:1 EPA:DHA per day) for two weeks, and 31 patients received **VASCAZEN®** for six weeks. The primary endpoint was the subjects' Omega-Score™, presented as a percentage of total whole blood fatty acids. Subjects in the study had an average age of 51 years. This study revealed a baseline Omega-3 Deficiency[2] in over 84.5% of the study group participants, irrespective of age or sex (Table 1, Figure 1). **VASCAZEN®** treatment resulted in a significant (p<0.0001) improvement in Omega-3 blood levels within two weeks, raising the mean Omega-Score™ from 3.4% to 5.7%, and to 7.5% (p<0.0001) within six weeks (Table 2, Figure 2).
[See table above]

TABLE 1.
Study Participant Baseline Characteristics:
The average age of patients was 50.9 years, with a slightly, but not significant age difference observed between the male (52.1 years) and female (46.9 years) groups. Mean Omega-Score™ values were in the "very high risk"[2] quartile and nearly identical between males and females. The vast majority of patients in the study had Omega-Score™ values less than 6.1%, signifying at least a moderate level of risk. Results showed 84.5% of patients were at risk, with similar trends in both the male and female populations. Confidence interval (CI), "±" (means ± standard deviation).

	Patient Group		
	Total N=143	Males N=106	Females N=37
Age (years)	46.9±15.0	50.9±14.6	52.1±13.6
Omega-Score™ Mean	3.4±1.3	3.4±1.4	3.5±1.19
Mean 95% CI	3.2 to 3.6 (±1.1 to 1.6)	3.2 to 3.7 (±1.1 to 1.6)	3.2 to 3.7 (±1.0 to 1.4)
% of Patients at Risk (<6.1% Omega-Score™)	84.5	82.1	89.2

FIGURE 1. Study Participant Baseline Omega-Score™ Values.

Out of 143 study participants, the majority of patients had a baseline Omega-Score™ of less than 6.1%, indicating an Omega-3 Deficiency, irrespective of sex.
[See first table at top of next page]
VASCAZEN® rapidly increases patient group Omega-Score™ means with significant improvements (P<0.0001) as early as two weeks after treatment (3.4 at baseline, to 5.7 after two weeks). After four weeks, Omega-Score™ means surpass 6.1% into the "low risk" quartile, and remain in this range through week 6 (P<0.0001). At the beginning of the study, 84.5% of patients were Omega-3 Deficient, and by week six, only 13.2% of study subjects were deficient, illustrating the efficacy of **VASCAZEN®** for use as an aid in the dietary management of Omega-3 Deficiency. Confidence interval (CI), "±" (means ± standard deviation).
[See figure 2 at top of next column]
Study subjects were administered four capsules per day of **VASCAZEN®**, supplying 3g EPA and DHA per day and were monitored for safety and efficacy of increasing Omega-Score™ values from baseline levels. A significant improvement was observed within two weeks, with 86.8% of subjects reaching the low risk Omega-Score™ quartile within six weeks.

VASCAZEN®-REVEAL Trial
VASCAZEN® safety and efficacy was evaluated in a multicenter, double-blind, randomized, placebo-controlled trial. The study screened 655 candidates for Omega-3 plasma levels, and 89% were found to be Omega-3 Deficient. Of the 655

FIGURE 2. Six Week Treatment with VASCAZEN®

Omega-Score™ Improvement

	Week			
	0	2	4	6
Omega-Score™ Mean	3.4±1.3	5.7±1.9	7.9±2.4	7.5±1.2
95% CI	3.1 to 3.7 (±0.9 to 3.7)	5.4 to 6.3 (±1.4 to 2.3)	6.6 to 9.1 (±1.2 to 3.7)	7.0 to 8.0 (±0.7 to 1.7)
% of Patients at Risk (<6.1% Omega-Score™)	84.5%	43.2%	15%	13.2%

TABLE 3: Median Baseline, Percent Change, and Placebo-Adjusted Differences in Blood Lipids.

Blood Lipids mg/dL	VASCAZEN® 4 capsules/day		Placebo 4 capsules/day		Placebo-Adjusted	
	Baseline mg/dL	% Change[c]	Baseline mg/dL	% Change[c]	Difference %[d]	P-Value
Cohort 1 (TG 90-199mg/dL)						
Omega-3 Index[a]	3.81	127	3.56	3	124	**p<0.0001***
Omega-Score™[b]	3.64	132	3.68	0	132	**p<0.0001***
AA/EPA[e]	21	-86	21	7	-93	**p<0.0001***
TG	155	-6	131	2	-8	p=0.1140
VLDL-C	26	-2	27	0	-2	p=0.3426
Total-C	187	2	180	2	0	p=0.5033
HDL-C	41	-2	46	-2	-2	p=0.4160
LDL-C	116	7	103	1	6	p=0.1197
ApoB-100	102	6	90	3	3	p=0.3232
Non-HDL-C	145	3	125	3	-1	p=0.2227
Cohort 2 (TG 200-500mg/dL)						
Omega-3 Index	3.34	109	3.54	-3	112	**p<0.0001***
Omega-Score™	3.15	119	3.36	-2	121	**p<0.0001***
AA/EPA[d]	16	-75	15	11	-87	**p<0.0001***
TG	275	-47	264	0	-48	**p=0.0005***
Total-C	185	4	186	3	2	p=0.3642
VLDL-C	185	-30	36	0	-30	**P=0.0023***
HDL-C	39	3	39	-6	9	**p=0.0069***
LDL-C	115	13	102	2	11	p=0.1164
ApoB-100	105	2	100	2	-2	p=0.7440
Non-HDL-C	148	2	143	4	-2	p=0.6757

[a]Omega-3 Index = EPA + DHA in red blood cells (rbc) expressed as a percentage of total rbc fatty acids levels. [b]Omega-Score™ =EPA+DHA+DPA expressed as a percentage of total plasma fatty acids levels. [c]% Change = Median % Change from baseline . [d]Difference = Median of (**VASCAZEN®** Percent Change) – (Placebo Percent Change). [e]Arachidonic Acid (AA) / EPA, both expressed as a percentage of total plasma fatty acids levels. TG (Triglycerides), Total-C (Total Cholesterol), VLDL-C (Very Low Density Lipoprotein Cholesterol), HDL-C (High Density Lipoprotein Cholesterol), LDL-C (Low Density Lipoprotein Cholesterol), ApoB-100 (Apolipoprotein B-100), Non-HDL-C (Non High Density Lipoprotein Cholesterol). [s]Statistically Significant

screened subjects, 110 met all study inclusion and exclusion criteria including the requirement for being Omega-3 Deficient, with one or more risk factors for CVD were enrolled in the trial. Patients with CVD risk factors included hypertension (32%), overweight or obesity (81%, BMI>25), diabetes (13%), elevated TG, (65%, >150mg/dL), low HDL cholesterol (Men: 64%,<40mg/dL; Women: 73% <50mg/dL), elevated LDL cholesterol (65%). The enrolled subjects were stratified by TG levels (Cohort 1: 90-199mg/dL, or Cohort 2: 200-500mg/dL), randomized and treated with four(4) capsules/day of **VASCAZEN®** (supplying 3g/day of EPA and DHA) or corn oil (placebo) for eight weeks.

The results show that **VASCAZEN®** effectively corrected the Omega-3 Deficiency by increasing Omega-3 blood levels from those associated with "moderate to very high risk" to those associated with "low risk" of sudden death from cardiac causes.[1,2] Specifically, **VASCAZEN®** treatment of subjects with high TG (Cohort 2) resulted in a significant improvement (121%, p<0.0001) in median Omega-Score™ levels (Figure 3) and Omega-3 Index levels (112%, p<0.0001) within eight weeks with a placebo-adjusted 48% reduction of TG (p=0.0005), a 30% reduction on VLDL-C (p=0.0023), and a 9% increase in HDL-C (p=0.0069) without a statistically significant increase in LDL-C (p=0.1164) or other secondary endpoints (Table 3). In the normal to moderately high-TG group (Cohort 1), **VASCAZEN®** treatment also significantly corrected the Omega 3 Deficiency and improved patients' Omega-Score™ by 132% (p<0.0001) with a TG reduction trend (-8%, p=0.1140), and non-significant changes in other blood lipid parameters (Table 3). Correction of the Omega-3 Deficiency in both cohorts brought subjects from very high CVD risk category to low risk quartile, as stipulated by Albert et. al., 2002[2].

FIGURE 3. Correction of Omega-3 Deficiency (OM3D) with VASCAZEN® Treatment.

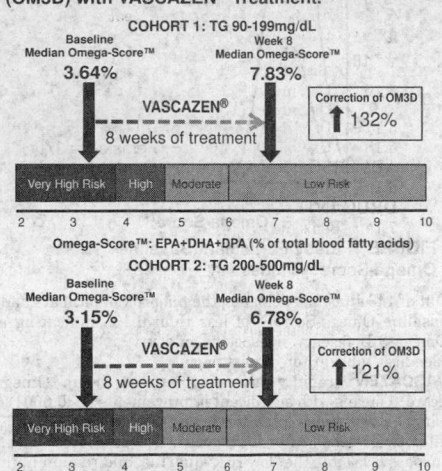

COHORT 1: TG 90-199mg/dL

Baseline Median Omega-Score™	Week 8 Median Omega-Score™
3.64%	7.83%

VASCAZEN®
8 weeks of treatment
Correction of OM3D ↑ 132%

Omega-Score™: EPA+DHA+DPA (% of total blood fatty acids)

COHORT 2: TG 200-500mg/dL

Baseline Median Omega-Score™	Week 8 Median Omega-Score™
3.15%	6.78%

VASCAZEN®
8 weeks of treatment
Correction of OM3D ↑ 121%

Omega-Score™: EPA+DHA+DPA (% of total blood fatty acids)

[See table 3 above]

ALLERGEN STATEMENT

VASCAZEN® contains fish oil and soy products. Patients with known hypersensitivity to fish or soy products should notify their physician.

ADVERSE REACTIONS

In an open label and a double-blind, randomized, placebo-controlled **VASCAZEN®**-REVEAL Trial, **VASCAZEN®** treatment for six to eight weeks was well-tolerated and adverse events were minimal and minor in degree with no severe adverse events reported. In the Open Label study, two subjects experienced a mild reflux/aftertaste, while an additional subject showed minor leg bruising that disappeared within three days. In the **VASCAZEN®**-REVEAL Trial, minor adverse reactions were reported: fishy burp (5% of patients),

flatulation (4% of patients), and nausea (4% of patients), although 5% of patients in the placebo group also experienced nausea.

FOOD EFFECTS

VASCAZEN® may be taken with or without other foods. Some patients may experience a fishy aftertaste/burp, and taking **VASCAZEN®** with food may help reduce this effect.

DRUG INTERACTIONS

Although clinical studies investigating the effect of **VASCAZEN®** plus anticoagulants have not been completed, caution should be taken when taking **VASCAZEN®** with anticoagulant drugs. Omega-3 fatty acids may extend bleeding time and patients receiving treatment with **VASCAZEN®** along with drugs that affect coagulation, should be monitored by a physician.

CAUTIONS

If you are pregnant, nursing or planning on becoming pregnant, ask your physician if **VASCAZEN®** is right for you. Safety studies have not yet been completed for the use of **VASCAZEN®** in pregnant or nursing women or pediatric pa-

tients (children under 18 years of age). Also, this product contains fish components and trace amounts of soy. Patients with a known hypersensitivity to any of the ingredients in **VASCAZEN®** should consult their physician prior to taking **VASCAZEN®**.

HOW SUPPLIED

VASCAZEN® capsules are supplied as transparent softgel capsules, filled with light yellow, ultra-purified fish oil. **VASCAZEN®** is manufactured according to Food and Drug Administration (FDA) current Good Manufacturing Practices (cGMP). Commercial product is supplied in 60-capsule cartons.

Commercial Product (60 Capsules)	27843-0172-46	Use Under Medical/ Physician Supervision.
Sample Product (15 Capsules)	27443-0172-48	Professional Samples (Not for sale)

PHYSICIAN SUPERVISION

VASCAZEN® is a Medical Food product dispensed by prescription only under ongoing physician supervision.

STORAGE

59-77°F (15-25°C). Keep from freezing. Protect from direct sunlight.

Manufactured by:

Captek Softgel Inc., Cerritos, CA, 90703

Manufactured for:

Pivotal Therapeutics (US), Inc.,

Boca Raton FL, 33431

P: 561-288-5231

Website: www.pivotaltherapeutics.us

REFERENCES

1. Siscovick DS, Raghunathan TE et. al. (1995). Dietary Intake and Cell Membrane Levels of Long-Chain n-3 Polyunsaturated Fatty Acids and the Risk of Primary Cardiac Arrest. JAMA. **274**:17;1363-1367.
2. Albert CM, Campos H, Stampfer MJ et al. (2002). Blood Levels of Long-Chain n-3 F atty Acids and the Risk of Sudden Death . New England Journal of Medicine **346**:1113-1118.
3. De Caterina R. (2011). N-3 Fatty Acids in Cardiovascular Disease. New England Journal of Medicine **364**:25;2439-2450.
4. Danaei G, Ding EL, Mozaffarian D. et al. (2009). The Preventable Causes of Death in the United States: Comparative Risk Assessment of Dietary, Lifestyle, and Metabolic Risk Factors. PLoS Medicine. 6(4):1-23.
5. Mozaffarian D, Lemaitre RN et. al. (2013) Plasma Phospholipid Long Chain Omega-3 Fatty Acids and Total and Cause-Specific Mortality in Older Adults: A Cohort Study. Annals of Internal Medicine 158(7):515-525.
6. Kris-Etherton PM, Harris WS et. al. (2002) Fish Consumption, Fish Oil, Omega-3 Fatty Acids, and Cardiovascular Disease. Circulation **106**:2747-2757.
7. Kris-Etherton PM, Taylor DS, et. al. (2000) Polyunsaturated fatty acid in the food chain in the United States. American Journal of Clinical Nutrition. **71(suppl)**:179S-88S.
8. Harris WS, Miller M. (2008) Omega-3 Fatty Acids and Coronary Heart Disease Risk: Clinical and Mechanistic Perspectives. Atherosclerosis. **197**:12-24.
9. GISSI-Prevenzione Investigators (1999). Dietary Supplementation with n-3 Polyunsaturated Fatty Acids and Vitamin E after Myocardial Infarction: Results of the GISSI-Prevenzione Trial. Lancet **354**:447-455.
10. Yokoyaa M, Origasa H, Matsuzaki M, et al. (2007). Effects of eicosapentaenoic acid on major coronary events in hypercholesterolaemic patients (JELIS): a randomised open- label, blinded endpoint analysis. Lancet. **369**:1090-1098.

VASCAZEN® is protected by a series of both issued and pending US and foreign patents.

Pivotal

THERAPEUTICS

Shown in Product Identification Guide, page 311

Purdue Pharma L.P.

ONE STAMFORD FORUM

STAMFORD, CT 06901-3431

For Medical Inquiries:

888-726-7535

Adverse Drug Experiences:

888-726-7535

Customer Service:

800-877-5666

FAX 800-877-3210

BUTRANS® ℞ Ⓒ

[*BYOO-trans*]

(buprenorphine)

Transdermal System for transdermal administration

HIGHLIGHTS OF PRESCRIBING INFORMATION

These highlights do not include all the information needed to use BUTRANS® safely and effectively. See full prescribing information for BUTRANS.

BUTRANS® (buprenorphine) Transdermal System for transdermal administration CIII

Initial U.S. Approval: 1981

WARNING: ADDICTION, ABUSE, and MISUSE; LIFE-THREATENING RESPIRATORY DEPRESSION; ACCIDENTAL EXPOSURE; and NEONATAL OPIOID WITH-

---

DRAWAL SYNDROME

See full prescribing information for complete boxed warning.

- BUTRANS exposes users to risks of addiction, abuse, and misuse, which can lead to overdose and death. Assess each patient's risk before prescribing, and monitor for development of these behaviors or conditions. (5.1, 10)
- Serious, life-threatening or fatal respiratory depression may occur. Monitor closely, especially upon initiation or following a dose increase. Instruct patients on proper administration of BUTRANS to reduce the risk. (5.2)
- Accidental exposure to BUTRANS, especially in children, can result in fatal overdose of buprenorphine. (5.2)
- Prolonged use of BUTRANS during pregnancy can result in neonatal opioid withdrawal syndrome, which may be life-threatening if not recognized and treated. If opioid use is required for a prolonged period in a pregnant woman, advise the patient of the risk of neonatal opioid withdrawal syndrome and ensure that appropriate treatment will be available. (5.3)

---RECENT MAJOR CHANGES---

Boxed Warning	04/2014
Indications and Usage (1)	04/2014
Dosage and Administration (2)	06/2014
Warnings and Precautions (5)	04/2014

---INDICATIONS AND USAGE---

BUTRANS is a partial opioid agonist product indicated for the management of pain severe enough to require daily, around-the-clock, long-term opioid treatment for which alternative treatment options are inadequate. (1)

Limitations of Use

- Because of the risks of addiction, abuse, and misuse with opioids, even at recommended doses, and because of the greater risks of overdose and death with extended-release opioid formulations, reserve BUTRANS for use in patients for whom alternative treatment options (e.g., non-opioid analgesics or immediate-release opioids) are ineffective, not tolerated, or would be otherwise inadequate to provide sufficient management of pain. (1)
- BUTRANS is not indicated as an as-needed (prn) analgesic. (1)

---DOSAGE AND ADMINISTRATION---

- BUTRANS doses of 7.5, 10, 15, and 20 mcg/hour are for opioid-experienced patients only. (2.1)
- For opioid-naïve patients, initiate with a 5 mcg/hour patch. (2.1)
- Instruct patients to wear BUTRANS for 7 days and to wait a minimum of 3 weeks before applying to the same site. (2.1)
- Do not abruptly discontinue BUTRANS in a physically dependent patient. (2.3)

---DOSAGE FORMS AND STRENGTHS---

Transdermal system: 5 mcg/hour, 7.5 mcg/hour, 10 mcg/hour, 15 mcg/hour, and 20 mcg/hour. (3)

---CONTRAINDICATIONS---

- Significant respiratory depression (4)
- Acute or severe bronchial asthma (4)
- Known or suspected paralytic ileus (4)
- Hypersensitivity to buprenorphine (4)

---WARNINGS AND PRECAUTIONS---

- Interactions with CNS depressants: Concomitant use may cause profound sedation, respiratory depression, and death. If coadministration is required, consider dose reduction of one or both drugs because of additive pharmacological effects. (5.4)
- Elderly, cachectic, debilitated patients, and those with chronic pulmonary disease: Monitor closely because of increased risk of respiratory depression. (5.5, 5.6)
- Avoid in patients with Long QT Syndrome, family history of Long QT Syndrome, or those taking Class IA or Class III antiarrhythmic medications. (5.7, 12.2)
- Hypotensive effects: Monitor during dose initiation and titration. (5.8)
- Patients with head injury or increased intracranial pressure: Monitor for sedation and respiratory depression and avoid use of BUTRANS in patients with impaired consciousness or coma susceptible to intracranial effects of CO_2 retention. (5.9)

---ADVERSE REACTIONS---

Most common adverse reactions (≥ 5%) include: nausea, headache, application site pruritus, dizziness, constipation, somnolence, vomiting, application site erythema, dry mouth, and application site rash. (6.1)

To report SUSPECTED ADVERSE REACTIONS, contact Purdue Pharma L.P. at 1-888-726-7535 or FDA at 1-800-FDA-1088 or *www.fda.gov/medwatch*.

---DRUG INTERACTIONS---

- Interaction with benzodiazepines: May increase buprenorphine-induced respiratory depression. Monitor patients on concurrent therapy closely. (7.1)
- CYP3A4 inhibitors/inducers: Initiating CYP3A4 inhibitors or discontinuing CYP3A4 inducers may result in an increase in buprenorphine plasma concentrations. Closely monitor patients starting CYP3A4 inhibitors or stopping CYP3A4 inducers for respiratory depression. (7.3)

---USE IN SPECIFIC POPULATIONS---

- Pregnancy: BUTRANS is not recommended for use during pregnancy. (8.1)
- Nursing Mothers: Buprenorphine has been detected in human milk. Closely monitor infants of nursing women receiving BUTRANS. (8.3)

See 17 for PATIENT COUNSELING INFORMATION and Medication Guide

Revised: 06/2014

FULL PRESCRIBING INFORMATION: CONTENTS*

WARNING: ADDICTION, ABUSE, and MISUSE; LIFE-THREATENING RESPIRATORY DEPRESSION; ACCIDENTAL EXPOSURE; and NEONATAL OPIOID WITHDRAWAL SYNDROME

FULL PRESCRIBING INFORMATION

WARNING: ADDICTION, ABUSE, and MISUSE; LIFE-THREATENING RESPIRATORY DEPRESSION; ACCIDENTAL EXPOSURE; and NEONATAL OPIOID WITHDRAWAL SYNDROME

Addiction, Abuse, and Misuse
BUTRANS® exposes patients and other users to the risks of opioid addiction, abuse, and misuse, which can lead to overdose and death. Assess each patient's risk prior to prescribing BUTRANS, and monitor all patients regularly for the development of these behaviors or conditions *[see Warnings and Precautions (5.1) and Overdosage (10)]*.

Life-Threatening Respiratory Depression
Serious, life-threatening, or fatal respiratory depression may occur with use of BUTRANS. Monitor for respiratory depression, especially during initiation of BUTRANS or following a dose increase. Misuse or abuse of BUTRANS by chewing, swallowing, snorting or injecting buprenorphine extracted from the transdermal system will result in the uncontrolled delivery of buprenorphine and pose a significant risk of overdose and death *[see Warnings and Precautions (5.2)]*.

Accidental Exposure
Accidental exposure to even one dose of BUTRANS, especially by children, can result in a fatal overdose of buprenorphine *[see Warnings and Precautions (5.2)]*.

Neonatal Opioid Withdrawal Syndrome
Prolonged use of BUTRANS during pregnancy can result in neonatal opioid withdrawal syndrome, which may be life-threatening if not recognized and treated, and requires management according to protocols developed by neonatology experts. If opioid use is required for a prolonged period in a pregnant woman, advise the patient of the risk of neonatal opioid withdrawal syndrome and ensure that appropriate treatment will be available *[see Warnings and Precautions (5.3)]*.

---

1 INDICATIONS AND USAGE

BUTRANS is indicated for the management of pain severe enough to require daily, around-the-clock, long-term opioid treatment and for which alternative treatment options are inadequate.
Limitations of Use
- Because of the risks of addiction, abuse and misuse with opioids, even at recommended doses, and because of the greater risk of overdose and death with extended-release opioid formulations, reserve BUTRANS for use in patients for whom alternative treatment options (e.g., non-opioid analgesics or immediate-release opioids) are ineffective, not tolerated, or would be otherwise inadequate to provide sufficient management of pain.
- BUTRANS is not indicated as an as-needed (prn) analgesic

2 DOSAGE AND ADMINISTRATION

2.1 Initial Dosing

BUTRANS should be prescribed only by healthcare professionals who are knowledgeable in the use of potent opioids for the management of chronic pain.
BUTRANS doses of 7.5, 10, 15, and 20 mcg/hour are for opioid-experienced patients only.
Initiate the dosing regimen for each patient individually; take into account the patient's prior analgesic treatment experience and risk factors for addiction, abuse, and misuse *[see Warnings and Precautions (5.1)]*. Monitor patients closely for respiratory depression, especially within the first 24-72 hours of initiating therapy with BUTRANS *[see Warnings and Precautions (5.2)]*.
BUTRANS is for transdermal use (on intact skin) only. Each BUTRANS patch is intended to be worn for 7 days.
Instruct patients not to use BUTRANS if the pouch seal is broken or the patch is cut, damaged, or changed in any way and not to cut BUTRANS.
Use of BUTRANS as the First Opioid Analgesic
Initiate treatment with BUTRANS with a 5 mcg/hour patch.
Conversion from Other Opioids to BUTRANS
Discontinue all other around-the-clock opioid drugs when BUTRANS therapy is initiated.
There is a potential for buprenorphine to precipitate withdrawal in patients who are already on opioids.
Prior Total Daily Dose of Opioid Less than 30 mg of Oral Morphine Equivalents per Day:
Initiate treatment with BUTRANS 5 mcg/hour at the next dosing interval (see Table 1 below, middle column).
Prior Total Daily Dose of Opioid Between 30 mg to 80 mg of Oral Morphine Equivalents per Day:

Taper the patient's current around-the-clock opioids for up to 7 days to no more than 30 mg of morphine or equivalent per day before beginning treatment with BUTRANS. Then initiate treatment with BUTRANS 10 mcg/hour at the next dosing interval (see Table 1 below, right column). Patients may use short-acting analgesics as needed until analgesic efficacy with BUTRANS is attained.
Prior Total Daily Dose of Opioid Greater than 80 mg of Oral Morphine Equivalents per Day:
BUTRANS 20 mcg/hour may not provide adequate analgesia for patients requiring greater than 80 mg/day oral morphine equivalents. Consider the use of an alternate analgesic.

Table 1: Initial BUTRANS Dose

Previous Opioid Analgesic Daily Dose (Oral Morphine Equivalent)	<30 mg	30-80 mg
Recommended BUTRANS Starting Dose	5 mcg/hour	10 mcg/hour

Conversion from Methadone to BUTRANS
Close monitoring is of particular importance when converting from methadone to other opioid agonists. The ratio between methadone and other opioid agonists may vary widely as a function of previous dose exposure. Methadone has a long half-life and can accumulate in the plasma.

2.2 Titration and Maintenance of Therapy

Individually titrate BUTRANS to a dose that provides adequate analgesia and minimizes adverse reactions. Continually reevaluate patients receiving BUTRANS to assess the maintenance of pain control and the relative incidence of adverse reactions, and monitor for the development of addiction, abuse, or misuse. Frequent communication is important among the prescriber, other members of healthcare team, the patient, and the caregiver/family during periods of changing analgesic requirements, including initial titration. During chronic therapy, periodically reassess the continued need for opioid analgesics.
The minimum BUTRANS titration interval is 72 hours, based on the pharmacokinetic profile and time to reach steady state levels *[see Clinical Pharmacology (12.3)]*.
The maximum BUTRANS dose is 20 mcg/hour. **Do not exceed a dose of one 20 mcg/hour BUTRANS system due to the risk of QTc interval prolongation.** In a clinical trial, BUTRANS 40 mcg/hour (given as two BUTRANS 20 mcg/hour systems) resulted in prolongation of the QTc interval *[see Warnings and Precautions (5.7) and Clinical Pharmacology (12.2)]*.
If the level of pain increases, attempt to identify the source of increased pain, while adjusting the BUTRANS dose to decrease the level of pain. Because steady-state plasma concentrations are achieved within 72 hours, BUTRANS dosage may be adjusted every 3 days. Dose adjustments may be made in 5 mcg/hour, 7.5 mcg/hour, or 10 mcg/hour increments by using no more than two patches of the 5 mcg/hour, 7.5 mcg/hour, or 10 mcg/hour system(s). The total dose from both patches should not exceed 20 mcg/hour. For the use of two patches, patients should be instructed to remove their current patch, and apply the two new patches at the same time, adjacent to one another at a different application site *[see Dosage and Administration (2.5)]*.
Patients who experience breakthrough pain may require dosage adjustment increase of BUTRANS, or may need rescue medication with an appropriate dose of an immediate-release analgesic. If the level of pain increases after dose stabilization, attempt to identify the source of increased pain before increasing the BUTRANS dose.
If unacceptable opioid-related adverse reactions are observed, the subsequent doses may be reduced. Adjust the dose to obtain an appropriate balance between the management of pain and opioid-related adverse reactions.

2.3 Cessation of Therapy

When the patient no longer requires therapy with BUTRANS, use a gradual downward titration of the dose every 7 days to prevent signs and symptoms of withdrawal in the physically dependent patient; consider introduction of an appropriate immediate-release opioid medication. Do not abruptly discontinue BUTRANS.

2.4 Patients with Hepatic Impairment

BUTRANS has not been evaluated in patients with severe hepatic impairment. As BUTRANS is only intended for 7-day application, consider use of an alternate analgesic that may permit more flexibility with the dosing in patients with severe hepatic impairment *[see Warnings and Precautions (5.10), Use in Specific Populations (8.6), and Clinical Pharmacology (12.3)]*.

2.5 Administration of BUTRANS

Instruct patients to apply immediately after removal from the individually sealed pouch. Instruct patients not to use BUTRANS if the pouch seal is broken or the patch is cut, damaged, or changed in any way. See the Instructions for Use for step-by-step instructions for applying BUTRANS.
Apply BUTRANS to the upper outer arm, upper chest, upper back or the side of the chest. These 4 sites (each present on both sides of the body) provide 8 possible application sites. Rotate BUTRANS among the 8 described skin sites. After BUTRANS removal, wait a minimum of 21 days before reapplying to the same skin site *[see Clinical Pharmacology (12.3)]*.
Apply BUTRANS to a hairless or nearly hairless skin site. If none are available, the hair at the site should be clipped, not shaven. Do not apply BUTRANS to irritated skin. If the application site must be cleaned, clean the site with water only. Do not use soaps, alcohol, oils, lotions, or abrasive devices. Allow the skin to dry before applying BUTRANS.
Incidental exposure of the BUTRANS patch to water, such as while bathing or showering is acceptable based on experience during clinical studies.
If problems with adhesion of BUTRANS occur, the edges may be taped with first aid tape. If problems with lack of adhesion continue, the patch may be covered with waterproof or semipermeable adhesive dressings suitable for 7 days of wear.
If BUTRANS falls off during the 7-day dosing interval, dispose of the transdermal system properly and place a new BUTRANS patch on at a different skin site.
When changing the system, instruct patients to remove BUTRANS and dispose of it properly *[see Dosage and Administration (2.6)]*.
If the buprenorphine-containing adhesive matrix accidentally contacts the skin, instruct patients or caregivers to wash the area with water and not to use soap, alcohol, or other solvents to remove the adhesive because they may enhance the absorption of the drug.

2.6 Disposal Instructions

Patients should refer to the Instructions for Use for proper disposal of BUTRANS. Dispose of used and unused patches by following the instructions on the Patch-Disposal Unit that is packaged with the BUTRANS patches.
Alternatively, patients can dispose of used patches by folding the adhesive side of the patch to itself, then flushing the patch down the toilet immediately upon removal. Unused patches should be removed from their pouches, the protective liners removed, the patches folded so that the adhesive side of the patch adheres to itself, and immediately flushed down the toilet.
Patients should dispose of any patches remaining from a prescription as soon as they are no longer needed.

3 DOSAGE FORMS AND STRENGTHS

BUTRANS is a rectangular or square, beige-colored system consisting of a protective liner and functional layers.
BUTRANS is available in five strengths:
- BUTRANS 5 mcg/hour Transdermal System (dimensions: 45 mm by 45 mm)
- BUTRANS 7.5 mcg/hour Transdermal System (dimensions: 58 mm by 45 mm)
- BUTRANS 10 mcg/hour Transdermal System (dimensions: 45 mm by 68 mm)
- BUTRANS 15 mcg/hour Transdermal System (dimensions: 59 mm by 72 mm)
- BUTRANS 20 mcg/hour Transdermal System (dimensions: 72 mm by 72 mm)

4 CONTRAINDICATIONS

BUTRANS is contraindicated in patients with:
- Significant respiratory depression
- Acute or severe bronchial asthma in an unmonitored setting or in the absence of resuscitative equipment
- Known or suspected paralytic ileus
- Hypersensitivity (e.g., anaphylaxis) to buprenorphine *[see Warnings and Precautions (5.12) and Adverse Reactions (6)]*

5 WARNINGS AND PRECAUTIONS

5.1 Addiction, Abuse, and Misuse

BUTRANS contains buprenorphine, a Schedule III controlled substance. As an opioid, BUTRANS exposes users to the risks of addiction, abuse, and misuse. As modified-release products such as BUTRANS deliver the opioid over an extended period of time, there is a greater risk for overdose and death, due to the larger amount of buprenorphine present.
Although the risk of addiction in any individual is unknown, it can occur in patients appropriately prescribed BUTRANS and in those who obtain the drug illicitly. Addiction can occur at recommended doses and if the drug is misused or abused *[see Drug Abuse and Dependence (9)]*.
Assess each patient's risk for opioid addiction, abuse, or misuse prior to prescribing BUTRANS, and monitor all patients receiving BUTRANS for the development of these behaviors or conditions. Risks are increased in patients with a personal or family history of substance abuse (including drug or alcohol abuse or addiction) or mental illness (e.g.,

major depression). The potential for these risks should not, however, prevent the proper management of pain in any given patient. Patients at increased risk may be prescribed modified-release opioid formulations such as BUTRANS, but use in such patients necessitates intensive counseling about the risks and proper use of BUTRANS, along with intensive monitoring for signs of addiction, abuse, or misuse. Abuse or misuse of BUTRANS by placing it in the mouth, chewing it, swallowing it, or using it in ways other than indicated may cause choking, overdose and death [see Overdosage (10)].

Opioid agonists such as BUTRANS are sought by drug abusers and people with addiction disorders and are subject to criminal diversion. Consider these risks when prescribing or dispensing BUTRANS. Strategies to reduce these risks include prescribing the drug in the smallest appropriate quantity and advising the patient on the proper disposal of unused drug [see Patient Counseling Information (17)]. Contact local state professional licensing board or state controlled substances authority for information on how to prevent and detect abuse or diversion of this product.

5.2   Life-Threatening Respiratory Depression
Serious, life-threatening, or fatal respiratory depression has been reported with the use of modified-release opioids, even when used as recommended. Respiratory depression, from opioid use, if not immediately recognized and treated, may lead to respiratory arrest and death. Management of respiratory depression may include close observation, supportive measures, and use of opioid antagonists, depending on the patient's clinical status [see Overdosage (10)]. Carbon dioxide (CO_2) retention from opioid-induced respiratory depression can exacerbate the sedating effects of opioids.

While serious, life-threatening, or fatal respiratory depression can occur at any time during the use of BUTRANS, the risk is greatest during the initiation of therapy or following a dose increase. Closely monitor patients for respiratory depression when initiating therapy with BUTRANS and following dose increases.

To reduce the risk of respiratory depression, proper dosing and titration of BUTRANS are essential [see Dosage and Administration (2)]. Overestimating the BUTRANS dose when converting patients from another opioid product can result in fatal overdose with the first dose.

Accidental exposure to BUTRANS, especially in children, can result in respiratory depression and death due to an overdose of buprenorphine.

5.3   Neonatal Opioid Withdrawal Syndrome
Prolonged use of BUTRANS during pregnancy can result in withdrawal signs in the neonate. Neonatal opioid withdrawal syndrome, unlike opioid withdrawal syndrome in adults, may be life-threatening if not recognized and treated, and requires management according to protocols developed by neonatology experts. If opioid use is required for a prolonged period in a pregnant woman, advise the patient of the risk of neonatal opioid withdrawal syndrome and ensure that appropriate treatment will be available.

Neonatal opioid withdrawal syndrome presents as irritability, hyperactivity and abnormal sleep pattern, high pitched cry, tremor, vomiting, diarrhea and failure to gain weight. The onset, duration, and severity of neonatal opioid withdrawal syndrome vary based on the specific opioid used, duration of use, timing and amount of last maternal use, and rate of elimination of the drug by the newborn.

5.4   Interactions with Central Nervous System Depressants
Hypotension, profound sedation, coma, respiratory depression, and death may result if BUTRANS is used concomitantly with alcohol or other (CNS) depressants (e.g., sedatives, anxiolytics, hypnotics, neuroleptics, other opioids).

When considering the use of BUTRANS in a patient taking a CNS depressant, assess the duration of use of the CNS depressant and the patient's response, including the degree of tolerance that has developed to CNS depression. Additionally, evaluate the patient's use of alcohol or illicit drugs that cause CNS depression. If the decision to begin BUTRANS therapy is made, start with BUTRANS 5 mcg/hour patch, monitor patients for signs of sedation and respiratory depression and consider using a lower dose of the concomitant CNS depressant [see Drug Interactions (7.2)].

5.5   Use in Elderly, Cachectic, and Debilitated Patients
Life-threatening respiratory depression is more likely to occur in elderly, cachectic, or debilitated patients as they may have altered pharmacokinetics or altered clearance compared to younger, healthier patients. Monitor such patients closely, particularly when initiating and titrating BUTRANS and when BUTRANS is given concomitantly with other drugs that depress respiration [see Warnings and Precautions (5.2)].

5.6   Use in Patients with Chronic Pulmonary Disease
Monitor patients with significant chronic obstructive pulmonary disease or cor pulmonale, and patients having a substantially decreased respiratory reserve, hypoxia, hypercapnia, or pre-existing respiratory depression for respira-

tory depression, particularly when initiating therapy and titrating with BUTRANS, as in these patients, even usual therapeutic doses of BUTRANS may decrease respiratory drive to the point of apnea [see Warnings and Precautions (5.2)]. Consider the use of alternative non-opioid analgesics in these patients if possible.

5.7   QTc Prolongation
A positive-controlled study of the effects of BUTRANS on the QTc interval in healthy subjects demonstrated no clinically meaningful effect at a BUTRANS dose of 10 mcg/hour; however, a BUTRANS dose of 40 mcg/hour (given as two BUTRANS 20 mcg/hour Transdermal Systems) was observed to prolong the QTc interval [see Dosage and Administration (2.2) and Clinical Pharmacology (12.2)].

Consider these observations in clinical decisions when prescribing BUTRANS to patients with hypokalemia or clinically unstable cardiac disease, including: unstable atrial fibrillation, symptomatic bradycardia, unstable congestive heart failure, or active myocardial ischemia. Avoid the use of BUTRANS in patients with a history of Long QT Syndrome or an immediate family member with this condition, or those taking Class IA antiarrhythmic medications (e.g., quinidine, procainamide, disopyramide) or Class III antiarrhythmic medications (e.g., sotalol, amiodarone, dofetilide).

5.8   Hypotensive Effects
BUTRANS may cause severe hypotension including orthostatic hypotension and syncope in ambulatory patients. There is an increased risk in patients whose ability to maintain blood pressure has already been compromised by a reduced blood volume or concurrent administration of certain CNS depressant drugs (e.g., phenothiazines or general anesthetics) [see Drug Interactions (7.2)]. Monitor these patients for signs of hypotension after initiating or titrating the dose of BUTRANS.

5.9   Use in Patients with Head Injury or Increased Intracranial Pressure
Monitor patients taking BUTRANS who may be susceptible to the intracranial effects of CO_2 retention (e.g., those with evidence of increased intracranial pressure or brain tumors) for signs of sedation and respiratory depression, particularly when initiating therapy with BUTRANS. BUTRANS may reduce respiratory drive, and the resultant CO_2 retention can further increase intracranial pressure. Opioids may also obscure the clinical course in a patient with a head injury.

Avoid the use of BUTRANS in patients with impaired consciousness or coma.

5.10   Hepatotoxicity
Although not observed in BUTRANS chronic pain clinical trials, cases of cytolytic hepatitis and hepatitis with jaundice have been observed in individuals receiving sublingual buprenorphine for the treatment of opioid dependence, both in clinical trials and in post-marketing adverse event reports. The spectrum of abnormalities ranges from transient asymptomatic elevations in hepatic transaminases to case reports of hepatic failure, hepatic necrosis, hepatorenal syndrome, and hepatic encephalopathy. In many cases, the presence of pre-existing liver enzyme abnormalities, infection with hepatitis B or hepatitis C virus, concomitant usage of other potentially hepatotoxic drugs, and ongoing injection drug abuse may have played a causative or contributory role. For patients at increased risk of hepatotoxicity (e.g., patients with a history of excessive alcohol intake, intravenous drug abuse or liver disease), obtain baseline liver enzyme levels and monitor periodically and during treatment with BUTRANS.

5.11   Application Site Skin Reactions
In rare cases, severe application site skin reactions with signs of marked inflammation including "burn," "discharge," and "vesicles" have occurred. Time of onset varies, ranging from days to months following the initiation of BUTRANS treatment. Instruct patients to promptly report the development of severe application site reactions and discontinue therapy.

5.12   Anaphylactic/Allergic Reactions
Cases of acute and chronic hypersensitivity to buprenorphine have been reported both in clinical trials and in the post-marketing experience. The most common signs and symptoms include rashes, hives, and pruritus. Cases of bronchospasm, angioneurotic edema, and anaphylactic shock have been reported. A history of hypersensitivity to buprenorphine is a contraindication to the use of BUTRANS.

5.13   Application of External Heat
Advise patients and their caregivers to avoid exposing the BUTRANS application site and surrounding area to direct external heat sources, such as heating pads or electric blankets, heat or tanning lamps, saunas, hot tubs, and heated water beds while wearing the system because an increase in absorption of buprenorphine may occur [see Clinical Pharmacology (12.3)]. Advise patients against exposure of the BUTRANS application site and surrounding area to hot water or prolonged exposure to direct sunlight. There is a po-

tential for temperature-dependent increases in buprenorphine released from the system resulting in possible overdose and death.

5.14   Patients with Fever
Monitor patients wearing BUTRANS systems who develop fever or increased core body temperature due to strenuous exertion for opioid side effects and adjust the BUTRANS dose if signs of respiratory or central nervous system depression occur.

5.15   Use in Patients with Gastrointestinal Conditions
BUTRANS is contraindicated in patients with paralytic ileus. Avoid the use of BUTRANS in patients with other GI obstruction.

The buprenorphine in BUTRANS may cause spasm of the sphincter of Oddi. Monitor patients with biliary tract disease, including acute pancreatitis, for worsening symptoms. Opioids may cause increases in the serum amylase.

5.16   Use in Patients with Convulsive or Seizure Disorders
The buprenorphine in BUTRANS may aggravate convulsions in patients with convulsive disorders, and may induce or aggravate seizures in some clinical settings. Monitor patients with a history of seizure disorders for worsened seizure control during BUTRANS therapy.

5.17   Driving and Operating Machinery
BUTRANS may impair the mental and physical abilities needed to perform potentially hazardous activities such as driving a car or operating machinery. Warn patients not to drive or operate dangerous machinery unless they are tolerant to the effects of BUTRANS and know how they will react to the medication.

5.18   Use in Addiction Treatment
BUTRANS has not been studied and is not approved for use in the management of addictive disorders.

6   ADVERSE REACTIONS
The following serious adverse reactions are described elsewhere in the labeling:
- Addiction, Abuse, and Misuse [see Warnings and Precautions (5.1)]
- Life-Threatening Respiratory Depression [see Warnings and Precautions (5.2)]
- QTc Prolongation [see Warnings and Precautions (5.7)]
- Neonatal Opioid Withdrawal Syndrome [see Warnings and Precautions (5.3)]
- Hypotensive Effects [see Warnings and Precautions (5.8)]
- Interactions with Other CNS Depressants [see Warnings and Precautions (5.4)]
- Application Site Skin Reactions [see Warnings and Precautions (5.11)]
- Anaphylactic/Allergic Reactions [see Warnings and Precautions (5.12)]
- Gastrointestinal Effects [see Warnings and Precautions (5.15)]
- Seizures [see Warnings and Precautions (5.16)]

6.1   Clinical Trial Experience
Because clinical trials are conducted under widely varying conditions, adverse reaction rates observed in the clinical trials of a drug cannot be directly compared to rates in the clinical trials of another drug and may not reflect the rates observed in practice.

A total of 5,415 patients were treated with BUTRANS in controlled and open-label chronic pain clinical trials. Nine hundred twenty-four subjects were treated for approximately six months and 183 subjects were treated for approximately one year. The clinical trial population consisted of patients with persistent moderate to severe pain.

The most common serious adverse drug reactions (all <0.1%) occurring during clinical trials with BUTRANS were: chest pain, abdominal pain, vomiting, dehydration, and hypertension/blood pressure increased.

The most common adverse events (≥ 2%) leading to discontinuation were: nausea, dizziness, vomiting, headache, and somnolence.

The most common adverse reactions (≥ 5%) reported by patients in clinical trials comparing BUTRANS 10 or 20 mcg/hour to placebo are shown in Table 2, and comparing BUTRANS 20 mcg/hour to BUTRANS 5 mcg/hour are shown in Table 3 below:

Table 2: Adverse Reactions Reported in ≥ 5% of Patients during the Open-Label Titration Period and Double-Blind Treatment Period: Opioid-Naïve Patients

MedDRA Preferred Term	Open-Label Titration Period BUTRANS (N = 1024)	Double-Blind Treatment Period BUTRANS (N = 256)	Placebo (N = 283)
Nausea	23%	13%	10%
Dizziness	10%	4%	1%

Headache	9%	5%	5%
Application site pruritus	8%	4%	7%
Somnolence	8%	2%	2%
Vomiting	7%	4%	1%
Constipation	6%	4%	1%

Table 3: Adverse Reactions Reported in ≥ 5% of Patients during the Open-Label Titration Period and Double-Blind Treatment Period: Opioid-Experienced Patients

MedDRA Preferred Term	Open-Label Titration Period BUTRANS	Double-Blind Treatment Period	
		BUTRANS 20	BUTRANS 5
	(N = 1160)	(N = 219)	(N = 221)
Nausea	14%	11%	6%
Application site pruritus	9%	13%	5%
Headache	9%	8%	3%
Somnolence	6%	4%	2%
Dizziness	5%	4%	2%
Constipation	4%	6%	3%
Application site erythema	3%	10%	5%
Application site rash	3%	8%	6%
Application site irritation	2%	6%	2%

The following table lists adverse reactions that were reported in at least 2.0% of patients in four placebo/active-controlled titration-to-effect trials.

Table 4: Adverse Reactions Reported in Titration-to-Effect Placebo/Active-Controlled Clinical Trials with Incidence ≥ 2%

MedDRA Preferred Term	BUTRANS (N = 392)	Placebo (N = 261)
Nausea	21%	6%
Application site pruritus	15%	12%
Dizziness	15%	7%
Headache	14%	9%
Somnolence	13%	4%
Constipation	13%	5%
Vomiting	9%	1%
Application site erythema	7%	2%
Application site rash	6%	6%
Dry mouth	6%	2%
Fatigue	5%	1%
Hyperhidrosis	4%	1%
Peripheral edema	3%	1%
Pruritus	3%	0%
Stomach discomfort	2%	0%

The adverse reactions seen in controlled and open-label studies are presented below in the following manner: most common (≥ 5%), common (≥ 1% to < 5%), and less common (< 1%).

The most common adverse reactions (≥ 5%) reported by patients treated with BUTRANS in the clinical trials were nausea, headache, application site pruritus, dizziness, constipation, somnolence, vomiting, application site erythema, dry mouth, and application site rash.

The common (≥ 1% to < 5%) adverse reactions reported by patients treated with BUTRANS in the clinical trials organized by MedDRA (Medical Dictionary for Regulatory Activities) System Organ Class were:

Gastrointestinal disorders: diarrhea, dyspepsia, and upper abdominal pain

General disorders and administration site conditions: fatigue, peripheral edema, application site irritation, pain, pyrexia, chest pain, and asthenia

Infections and infestations: urinary tract infection, upper respiratory tract infection, nasopharyngitis, influenza, sinusitis, and bronchitis

Injury, poisoning and procedural complications: fall

Metabolism and nutrition disorders: anorexia

Musculoskeletal and connective tissue disorders: back pain, arthralgia, pain in extremity, muscle spasms, musculoskeletal pain, joint swelling, neck pain, and myalgia

Nervous system disorders: hypoesthesia, tremor, migraine, and paresthesia

Psychiatric disorders: insomnia, anxiety, and depression

Respiratory, thoracic and mediastinal disorders: dyspnea, pharyngolaryngeal pain, and cough

Skin and subcutaneous tissue disorders: pruritus, hyperhidrosis, rash, and generalized pruritus

Vascular disorders: hypertension

Other less common adverse reactions, including those known to occur with opioid treatment, that were seen in < 1% of the patients in the BUTRANS trials include the following in alphabetical order:

Abdominal distention, abdominal pain, accidental injury, affect lability, agitation, alanine aminotransferase increased, angina pectoris, angioedema, apathy, application site dermatitis, asthma aggravated, bradycardia, chills, confusional state, contact dermatitis, coordination abnormal, dehydration, depersonalization, depressed level of consciousness, depressed mood, disorientation, disturbance in attention, diverticulitis, drug hypersensitivity, drug withdrawal syndrome, dry eye, dry skin, dysarthria, dysgeusia, dysphagia, euphoric mood, face edema, flatulence, flushing, gait disturbance, hallucination, hiccups, hot flush, hyperventilation, hypotension, hypoventilation, ileus, insomnia, libido decreased, loss of consciousness, malaise, memory impairment, mental impairment, mental status changes, miosis, muscle weakness, nervousness, nightmare, orthostatic hypotension, palpitations, psychotic disorder, respiration abnormal, respiratory depression, respiratory distress, respiratory failure, restlessness, rhinitis, sedation, sexual dysfunction, syncope, tachycardia, tinnitus, urinary hesitation, urinary incontinence, urinary retention, urticaria, vasodilatation, vertigo, vision blurred, visual disturbance, weight decreased, and wheezing.

7 DRUG INTERACTIONS

7.1 Benzodiazepines

There have been a number of reports regarding coma and death associated with the misuse and abuse of the combination of buprenorphine and benzodiazepines. In many, but not all of these cases, buprenorphine was misused by self-injection of crushed buprenorphine tablets. Preclinical studies have shown that the combination of benzodiazepines and buprenorphine altered the usual ceiling effect on buprenorphine-induced respiratory depression, making the respiratory effects of buprenorphine appear similar to those of full opioid agonists. Closely monitor patients with concurrent use of BUTRANS and benzodiazepines. Warn patients that it is extremely dangerous to self-administer benzodiazepines while taking BUTRANS, and warn patients to use benzodiazepines concurrently with BUTRANS only as directed by their physician.

7.2 CNS Depressants

The concomitant use of BUTRANS with other CNS depressants including sedatives, hypnotics, tranquilizers, general anesthetics, phenothiazines, other opioids, and alcohol can increase the risk of respiratory depression, profound sedation, coma and death. Monitor patients receiving CNS depressants and BUTRANS for signs of respiratory depression, sedation, and hypotension. When combined therapy with any of the above medications is considered, the dose of one or both agents should be reduced [see Dosage and Administration (2.2) and Warnings and Precautions (5.4)].

7.3 Drugs Affecting Cytochrome P450 Isoenzymes

Inhibitors of CYP3A4 and 2D6

Because the CYP3A4 isoenzyme plays a major role in the metabolism of buprenorphine, drugs that inhibit CYP3A4 activity may cause decreased clearance of buprenorphine which could lead to an increase in buprenorphine plasma concentrations and result in increased or prolonged opioid effects. These effects could be more pronounced with concomitant use of CYP2D6 and 3A4 inhibitors. If co-administration with BUTRANS is necessary, monitor patients for respiratory depression and sedation at frequent intervals and consider dose adjustments until stable drug effects are achieved [see Clinical Pharmacology (12.3)].

Inducers of CYP3A4

CYP450 3A4 inducers may induce the metabolism of buprenorphine and, therefore, may cause increased clearance of the drug which could lead to a decrease in buprenorphine plasma concentrations, lack of efficacy or, possibly, development of an abstinence syndrome in a patient who had developed physical dependence to buprenorphine.

After stopping the treatment of a CYP3A4 inducer, as the effects of the inducer decline, the buprenorphine plasma concentration will increase which could increase or prolong both the therapeutic and adverse effects, and may cause serious respiratory depression. If co-administration or discontinuation of a CYP3A4 inducer with BUTRANS is necessary, monitor for signs of opioid withdrawal and consider dose adjustments until stable drug effects are achieved [see Clinical Pharmacology (12.3)].

7.4 Muscle Relaxants

Buprenorphine may enhance the neuromuscular blocking action of skeletal muscle relaxants and produce an increased degree of respiratory depression. Monitor patients receiving muscle relaxants and BUTRANS for signs of respiratory depression that may be greater than otherwise expected.

7.5 Anticholinergics

Anticholinergics or other drugs with anticholinergic activity when used concurrently with opioid analgesics may result in increased risk of urinary retention and/or severe constipation, which may lead to paralytic ileus. Monitor patients for signs of urinary retention or reduced gastric motility when BUTRANS is used concurrently with anticholinergic drugs.

8 USE IN SPECIFIC POPULATIONS

8.1 Pregnancy

Clinical Considerations

Fetal/neonatal adverse reactions

Prolonged use of opioid analgesics during pregnancy for medical or nonmedical purposes can result in physical dependence in the neonate and neonatal opioid withdrawal syndrome shortly after birth. Observe newborns for symptoms of neonatal opioid withdrawal syndrome, such as poor feeding, diarrhea, irritability, tremor, rigidity, and seizures, and manage accordingly [see Warnings and Precautions (5.3)].

Teratogenic Effects - Pregnancy Category C

There are no adequate and well-controlled studies in pregnant women. BUTRANS should be used during pregnancy only if the potential benefit justifies the potential risk to the fetus.

In animal studies, buprenorphine caused an increase in the number of stillborn offspring, reduced litter size, and reduced offspring growth in rats at maternal exposure levels that were approximately 10 times that of human subjects who received one BUTRANS 20 mcg/hour, the maximum recommended human dose (MRHD).

Studies in rats and rabbits demonstrated no evidence of teratogenicity following BUTRANS or subcutaneous (SC) administration of buprenorphine during the period of major organogenesis. Rats were administered up to one BUTRANS 20 mcg/hour every 3 days (gestation days 6, 9, 12, & 15) or received daily SC buprenorphine up to 5 mg/kg (gestation days 6-17). Rabbits were administered four BUTRANS 20 mcg/hour every 3 days (gestation days 6, 9, 12, 15, 18, & 19) or received daily SC buprenorphine up to 5 mg/kg (gestation days 6-19). No teratogenicity was observed at any dose. AUC values for buprenorphine with BUTRANS application and SC injection were approximately 110 and 140 times, respectively, that of human subjects who received the MRHD of one BUTRANS 20 mcg/hour.

Non-Teratogenic Effects

In a peri- and post-natal study conducted in pregnant and lactating rats, administration of buprenorphine either as BUTRANS or SC buprenorphine was associated with toxicity to offspring. Buprenorphine was present in maternal milk. Pregnant rats were administered 1/4 of one BUTRANS 5 mcg/hour every 3 days or received daily SC buprenorphine at doses of 0.05, 0.5, or 5 mg/kg from gestation day 6 to lactation day 21 (weaning). Administration of BUTRANS or SC buprenorphine at 0.5 or 5 mg/kg caused maternal toxicity and an increase in the number of stillborns, reduced litter size, and reduced offspring growth at maternal exposure levels that were approximately 10 times that of human subjects who received the MRHD of one BUTRANS 20 mcg/hour. Maternal toxicity was also observed at the no observed adverse effect level (NOAEL) for offspring.

8.2 Labor and Delivery

Opioids cross the placenta and may produce respiratory depression in neonates. BUTRANS is not for use in women during and immediately prior to labor, when shorter acting analgesics or other analgesic techniques are more appropriate. Opioid analgesics can prolong labor through actions that temporarily reduce the strength, duration, and frequency of uterine contractions. However this effect is not consistent and may be offset by an increased rate of cervical dilatation, which tends to shorten labor.

8.3 Nursing Mothers

Buprenorphine is excreted in breast milk. The amount of buprenorphine received by the infant varies depending on the maternal plasma concentration, the amount of milk ingested by the infant, and the extent of first pass metabolism.

Withdrawal symptoms can occur in breast-feeding infants when maternal administration of buprenorphine is stopped. Because of the potential for adverse reactions in nursing infants from BUTRANS, a decision should be made whether to discontinue nursing or discontinue the drug, taking into account the importance of the drug to the mother.

8.4 Pediatric Use
The safety and efficacy of BUTRANS in patients under 18 years of age has not been established.

8.5 Geriatric Use
Of the total number of subjects in the clinical trials (5,415), BUTRANS was administered to 1,377 patients aged 65 years and older. Of those, 457 patients were 75 years of age and older. In the clinical program, the incidences of selected BUTRANS-related AEs were higher in older subjects. The incidences of application site AEs were slightly higher among subjects < 65 years of age than those ≥ 65 years of age for both BUTRANS and placebo treatment groups.

In a single-dose study of healthy elderly and healthy young subjects treated with BUTRANS 10 mcg/hour, the pharmacokinetics were similar. In a separate dose-escalation safety study, the pharmacokinetics in the healthy elderly and hypertensive elderly subjects taking thiazide diuretics were similar to those in the healthy young adults. In the elderly groups evaluated, adverse event rates were similar to or lower than rates in healthy young adult subjects, except for constipation and urinary retention, which were more common in the elderly. Although specific dose adjustments on the basis of advanced age are not required for pharmacokinetic reasons, use caution in the elderly population to ensure safe use [see Clinical Pharmacology (12.3)].

8.6 Hepatic Impairment
In a study utilizing intravenous buprenorphine, peak plasma levels (C_{max}) and exposure (AUC) of buprenorphine in patients with mild and moderate hepatic impairment did not increase as compared to those observed in subjects with normal hepatic function. BUTRANS has not been evaluated in patients with severe hepatic impairment. As BUTRANS is intended for 7-day dosing, consider the use of alternate analgesic therapy in patients with severe hepatic impairment [see Dosage and Administration (2.4) and Clinical Pharmacology (12.3)].

9 DRUG ABUSE AND DEPENDENCE
9.1 Controlled Substance
BUTRANS contains buprenorphine, a Schedule III controlled substance with an abuse potential similar to other Schedule III opioids. BUTRANS can be abused and is subject to misuse, addiction and criminal diversion [see Warnings and Precautions (5.1)].

9.2 Abuse
All patients treated with opioids require careful monitoring for signs of abuse and addiction, since use of opioid analgesic products carries the risk of addiction even under appropriate medical use.

Drug abuse is the intentional non-therapeutic use of an over-the-counter or prescription drug, even once, for its rewarding psychological or physiological effects. Drug abuse includes, but is not limited to the following examples: the use of a prescription or over-the-counter drug to get "high", or the use of steroids for performance enhancement and muscle build up.

Drug addiction is a cluster of behavioral, cognitive, and physiological phenomena that develop after repeated substance use and includes: a strong desire to take the drug, difficulties in controlling its use, persisting in its use despite harmful consequences, a higher priority given to drug use than to other activities and obligations, increased tolerance, and sometimes a physical withdrawal.

"Drug-seeking" behavior is very common to addicts and drug abusers. Drug-seeking tactics include emergency calls or visits near the end of office hours, refusal to undergo appropriate examination, testing or referral, repeated claims of loss of prescriptions, tampering with prescriptions and reluctance to provide prior medical records or contact information for other treating physician(s). "Doctor shopping" (visiting multiple prescribers) to obtain additional prescriptions is common among drug abusers and people suffering from untreated addiction. Preoccupation with achieving adequate pain relief can be appropriate behavior in a patient with poor pain control.

Abuse and addiction are separate and distinct from physical dependence and tolerance. Physicians should be aware that addiction may not be accompanied by concurrent tolerance and symptoms of physical dependence in all addicts. In addition, abuse of opioids can occur in the absence of true addiction.

BUTRANS, like other opioids, can be diverted for nonmedical use into illicit channels of distribution. Careful record-keeping of prescribing information, including quantity, frequency, and renewal requests, as required by state law, is strongly advised.

Proper assessment of the patient, proper prescribing practices, periodic re-evaluation of therapy, and proper dispensing and storage are appropriate measures that help to reduce abuse of opioid drugs.

Risks Specific to the Abuse of BUTRANS
BUTRANS is intended for transdermal use only. Abuse of BUTRANS poses a risk of overdose and death. This risk is increased with concurrent abuse of BUTRANS with alcohol and other substances including other opioids and benzodiazepines [see Warnings and Precautions (5.4) and Drug Interactions (7.2)]. Intentional compromise of the transdermal delivery system will result in the uncontrolled delivery of buprenorphine and pose a significant risk to the abuser that could result in overdose and death [see Warnings and Precautions (5.1)]. Abuse may occur by applying the transdermal system in the absence of legitimate purpose, or by swallowing, snorting, or injecting buprenorphine extracted from the transdermal system.

9.3 Dependence
Both tolerance and physical dependence can develop during chronic opioid therapy. Tolerance is the need for increasing doses of opioids to maintain a defined effect such as analgesia (in the absence of disease progression or other external factors). Tolerance may occur to both the desired and undesired effects of drugs, and may develop at different rates for different effects.

Physical dependence results in withdrawal symptoms after abrupt discontinuation or a significant dose reduction of a drug. Withdrawal also may be precipitated through the administration of drugs with opioid antagonist activity, e.g., naloxone, nalmefene, or mixed agonist/antagonist analgesics (pentazocine, butorphanol, nalbuphine). Physical dependence may not occur to a clinically significant degree until after several days to weeks of continued opioid usage.

BUTRANS should not be abruptly discontinued [see Dosage and Administration (2.3)]. If BUTRANS is abruptly discontinued in a physically-dependent patient, an abstinence syndrome may occur. Some or all of the following can characterize this syndrome: restlessness, lacrimation, rhinorrhea, yawning, perspiration, chills, myalgia, and mydriasis. Other signs and symptoms also may develop, including: irritability, anxiety, backache, joint pain, weakness, abdominal cramps, insomnia, nausea, anorexia, vomiting, diarrhea, or increased blood pressure, respiratory rate, or heart rate.

Infants born to mothers physically dependent on opioids will also be physically dependent and may exhibit respiratory difficulties and withdrawal symptoms [see Use in Specific Populations (8.1)].

10 OVERDOSAGE
Clinical Presentation
Acute overdosage with BUTRANS is manifested by respiratory depression, somnolence progressing to stupor or coma, skeletal muscle flaccidity, cold and clammy skin, constricted pupils, bradycardia, hypotension, partial or complete airway obstruction, atypical snoring and death. Marked mydriasis rather than miosis may be seen due to severe hypoxia in overdose situations.

Treatment of Overdose
In case of overdose, priorities are the re-establishment of a patent and protected airway and institution of assisted or controlled ventilation if needed. Employ other supportive measures (including oxygen, vasopressors) in the management of circulatory shock and pulmonary edema as indicated. Cardiac arrest or arrhythmias will require advanced life support techniques.

Naloxone may not be effective in reversing any respiratory depression produced by buprenorphine. High doses of naloxone, 10-35 mg/70 kg, may be of limited value in the management of buprenorphine overdose. The onset of naloxone effect may be delayed by 30 minutes or more. Doxapram hydrochloride (a respiratory stimulant) has also been used.

Remove BUTRANS immediately. Because the duration of reversal would be expected to be less than the duration of action of buprenorphine from BUTRANS, carefully monitor the patient until spontaneous respiration is reliably re-established. Even in the face of improvement, continued medical monitoring is required because of the possibility of extended effects as buprenorphine continues to be absorbed from the skin. After removal of BUTRANS, the mean buprenorphine concentrations decrease approximately 50% in 12 hours (range 10-24 hours) with an apparent terminal half-life of approximately 26 hours. Due to this long apparent terminal half-life, patients may require monitoring and treatment for at least 24 hours.

In an individual physically dependent on opioids, administration of an opioid receptor antagonist may precipitate an acute withdrawal. The severity of the withdrawal produced will depend on the degree of physical dependence and the dose of the antagonist administered. If a decision is made to treat serious respiratory depression in the physically dependent patient with an opioid antagonist, administration of the antagonist should be begun with care and by titration with smaller than usual doses of the antagonist.

11 DESCRIPTION
BUTRANS is a transdermal system providing systemic delivery of buprenorphine, a mu opioid partial agonist analge-

sic, continuously for 7 days. The chemical name of buprenorphine is 6,14-ethenomorphinan-7-methanol, 17-(cyclopropylmethyl)- α-(1,1-dimethylethyl)-4, 5-epoxy-18, 19-dihydro-3-hydroxy-6-methoxy-α-methyl-, [5α, 7α, (S)]. The structural formula is:

The molecular weight of buprenorphine is 467.6; the empirical formula is $C_{29}H_{41}NO_4$. Buprenorphine occurs as a white or almost white powder and is very slightly soluble in water, freely soluble in acetone, soluble in methanol and ether, and slightly soluble in cyclohexane. The pKa is 8.5 and the melting point is about 217°C.

System Components and Structure
Five different strengths of BUTRANS are available: 5, 7.5, 10, 15, and 20 mcg/hour (Table 5). The proportion of buprenorphine mixed in the adhesive matrix is the same in each of the five strengths. The amount of buprenorphine released from each system per hour is proportional to the active surface area of the system. The skin is the limiting barrier to diffusion from the system into the bloodstream.

Table 5: BUTRANS Product Specifications

Buprenorphine Delivery Rate (mcg/hour)	Active Surface Area (cm²)	Total Buprenorphine Content (mg)
BUTRANS 5	6.25	5
BUTRANS 7.5	9.375	7.5
BUTRANS 10	12.5	10
BUTRANS 15	18.75	15
BUTRANS 20	25	20

BUTRANS is a rectangular or square, beige-colored system consisting of a protective liner and functional layers. Proceeding from the outer surface toward the surface adhering to the skin, the layers are (1) a beige-colored web backing layer; (2) an adhesive rim without buprenorphine; (3) a separating layer over the buprenorphine-containing adhesive matrix; (4) the buprenorphine-containing adhesive matrix; and (5) a peel-off release liner. Before use, the release liner covering the adhesive layer is removed and discarded.

1. Backing Layer   2. Overlapping Adhesive Film   3. Separating Layer
4. Drug/Polymer Adhesive Matrix   5. Peel-off Release Liner

Figure 1: Cross-Section Diagram of BUTRANS (not to scale).

The active ingredient in BUTRANS is buprenorphine. The inactive ingredients in each system are: levulinic acid, oleyl oleate, povidone, and polyacrylate cross-linked with aluminum.

12 CLINICAL PHARMACOLOGY
12.1 Mechanism of Action
Buprenorphine is a partial agonist at mu opioid receptors. Buprenorphine is also an antagonist at kappa-opioid receptors, an agonist at delta-opioid receptors, and a partial agonist at ORL-1 (nociceptin) receptors. The contributions of these actions to its analgesic profile are unclear.

12.2 Pharmacodynamics
Effects on the Central Nervous System
The principal actions of therapeutic value of buprenorphine are analgesia and sedation. Specific CNS opiate receptors and endogenous compounds with morphine-like activity have been identified throughout the brain and spinal cord and are likely to play a role in the expression of analgesic effects.

Buprenorphine produces respiratory depression by direct action on brainstem respiratory centers. The mechanism of respiratory depression involves a reduction in the responsiveness of the brainstem respiratory centers to increases in carbon dioxide tension, and to electrical stimulation.

Buprenorphine causes miosis, even in total darkness, and little tolerance develops to this effect. Pinpoint pupils are a sign of opioid overdose but are not pathognomonic (e.g., pontine lesions of hemorrhagic or ischemic origins may produce similar findings). Marked mydriasis rather than miosis may be seen with worsening hypoxia in the setting of buprenorphine overdose.

Effects on the Gastrointestinal Tract and Other Smooth Muscle

Gastric, biliary, and pancreatic secretions are decreased by buprenorphine. Buprenorphine causes a reduction in motility associated with an increase in tone in the antrum of the stomach and duodenum. Digestion of food in the small intestine is delayed and propulsive contractions are decreased. Propulsive peristaltic waves in the colon are decreased, while tone is increased to the point of spasm. The end result is constipation. Buprenorphine can cause a marked increase in biliary tract pressure as a result of spasm of the sphincter of Oddi.

Effects on the Cardiovascular System

Buprenorphine may cause a reduction in blood pressure.

Effects on Cardiac Electrophysiology

The effect of BUTRANS 10 mcg/hour and 2 × BUTRANS 20 mcg/hour on QTc interval was evaluated in a double-blind (BUTRANS vs. placebo), randomized, placebo and active-controlled (moxifloxacin 400 mg, open label), parallel-group, dose-escalating, single-dose study in 132 healthy male and female subjects aged 18 to 55 years. The dose escalation sequence for BUTRANS during the titration period was: BUTRANS 5 mcg/hour for 3 days, then BUTRANS 10 mcg/hour for 3 days, then BUTRANS 20 mcg/hour for 3 days, then 2 × BUTRANS 20 mcg/hour for 4 days. The QTc evaluation was performed during the third day of BUTRANS 10 mcg/hour and the fourth day of 2 × BUTRANS 20 mcg/hour when the plasma levels of buprenorphine were at steady state for the corresponding doses [see Warnings and Precautions (5.7)].

There was no clinically meaningful effect on mean QTc with a BUTRANS dose of 10 mcg/hour. A BUTRANS dose of 40 mcg/hour (given as two 20 mcg/hour BUTRANS Transdermal Systems) prolonged mean QTc by a maximum of 9.2 (90% CI: 5.2-13.3) msec across the 13 assessment time points.

Effects on the Endocrine System

Opioids inhibit the secretion of ACTH, cortisol, and luteinizing hormone (LH) in humans. They also stimulate prolactin, growth hormone (GH) secretion, and pancreatic secretion of insulin and glucagon.

Effects on the Immune System

Opioids have been shown to have a variety of effects on components of the immune system in in vitro and animal models. The clinical significance of these findings is unknown. Overall, the effects of opioids appear to be modestly immunosuppressive.

12.3   Pharmacokinetics

Absorption

Each BUTRANS system provides delivery of buprenorphine for 7 days. Steady state was achieved during the first application by Day 3 (see Figure 2).

Figure 2 Mean (SD) Buprenorphine Plasma Concentrations Following Three Consecutive Applications of BUTRANS 10 mcg/hour (N = 36 Healthy Subjects)

BUTRANS 5, 10, and 20 mcg/hour provide dose-proportional total buprenorphine exposures (AUC) following 7-day applications. BUTRANS single 7-day application and steady-state pharmacokinetic parameters are summarized in Table 6. Plasma buprenorphine concentrations after titration showed no further change over the 60-day period studied.

Table 6: Pharmacokinetic Parameters of BUTRANS in Healthy Subjects, Mean (%CV)

Single 7-day Application	AUC_{inf} (pg.h/mL)	C_{max} (pg/mL)
BUTRANS 5 mcg/hour	12087 (37)	176 (67)
BUTRANS 10 mcg/hour	27035 (29)	191 (34)
BUTRANS 20 mcg/hour	54294 (36)	471 (49)
Multiple 7-day Applications	$AUC_{tau,ss}$ (pg.h/mL)	$C_{max,ss}$ (pg/mL)
BUTRANS 10 mcg/hour, steady-state	27543 (33)	224 (35)

Transdermal delivery studies showed that intact human skin is permeable to buprenorphine. In clinical pharmacol-

ogy studies, the median time for BUTRANS 10 mcg/hour to deliver quantifiable buprenorphine concentrations (≥ 25 pg/mL) was approximately 17 hours.

The absolute bioavailability of BUTRANS relative to IV administration, following a 7-day application, is approximately 15% for all doses (BUTRANS 5, 10, and 20 mcg/hour).

Effects of Application Site

A study in healthy subjects demonstrated that the pharmacokinetic profile of buprenorphine delivered by BUTRANS 10 mcg/hour is similar when applied to the upper outer arm, upper chest, upper back, or the side of the chest [see Dosage and Administration (2.5)].

The reapplication of BUTRANS 10 mcg/hour after various rest periods to the same application site in healthy subjects showed that the minimum rest period needed to avoid variability in drug absorption is 3 weeks (21 days) [see Dosage and Administration (2.5)].

Effects of Heat

In a study of healthy subjects, application of a heating pad directly on the BUTRANS 10 mcg/hour system caused a 26% - 55% increase in blood concentrations of buprenorphine. Concentrations returned to normal within 5 hours after the heat was removed. For this reason, instruct patients not to apply heating pads directly to the BUTRANS system during system wear [see Warnings and Precautions (5.13)].

Fever may increase the permeability of the skin, leading to increased buprenorphine concentrations during BUTRANS treatment. As a result, febrile patients are at increased risk for the possibility of BUTRANS-related reactions during treatment with BUTRANS. Monitor patients with febrile illness for adverse effects and consider dose adjustment [see Warnings and Precautions (5.14)]. In a crossover study of healthy subjects receiving endotoxin or placebo challenge during BUTRANS 10 mcg/hour wear, the AUC and C_{max} were similar despite a physiologic response of mild fever to endotoxin.

Distribution

Buprenorphine is approximately 96% bound to plasma proteins, mainly to alpha- and beta-globulin.

Studies of IV buprenorphine have shown a large volume of distribution (approximately 430 L), implying extensive distribution of buprenorphine.

CSF buprenorphine concentrations appear to be approximately 15-25% of concurrent plasma concentrations.

Metabolism

Buprenorphine metabolism in the skin following BUTRANS application is negligible.

Buprenorphine primarily undergoes N-dealkylation by CYP3A4 to norbuprenorphine and glucuronidation by UGT-isoenzymes (mainly UGT1A1 and 2B7) to buprenorphine 3β-O-glucuronide. Norbuprenorphine, the major metabolite, is also glucuronidated (mainly UGT1A3) prior to excretion. Norbuprenorphine is the only known active metabolite of buprenorphine. It has been shown to be a respiratory depressant in rats, but only at concentrations at least 50-fold greater than those observed following application to humans of BUTRANS 20 mcg/hour.

Elimination

Following IV administration, buprenorphine and its metabolites are secreted into bile and excreted in urine.

Following intramuscular administration of 2 mcg/kg dose of buprenorphine, approximately 70% of the dose was excreted in feces within 7 days. Approximately 27% was excreted in urine.

Following transdermal application, buprenorphine is eliminated via hepatic metabolism, with subsequent biliary excretion and renal excretion of soluble metabolites. After removal of BUTRANS, mean buprenorphine concentrations decrease approximately 50% within 10-24 hours, followed by decline with an apparent terminal half-life of approximately 26 hours. Since metabolism and excretion of buprenorphine occur mainly via hepatic elimination, reductions in hepatic blood flow induced by some general anesthetics (e.g., halothane) and other drugs may result in a decreased rate of hepatic elimination of the drug, leading to increased plasma concentrations.

The total clearance of buprenorphine is approximately 55 L/hour in postoperative patients.

Drug Interactions

Effect of CYP3A4 inhibitors

In a drug-drug interaction study, BUTRANS 10 mcg/hour (single dose × 7 days) was co-administered with 200 mg ketoconazole, a strong CYP3A4 inhibitor or ketoconazole placebo twice daily for 11 days and the pharmacokinetics of buprenorphine and its metabolites were evaluated. Plasma buprenorphine concentrations did not accumulate during co-medication with ketoconazole 200 mg twice daily. Based on the results from this study, metabolism during therapy with BUTRANS is not expected to be affected by co-administration of CYP3A4 inhibitors [see Drug Interactions (7.3)].

Antiretroviral agents have been evaluated for CYP3A4 mediated interactions with sublingual buprenorphine. Nucleoside reverse transcriptase inhibitors (NRTIs) and non-nucleoside reverse transcriptase inhibitors (NNRTIs) do not appear to have clinically significant interactions with buprenorphine. However, certain protease inhibitors (PIs) with CYP3A4 inhibitory activity such as atazanavir and atazanavir/ritonavir resulted in elevated levels of buprenorphine and norbuprenorphine when buprenorphine and naloxone were administered sublingually. C_{max} and AUC for buprenorphine increased by up to 1.6 and 1.9 fold, and C_{max} and AUC for norbuprenorphine increased by up to 1.6 and 2.0 fold respectively, when sublingual buprenorphine was administered with these PIs. Patients in this study reported increased sedation, and symptoms of opiate excess have been found in post-marketing reports of patients receiving buprenorphine and atazanavir with and without ritonavir concomitantly. It should be noted that atazanavir is both a CYP3A4 and UGT1A1 inhibitor. As such, the drug-drug interaction potential for buprenorphine with CYP3A4 inhibitors is likely to be dependent on the route of administration as well as the specificity of enzyme inhibition [see Drug Interactions (7.3)].

Effect of CYP3A4 Inducers

The interaction between buprenorphine and CYP3A4 inducers has not been studied.

Specific Populations

Geriatric Patients

Following a single application of BUTRANS 10 mcg/hour to 12 healthy young adults (mean age 32 years) and 12 healthy elderly subjects (mean age 72 years), the pharmacokinetic profile of BUTRANS was similar in healthy elderly and healthy young adult subjects, though the elderly subjects showed a trend toward higher plasma concentrations immediately after BUTRANS removal. Both groups eliminated buprenorphine at similar rates after system removal [see Use in Specific Populations (8.5)].

In a study of healthy young subjects, healthy elderly subjects, and elderly subjects treated with thiazide diuretics, BUTRANS at a fixed dose-escalation schedule (BUTRANS 5 mcg/hour for 3 days, followed by BUTRANS 10 mcg/hour for 3 days and BUTRANS 20 mcg/hour for 7 days) produced similar mean plasma concentration vs. time profiles for each of the three subject groups. There were no significant differences between groups in buprenorphine C_{max} or AUC [see Use in Specific Populations (8.5)].

Pediatric Patients

BUTRANS has not been studied in children and is not recommended for pediatric use.

Gender

In a pooled data analysis utilizing data from several studies that administered BUTRANS 10 mcg/hour to healthy subjects, no differences in buprenorphine C_{max} and AUC or body-weight normalized C_{max} and AUC were observed between males and females treated with BUTRANS.

Renal Impairment

No studies in patients with renal impairment have been performed with BUTRANS.

In an independent study, the effect of impaired renal function on buprenorphine pharmacokinetics after IV bolus and after continuous IV infusion administrations was evaluated. It was found that plasma buprenorphine concentrations were similar in patients with normal renal function and in patients with impaired renal function or renal failure. In a separate investigation of the effect of intermittent hemodialysis on buprenorphine plasma concentrations in chronic pain patients with end-stage renal disease who were treated with a transdermal buprenorphine product (marketed outside the US) up to 70 mcg/hour, no significant differences in buprenorphine plasma concentrations before or after hemodialysis were observed.

No notable relationship was observed between estimated creatinine clearance rates and steady-state buprenorphine concentrations among patients during BUTRANS therapy.

Hepatic Impairment

The pharmacokinetics of buprenorphine following an IV infusion of 0.3 mg of buprenorphine were compared in 8 patients with mild impairment (Child-Pugh A), 4 patients with moderate impairment (Child-Pugh B) and 12 subjects with normal hepatic function. Buprenorphine and norbuprenorphine exposure did not increase in the mild and moderate hepatic impairment patients.

BUTRANS has not been evaluated in patients with severe (Child-Pugh C) hepatic impairment [see Dosage and Administration (2.4), Warnings and Precautions (5.10), and Use in Specific Populations (8.6)].

13   NONCLINICAL TOXICOLOGY

13.1   Carcinogenesis, Mutagenesis, Impairment of Fertility

Carcinogenesis

Buprenorphine administered daily by skin painting to Sprague Dawley rats for 100 weeks at dosages (20, 60, or 200 mg/kg) produced systemic exposures (based on AUC) that ranged from approximately 130 to 350 times that of human subjects administered the maximum recommended human dose (MRHD) of BUTRANS 20 mcg/hour. An increased incidence of benign testicular interstitial cell tumors, considered buprenorphine treatment-related, was observed in male rats compared with concurrent controls. The tumor incidence was also above the highest incidence in the historical control database of the testing facility. These tumors were noted at 60 mg/kg/day and higher at approximately 220 times the proposed MRHD based on AUC. The no observed effect level (NOEL) was 20 mg/kg/day (approximately 140 times the proposed MRHD based on AUC). The mechanism leading to the tumor findings and the relevance to humans is unknown.

Buprenorphine was administered by skin painting to hemizygous Tg.AC mice over a 6-month study period. At the dosages administered daily (18.75, 37.5, 150, or 600 mg/kg/day), buprenorphine was not carcinogenic or tumorigenic at systemic exposure to buprenorphine, based on AUC, of up to approximately 1000 times that of human subjects administered BUTRANS 20 mcg/hour, the MRHD.

Mutagenesis

Buprenorphine was not genotoxic in 3 *in vitro* genetic toxicology studies (bacterial mutagenicity test, mouse lymphoma assay, chromosomal aberration assay in human peripheral blood lymphocytes), and in one *in vivo* mouse micronucleus test.

Impairment of Fertility

BUTRANS (1/4 of a BUTRANS 5 mcg/hour, one BUTRANS 5 mcg/hour, or one BUTRANS 20 mcg/hour every 3 days in males for 4 weeks prior to mating for a total of 10 weeks and in females for 2 weeks prior to mating through gestation day 7) had no effect on fertility or general reproductive performance of rats at AUC-based exposure levels as high as approximately 65 times (females) and 100 times (males) that for human subjects who received BUTRANS 20 mcg/hour, the MRHD.

14 CLINICAL STUDIES

The efficacy of BUTRANS has been evaluated in four 12-week double-blind, controlled clinical trials in opioid-naïve and opioid-experienced patients with moderate to severe chronic low back pain or osteoarthritis using pain scores as the primary efficacy variable. Two of these studies, described below, demonstrated efficacy in patients with low back pain. One study in low back pain and one study in osteoarthritis did not show a statistically significant pain reduction for either BUTRANS or the respective active comparators.

12-Week Study in Opioid-Naïve Patients with Chronic Low Back Pain

A total of 1,024 patients with chronic low back pain who were suboptimally responsive to their non-opioid therapy entered an open-label, dose-titration period for up to four weeks. Patients initiated therapy with three days of treatment with BUTRANS 5 mcg/hour. After three days, if adverse events were tolerated, the dose was increased to BUTRANS 10 mcg/hour. If adverse effects were tolerated but adequate analgesia was not reached, the dose was increased to BUTRANS 20 mcg/hour for an additional 10-12 days. Patients who achieved adequate analgesia and tolerable adverse effects on BUTRANS 10 or 20 mcg/hour were then randomized to remain on their titrated dose of BUTRANS or matching placebo. Fifty-three percent of the patients who entered the open-label titration period were able to titrate to a tolerable and effective dose and were randomized into a 12-week, double-blind treatment period. Twenty-three percent of patients discontinued due to an adverse event from the open-label titration period and 14% discontinued due to lack of a therapeutic effect. The remaining 10% of patients were dropped due to various administrative reasons.

During the first seven days of double-blind treatment patients were allowed up to two tablets per day of immediate-release oxycodone 5 mg as supplemental analgesia to minimize opioid withdrawal symptoms in patients randomized to placebo. Thereafter, the supplemental analgesia was limited to either acetaminophen 500 mg or ibuprofen 200 mg at a maximum of four tablets per day. Sixty-six percent of the patients treated with BUTRANS completed the 12-week treatment compared to 70% of the patients treated with placebo. Of the 256 patients randomized to BUTRANS, 9% discontinued due to lack of efficacy and 16% due to adverse events. Of the 283 patients randomized to placebo, 13% discontinued due to lack of efficacy and 7% due to adverse events.

Of the patients who were randomized, the mean pain (SE) NRS scores were 7.2 (0.08) and 7.2 (0.07) at screening and 2.6 (0.08) and 2.6 (0.07) at pre-randomization (beginning of double-blind phase) for the BUTRANS and placebo groups, respectively.

The score for average pain over the last 24 hours at the end of the study (Week 12/Early Termination) was statistically significantly lower for patients treated with BUTRANS compared with patients treated with placebo. The proportion of patients with various degrees of improvement, from screening to study endpoint, is shown in Figure 3 below.

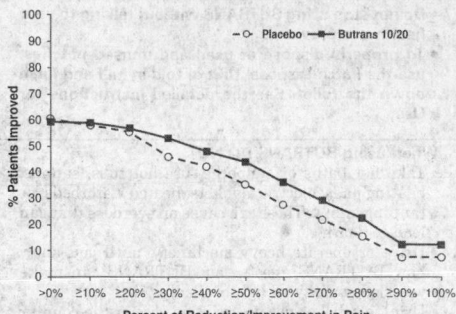

Figure 3: Percent Reduction in Pain Intensity

12-Week Study in Opioid-Experienced Patients with Chronic Low Back Pain

One thousand one hundred and sixty (1,160) patients on chronic opioid therapy (total daily dose 30-80 mg morphine equivalent) entered an open-label, dose-titration period with BUTRANS for up to 3 weeks, following taper of prior opioids. Patients initiated therapy with BUTRANS 10 mcg/hour for three days. After three days, if the patient tolerated the adverse effects, the dose was increased to BUTRANS 20 mcg/hour for up to 18 days. Patients with adequate analgesia and tolerable adverse effects on BUTRANS 20 mcg/hour were randomized to remain on BUTRANS 20 mcg/hour or were switched to a low-dose control (BUTRANS 5 mcg/hour) or an active control. Fifty-seven percent of the patients who entered the open-label titration period were able to titrate to and tolerate the adverse effects of BUTRANS 20 mcg/hour and were randomized into a 12-week double-blind treatment phase. Twelve percent of patients discontinued due to an adverse event and 21% discontinued due to lack of a therapeutic effect during the open-label titration period.

During the double-blind period, patients were permitted to take ibuprofen (200 mg tablets) or acetaminophen (500 mg tablets) every 4 hours as needed for supplemental analgesia (up to 3200 mg of ibuprofen and 4 grams of acetaminophen daily). Sixty-seven percent of patients treated with BUTRANS 20 mcg/hour and 58% of patients treated with BUTRANS 5 mcg/hour completed the 12-week treatment. Of the 219 patients randomized to BUTRANS 20 mcg/hour, 11% discontinued due to lack of efficacy and 13% due to adverse events. Of the 221 patients randomized to BUTRANS 5 mcg/hour, 24% discontinued due to lack of efficacy and 6% due to adverse events.

Of the patients who were able to be randomized in the double-blind period, the mean pain (SE) NRS scores were 6.4 (0.08) and 6.5 (0.08) at screening and were 2.8 (0.08) and 2.9 (0.08) at pre-randomization (beginning of Double-Blind Period) for the BUTRANS 5 mcg/hour and BUTRANS 20 mcg/hour, respectively.

The score for average pain over the last 24 hours at Week 12 was statistically significantly lower for subjects treated with BUTRANS 20 mcg/hour compared to subjects treated with BUTRANS 5 mcg/hour. A higher proportion of BUTRANS 20 mcg/hour patients (49%) had at least a 30% reduction in pain score from screening to study endpoint when compared to BUTRANS 5 mcg/hour patients (33%). The proportion of patients with various degrees of improvement from screening to study endpoint is shown in Figure 4 below.

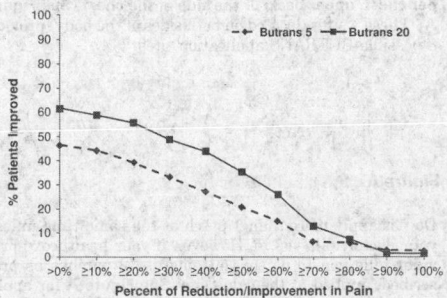

Figure 4: Percent Reduction in Pain Intensity

16 HOW SUPPLIED/STORAGE AND HANDLING

BUTRANS (buprenorphine) Transdermal System is supplied in cartons containing 4 individually-packaged systems and a pouch containing 4 Patch-Disposal Units.
BUTRANS 5 mcg/hour Transdermal System, 4-count carton
NDC 59011-750-04
BUTRANS 7.5 mcg/hour Transdermal System, 4-count carton
NDC 59011-757-04

BUTRANS 10 mcg/hour Transdermal System, 4-count carton
NDC 59011-751-04
BUTRANS 15 mcg/hour Transdermal System, 4-count carton
NDC 59011-758-04
BUTRANS 20 mcg/hour Transdermal System, 4-count carton
NDC 59011-752-04
Store at 25°C (77°F); excursions permitted between 15°C - 30°C (59°F - 86°F).

17 PATIENT COUNSELING INFORMATION

Advise the patient to read the FDA-approved patient labeling (Medication Guide and Instructions for Use).
Addiction, Abuse, and Misuse
Inform patients that the use of BUTRANS, even when taken as recommended, can result in addiction, abuse, and misuse, which could lead to overdose and death *[see Warnings and Precautions (5.1)]*. Instruct patients not to share BUTRANS with others and to take steps to protect BUTRANS from theft or misuse.
Life-Threatening Respiratory Depression
Inform patients of the risk of life-threatening respiratory depression, including information that the risk is greatest when starting BUTRANS or when the dose is increased, and that it can occur even at recommended doses *[see Warnings and Precautions (5.2)]*. Advise patients how to recognize respiratory depression and to seek medical attention if breathing difficulties develop.
Accidental Exposure
Inform patients that accidental exposure, especially in children, may result in respiratory depression or death *[see Warnings and Precautions (5.2)]*. Instruct patients to take steps to store BUTRANS securely and to dispose of unused BUTRANS by folding the patch in half and flushing it down the toilet.
Neonatal Opioid Withdrawal Syndrome
Inform female patients of reproductive potential that prolonged use of BUTRANS during pregnancy can result in neonatal opioid withdrawal syndrome, which may be life-threatening if not recognized and treated *[see Warnings and Precautions (5.3)]*.
Interaction with Alcohol and other CNS Depressants
Inform patients that potentially serious additive effects may occur if BUTRANS is used with alcohol or other CNS depressants, and not to use such drugs unless supervised by a health care provider.
Important Administration Instructions
Instruct patients how to properly use BUTRANS, including the following:
1. To carefully follow instructions for the application, removal, and disposal of BUTRANS. Each week, apply BUTRANS to a different site based on the 8 described skin sites, with a minimum of 3 weeks between applications to a previously used site.
2. To apply BUTRANS to a hairless or nearly hairless skin site. If none are available, instruct patients to clip the hair at the site and not to shave the area. Instruct patients not to apply to irritated skin. If the application site must be cleaned, use clear water only. Soaps, alcohol, oils, lotions, or abrasive devices should not be used. Allow the skin to dry before applying BUTRANS.
Hypotension
Inform patients that BUTRANS may cause orthostatic hypotension and syncope. Instruct patients how to recognize symptoms of low blood pressure and how to reduce the risk of serious consequences should hypotension occur (e.g., sit or lie down, carefully rise from a sitting or lying position).
Driving or Operating Heavy Machinery
Inform patients that BUTRANS may impair the ability to perform potentially hazardous activities such as driving a car or operating heavy machinery. Advise patients not to perform such tasks until they know how they will react to the medication.
Constipation
Advise patients of the potential for severe constipation, including management instructions and when to seek medical attention.
Anaphylaxis
Inform patients that anaphylaxis has been reported with ingredients contained in BUTRANS. Advise patients how to recognize such a reaction and when to seek medical attention.
Pregnancy
Advise female patients that BUTRANS can cause fetal harm and to inform the prescriber if they are pregnant or plan to become pregnant.
Disposal
Instruct patients to refer to the Instructions for Use for proper disposal of BUTRANS. Patients can dispose of used or unused BUTRANS patches in the trash by sealing them in the Patch-Disposal Unit, following the instructions on the unit.

Alternatively, instruct patients to dispose of used patches by folding the adhesive side of the patch to itself, then flushing the patch down the toilet immediately upon removal. Unused patches should be removed from their pouches, the protective liners removed, the patches folded so that the adhesive side of the patch adheres to itself, and immediately flushed down the toilet.

Instruct patients to dispose of any patches remaining from a prescription as soon as they are no longer needed.

Healthcare professionals can telephone Purdue Pharma's Medical Services Department (1-888-726-7535) for information on this product.

Distributed by: Purdue Pharma L.P., Stamford, CT 06901-3431

Manufactured by: LTS Lohmann Therapy Systems Corp., West Caldwell, NJ 07006

U.S. Patent Numbers 5681413; 5804215; 6264980; 6315854; 6344211; RE41408; RE41489; RE41571

© 2014, Purdue Pharma L.P.

Medication Guide

BUTRANS® (BYOO-trans) (buprenorphine) Transdermal System, CIII

BUTRANS is:
- A strong prescription pain medicine that contains an opioid (narcotic) that is used to manage pain severe enough to require daily, around-the-clock, long-term treatment with an opioid, when other pain treatments such as non-opioid pain medicines or immediate-release opioid medicines do not treat your pain well enough or you cannot tolerate them.
- A long-acting (extended-release) opioid pain medicine that can put you at risk for overdose and death. Even if you take your dose correctly as prescribed you are at risk for opioid addiction, abuse, and misuse that can lead to death.
- Not for use to treat pain that is not around-the-clock.

Important information about BUTRANS:
- **Get emergency help right away if you take too much BUTRANS (overdose).** When you first start taking BUTRANS, when your dose is changed, or if you take too much (overdose), serious or life-threatening breathing problems that can lead to death may occur.
- Never give anyone else your BUTRANS. They could die from taking it. Store BUTRANS away from children and in a safe place to prevent stealing or abuse. Selling or giving away BUTRANS is against the law.

Do not use BUTRANS if you have:
- severe asthma, trouble breathing, or other lung problems.
- a bowel blockage or have narrowing of the stomach or intestines.

Before applying BUTRANS, tell your healthcare provider if you have a history of:
- head injury, seizures
- liver, kidney, thyroid problems
- problems urinating
- pancreas or gallbladder problems
- heart rhythm problems (Long QT syndrome)
- abuse of street or prescription drugs, alcohol addiction, or mental health problems.

Tell your healthcare provider if you:
- have a fever
- **are pregnant or planning to become pregnant.** Prolonged use of BUTRANS during pregnancy can cause withdrawal symptoms in your newborn baby that could be life-threatening if not recognized and treated.
- **are breastfeeding.** BUTRANS passes into breast milk and may harm your baby.
- are taking prescription or over-the-counter medicines, vitamins, or herbal supplements. Taking BUTRANS with certain other medicines can cause serious side effects.

While using BUTRANS:
- Do not change your dose. Apply BUTRANS exactly as prescribed by your healthcare provider.
- See the detailed Instructions for Use for information about how to apply the BUTRANS patch.
- Do not apply a BUTRANS patch if the pouch seal is broken, or the patch is cut, damaged, or changed in any way.
- Do not apply more than 1 patch at the same time unless your healthcare provider tells you to.
- You should wear 1 BUTRANS patch continuously for 7 days.
- **Call your healthcare provider if the dose you are using does not control your pain.**

- Do not stop using BUTRANS without talking to your healthcare provider.
- To properly dispose of used and unused patches, use the Patch-Disposal Unit or fold in half and flush down the toilet. See the detailed Instructions for Use.

When using BUTRANS DO NOT:
- Take hot baths or sunbathe, use hot tubs, saunas, heating pads, electric blankets, heated waterbeds, or tanning lamps. These can cause an overdose that can lead to death.
- Drive or operate heavy machinery, until you know how BUTRANS affects you. BUTRANS can make you sleepy, dizzy, or lightheaded.
- Drink alcohol or use prescription or over-the-counter medicines containing alcohol. Using products containing alcohol during treatment with BUTRANS may cause you to overdose and die.

The possible side effects of BUTRANS are:
- constipation, nausea, sleepiness, vomiting, tiredness, headache, dizziness, itching, redness or rash where the patch is applied. Call your healthcare provider if you have any of these symptoms and they are severe.

Get emergency medical help if you have:
- trouble breathing, shortness of breath, fast heartbeat, chest pain, swelling of your face, tongue or throat, extreme drowsiness, light-headedness when changing positions, or you are feeling faint.

These are not all the possible side effects of BUTRANS. Call your doctor for medical advice about side effects. You may report side effects to FDA at 1-800-FDA-1088. **For more information go to dailymed.nlm.nih.gov**

Distributed by: Purdue Pharma L.P., Stamford, CT 06901-3431, **www.purduepharma.com or call 1-888-726-7535**

This Medication Guide has been approved by the U.S. Food and Drug Administration.   Revised: April 2014

Instructions for Use
BUTRANS® (BYOO-trans) CIII
(buprenorphine)
Transdermal System

Be sure that you read, understand, and follow these Instructions for Use before you use BUTRANS. Talk to your healthcare provider or pharmacist if you have any questions.

Before Applying BUTRANS:
- Do not use soap, alcohol, lotions, oils, or other products to remove any leftover adhesive from a patch because this may cause more BUTRANS to pass through the skin.
- Each patch is sealed in its own protective pouch. Do not remove a patch from the pouch until you are ready to use it.
- Do not use a patch if the seal on the protective pouch is broken or if the patch is cut, damaged or changed in any way.
- BUTRANS patches are available in different strengths and patch sizes. Make sure you have the right strength patch that has been prescribed for you.

Where to apply BUTRANS:
- BUTRANS should be applied to the **upper outer arm, upper chest, upper back, or the side of the chest (See Figure A).** These 4 sites (located on both sides of the body) provide 8 possible BUTRANS application sites.

Figure A

- Do not apply more than 1 patch at the same time unless your doctor tells you to. However, if your healthcare provider tells you to do so, you may use 2 patches as prescribed, applied at the same site (**See Figure A** for application sites) right next to each other (**See Figure B** for an example of patch position when applying 2 patches). Always apply and remove the two patches together at the same time.

Figure B

- You should change the skin site where you apply BUTRANS each week, making sure that at least 3 weeks (21 days) pass before you re-use the same skin site.
- Apply BUTRANS to **a hairless or nearly hairless skin site.** If needed, you can clip the hair at the skin site (**See Figure C**). Do not shave the area. The skin site should not be irritated. **Use only water to clean** the application site. You should not use soaps, alcohol, oils, lotions, or abrasive devices. Allow the skin to dry before you apply the patch.

Figure C

- The skin site should be free of cuts and irritation (rashes, swelling, redness, or other skin problems).

When to apply a new patch:
- When you apply a new patch, write down the date and time that the patch is applied. Use this to remember when the patch should be removed.
- Change the patch at the same time of day, one week (exactly 7 days) after you apply it.
- After removing and disposing of the patch, write down the time it was removed and how it was disposed.

How to apply BUTRANS:
- If you are wearing a patch, remember to remove it before applying a new one.
- Each patch is sealed in its own protective pouch.
- If you are using two patches, remember to apply them at the same site right next to each other. Always apply and remove the two patches together at the same time.
- Use scissors to cut open the pouch along the dotted line (**See Figure D**) and remove the patch. Do not remove the patch from the pouch until you are ready to use it. Do not use patches that have been cut or damaged in any way.

Figure D

- Hold the patch with the protective liner facing you.
- Gently bend the patch (**See Figures E and F**) along the faint line and slowly peel the larger portion of the liner, which covers the sticky surface of the patch.

Foil Backing
Patch
Foil Handle

Figure E

[See figure F at top of next column]
- Do not touch the sticky side of the patch with your fingers.
- Using the smaller portion of the protective liner as a handle (**See Figure G**), apply the sticky side of the patch to one

Figure F

of the 8 body locations described above (See **"Where to apply BUTRANS"**).

Figure G

• While still holding the sticky side down, gently fold back the smaller portion of the patch. Grasp an edge of the remaining protective liner and slowly peel it off (See **Figure H**).

Figure H

• Press the entire patch firmly into place with the palm (See **Figure I**) of your hand over the patch, for about 15 seconds. Do not rub the patch.

Figure I

• Make sure that the patch firmly sticks to the skin.
• Go over the edges with your fingers to assure good contact around the patch.
• If you are using two patches, follow the steps in this section to apply them right next to each other.
• Always wash your hands after applying or handling a patch.
• After the patch is applied, write down the date and time that the patch is applied. Use this to remember when the patch should be removed.
If the patch falls off right away after applying, throw it away and put a new one on at a different skin site (See **"Disposing of BUTRANS Patch"**).
If a patch falls off, do not touch the sticky side of the patch with your fingers. A new patch should be applied to a different site. **Patches that fall off should not be re-applied.** They must be thrown away correctly.
Short-term exposure of the BUTRANS patch to water, such as when bathing or showering, is permitted.

If the edges of the BUTRANS patch start to loosen:
• Apply first aid tape only to the edges of the patch.
• If problems with the patch not sticking continue, cover the patch with special see-through adhesive dressings (for example Bioclusive or Tegaderm).
  ○ Remove the backing from the transparent adhesive dressing and place it carefully and completely over the BUTRANS patch, smoothing it over the patch and your skin.
• **Never cover a BUTRANS patch with any other bandage or tape. It should only be covered with a special see-through adhesive dressing. Talk to your healthcare provider or pharmacist about the kinds of dressing that should be used.**
If your patch falls off later, but before 1 week (7 days) of use, throw it away properly (See **"Disposing of a BUTRANS Patch"**) and apply a new patch at a different skin site. Be sure to let your healthcare provider know that this has happened. Do not replace the new patch until 1 week (7 days) after you put it on (or as directed by your healthcare provider).
Disposing of BUTRANS Patch:
BUTRANS patches should be disposed of by using the Patch-Disposal Unit. Alternatively, the patches can be flushed down the toilet.
To dispose of BUTRANS patches in household trash using the Patch-Disposal Unit:
Remove your patch and follow the directions printed on the Patch-Disposal Unit (See **Figure J**) or see complete instructions below. **Use one Patch-Disposal Unit for each patch.**

Figure J

1. Peel back the disposal unit liner to show the sticky surface (See **Figure K**).

Figure K

2. Place the sticky side of the used or unused patch to the indicated area on the disposal unit (See **Figure L**).

Figure L

3. Close the disposal unit by folding the sticky sides together (See **Figure M**). Press firmly and smoothly over the entire disposal unit so that the patch is sealed within.
[See figure M at top of next column]
4. The closed disposal unit, with the patch sealed inside may be thrown away in the trash (See **Figure N**).
[See figure N at top of next column]
Do not put unused patches in household trash without first sealing them in the Patch-Disposal Unit.

Figure M

Figure N

Always remove the leftover patches from their protective pouch and remove the protective liner. The pouch and liner can be disposed of separately in the trash and should not be sealed in the Patch-Disposal Unit.
To flush your BUTRANS patches down the toilet:
Remove your BUTRANS patch, fold the sticky sides of a used patch together and flush it down the toilet right away (See **Figure O**).

Figure O

When disposing of unused BUTRANS patches you no longer need, remove the leftover patches from their protective pouch and remove the protective liner. Fold the patches in half with the sticky sides together, and flush the patches down the toilet.
Do not flush the pouch or the protective liner down the toilet. These items can be thrown away in the trash.
If you prefer not to flush the used patch down the toilet, you must use the Patch-Disposal Unit provided to you to discard the patch.
Never put used BUTRANS patches in the trash without first sealing them in the Patch-Disposal Unit.
This "Instructions for Use" has been approved by the U.S. Food and Drug Administration.

Distributed by: Purdue Pharma L.P., Stamford, CT 06901-3431
Revised: June 2014
©2014, Purdue Pharma L.P.
Bioclusive is a trademark of Systagenix Wound Management (US), Inc.
Tegaderm is a trademark of 3M.

Shown in Product Identification Guide, page 312

DILAUDID
[di-law-did]
(hydromorphone hydrochloride)
Oral Liquid
DILAUDID
(hydromorphone hydrochloride)
Tablets

℟ ℟

WARNING: DILAUDID ORAL LIQUID AND DILAUDID TABLETS CONTAIN HYDROMORPHONE, WHICH IS A POTENT SCHEDULE II CONTROLLED OPIOID AGONIST. SCHEDULE II OPIOID AGONISTS, INCLUDING MORPHINE, OXYMORPHONE, OXYCODONE, FENTANYL, AND METHADONE, HAVE THE HIGHEST POTENTIAL FOR ABUSE AND RISK OF PRODUCING RESPIRATORY DEPRESSION. ALCOHOL, OTHER OPIOIDS AND CENTRAL NERVOUS SYSTEM DEPRESSANTS (SEDATIVE-HYPNOTICS) POTENTIATE THE RESPIRATORY DEPRESSANT EFFECTS OF HYDROMORPHONE, INCREASING THE RISK OF RESPIRATORY DEPRESSION THAT MIGHT RESULT IN DEATH.

DESCRIPTION

DILAUDID (hydromorphone hydrochloride), a hydrogenated ketone of morphine, is an opioid analgesic.

The chemical name of DILAUDID (hydromorphone hydrochloride) is 4,5α-epoxy-3-hydroxy-17-methylmorphinan-6-one hydrochloride. The structural formula is:

M.W. 321.8

Each 5 mL (1 teaspoon) of DILAUDID ORAL LIQUID contains 5 mg of hydromorphone hydrochloride. In addition, other ingredients include purified water, methylparaben, propylparaben, sucrose, and glycerin. DILAUDID ORAL LIQUID may contain traces of sodium metabisulfite.

Color Coded Tablets (for oral administration) contain:

2 mg hydromorphone hydrochloride (orange tablet) and D&C red #30 Lake dye, D&C yellow #10 Lake dye, lactose, and magnesium stearate. DILAUDID 2 mg TABLET may contain traces of sodium metabisulfite.

4 mg hydromorphone hydrochloride (yellow tablet) and D&C yellow #10 Lake dye, lactose, and magnesium stearate. DILAUDID 4 mg TABLET may contain traces of sodium metabisulfite.

8 mg hydromorphone hydrochloride (white tablet) and lactose anhydrous, and magnesium stearate. DILAUDID 8 mg TABLET may contain traces of sodium metabisulfite.

CLINICAL PHARMACOLOGY

Hydromorphone hydrochloride is a pure opioid agonist with the principal therapeutic activity of analgesia. A significant feature of the analgesia is that it can occur without loss of consciousness. Opioid analgesics also suppress the cough reflex and may cause respiratory depression, mood changes, mental clouding, euphoria, dysphoria, nausea, vomiting and electroencephalographic changes. Many of the effects described below are common to this class of mu-opioid agonist analgesics which includes morphine, oxycodone, hydrocodone, codeine and fentanyl. In some instances, data may not exist to distinguish the effects of DILAUDID ORAL LIQUID and DILAUDID TABLETS from those observed with other opioid analgesics. However, in the absence of data to the contrary, it is assumed that DILAUDID ORAL LIQUID and DILAUDID TABLETS would possess all the actions of mu-agonist opioids.

Central Nervous System

The precise mode of analgesic action of opioid analgesics is unknown. However, specific CNS opiate receptors have been identified. Opioids are believed to express their pharmacological effects by combining with these receptors.

Hydromorphone depresses the cough reflex by direct effect on the cough center in the medulla.

Hydromorphone depresses the respiratory reflex by a direct effect on brain stem respiratory centers. The mechanism of respiratory depression also involves a reduction in the responsiveness of the brain stem respiratory centers to increases in carbon dioxide tension.

Hydromorphone causes miosis. Pinpoint pupils are a common sign of opioid overdose but are not pathognomonic (e.g., pontine lesions of hemorrhagic or ischemic origin may produce similar findings). Marked mydriasis rather than miosis may be seen with hypoxia in the setting of DILAUDID overdose.

Gastrointestinal Tract and Other Smooth Muscle

Gastric, biliary and pancreatic secretions are decreased by opioids such as hydromorphone. Hydromorphone causes a reduction in motility associated with an increase in tone in the gastric antrum and duodenum. Digestion of food in the small intestine is delayed and propulsive contractions are decreased. Propulsive peristaltic waves in the colon are decreased, and tone may be increased to the point of spasm. The end result is constipation. Hydromorphone can cause a marked increase in biliary tract pressure as a result of spasm of the sphincter of Oddi.

Cardiovascular System

Hydromorphone may produce hypotension as a result of either peripheral vasodilation or release of histamine, or both. Other manifestations of histamine release and/or peripheral vasodilation may include pruritus, flushing, and red eyes.

Pharmacokinetics and Metabolism

The analgesic activity of DILAUDID (hydromorphone hydrochloride) is due to the parent drug, hydromorphone. Hydromorphone is rapidly absorbed from the gastrointestinal tract after oral administration and undergoes extensive first-pass metabolism. Exposure of hydromorphone (C_{max} and AUC_{0-24}) is dose-proportional at a dose range of 2 and 8 mg. In vivo bioavailability following single-dose administration of the 8 mg tablet is approximately 24% (coefficient of variation 21%). Bioequivalence between the DILAUDID 8 mg TABLET and an equivalent dose of DILAUDID ORAL LIQUID has been demonstrated.

Absorption

After oral administration of DILAUDID 8 mg liquid or tablets, peak plasma hydromorphone concentrations are generally attained within ½ to 1-hour.

Mean (%cv) Dosage Form	C_{max} (ng)	T_{max} (hrs)	AUC (ng*hr/mL)	$T\frac{1}{2}$ (hrs)
8 mg Tablet	5.5 (33%)	0.74 (34%)	23.7 (28%)	2.6 (18%)
8 mg Oral Liquid	5.7 (31%)	0.73 (71%)	24.6 (29%)	2.8 (20%)

Food Effects

In a study conducted with a single 8 mg dose of hydromorphone (2 mg DILAUDID® IR tablets), food lowered C_{max} by 25%, prolonged T_{max} by 0.8 hour, and increased AUC by 35%. The effects may not be clinically relevant.

Distribution

At therapeutic plasma levels, hydromorphone is approximately 8-19% bound to plasma proteins. After an intravenous bolus dose, the steady state of volume distribution [mean (%cv)] is 302.9 (32%) liters.

Metabolism

Hydromorphone is extensively metabolized via glucuronidation in the liver, with greater than 95% of the dose metabolized to hydromorphone-3-glucuronide along with minor amounts of 6-hydroxy reduction metabolites.

Elimination

Only a small amount of the hydromorphone dose is excreted unchanged in the urine. Most of the dose is excreted as hydromorphone-3-glucuronide along with minor amounts of 6-hydroxy reduction metabolites. The systemic clearance is approximately 1.96 (20%) liters/minute. The terminal elimination half-life of hydromorphone after an intravenous dose is about 2.3 hours.

Special Populations

Hepatic Impairment

After oral administration of hydromorphone at a single 4 mg dose (2 mg Dilaudid IR Tablets), mean exposure to hydromorphone (C_{max} and AUC_∞) is increased 4-fold in patients with moderate (Child-Pugh Group B) hepatic impairment compared with subjects with normal hepatic function. Due to increased exposure of hydromorphone, patients with moderate hepatic impairment should be started at a lower dose and closely monitored during dose titration. Pharmacokinetics of hydromorphone in severe hepatic impairment patients has not been studied. Further increase in C_{max} and AUC of hydromorphone in this group is expected. As such, starting dose should be even more conservative. Use of oral liquid is recommended to adjust the dose (see **DOSAGE AND ADMINISTRATION**).

Renal Impairment

After oral administration of hydromorphone at a single 4 mg dose (2 mg Dilaudid IR Tablets), exposure to hydromorphone (C_{max} and AUC_{0-48}) is increased in patients with impaired renal function by 2-fold in moderate (CLcr = 40 - 60 mL/min) and 3-fold in severe (CLcr < 30 mL/min) renal impairment compared with normal subjects (CLcr > 80 mL/min). In addition, in patients with severe renal impairment hydromorphone appeared to be more slowly eliminated with longer terminal elimination half-life (40 hr) compared to patients with normal renal function (15 hr).

Patients with moderate renal impairment should be started on a lower dose. Starting doses for patients with severe renal impairment should be even lower. Patients with renal impairment should be closely monitored during dose titration. Use of oral liquid is recommended to adjust the dose (see **DOSAGE AND ADMINISTRATION**).

Pediatrics

Pharmacokinetics of hydromorphone have not been evaluated in children.

Geriatric

Age has no effect on the pharmacokinetics of hydromorphone.

Gender

Gender has little effect on the pharmacokinetics of hydromorphone. Females appear to have higher C_{max} (25%) than males with comparable AUC_{0-24} values. The difference observed in C_{max} may not be clinically relevant.

Pregnancy and Nursing Mothers

Hydromorphone crosses the placenta. Hydromorphone is also found in low levels in breast milk, and may cause respiratory compromise in newborns when administered during labor or delivery.

CLINICAL TRIALS

Analgesic effects of single doses of DILAUDID ORAL LIQUID administered to patients with post-surgical pain have been studied in double-blind controlled trials. In one study, both 5 mg and 10 mg of DILAUDID ORAL LIQUID provided significantly more analgesia than placebo. In another trial, 5 mg and 10 mg of DILAUDID ORAL LIQUID were compared to 30 mg and 60 mg of morphine sulfate oral liquid. The pain relief provided by 5 mg and 10 mg DILAUDID ORAL LIQUID was comparable to 30 mg and 60 mg oral morphine sulfate, respectively.

INDICATIONS AND USAGE

DILAUDID ORAL LIQUID and DILAUDID TABLETS are indicated for the management of pain in patients where an opioid analgesic is appropriate.

CONTRAINDICATIONS

DILAUDID ORAL LIQUID and DILAUDID TABLETS are contraindicated in: patients with known hypersensitivity to hydromorphone, patients with respiratory depression in the absence of resuscitative equipment, and in patients with status asthmaticus. DILAUDID ORAL LIQUID and DILAUDID TABLETS are also contraindicated for use in obstetrical analgesia.

WARNINGS

Respiratory Depression

Respiratory depression is the chief hazard of DILAUDID ORAL LIQUID and DILAUDID TABLETS. Respiratory depression is more likely to occur in the elderly, in the debilitated, and in those suffering from conditions accompanied by hypoxia or hypercapnia when even moderate therapeutic doses may dangerously decrease pulmonary ventilation.

DILAUDID ORAL LIQUID and DILAUDID TABLETS should be used with extreme caution in patients with chronic obstructive pulmonary disease or cor pulmonale, patients having a substantially decreased respiratory reserve, hypoxia, hypercapnia, or in patients with preexisting respiratory depression. In such patients even usual therapeutic doses of opioid analgesics may decrease respiratory drive while simultaneously increasing airway resistance to the point of apnea.

DILAUDID ORAL LIQUID and DILAUDID TABLETS contain hydromorphone, which is a potent Schedule II controlled opioid agonist. Schedule II opioid agonists, including morphine, oxymorphone, oxycodone, fentanyl, and methadone, have the highest potential for abuse and risk of producing respiratory depression. Alcohol, other opioids and central nervous system depressants (sedative-hypnotics) potentiate the respiratory depressant effects of hydromorphone, increasing the risk of respiratory depression that might result in death.

Misuse, Abuse, and Diversion of Opioids

Hydromorphone is an opioid agonist of the morphine-type. Such drugs are sought by drug abusers and people with addiction disorders and are subject to criminal diversion. DILAUDID can be abused in a manner similar to other opioid agonists, legal or illicit. This should be considered when prescribing or dispensing DILAUDID in situations where the physician or pharmacist is concerned about an increased risk of misuse, abuse, or diversion. Prescribers should monitor all patients receiving opioids for signs of abuse, misuse, and addiction. Furthermore, patients should be assessed for their potential for opioid abuse prior to being prescribed opioid therapy. Persons at increased risk for opioid abuse include those with a personal or family history of substance abuse (including drug or alcohol abuse) or mental illness (e.g., depression). Opioids may still be appropriate for use in these patients, however, they will require intensive monitoring for signs of abuse DILAUDID has been reported as being abused by crushing, chewing, snorting, or injecting the dissolved product. These practices pose a significant risk to the abuser that could result in overdose or death (see **WARNINGS** and **DRUG ABUSE AND DEPENDENCE**). Concerns about abuse, addiction, and diversion should not prevent the proper management of pain. Healthcare professionals should contact their State Professional Licensing Board or State Controlled Substances Authority for information on how to prevent and detect abuse or diversion of this product.

Interactions with Alcohol and Drugs of Abuse

Hydromorphone may be expected to have additive effects when used in conjunction with alcohol, other opioids, or illicit drugs that cause central nervous system depression.

Neonatal Withdrawal Syndrome

Infants born to mothers physically dependent on DILAUDID will also be physically dependent and may exhibit respiratory difficulties and withdrawal symptoms (see **DRUG ABUSE AND DEPENDENCE**).

Head Injury and Increased Intracranial Pressure

The respiratory depressant effects of DILAUDID ORAL LIQUID and DILAUDID TABLETS with carbon dioxide retention and secondary elevation of cerebrospinal fluid pressure may be markedly exaggerated in the presence of head injury, other intracranial lesions, or preexisting increase in intracranial pressure. Opioid analgesics including DILAUDID ORAL LIQUID and DILAUDID TABLETS (hydromorphone hydrochloride) may produce effects on pupillary response and consciousness which can obscure the clinical course and neurologic signs of further increase in intracranial pressure in patients with head injuries.

Hypotensive Effect

Opioid analgesics, including DILAUDID ORAL LIQUID and DILAUDID TABLETS, may cause severe hypotension in an individual whose ability to maintain blood pressure has already been compromised by a depleted blood volume, or a concurrent administration of drugs such as phenothiazines or general anesthetics (see **PRECAUTIONS - Drug Interactions**). Therefore, DILAUDID ORAL LIQUID and DILAUDID TABLETS should be administered with caution to patients in circulatory shock, since vasodilation produced by the drug may further reduce cardiac output and blood pressure.

Sulfites

Contains sodium metabisulfite, a sulfite that may cause allergic-type reactions including anaphylactic symptoms and life-threatening or less severe asthmatic episodes in certain susceptible people. The overall prevalence of sulfite sensitivity in the general population is unknown and probably low. Sulfite sensitivity is seen more frequently in asthmatic than in nonasthmatic people.

PRECAUTIONS

Special Risk Patients

DILAUDID ORAL LIQUID and DILAUDID TABLETS should be given with caution and the initial dose should be reduced in the elderly or debilitated and those with severe impairment of hepatic, pulmonary or renal functions; myxedema or hypothyroidism; adrenocortical insufficiency (e.g., Addison's Disease); CNS depression or coma; toxic psychoses; prostatic hypertrophy or urethral stricture; gall bladder disease; acute alcoholism; delirium tremens; kyphoscoliosis or following gastrointestinal surgery.

The administration of opioid analgesics including DILAUDID ORAL LIQUID and DILAUDID TABLETS may obscure the diagnoses or clinical course in patients with acute abdominal conditions and may aggravate preexisting convulsions in patients with convulsive disorders.

Reports of mild to severe seizures and myoclonus have been reported in severely compromised patients, administered high doses of parenteral hydromorphone, for cancer and severe pain. Opioid administration at very high doses is associated with seizures and myoclonus in a variety of diseases where pain control is the primary focus.

Use in Drug and Alcohol Dependent Patients

DILAUDID should be used with caution in patients with alcoholism and other drug dependencies due to the increased frequency of opioid tolerance, dependence, and the risk of addiction observed in these patient populations. Abuse of DILAUDID in combination with other CNS depressant drugs can result in serious risk to the patient.

Hydromorphone is an opioid with no approved use in the management of addictive disorders.

Use in Ambulatory Patients

DILAUDID ORAL LIQUID and DILAUDID TABLETS may impair mental and/or physical ability required for the performance of potentially hazardous tasks (e.g. driving, operating machinery). Patients should be cautioned accordingly. DILAUDID may produce orthostatic hypotension in ambulatory patients.

Use in Biliary Tract Disease

Opioid analgesics, including DILAUDID ORAL LIQUID and DILAUDID TABLETS, should also be used with caution in patients about to undergo surgery of the biliary tract since it may cause spasm of the sphincter of Oddi.

Tolerance and Physical Dependence

Tolerance is the need for increasing doses of opioids to maintain a defined effect such as analgesia (in the absence of disease progression or other external factors). Physical dependence is manifested by withdrawal symptoms after abrupt discontinuation of a drug or upon administration of an antagonist. Physical dependence and tolerance are not unusual during chronic opioid therapy.

The opioid abstinence or withdrawal syndrome is characterized by some or all of the following: restlessness, lacrimation, rhinorrhea, yawning, perspiration, chills, myalgia, mydriasis. Other symptoms also may develop, including: irritability, anxiety, backache, joint pain, weakness, abdominal cramps, insomnia, nausea, anorexia, vomiting, diarrhea, or increased blood pressure, respiratory rate, or heart rate.

In general, opioids used regularly should not be abruptly discontinued.

Information for Patients/Caregivers

Patients receiving DILAUDID (hydromorphone hydrochloride) ORAL LIQUID or DILAUDID TABLETS or their caregivers should be given the following information by the physician, nurse, or pharmacist:

1. Patients should be aware that DILAUDID tablets contain hydromorphone, which is a morphine-like substance and which could cause severe adverse effects including respiratory depression and even death if not taken according to the prescriber's directions.
2. Patients should be advised to report pain and adverse experiences occurring during therapy. Individualization of dosage is essential to make optimal use of this medication.
3. Patients should be advised not to adjust the dose of DILAUDID without consulting the prescribing professional.
4. Patients should be advised that DILAUDID may impair mental and/or physical ability required for the performance of potentially hazardous tasks (e.g., driving, operating heavy machinery).
5. Patients should not combine DILAUDID with alcohol or other central nervous system depressants (sleep aids, tranquilizers) except by the orders of the prescribing physician, because dangerous additive effects may occur, resulting in serious injury or death.
6. Women of childbearing potential who become, or are planning to become pregnant should be advised to consult their physician regarding the effects of analgesics and other drug use during pregnancy on themselves and their unborn child.
7. Patients should be advised that DILAUDID is a potential drug of abuse. They should protect it from theft, and it should never be given to anyone other than the individual for whom it was prescribed.
8. Patients should be advised that if they have been receiving treatment with DILAUDID for more than a few weeks and cessation of therapy is indicated, it may be appropriate to taper the DILAUDID dose, rather than abruptly discontinue it, due to the risk of precipitating withdrawal symptoms. Their physician can provide a dose schedule to accomplish a gradual discontinuation of the medication.
9. Patients should be instructed to keep DILAUDID in a secure place out of the reach of children. When DILAUDID is no longer needed, the unused tablets should be destroyed by flushing down the toilet.

Drug Interactions

Drug Interactions with Other CNS Depressants

The concomitant use of other central nervous system depressants including sedatives or hypnotics, general anesthetics, phenothiazines, tranquilizers and alcohol may produce additive depressant effects. Respiratory depression, hypotension and profound sedation or coma may occur. When such combined therapy is contemplated, the dose of one or both agents should be reduced. DILAUDID should not be taken with alcohol. Opioid analgesics, including DILAUDID ORAL LIQUID and DILAUDID TABLETS, may enhance the action of neuromuscular blocking agents and produce an excessive degree of respiratory depression.

Interactions with Mixed Agonist/Antagonist Opioid Analgesics

Agonist/antagonist analgesics (i.e., pentazocine, nalbuphine, butorphanol, and buprenorphine) should be administered with caution to a patient who has received or is receiving a course of therapy with a pure opioid agonist analgesic such as hydromorphone. In this situation, mixed agonist/antagonist analgesics may reduce the analgesic effect of hydromorphone and/or may precipitate withdrawal symptoms in these patients.

Carcinogenesis, Mutagenesis, Impairment of Fertility

No carcinogenicity studies have been conducted in animals. Hydromorphone was not mutagenic in the *in vitro* Ames reverse mutation assay or the human lymphocyte chromosome aberration assay. Hydromorphone was not clastogenic in the *in vivo* mouse micronucleus assay.

No effects on fertility, reproductive performance, or reproductive organ morphology were observed in male or female rats given oral doses up to 7 mg/kg/day, which is equivalent to the human dose of 2.5-10 mg every 3 to 6 hours for oral liquid, and 3-fold higher than the human dose of 2-4 mg every 4 to 6 hours for the tablet on a body surface area basis.

Pregnancy

Pregnancy Category C

No effects on teratogenicity or embryotoxicity were observed in female rats given oral doses up to 7 mg/kg/day, which is approximately equivalent to the human dose of 2.5-10 mg every 3 to 6 hours for oral liquid, and 3-fold higher than the human dose of 2-4 mg every 4 to 6 hours for the tablet on a body surface area basis. Hydromorphone produced skull malformations (exencephaly and cranioschisis) in Syrian hamsters given oral doses up to 20 mg/kg during the peak of organogenesis (gestation days 8-9). The skull malformations were observed at doses approximately 2-fold higher the human dose of 2.5-10 mg every 3 to 6 hours for oral liquid, and 7-fold higher than the human dose of 2-4 mg every 4 to 6 hours for the tablet on a body surface area basis. There are no adequate and well-controlled studies of DILAUDID in pregnant women.

Hydromorphone crosses the placenta, resulting in fetal exposure. DILAUDID ORAL LIQUID and DILAUDID TABLETS should be used in pregnant women only if the potential benefit justifies the potential risk to the fetus (see **Labor and Delivery** and **DRUG ABUSE AND DEPENDENCE**).

Nonteratogenic Effects

Babies born to mothers who have been taking opioids regularly prior to delivery will be physically dependent. The withdrawal signs include irritability and excessive crying, tremors, hyperactive reflexes, increased respiratory rate, increased stools, sneezing, yawning, vomiting, and fever. The intensity of the syndrome does not always correlate with the duration of maternal opioid use or dose. There is no consensus on the best method of managing withdrawal. Approaches to the treatment of this syndrome have included supportive care and, when indicated, drugs such as paregoric or phenobarbital.

Labor and Delivery

DILAUDID ORAL LIQUID and DILAUDID TABLETS are contraindicated in Labor and Delivery (see **CONTRAINDICATIONS**).

Nursing Mothers

Low levels of opioid analgesics have been detected in human milk. As a general rule, nursing should not be undertaken while a patient is receiving DILAUDID ORAL LIQUID and DILAUDID TABLETS since it, and other drugs in this class, may be excreted in the milk.

Pediatric Use

Safety and effectiveness in children have not been established.

Geriatric Use

Clinical studies of DILAUDID did not include sufficient numbers of subjects aged 65 and over to determine whether they respond differently from younger subjects. In general, dose selection for an elderly patient should be cautious, usually starting at the low end of the dosing range, reflecting the greater frequency of decreased hepatic, renal, or cardiac function, and of concomitant disease or other drug therapy (see **INDIVIDUALIZATION OF DOSAGE** and **PRECAUTIONS**).

ADVERSE REACTIONS

The major hazards of DILAUDID ORAL LIQUID and DILAUDID TABLETS include respiratory depression and apnea. To a lesser degree, circulatory depression, respiratory arrest, shock and cardiac arrest have occurred.

The most frequently observed adverse effects are lightheadedness, dizziness, sedation, nausea, vomiting, sweating, flushing, dysphoria, euphoria, dry mouth, and pruritus. These effects seem to be more prominent in ambulatory patients and in those not experiencing severe pain.

Less Frequently Observed Adverse Reactions

General and CNS

Weakness, headache, agitation, tremor, uncoordinated muscle movements, alterations of mood (nervousness, apprehension, depression, floating feelings, dreams), muscle rigidity, paresthesia, muscle tremor, blurred vision, nystagmus, diplopia and miosis, transient hallucinations and disorientation, visual disturbances, insomnia, increased intracranial pressure

Cardiovascular

Flushing of the face, chills, tachycardia, bradycardia, palpitation, faintness, syncope, hypotension, hypertension

Respiratory

Bronchospasm and laryngospasm

Gastrointestinal

Constipation, biliary tract spasm, ileus, anorexia, diarrhea, cramps, taste alteration

Genitourinary

Urinary retention or hesitancy, antidiuretic effects

Dermatologic
Urticaria, other skin rashes, diaphoresis

OVERDOSAGE

Serious overdosage with DILAUDID ORAL LIQUID and DILAUDID TABLETS is characterized by respiratory depression, somnolence progressing to stupor or coma, skeletal muscle flaccidity, cold and clammy skin, constricted pupils, and sometimes bradycardia and hypotension. In serious overdosage, particularly following intravenous injection, apnea, circulatory collapse, cardiac arrest and death may occur.

In the treatment of overdosage, primary attention should be given to the reestablishment of adequate respiratory exchange through provision of a patent airway and institution of assisted or controlled ventilation. A potentially serious oral ingestion, if recent, should be managed with gut decontamination. In unconscious patients with a secure airway, instill activated charcoal (30-100 g in adults, 1-2 g/kg in infants) via a nasogastric tube. A saline cathartic or sorbitol may be added to the first dose of activated charcoal.

Supportive measures (including oxygen, vasopressors) should be employed in the management of circulatory shock and pulmonary edema accompanying overdose as indicated. Cardiac arrest or arrhythmias may require cardiac massage or defibrillation.

The opioid antagonist, naloxone, is a specific antidote against respiratory depression which may result from overdosage, or unusual sensitivity to DILAUDID ORAL LIQUID and DILAUDID TABLETS. Therefore, an appropriate dose of this antagonist should be administered, preferably by the intravenous route, simultaneously with efforts at respiratory resuscitation. Naloxone should not be administered in the absence of clinically significant respiratory or circulatory depression. Naloxone should be administered cautiously to persons who are known, or suspected to be physically dependent on DILAUDID ORAL LIQUID and DILAUDID TABLETS. In such cases, an abrupt or complete reversal of narcotic effects may precipitate an acute withdrawal syndrome. Since the duration of action of DILAUDID ORAL LIQUID and DILAUDID TABLETS may exceed that of the antagonist, the patient should be kept under continued surveillance; repeated doses of the antagonist may be required to maintain adequate respiration. Apply other supportive measures when indicated.

DOSAGE AND ADMINISTRATION

Dilaudid Oral Liquid

The usual adult oral dosage of DILAUDID ORAL LIQUID is one-half (2.5 mL) to two teaspoonfuls (10 mL) (2.5 mg - 10 mg) every 3 to 6 hours as directed by the clinical situation. Oral dosages higher than the usual dosages may be required in some patients.

Dilaudid Tablets

The usual starting dose for DILAUDID tablets is 2 mg to 4 mg, orally, every 4 to 6 hours. Appropriate use of the DILAUDID TABLETS must be decided by careful evaluation of each clinical situation.

A gradual increase in dose may be required if analgesia is inadequate, as tolerance develops, or if pain severity increases. The first sign of tolerance is usually a reduced duration of effect. Patients with hepatic and renal impairment should be started on a lower starting dose (See CLINICAL PHARMACOLOGY - Pharmacokinetics and Metabolism).

INDIVIDUALIZATION OF DOSAGE

The dosage of opioid analgesics like hydromorphone hydrochloride should be individualized for any given patient, since adverse events can occur at doses that may not provide complete freedom from pain.

Safe and effective administration of opioid analgesics to patients with acute or chronic pain depends upon a comprehensive assessment of the patient. The nature of the pain (severity, frequency, etiology, and pathophysiology) as well as the concurrent medical status of the patient will affect selection of the starting dosage.

In non-opioid-tolerant patients, therapy with hydromorphone is typically initiated at an oral dose of 2-4 mg every four hours, but elderly patients may require lower doses (see PRECAUTIONS - Geriatric Use).

In patients receiving opioids, both the dose and duration of analgesia will vary substantially depending on the patient's opioid tolerance. The dose should be selected and adjusted so that at least 3-4 hours of pain relief may be achieved. In patients taking opioid analgesics, the starting dose of DILAUDID should be based on prior opioid usage. This should be done by converting the total daily usage of the previous opioid to an equivalent total daily dosage of oral DILAUDID using an equianalgesic table (see below). For opioids not in the table, first estimate the equivalent total daily usage of oral morphine, then use the table to find the equivalent total daily dosage of DILAUDID.

Once the total daily dosage of DILAUDID has been estimated, it should be divided into the desired number of doses. Since there is individual variation in response to different opioid drugs, only 1/2 to 2/3 of the estimated dose of DILAUDID calculated from equivalence tables should be given for the first few doses, then increased as needed according to the patient's response.

Since the pharmacokinetics of hydromorphone are affected in hepatic and renal impairment with a consequent increase in exposure, patients with hepatic and renal impairment should be started on a lower starting dose (See CLINICAL PHARMACOLOGY - Pharmacokinetics and Metabolism). In chronic pain, doses should be administered around-the-clock. A supplemental dose of 5-15% of the total daily usage may be administered every two hours on an "as-needed" basis.

Periodic reassessment after the initial dosing is always required. If pain management is not satisfactory and in the absence of significant opioid-induced adverse events, the hydromorphone dose may be increased gradually. If excessive opioid side effects are observed early in the dosing interval, the hydromorphone dose should be reduced. If this results in breakthrough pain at the end of the dosing interval, the dosing interval may need to be shortened. Dose titration should be guided more by the need for analgesia than the absolute dose of opioid employed.

OPIOID ANALGESIC EQUIVALENTS WITH APPROXIMATELY EQUIANALGESIC POTENCY*

Nonproprietary (Trade) Name	IM or SC Dose	ORAL Dose
Morphine sulfate	10 mg	40-60 mg
Hydromorphone HCl (DILAUDID)	1.3-2 mg	6.5-7.5 mg
Oxymorphone HCl (Numorphan)	1-1.1 mg	6.6 mg
Levorphanol tartrate (Levo-Dromoran)	2-2.3 mg	4 mg
Meperidine, pethidine HCl (Demerol)	75-100 mg	300-400 mg
Methadone HCl (Dolophine)	10 mg	10-20 mg

* Dosages, and ranges of dosages represented, are a compilation of estimated equipotent dosages from published references comparing opioid analgesics in cancer and severe pain.

DRUG ABUSE AND DEPENDENCE

DILAUDID ORAL LIQUID and DILAUDID TABLETS contain hydromorphone, a Schedule II controlled opioid agonist. Schedule II opioid substances which include morphine, oxycodone, oxymorphone, fentanyl, and methadone have the highest potential for abuse and risk of fatal overdose. Hydromorphone can be abused and is subject to criminal diversion.

Opioid analgesics may cause psychological and physical dependence. Physical dependence results in withdrawal symptoms in patients who abruptly discontinue the drug. Physical dependence usually does not occur to a clinically significant degree until after several weeks of continued opioid usage, but it may occur after as little as a week of opioid use. Physical dependence and tolerance are separate and distinct from abuse and addiction.

Addiction is a chronic, neurobiologic disease, with genetic, psychosocial, and environmental factors influencing its development and manifestations. It is characterized by behaviors that include one or more of the following: impaired control over drug use, compulsive use, continued use despite harm, and craving. Drug addiction is a treatable disease, utilizing a multidisciplinary approach, but relapse is common.

"Drug seeking" behavior is very common in addicts and drug abusers. Drug-seeking tactics include emergency calls or visits near the end of office hours, refusal to undergo appropriate examination, testing or referral, repeated "loss" of prescriptions, tampering with, forging or counterfeiting prescriptions and reluctance to provide prior medical records or contact information for other treating physician(s). "Doctor shopping" to obtain additional prescriptions is common among drug abusers, people suffering from untreated addiction and criminals seeking drugs to sell.

Physicians should be aware that addiction may not be accompanied by concurrent tolerance and symptoms of physical dependence in all addicts. In addition, abuse of opioids can occur in the absence of addiction and is characterized by misuse for non-medical purposes, often in combination with other psychoactive substances. Since DILAUDID ORAL LIQUID and DILAUDID TABLETS may be diverted for non-medical use, careful record keeping of prescribing information, including quantity, frequency, and renewal requests is strongly advised.

Proper assessment of the patient, proper prescribing practices, periodic re-evaluation of therapy, and proper dispensing and storage are appropriate measures that help to limit abuse of opioid drugs.

DILAUDID ORAL LIQUID and DILAUDID TABLETS are intended for oral use only. Misuse or abuse of DILAUDID ORAL LIQUID and DILAUDID TABLETS pose a risk of overdose and death. This risk is increased with concurrent abuse of alcohol and other CNS depressants. Parenteral drug abuse can potentially result in local tissue necrosis, infection, pulmonary granulomas, and increased risk of endocarditis and valvular heart injury. In addition, parenteral abuse is commonly associated with transmission of infectious diseases such as hepatitis and HIV.

SAFETY AND HANDLING INSTRUCTIONS

DILAUDID ORAL LIQUID and DILAUDID TABLETS pose little risk of direct exposure to health care personnel and should be handled and disposed of prudently in accordance with hospital or institutional policy. Significant absorption from dermal exposure is unlikely; accidental dermal exposure to DILAUDID ORAL LIQUID should be treated by removal of any contaminated clothing and rinsing the affected area with cool water. Patients and their families should be instructed to flush any DILAUDID ORAL LIQUID and DILAUDID TABLETS that are no longer needed.

Access to abuseable drugs such as DILAUDID ORAL LIQUID and DILAUDID TABLETS presents an occupational hazard for addiction in the health care industry. Routine procedures for handling controlled substances developed to protect the public may not be adequate to protect health care workers. Implementation of more effective accounting procedures and measures to restrict access to drugs of this class (appropriate to the practice setting) may minimize the risk of self-administration by health care providers.

HOW SUPPLIED

DILAUDID ORAL LIQUID is a clear, sweet, slightly viscous liquid. It is available in: Bottles of 1 pint (473 mL) - NDC# 59011-451-01

DILAUDID 2 mg TABLETS are light orange, round, flat-faced tablets, with beveled edges, debossed with a "P" on one side and the number "2" on the opposite side. They are available in:
Bottles of 100 - NDC # 59011-452-10
Unit Dose Packages of 100 (4×25) - NDC # 59011-452-01
DILAUDID 4 mg TABLETS are light yellow, round, flat-faced tablets, with beveled edges, debossed with a "P" on one side and the number "4" on the opposite side. They are available in:
Bottles of 100 - NDC # 59011-454-10
Unit Dose Packages of 100 (4×25) - NDC # 59011-454-01
Bottles of 500 - NDC # 59011-454-05
DILAUDID 8 mg TABLETS are white, triangular shaped tablets debossed with a "P" and an inverted "P" separated with a bisect on one side of the tablet and debossed with the number "8" on the other side of the tablet. They are available in:
Bottles of 100 - NDC# 59011-458-10
Healthcare professionals can telephone Purdue Pharma's Medical Services Department (1-888-726-7535) for information on this product.

Storage

Store at 25°C (77°F); excursions permitted to 15°-30°C (59°-86°F). [See USP Controlled Room Temperature]. Protect from light. A schedule CS-II Narcotic. DEA Order Form is Required.
Manufactured for Purdue Pharma L.P. Stamford, CT 06901-3431
By Halo Pharmaceutical, Inc.
Whippany, NJ 07981
Revised: 6/2013

Shown in Product Identification Guide, page 312

DILAUDID® and DILAUDID-HP® INJECTION   ℂ ℞

[Di-law-did]
DILAUDID® INJECTION (hydromorphone hydrochloride), CII
DILAUDID-HP® INJECTION (hydromorphone hydrochloride), CII
For intravenous, intramuscular and subcutaneous use

HIGHLIGHTS OF PRESCRIBING INFORMATION

These highlights do not include all the information needed to use DILAUDID® INJECTION and DILAUDID-HP® INJECTION safely and effectively. See full prescribing information for DILAUDID® INJECTION and DILAUDID-HP® INJECTION.

DILAUDID® INJECTION (hydromorphone hydrochloride)
DILAUDID-HP® INJECTION (hydromorphone hydrochloride)
CII

For intravenous, intramuscular and subcutaneous use
Initial U.S. Approval: January 1984

WARNING: RISK OF RESPIRATORY DEPRESSION, ABUSE, AND MEDICATION ERRORS
DILAUDID-HP® INJECTION IS FOR USE IN OPIOID-TOLERANT PATIENTS ONLY
See full prescribing information for complete boxed warning.
• Do not confuse DILAUDID-HP INJECTION with standard parenteral formulations of DILAUDID or other opioids, as overdose and death could result. (5)
• Hydromorphone is a potent Schedule II opioid agonist. Schedule II opioid agonists have the highest potential for abuse and risk of producing respiratory depression. Ethanol, other opioids, and other central nervous system depressants can potentiate the respiratory-depressant effects of hydromorphone and increase the risk of adverse outcomes, including death. (5.1, 7.1)

INDICATIONS AND USAGE

• DILAUDID INJECTION is an opioid analgesic indicated for the management of pain where an opioid analgesic is appropriate. (1)
• DILAUDID-HP INJECTION is indicated for the management of moderate-to-severe pain in opioid-tolerant patients who require higher doses of opioids. (1)

DOSAGE AND ADMINISTRATION

• DILAUDID INJECTION: The usual starting dose is 1 mg to 2 mg *subcutaneously* or *intramuscularly* every 2 to 3 hours as necessary. (2.3)
• DILAUDID-HP INJECTION should be used only if the amount of hydromorphone required can be delivered accurately with this formulation. (2.5)
• For patients already receiving opioids, use standard conversion ratio estimates. (2.4)
• The dose should be adjusted according to the severity of pain, as well as the patient's underlying disease state and age. (2.1, 2.2)
• Should intravenous administration be necessary, the injection should be given slowly, over at least 2 to 3 minutes and the usual starting dose is 0.2 to 1 mg. (2.3.2)

DOSAGE FORMS AND STRENGTHS

• DILAUDID INJECTION: 1 mg/mL, 2 mg/mL, or 4 mg/mL. (3)
• DILAUDID-HP INJECTION: 10 mg/mL in 1 mL or 5 mL ampule or 50 mL single-dose vial. (3)
• DILAUDID-HP INJECTION Sterile Lyophilized Powder: 250 mg of sterile, lyophilized hydromorphone hydrochloride to be reconstituted to provide a solution containing 10 mg/mL. (3)

CONTRAINDICATIONS

• Known hypersensitivity to hydromorphone, hydromorphone salts, any components of the product, or in any situation where opioids are contraindicated (4)
• Patients with respiratory depression in the absence of resuscitative equipment or in unmonitored settings; patients with status asthmaticus (4)
• Gastrointestinal obstruction, especially paralytic ileus (4)
• DILAUDID-HP INJECTION: Patients who are not opioid tolerant (4)

WARNINGS AND PRECAUTIONS

• DILAUDID-HP INJECTION is a concentrated formulation of hydromorphone. Do NOT confuse DILAUDID-HP INJECTION with DILAUDID INJECTION. Overdose and death could result. (5.1)
• May cause respiratory depression, use with extreme caution in patients at risk of respiratory depression, elderly, and debilitated patients. (5.2)
• Abuse of DILAUDID INJECTION and DILAUDID-HP INJECTION poses a hazard of overdose and death. (5.3)
• Risk of medication errors: Morphine does not convert to hydromorphone on a milligram per milligram basis. Use Table 1 to convert. (5.1)
• Alcohol, other opioids and central nervous system depressants potentiate the respiratory depressant effects of hydromorphone. (5.4)
• Infants born to mothers physically dependent on DILAUDID INJECTION or DILAUDID-HP INJECTION will also be physically dependent and may exhibit respiratory difficulties and withdrawal symptoms. (5.5)
• Respiratory depression may be markedly increased in patients with head injury, other intracranial lesions, or pre-existing increase in intracranial pressure. (5.6)
• May cause hypotension, use with caution in patients at increased risk of hypotension and in patients in circulatory shock. (5.7)
• DILAUDID INJECTION and DILAUDID-HP INJECTION contain sodium metabisulfite. There is a risk of anaphylactic symptoms and life-threatening asthmatic episodes in susceptible people. (5.8)

• Use with caution in patients with biliary tract disease including pancreatitis. (5.9)
• Use with caution and in reduced initial doses in the elderly, debilitated, or other patient populations with increased risk of adverse reactions from opioids. (5.10)
• Use with caution in patients with alcoholism or other drug dependencies. (5.11)
• May impair the mental and physical abilities needed to perform potentially hazardous activities such as driving a car or operating machinery. (5.12)

ADVERSE REACTIONS

Most common adverse reactions are lightheadedness, dizziness, sedation, nausea, vomiting, sweating, flushing, dysphoria, euphoria, dry mouth, and pruritus. (6)
To report Suspected Adverse Reactions, contact Purdue Pharma L.P. at 1-888-726-7535 or FDA at 1-800-FDA-1088 or www.fda.gov/medwatch.

DRUG INTERACTIONS

• Concurrent use of other CNS depressants may cause respiratory depression, hypotension, and profound sedation or coma. (7.1)
• Mixed agonist/antagonist analgesics may reduce the analgesic effect of hydromorphone and may precipitate withdrawal symptoms in these patients. (7.2)

USE IN SPECIFIC POPULATIONS

• Pregnancy: Based on animal data, may cause fetal harm. (8.1)
• Labor and Delivery: Use with caution during labor. (8.2)
• Nursing Mothers: Nursing should not be undertaken while a patient is receiving DILAUDID INJECTION or DILAUDID-HP INJECTION. (8.3)
• Pediatrics: Safety and effectiveness in pediatric patients have not been established. (8.4)
• Geriatrics: Use with caution in elderly patients, initiate dose at low end of dosing range. (8.5)
• Hepatic and Renal Impairment: Patients with hepatic and renal impairment should be started on a lower starting dose. (8.6, 8.7, 12.2)

Revised: 10/2011

FULL PRESCRIBING INFORMATION: CONTENTS*
BOX WARNING
1   INDICATIONS AND USAGE
2   DOSAGE AND ADMINISTRATION
     2.1   General Dosing Considerations
     2.2   Individualization of Dosing
     2.3   Initiation of Therapy in Opioid-Naïve Patients
     2.4   Conversion From Prior Opioid
     2.5   DILAUDID-HP Injection (for use in opioid-tolerant patients only)
     2.6   Administration and Reconstitution
3   DOSAGE FORMS AND STRENGTHS
4   CONTRAINDICATIONS
5   WARNINGS AND PRECAUTIONS
     5.1   Risk of Medication Errors
     5.2   Respiratory Depression
     5.3   Misuse, Abuse and Diversion of Opioids
     5.4   Interactions with Alcohol and other CNS Depressants
     5.5   Neonatal Withdrawal Syndrome
     5.6   Use in Increased Intracranial Pressure or Head Injury
     5.7   Hypotensive Effect
     5.8   Sulfites
     5.9   Use in Pancreatic/Biliary Tract Disease and Other Gastrointestinal Conditions
     5.10   Special Risk Patients
     5.11   Use in Drug and Alcohol Dependent Patients
     5.12   Use in Ambulatory Patients
     5.13   Parenteral Administration
6   ADVERSE REACTIONS
7   DRUG INTERACTIONS
     7.1   Drug Interactions with other CNS Depressants
     7.2   Interactions with Mixed Agonist/Antagonist Opioid Analgesics
     7.3   Monoamine Oxidase Inhibitors (MAOIs)
     7.4   Anticholinergics
8   USE IN SPECIFIC POPULATIONS
     8.1   Pregnancy
     8.2   Labor and Delivery
     8.3   Nursing Mothers
     8.4   Pediatric Use
     8.5   Geriatric Use
     8.6   Renal Impairment
     8.7   Hepatic Impairment
9   DRUG ABUSE AND DEPENDENCE
     9.1   Controlled Substance
     9.2   Abuse

     9.3   Dependence
10   OVERDOSAGE
     10.1   Signs and Symptoms
     10.2   Treatment
11   DESCRIPTION
12   CLINICAL PHARMACOLOGY
     12.1   Mechanism of Action
     12.2   Pharmacokinetics
13   NONCLINICAL TOXICOLOGY
     13.1   Carcinogenesis, Mutagenesis, Impairment of Fertility
14   CLINICAL STUDIES
16   HOW SUPPLIED/STORAGE AND HANDLING
     16.1   Safety and Handling Instructions
     16.2   How Supplied
     16.3   Storage
* Sections or subsections omitted from the full prescribing information are not listed

FULL PRESCRIBING INFORMATION
DILAUDID® INJECTION (hydromorphone hydrochloride), CII
DILAUDID-HP® INJECTION (hydromorphone hydrochloride), CII
For intravenous, intramuscular, and subcutaneous use

BOX WARNING
WARNING: RISK OF RESPIRATORY DEPRESSION, ABUSE, AND MEDICATION ERRORS
DILAUDID-HP INJECTION IS FOR USE IN OPIOID-TOLERANT PATIENTS ONLY
Patients considered opioid tolerant are those who are taking at least 60 mg oral morphine/day, 25 mcg transdermal fentanyl/hour, 30 mg oral oxycodone/day, 8 mg oral hydromorphone/day, 25 mg oral oxymorphone/day, or an equianalgesic dose of another opioid for one week or longer.
DILAUDID-HP INJECTION is a more concentrated solution of hydromorphone than DILAUDID INJECTION, and is for use in opioid-tolerant patients only. Do not confuse DILAUDID-HP INJECTION with standard parenteral formulations of DILAUDID INJECTION or other opioids, as overdose and death could result.
DILAUDID INJECTION and DILAUDID-HP INJECTION contain hydromorphone, an opioid agonist and a Schedule II controlled substance with an abuse liability similar to other opioid analgesics. DILAUDID INJECTION and DILAUDID-HP INJECTION can be abused in a manner similar to other opioid agonists, legal or illicit. These risks should be considered when administering, prescribing, or dispensing DILAUDID INJECTION and DILAUDID-HP INJECTION in situations where the healthcare professional is concerned about increased risk of misuse, abuse, or diversion.
Schedule II opioid agonists, including morphine, oxymorphone, hydromorphone, oxycodone, fentanyl and methadone, have the highest potential for abuse and risk of producing fatal overdose due to respiratory depression. Ethanol, other opioids, and other central nervous system depressants (e.g., sedative-hypnotics, skeletal muscle relaxants) can potentiate the respiratory-depressant effects of hydromorphone and increase the risk of adverse outcomes, including death.

1   INDICATIONS AND USAGE

DILAUDID INJECTION is indicated for the management of pain in patients where an opioid analgesic is appropriate. DILAUDID-HP INJECTION is indicated for the management of moderate-to-severe pain in opioid-tolerant patients who require higher doses of opioids.

2   DOSAGE AND ADMINISTRATION
2.1   General Dosing Considerations

Take care when prescribing and administering Dilaudid and Dilaudid-HP Injection to avoid dosing errors due to confusion between the different concentrations and between mg and mL, which could result in accidental overdose and death. Take care to ensure the proper dose is communicated and dispensed. When writing prescriptions, include both the total dose in mg and the total volume of the dose. Selection of patients and administration of Dilaudid and Dilaudid-HP injection should be governed by the same principles that apply to the use of similar opioid analgesics to treat patients with acute or chronic pain, and depends upon a comprehensive assessment of the patient. Individualize treatment in every case, using non-opioid analgesics, opioids on an as-needed basis and/or combination products, and chronic opioid therapy in a progressive plan of pain management such as outlined by the World Health Organization, the Agency for Healthcare Research and Quality, and the American Pain Society.

The nature of the pain (severity, frequency, etiology, and pathophysiology), as well as the medical status of the patient, will affect selection of the starting dosage. Opioid analgesics, including DILAUDID INJECTION and DILAUDID-HP INJECTION, have a narrow therapeutic index in certain patient populations, especially when combined with CNS depressant drugs, and should be reserved for cases where the benefits of opioid analgesia outweigh the known risks.

2.2 Individualization of Dosing

Initiate the dosing regimen for each patient individually, taking into account the patient's prior analgesic treatment. Give attention to the following:

- the age, general condition, and medical status of the patient;
- the patient's degree of opioid tolerance;
- the daily dose, potency, and specific characteristics of the opioid the patient has been taking previously;
- concurrent medications
- the type and severity of the patient's pain
- risk factors for abuse or addiction; including whether the patient has a previous or current substance abuse problem, a family history of substance abuse, or a history of mental illness or depression;
- the balance between pain control and adverse reactions.

Periodic reassessment after the initial dosing of DILAUDID INJECTION and DILAUDID-HP INJECTION is required. If pain management is not satisfactory, and opioid-induced adverse events are tolerable, the hydromorphone dose may be increased gradually. If excessive opioid side effects are observed early in the dosing interval, reduce the hydromorphone hydrochloride dose. If this results in breakthrough pain at the end of the dosing interval, the dosing interval may need to be shortened. Dose titration should be guided more by the need for analgesia and the severity of adverse events than the absolute dose of opioid employed.

2.3 Initiation of Therapy in Opioid-Naïve Patients

Always initiate dosing in opioid-naïve patients using Dilaudid Injection. Never administer Dilaudid-HP injection to opioid-naïve patients.

2.3.1 Subcutaneous or Intramuscular Administration

The usual starting dose of Dilaudid Injection is 1 mg to 2 mg every 2 to 3 hours as necessary. Depending on the clinical situation, the initial starting dose may be lowered in patients who are opioid naïve. Adjust the dose according to the severity of pain, the severity of adverse events, as well as the patient's underlying disease and age.

2.3.2 Intravenous Administration

The initial starting dose is 0.2 to 1 mg every 2 to 3 hours. Intravenous administration should be given **slowly**, over at least 2 to 3 minutes, depending on the dose. Titrate the dose to achieve acceptable analgesia and tolerable adverse events. The initial dose should be reduced in the elderly or debilitated and may be lowered to 0.2 mg.

2.3.3 Hepatic Impairment

Start patients with hepatic impairment on one-fourth to one-half the usual DILAUDID INJECTION starting dose depending on the extent of impairment [see CLINICAL PHARMACOLOGY, Pharmacokinetics (12.2)].

2.3.4 Renal Impairment

Start patients with renal impairment on one-fourth to one-half the usual DILAUDID INJECTION starting dose depending on the degree of impairment [see CLINICAL PHARMACOLOGY, Pharmacokinetics (12.2)].

2.4 Conversion From Prior Opioid

Use the equianalgesic dose table below (Table 1) as a guide to determine the appropriate dose of DILAUDID INJECTION. Convert the current total daily amount(s) of opioid(s) received to an equivalent total daily dose of DILAUDID INJECTION and reduce by one-half due to the possibility of incomplete cross tolerance. Divide the new total amount by the number of doses permitted based on dosing interval (e.g., 8 doses for every-three-hour dosing). Titrate the dose according to the patient's response. For opioids not in Table 1, first estimate the daily amount of morphine that is equivalent to the current total daily amount of other opioid(s) received, then use Table 1 to find the approximate equivalent total daily dose of DILAUDID INJECTION.

Table 1. OPIOID ANALGESIC EQUIVALENTS WITH APPROXIMATELY EQUIANALGESIC POTENCY FOR CONVERSION TO DILAUDID INJECTION*

DRUG SUBSTANCE	PARENTERAL DOSE	ORAL DOSE
Morphine sulfate	10 mg	40 – 60 mg
Hydromorphone HCl	1.3 – 2 mg	6.5 – 7.5 mg
Oxymorphone HCl	1 – 1.1 mg	6.6 mg
Levorphanol tartrate	2 – 2.3 mg	4 mg
Meperidine HCl (Pethidine HCl)	75 – 100 mg	300 – 400 mg
Methadone HCl	10 mg	10 – 20 mg
Nalbuphine HCl	10 – 12 mg	–
Butorphanol tartrate	1.5 – 2.5 mg	–

* Dosages, and ranges of dosages represented, are a compilation of estimated equipotent dosages from published references comparing opioid analgesics in cancer and severe pain.

2.5 DILAUDID-HP Injection (for use in opioid-tolerant patients only)

Do not use DILAUDID-HP for patients who are not tolerant to the respiratory depressant or sedating effects of opioids. Patients considered opioid tolerant are those who are taking at least 60 mg oral morphine/day, 25 mcg transdermal fentanyl/hour, 30 mg oral oxycodone/day, 8 mg oral hydromorphone/day, 25 mg oral oxymorphone/day, or an equianalgesic dose of another opioid for one week or longer. Use DILAUDID-HP ONLY for patients who require the higher concentration and lower total volume of DILAUDID-HP.

Because of its high concentration, the delivery of precise doses of DILAUDID-HP INJECTION may be difficult if low doses of hydromorphone are required. Therefore, use DILAUDID-HP INJECTION only if the amount of hydromorphone required can be delivered accurately with this formulation.

Base the starting dose for DILAUDID-HP INJECTION on the prior dose of DILAUDID INJECTION or on the prior dose of an alternate opioid as described above in Section 2.4 Conversion From Prior Opioid and Table 1.

2.6 Administration and Reconstitution

Inspect parenteral drug products visually for particulate matter and discoloration prior to administration, whenever solution and container permit. A slight yellowish discoloration may develop in DILAUDID INJECTION and DILAUDID-HP INJECTION ampules. No loss of potency has been demonstrated. DILAUDID INJECTION and DILAUDID-HP INJECTION are physically compatible and chemically stable for at least 24 hours at 25°C, protected from light in most common large-volume parenteral solutions.

500 mg/50 mL Vial

To use this single dose presentation, do not penetrate the stopper with a syringe. Instead, remove both the aluminum flipseal and rubber stopper in a suitable work area such as under a laminar flow hood (or equivalent clean air compounding area). The contents may then be withdrawn for preparation of a single, large-volume parenteral solution. Discard any unused portion in an appropriate manner.

Reconstitution of Sterile Lyophilized DILAUDID-HP INJECTION 250 mg

Reconstitute immediately prior to use with 25 mL of Sterile Water for Injection USP to provide a sterile solution containing 10 mg/mL of hydromorphone hydrochloride.

3 DOSAGE FORMS AND STRENGTHS

DILAUDID INJECTION:

Each 1 mL colorless ampule contains 1 mg/mL, 2 mg/mL, or 4 mg/mL of hydromorphone hydrochloride in a sterile, aqueous solution.

DILAUDID-HP INJECTION (for use in opioid-tolerant patients only):

Each amber ampule and amber single-dose vial contains 10 mg/mL of hydromorphone hydrochloride in a sterile, aqueous solution and is available in 1 mL or 5 mL ampules or in 50 mL single-dose vials[†].

DILAUDID-HP INJECTION Sterile Lyophilized Powder: Each amber, single-dose vial[†] contains 250 mg of sterile, lyophilized hydromorphone hydrochloride to be reconstituted with 25 mL of Sterile Water for Injection USP to provide a solution containing 10 mg/mL.

[†]**The Stoppers Of These Products Contain Natural Rubber Latex.**

4 CONTRAINDICATIONS

Both DILAUDID INJECTION and DILAUDID-HP INJECTION are contraindicated:

- In patients with known hypersensitivity to hydromorphone, hydromorphone salts, any other components of the product, or sulfite-containing medications [see WARNINGS AND PRECAUTIONS, Sulfites (5.8)].
- In any situation where opioids are contraindicated, e.g., in patients with respiratory depression in the absence of resuscitative equipment or in unmonitored settings; or patients with acute or severe bronchial asthma.
- In patients with, or at risk of developing, gastrointestinal obstruction, especially paralytic ileus because

hydromorphone diminishes the propulsive peristaltic wave in the gastrointestinal tract and may prolong the obstruction.

DILAUDID-HP INJECTION is contraindicated in patients who are not opioid tolerant [see WARNINGS AND PRECAUTIONS (5.1)].

5 WARNINGS AND PRECAUTIONS

5.1 Risk of Medication Errors

DILAUDID-HP INJECTION is a 10 mg/mL concentrated solution of hydromorphone, and is intended for use in opioid-tolerant patients only. Patients considered opioid tolerant are those who are taking at least 60 mg oral morphine/day, 25 mcg transdermal fentanyl/hour, 30 mg oral oxycodone/day, 8 mg oral hydromorphone/day, 25 mg oral oxymorphone/day, or an equianalgesic dose of another opioid for one week or longer.

Do not confuse DILAUDID-HP INJECTION with standard parenteral formulations of DILAUDID INJECTION (1 mg/mL, 2 mg/mL, 4 mg/mL) or other opioids, as overdose and death could result.

Morphine does not convert to hydromorphone on a mg per mg basis. Use Table 1 when converting a patient from morphine to hydromorphone to avoid errors that can lead to overdose or death.

5.2 Respiratory Depression

Respiratory depression is the chief hazard of DILAUDID INJECTION and DILAUDID-HP INJECTION. Respiratory depression occurs most frequently in the elderly, in the debilitated, and in those suffering from conditions accompanied by hypoxia or hypercapnia, or upper airway obstruction, in whom even moderate therapeutic doses may dangerously decrease pulmonary ventilation. Respiratory depression is also a particular problem following large initial doses in non opioid-tolerant patients or when opioids are given in conjunction with other agents that depress respiration.

Use DILAUDID INJECTION and DILAUDID-HP INJECTION with extreme caution in patients with chronic obstructive pulmonary disease or cor pulmonale, patients having a substantially decreased respiratory reserve, hypoxia, hypercapnia, or preexisting respiratory depression. In such patients, even usual therapeutic doses of opioid analgesics may decrease respiratory drive while simultaneously increasing airway resistance to the point of apnea. Consider using non-opioid analgesics, and administer DILAUDID only under careful medical supervision at the lowest effective dose in such patients.

5.3 Misuse, Abuse and Diversion of Opioids

DILAUDID INJECTION and DILAUDID-HP INJECTION contain hydromorphone, an opioid agonist with an abuse liability similar to morphine, and a Schedule II, controlled substance. Hydromorphone has the potential for being abused, is sought by drug abusers and people with addiction disorders, and is subject to criminal diversion. Diversion of Schedule II products is an act subject to criminal penalty.

Abuse of DILAUDID INJECTION and DILAUDID-HP INJECTION, poses a hazard of overdose and death. This risk is increased with concurrent abuse of alcohol and other substances. Schedule II opioid agonists have the highest potential for abuse and risk of fatal respiratory depression. DILAUDID INJECTION and DILAUDID-HP INJECTION can be abused in a manner similar to other opioid agonists, legal or illicit. This should be considered when prescribing or dispensing DILAUDID INJECTION and DILAUDID-HP INJECTION in situations where the physician or pharmacist is concerned about an increased risk of misuse, abuse or diversion.

Concerns about abuse, addiction, and diversion should not prevent the proper management of pain. Healthcare professionals should contact their State Professional Licensing Board or State Controlled Substances Authority for information on how to prevent and detect abuse or diversion of this product.

5.4 Interactions with Alcohol and other CNS Depressants

The concurrent use of DILAUDID INJECTION or DILAUDID-HP INJECTION with other central nervous system (CNS) depressants, including, but not limited to, other opioids, illicit drugs, sedatives, hypnotics, general anesthetics, phenothiazines, muscle relaxants, other tranquilizers, and alcohol, increases the risk of respiratory depression, hypotension, and profound sedation, potentially resulting in coma or death. Use with caution and in reduced dosages in patients taking CNS depressants.

5.5 Neonatal Withdrawal Syndrome

Infants born to mothers physically dependent on DILAUDID INJECTION or DILAUDID-HP INJECTION will also be physically dependent and may exhibit signs of withdrawal. The withdrawal signs include irritability and excessive crying, tremors, hyperactive reflexes, increased respiratory rate, increased stools, sneezing, yawning, vomiting, and fever. The intensity of the syndrome does not always correlate with the duration of maternal opioid use or dose. Neonatal opioid withdrawal syndrome may be life-threatening and should be treated according to protocols developed by neonatology experts [see DRUG ABUSE AND DEPENDENCE (9.3)].

5.6 Use in Increased Intracranial Pressure or Head Injury

The respiratory depressant effects of DILAUDID INJECTION and DILAUDID-HP INJECTION promote carbon dioxide retention which results in elevation of cerebrospinal fluid pressure. This increase in intracranial pressure may be markedly exaggerated in the presence of head injury, intracranial lesions, or other conditions that predispose patients to increased intracranial pressure.

DILAUDID INJECTION and DILAUDID-HP INJECTION may produce effects on pupillary response and consciousness which can obscure the clinical course and neurologic signs of further increase in pressure in patients with head injuries.

5.7 Hypotensive Effect

DILAUDID INJECTION and DILAUDID-HP INJECTION may cause severe hypotension in patients whose ability to maintain blood pressure is compromised by a depleted blood volume, or a concurrent administration of drugs such as phenothiazines, general anesthetics, or other agents which compromise vasomotor tone [see DRUG INTERACTIONS (7.1)].

DILAUDID INJECTION and DILAUDID-HP INJECTION may produce orthostatic hypotension in ambulatory patients.

Administer DILAUDID INJECTION and DILAUDID-HP INJECTION with caution to patients in circulatory shock, since vasodilation produced by the drug may further reduce cardiac output and blood pressure.

5.8 Sulfites

DILAUDID INJECTION and DILAUDID-HP INJECTION contain sodium metabisulfite, a sulfite that may cause allergic-type reactions including anaphylactic symptoms and life-threatening or less severe asthmatic episodes in certain susceptible people. The overall prevalence of sulfite sensitivity in the general population is unknown and probably low. Sulfite sensitivity is seen more frequently in asthmatic than in nonasthmatic people.

5.9 Use in Pancreatic/Biliary Tract Disease and Other Gastrointestinal Conditions

The administration of DILAUDID INJECTION or DILAUDID-HP INJECTION may obscure the diagnosis or clinical course in patients with acute abdominal conditions [see CONTRAINDICATIONS (4.0)].

Use DILAUDID INJECTION and DILAUDID-HP with caution in patients who are at risk of developing ileus.

Use DILAUDID INJECTION and DILAUDID-HP INJECTION with caution in patients with biliary tract disease, including acute pancreatitis, as hydromorphone may cause spasm of the sphincter of Oddi and diminish biliary and pancreatic secretions.

5.10 Special Risk Patients

Give DILAUDID INJECTION and DILAUDID-HP INJECTION with caution and the initial dose should be reduced in the elderly or debilitated and those with severe impairment of hepatic, pulmonary, or renal function; myxedema or hypothyroidism; adrenocortical insufficiency (e.g., Addison's Disease); CNS depression or coma; toxic psychoses; prostatic hypertrophy or urethral stricture; acute alcoholism; delirium tremens; or kyphoscoliosis associated with respiratory depression.

The administration of opioid analgesics including DILAUDID INJECTION and DILAUDID-HP INJECTION may aggravate preexisting convulsions in patients with convulsive disorders.

DILAUDID INJECTION and DILAUDID-HP INJECTION, as with other opioids, may aggravate convulsions in patients with convulsive disorders, and may induce or aggravate seizures in some clinical settings.

Reports of mild to severe seizures and myoclonus have been reported in severely compromised patients administered high doses of parenteral hydromorphone.

5.11 Use in Drug and Alcohol Dependent Patients

Use DILAUDID INJECTION and DILAUDID-HP INJECTION with caution in patients with alcoholism and other drug dependencies due to the increased frequency of opioid tolerance, dependence, and the risk of addiction observed in these patient populations. Abuse of DILAUDID INJECTION or DILAUDID-HP INJECTION in combination with other CNS depressant drugs can result in serious risk to the patient.

DILAUDID INJECTION and DILAUDID-HP INJECTION contain hydromorphone, an opioid with no approved use in the management of addiction disorders. Its proper usage in individuals with drug or alcohol dependence, either active or in remission, is for the management of pain requiring opioid analgesia.

5.12 Use in Ambulatory Patients

DILAUDID INJECTION and DILAUDID-HP INJECTION may impair mental and/or physical ability required for the performance of potentially hazardous tasks (e.g., driving, operating machinery). Patients should be cautioned accordingly. DILAUDID INJECTION and DILAUDID-HP INJECTION may produce orthostatic hypotension in ambulatory patients.

5.13 Parenteral Administration

DILAUDID INJECTION may be given intravenously, but the injection should be given very slowly. Rapid intravenous injection of opioid analgesics increases the possibility of side effects such as hypotension and respiratory depression [see DOSAGE AND ADMINSTRATION (2.3)].

6 ADVERSE REACTIONS

Because clinical trials are conducted under widely varying conditions, adverse reaction rates observed in the clinical trials of a drug cannot be directly compared to rates in the clinical trials of another drug and may not reflect the rates observed in clinical practice.

Serious adverse reactions associated with DILAUDID INJECTION and DILAUDID-HP INJECTION include respiratory depression and apnea and, to a lesser degree, circulatory depression, respiratory arrest, shock, and cardiac arrest.

The following serious adverse reactions described elsewhere in the labeling include:
- Respiratory depression and secondary effects on intracranial pressure [see WARNINGS AND PRECAUTIONS (5.2, 5.6)]
- Hypotension [see WARNINGS AND PRECAUTIONS (5.7)]
- Gastrointestinal effects and effects in sphincter of Oddi [see WARNINGS AND PRECAUTIONS (5.9)]
- Drug abuse, addiction, and dependence [see DRUG ABUSE AND DEPENDENCE (9.2, 9.3)]
- Effects on the ability to drive and operate machinery [see WARNINGS AND PRECAUTIONS (5.12)]

The most common adverse effects are lightheadedness, dizziness, sedation, nausea, vomiting, sweating, flushing, dysphoria, euphoria, dry mouth, and pruritus. These effects seem to be more prominent in ambulatory patients and in those not experiencing severe pain.

Less Frequently Observed Adverse Reactions

Cardiac disorders: tachycardia, bradycardia, palpitations

Eye disorders: vision blurred, diplopia, miosis, visual impairment

Gastrointestinal disorders: constipation, ileus, diarrhea, abdominal pain

General disorders and administration site conditions: weakness, feeling abnormal, chills, injection site urticaria

Hepatobiliary disorders: biliary colic

Metabolism and nutrition disorders: decreased appetite

Musculoskeletal and connective tissue disorders: muscle rigidity

Nervous system disorders: headache, tremor, paraesthesia, nystagmus, increased intracranial pressure, syncope, taste alteration, involuntary muscle contractions, presyncope

Psychiatric disorders: agitation, mood altered, nervousness, anxiety, depression, hallucination, disorientation, insomnia, abnormal dreams

Renal and urinary disorders: urinary retention, urinary hesitation, antidiuretic effects

Respiratory, thoracic, and mediastinal disorders: bronchospasm, laryngospasm

Skin and subcutaneous tissue disorders: injection site pain, urticaria, rash, hyperhidrosis

Vascular disorders: flushing, hypotension, hypertension

Postmarketing Experience

The following adverse reactions have been identified during post-approval use of hydromorphone. Because these events are reported voluntarily from a population of uncertain size, it is not always possible to reliably estimate their frequency or establish a causal relationship to drug exposure: anaphylactic reactions, confusional state, convulsions, drowsiness, dyskinesia, dyspnea, erectile dysfunction, fatigue, hepatic enzymes increased, hyperalgesia, hypersensitivity reaction, injection site reactions, lethargy, myoclonus, oropharyngeal swelling, peripheral edema, and somnolence.

7 DRUG INTERACTIONS

7.1 Drug Interactions with other CNS Depressants

DILAUDID INJECTION and DILAUDID-HP INJECTION should be used with caution and in reduced dosages when administered to patients concurrently receiving other central nervous system depressants including sedatives or hypnotics, general anesthetics, phenothiazines, centrally acting anti-emetics, tranquilizers, and alcohol because respiratory depression, hypotension, and profound sedation or coma may result.

When such combined therapy is contemplated, the dose of one or both agents should be reduced. Opioid analgesics, including DILAUDID INJECTION and DILAUDID-HP INJECTION, may enhance the action of neuromuscular blocking agents and produce an increased degree of respiratory depression.

7.2 Interactions with Mixed Agonist/Antagonist Opioid Analgesics

Agonist/antagonist analgesics (e.g., pentazocine, nalbuphine, and butorphanol) and partial agonist analgesics (buprenorphine) should be administered with caution to a patient who has received or is receiving a course of therapy with a pure opioid agonist analgesic such as DILAUDID INJECTION and DILAUDID-HP INJECTION. In this situation, mixed agonist/antagonist analgesics may reduce the analgesic effect of DILAUDID INJECTION and DILAUDID-HP INJECTION and/or may precipitate withdrawal symptoms in these patients.

7.3 Monoamine Oxidase Inhibitors (MAOIs)

MAOIs may potentiate the action of DILAUDID INJECTION and DILAUDID-HP INJECTION. Allow at least 14 days after stopping treatment with MAOIs before initiating treatment with DILAUDID INJECTION and DILAUDID-HP INJECTION.

7.4 Anticholinergics

Anticholinergics or other medications with anticholinergic activity when used concurrently with DILAUDID INJECTION and DILAUDID-HP INJECTION may result in increased risk of urinary retention and severe constipation, which may lead to paralytic ileus.

8 USE IN SPECIFIC POPULATIONS

8.1 Pregnancy

Teratogenic Effects

Pregnancy Category C: There are no adequate and well-controlled studies in pregnant women. Hydromorphone crosses the placenta. DILAUDID INJECTION or DILAUDID-HP INJECTION should be used during pregnancy only if the potential benefit justifies the potential risk to the fetus.

No effects on teratogenicity or embryotoxicity were observed in pregnant rats given oral doses up to 7 mg/kg/day which is 3-fold higher than the human dose of 24 mg DILAUDID INJECTION (4 mg every 4 hours), on a body surface area basis. Hydromorphone administration to pregnant Syrian hamsters and CF-1 mice during major organ development revealed teratogenic effects likely the result of maternal toxicity associated with sedation and hypoxia. In Syrian hamsters given single subcutaneous doses from 14 to 258 mg/kg during organogenesis (gestation days 8-10), doses ≥ 19 mg/kg of hydromorphone produced skull malformations (exencephaly and cranioschisis). In CF-1 mice, continuous infusion of hydromorphone (≥ 15 mg/kg over 24 hours) via implanted osmotic pumps during organogenesis (gestation days 7-10) produced soft tissue malformations (cryptorchidism, cleft palate, malformed ventricles and retina), and skeletal variations (split supraoccipital, checkerboard and split sternebrae, delayed ossification of the paws and ectopic ossification sites). The malformations and variations observed in the hamsters and mice were observed at doses approximately 6-fold and 3-fold higher, respectively, than the human dose of 24 mg DILAUDID INJECTION (4 mg every 4 hours) on a body surface area basis.

8.2 Labor and Delivery

DILAUDID should be used with caution during labor. Opioids cross the placenta and may produce respiratory depression and physiologic effects in neonates. Sinusoidal fetal heart rate patterns may occur with the use of opioid analgesics.

Occasionally, opioid analgesics, including DILAUDID INJECTION and DILAUDID-HP INJECTION, may prolong labor through actions which temporarily reduce the strength, duration, and frequency of uterine contractions. However, this effect is not consistent and may be offset by an increased rate of cervical dilatation, which tends to shorten labor.

Opioid analgesics, including DILAUDID INJECTION and DILAUDID-HP INJECTION, may cause respiratory depression in the newborn. Closely observe neonates whose mothers received opioid analgesics during labor for signs of respiratory depression. Have a specific opioid antagonist, such as naloxone or nalmefene, available for reversal of opioid-induced respiratory depression in the neonate.

Neonates whose mothers have been taking opioids chronically may also exhibit withdrawal signs, either at birth or in the nursery, because they have developed physical dependence. This is not, however, synonymous with addiction [see DRUG ABUSE AND DEPENDENCE (9.3)]. Neonatal opioid withdrawal syndrome, unlike opioid withdrawal syndrome in adults, may be life-threatening and should be treated according to protocols developed by neonatology experts [see WARNINGS AND PRECAUTIONS (5.3)].

The effect of DILAUDID, if any, on the later growth, development, and functional maturation of the child is unknown.

8.3 Nursing Mothers

Low levels of opioid analgesics have been detected in human milk. As a general rule, nursing should not be undertaken while a patient is receiving DILAUDID INJECTION or DILAUDID-HP INJECTION since it, and other drugs in this class, may be excreted in the milk.

8.4 Pediatric Use

The safety and effectiveness of DILAUDID INJECTION and DILAUDID-HP INJECTION in pediatric patients has not been established.

8.5 Geriatric Use

Clinical studies of DILAUDID INJECTION and DILAUDID-HP INJECTION did not include sufficient numbers of subjects aged 65 and over to determine whether they respond differently from younger subjects. In general, dose selection for an elderly patient should be cautious, usually starting at the low end of the dosing range, reflecting the greater frequency of decreased hepatic, renal, or cardiac function, and of concomitant disease or other drug therapy. Respiratory depression is the chief risk in elderly or debilitated patients, usually the result of large initial doses in non opioid-tolerant patients. Titration in these patients should proceed cautiously [see DOSAGE AND ADMINISTRATION (2.4) and WARNINGS AND PRECAUTIONS (5.10)].

8.6 Renal Impairment

The pharmacokinetics of hydromorphone following an oral administration of hydromorphone at a single 4 mg dose (2 mg hydromorphone immediate-release tablets) are affected by renal impairment. Mean exposure to hydromorphone (C_{max} and $AUC_{0-\infty}$) is increased by 2-fold in patients with moderate (CLcr = 40 - 60 mL/min) renal impairment and increased by 4-fold in patients with severe (CLcr < 30 mL/min) renal impairment compared with normal subjects (CLcr > 80 mL/min). In addition, in patients with severe renal impairment, hydromorphone appeared to be more slowly eliminated with a longer terminal elimination half-life (40 hr) compared to patients with normal renal function (15 hr). Start patients with renal impairment on one-fourth to one-half the usual starting dose depending on the degree of impairment. Patients with renal impairment should be closely monitored during dose titration [see CLINICAL PHARMACOLOGY (12.2)].

8.7 Hepatic Impairment

The pharmacokinetics of hydromorphone following an oral administration of hydromorphone at a single 4 mg dose (2 mg hydromorphone immediate-release tablets) are affected by hepatic impairment. Mean exposure to hydromorphone (C_{max} and AUC_{∞}) is increased 4-fold in patients with moderate (Child-Pugh Group B) hepatic impairment compared with subjects with normal hepatic function. Due to increased exposure of hydromorphone, patients with moderate hepatic impairment should be started at one-fourth to one-half the recommended starting dose depending on the degree of hepatic dysfunction and closely monitored during dose titration. The pharmacokinetics of hydromorphone in patients with severe hepatic impairment has not been studied. A further increase in C_{max} and AUC of hydromorphone in this group is expected and should be taken into consideration when selecting a starting dose [see CLINICAL PHARMACOLOGY (12.2)].

9 DRUG ABUSE AND DEPENDENCE

9.1 Controlled Substance

DILAUDID INJECTION and DILAUDID-HP INJECTION contain hydromorphone, which is a Schedule II controlled substance with an abuse liability similar to morphine. DILAUDID can be abused and is subject to criminal diversion.

9.2 Abuse

DILAUDID INJECTION and DILAUDID-HP INJECTION are intended for parenteral use only under the direct supervision of an appropriately licensed health care professional. Abuse of DILAUDID INJECTION and DILAUDID-HP INJECTION poses a hazard of overdose and death. This risk is increased with concurrent abuse of alcohol or other substances. Parenteral drug abuse is commonly associated with transmission of infectious diseases, such as hepatitis and HIV.

DILAUDID INJECTION and DILAUDID-HP INJECTION can be abused in a manner similar to other opioid agonists, legal or illicit. This should be considered when prescribing, dispensing, ordering, or administering DILAUDID INJECTION or DILAUDID-HP INJECTION in situations where the physician or pharmacist is concerned about an increased risk of misuse, abuse, or diversion. Prescribers should monitor all patients receiving opioids for signs of abuse, misuse, and addiction. Furthermore, patients should be assessed for their potential for opioid abuse prior to being prescribed opioid therapy. Persons at increased risk for opioid abuse include those with a personal or family history of substance abuse (including drug or alcohol abuse) or mental illness (e.g., depression). Opioids may still be appropriate for use in these patients, however, they will require intensive monitoring for indications of abuse.

Opioid drugs are sought by people with substance use disorders (abuse or addiction, the latter of which is also called "substance dependence") and criminals who supply them by diverting medicines out of legitimate distribution channels. DILAUDID INJECTION and DILAUDID-HP INJECTION are targets for diversion.

"Drug-seeking" behavior is very common in persons with substance use disorders. Drug-seeking tactics include, but are not limited to, emergency calls or visits near the end of office hours, refusal to undergo appropriate examination, testing or referral, repeated "loss" of prescriptions, altering or forging of prescriptions and reluctance to provide prior medical records or contact information for other treating physician(s). "Doctor shopping" to obtain additional prescriptions is common among people with untreated substance use disorders and criminals who divert controlled substances.

The risks of misuse and abuse should be considered when prescribing or dispensing DILAUDID INJECTION or DILAUDID-HP INJECTION. Concerns about abuse and addiction, should not prevent the proper management of pain, however. Treatment of pain should be individualized, balancing the potential benefits and risks for each patient.

Addiction is defined as a chronic, neurobiological disorder with genetic, psychosocial, and environmental aspects, characterized by one or more of the following: impaired control over drug use, compulsive use, continued use despite harm, and craving. Drug addiction is a treatable disease, utilizing a multidisciplinary approach, but relapse is common.

Abuse and addiction are separate and distinct from physical dependence and tolerance. Physicians should be aware that addiction may not be accompanied by concurrent tolerance and symptoms of physical dependence in all addicts. In addition, abuse of opioids can occur in the absence of addiction and is characterized by misuse for non-medical purposes, often in combination with other psychoactive substances. Careful record keeping of prescribing information, including quantity, frequency, and renewal requests is strongly advised.

Proper assessment of the patient, proper prescribing practices, periodic re-evaluation of therapy, proper dispensing and correct storage and handling are appropriate measures that help to limit misuse and abuse of opioid drugs. Careful record-keeping of prescribing information, including quantity, frequency, and renewal requests is strongly advised.

Healthcare professionals should contact their State Professional Licensing Board or State Controlled Substances Authority for information on how to prevent and detect abuse or diversion of this product.

9.3 Dependence

Tolerance to opioids is demonstrated by the need for increasing doses to maintain a defined effect such as analgesia (in the absence of disease progression or other external factors). Tolerance to different effects of opioids may develop to varying degrees and at varying rates in a given individual. There is also inter-patient variability in the rate and extent of tolerance that develops to various opioid effects, whether the effect is desirable (e.g., analgesia) or undesirable (e.g., nausea). In general, patients taking opioid analgesics that are appropriately titrated for pain control develop tolerance to the respiratory depressant effects fairly reliably. Conversely, tolerance to the constipating effects of opioids rarely develops, even when they are administered over long periods of time.

Physical dependence is manifested by withdrawal symptoms after abrupt discontinuation of a drug or upon administration of an antagonist. Physical dependence and tolerance are not unusual during chronic opioid therapy.

The opioid abstinence or withdrawal syndrome is characterized by some or all of the following: restlessness, lacrimation, rhinorrhea, yawning, perspiration, chills, myalgia, and mydriasis. Other signs and symptoms also may develop, including: irritability, anxiety, backache, joint pain, weakness, abdominal cramps, insomnia, nausea, anorexia, vomiting, diarrhea, or increased blood pressure, respiratory rate, or heart rate.

In general, opioids used regularly should not be abruptly discontinued.

10 OVERDOSAGE

10.1 Signs and Symptoms

Signs and symptoms of acute overdosage with DILAUDID INJECTION or DILAUDID-HP INJECTION include: respiratory depression, somnolence progressing to stupor or coma, skeletal muscle flaccidity, cold and clammy skin, constricted pupils, bradycardia, hypotension, partial or complete airway obstruction, atypical snoring, apnea, circulatory collapse, cardiac arrest, and death.

Hydromorphone may cause miosis, even in total darkness. Pinpoint pupils are a sign of opioid overdose but are not pathognomonic (pontine lesions of hemorrhagic or ischemic origin may produce similar findings). Marked mydriasis, rather than miosis, may be seen with hypoxia in overdose situations.

10.2 Treatment

In the treatment of overdosage, primary attention should be given to the reestablishment of a patent airway and institution of assisted or controlled ventilation. Supportive measures (including oxygen, vasopressors) should be employed in the management of circulatory shock and pulmonary edema accompanying overdose as indicated. Cardiac arrest or arrhythmias may require cardiac massage or defibrillation.

The opioid antagonist, naloxone, is a specific antidote against respiratory depression which may result from overdosage, or unusual sensitivity to DILAUDID INJECTION or DILAUDID-HP INJECTION. Therefore, an appropriate dose of this antagonist should be administered, preferably by the intravenous route, simultaneously with efforts at respiratory resuscitation. Naloxone should not be administered in the absence of clinically significant respiratory or circulatory depression. Naloxone should be administered cautiously to persons who are known, or suspected, to be physically dependent on DILAUDID INJECTION or DILAUDID-HP INJECTION. In such cases, an abrupt or complete reversal of opioid effects may precipitate an acute withdrawal syndrome.

Since the duration of action of DILAUDID INJECTION and DILAUDID-HP INJECTION may exceed that of the antagonist, the patient should be kept under continued surveillance; repeated doses of the antagonist may be required to maintain adequate respiration. Apply other supportive measures when indicated.

11 DESCRIPTION

DILAUDID (hydromorphone hydrochloride), a hydrogenated ketone of morphine, is an opioid analgesic. The chemical name of DILAUDID is 4,5α-epoxy-3-hydroxy-17-methylmorphinan-6-one hydrochloride. The structural formula is:

$C_{17}H_{19}NO_3 \cdot HCl$ 321.80

DILAUDID INJECTION is available as a sterile, aqueous solution in COLORLESS ampules for parenteral administration. Each 1 mL ampule contains 1 mg, 2 mg, or 4 mg of hydromorphone hydrochloride with 0.2% sodium citrate and 0.2% citric acid added as a buffer to maintain a pH between 3.5 and 5.5.

DILAUDID-HP INJECTION is available as a sterile, aqueous solution in AMBER ampules and in AMBER, single-dose vials for intravenous, subcutaneous, or intramuscular administration. Each ampule and single-dose vial contains 10 mg/mL of hydromorphone hydrochloride with 0.2% sodium citrate and 0.2% citric acid added as a buffer to maintain a pH of between 3.5 and 5.5. The single dose vials are capped with stoppers containing natural rubber latex.

DILAUDID-HP INJECTION is also available as sterile, lyophilized powder in an AMBER, single-dose vial for reconstitution for intravenous, subcutaneous, or intramuscular administration. Each single dose vial contains 250 mg sterile, lyophilized hydromorphone HCl with either hydrochloric acid or sodium hydroxide added to adjust the pH. Each vial is to be reconstituted with 25 mL of Sterile Water for Injection USP to provide a solution containing 10 mg/mL with a pH between 4.5 and 6.5. The single dose vials are capped with stoppers containing natural rubber latex.

12 CLINICAL PHARMACOLOGY

12.1 Mechanism of Action

The precise mode of analgesic action of opioid analgesics is unknown. However, specific CNS opiate receptors have been identified. Opioids are believed to express their pharmacological effects by combining with these receptors.

Hydromorphone hydrochloride is a mu-opioid receptor agonist whose principal therapeutic action is analgesia. Other members of the class known as opioid agonists include substances such as morphine, oxycodone, fentanyl, codeine, hydrocodone, and oxymorphone.

Central Nervous System

Pharmacological effects of opioid agonists include anxiolysis, euphoria, feelings of relaxation, and cough suppression, as well as analgesia.

Hydromorphone produces respiratory depression by direct effect on brain stem respiratory centers. The mechanism of respiratory depression also involves a reduction in the responsiveness of the brain stem respiratory centers to increases in carbon dioxide tension.

Hydromorphone causes miosis. Pinpoint pupils are a common sign of opioid overdose but are not pathognomonic (pontine lesions of hemorrhagic or ischemic origin may produce similar findings).

Gastrointestinal Tract and Other Smooth Muscle

Gastric, biliary and pancreatic secretions are decreased by opioids such as hydromorphone. Hydromorphone causes a reduction in motility associated with an increase in tone in the gastric antrum and duodenum. Digestion of food in the small intestine is delayed and propulsive contractions are decreased. Propulsive peristaltic waves in the colon are decreased, and tone may be increased to the point of spasm. The end result is constipation. Hydromorphone can cause a marked increase in biliary tract pressure as a result of spasm of the sphincter of Oddi.

Cardiovascular System
Hydromorphone may produce hypotension as a result of either peripheral vasodilation, release of histamine, or both. Other manifestations of histamine release and/or peripheral vasodilation may include pruritus, flushing, and red eyes. Effects on the myocardium after intravenous administration of opioids are not significant in normal persons, vary with different opioid analgesic agents and vary with the hemodynamic state of the patient, state of hydration and sympathetic drive.

Endocrine System
Opioids may influence the hypothalamic-pituitary-adrenal or -gonadal axes. Some changes that can be seen include an increase in serum prolactin, and decreases in plasma cortisol and testosterone. Clinical signs and symptoms may be manifest from these hormonal changes.

Immune System
In vitro and animal studies indicate that opioids have a variety of effects on immune functions. The clinical significance of these findings is unknown.

12.2 Pharmacokinetics
Distribution
At therapeutic plasma levels, hydromorphone is approximately 8-19% bound to plasma proteins. After an intravenous bolus dose, the steady state of volume of distribution [mean (%CV)] is 302.9 (32%) liters.

Metabolism
Hydromorphone is extensively metabolized via glucuronidation in the liver, with greater than 95% of the dose metabolized to hydromorphone-3-glucuronide along with minor amounts of 6-hydroxy reduction metabolites.

Elimination
Only a small amount of the hydromorphone dose is excreted unchanged in the urine. Most of the dose is excreted as hydromorphone-3-glucuronide along with minor amounts of 6-hydroxy reduction metabolites. The systemic clearance is approximately 1.96 (20%) liters/minute. The terminal elimination half-life of hydromorphone after an intravenous dose is about 2.3 hours.

Special Populations
Hepatic Impairment
After oral administration of hydromorphone at a single 4 mg dose (2 mg hydromorphone immediate-release tablets), mean exposure to hydromorphone (C_{max} and AUC_∞) is increased 4-fold in patients with moderate (Child-Pugh Group B) hepatic impairment compared with subjects with normal hepatic function. Patients with moderate hepatic impairment should be started at one-fourth to one-half the recommended starting dose and closely monitored during dose titration. The pharmacokinetics of hydromorphone in patients with severe hepatic impairment has not been studied. A further increase in C_{max} and AUC of hydromorphone in this group is expected and should be taken into consideration when selecting a starting dose *[see USE IN SPECIFIC POPULATIONS (8.7)]*.

Renal Impairment
The pharmacokinetics of hydromorphone following an oral administration of hydromorphone at a single 4 mg dose (2 mg hydromorphone immediate-release tablets) are affected by renal impairment. Mean exposure to hydromorphone (C_{max} and $AUC_{0-\infty}$) is increased by 2-fold in patients with moderate (CLcr = 40 - 60 mL/min) renal impairment and increased by 4-fold in patients with severe (CLcr < 30 mL/min) renal impairment compared with normal subjects (CLcr > 80 mL/min). In addition, in patients with severe renal impairment, hydromorphone appeared to be more slowly eliminated with a longer terminal elimination half-life (40 hr) compared to patients with normal renal function (15 hr). Start patients with renal impairment on one-fourth to one-half the usual starting dose depending on the degree of impairment. Patients with renal impairment should be closely monitored during dose titration *[see USE IN SPECIFIC POPULATIONS (8.6)]*.

Pediatrics
Pharmacokinetics of hydromorphone have not been evaluated in children.

Geriatric
In the geriatric population, age has no effect on the pharmacokinetics of hydromorphone.

Gender
Gender has little effect on the pharmacokinetics of hydromorphone. Females appear to have a higher C_{max} (25%) than males with comparable AUC_{0-24} values. The difference observed in C_{max} may not be clinically relevant.

Race
The effect of race on hydromorphone pharmacokinetics has not been studied.

Pregnancy and Nursing Mothers
Hydromorphone crosses the placenta. Hydromorphone is also found in low levels in breast milk, and may cause respiratory compromise in newborns when administered during labor or delivery.

13   NONCLINICAL TOXICOLOGY
13.1   Carcinogenesis, Mutagenesis, Impairment of Fertility
Carcinogenesis
Long term studies in animals to evaluate the carcinogenic potential of hydromorphone have not been conducted.
Mutagenesis
Hydromorphone was not mutagenic in the *in vitro* bacterial reverse mutation assay (Ames assay). Hydromorphone was not clastogenic in either the *in vitro* human lymphocyte chromosome aberration assay or the *in vivo* mouse micronucleus assay.
Impairment of Fertility
No effects on fertility, reproductive performance, or reproductive organ morphology were observed in male or female rats given oral doses up to 7 mg/kg/day which is 3-fold higher than the human dose of 24 mg DILAUDID INJECTION (4 mg every 4 hours), on a body surface area basis.

14   CLINICAL STUDIES
Analgesic effects of single doses of DILAUDID ORAL LIQUID administered to patients with post-surgical pain have been studied in double-blind controlled trials. In one study, both 5 mg and 10 mg of DILAUDID ORAL LIQUID provided significantly more analgesia than placebo.

16   HOW SUPPLIED/STORAGE AND HANDLING
16.1   Safety and Handling Instructions
DILAUDID INJECTION and DILAUDID-HP INJECTION pose little risk of direct exposure to health care personnel and should be handled and disposed of prudently in accordance with hospital or institutional policy. When DILAUDID INJECTION or DILAUDID-HP INJECTION is no longer needed, any unused liquid should be destroyed by flushing it down the toilet.
Access to drugs with a potential for abuse such as DILAUDID INJECTION and DILAUDID-HP INJECTION presents an occupational hazard for addiction in the health care industry. Routine procedures for handling controlled substances developed to protect the public may not be adequate to protect health care workers. Implementation of more effective accounting procedures and measures to restrict access to drugs of this class (appropriate to the practice setting) may minimize the risk of self-administration by health care providers.

16.2   How Supplied
DILAUDID INJECTION
DILAUDID INJECTION (hydromorphone hydrochloride) is supplied in COLORLESS ampules. Each 1 mL of sterile, aqueous solution contains 1 mg, 2 mg, or 4 mg hydromorphone hydrochloride with 0.2% sodium citrate and 0.2% citric acid solution. DILAUDID INJECTION contains no added preservative and is supplied as follows:
NDC 59011-441-10: Box of ten 1 mL (1 mg/mL) ampules
NDC 59011-442-10: Box of ten 1 mL (2 mg/mL) ampules
NDC 59011-442-25: Box of twenty-five 1 mL (2 mg/mL) ampules
NDC 59011-444-10: Box of ten 1 mL (4 mg/mL) ampules
DILAUDID-HP INJECTION
DILAUDID-HP   INJECTION   (hydromorphone hydrochloride) is supplied in AMBER ampules, and AMBER single-dose vials. Each ampule and single-dose vial of sterile aqueous solution contains 10 mg of hydromorphone hydrochloride with 0.2% sodium citrate and 0.2% citric acid solution.
DILAUDID-HP INJECTION Sterile Lyophilized Powder is supplied in an AMBER single-dose vial. Each vial contains 250 mg of sterile, lyophilized hydromorphone hydrochloride. DILAUDID-HP INJECTION contains no added preservative and is supplied as follows:
NDC 59011-445-01: Box of ten 1 mL (10 mg/mL) ampules
NDC 59011-445-05: Box of ten 5 mL (10 mg/mL) ampules
†**NDC** 59011-445-50: One 50 mL (10 mg/mL) single-dose vial with black rubber stopper and white flip-top/tear-off seal.
†**NDC** 59011-446-25: One 250 mg single-dose vial with black rubber stopper and black flip-top seal.
†**The Stoppers for These Products Contain Natural Rubber Latex**

16.3   Storage
PROTECT FROM LIGHT.
Keep covered in carton until time of use. Store at 20° to 25°C (68° to 77°F); excursions permitted to 15° to 30°C (59° to 86°F) [See USP Controlled Room Temperature].
Healthcare professionals can telephone Purdue Pharma L.P.'s Medical Services Department (1-888-726-7535) for information on this product.
CAUTION: DEA Order Form Required.
©2011 Purdue Pharma L.P.

Manufactured by
Hospira, Inc., Lake Forest, IL 60045, U.S.A.
For
Purdue Pharma L.P. Stamford, CT 06901-3431
U.S. Patent Number 6,589,960
302703-0A
Shown in Product Identification Guide, page 312

INTERMEZZO®   Ⓒ Ⓡ
[*in ter mét zoh*]
(zolpidem tartrate)
sublingual tablets

HIGHLIGHTS OF PRESCRIBING INFORMATION
These highlights do not include all the information needed to use INTERMEZZO® safely and effectively. See full prescribing information for INTERMEZZO.
INTERMEZZO® (zolpidem tartrate) sublingual tablets, CIV
Initial U.S. Approval: 1992

————————RECENT MAJOR CHANGES————————
Dosage and Administration (2)   02/2013

————————INDICATIONS AND USAGE————————
Intermezzo is a $GABA_A$ agonist indicated for use as needed for the treatment of insomnia when a middle-of-the-night awakening is followed by difficulty returning to sleep (1)
Limitation of Use: Not indicated for the treatment of middle-of-the night awakening when the patient has fewer than 4 hours of bedtime remaining before the planned time of waking (1)

————————DOSAGE AND ADMINISTRATION————————
• Take only if 4 hours of bedtime remain before the planned time of waking (2.1, 5.1)
• Intermezzo should be placed under the tongue and allowed to disintegrate completely before swallowing. The tablet should not be swallowed whole. (2.1)
• The effect of Intermezzo may be slowed if taken with or immediately after a meal (2.1)
• Recommended dose is 1.75 mg for women and 3.5 mg for men, taken only once per night if needed (2.2)
• Lower doses of CNS depressants may be necessary when taken concomitantly with Intermezzo (2.3)
• Co-administration with CNS depressants: Recommended dose is 1.75 mg for men and women (2.3)
• Geriatric patients and patients with hepatic impairment: Recommended dose is 1.75 mg for men and women (2.4, 2.5)

————————DOSAGE FORMS AND STRENGTHS————————
1.75 mg and 3.5 mg sublingual tablets (3)

————————CONTRAINDICATIONS————————
Known hypersensitivity to zolpidem (4)

————————WARNINGS AND PRECAUTIONS————————
• CNS depressant effects: Impairs alertness and motor coordination. Instruct patients on correct use (5.1)
• Evaluate for co-morbid diagnoses: Re-evaluate if insomnia persists after 7 to 10 days of use (5.2)
• Severe anaphylactic/anaphylactoid reactions: Angioedema and anaphylaxis have been reported. Do not re-challenge if such reactions occur (5.3)
• "Sleep-driving" and other complex behaviors while not fully awake. Risk increases with dose and use with other CNS depressants and alcohol. Immediately evaluate any new onset behavioral changes (5.4)
• Depression: Worsening of depression or suicidal thinking may occur. Prescribe the least number of tablets feasible to avoid intentional overdose (5.5)
• Respiratory Depression: Consider this risk before prescribing in patients with compromised respiratory function (5.6)

————————ADVERSE REACTIONS————————
Most commonly observed adverse reactions (> 1% in adult patients) are headache, nausea, and fatigue. (6.1)
To report SUSPECTED ADVERSE REACTIONS, contact Purdue Pharma at 1-888-726-7535 or FDA at 1-800-FDA-1088 or www.fda.gov/medwatch.

————————DRUG INTERACTIONS————————
• CNS depressants, including alcohol: Possible adverse additive CNS depressant effects (5.1, 7.1)
• Imipramine: Decreased alertness observed (7.1)
• Chlorpromazine: Impaired alertness and psychomotor performance observed (7.1)
• Rifampin: Combination use may decrease effects (7.2)
• Ketoconazole: Combination use may increase effects (7.2)

————————USE IN SPECIFIC POPULATIONS————————
• Pregnancy: Based on animal data, zolpidem may cause fetal harm. (8.1)

• Pediatric use: Safety and effectiveness of Intermezzo not established. With bedtime dosing of zolpidem, hallucinations observed (incidence 7%) (8.4).

See 17 for PATIENT COUNSELING INFORMATION and Medication Guide

Revised: 02/2013

FULL PRESCRIBING INFORMATION: CONTENTS*

FULL PRESCRIBING INFORMATION

1   INDICATIONS AND USAGE

Intermezzo® (zolpidem tartrate) sublingual tablet is indicated for use as needed for the treatment of insomnia when a middle-of-the-night awakening is followed by difficulty returning to sleep.

Limitations of Use: Intermezzo is not indicated for the treatment of middle-of-the-night insomnia when the patient has fewer than 4 hours of bedtime remaining before the planned time of waking.

2   DOSAGE AND ADMINISTRATION

2.1   Important Administration Instructions

Intermezzo is to be taken in bed when a patient wakes in the middle of the night and has difficulty returning to sleep. Intermezzo should only be taken if the patient has at least 4 hours of bedtime remaining before the planned time of waking [see Warnings and Precautions (5.1)].

Intermezzo should be placed under the tongue and allowed to disintegrate completely before swallowing. The tablet should not be swallowed whole. For optimal effect, Intermezzo should not be administered with or immediately after a meal. The tablet should be removed from the pouch just prior to dosing.

2.2   Basic Dosing Information

The recommended and maximum dose of Intermezzo is 1.75 mg for women and 3.5 mg for men, taken only once per night as needed if a middle-of-the-night awakening is followed by difficulty returning to sleep. The recommended doses for women and men are different because women clear zolpidem from the body at a lower rate than men [see Use in Specific Populations (8.6)].

2.3   Use with CNS Depressants

The recommended Intermezzo dose for men and women who are taking concomitant CNS depressants is 1.75 mg. Dose adjustment of concomitant CNS depressants may be necessary when co-administered with Intermezzo because of potentially additive effects. The use of Intermezzo with other sedative-hypnotics (including other zolpidem products) at bedtime or the middle of the night is not recommended [see Warnings and Precautions (5.1)].

2.4   Use in Geriatric Patients

Geriatric patients may be especially sensitive to the effects of zolpidem. The recommended dose of Intermezzo in men and women over 65 years old is 1.75 mg, taken only once per night if needed [see Use in Specific Populations (8.5)].

2.5   Use in Patients with Hepatic Impairment

The recommended dose of Intermezzo in patients with hepatic impairment is 1.75 mg, taken only once per night if needed [see Clinical Pharmacology (12.3)].

3   DOSAGE FORMS AND STRENGTHS

Intermezzo is available as 1.75 mg and 3.5 mg tablets for sublingual administration.

Intermezzo 1.75 mg tablets are yellow, round, uncoated, biconvex, debossed with ZZ on one side.

Intermezzo 3.5 mg tablets are beige, round, uncoated, biconvex, debossed with ZZ on one side.

4   CONTRAINDICATIONS

Intermezzo is contraindicated in patients with known hypersensitivity to zolpidem. Observed reactions with zolpidem include anaphylaxis and angioedema [see Warnings and Precautions (5.3)].

5   WARNINGS AND PRECAUTIONS

5.1   CNS Depressant Effects and Next-Day Impairment

Intermezzo, like other sedative-hypnotic drugs, has central nervous system (CNS) depressant effects. Co-administration with other CNS depressants (e.g., benzodiazepines, opioids, tricyclic antidepressants, alcohol) increases the risk of CNS depression. Dosage adjustments of Intermezzo and of other concomitant CNS depressants may be necessary when Intermezzo is administered with such agents because of the potentially additive effects. The use of Intermezzo with other sedative-hypnotics (including other zolpidem products) at bedtime or the middle of the night is not recommended [see Dosage and Administration (2.3)].

In a driving study, healthy subjects who received Intermezzo with fewer than four hours of bedtime remaining had evidence of impaired driving compared to subjects who received placebo [see Clinical Studies (14.2)]. The risk of next-day driving impairment (and psychomotor impairment) is increased if Intermezzo is taken with less than 4 hours of bedtime remaining, if higher than recommended dose is taken, if co-administered with other CNS depressants, or co-administered with other drugs that increase the blood levels of zolpidem.

5.2   Need to Evaluate for Co-morbid Diagnoses

Because sleep disturbances may be the presenting manifestation of a physical and/or psychiatric disorder, symptomatic treatment of insomnia should be initiated only after a careful evaluation of the patient. *The failure of insomnia to remit after 7 to 10 days of treatment may indicate the presence of a primary psychiatric and/or medical illness that should be evaluated.* Worsening of insomnia or the emergence of new thinking or behavior abnormalities may be the consequence of an unrecognized psychiatric or physical disorder. Such findings have emerged during the course of treatment with sedative-hypnotic drugs, including zolpidem.

5.3   Severe Anaphylactic and Anaphylactoid Reactions

Cases of angioedema involving the tongue, glottis, or larynx have been reported in patients after taking the first or subsequent doses of zolpidem. Some patients have had additional symptoms such as dyspnea, throat closing, or nausea and vomiting that suggest anaphylaxis. Some patients have required medical therapy in the emergency department. If angioedema involves the throat, glottis or larynx, airway obstruction may occur and be fatal. Patients who develop angioedema or anaphylaxis after treatment with zolpidem should not be rechallenged with Intermezzo.

5.4   Abnormal Thinking and Behavioral Changes

Abnormal thinking and behavior changes have been reported in patients treated with sedative-hypnotics including zolpidem. Some of these changes included decreased inhibition (e.g., aggressiveness and extroversion that seemed out of character), bizarre behavior, agitation, and depersonalization. Visual and auditory hallucinations have also been reported.

In controlled trials of zolpidem tartrate 10 mg taken at bedtime, < 1% of adults with insomnia who received zolpidem reported hallucinations. In a clinical trial, 7% of pediatric patients treated with zolpidem tartrate 0.25 mg/kg taken at bedtime, reported hallucinations, versus 0% treated with placebo [see Use in Specific Populations (8.4)].

Complex behaviors such as "sleep-driving" (i.e., driving while not fully awake after ingestion of a sedative-hypnotic, with amnesia for the event) have been reported in sedative-hypnotic-naive as well as in sedative-hypnotic-experienced persons. Although behaviors such as "sleep-driving" have occurred with zolpidem alone at therapeutic doses, the co-administration of zolpidem with alcohol and other CNS depressants increases the risk of such behaviors, as does the use of zolpidem at doses exceeding the maximum recommended dose. Due to the risk to the patient and the community, discontinuation of Intermezzo should be strongly considered for patients who report a "sleep-driving" episode. Other complex behaviors (e.g., preparing and eating food, making phone calls, or having sex) have been reported in patients who are not fully awake after taking a sedative-hypnotic. As with "sleep-driving," patients usually do not remember these events. Amnesia, anxiety and other neuropsychiatric symptoms may also occur.

The emergence of any new behavioral sign or symptom of concern requires careful and immediate evaluation.

5.5   Use in Patients with Depression

In primarily depressed patients treated with sedative-hypnotics, worsening of depression, and suicidal thoughts and actions (including completed suicides), have been reported. Suicidal tendencies may be present in such patients and protective measures may be required. Intentional overdosage is more common in this group of patients; therefore, the lowest number of tablets that is feasible should be prescribed for the patient at any one time.

5.6   Respiratory Depression

Although studies with 10 mg zolpidem tartrate did not reveal respiratory depressant effects at hypnotic doses in healthy subjects or in patients with mild-to-moderate chronic obstructive pulmonary disease (COPD), a reduction in the Total Arousal Index, together with a reduction in lowest oxygen saturation and increase in the times of oxygen desaturation below 80% and 90%, was observed in patients with mild-to-moderate sleep apnea when treated with zolpidem compared to placebo. Since sedative-hypnotics have the capacity to depress respiratory drive, precautions should be taken if Intermezzo is prescribed to patients with compromised respiratory function. Post-marketing reports of respiratory insufficiency in patients receiving 10 mg of zolpidem tartrate, most of whom had pre-existing respiratory impairment, have been reported. The risks of respiratory depression should be considered prior to prescribing Intermezzo in patients with respiratory impairment including sleep apnea and myasthenia gravis.

5.7   Withdrawal Effects

There have been reports of withdrawal signs and symptoms following the rapid dose decrease or abrupt discontinuation of zolpidem. Monitor patients for tolerance, abuse, and dependence [see Drug Abuse and Dependence (9.2) and (9.3)].

6   ADVERSE REACTIONS

The following serious adverse reactions in zolpidem-treated patients are discussed in greater detail in other sections of the labeling:

• CNS-depressant effects and next-day impairment [see Warnings and Precautions (5.1)]
• Serious anaphylactic and anaphylactoid reactions [see Warnings and Precautions (5.3)]
• Abnormal thinking and behavioral changes, and complex behaviors [see Warnings and Precautions (5.4)]
• Withdrawal effects [see Warnings and Precautions (5.7)]

6.1   Clinical Trials Experience

The safety data described below are based on two double-blind placebo-controlled trials of Intermezzo in adult patients with insomnia characterized by difficulty returning to sleep after a middle-of-the-night awakening [see Clinical Studies (14.1)]. These two trials included 230 and 82 patients treated with 3.5 mg and 1.75 mg of Intermezzo, respectively. The first study was a 3-way crossover sleep-laboratory study in 82 patients (58 female and 24 male; median age 47 years; 51% Caucasian, 44% African-American) of 1.75 mg and 3.5 mg of Intermezzo compared to placebo (Study 1). The second study was a 4-week, parallel-group at-home study in 295 patients (201 female and 94 male; median age 43 years) of 3.5 mg of Intermezzo compared to placebo, used on an as-needed basis after spontaneous middle-of-the-night awakenings (Study 2). In Study 2, patients took Intermezzo during the night on 62% of study nights.

Because clinical trials are conducted under widely varying conditions, adverse reaction rates observed in the clinical trials of a drug cannot be directly compared to rates in the clinical trials of another drug and may not reflect the rates observed in actual practice.

Table 1 shows the incidence of adverse reactions reported in Study 2 that occurred in 2% or more of Intermezzo-treated (3.5 mg) patients in which the incidence was greater than the incidence in placebo-treated patients. For women and other patients taking the 1.75 mg dose in Study 1, the incidence of adverse reactions was similar to the incidence seen with 3.5 mg of Intermezzo in Table 1.

The most commonly reported adverse reactions in all treatment groups were headache, nausea, and fatigue.

Table 1: Summary of Adverse Reactions (≥ 2%) in Outpatient, Double-Blind, Parallel-Group, Placebo-Controlled Study (Study 2)

MedDRA System Organ Class Preferred Term	3.5 mg Intermezzo (n=150)	Placebo (n=145)
Gastrointestinal Disorders	4%	2%
Nausea	1%	1%
General Disorders and Administration Site Conditions	3%	0%
Fatigue	1%	0%
Nervous System Disorders	5%	3%
Headache	3%	1%

7 DRUG INTERACTIONS

7.1 CNS-active Drugs

Co-administration of zolpidem with other CNS depressants increases the risk of CNS depression [see Warnings and Precautions (5.1)]. Zolpidem tartrate was evaluated in healthy volunteers in single-dose interaction studies for several CNS drugs.

Imipramine
Imipramine in combination with zolpidem produced no pharmacokinetic interaction other than a 20% decrease in peak levels of imipramine, but there was an additive effect of decreased alertness. Similarly, chlorpromazine in combination with zolpidem produced no pharmacokinetic interaction, but there was an additive effect of decreased alertness and psychomotor performance.

Haloperidol
A study involving haloperidol and zolpidem revealed no effect of haloperidol on the pharmacokinetics or pharmacodynamics of zolpidem. The lack of a drug interaction following single-dose administration does not predict the absence of an effect following chronic administration.

Alcohol
An additive adverse effect on psychomotor performance between alcohol and oral zolpidem was demonstrated [see Warnings and Precautions (5.1)].

Sertraline
Concomitant administration of zolpidem and sertraline increases exposure to zolpidem and may increase the pharmacodynamic effect of zolpidem.

Fluoxetine
After multiple doses of zolpidem tartrate and fluoxetine, an increase in the zolpidem half-life (17%) was observed. There was no evidence of an additive effect in psychomotor performance [see Clinical Pharmacology (12.3)].

7.2 Drugs that Affect Drug Metabolism via Cytochrome P450

Some compounds known to inhibit CYP3A may increase exposure to zolpidem. The effect of other P450 enzymes on the exposure to zolpidem is not known.

Rifampin
Rifampin, a CYP3A4 inducer, significantly reduced the exposure to and the pharmacodynamic effects of zolpidem. Use of rifampin in combination with zolpidem may decrease the efficacy of zolpidem.

Ketoconazole
Ketoconazole, a potent CYP3A4 inhibitor, increased the pharmacodynamic effects of zolpidem. Consideration should be given to using a lower dose of zolpidem when ketoconazole and zolpidem are given together.

8 USE IN SPECIFIC POPULATIONS

8.1 Pregnancy

Pregnancy Category C
There are no adequate and well-controlled studies of zolpidem in pregnant women. Studies in children to assess the effects of prenatal exposure to zolpidem have not been conducted; however, cases of severe neonatal respiratory depression have been reported when zolpidem was used at the end of pregnancy, especially when taken with other CNS-depressants. Children born to mothers taking sedative-hypnotic drugs may be at risk for withdrawal symptoms during the postnatal period. Neonatal flaccidity has also been reported in infants born to mothers who received sedative-hypnotic drugs during pregnancy. Intermezzo should be used during pregnancy only if the potential benefit outweighs the potential risk to the fetus.
Administration of zolpidem to pregnant rats and rabbits resulted in adverse effects on offspring at doses greater than the recommended human dose (RHD) of 3.5 mg/day (approximately 2.8 mg/day zolpidem base); however, teratogenicity was not observed.

When zolpidem was administered at oral doses of 4, 20, and 100 mg base/kg/day to pregnant rats during the period of organogenesis, dose-related decreases in fetal skull ossification were observed at all but the lowest dose, which is approximately 15 times the RHD on a mg/m² basis. In rabbits treated during organogenesis with zolpidem at oral doses of 1, 4, and 16 mg base/kg/day, increased embryo-fetal death and incomplete fetal skull ossification were seen at the highest dose tested. The no-effect dose for embryo-fetal toxicity in rabbits is approximately 30 times the RHD on a mg/m² basis. Administration of zolpidem to rats at oral doses of 4, 20, and 100 mg base/kg/day during the latter part of pregnancy and throughout lactation produced decreased offspring growth and survival at all but the lowest dose, which is approximately 15 times the RHD on a mg/m² basis.

8.3 Nursing Mothers

Zolpidem is excreted in human milk. The effect of zolpidem on the nursing infant is not known.

8.4 Pediatric Use

Intermezzo is not recommended for use in children. Safety and effectiveness of Intermezzo have not been established in pediatric patients below the age of 18.
In an 8-week study in pediatric patients (aged 6 to 17 years) with insomnia associated with ADHD, an oral solution of zolpidem tartrate dosed at 0.25 mg/kg at bedtime did not decrease sleep latency compared to placebo. Hallucinations were reported in 7% of the pediatric patients who received zolpidem; none of the pediatric patients who received placebo reported hallucinations.

8.5 Geriatric Use

Intermezzo dosage adjustment is necessary in geriatric patients. Sedating drugs may cause confusion and over-sedation in the elderly; elderly patients generally should be started on low doses of Intermezzo and observed closely [see Dosage and Administration (2.4), and Clinical Pharmacology (12.3)].
Clinical trial experience with other zolpidem formulations (5 mg to 10 mg oral zolpidem tartrate) given at bedtime:
A total of 154 patients in U.S.-controlled clinical trials and 897 patients in non-U.S. clinical trials who received oral zolpidem were ≥ 60 years of age. For a pool of U.S. patients receiving oral zolpidem tartrate at doses of ≤ 10 mg or placebo, there were three adverse reactions occurring at an incidence of at least 3% for zolpidem and for which the zolpidem incidence was at least twice the placebo incidence (see Table 2).

Table 2: Adverse Reactions in Geriatric Patients in Pooled Trials of 5 mg to 10 mg of Oral Zolpidem Tartrate Given at Bedtime

Adverse Reaction	5 to 10 mg Oral Zolpidem tartrate	Placebo
Dizziness	3%	0%
Drowsiness	5%	2%
Diarrhea	3%	1%

Falls in geriatric patients:
A total of 30/1,959 (2%) non-U.S. patients receiving other zolpidem formulations (5 mg to 10 mg oral zolpidem tartrate) reported falls, including 28/30 (93%) who were ≥ 70 years of age. Of these 28 patients, 23 (82%) were receiving zolpidem tartrate doses > 10 mg. A total of 24/1,959 (1%) non-U.S. patients receiving zolpidem reported confusion, including 18/24 (75%) who were ≥70 years of age. Of these 18 patients, 14 (78%) were receiving zolpidem tartrate doses >10 mg.
The dose of Intermezzo in elderly patients is 1.75 mg to minimize adverse effects related to impaired motor and/or cognitive performance and unusual sensitivity to sedative-hypnotic drugs.

8.6 Gender Differences in Pharmacokinetics

Women cleared zolpidem tartrate from the body after sublingual administration of a 3.5 mg dose of Intermezzo at a lower rate than men (2.7 mL/min/kg vs. 4.0 mL/min/kg). C_{max} and AUC parameters of zolpidem were approximately 45% higher at the same dose in female subjects compared with male subjects. Given the higher blood levels of zolpidem tartrate in women compared to men at a given dose, the recommended dose of Intermezzo for women is 1.75 mg, and the recommended dose for adult men is 3.5 mg.

9 DRUG ABUSE AND DEPENDENCE

9.1 Controlled Substance

Zolpidem tartrate is classified as a Schedule IV controlled substance by federal regulation.

9.2 Abuse

Abuse and addiction are separate and distinct from physical dependence and tolerance. Abuse is characterized by misuse of the drug for non-medical purposes, often in combination with other psychoactive substances. Tolerance is a state of adaptation in which exposure to a drug induces changes that result in diminution of one or more of the drug effects over time. Tolerance may occur to both desired and undesired effects of drugs and may develop at different rates for different effects.
Addiction is a primary, chronic, neurobiological disease with genetic, psychosocial, and environmental factors influencing its development and manifestations. It is characterized by behaviors that include one or more of the following: impaired control over drug use, compulsive use, continued use despite harm, and craving. Drug addiction is a treatable disease, using a multidisciplinary approach, but relapse is common.
Studies of abuse potential in former drug abusers found that the effects of single doses of 40 mg of oral zolpidem tartrate were similar, but not identical, to diazepam 20 mg, while 10 mg of oral zolpidem tartrate was difficult to distinguish from placebo.
Because persons with a history of addiction to or abuse of drugs or alcohol are at increased risk for misuse, abuse and addiction of zolpidem, they should be monitored carefully when receiving Intermezzo.

9.3 Dependence

Physical dependence is a state of adaptation that is manifested by a specific withdrawal syndrome that can be produced by abrupt cessation, rapid dose reduction, decreasing blood level of the drug, and/or administration of an antagonist.
Sedative-hypnotics have produced withdrawal signs and symptoms following abrupt discontinuation. These reported symptoms range from mild dysphoria and insomnia to a withdrawal syndrome that may include abdominal and muscle cramps, vomiting, sweating, tremors, and convulsions. The following adverse events which are considered to meet the DSM-III-R criteria for uncomplicated sedative-hypnotic withdrawal were reported during U.S. clinical trials with other oral zolpidem formulations following placebo substitution occurring within 48 hours following the last zolpidem treatment: fatigue, nausea, flushing, lightheadedness, uncontrolled crying, emesis, stomach cramps, panic attack, nervousness, and abdominal discomfort. These reported adverse events occurred at an incidence of 1% or less. However, available data cannot provide a reliable estimate of the incidence, if any, of dependence during treatment at recommended doses. Post-marketing reports of abuse, dependence, and withdrawal resulting from use of oral zolpidem tartrate have been received.

10 OVERDOSAGE

10.1 Signs and Symptoms

In post-marketing experience of overdose with oral zolpidem tartrate alone, or in combination with CNS-depressant agents, impairment of consciousness ranging from somnolence to coma, cardiovascular and/or respiratory compromise, and fatal outcomes have been reported.

10.2 Recommended Treatment

General symptomatic and supportive measures should be used along with immediate gastric lavage where appropriate. Intravenous fluids should be administered as needed. Zolpidem's sedative-hypnotic effect was shown to be reduced by flumazenil and therefore flumazenil may be useful; however, flumazenil administration may contribute to the appearance of neurological symptoms (convulsions). As in all cases of drug overdose, respiration, pulse, blood pressure, and other appropriate signs should be monitored and general supportive measures employed. Hypotension and CNS depression should be treated by appropriate medical intervention. Sedating drugs should be withheld following zolpidem overdosage, even if excitation occurs. The value of dialysis in the treatment of overdosage has not been determined, although hemodialysis studies in patients with renal failure receiving therapeutic doses have demonstrated that zolpidem is not dialyzable.
As with management of all overdosage, the possibility of multiple drug ingestion should be considered. The healthcare provider may wish to consider contacting a poison control center for up-to-date information on the management of hypnotic drug overdosage.

11 DESCRIPTION

Intermezzo contains zolpidem tartrate, a non-benzodiazepine hypnotic of the imidazopyridine class. Intermezzo is available in 1.75 mg and 3.5 mg strength tablets for sublingual administration. Intermezzo sublingual tablets are intended to be placed under the tongue where they will disintegrate.
Intermezzo sublingual tablets contain a bicarbonate-carbonate buffer.
Chemically, zolpidem tartrate is *N,N*-6-trimethyl-2-*p*-tolylimidazo[1,2-α]pyridine-3-acetamide L-(+)-tartrate (2:1). [See chemical structure at top of next column]
Zolpidem tartrate is a white to off-white crystalline powder that is sparingly soluble in water, alcohol, and propylene glycol. It has a molecular weight of 764.88.

Each Intermezzo tablet includes the following inactive ingredients: mannitol, sorbitol, crospovidone, silicon dioxide, sodium carbonate, sodium bicarbonate, croscarmellose sodium, sodium stearyl fumarate, silicon dioxide, natural and artificial spearmint flavor, silicon dioxide-colloidal, and sucralose. The 1.75 mg tablet also contains yellow iron oxide, and the 3.5 mg tablet contains beige iron oxide.

12 CLINICAL PHARMACOLOGY

12.1 Mechanism of Action

Zolpidem, the active moiety of zolpidem tartrate, is a hypnotic agent with a chemical structure unrelated to benzodiazepines, barbiturates, or other drugs with known hypnotic properties. It interacts with a GABA-BZ complex and shares some of the pharmacological properties of the benzodiazepines. In contrast to the benzodiazepines, which nonselectively bind to and activate all BZ receptor subtypes, zolpidem in vitro binds the BZ_1 receptor preferentially with a high affinity ratio of the $alpha_1/alpha_5$ subunits. This selective binding of zolpidem on the BZ_1 receptor is not absolute, but it may explain the relative absence of myorelaxant and anticonvulsant effects in animal studies as well as the preservation of deep sleep (stages 3 and 4) in human studies of zolpidem at hypnotic doses.

12.3 Pharmacokinetics

Absorption

Intermezzo disintegrates in the sublingual cavity after administration. On average, Intermezzo is rapidly absorbed in both genders, with a mean T_{max} across studies of about 35 minutes to about 75 minutes.

In healthy normal volunteers (age 21 to 45 years) dosed with 3.5 mg Intermezzo, the average C_{max} and AUC were 77 ng/mL and 296 ng•h/mL, respectively in women. The average C_{max} and AUC were 53 ng/mL and 198 ng•h/mL, respectively in men. In women, the average C_{max} and AUC of the 1.75 mg Intermezzo dose were 37 ng/mL and 151 ng•h/mL, respectively.

Food decreased the overall C_{max} and AUC of Intermezzo 3.5 mg by 42% and 19%, respectively, and increased the time to peak exposure (T_{max}) to nearly 3 hours. For optimal effect, Intermezzo should not be administered with or immediately after a meal.

Distribution

Based on data obtained with oral zolpidem, the total protein binding was found to be 93% ± 0.1% and remained constant independent of concentration between 40 ng/mL and 790 ng/mL.

Metabolism

Based on data obtained with oral zolpidem, zolpidem tartrate is converted to inactive metabolites that are eliminated primarily by renal excretion.

Elimination

The elimination half-life of a single dose of a 3.5 mg Intermezzo sublingual tablet is approximately 2.5 hours (range 1.4 to 3.6 hours).

Special Populations

Elderly: The recommended dose for Intermezzo is 1.75 mg. A pharmacokinetic study of 1.75 mg and 3.5 mg doses of Intermezzo showed that the plasma C_{max} and $AUC_{0-4 hr}$ in elderly subjects following the 3.5 mg dose was higher by 34% and 30%, respectively, than the non-elderly subjects. The C_{max} and AUC of 1.75 mg in elderly subjects were consistently lower than those observed for the 3.5 mg dose in non-elderly subjects but consistently higher than the 1.75 mg dose in non-elderly subjects. The elimination half-life remained unchanged.

Hepatic Impairment: The pharmacokinetics of oral zolpidem tartrate in eight patients with chronic hepatic insufficiency were compared to results in subjects with normal hepatic function. Following a single 20 mg oral zolpidem tartrate dose, mean C_{max} and AUC were found to be two times (250 ng/mL vs. 499 ng/mL) and five times (788 ng•hr/mL vs. 4203 ng•hr/mL) higher, respectively, in hepatically compromised patients compared to subjects with normal hepatic function. T_{max} did not change. The mean half-life in cirrhotic patients of 9.9 hr (range: 4.1 to 25.8 hr) was greater than that observed in subjects with normal hepatic function of 2.2 hr (range: 1.6 to 2.4 hr). Dosing should be modified accordingly in patients with hepatic insufficiency [see Dosage and Administration (2.5)].

Renal Impairment: The pharmacokinetics of zolpidem tartrate were studied in 11 patients with end-stage renal failure (mean Cl_{Cr}= 6.5 ± 1.5 mL/min) undergoing hemodialysis three times a week, who were dosed with zolpidem tartrate 10 mg orally each day for 14 or 21 days. No statistically significant differences were observed for C_{max}, T_{max},

half-life, and AUC between the first and last day of drug administration when baseline concentration adjustments were made. Zolpidem was not hemodialyzable. No accumulation of unchanged drug appeared after 14 or 21 days. Zolpidem pharmacokinetics were not significantly different in renally-impaired patients. No dosage adjustment is necessary in patients with renal impairment.

Drug Interactions

CNS-depressants

Co-administration of zolpidem with other CNS depressants increases the risk of CNS depression [see Warnings and Precautions (5.1)]. Zolpidem tartrate was evaluated in healthy volunteers in single-dose interaction studies for several CNS drugs. Imipramine in combination with zolpidem produced no pharmacokinetic interaction other than a 20% decrease in peak levels of imipramine, but there was an additive effect of decreased alertness. Similarly, chlorpromazine in combination with zolpidem produced no pharmacokinetic interaction, but there was an additive effect of decreased alertness and psychomotor performance.

A study involving haloperidol and zolpidem revealed no effect of haloperidol on the pharmacokinetics or pharmacodynamics of zolpidem. The lack of a drug interaction following single-dose administration does not predict the absence of an effect following chronic administration.

An additive adverse effect on psychomotor performance between alcohol and oral zolpidem was demonstrated [see Warnings and Precautions (5.1)].

Following five consecutive nightly doses at bedtime of oral zolpidem tartrate 10 mg in the presence of sertraline 50 mg (17 consecutive daily doses, at 7:00 am, in healthy female volunteers), zolpidem C_{max} was significantly higher (43%) and T_{max} was significantly decreased (-53%). Pharmacokinetics of sertraline and N-desmethylsertraline were unaffected by zolpidem.

A single-dose interaction study with zolpidem tartrate 10 mg and fluoxetine 20 mg at steady-state levels in male volunteers did not demonstrate any clinically significant pharmacokinetic or pharmacodynamic interactions. When multiple doses of zolpidem and fluoxetine were given at steady state and the concentrations evaluated in healthy females, an increase in the zolpidem half-life (17%) was observed. There was no evidence of an additive effect in psychomotor performance.

Drugs that Affect Drug Metabolism via Cytochrome P450

Some compounds known to inhibit CYP3A may increase exposure to zolpidem. The effect of inhibitors of other P450 enzymes on the pharmacokinetics of zolpidem is unknown.

A single-dose interaction study with zolpidem tartrate 10 mg and itraconazole 200 mg at steady-state levels in male volunteers resulted in a 34% increase in $AUC_{0-\infty}$ of zolpidem tartrate. There were no pharmacodynamic effects of zolpidem detected on subjective drowsiness, postural sway, or psychomotor performance.

A single-dose interaction study with zolpidem tartrate 10 mg and rifampin 600 mg at steady-state levels in female subjects showed significant reductions of the AUC (-73%), C_{max} (-58%), and $T_{1/2}$ (-36 %) of zolpidem together with significant reductions in the pharmacodynamic effects of zolpidem tartrate. Rifampin, a CYP3A4 inducer, significantly reduced the exposure to and the pharmacodynamic effects of zolpidem.

A single-dose interaction study with zolpidem tartrate 5 mg and ketoconazole, a potent CYP3A4 inhibitor, given as 200 mg twice daily for 2 days increased C_{max} of zolpidem (30%) and the total AUC of zolpidem (70%) compared to zolpidem alone and prolonged the elimination half-life (30%) along with an increase in the pharmacodynamic effects of zolpidem. Consideration should be given to using a lower dose of zolpidem when ketoconazole and zolpidem are given together.

Other Drugs with No Interactions with Zolpidem

A study involving cimetidine/zolpidem tartrate and ranitidine/zolpidem tartrate combinations revealed no effect of either drug on the pharmacokinetics or pharmacodynamics of zolpidem.

Zolpidem tartrate had no effect on digoxin pharmacokinetics and did not affect prothrombin time when given with warfarin in healthy subjects.

13 NONCLINICAL TOXICOLOGY

13.1 Carcinogenesis, Mutagenesis, Impairment of Fertility

Carcinogenesis: Zolpidem was administered in the diet to rats and mice for 2 years at doses of 4, 18, and 80 mg base/kg/day. In mice, these doses are approximately 7, 30, and 140 times, respectively, the recommended human dose (RHD) of 3.5 mg/day (approximately 2.8 mg zolpidem base) on a mg/m^2 basis. In rats, these doses are approximately 15, 60, and 280 times, respectively, the RHD on a mg/m^2 basis. No evidence of carcinogenic potential was observed in mice. In rats, renal tumors (lipoma, liposarcoma) were seen at the mid- and high doses.

Mutagenesis: Zolpidem was negative in in vitro (bacterial reverse mutation, mouse lymphoma, and chromosomal aberration) and in vivo (mouse micronucleus) genetic toxicology assays.

Impairment of fertility: Oral administration of zolpidem (doses of 4, 20, and 100 mg base/kg/day) to rats prior to and during mating, and continuing in females through postpartum day 25, resulted in irregular estrus cycles and prolonged precoital intervals at the highest dose tested. The no-effect dose for these findings is approximately 70 times the RHD on a mg/m^2 basis. There was no impairment of fertility at any dose tested.

14 CLINICAL STUDIES

14.1 Middle-of-the-Night Awakening Trials

Intermezzo was evaluated in two randomized, double-blind, placebo-controlled studies (Studies 1 and 2) in patients with insomnia characterized by difficulty returning to sleep after a middle-of-the-night (MOTN) awakening. In these studies, patients met the diagnosis for primary insomnia as defined by the Diagnostic and Statistical Manual of Mental Disorders (DSM-IV-TR) and had at least three prolonged MOTN awakenings per week that were at least 30 minutes in duration.

Sleep Laboratory Study (Scheduled Dosing)

Adult patients aged 19 to 64 years (N=82; 58 female, 24 male) with a history of difficulty returning to sleep after middle-of-the-night awakenings were evaluated in a double-blind, placebo-controlled, 3-period cross-over sleep laboratory study (Study 1). The primary outcome measure was latency to persistent sleep (LPS).

Doses of 3.5 mg and 1.75 mg of Intermezzo significantly decreased both objective (by polysomnography) and subjective (patient-estimated) sleep latency after a scheduled middle-of-the-night awakening as compared to placebo. The effect on sleep latency was similar for females receiving 1.75 mg of Intermezzo and males receiving 3.5 mg of Intermezzo.

Outpatient Study (As-needed Dosing)

Adult patients aged 18 to 64 years (N=295; 201 women, 94 men) with difficulty returning to sleep after middle-of-the-night awakenings were evaluated in a double-blind, placebo-controlled 4-week outpatient study of Intermezzo. Patients took study drug (3.5 mg of Intermezzo or placebo) on an as-needed (prn) basis, when they had difficulty returning to sleep after waking in the middle of the night, provided they had at least 4 hours time remaining in bed. Subjective (patient-estimated) time to fall back to sleep after middle-of-the-night awakening was significantly shorter for Intermezzo 3.5 mg compared to placebo.

14.2 Special Safety Studies

Driving Study

A randomized, double-blind, placebo-controlled, active-control, single-center, four-period, crossover study in 40 healthy subjects was conducted to evaluate the effects of middle-of-the-night administration of Intermezzo on next-morning driving performance. The four randomized treatments included Intermezzo 3.5 mg four hours before driving, Intermezzo 3.5 mg three hours before driving, placebo, and a positive control (an unapproved sedative-hypnotic) given nine hours before driving.

The primary outcome measure was the change in the standard deviation of lateral position (SDLP), a measure of driving impairment. The results were analyzed using a symmetry analysis, which determined the proportion of subjects whose change from their own SDLP in the placebo condition was statistically significantly above a threshold thought to reflect clinically meaningful driving impairment.

When driving began 3 hours after taking Intermezzo, testing had to be terminated for one subject (a 23-year old woman) due to somnolence. Overall, the symmetry analysis showed a statistically significant impairing effect at 3 hours. When driving began 4 hours after taking Intermezzo, statistically significant impairment was not found, but numerically Intermezzo was worse than placebo. Zolpidem blood levels were not measured in the driving study, and the study was not designed to correlate specific blood level with degree of impairment. However, the estimated blood level of zolpidem in patients whose SDLP worsened according to the symmetry analysis is considered to present a risk for driving impairment. In some women, the 3.5 mg dose of Intermezzo results in zolpidem blood levels that remain at or sometimes considerably above this level 4 or more hours after dosing. Therefore, the recommended dose for women is 1.75 mg. A small negative effect on SDLP may remain in some patients 4 hours after the 1.75 mg dose in women, and after the 3.5 mg dose in men, such that a potential negative effect on driving cannot be completely excluded.

Rebound effects

In studies performed with other zolpidem formulations (5 mg to 10 mg oral zolpidem tartrate) given at bedtime, there was no objective (polysomnographic) evidence of rebound insomnia at recommended doses seen in studies evaluating sleep on the nights following discontinuation. There was subjective evidence of impaired sleep in the elderly on the first post-treatment night at doses above the recommended elderly dose of 5 mg oral zolpidem tartrate.

Memory impairment in controlled studies

Controlled studies in adults utilizing objective measures of memory yielded no consistent evidence of next-day memory impairment following the administration at bedtime of 5 mg to 10 mg oral zolpidem tartrate. However, in one study involving zolpidem tartrate doses of 10 mg and 20 mg, there was a significant decrease in next-morning recall of information presented to subjects during peak drug effect (90 minutes post-dose), i.e., these subjects experienced anterograde amnesia. There was also subjective evidence from adverse event data for anterograde amnesia occurring in association with the administration of oral zolpidem tartrate, predominantly at doses above 10 mg.

16   HOW SUPPLIED/STORAGE AND HANDLING

Each sublingual tablet is individually packaged in a unit-dose pouch.

Intermezzo 1.75 mg tablets are yellow, round, uncoated, biconvex, debossed with ZZ on one side and supplied as:

NDC 59011-256-30:   Carton of 30 unit-dose pouches

Intermezzo 3.5 mg tablets are beige, round, uncoated, biconvex, debossed with ZZ on one side and supplied as:

NDC 59011-255-30:   Carton of 30 unit-dose pouches

Storage and Handling

Store between 20°C to 25°C (68°F to 77°F). Excursions permitted between 15°C and 30°C (59°F and 86°F). Protect from moisture.

The patient should be instructed not to remove the sublingual tablet from the unit-dose pouch until the patient is ready to consume it.

17   PATIENT COUNSELING INFORMATION

See FDA-approved patient labeling (Medication Guide).

Inform patients and their families about the benefits and risks of treatment with Intermezzo. Inform patients of the availability of a Medication Guide and instruct them to read the Medication Guide prior to initiating treatment with Intermezzo and with each prescription refill. Review the Intermezzo Medication Guide with every patient prior to initiation of treatment. Instruct patients or caregivers that Intermezzo should be taken only as prescribed.

CNS depressant Effects and Next-Day Impairment

Tell patients that Intermezzo has the potential to cause next-day impairment, and that this risk is increased if dosing instructions are not carefully followed. Tell patients to wait for at least 4 hours after dosing and until they feel fully awake before driving or engaging in other activities requiring full mental alertness.

Severe Anaphylactic and Anaphylactoid Reactions

Inform patients that severe anaphylactic and anaphylactoid reactions have occurred with zolpidem. Describe the signs/symptoms of these reactions and advise patients to seek medical attention immediately if any of them occur.

Sleep-driving and Other Complex Behaviors

Instruct patients to inform their families that zolpidem has been associated with "sleep-driving" and other complex behaviors while not being fully awake (preparing and eating food, making phone calls, or having sex), and tell patients and their families to call their healthcare providers immediately if they develop any of these symptoms.

Suicide

Tell patients to immediately report any suicidal thoughts.

Administration Instructions

For detailed instructions on how to use Intermezzo, tell patients to refer to the Patient Instructions for Use.

Tell patients that Intermezzo is to be taken only once per night if needed if they wake in the middle of the night and have difficulty returning to sleep. Tell patients that Intermezzo should only be taken if they have 4 hours of bedtime remaining before the planned time of waking.

Instruct the patient to place the tablet under the tongue, allowing it to disintegrate completely before swallowing. Tell the patient that Intermezzo should not be swallowed whole.

Tell patients that the effect of Intermezzo may be slowed if taken with or immediately after a meal.

Instruct patients to remove the tablet from the unit-dose pouch just prior to dosing.

Advise patients NOT to take Intermezzo if they drank alcohol that day or before bed.

Healthcare professionals can telephone Purdue Pharma's Medical Services Department (1-888-726-7535) for information on this product.

Distributed by:

Purdue Pharma L.P.

Stamford, CT 06901-3431

Manufactured by: Patheon Pharmaceuticals, Inc., Cincinnati, OH 45237

U.S. Patent Numbers 7658945; 7682628; 8,242,131; 8,252,809

©2013, Purdue Pharma L.P.

MEDICATION GUIDE

Intermezzo® (in ter mét zoh)

(zolpidem tartrate) sublingual tablet CIV

Read the Medication Guide that comes with Intermezzo® before you start taking it and each time you get a refill. There may be new information. This Medication Guide does not take the place of talking to your doctor about your medical condition or treatment.

What is the most important information I should know about Intermezzo?

Follow the Instructions for Use at the end of this Medication Guide when you take Intermezzo. If you do not follow the Instructions for Use, you might be drowsy in the morning without knowing it.

- **Only take one tablet a night, if needed.**
- **Only take Intermezzo if you have at least 4 hours of bedtime left.**

Intermezzo may cause serious side effects, including:

- **After taking Intermezzo, you may get up out of bed while not being fully awake and do an activity that you do not know you are doing. The next morning, you may not remember that you did anything during the night. You have a higher chance for doing these activities if you drank alcohol that day or take other medicines that make you sleepy with Intermezzo. Reported activities include:**
  ○ driving a car ("sleep-driving")
  ○ making and eating food
  ○ talking on the phone
  ○ having sex
  ○ sleep-walking

Call your healthcare provider right away if you find out that you have done any of the above activities after taking Intermezzo.

Important:

1. **Take Intermezzo exactly as prescribed**
2. **Do not take Intermezzo if you:**
   - drank alcohol that day or before bed.
   - took another medicine to help you sleep.
   - do not have at least 4 hours of bedtime remaining.

What is Intermezzo?

Intermezzo is a sedative-hypnotic (sleep) medicine. Intermezzo is used in adults for the treatment of a sleep problem called insomnia. Many people have difficulty returning to sleep after awakening in the middle of the night. Intermezzo is designed to specifically treat this problem.

It is not known if Intermezzo is safe and effective in children.

Intermezzo is a federally controlled substance (CIV) because it can be abused or lead to dependence. Keep Intermezzo in a safe place to prevent misuse and abuse. Selling or giving away Intermezzo may harm others, and is against the law. Tell your doctor if you have ever abused or have been dependent on alcohol, prescription medicines, or street drugs.

Who should not take Intermezzo?

- Do not take Intermezzo if you are allergic to zolpidem or any other ingredients in Intermezzo. See the end of this Medication Guide for a complete list of ingredients in Intermezzo.
- Do not take Intermezzo if you have had an allergic reaction to drugs containing zolpidem, such as Ambien, Ambien CR, Edluar, or Zolpimist.

Symptoms of a serious allergic reaction to Intermezzo can include:

- **swelling of your face, lips, and throat that may cause difficulty breathing or swallowing**
- **nausea and vomiting**

Intermezzo may not be right for you. Before starting Intermezzo, tell your doctor about all of your health conditions, including if you:

- have a history of depression, mental illness, or suicidal thoughts
- have a history of drug or alcohol abuse or addiction
- have kidney or liver disease
- have a lung disease or breathing problems
- are pregnant, planning to become pregnant, or breastfeeding

Tell your doctor about all of the medicines you take, including prescription and nonprescription medicines, vitamins, and herbal supplements. Medicines can interact with each other, sometimes causing serious side effects. Your doctor will tell you if you can take Intermezzo with your other medicines.

Know the medicines you take. Keep a list of your medicines with you to show your doctor and pharmacist each time you get a new medicine.

How should I take Intermezzo?

- See **"What is the most important information I should know about Intermezzo"**
- Read the **"Instructions for Use"** at the end of this Medication Guide for detailed instructions on how to take Intermezzo.
- Take Intermezzo exactly as prescribed. Only take one Intermezzo tablet per night if needed.

- Do not take Intermezzo if you drank alcohol that evening or before bed.
- While in bed, place the tablet under your tongue and allow it to break apart completely. Do not swallow it whole.
- You should not take Intermezzo with or right after a meal. Intermezzo may help you fall asleep faster when you take it on an empty stomach.
- Call your health care provider if your insomnia worsens or is not better within 7 to 10 days. This may mean that there is another condition causing your sleep problem.
- If you take too much Intermezzo or overdose, get emergency treatment.

What are the possible side effects of Intermezzo?

Intermezzo may cause serious side effects, including:

- **getting out of bed while not being fully awake and doing an activity that you do not know you are doing. (See "What is the most important information I should know about Intermezzo?")**
- **abnormal thoughts and behavior.** Symptoms include more outgoing or aggressive behavior than normal, confusion, agitation, hallucinations, worsening of depression, and suicidal thoughts or actions.
- **memory loss**
- **anxiety**
- **severe allergic reactions.** Symptoms include swelling of the tongue or throat, trouble breathing, and nausea and vomiting. Get emergency medical help if you get these symptoms after taking Intermezzo.

Call your health care provider right away if you have any of the above side effects or any other side effects that worry you while using Intermezzo.

The most common side effects of Intermezzo are:

- Headache
- Nausea
- Fatigue

Even if you follow the Instructions for Use, you may still feel drowsy in the morning after taking Intermezzo. Do not drive or do other dangerous activities after taking Intermezzo until you are fully awake.

These are not all the side effects of Intermezzo. Ask your health care provider or pharmacist for more information.

You may report side effects to FDA at 1-800-FDA-1088.

How should I store Intermezzo?

- Store Intermezzo at room temperature, 68° to 77°F (20° to 25°C). Protect from moisture.
- Only open the pouch when you are ready to use Intermezzo.

Keep Intermezzo and all medicines out of reach of children.

General Information about Intermezzo

Medicines are sometimes prescribed for purposes other than those listed in a Medication Guide. Do not use Intermezzo for a condition for which it was not prescribed. Do not give Intermezzo to other people, even if you think they have the same symptoms that you have. It may harm them and it is against the law.

This Medication Guide summarizes the most important information about Intermezzo. If you would like more information, talk with your doctor. You can ask your doctor or pharmacist for information about Intermezzo that is written for healthcare professionals. For more information about Intermezzo, call Purdue Pharma at 1-888-726-7535 or go to www.purduepharma.com or www.intermezzorx.com.

What are the ingredients in Intermezzo?

Active Ingredient: Zolpidem tartrate

Inactive Ingredients: Each Intermezzo tablet includes the following inactive ingredients: mannitol, sorbitol, crospovidone, silicon dioxide, sodium carbonate, sodium bicarbonate, croscarmellose sodium, sodium stearyl fumarate, silicon dioxide, natural and artificial spearmint flavor, silicon dioxide-colloidal, and sucralose. The 1.75 mg tablet also contains yellow iron oxide, and the 3.5 mg tablet contains beige iron oxide.

Rx only

This Medication Guide has been approved by the U.S. Food and Drug Administration.

Distributed by:

Purdue Pharma L.P.

Stamford, CT 06901-3431

Issued: February 2013

Instructions for Use

Intermezzo® (in ter mét zoh)

(zolpidem tartrate) sublingual tablet CIV

Read these Instructions for Use before you start taking Intermezzo and each time you get a refill. There may be new information. This information does not take the place of talking to your healthcare provider about your medical condition or your treatment.

What is the most important Information I should know about Intermezzo?

Follow these Instructions for Use when you take Intermezzo. If you do not follow these instructions, you might be drowsy in the morning without knowing it.

- Only take 1 tablet a night if needed
- Only take Intermezzo if you have at least 4 hours of bedtime left

Using Intermezzo the wrong way can make you drowsy in the morning.

Before you go to bed:
- Place only 1 Intermezzo pouch by your bed, and have a clock or watch nearby (see Figure A).

← only 1 pouch

Figure A

- Store all other unopened Intermezzo pouches with your other medicines away from your bedside.
- Only open the Intermezzo pouch when you are ready to use it.
- You can either use the **Intermezzo Dosing Time Chart** (see Figure B) or the **Dosing Time Tool** (see Figure C) that comes with Intermezzo to find the latest time during the night you can take Intermezzo.

Intermezzo Dosing Time Chart (see Figure B):
- You can take Intermezzo if you have at least 4 hours of bedtime left before you must be awake.
- Find the earliest time you have to be up and awake in the column on the left.
- Find the latest time you can take Intermezzo on the same line in the column on the right.

Intermezzo Dosing Time Chart

If you must be awake by:	Take Intermezzo before:
4 am	12 midnight
5 am	1 am
6 am	2 am
7 am	3 am
8 am	4 am
9 am	5 am

Figure B

Intermezzo Dosing Time Tool (see Figure C):
- Turn the Intermezzo Dosing Time Tool wheel to show the earliest time that you must be awake under the green arrow.
- Take Intermezzo before the time under the brown arrow.

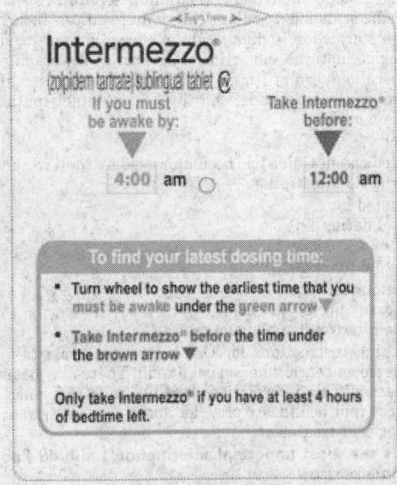

Intermezzo®
(zolpidem tartrate) sublingual tablet ℂ

If you must be awake by:	Take Intermezzo® before:
▼	▼
4:00 am ○	12:00 am

To find your latest dosing time:
- Turn wheel to show the earliest time that you must be awake under the green arrow ▼
- Take Intermezzo® before the time under the brown arrow ▼

Only take Intermezzo® if you have at least 4 hours of bedtime left.

Figure C

During the night when you take Intermezzo:
Step 1. Check the current time and use the Intermezzo Dosing Time Chart or the Intermezzo Dosing Time Tool to decide if you should take Intermezzo.
- Only take Intermezzo if you have at least 4 hours of bedtime left before you have to be awake (see Figure B).
Step 2. Open the Intermezzo pouch you placed by your bed.
- Fold the Intermezzo pouch along the dotted line. While the Intermezzo pouch is folded, tear the pouch open at the notch at the center of the dotted line (see Figure D).

TO OPEN POUCH

STEP ①: Fold along dotted line.

STEP ②: While folded, tear open at notch located at center of dotted line.

Figure D

Step 3. Remove the tablet from the Intermezzo pouch.
Step 4. Leave the empty Intermezzo pouch where you can see it. The empty pouch will help remind you that you already took your Intermezzo dose (see Figure E).

← empty pouch

Figure E

Step 5. While in bed, place the Intermezzo tablet under your tongue and allow it to break apart completely, then swallow. Do not swallow it whole (see Figure F).

Figure F

Step 6. Throw the empty Intermezzo pouch away in the morning.
When you wake up in the morning, be sure that at least 4 hours have passed since you have taken Intermezzo and you feel fully awake before driving. Do not do dangerous activities until you know how Intermezzo affects you.
This Medication Guide and Instructions for Use have been approved by the U.S. Food and Drug Administration.
Distributed by:
Purdue Pharma L.P.
Stamford, CT 06901-3431
Issued: February 2013
Shown in Product Identification Guide, page 312

OXYCONTIN®
[ŏks'ē-kŏn-tĭn]
(oxycodone hydrochloride controlled-release)
Tablets, for oral use

ℂ℞

HIGHLIGHTS OF PRESCRIBING INFORMATION
These highlights do not include all the information needed to use OXYCONTIN® safely and effectively. See full prescribing information for OXYCONTIN.
OXYCONTIN® (oxycodone hydrochloride extended-release tablets), for oral use, CII
Initial U.S. Approval: 1950

WARNING: ADDICTION, ABUSE and MISUSE; LIFE-THREATENING RESPIRATORY DEPRESSION; ACCIDENTAL INGESTION; NEONATAL OPIOID WITHDRAWAL SYNDROME; and CYTOCHROME P450 3A4 INTERACTION
See full prescribing information for complete boxed warning.
- OXYCONTIN exposes users to risks of addictions, abuse and misuse, which can lead to overdose and death. Assess each patient's risk before prescribing and monitor regularly for development of these behaviors and conditions. (5.1)
- Serious, life-threatening, or fatal respiratory depression may occur. Monitor closely, especially upon initiation or following a dose increase. Instruct patients to swallow OXYCONTIN tablets whole to avoid exposure to a potentially fatal dose of oxycodone. (5.2)
- Accidental ingestion of OXYCONTIN, especially in children, can result in a fatal overdose of oxycodone. (5.2)
- Prolonged use of OXYCONTIN during pregnancy can result in neonatal opioid withdrawal syndrome, which may be life-threatening if not recognized and treated. If opioid use is required for a prolonged period in a pregnant woman, advise the patient of the risk of neonatal opioid withdrawal syndrome and ensure that appropriate treatment will be available. (5.3)
- Initiation of CYP3A4 inhibitors (or discontinuation of CYP3A4 inducers) can result in a fatal overdose of oxycodone from OXYCONTIN. (5.14)

———RECENT MAJOR CHANGES———

Boxed Warning	04/2014
Indications and Usage (1)	04/2014
Dosage and Administration (2)	04/2014
Warnings and Precautions (5)	04/2014

———INDICATIONS AND USAGE———
OXYCONTIN is an opioid agonist product indicated for the management of pain severe enough to require daily, around-the-clock, long-term opioid treatment and for which alternative treatment options are inadequate. (1)
Limitations of Use
- Because of the risks of addiction, abuse and misuse with opioids, even at recommended doses, and because of the greater risks of overdose and death with extended-release formulations, reserve OXYCONTIN for use in patients for whom alternative treatment options (e.g. non-opioid analgesics or immediate-release opioids) are ineffective, not tolerated, or would be otherwise inadequate to provide sufficient management of pain. (1)
- OXYCONTIN is not indicated as an as-needed (prn) analgesic. (1)

———DOSAGE AND ADMINISTRATION———
- OXYCONTIN 60 mg and 80 mg tablets, a single dose greater than 40 mg, or a total daily dose greater than 80 mg are only for use in patients in whom tolerance to an opioid of comparable potency has been established. (2.1)
- For opioid-naïve and opioid non-tolerant patients, initiate with 10 mg tablets orally every 12 hours. (2.1)
- Do not abruptly discontinue OXYCONTIN in a physically dependent patient. (2.4)
- Tablets must be swallowed intact and are not to be cut, broken, chewed, crushed, or dissolved (risk of potentially fatal dose). (2.5, 5.1)
- OXYCONTIN tablets should be taken one tablet at a time, with enough water to ensure complete swallowing immediately after placing in the mouth. (2.5, 5.9, 17)

———DOSAGE FORMS AND STRENGTHS———
Extended-release tablets: 10 mg, 15 mg, 20 mg, 30 mg, 40 mg, 60 mg, and 80 mg (3)

———CONTRAINDICATIONS———
- Significant respiratory depression (4)
- Acute or severe bronchial asthma (4)

- Known or suspected paralytic ileus and GI obstruction (4)
- Hypersensitivity to oxycodone (4)

---WARNINGS AND PRECAUTIONS---

- Interactions with CNS depressants: Concomitant use may cause profound sedation, respiratory depression and death. If coadministration is required, consider dose reduction of one or both drugs. (5.4)
- Elderly, cachectic, debilitated patients, and those with chronic pulmonary disease: Monitor closely because of increased risk for life-threatening respiratory depression. (5.5, 5.6)
- Hypotensive effects: Monitor during dose initiation and titration. (5.7)
- Patients with head injury or increased intracranial pressure: Monitor for sedation and respiratory depression. Avoid use of OXYCONTIN in patients with impaired consciousness or coma susceptible to intracranial effects of CO_2 retention. (5.8)
- Use with caution in patients who have difficulty swallowing or have underlying GI disorders that may predispose them to obstruction. (5.9)
- Concomitant use of CYP3A4 inhibitors may increase opioid effects. (5.14)

---ADVERSE REACTIONS---

Most common adverse reactions (>5%) are constipation, nausea, somnolence, dizziness, vomiting, pruritus, headache, dry mouth, asthenia, and sweating. (6.1)

To report SUSPECTED ADVERSE REACTIONS, contact Purdue Pharma L.P. at 1-888-726-7535 or FDA at 1-800-FDA-1088 or www.fda.gov/medwatch.

---DRUG INTERACTIONS---

- Mixed agonist/antagonist and partial agonist opioid analgesics: Avoid use with OXYCONTIN because they may reduce analgesic effect of OXYCONTIN or precipitate withdrawal symptoms. (7.4)

---USE IN SPECIFIC POPULATIONS---

- Nursing mothers: Oxycodone has been detected in human milk. Closely monitor infants of nursing women receiving OXYCONTIN. (8.3)
- Geriatrics: The initial dose may need to be reduced to 1/3 to 1/2 of the usual doses. (8.5)
- Hepatic impairment: Initiate therapy at 1/3 to 1/2 the usual doses and titrate carefully. (8.6)

See 17 for PATIENT COUNSELING INFORMATION and Medication Guide

Revised: 04/2014

FULL PRESCRIBING INFORMATION

WARNING: ADDICTION, ABUSE and MISUSE; LIFE-THREATENING RESPIRATORY DEPRESSION; ACCIDENTAL INGESTION; NEONATAL OPIOID WITHDRAWAL SYNDROME; and CYTOCHROME P450 3A4 INTERACTION

Addiction, Abuse, and Misuse
OXYCONTIN® exposes patients and other users to the risks of opioid addiction, abuse and misuse, which can lead to overdose and death. Assess each patient's risk prior to prescribing OXYCONTIN and monitor all patients regularly for the development of these behaviors or conditions [see Warnings and Precautions (5.1)].

Life-Threatening Respiratory Depression
Serious, life-threatening, or fatal respiratory depression may occur with use of OXYCONTIN. Monitor for respiratory depression, especially during initiation of OXYCONTIN or following a dose increase. Instruct patients to swallow OXYCONTIN tablets whole; crushing, chewing, or dissolving OXYCONTIN tablets can cause rapid release and absorption of a potentially fatal dose of oxycodone [see Warnings and Precautions (5.2)].

Accidental Ingestion
Accidental ingestion of even one dose of OXYCONTIN, especially by children, can result in a fatal overdose of oxycodone [see Warnings and Precautions (5.2)].

Neonatal Opioid Withdrawal Syndrome
Prolonged use of OXYCONTIN during pregnancy can result in neonatal opioid withdrawal syndrome, which may be life-threatening if not recognized and treated, and requires management according to protocols developed by neonatology experts. If opioid use is required for a prolonged period in a pregnant woman, advise the patient of the risk of neonatal opioid withdrawal syndrome and ensure that appropriate treatment will be available [see Warnings and Precautions (5.3)].

Cytochrome P450 3A4 Interaction
The concomitant use of OXYCONTIN with all cytochrome P450 3A4 inhibitors may result in an increase in oxycodone plasma concentrations, which could increase or prolong adverse drug effects and may cause potentially fatal respiratory depression. In addition, discontinuation of a concomitantly used cytochrome P450 3A4 inducer may result in an increase in oxycodone plasma concentration. Monitor patients receiving OXYCONTIN and any CYP3A4 inhibitor or inducer [see Warnings and Precautions (5.14) and Clinical Pharmacology (12.3)].

1   INDICATIONS AND USAGE

OXYCONTIN is indicated for the management of pain severe enough to require daily, around-the-clock, long-term opioid treatment and for which alternative treatment options are inadequate.

Limitations of Use

- Because of the risks of addiction, abuse, and misuse with opioids, even at recommended doses, and because of the greater risks of overdose and death with extended-release opioid formulations, reserve OXYCONTIN for use in patients for whom alternative treatment options (e.g., nonopioid analgesics or immediate-release opioids) are ineffective, not tolerated, or would be otherwise inadequate to provide sufficient management of pain.
- OXYCONTIN is not indicated as an as-needed (prn) analgesic

2   DOSAGE AND ADMINISTRATION
2.1   Initial Dosing

OXYCONTIN should be prescribed only by healthcare professionals who are knowledgeable in the use of potent opioids for the management of chronic pain.

OXYCONTIN 60 mg and 80 mg tablets, a single dose greater than 40 mg, or a total daily dose greater than 80 mg are only for use in patients in whom tolerance to an opioid of comparable potency has been established. Patients considered opioid tolerant are those receiving, for one week or longer, at least 60 mg oral morphine/day, 25 mcg transdermal fentanyl/hour, 30 mg oral oxycodone/day, 8 mg oral hydromorphone/day, 25 mg oral oxymorphone/day, or an equianalgesic dose of another opioid.

Initiate the dosing regimen for each patient individually, taking into account the patient's prior analgesic treatment experience, and risk factors for addiction, abuse, and misuse [see Warnings and Precautions (5.1)]. Monitor patients closely for respiratory depression, especially within the first 24-72 hours of initiating therapy with OXYCONTIN [see Warnings and Precautions (5.2)].

OXYCONTIN tablets must be taken whole, one tablet at a time, with enough water to ensure complete swallowing immediately after placing in the mouth [see Patient Counseling Information (17)]. Crushing, chewing, or dissolving OXYCONTIN tablets will result in uncontrolled delivery of oxycodone and can lead to overdose or death [see Warnings and Precautions (5.1)].

Use of OXYCONTIN as the First Opioid Analgesic
Initiate treatment with OXYCONTIN with one 10 mg tablet orally every 12 hours.

Use of OXYCONTIN in Patients who are not Opioid Tolerant
The starting dose for patients who are not opioid tolerant is OXYCONTIN 10 mg orally every 12 hours. Patients who are opioid tolerant are those receiving, for one week or longer, at least 60 mg oral morphine per day, 25 mcg transdermal fentanyl per hour, 30 mg oral oxycodone per day, 8 mg oral hydromorphone per day, 25 mg oral oxymorphone per day, or an equianalgesic dose of another opioid. Use of higher starting doses in patients who are not opioid tolerant may cause fatal respiratory depression.

Conversion from other Oral Oxycodone Formulations to OXYCONTIN
Patients receiving other oral oxycodone formulations may be converted to OXYCONTIN by administering one-half of the patient's total daily oral oxycodone dose as OXYCONTIN every 12 hours.

Conversion from other Opioids to OXYCONTIN
Discontinue all other around-the-clock opioid drugs when OXYCONTIN therapy is initiated.

There are no established conversion ratios for conversion from other opioids to OXYCONTIN defined by clinical trials. Discontinue all other around-the-clock opioid drugs when OXYCONTIN therapy is initiated and initiate dosing using OXYCONTIN 10 mg orally every 12 hours.

It is safer to underestimate a patient's 24-hour oral oxycodone requirements and provide rescue medication (e.g., immediate-release opioid) than to overestimate the 24-hour oral oxycodone requirements which could result in adverse reactions. While useful tables of opioid equivalents are readily available, there is substantial inter-patient variability in the relative potency of different opioid drugs and products.

Conversion from Methadone to OXYCONTIN
Close monitoring is of particular importance when converting from methadone to other opioid agonists. The ratio between methadone and other opioid agonists may vary widely as a function of previous dose exposure. Methadone has a long half-life and can accumulate in the plasma.

Conversion from Transdermal Fentanyl to OXYCONTIN
Eighteen hours following the removal of the transdermal fentanyl patch, OXYCONTIN treatment can be initiated. Although there has been no systematic assessment of such conversion, a conservative oxycodone dose, approximately 10 mg every 12 hours of OXYCONTIN, should be initially substituted for each 25 mcg/hr fentanyl transdermal patch. Follow the patient closely during conversion from transdermal fentanyl to OXYCONTIN, as there is limited documented experience with this conversion.

2.2   Titration and Maintenance of Therapy
Individually titrate OXYCONTIN to a dose that provides adequate analgesia and minimizes adverse reactions. Con-

tinually reevaluate patients receiving OXYCONTIN to assess the maintenance of pain control and the relative incidence of adverse reactions, as well as monitoring for the development of addiction, abuse and misuse. Frequent communication is important among the prescriber, other members of the healthcare team, the patient, and the caregiver/family during periods of changing analgesic requirements, including initial titration. During chronic therapy, periodically reassess the continued need for the use of opioid analgesics.

Patients who experience breakthrough pain may require a dose increase of OXYCONTIN or may need rescue medication with an appropriate dose of an immediate-release analgesic. If the level of pain increases after dose stabilization, attempt to identify the source of increased pain before increasing the OXYCONTIN dose. Because steady-state plasma concentrations are approximated in 1 day, OXYCONTIN dosage may be adjusted every 1 to 2 days. If unacceptable opioid-related adverse reactions are observed, the subsequent dose may be reduced. Adjust the dose to obtain an appropriate balance between management of pain and opioid-related adverse reactions.

There are no well-controlled clinical studies evaluating the safety and efficacy with dosing more frequently than every 12 hours. As a guideline, the total daily oxycodone dose usually can be increased by 25% to 50% of the current dose, each time an increase is clinically indicated.

2.3 Patients with Hepatic Impairment
For patients with hepatic impairment, start dosing patients at 1/3 to 1/2 the usual starting dose followed by careful dose titration [see Clinical Pharmacology (12.3)].

2.4 Discontinuation of OXYCONTIN
When the patient no longer requires therapy with OXYCONTIN tablets, use a gradual downward titration of the dose to prevent signs and symptoms of withdrawal in the physically dependent patient. Do not abruptly discontinue OXYCONTIN.

2.5 Administration of OXYCONTIN
Instruct patients to swallow OXYCONTIN tablets intact. The tablets are not to be crushed, dissolved, or chewed due to the risk of rapid release and absorption of a potentially fatal dose of oxycodone [see Warnings and Precautions (5.1)]. Instruct patients to take OXYCONTIN one tablet at a time and with enough water to ensure complete swallowing immediately after placing in the mouth [see Warnings and Precautions (5.9) and Patient Counseling Information (17)].

3 DOSAGE FORMS AND STRENGTHS
- 10 mg film-coated extended-release tablets (round, white-colored, bi-convex tablets debossed with OP on one side and 10 on the other)
- 15 mg film-coated extended-release tablets (round, gray-colored, bi-convex tablets debossed with OP on one side and 15 on the other)
- 20 mg film-coated extended-release tablets (round, pink-colored, bi-convex tablets debossed with OP on one side and 20 on the other)
- 30 mg film-coated extended-release tablets (round, brown-colored, bi-convex tablets debossed with OP on one side and 30 on the other)
- 40 mg film-coated extended-release tablets (round, yellow-colored, bi-convex tablets debossed with OP on one side and 40 on the other)
- 60 mg film-coated extended-release tablets* (round, red-colored, bi-convex tablets debossed with OP on one side and 60 on the other)
- 80 mg film-coated extended-release tablets* (round, green-colored, bi-convex tablets debossed with OP on one side and 80 on the other)

* 60 mg and 80 mg tablets for use in opioid-tolerant patients only

4 CONTRAINDICATIONS
OXYCONTIN is contraindicated in patients with:
- Significant respiratory depression
- Acute or severe bronchial asthma in an unmonitored setting or in the absence of resuscitative equipment
- Known or suspected paralytic ileus and gastrointestinal obstruction
- Hypersensitivity (e.g., anaphylaxis) to oxycodone [see Adverse Reactions (6.2)]

5 WARNINGS AND PRECAUTIONS

5.1 Addiction, Abuse, and Misuse
OXYCONTIN contains oxycodone, a Schedule II controlled substance. As an opioid, OXYCONTIN exposes users to the risks of addiction, abuse, and misuse [see Drug Abuse and Dependence (9)]. As modified-release products such as OXYCONTIN deliver the opioid over an extended period of time, there is a greater risk for overdose and death due to the larger amount of oxycodone present [see Drug Abuse and Dependence (9)].

Although the risk of addiction in any individual is unknown, it can occur in patients appropriately prescribed OXYCONTIN. Addiction can occur at recommended doses and if the drug is misused or abused.

Assess each patient's risk for opioid addiction, abuse or misuse prior to prescribing OXYCONTIN, and monitor all patients receiving OXYCONTIN for the development of these behaviors or conditions. Risks are increased in patients with a personal or family history of substance abuse (including drug or alcohol abuse or addiction) or mental illness (e.g., major depression). The potential for these risks should not, however, prevent the proper management of pain in any given patient. Patients at increased risk may be prescribed modified-release opioid formulations such as OXYCONTIN, but use in such patients necessitates intensive counseling about the risks and proper use of OXYCONTIN along with intensive monitoring for signs of addiction, abuse, and misuse.

Abuse, or misuse of OXYCONTIN by crushing, chewing, snorting, or injecting the dissolved product will result in the uncontrolled delivery of oxycodone and can result in overdose and death [see Overdosage (10)].

Opioid agonists are sought by drug abusers and people with addiction disorders and are subject to criminal diversion. Consider these risks when prescribing or dispensing OXYCONTIN. Strategies to reduce these risks include prescribing the drug in the smallest appropriate quantity and advising the patient on the proper disposal of unused drug [see Patient Counseling Information (17)]. Contact local state professional licensing board or state controlled substances authority for information on how to prevent and detect abuse or diversion of this product.

5.2 Life-Threatening Respiratory Depression
Serious, life-threatening, or fatal respiratory depression has been reported with the use of modified-release opioids, even when used as recommended. Respiratory depression, if not immediately recognized and treated, may lead to respiratory arrest and death. Management of respiratory depression may include close observation, supportive measures, and use of opioid antagonists, depending on the patient's clinical status [see Overdosage (10)]. Carbon dioxide (CO_2) retention from opioid-induced respiratory depression can exacerbate the sedating effects of opioids.

While serious, life-threatening, or fatal respiratory depression can occur at any time during the use of OXYCONTIN, the risk is greatest during the initiation of therapy or following a dose increase. Closely monitor patients for respiratory depression when initiating therapy with OXYCONTIN and following dose increases.

To reduce the risk of respiratory depression, proper dosing and titration of OXYCONTIN are essential [see Dosage and Administration (2)]. Overestimating the OXYCONTIN dose when converting patients from another opioid product can result in a fatal overdose with the first dose.

Accidental ingestion of even one dose of OXYCONTIN, especially by children, can result in respiratory depression and death due to an overdose of oxycodone.

5.3 Neonatal Opioid Withdrawal Syndrome
Prolonged use of OXYCONTIN during pregnancy can result in withdrawal signs in the neonate. Neonatal opioid withdrawal syndrome, unlike opioid withdrawal syndrome in adults, may be life-threatening if not recognized and treated, and requires management according to protocols developed by neonatology experts. If opioid use is required for a prolonged period in a pregnant woman, advise the patient of the risk of neonatal opioid withdrawal syndrome and ensure that appropriate treatment will be available.

Neonatal opioid withdrawal syndrome presents as irritability, hyperactivity and abnormal sleep pattern, high pitched cry, tremor, vomiting, diarrhea and failure to gain weight. The onset, duration, and severity of neonatal opioid withdrawal syndrome vary based on the specific opioid used, duration of use, timing and amount of last maternal use, and rate of elimination of the drug by the newborn.

5.4 Interactions with Central Nervous System Depressants
Hypotension and profound sedation, coma, or respiratory depression may result if OXYCONTIN is used concomitantly with other central nervous system (CNS) depressants (e.g., sedatives, anxiolytics, hypnotics, neuroleptics, other opioids).

When considering the use of OXYCONTIN in a patient taking a CNS depressant, assess the duration of use of the CNS depressant and the patient's response, including the degree of tolerance that has developed to CNS depression. Additionally, evaluate the patient's use of alcohol or illicit drugs that can cause CNS depression. If the decision to begin OXYCONTIN therapy is made, start with 1/3 to 1/2 the usual dose of OXYCONTIN, monitor patients for signs of sedation and respiratory depression and consider using a lower dose of the concomitant CNS depressant [see Drug Interactions (7.1) and Dosage and Administration (2.2)].

5.5 Use in Elderly, Cachectic, and Debilitated Patients
Life-threatening respiratory depression is more likely to occur in elderly, cachectic, or debilitated patients as they may have altered pharmacokinetics or altered clearance compared to younger, healthier patients. Monitor such patients closely, particularly when initiating and titrating

OXYCONTIN and when OXYCONTIN is given concomitantly with other drugs that depress respiration [see Warnings and Precautions (5.2)].

5.6 Use in Patients with Chronic Pulmonary Disease
Monitor patients with significant chronic obstructive pulmonary disease or cor pulmonale, and patients having a substantially decreased respiratory reserve, hypoxia, hypercapnia, or pre-existing respiratory depression for respiratory depression, particularly when initiating therapy and titrating with OXYCONTIN, as in these patients, even usual therapeutic doses of OXYCONTIN may decrease respiratory drive to the point of apnea [see Warnings and Precautions (5.2)]. Consider the use of alternative non-opioid analgesics in these patients if possible.

5.7 Hypotensive Effects
OXYCONTIN may cause severe hypotension, including orthostatic hypotension and syncope in ambulatory patients. There is an increased risk in patients whose ability to maintain blood pressure has already been compromised by a reduced blood volume or concurrent administration of certain CNS depressant drugs (e.g., phenothiazines or general anesthetics) [see Drug Interactions (7.1)]. Monitor these patients for signs of hypotension after initiating or titrating the dose of OXYCONTIN. In patients with circulatory shock, OXYCONTIN may cause vasodilation that can further reduce cardiac output and blood pressure. Avoid the use of OXYCONTIN in patients with circulatory shock.

5.8 Use in Patients with Head Injury or Increased Intracranial Pressure
Monitor patients taking OXYCONTIN who may be susceptible to the intracranial effects of CO_2 retention (e.g., those with evidence of increased intracranial pressure or brain tumors) for signs of sedation and respiratory depression, particularly when initiating therapy with OXYCONTIN. OXYCONTIN may reduce respiratory drive, and the resultant CO_2 retention can further increase intracranial pressure. Opioids may also obscure the clinical course in a patient with a head injury.

Avoid the use of OXYCONTIN in patients with impaired consciousness or coma.

5.9 Difficulty in Swallowing and Risk for Obstruction in Patients at Risk for a Small Gastrointestinal Lumen
There have been post-marketing reports of difficulty in swallowing OXYCONTIN tablets. These reports included choking, gagging, regurgitation and tablets stuck in the throat. Instruct patients not to pre-soak, lick or otherwise wet OXYCONTIN tablets prior to placing in the mouth, and to take one tablet at a time with enough water to ensure complete swallowing immediately after placing in the mouth.

There have been rare post-marketing reports of cases of intestinal obstruction, and exacerbation of diverticulitis, some of which have required medical intervention to remove the tablet. Patients with underlying GI disorders such as esophageal cancer or colon cancer with a small gastrointestinal lumen are at greater risk of developing these complications. Consider use of an alternative analgesic in patients who have difficulty swallowing and patients at risk for underlying GI disorders resulting in a small gastrointestinal lumen.

5.10 Use in Patients with Gastrointestinal Conditions
OXYCONTIN is contraindicated in patients with GI obstruction, including paralytic ileus. The oxycodone in OXYCONTIN may cause spasm of the sphincter of Oddi. Monitor patients with biliary tract disease, including acute pancreatitis, for worsening symptoms. Opioids may cause increases in the serum amylase.

5.11 Use in Patients with Convulsive or Seizure Disorders
The oxycodone in OXYCONTIN may aggravate convulsions in patients with convulsive disorders, and may induce or aggravate seizures in some clinical settings. Monitor patients with a history of seizure disorders for worsened seizure control during OXYCONTIN therapy.

5.12 Avoidance of Withdrawal
Avoid the use of mixed agonist/antagonist (i.e., pentazocine, nalbuphine, and butorphanol) or partial agonist (buprenorphine) analgesics in patients who have received or are receiving a course of therapy with a full opioid agonist analgesic, including OXYCONTIN. In these patients, mixed agonist/antagonist and partial agonist analgesics may reduce the analgesic effect and/or may precipitate withdrawal symptoms.

When discontinuing OXYCONTIN, gradually taper the dose [see Dosage and Administration (2.4)]. Do not abruptly discontinue OXYCONTIN.

5.13 Driving and Operating Machinery
OXYCONTIN may impair the mental or physical abilities needed to perform potentially hazardous activities such as driving a car or operating machinery. Warn patients not to drive or operate dangerous machinery unless they are tolerant to the effects of OXYCONTIN and know how they will react to the medication.

5.14 Cytochrome P450 3A4 Inhibitors and Inducers

Since the CYP3A4 isoenzyme plays a major role in the metabolism of OXYCONTIN, drugs that alter CYP3A4 activity may cause changes in clearance of oxycodone which could lead to changes in oxycodone plasma concentrations. Inhibition of CYP3A4 activity by its inhibitors, such as macrolide antibiotics (e.g., erythromycin), azole-antifungal agents (e.g., ketoconazole), and protease inhibitors (e.g., ritonavir), may increase plasma concentrations of oxycodone and prolong opioid effects.

CYP450 inducers, such as rifampin, carbamazepine, and phenytoin, may induce the metabolism of oxycodone and, therefore, may cause increased clearance of the drug which could lead to a decrease in oxycodone plasma concentrations, lack of efficacy or, possibly, development of an abstinence syndrome in a patient who had developed physical dependence to oxycodone.

If co-administration is necessary, caution is advised when initiating OXYCONTIN treatment in patients currently taking, or discontinuing, CYP3A4 inhibitors or inducers. Evaluate these patients at frequent intervals and consider dose adjustments until stable drug effects are achieved [see Drug Interactions (7.3) and Clinical Pharmacology (12.3)].

5.15 Laboratory Monitoring

Not every urine drug test for "opioids" or "opiates" detects oxycodone reliably, especially those designed for in-office use. Further, many laboratories will report urine drug concentrations below a specified "cut-off" value as "negative". Therefore, if urine testing for oxycodone is considered in the clinical management of an individual patient, ensure that the sensitivity and specificity of the assay is appropriate, and consider the limitations of the testing used when interpreting results.

6 ADVERSE REACTIONS

The following serious adverse reactions are described elsewhere in the labeling:
- Addiction, Abuse, and Misuse [see Warnings and Precautions (5.1)]
- Life-Threatening Respiratory Depression [see Warnings and Precautions (5.2)]
- Neonatal Opioid Withdrawal Syndrome [see Warnings and Precautions (5.3)]
- Interactions with Other CNS Depressants [see Warnings and Precautions (5.4)]
- Hypotensive Effects [see Warnings and Precautions (5.7)]
- Gastrointestinal Effects [see Warnings and Precautions (5.9, 5.10)]
- Seizures [see Warnings and Precautions (5.11)]

6.1 Clinical Trial Experience

Because clinical trials are conducted under widely varying conditions, adverse reaction rates observed in the clinical trials of a drug cannot be directly compared to rates in the clinical trials of another drug and may not reflect the rates observed in practice.

The safety of OXYCONTIN was evaluated in double-blind clinical trials involving 713 patients with moderate to severe pain of various etiologies. In open-label studies of cancer pain, 187 patients received OXYCONTIN in total daily doses ranging from 20 mg to 640 mg per day. The average total daily dose was approximately 105 mg per day.

OXYCONTIN may increase the risk of serious adverse reactions such as those observed with other opioid analgesics, including respiratory depression, apnea, respiratory arrest, circulatory depression, hypotension, or shock [see Overdosage (10)].

The most common adverse reactions (>5%) reported by patients in clinical trials comparing OXYCONTIN with placebo are shown in Table 1 below:

TABLE 1: Common Adverse Reactions (>5%)

Adverse Reaction	OXYCONTIN (n=227) (%)	Placebo (n=45) (%)
Constipation	(23)	(7)
Nausea	(23)	(11)
Somnolence	(23)	(4)
Dizziness	(13)	(9)
Pruritus	(13)	(2)
Vomiting	(12)	(7)
Headache	(7)	(7)
Dry Mouth	(6)	(2)
Asthenia	(6)	-
Sweating	(5)	(2)

In clinical trials, the following adverse reactions were reported in patients treated with OXYCONTIN with an incidence between 1% and 5%:

Gastrointestinal disorders: abdominal pain, diarrhea, dyspepsia, gastritis

General disorders and administration site conditions: chills, fever

Metabolism and nutrition disorders: anorexia

Musculoskeletal and connective tissue disorders: twitching

Psychiatric disorders: abnormal dreams, anxiety, confusion, dysphoria, euphoria, insomnia, nervousness, thought abnormalities

Respiratory, thoracic and mediastinal disorders: dyspnea, hiccups

Skin and subcutaneous tissue disorders: rash

Vascular disorders: postural hypotension

The following adverse reactions occurred in **less than 1% of patients** involved in clinical trials:

Blood and lymphatic system disorders: lymphadenopathy

Ear and labyrinth disorders: tinnitus

Eye disorders: abnormal vision

Gastrointestinal disorders: dysphagia, eructation, flatulence, gastrointestinal disorder, increased appetite, stomatitis

General disorders and administration site conditions: withdrawal syndrome (with and without seizures), edema, peripheral edema, thirst, malaise, chest pain, facial edema

Injury, poisoning and procedural complications: accidental injury

Investigations: ST depression

Metabolism and nutrition disorders: dehydration

Nervous system disorders: syncope, migraine, abnormal gait, amnesia, hyperkinesia, hypesthesia, hypotonia, paresthesia, speech disorder, stupor, tremor, vertigo, taste perversion

Psychiatric disorders: depression, agitation, depersonalization, emotional lability, hallucination

Renal and urinary disorders: dysuria, hematuria, polyuria, urinary retention

Reproductive system and breast disorders: impotence

Respiratory, thoracic and mediastinal disorders: cough increased, voice alteration

Skin and subcutaneous tissue disorders: dry skin, exfoliative dermatitis

6.2 Postmarketing Experience

The following adverse reactions have been identified during post-approval use of controlled-release oxycodone: abuse, addiction, amenorrhea, cholestasis, death, dental caries, increased hepatic enzymes, hyperalgesia, hypogonadism, hyponatremia, ileus, muscular hypertonia, overdose, palpitations (in the context of withdrawal), seizures, syndrome of inappropriate antidiuretic hormone secretion, and urticaria. Anaphylaxis has been reported with ingredients contained in OXYCONTIN. Advise patients how to recognize such a reaction and when to seek medical attention.

In addition to the events listed above, the following have also been reported, potentially due to the swelling and hydrogelling property of the tablet: choking, gagging, regurgitation, tablets stuck in the throat and difficulty swallowing the tablet.

7 DRUG INTERACTIONS

7.1 CNS Depressants

The concomitant use of OXYCONTIN and other CNS depressants including sedatives, hypnotics, tranquilizers, general anesthetics, phenothiazines, other opioids, and alcohol can increase the risk of respiratory depression, profound sedation, coma, or death. Monitor patients receiving CNS depressants and OXYCONTIN for signs of respiratory depression, sedation, and hypotension.

When combined therapy with any of the above medications is considered, the dose of one or both agents should be reduced [see Dosage and Administration (2.2) and Warnings and Precautions (5.4)].

7.2 Muscle Relaxants

Oxycodone may enhance the neuromuscular blocking action of true skeletal muscle relaxants and produce an increased degree of respiratory depression. Monitor patients receiving muscle relaxants and OXYCONTIN for signs of respiratory depression that may be greater than otherwise expected.

7.3 Drugs Affecting Cytochrome P450 Isoenzymes

Inhibitors of CYP3A4 and 2D6

Because the CYP3A4 isoenzyme plays a major role in the metabolism of oxycodone, drugs that inhibit CYP3A4 activity may cause decreased clearance of oxycodone which could lead to an increase in oxycodone plasma concentrations and result in increased or prolonged opioid effects. These effects could be more pronounced with concomitant use of CYP2D6 and 3A4 inhibitors. If co-administration with OXYCONTIN is necessary, monitor patients for respiratory depression and sedation at frequent intervals and consider dose adjustments until stable drug effects are achieved [see Clinical Pharmacology (12.3)].

Inducers of CYP3A4

CYP450 3A4 inducers may induce the metabolism of oxycodone and, therefore, may cause increased clearance of the drug which could lead to a decrease in oxycodone plasma concentrations, lack of efficacy or, possibly, development of an abstinence syndrome in a patient who had developed physical dependence to oxycodone. If co-administration with OXYCONTIN is necessary, monitor for signs of opioid withdrawal and consider dose adjustments until stable drug effects are achieved.

After stopping the treatment of a CYP3A4 inducer, as the effects of the inducer decline, the oxycodone plasma concentration will increase which could increase or prolong both the therapeutic and adverse effects, and may cause serious respiratory depression [see Clinical Pharmacology (12.3)].

7.4 Mixed Agonist/Antagonist and Partial Agonist Opioid Analgesics

Mixed agonist/antagonist (i.e., pentazocine, nalbuphine, and butorphanol) and partial agonist (buprenorphine) analgesics may reduce the analgesic effect of oxycodone or precipitate withdrawal symptoms. Avoid the use of mixed agonist/antagonist and partial agonist analgesics in patients receiving OXYCONTIN.

7.5 Diuretics

Opioids can reduce the efficacy of diuretics by inducing the release of antidiuretic hormone. Opioids may also lead to acute retention of urine by causing spasm of the sphincter of the bladder, particularly in men with enlarged prostates.

7.6 Anticholinergics

Anticholinergics or other medications with anticholinergic activity when used concurrently with opioid analgesics may result in increased risk of urinary retention and/or severe constipation, which may lead to paralytic ileus. Monitor patients for signs of urinary retention or reduced gastric motility when OXYCONTIN is used concurrently with anticholinergic drugs.

8 USE IN SPECIFIC POPULATIONS

8.1 Pregnancy

Clinical Considerations

Fetal/neonatal adverse reactions

Prolonged use of opioid analgesics during pregnancy for medical or nonmedical purposes can result in physical dependence in the neonate and neonatal opioid withdrawal syndrome shortly after birth. Observe newborns for symptoms of neonatal opioid withdrawal syndrome, such as poor feeding, diarrhea, irritability, tremor, rigidity, and seizures, and manage accordingly [see Warnings and Precautions (5.3)].

Teratogenic Effects - Pregnancy Category C

There are no adequate and well-controlled studies in pregnant women. OXYCONTIN should be used during pregnancy only if the potential benefit justifies the risk to the fetus.

The effect of oxycodone in human reproduction has not been adequately studied. Studies with oral doses of oxycodone hydrochloride in rats up to 8 mg/kg/day and rabbits up to 125 mg/kg/day, equivalent to 0.5 and 15 times an adult human dose of 160 mg/day, respectively on a mg/m^2 basis, did not reveal evidence of harm to the fetus due to oxycodone. In a pre- and postnatal toxicity study, female rats received oxycodone during gestation and lactation. There were no long-term developmental or reproductive effects in the pups [see Nonclinical Toxicology (13.1)].

Non-Teratogenic Effects

Oxycodone hydrochloride was administered orally to female rats during gestation and lactation in a pre- and postnatal toxicity study. There were no drug-related effects on reproductive performance in these females or any long-term developmental or reproductive effects in pups born to these rats. Decreased body weight was found during lactation and the early post-weaning phase in pups nursed by mothers given the highest dose used (6 mg/kg/day, equivalent to approximately 0.4-times an adult human dose of 160 mg/day, on a mg/m^2 basis). However, body weight of these pups recovered.

8.2 Labor and Delivery

Opioids cross the placenta and may produce respiratory depression in neonates. OXYCONTIN is not recommended for use in women immediately prior to labor, when use of shorter-acting analgesics or other analgesic techniques are more appropriate. Opioid analgesics can prolong labor through actions which temporarily reduce the strength, duration and frequency of uterine contractions. However this effect is not consistent and may be offset by an increased rate of cervical dilatation, which tends to shorten labor.

8.3 Nursing Mothers

Oxycodone has been detected in breast milk. Instruct patients not to undertake nursing while receiving OXYCONTIN. Do not initiate OXYCONTIN therapy while nursing because of the possibility of sedation or respiratory depression in the infant.

Withdrawal signs can occur in breast-fed infants when maternal administration of an opioid analgesic is stopped, or when breast-feeding is stopped.

8.4 Pediatric Use

Safety and effectiveness of OXYCONTIN in pediatric patients below the age of 18 years have not been established.

8.5 Geriatric Use

In controlled pharmacokinetic studies in elderly subjects (greater than 65 years) the clearance of oxycodone was

Table 2: Summary of Maximum Drug Liking (E_{max}) Data Following Intranasal Administration

VAS Scale (100 mm)*		OXYCONTIN (finely crushed)	Original OXYCONTIN (finely crushed)	Oxycodone HCl (powdered)
Drug Liking	Mean (SE)	80.4 (3.9)	94.0 (2.7)	89.3 (3.1)
	Median (Range)	88 (36-100)	100 (51-100)	100 (50-100)
Take Drug Again	Mean (SE)	64.0 (7.1)	89.6 (3.9)	86.6 (4.4)
	Median (Range)	78 (0-100)	100 (20-100)	100 (0-100)

* Bipolar scales (0 = maximum negative response, 50 = neutral response, 100 = maximum positive response)

slightly reduced. Compared to young adults, the plasma concentrations of oxycodone were increased approximately 15% *[see Clinical Pharmacology (12.3)]*. Of the total number of subjects (445) in clinical studies of oxycodone hydrochloride controlled-release tablets, 148 (33.3%) were age 65 and older (including those age 75 and older) while 40 (9.0%) were age 75 and older. In clinical trials with appropriate initiation of therapy and dose titration, no untoward or unexpected adverse reactions were seen in the elderly patients who received oxycodone hydrochloride controlled-release tablets. Thus, the usual doses and dosing intervals may be appropriate for elderly patients. However, reduce the starting dose to 1/3 to 1/2 the usual dosage in debilitated, non-opioid-tolerant patients. Respiratory depression is the chief risk in elderly or debilitated patients, usually the result of large initial doses in patients who are not tolerant to opioids, or when opioids are given in conjunction with other agents that depress respiration. Titrate the dose of OXYCONTIN cautiously in these patients.

8.6 Hepatic Impairment
A study of OXYCONTIN in patients with hepatic impairment demonstrated greater plasma concentrations than those seen at equivalent doses in persons with normal hepatic function. Therefore, in the setting of hepatic impairment, start dosing patients at 1/3 to 1/2 the usual starting dose followed by careful dose titration *[see Clinical Pharmacology (12.3)]*.

8.7 Renal Impairment
In patients with renal impairment, as evidenced by decreased creatinine clearance (<60 mL/min), the concentrations of oxycodone in the plasma are approximately 50% higher than in subjects with normal renal function. Follow a conservative approach to dose initiation and adjust according to the clinical situation *[see Clinical Pharmacology (12.3)]*.

8.8 Gender Differences
In pharmacokinetic studies with OXYCONTIN, opioid-naïve females demonstrate up to 25% higher average plasma concentrations and greater frequency of typical opioid adverse events than males, even after adjustment for body weight. The clinical relevance of a difference of this magnitude is low for a drug intended for chronic usage at individualized dosages, and there was no male/female difference detected for efficacy or adverse events in clinical trials.

9 DRUG ABUSE AND DEPENDENCE

9.1 Controlled Substance
OXYCONTIN contains oxycodone, a Schedule II controlled substance with a high potential for abuse similar to other opioids including fentanyl, hydromorphone, methadone, morphine, and oxymorphone. OXYCONTIN can be abused and is subject to misuse, addiction, and criminal diversion *[see Warnings and Precautions (5.1)]*.
The high drug content in extended-release formulations adds to the risk of adverse outcomes from abuse and misuse.

9.2 Abuse
All patients treated with opioids require careful monitoring for signs of abuse and addiction, since use of opioid analgesic products carries the risk of addiction even under appropriate medical use.
Drug abuse is the intentional non-therapeutic use of an over-the-counter or prescription drug, even once, for its rewarding psychological or physiological effects. Drug abuse includes, but is not limited to, the following examples: the use of a prescription or over-the-counter drug to get "high," or the use of steroids for performance enhancement and muscle build up.
Drug addiction is a cluster of behavioral, cognitive, and physiological phenomena that develop after repeated substance use and include: a strong desire to take the drug, difficulties in controlling its use, persisting in its use despite harmful consequences, a higher priority given to drug use than to other activities and obligations, increased tolerance, and sometimes a physical withdrawal.
"Drug-seeking" behavior is very common to addicts and drug abusers. Drug-seeking tactics include emergency calls or visits near the end of office hours, refusal to undergo appropriate examination, testing or referral, repeated claims of loss of prescriptions, tampering with prescriptions and reluctance to provide prior medical records or contact information for other treating physician(s). "Doctor shopping" (visiting multiple prescribers) to obtain additional prescriptions is common among drug abusers and people suffering from untreated addiction. Preoccupation with achieving adequate pain relief can be appropriate behavior in a patient with poor pain control.
Abuse and addiction are separate and distinct from physical dependence and tolerance. Physicians should be aware that addiction may not be accompanied by concurrent tolerance and symptoms of physical dependence in all addicts. In addition, abuse of opioids can occur in the absence of true addiction.
OXYCONTIN, like other opioids, can be diverted for non-medical use into illicit channels of distribution. Careful recordkeeping of prescribing information, including quantity, frequency, and renewal requests as required by state law, is strongly advised.
Proper assessment of the patient, proper prescribing practices, periodic reevaluation of therapy, and proper dispensing and storage are appropriate measures that help to reduce abuse of opioid drugs.

Risks Specific to Abuse of OXYCONTIN
OXYCONTIN is for oral use only. Abuse of OXYCONTIN poses a risk of overdose and death. The risk is increased with concurrent use of OXYCONTIN with alcohol and other central nervous system depressants. Taking cut, broken, chewed, crushed, or dissolved OXYCONTIN enhances drug release and increases the risk of overdose and death.
With parenteral abuse, the inactive ingredients in OXYCONTIN can be expected to result in local tissue necrosis, infection, pulmonary granulomas, and increased risk of endocarditis and valvular heart injury. Parenteral drug abuse is commonly associated with transmission of infectious diseases, such as hepatitis and HIV.

Abuse Deterrence Studies
OXYCONTIN is formulated with inactive ingredients intended to make the tablet more difficult to manipulate for misuse and abuse. For the purposes of describing the results of studies of the abuse-deterrent characteristics of OXYCONTIN resulting from a change in formulation, in this section, the original formulation of OXYCONTIN, which is no longer marketed, will be referred to as "original OXYCONTIN" and the reformulated, currently marketed product will be referred to as "OXYCONTIN".

In Vitro Testing
In vitro physical and chemical tablet manipulation studies were performed to evaluate the success of different extraction methods in defeating the extended-release formulation. Results support that, relative to original OXYCONTIN, there is an increase in the ability of OXYCONTIN to resist crushing, breaking, and dissolution using a variety of tools and solvents. The results of these studies also support this finding for OXYCONTIN relative to an immediate-release oxycodone. When subjected to an aqueous environment, OXYCONTIN gradually forms a viscous hydrogel (i.e., a gelatinous mass) that resists passage through a needle.

Clinical Studies
In a randomized, double-blind, placebo-controlled 5-period crossover pharmacodynamic study, 30 recreational opioid users with a history of intranasal drug abuse received intranasally administered active and placebo drug treatments. The five treatment arms were finely crushed OXYCONTIN 30 mg tablets, coarsely crushed OXYCONTIN 30 mg tablets, finely crushed original OXYCONTIN 30 mg tablets, powdered oxycodone HCl 30 mg, and placebo. Data for finely crushed OXYCONTIN, finely crushed original OXYCONTIN, and powdered oxycodone HCl are described below.
Drug liking was measured on a bipolar drug liking scale of 0 to 100 where 50 represents a neutral response of neither liking nor disliking, 0 represents maximum disliking and 100 represents maximum liking. Response to whether the subject would take the study drug again was also measured on a bipolar scale of 0 to 100 where 50 represents a neutral response, 0 represents the strongest negative response

("definitely would not take drug again") and 100 represents the strongest positive response ("definitely would take drug again").
Twenty-seven of the subjects completed the study. Incomplete dosing due to granules falling from the subjects' nostrils occurred in 34% (n = 10) of subjects with finely crushed OXYCONTIN, compared with 7% (n = 2) of subjects with finely crushed original OXYCONTIN and no subjects with powdered oxycodone HCl.
The intranasal administration of finely crushed OXYCONTIN was associated with a numerically lower mean and median drug liking score and a lower mean and median score for take drug again, compared to finely crushed original OXYCONTIN or powdered oxycodone HCl as summarized in Table 2.
[See table 2 above]
Figure 1 demonstrates a comparison of drug liking for finely crushed OXYCONTIN compared to powdered oxycodone HCl in subjects who received both treatments. The Y-axis represents the percent of subjects attaining a percent reduction in drug liking for OXYCONTIN vs. oxycodone HCl powder greater than or equal to the value on the X-axis. Approximately 44% (n = 12) had no reduction in liking with OXYCONTIN relative to oxycodone HCl. Approximately 56% (n = 15) of subjects had some reduction in drug liking with OXYCONTIN relative to oxycodone HCl. Thirty-three percent (n = 9) of subjects had a reduction of at least 30% in drug liking with OXYCONTIN compared to oxycodone HCl, and approximately 22% (n = 6) of subjects had a reduction of at least 50% in drug liking with OXYCONTIN compared to oxycodone HCl.

Figure 1: Percent Reduction Profiles for E_{max} of Drug Liking VAS for OxyContin vs. oxycodone HCl, N=27 Following Intranasal Administration

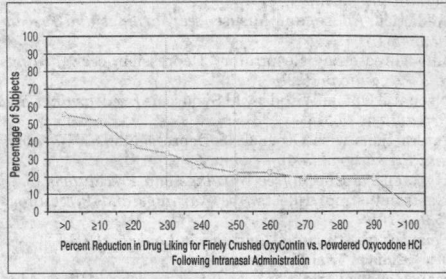

Percent Reduction in Drug Liking for Finely Crushed OxyContin vs. Powdered Oxycodone HCl Following Intranasal Administration

The results of a similar analysis of drug liking for finely crushed OXYCONTIN relative to finely crushed original OXYCONTIN were comparable to the results of finely crushed OXYCONTIN relative to powdered oxycodone HCl. Approximately 43% (n = 12) of subjects had no reduction in liking with OXYCONTIN relative to original OXYCONTIN. Approximately 57% (n = 16) of subjects had some reduction in drug liking, 36% (n = 10) of subjects had a reduction of at least 30% in drug liking, and approximately 29% (n = 8) of subjects had a reduction of at least 50% in drug liking with OXYCONTIN compared to original OXYCONTIN.

Summary
The in vitro data demonstrate that OXYCONTIN has physicochemical properties expected to make abuse via injection difficult. The data from the clinical study, along with support from the in vitro data, also indicate that OXYCONTIN has physicochemical properties that are expected to reduce abuse via the intranasal route. However, abuse of OXYCONTIN by these routes, as well as by the oral route, is still possible.
Additional data, including epidemiological data, when available, may provide further information on the impact of the current formulation of OXYCONTIN on the abuse liability of the drug. Accordingly, this section may be updated in the future as appropriate.
OXYCONTIN contains oxycodone, an opioid agonist and Schedule II controlled substance with an abuse liability similar to other opioid agonists, legal or illicit, including fentanyl, hydromorphone, methadone, morphine, and oxymorphone. OXYCONTIN can be abused and is subject to misuse, addiction, and criminal diversion *[see Warnings and Precautions (5.1) and Drug Abuse and Dependence (9.1)]*.

9.3 Dependence
Both tolerance and physical dependence can develop during chronic opioid therapy. Tolerance is the need for increasing doses of opioids to maintain a defined effect such as analgesia (in the absence of disease progression or other external factors). Tolerance may occur to both the desired and undesired effects of drugs, and may develop at different rates for different effects.
Physical dependence results in withdrawal symptoms after abrupt discontinuation or a significant dose reduction of a drug. Withdrawal also may be precipitated through the ad-

ministration of drugs with opioid antagonist activity, e.g., naloxone, nalmefene, mixed agonist/antagonist analgesics (pentazocine, butorphanol, nalbuphine), or partial agonists (buprenorphine). Physical dependence may not occur to a clinically significant degree until after several days to weeks of continued opioid usage.

OXYCONTIN should not be abruptly discontinued *[see Dosage and Administration (2.4)]*. If OXYCONTIN is abruptly discontinued in a physically-dependent patient, an abstinence syndrome may occur. Some or all of the following can characterize this syndrome: restlessness, lacrimation, rhinorrhea, yawning, perspiration, chills, myalgia, and mydriasis. Other signs and symptoms also may develop, including: irritability, anxiety, backache, joint pain, weakness, abdominal cramps, insomnia, nausea, anorexia, vomiting, diarrhea, or increased blood pressure, respiratory rate, or heart rate.

Infants born to mothers physically dependent on opioids will also be physically dependent and may exhibit respiratory difficulties and withdrawal signs *[see Use in Specific Populations (8.1)]*.

10   OVERDOSAGE

Clinical Presentation

Acute overdosage with OXYCONTIN can be manifested by respiratory depression, somnolence progressing to stupor or coma, skeletal muscle flaccidity, cold and clammy skin, constricted pupils, and in some cases, pulmonary edema, bradycardia, hypotension, partial or complete airway obstruction, atypical snoring and death. Marked mydriasis rather than miosis may be seen due to severe hypoxia in overdose situations.

Treatment of Overdose

In case of overdose, priorities are the reestablishment of a patent and protected airway and institution of assisted or controlled ventilation if needed. Employ other supportive measures (including oxygen, vasopressors) in the management of circulatory shock and pulmonary edema as indicated. Cardiac arrest or arrhythmias will require advanced life support techniques.

The opioid antagonists, naloxone or nalmefene, are specific antidotes to respiratory depression resulting from opioid overdose. Opioid antagonists should not be administered in the absence of clinically significant respiratory or circulatory depression secondary to oxycodone overdose. Such agents should be administered cautiously to persons who are known, or suspected to be physically dependent on OXYCONTIN. In such cases, an abrupt or complete reversal of opioid effects may precipitate an acute withdrawal syndrome.

Because the duration of reversal would be expected to be less than the duration of action of oxycodone in OXYCONTIN, carefully monitor the patient until spontaneous respiration is reliably reestablished. OXYCONTIN will continue to release oxycodone and add to the oxycodone load for 24 to 48 hours or longer following ingestion necessitating prolonged monitoring. If the response to opioid antagonists is suboptimal or not sustained, additional antagonist should be administered as directed in the product's prescribing information.

In an individual physically dependent on opioids, administration of the usual dose of the antagonist will precipitate an acute withdrawal syndrome. The severity of the withdrawal symptoms experienced will depend on the degree of physical dependence and the dose of the antagonist administered. If a decision is made to treat serious respiratory depression in the physically dependent patient, administration of the antagonist should be begun with care and by titration with smaller than usual doses of the antagonist.

11   DESCRIPTION

OXYCONTIN (oxycodone hydrochloride extended-release tablets) is an opioid analgesic supplied in 10 mg, 15 mg, 20 mg, 30 mg, 40 mg, 60 mg, and 80 mg tablets for oral administration. The tablet strengths describe the amount of oxycodone per tablet as the hydrochloride salt. The structural formula for oxycodone hydrochloride is as follows:

$C_{18}H_{21}NO_4 \cdot HCl$ MW 351.83

The chemical name is 4, 5α-epoxy-14-hydroxy-3-methoxy-17-methylmorphinan-6-one hydrochloride.

Oxycodone is a white, odorless crystalline powder derived from the opium alkaloid, thebaine. Oxycodone hydrochloride dissolves in water (1 g in 6 to 7 mL). It is slightly soluble in alcohol (octanol water partition coefficient 0.7).

The 10 mg, 15 mg, 20 mg, 30 mg, 40 mg, 60 mg and 80 mg tablets contain the following inactive ingredients: butylated hydroxytoluene (BHT), hypromellose, polyethylene glycol 400, polyethylene oxide, magnesium stearate, titanium dioxide.

The 10 mg tablets also contain hydroxypropyl cellulose.

The 15 mg tablets also contain black iron oxide, yellow iron oxide, and red iron oxide.

The 20 mg tablets also contain polysorbate 80 and red iron oxide.

The 30 mg tablets also contain polysorbate 80, red iron oxide, yellow iron oxide, and black iron oxide.

The 40 mg tablets also contain polysorbate 80 and yellow iron oxide.

The 60 mg tablets also contain polysorbate 80, red iron oxide and black iron oxide.

The 80 mg tablets also contain hydroxypropyl cellulose, yellow iron oxide and FD&C Blue #2/Indigo Carmine Aluminum Lake.

12   CLINICAL PHARMACOLOGY

Oxycodone hydrochloride is a full opioid agonist and is relatively selective for the mu receptor, although it can bind to other opioid receptors at higher doses. The principal therapeutic action of oxycodone is analgesia. Like all full opioid agonists, there is no ceiling effect to analgesia for oxycodone. Clinically, dosage is titrated to provide adequate analgesia and may be limited by adverse reactions, including respiratory and CNS depression.

12.1   Mechanism of Action

Central Nervous System

The precise mechanism of the analgesic action is unknown. However, specific CNS opioid receptors for endogenous compounds with opioid-like activity have been identified throughout the brain and spinal cord and are thought to play a role in the analgesic effects of this drug.

12.2   Pharmacodynamics

A single-dose, double-blind, placebo- and dose-controlled study was conducted using OXYCONTIN (10, 20, and 30 mg) in an analgesic pain model involving 182 patients with moderate to severe pain. OXYCONTIN doses of 20 mg and 30 mg produced statistically significant pain reduction compared to placebo.

Effects on the Central Nervous System

Oxycodone produces respiratory depression by direct action on brain stem respiratory centers. The respiratory depression involves both a reduction in the responsiveness of the brain stem respiratory centers to increases in CO_2 tension and to electrical stimulation.

Oxycodone depresses the cough reflex by direct effect on the cough center in the medulla. Antitussive effects may occur with doses lower than those usually required for analgesia. Oxycodone causes miosis, even in total darkness. Pinpoint pupils are a sign of opioid overdose but are not pathognomonic (e.g., pontine lesions of hemorrhagic or ischemic origin may produce similar findings). Marked mydriasis rather than miosis may be seen with hypoxia in the setting of oxycodone overdose *[see Overdosage (10)]*.

Effects on the Gastrointestinal Tract and Other Smooth Muscle

Oxycodone causes a reduction in motility associated with an increase in smooth muscle tone in the antrum of the stomach and duodenum. Digestion of food in the small intestine is delayed and propulsive contractions are decreased. Propulsive peristaltic waves in the colon are decreased, while tone may be increased to the point of spasm resulting in constipation. Other opioid-induced effects may include a reduction in gastric, biliary and pancreatic secretions, spasm of sphincter of Oddi, and transient elevations in serum amylase.

Effects on the Cardiovascular System

Oxycodone may produce release of histamine with or without associated peripheral vasodilation. Manifestations of histamine release and/or peripheral vasodilation may include pruritus, flushing, red eyes, sweating, and/or orthostatic hypotension.

Effects on the Endocrine System

Opioids inhibit the secretion of ACTH, cortisol, testosterone, and luteinizing hormone (LH) in humans. They also stimulate prolactin, growth hormone (GH) secretion, and pancreatic secretion of insulin and glucagon.

Effects on the Immune System

Opioids have been shown to have a variety of effects on components of the immune system in *in vitro* and animal models. The clinical significance of these findings is unknown. Overall, the effects of opioids appear to be modestly immunosuppressive.

Concentration –Efficacy Relationships

Studies in normal volunteers and patients reveal predictable relationships between oxycodone dosage and plasma oxycodone concentrations, as well as between concentration and certain expected opioid effects, such as pupillary constriction, sedation, overall subjective "drug effect", analgesia and feelings of relaxation.

The minimum effective analgesic concentration will vary widely among patients, especially among patients who have been previously treated with potent agonist opioids. As a result, patients must be treated with individualized titration of dosage to the desired effect. The minimum effective analgesic concentration of oxycodone for any individual patient may increase over time due to an increase in pain, the development of a new pain syndrome and/or the development of analgesic tolerance.

Concentration –Adverse Reaction Relationships

There is a relationship between increasing oxycodone plasma concentration and increasing frequency of dose-related opioid adverse reactions such as nausea, vomiting, CNS effects, and respiratory depression. In opioid-tolerant patients, the situation may be altered by the development of tolerance to opioid-related side effects.

The dose of OXYCONTIN must be individualized because the effective analgesic dose for some patients will be too high to be tolerated by other patients *[see Dosage and Administration (2.1)]*.

12.3   Pharmacokinetics

The activity of OXYCONTIN is primarily due to the parent drug oxycodone. OXYCONTIN is designed to provide delivery of oxycodone over 12 hours.

Cutting, breaking, chewing, crushing or dissolving OXYCONTIN impairs the controlled-release delivery mechanism and results in the rapid release and absorption of a potentially fatal dose of oxycodone.

Oxycodone release from OXYCONTIN is pH independent. The oral bioavailability of oxycodone is 60% to 87%. The relative oral bioavailability of oxycodone from OXYCONTIN to that from immediate-release oral dosage forms is 100%. Upon repeated dosing with OXYCONTIN in healthy subjects in pharmacokinetic studies, steady-state levels were achieved within 24-36 hours. Oxycodone is extensively metabolized and eliminated primarily in the urine as both conjugated and unconjugated metabolites. The apparent elimination half-life ($t_{½}$) of oxycodone following the administration of OXYCONTIN was 4.5 hours compared to 3.2 hours for immediate-release oxycodone.

Absorption

About 60% to 87% of an oral dose of oxycodone reaches the central compartment in comparison to a parenteral dose. This high oral bioavailability is due to low pre-systemic and/or first-pass metabolism.

Plasma Oxycodone Concentration over Time

Dose proportionality has been established for OXYCONTIN 10 mg, 15 mg, 20 mg, 30 mg, 40 mg, 60 mg, and 80 mg tablet strengths for both peak plasma concentrations (C_{max}) and extent of absorption (AUC) (see Table 3). Given the short elimination $t_{½}$ of oxycodone, steady-state plasma concentrations of oxycodone are achieved within 24-36 hours of initiation of dosing with OXYCONTIN. In a study comparing 10 mg of OXYCONTIN every 12 hours to 5 mg of immediate-release oxycodone every 6 hours, the two treatments were found to be equivalent for AUC and C_{max}, and similar for C_{min} (trough) concentrations.

TABLE 3

Mean [% coefficient of variation]

Regimen	Dosage Form	AUC (ng·hr/mL)*	C_{max} (ng/mL)	T_{max} (hr)
Single Dose†	10 mg	136 [27]	11.5 [27]	5.11 [21]
	15 mg	196 [28]	16.8 [29]	4.59 [19]
	20 mg	248 [25]	22.7 [25]	4.63 [22]
	30 mg	377 [24]	34.6 [21]	4.61 [19]
	40 mg	497 [27]	47.4 [30]	4.40 [22]
	60 mg	705 [22]	64.6 [24]	4.15 [26]
	80 mg	908 [21]	87.1 [29]	4.27 [26]

* for single-dose AUC = AUC_{0-inf}
† data obtained while subjects received naltrexone, which can enhance absorption

Food Effects

Food has no significant effect on the extent of absorption of oxycodone from OXYCONTIN.

Distribution

Following intravenous administration, the steady-state volume of distribution (Vss) for oxycodone was 2.6 L/kg. Oxycodone binding to plasma protein at 37°C and a pH of 7.4 was about 45%. Once absorbed, oxycodone is distributed to skeletal muscle, liver, intestinal tract, lungs, spleen, and brain. Oxycodone has been found in breast milk *[see Use in Specific Populations (8.3)]*.

Metabolism

Oxycodone is extensively metabolized by multiple metabolic pathways to produce noroxycodone, oxymorphone and noroxymorphone, which are subsequently glucuronidated. Noroxycodone and noroxymorphone are the major circulating metabolites. CYP3A mediated *N*-demethylation to noroxycodone is the primary metabolic pathway of oxycodone with a lower contribution from CYP2D6 mediated *O*-demethylation to oxymorphone. Therefore, the formation of these and related metabolites can, in theory, be affected by other drugs [see Drug Interactions (7.3)].

Noroxycodone exhibits very weak anti-nociceptive potency compared to oxycodone, however, it undergoes further oxidation to produce noroxymorphone, which is active at opioid receptors. Although noroxymorphone is an active metabolite and present at relatively high concentrations in circulation, it does not appear to cross the blood-brain barrier to a significant extent. Oxymorphone is present in the plasma only at low concentrations and undergoes further metabolism to form its glucuronide and noroxymorphone. Oxymorphone has been shown to be active and possessing analgesic activity but its contribution to analgesia following oxycodone administration is thought to be clinically insignificant. Other metabolites (α- and ß-oxycodol, noroxycodol and oxymorphol) may be present at very low concentrations and demonstrate limited penetration into the brain as compared to oxycodone. The enzymes responsible for keto-reduction and glucuronidation pathways in oxycodone metabolism have not been established.

Excretion

Oxycodone and its metabolites are excreted primarily via the kidney. The amounts measured in the urine have been reported as follows: free and conjugated oxycodone 8.9%, free noroxycodone 23%, free oxymorphone less than 1%, conjugated oxymorphone 10%, free and conjugated noroxymorphone 14%, reduced free and conjugated metabolites up to 18%. The total plasma clearance was approximately 1.4 L/min in adults.

Specific Populations
Geriatric Use
The plasma concentrations of oxycodone are only nominally affected by age, being 15% greater in elderly as compared to young subjects (age 21-45).
Gender
Across individual pharmacokinetic studies, average plasma oxycodone concentrations for female subjects were up to 25% higher than for male subjects on a body weight-adjusted basis. The reason for this difference is unknown [see Use in Specific Populations (8.8)].
Renal Impairment
Data from a pharmacokinetic study involving 13 patients with mild to severe renal dysfunction (creatinine clearance <60 mL/min) showed peak plasma oxycodone and noroxycodone concentrations 50% and 20% higher, respectively, and AUC values for oxycodone, noroxycodone, and oxymorphone 60%, 50%, and 40% higher than normal subjects, respectively. This was accompanied by an increase in sedation but not by differences in respiratory rate, pupillary constriction, or several other measures of drug effect. There was an increase in mean elimination $t_{1/2}$ for oxycodone of 1 hour.
Hepatic Impairment
Data from a study involving 24 patients with mild to moderate hepatic dysfunction show peak plasma oxycodone and noroxycodone concentrations 50% and 20% higher, respectively, than healthy subjects. AUC values are 95% and 65% higher, respectively. Oxymorphone peak plasma concentrations and AUC values are lower by 30% and 40%. These differences are accompanied by increases in some, but not other, drug effects. The mean elimination $t_{1/2}$ for oxycodone increased by 2.3 hours.
Drug-Drug Interactions
CYP3A4 Inhibitors
CYP3A4 is the major enzyme involved in noroxycodone formation. Co-administration of OXYCONTIN (10 mg single dose) and the CYP3A4 inhibitor ketoconazole (200 mg BID) increased oxycodone AUC and C_{max} by 170% and 100%, respectively [see Drug Interactions (7.3)].
CYP3A4 Inducers
A published study showed that the co-administration of rifampin, a drug metabolizing enzyme inducer, decreased oxycodone AUC and C_{max} values by 86% and 63%, respectively [see Drug Interactions (7.3)].
CYP2D6 Inhibitors
Oxycodone is metabolized in part to oxymorphone via CYP2D6. While this pathway may be blocked by a variety of drugs such as certain cardiovascular drugs (e.g., quinidine) and antidepressants (e.g., fluoxetine), such blockade has not been shown to be of clinical significance with OXYCONTIN [see Drug Interactions (7.3)].

13   NONCLINICAL TOXICOLOGY
13.1   Carcinogenesis, Mutagenesis, Impairment of Fertility
Carcinogenesis
No animal studies to evaluate the carcinogenic potential of oxycodone have been conducted.
Mutagenesis
Oxycodone was genotoxic in the mouse lymphoma assay at concentrations of 50 mcg/mL or greater with metabolic acti-

vation and at 400 mcg/mL or greater without metabolic activation. Clastogenicity was observed with oxycodone in the presence of metabolic activation in one chromosomal aberration assay in human lymphocytes at concentrations greater than or equal to 1250 mcg/mL at 24 but not 48 hours of exposure. In a second chromosomal aberration assay with human lymphocytes, no structural clastogenicity was observed either with or without metabolic activation; however, in the absence of metabolic activation, oxycodone increased numerical chromosomal aberrations (polyploidy). Oxycodone was not genotoxic in the following assays: Ames *S. typhimurium* and *E. coli* test with and without metabolic activation at concentrations up to 5000 µg/plate, chromosomal aberration test in human lymphocytes (in the absence of metabolic activation) at concentrations up to 1500 µg/mL, and with activation after 48 hours of exposure at concentrations up to 5000 µg/mL, and in the *in vivo* bone marrow micronucleus assay in mice (at plasma levels up to 48 µg/mL).

Impairment of Fertility
In a study of reproductive performance, rats were administered a once daily gavage dose of the vehicle or oxycodone hydrochloride (0.5, 2, and 8 mg/kg). Male rats were dosed for 28 days before cohabitation with females, during the cohabitation and until necropsy (2-3 weeks post-cohabitation). Females were dosed for 14 days before cohabitation with males, during cohabitation and up to gestation day 6. Oxycodone hydrochloride did not affect reproductive function in male or female rats at any dose tested (≤ 8 mg/kg/day).

14   CLINICAL STUDIES
A double-blind, placebo-controlled, fixed-dose, parallel group, two-week study was conducted in 133 patients with persistent, moderate to severe pain, who were judged as having inadequate pain control with their current therapy. In this study, OXYCONTIN 20 mg, but not 10 mg, was statistically significant in pain reduction compared with placebo.

16   HOW SUPPLIED/STORAGE AND HANDLING
OXYCONTIN (oxycodone hydrochloride extended-release tablets) 10 mg are film-coated, round, white-colored, bi-convex tablets debossed with OP on one side and 10 on the other and are supplied as child-resistant closure, opaque plastic bottles of 100 (**NDC 59011-410-10**) and unit dose packaging with 10 individually numbered tablets per card; two cards per glue end carton (**NDC 59011-410-20**).

OXYCONTIN (oxycodone hydrochloride extended-release tablets) 15 mg are film-coated, round, gray-colored, bi-convex tablets debossed with OP on one side and 15 on the other and are supplied as child-resistant closure, opaque plastic bottles of 100 (**NDC 59011-415-10**) and unit dose packaging with 10 individually numbered tablets per card; two cards per glue end carton (**NDC 59011-415-20**).

OXYCONTIN (oxycodone hydrochloride extended-release tablets) 20 mg are film-coated, round, pink-colored, bi-convex tablets debossed with OP on one side and 20 on the other and are supplied as child-resistant closure, opaque plastic bottles of 100 (**NDC 59011-420-10**) and unit dose packaging with 10 individually numbered tablets per card; two cards per glue end carton (**NDC 59011-420-20**).

OXYCONTIN (oxycodone hydrochloride extended-release tablets) 30 mg are film-coated, round, brown-colored, bi-convex tablets debossed with OP on one side and 30 on the other and are supplied as child-resistant closure, opaque plastic bottles of 100 (**NDC 59011-430-10**) and unit dose packaging with 10 individually numbered tablets per card; two cards per glue end carton (**NDC 59011-430-20**).

OXYCONTIN (oxycodone hydrochloride extended-release tablets) 40 mg are film-coated, round, yellow-colored, bi-convex tablets debossed with OP on one side and 40 on the other and are supplied as child-resistant closure, opaque plastic bottles of 100 (**NDC 59011-440-10**) and unit dose packaging with 10 individually numbered tablets per card; two cards per glue end carton (**NDC 59011-440-20**).

OXYCONTIN (oxycodone hydrochloride extended-release tablets) 60 mg are film-coated, round, red-colored, bi-convex tablets debossed with OP on one side and 60 on the other and are supplied as child-resistant closure, opaque plastic bottles of 100 (**NDC 59011-460-10**) and unit dose packaging with 10 individually numbered tablets per card; two cards per glue end carton (**NDC 59011-460-20**).

OXYCONTIN (oxycodone hydrochloride extended-release tablets) 80 mg are film-coated, round, green-colored, bi-convex tablets debossed with OP on one side and 80 on the other and are supplied as child-resistant closure, opaque plastic bottles of 100 (**NDC 59011-480-10**) and unit dose packaging with 10 individually numbered tablets per card; two cards per glue end carton (**NDC 59011-480-20**).

Store at 25°C (77°F); excursions permitted between 15°-30°C (59°-86°F).

Dispense in tight, light-resistant container.

CAUTION

DEA FORM REQUIRED

17   PATIENT COUNSELING INFORMATION
Advise the patient to read the FDA-approved patient labeling (Medication Guide).
Addiction, Abuse and Misuse
Inform patients that the use of OXYCONTIN, even when taken as recommended can result in addiction, abuse and misuse, which can lead to overdose and death [see Warnings and Precautions (5.1)]. Instruct patients not to share OXYCONTIN with others and to take steps to protect OXYCONTIN from theft or misuse.
Life-Threatening Respiratory Depression
Inform patients of the risk of life-threatening respiratory depression including information that the risk is greatest when starting OXYCONTIN or when the dose is increased and that it can occur even at recommended doses [see Warnings and Precautions (5.2)]. Advise patients how to recognize respiratory depression and to seek medical attention if breathing difficulties develop.
Accidental Ingestion
Inform patients that accidental ingestion, especially in children, may result in respiratory depression or death [see Warnings and Precautions (5.2)]. Instruct patients to take steps to store OXYCONTIN securely and to dispose of unused OXYCONTIN by flushing the tablets down the toilet.
Neonatal Opioid Withdrawal Syndrome
Inform female patients of reproductive potential that prolonged use of OXYCONTIN during pregnancy can result in neonatal opioid withdrawal syndrome, which may be life-threatening if not recognized and treated [see Warnings and Precautions (5.3)].
Interactions with Alcohol and other CNS Depressants
Inform patients that potentially serious additive effects may occur if OXYCONTIN is used with other CNS depressants, and not to use such drugs unless supervised by a health care provider.
Important Administration Instructions
Instruct patients how to properly take OXYCONTIN, including the following:
• OXYCONTIN is designed to work properly only if swallowed intact. Taking cut, broken, chewed, crushed, or dissolved OXYCONTIN tablets can result in a fatal overdose.
• OXYCONTIN tablets should be taken one tablet at a time.
• Do not pre-soak, lick or otherwise wet the tablet prior to placing in the mouth.
• Take each tablet with enough water to ensure complete swallowing immediately after placing in the mouth.
Hypotension
Inform patients that OXYCONTIN may cause orthostatic hypotension and syncope. Instruct patients how to recognize symptoms of low blood pressure and how to reduce the risk of serious consequences should hypotension occur (e.g., sit or lie down, carefully rise from a sitting or lying position).
Driving or Operating Heavy Machinery
Inform patients that OXYCONTIN may impair the ability to perform potentially hazardous activities such as driving a car or operating heavy machinery. Advise patients not to perform such tasks until they know how they will react to the medication.
Constipation
Advise patients of the potential for severe constipation, including management instructions and when to seek medical attention.
Anaphylaxis
Inform patients that anaphylaxis has been reported with ingredients contained in OXYCONTIN. Advise patients how to recognize such a reaction and when to seek medical attention.
Pregnancy
Advise female patients that OXYCONTIN can cause fetal harm and to inform the prescriber if they are pregnant or plan to become pregnant.
Disposal of Unused OXYCONTIN
Advise patients to flush the unused tablets down the toilet when OXYCONTIN is no longer needed.

Healthcare professionals can telephone Purdue Pharma's Medical Services Department (1-888-726-7535) for information on this product.

Purdue Pharma L.P.
Stamford, CT 06901-3431
©2014, Purdue Pharma L.P.
U.S. Patent Numbers 6,488,963; 7,129,248; 7,674,799; 7,674,800; 7,683,072; 7,776,314; 8,114,383; 8,309,060; and 8,337,888.

Medication Guide
OXYCONTIN®   (ox-e-KON-tin)   (oxycodone hydrochloride extended-release tablets), CII

OXYCONTIN is:
• A strong prescription pain medicine that contains an opioid (narcotic) that is used to manage pain severe enough to require daily around-the-clock, long-term

treatment with an opioid, when other pain treatments such as non-opioid pain medicines or immediate-release opioid pain medicines do not treat your pain well enough or you cannot tolerate them.
• A long-acting (extended-release) opioid pain medicine that can put you at risk for overdose and death. Even if you take your dose correctly as prescribed you are at risk for opioid addiction, abuse, and misuse that can lead to death.
• Not for use to treat pain that is not around-the-clock.

Important information about OXYCONTIN:
• **Get emergency help right away if you take too much OXYCONTIN (overdose).** When you first start taking OXYCONTIN, when your dose is changed, or if you take too much (overdose), serious or life-threatening breathing problems that can lead to death may occur.
• Never give anyone else your OXYCONTIN. They could die from taking it. Store OXYCONTIN away from children and in a safe place to prevent stealing or abuse. Selling or giving away OXYCONTIN is against the law.

Do not take OXYCONTIN if you have:
• severe asthma, trouble breathing, or other lung problems.
• a bowel blockage or have narrowing of the stomach or intestines.

Before taking OXYCONTIN, tell your healthcare provider if you have a history of:
• head injury, seizures
• liver, kidney, thyroid problems
• problems urinating
• pancreas or gallbladder problems
• abuse of street or prescription drugs, alcohol addiction, or mental health problems.

Tell your healthcare provider if you are:
• **pregnant or planning to become pregnant.** Prolonged use of OXYCONTIN during pregnancy can cause withdrawal symptoms in your newborn baby that could be life-threatening if not recognized and treated.
• **breastfeeding.** OXYCONTIN passes into breast milk and may harm your baby.
• taking prescription or over-the-counter medicines, vitamins, or herbal supplements. Taking OXYCONTIN with certain other medicines can cause serious side effects that could lead to death.

When taking OXYCONTIN:
• Do not change your dose. Take OXYCONTIN exactly as prescribed by your healthcare provider.
• Take your prescribed dose every 12 hours at the same time every day. Do not take more than your prescribed dose in 12 hours. If you miss a dose, take your next dose at your usual time.
• Swallow OXYCONTIN whole. Do not cut, break, chew, crush, dissolve, snort, or inject OXYCONTIN because this may cause you to overdose and die.
• OXYCONTIN should be taken 1 tablet at a time. Do not pre-soak, lick, or wet the tablet before placing in your mouth to avoid choking on the tablet.
• **Call your healthcare provider if the dose you are taking does not control your pain.**
• **Do not stop taking OXYCONTIN without talking to your healthcare provider.**
• After you stop taking OXYCONTIN, flush any unused tablets down the toilet.

While taking OXYCONTIN DO NOT:
• Drive or operate heavy machinery, until you know how OXYCONTIN affects you. OXYCONTIN can make you sleepy, dizzy, or lightheaded.
• Drink alcohol, or use prescription or over-the-counter medicines that contain alcohol. Using products containing alcohol during treatment with OXYCONTIN may cause you to overdose and die.

The possible side effects of OXYCONTIN are:
• constipation, nausea, sleepiness, vomiting, tiredness, headache, dizziness, abdominal pain. Call your healthcare provider if you have any of these symptoms and they are severe.

Get emergency medical help if you have:
• trouble breathing, shortness of breath, fast heartbeat, chest pain, swelling of your face, tongue or throat, extreme drowsiness, light-headedness when changing positions, or you are feeling faint.

These are not all the possible side effects of OXYCONTIN. Call your doctor for medical advice about side effects. You may report side effects to FDA at 1-800-FDA-1088. **For more information go to dailymed.nlm.nih.gov**

Manufactured by: Purdue Pharma L.P., Stamford, CT 06901-3431, **www.purduepharma.com or call 1-888-726-7535**

This Medication Guide has been approved by the U.S. Food and Drug Administration.   Revised: April 2014
Shown in Product Identification Guide, page 312

Ranbaxy Laboratories Inc.
**9431 FLORIDA MINING BOULEVARD EAST
JACKSONVILLE, FL 32257**

Main Phone: (609) 720-9200

ABSORICA   ℞
(isotretinoin)
capsules, for oral use

HIGHLIGHTS OF PRESCRIBING INFORMATION
These highlights do not include all the information needed to use ABSORICA safely and effectively. See full prescribing information for ABSORICA.
ABSORICA® (isotretinoin) capsules, for oral use
Initial U.S. Approval: 1982

WARNING: CAUSES BIRTH DEFECTS
See full prescribing information for complete boxed warning.
Pregnancy Category X.
• **ABSORICA must not be used by female patients who are or may become pregnant (5, 8.1, 8.6).**
• **There is an extremely high risk that severe birth defects will result if pregnancy occurs while taking ABSORICA in any amount, even for short periods of time. Potentially any fetus exposed during pregnancy can be affected (5.1, 8.1).**
• **There are no accurate means of determining whether an exposed fetus has been affected (5.1, 8.1).**
• **ABSORICA is available only through a restricted program called the iPLEDGE program. Prescribers, patients, pharmacies, and distributors must enroll in the program (5.2).**

INDICATIONS AND USAGE
ABSORICA is a retinoid indicated for the treatment of severe recalcitrant nodular acne in patients 12 years of age and older (1).
Limitations of Use
ABSORICA may only be administered to patients enrolled in the iPLEDGE program (1, 5.2).

DOSAGE AND ADMINISTRATION
• Recommended dosage of 0.5 to 1 mg/kg/day given in two divided doses without regards to meals for 15 to 20 weeks (2.1).
• Once daily dosing is **not** recommended (2.1).
• Perform pregnancy tests prior to prescribing, each month during therapy, end of therapy, and one month after discontinuation (2.4, 8.6).
• Prior to prescribing, perform fasting lipid profile and liver function tests (2.4).
• ABSORICA is not substitutable with other forms of isotretinoin (12.3).

DOSAGE FORMS AND STRENGTHS
Capsules: 10 mg, 20 mg, 25 mg, 30 mg, 35 mg and 40 mg (3)

CONTRAINDICATIONS
• Pregnancy (4.1, 8.1)
• Hypersensitivity to this product or any of its components (4.2, 5.14)

WARNINGS AND PRECAUTIONS
• Unacceptable Contraception: Micro-dosed progesterone preparations are not an acceptable method of contraception during ABSORICA therapy (5.3)
• Psychiatric Disorders: Depression, psychosis, suicidal thoughts and behavior, and aggressive and/or violent behaviors (5.4)
• Pseudotumor cerebri, some cases with concomitant tetracyclines (5.5)
• Serious skin reactions: Stevens-Johnson syndrome (SJS), toxic epidermal necrolysis (TEN) (5.6)

• Acute pancreatitis, rarely fatal hemorrhagic pancreatitis, in patients with either elevated or normal serum triglyceride levels (5.7)
• Lipid Abnormalities: Triglyceridemia low HDL and elevation of cholesterol. Monitor lipid levels at regular intervals (5.8, 5.15)
• Hearing Impairment (5.9)
• Hepatotoxicity: Monitor liver function tests at regular intervals (5.10, 5.15)
• Inflammatory Bowel Disease (5.11)
• Skeletal Abnormalities: Arthralgias, back pain, decreases in bone mineral density and premature epiphyseal closure (5.12)
• Ocular Abnormalities: corneal opacities, decreased night vision (5.13)
• Glucose and CPK Abnormalities (5.15)

ADVERSE REACTIONS
Most common adverse reactions (incidence ≥5%) are: lip dry, dry skin, back pain, dry eye, arthralgia, epistaxis, headache, nasopharyngitis, chapped lips, dermatitis, blood creatine kinase increased, cheilitis, musculoskeletal discomfort, upper respiratory tract infection, visual acuity reduced (6.1).
To report SUSPECTED ADVERSE REACTIONS, contact Ranbaxy, Inc. at 1-800-406-7984 or FDA at 1-800-FDA-1088 or www.fda.gov/medwatch or iPLEDGE at (1-866-495-0654).

DRUG INTERACTIONS
• Vitamin A: may cause additive adverse reactions (7.1)
• Tetracyclines: avoid concomitant use (7.2)
• St. John's Wort: may interfere with oral contraceptives (7.4)

See 17 for PATIENT COUNSELING INFORMATION and Medication Guide

                                    Revised: 08/2014

FULL PRESCRIBING INFORMATION

WARNING: CAUSES BIRTH DEFECTS

Pregnancy Category X.

- ABSORICA must not be used by female patients who are or may become pregnant [*see Warnings and Precautions* (5) *and Use in Specific Populations* (8.1, 8.6)].
- There is an extremely high risk that severe birth defects will result if pregnancy occurs while taking ABSORICA in any amount, even for short periods of time [*see Warnings and Precautions* (5.1) *and Use in Specific Populations* (8.1)].
- Potentially any fetus exposed during pregnancy can be affected [*see Use in Specific Populations* (8.1)].
- There are no accurate means of determining whether an exposed fetus has been affected [*see Warning and Precautions* (5.1) *and Use in Specific Populations* (8.1)].
- Birth defects which have been documented following isotretinoin exposure include abnormalities of the face, eyes, ears, skull, central nervous system, cardiovascular system, and thymus and parathyroid glands. Cases of IQ scores less than 85 with or without other abnormalities have been reported. There is an increased risk of spontaneous abortion and premature births have been reported [*see Use in Specific Populations* (8.1)].
- Documented external abnormalities include: skull abnormality; ear abnormalities (including anotia, micropinna, small or absent external auditory canals); eye abnormalities (including microphthalmia; facial dysmorphia; cleft palate). Documented internal abnormalities include: CNS abnormalities (including cerebral abnormalities, cerebellar malformation, hydrocephalus, microcephaly, cranial nerve deficit); cardiovascular abnormalities; thymus gland abnormality; parathyroid hormone deficiency. In some cases death has occurred with certain abnormalities previously noted [*see Use in Specific Populations* (8.1)].
- If pregnancy does occur during the treatment of a female patient who is taking ABSORICA, ABSORICA must be discontinued immediately and she should be referred to an Obstetrician-Gynecologist experienced in reproductive toxicity for further evaluation and counseling [*see Use in Specific Populations* (8.1)].

Special Prescribing Requirements

- Because of the risk of teratogenicity and to minimize fetal exposure, ABSORICA is available only through a restricted program under a Risk Evaluation and Mitigation Strategy (REMS) called iPLEDGE™. Under the ABSORICA REMS, prescribers, patients, pharmacies, and distributors must enroll and be registered in the program [*see Warnings and Precautions* (5.2)].

---

1 INDICATIONS AND USAGE

ABSORICA is a retinoid indicated for the treatment of severe recalcitrant nodular acne in patients 12 years of age and older. Nodules are inflammatory lesions with a diameter of 5 mm or greater. The nodules may become suppurative or hemorrhagic. "Severe," by definition, means "many" as opposed to "few or several" nodules. Because of significant adverse reactions associated with its use, ABSORICA should be reserved for patients with multiple severe nodular acne who are unresponsive to conventional therapy, including systemic antibiotics. In addition, ABSORICA is indicated only for those female patients who are not pregnant, because ABSORICA can cause severe birth defects [see *Contraindications* (4.1)].

Limitations of Use

A single course of therapy for 15 to 20 weeks has been shown to result in complete and prolonged remission of disease in many patients. If a second course of therapy is needed, it should not be initiated until at least 8 weeks after completion of the first course, because experience with isotretinoin has shown that patients may continue to improve following treatment with isotretinoin. The optimal interval before retreatment has not been defined for patients who have not completed skeletal growth [see *Warnings and Precautions* (5.12)].

As a part of the iPLEDGE program, ABSORICA may only be administered to patients enrolled in the program [see *Warnings and Precautions* (5.2)].

2 DOSAGE AND ADMINISTRATION

Healthcare professionals who prescribe ABSORICA must be certified in the iPLEDGE program and must comply with the required monitoring to ensure safe use of ABSORICA [see *Warnings and Precautions* (5.2)].

The required laboratory testing must be completed prior to dosing ABSORICA [see *Dosage and Administration* (2.4)]. Pregnancy Testing, and Contraceptive measures must be followed prior to dosing ABSORICA [see *Use in Specific Populations* (8.6)].

2.1 Recommended Dosage

The recommended dosage range for ABSORICA is 0.5 to 1 mg/kg/day given in two divided doses without regard to meals for 15 to 20 weeks (see Table 1). To decrease the risk of esophageal irritation, patients should swallow the capsules with a full glass of liquid [see *Patient Counseling Information* (17)].

The safety of once daily dosing with ABSORICA has not been established. Once daily dosing is **not** recommended.

Table 1: ABSORICA Dosing by Body Weight
(Based on Administration With or Without Food)

Body Weight		Total Daily (mg)		
Kilograms	Pounds	0.5 mg/kg	1 mg/kg	2 mg/kg
40	88	20	40	80
50	110	25	50	100
60	132	30	60	120
70	154	35	70	140
80	176	40	80	160
90	198	45	90	180
100	220	50	100	200

2.2 Dosage Range

In trials comparing 0.1, 0.5, and 1 mg/kg/day, it was found that all dosages provided initial clearing of disease, but there was a greater need for retreatment with the lower dosages. During treatment, the dose may be adjusted according to response of the disease and/or the appearance of clinical side effects, some of which may be dose-related. Adult patients whose disease is very severe with scarring or is primarily manifested on the trunk may require dose adjustments up to 2 mg/kg/day, as tolerated.

2.3 Duration of Use

A normal course of treatment is 15 – 20 weeks. If the total nodule count has been reduced by more than 70% prior to completing 15 to 20 weeks of treatment, the drug may be discontinued. After a period of 2 months or more off therapy, and if warranted by persistent or recurring severe nodular acne, a second course of therapy may be initiated. The optimal interval before retreatment has not been defined for patients who have not completed skeletal growth. Long-term use of ABSORICA, even in low doses, has not been studied, and is not recommended. It is important that ABSORICA be given at the recommended doses for no longer than the recommended duration. The effect of long-term use of ABSORICA on bone loss is unknown [see *Warnings and Precautions* (5.12)].

2.4 Laboratory Testing

Pregnancy Testing

[*See Use in Specific Populations* (8.6)]

Lipid Profile

Perform a fasting lipid profile including triglycerides prior to use of ABSORICA [see *Warnings and Precautions* (5.8, 5.15)].

Liver Function Test

Perform liver function tests prior to use of ABSORICA [see *Warnings and Precautions* (5.10, 5.15)].

3 DOSAGE FORMS AND STRENGTHS

ABSORICA is available in 10 mg, 20 mg, 25 mg, 30 mg, 35 mg and 40 mg capsules.

- **10 mg:** Dark yellow, opaque, capsule imprinted with black ink "G 240" on cap and "**10**" on the body
- **20 mg:** Red, opaque, capsule imprinted with black ink "G 241" on cap and "**20**" on the body
- **25 mg:** Green, opaque, capsule imprinted with white ink "G 342" on cap and "**25**" on the body
- **30 mg:** Brown, opaque, capsule imprinted with white ink "G 242" on cap and "**30**" on the body
- **35 mg:** Dark blue, opaque, capsule imprinted with white ink "G 343" on cap and "**35**" on the body
- **40 mg:** Brown and red, capsule imprinted with white ink "G 325" on cap and "**40**" on the body

4 CONTRAINDICATIONS

4.1 Pregnancy

ABSORICA can cause fetal harm when administered to a pregnant woman. Major congenital malformations, spontaneous abortions, and premature births have been documented following pregnancy exposure to isotretinoin in any amount and even for short periods of time. ABSORICA is contraindicated in females who are or may become pregnant. If this drug is used during pregnancy, or if the patient becomes pregnant while taking this drug, treatment should be discontinued and the patient should be apprised of the potential hazard to the fetus [see *Use in Specific Populations* (8.1)].

4.2 Hypersensitivity

Hypersensitivity to this product (or Vitamin A, given the chemical similarity to isotretinoin) or to any of its components [see *Warnings and Precautions* (5.14)].

5 WARNINGS AND PRECAUTIONS

ABSORICA must not be used by female patients who are or may become pregnant. There is an extremely high risk that severe birth defects will result if pregnancy occurs while taking ABSORICA in any amount, even for short periods of time.

5.1 Embryofetal Toxicity

Teratogenicity

Major congenital malformations, spontaneous abortions, and premature births have been documented following pregnancy exposure to isotretinoin [see *Use in Specific Populations* (8.1)]. Females of childbearing potential must comply with the pregnancy testing and contraception requirements described in the iPLEDGE program [see *Warnings and Precautions* (5.2) *and Use in Specific Populations* (8.6)]. There are no accurate means of determining whether an exposed fetus has been affected.

No Blood Donation

Patients must be informed not to donate blood during isotretinoin therapy and for 1 month following discontinuation of the drug because the blood might be given to a pregnant female patient whose fetus must not be exposed to isotretinoin.

5.2 iPLEDGE Program

Because of the risk of teratogenicity and to minimize fetal exposure, ABSORICA is available only through a restricted program under a REMS called iPLEDGE. Under the ABSORICA REMS, prescribers, patients, pharmacies, and distributors must enroll and be registered in the program. ABSORICA must not be prescribed, dispensed or otherwise obtained through the internet or any other means outside of the iPLEDGE program. Only FDA-approved isotretinoin products must be distributed, prescribed, dispensed, and used.

Required components of the iPLEDGE Program are:

- ABSORICA must only be prescribed by prescribers who are registered and activated with the iPLEDGE program and agree to comply with the REMS requirements described in the booklets entitled *The Guide to Best Practices for the iPLEDGE Program, The iPLEDGE Program Prescriber Contraception Counseling Guide*, and *Recognizing Psychiatric Disorders in Adolescents and Young Adults: A Guide for Prescribers of Isotretinoin*.
- Male patients and Female patients not of childbearing potential: To obtain ABSORICA, these patients must understand the risks and benefits of ABSORICA, comply with the REMS requirements described in the booklet entitled *The iPLEDGE Program Guide to Isotretinoin for Male Patients and Female Patients Who Cannot Get Pregnant*, and sign a Patient Information/Informed Consent form.
- Female patients of childbearing potential: ABSORICA is contraindicated in female patients who are or may become pregnant [see *Contraindications* (4.1)].
- Female patients of childbearing potential who are not pregnant must understand the risks and benefits, comply with the REMS requirements described in the booklet entitled *The iPLEDGE Program Guide to Isotretinoin for Female Patients Who Can Get Pregnant* and *The iPLEDGE Program Birth Control Workbook* (including the pregnancy testing and contraception requirements [see *Use in Specific Populations* (8.6) *and Patient Counseling Information* (17)]), and sign a Patient Information/Informed Consent form and Patient Information/ Informed Consent About Birth Defects form. Additionally, the patient must answer questions about the iPLEDGE program and pregnancy prevention monthly.
- Pharmacies that dispense ABSORICA must be registered and activated with iPLEDGE, must only dispense to patients who are authorized to receive ABSORICA, and agree to comply with the REMS requirements described in the booklet entitled *The Pharmacist Guide for the iPLEDGE Program*.
- Female patients of childbearing potential must fill and pick up the prescription within 7 days of the specimen collection for the pregnancy test; male patients and female patients not of childbearing potential must fill and pick up the prescription within 30 days of the office visit.
- ABSORICA must only be dispensed in no more than a 30-day supply with a Medication Guide. Refills require a new prescription and a new authorization from the iPLEDGE system.
- Wholesalers and distributors that distribute ABSORICA must be registered with iPLEDGE and agree to comply with the REMS requirements.

If a pregnancy does occur during ABSORICA treatment, ABSORICA must be discontinued immediately. The patient should be referred to an obstetrician-gynecologist experienced in reproductive toxicity for further evaluation and counseling. Any suspected fetal exposure during or 1 month after ABSORICA therapy must be reported immediately to the FDA via the MedWatch telephone number 1-800-FDA-1088 and also to the iPLEDGE pregnancy registry at 1-866-495-0654 or via the internet (www.ipledgeprogram.com).

Further information, including a list of qualified pharmacies, is available at www.ipledgeprogram.com or 1-866-495-0654.

5.3 Unacceptable Contraception
Micro-dosed Progesterone Preparations
Micro-dosed progesterone preparations ("minipills" that do not contain an estrogen) are an inadequate method of contraception during ABSORICA therapy.

5.4 Psychiatric Disorders
Isotretinoin may cause depression, psychosis and, rarely, suicidal ideation, suicide attempts, suicide, and aggressive and/or violent behaviors. No mechanism of action has been established for these reactions [see Adverse Reactions (6.1)]. Prescribers should read the brochure, *Recognizing Psychiatric Disorders in Adolescents and Young Adults: A Guide for Prescribers of Isotretinoin*. Prescribers should be alert to the warning signs of psychiatric disorders to guide patients to receive the help they need. Therefore, prior to initiation of ABSORICA therapy, patients and family members should be asked about any history of psychiatric disorder, and at each visit during therapy patients should be assessed for symptoms of depression, mood disturbance, psychosis, or aggression to determine if further evaluation may be necessary. Signs and symptoms of depression, as described in the brochure (*Recognizing Psychiatric Disorders in Adolescents and Young Adults*), include sad mood, hopelessness, feelings of guilt, worthlessness or helplessness, loss of pleasure or interest in activities, fatigue, difficulty concentrating, change in sleep pattern, change in weight or appetite, suicidal thoughts or attempts, restlessness, irritability, acting on dangerous impulses, and persistent physical symptoms unresponsive to treatment. Patients should stop ABSORICA and the patient or a family member should promptly contact their prescriber if the patient develops depression, mood disturbance, psychosis, or aggression, without waiting until the next visit. Discontinuation of ABSORICA therapy may be insufficient; further evaluation may be necessary. While such monitoring may be helpful, it may not detect all patients at risk. Patients may report mental health problems or family history of psychiatric disorders. These reports should be discussed with the patient and/or the patient's family. A referral to a mental health professional may be necessary. The physician should consider whether ABSORICA therapy is appropriate in this setting; for some patients the risks may outweigh the benefits of ABSORICA therapy.

5.5 Pseudotumor Cerebri
Isotretinoin use has been associated with cases of pseudotumor cerebri (benign intracranial hypertension), some of which involved concomitant use of tetracyclines. Concomitant treatment with tetracyclines should therefore be avoided. Early signs and symptoms of pseudotumor cerebri include papilledema, headache, nausea and vomiting, and visual disturbances. Patients with these symptoms should be screened for papilledema and, if present, they should be told to discontinue ABSORICA immediately and be referred to a neurologist for further diagnosis and care [see Adverse Reactions (6.1)].

5.6 Serious Skin Reactions
There have been post-marketing reports of erythema multiforme and severe skin reactions [e.g., Stevens-Johnson syndrome (SJS), toxic epidermal necrolysis (TEN)] associated with isotretinoin use. These reactions may be serious and result in death, life-threatening events, hospitalization, or disability. Patients should be monitored closely for severe skin reactions, and discontinuation of ABSORICA should be considered if warranted.

5.7 Pancreatitis
Acute pancreatitis has been reported in isotretinoin-treated patients with either elevated or normal serum triglyceride levels. In rare instances, fatal hemorrhagic pancreatitis has been reported. ABSORICA should be stopped if hypertriglyceridemia cannot be controlled at an acceptable level or if symptoms of pancreatitis occur.

5.8 Lipid Abnormalities
Elevations of serum triglycerides in excess of 800 mg/dL have been reported in patients treated with isotretinoin. Marked elevations of serum triglycerides were reported in approximately 25% of patients receiving isotretinoin in clinical trials. In addition, approximately 15% developed a decrease in high-density lipoproteins and about 7% showed an increase in cholesterol levels. In clinical trials, the effects of triglycerides, HDL and cholesterol were reversible upon cessation of isotretinoin therapy. Some patients have been able to reverse triglyceride elevation by reduction in weight, restriction of dietary fat and alcohol, and reduction in the dose while continuing isotretinoin.

Blood lipid determinations should be performed before ABSORICA is given and then at intervals until the lipid response to ABSORICA is established, which usually occurs within 4 weeks. Especially careful consideration must be given to risk/benefit for patients who may be at high risk of triglyceridemia during ABSORICA therapy (patients with diabetes, obesity, increased alcohol intake, lipid metabolism disorder or familial history of lipid metabolism disorder). If ABSORICA therapy is instituted, more frequent checks of serum values for lipids and/or blood sugar are recommended [see Warnings and Precautions (5.15)].

The cardiovascular consequences of hypertriglyceridemia associated with isotretinoin are unknown.

5.9 Hearing Impairment
Impaired hearing has been reported in patients taking isotretinoin; in some cases, the hearing impairment has been reported to persist after therapy has been discontinued. Mechanism(s) and causality for this reaction have not been established. Patients who experience tinnitus or hearing impairment should discontinue ABSORICA treatment and be referred for specialized care for further evaluation [see Adverse Reactions (6.1)].

5.10 Hepatotoxicity
Clinical hepatitis considered to be possibly or probably related to isotretinoin therapy has been reported. Additionally, mild to moderate elevations of liver enzymes have been observed in approximately 15% of individuals treated during clinical trials with isotretinoin, some of which normalized with dosage reduction or continued administration of the drug. If normalization does not readily occur or if hepatitis is suspected during treatment with ABSORICA, the drug should be discontinued and the etiology further investigated.

5.11 Inflammatory Bowel Disease
Isotretinoin has been associated with inflammatory bowel disease (including regional ileitis) in patients without a prior history of intestinal disorders. In some instances, symptoms have been reported to persist after isotretinoin treatment has been stopped. Patients experiencing abdominal pain, rectal bleeding or severe diarrhea should discontinue ABSORICA immediately [see Adverse Reactions (6.1)].

5.12 Skeletal Abnormalities
Bone Mineral Density Changes
Isotretinoin may have a negative effect on bone mineral density (BMD) in some patients. In a clinical trial of ABSORICA and a generic product of Accutane® (isotretinoin), 27/306 (8.8%) of adolescents had BMD declines, defined as ≥ 4% lumbar spine or total hip, or ≥ 5% femoral neck, during the 20 week treatment period. Repeat scans conducted within 2-3 months after the post-treatment scan showed no recovery of BMD. Longer term data at 4-11 months showed that 3 out of 7 patients had total hip and femoral neck BMD below pre-treatment baseline, and 2 others did not show the increase in BMD above baseline expected in this adolescent population. Therefore, physicians should use caution when prescribing ABSORICA to patients with a history of childhood osteoporosis conditions, osteomalacia, or other disorders of bone metabolism. This would include patients diagnosed with anorexia nervosa and those who are on chronic drug therapy that causes drug-induced osteoporosis/osteomalacia and/or affects vitamin D metabolism, such as systemic corticosteroids and any anticonvulsant [see Use in Specific Populations (8.4)].

Musculoskeletal Abnormalities
Approximately 16% of patients treated with isotretinoin in a clinical trial developed musculoskeletal symptoms (including arthralgia) during treatment. In general, these symptoms were mild to moderate, but occasionally required discontinuation of the drug.

In a trial of pediatric patients treated with isotretinoin, approximately 29% (104/358) developed back pain. Back pain was severe in 13.5% (14/104) of the cases and occurred at a higher frequency in female patients than male patients. Arthralgias were experienced in 22% (79/358) of pediatric patients. Arthralgias were severe in 7.6% (6/79) of patients. Appropriate evaluation of the musculoskeletal system should be done in patients who present with these symptoms during or after a course of ABSORICA. Consideration should be given to discontinuation of ABSORICA if any significant abnormality is found.

There have been spontaneous reports of osteoporosis, osteopenia, bone fractures and/or delayed healing of bone fractures in patients while on therapy with isotretinoin or following cessation of therapy with isotretinoin. While causality to isotretinoin has not been established, an effect cannot be ruled out.

Patients may be at an increased risk when participating in sports with repetitive impact where the risks of spondylolisthesis with and without pars fractures and hip growth plate injures in early and late adolescence are known.

Effects of multiple courses of isotretinoin on the developing musculoskeletal system are unknown. There is some evidence that long-term, high-dose, or multiple courses of therapy with isotretinoin have more of an effect than a single course of therapy on the musculoskeletal system.

Longer term effects have not been studied. It is important that ABSORICA be given at the recommended doses for no longer than the recommended duration.

Hyperostosis
A high prevalence of skeletal hyperostosis was noted in clinical trials for disorders of keratinization with a mean dose of 2.24 mg/kg/day of isotretinoin. Additionally, skeletal hyperostosis was noted in 6 of 8 patients in a prospective trial of disorders of keratinization. Minimal skeletal hyperostosis and calcification of ligaments and tendons have also been observed by x-ray in prospective trials of nodular acne patients treated with a single course of therapy at recommended doses. The skeletal effects of multiple isotretinoin treatment courses for acne are unknown.

In a clinical trial of 217 pediatric patients (12 to 17 years) with severe recalcitrant nodular acne, hyperostosis was not observed after 16 to 20 weeks of treatment with approximately 1 mg/kg/day of isotretinoin given in two divided doses. Hyperostosis may require a longer time frame to appear. The clinical course and significance remain unknown.

Premature Epiphyseal Closure
There are spontaneous literature reports of premature epiphyseal closure in acne patients receiving recommended doses of isotretinoin. The effect of multiple courses of isotretinoin on epiphyseal closure is unknown.

In a 20-week clinical trial that included 289 adolescents on ABSORICA or a generic product of Accutane® (isotretinoin) who had hand radiographs taken to assess bone age, a total of 9 (3.11%) patients had bone age changes that were clinically significant and for which a drug-related effect cannot be excluded.

5.13 Ocular Abnormalities
Visual problems should be carefully monitored. All ABSORICA patients experiencing visual difficulties should discontinue ABSORICA treatment and have an ophthalmological examination [see Adverse Reactions (6.1)].

Corneal Opacities
Corneal opacities have occurred in patients receiving isotretinoin for acne and more frequently when higher drug dosages were used in patients with disorders of keratinization. The corneal opacities that have been observed in clinical trial patients treated with isotretinoin have either completely resolved or were resolving at follow-up 6 to 7 weeks after discontinuation of the drug [see Adverse Reactions (6.1)].

Decreased Night Vision
Decreased night vision has been reported during isotretinoin therapy and in some instances the event has persisted after therapy was discontinued. Because the onset in some patients was sudden, patients should be advised of this potential problem and warned to be cautious when driving or operating any vehicle at night.

Dry Eye
Dry eye has been reported in subjects during isotretinoin therapy. Patients who wear contact lenses may have trouble wearing them while on ABSORICA treatment and afterwards.

5.14 Hypersensitivity
Anaphylactic reactions and other allergic reactions have been reported in isotretinoin-treated patients. Cutaneous allergic reactions and serious cases of allergic vasculitis, often with purpura (bruises and red patches) of the extremities and extracutaneous involvement (including renal) have been reported. Severe allergic reaction necessitates discontinuation of therapy and appropriate medical management.

5.15 Laboratory Monitoring for Adverse Reactions
Lipids Test
Pretreatment and follow-up blood lipids should be obtained under fasting conditions. After consumption of alcohol, at least 36 hours should elapse before these determinations are made. It is recommended that these tests be performed at weekly or biweekly intervals until the lipid response to ABSORICA is established. The incidence of hypertriglyceridemia is 1 patient in 4 on isotretinoin [see Warnings and Precautions (5.8)].

Liver Function Test
Since elevations of liver enzymes have been observed during clinical trials, and hepatitis has been reported in patients on isotretinoin, pretreatment and follow-up liver function tests should be performed at weekly or biweekly intervals until the response to ABSORICA has been established [see Warnings and Precautions (5.10)].

Glucose
Some patients receiving isotretinoin have experienced problems in the control of their blood sugar. In addition, new cases of diabetes have been diagnosed during isotretinoin therapy, although no causal relationship has been established.

CPK
Some patients undergoing vigorous physical activity while on isotretinoin therapy have experienced elevated CPK levels; however, the clinical significance is unknown. There have been rare postmarketing reports of rhabdomyolysis, some associated with strenuous physical activity. In an

isotretinoin clinical trial of 924 patients, marked elevations in CPK (≥350 U/L) were observed in approximately 24% of patients. In another clinical trial of 217 pediatric patients (12 – 17 years) elevations in CPK were observed in 12% of patients, including those undergoing strenuous physical activity in association with reported musculoskeletal adverse events such as back pain, arthralgia, limb injury, or muscle sprain. In these patients, approximately half of the CPK elevations returned to normal within 2 weeks and half returned to normal within 4 weeks. No cases of rhabdomyolysis were reported in this clinical trial.

6 ADVERSE REACTIONS

The following adverse reactions with ABSORICA or other isotretinoin products are described in more detail in other sections of the labeling:

- Embryofetal Toxicity [see Warnings and Precautions (5.1)]
- Psychiatric Disorders [see Warnings and Precautions (5.4)]
- Pseudotumor Cerebri [see Warnings and Precautions (5.5)]
- Serious Skin Reactions [see Warnings and Precautions (5.6)]
- Pancreatitis [see Warnings and Precautions (5.7)]
- Lipid Abnormalities [see Warnings and Precautions (5.8)]
- Hearing Impairment [see Warnings and Precautions (5.9)]
- Hepatotoxicity [see Warnings and Precautions (5.10)]
- Inflammatory Bowel Disease [see Warnings and Precautions (5.11)]
- Skeletal Abnormalities [see Warnings and Precautions (5.12)]
- Ocular Abnormalities [see Warnings and Precautions (5.13)]
- Hypersensitivity [see Warnings and Precautions (5.14)]

6.1 Clinical Trials Experience

Because clinical trials are conducted under widely varying conditions, adverse reaction rates observed in the clinical trials of ABSORICA cannot be directly compared to rates in clinical trials of other drugs and may not reflect the rates observed in practice.

The adverse reactions listed below reflect both clinical experience with ABSORICA, and consider other adverse reactions that are known from clinical trials and the post-marketing surveillance with oral isotretinoin. The relationship of some of these events to isotretinoin therapy is unknown. Many of the side effects and adverse events seen in patients receiving isotretinoin are similar to those described in patients taking very high doses of vitamin A (dryness of the skin and mucous membranes, e.g., of the lips, nasal passage, and eyes).

Dose Relationship

Cheilitis and hypertriglyceridemia are adverse reactions that are usually dose related. Most adverse reactions reported in clinical trials with isotretinoin were reversible when therapy was discontinued; however, some persisted after cessation of therapy.

Body as a Whole

The following adverse reactions have been reported in a clinical trial conducted with ABSORICA and a generic product of Accutane® (isotretinoin): fatigue, irritability, pain. In addition to the above adverse reactions, the following adverse reactions have been reported with isotretinoin: allergic reactions, including vasculitis, systemic hypersensitivity, edema, lymphadenopathy, weight loss.

Cardiovascular

The following adverse reactions have been reported with isotretinoin: vascular thrombotic disease, stroke, palpitation, tachycardia.

Endocrine/Metabolism and Nutritional

The following adverse reactions have been reported in a clinical trial conducted with ABSORICA and a generic product of Accutane® (isotretinoin): decreased appetite, weight fluctuation, hyperlipidaemia. In addition to the above adverse reactions, the following adverse reactions have been reported with isotretinoin: hypertriglyceridemia, alterations in blood sugar.

Gastrointestinal

The following adverse reactions have been reported in a clinical trial conducted with ABSORICA and a generic product of Accutane® (isotretinoin): lip dry, chapped lips, cheilitis, nausea, constipation, diarrhea, abdominal pain, vomiting. In addition to the above adverse reactions, the following adverse reactions have been reported with isotretinoin: inflammatory bowel disease, hepatitis, pancreatitis, bleeding and inflammation of the gums, colitis, esophagitis/esophageal ulceration, ileitis, and other nonspecific gastrointestinal symptoms.

Hematologic

The following adverse reactions have been reported with isotretinoin: allergic reactions, anemia, thrombocytopenia, neutropenia, rare reports of agranulocytosis.

Infections and infestations

The following adverse reactions have been reported in a clinical trial conducted with ABSORICA and a generic product of Accutane® (isotretinoin): nasopharyngitis, hordeolum, upper respiratory tract infection. In addition to the above adverse reactions, the following adverse reaction has been reported with isotretinoin: infections (including disseminated herpes simplex).

Laboratory Abnormalities

The following changes in laboratory tests have been noted in a clinical trial conducted with ABSORICA and a generic product of Accutane® (isotretinoin): blood creatine phosphokinase (CPK) increased, blood triglycerides increased, alanine aminotransferase (SGPT) increased, aspartate aminotransferase (SGOT) increased, gamma-glutamyltransferase (GGTP) increased, blood cholesterol increased, low density lipoprotein (LDL) increased, white blood cell count decreased, blood alkaline phosphatase increased, blood bilirubin increased, blood glucose increased, high density lipoprotein (HDL) decreased, bone mineral density decreased. In addition to the above adverse reactions, the following adverse reactions have been reported with isotretinoin: increased LDH, elevation of fasting blood sugar, hyperuricemia, decreases in red blood cell parameters, decreases in white blood cell counts (including severe neutropenia and rare reports of agranulocytosis), elevated sedimentation rates, elevated platelet counts, thrombocytopenia, white cells in the urine, proteinuria, microscopic or gross hematuria.

Musculoskeletal and Connective Tissue

The following adverse reactions have been reported in a clinical trial conducted with ABSORICA and a generic product of Accutane® (isotretinoin): decreases in bone mineral density, musculoskeletal symptoms (sometimes severe) including back pain, athralgia, musculoskeletal discomfort, musculoskeletal pain, neck pain, pain in extremity, myalgia, musculoskeletal stiffness [see Warnings and Precautions (5.12)]. In addition to the above adverse reactions, the following adverse reactions have been reported with isotretinoin: skeletal hyperostosis, calcification of tendons and ligaments, premature epiphyseal closure, tendonitis, arthritis, transient pain in the chest, and rare reports of rhabdomyolysis.

Neurological

The following adverse reactions have been reported in a clinical trial conducted with ABSORICA and a generic product of Accutane® (isotretinoin): headache, syncope. In addition to the above adverse reactions, other adverse reactions reported with isotretinoin include: pseudotumor cerebri, dizziness, drowsiness, lethargy, malaise, nervousness, paresthesias, seizures, stroke, weakness.

Psychiatric

The following adverse reactions have been reported in clinical trials conducted with ABSORICA and a generic product of Accutane® (isotretinoin): suicidal ideation, insomnia, anxiety, depression, irritability, panic attack, anger, euphoria, violent behaviors, emotional instability. In addition to the above adverse reactions, the following adverse reactions have been reported with isotretinoin: suicide attempts, suicide, aggression, psychosis and hallucination auditory. Of the patients reporting depression, some reported that the depression subsided with discontinuation of therapy and recurred with reinstitution of therapy.

Reproductive System

The following adverse reaction has been reported with isotretinoin: abnormal menses.

Respiratory

The following adverse reactions have been reported in a clinical trial conducted with ABSORICA and a generic product of Accutane® (isotretinoin): epistaxis, nasal dryness. In addition to the above adverse reactions, the following adverse reactions have been reported with isotretinoin: bronchospasms (with or without a history of asthma), respiratory infection, voice alteration.

Skin and Subcutaneous Tissue

The following adverse reactions have been reported in a clinical trial conducted with ABSORICA and a generic product of Accutane® (isotretinoin): dry skin, dermatitis, eczema, rash, dermatitis contact, alopecia, pruritus, sunburn, erythema. In addition to the above adverse reactions, the following adverse reactions have been reported with isotretinoin: acne fulminans, alopecia (which in some cases persists), bruising, dry nose, eruptive xanthomas, erythema multiforme, flushing, fragility of skin, hair abnormalities, hirsutism, hyperpigmentation and hypopigmentation, nail dystrophy, paronychia, peeling of palms and soles, photoallergic/photosensitizing reactions, pruritus, pyogenic granuloma, rash (including facial erythema, seborrhea, and eczema), Stevens-Johnson syndrome, sunburn susceptibility increased, sweating, toxic epidermal necrolysis, urticaria, vasculitis (including Wegener's granulomatosis), abnormal wound healing (delayed healing or exuberant granulation tissue with crusting).

Special Senses

Hearing: The following adverse reactions have been reported with isotretinoin: tinnitus and hearing impairment.
Ocular: The following adverse reactions have been reported in clinical trials conducted with ABSORICA and a generic product of Accutane® (isotretinoin): dry eye, visual acuity reduced, vision blurred, eye pruritis, eye irritation, asthenopia, decreased night vision, ocular hyperemia, increased lacrimation, and conjunctivitis. In addition to the above adverse reactions, the following adverse reactions have been reported with isotretinoin: corneal opacities, decreased night vision which may persist, cataracts, color vision disorder, conjunctivitis, eyelid inflammation, keratitis, optic neuritis, photobia, visual disturbances.

Renal and Urinary

The following adverse reactions have been reported in clinical trials conducted with isotretinoin: glomerulonephritis, nonspecific urogenital findings.

7 DRUG INTERACTIONS

7.1 Vitamin A

ABSORICA is closely related to vitamin A. Therefore, the use of both vitamin A and ABSORICA at the same time may lead to vitamin A side effects. Patients should be advised against taking vitamin supplements containing Vitamin A to avoid additive toxic effects.

7.2 Tetracyclines

Concomitant treatment with ABSORICA and tetracyclines should be avoided because isotretinoin use has been associated with a number of cases of pseudotumor cerebri (benign intracranial hypertension), some of which involved concomitant use of tetracyclines.

7.3 Phenytoin

Isotretinoin has not been shown to alter the pharmacokinetics of phenytoin in a trial in seven healthy volunteers. These results are consistent with the in vitro finding that neither isotretinoin nor its metabolites induce or inhibit the activity of the CYP2C9 human hepatic P450 enzyme. Phenytoin is known to cause osteomalacia. No formal clinical trials have been conducted to assess if there is an interactive effect on bone loss between phenytoin and isotretinoin. Therefore, caution should be exercised when using these drugs together.

7.4 St. John's Wort

Isotretinoin use is associated with depression in some patients. Patients should be prospectively cautioned not to self-medicate with the herbal supplement St. John's Wort because a possible interaction has been suggested with hormonal contraceptives based on reports of breakthrough bleeding on oral contraceptives shortly after starting St. John's Wort. Pregnancies have been reported by users of combined hormonal contraceptives who also used some form of St. John's Wort.

7.5 Systemic Corticosteroids

Systemic corticosteroids are known to cause osteoporosis. No formal clinical trials have been conducted to assess if there is an interactive effect on bone loss between systemic corticosteroids and isotretinoin. Therefore, caution should be exercised when using these drugs together.

7.6 Norethindrone/ethinyl estradiol

In a trial of 31 premenopausal female patients with severe recalcitrant nodular acne receiving Norethindrone/ethinyl estradiol as an oral contraceptive agent, isotretinoin at the recommended dose of 1 mg/kg/day, did not induce clinically relevant changes in the pharmacokinetics of ethinyl estradiol and norethindrone and in the serum levels of progesterone, follicle-stimulating hormone (FSH) and luteinizing hormone (LH). Prescribers are advised to consult the package insert of medication administered concomitantly with hormonal contraceptives, since some medications may decrease the effectiveness of these birth control products.

8 USE IN SPECIFIC POPULATIONS

8.1 Pregnancy

Pregnancy Category X [see Contraindications (4) and Warnings and Precautions (5.1)].

Risk Summary

ABSORICA is contraindicated during pregnancy because isotretinoin can cause can cause fetal harm when administered to a pregnant woman. There is an increased risk of major congenital malformations, spontaneous abortions, and premature births following isotretinoin exposure during pregnancy in humans. If this drug is used during pregnancy, or if the patient becomes pregnant while taking the drug, the patient should be apprised of the potential hazard to a fetus.

Clinical Considerations

If pregnancy does occur during treatment of a female patient who is taking ABSORICA, ABSORICA must be discontinued immediately and she should be referred to an obstetrician-gynecologist experienced in reproductive toxicity for further evaluation and counseling.

Human Data

Major congenital malformations that have been documented following isotretinoin exposure include malformations of the face, eyes, ears, skull, central nervous system, cardiovascular system, and thymus and parathyroid glands. External malformations include: skull; ear (including anotia, micropinna, small or absent external auditory canals); eye (including microphthalmia); facial dysmorphia and cleft palate. Internal abnormalities include: CNS (including cerebral and cerebellar malformations, hydrocephalus, microcephaly, cranial nerve deficit); cardiovascular; thymus gland; parathyroid hormone deficiency. In some cases death has occurred as a result of the malformations.

Isotretinoin is found in the semen of male patients taking isotretinoin, but the amount delivered to a female partner would be about one million times lower than an oral dose of 40 mg. While the no-effect limit for isotretinoin induced embryopathy is unknown and 20 years of post-marketing reports include four reports with isolated defects compatible with features of retinoid exposed fetuses, two of these reports were incomplete and two had other possible explanations for the defects observed.

Cases of IQ scores less than 85 with or without other abnormalities have been reported. An increased risk of spontaneous abortion and premature births have been documented with isotretinoin exposure during pregnancy.

8.3 Nursing Mothers
It is not known whether this drug is present in human milk. Because many drugs are present in human milk and because of the potential for serious adverse reactions in nursing infants from ABSORICA, a decision should be made whether to discontinue nursing or to discontinue the drug, taking into account the importance of the drug to the mother.

8.4 Pediatric Use
The use of ABSORICA in pediatric patients less than 12 years of age has not been studied. The use of ABSORICA for the treatment of severe recalcitrant nodular acne in pediatric patients ages 12 to 17 years should be given careful consideration, especially for those patients where a known metabolic or structural bone disease exists [see Warnings and Precautions (5.12)]. Use of ABSORICA in this age group for severe recalcitrant nodular acne is supported by evidence from a clinical trial of ABSORICA compared to a generic product of Accutane® (isotretinoin) in 397 pediatric patients (12 to 17 years). Results from this trial demonstrated that both ABSORICA and the other isotretinoin drug product, at a dose of 1 mg/kg/day given in two divided doses, was effective in treating severe recalcitrant nodular acne in pediatric patients.

In trials with isotretinoin, adverse reactions reported in pediatric patients were similar to those described in adults except for the increased incidence of back pain and arthralgia (both of which were sometimes severe) and myalgia in pediatric patients. In a trial of pediatric patients treated with isotretinoin, approximately 29% (104/358) developed back pain. Back pain was severe in 13.5% (14/104) of the cases and occurred at a higher frequency in female patients than male patients. Arthralgias were experienced in 22% (79/358) of pediatric patients. Arthralgias were severe in 7.6% (6/79) of patients. Appropriate evaluation of the musculoskeletal system should be done in patients who present with these symptoms during or after a course of ABSORICA. Consideration should be given to discontinuation of ABSORICA if any significant abnormality is found. The effect on bone mineral density (BMD) of a 20-week course of therapy with ABSORICA or a generic product of Accutane® (isotretinoin) was evaluated in a double-blind, randomized clinical trial involving 396 adolescents with severe recalcitrant nodular acne (mean age 15.4, range 12-17, 80% males). Following 20 weeks of treatment, there were no statistically significant differences between the treatment groups. The mean changes in BMD from baseline for the overall trial population were 1.8% for lumbar spine, -0.1% for total hip and -0.3% for femoral neck. Mean BMD Z-scores declined from baseline at each of these sites (-0.053, -0.109 and -0.104 respectively). Out of 306 adolescents, 27 (8.8%) had clinically significant BMD declines defined as ≥4% lumbar spine or total hip, or ≥5% femoral neck, including 2 subjects for lumbar spine, 17 for total hip and 20 for femoral neck. Repeat DXA scans within 2-3 months after the post treatment scan showed no recovery of BMD. Longer-term follow-up at 4-11 months showed that 3 out of 7 patients had total hip and femoral neck BMD below pre-treatment baseline, and 2 others did not show the increase in BMD above baseline expected in this adolescent population. The significance of these changes in regard to long-term bone health and future fracture risk is unknown [see Warnings and Precautions (5.12)].

In an open-label clinical trial (N=217) of a single course of therapy with isotretinoin for adolescents with severe recalcitrant nodular acne, bone density measurements at several skeletal sites were not significantly decreased (lumbar spine change >-4% and total hip change >-5%) or were increased in the majority of patients. One patient had a decrease in lumbar spine bone mineral density >4% based on unadjusted data. Sixteen (7.9%) patients had decreases in lumbar spine bone mineral density >4%, and all the other patients (92%) did not have significant decreases or had increases (adjusted for body mass index). Nine patients (4.5%) had a decrease in total hip bone mineral density >5% based on unadjusted data. Twenty-one (10.6%) patients had decreases in total hip bone mineral density >5%, and all the

other patients (89%) did not have significant decreases or had increases (adjusted for body mass index). Follow-up trials performed in 8 of the patients with decreased bone mineral density for up to 11 months thereafter demonstrated increasing bone density in 5 patients at the lumbar spine, while the other 3 patients had lumbar spine bone density measurements below baseline values. Total hip bone mineral densities remained below baseline (range −1.6% to −7.6%) in 5 of 8 patients (62.5%).

In a separate open-label extension trial of 10 patients, ages 13 to 18 years, who started a second course of isotretinoin 4 months after the first course, two patients showed a decrease in mean lumbar spine bone mineral density up to 3.25%.

There are spontaneous literature reports of premature epiphyseal closure in acne patients receiving recommended doses of isotretinoin. The effect of multiple courses of isotretinoin on epiphyseal closure is unknown. In a 20-week clinical trial that included 289 adolescents who had hand radiographs taken to assess bone age, a total of 9 patients had bone age changes that were clinically significant and for which a drug-related effect cannot be excluded [see Warnings and Precautions (5.12)].

8.5 Geriatric Use
Clinical trials of ABSORICA did not include sufficient numbers of subjects aged 65 years and over to determine whether they respond differently from younger subjects. Although reported clinical experience has not identified differences in responses between elderly and younger patients, effects of aging might be expected to increase some risks associated with ABSORICA therapy.

8.6 Females of Childbearing Potential
All females of childbearing potential must comply with the iPLEDGE program requirements [see Warnings and Precautions (5.2)].

Pregnancy Testing
ABSORICA must only be prescribed to female patients who are known not to be pregnant as confirmed by a negative CLIA-certified laboratory conducted pregnancy test. Female patients of childbearing potential must have two negative urine or serum pregnancy tests with a sensitivity of at least 25 mIU/mL before receiving the initial ABSORICA prescription. The first test (a screening test) is obtained by the prescriber when the decision is made to pursue qualification of the patient for ABSORICA. The second pregnancy test (a confirmation test) must be done in a CLIA-certified laboratory. The interval between the two tests must be at least 19 days.

• For patients with regular menstrual cycles, perform the second pregnancy test during the first 5 days of the menstrual period immediately preceding the beginning of ABSORICA therapy and after the patient has used 2 forms of contraception for 1 month.

• For patients with amenorrhea, irregular cycles, or using a contraceptive method that precludes withdrawal bleeding, perform the second pregnancy test immediately preceding the beginning of ABSORICA therapy and after the patient has used 2 forms of contraception for 1 month.

Each month of continued ABSORICA therapy, patients must have a negative result from a urine or serum pregnancy test. A pregnancy test must be repeated each month, in a CLIA-certified laboratory, prior to the female patient receiving each prescription. A pregnancy test must also be completed at the end of the entire course of isotretinoin therapy and 1 month after the discontinuation of isotretinoin.

Contraception
Females of childbearing potential must use 2 forms of effective contraception simultaneously, at least 1 of which must be a primary form, unless the patient commits to continuous abstinence from heterosexual contact, or the patient has undergone a hysterectomy or bilateral oophorectomy, or has been medically confirmed to be post-menopausal. Patients must use 2 forms of effective contraception for at least 1 month prior to initiation of ABSORICA therapy, during ABSORICA therapy, and for 1 month after discontinuing ABSORICA therapy. Micro-dosed progesterone preparations ("minipills") that do not contain an estrogen are an inadequate method of contraception during isotretinoin therapy [see Warnings and Precautions (5.3)].

Effective forms of contraception include both primary and secondary forms of contraception:

Primary forms	Secondary forms
• Tubal sterilization	Barrier:
• Partner's vasectomy	• male latex condom with or
• Intrauterine device	without spermicide
• Hormonal (combination	• diaphragm with
oral contraceptives,	spermicide
transdermal patch,	• cervical cap with
injectables, implantables,	spermicide
or vaginal ring)	Other:
	• Vaginal sponge (contains
	spermicide)

Any birth control method can fail. There have been reports of pregnancy from female patients who have used combination oral contraceptives, as well as transdermal patch/ injectable/ implantable/ vaginal ring hormonal birth control products; these pregnancies occurred while taking isotretinoin. These reports are more frequent for female patients who use only a single method of contraception. Therefore, it is critically important for female patients of childbearing potential use 2 effective forms of contraception simultaneously.

Using two forms of contraception simultaneously substantially reduces the chances that a female will become pregnant over the risk of pregnancy with either form alone. A drug interaction that decreases effectiveness of hormonal contraceptives has not been entirely ruled out for isotretinoin. Although hormonal contraceptives are highly effective, prescribers are advised to consult the package insert of any medication administered concomitantly with hormonal contraceptives, since some medications may decrease the effectiveness of these birth control products.

Patients should be prospectively cautioned not to self-medicate with the herbal supplement St. John's Wort because a possible interaction has been suggested with hormonal contraceptives based on reports of breakthrough bleeding on oral contraceptives shortly after starting St. John's Wort. Pregnancies have been reported by users of combined hormonal contraceptives who also used some form of St. John's Wort [see Drug Interactions (7.4)].

If the patient has unprotected heterosexual intercourse at any time 1 month before, during, or 1 month after therapy, she must:

a. Stop taking ABSORICA immediately, if on therapy
b. Have a pregnancy test at least 19 days after the last act of unprotected heterosexual intercourse
c. Start using 2 forms of effective contraception simultaneously again for 1 month before resuming ABSORICA therapy
d. Have a second pregnancy test after using 2 forms of effective contraception for 1 month as described above depending on whether she has regular menses or not.

If a pregnancy does occur during ABSORICA treatment, ABSORICA must be discontinued immediately. The patient should be referred to an Obstetrician-Gynecologist experienced in reproductive toxicity for further evaluation and counseling. Any suspected fetal exposure during or 1 month after ABSORICA therapy must be reported immediately to the FDA via the MedWatch number 1-800-FDA-1088 and also to the iPLEDGE pregnancy registry at 1-866-495-0654 or via the internet (www.ipledgeprogram.com) [see Warnings and Precautions (5.2)].

10 OVERDOSAGE

In humans, overdosage has been associated with vomiting, facial flushing, cheilosis, abdominal pain, headache, dizziness, and ataxia. These symptoms quickly resolve without apparent residual effects.

ABSORICA causes serious birth defects at any dosage (see Boxed CONTRAINDICATIONS AND WARNINGS). Female patients of childbearing potential who present with ABSORICA overdose must be evaluated for pregnancy. Patients who are pregnant should receive counseling about the risks to the fetus, as described in the Boxed CONTRAINDICATIONS AND WARNINGS. Non-pregnant patients must be warned to avoid pregnancy for at least one month and receive contraceptive counseling as described in Warnings and Precautions (5). Educational materials for such patients can be obtained by calling the manufacturer. Because an overdose would be expected to result in higher levels of isotretinoin in semen than found during a normal treatment course, male patients should use a condom, or avoid reproductive sexual activity with a female patient who is or might become pregnant, for 1 month after the overdose. All patients with ABSORICA overdose should not donate blood for at least 1 month.

11 DESCRIPTION

ABSORICA (isotretinoin) Capsules contain 10 mg, 20 mg, 25 mg, 30 mg, 35 mg or 40 mg of isotretinoin (a retinoid) in hard gelatin capsules for oral administration. In addition to the active ingredient, isotretinoin, each capsule contains the following inactive ingredients: propyl gallate, sorbitan monooleate, soybean oil and stearoyl polyoxylglycerides. The gelatin capsules contain the following dye systems:

• 10 mg – iron oxide (yellow) and titanium dioxide;
• 20 mg – iron oxide (red), and titanium dioxide;
• 25 mg – FD&C Blue #1, FD&C Yellow #5, FD&C Yellow #6 and titanium dioxide;
• 30 mg – iron oxide (black, red and yellow) and titanium dioxide;
• 35 mg – FD&C Blue #2, iron oxide (black, red and yellow) and titanium dioxide;
• 40 mg – iron oxide (black, red and yellow) and titanium dioxide.

Chemically, isotretinoin is 13-*cis*-retinoic acid and is related to both retinoic acid and retinol (vitamin A). It is a yellow to orange crystalline powder with a molecular weight of 300.44. It is practically insoluble in water, soluble in chloroform and sparingly soluble in alcohol and in isopropyl alcohol. The structural formula is:

Meets USP Dissolution Test 3

12 CLINICAL PHARMACOLOGY
12.1 Mechanism of Action
ABSORICA is a retinoid, which when administered in pharmacologic dosages of 0.5 to 1 mg/kg/day, inhibits sebaceous gland function and keratinization. Clinical improvement in nodular acne patients occurs in association with a reduction in sebum secretion. The decrease in sebum secretion is temporary and is related to the dose and duration of treatment with isotretinoin and reflects a reduction in sebaceous gland size and an inhibition of sebaceous gland differentiation. The exact mechanism of action of ABSORICA is unknown.
12.2 Pharmacodynamics
The pharmacodynamics of ABSORICA are unknown.
12.3 Pharmacokinetics
Absorption
Due to its high lipophilicity, oral absorption of isotretinoin is enhanced when given with a high-fat meal. ABSORICA is bioequivalent to Accutane® (isotretinoin) capsule when both drugs are taken with a high-fat meal. ABSORICA is more bioavailable than Accutane® (isotretinoin) capsules when both drugs are taken fasted; the AUC_{0-t} of ABSORICA is approximately 83% greater than that of Accutane®. ABSORICA is therefore not interchangeable with generic products of Accutane®.

A single dose two-way crossover pharmacokinetic trial was conducted in 14 healthy adult male subjects comparing ABSORICA 40 mg (1 × 40 mg capsules), dosed under fasted and fed conditions. Under fed conditions after a high-fat meal, it was observed that the mean AUC_{0-t} and C_{max} were approximately 50% and 26% higher, than that observed under fasting conditions (Table 2). The observed elimination half-life ($T_{1/2}$) was slightly lower in the fed state versus fasted. The time to peak concentration (T_{max}) increased with food and this may be related to a longer absorption phase.

Table 2: Pharmacokinetic parameters of ABSORICA mean (%CV) following administration of 40 mg strength, N=14

ABSORICA¶ (1 × 40 mg capsules)	AUC_{0-t} (ng × hr/mL)	C_{max} (ng/mL)	T_{max} (hr)	$T_{1/2}$ (hr)
Fed	6095 (26 %)	395 (39 %)	6.4 (47 %)	22 (25 %)
Fasted	4055 (20 %)	314 (26 %)	2.9 (34 %)	24 (28 %)

Published clinical literature has shown that there is no difference in the pharmacokinetics of isotretinoin between patients with nodular acne and healthy subjects with normal skin.

Distribution
Isotretinoin is more than 99.9% bound to plasma proteins, primarily albumin.

Metabolism
Following oral administration of isotretinoin, at least three metabolites have been identified in human plasma: 4-*oxo*-isotretinoin, retinoic acid (tretinoin), and 4-*oxo*-retinoic acid (4-*oxo*-tretinoin). Retinoic acid and 13-cis-retinoic acid are geometric isomers and show reversible interconversion. The administration of one isomer will give rise to the other. Isotretinoin is also irreversibly oxidized to 4-*oxo*-isotretinoin, which forms its geometric isomer 4-*oxo*-tretinoin.

After a single 40 mg oral dose of ABSORICA to 57 healthy adult subjects, concurrent administration of food increased the extent of formation of all metabolites in plasma when compared to the extent of formation under fasted conditions.

All of these metabolites possess retinoid activity that is in some in vitro models more than that of the parent isotretinoin. However, the clinical significance of these models is unknown.

In vitro studies indicate that the primary P450 isoforms involved in isotretinoin metabolism are 2C8, 2C9, 3A4, and 2B6. Isotretinoin and its metabolites are further metabolized into conjugates, which are then excreted in urine and feces.

Elimination
Following oral administration of an 80 mg dose of 14C-isotretinoin as a liquid suspension, 14C-activity in blood declined with a half-life of 90 hours. The metabolites of isotretinoin and any conjugates are ultimately excreted in the feces and urine in relatively equal amounts (total of 65% to 83%).

After a single 40 mg (2 × 20 mg) oral dose of ABSORICA to 57 healthy adult subjects under fed conditions, the mean ± SD elimination half-lives ($T_{1/2}$) of isotretinoin and 4-*oxo*-isotretinoin under fed states were 18 hours and 38 hours, respectively.

Special Patient Populations
The pharmacokinetics of isotretinoin were evaluated after single and multiple doses in 38 pediatric patients (12 to 15 years) and 19 adult patients (≥18 years) who received isotretinoin for the treatment of severe recalcitrant nodular acne. In both age groups, 4-*oxo*-isotretinoin was the major metabolite; tretinoin and 4-*oxo*-tretinoin were also observed. There were no statistically significant differences in the pharmacokinetics of isotretinoin between pediatric and adult patients.

13 NONCLINICAL TOXICOLOGY
13.1 Carcinogenesis, Mutagenesis and Impairment of Fertility
In male and female Fischer 344 rats given oral isotretinoin at dosages of 8 or 32 mg/kg/day (1.3 to 5.3 times the recommended clinical dose of 1 mg/kg/day, respectively, after normalization for total body surface area) for greater than 18 months, there was a dose-related increased incidence of pheochromocytoma relative to controls. The incidence of adrenal medullary hyperplasia was also increased at the higher dosage in both sexes. The relatively high level of spontaneous pheochromocytomas occurring in the male Fischer 344 rat makes it an equivocal model for study of this tumor; therefore, the relevance of this tumor to the human population is uncertain.

The Ames test was conducted with isotretinoin in two laboratories. The results of the tests in one laboratory were negative while in the second laboratory a weakly positive response (less than 1.6 × background) was noted in *S. typhimurium* TA100 when the assay was conducted with metabolic activation. No dose response effect was seen and all other strains were negative. Additionally, other tests designed to assess genotoxicity (Chinese hamster cell assay, mouse micronucleus test, *S. cerevisiae* D7 assay, in vitro clastogenesis assay with human-derived lymphocytes, and unscheduled DNA synthesis assay) were all negative.

In rats, no adverse effects on gonadal function, fertility, conception rate, gestation or parturition were observed at oral dosages of isotretinoin of 2, 8, or 32 mg/kg/day (0.3, 1.3, or 5.3 times the recommended clinical dose of 1 mg/kg/day, respectively, after normalization for total body surface area). In dogs, testicular atrophy was noted after treatment with oral isotretinoin for approximately 30 weeks at dosages of 20 or 60 mg/kg/day (10 or 30 times the recommended clinical dose of 1 mg/kg/day, respectively, after normalization for total body surface area). In general, there was microscopic evidence for appreciable depression of spermatogenesis but some sperm were observed in all testes examined and in no instance were completely atrophic tubules seen.

In trials of 66 men, 30 of whom were patients with nodular acne under treatment with oral isotretinoin, no significant changes were noted in the count or motility of spermatozoa in the ejaculate. In a study of 50 men (ages 17 to 32 years) receiving isotretinoin therapy for nodular acne, no significant effects were seen on ejaculate volume, sperm count, total sperm motility, morphology or seminal plasma fructose.

13.2 Animal Toxicology
In rats given 8 or 32 mg/kg/day of isotretinoin (1.3 to 5.3 times the recommended clinical dose of 1 mg/kg/day after normalization for total body surface area) for 18 months or longer, the incidences of focal calcification, fibrosis and inflammation of the myocardium, calcification of coronary, pulmonary and mesenteric arteries, and metastatic calcification of the gastric mucosa were greater than in control rats of similar age. Focal endocardial and myocardial calcifications associated with calcification of the coronary arteries were observed in two dogs after approximately 6 to 7 months of treatment with isotretinoin at a dosage of 60 to 120 mg/kg/day (30 to 60 times the recommended clinical dose of 1 mg/kg/day, respectively, after normalization for total body surface area).

14 CLINICAL STUDIES
A double-blind, randomized, parallel group trial (Study 1) was conducted in patients with severe recalcitrant nodular acne to evaluate the efficacy and safety of ABSORICA compared to a generic product of Accutane® under fed conditions. Enrolled patients had a weight of 40 to 110 kg with at least 10 nodular lesions on the face and/or trunk. A total of 925 patients were randomized 1:1 to receive ABSORICA or a generic product of Accutane® (isotretinoin). Study patients ranged from 12 to 54 years of age, were approximately 60% male, 40% female, and were 87% White, 4% Black, 6% Asian, and 3% Other. Patients were treated an initial dose of 0.5 mg/kg/day in two divided doses for the first 4 weeks followed by 1 mg/kg/day in two divided doses for the following 16 weeks.

Change from Baseline to Week 20 in total nodular lesion count and proportion of patients with at least a 90% reduction in total nodular lesion count from Baseline to Week 20 are presented in Table 3. Total nodular lesion counts by visit are presented in Figure 1.

Table 3: Efficacy Results at Week 20 (Study 1)

	ABSORICA¶ N=464	Isotretinoin* N=461
Nodular Lesions		
Mean Baseline Count	18.4	17.7
Mean Reduction	-15.68	-15.62
Patients Achieving 90% Reduction	324 (70%)	344 (75%)

*A generic product of Accutane®

Figure 1: Total Nodular (Facial and Truncal) Lesion Count by Visit in Study 1

* A generic product of Accutane®

16 HOW SUPPLIED/STORAGE AND HANDLING
ABSORICA (isotretinoin) Capsules are supplied as follows:
- **10 mg:** Dark yellow, opaque, capsule imprinted with black ink "G 240" on cap and "10" on the body
  Box of 30 capsules (3 × 10 Prescription Packs): NDC 10631-115-31
- **20 mg:** Red, opaque, capsule imprinted with black ink "G 241" on cap and "20" on the body
  Box of 30 capsules (3 × 10 Prescription Packs): NDC 10631-116-31
- **25 mg:** Green, opaque, capsule imprinted with white ink "G 342" on cap and "25" on the body
  Box of 30 capsules (3 × 10 Prescription Packs): NDC 10631-133-31
- **30 mg:** Brown, opaque, capsule imprinted with white ink "G 242" on cap and "30" on the body
  Box of 30 capsules (3 × 10 Prescription Packs): NDC 10631-117-31
- **35 mg:** Dark blue, opaque, capsule imprinted with white ink "G 343" on cap and "35" on the body
  Box of 30 capsules (3 × 10 Prescription Packs): NDC 10631-134-31
- **40 mg:** Brown and red, capsule imprinted with white ink "G 325" on cap and "40" on the body
  Box of 30 capsules (3 × 10 Prescription Packs): NDC 10631-118-31

Storage and Handling
Store at 20° C - 25° C (68° F - 77° F), excursion permitted between 15° C - 30° C (59° F - 86° F) [see USP controlled room temperature]. Protect from light.

17 PATIENT COUNSELING INFORMATION
See FDA-Approved Patient Labeling (Medication Guide) Advise the patient that ABSORICA is only available through a restricted program called iPLEDGE.
- As a component of the iPLEDGE program, prescribers must instruct patients to read the Medication Guide, the iPLEDGE program patient educational booklets, and watch the DVD with the following videos — "Be Prepared, Be Protected" and "Be Aware: The Risk of Pregnancy While on Isotretinoin". The DVD includes information about contraception, the most common reasons that contraception fails, and the importance of using 2 forms of effective contraception when taking teratogenic drugs and comprehensive information about types of potential birth defects which could occur if a female patient who is pregnant takes ABSORICA at any time during pregnancy.
- Male patients and Female patients not of childbearing potential must understand the risks and benefits of ABSORICA, comply with the REMS requirements described in the booklet entitled *The iPLEDGE Program Guide to Isotretinoin for Male Patients and Female Patients Who Cannot Get Pregnant,* and sign a Patient Information/Informed Consent form.
- Female patients of childbearing potential must be instructed that they must not be pregnant when ABSORICA

therapy is initiated or plan to become pregnant while receiving ABSORICA therapy. Additionally, they must use 2 forms of effective contraception simultaneously for 1 month before starting ABSORICA, while taking ABSORICA, and for 1 month after ABSORICA has been stopped, unless they commit to continuous abstinence from heterosexual intercourse. They should also sign a Patient Information/Informed Consent form and Patient Information/Informed Consent About Birth Defects (for female patients who can get pregnant) form prior to beginning ABSORICA therapy. Female patients should be seen by their prescribers monthly and have a urine or serum pregnancy test, in a CLIA-certified laboratory, performed each month during treatment to confirm negative pregnancy status before another ABSORICA prescription is written. Additionally, a pregnancy test must be completed at the end of the entire course of ABSORICA therapy and 1 month after discontinuation of therapy.

- Advise the patient that isotretinoin is found in the semen of male patients taking isotretinoin, but the amount delivered to a female partner would be about one million times lower than an oral dose of 40 mg. While the no-effect limit for isotretinoin induced embryopathy is unknown, 20 years of post-marketing reports include four with isolated defects compatible with features of retinoid exposed fetuses; however two of these reports were incomplete and two had other possible explanations for the defects observed.
- Advise the patient that ABSORICA is available only from pharmacies that are certified in the iPLEDGE program, and provide them with the telephone number (1-866-495-0654) and website (www.ipledgeprogram.com) for information on how to obtain.
- Advise patients that they may be requested to participate in a survey to evaluate the effectiveness of the iPLEDGE program.
- Prescribers should be alert to the warning signs of psychiatric disorders to guide patients to receive the help they need. Therefore, prior to initiation of ABSORICA treatment, patients and family members should be asked about any history of psychiatric disorder, and at each visit during treatment patients should be assessed for symptoms of depression, mood disturbance, psychosis, or aggression to determine if further evaluation may be necessary. Inform patients that **symptoms of depression include sad mood, hopelessness, feelings of guilt, worthlessness or helplessness, loss of pleasure or interest in activities, fatigue, difficulty concentrating, change in sleep pattern, change in weight or appetite, suicidal thoughts or attempts, restlessness, irritability, acting on dangerous impulses, and persistent physical symptoms unresponsive to treatment.** Patients should stop treatment and the patient or a family member should promptly contact their prescriber if the patient develops depression, mood disturbance, psychosis, or aggression, without waiting until the next visit. Discontinuation of ABSORICA treatment may be insufficient; further evaluation may be necessary. While such monitoring may be helpful, it may not detect all patients at risk. Patients may report mental health problems or family history of psychiatric disorders. These reports should be discussed with the patient and/or the patient's family. A referral to a mental health professional may be necessary. The physician should consider whether ABSORICA therapy is appropriate in this setting; for some patients the risks may outweigh the benefits of ABSORICA therapy.
- Patients must be informed that some patients, while taking isotretinoin or soon after stopping isotretinoin, have become depressed or developed other serious mental problems. Symptoms of depression include sad, "anxious" or empty mood, irritability, acting on dangerous impulses, anger, loss of pleasure or interest in social or sports activities, sleeping too much or too little, changes in weight or appetite, school or work performance going down, or trouble concentrating. Some patients taking isotretinoin have had thoughts about hurting themselves or putting an end to their own lives (suicidal thoughts), some have tried to end their own lives, and some have ended their own lives. There were reports that some of these people did not appear depressed. There have been reports of patients on isotretinoin becoming aggressive or violent. There have also been reports of psychotic symptoms, which indicate a loss of contact with reality. Psychotic symptoms include feelings of suspiciousness toward others, strange beliefs, hearing voices or other noises without an obvious source, and seeing unusual objects or people with no explanation. No one knows if isotretinoin caused these behaviors and symptoms or if they would have happened even if the person did not take isotretinoin. If any of these behaviors or symptoms occur, the patient should stop treatment and the patient or family member should contact the prescriber promptly without waiting until the next visit [see Warnings and Precautions (5.4)]. Some people have had other signs of depression while taking isotretinoin.

- Patients must be informed that they must not share ABSORICA with anyone else because of the risk of birth defects and other serious adverse reactions.
- Patients must be informed not to donate blood during therapy and for 1 month following discontinuation of the drug because the blood might be given to a pregnant female patient whose fetus must not be exposed to ABSORICA.
- ABSORICA may be taken without regard to meals [see Dosage and Administration (2.1)]. To decrease the risk of esophageal irritation, patients should swallow the capsules with a full glass of liquid.
- Patients should be informed that inflammatory bowel disease (including regional ileitis) may occur without a prior history of intestinal disorders. In rare instances, symptoms have been reported to persist after treatment has stopped. Patients should be informed that if they experience abdominal pain, rectal bleeding or severe diarrhea, they should discontinue ABSORICA immediately.
- Patients should be informed that transient exacerbation (flare) of acne has been seen, generally during the initial period of therapy.
- Wax epilation and skin resurfacing procedures (such as dermabrasion, laser) should be avoided during ABSORICA therapy and for at least 6 months thereafter due to the possibility of scarring.
- Patients should be advised to avoid prolonged exposure to UV rays or sunlight.
- Patients should be informed that they may experience dry eye, corneal opacities, and decreased night vision. Contact lens wearers may experience decreased tolerance to contact lenses during and after therapy.
- Patients should be informed that 16% of patients treated with isotretinoin in a clinical trial developed musculoskeletal symptoms (including arthralgia) during treatment. In general, these symptoms were mild to moderate, but occasionally required discontinuation of the drug. Transient pain in the chest has been reported less frequently. In the clinical trial, these symptoms generally cleared rapidly after discontinuation of therapy, but in some cases persisted.
- There have been rare postmarketing reports of rhabdomyolysis, some associated with strenuous physical activity.
- Pediatric patients and their caregivers should be informed that approximately 17% to 29% of pediatric patients treated with isotretinoin developed back pain. In a clinical trial, back pain was severe in 13.5% of the cases and occurred at a higher frequency in female patients than male patients. Arthralgias were experienced in 22% (79/358) of pediatric patients. Arthralgias were severe in 7.6% (6/79) of patients. Appropriate evaluation of the musculoskeletal system should be done in patients who present with these symptoms during or after a course of treatment. Consideration should be given to discontinuation of isotretinoin if any significant abnormality is found.
- Neutropenia and rare cases of agranulocytosis have been reported in patients treated with isotretinoin. ABSORICA should be discontinued if clinically significant decreases in white cell counts occur.
- Patients should be advised that severe skin reactions (Stevens-Johnson syndrome and toxic epidermal necrolysis) have been reported in post marketing data in patients treated with isotretinoin. Treatment with ABSORICA should be discontinued if clinically significant skin reactions occur.
- Adolescent patients who participate in sports with repetitive impact should be informed that isotretinoin use may increase their risk of spondylolisthesis or hip growth plate injuries. There are spontaneous reports of fractures and/or delayed healing in patients while on therapy with isotretinoin or following cessation of therapy with isotretinoin while involved in these activities [see Warnings and Precautions (5.12)].

MEDICATION GUIDE
ABSORICA® (AB-SORE-I-KAH)
(Isotretinoin Capsules)

Read the Medication Guide that comes with ABSORICA before you start taking it and each time you get a prescription. There may be new information. This information does not take the place of talking with your doctor about your medical condition or your treatment.

What is the most important information I should know about ABSORICA?
- ABSORICA is used to treat a type of severe acne (nodular acne) that has not been helped by other treatments, including antibiotics.
- Because ABSORICA can cause birth defects, ABSORICA is only for patients who can understand and agree to carry out all of the instructions in the iPLEDGE program.
- ABSORICA may cause serious mental health problems.

1. Birth defects (deformed babies), loss of a baby before birth (miscarriage), death of the baby, and early (premature) births. Female patients who are pregnant or who plan to become pregnant must not take ABSORICA. **Female patients must not get pregnant:**

- for 1 month before starting ABSORICA
- while taking ABSORICA
- for 1 month after stopping ABSORICA.

If you get pregnant while taking ABSORICA, stop taking it right away and call your doctor. Doctors and patients should report all cases of pregnancy to:
- FDA MedWatch at 1-800-FDA-1088, and
- the iPLEDGE pregnancy registry at 1-866-495-0654

2. Serious mental health problems. ABSORICA may cause:
- **depression**
- **psychosis** (seeing or hearing things that are not real)
- **suicide.** Some patients taking ABSORICA have had thoughts about hurting themselves or putting an end to their own lives (suicidal thoughts). Some people tried to end their own lives. And some people have ended their own lives.

Stop ABSORICA and call your doctor right away if you or a family member notices that you have any of the following signs and symptoms of depression or psychosis:
- start to feel sad or have crying spells
- lose interest in activities you once enjoyed
- sleep too much or have trouble sleeping
- become more irritable, angry, or aggressive than usual (for example, temper outbursts, thoughts of violence)
- have a change in your appetite or body weight
- have trouble concentrating
- withdraw from your friends or family
- feel like you have no energy
- have feelings of worthlessness or guilt
- start having thoughts about hurting yourself or taking your own life (suicidal thoughts)
- start acting on dangerous impulses
- start seeing or hearing things that are not real

After stopping ABSORICA, you may also need follow-up mental health care if you had any of these symptoms.

What is ABSORICA?
ABSORICA is a medicine taken by mouth to treat the most severe form of acne (nodular acne) that cannot be cleared up by any other acne treatments, including antibiotics. ABSORICA can cause serious side effects (see **"What is the most important information I should know about ABSORICA?"**). ABSORICA can only be:
- prescribed by doctors that are registered in the iPLEDGE program
- dispensed by a pharmacy that is registered with the iPLEDGE program
- given to patients who are registered in the iPLEDGE program and agree to do everything required in the program

What is severe nodular acne?
Severe nodular acne is when many red, swollen, tender lumps form in the skin. These can be the size of pencil erasers or larger. If untreated, nodular acne can lead to permanent scars.

Who should not take ABSORICA?
- **Do not take ABSORICA if you are pregnant, plan to become pregnant, or become pregnant during ABSORICA treatment.** ABSORICA causes severe birth defects. See **"What is the most important information I should know about ABSORICA?"**
- **Do not take ABSORICA if you are allergic to anything in it.** See the end of this Medication Guide for a complete list of ingredients in ABSORICA.

What should I tell my doctor before taking ABSORICA?
Tell your doctor if you or a family member has any of the following health conditions:
- mental problems
- asthma
- liver disease
- diabetes
- heart disease
- bone loss (osteoporosis) or weak bones
- an eating problem called anorexia nervosa (where people eat too little)
- food or medicine allergies

Tell your doctor if you are pregnant or breast-feeding. ABSORICA must not be used by women who are pregnant or breast-feeding.

Tell your doctor about all of the medicines you take including prescription and non-prescription medicines, vitamins and herbal supplements. ABSORICA and certain other medicines can interact with each other, sometimes causing serious side effects. Especially tell your doctor if you take:
- **Vitamin A supplements.** Vitamin A in high doses has many of the same side effects as ABSORICA. Taking them together may increase your chance of getting side effects.
- **Tetracycline antibiotics.** Tetracycline antibiotics taken with ABSORICA can increase the chances of getting increased pressure in the brain.
- **Progestin-only birth control pills (mini-pills).** They may not work while you take ABSORICA. Ask your doctor or pharmacist if you are not sure what type you are using.
- **Dilantin (phenytoin).** This medicine taken with ABSORICA may weaken your bones.

- **Corticosteroid medicines**. These medicines taken with ABSORICA may weaken your bones.
- **St. John's Wort**. This herbal supplement may make birth control pills work less effectively.

These medicines should not be used with ABSORICA unless your doctor tells you it is okay.

Know the medicines you take. Keep a list of them to show to your doctor and pharmacist. Do not take any new medicine without talking with your doctor.

How should I take ABSORICA?

- You must take ABSORICA exactly as prescribed. You must also follow all the instructions of the iPLEDGE program. Before prescribing ABSORICA, your doctor will:
  - explain the iPLEDGE program to you
  - have you sign the Patient Information/Informed Consent form (for all patients). Female patients who can get pregnant must also sign another consent form.

You will not be prescribed ABSORICA if you cannot agree to or follow all the instructions of the iPLEDGE program.

- You will get no more than a 30-day supply of ABSORICA at a time. This is to make sure you are following the ABSORICA iPLEDGE program. You should talk with your doctor each month about side effects.
- The amount of ABSORICA you take has been specially chosen for you. It is based on your body weight, and may change during treatment.
- Take ABSORICA 2 times a day without regard to meals, unless your doctor tells you otherwise. **Swallow your ABSORICA capsules whole with a full glass of liquid. Do not chew or suck on the capsule.** ABSORICA can hurt the tube that connects your mouth to your stomach (esophagus) if it is not swallowed whole.
- If you miss a dose, just skip that dose. Do **not** take two doses at the same time.
- If you take too much ABSORICA or overdose, call your doctor or poison control center right away.
- Your acne may get worse when you first start taking ABSORICA. This should last only a short while. Talk with your doctor if this is a problem for you.
- You must return to your doctor as directed to make sure you don't have signs of serious side effects. Your doctor may do blood tests to check for serious side effects from ABSORICA. Female patients who can get pregnant will get a pregnancy test each month.
- Female patients who can get pregnant must agree to use two separate forms of effective birth control at the same time one month before, while taking, and for one month after taking ABSORICA. **You must access the iPLEDGE system to answer questions about the program requirements and to enter your two chosen forms of birth control.** To access the iPLEDGE system, go to *www.ipledgeprogram.com* or call 1-866-495-0654.

You must talk about effective birth control methods with your doctor or go for a free visit to talk about birth control with another doctor or family planning expert. Your doctor can arrange this free visit, which will be paid for by the company that makes ABSORICA.

If you have sex at any time without using two forms of effective birth control, get pregnant, or miss your expected period, stop using ABSORICA and call your doctor right away.

What should I avoid while taking ABSORICA?

- **Do not get pregnant** while taking ABSORICA and for one month after stopping ABSORICA. See **"What is the most important information I should know about ABSORICA?"**
- **Do not breast-feed** while taking ABSORICA and for one month after stopping ABSORICA. We do not know if ABSORICA can pass through your milk and harm the baby.
- **Do not give blood** while you take ABSORICA and for one month after stopping ABSORICA. If someone who is pregnant gets your donated blood, her baby may be exposed to ABSORICA and may be born with birth defects.
- **Do not take other medicines or herbal products** with ABSORICA unless you talk to your doctor. See **"What should I tell my doctor before taking ABSORICA?"**
- **Do not drive at night until you know if ABSORICA has affected your vision.** ABSORICA may decrease your ability to see in the dark.
- **Do not have cosmetic procedures to smooth your skin, including waxing, dermabrasion, or laser procedures, while you are using ABSORICA and for at least 6 months after you stop.** ABSORICA can increase your chance of scarring from these procedures. Check with your doctor for advice about when you can have cosmetic procedures.
- **Avoid sunlight and ultraviolet lights** as much as possible. Tanning machines use ultraviolet lights. ABSORICA may make your skin more sensitive to light.

Do not share ABSORICA with other people. It can cause birth defects and other serious health problems.

What are the possible side effects of ABSORICA?

- ABSORICA can cause birth defects (deformed babies), loss of a baby before birth (miscarriage), death of the baby, and early (premature) births. See **"What is the most important information I should know about ABSORICA?"**

- **ABSORICA may cause serious mental health problems.** See **"What is the most important information I should know about ABSORICA?"**
- **serious brain problems.** ABSORICA can increase the pressure in your brain. This can lead to permanent loss of eyesight and, in rare cases, death. Stop taking ABSORICA and call your doctor right away if you get any of these signs of increased brain pressure:
  - bad headache
  - blurred vision
  - dizziness
  - nausea or vomiting
  - seizures (convulsions)
  - stroke
- **skin problems.** Skin rash can occur in patients taking ABSORICA. In some patients a rash can be serious. Stop using ABSORICA and call your doctor right away if you develop conjunctivitis (red or inflamed eyes, like "pink eye"), a rash with a fever, blisters on legs, arms or face and/or sores in your mouth, throat, nose, eyes, or if your skin begins to peel.
- **stomach area (abdomen) problems.** Certain symptoms may mean that your internal organs are being damaged. These organs include the liver, pancreas, bowel (intestines), and esophagus (connection between mouth and stomach). If your organs are damaged, they may not get better even after you stop taking ABSORICA. Stop taking ABSORICA and call your doctor if you get:
  - severe stomach, chest or bowel pain
  - trouble swallowing or painful swallowing
  - new or worsening heartburn
  - diarrhea
  - rectal bleeding
  - yellowing of your skin or eyes
  - dark urine
- **bone and muscle problems.** ABSORICA may affect bones, muscles, and ligaments and cause pain in your joints or muscles. Tell your doctor if you plan hard physical activity during treatment with ABSORICA. Tell your doctor if you get:
  - back pain
  - joint pain
  - broken bone. Tell all healthcare providers that you take ABSORICA if you break a bone.

  Stop ABSORICA and call your doctor right away if you have muscle weakness. Muscle weakness with or without pain can be a sign of serious muscle damage.

  ABSORICA may stop long bone growth in teenagers who are still growing.
- **hearing problems.** Stop using ABSORICA and call your doctor if your hearing gets worse or if you have ringing in your ears. Your hearing loss may be permanent.
- **vision problems.** ABSORICA may affect your ability to see in the dark. This condition usually clears up after you stop taking ABSORICA, but it may be permanent. Other serious eye effects can occur. Stop taking ABSORICA and call your doctor right away if you have any problems with your vision or dryness of the eyes that is painful or constant. If you wear contact lenses, you may have trouble wearing them while taking ABSORICA and after treatment.
- **lipid (fats and cholesterol in blood) problems.** ABSORICA can raise the level of fats and cholesterol in your blood. This can be a serious problem. Return to your doctor for blood tests to check your lipids and to get any needed treatment. These problems usually go away when ABSORICA treatment is finished.
- **serious allergic reactions.** Stop taking ABSORICA and get emergency care right away if you develop hives, a swollen face or mouth, or have trouble breathing. Stop taking ABSORICA and call your doctor if you get a fever, rash, or red patches or bruises on your legs.
- **blood sugar problems.** ABSORICA may cause blood sugar problems including diabetes. Tell your doctor if you are very thirsty or urinate a lot.
- **decreased red and white blood cells.** Call your doctor if you have trouble breathing, faint, or feel weak.
- **The common, less serious side effects of ABSORICA** are dry skin, chapped lips, dry eyes, and dry nose that may lead to nosebleeds. Call your doctor if you get any side effect that bothers you or that does not go away.

These are not all of the possible side effects with ABSORICA. Your doctor or pharmacist can give you more detailed information.

Call your doctor for medical advice about side effects. You may report side effects to FDA at 1-800-FDA-1088.

You may also report side effects to Ranbaxy Inc., the manufacturer of ABSORICA at 1-800-406-7984.

How should I store ABSORICA?

- Store ABSORICA at room temperature, 68° to 77° F (20° to 25° C). Protect from light.
- **Keep ABSORICA and all medicines out of the reach of children.**

General Information about ABSORICA

Medicines are sometimes prescribed for conditions that are not mentioned in Medication Guides. Do not use ABSORICA for a condition for which it was not prescribed. Do not give ABSORICA to other people, even if they have the same symptoms that you have. It may harm them.

This Medication Guide summarizes the most important information about ABSORICA. If you would like more information, talk with your doctor.

You can ask your doctor or pharmacist for information about ABSORICA that is written for health care professionals. You can also call iPLEDGE program at 1-866-495-0654 or visit www.ipledgeprogram.com.

What are the ingredients in ABSORICA?

Active ingredient: Isotretinoin, USP

Inactive ingredients: Propyl gallate, sorbitan monooleate, soybean oil and stearoyl polyoxylglycerides. Gelatin capsules contain the following dye systems: 10 mg – iron oxide (yellow), potassium hydroxide, propylene glycol, shellac and titanium dioxide; 20 mg – iron oxide (red), potassium hydroxide, propylene glycol, shellac and titanium dioxide; 25 mg – FD&C Blue #1, FD&C Yellow #5, FD&C Yellow #6, povidone, propylene glycol, shellac, sodium hydroxide and titanium dioxide; 30 mg – iron oxide (black, red and yellow), potassium hydroxide, povidone, propylene glycol, shellac, sodium hydroxide and titanium dioxide; 35 mg – FD&C Blue #2, iron oxide (black, red and yellow), povidone, propylene glycol, shellac, sodium hydroxide and titanium dioxide; and 40 mg – iron oxide (black, red and yellow), potassium hydroxide, povidone, propylene glycol, shellac, sodium hydroxide and titanium dioxide.

This Medication Guide has been approved by the U.S. Food and Drug Administration.

Dilantin is a registered trademark of Warner-Lambert Company LLC.

Distributed By:

Ranbaxy Laboratories Inc.

Ranbaxy Laboratories Inc.
Jacksonville, FL 32257 USA
GK-244 Revised: August 2014

Shown in Product Identification Guide, page 312

Recordati Rare Diseases, Inc.

**100 Corporate Dr
Lebanon, NJ 08833**

(908) 437-1210

CHEMET®
(succimer)
Capsule 100 mg

℞

R_x only

DESCRIPTION

CHEMET (succimer) is an orally active, heavy metal chelating agent. The chemical name for succimer is *meso* 2, 3-dimercaptosuccinic acid (DMSA). Its empirical formula is $C_4H_6O_4S_2$ and molecular weight is 182.2. The *meso*-structural formula is:

$$\begin{array}{c} COOH \\ | \\ H-C-SH \\ | \\ H-C-SH \\ | \\ COOH \end{array}$$

Succimer is a white crystalline powder with an unpleasant, characteristic mercaptan odor and taste.

Each CHEMET opaque white capsule for oral administration, contains beads coated with 100 mg of succimer and is imprinted black with CHEMET 100. Inactive ingredients in medicated beads are: povidone, sodium starch glycolate, starch and sucrose. Inactive ingredients in capsule are: gelatin, iron oxide, titanium dioxide and other ingredients.

CLINICAL PHARMACOLOGY

Succimer is a lead chelator; it forms water soluble chelates and, consequently, increases the urinary excretion of lead.

Preclinical Toxicology

CHEMET has low acute oral toxicity, with oral median lethal doses in rodents in excess of 3.6 g/kg. In a 28-day toxicity study, dogs receiving 30 and 100 mg/kg/day had lower urinary specific gravity and an increase in renal tubular regenerative hyperplasia. No renal toxicity was noted in dogs given 50 mg/kg/day orally for 14 consecutive days. In a chronic 6-month oral toxicity study, one male dog died (out of 7) at a dose of 200 mg/kg/day attributed to associated renal toxicity. Treatment related renal tubule epithelial changes in this study were observed in dogs after chronic (6-month) exposure to 110 and 200 mg/kg/day for 17 days then to 80 and 140 mg/kg/day for the remainder of the study. These changes were dose-dependent and correlated with increased kidney weights in male and female dogs at the 10 mg/kg/day dose. Nephropathy was not observed in dogs treated at 10 mg/kg/day. Reduced platelet counts were noted in 5 of 7 dogs receiving either 80 or 140 mg/kg/day for 3 or 6 months, although group means were not statistically different from concurrent controls. Platelets had not been quantified in earlier studies. Normal megakaryocytes in the bone marrow, plus the absence of fibrin degradation products or histologic evidence for DIC, suggested an autoimmune-mediated thrombocytopenia, a finding common in dogs but not in other species. However, serum antibody tests were inconclusive. Rats dosed chronically to 500 mg/kg/day developed no evidence for nephropathy or thrombocytopenia.

Pharmacokinetics

In a study performed in healthy adult volunteers, after a single dose of ^{14}C-succimer at 16, 32, or 48 mg/kg, absorption was rapid but variable with peak blood radioactivity levels between one and two hours. On average, 49% of the radiolabeled dose was excreted: 39% in the feces, 9% in the urine and 1% as carbon dioxide from the lungs. Since fecal excretion probably represented nonabsorbed drug, most of the absorbed drug was excreted by the kidneys. The apparent elimination half-life of the radiolabeled material in the blood was about two days.

In other studies of healthy adult volunteers receiving a single oral dose of 10 mg/kg, the chemical analysis of succimer and its metabolites in the urine showed that succimer was rapidly and extensively metabolized. Approximately 25% of the administered dose was excreted in the urine with the peak blood level and urinary excretion occurring between two and four hours. Of the total amount of drug eliminated in the urine, approximately 90% was eliminated in altered form as mixed succimer-cysteine disulfides; the remaining 10% was eliminated unchanged. The majority of mixed disulfides consisted of succimer in disulfide linkages with two molecules of L-cysteine, the remaining disulfides contained one L-cysteine per succimer molecule.

Pharmacodynamics

Dose ranging studies were performed in 18 men with blood lead levels of 44-96 mcg/dL. Three groups of 6 patients received either 10.0, 6.7 or 3.3 mg/kg succimer orally every 8 hours for 5 days. After five days the mean blood levels of the three groups decreased 72.5%, 58.3% and 35.5% respectively. The mean urinary lead excretions in the initial 24 hours were 28.6, 18.6 and 12.3 times the pretreatment 24 hour urinary lead excretion. As the chelatable pool was reduced during therapy, urinary lead output decreased. A mean of 19 mg of lead was excreted during a five-day course of 30 mg/kg/day succimer. Clinical symptoms, such as headache and colic, and biochemical indices of lead toxicity also improved. Decrease in urinary excretion of d-aminolevulinic acid (ALA) and coproporphyrin paralleled the improvement in erythrocyte d-aminolevulinic acid dehydratase (ALA-D). Three control patients with lead poisoning of similar severity received CaNa$_2$EDTA intravenously at a dose of 50 mg/kg/day for five days. The mean blood lead level decreased 47.4% and the mean urinary lead excretion was 21 mg in the control patients.

Effect on Essential Minerals

In the above studies succimer had no significant effect on the urinary elimination of iron, calcium or magnesium. Zinc excretion doubled during treatment. The effect of succimer on the excretion of essential minerals was small compared to that of CaNa$_2$EDTA, which can induce more than a tenfold increase in urinary excretion of zinc and doubling of copper and iron excretion.

Efficacy

A dose ranging study was performed in 15 pediatric patients aged 2 to 7 years with blood lead levels of 30-49 mcg/dL and positive CaNa$_2$EDTA lead mobilization tests. Each group of five patients received 350, 233 or 116 mg/m^2 succimer every 8 hours for 5 days. These doses corresponded to 10, 6.7 and 3.3 mg/kg. Six control patients received 1000 mg/m^2/day CaNa$_2$EDTA intravenously for 5 days. Following therapy, the mean blood lead levels decreased 78, 63 and 42% respectively in the three groups treated with succimer. The response of the 350 mg/m^2 every 8 hours (10 mg/kg every 8 hours) group was significantly better than that of the other succimer treated groups as well as that of the control group, whose mean blood lead level fell 48%. No adverse reactions or changes in essential mineral excretion were reported in the succimer treated groups. In the CaNa$_2$EDTA treated group, the cumulative amount of urinary lead excreted was slightly but significantly greater than in the succimer group. After CaNa$_2$EDTA, the urinary excretion of copper, zinc, iron and calcium were significantly increased.

As with other chelators, both adults and pediatric patients experienced a rebound in blood lead levels after discontinuation of CHEMET. In these studies, after treatment with a dose of 350 mg/m^2 (10 mg/kg) every 8 hours for five days, the mean lead level rebounded and plateaued at 60-85% of pretreatment levels two weeks after therapy. The rebound plateau was somewhat higher with lower doses of succimer and with intravenous CaNa$_2$EDTA.

In an attempt to control rebound of blood lead levels, 19 pediatric patients, ages 1-7 years, with blood lead levels of 42-67 mcg/dL, were treated with 350 mg/m^2 succimer every 8 hours for five days and then divided into three groups. One group was followed for two weeks with no further therapy, the second group was treated for two weeks with 350 mg/m^2 daily, and the third with 350 mg/m^2 every 12 hours. After the initial 5 days of therapy, the mean blood lead level in all subjects declined 61%. While the untreated group and the group treated with 350 mg/m^2 daily experienced rebound during the ensuing two weeks, the group who received the 350 mg/m^2 every 12 hours experienced no such rebound during the treatment period and less rebound following cessation of therapy.

In another study, ten pediatric patients, ages 21 to 72 months, with blood lead levels of 30-57 mcg/dL were treated with succimer 350 mg/m^2 every eight hours for five days followed by an additional 19-22 days of therapy at a dose of 350 mg/m^2 every 12 hours. The mean blood lead levels decreased and remained stable at under 15 mcg/dL during the extended dosing period.

In addition to the controlled studies, approximately 250 patients with lead poisoning have been treated with succimer either orally or parenterally in open U.S. and foreign studies with similar results reported. Succimer has been used for the treatment of lead poisoning in one patient with sickle cell anemia and in five patients with glucose-6-phosphodehydrogenase (G6PD) deficiency without adverse reactions.

Lead Encephalopathy

Three adults with lead encephalopathy have been reported in the literature to have improved with succimer therapy. However, data are not available regarding the use of succimer for the treatment of this rare and sometimes fatal complication of lead poisoning in pediatric patients.

Other Heavy Metal Poisoning

No controlled clinical studies have been conducted with succimer in poisoning with other heavy metals. A limited number of patients have received succimer for mercury or arsenic poisoning. These patients showed increased urinary excretion of the heavy metal and varying degrees of symptomatic improvement.

INDICATIONS AND USAGE

CHEMET is indicated for the treatment of lead poisoning in pediatric patients with blood lead levels above 45 mcg/dL. CHEMET is not indicated for prophylaxis of lead poisoning in a lead-containing environment; the use of CHEMET should always be accompanied by identification and removal of the source of the lead exposure.

CONTRAINDICATIONS

CHEMET should not be administered to patients with a history of allergy to the drug.

WARNINGS

Keep out of reach of pediatric patients. CHEMET is not a substitute for effective abatement of lead exposure.

Mild to moderate neutropenia has been observed in some patients receiving succimer. While a causal relationship to succimer has not been definitely established, neutropenia has been reported with other drugs in the same chemical class. A complete blood count with white blood cell differential and direct platelet counts should be obtained prior to and weekly during treatment with succimer. Therapy should either be withheld or discontinued if the absolute neutrophil count (ANC) is below 1200/mcL and the patient followed closely to document recovery of the ANC to above 1500/mcL or to the patient's baseline neutrophil count. There is limited experience with reexposure in patients who have developed neutropenia. Therefore, such patients should be rechallenged only if the benefit of succimer therapy clearly outweighs the potential risk of another episode of neutropenia and then only with careful patient monitoring.

Patients treated with succimer should be instructed to promptly report any signs of infection. If infection is suspected, the above laboratory tests should be conducted immediately.

PRECAUTIONS

The extent of clinical experience with CHEMET is limited. Therefore, patients should be carefully observed during treatment.

General

Elevated blood lead levels and associated symptoms may return rapidly after discontinuation of CHEMET because of redistribution of lead from bone stores to soft tissues and blood. After therapy, patients should be monitored for rebound of blood lead levels, by measuring blood lead levels at least once weekly until stable. However, the severity of lead intoxication (as measured by the initial blood lead level and the rate and degree of rebound of blood lead) should be used as a guide for more frequent blood lead monitoring.

All patients undergoing treatment should be adequately hydrated. Caution should be exercised in using CHEMET therapy in patients with compromised renal function. Limited data suggests that CHEMET is dialyzable, but that the lead chelates are not.

Transient mild elevations of serum transaminases have been observed in 6-10% of patients during the course of succimer therapy. Serum transaminases should be monitored before the start of therapy and at least weekly during therapy. Patients with a history of liver disease should be monitored closely. No data are available regarding the metabolism of succimer in patients with liver disease.

Clinical experience with repeated courses is limited. The safety of uninterrupted dosing longer than three weeks has not been established and it is not recommended.

The possibility of allergic or other mucocutaneous reactions to the drug must be borne in mind on readministration (as well as during initial courses). Patients requiring repeated courses of CHEMET should be monitored during each treatment course. One patient experienced recurrent mucocutaneous vesicular eruptions of increasing severity affecting the oral mucosa, the external urethral meatus and the perianal area on the third, fourth and fifth courses of the drug. The reaction resolved between courses and upon discontinuation of therapy.

Information for Patients

Patients should be instructed to maintain adequate fluid intake. If rash occurs, patients should consult their physician. Patients should be instructed to promptly report any indication of infection, which may be a sign of neutropenia (see WARNINGS and ADVERSE REACTIONS).

In young pediatric patients unable to swallow capsules, the contents of the capsule can be administered in a small amount of food (see DOSAGE AND ADMINISTRATION).

Drug Interaction

CHEMET is not known to interact with other drugs including iron supplements; interactions have not been systematically studied. Concomitant administration of CHEMET with other chelation therapy, such as CaNa$_2$EDTA is not recommended.

Drug/Laboratory Tests Interaction

Succimer may interfere with serum and urinary laboratory tests. In vitro studies have shown succimer to cause false positive results for ketones in urine using nitroprusside reagents such as Ketostix[1] and falsely decreased measurements of serum uric acid and CPK.

---

[1]Ketostix is a registered trademark of Bayer Diagnostics.

Carcinogenesis, Mutagenesis and Impairment of Fertility

CHEMET has not been tested for carcinogenic potential in long-term animal studies. CHEMET up to a dose of 510 mg/kg/day in males and 100 mg/kg/day in females did not show any adverse effect on fertility and reproductive performance. It was not mutagenic in the Ames bacterial assay and in the mammalian cell forward gene mutation assay.

Pregnancy

Teratogenic Effects

Pregnancy Category C.

CHEMET has been shown to be teratogenic and fetotoxic in pregnant mice when given subcutaneously in a dose range of 410 to 1640 mg/kg/day during the period of organogenesis. In a developmental study in rats, CHEMET produced maternal toxicity and deaths at the dose of 720 mg/kg/day or more during organogenesis.

The dose of 510 mg/kg/day was the highest tolerable dose in pregnant rats. Impaired development of reflexes was noted in pups of 720 mg/kg/day group dam. There are no adequate and well controlled studies in pregnant women. CHEMET should be used during pregnancy only if the potential benefit justifies the potential risk to the fetus.

Nursing Mothers

It is not known whether this drug is excreted in human milk. Because many drugs and heavy metals are excreted in human milk, nursing mothers requiring CHEMET therapy should be discouraged from nursing their infants.

Pediatric Use

Refer to the INDICATIONS and DOSAGE AND ADMINISTRATION sections. Safety and efficacy in pediatric patients less than 12 months of age have not been established.

ADVERSE REACTIONS

Clinical experience with CHEMET has been limited. Consequently, the full spectrum and incidence of adverse reactions including the possibility of hypersensitivity or idiosyncratic reactions have not been determined. The most common events attributable to succimer, i.e., gastrointestinal symptoms or increases in serum transaminases, have been observed in about 10% of patients (see PRECAUTIONS). Rashes, some necessitating discontinuation of therapy, have been reported in about 4% of patients. If rash occurs, other causes (e.g. measles) should be considered before ascribing the reaction to succimer. Rechallenge with succimer may be considered if lead levels are high enough to warrant retreatment. One allergic mucocutaneous reaction

TABLE I INCIDENCE OF ADVERSE EVENTS IN DOMESTIC STUDIES REGARDLESS OF ATTRIBUTION OR SUCCIMER DOSAGE

	Pediatric Patients (191)		Adults (134)	
	%	(n)	%	(n)
Digestive:	12.0	23	20.9	28
Nausea, vomiting, diarrhea, appetite loss, hemorrhoidal symptoms, loose stools, metallic taste in mouth.				
Body as a Whole:	5.2	10	15.7	21
Back pain, abdominal cramps, stomach pains, head pain, rib pain, chills, flank pain, fever, flu-like symptoms, heavy head/tired, head cold, headache, moniliasis.				
Metabolic:	4.2	8	10.4	14
Elevated SGPT, SGOT, alkaline phosphatase, elevated serum cholesterol.				
Nervous:	1.0	2	12.7	17
Drowsiness, dizziness, sensorimotor neuropathy, sleepiness, paresthesia.				
Skin and Appendages:	2.6	5	11.2	15
Papular rash, herpetic rash, rash, mucocutaneous eruptions, pruritus.				
Special Senses:	1.0	2	3.7	5
Cloudy film in eye, ears plugged, otitis media, eyes watery.				
Respiratory	3.7	7	0.7	1
Throat sore, rhinorrhea, nasal congestion, cough.				
Urogenital:	0.0		3.7	5
Decreased urination, voiding difficulty, proteinuria increased.				
Cardiovascular:	0.0		1.8	2
Arrhythmia				
Heme/Lymphatic:	0.5*	1	1.5*	2
Mild to moderate neutropenia, increased platelet count, intermittent eosinophilia.				
Musculoskeletal:	0.0		3.0	4
Kneecap pain, leg pains.				

*Does not include neutropenia - see WARNINGS.

has been reported on repeated administration of the drug (see PRECAUTIONS). Mild to moderate neutropenia has been observed in some patients receiving succimer (see WARNINGS). Table I presents adverse events reported with the administration of succimer for the treatment of lead and other heavy metal intoxication.

[See table 1 above]

To report SUSPECTED ADVERSE REACTIONS, contact Recordati Rare Diseases Inc. at 1-888-575-8344 or FDA at 1-800-FDA-1088 or www.fda.gov/medwatch.

OVERDOSAGE

Doses of 2300 mg/kg in the rat and 2400 mg/kg in the mouse produced ataxia, convulsions, labored respiration and frequently death. No case of overdosage has been reported in humans. Limited data indicate that succimer is dialyzable. In case of acute overdosage, induction of vomiting or gastric lavage followed by administration of an activated charcoal slurry and appropriate supportive therapy are recommended.

DOSAGE AND ADMINISTRATION

Start dosage at 10 mg/kg or 350 mg/m² every eight hours for five days. Initiation of therapy at higher doses is not recommended. (See Table II for Dosing chart and number of capsules.) Reduce frequency of administration to 10 mg/kg or 350 mg/m² every 12 hours (two-thirds of initial daily dosage) for an additional two weeks of therapy. A course of treatment lasts 19 days. Repeated courses may be necessary if indicated by weekly monitoring of blood lead concentration. A minimum of two weeks between courses is recommended unless blood lead levels indicate the need for more prompt treatment.

TABLE II CHEMET (SUCCIMER) PEDIATRIC DOSING CHART

LBS	KG	DOSE (MG)*	Number of CAPSULES*
18-35	8-15	100	1
36-55	16-23	200	2
56-75	24-34	300	3
76-100	35-44	400	4
> 100	> 45	500	5

*To be administered every 8 hours for 5 days, followed by dosing every 12 hours for 14 days.

In young pediatric patients who cannot swallow capsules, CHEMET can be administered by separating the capsule and sprinkling the medicated beads on a small amount of soft food or putting them in a spoon and following with fruit drink.

Identification of the source of lead in the pediatric patient's environment and its abatement are critical to a successful therapy outcome. Chelation therapy is not a substitute for preventing further exposure to lead and should not be used to permit continued exposure to lead.

Patients who have received CaNa₂EDTA with or without BAL may use CHEMET for subsequent treatment after an interval of four weeks. Data on the concomitant use of CHEMET with CaNa₂EDTA with or without BAL are not available, and such use is not recommended.

HOW SUPPLIED

100 mg capsules in bottle of 100 (NDC 55292-201-11). Store between 15°C and 25°C and avoid excessive heat.

Manufactured by:
Kremers Urban Pharmaceuticals Inc.
Seymour, IN 47274, USA
For: Recordati Rare Diseases Inc., Lebanon, NJ 08833, U.S.A.
® Trademark of Recordati Rare Diseases Inc.
Revised: February 2013
CIA72289C

Shown in Product Identification Guide, page 312

NEOPROFEN ℞

[ne-o-pro-fen]
(ibuprofen lysine)
Injection for intravenous use
Initial U.S. Approval: 2006

HIGHLIGHTS OF PRESCRIBING INFORMATION

These highlights do not include all the information needed to use NeoProfen safely and effectively. See full prescribing information for NeoProfen.
NeoProfen® (ibuprofen lysine) Injection for intravenous use
Initial U.S. Approval: 2006

RECENT MAJOR CHANGES

Dosage and Administration, Directions for Use (2.2) 12/2013

INDICATIONS AND USAGE

NeoProfen is indicated to close a clinically significant patent ductus arteriosus (PDA) in premature infants weighing between 500 and 1500 g, who are no more than 32 weeks gestational age when usual medical management is ineffective. The clinical trial was conducted among infants with an asymptomatic PDA. However, the consequences beyond 8 weeks after treatment have not been evaluated; therefore, treatment should be reserved for infants with clear evidence of a clinically significant PDA. (1)

DOSAGE AND ADMINISTRATION

- A course of therapy is three doses administered I.V. (2.1)
- An initial dose of 10 mg/kg (based on birth weight) is followed by two doses of 5 mg/kg each, after 24 and 48 hours (2.1)
- Do not administer if anuria or marked oliguria (<0.6 mL/kg/hr) is evident at the scheduled time of the second or third dose (2.1)

DOSAGE FORMS AND STRENGTHS

- 10 mg/mL as a clear sterile preservative-free solution of the L-lysine salt of ibuprofen in a 2 mL single-use vial (3)

CONTRAINDICATIONS

NeoProfen is contraindicated in preterm infants:
- With proven or suspected infection that is untreated (4)
- With congenital heart disease in whom patency of the PDA is necessary for satisfactory pulmonary or systemic blood flow (4)
- With impaired renal function (4)
- With thrombocytopenia, coagulation defects or who are bleeding (4)
- With or who are suspected of having necrotizing enterocolitis (4)

WARNINGS AND PRECAUTIONS

- NeoProfen has not been assessed for neurodevelopmental outcome and growth (5.1)
- NeoProfen may alter the usual signs of infection (5.2)
- NeoProfen can inhibit platelet aggregation, and has been shown to prolong bleeding time in normal adult subjects (5.3)
- Ibuprofen has been shown to displace bilirubin from albumin binding-sites (5.4)
- NeoProfen should be administered carefully to avoid extravascular injection or leakage (5.5)

ADVERSE REACTIONS

Most common adverse reactions (≥10%) are sepsis, anemia, intraventricular bleeding, apnea, gastrointestinal disorders, impaired renal function, respiratory infection, skin lesions, hypoglycemia, hypocalcemia, respiratory failure. (6)
To report SUSPECTED ADVERSE REACTIONS, contact Recordati Rare Diseases at 1-888-575-8344, or FDA at 1-800-FDA-1088 or FDA at 1-800-FDA-1088 or www.fda.gov/medwatch.

DRUG INTERACTIONS

Drug interactions in neonates have not been assessed. (7)
See 17 for PATIENT COUNSELING INFORMATION

Revised: 12/2013

FULL PRESCRIBING INFORMATION: CONTENTS*

* Sections or subsections omitted from the full prescribing information are not listed

FULL PRESCRIBING INFORMATION

1   INDICATIONS AND USAGE

NeoProfen is indicated to close a clinically significant patent ductus arteriosus (PDA) in premature infants weighing between 500 and 1500 g, who are no more than 32 weeks gestational age when usual medical management (e.g., fluid restriction, diuretics, respiratory support, etc.) is ineffective. The clinical trial was conducted among infants with an asymptomatic PDA. However, the consequences beyond 8 weeks after treatment have not been evaluated; therefore, treatment should be reserved for infants with clear evidence of a clinically significant PDA.

2   DOSAGE AND ADMINISTRATION

2.1   Recommended Dose

A course of therapy is three doses of NeoProfen administered intravenously (administration via an umbilical arterial line has not been evaluated). An initial dose of 10 mg per kilogram is followed by two doses of 5 mg per kilogram each, after 24 and 48 hours. All doses should be based on birth weight. If anuria or marked oliguria (urinary output <0.6 mL/kg/hr) is evident at the scheduled time of the second or third dose of NeoProfen, no additional dosage should be given until laboratory studies indicate that renal function has returned to normal. If the ductus arteriosus closes or is significantly reduced in size after completion of the first course of NeoProfen, no further doses are necessary. If during continued medical management the ductus arteriosus fails to close or reopens, then a second course of NeoProfen, alternative pharmacological therapy, or surgery may be necessary.

2.2 Directions for Use

For intravenous administration only. Parenteral drug products should be inspected visually for particulate matter and discoloration prior to administration whenever solution and container permit. Do not use NeoProfen if particulate matter is observed.

After the first withdrawal from the vial, any solution remaining must be discarded because NeoProfen contains no preservative.

For administration, NeoProfen should be diluted to an appropriate volume with dextrose or saline. NeoProfen should be prepared for infusion and administered within 30 minutes of preparation and infused continuously over a period of 15 minutes. The drug should be administered via the IV port that is nearest the insertion site. After the first withdrawal from the vial, any solution remaining must be discarded because NeoProfen contains no preservative.

Since NeoProfen is potentially irritating to tissues, it should be administered carefully to avoid extravasation.

NeoProfen should not be simultaneously administered in the same intravenous line with Total Parenteral Nutrition (TPN). If necessary, TPN should be interrupted for a 15-minute period prior to and after drug administration. Line patency should be maintained by using dextrose or saline.

3 DOSAGE FORMS AND STRENGTHS

10 mg/mL as a clear sterile preservative-free solution of the L-lysine salt of ibuprofen in a 2 mL single-use vial.

4 CONTRAINDICATIONS

NeoProfen is contraindicated in:

- Preterm infants with proven or suspected infection that is untreated;
- Preterm infants with congenital heart disease in whom patency of the PDA is necessary for satisfactory pulmonary or systemic blood flow (e.g., pulmonary atresia, severe tetralogy of Fallot, severe coarctation of the aorta);
- Preterm infants who are bleeding, especially those with active intracranial hemorrhage or gastrointestinal bleeding;
- Preterm infants with thrombocytopenia;
- Preterm infants with coagulation defects;
- Preterm infants with or who are suspected of having necrotizing enterocolitis;
- Preterm infants with significant impairment of renal function.

5 WARNINGS AND PRECAUTIONS

5.1 General

There are no long-term evaluations of the infants treated with ibuprofen at durations greater than the 36 weeks post-conceptual age observation period. Ibuprofen's effects on neurodevelopmental outcome and growth as well as disease processes associated with prematurity (such as retinopathy of prematurity and chronic lung disease) have not been assessed.

5.2 Infection

NeoProfen may alter the usual signs of infection. The physician must be continually on the alert and should use the drug with extra care in the presence of controlled infection and in infants at risk of infection.

5.3 Platelet Aggregation

NeoProfen, like other non-steroidal anti-inflammatory agents, can inhibit platelet aggregation. Preterm infants should be observed for signs of bleeding. Ibuprofen has been shown to prolong bleeding time (but within the normal range) in normal adult subjects. This effect may be exaggerated in patients with underlying hemostatic defects (see CONTRAINDICATIONS).

5.4 Bilirubin Displacement

Ibuprofen has been shown to displace bilirubin from albumin binding-sites; therefore, it should be used with caution in patients with elevated total bilirubin.

5.5 Administration

NeoProfen should be administered carefully to avoid extravascular injection or leakage, as solution may be irritating to tissue.

6 ADVERSE REACTIONS

6.1 Clinical Trials Experience

The most frequently reported adverse events with NeoProfen were as shown in Table 1.

Table 1. Adverse Events within 30 Days of Therapy in the Multicenter Study*

Adverse Event	% Incidence NeoProfen	Placebo
Sepsis	43	37
Anemia	32	25
Total Bleeding[†]	32	29
Intraventricular Hemorrhage, Grades 1/2	15	13
Intraventricular Hemorrhage, Grades 3/4	15	10
Other Bleeding	6	13
Intraventricular Hemorrhage, All Grades	29	24
Apnea	28	26
Gastrointestinal Disorders non-Necrotizing Enterocolitis	22	18
Total Renal Events[†]	21	15
Renal Failure	1	3
Renal Insufficiency, Impairment	6	4
Urine Output Reduced	3	1
Blood Creatinine Increased	3	1
Blood Urea Increased with Hematuria	1	0
Blood Urea Increased	7	4
Respiratory Infection	19	13
Skin Lesion/Irritation	16	6
Hypoglycemia	12	6
Hypocalcemia	12	9
Respiratory Failure	10	4
Urinary Tract Infection	9	4
Adrenal Insufficiency	7	1
Hypernatremia	7	4
Edema	4	0
Atelectasis	4	1

* Within 30 days of therapy, with an event rate greater on NeoProfen than on placebo, and greater than 2 events on NeoProfen.

[†] A given subject may have experienced more than one specific event within these adverse event categories. Only the most severe grade of IVH counted for a given subject.

6.2 Renal Function

Compared to placebo, there was a small decrease in urinary output in the ibuprofen group on days 2-6 of life, with a compensatory increase in urine output on day 9. In other studies, adverse events classified as renal insufficiency including oliguria, elevated BUN, elevated creatinine, or renal failure were reported in ibuprofen treated infants.

6.3 Additional Adverse Events

The adverse events reported in the multicenter study and of unknown association include tachycardia, cardiac failure, abdominal distension, gastroesophageal reflux, gastritis, ileus, inguinal hernia, injection site reactions, cholestasis, various infections, feeding problems, convulsions, jaundice, hypotension, and various laboratory abnormalities including neutropenia, thrombocytopenia, and hyperglycemia.

6.4 Post-marketing Experience

The following adverse reactions have been identified from spontaneous post-marketing reports or published literature: gastrointestinal perforation and necrotizing enterocolitis. Because these reactions are reported voluntarily from a population of uncertain size, it is not always possible to reliably estimate their frequency, or establish a causal relationship to drug exposure.

7 DRUG INTERACTIONS

Drug interactions of NeoProfen in neonates have not been assessed.

10 OVERDOSAGE

The following signs and symptoms have occurred in individuals (not necessarily in premature infants) following an overdose of oral ibuprofen: breathing difficulties, coma, drowsiness, irregular heartbeat, kidney failure, low blood pressure, seizures, and vomiting. There are no specific measures to treat acute overdosage with NeoProfen. The patient should be followed for several days because gastrointestinal ulceration and hemorrhage may occur.

11 DESCRIPTION

NeoProfen® is a clear sterile preservative-free solution of the L-lysine salt of (±)-ibuprofen which is the active ingredient. (±)-Ibuprofen is a nonsteroidal anti-inflammatory agent (NSAID). L-lysine is used to create a water-soluble drug product salt suitable for intravenous administration. Each mL of NeoProfen contains 17.1 mg of ibuprofen lysine (equivalent to 10 mg of (±)-ibuprofen) in Water for Injection, USP. The pH is adjusted to 7.0 with sodium hydroxide or hydrochloric acid.

The structural formula is:

$(CH_3)_2CHCH_2 \text{—} \bigcirc \text{—} \underset{\underset{CH_3}{|}}{CH}COOH \quad H_2N(CH_2)_4\underset{\underset{NH_2}{|}}{CH}COOH$

NeoProfen is designated chemically as α-methyl-4-(2-methyl propyl) benzeneacetic acid lysine salt. Its molecular weight is 352.48. Its empirical formula is $C_{19}H_{32}N_2O_4$. It occurs as a white crystalline solid which is soluble in water and slightly soluble in ethanol.

12 CLINICAL PHARMACOLOGY

12.1 Mechanism of Action

The mechanism of action through which ibuprofen causes closure of a patent ductus arteriosus (PDA) in neonates is not known. In adults, ibuprofen is an inhibitor of prostaglandin synthesis.

12.2 Pharmacokinetics and Bioavailability Studies

The pharmacokinetic data were obtained from 54 NeoProfen-treated premature infants included in a double-blind, placebo-controlled, randomized, multicenter study. Infants were less than 30 weeks gestational age, weighed between 500 and 1000 g, and exhibited asymptomatic PDA with evidence of echocardiographic documentation of ductal shunting. Dosing was initially 10 mg/kg followed by 5 mg/kg at 24 and 48 hours.

The population average clearance and volume of distribution values of racemic ibuprofen for premature infants at birth were 3 mL/kg/h and 320 mL/kg, respectively. Clearance increased rapidly with post-natal age (an average increase of approximately 0.5 mL/kg/h per day). Inter-individual variability in clearance and volume of distribution were 55% and 14%, respectively. In general, the half-life in infants is more than 10 times longer than in adults.

The metabolism and excretion of ibuprofen in premature infants have not been studied.

In adults, renal elimination of unchanged ibuprofen accounts for only 10-15% of the dose. The excretion of ibuprofen and metabolites occurs rapidly in both urine and feces. Approximately 80% of the dose administered orally is recovered in urine as hydroxyl and carboxyl metabolites, respectively, as a mixture of conjugated and unconjugated forms. Ibuprofen is eliminated primarily by metabolism in the liver where CYP2C9 mediates the 2- and 3-hydroxylations of R- and S-ibuprofen. Ibuprofen and its metabolites are further conjugated to acyl glucuronides.

In neonates, renal function and the enzymes associated with drug metabolism are underdeveloped at birth and substantially increase in the days after birth.

14 CLINICAL STUDIES

In a double-blind, multicenter clinical study premature infants of birth weight between 500 and 1000 g, less than 30 weeks post-conceptional age, and with echocardiographic evidence of a PDA were randomized to placebo or NeoProfen. These infants were asymptomatic from their PDA at the time of enrollment. The primary efficacy parameter was the need for rescue therapy (indomethacin, open-label ibuprofen, or surgery) to treat a hemodynamically significant PDA by study day 14. An infant was rescued if there was clinical evidence of a hemodynamically significant PDA that was echocardiographically confirmed. A hemodynamically significant PDA was defined by three of the following five criteria – bounding pulse, hyperdynamic precordium, pulmonary edema, increased cardiac silhouette, or systolic murmur – or hemodynamically significant ductus as determined by a neonatologist.

One hundred and thirty-six premature infants received either placebo or NeoProfen (10 mg/kg on the first dose and 5 mg/kg at 24 and 48 hours). Mean birth age was 1.5 days (range: 4.6 – 73.0 hours), mean gestational age was 26 weeks (range: 23 – 30 weeks), and mean weight was 798 g (range: 530 – 1015 g). All infants had a documented PDA with evidence of ductal shunting. As shown in Table 2, 25% of infants on NeoProfen required rescue therapy versus 48% of infants on placebo (p=0.003 from logistic regression controlling for site).

Table 2. Summary of Efficacy Results, n (%)

	NeoProfen N=68	Placebo N=68
Required rescue through study day 14		
Total	17 (25)	33 (48)
By age at treatment		
Birth to < 24 hours	3/14 (21)	8/16 (50)
24-48 hours	9/32 (28)	16/37 (43)
> 48 hours	5/22 (23)	9/15 (60)
Echocardiographically proven PDA prior to rescue	17 (100)	32 (97)
Reasons for Rescue		
Hemodynamically significant PDA per neonatologist	14 (82)	25 (76)
Bounding pulse	6 (35)	12 (36)
Systolic murmur	6 (35)	15 (45)
Pulmonary Edema	3 (18)	5 (15)
Hyperdynamic precordium	2 (12)	3 (9)
Increased cardiac silhouette	1 (6)	5 (15)

Of the infants requiring rescue within the first 14 days after the first dose of study drug, no statistically significant difference was observed between the NeoProfen and placebo groups for mean age at start of first rescue treatment (8.7 days, range 4-15 days, for the NeoProfen group and 6.9 days, range 2-15 days, for the placebo group).

The groups were similar in the number of deaths by day 14, the number of patients on a ventilator or requiring oxygenation at day 1, 4 and 14, the number of patients requiring surgical ligation of their PDA (12%), the number of cases of Pulmonary Hemorrhage and Pulmonary Hypertension by day 14, and Bronchopulmonary Dysplasia at day 28. In addition, no significant differences were noted in the incidences of Stage 2 and 3 Necrotizing Enterocolitis, Grades 3 and 4 Intraventricular Hemorrhage, Periventricular Leukomalacia and Retinopathy of Prematurity between groups as determined at 36±1 weeks adjusted gestational age.

Two supportive studies also determined that ibuprofen, either prophylactically (n=433, weight range: 400 – 2165 g) or as treatment (n=210, weight range: 400 – 2370 g), was superior to placebo (or no treatment) in preventing the need for rescue therapy for a symptomatic PDA.

16   HOW SUPPLIED/STORAGE AND HANDLING

How Supplied
NeoProfen (ibuprofen lysine) Injection is dispensed in clear glass single-use vials, each containing 2 mL of sterile solution (NDC 55292-122- 52). The solution is not buffered and contains no preservatives. Each milliliter contains 17.1 mg/mL (±)-ibuprofen L-lysine [equivalent to 10 mg/mL (±)-ibuprofen] dissolved in Water for Injection, USP. NeoProfen is supplied in a carton containing 3 single-use vials.

Storage and Handling
Store at 20 – 25°C (68 – 77°F); excursions permitted 15 – 30°C (59 – 86°F) [see USP Controlled Room Temperature]. Protect from light. Store vials in carton until contents have been used.

17   PATIENT COUNSELING INFORMATION

17.1   General
Patients' caregivers should be informed that the effects of ibuprofen on infants' neurodevelopmental outcome, growth and disease process with prematurity have not been assessed in long-term studies.

17.2   Infection
NeoProfen may alter signs of infection. Patients' caregivers should be informed that the infant will be carefully monitored for any signs of infection.

17.3   Platelet Aggregation
Patients' caregivers should be informed that like other NSAIDS, NeoProfen can inhibit clot formation therefore their infant will be monitored for any signs of bleeding.

17.4   Bilirubin Displacement
Patients' caregivers should be informed that the infants' blood will be tested for increased levels of total bilirubin.

17.5   Administration
Patients' caregivers should be informed that the infants' skin and tissues will be monitored as leakage from administration may be irritating to tissue.
Manufactured by: AAIPharma Services, Charleston, SC 29405, U.S.A.
For: Recordati Rare Diseases Inc., Lebanon, NJ 08833, U.S.A.

RECORDATI RARE DISEASES GROUP
® Trademark of Recordati Rare Diseases Inc.
Revised: December 2013
PC4477

PANHEMATIN®   ℞
Hemin For Injection
Rx only
For intravenous infusion only.

> PANHEMATIN (hemin for injection) should only be used by physicians experienced in the management of porphyrias in hospitals where the recommended clinical and laboratory diagnostic and monitoring techniques are available.
> PANHEMATIN therapy should be considered after an appropriate period of alternate therapy (i.e., 400 g glucose/day for 1 to 2 days). (See "WARNINGS", "PRECAUTIONS" and "DOSAGE AND ADMINISTRATION" sections.)

DESCRIPTION
PANHEMATIN (hemin for injection) is an enzyme inhibitor derived from processed red blood cells. Hemin for injection was known previously as hematin. The term hematin has been used to describe the chemical reaction product of hemin and sodium carbonate solution. Hemin is an iron containing metalloporphyrin. Chemically hemin is represented as chloro [7,12-diethenyl-3,8,13,17-tetramethyl-21H,23H-porphine-2,18-dipropanoato(2-)-N^{21},N^{22},N^{23},N^{24}] iron. The structural formula for hemin is:

PANHEMATIN is a sterile, lyophilized powder suitable for intravenous administration after reconstitution. Each dispensing vial of PANHEMATIN contains the equivalent of 313 mg hemin, 215 mg sodium carbonate and 300 mg of sorbitol. The pH may have been adjusted with hydrochloric acid; the product contains no preservatives. When mixed as directed with Sterile Water for Injection, USP, each 43 mL provides the equivalent of approximately 301 mg hematin (7 mg/mL).

CLINICAL PHARMACOLOGY
Heme acts to limit the hepatic and/or marrow synthesis of porphyrin. This action is likely due to the inhibition of δ-aminolevulinic acid synthetase, the enzyme which limits the rate of the porphyrin/heme biosynthetic pathway. The exact mechanism by which hematin produces symptomatic improvement in patients with acute episodes of the hepatic porphyrias has not been elucidated.[1,9]

Following intravenous administration of hematin in nonjaundiced human patients, an increase in fecal urobilinogen can be observed which is roughly proportional to the amount of hematin administered. This suggests an enterohepatic pathway as at least one route of elimination. Bilirubin metabolites are also excreted in the urine following hematin injections.[2]

PANHEMATIN (hemin for injection) therapy for the acute porphyrias is not curative. After discontinuation of PANHEMATIN treatment, symptoms generally return although in some cases remission is prolonged. Some neurological symptoms have improved weeks to months after therapy although little or no response was noted at the time of treatment.

Other aspects of human pharmacokinetics have not been defined.

INDICATIONS AND USAGE
PANHEMATIN (hemin for injection) is indicated for the amelioration of recurrent attacks of acute intermittent porphyria temporally related to the menstrual cycle in susceptible women.

Manifestations such as pain, hypertension, tachycardia, abnormal mental status and mild to progressive neurologic signs may be controlled in selected patients with this disorder.

Similar findings have been reported in other patients with acute intermittent porphyria, porphyria variegata and hereditary coproporphyria. PANHEMATIN is not indicated in porphyria cutanea tarda.

CONTRAINDICATIONS
PANHEMATIN is contraindicated in patients with known hypersensitivity to this drug.

WARNINGS
PANHEMATIN is made from human blood. Products made from human blood may contain infectious agents, such as viruses, that can cause disease. The risk that such products will transmit an infectious agent has been reduced by screening blood donors for prior exposure to certain viruses, by testing for the presence of certain current virus infections, and by inactivating certain viruses. Despite these measures, such products can still potentially transmit disease. There is also the possibility that unknown infectious agents may be present in such products. ALL infections thought by a physician possibly to have been transmitted by this product should be reported by the physician or other healthcare provider to Recordati Rare Diseases, (1-888-575-8344). The physician should discuss the risks and benefits of this product with the patient.

Because this product is made from human blood, it may carry a risk of transmitting infectious agents, e.g., viruses, and theoretically, the Creutzfeldt-Jakob disease (CJD) agent.

PANHEMATIN therapy is intended to limit the rate of porphyria/heme biosynthesis possibly by inhibiting the enzyme δ-aminolevulinic acid synthetase. For this reason, drugs such as estrogens, barbituric acid derivatives and steroid metabolites which increase the activity of δ-aminolevulinic acid synthetase should be avoided.

Also, because hemin for injection has exhibited transient, mild anticoagulant effects during clinical studies, concurrent anticoagulant therapy should be avoided.[9] The extent and duration of the hypocoagulable state induced by PANHEMATIN has not been established.

PRECAUTIONS
General
Clinical benefit from PANHEMATIN depends on prompt administration. Attacks of porphyria may progress to a point where irreversible neuronal damage has occurred. PANHEMATIN therapy is intended to prevent an attack from reaching the critical stage of neuronal degeneration. PANHEMATIN is not effective in repairing neuronal damage.[9]

Recommended dosage guidelines should be strictly followed. Reversible renal shutdown has been observed in a case where an excessive hematin dose (12.2 mg/kg) was administered in a single infusion. Oliguria and increased nitrogen retention occurred although the patient remained asymptomatic.[4] No worsening of renal function has been seen with administration of recommended dosages of hematin.[9]

A large arm vein or a central venous catheter should be utilized for the administration of PANHEMATIN to avoid the possibility of phlebitis.

Since reconstituted PANHEMATIN is not transparent, any undissolved particulate matter is difficult to see when inspected visually. Therefore, terminal filtration through a sterile 0.45 micron or smaller filter is recommended.

Because increased levels of iron and serum ferritin have been reported in post-marketing experience, physicians should monitor iron and serum ferritin in patients receiving multiple administrations of PANHEMATIN (See "ADVERSE REACTIONS" section).

Tests for Diagnosis and Monitoring of Therapy
Before PANHEMATIN therapy is begun, the presence of acute porphyria must be diagnosed using the following criteria:[9]
a. Presence of clinical symptoms.
b. Positive Watson-Schwartz or Hoesch test. (A negative Watson-Schwartz or Hoesch test indicates a porphyric attack is highly unlikely. When in doubt quantitative measures of δ-aminolevulinic acid and porphobilinogen in serum or urine may aid in diagnosis.)

Urinary concentrations of the following compounds may be *monitored* during PANHEMATIN therapy. Drug effect will be demonstrated by a decrease in one or more of the following compounds.[3-6]
  ALA - δ-aminolevulinic acid
  UPG - uroporphyrinogen
  PBG - porphobilinogen
  coproporphyrin

Carcinogenesis, Mutagenesis, Impairment of Fertility
PANHEMATIN was not mutagenic in bacteria systems *in vitro* and was not clastogenic in mammalian systems *in vitro* and *in vivo*. No data are available on potential for carcinogenicity or impairment of fertility in animals or humans.

Pregnancy
Teratogenic effects-Pregnancy Category C: Animal reproduction studies have not been conducted with hematin. It is also not known whether hematin can cause fetal harm when administered to a pregnant woman or can affect reproduction capacity. For this reason PANHEMATIN should not be given to a pregnant woman unless the expected benefits are sufficiently important to the health and welfare of the patient to outweigh the unknown hazard to the fetus.

Nursing Mothers
It is not known whether this drug is excreted in human milk. Because many drugs are excreted in human milk, caution should be exercised when PANHEMATIN is administered to a nursing woman.

Pediatric Use

Safety and effectiveness in pediatric patients under 16 years of age have not been established.

Geriatric Use

Clinical studies in PANHEMATIN did not include sufficient numbers of subjects aged 65 and over to determine whether they respond differently from younger subjects. Other reported clinical experience has not identified differences in response between the elderly and younger patients. In general, dose selection for an elderly patient should be cautious, usually starting at the low end of the dosing range, reflecting the greater frequency of decreased hepatic, renal, or cardiac function, and of concomitant disease or other drug therapy.

ADVERSE REACTIONS

Clinical Trials Experience

Phlebitis with or without leucocytosis and with or without mild pyrexia has occurred after administration of hematin through small arm veins.

Post-marketing Experience

Reversible renal shutdown has occurred with administration of excessive doses (See "PRECAUTIONS" section).

There have been post-marketing literature reports of thrombocytopenia and coagulopathy (including prolonged prothrombin time and prolonged partial thromboplastin time) in patients receiving PANHEMATIN.[8] Iron overload and serum ferritin increased have also been reported (See "PRECAUTIONS" section).

To report SUSPECTED ADVERSE REACTIONS, contact Recordati Rare Diseases at 1-888-575-8344 or FDA at 1-800-FDA-1088 or www.fda.gov/medwatch.

OVERDOSAGE

Reversible renal shutdown has been observed in a case where an excessive hematin dose (12.2 mg/kg) was administered in a single infusion. Treatment of this case consisted of ethacrynic acid and mannitol.[7]

DOSAGE AND ADMINISTRATION

Before administering PANHEMATIN, an appropriate period of alternate therapy (i.e., 400 g glucose/day for 1 to 2 days) must be considered. If improvement is unsatisfactory for the treatment of acute attacks of porphyria, an intravenous infusion of PANHEMATIN containing a dose of 1 to 4 mg/kg/day of hematin should be given over a period of 10 to 15 minutes for 3 to 14 days based on the clinical signs. In more severe cases this dose may be repeated no earlier than every 12 hours. No more than 6 mg/kg of hematin should be given in any 24 hour period.

After reconstitution each mL of PANHEMATIN contains the equivalent of approximately 7 mg of hematin. The drug may be administered directly from the vial.

Dosage Calculation Table

1 mg hematin equivalent = 0.14 mL PANHEMATIN
2 mg hematin equivalent = 0.28 mL PANHEMATIN
3 mg hematin equivalent = 0.42 mL PANHEMATIN
4 mg hematin equivalent = 0.56 mL PANHEMATIN

Since reconstituted PANHEMATIN is not transparent, any undissolved particulate matter is difficult to see when inspected visually. Therefore, terminal filtration through a sterile 0.45 micron or smaller filter is recommended.

Preparation of Solution:

Reconstitute PANHEMATIN by aseptically adding 43 mL of Sterile Water for Injection, USP, to the dispensing vial. Immediately after adding diluent, the product should be shaken well for a period of 2 to 3 minutes to aid dissolution.

NOTE: Because PANHEMATIN contains no preservative and because PANHEMATIN undergoes rapid chemical decomposition in solution, it should not be reconstituted until immediately before use. After the first withdrawal from the vial, any solution remaining must be discarded.

No drug or chemical agent should be added to a PANHEMATIN fluid admixture unless its effect on the chemical and physical stability has first been determined.

HOW SUPPLIED

PANHEMATIN is supplied as a sterile, lyophilized black powder in single dose dispensing vials (NDC 55292-701-54) in a carton (NDC 55292-701-55). When mixed as directed with Sterile Water for Injection, USP, each 43 mL provides the equivalent of approximately 301 mg hematin (7 mg/mL). Store lyophilized powder at 20-25°C (68-77°F). See USP controlled room temperature.

Caution: The packaging (vial stopper) of this product contains natural rubber latex which may cause allergic reactions.

REFERENCES

1. Bickers, D., Treatment of the Porphyrias: Mechanisms of Action, J Invest Dermatol 77(1):107-113, 1981.
2. Watson, C. J., Hematin and Porphyria, editorial, N Engl J Med 293(12): 605-607, September 18, 1975.
3. Lamon, J. M., Hematin Therapy for Acute Porphyria, Medicine 58(3): 252-269, 1979.
4. Dhar, G J., et al., Effects of Hematin in Hepatic Porphyria, Ann Intern Med 83: 20-30, 1975.
5. Watson, C. J., et al., Use of Hematin in the Acute Attack of the "Inducible" Hepatic Porphyrias, Adv Intern Med 23: 265-286, 1978.
6. McColl, K. E., et al., Treatment with Haematin in Acute Hepatic Porphyria, Q J Med, New Series L (198): 161-174, Spring, 1981.
7. Dhar, G. J., et al., Transitory Renal Failure Following Rapid Administration of a Relatively Large Amount of Hematin in a Patient with Acute Intermittent Porphyria in Clinical Remission, Acta Med Scand 203: 437-443, 1978.
8. Morris, D.L., et al., Coagulopathy Associated with Hematin Treatment for Acute Intermittent Porphyria, Ann Intern Med 95: 700-701, 1981.
9. Pierach, C. A., Hematin Therapy for the Porphyric Attack, Semin Liver Dis 2(2): 125-131, May, 1982.

Manufactured by: Fresenius Kabi USA, LLC
Raleigh, NC 27616
For: Recordati Rare Diseases Inc.
Lebanon, NJ 08833, U.S.A.
U.S. Lic. No. 1899
RECORDATI RARE DISEASES GROUP
® Trademark of Recordati Rare Diseases Inc.
Revised: February 2013
750-04243-7
Shown in Product Identification Guide, page 313

RLC Labs, Inc.
CAVE CREEK, AZ 85331

For Product Information:
(877) 797-7997
sales@rlclabs.com
For Customer Service & Ordering Information:
(877) 797-7997
(623) 879-8683 (Fax)
customerservice@rlclabs.com
www.rlclabs.com

NATURE-THROID®
(Thyroid USP) Tablets ℞

DESCRIPTION

Nature-Throid® (Thyroid USP) Tablets, micro-coated, easy to swallow with a reduced odor, for oral use are natural preparations derived from porcine thyroid glands (T3 liothyronine is approximately four times as potent as T4 levothyroxine on a microgram for microgram basis). They provide 38 mcg levothyroxine (T4) and 9 mcg liothyronine (T3) for each 65 mg (1 Grain) of the labeled content of thyroid.

INACTIVE INGREDIENTS

Colloidal Silicon Dioxide, Dicalcium Phosphate, Lactose Monohydrate[1], Magnesium Stearate, Microcrystalline Cellulose, Croscarmellose Sodium, Stearic Acid, Opadry II 85F19316 Clear.

The structural formulas of liothyronine (T3) and levothyroxine (T4) are as follows:

[1]Present in traceable amount as part of Thyroid USP (diluent)

CLINICAL PHARMACOLOGY

The steps in the synthesis of the thyroid hormones are controlled by thyrotropin (Thyroid Stimulating Hormone, TSH) secreted by the anterior pituitary. This hormone's secretion is in turn controlled by a feedback mechanism affected by the thyroid hormones themselves and by thyrotropin releasing hormone (TRH), a tripeptide of hypothalamic origin. En-

dogenous thyroid hormone secretion is suppressed when exogenous thyroid hormones are administered to euthyroid individuals in excess of the normal gland's secretion.

The mechanisms by which thyroid hormones exert their physiologic action are not well understood. These hormones enhance oxygen consumption by most tissues of the body, increase the basal metabolic rate, and the metabolism of carbohydrates, lipids, and proteins. Thus, they exert a profound influence on every organ system in the body and are of particular importance in the development of the central nervous system.

The normal thyroid gland contains approximately 200 mcg of levothyroxine (T4) per gram of gland, and 15 mcg of liothyronine (T3) per gram. The ratio of these two hormones in the circulation does not represent the ratio in the thyroid gland, since about 80 percent of peripheral liothyronine (T3) comes from monodeiodination of levothyroxine (T4). Peripheral monodeiodination of levothyroxine (T4) at the 5 position (inner ring) also results in the formation of reverse liothyronine (T3), which is calorigenically inactive. Liothyronine (T3) levels are low in the fetus and newborn, in old age, in chronic caloric deprivation, hepatic cirrhosis, renal failure, surgical stress, and chronic illnesses representing what has been called the "T3 thyronine syndrome".

Pharmacokinetics

Animal studies have shown that levothyroxine (T4) is only partially absorbed from the gastrointestinal tract. The degree of absorption is dependent on the vehicle used for its administration and by the character of the intestinal contents, the intestinal flora, including plasma protein, and soluble dietary factors, all of which bind thyroid, thereby making it unavailable for diffusion. Only 41 percent is absorbed when given in a gelatin capsule, as opposed to 74 percent absorption when given with an albumin carrier.

Depending on other factors, absorption has varied from 48 to 79 percent of the administered dose. Fasting increases absorption. Malabsorption syndromes, as well as dietary factors, (children's soybean formula, concomitant use of anionic exchange resins such as cholestyramine) cause excessive fecal loss. Liothyronine (T3) is almost totally absorbed, 95 percent in 4 hours. The hormones contained in the natural preparations are absorbed in a manner similar to the synthetic hormones.

More than 99 percent of circulating hormones are bound to serum proteins, including thyroid-binding globulin (TBg), thyroid-binding pre-albumin (TBPA), and albumin (TBa), whose capacities and affinities vary for the hormones. The higher affinity of levothyroxine (T4) for both TBg and TBPA, as compared to liothyronine (T3), partially explains the higher serum levels and longer half-life of the former hormone. Both protein-bound hormones exist in reverse equilibrium with minute amounts of free hormone, the latter accounting for the metabolic activity. Deiodination of levothyroxine (T4) occurs at a number of sites, including liver, kidney, and other tissues. The conjugated hormone, in the form of glucuronide or sulfate, is found in the bile and gut where it may complete an enterohepatic circulation. Eighty-five percent of levothyroxine (T4) metabolized daily is deiodinated.

INDICATIONS AND USAGE

1. As replacement of supplemental therapy in patients with hypothyroidism of any etiology, except transient hypothyroidism during the recovery phase of subacute thyroiditis. This category includes cretinism, myxedema, and ordinary hypothyroidism in patients of any age (children, adults, the elderly), or state (including pregnancy); primary hypothyroidism resulting from functional deficiency, primary atrophy, partial or total absence of thyroid gland, or the effects of surgery, radiation, or drugs, with or without the presence of goiter; and secondary (pituitary), or tertiary (hypothalamic) hypothyroidism (See WARNINGS).

2. As pituitary TSH suppressants, in the treatment or prevention of various types of euthyroid goiters, including thyroid nodules, subacute, or chronic lymphocytic thyroiditis (Hashimoto's), multinodular goiter, and in the management of thyroid cancer.

3. As diagnostic agents in suppression tests to differentiate suspected mild hyperthyroidism or thyroid gland anatomy.

CONTRAINDICATIONS

Thyroid hormone preparations are generally contraindicated in patients with diagnosed, but as yet, uncorrected adrenal cortical insufficiency, untreated thyrotoxicosis, and apparent hypersensitivity to any of their active or extraneous constituents. There is no well documented evidence in the literature of true allergic or idiosyncratic reactions to thyroid hormone.

WARNINGS

Drugs with thyroid hormone activity, alone or together with other therapeutic agents, have been used for the treatment of obesity. In euthyroid patients, doses within the range of daily hormonal requirements are ineffective for weight reduction. Larger doses may produce serious or even life-threatening manifestations of toxicity, particularly when given in association with sympathomimetic amines such as those used for their anorectic effects.

The use of thyroid hormones in the therapy of obesity, alone or combined with other drugs, is unjustified and has been shown to be ineffective. Neither is their use justified for the treatment of male or female infertility unless this condition is accompanied by hypothyroidism.

PRECAUTIONS

General: Thyroid hormones should be used with great caution in a number of circumstances where the integrity of the cardiovascular system, particularly the coronary arteries, is suspected. These include patients with angina pectoris or the elderly, whom have a greater likelihood of occult cardiac disease. With these patients, therapy should be initiated with low doses, i.e. 16.25 - 32.5 mg. When, in such patients, a euthyroid state can only be reached at the expense of an aggravation of the cardiovascular disease, thyroid hormone dosage should be reduced.

Thyroid hormone therapy in patients with concomitant diabetes mellitus or diabetes insipidus or adrenal cortical insufficiency aggravates the intensity of their symptoms. Appropriate adjustments of the various therapeutic measures directed at these concomitant endocrine diseases are required. The therapy of myxedema coma requires simultaneous administration of glucorticoids (See DOSAGE AND ADMINISTRATION).

Hypothyroidism decreases and hyperthyroidism increases the sensitivity to oral anticoagulants. Prothrombin time should be closely monitored in thyroid treated patients on oral anticoagulants and dosage of the latter agents should be adjusted on the basis of frequent prothrombin time determinations. In infants, excessive doses of thyroid hormone preparations may produce craniosynostosis.

Information for the Patient: Patients on thyroid hormone preparations and parents of children on thyroid therapy should be informed that:

1. Replacement therapy is to be taken essentially for life, with the exception of cases of transient hypothyroidism, usually associated with thyroiditis, and in those patients receiving a therapeutic trial of the drug.

2. They should immediately report, during the course of therapy, any signs or symptoms of thyroid hormone toxicity, e.g., chest pain, increased pulse rate, palpitations, excessive sweating, heat intolerance, nervousness, or any other unusual event.

3. In case of concomitant diabetes mellitus, the daily dosage of antidiabetic medication may need readjustment as thyroid hormone replacement is achieved. If thyroid medication is stopped, a downward readjustment of the dosage of insulin or oral hypoglycemic agent may be necessary to avoid hypoglycemia. At all times, close monitoring of urinary glucose levels is mandatory in such patients.

4. In case of concomitant oral anticoagulant therapy, the prothrombin time should be measured frequently to determine if the dosage of oral anticoagulants is to be readjusted.

5. Partial loss of hair may be experienced by children in the first few months of thyroid therapy, but this is usually a transient phenomenon and later recovery is usually the rule.

Laboratory Tests: Treatment of patients with thyroid hormones requires the periodic assessment of thyroid status by means of appropriate laboratory tests, besides the full clinical evaluation. The TSH suppression test can be used to test the effectiveness of any thyroid preparation, bearing in mind the relative insensitivity of the infant pituitary to the negative feedback effect of thyroid hormones. SerumT4 levels can be used to test the effectiveness of all thyroid medications except T3. When the total serum T4 is low but TSH is normal, a test specific to assess unbound (free) T4 levels is warranted. Specific measurements of T4 and T3 by competitive protein binding or radioimmunoassay are not influenced by blood levels of organic or inorganic iodine.

Drug Interactions: Oral Anticoagulants—Thyroid hormones appear to increase catabolism of vitamin K-dependent clotting factors. If oral anticoagulants are also being given, compensatory increases in clotting factor synthesis are impaired. Patients stabilized on oral anticoagulants that are found to require thyroid replacement therapy should be watched very closely when thyroid is started. If a patient is truly hypothyroid, it is likely that a reduction in anticoagulant dosage will be required. No special precautions appear to be necessary when oral anticoagulant therapy is begun in a patient already stabilized on maintenance thyroid replacement therapy.

Insulin or Oral Hypoglycemic—Initiating thyroid replacement therapy may cause increases in insulin or oral hypoglycemic requirements. The effects seen are poorly understood and depend upon a variety of factors such as dose and type of thyroid preparations and endocrine status of the patient. Patients receiving insulin or oral hypoglycemic should be closely watched during initiation of thyroid replacement therapy.

Cholestyramine or Colestipol—Cholestyramine or Colestipol binds both levothyroxine (T4) and liothyronine (T3) in the intestine, thus impairing absorption of these thyroid hormones. In vitro studies indicate that the binding is not easily removed. Therefore, four to five hours should elapse between administration of Cholestyramine or Colestipol and thyroid hormones.

Estrogen, Oral Contraceptives—Estrogens tend to increase serum thyroxine-binding globulin (TBg). In a patient with a nonfunctioning thyroid gland who is receiving thyroid replacement therapy, free levothyroxine (T4) may be decreased when estrogens are started thus increasing thyroid requirements. However, if the patient's thyroid gland has sufficient function, the decreased free levothyroxine (T4) will result in a compensatory increase in levothyroxine (T4) output by the thyroid. Therefore, patients without a functioning thyroid gland who are on thyroid replacement therapy, may need to increase their thyroid dose if estrogens or estrogen-containing oral contraceptives are given.

Drug/Laboratory Test Interactions: The following drugs or moieties are known to interfere with laboratory tests performed in patients on thyroid hormone therapy: androgens, corticosteroids, estrogens, oral contraceptives containing estrogens, iodine-containing preparations, and the numerous preparations containing salicylates.

1. Changes in TBg concentration should be taken into consideration in the interpretation of levothyroxine (T4) and liothyronine (T3) values. In such cases, the unbound (free) hormone should be measured. Pregnancy, estrogens, and estrogen-containing oral contraceptives increase TBg concentrations. TBg may also be increased during infectious hepatitis. Decreases in TBg concentrations are observed in nephrosis, acromegaly, and after androgen or corticosteroid therapy. Familial hyper or hypothyroxine-binding-globulinemias have been described. The incidence of TBg deficiency approximates 1 in 9,000. The binding of levothyroxine by TBPA is inhibited by salicylates.

2. Medicinal or dietary iodine interferes with all in vivo tests of radio-iodine uptake, producing low uptakes which may not be relative of a true decrease in hormone synthesis.

3. The persistence of clinical and laboratory evidence of hypothyroidism in spite of adequate dosage replacement indicates; either poor patient compliance, poor absorption, excessive fecal loss, or inactivity of the preparation. Intracellular resistance to thyroid hormone is quite rare.

Carcinogenesis, Mutagenesis, and Impairment of Fertility: A reportedly apparent association between prolonged thyroid therapy and breast cancer has not been confirmed and patients on thyroid for established indications should not discontinue therapy. No confirmatory long-term studies in animals have been performed to evaluate carcinogenic potential, mutagenicity, or impairment of fertility in either males or females.

Pregnancy-Category A: Thyroid hormones do not readily cross the placental barrier. The clinical experience to date does not indicate any adverse effect on fetuses when thyroid hormones are administered to pregnant women. On the basis of current knowledge, thyroid replacement therapy to hypothyroid women should not be discontinued during pregnancy.

Nursing Mothers: Minimal amounts of thyroid hormones are excreted in human milk. Thyroid is not associated with serious adverse reactions and does not have a known tumorigenic potential. However, caution should be exercised when thyroid is administered to a nursing woman.

Pediatric Use: Pregnant mothers provide little or no thyroid hormone to the fetus. The incidence of congenital hypothyroidism is relatively high (1:4,000) and the hypothyroid fetus would not derive any benefit from the small amounts of hormone crossing the placental barrier. Routine determination of serumT4 and/or TSH is strongly advised in neonates in view of the deleterious effects of thyroid deficiency on growth and development. Treatment should be initiated immediately upon diagnosis, and maintained for life, unless transient hypothyroidism is suspected; in which case, therapy may be interrupted for 2 to 8 weeks after the age of 3 years to reassess the condition. Cessation of therapy is justified in patients who have maintained a normal TSH during those 2 to 8 weeks.

Geriatric use: Clinical studies of Thyroid Tablets, USP did not include sufficient numbers of subjects aged 65 and over to determine whether they respond differently from younger subjects. Other reported clinical experience has not identified differences in responses between the elderly and younger patients. In general, dose selection for an elderly patient should be cautious, usually starting at the low end of the dosing range, reflecting the greater frequency of decreased hepatic, renal, or cardiac function, and of concomitant disease or other drug therapy.

ADVERSE REACTIONS

Adverse reactions other than those indicative of hyperthyroidism because of therapeutic overdosage, either initially or during the maintenance period, are rare (See OVERDOSAGE).

OVERDOSAGE

Signs and Symptoms: Excessive doses of thyroid result in a hypermetabolic state resembling in every respect the condition of endogenous origin. The condition may be self induced.

Treatment of Overdosage: Dosage should be reduced or therapy temporarily discontinued signs and symptoms of overdosage appear.

Treatment may be reinstituted at a lower dosage. In normal individuals, normal hypothalamic-pituitary-thyroid axis function is restored in 6 to 8 weeks after thyroid suppression.

Treatment of acute massive thyroid hormone overdosage is aimed at reducing gastrointestinal absorption of the drugs and counteracting central and peripheral effects, mainly those of increased sympathetic activity. Vomiting may be induced initially if further gastrointestinal absorption can reasonably be prevented and barring contraindications such as coma, convulsions, or loss of the gagging reflex. Treatment is symptomatic and supportive. Oxygen may be administered and ventilation maintained. Cardiac glycosides may be indicated if congestive heart failure develops. Measures to control fever, hypoglycemia, or fluid loss should be instituted if needed. Antiadrenergic agents, particularly propranolol, have been used advantageously in the treatment of increased sympathetic activity. Propranolol may be administered intravenously at a dosage of 1 to 3 mg, over a 10 minute period or orally, 80 to 160 mg/day, initially, especially when no contraindications exist for its use.

DOSAGE AND ADMINISTRATION

The dosage of thyroid hormones is determined by the indication and must in every case be individualized according to patient response and laboratory findings.

Thyroid hormones are given orally. In acute, emergency conditions, injectable levothyroxine sodium (T4) may be given intravenously when oral administration is not feasible or desirable (as in the treatment of myxedema coma, or during parenteral nutrition). Intramuscular administration is not advisable because of reported poor absorption.

Hypothyroidism: Therapy is usually instituted using low doses, with increments which depend on the cardiovascular status of the patient. The usual starting dose is 32.5 mg, with increment of 16.25 mg every 2 to 3 weeks. A lower starting dosage, 16.25 mg/day, is recommended in patients with longstanding myxedema, particularly if cardiovascular impairment is suspected, in which case extreme caution is recommended. The appearance of angina is an indication for reduction in dosage. Most patients require 65 - 130 mg/day. Failure to respond to doses of 195 mg suggests lack of compliance or malabsorption. Maintenance dosages 65 - 130 mg/day usually result in normal serum T4 and T3 levels. Adequate therapy usually results in normal TSH and T4 levels after 2 or 3 weeks of therapy.

Readjustment of thyroid hormone dosage should be made within the first four weeks of therapy, after proper clinical and laboratory evaluations, including serum levels of T4, bound and free, and TSH.

Liothyronine (T3) may be used in preference to levothyroxine (T4) during radio-isotope scanning procedures, since induction of hypothyroidism in those cases is more abrupt and can be of shorter duration. It may also be preferred when impairment of peripheral conversion of levothyroxine (T4) and liothyronine (T3) is suspected.

Myxedema Coma: Myxedema coma is usually precipitated in the hypothyroid patient of longstanding by intercurrent illness or drugs such as sedatives and anesthetics and should be considered a medical emergency. Therapy should be directed at the correction of electrolyte disturbances and possible infection, besides the administration of thyroid hormones. Corticosteroids should be administered routinely. Levothyroxine (T4) and Liothyronine (T3) may be administered via a nasogastric tube, but the preferred route of administration of both hormones is intravenous. Levothyroxine sodium (T4) is given at a starting dose of 400 mcg (100 mcg/mL) given rapidly, and is usually well tolerated, even in the elderly. This initial dose is followed by daily supplements of 100 to 200 mcg given IV. Normal T4 levels are achieved in 24 hours, followed in 3 days by threefold elevation of T3. Oral therapy with thyroid hormone would be resumed as soon as the clinical situation has been stabilized and the patient is able to take oral medication.

Thyroid Cancer: Exogenous thyroid hormone may produce regression of metastases from follicular and papillary carcinoma of the thyroid and is used as ancillary therapy of these conditions with radioactive iodine. TSH should be suppressed to low or undetectable levels. Therefore, larger amounts of thyroid hormone than those used for replacement therapy are required. Medullary carcinoma of the thyroid is usually unresponsive to this therapy.

Thyroid Suppression Therapy: Administration of thyroid hormone in doses higher than those produced physiologically by the gland results in suppression of the production of endogenous hormone. This is the basis for the thyroid suppression test and is used as an aid in the diagnosis of patients with signs of mild hyperthyroidism, in whom base line laboratory tests appear normal, or to demonstrate thyroid gland autonomy in patients with Grave's ophthalmopathy. 1 uptake is determined before and after the administration of the exogenous hormone. A fifty percent or greater suppression of uptake indicates a normal thyroid pituitary axis, and thus rules out thyroid gland autonomy.

For adults, the usual suppressive dose of levothyroxine (T4) is 1.56 mg/kg of body weight per day given for 7 to 10 days. These doses usually yield normal serum T4 and T3 levels and lack of response to TSH.

Thyroid hormones should be administered cautiously to patients in whom there is strong suspicion of thyroid gland autonomy, in view of the fact that the exogenous hormone effects will be additive to the endogenous source.

Pediatric Dosage: Pediatric dosage should follow the recommendations summarized in Table 1. In infants with congenital hypothyroidism, therapy with full doses should be instituted as soon as the diagnosis has been made.

TABLE 1. Recommended Pediatric Dosage for Congenital Hypothyroidism

Age	Dose per day	Daily dose per kg of body weight
0 - 6 months	16.25 - 32.5 mg	4.8-6.0 mg
6 - 12 months	32.5 - 48.75 mg	3.6-4.8 mg
1 - 5 years	48.75 - 65 mg	3.0-3.6 mg
6 - 12 years	65 - 97.5 mg	2.4-3.0 mg
Over 12 years	Over 97.5 mg	1.2-1.8 mg

HOW SUPPLIED

Nature-Throid® (Thyroid USP) Tablets are supplied as follows:

16.25 mg. (1/4 gr.) in bottles of 30 Count (NDC 64727-3298-4), 60 Count (NDC 64727-3298-5), 90 Count (NDC 64727-3298-6), 100 Count (NDC 64727-3298-1), 1,000 Count (NDC 64727-3298-2), 990 Count (NDC 64727-3298-3) & 1,008 Count (NDC 64727-3298-8)

32.5 mg. (1/2 gr.) in bottles of 30 Count (NDC 64727-3299-4), 60 Count (NDC 64727-3299-5), 90 Count (NDC 64727-3299-6), 100 Count (NDC 64727-3299-1), 1,000 Count (NDC 64727-3299-2), 990 Count (NDC 64727-3299-3) & 1,008 Count (NDC 64727-3299-8)

48.75 mg. (3/4 gr.) in bottles of 30 Count (NDC 64727-3302-4), 60 Count (NDC 64727-3302-5), 90 Count (NDC 64727-3302-6), 100 Count (NDC 64727-3302-1), 1,000 Count (NDC 64727-3302-2), 990 Count (NDC 64727-3302-3) & 1,008 Count (NDC 64727-3302-8)

65 mg. (1 gr.) in bottles of 30 Count (NDC 64727-3300-4), 60 Count (NDC 64727-3300-5), 90 Count (NDC 64727-3300-6), 100 Count (NDC 64727-3300-1), 1,000 Count (NDC 64727-3300-2), 990 Count (NDC 64727-3300-3) & 1,008 Count (NDC 64727-3300-8)

81.25 mg. (1 1/4 gr.) in bottles of 30 Count (NDC 64727-3303-4), 60 Count (NDC 64727-3303-5), 90 Count (NDC 64727-3303-6), 100 Count (NDC 64727-3303-1), 1,000 Count (NDC 64727-3303-2), 990 Count (NDC 64727-3303-3) & 1,008 Count (NDC 64727-3303-8)

97.5 mg. (1 1/2 gr.) in bottles of 30 Count (NDC 64727-3305-4), 60 Count (NDC 64727-3305-5), 90 Count (NDC 64727-3305-6), 100 Count (NDC 64727-3305-1), 1,000 Count (NDC 64727-3305-2), 990 Count (NDC 64727-3305-3) & 1,008 Count (NDC 64727-3305-8)

113.75 mg. (1 3/4 gr.) in bottles of 30 Count (NDC 64727-3307-4), 60 Count (NDC 64727-3307-5), 90 Count (NDC 64727-3307-6), 100 Count (NDC 64727-3307-1), 1,000 Count (NDC 64727-3307-2), 990 Count (NDC 64727-3307-3) & 1,008 Count (NDC 64727-3307-8)

130 mg. (2 gr.) in bottles of 30 Count (NDC 64727-3308-4), 60 Count (NDC 64727-3308-5), 90 Count (NDC 64727-3308-6), 100 Count (NDC 64727-3308-1), 1,000 Count (NDC 64727-3308-2), 990 Count (NDC 64727-3308-3) & 1,008 Count (NDC 64727-3308-8)

146.25 mg. (2 1/4 gr.) in bottles of 30 Count (NDC 64727-3309-4), 60 Count (NDC 64727-3309-5), 90 Count (NDC 64727-3309-6), 100 Count (NDC 64727-3309-1), 1,000 Count (NDC 64727-3309-2), 990 Count (NDC 64727-3309-3) & 1,008 Count (NDC 64727-3309-8)

162.5 mg. (2 1/2 gr.) in bottles of 30 Count (NDC 64727-3310-4), 60 Count (NDC 64727-3310-5), 90 Count (NDC 64727-3310-6), 100 Count (NDC 64727-3310-1), 1,000 Count (NDC 64727-3310-2), 990 Count (NDC 64727-3310-3) & 1,008 Count (NDC 64727-3310-8)

195 mg. (3 gr.) in bottles of 30 Count (NDC 64727-3312-4), 60 Count (NDC 64727-3312-5), 90 Count (NDC 64727-3312-6), 100 Count (NDC 64727-3312-1), 1,000 Count (NDC 64727-3312-2), 990 Count (NDC 64727-3312-3) & 1,008 Count (NDC 64727-3312-8)

260 mg. (4 gr.) in bottles of 30 Count (NDC 64727-3320-4), 60 Count (NDC 64727-3320-5), 90 Count (NDC 64727-3320-6), 100 Count (NDC 64727-3320-1), 1,000 Count (NDC 64727-3320-2), 990 Count (NDC 64727-3320-3) & 1,008 Count (NDC 64727-3320-8)

325 mg. (5 gr.) in bottles of 30 Count (NDC 64727-3340-4), 60 Count (NDC 64727-3340-

6), 100 Count (NDC 64727-3340-1), 1,000 Count (NDC 64727-3340-2), 990 Count (NDC 64727-3340-3) & 1,008 Count (NDC 64727-3340-8)

STORAGE: Store at controlled room temperature; 15°-30°C (59°-86°F)

Dispense in tight, light-resistant containers as defined in the USP/NF

Rx Only.

Distributed by:

RLC LABS

Cave Creek, AZ 85331

Rev051309/01   SCD#700809-1

Shown in Product Identification Guide, page 312

WP THYROID®
(Thyroid USP)
Tablets   Rx

DESCRIPTION

WP Thyroid® (Thyroid USP) Tablets, for oral use, are natural preparations derived from porcine thyroid glands (T3 liothyronine is approximately four times as potent as T4 levothyroxine on a microgram for microgram basis). They provide 38 mcg levothyroxine (T4) and 9 mcg liothyronine (T3) for each 65 mg (1 Grain) of the labeled content of thyroid.

INACTIVE INGREDIENTS

Inulin, Medium Chain Triglycerides, Lactose Monohydrate[1] The structural formulas of liothyronine (T3) and levothyroxine (T4) are as follows:

[1]Present in traceable amount as part of Thyroid USP (diluent)

CLINICAL PHARMACOLOGY

The steps in the synthesis of the thyroid hormones are controlled by thyrotropin (Thyroid Stimulating Hormone, TSH) secreted by the anterior pituitary. This hormone's secretion is in turn controlled by a feedback mechanism affected by the thyroid hormones themselves and by thyrotropin releasing hormone (TRH), a tripeptide of hypothalamic origin. Endogenous thyroid hormone secretion is suppressed when exogenous thyroid hormones are administered to euthyroid individuals in excess of the normal gland's secretion.

The mechanisms by which thyroid hormones exert their physiologic action are not well understood. These hormones enhance oxygen consumption by most tissues of the body, increase the basal metabolic rate, and the metabolism of carbohydrates, lipids, and proteins. Thus, they exert a profound influence on every organ system in the body and are of particular importance in the development of the central nervous system.

The normal thyroid gland contains approximately 200 mcg of levothyroxine (T4) per gram of gland, and 15 mcg of liothyronine (T3) per gram. The ratio of these two hormones in the circulation does not represent the ratio in the thyroid gland, since about 80 percent of peripheral liothyronine (T3) comes from monodeiodination of levothyroxine (T4). Peripheral monodeiodination of levothyroxine (T4) at the 5 position (inner ring) also results in the formation of reverse liothyronine (T3), which is calorigenically inactive. Liothyronine (T3) levels are low in the fetus and newborn, in old age, in chronic caloric deprivation, hepatic cirrhosis, renal failure, surgical stress, and chronic illnesses representing what has been called the "T3 thyronine syndrome".

Pharmacokinetics

Animal studies have shown that levothyroxine (T4) is only partially absorbed from the gastrointestinal tract. The degree of absorption is dependent on the vehicle used for its administration and by the character of the intestinal contents, the intestinal flora, including plasma protein, and soluble dietary factors, all of which bind thyroid, thereby making it unavailable for diffusion. Only 41 percent is absorbed when given in a gelatin capsule, as opposed to 74 percent absorption when given with an albumin carrier.

Depending on other factors, absorption has varied from 48 to 79 percent of the administered dose. Fasting increases absorption. Malabsorption syndromes, as well as dietary factors, (children's soybean formula, concomitant use of an-

ionic exchange resins such as cholestyramine) cause excessive fecal loss. Liothyronine (T3) is almost totally absorbed, 95 percent in 4 hours. The hormones contained in the natural preparations are absorbed in a manner similar to the synthetic hormones.

More than 99 percent of circulating hormones are bound to serum proteins, including thyroid-binding globulin (TBg), thyroid-binding pre-albumin (TBPA), and albumin (TBa), whose capacities and affinities vary for the hormones. The higher affinity of levothyroxine (T4) for both TBg and TBPA, as compared to liothyronine (T3), partially explains the higher serum levels and longer half-life of the former hormone. Both protein-bound hormones exist in reverse equilibrium with minute amounts of free hormone, the latter accounting for the metabolic activity. Deiodination of levothyroxine (T4) occurs at a number of sites, including liver, kidney, and other tissues. The conjugated hormone, in the form of glucuronide or sulfate, is found in the bile and gut where it may complete an enterohepatic circulation. Eighty-five percent of levothyroxine (T4) metabolized daily is deiodinated.

INDICATIONS AND USAGE

1. As replacement of supplemental therapy in patients with hypothyroidism of any etiology, except transient hypothyroidism during the recovery phase of subacute thyroiditis. This category includes cretinism, myxedema, and ordinary hypothyroidism in patients of any age (children, adults, the elderly), or state (including pregnancy); primary hypothyroidism resulting from functional deficiency, primary atrophy, partial or total absence of thyroid gland, or the effects of surgery, radiation, or drugs, with or without the presence of goiter; and secondary (pituitary), or tertiary (hypothalamic) hypothyroidism (See WARNINGS).

2. As pituitary TSH suppressants, in the treatment or prevention of various types of euthyroid goiters, including thyroid nodules, subacute, or chronic lymphocytic thyroiditis (Hashimoto's), multinodular goiter, and in the management of thyroid cancer.

3. As diagnostic agents in suppression tests to differentiate suspected mild hyperthyroidism or thyroid gland anatomy.

CONTRAINDICATIONS

Thyroid hormone preparations are generally contraindicated in patients with diagnosed, but as yet, uncorrected adrenal cortical insufficiency, untreated thyrotoxicosis, and apparent hypersensitivity to any of their active or extraneous constituents. There is no well documented evidence in the literature of true allergic or idiosyncratic reactions to thyroid hormone.

WARNINGS

Drugs with thyroid hormone activity, alone or together with other therapeutic agents, have been used for the treatment of obesity. In euthyroid patients, doses within the range of daily hormonal requirements are ineffective for weight reduction. Larger doses may produce serious or even life-threatening manifestations of toxicity, particularly when given in association with sympathomimetic amines such as those used for their anorectic effects.

The use of thyroid hormones in the therapy of obesity, alone or combined with other drugs, is unjustified and has been shown to be ineffective. Neither is their use justified for the treatment of male or female infertility unless this condition is accompanied by hypothyroidism.

PRECAUTIONS

General: Thyroid hormones should be used with great caution in a number of circumstances where the integrity of the cardiovascular system, particularly the coronary arteries, is suspected. These include patients with angina pectoris or the elderly, whom have a greater likelihood of occult cardiac disease. With these patients, therapy should be initiated with low doses, i.e. 16.25 - 32.5 mg. When, in such patients, a euthyroid state can only be reached at the expense of an aggravation of the cardiovascular disease, thyroid hormone dosage should be reduced.

Thyroid hormone therapy in patients with concomitant diabetes mellitus or diabetes insipidus or adrenal cortical insufficiency aggravates the intensity of their symptoms. Appropriate adjustments of the various therapeutic measures directed at these concomitant endocrine diseases are required. The therapy of myxedema coma requires simultaneous administration of glucorticoids (See DOSAGE AND ADMINISTRATION).

Hypothyroidism decreases and hyperthyroidism increases the sensitivity to oral anticoagulants. Prothrombin time should be closely monitored in thyroid treated patients on oral anticoagulants and dosage of the latter agents should be adjusted on the basis of frequent prothrombin time determinations. In infants, excessive doses of thyroid hormone preparations may produce craniosynostosis.

Information for the Patient: Patients on thyroid hormone preparations and parents of children on thyroid therapy should be informed that:

1. Replacement therapy is to be taken essentially for life, with the exception of cases of transient hypothyroidism, usually associated with thyroiditis, and in those patients receiving a therapeutic trial of the drug.

2. They should immediately report, during the course of therapy, any signs or symptoms of thyroid hormone toxicity, e.g., chest pain, increased pulse rate, palpitations, excessive sweating, heat intolerance, nervousness, or any other unusual event.

3. In case of concomitant diabetes mellitus, the daily dosage of antidiabetic medication may need readjustment as thyroid hormone replacement is achieved. If thyroid medication is stopped, a downward readjustment of the dosage of insulin or oral hypoglycemic agent may be necessary to avoid hypoglycemia. At all times, close monitoring of urinary glucose levels is mandatory in such patients.

4. In case of concomitant oral anticoagulant therapy, the prothrombin time should be measured frequently to determine if the dosage of oral anticoagulants is to be readjusted.

5. Partial loss of hair may be experienced by children in the first few months of thyroid therapy, but this is usually a transient phenomenon and later recovery is usually the rule.

Laboratory Tests: Treatment of patients with thyroid hormones requires the periodic assessment of thyroid status by means of appropriate laboratory tests, besides the full clinical evaluation. The TSH suppression test can be used to test the effectiveness of any thyroid preparation, bearing in mind the relative insensitivity of the infant pituitary to the negative feedback effect of thyroid hormones. Serum T4 levels can be used to test the effectiveness of all thyroid medications except T3. When the total serum T4 is low but TSH is normal, a test specific to assess unbound (free) T4 levels is warranted. Specific measurements of T4 and T3 by competitive protein binding or radioimmunoassay are not influenced by blood levels of organic or inorganic iodine.

Drug Interactions: Oral Anticoagulants-Thyroid hormones appear to increase catabolism of vitamin K- dependent clotting factors. If oral anticoagulants are also being given, compensatory increases in clotting factor synthesis are impaired. Patients stabilized on oral anticoagulants that are found to require thyroid replacement therapy should be watched very closely when thyroid is started. If a patient is truly hypothyroid, it is likely that a reduction in anticoagulant dosage will be required. No special precautions appear to be necessary when oral anticoagulant therapy is begun in a patient already stabilized on maintenance thyroid replacement therapy.

Insulin or Oral Hypoglycemic-Initiating thyroid replacement therapy may cause increases in insulin or oral hypoglycemic requirements. The effects seen are poorly understood and depend upon a variety of factors such as dose and type of thyroid preparations and endocrine status of the patient. Patients receiving insulin or oral hypoglycemic should be closely watched during initiation of thyroid replacement therapy.

Cholestyramine or Colestipol- Cholestyramine or Colestipol binds both levothyroxine (T4) and liothyronine (T3) in the intestine, thus impairing absorption of these thyroid hormones. In vitro studies indicate that the binding is not easily removed. Therefore, four to five hours should elapse between administration of Cholestyramine or Colestipol and thyroid hormones.

Estrogen, Oral Contraceptives- Estrogens tend to increase serum thyroxine-binding globulin (TBg). In a patient with a nonfunctioning thyroid gland who is receiving thyroid replacement therapy, free levothyroxine (T4) may be decreased when estrogens are started thus increasing thyroid requirements. However, if the patient's thyroid gland has sufficient function, the decreased free levothyroxine (T4) will result in a compensatory increase in levothyroxine (T4) output by the thyroid. Therefore, patients without a functioning thyroid gland who are on thyroid replacement therapy, may need to increase their thyroid dose if estrogens or estrogen-containing oral contraceptives are given.

Drug/Laboratory Test Interactions: The following drugs or moieties are known to interfere with laboratory tests performed in patients on thyroid hormone therapy: androgens, corticosteroids, estrogens, oral contraceptives containing estrogens, iodine-containing preparations, and the numerous preparations containing salicylates.

1. Changes in TBg concentration should be taken into consideration in the interpretation of levothyroxine (T4) and liothyronine (T3) values. In such cases, the unbound (free) hormone should be measured. Pregnancy, estrogens, and estrogen-containing oral contraceptives increase TBg concentrations. TBg may also be increased during infectious hepatitis. Decreases in TBg concentrations are observed in nephrosis, acromegaly, and after androgen or corticosteroid therapy. Familial hyper or hypothyroxine-binding-globulinemias have been described. The incidence of TBg deficiency approximates 1 in 9,000. The binding of levothyroxine by TBPA is inhibited by salicylates.

2. Medicinal or dietary iodine interferes with all in vivo tests of radio-iodine uptake, producing low uptakes which may not be relative of a true decrease in hormone synthesis.

3. The persistence of clinical and laboratory evidence of hypothyroidism in spite of adequate dosage replacement indicates; either poor patient compliance, poor absorption, excessive fecal loss, or inactivity of the preparation. Intracellular resistance to thyroid hormone is quite rare.

Carcinogenesis, Mutagenesis, and Impairment of Fertility: A reportedly apparent association between prolonged thyroid therapy and breast cancer has not been confirmed and patients on thyroid for established indications should not discontinue therapy. No confirmatory long-term studies in animals have been performed to evaluate carcinogenic potential, mutagenicity, or impairment of fertility in either males or females.

Pregnancy-Category A: Thyroid hormones do not readily cross the placental barrier. The clinical experience to date does not indicate any adverse effect on fetuses when thyroid hormones are administered to pregnant women. On the basis of current knowledge, thyroid replacement therapy to hypothyroid women should not be discontinued during pregnancy.

Nursing Mothers: Minimal amounts of thyroid hormones are excreted in human milk. Thyroid is not associated with serious adverse reactions and does not have a known tumorigenic potential. However, caution should be exercised when thyroid is administered to a nursing woman.

Pediatric Use: Pregnant mothers provide little or no thyroid hormone to the fetus. The incidence of congenital hypothyroidism is relatively high (1:4,000) and the hypothyroid fetus would not derive any benefit from the small amounts of hormone crossing the placental barrier. Routine determination of serum T4 and/or TSH is strongly advised in neonates in view of the deleterious effects of thyroid deficiency on growth and development. Treatment should be initiated immediately upon diagnosis, and maintained for life, unless transient hypothyroidism is suspected; in which case, therapy may be interrupted for 2 to 8 weeks after the age of 3 years to reassess the condition. Cessation of therapy is justified in patients who have maintained a normal TSH during those 2 to 8 weeks.

Geriatric use: Clinical studies of Thyroid Tablets, USP did not include sufficient numbers of subjects aged 65 and over to determine whether they respond differently from younger subjects. Other reported clinical experience has not identified differences in responses between the elderly and younger patients. In general, dose selection for an elderly patient should be cautious, usually starting at the low end of the dosing range, reflecting the greater frequency of decreased hepatic, renal, or cardiac function, and of concomitant disease or other drug therapy.

ADVERSE REACTIONS

Adverse reactions other than those indicative of hyperthyroidism because of therapeutic overdosage, either initially or during the maintenance period, are rare (See OVERDOSAGE).

OVERDOSAGE

Signs and Symptoms: Excessive doses of thyroid result in a hypermetabolic state resembling in every respect the condition of endogenous origin. The condition may be self induced.

Treatment of Overdosage: Dosage should be reduced or therapy temporarily discontinued signs and symptoms of overdosage appear.

Treatment may be reinstituted at a lower dosage. In normal individuals, normal hypothalamic-pituitary-thyroid axis function is restored in 6 to 8 weeks after thyroid suppression.

Treatment of acute massive thyroid hormone overdosage is aimed at reducing gastrointestinal absorption of the drugs and counteracting central and peripheral effects, mainly those of increased sympathetic activity. Vomiting may be induced initially if further gastrointestinal absorption can reasonably be prevented and barring contraindications such as coma, convulsions, or loss of the gagging reflex. Treatment is symptomatic and supportive. Oxygen may be administered and ventilation maintained. Cardiac glycosides may be indicated if congestive heart failure develops. Measures to control fever, hypoglycemia, or fluid loss should be instituted if needed. Antiadrenergic agents, particularly propranolol, have been used advantageously in the treatment of increased sympathetic activity. Propranolol may be administered intravenously at a dosage of 1 to 3 mg, over a 10 minute period or orally, 80 to 160 mg/day, initially, especially when no contraindications exist for its use.

DOSAGE AND ADMINISTRATION

The dosage of thyroid hormones is determined by the indication and must in every case be individualized according to patient response and laboratory findings.

Thyroid hormones are given orally. In acute, emergency conditions, injectable levothyroxine sodium (T4) may be given intravenously when oral administration is not feasible or desirable (as in the treatment of myxedema coma, or during parenteral nutrition). Intramuscular administration is not advisable because of reported poor absorption.

Hypothyroidism: Therapy is usually instituted using low doses, with increments which depend on the cardiovascular status of the patient. The usual starting dose is 32.5 mg, with increment of 16.25 mg every 2 to 3 weeks. A lower starting dosage, 16.25 mg/day, is recommended in patients with longstanding myxedema, particularly if cardiovascular impairment is suspected, in which case extreme caution is recommended. The appearance of angina is an indication for reduction in dosage. Most patients require 65 - 130 mg/day. Failure to respond to doses of 195 mg suggests lack of compliance or malabsorption. Maintenance dosages 65 - 130 mg/day usually result in normal serum T4 and T3 levels. Adequate therapy usually results in normal TSH and T4 levels after 2 or 3 weeks of therapy.

Readjustment of thyroid hormone dosage should be made within the first four weeks of therapy, after proper clinical and laboratory evaluations, including serum levels of T4, bound and free, and TSH.

Liothyronine (T3) may be used in preference to levothyroxine (T4) during radio-isotope scanning procedures, since induction of hypothyroidism in those cases is more abrupt and can be of shorter duration. It may also be preferred when impairment of peripheral conversion of levothyroxine (T4) and liothyronine (T3) is suspected.

Myxedema Coma: Myxedema coma is usually precipitated in the hypothyroid patient of longstanding by intercurrent illness or drugs such as sedatives and anesthetics and should be considered a medical emergency. Therapy should be directed at the correction of electrolyte disturbances and possible infection, besides the administration of thyroid hormones. Corticosteroids should be administered routinely. Levothyroxine (T4) and Liothyronine (T3) may be administered via a nasogastric tube, but the preferred route of administration of both hormones is intravenous. Levothyroxine sodium (T4) is given at a starting dose of 400 mcg (100 mcg/mL) given rapidly, and is usually well tolerated, even in the elderly. This initial dose is followed by daily supplements of 100 to 200 mcg given IV. Normal T4 levels are achieved in 24 hours, followed in 3 days by threefold elevation of T3. Oral therapy with thyroid hormone would be resumed as soon as the clinical situation has been stabilized and the patient is able to take oral medication.

Thyroid Cancer: Exogenous thyroid hormone may produce regression of metastases from follicular and papillary carcinoma of the thyroid and is used as ancillary therapy of these conditions with radioactive iodine. TSH should be suppressed to low or undetectable levels. Therefore, larger amounts of thyroid hormone than those used for replacement therapy are required. Medullary carcinoma of the thyroid is usually unresponsive to this therapy.

Thyroid Suppression Therapy: Administration of thyroid hormone in doses higher than those produced physiologically by the gland results in suppression of the production of endogenous hormone. This is the basis for the thyroid suppression test and is used as an aid in the diagnosis of patients with signs of mild hyperthyroidism, in whom base line laboratory tests appear normal, or to demonstrate thyroid gland autonomy in patients with Grave's ophthalmopathy. 131I uptake is determined before and after the administration of the exogenous hormone. A fifty percent or greater suppression of uptake indicates a normal thyroid pituitary axis, and thus rules out thyroid gland autonomy.

For adults, the usual suppressive dose of levothyroxine (T4) is 1.56 mg/kg of body weight per day given for 7 to 10 days. These doses usually yield normal serum T4 and T3 levels and lack of response to TSH.

Thyroid hormones should be administered cautiously to patients in whom there is strong suspicion of thyroid gland autonomy, in view of the fact that the exogenous hormone effects will be additive to the endogenous source.

Pediatric Dosage: Pediatric dosage should follow the recommendations summarized in Table 1. In infants with congenital hypothyroidism, therapy with full doses should be instituted as soon as the diagnosis has been made.

TABLE 1. Recommended Pediatric Dosage for Congenital Hypothyroidism

Age	Dose per day	Daily dose per kg of body weight
0 - 6 months	16.25 - 32.5 mg	4.8-6.0 mg
6 - 12 months	32.5 - 48.75 mg	3.6-4.8 mg
1 - 5 years	48.75 - 65 mg	3.0-3.6 mg
6 - 12 years	65 - 97.5 mg	2.4-3.0 mg
Over 12 years	Over 97.5 mg	1.2-1.8 mg

HOW SUPPLIED

WP Thyroid® (Thyroid USP) Tablets are supplied as follows: 16.25 mg. (1/4 gr.) in bottles of 30 Count (NDC 64727-5450-4), 60 Count (NDC 64727-5450-5), 90 Count (NDC 64727-5450-6), 100 Count (NDC 64727-5450-1) & 1,000 Count (NDC 64727-5450-2)

32.5 mg. (1/2 gr.) in bottles of 30 Count (NDC 64727-5550-4), 60 Count (NDC 64727-5550-5), 90 Count (NDC 64727-5550-6), 100 Count (NDC 64727-5550-1) & 1,000 Count (NDC 64727-5550-2)

48.75 mg. (3/4 gr.) in bottles of 30 Count (NDC 64727-5650-4), 60 Count (NDC 64727-5650-5), 90 Count (NDC 64727-5650-6), 100 Count (NDC 64727-5650-1) & 1,000 Count (NDC 64727-5650-2)

65 mg. (1 gr.) in bottles of 30 Count (NDC 64727-5750-4), 60 Count (NDC 64727-5750-5), 90 Count (NDC 64727-5750-6), 100 Count (NDC 64727-5750-1) & 1,000 Count (NDC 64727-5750-2)

81.25 mg. (1 1/4 gr.) in bottles of 30 Count (NDC 64727-6050-4), 60 Count (NDC 64727-6050-5), 90 Count (NDC 64727-6050-6), 100 Count (NDC 64727-6050-1) & 1,000 Count (NDC 64727-6050-2)

97.5 mg. (1 1/2 gr.) in bottles of 30 Count (NDC 64727-5850-4), 60 Count (NDC 64727-5850-5), 90 Count (NDC 64727-5850-6), 100 Count (NDC 64727-5850-1) & 1,000 Count (NDC 64727-5850-2)

113.75 mg. (1 3/4 gr.) in bottles of 30 Count (NDC 64727-6150-4), 60 Count (NDC 64727-6150-5), 90 Count (NDC 64727-6150-6), 100 Count (NDC 64727-6150-1) & 1,000 Count (NDC 64727-6150-2)

130 mg. (2 gr.) in bottles of 30 Count (NDC 64727-5950-4), 60 Count (NDC 64727-5950-5), 90 Count (NDC 64727-5950-6), 100 Count (NDC 64727-5950-1) & 1,000 Count (NDC 64727-5950-2)

146.25 mg. (2 1/4 gr.) in bottles of 30 Count (NDC 64727-6250-4), 60 Count (NDC 64727-6250-5), 90 Count (NDC 64727-6250-6), 100 Count (NDC 64727-6250-1) & 1,000 Count (NDC 64727-6250-2)

162.5 mg. (2 1/2 gr.) in bottles of 30 Count (NDC 64727-6350-4), 60 Count (NDC 64727-6350-5), 90 Count (NDC 64727-6350-6), 100 Count (NDC 64727-6350-1) & 1,000 Count (NDC 64727-6350-2)

195 mg. (3 gr.) in bottles of 30 Count (NDC 64727-6450-4), 60 Count (NDC 64727-6450-5), 90 Count (NDC 64727-6450-6), 100 Count (NDC 64727-6450-1) & 1,000 Count (NDC 64727-6450-2)

STORAGE: Store at controlled room temperature; 15°-30°C (59°-86°F)

Dispense in tight, light-resistant containers as defined in the USP/NF

Rx Only.

Distributed by:
RLC® LABS
Cave Creek, AZ 85331
Rev:063191/01
SCD#700809-3

Shown in Product Identification Guide, page 312

Salix Pharmaceuticals, Inc.
8510 COLONNADE CENTER DRIVE
RALEIGH, NC 27615

Direct Inquiries to:
(866) 669-7597 Phone
(919) 862-1817 Fax
www.salix.com

For adverse events, product quality complaints and patient information requests:
Product Information Center
(800) 508-0024 Phone
(510) 595-8183 Fax
E-mail: customerservice@salix.com

APRISO™ ℞
(mesalamine)
extended-release capsules

HIGHLIGHTS OF PRESCRIBING INFORMATION
These highlights do not include all the information needed to use APRISO safely and effectively. See full prescribing information for APRISO.
APRISO™ (mesalamine) extended-release capsules
Initial U.S. Approval: 1987

---INDICATIONS AND USAGE---
- APRISO is a locally-acting aminosalicylate indicated for the maintenance of remission of ulcerative colitis in adults (1)

---DOSAGE AND ADMINISTRATION---
- Four APRISO capsules once daily (1.5 g/day) in the morning with or without food. Do not co-administer with antacids (2)

---DOSAGE FORMS AND STRENGTHS---
- Extended-release capsules: 0.375 g (3)

---CONTRAINDICATIONS---
- Hypersensitivity to salicylates, aminosalicylates, or any component of APRISO capsules (4)

---WARNINGS AND PRECAUTIONS---
- Renal impairment may occur. Assess renal function at the beginning of treatment and periodically during therapy (5.1)
- Acute exacerbation of colitis symptoms can occur (5.2)
- Use caution with pre-existing liver disease (5.4)

---ADVERSE REACTIONS---
- The most common adverse reactions (incidence ≥3%) are headache, diarrhea, upper abdominal pain, nausea, nasopharyngitis, flu or flu-like illness, sinusitis (6.1)

To report SUSPECTED ADVERSE REACTIONS, contact Salix Pharmaceuticals, Inc. at 1-800-508-0024 or FDA at 1-800-FDA-1088 or www.fda.gov/medwatch.

---DRUG INTERACTIONS---
- Do not co-administer with antacids (7.1)

---USE IN SPECIFIC POPULATIONS---
- Use with caution in patients with renal disease (5.1)
- Monitor blood cell counts in geriatric patients (8.5)
- Advise patients with phenylketonuria that APRISO contains aspartame (17.1)

See 17 for PATIENT COUNSELING INFORMATION
Revised: 07/2009

FULL PRESCRIBING INFORMATION

1 INDICATIONS AND USAGE
APRISO capsules are indicated for the maintenance of remission of ulcerative colitis in patients 18 years of age and older.

2 DOSAGE AND ADMINISTRATION
The recommended dose for maintenance of remission of ulcerative colitis in adult patients is 1.5 g (four APRISO capsules) orally once daily in the morning. APRISO may be taken without regard to meals. APRISO should not be co-administered with antacids. An evaluation of renal function is recommended before initiating therapy with APRISO.

3 DOSAGE FORMS AND STRENGTHS
Extended-release capsules containing 0.375 g mesalamine.

4 CONTRAINDICATIONS
APRISO is contraindicated in patients with hypersensitivity to salicylates or aminosalicylates or to any of the components of APRISO capsules.

5 WARNINGS AND PRECAUTIONS
5.1 Renal Impairment
Renal impairment, including minimal change nephropathy, acute and chronic interstitial nephritis, and, rarely, renal failure, has been reported in patients given products such as APRISO that contain mesalamine or are converted to mesalamine.

It is recommended that patients have an evaluation of renal function prior to initiation of APRISO therapy and periodically while on therapy. Exercise caution when using APRISO in patients with known renal dysfunction or a history of renal disease.

In animal studies, the kidney was the principal organ for toxicity [See Nonclinical Toxicology (13.2)]

5.2 Mesalamine-Induced Acute Intolerance Syndrome
Mesalamine has been associated with an acute intolerance syndrome that may be difficult to distinguish from a flare of inflammatory bowel disease. Although the exact frequency of occurrence has not been determined, it has occurred in 3% of patients in controlled clinical trials of mesalamine or sulfasalazine. Symptoms include cramping, acute abdominal pain and bloody diarrhea, sometimes fever, headache, and rash. If acute intolerance syndrome is suspected, promptly discontinue treatment with APRISO.

5.3 Hypersensitivity
Some patients who have experienced a hypersensitivity reaction to sulfasalazine may have a similar reaction to APRISO capsules or to other compounds that contain or are converted to mesalamine.

5.4 Hepatic Impairment
There have been reports of hepatic failure in patients with pre-existing liver disease who have been administered mesalamine. Caution should be exercised when administering APRISO to patients with liver disease.

6 ADVERSE REACTIONS
6.1 Clinical Studies Experience
The data described below reflect exposure to APRISO in 557 patients, including 354 exposed for at least 6 months and 250 exposed for greater than one year. APRISO was studied in two placebo-controlled trials (n = 367 treated with APRISO) and in one open-label, long-term study (n = 190 additional patients). The population consisted of patients with ulcerative colitis; the mean age was 47 years, 54% were female, and 93% were white. Patients received doses of APRISO 1.5 g administered orally once per day for six months in the placebo-controlled trials and for up to 24 months in the open-label study.

Because clinical studies are conducted under widely varying conditions, adverse reaction rates observed in the clinical trials of a drug cannot be directly compared to rates in the clinical trials of another drug and may not reflect the rates observed in practice.

In the two placebo-controlled trials, 59% of APRISO-treated patients experienced an adverse reaction compared with 64% of placebo patients. Most adverse reactions with APRISO were mild or moderate in severity. Severe adverse reactions occurred in 6% of APRISO-treated patients and 5% of placebo-treated patients. Discontinuations due to adverse reactions occurred in 11% of APRISO-treated patients and 17% of placebo-treated patients; the most common adverse reaction resulting in study discontinuation was recurrence of ulcerative colitis (APRISO 6%, placebo 14%). The most common reactions reported with APRISO (≥3%) are shown in Table 1 below.

Table 1: Treatment-Emergent Adverse Reactions during Clinical Trials Occurring in at Least 3% of APRISO-Treated Patients and at a Greater Rate than with Placebo

MedDRA Preferred Term	APRISO 1.5g/day N=367	Placebo N=185
Headache	11%	8%
Diarrhea	8%	7%
Abdominal Pain Upper	5%	3%
Nausea	4%	3%
Nasopharyngitis	4%	3%
Influenza & Influenza-like illness	4%	4%
Sinusitis	3%	3%

The following adverse reactions, presented by body system, were reported at a frequency less than 3% in patients treated with APRISO for up to 24 months in controlled and open-label trials.

Ear and Labyrinth Disorders: tinnitus, vertigo
Dermatological Disorder: alopecia

Gastrointestinal: abdominal pain lower, rectal hemorrhage

Laboratory Abnormalities: increased triglycerides, decreased hematocrit and hemoglobin

General Disorders and Administration Site Disorders: fatigue

Hepatic: hepatitis cholestatic, transaminases increased

Renal Disorders: creatinine clearance decreased, hematuria

Musculoskeletal: pain, arthralgia

Respiratory: dyspnea

6.2 Adverse Reaction Information from Other Sources

The following adverse reactions have been identified during clinical trials of a product similar to APRISO and post approval use of other mesalamine-containing products such as APRISO. Because many of these reactions are reported voluntarily from a population of unknown size, it is not always possible to reliably estimate their frequency or establish a causal relationship to drug exposure.

Body as a Whole: lupus-like syndrome, drug fever

Cardiovascular: pericarditis, pericardial effusion, myocarditis

Gastrointestinal: pancreatitis, cholecystitis, gastritis, gastroenteritis, gastrointestinal bleeding, perforated peptic ulcer

Hepatic: jaundice, cholestatic jaundice, hepatitis, liver necrosis, liver failure, Kawasaki-like syndrome including changes in liver enzymes

Hematologic: agranulocytosis, aplastic anemia

Neurological/Psychiatric: peripheral neuropathy, Guillain-Barré syndrome, transverse myelitis

Respiratory/Pulmonary: eosinophilic pneumonia, interstitial pneumonitis

Skin: psoriasis, pyoderma gangrenosum, erythema nodosum

Renal/Urogenital: reversible oligospermia

7 DRUG INTERACTIONS

Based on in vitro studies, APRISO is not expected to inhibit the metabolism of drugs that are substrates of CYP1A2, CYP2C9, CYP2C19, CYP2D6, or CYP3A4.

7.1 Antacids

Because the dissolution of the coating of the granules in APRISO capsules depends on pH, APRISO capsules should not be co-administered with antacids.

8 USE IN SPECIFIC POPULATIONS

8.1 Pregnancy

Pregnancy Category B. Reproduction studies with mesalamine have been identified in rats at oral doses up to 320 mg/kg/day (about 1.7 times the recommended human dose based on a body surface area comparison) and rabbits at doses up to 495 mg/kg/day (about 5.4 times the recommended human dose based on a body surface area comparison) and have revealed no evidence of impaired fertility or harm to the fetus due to mesalamine. There are, however, no adequate and well-controlled studies in pregnant women. Because animal reproduction studies are not always predictive of human response, this drug should be used during pregnancy only if clearly needed.

Mesalamine is known to cross the placental barrier.

8.3 Nursing Mothers

Low concentrations of mesalamine and higher concentrations of its N-acetyl metabolite have been detected in human breast milk. The clinical significance of this has not been determined and there is limited experience of nursing women using mesalamine. Caution should be exercised when APRISO is administered to a nursing woman.

8.4 Pediatric Use

Safety and effectiveness of APRISO capsules in pediatric patients have not been established.

8.5 Geriatric Use

Clinical studies of APRISO did not include sufficient numbers of subjects aged 65 and over to determine whether they respond differently than younger subjects. Other reported clinical experience has not identified differences in responses between elderly and younger patients. In general, the greater frequency of decreased hepatic, renal, or cardiac function, and of concomitant disease or other drug therapy in elderly patients should be considered when prescribing APRISO.

Reports from uncontrolled clinical studies and postmarketing reporting systems suggested a higher incidence of blood dyscrasias, i.e., neutropenia, pancytopenia, in patients who were 65 years or older who were taking mesalamine-containing products such as APRISO. Caution should be taken to closely monitor blood cell counts during mesalamine therapy.

Mesalamine is known to be substantially excreted by the kidney, and the risk of adverse reactions to this drug may be greater in patients with impaired renal function. Because elderly patients are more likely to have decreased renal function, care should be taken when prescribing this drug therapy. [see Warnings and Precautions (5.1)].

10 OVERDOSAGE

APRISO is an aminosalicylate, and symptoms of salicylate toxicity include hematemesis, tachypnea, hyperpnea, tinnitus, deafness, lethargy, seizures, confusion, or dyspnea. Severe intoxication may lead to electrolyte and blood pH imbalance and potentially to other organ (e.g., renal and liver) involvement. There is no specific antidote for mesalamine overdose; however, conventional therapy for salicylate toxicity may be beneficial in the event of acute overdosage. This includes prevention of further gastrointestinal tract absorption by emesis and, if necessary, by gastric lavage. Fluid and electrolyte imbalance should be corrected by the administration of appropriate intravenous therapy. Adequate renal function should be maintained. APRISO is a pH-dependent delayed-release product and this factor should be considered when treating a suspected overdose.

11 DESCRIPTION

Each APRISO capsule is a delayed- and extended-release dosage form for oral administration. Each capsule contains 0.375 g of mesalamine USP (5-aminosalicylic acid, 5-ASA), an anti-inflammatory drug. The structural formula of mesalamine is:

Molecular Weight: 153.14

Molecular Formula: $C_7H_7NO_3$

Each APRISO capsule contains granules composed of mesalamine in a polymer matrix with an enteric coating that dissolves at pH 6 and above.

The inactive ingredients of APRISO capsules are colloidal silicon dioxide, magnesium stearate, microcrystalline cellulose, simethicone emulsion, ethylacrylate/methylmethacrylate copolymer nonoxynol 100 dispersion, hypromellose, methacrylic acid copolymer, talc, titanium dioxide, triethyl citrate, aspartame, anhydrous citric acid, povidone, vanilla flavor, and edible black ink.

12 CLINICAL PHARMACOLOGY

12.1 Mechanism of Action

The mechanism of action of mesalamine (5-ASA) is unknown, but appears to be local to the intestinal mucosa rather than systemic. Mucosal production of arachidonic acid metabolites, both through the cyclooxygenase pathways, i.e., prostanoids, and through the lipoxygenase pathways, i.e., leukotrienes and hydroxyeicosatetraenoic acids, is increased in patients with ulcerative colitis, and it is possible that 5-ASA diminishes inflammation by blocking production of arachidonic acid metabolites.

12.3 Pharmacokinetics

Absorption

The pharmacokinetics of 5-ASA and its metabolite, N-acetyl-5-aminosalicylic acid (N-Ac-5-ASA), were studied after a single and multiple oral doses of 1.5 g APRISO in a crossover study in healthy subjects under fasting conditions. In the multiple-dose period, each subject received APRISO 1.5 g (4 × 0.375 g capsules) every 24 hours (QD) for 7 consecutive days. Steady state was reached on Day 6 of QD dosing based on trough concentrations.

After single and multiple doses of APRISO, peak plasma concentrations were observed at about 4 hours post dose. At steady state, moderate increases (1.5-fold and 1.7-fold) in systemic exposure (AUC_{0-24}) to 5-ASA and N-Ac-5-ASA were observed when compared with a single-dose of APRISO.

Pharmacokinetic parameters after a single dose of 1.5 g APRISO and at steady state in healthy subjects under fasting condition are shown in Table 2.

Table 2: Single Dose and Multiple Dose Mean (±SD) Plasma Pharmacokinetic Parameters of Mesalamine (5-ASA) and N-Ac-5-ASA after 1.5 g APRISO Administration in Healthy Subjects

Mesalamine (5-ASA)	Single Dose (n=24)	Multiple Dose[c] (n=24)
AUC_{0-24} (µg*h/mL)	11 ± 5	17 ± 6
AUC_{0-inf} (µg*h/mL)	14 ± 5	-
C_{max} (µg/mL)	2.1 ± 1.1	2.7 ± 1.1
T_{max} (h) [a]	4 (2, 16)	4 (2, 8)
$t_{1/2}$ (h)[b]	9 ± 7	10 ± 8
N-Ac-5-ASA		
AUC_{0-24} (µg*h/mL)	26 ± 6	37 ± 9
AUC_{0-inf} (µg*h/mL)	51 ± 23	-
C_{max} (µg/mL)	2.8 ± 0.8	3.4 ± 0.9
T_{max} (h)[a]	4 (4, 12)	5 (2, 8)
$t_{1/2}$ (h)[b]	12 ± 11	14 ± 10

[a] Median (range); [b] Harmonic mean (pseudo SD); [c] after 7 days of treatment

In a separate study (n = 30), it was observed that under fasting conditions about 32% ± 11% (mean ± SD) of the administered dose was systemically absorbed based on the combined cumulative urinary excretion of 5-ASA and N-Ac-5-ASA over 96 hours post-dose.

The effect of a high fat meal intake on absorption of mesalamine granules (the same granules contained in APRISO capsules) was evaluated in 30 healthy subjects. Subjects received 1.6 g of mesalamine granules in sachet (2 × 0.8 g) following an overnight fast or a high fat meal in a crossover study. Under fed conditions, t_{max} for both 5-ASA and N-Ac-5-ASA was prolonged by 4 and 2 hours, respectively. A high fat meal did not affect C_{max} for 5-ASA, but a 27% increase in the cumulative urinary excretion of 5-ASA was observed with a high fat meal. The overall extent of absorption of N-Ac-5-ASA was not affected by a high fat meal. As APRISO and mesalamine granules in sachet were bioequivalent, APRISO can be taken without regard to food.

Distribution

In an *in vitro* study, at 2.5 µg/mL, mesalamine and N-Ac-5-ASA are 43 ± 6% and 78 ± 1% bound, respectively, to plasma proteins. Protein binding of N-Ac-5-ASA does not appear to be concentration dependent at concentrations ranging from 1 to 10 µg/mL.

Metabolism

The major metabolite of mesalamine is N-acetyl-5-aminosalicylic acid (N-Ac-5-ASA). It is formed by N-acetyltransferase activity in the liver and intestinal mucosa.

Elimination

Following single and multiple doses of APRISO, the mean half-lives were 9 to 10 hours for 5-ASA, and 12 to 14 hours for N-Ac-5-ASA. Of the approximately 32% of the dose absorbed, about 2% of the dose was excreted unchanged in the urine, compared with about 30% of the dose excreted as N-Ac-5-ASA.

In Vitro Drug-Drug Interaction Study

In an *in vitro* study using human liver microsomes, 5-ASA and its metabolite, N-Ac-5-ASA, were shown not to inhibit the major CYP enzymes evaluated (CYP1A2, CYP2C9, CYP2C19, CYP2D6, and CYP3A4). Therefore, mesalamine and its metabolite are not expected to inhibit the metabolism of other drugs that are substrates of CYP1A2, CYP2C9, CYP2C19, CYP2D6, or CYP3A4.

13 NONCLINICAL TOXICOLOGY

13.1 Carcinogenesis, Mutagenesis, Impairment of Fertility

Dietary mesalamine was not carcinogenic in rats at doses as high as 480 mg/kg/day, or in mice at 2000 mg/kg/day. These doses are about 2.6 and 5.4 times the recommended human dose of granulated mesalamine capsules of 1.5 g/day (30 mg/kg if 50 kg body weight assumed or 1110 mg/m², respectively, based on body surface area. Mesalamine was negative in the Ames test, the mouse lymphoma cell (L5178Y/TK+/-) forward mutation test, the sister chromatid exchange assay in the Chinese hamster bone marrow test, and the mouse bone marrow micronucleus test. Mesalamine at oral doses up to 320 mg/kg (about 1.7 times the recommended human dose based on body surface area) was found to have no effect on fertility or reproductive performance in rats.

13.2 Animal Toxicology and/or Pharmacology

Renal Toxicity

Animal studies with mesalamine (13-week and 26-week oral toxicity studies in rats, and 26-week and 52-week oral toxicity studies in dogs) have shown the kidney to be the major target organ of mesalamine toxicity. Oral doses of 40 mg/kg/day (about 0.20 times the human dose, on the basis of body surface area) produced minimal to slight tubular injury, and doses of 160 mg/kg/day (about 0.90 times the human dose, on the basis of body surface area) or higher in rats produced renal lesions including tubular degeneration, tubular mineralization, and papillary necrosis. Oral doses of 60 mg/kg/day (about 1.1 times the human dose, on the basis of body surface area) or higher in dogs also produced renal lesions including tubular atrophy, interstitial cell infiltration, chronic nephritis, and papillary necrosis.

Overdosage

Single oral doses of 800 mg/kg (about 2.2 times the recommended human dose, on the basis of body surface area) and 1800 mg/kg (about 9.7 times the recommended human dose, on the basis of body surface area) of mesalamine were lethal to mice and rats, respectively, and resulted in gastrointestinal and renal toxicity.

14 CLINICAL STUDIES

14.1 Ulcerative Colitis

Two similar, randomized, double-blind, placebo-controlled, multi-center studies were conducted in a total of 562 adult patients in remission from ulcerative colitis. The study populations had a mean age of 46 years (11% age 65 years or older), were 53% female, and were primarily white (92%). Ulcerative colitis disease activity was assessed using a modified Sutherland Disease Activity Index[1] (DAI), which is a sum of four subscores based on stool frequency, rectal bleeding, mucosal appearance on endoscopy, and physician's rating of disease activity. Each subscore can range from 0 to 3, for a total possible DAI score of 12.

At baseline, approximately 80% of patients had a total DAI score of 0 or 1.0. Patients were randomized 2:1 to receive either APRISO 1.5 g or placebo once daily in the morning for six months. Patients were assessed at baseline, 1 month, 3 months, and 6 months in the clinic, with endoscopy performed at baseline, at end of study, or if clinical symptoms developed. Relapse was defined as a rectal bleeding subscale score of 1 or more and a mucosal appearance subscale score of 2 or more using the DAI. The analysis of the intent-to-treat population was a comparison of the proportions of patients who remained relapse-free at the end of six months of treatment. For the table below (Table 3) all patients who prematurely withdrew from the study for any reason were counted as relapses.

In both studies, the proportion of patients who remained relapse-free at six months was greater for APRISO than for placebo.

Table 3: Percentage of Patients Relapse-Free* through 6 Months in APRISO Maintenance Studies

	APRISO 1.5 g/day % (# no relapse/N)	Placebo % (# no relapse/N)	Difference (95% C.I.)	P-value
Study 1	68% (143/209)	51% (49/96)	17% (5.5, 29.2)	<0.001
Study 2	71% (117/164)	59% (55/93)	12% (0, 24.5)	0.046

* Relapse counted as rectal bleeding score ≥1 and mucosal appearance score ≥ 2, or premature withdrawal from study.

Examination of gender subgroups did not identify difference in response to APRISO among these subgroups. There were too few elderly and too few African-American patients to adequately assess difference in effects in those populations. The use of APRISO for treating ulcerative colitis beyond six months has not been evaluated in controlled clinical trials.

15 REFERENCES

1. Sutherland LR, Martin F, Greer S, Robinson M, Greenberger N, Saibil F, et al. 5-Aminosalicylic acid enema in the treatment of distal ulcerative colitis, proctosigmoiditis, and proctitis. Gastroenterology 1987;92(6):1894-1898.

16 HOW SUPPLIED/STORAGE AND HANDLING

APRISO is available as light blue opaque hard gelatin capsules containing 0.375 g mesalamine and with the letters "G" and "M" on either side of a black band imprinted on the capsule.

NDC 65649-103-02 Bottles of 120 capsules
NDC 65649-103-01 Bottles of 4 capsules
Storage:
Store at 20° to 25°C (68° to 77°F); excursions permitted between 15° and 30°C (59° and 86°F). See USP Controlled Room Temperature.

17 PATIENT COUNSELING INFORMATION

17.1 Patients with Phenylketonuria
• Inform patients with phenylketonuria (PKU) or their caregivers that each APRISO capsule contains aspartame equivalent to 0.56 mg of phenylalanine, so that the recommended adult dosing provides an equivalent of 2.24 mg of phenylalanine per day.

17.2 General Counseling Information
• Instruct patients not to take APRISO capsules with antacids, because it could affect the way APRISO dissolves.
• Instruct patients to contact a health care provider if they experience a worsening of ulcerative colitis symptoms, because it could be due to a reaction to APRISO.

Manufactured by: Catalent Pharma Solutions
Manufactured for: Salix Pharmaceuticals, Inc., Raleigh, NC 27615
* APRISO™ is a trademark of Salix Pharmaceuticals, Inc.
Product protected by U.S. Patent No. 6,551,620 and U.S. Patent No. 7,547,451
Please see www.salix.com for patent information
VENART-113-2 / FEB 2012
Shown in Product Identification Guide, page 313

CYCLOSET®
(bromocriptine mesylate)
Tablets, oral

Rx

HIGHLIGHTS OF PRESCRIBING INFORMATION
These highlights do not include all the information needed to use CYCLOSET safely and effectively. See full prescribing information for CYCLOSET.
CYCLOSET® (bromocriptine mesylate) Tablets, oral
Initial U.S. Approval: 1978

———INDICATIONS AND USAGE———
CYCLOSET is a dopamine receptor agonist indicated as an adjunct to diet and exercise to improve glycemic control in adults with type 2 diabetes mellitus. (1.1)
Important Limitations of Use:
• Should not be used to treat type 1 diabetes or diabetic ketoacidosis (1.2)
• Limited efficacy data in combination with thiazolidinediones (1.2)
• Efficacy has not been confirmed in combination with insulin (1.2)

———DOSAGE AND ADMINISTRATION———
• Taken within two hours after waking in the morning with food (2.1)
• Initial dose is one tablet (0.8 mg) daily increased weekly by one tablet until maximal tolerated daily dose of 1.6 to 4.8 mg is achieved (2.2)

———DOSAGE FORMS AND STRENGTHS———
Tablets: 0.8 mg (3)

———CONTRAINDICATIONS———
• Do not use in patients with hypersensitivity to ergot-related drugs, bromocriptine or to any of the excipients in CYCLOSET (4)
• Do not use in patients with syncopal migraines. May precipitate hypotension (4)
• Do not use in nursing women. May inhibit lactation. Postmarketing reports of stroke in this patient population (4, 6.2, 8.3)

———WARNINGS AND PRECAUTIONS———
• Hypotension: Can cause orthostatic hypotension and syncope, particularly upon initiation or dose escalation. Use caution in patients taking anti-hypertensive medications. Assess orthostatic vital signs prior to initiation of CYCLOSET and periodically thereafter. Advise patients during early treatment to avoid situations that could lead to injury if syncope was to occur (5.1, 6.1)
• Psychosis: May exacerbate psychotic disorders or reduce the effectiveness of drugs that treat psychosis. Use in patients with severe psychotic disorders is not recommended (5.2)
• Somnolence: May cause somnolence. Advise patients not to operate heavy machinery if symptoms of somnolence occur (5.3)
• Interaction with dopamine antagonists: Concomitant use with dopamine antagonists such as neuroleptic agents may diminish the effectiveness of both drugs. Concomitant use is not recommended (5.4, 7)
• Other dopamine receptor agonists: Effectiveness and safety are unknown in patients already taking dopamine receptor agonists for other indications. Concomitant use is not recommended (5.5)
• Macrovascular outcomes: There have been no clinical studies establishing conclusive evidence of macrovascular risk reduction with CYCLOSET or any other antidiabetic drug. CYCLOSET does not increase the risk of macrovascular events (5.6, 6.1)

———ADVERSE REACTIONS———
In controlled clinical trials, adverse reactions reported in ≥ 5% of patients treated with CYCLOSET and reported more commonly than in patients treated with placebo, included nausea, fatigue, dizziness, vomiting, and headache. (6.1)
Postmarketing reports with higher doses of bromocriptine used for other indications include psychotic disorders, hallucinations, and fibrotic complications (6.2)
To report SUSPECTED ADVERSE REACTIONS, contact VeroScience, LLC at 1-877-757-0666 or FDA at 1-800-FDA-1088 or www.fda.gov/medwatch.

———DRUG INTERACTIONS———
• May increase the unbound fraction of highly protein-bound therapies, altering their effectiveness and safety profiles (7)
• May increase ergot-related side effects or reduce ergot effectiveness for migraines if co-administered within 6 hours of ergot-related drugs (7)
• Extensively metabolized by CYP3A4. Use caution when coadministering strong inhibitors, inducers, or substrates for CYP3A4 (7)

———USE IN SPECIFIC POPULATIONS———
Pediatrics: Safety and effectiveness have not been established (8.4)
See 17 for PATIENT COUNSELING INFORMATION and FDA-approved patient labeling

Revised: 09/2010

FULL PRESCRIBING INFORMATION

1 INDICATIONS AND USAGE
1.1 Type 2 diabetes mellitus
CYCLOSET is indicated as an adjunct to diet and exercise to improve glycemic control in adults with type 2 diabetes mellitus.
1.2 Important Limitations of Use
• CYCLOSET should not be used to treat type 1 diabetes or diabetic ketoacidosis.
• Limited efficacy data in combination with thiazolidinediones
• Efficacy has not been confirmed in combination with insulin.

2 DOSAGE AND ADMINISTRATION
2.1 Recommended Dosing
The recommended dose of CYCLOSET is 1.6 mg to 4.8 mg administered once daily within two hours after waking in the morning. CYCLOSET should be taken with food to potentially reduce gastrointestinal side effects such as nausea.
2.2 Titration
CYCLOSET should be initiated at one tablet (0.8 mg) and increased by one tablet per week until a maximum daily dose of 6 tablets (4.8 mg) or until the maximal tolerated number of tablets between 2 and 6 per day is reached.

3 DOSAGE FORMS AND STRENGTHS
0.8 mg tablets are white and round, imprinted with "C" on one side and "9" on the other.

4 CONTRAINDICATIONS
CYCLOSET is contraindicated in
• Patients with known hypersensitivity to bromocriptine, ergot-related drugs, or any of the excipients in CYCLOSET.
• Patients with syncopal migraine. Bromocriptine increases the likelihood of a hypotensive episode among patients with syncopal migraine. Loss of consciousness during a migraine may reflect dopamine receptor hypersensitivity. CYCLOSET is a dopamine receptor agonist, and may, therefore, potentiate the risk for syncope in these patients.

• Women who are nursing their children. CYCLOSET may inhibit lactation. There are postmarketing reports of stroke in this patient population although causality has not been proven [See Nursing Mothers (8.3)].

5 WARNINGS AND PRECAUTIONS

5.1 Hypotension

Hypotension, including orthostatic hypotension, can occur, particularly upon initiation of CYCLOSET therapy and with dose escalation. In a 52-week, randomized clinical trial of 3070 patients, hypotension was reported in 2.2% of patients randomized to CYCLOSET compared to 0.8% of patients randomized to placebo. Among CYCLOSET-treated patients reporting symptomatic hypotension, 98% were on at least one blood pressure medication compared to 73% on such medication in the total study population. In this trial, six CYCLOSET-treated patients (0.3%) reported an adverse event of orthostatic hypotension compared to 2 (0.2%) placebo-treated patients. All six patients were taking antihypertensive medications. Hypotension can result in syncope. In this trial, syncope due to any cause was reported in 1.6% of CYCLOSET-treated patients and 0.7% of placebo-treated patients [See Adverse Reactions (6.1)]. As a precaution, assessment of orthostatic vital signs is recommended prior to initiation of CYCLOSET and periodically thereafter. During early treatment with CYCLOSET, patients should be advised to make slow postural changes and to avoid situations that could lead to serious injury if syncope was to occur. Use caution in patients taking antihypertensive medications.

5.2 Psychotic disorders

In patients with severe psychotic disorders, treatment with a dopamine receptor agonist such as CYCLOSET may exacerbate the disorder or may diminish the effectiveness of drugs used to treat the disorder. Therefore, the use of CYCLOSET in patients with severe psychotic disorders is not recommended.

5.3 Somnolence

CYCLOSET may cause somnolence. In a 52-week, randomized clinical trial, 4.3% of CYCLOSET-treated patients and 1.3% of placebo-treated patients reported somnolence as an adverse event. None of these events were reported as serious and the majority of patients reported resolution of somnolence over time. Patients should be made aware of this potential side effect, particularly when initiating therapy with CYCLOSET. Patients experiencing somnolence should refrain from driving or operating heavy machinery.

5.4 Interaction with dopamine receptor antagonists

Dopamine receptor antagonists, including neuroleptic agents that have dopamine D2 receptor antagonist properties (e.g., Clozapine, Olanzapine, Ziprasidone), may reduce the effectiveness of CYCLOSET and CYCLOSET may reduce the effectiveness of these agents. CYCLOSET has not been studied in patients taking neuroleptic drugs. The concomitant use of CYCLOSET and dopamine receptor antagonists, including neuroleptic drugs, is not recommended.

5.5 Other dopamine receptor agonists

Other dopamine receptor agonists are indicated for the treatment of Parkinson's disease, hyperprolactinemia, restless leg syndrome, acromegaly, and other disorders. The effectiveness and safety of CYCLOSET in patients who are already taking one of these other dopamine receptor agonists is unknown. Concomitant use is not recommended.

5.6 Macrovascular outcomes

There have been no clinical studies establishing conclusive evidence of macrovascular risk reduction with CYCLOSET or any other anti-diabetic drug. In a 52-week, randomized clinical trial, CYCLOSET use was not associated with an increased risk for adverse cardiovascular events [See Adverse Reactions (6.1)].

6 ADVERSE REACTIONS

6.1 Clinical Trials Experience

Because clinical trials are conducted under widely varying conditions, the adverse reaction rates reported in one clinical trial may not be easily compared to those rates reported in another clinical trial, and may not reflect the rates actually observed in clinical practice.

In the pooled CYCLOSET phase 3 clinical trials (CYCLOSET N = 2298; placebo N = 1266), adverse events leading to discontinuation occurred in 539 (24%) CYCLOSET-treated patients and 118 (9%) placebo-treated patients. This between-group difference was driven mostly by gastrointestinal adverse events, particularly nausea.

The CYCLOSET safety trial was a 52-week, placebo-controlled study that included patients treated only with diet therapy or with other anti-diabetic medications. A total of 3,070 patients were randomized to CYCLOSET (titrated to 1.6 to 4.8 mg daily, as tolerated) or placebo. The study population had a mean baseline age of 60 years (range 27-80) and 33% were 65 years of age or older. Approximately 43% of the patients were female, 68% were Caucasian, 17% were Black, 13% were Hispanic, and 1% were Asian. The mean baseline body mass index was 32 kg/m². The mean duration of diabetes at baseline was 8 years and the mean baseline HbA1c was 7.0% with a mean baseline fasting plasma glucose of 142 mg/dL. At baseline, 12% of patients were treated with diet only, 40% were treated with one oral anti-diabetic agent, 33% were treated with two oral anti-diabetic agents, and 16% were treated with insulin alone or insulin in combination with an oral anti-diabetic agent. At baseline, 76% of patients reported a history of hypercholesterolemia, 75% reported a history of hypertension, 11% reported a history of revascularization surgery, 10% reported a history of myocardial infarction, 10% reported a history of angina, and 5% reported a history of stroke. Forty-seven percent of the CYCLOSET-treated patients and 32% of the placebo-treated patients prematurely discontinued treatment. Adverse events leading to discontinuation of study drug occurred among 24% of the CYCLOSET-treated patients and 15% of the placebo-treated patients. This between-group difference was driven mostly by gastrointestinal adverse events, particularly nausea.

Table 1 summarizes the adverse events reported in ≥5% of patients treated with CYCLOSET in the phase 3 clinical trials regardless of investigator assessment of causality. The most commonly reported adverse events (nausea, fatigue, vomiting, headache, dizziness) lasted a median of 14 days and were more likely to occur during the initial titration of CYCLOSET. None of the reports of nausea or vomiting were described as serious. There were no differences in the pattern of common adverse events across race groups or age groups (<65 years old vs. >65 years old). In the 52-week CYCLOSET safety trial, 11.5% of CYCLOSET-treated women compared to 3.6% of placebo-treated women reported vomiting. In this same trial, 5.4% of CYCLOSET-treated men compared to 2.8% of placebo-treated men reported vomiting.

Table 1: Adverse Events Reported in Phase 3 Clinical Trials of CYCLOSET (≥5% of Patients and Numerically More Frequent in CYCLOSET-Treated Patients than in Placebo-Treated Patients, Regardless of Investigator Assessment of Causality†)

Monotherapy	CYCLOSET 1.6 mg – 4.8 mg N (%)	Placebo N (%)
N = 159	N = 80	N = 79
Nausea	26 (32.5)	6 (7.6)
Rhinitis	11 (13.8)	3 (3.8)
Headache	10 (12.5)	7 (8.9)
Asthenia	10 (12.5)	5 (6.3)
Dizziness	10 (12.5)	6 (7.6)
Constipation	9 (11.3)	3 (3.8)
Sinusitis	8 (10.0)	2 (2.5)
Diarrhea	7 (8.8)	4 (5.1)
Amblyopia	6 (7.5)	1 (1.3)
Dyspepsia	6 (7.5)	2 (2.5)
Vomiting	5 (6.3)	1 (1.3)
Infection	5 (6.3)	4 (5.1)
Anorexia	4 (5.0)	1 (1.3)
Adjunct to Sulfonylurea (2 pooled 24 week studies)		
N = 494	N = 244	N = 250
Nausea	62 (25.4)	12 (4.8)
Asthenia	46 (18.9)	20 (8.0)
Headache	41 (16.8)	40 (16.0)
Flu syndrome	23 (9.4)	19 (7.6)
Constipation	24 (9.8)	11 (4.4)
Cold	20 (8.2)	20 (8.0)
Dizziness	29 (11.9)	14 (5.6)
Rhinitis	26 (10.7)	12 (4.8)
Sinusitis	18 (7.4)	16 (6.4)
Somnolence	16 (6.6)	5 (2.0)
Vomiting	13 (5.3)	8 (3.2)
Amblyopia	13 (5.3)	6 (2.4)
52-Week Safety Trial‡		
N=3070	N = 2054	N = 1016
Nausea	661 (32.2)	77 (7.6)
Dizziness	303 (14.8)	93 (9.2)
Fatigue	285 (13.9)	68 (6.7)
Headache	235 (11.4)	84 (8.3)
Vomiting	167 (8.1)	32 (3.1)
Diarrhea	167 (8.1)	81 (8.0)
Constipation	119 (5.8)	52 (5.1)

†All randomized subjects receiving at least one dose of study drug

‡ The Safety Trial enrolled patients treated with diet or no more than 2 anti-diabetic medications (metformin, insulin secretagogues such as a sulfonylurea, thiazolidinediones, alpha glucosidase inhibitors, and/or Insulin)

Hypoglycemia

In the monotherapy trial, hypoglycemia was reported in 2 CYCLOSET-treated patients (3.7%) and 1 placebo-treated patient (1.3%). In the add-on to sulfonylurea trials, the incidence of hypoglycemia was 8.6% among the CYCLOSET-treated patients and 5.2% among the placebo-treated patients. In the CYCLOSET safety trial, hypoglycemia was defined as any of the following: 1) symptoms suggestive of hypoglycemia that promptly resolved with appropriate intervention, 2) symptoms with a measured glucose <60 mg/dL or 3) measured glucose below 49 mg/dL regardless of symptoms. In the 52-week safety trial, the incidence of hypoglycemia was 6.9% among the CYCLOSET-treated patients and 5.3% among the placebo-treated patients. In the safety trial, severe hypoglycemia was defined as an inability to self-treat neurological symptoms consistent with hypoglycemia that occurred in the setting of a measured blood glucose < 50 mg/dl (or evidence of prompt resolution of these symptoms with administration of oral carbohydrates, subcutaneous glucagon, or intravenous glucose if blood glucose was not measured). In this trial, severe hypoglycemia was reported among 0.5% of CYCLOSET-treated patients and 1% of placebo-treated patients.

Syncope

In combined phase 2 and 3 clinical trials, syncope was reported in 1.4% of the 2,500 CYCLOSET-treated patients and 0.6% of the 1,454 placebo-treated patients. Among the 3,070 patients studied in the 52-week safety trial, 33 CYCLOSET-treated patients (1.6%) and 7 placebo-treated patients (0.7%) reported an adverse event of syncope. The cause of syncope is not known in all cases [See Warnings and Precautions (5.1)]. In this trial, electrocardiograms were not available at the time of these events, but an assessment of routine electrocardiograms obtained during the course of the trial did not identify arrhythmias or QTc interval prolongation among the CYCLOSET-treated patients reporting syncope.

Central Nervous System

In the 52-week safety trial, somnolence and hypoesthesia were the only adverse events within the nervous system organ class that occurred at a rate of < 5% and ≥ 1% and that occurred at a numerically greater frequency among CYCLOSET-treated patients (CYCLOSET 4.3% vs. Placebo 1.3% for somnolence; CYCLOSET 1.4% vs. Placebo 1.1% for hypoesthesia).

Serious Adverse Events and Cardiovascular Safety

The primary endpoint of the 52-week safety trial was the occurrence of all serious adverse events. A secondary endpoint was the occurrence of the composite of myocardial infarction, stroke, coronary revascularization, hospitalization for angina, and hospitalization for congestive heart failure. All serious adverse events and cardiovascular endpoints were adjudicated by an independent event adjudication committee. Serious adverse events occurred in 176/2054 (8.5%) CYCLOSET-treated patients and 98/1016 (9.6%) placebo-treated patients. The hazard ratio comparing CYCLOSET to placebo for the time to first occurrence of a serious adverse event was 1.02 (upper bound of one-sided 96% confidence interval, 1.27). None of the serious adverse events grouped by System-Organ-Class occurred more than 0.3 percentage points higher with CYCLOSET than with placebo. The composite cardiovascular endpoint occurred in 31 (1.5%) CYCLOSET-treated patients and 30 (3.0%) placebo-treated patients. The hazard ratio comparing

CYCLOSET to placebo for the time-to-first occurrence of the prespecified composite cardiovascular endpoint was 0.58 (two-sided 95% confidence interval, 0.35 – 0.96). Therefore, the incidence of this composite endpoint was not increased with CYCLOSET relative to placebo.

6.2 Postmarketing Experience

The active agent in CYCLOSET (bromocriptine mesylate) has been used in other formulations and often multiple times per day to treat hyperprolactinemia, acromegaly, and Parkinson's disease. The following adverse reactions have been identified during postapproval use of bromocriptine mesylate for these indications, generally at doses higher than those approved for the treatment of type 2 diabetes. Because these reactions are reported voluntarily from a population of uncertain size, it is generally not possible to reliably estimate their frequency or establish a causal relationship to drug exposure.

Hallucinations

Hallucinations and mental confusion including delusions have been reported with bromocriptine. To date, there have been no reported cases of hallucinations or delusions among CYCLOSET-treated patients (n=2500) in combined Phase 2 and 3 clinical trials of CYCLOSET.

Fibrotic - Related Complications

Fibrotic complications, including cases of retroperitoneal fibrosis, pulmonary fibrosis, pleural effusion, pleural thickening, pericarditis and pericardial effusions have been reported. These complications do not always resolve when bromocriptine is discontinued. Among several studies investigating a possible relation between bromocriptine exposure and cardiac valvulopathy, some events of cardiac valvulopathy have been reported, but no definitive association between bromocriptine mesylate use and clinically significant (moderate to severe) cardiac valvulopathy could be concluded.

To date, there have been no reported cases of retroperitoneal fibrosis, pulmonary infiltrates, pleural effusion, pleural thickening, pericarditis or pericardial effusions among the CYCLOSET–treated patients (n=2500) in combined Phase 2 and 3 controlled clinical trials of CYCLOSET. There was one unconfirmed case (0.04% event rate) of an adverse event of pulmonary fibrosis classified as nonserious in a CYCLOSET-treated patient.

No cases of cardiac valvulopathy have been reported in any of the clinical studies to date with CYCLOSET.

Psychotic and Psychiatric Disorders

Psychotic disorders have been reported with bromocriptine. Additionally, pathological gambling has been reported with bromocriptine used to treat patients with Parkinson's disease. To date, there have been no reported cases of psychoses or pathological gambling among the CYCLOSET-treated patients (N=2500) in combined Phase 2 and 3 controlled clinical trials of CYCLOSET.

Stroke

The indication for use of bromocriptine for inhibition of postpartum lactation was withdrawn based on postmarketing reports of stroke. Causality of bromocriptine use and the occurrence of stroke in this patient population has not been proven. Based on the CYCLOSET clinical trials, there is no evidence of increased risk for stroke when CYCLOSET is used to treat type 2 diabetes.

Neuroleptic - like malignant syndrome

A neuroleptic-like malignant syndrome (manifested by high fever and increase in creatinine phosphokinase) has been reported upon cessation of bromocriptine treatment in patients with advanced Parkinson's disease or patients with secondary Parkinsonism. To date, there have been no reported cases of neuroleptic-like malignant syndrome in combined Phase 2 and 3 controlled clinical trials of CYCLOSET, including the Safety Trial (N=2500). In the CYCLOSET Safety Trial, there were no reports of neuroleptic-like malignant syndrome during the 30 days of follow-up after cessation of CYCLOSET (N = 2054).

7 DRUG INTERACTIONS

• The active ingredient in CYCLOSET, bromocriptine mesylate, is highly bound to serum proteins. Therefore, CYCLOSET may increase the unbound fraction of other concomitantly used highly protein-bound therapies (e.g., salicylates, sulfonamides, chloramphenicol and probenecid), which may alter their risk for side effects.

• CYCLOSET is a dopamine receptor agonist. Concomitant use of dopamine receptor antagonists, such as neuroleptics (e.g., phenothiazines, butyrophenones, thioxanthenes), or metoclopramide may diminish the effectiveness of CYCLOSET and CYCLOSET may diminish the effectiveness of these other therapies. The concurrent use of CYCLOSET with these agents has not been studied in clinical trials and is not recommended [see *Warnings and Precautions 5.4*].

• CYCLOSET in combination with ergot-related drugs may cause an increase in the occurrence of ergot-related side effects such as nausea, vomiting, and fatigue, and may also reduce the effectiveness of these ergot therapies when used to treat migraine. The concurrent use of these ergot agents within 6 hours of CYCLOSET dosing is not recommended.

• CYCLOSET is extensively metabolized by the liver via CYP3A4. Therefore, potent inhibitors or inducers of CYP3A4 may increase or reduce the circulating levels of CYCLOSET, respectively. Use caution when co-administering drugs that are strong inhibitors, inducers, or substrates of CYP3A4 (e.g., azole antimycotics, HIV protease inhibitors) [See *Pharmacokinetics (12.3)*].

• There are postmarketing reports of hypertension and tachycardia when bromocriptine was co-administered with sympathomimetic drugs (e.g., phenylpropanolamine and isometheptene) in postpartum women. There are limited clinical trial data supporting the safety of co-administering sympathomimetic drugs and CYCLOSET for more than 10 days. Therefore, concomitant use of these agents with CYCLOSET for more than 10 days duration is not recommended. Also, there are limited clinical trial data supporting the safety of selective 5-hydroxytryptamine$_{1B}$ (5-HT$_{1B}$) agonists (e.g., sumatriptan) used concurrently with CYCLOSET and the concomitant use of these agents with CYCLOSET should be avoided.

8 USE IN SPECIFIC POPULATIONS

8.1 Pregnancy

Pregnancy Category B:

Two strains of pregnant rats were dosed orally with 3, 10, and 30 mg/kg/day (up to 72 times the human 4.8 mg daily dose, based on mg/m² comparison) from gestation day 6-15 and with a single dose of 10 mg/kg on gestation day 5. Implantation was inhibited at 10 and 30 mg/kg (24 and 72 times the human 4.8 mg daily dose, based on mg/m² comparison). When rats were dosed with 3, 10, and 30 mg/kg/day from gestation day 8-15 there was an increase in resorptions at 10 and 30 mg/kg. These effects were probably due to the dependence of implantation and the maintenance of gestation on prolactin in the rat and are not relevant for humans in which these events are not dependent on prolactin but on luteinizing hormone. There was no evidence of teratogenic effects in the rat.

In a small study in macaque monkeys given oral doses of 2 mg/kg/day (10 times the human 4.8 mg daily dose, based on mg/m² comparison) during organogenesis no embryotoxic or teratologic effects were observed.

When male rats given oral doses of 2, 10 or 50 mg/kg/day (up to 120 times the human 4.8 mg daily dose, based on mg/m² comparison) were mated with untreated females, there was a slight increase in pup loss in the 10 and 50 mg/kg/day groups (24-120 times the human 4.8 mg daily dose, based on mg/m² comparison).

In two strains of pregnant rabbits treated from gestation day 6-18 with oral doses of 3, 10, 30, 100, and 300 mg/kg/day (up to 1400 times the human 4.8 mg daily dose, based on mg/m² comparison) there was maternal toxicity and embryolethality at doses ≥10 mg/kg/day (48 times the human 4.8 mg daily dose, based on mg/m² comparison). Low incidences of fetal abnormalities were observed at maternally toxic doses of 100-300 mg/kg/day (480-1400 times the human 4.8 mg daily dose, based on mg/m² comparison). There were no treatment-related fetal abnormalities at doses ≤30 mg/kg/day (140 times the human 4.8 mg daily dose, based on mg/m² comparison). Implantation was not affected in rabbits treated from gestation day 1-6 with oral doses of 100-300 mg/kg/day (480-1400 times the human 4.8 mg daily dose, based on mg/m² comparison).

Studies in pregnant women have not shown that bromocriptine increases the risk of abnormalities when administered during pregnancy. Information concerning 1,276 pregnancies in women taking bromocriptine has been collected. In the majority of cases, bromocriptine was discontinued within the first 8 weeks of pregnancy (mean 29 days); however, 8 patients received the drug continuously throughout pregnancy. The mean daily dose for all patients was 5.8 mg (range 1-40 mg). Of these 1,276 pregnancies, there were 1,088 full-term deliveries (4 stillborn), 145 spontaneous abortions (11.4%), and 28 induced abortions (2.2%). Twelve extrauterine gravidities and 3 hydatidiform moles (twice in the same patient) caused early termination of pregnancy. These data compare favorably with the abortion rate (11-25%) cited for pregnancies induced by clomiphene citrate, menopausal gonadotropin, and chorionic gonadotropin. Although spontaneous abortions often go unreported, especially prior to 20 weeks of gestation, their frequency has been estimated to be 10-15% in the general population. The incidence of birth defects in the general population ranges from 2% to 4.5%. The incidence of birth defects in 1,109 live births from patients receiving bromocriptine was 3.3%. There is no suggestion that bromocriptine contributed to the type or incidence of birth defects in this group of infants.

A review of 4 different multicenter surveillance programs analyzed 2,351 pregnancies of 2,185 women treated with bromocriptine. In 583 children born of these women and followed for a minimum of 3-12 months, there was no suggestion of any adverse effect of intra-uterine exposure to bromocriptine on post-natal development. Most (≥75%) women had taken bromocriptine for 2-8 weeks and at 5-10 mg per day. Among 86 women having 93 pregnancies and treated with bromocriptine throughout pregnancy or from week 30 of pregnancy onwards (mostly for treatment of prolactinoma), there was only 1 spontaneous abortion. Similar results have been obtained in a Japanese hospital survey of 442 children born to 434 patients treated with bromocriptine during pregnancy and followed for at least one year.

Because the studies in humans cannot rule out the possibility of harm, CYCLOSET should be used during pregnancy only if clearly needed.

8.3 Nursing Mothers

CYCLOSET is contraindicated in women who are nursing their children. CYCLOSET contains bromocriptine which inhibits lactation. The indication for use of bromocriptine for inhibition of postpartum lactation was withdrawn based on postmarketing reports of stroke in this setting [See *Contraindications (4) and Adverse Reactions (6.2)*].

8.4 Pediatric Use

The safety and effectiveness of CYCLOSET in pediatric patients have not been established.

8.5 Geriatric Use

In the two clinical trials of CYCLOSET add-on to sulfonylurea therapy and in the monotherapy trial, a total of 54 patients randomized to CYCLOSET were ≥65 years old. In the 52-week safety trial, 601 of the 2,054 CYCLOSET-treated patients (29%) were ≥65 years old. No overall differences in safety or effectiveness were observed between the elderly and younger patients, but greater sensitivity of some older individuals cannot be ruled out. [See *Clinical Studies (14)*].

10 OVERDOSAGE

With another formulation of bromocriptine mesylate, the most commonly reported signs and symptoms associated with acute overdose were nausea, vomiting, constipation, diaphoresis, dizziness, pallor, severe hypotension, malaise, confusion, lethargy, drowsiness, delusions, hallucinations, and repetitive yawning. The lethal dose has not been established.

Treatment of overdose consists of removal of the drug by emesis (if conscious), gastric lavage, activated charcoal, or saline catharsis. Careful supervision and recording of fluid intake and output is essential. Hypotension should be treated by placing the patient in the Trendelenburg position and administering intravenous fluids. If satisfactory relief of hypotension cannot be achieved by using the above measures to their fullest extent, vasopressors should be considered.

11 DESCRIPTION

CYCLOSET Tablets contain bromocriptine mesylate, a dopamine receptor agonist. Bromocriptine mesylate is chemically designated [Ergotaman-3′,6′,18-trione, 2-bromo-12′-hydroxy-2′-(1-methylethyl)-5′-(2-methylpropyl)-, monomethanesulfonate (salt), (5′α)-]. CYCLOSET is a single enantiomer with absolute configuration 5R, 8R, 2′R, 5′S, 11′S, 12′S.

The structural formula of bromocriptine is shown below:

Bromocriptine mesylate is a white or slightly colored fine crystalline powder with a molecular formula of $C_{32}H_{40}BrN_5O_5 \cdot CH_4SO_3$ and a molecular weight of 750.72. CYCLOSET tablets contain bromocriptine mesylate USP in an amount equivalent to 0.8 of bromocriptine. Each tablet contains the following inactive ingredients: lactose, corn starch, magnesium stearate, colloidal silicon dioxide, and citric acid.

12 CLINICAL PHARMACOLOGY

12.1 Mechanism of Action

CYCLOSET contains bromocriptine mesylate, an ergot derivative that is a dopamine receptor agonist. The mechanism by which CYCLOSET improves glycemic control is unknown. Morning administration of CYCLOSET improves glycemic control in patients with type 2 diabetes without increasing plasma insulin concentrations.

Table 3: Changes in Glycemic Parameters for CYCLOSET versus Placebo in Two Add-on to Sulfonylurea Trials

	Study K†		Study L†	
	CYCLOSET Add-on to Sulfonylurea N = 122	Placebo Add-on to Sulfonylurea N = 123	CYCLOSET Add-on to Sulfonylurea N = 122	Placebo Add-on to Sulfonylurea N = 127
HbA1C (%)	n = 114	n =122	n = 114	n = 123
Baseline (mean)	9.3	9.4	9.3	9.4
Change from baseline (adj. mean)	-0.1	0.4	-0.4	0.3
Difference from placebo (adj. mean)	-0.5*		-0.6*	
Fasting plasma glucose (mg/dl)	n = 116	n = 119	n = 113	n = 123
Baseline (mean)	216	227	220	226
Change from baseline (adj. mean)	10	28	3	23
Difference from placebo (adj. mean)	-18**		-20‡	

† intent to treat population using last observation carried forward between group change from baseline in HbA1c
P-value calculated by ANOVA; *p≤ 0.001,**p=0.02; ‡ p = 0.006

Once daily morning administration of CYCLOSET to humans increases circulating levels of bromocriptine, a dopamine receptor agonist, for 4-5 hours after administration.

12.2 Pharmacodynamics
Postprandial Glucose and Insulin Response to a Meal
Patients with type 2 diabetes and inadequate glycemic control on diet alone were randomized to CYCLOSET or placebo in a 24-week monotherapy clinical trial. At baseline and study end, plasma samples for insulin and glucose were obtained before and 1 hour, and 2 hours after standardized meals for breakfast, lunch, and dinner. In this trial, once-daily (8 a.m.) CYCLOSET improved post-prandial glucose without increasing plasma insulin concentrations.

12.3 Pharmacokinetics
Absorption and Bioavailability
When administered orally, approximately 65-95% of the CYCLOSET dose of bromocriptine mesylate is absorbed. Due to extensive hepatic extraction and first-pass metabolism, approximately 7% of the dose reaches the systemic circulation. Under fasting conditions the time to maximum plasma concentration is 53 minutes. In contrast, following a standard high-fat meal, the time to maximum plasma concentration is increased to approximately 90-120 minutes. Also, the relative bioavailability of CYCLOSET is increased under fed as compared to fasting conditions by an average of approximately 55-65% (increase in AUCinf).

Distribution
Bromocriptine is 90-96% bound to plasma proteins. The volume of distribution is approximately 61 L.

Metabolism
Bromocriptine mesylate is extensively metabolized in the gastrointestinal tract and liver. Metabolism by CYP3A4 is the major metabolic pathway. Most of the absorbed dose (approximately 93%) undergoes first-pass metabolism. The remaining 7% reaches the systemic circulation.

Excretion
The major route of excretion of bromocriptine is in the bile with the remaining approximately 2-6% of an oral dose excreted via the urine. The elimination half-life is approximately 6 hours. Prior consumption of a standard high-fat meal has little to no effect on the elimination half-life of CYCLOSET.

Specific Populations
Renal Impairment
No pharmacokinetic studies have been conducted in patients with renal impairment. Although the kidney is a minor pathway for elimination of CYCLOSET, caution should be used in patients with renal impairment.

Hepatic Impairment
No pharmacokinetic studies have been conducted in patients with hepatic impairment. Because CYCLOSET is predominantly metabolized by the liver, caution should be used in patients with hepatic impairment.

Gender
The plasma exposure of CYCLOSET is increased 18-30% in females compared to males.

Geriatric
No pharmacokinetic studies have been conducted in geriatric subjects.

Pediatric
Studies characterizing the pharmacokinetics of CYCLOSET in pediatric patients have not been performed.

Race
Studies characterizing the pharmacokinetics of CYCLOSET among different ethnic groups have not been performed.

In Vitro Assessment of Drug Interactions
Results from in vitro studies demonstrate that CYP3A4 is the major enzyme responsible for the metabolism of bromocriptine. Bromocriptine is a competitive inhibitor of CYP3A4. The inhibitory potency for CYP3A4 is approximately 10,000-fold higher than the maximum plasma levels reached in vivo (Cmax of approximately 80-125 pg/mL) following a 4.8 mg oral dose of CYCLOSET.
Agents inducing CYP3A4 activity such as rifampin or dexamethasone would be expected to decrease CYCLOSET plasma levels. There was no significant in vitro inhibition of other major CYP450 enzymes (1A2, 2C9/19, 2D6) by bromocriptine.

In Vivo Assessment of Drug Interactions
The concomitant use of macrolide antibiotics such as erythromycin (250 mg four times a day), a known inhibitor of CYP3A4, along with bromocriptine (5 mg) was shown to increase the AUC (2.8 fold) and Cmax (4.6 fold) of bromocriptine. Therefore, use caution when co-administering drugs that are strong inhibitors or substrates of this enzyme, such as azole antimycotics and HIV protease inhibitors.

13 NONCLINICAL TOXICOLOGY
13.1 Carcinogenesis, Mutagenesis, Impairment of Fertility
Carcinogenesis
In a 74-week dietary study in mice at doses up to 50 mg/kg/day (56 times the human 4.8 mg daily dose, based on mg/m² comparison) there was no evidence of tumorigenicity.
In a 100-week dietary carcinogenicity study in rats at doses of 1.8, 9.9 and 44.5 mg/kg/day (up to 106 times the human 4.8 mg daily dose, based on mg/m² comparison) there was a significant increase in the incidence of malignant uterine neoplasms in the mid- and high dose groups (24-106 times the human 4.8 mg daily dose, based on mg/m² comparison). The increase in uterine neoplasms was probably due to the inhibition of prolactin-stimulated progesterone secretion resulting in estrogen domination and endometrial stimulation in the aging rat. Because prolactin does not play a role in human progesterone production this finding is unlikely to be clinically relevant.

Mutagenicity
Bromocriptine was not mutagenic in the in vitro Ames bacterial mutation assay, the V79 Chinese hamster fibroblast mutagenicity test, the in vivo bone marrow micronucleus test in mice and the in vivo Chinese hamster bone marrow chromosomal aberration test.

Impairment of Fertility
In female rats treated with oral doses of 1 and 3 mg/kg (2 to 7 times the human 4.8 mg daily dose, based on mg/m² comparison) from 2 weeks prior to mating through 2 weeks post mating or throughout lactation there was no effect on fertility. Postnatal pup weight gain was reduced dose-dependently in treated groups probably due to lactation inhibition.
In male rats treated with oral doses of 2, 10, and 50 mg/kg/day (up to 120 times the human 4.8 mg daily dose, based on mg/m² comparison) there was no effect on mating or fertility.

14 CLINICAL STUDIES
A total of 3,723 patients with type 2 diabetes were randomized across 4 double-blind, placebo-controlled clinical trials conducted to evaluate the safety and glycemic efficacy of CYCLOSET. In the pooled 24-week monotherapy trial and the two 24-week add-on to sulfonylurea trials (N = 653), the mean age of the CYCLOSET-treated patients (N=324) was 55 years, 71% were male and 73% Caucasian. In the 52-week safety trial (N=3,070), the mean age for the entire study population was 60 years and 43% of patients were female, 68% were Caucasian, 17% were Black, 13% were Hispanic, and 1% were Asian.
In all 4 clinical trials, patients assigned to treatment with CYCLOSET received an initial dose of 0.8 mg, which was increased by 0.8 mg each week for 6 weeks (4.8 mg/day final dose) if no intolerance occurred or until the maximum tolerated dose ≥ 1.6 mg/day was reached. In patients with type 2 diabetes, treatment with CYCLOSET produced clinically significant improvements in HbA1c and postprandial glucose (PPG).

14.1 Monotherapy
A total of 159 overweight (body mass index ≥26.0 kg/m² for males and ≥28.0 kg/m² for females) adults with type 2 diabetes and inadequate glycemic control (HbA1c 7.5-11%) participated in a 24-week placebo-controlled monotherapy trial that evaluated the efficacy and safety of CYCLOSET as an adjunct to diet and exercise. Mean body weight at baseline was 93 kg in the CYCLOSET group and 96 kg in the placebo group. Mean HbA1c at baseline was 9.0% in the CYCLOSET group and 8.8% in the placebo group. Mean duration of diabetes at baseline was 5 years in the CYCLOSET group and 4 years in the placebo group. Of the 80 patients in the CYLCOSET group, 69% (N=55) achieved the maximum daily dose of 4.8 mg. CYCLOSET improved HbA1c and fasting plasma glucose compared to placebo (Table 2). Mean change from baseline in body weight was +0.2 kg in the CYCLOSET group (N=78) and +0.5 kg in the placebo group (N=77).

Table 2: Changes in Glycemic Parameters in a 24-Week Placebo–Controlled Study of CYCLOSET as Monotherapy in Patients with Type 2 Diabetes†

	CYCLOSET N=80 (1.6-4.8 MG)	Placebo N=79
HbA1C (%)	N = 74	N = 74
Baseline (mean)	9.0	8.8
Change from baseline (adj. mean)	-0.1	0.3
Difference from placebo (adj. mean)	-0.4*	
Fasting Plasma Glucose (mg/dl)	N = 76	N = 75
Baseline (mean)	215	205
Change from baseline (adj. mean)	0	23
Difference from placebo (adj. mean)	-23**	

†intent to treat population with last observation carried forward
P-value calculated by ANOVA; *p=0.05, **p=0.005

14.2 Combination Therapy
CYCLOSET add-on to sulfonylurea therapy
Patients with type 2 diabetes and inadequate glycemic control (HbA1c 7.8-12.5%) on sulfonylurea therapy (mean HbA1c 9.4%) participated in Study L, a 24-week, randomized, double-blind, placebo-controlled trial that evaluated the safety and glycemic efficacy of CYCLOSET when added to stable sulfonylurea therapy. The mean duration of diabetes was 6 years in the CYCLOSET group and 8 years in the placebo group. The range of body mass index was 26-40 kg/m² for men and 28-40 kg/m² for women, with a mean of 32 kg/m² in both treatment groups. Of the 122 patients in the CYCLOSET group, 83 (68%) achieved the maximum dose of study drug. The mean change from baseline in body weight was +0.9 kg in the CYCLOSET group and +0.5 kg in the placebo group.
In another similarly designed trial, Study K, patients with type 2 diabetes and inadequate glycemic control (HbA1c 7.8-12.5 %) on stable sulfonylurea therapy were randomized to add-on therapy with either CYCLOSET (N = 122) or placebo (N = 123). The range of body mass index was 26-40 kg/m² for men and 28-40 kg/m² for women, with a

mean of 32 kg/m² in the CYCLOSET group and 33 kg/m² in the placebo group. Of the 122 patients in the CYCLOSET group, 91 (75%) achieved the maximum dose of study drug. Mean change from baseline in body weight was +1.4 kg in the CYCLOSET group and +0.5 kg in the placebo group. CYCLOSET improved HbA1c and fasting blood glucose concentrations compared to placebo (Table 3).

[See table 3 at top of previous page]

CYCLOSET add-on to various oral anti-diabetic agents

Patients with type 2 diabetes receiving various anti-diabetic therapies (mean baseline HbA1c 8.3%) participated in a 52-week randomized, double-blind, placebo-controlled safety trial *[See Adverse Reactions (6.1)]*. The daily CYCLOSET dose was initiated at 0.8 mg and increased by 0.8 mg each week for 6 weeks if no intolerance occurred or until the maximum tolerated dose ≥ 1.6 mg/day was reached. Approximately 70% of patients assigned to treatment with CYCLOSET reached the maximum daily dose of 4.8 mg. Physicians were instructed to adjust the dosage of concomitant diabetes therapies to avert hypoglycemia or uncontrolled hyperglycemia. Doses of background antidiabetic medications could be adjusted at any time during the trial and additional antidiabetic medications were permitted after Week 12, if needed to maintain ideal glycemic control. Mean baseline HbA1c was 7.0% in both treatment groups. The least-squares mean change in HbA1c from baseline to Week 24 was 0.0% with CYCLOSET (N=2049) and +0.2% with placebo (N=1015). Because many patients (60%) were already at treatment goal at baseline (HbA1c <7%), pre-specified subgroup analyses of glycemic efficacy (change in HbA1c from baseline to Week 24) were conducted for patients who had inadequate glycemic control (baseline HbA1c ≥7.5%) on 1-2 oral anti-diabetic therapies at the time of study entry. Patients receiving CYCLOSET, compared to placebo, experienced a significant improvement in HbA1c when used as adjunctive therapy to 1-2 oral antidiabetic medications, including the subgroup of patients treated only with background metformin + sulfonylurea (Table 4). The mean change in body weight for the glycemic efficacy subgroup (N = 559) from baseline to Week 24 was -0.1 kg with CYCLOSET and +0.1 kg. The mean change in body weight for the entire study population (N = 3070) from baseline to Week 52 was +0.2 kg with CYCLOSET and +0.1 kg with placebo.

Table 4: Changes in HbA1c from Baseline to Week 24 in the CYCLOSET Safety Trial Subgroup of Patients with Type 2 Diabetes and Inadequate Glycemic Control (Baseline HbA1c ≥7.5%) on 1-2 Oral Anti-Diabetic Medications†

	24-Week Intent to Treat	
	CYCLOSET	Placebo
Adjunct to 1-2 Oral Anti-Diabetic Medications	N = 376	N = 183
HbA1c (%)		
Baseline mean	8.3	8.4
Change from baseline (adjusted mean)	-0.4	0.0
Difference from placebo (adjusted mean)	-0.5*	
% Patients achieving HbA1c of ≤ 7.0	25	9
Adjunct to metformin + sulfonylurea only‡	N = 177	N = 90
HbA1c (%)		
Baseline mean	8.3	8.3
Change from baseline (adjusted mean)	-0.5	0.0
Difference from placebo (adjusted mean)	-0.5*	
% Patients achieving HbA1c of ≤ 7.0	27	9

†intent to treat population using last observation carried forward between group change from baseline in HbA1c
‡ patients in the "metformin + sulfonylurea only" subgroup are also counted in the "adjunct to 1-2 oral anti-diabetic medications" subgroup
P-value is based on an ANCOVA model with treatment and center as fixed effects, and baseline HbA1c as covariates; *p<0.001

14.3 Changes in Lipids and Blood Pressure

CYCLOSET does not have an unfavorable effect on fasting plasma lipids.

CYCLOSET has not demonstrated an unfavorable hypertensive effect on blood pressure. Hypotension has been reported with use of CYCLOSET in clinical trials *(See Warnings and Precautions).*

16 HOW SUPPLIED/STORAGE AND HANDLING

CYCLOSET 0.8 mg tablets are WHITE and round with "C" on one side and "9" on the other.

The tablets are supplied as follows:

NDC 68012-258-20 unit-of-use bottles of 200
NDC 68012-258-60 unit-of-use bottles of 600
NDC 68012-258-21 unit-of-use bottles of 21 (samples only).

Storage

Store at or below 25°C (77°F).

17 PATIENT COUNSELING INFORMATION

[See FDA-Approved Patient Labeling (17.2).]

17.1 Instructions

Patients should be informed of the potential risks and benefits of CYCLOSET and of alternative therapies. Patients should also be informed about the importance of adherence to dietary instructions, regular physical activity, periodic blood glucose monitoring and HbA1c testing, recognition and management of hypoglycemia and hyperglycemia, and assessment for diabetes complications. During periods of stress such as fever, trauma, infection, or surgery, medication requirements may change and patients should be advised to seek medical advice promptly.

Patients should be advised that they may develop postural (orthostatic) hypotension with or without symptoms such as dizziness, nausea, and diaphoresis. Hypotension and syncope may occur more frequently during initial therapy or with an increase in dose at any time. During early treatment with CYCLOSET, patients should be advised to make slow postural changes and to avoid situations that could predispose to serious injury if syncope was to occur.

Patients should be advised that CYCLOSET may cause somnolence. Advise patients not to operate heavy machinery if symptoms of somnolence occur.

Women who are nursing their children should be advised to not take CYCLOSET.

Physicians should instruct their patients to read the Patient Package Insert before starting CYCLOSET therapy and to reread it each time the prescription is renewed. Patients should be instructed to inform their healthcare provider if they develop any unusual symptoms or if any known symptom persists or worsens.

Manufactured for:
VeroScience, LLC
Tiverton, RI

Distributed and Marketed by:
Santarus, Inc., a wholly owned subsidiary of Salix Pharmaceuticals, inc.
Raleigh, NC 27615

Printed in USA

For information for health care professionals, call 1-888-778-0887

CYCLOSET is a registered trademark of VeroScience, LLC, Tiverton, RI 02878

This product is covered by one or more of the following: U.S. Patent Nos. 5,468,755; 5,679,685; 5,716,957; 5,756,513; 5,866,584

S0050A

17.2 FDA-Approved Patient Labeling

Patient Information
CYCLOSET® *[Si' klo' set]* (Bromocriptine Mesylate) **Tablets**

Read the Patient Information before you start taking CYCLOSET and each time you get a refill. There may be new information. This information does not take the place of talking with your healthcare provider about your medical condition or treatment.

What is CYCLOSET?

CYCLOSET is a prescription medicine used with diet and exercise to lower blood sugar in adults with type 2 diabetes. CYCLOSET may be taken alone or with other medicines that also help to control blood sugar.

CYCLOSET has not been studied in children.

Who should not take CYCLOSET?

Do not take CYCLOSET if you:

• are allergic to bromocriptine or any of the other ingredients in CYCLOSET
• take ergot medicines. Ask your healthcare provider for a list of these medicines, if you are not sure
• are breastfeeding
• have fainting (syncopal) migraine headaches

Talk to your healthcare provider before taking CYCLOSET if you have any of these conditions.

What should I tell my healthcare provider before taking CYCLOSET?

Before taking CYCLOSET, tell your healthcare provider about all of your medical conditions, including if you:

• have Type 1 diabetes mellitus
• have diabetic ketoacidosis
• have ever passed out or fainted
• have migraine headaches
• have or have had low blood pressure (hypotension)
• have or have had a mental health condition, especially a psychotic disorder
• are pregnant or plan to become pregnant. It is not known if CYCLOSET will harm your unborn baby. Talk with your healthcare provider if you are pregnant or plan to become pregnant.

Tell your healthcare provider about all the medicines you take, including prescription and non-prescription medicines, vitamins, and herbal supplements. Especially tell your healthcare provider if you take medicines for:

• mental health conditions, especially anti-psychotic medicines
• migraine or other types of headaches
• type 2 diabetes

Ask your healthcare provider or pharmacist for a list of medicines taken for these conditions, if you are not sure. CYCLOSET may affect the way other medicines work, and other medicines may affect how CYCLOSET works.

Know the medicines you take. Keep a list of your medicines and show it to your healthcare provider and pharmacist when you get a new medicine.

How should I take CYCLOSET?

• Take CYCLOSET exactly as your healthcare provider tells you to take it.
• Take CYCLOSET by mouth each day.
• Take CYCLOSET with food.
• Take CYCLOSET within 2 hours after waking in the morning.
• If you miss your morning dose, wait until the next morning to take your medication.
• Do not take a double dose of CYCLOSET.
• During periods of stress on the body, such as fever, trauma, infection, or surgery, your medication needs may change. Contact your healthcare provider right away.
• If you take too much CYCLOSET, call your healthcare provider or go to the nearest emergency department right away.
• While taking CYCLOSET:
  ○ check your blood sugar as your healthcare provider tells you to
  ○ stay on your prescribed diet and exercise program
  ○ learn to prevent, recognize, and manage low blood sugar (hypoglycemia), high blood sugar (hyperglycemia), and complications of diabetes
  ○ see your healthcare provider for regular blood tests, including your blood sugar levels and hemoglobin HbA1c

What are the possible side effects of CYCLOSET?

CYCLOSET may cause serious side effects, including:

• Low blood pressure
• Fainting
• Severe dizziness which can be caused by postural hypotension. This can happen when your blood pressure lowers rapidly after you stand up from a lying down position.

The most common side effects of CYCLOSET include:

• nausea
• headache
• fatigue (somnolence). If you have somnolence from CYCLOSET you should not drive or use other heavy machines until the somnolence is better.
• dizziness
• vomiting
• low blood sugar (hypoglycemia), especially when used with another type of diabetes medicine known as a sulfonylurea

Tell your healthcare provider if you have any side effect that bothers you or that does not go away.

These are not all the possible side effects of CYCLOSET. For more information, ask your healthcare provider or pharmacist.

Call your doctor for medical advice about side effects. You may report side effects to FDA at 1-800-FDA-1088

How Should I store CYCLOSET?

Store CYCLOSET at or below 77°F (25°C).

Keep CYCLOSET and all medicines out of the reach of children.

General information about the use of CYCLOSET

Medicines are sometimes prescribed for conditions that are not mentioned in patient information leaflets. Do not use CYCLOSET for a condition for which it was not prescribed. Do not give CYCLOSET to other people, even if they have the same symptoms you have. It may harm them.

This leaflet summarizes the most important information about CYCLOSET. If you would like more information, talk with your healthcare provider. You can ask your healthcare provider or pharmacist for additional information about CYCLOSET that is written for health professionals. For more information, go to www.CYCLOSET.com or call 1-888-778-0887.

What are the ingredients in CYCLOSET?
Active ingredient: bromocriptine mesylate
Inactive ingredients: lactose, corn starch, magnesium stearate, colloidal silicon dioxide, citric acid, and other inert ingredients
Issued September 2010
Manufactured for:
VeroScience, LLC
Tiverton, RI
Distributed and Marketed by:
Santarus, Inc., a wholly owned subsidiary of Salix Pharmaceuticals, Inc.
Raleigh, NC 27615
For information for health care professionals, call 1-888-778-0887
Revised 09/2010
CYCLOSET is a registered trademark of VeroScience, LLC, Tiverton, RI 02878
1-CYC10519

Shown in Product Identification Guide, page 313

FULYZAQ®   ℞
(crofelemer)
delayed-release tablets, for oral use

HIGHLIGHTS OF PRESCRIBING INFORMATION
These highlights do not include all the information needed to use FULYZAQ safely and effectively. See full prescribing information for FULYZAQ.
FULYZAQ® (crofelemer) delayed-release tablets, for oral use
Initial U.S. Approval: 2012

——————INDICATIONS AND USAGE——————
FULYZAQ is an anti-diarrheal indicated for the symptomatic relief of non-infectious diarrhea in adult patients with HIV/AIDS on anti-retroviral therapy. (1)

——————DOSAGE AND ADMINISTRATION——————
One 125 mg delayed-release tablet taken orally twice a day, with or without food. (2)

——————DOSAGE FORMS AND STRENGTHS——————
Delayed-Release Tablets: 125 mg (3)

——————CONTRAINDICATIONS——————
None. (4)

——————WARNINGS AND PRECAUTIONS——————
Rule out infectious etiologies of diarrhea before starting crofelemer. If infectious etiologies are not considered, there is a risk that patients with infectious etiologies will not receive the appropriate therapy and their disease may worsen. (5.1)

——————ADVERSE REACTIONS——————
Most common adverse reactions (incidence ≥ 3%) are upper respiratory tract infection, bronchitis, cough, flatulence and increased bilirubin. (6)

To report SUSPECTED ADVERSE REACTIONS, contact Salix Pharmaceuticals at 1-800-508-0024 or FDA at 1-800-FDA-1088 or *www.fda.gov/medwatch*

——————USE IN SPECIFIC POPULATIONS——————
• *Pregnancy:* Based on animal data, may cause fetal harm. (8.1)
• *Pediatric Use:* Safety and effectiveness of FULYZAQ has not been established in patients less than 18 years of age. (8.4)

See 17 for PATIENT COUNSELING INFORMATION
                                              Revised: 02/2013

FULL PRESCRIBING INFORMATION: CONTENTS*

FULL PRESCRIBING INFORMATION

1   INDICATIONS AND USAGE
FULYZAQ is indicated for symptomatic relief of non-infectious diarrhea in patients with HIV/AIDS on antiretroviral therapy.

2   DOSAGE AND ADMINISTRATION
The recommended dose of FULYZAQ is one 125 mg delayed-release tablet taken orally two times a day, with or without food. FULYZAQ tablets should **not be crushed or chewed**. Tablets should be swallowed whole.

3   DOSAGE FORMS AND STRENGTHS
FULYZAQ is a white, oval, enteric-coated 125 mg delayed-release tablet printed on one side with 125SLXP.

4   CONTRAINDICATIONS
None.

5   WARNINGS AND PRECAUTIONS
5.1   Risks of Treatment in Patients with Infectious Diarrhea
If infectious etiologies are not considered, and FULYZAQ is initiated based on a presumptive diagnosis of non-infectious diarrhea, then there is a risk that patients with infectious etiologies will not receive the appropriate treatments, and their disease may worsen. Before starting FULYZAQ, rule out infectious etiologies of diarrhea. FULYZAQ is not indicated for the treatment of infectious diarrhea.

6   ADVERSE REACTIONS
6.1   Clinical Trials Experience
Because clinical trials are conducted under widely varying conditions, adverse reaction rates observed in the clinical trials of a drug cannot be directly compared to rates in the clinical trials of another drug and may not reflect the rates observed in practice.
A total of 696 HIV-positive patients in three placebo-controlled trials received FULYZAQ for a mean duration of 78 days. Of the total population across the three trials, 229 patients received a dose of 125 mg twice a day for a mean duration of 141 days, 69 received a dose of 250 mg twice a day for a mean duration of 139 days, 102 patients received a dose of 250 mg four times a day for a mean duration of 14 days, 54 patients received a dose of 500 mg twice a day for a mean duration of 146 days, and 242 patients received a dose of 500 mg four times a day for a mean duration of 14 days.
Adverse reactions for FULYZAQ that occurred in at least 2% of patients and at a higher incidence than placebo are provided in Table 1.

Table 1: Adverse Reactions Occurring in at Least 2% of Patients in the 125 mg Twice Daily Group

Adverse Reaction	Crofelemer 125 mg BID* N = 229 n (%)	Placebo N = 274 n (%)
Upper respiratory tract infection	13 (5.7)	4 (1.5)
Bronchitis	9 (3.9)	0
Cough	8 (3.5)	3 (1.1)
Flatulence	7 (3.1)	3 (1.1)
Increased bilirubin	7 (3.1)	3 (1.1)
Nausea	6 (2.6)	4 (1.5)
Back pain	6 (2.6)	4 (1.5)
Arthralgia	6 (2.6)	0
Urinary tract infection	5 (2.2)	2 (0.7)
Nasopharyngitis	5 (2.2)	2 (0.7)
Musculoskeletal pain	5 (2.2)	1 (0.4)
Hemorrhoids	5 (2.2)	0
Giardiasis	5 (2.2)	0
Anxiety	5 (2.2)	1 (0.4)
Increased alanine aminotransferase	5 (2.2)	3 (1.1)
Abdominal distension	5 (2.2)	1 (0.4)

* Twice daily

Adverse reactions that occurred in between 1% and 2% of patients taking a 250 mg daily dose of FULYZAQ were abdominal pain, acne, increased aspartate aminotransferase, increased conjugated bilirubin, increased unconjugated blood bilirubin, constipation, depression, dermatitis, dizziness, dry mouth, dyspepsia, gastroenteritis, herpes zoster, nephrolithiasis, pain in extremity, pollakiuria, procedural pain, seasonal allergy, sinusitis and decreased white blood cell count.
Adverse reactions were similar in patients who received doses greater than 250 mg daily.

7   DRUG INTERACTIONS
7.1   Drug Interaction Potential
In vitro studies have shown that crofelemer has the potential to inhibit cytochrome P450 isoenzyme 3A and transporters MRP2 and OATP1A2 at concentrations expected in the gut. Due to the minimal absorption of crofelemer, it is unlikely to inhibit cytochrome P450 isoenzymes 1A2, 2A6, 2B6, 2C9, 2C19, 2D6, 2E1 and CYP3A4 systemically *[see Clinical Pharmacology (12.3)]*.
7.2   Nelfinavir, Zidovudine, and Lamivudine
FULYZAQ administration did not have a clinically relevant interaction with nelfinavir, zidovudine, or lamivudine in a drug-drug interaction trial.

8   USE IN SPECIFIC POPULATIONS
8.1   Pregnancy
Pregnancy Category C
Reproduction studies performed with crofelemer in rats at oral doses up to 177 times the recommended daily human dose of 4.2 mg/kg revealed no evidence of impaired fertility or harm to the fetus. In pregnant rabbits, crofelemer at an oral dose of about 96 times the recommended daily human dose of 4.2 mg/kg, caused abortions and resorptions of fetuses. However, it is not clear whether these effects are related to the maternal toxicity observed. A pre- and postnatal development study performed with crofelemer in rats at oral doses of up to 177 times the recommended daily human dose of 4.2 mg/kg revealed no evidence of adverse pre- and postnatal effects in offspring. There are, however, no adequate, well-controlled studies in pregnant women. Because animal reproduction studies are not always predictive of human response, this drug should be used during pregnancy only if clearly needed.
8.3   Nursing Mothers
It is not known whether crofelemer is excreted in human milk. Because many drugs are excreted in human milk and because of the potential for adverse reactions in nursing infants from FULYZAQ, a decision should be made whether to discontinue nursing or to discontinue the drug, taking into account the importance of the drug to the mother.
8.4   Pediatric Use
The safety and effectiveness of FULYZAQ have not been established in pediatric patients less than 18 years of age.
8.5   Geriatric Use
Clinical studies with crofelemer did not include sufficient numbers of patients aged 65 and over to determine whether they respond differently than younger patients.
8.6   Use in Patients with Low CD4 Counts and High Viral Loads
No dose modifications are recommended with respect to CD4 cell count and HIV viral load, based on the findings in subgroups of patients defined by CD4 cell count and HIV viral load.
The safety profile of crofelemer was similar in patients with baseline CD4 cell count less than 404 cells/µL (lower limit of normal range) (N=388) and patients with baseline CD4 cell counts greater than or equal to 404 cells/µL (N=289).
The safety profile of crofelemer was similar in patients with baseline HIV viral loads less than 400 copies/mL (N = 412) and patients with baseline HIV viral loads greater than or equal to 400 copies/mL (N = 278).

10   OVERDOSAGE
There has been no reported experience with overdosage of crofelemer.

11   DESCRIPTION
FULYZAQ (crofelemer) delayed-release tablets is an anti-diarrheal, enteric-coated drug product for oral administration. It contains 125 mg of crofelemer, a botanical drug substance that is derived from the red latex of *Croton lechleri* Müll. Arg. Crofelemer is an oligomeric proanthocyanidin mixture primarily composed of (+)-catechin, (-)-epicatechin, (+)-gallocatechin, and (-)-epigallocatechin monomer units linked in random sequence, as represented below. The average degree of polymerization for the oligomers ranges between 5 and 7.5, as determined by phloroglucinol degradation.

R = H or OH
range n = 3 to 5.5
Inactive ingredients: microcrystalline cellulose, croscarmellose sodium, colloidal silicon dioxide, and magnesium stearate.
Coating ingredients: ethylacrylate and methylacrylate copolymer dispersion, talc, triethyl citrate, and white dispersion which contains xanthan gum, titanium dioxide, propyl paraben, and methyl paraben.

12 CLINICAL PHARMACOLOGY

12.1 Mechanism of Action

Crofelemer is an inhibitor of both the cyclic adenosine monophosphate (cAMP)-stimulated cystic fibrosis transmembrane conductance regulator (CFTR) chloride ion (Cl⁻) channel, and the calcium-activated Cl⁻ channels (CaCC) at the luminal membrane of enterocytes. The CFTR Cl⁻ channel and CaCC regulate Cl⁻ and fluid secretion by intestinal epithelial cells. Crofelemer acts by blocking Cl⁻ secretion and accompanying high volume water loss in diarrhea, normalizing the flow of Cl⁻ and water in the GI tract.

12.2 Pharmacodynamics

Consistent with the mechanism of action of crofelemer (i.e., inhibition of CFTR and CaCC in the GI lumen), data suggest stool chloride concentrations decreased in patients treated with FULYZAQ (500 mg four times daily) (n=25) for four days relative to placebo (n=24); stool chloride concentrations decreased in both African American patients treated with FULYZAQ (n=3) relative to placebo (n=5) and non-African American patients treated with FULYZAQ (n=22) relative to placebo (n=19).
At a dose 10 times the maximum recommended dose, crofelemer does not prolong the QTc interval to any clinically relevant extent.

12.3 Pharmacokinetics

Absorption
The absorption of crofelemer is minimal following oral dosing in healthy adults and HIV-positive patients and concentrations of crofelemer in plasma are below the level of quantitation (50 ng/mL). Therefore, standard pharmacokinetic parameters such as area under the curve, maximum concentration, and half-life cannot be estimated.
Distribution
The distribution of crofelemer has not been determined.
Metabolism
No metabolites of crofelemer have been identified in healthy subjects or patients in clinical trials.
Elimination
The elimination route has not been identified in humans.
Food Effect
Administration of crofelemer with a high-fat meal was not associated with an increase in systemic exposure of crofelemer in healthy volunteers. In the clinical trial, a single 500 mg dose of crofelemer was administered one-half hour before the morning and evening meals. Therefore, crofelemer may be administered with or without a meal.
Drug-Drug Interactions
Results of a crossover study in healthy volunteers showed crofelemer 500 mg administered four times daily for five days had no effect on the exposure of zidovudine and nelfinavir when administered as a single dose. A 20% decrease in lamivudine exposure was also observed in the same study but was not considered to be clinically important.

13 NONCLINICAL TOXICOLOGY

13.1 Carcinogenesis, Mutagenesis, Impairment of Fertility

Carcinogenesis
Long-term studies in animals have not been performed to evaluate the carcinogenic potential of crofelemer.
Mutagenesis
Crofelemer was negative in the bacterial reverse mutation assay, chromosomal aberration assay, and rat bone marrow micronucleus assay.

Impairment of Fertility
Crofelemer, at oral doses of up to 738 mg/kg/day (177 times the recommended human daily dose of 4.2 mg/kg), had no effects on fertility or reproductive performance of male and female rats.

14 CLINICAL STUDIES

The efficacy of FULYZAQ 125 mg delayed-release tablets twice daily was evaluated in a randomized, double-blind, placebo-controlled (one month) and placebo-free (five month), multi-center study. The study enrolled 374 HIV-positive patients on stable anti-retroviral therapy (ART) with a history of diarrhea for one month or more. Diarrhea was defined as either persistently loose stools despite regular use of anti-diarrheal medication (ADM) (e.g., loperamide, diphenoxylate, and bismuth subsalicylate) or one or more watery bowel movements per day without regular ADM use.
Patients were excluded if they had a positive gastrointestinal (GI) biopsy, GI culture, or stool test for multiple bacteria (*Salmonella, Shigella, Campylobacter, Yersinia, Mycobacterium*), bacterial toxin (*Clostridium difficile*), ova and parasites (*Giardia, Entamoeba, Isospora, Cyclospora, Cryptosporidium, Microsporidium*), or viruses (*Cytomegalovirus*). Patients were also excluded if they had a history of ulcerative colitis, Crohn's disease, celiac sprue (gluten-enteropathy), chronic pancreatitis, malabsorption, or any other GI disease associated with diarrhea.
The study had a two-stage adaptive design. In both stages, patients received placebo for 10 days (screening period) followed by randomization to crofelemer or placebo for 31 days of treatment (double-blind period). Only patients with 1 or more watery bowel movements per day on at least 5 of the last 7 days in the screening period were randomized to the double-blind period. Each stage enrolled patients separately; the dose for the second stage was selected based on an interim analysis of data from the first stage. In the first stage, patients were randomized 1:1:1:1 to one of three crofelemer dose regimens (125, 250, or 500 mg twice daily) or placebo. In the second stage, patients were randomized 1:1 to crofelemer 125 mg twice daily or placebo. The efficacy analysis was based on results from the double-blind portion of both stages.
Each study stage also had a five month period (placebo-free period) that followed the double-blind period. Patients treated with crofelemer continued the same doses in the placebo-free period. In the first stage, patients that received placebo were re-randomized 1:1:1 to one of the three crofelemer dose regimens (125, 250, or 500 mg twice daily) in the placebo-free period. In the second stage, patients that received placebo were treated with crofelemer 125 mg twice daily in the placebo-free period.
The median time since diagnosis of HIV was 12 years. The percentage of patients with a CD4 cell count of less than 404 was 39%. The percentage of patients with a HIV viral load greater than or equal to 1000, 400 to 999, and less than 400 HIV copies/mL was 7%, 3%, and 9%, respectively; the remainder had a viral load that was not detectable. The median time since diarrhea started was 4 years. The median number of daily watery bowel movements was 2.5 per day. Most patients were male (85%). The percentage of patients that were Caucasian was 46%; the percentage of patients that were African-American was 32%. The median age was 45 years with a range of 21 to 68 years.
In the double-blind period of the study, 136 patients received crofelemer 125 mg twice daily, 54 patients received 250 mg twice daily, 47 patients received 500 mg twice daily, and 138 patients received placebo. The percentages of pa-

Table 2: Concomitant ART Use in the Double-Blind Period

	125 mg BID (N = 136) n (%)	250 mg BID (N = 54) n (%)	500 mg BID (N = 46) n (%)	Placebo BID (N = 138) n (%)
Any ART	135 (99)	53 (98)	45 (98)	134 (97)
Any PI	87 (64)	41 (76)	33 (72)	97 (70)
Tenofovir/Emtricitabine	45 (33)	22 (41)	16 (35)	52 (38)
Ritonavir	46 (34)	18 (33)	15 (33)	49 (36)
Lopinavir/Ritonavir	30 (22)	21 (39)	15 (33)	40 (29)
Efavirenz/Tenofovir/ Emtricitabine	30 (22)	7 (13)	7 (15)	21 (15)
Tenofovir disoproxil fumarate	18 (13)	8 (15)	5 (11)	14 (10)
Atazanavir sulfate	19 (14)	3 (6)	6 (13)	22 (16)
Abacavir w/ lamivudine	17 (13)	5 (9)	5 (11)	18 (13)
Darunavir	19 (14)	4 (7)	4 (9)	14 (10)
Raltegravir	16 (12)	4 (7)	5 (11)	11 (8)
Valaciclovir hydrochloride	12 (9)	8 (15)	5 (11)	16 (12)
Fosamprenavir	12 (9)	6 (11)	4 (9)	13 (9)
Zidovudine w/ lamivudine	12 (9)	3 (6)	3 (7)	15 (11)
Lamivudine	7 (5)	6 (11)	4 (9)	6 (4)
Nevirapine	8 (6)	6 (11)	3 (7)	9 (7)
Atazanavir	5 (4)	6 (11)	2 (4)	2 (1)

Abbreviations: ART = antiretroviral therapy; PI = Protease Inhibitor; BID = twice daily.

tients that completed the double-blind period were 92%, 100%, 85%, and 94% in the 125 mg, 250 mg, 500 mg, and placebo arms, respectively.
Most patients received concomitant protease inhibitors (PI) during the double-blind period (Table 2). The most frequently used ARTs in each group were tenofovir/emtricitabine, ritonavir, and lopinavir/ritonavir.
[See table 2 above]
The primary efficacy endpoint was the proportion of patients with a clinical response, defined as less than or equal to 2 watery bowel movements per week during at least 2 of the 4 weeks of the placebo-controlled phase. Patients who received concomitant ADMs or opiates were counted as clinical non-responders.
A significantly larger proportion of patients in the crofelemer 125 mg twice daily group experienced clinical response compared with patients in the placebo group (17.6% vs. 8.0%, 1-sided p < 0.01).
In the randomized clinical study, examination of duration of diarrhea, baseline number of daily watery bowel movements, use of protease inhibitors, CD4 cell count and age subgroups did not identify differences in the consistency of the crofelemer treatment effect among these subgroups. There were too few female subjects and subjects with an HIV viral load > 400 copies/mL to adequately assess differences in effects in these populations. Among race subgroups, there were no differences in the consistency of the crofelemer treatment effect except for the subgroup of African-Americans; crofelemer was less effective in African-Americans than non-African-Americans.
Although the CD4 cell count and HIV viral load did not appear to change over the one month placebo-controlled period, the clinical significance of this finding is unknown because of the short duration of the placebo-controlled period. Of the 24 clinical responders to crofelemer (125 mg twice daily), 22 entered the placebo-free period; 16 were responding at the end of month 3, and 14 were responding at the end of month 5.

16 HOW SUPPLIED/STORAGE AND HANDLING

Crofelemer delayed-release tablets, 125 mg, are white, oval enteric-coated tablets printed on one side with 125SLXP. They are available in the following package size:
Bottles of 60: NDC 65649-802-02
Store at 20°C-25°C (68°F-77°F); excursions permitted between 15°C-30°C (59°F-86°F). See USP Controlled Room Temperature.

17 PATIENT COUNSELING INFORMATION

• Instruct patients that FULYZAQ tablets may be taken with or without food.
• Instruct patients that FULYZAQ tablets should not be crushed or chewed. Tablets should be swallowed whole.
Rx Only
Manufactured by Patheon, Inc. for
Salix Pharmaceuticals, Inc., Raleigh, NC 27615
Copyright © Salix Pharmaceuticals, Inc.
US Patent Nos. 7,341,744 and 7,323,195.
FULYZAQ is distributed by Salix Pharmaceuticals, Inc. under license from Napo Pharmaceuticals, Inc.
The botanical drug substance of FULYZAQ is extracted from *Croton lechleri* (the botanical raw material) that is harvested from the wild in South America.
Shown in Product Identification Guide, page 313

MOVIPREP® ℞
(polyethylene glycol 3350, sodium sulfate, sodium chloride, potassium chloride, sodium ascorbate, and ascorbic acid for oral solution)

HIGHLIGHTS OF PRESCRIBING INFORMATION
These highlights do not include all the information needed to use MOVIPREP® safely and effectively. See full prescribing information for MOVIPREP.
MOVIPREP (polyethylene glycol 3350, sodium sulfate, sodium chloride, potassium chloride, sodium ascorbate, and ascorbic acid for oral solution)
Initial U.S. Approval: 2006

————RECENT MAJOR CHANGES————
Dosage and Administration (2)   11/2013

————INDICATIONS AND USAGE————
MoviPrep is an osmotic laxative indicated for cleansing of the colon as a preparation for colonoscopy in adults 18 years or older. (1)

————DOSAGE AND ADMINISTRATION————
• MoviPrep, supplied as powder for oral solution, must be mixed with water before use (2.1).
• Do not consume any food from the start of MoviPrep treatment until after the colonoscopy and do not consume any clear liquids at least 2 hours before your colonoscopy (2.1).
• There are two possible dosing regimens; each regimen requires different dosing times (2.1):
  • Split-dose (2-Day) regimen is the preferred method (2.2):
    • Dose 1: The evening before the colonoscopy (10 to 12 hours before Dose 2)
    • Dose 2: The next morning, on the day of the colonoscopy (start at least 3 ½ hours prior to the colonoscopy).
  • Evening only (1-Day) regimen is an alternative method (2.3):
    • Dose 1: Begin at least 3 ½ hours prior to bedtime the evening before the colonoscopy
    • Dose 2: Take Dose 2 approximately 1½ hours after starting Dose 1 the evening before the colonoscopy
• Consume additional clear liquids after every dose in either dosing regimen (2.2, 2.3).

————DOSAGE FORMS AND STRENGTHS————
• Powder for Oral Solution: 2 pouches labeled Pouch A and 2 pouches labeled Pouch B.
• Each pouch A contains 100 grams of polyethylene glycol (PEG) 3350, NF, 7.5 grams of sodium sulfate, USP, 2.691 grams of sodium chloride, USP, and 1.015 grams of potassium chloride, USP, plus the following excipients: aspartame, NF (sweetener), acesulfame potassium, NF (sweetener), and lemon flavoring (3).
• Each pouch B contains 4.7 grams of ascorbic acid, USP and 5.9 grams of sodium ascorbate, USP (3).

————CONTRAINDICATIONS————
• Gastrointestinal (GI) obstruction (4)
• Bowel perforation (4)
• Gastric retention (4)
• Ileus (4)
• Toxic colitis or toxic megacolon (4)
• Hypersensitivity to any components of MoviPrep (4)

————WARNINGS AND PRECAUTIONS————
• Risk of fluid and electrolyte abnormalities, arrhythmias, seizures and renal impairment – encourage adequate hydration, assess concurrent medications, and consider laboratory assessments prior to and after use (5.1, 5.2, 5.3)
• Patients with impaired renal function or patients taking concomitant medications that affect renal function – use caution, ensure adequate hydration and consider testing (5.4)
• Suspected GI obstruction or perforation – rule out the diagnosis before administration (5.6)
• Patients at risk for aspiration —observe during administration (5.7)
• Glucose-6-phosphate dehydrogenase deficiency (G-6-PD) – use with caution (5.8)
• Contains phenylalanine (5.9)

————ADVERSE REACTIONS————
Most common adverse reactions for split dosing (incidence ≥ 5%) are malaise, nausea, abdominal pain, vomiting, and upper abdominal pain (6). The most common adverse reactions for evening only dosing (incidence ≥ 5%) are abdominal distension, anal discomfort, thirst, nausea, abdominal pain, sleep disorder, rigors, hunger, malaise, vomiting, and dizziness (6).
To report SUSPECTED ADVERSE REACTIONS, contact Salix Pharmaceuticals, Inc. at 1-800-508-0024 or FDA at 1-800-FDA-1088 or www.fda.gov/medwatch.

————DRUG INTERACTIONS————
• Oral medications may not be absorbed when administered while taking MoviPrep (7).

————USE IN SPECIFIC POPULATIONS————
• Pregnancy: No human or animal data. Use only if clearly needed (8.1).
See 17 for PATIENT COUNSELING INFORMATION
Revised: 11/2013

FULL PRESCRIBING INFORMATION: CONTENTS*

FULL PRESCRIBING INFORMATION

1   INDICATIONS AND USAGE
MoviPrep is an osmotic laxative indicated for cleansing of the colon as a preparation for colonoscopy in adults 18 years of age or older.

2   DOSAGE AND ADMINISTRATION
2.1   Dosing Overview
There are two possible dosing regimens. Each regimen requires different dosing times:
• Split-dose (2-Day) [see Dosage and Administration (2.2)]
• Evening only (1-Day) [see Dosage and Administration (2.3)]
Both MoviPrep dosing regimens require administration of MoviPrep using the mixing container provided to dilute powder for oral solution (contents of Pouch A and B) with water to the Fill line. Preparation of MoviPrep solution (the contents of one Pouch A and one Pouch B) occurs twice in each dosing regimen. Additional fluids must be consumed in both dosing regimens [see Dosage and Administration (2.2, 2.3)]. Instruct patients to consume only clear liquids (no solid food) from the start of MoviPrep treatment until after the colonoscopy [see Warnings and Precautions (5.1)]. Additionally, instruct patients to not consume any clear liquids at least 2 hours before the colonoscopy.
2.2   Split-dose (2-Day) Regimen (Preferred Method)
The Split-Dose regimen is the preferred dosing method. Instruct patients to take two separate doses in conjunction with fluids, as follows:
Dose 1 – Take this dose the evening before the colonoscopy (10 to 12 hours before Dose 2)
1. Empty the contents of 1 pouch A and 1 pouch B into the container that comes with MoviPrep.
2. Add lukewarm water to the Fill line on the container.
3. Mix to completely dissolve the contents of pouch A and B into the lukewarm water.
4. Drink one 8 oz. (ounce) glass (240 mL) every 15 minutes. Be sure to drink all of the solution. This should take about 1 hour.

5. Fill the container with 16 oz. (two 8 oz. glasses) of clear liquid and drink all of this liquid before going to bed.
Dose 2 – Take this dose the next morning, on the day of the colonoscopy (start at least 3 ½ hours prior to colonoscopy)
1. Repeat steps 1 through 4 from Dose 1 of the Split-dose (2-Day) instructions.
2. Fill the container with 16 oz. (two 8 oz. glasses) of clear liquid and drink all of this liquid at least 2 hours before the colonoscopy.
3. Drink only clear liquids up to 2 hours before the colonoscopy or as prescribed by your healthcare provider. Then stop drinking liquids until after the colonoscopy.
2.3   Evening only (1-Day) Regimen (Alternative Method)
The Day-Before regimen is the alternative dosing method for patients for whom the Split-Dosing regimen is inappropriate. Instruct patients to take two separate doses in conjunction with fluids as follows:
Dose 1 – Take this dose at least 3 ½ hours before bedtime the evening before the colonoscopy:
1. Empty the contents of 1 pouch A and 1 pouch B into the container that comes with MoviPrep.
2. Add lukewarm water to the Fill Line on the container.
3. Mix to completely dissolve the contents of pouch A and B into the lukewarm water.
4. Drink one 8 oz. (ounce) glass (240 mL) every 15 minutes. Be sure to drink all of the solution. This should take about 1 hour.
Dose 2 – Take Dose 2 about 1 ½ hours after starting Dose 1 on the evening before the colonoscopy:
1. Repeat Steps 1 through 4 from Dose 1 of the Evening only (1-Day) instructions.
2. After you complete step 1 through 4, fill the container again to the Fill Line with clear liquid and drink all of this liquid before going to bed.
3. Drink only clear liquids up to 2 hours before the colonoscopy or as prescribed by your healthcare provider. Then stop drinking liquids until after the colonoscopy.
Additional Information:
MoviPrep solution may be refrigerated before drinking. Keep the mixed solution in an upright position and store in the refrigerator. MoviPrep should be taken within 24 hours after it is mixed in water. Do not add other ingredients to the MoviPrep solution.

3   DOSAGE FORMS AND STRENGTHS
Powder for Oral Solution: MoviPrep is available in a carton that contains 2 pouches labeled Pouch A and 2 pouches labeled Pouch B. Each pouch A contains 100 grams of polyethylene glycol (PEG) 3350, NF, 7.5 grams of sodium sulfate, USP, 2.691 grams of sodium chloride, USP, and 1.015 grams of potassium chloride, USP, plus the following excipients: aspartame, NF (sweetener), acesulfame potassium, NF (sweetener), and lemon flavoring. Each pouch B contains 4.7 grams of ascorbic acid, USP and 5.9 grams of sodium ascorbate, USP.

4   CONTRAINDICATIONS
MoviPrep is contraindicated in the following conditions:
• Gastrointestinal (GI) obstruction
• Bowel perforation
• Gastric retention
• Ileus
• Toxic colitis or toxic megacolon
• Hypersensitivity to any components of MoviPrep [see DESCRIPTION (11)]

5   WARNINGS AND PRECAUTIONS
5.1   Serious Fluid and Electrolyte Abnormalities
Advise patients to hydrate adequately before, during, and after the use of MoviPrep. If a patient develops significant vomiting or signs of dehydration after taking MoviPrep consider performing post-colonoscopy lab tests (electrolytes, creatinine, and BUN). Fluid and electrolyte disturbances can lead to serious adverse events including cardiac arrhythmias, seizures and renal impairment.
Patients with electrolyte abnormalities should have them corrected before treatment with MoviPrep. MoviPrep should be used with caution in patients using concomitant medications that increase the risk of electrolyte abnormalities [such as diuretics, angiotensin converting enzyme (ACE)-inhibitors or angiotensin receptor blockers (ARBs)] or in patients with known or suspected hyponatremia. Consider performing pre-dose and post-colonoscopy laboratory tests (sodium, potassium, calcium, creatinine, and BUN) in these patients. [See DRUG INTERACTIONS (7.1)]
5.2   Cardiac Arrhythmias
There have been rare reports of serious arrhythmias associated with the use of ionic osmotic laxative products for bowel preparation. Use caution when prescribing MoviPrep for patients at increased risk of arrhythmias (e.g., patients with a history of prolonged QT, uncontrolled arrhythmias, recent myocardial infarction, unstable angina, congestive heart failure, or cardiomyopathy). Pre-dose and post-colonoscopy ECGs should be considered in patients at increased risk of serious cardiac arrhythmias.

5.3 Seizures

There have been rare reports of generalized tonic-clonic seizures and/or loss of consciousness associated with use of bowel preparation products in patients with no prior history of seizures. The seizure cases were associated with electrolyte abnormalities (e.g., hyponatremia, hypokalemia, hypocalcemia, and hypomagnesemia) and low serum osmolality. The neurologic abnormalities resolved with correction of fluid and electrolyte abnormalities.

Use caution when prescribing MoviPrep for patients with a history of seizures and in patients at increased risk of seizure, such as patients taking medications that lower the seizure threshold (e.g., tricyclic antidepressants), patients withdrawing from alcohol or benzodiazepines, or patients with known or suspected hyponatremia.

5.4 Renal Impairment

Use with caution in patients with impaired renal function or patients taking concomitant medications that affect renal function (such as diuretics, angiotensin converting enzyme inhibitors, angiotensin receptor blockers, or non-steroidal anti-inflammatory drugs). Advise these patients of the importance of adequate hydration, and consider performing pre-dose and post-colonoscopy laboratory tests (electrolytes, creatinine, and BUN) in these patients.

5.5 (Colonic) Mucosal Ulceration, Ischemic Colitis and Ulcerative Colitis

Osmotic laxatives may produce colonic mucosal aphthous ulcerations and there have been reports of more serious cases of ischemic colitis requiring hospitalization. Concurrent use of stimulant laxatives and MoviPrep may increase the risk and is not recommended. The potential for mucosal ulcerations resulting from the bowel preparation should be considered when interpreting colonoscopy findings in patients with known or suspected inflammatory bowel disease.

5.6 Use in Patients with Significant Gastrointestinal Disease

If gastrointestinal obstruction or perforation is suspected, perform appropriate diagnostic studies to rule out these conditions before administering MoviPrep. If a patient experiences severe bloating, abdominal distension, or abdominal pain, administration should be slowed or temporarily discontinued until symptoms abate.

Use with caution in patients with severe ulcerative colitis.

5.7 Aspiration

Patients with impaired gag reflex and patients prone to regurgitation or aspiration should be observed during the administration of MoviPrep. Use with caution in these patients.

5.8 Glucose-6-phosphate Dehydrogenase (G-6-PD) Deficiency

Since MoviPrep contains sodium ascorbate and ascorbic acid, MoviPrep should be used with caution in patients with glucose-6-phosphate dehydrogenase (G-6-PD) deficiency, especially G-6-PD deficiency patients with an active infection, with a history of hemolysis, or taking concomitant medications known to precipitate hemolytic reactions.

5.9 Contains Phenylalanine

Phenylketonurics: Contains aspartame 233 mg per treatment which corresponds to 131 mg of phenylalanine per treatment (after hydrolysis of the aspartame molecule in-vivo to aspartic acid and phenylalanine).

6 ADVERSE REACTIONS

6.1 Clinical Studies Experience

Because clinical trials are conducted under widely varying conditions, adverse reaction rates observed in the clinical trials of a drug cannot be directly compared to rates in the clinical trials of another drug and may not reflect the rates observed in clinical practice.

In the MoviPrep trials, abdominal distension, anal discomfort, thirst, nausea, and abdominal pain were some of the most common adverse reactions to MoviPrep administration. Since diarrhea was considered as a part of the efficacy of MoviPrep, diarrhea was not defined as an adverse reaction in the clinical studies. Tables 1 and 2 display the most common drug-related adverse reactions of MoviPrep and its comparator in the controlled MoviPrep trials.

Table 1: The Most Common Drug-Related Adverse Reactions[1] (≥ 2%) in the Study of MoviPrep vs. 4 Liter Polyethylene Glycol plus Electrolytes Solution

	MoviPrep (split dose) N=180	4L PEG + E[2] N=179
	n (% = n/N)	n (% = n/N)
Malaise	35 (19.4)	32 (17.9)
Nausea	26 (14.4)	36 (20.1)
Abdominal pain	24 (13.3)	27 (15.1)
Vomiting	14 (7.8)	23 (12.8)
Upper abdominal pain	10 (5.6)	11 (6.1)
Dyspepsia	5 (2.8)	2 (1.1)

[1] Drug-related adverse reactions were adverse events that were possibly, probably, or definitely related to the study drug.

[2] 4L PEG + E is 4 liter Polyethylene Glycol plus Electrolytes Solution

Table 2: The Most Common Drug-Related Adverse Reactions[1] (≥ 5%) in the Study of MoviPrep vs. 90 mL Oral Sodium Phosphate Solution

	MoviPrep (evening-only) (full dose) N=169	90 mL OSPS[2] N=171
	n (% = n/N)	n (% = n/N)
Abdominal distension	101 (59.8)	70 (40.9)
Anal discomfort	87 (51.5)	89 (52.0)
Thirst	80 (47.3)	112 (65.5)
Nausea	80 (47.3)	80 (46.8)
Abdominal pain	66 (39.1)	55 (32.2)
Sleep disorder	59 (34.9)	49 (28.7)
Rigors	57 (33.7)	51 (29.8)
Hunger	51 (30.2)	121 (70.8)
Malaise	45 (26.6)	90 (52.6)
Vomiting	12 (7.1)	14 (8.2)
Dizziness	11 (6.5)	31 (18.1)
Headache	3 (1.8)	9 (5.3)
Hypokalemia	0 (0)	10 (5.8)
Hyperphosphatemia	0 (0)	10 (5.8)

[1] Drug-related adverse reactions were adverse events that were possibly, probably, or definitely related to the study drug. In addition to the recording of spontaneous adverse events, patients were also specifically asked about the occurrence of the following symptoms: shivering, anal irritations, abdominal bloating or fullness, sleep loss, nausea, vomiting, weakness, hunger sensation, abdominal cramps or pain, thirst sensation, and dizziness.

[2] OSPS is Oral Sodium Phosphate Solution

Isolated cases of urticaria, rhinorrhea, dermatitis, and anaphylactic reaction have been reported with PEG-based products and may represent allergic reactions.

Published literature contains isolated reports of serious adverse events following the administration of PEG-based products in patients over 60 years of age. These adverse events included upper gastrointestinal bleeding from a Mallory-Weiss tear, esophageal perforation, asystole, and acute pulmonary edema after aspirating PEG-based preparation.

6.2 Postmarketing Experience

In addition to adverse reactions reported from clinical trials, the following adverse events have been identified during post-approval use of MoviPrep. Because they are reported voluntarily from a population of uncertain size, it is not always possible to reliably estimate their frequency or establish a causal relationship to drug exposure. These events have been chosen for inclusion due to either their seriousness, frequency of reporting or causal connection to MoviPrep, or a combination of these factors.

Cardiovascular: Tachycardia, palpitations, hypertension, arrhythmia, atrial fibrillation, peripheral edema.

General: Hypersensitivity reactions including anaphylaxis (some of which were severe, including shock), rash, urticaria, pruritus, lip, tongue and facial swelling, dyspnea, chest tightness and throat tightness. Fever, chills and dehydration.

Nervous system: Syncope, tremor, seizure.

Renal: Renal impairment and/or failure.

7 DRUG INTERACTIONS

7.1 Drugs That May Increase Risks Due to Fluid and Electrolyte Abnormalities

Use caution when prescribing MoviPrep for patients with conditions, or who are using medications that increase the risk for fluid and electrolyte disturbances or may increase the risk of adverse events of seizure, arrhythmias, and prolonged QT in the setting of fluid and electrolyte abnormalities. Consider additional patient evaluations as appropriate. [See WARNINGS (5)]

7.2 Potential for Altered Drug Absorption

Oral medication administered within 1 hour of the start of administration of MoviPrep may be flushed from the gastrointestinal tract and the medication may not be absorbed.

8 USE IN SPECIFIC POPULATIONS

8.1 Pregnancy

Pregnancy Category C. Animal reproduction studies have not been performed with MoviPrep. It is also not known if MoviPrep can cause fetal harm when administered to a pregnant woman or can affect reproductive capacity. MoviPrep should be given to a pregnant woman only if clearly needed.

8.3 Nursing Mothers

It is not known whether this drug is excreted in human milk. Because many drugs are excreted in human milk, caution should be exercised when MoviPrep is administered to a nursing woman.

8.4 Pediatric Use

The safety and effectiveness of MoviPrep in pediatric patients has not been established.

8.5 Geriatric Use

Of the 413 patients in clinical studies receiving MoviPrep, 91 (22%) patients were aged 65 or older, while 25 (6%) patients were over 75 years of age. No overall differences in safety or effectiveness were observed between geriatric patients and younger patients, and other reported clinical experience has not identified differences in responses between geriatric patients and younger patients, but greater sensitivity of some older individuals cannot be ruled out.

10 OVERDOSAGE

There have been no reported cases of overdose with MoviPrep. Purposeful or gross accidental ingestion of more than the recommended dose of MoviPrep might be expected to lead to severe electrolyte disturbances, including hyponatremia and/or hypokalemia, as well as dehydration and hypovolemia, with signs and symptoms of these disturbances. The patient who has taken an overdose should be monitored carefully, and treated symptomatically for complications.

11 DESCRIPTION

MoviPrep (PEG-3350, sodium sulfate, sodium chloride, potassium chloride, sodium ascorbate, and ascorbic acid for oral solution) is an osmotic laxative consisting of 4 pouches (2 of pouch A and 2 of pouch B) containing white to yellow powder for reconstitution. Each pouch A contains 100 grams of polyethylene glycol (PEG) 3350, NF, 7.5 grams of sodium sulfate, USP, 2.691 grams of sodium chloride, USP, and 1.015 grams of potassium chloride, USP, plus the following excipients: aspartame, NF (sweetener), acesulfame potassium, NF (sweetener), and lemon flavoring. Each pouch B contains 4.7 grams of ascorbic acid, USP and 5.9 grams of sodium ascorbate, USP. When 1 pouch A and 1 pouch B are dissolved together in water to a volume of 1 liter, MoviPrep (PEG-3350, sodium sulfate, sodium chloride, potassium chloride, sodium ascorbate, and ascorbic acid) is an oral solution having a lemon taste.

The entire, reconstituted, 2-liter MoviPrep colon preparation contains 200 grams of PEG-3350, 15 grams of sodium sulfate, 5.38 grams of sodium chloride, 2.03 grams of potassium chloride, 9.4 grams of ascorbic acid, and 11.8 grams of sodium ascorbate plus the following excipients: aspartame (sweetener), acesulfame potassium (sweetener), and lemon flavoring.

A container for reconstitution is enclosed.

12 CLINICAL PHARMACOLOGY

12.1 Mechanism of Action

The primary mode of action is thought to be through the osmotic effect of polyethylene glycol 3350, sodium sulfate, sodium chloride, potassium chloride, sodium ascorbate, and ascorbic acid, which causes water to be retained in the colon and produces a watery stool.

12.3 Pharmacokinetics

The pharmacokinetics of MoviPrep have not been studied in patients with renal or hepatic insufficiency.

13 NONCLINICAL TOXICOLOGY

13.1 Carcinogenesis, Mutagenesis, Impairment of Fertility

Long-term studies in animals to evaluate the carcinogenic potential have not been performed with MoviPrep. Studies to evaluate potential for impairment of fertility or mutagenic potential have not been performed with MoviPrep.

14 CLINICAL STUDIES

The colon cleansing efficacy and safety of MoviPrep was evaluated in two randomized, actively-controlled, multicenter, investigator-blinded, phase 3 trials in patients scheduled to have an elective colonoscopy.

In the first study, patients were randomized to one of the following two colon preparation treatments: 1) 2 liters of MoviPrep with 1 additional liter of clear liquid split into two doses (during the evening before and the morning of the colonoscopy) and 2) 4 liters of polyethylene glycol plus electrolytes solution (4L PEG + E) split into two doses (during the evening before and the morning of the colonoscopy). Patients were allowed to have a morning breakfast, a light lunch, clear soup and/or plain yogurt for dinner. Dinner had to be completed at least one hour prior to initiation of the colon preparation administration.

The primary efficacy endpoint was the proportion of patients with effective colon cleansing as judged by blinded gastroenterologists on the basis of videotapes recorded during the colonoscopy.

The blinded gastroenterologists graded the colon cleansing twice (during introduction and withdrawal of the colonoscope) and the poorer of the two assessments was used in the primary efficacy analysis.

The efficacy analysis included 308 adult patients who had an elective colonoscopy. Patients ranged in age from 18 to 88 years old (mean age about 59 years old) with 52% female and 48% male patients. Table 3 displays the results.

Table 3: Effectiveness of Overall Colon Cleansing in the Study of MoviPrep vs. 4 Liter Polyethylene Glycol plus Electrolytes Solution

	Responders A[2] or B[3] (%)	C[4] (%)	D[5] (%)
MoviPrep (N=153)	88.9	9.8	1.3
4L PEG + E[1] (N=155)	94.8	4.5	0.6

[1] 4L PEG + E is 4 Liter Polyethylene Glycol plus Electrolytes Solution
[2] A: colon empty and clean or presence of clear liquid, but easily removed by suction
[3] B: brown liquid or semisolid remaining amounts of stool, fully removable by suction or displaceable, thus allowing a complete visualization of the gut mucosa
[4] C: semisolid amounts of stool, only partially removable with a risk of incomplete visualization of the gut mucosa
[5] D: semisolid or solid amounts of stool; consequently colonoscopy incomplete or needed to be terminated.

4 L PEG+E's responder rate was not significantly higher than MoviPrep's responder rate.

In the second study, patients were randomized to one of the following two colon preparation treatments: 1) 2 liters of MoviPrep with 1 additional liter of clear liquid in the evening prior to the colonoscopy and 2) 90 mL of oral sodium phosphate solution (90 mL OSPS) with at least 2 liters of additional clear liquid during the day and evening prior to the colonoscopy. Patients randomized to MoviPrep therapy were allowed to have a morning breakfast; a light lunch; and clear soup and/or plain yogurt for dinner. Dinner had to be completed at least one hour prior to initiation of the colon preparation administration.

The primary efficacy endpoint was the proportion of patients with effective colon cleansing as judged by the colonoscopist and one blinded gastroenterologist (on the basis of videotapes recorded during the colonoscopy). In case of a discrepancy between the colonoscopist and the blinded gastroenterologist, a second blinded gastroenterologist made the final efficacy determination.

The efficacy analysis included 280 adult patients who had an elective colonoscopy. Patients ranged in age from 21 to 76 years old (mean age about 53 years old) with 47% female and 53% male patients. Table 4 displays the results.

Table 4: Effectiveness of Overall Colon Cleansing in the Study of MoviPrep Vs. 90mL Oral Sodium Phosphate Solution

	Responders A[2] or B[3] (%)	C[4] (%)	D[5] (%)
MoviPrep (N=137)	73.0	23.4	3.6
90 mL OSPS[1] (N=143)	64.4	29.4	6.3

[1] OSPS is Oral Sodium Phosphate Solution
[2] A: empty and clean or clear liquid (transparent, yellow, or green)
[3] B: brown liquid or semisolid remaining small amounts of stool, fully removable by suction or displaceable allowing a complete visualization of the underlying mucosa

[4] C: semi solid only partially removable/displaceable stools; risk of incomplete examination of the underlying mucosa
[5] D: heavy and hard stool making the segment examination uninterpretable and, consequently, the colonoscopy needed to be terminated

MoviPrep's responder rate was not significantly higher than OSPS's responder rate.

16 HOW SUPPLIED/STORAGE AND HANDLING

MoviPrep is supplied as a white to yellow powder. MoviPrep is administered as an oral solution after reconstitution.
NDC 65649-201-75, MoviPrep, single use carton.
NDC 65649-201-76, MoviPrep, professional sample carton.
Each carton contains a disposable container for reconstitution of MoviPrep and 2 Pouches labeled Pouch A and 2 Pouches labeled Pouch B.

STORAGE

Store carton/container at room temperature, between 68°F to 77°F (20°C to 25°C); excursions permitted to 15-30°C (59-86°F). When reconstituted, store upright and keep solution refrigerated. Use within 24 hours.

17 PATIENT COUNSELING INFORMATION

• Advise patients who require a diet low in phenylalanine that MoviPrep contains aspartame – a maximum of 233 mg per treatment. This sweetener, after hydrolysis in the body, provides 131 mg of phenylalanine to the patient.
• Ask patients to inform you if they have trouble swallowing or are prone to regurgitation or aspiration.
• Instruct patients that each pouch needs to be diluted in water before ingestion and that they need to drink additional clear liquid. Examples of clear liquids are:
  • water
  • clear fruit juices without pulp including apple, white grape, or white cranberry
  • strained limeade or lemonade
  • coffee or tea (Do not use dairy or non-dairy creamer)
  • clear broth
  • clear soda
  • gelatin (without added fruit or topping)
  • popsicles (without pieces of fruit or fruit pulp)
• Inform patients that oral medications may not be absorbed properly if they are taken within one hour of starting each dose of MoviPrep.
• Tell patients not to take other laxatives while they are taking MoviPrep.
• Tell patients that MoviPrep produces a watery stool (diarrhea) which cleanses the colon before colonoscopy. Advise patients receiving MoviPrep to adequately hydrate before, during, and after the use of MoviPrep. Patients may have clear soup and/or plain yogurt for dinner, finishing the evening meal at least one hour prior to the start of MoviPrep treatment. No solid food should be taken from the start of MoviPrep treatment until after the colonoscopy.
• Tell patients that the first bowel movement may occur approximately 1 hour after the start of MoviPrep administration. Abdominal bloating and distention may occur before the first bowel movement. If severe abdominal discomfort or distention occurs, stop drinking MoviPrep temporarily or drink each portion at longer intervals until these symptoms diminish. If severe symptoms persist, notify your health provider.

Manufactured for:
Salix Pharmaceuticals, Inc.
Raleigh, NC 27615
2013 Salix Pharmaceuticals, Inc.
Rev NOV 2013
Product protected by U.S. Patent Nos. 7,169,381 and 7,658,914.
Please see www.salix.com for patent information

Medication Guide
MoviPrep® (moo-vee-prĕp)
(PEG 3350, sodium sulfate, sodium chloride, potassium chloride, sodium ascorbate, and ascorbic acid for oral solution)
Read this Medication Guide before you start taking MoviPrep. This information does not take the place of talking with your healthcare provider about your medical condition or your treatment.

What is the most important information I should know about MoviPrep?
MoviPrep can cause serious side effects, including:
Serious loss of body fluid (dehydration) and changes in blood salts (electrolytes) in your blood.
These changes can cause:
• **abnormal heartbeats that can cause death**
• **seizures.** This can happen even if you have never had a seizure
• **kidney problems**

Your risk of having fluid loss and changes in body salts with MoviPrep is higher if you:
• have heart problems
• have kidney problems
• take water pills (diuretics), high blood pressure medication, or non-steroidal anti-inflammatory drugs (NSAIDS)
Tell your healthcare provider right away if you have any of these symptoms of a loss of too much body fluid (dehydration) while taking MoviPrep:
• vomiting
• dizziness
• urinating less often than normal
• headache
See "What are the possible side effects of MoviPrep?" for more information about side effects.

What is MoviPrep?
MoviPrep is a prescription medicine used by adults 18 years of age and older to clean the colon before a colonoscopy. MoviPrep cleans your colon by causing you to have diarrhea.
Cleaning your colon helps your healthcare provider see the inside of your colon more clearly during your colonoscopy.
It is not known if MoviPrep is safe and effective in children.

Who should not take MoviPrep?
Do not take MoviPrep if your healthcare provider has told you that you have:
• a blockage in your intestine (bowel obstruction)
• an opening in the wall of your stomach or intestine (bowel perforation)
• problems with food and fluid emptying from your stomach (gastric retention)
• a very dilated intestine (toxic megacolon)
• an allergy to any of the ingredients in MoviPrep. See the end of this leaflet for a complete list of ingredients in MoviPrep.

What should I tell my healthcare provider before taking MoviPrep?
Before you take MoviPrep, tell your healthcare provider if you:
• have heart problems
• have a history of seizures
• have kidney problems
• have stomach or bowel problems, including ulcerative colitis
• have problems with swallowing or gastric reflux
• have a condition that destroys red blood cells called Glucose-6-phosphate dehydrogenase (G6PD) deficiency
• are withdrawing from drinking alcohol
• have a low blood salt (sodium) level
• are on a diet low in phenylalanine
• have any other medical conditions
• are pregnant or plan to become pregnant. It is not known if MoviPrep will harm your unborn baby.
• are breastfeeding or plan to breastfeed. It is not known if MoviPrep passes into your breast milk. You and your healthcare provider should decide if you will take MoviPrep while breastfeeding.
Tell your healthcare provider about all the medicines you take, including prescription and non-prescription medicines, vitamins, and herbal supplements.
MoviPrep may affect how other medicines work. Medicines taken by mouth may not be absorbed properly when taken within 1 hour before the start of MoviPrep.
Especially tell your healthcare provider if you take:
• medicines for blood pressure or heart problems
• medicines for kidney problems
• medicines for seizures
• water pills (diuretics)
• non-steroidal anti-inflammatory (NSAID) pain medicines
• laxatives
• medicines for depression or mental health problems
Ask your healthcare provider or pharmacist for a list of these medicines if you are not sure if you are taking any of the medicines listed above.
Know the medicines you take. Keep a list of them to show your healthcare provider and pharmacist when you get a new medicine.

How should I take MoviPrep?
See the Instructions for Use on the outer MoviPrep carton for dosing instructions. You must read, understand, and follow these instructions to take MoviPrep the right way.
• Take MoviPrep exactly as your healthcare provider tells you to take it. Your healthcare provider will prescribe the Split-dose (2-Day) option or the Evening only (1-Day) dosing option, depending on the scheduling of your colonoscopy.
• Do not take MoviPrep that has not been mixed with water.
• Drink clear liquids before, during, and after you take MoviPrep to help prevent fluid loss (dehydration). It is important for you to drink the additional prescribed amount of clear liquids listed in the Instructions for Use.

Examples of clear liquids are:
- water
- clear fruit juices without pulp including apple, white grape, or white cranberry
- strained limeade or lemonade
- coffee or tea (Do not use any dairy or non-dairy creamer)
- clear broth
- clear soda
- gelatin (without added fruit or topping)
- popsicles (without pieces of fruit or fruit pulp)
- **Do not eat or drink anything colored red or purple.**
- Do not take other laxatives while taking MoviPrep.
- You may eat clear broth and plain yogurt for dinner on the evening that you start taking MoviPrep. Finish eating this meal at least 1 hour before you start taking MoviPrep.
- **Do not eat solid foods while taking MoviPrep and until after your colonoscopy.**
- Drink only clear liquids:
  - while taking MoviPrep
  - after taking MoviPrep and until 2 hours before your colonoscopy
  Do not eat or drink anything 2 hours before your colonoscopy
- You may have stomach-area (abdomen) bloating before you have your first bowel movement.
- Stop drinking MoviPrep for a short time or wait a longer time between each dose of MoviPrep if you have severe stomach-area (abdomen) discomfort or bloating until your symptoms improve. If symptoms continue, tell your healthcare provider.
- Your first bowel movement may happen about 1 hour after you start taking MoviPrep.
- If you take too much MoviPrep, call your healthcare provider or go to the nearest hospital emergency room right away.

What are the possible side effects of MoviPrep?
MoviPrep can cause serious side effects, including:
- **See Section "What is the most important information I should know about MoviPrep?"**
- **changes in certain blood tests.** Your healthcare provider may do blood tests after you take MoviPrep to check your blood for changes. Tell your healthcare provider if you have any symptoms of too much fluid loss, including:
  - vomiting
  - nausea
  - bloating
  - dizziness
  - stomach-area (abdomen) cramping
  - headache
  - urinate less than usual
  - trouble drinking clear liquid
- **ulcers of the bowel or bowel problems (ischemic colitis).** Tell your healthcare provider right away if you have severe stomach-area (abdomen) pain or rectal bleeding.

The most common side effects of MoviPrep for split dosing include:
- discomfort
- nausea
- stomach-area (abdomen) pain
- vomiting
- indigestion

The most common side effects of MoviPrep for the Evening only (1-Day) dosing option include:
- stomach-area (abdominal) bloating
- anal discomfort
- thirst
- nausea
- stomach-area (abdomen) pain
- sleep problems
- chills
- hunger
- discomfort
- vomiting
- dizziness

Tell your healthcare provider if you have any side effect that bothers you or that does not go away.
These are not all the possible side effects of MoviPrep. For more information, ask your healthcare provider or pharmacist.
Call your doctor for medical advice about side effects. You may report side effects to FDA at 1-800-FDA-1088.

How should I store MoviPrep?
- Store MoviPrep that has not been mixed with water at room temperature, between 68°F to 77°F (20°C to 25°C).
- Store MoviPrep that has been mixed with water in an upright position in the refrigerator.
- MoviPrep should be taken within 24 hours after it has been mixed with water.

Keep MoviPrep and all medicines out of the reach of children.

General information about the safe and effective use of MoviPrep.
Medicines are sometimes prescribed for purposes other than those listed in a Medication Guide. Do not use MoviPrep for a condition for which it was not prescribed. Do not give MoviPrep to other people, even if they are going to have the same procedure you are. It may harm them.

This Medication Guide summarizes the most important information about MoviPrep. If you would like more information, talk with your healthcare provider. You can ask your pharmacist or healthcare provider for information that is written for health care professionals.
For more information, call 1-866-669-7597 or go to www.MoviPrep.com.

What are the ingredients in MoviPrep?
Active ingredients:
Pouch A: polyethylene glycol (PEG) 3350, sodium sulfate, sodium chloride, potassium chloride.
Pouch B: ascorbic acid and sodium ascorbate.
Inactive ingredients:
Pouch A: aspartame, acesulfame potassium, and lemon flavoring.
This Medication Guide has been approved by the U.S. Food and Drug Administration.
Manufactured for:
Salix Pharmaceuticals, Inc.
Raleigh, NC 27615
Product protected by U.S. Patent Nos. 7,169,381 and 7,658,914.
Please see www.salix.com for patent information
Revised: Nov 2013
Shown in Product Identification Guide, page 313

RELISTOR®
(methylnaltrexone bromide)
Subcutaneous Injection

℞

HIGHLIGHTS OF PRESCRIBING INFORMATION
These highlights do not include all the information needed to use RELISTOR safely and effectively. See full prescribing information for RELISTOR.
RELISTOR (methylnaltrexone bromide) Subcutaneous Injection
Initial U.S. Approval: 2008

RECENT MAJOR CHANGES

General Dosing Information (2.1)	[08/2013]
Dosing (2.2)	[08/2013]
Use in Patients with Severe Renal Impairment (2.3)	[08/2013]
Administration and Storage (2.4)	[08/2013]
Gastrointestinal Perforation (5.1)	[08/2013]
Severe or Persistent Diarrhea (5.2)	[08/2013]

INDICATIONS AND USAGE

RELISTOR is indicated for the treatment of opioid-induced constipation in patients with advanced illness who are receiving palliative care, when response to laxative therapy has not been sufficient. Use of RELISTOR beyond four months has not been studied. (1)

DOSAGE AND ADMINISTRATION

RELISTOR is administered as a subcutaneous injection. The usual schedule is one dose every other day, as needed, but no more frequently than one dose in a 24-hour period. (2.2)
The recommended dose of RELISTOR is 8 mg for patients weighing 38 to less than 62 kg or 12 mg for patients weighing 62 to 114 kg. Patients whose weights fall outside of these ranges should be dosed at 0.15 mg/kg. See the table below to determine the correct injection volume. (2.2)

Patient Weight	Injection Volume	Dose
Less than 38 kg	**See below***	0.15 mg/kg
38 kg to less than 62 kg	**0.4 mL**	8 mg
62 kg to 114 kg	**0.6 mL**	12 mg
More than 114 kg	**See below***	0.15 mg/kg

* The injection volume for these patients should be calculated using one of the following (2.2):
  - Multiply the patient weight in kilograms by 0.0075 and round up the volume to the nearest 0.1 mL.

Only patients requiring an 8 mg or 12 mg dose should be prescribed pre-filled syringes (2.2, 3).
In patients with severe renal impairment (creatinine clearance less than 30 mL/min), dose reductions of RELISTOR by one half is recommended. (8.6)

DOSAGE FORMS AND STRENGTHS

RELISTOR is available in the following dosage forms:
- Single-use vial containing 12 mg/0.6 mL solution for subcutaneous injection, for use with a 27 gauge × ½-inch needle and 1 mL syringe.

- Single-use vial containing 12 mg/0.6 mL solution for subcutaneous injection with one 1 mL syringe with retractable 27 gauge × ½-inch needle, two alcohol swabs.
- Single-use pre-filled syringe containing 8 mg/0.4 mL solution for subcutaneous injection.
- Single-use pre-filled syringe containing 12 mg/0.6 mL solution for subcutaneous injection.

CONTRAINDICATIONS

- RELISTOR is contraindicated in patients with known or suspected mechanical gastrointestinal obstruction. (4)

WARNINGS AND PRECAUTIONS

- Rare cases of gastrointestinal (GI) perforation have been reported in advanced illness patients. Use RELISTOR with caution in patients with known or suspected lesions of the GI tract. (5.1)
- If severe or persistent diarrhea occurs during treatment, advise patients to discontinue therapy with RELISTOR and consult their physician. (5.2)

ADVERSE REACTIONS

The most common (≥ 5%) adverse reactions reported with RELISTOR are abdominal pain, flatulence, nausea, dizziness, diarrhea and hyperhidrosis. (6.1)
To report SUSPECTED ADVERSE REACTIONS, contact Salix Pharmaceuticals Inc. at 1-800-508-0024 or FDA at 1-800-FDA-1088 or www.fda.gov/medwatch

DRUG INTERACTIONS

In an *in vivo* study RELISTOR did not significantly affect the metabolism of the CYP2D6 substrate, dextromethorphan. In vitro methylnaltrexone did not significantly inhibit or induce cytochrome P450 (CYP) isozymes including CYP 1A2, 2A6, 2B6, 2C9, 2C19, or 3A4 (7.1)

USE IN SPECIFIC POPULATIONS

Pediatric Use: Safety and efficacy of RELISTOR have not been established in pediatric patients. (8.4)
See 17 for PATIENT COUNSELING INFORMATION and FDA-approved patient labeling

Revised: 08/2013

FULL PRESCRIBING INFORMATION

1   INDICATIONS AND USAGE

RELISTOR® is indicated for the treatment of opioid-induced constipation in patients with advanced illness who are receiving palliative care, when response to laxative therapy has not been sufficient.

Limitation of use: Use of RELISTOR beyond four months has not been studied in the advanced illness population.

2 DOSAGE AND ADMINISTRATION

2.1 General Dosing Information
RELISTOR is for subcutaneous use only.

2.2 Dosing
For adult patients with opioid-induced constipation and advanced illness, the usual schedule is one dose every other day, as needed, but no more frequently than one dose in a 24-hour period [see Clinical Studies (14)].

The recommended dose of RELISTOR is 8 mg subcutaneously for opioid-induced constipation and advanced illness adult patients weighing 38 kg to less than 62 kg or 12 mg subcutaneously for patients weighing 62 kg to 114 kg. Adult patients whose weight falls outside of these ranges should be dosed at 0.15 mg/kg. See Table 1 to determine the correct injection volume. The prefilled syringe is designed to deliver a fixed dose; therefore, adult patients requiring dosing calculated on a mg/kg basis should not be prescribed pre-filled syringes.

Table 1: Weight of Adult Patient with Opioid-Induced Constipation and Advanced Illness	Injection Volume	Subcutaneous Dose
Less than 38 kg	See below*	0.15 mg/kg
38 kg to less than 62 kg	0.4 mL	8 mg
62 kg to 114 kg	0.6 mL	12 mg
More than 114 kg	See below*	0.15 mg/kg

* The injection volume for these patients should be calculated using the following method:
Multiply the patient weight in kilograms by 0.0075 and round up the volume to the nearest 0.1 mL.

2.3 Use in Patients with Severe Renal Impairment
In adult patients with severe renal impairment (creatinine clearance less than 30 mL/min as estimated by Cockcroft-Gault), dose reduction of RELISTOR by one-half is recommended [see Use in Specific Populations (8.6)]. No dosage adjustment is recommended for adult patients with mild to moderate renal impairment.

The pre-filled syringe is designed to deliver a fixed dose; therefore, adult patients with severe renal impairment should only be prescribed single-use vials to ensure correct dosing.

2.4 Administration and Storage
RELISTOR is a sterile, clear, and colorless to pale yellow aqueous solution. Inspect parenteral drug product visually for particulate matter and discoloration prior to administration, whenever solution and container permit. Do not use the vial if any of these are present.

Inject RELISTOR subcutaneously in the upper arm, abdomen or thigh. Do not inject at the same spot each time (rotate injection sites).

Single-use Vials
Once drawn into the 1 mL syringe with a 27-gauge × ½-inch needle, if immediate administration is not possible, store at ambient room temperature and administer within 24 hours. Discard any unused portion that remains in the vial. Advise patients concerning proper training in subcutaneous technique.

Single-use Pre-filled Syringes
Only adult patients requiring an 8 mg or 12 mg dose should be prescribed pre-filled syringes. Do not remove the pre-filled syringe from the tray until ready to administer.

3 DOSAGE FORMS AND STRENGTHS

- Single-use vial containing 12 mg/0.6 mL solution for subcutaneous injection, for use with a 27 gauge × ½-inch needle and 1 mL syringe.
- Single-use vial containing 12 mg/0.6 mL solution for subcutaneous injection, with one 1 mL syringe with retractable 27 gauge × ½-inch needle, two alcohol swabs
- Single-use pre-filled syringe containing 8 mg/0.4 mL solution for subcutaneous injection, with a 29-gauge × ½-inch fixed needle and a needle guard
- Single-use pre-filled syringe containing 12 mg/0.6 mL solution for subcutaneous injection, with a 29-gauge × ½-inch fixed needle and a needle guard

4 CONTRAINDICATIONS
RELISTOR is contraindicated in patients with known or suspected mechanical gastrointestinal obstruction.

5 WARNINGS AND PRECAUTIONS

5.1 Gastrointestinal Perforation
Cases of gastrointestinal (GI) perforation have been reported in adult patients with opioid-induced constipation and advanced illness with conditions that may be associated with localized or diffuse reduction of structural integrity in the wall of the GI tract (i.e., cancer, peptic ulcer, Ogilvie's syndrome). Perforations have involved varying regions of the GI tract (e.g., stomach, duodenum, or colon). Use RELISTOR with caution in patients with known or suspected lesions of the GI tract. Advise patients to discontinue therapy with RELISTOR and promptly notify their physician if they develop severe, persistent, or worsening abdominal symptoms.

5.2 Severe or Persistent Diarrhea
If severe or persistent diarrhea occurs during treatment, advise patients to discontinue therapy with RELISTOR and consult their physician.

6 ADVERSE REACTIONS

6.1 Clinical Trial Experience
Because clinical trials are conducted under widely varying conditions, adverse reaction rates observed in the clinical trials of a drug cannot be directly compared to rates in the clinical trials of another drug and may not reflect the rates observed in clinical practice.

The safety of RELISTOR was evaluated in two, double-blind, placebo-controlled trials in patients with advanced illness receiving palliative care: Study 1 included a single-dose, double-blind, placebo-controlled period, whereas Study 2 included a 14-day multiple dose, double-blind, placebo-controlled period [see Clinical Studies (14)]. The majority of patients had a primary diagnosis of incurable cancer; other primary diagnoses included end-stage COPD/emphysema, cardiovascular disease/heart failure, Alzheimer's disease/dementia, HIV/AIDS, or other advanced illnesses. Patients were receiving opioid therapy (median daily baseline oral morphine equivalent dose = 172 mg), and had opioid-induced constipation (either <3 bowel movements in the preceding week or no bowel movement for 2 days). Both the methylnaltrexone bromide and placebo patients were on a stable laxative regimen for at least 3 days prior to study entry and continued on their regimen throughout the study.

The most common (≥5%) adverse reactions in patients receiving RELISTOR are shown in Table 2 below.

Table 2: Adverse Reactions from all Doses in Double-Blind, Placebo-Controlled Clinical Studies of RELISTOR in Adult Patients with Opioid-Induced Constipation and Advanced Illness*		
Adverse Reaction	RELISTOR N = 165	Placebo N = 123
Abdominal Pain	47 (28.5%)	12 (9.8%)
Flatulence	22 (13.3%)	7 (5.7%)
Nausea	19 (11.5%)	6 (4.9%)
Dizziness	12 (7.3%)	3 (2.4%)
Diarrhea	9 (5.5%)	3 (2.4%)
Hyperhidrosis	11 (6.7%)	8 (6.5%)

* Doses: 0.075, 0.15, and 0.30 mg/kg/dose

The rates of discontinuation due to adverse events during the double-blind placebo controlled clinical trials (Study 1 and Study 2) were comparable between RELISTOR (1.2%) and placebo (2.4%).

6.2 Postmarketing Experience
The following additional adverse reactions have been identified during post-approval use of RELISTOR. Because they are reported voluntarily from a population of unknown size, estimates of frequency cannot be made. These events have been chosen for inclusion due to either their seriousness, frequency of reporting or causal connection to RELISTOR, or a combination of these factors.

Gastrointestinal
Perforation, cramping, vomiting
General Disorders and Administrative Site Disorders
Diaphoresis, flushing, malaise, pain. Cases of opioid withdrawal have been reported.

7 DRUG INTERACTIONS

7.1 Drugs Metabolized by Cytochrome P450 Isozymes
In healthy subjects, a subcutaneous dose of 0.30 mg/kg of methylnaltrexone did not significantly affect the metabolism of dextromethorphan, a CYP2D6 substrate.

In vitro methylnaltrexone did not significantly inhibit or induce the activity of cytochrome P450 (CYP) isozymes CYP1A2, CYP2A6, CYP2B6, CYP2C9, CYP2C19, or CYP3A4.

In vitro, methylnaltrexone did not induce the enzymatic activity of CYP2E1.

7.2 Drugs Renally Excreted
Methylnaltrexone is actively secreted in the kidney. The potential of drug interactions between methylnaltrexone bromide and other drugs that are inhibitors of transporters in the kidney has not been fully investigated [see Pharmacokinetics (12.3)].

7.3 Cimetidine
Cimetidine given 400 mg three times daily did not significantly affect the systemic exposure to methylnaltrexone. The effect of a higher cimetidine dose (e.g., 800 mg) on the systemic exposure of methylnaltrexone has not been evaluated.

8 USE IN SPECIFIC POPULATIONS

8.1 Pregnancy
Pregnancy Category B
Reproduction studies have been performed in pregnant rats at intravenous doses up to about 14 times the recommended maximum human subcutaneous dose of 0.3 mg/kg based on the body surface area and in pregnant rabbits at intravenous doses up to about 17 times the recommended maximum human subcutaneous dose based on the body surface area and have revealed no evidence of impaired fertility or harm to the fetus due to methylnaltrexone bromide. There are no adequate and well-controlled studies in pregnant women. Because animal reproduction studies are not always predictive of human response, methylnaltrexone bromide should be used during pregnancy only if clearly needed.

8.2 Labor and Delivery
Effects of RELISTOR on mother, fetus, duration of labor, and delivery are unknown. There were no effects on the mother, labor, delivery, or on offspring survival and growth in rats following subcutaneous injection of methylnaltrexone bromide at dosages up to 25 mg/kg/day.

8.3 Nursing Mothers
Results from an animal study using [³H]-labeled methylnaltrexone bromide indicate that methylnaltrexone bromide is excreted via the milk of lactating rats. It is not known whether this drug is excreted in human milk. Because many drugs are excreted in human milk, caution should be exercised when RELISTOR is administered to a nursing woman.

8.4 Pediatric Use
Safety and effectiveness of RELISTOR have not been established in pediatric patients.

8.5 Geriatric Use
In the phase 2 and 3 double-blind studies, a total of 77 (24%) patients aged 65-74 years (54 methylnaltrexone bromide, 23 placebo) and a total of 100 (31.2%) patients aged 75 years or older (61 methylnaltrexone bromide, 39 placebo) were enrolled. Pharmacokinetics of methylnaltrexone was similar between the elderly (mean age 72 years old) and young adults (mean age 30 years old). No overall differences in safety or effectiveness were observed between these patients and younger patients, and other reported clinical experience has not identified differences in responses between the elderly and younger patients, but greater sensitivity of some older individuals cannot be ruled out.

Based on pharmacokinetic data, and safety and efficacy data from controlled clinical trials, no dose adjustment based on age is recommended.

8.6 Renal Impairment
No dose adjustment is required in patients with mild or moderate renal impairment. Dose-reduction by one half is recommended in patients with severe renal impairment (creatinine clearance less than 30 mL/min as estimated by Cockcroft-Gault).

In a study of volunteers with varying degrees of renal impairment receiving a single dose of 0.30 mg/kg methylnaltrexone bromide, renal impairment had a marked effect on the renal excretion of methylnaltrexone bromide. Severe renal impairment decreased the renal clearance of methylnaltrexone bromide by 8- to 9-fold and resulted in a 2-fold increase in total methylnaltrexone bromide exposure (AUC). C_{max} was not significantly changed. No studies were performed in patients with end-stage renal impairment requiring dialysis.

8.7 Hepatic Impairment
No dose adjustment is required for patients with mild or moderate hepatic impairment. The effect of severe hepatic impairment on the pharmacokinetics of methylnaltrexone has not been studied.

10 OVERDOSAGE
During clinical trials of RELISTOR administered subcutaneously, no cases of methylnaltrexone bromide overdose were reported. A study of healthy volunteers noted orthostatic hypotension associated with a dose of 0.64 mg/kg administered as an intravenous bolus.

Signs or symptoms of orthostatic hypotension should be monitored, and treatment should be initiated, as appropriate.

11 DESCRIPTION

RELISTOR (methylnaltrexone bromide) injection, a peripherally-acting mu-opioid receptor antagonist, is a sterile, clear and colorless to pale yellow aqueous solution. The chemical name for methylnaltrexone bromide is (R)-N-(cyclopropylmethyl) noroxymorphone methobromide. The molecular formula is $C_{21}H_{26}NO_4Br$, and the molecular weight is 436.36.

Each 3 mL vial contains 12 mg of methylnaltrexone bromide in 0.6 mL of water. The excipients are 3.9 mg sodium chloride USP, 0.24 mg edetate calcium disodium USP, and 0.18 mg glycine hydrochloride. During manufacture, the pH may have been adjusted with hydrochloric acid and/or sodium hydroxide.

Each 8 mg/0.4 mL pre-filled syringe (1 mL syringe) contains 8 mg of methylnaltrexone bromide in 0.4 mL of water. The excipients are 2.6 mg sodium chloride USP, 0.16 mg edetate calcium disodium USP, and 0.12 mg glycine hydrochloride. Each 12 mg/0.6 mL pre-filled syringe (1 mL syringe) contains 12 mg of methylnaltrexone bromide in 0.6 mL of water. The excipients are 3.9 mg sodium chloride USP, 0.24 mg edetate calcium disodium USP, and 0.18 mg glycine hydrochloride.

The structural formula is:

12 CLINICAL PHARMACOLOGY

12.1 Mechanism of Action

Methylnaltrexone is a selective antagonist of opioid binding at the mu-opioid receptor. As a quaternary amine, the ability of methylnaltrexone to cross the blood-brain barrier is restricted. This allows methylnaltrexone to function as a peripherally-acting mu-opioid receptor antagonist in tissues such as the gastrointestinal tract, thereby decreasing the constipating effects of opioids without impacting opioid-mediated analgesic effects on the central nervous system.

12.2 Pharmacodynamics

Effect on Cardiac Repolarization

In a randomized, double-blind placebo- and (open-label) moxifloxacin-controlled 4-period crossover study, 56 healthy subjects were administered methylnaltrexone bromide 0.3 mg/kg and methylnaltrexone bromide 0.64 mg/kg by intravenous infusion over 20 minutes, placebo, and a single oral dose of moxifloxacin. At both the 0.3 mg/kg and 0.64 mg/kg methylnaltrexone bromide doses, no significant effect on the QTc interval was detected.

12.3 Pharmacokinetics

Absorption

Following subcutaneous administration, methylnaltrexone achieved peak concentrations (C_{max}) at approximately 0.5 hours. Across the range of doses from 0.15 mg/kg to 0.50 mg/kg, mean C_{max} and area under the plasma concentration-time curve (AUC) increased in a dose-proportional manner. There was no accumulation of methylnaltrexone following once-daily subcutaneous dosing of methylnaltrexone bromide 12 mg for seven consecutive days in healthy subjects.

Table 3: Pharmacokinetic Parameters of Methylnaltrexone Following Subcutaneous Doses

Parameter	0.15 mg/kg single dose	12 mg single dose	12 mg at steady-state
C_{max} (ng/mL) [i]	117 (32.7)	140 (35.6)	119 (27.2)
t_{max} (hr) [ii]	0.5 (0.25-0.75)	0.25 (0.25-0.5)	0.25 (0.25-0.5)
AUC_{24} (ng•hr/mL) [i]	175 (36.6)	218 (28.3)	223 (28.2)

[i] Expressed as mean (SD).
[ii] Expressed as median (range).

Distribution

The steady-state volume of distribution (Vss) of methylnaltrexone is approximately 1.1 L/kg. The fraction of methylnaltrexone bound to human plasma proteins is 11.0% to 15.3%, as determined by equilibrium dialysis.

Metabolism

In a mass balance study, approximately 44% of the administered radioactivity was recovered in the urine over 24 hours with 5 distinct metabolites and none of the detected metabolites was in amounts over 6% of administered radio-

activity. Conversion to methyl-6-naltrexol isomers (5% of total) and methylnaltrexone sulfate (1.3% of total) appear to be the primary pathways of metabolism. N-demethylation of methylnaltrexone to produce naltrexone is not significant.

After 12 mg once daily dosing the mean AUC_{0-24} ratio of metabolites to methylnaltrexone at steady-state was 30%, 19%, and 9% for methylnaltrexone sulfate, methyl-6α-naltrexol, and methyl-6β-naltrexol, respectively. Methyl-6α-naltrexol, and methyl-6β-naltrexol were active mu-opioid receptor antagonists and methylnaltrexone sulfate is a weak mu-opioid receptor antagonist.

Methylnaltrexone is conjugated by sulfotransferase SULT1E1 and SULT2A1 isoforms to methylnaltrexone sulfate. Conversion to methyl-6-naltrexol isomers is mediated by aldo-keto reductase 1C enzymes.

Excretion

After intravenous administration, approximately half of the dose was excreted in the urine (53.6%) and 17.3% of administered dose was excreted in the feces up to 168 hours postdose. Methylnaltrexone is excreted primarily as the unchanged drug in the urine and feces. The terminal half-life ($t_{1/2}$) is approximately 8 hours. Active renal secretion of methylnaltrexone is suggested by renal clearance of methylnaltrexone that is approximately 4-5 fold higher than creatinine clearance.

Specific Populations

Geriatric

A study was conducted to characterize the pharmacokinetics of methylnaltrexone after single dose of 24 mg methylnaltrexone via intravenous infusion over 20 min in healthy adults between 18 and 45 years of age and in healthy adults aged 65 years and older. In elderly subjects, mean clearance was about 20% lower (56 L/h versus 70 L/h) and AUC_∞ was 26% higher than in subjects between 18 and 45 years of age.

Renal impairment

In a study of volunteers with varying degrees of renal impairment receiving a single dose of 0.30 mg/kg methylnaltrexone bromide, renal impairment had a marked effect on the renal excretion of methylnaltrexone. Severe renal impairment decreased the renal clearance of methylnaltrexone by 8- to 9-fold and resulted in a 2-fold increase in total methylnaltrexone exposure (AUC). Mean C_{max} was not significantly changed.

Hepatic impairment

The effect of mild and moderate hepatic impairment on the systemic exposure to methylnaltrexone has been studied in 8 subjects each, with Child-Pugh Class A and B, compared to healthy subjects. Results showed no meaningful effect of hepatic impairment on the AUC or C_{max} of methylnaltrexone.

Drug Interactions

In vitro studies suggested that methylnaltrexone was a substrate of Organic Cation Transporter 1 but not a substrate of Organic Anion Transporter 1 or of P-glycoprotein.

Cimetidine

A clinical drug interaction study in healthy adult subjects evaluated the effects of cimetidine, a drug that inhibits the active renal secretion of organic cations, on the pharmacokinetics of methylnaltrexone (24 mg administered as an IV infusion over 20 minutes). A single dose of methylnaltrexone was administered before cimetidine dosing and with the last dose of cimetidine (400 mg every 8 hours for 6 days). Mean C_{max} and AUC of methylnaltrexone increased by 10% with concomitant cimetidine administration. The renal clearance of methylnaltrexone decreased about 40%.

13 NONCLINICAL TOXICOLOGY

13.1 Carcinogenesis, Mutagenesis, Impairment of Fertility

Carcinogenesis

Two-year oral carcinogenicity studies have been conducted with methylnaltrexone in CD-1 mice at doses up to 200 mg/kg/day (about 108 times the recommended human dose of 0.15 mg/kg based on body surface area) in males and 400 mg/kg/day (about 216 times the recommended human dose of 0.15 mg/kg based on body surface area) in females and in Sprague Dawley rats at oral doses up to 300 mg/kg/day (about 324 times the recommended human dose of 0.15 mg/kg based on body surface area). Oral administration of methylnaltrexone for 104 weeks did not produce tumors in mice and rats.

Mutagenesis

Methylnaltrexone bromide was negative in the Ames test, chromosome aberration tests in Chinese hamster ovary cells and human lymphocytes, in the mouse lymphoma cell forward mutation tests and in the *in vivo* mouse micronucleus test.

Impairment of Fertility

Methylnaltrexone bromide at subcutaneous doses up to 150 mg/kg/day (about 81 times the recommended maximum

human subcutaneous dose based on the body surface area) was found to have no adverse effect on fertility and reproductive performance of male and female rats.

13.2 Animal Toxicology and/or Pharmacology

In an *in vitro* human cardiac potassium ion channel (hERG) assay, methylnaltrexone bromide caused concentration-dependent inhibition of hERG current (1%, 12%, 13% and 40% inhibition at 30, 100, 300 and 1000 μM concentrations, respectively). Methylnaltrexone bromide had a hERG IC_{50} of > 1000 μM. In isolated dog Purkinje fibers, methylnaltrexone bromide caused prolongations in action potential duration (APD). The highest tested concentration (10 μM) in the dog Purkinje fiber study was about 18 and 37 times the C_{max} at human subcutaneous (SC) doses of 0.3 and 0.15 mg/kg, respectively. In isolated rabbit Purkinje fibers, methylnaltrexone bromide (up to 100 μM) did not have an effect on APD, compared to vehicle control. The highest methylnaltrexone bromide concentration (100 μM) tested was about 186 and 373 times the human C_{max} at SC doses of 0.3 and 0.15 mg/kg, respectively. In anesthetized dogs, methylnaltrexone bromide caused decreases in blood pressure, heart rate, cardiac output, left ventricular pressure, left ventricular end diastolic pressure, and +dP/dt at ≥ 1 mg/kg. In conscious dogs, methylnaltrexone bromide caused a dose-related increase in QTc interval. After a single intravenous dosage of 20 mg/kg to beagle dogs, predicted C_{max} and AUC values were approximately 482 and 144 times, respectively, the exposure at human SC dose of 0.15 mg/kg and 241 times and 66 times, respectively, the exposure at a human SC dose of 0.3 mg/kg. In conscious guinea pigs, methylnaltrexone caused mild prolongation of QTc (4% over baseline) at 20 mg/kg, intravenous. A thorough QTc assessment was conducted in humans [*see Clinical Pharmacology (12.2)*].

In juvenile rats administered intravenous methylnaltrexone bromide for 13 weeks, adverse clinical signs such as convulsions, tremors and labored breathing occurred at dosages of 3 and 10 mg/kg/day (about 3.2 and 11 times, respectively, the recommended human dose of 0.15 mg/kg based on the body surface area). Similar adverse clinical signs were seen in adult rats at 20 mg/kg/day (about 22 times the recommended human dose of 0.15 mg/kg based on the body surface area). Juvenile rats were found to be more sensitive to the toxicity of methylnaltrexone bromide when compared to adults. The no observed adverse effect levels (NOAELs) in juvenile and adult rats were 1 and 5 mg/kg/day, respectively (about 1.1 and 5.4 times respectively, the recommended human dose of 0.15 mg/kg based on the body surface area).

In juvenile dogs administered intravenous methylnaltrexone bromide for 13 weeks, juvenile dogs had a toxicity profile similar to adult dogs. Following intravenous administration of methylnaltrexone bromide for 13 weeks, decreased heart rate (13.2% reduction compared to pre-dose) in juvenile dogs and prolonged QTc interval in juvenile (9.6% compared to control) and adult (up to 15% compared to control) dogs occurred at 20 mg/kg/day (about 72 times the recommended human subcutaneous doses of 0.15 mg/kg based on the body surface area). Clinical signs consistent with effects on the CNS (including tremors and decreased activity) occurred in both juvenile and adult dogs. The NOAELs in juvenile and adult dogs were 5 mg/kg/day (about 18 times the recommended human subcutaneous doses of 0.15 mg/kg based on the body surface area).

14 CLINICAL STUDIES

The efficacy and safety of RELISTOR in the treatment of opioid-induced constipation in advanced illness patients receiving palliative care was demonstrated in two randomized, double-blind, placebo-controlled studies. In these studies, the median age was 68 years (range 21-100); 51% were females. The majority of patients had a primary diagnosis of incurable cancer; other primary diagnoses included end-stage COPD/emphysema, cardiovascular disease/heart failure, Alzheimer's disease/dementia, HIV/AIDS, or other advanced illnesses. Prior to screening, patients had been receiving palliative opioid therapy (median daily baseline oral morphine equivalent dose = 172 mg), and had opioid-induced constipation (either <3 bowel movements in the preceding week or no bowel movement for >2 days). Patients were on a stable opioid regimen ≥ 3 days prior to randomization (not including PRN or rescue pain medication) and received their opioid medication during the study as clinically needed. Patients maintained their regular laxative regimen for at least 3 days prior to study entry, and throughout the study. Rescue laxatives were prohibited from 4 hours before to 4 hours after taking an injection of study medication.

Study 1 compared a single, double-blind, subcutaneous dose of RELISTOR 0.15 mg/kg, or RELISTOR 0.3 mg/kg versus placebo. The double-blind dose was followed by an open-label 4-week dosing period, where RELISTOR could be used as needed, no more frequently than 1 dose in a 24 hour period. Throughout both study periods, patients maintained

NDC NUMBER	PACK SIZE	CONTENTS
65649-551-02	1 vial per carton	one 12 mg/0.6 mL single-use vial
65649-553-05	7 trays per kit	Each tray contains: one 12 mg/0.6 mL single-use vial, one 1 cc (mL) syringe with retractable (27-gauge × ½-inch) needle (VanishPoint®), two alcohol swabs
65649-552-04	7 pre-filled syringes per carton	seven 8 mg/0.4 mL single-use pre-filled syringes with needle guard system
65649-551-03	7 pre-filled syringes per carton	seven 12 mg/0.6 mL single-use pre-filled syringes with needle guard system
65649-551-07	1 pre-filled syringe per carton	one 12 mg/0.6 mL single-use pre-filled syringe with needle guard system

their regular laxative regimen. A total of 154 patients (47 RELISTOR 0.15 mg/kg, 55 RELISTOR 0.3 mg/kg, 52 placebo) were enrolled and treated in the double-blind period. The primary endpoint was the proportion of patients with a rescue-free laxation within 4 hours of the double-blind dose of study medication. RELISTOR-treated patients had a significantly higher rate of laxation within 4 hours of the double-blind dose (62% for 0.15 mg/kg and 58% for 0.3 mg/kg) than did placebo-treated patients (14%); p < 0.0001 for each dose versus placebo (Figure 1).

Study 2 compared double-blind, subcutaneous doses of RELISTOR given every other day for 2 weeks versus placebo. Patients received opioid medication ≥ 2 weeks prior to receiving study medication. During the first week (days 1, 3, 5, 7) patients received either 0.15 mg/kg RELISTOR or placebo. In the second week the patient's assigned dose could be increased to 0.30 mg/kg if the patient had 2 or fewer rescue-free laxations up to day 8. At any time, the patient's assigned dose could be reduced based on tolerability. Data from 133 (62 RELISTOR, 71 placebo) patients were analyzed. There were 2 primary endpoints: proportion of patients with a rescue-free laxation within 4 hours of the first dose of study medication and proportion of patients with a rescue-free laxation within 4 hours after at least 2 of the first 4 doses of study medication. RELISTOR-treated patients had a higher rate of laxation within 4 hours of the first dose (48%) than placebo-treated patients (16%); p < 0.0001 (Figure 1). RELISTOR-treated patients also had significantly higher rates of laxation within 4 hours after at least 2 of the first 4 doses (52%) than did placebo-treated patients (9%); p < 0.0001. In both studies, in approximately 30% of patients, laxation was reported within 30 minutes of a dose of RELISTOR.

*p < 0.0001 vs. Placebo

Figure 1. Laxation Response Within 4 Hours of the First Dose

In both studies, there was no evidence of differential effects of age or gender on safety or efficacy. No meaningful subgroup analysis could be conducted on race because the study population was predominantly Caucasian (88%).

Durability of Response
Durability of response was explored in Study 2 and the laxation response rate was consistent from dose 1 through dose 7 over the course of the 2-week, double-blind period.
The efficacy and safety of methylnaltrexone bromide was also demonstrated in open-label treatment administered from Day 2 through Week 4 in Study 1, and in two open-label extension studies (Study 1EXT and Study 2EXT) in which RELISTOR was given as needed for up to 4 months. During open-label treatment, patients maintained their regular laxative regimen. A total of 136, 21, and 82 patients received at least 1 open-label dose in studies 1, 1EXT, and 2EXT, respectively. Laxation response was also explored in this open-label setting and appeared to be maintained over the course of 3 to 4 months of open-label treatment.

Opioid Use and Pain Scores
No relationship between baseline opioid dose and laxation response in methylnaltrexone bromide-treated patients was identified in exploratory analyses of these studies. In addition, median daily opioid dose did not vary meaningfully

from baseline in either RELISTOR -treated patients or in placebo-treated patients. There were no clinically relevant changes in pain scores from baseline in either the methylnaltrexone bromide or placebo-treated patients.

16   HOW SUPPLIED/STORAGE AND HANDLING
How Supplied
[See table above]
16.1   Storage
RELISTOR should be stored at 20°C to 25°C (68°F to 77°F); excursions permitted to 15°C to 30°C (59°F to 86°F) [see USP Controlled Room Temperature]. Do not freeze. **Protect from light.**

17   PATIENT COUNSELING INFORMATION
See FDA-approved patient labeling (Patient Information and Instructions for Use)
- Instruct patients not to continue taking RELISTOR and to promptly notify their physician if they experience severe, persistent, or worsening abdominal symptoms because these could be symptoms of gastrointestinal perforation [*see Warnings and Precautions (5.1)*].
- Instruct patients not to continue taking RELISTOR if they experience severe or persistent diarrhea. Inform patients that common side effects of RELISTOR include abdominal pain, flatulence, nausea, dizziness, and diarrhea.
- Advise patients to be within close proximity to toilet facilities once the drug is administered.
- Instruct patients with opioid-induced constipation and advanced illness to administer one dose subcutaneously every other day, as needed, but no more frequently than one dose in a 24-hour period.
- Instruct patients to discontinue RELISTOR if they stop taking their opioid pain medication.
- Instruct patients to use the RELISTOR single-use vial with a 27 gauge × ½-inch needle and 1 mL syringe.

Patient Information
RELISTOR® (rel - *i* – store)
(methylnaltrexone bromide)
Subcutaneous Injection
Read this Patient Information that comes with RELISTOR before you start using it and each time you get a refill. There may be new information. This leaflet does not take the place of talking with your healthcare provider about your medical condition or your treatment.

What is RELISTOR?
RELISTOR is a prescription medicine used to treat constipation that is caused by prescription pain medicines, called opioids, in patients receiving supportive care for their advanced illness, when other medicines for constipation, called laxatives, have not worked well enough.
It is not known if RELISTOR is safe and effective if used for longer than 4 months in people with advanced illness.
It is not known if RELISTOR is safe and effective in children.

Who should not use RELISTOR?
Do not use RELISTOR if you have or may have a blockage in your intestines called a mechanical bowel obstruction. Symptoms of this blockage are vomiting, stomach pain, and swelling of your stomach-area (abdomen). Talk to your healthcare provider if you have any of these symptoms before using RELISTOR.

What should I tell my healthcare provider before using RELISTOR?
Before you start using RELISTOR, tell your healthcare provider if you:
- have kidney problems
- have or had cancer of the stomach or intestine
- have or had a stomach ulcer
- have had a blockage in your intestine
- have any other medical condition
- are pregnant or plan to become pregnant. It is not known if RELISTOR can harm your unborn baby.
- are breast-feeding or plan to breast-feed. It is not known if RELISTOR passes into your breast milk.

Tell your healthcare provider about all medicines you take, including prescription and non-prescription medicines, vitamins, and herbal supplements. Continue taking your other medicines for constipation unless your healthcare provider tells you to stop taking them.
How should I use RELISTOR?
- RELISTOR is injected under the skin (subcutaneous injection) of the upper arm, abdomen, or thigh.
- Inject RELISTOR exactly as your healthcare provider tells you.
- RELISTOR is usually used every other day. Do not inject more than one dose of RELISTOR in a 24-hour period.
- Stay close to a toilet after using RELISTOR.
- Stop using RELISTOR if you stop taking your prescription opioid pain medicine.
- If you inject more RELISTOR than prescribed, talk to your healthcare provider right away.
See the detailed Instructions for Use that comes with RELISTOR for information about how to prepare and inject RELISTOR, and properly throw away (dispose of) used needles and syringes the right way.
What are the possible side effects of RELISTOR?
RELISTOR can cause serious side effects, including:
- **Tear in your stomach or intestinal wall (perforation). Stop using RELISTOR and call your healthcare provider right away** if you develop swelling or pain in your stomach-area (abdomen) that is severe, gets worse, or that does not go away, nausea or vomiting that does not go away, or if you vomit blood or have black sticky stools.
- **Diarrhea that is severe or that will not go away.** Stop using RELISTOR and call your healthcare provider if you get diarrhea that is severe or that does not go away during treatment with RELISTOR.

The most common side effects of RELISTOR include:
- stomach-area (abdomen) pain
- gas
- nausea
- dizziness
- diarrhea
- sweating

Tell your healthcare provider if you have any side effect that bothers you or that does not go away.
These are not all of the possible side effects of RELISTOR. Call your doctor for medical advice about side effects. You may report side effects to FDA at 1-800-FDA-1088.
How should I store RELISTOR?
- Store RELISTOR vials and pre-filled syringes at room temperature between 68°F to 77°F (20°C to 25°C).
- Do not freeze RELISTOR.
- Keep RELISTOR away from light until you are ready to use it.
- If RELISTOR has been drawn into a syringe and you are unable to use the medicine right away, keep the syringe at room temperature for up to 24 hours. The syringe does not need to be kept away from light during the 24-hour period.
Keep RELISTOR and all medicines, needles and syringes out of the reach of children.
General information about RELISTOR
Medicines are sometimes prescribed for purposes other than those listed in a Patient Information leaflet. Do not use RELISTOR for a condition for which it was not prescribed. Do not give RELISTOR to other people, even if they have the same symptoms that you have. It may harm them.
This leaflet summarizes the most important information about RELISTOR. If you would like more information, talk with your healthcare provider. You can ask your pharmacist or healthcare provider for information about RELISTOR that is written for health professionals.
For more information, go to WWW.RELISTOR.COM.
What are the ingredients in RELISTOR?
Active ingredient: methylnaltrexone bromide
Inactive ingredients: sodium chloride, edetate calcium disodium USP, glycine hydrochloride.
During manufacture, the pH may have been adjusted with hydrochloric acid and/or sodium hydroxide.
This Patient Information has been approved by the U.S. Food and Drug Administration.
Manufactured for:
Salix Pharmaceuticals, Inc.
Raleigh, NC 27615
Under license from:
Progenics Pharmaceuticals, Inc.
Tarrytown, NY 10591
Revised: AUG 2013
Product protected by U.S. Patent Nos. 6,559,158, 8,247,425, and 8,420,663.
Please see www.salix.com for patent information
Instructions for Use
RELISTOR® (rel-i-store)
(methylnaltrexone bromide)
Pre-filled Syringe
Read this Instructions for Use before you start using RELISTOR and each time you get a refill. There may be new information. This information does not take the place of talking with your healthcare provider about your medical condition or your treatment.

The following instructions explain how to prepare and give an injection of RELISTOR the right way, when using a pre-filled syringe of RELISTOR.

Important information:

- **Do not** use a RELISTOR pre-filled syringe and attached needle more than one time, even if there is medicine left in the syringe. **See Step 4 "Dispose of used pre-filled syringes and needles."**
- Safely throw away RELISTOR pre-filled syringes and attached needle after use.
- To avoid needle-stick injuries, **do not** recap used needles.
- Avoid touching the trigger fingers of the RELISTOR pre-filled syringe to keep from activating the needle guard (safety device) too soon. The needle guard is activated by pressure from the plunger on the trigger fingers (See Figure A).

Gather the supplies you will need for your injection (See Figure A). These include:

- 1 RELISTOR pre-filled syringe with attached needle
- 1 alcohol swab
- 1 cotton ball or gauze
- 1 adhesive bandage
- a container to dispose of used pre-filled syringes and needles. See Step 4: "Dispose of used pre-filled syringes and needles."

Pre-filled Syringe Parts

Figure A

Step 1: Choose and prepare the injection site

- Choose an injection site on your abdomen, thighs, or upper arms. See the shaded areas in Figures B and C below. Do not inject at the exact same spot each time (rotate injection sites). Do not inject into areas where the skin is tender, bruised, red or hard. Avoid areas with scars or stretch marks.

Figure B Abdomen or thigh – use these sites when injecting yourself or another person.

Figure C Upper arm – use this site only when injecting another person.

Figure B   Figure C

- Clean the injection site with an alcohol swab and let it air dry. Do not touch this area again before giving the injection (See Figure D).

Figure D

Step 2: Prepare the pre-filled syringe

- Choose a flat, clean, well-lit work surface.
- Wash your hands with soap and water before preparing for the injection.
- Look at the pre-filled syringe of RELISTOR (See Figure E). Make sure that the dose prescribed by your healthcare provider matches the dose on the pre-filled syringe label. Look at the plunger rod of the syringe. If the dose prescribed by your healthcare provider is 8 mg, the plunger rod will be yellow; if the prescribed dose is 12 mg, the plunger rod of the syringe will be dark blue (See Figure E). [See figure E at top of next column]
- The liquid in the pre-filled syringe should be clear and colorless to pale yellow, and should not have any particles in it. Do not use the pre-filled syringe if it looks discolored, cloudy, or has any particles.
- Use one hand to firmly hold the barrel of the pre-filled syringe. Use your other hand to pull the needle cap straight off (Figure F). Do not touch the needle or allow it to touch anything. [See figure F at top of next column]

Figure E

Figure F

Step 3: Inject RELISTOR

- Use one hand to pinch the skin around the injection site (See Figure G).

Figure G

- Use your other hand to hold the pre-filled syringe. Insert the full length of the needle into the skin at a 45-degree angle with a quick "dart-like" motion (See Figure H).

Figure H

- Let go of the skin and slowly push the plunger in with your thumb until the pre-filled syringe is empty (See Figure I). This will release the needle guard (safety device).

Figure I

- Continue to hold pressure on the plunger with your thumb and quickly pull the needle out of the skin. Be careful to keep the needle at the same angle as it was inserted. Remove your thumb from the plunger to allow the protective sleeve to cover the needle (See Figure J). There may be a little bleeding at the injection site.

Figure J

- Hold a cotton ball or gauze over the injection site (See Figure K). Do not rub the injection site. Apply an adhesive bandage to the injection site if needed.

Figure K

Step 4: Dispose of used pre-filled syringes and needles

- **Do not** re-use the pre-filled syringe and attached needle.
- To avoid needle-stick injuries, **do not** recap used needles.
- Put your used pre-filled syringes and attached needles **in a FDA-cleared sharps disposal container** right away after use. **Do not throw away (dispose of) loose needles and syringes in your household trash.**
- If you do not have a FDA-cleared sharps disposal container, you may use a household container that is:
  ○ made of a heavy-duty plastic,
  ○ can be closed with a tight-fitting, puncture-resistant lid, without sharps being able to come out,
  ○ upright and stable during use,
  ○ leak-resistant, and
  ○ properly labeled to warn of hazardous waste inside the container.
- When your sharps disposal container is almost full, you will need to follow your community guidelines for the right way to dispose of your sharps disposal container. There may be state or local laws about how you should throw away used needles and syringes. For more information about safe sharps disposal, and for specific information about sharps disposal in the state that you live in, go to the FDA's website at: http://www.fda.gov/safesharpsdisposal
- Do not dispose of your used sharps disposal container in your household trash unless your community guidelines permit this. Do not recycle your used sharps disposal container.
- If you have any questions, talk to your healthcare provider or pharmacist.

How should i store RELISTOR?

- Store pre-filled syringes at room temperature between 68°F to 77°F (20°C to 25°C).
- Do not freeze RELISTOR.
- Keep RELISTOR away from light until you are ready to use it.

Keep RELISTOR and all medicines, needles and syringes out of the reach of children.

This Instructions for Use has been approved by the U.S. Food and Drug Administration.

Manufactured for:
Salix Pharmaceuticals, Inc.
Raleigh, NC 27615
Under license from:
Progenics Pharmaceuticals, Inc.
Tarrytown, NY 10591
Revised AUG 2013
Product protected by U.S. Patent Nos. 6,559,158, 8,247,425, and 8,420,663.
See www.salix.com for patent information

Instructions for Use
RELISTOR® (rel-i-store)
(methylnaltrexone bromide)
Vial and Syringe with Retractable Needle in Tray

Read this Instructions for Use before you start using RELISTOR and each time you get a refill. There may be new information. This information does not take the place of talking to your healthcare provider about your medical condition or your treatment.

The following instructions explain how to prepare and give an injection of RELISTOR the right way, when using a RELISTOR tray containing a syringe with a retractable needle. A retractable needle is one that is pulled back so that it is covered after use, to prevent needle-stick injury.

Important information:

- **Do not** use a RELISTOR vial more than one time, even if there is medicine left in the vial.
- If RELISTOR has been drawn into a syringe and you are unable to use the medicine right away, carefully recap the needle and keep the syringe at room temperature for up to 24 hours. The syringe does not need to be kept away from light during the 24-hour period. For more information about how to store RELISTOR, see the section called "How should I store RELISTOR?" at the end of this Instructions for Use.
- Safely throw away RELISTOR vials after use.
- **Do not** reuse syringes and needles. **See Step 5: "Dispose of used syringes and needles"** for information about how to safely throw away used needles and syringes.
- To avoid needle-stick injuries, **do not** recap used needles.

Your tray should include (See Figure A):
- 1 RELISTOR vial
- 1 1 mL syringe with retractable needle (VanishPoint®)
- 2 alcohol swabs

You will also need:
- 1 cotton ball or gauze
- 1 adhesive bandage
- a container to dispose of your used syringes and needles. See Step 5: "Dispose of used syringes and needles."

Vial and Syringe Parts

Cap
Rubber Stopper
Barrel
Needle Cap
Plunger
Retractable Needle

Figure A

Step 1: Choose and prepare the injection site
- Choose an injection site on your abdomen, thighs, or upper arms. See the shaded areas in B and C below. Do not inject at the exact same spot each time (rotate injection sites). Do not inject into areas where the skin is tender, bruised, red, or hard. Avoid areas with scars or stretch marks.
  Figure B Abdomen or thigh – use these sites when injecting yourself or another person.
  Figure C Upper arm – use this site only when injecting another person.

Figure B   **Figure C**

- Clean the injection site with an alcohol swab and let it air dry. Do not touch this area again before giving the injection (See Figure D).

Figure D

Step 2: Prepare the injection
- Choose a flat, clean, well-lit work surface.
- Wash your hands with soap and water before preparing for the injection.
- Look at the vial of RELISTOR (See Figure E). The liquid in the vial should be clear and colorless to pale yellow, and should not have any particles in it. Do not use the vial if it looks discolored, cloudy, or has any particles.

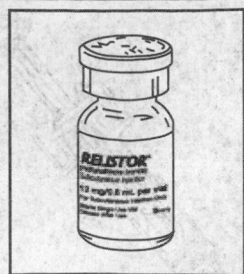

Figure E

Step 3: Prepare the syringe
- Remove the cap from the vial containing RELISTOR (See Figure F).

Figure F

- Wipe the rubber stopper with an alcohol swab (See Figure G).

Figure G

- Firmly hold the barrel of the syringe with one hand. With your other hand, pull the needle cap straight off (See Figure H). Do not touch the needle or allow it to touch anything

Figure H

- Carefully pull back on the plunger to the line that matches the dose prescribed by your healthcare provider (See Figures I and J). For most people, this will be the 0.4 mL mark which is an 8 mg dose or the 0.6 mL mark which is a 12 mg dose.

Figure I

Plunger tip lined up with dose mark on syringe barrel

Figure J

- Use one hand to hold the vial steady. Use your other hand to insert the needle straight down into the rubber top of the RELISTOR vial (See Figure K). Do not insert it at an angle. This may cause the needle to bend or break. You will feel some resistance as the needle passes through the rubber top.

Figure K

- Gently push down on the plunger until you feel resistance, and most of the air has gone from the syringe into the vial (See Figure L). Stop pushing down on the plunger when you feel resistance. If you continue to push down on the plunger when you feel resistance, the needle will pull back (retract) into the syringe barrel.

Figure L

- With the needle still in the vial, turn the vial and syringe upside down. Hold the syringe at eye level. Make sure the tip of the needle is in the fluid. Slowly pull back on the plunger (See Figure M) until the tip lines up with the mark that matches your prescribed dose. For most people, this will be the 0.4 mL mark which is an 8 mg dose or the 0.6 mL mark which is a 12 mg dose.

Figure M

- You may see some fluid or bubbles inside the vial when the syringe is filled. This is normal.
- With the needle still in the vial, gently tap the syringe to make any air bubbles rise to the top (See Figure N).

Figure N

- Gently push the plunger up until all air bubbles are out of the syringe (See Figure O). A small air bubble may stay in the syringe. This is okay and it will not affect the dose of medicine in the syringe.

Figure O

- Make sure the tip of the needle is in the fluid. Slowly pull back the plunger to draw the right amount of liquid back into the syringe (See Figure P).

Figure P

Check to be sure that you have the right dose of RELISTOR in the syringe.
- Slowly withdraw the needle from the vial. Do not touch the needle or allow it to touch anything). Safely throw away the vial with any unused medicine.

Step 4: Inject RELISTOR
- Use one hand to pinch the skin around the injection site (See Figure Q).

Figure Q

- Use your other hand to hold the syringe. Insert the full length of the needle into the skin at a 45-degree angle with a "quick dart-like" motion (See Figure R).

Figure R

- Let go of the skin and slowly push in on the plunger past the resistance point, until the syringe is empty and you hear a click (See Figure S).

Figure S

- The click sound means that the needle (T) has been pulled back (retracted) into the syringe barrel (See Figure U). You can now remove the syringe from your skin.

Figure T   **Figure U**

- Hold a cotton ball or gauze over the injection site (See Figure V). Do not rub the injection site. Apply an adhesive bandage to the injection site if needed.

Figure V

Step 5: Dispose of used syringes and needles
- **Do not** re-use syringes or needles.
- To avoid needle-stick injuries, **do not** recap used needles.
- Put your used needles and syringes in a FDA-cleared sharps disposal container right away after use. **Do not throw away (dispose of) loose needles and syringes in your household trash.**
- If you do not have a FDA-cleared sharps disposal container, you may use a household container that is:
  - made of a heavy-duty plastic,
  - can be closed with a tight-fitting, puncture-resistant lid, without sharps being able to come out,
  - upright and stable during use,
  - leak-resistant, and
  - properly labeled to warn of hazardous waste inside the container.
- When your sharps disposal container is almost full, you will need to follow your community guidelines for the right way to dispose of your sharps disposal container. There may be state or local laws about how you should throw away used needles and syringes. For more information about safe sharps disposal, and for specific information about sharps disposal in the state that you live in, go to the FDA's website at: http://www.fda.gov/safesharpsdisposal.
- Do not dispose of your used sharps disposal container in your household trash unless your community guidelines permit this. Do not recycle your used sharps disposal container.
- If you have any questions, talk to your healthcare provider or pharmacist.

How should I store RELISTOR?
- Store RELISTOR vials at room temperature between 68°F to 77°F (20 °C to 25°C).
- Do not freeze RELISTOR.
- Keep RELISTOR away from light until you are ready to use it.
- If RELISTOR has been drawn into a syringe and you are unable to use the medicine right away, keep the syringe at room temperature for up to 24 hours. The syringe does not need to be kept away from light during the 24-hour period.

Keep RELISTOR and all medicines, needles and syringes out of the reach of children.

This Instructions for Use has been approved by the U.S. Food and Drug Administration.
Manufactured for:
Salix Pharmaceuticals, Inc.
Raleigh, NC 27615
Under license from:
Progenics Pharmaceuticals, Inc.
Tarrytown, NY 10591
Revised AUG 2013
Product protected by U.S. Patent Nos. 6,559,158, 8,247,425, and 8,420,663.
See www.salix.com for patent information

Instructions for Use
RELISTOR® (rel-i-store)
(methylnaltrexone bromide)
Subcutaneous Injection
Vial
Read this Instructions for Use before you start using RELISTOR and each time you get a refill. There may be new information. This information does not take the place of talking to your healthcare provider about your medical condition or your treatment.
The following instructions explain how to prepare and give an injection of RELISTOR the right way, when using a vial of RELISTOR.

Important information:
- Use the syringes and needles prescribed by your healthcare provider.
- **Do not** use a RELISTOR vial more than one time, even if there is medicine left in the vial.
- If RELISTOR has been drawn into a syringe and you are unable to use the medicine right away, carefully recap the needle and keep the syringe at room temperature for up to 24 hours. The syringe does not need to be kept away from light during the 24-hour period. For more information about how to store RELISTOR, see the section **"How should I store RELISTOR?"** at the end of this Instructions for Use.
- Safely throw away RELISTOR vials after use.
- **Do not** re-use syringes or needles. **See Step 5 "Dispose of used syringes and needles"** for information about how to safely throw away used needles and syringes.
- To avoid needle-stick injuries, **do not** recap used needles. Gather the supplies you will need for your injection (See Figure A). These include:
- 1 RELISTOR vial
- 1 1 mL syringe with a 27-gauge, ½ inch needle for subcutaneous use
- 2 alcohol swabs
- 1 cotton ball or gauze
- 1 adhesive bandage
- a container to dispose of used syringes and needles. See Step 5: "Dispose of used syringes and needles."

Vial and Syringe Parts

Figure A

Step 1: Choose and prepare the injection site
- Choose an injection site on your abdomen, thighs, or upper arms. See the shaded areas in Figures B and C below. Do not inject at the exact same spot each time (rotate injection sites). Do not inject into areas where the skin is tender, bruised, red or hard. Avoid areas with scars or stretch marks.
  Figure B Abdomen or thigh – use these sites when injecting yourself or another person.
  Figure C Upper arm – use this site only when injecting another person.

Figure B   Figure C

- Clean the injection site with an alcohol swab and let it air dry. Do not touch this area again before giving the injection (See Figure D).

Figure D

Step 2: Prepare the injection
- Choose a flat, clean, well-lit work surface.
- Wash your hands with soap and water before preparing for the injection.

- Look at the vial of RELISTOR (See Figure E). The liquid in the vial should be clear and colorless to pale yellow, and should not have any particles in it. Do not use the vial if it looks discolored, cloudy, or has any particles.

Figure E

Step 3: Prepare the syringe
- Remove the cap from the RELISTOR vial (See Figure F).

Figure F

- Wipe the rubber stopper with an alcohol swab (See Figure G).

Figure G

- Firmly hold the barrel of the syringe with one hand. With your other hand, pull the needle cap straight off (See Figure H). Do not touch the needle or allow it to touch anything.

Figure H

- Carefully pull back on the plunger to the line that matches the dose prescribed by your healthcare provider (See Figures I and J). For most people, this will be the 0.4 mL mark which is an 8 mg dose or the 0.6 mL mark which is a 12 mg dose.

Figure I

Plunger tip lined up with dose mark on syringe barrel

Figure J

- Use one hand to hold the vial steady. Use your other hand to insert the needle straight down into the rubber top of the vial (See Figure K). Do not insert it at an angle. This may cause the needle to bend or break. You will feel some resistance as the needle passes through the rubber top.

Figure K

- Gently push down the plunger until all of the air has gone from the syringe into the vial (See Figure L).

Figure L

- With the needle still in the vial, turn the vial and syringe upside down. Hold the syringe at eye level. Make sure the tip of the needle is in the fluid. Slowly pull back on the plunger (See Figure M) until the tip lines up with the mark that matches your prescribed dose. For most people, this will be the 0.4 mL mark which is an 8 mg dose or the 0.6 mL mark which is a 12 mg dose.

Figure M

- You may see some fluid or bubbles inside the vial when the syringe is filled. This is normal.
- With the needle still in the vial, gently tap the side of the syringe to make any air bubbles rise to the top (See Figure N).
[See figure N at top of next column]
- Slowly push the plunger up until all air bubbles are out of the syringe (See Figure O). A small air bubble may stay in the syringe. This is okay and it will not affect the dose of medicine in the syringe.
[See figure O at top of next column]

Figure N

Figure O

- Make sure the tip of the needle is in the fluid. Slowly pull back the plunger to draw the right amount of liquid back into the syringe (See Figure P).

Figure P

Check to be sure that you have the right dose of RELISTOR in the syringe.
- Slowly withdraw the needle from the vial. Do not touch the needle or allow it to touch anything. Safely throw away the vial with any unused medicine.

Step 4: Inject RELISTOR
- Use one hand to pinch the skin around the injection site (See Figure Q).

Figure Q

- Use your other hand to hold the syringe. Insert the full length of the needle into the skin at a 45-degree angle with a quick "dart-like" motion (See Figure R).
[See figure R at top of next column]
- Let go of the skin and slowly push in on the plunger until the syringe is empty (Figure S).
[See figure S at top of next column]

Figure R

Figure S

- When the syringe is empty, quickly pull the needle out of the skin, being careful to keep it at the same angle as it was inserted. There may be a little bleeding at the injection site.
- Hold a cotton ball or gauze over the injection site (Figure T). Do not rub the injection site. Apply an adhesive bandage to the injection site if needed.

Figure T

Step 5: Dispose of used syringes and needles
- **Do not** re-use a syringe or needle.
- To avoid needle-stick injuries, **do not** recap a used needle.
- Put your used needles and syringes in a FDA-cleared sharps disposal container right away after use. **Do not throw away (dispose of) loose needles and syringes in your household trash.**
- If you do not have a FDA-cleared sharps disposal container, you may use a household container that is:
  - made of a heavy-duty plastic,
  - can be closed with a tight-fitting, puncture-resistant lid, without sharps being able to come out,
  - upright and stable during use,
  - leak-resistant, and
  - properly labeled to warn of hazardous waste inside the container.
- When your sharps disposal container is almost full, you will need to follow your community guidelines for the right way to dispose of your sharps disposal container. There may be state or local laws about how you should throw away used needles and syringes. For more information about safe sharps disposal, and for specific information about sharps disposal in the state that you live in, go to the FDA's website at: http://www.fda.gov/safesharpsdisposal.
- Do not dispose of your used sharps disposal container in your household trash unless your community guidelines permit this. Do not recycle your used sharps disposal container.
- If you have any questions, talk to your healthcare provider or pharmacist.

How should I store RELISTOR?
- Store RELISTOR vials at room temperature between 68°F to 77°F (20°C to 25°C).
- Do not freeze RELISTOR.
- Keep RELISTOR away from light until you are ready to use it.
- If RELISTOR has been drawn into a syringe and you are unable to use the medicine right away, keep the syringe at room temperature for up to 24 hours. The syringe does not need to be kept away from light during the 24-hour period.

Keep RELISTOR and all medicines, needles and syringes out of the reach of children.

This Instructions for Use has been approved by the U.S. Food and Drug Administration.

Manufactured for:
Salix Pharmaceuticals, Inc.
Raleigh, NC 27615
Under license from:
Progenics Pharmaceuticals, Inc.
Tarrytown, NY 10591
Revised AUG 2013

Product protected by U.S. Patent Nos. 6,559,158, 8,247,425, and 8,420,663.
See www.salix.com for patent information
Shown in Product Identification Guide, page 313

UCERIS®   ℞
(budesonide)
extended release tablets, for oral use

HIGHLIGHTS OF PRESCRIBING INFORMATION
These highlights do not include all the information needed to use UCERIS safely and effectively. See full prescribing information for UCERIS.
UCERIS (budesonide) extended release tablets, for oral use
Initial U.S. approval: 1997

————————**INDICATIONS AND USAGE**————————

UCERIS (budesonide) is a glucocorticosteroid indicated for the induction of remission in patients with active, mild to moderate ulcerative colitis. (1)

————————**DOSAGE AND ADMINISTRATION**————————

The recommended dosage for the induction of remission in adult patients with active, mild to moderate ulcerative colitis is one 9 mg tablet to be taken once daily in the morning with or without food for up to 8 weeks. (2.1)

————————**DOSAGE FORMS AND STRENGTHS**————————

- extended release tablets: 9 mg (3)

————————**CONTRAINDICATIONS**————————

- Known hypersensitivity to budesonide or any of the ingredients in UCERIS tablets (4)

————————**WARNINGS AND PRECAUTIONS**————————

- Hypercorticism and adrenal suppression: Since UCERIS is a glucocorticosteroid, follow general warnings concerning glucocorticoids. (5.1)
- Transferring patients from systemic glucocorticoids: Risk of impaired adrenal function when transferring from glucocorticoid treatment with higher systemic effects to glucocorticoid treatment with lower systemic effects, such as UCERIS. Taper patients slowly from systemic corticosteroids if transferring to UCERIS. (5.2)
- Immunosuppression: Potential worsening of infections (e.g., existing tuberculosis, fungal, bacterial, viral, or parasitic infection; or ocular herpes simplex). Use with caution in patients with these infections. More serious or even fatal course of chickenpox or measles can occur in susceptible patients. (5.3)

————————**ADVERSE REACTIONS**————————

Most common adverse reactions (incidence ≥ 2%) are headache, nausea, decreased blood cortisol, upper abdominal pain, fatigue, flatulence, abdominal distension, acne, urinary tract infection, arthralgia, and constipation. (6)
To report SUSPECTED ADVERSE REACTIONS, contact Salix Pharmaceuticals Inc. at 1-800-508-0024 or FDA at 1-800-FDA-1088 or *www.fda.gov/medwatch*.

————————**DRUG INTERACTIONS**————————

- Avoid Cytochrome P450 3A4 inhibitors (e.g., ketoconazole, grapefruit juice). May cause increased systemic corticosteroid effects. (2.2, 7, 12.3)

————————**USE IN SPECIFIC POPULATIONS**————————

- Hepatic Impairment: Monitor patients for signs and/or symptoms of hypercorticism. (5.4, 8.6)

--PATIENT COUNSELING INFORMATION STATEMENT--
See 17 for PATIENT COUNSELING INFORMATION and FDA-approved patient labeling

Revised: 01/2013

FULL PRESCRIBING INFORMATION

1   INDICATIONS AND USAGE
UCERIS (budesonide) extended release tablets are indicated for the induction of remission in patients with active, mild to moderate ulcerative colitis.

2   DOSAGE AND ADMINISTRATION
2.1   Mild to Moderate Ulcerative Colitis
The recommended dosage for the induction of remission in adult patients with active, mild to moderate ulcerative colitis is 9 mg taken orally once daily in the morning with or without food for up to 8 weeks. UCERIS should be swallowed whole and not chewed, crushed or broken.
2.2   CYP3A4 Inhibitors
If concomitant administration with ketoconazole, or any other CYP3A4 inhibitor, is indicated, patients should be closely monitored for increased signs and/or symptoms of hypercorticism. Avoid grapefruit juice, which is known to inhibit CYP3A4, when taking UCERIS. In these cases, discontinuation of UCERIS or the CYP3A4 inhibitor should be considered [See *Drug Interactions* (7) *and Clinical Pharmacology* (12.3)].

3   DOSAGE FORMS AND STRENGTHS
White, round, biconvex extended release tablets debossed with "MX9". Each extended release tablet contains 9 mg budesonide.

4   CONTRAINDICATIONS
UCERIS is contraindicated in patients with hypersensitivity to budesonide or any of the ingredients of UCERIS. Anaphylactic reactions have occurred with other budesonide formulations [See *Adverse Reactions* (6.2)].

5   WARNINGS AND PRECAUTIONS
5.1   Hypercorticism and Adrenal Axis Suppression
When glucocorticosteroids are used chronically, systemic effects such as hypercorticism and adrenal suppression may occur. Glucocorticosteroids can reduce the response of the hypothalamus-pituitary-adrenal (HPA) axis to stress. In situations where patients are subject to surgery or other stress situations, supplementation with a systemic glucocorticosteroid is recommended. Since UCERIS is a glucocorticosteroid, general warnings concerning glucocorticoids should be followed.
5.2   Transferring Patients from Systemic Glucocorticosteroid Therapy
Care is needed in patients who are transferred from glucocorticosteroid treatment with higher systemic effects to glucocorticosteroids with lower systemic effects, such as UCERIS, since symptoms attributed to withdrawal of steroid therapy, including those of acute adrenal suppression or benign intracranial hypertension, may develop. Adrenocortical function monitoring may be required in these patients and the dose of glucocorticosteroid treatment with high systemic effects should be reduced cautiously.
5.3   Immunosuppression
Patients who are on drugs that suppress the immune system are more susceptible to infection than healthy individuals. Chicken pox and measles, for example, can have a more serious or even fatal course in susceptible patients or patients on immunosuppressant doses of glucocorticosteroids. In patients who have not had these diseases, particular care should be taken to avoid exposure.
How the dose, route, and duration of glucocorticosteroid administration affect the risk of developing a disseminated infection is not known. The contribution of the underlying disease and/or prior glucocorticosteroid treatment to the risk is also not known. If exposed, therapy with varicella zoster immune globulin (VZIG) or pooled intravenous immunoglobulin (IVIG), as appropriate, may be indicated. If exposed to measles, prophylaxis with pooled intramuscular immunoglobulin (IG) may be indicated. (See prescribing information

for VZIG and IG.) If chicken pox develops, treatment with antiviral agents may be considered.

Glucocorticosteroids should be used with caution, if at all, in patients with active or quiescent tuberculosis infection, untreated fungal, bacterial, systemic viral or parasitic infections.

Replacement of systemic glucocorticosteroids with UCERIS tablets may unmask allergies (e.g., rhinitis and eczema), which were previously controlled by the systemic drug.

5.4 Increased Systemic Glucocorticoid Susceptibility

Reduced liver function affects the elimination of glucocorticosteroids, and increased systemic availability of oral budesonide has been demonstrated in patients with liver cirrhosis [See Use in Specific Populations (8.6)].

5.5 Other Glucocorticosteroid Effects

Caution should be taken in patients with hypertension, diabetes mellitus, osteoporosis, peptic ulcer, glaucoma or cataracts, or with a family history of diabetes or glaucoma, or with any other condition where glucocorticosteroids may have unwanted effects.

6 ADVERSE REACTIONS

Systemic glucocorticosteroid use may result in the following:

- Hypercorticism and Adrenal Suppression [See Warnings and Precautions (5.1)]
- Symptoms of steroid withdrawal in those patients transferring from Systemic Glucocorticosteroid Therapy [See Warnings and Precautions (5.2)]
- Immunosuppression [See Warnings and Precautions (5.3)]
- Increased Systemic Glucocorticosteroid Susceptibility [See Warnings and Precautions (5.4)]
- Other Glucocorticosteroid Effects [See Warnings and Precautions (5.5)]

6.1 Clinical Trials Experience

Because clinical trials are conducted under widely varying conditions, adverse reaction rates observed in the clinical trials of a drug cannot be directly compared to rates in the clinical trials of another drug and may not reflect the rates observed in practice.

The safety of UCERIS has been evaluated in controlled and open-label clinical trials which enrolled a combined total of 1,105 patients with ulcerative colitis.

In two 8-week, placebo-controlled studies in patients with active disease (Study 1 and Study 2), a total of 255 patients received UCERIS 9 mg, 254 patients received UCERIS 6 mg, and 258 patients received placebo. They ranged in age from 18-77 years (mean 43), 56% were male, and 75% were Caucasian. The most common adverse reactions were headache, nausea, decreased blood cortisol, upper abdominal pain, fatigue, flatulence, abdominal distension, acne, urinary tract infection, arthralgia, and constipation. The adverse reactions occurring in 2% or more of patients on therapy with UCERIS 9 mg are summarized in Table 1.

Table 1. Summary of Adverse Reactions in Two Placebo-Controlled Trials Experienced by at Least 2% of the UCERIS 9 mg Group (Studies 1 and 2)

	UCERIS 9 mg (N = 255) n (%)	UCERIS 6 mg (N = 254) n (%)	Placebo (N = 258) n (%)
Headache	29 (11.4)	37 (14.6)	27 (10.5)
Nausea	13 (5.1)	12 (4.7)	11 (4.3)
Decreased Blood Cortisol	11 (4.3)	6 (2.4)	1 (0.4)
Upper Abdominal Pain	10 (3.9)	8 (3.1)	5 (1.9)
Fatigue	8 (3.1)	5 (2.0)	5 (1.9)
Flatulence	6 (2.4)	8 (3.1)	5 (1.9)
Abdominal Distension	6 (2.4)	4 (1.6)	2 (0.8)
Acne	6 (2.4)	2 (0.8)	5 (1.9)
Urinary Tract Infection	5 (2.0)	1 (0.4)	1 (0.4)
Arthralgia	5 (2.0)	5 (2.0)	4 (1.6)
Constipation	5 (2.0)	1 (0.4)	2 (0.8)

Of UCERIS 9 mg patients, a total of 15% discontinued treatment due to any adverse event (including adverse reactions) compared with 17% in the placebo group.

Table 2 summarizes the percentages of patients reporting glucocorticoid related effects in the 2 placebo-controlled studies.

Table 2. Summary of Glucocorticoid Related Effects in Two Placebo-Controlled Trials (Studies 1 and 2)

	UCERIS 9 mg (N = 255) n (%)	UCERIS 6 mg (N = 254) n (%)	Placebo (N = 258) n (%)
Overall	26 (10.2)	19 (7.5)	27 (10.5)
Mood changes	9 (3.5)	10 (3.9)	11 (4.3)
Sleep changes	7 (2.7)	10 (3.9)	12 (4.7)
Insomnia	6 (2.4)	6 (2.4)	8 (3.1)
Acne	6 (2.4)	2 (0.8)	5 (1.9)
Moon face	3 (1.2)	3 (1.2)	4 (1.6)
Fluid retention	2 (0.8)	3 (1.2)	3 (1.2)
Hirsutism	1 (0.4)	0	0
Striae rubrae	0	0	2 (0.8)
Flushing	0	1 (0.4)	3 (1.2)

No clinically significant differences were observed with respect to the overall percentages of patients with any glucocorticoid related effects between UCERIS and placebo after 8 weeks of induction therapy.

Study 3 was an open-label study evaluating UCERIS 9 mg once daily for 8 weeks in 60 patients who had previously completed an 8-week induction study (Study 1), but had not achieved remission. Among patients who took UCERIS 9 mg up to 16 weeks cumulatively across Study 1 and Study 3 combined, similar rates of adverse reactions and glucocorticoid-related effects were seen compared to those who took UCERIS 9 mg for 8 weeks in Study 1.

In Study 4, the safety of long-term treatment with UCERIS 6 mg was evaluated in a placebo-controlled 12-month maintenance study of 123 patients. Patients who had previously completed 8 weeks of therapy in any induction study (Study 1, 2, or 3) and were in remission were randomized to UCERIS 6 mg or placebo once daily for 12 months. In patients who took UCERIS 6 mg for up to 12 months, similar rates of adverse reactions were seen between placebo and UCERIS 6 mg. After up to 12 months of study treatment, 77% (27/35) of the patients in the UCERIS 6 mg and 74% (29/39) of the patients in the placebo treatment groups had normal bone density scans.

In Study 4, the glucocorticoid related effects were similar in patients with up to 12 months of therapy with UCERIS 6 mg and placebo (Table 3).

Table 3. Summary of Glucocorticoid Related Effects Over 12-month Treatment (Study 4)

	UCERIS 6 mg (N = 62) n (%)	Placebo (N = 61) n (%)
Overall	9 (14.5)	7 (11.5)
Insomnia	4 (6.5)	4 (6.6)
Mood changes	4 (6.5)	2 (3.3)
Moon face	3 (4.8)	3 (4.9)
Sleep changes	3 (4.8)	3 (4.9)
Acne	3 (4.8)	0
Hirsutism	3 (4.8)	0
Flushing	1 (1.6)	1 (1.6)
Fluid retention	1 (1.6)	1 (1.6)

6.2 Postmarketing Experience

The following adverse reactions have been identified during postapproval use of oral budesonide. Because these reactions are reported voluntarily from a population of uncertain size, it is not always possible to reliably estimate their frequency or establish a causal relationship to drug exposure.

Immune System Disorders: anaphylactic reactions
Nervous System Disorders: benign intracranial hypertension
Psychiatric Disorders: mood swings

7 DRUG INTERACTIONS

7.1 Interaction with CYP3A4 inhibitors

Concomitant oral administration of ketoconazole (a known inhibitor of CYP3A4 activity in the liver and in the intestinal mucosa) caused an eight-fold increase of the systemic exposure to oral budesonide. If treatment with inhibitors of CYP3A4 activity (such as ketoconazole, itraconazole, ritonavir, indinavir, saquinavir, erythromycin) is indicated, discontinuation of the UCERIS should be considered. After extensive intake of grapefruit juice (which inhibits CYP3A4 activity predominantly in the intestinal mucosa), the systemic exposure for oral budesonide increased about two times. Ingestion of grapefruit or grapefruit juice should be avoided in connection with UCERIS administration [See Dosage and Administration (2) and Clinical Pharmacology (12.3)].

7.2 Inhibitors of Gastric Acid Secretion

Since the dissolution of the coating of UCERIS is pH dependent, the release properties and uptake of the compound may be altered when UCERIS is used after treatment with gastric acid reducing agents (e.g., PPIs, H_2-blockers and antacids).

8 USE IN SPECIFIC POPULATIONS

8.1 Pregnancy

Teratogenic Effects: Pregnancy Category C

Budesonide was teratogenic and embryocidal in rabbits and rats. Budesonide produced fetal loss, decreased pup weights, and skeletal abnormalities at subcutaneous doses of 25 mcg/kg in rabbits (approximately 0.05 times the maximum recommended human dose on a body surface area basis) and 500 mcg/kg in rats (approximately 0.5 times the maximum recommended human dose on a body surface area basis).

There are no adequate and well-controlled studies in pregnant women. Budesonide should be used during pregnancy only if the potential benefit justifies the potential risk to the fetus.

Nonteratogenic Effects: Hypoadrenalism may occur in infants born of mothers receiving glucocorticosteroids during pregnancy. Such infants should be carefully observed.

8.3 Nursing Mothers

The disposition of budesonide when delivered by inhalation from a dry powder inhaler at doses of 200 or 400 mcg twice daily for at least 3 months was studied in eight lactating women with asthma from 1 to 6 months postpartum.[1] Systemic exposure to budesonide in these women appears to be comparable to that in non-lactating women with asthma from other studies. Breast milk obtained over eight hours post-dose revealed that the maximum budesonide concentration for the 400 and 800 mcg total daily doses was 0.39 and 0.78 nmol/L, respectively, and occurred within 45 minutes after inhalation. The estimated oral daily dose of budesonide from breast milk to the infant is approximately 0.007 and 0.014 mcg/kg/day for the two dose regimens used in this study, which represents approximately 0.3% to 1% of the dose inhaled by the mother. Budesonide plasma concentrations obtained from five infants at about 90 minutes after breast feeding (and about 140 minutes after drug administration to the mother) were below quantifiable levels (<0.02 nmol/L in four infants and <0.04 nmol/L in one infant).

The recommended daily dose of UCERIS extended release tablets is higher (9 mg daily) compared with inhaled budesonide (up to 800 µg daily) given to mothers in the above study. The maximum budesonide plasma concentration following a 9 mg daily dose (in both single- and repeated-dose pharmacokinetic studies) of oral budesonide is approximately 5-10 nmol/L which is up to 10 times higher than the 1-2 nmol/L for a 800 mcg daily dose of inhaled budesonide at steady state in the above inhalation study. Since there are no data from controlled trials on the use of UCERIS by nursing mothers or their infants, and because of the potential for serious adverse reactions in nursing infants from UCERIS, a decision should be made whether to discontinue nursing or to discontinue UCERIS, taking into account the clinical importance of UCERIS to the mother. Budesonide is secreted in human milk. Data from budesonide delivered via dry powder inhaler indicates that the total daily oral dose of budesonide available in breast milk to the infant is approximately 0.3% to 1% of the dose inhaled by the mother. Assuming the coefficient of extrapolation between the inhaled and oral doses is constant across all dose levels, at therapeutic doses of UCERIS, budesonide exposure to the nursing child may be up to 10 times higher than that by budesonide inhalation.

8.4 Pediatric Use

Safety and effectiveness of UCERIS in pediatric patients have not been established. Glucocorticosteroids, such as UCERIS may cause a reduction of growth velocity in pediatric patients.

8.5 Geriatric Use

Clinical studies of UCERIS did not include sufficient numbers of subjects aged 65 and over to determine whether they respond differently from younger subjects. Other reported clinical experience has not identified differences in responses between the elderly and younger patients. In general, UCERIS should be used cautiously in elderly patients due to the potential for decreased hepatic, renal, or cardiac function, and of concomitant disease or other drug therapy.

8.6 Hepatic Impairment

Patients with moderate to severe liver disease should be monitored for increased signs and/or symptoms of hypercorticism. Discontinuing the use of UCERIS tablets should be considered in these patients [See *Warnings and Precautions* (5.4)].

10 OVERDOSAGE

Reports of acute toxicity and/or death following overdosage of glucocorticosteroids are rare. Treatment consists of immediate gastric lavage or emesis followed by supportive and symptomatic therapy.

If glucocorticosteroids are used at excessive doses for prolonged periods, systemic glucocorticosteroid effects such as hypercorticism and adrenal suppression may occur. For chronic overdosage in the face of severe disease requiring continuous steroid therapy, the dosage may be reduced temporarily.

Single oral budesonide doses of 200 and 400 mg/kg were lethal in female and male mice, respectively. The signs of acute toxicity were decreased motor activity, piloerection and generalized edema.

11 DESCRIPTION

UCERIS (budesonide) extended release tablets, for oral administration, contain budesonide, a synthetic corticosteroid, as the active ingredient. Budesonide is designated chemically as (RS)-11β, 16α, 17,21 tetrahydroxypregna-1,4-diene-3,20-dione cyclic 16,17-acetal with butyraldehyde.

Budesonide is provided as a mixture of two epimers (22R and 22S). The empirical formula of budesonide is $C_{25}H_{34}O_6$ and its molecular weight is 430.5. Its structural formula is:

Budesonide is a white to off-white, tasteless, odorless powder that is practically insoluble in water, sparingly soluble in alcohol, and freely soluble in chloroform.

UCERIS, a delayed and extended-release tablet, is coated with a polymer film, which breaks down at or above pH 7.0. The tablet core contains budesonide with polymers that provide for extended release of budesonide.

Each tablet contains the following inactive ingredients: stearic acid, lecithin, microcrystalline cellulose, hydroxypropylcellulose, lactose, silicon dioxide, magnesium stearate, methacrylic acid copolymer types A and B, talc, triethylcitrate, and titanium dioxide.

12 CLINICAL PHARMACOLOGY

12.1 Mechanism of Action

Budesonide has a high topical glucocorticosteroid (GCS) activity and substantial first-pass elimination. The formulation contains budesonide in an extended release tablet core. The tablet core is enteric coated to protect dissolution in gastric juice which delays budesonide release until exposure to a pH $\geq$ 7 in the small intestine. Upon disintegration of the coating, the core matrix provides extended release of budesonide in a time dependent manner.

12.2 Pharmacodynamics

Budesonide has a high glucocorticoid effect and a weak mineralocorticoid effect, and the affinity of budesonide to GCS receptors, which reflects the intrinsic potency of the drug, is about 200-fold that of cortisol and 15-fold that of prednisolone.

Treatment with systemically active GCS, including UCERIS, is associated with a suppression of endogenous cortisol concentrations and an impairment of the hypothalamus-pituitary-adrenal (HPA) axis function. Markers, indirect and direct, of this are cortisol levels in plasma or urine and response to ACTH stimulation.

In a study assessing the response to ACTH stimulation test in patients treated with UCERIS 9 mg once daily, the proportion of patients with abnormal response was 47% at 4 weeks and 79% at 8 weeks.

12.3 Pharmacokinetics

Absorption

Following single oral administration of UCERIS 9 mg in healthy subjects, peak plasma concentration (C_{max}) was 1.35 ± 0.96 ng/mL, the time to peak concentration (T_{max}) on average was 13.3 ± 5.9 hours, although it varied across different individual patients, and the area under the plasma concentration time curve (AUC) was approximately 16.43 ± 10.52 ng·hr/mL. The pharmacokinetic parameters of UCERIS 9 mg have a high degree of variability among subjects. There was no accumulation of budesonide with respect to both AUC and C_{max} following 7 days of UCERIS 9 mg once daily dosing.

Food Effect

A food-effect study involving administration of UCERIS to healthy volunteers under fasting conditions and with a high-fat meal indicated that the C_{max} was decreased by 27% while there was no significant decrease in AUC. Additionally, a mean delay in absorption lag time of 2.4 hours is observed under fed conditions.

Distribution

The mean volume of distribution (V_{SS}) of budesonide varies between 2.2 and 3.9 L/kg in healthy subjects and in patients. Plasma protein binding is estimated to be 85 to 90% in the concentration range 1 to 230 nmol/L, independent of gender. The erythrocyte/plasma partition ratio at clinically relevant concentrations is about 0.8.

Metabolism

Following absorption, budesonide is subject to high first-pass metabolism (80-90%). *In vitro* experiments in human liver microsomes demonstrate that budesonide is rapidly and extensively biotransformed, mainly by CYP3A4, to its 2 major metabolites, 6β-hydroxy budesonide and 16α-hydroxy prednisolone. The glucocorticoid activity of these metabolites is negligible (< 1/100) in relation to that of the parent compound.

In vivo investigations with intravenous doses in healthy subjects are in agreement with the *in vitro* findings and demonstrate that budesonide has a high plasma clearance, 0.9-1.8 L/min. These high plasma clearance values approach the estimated liver blood flow, and, accordingly, suggest that budesonide is a high hepatic clearance drug. The plasma elimination half-life, $t_{1/2}$, after administration of intravenous doses ranges between 2.0 and 3.6 hours.

Excretion

Budesonide is excreted in urine and feces in the form of metabolites. After oral as well as intravenous administration of micronized [^{3}H]-budesonide, approximately 60% of the recovered radioactivity is found in urine. The major metabolites, including 6β-hydroxy budesonide and 16α-hydroxy prednisolone, are mainly renally excreted, intact or in conjugated forms. No unchanged budesonide is detected in urine.

Special Populations

Hepatic Impairment

In patients with liver cirrhosis, systemic availability of orally administered budesonide correlates with disease severity and is, on average, 2.5-fold higher compared with healthy controls. Patients with mild liver disease are minimally affected. Patients with severe liver dysfunction were not studied. Absorption parameters are not altered, and for the intravenous dose, no significant differences in CL or V_{SS} are observed.

Renal Impairment

The pharmacokinetics of budesonide in patients with renal impairment has not been studied. Intact budesonide is not renally excreted, but metabolites are to a large extent, and might therefore reach higher levels in patients with impaired renal function. However, these metabolites have negligible corticosteroid activity as compared with budesonide (< 1/100).

Drug-Drug Interactions

Budesonide is metabolized via CYP3A4. Potent inhibitors of CYP3A4 can increase the plasma levels of budesonide several-fold. Co-administration of ketoconazole results in an eight-fold increase in AUC of budesonide, compared to budesonide alone. Grapefruit juice, an inhibitor of gut mucosal CYP3A, approximately doubles the systemic exposure of oral budesonide.

Conversely, induction of CYP3A4 can result in the lowering of budesonide plasma levels [See *Dosage and Administration* (2) and *Drug Interactions* (7)].

Oral contraceptives containing ethinyl estradiol, which are also metabolized by CYP3A4, do not affect the pharmacokinetics of budesonide. Budesonide does not affect the plasma levels of oral contraceptives (i.e., ethinyl estradiol).

13 NONCLINICAL TOXICOLOGY

13.1 Carcinogenesis, Mutagenesis, Impairment of Fertility

Carcinogenicity

Carcinogenicity studies with budesonide were conducted in rats and mice. In a two-year study in Sprague-Dawley rats, budesonide caused a statistically significant increase in the incidence of gliomas in male rats at an oral dose of 50 mcg/kg (approximately 0.05 times the maximum recommended human dose on a body surface area basis). In addition, there were increased incidences of primary hepatocellular tumors in male rats at 25 mcg/kg (approximately 0.023 times the maximum recommended human dose on a body surface area basis) and above. No tumorigenicity was seen in female rats at oral doses up to 50 mcg/kg (approximately 0.05 times the maximum recommended human dose on a body surface area basis). In an additional two-year study in male Sprague-Dawley rats, budesonide caused no gliomas at an oral dose of 50 mcg/kg (approximately 0.05 times the maximum recommended human dose on a body surface area basis). However, it caused a statistically significant increase in the incidence of hepatocellular tumors at an oral dose of 50 mcg/kg (approximately 0.05 times the maximum recommended human dose on a body surface area basis). The concurrent reference glucocorticosteroids (prednisolone and triamcinolone acetonide) showed similar findings. In a 91-week study in mice, budesonide caused no treatment-related carcinogenicity at oral doses up to 200 mcg/kg (approximately 0.1 times the maximum recommended human dose on a body surface area basis).

Mutagenesis

Budesonide was not genotoxic in the Ames test, the mouse lymphoma cell forward gene mutation (TK$^{+/-}$) test, the human lymphocyte chromosome aberration test, the *Drosophila melanogaster* sex-linked recessive lethality test, the rat hepatocyte UDS test and the mouse micronucleus test.

Impairment of Fertility

In rats, budesonide had no effect on fertility at subcutaneous doses up to 80 mcg/kg (approximately 0.07 times the maximum recommended human dose on a body surface area basis). However, it caused a decrease in prenatal viability and viability in pups at birth and during lactation, along with a decrease in maternal body-weight gain, at subcutaneous doses of 20 mcg/kg (approximately 0.02 times the maximum recommended human dose on a body surface area basis) and above. No such effects were noted at 5 mcg/kg (approximately 0.005 times the maximum recommended human dose on a body surface area basis).

14 CLINICAL STUDIES

Induction of Remission in Active Mild to Moderate Ulcerative Colitis

Two similarly-designed, randomized, double-blind, placebo-controlled studies were conducted in a total of 970 adult patients with active, mild to moderate ulcerative colitis (UC) which was defined as an Ulcerative Colitis Disease Activity Index (UCDAI of ≥ 4 and ≤ 10). Eight-hundred ninety-nine of these patients had histology consistent with active UC; this was considered the primary analysis population. UCDAI is a four-component scale (total score of 0 to 12) that encompasses the clinical assessments of stool frequency, rectal bleeding, mucosal appearance and physician's rating of disease activity (score of 0 to 3 for each of the components).

The baseline median UCDAI score in both studies was 7. In Study 1, 56% of patients were male, and the median age was 42 years. In Study 2, 57% of patients were male, and the median age was 44 years. In Study 1, 50% of patients were Caucasian, 7% were African American, and 34% were Asian. In Study 2, more than 99% were Caucasian.

Both studies compared UCERIS 9 mg and 6 mg with placebo and included an active reference arm (a mesalamine 2.4 g in Study 1; and a budesonide* 9 mg not approved for the treatment of UC in Study 2)*. The primary endpoint was induction of remission after 8 weeks of treatment. Remission was defined as a UCDAI score of ≤ 1 with subscores of 0 for rectal bleeding, stool frequency, and mucosal appearance and with a ≥ 1 point reduction in an endoscopy-only score.[2] In both studies, UCERIS 9 mg extended release tablets demonstrated superiority to placebo in inducing remission (Table 4).

Table 4. Induction of Remission in Studies 1 and 2

Treatment Group	Study 1 n/N (%)	Study 2 n/N (%)
UCERIS 9 mg	22/123 (17.9)	19/109 (17.4)
UCERIS 6 mg	16/121 (13.2)	9/109 (8.3)
Reference Arm*	15/124 (12.1)	13/103 (12.6)
Placebo	9/121 (7.4)	4/89 (4.5)
Treatment Difference between UCERIS 9 mg and Placebo (95% CI)[†]	10.4% (2.2%, 18.7%)	12.9% (4.6%, 21.3%)

Remission is defined as a UCDAI score of ≤ 1, with subscores of 0 for rectal bleeding, stool frequency, and mucosal appearance and with a ≥ 1 point reduction in an endoscopy-only score.[2]

The primary analysis population included only patients that had histology consistent with active UC.

CI=Confidence Interval

*The reference arm in Study 1 is a delayed release mesalamine 2.4 g; the reference arm in Study 2 is a budesonide 9 mg not approved for the treatment of UC.

[†]p<0.025 for UCERIS 9 mg vs. placebo in both Studies 1 and 2 based on the Chi-square test (alpha = 0.025)

15 REFERENCES

1. Falt A, Bengtsson T, Kennedy B, et al. Exposure of infants to budesonide through breast milk of asthmatic mothers. *J. Allergy Clin Immunol.* 2007;120(4):798-802.

2. Rachmilewitz D. Coated mesalazine (5-aminosalicylic acid) versus sulphasalazine in the treatment of active ulcerative colitis: a randomised trial. *BMJ.* 1989;298: 82-6.

16   HOW SUPPLIED/STORAGE AND HANDLING

UCERIS (budesonide) extended release tablets 9 mg, are white, round, biconvex tablets and debossed with "MX9". They are supplied as follows:

NDC (68012-309-30):   Bottles of 30 tablets.

Store at 25°C (77°F); excursions permitted to 15 - 30°C (59 - 86°F). [See USP Controlled Room Temperature].

Keep container tightly closed. Protect from light and moisture.

17   PATIENT AND COUNSELING INFORMATION

See FDA-Approved Patient Labeling (Patient Information). Patients being treated with UCERIS extended release tablets should receive the following information and instructions. This information is intended to aid the patient in the safe and effective use of UCERIS.

17.1   Hypercorticism and Adrenal Suppression

Patients should be advised that UCERIS extended release tablets may cause systemic glucocorticosteroid effects of hypercorticism and adrenal suppression. Patients should taper slowly from systemic corticosteroids if transferring to UCERIS extended release tablets [*See Warnings and Precautions* (5.1) and (5.2)].

17.2   Immunosuppression

Patients who are on immunosuppressant doses of glucocorticosteroids should be warned to avoid exposure to chickenpox or measles and, if exposed, to consult their physician immediately. If exposure to such a person occurs, and the patient has not had chicken pox or been properly vaccinated, a physician should be consulted immediately. Patients should be informed of potential worsening of existing tuberculosis, fungal, bacterial, viral, or parasitic infections, or ocular herpes simplex [See *Warnings and Precautions* (5.3)].

17.3   How to Take UCERIS extended release tablets

UCERIS extended release tablets should be swallowed whole with water and NOT CHEWED, CRUSHED, OR BROKEN. Patients should be advised to avoid the consumption of grapefruit juice for the duration of their UCERIS therapy [See *Dosage and Administration* (2)].

Manufactured for Santarus, Inc., Raleigh, NC 27615 • 1-888-778-0887

Manufactured by: Cosmo S.p.A., Milan, Italy.

Santarus, Inc.®

Salix Pharmaceuticals, Inc.

UCERIS® is a trademark of Santarus, Inc., a wholly owned subsidiary of Salix Pharmaceuticals, Inc. Raleigh, NC 27615

U.S. Patent Nos: 7,410,651; 7,431,943; RE43799; 8,293,273.

© 2013 Santarus, Inc

Revised: March 2014

FDA-approved Patient Labeling

UCERIS (u SAIR us)

(budesonide) (bew DEH so nide)

extended release tablets

What is UCERIS extended release tablets?

UCERIS is a prescription corticosteroid medicine used to help get mild to moderate ulcerative colitis (UC) under control (induce remission).

It is not known if UCERIS is safe and effective in children.

Who should not take UCERIS extended release tablets?

Do not take UCERIS extended release tablets if:

• you are allergic to budesonide or any of the ingredients in UCERIS extended release tablets. See the end of this leaflet for a complete list of ingredients in UCERIS extended release tablets.

What should I tell my healthcare provider before taking UCERIS extended release tablets?

Before you take UCERIS extended release tablets tell your healthcare provider if you:

• have liver problems

• are planning to have surgery

• have chicken pox or measles or have recently been near anyone with chicken pox or measles

• have an infection

• have or had a family history of diabetes, cataracts or glaucoma

• have or had tuberculosis

• have high blood pressure (hypertension)

• have decreased bone mineral density (osteoporosis)

• stomach ulcers

• any other medical condition

• are pregnant or plan to become pregnant. It is not known if UCERIS extended release tablets will harm your unborn baby.

• are breastfeeding or plan to breastfeed. UCERIS extended release tablets can pass into your breast milk and may harm your baby. You and your healthcare provider should decide if you will take UCERIS extended release tablets or breastfeed. You should not do both.

Tell your healthcare provider about all the medicines you take, including prescription and over-the-counter vitamins, and herbal supplements. UCERIS extended release tablets and other medicines may affect each other causing side effects.

Know the medicines you take. Keep a list of them to show your healthcare provider and pharmacist when you get a new medicine.

How should I take UCERIS extended release tablets?

• Take UCERIS extended release tablets exactly as your healthcare provider tells you to take it.

• Your healthcare provider will tell you how many UCERIS extended release tablets to take.

• Take UCERIS extended release tablets in the morning.

• Take UCERIS extended release tablets whole with water. Do not chew, crush, or break UCERIS extended release tablets before swallowing.

• If you take too much of UCERIS, call your healthcare provider right away or go to the nearest hospital emergency room.

What should I avoid while taking UCERIS extended release tablets?

• Do not eat grapefruit or drink grapefruit juice while taking UCERIS extended release tablets. Eating grapefruit or drinking grapefruit juice can increase the level of UCERIS extended release tablets in your blood.

What are the possible side effects of UCERIS extended release tablets?

UCERIS can cause some serious side effects, including:

• **Effects of having too much corticosteroid medicine in your blood (hypercorticism).**

Long-time use of UCERIS extended release tablets can cause you to have too much glucocorticosteroid medicine in your blood. Tell your healthcare provider if you have any of the following signs and symptoms of hypercorticism:

• acne

• bruise easily

• rounding of your face (moon face)

• ankle swelling

• thicker or more hair on your body and face

• a fatty pad or hump between your shoulders (buffalo hump)

• pink or purple stretch marks on the skin of your abdomen, thighs, breasts and arms

• **Adrenal suppression.** When UCERIS extended release tablets is taken for a long period of time (chronic use), the adrenal glands do not make enough steroid hormones (adrenal suppression). Tell your healthcare provider if you are under stress or have any symptoms of adrenal suppression during treatment with UCERIS extended release tablets including:

• tiredness	• vomiting
• weakness	• low blood pressure
• nausea	

• **Immune system effects and a higher chance of infections.** UCERIS extended release tablets weaken your immune system. Taking medicines that weaken your immune system makes you more likely to get infections. Avoid contact with people who have contagious diseases such as chicken pox or measles, while taking UCERIS extended release tablets.

Tell your health care provider about any signs or symptoms of infection during treatment with UCERIS extended release tablets, including:

• fever	• chills
• pain	• feeling tired
• aches	• nausea and vomiting

• **Worsening of allergies.** If you take certain other corticosteroid medicines to treat allergies, switching to UCERIS extended release tablets may cause your allergies to come back. These allergies may include eczema (a skin disease) or rhinitis (inflammation inside your nose). Tell your healthcare provider if any of your allergies become worse while taking UCERIS extended release tablets.

The most common side effects of UCERIS extended release tablets include:

• headache	• bloating
• nausea	• acne
• decreased blood cortisol levels	• urinary tract infection
• stomach-area pain	
• tiredness	• joint pain
• stomach or intestinal gas	• constipation

Tell your healthcare provider if you have any side effect that bothers you or that does not go away.

These are not all the possible side effects of UCERIS extended release tablets. For more information, ask your healthcare provider or pharmacist.

Call your doctor for medical advice about side effects. You may report side effects to FDA at 1-800-FDA-1088.

How should I store UCERIS extended release tablets?

• Store UCERIS extended release tablets at room temperature, between 68°F to 77°F (20°C to 25°C)

• Keep the bottle tightly closed to protect UCERIS from light and moisture.

Keep UCERIS extended release tablets and all medicines out of the reach of children.

General Information about UCERIS extended release tablets

Medicines are sometimes prescribed for purposes other than those listed in a patient information leaflet. Do not use UCERIS for a condition for which it was not prescribed. Do not give UCERIS to other people, even if they have the same symptoms you have. It may harm them.

If you would like more information, talk with your healthcare provider. You can ask your healthcare provider or pharmacist for information about UCERIS that is written for health professionals.

For more information go to www.UCERIS.com or call (1-888-778-0887).

What are the ingredients in UCERIS extended release tablets?

Active Ingredients: budesonide

Inactive ingredients: stearic acid, lecithin, microcrystalline cellulose, hydroxypropylcellulose, lactose, silicon dioxide, magnesium stearate, methacrylic acid copolymer types A and B, talc, triethylcitrate, and titanium dioxide.

This Patient Information has been approved by the U.S. Food and Drug Administration.

UCERIS (budesonide) Tablets are manufactured for Santarus, Inc., a wholly owned subsidiary of Salix Pharmaceuticals, Inc., 8510 Colonnade Center Drive, Raleigh, NC 27615, USA by: Cosmo S.p.A., Milan, Italy.

UCERIS® is a trademark of Santarus, Inc.,a wholly owned subsidiary of Salix Pharmaceuticals, Inc. Raleigh, NC 27615

© 2013 Santarus, Inc., a wholly owned subsidiary of Salix Pharmaceuticals, Inc.

Revised: March 2014

Shown in Product Identification Guide, page 313

XIFAXAN®
(rifaximin)
Tablets   ℞

HIGHLIGHTS OF PRESCRIBING INFORMATION
These highlights do not include all the information needed to use XIFAXAN safely and effectively. See full prescribing information for XIFAXAN.
XIFAXAN® (rifaximin) Tablets
Initial U.S. Approval: 2004

To reduce the development of drug-resistant bacteria and maintain the effectiveness of XIFAXAN and other antibacterial drugs, XIFAXAN should be used only to treat or prevent infections that are proven or strongly suspected to be caused by bacteria.

————RECENT MAJOR CHANGES————

Indications and Usage, Hepatic Encephalopathy (1.2)	03/2010
Dosage and Administration, Hepatic Encephalopathy (2.2)	03/2010

————INDICATIONS AND USAGE————

XIFAXAN is a rifamycin antibacterial indicated for:

• The treatment of patients (≥ 12 years of age) with travelers' diarrhea (TD) caused by noninvasive strains of *Escherichia coli* (1.1)

• Reduction in risk of overt hepatic encephalopathy (HE) recurrence in patients ≥ 18 years of age (1.2)

Limitations of Use

• TD: Do not use in patients with diarrhea complicated by fever or blood in the stool or diarrhea due to pathogens other than *Escherichia coli* (1.1)

————DOSAGE AND ADMINISTRATION————

• Travelers' diarrhea: One 200 mg tablet taken orally three times a day for 3 days, with or without food (2.1)

• Hepatic encephalopathy: One 550 mg tablet taken orally two times a day, with or without food (2.2)

————DOSAGE FORMS AND STRENGTHS————

• 200 mg and 550 mg tablets (3)

————CONTRAINDICATIONS————

History of hypersensitivity to rifaximin, rifamycin antimicrobial agents, or any of the components of XIFAXAN (4.1)

————WARNINGS AND PRECAUTIONS————

• Travelers' Diarrhea Not Caused by *E. coli*:   XIFAXAN was not effective in diarrhea complicated by fever and/or blood in the stool or diarrhea due to pathogens other than *E. coli*. If diarrhea symptoms get worse or persist for more than 24-48 hours, discontinue XIFAXAN and consider alternative antibiotics (5.1)

- *Clostridium difficile*-Associated Diarrhea: Evaluate if diarrhea occurs after therapy or does not improve or worsens during therapy (5.2)
- Hepatic Impairment: Use with caution in patients with severe (Child-Pugh C) hepatic impairment (5.4, 8.7)
- Concomitant P-glycoprotein inhibitor: Caution should be exercised when concomitant use of rifaximin and a P-glycoprotein inhibitor is needed (5.5,7.2)

---ADVERSE REACTIONS---

- Most common adverse reactions in travelers' diarrhea (≥ 5%): Flatulence, headache, abdominal pain, rectal tenesmus, defecation urgency and nausea (6.1)
- Most common adverse reactions in HE (≥ 10%): Peripheral edema, nausea, dizziness, fatigue, and ascites (6.1)

To report suspected adverse reactions, contact Salix Pharmaceuticals at 1-800-508-0024 and www.Salix.com or FDA at 1-800-FDA-1088 or *www.fda.gov/medwatch*

---USE IN SPECIFIC POPULATIONS---

- Pregnancy: Based on animal data, may cause fetal harm (8.1)
- Nursing Mothers: Discontinue nursing or drug, taking into account the importance of the drug to the mother (8.3)

See 17 for PATIENT COUNSELING INFORMATION

Revised: 03/2014

FULL PRESCRIBING INFORMATION: CONTENTS*

FULL PRESCRIBING INFORMATION

1   INDICATIONS AND USAGE

To reduce the development of drug-resistant bacteria and maintain the effectiveness of XIFAXAN and other antibacterial drugs, XIFAXAN when used to treat infection should be used only to treat or prevent infections that are proven or strongly suspected to be caused by susceptible bacteria. When culture and susceptibility information are available, they should be considered in selecting or modifying antibacterial therapy. In the absence of such data, local epidemiology and susceptibility patterns may contribute to the empiric selection of therapy.

1.1   Travelers' Diarrhea

XIFAXAN 200 mg is indicated for the treatment of patients (≥ 12 years of age) with travelers' diarrhea caused by non-invasive strains of *Escherichia coli* [see *Warnings and Precautions (5), Clinical Pharmacology (12.4) and Clinical Studies (14.1)*].

Limitations of Use

XIFAXAN should not be used in patients with diarrhea complicated by fever or blood in the stool or diarrhea due to pathogens other than *Escherichia coli.*

1.2   Hepatic Encephalopathy

XIFAXAN 550 mg is indicated for reduction in risk of overt hepatic encephalopathy (HE) recurrence in patients ≥ 18 years of age.

In the trials of XIFAXAN for HE, 91% of the patients were using lactulose concomitantly. Differences in the treatment effect of those patients not using lactulose concomitantly could not be assessed.

XIFAXAN has not been studied in patients with MELD (Model for End-Stage Liver Disease) scores > 25, and only 8.6% of patients in the controlled trial had MELD scores over 19. There is increased systemic exposure in patients with more severe hepatic dysfunction [see *Warnings and Precautions (5.4), Use in Specific Populations (8.7), Clinical Pharmacology (12.3)*].

2   DOSAGE AND ADMINISTRATION

2.1   Dosage for Travelers' Diarrhea

The recommended dose of XIFAXAN is one 200 mg tablet taken orally three times a day for 3 days. XIFAXAN can be administered orally, with or without food [see *Clinical Pharmacology (12.3)*].

2.2   Dosage for Hepatic Encephalopathy

The recommended dose of XIFAXAN is one 550 mg tablet taken orally two times a day, with or without food [see *Clinical Pharmacology (12.3)*].

3   DOSAGE FORMS AND STRENGTHS

XIFAXAN is a pink-colored biconvex tablet and is available in the following strengths:
- 200 mg – a round tablet debossed with "Sx" on one side.
- 550 mg – an oval tablet debossed with "rfx" on one side.

4   CONTRAINDICATIONS

4.1   Hypersensitivity

XIFAXAN is contraindicated in patients with a hypersensitivity to rifaximin, any of the rifamycin antimicrobial agents, or any of the components in XIFAXAN. Hypersensitivity reactions have included exfoliative dermatitis, angioneurotic edema, and anaphylaxis [see *Adverse Reactions (6.2)*].

5   WARNINGS AND PRECAUTIONS

5.1   Travelers' Diarrhea Not Caused by *Escherichia coli*

XIFAXAN was not found to be effective in patients with diarrhea complicated by fever and/or blood in the stool or diarrhea due to pathogens other than *Escherichia coli.*

Discontinue XIFAXAN if diarrhea symptoms get worse or persist more than 24-48 hours and alternative antibiotic therapy should be considered.

XIFAXAN is not effective in cases of travelers' diarrhea due to *Campylobacter jejuni*. The effectiveness of XIFAXAN in travelers' diarrhea caused by *Shigella* spp. and *Salmonella* spp. has not been proven. XIFAXAN should not be used in patients where *Campylobacter jejuni*, *Shigella* spp., or *Salmonella* spp. may be suspected as causative pathogens.

5.2   *Clostridium difficile*-Associated Diarrhea

Clostridium difficile-associated diarrhea (CDAD) has been reported with use of nearly all antibacterial agents, including XIFAXAN, and may range in severity from mild diarrhea to fatal colitis. Treatment with antibacterial agents alters the normal flora of the colon which may lead to overgrowth of *C. difficile.*

C. difficile produces toxins A and B which contribute to the development of CDAD. Hypertoxin producing strains of *C. difficile* cause increased morbidity and mortality, as these infections can be refractory to antimicrobial therapy and may require colectomy. CDAD must be considered in all patients who present with diarrhea following antibiotic use. Careful medical history is necessary since CDAD has been reported to occur over two months after the administration of antibacterial agents.

If CDAD is suspected or confirmed, ongoing antibiotic use not directed against *C. difficile* may need to be discontinued. Appropriate fluid and electrolyte management, protein supplementation, antibiotic treatment of *C. difficile*, and surgical evaluation should be instituted as clinically indicated.

5.3   Development of Drug Resistant Bacteria

Prescribing XIFAXAN for travelers' diarrhea in the absence of a proven or strongly suspected bacterial infection or a prophylactic indication is unlikely to provide benefit to the patient and increases the risk of the development of drug-resistant bacteria.

5.4   Severe (Child-Pugh C) Hepatic Impairment

There is increased systemic exposure in patients with severe hepatic impairment. Animal toxicity studies did not achieve systemic exposures that were seen in patients with severe hepatic impairment. The clinical trials were limited to patients with MELD scores <25. Therefore, caution should be exercised when administering XIFAXAN to patients with severe hepatic impairment (Child-Pugh C) [see *Use in Specific Populations (8.7) and Clinical Studies (14.2)*].

5.5   Concomitant use with P-glycoprotein Inhibitors

Concomitant administration of drugs that are P-glycoprotein inhibitors with rifaximin can substantially increase the systemic exposure to rifaximin. Caution should be exercised when concomitant use of rifaximin and a P-glycoprotein inhibitor such as cyclosporine is needed. In patients with hepatic impairment, a potential additive effect of reduced metabolism and concomitant P-glycoprotein inhibitors may further increase the systemic exposure to rifaximin [see *Drug Interactions (7.2) and Pharmacokinetics (12.3)*].

6   ADVERSE REACTIONS

6.1   Clinical Studies Experience

Because clinical trials are conducted under widely varying conditions, adverse reaction rates observed in the clinical trials of a drug cannot be directly compared to rates in the clinical trials of another drug and may not reflect the rates observed in practice.

Travelers' Diarrhea

The safety of XIFAXAN 200 mg taken three times a day was evaluated in patients with travelers' diarrhea consisting of 320 patients in two placebo-controlled clinical trials with 95% of patients receiving three or four days of treatment with XIFAXAN. The population studied had a mean age of 31.3 (18-79) years of which approximately 3% were ≥ 65 years old, 53% were male and 84% were White, 11% were Hispanic.

Discontinuations due to adverse reactions occurred in 0.4% of patients. The adverse reactions leading to discontinuation were taste loss, dysentery, weight decrease, anorexia, nausea and nasal passage irritation.

All adverse reactions for XIFAXAN 200 mg three times daily that occurred at a frequency ≥ 2% in the two placebo-controlled trials combined are provided in Table 1. (These include adverse reactions that may be attributable to the underlying disease.)

Table 1. All Adverse Reactions With an Incidence ≥ 2% Among Patients Receiving XIFAXAN Tablets, 200 mg Three Times Daily, in Placebo-Controlled Studies

MedDRA Preferred Term	Number (%) of Patients	
	XIFAXAN Tablets, 600 mg/day N = 320	Placebo N = 228
Flatulence	36 (11%)	45 (20%)
Headache	31 (10%)	21 (9%)
Abdominal Pain NOS*	23 (7%)	23 (10%)
Rectal Tenesmus	23 (7%)	20 (9%)
Defecation Urgency	19 (6%)	21 (9%)
Nausea	17 (5%)	19 (8%)
Constipation	12 (4%)	8 (4%)
Pyrexia	10 (3%)	10 (4%)
Vomiting NOS	7 (2%)	4 (2%)

* NOS: Not otherwise specified

The following adverse reactions, presented by body system, have also been reported in <2% of patients taking XIFAXAN in the two placebo-controlled clinical trials where the 200 mg tablet was taken three times a day for travelers' diarrhea. The following includes adverse reactions regardless of causal relationship to drug exposure.

Blood and Lymphatic System Disorders: Lymphocytosis, monocytosis, neutropenia

Ear and Labyrinth Disorders: Ear pain, motion sickness, tinnitus

Gastrointestinal Disorders: Abdominal distension, diarrhea NOS, dry throat, fecal abnormality NOS, gingival disorder NOS, inguinal hernia NOS, dry lips, stomach discomfort

General Disorders and Administration Site Conditions: Chest pain, fatigue, malaise, pain NOS, weakness

Infections and Infestations: Dysentery NOS, respiratory tract infection NOS, upper respiratory tract infection NOS

Injury and Poisoning: Sunburn

Investigations: Aspartate aminotransferase increased, blood in stool, blood in urine, weight decreased

Metabolic and Nutritional Disorders: Anorexia, dehydration

Musculoskeletal, Connective Tissue, and Bone Disorders: Arthralgia, muscle spasms, myalgia, neck pain

Nervous System Disorders: Abnormal dreams, dizziness, migraine NOS, syncope, loss of taste

Psychiatric Disorders: Insomnia

Renal and Urinary Disorders: Choluria, dysuria, hematuria, polyuria, proteinuria, urinary frequency

Respiratory, Thoracic, and Mediastinal Disorders: Dyspnea NOS, nasal passage irritation, nasopharyngitis, pharyngitis, pharyngolaryngeal pain, rhinitis NOS, rhinorrhea

Skin and Subcutaneous Tissue Disorders: Clamminess, rash NOS, sweating increased

Vascular Disorders: Hot flashes NOS

Hepatic Encephalopathy

The data described below reflect exposure to XIFAXAN 550 mg in 348 patients, including 265 exposed for 6 months and 202 exposed for more than a year (mean exposure was 364 days). The safety of XIFAXAN 550 mg taken two times a day for reducing the risk of overt hepatic encephalopathy recurrence in adult patients was evaluated in a 6-month placebo-controlled clinical trial (n = 140) and in a long term follow-up study (n = 280). The population studied had a mean age of 56.26 (range: 21-82) years; approximately 20% of the patients were ≥ 65 years old, 61% were male, 86% were White, and 4% were Black. Ninety-one percent of patients in the trial were taking lactulose concomitantly. All adverse reactions that occurred at an incidence ≥ 5% and at a higher incidence in XIFAXAN 550 mg-treated subjects than in the placebo group in the 6-month trial are provided in Table 2. (These include adverse events that may be attributable to the underlying disease).

Table 2: Adverse Reactions Occurring in ≥ 5% of Patients Receiving XIFAXAN and at a Higher Incidence Than Placebo

MedDRA Preferred Term	Number (%) of Patients	
	XIFAXAN Tablets 550 mg TWICE DAILY N = 140	Placebo N = 159
Edema peripheral	21 (15%)	13 (8%)
Nausea	20 (14%)	21 (13%)
Dizziness	18 (13%)	13 (8%)
Fatigue	17 (12%)	18 (11%)
Ascites	16 (11%)	15 (9%)
Muscle spasms	13 (9%)	11 (7%)
Pruritus	13 (9%)	10 (6%)
Abdominal pain	12 (9%)	13 (8%)
Abdominal distension	11 (8%)	12 (8%)
Anemia	11 (8%)	6 (4%)
Cough	10 (7%)	11 (7%)
Depression	10 (7%)	8 (5%)
Insomnia	10 (7%)	11 (7%)
Nasopharyngitis	10 (7%)	10 (6%)
Abdominal pain upper	9 (6%)	8 (5%)
Arthralgia	9 (6%)	4 (3%)
Back pain	9 (6%)	10 (6%)
Constipation	9 (6%)	10 (6%)
Dyspnea	9 (6%)	7 (4%)
Pyrexia	9 (6%)	5 (3%)
Rash	7 (5%)	6 (4%)

The following adverse reactions, presented by body system, have also been reported in the placebo-controlled clinical trial in greater than 2% but less than 5% of patients taking XIFAXAN 550 mg taken orally two times a day for hepatic encephalopathy. The following includes adverse events occurring at a greater incidence than placebo, regardless of causal relationship to drug exposure.

Ear and Labyrinth Disorders: Vertigo

Gastrointestinal Disorders: Abdominal pain lower, abdominal tenderness, dry mouth, esophageal variceal bleed, stomach discomfort

General Disorders and Administration Site Conditions: Chest pain, generalized edema, influenza like illness, pain NOS

Infections and Infestations: Cellulitis, pneumonia, rhinitis, upper respiratory tract infection NOS

Injury, Poisoning and Procedural Complications: Contusion, fall, procedural pain

Investigations: Weight increased

Metabolic and Nutritional Disorders: Anorexia, dehydration, hyperglycemia, hyperkalemia, hypoglycemia, hyponatremia

Musculoskeletal, Connective Tissue, and Bone Disorders: Myalgia, pain in extremity

Nervous System Disorders: Amnesia, disturbance in attention, hypoesthesia, memory impairment, tremor

Psychiatric Disorders: Confusional state

Respiratory, Thoracic, and Mediastinal Disorders: Epistaxis

Vascular Disorders: Hypotension

6.2   Postmarketing Experience

The following adverse reactions have been identified during post approval use of XIFAXAN. Because these reactions are reported voluntarily from a population of unknown size, estimates of frequency cannot be made. These reactions have been chosen for inclusion due to either their seriousness, frequency of reporting or causal connection to XIFAXAN.

Infections and Infestations

Cases of *C. difficile*-associated colitis have been reported *[see Warnings and Precautions (5.2)]*.

General

Hypersensitivity reactions, including exfoliative dermatitis, rash, angioneurotic edema (swelling of face and tongue and difficulty swallowing), urticaria, flushing, pruritus and anaphylaxis have been reported. These events occurred as early as within 15 minutes of drug administration.

7   DRUG INTERACTIONS

7.1   Effects of rifaximin on cytochrome P450 enzymes

In vitro studies have shown that rifaximin did not inhibit cytochrome P450 isoenzymes 1A2, 2A6, 2B6, 2C9, 2C19, 2D6, 2E1 and CYP3A4 at concentrations ranging from 2 to 200 ng/mL *[see Clinical Pharmacology (12.3)]*. Rifaximin is not expected to inhibit these enzymes in clinical use.

An *in vitro* study has suggested that rifaximin induces CYP3A4 *[see Clinical Pharmacology (12.3)]*. However, in patients with normal liver function, rifaximin at the recommended dosing regimen is not expected to induce CYP3A4. It is unknown whether rifaximin can have a significant effect on the pharmacokinetics of concomitant CYP3A4 substrates in patients with reduced liver function who have elevated rifaximin concentrations.

7.2   Concomitant P-glycoprotein inhibitors

An *in vitro* study suggested that rifaximin is a substrate of P-glycoprotein. Co-administration of cyclosporine, a potent P-glycoprotein inhibitor, with rifaximin resulted in 83-fold and 124-fold increases in rifaximin mean C_{max} and $AUC_∞$ in healthy subjects. The clinical significance of this increase in systemic exposure is unknown *[see Clinical Pharmacology (12.3)]*.

8   USE IN SPECIFIC POPULATIONS

8.1   Pregnancy

Pregnancy Category C

There are no adequate and well controlled studies in pregnant women. Rifaximin has been shown to be teratogenic in rats and rabbits at doses that caused maternal toxicity. XIFAXAN tablets should be used during pregnancy only if the potential benefit justifies the potential risk to the fetus. Administration of rifaximin to pregnant rats and rabbits at dose levels that caused reduced body weight gain resulted in eye malformations in both rat and rabbit fetuses. Additional malformations were observed in fetal rabbits that included cleft palate, lumbar scoliosis, brachygnathia, interventricular septal defect, and large atrium.

The fetal rat malformations were observed in a study of pregnant rats administered a high dose that resulted in 16 times the therapeutic dose to diarrheic patients or 1 times the therapeutic dose to patients with hepatic encephalopathy (based upon plasma AUC comparisons). Fetal rabbit malformations were observed from pregnant rabbits administered mid and high doses that resulted in 1 or 2 times the therapeutic dose to diarrheic patients or less than 0.1 times the dose in patients with hepatic encephalopathy, based upon plasma AUC comparisons.

Post-natal developmental effects were not observed in rat pups from pregnant/lactating female rats dosed during the period from gestation to Day 20 post-partum at the highest dose which resulted in approximately 16 times the human therapeutic dose for travelers' diarrhea (based upon AUCs) or approximately 1 times the AUCs derived from therapeutic doses to patients with hepatic encephalopathy.

8.3   Nursing Mothers

It is not known whether rifaximin is excreted in human milk. Because many drugs are excreted in human milk and because of the potential for adverse reactions in nursing infants from XIFAXAN, a decision should be made whether to discontinue nursing or to discontinue the drug, taking into account the importance of the drug to the mother.

8.4   Pediatric Use

The safety and effectiveness of XIFAXAN 200 mg in pediatric patients with travelers' diarrhea less than 12 years of age have not been established.

The safety and effectiveness of XIFAXAN 550 mg for HE have not been established in patients < 18 years of age.

8.5   Geriatric Use

Clinical studies with rifaximin 200 mg for travelers' diarrhea did not include sufficient numbers of patients aged 65 and over to determine whether they respond differently than younger subjects.

In the controlled trial with XIFAXAN 550 mg for hepatic encephalopathy, 19.4% were 65 and over, while 2.3% were 75 and over. No overall differences in safety or effectiveness were observed between these subjects and younger subjects, and other reported clinical experience has not identified differences in responses between the elderly and younger patients, but greater sensitivity of some older individuals cannot be ruled out.

8.6   Renal Impairment

The pharmacokinetics of rifaximin in patients with impaired renal function has not been studied.

8.7   Hepatic Impairment

Following administration of XIFAXAN 550 mg twice daily to patients with a history of hepatic encephalopathy, the systemic exposure (i.e., $AUC_τ$) of rifaximin was about 10-, 13-, and 20-fold higher in those patients with mild (Child-Pugh A), moderate (Child-Pugh B) and severe (Child-Pugh C) hepatic impairment, respectively, compared to that in healthy volunteers. No dosage adjustment is recommended because rifaximin is presumably acting locally. Nonetheless, caution should be exercised when XIFAXAN is administered to patients with severe hepatic impairment *[see Warnings and Precautions (5.4), Clinical Pharmacology (12.3), and Clinical Studies (14.2)]*.

10   OVERDOSAGE

No specific information is available on the treatment of overdosage with XIFAXAN. In clinical studies at doses higher than the recommended dose (> 600 mg/day for travelers' diarrhea or > 1100 mg/day for hepatic encephalopathy), adverse reactions were similar in subjects who received doses higher than the recommended dose and placebo. In the case of overdosage, discontinue XIFAXAN, treat symptomatically, and institute supportive measures as required.

11   DESCRIPTION

XIFAXAN tablets contain rifaximin, a non-aminoglycoside semi-synthetic, nonsystemic antibiotic derived from rifamycin SV. Rifaximin is a structural analog of rifampin. The chemical name for rifaximin is (2S,16Z,18E,20S, 21S,22R,23R,24R,25S,26S,27S,28E)-5,6,21,23,25-pentahydroxy-27-methoxy-2,4,11,16,20,22,24,26-octamethyl-2,7-(epoxypentadeca-[1,11,13]trienimino)benzofuro[4,5-e]pyrido[1,2-á]-benzimidazole-1,15(2H)-dione,25-acetate. The empirical formula is $C_{43}H_{51}N_3O_{11}$ and its molecular weight is 785.9. The chemical structure is represented below:

XIFAXAN tablets for oral administration are film-coated and contain 200 mg or 550 mg of rifaximin.

Inactive ingredients:

Each 200 mg tablet contains colloidal silicon dioxide, disodium edetate, glycerol palmitostearate, hypromellose, microcrystalline cellulose, propylene glycol, red iron oxide, sodium starch glycolate, talc, and titanium dioxide.

Each 550 mg tablet contains colloidal silicon dioxide, glycerol palmitostearate, microcrystalline cellulose, polyethylene glycol/macrogol, polyvinyl alcohol, red iron oxide, sodium starch glycolate, talc, and titanium dioxide.

12   CLINICAL PHARMACOLOGY

12.1   Mechanism of Action

Rifaximin is an antibacterial drug *[see Clinical Pharmacology (12.4)]*.

12.3   Pharmacokinetics

Absorption

Travelers' Diarrhea

Systemic absorption of rifaximin (200 mg three times daily) was evaluated in 13 subjects challenged with shigellosis on Days 1 and 3 of a three-day course of treatment. Rifaximin plasma concentrations and exposures were low and variable. There was no evidence of accumulation of rifaximin following repeated administration for 3 days (9 doses). Peak plasma rifaximin concentrations after 3 and 9 consecutive doses ranged from 0.81 to 3.4 ng/mL on Day 1 and 0.68 to 2.26 ng/mL on Day 3. Similarly, AUC_{0-last} estimates were 6.95 ± 5.15 ng•h/mL on Day 1 and 7.83 ± 4.94 ng•h/mL on Day 3. XIFAXAN is not suitable for treating systemic bacterial infections because of limited systemic exposure after oral administration *[see Warnings and Precautions (5.1)]*.

Hepatic Encephalopathy

After a single dose and multiple doses of rifaximin 550 mg in healthy subjects, the mean time to reach peak plasma concentrations was about an hour. The pharmacokinetic (PK) parameters were highly variable and the accumulation ratio based on AUC was 1.37.

The PK of rifaximin in patients with a history of HE was evaluated after administration of XIFAXAN, 550 mg two times a day. The PK parameters were associated with a high variability and mean rifaximin exposure ($AUC_τ$) in patients with a history of HE (147 ng•h/mL) was approximately 12-

fold higher than that observed in healthy subjects following the same dosing regimen (12.3 ng•h/mL). When PK parameters were analyzed based on Child-Pugh Class A, B, and C, the mean AUC_τ was 10-, 13-, and 20-fold higher, respectively, compared to that in healthy subjects (Table 3). [See table 3 above]

Food Effect in Healthy Subjects
A high-fat meal consumed 30 minutes prior to XIFAXAN dosing in healthy subjects delayed the mean time to peak plasma concentration from 0.75 to 1.5 hours and increased the systemic exposure (AUC) of rifaximin by 2-fold (Table 4).

Table 4. Mean (± SD) Pharmacokinetic Parameters After Single-Dose Administration of XIFAXAN Tablets 550 mg in Healthy Subjects Under Fasting and Fed Conditions (N = 12)

Parameter	Fasting	Fed
C_{max} (ng/mL)	4.1 ± 1.5	4.8 ± 4.3
T_{max}[1] (h)	0.8 (0.5, 2.1)	1.5 (0.5, 4.1)
Half-Life (h)	1.8 ± 1.4	4.8 ± 1.3
AUC (ng•h/mL)	11.1 ± 4.2	22.5 ± 12

[1] Median (range)

XIFAXAN can be administered with or without food *[see Dosage and Administration (2.1 and 2.2)]*.

Distribution
Rifaximin is moderately bound to human plasma proteins. *In vivo*, the mean protein binding ratio was 67.5% in healthy subjects and 62% in patients with hepatic impairment when XIFAXAN 550 mg was administered.

Metabolism and Excretion
In a mass balance study, after administration of 400 mg ^{14}C-rifaximin orally to healthy volunteers, of the 96.94% total recovery, 96.62% of the administered radioactivity was recovered in feces almost exclusively as the unchanged drug and 0.32% was recovered in urine mostly as metabolites with 0.03% as the unchanged drug. Rifaximin accounted for 18% of radioactivity in plasma. This suggests that the absorbed rifaximin undergoes metabolism with minimal renal excretion of the unchanged drug. The enzymes responsible for metabolizing rifaximin are unknown.

In a separate study, rifaximin was detected in the bile after cholecystectomy in patients with intact gastrointestinal mucosa, suggesting biliary excretion of rifaximin.

Specific Populations
Hepatic Impairment
The systemic exposure of rifaximin was markedly elevated in patients with hepatic impairment compared to healthy subjects. The mean AUC in patients with Child-Pugh Class C hepatic impairment was 2-fold higher than in patients with Child-Pugh Class A hepatic impairment (see Table 3), *[see Warnings and Precautions (5.4) and Use in Specific Populations (8.7)]*.

Renal Impairment
The pharmacokinetics of rifaximin in patients with impaired renal function has not been studied.

Drug Interactions
In vitro drug interaction studies have shown that rifaximin, at concentrations ranging from 2 to 200 ng/mL, did not inhibit human hepatic cytochrome P450 isoenzymes 1A2, 2A6, 2B6, 2C9, 2C19, 2D6, 2E1, and 3A4.
In an *in vitro* study, rifaximin was shown to induce CYP3A4 at the concentration of 0.2 μM.
An *in vitro* study suggests that rifaximin is a substrate of P-glycoprotein. In the presence of P-glycoprotein inhibitor verapamil, the efflux ratio of rifaximin was reduced greater than 50% *in vitro*. Following co-administration of a single 600-mg dose of cyclosporine, a potent inhibitor of P-glycoprotein and a weak inhibitor of CYP3A4, OATP, and BCRP, with a single dose of rifaximin 550 mg, rifaximin mean C_{max} was increased 83-fold, from 0.48 to 40.0 ng/mL; mean AUC_∞ was increased 124-fold, from 2.54 to 314 ng•h/mL.
The inhibitory effect of rifaximin on P-gp transport was observed in an *in vitro* study. The effect of rifaximin on P-gp transporter was not evaluated *in vivo*.

Midazolam
The effect of rifaximin 200 mg administered orally every 8 hours for 3 days and for 7 days on the pharmacokinetics of a single dose of either midazolam 2 mg intravenous or midazolam 6 mg orally was evaluated in healthy subjects. No significant difference was observed in the metrics of systemic exposure or elimination of intravenous or oral midazolam or its major metabolite, 1'-hydroxymidazolam, between midazolam alone or together with rifaximin. Therefore, rifaximin was not shown to significantly affect intestinal or hepatic CYP3A4 activity for the 200 mg three times a day dosing regimen.
After XIFAXAN 550 mg was administered three times a day for 7 days and 14 days to healthy subjects, the mean AUC of single midazolam 2 mg orally was 3.8% and 8.8% lower, re-

spectively, than when midazolam was administered alone. The mean C_{max} of midazolam was also decreased by 4-5% when XIFAXAN was administered for 7-14 days prior to midazolam administration. This degree of interaction is not considered clinically meaningful.
The effect of rifaximin on CYP3A4 in patients with impaired liver function who have elevated systemic exposure is not known.

Oral Contraceptives Containing 0.07 mg Ethinyl Estradiol and 0.5 mg Norgestimate
The oral contraceptive study utilized an open-label, crossover design in 28 healthy female subjects to determine if rifaximin 200 mg orally administered three times a day for 3 days (the dosing regimen for travelers' diarrhea) altered the pharmacokinetics of a single dose of an oral contraceptive containing 0.07 mg ethinyl estradiol and 0.5 mg norgestimate. Results showed that the pharmacokinetics of single doses of ethinyl estradiol and norgestimate were not altered by rifaximin.
Effect of rifaximin on oral contraceptives was not studied for XIFAXAN 550 mg twice a day, the dosing regimen for hepatic encephalopathy.

12.4 Microbiology
Mechanism of Action
Rifaximin is a non-aminoglycoside semi-synthetic antibacterial derived from rifamycin SV. Rifaximin acts by binding to the beta-subunit of bacterial DNA-dependent RNA polymerase resulting in inhibition of bacterial RNA synthesis.
Drug Resistance and Cross-Resistance
Escherichia coli has been shown to develop resistance to rifaximin *in vitro*. However, the clinical significance of such an effect has not been studied.
Rifaximin is a structural analog of rifampin. Organisms with high rifaximin minimum inhibitory concentration (MIC) values also have elevated MIC values against rifampin. Cross-resistance between rifaximin and other classes of antimicrobials has not been studied.
Activity In Vitro and in Critical Infections
Rifaximin has been shown to be active against the following pathogen in clinical studies of infectious diarrhea as described in the *Indications and Usage (1)* section: *Escherichia coli* (enterotoxigenic and enteroaggregative strains).
For HE, rifaximin is thought to have an effect on the gastrointestinal flora.
Susceptibility Tests
In vitro susceptibility testing was performed according to the National Committee for Clinical Laboratory Standards (NCCLS) agar dilution method M7-A6 *[see References (15)]*. However, the correlation between susceptibility testing and clinical outcome has not been determined.

13 NONCLINICAL TOXICOLOGY
13.1 Carcinogenesis, Mutagenesis, Impairment of Fertility
Malignant schwannomas in the heart were significantly increased in male Crl:CD® (SD) rats that received rifaximin by oral gavage for two years at 150 to 250 mg/kg/day (doses equivalent to 2.4 to 4 times the recommended dose of 200 mg three times daily for travelers' diarrhea, and equivalent to 1.3 to 2.2 times the recommended dose of 550 mg twice daily for hepatic encephalopathy, based on relative body surface area comparisons). There was no increase in tumors in Tg.rasH2 mice dosed orally with rifaximin for 26 weeks at 150 to 2000 mg/kg/day (doses equivalent to 1.2 to 16 times the recommended daily dose for travelers' diarrhea and equivalent to 0.7 to 9 times the recommended daily dose for hepatic encephalopathy, based on relative body surface area comparisons).
Rifaximin was not genotoxic in the bacterial reverse mutation assay, chromosomal aberration assay, rat bone marrow micronucleus assay, rat hepatocyte unscheduled DNA synthesis assay, or the CHO/HGPRT mutation assay. There was no effect on fertility in male or female rats following the administration of rifaximin at doses up to 300 mg/kg (approximately 5 times the clinical dose of 600 mg/day, and approximately 2.6 times the clinical dose of 1100 mg/day, adjusted for body surface area).

Table 3. Mean (± SD) Pharmacokinetic Parameters of Rifaximin at Steady-State in Patients with a History of Hepatic Encephalopathy by Child-Pugh Class[1]

	Healthy Subjects (n = 14)	Child-Pugh Class		
		A (n = 18)	B (n = 7)	C (n = 4)
AUC_{tau} (ng•h/mL)	12.3 ± 4.8	118 ± 67.8	161 ± 101	246 ± 120
C_{max} (ng/mL)	3.4 ± 1.6	19.5 ± 11.4	25.1 ± 12.6	35.5 ± 12.5
T_{max}[2] (h)	0.8 (0.5, 4.0)	1 (0.9, 10)	1 (0.97, 1)	1 (0, 2)

[1] Cross-study comparison with PK parameters in healthy subjects
[2] Median (range)

14 CLINICAL STUDIES
14.1 Travelers' Diarrhea
The efficacy of XIFAXAN given as 200 mg orally taken three times a day for 3 days was evaluated in 2 randomized, multi-center, double-blind, placebo-controlled studies in adult subjects with travelers' diarrhea. One study was conducted at clinical sites in Mexico, Guatemala, and Kenya (Study 1). The other study was conducted in Mexico, Guatemala, Peru, and India (Study 2). Stool specimens were collected before treatment and 1 to 3 days following the end of treatment to identify enteric pathogens. The predominant pathogen in both studies was *Escherichia coli*.
The clinical efficacy of XIFAXAN was assessed by the time to return to normal, formed stools and resolution of symptoms. The primary efficacy endpoint was time to last unformed stool (TLUS) which was defined as the time to the last unformed stool passed, after which clinical cure was declared. Table 5 displays the median TLUS and the number of patients who achieved clinical cure for the intent to treat (ITT) population of Study 1. The duration of diarrhea was significantly shorter in patients treated with XIFAXAN than in the placebo group. More patients treated with XIFAXAN were classified as clinical cures than were those in the placebo group.

Table 5. Clinical Response in Study 1 (ITT population)

	XIFAXAN (n=125)	Placebo (n=129)	Estimate (97.5% CI)	P-Value
Median TLUS (hours)	32.5	58.6	1.78[a] (1.26, 2.50)	0.0002
Clinical cure, n (%)	99 (79.2)	78 (60.5)	18.7[b] (5.3, 32.1)	0.001

[a] Hazard Ratio
[b] Difference in rates

Microbiological eradication (defined as the absence of a baseline pathogen in culture of stool after 72 hours of therapy) rates for Study 1 are presented in Table 6 for patients with any pathogen at baseline and for the subset of patients with *Escherichia coli* at baseline. *Escherichia coli* was the only pathogen with sufficient numbers to allow comparisons between treatment groups.
Even though XIFAXAN had microbiologic activity similar to placebo, it demonstrated a clinically significant reduction in duration of diarrhea and a higher clinical cure rate than placebo. Therefore, patients should be managed based on clinical response to therapy rather than microbiologic response.

Table 6. Microbiologic Eradication Rates in Study 1 Subjects with a Baseline Pathogen

	XIFAXAN	Placebo
Overall	48/70 (68.6)	41/61 (67.2)
E. coli	38/53 (71.7)	40/54 (74.1)

The results of Study 2 supported the results presented for Study 1. In addition, this study provided evidence that subjects treated with XIFAXAN with fever and/or blood in the stool at baseline had prolonged TLUS. These subjects had lower clinical cure rates than those without fever or blood in the stool at baseline. Many of the patients with fever and/or blood in the stool (dysentery-like diarrheal syndromes) had invasive pathogens, primarily *Campylobacter jejuni*, isolated in the baseline stool.
Also in this study, the majority of the subjects treated with XIFAXAN who had *Campylobacter jejuni* isolated as a sole pathogen at baseline failed treatment and the resulting clinical cure rate for these patients was 23.5% (4/17). In addition to not being different from placebo, the microbiologic

eradication rates for subjects with *Campylobacter jejuni* isolated at baseline were much lower than the eradication rates seen for *Escherichia coli*.

In an unrelated open-label, pharmacokinetic study of oral XIFAXAN 200 mg taken every 8 hours for 3 days, 15 adult subjects were challenged with *Shigella flexneri* 2a, of whom 13 developed diarrhea or dysentery and were treated with XIFAXAN. Although this open-label challenge trial was not adequate to assess the effectiveness of XIFAXAN in the treatment of shigellosis, the following observations were noted: eight subjects received rescue treatment with ciprofloxacin either because of lack of response to XIFAXAN treatment within 24 hours (2), or because they developed severe dysentery (5), or because of recurrence of *Shigella flexneri* in the stool (1); five of the 13 subjects received ciprofloxacin although they did not have evidence of severe disease or relapse.

14.2 Hepatic Encephalopathy

The efficacy of XIFAXAN 550 mg taken orally two times a day was evaluated in a randomized, placebo-controlled, double-blind, multi-center 6-month trial of adult subjects from the U.S., Canada and Russia who were defined as being in remission (Conn score of 0 or 1) from hepatic encephalopathy (HE). Eligible subjects had ≥ 2 episodes of HE associated with chronic liver disease in the previous 6 months. A total of 299 subjects were randomized to receive either XIFAXAN (n=140) or placebo (n=159) in this study. Patients had a mean age of 56 years (range, 21-82 years), 81% < 65 years of age, 61% were male and 86% White. At baseline, 67% of patients had a Conn score of 0 and 68% had an asterixis grade of 0. Patients had MELD scores of either ≤ 10 (27%) or 11 to 18 (64%) at baseline. No patients were enrolled with a MELD score of > 25. Nine percent of the patients were Child-Pugh Class C. Lactulose was concomitantly used by 91% of the patients in each treatment arm of the study. Per the study protocol, patients were withdrawn from the study after experiencing a breakthrough HE episode. Other reasons for early study discontinuation included: adverse reactions (XIFAXAN 6%; placebo 4%), patient request to withdraw (XIFAXAN 4%; placebo 6%) and other (XIFAXAN 7%; placebo 5%).

The primary endpoint was the time to first breakthrough overt HE episode. A breakthrough overt HE episode was defined as a marked deterioration in neurological function and an increase of Conn score to Grade ≥ 2. In patients with a baseline Conn score of 0, a breakthrough overt HE episode was defined as an increase in Conn score of 1 and asterixis grade of 1.

Breakthrough overt HE episodes were experienced by 31 of 140 subjects (22%) in the XIFAXAN group and by 73 of 159 subjects (46%) in the placebo group during the 6-month treatment period. Comparison of Kaplan-Meier estimates of event-free curves showed XIFAXAN significantly reduced the risk of HE breakthrough by 58% during the 6-month treatment period. Presented below in Figure 1 is the Kaplan-Meier event-free curve for all subjects (n = 299) in the study.

Figure 1: Kaplan-Meier Event-Free Curves[1] in HE Study (Time to First Breakthrough-HE Episode up to 6 Months of Treatment, Day 170) (ITT Population)

Note: Open diamonds and open triangles represent censored subjects.
[1] Event-free refers to non-occurrence of breakthrough HE.

When the results were evaluated by the following demographic and baseline characteristics, the treatment effect of XIFAXAN 550 mg in reducing the risk of breakthrough overt HE recurrence was consistent for: sex, baseline Conn score, duration of current remission and diabetes. The differences in treatment effect could not be assessed in the following subpopulations due to small sample size: non-White (n=42), baseline MELD > 19 (n=26), Child-Pugh C (n=31), and those without concomitant lactulose use (n=26).

HE-related hospitalizations (hospitalizations directly resulting from HE, or hospitalizations complicated by HE) were reported for 19 of 140 subjects (14%) and 36 of 159 subjects (23%) in the XIFAXAN and placebo groups respectively. Comparison of Kaplan-Meier estimates of event-free curves showed XIFAXAN significantly reduced the risk of

HE-related hospitalizations by 50% during the 6-month treatment period. Comparison of Kaplan-Meier estimates of event-free curves is shown in Figure 2.

Figure 2: Kaplan-Meier Event-Free Curves[1] in Pivotal HE Study (Time to First HE-Related Hospitalization in HE Study up to 6 Months of Treatment, Day 170) (ITT Population)

Note: Open diamonds and open triangles represent censored subjects.
[1] Event-free refers to non-occurrence of HE-related hospitalization.

15 REFERENCES

Clinical and Laboratory Standards Institute (CLSI). Methods for Dilution Antimicrobial Susceptibility Tests for Bacteria that Grow Aerobically; Approved Standard - Ninth Edition. CLSI document M07-A9, Clinical and Laboratory Standards Institute, 950 West Valley Road, Suite 2500, Wayne, Pennsylvania 19087, USA, 2012.

16 HOW SUPPLIED/STORAGE AND HANDLING

The 200 mg tablet is a pink-colored, round, biconvex tablet with "Sx" debossed on one side. It is available in the following presentations:

• NDC 65649-301-03, bottles of 30 tablets
• NDC 65649-301-41, bottles of 100 tablets
• NDC 65649-301-05, carton of 100 tablets, Unit Dose

The 550 mg tablet is a pink-colored, oval, biconvex tablet with "rfx" debossed on one side. It is available in the following presentations:

• NDC 65649-303-02, bottles of 60 tablets
• NDC 65649-303-03, carton of 60 tablets, Unit Dose

Storage

Store XIFAXAN Tablets at 20–25°C (68–77°F); excursions permitted to 15–30°C (59-86°F). See USP Controlled Room Temperature.

17 PATIENT COUNSELING INFORMATION

17.1 Persistent Diarrhea

For those patients being treated for travelers' diarrhea, discontinue XIFAXAN if diarrhea persists more than 24-48 hours or worsens. Advise the patient to seek medical care for fever and/or blood in the stool *[see Warnings and Precautions (5.1)]*.

17.2 *Clostridium difficile*-Associated Diarrhea

Clostridium difficile-associated diarrhea (CDAD) has been reported with use of nearly all antibacterial agents, including XIFAXAN, and may range in severity from mild diarrhea to fatal colitis. Treatment with antibiotics alters the normal flora of the colon which may lead to *C. difficile*. Patients can develop watery and bloody stools (with or without stomach cramps and fever) even as late as two or more months after having taken the last dose of the antibiotic. If diarrhea occurs after therapy or does not improve or worsens during therapy, advise patients to contact a physician as soon as possible *[see Warnings and Precautions (5.4)]*.

17.3 Administration with Food

Inform patients that XIFAXAN may be taken with or without food.

17.4 Antibacterial Resistance

Counsel patients that antibacterial drugs including XIFAXAN should only be used to treat bacterial infections. They do not treat viral infections (e.g., the common cold). When XIFAXAN is prescribed to treat a bacterial infection, patients should be told that although it is common to feel better early in the course of therapy, the medication should be taken exactly as directed. Skipping doses or not completing the full course of therapy may (1) decrease the effectiveness of the immediate treatment and (2) increase the likelihood that bacteria will develop resistance and will not be treatable by XIFAXAN or other antibacterial drugs in the future.

17.5 Severe Hepatic Impairment

Patients should be informed that in patients with severe hepatic impairment (Child-Pugh C) there is an increase in systemic exposure to XIFAXAN *[see Warnings and Precautions (5.4)]*.

Manufactured for:
Salix Pharmaceuticals, Inc.
Raleigh, NC 27615

XIFAXAN® is a trademark of Alfa Wassermann S.p.A. used under license by Salix Pharmaceuticals, Inc.
Copyright © Salix Pharmaceuticals, Inc.
Rifaximin for Travelers' Diarrhea and Hepatic encephalopathy is protected by US Patent Nos. 7,045,620; 7,612,199; 7,902,206; 7,906,542; 8,158,781; 8,158,644; 8,193,196; and 8,518,949. Rifaximin for Travelers' Diarrhea is also protected by US Patent No. 7,928,115. Rifaximin for Hepatic encephalopathy is also protected by US Patent No. 8,642,573.
Web site: www.Salix.com
All rights reserved.
VENART-185-2
MAR 2014
Shown in Product Identification Guide, page 313

Schering Corporation
for product information, please see Merck

Smith & Nephew, Inc.
Biotherapeutics
3909 Hulen Street
Fort Worth TX 76107

Direct Inquiries to:
800-441-8227

COLLAGENASE SANTYL® OINTMENT℞
250 units/g

Rx only

DESCRIPTION

Collagenase Santyl® Ointment is a sterile enzymatic debriding ointment which contains 250 collagenase units per gram of white petrolatum USP. The enzyme collagenase is derived from the fermentation by *Clostridium histolyticum*. It possesses the unique ability to digest collagen in necrotic tissue.

CLINICAL PHARMACOLOGY

Since collagen accounts for 75% of the dry weight of skin tissue, the ability of collagenase to digest collagen in the physiological pH and temperature range makes it particularly effective in the removal of detritus.[1] Collagenase thus contributes towards the formation of granulation tissue and subsequent epithelization of dermal ulcers and severely burned areas.[2,3,4,5,6] Collagen in healthy tissue or in newly formed granulation tissue is not attacked.[2,3,4,5,6,7,8] There is no information available on collagenase absorption through skin or its concentration in body fluids associated with therapeutic and/or toxic effects, degree of binding to plasma proteins, degree of uptake by a particular organ or in the fetus, and passage across the blood brain barrier.

INDICATIONS AND USAGE

Collagenase Santyl® Ointment is indicated for debriding chronic dermal ulcers[2,3,4,5,6,8,9,10,11,12,13,14,15,16,17,18] and severely burned areas.[3,4,5,7,16,19,20,21]

CONTRAINDICATIONS

Collagenase Santyl® Ointment is contraindicated in patients who have shown local or systemic hypersensitivity to collagenase.

PRECAUTIONS

The optimal pH range of collagenase is 6 to 8. Higher or lower pH conditions will decrease the enzyme's activity and appropriate precautions should be taken. The enzymatic activity is also adversely affected by certain detergents, and heavy metal ions such as mercury and silver which are used in some antiseptics. When it is suspected such materials have been used, the site should be carefully cleansed by repeated washings with normal saline before Collagenase Santyl® Ointment is applied. Soaks containing metal ions or acidic solutions should be avoided because of the metal ion and low pH. Cleansing materials such as Dakin's solution and normal saline are compatible with Collagenase Santyl® Ointment.

Debilitated patients should be closely monitored for systemic bacterial infections because of the theoretical possibility that debriding enzymes may increase the risk of bacteremia.

A slight transient erythema has been noted occasionally in the surrounding tissue, particularly when Collagenase Santyl® Ointment was not confined to the wound. Therefore, the ointment should be applied carefully within the area of the wound. Safety and effectiveness in pediatric patients have not been established.

ADVERSE REACTIONS

No allergic sensitivity or toxic reactions have been noted in clinical use when used as directed. However, one case of systemic manifestations of hypersensitivity to collagenase in a patient treated for more than one year with a combination of collagenase and cortisone has been reported.

OVERDOSAGE

No systemic or local reaction attributed to overdose has been observed in clinical investigations and clinical use. If deemed necessary the enzyme may be inactivated by washing the area with povidone iodine.

DOSAGE AND ADMINISTRATION

Collagenase Santyl® Ointment should be applied once daily (or more frequently if the dressing becomes soiled, as from incontinence). When clinically indicated, crosshatching thick eschar with a #10 blade allows Collagenase Santyl® Ointment more surface contact with necrotic debris. It is also desirable to remove, with forceps and scissors, as much loosened detritus as can be done readily. Use Collagenase Santyl® Ointment in the following manner:

1 - Prior to application the wound should be cleansed of debris and digested material by gently rubbing with a gauze pad saturated with normal saline solution, or with the desired cleansing agent compatible with Collagenase Santyl® Ointment (See PRECAUTIONS), followed by a normal saline solution rinse.

2 - Whenever infection is present, it is desirable to use an appropriate topical antibiotic powder. The antibiotic should be applied to the wound prior to the application of Collagenase Santyl® Ointment. Should the infection not respond, therapy with Collagenase Santyl® Ointment should be discontinued until remission of the infection.

3 - Collagenase Santyl® Ointment may be applied directly to the wound or to a sterile gauze pad which is then applied to the wound and properly secured.

4 - Use of Collagenase Santyl® Ointment should be terminated when debridement of necrotic tissue is complete and granulation tissue is well established.

HOW SUPPLIED

Collagenase Santyl® Ointment contains 250 units of collagenase enzyme per gram of white petrolatum USP.
Do not store above 25°C (77°F). Sterility guaranteed until tube is opened.
Collagenase Santyl® Ointment is available in 15 gram and 30 gram tubes, and 90 gram tubes.

REFERENCES

1 - Mandl, I., Adv Enzymol. 23:163, 1961.
2 - Boxer, A.M., Gottesman, N., Bernstein, H., & Mandl, I., Geriatrics. 24:75, 1969.
3 - Mazurek, I., Med. Welt. 22:150, 1971.
4 - Zimmerman, WE., in "Collagenase," Mandl, I., ed., Gordon & Breach, Science Publishers, New York, 1971, p. 131, p. 185.
5 - Vetra, H., & Whittaker, D., Geriatrics. 30:53, 1975.
6 - Rao, D.B., Sane, P.G., & Georgiev, E.L., J. Am. Geriatrics Soc. 23:22, 1975.
7 - Vrabec, R., Moserova, J., Konickova, Z., Behounkova, E., & Blaha, J., J. Hyg. Epidemiol. Microbiol. Immunol. 18:496, 1974.
8 - Lippmann, H.I., Arch. Phys. Med. Rehabil. 54:588, 1973.
9 - German, F. M., in "Collagenase," Mandl, I., ed., Gordon & Breach, Science Publishers, New York, 1971, p. 165.
10 - Haimovici, H. & Strauch, B., in "Collagenase," Mandl, I., ed., Gordon & Breach, Science Publishers, New York, 1971, p. 177.
11 - Lee, L.K., & Ambrus, J.L., Geriatrics. 30:91, 1975.
12 - Locke, R.K., & Heifitz, N.M., J. Am. Pod. Assoc. 65:242, 1975.
13 - Varma, A.O., Bugatch, E., & German, F.M., Surg. Gynecol. Obstet. 136:281, 1973.
14 - Barrett, D., Jr., & Klibanski, A., Am. J. Nurs. 73:849, 1973.
15 - Bardfeld, L.A., J. Pod. Ed. 1:41, 1970.
16 - Blum, G., Schweiz, Rundschau Med Praxis. 62:820, 1973. Abstr. in Dermatology Digest, Feb. 1974, p. 36.
17 - Zaruba, F., Lettl, A., Brozkova, L., Skrdlantova, H., & Krs, V., J. Hyg. Epidemiol. Microbiol. Immunol. 18:499, 1974.
18 - Altman, M.I., Goldstein, L., & Horwitz, S., J. Am. Pod. Assoc. 68:11, 1978.
19 - Rehn, V.J., Med. Klin. 58:799, 1963.
20 - Krauss, H., Koslowski, L., & Zimmermann, W. E., Langenbecks Arch. Klin. Chir. 303:23, 1963.
21 - Gruenagel, H.H., Med. Klin. 58:442, 1963.
Manufactured by: Healthpoint, Ltd., Fort Worth, Texas 76107
US Gov't License #1885

Marketed by: Healthpoint Biotherapeutics®
1-800-441-8227
Healthpoint Biotherapeutics, Fort Worth, Texas 76107
Distributed by: DPT Laboratories, Ltd., San Antonio, Texas 78215
Reorder Nos.: 0064-5010-15 (15 g tube), 0064-5010-30 (30 g tube), and 0064-5010-90 (90 g tube)
© 2013 Healthpoint, Ltd.
SANTYL is a registered trademark of Healthpoint, Ltd.
140163-0713
Shown in Product Identification Guide, page 313

Stiefel Laboratories, Inc.
RESEARCH TRIANGLE PARK, NC 27709

For all inquiries, including adverse event and quality assurance reporting, contact the GSK Response Center at 1-888-825-5249.
For updates to the product information listed below, also consult www.gsk.com.

ALTABAX   Rx
(retapamulin ointment)
1%
For Dermatological use only

HIGHLIGHTS OF PRESCRIBING INFORMATION
These highlights do not include all the information needed to use ALTABAX safely and effectively. See full prescribing information for ALTABAX.
ALTABAX (retapamulin ointment), 1%
For Dermatological use only
Initial U.S. Approval: 2007

──────INDICATIONS AND USAGE──────
ALTABAX, a pleuromutilin antibacterial, is indicated for the topical treatment of impetigo due to *Staphylococcus aureus* (methicillin-susceptible isolates only) or *Streptococcus pyogenes* in patients aged 9 months or older. Safety in patients younger than 9 months has not been established.

──────DOSAGE AND ADMINISTRATION──────
• Apply a thin layer of ALTABAX to the affected area (up to 100 cm^2 in total area in adults or 2% total body surface area in pediatric patients aged 9 months or older) twice daily for 5 days. (2)
• The treated area may be covered with a sterile bandage or gauze dressing if desired. (2)

──────DOSAGE FORMS AND STRENGTHS──────
10 mg retapamulin/1g of ointment in 15-, and 30-gram tubes

──────CONTRAINDICATIONS──────
None.

──────WARNINGS AND PRECAUTIONS──────
• Discontinue in the event of sensitization or severe local irritation. (5.1)
• Not intended for ingestion. Not for intraoral, intranasal, ophthalmic, or intravaginal use. (5.2)

──────ADVERSE REACTIONS──────
The most common drug-related adverse reaction was application site irritation (≤2% of subjects). (6.1)
To report SUSPECTED ADVERSE REACTIONS, contact GlaxoSmithKline at 1-888-825-5249 or FDA at 1-800-FDA-1088 or www.fda.gov/medwatch
See 17 for PATIENT COUNSELING INFORMATION
                                              Revised: 07/2013

FULL PRESCRIBING INFORMATION: CONTENTS*

FULL PRESCRIBING INFORMATION

1   INDICATIONS AND USAGE
ALTABAX® is indicated for use in adults and pediatric patients aged 9 months and older for the topical treatment of impetigo (up to 100 cm^2 in total area in adults or 2% total body surface area in pediatric patients aged 9 months or older) due to *Staphylococcus aureus* (methicillin-susceptible isolates only) or *Streptococcus pyogenes[see Clinical Studies (14)]*. Safety in patients younger than 9 months has not been established.
To reduce the development of drug-resistant bacteria and maintain the effectiveness of ALTABAX and other antibacterial drugs, ALTABAX should be used only to treat or prevent infections that are proven or strongly suspected to be caused by susceptible bacteria.

2   DOSAGE AND ADMINISTRATION
A thin layer of ALTABAX should be applied to the affected area (up to 100 cm^2 in total area in adults or 2% total body surface area in pediatric patients aged 9 months or older) twice daily for 5 days. The treated area may be covered with a sterile bandage or gauze dressing if desired *[see Patient Counseling Information (17)]*.

3   DOSAGE FORMS AND STRENGTHS
10 mg retapamulin/1g of ointment in 15- and 30 gram tubes.

4   CONTRAINDICATIONS
None.

5   WARNINGS AND PRECAUTIONS
5.1   Local Irritation
In the event of sensitization or severe local irritation from ALTABAX, usage should be discontinued, the ointment wiped off, and appropriate alternative therapy for the infection instituted *[see Patient Counseling Information (17)]*.
5.2   Not for Systemic or Mucosal Use
ALTABAX is not intended for ingestion or for oral, intranasal, ophthalmic, or intravaginal use. The efficacy and safety of ALTABAX on mucosal surfaces have not been established. Epistaxis has been reported with the use of ALTABAX on nasal mucosa.
5.3   Potential for Microbial Overgrowth
The use of antibiotics may promote the selection of nonsusceptible organisms. Should superinfection occur during therapy, appropriate measures should be taken.
Prescribing ALTABAX in the absence of a proven or strongly suspected bacterial infection is unlikely to provide benefit to the patient and increases the risk of the development of drug-resistant bacteria.

6   ADVERSE REACTIONS
6.1   Clinical Studies Experience
Because clinical trials are conducted under varying conditions, adverse reaction rates observed in the clinical trials of a drug cannot be directly compared with rates in the clinical trials of another drug and may not reflect the rates observed in practice. The adverse reaction information from the clinical trials does, however, provide a basis for identifying the adverse events that appear to be related to drug use and for approximating rates.
The safety profile of ALTABAX was assessed in 2,115 adult and pediatric subjects ≥9 months who used at least one dose from a 5-day, twice a day regimen of retapamulin ointment. Control groups included 819 adult and pediatric subjects who used at least one dose of the active control (oral cephalexin), 172 subjects who used an active topical comparator (not available in the US), and 71 subjects who used placebo. Adverse events rated by investigators as drug-related occurred in 5.5% (116/2,115) of subjects treated with retapamulin ointment, 6.6% (54/819) of subjects receiving cephalexin, and 2.8% (2/71) of subjects receiving placebo. The most common drug-related adverse events (≥1% of subjects) were application site irritation (1.4%) in the retapamulin group, diarrhea (1.7%) in the cephalexin group, and application site pruritus (1.4%) and application site paresthesia (1.4%) in the placebo group.

Adults:

The adverse events, regardless of attribution, reported in at least 1% of adults (aged 18 years and older) who received ALTABAX or comparator are presented in Table 1.

Table 1. Adverse Events Reported by ≥1% of Adult Subjects Treated With ALTABAX or Comparator in Phase 3 Clinical Trials

Adverse Event	ALTABAX N = 1,527 %	Cephalexin N = 698 %
Headache	2.0	2.0
Application site irritation	1.6	<1.0
Diarrhea	1.4	2.3
Nausea	1.2	1.9
Nasopharyngitis	1.2	<1.0
Creatinine phosphokinase increased	<1.0	1.0

Pediatrics:

The adverse events, regardless of attribution, reported in at least 1% of pediatric subjects aged 9 months to 17 years who received ALTABAX are presented in Table 2.

Table 2. Adverse Events Reported by ≥1% in Pediatric Subjects Aged 9 Months to 17 Years Treated With ALTABAX in Phase 3 Clinical Trials

Adverse Event	ALTABAX N = 588 %	Cephalexin N = 121 %	Placebo N = 64 %
Application site pruritus	1.9	0	0
Diarrhea	1.7	5.0	0
Nasopharyngitis	1.5	1.7	0
Pruritus	1.5	0	1.6
Eczema	1.0	0	0
Headache	1.2	1.7	0
Pyrexia	1.2	<1.0	1.6

Other Adverse Events:

Application site pain, erythema, and contact dermatitis were reported in less than 1% of subjects in clinical trials.

6.2 Postmarketing Experience

In addition to reports in clinical trials, the following events have been identified during postmarketing use of ALTABAX. Because these events are reported voluntarily from a population of uncertain size, it is not possible to reliably estimate their frequency or establish a causal relationship to drug exposure.

General Disorders and Administration Site Conditions: Application site burning.

Immune System Disorders: Hypersensitivity including angioedema.

7 DRUG INTERACTIONS

Coadministration of oral ketoconazole 200 mg twice daily increased retapamulin geometric mean $AUC_{(0-24)}$ and C_{max} by 81% after topical application of retapamulin ointment, 1% on the abraded skin of healthy adult males. Due to low systemic exposure to retapamulin following topical application in adults and pediatric patients aged 2 years and older, dosage adjustments for retapamulin are unnecessary when coadministered with CYP3A4 inhibitors, such as ketoconazole. Based on in vitro P450 inhibition studies and the low systemic exposure observed following topical application of ALTABAX, retapamulin is unlikely to affect the metabolism of other P450 substrates.

Concomitant administration of retapamulin and CYP3A4 inhibitors, such as ketoconazole, has not been studied in pediatric patients. In pediatric subjects aged 2 to 24 months, systemic exposure of retapamulin was higher compared with subjects aged 2 years and older after topical application [see Pharmacokinetics (12.3)]. Based on the higher exposure of retapamulin, it is not recommended to coadminister ALTABAX with strong CYP3A4 inhibitors in patients younger than 24 months.

The effect of concurrent application of ALTABAX and other topical products to the same area of skin has not been studied.

8 USE IN SPECIFIC POPULATIONS

8.1 Pregnancy

Pregnancy Category B

Effects on embryo-fetal development were assessed in pregnant rats given 50, 150, or 450 mg/kg/day by oral gavage on days 6 to 17 postcoitus. Maternal toxicity (decreased body weight gain and food consumption) and developmental toxicity (decreased fetal body weight and delayed skeletal ossification) were evident at doses ≥150 mg/kg/day. There were no treatment-related malformations observed in fetal rats. Retapamulin was given as a continuous intravenous infusion to pregnant rabbits at dosages of 2.4, 7.2, or 24 mg/kg/day from day 7 to 19 of gestation. Maternal toxicity (decreased body weight gain, food consumption, and abortions) was demonstrated at dosages ≥7.2 mg/kg/day (8-fold the estimated maximum achievable human exposure, based on AUC, at 7.2 mg/kg/day). There was no treatment-related effect on embryo-fetal development.

There are no adequate and well-controlled trials in pregnant women. Because animal reproduction studies are not always predictive of human response, ALTABAX should be used in pregnancy only when the potential benefits outweigh the potential risk.

8.3 Nursing Mothers

It is not known whether retapamulin is excreted in human milk. Because many drugs are excreted in human milk, caution should be exercised when ALTABAX is administered to a nursing woman. The safe use of retapamulin during breastfeeding has not been established.

8.4 Pediatric Use

The safety and effectiveness of ALTABAX in the treatment of impetigo have been established in pediatric patients aged 9 months to 17 years. Use of ALTABAX in pediatric patients (9 months to 17 years) is supported by evidence from adequate and well-controlled trials of ALTABAX in which 588 pediatric subjects received at least one dose of retapamulin ointment, 1% [see Adverse Reactions (6.1), Clinical Studies (14)]. The magnitude of efficacy and the safety profile of ALTABAX in pediatric subjects 9 months and older were similar to those in adults.

The safety and effectiveness of ALTABAX in pediatric patients younger than 9 months of age have not been established. An open-label clinical trial of topical treatment with ALTABAX (twice daily for 5 days) was conducted in patients aged 2 to 24 months. Plasma samples were obtained from 79 subjects. In these pediatric subjects, systemic exposure of retapamulin was higher compared with subjects aged 2 to 17 years. Furthermore, a higher proportion of pediatric subjects aged 2 to 9 months had measurable concentrations (>0.5 ng/mL) of retapamulin compared with subjects aged 9 to 24 months [see Pharmacokinetics (12.3)]. The highest levels were seen in subjects aged 2 to 6 months [see Pharmacokinetics (12.3)]. The use of retapamulin is not indicated in pediatric patients younger than 9 months.

8.5 Geriatric Use

Of the total number of subjects in the adequate and well-controlled trials of ALTABAX, 234 subjects were 65 years of age and older, of whom 114 subjects were 75 years of age and older. No overall differences in effectiveness or safety were observed between these subjects and younger adult subjects.

10 OVERDOSAGE

Overdosage with ALTABAX has not been reported. Any signs or symptoms of overdose, either topically or by accidental ingestion, should be treated symptomatically consistent with good clinical practice.

There is no known antidote for overdoses of ALTABAX.

11 DESCRIPTION

ALTABAX contains retapamulin, a semisynthetic pleuromutilin antibiotic. The chemical name of retapamulin is acetic acid, [[(3-exo)-8-methyl-8-azabicyclo[3.2.1]oct-3-yl]thio]-, (3aS,4R,5S,6S,8R,9R,9aR,10R)-6-ethenyldecahydro-5-hydroxy-4,6,9,10-tetramethyl-1-oxo-3a,9-propano-3aH-cyclopentacycloocten-8-yl ester. Retapamulin, a white to pale-yellow crystalline solid, has a molecular formula of $C_{30}H_{47}NO_4S$, and a molecular weight of 517.78. The chemical structure is:

Each gram of ointment for dermatological use contains 10 mg of retapamulin in white petrolatum.

12 CLINICAL PHARMACOLOGY

12.1 Mechanism of Action

ALTABAX is an antibacterial agent [see Clinical Pharmacology (12.4)].

12.2 Pharmacodynamics

In post-hoc analyses of manually over-read 12-lead ECGs from healthy subjects (N = 103), no significant effects on QT/QTc intervals were observed after topical application of retapamulin ointment on intact and abraded skin. Due to the low systemic exposure to retapamulin with topical application, QT prolongation in patients is unlikely [see Clinical Pharmacology (12.3)].

12.3 Pharmacokinetics

Absorption:

In a trial of healthy adult subjects, retapamulin ointment, 1% was applied once daily to intact skin (800 cm² surface area) and to abraded skin (200 cm² surface area) under occlusion for up to 7 days. Systemic exposure following topical application of retapamulin through intact and abraded skin was low. Three percent of blood samples obtained on Day 1 after topical application to intact skin had measurable retapamulin concentrations (lower limit of quantitation 0.5 ng/mL); thus C_{max} values on Day 1 could not be determined. Eighty-two percent of blood samples obtained on Day 7 after topical application to intact skin and 97% and 100% of blood samples obtained after topical application to abraded skin on Days 1 and 7, respectively, had measurable retapamulin concentrations. The median C_{max} value in plasma after application to 800 cm² of intact skin was 3.5 ng/mL on Day 7 (range: 1.2 to 7.8 ng/mL). The median C_{max} value in plasma after application to 200 cm² of abraded skin was 11.7 ng/mL on Day 1 (range: 5.6 to 22.1 ng/mL) and 9.0 ng/mL on Day 7 (range: 6.7 to 12.8 ng/mL).

Plasma samples were obtained from 380 adult subjects and 136 pediatric subjects (aged 2 to 17 years) who were receiving topical treatment with ALTABAX topically twice daily. Eleven percent had measurable retapamulin concentrations (lower limit of quantitation 0.5 ng/mL), of which the median concentration was 0.8 ng/mL. The maximum measured retapamulin concentration in adults was 10.7 ng/mL and in pediatric subjects (aged 2 to 17 years) was 18.5 ng/mL.

A single plasma sample was obtained from 79 pediatric subjects (aged 2 to 24 months) who were receiving topical treatment with ALTABAX twice daily. Forty-six percent had measurable retapamulin concentrations (>0.5 ng/mL) compared with 7% in pediatric subjects aged 2 to 17 years. A higher proportion (69%) of pediatric subjects aged 2 to 9 months had measurable concentrations of retapamulin compared with subjects aged 9 to 24 months (32%). Among pediatric subjects aged 2 to 9 months (n = 29), 4 subjects had retapamulin concentrations that were higher (≥26.9 ng/mL) than the maximum concentration observed in pediatric subjects aged 2 to 17 years (18.5 ng/mL). Among pediatric subjects aged 9 to 24 months (n = 50), 1 subject had a retapamulin concentration that was higher (95.1 ng/mL) than the maximum level observed in pediatric subjects aged 2 to 17 years.

Distribution:

Retapamulin is approximately 94% bound to human plasma proteins, and the protein binding is independent of concentration. The apparent volume of distribution of retapamulin has not been determined in humans.

Metabolism:

In vitro studies with human hepatocytes showed that the main routes of metabolism were mono-oxygenation and di-oxygenation. In vitro studies with human liver microsomes demonstrated that retapamulin is extensively metabolized to numerous metabolites, of which the predominant routes of metabolism were mono-oxygenation and N-demethylation. The major enzyme responsible for metabolism of retapamulin in human liver microsomes was cytochrome P450 3A4 (CYP3A4).

Elimination:

Retapamulin elimination in humans has not been investigated due to low systemic exposure after topical application.

12.4 Microbiology

Retapamulin is a semisynthetic derivative of the compound pleuromutilin, which is isolated through fermentation from Clitopiluspasseckerianus (formerly Pleurotuspasseckerianus). In vitro activity of retapamulin against isolates of Staphylococcus aureus as well as Streptococcus pyogenes has been demonstrated.

Antimicrobial Mechanism of Action:

Retapamulin selectively inhibits bacterial protein synthesis by interacting at a site on the 50S subunit of the bacterial ribosome through an interaction that is different from that of other antibiotics. This binding site involves ribosomal protein L3 and is in the region of the ribosomal P site and peptidyl transferase center. By virtue of binding to this site, pleuromutilins inhibit peptidyl transfer, block P-site interactions, and prevent the normal formation of active 50S ribosomal subunits. Retapamulin is bacteriostatic against Staphylococcus aureus and Streptococcus pyogenes at the retapamulin in vitro minimum inhibitory concentration (MIC) for these organisms. At concentrations 1,000× the in vitro MIC, retapamulin is bactericidal against these same organisms. Although cross-resistance between retapamulin and other antibacterial classes (such as clindamycin and oxazolidones) exist, isolates resistant to these classes may be susceptible to retapamulin.

Mechanisms of Decreased Susceptibility to Retapamulin:
In vitro, 2 mechanisms that cause reduced susceptibility to retapamulin have been identified, specifically, mutations in ribosomal protein L3, the presence of Cfr rRNA methyltransferase or the presence of an efflux mechanism. Decreased susceptibility of *S. aureus* to retapamulin (highest retapamulin MIC was 2 mcg/mL) develops slowly in vitro via multistep mutations in L3 after serial passage in subinhibitory concentrations of retapamulin. There was no apparent treatment-associated reduction in susceptibility to retapamulin in the Phase 3 clinical program. The clinical significance of these findings is not known.

Other:
Based on in vitro broth microdilution susceptibility testing, no differences were observed in susceptibility of *S. aureus* to retapamulin whether the isolates were methicillin-resistant or methicillin-susceptible. Retapamulin susceptibility did not correlate with clinical success rates in patients with methicillin-resistant *S.aureus*. The reason for this is not known but may have been influenced by the presence of particular strains of *S. aureus* possessing certain virulence factors, such as Panton-Valentine Leukocidin (PVL). In the case of treatment failure associated with *S. aureus* (regardless of methicillin susceptibility), the presence of strains possessing additional virulence factors (such as PVL) should be considered.

Retapamulin has been shown to be active against the following microorganisms, both in vitro and in clinical trials *[see Indications and Usage (1)].*

Aerobic and Facultative Gram-Positive Bacteria:
Staphylococcus aureus (methicillin-susceptible isolates only)
Streptococcus pyogenes

Susceptibility Testing:
The clinical microbiology laboratory should provide cumulative results of the in vitro susceptibility test results for antimicrobial drugs used in local hospitals and practice areas to the physician as periodic reports that describe the susceptibility profile of nosocomial and community-acquired pathogens. These reports should aid the physician in selecting the most effective antimicrobial.

Susceptibility Testing Techniques:
Dilution Techniques:
Quantitative methods can be used to determine the MIC of retapamulin that will inhibit the growth of the bacteria being tested. The MIC provides an estimate of the susceptibility of bacteria to retapamulin. The MIC should be determined using a standardized procedure.[1,2] Standardized procedures are based on a dilution method (broth or agar) or equivalent with standardized inoculum concentrations and standardized concentrations of retapamulin powder.

Diffusion Techniques:
Quantitative methods that require measurement of zone diameters also provide reproducible estimates of the susceptibility of bacteria to antimicrobial compounds. One such standardized procedure requires the use of standardized inoculum concentrations.[2,3] This procedure uses paper disks impregnated with 2 mcg of retapamulin to test the susceptibility of microorganisms to retapamulin.

Susceptibility Test Interpretive Criteria:
In vitro susceptibility test interpretive criteria for retapamulin have not been determined for this topical antimicrobial. The relation of the in vitro MIC and/or disk diffusion susceptibility test results to clinical efficacy of retapamulin against the bacteria tested should be monitored.

Quality Control Parameters for Susceptibility Testing:
In vitro susceptibility test quality control parameters were developed for retapamulin so that laboratories that test the susceptibility of bacterial isolates to retapamulin can determine if the susceptibility test is performing correctly. Standardized dilution techniques and diffusion methods require the use of laboratory control microorganisms to monitor the technical aspects of the laboratory procedures. Standard retapamulin powder should provide the following MIC and a 2 mcg retapamulin disk should produce the following zone diameters with the indicated quality control strains in Table 3.

Table 3. Acceptable Quality Control Ranges for Retapamulin

Microorganism	MIC Range (mcg/mL)	Disk Diffusion Zone Diameter (mm)
Staphylococcus aureus ATCC 29213	0.06-0.25	NA
Staphylococcus aureus ATCC 25923	NA	23-30
Streptococcus pneumoniae ATCC 49619	0.06-0.5[a]	13-19[b]

NA = Not applicable.
[a] This quality control range is applicable using cation-adjusted Mueller-Hinton broth with 2% to 5% lysed horse blood.
[b] This quality control limit is applicable using Mueller-Hinton agar with 5% sheep blood.

Table 4. Clinical Response at End of Therapy and at Follow-Up by Analysis Population

Analysis Population	ALTABAX		Placebo		Difference in Success Rates (%)	95% CI (%)
	n/N	Success Rate (%)	n/N	Success Rate (%)		
End of Therapy						
PPC	111/124	89.5	33/62	53.2	36.3	(22.8, 49.8)
ITTC	119/139	85.6	37/71	52.1	33.5	(20.5, 46.5)
PPB	96/107	89.7	26/52	50.0	39.7	(25.0, 54.5)
ITTB	101/114	88.6	28/57	49.1	39.5	(25.2, 53.7)
Follow-Up						
PPC	98/119	82.4	25/58	43.1	39.2	(24 8, 53.7)
ITTC	105/139	75.5	28/71	39.4	36.1	(22.7, 49.5)
PPB	86/102	84.3	18/48	37.5	46.8	(31.4, 62.2)
ITTB	91/114	79.8	19/57	33.3	46.5	(32.2, 60.8)

n = number with clinical success outcome, N = number in analysis population, PPC = Clinical Per Protocol Population, ITTC = Clinical Intent to Treat Population, PPB = Bacteriological Per Protocol Population, ITTB = Bacteriological Intent to Treat Population.

Table 5. Clinical Response at End of Therapy and Follow-Up for Subjects With Staphylococcus aureus and Streptococcus pyogenes at Baseline in the Per Protocol Bacteriological Population (PPB)

Pathogen	ALTABAX		Placebo	
	n/N	Success Rate (%)	n/N	Success Rate (%)
End of Therapy				
Staphylococcus aureus (Methicillin-susceptible)	79/88	89.8	25/48	52.1
Streptococcus pyogenes	29/32	90.6	3/7	42.9
Follow-Up				
Staphylococcus aureus (Methicillin-susceptible)	71/84	84.5	19/44	43.2
Streptococcus pyogenes	29/32	90.6	2/6	33.3

n/N = Number of clinical successes/number of pathogens isolated at baseline.

13 NONCLINICAL TOXICOLOGY
13.1 Carcinogenesis, Mutagenesis, Impairment of Fertility
Long-term studies in animals to evaluate carcinogenic potential have not been conducted with retapamulin.
Retapamulin showed no genotoxicity when evaluated in vitro for gene mutation and/or chromosomal effects in the mouse lymphoma cell assay, in cultured human peripheral blood lymphocytes, or when evaluated in vivo in a rat micronucleus test.
No evidence of impaired fertility was found in male or female rats given retapamulin 50, 150, or 450 mg/kg/day orally.

14 CLINICAL STUDIES
ALTABAX was evaluated in a placebo-controlled trial that enrolled adult and pediatric subjects aged 9 months and older for treatment of impetigo up to 100 cm² in total area (up to 10 lesions) or a total body surface area not exceeding 2%. The majority of subjects enrolled (164/210, 78%) were under the age of 13. The trial was a double-blind, randomized, multi-center, parallel-group comparison of the safety of ALTABAX and placebo ointment, both applied twice daily for 5 days. Patients were randomized to ALTABAX or placebo (2:1). Subjects with underlying skin disease (e.g., pre-existing eczematous dermatitis) or skin trauma, with clinical evidence of secondary infection were excluded from the trial. In addition, subjects with any systemic signs and symptoms of infection (such as fever) were excluded from the trial. Clinical success was defined as the absence of treated lesions, or treated lesions had become dry without crusts with or without erythema compared with baseline, or had improved (defined as a decline in the size of the affected area, number of lesions or both) such that no further antimicrobial therapy was required. The intent-to-treat clinical (ITTC) population consisted of all randomized subjects who took at least 1 dose of trial medication. The clinical per protocol (PPC) population included all ITTC subjects who satisfied the inclusion/exclusion criteria and subsequently adhered to the protocol. The intent-to-treat bacteriological (ITTB) population consisted of all randomized subjects who took at least 1 dose of trial medication and had a pathogen identified at trial entry. The bacteriological per protocol (PPB) population included all ITTB subjects who satisfied the inclusion/exclusion criteria and subsequently adhered to the protocol.
Table 4 presents the results for clinical response at end of therapy (2 days after treatment) and follow-up (9 days after treatment), by analysis population:
[See table 4 above]
Table 5 presents the clinical success at end of therapy and follow-up by baseline pathogen:
[See table 5 above]
Examination of age and gender subgroups did not identify differences in response to ALTABAX among these groups. The majority of subjects entered into this trial were classified as White/Caucasian or of Asian heritage; when response rates by racial subgroups were viewed across trials, differences in response to ALTABAX were not identified.

15 REFERENCES
1. Clinical and Laboratory Standards Institute (CLSI) Methods for Dilution Antimicrobial Susceptibility Tests for Bacteria that Grow Aerobically: Approved Standard-Eighth Edition. CLSI Document M07-A9, Vol. 32, No. 2. CLSI, Wayne, PA, Jan. 2012.
2. Clinical and Laboratory Standards Institute (CLSI). Performance Standards for Antimicrobial Susceptibility Testing: Nineteenth Informational Supplement. CLSI Document M100-S22. Vol. 32, No. 3. CLSI, Wayne, PA, Jan. 2012.

3. Clinical and Laboratory Standards Institute (CLSI). Performance Standards for Antimicrobial Disk Susceptibility Tests. Approved Standard-Tenth Edition. CLSI Document M02-A11, Vol. 32, No. 1. CLSI, Wayne, PA, Jan. 2012.

16 HOW SUPPLIED/STORAGE AND HANDLING

ALTABAX is supplied in 15-, and 30-gram tubes.
NDC 0007-5180-22 (15 gram tube)
NDC 0007-5180-25 (30 gram tube)
Store at 25°C (77°F) with excursions permitted to 15°-30°C (59°-86°F).

17 PATIENT COUNSELING INFORMATION

Patients using ALTABAX and/or their guardians should receive the following information and instructions:

- Use ALTABAX as directed by the healthcare practitioner. As with any topical medication, patients and caregivers should wash their hands after application if the hands are not the area for treatment.
- ALTABAX is for external use only. Do not swallow ALTABAX or use it in the eyes, on the mouth or lips, inside the nose, or inside the female genital area.
- The treated area may be covered by a sterile bandage or gauze dressing, if desired. This may also be helpful for infants and young children who accidentally touch or lick the lesion site. A bandage will protect the treated area and avoid accidental transfer of ointment to the eyes or other areas.
- Use the medication for the full time recommended by the healthcare practitioner, even though symptoms may have improved.
- Notify the healthcare practitioner if there is no improvement in symptoms within 3 to 4 days after starting use of ALTABAX.
- ALTABAX may cause reactions at the site of application of the ointment. Inform the healthcare practitioner if the area of application worsens in irritation, redness, itching, burning, swelling, blistering, or oozing.

ALTABAX is a registered trademark of GlaxoSmithKline.
GlaxoSmithKline
Research Triangle Park, NC 27709
©2013, GlaxoSmithKline. All rights reserved.
ALX:5PI

BACTROBAN CREAM®
(mupirocin calcium cream, 2%)
For Dermatologic Use

℞

DESCRIPTION

BACTROBAN CREAM (mupirocin calcium cream, 2%) contains the dihydrate crystalline calcium hemi-salt of the antibiotic mupirocin. Chemically, it is ($\alpha E,2S,3R,4R,5S$)-5-[(2S,3S,4S,5S)-2,3-Epoxy-5-hydroxy-4-methylhexyl]tetrahydro-3,4-dihydroxy-β-methyl-2H-pyran-2-crotonic acid, ester with 9-hydroxynonanoic acid, calcium salt (2:1), dihydrate.

The molecular formula of mupirocin calcium is ($C_{26}H_{43}O_9$)$_2$Ca•2H$_2$O, and the molecular weight is 1075.3. The molecular weight of mupirocin free acid is 500.6. The structural formula of mupirocin calcium is:

BACTROBAN CREAM is a white cream that contains 2.15% w/w mupirocin calcium (equivalent to 2.0% mupirocin free acid) in an oil and water-based emulsion. The inactive ingredients are benzyl alcohol, cetomacrogol 1000, cetyl alcohol, mineral oil, phenoxyethanol, purified water, stearyl alcohol, and xanthan gum.

CLINICAL PHARMACOLOGY
Pharmacokinetics

Systemic absorption of mupirocin through intact human skin is minimal. The systemic absorption of mupirocin was studied following application of BACTROBAN CREAM 3 times daily for 5 days to various skin lesions (>10 cm in length or 100 cm² in area) in 16 adults (aged 29 to 60 years) and 10 children (aged 3 to 12 years). Some systemic absorption was observed as evidenced by the detection of the metabolite, monic acid, in urine. Data from this study indicated more frequent occurrence of percutaneous absorption in children (90% of patients) compared to adults (44% of patients); however, the observed urinary concentrations in children (0.07 - 1.3 mcg/mL [1 pediatric patient had no detectable level]) are within the observed range (0.08 - 10.03 mcg/mL [9 adults had no detectable level]) in the adult population. In general, the degree of percutaneous absorption following multiple dosing appears to be minimal

in adults and children. Any mupirocin reaching the systemic circulation is rapidly metabolized, predominantly to inactive monic acid, which is eliminated by renal excretion.

Microbiology

Mupirocin is an antibacterial agent produced by fermentation using the organism *Pseudomonas fluorescens*. It is active against a wide range of gram-positive bacteria including methicillin-resistant *Staphylococcus aureus* (MRSA). It is also active against certain gram-negative bacteria. Mupirocin inhibits bacterial protein synthesis by reversibly and specifically binding to bacterial isoleucyl transfer-RNA synthetase. Due to this unique mode of action, mupirocin demonstrates no in vitro cross-resistance with other classes of antimicrobial agents.

Resistance occurs rarely; however, when mupirocin resistance does occur, it appears to result from the production of a modified isoleucyl-tRNA synthetase. High-level plasmid-mediated resistance (MIC >1024 mcg/mL) has been reported in some strains of *Staphylococcus aureus* and coagulase-negative staphylococci.

Mupirocin is bactericidal at concentrations achieved by topical application. The minimum bactericidal concentration (MBC) against relevant pathogens is generally 8-fold to 30-fold higher than the minimum inhibitory concentration (MIC). In addition, mupirocin is highly protein bound (>97%), and the effect of wound secretions on the MICs of mupirocin has not been determined.

Mupirocin has been shown to be active against most strains of *S. aureus* and *Streptococcus pyogenes*, both in vitro and in clinical studies. (See INDICATIONS AND USAGE.) The following in vitro data are available, BUT THEIR CLINICAL SIGNIFICANCE IS UNKNOWN. Mupirocin is active against most strains of *Staphylococcus epidermidis* and *Staphylococcus saprophyticus*.

INDICATIONS AND USAGE

BACTROBAN CREAM is indicated for the treatment of secondarily infected traumatic skin lesions (up to 10 cm in length or 100 cm² in area) due to susceptible strains of *S. aureus* and *S. pyogenes*.

CONTRAINDICATIONS

BACTROBAN CREAM is contraindicated in patients with known hypersensitivity to any of the constituents of the product.

WARNINGS

Avoid contact with the eyes.
In the event of a sensitization or severe local irritation from BACTROBAN CREAM, usage should be discontinued, and appropriate alternative therapy for the infection instituted.

PRECAUTIONS
General

As with other antibacterial products, prolonged use may result in overgrowth of nonsusceptible microorganisms, including fungi. (See DOSAGE AND ADMINISTRATION.) BACTROBAN CREAM is not formulated for use on mucosal surfaces.

Information for Patients

- Use this medication only as directed by your healthcare provider. It is for external use only. Avoid contact with the eyes.
- The treated area may be covered by gauze dressing if desired.
- Report to your healthcare provider any signs of local adverse reactions. The medication should be stopped and your healthcare provider contacted if irritation, severe itching, or rash occurs.
- If no improvement is seen in 3 to 5 days, contact your healthcare provider.

Drug Interactions

The effect of the concurrent application of topical mupirocin calcium cream and other topical products has not been studied.

Carcinogenesis, Mutagenesis, Impairment of Fertility

Long-term studies in animals to evaluate carcinogenic potential of mupirocin calcium have not been conducted. Results of the following studies performed with mupirocin calcium or mupirocin sodium in vitro and in vivo did not indicate a potential for mutagenicity: Rat primary hepatocyte unscheduled DNA synthesis, sediment analysis for DNA strand breaks, *Salmonella* reversion test (Ames), *Escherichia coli* mutation assay, metaphase analysis of human lymphocytes, mouse lymphoma assay, and bone marrow micronuclei assay in mice.

Fertility studies were performed in rats with mupirocin administered subcutaneously at doses up to 49 times a human topical dose of 1 gram/day (approximately 20 mg mupirocin per day) on a mg/m² basis and revealed no evidence of impaired fertility from mupirocin sodium.

Pregnancy

Teratogenic Effects: Pregnancy Category B. Teratology studies have been performed in rats and rabbits with mupirocin administered subcutaneously at doses up to 78

and 154 times, respectively, a human topical dose of 1 gram/day (approximately 20 mg mupirocin per day) on a mg/m² basis and revealed no evidence of harm to the fetus due to mupirocin. There are, however, no adequate and well-controlled studies in pregnant women. Because animal reproduction studies are not always predictive of human response, this drug should be used during pregnancy only if clearly needed.

Nursing Mothers

It is not known whether this drug is excreted in human milk. Because many drugs are excreted in human milk, caution should be exercised when BACTROBAN CREAM is administered to a nursing woman.

Pediatric Use

The safety and effectiveness of BACTROBAN CREAM have been established in the age groups 3 months to 16 years. Use of BACTROBAN CREAM in these age groups is supported by evidence from adequate and well-controlled studies of BACTROBAN CREAM in adults with additional data from 93 pediatric patients studied as part of the pivotal trials in adults. (See CLINICAL STUDIES.)

Geriatric Use

In 2 well-controlled studies, 30 patients older than 65 years were treated with BACTROBAN CREAM. No overall difference in the efficacy or safety of BACTROBAN CREAM was observed in this patient population when compared to that observed in younger patients.

ADVERSE REACTIONS

In 2 randomized, double-blind, double-dummy trials, 339 patients were treated with topical BACTROBAN CREAM plus oral placebo. Adverse events thought to be possibly or probably drug-related occurred in 28 (8.3%) patients. The incidence of those events that were reported in at least 1% of patients enrolled in these trials were: Headache (1.7%), rash, and nausea (1.1% each).

Other adverse events thought to be possibly or probably drug-related which occurred in less than 1% of patients were: Abdominal pain, burning at application site, cellulitis, dermatitis, dizziness, pruritus, secondary wound infection, and ulcerative stomatitis.

In a supportive study in the treatment of secondarily infected eczema, 82 patients were treated with BACTROBAN CREAM. The incidence of adverse events thought to be possibly or probably drug-related was as follows: Nausea (4.9%), headache, and burning at application site (3.6% each), pruritus (2.4%) and 1 report each of abdominal pain, bleeding secondary to eczema, pain secondary to eczema, hives, dry skin, and rash.

OVERDOSAGE

Intravenous infusions of 252 mg, as well as single oral doses of 500 mg of mupirocin, have been well tolerated in healthy adult subjects. There is no information regarding overdose of BACTROBAN CREAM.

DOSAGE AND ADMINISTRATION

A small amount of BACTROBAN CREAM should be applied to the affected area 3 times daily for 10 days. The area treated may be covered with gauze dressing if desired. Patients not showing a clinical response within 3 to 5 days should be re-evaluated.

CLINICAL STUDIES

The efficacy of topical BACTROBAN CREAM for the treatment of secondarily infected traumatic skin lesions (e.g., lacerations, sutured wounds, and abrasions not more than 10 cm in length or 100 cm² in total area) was compared to that of oral cephalexin in 2 randomized, double-blind, double-dummy clinical trials. Clinical efficacy rates at follow-up in the per protocol populations (adults and pediatric patients included) were 96.1% for BACTROBAN CREAM (n = 231) and 93.1% for oral cephalexin (n = 219). Pathogen eradication rates at follow-up in the per protocol populations were 100% for both BACTROBAN CREAM and oral cephalexin.

Pediatrics: There were 93 pediatric patients aged 2 weeks to 16 years enrolled per protocol in the secondarily infected skin lesion studies, although only 3 were less than 2 years of age in the population treated with BACTROBAN CREAM. Patients were randomized to either 10 days of topical BACTROBAN CREAM 3 times daily or 10 days of oral cephalexin (250 mg 4 times daily for patients >40 kg or 25 mg/kg/day oral suspension in 4 divided doses for patients ≤40 kg). Clinical efficacy at follow-up (7 to 12 days posttherapy) in the per protocol populations was 97.7% (43/44) for BACTROBAN CREAM and 93.9% (46/49) for cephalexin. Only 1 adverse event (headache) was thought to be possibly or probably related to drug therapy with BACTROBAN CREAM in the intent-to-treat pediatric population of 70 children (1.4%).

HOW SUPPLIED

BACTROBAN CREAM is supplied in 15-gram and 30-gram tubes.
NDC 0029-1527-22 (15-gram tube)
NDC 0029-1527-25 (30-gram tube)
Store at or below 25°C (77°F). Do not freeze.
GlaxoSmithKline
Research Triangle Park, NC 27709
BACTROBAN CREAM is a registered trademark of GlaxoSmithKline.
©2005, GlaxoSmithKline. All rights reserved.
May 2005 BB:L7B

BACTROBAN NASAL®
(mupirocin calcium ointment, 2%)
for intranasal use only

℞

DESCRIPTION

BACTROBAN NASAL (mupirocin calcium ointment, 2%) contains the dihydrate crystalline calcium hemi-salt of the antibiotic mupirocin. Chemically, it is $(\alpha E, 2S, 3R, 4R, 5S)$-5-[(2S,3S,4S,5S)-2,3-Epoxy-5-hydroxy-4-methylhexyl]tetrahydro-3,4-dihydroxy-β-methyl-2H-pyran-2-crotonic acid, ester with 9-hydroxynonanoic acid, calcium salt (2:1), dihydrate.
The molecular formula of mupirocin calcium is $(C_{26}H_{43}O_9)_2Ca \cdot 2H_2O$, and the molecular weight is 1075.3. The molecular weight of mupirocin free acid is 500.6. The structural formula of mupirocin calcium is:

BACTROBAN NASAL is a white to off-white ointment that contains 2.15% w/w mupirocin calcium (equivalent to 2.0% pure mupirocin free acid) in a soft white ointment base. The inactive ingredients are paraffin and a mixture of glycerin esters (SOFTISAN® 649).

CLINICAL PHARMACOLOGY

Pharmacokinetics

Following single or repeated intranasal applications of 0.2 gram of BACTROBAN NASAL 3 times daily for 3 days to 5 healthy adult male subjects, no evidence of systemic absorption of mupirocin was demonstrated. The dosage regimen used in this study was for pharmacokinetic characterization only. (See DOSAGE AND ADMINISTRATION for proper clinical dosing information.)
In this study, the concentrations of mupirocin in urine and of monic acid in urine and serum were below the limit of determination of the assay for up to 72 hours after the applications. The lowest levels of determination of the assay used were 50 ng/mL of mupirocin in urine, 75 ng/mL of monic acid in urine, and 10 ng/mL of monic acid in serum. Based on the detectable limit of the urine assay for monic acid, one can extrapolate that a mean of 3.3% (range: 1.2 to 5.1%) of the applied dose could be systemically absorbed from the nasal mucosa of **adults**.
Data from a report of a pharmacokinetic study in neonates and premature infants indicate that, unlike in adults, significant systemic absorption occurred following intranasal administration of BACTROBAN NASAL in this population. **At this time, the pharmacokinetic properties of mupirocin following intranasal application of BACTROBAN NASAL have not been adequately characterized in neonates or other children less than 12 years of age, and in addition, the safety of the product in children less than 12 years of age has not been established.**
The effect of the concurrent application of intranasal mupirocin calcium ointment, 2% with other intranasal products has not been studied. (See PRECAUTIONS, Drug Interactions.)
Following intravenous or oral administration, mupirocin is rapidly metabolized. The principal metabolite, monic acid, demonstrates no antibacterial activity. In a study conducted in 7 healthy adult male subjects, the elimination half-life after intravenous administration of mupirocin was 20 to 40 minutes for mupirocin and 30 to 80 minutes for monic acid. Monic acid is predominantly eliminated by renal excretion. The pharmacokinetics of mupirocin has not been studied in individuals with renal insufficiency.

Microbiology

Mupirocin is an antibacterial agent produced by fermentation using the organism Pseudomonas fluorescens. Mupirocin inhibits bacterial protein synthesis by reversibly and specifically binding to bacterial isoleucyl transfer-RNA synthetase. Due to this mode of action, mupirocin demonstrates no in vitro cross-resistance with other classes of antimicrobial agents.
When mupirocin resistance does occur, it appears to result from the production of a modified isoleucyl-tRNA synthetase. High-level plasmid-mediated resistance (MIC >1,024 mcg/mL) has been reported in some strains of Staphylococcus aureus and coagulase-negative staphylococci.
Mupirocin is bactericidal at concentrations achieved topically by intranasal administration. However, the minimum bactericidal concentration (MBC) against relevant intranasal pathogens is generally 8-fold to 30-fold higher than the minimum inhibitory concentration (MIC). In addition, mupirocin is highly protein bound (>97%), and the effect of nasal secretions on the MICs of intranasally applied mupirocin has not been determined.
Mupirocin has been shown to be active against most strains of methicillin-resistant S. aureus, both in vitro and in clinical studies of the eradication of nasal colonization. BACTROBAN NASAL only has established clinical utility in nasal eradication as part of a comprehensive program to curtail institutional outbreaks of infections with methicillin-resistant S. aureus. (See INDICATIONS AND USAGE.)
The following in vitro data are available, **but their clinical significance is unknown.** Mupirocin exhibits in vitro MICs of 1 mcg/mL or less against most (>90%) strains of methicillin-susceptible S. aureus; however, the safety and effectiveness of mupirocin calcium in eradicating nasal colonization of and preventing subsequent infections due to methicillin-susceptible S. aureus have not been established.

INDICATIONS AND USAGE

BACTROBAN NASAL is indicated for the eradication of nasal colonization with methicillin-resistant S. aureus in adult patients and health care workers as part of a comprehensive infection control program to reduce the risk of infection among patients at high risk of methicillin-resistant S. aureus infection during institutional outbreaks of infections with this pathogen.

NOTE:

1. There are insufficient data at this time to establish that this product is safe and effective as part of an intervention program to prevent autoinfection of high-risk patients from their own nasal colonization with S. aureus.
2. There are insufficient data at this time to recommend use of BACTROBAN NASAL for general prophylaxis of any infection in any patient population.
3. Greater than 90% of subjects/patients in clinical trials had eradication of nasal colonization 2 to 4 days after therapy was completed. Approximately 30% recolonization was reported in 1 domestic study within 4 weeks after completion of therapy. These eradication rates were clinically and statistically superior to those reported in subjects/patients in the vehicle-treated arms of the adequate and well-controlled studies. Those treated with vehicle had eradication rates of 5% to 30% at 2 to 4 days post-therapy with 85% to 100% recolonization within 4 weeks.

All adequate and well-controlled trials of this product were vehicle-controlled; therefore, no data from direct, head-to-head comparisons with other products are available at this time.

CONTRAINDICATIONS

BACTROBAN NASAL is contraindicated in patients with known hypersensitivity to any of the constituents of the product.

WARNINGS

AVOID CONTACT WITH THE EYES. Application of BACTROBAN NASAL to the eye under testing conditions has caused severe symptoms such as burning and tearing. These symptoms resolved within days to weeks after discontinuation of the ointment.
In the event of a sensitization or severe local irritation from BACTROBAN NASAL, usage should be discontinued.

PRECAUTIONS

General

As with other antibacterial products, prolonged use may result in overgrowth of nonsusceptible microorganisms, including fungi. (See DOSAGE AND ADMINISTRATION.)

Information for Patients

Patients should be given the following instructions:
• Apply approximately one-half of the ointment from the single-use tube directly into 1 nostril and the other half into the other nostril;
• Avoid contact of the medication with the eyes;
• Discard the tube after using, do not re-use;
• Press the sides of the nose together and gently massage after application to spread the ointment throughout the inside of the nostrils; and
• Discontinue usage of the medication and call your healthcare practitioner if sensitization or severe local irritation occurs.

Drug Interactions

The effect of the concurrent application of intranasal mupirocin calcium and other intranasal products has not been studied. Until further information is known, mupirocin calcium ointment, 2% should not be applied concurrently with any other intranasal products.

Carcinogenesis, Mutagenesis, Impairment of Fertility

Long-term studies in animals to evaluate carcinogenic potential of mupirocin calcium have not been conducted. Results of the following studies performed with mupirocin calcium or mupirocin sodium in vitro and in vivo did not indicate a potential for mutagenicity: Rat primary hepatocyte unscheduled DNA synthesis, sediment analysis for DNA strand breaks, Salmonella reversion test (Ames), Escherichia coli mutation assay, metaphase analysis of human lymphocytes, mouse lymphoma assay, and bone marrow micronuclei assay in mice.
Reproduction studies were performed in rats with mupirocin administered subcutaneously at doses up to **40** times the human intranasal dose (approximately 20 mg mupirocin per day) on a mg/m² basis and revealed no evidence of impaired fertility from mupirocin sodium.

Pregnancy

Teratogenic Effects: Pregnancy Category B
Reproduction studies have been performed in rats and rabbits with mupirocin administered subcutaneously at doses up to 65 and 130 times, respectively, the human intranasal dose (approximately 20 mg mupirocin per day) on a mg/m2 basis and revealed no evidence of harm to the fetus due to mupirocin. There are, however, no adequate and well-controlled studies in pregnant women. Because animal reproduction studies are not always predictive of human response, this drug should be used during pregnancy only if clearly needed.

Nursing Mothers

It is not known whether this drug is excreted in human milk. Because many drugs are excreted in human milk, caution should be exercised when BACTROBAN NASAL is administered to a nursing woman.

Pediatric Use

Safety in children under the age of 12 years has not been established. (See CLINICAL PHARMACOLOGY.)

ADVERSE REACTIONS

Clinical Trials

In clinical trials, 210 domestic and 2,130 foreign adult subjects/patients received BACTROBAN NASAL ointment. Less than 1% of domestic or foreign subjects and patients in clinical trials were withdrawn due to adverse events.
The most frequently reported adverse events in foreign clinical trials were as follows: Rhinitis (1.0%), taste perversion (0.8%), pharyngitis (0.5%).
In domestic clinical trials, 17% (36/210) of adults treated with BACTROBAN NASAL ointment reported adverse events thought to be at least possibly drug-related. The incidence of adverse events that were reported in at least 1% of adults enrolled in domestic clinical trials were as follows:

ADVERSE EVENTS (≥1% INCIDENCE)-ADULTS IN US TRIALS

	% of Subjects/Patients Experiencing Event BACTROBAN NASAL (n=210)
Headache	9%
Rhinitis	6%
Respiratory disorder, including upper respiratory tract congestion	5%
Pharyngitis	4%
Taste perversion	3%
Burning/stinging	2%
Cough	2%
Pruritus	1%

The following events thought possibly drug-related were reported in less than 1% of adults enrolled in domestic clinical trials: Blepharitis, diarrhea, dry mouth, ear pain, epistaxis, nausea, and rash.
All adequate and well-controlled clinical trials have been performed using BACTROBAN NASAL ointment, 2% in 1 arm and the vehicle ointment in the other arm of the study. No adequate and well-controlled safety data are available from direct, head-to-head comparative studies of this product and other products for this indication.

OVERDOSAGE

Following single or repeated intranasal applications of BACTROBAN NASAL to adults, no evidence for systemic absorption of mupirocin was obtained. Intravenous infusions of 252 mg, as well as single oral doses of 500 mg of mupirocin, have been well tolerated in healthy adult subjects. There is no information regarding local overdose of BACTROBAN NASAL or regarding oral ingestion of the nasal ointment formulation.

DOSAGE AND ADMINISTRATION

(See INDICATIONS AND USAGE.)

Adults (12 years of age and older): Approximately one-half of the ointment from the single-use tube should be applied into 1 nostril and the other half into the other nostril twice daily (morning and evening) for 5 days.

After application, the nostrils should be closed by pressing together and releasing the sides of the nose repetitively for approximately 1 minute. This will spread the ointment throughout the nares.

The single-use 1.0 gram tube will deliver a total of approximately 0.5 grams of the ointment (approximately 0.25 grams/nostril).

The tube should be discarded after usage; it should not be re-used.

The safety and effectiveness of applications of this medication for greater than 5 days have not been established. There are no human clinical or pre-clinical animal data to support the use of this product in a chronic manner or in manners other than those described in this package insert. Until further information is known, BACTROBAN NASAL should not be applied concurrently with any other intranasal products.

HOW SUPPLIED

BACTROBAN NASAL is supplied in 1.0-gram tubes.
NDC 0029-1526-11 (package of 10 single-tube cartons).
Store between 20° and 25°C (68° and 77°F); excursions permitted to 15°-30°C (59°-86°F). Do not refrigerate.

REFERENCE

1. Clinical and Laboratory Standards Institute (CLSI). Methods for Dilution Antimicrobial Susceptibility Tests for Bacteria That Grow Aerobically. Approved Standard. CLSI Document M7-A7. CLSI, Wayne, PA, January 2006.
BACTROBAN NASAL is a registered trademark of GlaxoSmithKline.
SOFTISAN is a registered trademark of Sasol Olefins & Surfactants GmbH.
GlaxoSmithKline
Research Triangle Park, NC 27709
©2009, GlaxoSmithKline. All rights reserved.
April 2009
BBN:2PI

BACTROBAN OINTMENT®   ℞
(mupirocin ointment, 2%)
For Dermatologic Use

DESCRIPTION

Each gram of BACTROBAN OINTMENT (mupirocin ointment, 2%) contains 20 mg mupirocin in a bland water miscible ointment base (polyethylene glycol ointment, N.F.) consisting of polyethylene glycol 400 and polyethylene glycol 3350. Mupirocin is a naturally occurring antibiotic. The chemical name is (E)-$(2S,3R,4R,5S)$-5-[$(2S,3S,4S,5S)$-2,3-Epoxy-5-hydroxy-4-methylhexyl]tetrahydro-3,4-dihydroxy-β-methyl-$2H$-pyran-2-crotonic acid, ester with 9-hydroxynonanoic acid. The molecular formula of mupirocin is $C_{26}H_{44}O_9$, and the molecular weight is 500.63. The chemical structure is:

CLINICAL PHARMACOLOGY

Application of ^{14}C-labeled mupirocin ointment to the lower arm of normal male subjects followed by occlusion for 24 hours showed no measurable systemic absorption (<1.1 nanogram mupirocin per milliliter of whole blood). Measurable radioactivity was present in the stratum corneum of these subjects 72 hours after application.

Following intravenous or oral administration, mupirocin is rapidly metabolized. The principal metabolite, monic acid, is eliminated by renal excretion, and demonstrates no antibacterial activity. In a study conducted in 7 healthy adult male subjects, the elimination half-life after intravenous administration of mupirocin was 20 to 40 minutes for mupirocin and 30 to 80 minutes for monic acid. The pharmacokinetics of mupirocin has not been studied in individuals with renal insufficiency.

Microbiology

Mupirocin is an antibacterial agent produced by fermentation using the organism *Pseudomonas fluorescens*. It is active against a wide range of gram-positive bacteria including methicillin-resistant *Staphylococcus aureus* (MRSA). It is also active against certain gram-negative bacteria. Mupirocin inhibits bacterial protein synthesis by reversibly and specifically binding to bacterial isoleucyl transfer-RNA synthetase. Due to this unique mode of action, mupirocin demonstrates no in vitro cross-resistance with other classes of antimicrobial agents.

Resistance occurs rarely. However, when mupirocin resistance does occur, it appears to result from the production of a modified isoleucyl-tRNA synthetase. High-level plasmid-mediated resistance (MIC >1024 mcg/mL) has been reported in some strains of *S. aureus* and coagulase-negative staphylococci.

Mupirocin is bactericidal at concentrations achieved by topical administration. However, the minimum bactericidal concentration (MBC) against relevant pathogens is generally 8-fold to 30-fold higher than the minimum inhibitory concentration (MIC). In addition, mupirocin is highly protein-bound (>97%), and the effect of wound secretions on the MICs of mupirocin has not been determined.

Mupirocin has been shown to be active against most strains of *S. aureus* and *Streptococcus pyogenes*, both in vitro and in clinical studies (see INDICATIONS AND USAGE). The following in vitro data are available, BUT THEIR CLINICAL SIGNIFICANCE IS UNKNOWN. Mupirocin is active against most strains of *Staphylococcus epidermidis* and *Staphylococcus saprophyticus*.

INDICATIONS AND USAGE

BACTROBAN OINTMENT is indicated for the topical treatment of impetigo due to: *S. aureus* and *S. pyogenes*.

CONTRAINDICATIONS

This drug is contraindicated in individuals with a history of sensitivity reactions to any of its components.

WARNINGS

BACTROBAN OINTMENT is not for ophthalmic use.

PRECAUTIONS

If a reaction suggesting sensitivity or chemical irritation should occur with the use of BACTROBAN OINTMENT, treatment should be discontinued and appropriate alternative therapy for the infection instituted.

As with other antibacterial products, prolonged use may result in overgrowth of nonsusceptible organisms, including fungi.

BACTROBAN OINTMENT is not formulated for use on mucosal surfaces. Intranasal use has been associated with isolated reports of stinging and drying. A paraffin-based formulation — BACTROBAN NASAL® (mupirocin calcium ointment)— is available for intranasal use.

Polyethylene glycol can be absorbed from open wounds and damaged skin and is excreted by the kidneys. In common with other polyethylene glycol-based ointments, BACTROBAN OINTMENT should not be used in conditions where absorption of large quantities of polyethylene glycol is possible, especially if there is evidence of moderate or severe renal impairment.

Information for Patients

Use this medication only as directed by your healthcare provider. It is for external use only. Avoid contact with the eyes. The medication should be stopped and your healthcare practitioner contacted if irritation, severe itching, or rash occurs.

If impetigo has not improved in 3 to 5 days, contact your healthcare practitioner.

Drug Interactions

The effect of the concurrent application of BACTROBAN OINTMENT and other drug products has not been studied.

Carcinogenesis, Mutagenesis, Impairment of Fertility

Long-term studies in animals to evaluate carcinogenic potential of mupirocin have not been conducted.

Results of the following studies performed with mupirocin calcium or mupirocin sodium in vitro and in vivo did not indicate a potential for genotoxicity: Rat primary hepatocyte unscheduled DNA synthesis, sediment analysis for DNA strand breaks, *Salmonella* reversion test (Ames), *Escherichia coli* mutation assay, metaphase analysis of human lymphocytes, mouse lymphoma assay, and bone marrow micronuclei assay in mice.

Reproduction studies were performed in male and female rats with mupirocin administered subcutaneously at doses up to 14 times a human topical dose (approximately 60 mg mupirocin per day) on a mg/m^2 basis and revealed no evidence of impaired fertility and reproductive performance from mupirocin.

Pregnancy

Teratogenic Effects

Reproduction studies have been performed in rats and rabbits with mupirocin administered subcutaneously at doses up to 22 and 43 times, respectively, the human topical dose (approximately 60 mg mupirocin per day) on a mg/m^2 basis and revealed no evidence of harm to the fetus due to mupirocin. There are, however, no adequate and well-controlled studies in pregnant women. Because animal studies are not always predictive of human response, this drug should be used during pregnancy only if clearly needed.

Nursing Mothers

It is not known whether this drug is excreted in human milk. Because many drugs are excreted in human milk, caution should be exercised when BACTROBAN OINTMENT is administered to a nursing woman.

Pediatric Use

The safety and effectiveness of BACTROBAN OINTMENT have been established in the age range of 2 months to 16 years. Use of BACTROBAN OINTMENT in these age groups is supported by evidence from adequate and well-controlled studies of BACTROBAN OINTMENT in impetigo in pediatric patients studied as a part of the pivotal clinical trials (see CLINICAL STUDIES).

ADVERSE REACTIONS

The following local adverse reactions have been reported in connection with the use of BACTROBAN OINTMENT: Burning, stinging, or pain in 1.5% of patients; itching in 1% of patients; rash, nausea, erythema, dry skin, tenderness, swelling, contact dermatitis, and increased exudate in less than 1% of patients. Systemic reactions to BACTROBAN OINTMENT have occurred rarely.

DOSAGE AND ADMINISTRATION

A small amount of BACTROBAN OINTMENT should be applied to the affected area 3 times daily. The area treated may be covered with a gauze dressing if desired. Patients not showing a clinical response within 3 to 5 days should be re-evaluated.

CLINICAL STUDIES

The efficacy of topical BACTROBAN OINTMENT in impetigo was tested in 2 studies. In the first, patients with impetigo were randomized to receive either BACTROBAN OINTMENT or vehicle placebo 3 times daily for 8 to 12 days. Clinical efficacy rates at end of therapy in the evaluable populations (adults and pediatric patients included) were 71% for BACTROBAN OINTMENT (n = 49) and 35% for vehicle placebo (n = 51). Pathogen eradication rates in the evaluable populations were 94% for BACTROBAN OINTMENT and 62% for vehicle placebo. There were no side effects reported in the group receiving BACTROBAN OINTMENT.

In the second study, patients with impetigo were randomized to receive either BACTROBAN OINTMENT 3 times daily or 30 to 40 mg/kg oral erythromycin ethylsuccinate per day (this was an unblinded study) for 8 days. There was a follow-up visit 1 week after treatment ended. Clinical efficacy rates at the follow-up visit in the evaluable populations (adults and pediatric patients included) were 93% for BACTROBAN OINTMENT (n = 29) and 78.5% for erythromycin (n = 28). Pathogen eradication rates in the evaluable patient populations were 100% for both test groups. There were no side effects reported in the group receiving BACTROBAN OINTMENT.

Pediatrics

There were 91 pediatric patients aged 2 months to 15 years in the first study described above. Clinical efficacy rates at end of therapy in the evaluable populations were 78% for BACTROBAN OINTMENT (n = 42) and 36% for vehicle placebo (n = 49). In the second study described above, all patients were pediatric except 2 adults in the group receiving BACTROBAN OINTMENT. The age range of the pediatric patients was 7 months to 13 years. The clinical efficacy rate for BACTROBAN OINTMENT (n = 27) was 96%, and for erythromycin it was unchanged (78.5%).

HOW SUPPLIED

BACTROBAN OINTMENT is supplied in 22-gram tubes.
NDC 0029-1525-44 (22-gram tube)
Store at controlled room temperature 20° to 25°C (68° to 77°F).
GlaxoSmithKline
Research Triangle Park, NC 27709
BACTROBAN OINTMENT and BACTROBAN NASAL are registered trademarks of GlaxoSmithKline.
©2005, GlaxoSmithKline. All rights reserved.
MAY 2005 BC:L13C

DUAC®   ℞
[dū-ăk]
(clindamycin phosphate and benzoyl peroxide)
Gel, 1.2%/5%
for topical use

HIGHLIGHTS OF PRESCRIBING INFORMATION

These highlights do not include all the information needed to use DUAC Gel safely and effectively. See full prescribing information for DUAC Gel.

DUAC (clindamycin phosphate and benzoyl peroxide) Gel, 1.2%/5%
for topical use
Initial U.S. Approval: 2000

INDICATIONS AND USAGE

DUAC Gel is a combination of clindamycin phosphate (a lincosamide antibacterial) and benzoyl peroxide indicated for the topical treatment of inflammatory acne vulgaris. (1.1)
Limitation of Use:
DUAC Gel has not been demonstrated to have any additional benefit when compared with benzoyl peroxide alone in the same vehicle when used for the treatment of non-inflammatory acne. (1.2)

DOSAGE AND ADMINISTRATION

- Apply a thin layer of DUAC Gel to the face once daily, in the evening. (2)
- Not for oral, ophthalmic, or intravaginal use. (2)

DOSAGE FORMS AND STRENGTHS

Gel, 1.2%/5%: Each gram of DUAC Gel contains 12 mg clindamycin phosphate (equivalent to 10 mg of clindamycin) and 50 mg benzoyl peroxide. (3)

CONTRAINDICATIONS

DUAC Gel is contraindicated in:
- Patients who have a demonstrated hypersensitivity (e.g., anaphylaxis) to clindamycin, benzoyl peroxide, any components of the formulation, or lincomycin. (4)
- Patients with a history of regional enteritis, ulcerative colitis, or antibiotic-associated colitis (including pseudomembranous colitis). (4)

WARNINGS AND PRECAUTIONS

- Colitis: Clindamycin can cause severe colitis, which may result in death. Diarrhea, bloody diarrhea, and colitis (including pseudomembranous colitis) have been reported with the use of clindamycin. DUAC Gel should be discontinued if significant diarrhea occurs. (5.1)
- Ultraviolet light and environmental exposure (including use of tanning beds or sun lamps): Minimize sun exposure following drug application. (5.2)

ADVERSE REACTIONS

- The most common local adverse reactions (≥5%) are erythema, peeling, dryness and burning. (6.1)

To report SUSPECTED ADVERSE REACTIONS, contact Stiefel Laboratories, Inc. at 1-888-784-3335 or FDA at 1-800-FDA-1088 or www.fda.gov/medwatch.

DRUG INTERACTIONS

- DUAC Gel should not be used in combination with erythromycin-containing products because of its clindamycin component. (7.1)

See 17 for PATIENT COUNSELING INFORMATION and FDA-approved patient labeling

Revised: 01/2014

FULL PRESCRIBING INFORMATION: CONTENTS*

* Sections or subsections omitted from the full prescribing information are not listed

Table 1: Local Skin Reactions With Use of DUAC Gel Combined Results From Five Trials (n = 397

| | % of Subjects Using DUAC Gel With Symptom Present | | | | | |
| Symptom | Before Treatment (Baseline) | | | During Treatment | | |
	Mild	Moderate	Severe	Mild	Moderate	Severe
Erythema	28%	3%	0	26%	5%	0
Peeling	6%	<1%	0	17%	2%	0
Burning	3%	<1%	0	5%	<1%	0
Dryness	6%	<1%	0	15%	1%	0

FULL PRESCRIBING INFORMATION

1 INDICATIONS AND USAGE

1.1 Indication

DUAC® (clindamycin phosphate and benzoyl peroxide) Gel, 1.2%/5% is indicated for the topical treatment of inflammatory acne vulgaris in patients 12 years and older.

1.2 Limitations of Use

DUAC Gel has not been demonstrated to have any additional benefit when compared with benzoyl peroxide alone in the same vehicle when used for the treatment of noninflammatory acne.

2 DOSAGE AND ADMINISTRATION

Apply a thin layer of DUAC Gel to the face once daily, in the evening or as directed by the physician. The skin should be gently washed, rinsed with warm water, and patted dry before applying DUAC Gel. Avoid the eyes, mouth, lips, mucous membranes, or areas of broken skin.
DUAC Gel is not for oral, ophthalmic, or intravaginal use.

3 DOSAGE FORMS AND STRENGTHS

Gel, 1.2%/5%
DUAC Gel is a white to slightly yellow, opaque gel. Each gram of DUAC Gel contains 12 mg clindamycin phosphate (equivalent to 10 mg of clindamycin) and 50 mg benzoyl peroxide.

4 CONTRAINDICATIONS

4.1 Hypersensitivity

DUAC Gel is contraindicated in those individuals who have shown hypersensitivity to clindamycin, benzoyl peroxide, any components of the formulation, or lincomycin. Anaphylaxis, as well as allergic reactions leading to hospitalization, has been reported in postmarketing use with DUAC Gel. [See Postmarketing Experience (6.2).]

4.2 Colitis/Enteritis

DUAC Gel is contraindicated in those individuals with a history of regional enteritis, ulcerative colitis, pseudomembranous colitis, or antibiotic-associated colitis. [see Warnings and Precautions (5.1)].

5 WARNINGS AND PRECAUTIONS

5.1 Colitis

Systemic absorption of clindamycin has been demonstrated following topical use of clindamycin. Diarrhea, bloody diarrhea, and colitis (including pseudomembranous colitis) have been reported with the use of topical and systemic clindamycin. If significant diarrhea occurs, DUAC Gel should be discontinued.
Severe colitis has occurred following oral and parenteral administration of clindamycin with an onset of up to several weeks following cessation of therapy. Antiperistaltic agents such as opiates and diphenoxylate with atropine may prolong and/or worsen severe colitis. Severe colitis may result in death.
Studies indicate a toxin(s) produced by Clostridia is one primary cause of antibiotic-associated colitis. The colitis is usually characterized by severe persistent diarrhea and severe abdominal cramps and may be associated with the passage of blood and mucus. Stool cultures for *Clostridium difficile* and stool assay for *C. difficile* toxin may be helpful diagnostically.

5.2 Ultraviolet Light and Environmental Exposure

Benzoyl peroxide, a component of DUAC Gel, may cause increased sensitivity to sunlight. Minimize sun exposure (including use of tanning beds or sun lamps) following drug application. [See Nonclinical Toxicology (13.1).] Patients who may be required to have considerable sun exposure due to occupation and those with inherent sensitivity to the sun should exercise particular caution.

6 ADVERSE REACTIONS

The following adverse reaction is described in more detail in the *Warnings and Precautions* section of the label:
- Colitis [see Warnings and Precautions (5.1)].

6.1 Clinical Trials Experience

Because clinical trials are conducted under widely varying conditions, adverse reaction rates observed in the clinical trials of a drug cannot be directly compared with rates in the clinical trials of another drug and may not reflect the rates observed in practice.
During clinical trials, 397 subjects used DUAC Gel once daily for 11 weeks for the treatment of moderate to moderately severe facial acne vulgaris. All subjects were graded for facial local skin reactions (erythema, peeling, burning, and dryness) on the following scale: 0 = absent, 1 = mild, 2 = moderate, and 3 = severe. The percentage of subjects that had symptoms present before treatment (at baseline) and during treatment is presented in Table 1.
[See table 1 above]
(Percentages derived by number of subjects receiving DUAC Gel with symptom score/number of enrolled subjects receiving DUAC Gel).

6.2 Postmarketing Experience

The following adverse reactions have been identified during post approval use of DUAC Gel. Because these reactions are reported voluntarily from a population of uncertain size, it is not always possible to reliably estimate their frequency or establish a causal relationship to drug exposure.
Anaphylaxis, as well as allergic reactions leading to hospitalization, has been reported in postmarketing use with DUAC Gel.

7 DRUG INTERACTIONS

7.1 Erythromycin

Avoid using DUAC Gel in combination with erythromycin-containing products due to its clindamycin component. In vitro studies have shown antagonism between erythromycin and clindamycin. The clinical significance of this in vitro antagonism is not known.

7.2 Concomitant Topical Medications

Concomitant topical acne therapies should be used with caution since a possible cumulative irritancy effect may occur, especially with the use of peeling, desquamating, or abrasive agents. If irritancy or dermatitis occurs, reduce frequency of application or temporarily interrupt treatment and resume once the irritation subsides. Treatment should be discontinued if the irritation persists.

7.3 Neuromuscular Blocking Agents

Clindamycin has been shown to have neuromuscular blocking properties that may enhance the action of other neuromuscular blocking agents. DUAC Gel should be used with caution in patients receiving such agents.

8 USE IN SPECIFIC POPULATIONS

8.1 Pregnancy

Pregnancy Category C.
There are no adequate and well-controlled studies in pregnant women treated with DUAC Gel. DUAC Gel should be used during pregnancy only if the potential benefit justifies the potential risk to the fetus.
Developmental toxicity studies performed in rats and mice using oral doses of clindamycin up to 600 mg/kg/day (240 and 120 times the amount of clindamycin in the highest recommended adult human dose based on mg/m², respectively) or subcutaneous doses of clindamycin up to 250 mg/kg/day (100 and 50 times the amount of clindamycin in the highest recommended adult human dose based on mg/m², respectively) revealed no evidence of teratogenicity.

8.3 Nursing Mothers

It is not known whether DUAC Gel is excreted into human milk after topical application. However, orally and parenterally administered clindamycin has been reported to appear in breast milk. Because of the potential for serious adverse reactions in nursing infants, a decision should be made whether to discontinue nursing or to discontinue the drug,

Table 2. Mean Percent Reduction in Inflammatory Lesion Counts

Treatment	Trial 1 (n = 120)	Trial 2 (n = 273)	Trial 3 (n = 280)	Trial 4 (n = 288)	Trial 5 (n = 358)
DUAC Gel	65%	56%	42%	57%	52%
Benzoyl Peroxide	36%	37%	32%	57%	41%
Clindamycin	34%	30%	38%	49%	33%
Vehicle	19%	-0.4%	29%		29%

taking into account the importance of the drug to the mother. Because many drugs are excreted in human milk, caution should be exercised when DUAC Gel is administered to a nursing woman.

8.4 Pediatric Use
Safety and effectiveness of DUAC Gel in pediatric patients below the age of 12 have not been established.

8.5 Geriatric Use
Clinical studies of DUAC Gel did not include sufficient numbers of subjects ages 65 and over to determine whether they respond differently from younger subjects.

11 DESCRIPTION
DUAC (clindamycin phosphate and benzoyl peroxide) Gel, 1.2%/5% is a fixed combination product with two active ingredients in a white to slightly yellow, opaque, aqueous gel formulation.

Clindamycin phosphate is a water soluble ester of the semi-synthetic antibiotic produced by a 7(S)-chloro-substitution of the 7(R)-hydroxyl group of the parent antibiotic lincomycin.

Clindamycin phosphate is $C_{18}H_{34}ClN_2O_8PS$. The structural formula for clindamycin phosphate is represented below:

Clindamycin phosphate has a molecular weight of 504.97 and its chemical name is methyl 7-chloro-6,7,8-trideoxy-6-(1-methyl-*trans*-4-propyl-L-2-pyrrolidinecarboxamido)-1-thio-L-*threo*-α-D-*galacto*-octopyranoside 2-(dihydrogen phosphate).

Benzoyl peroxide is $C_{14}H_{10}O_4$. It has the following structural formula:

Benzoyl peroxide has a molecular weight of 242.23.

Each gram of DUAC Gel contains 10 mg (1%) clindamycin, as clindamycin phosphate, and 50 mg (5%) benzoyl peroxide in a base consisting of carbomer homopolymer (type C), dimethicone, disodium lauryl sulfosuccinate, edetate disodium, glycerin, methylparaben, poloxamer 182, purified water, silicon dioxide, and sodium hydroxide.

12 CLINICAL PHARMACOLOGY
12.1 Mechanism of Action
Clindamycin: Clindamycin is a lincosamide antibacterial [see Clinical Pharmacology (12.4)].
Benzoyl Peroxide: Benzoyl peroxide is an oxidizing agent with bacteriocidal and keratolytic effects, but the precise mechanism of action is unknown.

12.3 Pharmacokinetics
A comparative trial of the pharmacokinetics of DUAC Gel and 1% clindamycin solution alone in 78 subjects indicated that mean plasma clindamycin levels during the 4-week dosing period were <0.5 ng/mL for both treatment groups. Benzoyl peroxide has been shown to be absorbed by the skin where it is converted to benzoic acid. Less than 2% of the dose enters systemic circulation as benzoic acid.

12.4 Microbiology
Clindamycin binds to the 50S ribosomal subunits of susceptible bacteria and prevents elongation of peptide chains by interfering with peptidyl transfer, thereby suppressing protein synthesis.
In Vivo Activity: No microbiology studies were conducted in the clinical trials with this product.
In Vitro Activity: The clindamycin and benzoyl peroxide components individually have been shown to have in vitro activity against *Propionibacterium acnes*, an organism

which has been associated with acne vulgaris; however, the clinical significance of this in vitro activity is not known.
Drug Resistance: There are reports of an increase of *P. acnes* resistance to clindamycin in the treatment of acne. In patients with *P. acnes* resistant to clindamycin, the clindamycin component may provide no additional benefit beyond benzoyl peroxide alone.

13 NONCLINICAL TOXICOLOGY
13.1 Carcinogenesis, Mutagenesis, Impairment of Fertility
Benzoyl peroxide has been shown to be a tumor promoter and progression agent in a number of animal studies. Benzoyl peroxide in acetone at doses of 5 and 10 mg administered twice per week induced squamous cell skin tumors in transgenic TgAC mice in a study using 20 weeks of topical treatment. The clinical significance of this is unknown.
In a 2-year dermal carcinogenicity study in mice, treatment with DUAC Gel at doses up to 8,000 mg/kg/day (16 times the highest recommended adult human dose of 2.5 g DUAC Gel, based on mg/m²) did not cause an increase in skin tumors. However, topical treatment with another formulation containing 1% clindamycin and 5% benzoyl peroxide at doses of 100, 500, or 2,000 mg/kg/day caused a dose-dependent increase in the incidence of keratoacanthoma at the treated skin site of male rats in a 2–year dermal carcinogenicity study in rats.
In a 52-week photocarcinogenicity study in hairless mice (40 weeks of treatment followed by 12 weeks of observation), the median time to onset of skin tumor formation decreased and the number of tumors per mouse increased relative to controls following chronic concurrent topical treatment with DUAC Gel and exposure to ultraviolet radiation.
Genotoxicity studies were not conducted with DUAC Gel. Clindamycin phosphate was not genotoxic in *Salmonella typhimurium* or in a rat micronucleus test. Benzoyl peroxide has been found to cause DNA strand breaks in a variety of mammalian cell types, to be mutagenic in *Salmonella typhimurium* tests by some but not all investigators, and to cause sister chromatid exchanges in Chinese hamster ovary cells. Studies have not been performed with DUAC Gel or benzoyl peroxide to evaluate the effect on fertility. Fertility studies in rats treated orally with up to 300 mg/kg/day of clindamycin (approximately 120 times the amount of clindamycin in the highest recommended adult human dose of 2.5 g DUAC Gel, based on mg/m²) revealed no effects on fertility or mating ability.

14 CLINICAL STUDIES
In five randomized, double-blind clinical trials of 1,319 subjects, 397 used DUAC Gel, 396 used benzoyl peroxide, 349 used clindamycin, and 177 used vehicle. Subjects were instructed to wash the face, wait 10 to 20 minutes, and then apply medication to the entire face, once daily in the evening before retiring. DUAC Gel applied once daily for 11 weeks was significantly more effective than vehicle, benzoyl peroxide, and clindamycin in the treatment of inflammatory lesions of moderate to moderately severe facial acne vulgaris in three of the five trials (Trials 1, 2, and 5).
Subjects were evaluated and acne lesions counted at each clinical visit at Weeks 2, 5, 8, 11. The primary efficacy measures were the lesion counts and the investigator's global assessment evaluated at Week 11. Percent reductions in inflammatory lesion counts after treatment for 11 weeks in these 5 trials are shown in Table 2.
[See table 2 above]
The group treated with DUAC Gel showed greater overall improvement in the investigator's global assessment than the benzoyl peroxide, clindamycin, and vehicle groups in three of the five trials (Trials 1, 2, and 5).
Clinical trials have not adequately demonstrated the effectiveness of DUAC Gel versus benzoyl peroxide alone in the treatment of non-inflammatory lesions of acne.

16 HOW SUPPLIED/STORAGE AND HANDLING
16.1 How Supplied
DUAC Gel is a white to slightly yellow, opaque gel. It is supplied as follows:
• 45 gram tube NDC 0145-2371-05

16.2 Storage and Handling
Pharmacist:
• Prior to Dispensing: Store in a cold place, preferably in a refrigerator, between 2°C and 8°C (36°F and 46°F). Do not freeze.
16.3 Dispensing Instructions for the Pharmacist
• Dispense DUAC Gel with a 60 day expiration date.
• Specify "Store at room temperature up to 25°C (77°F). Do not freeze."
• Keep tube tightly closed.
• Keep out of the reach of small children.

17 PATIENT COUNSELING INFORMATION
See FDA-approved patient labeling (Patient Information).
• Patients who develop allergic reactions such as severe swelling or shortness of breath should discontinue use and contact their physician immediately.
• DUAC Gel may cause irritation such as erythema, scaling, itching, or burning, especially when used in combination with other topical acne therapies.
• Excessive or prolonged exposure to sunlight should be limited. To minimize exposure to sunlight, a hat or other clothing should be worn. Sunscreen may also be used.
• DUAC Gel may bleach hair or colored fabric.
DUAC is a registered trademark of Stiefel Laboratories, Inc.
Stiefel Laboratories, Inc.
Research Triangle Park, NC 27709
©2013, Stiefel Laboratories, Inc.
DUA:6PI
PHARMACIST – DETACH HERE AND GIVE INSTRUCTIONS TO PATIENT
PATIENT INFORMATION
DUAC® (Doo-ack)
(clindamycin phosphate and benzoyl peroxide) Gel, 1.2%/5%

IMPORTANT: For use on skin only (topical use). Do not get DUAC Gel in your mouth, eyes, vagina, or on your lips.

Read this Patient Information before you start using DUAC Gel and each time you get a refill. There may be new information. This informationn does not take the place of talking with your healthcare provider about your medical condition or your treatment.
What is DUAC Gel?
DUAC Gel is a prescription medicine used on the skin (topical) to treat inflamed acne in people 12 years and older.
Who should not use DUAC Gel?
Do not use DUAC Gel if you have:
• had an allergic reaction to clindamycin, lincomycin, benzoyl peroxide, or any of the ingredients in DUAC Gel. See the end of this leaflet for a complete list of ingredients in DUAC Gel.
• Crohn's disease or ulcerative colitis.
• had inflammation of the colon (colitis) with past antibiotic use.
What should I tell my healthcare provider before using DUAC Gel?
Before using DUAC Gel, tell your healthcare provider about all of your medical conditions, including if you:
• plan to have surgery with general anesthesia.
• are sensitive to sunlight.
• are pregnant or plan to become pregnant.It is not known if DUAC Gel will harm your unborn baby.
• are breastfeeding or plan to breastfeed. It is not known if DUAC Gel passes into your breast milk. One of the medicines in DUAC Gel is clindamycin. Clindamycin when taken by mouth or by injection has been reported to appear in breast milk. You and your healthcare provider should decide if you will use DUAC Gel while breastfeeding.
Tell your healthcare provider about all the medicines you take, including prescription or over-the-counter medicines, vitamins, herbal supplements, and skin products you use. Using other topical acne products may increase the irritation of your skin when used with DUAC Gel.
• Especially tell your healthcare provider if you take a medicine that contains erythromycin. DUAC Gel should not be used with products that contain erythromycin.
How should I use DUAC Gel?
• Use DUAC Gel exactly as your healthcare provider tells you to use it.
• Before you apply DUAC Gel, wash your face gently with a mild soap, rinse with warm water, and pat the skin dry.
• Apply a thin layer of DUAC Gel to your face 1 time a day, in the evening or as directed by your healthcare provider. Wash your hands with soap and water after applying DUAC Gel.
• Do not get DUAC Gel in your mouth, eyes, nose, vagina, or on your lips. Do not get DUAC Gel on cuts or open wounds.
What should I avoid while using DUAC Gel?
• Limit your time in sunlight. Avoid using tanning beds or sun lamps. If you have to be in sunlight, wear a wide-brimmed hat or other protective clothing. Sunscreen may also be used.

- Talk to your healthcare provider if you spend a lot of time in the sun.
- DUAC Gel may bleach hair or colored fabric.

What are the possible side effects with DUAC Gel?
DUAC Gel may cause serious side effects, including:
- **Inflammation of the colon (colitis).** Stop using DUAC Gel and call your healthcare provider right away if you have severe watery diarrhea, or bloody diarrhea.
- **Allergic reactions.** Stop using DUAC Gel and call your healthcare provider or get help right away if you have any of the following symptoms:
  ○ severe itching
  ○ swelling of your face, eyes, lips, tongue, or throat
  ○ trouble breathing

The most common side effects with DUAC Gel are skin reactions and may include redness, peeling, dryness, and burning. These are not all the possible side effects with DUAC Gel.
Call your doctor for medical advice about side effects. You may report side effects to FDA at 1-800-FDA-1088.

How should I store DUAC Gel?
- Store DUAC Gel at room temperature up to 25°C (77°F). Do not freeze DUAC Gel.
- The expiration date of DUAC Gel is 60 days from the date when you fill your prescription.
- Safely throw away expired DUAC Gel.
- Keep the tube tightly closed.

Keep DUAC Gel and all medicines out of the reach of children.

General information about DUAC Gel
Medicines are sometimes prescribed for purposes other than those listed in a Patient Information leaflet. Do not use DUAC Gel for a condition for which it was not prescribed. Do not give DUAC Gel to other people, even if they have the same symptoms you have. It may harm them.
If you would like more information, talk with your healthcare provider. You can also ask your pharmacist or healthcare provider for information about DUAC Gel that is written for healthcare professionals.
For more information, call 1-888-784-3335.

What are the ingredients in DUAC Gel?
Active Ingredients: clindamycin phosphate 1.2% and benzoyl peroxide 5%
Inactive Ingredients: carbomer homopolymer (type C), dimethicone, disodium lauryl sulfosuccinate, edetate disodium, glycerin, methylparaben, poloxamer 182, purified water, silicon dioxide, and sodium hydroxide.
This Patient Information Leaflet has been approved by the U.S. Food and Drug Administration.
DUAC is a registered trademark of Stiefel Laboratories, Inc.
Stiefel Laboratories, Inc.
Research Triangle Park, NC 27709
©2013, Stiefel Laboratories, Inc.
December 2013
DUA:1PIL

FABIOR™

(tazarotene)
Foam, 0.1%, for topical use

℞

HIGHLIGHTS OF PRESCRIBING INFORMATION
These highlights do not include all the information needed to use FABIOR Foam safely and effectively. See full prescribing information for FABIOR Foam.
FABIOR (tazarotene) Foam, 0.1%, for topical use
Initial U.S. Approval: 1997

---INDICATIONS AND USAGE---
- FABIOR Foam is a retinoid indicated for the topical treatment of acne vulgaris in patients 12 years of age or older. (1)

---DOSAGE AND ADMINISTRATION---
- Apply a thin layer to the entire affected areas of the face and/or upper trunk once daily in the evening. Avoid the eyes, lips, and mucous membranes. Wash hands after application. (2)

---DOSAGE FORMS AND STRENGTHS---
- 0.1%, foam. (3)

---CONTRAINDICATIONS---
- Pregnancy. (4, 8.1)

---WARNINGS AND PRECAUTIONS---
- Fetal Risk: FABIOR Foam contains tazarotene, which is a teratogenic substance. FABIOR Foam is contraindicated in pregnancy. Females of childbearing potential should have a negative pregnancy test within 2 weeks prior to initiating treatment and use an effective method of contraception during treatment. (5.1)

- Local Irritation: Use with caution in patients with a history of local tolerability reactions or local hypersensitivity. (5.2)
- Potential Irritant Effect with Concomitant Topical Medications: Use with caution because a cumulative irritant effect may occur. (5.3)
- Photosensitivity and Risk for Sunburn: Avoid exposure to sunlight, sunlamps, and weather extremes. Wear sunscreen daily. (5.4)
- Contents are flammable. Instruct the patient to avoid fire, flame, and smoking during and immediately following application. (5.5)

---ADVERSE REACTIONS---
- Most common adverse reactions reported at an incidence ≥6% are application site irritation, application site dryness, application site erythema, and application site exfoliation. (6.1)
To report SUSPECTED ADVERSE REACTIONS, contact Stiefel Laboratories, Inc at 1-888-784-3335 (1-888-STIEFEL) or FDA at 1-800-FDA-1088 or www.fda.gov/medwatch

---DRUG INTERACTIONS---
- Avoid concomitant dermatologic medications and cosmetics that have a strong drying effect. (7)
See 17 for PATIENT COUNSELING INFORMATION and FDA-approved patient labeling

Revised: 01/2014

FULL PRESCRIBING INFORMATION

1   INDICATIONS AND USAGE

FABIOR® (tazarotene) Foam, 0.1% is indicated for the topical treatment of acne vulgaris in patients 12 years of age or older.

2   DOSAGE AND ADMINISTRATION

FABIOR Foam is for topical use only. FABIOR Foam is not for oral, ophthalmic, or intravaginal use.
FABIOR Foam should be applied once daily in the evening after washing with a mild cleanser and fully drying the affected area. Dispense a small amount of foam into the palm of the hand. Using fingertips, apply only enough foam to lightly cover the entire affected areas of the face and/or upper trunk with a thin layer; gently massage the foam into the skin until the foam disappears. Avoid the eyes, lips, and mucous membranes. Wash hands after application.
Patients may use moisturizer as needed.
If undue irritation (redness, peeling, or discomfort) occurs, patients should reduce frequency of application or temporarily interrupt treatment. Treatment may be resumed once irritation subsides. Treatment should be discontinued if irritation persists.

3   DOSAGE FORMS AND STRENGTHS

0.1%, white to off-white foam

4   CONTRAINDICATIONS

FABIOR Foam is contraindicated in pregnancy.
FABIOR Foam may cause fetal harm when administered to a pregnant woman. Tazarotene elicits teratogenic and de-

velopmental effects associated with retinoids after topical or systemic administration in rats and rabbits [see Use in Specific Populations (8.1)].
If this drug is used during pregnancy, or if the patient becomes pregnant while taking this drug, treatment should be discontinued and the patient apprised of the potential hazard to the fetus [see Warnings and Precautions (5.1), Use in Specific Populations (8.1)].

5   WARNINGS AND PRECAUTIONS

5.1   Fetal Risk

Systemic exposure to tazarotenic acid is dependent upon the extent of the body surface area treated. In patients treated topically over sufficient body surface area, exposure could be in the same order of magnitude as in orally treated animals. Tazarotene is a teratogenic substance, and it is not known what level of exposure is required for teratogenicity in humans [see Clinical Pharmacology (12)].
There were 5 reported pregnancies in subjects who participated in clinical trials for topical tazarotene foam. One of the subjects was found to have been treated with topical tazarotene for 25 days, 2 were treated with vehicle foam, and the other 2 did not receive either tazarotene foam or vehicle foam. The subjects were discontinued from the trials when their pregnancy was reported. The one pregnant woman who was inadvertently exposed to topical tazarotene during the clinical trial delivered a full-term healthy infant.
Females of Childbearing Potential:
Females of child-bearing potential should be warned of the potential risk and use adequate birth-control measures when tazarotene foam is used. The possibility of pregnancy should be considered in females of child-bearing potential at the time of institution of therapy.
A negative serum or urine result for pregnancy test having a sensitivity down to at least 25 mIU/mL for human chorionic gonadotropin (hCG) should be obtained within 2 weeks prior to therapy with FABIOR Foam, which should begin during a normal menstrual period for females of childbearing potential. Advise patients of the need to use an effective method of contraception to avoid pregnancy [see Use in Specific Populations (8.1)].

5.2   Local Irritation

FABIOR Foam should be used with caution in patients with a history of local tolerability reactions or local hypersensitivity. Retinoids should not be used on abraded or eczematous skin, as they may cause severe irritation. Contact with the mouth, eyes, and mucous membranes should be avoided. In case of accidental contact, rinse well with water. Some individuals may experience skin redness, peeling, burning or excessive pruritus. If these effects occur, the medication should either be discontinued until the integrity of the skin is restored, or the dosing should be reduced to an interval the patient can tolerate. However, efficacy at reduced frequency of application has not been established. Weather extremes, such as wind or cold, may be more irritating to patients using FABIOR Foam.

5.3   Potential Irritant Effect With Concomitant Topical Medications

Concomitant topical acne therapy should be used with caution because a cumulative irritant effect may occur. If irritancy or dermatitis occurs, reduce frequency of application or temporarily interrupt treatment and resume once the irritation subsides. Treatment should be discontinued if irritation persists.

5.4   Photosensitivity and Risk for Sunburn

Because of heightened burning susceptibility, exposure to sunlight (including sunlamps) should be avoided. Patients must be warned to use sunscreens and protective clothing when using Fabior Foam. Patients with sunburn should be advised not to use FABIOR Foam until fully recovered. Patients who may have considerable sun exposure due to their occupation and those patients with inherent sensitivity to sunlight should exercise particular caution when using FABIOR Foam and ensure that the precautions are observed [see FDA-approved patient labeling]. Due to the potential for photosensitivity resulting in greater risk for sunburn, FABIOR Foam should be used with caution in patients with a personal or family history of skin cancer.
FABIOR Foam should be administered with caution if the patient is also taking drugs known to be photosensitizers (e.g., thiazides, tetracyclines, fluoroquinolones, phenothiazines, sulfonamides) because of the increased possibility of augmented photosensitivity.

5.5   Flammability

The propellant in FABIOR Foam is flammable. Instruct the patient to avoid fire, flame, and/or smoking during and immediately following application.

6   ADVERSE REACTIONS

6.1   Clinical Trials Experience

Because clinical trials are conducted under widely varying conditions, adverse reaction rates observed in clinical trials of a drug cannot be directly compared with rates in the clinical trials of another drug and may not reflect the rates observed in clinical practice.

The safety data reflect exposure to FABIOR Foam in 744 subjects with acne vulgaris. Subjects were aged 12 to 45 years and were treated once daily in the evening for 12 weeks. Adverse reactions reported in ≥ 1% of subjects treated with FABIOR Foam are presented in Table 1. Most adverse reactions were mild to moderate in severity. Severe adverse reactions represented 3.0% of the subjects treated. Overall, 2.6% (20/744) of subjects discontinued FABIOR Foam because of local skin reactions.

Table 1. Incidence of Adverse Reactions in ≥1 % of Subjects Treated With FABIOR Foam

	FABIOR Foam N = 744	Vehicle Foam N = 741
Patients with any treatment-related adverse reaction, n (%)	163 (22)	19 (3)
Application site irritation	107 (14)	9 (1)
Application site dryness	50 (7)	8 (1)
Application site erythema	48 (6)	3 (<1)
Application site exfoliation	44 (6)	3 (<1)
Application site pain	9 (1)	0
Application site pruritus	7 (1)	3 (<1)
Application site dermatitis	6 (1)	1 (<1)

Additional adverse reactions that were reported in <1% of subjects treated with FABIOR Foam included application site reactions (including discoloration, discomfort, edema, rash, and swelling), dermatitis, impetigo, and pruritus.

Local skin reactions, dryness, erythema, and peeling actively assessed by the investigator and burning/stinging and itching reported by the subject were evaluated at baseline, during treatment, and end of treatment. During the 12 weeks of treatment, each local skin reaction peaked at Week 2 and gradually reduced thereafter with the continued use of FABIOR Foam.

7   DRUG INTERACTIONS

No formal drug-drug interaction studies were conducted with FABIOR Foam.

Concomitant dermatologic medications and cosmetics that have a strong drying effect should be avoided. It is recommended to postpone treatment until the effects of these products subside before use of FABIOR Foam is started.

Concomitant use with oxidizing agents, such as benzoyl peroxide, may cause degradation of tazarotene and may reduce the clinical efficacy of tazarotene. If combination therapy is required, they should be applied at different times of the day (e.g. one in the morning and the other in the evening).

The impact of tazarotene on the pharmacokinetics of progestin-only oral contraceptives (i.e., minipills) has not been evaluated.

In a trial of 27 healthy female subjects between the ages of 20 to 55 years receiving a combination oral contraceptive tablet containing 1 mg norethindrone and 35 mcg ethinyl estradiol, concomitant use of tazarotene did not affect the pharmacokinetics of norethindrone and ethinyl estradiol over a complete cycle.

8   USE IN SPECIFIC POPULATIONS
8.1   Pregnancy
Pregnancy Category X.

FABIOR Foam is contraindicated in pregnancy [see Contraindications (4)].

There are no adequate and well-controlled studies with FABIOR Foam in pregnant women. FABIOR Foam is contraindicated in females who are or may become pregnant [see Contraindications (4)]. Females of child-bearing potential should be warned of the potential risk and use adequate birth-control measures when FABIOR Foam is used. The possibility that a female of child-bearing potential is pregnant at the time of institution of therapy should be considered. A negative serum or urine result for pregnancy test having a sensitivity down to at least 25 mIU/mL for hCG should be obtained within 2 weeks prior to therapy with FABIOR Foam, which should begin during a normal menstrual period for females of childbearing potential.

In rats, tazarotene 0.05% gel administered topically during gestation days 6 through 17 at 0.25 mg/kg/day resulted in reduced fetal body weights and reduced skeletal ossification. Rabbits dosed topically with 0.25 mg/kg/day tazarotene gel during gestation days 6 through 18 were noted with single incidences of known retinoid malformations, including spina bifida, hydrocephaly, and heart anomalies.

Systemic exposure (AUC) to tazarotenic acid at topical doses of 0.25 mg/kg/day tazarotene in a gel formulation in rats and rabbits were 15 and 166 times, respectively, the AUC in acne patients treated with 2 mg/cm^2 of FABIOR Foam 0.1% over a 15% body surface area.

As with other retinoids, when tazarotene was administered orally to experimental animals, developmental delays were seen in rats, and teratogenic effects and post-implantation loss were observed in rats and rabbits at doses 13 and 325 times, respectively, the AUC to tazarotenic acid in acne patients treated with 2 mg/cm^2 of FABIOR Foam 0.1% over a 15% body surface area.

In female rats orally administered 2 mg/kg/day tazarotene from 15 days before mating through gestation day 7, a number of classic developmental effects of retinoids were observed including decreased number of implantation sites, decreased litter size, decreased numbers of live fetuses, and decreased fetal body weights. A low incidence of retinoid-related malformations was also observed. AUC in rats was 42 times the AUC in acne patients treated with 2 mg/cm^2 of FABIOR Foam 0.1% over a 15% body surface area.

8.3   Nursing Mothers
After single topical doses of ^{14}C-tazarotene to the skin of lactating rats, radioactivity was detected in milk, suggesting that there would be transfer of drug-related material to the offspring via milk. It is not known whether this drug is excreted in human milk. The safe use of FABIOR Foam during lactation has not been established. A decision should be made whether to discontinue breastfeeding or to discontinue therapy with FABIOR Foam taking into account the benefit of breastfeeding for the child and the benefit of therapy for the woman.

8.4   Pediatric Use
The safety and effectiveness of FABIOR Foam in pediatric patients younger than 12 years have not been established. Clinical studies of FABIOR Foam included 860 patients aged 12 to 17 years with acne vulgaris.

8.5   Geriatric Use
FABIOR Foam for the treatment of acne has not been clinically evaluated in persons over the age of 65.

10   OVERDOSAGE

Excessive topical application of FABIOR Foam may lead to marked redness, peeling, or discomfort. [see Warnings and Precautions (5.3).] Management of accidental ingestion or excessive application to the skin should be as clinically indicated.

11   DESCRIPTION

FABIOR (tazarotene) Foam, 0.1% contains the compound tazarotene, a member of the acetylenic class of retinoids. It is for topical use only.

Chemically, tazarotene is ethyl 6-[(4,4-dimethylthiochroman-6-yl)ethynyl]nicotinate. The structural formula is represented below:

Molecular Formula: C$_{21}$H$_{21}$NO$_2$S Molecular Weight: 351.46

Tazarotene is a pale yellow to yellow substance. FABIOR Foam contains tazarotene, 1 mg/g, in aqueous-based white to off-white foam vehicle consisting of butylated hydroxytoluene, ceteareth-12, citric acid anhydrous, diisopropyl adipate, light mineral oil, potassium citrate monohydrate, potassium sorbate, purified water, and sorbic acid. FABIOR Foam is dispensed from an aluminum can pressurized with a hydrocarbon (propane/n-butane/isobutane) propellant.

12   CLINICAL PHARMACOLOGY
12.1   Mechanism of Action
Tazarotene is a retinoid prodrug that is converted to its active form, the cognate carboxylic acid of tazarotene, by rapid deesterification in animals and man. Tazarotenic acid binds to all 3 members of the retinoic acid receptor (RAR) family: RARα, RARβ, and RARγ but shows relative selectivity for RARβ and RARγ and may modify gene expression. The clinical significance of these findings is unknown.

The mechanism of tazarotene action in acne vulgaris is not defined. However, the basis of tazarotene's therapeutic effect in acne may be due to its anti-hyperproliferative, normalizing-of-differentiation and anti-inflammatory effects. Tazarotene inhibited corneocyte accumulation in rhino mouse skin and cross-linked envelope formation in cultured human keratinocytes. The clinical significance of these findings is unknown.

12.2   Pharmacodynamics
The pharmacodynamics of FABIOR Foam are unknown.

12.3   Pharmacokinetics
Following topical application, tazarotene undergoes esterase hydrolysis to form its active metabolite, tazarotenic acid. Tazarotenic acid was highly bound to plasma proteins (greater than 99%). Tazarotene and tazarotenic acid were metabolized to sulfoxides, sulfones, and other polar metabolites which were eliminated through urinary and fecal pathways.

Systemic exposure following topical application of FABIOR Foam 0.1% was evaluated in one trial. Patients aged 15 years and older with moderate-to-severe acne applied approximately 3.7 grams of FABIOR Foam 0.1% (N = 13) to approximately 15% body surface area (face, upper chest, upper back, and shoulders) once daily for 22 days. On Day 22, the mean (±SD) tazarotenic acid C_{max} was 0.43 (±0.19) ng/mL, the AUC$_{0-24h}$ was 6.98 (±3.56) ng•h/mL, and the half-life was 21.7 (±15.7) hours. The median T_{max} was 6 hours (range: 4.4 to 12 hours). The AUC$_{0-24h}$ for tazarotenic acid was approximately 50-fold higher compared with the parent compound tazarotene. The mean (±SD) half-life of tazarotene was 8.1 (±3.7) hours.

Accumulation was observed upon repeated once-daily dosing as the tazarotenic acid predose concentrations were measurable in the majority of subjects. Steady state was attained within 22 days of daily application. Once-daily dosing resulted in little to no accumulation of tazarotene as predose concentrations were mostly below the quantitation limit throughout the study.

13   NONCLINICAL TOXICOLOGY
13.1   Carcinogenesis, Mutagenesis, Impairment of Fertility
Carcinogenesis:
A long-term study of tazarotene following oral administration of 0.025, 0.050, and 0.125 mg/kg/day to rats showed no indications of increased carcinogenic risk. Based on pharmacokinetic data from a shorter-term study in rats, the highest dose of 0.125 mg/kg/day was anticipated to give systemic exposure in rats approximately 2 times the AUC in acne patients treated with 2 mg/cm^2 of FABIOR Foam 0.1% over a 15% body surface area.

A long-term topical application study of up to 0.1% tazarotene in a gel formulation in mice terminated at 88 weeks showed that dose levels of 0.05, 0.125, 0.25, and 1 mg/kg/day (reduced to 0.5 mg/kg/day for males after 41 weeks due to severe dermal irritation) revealed no apparent carcinogenic effects when compared with vehicle control animals. AUC at the highest dose in mice was 49 times the AUC in acne patients treated with 2 mg/cm^2 of FABIOR Foam 0.1% over a 15% body surface area.

In evaluation of photocarcinogenicity, median time to onset of tumors was decreased and the number of tumors increased in hairless mice following chronic topical dosing with exposure to ultraviolet radiation at tazarotene concentrations of 0.001%, 0.005%, and 0.01% in a gel formulation for up to 40 weeks.

Mutagenesis:
Tazarotene was non-mutagenic in the Ames assay and did not produce structural chromosomal aberrations in a human lymphocyte assay. Tazarotene was non-mutagenic in the CHO/HGPRT mammalian cell forward gene mutation assay and was non-clastogenic in the in vivo mouse micronucleus test.

Impairment of Fertility:
No impairment of fertility was observed in rats when male animals were treated for 70 days prior to mating and female animals were treated for 14 days prior to mating and continuing through gestation and lactation with topical doses of tazarotene gel up to 0.125 mg/kg/day. Based on data from another study, the systemic drug exposure at the 0.125 mg/kg/day dose in rats would be equivalent to 7.6 times the AUC in acne patients treated with 2 mg/cm^2 of FABIOR Foam 0.1% over a 15% body surface area.

No impairment of mating performance or fertility was observed in male rats treated for 70 days prior to mating with oral doses of up to 1 mg/kg/day tazarotene. AUC at the highest dose in rats was 23 times the AUC in acne patients treated with 2 mg/cm^2 of FABIOR Foam 0.1% over a 15% body surface area.

No effect on parameters of mating performance or fertility was observed in female rats treated for 15 days prior to mating and continuing through gestation day 7 with oral doses of tazarotene up to 2 mg/kg/day. However, there was a significant decrease in the number of estrous stages and an increase in developmental effects at that dose [see Pregnancy (8.1)]. AUC at the highest dose in rats was 42 times the AUC in acne patients treated with 2 mg/cm^2 of FABIOR Foam 0.1% over a 15% body surface area.

Reproductive capabilities of F1 animals, including F2 survival and development, were not affected by topical administration of tazarotene gel to female F0 parental rats from gestation day 16 through lactation day 20 at the maximum tolerated dose of 0.125 mg/kg/day. Based on data from another study, AUC in rats would be equivalent to 7.6 times the AUC in acne patients treated with 2 mg/cm^2 of FABIOR Foam 0.1% over a 15% body surface area.

14   CLINICAL STUDIES

In 2 multi-center, randomized, double-blind, vehicle-controlled studies, a total of 1,485 subjects with moderate-to-severe acne vulgaris were randomized 1:1 to FABIOR Foam or vehicle applied once daily for 12 weeks. Acne severity was evaluated using lesion counts and the 6-point Investigator's Global Assessment (IGA) scale (see Table 2). At baseline, 80% of subjects were graded as "moderate" or Grade 3 and 20% were graded as "severe"-or Grade 4 on the IGA scale. At baseline, subjects had an average of 79.8 total lesions of which the mean number of inflammatory lesions was 31.9 and the mean number of non-inflammatory lesions was 47.8. Subjects ranged in age from 12 to 45 years, with 860 (58%) subjects aged 12 to 17 years; 428 (29%) subjects aged 18 to 25 years; 143 (10%) subjects aged 26 to 35 years and 54 (4%) subjects aged 36 to 45 years. Subjects enrolled in the studies by race were white (77%), black (15%), Asian (4%), and other (4%). Hispanics comprised 18% of the population. An equal number of males (49%) and females (51%) were enrolled. Treatment success was defined as a score of "clear" (Grade 0) or "almost clear" (Grade 1) and at least 2-grade improvement from the baseline score to Week 12.

Table 2. Investigator's Global Assessment Scale

Grade		Description
0	Clear	Clear skin with no inflammatory or non-inflammatory lesions.
1	Almost clear	Rare non-inflammatory lesions with no more than rare papules.
2	Mild	Greater than Grade 1, some non-inflammatory lesions with no more than a few inflammatory lesions (papules/pustules only, no nodular lesions).
3	Moderate	Greater than Grade 2, up to many non-inflammatory lesions and may have some inflammatory lesions, but no more than one small nodular lesion.
4	Severe	Greater than Grade 3, up to many non-inflammatory and inflammatory lesions, but no more than a few nodular lesions.
5	Very severe	Many non-inflammatory and inflammatory lesions and more than a few nodular lesions. May have cystic lesions.

Absolute and percent reductions in lesion counts and the IGA scale after 12 weeks of treatment in these 2 trials are shown in Table 3. Each trial needed to have a statistically significant reduction in 2 out of 3 lesion counts at Week 12. [See table 3 above]

16 HOW SUPPLIED/STORAGE AND HANDLING
How Supplied:
FABIOR Foam, 0.1% (1 mg/g) is a white to off-white foam, supplied as follows:
50-g aluminum can NDC 0145-0020-03
100-g aluminum can NDC 0145-0020-02
Storage and Handling:
- Store at 20°C to 25°C (68°F to 77°F); excursions permitted to 15°C to 30°C (59°F to 86°F). See USP-controlled room temperature.
- Store upright.
- Protect from freezing.
- Flammable. Avoid fire, flame, or smoking during and immediately following application. Contents under pressure. Do not puncture or incinerate. Do not expose to heat or store at temperatures above 120°F (49°C).
- Shake can before use. Hold can at an upright angle and press firmly to dispense.

17 PATIENT COUNSELING INFORMATION
See FDA-Approved Patient Labeling (Patient Information).
Inform the patient of the following:
- Fetal risk associated with FABIOR Foam for females of childbearing potential. Advise patients to use an effective method of contraception during treatment to avoid pregnancy. Advise the patient to stop medication if she becomes pregnant and call her doctor.
- If undue irritation (redness, peeling, or discomfort) occurs, reduce frequency of application or temporarily interrupt treatment. Treatment may be resumed once irritation subsides.
- Do not place FABIOR Foam in the freezer.
- Avoid exposure of the treated areas to either natural or artificial sunlight, including tanning beds and sun lamps.
- Avoid contact with the eyes. If FABIOR Foam gets in or near their eyes, to rinse thoroughly with water.
- Wash their hands after applying FABIOR Foam.

Table 3. Reductions in Lesion Counts and Improvements in Investigator's Global Assessment at Week 12

	Trial 1		Trial 2	
	FABIOR Foam N = 371	Vehicle Foam N = 372	FABIOR Foam N = 373	Vehicle Foam N = 369
Inflammatory Lesions				
Mean absolute reduction from Baseline	18.0	14.0	18.0	15.0
Mean percent reduction from Baseline	58%	45%	55%	45%
Non-inflammatory Lesions				
Mean absolute reduction from Baseline	28.0	17.0	26.0	18.0
Mean percent reduction from Baseline	55%	33%	57%	41%
Total Lesions				
Mean absolute reduction from Baseline	46.0	31.0	43.0	33.0
Mean percent reduction from Baseline	56%	39%	56%	43%
Investigator's Global Assessment (IGA), n (%) Minimum 2-grade improvement *and* IGA of 0 or 1	107 (29%)	60 (16%)	103 (28%)	49 (13%)

- Avoid fire, flame, or smoking during and immediately following application since FABIOR Foam is flammable.
- Keep out of the reach of children.
- Not for ophthalmic, oral, or intravaginal use.
FABIOR is a registered trademark of the GlaxoSmithKline group of companies, used under license by Stiefel Laboratories, Inc.
Manufactured for
Stiefel Laboratories, Inc.
Research Triangle Park, NC 27709
Licensed from Allergan, Inc.
©2013, Stiefel Laboratories, Inc.
FAB:3PI
Pharmacist-Detach here and Give Instructions to Patient
Patient Information
FABIOR
(fab′ ee ore)
(tazarotene)
Foam
IMPORTANT: For skin use only. Do not get FABIOR Foam in your eyes, mouth or vagina.
Read the Patient Information that comes with FABIOR Foam before you start using it and each time you get a refill. There may be new information. This leaflet does not take the place of talking with your doctor about your condition or treatment.
What is FABIOR Foam?
FABIOR Foam is a prescription medicine used on the skin (topical) to treat acne in people 12 years and older.
It is not known if FABIOR Foam is safe and effective in children under 12 years of age.
Who should not use FABIOR Foam?
Do not use FABIOR Foam if you are pregnant or plan to become pregnant. FABIOR Foam may harm your unborn baby, if used during pregnancy.
If you are a female who can become pregnant:
- Use an effective method of birth control during treatment with FABIOR Foam. Talk with your doctor about birth control methods that are right for you during treatment with FABIOR Foam.
- Your doctor should do a blood or urine pregnancy test within 2 weeks before you begin to use FABIOR Foam to be sure you are not pregnant.
- If you have menstrual periods, begin using FABIOR Foam during a normal menstrual period to help assure that you are not pregnant when you begin use.
Stop using FABIOR Foam and call your doctor right away if you become pregnant during treatment with FABIOR Foam.
What should I tell my doctor before using FABIOR Foam?
Before you use FABIOR Foam, tell your doctor if you:
- or a family member have or had skin cancer.
- have eczema.
- have had a reaction to topical products in the past.
- have any condition that makes you sensitive to light.
- have any other medical conditions.
- are pregnant or plan to become pregnant. **See "Who should not use FABIOR Foam?"**
- are breastfeeding or plan to breastfeed. It is not known if tazarotene passes into your breast milk. You and your doctor should decide if you will use FABIOR Foam or breastfeed. You should not do both. Talk to your doctor about the best way to feed your baby if you use FABIOR Foam.
Tell your doctor about all the medicines you take including prescription and nonprescription medicines, vitamins, and herbal supplements.
Especially tell your doctor if you:
- use other medicines or products that make your skin dry
- take other medicines that may increase your sensitivity to sunlight

Ask your doctor or pharmacist if you are not sure if your medicine is one that is listed above.
Know the medicines you take. Keep a list of your medicines and show it to your doctor and pharmacist when you get a new medicine.
How should I use FABIOR Foam?
- Use FABIOR Foam exactly as your doctor tells you to. Do not use more FABIOR Foam than prescribed and do not use it more often than your doctor tells you to.
- If you are a female and have menstrual periods, begin using FABIOR Foam during a normal menstrual period to help assure that you are not pregnant when you begin use. **See "Who should not use FABIOR Foam?"**
- FABIOR Foam is flammable. Avoid fire, flame, and smoking during and right after you apply FABIOR Foam.
- Gently clean the affected area (face and/or upper trunk) with a mild cleanser and dry completely before using FABIOR Foam.
- Apply FABIOR Foam one time each day, before going to bed, to the affected areas (face and/or upper trunk) where you have acne lesions. Use enough foam to cover the entire affected area with a thin film of FABIOR Foam.
- Keep FABIOR Foam away from your eyes, eyelids, mouth, and vagina. If FABIOR Foam comes into contact with your eyes, rinse them well with water.
- Wash your hands after applying FABIOR Foam.
- If you use too much FABIOR Foam, you may get redness, peeling, or skin irritation in the treated area. Call your doctor if this happens, or if you accidently swallow FABIOR Foam.
- Follow your doctor's directions for other routine skin care and the use of make-up.
- You may also use a moisturizer as needed.
Instructions for applying FABIOR Foam
1. Shake the FABIOR Foam can before use.
2. Remove cap from can. Nozzle should be lined up with black mark on rim of can. If black mark is not lined up with the nozzle, twist nozzle to line up with black mark. See Figure A.

Figure A

3. Hold the FABIOR Foam can upright at a slight angle and press the nozzle. See Figure B.

Figure B

4. Dispense a small amount of FABIOR Foam into the palm of your hand. See Figure C.
[See figure C at top of next column]
5. Use the fingertips of your other hand to apply enough FABIOR Foam to cover the affected area with a thin layer.

Figure C

Gently rub the foam into the affected area until it disappears into the skin. See Figure D.

Figure D

6. Wash hands after applying FABIOR Foam. See Figure E.

Figure E

Avoid getting FABIOR Foam in your eyes, mouth, or vagina.

What should I avoid while using FABIOR Foam?
• Avoid using abrasive soaps or cleansers that might dry or irritate your skin, unless your doctor tells you it is ok.
• Avoid sunlight. FABIOR Foam can make your skin sensitive to sunlight and the light from sunlamps or tanning beds. You could get a sunburn. Use sunscreen and protective clothing during the day if you must be in sunlight.
• Avoid using FABIOR Foam if you have a sunburn. If you have a sunburn, wait until it is fully healed before using FABIOR Foam.
• Talk to your doctor before using FABIOR Foam if you are sensitive to sunlight, take medications that increase your sensitivity to sunlight, or you must spend a lot of time in the sun for your job.
• Avoid weather extremes, such as wind and cold, because they may irritate your skin more while you are using FABIOR Foam.

What are the possible side effects of FABIOR Foam?
FABIOR Foam may harm your unborn baby, if used during pregnancy.
• Do not use FABIOR Foam during pregnancy. See "Who should not use FABIOR Foam?"
The most common side effects of FABIOR Foam are:
• burning or stinging
• dry skin
• red skin
• peeling or flaking skin
Sometimes these symptoms can become severe and may be uncomfortable. Tell your doctor if these side effects become uncomfortable for you. Your doctor may tell you to stop using FABIOR Foam until your skin heals and your symptoms improve, or to use FABIOR Foam less often to help you tolerate it better.
These are not all the possible side effects of FABIOR Foam. For more information, ask your doctor or pharmacist.
Call your doctor for medical advice about side effects. You may report side effects to FDA at 1-800-FDA-1088.
You may also report side effects to Stiefel Laboratories, Inc at 1-888-784-3335.

How should I store FABIOR Foam?
• Store FABIOR Foam at room temperature, between 68°F to 77°F (20°C to 25°C).
• Store FABIOR Foam upright.
• Do not freeze FABIOR Foam.
• FABIOR Foam is flammable. Keep the can away from fire and heat. Do not spray FABIOR Foam near fire or direct heat.
• Do not puncture the can or throw it into a fire, even if the can is empty.

Keep FABIOR Foam and all medicines out of the reach of children.

General Information about FABIOR Foam
Medicines are sometimes prescribed for purposes other than those listed in Patient Information leaflets. Do not use FABIOR Foam for a condition for which it was not prescribed. Do not give FABIOR Foam to other people even if they have the same symptoms that you have. It may harm them.

This Patient Information leaflet summarizes the most important information about FABIOR Foam. If you would like more information, talk with your doctor. You can ask your doctor or pharmacist for information about FABIOR Foam that is written for health professionals.

What are the ingredients in FABIOR Foam?
Active ingredient: tazarotene
Inactive ingredients: butylated hydroxytoluene, ceteareth-12, citric acid anhydrous, diisopropyl adipate, light mineral oil, potassium citrate monohydrate, potassium sorbate, purified water, and sorbic acid. The foam is dispensed from an aluminum can pressurized with a hydrocarbon (propane/n-butane/isobutane) propellant.
The Patient Information leaflet has been approved by the U.S. Food and Drug Administration
FABIOR is a registered trademark of the GlaxoSmithKline group of companies, used under license by Stiefel Laboratories, Inc.
Licensed from Allergan, Inc.
Manufactured for:
Stiefel Laboratories, Inc.
Research Triangle Park, NC 27709
©2013 Stiefel Laboratories, Inc.
December 2013
FAB:3PIL

SORIATANE® ℞
[sŏr-ĭ-ă-tēn]
(acitretin)
CAPSULES

SORIATANE®
(acitretin)
Capsules

CAUSES BIRTH DEFECTS

DO NOT GET PREGNANT

CONTRAINDICATIONS AND WARNINGS: Pregnancy
SORIATANE must not be used by females who are pregnant, or who intend to become pregnant during therapy or at any time for at least 3 years following discontinuation of therapy. SORIATANE also must not be used by females who may not use reliable contraception while undergoing treatment and for at least 3 years following discontinuation of treatment. Acitretin is a metabolite of etretinate (TEGISON®), and major human fetal abnormalities have been reported with the administration of acitretin and etretinate. Potentially, any fetus exposed can be affected. Clinical evidence has shown that concurrent ingestion of acitretin and ethanol has been associated with the formation of etretinate, which has a significantly longer elimination half-life than acitretin. Because the longer elimination half-life of etretinate would increase the duration of teratogenic potential for female patients, ethanol must not be ingested by female patients either during treatment with SORIATANE or for 2 months after cessation of therapy. This allows for elimination of acitretin, thus removing the substrate for transesterification to etretinate. The mechanism of the metabolic process for conversion of acitretin to etretinate has not been fully defined. It is not known whether substances other than ethanol are associated with transesterification. Acitretin has been shown to be embryotoxic and/or teratogenic in rabbits, mice, and rats at oral doses of 0.6, 3, and 15 mg/kg, respectively. These doses are approximately 0.2, 0.3, and 3 times the maximum recommended therapeutic dose, respectively, based on a mg/m^2 comparison.
Major human fetal abnormalities associated with acitretin and/or etretinate administration have been reported including meningomyelocele; meningoencephalocele; multiple synostoses; facial dysmorphia; syndactyly; absence of terminal phalanges; malformations of hip, ankle, and forearm; low-set ears; high palate; decreased cranial volume; cardiovascular malformation; and alterations of the skull and cervical vertebrae.
SORIATANE should be prescribed only by those who have special competence in the diagnosis and treat-

---

ment of severe psoriasis, are experienced in the use of systemic retinoids, and understand the risk of teratogenicity.
Because of the teratogenicity of SORIATANE, a program called the *Do Your P.A.R.T* program, Pregnancy Prevention Actively Required During and After Treatment, has been developed to educate women of childbearing potential and their healthcare providers about the serious risks associated with acitretin and to help prevent pregnancies from occurring with the use of this drug and for 3 years after its discontinuation. The *Do Your P.A.R.T.* program requirements are described below and program materials are available at www.soriatane.com/doyour-part-Program.html or may be requested by calling 1-888-784-3335 (1-888-STIEFEL). (see also PRECAUTIONS section).
Important Information for Women of Childbearing Potential:
SORIATANE should be considered only for women with severe psoriasis unresponsive to other therapies or whose clinical condition contraindicates the use of other treatments.
Females of reproductive potential must not be given a prescription for SORIATANE until pregnancy is excluded. SORIATANE is contraindicated in females of reproductive potential unless the patient meets ALL of the following conditions:
• Must have had 2 negative urine or serum pregnancy tests with a sensitivity of at least 25 mIU/mL before receiving the initial prescription for SORIATANE. The first test (a screening test) is obtained by the prescriber when the decision is made to pursue therapy with SORIATANE. The second pregnancy test (a confirmation test) should be done during the first 5 days of the menstrual period immediately preceding the beginning of therapy with SORIATANE. For patients with amenorrhea, the second test should be done at least 11 days after the last act of unprotected sexual intercourse (without using 2 effective forms of contraception [birth control] simultaneously).
• Must have a pregnancy test repeated every month during treatment with SORIATANE. The patient must have a negative result from a urine or serum pregnancy test before receiving a prescription for SORIATANE. To encourage compliance with this recommendation, a limited supply of the drug should be prescribed. For at least 3 years after discontinuing therapy with SORIATANE, a pregnancy test must be repeated every 3 months.
• Must have selected and have committed to use 2 effective forms of contraception (birth control) simultaneously, at least 1 of which must be a primary form, unless absolute abstinence is the chosen method, or the patient has undergone a hysterectomy or is clearly postmenopausal.
• Patients must use 2 effective forms of contraception (birth control) simultaneously for at least 1 month prior to initiation of therapy with SORIATANE, during therapy with SORIATANE, and for at least 3 years after discontinuing therapy with SORIATANE. A SORIATANE Referral Form is available so that patients can receive an initial free contraceptive counseling session and pregnancy testing. Counseling about contraception and behaviors associated with an increased risk of pregnancy must be repeated on a monthly basis by the prescriber during therapy with SORIATANE and every 3 months for at least 3 years following discontinuation of SORIATANE.
Effective forms of contraception include both primary and secondary forms of contraception. Primary forms of contraception include: tubal ligation, partner's vasectomy, intrauterine devices, birth control pills, and injectable/implantable/insertable/topical hormonal birth control products. Secondary forms of contraception include latex condoms (with or without spermicide), diaphragms and cervical caps (which must be used with a spermicide).
Any birth control method can fail. Therefore, it is critically important that women of childbearing potential use 2 effective forms of contraception (birth control) simultaneously. It has not been established if there is a pharmacokinetic interaction between acitretin and combined oral contraceptives. However, it has been established that acitretin interferes with the contraceptive effect of microdosed progestin preparations.[1] Microdosed "minipill" progestin preparations are not recommended for use with SORIATANE. *It is not known whether other progestational contraceptives, such as implants and injectables, are adequate methods of contraception during acitretin therapy.*
Prescribers are advised to consult the package insert of any medication administered concomitantly with hormonal contraceptives, since some medications may decrease the effectiveness of these birth control products. Patients should be prospectively cautioned not to self-medicate with the herbal supplement St. John's wort because a possible interaction has been suggested with hormonal contraceptives based on

reports of breakthrough bleeding on oral contraceptives shortly after starting St. John's wort. Pregnancies have been reported by users of combined hormonal contraceptives who also used some form of St. John's wort (see PRECAUTIONS).

- **Must have signed a Patient Agreement/Informed Consent for Female Patients** that contains warnings about the risk of potential birth defects if the fetus is exposed to SORIATANE, about contraceptive failure, about the fact that they must not ingest beverages or products containing ethanol while taking SORIATANE and for 2 months after SORIATANE treatment has been discontinued, and about preventing pregnancy while taking SORIATANE and for at least 3 years after discontinuing SORIATANE.

If pregnancy does occur during therapy with SORIATANE or at any time for at least 3 years following discontinuation of SORIATANE, the prescriber and patient should discuss the possible effects on the pregnancy. The available information is as follows:

Acitretin, the active metabolite of etretinate, is teratogenic and is contraindicated during pregnancy. The risk of severe fetal malformations is well established when systemic retinoids are taken during pregnancy. Pregnancy must also be prevented after stopping acitretin therapy, while the drug is being eliminated to below a threshold blood concentration that would be associated with an increased incidence of birth defects. Because this threshold has not been established for acitretin in humans and because elimination rates vary among patients, the duration of posttherapy contraception to achieve adequate elimination cannot be calculated precisely. It is strongly recommended that contraception be continued for at least 3 years after stopping treatment with acitretin, based on the following considerations:

- **In the absence of transesterification to form etretinate**, greater than 98% of the acitretin would be eliminated within 2 months, assuming a mean elimination half-life of 49 hours.
- **In cases where etretinate is formed, as has been demonstrated with concomitant administration of acitretin and ethanol,**
  - greater than 98% of the etretinate formed would be eliminated in 2 years, assuming a mean elimination half-life of 120 days.
  - greater than 98% of the etretinate formed would be eliminated in 3 years, based on the longest demonstrated elimination half-life of 168 days.

However, etretinate was found in plasma and subcutaneous fat in one patient reported to have had sporadic alcohol intake, 52 months after she stopped acitretin therapy.[2]

- Severe birth defects have been reported where conception occurred during the time interval when the patient was being treated with acitretin and/or etretinate. In addition, severe birth defects have also been reported when conception occurred after the mother completed therapy. These cases have been reported both prospectively (before the outcome was known) and retrospectively (after the outcome was known). The events below are listed without distinction as to whether the reported birth defects are consistent with retinoid-induced embryopathy or not.
  - There have been 318 prospectively reported cases involving pregnancies and the use of etretinate, acitretin or both. In 238 of these cases, the conception occurred after the last dose of etretinate (103 cases), acitretin (126 cases), or both (9). Fetal outcome remained unknown in approximately one-half of these cases, of which 62 were terminated and 14 were spontaneous abortions. Fetal outcome is known for the other 118 cases and 15 of the outcomes were abnormal (including cases of absent hand/wrist, clubfoot, GI malformation, hypocalcemia, hypotonia, limb malformation, neonatal apnea/anemia, neonatal ichthyosis, placental disorder/death, undescended testicle, and 5 cases of premature birth). In the 126 prospectively reported cases where conception occurred after the last dose of acitretin only, 43 cases involved conception at least 1 year but less than 2 years after the last dose. There were 3 reports of abnormal outcomes out of these 43 cases (involving limb malformation, GI tract malformations, and premature birth). There were only 4 cases where conception occurred at least 2 years after the last dose but there were no reports of birth defects in these cases.

- There is also a total of 35 retrospectively reported cases where conception occurred at least 1 year after the last dose of etretinate, acitretin or both. From these cases there are 3 reports of birth defects when the conception occurred at least 1 year but less than 2 years after the last dose of acitretin (including heart malformations, Turner's Syndrome, and unspecified congenital malformations) and 4 reports of birth defects when conception occurred 2 or more years after the last dose of acitretin (including foot malformation, cardiac malformations [2 cases], and unspecified neonatal and infancy disorder). There were 3 additional abnormal outcomes in cases where conception occurred 2 or more years after the last dose of etretinate (including chromosome disorder, forearm aplasia, and stillbirth).

- **Females who have taken TEGISON (etretinate) must continue to follow the contraceptive recommendations for TEGISON.** TEGISON is no longer marketed in the US; for information, call Stiefel at 1-888-784-3335 (1-888-STIEFEL).

- Patients should not donate blood during and for at least 3 years following the completion of therapy with SORIATANE because women of childbearing potential must not receive blood from patients being treated with SORIATANE.

Important Information For Males Taking SORIATANE:

- Patients should not donate blood during and for at least 3 years following therapy with SORIATANE because women of childbearing potential must not receive blood from patients being treated with SORIATANE.

- Samples of seminal fluid from 3 male patients treated with acitretin and 6 male patients treated with etretinate have been assayed for the presence of acitretin. The maximum concentration of acitretin observed in the seminal fluid of these men was 12.5 ng/mL. Assuming an ejaculate volume of 10 mL, the amount of drug transferred in semen would be 125 ng, which is 1/200,000 of a single 25 mg capsule. Thus, although it appears that residual acitretin in seminal fluid poses little, if any, risk to a fetus while a male patient is taking the drug or after it is discontinued, the no-effect limit for teratogenicity is unknown and there is no registry for birth defects associated with acitretin. The available data are as follows:

There have been 25 cases of reported conception when the male partner was taking acitretin. The pregnancy outcome is known in 13 of these 25 cases. Of these, 9 reports were retrospective and 4 were prospective (meaning the pregnancy was reported prior to knowledge of the outcome)[3].

Timing of Paternal Acitretin Treatment Relative to Conception	Delivery of Healthy Neonate	Spontaneous Abortion	Induced Abortion	Total
At time of conception	5[a]	5	1	11
Discontinued ~4 weeks prior	0	0	1[b]	1
Discontinued ~6 to 8 months prior	0	1	0	1

[a] Four of 5 cases were prospective.
[b] With malformation pattern not typical of retinoid embryopathy (bilateral cystic hygromas of neck, hypoplasia of lungs bilateral, pulmonary atresia, VSD with overriding truncus arteriosus).

For All Patients: A SORIATANE MEDICATION GUIDE MUST BE GIVEN TO THE PATIENT EACH TIME SORIATANE IS DISPENSED, AS REQUIRED BY LAW.

DESCRIPTION

SORIATANE (acitretin), a retinoid, is available in 10 mg, 17.5 mg, and 25 mg gelatin capsules for oral administration. Chemically, acitretin is all-trans-9-(4-methoxy-2,3,6-trimethylphenyl)-3,7-dimethyl-2,4,6,8-nonatetraenoic acid. It is a metabolite of etretinate and is related to both retinoic acid and retinol (vitamin A). It is a yellow to greenish-yellow powder with a molecular weight of 326.44. The structural formula is:

Each capsule contains acitretin, black monogramming ink, gelatin, maltodextrin (a mixture of polysaccharides), microcrystalline cellulose, and sodium ascorbate.

Gelatin capsule shells contain gelatin, iron oxide (yellow, black, and red), and titanium dioxide. They may also contain benzyl alcohol, carboxymethylcellulose sodium, edetate calcium disodium.

CLINICAL PHARMACOLOGY

The mechanism of action of SORIATANE is unknown.

Pharmacokinetics:

Absorption:

Oral absorption of acitretin is optimal when given with food. For this reason, acitretin was given with food in all of the following trials. After administration of a single 50 mg oral dose of acitretin to 18 healthy subjects, maximum plasma concentrations ranged from 196 to 728 ng/mL (mean: 416 ng/mL) and were achieved in 2 to 5 hours (mean: 2.7 hours). The oral absorption of acitretin is linear and proportional with increasing doses from 25 to 100 mg. Approximately 72% (range: 47% to 109%) of the administered dose was absorbed after a single 50 mg dose of acitretin was given to 12 healthy subjects.

Distribution:

Acitretin is more than 99.9% bound to plasma proteins, primarily albumin.

Metabolism

(See Pharmacokinetic Drug Interactions: Ethanol.)

Following oral absorption, acitretin undergoes extensive metabolism and interconversion by simple isomerization to its 13-cis form (cis-acitretin). The formation of cis-acitretin relative to parent compound is not altered by dose or fed/fast conditions of oral administration of acitretin. Both parent compound and isomer are further metabolized into chain-shortened breakdown products and conjugates, which are excreted. Following multiple-dose administration of acitretin, steady-state concentrations of acitretin and cis-acitretin in plasma are achieved within approximately 3 weeks.

Elimination:

The chain-shortened metabolites and conjugates of acitretin and cis-acitretin are ultimately excreted in the feces (34% to 54%) and urine (16% to 53%). The terminal elimination half-life of acitretin following multiple-dose administration is 49 hours (range: 33 to 96 hours), and that of cis-acitretin under the same conditions is 63 hours (range: 28 to 157 hours). The accumulation ratio of the parent compound is 1.2; that of cis-acitretin is 6.6.

Special Populations:

Psoriasis:

In an 8-week trial of acitretin pharmacokinetics in subjects with psoriasis, mean steady-state trough concentrations of acitretin increased in a dose-proportional manner with dosages ranging from 10 to 50 mg daily. Acitretin plasma concentrations were nonmeasurable (<4 ng/mL) in all subjects 3 weeks after cessation of therapy.

Elderly:

In a multiple-dose trial in healthy young (n = 6) and elderly (n = 8) subjects, a 2-fold increase in acitretin plasma concentrations were seen in elderly subjects, although the elimination half-life did not change.

Renal Failure:

Plasma concentrations of acitretin were significantly (59.3%) lower in subjects with end-stage renal failure (n = 6) when compared with age-matched controls, following single 50 mg oral doses. Acitretin was not removed by hemodialysis in these subjects.

Pharmacokinetic Drug Interactions

(see also boxed CONTRAINDICATIONS AND WARNINGS and PRECAUTIONS: Drug Interactions): In studies of in vivo pharmacokinetic drug interactions, no interaction was seen between acitretin and cimetidine, digoxin, phenprocoumon, or glyburide.

Ethanol:

Clinical evidence has shown that etretinate (a retinoid with a much longer half-life, see below) can be formed with concurrent ingestion of acitretin and ethanol. In a 2-way crossover trial, all 10 subjects formed etretinate with concurrent ingestion of a single 100 mg oral dose of acitretin during a 3-hour period of ethanol ingestion (total ethanol, approximately 1.4 g/kg body weight). A mean peak etretinate concentration of 59 ng/mL (range: 22 to 105 ng/mL) was observed, and extrapolation of AUC values indicated that the formation of etretinate in this trial was comparable to a single 5 mg oral dose of etretinate. There was no detectable formation of etretinate when a single 100 mg oral dose of acitretin was administered without concurrent ethanol ingestion, although the formation of etretinate without concurrent ethanol ingestion cannot be excluded (see boxed CONTRAINDICATIONS AND WARNINGS). Of 93 evaluable psoriatic subjects on acitretin therapy in several foreign trials (10 to 80 mg/day), 16% had measurable etretinate levels (>5 ng/mL).

Etretinate has a much longer elimination half-life compared with that of acitretin. In one trial the apparent mean terminal half-life after 6 months of therapy was approximately 120 days (range: 84 to 168 days). In another trial of 47 subjects treated chronically with etretinate, 5 had detectable serum drug levels (in the range of 0.5 to 12 ng/mL) 2.1 to 2.9 years after therapy was discontinued. The long half-life appears to be due to storage of etretinate in adipose tissue.

Progestin-only Contraceptives:

It has not been established if there is a pharmacokinetic interaction between acitretin and combined oral contraceptives. However, it has been established that acitretin interferes with the contraceptive effect of microdosed progestin preparations.[1] Microdosed "minipill" progestin preparations are *not* recommended for use with SORIATANE. *It is not known whether other progestational contraceptives, such as implants and injectables, are adequate methods of contraception during acitretin therapy.*

CLINICAL STUDIES

In 2 double-blind, placebo-controlled trials, SORIATANE was administered once daily to subjects with severe psoriasis (e.g., covering at least 10% to 20% of the body surface area). At 8 weeks (see Table 1) subjects treated in Trial A with 50 mg of SORIATANE per day showed significant improvements ($P \leq 0.05$) relative to baseline and to placebo in the physician's global evaluation and in the mean ratings of severity of psoriasis (scaling, thickness, and erythema). In Trial B, differences from baseline and from placebo were statistically significant ($P \leq 0.05$) for all variables at both the 25 mg and 50 mg doses; it should be noted for Trial B that no statistical adjustment for multiplicity was carried out. [See table 1 above]

A subset of 141 subjects from both pivotal Trials A and B continued to receive SORIATANE in an open fashion for up to 24 weeks. At the end of the treatment period, all efficacy variables, as indicated in Table 2, were significantly improved ($P \leq 0.01$) from baseline, including extent of psoriasis, mean ratings of psoriasis severity, and physician's global evaluation.

Table 2. Summary of the First Course of Therapy With SORIATANE (24 Weeks)

Variables	Trial A	Trial B
Mean Total Daily Dose of SORIATANE (mg)	42.8	43.1
Mean Duration of Therapy (Weeks)	21.1	22.6
Physician's Global Evaluation	N = 39	N = 98
Baseline	4.51	4.43
Mean Change From Baseline	-2.26[a]	-2.60[a]
Scaling	N = 59	N = 132
Baseline	3.97	4.07
Mean Change From Baseline	-2.15[a]	-2.42[a]
Thickness	N = 59	N = 132
Baseline	4.00	4.12
Mean Change From Baseline	-2.44[a]	-2.66[a]
Erythema	N = 59	N = 132
Baseline	4.35	4.33
Mean Change From Baseline	-2.31[a]	-2.29[a]

[a] Indicates that the difference from baseline was statistically significant ($P < 0.01$).
The efficacy variables consisted of: the mean severity rating of scale, lesion thickness, erythema, and the physician's global evaluation of the current status of the disease. Ratings of scaling, erythema, and lesion thickness, and the ratings of the global assessments were made using a 7-point scale (0 = none, 1 = trace, 2 = mild, 3 = mild-moderate, 4 = moderate, 5 = moderate-severe, 6 = severe).

Table 1. Summary of the Efficacy Results of the 8-Week Double-Blind Phase of Trials A and B of SORIATANE

Efficacy Variables	Trial A		Trial B		
	Total Daily Dose		Total Daily Dose		
	Placebo (N = 29)	50 mg (N = 29)	Placebo (N = 72)	25 mg (N = 74)	50 mg (N = 71)
Physician's Global Evaluation					
Baseline	4.62	4.55	4.43	4.37	4.49
Mean Change After 8 Weeks	-0.29	-2.00[a]	-0.06	-1.06[a]	-1.57[a]
Scaling					
Baseline	4.10	3.76	3.97	4.11	4.10
Mean Change After 8 Weeks	-0.22	-1.62[a]	-0.21	-1.50[a]	-1.78[a]
Thickness					
Baseline	4.10	4.10	4.03	4.11	4.20
Mean Change After 8 Weeks	-0.39	-2.10[a]	-0.18	-1.43[a]	-2.11[a]
Erythema					
Baseline	4.21	4.59	4.42	4.24	4.45
Mean Change After 8 Weeks	-0.33	-2.10[a]	-0.37	-1.12[a]	-1.65[a]

[a] Values were statistically significantly different from placebo and from baseline ($P < 0.05$). No adjustment for multiplicity was done for Trial B.
The efficacy variables consisted of: the mean severity rating of scale, lesion thickness, erythema, and the physician's global evaluation of the current status of the disease. Ratings of scaling, erythema, and lesion thickness, and the ratings of the global assessments were made using a 7-point scale (0 = none, 1 = trace, 2 = mild, 3 = mild-moderate, 4 = moderate, 5 = moderate-severe, 6 = severe).

All efficacy variables improved significantly in a subset of 55 subjects from Trial A treated for a second, 6-month maintenance course of therapy (for a total of 12 months of treatment); a small subset of subjects (n = 4) from Trial A continued to improve after a third 6-month course of therapy (for a total of 18 months of treatment).

INDICATIONS AND USAGE

SORIATANE is indicated for the treatment of severe psoriasis in adults. Because of significant adverse effects associated with its use, SORIATANE should be prescribed only by those knowledgeable in the systemic use of retinoids. In females of reproductive potential, SORIATANE should be reserved for non-pregnant patients who are unresponsive to other therapies or whose clinical condition contraindicates the use of other treatments (see boxed CONTRAINDICATIONS AND WARNINGS — SORIATANE can cause severe birth defects).

Most patients experience relapse of psoriasis after discontinuing therapy. Subsequent courses, when clinically indicated, have produced efficacy results similar to the initial course of therapy.

CONTRAINDICATIONS
Pregnancy Category X:
(See boxed CONTRAINDICATIONS AND WARNINGS.)
SORIATANE is contraindicated in patients with severely impaired liver or kidney function and in patients with chronic abnormally elevated blood lipid values (see boxed WARNINGS:Hepatotoxicity, WARNINGS:Lipids and Possible Cardiovascular Effects, and PRECAUTIONS).

An increased risk of hepatitis has been reported to result from combined use of methotrexate and etretinate. Consequently, the combination of methotrexate with SORIATANE is also contraindicated (see PRECAUTIONS: Drug Interactions).

Since both SORIATANE and tetracyclines can cause increased intracranial pressure, their combined use is contraindicated (see WARNINGS: Pseudotumor Cerebri).

SORIATANE is contraindicated in cases of hypersensitivity (e.g., angioedema, urticaria) to the preparation (acitretin or excipients) or to other retinoids.

WARNINGS
(See also boxed CONTRAINDICATIONS AND WARNINGS.)

Hepatotoxicity: Of the 525 subjects treated in US clinical trials, 2 had clinical jaundice with elevated serum bilirubin and transaminases considered related to treatment with SORIATANE. Liver function test results in these subjects returned to normal after SORIATANE was discontinued. Two of the 1,289 subjects treated in European clinical trials developed biopsy-confirmed toxic hepatitis. A second biopsy in one of these subjects revealed nodule formation suggestive of cirrhosis. One subject in a Canadian clinical trial of 63 subjects developed a 3-fold increase of transaminases. A liver biopsy of this subject showed mild lobular disarray, multifocal hepatocyte loss, and mild triaditis of the portal tracts compatible with acute reversible hepatic injury. The subject's transaminase levels returned to normal 2 months after SORIATANE was discontinued.

The potential of therapy with SORIATANE to induce hepatotoxicity was prospectively evaluated using liver biopsies in an open-label trial of 128 subjects. Pretreatment and posttreatment biopsies were available for 87 subjectss. A comparison of liver biopsy findings before and after therapy revealed 49 (58%) subjects showed no change, 21 (25%) improved, and 14 (17%) subjects had a worsening of their liver biopsy status. For 6 subjects, the classification changed from class 0 (no pathology) to class I (normal fatty infiltration; nuclear variability and portal inflammation; both mild); for 7 subjects, the change was from class I to class II (fatty infiltration, nuclear variability, portal inflammation, and focal necrosis; all moderate to severe); and for 1 subject, the change was from class II to class IIIb (fibrosis, moderate to severe). No correlation could be found between liver function test result abnormalities and the change in liver biopsy status, and no cumulative dose relationship was found.

Elevations of AST (SGOT), ALT (SGPT), GGT (GGTP) or LDH have occurred in approximately 1 in 3 subjects treated with SORIATANE. Of the 525 subjectss treated in clinical trials in the US, treatment was discontinued in 20 (3.8%) due to elevated liver function test results. If hepatotoxicity is suspected during treatment with SORIATANE, the drug should be discontinued and the etiology further investigated.

Ten of 652 subjects treated in US clinical trials of etretinate, of which acitretin is the active metabolite, had clinical or histologic hepatitis considered to be possibly or probably related to etretinate treatment. There have been reports of hepatitis-related deaths worldwide; a few of these subjects had received etretinate for a month or less before presenting with hepatic symptoms or signs.

Hyperostosis:
In adults receiving long-term treatment with SORIATANE, appropriate examinations should be periodically performed in view of possible ossification abnormalities (see ADVERSE REACTIONS). Because the frequency and severity of iatrogenic bony abnormality in adults is low, periodic radiography is only warranted in the presence of symptoms or long-term use of SORIATANE. If such disorders arise, the continuation of therapy should be discussed with the patient on the basis of a careful risk/benefit analysis. In clinical trials with SORIATANE, subjects were prospectively evaluated for evidence of development or change in bony abnormalities of the vertebral column, knees, and ankles.

Vertebral Results:
Of 380 subjects treated with SORIATANE, 15% had pre-existing abnormalities of the spine which showed new changes or progression of preexisting findings. Changes included degenerative spurs, anterior bridging of spinal vertebrae, diffuse idiopathic skeletal hyperostosis, ligament calcification, and narrowing and destruction of a cervical disc space. De novo changes (formation of small spurs) were seen in 3 subjects after 1½ to 2½ years.
Skeletal Appendicular Results:
Six of 128 subjects treated with SORIATANE showed abnormalities in the knees and ankles before treatment that progressed during treatment. In 5, these changes involved the formation of additional spurs or enlargement of existing spurs. The sixth subject had degenerative joint disease which worsened. No subjects developed spurs de novo. Clinical complaints did not predict radiographic changes.
Lipids and Possible Cardiovascular Effects:
Blood lipid determinations should be performed before SORIATANE is administered and again at intervals of 1 to 2 weeks until the lipid response to the drug is established, usually within 4 to 8 weeks. In subjects receiving SORIATANE during clinical trials, 66% and 33% experienced elevation in triglycerides and cholesterol, respectively. Decreased high density lipoproteins (HDL) occurred in 40% of subjects. These effects of SORIATANE were generally reversible upon cessation of therapy.
Subjects with an increased tendency to develop hypertriglyceridemia included those with disturbances of lipid metabolism, diabetes mellitus, obesity, increased alcohol intake, or a familial history of these conditions. Because of the risk of hypertriglyceridemia, serum lipids must be more closely monitored in high-risk patients and during long-term treatment.
Hypertriglyceridemia and lowered HDL may increase a patient's cardiovascular risk status. Although no causal relationship has been established, there have been post-marketing reports of acute myocardial infarction or thromboembolic events in patients on therapy with SORIATANE. In addition, elevation of serum triglycerides to greater than 800 mg/dL has been associated with fatal fulminant pancreatitis. Therefore, dietary modifications, reduction in dose of SORIATANE, or drug therapy should be employed to control significant elevations of triglycerides. If, despite these measures, hypertriglyceridemia and low HDL levels persist, the discontinuation of SORIATANE should be considered.
Ophthalmologic Effects:
The eyes and vision of 329 subjects treated with SORIATANE were examined by ophthalmologists. The findings included dry eyes (23%), irritation of eyes (9%), and brow and lash loss (5%). The following were reported in less than 5% of patients: Bell's Palsy, blepharitis and/or crusting of lids, blurred vision, conjunctivitis, corneal epithelial abnormality, cortical cataract, decreased night vision, diplopia, itchy eyes or eyelids, nuclear cataract, pannus, papilledema, photophobia, posterior subcapsular cataract, recurrent sties, and subepithelial corneal lesions.
Any patient treated with SORIATANE who is experiencing visual difficulties should discontinue the drug and undergo ophthalmologic evaluation.
Pancreatitis:
Lipid elevations occur in 25% to 50% of patients treated with SORIATANE. Triglyceride increases sufficient to be associated with pancreatitis are much less common, although fatal fulminant pancreatitis has been reported. There have been rare reports of pancreatitis during therapy with SORIATANE in the absence of hypertriglyceridemia.
Pseudotumor Cerebri:
SORIATANE and other retinoids administered orally have been associated with cases of pseudotumor cerebri (benign intracranial hypertension). Some of these events involved concomitant use of isotretinoin and tetracyclines. However,

the event seen in a single patient receiving SORIATANE was not associated with tetracycline use. Early signs and symptoms include papilledema, headache, nausea and vomiting, and visual disturbances. Patients with these signs and symptoms should be examined for papilledema and, if present, should discontinue SORIATANE immediately and be referred for neurological evaluation and care. Since both SORIATANE and tetracyclines can cause increased intracranial pressure, their combined use is contraindicated (see CONTRAINDICATIONS).
Capillary Leak Syndrome:
Capillary leak syndrome, a potential manifestation of retinoic acid syndrome, has been reported in patients receiving SORIATANE. Features of this syndrome may include localized or generalized edema with secondary weight gain, fever, and hypotension. Rhabdomyolysis and myalgias have been reported in association with capillary leak syndrome, and laboratory tests may reveal neutrophilia, hypoalbuminemia, and an elevated hematocrit. Discontinue SORIATANE if capillary leak syndrome develops during therapy.
Exfoliative Dermatitis/Erythroderma:
Exfoliative dermatitis/erythroderma has been reported in patients receiving SORIATANE. Discontinue SORIATANE if exfoliative dermatitis/erythroderma occurs during therapy.

PRECAUTIONS
A description of the *Do Your P.A.R.T.* materials is provided below. The main goals of the materials are to explain the program requirements, to reinforce the educational messages, and to assess program effectiveness.
The *Do Your P.A.R.T.* booklet includes:
• The *Do Your P.A.R.T. Patient Brochure:* information on the program requirements, risks of acitretin, and the types of contraceptive methods
• The Contraceptive Counseling Referral Form for female patients who want to receive free contraception counseling reimbursed by the manufacturer
• The Patient Agreement/Informed Consent Form for female patients
• Medication Guide
The *Do Your P.A.R.T.* program also includes a voluntary patient survey for women of childbearing potential to assess the effectiveness of the SORIATANE Pregnancy Prevention Program *Do Your P.A.R.T. Do Your P.A.R.T* Program materials are available at www.soriatane.com/doyour-part-Program.html or may be requested by calling 1-888-784-3335 (1-888-STIEFEL).
Information for Patients:
   (See Medication Guide for all patients and Patient Agreement/Informed Consent for Female Patients at end of professional labeling.)
Patients should be instructed to read the Medication Guide supplied as required by law when SORIATANE is dispensed.
Females of Reproductive Potential:
SORIATANE can cause severe birth defects. Female patients must not be pregnant when therapy with SORIATANE is initiated, they must not become pregnant while taking SORIATANE and for at least 3 years after stopping SORIATANE, so that the drug can be eliminated to below a blood concentration that would be associated with an increased incidence of birth defects. Because this threshold has not been established for acitretin in humans and because elimination rates vary among patients, the duration of posttherapy contraception to achieve adequate elimination cannot be calculated precisely (see boxed CONTRAINDICATIONS AND WARNINGS).

Females of reproductive potential should also be advised that they must not ingest beverages or products containing ethanol while taking SORIATANE and for 2 months after SORIATANE has been discontinued. This allows for elimination of the acitretin which can be converted to etretinate in the presence of alcohol.
Female patients should be advised that any method of birth control can fail, including tubal ligation, and that microdosed progestin "minipill" preparations are *not* recommended for use with SORIATANE (see CLINICAL PHARMACOLOGY: Pharmacokinetic Drug Interactions). Data from one patient who received a very low-dosed progestin contraceptive (levonorgestrel 0.03 mg) had a significant increase of the progesterone level after 3 menstrual cycles during acitretin treatment.[2]
Female patients should sign a consent form prior to beginning therapy with SORIATANE (see boxed CONTRAINDICATIONS AND WARNINGS).
Nursing Mothers:
Studies on lactating rats have shown that etretinate is excreted in the milk. There is one prospective case report where acitretin is reported to be excreted in human milk. Therefore, nursing mothers should not receive SORIATANE prior to or during nursing because of the potential for serious adverse reactions in nursing infants.

All Patients:
Depression and/or other psychiatric symptoms such as aggressive feelings or thoughts of self-harm have been reported. These events, including self-injurious behavior, have been reported in patients taking other systemically administered retinoids, as well as in patients taking SORIATANE. Since other factors may have contributed to these events, it is not known if they are related to SORIATANE. Patients should be counseled to stop taking SORIATANE and notify their prescriber immediately if they experience psychiatric symptoms.
Patients should be advised that a transient worsening of psoriasis is sometimes seen during the initial treatment period. Patients should be advised that they may have to wait 2 to 3 months before they get the full benefit of SORIATANE, although some patients may achieve significant improvements within the first 8 weeks of treatment as demonstrated in clinical trials.
Decreased night vision has been reported during therapy with SORIATANE. Patients should be advised of this potential problem and warned to be cautious when driving or operating any vehicle at night. Visual problems should be carefully monitored (see WARNINGS and ADVERSE REACTIONS). Patients should be advised that they may experience decreased tolerance to contact lenses during the treatment period and sometimes after treatment has stopped.
Patients should not donate blood during and for at least 3 years following therapy because SORIATANE can cause birth defects and women of childbearing potential must not receive blood from patients being treated with SORIATANE.
Because of the relationship of SORIATANE to vitamin A, patients should be advised against taking vitamin A supplements in excess of minimum recommended daily allowances to avoid possible additive toxic effects.
Patients should avoid the use of sun lamps and excessive exposure to sunlight (non-medical UV exposure) because the effects of UV light are enhanced by retinoids.
Patients should be advised that they must not give their SORIATANE to any other person.
For Prescribers:
SORIATANE has not been studied in and is not indicated for treatment of acne.
Phototherapy:
Significantly lower doses of phototherapy are required when SORIATANE is used because effects on the stratum corneum induced by SORIATANE can increase the risk of erythema (burning) (see DOSAGE AND ADMINISTRATION).
Drug Interactions:
Ethanol:
Clinical evidence has shown that etretinate can be formed with concurrent ingestion of acitretin and ethanol (see boxed CONTRAINDICATIONS AND WARNINGS and CLINICAL PHARMACOLOGY: Pharmacokinetics).
Glyburide:
In a trial of 7 healthy male volunteers, acitretin treatment potentiated the blood glucose-lowering effect of glyburide (a sulfonylurea similar to chlorpropamide) in 3 of the 7 subjects. Repeating the trial with 6 healthy male volunteers in the absence of glyburide did not detect an effect of acitretin on glucose tolerance. Careful supervision of diabetic patients under treatment with SORIATANE is recommended (see CLINICAL PHARMACOLOGY: Pharmacokinetics and DOSAGE AND ADMINISTRATION).
Hormonal Contraceptives:
It has not been established if there is a pharmacokinetic interaction between acitretin and combined oral contraceptives. However, it has been established that acitretin interferes with the contraceptive effect of microdosed progestin "minipill" preparations. Microdosed "minipill" progestin preparations are *not* recommended for use with SORIATANE (see CLINICAL PHARMACOLOGY: Pharmacokinetic Drug Interactions). *It is not known whether other progestational contraceptives, such as implants and injectables, are adequate methods of contraception during acitretin therapy.*
Methotrexate:
An increased risk of hepatitis has been reported to result from combined use of methotrexate and etretinate. Consequently, the combination of methotrexate with acitretin is also contraindicated (see CONTRAINDICATIONS).
Phenytoin:
If acitretin is given concurrently with phenytoin, the protein binding of phenytoin may be reduced.
Tetracyclines:
Since both acitretin and tetracyclines can cause increased intracranial pressure, their combined use is contraindicated (see CONTRAINDICATIONS and WARNINGS: Pseudotumor Cerebri).
Vitamin A and Oral Retinoids:
Concomitant administration of vitamin A and/or other oral retinoids with acitretin must be avoided because of the risk of hypervitaminosis A.

Table 3. Adverse Events Frequently Reported During Clinical Trials Percent of Subjects Reporting (N = 525)

Body System	>75%	50% to 75%	25% to 50%	10% to 25%
CNS				Rigors
Eye Disorders				Xerophthalmia
Mucous Membranes	Cheilitis		Rhinitis	Dry mouth Epistaxis
Musculoskeletal				Arthralgia Spinal hyperostosis (progression of existing lesions)
Skin and Appendages		Alopecia Skin peeling	Dry skin Nail disorder Pruritus	Erythematous rash Hyperesthesia Paresthesia Paronychia Skin atrophy Sticky skin

Other:
There appears to be no pharmacokinetic interaction between acitretin and cimetidine, digoxin, or glyburide. Investigations into the effect of acitretin on the protein binding of anticoagulants of the coumarin type (warfarin) revealed no interaction.

Laboratory Tests:
If significant abnormal laboratory results are obtained, either dosage reduction with careful monitoring or treatment discontinuation is recommended, depending on clinical judgment.

Blood Sugar:
Some patients receiving retinoids have experienced problems with blood sugar control. In addition, new cases of diabetes have been diagnosed during retinoid therapy, including diabetic ketoacidosis. In diabetics, blood-sugar levels should be monitored very carefully.

Lipids:
In clinical trials, the incidence of hypertriglyceridemia was 66%, hypercholesterolemia was 33%, and that of decreased HDL was 40%. Pretreatment and follow-up measurements should be obtained under fasting conditions. It is recommended that these tests be performed weekly or every other week until the lipid response to SORIATANE has stabilized (see WARNINGS).

Liver Function Tests:
Elevations of AST (SGOT), ALT (SGPT), or LDH were experienced by approximately 1 in 3 patients treated with SORIATANE. It is recommended that these tests be performed prior to initiation of therapy with SORIATANE, at 1- to 2-week intervals until stable, and thereafter at intervals as clinically indicated (see CONTRAINDICATIONS and boxed WARNINGS).

Carcinogenesis, Mutagenesis, Impairment of Fertility:
Carcinogenesis:
A carcinogenesis study of acitretin in Wistar rats, at doses up to 2 mg/kg/day administered 7 days/week for 104 weeks, has been completed. There were no neoplastic lesions observed that were considered to have been related to treatment with acitretin. An 80-week carcinogenesis study in mice has been completed with etretinate, the ethyl ester of acitretin. Blood level data obtained during this study demonstrated that etretinate was metabolized to acitretin and that blood levels of acitretin exceeded those of etretinate at all times studied. In the etretinate study, an increased incidence of blood vessel tumors (hemangiomas and hemangiosarcomas at several different sites) was noted in male, but not female, mice at doses approximately one-half the maximum recommended human therapeutic dose based on a mg/m² comparison.
Mutagenesis:
Acitretin was evaluated for mutagenic potential in the Ames test, in the Chinese hamster (V79/HGPRT) assay, in unscheduled DNA synthesis assays using rat hepatocytes and human fibroblasts, and in an in vivo mouse micronucleus assay. No evidence of mutagenicity of acitretin was demonstrated in any of these assays.
Impairment of Fertility:
In a fertility study in rats, the fertility of treated animals was not impaired at the highest dosage of acitretin tested, 3 mg/kg/day (approximately one-half the maximum recommended therapeutic dose based on a mg/m² comparison). Chronic toxicity studies in dogs revealed testicular changes (reversible mild to moderate spermatogenic arrest and appearance of multinucleated giant cells) in the highest dosage group (50 then 30 mg/kg/day).
No decreases in sperm count or concentration and no changes in sperm motility or morphology were noted in 31 men (17 psoriatic subjects, 8 subjects with disorders of keratinization, and 6 healthy volunteers) given 30 to 50 mg/day of acitretin for at least 12 weeks. In these trials, no del-

eterious effects were seen on either testosterone production, LH, or FSH in any of the 31 men.[4-6] No deleterious effects were seen on the hypothalamic-pituitary axis in any of the 18 men where it was measured.[4,5]

Pregnancy:
Teratogenic Effects:
Pregnancy Category X
(see boxed CONTRAINDICATIONS AND WARNINGS).
In a study in which acitretin was administered to male rats only at a dosage of 5 mg/kg/day for 10 weeks (approximate duration of one spermatogenic cycle) prior to and during mating with untreated female rats, no teratogenic effects were observed in the progeny (see boxed CONTRAINDICATIONS AND WARNINGS for information about male use of SORIATANE).
Nonteratogenic Effects:
In rats dosed at 3 mg/kg/day (approximately one-half the maximum recommended therapeutic dose based on a mg/m² comparison), slightly decreased pup survival and delayed incisor eruption were noted. At the next lowest dose tested, 1 mg/kg/day, no treatment-related adverse effects were observed.

Pediatric Use:
Safety and effectiveness in pediatric patients have not been established. No clinical trials have been conducted in pediatric subjects. Ossification of interosseous ligaments and tendons of the extremities, skeletal hyperostoses, decreases in bone mineral density, and premature epiphyseal closure have been reported in children taking other systemic retinoids, including etretinate, a metabolite of SORIATANE. A causal relationship between these effects and SORIATANE has not been established. While it is not known that these occurrences are more severe or more frequent in children, there is special concern in pediatric patients because of the implications for growth potential (see WARNINGS: Hyperostosis).

Geriatric Use:
Clinical trials of SORIATANE did not include sufficient numbers of subjects aged 65 and over to determine whether they respond differently than younger subjects. Other reported clinical experience has not identified differences in responses between the elderly and younger subjects. In general, dose selection for an elderly patient should be cautious, usually starting at the low end of the dosing range, reflecting the greater frequency of decreased hepatic, renal, or cardiac function, and of concomitant disease or other drug therapy. A 2-fold increase in acitretin plasma concentrations was seen in healthy elderly subjects compared with young subjects, although the elimination half-life did not change (see CLINICAL PHARMACOLOGY: Special Populations).

ADVERSE REACTIONS
Hypervitaminosis A produces a wide spectrum of signs and symptoms primarily of the mucocutaneous, musculoskeletal, hepatic, neuropsychiatric, and central nervous systems. Many of the clinical adverse reactions reported to date with administration of SORIATANE resemble those of the hypervitaminosis A syndrome.

Adverse Events/Postmarketing Reports:
In addition to the events listed in the tables for the clinical trials, the following adverse events have been identified during postapproval use of SORIATANE. Because these events are reported voluntarily from a population of uncertain size, it is not always possible to reliably estimate their frequency or establish a causal relationship to drug exposure.
Cardiovascular:
Acute myocardial infarction, thromboembolism (see WARNINGS), stroke
Immune System Disorders:
Hypersensitivity, including angioedema and urticaria (see CONTRAINDICATIONS).

Nervous System:
Myopathy with peripheral neuropathy has been reported during therapy with SORIATANE. Both conditions improved with discontinuation of the drug.
Psychiatric:
Aggressive feelings and/or suicidal thoughts have been reported. These events, including self-injurious behavior, have been reported in patients taking other systemically administered retinoids, as well as in patients taking SORIATANE. Since other factors may have contributed to these events, it is not known if they are related to SORIATANE (see PRECAUTIONS).
Reproductive:
Vulvo-vaginitis due to *Candida albicans*.
Skin and Appendages:
Thinning of the skin, skin fragility, and scaling may occur all over the body, particularly on the palms and soles; nail fragility is frequently observed. Madarosis and exfoliative dermatitis/erythroderma have been reported (see WARNINGS).
Vascular Disorders:
Capillary leak syndrome (see WARNINGS).
Clinical Trials:
During clinical trials with SORIATANE, 513/525 (98%) of subjects reported a total of 3,545 adverse events. One-hundred sixteen subjects (22%) left trials prematurely, primarily because of adverse experiences involving the mucous membranes and skin. Three subjects died. Two of the deaths were not drug-related (pancreatic adenocarcinoma and lung cancer); the other subject died of an acute myocardial infarction, considered remotely related to drug therapy. In clinical trials, SORIATANE was associated with elevations in liver function test results or triglyceride levels and hepatitis.
The tables below list by body system and frequency the adverse events reported during clinical trials of 525 subjects with psoriasis.
[See table 3 above]
[See table 4 at top of next page]
Laboratory:
Therapy with SORIATANE induces changes in liver function tests in a significant number of patients. Elevations of AST (SGOT), ALT (SGPT) or LDH were experienced by approximately 1 in 3 subjects treated with SORIATANE. In most subjects, elevations were slight to moderate and returned to normal either during continuation of therapy or after cessation of treatment. In subjects receiving SORIATANE during clinical trials, 66% and 33% experienced elevation in triglycerides and cholesterol, respectively. Decreased high density lipoproteins (HDL) occurred in 40% (see WARNINGS). Transient, usually reversible elevations of alkaline phosphatase have been observed.
Table 5 lists the laboratory abnormalities reported during clinical trials.
[See table 5 at top of page 2190]

OVERDOSAGE
In the event of acute overdosage, SORIATANE must be withdrawn at once. Symptoms of overdose are identical to acute hypervitaminosis A (e.g., headache and vertigo). The acute oral toxicity (LD$_{50}$) of acitretin in both mice and rats was greater than 4,000 mg/kg.
In one reported case of overdose, a 32-year-old male with Darier's disease took 21 × 25 mg capsules (525 mg single dose). He vomited several hours later but experienced no other ill effects.
All female patients of childbearing potential who have taken an overdose of SORIATANE must:
1) Have a pregnancy test at the time of overdose; 2) Be counseled as per the boxed CONTRAINDICATIONS AND WARNINGS and PRECAUTIONS sections regarding birth defects and contraceptive use for at least 3 years' duration after the overdose.

DOSAGE AND ADMINISTRATION
There is intersubject variation in the pharmacokinetics, clinical efficacy, and incidence of side effects with SORIATANE. A number of the more common side effects are dose-related. Individualization of dosage is required to achieve sufficient therapeutic response while minimizing side effects. Therapy with SORIATANE should be initiated at 25 to 50 mg per day, given as a single dose with the main meal. Maintenance doses of 25 to 50 mg per day may be given dependent upon an individual patient's response to initial treatment. Relapses may be treated as outlined for initial therapy.
When SORIATANE is used with phototherapy, the prescriber should decrease the phototherapy dose, dependent on the patient's individual response (see PRECAUTIONS: General).
Females who have taken TEGISON (etretinate) must continue to follow the contraceptive recommendations for TEGISON. TEGISON is no longer marketed in the US; for information, call Stiefel at 1-888-784-3335 (1-888-STIEFEL).

Information for Pharmacists:

A SORIATANE Medication Guide must be given to the patient each time SORIATANE is dispensed, as required by law.

HOW SUPPLIED:

Brown and white capsules, 10 mg, imprinted "A-10 mg"; bottles of 30 (NDC 0145-0090-25).
Rich yellow capsules, 17.5 mg, imprinted "A-17.5 mg"; bottles of 30 (NDC 0145-3817-03).
Brown and yellow capsules, 25 mg, imprinted "A-25 mg"; bottles of 30 (NDC 0145-0091-25).
Store between 15° and 25°C (59° and 77°F). Protect from light. Avoid exposure to high temperatures and humidity after the bottle is opened.

REFERENCES:

1. Berbis Ph, et al.: *Arch Dermatol Res* (1988) 280:388-389.
2. Maier H, Honigsmann H: Concentration of etretinate in plasma and subcutaneous fat after long-term acitretin. *Lancet* 348:1107, 1996.
3. Geiger JM, Walker M: Is there a reproductive safety risk in male patients treated with acitretin (Neotigason®/ Soriatane®)? *Dermatology* 205:105-107, 2002.
4. Sigg C, et al.: Andrological investigations in patients treated with etretin. *Dermatologica* 175:48-49, 1987.
5. Parsch EM, et al.: Andrological investigation in men treated with acitretin (Ro 10-1670). *Andrologia* 22:479-482, 1990.
6. Kadar L, et al.: Spermatological investigations in psoriatic patients treated with acitretin. In: Pharmacology of Retinoids in the Skin; Reichert U. et al., ed, KARGER, Basel, vol. 3, pp 253-254, 1988.

PATIENT AGREEMENT/INFORMED CONSENT FOR FEMALE PATIENTS

To be completed by the patient* and signed by her prescriber

CAUSES BIRTH DEFECTS

DO NOT GET PREGNANT

*Must also be initialed by the parent or guardian of a minor patient (under age 18)
Read each item below and initial in the space provided to show that you understand each item. **Do not sign this consent and do not take SORIATANE® (acitretin) if there is anything that you do not understand.**

_____
(Patient's name)
1. I understand that there is a very high risk that my unborn baby could have severe birth defects if I am pregnant or become pregnant while taking SORIATANE in any amount even for short periods of time. Birth defects have also happened in babies of women who became pregnant after stopping treatment with SORIATANE.
INITIAL: _____
2. I understand that I must not become pregnant while taking SORIATANE and for at least 3 years after the end of my treatment with SORIATANE.
INITIAL: _____
3. I know that I must avoid all alcohol, including drinks, food, medicines, and over-the-counter products that contain alcohol. I understand that the risk of birth defects may last longer than 3 years if I swallow any form of alcohol during therapy with SORIATANE, and for 2 months after I stop taking SORIATANE.
INITIAL: _____
4. I understand that I must not have sexual intercourse, or I must use 2 separate, effective forms of birth control **at the same time.** The only exceptions are if I have had surgery to remove the womb (a hysterectomy) or my prescriber has told me I have gone completely through menopause.
INITIAL: _____
5. I understand that I have to use 2 effective forms of birth control (contraception) at the same time for at least one month before starting SORIATANE, for the entire time of therapy with SORIATANE, and for at least 3 years after stopping SORIATANE.
INITIAL: _____
6. I understand that any form of birth control can fail. Therefore, I must use 2 different methods at the same time, every time I have sexual intercourse.
INITIAL: _____
7. I understand that the following are considered effective forms of birth control: Primary: Tubal ligation (having my tubes tied), partner's vasectomy, birth control pills, injectable/implantable/insertable/topical (patch) hormonal birth control products, and IUDs (intrauterine devices). Secondary: Latex condoms (with or without spermicide, which is a special cream or jelly that kills sperm), diaphragms and cervical caps (which must be used with a spermicide). I understand that at least 1 of my 2 methods of birth control must be a primary method.
INITIAL: _____
8. I will talk with my prescriber about any medicines or dietary supplements I plan to take while taking SORIATANE because certain birth control methods may not work if I am

Table 4. Adverse Events Less Frequently Reported During Clinical Trials (Some of Which May Bear No Relationship to Therapy) Percent of Subjects Reporting (N = 525)

Body System	1% to 10%		<1%	
Body as a Whole	Anorexia Edema Fatigue Hot flashes Increased appetite		Alcohol intolerance Dizziness Fever Influenza-like symptoms	Malaise Moniliasis Muscle weakness Weight increase
Cardiovascular	Flushing		Chest pain Cyanosis Increased bleeding time	Intermittent claudication Peripheral ischemia
CNS (also see Psychiatric)	Headache Pain		Abnormal gait Migraine Neuritis	Pseudotumor cerebri (intracranial hypertension)
Eye Disorders	Abnormal/ blurred vision Blepharitis Conjunctivitis/ irritation Corneal epithelial abnormality	Decreased night vision/night blindness Eye abnormality Eye pain Photophobia	Abnormal lacrimation Chalazion Conjunctival hemorrhage Corneal ulceration Diplopia Ectropion	Itchy eyes and lids Papilledema Recurrent sties Subepithelial corneal lesions
Gastrointestinal	Abdominal pain Diarrhea Nausea Tongue disorder		Constipation Dyspepsia Esophagitis Gastritis Gastroenteritis	Glossitis Hemorrhoids Melena Tenesmus Tongue ulceration
Liver and Biliary			Hepatic function abnormal Hepatitis Jaundice	
Mucous Membranes	Gingival bleeding Gingivitis Increased saliva	Stomatitis Thirst Ulcerative stomatitis	Altered saliva Anal disorder Gum hyperplasia	Hemorrhage Pharyngitis
Musculoskeletal	Arthritis Arthrosis Back pain Hypertonia Myalgia	Osteodynia Peripheral joint hyperostosis (progression of existing lesions)	Bone disorder Olecranon bursitis Spinal hyperostosis (new lesions) Tendonitis	
Psychiatric	Depression Insomnia Somnolence		Anxiety Dysphonia Libido decreased Nervousness	
Reproductive			Atrophic vaginitis Leukorrhea	
Respiratory	Sinusitis		Coughing Increased sputum Laryngitis	
Skin and Appendages	Abnormal skin odor Abnormal hair texture Bullous eruption Cold/clammy skin Dermatitis Increased sweating Infection	Psoriasiform rash Purpura Pyogenic granuloma Rash Seborrhea Skin fissures Skin ulceration Sunburn	Acne Breast pain Cyst Eczema Fungal infection Furunculosis Hair discoloration Herpes simplex Hyperkeratosis Hypertrichosis Hypoesthesia Impaired healing Otitis media	Otitis externa Photosensitivity reaction Psoriasis aggravated Scleroderma Skin nodule Skin hypertrophy Skin disorder Skin irritation Sweat gland disorder Urticaria Verrucae
Special Senses/ Other	Earache Taste perversion Tinnitus		Ceruminosis Deafness Taste loss	
Urinary			Abnormal urine Dysuria Penis disorder	

taking certain medicines or herbal products (for example, St. John's wort).
INITIAL: _____

9. Unless I have had a hysterectomy or my prescriber says I have gone completely through menopause, I understand that I must have 2 negative pregnancy test results before I can get a prescription to start SORIATANE. I will then have pregnancy tests on a monthly basis during therapy with SORIATANE as instructed by my prescriber. In addition, for at least 3 years after I stop taking SORIATANE, I will have a pregnancy test every 3 months.
INITIAL: _____

10. I understand that I should not start taking SORIATANE until I am *sure* that I am not pregnant and have negative results from 2 pregnancy tests.
INITIAL: _____

11. I have received information on emergency contraception (birth control).
INITIAL: _____

12. I understand that my prescriber can give me a referral for a free contraceptive (birth control) counseling session and pregnancy testing.
INITIAL: _____

13. I understand that on a monthly basis during therapy with SORIATANE and every 3 months for at least 3 years after stopping SORIATANE that I should receive counseling from my prescriber about contraception (birth control) and behaviors associated with an increased risk of pregnancy.
INITIAL: _____

14. I understand that I must stop taking SORIATANE right away and call my prescriber if I get pregnant, miss my menstrual period, stop using birth control, or have sexual intercourse without using my 2 birth control methods during and at least 3 years after stopping SORIATANE.
INITIAL: _____

15. If I do become pregnant while on SORIATANE or at any time within 3 years of stopping SORIATANE, I understand that I should report my pregnancy to Stiefel at 1-888-784-3335 (1-888-STIEFEL) or to the Food and Drug Administration (FDA) MedWatch program at 1-800-FDA-1088. The information I share will be kept confidential (private) and will help the company and the FDA evaluate the pregnancy prevention program to prevent birth defects.
INITIAL: _____

I have received a copy of the Do Your P.A.R.T™ brochure. My prescriber has answered all my questions about SORIATANE. I understand that it is my responsibility to follow my doctor's instructions, and not to get pregnant during treatment with SORIATANE or for at least 3 years after I stop taking SORIATANE.

I now authorize my prescriber, _____, to begin my treatment with SORIATANE.
Patient signature: _____
Date: _____
Parent/guardian signature (if under age 18): _____
Date: _____
Please print: Patient name and address:
_____
_____
Telephone: _____
I have fully explained to the patient, _____, the nature and purpose of the treatment described above and the risks to females of childbearing potential. I have asked the patient if she has any questions regarding her treatment with SORIATANE and have answered those questions to the best of my ability.
Prescriber signature: _____
Date: _____
Revised 05/2014
SRN:4PI

MEDICATION GUIDE
SORIATANE®
(sor-RYE-uh-tane)
(acitretin)
Capsules
Read this Medication Guide carefully before you start taking SORIATANE and read it each time you get more SORIATANE. There may be new information.
The first information in this Guide is about birth defects and how to avoid pregnancy. **After this section there is important safety information about possible effects for any patient taking SORIATANE.** ALL patients should read this entire Medication Guide carefully.
This information does not take the place of talking with your prescriber about your medical condition or treatment.
What is the most important information I should know about SORIATANE?
SORIATANE can cause serious side effects, including:
1. Severe birth defects. If you are a female who can get pregnant, you should use SORIATANE only if you are not pregnant now, can avoid becoming pregnant for at least 3 years, and other medicines do not work for your severe pso-

riasis or you cannot use other psoriasis medicines. Information about effects on unborn babies and about how to avoid pregnancy is found in the next section: "What are the important warnings and instructions for females taking SORIATANE?"

CAUSES BIRTH DEFECTS

DO NOT GET PREGNANT

2. Liver problems, including abnormal liver function tests and inflammation of your liver (hepatitis). Your prescriber should do blood tests to check how your liver is working before you start taking and during treatment with SORIATANE. Stop taking SORIATANE and call your prescriber right away if you have any of the following signs or symptoms of a serious liver problem:
• yellowing of your skin or the whites of your eyes
• nausea and vomiting
• loss of appetite
• dark urine
What are the important warnings and instructions for females taking SORIATANE?
• Before you receive your first prescription for SORIATANE, you should have discussed and signed a Patient Information/Consent form with your prescriber. This is to help make sure you understand the risk of birth defects and how to avoid getting pregnant. If you did not talk to your prescriber about this and sign the form, contact your prescriber.

• **You must not take SORIATANE if you are pregnant or might become pregnant during treatment or at any time for at least 3 years after you stop treatment because SORIATANE can cause severe birth defects.**
• **During treatment with SORIATANE and for 2 months after you stop treatment with SORIATANE, you must avoid drinks, foods, and all medicines that contain alcohol. This includes over-the-counter products that contain alcohol.** Avoiding alcohol is very important, because alcohol changes SORIATANE into a drug that may take longer than 3 years to leave your body. The chance of birth defects may last longer than 3 years if you swallow any form of alcohol during treatment with SORIATANE and for 2 months after you stop taking SORIATANE.
• **You and your prescriber must be sure you are not pregnant before you start therapy with SORIATANE. You must have negative results from 2 pregnancy tests before you start treatment with SORIATANE.** A negative result shows you are not pregnant. Because it takes a few days after pregnancy begins for a test to show that you are pregnant, the first negative test may not ensure you are not pregnant. Do not start SORIATANE until you have negative results from 2 pregnancy tests.
• The **first pregnancy test** will be done at the time you and your prescriber decide if SORIATANE might be right for you.
• The **second pregnancy test** will usually be done during the first 5 days of your menstrual period, right before you plan to start SORIATANE. Your prescriber may suggest another time.
• After you start taking SORIATANE, you must have a pregnancy test repeated each month that you are taking SORIATANE. This is to be sure that you are not pregnant during treatment because SORIATANE can cause birth defects.
• For at least 3 years after stopping treatment with SORIATANE, you must have a pregnancy test repeated every 3 months to make sure that you are not pregnant.

Body System	50% to 75%	25% to 50%	10% to 25%	1% to 10%
Electrolytes			Increased: –Phosphorus –Potassium –Sodium Increased and decreased: –Magnesium	Decreased: –Phosphorus –Potassium –Sodium Increased and decreased: –Calcium –Chloride
Hematologic		Increased: –Reticulocytes	Decreased: –Hematocrit –Hemoglobin –WBC Increased: –Haptoglobin –Neutrophils –WBC	Increased: –Bands –Basophils –Eosinophils –Hematocrit –Hemoglobin –Lymphocytes –Monocytes Decreased: –Haptoglobin –Lymphocytes –Neutrophils –Reticulocytes Increased or decreased: –Platelets –RBC
Hepatic		Increased: –Cholesterol –LDH –SGOT –SGPT Decreased: –HDL cholesterol	Increased: –Alkaline phosphatase –Direct bilirubin –GGTP	Increased: –Globulin –Total bilirubin –Total protein Increased and decreased: –Serum albumin
Miscellaneous	Increased: –Triglycerides	Increased: –CPK –Fasting blood sugar	Decreased: –Fasting blood sugar –High occult blood	Increased and decreased: –Iron
Renal			Increased: –Uric acid	Increased: –BUN –Creatinine
Urinary		WBC in urine	Acetonuria Hematuria RBC in urine	Glycosuria Proteinuria

Table 5. Abnormal Laboratory Test Results Reported During Clinical Trials Percent of Subjects Reporting

- Discuss effective birth control (contraception) with your prescriber. You must use 2 effective forms of birth control (contraception) at the same time during all of the following:
  - for at least 1 month before beginning treatment with SORIATANE
  - during treatment with SORIATANE
  - for at least 3 years after stopping treatment with SORIATANE
- If you are sexually active, you must use 2 effective forms of birth control (contraception) at the same time even if you think you cannot become pregnant, unless 1 of the following is true for you:
  - You had your womb (uterus) removed during an operation (a hysterectomy).
  - Your prescriber said you have gone completely through menopause (the "change of life").
- You can get a free birth control counseling session and pregnancy testing from a prescriber or family planning expert. Your prescriber can give you a SORIATANE Patient Referral Form for this free session.
- You must use 2 effective forms of birth control (contraception) at the same time while you are on treatment with SORIATANE. You must use birth control for at least 1 month before you start taking SORIATANE, during treatment, and at least 3 years after you stop treatment with SORIATANE.

The following are considered effective forms of birth control:

Primary Forms:
- having your tubes tied (tubal ligation)
- partner's vasectomy
- IUD (Intrauterine device)
- birth control pills that contain both estrogen and progestin (combination oral contraceptives)
- hormonal birth control products that are injected, implanted, or inserted in your body
- birth control patch

Secondary Forms (use with a Primary Form):
- diaphragms with spermicide
- latex condoms (with or without spermicide)
- cervical caps with spermicide

At least 1 of your 2 methods of birth control must be a primary form.

- If you have sex at any time without using 2 effective forms of birth control (contraception) at the same time, or if you get pregnant or miss your period, stop using SORIATANE and call your prescriber right away.
- Consider "Emergency Contraception" (EC) if you have sex with a male without correctly using 2 effective forms of birth control (contraception) at the same time. EC is also called "emergency birth control" or the "morning after" pill. Contact your prescriber **as soon as possible** if you have sex without using 2 effective forms of birth control (contraception) at the same time, because EC works best if it is used within 1 or 2 days after sex. EC is not a replacement for your usual 2 effective forms of birth control (contraception) because it is not as effective as regular birth control methods.

You can get EC from private doctors or nurse practitioners, women's health centers, or hospital emergency rooms. You can get the name and phone number of EC providers nearest you by calling the free Emergency Contraception Hotline at 1-888-668-2528 (1-888-NOT-2-LATE).

- Stop taking SORIATANE right away and contact your prescriber if you get pregnant while taking SORIATANE or at any time for at least 3 years after treatment has stopped. You need to discuss the possible effects on the unborn baby with your prescriber.
- If you do become pregnant while taking SORIATANE or at any time for at least 3 years after stopping SORIATANE, you should report your pregnancy to Stiefel Laboratories, Inc. at 1-888-784-3335 (1-888-STIEFEL) or directly to the Food and Drug Administration (FDA) MedWatch program at 1-800-FDA-1088. Your name will be kept in private (confidential). The information you share will help the FDA and the manufacturer evaluate the Pregnancy Prevention Program for SORIATANE.
- Do not take SORIATANE if you are breastfeeding. SORIATANE can pass into your milk and may harm your baby. You will need to choose either to breast feed or take SORIATANE, but not both.

What should males know before taking SORIATANE?
Small amounts of SORIATANE are found in the semen of males taking SORIATANE. Based upon available information, it appears that these small amounts of SORIATANE in semen pose little, if any, risk to an unborn child while a male patient is taking the drug or after it is discontinued. Discuss any concerns you have about this with your prescriber.

All patients should read the rest of this Medication Guide.
What is SORIATANE?
SORIATANE is a medicine used to treat severe forms of psoriasis in adults. Psoriasis is a skin disease that causes cells in the outer layer of the skin to grow faster than normal and

pile up on the skin's surface. In the most common type of psoriasis, the skin becomes inflamed and produces red, thickened areas, often with silvery scales.

Because SORIATANE can have serious side effects, you should talk with your prescriber about whether possible benefits of SORIATANE outweigh its possible risks. SORIATANE may not work right away. You may have to wait 2 to 3 months before you get the full benefit of SORIATANE. Psoriasis gets worse for some patients when they first start treatment with SORIATANE.
SORIATANE has not been studied in children.

Who should not take SORIATANE?
- **Do NOT take SORIATANE if you can get pregnant.** Do not take SORIATANE if you are pregnant or might get pregnant during SORIATANE treatment or at any time for **at least 3 years** after you stop SORIATANE treatment (see "What are the important warnings and instructions for females taking SORIATANE?").
- **Do NOT take SORIATANE if you are breastfeeding.** SORIATANE can pass into your milk and may harm your baby. You will need to choose either to breast feed or take SORIATANE, but not both.
- **Do NOT take SORIATANE if you have severe liver or kidney disease.**
- **Do NOT take SORIATANE if you have repeated high blood lipids (fat in the blood).**
- **Do NOT take SORIATANE if you take these medicines:**
  - methotrexate
  - tetracyclines

The use of these medicines with SORIATANE may cause serious side effects.
- **Do NOT take SORIATANE if you are allergic to acitretin,** the active ingredient in SORIATANE, to any of the other ingredients in SORIATANE (see the end of this Medication Guide for a list of all the ingredients in SORIATANE), or to any medicines that are like SORIATANE. Ask your prescriber or pharmacist if any medicines you are allergic to are like SORIATANE.

Tell your prescriber if you have or ever had:
- diabetes or high blood sugar
- liver problems
- kidney problems
- high cholesterol or high triglycerides (fat in the blood)
- heart disease
- depression
- alcoholism
- an allergic reaction to a medication

Your prescriber needs this information to decide if SORIATANE is right for you and to know what dose is best for you.

Tell your prescriber about all the medicines you take, including prescription and over-the-counter medicines, vitamins, and herbal supplements. Some medicines can cause serious side effects if taken while you also take SORIATANE. Some medicines may affect how SORIATANE works, or SORIATANE may affect how your other medicines work. **Be especially sure to tell your prescriber if you are taking the following medicines:**
- methotrexate
- tetracyclines
- glyburide
- phenytoin
- vitamin A supplements
- progestin-only oral contraceptives ("minipills")
- TEGISON® or TIGASON (etretinate). Tell your prescriber if you have ever taken this medicine in the past.
- St. John's wort herbal supplement

Tell your prescriber if you are getting phototherapy treatment. Your doses of phototherapy may need to be changed to prevent a burn.

How should I take SORIATANE?
- Take SORIATANE with food.
- Be sure to take your medicine as prescribed by your prescriber. The dose of SORIATANE varies from patient to patient. The number of capsules you must take is chosen specially for you by your prescriber. This dose may change during treatment.
- If you miss a dose, do not double the next dose. Skip the missed dose and resume your normal schedule.
- If you take too much SORIATANE (overdose), call your local poison control center or emergency room.

You should have blood tests for liver function, cholesterol, and triglycerides before starting treatment and during treatment to check your body's response to SORIATANE. Your prescriber may also do other tests.
Once you stop taking SORIATANE, your psoriasis may return. Do *not* treat this new psoriasis with leftover SORIATANE. It is important to see your prescriber again for treatment recommendations because your situation may have changed.

What should I avoid while taking SORIATANE?
- **Avoid pregnancy.** See "What is the most important information I should know about SORIATANE?", and "What are the important warnings and instructions for females taking SORIATANE?".

- **Avoid breastfeeding.** See "What are the important warnings and instructions for females taking SORIATANE?"
- **Avoid alcohol.** Females must avoid drinks, foods, medicines, and over-the-counter products that contain alcohol. The risk of birth defects may continue for longer than 3 years if you swallow any form of alcohol during treatment with SORIATANE and for 2 months after stopping SORIATANE (see "What are the important warnings and instructions for females taking SORIATANE?").
- **Avoid giving blood. Do not donate blood** while you are taking SORIATANE and **for at least 3 years after stopping** treatment with SORIATANE. SORIATANE in your blood can harm an unborn baby if your blood is given to a pregnant woman. SORIATANE does not affect your ability to receive a blood transfusion.
- **Avoid progestin-only birth control pills ("minipills").** This type of birth control pill may not work while you take SORIATANE. Ask your prescriber if you are not sure what type of pills you are using.
- **Avoid night driving if you develop any sudden vision problems.** Stop taking SORIATANE and call your prescriber if this occurs (see "Serious side effects").
- **Avoid non-medical ultraviolet (UV) light.** SORIATANE can make your skin more sensitive to UV light. Do not use sunlamps, and avoid sunlight as much as possible. If you are taking light treatment (phototherapy), your prescriber may need to change your light dosages to avoid burns.
- **Avoid dietary supplements containing vitamin A.** SORIATANE is related to vitamin A. Therefore, do not take supplements containing vitamin A, because they may add to the unwanted effects of SORIATANE. Check with your prescriber or pharmacist if you have any questions about vitamin supplements.
- **DO NOT SHARE SORIATANE with anyone else, even if they have the same symptoms.** Your medicine may harm them or their unborn child.

What are the possible side effects of SORIATANE?
SORIATANE can cause serious side effects. **See "What is the most important information I should know about SORIATANE?" and "What are the important warnings and instructions for females taking SORIATANE?"**
Stop taking SORIATANE and call your prescriber right away if you get the following signs or symptoms of possible serious side effects:
- **Bad headaches, nausea, vomiting, blurred vision.** These symptoms can be signs of increased brain pressure that can lead to blindness or even death.
- **Vision problems. Decreased vision in the dark (night blindness).** Since this can start suddenly, you should be very careful when driving at night. This problem usually goes away when SORIATANE treatment stops. Stop taking SORIATANE and call your prescriber if you develop any vision problems or eye pain.
- **Depression.** There have been some reports of patients developing mental problems including a depressed mood, aggressive feelings, or thoughts of ending their own life (suicide). These events, including suicidal behavior, have been reported in patients taking other drugs similar to SORIATANE as well as patients taking SORIATANE. Since other things may have contributed to these problems, it is not known if they are related to SORIATANE.
- **Aches or pains in your bones, joints, muscles, or back, trouble moving, or loss of feeling in your hands or feet.** These can be signs of abnormal changes to your bones or muscles.
- **Frequent urination, great thirst or hunger.** SORIATANE can affect blood sugar control, even if you do not already have diabetes. These are some of the signs of high blood sugar.
- **Shortness of breath, dizziness, nausea, chest pain, weakness, trouble speaking, or swelling of a leg. These may be signs of a heart attack, blood clots, or stroke.** SORIATANE can cause serious changes in blood fats (lipids). It is possible for these changes to cause blood vessel blockages that lead to heart attacks, strokes, or blood clots.
- **Blood vessel problems.** SORIATANE can cause fluid to leak out of your blood vessels into your body tissues. **Call your prescriber right away if you have any of the following symptoms:** sudden swelling in one part of your body or all over your body, rapid weight gain, fever, lightheadedness or feeling faint, or muscle aches. If this happens, your prescriber will tell you to stop taking SORIATANE.
- **Serious allergic reactions.** See "Who should not take SORIATANE?" Serious allergic reactions can happen during treatment with SORIATANE. **Call your prescriber right away if you get any of the following symptoms of an allergic reaction:** hives, itching, swelling of your face, mouth, or tongue, or problems breathing. **If this happens, stop taking SORIATANE and do not take it again.**
- **Serious skin problems.** SORIATANE can cause skin problems that can begin in a small area and then spread over large areas of your body. **Call your prescriber right away if your skin becomes red and swollen (inflamed), you have peeling of your skin, or your skin becomes itchy and painful. You should stop SORIATANE if this happens.**

Common side effects

If you develop any of these side effects or any unusual reaction, check with your prescriber to find out if you need to change the amount of SORIATANE you take. These side effects usually get better if the dose of SORIATANE is reduced or SORIATANE is stopped.

- **Chapped lips, peeling fingertips, palms, and soles, itching, scaly skin all over, weak nails, sticky or fragile (weak) skin, runny or dry nose, or nosebleeds.** Your prescriber or pharmacist can recommend a lotion or cream to help treat drying or chapping.
- **Dry mouth**
- **Joint pain**
- **Tight muscles**
- **Hair loss.** Most patients have some hair loss, but this condition varies among patients. No one can tell if you will lose hair, how much hair you may lose or if and when it may grow back. You may also lose your eyelashes.
- **Dry eyes.** SORIATANE may dry your eyes. Wearing **contact lenses** may be uncomfortable during and after treatment with SORIATANE because of the dry feeling in your eyes. If this happens, remove your contact lenses and call your prescriber. Also read the section about vision under "Serious side effects".
- **Rise in blood fats (lipids).** SORIATANE can cause your blood fats (lipids) to rise. Most of the time this is not serious. But sometimes the increase can become a serious problem (see information under "Serious side effects"). You should have blood tests as directed by your prescriber.

Psoriasis gets worse for some patients when they first start treatment with SORIATANE. Some patients have more redness or itching. If this happens, tell your prescriber. These symptoms usually get better as treatment continues, but your prescriber may need to change the amount of your medicine.

These are not all the possible side effects of SORIATANE. For more information, ask your prescriber or pharmacist. Call your doctor for medical advice about side effects. You may report side effects to FDA at 1-800-FDA-1088.

How should I store SORIATANE?

- Keep SORIATANE away from sunlight, high temperature, and humidity.
- Keep SORIATANE and all medicines out of the reach of children.

What are the ingredients in SORIATANE?

Active ingredient: acitretin.

Inactive ingredients: black monogramming ink, gelatin, maltodextrin (a mixture of polysaccharides), microcrystalline cellulose, and sodium ascorbate. Gelatin capsule shells contain gelatin, iron oxide (yellow, black, and red), and titanium dioxide. They may also contain benzyl alcohol, carboxymethylcellulose sodium, edetate calcium disodium.

General information about the safe and effective use of SORIATANE

Medicines are sometimes prescribed for purposes other than those listed in a Medication Guide. Do not use SORIATANE for a condition for which it was not prescribed. Do not give SORIATANE to other people, even if they have the same symptoms that you have.

This Medication Guide summarizes the most important information about SORIATANE. If you would like more information, talk with your prescriber. You can ask your pharmacist or prescriber for information about SORIATANE that is written for health professionals.

For more information about SORIATANE call 1-888-784-3335 or go to www.soriatane.com.

This Medication Guide has been approved by the U.S. Food and Drug Administration.

Manufactured for
Stiefel Laboratories, Inc.
Research Triangle Park, NC 27709
Revised 05/2014
TEGISON® is a registered trademark of Hoffmann-La Roche Inc.
Do Your P.A.R.T. is a trademark and SORIATANE is a registered trademark of Stiefel Laboratories, Inc.
©2014, Stiefel Laboratories, Inc.
SRN:4MG

SORILUX℞
[SOR-i-lux]
(calcipotriene)
foam, 0.005%, for topical use

HIGHLIGHTS OF PRESCRIBING INFORMATION
These highlights do not include all the information needed to use SORILUX safely and effectively. See full prescribing information for SORILUX.

SORILUX (calcipotriene) foam, 0.005%, for topical use
Initial U.S. Approval: 1993

---INDICATIONS AND USAGE---
SORILUX™ Foam is a vitamin D analog indicated for the topical treatment of plaque psoriasis of the scalp and body in patients 18 years and older. (1)

---DOSAGE AND ADMINISTRATION---
- For topical use only; not for oral, ophthalmic, or intravaginal use. (2)
- Apply twice daily. (2)

---DOSAGE FORMS AND STRENGTHS---
- 0.005%, foam

---CONTRAINDICATIONS---
- Do not use in patients with known hypercalcemia. (4)

---WARNINGS AND PRECAUTIONS---
- Contents are flammable. Instruct the patient to avoid fire, flame, and smoking during and immediately following application. (5.1)
- If elevation of serum calcium occurs, instruct patients to discontinue treatment until normal calcium levels are restored. (5.2)
- Avoid excessive exposure of the treated areas to natural or artificial sunlight. (5.3)

---ADVERSE REACTIONS---
Adverse reactions reported in ≥1% of subjects treated with SORILUX Foam and at a higher incidence than subjects treated with vehicle were application site erythema and application site pain. (6.1)

To report SUSPECTED ADVERSE REACTIONS, contact Stiefel Laboratories, Inc. at 1-888-784-3335 (1-888-STIEFEL) or FDA at 1-800-FDA-1088 or www.fda.gov/medwatch.

See 17 for PATIENT COUNSELING INFORMATION and FDA-approved patient labeling

Revised: 09/2013

FULL PRESCRIBING INFORMATION

1 INDICATIONS AND USAGE

SORILUX Foam is indicated for the topical treatment of plaque psoriasis of the scalp and body in patients 18 years and older.

2 DOSAGE AND ADMINISTRATION

SORILUX Foam is for topical use only. SORILUX Foam is not for oral, ophthalmic, or intravaginal use.

Apply a thin layer of SORILUX Foam twice daily to the affected areas and rub in gently and completely. Avoid contact with the face and eyes.

3 DOSAGE FORMS AND STRENGTHS

0.005%, white foam

4 CONTRAINDICATIONS

SORILUX Foam should not be used by patients with known hypercalcemia.

5 WARNINGS AND PRECAUTIONS

5.1 Flammability

The propellant in SORILUX Foam is flammable. Instruct the patient to avoid fire, flame, and smoking during and immediately following application.

5.2 Effects on Calcium Metabolism

Transient, rapidly reversible elevation of serum calcium has occurred with use of calcipotriene. If elevation in serum calcium outside the normal range should occur, discontinue treatment until normal calcium levels are restored.

5.3 Risk of Ultraviolet Light Exposure

Instruct the patient to avoid excessive exposure of the treated areas to either natural or artificial sunlight, including tanning booths and sun lamps. Physicians may wish to limit or avoid use of phototherapy in patients who use SORILUX Foam. [See Nonclinical Toxicology (13.1).]

6 ADVERSE REACTIONS

6.1 Clinical Trials Experience

Because clinical trials are conducted under widely varying conditions, adverse reaction rates observed in clinical trials of a drug cannot be directly compared with rates in the clinical trials of another drug and may not reflect the rates observed in clinical practice.

SORILUX Foam was studied in four vehicle-controlled trials. A total of 1094 subjects with plaque psoriasis, including 654 exposed to SORILUX Foam, were treated twice daily for 8 weeks.

Adverse reactions reported in ≥1% of subjects treated with SORILUX Foam and at a higher incidence than subjects treated with vehicle were application site erythema (2%) and application site pain (3%). The incidence of these adverse reactions was similar between the body and scalp.

7 DRUG INTERACTIONS

No drug interaction studies were conducted with SORILUX Foam.

8 USE IN SPECIFIC POPULATIONS

8.1 Pregnancy

Teratogenic Effects, Pregnancy Category C:

There are no adequate and well-controlled trials in pregnant women. Therefore, SORILUX Foam should be used during pregnancy only if the potential benefit justifies the potential risk to the fetus.

Studies of teratogenicity were done by the oral route where bioavailability is expected to be approximately 40-60% of the administered dose. Increased rabbit maternal and fetal toxicity was noted at 12 mcg/kg/day (132 mcg/m²/day). Rabbits administered 36 mcg/kg/day (396 mcg/m²/day) resulted in fetuses with a significant increase in the incidences of incomplete ossification of pubic bones and forelimb phalanges. In a rat study, doses of 54 mcg/kg/day (318 mcg/m²/day) resulted in a significantly higher incidence of skeletal abnormalities consisting primarily of enlarged fontanelles and extra ribs. The enlarged fontanelles are most likely due to calcitriene's effect upon calcium metabolism. The maternal and fetal no-effect exposures in the rat (43.2 mcg/m²/day) and rabbit (17.6 mcg/m²/day) studies are approximately equal to the expected human systemic exposure level (18.5 mcg/m²/day) from dermal application.

8.3 Nursing Mothers

It is not known whether calcipotriene is excreted in human milk. Because many drugs are excreted in human milk, caution should be exercised when SORILUX Foam is administered to a nursing woman.

8.4 Pediatric Use

Safety and effectiveness of SORILUX Foam in pediatric patients less than 18 years of age have not been established.

8.5 Geriatric Use

Clinical trials of SORILUX Foam did not include sufficient numbers of subjects aged 65 and over to determine whether they respond differently from younger subjects. Other reported clinical experience has not identified differences in responses between the elderly and younger patients.

8.6 Unevaluated Uses

SORILUX Foam has not been evaluated in patients with erythrodermic, exfoliative, or pustular psoriasis.

10 OVERDOSAGE

Topically applied calcipotriene can be absorbed in sufficient amounts to produce systemic effects. Elevated serum calcium has been observed with use of topical calcipotriene [See Warnings and Precautions (5.2).]

11 DESCRIPTION

SORILUX Foam contains the compound calcipotriene, a synthetic vitamin D_3 analog.

Chemically, calcipotriene is (5Z,7E,22E,24S)-24-cyclopropyl-9,10-secochola-5,7,10(19), 22-tetraene-1α,3β,24-triol. The structural formula is represented below:

[See chemical structure at top of next column]

Calcipotriene is a white or off-white crystalline substance. SORILUX Foam contains calcipotriene 50 mcg/g in an aqueous-based emulsion foam vehicle consisting of cetyl alcohol, dibasic sodium phosphate, dl-α-tocopherol, edetate disodium, isopropyl myristate, light mineral oil, polyoxyl 20 cetostearyl ether, propylene glycol, purified water, stearyl alcohol, and white petrolatum. SORILUX Foam is dispensed from an aluminum can pressurized with a hydrocarbon (propane/n-butane/isobutane) propellant.

Molecular Formula: $C_{27}H_{40}O_3$ Molecular Weight: 412.6

12 CLINICAL PHARMACOLOGY

12.1 Mechanism of Action

Calcipotriene is a synthetic vitamin D_3 analog that has a similar receptor binding affinity as natural vitamin D_3. However, the exact mechanism of action contributing to the clinical efficacy in the treatment of psoriasis is unknown.

12.2 Pharmacodynamics

The pharmacodynamics of SORILUX Foam are unknown.

12.3 Pharmacokinetics

The systemic absorption of calcipotriene in subjects with psoriasis of the body was evaluated at steady state following application of either SORILUX Foam or calcipotriene ointment to a body surface area of 5% to 10%. In the SORILUX Foam treatment group, 15 out of 16 subjects had calcipotriene plasma concentrations below the limit of quantitation (10 pg/mL), while in the calcipotriene ointment treated group, 5 out of 16 subjects had measurable calcipotriene plasma concentrations at various time points. All measurable plasma calcipotriene concentrations were below 25 pg/mL.

The systemic disposition of calcipotriene is expected to be similar to that of the naturally occurring vitamin D. Absorbed calcipotriene is known to be converted to inactive metabolites within 24 hours of application and the metabolism occurs via a similar pathway to the natural hormone.

13 NONCLINICAL TOXICOLOGY

13.1 Carcinogenesis, Mutagenesis, Impairment of Fertility

Carcinogenesis: Calcipotriene topically administered to mice for up to 24 months at dose levels of 3, 10, or 30 mcg /kg/day (corresponding to 9, 30, or 90 mcg /m^2/day) showed no significant changes in tumor incidence when compared with controls. In a study in which albino hairless mice were exposed to both UVR and topically applied calcipotriene, a reduction in the time required for UVR to induce the formation of skin tumors was observed (statistically significant in males only), suggesting that calcipotriene may enhance the effect of UVR to induce skin tumors [See Warnings and Precautions (5.3).]

Mutagenesis: The genotoxic potential of calcipotriene was evaluated in an Ames assay, a mouse lymphoma TK locus assay, a human lymphocyte chromosome aberration assay, and a mouse micronucleus assay. All assay results were negative.

Impairment of Fertility: Studies in rats at doses up to 54 mcg /kg/day (318 mcg /m^2/day) of calcipotriene indicated no impairment of fertility or general reproductive performance.

14 CLINICAL STUDIES

In two multi-center, randomized, double-blind, vehicle-controlled clinical trials a total of 659 subjects with psoriasis were randomized 2:1 to SORILUX Foam or vehicle; subjects applied the assigned treatment twice daily for 8 weeks. Baseline disease severity was graded using a 5-point Investigator Static Global Assessment scale (ISGA), on which subjects scored either "mild" or "moderate" as shown in Table 1.

Table 1. Investigator Static Global Assessment (ISGA) Scale for Body

Disease Severity	Grade	Definition
Clear	0	No evidence of scaling, erythema, or plaque thickness
Almost clear	1	Occasional fine scale, faint erythema, and barely perceptible plaque thickness
Mild	2	Fine scale with light coloration and mild plaque elevation
Moderate	3	Coarse scale with moderate red coloration and moderate plaque thickness
Severe	4	Thick tenacious scale with deep coloration and severe plaque thickness

Efficacy evaluation was carried out at Week 8 with treatment success being defined as a score of "clear" (grade 0) or "almost clear" (grade 1) and at least 2 grade improvement from the baseline score. Approximately 30% of enrolled subjects were graded as "mild" on the ISGA scale. The study population ranged in age from 12 to 89 years with 10 subjects less than 18 years of age at baseline. The subjects were 54% male and 88% Caucasian. Table 2 presents the efficacy results for each trial.

[See table 2 above]

In one trial, subjects graded as "mild" at baseline showed a greater response to vehicle than SORILUX Foam.

Table 3 presents the success rates by disease severity at baseline for each trial.

[See table 3 above]

In another multi-center, randomized, double-blind, vehicle-controlled clinical trial, a total of 363 subjects with moderate plaque psoriasis of the scalp and body were randomized 1:1 to SORILUX Foam or vehicle. Subjects applied the assigned treatment to the affected areas twice daily for 8 weeks. Baseline disease severity of the scalp was graded using a 6-point ISGA; a score of "moderate" corresponded to grade 3.

The primary efficacy evaluation for scalp involvement was carried out at Week 8 with treatment success being defined as a score of "clear" (grade 0) or "almost clear" (grade 1). The study population ranged in age from 12 to 97 years with 11 subjects less than 18 years of age at baseline. The subjects were 60% male and 87% Caucasian. Table 4 presents the efficacy results for the trial.

Table 2. Number and Percent of Subjects Achieving Success for Body at Week 8 in Each Trial

	Trial 1		Trial 2	
	SORILUX Foam N = 223	Vehicle Foam N = 113	SORILUX Foam N = 214	Vehicle Foam N = 109
Number (%) of Subjects with Treatment Success	31 (14%)	8 (7%)	58 (27%)	17 (16%)

Table 3. Number and Percent of Subjects Achieving Success for Body by Baseline ISGA Score and by Trial

	Trial 1		Trial 2	
ISGA Scores at Baseline	SORILUX Foam (N = 223)	Vehicle Foam (N = 113)	SORILUX Foam (N = 214)	Vehicle Foam (N = 109)
Mild	2/73 (2.7%)	3/34 (8.8%)	8/56 (14.3%)	4/31 (12.9%)
Moderate	29/150 (19.3%)	5/79 (6.3%)	50/158 (31.6%)	13/78 (16.7%)

Table 4. Number and Percent of Subjects Achieving Success for Scalp at Week 8

	Trial 3	
	SORILUX Foam N = 181	Vehicle Foam N = 182
Number (%) of Subjects with Treatment Success	74 (41%)	44 (24%)

The contribution to efficacy of individual components of the vehicle has not been established.

16 HOW SUPPLIED/STORAGE AND HANDLING

16.1 How Supplied

SORILUX (calcipotriene) Foam, 0.005%, is supplied as follows:

60 g aluminum can	NDC 0145-2130-06
120 g aluminum can	NDC 0145-2130-07

16.2 Storage and Handling

• Store at 20°C to 25°C (68°F to 77°F); excursions permitted to 15°C – 30°C (59°F –86°F).
• Flammable. Contents under pressure. Do not puncture or incinerate. Do not expose to heat or store at temperatures above 120°F (49°C).
• Keep out of reach of children.

17 PATIENT COUNSELING INFORMATION

See FDA-approved patient labeling (Patient Information)
Inform the patient to adhere to the following instructions:
• Avoid excessive exposure of the treated areas to either natural or artificial sunlight, including tanning beds and sun lamps.
• Avoid contact with the face and eyes. If SORILUX Foam gets on the face or in or near their eyes, rinse thoroughly with water.
• Apply SORILUX Foam to the scalp when the hair is dry.
• Talk to your doctor if your skin does not improve after treatment with SORILUX Foam for 8 weeks.
• Wash your hands after applying SORILUX Foam unless your hands are the affected site.
• Avoid fire, flame, and smoking during and immediately following application since SORILUX Foam is flammable.
• Do not place SORILUX Foam in the refrigerator or freezer.
SORILUX is a trademark of Stiefel Laboratories, Inc.
Manufactured for
Stiefel Laboratories, Inc.
Research Triangle Park, NC 27709
©2013, Stiefel Laboratories, Inc.
SOR:6PI

PHARMACIST—DETACH HERE AND GIVE INSTRUCTIONS TO PATIENT

Patient Information
SORILUX (SOR-i-lux)
(calcipotriene)
Foam

Important: For skin use only. Do not get SORILUX Foam on your face or in your eyes, mouth, or vagina.

Read the Patient Information before you start using SORILUX Foam and each time you get a refill. There may be new information. This information does not take the place of talking with your doctor about your medical condition or treatment.

What is SORILUX Foam?

SORILUX Foam is a prescription medicine used on the skin (topical) to treat plaque psoriasis of the scalp and body in people 18 years and older.

It is not known if SORILUX Foam is safe and effective in people under 18 years old.

Who should not use SORILUX Foam?

Do not use SORILUX Foam if you have been told by your doctor that you have a high level of calcium in your blood (hypercalcemia).

What should I tell my doctor before using SORILUX Foam?

Before you use SORILUX Foam, tell your doctor if you:
• are getting light therapy for your psoriasis
• have any other medical conditions
• are pregnant or planning to become pregnant. It is not known if SORILUX Foam can harm your unborn baby. Talk to your doctor if you are pregnant or plan to become pregnant.
• are breastfeeding. It is not known if SORILUX Foam passes into breast milk. Do not apply SORILUX Foam to the chest area if you are breastfeeding a baby. This will help to prevent the baby from accidentally getting SORILUX Foam into their mouth.

Tell your doctor about all the medicines you take, including prescription and nonprescription medicines, vitamins, and herbal supplements.

Know the medicines you take. Keep a list of your medicines with you to show your doctor and pharmacist when you get a new medicine.

How should I use SORILUX Foam?

• Apply SORILUX Foam exactly as prescribed. SORILUX Foam is usually applied to the affected skin areas two times each day.
• SORILUX Foam is for use on the skin only. Do not get SORILUX Foam in your eyes, mouth, or vagina.
• SORILUX Foam is flammable. Avoid fire, flame, or smoking during and right after you apply SORILUX Foam to your skin.

- Avoid excessive natural or artificial sunlight including tanning booths and sunlamps. Wear a hat and clothes that cover the treated areas of your skin if you have to be in sunlight.

Instructions for applying SORILUX Foam

1. Before applying SORILUX Foam for the first time, break the tiny plastic piece at the base of the can's rim by gently pushing back (away from the piece) on the nozzle. See Figure A.

Figure A

2. Shake the can of SORILUX Foam before use. See Figure B.

Figure B

3. Turn the can of SORILUX Foam upside down and press the nozzle. See Figure C.

Figure C

4. Dispense a small amount of SORILUX Foam into the palm of your hand. See Figure D.

Figure D

5. Use enough SORILUX Foam to cover the affected area with a thin layer. Apply SORILUX Foam to your scalp when your hair is dry. Part your hair and apply directly on the affected area. Gently rub the foam into the affected area until it disappears into the skin. See Figures E, F and G.

Figure E

Figure F

Figure G

6. Avoid getting SORILUX Foam on your face or in or near the eyes, mouth, or vagina. If SORILUX Foam gets on your face or in or near your eyes, rinse with water. Wash hands after applying SORILUX Foam unless your hands are a treated area.

What are the possible side effects of SORILUX Foam?

The most common side effects of SORILUX Foam are redness and pain of the treated skin areas.

Tell your doctor if you have any side effect that bothers you or that does not go away.

These are not all the possible side effects of SORILUX Foam. Ask your doctor or pharmacist for more information. Call your doctor for medical advice about side effects. You may report side effects to FDA at 1-800-FDA-1088.

You may also report side effects to Stiefel Laboratories, Inc. at 1-888-784-3335.

How should I store SORILUX Foam?

- Store SORILUX Foam at room temperature, between 68°F to 77°F (20C° to 25°C).
- SORILUX Foam is flammable. Keep the can away from all sources of fire and heat.
- Do not spray SORILUX Foam near fire or direct heat. Never throw the can into a fire, even if the can is empty.
- Do not puncture the can of SORILUX Foam.

Keep SORILUX Foam and all medicines out of the reach of children.

General Information about SORILUX Foam

Medicines are sometimes prescribed for purposes other than those listed in Patient Information leaflets. Do not use SORILUX Foam for a condition for which it was not prescribed. Do not give SORILUX Foam to other people even if they have the same symptoms that you have. It may harm them.

This Patient Information leaflet summarizes the most important information about SORILUX Foam. If you would like more information, talk with your doctor. You can ask your doctor or pharmacist for information about SORILUX Foam that is written for health professionals.

What are the ingredients of SORILUX Foam?

Active ingredient: calcipotriene

Inactive ingredients: cetyl alcohol, dibasic sodium phosphate, dl-α-tocopherol, edetate disodium, isopropyl myristate, light mineral oil, polyoxyl 20 cetostearyl ether, propylene glycol, purified water, stearyl alcohol, and white petrolatum. The foam is dispensed from an aluminum can pressurized with a hydrocarbon (propane/n-butane/isobutane) propellant.

This Patient Information has been approved by the U.S. Food and Drug Administration.

SORILUX is a trademark of Stiefel Laboratories, Inc.

Manufactured for:
Stiefel Laboratories, Inc.
Research Triangle Park, NC 27709
©2013, Stiefel Laboratories, Inc
September 2013
SOR:6PIL

VELTIN®   ℞
[vel-tin]
(clindamycin phosphate and tretinoin)
Gel 1.2%/0.025%
For topical use only

HIGHLIGHTS OF PRESCRIBING INFORMATION
These highlights do not include all the information needed to use VELTIN Gel safely and effectively. See full prescribing information for VELTIN Gel.
VELTIN (clindamycin phosphate and tretinoin) Gel 1.2%/0.025%
For topical use only
Initial U.S. Approval: 2006

————INDICATIONS AND USAGE————
- VELTIN Gel is a lincosamide antibiotic and retinoid combination product indicated for the topical treatment of acne vulgaris in patients 12 years and older. (1)

————DOSAGE AND ADMINISTRATION————
- Apply a pea-sized amount once daily in the evening lightly covering the entire affected area. Avoid the eyes, lips, and mucous membranes. (2)

- Not for oral, ophthalmic, or intravaginal use. (2)

————DOSAGE FORMS AND STRENGTHS————
- Topical gel: clindamycin phosphate 1.2% and tretinoin 0.025% in 30-gram and 60-gram tubes. (3)

————CONTRAINDICATIONS————
- VELTIN Gel is contraindicated in patients with regional enteritis, ulcerative colitis, or history of antibiotic-associated colitis. (4)

————WARNINGS AND PRECAUTIONS————
- Colitis: Clindamycin can cause severe colitis, which may result in death. Diarrhea, bloody diarrhea, and colitis (including pseudomembranous colitis) have been reported with the use of clindamycin. VELTIN Gel should be discontinued if significant diarrhea occurs. (5.1)
- Ultraviolet Light and Environmental Exposure: Avoid exposure to sunlight, sunlamps, and weather extremes. Wear sunscreen daily. (5.2)

————ADVERSE REACTIONS————
Observed local treatment-related adverse reactions (≥ 1%) in clinical trials with VELTIN Gel were application site reactions, including dryness, irritation, exfoliation, erythema, pruritus, and dermatitis. Sunburn was also reported. (6.1)
To report SUSPECTED ADVERSE REACTIONS, contact Stiefel Laboratories, Inc. at 1-888-784-3335 or FDA at 1-800-FDA-1088 or www.fda.gov/medwatch.

————DRUG INTERACTIONS————
- VELTIN Gel should not be used in combination with erythromycin-containing products because of its clindamycin component. (7.1)

————USE IN SPECIFIC POPULATIONS————
- Pediatric Use: The efficacy and safety have not been established in pediatric patients younger than 12 years. (8.4)

See 17 for PATIENT COUNSELING INFORMATION and FDA-approved patient labeling

Revised: 03/2014

FULL PRESCRIBING INFORMATION

1   INDICATIONS AND USAGE

VELTIN® (clindamycin phosphate and tretinoin) Gel, 1.2%/0.025% is indicated for the topical treatment of acne vulgaris in patients 12 years and older.

2   DOSAGE AND ADMINISTRATION

VELTIN Gel should be applied once daily in the evening, gently rubbing the medication to lightly cover the entire affected area. Approximately a pea-sized amount will be needed for each application. Avoid the eyes, lips, and mucous membranes.
VELTIN Gel is not for oral, ophthalmic, or intravaginal use.

3   DOSAGE FORMS AND STRENGTHS

VELTIN Gel, containing clindamycin phosphate 1.2% and tretinoin 0.025%, is a yellow, opaque topical gel. Each gram of VELTIN Gel contains, as dispensed, 10 mg (1%) clindamycin as clindamycin phosphate, and 0.25 mg (0.025%) tretinoin solubilized in an aqueous-based gel.

4 CONTRAINDICATIONS

VELTIN Gel is contraindicated in patients with regional enteritis, ulcerative colitis, or history of antibiotic-associated colitis.

5 WARNINGS AND PRECAUTIONS

5.1 Colitis

Systemic absorption of clindamycin has been demonstrated following topical use. Diarrhea, bloody diarrhea, and colitis (including pseudomembranous colitis) have been reported with the use of topical clindamycin. If significant diarrhea occurs, VELTIN Gel should be discontinued.

Severe colitis has occurred following oral or parenteral administration of clindamycin with an onset of up to several weeks following cessation of therapy. Antiperistaltic agents such as opiates and diphenoxylate with atropine may prolong and/or worsen severe colitis. Severe colitis may result in death.

Studies indicate a toxin(s) produced by clostridia is one primary cause of antibiotic-associated colitis. The colitis is usually characterized by severe persistent diarrhea and severe abdominal cramps and may be associated with the passage of blood and mucus. Stool cultures for *Clostridium difficile* and stool assay for *C. difficile* toxin may be helpful diagnostically.

5.2 Ultraviolet Light and Environmental Exposure

Exposure to sunlight, including sunlamps, should be avoided during the use of VELTIN Gel. Patients with sunburn should be advised not to use the product until fully recovered because of heightened susceptibility to sunlight as a result of the use of tretinoin. Patients who are required to have considerable sun exposure due to occupation and those with inherent sensitivity to the sun should exercise particular caution. For purposes of comparison of the sun should exercise particular caution. Daily use of sunscreen products and protective apparel (e.g., a hat) are recommended. Weather extremes, such as wind or cold, also may be irritating to patients under treatment with VELTIN Gel.

6 ADVERSE REACTIONS

6.1 Adverse Reactions in Clinical Trials

Because clinical trials are conducted under widely varying conditions, adverse reaction rates observed in clinical trials of a drug cannot be directly compared with rates in the clinical trials of another drug and may not reflect the rates observed in clinical practice.

The safety data reflect exposure to VELTIN Gel in 1,104 subjects with acne vulgaris. Subjects were 12 years and older and were treated once daily in the evening for 12 weeks. Adverse reactions that were reported in ≥1% of subjects treated with VELTIN Gel are presented in Table 1.
[See table 1 above]

Local skin reactions actively assessed at baseline and end of treatment with a score >0 are presented in Table 2.
[See table 2 above]

During the 12 weeks of treatment, each local skin reaction peaked at Week 2 and gradually reduced thereafter.

7 DRUG INTERACTIONS

7.1 Erythromycin

VELTIN Gel should not be used in combination with erythromycin-containing products due to possible antagonism to the clindamycin component. In vitro studies have shown antagonism between these 2 antimicrobials. The clinical significance of this in vitro antagonism is not known.

7.2 Neuromuscular Blocking Agents

Clindamycin has been shown to have neuromuscular blocking properties that may enhance the action of other neuromuscular blocking agents. Therefore, VELTIN Gel should be used with caution in patients receiving such agents.

8 USE IN SPECIFIC POPULATIONS

8.1 Pregnancy

Pregnancy Category C.

There are no well-controlled studies in pregnant women treated with VELTIN Gel. VELTIN Gel should be used during pregnancy only if the potential benefit justifies the potential risk to the fetus. A limit teratology study performed in Sprague Dawley rats treated topically with VELTIN Gel or 0.025% tretinoin gel at a dose of 2 mL/kg during gestation days 6 to 15 did not result in teratogenic effects. Although no systemic levels of tretinoin were detected, craniofacial and heart abnormalities were described in drug-treated groups. These abnormalities are consistent with retinoid effects and occurred at 16 times the recommended clinical dose assuming 100% absorption and based on body surface area comparison. For purposes of comparison of the animal exposure to human exposure, the recommended clinical dose is defined as 1 g of VELTIN Gel applied daily to a 50-kg person.

Clindamycin: Reproductive developmental toxicity studies performed in rats and mice using oral doses of clindamycin up to 600 mg/kg/day (480 and 240 times the recommended clinical dose based on body surface area comparison, respectively) or subcutaneous doses of clindamycin up to 180 mg/kg/day (140 and 70 times the recommended clinical dose based on body surface area comparison, respectively) revealed no evidence of teratogenicity.

Tretinoin: Oral tretinoin has been shown to be teratogenic in mice, rats, hamsters, rabbits, and primates. It was teratogenic and fetotoxic in Wistar rats when given orally at doses greater than 1 mg/kg/day (32 times the recommended clinical dose based on body surface area comparison). However, variations in teratogenic doses among various strains of rats have been reported. In the cynomologous monkey, a species in which tretinoin metabolism is closer to humans than in other species examined, fetal malformations were reported at oral doses of 10 mg/kg/day or greater, but none were observed at 5 mg/kg/day (324 times the recommended clinical dose based on body surface area comparison), although increased skeletal variations were observed at all doses. Dose-related teratogenic effects and increased abortion rates were reported in pigtail macaques.

With widespread use of any drug, a small number of birth defect reports associated temporally with the administration of the drug would be expected by chance alone. Thirty cases of temporally associated congenital malformations have been reported during 2 decades of clinical use of another formulation of topical tretinoin. Although no definite pattern of teratogenicity and no causal association have been established from these cases, 5 of the reports describe the rare birth defect category, holoprosencephaly (defects associated with incomplete midline development of the forebrain). The significance of these spontaneous reports in terms of risk to fetus is not known.

8.3 Nursing Mothers

It is not known whether clindamycin is excreted in human milk following use of VELTIN Gel. However, orally and parenterally administered clindamycin has been reported to appear in breast milk. Because of the potential for serious adverse reactions in nursing infants, a decision should be made whether to discontinue nursing or to discontinue the drug, taking into account the importance of the drug to the mother. It is not known whether tretinoin is excreted in human milk. Because many drugs are excreted in human milk, caution should be exercised when VELTIN Gel is administered to a nursing woman.

8.4 Pediatric Use

Safety and effectiveness of VELTIN Gel in pediatric patients younger than 12 years have not been established.

Clinical trials of VELTIN Gel included 2,086 subjects aged 12 through 17 years with acne vulgaris. [See Clinical Studies (14).]

8.5 Geriatric Use

Clinical trials of VELTIN Gel did not include sufficient numbers of subjects aged 65 and older to determine whether they respond differently from younger subjects.

11 DESCRIPTION

VELTIN (clindamycin phosphate and tretinoin) Gel, 1.2%/0.025%, is a fixed combination of 2 solubilized active ingredients in an aqueous-based gel. Clindamycin phosphate is a water soluble ester of the semi-synthetic antibiotic produced by a 7(S)-chloro-substitution of the 7(R)-hydroxyl group of the parent antibiotic lincomycin.

The chemical name for clindamycin phosphate is methyl 7-chloro-6,7,8-trideoxy-6-(1-methyl-*trans*-4-propyl-L-2-pyrrolidinecarboxamido)-1-thio-L-*threo*-α-D-*galacto*-octopyranoside 2-(dihydrogen phosphate). The structural formula for clindamycin phosphate is represented below:

Molecular Formula: $C_{18}H_{34}ClN_2O_8PS$
Molecular Weight: 504.97

The chemical name for tretinoin is all-*trans* 3,7-dimethyl-9-(2,6,6-trimethyl-1-cyclohexen-1-yl)-2,4,6,8-nonatetraenoic acid. It is a member of the retinoid family of compounds. The structural formula for tretinoin is represented below:

Molecular Formula: $C_{20}H_{28}O_2$
Molecular Weight: 300.44

VELTIN Gel contains the following inactive ingredients: anhydrous citric acid, butylated hydroxytoluene, carbomer homopolymer (type C), edetate disodium, laureth 4, methylparaben, propylene glycol, purified water, and tromethamine.

Table 1. Treatment-Related Adverse Reactions Reported by ≥1% of Subjects

	VELTIN Gel N = 1,104 n (%)	Clindamycin Gel N = 1,091 n (%)	Tretinoin Gel N = 1,084 n (%)	Vehicle Gel N = 552 n (%)
Patients with at least one adverse reaction	140 (13)	38 (3)	141 (13)	17 (3)
Application site dryness	64 (6)	12 (1)	62 (6)	3 (1)
Application site irritation	50 (5)	4 (<1)	57 (5)	5 (1)
Application site exfoliation	50 (5)	2 (<1)	56 (5)	2 (<1)
Application site erythema	40 (4)	6 (1)	39 (4)	3 (1)
Application site pruritus	26 (2)	7 (1)	23 (2)	6 (1)
Sunburn	11 (1)	6 (1)	7 (1)	3 (1)
Application site dermatitis	6 (1)	0 (0)	8 (1)	1 (<1)

Table 2. Local Skin Reactions in Subjects Treated With VELTIN Gel

Local Reaction	VELTIN Gel		Vehicle Gel	
	Baseline N = 476 (%)	End of Treatment N = 409 (%)	Baseline N = 219 (%)	End of Treatment N = 209 (%)
Erythema	24%	21%	31%	35%
Scaling	8%	19%	14%	12%
Dryness	11%	22%	18%	13%
Burning	8%	13%	8%	4%
Itching	17%	15%	22%	14%

Table 3. Efficacy Results at Week 12

Trial 1	VELTIN Gel N = 476	Clindamycin Gel N = 467	Tretinoin Gel N = 464	Vehicle Gel N = 242
Investigator's Global Assessment				
Percentage of subjects achieving 2-Grade Improvement	36.3%	26.6%	26.1%	20.2%
Percentage of subjects achieving an IGA of 0 or 1 with a 2-Grade Improvement	33.2%	24.0%	22.6%	17.8%
Inflammatory Lesions:				
Mean absolute reduction	15.5	14.5	13.9	11.1
Mean percentage (%) reduction	60.4%	56.5%	54.5%	43.3%
Non-inflammatory Lesions:				
Mean absolute reduction	23.2	19.5	22.1	17.0
Mean percentage (%) reduction	51.0%	42.9%	47.3%	36.0%
Total Lesions:				
Mean absolute reduction	38.7	34.0	36.0	28.1
Mean percentage (%) reduction	55.0%	49.0%	50.5%	39.1%

12 CLINICAL PHARMACOLOGY

12.1 Mechanism of Action

Clindamycin: *[See Microbiology (12.4).]*

Tretinoin: Although the exact mode of action of tretinoin is unknown, current evidence suggests that topical tretinoin decreases cohesiveness of folliculare epithelial cells with decreased microcomedone formation. Additionally, tretinoin stimulates mitotic activity and increased turnover of follicular epithelial cells causing extrusion of the comedones.

12.3 Pharmacokinetics

In an open-label trial of 17 subjects with moderate-to-severe acne vulgaris, topical administration of approximately 3 grams of VELTIN Gel once daily for 5 days, clindamycin concentrations were quantifiable in all 17 subjects starting from 1 hour post-dose. All plasma clindamycin concentrations were ≤5.56 ng/mL on Day 5, with the exception of 1 subject who had a maximum clindamycin concentration of 8.73 ng/mL at 4 hours post-dose. There was no appreciable increase in systemic exposure to tretinoin, as compared with the baseline value. The average tretinoin concentration across all sampling times on Day 5 ranged from 1.19 to 1.23 ng/mL compared with the corresponding baseline mean tretinoin concentration range of 1.16 to 1.30 ng/mL.

12.4 Microbiology

No microbiology studies were conducted in the clinical trials with this product.

Mechanism of Action: Clindamycin binds to the 50S ribosomal subunit of susceptible bacteria and prevents elongation of peptide chains by interfering with peptidyl transfer, thereby suppressing protein synthesis. Clindamycin has been shown to have *in vitro* activity against *Propionibacterium acnes (P. acnes)*, an organism that has been associated with acne vulgaris; however, the clinical significance of this activity against *P. acnes* was not examined in clinical trials with VELTIN Gel. *P. acnes* resistance to clindamycin has been documented.

Inducible Clindamycin Resistance: The treatment of acne with antimicrobials is associated with the development of antimicrobial resistance in *P. acnes* as well as other bacteria (e.g., *Staphylococcus aureus*, *Streptococcus pyogenes*). The use of clindamycin may result in developing inducible resistance in these organisms. This resistance is not detected by routine susceptibility testing.

Cross Resistance: Resistance to clindamycin is often associated with resistance to erythromycin.

13 NONCLINICAL TOXICOLOGY

13.1 Carcinogenesis, Mutagenesis, Impairment of Fertility

Long-term animal studies have not been performed to evaluate the carcinogenic potential of VELTIN Gel or the effect of VELTIN Gel on fertility. VELTIN Gel was negative for mutagenic potential when evaluated in an *in vitro* Ames *Salmonella* reversion assay. VELTIN Gel was equivocal for clastogenic potential in the absence of metabolic activation when tested in an *in vitro* chromosomal aberration assay.

Clindamycin: Once-daily dermal administration of 1% clindamycin as clindamycin phosphate in the gel vehicle (32 mg/kg/day, 13 times the recommended clinical dose based on body surface area comparison) to mice for up to 2 years did not produce evidence of tumorigenicity.

Fertility studies in rats treated orally with up to 300 mg/kg/day of clindamycin (240 times the recommended clinical dose based on body surface area comparison) revealed no effects on fertility or mating ability.

Tretinoin: In 2 independent mouse studies where tretinoin was administered topically (0.025% or 0.1%) 3 times per week for up to 2 years no carcinogenicity was observed, with maximum effects of dermal amyloidosis. However, in a dermal carcinogenicity study in mice, tretinoin applied at a dose of 5.1 mcg (1.4 times the recommended clinical dose based on body surface area comparison) 3 times per week for 20 weeks acted as a weak promoter of skin tumor formation following a single application of dimethylbenz[α]anthracene (DMBA).

In a study in female SENCAR mice, papillomas were induced by topical exposure to DMBA followed by promotion with 12-O-tetradecanoylphorbol-13-acetate or mezerein for up to 20 weeks. Topical application of tretinoin prior to each application of promoting agent resulted in a reduction in the number of papillomas per mouse. However, papillomas resistant to topical tretinoin suppression were at higher risk for pre-malignant progression.

Tretinoin has been shown to enhance photocarcinogenicity in properly performed specific studies, employing concurrent or intercurrent exposure to tretinoin and UV radiation. The photocarcinogenic potential of the clindamycin tretinoin combination is unknown. Although the significance of these studies to humans is not clear, patients should avoid exposure to sun.

The genotoxic potential of tretinoin was evaluated in an *in vitro* Ames *Salmonella* reversion test and an *in vitro* chromosomal aberration assay in Chinese hamster ovary cells. Both tests were negative.

In oral fertility studies in rats treated with tretinoin, the no-observed-effect-level was 2 mg/kg/day (64 times the recommended clinical dose based on body surface area comparison).

14 CLINICAL STUDIES

The safety and efficacy of VELTIN Gel, applied once daily for the treatment of acne vulgaris, was evaluated in 12-week multi-center, randomized, blinded trials in subjects 12 years and older.

Treatment response was defined as the percent of subjects who had a 2-grade improvement from baseline to Week 12 based on the Investigator's Global Assessment (IGA) and a mean absolute change from baseline to Week 12 in 2 out of 3 (total, inflammatory and non-inflammatory) lesion counts. The IGA scoring scale used in all the clinical trials for VELTIN Gel is as follows:

0	Clear	Normal, clear skin with no evidence of acne vulgaris.
1	Almost Clear	Skin almost clear; rare non-inflammatory lesions present, with rare non-inflamed papules (papules must be resolving and may be hyperpigmented, though not pink-red) requiring no further treatment in the Investigator's opinion.
2	Mild	Some non-inflammatory lesions are present, with few inflammatory lesions (papules/pustules only, no nodulo-cystic lesions).
3	Moderate	Non-inflammatory lesions predominate, with multiple inflammatory lesions evident; several-to-many comedones and papules/pustules, and there may or may not be 1 small nodulo-cystic lesion.
4	Severe	Inflammatory lesions are more apparent; many comedones and papules/pustules, there may or may not be a few nodulo-cystic lesions.
5	Very Severe	Highly inflammatory lesions predominate; variable numbers of comedones, many papules/pustules and nodulo-cystic lesions.

In Trial 1, 1,649 subjects were randomized to VELTIN Gel, clindamycin gel, tretinoin gel, and vehicle gel. The median age of subjects was 17 years and 58% were females. At baseline, subjects had an average of 71 total lesions of which the mean number of inflammatory lesions was 25.5 lesions and the mean number of non-inflammatory lesions was 45.1 lesions. The majority of subjects enrolled with a baseline IGA score of 3. The efficacy results at Week 12 are presented in Table 3.

[See table 3 above]

The safety and efficacy of clindamycin-tretinoin gel was also evaluated in 2 additional 12-week, multi-centered, randomized, blinded trials in subjects 12 years and older. A total of 2,219 subjects with mild-to-moderate acne vulgaris were treated once daily for 12 weeks. Of the 2,219 subjects, 634 subjects were treated with clindamycin-tretinoin gel. These trials demonstrated consistent outcomes.

16 HOW SUPPLIED/STORAGE AND HANDLING

How Supplied

VELTIN Gel is supplied as follows:

- 30 g aluminum tubes NDC 0145-0071-30
- 60 g aluminum tubes NDC 0145-0071-60

Storage and Handling

- Store at 25°C (77°F); excursions permitted from 15°C to 30°C (59°F to 86°F).
- Protect from heat.
- Protect from light.
- Protect from freezing.
- Keep out of reach of children.
- Keep tube tightly closed.

17 PATIENT COUNSELING INFORMATION

See FDA-approved patient labeling (Patient Information).

Instructions for Use

- At bedtime, the face should be gently washed with a mild soap and water. After patting the skin dry, apply VELTIN Gel as a thin layer over the entire affected area (excluding the eyes and lips).
- Patients should be advised not to use more than a pea-sized amount to cover the face and not to apply more often than once daily (at bedtime) as this will not make for faster results and may increase irritation.
- A sunscreen should be applied every morning and reapplied over the course of the day as needed. Patients should be advised to avoid exposure to sunlight, sunlamp, ultraviolet light, and other medicines that may increase sensitivity to sunlight.
- Other topical products with a strong drying effect such as abrasive soaps or cleansers may cause an increase in skin irritation with VELTIN Gel.

Skin Irritation

VELTIN Gel may cause irritation such as erythema, scaling, itching, burning, or stinging.

Colitis

In the event a patient treated with VELTIN Gel experiences severe diarrhea or gastrointestinal discomfort, VELTIN Gel should be discontinued and a physician should be contacted.

VELTIN is a registered trademark of Astellas Pharma Europe B.V.

Stiefel Laboratories, Inc.
Research Triangle Park, NC 27709
©2014, Stiefel Laboratories, Inc.
VEL:4PI

PATIENT INFORMATION

VELTIN® (vel-tin)

(clindamycin phosphate and tretinoin) Gel, 1.2%/0.025%

IMPORTANT: For use on skin only (topical use). Do not get VELTIN Gel in your mouth, eyes, or vagina.

Read the Patient Information that comes with VELTIN Gel before you start using it and each time you get a refill. There may be new information. This leaflet does not take the place of talking with your doctor about your medical condition or your treatment.

What is VELTIN Gel?

VELTIN Gel is prescription medicine used on the skin to treat acne in people 12 years and older.

It is not known if VELTIN Gel is safe and effective in children younger than 12 years.

Who should not use VELTIN Gel?

Do not use VELTIN Gel if you have:

- Crohn's disease
- ulcerative colitis
- had inflammation of the colon (colitis) with past antibiotic use

Talk to your doctor if you are not sure if you have one of these conditions.

What should I tell my doctor before using VELTIN Gel?
Before using VELTIN Gel, tell your doctor if you:
• have any allergies
• **plan to have surgery with general anesthesia.** One of the medicines in VELTIN Gel can affect how certain anesthesia medicines work.
• **have any other medical conditions**
• **are pregnant or plan to become pregnant.** It is not known if VELTIN Gel may harm your unborn baby.
• **are breastfeeding or plan to breastfeed.** It is not known if VELTIN Gel passes into your breast milk. One of the medicines in VELTIN Gel contains clindamycin. When clindamycin is taken by mouth or injection, it may pass into breast milk. You and your doctor should decide if you will take VELTIN Gel or breastfeed. You should not do both.

Tell your doctor about all the medicines and skin products you use. Especially tell your doctor if you take medicine that contains erythromycin. VELTIN Gel should not be used with products that contain erythromycin.

Know the medicines you take. Keep a list of your medicines and show it to your doctor and pharmacist when you get a new medicine.

How should I use VELTIN Gel?
• Use VELTIN Gel exactly as prescribed.
• Your doctor will tell you how long to use VELTIN Gel.
• **Do not** apply VELTIN Gel more than one time each day.
• **Do not** use too much VELTIN Gel, because it may irritate your skin.

Instructions for applying VELTIN Gel:
1. At bedtime, wash your face gently with a mild soap; rinse with water.
2. Pat the skin dry.
3. Squeeze a pea-sized amount of medication onto one fingertip. Then, gently rub over the entire affected area. **Do not get VELTIN Gel in your eyes, mouth, or on your lips.**

What should I avoid while using VELTIN Gel?
• Limit your time in sunlight. Avoid using tanning beds or sun lamps. If you have to be in sunlight, wear a wide-brimmed hat or other protective clothing. Apply a sunscreen every morning and re-apply during the day as needed.
• Avoid wind and cold weather during treatment with VELTIN Gel. These may be irritating to your skin.
• Avoid using abrasive soaps and cleansers. These may cause increased skin irritation with VELTIN Gel.

What are the possible side effects of VELTIN Gel?
VELTIN Gel may cause serious side effects, including:
• **Inflammation of the colon (colitis).** Clindamycin, one of the ingredients in VELTIN Gel, can cause severe colitis that may lead to death. Stop taking VELTIN Gel and call your doctor if you develop severe watery diarrhea, or bloody diarrhea.
• **Sunburn.** VELTIN Gel may cause your skin to become sunburned more easily. If your face is sunburned, do not use VELTIN Gel until your sunburn is completely healed. Tretinoin, one of the medicines in VELTIN Gel, makes your skin more sensitive to sunlight. See **"What should I avoid while using VELTIN Gel?"**

Common side effects of VELTIN Gel include:
• **Skin irritation.** VELTIN Gel may cause skin irritation such as dryness, peeling, burning, or itching.

Talk to your doctor about any side effect that bothers you or that does not go away.

These are not all the side effects with VELTIN Gel. Ask your doctor or pharmacist for more information.

Call your doctor for medical advice about side effects. You may report side effects to FDA at 1-800-FDA-1088.

How should I store VELTIN Gel?
• **Store VELTIN Gel** at room temperature, between 59°F to 86°F (15°C to 30°C).
• Protect from freezing.
• Keep VELTIN Gel away from heat and light.
• **Keep VELTIN Gel and all medicines out of the reach of children.**

General information about VELTIN Gel
Medicines are sometimes prescribed for purposes other than those listed in the patient information leaflet. Do not use VELTIN Gel for a condition for which it was not prescribed. **Do not give VELTIN Gel to other people, even if they have the same symptoms you have. It may harm them.**

This patient information leaflet summarizes the most important information about VELTIN Gel. If you would like more information, talk with your doctor. You can also ask your pharmacist or doctor for information about VELTIN Gel that is written for healthcare professionals. For more information call 1-888-784-3335.

What are the ingredients in VELTIN Gel?
Active Ingredients: clindamycin phosphate and tretinoin
Inactive ingredients: anhydrous citric acid, butylated hydroxytoluene, carbomer homopolymer (type C), edetate disodium, laureth 4, methylparaben, propylene glycol, purified water, and tromethamine.

This Patient Information has been approved by the U.S. Food and Drug Administration.
VELTIN is a registered trademark of Astellas Pharma Europe B.V.
Stiefel Laboratories, Inc.
Research Triangle Park, NC 27709
©2014, Stiefel Laboratories, Inc.
March 2014
VEL:3PIL

Sunovion Pharmaceuticals Inc.
84 WATERFORD DRIVE
MARLBOROUGH, MA 01752
(508) 481-6700

For Medical Information Inquiries:
Medical Information
(800) 739-0565
minfo@sunovion.com
www.SunovionMedical.com
For Adverse Event Reporting
(877) 737-7226
For Customer Service
(888) 394-7377
CAC@sunovion.com

APTIOM®   ℞
[ap tee' om]
(eslicarbazepine acetate)
tablets, for oral use

HIGHLIGHTS OF PRESCRIBING INFORMATION
These highlights do not include all the information needed to use APTIOM safely and effectively. See full prescribing information for APTIOM.
APTIOM® (eslicarbazepine acetate) tablets, for oral use
Initial U.S. Approval: 2013

─────────INDICATIONS AND USAGE─────────
APTIOM is indicated as adjunctive treatment of partial-onset seizures. (1.1)

──────DOSAGE AND ADMINISTRATION──────
• Start treatment at 400 mg once daily. After one week, increase dosage to 800 mg once daily (recommended maintenance dosage). Maximum recommended maintenance dosage is 1200 mg once daily (after a minimum of one week at 800 mg once daily). (2.2)
• Patients with moderate to severe renal impairment: Start treatment at 200 mg once daily. After two weeks, increase dosage to 400 mg once daily. Maximum recommended maintenance dosage is 600 mg once daily. (2.4)

──────DOSAGE FORMS AND STRENGTHS──────
Tablets: 200 mg, 400 mg, 600 mg, 800 mg (3)

─────────CONTRAINDICATIONS─────────
Hypersensitivity to eslicarbazepine acetate or oxcarbazepine. (4)

──────WARNINGS AND PRECAUTIONS──────
• *Suicidal Behavior and Ideation:* Monitor for suicidal thoughts or behavior. (5.1)
• *Serious Dermatologic Reactions:* Monitor for dermatologic reactions and discontinue in the case of serious dermatologic reaction. (5.2)
• *Drug Reaction with Eosinophilia and Systemic Symptoms:* Monitor for hypersensitivity. Discontinue if another cause cannot be established. (5.3)
• *Anaphylactic Reactions and Angioedema:* Monitor for breathing difficulties or swelling. Discontinue if another cause cannot be established. (5.4)
• *Hyponatremia:* Monitor sodium levels in patients at risk or patients experiencing hyponatremia symptoms. (5.5)
• *Neurological Adverse Reactions:* Monitor for dizziness, disturbance in gait and coordination, somnolence, fatigue, cognitive dysfunction, and visual changes. Use caution when driving or operating machinery. (5.6)
• *Withdrawal of APTIOM:* Withdraw APTIOM gradually to minimize the risk of increased seizure frequency and status epilepticus. (2.6, 5.7)
• *Drug Induced Liver Injury:* Discontinue APTIOM in patients with jaundice or evidence of significant liver injury. (5.8)

─────────ADVERSE REACTIONS─────────
The most common adverse reactions in patients receiving APTIOM (≥4% and ≥2% greater than placebo) were dizziness, somnolence, nausea, headache, diplopia, vomiting, fatigue, vertigo, ataxia, blurred vision, and tremor. (6.1)
To report SUSPECTED ADVERSE REACTIONS, contact Sunovion at 1-877-737-7226 or FDA at 1-800-FDA-1088 or www.fda.gov/medwatch.

─────────DRUG INTERACTIONS─────────
• *Carbamazepine:* May need dose adjustment for APTIOM or carbamazepine. (2.3, 5.6, 7.2, 7.3)
• *Phenytoin:* Higher dosage of APTIOM may be necessary and dose adjustment may be needed for phenytoin based on clinical response and serum levels of phenytoin. (2.3, 7.2, 7.3)
• *Phenobarbital or Primidone:* Higher dosage of APTIOM may be necessary. (2.3, 7.2)
• *Hormonal Contraceptives:* APTIOM may decrease the effectiveness of hormonal contraceptives. Females of reproductive potential should use additional or alternative non-hormonal birth control. (7.3, 7.4, 8.9)

──────USE IN SPECIFIC POPULATIONS──────
Pregnancy: Based on animal data, may cause fetal harm. (8.1)
See 17 for PATIENT COUNSELING INFORMATION and Medication Guide

                                    Revised: 11/2013

─────────────────────────────
FULL PRESCRIBING INFORMATION: CONTENTS*

FULL PRESCRIBING INFORMATION

1 INDICATIONS AND USAGE

1.1 Partial-Onset Seizures

APTIOM (eslicarbazepine acetate) is indicated as adjunctive treatment of partial-onset seizures.

2 DOSAGE AND ADMINISTRATION

2.1 Important Administration Instructions

Instruct patients to administer APTIOM either as whole or as crushed tablets. Instruct patients to take APTIOM either with or without food.

2.2 Dosage for Partial-Onset Seizures

Start treatment at 400 mg once daily. After one week, increase dosage to 800 mg once daily, which is the recommended maintenance dosage. Some patients may benefit from the maximum recommended maintenance dosage of 1200 mg once daily, although this dosage is associated with an increase in adverse reactions. A maximum dose of 1200 mg daily should only be initiated after the patient has tolerated 800 mg daily for at least a week. For some patients, treatment may be initiated at 800 mg once daily if the need for additional seizure reduction outweighs an increased risk of adverse reactions during initiation [see Adverse Reactions (6.1)].

2.3 Dosage Modifications with Other Antiepileptic Drugs

APTIOM should not be taken as an adjunctive therapy with oxcarbazepine.

Some adverse reactions occur more frequently when patients take APTIOM with carbamazepine [see Warnings and Precautions (5.6)]. However, carbamazepine reduces the plasma concentration of eslicarbazepine [see Drug Interactions (7.2)]. When APTIOM and carbamazepine are taken concomitantly, the dose of APTIOM or carbamazepine may need to be adjusted based on efficacy and tolerability. For patients taking other enzyme-inducing antiepileptic drugs (AEDs) (i.e., phenobarbital, phenytoin, and primidone), higher doses of APTIOM may be needed [see Drug Interactions (7.2)].

2.4 Dosage Modifications in Patients with Renal Impairment

A dose reduction is recommended in patients with moderate and severe renal impairment (i.e., creatinine clearance < 50 mL/min). Start treatment at 200 mg once daily. After two weeks, increase dosage to 400 mg once daily, which is the recommended maintenance dosage. Some patients may benefit from the maximum recommended maintenance dosage of 600 mg once daily [see Use in Specific Populations (8.6) and Clinical Pharmacology (12.3)].

2.5 Patients with Hepatic Impairment

Dose adjustments are not required in patients with mild to moderate hepatic impairment. Use of APTIOM in patients with severe hepatic impairment has not been studied, and use in these patients is not recommended [see Use in Specific Populations (8.7) and Clinical Pharmacology (12.3)].

2.6 Discontinuation of APTIOM

When discontinuing APTIOM, reduce the dosage gradually and avoid abrupt discontinuation in order to minimize the risk of increased seizure frequency and status epilepticus [see Warnings and Precautions (5.7)].

3 DOSAGE FORMS AND STRENGTHS

APTIOM tablets are available in the following shapes and color (Table 1) with respective one-sided engraving:

Table 1: APTIOM Tablet Presentations

Tablet Strength	Tablet Color/ Shape	Tablet Markings	Functional Score
200 mg	White oblong	ESL 200	Yes
400 mg	White circular bi-convex	ESL 400	No
600 mg	White oblong	ESL 600	Yes
800 mg	White oblong	ESL 800	Yes

4 CONTRAINDICATIONS

APTIOM is contraindicated in patients with a hypersensitivity to eslicarbazepine acetate or oxcarbazepine [see Warnings and Precautions (5.2, 5.3, and 5.4)].

5 WARNINGS AND PRECAUTIONS

5.1 Suicidal Behavior and Ideation

Antiepileptic drugs (AEDs), including APTIOM, increase the risk of suicidal thoughts or behavior in patients taking these drugs for any indication. Patients treated with any AED for any indication should be monitored for the emergence or worsening of depression, suicidal thoughts or behavior, and/or any unusual changes in mood or behavior. Pooled analyses of 199 placebo-controlled clinical trials (mono- and adjunctive therapy) of 11 different AEDs showed that patients randomized to one of the AEDs had approximately twice the risk (adjusted Relative Risk 1.8, 95% confidence interval [CI]: 1.2, 2.7) of suicidal thinking or behavior compared to patients randomized to placebo. In these trials, which had a median treatment duration of 12 weeks, the estimated incidence of suicidal behavior or ideation among 27,863 AED-treated patients was 0.43%, compared to 0.24% among 16,029 placebo-treated patients, representing an increase of approximately one case of suicidal thinking or behavior for every 530 patients treated. There were four suicides in drug-treated patients in the trials and none in placebo-treated patients, but the number of events is too small to allow any conclusion about drug effect on suicide. The increased risk of suicidal thoughts or behavior with AEDs was observed as early as one week after starting treatment with AEDs and persisted for the duration of treatment assessed. Because most trials included in the analysis did not extend beyond 24 weeks, the risk of suicidal thoughts or behavior beyond 24 weeks could not be assessed.

The risk of suicidal thoughts or behavior was generally consistent among drugs in the data analyzed. The finding of increased risk with AEDs of varying mechanisms of action and across a range of indications suggests that the risk applies to all AEDs used for any indication. The risk did not vary substantially by age (5-100 years) in the clinical trials analyzed.

Table 2 shows absolute and relative risk by indication for all evaluated AEDs.

[See table 2 below]

The relative risk for suicidal thoughts or behavior was higher in clinical trials in patients with epilepsy than in clinical trials in patients with psychiatric or other conditions, but the absolute risk differences were similar for epilepsy and psychiatric indications.

Anyone considering prescribing APTIOM or any other AED must balance this risk with the risk of untreated illness. Epilepsy and many other illnesses for which AEDs are prescribed are themselves associated with morbidity and mortality and an increased risk of suicidal thoughts and behavior. Should suicidal thoughts and behavior emerge during treatment, the prescriber needs to consider whether the emergence of these symptoms in any given patient may be related to the illness being treated.

Patients, their caregivers, and families should be informed that AEDs increase the risk of suicidal thoughts and behavior and should be advised of the need to be alert for the emergence or worsening of the signs and symptoms of depression; any unusual changes in mood or behavior; or the emergence of suicidal thoughts, behavior, or thoughts about self-harm. Behaviors of concern should be reported immediately to healthcare providers.

5.2 Serious Dermatologic Reactions

Serious dermatologic reactions including Stevens-Johnson Syndrome (SJS) have been reported in association with APTIOM use. Serious and sometimes fatal dermatologic reactions, including toxic epidermal necrolysis (TEN) and SJS, have been reported in patients using oxcarbazepine or carbamazepine which are chemically related to APTIOM. The reporting rate of these reactions associated with oxcarbazepine use exceeds the background incidence rate estimates by a factor of 3- to 10-fold. Risk factors for development of serious dermatologic reactions with APTIOM use have not been identified.

If a patient develops a dermatologic reaction while taking APTIOM, discontinue APTIOM use, unless the reaction is clearly not drug-related. Patients with a prior dermatologic reaction with either oxcarbazepine or APTIOM should not be treated with APTIOM [see Contraindications (4)].

5.3 Drug Reaction with Eosinophilia and Systemic Symptoms (DRESS)/Multiorgan Hypersensitivity

Drug Reaction with Eosinophilia and Systemic Symptoms (DRESS), also known as Multiorgan Hypersensitivity, has been reported in patients taking APTIOM. DRESS may be fatal or life-threatening. DRESS typically, although not exclusively, presents with fever, rash, and/or lymphadenopathy, in association with other organ system involvement, such as hepatitis, nephritis, hematological abnormalities, myocarditis, or myositis sometimes resembling an acute viral infection. Eosinophilia is often present. Because this disorder is variable in its expression, other organ systems not noted here may be involved. It is important to note that early manifestations of hypersensitivity, such as fever or lymphadenopathy, may be present even though rash is not evident. If such signs or symptoms are present, the patient should be evaluated immediately. APTIOM should be discontinued and not be resumed if an alternative etiology for the signs or symptoms cannot be established. Patients with a prior DRESS reaction with either oxcarbazepine or APTIOM should not be treated with APTIOM [see Contraindications (4)].

5.4 Anaphylactic Reactions and Angioedema

Rare cases of anaphylaxis and angioedema have been reported in patients taking APTIOM. Anaphylaxis and angioedema associated with laryngeal edema can be fatal. If a patient develops any of these reactions after treatment with APTIOM, the drug should be discontinued. Patients with a prior anaphylactic-type reaction with either oxcarbazepine or APTIOM should not be treated with APTIOM [see Contraindications (4)].

5.5 Hyponatremia

Clinically significant hyponatremia (sodium <125 mEq/L) can develop in patients taking APTIOM. In the controlled epilepsy trials, 4/415 patients (1.0%) treated with 800 mg and 6/410 (1.5%) patients treated with 1200 mg of APTIOM had at least one serum sodium value less than 125 mEq/L, compared to none of the patients assigned to placebo. A higher percentage of APTIOM-treated patients (5.1%) than placebo-treated patients (0.7%) experienced decreases in sodium values of more than 10 mEq/L. These effects were dose-related and generally appeared within the first 8 weeks of treatment (as early as after 3 days). Serious, life-threatening complications were reported with APTIOM-associated hyponatremia (as low as 112 mEq/L) including seizures, severe nausea/vomiting leading to dehydration, severe gait instability, and injury. Some patients required hospitalization and discontinuation of APTIOM. Concurrent hypochloremia was also present in patients with hyponatremia. Depending on the severity of hyponatremia, the dose of APTIOM may need to be reduced or discontinued.

Measurement of serum sodium and chloride levels should be considered during maintenance treatment with APTIOM, particularly if the patient is receiving other medications known to decrease serum sodium levels and should be performed if symptoms of hyponatremia develop (e.g., nausea/vomiting, malaise, headache, lethargy, confusion, irritability, muscle weakness/spasms, obtundation, or increase in seizure frequency or severity).

5.6 Neurological Adverse Reactions

Dizziness and Disturbance in Gait and Coordination

APTIOM causes dose-related increases in adverse reactions related to dizziness and disturbance in gait and coordination (dizziness, ataxia, vertigo, balance disorder, gait disturbance, nystagmus, and abnormal coordination) [see Adverse Reactions (6.1)]. In controlled epilepsy trials, these events were reported in 26% and 38% of patients randomized to receive APTIOM at doses of 800 mg and 1200 mg/day, respectively, compared to 12% of placebo-treated patients. Events related to dizziness and disturbance in gait and coordination were more often serious in APTIOM-treated patients than in placebo-treated patients (2% vs. 0%), and more often led to study withdrawal in APTIOM-treated patients than in placebo-treated patients (9% vs. 0.7%). There was an increased risk of these adverse reactions during the titration period (compared to the maintenance period) and there also may be an increased risk of these adverse reactions in patients 60 years of age and older compared to younger adults. Nausea and vomiting also occurred with these events.

The incidence of dizziness was greater with the concomitant use of APTIOM and carbamazepine compared to the use of APTIOM without carbamazepine (up to 37% vs. 19%, respectively). Therefore, consider dosage modifications of both APTIOM and carbamazepine if these drugs are used concomitantly [see Dosage and Administration (2.3)].

Somnolence and Fatigue

APTIOM causes dose-dependent increases in somnolence and fatigue-related adverse reactions (fatigue, asthenia,

Table 2: Risk of Suicidal Thoughts or Behaviors by Indication for Antiepileptic Drugs in the Pooled Analysis

Indication	Placebo Patients with Events Per 1000 Patients	Drug Patients with Events Per 1000 Patients	Relative Risk: Incidence of Events in Drug Patients/ Incidence in Placebo Patients	Risk Differences: Additional Drug Patients with Events Per 1000 Patients
Epilepsy	1.0	3.4	3.5	2.4
Psychiatric	5.7	8.5	1.5	2.9
Other	1.0	1.8	1.9	0.9
Total	2.4	4.3	1.8	1.9

Figure 1: Potential Impact of Other AEDs on AUC of Eslicarbazepine

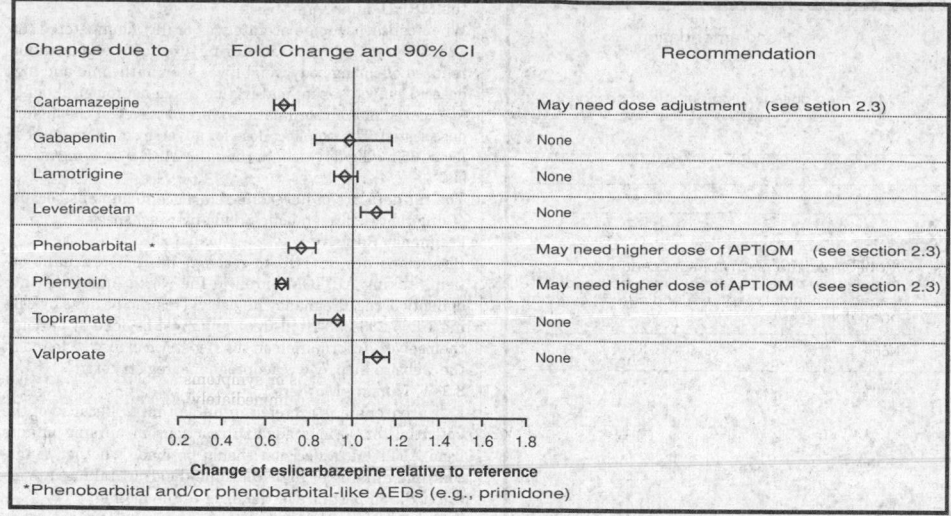

Change due to	Fold Change and 90% CI	Recommendation
Carbamazepine		May need dose adjustment (see setion 2.3)
Gabapentin		None
Lamotrigine		None
Levetiracetam		None
Phenobarbital *		May need higher dose of APTIOM (see section 2.3)
Phenytoin		May need higher dose of APTIOM (see section 2.3)
Topiramate		None
Valproate		None

0.2 0.4 0.6 0.8 1.0 1.2 1.4 1.6 1.8

Change of eslicarbazepine relative to reference

*Phenobarbital and/or phenobarbital-like AEDs (e.g., primidone)

---

malaise, hypersomnia, sedation, and lethargy). In the controlled epilepsy trials, these events were reported in 13% of placebo patients, 16% of patients randomized to receive 800 mg/day APTIOM, and 28% of patients randomized to receive 1200 mg/day APTIOM. Somnolence and fatigue-related events were serious in 0.3% of APTIOM-treated patients (and 0 placebo patients) and led to discontinuation in 3% of APTIOM-treated patients (and 0.7% of placebo-treated patients).

Cognitive Dysfunction

APTIOM causes dose-dependent increases in cognitive dysfunction-related events (memory impairment, disturbance in attention, amnesia, confusional state, aphasia, speech disorder, slowness of thought, disorientation, and psychomotor retardation). In the controlled epilepsy trials, these events were reported in 1% of placebo patients, 4% of patients randomized to receive 800 mg/day APTIOM, and 7% of patients randomized to receive 1200 mg/day APTIOM. Cognitive dysfunction-related events were serious in 0.2% of APTIOM-treated patients (and 0.2% of placebo patients) and led to discontinuation in 1% of APTIOM-treated patients (and 0.5% of placebo-treated patients).

Visual Changes

APTIOM causes dose-dependent increases in events related to visual changes including diplopia, blurred vision, and impaired vision. In the controlled epilepsy trials, these events were reported in 16% of patients randomized to receive APTIOM compared to 6% of placebo patients. Eye events were serious in 0.7% of APTIOM-treated patients (and 0 placebo patients) and led to discontinuation in 4% of APTIOM-treated patients (and 0.2% of placebo-treated patients). There was an increased risk of these adverse reactions during the titration period (compared to the maintenance period) and also in patients 60 years of age and older (compared to younger adults). The incidence of diplopia was greater with the concomitant use of APTIOM and carbamazepine compared to the use of APTIOM without carbamazepine (up to 16% vs. 6%, respectively) [see Dosage and Administration (2.3)].

Hazardous Activities

Prescribers should advise patients against engaging in hazardous activities requiring mental alertness, such as operating motor vehicles or dangerous machinery, until the effect of APTIOM is known.

5.7   Withdrawal of AEDs

As with all antiepileptic drugs, APTIOM should be withdrawn gradually because of the risk of increased seizure frequency and status epilepticus.

5.8   Drug Induced Liver Injury

Hepatic effects, ranging from mild to moderate elevations in transaminases (>3 times the upper limit of normal) to rare cases with concomitant elevations of total bilirubin (>2 times the upper limit of normal) have been reported with APTIOM use. Baseline evaluations of liver laboratory tests are recommended. The combination of transaminase elevations and elevated bilirubin without evidence of obstruction is generally recognized as an important predictor of severe liver injury. APTIOM should be discontinued in patients with jaundice or other evidence of significant liver injury (e.g., laboratory evidence).

5.9   Abnormal Thyroid Function Tests

Dose-dependent decreases in serum T3 and T4 (free and total) values have been observed in patients taking APTIOM. These changes were not associated with other abnormal thyroid function tests suggesting hypothyroidism. Abnormal thyroid function tests should be clinically evaluated.

6   ADVERSE REACTIONS

The following adverse reactions are described in more detail in the Warnings and Precautions section of the label:

- Suicidal Behavior and Ideation [see Warnings and Precautions (5.1)]
- Serious Dermatologic Reactions [see Warnings and Precautions (5.2)]
- Drug Reaction with Eosinophilia and Systemic Symptoms (DRESS)/Multiorgan Hypersensitivity [see Warnings and Precautions (5.3)]
- Anaphylactic Reactions and Angioedema [see Warnings and Precautions (5.4)]
- Hyponatremia [see Warnings and Precautions (5.5)]
- Neurological Adverse Reactions [see Warnings and Precautions (5.6)]
- Drug Induced Liver Injury [see Warnings and Precautions (5.8)]
- Abnormal Thyroid Function Tests [see Warnings and Precautions (5.9)]

6.1   Clinical Trials Experience

Because clinical trials are conducted under widely varying conditions, adverse reaction rates observed in the clinical trials of a drug cannot be directly compared to rates in the clinical trials of another drug and may not reflect the rates observed in practice.

In all controlled and uncontrolled trials in patients with partial-onset seizures, 1195 patients received APTIOM of whom 586 were treated for longer than 6 months and 462 for longer than 12 months. In the placebo controlled trials in patients with partial-onset seizures, 1021 patients received APTIOM. Of the patients in those trials, approximately 95% were between 18 and 60 years old, approximately 50% were male, and approximately 80% were Caucasian.

Adverse Reactions Leading to Discontinuation

In the controlled epilepsy trials (Studies 1, 2, and 3) [see Clinical Studies (14.1)], the rate of discontinuation as a result of any adverse reaction was 14% for the 800 mg dose, 25% for the 1200 mg dose, and 7% in subjects randomized to placebo. The adverse reactions most commonly (≥1% in any APTIOM treatment group, and greater than placebo) leading to discontinuation, in descending order of frequency, were dizziness, nausea, vomiting, ataxia, diplopia, somnolence, headache, blurred vision, vertigo, asthenia, fatigue, rash, dysarthria, and tremor.

Most Common Adverse Reactions

The most frequently reported adverse reactions in patients receiving APTIOM at doses of 800 mg or 1200 mg (≥4% and ≥2% greater than placebo) were dizziness, somnolence, nausea, headache, diplopia, vomiting, fatigue, vertigo, ataxia, blurred vision, and tremor.

Table 3 gives the incidence of adverse reactions that occurred in ≥2% of subjects with partial-onset seizures in any APTIOM treatment group and for which the incidence was greater than placebo during the controlled clinical trials. Adverse reactions during titration were less frequent for patients who began therapy at an initial dose of 400 mg for 1 week and then increased to 800 mg compared to patients who initiated therapy at 800 mg.

Table 3: Adverse Reactions Incidence in Pooled Controlled Clinical Trials of Adjunctive Therapy in Adults (Events ≥2% of Patients in the APTIOM 800 mg or 1200 mg Dose Group and More Frequent Than in the Placebo Group)

	Placebo	APTIOM	
		800 mg	1200 mg
	(N=426) %	(N=415) %	(N=410) %
Ear and labyrinth disorders			
Vertigo	<1	2	6
Eye disorders			
Diplopia	2	9	11
Blurred vision	1	6	5
Visual impairment	1	2	1
Gastrointestinal disorders			
Nausea	5	10	16
Vomiting	3	6	10
Diarrhea	3	4	2
Constipation	1	2	2
Abdominal pain	1	2	2
Gastritis	<1	2	<1
General disorders and administration site conditions			
Fatigue	4	4	7
Asthenia	2	2	3
Gait disturbance	<1	2	2
Peripheral edema	1	2	1
Infections and Infestations			
Urinary tract infections	1	2	2
Injury, poisoning and procedural complications			
Fall	1	3	1
Metabolism and nutrition disorders			
Hyponatremia	<1	2	2
Nervous system disorders			
Dizziness	9	20	28
Somnolence	8	11	18
Headache	9	13	15
Ataxia	2	4	6
Balance disorder	<1	3	3
Tremor	1	2	4
Dysarthria	0	1	2
Memory impairment	<1	1	2
Nystagmus	<1	1	2
Psychiatric disorders			
Depression	2	1	3
Insomnia	1	2	2
Respiratory, thoracic and mediastinal disorders			
Cough	1	2	1
Skin and subcutaneous tissue disorders			
Rash	1	2	3
Vascular disorders			
Hypertension	1	1	2

Other Adverse Reactions with APTIOM Use

Compared to placebo, APTIOM use was associated with slightly higher frequencies of decreases in hemoglobin and hematocrit, increases in total cholesterol, triglycerides, and LDL, and increases in creatine phosphokinase.

Adverse Reactions Based on Gender and Race

No significant gender differences were noted in the incidence of adverse reactions. Although there were few non-Caucasian patients, no differences in the incidences of adverse reactions compared to Caucasian patients were observed.

Figure 2a: Potential Impact of APTIOM on the AUC of AEDs

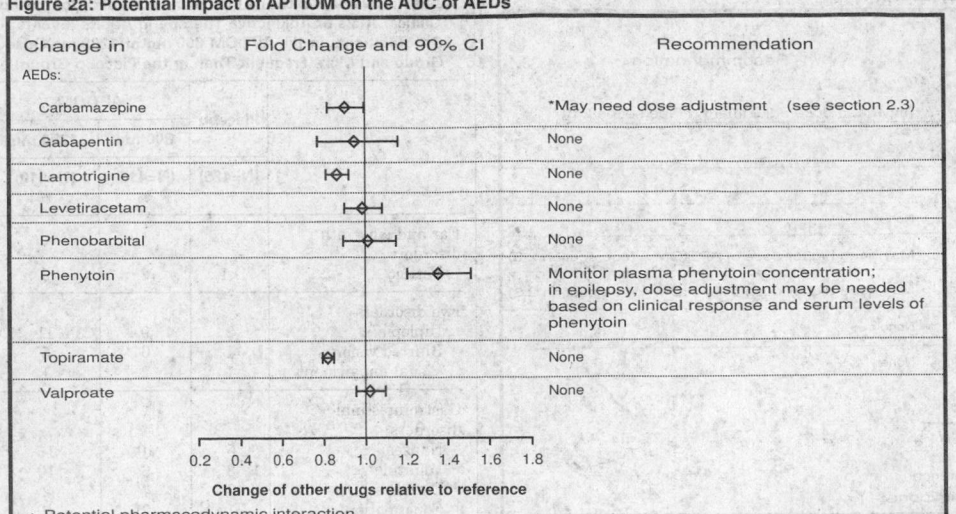

Figure 2a shows Change in AEDs, Fold Change and 90% CI, and Recommendation:

Change in AEDs:	Fold Change and 90% CI	Recommendation
Carbamazepine		*May need dose adjustment (see section 2.3)
Gabapentin		None
Lamotrigine		None
Levetiracetam		None
Phenobarbital		None
Phenytoin		Monitor plasma phenytoin concentration; in epilepsy, dose adjustment may be needed based on clinical response and serum levels of phenytoin
Topiramate		None
Valproate		None

Change of other drugs relative to reference (0.2 0.4 0.6 0.8 1.0 1.2 1.4 1.6 1.8)

* Potential pharmacodynamic interaction

Figure 2b: Potential Impact of APTIOM on the AUC of Non-AEDs

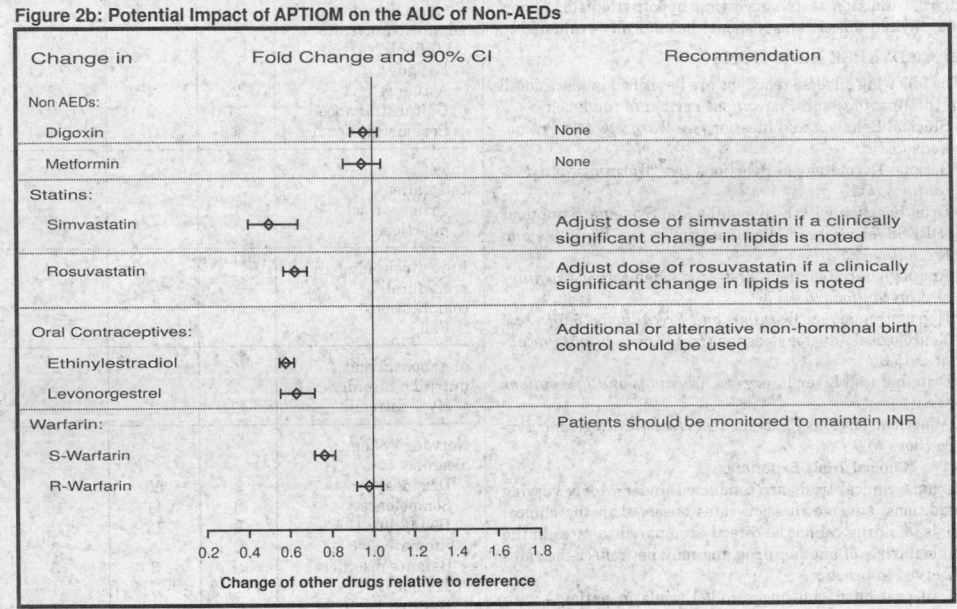

Change in Non AEDs:	Fold Change and 90% CI	Recommendation
Digoxin		None
Metformin		None
Statins:		
Simvastatin		Adjust dose of simvastatin if a clinically significant change in lipids is noted
Rosuvastatin		Adjust dose of rosuvastatin if a clinically significant change in lipids is noted
Oral Contraceptives:		Additional or alternative non-hormonal birth control should be used
Ethinylestradiol		
Levonorgestrel		
Warfarin:		Patients should be monitored to maintain INR
S-Warfarin		
R-Warfarin		

Change of other drugs relative to reference (0.2 0.4 0.6 0.8 1.0 1.2 1.4 1.6 1.8)

7 DRUG INTERACTIONS

7.1 General Information

Several AEDs (e.g., carbamazepine, phenobarbital, phenytoin, and primidone) can induce enzymes that metabolize APTIOM and can cause decreased plasma concentrations of eslicarbazepine (see Figure 1).

APTIOM can inhibit CYP2C19, which can cause increased plasma concentrations of drugs that are metabolized by this isoenzyme (e.g., phenytoin, clobazam, and omeprazole). In vivo studies suggest that APTIOM can induce CYP3A4, decreasing plasma concentrations of drugs that are metabolized by this isoenzyme (e.g., simvastatin) (see Figure 2).

7.2 Potential for Other AEDs to Affect Eslicarbazepine

The potential impact of other AEDs on the systemic exposure (area under the curve, AUC) of eslicarbazepine, the active metabolite of APTIOM, is shown in Figure 1:

[See figure 1 at top of previous page]

7.3 Potential for APTIOM to Affect Other Drugs

The potential impact of APTIOM on the systemic exposure (AUC) of other drugs (including AEDs) is shown in Figure 2:

[See figure 2a above]
[See figure 2b above]

7.4 Oral Contraceptives

Because concomitant use of APTIOM and ethinylestradiol and levonorgestrel is associated with lower plasma levels of these hormones, females of reproductive potential should use additional or alternative non-hormonal birth control.

8 USE IN SPECIFIC POPULATIONS

8.1 Pregnancy

Pregnancy Category C

There are no adequate and well-controlled studies in pregnant women. In oral studies conducted in pregnant mice, rats, and rabbits, eslicarbazepine acetate demonstrated developmental toxicity, including teratogenicity (mice), embryolethality (rats), and fetal growth retardation, at clinically relevant doses. APTIOM should be used during pregnancy only if the potential benefit justifies the potential risk to the fetus.

When eslicarbazepine acetate was orally administered (150, 350, 650 mg/kg/day) to pregnant mice throughout organogenesis, increased incidences of fetal malformations was observed at all doses and fetal growth retardation was observed at the mid and high doses. A no-effect dose for adverse developmental effects was not identified. At the lowest dose tested, plasma eslicarbazepine exposure (C_{max}, AUC) is less than that in humans at the maximum recommended human dose (MRHD) of 1200 mg/day.

Oral administration of eslicarbazepine acetate (40, 160, 320 mg/kg/day) to pregnant rabbits throughout organogenesis resulted in fetal growth retardation and increased incidences of skeletal variations at the mid and high doses. The no-effect dose (40 mg/kg/day) is less than the MRHD on a mg/m² basis.

Oral administration to pregnant rats (65, 125, 250 mg/kg/day) throughout organogenesis resulted in embryolethality at all doses, increased incidences of skeletal variations at the mid and high doses, and fetal growth retardation at the high dose. The lowest dose tested (65 mg/kg/day) is less than the MRHD on a mg/m² basis.

When eslicarbazepine acetate was orally administered to female mice during pregnancy and lactation (150, 350, 650 mg/kg/day), the gestation period was prolonged at the highest dose tested. In offspring, a persistent reduction in offspring body weight and delayed physical development and sexual maturation were observed at the mid and high doses. The lowest dose tested (150 mg/kg/day) is less than the MRHD on a mg/m² basis.

When eslicarbazepine acetate was orally administered (65, 125, 250 mg/kg/day) to rats during pregnancy and lactation, reduced offspring body weight was seen at the mid and high doses. Delayed sexual maturation and a neurological deficit (decreased motor coordination) were observed at the highest dose tested. The no-effect dose for adverse developmental effects (65 mg/kg/day) is less than the MRHD on a mg/m² basis.

The rat data are of uncertain relevance to humans because of differences in metabolic profile between species.

Pregnancy Registry

Physicians are advised to recommend that pregnant patients taking APTIOM enroll in the North American Antiepileptic Drug Pregnancy Registry. This can be done by calling 1-888-233-2334 (toll-free), and must be done by patients themselves. Information on the registry can also be found at the website http://www.aedpregnancyregistry.org/.

8.3 Nursing Mothers

Eslicarbazepine is excreted in human milk. Because of the potential for serious adverse reactions in nursing infants from APTIOM, a decision should be made whether to discontinue nursing or to discontinue the drug, taking into account the importance of the drug to the mother.

8.4 Pediatric Use

Safety and effectiveness in patients below 18 years of age have not been established.

In a juvenile animal study in which eslicarbazepine acetate (40, 60, 160 mg/kg/day) was orally administered to young dogs for 10 months starting on postnatal day 21, mortality and evidence of immunotoxicity (bone marrow hypocellularity and lymphoid tissue depletion) were observed at all doses. Convulsions were seen at the highest dose tested. Adverse effects on bone growth (decreased bone mineral content and density) were seen in females at all doses at the end of the dosing period, but not at the end of a 2-month recovery period. None of these findings were reported in adult dogs dosed with eslicarbazepine acetate for up to 12 months in duration. A no-effect dose for adverse effects on juvenile dogs was not identified.

8.5 Geriatric Use

There were insufficient numbers of patients ≥65 years old enrolled in the controlled epilepsy trials (N=15) to determine the efficacy of APTIOM in this patient population. The pharmacokinetics of APTIOM were evaluated in elderly healthy subjects (N=12) (Figure 3). Although the pharmacokinetics of eslicarbazepine are not affected by age independently, dose selection should take in consideration the greater frequency of renal impairment and other concomitant medical conditions and drug therapies in the elderly patient. Dose adjustment is necessary if CrCl <50 mL/min [see Clinical Pharmacology (12.3)].

8.6 Patients with Renal Impairment

Clearance of eslicarbazepine is decreased in patients with impaired renal function and is correlated with creatinine clearance. Dosage adjustment is necessary in patients with CrCl<50 mL/min (Figure 3) [see Dosage and Administration (2.4) and Clinical Pharmacology (12.3)].

8.7 Patients with Hepatic Impairment

Dose adjustments are not required in patients with mild to moderate hepatic impairment (Figure 3). Use of APTIOM in patients with severe hepatic impairment has not been evaluated, and use in these patients is not recommended [see Clinical Pharmacology (12.3)].

8.8 Gender

No dosage adjustment is recommended on the basis of gender (Figure 3) [see Clinical Pharmacology (12.3)].

[See figure 3 at top of next page]

8.9 Females of Reproductive Potential

Because concomitant use of APTIOM and ethinylestradiol and levonorgestrel is associated with lower plasma levels of these hormones, females of reproductive potential should use additional or alternative non-hormonal birth control [see Drug Interactions (7.3, 7.4)].

9 DRUG ABUSE AND DEPENDENCE

9.1 Controlled Substance

APTIOM is not a controlled substance.

9.2 Abuse

Prescription drug abuse is the intentional non-therapeutic use of a drug, even once, for its rewarding psychological or physiological effects. Drug addiction, which develops after repeated drug abuse, is characterized by a strong desire to take a drug despite harmful consequences, difficulty in controlling its use, giving a higher priority to drug use than to obligations, increased tolerance, and sometimes physical withdrawal. Drug abuse and drug addiction are separate and distinct from physical dependence (for example, abuse may not be accompanied by physical dependence) [see Drug Abuse and Dependence (9.3)].

In a human abuse study in recreational sedative abusers APTIOM showed no evidence of abuse. In Phase 1, 1.5% of the healthy volunteers taking APTIOM reported euphoria compared to 0.4% taking placebo.

9.3 Dependence
Physical dependence is characterized by withdrawal symptoms after abrupt discontinuation or a significant dose reduction of a drug.

The potential for APTIOM to produce withdrawal symptoms has not been adequately evaluated. In general, antiepileptic drugs should not be abruptly discontinued in patients with epilepsy because of the risk of increased seizure frequency and status epilepticus.

10 OVERDOSAGE
10.1 Signs, Symptoms, and Laboratory Findings of Acute Overdose in Humans
Symptoms of overdose are consistent with the known adverse reactions of APTIOM and include hyponatremia (sometimes severe), dizziness, nausea, vomiting, somnolence, euphoria, oral paraesthesia, ataxia, walking difficulties, and diplopia.

10.2 Treatment or Management of Overdose
There is no specific antidote for overdose with APTIOM. Symptomatic and supportive treatment should be administered as appropriate. Removal of the drug by gastric lavage and/or inactivation by administering activated charcoal should be considered.

Standard hemodialysis procedures result in partial clearance of APTIOM. Hemodialysis may be considered based on the patient's clinical state or in patients with significant renal impairment.

11 DESCRIPTION
The chemical name of APTIOM (eslicarbazepine acetate) is (S)-10-Acetoxy-10,11-dihydro-5H-dibenz[b,f]azepine-5-carboxamide. APTIOM is a dibenz[b,f]azepine-5-carboxamide derivative. Its molecular formula is $C_{17}H_{16}N_2O_3$ and its molecular weight is 296.32. The chemical structure is:

APTIOM is a white to off-white, odorless crystalline solid. It is insoluble in hexane, very slightly soluble in aqueous solvents and soluble in organic solvents such as acetone, acetonitrile, and methanol.

Each APTIOM tablet contains 200 mg, 400 mg, 600 mg or 800 mg of eslicarbazepine acetate and the following inactive ingredients: povidone, croscarmellose sodium, and magnesium stearate.

12 CLINICAL PHARMACOLOGY
12.1 Mechanism of Action
APTIOM is extensively converted to eslicarbazepine, which is considered to be responsible for therapeutic effects in humans. The precise mechanism(s) by which eslicarbazepine exerts anticonvulsant activity is unknown but is thought to involve inhibition of voltage-gated sodium channels.

12.2 Pharmacodynamics
The effect of APTIOM on cardiac repolarization was evaluated in a randomized, double-blind, placebo- and active-controlled 4-period crossover trial in healthy adult men and women. Subjects received APTIOM 1200 mg once daily × 5 days, APTIOM 2400 mg once daily × 5 days, an active-control, moxifloxacin 400 mg × 1 dose on Day 5, and placebo once daily × 5 days. At both doses of APTIOM, no significant effect on the QTc interval was detected.

12.3 Pharmacokinetics
The pharmacokinetics of eslicarbazepine is linear and dose-proportional in the dose range of 400 mg to 1200 mg once daily, both in healthy subjects and patients. The apparent half-life of eslicarbazepine in plasma was 13 -20 hours in epilepsy patients. Steady-state plasma concentrations are attained after 4 to 5 days of once daily dosing.

Absorption, Distribution, Metabolism, and Excretion

Absorption

APTIOM is mostly undetectable (0.01% of the systemic exposure) after oral administration. Eslicarbazepine, the major metabolite, is primarily responsible for the pharmacological effect of APTIOM. Peak plasma concentrations (C_{max}) of eslicarbazepine are attained at 1-4 hours post-dose. Eslicarbazepine is highly bioavailable, because the amount of eslicarbazepine and glucuronide metabolites recovered in urine corresponded to more than 90% of an APTIOM dose. Food has no effect on the pharmacokinetics of eslicarbazepine after oral administration of APTIOM.

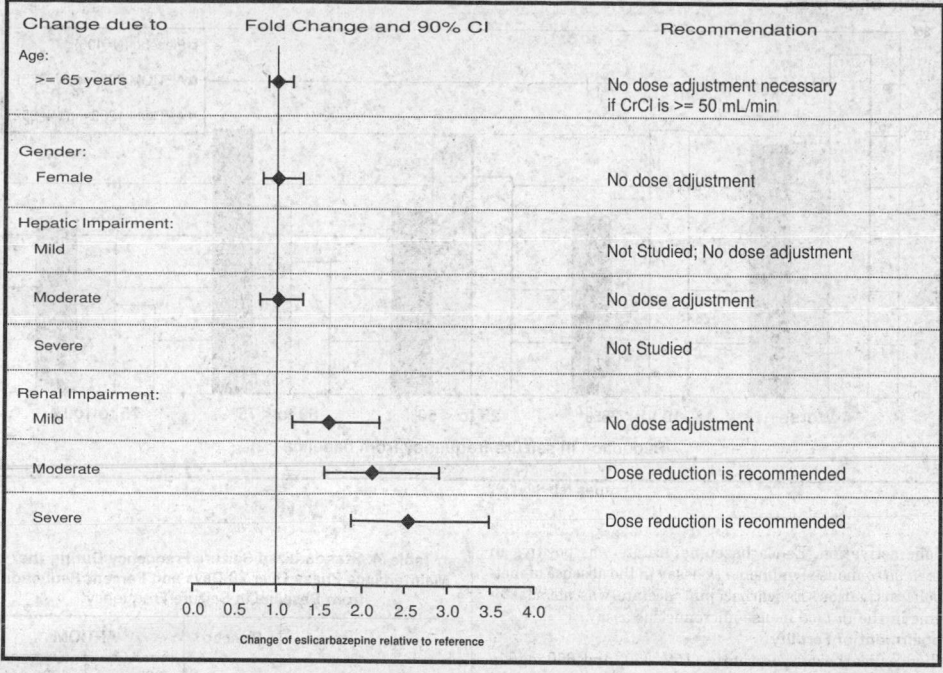

Figure 3: Impact of Intrinsic Factors on AUC of Eslicarbazepine

Change due to	Fold Change and 90% CI	Recommendation
Age:		
>= 65 years		No dose adjustment necessary if CrCl is >= 50 mL/min
Gender:		
Female		No dose adjustment
Hepatic Impairment:		
Mild		Not Studied; No dose adjustment
Moderate		No dose adjustment
Severe		Not Studied
Renal Impairment:		
Mild		No dose adjustment
Moderate		Dose reduction is recommended
Severe		Dose reduction is recommended

Change of eslicarbazepine relative to reference

Distribution

The binding of eslicarbazepine to plasma proteins is relatively low (<40%) and independent of concentration. *In vitro* studies have shown that plasma protein binding was not relevantly affected by the presence of warfarin, diazepam, digoxin, phenytoin, or tolbutamide. Similarly, the binding of warfarin, diazepam, digoxin, phenytoin or tolbutamide was not significantly affected by the presence of eslicarbazepine. The apparent volume of distribution of eslicarbazepine is 61 L for body weight of 70 kg based on population PK analysis.

Metabolism

APTIOM is rapidly and extensively metabolized to its major active metabolite eslicarbazepine by hydrolytic first-pass metabolism. Eslicarbazepine corresponds to 91% of systemic exposure. The systemic exposure to minor active metabolites of (R)-licarbazepine is 5% and oxcarbazepine is 1%. The inactive glucuronides of these active metabolites correspond to approximately 3% of systemic exposure.

In *in vitro* studies in human liver microsomes, eslicarbazepine had no clinically relevant inhibitory effect on the activity of CYP1A2, CYP2A6, CYP2B6, CYP2D6, CYP2E1, and CYP3A4, and only a moderate inhibitory effect on CYP2C19. Studies with eslicarbazepine in fresh human hepatocytes showed no induction of enzymes involved in glucuronidation and sulfation of 7-hydroxy-coumarin. A mild activation of UGT1A1- mediated glucuronidation was observed in human hepatic microsomes.

No apparent autoinduction of metabolism has been observed with APTIOM in humans.

Excretion

APTIOM metabolites are eliminated from the systemic circulation primarily by renal excretion, in the unchanged and glucuronide conjugate forms. In total, eslicarbazepine and its glucuronide account for more than 90% of total metabolites excreted in urine, approximately two thirds in the unchanged form and one third as glucuronide conjugate. Other minor metabolites account for the remaining 10% excreted in the urine. In healthy subjects with normal renal function, the renal clearance of eslicarbazepine (approximately 20 mL/min) is substantially lower than glomerular filtration rate (80-120 mL/min), suggesting that renal tubular reabsorption occurs. The apparent plasma half-life of eslicarbazepine was 13-20 hours in epilepsy patients *[see Dosage and Administration (2.4) and Use in Specific Populations (8.6)]*.

Specific Populations

Elderly (≥65 years of age)

The pharmacokinetic profile of eslicarbazepine was unaffected in elderly subjects with creatinine clearance >60 mL/min compared to healthy subjects (18-40 years) after single and repeated doses of 600 mg APTIOM during 8 days of dosing. No dose adjustment is necessary in adults based on age, if CrCl is ≥50 mL/min.

Gender

Studies in healthy subjects and patients showed that pharmacokinetics of eslicarbazepine was not affected by gender.

Race

No clinically significant effect of race (Caucasian N=849, Black N=53, Asian N=65, and Other N=51) on the pharmacokinetics of eslicarbazepine was noted in a population pharmacokinetic analysis of pooled data from the clinical studies.

Renal Impairment

APTIOM metabolites are eliminated from the systemic circulation primarily by renal excretion. The extent of systemic exposure of eslicarbazepine following an 800 mg single dose was increased by 62% in patients with mild renal impairment (CrCl 50-80 mL/min), by 2-fold in patients with moderate renal impairment (CrCl 30-49 mL/min) and by 2.5-fold in patients with severe renal impairment (CrCl <30 mL/min) in comparison to the healthy subjects (CrCl >80 mL/min). Dosage adjustment is recommended in patients with creatinine clearance below 50 mL/min *[see Dosage and Administration (2.4) and Use in Specific Populations (8.6)]*.

In patients with end stage renal disease, repeated hemodialysis removed APTIOM metabolites from systemic circulation.

Hepatic Impairment

The pharmacokinetics and metabolism of APTIOM was evaluated in healthy subjects and patients with moderate liver impairment (7-9 points on the Child-Pugh assessment) after multiple oral doses. Moderate hepatic impairment did not affect the pharmacokinetics of APTIOM. No dose adjustment is recommended in patients with mild to moderate liver impairment.

The pharmacokinetics of APTIOM has not been studied in patients with severe hepatic impairment.

13 NONCLINICAL TOXICOLOGY
13.1 Carcinogenesis, Mutagenesis, Impairment of Fertility

Carcinogenesis

In a two-year carcinogenicity study in mice, eslicarbazepine acetate was administered orally at doses of 100, 250, and 600 mg/day. An increase in the incidence of hepatocellular adenomas and carcinomas was observed at 250 and 600 mg/kg/day in males and at 600 mg/kg/day in females. The dose not associated with an increase in tumors (100 mg/kg/day) is less than the maximum recommended human dose of 1200 mg/day on a mg/m² basis.

Mutagenesis

Eslicarbazepine acetate and eslicarbazepine were not mutagenic in the *in vitro* Ames assay. In *in vitro* assays in mammalian cells, eslicarbazepine acetate and eslicarbazepine were not clastogenic in human peripheral blood lymphocytes; however, eslicarbazepine acetate was clastogenic in Chinese hamster ovary (CHO) cells, with and without met-

Figure 4: Proportion of Patients by Category of Seizure Reduction for APTIOM and Placebo Across All Three Double-blind Trials

Figure 4: Proportion of Patients by Category of Seizure Reduction for APTIOM and Placebo Across All Three Double-blind Trials

fied with strength-specific one-sided engraving on the other side, "ESL 200" (200 mg), "ESL 400" (400 mg), "ESL 600" (600 mg), or "ESL 800" (800 mg). Tablets are supplied in the following strengths and package configurations (Table 5):

Table 5: Package Configuration for APTIOM Tablets

Tablet Strength	Package Configuration	NDC Code
200 mg	Bottles of 30	63402-202-30
400 mg	Bottles of 30	63402-204-30
600 mg	Bottles of 60	63402-206-60
	Bottles of 90	63402-206-90
800 mg	Bottles of 30	63402-208-30
	Bottles of 90	63402-208-90

Storage
Store APTIOM tablets at 20°C to 25°C (68°F to 77°F); excursions permitted to 15°C to 30°C (59°F to 86°F) [see USP Controlled Room Temperature].

17   PATIENT COUNSELING INFORMATION
See FDA-approved patient labeling (Medication Guide). Inform patients of the availability of a Medication Guide, and instruct them to read the Medication Guide prior to taking APTIOM. Instruct patients to take APTIOM only as prescribed.

Suicidal Behavior and Ideation
Counsel patients, their caregivers, and families that AEDs, including APTIOM, may increase the risk of suicidal thoughts and behavior and advise them of the need to be alert for the emergence or worsening of symptoms of depression, any unusual changes in mood or behavior, or the emergence of suicidal thoughts, behavior, or thoughts about self-harm. Instruct patients, caregivers, and families to report behaviors of concern immediately to healthcare providers [see Warnings and Precautions (5.1)].

Serious Dermatologic Reactions
Advise patients and caregivers about the risk of potentially fatal serious skin reactions. Educate patients about the signs and symptoms that may signal a serious skin reaction. Instruct patients to consult with their healthcare provider immediately if a skin reaction occurs during treatment with APTIOM [see Warnings and Precautions (5.2)].

DRESS/Multiorgan Hypersensitivity
Instruct patients that a fever associated with signs of other organ system involvement (e.g., rash, lymphadenopathy, hepatic dysfunction) may be drug-related and should be reported to their healthcare provider immediately [see Warnings and Precautions (5.3)].

Anaphylactic Reactions and Angioedema
Advise patients of life threatening symptoms suggesting anaphylaxis or angioedema (swelling of the face, eyes, lips, tongue, or difficulty in swallowing or breathing) that can occur with APTIOM. Instruct them to immediately report these symptoms to their healthcare provider [see Warnings and Precautions (5.4)].

Hyponatremia
Advise patients that APTIOM may reduce serum sodium concentrations, especially if they are taking other medications that can lower sodium. Advise patients to report symptoms of low sodium such as nausea, tiredness, lack of energy, irritability, confusion, muscle weakness/spasms, or more frequent or more severe seizures [see Warnings and Precautions (5.5)].

Neurological Adverse Reactions
Counsel patients that APTIOM may cause dizziness, gait disturbance, somnolence/fatigue, cognitive dysfunction, and visual changes. These adverse reactions, if observed, are more likely to occur during the titration period compared to the maintenance period. Advise patients not to drive or operate machinery until they have gained sufficient experience on APTIOM to gauge whether it adversely affects their ability to drive or operate machinery [see Warnings and Precautions (5.6)].

Withdrawal of APTIOM
Advise patients not to discontinue use of APTIOM without consulting with their healthcare provider. APTIOM should be gradually withdrawn to minimize the potential of increased seizure frequency and status epilepticus [see Warnings and Precautions (5.7)].

Interaction with Oral Contraceptives
Inform patients that APTIOM can significantly decrease the effectiveness of hormonal contraceptives. Recommend that female patients of childbearing potential use additional or alternative non-hormonal forms of contraception during treatment with APTIOM and after treatment has been dis-

abolic activation. Eslicarbazepine acetate was positive in the *in vitro* mouse lymphoma *tk* assay in the absence of metabolic activation. Eslicarbazepine acetate was not clastogenic in the *in vivo* mouse micronucleus assay.

Impairment of Fertility
When eslicarbazepine acetate (150, 350, and 650 mg/kg/day) was orally administered to male and female mice prior to and throughout the mating period, and continuing in females to gestation day 6, there was an increase in embryolethality at all doses. The lowest dose tested is less than the maximum recommended human dose (1200 mg/day) on a mg/m² basis.
When eslicarbazepine acetate (65, 125, 250 mg/kg/day) was orally administered to male and female rats prior to and throughout the mating period, and continuing in females to implantation, lengthening of the estrus cycle was observed at the highest dose tested. The data in rats are of uncertain relevance to humans because of differences in metabolic profile between species.

14   CLINICAL STUDIES
14.1   Clinical Studies in Adults with Partial-Onset Seizures
The efficacy of APTIOM as adjunctive therapy in partial-onset seizures was established in three randomized, double-blind, placebo-controlled, multicenter trials in adult patients with epilepsy (Studies 1, 2, and 3). Patients enrolled had partial-onset seizures with or without secondary generalization and were not adequately controlled with 1 to 3 concomitant AEDs. During an 8-week baseline period, patients were required to have an average of ≥4 partial-onset seizures per 28 days with no seizure-free period exceeding 21 days. In these three trials, patients had a median duration of epilepsy of 19 years and a median baseline seizure frequency of 8 seizures per 28 days. Two-thirds (69%) of subjects used 2 concomitant AEDs and 28% used 1 concomitant AED. The most commonly used AEDs were carbamazepine (50%), lamotrigine (24%), valproic acid (21%), and levetiracetam (18%). Oxcarbazepine was not allowed as a concomitant AED.
Studies 1 and 2 compared dosages of APTIOM 400, 800, and 1200 mg once daily with placebo. Study 3 compared dosages of APTIOM 800 and 1200 mg once daily with placebo. In all three trials, following an 8-week Baseline Phase, which established a baseline seizure frequency, subjects were randomized to a treatment arm. Patients entered a treatment period consisting of an initial titration phase (2 weeks), and a subsequent maintenance phase (12 weeks). The specific titration schedule differed amongst the three studies. Thus, patients were started on a daily dose of 400 mg or 800 mg and subsequently increased by 400 mg/day following one or two weeks, until the final daily target dose was achieved.
The standardized seizure frequency during the Maintenance Phase over 28 days was the primary efficacy endpoint in all three trials. Table 4 presents the results for the primary endpoint, as well as the secondary endpoint of percent reduction from baseline in seizure frequency. The APTIOM treatment at 400 mg/day was studied in Studies 1 and 2 and did not show significant treatment effect. A statistically significant effect was observed with APTIOM treatment at doses of 800 mg/day in Studies 1 and 2 but not in Study 3, and at doses of 1200 mg/day in all 3 studies.

Table 4: Standardized Seizure Frequency During the Maintenance Phase Over 28 Days and Percent Reduction from Baseline in Seizure Frequency

	Placebo	APTIOM 800 mg	APTIOM 1200 mg
Study 1			
N	95	88	87
Seizure Frequency (LS Mean seizures per 28 days) (p-value)	6.6	5.0 (0.047*)	4.3 (0.001*)
Median Percent Reduction from Baseline in Seizure Frequency (%)	-15	-36	-39
Study 2			
N	99	87	81
Seizure Frequency (LS Mean seizures per 28 days) (p-value)	8.6	6.2 (0.006*)	6.6 (0.042*)
Median Percent Reduction from Baseline in Seizure Frequency (%)	-6	-33	-28
Study 3			
N	212	200	184
Seizure Frequency (LS Mean seizures per 28 days) (p-value)	7.9	6.5 (0.058)	6.0 (0.004*)
Median Percent Reduction from Baseline in Seizure Frequency (%)	-22	-30	-36

*statistically significant compared to placebo

Figure 4 shows changes from baseline in the 28-day total partial seizure frequency by category of reduction in seizure frequency from baseline for patients treated with APTIOM and placebo in an integrated analysis across the three clinical trials. Patients in whom the seizure frequency increased are shown to the left as "Worse." Patients in whom the seizure frequency decreased are shown in four categories.
[See figure 4 above]

16   HOW SUPPLIED/STORAGE AND HANDLING
APTIOM tablets are white, oblong and with functional scoring on one side (200 mg, 600 mg, and 800 mg) or white, circular bi-convex and plain on one side (400 mg) and identi-

continued for at least one menstrual cycle or until otherwise instructed by their healthcare provider [see Drug Interactions (7.3, 7.4)].

Pregnancy Registry

Encourage patients to enroll in the North American Antiepileptic Drug Pregnancy Registry if they become pregnant. This Registry is collecting information about the safety of AEDs during pregnancy. To enroll, patients can call 1-888-233-2334 (toll-free) [see Use in Specific Populations (8.1)].

SUNOVION

Manufactured for:

Sunovion Pharmaceuticals Inc.

Marlborough, MA 01752 USA

Under license from   Bial

© 2013 Sunovion Pharmaceuticals Inc. All rights reserved.

901716R00

MEDICATION GUIDE

APTIOM (ap tee' om)

(eslicarbazepine acetate)

tablets

Read this Medication Guide before you start taking APTIOM and each time you get a refill. There may be new information. This information does not take the place of talking to your healthcare provider about your medical condition or treatment.

What is the most important information I should know about APTIOM?

Do not stop taking APTIOM without first talking to your healthcare provider.

Stopping APTIOM suddenly can cause serious problems.

1. **Like other antiepileptic drugs, APTIOM may cause suicidal thoughts or actions in a very small number of people, about 1 in 500.**

   Call a healthcare provider right away if you have any of these symptoms, especially if they are new, worse, or worry you:
   * thoughts about suicide or dying
   * attempt to commit suicide
   * new or worse depression
   * new or worse anxiety
   * feeling agitated or restless
   * panic attacks
   * trouble sleeping (insomnia)
   * new or worse irritability
   * acting aggressive, being angry, or violent
   * acting on dangerous impulses
   * an extreme increase in activity and talking (mania)
   * other unusual changes in behavior or mood

   How can I watch for early symptoms of suicidal thoughts and actions?
   * Pay attention to any changes, especially sudden changes, in mood, behaviors, thoughts, or feelings.
   * Keep all follow-up visits with your healthcare provider as scheduled.

   Call your healthcare provider between visits as needed, especially if you are worried about symptoms.

   Do not stop taking APTIOM without first talking to a healthcare provider.

   Stopping APTIOM suddenly can cause serious problems. Stopping a seizure medicine suddenly in a patient who has epilepsy may cause seizures that will not stop (status epilepticus).

   Suicidal thoughts or actions may be caused by things other than medicines. If you have suicidal thoughts or actions, your healthcare provider may check for other causes.

2. APTIOM may cause allergic reactions or serious problems which may affect organs and other parts of your body like the liver or blood cells. You may or may not have a rash with these types of reactions.

   Call your healthcare provider right away if you have any of the following:
   * swelling of your face, eyes, lips, or tongue
   * trouble swallowing or breathing
   * a skin rash
   * hives
   * fever, swollen glands, or sore throat that do not go away or come and go
   * painful sores in the mouth or around your eyes
   * yellowing of your skin or eyes
   * unusual bruising or bleeding
   * severe fatigue or weakness
   * severe muscle pain
   * frequent infections or infections that do not go away

3. APTIOM may cause the level of sodium in your blood to be low. Symptoms of low blood sodium include:
   * nausea
   * tiredness, lack of energy
   * irritability
   * confusion
   * muscle weakness or muscle spasms
   * more frequent or more severe seizures

Some medicines can also cause low sodium in your blood. Be sure to tell your healthcare provider about all the other medicines that you are taking.

What is APTIOM?

APTIOM is a prescription medicine used with other medicines to treat partial-onset seizures.

It is not known if APTIOM is safe and effective in children under 18 years of age.

Who should not take APTIOM?

Do not take APTIOM if you are allergic to eslicarbazepine acetate, any of the other ingredients in APTIOM, or oxcarbazepine. See the end of this Medication Guide for a complete list of ingredients in APTIOM.

What should I tell my healthcare provider before taking APTIOM?

Before taking APTIOM, tell your healthcare provider about all your medical conditions, including if you:
* have or have had suicidal thoughts or actions, depression or mood problems
* have liver problems
* have kidney problems
* are allergic to oxcarbazepine. Some people who are allergic to oxcarbazepine may also be allergic to APTIOM.
* use birth control medicine. APTIOM may cause your birth control medicine to be less effective. Talk to your healthcare provider about the best birth control method to use.
* are pregnant or plan to become pregnant. APTIOM may harm your unborn baby. Tell your healthcare provider right away if you become pregnant while taking APTIOM. You and your healthcare provider will decide if you should take APTIOM while you are pregnant.
  ◦ If you become pregnant while taking APTIOM, talk to your healthcare provider about registering with the North American Antiepileptic Drug (NAAED) Pregnancy Registry. The purpose of this registry is to collect information about the safety of antiepileptic medicine during pregnancy. You can enroll in this registry by calling 1-888-233-2334.
* are breastfeeding or plan to breastfeed. APTIOM passes into breast milk. You and your healthcare provider should discuss whether you should take APTIOM or breastfeed.

Tell your healthcare provider about all the medicines you take, including prescription and over-the-counter medicines, vitamins, and herbal supplements.

Taking APTIOM with certain other medicines may cause side effects or affect how well they work. Do not start or stop other medicines without talking to your healthcare provider.

Especially tell your healthcare provider if you take:

• oxcarbazepine	• omeprazole
• carbamazepine	• simvastatin
• phenobarbital	• rosuvastatin
• phenytoin	• birth control
• primidone	medicine
• clobazam	

Ask your healthcare provider or pharmacist for a list of these medicines, if you are not sure.

Know the medicines you take. Keep a list of them and show it to your healthcare provider and pharmacist when you get a new medicine.

How should I take APTIOM?
* Do not stop taking APTIOM without talking to your healthcare provider. Stopping APTIOM suddenly can cause serious problems, including seizures that will not stop (status epilepticus).
* Take APTIOM exactly as prescribed.
* Your healthcare provider may change your dose.
* Your healthcare provider will tell you how much APTIOM to take.
* APTIOM can be taken with or without food.
* APTIOM can be taken as a whole tablet or crushed.
* If you take too much APTIOM, call your healthcare provider or go to the nearest hospital emergency room right away.
* Talk with your healthcare provider about what you should do if you miss a dose.

What should I avoid while taking APTIOM?
* Do not drive, operate heavy machinery, or do dangerous activities until you know how APTIOM affects you. APTIOM may slow your thinking and motor skills.

What are the possible side effects of APTIOM?

See "What is the most important information I should know about APTIOM?"

APTIOM may cause other serious side effects including:
* **Nervous system problems.** APTIOM may cause problems that can affect your nervous system. Symptoms of nervous system problems include:
  ◦ dizziness
  ◦ trouble walking or with coordination
  ◦ feeling sleepy and tired
  ◦ trouble concentrating
  ◦ vision problems

* **Liver problems.** APTIOM may affect your liver. Symptoms of liver problems include:
  * yellowing of your skin or the whites of your eyes
  * nausea or vomiting
  * loss of appetite
  * stomach pain
  * dark urine

Get medical help right away if you have any of the symptoms listed above or listed in "What is the most important information I should know about APTIOM?"

The most common side effects of APTIOM include:

• dizziness	• vomiting
• sleepiness	• feeling tired
• nausea	• problems with
• headache	coordination
• double vision	• blurred vision
	• shakiness

Tell your healthcare provider if you have any side effect that bothers you or that does not go away.

These are not all the possible side effects of APTIOM. For more information, ask your healthcare provider or pharmacist.

Call your doctor for medical advice about side effects. You may report side effects to FDA at 1-800-FDA-1088.

How should I store APTIOM?
* Store APTIOM at 68°F to 77°F (20°C to 25°C).
* Safely throw away medicine that is out of date or no longer needed.

Keep APTIOM and all medicines out of reach of children.

General information about the safe and effective use of APTIOM.

Medicines are sometimes prescribed for purposes other than those listed in a Medication Guide. Do not use APTIOM for a condition for which it was not prescribed. Do not give APTIOM to other people, even if they have the same symptoms that you have. It may harm them.

This Medication Guide summarizes the most important information about APTIOM. If you would like more information, talk with your healthcare provider. You can ask your pharmacist or healthcare provider for information about APTIOM that is written for health professionals.

For more information, go to www.aptiom.com or call 1-888-394-7377.

What are the ingredients in APTIOM?

Active ingredient: eslicarbazepine acetate

Inactive ingredients: povidone, croscarmellose sodium, and magnesium stearate.

This Medication Guide has been approved by the U.S. Food and Drug Administration.

SUNOVION

Manufactured for:

Sunovion Pharmaceuticals Inc.

Marlborough, MA 01752 USA

Under license from   Bial

© 2013 Sunovion Pharmaceuticals Inc. All rights reserved.

November 2013

Shown in Product Identification Guide, page 313

BROVANA®   ℞

(arformoterol tartrate)

Inhalation Solution

HIGHLIGHTS OF PRESCRIBING INFORMATION

These highlights do not include all the information needed to use BROVANA® safely and effectively. See full prescribing information for BROVANA.

BROVANA® (arformoterol tartrate) Inhalation Solution

Initial U.S. Approval: 2006

WARNING: ASTHMA-RELATED DEATH

See full prescribing information for complete boxed warning.

* **Long-acting beta$_2$-adrenergic agonists (LABA) increase the risk of asthma-related death. (5.1)**
* **A placebo-controlled study with another long-acting beta$_2$-adrenergic agonist (salmeterol) showed an increase in asthma related deaths in patients receiving salmeterol. (5.1)**
* **The finding of an increase in the risk of asthma-related deaths with salmeterol is considered a class effect of LABA, including arformoterol, the active ingredient in BROVANA Inhalation Solution. The safety and efficacy of BROVANA Inhalation Solution in patients with asthma have not been established. All LABA, including BROVANA Inhalation Solution, are contraindicated in patients with asthma without use of a long-term asthma control medication. (4, 5.1)**

——————INDICATIONS AND USAGE——————

BROVANA Inhalation Solution is a long-acting beta$_2$-adrenergic agonist (beta$_2$-agonist) indicated for:

- Long-term, twice daily (morning and evening) administration in the maintenance treatment of bronchoconstriction in patients with chronic obstructive pulmonary disease (COPD), including chronic bronchitis and emphysema. (1.1)

Important limitations of use:
- BROVANA Inhalation Solution is not indicated to treat acute deteriorations of chronic obstructive pulmonary disease. (1.2, 5.2)
- BROVANA Inhalation Solution is not indicated to treat asthma. (1.2)

——————DOSAGE AND ADMINISTRATION——————

For oral inhalation only.
- A total daily dose of greater than 30 mcg is not recommended. (2)
- One 15 mcg/2 mL vial every 12 hours. (2)
- For use with a standard jet nebulizer (with a face mask or mouthpiece) connected to an air compressor. (2)

——————DOSAGE FORMS AND STRENGTHS——————

Inhalation Solution (unit-dose vial for nebulization): 15 mcg/2 mL solution (3)

——————CONTRAINDICATIONS——————

- BROVANA Inhalation Solution is contraindicated in patients with a history of hypersensitivity to arformoterol, racemic formoterol or to any other components of this product. (4)
- All LABA, including BROVANA Inhalation Solution, are contraindicated in patients with asthma without use of a long-term asthma control medication. (4)

——————WARNINGS AND PRECAUTIONS——————

- Do not initiate BROVANA Inhalation Solution in acutely deteriorating patients. (5.2)
- Do not use for relief of acute symptoms. Concomitant short-acting beta₂-agonists can be used as needed for acute relief. (5.2)
- Do not exceed the recommended dose. Excessive use of BROVANA Inhalation Solution, or use in conjunction with other medications containing long-acting beta₂-agonists, can result in clinically significant cardiovascular effects, and may be fatal. (5.3, 5.5)
- Life-threatening paradoxical bronchospasm can occur. Discontinue BROVANA Inhalation Solution immediately. (5.4)
- Use with caution in patients with cardiovascular or convulsive disorders, thyrotoxicosis, or with sensitivity to sympathomimetic drugs. (5.6, 5.7)

——————ADVERSE REACTIONS——————

Most common adverse reactions (≥2% incidence and more common than placebo) are pain, chest pain, back pain, diarrhea, sinusitis, leg cramps, dyspnea, rash, flu syndrome, peripheral edema and lung disorder. (6.2)

To report SUSPECTED ADVERSE REACTIONS, contact Sunovion Pharmaceuticals Inc. at 1-877-737-7226 or FDA at 1-800-FDA-1088 or www.fda.gov/medwatch.

——————DRUG INTERACTIONS——————

- Other adrenergic drugs may potentiate effect. Use with caution. (5.3, 7.1)
- Xanthine derivatives, steroids, diuretics, or non-potassium sparing diuretics may potentiate hypokalemia or ECG changes. Use with caution. (5.7, 7.2, 7.3)
- MAO inhibitors, tricyclic antidepressants and drugs that prolong the QTc interval may potentiate effect on the cardiovascular system. Use with extreme caution. (7.4)
- Beta-blockers may decrease effectiveness. May block bronchodilatory effects of beta-agonists. Use with caution and only when medically necessary. (7.5)

——————USE IN SPECIFIC POPULATIONS——————

- Hepatic Impairment
Use with caution in patients with hepatic impairment. (8.6)

See 17 for PATIENT COUNSELING INFORMATION and Medication Guide

Revised: 02/2014

FULL PRESCRIBING INFORMATION: CONTENTS*
WARNING: ASTHMA RELATED DEATH
1   INDICATIONS AND USAGE
     1.1   Maintenance Treatment of COPD
     1.2   Important Limitations of Use
2   DOSAGE AND ADMINISTRATION
3   DOSAGE FORMS AND STRENGTHS
4   CONTRAINDICATIONS
5   WARNINGS AND PRECAUTIONS
     5.1   Asthma-Related Deaths
     5.2   Deterioration of Disease and Acute Episodes
     5.3   Excessive Use of BROVANA Inhalation Solution and Use with Other Long-Acting Beta₂-Agonists

     5.4   Paradoxical Bronchospasm
     5.5   Cardiovascular Effects
     5.6   Coexisting Conditions
     5.7   Hypokalemia and Hyperglycemia
     5.8   Immediate Hypersensitivity Reactions
6   ADVERSE REACTIONS
     6.1   Beta₂-Agonist Adverse Reaction Profile
     6.2   Clinical Trials Experience
7   DRUG INTERACTIONS
     7.1   Adrenergic Drugs
     7.2   Xanthine Derivatives, Steroids, or Diuretics
     7.3   Non-potassium Sparing Diuretics
     7.4   MAO Inhibitors, Tricyclic Antidepressants, QTc Prolonging Drugs
     7.5   Beta-Blockers
8   USE IN SPECIFIC POPULATIONS
     8.1   Pregnancy
     8.2   Labor and Delivery
     8.3   Nursing Mothers
     8.4   Pediatric Use
     8.5   Geriatric Use
     8.6   Hepatic Impairment
     8.7   Renal Impairment
9   DRUG ABUSE AND DEPENDENCE
10   OVERDOSAGE
11   DESCRIPTION
12   CLINICAL PHARMACOLOGY
     12.1   Mechanism of Action
     12.2   Pharmacodynamics
     12.3   Pharmacokinetics
     12.5   Pharmacogenetics
13   NONCLINICAL TOXICOLOGY
     13.1   Carcinogenesis, Mutagenesis, Impairment of Fertility
     13.2   Animal Toxicology and/or Pharmacology
14   CLINICAL STUDIES
     14.1   Adult COPD Trials
16   HOW SUPPLIED/STORAGE AND HANDLING
17   PATIENT COUNSELING INFORMATION
* Sections or subsections omitted from the full prescribing information are not listed

FULL PRESCRIBING INFORMATION

WARNING: ASTHMA RELATED DEATH

Long-acting beta₂-adrenergic agonists (LABA) increase the risk of asthma-related death. Data from a large placebo-controlled US study that compared the safety of another long-acting beta₂-adrenergic agonist (salmeterol) or placebo added to usual asthma therapy showed an increase in asthma-related deaths in patients receiving salmeterol. This finding with salmeterol is considered a class effect of LABA, including arformoterol, the active ingredient in BROVANA Inhalation Solution [see WARNINGS AND PRECAUTIONS (5.1)]. The safety and efficacy of BROVANA Inhalation Solution in patients with asthma have not been established. All LABA, including BROVANA Inhalation Solution, are contraindicated in patients with asthma without use of a long-term asthma control medication [see CONTRAINDICATIONS (4), WARNINGS AND PRECAUTIONS (5.1)].

---

1   INDICATIONS AND USAGE
1.1   Maintenance Treatment of COPD
BROVANA (arformoterol tartrate) Inhalation Solution is indicated for the long-term, twice daily (morning and evening) maintenance treatment of bronchoconstriction in patients with chronic obstructive pulmonary disease (COPD), including chronic bronchitis and emphysema. BROVANA Inhalation Solution is for use by nebulization only.
1.2   Important Limitations of Use
BROVANA Inhalation Solution is not indicated to treat acute deteriorations of chronic obstructive pulmonary disease [see WARNINGS AND PRECAUTIONS (5.2)].
BROVANA Inhalation Solution is not indicated to treat asthma. The safety and effectiveness of BROVANA Inhalation Solution in asthma have not been established.

2   DOSAGE AND ADMINISTRATION

The recommended dose of BROVANA (arformoterol tartrate) Inhalation Solution is one 15 mcg unit-dose vial administered twice daily (morning and evening) by nebulization. A total daily dose of greater than 30 mcg (15 mcg twice daily) is not recommended.
BROVANA Inhalation Solution should be administered by the orally inhaled route via a standard jet nebulizer connected to an air compressor (see the accompanying **Medication Guide**). BROVANA Inhalation Solution should not be swallowed. BROVANA Inhalation Solution should be stored refrigerated in foil pouches. After opening the pouch, un-

used unit-dose vials should be returned to, and stored in, the pouch. An opened unit-dose vial should be used right away.
If the recommended maintenance treatment regimen fails to provide the usual response, medical advice should be sought immediately, as this is often a sign of destabilization of COPD. Under these circumstances, the therapeutic regimen should be reevaluated and additional therapeutic options should be considered.
No dose adjustment is required for patients with renal or hepatic impairment. However, since the clearance of BROVANA Inhalation Solution is prolonged in patients with hepatic impairment, they should be monitored closely. The drug compatibility (physical and chemical), efficacy, and safety of BROVANA Inhalation Solution when mixed with other drugs in a nebulizer have not been established.
The safety and efficacy of BROVANA Inhalation Solution have been established in clinical trials when administered using the PARI LC® Plus nebulizer (with a face mask or mouthpiece) and the PARI DURA NEB™ 3000 compressor. The safety and efficacy of BROVANA Inhalation Solution delivered from non-compressor based nebulizer systems have not been established.

3   DOSAGE FORMS AND STRENGTHS
BROVANA (arformoterol tartrate) Inhalation Solution is supplied as a sterile solution for nebulization in low-density polyethylene unit-dose vials. Each 2 mL vial contains 15 mcg of arformoterol equivalent to 22 mcg of arformoterol tartrate.

4   CONTRAINDICATIONS
BROVANA Inhalation Solution is contraindicated in patients with a history of hypersensitivity to arformoterol, racemic formoterol or to any other components of this product.
All LABA, including BROVANA Inhalation Solution, are contraindicated in patients with asthma without use of a long-term asthma control medication [see WARNINGS AND PRECAUTIONS (5)].

5   WARNINGS AND PRECAUTIONS
5.1   Asthma-Related Deaths
[see BOXED WARNING]
Data from a large placebo-controlled study in asthma patients showed that long-acting beta₂-adrenergic agonists (LABA) increase the risk of asthma-related death. This finding is considered a class effect of LABA, including arformoterol, the active ingredient in BROVANA Inhalation Solution. The safety and efficacy of BROVANA Inhalation Solution in patients with asthma have not been established. All LABA, including BROVANA Inhalation Solution, are contraindicated in patients with asthma without use of a long-term asthma control medication [see CONTRAINDICATIONS (4)]. Data are not available to determine whether the rate of deaths in patients with COPD is increased by long-acting beta₂-adrenergic agonists.
A 28-week, placebo-controlled US study comparing the safety of salmeterol with placebo, each added to usual asthma therapy, showed an increase in asthma-related deaths in patients receiving salmeterol (13/13,176 in patients treated with salmeterol vs. 3/13,179 in patients treated with placebo; RR 4.37, 95% CI 1.25, 15.34). The increased risk of asthma-related death is considered a class effect of the long-acting beta₂-adrenergic agonists, including BROVANA Inhalation Solution. No study adequate to determine whether the rate of asthma-related death is increased in patients treated with BROVANA Inhalation Solution has been conducted.
Clinical studies with racemic formoterol suggested a higher incidence of serious asthma exacerbations in patients who received racemic formoterol than in those who received placebo. The sizes of these studies were not adequate to precisely quantify the differences in serious asthma exacerbation rates between treatment groups.
5.2   Deterioration of Disease and Acute Episodes
BROVANA Inhalation Solution should not be initiated in patients with acutely deteriorating COPD, which may be a life-threatening condition. The use of BROVANA Inhalation Solution in this setting is inappropriate.
BROVANA Inhalation Solution is not indicated for the treatment of acute episodes of bronchospasm, i.e., as rescue therapy and acute doses should not be used for that purpose. Acute symptoms should be treated with an inhaled short-acting beta₂-agonist.
When beginning BROVANA Inhalation Solution, patients who have been taking inhaled short-acting beta₂-agonists on a regular basis (e.g., four times a day) should be instructed to discontinue the regular use of these drugs and use them only for symptomatic relief of acute respiratory symptoms. When prescribing BROVANA Inhalation Solution, the healthcare provider should also prescribe an inhaled, short-acting beta₂-agonist and instruct the patient how it should be used. Increasing inhaled beta₂-agonist use is a signal of deteriorating disease for which prompt medical attention is indicated. COPD may deteriorate acutely over a

period of hours or chronically over several days or longer. If BROVANA Inhalation Solution no longer controls the symptoms of bronchoconstriction, or the patient's inhaled, short-acting beta$_2$-agonist becomes less effective or the patient needs more inhalation of short-acting beta$_2$-agonist than usual, these may be markers of deterioration of disease. In this setting, a reevaluation of the patient and the COPD treatment regimen should be undertaken at once. Increasing the daily dosage of BROVANA Inhalation Solution beyond the recommended 15 mcg twice daily dose is not appropriate in this situation.

5.3 Excessive Use of BROVANA Inhalation Solution and Use with Other Long-Acting Beta$_2$-Agonists

Fatalities have been reported in association with excessive use of inhaled sympathomimetic drugs. As with other inhaled beta$_2$-adrenergic drugs, BROVANA Inhalation Solution should not be used more often, at higher doses than recommended, or in conjunction with other medications containing long-acting beta$_2$-agonists.

5.4 Paradoxical Bronchospasm

As with other inhaled beta$_2$-agonists, BROVANA Inhalation Solution can produce paradoxical bronchospasm that may be life-threatening. If paradoxical bronchospasm occurs, BROVANA Inhalation Solution should be discontinued immediately and alternative therapy instituted.

5.5 Cardiovascular Effects

BROVANA Inhalation Solution, like other beta$_2$-agonists, can produce a clinically significant cardiovascular effect in some patients as measured by increases in pulse rate, systolic and/or diastolic blood pressure, and/or symptoms. If such effects occur, the drug may need to be discontinued. In addition, beta-agonists have been reported to produce ECG changes, such as flattening of the T-wave, prolongation of the QTc interval, and ST segment depression. The clinical significance of these findings is unknown. BROVANA Inhalation Solution, as with other sympathomimetic amines, should be used with caution in patients with cardiovascular disorders, especially coronary insufficiency, cardiac arrhythmias, and hypertension.

5.6 Coexisting Conditions

BROVANA Inhalation Solution, like other sympathomimetic amines, should be used with caution in patients with cardiovascular disorders, especially coronary insufficiency, cardiac arrhythmias, and hypertension; in patients with convulsive disorders or thyrotoxicosis, and in patients who are unusually responsive to sympathomimetic amines. In two pooled, 12-week, placebo-controlled trials investigating BROVANA Inhalation Solution doses of 15 µg BID, 25 µg BID, and 50 µg QD, changes in mean predose and 2-hour post dose systolic and/or diastolic blood pressure were seen as a general fall of 2-4 mm/Hg; for pulse rate the mean of maximal increases were 8.8-12.0 beats/min. Over the course of a one-year study measuring serial electrocardiograms while receiving a dose of 50 mcg BID of BROVANA Inhalation Solution resulted in an approximately 3.0 ms increase in QT_{C-F} compared to the active comparator, salmeterol. Doses of the related beta$_2$-agonist albuterol, when administered intravenously, have been reported to aggravate preexisting diabetes mellitus and ketoacidosis.

5.7 Hypokalemia and Hyperglycemia

Beta-agonist medications may produce significant hypokalemia in some patients, possibly through intracellular shunting, which has the potential to produce adverse cardiovascular effects [see *CLINICAL PHARMACOLOGY (12.2)*]. The decrease in serum potassium is usually transient, not requiring supplementation. Beta-agonist medications may produce transient hyperglycemia in some patients.

Clinically significant and dose-related changes in serum potassium and blood glucose were infrequent during clinical trials with long-term administration of BROVANA Inhalation Solution at the recommended dose.

5.8 Immediate Hypersensitivity Reactions

Immediate hypersensitivity reactions may occur after administration of BROVANA Inhalation Solution as demonstrated by cases of anaphylactic reaction, urticaria, angioedema, rash and bronchospasm.

6 ADVERSE REACTIONS

Long-acting beta$_2$-adrenergic agonists increase the risk of asthma-related death [see BOXED WARNING and WARNINGS AND PRECAUTIONS (5.1)].

6.1 Beta$_2$-Agonist Adverse Reaction Profile

Adverse reactions to BROVANA Inhalation Solution are expected to be similar in nature to other beta$_2$-adrenergic receptor agonists including: angina, hypertension or hypotension, tachycardia, arrhythmias, nervousness, headache, tremor, dry mouth, palpitation, muscle cramps, nausea, dizziness, fatigue, malaise, hypokalemia, hyperglycemia, metabolic acidosis and insomnia.

6.2 Clinical Trials Experience

Because clinical trials are conducted under widely varying conditions, adverse reaction rates observed in clinical trials of a drug cannot be directly compared to rates in the clinical trials of another drug and may not reflect the rates observed in clinical practice.

Adults with COPD in Short-Term Trials (12 weeks)

The safety data described below for adults ≥35 years of age are based on 2 clinical trials of 12 weeks. In the 2 trials of 12 weeks duration, 1456 patients (860 males and 596 females, ages 34 to 89 years old) with COPD were treated with BROVANA Inhalation Solution 15 mcg twice daily, 25 mcg twice daily, 50 mcg once daily, salmeterol 42 mcg twice daily, or placebo. The racial/ethnic distribution in these two trials included 1383 Caucasians, 49 Blacks, 10 Asians, and 10 Hispanics, and 4 patients classified as Other. Among the 1,456 COPD patients in two 12-week, placebo-controlled trials, 288 were treated with BROVANA Inhalation Solution 15 mcg twice daily and 293 were treated with placebo. Doses of 25 mcg twice daily and 50 mcg once daily were also evaluated.

Table 1 shows adverse reaction rates among patients from these two trials where the frequency was greater than or equal to 2% in the BROVANA Inhalation Solution 15 mcg twice daily group and where the rate in the BROVANA Inhalation Solution 15 mcg twice daily group exceeded the rate in the placebo group. The total number and percent of patients who reported adverse events were 202 (70%) in the 15 mcg twice daily and 219 (75%) in the placebo groups. Ten adverse events demonstrated a dose relationship: asthenia, fever, bronchitis, COPD, headache, vomiting, hyperkalemia, leukocytosis, nervousness, and tremor.

Table 1: Number of Patients Experiencing Adverse Events from Two 12-Week, Double-Blind, Placebo-Controlled Clinical Trials

	BROVANA Inhalation Solution 15 mcg twice daily		Placebo	
	n	(%)	n	(%)
Total Patients	288	(100)	293	(100)
Pain	23	(8)	16	(5)
Chest Pain	19	(7)	19	(6)
Back Pain	16	(6)	6	(2)
Diarrhea	16	(6)	13	(4)
Sinusitis	13	(5)	11	(4)
Leg Cramps	12	(4)	6	(2)
Dyspnea	11	(4)	7	(2)
Rash	11	(4)	5	(2)
Flu Syndrome	10	(3)	4	(1)
Peripheral Edema	8	(3)	7	(2)
Lung Disorder*	7	(2)	2	(1)

* Reported terms coded to "Lung Disorder" were predominantly pulmonary or chest congestion.

Adverse events occurring in patients treated with BROVANA Inhalation Solution 15 mcg twice daily with a frequency of <2%, but greater than placebo, were as follows:

Body as a Whole: abscess, allergic reaction, digitalis intoxication, fever, hernia, injection site pain, neck rigidity, neoplasm, pelvic pain, retroperitoneal hemorrhage

Cardiovascular: arteriosclerosis, atrial flutter, AV block, congestive heart failure, heart block, myocardial infarct, QT interval prolonged, supraventricular tachycardia, inverted T-wave

Digestive: constipation, gastritis, melena, oral moniliasis, periodontal abscess, rectal hemorrhage

Metabolic and Nutritional Disorders: dehydration, edema, glucose tolerance decreased, gout, hyperglycemia, hyperlipemia, hypoglycemia, hypokalemia

Musculoskeletal: arthralgia, arthritis, bone disorder, rheumatoid arthritis, tendinous contracture

Nervous: agitation, cerebral infarct, circumoral paresthesia, hypokinesia, paralysis, somnolence, tremor

Respiratory: carcinoma of the lung, respiratory disorder, voice alteration

Skin and Appendages: dry skin, herpes simplex, herpes zoster, skin discoloration, skin hypertrophy

Special Senses: abnormal vision, glaucoma

Urogenital: breast neoplasm, calcium crystalluria, cystitis, glycosuria, hematuria, kidney calculus, nocturia, PSA increase, pyuria, urinary tract disorder, urine abnormality.

In these trials, the overall frequency of all cardiovascular adverse events was 6.9% in BROVANA Inhalation Solution 15 mcg twice daily and 13.3% in the placebo group. There were no frequently occurring specific cardiovascular adverse events for BROVANA Inhalation Solution (frequency ≥1% and greater than placebo). The rate of COPD exacerbations was also comparable between the BROVANA Inhalation Solution 15 mcg twice daily and placebo groups, 12.2% and 15.1%, respectively.

Adults with COPD in Long-Term (52-week) Safety Trial

BROVANA Inhalation Solution was evaluated in one 52 week double-blind, randomized, placebo-controlled, safety trial conducted in patients with moderate to severe COPD. The primary endpoint was time to either respiratory death or first COPD exacerbation-related hospitalization, whichever occurred first. The event had to be a death or hospitalization for which the patient's respiratory status was predominant and/or inciting contributor, as determined by the clinical investigator. The objective of the trial was to demonstrate that the risk of respiratory death or COPD exacerbation-related hospitalization for patients treated with BROVANA Inhalation Solution was not greater than 40% more than the risk for patient treated with placebo. A total of 841 patients (479 males and 361 females, ages 41 to 94 years old) with COPD were randomized: 420 to BROVANA Inhalation Solution 15 mcg twice daily and 421 to placebo. Of the randomized patients, 255 (61%) in the BROVANA Inhalation Solution group and 211 (50%) in the placebo group, completed one year of treatment. The trial objective was met demonstrating that COPD patients treated with BROVANA Inhalation Solution are not at an increased risk of respiratory death or COPD exacerbation-related hospitalizations compared to placebo.

7 DRUG INTERACTIONS

7.1 Adrenergic Drugs

If additional adrenergic drugs are to be administered by any route, they should be used with caution because the sympathetic effects of arformoterol may be potentiated [see *WARNINGS AND PRECAUTIONS (5.3, 5.5, 5.6, 5.7)*].

7.2 Xanthine Derivatives, Steroids, or Diuretics

Concomitant treatment with methylxanthine (aminophylline, theophylline), steroids, or diuretics may potentiate any hypokalemic effect of adrenergic agonists including BROVANA Inhalation Solution [see *WARNINGS AND PRECAUTIONS (5.7)*].

The concurrent use of intravenously or orally administered methylxanthines (e.g., aminophylline, theophylline) by patients receiving BROVANA Inhalation Solution has not been completely evaluated. In two combined 12-week, placebo-controlled trials that included BROVANA Inhalation Solution doses of 15 mcg twice daily, 25 mcg twice daily, and 50 mcg once daily, 54 of 873 BROVANA Inhalation Solution-treated subjects received concomitant theophylline at study entry. In a 12-month controlled trial that included a 50 mcg once daily BROVANA Inhalation Solution dose, 30 of the 528 BROVANA Inhalation Solution-treated subjects received concomitant theophylline at study entry. In these trials, heart rate and systolic blood pressure were approximately 2-3 bpm and 6-8 mm Hg higher, respectively, in subjects on concomitant theophylline compared with the overall population.

7.3 Non-potassium Sparing Diuretics

The ECG changes and/or hypokalemia that may result from the administration of non-potassium sparing diuretics (such as loop or thiazide diuretics) can be acutely worsened by beta-agonists, especially when the recommended dose of the beta-agonist is exceeded. Although the clinical significance of these effects is not known, caution is advised in the co-administration of beta-agonists, including BROVANA Inhalation Solution, with non-potassium sparing diuretics.

7.4 MAO Inhibitors, Tricyclic Antidepressants, QTc Prolonging Drugs

BROVANA Inhalation Solution, as with other beta-agonists, should be administered with extreme caution to patients being treated with monoamine oxidase inhibitors, tricyclic antidepressants, or drugs known to prolong the QTc interval because of the effect of adrenergic agonists on the cardiovascular system may be potentiated by these agents. Drugs that are known to prolong the QTc interval have an increased risk of ventricular arrhythmias.

7.5 Beta-Blockers

Beta-adrenergic receptor antagonists (beta-blockers) and BROVANA Inhalation Solution may inhibit the effect of each other when administered concurrently. Beta-blockers not only block the therapeutic effects of beta-agonists, but may produce severe bronchospasm in COPD patients. Therefore, patients with COPD should not normally be treated with beta-blockers. However, under certain circumstances, e.g., as prophylaxis after myocardial infarction, there may be no acceptable alternatives to the use of beta-blockers in patients with COPD. In this setting, cardioselective beta-blockers could be considered, although they should be administered with caution.

8 USE IN SPECIFIC POPULATIONS

8.1 Pregnancy

Teratogenic Effects: Pregnancy Category C

There are no adequate and well-controlled studies of BROVANA Inhalation Solution in pregnant women. Arformoterol has been shown to be teratogenic in rats and rabbits. Arformoterol also caused neonatal mortality and developmental delays in rats. Because animal reproduction studies are not always predictive of human response, BROVANA Inhalation Solution should be used during pregnancy, only if the potential benefit justifies the potential risk to the fetus.

Arformoterol has been shown to be teratogenic in rats based upon findings of omphalocele (umbilical hernia), a malformation, at oral doses equal to and greater than approximately 370 times adult exposure at the maximum recommended daily inhalation dose. Increased pup loss at birth and during lactation and decreased pup weights were observed in rats at oral doses equal to and greater than approximately 1100 times adult exposure at the maximum recommended daily inhalation dose. Delays in development were evident with an oral dose approximately 2400 times adult exposure at the maximum recommended daily inhalation dose.

Arformoterol has been shown to be teratogenic in rabbits based upon findings of malpositioned right kidney, a malformation, at oral doses equal to and greater than approximately 8400 times adult exposure at the maximum recommended daily inhalation dose. Malformations including brachydactyly, bulbous aorta, and liver cysts were observed at oral doses equal to and greater than approximately 22,000 times the maximum recommended daily inhalation dose in adults on a mg/m^2 basis. Malformations including adactyly, lobular dysgenesis of the lung, and interventricular septal defect were observed at an oral dose approximately 43,000 times the maximum recommended daily inhalation dose in adults on a mg/m^2 basis. Embryolethality was observed at an oral dose approximately 43,000 times the maximum recommended daily inhalation dose in adults on a mg/m^2 basis. Decreased pup body weights were observed at oral doses equal to and greater than approximately 22,000 times the maximum recommended daily inhalation dose in adults on a mg/m^2 basis. There were no teratogenic findings in rabbits with oral doses equal to or less than approximately 4900 times adult exposure at the maximum recommended daily inhalation dose.

8.2 Labor and Delivery

There are no human studies that have investigated the effects of BROVANA Inhalation Solution on preterm labor or labor at term.

Because beta-agonists may potentially interfere with uterine contractility, BROVANA Inhalation Solution should be used during labor and delivery only if the potential benefit justifies the potential risk.

8.3 Nursing Mothers

In reproductive studies in rats, arformoterol was excreted in the milk. It is not known whether arformoterol is excreted in human milk. Because many drugs are excreted in human milk, caution should be exercised when BROVANA Inhalation Solution is administered to a nursing woman.

8.4 Pediatric Use

BROVANA Inhalation Solution is approved for use in the long-term maintenance treatment of bronchoconstriction associated with chronic obstructive pulmonary disease, including chronic bronchitis and emphysema. This disease does not occur in children. The safety and efficacy of BROVANA Inhalation Solution in pediatric patients have not been established.

8.5 Geriatric Use

Of the 873 patients who received BROVANA Inhalation Solution in two placebo-controlled clinical studies in adults with COPD, 391 (45%) were 65 years of age or older while 96 (11%) were 75 years of age or older. No overall differences in safety or effectiveness were observed between these subjects and younger subjects. Among subjects age 65 years and older, 129 (33%) received BROVANA Inhalation Solution at the recommended dose of 15 mcg twice daily, while the remainder received higher doses. ECG alerts for ventricular ectopy in patients 65 to ≤75 years of age were comparable among patients receiving 15 mcg twice daily, 25 mcg twice daily, and placebo (3.9%, 5.2%, and 7.1%, respectively). A higher frequency (12.4%) was observed when BROVANA Inhalation Solution was dosed at 50 mcg once daily. The clinical significance of this finding is not known. Other reported clinical experience has not identified differences in responses between the elderly and younger patients, but greater sensitivity of some older individuals cannot be ruled out.

8.6 Hepatic Impairment

BROVANA Inhalation Solution should be used cautiously in patients with hepatic impairment due to increased systemic exposure in these patients [see *Clinical Pharmacology (12.3)*].

8.7 Renal Impairment

The systemic exposure to arformoterol was similar to renally impaired patients compared with demographically matched healthy control subjects [see *Clinical Pharmacology (12.3)*].

9 DRUG ABUSE AND DEPENDENCE

There were no reported cases of abuse or evidence of drug dependence with the use of BROVANA Inhalation Solution in the clinical trials.

10 OVERDOSAGE

The expected signs and symptoms associated with overdosage of BROVANA (arformoterol tartrate) Inhalation Solution are those of excessive beta-adrenergic stimulation and/or occurrence or exaggeration of any of the signs and symptoms listed under **ADVERSE REACTIONS**. Signs and symptoms may include angina, hypertension or hypotension, tachycardia, with rates up to 200 beats/min, arrhythmias, nervousness, headache, tremor, dry mouth, palpitation, muscle cramps, nausea, dizziness, fatigue, malaise, hypokalemia, hyperglycemia, metabolic acidosis and insomnia. As with all inhaled sympathomimetic medications, cardiac arrest and even death may be associated with an overdose of BROVANA Inhalation Solution.

Treatment of overdosage consists of discontinuation of BROVANA Inhalation Solution together with institution of appropriate symptomatic and/or supportive therapy. The judicious use of a cardioselective beta-receptor blocker may be considered, bearing in mind that such medication can produce bronchospasm. There is insufficient evidence to determine if dialysis is beneficial for overdosage of BROVANA Inhalation Solution. Cardiac monitoring is recommended in cases of overdosage.

Clinical signs in dogs included flushing of the body surface and facial area, reddening of the ears and gums, tremor, and increased heart rate. A death was reported in dogs after a single oral dose of 5 mg/kg (approximately 4500 times the maximum recommended daily inhalation dose in adults on a mg/m^2 basis). Death occurred for a rat that received arformoterol at a single inhalation dose of 1600 mcg/kg (approximately 430 times the maximum recommended daily inhalation dose in adults on a mg/m^2 basis).

11 DESCRIPTION

BROVANA (arformoterol tartrate) Inhalation Solution is a sterile, clear, colorless, aqueous solution of the tartrate salt of arformoterol, the (R,R)-enantiomer of formoterol.

Arformoterol is a selective beta$_2$-adrenergic bronchodilator. The chemical name for arformoterol tartrate is formamide, N-[2-hydroxy-5-[(1R)-1-hydroxy-2-[[(1R)-2-(4-methoxyphenyl)-1-methylethyl]amino]ethyl]phenyl]-, (2R,3R)-2,3-dihydroxybutanedioate (1:1 salt), and its established structural formula is as follows:

The molecular weight of *arformoterol tartrate* is 494.5 g/mol, and its empirical formula is $C_{19}H_{24}N_2O_4 \cdot C_4H_6O_6$ (1:1 salt). It is a white to off-white solid that is slightly soluble in water.

Arformoterol tartrate is the United States Adopted Name (USAN) for (R,R)-formoterol L-tartrate.

BROVANA (arformoterol tartrate) Inhalation Solution is supplied as 2 mL of arformoterol tartrate solution packaged in 2.1 mL unit-dose, low-density polyethylene (LDPE) unit-dose vials. Each unit-dose vial contains 15 mcg of arformoterol (equivalent to 22 mcg of arformoterol tartrate) in a sterile, isotonic saline solution, pH-adjusted to 5.0 with citric acid and sodium citrate.

BROVANA Inhalation Solution requires no dilution before administration by nebulization. Like all other nebulized treatments, the amount delivered to the lungs will depend upon patient factors, the nebulizer used, and compressor performance. Using the PARI LC® Plus nebulizer (with mouthpiece) connected to a PARI DURA NEB™ 3000 compressor under *in vitro* conditions, the mean delivered dose from the mouthpiece (% nominal) was approximately 4.1 mcg (27.6%) at a mean flow rate of 3.3 L/min. The mean nebulization time was 6 minutes or less. BROVANA Inhalation Solution should be administered from a standard jet nebulizer at adequate flow rates via face mask or mouthpiece.

Patients should be carefully instructed on the correct use of this drug product (please refer to the accompanying **Medication Guide**).

12 CLINICAL PHARMACOLOGY

12.1 Mechanism of Action

Arformoterol, the (R,R)-enantiomer of formoterol, is a selective long-acting beta$_2$-adrenergic receptor agonist (beta$_2$-agonist) that has two-fold greater potency than racemic formoterol (which contains both the (S,S) and (R,R)-enantiomers). The (S,S)-enantiomer is about 1,000-fold less potent as a beta$_2$-agonist than the (R,R)-enantiomer. While it is recognized that beta$_2$-receptors are the predominant adrenergic receptors in bronchial smooth muscle and beta$_1$-receptors are the predominant receptors in the heart, data indicate that there are also beta$_2$-receptors in the human heart comprising 10% to 50% of the total beta-adrenergic receptors. The precise function of these receptors has not been established, but they raise the possibility that even highly selective beta$_2$-agonists may have cardiac effects.

The pharmacologic effects of beta$_2$-adrenoceptor agonist drugs, including arformoterol, are at least in part attributable to stimulation of intracellular adenyl cyclase, the enzyme that catalyzes the conversion of adenosine triphosphate (ATP) to cyclic-3',5'-adenosine monophosphate (cyclic AMP). Increased intracellular cyclic AMP levels cause relaxation of bronchial smooth muscle and inhibition of release of mediators of immediate hypersensitivity from cells, especially from mast cells.

In vitro tests show that arformoterol is an inhibitor of the release of mast cell mediators, such as histamine and leukotrienes, from the human lung. Arformoterol also inhibits histamine-induced plasma albumin extravasation in anesthetized guinea pigs and inhibits allergen-induced eosinophil influx in dogs with airway hyper-responsiveness. The relevance of these *in vitro* and animal findings to humans is unknown.

12.2 Pharmacodynamics

Systemic Safety and Pharmacokinetic/Pharmacodynamic Relationships

The predominant adverse effects of inhaled beta$_2$-agonists occur as a result of excessive activation of systemic beta-adrenergic receptors. The most common adverse effects may include skeletal muscle tremor and cramps, insomnia, tachycardia, decreases in plasma potassium, and increases in plasma glucose.

Effects on Serum Potassium and Serum Glucose Levels

Changes in serum potassium and serum glucose were evaluated in a dose-ranging study of twice daily (5 mcg, 15 mcg, or 25 mcg; 215 patients with COPD) and once daily (15 mcg, 25 mcg, or 50 mcg; 191 patients with COPD) BROVANA Inhalation Solution in COPD patients. At 2 and 6 hours post dose at week 0 (after the first dose), mean changes in serum potassium ranging from 0 to -0.3 mEq/L were observed in the BROVANA Inhalation Solution groups with similar changes observed after 2 weeks of treatment. Changes in mean serum glucose levels, ranging from a decrease of 1.2 mg/dL to an increase of 32.8 mg/dL were observed for BROVANA Inhalation Solution dose groups at both 2 and 6 hours post dose, both after the first dose and 14 days of daily treatment.

Electrophysiology

The effect of BROVANA Inhalation Solution on QT interval was evaluated in a dose-ranging study following multiple doses of BROVANA Inhalation Solution 5 mcg, 15 mcg, or 25 mcg twice daily or 15 mcg, 25 mcg, or 50 mcg once daily for 2 weeks in patients with COPD. ECG assessments were performed at baseline, time of peak plasma concentration and throughout the dosing interval. Different methods of correcting for heart rate were employed, including a subject-specific method and the Fridericia method.

Relative to placebo, the mean change in subject-specific QTc averaged over the dosing interval ranged from -1.8 to 2.7 msec, indicating little effect of BROVANA Inhalation Solution on cardiac repolarization after 2 weeks of treatment. The maximum mean change in subject-specific QTc for the BROVANA Inhalation Solution 15 mcg twice daily dose was 17.3 msec, compared with 15.4 msec in the placebo group. No apparent correlation of QTc with arformoterol plasma concentration was observed.

Electrocardiographic Monitoring in Patients with COPD

The effect of different doses of BROVANA Inhalation Solution on cardiac rhythm was assessed using 24-hour Holter monitoring in two 12-week, double-blind, placebo-controlled studies of 1,456 patients with COPD (873 received BROVANA Inhalation Solution at 15 or 25 mcg twice daily or 50 mcg once daily doses; 293 received placebo; 290 received salmeterol). The 24-hour Holter monitoring occurred once at baseline, and up to 3 times during the 12-week treatment period. The rates of new-onset cardiac arrhythmias not present at baseline over the double-blind 12-week treatment period were similar (approximately 33-34%) for patients who received BROVANA Inhalation Solution 15 mcg twice daily to those who received placebo. There was a dose-related increase in new, treatment-emergent arrhythmias seen in patients who received BROVANA Inhalation Solution 25 mcg twice daily and 50 mcg once daily, 37.6% and 40.1%, respectively. The frequencies of new treatment-emergent events of non-sustained (3-10 beat run) and sustained (>10 beat run) ventricular tachycardia were 7.4% and 1.1% in BROVANA Inhalation Solution 15 mcg twice daily and 6.9% and 1.0% in placebo. In patients who received BROVANA Inhalation Solution 25 mcg twice daily and 50 mcg once daily, the frequencies of non-sustained (6.2% and 8.2%, respectively) and sustained ventricular tachycardia (1.0% and 1.0%, respectively) were similar. Five cases of ventricular tachycardia were reported as adverse events (1 in BROVANA Inhalation Solution 15 mcg twice daily and 4 in placebo), with two of these events leading to discontinuation of treatment (2 in placebo).

There were no baseline occurrences of atrial fibrillation/flutter observed on 24-hour Holter monitoring in patients treated with BROVANA Inhalation Solution 15 mcg twice daily or placebo. New, treatment-emergent atrial fibrillation/flutter occurred in 0.4% of patients who received BROVANA Inhalation Solution 15 mcg twice daily and 0.3% of patients who received placebo. There was a dose-related increase in the frequency of atrial fibrillation/flutter reported in the BROVANA Inhalation Solution 25 mcg twice daily and 50 mcg once daily dose groups of 0.7% and 1.4%, respectively. Two cases of atrial fibrillation/flutter were reported as adverse events (1 in BROVANA Inhalation Solution 15 mcg twice daily and 1 in placebo).

Dose-related increases in mean maximum change in heart rate in the 12 hours after dosing were also observed following 12 weeks of dosing with BROVANA Inhalation Solution 15 mcg twice daily (8.8 bpm), 25 mcg twice daily (9.9 bpm) and 50 mcg once daily (12 bpm) versus placebo (8.5 bpm).

Tachyphylaxis/Tolerance
Tolerance to the effects of inhaled beta-agonists can occur with regularly-scheduled, chronic use.
In two placebo-controlled clinical trials in patients with COPD involving approximately 725 patients in each, the overall efficacy of BROVANA Inhalation Solution was maintained throughout the 12-week trial duration. However, tolerance to the bronchodilator effect of BROVANA Inhalation Solution was observed after 6 weeks of dosing, as measured by a decrease in trough FEV_1. FEV_1 improvement at the end of the 12-hour dosing interval decreased by approximately one-third (22.1% mean improvement after the first dose compared to 14.6% at week 12). Tolerance to the trough FEV_1 bronchodilator effect of BROVANA Inhalation Solution was not accompanied by other clinical manifestations of tolerance in these trials.

12.3 Pharmacokinetics
The pharmacokinetics (PK) of arformoterol have been investigated in healthy subjects, elderly subjects, renally and hepatically impaired subjects, and COPD patients following the nebulization of the recommended therapeutic dose and doses up to 96 mcg.

Absorption
In COPD patients administered 15 mcg arformoterol every 12 hours for 14 days, the mean steady-state peak (R,R)-formoterol plasma concentration (C_{max}) and systemic exposure (AUC_{0-12h}) were 4.3 pg/mL and 34.5 pg.hr/mL, respectively. The median steady-state peak (R,R)-formoterol plasma concentration time (t_{max}) was observed approximately one-half hour after drug administration.
Systemic exposure to (R,R)-formoterol increased linearly with dose in COPD patients following arformoterol doses of 5 mcg, 15 mcg, or 25 mcg twice daily for 2 weeks or 15 mcg, 25 mcg, or 50 mcg once daily for 2 weeks.
In a crossover study in patients with COPD, when arformoterol 15 mcg inhalation solution and 12 and 24 mcg formoterol fumarate inhalation powder (Foradil® Aerolizer®) was administered twice daily for 2 weeks, the accumulation index was approximately 2.5 based on the plasma (R,R)-formoterol concentrations in all three treatments. At steady-state, geometric means of systemic exposure (AUC_{0-12h}) to (R,R)-formoterol following 15 mcg of arformoterol inhalation solution and 12 mcg of formoterol fumarate inhalation powder were 39.33 pg.hr/mL and 33.93 pg.hr/mL, respectively (ratio 1.16; 90% CI 1.00, 1.35), while the geometric means of the C_{max} were 4.30 pg/mL and 4.75 pg/mL, respectively (ratio 0.91; 90% CI 0.76, 1.09).
In a study in patients with asthma, treatment with arformoterol 50 mcg with pre- and post-treatment with activated charcoal resulted in a geometric mean decrease in (R,R)-formoterol AUC_{0-6h} by 27% and C_{max} by 23% as compared to treatment with arformoterol 50 mcg alone. This suggests that a substantial portion of systemic drug exposure is due to pulmonary absorption.

Distribution
The binding of arformoterol to human plasma proteins *in vitro* was 52-65% at concentrations of 0.25, 0.5 and 1.0 ng/mL of radiolabeled arformoterol. The concentrations of arformoterol used to assess the plasma protein binding were higher than those achieved in plasma following inhalation of multiple doses of 50 mcg arformoterol.

Metabolism
In vitro profiling studies in hepatocytes and liver microsomes have shown that arformoterol is primarily metabolized by direct conjugation (glucuronidation) and secondarily by O-demethylation. At least five human uridine diphosphoglucuronosyltransferase (UGT) isozymes catalyze arformoterol glucuronidation *in vitro*. Two cytochrome P450 isozymes (CYP2D6 and secondarily CYP2C19) catalyze the O-demethylation of arformoterol.
Arformoterol was almost entirely metabolized following oral administration of 35 mcg of radiolabeled arformoterol in eight healthy subjects. Direct conjugation of arformoterol with glucuronic acid was the major metabolic pathway. Most of the drug-related material in plasma and urine was in the form of glucuronide or sulfate conjugates of arformoterol. O-Desmethylation and conjugates of the O-desmethyl metabolite were relatively minor metabolites accounting for less than 17% of the dose recovered in urine and feces.

Elimination
After administration of a single oral dose of radiolabeled arformoterol to eight healthy male subjects, 63% of the total radioactive dose was recovered in urine and 11% in feces within 48 hours. A total of 89% of the total radioactive dose was recovered within 14 days, with 67% in urine and 22% in feces. Approximately 1% of the dose was recovered as unchanged arformoterol in urine over 14 days. Renal clearance was 8.9 L/hr for unchanged arformoterol in these subjects. In COPD patients given 15 mcg inhaled arformoterol twice a day for 14 days, the mean terminal half-life of arformoterol was 26 hours.
Special Populations:
Gender
A population PK analysis indicated that there was no effect of gender upon the pharmacokinetics of arformoterol.
Race
The influence of race on arformoterol pharmacokinetics was assessed using a population PK analysis and data from healthy subjects. There was no clinically significant impact of race upon the pharmacokinetic profile of arformoterol.
Geriatric
The pharmacokinetic profile of arformoterol in 24 elderly subjects (aged 65 years or older) was compared to a younger cohort of 24 subjects (18-45 years) that were matched for body weight and gender. No significant differences in systemic exposure (AUC and C_{max}) were observed when the two groups were compared.
Pediatric
The pharmacokinetics of arformoterol have not been studied in pediatric subjects.
Hepatic Impairment
The pharmacokinetic profile of arformoterol was assessed in 24 subjects with mild, moderate, and severe hepatic impairment. The systemic exposure (C_{max} and AUC) to arformoterol increased 1.3 to 2.4-fold in subjects with hepatic impairment compared to 16 demographically matched healthy control subjects. No clear relationship between drug exposure and the severity of hepatic impairment was observed. BROVANA Inhalation Solution should be used cautiously in patients with hepatic impairment.
Renal Impairment
The impact of renal disease upon the pharmacokinetics of arformoterol was studied in 24 subjects with mild, moderate, or severe renal impairment. Systemic exposure (AUC and C_{max}) to arformoterol was similar in renally impaired patients compared with demographically matched healthy control subjects.
Drug-Drug Interaction
When paroxetine, a potent inhibitor of CYP2D6, was co-administered with BROVANA Inhalation Solution at steady-state, exposure to either drug was not altered. Dosage adjustments of BROVANA Inhalation Solution are not necessary when the drug is given concomitantly with potent CYP2D6 inhibitors.
Arformoterol did not inhibit CYP1A2, CYP2A6, CYP2C9/10, CYP2C19, CYP2D6, CYP2E1, CYP3A4/5, or CYP4A9/11 enzymes at >1,000-fold higher concentrations than the expected peak plasma concentrations following a therapeutic dose.

12.5 Pharmacogenetics
Arformoterol is eliminated through the action of multiple drug metabolizing enzymes. Direct glucuronidation of arformoterol is mediated by several UGT enzymes and is the primary elimination route. O-Desmethylation is a secondary route catalyzed by the CYP enzymes CYP2D6 and CYP2C19. In otherwise healthy subjects with reduced CYP2D6 and/or UGT1A1 enzyme activity, there was no impact on systemic exposure to arformoterol compared to subjects with normal CYP2D6 and/or UGT1A1 enzyme activities.

13 NONCLINICAL TOXICOLOGY
13.1 Carcinogenesis, Mutagenesis, Impairment of Fertility
Long-term studies were conducted in mice using oral administration and rats using inhalation administration to evaluate the carcinogenic potential of arformoterol.

In a 24-month carcinogenicity study in CD-1 mice, arformoterol caused a dose-related increase in the incidence of uterine and cervical endometrial stromal polyps and stromal cell sarcoma in female mice at oral doses of 1 mg/kg and above (AUC exposure approximately 70 times adult exposure at the maximum recommended daily inhalation dose). In a 24-month carcinogenicity study in Sprague-Dawley rats, arformoterol caused a statistically significant increase in the incidence of thyroid gland c-cell adenoma and carcinoma in female rats at an inhalation dose of 200 mcg/kg (AUC exposure approximately 130 times adult exposure at the maximum recommended daily inhalation dose). There were no tumor findings with an inhalation dose of 40 mcg/kg (AUC exposure approximately 55 times adult exposure at the maximum recommended daily inhalation dose).
Arformoterol was not mutagenic or clastogenic in the following tests: mutagenicity tests in bacteria, chromosome aberration analyses in mammalian cells, and micronucleus test in mice.
Arformoterol had no effects on fertility and reproductive performance in rats at oral doses up to 10 mg/kg (approximately 2700 times the maximum recommended daily inhalation dose in adults on a mg/m² basis).

13.2 Animal Toxicology and/or Pharmacology
Animal Pharmacology
In animal studies investigating its cardiovascular effects, arformoterol induced dose-dependent increases in heart rate and decreases in blood pressure consistent with its pharmacology as a beta-adrenergic agonist. In dogs, at systemic exposures higher than anticipated clinically, arformoterol also induced exaggerated pharmacologic effects of a beta-adrenergic agonist on cardiac function as measured by electrocardiogram (sinus tachycardia, atrial premature beats, ventricular escape beats, PVCs).
Studies in laboratory animals (minipigs, rodents, and dogs) have demonstrated the occurrence of arrhythmias and sudden death (with histologic evidence of myocardial necrosis) when beta-agonists and methylxanthines are administered concurrently. The clinical significance of these findings is unknown.
Reproductive Toxicology Studies
Arformoterol has been shown to be teratogenic in rats based upon findings of omphalocele (umbilical hernia), a malformation, at oral doses of 1 mg/kg and above (AUC exposure approximately 370 times adult exposure at the maximum recommended daily inhalation dose). Increased pup loss at birth and during lactation and decreased pup weights were observed in rats at oral doses of 5 mg/kg and above (AUC exposure approximately 1100 times adult exposure at the maximum recommended daily inhalation dose). Delays in development were evident with an oral dose of 10 mg/kg (AUC exposure approximately 2400 times adult exposure at the maximum recommended daily inhalation dose).
Arformoterol has been shown to be teratogenic in rabbits based upon findings of malpositioned right kidney, a malformation, at oral doses of 20 mg/kg and above (AUC exposure approximately 8400 times adult exposure at the maximum recommended daily inhalation dose). Malformations including brachydactyly, bulbous aorta, and liver cysts were observed at doses of 40 mg/kg and above (approximately 22,000 times the maximum recommended daily inhalation dose in adults on a mg/m² basis). Malformations including adactyly, lobular dysgenesis of the lung, and interventricular septal defect were observed at 80 mg/kg (approximately 43,000 times the maximum recommended daily inhalation dose in adults on a mg/m² basis). Embryolethality was observed at 80 mg/kg/day (approximately 43,000 times the maximum recommended daily inhalation dose in adults on a mg/m² basis). Decreased pup body weights were observed at doses of 40 mg/kg/day and above (approximately 22,000 times the maximum recommended daily inhalation dose in adults on a mg/m² basis). There were no teratogenic findings in rabbits with oral dose of 10 mg/kg and lower (AUC exposure approximately 4900 times adult exposure at the maximum recommended daily inhalation dose).

14 CLINICAL STUDIES
14.1 Adult COPD Trials
BROVANA (arformoterol tartrate) Inhalation Solution was studied in two identical, 12-week, double-blind, placebo- and active-controlled, randomized, multi-center, parallel group trials conducted in the United States (Clinical Trial A and Clinical Trial B). A total of 1,456 adult patients (age range: 34 to 89 years; mean age: 63 years; gender: 860 males and 596 females) with COPD who had a mean FEV_1 of 1.3 L (42% of predicted) were enrolled in the two clinical trials. The racial/ethnic distribution in these two trials included 1383 Caucasians, 49 Blacks, 10 Asians, and 10 Hispanics, and 4 patients classified as Other. The diagnosis of COPD was based on a prior clinical diagnosis of COPD, a smoking history (greater than 15 pack-years), age (at least 35 years), spirometry results (baseline FEV_1 ≤65% of predicted value and >0.70 L, and a FEV_1/forced vital capacity

(FVC) ratio ≤70%). About 80% of patients in these studies had bronchodilator reversibility, defined as a 10% or greater increase in FEV_1 after inhalation of 2 actuations (180 mcg racemic albuterol from a metered dose inhaler). Both trials compared BROVANA Inhalation Solution 15 mcg twice daily (288 patients), 25 mcg twice daily (292 patients), 50 mcg once daily (293 patients) with placebo (293 subjects). Both trials included salmeterol inhalation aerosol, 42 mcg twice daily as an active comparator (290 patients).

In both 12-week trials, BROVANA Inhalation Solution 15 mcg twice daily resulted in a statistically significant change of approximately 11% in mean FEV_1 (as measured by percent change from study baseline FEV_1 at the end of the dosing interval over the 12 weeks of treatment, the primary efficacy endpoint) compared to placebo. Compared to BROVANA Inhalation Solution 15 mcg twice daily, BROVANA Inhalation Solution 25 mcg twice daily and 50 mcg once daily did not provide sufficient additional benefit on a variety of endpoints, including FEV_1, to support the use of higher doses. Plots of the mean change in FEV_1 values obtained over the 12 hours after dosing for the BROVANA Inhalation Solution 15 mcg twice daily dose group and for the placebo group are provided in Figures 1 and 2 for Clinical Trial A, below. The plots include mean FEV_1 change observed after the first dose and after 12 weeks of treatment. The results from Clinical Trial B were similar.

Figure 1 Mean Change in FEV_1 Over Time for Clinical Trial A at Week 0 (Day 1)

- Placebo (ITT n=143) Baseline FEV1=1.20 (L)
- 15 mcg BROVANA BID (ITT n=141) Baseline FEV1=1.15 (L)

Figure 2 Mean Change in FEV_1 Over Time for Clinical Trial A at Week 12

- Placebo (ITT n=143) Baseline FEV1=1.20 (L)
- 15 mcg BROVANA BID (ITT n=141) Baseline FEV1=1.15 (L)

BROVANA Inhalation Solution 15 mcg twice daily significantly improved bronchodilation compared to placebo over the 12 hours after dosing (FEV_1 AUC_{0-12h}). This improvement was maintained over the 12-week study period.

Following the first dose of BROVANA Inhalation Solution 15 mcg, the median time to onset of bronchodilation, defined by an FEV_1 increase of 15%, occurred at 6.7 min. When defined as an increase in FEV_1 of 12% and 200 mL, the time to onset of bronchodilation was 20 min after dosing. Peak bronchodilator effect was generally seen within 1-3 hours of dosing.

In both clinical trials, compared to placebo, patients treated with BROVANA Inhalation Solution demonstrated improvements in peak expiratory flow rates, supplemental ipratropium and rescue albuterol use.

16   HOW SUPPLIED/STORAGE AND HANDLING

BROVANA (arformoterol tartrate) Inhalation Solution is supplied in a single strength (15 mcg of arformoterol, equivalent to 22 mcg of arformoterol tartrate) as 2 mL of a sterile solution in low-density polyethylene (LDPE) unit-dose vials overwrapped in foil. BROVANA Inhalation Solution is available in a shelf-carton containing 30 or 60 unit-dose vials.

NDC 63402-911-30: carton of 30 individually pouched unit-dose vials.

NDC 63402-911-64: carton of 60 unit-dose vials (15×4 unit-dose vial pouches).

Storage and Handling

Store BROVANA Inhalation Solution in the protective foil pouch under refrigeration at 36°-46°F (2°-8°C). Protect from light and excessive heat. After opening the pouch, unused unit-dose vials should be returned to, and stored in, the pouch. An opened unit-dose vial should be used right away. Discard any unit-dose vial if the solution is not colorless. Unopened foil pouches of BROVANA Inhalation Solution can also be stored at room temperature 68°-77°F (20°-25°C) for up to 6 weeks. If stored at room temperature, discard if not used after 6 weeks or if past the expiration date, whichever is sooner.

17   PATIENT COUNSELING INFORMATION

Advise the patient to read the FDA-approved patient labeling (Medication Guide and Instructions for Use) with each new prescription and refill.

The complete text of the Medication Guide is reprinted at the end of this document. Patients should be given the following information:

Asthma-Related Deaths, Acute Exacerbations or Deteriorations

Patients should be informed that long-acting beta₂-adrenergic agonists, such as BROVANA Inhalation Solution, increase risk of asthma-related death in patients with asthma.

BROVANA Inhalation Solution is not indicated to relieve acute respiratory symptoms and extra doses should not be used for that purpose. Acute symptoms should be treated with an inhaled, short-acting beta₂-agonist (the healthcare provider should prescribe the patient with such medication and instruct the patient in how it should be used). Patients should be instructed to seek medical attention if their symptoms worsen despite recommended doses of BROVANA Inhalation Solution, if BROVANA Inhalation Solution treatment becomes less effective, or if they need more inhalations of a short-acting beta₂-agonist than usual.

Appropriate Dosing

Patients should not stop using BROVANA Inhalation Solution unless told to do so by a healthcare provider because symptoms may get worse. Patients should not inhale more than one dose at any one time. The daily dosage of BROVANA Inhalation Solution should not exceed one unit-dose vial (15 mcg) by inhalation twice daily (30 mcg total daily dose). Excessive use of sympathomimetics may cause significant cardiovascular effects, and may be fatal.

Concomitant Therapy

Patients who have been taking inhaled, short-acting beta₂-agonists (e.g., levalbuterol) on a regular basis should be instructed to discontinue the regular use of these products and use them only for the symptomatic relief of acute symptoms.

BROVANA Inhalation Solution should not be used in conjunction with other inhaled medications containing long-acting beta₂-agonists. Patients should be warned not to stop or change the dose of other concomitant COPD therapy without medical advice, even if symptoms improve after initiating treatment with BROVANA Inhalation Solution.

Common Adverse Reactions with Beta₂-agonists

Patients should be informed that treatment with beta₂-agonists may lead to adverse reactions that include palpitations, chest pain, rapid heart rate, increased or decreased blood pressure, headache, tremor, nervousness, dry mouth, muscle cramps, nausea, dizziness, fatigue, malaise, low blood potassium, high blood sugar, high blood acid, or trouble sleeping [see ADVERSE REACTIONS (6.1)].

Instructions for Administration

It is important that patients understand how to use BROVANA Inhalation Solution with a nebulizer appropriately and how it should be used in relation to other medications to treat COPD they are taking [see the accompanying **Medication Guide**]. Patients should be instructed not to mix other medications with BROVANA Inhalation Solution and not to inject or swallow BROVANA Inhalation Solution. Patients should throw the plastic dispensing vials away immediately after use. Due to their small size, the vials pose a danger of choking to young children.

Women should be advised to contact their physician if they become pregnant or if they are nursing.

FDA-Approved Medication Guide

See the accompanying **Medication Guide**.

SUNOVION

Manufactured for:

Sunovion Pharmaceuticals Inc.

Marlborough, MA 01752 USA

© 2011, 2014 Sunovion Pharmaceuticals Inc. All rights reserved.

For customer service, call 1-888-394-7377.
To report adverse events, call 1-877-737-7226.
For medical information, call 1-800-739-0565.
901552R02

MEDICATION GUIDE

BROVANA® [Brō vă '-nah]
(arformoterol tartrate) Inhalation Solution

BROVANA is only for use with a nebulizer.

Read the Medication Guide that comes with BROVANA before you start using it and each time you get a refill. There may be new information. This Medication Guide does not take the place of talking to your healthcare provider about your medical condition or treatment.

What is the most important information I should know about BROVANA?

BROVANA can cause serious side effects, including:

- **People with asthma, who take long-acting beta₂-adrenergic agonist (LABA) medicines, such as BROVANA, have an increased risk of death from asthma problems.**
- It is not known if LABA medicines, such as BROVANA, increase the risk of death in people with chronic obstructive pulmonary disease (COPD).
- Get emergency medical care if:
  - breathing problems worsen quickly
  - you use your rescue inhaler medicine, but it does not relieve your breathing problems

What is BROVANA?

BROVANA is used long term, 2 times each day (morning and evening), in controlling symptoms of chronic obstructive pulmonary disease (COPD) in adults with COPD.

BROVANA is only for use with a nebulizer.

LABA medicines such as BROVANA help the muscles around the airways in your lungs stay relaxed to prevent symptoms, such as wheezing, cough, chest tightness, and shortness of breath.

BROVANA should not be used in children. It is not known if BROVANA is safe and effective in children.

It is not known if BROVANA is safe and effective in people with asthma.

Who should not use BROVANA?

Do not use BROVANA if you:

- have had a serious allergic reaction to arformoterol, formoterol, or any of the ingredients in BROVANA. Ask your healthcare provider if you are not sure. See the end of this Medication Guide for a complete list of ingredients in BROVANA.
- have asthma without using a long-term asthma control medicine.

What should I tell my healthcare provider before using BROVANA?

Tell your healthcare provider about all of your health conditions, including if you:

- have heart problems
- have high blood pressure
- have seizures
- have thyroid problems
- have diabetes
- have liver problems
- are pregnant or planning to become pregnant. It is not known if BROVANA can harm your unborn baby.
- are breastfeeding. It is not known if BROVANA passes into your milk and if it can harm your baby.

Tell your healthcare provider about all the medicines you take including prescription and non-prescription medicines, vitamins and herbal supplements. BROVANA and certain other medicines may interact with each other. This may cause serious side effects.

Know the medicines you take. Keep a list of them to show your healthcare provider and pharmacist each time you get a new medicine.

How should I use BROVANA?

Read the step-by-step instructions for using BROVANA at the end of this Medication Guide.

- Use BROVANA exactly as prescribed. One ready-to-use vial of BROVANA is one dose. The usual dose of BROVANA is 1 ready-to-use vial, twice a day (morning and evening) breathed in through your nebulizer machine. The 2 doses should be about 12 hours apart. **Do not use more than 2 ready-to-use vials of BROVANA a day.**
- Do not swallow or inject BROVANA.
- BROVANA is for use with a standard jet nebulizer machine connected to an air compressor. Read the complete instructions for use at the end of this Medication Guide before starting BROVANA.
- Do not mix other medicines with BROVANA in your nebulizer machine.
- If you miss a dose of BROVANA, just skip that dose. Take your next dose at your usual time. Do not take 2 doses at one time.
- While you are using BROVANA 2 times each day:
  - **do not use** other medicines that contain a long-acting beta₂-agonist (LABA) for any reason.
  - **do not use** your short-acting beta₂-agonist medicine on a regular basis (four times a day).
- BROVANA does not relieve sudden symptoms of COPD. Always have a rescue inhaler medicine with you to treat sudden symptoms. If you do not have a rescue inhaler medicine, call your healthcare provider to have one prescribed for you.
- Do not stop using BROVANA or other medicines to control or treat your COPD unless told to do so by your healthcare provider because your symptoms might get worse. Your healthcare provider will change your medicines as needed.

- Do not use BROVANA:
  - **more often than prescribed**
  - **more medicine than prescribed to you**
  - **with other LABA medicines**

Call your healthcare provider or get emergency medical care right away if:
- your breathing problems worsen with BROVANA
- you need to use your rescue inhaler medicine more often than usual
- your rescue inhaler medicine does not work as well for you at relieving symptoms

What are the possible side effects with BROVANA?
BROVANA can cause serious side effects, including:
- See "What is the most important information I should know about BROVANA?"
- Sudden shortness of breath immediately after use of BROVANA
- If your COPD symptoms worsen over time, do not increase your dose of BROVANA; instead, call your healthcare provider.
- Increased blood pressure
- Fast or irregular heartbeat
- serious allergic reactions including rash, hives, swelling of the face, mouth, and tongue, and breathing problems. Call your healthcare provider or get emergency medical care if you get any symptoms of a serious allergic reaction.

Common side effects of BROVANA include:
- chest or back pain
- diarrhea
- sinus congestion
- headache
- tremor
- nervousness
- leg cramps
- high blood potassium
- shortness of breath
- rash
- fever
- increased white blood cells
- vomiting
- tiredness
- leg swelling
- chest congestion or bronchitis

Tell your healthcare provider if you get any side effect that bothers you or that does not go away.

These are not all the side effects with BROVANA. Ask your healthcare provider or pharmacist for more information. Call your doctor for medical advice about side effects. You may report side effects to FDA at 1-800-FDA-1088.

How should I store BROVANA?
- Store BROVANA in a refrigerator between 36° to 46°F (2° to 8°C) in the protective foil pouch. Protect from light and excessive heat. **Do not open a sealed pouch until you are ready to use a dose of BROVANA. After opening the pouch, unused ready-to-use vials should be returned to, and stored in, the pouch. An opened ready-to-use vial should be used right away.** BROVANA may be used directly from the refrigerator.
- BROVANA may also be stored at room temperature between 68° to 77°F (20° to 25°C) for up to 6 weeks (42 days). If stored at room temperature, discard BROVANA if it is not used after 6 weeks or if past the expiration date, whichever is sooner. Space is provided on the packaging to record room temperature storage times.
- Do not use BROVANA after the expiration date provided on the foil pouch and ready-to-use vial.
- BROVANA should be colorless. Discard BROVANA if it is not colorless.
- **Keep BROVANA and all medicines out of the reach of children.**

General Information about BROVANA
Medicines are sometimes prescribed for purposes not mentioned in a Medication Guide. Do not use BROVANA for a condition for which it was not prescribed. Do not give BROVANA to other people, even if they have the same condition. It may harm them.
This Medication Guide summarizes the most important information about BROVANA. If you would like more information, talk with your healthcare provider. You can ask your healthcare provider or pharmacist for information about BROVANA that was written for healthcare professionals.
- For customer service, call 1-888-394-7377.
- To report side effects, call 1-877-737-7226.
- For medical information, call 1-800-739-0565.

Instructions for Using BROVANA (arformoterol tartrate) Inhalation Solution

BROVANA is used only in a standard jet nebulizer machine connected to an air compressor. Make sure you know how to use your nebulizer machine before you use it to breathe in BROVANA or other medicines.

Do not mix BROVANA with other medicines in your nebulizer machine.

BROVANA comes sealed in a foil pouch. Do not open a sealed pouch until you are ready to use a dose of BROVANA. After opening the pouch, unused ready-to-use vials should be returned to, and stored in, the pouch. An opened ready-to-use vial should be used right away.
1. Open the foil pouch by tearing on the rough edge along the seam of the pouch. Remove a ready-to-use vial of BROVANA.
2. Carefully twist open the top of the ready-to-use vial and use it right away (**Figure 1**).

Figure 1

3. Squeeze all of the medicine from the ready-to-use vial into the nebulizer medicine cup (reservoir) (**Figure 2**).

RESERVOIR

Figure 2

4. Connect the nebulizer reservoir to the mouthpiece (**Figure 3**) or face mask (**Figure 4**).

MOUTHPIECE

Figure 3

FACE MASK

Figure 4

5. Connect the nebulizer to the compressor (**Figure 5**).

COMPRESSOR

TUBING

Figure 5

6. Sit in a comfortable, upright position. Place the mouthpiece in your mouth (**Figure 6**) (or put on the face mask) and turn on the compressor.

Figure 6

7. Breathe as calmly, deeply, and evenly as possible until no more mist is formed in the nebulizer reservoir. It takes about 5 to 10 minutes for each treatment.
8. Clean the nebulizer (see manufacturer's instructions).

Rx Only
This Medication Guide has been approved by the Food and Drug Administration.
SUNOVION
Manufactured for:
Sunovion Pharmaceuticals Inc.
Marlborough, MA 01752 USA
© 2011, 2014 Sunovion Pharmaceuticals Inc. All rights reserved.
February 2014
901552R02
Shown in Product Identification Guide, page 313

LATUDA
(lurasidone hydrochloride)
tablets, for oral use   ℞

HIGHLIGHTS OF PRESCRIBING INFORMATION
These highlights do not include all the information needed to use LATUDA safely and effectively. See full prescribing information for LATUDA.
LATUDA (lurasidone hydrochloride) tablets, for oral use
Initial U.S. Approval: 2010

> **WARNINGS: INCREASED MORTALITY IN ELDERLY PATIENTS WITH DEMENTIA-RELATED PSYCHOSIS; AND SUICIDAL THOUGHTS AND BEHAVIORS**
> *See full prescribing information for complete boxed warning.*
> - **Elderly patients with dementia-related psychosis treated with antipsychotic drugs are at an increased risk of death.**
> - **LATUDA is not approved for the treatment of patients with dementia-related psychosis (5.1).**
> - **Increased risk of suicidal thinking and behavior in children, adolescents, and young adults taking antidepressants (5.2).**
> - **Monitor for worsening and emergence of suicidal thoughts and behaviors (5.2)**

————**RECENT MAJOR CHANGES**————
Boxed Warnings, Suicidal Thoughts and Behaviors (5.2) 6/2013
Indications and Usage, Bipolar Depression (1.2) 6/2013
Dosage and Administration, Bipolar Depression (2.1) 6/2013
Dosage Forms and Strengths (3) 7/2013
Warnings and Precautions (5.2, 5.6, 5.7, 5.9, 5.10, 5.11, 5.13, 5.14) 6/2013

————**INDICATIONS AND USAGE**————
LATUDA is an atypical antipsychotic for the treatment of:
- Schizophrenia (1.1, 14.1)
- Depressive episodes associated with Bipolar I Disorder (bipolar depression), as monotherapy and as adjunctive therapy with lithium or valproate (1.2, 14.2).

————**DOSAGE AND ADMINISTRATION**————
LATUDA should be taken with food (at least 350 calories). Administration with food substantially increases the absorption of LATUDA (2.3, 12.3).

Indication	Starting Dose	Recommended Dose
Schizophrenia (2.1)	40 mg per day	40 mg to 160 mg per day
Bipolar Depression (2.2)	20 mg per day	20 mg to 120 mg per day

- Moderate and Severe Renal Impairment: Recommended starting dose is 20 mg per day, and the maximum recommended dose is 80 mg per day (2.4, 8.6).
- Moderate and Severe Hepatic Impairment: Recommended starting dose is 20 mg per day. The maximum recommended dose is 80 mg per day in moderate hepatic impairment and 40 mg per day in severe hepatic impairment (2.4, 8.6).
- Concomitant Use of a Moderate CYP3A4 inhibitor (e.g., diltiazem): LATUDA dose should be reduced to half of the original dose level. Recommended starting dose is 20 mg per day. Maximum recommended dose is 80 mg per day (2.5, 7.1)
- Concomitant Use of a Moderate CYP3A4 Inducer: It may be necessary to increase the dose of LATUDA (2.5, 7.1).

DOSAGE FORMS AND STRENGTHS
Tablets: 20 mg, 40 mg, 60 mg, 80 mg and 120 mg (3)

CONTRAINDICATIONS
- Known hypersensitivity to LATUDA or any components in the formulation (4).
- Concomitant use with a strong CYP3A4 inhibitor (e.g., ketoconazole) (2.5, 4, 7.1).
- Concomitant use with a strong CYP3A4 inducer (e.g., rifampin) (2.5, 4, 7.1).

WARNINGS AND PRECAUTIONS
- Cerebrovascular Adverse Reactions in Elderly Patients with Dementia-Related Psychosis: Increased incidence of cerebrovascular adverse events (e.g., stroke, transient ischemic attack) (5.2).
- Neuroleptic Malignant Syndrome: Manage with immediate discontinuation and close monitoring (5.4).
- Tardive Dyskinesia: Discontinue if clinically appropriate (5.5).
- Metabolic Changes: Atypical antipsychotic drugs have been associated with metabolic changes that may increase cardiovascular/cerebrovascular risk. These metabolic changes include hyperglycemia, dyslipidemia, and weight gain (5.6).
  - Hyperglycemia and Diabetes Mellitus: Monitor patients for symptoms of hyperglycemia including polydipsia, polyuria, polyphagia, and weakness. Monitor glucose regularly in patients with diabetes or at risk for diabetes.
  - Dyslipidemia: Undesirable alterations have been observed in patients treated with atypical antipsychotics.
  - Weight Gain: Gain in body weight has been observed. Monitor weight.
- Hyperprolactinemia: Prolactin elevations may occur (5.7).
- Leukopenia, Neutropenia, and Agranulocytosis: Perform complete blood counts (CBC) in patients with a pre-existing low white blood cell count (WBC) or a history of leukopenia or neutropenia. Consider discontinuing LATUDA if a clinically significant decline in WBC occurs in the absence of other causative factors (5.8).
- Orthostatic Hypotension and Syncope: Dizziness, tachycardia or bradycardia, and syncope may occur, especially early in treatment. In patients with known cardiovascular or cerebrovascular disease, and in antipsychotic-naïve patients, consider a lower starting dose and slower titration (5.9).

ADVERSE REACTIONS
Commonly observed adverse reactions (incidence ≥ 5% and at least twice the rate for placebo) were (6.1):
- Schizophrenia: somnolence, akathisia, extrapyramidal symptoms, and nausea
- Bipolar depression: akathisia, extrapyramidal symptoms, and somnolence

To report SUSPECTED ADVERSE REACTIONS, contact Sunovion Pharmaceuticals Inc. at 1-877-737-7226 or FDA at 1-800-FDA-1088 or www.fda.gov/medwatch.

USE IN SPECIFIC POPULATIONS
- Pregnancy: Use LATUDA during pregnancy only if the potential benefit justifies the potential risk (8.1).
- Nursing Mothers: Discontinue drug or nursing, considering risk of drug discontinuation to the mother (8.3).

See 17 for PATIENT COUNSELING INFORMATION and Medication Guide

Revised: 07/2013

FULL PRESCRIBING INFORMATION: CONTENTS*
WARNINGS: INCREASED MORTALITY IN ELDERLY PATIENTS WITH DEMENTIA-RELATED PSYCHOSIS; AND SUICIDAL THOUGHTS AND BEHAVIORS

1   INDICATIONS AND USAGE
     1.1   Schizophrenia
     1.2   Depressive Episodes Associated with Bipolar I Disorder

FULL PRESCRIBING INFORMATION

WARNINGS: INCREASED MORTALITY IN ELDERLY PATIENTS WITH DEMENTIA-RELATED PSYCHOSIS; AND SUICIDAL THOUGHTS AND BEHAVIORS
- Elderly patients with dementia-related psychosis treated with antipsychotic drugs are at an increased risk of death [see Warnings and Precautions (5.1)].
- LATUDA is not approved for use in patients with dementia-related psychosis [see Warnings and Precautions (5.1)].
- Antidepressants increased the risk of suicidal thoughts and behavior in children, adolescents, and young adults in short-term studies. These studies did not show an increase in the risk of suicidal thoughts and behavior with antidepressant use in patients over age 24; there was a reduction in risk with antidepressant use in patients aged 65 and older [see Warnings and Precautions (5.2)].
- In patients of all ages who are started on antidepressant therapy, monitor closely for worsening, and for emergence of suicidal thoughts and behaviors. Advise families and caregivers of the need for close observation and communication with the prescriber [see Warnings and Precautions (5.2)].

1   INDICATIONS AND USAGE
1.1   Schizophrenia
LATUDA is indicated for the treatment of patients with schizophrenia.
The efficacy of LATUDA in schizophrenia was established in five 6-week controlled studies of adult patients with schizophrenia [see Clinical Studies (14.1)].
The effectiveness of LATUDA for longer-term use, that is, for more than 6 weeks, has not been established in controlled studies. Therefore, the physician who elects to use LATUDA for extended periods should periodically re-evaluate the long-term usefulness of the drug for the individual patient [see Dosage and Administration (2)].
1.2   Depressive Episodes Associated with Bipolar I Disorder
Monotherapy: LATUDA is indicated as monotherapy for the treatment of patients with major depressive episodes associated with bipolar I disorder (bipolar depression). The efficacy of LATUDA was established in a 6-week monotherapy study in adult patients with bipolar depression [see Clinical Studies (14.2)].
Adjunctive Therapy with Lithium or Valproate: LATUDA is indicated as adjunctive therapy with either lithium or valproate for the treatment of patients with major depressive episodes associated with bipolar I disorder (bipolar depression). The efficacy of LATUDA as adjunctive therapy was established in a 6-week study in adult patients with bipolar depression who were treated with lithium or valproate [see Clinical Studies (14.2)].
The effectiveness of LATUDA for longer-term use, that is, for more than 6 weeks, has not been established in controlled studies. Therefore, the physician who elects to use LATUDA for extended periods should periodically re-evaluate the long-term usefulness of the drug for the individual patient [see Dosage and Administration (2.2)].
The efficacy of LATUDA in the treatment of mania associated with bipolar disorder has not been established.

2   DOSAGE AND ADMINISTRATION
2.1   Schizophrenia
The recommended starting dose of LATUDA is 40 mg once daily. Initial dose titration is not required. LATUDA has been shown to be effective in a dose range of 40 mg per day to 160 mg per day [see Clinical Studies (14.1)]. The maximum recommended dose is 160 mg per day.
2.2   Depressive Episodes Associated with Bipolar I Disorder
The recommended starting dose of LATUDA is 20 mg given once daily as monotherapy or as adjunctive therapy with lithium or valproate. Initial dose titration is not required. LATUDA has been shown to be effective in a dose range of 20 mg per day to 120 mg per day as monotherapy or as adjunctive therapy with lithium or valproate [see Clinical Studies (14.2)]. The maximum recommended dose, as monotherapy or as adjunctive therapy with lithium or valproate, is 120 mg per day. In the monotherapy study, the higher dose range (80 mg to 120 mg per day) did not provide additional efficacy, on average, compared to the lower dose range (20 to 60 mg per day) [see Clinical Studies (14.2)].
2.3   Administration Instructions
LATUDA should be taken with food (at least 350 calories). Administration with food substantially increases the absorption of LATUDA. Administration with food increases the AUC approximately 2-fold and increases the Cmax approximately 3-fold. In the clinical studies, LATUDA was administered with food [see Clinical Pharmacology (12.3)].
2.4   Dose Modifications in Special Populations
Renal Impairment
Dose adjustment is recommended in moderate (creatinine clearance: 30 to <50 mL/min) and severe renal impairment (creatinine clearance <30 mL/min) patients. The recommended starting dose is 20 mg per day. The dose in these patients should not exceed 80 mg per day [see Use in Specific Populations (8.6)].
Hepatic Impairment
Dose adjustment is recommended in moderate (Child-Pugh Score = 7 to 9) and severe hepatic impairment (Child-Pugh Score = 10 to 15) patients. The recommended starting dose

is 20 mg per day. The dose in moderate hepatic impairment patients should not exceed 80 mg per day and the dose in severe hepatic impairment patients should not exceed 40 mg/day *[see Use in Specific Populations (8.6)].*

2.5 Dose Modifications Due to Drug Interactions

Concomitant Use with CYP3A4 Inhibitors

LATUDA should not be used concomitantly with a strong CYP3A4 inhibitor (e.g., ketoconazole, clarithromycin, ritonavir, voriconazole, mibefradil, etc.) *[see Contraindications (4)].*

If LATUDA is being prescribed and a moderate CYP3A4 inhibitor (e.g. diltiazem, atazanavir, erythromycin, fluconazole, verapamil etc.) is added to the therapy, the LATUDA dose should be reduced to half of the original dose level. Similarly, if a moderate CYP3A4 inhibitor is being prescribed and LATUDA is added to the therapy, the recommended starting dose of LATUDA is 20 mg per day, and the maximum recommended dose of LATUDA is 80 mg per day *[see Contraindications (4); Drug Interactions (7.1)].*

Grapefruit and grapefruit juice should be avoided in patients taking LATUDA, since these may inhibit CYP3A4 and alter LATUDA concentrations *[see Drug Interactions (7.1)].*

Concomitant Use with CYP3A4 Inducers

LATUDA should not be used concomitantly with a strong CYP3A4 inducer (e.g., rifampin, avasimibe, St. John's wort, phenytoin, carbamazepine, etc.) *[see Contraindications (4); Drug Interactions (7.1)].* If LATUDA is used concomitantly with a moderate CYP3A4 inducer, it may be necessary to increase the LATUDA dose after chronic treatment (7 days or more) with the CYP3A4 inducer.

3 DOSAGE FORMS AND STRENGTHS

LATUDA tablets are available in the following shape and color (Table 1) with respective one-sided debossing:

Table 1: LATUDA Tablet Presentations

Tablet Strength	Tablet Color/Shape	Tablet Markings
20 mg	white to off-white round	L20
40 mg	white to off-white round	L40
60 mg	white to off white oblong	L60
80 mg	pale green oval	L80
120 mg	white to off-white oval	L120

4 CONTRAINDICATIONS

- Known hypersensitivity to lurasidone HCl or any components in the formulation. Angioedema has been observed with lurasidone *[see Adverse Reactions (6.1)].*
- Strong CYP3A4 inhibitors (e.g., ketoconazole, clarithromycin, ritonavir, voriconazole, mibefradil, etc.) *[see Drug Interactions (7.1)].*
- Strong CYP3A4 inducers (e.g., rifampin, avasimibe, St. John's wort, phenytoin, carbamazepine, etc.) *[see Drug Interactions (7.1)].*

5 WARNINGS AND PRECAUTIONS

5.1 Increased Mortality in Elderly Patients with Dementia-Related Psychosis

Elderly patients with dementia-related psychosis treated with antipsychotic drugs are at an increased risk of death. Analyses of 17 placebo-controlled trials (modal duration of 10 weeks), largely in patients taking atypical antipsychotic drugs, revealed a risk of death in drug-treated patients of between 1.6- to 1.7-times the risk of death in placebo-treated patients. Over the course of a typical 10-week controlled trial, the rate of death in drug-treated patients was about 4.5%, compared to a rate of about 2.6% in the placebo group. Although the causes of death were varied, most of the deaths appeared to be either cardiovascular (e.g., heart failure, sudden death) or infectious (e.g., pneumonia) in nature. Observational studies suggest that, similar to atypical antipsychotic drugs, treatment with conventional antipsychotic drugs may increase mortality. The extent to which the findings of increased mortality in observational studies may be attributed to the antipsychotic drug as opposed to some characteristic(s) of the patients is not clear. LATUDA is not approved for the treatment of patients with dementia-related psychosis *[see Boxed Warning].*

5.2 Suicidal Thoughts and Behaviors in Adolescents and Young Adults

Patients with major depressive disorder (MDD), both adult and pediatric, may experience worsening of their depression and/or the emergence of suicidal ideation and behavior (sui-cidality) or unusual changes in behavior, whether or not they are taking antidepressant medications, and this risk may persist until significant remission occurs. Suicide is a known risk of depression and certain other psychiatric disorders, and these disorders themselves are the strongest predictors of suicide. There has been a long-standing concern, however, that antidepressants may have a role in inducing worsening of depression and the emergence of suicidality in certain patients during the early phases of treatment.

Pooled analyses of short-term placebo-controlled trials of antidepressant drugs (SSRIs and others) showed that these drugs increase the risk of suicidal thinking and behavior (suicidality) in children, adolescents, and young adults (ages 18-24) with major depressive disorder (MDD) and other psychiatric disorders. Short-term studies did not show an increase in the risk of suicidality with antidepressants compared to placebo in adults beyond age 24; there was a reduction with antidepressants compared to placebo in adults aged 65 and older.

The pooled analyses of placebo-controlled trials in children and adolescents with MDD, obsessive compulsive disorder (OCD), or other psychiatric disorders included a total of 24 short-term trials of 9 antidepressant drugs in over 4400 patients. The pooled analyses of placebo-controlled trials in adults with MDD or other psychiatric disorders included a total of 295 short-term trials (median duration of 2 months) of 11 antidepressant drugs in over 77,000 patients. There was considerable variation in risk of suicidality among drugs, but a tendency toward an increase in the younger patients for almost all drugs studied. There were differences in absolute risk of suicidality across the different indications, with the highest incidence in MDD. The risk of differences (drug vs. placebo), however, were relatively stable within age strata and across indications. These risk differences (drug-placebo difference in the number of cases of suicidality per 1000 patients treated) are provided in Table 2.

Table 2

Age Range	Drug-Placebo Difference in Number of Cases of Suicidality per 1000 Patients Treated
	Increases Compared to Placebo
<18	14 additional cases
18-24	5 additional cases
	Decreases Compared to Placebo
25-64	1 fewer case
>65	6 fewer cases

No suicides occurred in any of the pediatric trials. There were suicides in the adult trials, but the number was not sufficient to reach any conclusion about drug effect on suicide.

It is unknown whether the suicidality risk extends to longer-term use, i.e., beyond several months. However, there is substantial evidence from placebo-controlled maintenance trials in adults with depression that the use of antidepressants can delay the recurrence of depression.

All patients being treated with antidepressants for any indication should be monitored appropriately and observed closely for clinical worsening, suicidality, and unusual changes in behavior, especially during the initial few months of a course of drug therapy, or at times of dose changes, either increases or decreases.

The following symptoms, anxiety, agitation, panic attacks, insomnia, irritability, hostility, aggressiveness, impulsivity, akathisia (psychomotor restlessness), hypomania, and mania, have been reported in adult and pediatric patients being treated with antidepressants for major depressive disorder as well as for other indications, both psychiatric and nonpsychiatric. Although a causal link between the emergence of such symptoms and either the worsening of depression and/or the emergence of suicidal impulses has not been established, there is concern that such symptoms may represent precursors to emerging suicidality.

Consideration should be given to changing the therapeutic regimen, including possibly discontinuing the medication, in patients whose depression is persistently worse, or who are experiencing emergent suicidality or symptoms that might be precursors to worsening depression or suicidality, especially if these symptoms are severe, abrupt in onset, or were not part of the patient's presenting symptoms.

Families and caregivers of patients being treated with antidepressants for major depressive disorder or other indications, both psychiatric and nonpsychiatric, should be alerted about the need to monitor patients for the emergence of agitation, irritability, unusual changes in behavior, and the other symptoms described above, as well as the emergence of suicidal thoughts and behaviors, and to report such symptoms immediately to health care providers. Such monitoring should include daily observation by families and caregivers. Prescriptions for LATUDA should be written for the smallest quantity of capsules consistent with good patient management, in order to reduce the risk of overdose.

5.3 Cerebrovascular Adverse Reactions, Including Stroke in Elderly Patients with Dementia-Related Psychosis

In placebo-controlled trials with risperidone, aripiprazole, and olanzapine in elderly subjects with dementia, there was a higher incidence of cerebrovascular adverse reactions (cerebrovascular accidents and transient ischemic attacks), including fatalities, compared to placebo-treated subjects. LATUDA is not approved for the treatment of patients with dementia-related psychosis *[see also Boxed Warning and Warnings and Precautions (5.1)].*

5.4 Neuroleptic Malignant Syndrome

A potentially fatal symptom complex sometimes referred to as Neuroleptic Malignant Syndrome (NMS) has been reported in association with administration of antipsychotic drugs, including LATUDA.

Clinical manifestations of NMS are hyperpyrexia, muscle rigidity, altered mental status, and evidence of autonomic instability (irregular pulse or blood pressure, tachycardia, diaphoresis, and cardiac dysrhythmia). Additional signs may include elevated creatine phosphokinase, myoglobinuria (rhabdomyolysis), and acute renal failure.

The diagnostic evaluation of patients with this syndrome is complicated. It is important to exclude cases where the clinical presentation includes both serious medical illness (e.g., pneumonia, systemic infection) and untreated or inadequately treated extrapyramidal signs and symptoms (EPS). Other important considerations in the differential diagnosis include central anticholinergic toxicity, heat stroke, drug fever, and primary central nervous system pathology.

The management of NMS should include: 1) immediate discontinuation of antipsychotic drugs and other drugs not essential to concurrent therapy; 2) intensive symptomatic treatment and medical monitoring; and 3) treatment of any concomitant serious medical problems for which specific treatments are available. There is no general agreement about specific pharmacological treatment regimens for NMS.

If a patient requires antipsychotic drug treatment after recovery from NMS, the potential reintroduction of drug therapy should be carefully considered. If reintroduced, the patient should be carefully monitored, since recurrences of NMS have been reported.

5.5 Tardive Dyskinesia

Tardive dyskinesia is a syndrome consisting of potentially irreversible, involuntary, dyskinetic movements that can develop in patients treated with antipsychotic drugs. Although the prevalence of the syndrome appears to be highest among the elderly, especially elderly women, it is impossible to rely upon prevalence estimates to predict, at the inception of antipsychotic treatment, which patients are likely to develop the syndrome. Whether antipsychotic drug products differ in their potential to cause tardive dyskinesia is unknown.

The risk of developing tardive dyskinesia and the likelihood that it will become irreversible are believed to increase as the duration of treatment and the total cumulative dose of antipsychotic drugs administered to the patient increase. However, the syndrome can develop, although much less commonly, after relatively brief treatment periods at low doses.

There is no known treatment for established cases of tardive dyskinesia, although the syndrome may remit, partially or completely, if antipsychotic treatment is withdrawn. Antipsychotic treatment, itself, however, may suppress (or partially suppress) the signs and symptoms of the syndrome and thereby may possibly mask the underlying process. The effect that symptomatic suppression has upon the long-term course of the syndrome is unknown.

Given these considerations, LATUDA should be prescribed in a manner that is most likely to minimize the occurrence of tardive dyskinesia. Chronic antipsychotic treatment should generally be reserved for patients who suffer from a chronic illness that (1) is known to respond to antipsychotic drugs, and (2) for whom alternative, equally effective, but potentially less harmful treatments are not available or appropriate. In patients who do require chronic treatment, the smallest dose and the shortest duration of treatment producing a satisfactory clinical response should be sought. The need for continued treatment should be reassessed periodically.

If signs and symptoms of tardive dyskinesia appear in a patient on LATUDA, drug discontinuation should be considered. However, some patients may require treatment with LATUDA despite the presence of the syndrome.

5.6 Metabolic Changes

Atypical antipsychotic drugs have been associated with metabolic changes that may increase cardiovascular/cere-

Table 3: Change in Fasting Glucose in Schizophrenia Studies

	Placebo	LATUDA 20 mg/day	40 mg/day	80 mg/day	120 mg/day	160 mg/day
Mean Change from Baseline (mg/dL)						
	n=680	n=71	n=478	n=508	n=283	n=113
Serum Glucose	-0.0	-0.6	+2.6	-0.4	+2.5	+ 2.5
Proportion of Patients with Shifts to ≥ 126 mg/dL						
Serum Glucose (≥ 126 mg/dL)	8.3% (52/628)	11.7% (7/60)	12.7% (57/449)	6.8% (32/472)	10.0% (26/260)	5.6% (6/108)

Table 4: Change in Fasting Glucose in the Monotherapy Bipolar Depression Study

	Placebo	LATUDA 20 to 60 mg/day	80 to 120 mg/day
Mean Change from Baseline (mg/dL)			
	n=148	n=140	n=143
Serum Glucose	+1.8	-0.8	+1.8
Proportion of Patients with Shifts to ≥ 126 mg/dL			
Serum Glucose (≥ 126 mg/dL)	4.3% (6/141)	2.2% (3/138)	6.4% (9/141)

Patients were randomized to flexibly dosed LATUDA 20 to 60 mg/day, LATUDA 80 to 120 mg/day, or placebo

Table 6: Change in Fasting Lipids in Schizophrenia Studies

	Placebo	LATUDA 20 mg/day	40 mg/day	80 mg/day	120 mg/day	160 mg/day
Mean Change from Baseline (mg/dL)						
	n=660	n=71	n=466	n=499	n=268	n=115
Total Cholesterol	-5.8	-12.3	-5.7	-6.2	-3.8	-6.9
Triglycerides	-13.4	-29.1	-5.1	-13.0	-3.1	-10.6
Proportion of Patients with Shifts						
Total Cholesterol (≥ 240 mg/dL)	5.3% (30/571)	13.8% (8/58)	6.2% (25/402)	5.3% (23/434)	3.8% (9/238)	4.0% (4/101)
Triglycerides (≥ 200 mg/dL)	10.1% (53/526)	14.3% (7/49)	10.8% (41/379)	6.3% (25/400)	10.5% (22/209)	7.0% (7/100)

Table 7: Change in Fasting Lipids in the Monotherapy Bipolar Depression Study

	Placebo	LATUDA 20 to 60 mg/day	80 to 120 mg/day
Mean Change from Baseline (mg/dL)			
	n=147	n=140	n=144
Total cholesterol	-3.2	+1.2	-4.6
Triglycerides	+6.0	+5.6	+0.4
Proportion of Patients with Shifts			
Total cholesterol (≥ 240 mg/dL)	4.2% (5/118)	4.4% (5/113)	4.4% (5/114)
Triglycerides (≥ 200 mg/dL)	4.8% (6/126)	10.1% (12/119)	9.8% (12/122)

Patients were randomized to flexibly dosed LATUDA 20 to 60 mg/day, LATUDA 80 to 120 mg/day, or placebo

brovascular risk. These metabolic changes include hyperglycemia, dyslipidemia, and body weight gain. While all of the drugs in the class have been shown to produce some metabolic changes, each drug has its own specific risk profile.

Hyperglycemia and Diabetes Mellitus
Hyperglycemia, in some cases extreme and associated with ketoacidosis or hyperosmolar coma or death, has been reported in patients treated with atypical antipsychotics. Assessment of the relationship between atypical antipsychotic use and glucose abnormalities is complicated by the possibility of an increased background risk of diabetes mellitus in patients with schizophrenia and the increasing incidence of diabetes mellitus in the general population. Given these confounders, the relationship between atypical antipsychotic use and hyperglycemia-related adverse events is not completely understood. However, epidemiological studies suggest an increased risk of treatment-emergent hyperglycemia-related adverse events in patients treated with the atypical antipsychotics. Because LATUDA was not marketed at the time these studies were performed, it is not known if LATUDA is associated with this increased risk. Patients with an established diagnosis of diabetes mellitus who are started on atypical antipsychotics should be monitored regularly for worsening of glucose control. Patients with risk factors for diabetes mellitus (e.g., obesity, family history of diabetes) who are starting treatment with atypical antipsychotics should undergo fasting blood glucose testing at the beginning of treatment and periodically during treatment. Any patient treated with atypical antipsychotics should be monitored for symptoms of hyperglycemia including polydipsia, polyuria, polyphagia, and weakness. Patients who develop symptoms of hyperglycemia during treatment with atypical antipsychotics should undergo fasting blood glucose testing. In some cases, hyperglycemia has resolved when the atypical antipsychotic was discontinued; however, some patients required continuation of antidiabetic treatment despite discontinuation of the suspect drug.

Schizophrenia
Pooled data from short-term, placebo-controlled schizophrenia studies are presented in Table 3.
[See table 3 above]
In the uncontrolled, longer-term schizophrenia studies (primarily open-label extension studies), LATUDA was associated with a mean change in glucose of +1.8 mg/dL at week 24 (n=355), +0.8 mg/dL at week 36 (n=299) and +2.3 mg/dL at week 52 (n=307).

Bipolar Depression
Monotherapy
Data from the short-term, flexible-dose, placebo-controlled monotherapy bipolar depression study are presented in Table 4.
[See table 4 above]
In the uncontrolled, open-label, longer-term bipolar depression study, patients who received LATUDA as monotherapy in the short-term study and continued in the longer-term study, had a mean change in glucose of +1.2 mg/dL at week 24 (n=129).

Adjunctive Therapy with Lithium or Valproate
Data from the short-term, flexible-dosed, placebo-controlled adjunctive therapy bipolar depression studies are presented in Table 5.

Table 5: Change in Fasting Glucose in the Adjunctive Therapy Bipolar Depression Studies

	Placebo	LATUDA 20 to 120 mg/day
Mean Change from Baseline (mg/dL)		
	n=302	n=319
Serum Glucose	-0.9	+1.2
Proportion of Patients with Shifts to ≥ 126 mg/dL		
Serum Glucose (≥ 126 mg/dL)	1.0% (3/290)	1.3% (4/316)

Patients were randomized to flexibly dosed LATUDA 20 to 120 mg/day or placebo as adjunctive therapy with lithium or valproate.

In the uncontrolled, open-label, longer-term bipolar depression study, patients who received LATUDA as adjunctive therapy with either lithium or valproate in the short-term study and continued in the longer-term study, had a mean change in glucose of +1.7 mg/dL at week 24 (n=88).

Dyslipidemia
Undesirable alterations in lipids have been observed in patients treated with atypical antipsychotics.

Schizophrenia
Pooled data from short-term, placebo-controlled schizophrenia studies are presented in Table 6.
[See table 6 above]
In the uncontrolled, longer-term schizophrenia studies (primarily open-label extension studies), LATUDA was associated with a mean change in total cholesterol and triglycerides of -3.8 (n=356) and -15.1 (n=357) mg/dL at week 24, -3.1 (n=303) and -4.8 (n=303) mg/dL at week 36 and -2.5 (n=307) and -6.9 (n=307) mg/dL at week 52, respectively.

Bipolar Depression
Monotherapy
Data from the short-term, flexible-dosed, placebo-controlled, monotherapy bipolar depression study are presented in Table 7.
[See table 7 above]
In the uncontrolled, open-label, longer-term bipolar depression study, patients who received LATUDA as monotherapy in the short-term and continued in the longer-term study had a mean change in total cholesterol and triglycerides of -0.5 (n=130) and -1.0 (n=130) mg/dL at week 24, respectively.

Adjunctive Therapy with Lithium or Valproate
Data from the short-term, flexible-dosed, placebo-controlled, adjunctive therapy bipolar depression studies are presented in Table 8.

Table 8: Change in Fasting Lipids in the Adjunctive Therapy Bipolar Depression Studies

	Placebo	LATUDA 20 to 120 mg/day
Mean Change from Baseline (mg/dL)		
	n=303	n=321
Total cholesterol	-2.9	-3.1
Triglycerides	-4.6	+4.6
Proportion of Patients with Shifts		
Total cholesterol (≥ 240 mg/dL)	5.7% (15/263)	5.4% (15/276)
Triglycerides (≥ 200 mg/dL)	8.6% (21/243)	10.8% (28/260)

Patients were randomized to flexibly dosed LATUDA 20 to 120 mg/day or placebo as adjunctive therapy with lithium or valproate.

In the uncontrolled, open-label, longer-term bipolar depression study, patients who received LATUDA, as adjunctive therapy with either lithium or valproate in the short-term study and continued in the longer-term study, had a mean change in total cholesterol and triglycerides of -0.9 (n=88) and +5.3 (n=88) mg/dL at week 24, respectively.

Weight Gain
Weight gain has been observed with atypical antipsychotic use. Clinical monitoring of weight is recommended.

Schizophrenia
Pooled data from short-term, placebo-controlled schizophrenia studies are presented in Table 9. The mean weight gain was +0.43 kg for LATUDA-treated patients compared to -0.02 kg for placebo-treated patients. Change in weight from baseline for olanzapine was +4.15 kg and for quetiapine extended-release was +2.09 kg in Studies 3 and 5 *[see Clinical Studies (14.1)]*, respectively. The proportion of patients with a ≥ 7% increase in body weight (at Endpoint) was 4.8% for LATUDA-treated patients versus 3.3% for placebo-treated patients.
[See table 9 above]
In the uncontrolled, longer-term schizophrenia studies (primarily open-label extension studies), LATUDA was associated with a mean change in weight of -0.69 kg at week 24 (n=755), -0.59 kg at week 36 (n=443) and -0.73 kg at week 52 (n=377).

Bipolar Depression
Monotherapy
Data from the short-term, flexible-dosed, placebo-controlled monotherapy bipolar depression study are presented in Table 10. The mean weight gain was +0.29 kg for LATUDA-treated patients compared to -0.04 kg for placebo-treated patients. The proportion of patients with a ≥ 7% increase in body weight (at Endpoint) was 2.4% for LATUDA-treated patients versus 0.7% for placebo-treated patients.

Table 10: Mean Change in Weight (kg) from Baseline in the Monotherapy Bipolar Depression Study

	Placebo (n=151)	LATUDA 20 to 60 mg/day (n=143)	LATUDA 80 to 120 mg/day (n=147)
All Patients	-0.04	+0.56	+0.02

Patients were randomized to flexibly dosed LATUDA 20 to 60 mg/day, LATUDA 80 to 120 mg/day, or placebo

In the uncontrolled, open-label, longer-term bipolar depression study, patients who received LATUDA as monotherapy in the short-term and continued in the longer-term study had a mean change in weight of -0.02 kg at week 24 (n=130).
Adjunctive Therapy with Lithium or Valproate
Data from the short-term, flexible-dosed, placebo-controlled adjunctive therapy bipolar depression studies are presented in Table 11. The mean weight gain was +0.11 kg for LATUDA-treated patients compared to +0.16 kg for placebo-treated patients. The proportion of patients with a ≥ 7% increase in body weight (at Endpoint) was 3.1% for LATUDA-treated patients versus 0.3% for placebo-treated patients.

Table 9: Mean Change in Weight (kg) from Baseline in Schizophrenia Studies

	Placebo (n=696)	LATUDA 20 mg/day (n=71)	LATUDA 40 mg/day (n=484)	LATUDA 80 mg/day (n=526)	LATUDA 120 mg/day (n=291)	LATUDA 160 mg/day (n=114)
All Patients	-0.02	-0.15	+0.22	+0.54	+0.68	+0.60

Table 12: Median Change in Prolactin (ng/mL) from Baseline in Schizophrenia Studies

	Placebo	LATUDA 20 mg/day	LATUDA 40 mg/day	LATUDA 80 mg/day	LATUDA 120 mg/day	LATUDA 160 mg/day
All Patients	-1.9 (n=672)	-1.1 (n=70)	-1.4 (n=476)	-0.2 (n=495)	+3.3 (n=284)	+3.3 (n=115)
Females	-5.1 (n=200)	-0.7 (n=19)	-4.0 (n=149)	-0.2 (n=150)	+6.7 (n=70)	+7.1 (n=36)
Males	-1.3 (n=472)	-1.2 (n=51)	-0.7 (n=327)	-0.2 (n=345)	+3.1 (n=214)	+2.4 (n=79)

Table 13: Median Change in Prolactin (ng/mL) from Baseline in the Monotherapy Bipolar Depression Study

	Placebo	LATUDA 20 to 60 mg/day	LATUDA 80 to 120 mg/day
All Patients	+0.3 (n=147)	+1.7 (n=140)	+3.5 (n=144)
Females	0.0 (n=82)	+1.8 (n=78)	+5.3 (n=88)
Males	+0.4 (n=65)	+1.2 (n=62)	+1.9 (n=56)

Patients were randomized to flexibly dosed LATUDA 20 to 60 mg/day, LATUDA 80 to 120 mg/day, or placebo

Table 11: Mean Change in Weight (kg) from Baseline in the Adjunctive Therapy Bipolar Depression Studies

	Placebo (n=307)	LATUDA 20 to 120 mg/day (n=327)
All Patients	+0.16	+0.11

Patients were randomized to flexibly dosed LATUDA 20 to 120 mg/day or placebo as adjunctive therapy with lithium or valproate.

In the uncontrolled, open-label, longer-term bipolar depression study, patients who were treated with LATUDA, as adjunctive therapy with either lithium or valproate in the short-term and continued in the longer-term study, had a mean change in weight of +1.28 kg at week 24 (n=86).

5.7   Hyperprolactinemia
As with other drugs that antagonize dopamine D_2 receptors, LATUDA elevates prolactin levels.
Hyperprolactinemia may suppress hypothalamic GnRH, resulting in reduced pituitary gonadotrophin secretion. This, in turn, may inhibit reproductive function by impairing gonadal steroidogenesis in both female and male patients. Galactorrhea, amenorrhea, gynecomastia, and impotence have been reported with prolactin-elevating compounds. Long-standing hyperprolactinemia, when associated with hypogonadism, may lead to decreased bone density in both female and male patients *[see Adverse Reactions (6)]*.
Tissue culture experiments indicate that approximately one-third of human breast cancers are prolactin-dependent *in vitro*, a factor of potential importance if the prescription of these drugs is considered in a patient with previously detected breast cancer. As is common with compounds which increase prolactin release, an increase in mammary gland neoplasia was observed in a LATUDA carcinogenicity study conducted in rats and mice *[see Nonclinical Toxicology (13)]*. Neither clinical studies nor epidemiologic studies conducted to date have shown an association between chronic administration of this class of drugs and tumorigenesis in humans, but the available evidence is too limited to be conclusive.
Schizophrenia
In short-term, placebo-controlled schizophrenia studies, the median change from baseline to endpoint in prolactin levels for LATUDA-treated patients was +0.4 ng/mL and was -1.9 ng/mL in the placebo-treated patients. The median change from baseline to endpoint for males was +0.5 ng/mL

and for females was -0.2 ng/mL. Median changes for prolactin by dose are shown in Table 12.
[See table 12 above]
The proportion of patients with prolactin elevations ≥ 5× upper limit of normal (ULN) was 2.8% for LATUDA-treated patients versus 1.0% for placebo-treated patients. The proportion of female patients with prolactin elevations ≥ 5× ULN was 5.7% for LATUDA-treated patients versus 2.0% for placebo-treated female patients. The proportion of male patients with prolactin elevations ≥ 5× ULN was 1.6% versus 0.6% for placebo-treated male patients.
In the uncontrolled longer-term schizophrenia studies (primarily open-label extension studies), LATUDA was associated with a median change in prolactin of -0.9 ng/mL at week 24 (n=357), -5.3ng/mL at week 36 (n=190) and -2.2 ng/mL at week 52 (n=307).
Bipolar Depression
Monotherapy
The median change from baseline to endpoint in prolactin levels, in the short-term, flexible-dosed, placebo-controlled monotherapy bipolar depression study, was +1.7 ng/mL and +3.5 ng/mL with LATUDA 20 to 60 mg/day and 80 to 120 mg/day, respectively compared to +0.3 ng/mL with placebo-treated patients. The median change from baseline to endpoint for males was +1.5 ng/mL and for females was +3.1 ng/mL. Median changes for prolactin by dose range are shown in Table 13.
[See table 13 above]
The proportion of patients with prolactin elevations ≥ 5× upper limit of normal (ULN) was 0.4% for LATUDA-treated patients versus 0.0% for placebo-treated patients. The proportion of female patients with prolactin elevations ≥ 5× ULN was 0.6% for LATUDA-treated patients versus 0% for placebo-treated female patients. The proportion of male patients with prolactin elevations ≥ 5× ULN was 0% versus 0% for placebo-treated male patients.
In the uncontrolled, open-label, longer-term bipolar depression study, patients who were treated with LATUDA as monotherapy in the short-term and continued in the longer-term study, had a median change in prolactin of -1.15 ng/mL at week 24 (n=130).
Adjunctive Therapy with Lithium or Valproate
The median change from baseline to endpoint in prolactin levels, in the short-term, flexible-dosed, placebo-controlled adjunctive therapy bipolar depression studies was +2.8 ng/mL with LATUDA 20 to 120 mg/day compared to 0.0 ng/mL with placebo-treated patients. The median change from baseline to endpoint for males was +2.4 ng/mL and for females was +3.2 ng/mL. Median changes for prolactin across the dose range are shown in Table 14.

Table 14: Median Change in Prolactin (ng/mL) from Baseline in the Adjunctive Therapy Bipolar Depression Studies

	Placebo	LATUDA 20 to 120 mg/day
All Patients	0.0 (n=301)	+2.8 (n=321)
Females	+0.4 (n=156)	+3.2 (n=162)
Males	-0.1 (n=145)	+2.4 (n=159)

Patients were randomized to flexibly dosed LATUDA 20 to 120 mg/day or placebo as adjunctive therapy with lithium or valproate.

The proportion of patients with prolactin elevations ≥ 5× upper limit of normal (ULN) was 0.0% for LATUDA-treated patients versus 0.0% for placebo-treated patients. The proportion of female patients with prolactin elevations ≥ 5× ULN was 0% for LATUDA-treated patients versus 0% for placebo-treated female patients. The proportion of male patients with prolactin elevations ≥ 5× ULN was 0% versus 0% for placebo-treated male patients.

In the uncontrolled, open-label, longer-term bipolar depression study, patients who were treated with LATUDA, as adjunctive therapy with either lithium or valproate, in the short-term and continued in the longer-term study, had a median change in prolactin of -2.9 ng/mL at week 24 (n=88).

5.8 Leukopenia, Neutropenia and Agranulocytosis
Leukopenia/neutropenia has been reported during treatment with antipsychotic agents. Agranulocytosis (including fatal cases) has been reported with other agents in the class. Possible risk factors for leukopenia/neutropenia include pre-existing low white blood cell count (WBC) and history of drug-induced leukopenia/neutropenia. Patients with a pre-existing low WBC or a history of drug-induced leukopenia/neutropenia should have their complete blood count (CBC) monitored frequently during the first few months of therapy and LATUDA should be discontinued at the first sign of decline in WBC, in the absence of other causative factors. Patients with neutropenia should be carefully monitored for fever or other symptoms or signs of infection and treated promptly if such symptoms or signs occur. Patients with severe neutropenia (absolute neutrophil count < 1000/mm³) should discontinue LATUDA and have their WBC followed until recovery.

5.9 Orthostatic Hypotension and Syncope
LATUDA may cause orthostatic hypotension and syncope, perhaps due to its α1-adrenergic receptor antagonism. Associated adverse reactions can include dizziness, lightheadedness, tachycardia, and bradycardia. Generally, these risks are greatest at the beginning of treatment and during dose escalation. Patients at increased risk of these adverse reactions or at increased risk of developing complications from hypotension include those with dehydration, hypovolemia, treatment with antihypertensive medication, history of cardiovascular disease (e.g., heart failure, myocardial infarction, ischemia, or conduction abnormalities), history of cerebrovascular disease, as well as patients who are antipsychotic-naïve. In such patients, consider using a lower starting dose and slower titration, and monitor orthostatic vital signs.
Orthostatic hypotension, as assessed by vital sign measurement, was defined by the following vital sign changes: ≥ 20 mm Hg decrease in systolic blood pressure and ≥ 10 bpm increase in pulse from sitting to standing or supine to standing position.
Schizophrenia
The incidence of orthostatic hypotension and syncope reported as adverse events from short-term, placebo-controlled schizophrenia studies was (LATUDA incidence, placebo incidence): orthostatic hypotension [0.3% (5/1508), 0.1% (1/708)] and syncope [0.1% (2/1508), 0% (0/708)].
In short-term schizophrenia clinical studies, orthostatic hypotension, as assessed by vital signs, occurred with a frequency of 0.8% with LATUDA 40 mg, 2.1% with LATUDA 80 mg, 1.7% with LATUDA 120 mg and 0.8% with LATUDA 160 mg compared to 0.7% with placebo.
Bipolar Depression
Monotherapy
In the short-term, flexible-dose, placebo-controlled monotherapy bipolar depression study, there were no reported adverse events of orthostatic hypotension and syncope.
Orthostatic hypotension, as assessed by vital signs, occurred with a frequency of 0.6% with LATUDA 20 to 60 mg and 0.6% with LATUDA 80 to 120 mg compared to 0% with placebo.
Adjunctive Therapy with Lithium or Valproate
In the short-term, flexible-dose, placebo-controlled adjunctive therapy bipolar depression therapy studies, there were

no reported adverse events of orthostatic hypotension and syncope. Orthostatic hypotension, as assessed by vital signs, occurred with a frequency of 1.1% with LATUDA 20 to 120 mg compared to 0.9% with placebo.
5.10 Seizures
As with other antipsychotic drugs, LATUDA should be used cautiously in patients with a history of seizures or with conditions that lower the seizure threshold, e.g., Alzheimer's dementia. Conditions that lower the seizure threshold may be more prevalent in patients 65 years or older.
Schizophrenia
In short-term, placebo-controlled schizophrenia studies, seizures/convulsions occurred in 0.1% (2/1508) of patients treated with LATUDA compared to 0.1% (1/708) placebo-treated patients.
Bipolar Depression
Monotherapy
In the short-term, flexible-dose, placebo-controlled monotherapy bipolar depression study, no patient experienced seizures/convulsions.
Adjunctive Therapy with Lithium or Valproate
In the short-term, flexible-dose, placebo-controlled adjunctive therapy bipolar depression studies, no patient experienced seizures/convulsions.
5.11 Potential for Cognitive and Motor Impairment
LATUDA, like other antipsychotics, has the potential to impair judgment, thinking or motor skills. Caution patients about operating hazardous machinery, including motor vehicles, until they are reasonably certain that therapy with LATUDA does not affect them adversely.
In clinical studies with LATUDA, somnolence included: hypersomnia, hypersomnolence, sedation and somnolence.
Schizophrenia
In short-term, placebo-controlled schizophrenia studies, somnolence was reported by 17.0% (256/1508) of patients treated with LATUDA (15.5% LATUDA 20 mg, 15.6% LATUDA 40 mg, 15.2% LATUDA 80 mg, 26.5% LATUDA 120 mg and 8.3% LATUDA 160 mg/day) compared to 7.1% (50/708) of placebo patients.
Bipolar Depression
Monotherapy
In the short-term, flexible-dosed, placebo-controlled monotherapy bipolar depression study, somnolence was reported by 7.3% (12/164) and 13.8% (23/167) with LATUDA 20 to 60 mg and 80 to120 mg, respectively compared to 6.5% (11/168) of placebo patients.
Adjunctive Therapy with Lithium or Valproate
In the short-term, flexible-dosed, placebo-controlled adjunctive therapy bipolar depression studies, somnolence was reported by 11.4% (41/360) of patients treated with LATUDA 20-120 mg compared to 5.1% (17/334) of placebo patients.
5.12 Body Temperature Dysregulation
Disruption of the body's ability to reduce core body temperature has been attributed to antipsychotic agents. Appropriate care is advised when prescribing LATUDA for patients who will be experiencing conditions that may contribute to an elevation in core body temperature, e.g., exercising strenuously, exposure to extreme heat, receiving concomitant medication with anticholinergic activity, or being subject to dehydration [see Patient Counseling Information (17.9)].
5.13 Suicide
The possibility of a suicide attempt is inherent in psychotic illness and close supervision of high-risk patients should accompany drug therapy. Prescriptions for LATUDA should be written for the smallest quantity of tablets consistent with good patient management in order to reduce the risk of overdose.
Schizophrenia
In short-term, placebo-controlled schizophrenia studies, the incidence of treatment-emergent suicidal ideation was 0.4% (6/1508) for LATUDA-treated patients compared to 0.8% (6/708) on placebo. No suicide attempts or completed suicides were reported in these studies.
Bipolar Depression
Monotherapy
In the short-term, flexible-dose, placebo-controlled monotherapy bipolar depression study, the incidence of treatment-emergent suicidal ideation was 0.0% (0/331) with LATUDA-treated patients compared to 0.0% (0/168) with placebo-treated patients. No suicide attempts or completed suicides were reported in this study.
Adjunctive Therapy with Lithium or Valproate
In the short-term, flexible-dose, placebo-controlled adjunctive therapy bipolar depression studies, the incidence of treatment-emergent suicidal ideation was 1.1% (4/360) for LATUDA-treated patients compared to 0.3% (1/334) on placebo. No suicide attempts or completed suicides were reported in these studies.
5.14 Activation of Mania/Hypomania
Antidepressant treatment can increase the risk of developing a manic or hypomanic episode, particularly in patients with bipolar disorder. Monitor patients for the emergence of such episodes.
In the bipolar depression monotherapy and adjunctive therapy (with lithium or valproate) studies, less than 1% of subjects in the LATUDA and placebo groups developed manic or hypomanic episodes.

5.15 Dysphagia
Esophageal dysmotility and aspiration have been associated with antipsychotic drug use. Aspiration pneumonia is a common cause of morbidity and mortality in elderly patients, in particular those with advanced Alzheimer's dementia. LATUDA and other antipsychotic drugs should be used cautiously in patients at risk for aspiration pneumonia.
5.16 Neurological Adverse Reactions in Patients with Parkinson's Disease or Dementia with Lewy Bodies
Patients with Parkinson's Disease or Dementia with Lewy Bodies are reported to have an increased sensitivity to antipsychotic medication. Manifestations of this increased sensitivity include confusion, obtundation, postural instability with frequent falls, extrapyramidal symptoms, and clinical features consistent with the neuroleptic malignant syndrome.

6 ADVERSE REACTIONS
The following adverse reactions are discussed in more detail in other sections of the labeling:
- Increased Mortality in Elderly Patients with Dementia-Related Psychosis [see Boxed Warning and Warnings and Precautions (5.1)]
- Suicidal Thoughts and Behaviors [see Boxed Warning and Warnings and Precautions (5.2)]
- Cerebrovascular Adverse Reactions, Including Stroke, in Elderly Patients with Dementia-related Psychosis [see Warnings and Precautions (5.23)]
- Neuroleptic Malignant Syndrome [see Warnings and Precautions (5.4)]
- Tardive Dyskinesia [see Warnings and Precautions (5.5)]
- Metabolic Changes (Hyperglycemia and Diabetes Mellitus, Dyslipidemia, and Weight Gain) [see Warnings and Precautions (5.6)]
- Hyperprolactinemia [see Warnings and Precautions (5.7)]
- Leukopenia, Neutropenia, and Agranulocytosis [see Warnings and Precautions (5.8)]
- Orthostatic Hypotension and Syncope [see Warnings and Precautions (5.9)]
- Seizures [see Warnings and Precautions (5.10)]
- Potential for Cognitive and Motor Impairment [see Warnings and Precautions (5.11)]
- Body Temperature Dysregulation [see Warnings and Precautions (5.12)]
- Suicide [see Warnings and Precautions (5.13)]
- Activation of Mania/Hypomania [see Warnings and Precautions (5.14)]
- Dysphagia [see Warnings and Precautions (5.15)]
- Neurological Adverse Reactions in Patients with Parkinson's Disease or Dementia with Lewy Bodies [see Warnings and Precautions (5.16)]
6.1 Clinical Trials Experience
Because clinical trials are conducted under widely varying conditions, adverse reaction rates observed in clinical trials of a drug cannot be directly compared to rates in the clinical trials of another drug and may not reflect the rates observed in clinical practice.
The information below is derived from an integrated clinical study database for LATUDA consisting of 3799 patients exposed to one or more doses of LATUDA for the treatment of schizophrenia and bipolar depression in placebo-controlled studies. This experience corresponds with a total experience of 1250.9 patient-years. A total of 1106 LATUDA-treated patients had at least 24 weeks and 371 LATUDA-treated patients had at least 52 weeks of exposure.
Adverse events during exposure to study treatment were obtained by general inquiry and voluntarily reported adverse experiences, as well as results from physical examinations, vital signs, ECGs, weights and laboratory investigations. Adverse experiences were recorded by clinical investigators using their own terminology. In order to provide a meaningful estimate of the proportion of individuals experiencing adverse events, events were grouped in standardized categories using MedDRA terminology.
Schizophrenia
The following findings are based on the short-term, placebo-controlled premarketing studies for schizophrenia in which LATUDA was administered at daily doses ranging from 20 to 160 mg (n=1508).
Commonly Observed Adverse Reactions: The most common adverse reactions (incidence ≥ 5% and at least twice the rate of placebo) in patients treated with LATUDA were somnolence, akathisia, extrapyramidal symptoms, and nausea.
Adverse Reactions Associated with Discontinuation of Treatment: A total of 9.5% (143/1508) LATUDA-treated patients and 9.3% (66/708) of placebo-treated patients discontinued due to adverse reactions. There were no adverse reactions associated with discontinuation in subjects treated with LATUDA that were at least 2% and at least twice the placebo rate.

Table 15: Adverse Reactions in 2% or More of LATUDA-Treated Patients and That Occurred at Greater Incidence than in the Placebo-Treated Patients in Short-term Schizophrenia Studies

Percentage of Patients Reporting Reaction

Body System or Organ Class	Placebo (N=708) (%)	20 mg/day (N=71) (%)	40 mg/day (N=487) (%)	80 mg/day (N=538) (%)	120 mg/day (N=291) (%)	160 mg/day (N=121) (%)	All LATUDA (N=1508) (%)
Gastrointestinal Disorders							
Nausea	5	11	10	9	13	7	10
Vomiting	6	7	6	9	9	7	8
Dyspepsia	5	11	6	5	8	6	6
Salivary Hypersecretion	<1	1	1	2	4	2	2
Musculoskeletal and Connective Tissue Disorders							
Back Pain	2	0	4	3	4	0	3
Nervous System Disorders							
Somnolence*	7	15	16	15	26	8	17
Akathisia	3	6	11	12	22	7	13
Extrapyramidal Disorder**	6	6	11	12	22	13	14
Dizziness	2	6	4	4	5	6	4
Psychiatric Disorders							
Insomnia	8	8	10	11	9	7	10
Agitation	4	10	7	3	6	5	5
Anxiety	4	3	6	4	7	3	5
Restlessness	1	1	3	1	3	2	2

Note: Figures rounded to the nearest integer

* Somnolence includes adverse event terms: hypersomnia, hypersomnolence, sedation, and somnolence

** Extrapyramidal symptoms includes adverse event terms: bradykinesia, cogwheel rigidity, drooling, dystonia, extrapyramidal disorder, hypokinesia, muscle rigidity, oculogyric crisis, oromandibular dystonia, parkinsonism, psychomotor retardation, tongue spasm, torticollis, tremor, and trismus

---

Table 16: Adverse Reactions in 2% or More of LATUDA-Treated Patients and That Occurred at Greater Incidence than in the Placebo-Treated Patients in a Short-term Monotherapy Bipolar Depression Study

Percentage of Patients Reporting Reaction

Body System or Organ Class Dictionary-derived Term	Placebo (N=168) (%)	LATUDA 20-60 mg/day (N=164) (%)	LATUDA 80-120 mg/day (N=167) (%)	All LATUDA (N=331) (%)
Gastrointestinal Disorders				
Nausea	8	10	17	14
Dry Mouth	4	6	4	5
Vomiting	2	2	6	4
Diarrhea	2	5	3	4
Infections and Infestations				
Nasopharyngitis	1	4	4	4
Influenza	1	<1	2	2
Urinary Tract Infection	<1	2	2	2
Musculoskeletal and Connective Tissue Disorders				
Back Pain	<1	3	<1	2
Nervous System Disorders				
Extrapyramidal Symptoms*	2	5	9	7
Akathisia	2	8	11	9
Somnolence**	7	7	14	11
Psychiatric Disorders				
Anxiety	1	4	5	4

Note: Figures rounded to the nearest integer

*Extrapyramidal symptoms includes adverse event terms: bradykinesia, cogwheel rigidity, drooling, dystonia, extrapyramidal disorder, glabellar reflex abnormal, hypokinesia, muscle rigidity, oculogyric crisis, oromandibular dystonia, parkinsonism, psychomotor retardation, tongue spasm, torticollis, tremor, and trismus

** Somnolence includes adverse event terms: hypersomnia, hypersomnolence, sedation, and somnolence

---

Adverse Reactions Occurring at an Incidence of 2% or More in LATUDA-Treated Patients: Adverse reactions associated with the use of LATUDA (incidence of 2% or greater, rounded to the nearest percent and LATUDA incidence greater than placebo) that occurred during acute therapy (up to 6 weeks in patients with schizophrenia) are shown in Table 15.

[See table 15 above]

Dose-Related Adverse Reactions in the Schizophrenia Studies

Akathisia and extrapyramidal symptoms were dose-related. The frequency of akathisia increased with dose up to 120 mg/day (5.6% for LATUDA 20 mg, 10.7% for LATUDA 40 mg, 12.3% for LATUDA 80 mg, and 22.0% for LATUDA 120 mg). Akathisia was reported by 7.4% (9/121) of patients receiving 160 mg/day. Akathisia occurred in 3.0% of subjects receiving placebo. The frequency of extrapyramidal symp-

toms increased with dose up to 120 mg/day (5.6% for LATUDA 20 mg, 11.5% for LATUDA 40 mg, 11.9% for LATUDA 80 mg, and 22.0% for LATUDA 120 mg).

Bipolar Depression (Monotherapy)

The following findings are based on the short-term, placebo-controlled premarketing study for bipolar depression in which LATUDA was administered at daily doses ranging from 20 to 120 mg (n=331).

Commonly Observed Adverse Reactions: The most common adverse reactions (incidence ≥ 5%, in either dose group, and at least twice the rate of placebo) in patients treated with LATUDA were akathisia, extrapyramidal symptoms, somnolence, nausea, vomiting, diarrhea, and anxiety.

Adverse Reactions Associated with Discontinuation of Treatment: A total of 6.0% (20/331) LATUDA-treated patients and 5.4% (9/168) of placebo-treated patients discontinued due to adverse reactions. There were no adverse reactions

associated with discontinuation in subjects treated with LATUDA that were at least 2% and at least twice the placebo rate.

Adverse Reactions Occurring at an Incidence of 2% or More in LATUDA-Treated Patients: Adverse reactions associated with the use of LATUDA (incidence of 2% or greater, rounded to the nearest percent and LATUDA incidence greater than placebo) that occurred during acute therapy (up to 6 weeks in patients with bipolar depression) are shown in Table 16.

[See table 16 above]

Dose-Related Adverse Reactions in the Monotherapy Study: In the short-term, placebo-controlled study (involving lower and higher LATUDA dose ranges) [see Clinical Studies (14.2)] the adverse reactions that occurred with a greater than 5% incidence in the patients treated with LATUDA in any dose group and greater than placebo in both groups were nausea (10.4%, 17.4%), somnolence (7.3%, 13.8%), akathisia (7.9%, 10.8%), and extrapyramidal symptoms (4.9%, 9.0%) for LATUDA 20 to 60 mg/day and LATUDA 80 to 120 mg/day, respectively.

Bipolar Depression

Adjunctive Therapy with Lithium or Valproate

The following findings are based on two short-term, placebo-controlled premarketing studies for bipolar depression in which LATUDA was administered at daily doses ranging from 20 to 120 mg as adjunctive therapy with lithium or valproate (n=360).

Commonly Observed Adverse Reactions: The most common adverse reactions (incidence ≥ 5% and at least twice the rate of placebo) in subjects treated with LATUDA were akathisia and somnolence.

Adverse Reactions Associated with Discontinuation of Treatment: A total of 5.8% (21/360) LATUDA-treated patients and 4.8% (16/334) of placebo-treated patients discontinued due to adverse reactions. There were no adverse reactions associated with discontinuation in subjects treated with LATUDA that were at least 2% and at least twice the placebo rate.

Adverse Reactions Occurring at an Incidence of 2% or More in LATUDA-Treated Patients: Adverse reactions associated with the use of LATUDA (incidence of 2% or greater, rounded to the nearest percent and LATUDA incidence greater than placebo) that occurred during acute therapy (up to 6 weeks in patients with bipolar depression) are shown in Table 17.

[See table 17 at top of next page]

Extrapyramidal Symptoms

Schizophrenia

In the short-term, placebo-controlled schizophrenia studies, for LATUDA-treated patients, the incidence of reported events related to extrapyramidal symptoms (EPS), excluding akathisia and restlessness, was 13.5% versus 5.8% for placebo-treated patients. The incidence of akathisia for LATUDA-treated patients was 12.9% versus 3.0% for placebo-treated patients. Incidence of EPS by dose is provided in Table 18.

[See table 18 at top of next page]

Bipolar Depression

Monotherapy

In the short-term, placebo-controlled monotherapy bipolar depression study, for LATUDA-treated patients, the incidence of reported events related to EPS, excluding akathisia and restlessness was 6.9% versus 2.4% for placebo-treated patients. The incidence of akathisia for LATUDA-treated patients was 9.4% versus 2.4% for placebo-treated patients. Incidence of EPS by dose groups is provided in Table 19.

[See table 19 at top of next page]

Adjunctive Therapy with Lithium or Valproate

In the short-term, placebo-controlled adjunctive therapy bipolar depression studies, for LATUDA-treated patients, the incidence of EPS, excluding akathisia and restlessness, was 13.9% versus 8.7% for placebo. The incidence of akathisia for LATUDA-treated patients was 10.8% versus 4.8% for placebo-treated patients. Incidence of EPS is provided in Table 20.

Table 20: Incidence of EPS Compared to Placebo in the Adjunctive Therapy Bipolar Depression Studies

Adverse Event Term	Placebo (N=334) (%)	LATUDA 20 to 120 mg/day (N=360) (%)
All EPS events	13	24
All EPS events, excluding Akathisia/Restlessness	9	14
Akathisia	5	11
Dystonia*	<1	1

Parkinsonism**	8	13
Restlessness	<1	4

Note: Figures rounded to the nearest integer
* Dystonia includes adverse event terms: dystonia, oculogyric crisis, oromandibular dystonia, tongue spasm, torticollis, and trismus
** Parkinsonism includes adverse event terms: bradykinesia, cogwheel rigidity, drooling, extrapyramidal disorder, glabellar reflex abnormal, hypokinesia, muscle rigidity, parkinsonism, psychomotor retardation, and tremor

In the short-term, placebo-controlled schizophrenia and bipolar depression studies, data was objectively collected on the Simpson Angus Rating Scale (SAS) for extrapyramidal symptoms (EPS), the Barnes Akathisia Scale (BAS) for akathisia and the Abnormal Involuntary Movement Scale (AIMS) for dyskinesias.

Schizophrenia
The mean change from baseline for LATUDA-treated patients for the SAS, BAS and AIMS was comparable to placebo-treated patients, with the exception of the Barnes Akathisia Scale global score (LATUDA, 0.1; placebo, 0.0). The percentage of patients who shifted from normal to abnormal was greater in LATUDA-treated patients versus placebo for the BAS (LATUDA, 14.4%; placebo, 7.1%), the SAS (LATUDA, 5.0%; placebo, 2.3%) and the AIMS (LATUDA, 7.4%; placebo, 5.8%).

Bipolar Depression
Monotherapy
The mean change from baseline for LATUDA-treated patients for the SAS, BAS and AIMS was comparable to placebo-treated patients. The percentage of patients who shifted from normal to abnormal was greater in LATUDA-treated patients versus placebo for the BAS (LATUDA, 8.4%; placebo, 5.6%), the SAS (LATUDA, 3.7%; placebo, 1.9%) and the AIMS (LATUDA, 3.4%; placebo, 1.2%).

Adjunctive Therapy with Lithium or Valproate
The mean change from baseline for LATUDA-treated patients for the SAS, BAS and AIMS was comparable to placebo-treated patients. The percentage of patients who shifted from normal to abnormal was greater in LATUDA-treated patients versus placebo for the BAS (LATUDA, 8.7%; placebo, 2.1%), the SAS (LATUDA, 2.8%; placebo, 2.1%) and the AIMS (LATUDA, 2.8%; placebo, 0.6%).

Dystonia
Class Effect: Symptoms of dystonia, prolonged abnormal contractions of muscle groups, may occur in susceptible individuals during the first few days of treatment. Dystonic symptoms include: spasm of the neck muscles, sometimes progressing to tightness of the throat, swallowing difficulty, difficulty breathing, and/or protrusion of the tongue. While these symptoms can occur at low doses, they occur more frequently and with greater severity with high potency and at higher doses of first-generation antipsychotic drugs. An elevated risk of acute dystonia is observed in males and younger age groups.

Schizophrenia
In the short-term, placebo-controlled schizophrenia clinical studies, dystonia occurred in 4.2% of LATUDA-treated subjects (0.0% LATUDA 20 mg, 3.5% LATUDA 40 mg, 4.5% LATUDA 80 mg, 6.5% LATUDA 120 mg and 2.5% LATUDA 160 mg) compared to 0.8% of subjects receiving placebo. Seven subjects (0.5%, 7/1508) discontinued clinical trials due to dystonic events – four were receiving LATUDA 80 mg/day and three were receiving LATUDA 120 mg/day.

Bipolar Depression
Monotherapy
In the short-term, flexible-dose, placebo-controlled monotherapy bipolar depression study, dystonia occurred in 0.9% of LATUDA-treated subjects (0.0% and 1.8% for LATUDA 20 to 60 mg/day and LATUDA 80 to 120 mg/day, respectively) compared to 0.0% of subjects receiving placebo. No subject discontinued the clinical study due to dystonic events.

Adjunctive Therapy with Lithium or Valproate
In the short-term, flexible-dose, placebo-controlled adjunctive therapy bipolar depression studies, dystonia occurred in 1.1% of LATUDA-treated subjects (20 to 120 mg) compared to 0.6% of subjects receiving placebo. No subject discontinued the clinical study due to dystonic events.

Other Adverse Reactions Observed During the Premarketing Evaluation of LATUDA
Following is a list of adverse reactions reported by patients treated with LATUDA at multiple doses of ≥ 20 mg once daily within the premarketing database of 2905 patients with schizophrenia. The reactions listed are those that could be of clinical importance, as well as reactions that are plausibly drug-related on pharmacologic or other grounds. Reactions listed in Table 15 or those that appear elsewhere

Table 17: Adverse Reactions in 2% or More of LATUDA-Treated Patients and That Occurred at Greater Incidence than in the Placebo-Treated Patients in the Short-term Adjunctive Therapy Bipolar Depression Studies

Body System or Organ Class Dictionary-derived Term	Percentage of Patients Reporting Reaction	
	Placebo (N=334) (%)	LATUDA 20 to 120 mg/day (N=360) (%)
Gastrointestinal Disorders		
Nausea	10	14
Vomiting	1	4
General Disorders		
Fatigue	1	3
Infections and Infestations		
Nasopharyngitis	2	4
Investigations		
Weight Increased	<1	3
Metabolism and Nutrition Disorders		
Increased Appetite	1	3
Nervous System Disorders		
Extrapyramidal Symptoms*	9	14
Somnolence**	5	11
Akathisia	5	11
Psychiatric Disorders		
Restlessness	<1	4

Note: Figures rounded to the nearest integer
*Extrapyramidal symptoms includes adverse event terms: bradykinesia, cogwheel rigidity, drooling, dystonia, extrapyramidal disorder, glabellar reflex abnormal, hypokinesia, muscle rigidity, oculogyric crisis, oromandibular dystonia, parkinsonism, psychomotor retardation, tongue spasm, torticollis, tremor, and trismus
** Somnolence includes adverse event terms: hypersomnia, hypersomnolence, sedation, and somnolence

Table 18: Incidence of EPS Compared to Placebo in Schizophrenia Studies

Adverse Event Term	Placebo (N=708) (%)	LATUDA				
		20 mg/day (N=71) (%)	40 mg/day (N=487) (%)	80 mg/day (N=538) (%)	120 mg/day (N=291) (%)	160 mg/day (N=121) (%)
All EPS events	9	10	21	23	39	20
All EPS events, excluding Akathisia/Restlessness	6	6	11	12	22	13
Akathisia	3	6	11	12	22	7
Dystonia*	<1	0	4	5	7	2
Parkinsonism**	5	6	9	8	17	11
Restlessness	1	1	3	1	3	2

Note: Figures rounded to the nearest integer
* Dystonia includes adverse event terms: dystonia, oculogyric crisis, oromandibular dystonia, tongue spasm, torticollis, and trismus
** Parkinsonism includes adverse event terms: bradykinesia, cogwheel rigidity, drooling, extrapyramidal disorder, hypokinesia, muscle rigidity, parkinsonism, psychomotor retardation, and tremor

Table 19: Incidence of EPS Compared to Placebo in the Monotherapy Bipolar Depression Study

Adverse Event Term	Placebo (N=168) (%)	LATUDA	
		20 to 60 mg/day (N=164) (%)	80 to 120 mg/day (N=167) (%)
All EPS events	5	12	20
All EPS events, excluding Akathisia/Restlessness	2	5	9
Akathisia	2	8	11
Dystonia*	0	0	2
Parkinsonism**	2	5	8
Restlessness	<1	0	3

Note: Figures rounded to the nearest integer
* Dystonia includes adverse event terms: dystonia, oculogyric crisis, oromandibular dystonia, tongue spasm, torticollis, and trismus
** Parkinsonism includes adverse event terms: bradykinesia, cogwheel rigidity, drooling, extrapyramidal disorder, glabellar reflex abnormal, hypokinesia, muscle rigidity, parkinsonism, psychomotor retardation, and tremor

in the LATUDA label are not included. Although the reactions reported occurred during treatment with LATUDA, they were not necessarily caused by it.

Reactions are further categorized by organ class and listed in order of decreasing frequency according to the following definitions: those occurring in at least 1/100 patients (frequent) (only those not already listed in the tabulated results from placebo-controlled studies appear in this listing); those occurring in 1/100 to 1/1000 patients (infrequent); and those occurring in fewer than 1/1000 patients (rare).

Blood and Lymphatic System Disorders: **Infrequent:** *anemia*

Cardiac Disorders: **Frequent:** *tachycardia;* **Infrequent:** *AV block 1st degree, angina pectoris, bradycardia*

Ear and Labyrinth Disorders: **Infrequent:** *vertigo*

Eye Disorders: **Frequent:** *blurred vision*

Gastrointestinal Disorders: **Frequent:** *abdominal pain, diarrhea;* **Infrequent:** *gastritis*

General Disorders and Administrative Site Conditions: **Rare:** *sudden death*

Investigations: **Frequent:** *CPK increased*

Metabolism and Nutritional System Disorders: **Frequent:** *decreased appetite*

Musculoskeletal and Connective Tissue Disorders: **Rare:** *rhabdomyolysis*

Nervous System Disorders: **Infrequent:** *cerebrovascular accident, dysarthria*

Psychiatric Disorders: **Infrequent:** *abnormal dreams, panic attack, sleep disorder*

Renal and Urinary Disorders: **Infrequent:** *dysuria;* **Rare:** *renal failure*

Reproductive System and Breast Disorders: **Infrequent:** *amenorrhea, dysmenorrhea;* **Rare:** *breast enlargement, breast pain, galactorrhea, erectile dysfunction*

Skin and Subcutaneous Tissue Disorders: **Frequent:** *rash, pruritus;* **Rare:** *angioedema*

Vascular Disorders: **Frequent:** *hypertension*

Clinical Laboratory Changes

Schizophrenia

Serum Creatinine: In short-term, placebo-controlled trials, the mean change from Baseline in serum creatinine was +0.05 mg/dL for LATUDA-treated patients compared to +0.02 mg/dL for placebo-treated patients. A creatinine shift from normal to high occurred in 3.0% (43/1453) of LATUDA-treated patients and 1.6% (11/681) on placebo. The threshold for high creatinine value varied from > 0.79 to > 1.3 mg/dL based on the centralized laboratory definition for each study (Table 21).

[See table 21 above]

Bipolar Depression

Monotherapy

Serum Creatinine: In the short-term, flexible-dose, placebo-controlled monotherapy bipolar depression study, the mean change from Baseline in serum creatinine was +0.01 mg/dL for LATUDA-treated patients compared to -0.02 mg/dL for placebo-treated patients. A creatinine shift from normal to high occurred in 2.8% (9/322) of LATUDA-treated patients and 0.6% (1/162) on placebo (Table 22).

Table 22: Serum Creatinine Shifts from Normal at Baseline to High at Study End-Point in a Monotherapy Bipolar Depression Study

Laboratory Parameter	Placebo (N=168)	LATUDA 20 to 60 mg/day (N=164)	LATUDA 80 to 120 mg/day (N=167)
Serum Creatinine Elevated	<1%	2%	4%

Adjunctive Therapy with Lithium or Valproate

Serum Creatinine: In short-term, placebo-controlled pre-marketing adjunctive studies for bipolar depression, the mean change from Baseline in serum creatinine was +0.04 mg/dL for LATUDA-treated patients compared to -0.01 mg/dL for placebo-treated patients. A creatinine shift from normal to high occurred in 4.3% (15/360) of LATUDA-treated patients and 1.6% (5/334) on placebo (Table 23).

Table 23: Serum Creatinine Shifts from Normal at Baseline to High at Study End-Point in the Adjunctive Therapy Bipolar Depression Studies

Laboratory Parameter	Placebo (N=334)	LATUDA 20 to 120 mg/day (N=360)
Serum Creatinine Elevated	2%	4%

7 DRUG INTERACTIONS
7.1 Potential for Other Drugs to Affect LATUDA

LATUDA is predominantly metabolized by CYP3A4. LATUDA should not be used concomitantly with strong CYP3A4 inhibitors (e.g., ketoconazole, clarithromycin, ritonavir, voriconazole, mibefradil, etc.) or strong CYP3A4 inducers (e.g., rifampin, avasimibe, St. John's wort, phenytoin, carbamazepine, etc.) *[see Contraindications (4)].* The LATUDA dose should be reduced to half of the original level when used concomitantly with moderate inhibitors of

Table 21: Serum Creatinine Shifts from Normal at Baseline to High at Study End-Point in Schizophrenia Studies

Laboratory Parameter	Placebo (N=708)	LATUDA 20 mg/day (N=71)	LATUDA 40 mg/day (N=487)	LATUDA 80 mg/day (N=538)	LATUDA 120 mg/day (N=291)	LATUDA 160 mg/day (N=121)
Serum Creatinine Elevated	2%	1%	2%	2%	5%	7%

Figure 1: Impact of Other Drugs on LATUDA Pharmacokinetics

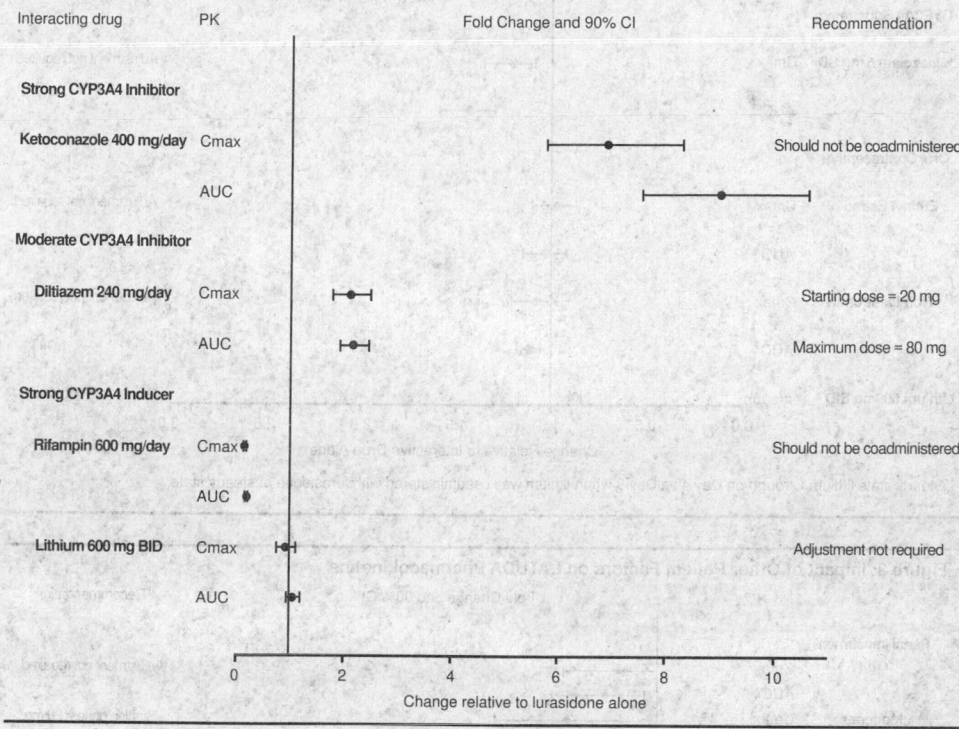

CYP3A4 (e.g., diltiazem, atazanavir, erythromycin, fluconazole, verapamil, etc.). If LATUDA is used concomitantly with a moderate CYP3A4 inducer, it may be necessary to increase the LATUDA dose *[see Dosage and Administration (2.5)].*

Lithium: It is not necessary to adjust the LATUDA dose when used concomitantly with lithium (Figure 1).

Valproate: It is not necessary to adjust the LATUDA dose when used concomitantly with valproate. A dedicated drug-drug interaction study has not been conducted with valproate and LATUDA. Based on pharmacokinetic data from the bipolar depression studies valproate levels were not affected by lurasidone, and lurasidone concentrations were not affected by valproate.

Grapefruit: Grapefruit and grapefruit juice should be avoided in patients taking LATUDA, since these may inhibit CYP3A4 and alter LATUDA concentrations *[see Dosage and Administration (2.5)].*

[See figure 1 above]

7.2 Potential for LATUDA to Affect Other Drugs

No dose adjustment is needed for lithium, substrates of P-gp, CYP3A4 (Figure 2) or valproate when coadministered with LATUDA.).

[See figure 2 at top of next page]

8 USE IN SPECIFIC POPULATIONS
8.1 Pregnancy
Pregnancy Category B
Risk Summary

There are no adequate and well controlled studies of LATUDA use in pregnant women. Neonates exposed to antipsychotic drugs during the third trimester of pregnancy are at risk for extrapyramidal and/or withdrawal symptoms following delivery. There have been reports of agitation, hypertonia, hypotonia, tremor, somnolence, respiratory distress and feeding disorder in these neonates. These complications have varied in severity; while in some cases symptoms have been self-limited, in other cases neonates have required intensive care unit support and prolonged hospitalization.

LATUDA should be used during pregnancy only if the potential benefit justifies the potential risk to the fetus.

Human Data

Safe use of LATUDA during pregnancy or lactation has not been established; therefore, use of LATUDA in pregnancy,

in nursing mothers, or in women of childbearing potential requires that the benefits of treatment be weighed against the possible risks to mother and child.

Animal Data

No adverse developmental effects were observed in a study in which pregnant rats were given lurasidone during the period of organogenesis and continuing through weaning at doses up to 10 mg/kg/day, which is approximately half of the maximum recommended human dose (MRHD) of 160 mg/day, based on mg/m² body surface area.

No teratogenic effects were seen in studies in which pregnant rats and rabbits were given lurasidone during the period of organogenesis at doses up to 25 and 50 mg/kg/day, respectively. These doses are 1.5- and 6-times, in rats and rabbits, respectively, the MRHD of 160 mg/day based on mg/m² body surface area.

8.3 Nursing Mothers

LATUDA was excreted in milk of rats during lactation. It is not known whether LATUDA or its metabolites are excreted in human milk. Because of the potential for serious adverse reactions in nursing infants, a decision should be made whether to discontinue nursing or to discontinue the drug, considering the risk of drug discontinuation to the mother.

8.4 Pediatric Use

Safety and effectiveness in pediatric patients have not been established.

8.5 Geriatric Use

Clinical studies with LATUDA did not include sufficient numbers of patients aged 65 and older to determine whether or not they respond differently from younger patients. In elderly patients with psychosis (65 to 85), LATUDA concentrations (20 mg/day) were similar to those in young subjects. It is unknown whether dose adjustment is necessary on the basis of age alone.

Elderly patients with dementia-related psychosis treated with LATUDA are at an increased risk of death compared to placebo. LATUDA is not approved for the treatment of patients with dementia-related psychosis *[see Boxed Warning].*

8.6 Other Patient Factors

The effect of intrinsic patient factors on the pharmacokinetics of LATUDA is presented in Figure 3.

[See figure 3 at top of next page]

Figure 2: Impact of LATUDA on Other Drugs

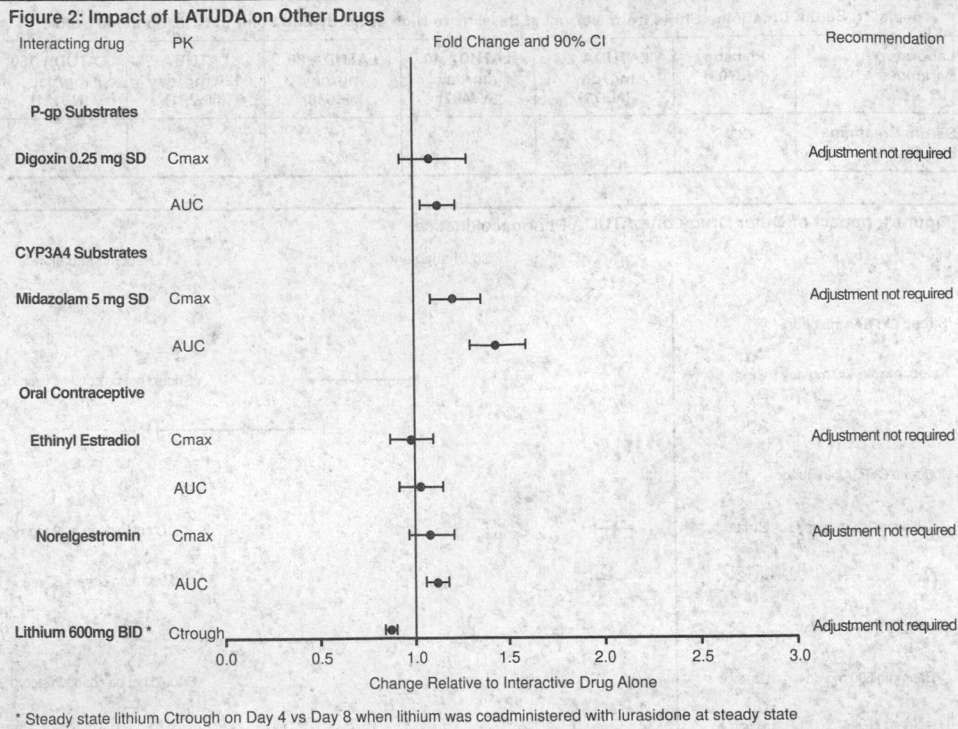

* Steady state lithium Ctrough on Day 4 vs Day 8 when lithium was coadministered with lurasidone at steady state

Figure 3: Impact of Other Patient Factors on LATUDA Pharmacokinetics

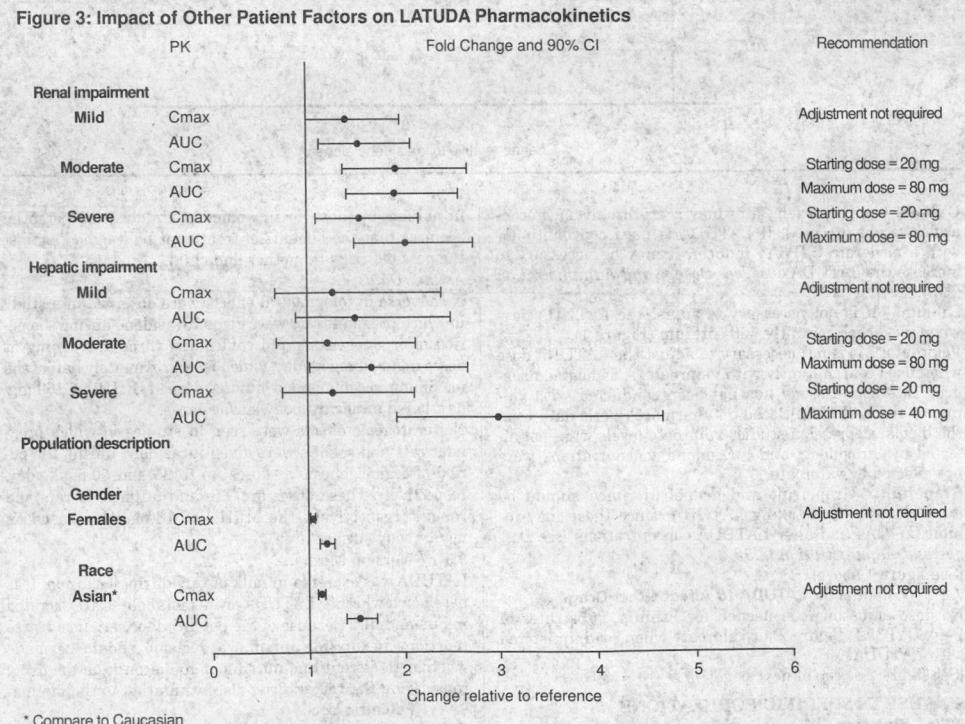

* Compare to Caucasian

9   DRUG ABUSE AND DEPENDENCE

9.1   Controlled Substance

LATUDA is not a controlled substance.

9.2   Abuse

LATUDA has not been systematically studied in humans for its potential for abuse or physical dependence or its ability to induce tolerance. While clinical studies with LATUDA did not reveal any tendency for drug-seeking behavior, these observations were not systematic and it is not possible to predict the extent to which a CNS-active drug will be misused, diverted and/or abused once it is marketed. Patients should be evaluated carefully for a history of drug abuse, and such patients should be observed carefully for signs of LATUDA misuse or abuse (e.g., development of tolerance, drug-seeking behavior, increases in dose).

10   OVERDOSAGE

10.1   Human Experience

In premarketing clinical studies, accidental or intentional overdosage of LATUDA was identified in one patient who ingested an estimated 560 mg of LATUDA. This patient recovered without sequelae. This patient resumed LATUDA treatment for an additional two months.

10.2   Management of Overdosage

Consult a Certified Poison Control Center for up-to-date guidance and advice. There is no specific antidote to LATUDA, therefore, appropriate supportive measures should be instituted and close medical supervision and monitoring should continue until the patient recovers. Consider the possibility of multiple-drug overdose.

Cardiovascular monitoring should commence immediately, including continuous electrocardiographic monitoring for possible arrhythmias. If antiarrhythmic therapy is administered, disopyramide, procainamide, and quinidine carry a theoretical hazard of additive QT-prolonging effects when administered in patients with an acute overdose of LATUDA. Similarly, the alpha-blocking properties of bretylium might be additive to those of LATUDA, resulting in problematic hypotension.

Hypotension and circulatory collapse should be treated with appropriate measures. Epinephrine and dopamine should not be used, or other sympathomimetics with beta-agonist activity, since beta stimulation may worsen hypotension in the setting of LATUDA-induced alpha blockade. In case of severe extrapyramidal symptoms, anticholinergic medication should be administered.

Gastric lavage (after intubation if patient is unconscious) and administration of activated charcoal together with a laxative should be considered.

The possibility of obtundation, seizures, or dystonic reaction of the head and neck following overdose may create a risk of aspiration with induced emesis.

11   DESCRIPTION

LATUDA is an atypical antipsychotic belonging to the chemical class of benzisothiazol derivatives.

Its chemical name is $(3aR,4S,7R,7aS)$-2-[(1R,2R)-2-[4-(1,2-benzisothiazol-3-yl)piperazin-1-ylmethyl] cyclohexylmethyl]hexahydro-4,7-methano-2H-isoindole-1,3-dione hydrochloride. Its molecular formula is $C_{28}H_{36}N_4O_2S \cdot HCl$ and its molecular weight is 529.14.

The chemical structure is:

Lurasidone hydrochloride is a white to off-white powder. It is very slightly soluble in water, practically insoluble or insoluble in 0.1 N HCl, slightly soluble in ethanol, sparingly soluble in methanol, practically insoluble or insoluble in toluene and very slightly soluble in acetone.

LATUDA tablets are intended for oral administration only. Each tablet contains 20 mg, 40 mg, 60 mg, 80 mg, or 120 mg of lurasidone hydrochloride.

Inactive ingredients are mannitol, pregelatinized starch, croscarmellose sodium, hypromellose, magnesium stearate, Opadry® and carnauba wax. Additionally, the 80 mg tablet contains yellow ferric oxide and FD&C Blue No. 2 Aluminum Lake.

12   CLINICAL PHARMACOLOGY

12.1   Mechanism of Action

The mechanism of action of LATUDA in the treatment of schizophrenia and bipolar depression is unknown. However, its efficacy in schizophrenia and bipolar depression could be mediated through a combination of central dopamine Type 2 (D_2) and serotonin Type 2 ($5HT_{2A}$) receptor antagonism.

12.2   Pharmacodynamics

LATUDA is an antagonist with high affinity binding at the dopamine D_2 receptors (Ki=1 nM) and the 5-hydroxytryptamine (5-HT, serotonin) receptors 5-HT$_{2A}$ (Ki=0.5 nM) and 5-HT$_7$ (Ki=0.5 nM) receptors. It also binds with moderate affinity to the human α_{2C} adrenergic receptors (Ki=11 nM), is a partial agonist at serotonin 5-HT$_{1A}$ (Ki=6.4 nM) receptors, and is an antagonist at the α_{2A} adrenergic receptors (Ki=41 nM). LATUDA exhibits little or no affinity for histamine H$_1$ and muscarinic M$_1$ receptors (IC$_{50}$ > 1,000 nM).

ECG Changes

The effects of LATUDA on the QTc interval were evaluated in a randomized, double-blind, multiple-dose, parallel-dedicated thorough QT study in 43 patients with schizophrenia or schizoaffective disorder, who were treated with LATUDA doses of 120 mg daily, 600 mg daily and completed the study. The maximum mean (upper 1-sided, 95% CI) increase in baseline-adjusted QTc intervals based on individual correction method (QTcI) was 7.5 (11.7) ms and 4.6 (9.5) ms, for the 120 mg and 600 mg dose groups respectively, observed at 2 to 4 hours after dosing. In this study, there was no apparent dose (exposure)-response relationship.

In short-term, placebo-controlled studies in schizophrenia and bipolar depression, no post-baseline QT prolongations exceeding 500 msec were reported in patients treated with LATUDA or placebo.

12.3   Pharmacokinetics

The activity of LATUDA is primarily due to the parent drug. The pharmacokinetics of LATUDA is dose-proportional within a total daily dose range of 20 mg to 160 mg. Steady-state concentrations of LATUDA are reached within 7 days of starting LATUDA.

Following administration of 40 mg of LATUDA, the mean (%CV) elimination half-life was 18 (7) hours.

Absorption and Distribution: LATUDA is absorbed and reaches peak serum concentrations in approximately 1-3 hours. It is estimated that 9-19% of an administered dose is absorbed. Following administration of 40 mg of LATUDA, the mean (%CV) apparent volume of distribution was 6173 (17.2) L. LATUDA is highly bound (~99%) to serum proteins.

In a food effect study, LATUDA mean C_{max} and AUC were about 3-times and 2-times, respectively, when administered with food compared to the levels observed under fasting conditions. LATUDA exposure was not affected as meal size was increased from 350 to 1000 calories and was independent of meal fat content [see *Dosage and Administration (2.3)*].

In clinical studies, establishing the safety and efficacy of LATUDA, patients were instructed to take their daily dose with food [see *Dosage and Administration (2.3)*].

Metabolism and Elimination: LATUDA is metabolized mainly via CYP3A4. The major biotransformation pathways are oxidative *N*-dealkylation, hydroxylation of norbornane ring, and *S*-oxidation. LATUDA is metabolized into two active metabolites (ID-14283 and ID-14326) and two major non-active metabolites (ID-20219 and ID-20220). Based on *in vitro* studies, LATUDA is not a substrate of CYP1A1, CYP1A2, CYP2A6, CYP4A11, CYP2B6, CYP2C8, CYP2C9, CYP2C19, CYP2D6 or CYP2E1 enzymes. Because LATUDA is not a substrate for CYP1A2, smoking is not expected to have an effect on the pharmacokinetics of LATUDA.

Total excretion of radioactivity in urine and feces combined was approximately 89%, with about 80% recovered in feces and 9% recovered in urine, after a single dose of [^{14}C]-labeled LATUDA.

Following administration of 40 mg of LATUDA, the mean (%CV) apparent clearance was 3902 (18.0) mL/min.

13   NONCLINICAL TOXICOLOGY

13.1   Carcinogenesis, Mutagenesis, Impairment of Fertility

Carcinogenesis: LATUDA increased incidences of malignant mammary gland tumors and pituitary gland adenomas in female mice orally dosed with 30, 100, 300, or 650 mg/kg/day. The lowest dose produced plasma levels (AUC) approximately equal to those in humans receiving the MRHD of 160 mg/day. No increases in tumors were seen in male mice up to the highest dose tested, which produced plasma levels (AUC) 14-times those in humans receiving the MRHD.

LATUDA increased the incidence of mammary gland carcinomas in females rats orally dosed at 12 and 36 mg/kg/day; the lowest dose; 3 mg/kg/day is the no-effect dose which produced plasma levels (AUC) 0.4-times those in humans receiving the MRHD. No increases in tumors were seen in male rats up to the highest dose tested, which produced plasma levels (AUC) 6-times those in humans receiving the MRHD.

Proliferative and/or neoplastic changes in the mammary and pituitary glands of rodents have been observed following chronic administration of antipsychotic drugs and are considered to be prolactin-mediated. The relevance of this increased incidence of prolactin-mediated pituitary or mammary gland tumors in rodents to humans is unknown [see *Warnings and Precautions (5.7)*].

Mutagenesis: LATUDA did not cause mutation or chromosomal aberration when tested *in vitro* and *in vivo*. LATUDA was negative in the Ames gene mutation test, the Chinese Hamster Lung (CHL) cells, and in the *in vivo* mouse bone marrow micronucleus test up to 2000 mg/kg (61 times the MRHD of 160 mg/day based on mg/m^2 body surface area).

Impairment of Fertility: Estrus cycle irregularities were seen in rats orally administered LATUDA at 1.5, 15 and 150 mg/kg/day for 15 consecutive days prior to mating, during the mating period, and through day 7 of gestation. The no-effect dose is 0.1 mg/kg which is approximately 0.006-times the MRHD of 160 mg/day based on body surface area. Fertility was reduced only at the highest dose, which was reversible after a 14-day drug-free period. The no-effect dose for reduced fertility was 15 mg/kg, which is approximately equal to the MRHD based on body surface area.

LATUDA had no effect on fertility in male rats treated orally with LATUDA for 64 consecutive days prior to mating and during the mating period at doses up to 150 mg/kg/day (9-times the MRHD based on mg/m^2 body surface area).

14   CLINICAL STUDIES

14.1   Schizophrenia

The efficacy of LATUDA for the treatment of schizophrenia was established in five short-term (6-week), placebo-controlled studies in adult patients (mean age of 38.4 years, range 18-72) who met DSM-IV criteria for schizophrenia.

Table 24: Primary Efficacy Results for Studies in Schizophrenia (BPRSd or PANSS Scores)

| Study | Treatment Group | Primary Efficacy Measure: BPRSd | | |
		Mean Baseline Score (SD)	LS Mean Change from Baseline (SE)	Placebo-subtracted Difference[a] (95% CI)
1	LATUDA (40 mg/day)*	54.2 (8.8)	-9.4 (1.6)	-5.6 (-9.8, -1.4)
	LATUDA (120 mg/day)*	52.7 (7.6)	-11.0 (1.6)	-6.7 (-11.0, -2.5)
	Placebo	54.7 (8.1)	-3.8 (1.6)	--
2	LATUDA (80 mg/day)*	55.1 (6.0)	-8.9 (1.3)	-4.7 (-8.3, -1.1)
	Placebo	56.1 (6.8)	-4.2 (1.4)	--

| Study | Treatment Group | Primary Efficacy Measure: PANSS | | |
		Mean Baseline Score (SD)	LS Mean Change from Baseline (SE)	Placebo-subtracted Difference[a] (95% CI)
3	LATUDA (40 mg/day)*	96.6 (10.7)	-25.7 (2.0)	-9.7 (-15.3, -4.1)
	LATUDA (120 mg/day)*	97.9 (11.3)	-23.6 (2.1)	-7.5 (-13.4, -1.7)
	Olanzapine (15 mg/day)*[b]	96.3 (12.2)	-28.7 (1.9)	-12.6 (-18.2, -7.9)
	Placebo	95.8 (10.8)	-16.0 (2.1)	--
4	LATUDA (40 mg/day)	96.5 (11.5)	-19.2 (1.7)	-2.1 (-7.0, 2.8)
	LATUDA (80 mg/day)	96.0 (10.8)	-23.4 (1.8)	-6.4 (-11.3, -1.5)
	LATUDA (120 mg/day)	96.0 (9.7)	-20.5 (1.8)	-3.5 (-8.4, 1.4)
	Placebo	96.8 (11.1)	-17.0 (1.8)	--
5	LATUDA (80 mg/day)*	97.7 (9.7)	-22.2 (1.8)	-11.9 (-16.9, -6.9)
	LATUDA (160 mg/day)*	97.5 (11.8)	-26.5 (1.8)	-16.2 (-21.2, -11.2)
	Quetiapine Extended-release (600 mg/day)*[b]	97.7 (10.2)	-27.8 (1.8)	-17.5 (-22.5, -12.4)
	Placebo	96.6 (10.2)	-10.3 (1.8)	--

SD: standard deviation; SE: standard error; LS Mean: least-squares mean; CI: confidence interval, unadjusted for multiple comparisons.
[a] Difference (drug minus placebo) in least-squares mean change from baseline.
[b] Included for assay sensitivity.
* Doses statistically significantly superior to placebo.

An active-control arm (olanzapine or quetiapine extended-release) was included in two studies to assess assay sensitivity.

Several instruments were used for assessing psychiatric signs and symptoms in these studies:
1. Positive and Negative Syndrome Scale (PANSS), is a multi-item inventory of general psychopathology used to evaluate the effects of drug treatment in schizophrenia. PANSS total scores may range from 30 to 210.
2. Brief Psychiatric Rating Scale derived (BPRSd), derived from the PANSS, is a multi-item inventory primarily focusing on positive symptoms of schizophrenia, whereas the PANSS includes a wider range of positive, negative and other symptoms of schizophrenia. The BPRSd consists of 18 items rated on a scale of 1 (not present) to 7 (severe). BPRSd scores may range from 18 to 126.
3. The Clinical Global Impression severity scale (CGI-S) is a clinician-rated scale that measures the subject's current illness state on a 1- to 7-point scale.

The endpoint associated with each instrument is change from baseline in the total score to the end of week 6. These changes are then compared to placebo changes for the drug and control groups.

The results of the studies follow:
1. Study 1: In a 6-week, placebo-controlled trial (N=145) involving two fixed doses of LATUDA (40 or 120 mg/day), both doses of LATUDA at Endpoint were superior to placebo on the BPRSd total score, and the CGI-S.
2. Study 2: In a 6-week, placebo-controlled trial (N=180) involving a fixed dose of LATUDA (80 mg/day), LATUDA at Endpoint was superior to placebo on the BPRSd total score, and the CGI-S.
3. Study 3: In a 6-week, placebo- and active-controlled trial (N=473) involving two fixed doses of LATUDA (40 or 120 mg/day) and an active control (olanzapine), both LATUDA doses and the active control at Endpoint were superior to placebo on the PANSS total score, and the CGI-S.
4. Study 4: In a 6-week, placebo-controlled trial (N=489) involving three fixed doses of LATUDA (40, 80 or 120 mg/day), only the 80 mg/day dose of LATUDA at Endpoint was superior to placebo on the PANSS total score, and the CGI-S.
5. Study 5: In a 6-week, placebo- and active-controlled trial (N=482) involving two fixed doses of LATUDA (80 or 160 mg/day) and an active control (quetiapine extended-release), both LATUDA doses and the active control at Endpoint were superior to placebo on the PANSS total score, and the CGI-S.

Thus, the efficacy of LATUDA at doses of 40, 80, 120 and 160 mg/day has been established (Table 24).
[See table 24 above]

Examination of population subgroups based on age (there were few patients over 65), gender and race did not reveal any clear evidence of differential responsiveness.

14.2   Depressive Episodes Associated with Bipolar I Disorder

Monotherapy

The efficacy of LATUDA, as monotherapy, was established in a 6-week, multicenter, randomized, double-blind, placebo-controlled study of adult patients (mean age of 41.5 years, range 18 to 74) who met DSM-IV-TR criteria for major depressive episodes associated with bipolar I disorder, with or without rapid cycling, and without psychotic features (N=485). Patients were randomized to one of two flexible-dose ranges of LATUDA (20 to 60 mg/day, or 80 to 120 mg/day) or placebo.

The primary rating instrument used to assess depressive symptoms in this study was the Montgomery-Asberg Depression Rating Scale (MADRS), a 10-item clinician-rated scale with total scores ranging from 0 (no depressive features) to 60 (maximum score). The primary endpoint was the change from baseline in MADRS score at Week 6. The key secondary instrument was the Clinical Global Impression-Bipolar-Severity of Illness scale (CGI-BP-S), a clinician-rated scale that measures the subject's current illness state on a 7-point scale, where a higher score is associated with greater illness severity.

For both dose groups, LATUDA was superior to placebo in reduction of MADRS and CGI-BP-S scores at Week 6. The primary efficacy results are provided in Table 25. The high dose range (80 to 120 mg per day) did not provide additional efficacy on average, compared to the low dose range (20 to 60 mg per day).

Adjunctive Therapy with Lithium or Valproate

The efficacy of LATUDA, as an adjunctive therapy with lithium or valproate, was established in a 6-week, multicenter, randomized, double-blind, placebo-controlled study of adult patients (mean age of 41.7 years, range 18 to 72) who met DSM-IV-TR criteria for major depressive episodes associated with bipolar I disorder, with or without rapid cycling, and without psychotic features (N=340). Patients who remained symptomatic after treatment with lithium or valproate were randomized to flexibly dosed LATUDA 20 to 120 mg/day or placebo.

The primary rating instrument used to assess depressive symptoms in this study was the MADRS. The primary endpoint was the change from baseline in MADRS score at Week 6. The key secondary instrument was the CGI-BP-S scale.

LATUDA was superior to placebo in reduction of MADRS and CGI-BP-S scores at Week 6, as an adjunctive therapy with lithium or valproate (Table 25).

[See table 25 at top of next page]

Table 25: Primary Efficacy Results for Studies in Depressive Episodes Associated with Bipolar I Disorder (MADRS Scores)

Study	Treatment Group	Primary Efficacy Measure: MADRS		
		Mean Baseline Score (SD)	LS Mean Change from Baseline (SE)	Placebo-subtracted Difference[a] (95% CI)
Monotherapy study	LATUDA (20-60 mg/day)*	30.3 (5.0)	-15.4 (0.8)	-4.6 (-6.9, -2.3)
	LATUDA (80-120 mg/day)*	30.6 (4.9)	-15.4 (0.8)	-4.6 (-6.9, -2.3)
	Placebo	30.5 (5.0)	-10.7 (0.8)	--
Adjunctive Therapy study	LATUDA (20-120 mg/day)* + lithium or valproate	30.6 (5.3)	-17.1 (0.9)	-3.6 (-6.0, -1.1)
	Placebo + lithium or valproate	30.8 (4.8)	-13.5 (0.9)	--

SD: standard deviation; SE: standard error; LS Mean: least-squares mean; CI: confidence interval, unadjusted for multiple comparisons.
[a] Difference (drug minus placebo) in least-squares mean change from baseline. * Treatment group statistically significantly superior to placebo.

16   HOW SUPPLIED/STORAGE AND HANDLING

LATUDA tablets are white to off-white, round (20 mg or 40 mg), white to off-white, oblong (60 mg), pale green, oval (80 mg) or white to off-white, oval (120 mg) and identified with strength-specific one-sided debossing, "L20" (20 mg), "L40" (40 mg), "L80" (80 mg) or "L120" (120 mg). Tablets are supplied in the following strengths and package configurations (Table 26):

Table 26: Package Configuration for LATUDA Tablets

Tablet Strength	Package Configuration	NDC Code
20 mg	Bottles of 30	63402-302-30
	Bottles of 90	63402-302-90
	Bottles of 500	63402-302-50
	Box of 100 (Hospital Unit Dose) 10 blister cards, 10 tablets each	63402-302-10 Carton 63402-302-01 Blister
40 mg	Bottles of 30	63402-304-30
	Bottles of 90	63402-304-90
	Bottles of 500	63402-304-50
	Box of 100 (Hospital Unit Dose) 10 blister cards, 10 tablets each	63402-304-10 Carton 63402-304-01 Blister
60 mg	Bottles of 30	63402-306-30
	Bottles of 90	63402-306-90
	Bottles of 500	63402-306-50
	Box of 100 (Hospital Unit Dose) 10 blister cards, 10 tablets each	63402-306-10 Carton 63402-306-01 Blister
80 mg	Bottles of 30	63402-308-30
	Bottles of 90	63402-308-90
	Bottles of 500	63402-308-50
	Box of 100 (Hospital Unit Dose) 10 blister cards, 10 tablets each	63402-308-10 Carton 63402-308-01 Blister
120 mg	Bottles of 30	63402-312-30
	Bottles of 90	63402-312-90
	Bottles of 500	63402-312-50
	Box of 100 (Hospital Unit Dose) 10 blister cards, 10 tablets each	63402-312-10 Carton 63402-312-01 Blister

Storage
Store LATUDA tablets at 25°C (77°F); excursions permitted to 15° - 30°C (59° - 86°F) [See USP Controlled Room Temperature].

17   PATIENT COUNSELING INFORMATION

Physicians are advised to discuss with patients for whom they prescribe LATUDA all relevant safety information including, but not limited to, the following:

17.1   Increased Mortality in Elderly Patients with Dementia-Related Psychosis

Advise patients and caregivers that elderly patients with dementia-related psychoses treated with atypical antipsychotic drugs are at increased risk of death compared with placebo. LATUDA is not approved for elderly patients with dementia-related psychosis [see Boxed Warning; Warnings and Precautions (5.1)].

17.2   Suicidal Thoughts and Behaviors; and Activation of Mania or Hypomania

Educate patients, families, and caregivers about the risk of suicidal thoughts and behaviors with antidepressant treatment, as well as the risk of mania and hypomania. Advise them about monitoring for the emergence of suicidal thoughts and behavior, manic/hypomanic symptoms, irritability, agitation, or unusual changes in behavior. Instruct patients, families, and caregivers to report such symptoms to the healthcare provider [see Warnings and Precautions (5.2 and 5.14)].

17.3   Neuroleptic Malignant Syndrome

Advise patients and caregivers that a potentially fatal symptom complex sometimes referred to as NMS has been reported in association with administration of antipsychotic drugs. Signs and symptoms of NMS include hyperpyrexia, muscle rigidity, altered mental status, and evidence of autonomic instability (irregular pulse or blood pressure, tachycardia, diaphoresis, and cardiac dysrhythmia) [see Warnings and Precautions (5.4)].

17.4   Metabolic Changes (Hyperglycemia and Diabetes Mellitus, Dyslipidemia, and Weight Gain)

Educate patients and caregivers about the risk of metabolic changes and the need for specific monitoring. The risks include hyperglycemia and diabetes mellitus, dyslipidemia, weight gain, and cardiovascular reactions. Educate patients and caregivers about the symptoms of hyperglycemia (high blood sugar) and diabetes mellitus (e.g., polydipsia, polyuria, polyphagia, and weakness). Monitor all patients for these symptoms. Patients who are diagnosed with diabetes or have risk factors for diabetes (obesity, family history of diabetes) should have their fasting blood glucose monitored before beginning treatment and periodically during treatment. Patients who develop symptoms of hyperglycemia should have assessments of fasting glucose. Clinical monitoring of weight is recommended [see Warnings and Precautions (5.6)].

17.5   Orthostatic Hypotension

Educate patients about the risk of orthostatic hypotension, particularly at the time of initiating treatment, re-initiating treatment, or increasing the dose [see Warnings and Precautions (5.9)].

17.6   Leukopenia/Neutropenia

Advise patients with a pre-existing low WBC or a history of drug-induced leukopenia/neutropenia that they should have their CBC monitored while taking LATUDA [see Warnings and Precautions (5.8)].

17.7   Interference with Cognitive and Motor Performance

Caution patients about performing activities requiring mental alertness, such as operating hazardous machinery or operating a motor vehicle, until they are reasonably certain that LATUDA therapy does not affect them adversely [see Warnings and Precautions (5.11)].

17.8   Pregnancy and Nursing

Instruct patients to notify their physician if they become pregnant or intend to become pregnant during therapy with LATUDA [see Use in Specific Populations (8.1)].

17.9   Concomitant Medication and Alcohol

Instruct patients to inform their physicians if they are taking, or plan to take, any prescription or over-the-counter drugs, because there is a potential for drug interactions. Advise patients to avoid alcohol while taking LATUDA [see Drug Interactions (7)].

17.10   Heat Exposure and Dehydration

Educate patients regarding appropriate care in avoiding overheating and dehydration [see Warnings and Precautions (5.12)].

SUNOVION
Manufactured for:
Sunovion Pharmaceuticals Inc.
Marlborough, MA 01752 USA
For Customer Service, call 1-888-394-7377.
For Medical Information, call 1-800-739-0565.
To report suspected adverse reactions, call 1-877-737-7226.
Revised: Month Year
901456RXX
LATUDA is a registered trademark of Dainippon Sumitomo Pharma Co. Ltd.,
Sunovion Pharmaceuticals Inc. is a U.S. subsidiary of Dainippon Sumitomo Pharma Co. Ltd.,
© 20XX Sunovion Pharmaceuticals Inc.

Medication Guide
LATUDA (luh-TOO-duh)
(lurasidone hydrochloride)
Tablets

What is the most important information I should know about LATUDA?

LATUDA may cause serious side effects, including:

1. **Increased risk of death in elderly people who are confused, have memory loss and have lost touch with reality (dementia-related psychosis).** Medicines like LATUDA can increase the risk of death in elderly people who are confused, have memory loss and have lost touch with reality (dementia-related psychosis). LATUDA should not be used to treat people with dementia-related psychosis.

2. **Increased risk of suicidal thoughts or actions (antidepressant medicines, depression and other serious mental illnesses, and suicidal thoughts or actions).**
   - **Talk to your, or your family member's, healthcare provider about:**
     ○ all risks and benefits of treatment with antidepressant medicines.
     ○ all treatment choices for depression or other serious mental illness.
   - **Antidepressant medicines may increase suicidal thoughts or actions in some children, teenagers, and young adults within the first few months of treatment.**
   - **Depression and other serious mental illnesses are the most important causes of suicidal thoughts and actions. Some people may have a particularly high risk of having suicidal thoughts or actions.** These include people who have (or have a family history of) depression, bipolar illness (also called manic-depressive illness), or a history of suicidal thoughts or actions.
   - **How can I watch for and try to prevent suicidal thoughts and actions in myself or a family member?**
     ○ Pay close attention to any changes, especially sudden changes, in mood, behaviors, thoughts, or feelings. This is very important when an antidepressant medicine is started or when the dose is changed.
     ○ Call the healthcare provider right away to report new or sudden changes in mood, behavior, thoughts, or feelings.
     ○ Keep all follow-up visits with the healthcare provider as scheduled. Call the healthcare provider between visits as needed, especially if you have concerns about symptoms.

Call a healthcare provider right away if you or your family member has any of the following symptoms, especially if they are new, worse, or worry you:
- thoughts about suicide or dying
- attempts to commit suicide
- new or worse depression
- new or worse anxiety
- feeling very agitated or restless
- panic attacks
- trouble sleeping (insomnia)
- new or worse irritability
- acting aggressive, being angry, or violent
- acting on dangerous impulses
- an extreme increase in activity and talking (mania)
- other unusual changes in behavior or mood

What else do I need to know about antidepressant medicines?
- **Never stop an antidepressant medicine without first talking to your healthcare provider.** Stopping an antidepressant medicine suddenly can cause other symptoms.
- **Antidepressants are medicines used to treat depression and other illnesses.** It is important to discuss all the risks of treating depression and also the risks of not treating it. Patients and their families or other caregivers should discuss all treatment choices with the healthcare provider, not just the use of antidepressants.

- **Antidepressant medicines have other side effects.** Talk to the healthcare provider about the side effects of the medicine prescribed for you or your family member.
- **Antidepressant medicines can interact with other medicines.** Know all of the medicines that you or your family member takes. Keep a list of all medicines to show the healthcare provider. Do not start new medicines without first checking with your healthcare provider.
- **Not all antidepressant medicines prescribed for children are FDA approved for use in children.** Talk to your child's healthcare provider for more information.

What is LATUDA?
LATUDA is a prescription medicine used to treat adults with:
- schizophrenia
- depressive episodes associated with bipolar I disorder, alone or with lithium or valproate

It is not known if LATUDA is safe and effective in children.

Who should not take LATUDA?
Do not take LATUDA if you:
- are allergic to lurasidone hydrochloride or any of the ingredients in LATUDA. See the end of this Medication Guide for a complete list of ingredients in LATUDA.
- are taking certain other medicines called CYP3A4 inhibitors or inducers including ketoconazole, clarithromycin, ritonavir, voriconazole, mibefradil, rifampin, avasimibe, St. John's wort, phenytoin, or carbamazepine. Ask your healthcare provider if you are not sure if you are taking any of these medicines.

What should I tell my healthcare provider before taking LATUDA?
Before you take LATUDA, tell your healthcare provider if you:
- have or have had diabetes or high blood sugar in you or your family. Your healthcare provider should check your blood sugar before you start LATUDA and also during therapy.
- have or have had high levels of total cholesterol, triglycerides or LDL-cholesterol or low levels of HDL-cholesterol
- have or have had low or high blood pressure
- have or have had low white blood cell count
- have or have had seizures
- have or have had abnormal thyroid tests
- have or have had high prolactin levels
- have or have had heart problems
- have or have had liver problems
- have or have had any other medical conditions
- are pregnant or plan to become pregnant. It is not known if LATUDA will harm your unborn baby.
- are breastfeeding or plan to breastfeed. It is not known if LATUDA passes into your breast milk. You and your healthcare provider should decide if you will take LATUDA or breastfeed. You should not do both.

Tell the healthcare provider about all the medicines that you take or recently have taken including prescription medicines, over-the-counter medicines, herbal supplements and vitamins.

LATUDA and other medicines may affect each other causing serious side effects. LATUDA may affect the way other medicines work, and other medicines may affect how LATUDA works.

Especially tell your healthcare provider if you take or plan to take medicines for:
- depression
- high blood pressure
- Parkinson's disease
- trouble sleeping
- abnormal heart beats or rhythm
- epilepsy
- inflammation
- psychosis

Know the medicines you take. Keep a list of your medicines to show your healthcare provider and pharmacist when you get a new medicine.

How should I take LATUDA?
- Take LATUDA exactly as your healthcare provider tells you to take it. Do not change the dose yourself.
- Take LATUDA by mouth, with food (at least 350 calories).
- If you take too much LATUDA, call your healthcare provider or poison control center at 1-800-222-1222 right away, or go to the nearest hospital emergency room.

What should I avoid while taking LATUDA?
- Avoid eating grapefruit or drinking grapefruit juice while you take LATUDAsince these can affect the amount of LATUDA in the blood. Do not drive, operate machinery, or do other dangerous activities until you know how LATUDA affects you. LATUDA may make you drowsy.
- Avoid getting overheated or dehydrated.
- Do not over-exercise.
- In hot weather, stay inside in a cool place if possible.
- Stay out of the sun. Do not wear too much or heavy clothing.
- Drink plenty of water.

- Do not drink alcohol while taking LATUDA. It may make some side effects of LATUDA worse.

What are possible side effects of LATUDA?
LATUDA can cause serious side effects, including:
- See "What is the most important information I should know about LATUDA?"
- **stroke that can lead to death can happen in elderly people with dementia who take medicines like LATUDA**
- **neuroleptic malignant syndrome (NMS).** NMS is a rare but very serious condition that can happen in people who take antipsychotic medicines, including LATUDA. NMS can cause death and must be treated in a hospital. Call your healthcare provider right away if you become severely ill and have some or all of these symptoms:
  - high fever
  - excessive sweating
  - rigid muscles
  - confusion
  - changes in your breathing, heartbeat, and blood pressure
- **movements you cannot control in your face, tongue, or other body parts (tardive dyskinesia).** These may be signs of a serious condition. Tardive dyskinesia may not go away, even if you stop taking LATUDA. Tardive dyskinesia may also start after you stop taking LATUDA.
- **high blood sugar (hyperglycemia).** High blood sugar can happen if you have diabetes already or if you have never had diabetes. High blood sugar could lead to:
  - build-up of acid in your blood due to ketones (ketoacidosis)
  - coma
  - death

Increases in blood sugar can happen in some people who take LATUDA. Extremely high blood sugar can lead to coma or death. If you have diabetes or risk factors for diabetes (such as being overweight or a family history of diabetes) your healthcare provider should check your blood sugar before you start LATUDA and during therapy.

Call your healthcare provider if you have any of these symptoms of high blood sugar (hyperglycemia) while taking LATUDA:
  - feel very thirsty
  - need to urinate more than usual
  - feel very hungry
  - feel weak or tired
  - feel sick to your stomach
  - feel confused, or your breath smells fruity
- **high fat levels in your blood (increased cholesterol and triglycerides).** High fat levels may happen in people treated with LATUDA. You may not have any symptoms, so your healthcare provider may decide to check your cholesterol and triglycerides during your treatment with LATUDA.
- **increase in weight (weight gain).** Weight gain has been reported in patients taking medicines like LATUDA. You and your healthcare provider should check your weight regularly. Talk to your healthcare provider about ways to control weight gain, such as eating a healthy, balanced diet, and exercising.
- **increases in prolactin levels.** Your healthcare provider may do blood tests to check your prolactin levels.
- **low white blood cell count**
- **decreased blood pressure (orthostatic hypotension),** including lightheadedness or fainting caused by a sudden change in heart rate and blood pressure when rising too quickly from a sitting or lying position.
- **seizures**
- **difficulty swallowing**

The most common side effects of LATUDA include:
- sleepiness or drowsiness
- restlessness and feeling like you need to move around (akathisia)
- difficulty moving, slow movements, muscle stiffness, or tremor
- nausea

These are not all the possible side effects of LATUDA. For more information, ask your healthcare provider or pharmacist.

Call your doctor for medical advice about side effects. You may report side effects to FDA at 1-800-FDA-1088.

How should I store LATUDA?
- Store LATUDA tablets at room temperature between 68°F to 77°F (20°C to 25°C).
- Keep LATUDA and all medicines out of the reach of children.

General information about the safe and effective use of LATUDA.
Medicines are sometimes prescribed for purposes other than those listed in a Medication Guide. Do not use LATUDA for a condition for which it was not prescribed. Do not give LATUDA to other people, even if they have the same symptoms you have. It may harm them.

This Medication Guide summarizes the most important information about LATUDA. If you would like more informa-

tion, talk with your healthcare provider. You can ask your pharmacist or healthcare provider for information about LATUDA that is written for health professionals.

For more information, go to www.LATUDA.com or call 1-888-394-7377.

What are the ingredients in LATUDA?
Active ingredient: lurasidone hydrochloride
Inactive ingredients: mannitol, pregelatinized starch, croscarmellose sodium, hypromellose, magnesium stearate, Opadry® and carnauba wax. Additionally, the 80 mg tablet contains yellow ferric oxide and FD&C Blue No. 2 Aluminum Lake

This Medication Guide has been approved by the U.S. Food and Drug Administration.

Manufactured for:
Sunovion Pharmaceuticals Inc.
Marlborough, MA 01752 USA
LATUDA is a registered trademark of Dainippon Sumitomo Pharma Co. Ltd.,
Sunovion Pharmaceuticals Inc. is a U.S. subsidiary of Dainippon Sumitomo Pharma Co. Ltd.,
© 2013 Sunovion Pharmaceuticals Inc.
Issued: July/2013

Shown in Product Identification Guide, page 313

Supernus Pharmaceuticals, Inc.
1550 E GUDE DR
ROCKVILLE, MD 20850

Direct Inquiries: 1-866-398-0833

OXTELLAR XR ℞
(oxcarbazepine)
extended-release tablets, for oral use

HIGHLIGHTS OF PRESCRIBING INFORMATION
These highlights do not include all the information needed to use OXTELLAR XR safely and effectively. See full prescribing information for OXTELLAR XR.
OXTELLAR XR (oxcarbazepine) extended-release tablets, for oral use
Initial U.S. Approval: 2000

---INDICATIONS AND USAGE---
Oxtellar XR™ is an antiepileptic drug (AED) indicated for:
- Adults: Adjunctive therapy in the treatment of partial seizures
- Children: Adjunctive therapy in the treatment of partial seizures in children 6 to 17 years (1)

---DOSAGE AND ADMINISTRATION---
- Recommended daily dose is 1,200 mg to 2,400 mg once per day (2.2)
- Adults: Initiate with a dose of 600 mg once per day. Dose increases can be made at weekly intervals in 600 mg per day increments to achieve the recommended daily dose (2.2)
- Children: Target dose is based upon weight. Titrate to target dose over two to three weeks. Initiate with 8 mg/kg to 10 mg/kg once per day. Increase in weekly increments of 8 mg/kg to 10 mg/kg once daily, not to exceed 600 mg, to achieve target daily dose (2.3)
- Patients with creatinine clearance less than 30mL/minute: Start at 300 mg per day and increase slowly (2.4)
- Geriatric Patients: Start at lower dose (300 mg or 450 mg per day) and increase slowly (2.5)
- In conversion of oxcarbazepine immediate-release to Oxtellar XR™, higher doses of Oxtellar XR™ may be necessary (2.8, 12.3)

---DOSAGE FORMS AND STRENGTHS---
Extended-release tablets: 150 mg, 300 mg and 600 mg (3)

---CONTRAINDICATIONS---
- Known hypersensitivity to oxcarbazepine or to any of its components (4)

---WARNINGS AND PRECAUTIONS---
- *Hyponatremia:* Monitor sodium as recommended. (5.1)
- *Anaphylactic Reactions and Angioedema.* Discontinue if occurs (5.2)
- *Patients with a Past History of Hypersensitivity Reaction to Carbamazepine:* Only use based upon risk benefit (5.3)
- *Serious Dermatological Reactions:* Discontinue if observed (5.4)
- *Suicidal Behavior and Ideation:* Monitor for symptoms (5.5)
- *Withdrawal of Oxtellar XR™:* Withdrawal gradually (5.6)

- *Multi-Organ Hypersensitivity:* Discontinue if suspected (5.7)
- *Hematologic Reactions:* Discontinue if suspected (5.8)

ADVERSE REACTIONS

Most commonly observed (≥5%) and more frequent than placebo adverse reactions were: dizziness, somnolence, headache, balance disorder, tremor, vomiting, diplopia, asthenia, and fatigue (6.1).

To report SUSPECTED ADVERSE REACTIONS, contact Supernus, Inc. at (1-866-398-0833) or contact FDA at 1-800-FDA-1088 or www.fda.gov/medwatch

---

DRUG INTERACTIONS

- *Phenytoin, Carbamazepine, and Phenobarbital:* Coadministration decreased blood levels of an active metabolite of Oxtellar XR™: Greater dose of Oxtellar XR™ may be required (2.6, 7.1).
- *Oral Contraceptives:* Advise patients that Oxtellar XR™ may decrease the effectiveness of hormonal contraceptives. Additional non-hormonal forms of contraception are recommended. (7.2)

USE IN SPECIFIC POPULATIONS

- *Pregnancy:* Plasma levels of active metabolite may be decreased. Monitor patients. Based on animal data, may cause fetal harm. (5.9, 8.1).
- *Severe Hepatic Impairment:* Not recommended (8.6).

See 17 for PATIENT COUNSELING INFORMATION and Medication Guide

Revised: 10/2012

FULL PRESCRIBING INFORMATION

1 INDICATIONS AND USAGE

Oxtellar XR™ is indicated as adjunctive therapy of partial seizures in adults and in children 6 years to 17 years of age.

2 DOSAGE AND ADMINISTRATION

2.1 Important Administration Instructions

Administer Oxtellar XR™ as a single daily dose taken on an empty stomach (at least 1 hour before or at least 2 hours after meals) [see *Clinical Pharmacology (12.3)*]. If Oxtellar XR™ is taken with food, adverse reactions are more likely to occur because of increased peak levels [see *Clinical Pharmacology (12.3)*].

Swallow Oxtellar XR™ tablets whole. Do not cut, crush, or chew the tablets. For ease of swallowing in pediatric patients or patients with difficulty swallowing, achieve daily dosages with multiples of appropriate lower strength tablets (e.g., 150 mg tablets).

2.2 Dosing for Adults in Adjunctive Therapy

The recommended daily dose of Oxtellar XR™ is 1,200 mg to 2,400 mg per day, given once daily. The dose of 2,400 mg per day showed slightly greater efficacy than 1,200 mg per day, but was associated with an increase in adverse reactions.

Initiate treatment at a dose of 600 mg per day given once daily for one week. Subsequent dose increases can be made at weekly intervals in 600 mg per day increments to achieve the recommended daily dose.

2.3 Dosing for Children (6 to 17 years of age) in Adjunctive Therapy

In pediatric patients 6 years to 17 years of age, initiate treatment at a daily dose of 8 mg/kg to 10 mg/kg once daily, not to exceed 600 mg per day in the first week.

Subsequent dose increases can be made at weekly intervals in 8 mg/kg to 10 mg/kg increments once daily, not to exceed 600 mg, to achieve the target daily dose. The target maintenance dose, achieved over two to three weeks, is displayed in Table 1.

Table 1: Target Daily Dose in Pediatric Patients Aged 6 to 17 Years Old

Weight	Target Daily Dose
20 kg to 29 kg	900 mg per day
29.1 kg to 39 kg	1200 mg per day
Greater than 39 kg	1800 mg per day

2.4 Dosage Modifications in Patients with Renal Impairment

In patients with severe renal impairment (creatinine clearance less than 30 mL/minute), initiate Oxtellar XR™ at one-half the usual starting dose (300 mg per day). Subsequent dose increases can be made at weekly intervals in increments of 300 mg to 450 mg per day to achieve the desired clinical response. [see *Use in Specific Populations (8.5)*].

2.5 Dosage Modifications in Geriatric Patients

In geriatric patients, consider starting at a lower dose (300 mg or 450 mg per day). Subsequent dose increases can be made at weekly intervals in increments of 300 mg to 450 mg per day to achieve the desired clinical effect [see *Use in Specific Populations (8.4)*].

2.6 Dosage Modification for use with Concomitant Antiepileptic Drugs

Enzyme inducing antiepileptic drugs such as carbamazepine, phenobarbital, and phenytoin decrease exposure to 10-monohydroxy derivative (MHD), the active metabolite. Dosage increases may be necessary. Consider initiating dose at 900 mg once per day [see *Drug Interactions (7.1)*].

2.7 Withdrawal of AEDs

As with all antiepileptic drugs, Oxtellar XR™ should be withdrawn gradually to minimize the potential of increased seizure frequency [see *Warnings and Precautions (5.6)*].

2.8 Conversion from Immediate-Release Oxcarbazepine to Oxtellar XR™

In conversion of oxcarbazepine immediate-release to Oxtellar XR™, higher doses of Oxtellar XR™ may be necessary [see *Clinical Pharmacology (12.3)*].

3 DOSAGE FORMS AND STRENGTHS

Extended-release tablets:
150 mg: yellow modified-oval shaped with "150" printed on one side
300 mg: brown modified-oval shaped with "300" printed on one side
600 mg: brownish red modified-oval shaped with "600" printed on one side

4 CONTRAINDICATIONS

Oxtellar XR™ is contraindicated in patients with a known hypersensitivity to oxcarbazepine or to any of its components [see *Warnings and Precautions (5.2, 5.3)*].

5 WARNINGS AND PRECAUTIONS

5.1 Hyponatremia

Clinically significant hyponatremia (sodium <125 mmol/L) may develop during Oxtellar XR™ use. Serum sodium levels less than 125 mmol/L have occurred in immediate-release oxcarbazepine-treated patients generally in the first three months of treatment. However, clinically significant hyponatremia may develop more than a year after initiating therapy.

Most immediate-release oxcarbazepine-treated patients who developed hyponatremia were asymptomatic in clinical trials. However, some of these patients had their dose reduced, discontinued, or had their fluid intake restricted for hyponatremia. Serum sodium levels returned toward normal when the dosage was reduced or discontinued, or when the patient was treated conservatively (e.g., fluid restriction). Post-marketing cases of symptomatic hyponatremia have been reported during post-marketing use of immediate-release oxcarbazepine.

Among treated patients in a controlled trial of adjunctive therapy with Oxtellar XR™ in 366 adults with complex partial seizures, 1 patient receiving 2400 mg experienced a severe reduction in serum sodium (117 mEq/L) requiring discontinuation from treatment, while 2 other patients receiving 1200 mg experienced serum sodium concentrations low enough (125 and 126 mEq/L) to require discontinuation from treatment. The overall incidence of clinically significant hyponatremia in patients treated with Oxtellar XR™ was 1.2%, although slight shifts in serum sodium concentrations from Normal to Low (<135 mEq/L) were observed for the 2400 mg (6.5%) and 1200 mg (9.8%) groups compared to placebo (1.7%). Measure serum sodium concentrations if patients develop symptoms of hyponatremia (e.g., nausea, malaise, headache, lethargy, confusion, obtunded consciousness, or increase in seizure frequency or severity). Consider measurement of serum sodium concentrations during treatment with Oxtellar XR™, particularly if the patient receives concomitant medications known to decrease serum sodium levels (for example, drugs associated with inappropriate ADH secretion).

5.2 Anaphylactic Reactions and Angioedema

Rare cases of anaphylaxis and angioedema involving the larynx, glottis, lips and eyelids have been reported in patients after taking the first or subsequent doses of immediate-release oxcarbazepine. Angioedema associated with laryngeal edema can be fatal. If a patient develops any of these reactions after treatment with Oxtellar XR™, discontinue the drug and initiate an alternative treatment. Do not rechallenge these patients with Oxtellar XR™.

5.3 Hypersensitivity Reactions in Patients with Hypersensitivity to Carbamazepine

Inform patients who have had hypersensitivity reactions to carbamazepine that approximately 25%-30% of them will experience hypersensitivity reactions with Oxtellar XR™. Question patients about any prior adverse reactions with carbamazepine. Patients with a history of hypersensitivity reactions to carbamazepine should ordinarily be treated with Oxtellar XR™ only if the potential benefit justifies the potential risk. Discontinue Oxtellar XR™ immediately if signs or symptoms of hypersensitivity develop [see *Warnings and Precautions (5.8)*].

5.4 Serious Dermatological Reactions

Serious dermatological reactions, including Stevens-Johnson syndrome (SJS) and toxic epidermal necrolysis (TEN), have occurred in both children and adults in treated with immediate-release oxcarbazepine use. The median time of onset for reported cases was 19 days. Such serious skin reactions may be life threatening, and some patients have required hospitalization with very rare reports of fatal outcome. Recurrence of the serious skin reactions following rechallenge with immediate-release oxcarbazepine has also been reported.

The reporting rate of TEN and SJS associated with immediate-release oxcarbazepine use, which is generally accepted to be an underestimate due to underreporting, exceeds the background incidence rate estimates by a factor of 3- to 10-fold. Estimates of the background incidence rate for these serious skin reactions in the general population range between 0.5 to 6 cases per million-person years. Therefore, if a patient develops a skin reaction while taking Oxtellar XR™, consider discontinuing Oxtellar XR™ use and prescribing another AED.

5.5 Suicidal Behavior and Ideation

Antiepileptic drugs (AEDs), including Oxtellar XR™, increase the risk of suicidal thoughts or behavior in patients taking these drugs for any indication. Monitor patients treated with any AED for any indication for the emergence or worsening of depression, suicidal thoughts or behavior, and/or any unusual changes in mood or behavior.

Pooled analyses of 199 placebo-controlled clinical trials (mono- and adjunctive therapy) of 11 different AEDs showed that patients randomized to one of the AEDs had approximately twice the risk (adjusted Relative Risk 1.8, 95% CI:1.2, 2.7) of suicidal thinking or behavior compared to patients randomized to placebo. In these trials, which had a median treatment duration of 12 weeks, the estimated incidence rate of suicidal behavior or ideation among 27,863 AED-treated patients was 0.43%, compared to 0.24% among 16,029 placebo-treated patients, representing an increase of approximately one case of suicidal thinking or behavior for every 530 patients treated. There were four suicides in drug-treated patients in the trials and none in placebo-treated patients, but the number is too small to allow any conclusion about drug effect on suicide.

The increased risk of suicidal thoughts or behavior with AEDs was observed as early as one week after starting drug treatment with AEDs and persisted for the duration of treatment assessed. Because most trials included in the analysis did not extend beyond 24 weeks, the risk of suicidal thoughts or behavior beyond 24 weeks could not be assessed.

The risk of suicidal thoughts or behavior was generally consistent among drugs in the data analyzed. The finding of increased risk with AEDs of varying mechanisms of action and across a range of indications suggests that the risk applies to all AEDs used for any indication. The risk did not vary substantially by age (5-100 years) in the clinical trials analyzed. Table 2 shows absolute and relative risk by indication for all evaluated AEDs.

[See table 2 above]

The relative risk for suicidal thoughts or behavior was higher in clinical trials for epilepsy than in clinical trials for psychiatric or other conditions, but the absolute risk differences were similar for the epilepsy and psychiatric indications.

Anyone considering prescribing Oxtellar XR™ or any other AED must balance the risk of suicidal thoughts or behavior with the risk of untreated illness. Epilepsy and many other illnesses for which AEDs are prescribed are themselves associated with morbidity and mortality and an increased risk of suicidal thoughts and behavior. Should suicidal thoughts and behavior emerge during Oxtellar XR™ treatment, the prescriber needs to consider whether the emergence of these symptoms in any given patient may be related to the illness being treated.

Patients, their caregivers, and families should be informed that AEDs increase the risk of suicidal thoughts and behavior and should be advised of the need to be alert for the emergence or worsening of the signs and symptoms of depression, any unusual changes in mood or behavior, or the emergence of suicidal thoughts, behavior, or thoughts about self-harm. Behaviors of concern should be reported immediately to healthcare providers.

5.6 Withdrawal of AEDs

As with all AEDs, Oxtellar XR™ should be withdrawn gradually to minimize the potential of increased seizure frequency.

5.7 Multi-Organ Hypersensitivity

Multi-organ hypersensitivity reactions have occurred in close temporal association (median time to detection 13 days: range 4-60) to the initiation of immediate-release oxcarbazepine therapy in adult and pediatric patients. Although there have been a limited number of reports, many of these cases resulted in hospitalization and some were life-threatening. Signs and symptoms of this disorder were diverse; however, patients typically, although not exclusively, presented with fever and rash associated with other organ system involvement. These included the following: hematologic and lymphatic (e.g., eosinophilia, thrombocytopenia, lymphadenopathy, leukopenia, neutropenia, splenomegaly), hepatobiliary (e.g., hepatitis, liver function test abnormalities), renal (e.g., proteinuria, nephritis, oliguria, renal failure), muscles and joints (e.g., joint swelling, myalgia, arthralgia, asthenia), nervous system (e.g., hepatic encephalopathy), respiratory (e.g., dyspnea, pulmonary edema, asthma, bronchospasm, interstitial lung disease), hepatorenal syndrome, pruritus, and angioedema. Because the disorder is variable in its expression, other organ system symptoms and signs, not noted here, may occur. If this reaction is suspected, discontinue Oxtellar XR™ and initiate an alternative treatment.

5.8 Hematologic Reactions

Rare reports of pancytopenia, agranulocytosis, and leukopenia have been seen in patients treated with immediate-release oxcarbazepine during post-marketing experience. Discontinuation of Oxtellar XR™ should be considered if any evidence of these hematologic reactions develops.

5.9 Risk of Seizures in the Pregnant Patient

Due to physiological changes during pregnancy, plasma concentrations of the active metabolite of oxcarbazepine, the 10-monohydroxy derivative (MHD), may gradually decrease throughout pregnancy. Monitor patients carefully during pregnancy and through the postpartum period because MHD concentrations may increase after delivery.

Table 2: Risk by Indication for Antiepileptic Drugs in the Pooled Analysis

Indication	Placebo Patients with Events per 1,000 Patients	Drug Patients with Events per 1,000 Patients	Relative Risk: Incidence of Events in Drug Patients/Incidence in Placebo Patients	Risk Difference: Additional Drug Patients with Events per 1,000 Patients
Epilepsy	1.0	3.4	3.5	2.4
Psychiatric	5.7	8.5	1.5	2.9
Other	1.0	1.8	1.9	0.9
Total	2.4	4.3	1.8	1.9

Table 3: Adverse Reaction Incidence in a Controlled Clinical Study of Oxtellar XR™ with Concomitant AEDs in Adults*

	Oxtellar XR 2400 mg/day N=123 %	Oxtellar XR 1200 mg/day N=122 %	Placebo N=121 %
Any System / Any Term	69	57	55
Nervous System Disorders			
Dizziness	41	20	15
Somnolence	14	12	9
Headache	15	8	7
Balance Disorder	7	5	5
Tremor	1	5	2
Nystagmus	3	3	1
Ataxia	1	3	1
Gastrointestinal Disorders			
Vomiting	15	6	9
Abdominal Pain Upper	0	3	1
Dyspepsia	0	3	1
Gastritis	0	3	2
Eye Disorders			
Diplopia	13	10	4
Vision Blurred	1	4	3
Visual Impairment	1	3	0
General Disorders And Administration Site Conditions			
Asthenia	7	3	1
Fatigue	3	6	1
Gait Disturbance	0	3	1
Drug Intolerance	2	0	0
Infections And Infestations			
Nasopharyngitis	0	3	0
Sinusitis	0	3	2

* Reported by ≥ 2% of Patients Treated with Oxtellar XR™ and Numerically More Frequent than in the Placebo Group

5.10 Laboratory Tests

Laboratory data from clinical trials suggest that immediate-release oxcarbazepine may be associated with decreases in T4, without changes in T3 or TSH.

6 ADVERSE REACTIONS

The following adverse reactions are described in other sections of the labeling:

- Hyponatremia [see *Warnings and Precautions (5.1)*]
- Anaphylactic Reactions and Angioedema [see *Warnings and Precautions (5.2)*]
- Hypersensitivity Reactions in Patients with Hypersensitivity to Carbamazepine [see *Warnings and Precautions (5.3)*]
- Serious Dermatological Reactions [see *Warnings and Precautions (5.4)*]
- Suicidal Behavior and Ideation [see *Warnings and Precautions (5.5)*]
- Withdrawal of AEDs [see *Warnings and Precautions (5.6)*]
- Multi-Organ Hypersensitivity [see *Warnings and Precautions (5.7)*]
- Hematologic Reactions [see *Warnings and Precautions (5.8)*]
- Risk of Seizures in the Pregnant Patient [see *Warnings and Precautions (5.9)*]
- Laboratory Tests [see *Warnings and Precautions (5.10)*]

Table 4: Adverse Reaction Incidence in a Controlled Clinical Study of Immediate Release Oxcarbazepine with Concomitant AEDs in Adults*

	Immediate-Release Oxcarbazepine Dosage (mg/day)			Placebo N = 166%
	OXC 600 N = 163%	OXC 1200 N = 171%	OXC 2400 N = 126%	
Body as a Whole				
Fatigue	15	12	15	7
Asthenia	6	3	6	5
Edema Legs	2	1	2	1
Weight Increase	1	2	2	1
Feeling Abnormal	0	1	2	0
Cardiovascular System				
Hypotension	0	1	2	0
Digestive System				
Nausea	15	25	29	10
Vomiting	13	25	36	5
Pain Abdominal	10	13	11	5
Diarrhea	5	6	7	6
Dyspepsia	5	5	6	2
Constipation	2	2	6	4
Gastritis	2	1	2	1
Metabolic and Nutritional Disorders				
Hyponatremia	3	1	2	1
Musculoskeletal System				
Muscle Weakness	1	2	2	0
Sprains and Strains	0	2	2	1
Nervous System				
Headache	32	28	26	23
Dizziness	36	32	49	13
Somnolence	20	28	36	12
Ataxia	9	17	31	5
Nystagmus	7	20	26	5
Gait Abnormal	5	10	17	1
Insomnia	4	2	3	1
Tremor	3	8	16	5
Nervousness	2	4	2	1
Agitation	1	1	2	1
Coordination Abnormal	1	3	2	1
EEG Abnormal	0	0	2	0
Speech Disorder	1	1	3	0
Confusion	1	1	2	1
Cranial Injury NOS	1	0	2	1
Dysmetria	1	2	3	0
Thinking Abnormal	0	2	4	0

(Table continued on next page)

The safety data presented below are from 384 patients with partial epilepsy who received Oxtellar XR™ (366 adults and 18 children) with concomitant AEDs.

In addition, safety data presented below are from a total of 2,288 patients with seizure disorders treated with immediate-release oxcarbazepine; 1,832 were adults and 456 were children.

Most Common Adverse Reactions Reported by Adult Patients Receiving Concomitant AEDs in Oxtellar XR™ Clinical Studies

Table 3 lists adverse reactions that occurred in at least 2% of adult patients with epilepsy treated with Oxtellar XR™ or placebo and concomitant AEDs and that were numerically more common in the patients treated with any dose of Oxtellar XR™ than in patients receiving placebo.

The overall incidence of adverse reactions appeared to be dose related, particularly during the Titration Period. The most commonly observed (≥ 5%) adverse reactions seen in association with Oxtellar XR™ and more frequent than in placebo-treated patients were: dizziness, somnolence, headache, balance disorder, tremor, vomiting, diplopia, and asthenia.

[See table 3 at top of previous page]

Adverse Reactions Associated with Discontinuation of Oxtellar XR™ Treatment: Approximately 23.3% of the 366 adult patients receiving Oxtellar XR™ in clinical studies discontinued treatment because of an adverse reaction. The adverse reactions most commonly associated with discontinuation of Oxtellar XR™ (reported by ≥2%) were: dizziness (9.8%), vomiting (5.3%), nausea (3.7%), diplopia (3.2%), and somnolence (2.4%).

Adjunctive Therapy with Oxtellar XR™ in Pediatric Patients 4 to 16 Years Old Previously Treated with other AEDs

In a pharmacokinetic study in 18 children (age 4-16 years) with partial seizures treated with different doses of Oxtellar XR™, the observed adverse reactions seen in association with Oxtellar XR™ were similar to those seen in adults.

Most Common Adverse Reactions in Immediate-Release Oxcarbazepine Controlled Clinical Studies

Controlled Clinical Studies of Adjunctive Therapy with Immediate-Release Oxcarbazepine in Adults Previously Treated with other AEDs: Table 4 lists adverse reactions that occurred in at least 2% of adult patients with epilepsy treated with immediate-release oxcarbazepine or placebo with concomitant AEDs and that were numerically more common in the patients treated with any dose of immediate-release oxcarbazepine than in placebo. As immediate-release oxcarbazepine and Oxtellar XR™ were not examined in the same trial, adverse event frequencies cannot be directly compared between the two formulations.

[See table 4 above and on next page]

Other Reactions Observed in Association with the Administration of Immediate-Release Oxcarbazepine

In the paragraphs that follow, the adverse reactions, other than those in the preceding tables or text, that occurred in a total of 565 children and 1,574 adults exposed to immediate-release oxcarbazepine and that are reasonably likely to be related to drug use are presented. Events common in the population, events reflecting chronic illness and events likely to reflect concomitant illness are omitted particularly if minor. They are listed in order of decreasing frequency. Because the reports cite reactions observed in open label and uncontrolled trials, the role of immediate-release oxcarbazepine in their causation cannot be reliably determined.

Body as a Whole: fever, malaise, pain chest precordial, rigors, weight decrease.

Cardiovascular System: bradycardia, cardiac failure, cerebral hemorrhage, hypertension, hypotension postural, palpitation, syncope, tachycardia.

Digestive System: appetite increased, blood in stool, cholelithiasis, colitis, duodenal ulcer, dysphagia, enteritis, eructation, esophagitis, flatulence, gastric ulcer, gingival bleeding, gum hyperplasia, hematemesis, hemorrhage rectum, hemorrhoids, hiccup, mouth dry, pain biliary, pain right hypochondrium, retching, sialoadenitis, stomatitis, stomatitis ulcerative.

Hematologic and Lymphatic System: thrombocytopenia.

Laboratory Abnormality: gamma-GT increased, hyperglycemia, hypocalcemia, hypoglycemia, hypokalemia, liver enzymes elevated, serum transaminase increased.

Musculoskeletal System: hypertonia muscle.

Nervous System: aggressive reaction, amnesia, anguish, anxiety, apathy, aphasia, aura, convulsions aggravated, delirium, delusion, depressed level of consciousness, dysphonia, dystonia, emotional lability, euphoria, extrapyramidal disorder, feeling drunk, hemiplegia, hyperkinesia, hyperreflexia, hypoesthesia, hypokinesia, hyporeflexia, hypotonia, hysteria, libido decreased, libido increased, manic reaction, migraine, muscle contractions involuntary, nervousness, neuralgia, oculogyric crisis, panic disorder, paralysis, paroniria, personality disorder, psychosis, ptosis, stupor, tetany.

Respiratory System: asthma, bronchitis, coughing, dyspnea, epistaxis, laryngismus, pleurisy.

6.1   Clinical Trials Experience

Because clinical trials are conducted under widely varying conditions, adverse reaction rates observed in the clinical trials of a drug cannot be directly compared to rates in the clinical trials of another drug and may not reflect the rates observed in clinical practice.

Skin and Appendages: acne, alopecia, angioedema, bruising, dermatitis contact, eczema, facial rash, flushing, folliculitis, heat rash, hot flushes, photosensitivity reaction, pruritus genital, psoriasis, purpura, rash erythematous, rash maculopapular, vitiligo, urticaria.

Special Senses: accommodation abnormal, cataract, conjunctival hemorrhage, edema eye, hemianopia, mydriasis, otitis externa, photophobia, scotoma, taste perversion, tinnitus, xerophthalmia.

Urogenital and Reproductive System: dysuria, hematuria, intermenstrual bleeding, leukorrhea, menorrhagia, micturition frequency, pain renal, pain urinary tract, polyuria, priapism, renal calculus, urinary tract infection.

Other: Systemic lupus erythematosus.

6.2 Postmarketing and Other Experience

The following adverse reactions have been identified during post-approval use of immediate-release oxcarbazepine. Because these reactions are reported voluntarily from a population of uncertain size, it is not always possible to reliably estimate their frequency or establish a causal relationship to drug exposure.

Body as a Whole: multi-organ hypersensitivity disorders characterized by features such as rash, fever, lymphadenopathy, abnormal liver function tests, eosinophilia and arthralgia [see *Warnings and Precautions (5.7)*]

Anaphylaxis: [see *Warnings and Precautions (5.2)*]

Digestive System: pancreatitis and/or lipase and/or amylase increase

Hematologic and Lymphatic Systems: aplastic anemia [see *Warnings and Precautions (5.8)*]

Skin and Appendages: erythema multiforme, Stevens-Johnson syndrome, toxic epidermal necrolysis [see *Warnings and Precautions (5.4)*]

7 DRUG INTERACTIONS

Oxcarbazepine and MHD induce a subgroup of the cytochrome P450 3A family (CYP3A4 and CYP3A5).

In addition, several AEDs that are cytochrome P450 inducers can decrease plasma concentrations of oxcarbazepine and MHD.

These interactions have implications when Oxtellar XR™ is used with other AEDs or hormonal contraceptives.

7.1 Other Antiepileptic Drugs

Potential interactions between immediate-release oxcarbazepine and other AEDs were assessed in clinical studies. Oxtellar XR™ would be expected to have the same effects on coadministered AEDs as immediate-release oxcarbazepine.

[See table 5 above]

7.2 Hormonal Contraceptives

Coadministration of immediate-release oxcarbazepine with an oral contraceptive decreased the plasma concentrations of two components of hormonal contraceptives, ethinylestradiol and levonorgestrel. Therefore, concurrent use of Oxtellar XR™ with these hormonal contraceptives and other oral or implant contraceptives may render these contraceptives less effective [see *Clinical Pharmacology (12.3)*]. Additional non-hormonal forms of contraception are recommended.

8 USE IN SPECIFIC POPULATIONS

8.1 Pregnancy

Oxtellar XR™ plasma concentrations may decrease during pregnancy [see *Warnings and Precautions (5.9)*]

Pregnancy Category C

There are no adequate and well-controlled clinical studies of Oxtellar XR™ in pregnant women; however, Oxtellar XR™ is closely related structurally to carbamazepine, which is considered to be teratogenic in humans. Given this fact, and the results of the animal studies described, it is likely that Oxtellar XR™ is a human teratogen. Oxtellar XR™ should be used during pregnancy only if the potential benefit justifies the potential risk to the fetus.

Increased incidences of fetal structural abnormalities and other manifestations of developmental toxicity (embryolethality, growth retardation) were observed in the offspring of animals treated with either oxcarbazepine or its active 10-hydroxy metabolite (MHD) during pregnancy at doses similar to the maximum recommended human dose.

When pregnant rats were given oxcarbazepine (30, 300, or 1000 mg/kg) orally throughout the period of organogenesis, increased incidences of fetal malformations (craniofacial, cardiovascular, and skeletal) and variations were observed at the intermediate and high doses (approximately 1.2 and 4 times, respectively, the maximum recommended human dose [MRHD] on a mg/m² basis). Increased embryofetal death and decreased fetal body weights were seen at the high dose. Doses ≥ 300 mg/kg were also maternally toxic (decreased body weight gain, clinical signs), but there is no evidence to suggest that teratogenicity was secondary to the maternal effects.

In a study in which pregnant rabbits were orally administered MHD (20, 100, or 200 mg/kg) during organogenesis, embryofetal mortality was increased at the highest dose (1.5 times the MRHD on a mg/m² basis). This dose produced only minimal maternal toxicity.

Table 4 (cont.): Adverse Reaction Incidence in a Controlled Clinical Study of Immediate Release Oxcarbazepine with Concomitant AEDs in Adults*

	Immediate-Release Oxcarbazepine Dosage (mg/day)			Placebo N = 166%
	OXC 600 N = 163%	OXC 1200 N = 171%	OXC 2400 N = 126%	
Respiratory System				
Rhinitis	2	4	5	4
Skin and Appendages				
Acne	1	2	2	0
Special Senses				
Diplopia	14	30	40	5
Vertigo	6	12	15	2
Vision Abnormal	6	14	13	4
Accommodation Abnormal	0	0	2	0

* Events in at Least 2% of Patients Treated with 2400mg/day of Immediate-Release Oxcarbazepine and Numerically More Frequent than in the Placebo Group

---

Table 5: AED Drug Interactions with Oxcarbazepine

AED Coadministered (daily dose)	IR-Oxcarbazepine (daily dose)	Influence of IR-Oxcarbazepine on AED Concentration Mean Change [90% Confidence Interval]	Influence of AED on MHD Concentration (Mean Change, 90% Confidence Interval)	Recommendation
Carbamazepine (400 – 2000 mg)	900 mg	nc[1]	40% decrease [CI: 17% decrease, 57% decrease]	Consider initiating Oxtellar XR™ at a higher dose. Monitor and titrate dose to desired clinical effect (see 2.6)
Phenobarbital (100 – 150 mg)	600 – 1800 mg	14% increase [CI: 2% increase, 24% increase]	25% decrease [CI: 12% decrease, 51% decrease]	
Phenytoin (250 – 500 mg)	600 – 1800 >1200-2400	nc[1,2] up to 40% increase[3] [CI: 12% increase, 60% increase]	30% decrease [CI: 3% decrease, 48% decrease]	
Valproic Acid (400 – 2800 mg)	600-1800	nc[1]	18% decrease [CI: 13% decrease, 40% decrease]	Monitor. Dose adjustment of Oxtellar XR™ may not be needed.

[1]nc denotes a mean change of less than 10%
[2]Pediatrics
[3]Mean increase in adults at high doses of immediate-release oxcarbazepine

---

In a study in which female rats were dosed orally with oxcarbazepine (25, 50, or 150 mg/kg) during the latter part of gestation and throughout the lactation period, a persistent reduction in body weights and altered behavior (decreased activity) were observed in offspring exposed to the highest dose (0.6 times the MRHD on a mg/m² basis). Oral administration of MHD (25, 75, or 250 mg/kg) to rats during gestation and lactation resulted in a persistent reduction in offspring weights at the highest dose (equivalent to the MRHD on a mg/m² basis).

To provide information regarding the effects of in utero exposure to Oxtellar XR™, physicians are advised to recommend that pregnant patients taking Oxtellar XR™ enroll in the NAAED Pregnancy Registry. This can be done by calling the toll free number 1-888-233-2334, and must be done by patients themselves. Information on the registry can also be found at the website http://www.aedpregnancyregistry.org/.

8.2 Nursing Mothers

Oxcarbazepine and its active metabolite (MHD) are excreted in human milk. A milk-to-plasma concentration ratio of 0.5 was found for both. Because of the potential for serious adverse reactions to Oxtellar XR™ in nursing infants, a decision should be made about whether to discontinue nursing or to discontinue the drug in nursing women, taking into account the importance of the drug to the mother.

8.3 Pediatric Use

The short term safety and effectiveness of Oxtellar XR™ in pediatric patients ages 6 to 16 years with partial onset seizures is supported by:

1) An adequate and well-controlled short term safety and efficacy study of Oxtellar XR™ in adults that included pharmacokinetic sampling [see *Clinical Studies (14.1)*],

2) A pharmacokinetic study of Oxtellar XR™ in pediatric patients ages 4 to 16 years [see *Clinical Pharmacology (12.3)*], and

3) Safety and efficacy studies with the immediate-release formulation in adults and pediatric patients [see *Clinical Studies (14.2)* and *Adverse Reactions (6.1)*].

Oxtellar XR™ is not approved for pediatric patients less than 6 years of age because the size of the tablets are inappropriate for younger children, and has not been studied in patients younger than 4 years of age.

8.4 Geriatric Use

Following administration of single (300 mg) and multiple (600 mg/day) doses of immediate-release oxcarbazepine to elderly volunteers (60-82 years of age), the maximum plasma concentrations and AUC values of MHD were 30%-60% higher than in younger volunteers (18-32 years of age). Comparisons of creatinine clearance in young and elderly volunteers indicate that the difference was due to age-related reductions in creatinine clearance. Consider starting at a lower dose and lower titration [see *Dosage and Administration (2.5)*].

8.5 Renal Impairment

There is a linear correlation between creatinine clearance and the renal clearance of MHD. [see *Clinical Pharmacology (12.3)* and *Dosage and Administration (2.4)*].

The pharmacokinetics of Oxtellar XR™ has not been evaluated in patients with renal impairment. In patients with severe renal impairment (creatinine clearance <30 mL/min) given immediate release oxcarbazepine, the elimination half-life of MHD was prolonged with a corresponding two-fold increase in AUC [see *Clinical Pharmacology (12.3)*]. In these patients initiate Oxtellar XR™ at a lower starting dose and increase, if necessary, at a slower than usual rate until the desired clinical response is achieved [see *Dosage and Administration (2.4)*].

In patients with end-stage renal disease on dialysis, it is recommended that immediate release oxcarbazepine be used instead of Oxtellar XR™.

8.6 Hepatic Impairment

The pharmacokinetics of oxcarbazepine and MHD has not been evaluated in severe hepatic impairment, and therefore is not recommended in these patients. [see *Clinical Pharmacology (12.3)*].

9 DRUG ABUSE AND DEPENDENCE

9.2 Abuse

The abuse potential of Oxtellar XR™ has not been evaluated in human studies. Oxtellar XR™ is not habit forming, and is not expected to encourage abuse.

9.3 Dependence

Intragastric injections of oxcarbazepine to four cynomolgus monkeys demonstrated no signs of physical dependence as measured by the desire to self-administer oxcarbazepine by lever pressing activity.

10 OVERDOSAGE

Human Overdose Experience

Isolated cases of overdose with immediate-release oxcarbazepine have been reported. The maximum dose taken was approximately 24,000 mg. All patients recovered with symptomatic treatment.

Treatment and Management

There is no specific antidote for Oxtellar XR™ overdose. Administer symptomatic and supportive treatment as appropriate. Options include removal of the drug by gastric lavage and/or inactivation by administering activated charcoal.

11 DESCRIPTION

Oxtellar XR™ is an antiepileptic drug (AED). Oxtellar XR™ extended-release tablets contain oxcarbazepine for once-a-day oral administration.

Oxcarbazepine is 10,11-Dihydro-10-oxo-5H-dibenz[b,f]-azepine-5-carboxamide, and its structural formula is

Oxcarbazepine is off-white to yellow crystalline powder. Oxcarbazepine is sparingly soluble in chloroform (30-100 g/L). In aqueous media over pH range 1 to 8, oxcarbazepine is practically insoluble and its solubility is 40 mg/L (0.04 g/L) at pH 7.0, 25°C. The molecular formula is $C_{15}H_{12}N_2O_2$ and its molecular weight is 252.27.

Oxtellar XR™ tablets contain the following inactive ingredients: colloidal silicon dioxide, hypromellose, yellow iron oxide (150 mg, 300 mg tablets only), red iron oxide (300 mg, 600 mg tablets only), black iron oxide (300 mg tablet only), magnesium stearate, methacrylic acid copolymer, microcrystalline cellulose, polyethylene glycol, polyvinyl alcohol, povidone, sodium lauryl sulfate, talc, and titanium dioxide. Each tablet is printed on one side with edible black ink.

12 CLINICAL PHARMACOLOGY

12.1 Mechanism of Action

The pharmacological activity of Oxtellar XR™ is primarily exerted through the 10-monohydroxy metabolite (MHD) of oxcarbazepine [see *Clinical Pharmacology (12.3)*]. The precise mechanism by which oxcarbazepine and MHD exert their antiseizure effect is unknown; however, in vitro electrophysiological studies indicate that they produce blockade of voltage-sensitive sodium channels, resulting in stabilization of hyperexcited neural membranes, inhibition of repetitive neuronal firing, and diminution of propagation of synaptic impulses. These actions are thought to be important in the prevention of seizure spread in the intact brain. In addition, increased potassium conductance and modulation of high-voltage activated calcium channels may contribute to the anticonvulsant effects of the drug. No significant interactions of oxcarbazepine or MHD with brain neurotransmitter or modulator receptor sites have been demonstrated.

12.2 Pharmacodynamics

Oxcarbazepine and its active metabolite (MHD) exhibit anticonvulsant properties in animal seizure models. They protected rodents against electrically induced tonic extension seizures and, to a lesser degree, chemically induced clonic seizures, and abolished or reduced the frequency of chronically recurring focal seizures in Rhesus monkeys with aluminum implants. No development of tolerance (i.e., attenuation of anticonvulsive activity) was observed in the maximal electroshock test when mice and rats were treated daily for five days and four weeks, respectively, with oxcarbazepine or MHD.

12.3 Pharmacokinetics

Following oral administration, oxcarbazepine is absorbed and extensively metabolized to its pharmacologically active 10-monohydroxy metabolite (MHD), which is responsible for most antiepileptic activity.

In clinical studies of Oxtellar XR™, the elimination half-life of oxcarbazepine is between 7 and 11 hours; the elimination half-life of MHD is between 9 and 11 hours.

In a mass balance study in human, only 2% of total radioactivity in plasma after administration of immediate-release oxcarbazepine was due to unchanged oxcarbazepine, with approximately 70% present as MHD, and the remainder attributable to minor metabolites.

Absorption

Oxtellar XR™ administered as a once daily dose is not bioequivalent to the same total dose of the immediate release formulation given twice daily at steady state. Steady state plasma concentrations of MHD are reached within 5 days when Oxtellar XR™ is given once daily. At steady state, when 1200 mg Oxtellar XR™ was given once daily, MHD C_{max} occurred 7 hours post-dose. At steady state, Oxtellar XR™ given once daily produced MHD exposures (AUC and C_{max}) about 19% lower and MHD minimum concentrations (C_{min}) about 16% lower than the immediate-release oxcarbazepine given twice daily when administered at the same 1200 mg total daily dose. When Oxtellar XR™ was administered at an equivalent 600 mg single dose (4×150 mg tablets, 2×300 mg tablets, or 1×600 mg tablet), equivalent MHD exposures (AUC) were observed.

Following a single dose of Oxtellar XR™ (1×150 mg tablets, 1×300 mg tablets, or 1×600 mg tablet), the pharmacokinetics of MHD are not linear and show greater than dose proportional increase in AUC and less than proportional increase in C_{max}: AUC increases 2.4-fold and C_{max} increases 1.9-fold with a 2-fold increase in dose.

Effect of Food: Single dose administration of 600 mg Oxtellar XR™ following a high fat meal (800 – 1000 calories) produced MHD exposure (AUC) equivalent to that produced under fasting conditions. Peak MHD concentration (C_{max}) was about 60% higher and occurred 2 hours earlier under fed conditions than under fasting conditions.

The increase in C_{max}, even without a significant change in the overall exposure, should be considered by the prescriber especially during the titration phase, when some adverse reactions are most likely to occur coincidentally with peak levels.

Distribution

The apparent volume of distribution of MHD is 49 L. Approximately 40% of MHD is bound to serum proteins, predominantly to albumin. Binding is independent of the serum concentration within the therapeutically relevant range. Oxcarbazepine and MHD do not bind to alpha-1-acid glycoprotein.

Metabolism

Oxcarbazepine is rapidly reduced by cytosolic enzymes in the liver to MHD, which is primarily responsible for the pharmacological effect of Oxtellar XR™. MHD is metabolized further by conjugation with glucuronic acid. Minor amounts (4% of the dose) are oxidized to the pharmacologically inactive 10,11-dihydroxy metabolite (DHD).

Elimination

Oxcarbazepine is cleared from the body mostly in the form of metabolites which are predominantly excreted by the kidneys. More than 95% of a dose of immediate-release oxcarbazepine appears in the urine, with less than 1% as unchanged oxcarbazepine. Fecal excretion accounts for less than 4% of an administered dose. Approximately 80% of the dose is excreted in the urine either as glucuronides of MHD (49%) or as unchanged MHD (27%); the inactive DHD accounts for approximately 3% and conjugates of MHD and oxcarbazepine account for 13% of the dose.

The half-life of the parent was about two hours, while the half-life of MHD was about nine hours after the immediate release formulation. A population pharmacokinetic model for Oxtellar XR™ was developed in healthy normal adults and applied to pharmacokinetic data in patients with epilepsy. For oxcarbazepine, systemic parameters were scaled allometrically, suggesting that steady state oxcarbazepine exposure will vary inversely with weight.

Special Populations

Elderly

No studies with Oxtellar XR™ in elderly patients have been completed [see *Use in Specific Populations (8.4)*].

Following administration of single (300 mg) and multiple (600 mg/day) doses of immediate-release oxcarbazepine to elderly volunteers (60-82 years of age), the maximum plasma concentrations and AUC values of MHD were 30%-60% higher than in younger volunteers (18-32 years of age). Comparisons of creatinine clearance in young and elderly volunteers indicate that the difference was due to age-related reductions in creatinine clearance.

Pediatric

Oxtellar XR™ is not approved for pediatric patients less than 6 years of age because the size of the tablets are inappropriate for younger children, and has not been studied in patients younger than 4 years of age. A pharmacokinetic study of Oxtellar XR™ was performed in 18 pediatric patients with epilepsy, 4 to 16 years of age, after multiple doses. The population pharmacokinetic model suggested that dosing of pediatric patients with Oxtellar XR™ can be determined based on body weight. Weight-normalized doses in pediatric patients should produce MHD exposures (AUC) comparable to that in typical adults, with oxcarbazepine exposures ~40% higher in children than in adults [see *Use in Specific Populations (8.3)*].

Gender

The effects of gender have not been studied for Oxtellar XR™.

No gender-related pharmacokinetic differences have been observed in children, adults, or the elderly with immediate-release oxcarbazepine.

Race

The effects of race have not been studied for Oxtellar XR™.

Renal or Hepatic Impairment

The effects of renal or hepatic impairment have not been studied for Oxtellar XR™ [see *Use in Specific Populations (8.5, 8.6)*].

Based on investigations with immediate-release oxcarbazepine, there is a linear correlation between creatinine clearance and the renal clearance of MHD. When immediate-release oxcarbazepine is administered as a single 300 mg dose in renally-impaired patients (creatinine clearance <30 mL/min), the elimination half-life of MHD is prolonged to 19 hours, with a two-fold increase in AUC. Dose adjustment is recommended in these patients [see *Dosage and Administration (2.4)* and *Use in Special Populations (8.5)*].

The pharmacokinetics and metabolism of immediate-release oxcarbazepine and MHD were evaluated in healthy volunteers and hepatically impaired subjects after a single 900 mg oral dose. Mild-to-moderate hepatic impairment did not affect the pharmacokinetics of immediate-release oxcarbazepine and MHD. The pharmacokinetics of oxcarbazepine and MHD have not been evaluated in severe hepatic impairment, and therefore it is not recommended in these patients [see *Use in Specific Populations (8.6)*].

Pregnancy

Due to physiological changes during pregnancy, MHD plasma levels may gradually decrease throughout pregnancy [see *Use in Specific Populations (8.1)*]

Drug Interaction Studies

In Vitro: Oxcarbazepine can inhibit CYP2C19 and induce CYP3A4/5 with potentially important effects on plasma concentrations of other drugs. In addition, several AEDs that are cytochrome P450 inducers can decrease plasma concentrations of oxcarbazepine and MHD.

Oxcarbazepine was evaluated in human liver microsomes to determine its capacity to inhibit the major cytochrome P450 enzymes responsible for the metabolism of other drugs. Results demonstrate that oxcarbazepine and its pharmacologically active 10-monohydroxy metabolite (MHD) have little or no capacity to function as inhibitors for most of the human cytochrome P450 enzymes evaluated (CYP1A2, CYP2A6, CYP2C9, CYP2D6, CYP2E1, CYP4A9 and CYP4A11) with the exception of CYP2C19 and CYP3A4/5. Although inhibition of CYP3A4/5 by oxcarbazepine and MHD did occur at high concentrations, it is not likely to be of clinical significance. The inhibition of CYP2C19 by oxcarbazepine and MHD, is clinically relevant.

In vitro, the UDP-glucuronyl transferase level was increased, indicating induction of this enzyme. Increases of 22% with MHD and 47% with oxcarbazepine were observed. As MHD, the predominant plasma substrate, is only a weak inducer of UDP-glucuronyl transferase, it is unlikely to have an effect on drugs that are mainly eliminated by conjugation through UDPglucuronyl transferase (e.g., valproic acid, lamotrigine).

In addition, oxcarbazepine and MHD induce a subgroup of the cytochrome P450 3A family (CYP3A4 and CYP3A5) responsible for the metabolism of dihydropyridine calcium antagonists, oral contraceptives and cyclosporine resulting in a lower plasma concentration of these drugs.

Several AEDs that are cytochrome P450 inducers can decrease plasma concentrations of oxcarbazepine and MHD. No autoinduction has been observed with immediate-release oxcarbazepine.

As binding of MHD to plasma proteins is low (40%), clinically significant interactions with other drugs through competition for protein binding sites are unlikely.

In Vivo:

Hormonal Contraceptives

Coadministration of immediate-release oxcarbazepine with an oral contraceptive has been shown to influence the plasma concentrations of two components of hormonal contraceptives, ethinylestradiol (EE) and levonorgestrel (LNG). The mean AUC values of EE were decreased by 48% [90% CI: 22-65] in one study and 52% [90% CI: 38-52] in another study. The mean AUC values of LNG were decreased by 32% [90% CI: 20-45] in one study and 52% [90% CI: 42-52] in another study. Therefore, concurrent use of oxcarbazepine with hormonal contraceptives may render these contraceptives less effective.

Calcium Channel Antagonists

After repeated coadministration of immediate-release oxcarbazepine, the AUC of felodipine was lowered by 28% [90% CI: 20-33]. Verapamil produced a decrease of 20% [90% CI: 18-27] of the plasma levels of MHD after coadministration with immediate-release oxcarbazepine.

Other Interactions

Cimetidine, erythromycin and dextropropoxyphene had no effect on the pharmacokinetics of MHD after coadministration with immediate-release oxcarbazepine. Results with warfarin show no evidence of interaction with either single or repeated doses of immediate-release oxcarbazepine.

13 NONCLINICAL TOXICOLOGY

13.1 Carcinogenesis, Mutagenesis, Impairment of Fertility

Carcinogenesis

In two-year carcinogenicity studies, oxcarbazepine was administered in the diet at doses of up to 100 mg/kg/day to mice and by gavage at doses of up to 250 mg/kg/day to rats, and the pharmacologically active 10-hydroxy metabolite (MHD) was administered orally at doses of up to 600 mg/kg/day to rats.

In mice, a dose-related increase in the incidence of hepatocellular adenomas was observed at oxcarbazepine doses ≥ 70 mg/kg/day or approximately 0.1 times the maximum recommended human dose (MRHD) on a mg/m^2 basis.

In rats, the incidence of hepatocellular carcinomas was increased in females treated with oxcarbazepine at doses ≥25 mg/kg/day (0.1 times the MRHD on a mg/m^2 basis), and incidences of hepatocellular adenomas and/or carcinomas were increased in males and females treated with MHD at doses of 600 mg/kg/day (2.4 times the MRHD on a mg/m^2 basis) and ≥ 250 mg/kg/day (equivalent to the MRHD on a mg/m^2 basis), respectively.

There was an increase in the incidence of benign testicular interstitial cell tumors in rats at 250 mg oxcarbazepine/kg/day and at ≥ 250 mg MHD/kg/day, and an increase in the incidence of granular cell tumors in the cervix and vagina in rats at 600 mg MHD/kg/day.

Mutagenesis

Oxcarbazepine increased mutation frequencies in the Ames test in vitro in the absence of metabolic activation in one of five bacterial strains. Both oxcarbazepine and MHD produced increases in chromosomal aberrations and polyploidy in the Chinese hamster ovary assay in vitro in the absence of metabolic activation. MHD was negative in the Ames test, and no mutagenic or clastogenic activity was found with either oxcarbazepine or MHD in V79 Chinese hamster cells in vitro. Oxcarbazepine and MHD were both negative for clastogenic or aneugenic effects (micronucleus formation) in an in vivo rat bone marrow assay.

Impairment of Fertility

In a fertility study in which rats were administered MHD (50, 150, or 450 mg/kg) orally prior to and during mating and early gestation, estrous cyclicity was disrupted and numbers of corpora lutea, implantations, and live embryos were reduced in females receiving the highest dose (approximately two times the MRHD on a mg/m^2 basis).

14 CLINICAL STUDIES

Oxtellar XR™ has been evaluated as adjunctive therapy for partial seizures in adults. The use of Oxtellar XR™ for the treatment of partial seizures in children is based on adequate and well-controlled studies of Oxtellar XR™ in adults, along with clinical trials of immediate-release oxcarbazepine in children, and on pharmacokinetic evaluations of the use of Oxtellar XR™ in children.

14.1 Oxtellar XR™ Primary Trial

A multicenter, randomized, double-blind, placebo-controlled, three-arm, parallel-group study (Study 1) in male and female adults with refractory partial epilepsy (18 to 65 years of age, inclusive) was performed to examine the safety and efficacy of Oxtellar XR™.

Patients had at least three partial seizures per 28 days during an 8 week Baseline Period. Subjects were receiving treatment with at least one to three antiepileptic drugs and were on stable treatment for a minimum of 4 weeks. Subjects with a diagnosis other than partial epilepsy were excluded.

Table 6: Primary Efficacy Results in Study 1: Percent Change from Baseline in Partial Seizure Frequency in the 16-week Treatment Period

	Median seizure frequency during 8-week baseline period (per 28 days)	Median seizure frequency during 16-week treatment period (per 28 days)	Median percent change in seizure frequency	Seizure frequency percent change effect size	P value vs placebo*
Placebo (N=121)	7.0	5.0	-28.7 %		
Oxtellar XR™ 1200mg/day (N=122)	6.0	4.3	-38.2 %	9.5%	0.078
Oxtellar XR™ 2400mg/day (N=123)	6.0	3.7	-42.9 %	14.2%	0.003

*Wilcoxon rank-sum test of the median percentage change in partial seizure frequency per 28 days during the 16-week Treatment Phase (Titration + Maintenance Periods) relative to the 8-week Baseline Phase.

The study included an 8 week Baseline Period, followed by a Treatment Period, which included a 4 week Titration Phase followed by a 12 week Maintenance Phase. The primary endpoint of the study was median percentage change from baseline in seizure frequency per 28 days during the treatment period relative to the baseline period. The criterion for statistical significance was p < 0.05. A total of 366 patients were enrolled at 88 sites in North America and Eastern Europe. Subjects were randomized to one of three treatment groups and took Oxtellar XR™ (1200 or 2400 mg/day) or placebo.

Table 6 presents the primary efficacy results by treatment group.

[See table 6 above]

Although the 1200 mg/day-placebo contrast did not reach statistical significance, concentration-response analyses reveal that the 1200 mg/day dose is an effective dose.

14.2 Immediate-Release Oxcarbazepine Adjunctive Therapy Trials

The effectiveness of immediate-release oxcarbazepine as an adjunctive therapy for partial seizures in adults was demonstrated at doses of 600mg per day, 1200mg per day and 2400mg per day (divided twice daily) in a randomized, double-blind, placebo-controlled trial. All doses resulted in a statistically significant reduction in seizure frequency when compared to placebo (p<0.05).

The effectiveness of immediate-release oxcarbazepine in doses of 30-46 mg/kg/day, depending on baseline weight, as an adjunctive therapy for partial seizures in children 3 years to 17 years of age was studied in a randomized, double-blind, placebo-controlled trial. Oxcarbazepine in the single weight based dose group resulted in a statistically significant reduction in seizure frequency when compared to placebo (p<0.05).

16 HOW SUPPLIED/STORAGE AND HANDLING

16.1 Dosage Form Supplied

150 mg (yellow modified-oval shaped tablet printed "150" on one side with edible black ink).

Bottles of 100 tablets   NDC 17772-121-01

300 mg (brown modified-oval shaped tablet printed "300" on one side with edible black ink).

Bottles of 100 tablets   NDC 17772-122-01

600 mg (brownish red modified-oval shaped tablet printed "600" on one side with edible black ink).

Bottles of 100 tablets   NDC 17772-123-01

16.2 Storage and Handling

Store at 25°C (77°F); excursions permitted between 15°C and 30°C (59°F to 86°F) [See USP controlled room temperature]. Protect from light and moisture. Dispense in a tight, light-resistant container.

17 PATIENT COUNSELING INFORMATION

See FDA-Approved patient labeling (Medication Guide). Inform patients and caregivers of the availability of a Medication Guide. Instruct patients and caregivers to read the Medication Guide prior to taking Oxtellar XR™.

- Advise patients to take the tablet whole with water or other liquid, and not to cut, chew or crush the tablet. Cutting, chewing or crushing Oxtellar XR™ tablet could affect its performance.
- Advise patients to take Oxtellar XR™ on an empty stomach. This means they should take Oxtellar XR™ at least one hour before food or at least two hours after food [see Clinical Pharmacology (12.3)].
- Advise patients that Oxtellar XR™ may reduce serum sodium concentrations especially if they are taking other medications that can lower sodium. Advise patients to report symptoms of low sodium like nausea, tiredness, lack of energy, confusion, and more frequent or more severe seizures [see Warnings and Precautions (5.1)].
- Anaphylactic reactions and angioedema may occur during treatment with Oxtellar XR™. Advise patients to immediately report signs and symptoms suggesting angioedema (swelling of the face, eyes, lips, tongue or difficulty in swallowing or breathing) and to stop taking the drug until they have consulted with their physician [see Warnings and Precautions (5.2)].
- Inform patients who have exhibited hypersensitivity reactions to carbamazepine that approximately 25%-30% of these patients may also experience hypersensitivity reactions with Oxtellar XR™. If patients experience a hypersensitivity reaction while taking Oxtellar XR™, advise them to consult with their physician immediately [see Warnings and Precautions (5.3)].
- Advise patients that serious skin reactions have been reported in association with immediate-release oxcarbazepine. If patients experience a skin reaction while taking Oxtellar XR™, advise patients to consult with their physician immediately [see Warnings and Precautions (5.4)].
- Instruct patients that a fever associated with other organ system involvement (rash, lymphadenopathy, etc.) occurring during treatment with Oxtellar XR™ may be drug-related and advise them to consult their physician immediately [see Warnings and Precautions (5.7)].
- Advise patients that there have been rare reports of blood disorders reported in patients treated with immediate-release oxcarbazepine. Instruct patients to immediately consult with their physician if they experience symptoms suggestive of blood disorders during treatment with Oxtellar XR™ [see Warnings and Precautions (5.8)].
- Warn female patients of childbearing age that the concurrent use of Oxtellar XR™ with hormonal contraceptives may render this method of contraception less effective [see Drug Interactions (7.2)]. Additional non-hormonal forms of contraception are recommended when using Oxtellar XR™.
- Counsel patients, their caregivers, and families that AEDs, including Oxtellar XR™, may increase the risk of suicidal thoughts and behavior and that they need to be alert for the emergence or worsening of symptoms of depression, any unusual changes in mood or behavior, or the emergence of suicidal thoughts, behavior, or thoughts about self-harm. Advise them to immediately report behaviors of concern to healthcare providers.
- Advise patients to exercise caution if alcohol is taken in combination with Oxtellar XR™ therapy, due to a possible additive sedative effect.
- Advise patients that Oxtellar XR™ may cause dizziness and somnolence. Accordingly, advise patients not to drive or operate machinery until they have gained sufficient experience on Oxtellar XR™ to gauge whether it adversely affects their ability to drive or operate machinery.
- Encourage patients to enroll in the North American Antiepileptic Drug (NAAED) Pregnancy Registry if they become pregnant. This registry is collecting information about the safety of antiepileptic drugs during pregnancy. To enroll, patients can call the toll free number 1-888-233-2334 [see Use in Specific Populations (8.1)].
- Advise patients that they should call their healthcare provider or poison control center (phone number 1-800-222-1222) if they take too much Oxtellar XR™.
- Discuss with your patient what they should do if they miss a dose.

Oxtellar XR™ is manufactured by:
Patheon Inc.
Whitby, Ontario L1N 5Z5 CANADA
Distributed by:
Supernus Pharmaceuticals, Inc.
Rockville, MD 20850 USA
Oxtellar XR™ is a trademark of Supernus Pharmaceuticals, Inc.
Revised: October 2012

MEDICATION GUIDE
Oxtellar XR™((ahks-TEH-lahr eks ahr))
(oxcarbazepine)
Extended-Release Tablets
Read this Medication Guide before you start taking Oxtellar XR™ and each time you get a refill. There may be new information. This information does not take the place of talking to your healthcare provider about your medical condition or treatment.

What is the most important information I should know about Oxtellar XR™?
Do not stop taking Oxtellar XR™ without first talking to your healthcare provider.
Stopping Oxtellar XR™ suddenly can cause serious problems.
Oxtellar XR™ can cause serious side effects, including:
1. Oxtellar XR™ may cause the level of sodium in your blood to be low. Symptoms of low blood sodium include:
• nausea
• tiredness, lack of energy
• headache
• confusion
• more frequent or more severe seizures.
Similar symptoms that are not related to low sodium may occur from taking Oxtellar XR™. You should tell your healthcare provider if you have any of these side effects and if they bother you or they do not go away.
Some other medicines can also cause low sodium in your blood. Be sure to tell your healthcare provider about all the other medicines that you are taking.
2. Oxtellar XR™ may also cause allergic reactions or serious problems which may affect organs and other parts of your body like the liver or blood cells. You may or may not have a rash with these types of reactions.
Call your healthcare provider right away if you have any of the following:
• swelling of your face, eyes, lips, or tongue
• trouble swallowing or breathing
• a skin rash
• hives
• fever, swollen glands, or sore throat that do not go away or come and go
• painful sores in the mouth or around your eyes
• yellowing of your skin or eyes
• unusual bruising or bleeding
• severe fatigue or weakness
• severe muscle pain
• frequent infections or infections that do not go away
Many people who are allergic to carbamazepine are also allergic to Oxtellar XR™. Tell your healthcare provider if you are allergic to carbamazepine.
3. Like other antiepileptic drugs, Oxtellar XR™ may cause suicidal thoughts or actions in a very small number of people, about 1 in 500.
Call your healthcare provider right away if you have any of these symptoms, especially if they are new, worse, or worry you:
• thoughts about suicide or dying
• attempts to commit suicide
• new or worse depression
• new or worse anxiety
• feeling agitated or restless
• panic attacks
• trouble sleeping (insomnia)
• new or worse irritability
• acting aggressive, being angry, or violent
• acting on dangerous impulses
• an extreme increase in activity and talking (mania)
• other unusual changes in behavior or mood
How can I watch for early symptoms of suicidal thoughts and actions?
• Pay attention to any changes, especially sudden changes, in mood, behaviors, thoughts, or feelings.
• Keep all follow-up visits with your healthcare provider as scheduled.
Call your healthcare provider between visits as needed, especially if you are worried about symptoms.
Do not stop taking Oxtellar XR™ without first talking to a healthcare provider.
Stopping Oxtellar XR™ suddenly can cause serious problems. Stopping a seizure medicine suddenly in a patient who has epilepsy may cause seizures that will not stop (status epilepticus).

Suicidal thoughts or actions may be caused by things other than medicines. If you have suicidal thoughts or actions, your healthcare provider may check for other causes.
What is Oxtellar XR™?
Oxtellar XR™ is a prescription medicine used:
• with other medicines to treat partial seizures in adults
• with other medicines to treat partial seizures in children 6 to 17 years of age.
It is not known if Oxtellar XR™ is safe and effective in children under 6 years of age.
Who should not take Oxtellar XR™?
• Do not take Oxtellar XR™ if you are allergic to oxcarbazepine or any of the other ingredients in Oxtellar XR™. See the end of this leaflet for a complete list of ingredients in Oxtellar XR™.
What should I tell my healthcare provider before taking Oxtellar XR™?
Before taking Oxtellar XR™, tell your healthcare provider about all your medical conditions, including if you:
• have or have had suicidal thoughts or actions, depression or mood problems
• have liver problems
• have kidney problems
• use birth control medicine. Oxtellar XR™ may cause your birth control medicine to be less effective. Talk to your healthcare provider about the best birth control method to use.
• are pregnant or plan to become pregnant. Oxtellar XR™ may harm your unborn baby. Tell your healthcare provider right away if you become pregnant while taking Oxtellar XR™. You and your healthcare provider will decide if you should take Oxtellar XR™ while you are pregnant.
• If you become pregnant while taking Oxtellar XR™, talk to your healthcare provider about registering with the North American Antiepileptic Drug (NAAED) Pregnancy Registry. The purpose of this registry is to collect information about the safety of antiepileptic medicine during pregnancy. You can enroll in this registry by calling 1-888-233-2334.
• are breastfeeding or plan to breastfeed. Oxtellar XR™ passes into breast milk. You and your healthcare provider should discuss whether you should take Oxtellar XR™ or breastfeed. You should not do both.
Tell your healthcare provider about all the medicines you take, including prescription and non-prescription medicines, vitamins, and herbal supplements.
Taking Oxtellar XR™ with certain other medicines may cause side effects or affect how well they work. Do not start or stop other medicines without talking to your healthcare provider.
Especially tell your healthcare provider if you take: carbamazepine, phenobarbital, phenytoin, or birth control medicine.
Ask your healthcare provider or pharmacist for a list of these medicines, if you are not sure.
Know the medicines you take. Keep a list of them and show it to your healthcare provider and pharmacist when you get a new medicine.
How should I take Oxtellar XR™?
Do not stop taking Oxtellar XR™ without talking to your healthcare provider. Stopping Oxtellar XR™ suddenly can cause serious problems, including seizures that will not stop (status epilepticus).Take Oxtellar XR™ exactly as prescribed. Your healthcare provider may change your dose. Your healthcare provider will tell you how much Oxtellar XR™ to take.
Take Oxtellar XR™ 1 time each day.
Take Oxtellar XR™ on an empty stomach. This means you should take Oxtellar XR™ at least 1 hour before or at least 2 hours after a meal. Take Oxtellar XR™ tablets whole with water or other liquid.
Do not cut, crush, or chew the tablets before swallowing.
If you take too much Oxtellar XR™ call your healthcare provider or call the poison control center at 1-800-222-1222.
Take Oxtellar XR™ at the same time each day.
Talk with your healthcare provider about what you should do if you miss a dose.
What should I avoid while taking Oxtellar XR™?
• Do not drive, operate heavy machinery, or do other dangerous activities until you know how Oxtellar XR™ affects you. Oxtellar XR™ may slow your thinking and motor skills.
• Do not drink alcohol or take other drugs that make you sleepy or dizzy while taking Oxtellar XR™ until you talk to your healthcare provider. Oxtellar XR™ taken with alcohol or drugs that cause sleepiness or dizziness may make your sleepiness or dizziness worse.
What are the possible side effects of Oxtellar XR™?
See "What is the most important information I should know about Oxtellar XR™?"
Oxtellar XR™ may cause other serious side effects including:
• your seizures can happen more often or become worse
• trouble concentrating

• problems with your speech and language
• feeling confused
• feeling sleepy and tired
• trouble walking and with coordination
Get medical help right away if you have any of the symptoms listed above or listed in "What is the most important information I should know about Oxtellar XR™?"
The most common side effects of Oxtellar XR™ include:
• dizziness
• sleepiness
• headache
• problems with walking and coordination (unsteadiness)
• shakiness
• nausea
• vomiting
• double vision
• weakness
• tiredness
These are not all the possible side effects of Oxtellar XR™. For more information, ask your healthcare provider or pharmacist.
Tell your healthcare provider if you have any side effect that bothers you or does not go away.
Call your doctor for medical advice about side effects. You may report side effects to FDA at 1-800-FDA-1088.
How should I store Oxtellar XR™?
• Store Oxtellar XR™ at room temperature 68°F to 77°F (20°C and 25°C)
• Keep Oxtellar XR™ in a tightly closed container, and keep Oxtellar XR™ out of the light.
• Keep Oxtellar XR™ tablets dry.
Keep Oxtellar XR™ and all medicines out of the reach of children.
General Information about the safe and effective use of Oxtellar XR™
Medicines are sometimes prescribed for purposes other than those listed in a Medication Guide. Do not use Oxtellar XR™ for a condition for which it was not prescribed. Do not give Oxtellar XR™ to other people, even if they have the same symptoms that you have. It may harm them.
This Medication Guide summarizes the most important information about Oxtellar XR™. If you would like more information, talk with your healthcare provider. You can ask your pharmacist or healthcare provider for the full prescribing information about Oxtellar XR™ that is written for health professionals.
For more information, go to www.supernus.com or call 1-866-398-0833.
What are the ingredients in Oxtellar XR™?
Active ingredient: oxcarbazepine
Inactive ingredients:
150 mg tablets: colloidal silicon dioxide, hypromellose, yellow iron oxide, magnesium stearate, methacrylic acid copolymer, microcrystalline cellulose, polyethylene glycol, polyvinyl alcohol, povidone, sodium lauryl sulfate, talc, and titanium dioxide.
300 mg tablets: colloidal silicon dioxide, hypromellose, yellow iron oxide, red iron oxide, black iron oxide, magnesium stearate, methacrylic acid copolymer, microcrystalline cellulose, polyethylene glycol, polyvinyl alcohol, povidone, sodium lauryl sulfate, talc, and titanium dioxide.
600 mg tablets: red iron oxide, magnesium stearate, methacrylic acid copolymer, microcrystalline cellulose, polyethylene glycol, polyvinyl alcohol, povidone, sodium lauryl sulfate, talc, and titanium dioxide.
This Medication Guide has been approved by the U.S. Food and Drug Administration.
Distributed by:
Supernus Pharmaceuticals, Inc.
© Supernus Pharmaceuticals Inc.
Issued October 2012.
Shown in Product Identification Guide, page 313

TROKENDI XR   ℞
(topiramate)
extended-release capsules for oral use

HIGHLIGHTS OF PRESCRIBING INFORMATION
These highlights do not include all the information needed to use TROKENDI XR safely and effectively. See full prescribing information for TROKENDI XR.
Trokendi XR (topiramate) extended-release capsules for oral use
Initial U.S. Approval: 1996

―――――――INDICATIONS AND USAGE―――――――
Trokendi XR™ is an antiepileptic drug indicated for:
• Partial Onset Seizure and Primary Generalized Tonic-Clonic Seizures - initial monotherapy in patients 10 years of age and older with partial onset or primary generalized tonic-clonic seizures and adjunctive therapy in patients 6 years of age and older with partial onset or primary generalized tonic-clonic seizures (1.1)
• Lennox-Gastaut Syndrome (LGS) - adjunctive therapy in patients 6 years of age and older with seizures associated with Lennox-Gastaut syndrome (1.2)

	Initial Dose	Titration	Recommended Dose
Monotherapy Therapy: Partial Onset or Primary Generalized Tonic-Clonic Seizures			
Adults and pediatric patients 10 years and older (2.1)	50 mg orally once daily	Increase dose weekly by increments of 50 mg for first 4 weeks then 100 mg for weeks 5 to 6	400 mg once daily
Adjunctive Therapy			
Adults with partial onset seizures or LGS (2.2)	25 mg to 50 mg orally once daily	Increase dose weekly by increments of 25 mg to 50 mg to achieve an effective dose	200 mg to 400 mg once daily
Adults with primary generalized tonic-clonic seizures (2.2)	25 mg to 50 mg orally once daily	Increase dose weekly to an effective dose by increments of 25 mg to 50 mg	400 mg once daily
Pediatric patients 6 years and older with partial onset seizures, primary generalized tonic-clonic seizures or LGS (2.2)	25 mg once at night-time (based on a range of 1 mg/kg to 3 mg/kg once daily) for first week	Increase dosage at 1- or 2-week intervals by increments of 1 mg/kg to 3 mg/kg. Dose titration should be guided by clinical outcome	5 mg/kg to 9 mg/kg once daily

DOSAGE AND ADMINISTRATION

[See table above]

Swallow capsule whole and intact. Do not sprinkle on food, chew or crush (2.9)

DOSAGE FORMS AND STRENGTHS

- Extended-release capsules: 25 mg, 50 mg, 100 mg, and 200 mg (3)

CONTRAINDICATIONS

- With recent alcohol use (i.e., within 6 hours prior to and 6 hours after Trokendi XR use [(4), (5.4)]
- In patients with metabolic acidosis taking concomitant metformin [(4), (5.3)]

WARNINGS AND PRECAUTIONS

- *Acute myopia and secondary angle closure glaucoma:* Untreated elevated intraocular pressure can lead to permanent visual loss. Discontinue Trokendi XR™ if it occurs (5.1)
- *Oligohydrosis and hyperthermia:* Monitor decreased sweating and increased body temperature, especially in pediatric patients (5.2)
- *Metabolic acidosis:* Measure baseline and periodic measurement of serum bicarbonate. Consider dose reduction or discontinuation of Trokendi XR™ if clinically appropriate (5.3)
- *Suicidal behavior and ideation:* Antiepileptic drugs increase the risk of suicidal behavior or ideation (5.5)
- *Cognitive/neuropsychiatric:* Trokendi XR™ may cause cognitive dysfunction. Use caution when operating machinery including automobiles. Depression and mood problems may occur (5.6)
- *Fetal toxicity:* Topiramate use during pregnancy can cause cleft lip and/or palate (5.7)
- *Withdrawal of AEDs:* Withdrawal of Trokendi XR™ should be done gradually (5.8)
- *Hyperammonemia and encephalopathy:* Patients with inborn errors of metabolism or reduced mitochondrial activity may have an increased risk of hyper-ammonemia. Measure ammonia if encephalopathic symptoms occur (5.9)
- *Kidney stones:* Avoid use with other carbonic anhydrase inhibitors, other drugs causing metabolic acidosis, or in patients on a ketogenic diet (5.10)
- *Hypothermia:* Reported with concomitant valproic acid use (5.11)

ADVERSE REACTIONS

The most common (greater than 5% more frequent than placebo or low-dose topiramate in monotherapy) adverse reactions were paresthesia, anorexia, weight decrease, fatigue, dizziness, somnolence, nervousness, psychomotor slowing, difficulty with memory, difficulty with concentration/attention, cognitive problem, confusion, mood problems, fever, infection, and flushing (6.1)

To report SUSPECTED ADVERSE REACTIONS, contact Supernus Pharmaceuticals at 1-866-398-0833- or FDA at 1-800-FDA-1088 or www.fda.gov/medwatch.

DRUG INTERACTIONS

- *Oral contraceptives:* Decreased contraceptive efficacy and increased breakthrough bleeding, especially at doses greater than 200 mg per day (7.2)
- *Phenytoin or carbamazepine:* Concomitant administration with topiramate decreased plasma concentrations of topiramate (7.3)
- *Other carbonic anhydrase inhibitors:* Monitor for the appearance or worsening of metabolic acidosis (7.5)
- *Lithium:* Monitor lithium levels when co-administered with high-dose topiramate (7.7)

USE IN SPECIFIC POPULATIONS

- *Renal Impairment:* (creatinine clearance less than 70 mL/min/1.73m2), one-half of the adult dose is recommended (8.7)
- *Patients undergoing hemodialysis:* Topiramate is cleared by hemodialysis. Dosage adjustment is necessary to avoid rapid drops in topiramate plasma concentration during hemodialysis (8.8)
- *Pregnancy:* Increased risk of cleft lip and/or palate. Pregnancy registry available (8.1)
- *Nursing mothers:* Caution should be exercised when administered to a nursing mother (8.3)
- *Pediatric Use:* Because the capsule must be swallowed whole, and may not be sprinkled on food, crushed or chewed, Trokendi XR™ is recommended only for children ages 6 years and older (8.4)

See 17 for PATIENT COUNSELING INFORMATION and Medication Guide

Revised: 08/2013

FULL PRESCRIBING INFORMATION

1   INDICATIONS AND USAGE

1.1   Partial Onset Seizure and Primary Generalized Tonic-Clonic Seizures

Trokendi XR™ (topiramate) extended-release capsules are indicated as initial monotherapy in patients 10 years of age and older with partial onset or primary generalized tonic-clonic seizures and adjunctive therapy in patients 6 years of age and older with partial onset or primary generalized tonic-clonic seizures [see Clinical Studies (14.2, 14.3, 14.4)]. Safety and effectiveness in patients who were converted to monotherapy from a previous regimen of other anticonvulsant drugs have not been established in controlled trials [see Clinical Studies (14.2)].

1.2   Lennox-Gastaut Syndrome

Trokendi XR™ (topiramate) extended-release capsules are indicated as adjunctive therapy in patients 6 years of age and older with seizures associated with Lennox-Gastaut syndrome [see Clinical Studies (14.5)].

2   DOSAGE AND ADMINISTRATION

2.1   Monotherapy Use

Adults and Pediatric Patients 10 Years and Older with Partial Onset or Primary Generalized Tonic-Clonic Seizures

The recommended dose for topiramate monotherapy in adults and pediatric patients 10 years of age and older is 400 mg orally once daily. Titrate Trokendi XR™ according to the following schedule:

Week 1	50 mg once daily
Week 2	100 mg once daily
Week 3	150 mg once daily
Week 4	200 mg once daily
Week 5	300 mg once daily
Week 6	400 mg once daily

2.2   Adjunctive Therapy Use

Adults (17 Years of Age and Older) - Partial Onset Seizures, Primary Generalized Tonic-Clonic Seizures, or Lennox-Gastaut Syndrome

The recommended total daily dose of Trokendi XR™ as adjunctive therapy in adults with partial onset seizures or Lennox-Gastaut Syndrome is 200 mg to 400 mg orally once daily with primary generalized tonic-clonic seizures is 400 mg orally once daily.

Initiate therapy at 25 mg to 50 mg once daily followed by titration to an effective dose in increments of 25 mg to 50mg every week. Daily topiramate doses above 1,600 mg have not been studied.

In the study of primary generalized tonic-clonic seizures using topiramate, the assigned dose was reached at the end of 8 weeks [see Clinical Studies (14.4)].

Pediatric Patients (Ages 6 years to 16 Years) - Partial Onset Seizures, Primary Generalized Tonic-Clonic Seizures, or Lennox-Gastaut Syndrome

The recommended total daily dose of Trokendi XR™ as adjunctive therapy for pediatric patients with partial onset seizures, primary generalized tonic-clonic seizures, or seizures associated with Lennox-Gastaut syndrome is approximately 5 mg/kg to 9 mg/kg orally once daily. Begin titration at 25 mg once daily (based on a range of 1 mg/kg/day to 3 mg/kg/day) given nightly for the first week. Subsequently, increase the dosage at 1- or 2-week intervals by increments of 1 mg/kg to 3 mg/kg to achieve optimal clinical response. Dose titration should be guided by clinical outcome. If required, longer intervals between dose adjustments can be used.

In the study of primary generalized tonic-clonic seizures, the assigned dose of 6 mg/kg once daily was reached at the end of 8 weeks [see Clinical Studies (14.4)].

2.3 Administration with Alcohol

Alcohol use should be completely avoided within 6 hours prior to and 6 hours after Trokendi XR™ administration [see Warnings and Precautions (5.4)].

2.4 Dose Modifications in Patients with Renal Impairment

In patients with renal impairment (creatinine clearance less than 70 mL/min/1.73 m²), one-half of the usual adult dose is recommended. Such patients will require a longer time to reach steady-state at each dose.

Prior to dosing, obtain an estimated GFR measurement in patients at high risk for renal insufficiency (e.g., older patients, or those with diabetes mellitus, hypertension, or autoimmune disease).

2.5 Dosage Modifications in Patients Undergoing Hemodialysis

Topiramate is cleared by hemodialysis at a rate that is 4 to 6 times greater than in patients with normal renal function. Accordingly, a prolonged period of dialysis may cause topiramate concentration to fall below that required to maintain an anti-seizure effect. To avoid rapid drops in topiramate plasma concentration during hemodialysis, a supplemental dose of topiramate may be required. The actual adjustment should take into account the:

- duration of dialysis period
- clearance rate of the dialysis system being used
- effective renal clearance of topiramate in the patient being dialyzed.

2.6 Laboratory Testing Prior to Treatment Initiation

Measurement of baseline and periodic serum bicarbonate during Trokendi XR™ treatment is recommended [see Warnings and Precautions (5.3)].

2.7 Dosing Modifications in Patients Taking Phenytoin and/or Carbamazepine

The co-administration of Trokendi XR™ with phenytoin may require an adjustment of the dose of phenytoin to achieve optimal clinical outcome. Addition or withdrawal of phenytoin and/or carbamazepine during adjunctive therapy with Trokendi XR™ may require adjustment of the dose of Trokendi XR™.

2.8 Monitoring for Therapeutic Blood Levels

It is not necessary to monitor topiramate plasma concentrations to optimize Trokendi XR™ therapy.

2.9 Administration Instructions

Trokendi XR™ can be taken without regard to meals. Swallow capsule whole and intact. Do not sprinkle on food, chew or crush.

3 DOSAGE FORMS AND STRENGTHS

Trokendi XR™ (topiramate) extended-release capsules are available in the following strengths and colors:

25 mg: Size 2 capsules, light green opaque body/yellow opaque cap (printed "SPN" on the cap, "25" on the body)

50 mg: Size 0 capsules, light green opaque body/orange opaque cap (printed "SPN" on the cap, "50" on the body)

100 mg: Size 00 capsules, green opaque body/blue opaque cap (printed "SPN" on the cap, "100" on the body)

200 mg: Size 00 capsules, pink opaque body/blue opaque cap (printed "SPN" on the cap, "200" on the body)

4 CONTRAINDICATIONS

Trokendi XR™ is contraindicated in patients:

- With recent alcohol use (i.e., within 6 hours prior to and 6 hours after Trokendi XR™ use) [see Warnings and Precautions (5. 4)]
- With metabolic acidosis who are taking concomitant metformin [see Warnings and Precautions (5.3) and Drug Interactions (7.6)]

5 WARNINGS AND PRECAUTIONS

5.1 Acute Myopia and Secondary Angle Closure Glaucoma

A syndrome consisting of acute myopia associated with secondary angle closure glaucoma has been reported in patients receiving topiramate. Symptoms include acute onset of decreased visual acuity and/or ocular pain. Ophthalmologic findings can include myopia, anterior chamber shallowing, ocular hyperemia (redness) and increased intraocular pressure. Mydriasis may or may not be present. This syndrome may be associated with supraciliary effusion resulting in anterior displacement of the lens and iris, with secondary angle closure glaucoma. Symptoms typically occur within 1 month of initiating topiramate therapy. In contrast to primary narrow angle glaucoma, which is rare under 40 years of age, secondary angle closure glaucoma associated with topiramate has been reported in pediatric patients as well as adults. The primary treatment to reverse symptoms is discontinuation of Trokendi XR™ as rapidly as possible, according to the judgment of the treating physician. Other measures, in conjunction with discontinuation of Trokendi XR™, may be helpful.

Elevated intraocular pressure of any etiology, if left untreated, can lead to serious sequelae including permanent vision loss.

5.2 Oligohydrosis and Hyperthermia

Oligohydrosis (decreased sweating), resulting in hospitalization in some cases, has been reported in association with topiramate use. Decreased sweating and an elevation in body temperature above normal characterized these cases. Some of the cases were reported after exposure to elevated environmental temperatures.

The majority of the reports have been in pediatric patients. Patients, especially pediatric patients, treated with Trokendi XR™ should be monitored closely for evidence of decreased sweating and increased body temperature, especially in hot weather. Caution should be used when Trokendi XR™ is prescribed with other drugs that predispose patients to heat-related disorders; these drugs include, but are not limited to, other carbonic anhydrase inhibitors and drugs with anticholinergic activity.

5.3 Metabolic Acidosis

Hyperchloremic, non-anion gap, metabolic acidosis (i.e., decreased serum bicarbonate below the normal reference range in the absence of chronic respiratory alkalosis) is associated with topiramate, and can be expected with treatment with Trokendi XR™. This metabolic acidosis is caused by renal bicarbonate loss due to the inhibitory effect of topiramate on carbonic anhydrase. Such electrolyte imbalance has been observed with the use of topiramate in placebo-controlled clinical trials and in the post-marketing period. Generally, topiramate-induced metabolic acidosis occurs early in treatment although cases can occur at any time during treatment. Bicarbonate decrements are usually mild-moderate (average decrease of 4 mEq/L at daily doses of 400 mg in adults and at approximately 6 mg/kg/day in pediatric patients); rarely, patients can experience severe decrements to values below 10 mEq/L. Conditions or therapies that predispose patients to acidosis (such as renal disease, severe respiratory disorders, status epilepticus, diarrhea, ketogenic diet or specific drugs) may be additive to the bicarbonate lowering effects of topiramate.

Adults

In adults, the incidence of persistent treatment-emergent decreases in serum bicarbonate (levels of less than 20 mEq/L at two consecutive visits or at the final visit) in controlled clinical trials for adjunctive treatment of epilepsy was 32% for 400 mg per day, and 1% for placebo. Metabolic acidosis has been observed at doses as low as 50 mg per day. The incidence of persistent treatment-emergent decreases in serum bicarbonate in adults in the epilepsy controlled clinical trial for monotherapy was 15% for 50 mg per day and 25% for 400 mg per day. The incidence of a markedly abnormally low serum bicarbonate (i.e., absolute value less than 17 mEq/L and greater than 5 mEq/L decrease from pretreatment) in the adjunctive therapy trials was 3% for 400 mg per day, and 0% for placebo and in the monotherapy trial was 1% for 50 mg per day and 7% for 400 mg per day. Serum bicarbonate levels have not been systematically evaluated at daily doses greater than 400 mg per day.

Pediatric Patients (2 years to 16 years of age)

Although Trokendi XR™ is not approved for use in patients below the age of 6, the incidence of persistent treatment-emergent decreases in serum bicarbonate in placebo-controlled trials for adjunctive treatment of Lennox-Gastaut syndrome or refractory partial onset seizures in patients age 2 years to 16 years was 67% for topiramate (at approximately 6 mg/kg/day), and 10% for placebo. The incidence of a markedly abnormally low serum bicarbonate (i.e., absolute value less than17 mEq/L and greater than 5 mEq/L decrease from pretreatment) in these trials was 11% for topiramate and 0% for placebo. Cases of moderately severe metabolic acidosis have been reported in patients as young as 5 months old, especially at daily doses above 5 mg/kg/day.

In pediatric patients (6 years to 15 years of age), the incidence of persistent treatment-emergent decreases in serum bicarbonate in the epilepsy controlled clinical trial for monotherapy performed with topiramate was 9% for 50 mg per day and 25% for 400 mg per day. The incidence of a markedly abnormally low serum bicarbonate (i.e., absolute value less than 17 mEq/L and greater than 5 mEq/L decrease from pretreatment) in this trial was 1% for 50 mg per day and 6% for 400 mg per day.

Pediatric Patients (under 2 years of age)

Although Trokendi XR™ is not approved for use in patients less than 6 years of age with partial onset seizures, a study of topiramate as adjunctive use in patients under 2 years of age revealed that topiramate produced a metabolic acidosis that is notably greater in magnitude than that observed in controlled trials in older children and adults. The mean treatment difference (25 mg/kg/day topiramate-placebo) was -5.9 mEq/L for bicarbonate. The incidence of metabolic acidosis (defined by a serum bicarbonate less than 20 mEq/L) was 0% for placebo, 30% for 5 mg/kg/day, 50% for 15 mg/kg/day, and 45% for 25 mg/kg/day [see Use in Specific Populations(8.4)].

Manifestations of Metabolic Acidosis

Some manifestations of acute or chronic metabolic acidosis may include hyperventilation, nonspecific symptoms such as fatigue and anorexia, or more severe sequelae including cardiac arrhythmias or stupor. Chronic, untreated metabolic acidosis may increase the risk for nephrolithiasis or nephrocalcinosis, and may also result in osteomalacia (referred to as rickets in pediatric patients) and/or osteoporosis with an increased risk for fractures. Chronic metabolic acidosis in pediatric patients may also reduce growth rates. A reduction in growth rate may eventually decrease the maximal height achieved. The effect of topiramate on growth and bone-related sequelae has not been systematically investigated in long-term, placebo-controlled trials. Longterm, open-label treatment of infants/toddlers, with intractable partial epilepsy, for up to 1 year, showed reductions from baseline in Z SCORES for length, weight, and head circumference compared to age and sex-matched normative data, although these patients with epilepsy are likely to have different growth rates than normal infants. Reductions in Z SCORES for length and weight were correlated to the degree of acidosis [see Pediatric Use (8.4)]. Topiramate treatment that causes metabolic acidosis during pregnancy can possibly produce adverse effects on the fetus and might also cause metabolic acidosis in the neonate from possible transfer of topiramate to the fetus [see Warnings and Precautions (5.7) and Use in Specific Populations (8.1)].

Risk Mitigation Strategies

Measurement of baseline and periodic serum bicarbonate during topiramate treatment is recommended. If metabolic acidosis develops and persists, consideration should be given to reducing the dose or discontinuing topiramate (using dose tapering). If the decision is made to continue patients on topiramate in the face of persistent acidosis, alkali treatment should be considered.

5.4 Interaction with Alcohol

In vitro data show that, in the presence of alcohol, the pattern of topiramate release from Trokendi XR™ capsules is significantly altered. As a result, plasma levels of topiramate with Trokendi XR™ may be markedly higher soon after dosing and subtherapeutic later in the day. Therefore, alcohol use should be completely avoided within 6 hours prior to and 6 hours after Trokendi XR™ administration.

5.5 Suicidal Behavior and Ideation

Antiepileptic drugs (AEDs) increase the risk of suicidal thoughts or behavior in patients taking these drugs for any indication. Patients treated with any AED, including Trokendi XR™ for any indication should be monitored for the emergence or worsening of depression, suicidal thoughts or behavior, and/or any unusual changes in mood or behavior.

Pooled analyses of 199 placebo-controlled clinical trials (mono- and adjunctive therapy) of 11 different AEDs showed that patients randomized to one of the AEDs had approximately twice the risk (adjusted Relative Risk 1.8, 95% CI:1.2, 2.7) of suicidal thinking or behavior compared to patients randomized to placebo. In these trials, which had a median treatment duration of 12 weeks, the estimated incidence rate of suicidal behavior or ideation among 27,863 AED-treated patients was 0.43%, compared to 0.24% among 16,029 placebo-treated patients, representing an increase of approximately one case of suicidal thinking or behavior for every 530 patients treated. There were four suicides in drug-treated patients in the trials and none in placebo-treated patients, but the number is too small to allow any conclusion about drug effect on suicide.

The increased risk of suicidal thoughts or behavior with AEDs was observed as early as one week after starting drug treatment with AEDs and persisted for the duration of treatment assessed. Because most trials included in the analysis did not extend beyond 24 weeks, the risk of suicidal thoughts or behavior beyond 24 weeks could not be assessed.

The risk of suicidal thoughts or behavior was generally consistent among drugs in the data analyzed. The finding of increased risk with AEDs of varying mechanisms of action and across a range of indications suggests that the risk applies to all AEDs used for any indication. The risk did not vary substantially by age (5 to 100 years) in the clinical trials analyzed.

Table 1 shows absolute and relative risk by indication for all evaluated AEDs.

[See table 1 above]

The relative risk for suicidal thoughts or behavior was higher in clinical trials for epilepsy than in clinical trials for psychiatric or other conditions, but the absolute risk differences were similar for the epilepsy and psychiatric indications.

Anyone considering prescribing Trokendi XR™ or any other AED must balance the risk of suicidal thoughts or behavior with the risk of untreated illness. Epilepsy and many other illnesses for which AEDs are prescribed are themselves associated with morbidity and mortality and an increased risk of suicidal thoughts and behavior. Should suicidal thoughts and behavior emerge during treatment, the prescriber needs to consider whether the emergence of these symptoms in any given patient may be related to the illness being treated.

Patients, their caregivers, and families should be informed that AEDs increase the risk of suicidal thoughts and behavior and should be advised of the need to be alert for the emergence or worsening of the signs and symptoms of depression, any unusual changes in mood or behavior or the emergence of suicidal thoughts, behavior or thoughts about self-harm. Behaviors of concern should be reported immediately to healthcare providers.

5.6 Cognitive/Neuropsychiatric Adverse Reactions

Adverse reactions most often associated with the use of topiramate, and therefore expected to be associated with the use of Trokendi XR™ were related to the central nervous system and were observed in the epilepsy population. In adults, the most frequent of these can be classified into three general categories: 1) Cognitive-related dysfunction (e.g. confusion, psychomotor slowing, difficulty with concentration/attention, difficulty with memory, speech or language problems, particularly word-finding difficulties), 2) Psychiatric/behavioral disturbances (e.g. depression or mood problems), and 3) Somnolence or fatigue.

Adult Patients
Cognitive Related Dysfunction
The majority of cognitive-related adverse reactions were mild to moderate in severity, and they frequently occurred in isolation. Rapid titration rate and higher initial dose were associated with higher incidences of these reactions. Many of these reactions contributed to withdrawal from treatment [*see Adverse Reactions (6.1)*].

In the adjunctive epilepsy controlled trials conducted with topiramate (using rapid titration such as 100 mg per day to 200mg per day weekly increments), the proportion of patients who experienced one or more cognitive-related adverse reactions was 42% for 200mg per day, 41% for 400mg per day, 52% for 600mg per day, 56% for 800 and 1,000 mg per day, and 14% for placebo. These dose-related adverse reactions began with a similar frequency in the titration or in the maintenance phase, although in some patients the events began during titration and persisted into the maintenance phase. Some patients who experienced one or more cognitive-related adverse reactions in the titration phase had a dose-related recurrence of these reactions in the maintenance phase.

In the monotherapy epilepsy controlled trial conducted with topiramate, the proportion of patients who experienced one or more cognitive-related adverse reactions was 19% for topiramate 50mg per day and 26% for 400mg per day.
Psychiatric/Behavioral Disturbances
Psychiatric/behavioral disturbances (depression or mood) were dose-related for the epilepsy population treated with topiramate [*see Warnings and Precautions (5.6)*].
Somnolence/Fatigue
Somnolence and fatigue were the adverse reactions most frequently reported during clinical trials of topiramate for adjunctive epilepsy. For the adjunctive epilepsy population, the incidence of somnolence did not differ substantially between 200 mg per day and 1,000 mg per day, but the incidence of fatigue was dose-related and increased at dosages above 400 mg per day. For the monotherapy epilepsy population in the 50 mg per day and 400 mg per day groups, the incidence of somnolence was dose-related (9% for the 50 mg per day group and 15% for the 400 mg per day group) and the incidence of fatigue was comparable in both treatment

groups (14% each). For other uses not approved for Trokendi XR™, somnolence and fatigue were more common in the titration phase.

Additional nonspecific CNS events commonly observed with topiramate in the adjunctive epilepsy population include dizziness or ataxia.
Pediatric Patients
In double-blind adjunctive therapy and monotherapy epilepsy clinical studies conducted with topiramate, the incidences of cognitive/neuropsychiatric adverse reactions in pediatric patients were generally lower than observed in adults. These reactions included psychomotor slowing, difficulty with concentration/attention, speech disorders/related speech problems and language problems. The most frequently reported neuropsychiatric reactions in pediatric patients during adjunctive therapy double-blind studies were somnolence and fatigue. The most frequently reported neuropsychiatric reactions in pediatric patients in the 50 mg per day and 400 mg per day groups during the monotherapy double-blind study were headache, dizziness, anorexia, and somnolence.

No patients discontinued treatment due to any adverse events in the adjunctive epilepsy double-blind trials. In the monotherapy epilepsy double-blind trial conducted with immediate-release topiramate product, 1 pediatric patient (2%) in the 50 mg per day group and 7 pediatric patients (12%) in the 400 mg per day group discontinued treatment due to any adverse events. The most common adverse reaction associated with discontinuation of therapy was difficulty with concentration/attention; all occurred in the 400 mg per day group.
5.7 Fetal Toxicity
Topiramate can cause fetal harm when administered to a pregnant woman. Data from pregnancy registries indicate that infants exposed to topiramate *in utero* have an increased risk for cleft lip and/or cleft palate (oral clefts). When multiple species of pregnant animals received topiramate at clinically relevant doses, structural malformations, including craniofacial defects, and reduced fetal weights occurred in offspring [*see Use in Specific Populations (8.1)*].

Consider the benefits and risks of topiramate when administering the drug in women of childbearing potential, particularly when topiramate is considered for a condition not usually associated with permanent injury or death [*see Use in Specific Populations (8.9)*]. Topiramate should be used during pregnancy only if the potential benefit outweighs the potential risk. If this drug is used during pregnancy, or if the patient becomes pregnant while taking this drug, the patient should be informed of the potential hazard to a fetus [*see Use in Specific Populations (8.1) and (8.9)*].
5.8 Withdrawal of Antiepileptic Drugs
In patients with or without a history of seizures or epilepsy, antiepileptic drugs including Trokendi XR™ should be gradually withdrawn to minimize the potential for seizures or increased seizure frequency [*see Clinical Studies (14)*]. In situations where rapid withdrawal of Trokendi XR™ is medically required, appropriate monitoring is recommended.
5.9 Hyperammonemia and Encephalopathy
Hyperammonemia/Encephalopathy Without Concomitant Valproic Acid (VPA)
Topiramate treatment has produced hyperammonemia (in some instances dose-related) in clinical investigational programs in very young pediatric patients (1 month to 24 months) who were treated with adjunctive topiramate for partial onset epilepsy (8% for placebo, 10% for 5 mg/kg/day, 0% for 15 mg/kg/day, 9 % for 25 mg/kg/day). Trokendi XR™ is not approved as adjunctive treatment of partial onset seizures in pediatric patients less than 6 years old. In some patients, ammonia was markedly increased (greater than 50 % above upper limit of normal). The hyperammonemia associated with topiramate treatment occurred with and without encephalopathy in placebo-controlled trials, and in an open-label, extension trial. Dose-related hyperammonemia was also observed in the extension trial in pediatric patients up to 2 years old. Clinical symptoms of hyperammo-

nemic encephalopathy often include acute alterations in level of consciousness and/or cognitive function with lethargy or vomiting.

Hyperammonemia with and without encephalopathy has also been observed in post-marketing reports in patients who were taking topiramate without concomitant valproic acid (VPA).
Hyperammonemia/Encephalopathy With Concomitant Valproic Acid (VPA)
Concomitant administration of topiramate and valproic acid (VPA) has been associated with hyperammonemia with or without encephalopathy in patients who have tolerated either drug alone based upon post-marketing reports. Although hyperammonemia may be asymptomatic, clinical symptoms of hyperammonemic encephalopathy often include acute alterations in level of consciousness and/or cognitive function with lethargy or vomiting. In most cases, symptoms and signs abated with discontinuation of either drug. This adverse reaction is not due to a pharmacokinetic interaction.

Although Trokendi XR™ is not indicated for use in infants/toddlers (1month to 24 months), topiramate with concomitant VPA clearly produced a dose-related increase in the incidence of treatment-emergent hyperammonemia (above the upper limit of normal, 0% for placebo, 12% for 5 mg/kg/day, 7% for 15 mg/kg/day, 17% for 25 mg/kg/day) in an investigational program using topiramate. Markedly increased, dose-related hyperammonemia (0% for placebo and 5 mg/kg/day, 7% for 15 mg/kg/day, and 8% for 25 mg/kg/day) also occurred in these infants/toddlers. Dose-related hyperammonemia was similarly observed in a long-term, extension trial utilizing topiramate in these very young, pediatric patients [*see Use in Specific Populations (8.4)*].

Hyperammonemia with and without encephalopathy has also been observed in post-marketing reports in patients taking topiramate with valproic acid (VPA).

The hyperammonemia associated with topiramate treatment appears to be more common when used concomitantly with VPA.
Monitoring for Hyperammonemia
Patients with inborn errors of metabolism or reduced hepatic mitochondrial activity may be at an increased risk for hyperammonemia with or without encephalopathy. Although not studied, topiramate or Trokendi XR™ treatment or an interaction of concomitant topiramate-based product and valproic acid treatment may exacerbate existing defects or unmask deficiencies in susceptible persons.

In patients who develop unexplained lethargy, vomiting, or changes in mental status associated with any topiramate treatment, hyperammonemic encephalopathy should be considered and an ammonia level should be measured.
5.10 Kidney Stones
A total of 32/2086 (1.5%) of adults exposed to topiramate during its adjunctive epilepsy therapy development reported the occurrence of kidney stones, an incidence about 2 to 4 times greater than expected in a similar, untreated population. In the double-blind monotherapy epilepsy study, a total of 4/319 (1.3%) of adults exposed to topiramate reported the occurrence of kidney stones. As in the general population, the incidence of stone formation among topiramate treated patients was higher in men. Kidney stones have also been reported in pediatric patients. During long-term (up to 1 year) topiramate treatment in an open-label extension study of 284 pediatric patients 1 month to 24 months old with epilepsy, 7% developed kidney or bladder stones that were diagnosed clinically or by sonogram. Trokendi XR™ is not approved for pediatric patients less than 6 years old [*see Use in Specific Populations (8.4)*].

Trokendi XR™ would be expected to have the same effect as topiramate on the formation of kidney stones. An explanation for the association of topiramate and kidney stones may lay in the fact that topiramate is a carbonic anhydrase inhibitor. Carbonic anhydrase inhibitors (e.g., zonisamide, acetazolamide or dichlorphenamide) can promote stone formation by reducing urinary citrate excretion and by increasing urinary pH [*see Warnings and Precautions (5.9)*]. The concomitant use of Trokendi XR™ with any other drug produc-

Table 1: Risk by Indication for Antiepileptic Drugs in the Pooled Analysis

Indication	Placebo Patients with Events per 1,000 Patients	Drug Patients with Events per 1,000 Patients	Relative Risk: Incidence of Events in Drug Patients/ Incidence in Placebo Patients	Risk Difference: Additional Drug Patients with Events per 1,000 patients
Epilepsy	1.0	3.4	3.5	2.4
Psychiatric	5.7	8.5	1.5	2.9
Other	1.0	1.8	1.9	0.9
Total	2.4	4.3	1.8	1.9

ing metabolic acidosis, or potentially in patients on a keto-genic diet may create a physiological environment that increases the risk of kidney stone formation, and should therefore be avoided.

Increased fluid intake increases the urinary output, lowering the concentration of substances involved in stone formation. Hydration is recommended to reduce new stone formation.

5.11 Hypothermia with Concomitant Valproic Acid Use

Hypothermia, defined as an unintentional drop in body core temperature to less than 35°C (95°F) has been reported in association with topiramate use with concomitant valproic acid (VPA) both in the presence and in the absence of hyperammonemia. This adverse reaction in patients using concomitant topiramate and valproate can occur after starting topiramate treatment or after increasing the daily dose of topiramate [see Drug Interactions (7.5)]. Consideration should be given to stopping topiramate or valproate in patients who develop hypothermia, which may be manifested by a variety of clinical abnormalities including lethargy, confusion, coma, and significant alterations in other major organ systems such as the cardiovascular and respiratory systems. Clinical management and assessment should include examination of blood ammonia levels.

5.12 Paresthesia

Paresthesia (usually tingling of the extremities), an effect associated with the use of other carbonic anhydrase inhibitors, appears to be a common effect of topiramate. Paresthesia was more frequently reported in the monotherapy epilepsy trials conducted with topiramate than in the adjunctive therapy epilepsy trials conducted with the same product. In the majority of instances, paresthesia did not lead to treatment discontinuation.

5.13 Interaction with Other CNS Depressants

Topiramate is a CNS depressant. Concomitant administration of topiramate with other CNS depressant drugs can result in significant CNS depression. Patients should be watched carefully when Trokendi XR™ is co-administered with other CNS depressant drugs.

6 ADVERSE REACTIONS

The following adverse reactions are discussed in more detail in other sections of the labeling:
- Acute Myopia and Secondary Angle Closure [see Warnings and Precautions (5.1)]
- Oligohydrosis and Hyperthermia [see Warnings and Precautions (5.2)]
- Metabolic Acidosis [see Warnings and Precautions (5.3)]
- Suicidal Behavior and Ideation [see Warnings and Precautions (5.5)]
- Cognitive/Neuropsychiatric Adverse Reactions [see Warnings and Precautions (5.6)]
- Fetal Toxicity [see Warnings and Precautions (5.7)]
- Withdrawal of Antiepileptic Drugs [see Warnings and Precautions (5.8)]
- Hyperammonemia and Encephalopathy (Without and With Concomitant Valproic Acid Use [see Warnings and Precautions (5.9)]
- Kidney Stones [see Warnings and Precautions (5.10)]
- Hypothermia with Concomitant Valproic Acid Use [see Warnings and Precautions (5.11)]
- Paresthesia [see Warnings and Precautions (5.12)]

The data described in the following sections were obtained using immediate-release topiramate tablets in studies of patients with epilepsy. Trokendi XR™ has not been studied in a randomized, placebo-controlled Phase III clinical study in the epilepsy patient population. However, it is expected that Trokendi XR™ would produce a similar adverse reaction profile as immediate-release topiramate.

6.1 Clinical Trials Experience

Because clinical trials are conducted under widely varying conditions, adverse reaction rates observed in the clinical trials of a drug cannot be directly compared to rates in the clinical trials of another drug and may not reflect the rates observed in clinical practice.

Adverse Reactions Observed in Monotherapy Trial
Adults 17 Years and Older
The adverse reactions in the controlled trial (Study 1) that occurred most commonly in adults in the 400 mg per day group (incidence greater than or equal to 5%) and at a rate higher than the 50 mg per day group were paresthesia, weight decrease, somnolence, anorexia, dizziness, and difficulty with memory (see Table 2) [see Clinical Studies (14.2)]. Approximately 21% of the 159 adult patients in the 400 mg per day group who received topiramate as monotherapy in Study 1 discontinued therapy due to adverse reactions. The most common (greater than or equal to 2% more frequent than low-dose 50 mg per day topiramate) adverse reactions causing discontinuation in this trial were difficulty with memory, fatigue, asthenia, insomnia, somnolence and paresthesia.

Pediatric Patients 10 Years to 16 Years of Age
The adverse reactions in the controlled trial (Study 1) that occurred most commonly in children (10 years up to 16

years of age) in the 400 mg per day topiramate group (incidence greater than or equal to 5%) and at a rate higher than in the 50 mg per day group were weight decrease, upper respiratory tract infection, paresthesia, anorexia, diarrhea, and mood problems (see Table 3) [see Clinical Studies (14.2)].

Approximately 12% of the 57 pediatric patients in the 400 mg per day group who received topiramate as monotherapy in the controlled clinical trial discontinued therapy due to adverse reactions. The most common (greater than 5%) adverse reactions resulting in discontinuation in this trial were difficulty with concentration/attention.

Table 2: Incidence of Treatment-Emergent Adverse Reaction in the Monotherapy Epilepsy Trial in Adults* Where Incidence Was at Least 2% in the 400 mg/day Immediate-Release Topiramate Group and Greater Than the Rate in the 50 mg/day Immediate-Release Topiramate Group

Body System/	Immediate-release topiramate Dosage (mg/day)	
	50	400
Adverse Reaction	(N=160)	(N=159)
Body as a Whole-General Disorders		
Asthenia	4	6
Leg Pain	2	3
Chest Pain	1	2
Central & Peripheral Nervous System Disorders		
Paresthesia	21	40
Dizziness	13	14
Hypoasthesia	4	5
Ataxia	3	4
Hypertonia	0	3
Gastro-intestinal System Disorders		
Diarrhea	5	6
Constipation	1	4
Gastritis	0	3
Dry Mouth	1	3
Gastroesophogeal Reflux	1	2
Liver and Biliary System Disorders		
Gamma-GT Increased	1	3
Metabolic and Nutritional Disorders		
Weight Decrease	6	16
Psychiatric Disorders		
Somnolence	9	15
Anorexia	4	14
Difficulty with Memory NOS	5	10
Insomnia	8	9
Depression	7	9
Difficulty with Concentration/Attention	7	8
Anxiety	4	6
Pychomotor Slowing	3	5
Mood Problems	2	5
Confusion	3	4
Cognitive Problem NOS	1	4
Libido Decreased	0	3

Body System/	50	400
Reproductive Disorders, Female		
Vaginal Hemorrhage	0	3
Red Blood Cell Disorders		
Anemia	1	2
Resistance Mechanism Disorders		
Infection Viral	6	8
Infection	2	3
Respiratory System Disorders		
Bronchitis	3	4
Rhinitis	2	4
Dyspnea	1	2
Skin and Appendages Disorders		
Rash	1	4
Pruritus	1	4
Acne	2	3
Special Senses Other, Disorders		
Taste Perversion	3	5
Urinary System Disorders		
Cystitis	1	3
Renal Calculus	0	3
Urinary Tract Infection	1	2
Dysuria	0	2
Micturition Frequency	0	2

* Values represent the percentage of patients reporting a given adverse reaction. Patients may have reported more than one adverse reaction during the study and can be included in more than one adverse reaction category

Table 3: Incidence of Treatment-Emergent Adverse Reactions in the Monotherapy Epilepsy Trial in Pediatric Patients (Ages 10 up to 16 Years)* Where Incidence Was at Least 5% in the 400 mg/day Immediate-Release Topiramate Group and Greater than the Rate in the 50mg/day Immediate-Release Topiramate Group

Body System/	Immediate-release topiramate Dosage (mg/day)	
	50	400
Adverse Reaction	(N=57)	(N=57)
Body as a Whole-General Disorders		
Fever	0	9
Central & Peripheral Nervous System Disorders		
Paresthesia	2	16
Gastro-Intestinal System Disorders		
Diarrhea	5	11
Metabolic and Nutritional Disorders		
Weight Decrease	7	21
Psychiatric Disorders		
Anorexia	11	14
Mood Problems	2	11
Difficulty with Concentration/Attention	4	9
Cognitive Problem NOS	0	7
Nervousness	4	5

Resistance Mechanism Disorders

Infection Viral	4	9
Infection	2	7

Respiratory System Disorders

Upper Respiratory Tract Infection	16	18
Rhinitis	2	7
Bronchitis	2	7
Sinusitis	2	5

Skin and Appendages Disorders

Alopecia	2	5

* Values represent the percentage of patients reporting a given adverse event. Patients may have reported more than one adverse event during the study and can be included in more than one adverse event category

Adverse Reactions Observed in Adjunctive Therapy Epilepsy Trials

The most commonly observed adverse reactions associated with the use of topiramate at dosages of 200 to 400 mg per day in controlled trials in adults with partial onset seizures, primary generalized tonic-clonic seizures, or Lennox-Gastaut syndrome that were seen at greater frequency in topiramate-treated patients and did not appear to be dose-related were: somnolence, ataxia, speech disorders and related speech problems, psychomotor slowing, abnormal vision, difficulty with memory, paresthesia and diplopia [see Table 4] [see Clinical Studies (14.3, 14.4, and 14.5)]. The most common dose-related adverse reactions at dosages of 200 mg to 1,000 mg per day were: fatigue, nervousness, difficulty with concentration or attention, confusion, depression, anorexia, language problems, anxiety, mood problems, and weight decrease [see Table 6].

Adverse reactions associated with the use of topiramate at dosages of 5 mg/kg/day to 9 mg/kg/day in controlled trials in pediatric patients with partial onset seizures, primary generalized tonic-clonic seizures, or Lennox-Gastaut syndrome that were seen at greater frequency in topiramate-treated patients were: fatigue, somnolence, anorexia, nervousness, difficulty with concentration/attention, difficulty with memory, aggressive reaction [see Table 7]. In controlled clinical trials in adults, 11% of patients receiving topiramate 200 to 400mg per day as adjunctive therapy discontinued due to adverse reactions. This rate appeared to increase at dosages above 400mg per day. Adverse events associated with discontinuing therapy included somnolence, dizziness, anxiety, difficulty with concentration or attention, fatigue, and paresthesia at dosages above 400 mg per day. None of the pediatric patients who received topiramate adjunctive therapy at 5 mg/kg/day to 9 mg/kg/day in controlled clinical trials discontinued due to adverse reactions.

Approximately 28% of the 1757 adults with epilepsy who received topiramate at dosages of 200 mg to 1,600 mg per day in clinical studies discontinued treatment because of adverse reactions; an individual patient could have reported more than one adverse reaction. These adverse reactions were: psychomotor slowing (4.0%), difficulty with memory (3.2%), fatigue (3.2%), confusion (3.1%), somnolence (3.2%), difficulty with concentration/attention (2.9%), anorexia (2.7%), depression (2.6%), dizziness (2.5%), weight decrease (2.5%), nervousness (2.3%), ataxia (2.1%), and paresthesia (2.0%). Approximately 11% of the 310 pediatric patients who received topiramate at dosages up to 30 mg/kg/day discontinued due to adverse reactions. Adverse reactions associated with discontinuing therapy included aggravated convulsions (2.3%), difficulty with concentration/attention (1.6%), language problems (1.3%), personality disorder (1.3%), and somnolence (1.3%).

Incidence in Epilepsy Controlled Clinical Trials – Adjunctive Therapy – Partial Onset Seizures, Primary Generalized Tonic-Clonic Seizures, and Lennox-Gastaut Syndrome
Table 4 lists adverse reactions that occurred in at least 1% of adults treated with 200 to 400 mg per day topiramate in controlled trials that were numerically more common at this dose than in the patients treated with placebo. In general, most patients who experienced adverse reactions during the first eight weeks of these trials no longer experienced them by their last visit. Table 7 lists adverse reactions that occurred in at least 1% of pediatric patients treated with 5 mg/kg to 9 mg/kg topiramate in controlled trials that were numerically more common than in patients treated with placebo.

Other Adverse Reactions Observed During Double-Blind Epilepsy Adjunctive Therapy Trials
Other adverse reactions that occurred in more than 1% of adults treated with 200 mg to 400 mg of topiramate in placebo-controlled epilepsy trials but with equal or greater frequency in the placebo group were headache, injury, anxiety, rash, pain, convulsions aggravated, coughing, fever, diarrhea, vomiting, muscle weakness, insomnia, personality disorder, dysmenorrhea, upper respiratory tract infection, and eye pain.

Table 4: Incidence of Adverse Reactions in Placebo-Controlled, Adjunctive Epilepsy Trials in Adults *,†,‡

Body System/	Placebo	200-400	600-1,000
Adverse Reaction‡	(N=291)	(N=183)	(N=414)
Body as a Whole-General Disorders			
Fatigue	13	15	30
Asthenia	1	6	3
Back pain	4	5	3
Chest pain	3	4	2
Influenza-like symptoms	2	3	4
Leg pain	2	2	4
Hot flushes	1	2	1
Allergy	1	2	3
Edema	1	2	1
Body odor	0	1	0
Rigors	0	1	<1
Central & Peripheral Nervous System Disorders			
Dizziness	15	25	32
Ataxia	7	16	14
Speech disorders/Related speech problems	2	13	11
Paresthesia	4	11	19
Nystagmus	7	10	11
Tremor	6	9	9
Language problems	1	6	10
Coordination abnormal	2	4	4
Hypoaesthesia	1	2	1
Gait abnormal	1	3	2
Muscle contractions involuntary	1	2	2
Stupor	0	2	1
Vertigo	1	1	2
Gastro-intestinal System Disorders			
Nausea	8	10	12
Dyspepsia	6	7	6
Abdominal pain	4	6	7
Constipation	2	4	3
Gastroenteritis	1	2	1
Dry mouth	1	2	4
Gingivitis	<1	1	1
GI disorder	<1	1	0
Hearing and Vestibular Disorders			
Hearing decreased	1	2	1
Metabolic and Nutritional Disorders			
Weight decrease	3	9	13
Musculo-Skeletal System Disorders			
Myalgia	1	2	2
Skeletal pain	0	1	0
Platelet, Bleeding & Clotting Disorders			
Epistaxis	1	2	1
Psychiatric Disorders			
Somnolence	12	29	28
Nervousness	6	16	19
Psychomotor slowing	2	13	21
Difficulty with memory	3	12	14
Anorexia	4	10	12
Confusion	5	11	14
Depression	5	5	13
Difficulty with concentration/attention	2	6	14
Mood problems	2	4	9
Agitation	2	3	3
Aggressive reaction	2	3	3
Emotional liability	1	3	3
Cognitive problems	1	3	3
Libido decreased	1	2	<1
Apathy	1	1	3
Depersonalization	1	1	2
Reproductive Disorders, Female			
Breast pain	2	4	0
Amenorrhea	1	2	2
Menorrhagia	0	2	1
Menstrual disorder	1	2	1
Reproductive Disorders, Male			
Prostatic disorder	<1	2	0
Resistance Mechanism Disorders			
Infection	1	2	1
Infection viral	1	2	<1
Moniliasis	<1	1	0
Respiratory System Disorders			
Pharyngitis	2	6	3
Rhinitis	6	7	6
Sinusitis	4	5	6
Dyspnea	1	1	2
Skin and Appendages Disorders			
Skin disorder	<1	2	1
Sweating increased	<1	1	<1
Rash, erythematous	<1	1	<1
Special Senses Other, Disorders			
Taste perversion	0	2	4
Urinary System Disorders			
Hematuria	1	2	<1

Table 6: Incidence (%) of Dose-Related Adverse Reactions From Placebo-Controlled, Adjunctive Trials in Adults With Partial Onset Seizures (Studies 2 through 7)*

Adverse Reaction	Placebo	(Topiramate) Dosage (mg per day) 200	400	600-1,000
	(N=216)	(N=45)	(N=68)	(N=414)
Fatigue	13	11	12	30
Nervousness	7	13	18	19
Difficulty with concentration/attention	1	7	9	14
Confusion	4	9	10	14
Depression	6	9	7	13
Anorexia	4	4	6	12
Language Problems	<1	2	9	10
Anxiety	6	2	3	10
Mood Problems	2	0	6	9
Weight Decrease	3	4	9	13

* Dose-response studies were not conducted for other adult indications or for pediatric indications

Urinary tract infection	1	2	3
Micturition frequency	1	1	2
Urinary incontinence	<1	2	1
Urine abnormal	0	1	<1

Vision Disorders

Vision abnormal	2	13	10
Diplopia	5	10	10

White Cell and RES Disorders

Leukopenia	1	2	1

* Patients in these adjunctive trials were receiving 1 to 2 concomitant antiepileptic drugs in addition to topiramate or placebo
† Values represent the percentage of patients reporting a given reaction. Patient may have reported more than one adverse reaction during the study and can be included in more than one adverse reaction category.
‡ Adverse reactions reported by at least 1% of patients in the topiramate 200 mg to 400 mg per day group and more common than in the placebo group

Adverse Reactions Observed in Adjunctive Therapy Trial in Adults with Partial Onset Seizures (Study 7)
Study 7 was a randomized, double-blind, adjunctive, placebo-controlled, parallel group study with 3 treatment arms: 1) placebo; 2) topiramate 200 mg per day with a 25 mg per day starting dose, increased by 25 mg per day each week for 8 weeks until the 200 mg per day maintenance dose was reached; and 3) topiramate 200 mg per day with a 50 mg per day starting dose, increased by 50 mg per day each week for 4 weeks until the 200 mg per day maintenance dose was reached. All patients were maintained on concomitant carbamazepine with or without another concomitant antiepileptic drug.
The incidence of adverse reactions (Table 5) did not differ significantly between the 2 topiramate regimens. Because the frequencies of adverse reactions reported in this study were markedly lower than those reported in the previous epilepsy studies, they cannot be directly compared with data obtained in other studies.

Table 5: Incidence of Adverse Reactions in Study 7*,†,‡

Body System/ Adverse Reaction‡	Placebo	Topiramate Dosage (mg per day) 200
	(N=92)	(N=171)
Body as a Whole-General Disorders		
Fatigue	4	9

Chest pain	1	2
Cardiovasular Disorders, General		
Hypertension	0	2
Central & Peripheral Nervous System Disorders		
Paresthesia	2	9
Dizziness	4	7
Tremor	2	3
Hypoesthesia	0	2
Leg cramps	0	2
Language problems	0	2
Gastro-intestinal System Disorders		
Abdominal pain	3	5
Constipation	0	4
Diarrhea	1	2
Dyspepsia	0	2
Dry mouth	0	2
Hearing and Vestibular Disorders		
Tinnitus	0	2
Metabolic and Nutritional Disorders		
Weight decrease	4	8
Psychiatric Disorders		
Somnolence	9	15
Anorexia	7	9
Nervousness	2	9
Difficulty with concentration/attention	0	5
Insomnia	3	4
Difficulty with memory	1	2
Aggressive reaction	0	2
Respiratory System Disorders		
Rhinitis	0	4

Urinary System Disorders		
Cystitis	0	2
Vision Disorder		
Diplopia	0	2
Vision abnormal	0	2

* Patients in these adjunctive trials were receiving 1 to 2 concomitant antiepileptic drugs in addition to topiramate or placebo
† Values represent the percentage of patients reporting a given adverse reaction. Patients may have reported more than one adverse reaction during the study and can be included in more than one adverse reaction category
‡ Adverse reactions reported by at least 2% of patients in the topiramate 200 mg per day group and more common than in the placebo group

[See table 6 above]

Table 7: Incidence (%) of Adverse Reaction in Placebo-Controlled, Adjunctive Epilepsy Trial in Pediatric Patients (Ages 2 Years to 16 Years)*,†,‡ (Study 8)

Body System/ Adverse Reaction	Placebo (N=101)	Topiramate (N=98)
Body as a Whole-General Disorders		
Fatigue	5	16
Injury	13	14
Allergic reaction	1	2
Back pain	0	1
Pallor	0	1
Cardiovascular Disorders, General		
Hypertension	0	1
Central & Peripheral Nervous System Disorders		
Gait abnormal	5	8
Ataxia	2	6
Hyperkinesia	4	5
Dizziness	2	4
Speech disorders/Related speech problems	2	4
Hyporeflexia	0	2
Convulsions grand mal	0	1
Fecal incontinence	0	1
Paresthesia	0	1
Gastro-Intestinal System Disorders		
Nausea	5	6
Saliva increased	4	6
Constipation	4	5
Gastroenteritis	2	3
Dysphagia	0	1
Flatulence	0	1
Gastroesophageal reflux	0	1
Glossitis	0	1
Gum hyperplasia	0	1
Heart Rate and Rhythm Disorders		
Bradycardia	0	1
Metabolic and Nutritional Disorders		
Weight decrease	1	9

Thirst	1	2
Hypoglycemia	0	1
Weight increase	0	1
Platelet, Bleeding & Clotting Disorders		
Purpura	4	8
Epistaxis	1	4
Hematoma	0	1
Prothrombin increased	0	1
Thrombocytopenia	0	1
Psychiatric Disorders		
Somnolence	16	26
Anorexia	15	24
Nervousness	7	14
Personality disorder (Behavior Problems)	9	11
Difficulty with concentration/attention	2	10
Aggressive reaction	4	9
Insomnia	7	8
Difficulty with memory	0	5
Confusion	3	4
Psychomotor slowing	2	3
Appetite increased	0	1
Neurosis	0	1
Reproductive Disorders, Female		
Leukorrhea	0	2
Resistance Mechanism Disorders		
Infection viral	3	7
Respiratory System Disorders		
Pneumonia	1	5
Respiratory disorder	0	1
Skin and Appendages Disorders		
Skin Disorder	2	3
Alopecia	1	2
Dermatitis	0	2
Hypertrichosis	1	2
Rash erythematous	0	2
Eczema	0	1
Seborrhea	0	1
Skin discoloration	0	1
Urinary System Disorders		
Urinary incontinence	2	4
Nocturia	0	1
Vision Disorders		
Eye abnormality	1	2
Vision abnormal	1	2
Diplopia	0	1
Lacrimation abnormal	0	1
Myopia	0	1

White Cell and RES Disorders

Leukopenia	0	2

* Patients in these adjunctive trials were receiving 1 to 2 concomitant antiepileptic drugs in addition to topiramate or placebo

† Values represent the percentage of patients reporting a given adverse reaction. Patients may have reported more than one adverse reaction during the study and can be included in more than one adverse reaction category

‡ Reactions that Occurred in at Least 1% of Topiramate-Treated Patients and Occurred More Frequently in Topiramate-Treated Than Placebo-Treated Patients

Laboratory Abnormalities
Topiramate decreases serum bicarbonate [*see Warnings and Precautions (5.3)*]
Immediate-release topiramate treatment was associated with changes in several clinical laboratory analytes in randomized, double-blind, placebo-controlled studies. Similar effects should be anticipated with use of Trokendi XR™.
Controlled trials of adjunctive topiramate treatment of adults for partial onset seizures showed an increased incidence of markedly decreased serum phosphorus (6% topiramate, 2% placebo), markedly increased serum alkaline phosphatase (3% topiramate, 1% placebo), and decreased serum potassium (0.4 % topiramate, 0.1 % placebo). The clinical significance of these abnormalities has not been clearly established.
Changes in several clinical laboratory results (increased creatinine, BUN, alkaline phosphatase, total protein, total eosinophil count and decreased potassium) have been observed in a clinical investigational program in very young (2 years and younger) pediatric patients who were treated with adjunctive topiramate for partial onset seizures [*see Use in Specific Populations (8.4)*].
Topiramate treatment produced a dose-related increased shift in serum creatinine from normal at baseline to an increased value at the end of 4 months treatment in adolescent patients (ages 12 years to 16 years) in a double-blind, placebo-controlled study. The incidence of these abnormal shifts was 4% for placebo, 4% for 50 mg, and 18% for 100 mg.
Topiramate treatment with or without concomitant valproic acid (VPA) can cause hyperammonemia with or without encephalopathy [*see Warnings and Precautions (5.9)*].

6.2   Postmarketing Experience
The following adverse reactions have been identified during post-approval use of topiramate. Because these reactions are reported voluntarily from a population of uncertain size, it is not always possible to reliably estimate their frequency or establish a causal relationship to drug exposure. The listing is alphabetized: bullous skin reactions (including erythema multiforme, Stevens-Johnson syndrome, toxic epidermal necrolysis), hepatic failure (including fatalities), hepatitis, maculopathy, pancreatitis, and pemphigus.

7   DRUG INTERACTIONS
7.1   Alcohol
Alcohol use is contraindicated within 6 hours prior to and 6 hours after Trokendi XR™ administration [*see Contraindications (4) and Warnings and Precautions (5.4)*].
7.2   Oral Contraceptives
Exposure to ethinyl estradiol was statistically significantly decreased when topiramate (at doses above 200 mg) was given as adjunctive therapy in patients taking valproic acid. However, norethindrone exposure was not significantly affected.
In another pharmacokinetic interaction study in healthy volunteers with a concomitantly administered combination oral contraceptive product containing 1 mg norethindrone (NET) plus 35 mcg ethinyl estradiol (EE), topiramate, given in the absence of other medications at doses of 50 to 200 mg per day, was not associated with statistically significant changes in mean exposure to either component of the oral contraceptive.
The possibility of decreased contraceptive efficacy and increased breakthrough bleeding should be considered in patients taking combination oral contraceptive products with Trokendi XR™. Patients taking estrogen-containing contraceptives should be asked to report any change in their bleeding patterns. Contraceptive efficacy can be decreased even in the absence of breakthrough bleeding [*see Clinical Pharmacology (12.3)*].
7.3   Antiepileptic Drugs
Concomitant administration of phenytoin or carbamazepine with topiramate decreased plasma concentrations of topiramate [*see Clinical Pharmacology (12.3)*].
Concomitant administration of valproic acid and topiramate has been associated with hyperammonemia with and with-

out encephalopathy. Concomitant administration of topiramate with valproic acid has also been associated with hypothermia (with and without hyperammonemia) in patients who have tolerated either drug alone. It may be prudent to examine blood ammonia levels in patients in whom the onset of hypothermia has been reported [*see Warnings and Precautions (5.8), (5.10)and Clinical Pharmacology (12.3)*].
Numerous AEDs are substrates of the CYP enzyme system. *In vitro* studies indicate that topiramate does not inhibit enzyme activity for CYP1A2, CYP2A6, CYP2B6, CYP2C9, CYP2D6, CYP2E1, and CYP3A4/5 isozymes. *In vitro* studies indicate that immediate-release topiramate is a mild inhibitor of CYP2C19 and a mild inducer of CYP3A4. The same drug interactions can be expected with the use of Trokendi XR™.
7.4   CNS Depressants
Topiramate is a CNS depressant. Concomitant administration of topiramate with other CNS depressant drugs or alcohol can result in significant CNS depression [*see Warnings and Precautions (5.13)*].
7.5   Other Carbonic Anhydrase Inhibitors
Concomitant use of topiramate, a carbonic anhydrase inhibitor, with any other carbonic anhydrase inhibitor (e.g., zonisamide, acetazolamide or dichlorphenamide), may increase the severity of metabolic acidosis and may also increase the risk of kidney stone formation. Patient should be monitored for the appearance or worsening of metabolic acidosis when Trokendi XR™ is given concomitantly with another carbonic anhydrase inhibitor [*see Clinical Pharmacology (12.3)*].
7.6   Metformin
Topiramate treatment can frequently cause metabolic acidosis, a condition for which the use of metformin is contraindicated. The concomitant use of Trokendi XR™ and metformin is contraindicated in patients with metabolic acidosis. [*see Clinical Pharmacology (12.3)*].
7.7   Lithium
In patients, there was an observed increase in systemic exposure of lithium following topiramate doses of up to 600 mg per day. Lithium levels should be monitored when co-administered with high-dose Trokendi XR™ [*see Clinical Pharmacology (12.3)*].

8   USE IN SPECIFIC POPULATIONS
8.1   Pregnancy
Pregnancy Category D [*see Warnings and Precautions (5.7)*]
Topiramate can cause fetal harm when administered to a pregnant woman. Data from pregnancy registries indicate that infants exposed to topiramate *in utero* have increased risk for cleft lip and/or cleft palate (oral clefts). When multiple species of pregnant animals received topiramate at clinically relevant doses, structural malformations, including craniofacial defects, and reduced fetal weights occurred in offspring. Topiramate should be used during pregnancy only if the potential benefit outweighs the potential risk. If this drug is used during pregnancy, or if the patient becomes pregnant while taking this drug, the patient should be informed of the potential hazard to the fetus [*see Use in Specific Populations (8.9)*].
Pregnancy Registry
Patients should be encouraged to enroll in the North American Antiepileptic Drug (NAAED) Pregnancy Registry if they become pregnant. This registry is collecting information about the safety of antiepileptic drugs during pregnancy. To enroll, patients can call the toll-free number 1-888-233-2334. Information about the North American Drug Pregnancy Registry can be found at *http://www.massgeneral.org/aed/*.
Human Data
Data from the NAAED Pregnancy Registry indicate an increased risk of oral clefts in infants exposed to topiramate monotherapy during the first trimester of pregnancy. The prevalence of oral clefts was 1.2% compared to a prevalence of 0.39% - 0.46% in infants exposed to other AEDs, and a prevalence of 0.12% in infants of mothers without epilepsy, or treatment with other AEDs. For comparison, the Centers for Disease Control and Prevention (CDC) reviewed available data on oral clefts in the United States and found a similar background rate of 0.17%. The relative risk of oral clefts in topiramate-exposed pregnancies in the NAAED Pregnancy Registry was 9.6 (95% Confidence Interval=CI 3.6-25.7) as compared to the risk in a background population of untreated women. The UK Epilepsy and Pregnancy Register reported a similarly increased prevalence of oral clefts of 3.2% among infants exposed to topiramate monotherapy. The observed rate of oral clefts was 16 times higher than the background rate in the UK, which is approximately 0.2%.
Topiramate treatment can cause metabolic acidosis (*see Warnings and Precautions (5.3)*). The effect of topiramate-induced metabolic acidosis has not been studied in pregnancy; however, metabolic acidosis in pregnancy (due to other causes) can cause decreased fetal growth, decreased fetal oxygenation, and fetal death, and may affect the fetus' ability to tolerate labor. Pregnant patients should be monitored for metabolic acidosis and treated as in the nonpregnant state [*see Warnings and Precautions (5.3)*]. Newborns

of mothers treated with topiramate should be monitored for metabolic acidosis because of transfer of topiramate to the fetus and possible occurrence of transient metabolic acidosis following birth.

Animal Data

Topiramate has demonstrated selective developmental toxicity, including teratogenicity, in multiple animal species at clinically relevant doses. When oral doses of 20 mg/kg, 100 mg/kg, or 500 mg/kg were administered to pregnant mice during the period of organogenesis, the incidence of fetal malformations (primarily craniofacial defects) was increased at all doses. The low dose is approximately 0.2 times the recommended human dose (RHD) 400mg per day on a mg/m² basis. Fetal body weights and skeletal ossification were reduced at 500 mg/kg in conjunction with decreased maternal body weight gain.

In rat studies (oral doses of 20 mg/kg, 100 mg/kg, and 500 mg/kg or 0.2 mg/kg, 2.5 mg/kg, 30 mg/kg, and 400 mg/kg), the frequency of limb malformations (ectrodactyly, micromelia, and amelia) was increased among the offspring of dams treated with 400 mg/kg (10 times the RHD on a mg/m² basis) or greater during the organogenesis period of pregnancy. Embryotoxicity (reduced fetal body weights, increased incidence of structural variations) was observed at doses as low as 20 mg/kg (0.5 times the RHD on a mg/m² basis). Clinical signs of maternal toxicity were seen at 400 mg/kg and above, and maternal body weight gain was reduced during treatment with 100 mg/kg or greater.

In rabbit studies (20 mg/kg, 60 mg/kg, and 180 mg/kg or 10 mg/kg, 35 mg/kg, and 120 mg/kg orally during organogenesis), embryo/fetal mortality was increased at 35 mg/kg (2 times the RHD on a mg/m² basis) or greater, and teratogenic effects (primarily rib and vertebral malformations) were observed at 120 mg/kg (6 times the RHD on a mg/m² basis). Evidence of maternal toxicity (decreased body weight gain, clinical signs, and/or mortality) was seen at 35 mg/kg and above.

When female rats were treated during the latter part of gestation and throughout lactation (0.2 mg/kg, 4 mg/kg, 20 mg/kg, and 100 mg/kg or 2, 20, and 200 mg/kg), offspring exhibited decreased viability and delayed physical development at 200 mg/kg (5 times the RHD on a mg/m² basis) and reductions in pre-and/or postweaning body weight gain at 2mg/kg (0.05 times the RHD on a mg/m² basis) and above. Maternal toxicity (decreased body weight gain, clinical signs) was evident at 100 mg/kg or greater.

In a rat embryo/fetal development study with a postnatal component (0.2 mg/kg, 2.5 mg/kg, 30 mg/kg, or 400mg/kg during organogenesis; noted above), pups exhibited delayed physical development at 400 mg/kg (10 times the RHD on a mg/m² basis) and persistent reductions in body weight gain at 30 mg/kg (1 times the RHD on a mg/m² basis) and higher.

8.2   Labor and Delivery

Although the effect of topiramate on labor and delivery in humans has not been established, the development of topiramate-induced metabolic acidosis in the mother and/or in the fetus might affect the fetus' ability to tolerate labor [*see Use in Specific Populations (8.1)*].

8.3   Nursing Mothers

Limited data on 5 breastfeeding infants exposed to topiramate showed infant plasma topiramate levels equal to 10-20% of the maternal plasma level. The effects of this exposure on infants are unknown. Caution should be exercised when Trokendi XR™ is administered to a nursing woman.

8.4   Pediatric Use

Seizures in Pediatric Patients 6 Years of Age and Older

Because the capsule must be swallowed whole, and may not be sprinkled on food, crushed or chewed, Trokendi XR™ is recommended only for children age 6 or older.

The safety and effectiveness of Trokendi XR™ in pediatric patients is based on controlled trials with immediate-release topiramate [*see Clinical Studies (14)*].

The adverse reactions (both common and serious) in pediatric patients are similar to those seen in adults [*see Warnings and Precautions (5) and Adverse Reactions (6)*].

These include, but are not limited to:

- oligohydrosis and hyperthermia [*see Warnings and Precautions (5.2)*].
- dose-related increased incidence of metabolic acidosis [*see Warnings and Precautions (5.3)*].
- dose-related increased incidence of hyperammonemia [*see Warnings and Precautions (5.9)*].

Adjunctive Treatment for Partial Onset Epilepsy in Infants and Toddlers (1 to 24 months)

The following pediatric use information is based on studies conducted with immediate-release topiramate.

Safety and effectiveness in patients below the age of 2 years have not been established for the adjunctive therapy treatment of partial onset seizures, primary generalized tonic-clonic seizures, or seizures associated with Lennox-Gastaut syndrome. In a single randomized, double-blind, placebo-controlled investigational trial, the efficacy, safety, and tolerability of immediate-release topiramate oral liquid and

sprinkle formulations as an adjunct to concurrent antiepileptic drug therapy in infants 1 to 24 months of age with refractory partial onset seizures, was assessed. After 20 days of double-blind treatment, immediate-release topiramate (at fixed doses of 5 mg/kg, 15 mg/kg, and 25 mg/kg per day) did not demonstrate efficacy compared with placebo in controlling seizures.

In general, the adverse reaction profile in this population was similar to that of older pediatric patients, although results from the above controlled study, and an open-label, long-term extension study in these infants/toddlers (1 to 24 months old) suggested some adverse reactions not previously observed in older pediatric patients and adults; i.e., growth/length retardation, certain clinical laboratory abnormalities, and other adverse reactions that occurred with a greater frequency and/or greater severity than had been recognized previously from studies in older pediatric patients or adults for various indications.

These very young pediatric patients appeared to experience an increased risk for infections (any topiramate dose 12%, placebo 0%) and of respiratory disorders (any topiramate dose 40%, placebo 16%). The following adverse reactions were observed in at least 3% of patients on immediate-release topiramate and were 3% to 7% more frequent than in patients on placebo: viral infection, bronchitis, pharyngitis, rhinitis, otitis media, upper respiratory infection, cough, and bronchospasm. A generally similar profile was observed in older children [*see Adverse Reactions (6)*].

Immediate-release topiramate resulted in an increased incidence of patients with increased creatinine (any topiramate dose 5%, placebo 0%), BUN (any topiramate dose 3%, placebo 0%), and protein (any topiramate dose 34%, placebo 6%), and an increased incidence of decreased potassium (any topiramate dose 7%, placebo 0%). This increased frequency of abnormal values was not dose related. Creatinine was the only analyte showing a noteworthy increased incidence (topiramate 25 mg/kg/day 5%, placebo 0%) of a markedly abnormal increase [*see Adverse Reactions (6.1)*]. The significance of these findings is uncertain. Immediate-release topiramate treatment also produced a dose-related increase in the percentage of patients who had a shift from normal at baseline to high/increased (above the normal reference range) in total eosinophil count at the end of treatment. The incidence of these abnormal shifts was 6 % for placebo, 10% for 5 mg/kg/day, 9% for 15 mg/kg/day, 14% for 25 mg/kg/day, and 11% for any topiramate dose [*see Adverse Reactions (6.1)*]. There was a mean dose-related increase in alkaline phosphatase. The significance of these findings is uncertain.

Treatment with immediate-release topiramate for up to 1 year was associated with reductions in Z SCORES for length, weight, and head circumference [*see Warnings and Precautions (5.3) and Adverse Reactions (6)*].

In open-label, uncontrolled experience, increasing impairment of adaptive behavior was documented in behavioral testing over time in this population. There was a suggestion that this effect was dose-related. However, because of the absence of an appropriate control group, it is not known if this decrement in function was treatment related or reflects the patient's underlying disease (e.g., patients who received higher doses may have more severe underlying disease) [*see Warnings and Precautions (5.6)*].

In this open-label, uncontrolled study, the mortality was 37 deaths/1000 patient years. It is not possible to know whether this mortality rate is related to immediate-release topiramate treatment, because the background mortality rate for a similar, significantly refractory, young pediatric population (1month to 24 months) with partial epilepsy is not known.

Other Pediatric Studies

Topiramate treatment produced a dose-related increased shift in serum creatinine from normal at baseline to an increased value at the end of 4 months treatment in adolescent patients (ages 12 years to 16 years) in a double-blind, placebo-controlled study [*see Adverse Reactions (6.1)*].

Juvenile Animal Studies

When topiramate (30 mg/kg/day, 90 mg/kg/day or 300 mg/kg/day) was administered orally to rats during the juvenile period of development (postnatal days 12 to 50), bone growth plate thickness was reduced in males at the highest dose, which is approximately 5 to 8 times the maximum recommended pediatric dose 9 mg/kg/day) on a body surface area (mg/m²) basis.

8.5   Geriatric Use

Clinical studies of immediate-release topiramate did not include sufficient numbers of subjects aged 65 and over to determine whether they respond differently than younger subjects. Dosage adjustment is necessary for elderly with creatinine clearance less than 70 mL/min/1.73 m². Estimate GFR should be measured prior to dosing [*see Dosage and Administration (2) and Clinical Pharmacology (12.3)*].

8.6   Race and Gender Effects

Evaluation of effectiveness and safety of topiramate in clinical trials has shown no race- or gender-related effects.

8.7   Renal Impairment

The clearance of topiramate was reduced by 42% in moderately renally impaired (creatinine clearance 30 to 69 mL/min/1.73m²) and by 54% in severely renally impaired subjects (creatinine clearance less than 30 mL/min/1.73m²) compared to normal renal function subjects (creatinine clearance greater than70 mL/min/1.73m²). One-half the usual starting and maintenance dose is recommended in patients with moderate or severe renal impairment [*see Dosage and Administration (2.4) and Clinical Pharmacology (12.3)*].

8.8   Patients Undergoing Hemodialysis

Topiramate is cleared by hemodialysis at a rate that is 4 to 6 times greater than a normal individual. Accordingly, a prolonged period of dialysis may cause topiramate concentration to fall below that required to maintain an anti-seizure effect. To avoid rapid drops in topiramate plasma concentration during hemodialysis, a supplemental dose of topiramate may be required. The actual adjustment should take into account the duration of dialysis period, the clearance rate of the dialysis system being used, and the effective renal clearance of topiramate in the patient being dialyzed [*see Dosage and Administration (2.5) and Clinical Pharmacology (12.3)*].

8.9   Women of Childbearing Potential

Data from pregnancy registries indicate that infants exposed to topiramate *in utero* have an increased risk for cleft lip and/or cleft palate (oral clefts) [*see Warnings and Precautions (5.7) and Use in Specific Populations (8.1)*]. Consider the benefits and risks of topiramate when prescribing this drug to women of childbearing potential, particularly when topiramate is considered for a condition not usually associated with permanent injury or death. Because of the risk of oral clefts to the fetus, which occur in the first trimester of pregnancy before many women know they are pregnant, all women of childbearing potential should be apprised of the potential hazard to the fetus from exposure to topiramate. If the decision is made to use topiramate, women who are not planning a pregnancy would use effective contraception [*see Drug Interactions (7.2)*] Women who are planning a pregnancy would be counseled regarding the relative risks and benefits of topiramate use during pregnancy, and alternative therapeutic options should be considered for these patients.

9   DRUG ABUSE AND DEPENDENCE

9.1   Controlled Substance

Trokendi XR™ (topiramate) extended-release capsule is not a controlled substance.

9.2   Abuse

The abuse and dependence potential of Trokendi XR™ has not been evaluated in human studies.

9.3   Dependence

Trokendi XR™ has not been systematically studied in animals or humans for its potential for tolerance or physical dependence.

10   OVERDOSAGE

Overdoses of topiramate resulted in signs and symptoms which included convulsions, drowsiness, speech disturbance, blurred vision, diplopia, mentation impaired, lethargy, abnormal coordination, stupor, hypotension, abdominal pain, agitation, dizziness and depression. The clinical consequences were not severe in most cases, but deaths have been reported after polydrug overdoses involving topiramate.

Topiramate overdose has resulted in severe metabolic acidosis [*see Warnings and Precautions (5.3)*].

A patient who ingested a dose between 96 g and 110 g of topiramate was admitted to hospital with coma lasting 20 to 24 hours followed by full recovery after 3 to 4 days.

Similar signs, symptoms, and clinical consequences are expected to occur with overdosage of Trokendi XR™. Therefore, in acute Trokendi XR™ overdose, if the ingestion is recent, the stomach should be emptied immediately by lavage or by induction of emesis. Activated charcoal has been shown to adsorb topiramate *in vitro*. Treatment should be appropriately supportive. Hemodialysis is an effective means of removing topiramate from the body.

11   DESCRIPTION

Topiramate, USP, is a sulfamate-substituted monosaccharide. Trokendi XR™ (topiramate) extended-release capsules are available as 25 mg, 50 mg, 100 mg and 200 mg capsules for oral administration.

Topiramate is a white to off-white powder. Topiramate is freely soluble in polar organic solvents such as acetonitrile and acetone; and very slightly soluble to practically insoluble in non-polar organic solvents such as hexanes. Topiramate has the molecular formula $C_{12}H_{21}NO_8S$ and a molecular weight of 339.4. Topiramate is designated chemically as 2,3:4,5-Di-*O*-isopropylidene-β-D-fructopyranose sulfamate and has the following structural formula:

Trokendi XR™ (topiramate) is an extended-release capsule. Trokendi XR™ capsules contain the following inactive ingredients:

Sugar Spheres, NF
Hypromellose (Type 2910), USP
Mannitol, USP
Docusate Sodium, USP
Sodium Benzoate, NF
Ethylcellulose, NF
Oleic Acid, NF
Medium Chain Triglycerides, NF
Polyethylene Glycol, NF
Polyvinyl Alcohol, USP
Titanium Dioxide, USP
Talc, USP
Lecithin, NF
Xanthan Gum, NF

The capsule shells contain gelatin, USP; Titanium Dioxide, USP; and Colorants.

The colorants are:
FD&C Blue #1 (all strength capsules)
Yellow Iron Oxide, USP (25 mg and 50 mg capsules)
FD&C Red #3 (50 mg, 100 mg and 200 mg capsules)
FD&C Yellow #6 (50 mg, 100 mg and 200 mg capsules)
Riboflavin, USP (25 mg capsules)

All capsule shells are imprinted with black print that contains shellac, NF, and black iron oxide, NF.

12 CLINICAL PHARMACOLOGY

12.1 Mechanism of Action

The precise mechanisms by which topiramate exerts its anticonvulsant effects are unknown; however, preclinical studies have revealed four properties that may contribute to topiramate's efficacy for epilepsy. Electrophysiological and biochemical evidence suggests that topiramate, at pharmacologically relevant concentrations, blocks voltage-dependent sodium channels, augments the activity of the neurotransmitter gamma-aminobutyrate at some subtypes of the GABA-A receptor, antagonizes the AMPA/kainate subtype of the glutamate receptor, and inhibits the carbonic anhydrase enzyme, particularly isozymes II and IV.

12.2 Pharmacodynamics

Topiramate has anticonvulsant activity in rat and mouse maximal electroshock seizure (MES) tests. Topiramate is only weakly effective in blocking clonic seizures induced by the GABAA receptor antagonist, pentylenetetrazole. Topiramate is also effective in rodent models of epilepsy, which include tonic and absence-like seizures in the spontaneous epileptic rat (SER) and tonic and clonic seizures induced in rats by kindling of the amygdala or by global ischemia.

12.3 Pharmacokinetics

Absorption and Distribution

Linear pharmacokinetics of topiramate from Trokendi XR™ were observed following a single oral dose over the range of 50 mg to 200 mg. At 25 mg, the pharmacokinetics of Trokendi XR™ is nonlinear possibly due to the binding of topiramate to carbonic anhydrase in red blood cells.

The peak plasma concentrations (C_{max}) of topiramate occurred at approximately 24 hours following a single 200 mg oral dose of Trokendi XR™. At steady-state, the (AUC_{0-24hr}, C_{max}, and C_{min}) of topiramate from Trokendi XR™ administered once-daily and the immediate-release tablet administered twice-daily were shown to be bioequivalent. Fluctuation of topiramate plasma concentrations at steady-state for Trokendi XR™ administered once-daily was approximately 26% and 42% in healthy subjects and in epileptic patients, respectively, compared to approximately 40% and 51%, respectively, for immediate-release topiramate [see *Clinical Pharmacology (12.6)*].

Compared to the fasted state, high-fat meal increased the C_{max} of topiramate by 37% and shortened the T_{max} to approximately 8 hour following a single dose of Trokendi XR™, while having no effect on the AUC. Modeling of the observed single dose fed data with simulation to steady state showed that the effect on C_{max} is significantly reduced following repeat administrations. Trokendi XR™ can be taken without regard to meals.

Topiramate is 15% to 41% bound to human plasma proteins over the blood concentration range of 0.5 mcg/mL to 250 mcg/mL. The fraction bound decreased as blood concentration increased.

Carbamazepine and phenytoin do not alter the binding of immediate-release topiramate. Sodium valproate, at 500 mcg/mL (a concentration 5 to 10 times higher than considered therapeutic for valproate) decreased the protein binding of immediate-release topiramate from 23% to 13%. Immediate-release topiramate does not influence the binding of sodium valproate.

Metabolism and Excretion

Topiramate is not extensively metabolized and is primarily eliminated unchanged in the urine (approximately 70% of an administered dose). Six metabolites have been identified in humans, none of which constitutes more than 5% of an administered dose. The metabolites are formed via hydroxylation, hydrolysis, and glucuronidation. There is evidence of renal tubular reabsorption of topiramate. In rats, given probenecid to inhibit tubular reabsorption, along with topiramate, a significant increase in renal clearance of topiramate was observed. This interaction has not been evaluated in humans. Overall, oral plasma clearance (CL/F) is approximately 20 mL/min to 30 mL/min in adults following oral administration. The mean elimination half-life of topiramate was approximately 31 hours following repeat administration of Trokendi XR™.

Specific Populations

Renal Impairment

The clearance of topiramate was reduced by 42% in moderately renally impaired (creatinine clearance 30 to 69 mL/min/1.73m²) and by 54% in severely renally impaired subjects (creatinine clearance less than 30 mL/min/1.73m²) compared to normal renal function subjects (creatinine clearance greater than70 mL/min/1.73m²). Since topiramate is presumed to undergo significant tubular reabsorption, it is uncertain whether this experience can be generalized to all situations of renal impairment. It is conceivable that some forms of renal disease could differentially affect glomerular filtration rate and tubular reabsorption resulting in a clearance of topiramate not predicted by creatinine clearance. In general, however, use of one-half the usual starting and maintenance dose is recommended in patients with creatinine clearance less than 70 mL/min/1.73 m² [see *Dosage and Administration (2.3), (2.4)*].

Hemodialysis

Topiramate is cleared by hemodialysis. Using a high-efficiency, counterflow, single pass-dialysate hemodialysis procedure, topiramate dialysis clearance was 120 mL/min with blood flow through the dialyzer at 400 mL/min. This high clearance (compared to 20 mL/min to 30 mL/min total oral clearance in healthy adults) will remove a clinically significant amount of topiramate from the patient over the hemodialysis treatment period. Therefore, a supplemental dose may be required [see *Dosage and Administration (2.5)*].

Hepatic Impairment

In hepatically impaired subjects, the clearance of topiramate may be decreased; the mechanism underlying the decrease is not well understood.

Age, Gender and Race

The pharmacokinetics of topiramate in elderly subjects (65 to 85 years of age, N=16) were evaluated in a controlled clinical study. The elderly subject population had reduced renal function (creatinine clearance [-20%]) compared to young adults. Following a single oral 100 mg dose, maximum plasma concentration for elderly and young adults was achieved at approximately 1 to 2 hours. Reflecting the primary renal elimination of topiramate, topiramate plasma and renal clearance were reduced 21% and 19%, respectively, in elderly subjects, compared to young adults. Similarly, topiramate half-life was longer (13%) in the elderly. Reduced topiramate clearance resulted in slightly higher maximum plasma concentration (23%) and AUC (25%) in elderly subjects than observed in young adults. Topiramate clearance is decreased in the elderly only to the extent that renal function is reduced.

In a study of 13 healthy elderly subjects and 18 healthy young adults who received Trokendi XR™, 30% higher mean C_{max} and 44% higher AUC values were observed in elderly compared to young subjects. Elderly subjects exhibited shorter median T_{max} at 16 hours versus 24 hours in young subjects. The apparent elimination half-life was similar across age groups. As recommended for all patients, dosage adjustment is indicated in elderly patients with a creatinine clearance rate less than 70 mL/min/1.73 m²) [see *Dosage and Administration (2.4)*].

Clearance of topiramate in adults was not affected by gender or race.

Pediatric Pharmacokinetics

Pharmacokinetics of immediate-release topiramate were evaluated in patients ages 2 years to less than 16 years. Patients received either no or a combination of other antiepileptic drugs. A population pharmacokinetic model was developed on the basis of pharmacokinetic data from relevant topiramate clinical studies. This dataset contained data from 1217 subjects including 258 pediatric patients aged 2 years to less than 16 years (95 pediatric patients less than 10 years of age). Pediatric patients on adjunctive treatment exhibited a higher oral clearance (L/h) of topiramate compared to patients on monotherapy, presumably because of increased clearance from concomitant enzyme-inducing antiepileptic drugs. In comparison, topiramate clearance per kg is greater in pediatric patients than in adults and in young pediatric patients (down to 2 years) than in older pediatric patients. Consequently, the plasma drug concentration for the same mg/kg/day dose would be lower in pediatric patients compared to adults and also in younger pediatric patients compared to older pediatric patients. Clearance was independent of dose.

As in adults, hepatic enzyme-inducing antiepileptic drugs decrease the steady state plasma concentrations of topiramate.

Drug-Drug Interaction Studies

Antiepileptic Drugs

Potential interactions between immediate-release topiramate and standard AEDs were assessed in controlled clinical pharmacokinetic studies in patients with epilepsy. The effects of these interactions on mean plasma AUCs are summarized in Table 8. Interaction of Trokendi XR™ and standard AEDs is not expected to differ from the experience with immediate-release topiramate products.

In Table 8, the second column (AED concentration) describes what happened to the concentration of the AED listed in the first column when topiramate was added. The third column (topiramate concentration) describes how the co-administration of a drug listed in the first column modified the concentration of topiramate in experimental settings when topiramate was given alone.

Table 8: Summary of AED Interactions with topiramate

AED Coadministered	AED Concentration	Topiramate Concentration
Phenytoin	NC or 25% increase*	48% decrease
Carbamazepine (CBZ)	NC	40% decrease
CBZ epoxide†	NC	NE
Valproic acid	11% decrease	14% decrease
Phenobarbital	NC	NE
Primidone	NC	NE
Lamotrigine	NC at TPM doses up to 400mg per day	13% decrease

NC=Less than 10% change in plasma concentration
AED=Antiepileptic drug
NE=Not evaluated
TPM=topiramate
* =Plasma concentration increased 25% in some patients, generally those on a twice a day dosing regimen of phenytoin
† =Is not administered but is an active metabolite of carbamazepine

In addition to the pharmacokinetic interaction described in the above table, concomitant administration of valproic acid and topiramate has been associated with hyperammonemia with and without encephalopathy and hypothermia [see *Warnings and Precautions (5.9), (5.11) and Drug Interactions (7.5)*].

CNS Depressants or Alcohol

Concomitant administration of Trokendi XR™ and other CNS depressant drugs or alcohol has not been evaluated in clinical studies. [see *Contraindications (4), Warnings and Precautions (5.4), (5.13), and Drug Interactions (7.1),(7.4)*].

Oral Contraceptives

In a pharmacokinetic interaction study in healthy volunteers with a concomitantly administered combination oral contraceptive product containing 1 mg norethindrone (NET) plus 35 mcg ethinyl estradiol (EE), topiramate, given in the absence of other medications at doses of 50 to 200 mg per day, was not associated with statistically significant changes in mean exposure (AUC) to either component of the oral contraceptive. In another study, exposure to EE was statistically significantly decreased at doses of 200, 400, and 800 mg per day (18%, 21%, and 30%, respectively) when given as adjunctive therapy in patients taking valproic acid. In both studies, topiramate (50 mg per day to 800 mg per day) did not significantly affect exposure to NET. Although there was a dose-dependent decrease in EE exposure for doses between 200 to 800 mg per day, there was no significant dose-dependent change in EE exposure for doses of 50 to 200 mg per day. The clinical significance of the changes observed is not known. The possibility of decreased contraceptive efficacy and increased breakthrough bleeding should be considered in patients taking combination oral contraceptive products with Trokendi XR™. Patients taking estrogen-containing contraceptives should be asked to report any change in their bleeding patterns. Contraceptive efficacy can be decreased even in the absence of breakthrough bleeding [see *Drug Interactions (7.2)*].

Digoxin
In a single-dose study, serum digoxin AUC was decreased by 12% with concomitant topiramate administration. The clinical relevance of this observation has not been established.

Hydrochlorothiazide
A drug-drug interaction study conducted in healthy volunteers evaluated the steady-state pharmacokinetics of hydrochlorothiazide (HCTZ) (25 mg every 24 hours) and topiramate (96 mg every 12 hours) when administered alone and concomitantly. The results of this study indicate that topiramate C_{max} increased by 27% and AUC increased by 29% when HCTZ was added to topiramate. The clinical significance of this change is unknown. The addition of HCTZ to Trokendi XR™ therapy may require an adjustment of the Trokendi XR™ dose. The steady-state pharmacokinetics of HCTZ were not significantly influenced by the concomitant administration of topiramate. Clinical laboratory results indicated decreases in serum potassium after topiramate or HCTZ administration, which were greater when HCTZ and topiramate were administered in combination.

Metformin
Topiramate treatment can frequently cause metabolic acidosis, a condition for which the use of metformin is contraindicated. Trokendi XR™ is expected to exhibit the same degree of metabolic acidosis as topiramate.
A drug-drug interaction study conducted in healthy volunteers evaluated the steady-state pharmacokinetics of metformin (500 mg every 12 hr) and topiramate in plasma when metformin was given alone and when metformin and topiramate (100 mg every 12 hr) were given simultaneously. The results of this study indicated that the mean metformin C_{max} and AUC_{0-12h} increased by 17% and 25%, respectively, when topiramate was added. Topiramate did not affect metformin tmax. The clinical significance of the effect of topiramate on metformin pharmacokinetics is not known. Oral plasma clearance of topiramate appears to be reduced when administered with metformin. The clinical significance of the effect of metformin on topiramate or Trokendi XR™ pharmacokinetics is unclear. [see Drug Interactions (7.6)].

Pioglitazone
A drug-drug interaction study conducted in healthy volunteers evaluated the steady-state pharmacokinetics of topiramate and pioglitazone when administered alone and concomitantly. A 15% decrease in the $AUC_{\tau,ss}$ of pioglitazone with no alteration in $C_{max,ss}$ was observed. This finding was not statistically significant. In addition, a 13% and 16% decrease in $C_{max,ss}$ and $AUC_{\tau,ss}$, respectively, of the active hydroxy-metabolite was noted as well as a 60% decrease in $C_{max,ss}$ and $AUC_{\tau,ss}$ of the active keto-metabolite. The clinical significance of these findings is not known.
When Trokendi XR™ is added to pioglitazone therapy or pioglitazone is added to Trokendi XR™ therapy, careful attention should be given to the routine monitoring of patients for adequate control of their diabetic disease state.

Glyburide
A drug-drug interaction study conducted in patients with type 2 diabetes evaluated the steady-state pharmacokinetics of glyburide (5mg per day) alone and concomitantly with topiramate (150 mg per day). There was a 22% decrease in C_{max} and 25% reduction in AUC_{24} for glyburide during topiramate administration. Systemic exposure (AUC) of the active metabolites, 4-trans-hydroxy glyburide (M1) and 3-cis-hydroxyglyburide (M2), was also reduced by 13% and 15%, reduced C_{max} by 18% and 25%, respectively. The steady-state pharmacokinetics of topiramate were unaffected by concomitant administration of glyburide.

Lithium
In patients, the pharmacokinetics of lithium were unaffected during treatment with topiramate at doses of 200 mg per day; however, there was an observed increase in systemic exposure of lithium (27% for C_{max} and 26% for AUC) following topiramate doses up to 600 mg per day. Lithium levels should be monitored when co-administered with high-dose Trokendi XR™ [see Drug Interactions (7.7)].

Haloperidol
The pharmacokinetics of a single dose of haloperidol (5 mg) were not affected following multiple dosing of topiramate (100 mg every 12 hr) in 13 healthy adults (6 males, 7 females).

Amitriptyline
There was a 12% increase in AUC and C_{max} for amitriptyline (25 mg per day) in 18 normal subjects (9 males, 9 females) receiving 200 mg per day of topiramate. Some subjects may experience a large increase in amitriptyline concentration in the presence of Trokendi XR™ and any adjustments in amitriptyline dose should be made according to the patient's clinical response and not on the basis of plasma levels.

Sumatriptan
Multiple dosing of topiramate (100 mg every 12 hrs) in 24 healthy volunteers (14 males, 10 females) did not affect the pharmacokinetics of single-dose sumatriptan either orally (100 mg) or subcutaneously (6 mg).

Risperidone
When administered concomitantly with topiramate at escalating doses of 100, 250, and 400 mg per day, there was a reduction in risperidone systemic exposure (16% and 33% for steady-state AUC at the 250 and 400 mg per day doses of topiramate). No alterations of 9-hydroxyrisperidone levels were observed. Coadministration of topiramate 400 mg per day with risperidone resulted in a 14% increase in C_{max} and a 12% increase in AUC_{12} of topiramate. There were no clinically significant changes in the systemic exposure of risperidone plus 9-hydroxyrisperidone or of topiramate; therefore, this interaction is not likely to be of clinical significance.

Propranolol
Multiple dosing of topiramate (200 mg per day) in 34 healthy volunteers (17 males, 17 females) did not affect the pharmacokinetics of propranolol following daily 160 mg doses. Propranolol doses of 160 mg per day in 39 volunteers (27 males, 12 females) had no effect on the exposure to topiramate at a dose of 200 mg per day of topiramate.

Dihydroergotamine
Multiple dosing of topiramate (200 mg per day) in 24 healthy volunteers (12 males, 12 females) did not affect the pharmacokinetics of a 1 mg subcutaneous dose of dihydroergotamine. Similarly, a 1 mg subcutaneous dose of dihydroergotamine did not affect the pharmacokinetics of a 200 mg per day dose of topiramate in the same study.

Diltiazem
Co-administration of diltiazem (240 mg Cardizem CD®) with topiramate (150 mg per day) resulted in a 10% decrease in C_{max} and 25% decrease in diltiazem AUC, 27% decrease in C_{max} and 18% decrease in des-acetyl diltiazem AUC, and no effect on N-desmethyl diltiazem. Co-administration of topiramate with diltiazem resulted in a 16% increase in C_{max} and a 19% increase in AUC_{12} of topiramate.

Venlafaxine
Multiple dosing of topiramate (150 mg per day) in healthy volunteers did not affect the pharmacokinetics of venlafaxine or O-desmethyl venlafaxine. Multiple dosing of venlafaxine (150 mg) did not affect the pharmacokinetics of topiramate.

Other Carbonic Anhydrase Inhibitors
Concomitant use of Trokendi XR™, a carbonic anhydrase inhibitor, with any other carbonic anhydrase inhibitor (e.g., zonisamide, acetazolamide, or dichlorphenamide), may increase the severity of metabolic acidosis and may also increase the risk of kidney stone formation. Therefore, if Trokendi XR™ is given concomitantly with another carbonic anhydrase inhibitor, the patient should be monitored for the appearance or worsening of metabolic acidosis [see Drug Interactions (7.5)].

Drug/Laboratory Tests Interactions
There are no known interactions of Trokendi XR™ with commonly used laboratory tests.

12.6   Relative Bioavailability of Trokendi XR™ Compared to Immediate-Release Topiramate
Study in Healthy Normal Volunteers
Trokendi XR™ taken once a day provides steady state plasma levels comparable to immediate-release topiramate taken every 12 hours, when administered at the same total 200 mg daily dose. In a crossover study, 33 healthy subjects were titrated to a 200mg dose of either Trokendi XR™ or immediate-release topiramate and were maintained at 200mg per day for 10 days.
The 90% CI for the ratios of AUC_{0-24}, C_{max} and C_{min}, as well as partial AUC (the area under the concentration-time curve from time 0 to time p (post dose) for multiple time points were within the 80 to 125% bioequivalence limits, indicating no clinically significant difference between the two formulations. In addition, the 90% CI for the ratios of topiramate plasma concentration at each of multiple time points over 24 hours for the two formulations were within the 80 to 125% bioequivalence limits, except for the initial time points before 1.5 hour post-dose.
Study in Patients with Epilepsy
In a study in epilepsy patients treated with immediate-release topiramate alone or in combination with either enzyme-inducing or neutral AEDs who were switched to an equivalent daily dose of Trokendi XR™, there was a 10% decrease in AUC_{0-24}, C_{max}, and C_{min} on the first day after the switch in all patients. At steady state, AUC_{0-24} and C_{max} were comparable to immediate-release topiramate in all patients. While patients treated with Trokendi XR™ alone or in combination with neutral AEDs showed comparable C_{min} at steady state, patients treated with enzyme-inducers showed a 10% decrease in C_{min}. This difference is likely not clinically significant and probably due to the small number of patients on enzyme-inducers.

13   NON-CLINICAL TOXICOLOGY
13.1   Carcinogenesis, Mutagenesis, and Impairment of Fertility
Carcinogenesis
An increase in urinary bladder tumors was observed in mice given topiramate (20 mg/kg, 75 mg/kg, and 300 mg/kg) in

the diet for 21 months. The elevated bladder tumor incidence, which was statistically significant in males and females receiving 300 mg/kg, was primarily due to the increased occurrence of a smooth muscle tumor considered histomorphologically unique to mice. Plasma exposures in mice receiving 300 mg/kg were approximately 0.5 to 1 times steady-state exposures measured in patients receiving topiramate monotherapy at the recommended human dose (RHD) of 400 mg, and 1.5 to 2 times steady-state topiramate exposures in patients receiving 400 mg of topiramate plus phenytoin. The relevance of this finding to human carcinogenic risk is uncertain.
No evidence of carcinogenicity was seen in rats following oral administration of topiramate for 2 years at doses up to 120 mg/kg (approximately 3 times the RHD on a mg/m² basis).

Mutagenesis
Topiramate did not demonstrate genotoxic potential when tested in a battery of in vitro and in vivo assays. Topiramate was not mutagenic in the Ames test or the in vitro mouse lymphoma assay; it did not increase unscheduled DNA synthesis in rat hepatocytes in vitro; and it did not increase chromosomal aberrations in human lymphocytes in vitro or in rat bone marrow in vivo.

Impairment of Fertility
No adverse effects on male or female fertility were observed in rats at doses up to 100 mg/kg (2.5 times the RHD on a mg/m² basis).

14   CLINICAL STUDIES
14.1   Bridging Study to Demonstrate Pharmacokinetic Equivalence between Extended-Release and Immediate-Release Topiramate Formulations
The basis for approval of the extended-release formulation (Trokendi XR™) included the studies described below using an immediate-release formulation and the demonstration of the pharmacokinetic equivalence of Trokendi XR™ to immediate-release topiramate through the analysis of concentrations and cumulative AUCs at multiple time points [see Clinical Pharmacology (12.6)].
The clinical studies described in the following sections were conducted using immediate-release topiramate.

14.2   Monotherapy Treatment in Patients with Partial Onset or Primary Generalized Tonic-Clonic Seizures
Adults and Pediatric Patients 10 Years of Age and Older
The effectiveness of topiramate as initial monotherapy in adults and children 10 years of age and older with partial onset or primary generalized tonic-clonic seizures was established in a multicenter, randomized, double-blind, dose-controlled, parallel-group trial (Study 1).
Study 1 was conducted in 487 patients diagnosed with epilepsy (6 to 83 years of age) who had 1 or 2 well-documented seizures during the 3-month retrospective baseline phase who then entered the study and received topiramate 25 mg per day for 7 days in an open-label fashion. Forty-nine percent of subjects had no prior AED treatment and 17% had a diagnosis of epilepsy for greater than 24 months. Any AED therapy used for temporary or emergency purposes was discontinued prior to randomization. In the double-blind phase, 470 patients were randomized to titrate up to 50 mg per day or 400 mg per day of topiramate. If the target dose could not be achieved, patients were maintained on the maximum tolerated dose. Fifty eight percent of patients achieved the maximal dose of 400 mg per day for greater than 2 weeks, and patients who did not tolerate 150 mg per day were discontinued.
The primary efficacy assessment was a between-group comparison of time to first seizure during the double-blind phase. Comparison of the Kaplan-Meier survival curves of time to first seizure favored the topiramate 400 mg per day group over the topiramate 50 mg per day group (p=0.0002, log rank test; Figure 1). The treatment effects with respect to time to first seizure were consistent across various patient subgroups defined by age, sex, geographic region, baseline body weight, baseline seizure type, time since diagnosis, and baseline AED use.
[See figure 1 at top of next column]

14.3   Adjunctive Therapy in Patients with Partial Onset Seizures
Adult Patients with Partial Onset Seizures
The effectiveness of topiramate as an adjunctive treatment for adults with partial onset seizures was established in six multicenter, randomized, double-blind, placebo-controlled trials (Studies 2, 3, 4, 5, 6, and 7), two comparing several dosages of topiramate and placebo and four comparing a single dosage with placebo, in patients with a history of partial onset seizures, with or without secondarily generalized seizures.
Patients in these studies were permitted a maximum of two antiepileptic drugs (AEDs) in addition to topiramate tablets or placebo. In each study, patients were stabilized on optimum dosages of their concomitant AEDs during baseline phase lasting between 4 and 12 weeks. Patients who expe-

Figure 1: Kaplan-Meier Estimates of Cumulative Rates for Time to First Seizure in Study 1

rienced a prespecified minimum number of partial onset seizures, with or without secondary generalization, during the baseline phase (12 seizures for 12-week baseline, 8 for 8-week baseline or 3 for 4-week baseline) were randomly assigned to placebo or a specified dose of topiramate tablets in addition to their other AEDs.

Following randomization, patients began the double-blind phase of treatment. In five of the six studies, patients received active drug beginning at 100 mg per day; the dose was then increased by 100 mg or 200 mg per day increments weekly or every other week until the assigned dose was reached, unless intolerance prevented increases. In Study 7, the 25 or 50 mg per day initial doses of topiramate were followed by respective weekly increments of 25 or 50 mg per day until the target dose of 200 mg per day was reached. After titration, patients entered a 4, 8 or 12-week stabilization period. The numbers of patients randomized to each dose, and the actual mean and median doses in the stabilization period are shown in Table 9.

[See table 9 above]

Pediatric Patients Ages 2 to 16 Years with Partial Onset Seizures

The effectiveness of topiramate as an adjunctive treatment for pediatric patients ages 2 to 16 years with partial onset seizures was established in a multicenter, randomized, double-blind, placebo-controlled trial (Study 8), comparing topiramate and placebo in patients with a history of partial onset seizures, with or without secondarily generalized seizures.

Patients in Study 8 were permitted a maximum of two antiepileptic drugs (AEDs) in addition to topiramate tablets or placebo. In Study 8, patients were stabilized on optimum dosages of their concomitant AEDs during an 8-week baseline phase. Patients who experienced at least six partial onset seizures, with or without secondarily generalized seizures, during the baseline phase were randomly assigned to placebo or topiramate in addition to their other AEDs.

Following randomization, patients began the double-blind phase of treatment. Patients received active drug beginning at 25 or 50 mg per day; the dose was then increased by 25 mg to 150 mg per day increments every other week until the assigned dosage of 125, 175, 225 or 400 mg per day based on patients' weight to approximate a dosage of 6 mg/kg/day per day was reached, unless intolerance prevented increases. After titration, patients entered an 8-week stabilization period.

14.4 Adjunctive Therapy in Patients With Primary Generalized Tonic-Clonic Seizures

The effectiveness of topiramate as an adjunctive treatment for primary generalized tonic-clonic seizures in patients 2 years old and older was established in a multicenter, randomized, double-blind, placebo-controlled trial (Study 9), comparing a single dosage of topiramate and placebo.

Patients in Study 9 were permitted a maximum of two antiepileptic drugs (AEDs) in addition to topiramate or placebo. Patients were stabilized on optimum dosages of their concomitant AEDs during an 8-week baseline phase. Patients who experienced at least three primary generalized tonic-clonic seizures during the baseline phase were randomly assigned to placebo or topiramate in addition to their other AEDs.

Following randomization, patients began the double-blind phase of treatment. Patients received active drug beginning at 50 mg per day for four weeks; the dose was then increased by 50 mg to 150 mg per day increments every other week until the assigned dose of 175, 225 or 400 mg per day based on patients' body weight to approximate a dosage of 6 mg/kg/day was reached, unless intolerance prevented increases. After titration, patients entered a 12-week stabilization period.

14.5 Adjunctive Therapy in Patients With Lennox-Gastaut Syndrome

The effectiveness of topiramate as an adjunctive treatment for seizures associated with Lennox-Gastaut syndrome was established in a multicenter, randomized, double-blind,

placebo-controlled trial comparing a single dosage of topiramate with placebo in patients 2 years of age and older (Study 10).

Patients in Study 10 were permitted a maximum of two antiepileptic drugs (AEDs) in addition to topiramate or placebo. Patients who were experiencing at least 60 seizures per month before study entry were stabilized on optimum dosages of their concomitant AEDs during a 4 week baseline phase. Following baseline, patients were randomly assigned to placebo or topiramate in addition to their other AEDs. Active drug was titrated beginning at 1 mg/kg/day for a week; the dose was then increased to 3 mg/kg/day for one week then to 6 mg/kg/day. After titration, patients entered an 8-week stabilization period. The primary measures of effectiveness were the percent reduction in drop attacks and a parental global rating of seizure severity.

In all adjunctive topiramate trials, the reduction in seizure rate from baseline during the entire double-blind phase was measured. The median percent reductions in seizure rates and the responder rates (fraction of patients with at least a 50% reduction) by treatment group for each study are shown below in Table 10. As described above, a global improvement in seizure severity was also assessed in the Lennox-Gastaut trial.

[See table 10 at top of next page]

Subset analyses of the antiepileptic efficacy of topiramate tablets in these studies showed no differences as a function of gender, race, age, baseline seizure rate, or concomitant AED.

In clinical trials for epilepsy, daily dosages were decreased in weekly intervals by 50 mg per day to 100 mg per day in adults and over a 2- to 8-week period in children; transition was permitted to a new antiepileptic regimen when clinically indicated.

16 HOW SUPPLIED/STORAGE AND HANDLING

16.1 Trokendi XR™ Capsules

Trokendi XR™ (topiramate) extended-release capsules are available as extended-release capsules in the following strengths and colors:

Bottles

25 mg (light green opaque body/yellow opaque cap) topiramate extended-release capsules (black print "SPN" and "25") - bottles of 100 count (NDC-17772-101-01)

50 mg (light green opaque body/orange opaque cap) topiramate extended-release capsules (black print "SPN" and "50") - bottles of 100 count (NDC-17772-102-01)

100 mg (green opaque body/blue opaque cap) topiramate extended-release capsules (black print "SPN" and "100") - bottles of 100 count (NDC-17772-103-01)

200 mg (pink opaque body/blue opaque cap) topiramate extended-release capsules (black print "SPN" and "200") - bottles of 100 count (NDC-17772-104-01)

Blister package

25 mg (light green opaque body/yellow opaque cap) topiramate extended-release capsules (black print "SPN" and "25") – blister packages of 30-count (NDC-17772-101-15)

50 mg (light green opaque body/orange opaque cap) topiramate extended-release capsules (black print "SPN" and "50") – blister packages of 30-count (NDC-17772-102-15)

100 mg (green opaque body/blue opaque cap) topiramate extended-release capsules (black print "SPN" and "100") – blister packages of 30-count (NDC-17772-103-15)

200 mg (pink opaque body/blue opaque cap) topiramate extended-release capsules (black print "SPN" and "200") – blister packages of 30-count (NDC-17772-104-15)

16.2 Storage and Handling

Trokendi XR™ (topiramate) extended-release capsules should be stored in well closed containers at controlled room temperature [25°C (77°F); excursions 15°C-30°C (59°F-86°F)]. Protect from moisture and light.

17 PATIENT COUNSELING INFORMATION

See FDA-approved patient labeling (Medication Guide)

Administration Instructions

Counsel patients to swallow Trokendi XR™ capsules whole and intact. Trokendi XR™ should not be sprinkled on food, chewed or crushed. *[See Dosage and Administration (2.9)].*

Consumption of Alcohol

Advise patients to completely avoid consumption of alcohol at least 6 hours prior to and 6 hours after taking Trokendi XR™*[see Warnings and Precautions (5.4)].*

Acute Myopia and Secondary Angle Closure Glaucoma

Advise patients taking Trokendi XR™ to seek immediate medical attention if they experience blurred vision, visual disturbances or periorbital pain *[see Warnings and Precautions (5.1)].*

Oligohydrosis and Hyperthermia

Counsel patients that Trokendi XR™, especially pediatric patients, can cause decreased sweating and increased body

Table 9: Immediate Release Topiramate Dose Summary During the Stabilization Periods of Each of Six Double-Blind, Placebo-Controlled, Adjunctive Trials in Adults with Partial Onset Seizures*

Study	Stabilization Dose	Placebo†	200	400	600	800	1,000
				Target Topiramate Dosage (mg per day)			
2	N	42	42	40	41	--	--
	Mean Dose	5.9	200	390	556	--	--
	Median Dose	6.0	200	400	600	--	--
3	N	44	--	--	40	45	40
	Mean Dose	9.7	--	--	544	739	796
	Median Dose	10.0	--	--	600	800	1,000
4	N	23	--	19	--	--	--
	Mean Dose	3.8	--	395	--	--	--
	Median Dose	4.0	--	400	--	--	--
5	N	30	--	--	28	--	--
	Mean Dose	5.7	--	--	522	--	--
	Median Dose	6.0	--	--	600	--	--
6	N	28	--	--	--	25	--
	Mean Dose	8.0	--	--	--	568	--
	Median Dose	8.0	--	--	--	600	--
7	N	90	157	--	--	--	--
	Mean Dose	8	200	--	--	--	--
	Median Dose	8	200	--	--	--	--

* Dose-response studies were not conducted for other indications or pediatric partial-onset seizures
† Placebo dosages are given as the number of tablets. Placebo target dosages were as follows: Study 4 (4 tablets/day); Studies 2 and 5 (6 tablets/day); Studies 6 and 7 (8 tablets/day); Study 3 (10 tablets/day)

Table 10: Efficacy Results in Double-Blind, Placebo-Controlled, Adjunctive Epilepsy Trials

Target Topiramate Dosage (mg per day)

Study #	#	Placebo	200	400	600	800	1,000	≈6mg/kg/day*
Partial Onset Seizures Studies in Adults								
2	N	45	45	45	46	--	--	--
	Median % Reduction	11.6	27.2†	47.5‡	44.7§	--	--	--
	% Responders	18	24	44¶	46¶	--	--	--
3	N	47	--	--	48	48	47	--
	Median % Reduction	1.7	--	--	40.8§	41.0§	36.0§	--
	% Responders	9	--	--	40§	41§	36¶	--
4	N	24	--	23	--	--	--	--
	Median % Reduction	1.1	--	40.7#	--	--	--	--
	% Responders	8	--	35¶	--	--	--	--
5	N	30	--	--	30	--	--	--
	Median % Reduction	-12.2	--	--	46.4Þ	--	--	--
	% Responders	10	--	--	47§	--	--	--
6	N	28	--	--	--	28	--	--
	Median % Reduction	-20.6	--	--	--	24.3§	--	--
	% Responders	0	--	--	--	43§	--	--
7	N	91	168	--	--	--	--	--
	Median % Reduction	20.0	44.2§	--	--	--	--	--
	% Responders	24	45§	--	--	--	--	--
Studies in Pediatric Patients								
8	N	45	--	--	--	--	--	41
	Median % Reduction	10.5	--	--	--	--	--	33.1¶
	% Responders	20	--	--	--	--	--	39
Primary Generalized Tonic-Clonicß								
9	N	40	--	--	--	--	--	39
	Median % Reduction	9.0	--	--	--	--	--	56.7¶
	% Responders	20	--	--	--	--	--	56§
Lennox-Gastaut Syndromeà								
10	N	49	--	--	--	--	--	46
	Median % Reduction	-5.1	--	--	--	--	--	14.8¶
	% Responders	14	--	--	--	--	--	28è
	Improvement in Seizure Severityð	28	--	--	--	--	--	52¶

* For Studies 8 and 9, specified target dosages (less than 9.3 mg/kg/day) were assigned based on subject's weight to approximate a dosage of 6mg/kg per day; these dosages corresponded to mg per day dosages of 125 mg per day, 175 mg per day, 225 mg per day, and 400 mg per day
† Comparisons with placebo: p=0.080;
‡ p ≤ 0.010;
§ p ≤ 0.001;
¶ p ≤ 0.050;
# p=0.065;
Þ p ≤0.005;
ß Median % reduction and % responders are reported for PGTC seizures;
à Median % reduction and % responders for drop attacks, i.e., tonic or atonic seizures
è p=0.071;
ð Percent of subjects who were minimally, much, or very much improved from baseline.

temperature, especially in hot weather, and they should seek medical attention if this is noticed [see *Warnings and Precautions (5.2)*].

Metabolic Acidosis
Inform patients about the potentially significant risk for metabolic acidosis that may be asymptomatic and may be associated with adverse effects on kidneys (e.g., kidney stones, nephrocalcinosis), bones (e.g., osteoporosis, osteomalacia, and/or rickets in children), and growth (e.g., growth delay/retardation) in pediatric patients, and on the fetus [see *Warnings and Precautions (5.3)*]

Suicidal Behavior and Ideation
Counsel patients, their caregivers, and families that AEDs, including Trokendi XR™, may increase the risk of suicidal thoughts and behavior and they should be advised of the need to be alert for the emergence or worsening of the signs and symptoms of depression, any unusual changes in mood or behavior or the emergence of suicidal thoughts, behavior or thoughts about self-harm. Behaviors of concern should be reported immediately to healthcare providers. [see *Warnings and Precautions (5.5)*].

Interference with Cognitive and Motor Performance
Warn patients about the potential for somnolence, dizziness, confusion, difficulty concentrating, visual effects and advise them not to drive or operate machinery until they have gained sufficient experience on Trokendi XR™ to gauge whether it adversely affects their mental performance, motor performance, and/or vision. [see *Warnings and Precautions (5.6)*].

Advise patients that even when taking Trokendi XR™ or other anticonvulsants, some patients with epilepsy will continue to have unpredictable seizures. Therefore, counsel all patients taking Trokendi XR™ for epilepsy to exercise appropriate caution when engaging in any activities where loss of consciousness could result in serious danger to themselves or those around them (including swimming, driving a car, climbing in high places, etc.). Some patients with refractory epilepsy will need to avoid such activities altogether. Physicians should discuss the appropriate level of caution with their patients, before patients with epilepsy engage in such activities.

Fetal Toxicity
Counsel pregnant women and women of childbearing potential that use of topiramate during pregnancy can cause fetal harm, including an increased risk for cleft lip and/or cleft palate (oral clefts), which occur early in pregnancy before many women know they are pregnant. When appropriate, prescribers should counsel pregnant women and women of childbearing potential about alternative therapeutic options.

Advise women of childbearing potential who are not planning a pregnancy to use effective contraception while using topiramate, keeping in mind that there is a potential for decreased contraceptive efficacy when using estrogen-containing birth control with topiramate [see *Warnings and Precautions (5.7) and Drug Interactions (7.2)*].

Encourage pregnant women using topiramate to enroll in the North American Antiepileptic Drug (NAAED) Pregnancy Registry. The registry is collecting information about the safety of antiepileptic drugs during pregnancy. To enroll, patients can call the toll free number, 1-888-233-2334. Information about the North American Drug Pregnancy Registry can be found at http://www.massgeneral.org/aed/ [see *Use in Specific Populations (8.1)*].

Hyperammonemia and Encephalopathy
Warn patients about the possible development of hyperammonemia with or without encephalopathy. Although hyperammonemia may be asymptomatic, clinical symptoms of hyperammonemic encephalopathy often include acute alterations in level of consciousness and/or cognitive function with lethargy or vomiting. This hyperammonemia and encephalopathy can develop with topiramate treatment alone or with topiramate treatment with concomitant valproic acid (VPA). Patients should be instructed to contact their physician if they develop unexplained lethargy, vomiting, or changes in mental status [see *Warnings and Precautions (5.9)*].

Kidney Stones
Instruct patients, particularly those with predisposing factors, to maintain an adequate fluid intake in order to minimize the risk of kidney stone formation [see *Warnings and Precautions (5.10)*].

Hypothermia
Counsel patients that Trokendi XR™ can cause a reduction in body temperature, which can lead to alterations in mental status. If they note such changes, they should call their health care professional and measure their body temperature. Patients taking concomitant valproic acid should be specifically counseled on this potential adverse reaction [see *Warnings and Precautions (5.11)*].

Paresthesia
Counsel patients that they may experience tingling in the arms and legs. If this symptom occurs, they should consult with their physician [see *Warnings and Precautions (5.12)*].

Manufactured by: Catalent Pharma Solutions, Winchester, Kentucky 40391

Manufactured for: Supernus Pharmaceuticals, Inc., Rockville, Maryland 20850

RA-TRO-V1
Revised: August 2013

MEDICATION GUIDE
Trokendi XR™ (tro-KEN-dee eks ahr)
(topiramate)
Extended-release Capsules

Read this Medication Guide before you start taking Trokendi XR™ and each time you get a refill. There may be new information. This information does not take the place of talking to your healthcare provider about your medical condition or treatment. If you have any questions about Trokendi XR™, talk to your healthcare provider or pharmacist.

What is the most important information I should know about Trokendi XR™?

Take Trokendi XR™ capsules whole. Do not sprinkle Trokendi XR™ on food, or break, crush, dissolve, or chew Trokendi XR™ capsules before swallowing. If you cannot swallow Trokendi XR™ capsules whole, tell your healthcare provider. You may need a different medicine.

Do not drink alcohol within 6 hours prior to and 6 hours after Trokendi XR™ administration.

Trokendi XR™ may cause eye problems. Serious eye problems include:

• any sudden decrease in vision with or without eye pain and redness,

• a blockage of fluid in the eye causing increased pressure in the eye (secondary angle closure glaucoma).

• These eye problems can lead to permanent loss of vision if not treated. You should call your healthcare provider right away if you have any new eye symptoms.

Trokendi XR™ may cause decreased sweating and increased body temperature (fever). People, especially children, should be watched for signs of decreased sweating and fever, especially in hot temperatures. Some people may need to be hospitalized for this condition.

Trokendi XR™ can increase the level of acid in your blood (metabolic acidosis). If left untreated, metabolic acidosis can cause brittle or soft bones (osteoporosis, osteomalacia, osteopenia), kidney stones, can slow the rate of growth in children, and may possibly harm your baby if you are pregnant. Metabolic acidosis can happen with or without symptoms. Sometimes people with metabolic acidosis will:

• feel tired

• not feel hungry (loss of appetite)

• feel changes in heartbeat

• have trouble thinking clearly

Your healthcare provider should do a blood test to measure the level of acid in your blood before and during your treatment with Trokendi XR™. If you are pregnant, you should talk to your healthcare provider about whether you have metabolic acidosis.

Like other antiepileptic drugs, Trokendi XR™ may cause suicidal thoughts or actions in a very small number of people, about 1 in 500.

Call a healthcare provider right away if you have any of these symptoms, especially if they are new, worse, or worry you:

• thoughts about suicide or dying

• attempts to commit suicide

• new or worse depression

• new or worse anxiety

• feeling agitated or restless

• panic attacks

• trouble sleeping (insomnia)

• new or worse irritability

• acting aggressive, being angry, or violent

• acting on dangerous impulses

• an extreme increase in activity and talking (mania)

• other unusual changes in behavior or mood

Do not stop taking Trokendi XR™ without first talking to a healthcare provider.

• Stopping Trokendi XR™ suddenly can cause serious problems.

• Suicidal thoughts or actions can be caused by things other than medicines. If you have suicidal thoughts or actions, your healthcare provider may check for other causes.

How can I watch for early symptoms of suicidal thoughts and actions?

• Pay attention to any changes, especially sudden changes, in mood, behaviors, thoughts, or feelings.

• Keep all follow-up visits with your healthcare provider as scheduled.

• Call your healthcare provider between visits as needed, especially if you are worried about symptoms.

Trokendi XR™ can harm your unborn baby.

• If you take Trokendi XR™ during pregnancy, your baby has a higher risk for birth defects called cleft lip and cleft palate. These defects can begin early in pregnancy, even before you know you are pregnant.

• Cleft lip and cleft palate may happen even in children born to women who are not taking any medicines and do not have other risk factors.

• There may be other medicines to treat your condition that have a lower chance of birth defects.

• All women of childbearing age should talk to their healthcare providers about using other possible treatments instead of Trokendi XR™. If the decision is made to use Trokendi XR™, you should use effective birth control (contraception) unless you are planning to become pregnant. You should talk to your doctor about the best kind of birth control to use while you are taking Trokendi XR™.

• Tell your healthcare provider right away if you become pregnant while taking Trokendi XR™. You and your healthcare provider should decide if you will continue to take Trokendi XR™ while you are pregnant.

• Metabolic acidosis may have harmful affects on your baby. Talk to your healthcare provider if Trokendi XR™ has caused metabolic acidosis during your pregnancy.

• Pregnancy Registry: If you become pregnant while taking Trokendi XR™, talk to your healthcare provider about registering with the North American Antiepileptic Drug Pregnancy Registry. You can enroll in this registry by calling 1-888-233-2334. The purpose of this registry is to collect information about the safety of Trokendi XR™ and other antiepileptic drugs during pregnancy.

What is Trokendi XR™?

Trokendi XR™ is a prescription medicine used:

• to treat certain types of seizures (partial onset seizures and primary generalized tonic-clonic seizures) in people 10 years and older,

• with other medicines to treat certain types of seizures (partial onset seizures, primary generalized tonic-clonic seizures, and seizures associated with Lennox-Gastaut syndrome) in adults and children 6 years and older.

What should I tell my healthcare provider before taking Trokendi XR™?

Before taking Trokendi XR™, tell your healthcare provider about all your medical conditions, including if you:

• have or have had depression, mood problems or suicidal thoughts or behavior

• have kidney problems, kidney stones or are getting kidney dialysis

• have a history of metabolic acidosis (too much acid in the blood)

• have liver problems

• have weak, brittle or soft bones (osteomalacia, osteoporosis, osteopenia, or decreased bone density)

• have lung or breathing problems

• have eye problems, especially glaucoma

• have diarrhea

• have a growth problem

• are on a diet high in fat and low in carbohydrates, which is called a ketogenic diet

• are having surgery

• are pregnant or plan to become pregnant

• are breastfeeding. Trokendi XR™ passes into your breast milk. It is not known if the Trokendi XR™ that passes into breast milk can harm your baby. Talk to your healthcare provider about the best way to feed your baby if you take Trokendi XR™.

Tell your healthcare provider about all the medicines you take, including prescription and non-prescription medicines, vitamins, and herbal supplements. Trokendi XR™ and other medicines may affect each other causing side effects.

Especially, tell your healthcare provider if you take:

• Metformin (such as Glucophage)

• Valproic acid (such as DEPAKENE® or DEPAKOTE®)

• any medicines that impair or decrease your thinking, concentration, or muscle coordination

• birth control pills. Trokendi XR™ may make your birth control pills less effective. Tell your healthcare provider if your menstrual bleeding changes while you are taking birth control pills and Trokendi XR™.

Ask your healthcare provider if you are not sure if your medicine is listed above.

Know the medicines you take. Keep a list of them to show your healthcare provider and pharmacist each time you get a new medicine. Do not start a new medicine without talking with your healthcare provider.

How should I take Trokendi XR™?

• Take Trokendi XR™ exactly as prescribed.

• Your healthcare provider may change your dose. **Do not** change your dose without talking to your healthcare provider.

• **Take Trokendi XR™ capsules whole. Do not** sprinkle Trokendi XR™ on food, or break, crush, dissolve, or chew Trokendi XR™ capsules before swallowing.

• Trokendi XR™ can be taken before, during, or after a meal. Drink plenty of fluids during the day. This may help prevent kidney stones while taking Trokendi XR™.

• If you take too much Trokendi XR™, call your healthcare provider or poison control center right away or go to the nearest emergency room.

• If you miss a single dose of Trokendi XR™, take it as soon as you can. Do not double your dose. If you have missed more than one dose, you should call your healthcare professional for advice.

• Do not stop taking Trokendi XR™ without talking to your healthcare provider. Stopping Trokendi XR™ suddenly may cause serious problems. If you have epilepsy and you stop taking Trokendi XR™ suddenly, you may have seizures that do not stop. Your healthcare provider will tell you how to stop taking Trokendi XR™ slowly.

• Your healthcare provider may do blood tests while you take Trokendi XR™.

What should I avoid while taking Trokendi XR™?

• Do not drink alcohol within 6 hours before or 6 hours after taking Trokendi XR™ capsules. Trokendi XR and alcohol can cause serious side effects such as severe sleepiness and dizziness and an increase in seizures.

• Do not drive a car or operate heavy machinery until you know how Trokendi XR™ affects you. Trokendi XR™ can slow your thinking and motor skills, and may affect vision.

What are the possible side effects of Trokendi XR™?

Trokendi XR™ may cause serious side effects including:

See "What is the most important information I should know about Trokendi XR™?"

• **High blood ammonia levels.** High ammonia in the blood can affect your mental activities, slow your alertness, make you feel tired, or cause vomiting. This has happened when Trokendi XR™ is taken with a medicine called valproic acid (DEPAKENE ® and DEPAKOTE®).

• **Kidney stones.** Drink plenty of fluids when taking Trokendi XR™ to decrease your chances of getting kidney stones.

• **Low body temperature.** Taking Trokendi XR™ when you are also taking valproic acid cause a drop in body temperature to less than 95°F, feeling tired, confusion, or coma.

• **Effects on thinking and alertness.** Trokendi XR™ may affect how you think, and cause confusion, problems with concentration, attention, memory, or speech. Trokendi XR™ may cause depression or mood problems, tiredness, and sleepiness.

• **Dizziness or loss of muscle coordination.**

Call your healthcare provider right away if you have any of the symptoms above.

The most common side effects of Trokendi XR™ include:

• tingling of the arms and legs (paresthesia)

• not feeling hungry

• nausea

• a change in the way foods taste

• diarrhea

• weight loss

• nervousness

• upper respiratory tract infection

Tell your healthcare provider about any side effect that bothers you or that does not go away.

These are not all the possible side effects of Trokendi XR™. For more information, ask your healthcare provider or pharmacist.

Call your doctor for medical advice about side effects. You may report side effects to FDA at 1 800-FDA-1088.

You may also report side effects to Supernus Pharmaceuticals, Inc. at 1-866-398-0833.

How should I store Trokendi XR™?

• Store Trokendi XR™ tablets at room temperature between 59°F to 86°F (15°C to 30°C).

• Keep Trokendi XR™ in a tightly closed container.

• Keep Trokendi XR™ dry and away from moisture and light.

• **Keep Trokendi XR™ and all medicines out of the reach of children.**

General information about Trokendi XR™

Medicines are sometimes prescribed for purposes other than those listed in a Medication Guide. Do not use Trokendi XR™ for a condition for which it was not prescribed. Do not give Trokendi XR™ to other people, even if they have the same symptoms that you have. It may harm them.

This Medication Guide summarizes the most important information about Trokendi XR™. If you would like more information, talk with your healthcare provider. You can ask your pharmacist or healthcare provider for information about Trokendi XR™ that is written for health professionals.

For more information, go to www.trokendixrcom or call 1-866-398-0833.

What are the ingredients in Trokendi XR™?

Active ingredient: topiramate

Inactive ingredients:

Sugar Spheres, NF, Hypromellose (Type 2910), USP, mannitol, USP, docusate sodium, USP, sodium benzoate, NF,, ethylcellulose, NF, oleic acid, NF, medium chain triglycerides, NF, polyethylene glycol, NF, polyvinyl alcohol, USP titanium dioxide, USP, talc, USP, lecithin, NF, xanthan gum, NF

Capsule shells: Gelatin, USP; titanium Dioxide, USP, and Colorants.

Colorants:

FD&C Blue #1 (all strength capsules)

Yellow iron oxide, USP (25 mg and 50 mg capsules)

FD&C red #3 (50 mg, 100 mg and 200 mg capsules)

FD&C yellow #6 (50 mg, 100 mg and 200 mg capsules)

Riboflavin, USP (25 mg capsules)

All capsule shells are imprinted with black print that contains shellac, NF, and black iron oxide, NF.

This Medication Guide has been approved by the U.S. Food and Drug Administration.

Manufactured by: Catalent Pharma Solutions, Winchester, KY USA 40391

Manufactured for: Supernus Pharmaceuticals, Inc. Rockville, MD USA 20850

© Supernus Pharmaceuticals, June 2013

RA-TRO-MGV1

Issued: August 2013

Shown in Product Identification Guide, page 313

Takeda Pharmaceuticals U.S.A., Inc.
ONE TAKEDA PARKWAY
DEERFIELD, IL 60015

Direct Inquiries to:
Sales and Ordering:
Customer Service
(877) TAKEDA7
(877) 825-3327
For Medical Information:
(877) TAKEDA7
(877) 825-3327
To Report Adverse Drug Experiences:
(877) TAKEDA7
(877) 825-3327

AMITIZA ℞
[ahm-i-TEE-za]
(lubiprostone)
capsules, for oral use

HIGHLIGHTS OF PRESCRIBING INFORMATION
These highlights do not include all the information needed to use AMITIZA safely and effectively. See full prescribing information for AMITIZA.
AMITIZA (lubiprostone) capsules, for oral use
Initial U.S. Approval: 2006

————RECENT MAJOR CHANGES————

Indications and Usage (1.2)	04/2013
Dosage and Administration (2.1)	04/2013
Warnings and Precautions, Pregnancy (5.1)	removed 11/2012

————INDICATIONS AND USAGE————
Amitiza is a chloride channel activator indicated for:
• Treatment of chronic idiopathic constipation in adults (1.1)
• Treatment of opioid-induced constipation in adults with chronic, non-cancer pain (1.2)
• Treatment of irritable bowel syndrome with constipation in women ≥ 18 years old (1.3)
Limitations of Use:
Effectiveness of Amitiza in the treatment of opioid-induced constipation in patients taking diphenylheptane opioids (e.g., methadone) has not been established (1) (14.2)

————DOSAGE AND ADMINISTRATION————
Capsules should be swallowed whole and should not be broken apart or chewed (2)
Chronic Idiopathic Constipation and Opioid-induced Constipation
• 24 mcg taken twice daily orally with food and water (2.1)
Reduce the dosage in patients with moderate and severe hepatic impairment (2.1)
Irritable Bowel Syndrome with Constipation
• 8 mcg taken twice daily orally with food and water (2.2)
Reduce the dosage in patients with severe hepatic impairment (2.2)

————DOSAGE FORMS AND STRENGTHS————
• Capsules: 8 mcg and 24 mcg (3)

————CONTRAINDICATIONS————
• Amitiza is contraindicated in patients with known or suspected mechanical gastrointestinal obstruction. (4)

————WARNINGS AND PRECAUTIONS————
• Patients may experience nausea; concomitant administration of food may reduce this symptom (5.1)
• Do not prescribe for patients that have severe diarrhea (5.2)
• Patients taking Amitiza may experience dyspnea within an hour of first dose. This symptom generally resolves within 3 hours, but may recur with repeat dosing (5.3)
• Evaluate patients with symptoms suggestive of mechanical gastrointestinal obstruction prior to initiating treatment with Amitiza (5.4)

————ADVERSE REACTIONS————
• Most common adverse reactions (incidence > 4%) in chronic idiopathic constipation are nausea, diarrhea, headache, abdominal pain, abdominal distension, and flatulence (6.1)
• Most common adverse reactions (incidence > 4%) in opioid-induced constipation are nausea and diarrhea (6.1)

• Most common adverse reactions (incidence > 4%) in irritable bowel syndrome with constipation are nausea, diarrhea, and abdominal pain (6.1)
To report SUSPECTED ADVERSE REACTIONS, contact Takeda Pharmaceuticals at 1-877-825-3327 or FDA at 1-800-FDA-1088 or www.fda.gov/medwatch.

————DRUG INTERACTIONS————
• Concomitant use of diphenylheptane opioids (e.g., methadone) may interfere with the efficacy of Amitiza (7)

————USE IN SPECIFIC POPULATIONS————
• Pregnancy: Based on animal data, may cause fetal harm (8.1)
• Nursing Mothers: Caution should be exercised when administering to a nursing woman (8.3)
See 17 for PATIENT COUNSELING INFORMATION
Revised: 04/2013

FULL PRESCRIBING INFORMATION: CONTENTS*
1 **INDICATIONS AND USAGE**
  1.1 Chronic Idiopathic Constipation
  1.2 Opioid-induced Constipation
  1.3 Irritable Bowel Syndrome with Constipation
2 **DOSAGE AND ADMINISTRATION**
  2.1 Chronic Idiopathic Constipation and Opioid-induced Constipation
  2.2 Irritable Bowel Syndrome with Constipation
3 **DOSAGE FORMS AND STRENGTHS**
4 **CONTRAINDICATIONS**
5 **WARNINGS AND PRECAUTIONS**
  5.1 Nausea
  5.2 Diarrhea
  5.3 Dyspnea
  5.4 Bowel Obstruction
6 **ADVERSE REACTIONS**
  6.1 Clinical Studies Experience
  6.2 Postmarketing Experience
7 **DRUG INTERACTIONS**
8 **USE IN SPECIFIC POPULATIONS**
  8.1 Pregnancy
  8.3 Nursing Mothers
  8.4 Pediatric Use
  8.5 Geriatric Use
  8.6 Renal Impairment
  8.7 Hepatic Impairment
10 **OVERDOSAGE**
11 **DESCRIPTION**
12 **CLINICAL PHARMACOLOGY**
  12.1 Mechanism of Action
  12.2 Pharmacodynamics
  12.3 Pharmacokinetics
13 **NONCLINICAL TOXICOLOGY**
  13.1 Carcinogenesis, Mutagenesis, Impairment of Fertility
14 **CLINICAL STUDIES**
  14.1 Chronic Idiopathic Constipation
  14.2 Opioid-induced Constipation
  14.3 Irritable Bowel Syndrome with Constipation
16 **HOW SUPPLIED/STORAGE AND HANDLING**
17 **PATIENT COUNSELING INFORMATION**
  17.1 Nausea, Dyspnea or Diarrhea
  17.2 Nursing Mothers
* Sections or subsections omitted from the full prescribing information are not listed

FULL PRESCRIBING INFORMATION

1 INDICATIONS AND USAGE
1.1 Chronic Idiopathic Constipation
Amitiza® is indicated for the treatment of chronic idiopathic constipation in adults.
1.2 Opioid-induced Constipation
Amitiza is indicated for the treatment of opioid-induced constipation (OIC) in adults with chronic non-cancer pain.
Limitations of Use:
• Effectiveness of Amitiza in the treatment of opioid-induced constipation in patients taking diphenylheptane opioids (e.g., methadone) has not been established. [see Clinical Studies (14.2)]
1.3 Irritable Bowel Syndrome with Constipation
Amitiza is indicated for the treatment of irritable bowel syndrome with constipation (IBS-C) in women ≥ 18 years old.

2 DOSAGE AND ADMINISTRATION
Take Amitiza orally with food and water. Swallow capsules whole and do not break apart or chew. Physicians and patients should periodically assess the need for continued therapy.
2.1 Chronic Idiopathic Constipation and Opioid-induced Constipation
The recommended dose is 24 mcg twice daily orally with food and water.

Dosage in patients with hepatic impairment
For patients with moderately impaired hepatic function (Child-Pugh Class B), the recommended starting dose is 16 mcg twice daily. For patients with severely impaired hepatic function (Child-Pugh Class C), the recommended starting dose is 8 mcg twice daily. If this dose is tolerated and an adequate response has not been obtained after an appropriate interval, doses can then be escalated to full dosing with appropriate monitoring of patient response [see Use in Specific Populations (8.7) and Clinical Pharmacology (12.3)].
2.2 Irritable Bowel Syndrome with Constipation
The recommended dose is 8 mcg twice daily orally with food and water.
Dosage in patients with hepatic impairment
For patients with severely impaired hepatic function (Child-Pugh Class C), the recommended starting dose is 8 mcg once daily. If this dose is tolerated and an adequate response has not been obtained after an appropriate interval, doses can then be escalated to full dosing with appropriate monitoring of patient response. Dosage adjustment is not required for patients with moderately impaired hepatic function (Child-Pugh Class B) [see Use in Specific Populations (8.7) and Clinical Pharmacology (12.3)].

3 DOSAGE FORMS AND STRENGTHS
Amitiza is available as an oval, gelatin capsule containing 8 mcg or 24 mcg of lubiprostone.
• 8 mcg capsules are pink and are printed with "SPI" on one side
• 24 mcg capsules are orange and are printed with "SPI" on one side

4 CONTRAINDICATIONS
Amitiza is contraindicated in patients with known or suspected mechanical gastrointestinal obstruction.

5 WARNINGS AND PRECAUTIONS
5.1 Nausea
Patients taking Amitiza may experience nausea. Concomitant administration of food with Amitiza may reduce symptoms of nausea [see Adverse Reactions (6.1)].
5.2 Diarrhea
Amitiza should not be prescribed to patients that have severe diarrhea. Patients should be aware of the possible occurrence of diarrhea during treatment. Patients should be instructed to discontinue Amitiza and inform their physician if severe diarrhea occurs [see Adverse Reactions (6.1)].
5.3 Dyspnea
In clinical trials, dyspnea was reported by 3%, 1%, and < 1% of the treated CIC, OIC, and IBS-C populations receiving Amitiza, respectively, compared to 0%, 1%, and < 1% of placebo-treated patients. There have been postmarketing reports of dyspnea when using Amitiza 24 mcg twice daily. Some patients have discontinued treatment because of dyspnea. These events have usually been described as a sensation of chest tightness and difficulty taking in a breath, and generally have an acute onset within 30–60 minutes after taking the first dose. They generally resolve within a few hours after taking the dose, but recurrence has been frequently reported with subsequent doses.
5.4 Bowel Obstruction
In patients with symptoms suggestive of mechanical gastrointestinal obstruction, perform a thorough evaluation to confirm the absence of an obstruction prior to initiating therapy with Amitiza.

6 ADVERSE REACTIONS
The following adverse reactions are described below and elsewhere in labeling:
• Nausea [see Warnings and Precautions (5.1)]
• Diarrhea [see Warnings and Precautions (5.2)]
• Dyspnea [see Warnings and Precautions (5.3)]
6.1 Clinical Studies Experience
Because clinical studies are conducted under widely varying conditions, adverse reaction rates observed in the clinical studies of a drug cannot be directly compared to rates in the clinical studies of another drug and may not reflect the rates observed in practice.
During clinical development of Amitiza for CIC, OIC, and IBS-C, 1234 patients were treated with Amitiza for 6 months and 524 patients were treated for 1 year (not mutually exclusive).
Chronic Idiopathic Constipation
Adverse reactions in dose-finding, efficacy, and long-term clinical studies: The data described below reflect exposure to Amitiza 24 mcg twice daily in 1113 patients with chronic idiopathic constipation over 3- or 4-week, 6-month, and 12-month treatment periods; and from 316 patients receiving placebo over short-term exposure (≤ 4 weeks). The placebo population (N = 316) had a mean age of 47.8 (range 21–81) years; 87.3% female; 80.7% Caucasian, 10.1% African American, 7.3% Hispanic, 0.9% Asian; and 11.7% elderly (≥ 65 years of age). Of those patients treated with Amitiza 24 mcg twice daily (N=1113), the mean age was 50.3 (range 19-86) years; 86.9% were female; 86.1% Caucasian, 7.6% Af-

rican American, 4.7% Hispanic, 1.0% Asian; and 16.7% elderly (≥ 65 years of age). Table 1 presents data for the adverse reactions that occurred in at least 1% of patients who received Amitiza 24 mcg twice daily and that occurred more frequently with study drug than placebo.

Table 1: Percent of Patients with Adverse Reactions (Chronic Idiopathic Constipation)

System/Adverse Reaction*	Placebo N = 316 %	Amitiza 24 mcg Twice Daily N = 1113 %
Gastrointestinal disorders		
Nausea	3	29
Diarrhea	1	12
Abdominal pain	3	8
Abdominal distension	2	6
Flatulence	2	6
Vomiting	0	3
Loose stools	0	3
Abdominal discomfort†	1	3
Dyspepsia	< 1	2
Dry mouth	< 1	1
Nervous system disorders		
Headache	5	11
Dizziness	1	3
General disorders and site administration conditions		
Edema	< 1	3
Fatigue	1	2
Chest discomfort/pain	0	2
Respiratory, thoracic, and mediastinal disorders		
Dyspnea	0	2

* Includes only those events associated with treatment (possibly, probably, or definitely related, as assessed by the investigator).
† This term combines "abdominal tenderness," "abdominal rigidity," "gastrointestinal discomfort," "stomach discomfort", and "abdominal discomfort."

The most common adverse reactions (incidence > 4%) in CIC were nausea, diarrhea, headache, abdominal pain, abdominal distension, and flatulence.

Nausea: Approximately 29% of patients who received Amitiza 24 mcg twice daily experienced nausea; 4% of patients had severe nausea and 9% of patients discontinued treatment due to nausea. The rate of nausea associated with Amitiza 24 mcg twice daily was lower among male (8%) and elderly (19%) patients. No patients in the clinical studies were hospitalized due to nausea.

Diarrhea: Approximately 12% of patients who received Amitiza 24 mcg twice daily experienced diarrhea; 2% of patients had severe diarrhea and 2% discontinued treatment due to diarrhea.

Electrolytes: No serious adverse reactions of electrolyte imbalance were reported in clinical studies, and no clinically significant changes were seen in serum electrolyte levels in patients receiving Amitiza.

Less common adverse reactions: The following adverse reactions (assessed by investigator as probably or definitely related to treatment) occurred in less than 1% of patients receiving Amitiza 24 mcg twice daily in clinical studies, occurred in at least two patients, and occurred more frequently in patients receiving study drug than those receiving placebo: fecal incontinence, muscle cramp, defecation urgency, frequent bowel movements, hyperhidrosis, pharyngolaryngeal pain, intestinal functional disorder, anxiety, cold sweat, constipation, cough, dysgeusia, eructation, influenza, joint swelling, myalgia, pain, syncope, tremor, decreased appetite.

Opioid-induced Constipation
Adverse reactions in efficacy and long-term clinical studies: The data described below reflect exposure to Amitiza 24 mcg twice daily in 860 patients with OIC for up to 12 months and from 632 patients receiving placebo twice daily for up to 12 weeks. The total population (N = 1492) had a mean age of 50.4 (range 20–89) years; was 62.7% female; 82.7% Caucasian, 14.2% African American, 0.8% American Indian/Alaska Native, 0.8% Asian; 5.2% were of Hispanic ethnicity; and 8.8% were elderly (≥ 65 years of age). Table 2 presents data for the adverse reactions that occurred in at least 1% of patients who received Amitiza 24 mcg twice daily and that occurred more frequently with study drug than placebo.

Table 2: Percent of Patients with Adverse Reactions (OIC Studies)

System/Adverse Reaction*	Placebo N = 632 %	Amitiza 24 mcg Twice Daily N = 860 %
Gastrointestinal disorders		
Nausea	5	11
Diarrhea	2	8
Abdominal pain	1	4
Flatulence	3	4
Abdominal distension	2	3
Vomiting	2	3
Abdominal discomfort†	1	1
Nervous system disorders		
Headache	1	2
General disorders and site administration conditions		
Peripheral edema	< 1	1

* Includes only those events associated with treatment (possibly, probably, or definitely related, as assessed by the investigator).
† This term combines "abdominal tenderness," "abdominal rigidity," "gastrointestinal discomfort," "stomach discomfort", and "abdominal discomfort."

The most common adverse reactions (incidence > 4%) in OIC were nausea and diarrhea.
Nausea: Approximately 11% of patients who received Amitiza 24 mcg twice daily experienced nausea; 1% of patients had severe nausea and 2% of patients discontinued treatment due to nausea.
Diarrhea: Approximately 8% of patients who received Amitiza 24 mcg twice daily experienced diarrhea; 2% of patients had severe diarrhea and 1% of patients discontinued treatment due to diarrhea.
Less common adverse reactions: The following adverse reactions (assessed by investigator as probably or definitely related to treatment) occurred in less than 1% of patients receiving Amitiza 24 mcg twice daily in clinical studies, occurred in at least two patients, and occurred more frequently in patients receiving study drug than those receiving placebo: fecal incontinence, blood potassium decreased.

Irritable Bowel Syndrome with Constipation
Adverse reactions in dose-finding, efficacy, and long-term clinical studies: The data described below reflect exposure to Amitiza 8 mcg twice daily in 1011 patients with IBS-C for up to 12 months and from 435 patients receiving placebo twice daily for up to 16 weeks. The total population (N = 1267) had a mean age of 46.5 (range 18–85) years; was 91.6% female; 77.5% Caucasian, 12.9% African American, 8.6% Hispanic, 0.4% Asian; and 8.0% elderly (≥ 65 years of age). Table 3 presents data for the adverse reactions that occurred in at least 1% of patients who received Amitiza 8 mcg twice daily and that occurred more frequently with study drug than placebo.

Table 3: Percent of Patients with Adverse Reactions (IBS-C Studies)

System/Adverse Reaction*	Placebo N = 435 %	Amitiza 8 mcg Twice Daily N = 1011 %
Gastrointestinal disorders		
Nausea	4	8
Diarrhea	4	7
Abdominal pain	5	5
Abdominal distension	2	3

* Includes only those events associated with treatment (possibly or probably related, as assessed by the investigator).

The most common adverse reactions (incidence > 4%) in IBS-C were nausea, diarrhea, and abdominal pain.
Nausea: Approximately 8% of patients who received Amitiza 8 mcg twice daily experienced nausea; 1% of patients had severe nausea and 1% of patients discontinued treatment due to nausea.
Diarrhea: Approximately 7% of patients who received Amitiza 8 mcg twice daily experienced diarrhea; <1% of patients had severe diarrhea and <1% of patients discontinued treatment due to diarrhea.
Less common adverse reactions: The following adverse reactions (assessed by investigator as probably related to

treatment) occurred in less than 1% of patients receiving Amitiza 8 mcg twice daily in clinical studies, occurred in at least two patients, and occurred more frequently in patients receiving study drug than those receiving placebo: dyspepsia, loose stools, vomiting, fatigue, dry mouth, edema, increased alanine aminotransferase, increased aspartate aminotransferase, constipation, eructation, gastroesophageal reflux disease, dyspnea, erythema, gastritis, increased weight, palpitations, urinary tract infection, anorexia, anxiety, depression, fecal incontinence, fibromyalgia, hard feces, lethargy, rectal hemorrhage, pollakiuria.

6.2   Postmarketing Experience
The following additional adverse reactions have been identified during post-approval use of Amitiza. Because these reactions are reported voluntarily from a population of uncertain size, it is not always possible to reliably estimate their frequency or establish a causal relationship to drug exposure.
Voluntary reports of adverse reactions occurring with the use of Amitiza include the following: syncope, ischemic colitis, hypersensitivity/allergic-type reactions (including rash, swelling, and throat tightness), malaise, tachycardia, muscle cramps or muscle spasms, and asthenia.

7   DRUG INTERACTIONS
No *in vivo* drug-drug interaction studies have been performed with Amitiza.
Based upon the results of *in vitro* human microsome studies, there is low likelihood of pharmacokinetic drug-drug interactions. *In vitro* studies using human liver microsomes indicate that cytochrome P450 isoenzymes are not involved in the metabolism of lubiprostone. Further *in vitro* studies indicate microsomal carbonyl reductase may be involved in the extensive biotransformation of lubiprostone to the metabolite M3 [see *Clinical Pharmacology (12.3)*]. Additionally, *in vitro* studies in human liver microsomes demonstrate that lubiprostone does not inhibit cytochrome P450 isoforms 3A4, 2D6, 1A2, 2A6, 2B6, 2C9, 2C19, or 2E1, and *in vitro* studies of primary cultures of human hepatocytes show no induction of cytochrome P450 isoforms 1A2, 2B6, 2C9, and 3A4 by lubiprostone. Based on the available information, no protein binding–mediated drug interactions of clinical significance are anticipated.
Interaction potential with diphenylheptane opioids (e.g. methadone): Non-clinical studies have shown opioids of the diphenylheptane chemical class (e.g., methadone) to dose-dependently reduce the activation of ClC-2 by lubiprostone in the gastrointestinal tract. There is a possibility of a dose-dependent decrease in the efficacy of Amitiza in patients using diphenylheptane opioids.

8   USE IN SPECIFIC POPULATIONS
8.1   Pregnancy
Pregnancy Category C.
Risk Summary
There are no adequate and well-controlled studies with Amitiza in pregnant women. A dose dependent increase in fetal loss was observed in pregnant guinea pigs that received lubiprostone doses equivalent to 0.2 to 6 times the maximum recommended human dose (MRHD) based on body surface area (mg/m²). Animal studies did not show an increase in structural malformations. Amitiza should be used during pregnancy only if the potential benefit justifies the potential risk to the fetus.
Clinical Considerations
Current available data suggest that miscarriage occurs in 15-18% of clinically recognized pregnancies, regardless of any drug exposure. Consider the risks and benefits of available therapies when treating a pregnant woman for chronic idiopathic constipation, opioid-induced constipation or irritable bowel syndrome with constipation.
Animal Data
In developmental toxicity studies, pregnant rats and rabbits received oral lubiprostone during organogenesis at doses up to approximately 338 times (rats) and approximately 34 times (rabbits) the maximum recommended human dose (MHRD) based on body surface area (mg/m²). Maximal animal doses were 2000 mcg/kg/day (rats) and 100 mcg/kg/day (rabbits). In rats, there were increased incidences of early resorptions and soft tissue malformations (*situs inversus*, cleft palate) at the 2000 mcg/kg/day dose; however, these effects were probably secondary to maternal toxicity. A dose-dependent increase in fetal loss occurred when guinea pigs received lubiprostone after the period of organogenesis, on days 40 to 53 of gestation, at daily oral doses of 1, 10, and 25 mcg/kg/day (approximately 0.2, 2 and 6 times the MRHD based on body surface area (mg/m²)). The potential of lubiprostone to cause fetal loss was also examined in pregnant Rhesus monkeys. Monkeys received lubiprostone post-organogenesis on gestation days 110 through 130 at daily oral doses of 10 and 30 mcg/kg/day (approximately 3 and 10 times the MHRD based on body surface area (mg/m²)). Fetal loss was noted in one monkey from the 10-mcg/kg dose group, which is within normal historical rates for this species. There was no drug-related adverse effect seen in monkeys.

8.3   Nursing Mothers
It is not known whether lubiprostone is excreted in human milk. In rats, neither lubiprostone nor its active metabolites

were detectable in breast milk following oral administration of lubiprostone. Because lubiprostone increases fluid secretion in the intestine and intestinal motility, human milk-fed infants should be monitored for diarrhea. Caution should be exercised when Amitiza is administered to a nursing woman.

8.4 Pediatric Use
Safety and effectiveness in pediatric patients have not been established.

8.5 Geriatric Use

Chronic Idiopathic Constipation

The efficacy of Amitiza in the elderly (≥ 65 years of age) subpopulation was consistent with the efficacy in the overall study population. Of the total number of constipated patients treated in the dose-finding, efficacy, and long-term studies of Amitiza, 15.5% were ≥ 65 years of age, and 4.2% were ≥ 75 years of age. Elderly patients taking Amitiza 24 mcg twice daily experienced a lower rate of associated nausea compared to the overall study population taking Amitiza (19% vs. 29%, respectively).

Opioid-induced Constipation

The safety profile of Amitiza in the elderly (≥ 65 years of age) subpopulation (8.8% were ≥ 65 years of age and 1.6% were ≥ 75 years of age) was consistent with the safety profile in the overall study population. Clinical studies of Amitiza did not include sufficient numbers of patients aged 65 years and over to determine whether they respond differently from younger patients.

Irritable Bowel Syndrome with Constipation

The safety profile of Amitiza in the elderly (≥ 65 years of age) subpopulation (8.0% were ≥ 65 years of age and 1.8% were ≥ 75 years of age) was consistent with the safety profile in the overall study population. Clinical studies of Amitiza did not include sufficient numbers of patients aged 65 years and over to determine whether they respond differently from younger patients.

8.6 Renal Impairment
No dosage adjustment is required in patients with renal impairment [see *Clinical Pharmacology (12.3)*].

8.7 Hepatic Impairment
Patients with moderate hepatic impairment (Child-Pugh Class B) and severe hepatic impairment (Child-Pugh Class C) experienced markedly higher systemic exposure of lubiprostone active metabolite M3, when compared to normal subjects [see *Clinical Pharmacology (12.3)*]. Clinical safety results demonstrated an increased incidence and severity of adverse events in subjects with greater severity of hepatic impairment.

In case of chronic idiopathic constipation or opioid-induced constipation indications, the starting dosage of Amitiza should be reduced in patients with moderate hepatic impairment. The starting dose of Amitiza should be reduced in all patients with severe hepatic impairment, regardless of the indication [see *Dosage and Administration (2.1, 2.2)*]. No dosing adjustment is required in patients with mild hepatic impairment (Child-Pugh Class A).

10 OVERDOSAGE

There have been two confirmed reports of overdosage with Amitiza. The first report involved a 3-year-old child who accidentally ingested 7 or 8 capsules of 24 mcg of Amitiza and fully recovered. The second report was a study patient who self-administered a total of 96 mcg of Amitiza per day for 8 days. The patient experienced no adverse reactions during this time. Additionally, in a Phase 1 cardiac repolarization study, 38 of 51 healthy volunteers given a single oral dose of 144 mcg of Amitiza (6 times the highest recommended dose) experienced an adverse event that was at least possibly related to the study drug. Adverse reactions that occurred in at least 1% of these volunteers included the following: nausea (45%), diarrhea (35%), vomiting (27%), dizziness (14%), headache (12%), abdominal pain (8%), flushing/hot flash (8%), retching (8%), dyspnea (4%), pallor (4%), stomach discomfort (4%), anorexia (2%), asthenia (2%), chest discomfort (2%), dry mouth (2%), hyperhidrosis (2%), and syncope (2%).

11 DESCRIPTION

Amitiza (lubiprostone) is a chloride channel activator for oral use.

The chemical name for lubiprostone is (−)-7-[(2R,4aR,5R,7aR)-2-(1,1-difluoropentyl)-2-hydroxy-6-oxooctahydrocyclopenta[b]pyran-5-yl]heptanoic acid. The

molecular formula of lubiprostone is $C_{20}H_{32}F_2O_5$ with a molecular weight of 390.46 and a chemical structure as follows:

Lubiprostone drug substance occurs as white, odorless crystals or crystalline powder, is very soluble in ether and ethanol, and is practically insoluble in hexane and water. Amitiza is available as an imprinted, oval, soft gelatin capsule in two strengths. Pink capsules contain 8 mcg of lubiprostone and the following inactive ingredients: medium-chain triglycerides, gelatin, sorbitol, ferric oxide, titanium dioxide, and purified water. Orange capsules contain 24 mcg of lubiprostone and the following inactive ingredients: medium-chain triglycerides, gelatin, sorbitol, FD&C Red #40, D&C Yellow #10, and purified water.

12 CLINICAL PHARMACOLOGY

12.1 Mechanism of Action
Lubiprostone is a locally acting chloride channel activator that enhances a chloride-rich intestinal fluid secretion without altering sodium and potassium concentrations in the serum. Lubiprostone acts by specifically activating ClC-2, which is a normal constituent of the apical membrane of the human intestine, in a protein kinase A–independent fashion.

By increasing intestinal fluid secretion, lubiprostone increases motility in the intestine, thereby facilitating the passage of stool and alleviating symptoms associated with chronic idiopathic constipation. Patch clamp cell studies in human cell lines have indicated that the majority of the beneficial biological activity of lubiprostone and its metabolites is observed only on the apical (luminal) portion of the gastrointestinal epithelium.

Lubiprostone, via activation of apical ClC-2 channels in intestinal epithelial cells, bypasses the antisecretory action of opiates that results from suppression of secretomotor neuron excitability.

Activation of ClC-2 by lubiprostone has also been shown to stimulate recovery of mucosal barrier function and reduce intestinal permeability via the restoration of tight junction protein complexes in *ex vivo* studies of ischemic porcine intestine.

12.2 Pharmacodynamics
Although the pharmacologic effects of lubiprostone in humans have not been fully evaluated, animal studies have shown that oral administration of lubiprostone increases chloride ion transport into the intestinal lumen, enhances fluid secretion into the bowels, and improves fecal transit.

12.3 Pharmacokinetics
Lubiprostone has low systemic availability following oral administration and concentrations of lubiprostone in plasma are below the level of quantitation (10 pg/mL). Therefore, standard pharmacokinetic parameters such as area under the curve (AUC), maximum concentration (C_{max}), and half-life ($t_{1/2}$) cannot be reliably calculated. However, the pharmacokinetic parameters of M3 (only measurable active metabolite of lubiprostone) have been characterized. Gender has no effect on the pharmacokinetics of M3 following the oral administration of lubiprostone.

Absorption

Concentrations of lubiprostone in plasma are below the level of quantitation (10 pg/mL) because lubiprostone has a low systemic availability following oral administration. Peak plasma levels of M3, after a single oral dose with 24 mcg of lubiprostone, occurred at approximately 1.10 hours. The C_{max} was 41.5 pg/mL and the mean AUC_{0-t} was 57.1 pg·hr/mL. The AUC_{0-t} of M3 increases dose proportionally after single 24-mcg and 144-mcg doses of lubiprostone.

Distribution

In vitro protein binding studies indicate lubiprostone is approximately 94% bound to human plasma proteins. Studies in rats given radiolabeled lubiprostone indicate minimal

distribution beyond the gastrointestinal tissues. Concentrations of radiolabeled lubiprostone at 48 hours post-administration were minimal in all tissues of the rats.

Metabolism

The results of both human and animal studies indicate that lubiprostone is rapidly and extensively metabolized by 15-position reduction, α-chain β-oxidation, and ω-chain ω-oxidation. These biotransformations are not mediated by the hepatic cytochrome P450 system but rather appear to be mediated by the ubiquitously expressed carbonyl reductase. M3, a metabolite of lubiprostone found in both humans and animals, is formed by the reduction of the carbonyl group at the 15-hydroxy moiety that consists of both α-hydroxy and β-hydroxy epimers. M3 makes up less than 10% of the dose of radiolabeled lubiprostone. Animal studies have shown that metabolism of lubiprostone rapidly occurs within the stomach and jejunum, most likely in the absence of any systemic absorption.

Elimination

Lubiprostone could not be detected in plasma; however, M3 has a $t_{1/2}$ ranging from 0.9 to 1.4 hours. After a single oral dose of 72 mcg of [3H]-labeled lubiprostone, 60% of total administered radioactivity was recovered in the urine within 24 hours and 30% of total administered radioactivity was recovered in the feces by 168 hours. Lubiprostone and M3 are only detected in trace amounts in human feces.

Food Effect

A study was conducted with a single 72-mcg dose of [3H]-labeled lubiprostone to evaluate the potential of a food effect on lubiprostone absorption, metabolism, and excretion. Pharmacokinetic parameters of total radioactivity demonstrated that C_{max} decreased by 55% while $AUC_{0-∞}$ was unchanged when lubiprostone was administered with a high-fat meal. The clinical relevance of the effect of food on the pharmacokinetics of lubiprostone is not clear. However, lubiprostone was administered with food and water in a majority of clinical trials.

Special Populations

Renal Impairment

Sixteen subjects, 34–47 years old (8 severe renally impaired subjects [creatinine clearance (CrCl) < 20 mL/min] who required hemodialysis and 8 control subjects with normal renal function [CrCl > 80 mL/min]), received a single oral 24-mcg dose of Amitiza. Following administration, lubiprostone plasma concentrations were below the limit of quantitation (10 pg/mL). Plasma concentrations of M3 were within the range of exposure from previous clinical experience with Amitiza.

Hepatic Impairment

Twenty-five subjects, 38–78 years old (9 with severe hepatic impairment [Child-Pugh Class C], 8 with moderate impairment [Child-Pugh Class B], and 8 with normal liver function), received either 12 mcg or 24 mcg of Amitiza under fasting conditions. Following administration, lubiprostone plasma concentrations were below the limit of quantitation (10 pg/mL) except for two subjects. In moderately and severely impaired subjects, the C_{max} and AUC_{0-t} of the active lubiprostone metabolite M3 were increased, as shown in Table 4.

[See table 4 below]

These results demonstrate that there is a correlation between increased exposure of M3 and severity of hepatic impairment. *[see Use in Specific Populations (8.7)]*

13 NONCLINICAL TOXICOLOGY

13.1 Carcinogenesis, Mutagenesis, Impairment of Fertility

Carcinogenesis

Two 2-year oral (gavage) carcinogenicity studies (one in Crl:B6C3F1 mice and one in Sprague-Dawley rats) were conducted with lubiprostone. In the 2-year carcinogenicity study in mice, lubiprostone doses of 25, 75, 200, and 500 mcg/kg/day (approximately 2, 6, 17, and 42 times the highest recommended human dose, respectively, based on body surface area) were used. In the 2-year rat carcinogenicity study, lubiprostone doses of 20, 100, and 400 mcg/kg/day (approximately 3, 17, and 68 times the highest recommended human dose, respectively, based on body surface area) were used. In the mouse carcinogenicity study, there was no significant increase in any tumor incidences. There was a significant increase in the incidence of interstitial cell adenoma of the testes in male rats at the 400 mcg/kg/day dose. In female rats, treatment with lubiprostone produced hepatocellular adenoma at the 400 mcg/kg/day dose.

Mutagenesis

Lubiprostone was not genotoxic in the *in vitro* Ames reverse mutation assay, the *in vitro* mouse lymphoma (L5178Y TK +/−) forward mutation assay, the *in vitro* Chinese hamster lung (CHL/IU) chromosomal aberration assay, and the *in vivo* mouse bone marrow micronucleus assay.

Impairment of Fertility

Lubiprostone, at oral doses of up to 1000 mcg/kg/day, had no effect on the fertility and reproductive function of male and

Table 4: Pharmacokinetic Parameters of the Metabolite M3 for Subjects with Normal or Impaired Liver Function following Dosing with Amitiza

Liver Function Status	Mean (SD) AUC_{0-t} (pg·hr/mL)	% Change vs. Normal	Mean (SD) C_{max} (pg/mL)	% Change vs. Normal
Normal (n=8)	39.6 (18.7)	n.a.	37.5 (15.9)	n.a.
Child-Pugh Class B (n=8)	119 (104)	+119	70.9 (43.5)	+66
Child-Pugh Class C (n=8)	234 (61.6)	+521	114 (59.4)	+183

female rats. However, the number of implantation sites and live embryos were significantly reduced in rats at the 1000 mcg/kg/day dose as compared to control. The number of dead or resorbed embryos in the 1000 mcg/kg/day group was higher compared to the control group, but was not statistically significant. The 1000 mcg/kg/day dose in rats is approximately 169 times the highest recommended human dose of 48 mcg/day, based on body surface area.

14 CLINICAL STUDIES

14.1 Chronic Idiopathic Constipation

Two double-blinded, placebo-controlled studies of identical design were conducted in patients with chronic idiopathic constipation. Chronic idiopathic constipation was defined as, on average, less than 3 spontaneous bowel movements (SBMs) per week (a SBM is a bowel movement occurring in the absence of laxative use) along with one or more of the following symptoms of constipation for at least 6 months prior to randomization: 1) very hard stools for at least a quarter of all bowel movements; 2) sensation of incomplete evacuation following at least a quarter of all bowel movements; and 3) straining with defecation at least a quarter of the time.

Following a 2-week baseline/washout period, a total of 479 patients (mean age 47.2 [range 20–81] years; 88.9% female; 80.8% Caucasian, 9.6% African American, 7.3% Hispanic, 1.5% Asian; 10.9% ≥ 65 years of age) were randomized and received Amitiza 24 mcg twice daily or placebo twice daily for 4 weeks. The primary endpoint of the studies was SBM frequency. The studies demonstrated that patients treated with Amitiza had a higher frequency of SBMs during Week 1 than the placebo patients. In both studies, results similar to those in Week 1 were also observed in Weeks 2, 3, and 4 of therapy (Table 5).

[See table 5 above]

In both studies, Amitiza demonstrated increases in the percentage of patients who experienced SBMs within the first 24 hours after administration when compared to placebo (56.7% vs. 36.9% in Study 1 and 62.9% vs. 31.9% in Study 2, respectively). Similarly, the time to first SBM was shorter for patients receiving Amitiza than for those receiving placebo.

Signs and symptoms related to constipation, including abdominal bloating, abdominal discomfort, stool consistency, and straining, as well as constipation severity ratings, were also improved with Amitiza versus placebo. The results were consistent in subpopulation analyses for gender, race, and elderly patients (≥ 65 years of age).

During a 7-week randomized withdrawal study, patients who received Amitiza during a 4-week treatment period were then randomized to receive either placebo or to continue treatment with Amitiza. In Amitiza-treated patients randomized to placebo, SBM frequency rates returned toward baseline within 1 week and did not result in worsening compared to baseline. Patients who continued on Amitiza maintained their response to therapy over the additional 3 weeks of treatment.

14.2 Opioid-induced Constipation

The efficacy of Amitiza in the treatment of opioid-induced constipation in patients receiving opioid therapy for chronic, non-cancer-related pain was assessed in three randomized, double-blinded, placebo-controlled studies. In Study 1, the median age was 52 years (range 20–82) and 63.1% were female. In Study 2, the median age was 50 years (range 21–77) and 64.4% were female. In Study 3, the median age was 50 years (range 21–89) and 60.1% were female. Patients had been receiving stable opioid therapy for at least 30 days prior to screening, which was to continue throughout the 12-week treatment period. At baseline, mean oral morphine equivalent daily doses (MEDDs) were 99 mg and 130 mg for placebo-treated and Amitiza-treated patients, respectively, in Study 1. Baseline mean MEDDs were 237 mg and 265 mg for placebo-treated and Amitiza-treated patients, respectively, in Study 2. In Study 3, baseline mean MEDDs were 330 mg and 373 mg for placebo-treated and Amitiza-treated patients, respectively. The Brief Pain Inventory-Short Form (BPI-SF) questionnaire was administered to patients at baseline and monthly during the treatment period to assess pain control. Patients had documented opioid-induced constipation at baseline, defined as having less than 3 spontaneous bowel movements (SBMs) per week, with at least 25% of SBMs associated with one or more of the following conditions: (1) hard to very hard stool consistency; (2) moderate to very severe straining; and/or (3) having a sensation of incomplete evacuation. Laxative use was discontinued at the beginning of the screening period and throughout the study. With the exception of the 48-hour period prior to first dose and for at least 72 hours (Study 1) or 1 week (Study 2 and Study 3) following first dose, use of rescue medication was allowed in cases where no bowel movement had occurred in a 3-day period. Median weekly SBM frequencies at baseline were 1.5 for placebo patients and 1.0 for Amitiza patients in Study 1 and, for both Study 2 and Study 3, median weekly SBM frequencies at baseline were 1.5 for both treatment groups.

In Study 1, patients receiving non-diphenylheptane (e.g., non-methadone) opioids (n = 431) were randomized to receive placebo (n = 217) or Amitiza 24 mcg twice daily (n = 214) for 12 weeks. The primary efficacy analysis was a comparison of the proportion of "overall responders" in each treatment arm. A patient was considered an "overall responder" if ≥1 SBM improvement over baseline was reported for all treatment weeks for which data were available *and* ≥3 SBMs/week were reported for at least 9 of 12 treatment weeks. The proportion of patients in Study 1 qualifying as an "overall responder" was 27.1% in the group receiving Amitiza 24 mcg twice daily compared to 18.9% of patients receiving placebo twice daily (treatment difference = 8.2%; p-value = 0.03). Examination of gender and race subgroups did not identify differences in response to Amitiza among these subgroups. There were too few elderly patients (≥ 65 years of age) to adequately assess differences in effects in that population.

In Study 2, patients receiving opioids (N = 418) were randomized to receive placebo (n = 208) or Amitiza 24 mcg twice daily (n = 210) for 12 weeks. Study 2 did not exclude patients receiving diphenylheptane opioids (e.g., methadone). The primary efficacy endpoint was the mean change from baseline in SBM frequency at Week 8; 3.3 vs. 2.4 for Amitiza and placebo-treated patients, respectively; treatment difference = 0.9; p-value = 0.004. The proportion of patients in Study 2 qualifying as an "overall responder," as prespecified in Study 1, was 24.3% in the group receiving Amitiza compared to 15.4% of patients receiving placebo. In the subgroup of patients in Study 2 taking diphenylheptane opioids (baseline mean [median] MEDDs of 691 [403] mg and 672 [450] mg for placebo and Amitiza patients, respectively), the proportion of patients qualifying as an "overall responder" was 20.5% (8/39) in the group receiving Amitiza compared to 6.3% (2/32) of patients receiving placebo. Examination of gender and race subgroups did not identify differences in response to Amitiza among these subgroups. There were too few elderly patients (≥ 65 years of age) to adequately assess differences in effects in that population.

In Study 3, patients receiving opioids (N = 451) were randomized to placebo (n = 216) or Amitiza 24 mcg twice daily (n = 235) for 12 weeks. Study 3 did not exclude patients receiving diphenylheptane opioids (e.g., methadone). The primary efficacy endpoint was the change from baseline in SBM frequency at Week 8. The study did not demonstrate a statistically significant improvement in SBM frequency rates at Week 8 (mean change from baseline of 2.7 vs. 2.5 for Amitiza and placebo-treated patients, respectively; treatment difference = 0.2; p-value = 0.76). The proportion of patients in Study 3 qualifying as an "overall responder," as prespecified in Study 1, was 15.3% in the patients receiving Amitiza compared to 13.0% of patients receiving placebo. In the subgroup of patients in Study 3 taking diphenylheptane opioids (baseline mean [median] MEDDs of 730 [518] mg and 992 [480] mg for placebo and Amitiza patients, respectively), the proportion of patients qualifying as an "overall responder" was 2.1% (1/47) in the group receiving Amitiza compared to 12.2% (5/41) of patients receiving placebo.

14.3 Irritable Bowel Syndrome with Constipation

Two double-blinded, placebo-controlled studies of similar design were conducted in patients with IBS-C. IBS was defined as abdominal pain or discomfort occurring over at least 6 months with two or more of the following: 1) relieved with defecation; 2) onset associated with a change in stool frequency; and 3) onset associated with a change in stool form. Patients were sub-typed as having IBS-C if they also experienced two of three of the following: 1) < 3 spontaneous bowel movements (SBMs) per week, 2) > 25% hard stools, and 3) > 25% SBMs associated with straining.

Following a 4-week baseline/washout period, a total of 1154 patients (mean age 46.6 [range 18–85] years; 91.6% female; 77.4% Caucasian, 13.2% African American, 8.5% Hispanic, 0.4% Asian; 8.3% ≥ 65 years of age) were randomized and received Amitiza 8 mcg twice daily (16 mcg/day) or placebo twice daily for 12 weeks. The primary efficacy endpoint was assessed weekly utilizing the patient's response to a global symptom relief question based on a 7-point, balanced scale ("significantly worse" to "significantly relieved"): "How would you rate your relief of IBS symptoms (abdominal discomfort/pain, bowel habits, and other IBS symptoms) over the past week compared to how you felt before you entered the study?"

The primary efficacy analysis was a comparison of the proportion of "overall responders" in each arm. A patient was considered an "overall responder" if the criteria for being designated a "monthly responder" were met in at least 2 of the 3 months on study. A "monthly responder" was defined as a patient who had reported "significantly relieved" for at least 2 weeks of the month or at least "moderately relieved" in all 4 weeks of that month. During each monthly evaluation period, patients reporting "moderately worse" or "significantly worse" relief, an increase in rescue medication use, or those who discontinued due to lack of efficacy, were deemed non-responders.

The percentage of patients in Study 1 qualifying as an "overall responder" was 13.8% in the group receiving Amitiza 8 mcg twice daily compared to 7.8% of patients receiving placebo twice daily. In Study 2, 12.1% of patients in the Amitiza 8 mcg group were "overall responders" versus 5.7% of patients in the placebo group. In both studies, the treatment differences between the placebo and Amitiza groups were statistically significant.

Results in men: The two randomized, placebo-controlled, double-blinded studies comprised 97 (8.4%) male patients, which is insufficient to determine whether men with IBS-C respond differently to Amitiza from women.

During a 4-week randomized withdrawal period following Study 1, patients who received Amitiza during the 12-week treatment period were re-randomized to receive either placebo or to continue treatment with Amitiza. In Amitiza-treated patients who were "overall responders" during Study 1 and who were re-randomized to placebo, SBM frequency rates did not result in worsening compared to baseline.

16 HOW SUPPLIED/STORAGE AND HANDLING

Amitiza is available as an oval, soft gelatin capsule containing 8 mcg or 24 mcg of lubiprostone with "SPI" printed on one side. Amitiza is available as follows:
8 mcg pink capsule
• Bottles of 60 (NDC 64764-080-60)
24 mcg orange capsule
• Bottles of 60 (NDC 64764-240-60)
• Bottles of 100 (NDC 64764-240-10)
Store at 25°C (77°F); excursions permitted to 15° to 30°C (59° to 86°F).
Protect from light and extreme temperatures.

17 PATIENT COUNSELING INFORMATION

Physicians and patients should periodically assess the need for continued therapy.

17.1 Nausea, Dyspnea or Diarrhea

Instruct patients to take Amitiza twice daily with food and water to reduce the occurrence of nausea. Patients taking

Table 5: Spontaneous Bowel Movement Frequency Rates* (Efficacy Studies)

Trial	Study Arm	Baseline *Mean ± SD* *Median*	Week 1 *Mean ± SD* *Median*	Week 2 *Mean ± SD* *Median*	Week 3 *Mean ± SD* *Median*	Week 4 *Mean ± SD* *Median*	Week 1 Change from Baseline *Mean ± SD* *Median*	Week 4 Change from Baseline *Mean ± SD* *Median*
Study 1	Placebo	1.6 ± 1.3 1.5	3.5 ± 2.3 3.0	3.2 ± 2.5 3.0	2.8 ± 2.2 2.0	2.9 ± 2.4 2.3	1.9 ± 2.2 1.5	1.3 ± 2.5 1.0
	Amitiza 24 mcg Twice Daily	1.4 ± 0.8 1.5	5.7 ± 4.4 5.0	5.1 ± 4.1 4.0	5.3 ± 4.9 5.0	5.3 ± 4.7 4.0	4.3 ± 4.3 3.5	3.9 ± 4.6 3.0
Study 2	Placebo	1.5 ± 0.8 1.5	4.0 ± 2.7 3.5	3.6 ± 2.7 3.0	3.4 ± 2.8 3.0	3.5 ± 2.9 3.0	2.5 ± 2.6 1.5	1.9 ± 2.7 1.5
	Amitiza 24 mcg Twice Daily	1.3 ± 0.9 1.5	5.9 ± 4.0 5.0	5.0 ± 4.2 4.0	5.6 ± 4.6 5.0	5.4 ± 4.8 4.3	4.6 ± 4.1 3.8	4.1 ± 4.8 3.0

* Frequency rates are calculated as 7 times (number of SBMs) / (number of days observed for that week).

Amitiza may experience dyspnea within an hour of the first dose. Dyspnea generally resolves within 3 hours, but may recur with repeat dosing. Patients on treatment who experience severe nausea, dyspnea, or diarrhea should notify their physician.

17.2 Nursing Mothers
Advise lactating women to monitor their human milk-fed infants for diarrhea while taking Amitiza [see *Use in Specific Populations (8.3)*].

Marketed by:
Sucampo Pharma Americas, LLC
Bethesda, MD 20814
and
Takeda Pharmaceuticals America, Inc.
Deerfield, IL 60015
Amitiza® is a registered trademark of Sucampo AG.
Shown in Product Identification Guide, page 313

BRINTELLIX   ℞
(vortioxetine)
tablets, for oral use

HIGHLIGHTS OF PRESCRIBING INFORMATION
These highlights do not include all the information needed to use BRINTELLIX safely and effectively. See full prescribing information for BRINTELLIX.
BRINTELLIX (vortioxetine) tablets, for oral use
Initial U.S. Approval: 2013

> **WARNING: SUICIDAL THOUGHTS AND BEHAV-IORS**
> *See full prescribing information for complete boxed warning.*
> - Increased risk of suicidal thinking and behavior in children, adolescents, and young adults taking antidepressants (5.1).
> - Monitor for worsening and emergence of suicidal thoughts and behaviors (5.1).
> - BRINTELLIX has not been evaluated for use in pediatric patients (8.4).

―――――RECENT MAJOR CHANGES―――――
Warnings and Precautions (5.5)   7/2014
―――――INDICATIONS AND USAGE―――――
BRINTELLIX is indicated for the treatment of major depressive disorder (MDD) (1, 14).
―――――DOSAGE AND ADMINISTRATION―――――
- The recommended starting dose is 10 mg administered orally once daily without regard to meals (2.1).
- The dose should then be increased to 20 mg/day, as tolerated (2.1).
- Consider 5 mg/day for patients who do not tolerate higher doses (2.1).
- BRINTELLIX can be discontinued abruptly. However, it is recommended that doses of 15 mg/day or 20 mg/day be reduced to 10 mg/day for one week prior to full discontinuation if possible (2.3).
- The maximum recommended dose is 10 mg/day in known CYP2D6 poor metabolizers (2.6).
―――――DOSAGE FORMS AND STRENGTHS―――――
BRINTELLIX is available as 5 mg, 10 mg, 15 mg, and 20 mg immediate release tablets (3).
―――――CONTRAINDICATIONS―――――
- Hypersensitivity to vortioxetine or any components of the BRINTELLIX formulation (4).
- Monoamine Oxidase Inhibitors (MAOIs): Do not use MAOIs intended to treat psychiatric disorders with BRINTELLIX or within 21 days of stopping treatment with BRINTELLIX. Do not use BRINTELLIX within 14 days of stopping an MAOI intended to treat psychiatric disorders. In addition, do not start BRINTELLIX in a patient who is being treated with linezolid or intravenous methylene blue (4).
―――――WARNINGS AND PRECAUTIONS―――――
- Serotonin Syndrome has been reported with serotonergic antidepressants (SSRIs, SNRIs, and others), including with BRINTELLIX, both when taken alone, but especially when co-administered with other serotonergic agents (including triptans, tricyclic antidepressants, fentanyl, lithium, tramadol, tryptophan, buspirone, and St. John's Wort). If such symptoms occur, discontinue BRINTELLIX and initiate supportive treatment. If concomitant use of BRINTELLIX with other serotonergic drugs is clinically warranted, patients should be made aware of a potential increased risk for serotonin syndrome, particularly during treatment initiation and dose increases (5.2).
- Treatment with serotonergic antidepressants (SSRIs, SNRIs, and others) may increase the risk of abnormal bleeding. Patients should be cautioned about the increased risk of bleeding when BRINTELLIX is coadministered with nonsteroidal anti-inflammatory drugs (NSAIDs), aspirin, or other drugs that affect coagulation (5.3).

- Activation of Mania/Hypomania can occur with antidepressant treatment. Screen patients for bipolar disorder (5.4).
- Angle Closure Glaucoma: Angle closure glaucoma has occurred in patients with untreated anatomically narrow angles treated with antidepressants (5.5).
- Hyponatremia can occur in association with the syndrome of inappropriate antidiuretic hormone secretion (SIADH) (5.6).
―――――ADVERSE REACTIONS―――――
Most common adverse reactions (incidence ≥5% and at least twice the rate of placebo) were: nausea, constipation and vomiting (6).
To report SUSPECTED ADVERSE REACTIONS, contact Takeda Pharmaceuticals at 1-877-TAKEDA-7 (1-877-825-3327) or FDA at 1-800-FDA-1088 or www.fda.gov/medwatch.
―――――DRUG INTERACTIONS―――――
- Strong inhibitors of CYP2D6: Reduce BRINTELLIX dose by half when a strong CYP2D6 inhibitor (e.g., bupropion, fluoxetine, paroxetine, or quinidine) is coadministered (2.6 and 7.3).
- Strong CYP Inducers: Consider increasing BRINTELLIX dose when a strong CYP inducer (e.g., rifampin, carbamazepine, or phenytoin) is coadministered for more than 14 days. The maximum recommended dose should not exceed 3 times the original dose (2.7 and 7.3).
―――――USE IN SPECIFIC POPULATIONS―――――
- Pregnancy: Based on animal data, BRINTELLIX may cause fetal harm (8.1).
- Nursing Mothers: Discontinue BRINTELLIX or nursing (8.3).
See 17 for PATIENT COUNSELING INFORMATION and Medication Guide

Revised: 07/2014

―――――FULL PRESCRIBING INFORMATION: CONTENTS*
WARNING: SUICIDAL THOUGHTS AND BEHAVIORS

FULL PRESCRIBING INFORMATION

> **WARNING: SUICIDAL THOUGHTS AND BE-HAVIORS**
> Antidepressants increased the risk of suicidal thoughts and behavior in children, adolescents, and young adults in short-term studies. These studies did not show an increase in the risk of suicidal thoughts and behavior with antidepressant use in patients over age 24; there was a trend toward reduced risk with antidepressant use in patients aged 65 and older [see *Warnings and Precautions (5.1)*].
> In patients of all ages who are started on antidepressant therapy, monitor closely for worsening, and for emergence of suicidal thoughts and behaviors. Advise families and caregivers of the need for close observation and communication with the prescriber [see *Warnings and Precautions (5.1)*].
> BRINTELLIX has not been evaluated for use in pediatric patients [see *Use in Specific Populations (8.4)*].

1 INDICATIONS AND USAGE
1.1 Major Depressive Disorder
BRINTELLIX is indicated for the treatment of major depressive disorder (MDD). The efficacy of BRINTELLIX was established in six 6 to 8 week studies (including one study in the elderly) and one maintenance study in adults [see *Clinical Studies (14)*].

2 DOSAGE AND ADMINISTRATION
2.1 General Instruction for Use
The recommended starting dose is 10 mg administered orally once daily without regard to meals. Dosage should then be increased to 20 mg/day, as tolerated, because higher doses demonstrated better treatment effects in trials conducted in the United States. The efficacy and safety of doses above 20 mg/day have not been evaluated in controlled clinical trials. A dose decrease down to 5 mg/day may be considered for patients who do not tolerate higher doses [see *Clinical Studies (14)*].
2.2 Maintenance/Continuation/Extended Treatment
It is generally agreed that acute episodes of major depression should be followed by several months or longer of sustained pharmacologic therapy. A maintenance study of BRINTELLIX demonstrated that BRINTELLIX decreased the risk of recurrence of depressive episodes compared to placebo.
2.3 Discontinuing Treatment
Although BRINTELLIX can be abruptly discontinued, in placebo-controlled trials patients experienced transient adverse reactions such as headache and muscle tension following abrupt discontinuation of BRINTELLIX 15 mg/day or 20 mg/day. To avoid these adverse reactions, it is recommended that the dose be decreased to 10 mg/day for one week before full discontinuation of BRINTELLIX 15 mg/day or 20 mg/day [see *Adverse Reactions (6)*].
2.4 Switching a Patient To or From a Monoamine Oxidase Inhibitor (MAOI) Intended to Treat Psychiatric Disorders
At least 14 days should elapse between discontinuation of a MAOI intended to treat psychiatric disorders and initiation of therapy with BRINTELLIX to avoid the risk of Serotonin Syndrome [see *Warnings and Precautions (5.2)*]. Conversely, at least 21 days should be allowed after stopping BRINTELLIX before starting an MAOI intended to treat psychiatric disorders [see *Contraindications (4)*].
2.5 Use of BRINTELLIX with Other MAOIs such as Linezolid or Methylene Blue
Do not start BRINTELLIX in a patient who is being treated with linezolid or intravenous methylene blue because there is an increased risk of serotonin syndrome. In a patient who requires more urgent treatment of a psychiatric condition, other interventions, including hospitalization, should be considered [see *Contraindications (4)*].
In some cases, a patient already receiving BRINTELLIX therapy may require urgent treatment with linezolid or intravenous methylene blue. If acceptable alternatives to linezolid or intravenous methylene blue treatment are not available and the potential benefits of linezolid or intravenous methylene blue treatment are judged to outweigh the risks of serotonin syndrome in a particular patient, BRINTELLIX should be stopped promptly, and linezolid or intravenous methylene blue can be administered. The patient should be monitored for symptoms of serotonin syndrome for 21 days or until 24 hours after the last dose of linezolid or intravenous methylene blue, whichever comes first. Therapy with BRINTELLIX may be resumed 24 hours after the last dose of linezolid or intravenous methylene blue [see *Warnings and Precautions (5.2)*].

The risk of administering methylene blue by non-intravenous routes (such as oral tablets or by local injection) or in intravenous doses much lower than 1 mg/kg with BRINTELLIX is unclear. The clinician should, nevertheless, be aware of the possibility of emergent symptoms of serotonin syndrome with such use *[see Warnings and Precautions (5.2)]*.

2.6 Use of BRINTELLIX in Known CYP2D6 Poor Metabolizers or in Patients Taking Strong CYP2D6 Inhibitors

The maximum recommended dose of BRINTELLIX is 10 mg/day in known CYP2D6 poor metabolizers. Reduce the dose of BRINTELLIX by one-half when patients are receiving a CYP2D6 strong inhibitor (e.g., bupropion, fluoxetine, paroxetine, or quinidine) concomitantly. The dose should be increased to the original level when the CYP2D6 inhibitor is discontinued *[see Drug Interactions (7.3)]*.

2.7 Use of BRINTELLIX in Patients Taking Strong CYP Inducers

Consider increasing the dose of BRINTELLIX when a strong CYP inducer (e.g., rifampin, carbamazepine, or phenytoin) is coadministered for greater than 14 days. The maximum recommended dose should not exceed three times the original dose. The dose of BRINTELLIX should be reduced to the original level within 14 days, when the inducer is discontinued *[see Drug Interactions (7.3)]*.

3 DOSAGE FORMS AND STRENGTHS

BRINTELLIX is available as immediate-release, film-coated tablets in the following strengths:
- 5 mg: pink, almond shaped biconvex film coated tablet, debossed with "5" on one side and "TL" on the other side
- 10 mg: yellow, almond shaped biconvex film coated tablet, debossed with "10" on one side and "TL" on the other side
- 15 mg: orange, almond shaped biconvex film coated tablet, debossed with "15" on one side and "TL" on the other side
- 20 mg: red, almond shaped biconvex film coated tablet, debossed with "20" on one side and "TL" on the other side

4 CONTRAINDICATIONS

- Hypersensitivity to vortioxetine or any components of the formulation. Angioedema has been reported in patients treated with BRINTELLIX.
- The use of MAOIs intended to treat psychiatric disorders with BRINTELLIX or within 21 days of stopping treatment with BRINTELLIX is contraindicated because of an increased risk of serotonin syndrome. The use of BRINTELLIX within 14 days of stopping an MAOI intended to treat psychiatric disorders is also contraindicated *[see Dosage and Administration (2.4) and Warnings and Precautions (5.2)]*.

Starting BRINTELLIX in a patient who is being treated with MAOIs such as linezolid or intravenous methylene blue is also contraindicated because of an increased risk of serotonin syndrome *[see Dosage and Administration (2.5) and Warnings and Precautions (5.2)]*.

5 WARNINGS AND PRECAUTIONS

5.1 Clinical Worsening and Suicide Risk

Patients with major depressive disorder (MDD), both adult and pediatric, may experience worsening of their depression and/or the emergence of suicidal ideation and behavior (suicidality) or unusual changes in behavior, whether or not they are taking antidepressant medications, and this risk may persist until significant remission occurs. Suicide is a known risk of depression and certain other psychiatric disorders, and these disorders themselves are the strongest predictors of suicide. There has been a long-standing concern, however, that antidepressants may have a role in inducing worsening of depression and the emergence of suicidality in certain patients during the early phases of treatment. Pooled analyses of short-term placebo-controlled studies of antidepressant drugs (selective serotonin reuptake inhibitors [SSRIs] and others) showed that these drugs increase the risk of suicidal thinking and behavior (suicidality) in children, adolescents, and young adults (ages 18 to 24) with MDD and other psychiatric disorders. Short-term studies did not show an increase in the risk of suicidality with antidepressants compared to placebo in adults beyond age 24; there was a trend toward reduction with antidepressants compared to placebo in adults aged 65 and older.

The pooled analyses of placebo-controlled studies in children and adolescents with MDD, obsessive-compulsive disorder (OCD), or other psychiatric disorders included a total of 24 short-term studies of nine antidepressant drugs in over 4,400 patients. The pooled analyses of placebo-controlled studies in adults with MDD or other psychiatric disorders included a total of 295 short-term studies (median duration of two months) of 11 antidepressant drugs in over 77,000 patients. There was considerable variation in risk of suicidality among drugs, but a tendency toward an increase in the younger patients for almost all drugs studied. There were differences in absolute risk of suicidality across the different indications, with the highest incidence in MDD. The

risk differences (drug vs. placebo), however, were relatively stable within age strata and across indications. These risk differences (drug-placebo difference in the number of cases of suicidality per 1000 patients treated) are provided in *Table 1*.

Table 1. Drug-Placebo Difference in Number of Cases of Suicidality per 1000 Patients Treated

Age Range	
Increases Compared to Placebo	
<18	14 additional cases
18-24	5 additional cases
Decreases Compared to Placebo	
25-64	1 fewer case
≥65	6 fewer cases

No suicides occurred in any of the pediatric studies. There were suicides in the adult studies, but the number was not sufficient to reach any conclusion about drug effect on suicide.

It is unknown whether the suicidality risk extends to longer-term use, i.e., beyond several months. However, there is substantial evidence from placebo-controlled maintenance studies in adults with depression that the use of antidepressants can delay the recurrence of depression.

All patients being treated with antidepressants for any indication should be monitored appropriately and observed closely for clinical worsening, suicidality, and unusual changes in behavior, especially during the initial few months of a course of drug therapy, or at times of dose changes, either increases or decreases.

The following symptoms anxiety, agitation, panic attacks, insomnia, irritability, hostility, aggressiveness, impulsivity, akathisia (psychomotor restlessness), hypomania, and mania have been reported in adult and pediatric patients being treated with antidepressants for MDD as well as for other indications, both psychiatric and nonpsychiatric. Although a causal link between the emergence of such symptoms and either the worsening of depression and/or the emergence of suicidal impulses has not been established, there is concern that such symptoms may represent precursors to emerging suicidality.

Consideration should be given to changing the therapeutic regimen, including possibly discontinuing the medication, in patients whose depression is persistently worse, or who are experiencing emergent suicidality or symptoms that might be precursors to worsening depression or suicidality, especially if these symptoms are severe, abrupt in onset, or were not part of the patient's presenting symptoms.

Families and caregivers of patients being treated with antidepressants for MDD or other indications, both psychiatric and nonpsychiatric, should be alerted about the need to monitor patients for the emergence of agitation, irritability, unusual changes in behavior, and the other symptoms described above, as well as the emergence of suicidality, and to report such symptoms immediately to healthcare providers. Such monitoring should include daily observation by families and caregivers.

Screening Patients for Bipolar Disorder

A major depressive episode may be the initial presentation of bipolar disorder. It is generally believed (though not established in controlled studies) that treating such an episode with an antidepressant alone may increase the likelihood of precipitation of a mixed/manic episode in patients at risk for bipolar disorder. Whether any of the symptoms described above represent such a conversion is unknown. However, prior to initiating treatment with an antidepressant, patients with depressive symptoms should be adequately screened to determine if they are at risk for bipolar disorder; such screening should include a detailed psychiatric history, including a family history of suicide, bipolar disorder, and depression. It should be noted that BRINTELLIX is not approved for use in treating bipolar depression.

5.2 Serotonin Syndrome

The development of a potentially life-threatening serotonin syndrome has been reported with serotonergic antidepressants including BRINTELLIX, when used alone but more often when used concomitantly with other serotonergic drugs (including triptans, tricyclic antidepressants, fentanyl, lithium, tramadol, tryptophan, buspirone, and St. John's Wort), and with drugs that impair metabolism of serotonin (in particular, MAOIs, both those intended to treat psychiatric disorders and also others, such as linezolid and intravenous methylene blue).

Serotonin syndrome symptoms may include mental status changes (e.g., agitation, hallucinations, delirium, and coma), autonomic instability (e.g., tachycardia, labile blood pressure, dizziness, diaphoresis, flushing, hyperthermia), neuromuscular symptoms (e.g., tremor, rigidity, myoclonus, hyperreflexia, incoordination), seizures, and/or gastrointestinal symptoms (e.g., nausea, vomiting, diarrhea). Patients should be monitored for the emergence of serotonin syndrome.

The concomitant use of BRINTELLIX with MAOIs intended to treat psychiatric disorders is contraindicated. BRINTELLIX should also not be started in a patient who is being treated with MAOIs such as linezolid or intravenous methylene blue. All reports with methylene blue that provided information on the route of administration involved intravenous administration in the dose range of 1 mg/kg to 8 mg/kg. No reports involved the administration of methylene blue by other routes (such as oral tablets or local tissue injection) or at lower doses. There may be circumstances when it is necessary to initiate treatment with a MAOI such as linezolid or intravenous methylene blue in a patient taking BRINTELLIX. BRINTELLIX should be discontinued before initiating treatment with the MAOI *[see Contraindications (4) and Dosage and Administration (2.4)]*.

If concomitant use of BRINTELLIX with other serotonergic drugs, including triptans, tricyclic antidepressants, fentanyl, lithium, tramadol, buspirone, tryptophan, and St. John's Wort is clinically warranted, patients should be made aware of a potential increased risk for serotonin syndrome, particularly during treatment initiation and dose increases.

Treatment with BRINTELLIX and any concomitant serotonergic agents should be discontinued immediately if the above events occur and supportive symptomatic treatment should be initiated.

5.3 Abnormal Bleeding

The use of drugs that interfere with serotonin reuptake inhibition, including BRINTELLIX, may increase the risk of bleeding events. Concomitant use of aspirin, nonsteroidal anti-inflammatory drugs (NSAIDs), warfarin, and other anticoagulants may add to this risk. Case reports and epidemiological studies (case-control and cohort design) have demonstrated an association between use of drugs that interfere with serotonin reuptake and the occurrence of gastrointestinal bleeding. Bleeding events related to drugs that inhibit serotonin reuptake have ranged from ecchymosis, hematoma, epistaxis, and petechiae to life-threatening hemorrhages.

Patients should be cautioned about the increased risk of bleeding when BRINTELLIX is coadministered with NSAIDs, aspirin, or other drugs that affect coagulation or bleeding *[see Drug Interactions (7.2)]*.

5.4 Activation of Mania/Hypomania

Symptoms of mania/hypomania were reported in <0.1% of patients treated with BRINTELLIX in pre-marketing clinical studies. Activation of mania/hypomania has been reported in a small proportion of patients with major affective disorder who were treated with other antidepressants. As with all antidepressants, use BRINTELLIX cautiously in patients with a history or family history of bipolar disorder, mania, or hypomania.

5.5 Angle Closure Glaucoma

Angle Closure Glaucoma: The pupillary dilation that occurs following use of many antidepressant drugs, including BRINTELLIX, may trigger an angle closure attack in a patient with anatomically narrow angles who does not have a patent iridectomy.

5.6 Hyponatremia

Hyponatremia has occurred as a result of treatment with serotonergic drugs. In many cases, hyponatremia appears to be the result of the syndrome of inappropriate antidiuretic hormone secretion (SIADH). One case with serum sodium lower than 110 mmol/L was reported in a subject treated with BRINTELLIX in a pre-marketing clinical study. Elderly patients may be at greater risk of developing hyponatremia with a serotonergic antidepressant. Also, patients taking diuretics or who are otherwise volume depleted can be at greater risk. Discontinuation of BRINTELLIX in patients with symptomatic hyponatremia and appropriate medical intervention should be instituted. Signs and symptoms of hyponatremia include headache, difficulty concentrating, memory impairment, confusion, weakness, and unsteadiness, which can lead to falls. More severe and/or acute cases have included hallucination, syncope, seizure, coma, respiratory arrest, and death.

6 ADVERSE REACTIONS

The following adverse reactions are discussed in greater detail in other sections of the label.
- Hypersensitivity *[see Contraindications (4)]*
- Clinical Worsening and Suicide Risk *[see Warnings and Precautions (5.1)]*
- Serotonin Syndrome *[see Warnings and Precautions (5.2)]*
- Abnormal Bleeding *[see Warnings and Precautions (5.3)]*
- Activation of Mania/Hypomania *[see Warnings and Precautions (5.4)]*
- Hyponatremia *[see Warnings and Precautions (5.6)]*

Table 2. Common Adverse Reactions Occurring in ≥2% of Patients Treated with any BRINTELLIX Dose and at Least 2% Greater than the Incidence in Placebo-treated Patients

System Organ Class Preferred Term	BRINTELLIX 5 mg/day N=1013 %	BRINTELLIX 10 mg/day N=699 %	BRINTELLIX 15 mg/day N=449 %	BRINTELLIX 20 mg/day N=455 %	Placebo N=1621 %
Gastrointestinal disorders					
Nausea	21	26	32	32	9
Diarrhea	7	7	10	7	6
Dry mouth	7	7	6	8	6
Constipation	3	5	6	6	3
Vomiting	3	5	6	6	1
Flatulence	1	3	2	1	1
Nervous system disorders					
Dizziness	6	6	8	9	6
Psychiatric disorders					
Abnormal dreams	<1	<1	2	3	1
Skin and subcutaneous tissue disorders					
Pruritus*	1	2	3	3	1

*includes pruritus generalized

Table 3. ASEX Incidence of Treatment Emergent Sexual Dysfunction*

	BRINTELLIX 5 mg/day N=65:67[†]	BRINTELLIX 10 mg/day N=94:86[†]	BRINTELLIX 15 mg/day N=57:67[†]	BRINTELLIX 20 mg/day N=67:59[†]	Placebo N=135:162[†]
Females	22%	23%	33%	34%	20%
Males	16%	20%	19%	29%	14%

* Incidence based on number of subjects with sexual dysfunction during the study / number of subjects without sexual dysfunction at baseline. Sexual dysfunction was defined as a subject scoring any of the following on the ASEX scale at two consecutive visits during the study: 1) total score ≥19; 2) any single item ≥5; 3) three or more items each with a score ≥4
[†] Sample size for each dose group is the number of patients (females:males) without sexual dysfunction at baseline

6.1 Clinical Studies Experience

Because clinical trials are conducted under widely varying conditions, adverse reaction rates observed in the clinical trials of a drug cannot be directly compared to rates in the clinical studies of another drug and may not reflect the rates observed in clinical practice.

Patient Exposure

BRINTELLIX was evaluated for safety in 4746 patients (18 years to 88 years of age) diagnosed with MDD who participated in pre-marketing clinical studies; 2616 of those patients were exposed to BRINTELLIX in 6 to 8 week, placebo-controlled studies at doses ranging from 5 mg to 20 mg once daily and 204 patients were exposed to BRINTELLIX in a 24 week to 64 week placebo-controlled maintenance study at doses of 5 mg to 10 mg once daily. Patients from the 6 to 8 week studies continued into 12-month open-label studies. A total of 2586 patients were exposed to at least one dose of BRINTELLIX in open-label studies, 1727 were exposed to BRINTELLIX for six months and 885 were exposed for at least one year.

Adverse Reactions Reported as Reasons for Discontinuation of Treatment

In pooled 6 to 8 week placebo-controlled studies the incidence of patients who received BRINTELLIX 5 mg/day, 10 mg/day, 15 mg/day and 20 mg/day and discontinued treatment because of an adverse reaction was 5%, 6%, 8% and 8%, respectively, compared to 4% of placebo-treated patients. Nausea was the most common adverse reaction reported as a reason for discontinuation.

Common Adverse Reactions in Placebo-Controlled MDD Studies

The most commonly observed adverse reactions in MDD patients treated with BRINTELLIX in 6 to 8 week placebo-controlled studies (incidence ≥5% and at least twice the rate of placebo) were nausea, constipation and vomiting.

Table 2 shows the incidence of common adverse reactions that occurred in ≥2% of MDD patients treated with any

BRINTELLIX dose and at least 2% more frequently than in placebo-treated patients in the 6 to 8 week placebo-controlled studies.

[See table 2 above]

Nausea

Nausea was the most common adverse reaction and its frequency was dose-related *(Table 2)*. It was usually considered mild or moderate in intensity and the median duration was 2 weeks. Nausea was more common in females than males. Nausea most commonly occurred in the first week of BRINTELLIX treatment with 15 to 20% of patients experiencing nausea after 1 to 2 days of treatment. Approximately 10% of patients taking BRINTELLIX 10 mg/day to 20 mg/day had nausea at the end of the 6 to 8 week placebo-controlled studies.

Sexual Dysfunction

Difficulties in sexual desire, sexual performance and sexual satisfaction often occur as manifestations of psychiatric disorders, but they may also be consequences of pharmacologic treatment.

In the MDD 6 to 8 week controlled trials of BRINTELLIX, voluntarily reported adverse reactions related to sexual dysfunction were captured as individual event terms. These event terms have been aggregated and the overall incidence was as follows. In male patients the overall incidence was 3%, 4%, 4%, 5% in BRINTELLIX 5 mg/day, 10 mg/day, 15 mg/day, 20 mg/day, respectively, compared to 2% in placebo. In female patients, the overall incidence was <1%, 1%, <1%, 2% in BRINTELLIX 5 mg/day, 10 mg/day, 15 mg/day, 20 mg/day, respectively, compared to <1% in placebo.

Because voluntarily reported adverse sexual reactions are known to be underreported, in part because patients and physicians may be reluctant to discuss them, the Arizona Sexual Experiences Scale (ASEX), a validated measure designed to identify sexual side effects, was used prospectively in seven placebo-controlled trials. The ASEX scale includes five questions that pertain to the following aspects of sexual

function: 1) sex drive, 2) ease of arousal, 3) ability to achieve erection (men) or lubrication (women), 4) ease of reaching orgasm, and 5) orgasm satisfaction.

The presence or absence of sexual dysfunction among patients entering clinical studies was based on their ASEX scores. For patients without sexual dysfunction at baseline (approximately 1/3 of the population across all treatment groups in each study), *Table 3* shows the incidence of patients that developed treatment-emergent sexual dysfunction when treated with BRINTELLIX or placebo in any fixed dose group. Physicians should routinely inquire about possible sexual side effects.

[See table 3 above]

Adverse Reactions Following Abrupt Discontinuation of BRINTELLIX Treatment

Discontinuation symptoms have been prospectively evaluated in patients taking BRINTELLIX 10 mg/day, 15 mg/day, and 20 mg/day using the Discontinuation-Emergent Signs and Symptoms (DESS) scale in clinical trials. Some patients experienced discontinuation symptoms such as headache, muscle tension, mood swings, sudden outbursts of anger, dizziness, and runny nose in the first week of abrupt discontinuation of BRINTELLIX 15 mg/day and 20 mg/day.

Laboratory Tests

BRINTELLIX has not been associated with any clinically important changes in laboratory test parameters in serum chemistry (except sodium), hematology and urinalysis as measured in the 6 to 8 week placebo-controlled studies. Hyponatremia has been reported with the treatment of BRINTELLIX *[see Warnings and Precautions (5.6)]*. In the 6-month, double-blind, placebo-controlled phase of a long-term study in patients who had responded to BRINTELLIX during the initial 12-week, open-label phase, there were no clinically important changes in lab test parameters between BRINTELLIX and placebo-treated patients.

Weight

BRINTELLIX had no significant effect on body weight as measured by the mean change from baseline in the 6 to 8 week placebo-controlled studies. In the 6-month, double-blind, placebo-controlled phase of a long-term study in patients who had responded to BRINTELLIX during the initial 12-week, open-label phase, there was no significant effect on body weight between BRINTELLIX and placebo-treated patients.

Vital Signs

BRINTELLIX has not been associated with any clinically significant effects on vital signs, including systolic and diastolic blood pressure and heart rate, as measured in placebo-controlled studies.

Other Adverse Reactions Observed in Clinical Studies

The following listing does not include reactions: 1) already listed in previous tables or elsewhere in labeling, 2) for which a drug cause was remote, 3) which were so general as to be uninformative, 4) which were not considered to have significant clinical implications, or 5) which occurred at a rate equal to or less than placebo.

Ear and labyrinth disorders — vertigo
Gastrointestinal disorders — dyspepsia
Nervous system disorders — dysgeusia
Vascular disorders — flushing

7 DRUG INTERACTIONS

7.1 CNS Active Agents

Monoamine Oxidase Inhibitors

Adverse reactions, some of which are serious or fatal, can develop in patients who use MAOIs or who have recently been discontinued from an MAOI and started on a serotonergic antidepressant(s) or who have recently had SSRI or SNRI therapy discontinued prior to initiation of an MAOI *[see Dosage and Administration (2.4), Contraindications (4) and Warnings and Precautions (5.2)]*.

Serotonergic Drugs

Based on the mechanism of action of BRINTELLIX and the potential for serotonin toxicity, serotonin syndrome may occur when BRINTELLIX is coadministered with other drugs that may affect the serotonergic neurotransmitter systems (e.g., SSRIs, SNRIs, triptans, buspirone, tramadol, and tryptophan products etc.). Closely monitor symptoms of serotonin syndrome if BRINTELLIX is co-administered with other serotonergic drugs. Treatment with BRINTELLIX and any concomitant serotonergic agents should be discontinued immediately if serotonin syndrome occurs *[see Warnings and Precautions (5.2)]*.

Other CNS Active Agents

No clinically relevant effect was observed on steady state lithium exposure following coadministration with multiple daily doses of BRINTELLIX. Multiple doses of BRINTELLIX did not affect the pharmacokinetics or pharmacodynamics (composite cognitive score) of diazepam. A clinical study has shown that BRINTELLIX (single dose of 20 or 40 mg) did not increase the impairment of mental and motor skills caused by alcohol (single dose of 0.6 g/kg). Details on the potential pharmacokinetic interactions between BRINTELLIX and bupropion can be found in Section 7.3.

7.2 Drugs that Interfere with Hemostasis (e.g., NSAIDs, Aspirin, and Warfarin)

Serotonin release by platelets plays an important role in hemostasis. Epidemiological studies of case-control and cohort design have demonstrated an association between use of psychotropic drugs that interfere with serotonin reuptake and the occurrence of upper gastrointestinal bleeding. These studies have also shown that concurrent use of an NSAID or aspirin may potentiate this risk of bleeding. Altered anticoagulant effects, including increased bleeding, have been reported when SSRIs and SNRIs are coadministered with warfarin.

Following coadministration of stable doses of warfarin (1 to 10 mg/day) with multiple daily doses of BRINTELLIX, no significant effects were observed in INR, prothrombin values or total warfarin (protein bound plus free drug) pharmacokinetics for both R- and S-warfarin *[see Drug Interactions (7.4)]*. Coadministration of aspirin 150 mg/day with multiple daily doses of BRINTELLIX had no significant inhibitory effect on platelet aggregation or pharmacokinetics of aspirin and salicylic acid *[see Drug Interactions (7.4)]*. Patients receiving other drugs that interfere with hemostasis should be carefully monitored when BRINTELLIX is initiated or discontinued *[see Warnings and Precautions (5.3)]*.

7.3   Potential for Other Drugs to Affect BRINTELLIX

Reduce BRINTELLIX dose by half when a strong CYP2D6 inhibitor (e.g., bupropion, fluoxetine, paroxetine, quinidine) is coadministered. Consider increasing the BRINTELLIX dose when a strong CYP inducer (e.g., rifampicin, carbamazepine, phenytoin) is coadministered. The maximum dose is not recommended to exceed three times the original dose *[see Dosage and Administration (2.5 and 2.6)]* (Figure 1).

[See figure 1 above]

7.4   Potential for BRINTELLIX to Affect Other Drugs

No dose adjustment for the comedications is needed when BRINTELLIX is coadministered with a substrate of CYP1A2 (e.g., duloxetine), CYP2A6, CYP2B6 (e.g., bupropion), CYP2C8 (e.g., repaglinide), CYP2C9 (e.g., S-warfarin), CYP2C19 (e.g., diazepam), CYP2D6 (e.g., venlafaxine), CYP3A4/5 (e.g., budesonide), and P-gp (e.g., digoxin). In addition, no dose adjustment for lithium, aspirin, and warfarin is necessary.

Vortioxetine and its metabolites are unlikely to inhibit the following CYP enzymes and transporter based on *in vitro* data: CYP1A2, CYP2A6, CYP2B6, CYP2C8, CYP2C9, CYP2C19, CYP2D6, CYP2E1, CYP3A4/5, and P-gp. As such, no clinically relevant interactions with drugs metabolized by these CYP enzymes would be expected.

In addition, vortioxetine did not induce CYP1A2, CYP2A6, CYP2B6, CYP2C8, CYP2C9, CYP2C19, and CYP3A4/5 in an *in vitro* study in cultured human hepatocytes. Chronic administration of BRINTELLIX is unlikely to induce the metabolism of drugs metabolized by these CYP isoforms. Furthermore, in a series of clinical drug interaction studies, coadministration of BRINTELLIX with substrates for CYP2B6 (e.g., bupropion), CYP2C9 (e.g., warfarin), and CYP2C19 (e.g., diazepam), had no clinical meaningful effect on the pharmacokinetics of these substrates *(Figure 2)*.

Because vortioxetine is highly bound to plasma protein, coadministration of BRINTELLIX with another drug that is highly protein bound may increase free concentrations of the other drug. However, in a clinical study with coadministration of BRINTELLIX (10 mg/day) and warfarin (1 mg/day to 10 mg/day), a highly protein-bound drug, no significant change in INR was observed *[see Drug Interactions (7.2)]*.

[See figure 2 above]

8   USE IN SPECIFIC POPULATIONS

8.1   Pregnancy

Pregnancy Category C

Risk Summary

There are no adequate and well-controlled studies of BRINTELLIX in pregnant women. Vortioxetine caused developmental delays when administered during pregnancy to rats and rabbits at doses 15 and 10 times the maximum recommended human dose (MRHD) of 20 mg, respectively. Developmental delays were also seen after birth in rats at doses 20 times the MRHD of vortioxetine given during pregnancy and through lactation. There were no teratogenic effects in rats or rabbits at doses up to 77 and 58 times, the MRHD of vortioxetine, given during organogenesis. The incidence of malformations in human pregnancies has not been established for BRINTELLIX. All human pregnancies, regardless of drug exposure, have a background rate of 2 to 4% for major malformations, and 15 to 20% for pregnancy loss. BRINTELLIX should be used during pregnancy only if the potential benefit justifies the potential risk to the fetus.

Clinical Considerations

Neonates exposed to SSRIs or SNRIs, late in the third trimester have developed complications requiring prolonged hospitalization, respiratory support and tube feeding. Such complications can arise immediately upon delivery. Reported clinical findings have included respiratory distress, cyanosis, apnea, seizures, temperature instability, feeding difficulty, vomiting, hypoglycemia, hypotonia, hypertonia, hyperreflexia, tremor, jitteriness, irritability and constant crying. These features are consistent with either a direct

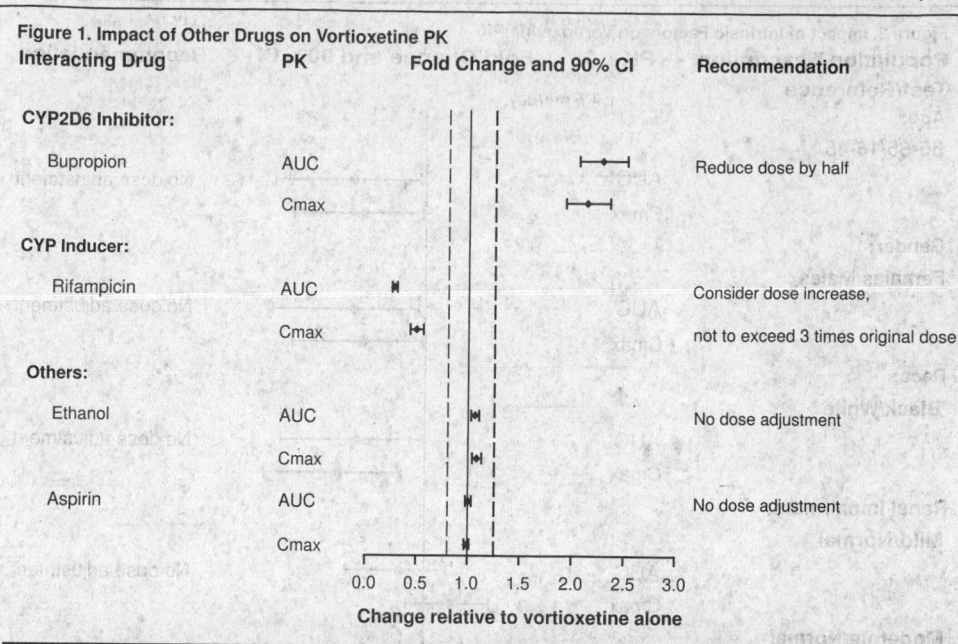

Figure 1. Impact of Other Drugs on Vortioxetine PK

Interacting Drug	PK	Fold Change and 90% CI	Recommendation
CYP2D6 Inhibitor:			
Bupropion	AUC		Reduce dose by half
	Cmax		
CYP Inducer:			
Rifampicin	AUC		Consider dose increase,
	Cmax		not to exceed 3 times original dose
Others:			
Ethanol	AUC		No dose adjustment
	Cmax		
Aspirin	AUC		No dose adjustment
	Cmax		

Change relative to vortioxetine alone

Figure 2. Impact of Vortioxetine on PK of Other Drugs

Interacting Drug	PK	Fold Change and 90% CI	Recommendation
CYP2B6 substrate:			
Bupropion	AUC		No dose adjustment
	Cmax		
CYP2C9 Substrate:			
(S)-Warfarin	AUC		No dose adjustment
	Cmax		
CYP2C19 Substrate:			
Diazepam	AUC		No dose adjustment
	Cmax		
Others:			
(R)-Warfarin	AUC		No dose adjustment
	Cmax		
Aspirin	AUC		No dose adjustment
	Cmax		
Ethanol	AUC		No dose adjustment
	Cmax		
Lithium	AUC		No dose adjustment
	Cmax		

Change relative to interacting drug alone

toxic effect of these classes of drugs or possibly, a drug discontinuation syndrome. It should be noted that in some cases, the clinical picture is consistent with serotonin syndrome *[see Warnings and Precautions (5.2)]*. When treating a pregnant woman with BRINTELLIX during the third trimester, the physician should carefully consider the potential risks and benefits of treatment.

Neonates exposed to SSRIs in pregnancy may have an increased risk for persistent pulmonary hypertension of the newborn (PPHN). PPHN occurs in one to two per 1,000 live births in the general population and is associated with sub-

stantial neonatal morbidity and mortality. Several recent epidemiologic studies suggest a positive statistical association between SSRI use in pregnancy and PPHN. Other studies do not show a significant statistical association. A prospective longitudinal study was conducted of 201 pregnant women with a history of major depression, who were either on antidepressants or had received antidepressants less than 12 weeks prior to their last menstrual period, and were in remission. Women who discontinued antidepressant medication during pregnancy showed a significant increase in relapse of their major depression compared to those

Figure 3. Impact of Intrinsic Factors on Vortioxetine PK

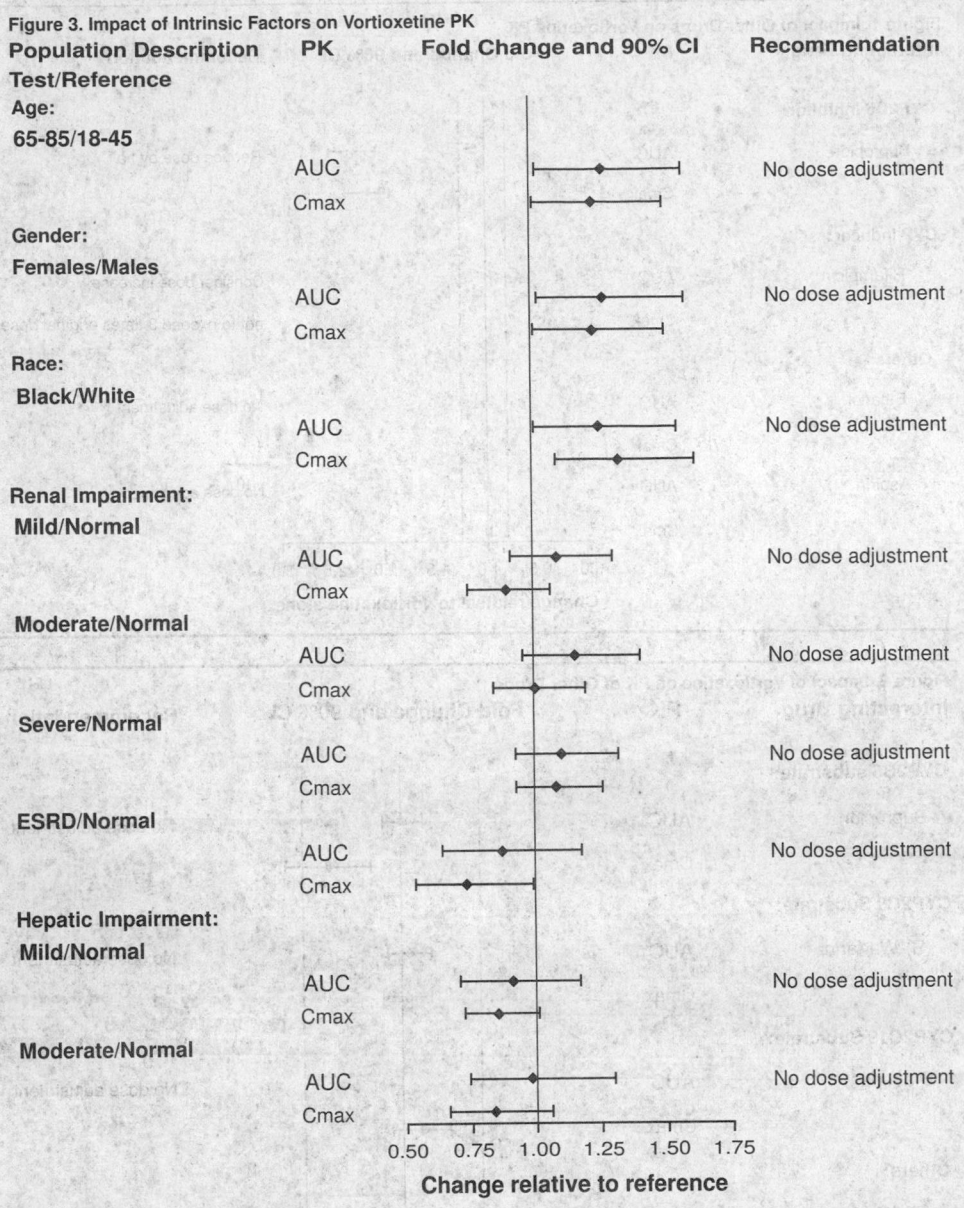

Population Description Test/Reference	PK	Fold Change and 90% CI	Recommendation
Age: 65-85/18-45	AUC / Cmax		No dose adjustment
Gender: Females/Males	AUC / Cmax		No dose adjustment
Race: Black/White	AUC / Cmax		No dose adjustment
Renal Impairment: Mild/Normal	AUC / Cmax		No dose adjustment
Moderate/Normal	AUC / Cmax		No dose adjustment
Severe/Normal	AUC / Cmax		No dose adjustment
ESRD/Normal	AUC / Cmax		No dose adjustment
Hepatic Impairment: Mild/Normal	AUC / Cmax		No dose adjustment
Moderate/Normal	AUC / Cmax		No dose adjustment

0.50 0.75 1.00 1.25 1.50 1.75
Change relative to reference

women who remained on antidepressant medication throughout pregnancy. When treating a pregnant woman with BRINTELLIX, the physician should carefully consider both the potential risks of taking a serotonergic antidepressant, along with the established benefits of treating depression with an antidepressant.

Animal Data
In pregnant rats and rabbits, no teratogenic effects were seen when vortioxetine was given during the period of organogenesis at oral doses up to 160 and 60 mg/kg/day, respectively. These doses are 77 and 58 times, in rats and rabbits, respectively, the maximum recommended human dose (MRHD) of 20 mg on a mg/m² basis. Developmental delay, seen as decreased fetal body weight and delayed ossification, occurred in rats and rabbits at doses equal to and greater than 30 and 10 mg/kg (15 and 10 times the MRHD, respectively) in the presence of maternal toxicity (decreased food consumption and decreased body weight gain). When vortioxetine was administered to pregnant rats at oral doses up to 120 mg/kg (58 times the MRHD) throughout pregnancy and lactation, the number of live-born pups was decreased and early postnatal pup mortality was increased at 40 and 120 mg/kg. Additionally, pup weights were decreased at birth to weaning at 120 mg/kg and development (specifically eye opening) was slightly delayed at 40 and 120 mg/kg. These effects were not seen at 10 mg/kg (5 times the MRHD).

8.3   Nursing Mothers
It is not known whether vortioxetine is present in human milk. Vortioxetine is present in the milk of lactating rats. Because many drugs are present in human milk and because of the potential for serious adverse reactions in nurs-

ing infants from BRINTELLIX, a decision should be made whether to discontinue nursing or to discontinue the drug, taking into account the importance of the drug to the mother.

8.4   Pediatric Use
Clinical studies on the use of BRINTELLIX in pediatric patients have not been conducted; therefore, the safety and effectiveness of BRINTELLIX in the pediatric population have not been established.

8.5   Geriatric Use
No dose adjustment is recommended on the basis of age (Figure 3). Results from a single-dose pharmacokinetic study in elderly (>65 years old) vs. young (24 to 45 years old) subjects demonstrated that the pharmacokinetics were generally similar between the two age groups.
Of the 2616 subjects in clinical studies of BRINTELLIX, 11% (286) were 65 and over, which included subjects from a placebo-controlled study specifically in elderly patients [see Clinical Studies (14)]. No overall differences in safety or effectiveness were observed between these subjects and younger subjects, and other reported clinical experience has not identified differences in responses between the elderly and younger patients.
Serotonergic antidepressants have been associated with cases of clinically significant hyponatremia in elderly patients, who may be at greater risk for this adverse event [see Warnings and Precautions (5.6)].

8.6   Use in Other Patient Populations
No dose adjustment of BRINTELLIX on the basis of race, gender, ethnicity, or renal function (from mild renal impairment to end-stage renal disease) is necessary. In addition, the same dose can be administered in patients with mild to

moderate hepatic impairment (Figure 3). BRINTELLIX has not been studied in patients with severe hepatic impairment. Therefore, BRINTELLIX is not recommended in patients with severe hepatic impairment.
[See figure 3 above]

9   DRUG ABUSE AND DEPENDENCE
BRINTELLIX is not a controlled substance.

10   OVERDOSAGE
10.1   Human Experience
There is limited clinical trial experience regarding human overdosage with BRINTELLIX. In pre-marketing clinical studies, cases of overdose were limited to patients who accidentally or intentionally consumed up to a maximum dose of 40 mg of BRINTELLIX. The maximum single dose tested was 75 mg in men. Ingestion of BRINTELLIX in the dose range of 40 to 75 mg was associated with increased rates of nausea, dizziness, diarrhea, abdominal discomfort, generalized pruritus, somnolence, and flushing.

10.2   Management of Overdose
No specific antidotes for BRINTELLIX are known. In managing over dosage, consider the possibility of multiple drug involvement. In case of overdose, call Poison Control Center at 1-800-222-1222 for latest recommendations.

11   DESCRIPTION
BRINTELLIX is an immediate-release tablet for oral administration that contains the beta (β) polymorph of vortioxetine hydrobromide (HBr), an antidepressant. Vortioxetine HBr is known chemically as 1-[2-(2,4-Dimethyl-phenylsulfanyl)-phenyl]-piperazine, hydrobromide. The empirical formula is $C_{18} H_{22} N_2 S$, HBr with a molecular weight of 379.36 g/mol. The structural formula is:

Vortioxetine HBr is a white to very slightly beige powder that is slightly soluble in water.
Each BRINTELLIX tablet contains 6.355 mg, 12.71 mg, 19.065 mg, or 25.42 mg of vortioxetine HBr equivalent to 5 mg, 10 mg, 15 mg, or 20 mg of vortioxetine, respectively. The inactive ingredients in BRINTELLIX tablets include mannitol, microcrystalline cellulose, hydroxypropyl cellulose, sodium starch glycolate, magnesium stearate and film coating which consists of hypromellose, titanium dioxide, polyethylene glycol 400, iron oxide red (5 mg, 15 mg, and 20 mg) and iron oxide yellow (10 mg and 15 mg).

12   CLINICAL PHARMACOLOGY
12.1   Mechanism of Action
The mechanism of the antidepressant effect of vortioxetine is not fully understood, but is thought to be related to its enhancement of serotonergic activity in the CNS through inhibition of the reuptake of serotonin (5-HT). It also has several other activities including 5-HT3 receptor antagonism and 5-HT1A receptor agonism. The contribution of these activities to vortioxetine's antidepressant effect has not been established.

12.2   Pharmacodynamics
Vortioxetine binds with high affinity to the human serotonin transporter (Ki=1.6 nM), but not to the norepinephrine (Ki=113 nM) or dopamine (Ki>1000 nM) transporters. Vortioxetine potently and selectively inhibits reuptake of serotonin (IC50=5.4 nM). Vortioxetine binds to 5-HT3 (Ki=3.7 nM), 5-HT1A (Ki=15 nM), 5-HT7 (Ki=19 nM), 5-HT1D (Ki=54 nM), and 5-HT1B (Ki=33 nM), receptors and is a 5-HT3, 5-HT1D, and 5-HT7 receptor antagonist, 5-HT1B receptor partial agonist, and 5-HT1A receptor agonist.
In humans, the mean 5-HT transporter occupancy, based on the results from 2 clinical PET studies using 5-HTT ligands ([¹¹C]-MADAM or [¹¹C]-DASB), was approximately 50% at 5 mg/day, 65% at 10 mg/day and approximately 80% at 20 mg/day in the regions of interest.

Effect on Cardiac Repolarization
The effect of vortioxetine 10 mg and 40 mg administered once daily on QTc interval was evaluated in a randomized, double-blind, placebo-, and active-controlled (moxifloxacin 400 mg), four-treatment-arm parallel study in 340 male subjects. In the study the upper bound of the one-sided 95% confidence interval for the QTc was below 10 ms, the threshold for regulatory concern. The oral dose of 40 mg is sufficient to assess the effect of metabolic inhibition.

Effect on Driving Performance
In a clinical study in healthy subjects, BRINTELLIX did not impair driving performance, or have adverse psychomotor or cognitive effects following single and multiple doses of 10 mg/day. Because any psychoactive drug may impair judgment, thinking, or motor skills, however, patients should be cautioned about operating hazardous machinery, including

automobiles, until they are reasonably certain that BRINTELLIX therapy does not affect their ability to engage in such activities.

12.3 Pharmacokinetics

Vortioxetine pharmacological activity is due to the parent drug. The pharmacokinetics of vortioxetine (2.5 mg to 60 mg) are linear and dose-proportional when vortioxetine is administered once daily. The mean terminal half-life is approximately 66 hours, and steady-state plasma concentrations are typically achieved within two weeks of dosing.

Absorption

The maximal plasma vortioxetine concentration (C_{max}) after dosing is reached within 7 to 11 hours postdose (T_{max}). Steady-state mean C_{max} values were 9, 18, and 33 ng/mL following doses of 5, 10, and 20 mg/day. Absolute bioavailability is 75%. No effect of food on the pharmacokinetics was observed.

Distribution

The apparent volume of distribution of vortioxetine is approximately 2600 L, indicating extensive extravascular distribution. The plasma protein binding of vortioxetine in humans is 98%, independent of plasma concentrations. No apparent difference in the plasma protein binding between healthy subjects and subjects with hepatic (mild, moderate) or renal (mild, moderate, severe, ESRD) impairment is observed.

Metabolism and Elimination

Vortioxetine is extensively metabolized primarily through oxidation via cytochrome P450 isozymes CYP2D6, CYP3A4/5, CYP2C19, CYP2C9, CYP2A6, CYP2C8 and CYP2B6 and subsequent glucuronic acid conjugation. CYP2D6 is the primary enzyme catalyzing the metabolism of vortioxetine to its major, pharmacologically inactive, carboxylic acid metabolite, and poor metabolizers of CYP2D6 have approximately twice the vortioxetine plasma concentration of extensive metabolizers.

Following a single oral dose of [^{14}C]-labeled vortioxetine, approximately 59% and 26% of the administered radioactivity was recovered in the urine and feces, respectively as metabolites. Negligible amounts of unchanged vortioxetine were excreted in the urine up to 48 hours. The presence of hepatic (mild or moderate) or renal impairment (mild, moderate, severe and ESRD) did not affect the apparent clearance of vortioxetine.

13 NONCLINICAL TOXICOLOGY

13.1 Carcinogenesis, Mutagenesis, Impairment of Fertility

Carcinogenesis

Carcinogenicity studies were conducted in which CD-1 mice and Wistar rats were given oral doses of vortioxetine up to 50 and 100 mg/kg/day for male and female mice, respectively, and 40 and 80 mg/kg/day for male and female rats, respectively, for 2 years. The doses in the two species were approximately 12, 24, 20, and 39 times, respectively, the maximum recommended human dose (MRHD) of 20 mg on a mg/m² basis.

In rats, the incidence of benign polypoid adenomas of the rectum was statistically significantly increased in females at doses 39 times the MRHD, but not at 15 times the MRHD. These were considered related to inflammation and hyperplasia and possibly caused by an interaction with a vehicle component of the formulation used for the study. The finding did not occur in male rats at 20 times the MRHD.

In mice, vortioxetine was not carcinogenic in males or females at doses up to 12 and 24 times, respectively, the MRHD.

Mutagenicity

Vortioxetine was not genotoxic in the *in vitro* bacterial reverse mutation assay (Ames test), an *in vitro* chromosome aberration assay in cultured human lymphocytes, and an *in vivo* rat bone marrow micronucleus assay.

Impairment of Fertility

Treatment of rats with vortioxetine at doses up to 120 mg/kg/day had no effect on male or female fertility, which is 58 times the maximum recommended human dose (MRHD) of 20 mg on a mg/m² basis.

14 CLINICAL STUDIES

The efficacy of BRINTELLIX in treatment for MDD was established in six 6 to 8 week randomized, double-blind, placebo-controlled, fixed-dose studies (including one study in the elderly) and one maintenance study in adult inpatients and outpatients who met the Diagnostic and Statistical Manual of Mental Disorders (DSM-IV-TR) criteria for MDD.

Adults (aged 18 years to 75 years)

The efficacy of BRINTELLIX in patients aged 18 years to 75 years was demonstrated in five 6 to 8 week, placebo-controlled studies (Studies 1 to 5 in *Table 4*). In these studies, patients were randomized to BRINTELLIX 5 mg, 10 mg, 15 mg or 20 mg or placebo once daily. For patients

Table 4. Primary Efficacy Results of 6 Week to 8 Week Clinical Trials

Study No. [Primary Measure]	Treatment Group	Number of Patients	Mean Baseline Score (SD)	LS Mean Change from Baseline (SE)	Placebo-subtracted Difference* (95% CI)
Study 1 [MADRS] Non-US Study	BRINTELLIX (5 mg/day)†	108	34.1 (2.6)	-20.4 (1.0)	-5.9 (-8.6, -3.2)
	BRINTELLIX (10 mg/day)†	100	34.0 (2.8)	-20.2 (1.0)	-5.7 (-8.5, -2.9)
	Placebo	105	33.9 (2.7)	-14.5 (1.0)	--
Study 2 [HAMD-24] Non-US Study	BRINTELLIX (5 mg/day)	139	32.2 (5.0)	-15.4 (0.7)	-4.1 (-6.2, -2.1)
	BRINTELLIX (10 mg/day)†	139	33.1 (4.8)	-16.2 (0.8)	-4.9 (-7.0, -2.9)
	Placebo	139	32.7 (4.4)	-11.3 (0.7)	--
Study 3 [MADRS] Non-US Study	BRINTELLIX (15 mg/day)†	149	31.8 (3.4)	-17.2 (0.8)	-5.5 (-7.7, -3.4)
	BRINTELLIX (20 mg/day)†	151	31.2 (3.4)	-18.8 (0.8)	-7.1 (-9.2, -5.0)
	Placebo	158	31.5 (3.6)	-11.7 (0.8)	--
Study 4 [MADRS] US Study	BRINTELLIX (15 mg/day)	145	31.9 (4.1)	-14.3 (0.9)	-1.5 (-3.9, 0.9)
	BRINTELLIX (20 mg/day)†	147	32.0 (4.4)	-15.6 (0.9)	-2.8 (-5.1, -0.4)
	Placebo	153	31.5 (4.2)	-12.8 (0.8)	--
Study 5 [MADRS] US Study	BRINTELLIX (10 mg/day)	154	32.2 (4.5)	-13.0 (0.8)	-2.2 (-4.5, 0.1)
	BRINTELLIX (20 mg/day)†	148	32.5 (4.3)	-14.4 (0.9)	-3.6 (-5.9, -1.4)
	Placebo	155	32.0 (4.0)	-10.8 (0.8)	--
Study 6 (elderly) [HAMD-24] US and Non-US	BRINTELLIX (5 mg/day)†	155	29.2 (5.0)	-13.7 (0.7)	-3.3 (-5.3, -1.3)
	Placebo	145	29.4 (5.1)	-10.3 (0.8)	--

SD: standard deviation; SE: standard error; LS Mean: least-squares mean; CI: unadjusted confidence interval.

* Difference (drug minus placebo) in least-squares mean change from baseline.
† Doses that are statistically significantly superior to placebo after adjusting for multiplicity.

who were randomized to BRINTELLIX 15 mg/day or 20 mg/day, the final doses were titrated up from 10 mg/day after the first week.

The primary efficacy measures were the Hamilton Depression Scale (HAMD-24) total score in Study 2 and the Montgomery-Asberg Depression Rating Scale (MADRS) total score in all other studies. In each of these studies, at least one dose group of BRINTELLIX was superior to placebo in improvement of depressive symptoms as measured by mean change from baseline to endpoint visit on the primary efficacy measurement *(see Table 4)*. Subgroup analysis by age, gender or race did not suggest any clear evidence of differential responsiveness. Two studies of the 5 mg dose in the U.S. (not represented in *Table 4*) failed to show show effectiveness.

Elderly Study (aged 64 years to 88 years)

The efficacy of BRINTELLIX for the treatment of MDD was also demonstrated in a randomized, double-blind, placebo-controlled, fixed-dose study of BRINTELLIX in elderly patients (aged 64 years to 88 years) with MDD (Study 6 in *Table 4*). Patients meeting the diagnostic criteria for recurrent MDD with at least one previous major depressive episode before the age of 60 years and without comorbid cognitive impairment (Mini Mental State Examination score <24) received BRINTELLIX 5 mg or placebo.

[See table 4 above]

Time Course of Treatment Response

In the 6 to 8 week placebo-controlled studies, an effect of BRINTELLIX based on the primary efficacy measure was generally observed starting at week 2 and increased in subsequent weeks with the full antidepressant effect of BRINTELLIX generally not seen until Study week 4 or later. *Figure 4* depicts time course of response in U.S. based on the primary efficacy measure (MADRS) in Study 5.

[See figure 4 at top of next column]
[See figure 5 at top of next column]

Maintenance Study

In a non-US maintenance study (Study 7 in *Figure 6*), 639 patients meeting DSM-IV-TR criteria for MDD received flexible doses of BRINTELLIX (5 mg or 10 mg) once daily during an initial 12 week open-label treatment phase; the dose of BRINTELLIX was fixed during Weeks 8 to 12. Three hundred ninety six (396) patients who were in remission (MADRS total score ≤10 at both Weeks 10 and 12) after open-label treatment were randomly assigned to continuation of a fixed dose of BRINTELLIX at the final dose they responded to (about 75% of patients were on 10 mg/day) during the open-label phase or to placebo for 24 to 64 weeks.

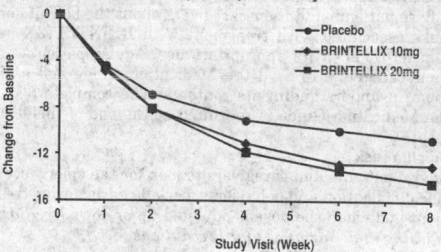

Figure 4. Change from Baseline in MADRS Total Score by Study Visit (Week) in Study 5

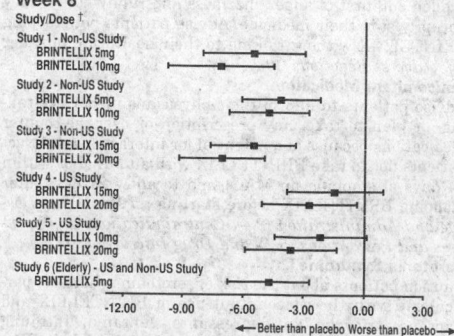

Figure 5. Difference from Placebo in Mean Change from Baseline in MADRS Total Score at Week 6 or Week 8

†Results (point estimate and unadjusted 95% confidence interval) are from mixed model for repeated measures (MMRM) analysis. In Studies 1 and 6, the primary analysis was not based on MMRM and in Studies 2 and 6 the primary efficacy measure was not based on MADRS.

Approximately 61% of randomized patients satisfied remission criterion (MADRS total score ≤10) for at least 4 weeks (since Week 8), and 15% for at least 8 weeks (since Week 4). Patients on BRINTELLIX experienced a statistically significantly longer time to have recurrence of depressive epi-

Features	Strengths			
	5 mg	10 mg	15 mg	20 mg
Color	pink	yellow	orange	red
Debossment	"5" on one side of tablet "TL" on other side of tablet	"10" on one side of tablet "TL" on other side of tablet	"15" on one side of tablet "TL" on other side of tablet	"20" on one side of tablet "TL" on other side of tablet

Presentations and NDC Codes

Bottles of 30*	64764-550-30	64764-560-30	64764-570-30	64764-580-30
Bottles of 90*	64764-550-90	64764-560-90	64764-570-90	64764-580-90
Bottles of 500	64764-550-77	64764-560-77	64764-570-77	64764-580-77

*The unit-of-use package is intended to be dispensed as a unit.

sodes than did patients on placebo. Recurrence of depressive episode was defined as a MADRS total score ≥22 or lack of efficacy as judged by the investigator.

Figure 6. Kaplan-Meier Estimates of Proportion of Patients with Recurrence (Study 7)

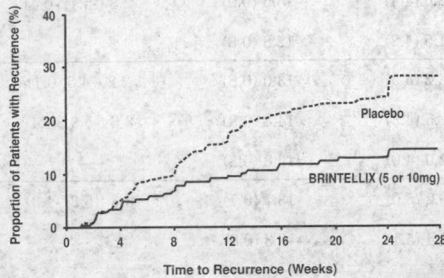

16   HOW SUPPLIED/STORAGE AND HANDLING

BRINTELLIX tablets are available as follows:
[See table above]
Storage: Store at 77°F (25°C); excursions permitted to 59°F to 86°F (15°C to 30°C) [see USP Controlled Room Temperature].

17   PATIENT COUNSELING INFORMATION

See FDA-approved patient labeling (Medication Guide)
Advise patients and their caregivers about the benefits and risks associated with treatment with BRINTELLIX and counsel them in its appropriate use. Advise patients and their caregivers to read the Medication Guide and assist them in understanding its contents. The complete text of the Medication Guide is reprinted at the end of this document.

Suicide Risk
Advise patients and caregivers to look for the emergence of suicidal ideation and behavior, especially early during treatment and when the dose is adjusted up or down [see Boxed Warning and Warnings and Precautions (5.1)].

Discontinuation of Treatment
Patients who are on BRINTELLIX 15 mg/day or 20 mg/day may experience headache, muscle tension, mood swings, sudden outburst of anger, dizziness and runny nose if they abruptly stop their medicine. Advise patients not stopping BRINTELLIX without talking to their healthcare provider [see Adverse Reactions (6)].

Concomitant Medication
Advise patients to inform their physicians if they are taking, or plan to take, any prescription or over-the-counter medications because of a potential for interactions. Instruct patients not to take BRINTELLIX with an MAOI or within 14 days of stopping an MAOI and to allow 21 days after stopping BRINTELLIX before starting an MAOI [see Dosage and Administration (2.4), Contraindications (4), Warnings and Precautions (5.2), and Drug Interactions (7.1)].

Serotonin Syndrome
Caution patients about the risk of serotonin syndrome, particularly with the concomitant use of BRINTELLIX and triptans, tricyclic antidepressants, fentanyl, Lithium, tramadol, tryptophan supplements, and St. John's Wort supplements [see Warnings and Precautions (5.2) and Drug Interactions (7.1, 7.2)].

Abnormal Bleeding
Caution patients about the increased risk of abnormal bleeding when BRINTELLIX is given with NSAIDs, aspirin, warfarin, or other drugs that affect coagulation [see Warnings and Precautions (5.3)].

Activation of Mania/Hypomania
Advise patients and their caregivers to look for signs of activation of mania/hypomania [see Warnings and Precautions (5.4)].

Angle Closure Glaucoma
Patients should be advised that taking BRINTELLIX can cause mild pupillary dilation, which in susceptible individuals, can lead to an episode of angle closure glaucoma. Pre-existing glaucoma is almost always open-angle glaucoma because angle closure glaucoma, when diagnosed, can be treated definitively with iridectomy. Open-angle glaucoma is not a risk factor for angle closure glaucoma. Patients may wish to be examined to determine whether they are susceptible to angle closure, and have a prophylactic procedure (e.g., iridectomy), if they are susceptible [see Warnings and Precautions (5.5)].

Hyponatremia
Advise patients that if they are treated with diuretics, or are otherwise volume depleted, or are elderly, they may be at greater risk of developing hyponatremia while taking BRINTELLIX [see Warnings and Precautions (5.6)].

Nausea
Advise patients that nausea is the most common adverse reaction, and is dose related. Nausea commonly occurs within the first week of treatment, then decreases in frequency but can persist in some patients.

Alcohol
A clinical study has shown that BRINTELLIX (single dose of 20 or 40 mg/day) did not increase the impairment of mental and motor skills caused by alcohol.

Allergic Reactions
Advise patients to notify their healthcare provider if they develop an allergic reaction such as rash, hives, swelling, or difficulty breathing.

Pregnancy
Advise patients to notify their healthcare provider if they become pregnant or intend to become pregnant during therapy with BRINTELLIX [see Use in Specific Populations (8.1)].

Nursing Mothers
Advise patients to notify their healthcare provider if they are breast-feeding an infant and would like to continue or start BRINTELLIX [see Use in Specific Populations (8.3)].

Distributed and marketed by:
Takeda Pharmaceuticals America, Inc.
Deerfield, IL 60015
Marketed by:
Lundbeck
Deerfield, IL 60015
BRINTELLIX is a trademark of H. Lundbeck A/S and is used under license by Takeda Pharmaceuticals America, Inc.
©2013, 2014 Takeda Pharmaceuticals America, Inc.
LUN205 R3 July 2014

MEDICATION GUIDE
BRINTELLIX [brin'-tel-ix]
(vortioxetine) Tablets

Read this Medication Guide before you start taking BRINTELLIX and each time you get a refill. There may be new information. This information does not take the place of talking to your healthcare provider about your medical condition or your treatment.

What is the most important information I should know about BRINTELLIX?

BRINTELLIX and other antidepressant medicines may cause serious side effects.

1. **Antidepressant medicines may increase suicidal thoughts or actions in some children, teenagers, or young adults within the first few months of treatment.**
2. **Depression or other serious mental illnesses are the most important causes of suicidal thoughts or actions. Some people may have a particularly high risk of having suicidal thoughts or actions. These include people who have (or have a family history of) bipolar illness (also called manic-depressive illness) or suicidal thoughts or actions.**

3. **How can I watch for and try to prevent suicidal thoughts and actions?**
- Pay close attention to any changes, especially sudden changes in mood, behavior, thoughts, or feelings. This is very important when an antidepressant medicine is started or when the dose is changed.
- Call your healthcare provider right away to report new or sudden changes in mood, behavior, thoughts, or feelings.
- Keep all follow-up visits with your healthcare provider as scheduled. Call your healthcare provider between visits as needed, especially if you have concerns about symptoms.

Call your healthcare provider right away if you have any of the following symptoms, especially if they are new, worse, or worry you:
- attempts to commit suicide
- acting on dangerous impulses
- acting aggressive, being angry or violent
- thoughts about suicide or dying
- new or worse depression
- new or worse anxiety
- feeling agitated, restless, angry or irritable
- trouble sleeping
- an extreme increase in activity or talking (mania)
- other unusual changes in behavior or mood
- panic attacks
- new or worse irritability

What is BRINTELLIX?
BRINTELLIX is a prescription medicine used to treat a certain type of depression called Major Depressive Disorder (MDD).
It is important to talk with your healthcare provider about the risks of treating depression and also the risk of not treating it. You should discuss all treatment choices with your healthcare provider.
- Talk to your healthcare provider if you do not think that your condition is getting better with BRINTELLIX treatment.

Who should not take BRINTELLIX?
Do not take BRINTELLIX if you:
- are allergic to vortioxetine, or any of the ingredients in BRINTELLIX. See the end of this Medication Guide for a complete list of ingredients in BRINTELLIX.
- take a Monoamine Oxidase Inhibitor (MAOI). Ask your healthcare provider or pharmacist if you are not sure if you take an MAOI, including the antibiotic linezolid.
- Do not take an MAOI within 21 days of stopping BRINTELLIX.
- Do not start BRINTELLIX if you stopped taking an MAOI in the last 14 days.

What should I tell my healthcare provider before taking BRINTELLIX?
Tell your healthcare provider if you:
- have liver problems
- have or had seizures or convulsions
- have mania or bipolar disorder (manic depression)
- have low salt (sodium) levels in your blood
- have or had bleeding problems
- drink alcohol
- have any other medical conditions
- are pregnant or plan to become pregnant. It is not known if BRINTELLIX will harm your unborn baby.
- are breastfeeding or plan to breastfeed. It is not known if BRINTELLIX passes into breast milk. Talk to your healthcare provider about the best way to feed your baby if you take BRINTELLIX.

Tell your healthcare provider about all the medicines that you take, including prescription and over-the-counter medicines, vitamins, and herbal supplements. BRINTELLIX and some medicines may interact with each other, may not work as well, or may cause serious side effects when taken together.

Especially tell your healthcare provider if you take:
- medicines used to treat migraine headache (e.g. triptans)
- medicines used to treat mood, anxiety, psychotic or thought disorders, including tricyclics, lithium, selective serotonin reuptake inhibitors (SSRIs), serotonin norepinephrine reuptake inhibitors (SNRIs), buspirone, or antipsychotics
- MAOIs (including linezolid, an antibiotic)
- Tramadol or fentanyl
- over-the-counter supplements such as tryptophan or St. John's Wort
- nonsteroidal anti-inflammatory drugs (NSAIDs)
- aspirin
- warfarin (Coumadin, Jantoven)
- diuretics
- rifampicin
- carbamazepine
- phenytoin
- quinidine
Ask your healthcare provider if you are not sure if you are taking any of these medicines.

Before you take BRINTELLIX with any of these medicines, talk to your healthcare provider about serotonin syndrome. See "What are the possible side effects of BRINTELLIX?" Know the medicines you take. Keep a list of them to show your healthcare provider or pharmacist when you get new medicine.

How should I take BRINTELLIX?
• Take BRINTELLIX exactly as your healthcare providers tells you to take it.
• Take BRINTELLIX at about the same time each day.
• Your healthcare provider may need to change the dose of BRINTELLIX until it is the right dose for you.
• Do not start or stop taking BRINTELLIX without talking to your healthcare provider first. Suddenly stopping BRINTELLIX when you take higher doses may cause you to have side effects, including:
  • headache
  • stiff muscles
  • mood swings
  • sudden outburst of anger
  • dizziness or feeling lightheaded
  • runny nose
• BRINTELLIX may be taken with or without food.
• If you take too much BRINTELLIX, call the Poison Control Center at 1-800-222-1222 or go to the nearest hospital emergency room right away.

What should I avoid while taking BRINTELLIX?
• Do not drive, operate heavy machinery, or do other dangerous activities until you know how BRINTELLIX affects you.
• Avoid drinking alcohol while taking BRINTELLIX.

What are the possible side effects of BRINTELLIX?
BRINTELLIX may cause serious side effects, including:
• See "What is the most important information I should know about BRINTELLIX?"
• serotonin syndrome. A potentially life-threatening problem called serotonin syndrome can happen when medicines such as BRINTELLIX are taken with certain other medicines. Symptoms of serotonin syndrome may include:
  • agitation, hallucinations, coma or other changes in mental status
  • problems controlling your movements or muscle twitching
  • fast heartbeat
  • high or low blood pressure
  • sweating or fever
  • nausea or vomiting
  • diarrhea
  • muscle stiffness or tightness
• **abnormal bleeding or bruising.** BRINTELLIX may increase your risk of bleeding or bruising, especially if you take the blood thinner warfarin (Coumadin®, Jantoven®), a non-steroidal anti-inflammatory drug (NSAID), or aspirin.
• **hypomania** (manic episodes). Symptoms of manic episodes include:
  • greatly increased energy
  • severe problems sleeping
  • racing thoughts
  • reckless behavior
  • unusually grand ideas
  • excessive happiness or irritability
  • talking more or faster than usual
• **visual problems**
  • eye pain
  • changes in vision
  • swelling or redness in or around the eye
Only some people are at risk for these problems. You may want to undergo an eye examination to see if you are at risk and receive preventative treatment if you are.
• **low levels of salt (sodium) in your blood.** Symptoms of this may include: headache, difficulty concentrating, memory changes, confusion, weakness and unsteadiness on your feet. Symptoms of severe or sudden cases of low salt levels in your blood may include: hallucinations (seeing or hearing things that are not real), fainting, seizures and coma. If not treated, severe low sodium levels can cause death.
Common side effects in people who take BRINTELLIX include:
• nausea
• constipation
• vomiting
Tell your healthcare provider if you have any side effect that bothers you or that does not go away. These are not all the possible side effects of BRINTELLIX. For more information, ask your healthcare provider or pharmacist.
Call your doctor for medical advice about side effects. You may report side effects to FDA at 1-800-FDA-1088.
How should I store BRINTELLIX?
Store BRINTELLIX at room temperature between 59°F to 86°F (15°C to 30°C).
Keep BRINTELLIX and all medicines out of the reach of children.

General information about the safe and effective use of BRINTELLIX.
Medicines are sometimes prescribed for purposes other than those listed in a Medication Guide. Do not use BRINTELLIX for a condition for which it was not prescribed. Do not give BRINTELLIX to other people, even if they have the same condition. It may harm them.
This Medication Guide summarizes the most important information about BRINTELLIX. If you would like more information, talk with your healthcare provider. You may ask your healthcare provider or pharmacist for information about BRINTELLIX that is written for healthcare professionals.
For more information, go to www.BRINTELLIX.com or call 1-877-TAKEDA-7 (1-877-825-3327).
What are the ingredients in BRINTELLIX?
Active ingredient: vortioxetine hydrobromide
Inactive ingredients: mannitol, microcrystalline cellulose, hydroxypropyl cellulose, sodium starch glycolate, magnesium stearate and film coating consisting of hypromellose, titanium dioxide, polyethylene glycol 400, iron oxide red (5 mg, 15 mg, and 20 mg) and iron oxide yellow (10 mg and 15 mg)
This Medication Guide has been approved by the U.S. Food and Drug Administration.
Distributed and Marketed by:
Takeda Pharmaceuticals America, Inc.
Deerfield, IL 60015
Marketed by:
Lundbeck
Deerfield, IL 60015
BRINTELLIX is a trademark of H. Lundbeck A/S and is used under license by Takeda Pharmaceuticals America, Inc.
All other trademarks are the property of their respective owners.
©2013, 2014 Takeda Pharmaceuticals America, Inc.
LUN205 R3 July 2014
Shown in Product Identification Guide, page 313

COLCRYS®   ℞
(colchicine, USP)
tablets for Oral use

HIGHLIGHTS OF PRESCRIBING INFORMATION
These highlights do not include all the information needed to use colchicine safely and effectively. See full prescribing information for COLCRYS®.
COLCRYS® (colchicine, USP) tablets for Oral use
Initial U.S. Approval: 1961

———————INDICATIONS AND USAGE———————
COLCRYS (colchicine, USP) tablets are an alkaloid indicated for:
• Prophylaxis and Treatment of Gout Flares in adults (1.1).
• Familial Mediterranean fever (FMF) in adults and children 4 years or older (1.2).
COLCRYS is not an analgesic medication and should not be used to treat pain from other causes.

—————DOSAGE AND ADMINISTRATION—————
• **Gout Flares:**
  Prophylaxis of Gout Flares: 0.6 mg once or twice daily in adults and adolescents older than 16 years of age (2.1). Maximum dose 1.2 mg/day.
  Treatment of Gout Flares: 1.2 mg (2 tablets) at the first sign of a gout flare followed by 0.6 mg (1 tablet) one hour later (2.1).
• **FMF:** Adults and Children older than 12 years 1.2 – 2.4 mg; Children 6 to 12 years 0.9 – 1.8 mg; Children 4 to 6 years 0.3 – 1.8 mg (2.2, 2.3).
  ○ Give total daily dose in one or two divided doses (2.2).
  ○ Increase or decrease the dose as indicated and as tolerated in increments of 0.3 mg/day, not to exceed the maximum recommended daily dose (2.2).
Colchicine tablets are administered orally, without regard to meals.
See full prescribing information for dose adjustment regarding patients with impaired renal function (2.5), impaired hepatic function (2.6), the patient's age (2.3, 8.5), or use of co-administered drugs (2.4).

————DOSAGE FORMS AND STRENGTHS————
• 0.6 mg tablets (3).

———————CONTRAINDICATIONS———————
Patients with renal or hepatic impairment should not be given COLCRYS in conjunction with P-gp or strong

CYP3A4 inhibitors (5.3). In these patients, life-threatening and fatal colchicine toxicity has been reported with colchicine taken in therapeutic doses (7).

————WARNINGS AND PRECAUTIONS————
• *Fatal overdoses* have been reported with colchicine in adults and children. Keep COLCRYS out of the reach of children (5.1, 10).
• *Blood dyscrasias:* myelosuppression, leukopenia, granulocytopenia, thrombocytopenia, and aplastic anemia have been reported (5.2).
• Monitor for toxicity and if present consider temporary interruption or discontinuation of colchicine (5.2, 5.3, 5.4, 6, 10).
• *Drug interaction P-gp and/or CYP3A4 inhibitors:* Co-administration of colchicine with P-gp and/or strong CYP3A4 inhibitors has resulted in life-threatening interactions and death (5.3, 7).
• *Neuromuscular toxicity:* Myotoxicity including rhabdomyolysis may occur, especially in combination with other drugs known to cause this effect. Consider temporary interruption or discontinuation of COLCRYS (5.4, 7).

————————ADVERSE REACTIONS————————
Prophylaxis of Gout Flares: The most commonly reported adverse reaction in clinical trials for the prophylaxis of gout was diarrhea.
Treatment of Gout Flares: The most common adverse reactions reported in the clinical trial for gout were diarrhea (23%) and pharyngolaryngeal pain (3%).
FMF: Most common adverse reactions (up to 20%) are abdominal pain, diarrhea, nausea, and vomiting. These effects are usually mild, transient, and reversible upon lowering the dose (6).
To report SUSPECTED ADVERSE REACTIONS, contact Takeda Pharmaceuticals America, Inc. at 1-877-825-3327 or FDA at 1-800-FDA-1088 or www.fda.gov/medwatch.

————————DRUG INTERACTIONS————————
Co-administration of P-gp and/or CYP3A4 inhibitors (*e.g.*, clarithromycin or cyclosporine) have been demonstrated to alter the concentration of colchicine. The potential for drug-drug interactions must be considered prior to and during therapy. See full prescribing information for a complete list of reported and potential interactions (2.4, 5.3, 7).

————USE IN SPECIFIC POPULATIONS————
• In the presence of mild to moderate renal or hepatic impairment, adjustment of dosing is not required for treatment of gout flare, prophylaxis of gout flare, and FMF but patients should be monitored closely (2.5, 8.6).
• In patients with severe renal impairment the starting dose should be 0.3 mg/day, for gout flares no dose adjustment is required but a treatment course should be repeated no more than once every 2 weeks. In FMF patients, start with 0.3 mg/day and any increase in dose should be done with close monitoring (2.5, 8.6).
• In patients with severe hepatic impairment, a dose reduction may be needed in prophylaxis of gout flares and FMF patients; while a dose reduction may not be needed in gout flares, a treatment course should be repeated no more than once every 2 weeks (2.5, 2.6, 8.6, 8.7).
• For patients undergoing dialysis, the total recommended dose for prophylaxis of gout flares should be 0.3 mg given twice a week with close monitoring. For treatment of gout flares, the total recommended dose should be reduced to 0.6 mg (1 tablet) × 1 dose and the treatment course should not be repeated more than once every two weeks. For FMF patients the starting dose should be 0.3 mg per day and dosing can be increased with close monitoring (2.5, 8.6).
• Pregnancy: Use only if the potential benefit justifies the potential risk to the fetus (8.1).
• Nursing Mothers: Caution should be exercised when administered to a nursing woman (8.3).
• Geriatric Use: The recommended dose of colchicine should be based on renal function (2.5, 8.5).
See 17 for PATIENT COUNSELING INFORMATION and Medication Guide

Revised: 01/2014

FULL PRESCRIBING INFORMATION: CONTENTS*

FULL PRESCRIBING INFORMATION

1   INDICATIONS AND USAGE

1.1   Gout Flares

COLCRYS® (colchicine, USP) tablets are indicated for prophylaxis and the treatment of acute gout flares.

Prophylaxis of Gout Flares:
COLCRYS is indicated for prophylaxis of gout flares.

Treatment of Gout Flares:
COLCRYS tablets are indicated for treatment of acute gout flares when taken at the first sign of a flare.

1.2   Familial Mediterranean fever (FMF)

COLCRYS® (colchicine, USP) tablets are indicated in adults and children 4 years or older for treatment of familial Mediterranean fever (FMF).

2   DOSAGE AND ADMINISTRATION

The long term use of colchicine is established for FMF and the prophylaxis of gout flares but the safety and efficacy of repeat treatment for gout flares has not been evaluated. The dosing regimens for COLCRYS are different for each indication and must be individualized.

The recommended dosage of COLCRYS depends on the patient's age, renal function, hepatic function, and use of coadministered drugs [see Dose Modification for Coadministration of Interacting Drugs (2.4)].

COLCRYS tablets are administered orally, without regard to meals.

COLCRYS is not an analgesic medication and should not be used to treat pain from other causes.

2.1   Gout Flares

Prophylaxis of Gout Flares:
The recommended dosage of COLCRYS for prophylaxis of gout flares for adults and adolescents older than 16 years of age is 0.6 mg once or twice daily. The maximum recommended dose for prophylaxis of gout flares is 1.2 mg/day.

Treatment of Gout Flares:
The recommended dose of COLCRYS for treatment of a gout flare is 1.2 mg (2 tablets) at the first sign of the flare followed by 0.6 mg (1 tablet) one hour later. Higher doses have not been found to be more effective. The maximum recommended dose for treatment of gout flares is 1.8 mg over a 1 hour period. COLCRYS may be administered for treatment of a gout flare during prophylaxis at doses not to exceed 1.2 mg (2 tablets) at the first sign of the flare followed by 0.6 mg (1 tablet) one hour later. Wait 12 hours and then resume the prophylactic dose.

2.2   FMF

The recommended dosage of COLCRYS for FMF in adults is 1.2 mg to 2.4 mg daily.

COLCRYS should be increased as needed to control disease and as tolerated in increments of 0.3 mg/day to a maximum

Table 1 COLCRYS Dose Adjustment for Co-administration with Interacting Drugs if no Alternative Available*

Strong CYP3A4 Inhibitors[†]

| Drug | Noted or Anticipated Outcome | Gout Flares | | | | FMF | |
| | | Prophylaxis of Gout Flares | | Treatment of Gout Flares | | Original Intended Dosage | Adjusted Dose |
		Original Intended Dosage	Adjusted Dose	Original Intended Dosage	Adjusted Dose		
Atazanavir Clarithromycin Darunavir/ Ritonavir[‡] Indinavir Itraconazole Ketoconazole Lopinavir/ Ritonavir[‡] Nefazodone Nelfinavir Ritonavir Saquinavir Telithromycin Tipranavir/ Ritonavir[‡]	Significant increase in colchicine plasma levels*; fatal colchicine toxicity has been reported with clarithromycin, a strong CYP3A4 inhibitor. Similarly, significant increase in colchicine plasma levels is anticipated with other strong CYP3A4 inhibitors.	0.6 mg twice a day 0.6 mg once a day	0.3 mg once a day 0.3 mg once every other day	1.2 mg (2 tablets) followed by 0.6 mg (1 tablet) 1 hour later. Dose to be repeated no earlier than 3 days.	0.6 mg (1 tablet) × 1 dose, followed by 0.3 mg (1/2 tablet) 1 hour later. Dose to be repeated no earlier than 3 days.	Maximum daily dose of 1.2 – 2.4 mg	Maximum daily dose of 0.6 mg (may be given as 0.3 mg twice a day)

Moderate CYP3A4 Inhibitors

| Drug | Noted or Anticipated Outcome | Gout Flares | | | | FMF | |
| | | Prophylaxis of Gout Flares | | Treatment of Gout Flares | | Original Intended Dosage | Adjusted Dose |
		Original Intended Dosage	Adjusted Dose	Original Intended Dosage	Adjusted Dose		
Amprenavir[‡] Aprepitant Diltiazem Erythromycin Fluconazole Fosamprenavir[‡] (pro-drug of Amprenavir) Grapefruit Juice Verapamil	Significant increase in colchicine plasma concentration is anticipated. Neuromuscular toxicity has been reported with diltiazem and verapamil interactions.	0.6 mg twice a day 0.6 mg once a day	0.3 mg twice a day or 0.6 mg once a day 0.3 mg once a day	1.2 mg (2 tablets) followed by 0.6 mg (1 tablet) 1 hour later. Dose to be repeated no earlier than 3 days.	1.2 mg (2 tablets) × 1 dose. Dose to be repeated no earlier than 3 days.	Maximum daily dose of 1.2 – 2.4 mg.	Maximum daily dose of 1.2 mg (may be given as 0.6 mg twice a day)

P-gp Inhibitors[†]

| Drug | Noted or Anticipated Outcome | Gout Flares | | | | FMF | |
| | | Prophylaxis of Gout Flares | | Treatment of Gout Flares | | Original Intended Dosage | Adjusted Dose |
		Original Intended Dosage	Adjusted Dose	Original Intended Dosage	Adjusted Dose		
Cyclosporine Ranolazine	Significant increase in colchicine plasma levels*; fatal colchicine toxicity has been reported with cyclosporine, a P-gp inhibitor. Similarly, significant increase in colchicine plasma levels is anticipated with other P-gp inhibitors.	0.6 mg twice a day 0.6 mg once a day	0.3 mg once a day 0.3 mg once every other day	1.2 mg (2 tablets) followed by 0.6 mg (1 tablet) 1 hour later. Dose to be repeated no earlier than 3 days.	0.6 mg (1 tablet) × 1 dose. Dose to be repeated no earlier than 3 days.	Maximum daily dose of 1.2 – 2.4 mg	Maximum daily dose of 0.6 mg (may be given as 0.3 mg twice a day)

* For magnitude of effect on colchicine plasma concentrations [see Pharmacokinetics (12.3)]
† Patients with renal and hepatic impairment should not be given COLCRYS in conjunction with strong CYP3A4 or P-gp inhibitors [see CONTRAINDICATIONS (4)].
‡ When used in combination with Ritonavir, see dosing recommendations for strong CYP3A4 inhibitors [see CONTRAINDICATIONS (4)].

recommended daily dose. If intolerable side effects develop, the dose should be decreased in increments of 0.3 mg/day. The total daily COLCRYS dose may be administered in one to two divided doses.

2.3   Recommended Pediatric Dosage

Prophylaxis and Treatment of Gout Flares:
COLCRYS is not recommended for pediatric use in prophylaxis or treatment of gout flares.

FMF:
The recommended dosage of COLCRYS for FMF in pediatric patients 4 years of age and older is based on age. The following daily doses may be given as a single or divided dose twice daily:
• Children 4 – 6 years: 0.3 mg to 1.8 mg daily
• Children 6 – 12 years: 0.9 mg to 1.8 mg daily
• Adolescents older than 12 years: 1.2 mg to 2.4 mg daily

2.4 Dose Modification for Co-administration of Interacting Drugs

Concomitant Therapy:

Co-administration of COLCRYS with drugs known to inhibit CYP3A4 and/or P-glycoprotein (P-gp) increases the risk of colchicine-induced toxic effects (Table 1). If patients are taking or have recently completed treatment with drugs listed in Table 1 within the prior 14 days, the dose adjustments are as shown on the table below [*see DRUG INTERACTIONS (7)*].

[See table 1 at top of previous page]

[See table 2 above and on next page]

Treatment of gout flares with COLCRYS is not recommended in patients receiving prophylactic dose of COLCRYS and CYP3A4 inhibitors.

2.5 Dose Modification in Renal Impairment

Colchicine dosing must be individualized according to the patient's renal function [*see Renal Impairment (8.6)*].

Clcr in mL/minute may be estimated from serum creatinine (mg/dL) determination using the following formula:

[See second table at top of next page]

Gout Flares:

Prophylaxis of Gout Flares:

For prophylaxis of gout flares in patients with mild (estimated creatinine clearance Clcr 50 – 80 mL/min) to moderate (Clcr 30 – 50 mL/min) renal function impairment, adjustment of the recommended dose is not required, but patients should be monitored closely for adverse effects of colchicine. However, in patients with severe impairment, the starting dose should be 0.3 mg per day and any increase in dose should be done with close monitoring. For the prophylaxis of gout flares in patients undergoing dialysis, the starting doses should be 0.3 mg given twice a week with close monitoring [*see Clinical Pharmacology (12.3) and Renal Impairment (8.6)*].

Treatment of Gout Flares:

For treatment of gout flares in patients with mild (Clcr 50 – 80 mL/min) to moderate (Clcr 30 – 50 mL/min) renal function impairment, adjustment of the recommended dose is not required, but patients should be monitored closely for adverse effects of colchicine. However, in patients with severe impairment, while the dose does not need to be adjusted for the treatment of gout flares, a treatment course should be repeated no more than once every 2 weeks. For patients with gout flares requiring repeated courses consideration should be given to alternate therapy. For patients undergoing dialysis, the total recommended dose for the treatment of gout flares should be reduced to a single dose of 0.6 mg (1 tablet). For these patients, the treatment course should not be repeated more than once every 2 weeks [*see Clinical Pharmacology (12.3) and Renal Impairment (8.6)*]. Treatment of gout flares with COLCRYS is not recommended in patients with renal impairment who are receiving COLCRYS for prophylaxis.

FMF:

Caution should be taken in dosing patients with moderate and severe renal impairment and in patients undergoing dialysis. For these patients, the dosage should be reduced [*see Clinical Pharmacology (12.3)*]. Patients with mild (Clcr 50 – 80 mL/min) and moderate (Clcr 30 – 50 mL/min) renal impairment should be monitored closely for adverse effects of COLCRYS. Dose reduction may be necessary. For patients with severe renal failure (Clcr less than 30 mL/minute), start with 0.3 mg/day; any increase in dose should be done with adequate monitoring of the patient for adverse effects of colchicine [*see Renal Impairment (8.6)*]. For patients undergoing dialysis, the total recommended starting dose should be 0.3 mg (half tablet) per day. Dosing can be increased with close monitoring. Any increase in dose should be done with adequate monitoring of the patient for adverse effects of colchicine [*see Clinical Pharmacology (12.3) and Renal Impairment (8.6)*].

2.6 Dose Modification in Hepatic Impairment

Gout Flares

Prophylaxis of Gout Flares:

For prophylaxis of gout flares in patients with mild to moderate hepatic function impairment, adjustment of the recommended dose is not required, but patients should be monitored closely for adverse effects of colchicine. Dose reduction should be considered for the prophylaxis of gout flares in patients with severe hepatic impairment [*see Hepatic Impairment (8.7)*].

Treatment of Gout Flares:

For treatment of gout flares in patients with mild to moderate hepatic function impairment, adjustment of the recommended dose is not required, but patients should be monitored closely for adverse effects of colchicine. However, for the treatment of gout flares in patients with severe impairment while the dose does not need to be adjusted, but a treatment course should be repeated no more than once every 2 weeks. For these patients, requiring repeated courses for the treatment of gout flares, consideration should be given to alternate therapy [*see Hepatic Impairment (8.7)*].

Treatment of gout flares with COLCRYS is not recommended in patients with hepatic impairment who are receiving COLCRYS for prophylaxis.

FMF:

Patients with mild to moderate hepatic impairment should be monitored closely for adverse effects of colchicine. Dose reduction should be considered in patients with severe hepatic impairment [*see Hepatic Impairment (8.7)*].

3 DOSAGE FORMS AND STRENGTHS

0.6 mg tablets — purple capsule-shaped, film-coated with AR 374 debossed on one side and scored on the other side.

4 CONTRAINDICATIONS

Patients with renal or hepatic impairment should not be given COLCRYS in conjunction with P-gp or strong CYP3A4 inhibitors (this includes all protease inhibitors, except fosamprenavir). In these patients, life-threatening and fatal colchicine toxicity has been reported with colchicine taken in therapeutic doses.

5 WARNINGS AND PRECAUTIONS

5.1 Fatal Overdose

Fatal overdoses, both accidental and intentional, have been reported in adults and children who have ingested colchicine [*see OVERDOSAGE (10)*]. COLCRYS should be kept out of the reach of children.

5.2 Blood Dyscrasias

Myelosuppression, leukopenia, granulocytopenia, thrombocytopenia, pancytopenia, and aplastic anemia have been reported with colchicine used in therapeutic doses.

5.3 Drug Interactions

Colchicine is a P-gp and CYP3A4 substrate. Life-threatening and fatal drug interactions have been reported in patients treated with colchicine given with P-gp and strong CYP3A4 inhibitors. If treatment with a P-gp or strong CYP3A4 inhibitor is required in patients with normal renal and hepatic function, the patient's dose of colchicine may need to be reduced or interrupted [*see DRUG INTERACTIONS (7)*]. Use of COLCRYS in conjunction with P-gp or strong CYP3A4 inhibitors (this includes all protease

Table 2 COLCRYS Dose Adjustment for Co-administration with Protease Inhibitors

Protease Inhibitor	Clinical Comment	w/Colchicine – Prophylaxis of Gout Flares		w/Colchicine – Treatment of Gout Flares	w/Colchicine – Treatment of FMF
Atazanavir sulfate (Reyataz)	Patients with renal or hepatic impairment should not be given colchicine with Reyataz.	Original dose	Adjusted dose	0.6 mg (1 tablet) × 1 dose, followed by 0.3 mg (1/2 tablet) 1 hour later. Dose to be repeated no earlier than 3 days.	Maximum daily dose of 0.6 mg (may be given as 0.3 mg twice a day)
		0.6 mg twice a day	0.3 mg once a day		
		0.6 mg once a day	0.3 mg once every other day		
Darunavir (Prezista)	Patients with renal or hepatic impairment should not be given colchicine with Prezista/ritonavir.	Original dose	Adjusted dose	0.6 mg (1 tablet) × 1 dose, followed by 0.3 mg (1/2 tablet) 1 hour later. Dose to be repeated no earlier than 3 days.	Maximum daily dose of 0.6 mg (may be given as 0.3 mg twice a day)
		0.6 mg twice a day	0.3 mg once a day		
		0.6 mg once a day	0.3 mg once every other day		
Fosamprenavir (Lexiva) with Ritonavir	Patients with renal or hepatic impairment should not be given colchicine with Lexiva/ritonavir.	Original dose	Adjusted dose	0.6 mg (1 tablet) × 1 dose, followed by 0.3 mg (1/2 tablet) 1 hour later. Dose to be repeated no earlier than 3 days.	Maximum daily dose of 0.6 mg (may be given as 0.3 mg twice a day)
		0.6 mg twice a day	0.3 mg once a day		
		0.6 mg once a day	0.3 mg once every other day		
Fosamprenavir (Lexiva)	Patients with renal or hepatic impairment should not be given colchicine with Lexiva/ritonavir.	Original dose	Adjusted dose	1.2 mg (2 tablets) × 1 dose. Dose to be repeated no earlier than 3 days.	Maximum daily dose of 1.2 mg (may be given as 0.6 mg twice a day)
		0.6 mg twice a day	0.3 mg twice a day or 0.6 mg once a day		
		0.6 mg once a day	0.3 mg once a day		
Indinavir (Crixivan)	Patients with renal or hepatic impairment should not be given colchicine with Crixivan.	Original dose	Adjusted dose	0.6 mg (1 tablet) × 1 dose, followed by 0.3 mg (1/2 tablet) 1 hour later. Dose to be repeated no earlier than 3 days.	Maximum daily dose of 0.6 mg (may be given as 0.3 mg twice a day)
		0.6 mg twice a day	0.3 mg once a day		
		0.6 mg once a day	0.3 mg once every other day		
Lopinavir/Ritonavir (Kaletra)	Patients with renal or hepatic impairment should not be given colchicine with Kaletra.	Original dose	Adjusted dose	0.6 mg (1 tablet) × 1 dose, followed by 0.3 mg (1/2 tablet) 1 hour later. Dose to be repeated no earlier than 3 days.	Maximum daily dose of 0.6 mg (may be given as 0.3 mg twice a day)
		0.6 mg twice a day	0.3 mg once a day		
		0.6 mg once a day	0.3 mg once every other day		
Nelfinavir mesylate (Viracept)	Patients with renal or hepatic impairment should not be given colchicine with Viracept.	Original dose	Adjusted dose	0.6 mg (1 tablet) × 1 dose, followed by 0.3 mg (1/2 tablet) 1 hour later. Dose to be repeated no earlier than 3 days.	Maximum daily dose of 0.6 mg (may be given as 0.3 mg twice a day)
		0.6 mg twice a day	0.3 mg once a day		
		0.6 mg once a day	0.3 mg once every other day		

(Table continued on next page)

Table 2 (cont.) COLCRYS Dose Adjustment for Co-administration with Protease Inhibitors

Protease Inhibitor	Clinical Comment	w/Colchicine – Prophylaxis of Gout Flares		w/Colchicine – Treatment of Gout Flares	w/Colchicine – Treatment of FMF
Ritonavir (Norvir)	Patients with renal or hepatic impairment should not be given colchicine with Norvir.	**Original dose** 0.6 mg twice a day 0.6 mg once a day	**Adjusted dose** 0.3 mg once a day 0.3 mg once every other day	0.6 mg (1 tablet) × 1 dose, followed by 0.3 mg (1/2 tablet) 1 hour later. Dose to be repeated no earlier than 3 days.	Maximum daily dose of 0.6 mg (may be given as 0.3 mg twice a day)
Saquinavir mesylate (Invirase)	Patients with renal or hepatic impairment should not be given colchicine with Invirase/ritonavir.	**Original dose** 0.6 mg twice a day 0.6 mg once a day	**Adjusted dose** 0.3 mg once a day 0.3 mg once every other day	0.6 mg (1 tablet) × 1 dose, followed by 0.3 mg (1/2 tablet) 1 hour later. Dose to be repeated no earlier than 3 days.	Maximum daily dose of 0.6 mg (may be given as 0.3 mg twice a day)
Tipranavir (Aptivus)	Patients with renal or hepatic impairment should not be given colchicine with Aptivus/ritonavir.	**Original dose** 0.6 mg twice a day 0.6 mg once a day	**Adjusted dose** 0.3 mg once a day 0.3 mg once every other day	0.6 mg (1 tablet) × 1 dose, followed by 0.3 mg (1/2 tablet) 1 hour later. Dose to be repeated no earlier than 3 days.	Maximum daily dose of 0.6 mg (may be given as 0.3 mg twice a day)

$$Clcr = \frac{[140 - age\ (years) \times weight\ (kg)]}{72 \times serum\ creatinine\ (mg/dL)} \times 0.85\ for\ female\ patients$$

Table 3 Number (%) of Patients with at Least One Drug-Related Treatment Emergent Adverse Events with an Incidence of ≥ 2% of Patients in Any Treatment Group

MedDRA System Organ Class MedDRA Preferred Term	COLCRYS Dose		Placebo (N=59) n (%)
	High (N=52) n (%)	Low (N=74) n (%)	
Number of Patients with at Least One Drug-Related TEAE	40 (77)	27 (37)	16 (27)
Gastrointestinal Disorders	40 (77)	19 (26)	12 (20)
Diarrhea	40 (77)	17 (23)	8 (14)
Nausea	9 (17)	3 (4)	3 (5)
Vomiting	9 (17)	0	0
Abdominal Discomfort	0	0	2 (3)
General Disorders and Administration Site Conditions	4 (8)	1 (1)	1 (2)
Fatigue	2 (4)	1 (1)	1 (2)
Metabolic and Nutrition Disorders	0	3 (4)	2 (3)
Gout	0	3 (4)	1 (2)
Nervous System Disorders	1 (2)	1 (1.4)	2 (3)
Headache	1 (2)	1 (1)	2 (3)
Respiratory Thoracic Mediastinal Disorders	1 (2)	2 (3)	0
Pharyngolaryngeal Pain	1 (2)	2 (3)	0

inhibitors, except fosamprenavir) is contraindicated in patients with renal or hepatic impairment [see CONTRAINDICATIONS (4)].

5.4   Neuromuscular Toxicity
Colchicine-induced neuromuscular toxicity and rhabdomyolysis have been reported with chronic treatment in therapeutic doses. Patients with renal dysfunction and elderly patients, even those with normal renal and hepatic function, are at increased risk. Concomitant use of atorvastatin, simvastatin, pravastatin, fluvastatin, lovastatin, gemfibrozil, fenofibrate, fenofibric acid, or benzafibrate (themselves associated with myotoxicity) or cyclosporine with COLCRYS may potentiate the development of myopathy [see DRUG INTERACTIONS (7)]. Once colchicine is stopped, the symptoms generally resolve within 1 week to several months.

6   ADVERSE REACTIONS
Prophylaxis of Gout Flares:
The most commonly reported adverse reaction in clinical trials of colchicine for the prophylaxis of gout was diarrhea.

Treatment of Gout Flares:
The most common adverse reactions reported in the clinical trial with COLCRYS for treatment of gout flares were diarrhea (23%) and pharyngolaryngeal pain (3%).
FMF:
Gastrointestinal tract adverse effects are the most frequent side effects in patients initiating COLCRYS, usually presenting within 24 hours, and occurring in up to 20% of patients given therapeutic doses. Typical symptoms include cramping, nausea, diarrhea, abdominal pain, and vomiting. These events should be viewed as dose-limiting if severe as they can herald the onset of more significant toxicity.
6.1   Clinical Trials Experience in Gout
Because clinical studies are conducted under widely varying and controlled conditions, adverse reaction rates observed in clinical studies of a drug cannot be directly compared to rates in the clinical studies of another drug, and may not predict the rates observed in a broader patient population in clinical practice.

In a randomized, double-blind, placebo-controlled trial in patients with a gout flare, gastrointestinal adverse reactions occurred in 26% of patients using the recommended dose (1.8 mg over 1 hour) of COLCRYS compared to 77% of patients taking a non-recommended high-dose (4.8 mg over 6 hours) of colchicine and 20% of patients taking placebo. Diarrhea was the most commonly reported drug-related gastrointestinal adverse event. As shown in Table 3, diarrhea is associated with COLCRYS treatment. Diarrhea was more likely to occur in patients taking the high-dose regimen than the low-dose regimen. Severe diarrhea occurred in 19% and vomiting occurred in 17% of patients taking the non-recommended high-dose colchicine regimen but did not occur in the recommended low-dose COLCRYS regimen. [See table 3 above]
6.2   Postmarketing Experience
Serious toxic manifestations associated with colchicine include myelosuppression, disseminated intravascular coagulation, and injury to cells in the renal, hepatic, circulatory, and central nervous systems.
These most often occur with excessive accumulation or overdosage [see OVERDOSAGE (10)].
The following adverse reactions have been reported with colchicine. These have been generally reversible upon temporarily interrupting treatment or lowering the dose of colchicine.
Neurological: sensory motor neuropathy
Dermatological: alopecia, maculopapular rash, purpura, rash
Digestive: abdominal cramping, abdominal pain, diarrhea, lactose intolerance, nausea, vomiting
Hematological: leukopenia, granulocytopenia, thrombocytopenia, pancytopenia, aplastic anemia
Hepatobiliary: elevated AST, elevated ALT
Musculoskeletal: myopathy, elevated CPK, myotonia, muscle weakness, muscle pain, rhabdomyolysis
Reproductive: azoospermia, oligospermia

7   DRUG INTERACTIONS
COLCRYS (colchicine) is a substrate of the efflux transporter P-glycoprotein (P-gp). Of the cytochrome P450 enzymes tested, CYP3A4 was mainly involved in the metabolism of colchicine. If COLCRYS is administered with drugs that inhibit P-gp, most of which also inhibit CYP3A4, increased concentrations of colchicine are likely. Fatal drug interactions have been reported.
Physicians should ensure that patients are suitable candidates for treatment with COLCRYS and remain alert for signs and symptoms of toxicities related to increased colchicine exposure as a result of a drug interaction. Signs and symptoms of COLCRYS toxicity should be evaluated promptly and, if toxicity is suspected, COLCRYS should be discontinued immediately.
Table 4 provides recommendations as a result of other potentially significant drug interactions. Table 1 provides recommendations for strong and moderate CYP3A4 inhibitors and P-gp inhibitors.
[See table 4 at top of next page]

8   USE IN SPECIFIC POPULATIONS
8.1   Pregnancy
Pregnancy Category C
There are no adequate and well-controlled studies with colchicine in pregnant women. Colchicine crosses the human placenta. While not studied in the treatment of gout flares, data from a limited number of published studies found no evidence of an increased risk of miscarriage, stillbirth, or teratogenic effects among pregnant women using colchicine to treat familial Mediterranean fever (FMF). Although animal reproductive and developmental studies were not conducted with COLCRYS, published animal reproduction and development studies indicate that colchicine causes embryofetal toxicity, teratogenicity, and altered postnatal development at exposures within or above the clinical therapeutic range. COLCRYS should be used during pregnancy only if the potential benefit justifies the potential risk to the fetus.
8.2   Labor and Delivery
The effect of colchicine on labor and delivery is unknown.
8.3   Nursing Mothers
Colchicine is excreted into human milk. Limited information suggests that exclusively breast-fed infants receive less than 10 percent of the maternal weight-adjusted dose. While there are no published reports of adverse effects in breast-feeding infants of mothers taking colchicine, colchicine can affect gastrointestinal cell renewal and permeability. Caution should be exercised and breast-feeding infants should be observed for adverse effects when COLCRYS is administered to a nursing woman.
8.4   Pediatric Use
The safety and efficacy of colchicine in children of all ages with FMF has been evaluated in uncontrolled studies. There does not appear to be an adverse effect on growth in children with FMF treated long-term with colchicine. Gout is rare in pediatric patients, safety and effectiveness of colchicine in pediatric patients has not been established.
8.5   Geriatric Use
Clinical studies with colchicine for prophylaxis and treatment of gout flares and for treatment of FMF did not in-

clude sufficient numbers of patients aged 65 years and older to determine whether they respond differently from younger patients. In general, dose selection for an elderly patient with gout should be cautious, reflecting the greater frequency of decreased renal function, concomitant disease, or other drug therapy [see Dose Modification for Co-administration of Interacting Drugs (2.4)].

8.6 Renal Impairment

Colchicine is significantly excreted in urine in healthy subjects. Clearance of colchicine is decreased in patients with impaired renal function. Total body clearance of colchicine was reduced by 75% in patients with end-stage renal disease undergoing dialysis.

Prophylaxis of Gout Flares:

For prophylaxis of gout flares in patients with mild (estimated creatinine clearance Clcr 50 – 80 mL/min) to moderate (Clcr 30 – 50 mL/min) renal function impairment, adjustment of the recommended dose is not required, but patients should be monitored closely for adverse effects of colchicine. However, in patients with severe impairment, the starting dose should be 0.3 mg per day and any increase in dose should be done with close monitoring. For the prophylaxis of gout flares in patients undergoing dialysis, the starting doses should be 0.3 mg given twice a week with close monitoring [see Dose Modification in Renal Impairment (2.5)].

Treatment of Gout Flares:

For treatment of gout flares in patients with mild (Clcr 50 – 80 mL/min) to moderate (Clcr 30 – 50 mL/min) renal function impairment, adjustment of the recommended dose is not required, but patients should be monitored closely for adverse effects of COLCRYS. However, in patients with severe impairment, while the dose does not need to be adjusted for the treatment of gout flares, a treatment course should be repeated no more than once every 2 weeks. For patients with gout flares requiring repeated courses consideration should be given to alternate therapy. For patients undergoing dialysis, the total recommended dose for the treatment of gout flares should be reduced to a single dose of 0.6 mg (1 tablet). For these patients, the treatment course should not be repeated more than once every 2 weeks [see Dose Modification in Renal Impairment (2.5)].

FMF

Although, pharmacokinetics of colchicine in patients with mild (Clcr 50 – 80 mL/min) and moderate (Clcr 30 – 50 mL/min) renal impairment is not known, these patients should be monitored closely for adverse effects of colchicine. Dose reduction may be necessary. In patients with severe renal failure (Clcr less than 30 mL/minute) and end-stage renal disease requiring dialysis, COLCRYS may be started at the dose of 0.3 mg/day. Any increase in dose should be done with adequate monitoring of the patient for adverse effects of COLCRYS [see Pharmacokinetics (12.3) and Dose Modification in Renal Impairment (2.5)].

8.7 Hepatic Impairment

The clearance of colchicine may be significantly reduced and plasma half-life prolonged in patients with chronic hepatic impairment, compared to healthy subjects [see Pharmacokinetics (12.3)].

Prophylaxis of Gout Flares:

For prophylaxis of gout flares in patients with mild to moderate hepatic function impairment, adjustment of the recommended dose is not required, but patients should be monitored closely for adverse effects of colchicine. Dose reduction should be considered for the prophylaxis of gout flares in patients with severe hepatic impairment [see Dose Modification in Hepatic Impairment (2.6)].

Treatment of Gout Flares:

For treatment of gout flares in patients with mild to moderate hepatic function impairment, adjustment of the recommended COLCRYS dose is not required, but patients should be monitored closely for adverse effects of COLCRYS. However, for the treatment of gout flares in patients with severe impairment while the dose does not need to be adjusted, the treatment course should be repeated no more than once every 2 weeks. For these patients, requiring repeated courses for the treatment of gout flares, consideration should be given to alternate therapy [see Dose Modification in Hepatic Impairment (2.6)].

FMF

In patients with severe hepatic disease, dose reduction should be considered with careful monitoring [see Pharmacokinetics (12.3) and Dose Modification in Hepatic Impairment (2.6)].

9 DRUG ABUSE AND DEPENDENCE

Tolerance, abuse, or dependence with colchicine has not been reported.

10 OVERDOSAGE

The exact dose of colchicine that produces significant toxicity is unknown. Fatalities have occurred after ingestion of a dose as low as 7 mg over a 4-day period, while other patients have survived after ingesting more than 60 mg. A re-view of 150 patients who overdosed on colchicine found that those who ingested less than 0.5 mg/kg survived and tended to have milder toxicities, such as gastrointestinal symptoms, whereas those who took 0.5 to 0.8 mg/kg had more severe reactions, such as myelosuppression. There was 100% mortality in those who ingested more than 0.8 mg/kg.

The first stage of acute colchicine toxicity typically begins within 24 hours of ingestion and includes gastrointestinal symptoms, such as abdominal pain, nausea, vomiting, diarrhea, and significant fluid loss, leading to volume depletion. Peripheral leukocytosis may also be seen. Life-threatening complications occur during the second stage, which occurs 24 to 72 hours after drug administration, attributed to multi-organ failure and its consequences. Death is usually a result of respiratory depression and cardiovascular collapse. If the patient survives, recovery of multi-organ injury may be accompanied by rebound leukocytosis and alopecia starting about 1 week after the initial ingestion.

Treatment of colchicine poisoning should begin with gastric lavage and measures to prevent shock. Otherwise, treatment is symptomatic and supportive. No specific antidote is known. Colchicine is not effectively removed by dialysis [see Pharmacokinetics (12.3)].

11 DESCRIPTION

Colchicine is an alkaloid chemically described as (S)N-(5,6,7,9-tetrahydro- 1,2,3, 10-tetramethoxy-9-oxobenzo [alpha] heptalen-7-yl) acetamide with a molecular formula of $C_{22}H_{25}NO_6$ and a molecular weight of 399.4. The structural formula of colchicine is given below.

Colchicine occurs as a pale yellow powder that is soluble in water.

COLCRYS® (colchicine, USP) tablets are supplied for oral administration as purple, film-coated, capsule-shaped tablets (0.1575″ × 0.3030″), debossed with 'AR 374' on one side and scored on the other, containing 0.6 mg of the active ingredient colchicine USP. Inactive ingredients: carnauba wax, FD&C blue #2, FD&C red #40, hypromellose, lactose monohydrate, magnesium stearate, microcrystalline cellulose, polydextrose, polyethylene glycol, pregelatinized starch, sodium starch glycolate, titanium dioxide, and triacetin.

12 CLINICAL PHARMACOLOGY

12.1 Mechanism of Action

The mechanism by which COLCRYS exerts its beneficial effect in patients with FMF has not been fully elucidated; however, evidence suggests that colchicine may interfere with the intracellular assembly of the inflammasome com-plex present in neutrophils and monocytes that mediates activation of interleukin-1β. Additionally, colchicine disrupts cytoskeletal functions through inhibition of β-tubulin polymerization into microtubules, and consequently prevents the activation, degranulation, and migration of neutrophils thought to mediate some gout symptoms.

12.3 Pharmacokinetics

Absorption

In healthy adults, COLCRYS is absorbed when given orally, reaching a mean C_{max} of 2.5 ng/mL (range 1.1 to 4.4 ng/mL) in 1 to 2 hours (range 0.5 to 3 hours) after a single dose administered under fasting conditions.

Following oral administration of COLCRYS given as 1.8 mg colchicine over 1 hour to healthy, young adults under fasting conditions, colchicine appears to be readily absorbed, reaching mean maximum plasma concentrations of 6.2 ng/mL at a median 1.81 hours (range: 1.0 to 2.5 hours). Following administration of the non-recommended high-dose regimen (4.8 mg over 6 hours), mean maximal plasma concentrations were 6.8 ng/mL, at a median 4.47 hours (range: 3.1 to 7.5 hours).

After 10 days on a regimen of 0.6 mg twice daily, peak concentrations are 3.1 to 3.6 ng/mL (range 1.6 to 6.0 ng/mL), occurring 1.3 to 1.4 hours post-dose (range 0.5 to 3.0 hours). Mean pharmacokinetic parameter values in healthy adults are shown in Table 5 below.

[See table 5 above]

In some subjects, secondary colchicine peaks are seen, occurring between 3 and 36 hours post-dose and ranging from 39% to 155% of the height of the initial peak. These observations are attributed to intestinal secretion and reabsorption and/or biliary recirculation.

Absolute bioavailability is reported to be approximately 45%.

Administration of COLCRYS with food has no effect on the rate of colchicine absorption, but did decrease the extent of colchicine by approximately 15%. This is without clinical significance.

Distribution

The mean apparent volume of distribution in healthy young volunteers was approximately 5 to 8 L/kg.

Colchicine binding to serum protein is low, 39 ± 5%, primarily to albumin regardless of concentration.

Colchicine crosses the placenta (plasma levels in the fetus are reported to be approximately 15% of the maternal concentration). Colchicine also distributes into breast milk at concentrations similar to those found in the maternal serum [see Pregnancy (8.1) and Nursing Mothers (8.3)].

Metabolism

Colchicine is demethylated to two primary metabolites, 2-O-demethylcolchicine and 3-O-demethylcolchicine (2- and 3-DMC, respectively), and one minor metabolite, 10-O-demethylcolchicine (also known as colchiceine). In vitro studies using human liver microsomes have shown that CYP3A4 is involved in the metabolism of colchicine to 2-and 3-DMC. Plasma levels of these metabolites are minimal (less than 5% of parent drug).

Elimination/Excretion

In healthy volunteers (n=12) 40 – 65% of 1 mg orally administered colchicine was recovered unchanged in urine. Enterohepatic recirculation and biliary excretion are also postulated to play a role in colchicine elimination. Following multiple oral doses (0.6 mg twice daily), the mean elimina-

Table 4 Other Potentially Significant Drug Interactions

Concomitant Drug Class or Food	Noted or anticipated Outcome	Clinical Comment
HMG-Co A Reductase Inhibitors: atorvastatin, fluvastatin, lovastatin, pravastatin, simvastatin	Pharmacokinetic and/or pharmacodynamic interaction: the addition of one drug to a stable long-term regimen of the other has resulted in myopathy and rhabdomyolysis (including a fatality)	Weigh the potential benefits and risks and carefully monitor patients for any signs or symptoms of muscle pain, tenderness, or weakness, particularly during initial therapy; monitoring CPK (creatine phosphokinase) will not necessarily prevent the occurrence of severe myopathy.
Other Lipid Lowering Drugs: fibrates, gemfibrozil		
Digitalis Glycosides: digoxin	P-gp substrate; rhabdomyolysis has been reported	

Table 5 Mean (%CV) Pharmacokinetic Parameters in Healthy Adults Given COLCRYS

C_{max} (colchicine ng/mL)	T_{max}* (h)	Vd/F (L)	CL/F (L/hr)	$t_{1/2}$ (h)
COLCRYS 0.6 mg Single Dose (N=13)				
2.5 (28.7)	1.5 (1.0 – 3.0)	341.5 (54.4)	54.1 (31.0)	--
COLCRYS 0.6 mg b.i.d. × 10 days (N=13)				
3.6 (23.7)	1.3 (0.5 – 3.0)	1150 (18.7)	30.3 (19.0)	26.6 (16.3)

CL= Dose/AUC$_{0-t}$ (Calculated from mean values)
Vd = CL/Ke (Calculated from mean values)

* T_{max} mean (range)

Table 6 Drug Interactions: Pharmacokinetic Parameters for COLCRYS (colchicine, USP) tablets in the Presence of the Co-Administered Drug

Co-administered Drug	Dose of Co-administered Drug (mg)	Dose of COLCRYS (mg)	N	% Change in Colchicine Concentrations from Baseline (Range: Min - Max)	
				C_{max}	AUC_{0-t}
Cyclosporine	100 mg single-dose	0.6 mg single-dose	23	270.0 (62.0 to 606.9)	259.0 (75.8 to 511.9)
Clarithromycin	250 mg BID, 7 days	0.6 mg single-dose	23	227.2 (65.7 to 591.1)	281.5 (88.7 to 851.6)
Ketoconazole	200 mg BID, 5 days	0.6 mg single-dose	24	101.7 (19.6 to 219.0)	212.2 (76.7 to 419.6)
Ritonavir	100 mg BID, 5 days	0.6 mg single-dose	18	184.4 (79.2 to 447.4)	296.0 (53.8 to 924.4)
Verapamil	240 mg daily, 5 days	0.6 mg single-dose	24	40.1 (-47.1 to 149.5)	103.3 (-9.8 to 217.2)
Diltiazem	240 mg daily, 7 days	0.6 mg single-dose	20	44.2 (-46.0 to 318.3)	93.4 (-30.2 to 338.6)
Azithromycin	500 mg × 1 day, then 250 mg × 4 days	0.6 mg single-dose	21	21.6 (-41.7 to 222.0)	57.1 (-24.3 to 241.1)
Grapefruit Juice	240 mL BID, 4 days	0.6 mg single-dose	21	-2.55 (-53.4 to 55.0)	-2.36 (-46.4 to 62.2)

Table 7 Drug Interactions: Pharmacokinetic Parameters for Co-Administration of Drug in the Presence of COLCRYS (colchicine, USP) tablets

Co-administered Drug	Dose of Co-administered Drug (mg)	Dose of COLCRYS (mg)	N	% Change in Co-Administered Drug Concentrations from Baseline (Range: Min - Max)	
				C_{max}	AUC_{0-t}
Theophylline	300 mg (elixir) single-dose	0.6 mg BID × 14 days	27	1.6 (-30.4 to 23.1)	1.6 (-28.5 to 27.1)
Ethinyl Estradiol (Ortho-Novum® 1/35)	21-Day Cycle (Active Treatment) + 7-Day Placebo	0.6 mg BID × 14 days	27*	-6.7 (-40.3 to 44.7)	-3.0† (-25.3 to 24.9)
Norethindrone (Ortho-Novum® 1/35)				0.94 (-37.3 to 59.4)	-1.6† (-32.0 to 33.7)

* Conducted in healthy adult females
† $AUC\tau$

Table 8 Number (%) of Responders Based on Target Joint Pain Score at 24 Hours Post First Dose

COLCRYS Dose Responders n (%)		Placebo n (%) (n=58)	% Differences in Proportion	
Low-dose (n=74)	High-dose (n=52)		Low-dose vs Placebo (95% CI)	High-dose vs Placebo (95% CI)
28 (38%)	17 (33%)	9 (16%)	22 (8, 37)	17 (1, 33)

tion half-lives in young healthy volunteers (mean age 25 to 28 years of age) is 26.6 to 31.2 hours. Colchicine is a substrate of P-gp.

Extracorporeal Elimination: Colchicine is not removed by hemodialysis.

Special Populations
There is no difference between men and women in the pharmacokinetic disposition of colchicine.

Pediatric Patients: Pharmacokinetics of colchicine was not evaluated in pediatric patients.

Elderly: Pharmacokinetics of colchicine has not been determined in elderly patients. A published report described the pharmacokinetics of 1 mg oral colchicine tablet in four elderly women compared to six young healthy males. The mean age of the four elderly women was 83 years (range 75 – 93), mean weight was 47 kg (38 – 61 kg) and mean creatinine clearance was 46 mL/min (range 25 – 75 mL/min). Mean peak plasma levels and AUC of colchicine were two times higher in elderly subjects compared to young healthy males. However, it is possible that the higher exposure in the elderly subjects was due to decreased renal function.

Renal impairment: Pharmacokinetics of colchicine in patients with mild and moderate renal impairment is not known. A published report described the disposition of colchicine (1 mg) in young adult men and women with FMF who had normal renal function or end-stage renal disease requiring dialysis. Patients with end-stage renal disease had 75% lower colchicine clearance (0.17 vs 0.73 L/hr/kg)

and prolonged plasma elimination half-life (18.8 hrs vs 4.4 hrs) as compared to subjects with FMF and normal renal function [see Dose Modification in Renal Impairment (2.5) and Renal Impairment (8.6)].

Hepatic impairment: Published reports on the pharmacokinetics of IV colchicine in patients with severe chronic liver disease, as well as those with alcoholic or primary biliary cirrhosis, and normal renal function suggest wide interpatient variability. In some subjects with mild to moderate cirrhosis, the clearance of colchicine is significantly reduced and plasma half-life prolonged compared to healthy subjects. In subjects with primary biliary cirrhosis, no consistent trends were noted [see Dose Modification in Hepatic Impairment (2.6) and Hepatic Impairment (8.7)]. No pharmacokinetic data are available for patients with severe hepatic impairment (Child-Pugh C).

Drug interactions:
In vitro drug interactions:
In vitro studies in human liver microsomes have shown that colchicine is not an inhibitor or inducer of CYP1A2, CYP2A6, CYP2B6, CYP2C8, CYP2C9, CYP2C19, CYP2D6, CYP2E1, or CYP3A4 activity.
In vivo drug interactions:
The effects of co-administration of other drugs with COLCRYS on C_{max}, AUC, and C_{min} are summarized in Table 6 (effect of other drugs on colchicine) and Table 7 (effect of colchicine on other drugs). For information regarding clini-

cal recommendations, see Table 1 in Dose Modification for Co-administration of Interacting Drugs [see Dose Modification for Co-administration of Interacting Drugs (2.4)].
[See table 6 above]
Estrogen-containing oral contraceptives: In healthy female volunteers given ethinyl estradiol and norethindrone (Ortho-Novum® 1/35) co-administered with COLCRYS (0.6 mg b.i.d. × 14 days), hormone concentrations are not affected.
In healthy volunteers given theophylline co-administered with COLCRYS (0.6 mg b.i.d. × 14 days), theophylline concentrations were not affected.
[See table 7 above]

13   NONCLINICAL TOXICOLOGY
13.1   Carcinogenesis, Mutagenesis, Impairment of Fertility
Carcinogenesis
Carcinogenicity studies of colchicine have not been conducted. Due to the potential for colchicine to produce aneuploid cells (cells with an unequal number of chromosomes), there is theoretically an increased risk of malignancy.
Mutagenesis
Colchicine was negative for mutagenicity in the bacterial reverse mutation assay. In a chromosomal aberration assay in cultured human white blood cells, colchicine treatment resulted in the formation of micronuclei. Since published studies demonstrated that colchicine induces aneuploidy from the process of mitotic nondisjunction without structural DNA changes, colchicine is not considered clastogenic, although micronuclei are formed.
Impairment of Fertility
No studies of colchicine effects on fertility were conducted with COLCRYS. However, published nonclinical studies demonstrated that colchicine-induced disruption of microtubule formation affects meiosis and mitosis. Reproductive studies also reported abnormal sperm morphology and reduced sperm counts in males, and interference with sperm penetration, second meiotic division, and normal cleavage in females when exposed to colchicine. Colchicine administered to pregnant animals resulted in fetal death and teratogenicity. These effects were dose dependent, with the timing of exposure critical for the effects on embryofetal development. The nonclinical doses evaluated were generally higher than an equivalent human therapeutic dose, but safety margins for reproductive and developmental toxicity could not be determined.
Case reports and epidemiology studies in human male subjects on colchicine therapy indicated that infertility from colchicine is rare. A case report indicated that azoospermia was reversed when therapy was stopped. Case reports and epidemiology studies in female subjects on colchicine therapy have not established a clear relationship between colchicine use and female infertility. However, since the progression of FMF without treatment may result in infertility, the use of colchicine needs to be weighed against the potential risks.

14   CLINICAL STUDIES
The evidence for the efficacy of colchicine in patients with chronic gout is derived from the published literature. Two randomized clinical trials assessed the efficacy of colchicine 0.6 mg twice a day for the prophylaxis of gout flares in patients with gout initiating treatment with urate lowering therapy. In both trials, treatment with colchicine decreased the frequency of gout flares.
The efficacy of a low dosage regimen of oral colchicine (COLCRYS total dose 1.8 mg over 1 hour) for treatment of gout flares was assessed in a multicenter, randomized, double-blind, placebo-controlled, parallel group, 1 week, dose comparison study. Patients meeting American College of Rheumatology criteria for gout were randomly assigned to three groups: high-dose colchicine (1.2 mg, then 0.6 mg hourly × 6 hours [4.8 mg total]); low-dose colchicine (1.2 mg, then 0.6 mg in 1 hour [1.8 mg total] followed by 5 placebo doses hourly); or placebo (2 capsules, then 1 capsule hourly × 6 hours). Patients took the first dose within 12 hours of the onset of the flare and recorded pain intensity (11-point Likert scale) and adverse events over 72 hours. The efficacy of colchicine was measured based on response to treatment in the target joint, using patient self assessment of pain at 24 hours following the time of first dose as recorded in the diary. A responder was one who achieved at least a 50% reduction in pain score at the 24-hour post-dose assessment relative to the pre-treatment score and did not use rescue medication prior to the actual time of 24-hour post-dose assessment.
Rates of response were similar for the recommended low-dose treatment group (38%) and the non-recommended high-dose group (33%) but were higher as compared to the placebo group (16%) as shown in Table 8.
[See table 8 above]
Figure 1 below shows the percentage of patients achieving varying degrees of improvement in pain from baseline at 24 hours.

Figure 1
Pain Relief on Low and High Doses of COLCRYS and Placebo (Cumulative)

The evidence for the efficacy of colchicine in patients with FMF is derived from the published literature. Three randomized, placebo-controlled studies were identified. The three placebo-controlled studies randomized a total of 48 adult patients diagnosed with FMF and reported similar efficacy endpoints as well as inclusion and exclusion criteria. One of the studies randomized 15 patients with FMF to a 6-month crossover study during which 5 patients discontinued due to study non-compliance. The 10 patients completing the study experienced 5 attacks over the course of 90 days while treated with colchicine compared to 59 attacks over the course of 90 days while treated with placebo. Similarly, the second study randomized 22 patients with FMF to a 4-month crossover study during which 9 patients discontinued due to lack of efficacy while receiving placebo or study non-compliance. The 13 patients completing the study experienced 18 attacks over the course of 60 days while treated with colchicine compared to 68 attacks over the course of 60 days while treated with placebo. The third study was discontinued after an interim analysis of 6 of the 11 patients enrolled had completed the study; results could not be confirmed.

Open-label experience with colchicine in adults and children with FMF is consistent with the randomized, controlled trial experience, and was utilized to support information on the safety profile of colchicine and for dosing recommendations.

16 HOW SUPPLIED/STORAGE AND HANDLING

16.1 How Supplied

COLCRYS® (colchicine, USP) tablets 0.6 mg, are purple, film-coated, capsule-shaped tablets, debossed with 'AR 374' on one side and scored on the other side.

Bottles of 30	NDC 64764-119-07
Bottles of 60	NDC 64764-119-06
Bottles of 100	NDC 64764-119-01
Bottles of 250	NDC 64764-119-03
Bottles of 500	NDC 64764-119-05
Bottles of 1000	NDC 64764-119-10

16.2 Storage

Store at 20° to 25°C (68° to 77°F).
[See USP Controlled Room Temperature]
Protect from light.
DISPENSE IN TIGHT, LIGHT-RESISTANT CONTAINER.

17 PATIENT COUNSELING INFORMATION

[See Medication Guide]

17.1 Dosing Instructions

Patients should be advised to take COLCRYS as prescribed, even if they are feeling better. Patients should not alter the dose or discontinue treatment without consulting with their doctor. If a dose of COLCRYS is missed:
- For treatment of a gout flare when the patient is not being dosed for prophylaxis, take the missed dose as soon as possible.
- For treatment of a gout flare during prophylaxis, take the missed dose immediately, wait twelve hours, then resume the previous dosing schedule.
- For prophylaxis without treatment for a gout flare, or FMF, take the dose as soon as possible and then return to the normal dosing schedule. However, if a dose is skipped the patient should not double the next dose.

17.2 Fatal Overdose

Instruct patient that fatal overdoses, both accidental and intentional, have been reported in adults and children who have ingested colchicine. COLCRYS should be kept out of the reach of children.

17.3 Blood Dyscrasias

Patients should be informed that bone marrow depression with agranulocytosis, aplastic anemia, and thrombocytopenia may occur with COLCRYS.

17.4 Drug and Food Interactions

Patients should be advised that many drugs or other substances may interact with COLCRYS and some interactions could be fatal. Therefore, patients should report to their healthcare provider all of the current medications they are taking, and check with their healthcare provider before starting any new medications, particularly antibiotics. Patients should also be advised to report the use of non-prescription medication or herbal products. Grapefruit and grapefruit juice may also interact and should not be consumed during COLCRYS treatment.

17.5 Neuromuscular Toxicity

Patients should be informed that muscle pain or weakness, tingling or numbness in fingers or toes may occur with COLCRYS alone or when it is used with certain other drugs. Patients developing any of these signs or symptoms must discontinue COLCRYS and seek medical evaluation immediately.

17.6 Medication Guide

All trademarks are the property of their respective owners.
Distributed by:
Takeda Pharmaceuticals America, Inc.
Deerfield, IL 60015
Rev 01, June 2012
MEDICATION GUIDE
COLCRYS
(KOL-kris)
(colchicine) tablets

Read the Medication Guide that comes with COLCRYS before you start taking it and each time you get a refill. There may be new information. This Medication Guide does not take the place of talking to your healthcare provider about your medical condition or treatment. You and your healthcare provider should talk about COLCRYS when you start taking it and at regular checkups.

What is the most important information I should know about COLCRYS?

COLCRYS can cause serious side effects or death if levels of COLCRYS are too high in your body.
- Taking certain medicines with COLCRYS can cause your level of COLCRYS to be too high, especially if you have kidney or liver problems.
- Tell your healthcare provider about all your medical conditions, including if you have kidney or liver problems. Your dose of COLCRYS may need to be changed.
- Tell your healthcare provider about all the medicines you take, including prescription and non-prescription medicines, vitamins and herbal supplements.
- Even medicines that you take for a short period of time, such as antibiotics, can interact with COLCRYS and cause serious side effects or death.
- Talk to your healthcare provider or pharmacist before taking any new medicine.
- Especially tell your healthcare provider if you take:

• atazanavir sulfate (Reyataz®)	• clarithromycin (Biaxin®)
• cyclosporine (Neoral®, Gengraf®, Sandimmune®)	• darunavir (Prezista®)
	• fosamprenavir (Lexiva®)
• fosamprenavir (Lexiva®) with ritonavir	• itraconazole (Sporanox®)
	• lopinavir/ritonavir (Kaletra®)
• indinavir (Crixivan®)	• nelfinavir mesylate (Viracept®)
• ketoconazole (Nizoral®)	
• nefazodone (Serzone®)	• saquinavir mesylate (Invirase®)
• ritonavir (Norvir®)	
• telithromycin (Ketek®)	• tipranavir (Aptivus®)

Ask your healthcare provider or pharmacist if you are not sure if you take any of the medicines listed above. This is not a complete list of all the medicines that can interact with COLCRYS.
- Know the medicines you take. Keep a list of them and show it to your healthcare provider and pharmacist when you get a new medicine.
- Keep COLCRYS out of the reach of children.

What is COLCRYS?

COLCRYS is a prescription medicine used to:
- prevent and treat gout flares in adults
- treat familial Mediterranean fever (FMF) in adults and children age four or older

COLCRYS is not a pain medicine and it should not be taken to treat pain related to other conditions unless specifically prescribed for those conditions.

Who should not take COLCRYS?

Do not take COLCRYS if you have liver or kidney problems and you take certain other medicines. Serious side effects, including death, have been reported in these patients even when taken as directed. See "What is the most important information I should know about COLCRYS?"

What should I tell my healthcare provider before starting COLCRYS?

See "What is the most important information I should know about COLCRYS?"
Before you take COLCRYS tell your healthcare provider about all your medical conditions including if you:
- have liver or kidney problems
- are pregnant or plan to become pregnant. It is not known if COLCRYS will harm your unborn baby. Talk to your healthcare provider if you are pregnant or plan to become pregnant.
- are breast-feeding or plan to breast-feed. COLCRYS passes into your breast milk. You and your healthcare provider should decide if you will take COLCRYS or breast-feed. If you take COLCRYS and breast-feed, you should talk to your child's healthcare provider about how to watch for side effects in your child.

Tell your healthcare provider about all the medicines you take, including ones that you may only be taking for a short time, such as antibiotics. See "What is the most important information I should know about COLCRYS?" Do not start a new medicine without talking to your healthcare provider. Using COLCRYS with certain other medicines, such as cholesterol-lowering medications and digoxin, can affect each other causing serious side effects. Your healthcare provider may need to change your dose of COLCRYS. Talk to your healthcare provider about whether the medications you are taking might interact with COLCRYS, and what side effects to look for.

How should I take COLCRYS?

- Take COLCRYS exactly as your healthcare provider tells you to take it. **If you are not sure about your dosing,** call your healthcare provider.
- COLCRYS can be taken with or without food.
- If you take too much COLCRYS go to the nearest hospital emergency room right away.
- Do not stop taking COLCRYS even if you start to feel better, unless your healthcare provider tells you.
- Your healthcare provider may do blood tests while you take COLCRYS.
- If you take COLCRYS daily and you miss a dose, then take it as soon as you remember. If it is almost time for your next dose, just skip the missed dose. Take the next dose at your regular time. Do not take 2 doses at the same time.
- If you have a gout flare while taking COLCRYS daily, report this to your healthcare provider.

What should I avoid while taking COLCRYS?

- Avoid eating grapefruit or drinking grapefruit juice while taking COLCRYS. It can increase your chances of getting serious side effects.

What are the possible side effects of COLCRYS?

COLCRYS can cause serious side effects or even cause death. See "What is the most important information I should know about COLCRYS?"
Get medical help right away, if you have:
- Muscle weakness or pain
- Numbness or tingling in your fingers or toes
- Unusual bleeding or bruising
- Increased infections
- Feel weak or tired
- Pale or gray color to your lips, tongue, or palms of your hands
- Severe diarrhea or vomiting

Gout Flares: The most common side effect of COLCRYS in people who have gout flares is diarrhea.

FMF: The most common side effects of COLCRYS in people who have FMF are abdominal pain, diarrhea, nausea and vomiting.
Tell your healthcare provider if you have any side effect that bothers you or that does not go away.
These are not all of the possible side effects of COLCRYS. For more information, ask your healthcare provider or pharmacist.
Call your doctor for medical advice about side effects. You may report side effects to FDA at 1-800-FDA-1088.

How should I store COLCRYS?

- Store COLCRYS at room temperature between 68° and 77°F (20° to 25°C).
- Keep COLCRYS in a tightly closed container.
- Keep COLCRYS out of the light.

Keep COLCRYS and all medicines out of the reach of children.

General Information about COLCRYS

Medicines are sometimes prescribed for purposes other than those listed in a Medication Guide. Do not use COLCRYS for a condition for which it was not prescribed. Do not give COLCRYS to other people, even if they have the same symptoms that you have. It may harm them. This Medication Guide summarizes the most important information about COLCRYS. If you would like more information, talk with your healthcare provider. You can ask your healthcare provider or pharmacist for information about COLCRYS that is written for healthcare professionals.
For more information, go to www.COLCRYS.com or call 1-877-825-3327.

Help Patients Save on Rx Drugs: PDR.net/PharmacyDiscountCard

What are the ingredients in COLCRYS?

Active Ingredient: Colchicine

Inactive Ingredients: carnauba wax, FD&C blue #2, FD&C red #40, hypromellose, lactose monohydrate, magnesium stearate, microcrystalline cellulose, polydextrose, polyethylene glycol, pregelatinized starch, sodium starch glycolate, titanium dioxide, and triacetin.

This Medication Guide has been approved by the U.S. Food and Drug Administration.

All trademarks are the property of their respective owners.

Distributed by:
Takeda Pharmaceuticals America, Inc.
Deerfield, IL 60015
Rev 01, June 2012

Shown in Product Identification Guide, page 313

CONTRAVE®   ℞

[CON-trayv]
(naltrexone HCl and bupropion HCl)
Extended-Release Tablets

HIGHLIGHTS OF PRESCRIBING INFORMATION

These highlights do not include all the information needed to use CONTRAVE® safely and effectively.
See full prescribing information for CONTRAVE.
CONTRAVE (naltrexone HCl and bupropion HCl)
Extended-Release Tablets
Initial U.S. Approval: 2014

> **WARNING: SUICIDAL THOUGHTS AND BEHAVIORS; AND NEUROPSYCHIATRIC REACTIONS**
> *See full prescribing information for complete boxed warning*
> - Increased risk of suicidal thinking and behavior in children, adolescents, and young adults taking antidepressants for major depressive disorder and other psychiatric disorders. (5.1)
> - Monitor for worsening and emergence of suicidal thoughts and behaviors. (5.1)
> - Serious neuropsychiatric events have been reported in patients taking bupropion for smoking cessation. (5.2)
> - CONTRAVE has not been studied in pediatric patients. (5.1)

INDICATIONS AND USAGE

CONTRAVE is a combination of naltrexone, an opioid antagonist, and bupropion, an aminoketone antidepressant, indicated as an adjunct to a reduced-calorie diet and increased physical activity for chronic weight management in adults with an initial body mass index (BMI) of:
- 30 kg/m² or greater (obese) or
- 27 kg/m² or greater (overweight) in the presence of at least one weight-related comorbidity (e.g., hypertension, type 2 diabetes mellitus, or dyslipidemia). (1)

Limitations of Use:
- The effect of CONTRAVE on cardiovascular morbidity and mortality has not been established. (1)
- The safety and effectiveness of CONTRAVE in combination with other products intended for weight loss, including prescription and over-the-counter drugs, and herbal preparations, have not been established. (1)

DOSAGE AND ADMINISTRATION

CONTRAVE dose escalation schedule (2.1):

	Morning Dose	Evening Dose
Week 1	1 tablet	None
Week 2	1 tablet	1 tablet
Week 3	2 tablets	1 tablet
Week 4 – Onward	2 tablets	2 tablets

DOSAGE FORMS AND STRENGTHS

Extended-Release Tablets: 8 mg naltrexone HCl /90 mg bupropion HCl (3)

CONTRAINDICATIONS

- Uncontrolled hypertension (4)
- Seizure disorders, anorexia nervosa or bulimia, or undergoing abrupt discontinuation of alcohol, benzodiazepines, barbiturates, and antiepileptic drugs (4)
- Use of other bupropion-containing products (4)
- Chronic opioid use (4)
- During or within 14 days of taking monoamine oxidase inhibitors (MAOI) (4)
- Known allergy to any of the ingredients in CONTRAVE (4)
- Pregnancy (4)

WARNINGS AND PRECAUTIONS

- Suicidal Behavior and Ideation: Monitor for depression or suicidal thoughts. Discontinue CONTRAVE if symptoms develop. (5.1)
- Risk of seizure may be minimized by adhering to the recommended dosing schedule and avoiding coadministration with high-fat meal. (5.3)
- Increase in Blood Pressure and Heart Rate: Monitor blood pressure and heart rate in all patients, especially those with cardiac or cerebrovascular disease. (5.5)
- Hepatotoxicity: Cases of hepatitis and clinically significant liver dysfunction observed with naltrexone exposure. (5.7)
- Angle-closure glaucoma: Angle-closure glaucoma has occurred in patients with untreated anatomically narrow angles treated with antidepressants. (5.9)
- Use of Antidiabetic Medications: Weight loss may cause hypoglycemia. Monitor blood glucose. (5.10)

ADVERSE REACTIONS

- Most common adverse reactions (greater than or equal to 5%): nausea, constipation, headache, vomiting, dizziness, insomnia, dry mouth and diarrhea. (6.1)

To report SUSPECTED ADVERSE REACTIONS, contact Takeda Pharmaceuticals America, Inc. at 1-877-TAKEDA-7 (1-877-825-3327) or FDA at 1-800-FDA-1088 or *www.fda.gov/medwatch*.

DRUG INTERACTIONS

- MAOIs: Increased risk of hypertensive reactions can occur when used concomitantly. (7.1)
- Drugs Metabolized by CYP2D6: Bupropion inhibits CYP2D6 and can increase concentrations of: antidepressants, (e.g., selective serotonin reuptake inhibitors and many tricyclics), antipsychotics (e.g., haloperidol, risperidone and thioridazine), beta-blockers (e.g., metoprolol) and Type 1C antiarrhythmics (e.g., propafenone and flecainide): Consider dose reduction when using with CONTRAVE. (7.3)
- Concomitant Treatment with CYP2B6 Inhibitors (e.g., ticlopidine or clopidogrel) can increase bupropion exposure. Do not exceed one tablet twice daily when taken with CYP2B6 inhibitors. (2.5, 7.4)
- CYP2B6 Inducers (e.g., ritonavir, lopinavir, efavirenz, carbamazepine, phenobarbital, and phenytoin) may reduce efficacy by reducing bupropion exposure, avoid concomitant use. (7.4)
- Drugs that Lower Seizure Threshold: Dose CONTRAVE with caution. (5.3, 7.5)
- Dopaminergic Drugs (levodopa and amantadine): CNS toxicity can occur when used concomitantly with CONTRAVE. (7.6)
- Drug-Laboratory Test Interactions: CONTRAVE can cause false-positive urine test results for amphetamines. (7.8)

USE IN SPECIFIC POPULATIONS

- Nursing Mothers: Discontinue drug or nursing. (8.3)
- Pediatric Use: Safety and effectiveness not established and use not recommended. (8.4)

See 17 for PATIENT COUNSELING INFORMATION and Medication Guide.

Revised: 09/2014

FULL PRESCRIBING INFORMATION: CONTENTS*
WARNING: SUICIDAL THOUGHTS AND BEHAVIORS; AND NEUROPSYCHIATRIC REACTIONS:
1 INDICATIONS AND USAGE
2 DOSAGE AND ADMINISTRATION
  2.1 Recommended Dosing
  2.2 Dose Adjustment in Patients with Renal Impairment
  2.3 Dose Adjustment in Patients with Hepatic Impairment
  2.4 Switching a Patient To or From a Monoamine Oxidase Inhibitor (MAOI) Antidepressant
  2.5 Concomitant Use with CYP2B6 Inhibitors
3 DOSAGE FORMS AND STRENGTHS
4 CONTRAINDICATIONS
5 WARNINGS AND PRECAUTIONS
  5.1 Suicidal Behavior and Ideation
  5.2 Neuropsychiatric Symptoms and Suicide Risk in Smoking Cessation Treatment
  5.3 Seizures
  5.4 Patients Receiving Opioid Analgesics
  5.5 Increase in Blood Pressure and Heart Rate
  5.6 Allergic Reactions
  5.7 Hepatotoxicity
  5.8 Activation of Mania
  5.9 Angle-Closure Glaucoma
  5.10 Potential Risk of Hypoglycemia in Patients with Type 2 Diabetes Mellitus on Antidiabetic Therapy
6 ADVERSE REACTIONS
  6.1 Clinical Trials Experience
7 DRUG INTERACTIONS
  7.1 Monoamine Oxidase Inhibitors (MAOI)
  7.2 Opioid Analgesics
  7.3 Potential for CONTRAVE to Affect Other Drugs
  7.4 Potential for Other Drugs to Affect CONTRAVE
  7.5 Drugs That Lower Seizure Threshold
  7.6 Dopaminergic Drugs (Levodopa and Amantadine)
  7.7 Use with Alcohol
  7.8 Drug-Laboratory Test Interactions
  7.9 Drug-Transporter Interactions
8 USE IN SPECIFIC POPULATIONS
  8.1 Pregnancy
  8.3 Nursing Mothers
  8.4 Pediatric Use
  8.5 Geriatric Use
  8.6 Renal Impairment
  8.7 Hepatic Impairment
9 DRUG ABUSE AND DEPENDENCE
  9.2 Abuse
10 OVERDOSAGE
12 CLINICAL PHARMACOLOGY
  12.1 Mechanism of Action
  12.2 Pharmacodynamics
  12.3 Pharmacokinetics
13 NONCLINICAL TOXICOLOGY
  13.1 Carcinogenesis, Mutagenesis, Impairment of Fertility
14 CLINICAL STUDIES
16 HOW SUPPLIED/STORAGE AND HANDLING
17 PATIENT COUNSELING INFORMATION
* Sections or subsections omitted from the full prescribing information are not listed

---

FULL PRESCRIBING INFORMATION

> **WARNING: SUICIDAL THOUGHTS AND BEHAVIORS; AND NEUROPSYCHIATRIC REACTIONS**
>
> **SUICIDALITY AND ANTIDEPRESSANT DRUGS**
> CONTRAVE® is not approved for use in the treatment of major depressive disorder or other psychiatric disorders. CONTRAVE contains bupropion, the same active ingredient as some other antidepressant medications (including, but not limited to, WELLBUTRIN, WELLBUTRIN SR, WELLBUTRIN XL and APLENZIN). Antidepressants increased the risk of suicidal thoughts and behavior in children, adolescents, and young adults in short-term trials. These trials did not show an increase in the risk of suicidal thoughts and behavior with antidepressant use in subjects over age 24; there was a reduction in risk with antidepressant use in subjects aged 65 and older. In patients of all ages who are started on CONTRAVE, monitor closely for worsening, and for the emergence of suicidal thoughts and behaviors. Advise families and caregivers of the need for close observation and communication with the prescriber. CONTRAVE is not approved for use in pediatric patients *[see Warnings and Precautions (5.1), Use in Specific Populations (8.4)]*.
>
> **NEUROPSYCHIATRIC REACTIONS IN PATIENTS TAKING BUPROPION FOR SMOKING CESSATION**
> Serious neuropsychiatric reactions have occurred in patients taking bupropion for smoking cessation *[see Warnings and Precautions (5.2)]*. The majority of these reactions occurred during bupropion treatment, but some occurred in the context of discontinuing treatment. In many cases, a causal relationship to bupropion treatment is not certain, because depressed mood may be a symptom of nicotine withdrawal. However, some of the cases occurred in patients taking bupropion who continued to smoke. Although CONTRAVE is not approved for smoking cessation, observe all patients for neuropsychiatric reactions. Instruct the patient to contact a healthcare provider if such reactions occur *[see Warnings and Precautions (5.2)]*.

1 INDICATIONS AND USAGE

CONTRAVE is indicated as an adjunct to a reduced-calorie diet and increased physical activity for chronic weight management in adults with an initial body mass index (BMI) of:
- 30 kg/m² or greater (obese) or
- 27 kg/m² or greater (overweight) in the presence of at least one weight-related comorbid condition (e.g., hypertension, type 2 diabetes mellitus, or dyslipidemia).

Limitations of Use:
- The effect of CONTRAVE on cardiovascular morbidity and mortality has not been established.
- The safety and effectiveness of CONTRAVE in combination with other products intended for weight loss, including prescription drugs, over-the-counter drugs, and herbal preparations, have not been established.

Weight (lb)	125	130	135	140	145	150	155	160	165	170	175	180	185	190	195	200	205	210	215	220	225
(kg)	56.8	59.1	61.4	63.6	65.9	68.2	70.5	72.7	75.0	77.3	79.5	81.8	84.1	86.4	88.6	90.9	93.2	95.5	97.7	100.0	102.3
Height (in) / (cm)																					
58 / 147.3	26	27	28	29	30	31	32	34	35	36	37	38	39	40	41	42	43	44	45	46	47
59 / 149.9	25	26	27	28	29	30	31	32	33	34	35	36	37	38	39	40	41	43	44	45	46
60 / 152.4	24	25	26	27	28	29	30	31	32	33	34	35	36	37	38	39	40	41	42	43	44
61 / 154.9	24	25	26	27	27	28	29	30	31	32	33	34	35	36	37	38	39	40	41	42	43
62 / 157.5	23	24	25	26	27	27	28	29	30	31	32	33	34	35	36	37	38	38	39	40	41
63 / 160.0	22	23	24	24	25	26	27	28	29	30	31	32	33	34	35	36	36	37	38	39	40
64 / 162.6	22	22	23	24	25	26	27	28	28	29	30	31	32	33	34	34	35	36	37	38	39
65 / 165.1	21	22	22	23	24	25	26	27	28	29	30	30	31	32	33	33	34	35	36	37	38
66 / 167.6	20	21	22	23	23	24	25	26	27	27	28	29	30	31	32	32	33	34	35	36	36
67 / 170.2	20	20	21	22	23	24	24	25	26	27	27	28	29	30	31	31	32	33	34	35	35
68 / 172.7	19	20	21	21	22	23	24	24	25	26	27	27	28	29	30	30	31	32	33	34	34
69 / 175.3	18	19	20	21	21	22	23	24	24	25	26	27	27	28	29	30	30	31	32	33	33
70 / 177.8	18	19	19	20	21	22	22	23	24	24	25	26	27	27	28	29	29	30	31	32	32
71 / 180.3	17	18	19	20	20	21	22	22	23	24	24	25	26	27	27	28	29	29	30	31	31
72 / 182.9	17	18	18	19	20	20	21	22	22	23	24	24	25	26	27	27	28	29	29	30	31
73 / 185.4	17	17	18	19	19	20	20	21	22	22	23	24	24	25	26	26	27	28	28	29	30
74 / 188.0	16	17	17	18	19	19	20	21	21	22	23	23	24	24	25	26	26	27	28	28	29
75 / 190.5	16	16	17	18	18	19	19	20	21	21	22	23	23	24	24	25	26	26	27	28	28
76 / 193.0	15	16	16	17	18	18	19	20	20	21	21	22	23	23	24	24	25	26	26	27	27

2 DOSAGE AND ADMINISTRATION

2.1 Recommended Dosing

CONTRAVE dosing should be escalated according to the following schedule:

	Morning Dose	Evening Dose
Week 1	1 tablet	None
Week 2	1 tablet	1 tablet
Week 3	2 tablets	1 tablet
Week 4 – Onward	2 tablets	2 tablets

A total daily dosage of two CONTRAVE 8 mg/90 mg tablets twice daily (32 mg/360 mg) is reached at the start of Week 4. CONTRAVE should be taken by mouth in the morning and in the evening. The tablets should not be cut, chewed, or crushed. Total daily doses greater than 32 mg/360 mg per day (two tablets twice daily) are not recommended. In clinical trials, CONTRAVE was administered with meals. However, CONTRAVE should not be taken with a high-fat meal because of a resulting significant increase in bupropion and naltrexone systemic exposure [see Warnings and Precautions (5.3) and Clinical Pharmacology (12.3)].

Patients may develop elevated blood pressure or heart rate during CONTRAVE treatment; the risk may be greater during the initial three months of therapy [see Warnings and Precautions (5.6)]. Because patients with hypertension may be at increased risk for developing blood pressure elevations, such patients should be monitored for this potential effect when initiating treatment with CONTRAVE.

Response to therapy should be evaluated after 12 weeks at the maintenance dosage. If a patient has not lost at least 5% of baseline body weight, discontinue CONTRAVE, as it is unlikely that the patient will achieve and sustain clinically meaningful weight loss with continued treatment.

BMI is calculated by dividing weight (in kg) by height (in meters) squared. A BMI chart for determining BMI based on height and weight is provided in Table 1.

Table 1. BMI Conversion Chart

[See table above]

2.2 Dose Adjustment in Patients with Renal Impairment

In patients with moderate or severe renal impairment, the maximum recommended daily dose for CONTRAVE is two tablets (one tablet each morning and evening). CONTRAVE is not recommended for use in patients with end-stage renal disease. There is a lack of adequate information to guide dosing in patients with mild renal impairment [see Use in Specific Population (8.6) and Clinical Pharmacology (12.3)].

2.3 Dose Adjustment in Patients with Hepatic Impairment

In patients with hepatic impairment, the maximum recommended daily dose of CONTRAVE is one tablet in the morning [see Use in Specific Population (8.7) and Clinical Pharmacology (12.3)].

2.4 Switching a Patient To or From a Monoamine Oxidase Inhibitor (MAOI) Antidepressant

At least 14 days should elapse between discontinuation of an MAOI intended to treat depression and initiation of therapy with CONTRAVE. Conversely, at least 14 days should be allowed after stopping CONTRAVE before starting an MAOI antidepressant [see Contraindications (4) and Drug Interactions (7.1)].

2.5 Concomitant Use with CYP2B6 Inhibitors

During concomitant use with CYP2B6 inhibitors (e.g., ticlopidine or clopidogrel), the maximum recommended daily dose of CONTRAVE is two tablets (one tablet each morning and evening) [see Drug Interactions (7.4) and Clinical Pharmacology (12.3)].

3 DOSAGE FORMS AND STRENGTHS

CONTRAVE extended-release tri-layer tablets, 8 mg/90 mg, are blue, round, bi-convex, film-coated, and debossed with "NB-890" on one side.

4 CONTRAINDICATIONS

CONTRAVE is contraindicated in
• Uncontrolled hypertension [see Warnings and Precautions (5.5)]
• Seizure disorder or a history of seizures [see Warnings and Precautions (5.3)]
• Use of other bupropion-containing products (including, but not limited to, Wellbutrin, Wellbutrin SR, Wellbutrin XL, and Aplenzin)
• Bulimia or anorexia nervosa, which increase the risk for seizure [see Warnings and Precautions (5.3)]
• Chronic opioid or opiate agonist (e.g., methadone) or partial agonists (e.g., buprenorphine) use, or acute opiate withdrawal [see Warnings and Precautions (5.4) and Drug Interactions (7.2)]
• Patients undergoing an abrupt discontinuation of alcohol, benzodiazepines, barbiturates, and antiepileptic drugs [see Warnings and Precautions (5.3) and Drug Interactions (7.7)]
• Concomitant administration of monoamine oxidase inhibitors (MAOI). At least 14 days should elapse between discontinuation of MAOI and initiation of treatment with CONTRAVE. There is an increased risk of hypertensive reactions when CONTRAVE is used concomitantly with MAOIs. Starting CONTRAVE in a patient treated with reversible MAOIs such as linezolid or intravenous methylene blue is also contraindicated [see Dosage and Administration (2.4), Drug Interactions (7.1)]
• Known allergy to bupropion, naltrexone or any other component of CONTRAVE.
Anaphylactoid/anaphylactic reactions and Stevens-Johnson syndrome have been reported with bupropion [see Warnings and Precautions (5.6)]
• Pregnancy [see Use in Specific Populations (8.1)]

5 WARNINGS AND PRECAUTIONS

5.1 Suicidal Behavior and Ideation

CONTRAVE contains bupropion, a dopamine and norepinephrine re-uptake inhibitor that is similar to some drugs used for the treatment of depression; therefore, the following precautions pertaining to these products should be considered when treating patients with CONTRAVE.

Patients with major depressive disorder, both adult and pediatric, may experience worsening of their depression and/or the emergence of suicidal ideation and behavior (suicidality) or unusual changes in behavior, whether or not they are taking antidepressant medications, and this risk may persist until significant remission occurs. Suicide is a known risk of depression and certain other psychiatric disorders, and these disorders themselves are the strongest predictors of suicide. There has been a long-standing concern that antidepressants may have a role in inducing worsening of depression and the emergence of suicidality in certain patients during the early phases of treatment.

In placebo-controlled clinical trials with CONTRAVE for the treatment of obesity in adult patients, no suicides or suicide attempts were reported in studies up to 56 weeks duration with CONTRAVE (equivalent to bupropion doses of 360 mg/day). In these same studies, suicidal ideation was reported by 3 (0.20%) of 1,515 patients treated with placebo compared with 1 (0.03%) of 3,239 treated with CONTRAVE.

Pooled analyses of short-term placebo-controlled trials of antidepressant drugs (selective serotonin re-uptake inhibitors [SSRIs] and others) show that these drugs increase the risk of suicidal thinking and behavior (suicidality) in children, adolescents, and young adults (ages 18 to 24) with major depressive disorder (MDD) and other psychiatric disorders. Short-term clinical trials did not show an increase in the risk of suicidality with antidepressants compared with placebo in adults beyond age 24; there was a reduction with antidepressants compared with placebo in adults aged 65 and older.

The pooled analyses of placebo-controlled trials of antidepressant drugs in children and adolescents with MDD, obsessive compulsive disorder (OCD), or other psychiatric disorders included a total of 24 short-term trials of nine antidepressant drugs in over 4,400 patients. The pooled analyses of placebo-controlled trials in adults with MDD or other psychiatric disorders included a total of 295 short-term trials (median duration of two months) of 11 antidepressant drugs in over 77,000 patients. There was considerable variation in risk of suicidality among drugs, but a tendency toward an increase in the younger patients for almost all drugs studied. There were differences in absolute risk of suicidality across the different indications, with the highest incidence in MDD. The risk differences (drug vs placebo), however, were relatively stable within age strata and across indications. These risk differences (drug-placebo difference in the number of cases of suicidality per 1,000 patients treated) are provided in *Table 2*.

Table 2. Risk Differences in the Number of Suicidality Cases by Age Group in the Pooled Placebo-Controlled Trials of Antidepressants in Pediatric and Adult Subjects

Age Range	Drug-Placebo Difference in Number of Cases of Suicidality per 1,000 Patients Treated
	Increases Compared to Placebo
<18	14 additional cases
18 to 24	5 additional cases
	Decreases Compared to Placebo
25 to 64	1 fewer case
≥65	6 fewer cases

No suicides occurred in any of the antidepressant pediatric trials. There were suicides in the adult antidepressant trials, but the number was not sufficient to reach any conclusion about drug effect on suicide.

It is unknown whether the suicidality risk extends to longer-term use, i.e., beyond several months. However, there is substantial evidence from placebo-controlled trials in adults with depression that the use of antidepressants can delay the recurrence of depression.

All patients being treated with antidepressants for any indication should be monitored appropriately and observed closely for clinical worsening, suicidality, and unusual changes in behavior, especially during the initial few months of a course of drug therapy, or at times of dose changes, either increases or decreases. This warning applies to CONTRAVE because one of its components, bupropion, is a member of an antidepressant class.

The following symptoms, anxiety, agitation, panic attacks, insomnia, irritability, hostility, aggressiveness, impulsivity, akathisia (psychomotor restlessness), hypomania, and mania, have been reported in adult and pediatric patients being treated with antidepressants for major depressive disorder as well as for other indications, both psychiatric and nonpsychiatric. Although a causal link between the emergence of such symptoms and either the worsening of depression and/or the emergence of suicidal impulses has not been established, there is concern that such symptoms may represent precursors to emerging suicidality.

Consideration should be given to changing the therapeutic regimen, including possibly discontinuing the medication, in patients whose depression is persistently worse, or who are experiencing emergent suicidality or symptoms that might be precursors to worsening depression or suicidality, especially if these symptoms are severe, abrupt in onset, or were not part of the patient's presenting symptoms.

Families and caregivers of patients being treated with antidepressants for major depressive disorder or other indications, both psychiatric and nonpsychiatric, should be alerted about the need to monitor patients for the emergence of anxiety, agitation, irritability, unusual changes in behavior, and the other symptoms described above, as well as the emergence of suicidality, and to report such symptoms immediately to healthcare providers. Such monitoring should include daily observation by families and caregivers. Prescriptions for CONTRAVE should be written for the smallest quantity of tablets consistent with good patient management, in order to reduce the risk of overdose.

5.2   Neuropsychiatric Symptoms and Suicide Risk in Smoking Cessation Treatment

CONTRAVE is not approved for smoking cessation treatment, but serious neuropsychiatric symptoms have been reported in patients taking bupropion for smoking cessation. These have included changes in mood (including depression and mania), psychosis, hallucinations, paranoia, delusions, homicidal ideation, hostility, agitation, aggression, anxiety, and panic, as well as suicidal ideation, suicide attempt, and completed suicide *[see Warnings and Precautions (5.1)]*. Observe patients for the occurrence of neuropsychiatric reactions. Instruct patients to contact a healthcare professional if such reactions occur.

In many of these cases, a causal relationship to bupropion treatment is not certain, because depressed mood can be a symptom of nicotine withdrawal. However, some of the cases occurred in patients taking bupropion who continued to smoke.

Depression, suicide, attempted suicide and suicidal ideation have been reported in the postmarketing experience with naltrexone used in the treatment of opioid dependence. No causal relationship has been demonstrated.

5.3   Seizures

Bupropion, a component of CONTRAVE, can cause seizures. The risk of seizure is dose-related. The incidence of seizure in patients receiving CONTRAVE in clinical trials was approximately 0.1% vs 0% on placebo. CONTRAVE should be discontinued and not restarted in patients who experience a seizure while being treated with CONTRAVE.

The risk of seizures is also related to patient factors, clinical situations, and concomitant medications that lower the seizure threshold. Consider these risks before initiating treatment with CONTRAVE. CONTRAVE is contraindicated in patients with a seizure disorder, current or prior diagnosis of anorexia nervosa or bulimia, or undergoing abrupt discontinuation of alcohol, benzodiazepines, barbiturates, and antiepileptic drugs. Caution should be used when prescribing CONTRAVE to patients with predisposing factors that may increase the risk of seizure including:

- history of head trauma or prior seizure, severe stroke, arteriovenous malformation, central nervous system tumor or infection, or metabolic disorders (e.g., hypoglycemia, hyponatremia, severe hepatic impairment, and hypoxia)
- excessive use of alcohol or sedatives, addiction to cocaine or stimulants, or withdrawal from sedatives
- patients with diabetes treated with insulin and/or oral diabetic medications (sulfonylureas and meglitinides) that may cause hypoglycemia
- concomitant administration of medications that may lower the seizure threshold, including other bupropion products, antipsychotics, tricyclic antidepressants, theophylline, systemic steroids

Recommendations for Reducing the Risk of Seizure: Clinical experience with bupropion suggests that the risk of seizure may be minimized by adhering to the recommended dosing recommendations *[see Dosage and Administration (2)]*, in particular:

- the total daily dose of CONTRAVE does not exceed 360 mg of the bupropion component (i.e., four tablets per day)
- the daily dose is administered in divided doses (twice daily)
- the dose is escalated gradually
- no more than two tablets are taken at one time
- coadministration of CONTRAVE with high-fat meals is avoided *[see Dosage and Administration (2.1) and Clinical Pharmacology (12.3)]*
- if a dose is missed, a patient should wait until the next scheduled dose to resume the regular dosing schedule

5.4   Patients Receiving Opioid Analgesics

Vulnerability to Opioid Overdose: CONTRAVE should not be administered to patients receiving chronic opioids, due to the naltrexone component, which is an opioid receptor antagonist *[see Contraindications (4)]*. If chronic opiate therapy is required, CONTRAVE treatment should be stopped. In patients requiring intermittent opiate treatment, CONTRAVE therapy should be temporarily discontinued and lower doses of opioids may be needed. Patients should be alerted that they may be more sensitive to opioids, even at lower doses, after CONTRAVE treatment is discontinued. An attempt by a patient to overcome any naltrexone opioid blockade by administering large amounts of exogenous opioids is especially dangerous and may lead to a fatal overdose or life-threatening opioid intoxication (e.g., respiratory arrest, circulatory collapse). Patients should be told of the serious consequences of trying to overcome the opioid blockade.

Precipitated Opioid Withdrawal: The symptoms of spontaneous opioid withdrawal, which are associated with the discontinuation of opioid in a dependent individual, are uncomfortable, but they are not generally believed to be severe or necessitate hospitalization. However, when withdrawal is precipitated abruptly, the resulting withdrawal syndrome can be severe enough to require hospitalization. To prevent occurrence of either precipitated withdrawal in patients dependent on opioids or exacerbation of a pre-existing subclinical withdrawal symptoms, opioid-dependent patients, including those being treated for alcohol dependence, should be opioid-free (including tramadol) before starting CONTRAVE treatment. An opioid-free interval of a minimum of 7 to 10 days is recommended for patients previously dependent on short-acting opioids, and those patients transitioning from buprenorphine or methadone may need as long as two weeks. Patients should be made aware of the risks associated with precipitated withdrawal and encouraged to give an accurate account of last opioid use.

5.5   Increase in Blood Pressure and Heart Rate

CONTRAVE can cause an increase in systolic and/or diastolic blood pressure as well as an increase in resting heart rate. In clinical practice with other bupropion-containing products, hypertension, in some cases severe and requiring acute treatment, has been reported. The clinical significance of the increases in blood pressure and heart rate observed with CONTRAVE treatment is unclear, especially for patients with cardiac and cerebrovascular disease, since patients with a history of myocardial infarction or stroke in the previous 6 months, life-threatening arrhythmias, or congestive heart failure were excluded from CONTRAVE clinical trials. Blood pressure and pulse should be measured prior to starting therapy with CONTRAVE and should be monitored at regular intervals consistent with usual clinical practice, particularly among patients with controlled hypertension prior to treatment *[see Dosage and Administration (2.1)]*. CONTRAVE should not be given to patients with uncontrolled hypertension *[see Contraindications (4)]*.

Among patients treated with CONTRAVE in placebo-controlled clinical trials, mean systolic and diastolic blood pressure was approximately 1 mmHg higher than baseline at Weeks 4 and 8, similar to baseline at Week 12, and approximately 1 mmHg below baseline between Weeks 24 and 56. In contrast, among patients treated with placebo, mean blood pressure was approximately 2 to 3 mmHg below baseline throughout the same time points, yielding statistically significant differences between the groups at every assessment during this period. The largest mean differences between the groups were observed during the first 12 weeks (treatment difference +1.8 to +2.4 mmHg systolic, all p<0.001; +1.7 to +2.1 mmHg diastolic, all p<0.001).

For heart rate, at both Weeks 4 and 8, mean heart rate was statistically significantly higher (2.1 bpm) in the CONTRAVE group compared with the placebo group; at Week 52, the difference between groups was +1.7 bpm (p<0.001).

In an ambulatory blood pressure monitoring substudy of 182 patients, the mean change from baseline in systolic blood pressure after 52 weeks of treatment was -0.2 mmHg for the CONTRAVE group and -2.8 mmHg for the placebo group (treatment difference, +2.6 mmHg, p=0.08); the mean change in diastolic blood pressure was +0.8 mmHg for the CONTRAVE group and -2.1 mmHg for the placebo group (treatment difference, +2.9 mmHg, p=0.004).

A greater percentage of subjects had adverse reactions related to blood pressure or heart rate in the CONTRAVE group compared to the placebo group (6.3% vs 4.2%, respectively), primarily attributable to adverse reactions of Hypertension/Blood Pressure Increased (5.9% vs 4.0%, respectively). These events were observed in both patients with and without evidence of preexisting hypertension. In a trial that enrolled individuals with diabetes, 12.0% of patients in the CONTRAVE group and 6.5% in the placebo group had a blood pressure-related adverse reaction.

5.6   Allergic Reactions

Anaphylactoid/anaphylactic reactions characterized by symptoms such as pruritus, urticaria, angioedema, and dyspnea requiring medical treatment have been reported in clinical trials with bupropion. In addition, there have been rare spontaneous postmarketing reports of erythema multiforme, Stevens-Johnson syndrome, and anaphylactic shock associated with bupropion. Instruct patients to discontinue CONTRAVE and consult a healthcare provider if they develop an allergic or anaphylactoid/anaphylactic reaction (e.g., skin rash, pruritus, hives, chest pain, edema, or shortness of breath) during treatment.

Arthralgia, myalgia, fever with rash, and other symptoms suggestive of delayed hypersensitivity have been reported in association with bupropion. These symptoms may resemble serum sickness.

5.7   Hepatotoxicity

Cases of hepatitis and clinically significant liver dysfunction were observed in association with naltrexone exposure during naltrexone clinical trials and in postmarketing reports for patients using naltrexone. Transient, asymptomatic hepatic transaminase elevations were also observed. When patients presented with elevated transaminases, there were often other potential causative or contributory etiologies identified, including pre-existing alcoholic liver disease, hepatitis B and/or C infection, and concomitant usage of other potentially hepatotoxic drugs. Although clinically significant liver dysfunction is not typically recognized as a manifestation of opioid withdrawal, opioid withdrawal that is precipitated abruptly may lead to systemic sequelae, including acute liver injury.

Patients should be warned of the risk of hepatic injury and advised to seek medical attention if they experience symptoms of acute hepatitis. Use of CONTRAVE should be discontinued in the event of symptoms and/or signs of acute hepatitis.

In CONTRAVE clinical trials, there were no cases of elevated transaminases greater than three times the upper limit of normal (ULN) in conjunction with an increase in bilirubin greater than two times ULN.

5.8 Activation of Mania

Bupropion, a component of CONTRAVE, is a drug used for the treatment of depression. Antidepressant treatment can precipitate a manic, mixed, or hypomanic episode. The risk appears to be increased in patients with bipolar disorder or who have risk factors for bipolar disorder. Prior to initiating CONTRAVE, screen patients for a history of bipolar disorder and the presence of risk factors for bipolar disorder (e.g., family history of bipolar disorder, suicide, or depression). CONTRAVE is not approved for use in treating bipolar depression. No activation of mania or hypomania was reported in the clinical trials evaluating effects of CONTRAVE in obese patients; however, patients receiving antidepressant medications and patients with a history of bipolar disorder or recent hospitalization because of psychiatric illness were excluded from CONTRAVE clinical trials.

5.9 Angle-Closure Glaucoma

The pupillary dilation that occurs following use of many antidepressant drugs including bupropion, a component of CONTRAVE, may trigger an angle-closure attack in a patient with anatomically narrow angles who does not have a patent iridectomy.

5.10 Potential Risk of Hypoglycemia in Patients with Type 2 Diabetes Mellitus on Antidiabetic Therapy

Weight loss may increase the risk of hypoglycemia in patients with type 2 diabetes mellitus treated with insulin and/or insulin secretagogues (e.g., sulfonylureas). Measurement of blood glucose levels prior to starting CONTRAVE and during CONTRAVE treatment is recommended in patients with type 2 diabetes. Decreases in medication doses for antidiabetic medications which are non-glucose-dependent should be considered to mitigate the risk of hypoglycemia. If a patient develops hypoglycemia after starting CONTRAVE, appropriate changes should be made to the antidiabetic drug regimen.

6 ADVERSE REACTIONS

The following adverse reactions are discussed in other sections of the labeling:

- Suicidal Behavior and Ideation *[see Warnings and Precautions (5.1)]*
- Neuropsychiatric Symptoms *[see Warnings and Precautions (5.2)]*
- Seizures *[see Contraindications (4), Warnings and Precautions (5.3)]*
- Increase in Blood Pressure and Heart Rate *[see Warnings and Precautions (5.5)]*
- Allergic Reactions *[see Warnings and Precautions (5.6)]*
- Angle-Closure Glaucoma *[see Warnings and Precautions (5.9)]*

6.1 Clinical Trials Experience

Because clinical trials are conducted under widely varying conditions, the adverse reaction rates observed in the clinical trials of a drug cannot be directly compared to rates in the clinical trials of another drug and may not reflect the rates observed in practice.

CONTRAVE was evaluated for safety in five double-blind placebo controlled trials in 4,754 overweight or obese patients (3,239 patients treated with CONTRAVE and 1,515 patients treated with placebo) for a treatment period up to 56 weeks. The majority of patients were treated with CONTRAVE 32 mg/360 mg total daily dose. In addition, some patients were treated with other combination daily doses including naltrexone up to 50 mg and bupropion up to 400 mg. All subjects received study drug in addition to diet and exercise counseling. One trial (N=793) evaluated patients participating in an intensive behavioral modification program and another trial (N=505) evaluated patients with type 2 diabetes. In these randomized, placebo-controlled trials, 2,545 patients received CONTRAVE 32 mg/360 mg for a mean treatment duration of 36 weeks (median, 56 weeks). Baseline patient characteristics included a mean age of 46 years, 82% women, 78% white, 25% with hypertension, 13% with type 2 diabetes, 56% with dyslipidemia, 25% with BMI greater than 40 kg/m², and less than 2% with coronary artery disease. Dosing was initiated and increased weekly to reach the maintenance dose within 4 weeks.

In CONTRAVE clinical trials, 24% of subjects receiving CONTRAVE and 12% of subjects receiving placebo discontinued treatment because of an adverse event. The most frequent adverse reactions leading to discontinuation with CONTRAVE were nausea (6.3%), headache (1.7%) and vomiting (1.1%).

Common Adverse Reactions

Adverse reactions that were reported by greater than or equal to 2% of patients, and were more frequently reported by patients treated with CONTRAVE compared to placebo, are summarized in *Table 3*.

Table 3. Adverse Reactions Reported by Obese or Overweight Patients With an Incidence (%) of at Least 2% Among Patients Treated with CONTRAVE and More Common than with Placebo

Adverse Reaction	CONTRAVE 32 mg/360 mg N=2545 %	Placebo N=1515 %
Nausea	32.5	6.7
Constipation	19.2	7.2
Headache	17.6	10.4
Vomiting	10.7	2.9
Dizziness	9.9	3.4
Insomnia	9.2	5.9
Dry mouth	8.1	2.3
Diarrhea	7.1	5.2
Anxiety	4.2	2.8
Hot flush	4.2	1.2
Fatigue	4.0	3.4
Tremor	4.0	0.7
Upper abdominal pain	3.5	1.3
Viral gastroenteritis	3.5	2.6
Influenza	3.4	3.2
Tinnitus	3.3	0.6
Urinary tract infection	3.3	2.8
Hypertension	3.2	2.2
Abdominal pain	2.8	1.4
Hyperhidrosis	2.6	0.6
Irritability	2.6	1.8
Blood pressure increased	2.4	1.5
Dysgeusia	2.4	0.7
Rash	2.4	2.0
Muscle strain	2.2	1.7
Palpitations	2.1	0.9

Other Adverse Reactions

The following additional adverse reactions were reported in less than 2% of patients treated with CONTRAVE but with an incidence at least twice that of placebo:

Cardiac Disorders: tachycardia, myocardial infarction

Ear and Labyrinth Disorders: vertigo, motion sickness

Gastrointestinal Disorders: lower abdominal pain, eructation, lip swelling, hematochezia, hernia

General Disorders and Administration Site Conditions: feeling jittery, feeling abnormal, asthenia, thirst, feeling hot

Hepatobiliary Disorders: cholecystitis

Infections and Infestations: pneumonia, staphylococcal infection, kidney infection

Investigations: increased blood creatinine, increased hepatic enzymes, decreased hematocrit

Metabolism and Nutrition Disorders: dehydration

Musculoskeletal and Connective Tissue Disorders: intervertebral disc protrusion, jaw pain

Nervous System Disorders: disturbance in attention, lethargy, intention tremor, balance disorder, memory impairment, amnesia, mental impairment, presyncope

Psychiatric Disorders: abnormal dreams, nervousness, dissociation (feeling spacey), tension, agitation, mood swings

Renal and Urinary Disorders: micturition urgency

Reproductive System and Breast Disorders: vaginal hemorrhage, irregular menstruation, erectile dysfunction, vulvovaginal dryness

Skin and Subcutaneous Tissue Disorders: alopecia

Psychiatric and Sleep Disorders

In the one-year controlled trials of CONTRAVE, the proportion of patients reporting one or more adverse reactions related to psychiatric and sleep disorders was higher in the CONTRAVE 32/360 mg group than the placebo group (22.2% and 15.5%, respectively). These events were further categorized into sleep disorders (13.8% CONTRAVE, 8.4% placebo), depression (6.3% CONTRAVE, 5.9% placebo), and anxiety (6.1% CONTRAVE, 4.4% placebo). Patients who were 65 years or older experienced more psychiatric and sleep disorder adverse reactions in the CONTRAVE group (28.6%) compared to placebo (6.3%), although the sample size in this subgroup was small (56 CONTRAVE, 32 placebo); the majority of these events were insomnia (10.7% CONTRAVE, 3.1% placebo) and depression (7.1% CONTRAVE, 3.1% placebo).

Neurocognitive Adverse Reactions

Adverse reactions involving attention, dizziness, and syncope occurred more often in individuals randomized to CONTRAVE 32/360 mg group compared to placebo (15.0% and 5.5%, respectively). The most common cognitive-related adverse reactions were attention disorders (2.5% CONTRAVE, 0.6% placebo). Adverse reactions involving dizziness and syncope were more common in patients treated with CONTRAVE (10.6%) than in placebo-treated patients (3.6%); dizziness accounted for almost all of these reported events (10.4% CONTRAVE, 3.4% placebo). Dizziness was the primary reason for discontinuation for 0.9% and 0.3% of patients in the CONTRAVE and placebo groups, respectively.

Increases in Serum Creatinine

In the one-year controlled trials of CONTRAVE, larger mean increases in serum creatinine from baseline to trial endpoint were observed in the CONTRAVE group compared with the placebo group (0.07 mg/dL and 0.01 mg/dL, respectively) as well as from baseline to the maximum value during follow-up (0.15 mg/dL and 0.07 mg/dL, respectively). Increases in serum creatinine that exceeded the upper limit of normal and were also greater than or equal to 50% higher than baseline occurred in 0.6% of subjects receiving CONTRAVE compared to 0.1% receiving placebo. An *in vitro* drug-drug interaction study demonstrated that bupropion and its metabolites inhibit organic cation transporter 2 (OCT2), which is involved in the tubular secretion of creatinine, suggesting that the observed increase in serum creatinine may be the result of OCT2 inhibition.

Based on *in vitro* results and FDA guidance for Drug Interaction Studies, the ratios of the free (unbound) C_{max} and IC50 value of bupropion and hydroxybupropion were well below 0.1 suggesting a drug-drug interaction between CONTRAVE and OCT2 substrate due to bupropion and hydroxybupropion is unlikely. The ratio for the threohydrobupropion and erythrohydrobupropion metabolite mixture was 0.29, suggesting a drug-drug interaction between CONTRAVE and OCT2 due to threohydrobupropion and erythrohydrobupropion is possible.

7 DRUG INTERACTIONS

7.1 Monoamine Oxidase Inhibitors (MAOI)

Concomitant use of MAOIs and bupropion is contraindicated. Bupropion inhibits the re-uptake of dopamine and norepinephrine and can increase the risk for hypertensive reactions when used concomitantly with drugs that also inhibit the re-uptake of dopamine or norepinephrine, including MAOIs. Studies in animals demonstrate that the acute toxicity of bupropion is enhanced by the MAOI phenelzine. At least 14 days should elapse between discontinuation of an MAOI and initiation of treatment with CONTRAVE. Conversely, at least 14 days should be allowed after stopping CONTRAVE before starting an MAOI *[see Contraindications (4)].*

7.2 Opioid Analgesics

Patients taking CONTRAVE may not fully benefit from treatment with opioid-containing medicines, such as cough and cold remedies, antidiarrheal preparations, and opioid analgesics. In patients requiring intermittent opiate treatment, CONTRAVE therapy should be temporarily discontinued and opiate dose should not be increased above the standard dose. CONTRAVE may be used with caution after chronic opioid use has been stopped for 7 to 10 days in order to prevent precipitation of withdrawal *[see Contraindications (4) and Warnings and Precautions (5.4)].*

During CONTRAVE clinical studies, the use of concomitant opioid or opioid-like medications, including analgesics or antitussives, were excluded.

7.3 Potential for CONTRAVE to Affect Other Drugs Metabolized by CYP2D6

In a clinical study, CONTRAVE (32 mg naltrexone/360 mg bupropion) daily was coadministered with a 50 mg dose of metoprolol (a CYP2D6 substrate). CONTRAVE increased metoprolol AUC and C_{max} by approximately 4- and 2-fold, respectively, relative to metoprolol alone. Similar clinical drug interactions resulting in increased pharmacokinetic exposure of CYP2D6 substrates have also been observed with bupropion as a single agent with desipramine or venlafaxine.

Coadministration of CONTRAVE with drugs that are metabolized by CYP2D6 isozyme including certain antidepressants (SSRIs and many tricyclics), antipsychotics (e.g., haloperidol, risperidone and thioridazine), beta-blockers (e.g., metoprolol) and Type 1C antiarrhythmics (e.g., propafenone and flecainide), should be approached with caution and should be initiated at the lower end of the dose range of the concomitant medication. If CONTRAVE is added to the treatment regimen of a patient already receiving a drug metabolized by CYP2D6, the need to decrease the dose of the original medication should be considered, particularly for those concomitant medications with a narrow therapeutic index [see Clinical Pharmacology (12.3)].

7.4 Potential for Other Drugs to Affect CONTRAVE
Bupropion is primarily metabolized to hydroxybupropion by CYP2B6. Therefore, the potential exists for drug interactions between CONTRAVE and drugs that are inhibitors or inducers of CYP2B6.

Inhibitors of CYP2B6: Ticlopidine and Clopidogrel: Concomitant treatment with these drugs can increase bupropion exposure but decrease hydroxybupropion exposure. During concomitant use with CYP2B6 inhibitors (e.g., ticlopidine or clopidogrel), the CONTRAVE daily dose should not exceed two tablets (one tablet each morning and evening) [see Dosage and Administration (2.5) and Clinical Pharmacology (12.3)].

Inducers of CYP2B6: Ritonavir, Lopinavir, and Efavirenz: Concomitant treatment with these drugs can decrease bupropion and hydroxybupropion exposure and may reduce efficacy. Avoiding concomitant use with ritonavir, lopinavir, or efavirenz is recommended [see Clinical Pharmacology (12.3)].

7.5 Drugs That Lower Seizure Threshold
Use extreme caution when coadministering CONTRAVE with other drugs that lower seizure threshold (e.g., antipsychotics, antidepressants, theophylline, or systemic corticosteroids). Use low initial doses and increase the dose gradually. Concomitant use of other bupropion-containing products is contraindicated [see Contraindications (4) and Warnings and Precautions (5.3)].

7.6 Dopaminergic Drugs (Levodopa and Amantadine)
Bupropion, levodopa, and amantadine have dopamine agonist effects. CNS toxicity has been reported when bupropion was coadministered with levodopa or amantadine. Adverse reactions have included restlessness, agitation, tremor, ataxia, gait disturbance, vertigo, and dizziness. It is presumed that the toxicity results from cumulative dopamine agonist effects. Use caution and monitor for such adverse reactions when administering CONTRAVE concomitantly with these drugs.

7.7 Use with Alcohol
In postmarketing experience, there have been rare reports of adverse neuropsychiatric events or reduced alcohol tolerance in patients who were drinking alcohol during treatment with bupropion. The consumption of alcohol during treatment with CONTRAVE should be minimized or avoided.

7.8 Drug-Laboratory Test Interactions
False-positive urine immunoassay screening tests for amphetamines have been reported in patients taking bupropion. This is due to lack of specificity of some screening tests. False-positive test results may result even following discontinuation of bupropion therapy. Confirmatory tests, such as gas chromatography/mass spectrometry, will distinguish bupropion from amphetamines.

7.9 Drug-Transporter Interactions
In vitro, CONTRAVE constituents inhibited the renal organic cation transporter OCT2 to a clinically relevant level. The systemic concentrations of substrate drugs transported by OCT2 (such as amantadine, amiloride, cimetidine, dopamine, famotidine, memantine, metformin, pindolol, procainamide, ranitidine, varenicline, oxaliplatin) are likely to increase as a result of reduced renal clearance when coadministered with CONTRAVE. Coadministration of CONTRAVE with such drugs should be approached with caution and patients should be monitored for adverse effects.

8 USE IN SPECIFIC POPULATIONS

8.1 Pregnancy
Pregnancy Category X
Risk Summary
CONTRAVE is contraindicated during pregnancy, because weight loss offers no potential benefit to a pregnant woman and may result in fetal harm. If this drug is used during pregnancy, or if the patient becomes pregnant while taking this drug, the patient should be apprised of the potential hazard of maternal weight loss to the fetus.

Clinical Considerations
A minimum weight gain, and no weight loss, is currently recommended for all pregnant women, including those who are already overweight or obese, due to the obligatory weight gain that occurs in maternal tissues during pregnancy.

Human Data
There are no adequate and well-controlled studies of CONTRAVE in pregnant women. In clinical studies, 21 (0.7%) of 3,024 women became pregnant while taking CONTRAVE: 11 carried to term and gave birth to a healthy infant, three had elective abortions, four had spontaneous abortions, and the outcome of three pregnancies were unknown.

Data from the international bupropion Pregnancy Registry (675 first trimester exposures) and a retrospective cohort study using the United Healthcare database (1,213 first-trimester exposures) did not show an increased risk for malformations overall.

No increased risk for cardiovascular malformations overall has been observed after bupropion exposure during the first trimester. The prospectively observed rate of cardiovascular malformations in pregnancies with exposure to bupropion in the first trimester from the international Pregnancy Registry was 1.3% (9 cardiovascular malformations out of 675 first-trimester maternal bupropion exposures), which is similar to the background rate of cardiovascular malformations (approximately 1%). Data from the United Healthcare database and a case-control study (6,853 infants with cardiovascular malformations and 5,763 with non-cardiovascular malformations) from the National Birth Defects Prevention Study (NBDPS) did not show an increased risk for cardiovascular malformations overall after bupropion exposure during the first trimester.

Study findings on bupropion exposure during the first trimester and risk for left ventricular outflow tract obstruction (LVOTO) are inconsistent and do not allow conclusions regarding a possible association. The United Healthcare database lacked sufficient power to evaluate this association; the NBDPS found increased risk for LVOTO (n = 10; adjusted odds ratio [OR] = 2.6; 95% CI: 1.2, 5.7), and the Slone Epidemiology case control study did not find increased risk for LVOTO.

Study findings on bupropion exposure during the first trimester and risk for ventricular septal defect (VSD) are inconsistent and do not allow conclusions regarding a possible association. The Slone Epidemiology Study found an increased risk for VSD following first trimester maternal bupropion exposure (n = 17; adjusted OR = 2.5; 95% CI: 1.3, 5.0) but did not find increased risk for any other cardiovascular malformations studied (including LVOTO as above). The NBDPS and United Healthcare database study did not find an association between first trimester maternal bupropion exposure and VSD.

For the findings of LVOTO and VSD, the studies were limited by the small number of exposed cases, inconsistent findings among studies, and the potential for chance findings from multiple comparisons in case control studies.

Animal Data
Reproduction and developmental studies have not been conducted for the combined products naltrexone and bupropion in CONTRAVE. Safety margins were estimated using body surface area exposure (mg/m^2) based on a body weight of 100 kg.

Separate studies with bupropion and naltrexone have been conducted in pregnant rats and rabbits.

Naltrexone administered orally has also been shown to increase the incidence of early fetal loss in rats administered ≥30 mg/kg/day (180 mg/m^2/day) and rabbits administered ≥60 mg/kg/day (720 mg/m^2/day), doses at least 15 and 60 times, respectively, the maximum recommended human dose [MRHD] of the naltrexone component in CONTRAVE on a mg/m^2 basis. There was no evidence of teratogenicity when naltrexone was administered orally to rats and rabbits during the period of major organogenesis at doses up to 200 mg/kg/day (approximately 100 and 200 times the recommended therapeutic dose, respectively, on a mg/m^2 basis). Rats do not form appreciable quantities of the major human metabolite, 6-beta-naltrexol; therefore, the potential reproductive toxicity of the metabolite in rats is not known. Bupropion was administered orally in studies conducted in rats and rabbits at doses up to 450 and 150 mg/kg/day, respectively (approximately 20 and 15 times the MRHD, respectively, of the bupropion component in CONTRAVE on a mg/m^2 basis), during the period of organogenesis. No clear evidence of teratogenic activity was found in either species; however, in rabbits, slightly increased incidences of fetal malformations and skeletal variations were observed at the lowest dose tested (25 mg/kg/day, approximately 2 times the MRHD on a mg/m^2 basis) and greater. Decreased fetal weights were seen at 50 mg/kg and greater (approximately 5 times the MRHD of the bupropion component in CONTRAVE on a mg/m^2 basis). When rats were administered bupropion at oral doses of up to 300 mg/kg/day (ap-

proximately 15 times the MRHD of the bupropion component in CONTRAVE on a mg/m^2 basis) prior to mating and throughout pregnancy and lactation, there were no apparent adverse effects on offspring development.

8.3 Nursing Mothers
The constituents and metabolites of CONTRAVE have been shown to be secreted in human milk. Transfer of naltrexone and 6-beta-naltrexol into human milk has been reported with oral naltrexone. Bupropion and its metabolites are also secreted in human milk. CONTRAVE is not recommended for nursing mothers.

8.4 Pediatric Use
The safety and effectiveness of CONTRAVE in pediatric patients below the age of 18 have not been established, and the use of CONTRAVE is not recommended in pediatric patients.

8.5 Geriatric Use
Of the 3,239 subjects who participated in clinical trials with CONTRAVE, 62 (2%) were 65 years and older and none were 75 years and older. Clinical studies of CONTRAVE did not include sufficient numbers of subjects aged 65 and over to determine whether they respond differently from younger subjects. Older individuals may be more sensitive to the central nervous system adverse effects of CONTRAVE. Naltrexone and bupropion are known to be substantially excreted by the kidney, and the risk of adverse reactions to CONTRAVE may be greater in patients with impaired renal function. Because elderly patients are more likely to have decreased renal function, care should be taken in dose selection, and it may be useful to monitor renal function. CONTRAVE should be used with caution in patients over 65 years of age.

8.6 Renal Impairment
A dedicated pharmacokinetic study has not been conducted for CONTRAVE in subjects with renal impairment. Based on information available for the individual constituents, systemic exposure is significantly higher for bupropion and metabolites (two- to three-fold), and naltrexone and their metabolites in subjects with moderate-to-severe renal impairment. Therefore, the maximum recommended daily maintenance dose for CONTRAVE is two tablets (one tablet each morning and evening) in patients with moderate or severe renal impairment. CONTRAVE is not recommended for use in patients with end-stage renal disease. There is a lack of adequate information to guide CONTRAVE dosing in patients with mild renal impairment [see Dosage and Administration (2.2) and Clinical Pharmacology (12.3)].

8.7 Hepatic Impairment
CONTRAVE has not been evaluated in subjects with hepatic impairment. Based on information available for the individual constituents, systemic exposure is significantly higher for bupropion and metabolites (two- to three-fold), and naltrexone and their metabolites (up to 10-fold higher) in subjects with moderate-to-severe hepatic impairment. Therefore, the maximum recommended daily dose of CONTRAVE is one tablet in the morning in patients with hepatic impairment [see Dosage and Administration (2.3) and Clinical Pharmacology (12.3)].

9 DRUG ABUSE AND DEPENDENCE

9.2 Abuse
Humans
CONTRAVE (naltrexone HCl and bupropion HCl) has not been systematically studied in humans for its potential for abuse, tolerance, or physical dependence. However, in outpatient clinical studies of up to 56 weeks in duration, there was no evidence of euphoric drug intoxication, physical dependence, diversion, or abuse. There was no evidence of an abstinence syndrome following abrupt or tapered drug discontinuation after 56 weeks of double-blind, placebo-controlled, randomized treatment.

Naltrexone is a pure opioid antagonist. It does not lead to physical or psychological dependence. Tolerance to the opioid antagonistic effect is not known to occur.

Controlled clinical trials of bupropion (immediate-release formulation) conducted in normal volunteers, in subjects with a history of multiple drug abuse, and in depressed subjects showed some increase in motor activity and agitation/excitement. In a population of individuals experienced with drugs of abuse, a single dose of 400 mg of bupropion produced mild amphetamine-like activity as compared with placebo on the Morphine-Benzedrine Subscale of the Addiction Research Center Inventories (ARCI) and a score intermediate between placebo and amphetamine on the Liking Scale of the ARCI. These scales measure general feelings of euphoria and drug desirability.

Findings in clinical trials, however, are not known to reliably predict the abuse potential of drugs. Nonetheless, evidence from single-dose studies does suggest that the recommended daily dosage of bupropion when administered in divided doses is not likely to be significantly reinforcing to amphetamine or CNS stimulant abusers.

Animals
Studies in rodents and primates have shown that bupropion exhibits some pharmacologic actions common to psycho-

stimulants. In rodents, it has been shown to increase loco-motor activity, elicit a mild stereotyped behavioral response, and increased rates of responding in several schedule-controlled behavior paradigms. In primate models assessing the positive reinforcing effects of psychoactive drugs, bupropion was self-administered intravenously. In rats, bupropion produced amphetamine-like and cocaine-like dis-criminative stimulus effects in drug discrimination para-digms used to characterize the subjective effects of psycho-active drugs.

10 OVERDOSAGE

Human Experience
There is no clinical experience with overdosage with CONTRAVE. The maximum dose of CONTRAVE ad-ministered in clinical trials contained 50 mg naltrexone and 400 mg bupropion. The most serious clinical implications of CONTRAVE overdose are likely those related to overdose of bupropion.

Overdoses of up to 30 grams or more of bupropion (equiva-lent of up to 83 times the recommended daily dose of CONTRAVE 32 mg/360 mg) have been reported. Seizure was reported in approximately one-third of all cases. Other serious reactions reported with overdoses of bupropion alone included hallucinations, loss of consciousness, sinus tachycardia, and ECG changes such as conduction distur-bances (including QRS prolongation) or arrhythmias. Fever, muscle rigidity, rhabdomyolysis, hypotension, stupor, coma, and respiratory failure have been reported mainly when bupropion was part of multiple drug overdoses.

Although most patients recovered without sequelae, deaths associated with overdoses of bupropion alone have been re-ported in patients ingesting large doses of the drug. Multi-ple uncontrolled seizures, bradycardia, cardiac failure, and cardiac arrest prior to death were reported in these pa-tients.

There is limited experience with overdose of naltrexone monotherapy in humans. In one study, subjects who re-ceived 800 mg naltrexone daily (equivalent to 25 times the recommended daily dose of CONTRAVE 32 mg/360 mg) for up to one week showed no evidence of toxicity.

Animal Experience
In the mouse, rat, and guinea pig, the oral LD50s for naltrexone were 1,100 to 1,550 mg/kg; 1,450 mg/kg; and 1,490 mg/kg; respectively. High doses of naltrexone (gener-ally greater than or equal to 1,000 mg/kg) produced saliva-tion, depression/reduced activity, tremors, and convulsions. Mortality in animals due to high-dose naltrexone adminis-tration usually was due to clonic-tonic convulsions and/or respiratory failure.

Overdosage Management
If over-exposure occurs, call your poison control center at 1-800-222-1222. There are no known antidotes for CONTRAVE. In case of an overdose, provide supportive care, including close medical supervision and monitoring. Consider the possibility of multiple drug overdose. Ensure an adequate airway, oxygenation, and ventilation. Monitor cardiac rhythm and vital signs. Induction of emesis is not recommended.

11 DESCRIPTION
CONTRAVE extended-release tablets contain naltrexone hydrochloride and bupropion hydrochloride.

Naltrexone hydrochloride, USP, an opioid antagonist, is a synthetic congener of oxymorphone with no opioid agonist properties. Naltrexone differs in structure from oxymor-phone in that the methyl group on the nitrogen atom is re-placed by a cyclopropylmethyl group. Naltrexone hydrochloride is also related to the potent opioid antagonist, naloxone, or n-allylnoroxymorphone.

Naltrexone hydrochloride has the chemical name of morphinan-6-one, 17-(cyclopropylmethyl)-4,5-epoxy-3,14-dihydroxy-, hydrochloride, (5α)-. The empirical formula is $C_{20}H_{23}NO_4 \cdot HCl$ and the molecular weight is 377.86. The structural formula is:

Naltrexone hydrochloride is a white to yellowish, crystalline compound. It is soluble in water to the extent of about 100 mg/mL.

Bupropion hydrochloride is an antidepressant of the ami-noketone class. Bupropion hydrochloride closely resembles the structure of diethylpropion. It is designated as (±)-1-(3 chlorophenyl)-2-[(1,1-dimethylethyl)amino]-1-propranone hydrochloride. It is related to phenylethylamines. The empirical formula is $C_{13}H_{18}ClNO \cdot HCl$ and the molecular weight is 276.2. The structural formula is:

Bupropion hydrochloride powder is white, crystalline, and highly soluble in water.

CONTRAVE is available for oral administration as a round, bi-convex, film-coated, extended-release tablet. Each tablet has a trilayer core composed of two drug layers, containing the drug and excipients, separated by a more rapidly dis-solving inert layer. Each tablet contains 8 mg of naltrexone hydrochloride and 90 mg of bupropion hydrochloride. Tab-lets are blue and are debossed with NB-890 on one side. Each tablet contains the following inactive ingredients: mi-crocrystalline cellulose, hydroxypropyl cellulose, lactose an-hydrous, L-cysteine hydrochloride, crospovidone, magne-sium stearate, hypromellose, edetate disodium, lactose monohydrate, colloidal silicon dioxide, Opadry II Blue and FD&C Blue #2 aluminum lake.

12 CLINICAL PHARMACOLOGY

12.1 Mechanism of Action
CONTRAVE has two components: naltrexone, an opioid an-tagonist, and bupropion, a relatively weak inhibitor of the neuronal reuptake of dopamine and norepinephrine. Non-clinical studies suggest that naltrexone and bupropion have effects on two separate areas of the brain involved in the regulation of food intake: the hypothalamus (appetite regu-latory center) and the mesolimbic dopamine circuit (reward system). The exact neurochemical effects of CONTRAVE leading to weight loss are not fully understood.

12.2 Pharmacodynamics
Combined, bupropion and naltrexone increased the firing rate of hypothalamic pro-opiomelanocortin (POMC) neurons in vitro, which are associated with regulation of appetite. The combination of bupropion and naltrexone also reduced food intake when injected directly into the ventral tegmen-tal area of the mesolimbic circuit in mice, an area associated with regulation of reward pathways.

12.3 Pharmacokinetics

Absorption

Naltrexone
Following single oral administration of CONTRAVE (two 8 mg naltrexone/90 mg bupropion tablets) to healthy sub-jects, mean peak naltrexone concentration (C_{max}) was 1.4 ng/mL, time to peak concentration (T_{max}) was 2 hours, and extent of exposure (AUC_{0-inf}) was 8.4 ng•hr/mL.

Bupropion
Following single oral administration of CONTRAVE (two 8 mg naltrexone/90 mg bupropion tablets) to healthy subjects, mean peak bupropion concentration (C_{max}) was 168 ng/mL, time to peak concentration (T_{max}) was three hours, and extent of exposure (AUC_{0-inf}) was 1,607 ng•hr/mL.

Food Effect on Absorption
When CONTRAVE was administered with a high-fat meal, the AUC and C_{max} for naltrexone increased 2.1-fold and 3.7-fold, respectively, and the AUC and C_{max} for bupropion in-creased 1.4-fold and 1.8-fold, respectively. At steady state, the food effect increased AUC and C_{max} for naltrexone by 1.7-fold and 1.9-fold, respectively, and increased AUC and C_{max} for bupropion by 1.1-fold and 1.3-fold, respectively. Thus, CONTRAVE should not be taken with high-fat meals because of the resulting significant increases in bupropion and naltrexone systemic exposure.

Distribution

Naltrexone
Naltrexone is 21% plasma protein bound. The mean appar-ent volume of distribution at steady state for naltrexone (V_{ss}/F) is 5,697 liters.

Bupropion
Bupropion is 84% plasma protein bound. The mean appar-ent volume of distribution at steady state for bupropion (V_{ss}/F) is 880 liters.

Metabolism and Excretion

Naltrexone
The major metabolite of naltrexone is 6-beta-naltrexol. The activity of naltrexone is believed to be the result of both the parent and the 6-beta-naltrexol metabolite. Though less po-tent, 6-beta-naltrexol is eliminated more slowly and thus circulates at much higher concentrations than naltrexone. Naltrexone and 6-beta-naltrexol are not metabolized by cy-tochrome P450 enzymes and in vitro studies indicate that there is no potential for inhibition or induction of important isozymes.

Naltrexone and its metabolites are excreted primarily by the kidney (53% to 79% of the dose). Urinary excretion of unchanged naltrexone accounts for less than 2% of an oral dose. Urinary excretion of unchanged and conjugated 6-beta-naltrexol accounts for 43% of an oral dose. The renal clearance for naltrexone ranges from 30 to 127 mL/min, suggesting that renal elimination is primarily by glomeru-lar filtration. The renal clearance for 6-beta-naltrexol

ranges from 230 to 369 mL/min suggesting an additional re-nal tubular secretory mechanism. Fecal excretion is a minor elimination pathway.

Following single oral administration of CONTRAVE tablets to healthy subjects, mean elimination half-life ($T_{1/2}$) was ap-proximately 5 hours for naltrexone. Following twice daily administration of CONTRAVE, naltrexone did not accumu-late and its kinetics appeared linear. However, in compari-son to naltrexone, 6-beta-naltrexol accumulates to a larger extent (accumulation ratio ~3).

Bupropion
Bupropion is extensively metabolized with three active me-tabolites: hydroxybupropion, threohydrobupropion and erythrohydrobupropion. The metabolites have longer elimi-nation half-lives than bupropion and accumulate to a greater extent. Following bupropion administration, more than 90% of the exposure is a result of metabolites. In vitro findings suggest that CYP2B6 is the principal isozyme in-volved in the formation of hydroxybupropion whereas cyto-chrome P450 isozymes are not involved in the formation of the other active metabolites. Bupropion and its metabolites inhibit CYP2D6. Plasma protein binding of hydroxybupro-pion is similar to that of bupropion (84%) whereas the other two metabolites have approximately half the binding.

Following oral administration of 200 mg of ^{14}C-bupropion in humans, 87% and 10% of the radioactive dose were recov-ered in the urine and feces, respectively. The fraction of the oral dose of bupropion excreted unchanged was 0.5%, a find-ing consistent with the extensive metabolism of bupropion. Following single oral administration of CONTRAVE tablets to healthy subjects, mean elimination half-life ($T_{1/2}$) was ap-proximately 21 hours for bupropion. Following twice daily administration of CONTRAVE, metabolites of bupropion, and to a lesser extent unchanged bupropion, accumulate and reach steady-state concentrations in approximately one week.

Specific Populations

Gender
Pooled analysis of CONTRAVE data suggested no clinically meaningful differences in the pharmacokinetic parameters of bupropion or naltrexone based on gender.

Race
Pooled analysis of CONTRAVE data suggested no clinically meaningful differences in the pharmacokinetic parameters of bupropion or naltrexone based on race.

Elderly
The pharmacokinetics of CONTRAVE have not been evalu-ated in the geriatric population. The effects of age on the pharmacokinetics of naltrexone or bupropion and their me-tabolites have not been fully characterized. An exploration of steady-state bupropion concentrations from several de-pression efficacy studies involving patients dosed in a range of 300 to 750 mg/day, on a three times daily schedule, re-vealed no relationship between age (18 to 83 years) and plasma concentration of bupropion. A single-dose pharma-cokinetic study demonstrated that the disposition of bupropion and its metabolites in elderly subjects was simi-lar to that of younger subjects. These data suggest there is no prominent effect of age on bupropion concentration; how-ever, another pharmacokinetic study, single and multiple dose, has suggested that the elderly are at increased risk for accumulation of bupropion and its metabolites [see Use in Specific Populations (8.5)].

Smokers
Pooled analysis of CONTRAVE data revealed no meaningful differences in the plasma concentrations of bupropion or naltrexone in smokers compared with nonsmokers. The ef-fects of cigarette smoking on the pharmacokinetics of bupropion were studied in 34 healthy male and female vol-unteers; 17 were chronic cigarette smokers and 17 were nonsmokers. Following oral administration of a single 150 mg dose of bupropion, there was no statistically signif-icant difference in C_{max}, half-life, T_{max}, AUC, or clearance of bupropion or its active metabolites between smokers and nonsmokers.

Hepatic Impairment
Pharmacokinetic data are not available with CONTRAVE in patients with hepatic impairment. The following informa-tion is available for individual constituents.

Naltrexone
An increase in naltrexone AUC of approximately 5- and 10-fold in patients with compensated and decompensated liver cirrhosis, respectively, compared with subjects with normal liver function, has been reported. These data also suggest that alterations in naltrexone bioavailability are related to liver disease severity.

Bupropion
The effect of hepatic impairment on the pharmacokinetics of bupropion was characterized in two single-dose trials, one trial in patients with alcoholic liver disease and a second trial in patients with mild-to-severe cirrhosis.

The first trial showed that the half-life of hydroxybupropion was significantly longer in eight patients with alcoholic liver disease than in eight healthy volunteers (32±14 hours

Table 4. Pharmacokinetics of Bupropion and Metabolites in Patients With Severe Hepatic Cirrhosis: Ratio Relative to Healthy Matched Controls

	C_{max}	AUC	$t\frac{1}{2}$	T_{max}*
Bupropion	1.69	3.12	1.43	0.5 h
Hydroxybupropion	0.31	1.28	3.88	19 h
Threo/erythrohydrobupropion amino alcohol	0.69	2.48	1.96	20 h

*= Difference

vs 21±5 hours, respectively). Although not statistically significant, the AUCs for bupropion and hydroxybupropion were more variable and tended to be greater (by 53% to 57%) in patients with alcoholic liver disease. The differences in half-life for bupropion and the other metabolites in the two patient groups were minimal.

The second trial demonstrated no statistically significant differences in the pharmacokinetics of bupropion and its active metabolites in nine subjects with mild-to-moderate hepatic cirrhosis compared with eight healthy volunteers. However, more variability was observed in some of the pharmacokinetic parameters for bupropion (AUC, C_{max}, and T_{max}) and its active metabolites ($t\frac{1}{2}$) in subjects with mild-to-moderate hepatic cirrhosis. In subjects with severe hepatic cirrhosis, significant alterations in the pharmacokinetics of bupropion and its metabolites were seen *(Table 4)*. [See table 4 above]

The dose of CONTRAVE should be reduced in patients with hepatic impairment *[see Dosage and Administration (2.3) and Use in Specific Populations (8.7)]*.

Renal Impairment
A dedicated pharmacokinetic study has not been conducted for CONTRAVE in subjects with renal impairment. The following information is available for the individual constituents:

Naltrexone
Limited information is available for naltrexone in patients with moderate to severe renal impairment. In a study of seven patients with end-stage renal disease requiring dialysis, peak plasma concentrations of naltrexone were elevated at least 6-fold compared to healthy subjects.

Bupropion
Limited information is available for bupropion in patients with moderate to severe renal impairment. An inter-trial comparison between normal subjects and patients with end-stage renal failure demonstrated that the bupropion C_{max} and AUC values were comparable in the two groups, whereas the hydroxybupropion and threohydrobupropion metabolites had a 2.3- and 2.8-fold increase, respectively, in AUC for patients with end-stage renal failure. A second trial, comparing normal subjects and patients with moderate-to-severe renal impairment (GFR 30.9 ± 10.8 mL/min) showed that exposure after a single 150 mg dose of sustained-release bupropion was approximately 2-fold higher in patients with impaired renal function while levels of the hydroxybupropion and threo/erythrohydrobupropion (combined) metabolites were similar in the two groups. The elimination of bupropion and/or the major metabolites of bupropion may be reduced by impaired renal function.

The dose of CONTRAVE should be reduced in patients with moderate or severe renal impairment. CONTRAVE is not recommended for use in patients with end-stage renal disease *[see Dosage and Administration (2.2) and Use in Specific Populations(8.6)]*.

Drug Interactions
In Vitro Assessment of Drug Interactions
At therapeutically relevant concentrations, naltrexone and 6-beta-naltrexol are not major inhibitors of CYP isoforms CYP1A2, CYP2B6, CYP2C8, CYP2E1, CYP2C9, CYP2C19, CYP2D6 or CYP3A4. Both naltrexone and 6-beta-naltrexol are not major inducers of CYP isoforms CYP1A2, CYP2B6, or CYP3A4.

Bupropion and its metabolites (hydroxybupropion, erythrohydrobupropion, threohydrobupropion) are inhibitors of CYP2D6.

In vitro studies suggest that paroxetine, sertraline, norfluoxetine, fluvoxamine, and nelfinavir inhibit the hydroxylation of bupropion.

Bupropion (IC_{50} 9.3 mcM) and its metabolites, hydroxybupropion (IC_{50} 82 mcM) and threohydrobupropion and erythrohydrobupropion (1:1 mixture; IC_{50} 7.8 mcM), inhibited the renal organic transporter OCT2 to a clinically relevant level. The systemic concentrations of substrate drugs transported by OCT2 are likely to increase as a result of reduced renal clearance when coadministered with CONTRAVE.

Effects of Naltrexone/Bupropion on the Pharmacokinetics of Other Drugs
Drug interaction between CONTRAVE and CYP2D6 substrates (metoprolol) or other drugs (atorvastatin, glyburide, lisinopril, nifedipine, valsartan) has been evaluated. In addition, drug interaction between bupropion, a component of CONTRAVE, and CYP2D6 substrates (desipramine) or other drugs (citalopram, lamotrigine) has also been evaluated.

Table 5. Effect of Naltrexone/Bupropion Coadministration on Systemic Exposure of Other Drugs

Naltrexone/ Bupropion Dosage	Coadministered Drug		Change in Systemic Exposure
	Name and Dose Regimens		
Initiate the following drugs at the lower end of the dose range during concomitant use with CONTRAVE *[see Drug Interactions 7]:*			
Bupropion 150 mg twice daily for 10 days	Desipramine 50 mg single dose		↑5-fold AUC, ↑2-fold C_{max}
Bupropion 300 mg (as XL) once daily for 14 days	Citalopram 40 mg once daily for 14 days		↑40% AUC, ↑30% C_{max}
Naltrexone/ Bupropion 16 mg/180 mg twice daily for 7 days	Metoprolol 50 mg single dose		↑4-fold AUC, ↑2-fold C_{max}
No dose adjustment needed for the following drugs during concomitant use with CONTRAVE:			
Naltrexone/ Bupropion 16 mg/180 mg single dose	Atorvastatin 80 mg single dose		No Effect
Naltrexone/ Bupropion 16 mg/180 mg single dose	Glyburide 6 mg single dose		No Effect
Naltrexone/ Bupropion 16 mg/180 mg single dose	Lisinopril 40 mg single dose		No Effect
Naltrexone/ Bupropion 16 mg/180 mg single dose	Nifedipine 90 mg single dose		No Effect
Naltrexone/ Bupropion 16 mg/180 mg single dose	Valsartan 320 mg single dose		No Effect
Bupropion 150 mg twice daily for 12 days	Lamotrigine 100 mg single dose		No Effect

Effects of Other Drugs on the Pharmacokinetics of Naltrexone/Bupropion
Drug interactions between CYP2B6 inhibitors (ticlopidine, clopidogrel, prasugrel), CYP2B6 inducers (ritonavir, lopinavir) and bupropion (one of the CONTRAVE components), or between other drugs (atorvastatin, glyburide, metoprolol, lisinopril, nifedipine, valsartan) and CONTRAVE have been evaluated. While not systematically studied, carbamazepine, phenobarbital, or phenytoin may induce the metabolism of bupropion.
[See table 6 at top of next page]

13   NONCLINICAL TOXICOLOGY
13.1   Carcinogenesis, Mutagenesis, Impairment of Fertility
Studies to evaluate carcinogenesis, mutagenesis, or impairment of fertility with the combined products in CONTRAVE have not been conducted. The following findings are from studies performed individually with naltrexone and bupropion. The potential carcinogenic, mutagenic and fertility effects of the metabolite 6-beta-naltrexol are unknown. Safety margins were estimated using body surface area exposure (mg/m^2) based on a body weight of 100 kg.

In a two-year carcinogenicity study in rats with naltrexone, there were small increases in the numbers of testicular mesotheliomas in males and tumors of vascular origin in males and females. The incidence of mesothelioma in males given naltrexone at a dietary dose of 100 mg/kg/day (approximately 50 times the recommended therapeutic dose on a mg/m^2 basis for the naltrexone maintenance dose for CONTRAVE) was 6%, compared with a maximum historical incidence of 4%. The incidence of vascular tumors in males and females given dietary doses of 100 mg/kg/day was 4%, but only the incidence in females was increased compared with a maximum historical control incidence of 2%. There was no evidence of carcinogenicity in a two-year dietary study with naltrexone in male and female mice.

Lifetime carcinogenicity studies of bupropion were performed in rats and mice at doses up to 300 and 150 mg/kg/day, respectively. These doses are approximately 15 and 3 times the maximum recommended human dose (MRHD) of the bupropion component in CONTRAVE, respectively, on a mg/m^2 basis. In the rat study there was an increase in nodular proliferative lesions of the liver at doses of 100 to 300 mg/kg/day (approximately 5 to 15 times the MRHD of the bupropion component in CONTRAVE on a mg/m^2 basis); lower doses were not tested. The question of whether or not such lesions may be precursors of neoplasms of the liver is currently unresolved. Similar liver lesions were not seen in the mouse study, and no increase in malignant tumors of the liver and other organs was seen in either study.

There was limited evidence of a weak genotoxic effect of naltrexone in one gene mutation assay in a mammalian cell line, in the Drosophila recessive lethal assay, and in nonspecific DNA repair tests with *E. coli*. However, no evidence of genotoxic potential was observed in a range of other *in vitro* tests, including assays for gene mutation in bacteria, yeast, or in a second mammalian cell line, a chromosomal aberration assay, and an assay for DNA damage in human cells. Naltrexone did not exhibit clastogenicity in an *in vivo* mouse micronucleus assay.

Bupropion produced a positive response (two to three times control mutation rate) in two of five strains in the Ames bacterial mutagenicity test and an increase in chromosomal aberrations in one of three *in vivo* rat bone marrow cytogenetic studies.

Naltrexone administered orally to rats caused a significant increase in pseudopregnancy and a decrease in pregnancy rates in rats at 100 mg/kg/day (approximately 50 times the MRHD of the naltrexone component in CONTRAVE on a mg/m^2 basis). There was no effect on male fertility at this dose level. The relevance of these observations to human fertility is not known.

A fertility study of bupropion in rats at doses up to 300 mg/kg/day (approximately 15 times the MRHD of the bupropion component in CONTRAVE on a mg/m^2 basis) revealed no evidence of impaired fertility.

14   CLINICAL STUDIES
The effects of CONTRAVE on weight loss in conjunction with reduced caloric intake and increased physical activity was studied in double-blind, placebo-controlled trials (BMI range 27 to 45 kg/m^2) with study durations of 16 to 56 weeks randomized to naltrexone (16 to 50 mg/day) and/or bupropion (300 to 400 mg/day) or placebo.

Effect on Weight Loss and Weight Maintenance
Four 56-week multicenter, double-blind, placebo-controlled obesity trials (CONTRAVE Obesity Research, or COR-I, COR-II, COR-BMOD, and COR-Diabetes) were conducted to evaluate the effect of CONTRAVE in conjunction with lifestyle modification in 4,536 patients randomized to CONTRAVE or placebo. The COR-I, COR-II, and COR-BMOD trials enrolled patients with obesity (BMI 30 kg/m^2 or greater) or overweight (BMI 27 kg/m^2 or greater) and at least one comorbidity (hypertension or dyslipidemia). The COR-Diabetes trial enrolled patients with BMI greater than 27 kg/m^2 with type 2 diabetes with or without hypertension and/or dyslipidemia.

Treatment was initiated with a three-week dose-escalation period followed by approximately 1 year of continued ther-

Table 6. Effect of Coadministered Drugs on Systemic Exposure of Naltrexone/Bupropion

Name and Dose Regimens	CONTRAVE Components	Change in Systemic Exposure
Do not exceed one tablet twice daily dose of CONTRAVE with the following drugs:		
Ticlopidine 250 mg twice daily for 4 days	Bupropion Hydroxybupropion	↑85% AUC, ↑38% C_{max} ↓84% AUC, ↓78% C_{max}
Clopidogrel 75 mg once daily for 4 days	Bupropion Hydroxybupropion	↑60% AUC, ↑40% C_{max} ↓52% AUC, ↓50% C_{max}
No dose adjustment needed for CONTRAVE with the following drugs:		
Atorvastatin 80 mg single dose	Naltrexone 6-beta naltrexol Bupropion Hydroxybupropion Threohydrobupropion Erythrohydrobupropion	No Effect No Effect No Effect No Effect No Effect No Effect
Lisinopril 40 mg single dose	Naltrexone 6-beta naltrexol Bupropion Hydroxybupropion Threohydrobupropion Erythrohydrobupropion	No Effect No Effect No Effect No Effect No Effect No Effect
Valsartan 320 mg single dose	Naltrexone 6-beta naltrexol Bupropion Hydroxybupropion Threohydrobupropion Erythrohydrobupropion	No Effect No Effect No Effect ↓14% AUC, No Effect on C_{max} No Effect No Effect
Cimetidine 800 mg single dose	Bupropion Hydroxybupropion Threo/Erythrohydrobupropion	No Effect No Effect ↑16% AUC, ↑32% C_{max}
Citalopram 40 mg once daily for 14 days	Bupropion Hydroxybupropion Threohydrobupropion Erythrohydrobupropion	No Effect No Effect No Effect No Effect
Metoprolol 50 mg single dose	Naltrexone 6-beta naltrexol Bupropion Hydroxybupropion Threohydrobupropion Erythrohydrobupropion	↓25% AUC, ↓29% C_{max} No Effect No Effect No Effect No Effect No Effect
Nifedipine 90 mg single dose	Naltrexone 6-beta naltrexol Bupropion Hydroxybupropion Threohydrobupropion Erythrohydrobupropion	↑24% AUC, ↑58% C_{max} No Effect No Effect on AUC, ↑22% C_{max} No Effect No Effect No Effect
Prasugrel 10 mg once daily for 6 days	Bupropion Hydroxybupropion	↑18% AUC, ↑14% C_{max} ↓24%AUC, ↓32% C_{max}
Use CONTRAVE with caution with the following drugs:		
Glyburide 6 mg single dose*	Naltrexone 6-beta naltrexol Bupropion Hydroxybupropion Threohydrobupropion Erythrohydrobupropion	↑2-fold AUC, ↑2-fold C_{max} No Effect ↑36% AUC, ↑18% C_{max} ↑22% AUC, ↑21% C_{max} No Effect on AUC, ↑15% C_{max} No Effect
Avoid concomitant use of CONTRAVE with following drugs:		
Ritonavir 100 mg twice daily for 17 days	Bupropion Hydroxybupropion Threohydrobupropion Erythrohydrobupropion	↓22% AUC, ↓21 % C_{max} ↓23% AUC, No Effect on C_{max} ↓38% AUC, ↓39 % C_{max} ↓48% AUC, ↓28 % C_{max}
600 mg twice daily for 8 days	Bupropion Hydroxybupropion Threohydrobupropion Erythrohydrobupropion	↓66% AUC, ↓62 % C_{max} ↓78% AUC, ↓42 % C_{max} ↓50% AUC, ↓58 % C_{max} ↓68% AUC, ↓48 % C_{max}
Lopinavir/Ritonavir 400 mg/100 mg twice daily for 14 days	Bupropion Hydroxybupropion	↓57% AUC, ↓57% C_{max} ↓50% AUC, ↓31% C_{max}
Efavirenz 600 mg once daily for 2 weeks	Bupropion Hydroxybupropion	↓55% AUC, ↓34% C_{max} No Effect on AUC, ↑50% C_{max}

*Results were confounded by the food-effect due to oral glucose coadministered with the treatment.

apy. Patients were instructed to take CONTRAVE with food. COR–I and COR–II included a program consisting of a reduced-calorie diet resulting in an approximate 500 kcal/day decrease in caloric intake, behavioral counseling, and increased physical activity. COR-BMOD included an intensive behavioral modification program consisting of

28 group counseling sessions over 56 weeks as well as a prescribed diet and exercise regimen. COR-Diabetes evaluated patients with type 2 diabetes not achieving glycemic goal of a HbA1c less than 7% either with oral antidiabetic agents or with diet and exercise alone. Of the overall population from these four trials, 24% had hypertension, 54% had dyslipidemia at study entry, and 10% had type 2 diabetes.

Apart from COR-Diabetes, which only enrolled patients with type 2 diabetes, the demographic characteristics of patients were similar across all four trials. For the four trial populations combined, the mean age was 46 years, 83% were female, 77% were Caucasian, 18% were black, and 5% were other races. At baseline, mean BMI was 36 kg/m^2 and mean waist circumference was 110 cm.

A substantial percentage of randomized patients withdrew from the trials prior to Week 56: 45% for the placebo group and 46% for the CONTRAVE group. The majority of these patients discontinued within the first 12 weeks of treatment. Approximately 24% of patients treated with CONTRAVE and 12% of patients treated with placebo discontinued treatment because of an adverse reaction *[see Adverse Reactions (6.1)]*.

The co-primary endpoints were percent change from baseline body weight and the proportion of patients achieving at least a 5% reduction in body weight. In the 56-week COR-I trial, the mean change in body weight was −5.4% among patients assigned to CONTRAVE 32 mg/360 mg compared with −1.3% among patients assigned to placebo (Intent-To-Treat [ITT] population), as shown in Table 7 and Figure 1. In this trial, the achievement of at least a 5% reduction in body weight from baseline occurred more frequently for patients treated with CONTRAVE 32 mg/360 mg compared with placebo (42% vs 17%; *Table 7*). Results from COR-BMOD and COR-Diabetes are shown in Table 7 and Figures 2 and 3.

[See table 7 at top of next page]
[See figures 1 and 2 at top of next page]

Figure 3. Weight Loss Over Time in Completer Population: COR-Diabetes Trial

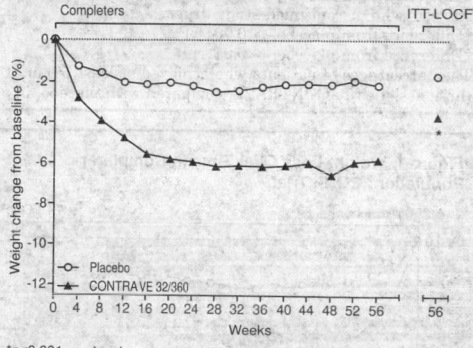

*p<0.001 vs placebo
COR-Diabetes trial: 41.2% in the placebo group and 47.8% in the CONTRAVE group discontinued study drug.

Effect on Cardiovascular and Metabolic Parameters
Changes in cardiovascular and metabolic parameters associated with obesity are presented for COR-I and COR-BMOD *(Table 8)*. Changes in mean blood pressure and heart rate are further described elsewhere *[see Warnings and Precautions (5.5)]*.
[See table 8 at top of page 2269]

Effect of CONTRAVE on Cardiometabolic Parameters and Anthropometry in Patients with Type 2 Diabetes Mellitus
Changes in glycemic control observed from baseline to Week 56 among patients with type 2 diabetes and obesity assigned to either CONTRAVE 32 mg/360 mg or placebo are shown in *Table 9*.
[See table 9 at top of page 2270]

Effect on Body Composition
In a subset of 124 patients (79 CONTRAVE, 45 placebo), body composition was measured using dual energy X-ray absorptiometry (DEXA). The DEXA assessment showed that mean total body fat mass decreased by 4.7 kg (11.7%) in the CONTRAVE group vs 1.4 kg (4.3%) in the placebo group at Week 52/LOCF (treatment difference, -3.3 kg [-7.4%], p<0.01).

16 HOW SUPPLIED/STORAGE AND HANDLING
CONTRAVE 8 mg/90 mg (naltrexone HCl 8 mg and bupropion HCl 90 mg) extended-release tri-layer tablets are blue, round, bi-convex, film-coated tablets debossed with "NB-890" on one side. CONTRAVE tablets are available as follows:

NDC 64764-890-99	Bottles of 120 tablets

Table 7. Changes in Weight in 56-Week Trials with CONTRAVE (ITT/LOCF*)

	COR-I		COR-BMOD		COR-Diabetes	
	CONTRAVE 32 mg/ 360 mg	Placebo	CONTRAVE 32 mg/ 360 mg	Placebo	CONTRAVE 32 mg/ 360 mg	Placebo
N	538	536	565	196	321	166
Weight (kg)						
Baseline mean (SD)	99.8 (16.1)	99.5 (14.4)	100.3 (15.5)	101.8 (15.0)	104.2 (19.1)	105.3 (16.9)
LS Mean % Change From Baseline (SE)	-5.4 (0.3)	-1.3 (0.3)	-8.1 (0.4)	-4.9 (0.6)	-3.7 (0.3)	-1.7 (0.4)
Difference from placebo (95% CI)	-4.1[†] (-4.9, -3.3)		-3.2[†] (-4.5, -1.8)		-2.0[†] (-3.0, -1.0)	
Percentage of patients losing greater than or equal to 5% body weight	42	17	57	43	36	18
Risk difference vs placebo (95% CI)	25[†] (19, 30)		14[†] (6, 22)		18[†] (9, 25)	
Percentage of patients losing greater than or equal to 10% body weight	21	7	35	21	15	5
Risk difference vs placebo (95% CI)	14[†] (10, 18)		14[†] (7, 21)		10[‡] (4, 15)	

Type 1 error was controlled across all 3 endpoints

*Based on last observation carried forward (LOCF) in all randomized subjects who had a baseline body weight measurement and at least one post baseline body weight measurement during the defined treatment phase. All available body weight data during the double-blind treatment phase are included in the analysis, including data collected from subjects who discontinued study drug.
[†]Difference from placebo, p<0.001
[‡]Difference from placebo, p<0.01
The percentages of patients who achieved at least 5% or at least 10% body weight loss from baseline were greater among those assigned to CONTRAVE, compared with placebo, in all four obesity trials (Table 7).

Figure 1. Weight Loss Over Time in Completer Population: COR-I Trial

*p<0.001 vs placebo
COR-I trial: 50.1% in the placebo group and 49.2% in the CONTRAVE group discontinued study drug.

Figure 2. Weight Loss Over Time in Completer Population: COR-BMOD Trial

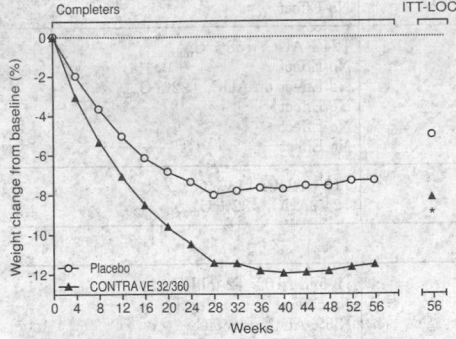

*p<0.001 vs placebo
COR-BMOD trial: 41.6% in the placebo group and 42.1% in the CONTRAVE group discontinued study drug.

Storage
Store at 25°C (77°F); excursions permitted to 15° to 30°C (59° to 86°F) [see USP Controlled Room Temperature].

17   PATIENT COUNSELING INFORMATION
See FDA-Approved Patient Labeling (Medication Guide)
Patient information is printed at the end of this insert. This information and the instructions provided in the Medication Guide should be discussed with patients.
Patients should be advised to take CONTRAVE exactly as prescribed. Patients should be instructed to follow the dose escalation schedule and not to take more than the recommended dose of CONTRAVE.
Patients should be made aware that CONTRAVE contains the same active ingredient (bupropion) found in certain antidepressants and smoking cessation products (including, but not limited to, WELLBUTRIN, WELLBUTRIN SR, WELLBUTRIN XL, and APLENZIN) and that CONTRAVE should not be used in combination with any other medications that contain bupropion.
Patients should be advised that some patients have experienced changes in mood (including depression and mania), psychosis, hallucinations, paranoia, delusions, homicidal ideation, aggression, anxiety, and panic, as well as suicidal ideation, suicide attempt, and completed suicide when attempting to quit smoking while taking bupropion. If patients develop agitation, hostility, depressed mood, or changes in thinking or behavior that are not typical for them, or if patients develop suicidal ideation or behavior, they should be urged to report these symptoms to their healthcare provider immediately.
Patients should be advised of the potential serious risks associated with the use of CONTRAVE, including suicidality, seizures, and increases in blood pressure or heart rate.
Patients should be advised to call their healthcare provider to report new or sudden changes in mood, behavior, thoughts, or feelings.
Patients should be advised that taking CONTRAVE can cause mild pupillary dilation, which in susceptible individuals, can lead to an episode of angle-closure glaucoma. Pre-existing glaucoma is almost always open-angle glaucoma because angle-closure glaucoma, when diagnosed, can be treated definitively with iridectomy. Open-angle glaucoma is not a risk factor for angle-closure glaucoma. Patients may wish to be examined to determine whether they are susceptible to angle closure, and have a prophylactic procedure (e.g., iridectomy), if they are susceptible.
Patients should be educated on the symptoms of hypersensitivity and to discontinue CONTRAVE if they have a severe allergic reaction to CONTRAVE.
Patients should be told that CONTRAVE should be discontinued and not restarted if they experience a seizure while on treatment.
Patients should be advised that the excessive use or abrupt discontinuation of alcohol, benzodiazepines, antiepileptic drugs, or sedatives/hypnotics can increase the risk of seizure. Patients should be advised to minimize or avoid use of alcohol.
Patients should be advised that if they previously used opioids, they may be more sensitive to lower doses of opioids and at risk of accidental overdose should they use opioids after CONTRAVE treatment is discontinued or temporarily interrupted.
Patients should be advised that because naltrexone, a component of CONTRAVE, can block the effects of opioids, they will not perceive any effect if they attempt to self-administer any opioid drug in small doses while on CONTRAVE. Further advise patients that the attempt to administer large doses of any opioid or to bypass the blockade while on CONTRAVE may lead to serious injury, coma, or death.
Patients should be off all opioids for a minimum of 7 to 10 days before starting CONTRAVE in order to avoid precipitation of withdrawal. Advise patients they should not take CONTRAVE if they have any symptoms of opioid withdrawal.
Patients should be advised to call their healthcare provider if they experience increased blood pressure or heart rate.
Patients should be advised to notify their healthcare provider if they are taking, or plan to take, any prescription or over-the-counter drugs. Concern is warranted because CONTRAVE and other drugs may affect each other's metabolism.
Patients should be advised to notify their healthcare provider if they become pregnant, intend to become pregnant, or are breastfeeding during therapy.
Patients with type 2 diabetes mellitus on antidiabetic therapy should be advised to monitor their blood glucose levels and report symptoms of hypoglycemia to their healthcare provider(s).
Patients should be advised to swallow CONTRAVE tablets whole so that the release rate is not altered. Do not chew, divide, or crush tablets.
Distributed by:
Takeda Pharmaceuticals America, Inc.
Deerfield, IL 60015
Manufactured for:
Orexigen Therapeutics, Inc.
La Jolla, CA 92037
CONTRAVE® is a trademark of Orexigen Therapeutics, Inc. registered with the U.S. Patent and Trademark Office and used under license by Takeda Pharmaceuticals America, Inc.
All other trademarks are the property of their respective owners.
©2014 Takeda Pharmaceuticals America, Inc.
CON067 R1
Medication Guide
CONTRAVE® (CON-trayv)
(naltrexone HCl and bupropion HCl)
Extended-Release Tablets
Read this Medication Guide before you start taking CONTRAVE and each time you get a refill. There may be new information. This information does not take the place of talking with your healthcare provider about your medical problems or treatment.
What is the most important information I should know about CONTRAVE?
CONTRAVE can cause serious side effects, including:
• **Suicidal thoughts or actions.** One of the ingredients in CONTRAVE is bupropion. Bupropion has caused some people to have suicidal thoughts or actions or unusual changes in behavior, whether or not they are taking medicines used to treat depression.
Bupropion may increase suicidal thoughts or actions in some children, teenagers, and young adults within the first few months of treatment.
If you already have depression or other mental illnesses, taking bupropion may cause it to get worse, especially within the first few months of treatment.
Stop taking CONTRAVE and call a healthcare provider right away if you, or your family member, have any of the following symptoms, especially if they are new, worse, or worry you:

- thoughts about suicide or dying
- attempts to commit suicide
- new or worse depression
- new or worse anxiety
- feeling very agitated or restless
- panic attacks
- trouble sleeping (insomnia)

- new or worse irritability
- acting aggressive, being angry, or violent
- acting on dangerous impulses
- an extreme increase in activity and talking (mania)
- other unusual changes in behavior or mood

While taking CONTRAVE, you or your family members should:

- Pay close attention to any changes, especially sudden changes, in mood, behaviors, thoughts, or feelings. This is very important when you start taking CONTRAVE or when your dose changes.
- Keep all follow-up visits with your healthcare provider as scheduled. Call your healthcare provider between visits as needed, especially if you have concerns about symptoms.

CONTRAVE has not been studied in and is not approved for use in children under the age of 18.

What is CONTRAVE?

CONTRAVE is a prescription medicine which contains 2 medicines (naltrexone and bupropion) that may help some obese or overweight adults, who also have weight related medical problems, lose weight and keep the weight off.

- CONTRAVE should be used with a reduced calorie diet and increased physical activity.
- It is not known if CONTRAVE changes your risk of heart problems or stroke or of death due to heart problems or stroke.
- It is not known if CONTRAVE is safe and effective when taken with other prescription, over-the-counter, or herbal weight loss products.
- It is not known if CONTRAVE is safe and effective in children under 18 years of age.
- CONTRAVE is not approved to treat depression or other mental illnesses, or to help people quit smoking (smoking cessation). One of the ingredients in CONTRAVE, bupropion, is the same ingredient in some other medicines used to treat depression and to help people quit smoking.

Who should not take CONTRAVE?

Do not take CONTRAVE if you:

- have uncontrolled hypertension
- have or have had seizures
- use other medicines that contain bupropion such as WELLBUTRIN, WELLBUTRIN SR, WELLBUTRIN XL and APLENZIN
- have or have had an eating disorder called anorexia (eating very little) or bulimia (eating too much and vomiting to avoid gaining weight)
- are dependent on opioid pain medicines or use medicines to help stop taking opioids such as methadone or buprenorphine, or are in opiate withdrawal
- drink a lot of alcohol and abruptly stop drinking, or use medicines called sedatives (these make you sleepy), benzodiazepines, or anti-seizure medicines and you stop using them all of a sudden
- are taking medicines called monoamine oxidase inhibitors (MAOIs). Ask your healthcare provider or pharmacist if you are not sure if you take an MAOI, including linezolid. **Do not** start CONTRAVE until you have stopped taking your MAOI for at least 14 days.
- are allergic to naltrexone or bupropion or any of the ingredients in CONTRAVE. See the end of this Medication Guide for a complete list of ingredients in CONTRAVE.
- are pregnant or planning to become pregnant. Tell your healthcare provider right away if you become pregnant while taking CONTRAVE.

What should I tell my healthcare provider before taking CONTRAVE?

Before you take CONTRAVE, tell your healthcare provider if you:

- have or have had depression or other mental illnesses (such as bipolar disorder)
- have attempted suicide in the past
- have or have had seizures
- have had a head injury
- have had a tumor or infection of your brain or spine (central nervous system)
- have had a problem with low blood sugar (hypoglycemia) or low levels of sodium in your blood (hyponatremia)
- have or have had liver problems
- have high blood pressure
- have or have had a heart attack, heart problems, or have had a stroke
- have kidney problems

- are diabetic taking insulin or other medicines to control your blood sugar
- have or have had an eating disorder
- drink a lot of alcohol
- abuse prescription medicines or street drugs
- are over the age of 65
- have any other medical conditions
- are breastfeeding or plan to breastfeed. CONTRAVE can pass into your breast milk and may harm your baby. You and your healthcare provider should decide if you should take CONTRAVE or breastfeed. You should not do both.
- **Tell your healthcare provider about all the medicines you take** including prescription and over-the-counter medicines, vitamins, and herbal supplements.

CONTRAVE may affect the way other medicines work and other medicines may affect the way CONTRAVE works causing side effects.

Ask your healthcare provider for a list of these medicines if you are not sure.

Know the medicines you take. Keep a list of them to show your healthcare provider or pharmacist when you get a new medicine.

Table 8. Change in Markers of Cardiovascular and Metabolic Parameters from Baseline in 56 Week Trials with CONTRAVE 32 mg/360 mg (COR-I and COR-BMOD)*

Parameter	COR-I			COR-BMOD		
	CONTRAVE 32 mg/360 mg N=471	Placebo N=511	CONTRAVE minus Placebo (LS Mean)	CONTRAVE 32 mg/360 mg N=482	Placebo N=193	CONTRAVE minus Placebo (LS Mean)
Triglycerides, mg/dL						
Baseline median (Q1, Q3)	113 (86, 158)	112 (78, 157)	-10.7†	110 (78, 162)	103 (76, 144)	-9.9†
Median % change	-11.6	1.7		-17.8	-7.4	
HDL-C, mg/dL						
Baseline mean (SD)	51.9 (13.6)	52.0 (13.6)	7.2	53.6 (13.5)	55.3 (12.9)	6.6
LS Mean % change (SE)	8.0 (0.9)	0.8 (0.9)		9.4 (1.0)	2.8 (1.6)	
LDL-C, mg/dL						
Baseline mean (SD)	118.8 (32.6)	119.7 (34.8)	-1.5	109.5 (27.5)	109.2 (27.3)	-2.9
LS Mean % change (SE)	-2.0 (1.0)	-0.5 (1.1)		7.1 (1.4)	10.0 (2.2)	
Waist circumference, cm						
Baseline mean (SD)	108.8 (11.3)	110.0 (12.2)	-3.8‡	109.3 (11.4)	109.0 (11.8)	-3.2‡
LS Mean change (SE)	-6.2 (0.4)	-2.5 (0.4)		-10.0 (0.5)	-6.8 (0.8)	
Heart rate, bpm						
Baseline mean (SD)	72.1 (8.7)	71.8 (8.0)	1.2	70.7 (8.3)	70.4 (9.0)	0.9
LS Mean change (SE)	1.0 (0.3)	-0.2 (0.3)		1.1 (0.4)	0.2 (0.5)	
Systolic blood pressure, mmHg						
Baseline mean (SD)	118.9 (9.8)	119.0 (9.8)	1.8	116.9 (9.9)	116.7 (10.9)	2.6
LS Mean change (SE)	-0.1 (0.4)	-1.9 (0.4)		-1.3 (0.5)	-3.9 (0.7)	
Diastolic blood pressure, mmHg						
Baseline mean (SD)	77.1 (7.2)	77.3 (6.6)	0.9	78.2 (7.2)	77.2 (7.4)	1.4
LS Mean change (SE)	0.0 (0.3)	-0.9 (0.3)		-1.4 (0.3)	-2.8 (0.5)	

Q1: first quartile; Q3: third quartile

*Based on last observation carried forward (LOCF) while on study drug
†Hodges-Lehmann estimate of treatment difference
‡Statistically significant vs placebo (p<0.001) based on the pre-specified closed testing procedure method for controlling Type I error

How should I take CONTRAVE?

How to take CONTRAVE

	Morning Dose	Evening Dose
Starting: Week 1	1 tablet	None
Week 2	1 tablet	1 tablet
Week 3	2 tablets	1 tablet
Week 4 Onward	2 tablets	2 tablets

- Take CONTRAVE exactly as your healthcare provider tells you to.
- **Do not** change your CONTRAVE dose without talking with your healthcare provider.
- Your healthcare provider will change your dose if needed.

Table 9. Changes in Cardiometabolic Parameters and Waist Circumference in Patients with Type 2 Diabetes Mellitus in a 56 Week Trial with CONTRAVE 32 mg/360 mg (COR-Diabetes)

	CONTRAVE 32 mg/360 mg N=265		Placebo N=159		CONTRAVE minus Placebo (LS Mean)
	Baseline	Change from Baseline (LS Mean)	Baseline	Change from Baseline (LS Mean)	
HbA1c (%)	8.0	-0.6	8.0	-0.1	-0.5*
Fasting Glucose (mg/dL)	160.0	-11.9	163.9	-4.0	-7.9
Waist Circumference (cm)	115.6	-5.0	114.3	-2.9	-2.1
Systolic blood pressure (mmHg)	125.0	0.0	124.5	-1.1	1.2
Diastolic blood pressure (mmHg)	77.5	-1.1	77.4	-1.5	0.4
Heart rate (bpm)	72.9	0.7	73.1	-0.2	0.9
	Baseline	% Change from Baseline (LS Mean)	Baseline	% Change from Baseline (LS Mean)	CONTRAVE minus Placebo (LS Mean)
Triglycerides (mg/dL)†	147 (98, 200)	-7.7	168 (114, 236)	-8.6	-3.3
HDL Cholesterol (mg/dL)	46.2	7.4	46.1	-0.2	7.6
LDL Cholesterol (mg/dL)	100.2	2.4	101.0	4.2	-1.9

Based on last observation carried forward (LOCF) while on study drug

*Statistically significant vs placebo (p<0.001) based on the pre-specified closed testing procedure method for controlling Type I error
†Values are baseline median (first and third quartiles), median % change, and the Hodges-Lehmann estimate of the median treatment difference

- Your healthcare provider should tell you to stop taking CONTRAVE if you have not lost a certain amount of weight after 16 weeks of treatment.
- **Swallow CONTRAVE tablets whole. Do not cut, chew, or crush CONTRAVE tablets.** Tell your healthcare provider if you cannot swallow CONTRAVE tablets whole.
- **Do not** take more than 2 tablets in the morning and 2 tablets in the evening.
- **Do not** take more than 2 tablets at the same time or more than 4 tablets in 1 day.
- **Do not** take CONTRAVE with high-fat meals. It may increase your risk of seizures.
- If you miss a dose of CONTRAVE, wait until your next regular time to take it. **Do not** take more than 1 dose of CONTRAVE at a time.
- If you take too much CONTRAVE, call your healthcare provider or go to the nearest emergency room right away.

What should I avoid while taking CONTRAVE?
- **Do not** drink a lot of alcohol while taking CONTRAVE. If you drink a lot of alcohol, talk with your healthcare provider before suddenly stopping. If you suddenly stop drinking alcohol, you may increase your chance of having a seizure.

What are the possible side effects of CONTRAVE?
CONTRAVE may cause serious side effects, including:
- See "What is the most important information I should know about CONTRAVE?"
- **Seizures.** There is a risk of having a seizure when you take CONTRAVE. The risk of seizure is higher in people who:
  - take higher doses of CONTRAVE
  - have certain medical conditions
  - take CONTRAVE with certain other medicines
Do not take any other medicines while you are taking CONTRAVE unless your healthcare provider has said it is okay to take them.
If you have a seizure while taking CONTRAVE, stop taking CONTRAVE and call your healthcare provider right away. You should not take CONTRAVE again if you have a seizure.
- **Risk of opioid overdose.** One of the ingredients in CONTRAVE (naltrexone) can increase your chance of having an opioid overdose if you take opioid medicines while taking CONTRAVE.
You can accidentally overdose in 2 ways:
- Naltrexone blocks the effects of opioids, such as heroin, methadone or opioid pain medicines. **Do not** take large amounts of opioids, including opioid-containing medicines, such as heroin or prescription pain pills, to try to overcome the opioid-blocking effects of naltrexone. This can lead to serious injury, coma, or death.
- After you take naltrexone, its blocking effect slowly decreases and completely goes away over time. If you have used opioid street drugs or opioid-containing medicines in the past, using opioids in amounts that you used before

treatment with naltrexone can lead to overdose and death. You may also be more sensitive to the effects of lower amounts of opioids:
- after you have gone through detoxification
- when your next dose of CONTRAVE is due
- if you miss a dose of CONTRAVE
- after you stop CONTRAVE treatment
It is important that you tell your family and the people closest to you of this increased sensitivity to opioids and the risk of overdose.
You or someone close to you should get emergency medical help right away if you:
- have trouble breathing
- become very drowsy with slowed breathing
- have slow, shallow breathing (little chest movement with breathing)
- feel faint, very dizzy, confused, or have unusual symptoms
- **Sudden opioid withdrawal.** People who take CONTRAVE must not use any type of opioid (must be opioid-free) including street drugs, prescription pain medicines (including tramadol), cough, cold, or diarrhea medicines that contain opioids, or opioid dependence treatments, buprenorphine or methadone, **for at least 7 to 10 days before starting CONTRAVE.** Using opioids in the 7 to 10 days before you start taking CONTRAVE may cause you to suddenly have symptoms of opioid withdrawal when you take it. Sudden opioid withdrawal can be severe, and you may need to go to the hospital. Tell your healthcare provider you are taking CONTRAVE before a medical procedure or surgery.
- **Severe allergic reactions.** Some people have had a severe allergic reaction to bupropion, one of the ingredients in CONTRAVE. **Stop taking CONTRAVE and call your healthcare provider or go to the nearest hospital emergency room right away** if you have any of the following signs and symptoms of an allergic reaction:

- rash
- itching
- hives
- fever
- swollen lymph glands
- painful sores in your mouth or around your eyes
- swelling of your lips or tongue
- chest pain
- trouble breathing

- **Increases in blood pressure or heart rate.** Some people may get high blood pressure or have a higher heart rate when taking CONTRAVE. Your healthcare provider should check your blood pressure and heart rate before you start taking, and while you take CONTRAVE.
- **Liver damage or hepatitis.** One of the ingredients in CONTRAVE, naltrexone can cause liver damage or hepatitis. Stop taking CONTRAVE and tell your healthcare provider if you have any of the following symptoms of liver problems:

- stomach area pain lasting more than a few days
- dark urine
- yellowing of the whites of your eyes
- tiredness
Your healthcare provider may need to stop treating you with CONTRAVE if you get signs or symptoms of a serious liver problem.
- **Manic episodes.** One of the ingredients in CONTRAVE, bupropion can cause some people who were manic or depressed in the past to become manic or depressed again.
- **Visual problems (angle-closure glaucoma).** One of the ingredients in CONTRAVE, bupropion, can cause some people to have visual problems (angle-closure glaucoma). Signs and symptoms of angle-closure glaucoma may include:
  - eye pain
  - changes in vision
  - swelling or redness in or around the eye
Talk with your healthcare provider to find out if you are at risk for angle-closure glaucoma and to get treatment to prevent it if you are at risk.
- **Increased risk of low blood sugar (hypoglycemia) in people with type 2 diabetes mellitus who also take medicines to treat their diabetes.** Weight loss can cause low blood sugar in people with type 2 diabetes mellitus who also take medicines used to treat type 2 diabetes mellitus (such as insulin or sulfonylureas). You should check your blood sugar before you start taking CONTRAVE and while you take CONTRAVE.
The most common side effects of CONTRAVE include:

- nausea
- constipation
- headache
- vomiting
- dizziness
- trouble sleeping
- dry mouth
- diarrhea

Tell your healthcare provider about any side effect that bothers you or does not go away. These are not all the possible side effects of CONTRAVE. For more information, ask your healthcare provider or pharmacist.
Call your doctor for medical advice about side effects. You may report side effects to FDA at 1–800-FDA-1088.
How should I store CONTRAVE?
Store CONTRAVE at room temperature between 59°F to 86°F (15°C to 30°C).
Keep CONTRAVE and all medicines out of the reach of children.
General information about the safe and effective use of CONTRAVE.
Medicines are sometimes prescribed for purposes other than those listed in a Medication Guide. Do not use CONTRAVE for a condition for which it was not prescribed. Do not give CONTRAVE to other people, even if they have the same symptoms or condition that you have. It may harm them.
If you take a urine drug screening test, CONTRAVE may make the test result positive for amphetamines. If you tell the person giving you the drug screening test that you are taking CONTRAVE, they can do a more specific drug screening test that should not have this problem.
This Medication Guide summarizes the most important information about CONTRAVE. If you would like more information, talk with your healthcare provider. You can ask your pharmacist or healthcare provider for information about CONTRAVE that is written for health professionals. For more information, go to www.contrave.com or call 1-877-825-3327.
What are the ingredients in CONTRAVE?
Active ingredients: naltrexone hydrochloride and bupropion hydrochloride
Inactive ingredients: microcrystalline cellulose, hydroxypropyl cellulose, lactose anhydrous, L-cysteine hydrochloride, crospovidone, magnesium stearate, hypromellose, edetate disodium, lactose monohydrate, colloidal silicon dioxide, Opadry II Blue and FD&C Blue #2 aluminum lake
This Medication Guide has been approved by the U.S. Food and Drug Administration.
Distributed by:
Takeda Pharmaceuticals America, Inc.
Deerfield, IL 60015
Manufactured for:
Orexigen Therapeutics, Inc.
La Jolla, CA 92037
CONTRAVE® is a trademark of Orexigen Therapeutics, Inc. registered with the U.S. Patent and Trademark Office and used under license by Takeda Pharmaceuticals America, Inc.
All other trademarks are the property of their respective owners.
©2014 Takeda Pharmaceuticals America, Inc.
Approved: 2014
Shown in Product Identification Guide, page 313

DEXILANT ℞
[decks-ī-launt]
(dexlansoprazole)
delayed-release capsules for oral use

HIGHLIGHTS OF PRESCRIBING INFORMATION
These highlights do not include all the information needed to use DEXILANT safely and effectively. See full prescribing information for DEXILANT.

DEXILANT (dexlansoprazole) delayed-release capsules for oral use.

Initial U.S. Approval: 1995 (lansoprazole)

————RECENT MAJOR CHANGES————
Dosage and Administration:
• Important Administration Information (2.3)   8/2013
Warnings and Precautions
• *Clostridium difficile* associated diarrhea (5.2)   9/2012

————INDICATIONS AND USAGE————
DEXILANT is a proton pump inhibitor (PPI) indicated for:
• Healing of all grades of erosive esophagitis (EE). (1.1)
• Maintaining healing of EE and relief of heartburn. (1.2)
• Treating heartburn associated with symptomatic non-erosive gastroesophageal reflux disease (GERD). (1.3)

————DOSAGE AND ADMINISTRATION————
• Healing of EE: 60 mg once daily for up to 8 weeks. (2.1)
• Maintenance of healed EE: 30 mg once daily for up to 6 months. (2.1)
• Symptomatic non-erosive GERD: 30 mg once daily for 4 weeks. (2.1)
• Hepatic impairment: Consider 30 mg maximum daily dose for patients with moderate hepatic impairment (Child-Pugh Class B). No studies were conducted in patients with severe hepatic impairment (Child-Pugh Class C). (2.2, 8.7)
• DEXILANT can be taken without regard to food. (2.3)
• DEXILANT should be swallowed whole. See full prescribing information for administration options. (2.3)

————DOSAGE FORMS AND STRENGTHS————
• Delayed-Release Capsules: 30 mg and 60 mg. (3)

————CONTRAINDICATIONS————
• Patients with known hypersensitivity to any component of the formulation. (4)

————WARNINGS AND PRECAUTIONS————
• Gastric Malignancy: Symptomatic response with DEXILANT does not preclude the presence of gastric malignancy. (5.1)
• *Clostridium difficile* associated diarrhea: PPI therapy may be associated with increased risk of *Clostridium difficile* associated diarrhea. (5.2)
• Bone Fracture: Long-term and multiple daily dose PPI therapy may be associated with an increased risk for osteoporosis-related fractures of the hip, wrist or spine. (5.3)
• Hypomagnesemia: Hypomagnesemia has been reported rarely with prolonged treatment with PPIs. (5.4)

————ADVERSE REACTIONS————
Most commonly reported adverse reactions (≥2%): diarrhea, abdominal pain, nausea, upper respiratory tract infection, vomiting, and flatulence. (6.1)

To report SUSPECTED ADVERSE REACTIONS, contact Takeda Pharmaceuticals America, Inc. at 1-877-TAKEDA-7 (1-877-825-3327) or FDA at 1-800-FDA-1088 or www.fda.gov/medwatch.

————DRUG INTERACTIONS————
• Atazanavir: Do not co-administer with DEXILANT because atazanavir systemic concentrations may be substantially decreased. (7.1)
• Drugs with pH-dependent absorption (e.g., Ampicillin esters, Digoxin, iron salts, ketoconazole, erlotinib): DEXILANT may interfere with absorption of drugs for which gastric pH is important for bioavailability. (7.1)
• Warfarin: Patients taking concomitant warfarin may require monitoring for increases in international normalized ratio (INR) and prothrombin time. (7.2)
• Tacrolimus: Concomitant tacrolimus use may increase tacrolimus whole blood concentrations. (7.3)
• Methotrexate: DEXILANT may increase serum levels of methotrexate. (7.5)

See 17 for PATIENT COUNSELING INFORMATION and Medication Guide

Revised: 08/2013

FULL PRESCRIBING INFORMATION: CONTENTS*

FULL PRESCRIBING INFORMATION

1   INDICATIONS AND USAGE
1.1   Healing of Erosive Esophagitis
DEXILANT is indicated for healing of all grades of erosive esophagitis (EE) for up to eight weeks.

1.2   Maintenance of Healed Erosive Esophagitis
DEXILANT is indicated to maintain healing of EE and relief of heartburn for up to six months.

1.3   Symptomatic Non-Erosive Gastroesophageal Reflux Disease
DEXILANT is indicated for the treatment of heartburn associated with symptomatic non-erosive gastroesophageal reflux disease (GERD) for four weeks.

2   DOSAGE AND ADMINISTRATION
2.1   Recommended Dose
DEXILANT is available as capsules in 30 mg and 60 mg strengths for adult use. Directions for use in each indication are summarized in Table 1.

Table 1. DEXILANT Dosing Recommendations

Indication	Recommended Dose	Frequency
Healing of EE	60 mg	Once daily for up to 8 weeks
Maintenance of Healed EE and relief of heartburn	30 mg	Once daily*
Symptomatic Non-Erosive GERD	30 mg	Once daily for 4 weeks

*Controlled studies did not extend beyond 6 months.

2.2   Hepatic Impairment
No adjustment for DEXILANT is necessary for patients with mild hepatic impairment (Child-Pugh Class A). Consider a maximum daily dose of 30 mg for patients with moderate hepatic impairment (Child-Pugh Class B). No studies have been conducted in patients with severe hepatic impairment (Child-Pugh Class C) [see Use in Specific Populations (8.7) and Clinical Pharmacology (12.3)].

2.3   Important Administration Information
• DEXILANT can be taken without regard to food.
• DEXILANT should be swallowed whole.
• DEXILANT should not be chewed.

For patients who have difficulty swallowing capsules, follow the instructions below for administration:
Administration with Applesauce
1. Place one tablespoon of applesauce into a clean container.
2. Open capsule.
3. Sprinkle intact granules on applesauce.
4. Swallow applesauce and granules immediately. Do not chew granules. Do not save the applesauce and granules for later use.

Administration with Water in an Oral Syringe
1. Open the capsule and empty the granules into a clean container with 20 mL of water.
2. Withdraw the entire mixture into a syringe.
3. Gently swirl the syringe in order to keep granules from settling.
4. Administer the mixture immediately into the mouth. Do not save the water and granule mixture for later use.
5. Refill the syringe with 10 mL of water, swirl gently, and administer.
6. Refill the syringe again with 10 mL of water, swirl gently, and administer.

Administration with Water via a Nasogastric Tube (≥16 French)
1. Open the capsule and empty the granules into a clean container with 20 mL of water.
2. Withdraw the entire mixture into a catheter-tip syringe.
3. Swirl the syringe gently in order to keep the granules from settling, and immediately inject the mixture through the nasogastric tube into the stomach. Do not save the water and granule mixture for later use.
4. Refill the syringe with 10 mL of water, swirl gently, and flush the tube.
5. Refill the syringe again with 10 mL of water, swirl gently, and administer.

3   DOSAGE FORMS AND STRENGTHS
• 30 mg delayed-release capsules are opaque, blue and gray with TAP and "30" imprinted on the capsule.
• 60 mg delayed-release capsules are opaque, blue with TAP and "60" imprinted on the capsule.

4   CONTRAINDICATIONS
DEXILANT is contraindicated in patients with known hypersensitivity to any component of the formulation [see Description (11)]. Hypersensitivity and anaphylaxis have been reported with DEXILANT use [see Adverse Reactions (6.1)].

5   WARNINGS AND PRECAUTIONS
5.1   Gastric Malignancy
Symptomatic response with DEXILANT does not preclude the presence of gastric malignancy.

5.2   *Clostridium Difficile* Associated Diarrhea
Published observational studies suggest that PPI therapy like DEXILANT may be associated with an increased risk of *Clostridium difficile* associated diarrhea, especially in hospitalized patients. This diagnosis should be considered for diarrhea that does not improve [see Adverse Reactions (6.2)]. Patients should use the lowest dose and shortest duration of PPI therapy appropriate to the condition being treated.

5.3   Bone Fracture
Several published observational studies suggest that PPI therapy may be associated with an increased risk for osteoporosis-related fractures of the hip, wrist or spine. The risk of fracture was increased in patients who received high-dose, defined as multiple daily doses, and long-term PPI therapy (a year or longer). Patients should use the lowest dose and shortest duration of PPI therapy appropriate to the conditions being treated. Patients at risk for osteoporosis-related fractures should be managed according to established treatment guidelines [see Dosage and Administration (2) and Adverse Reactions (6)].

5.4   Hypomagnesemia
Hypomagnesemia, symptomatic and asymptomatic, has been reported rarely in patients treated with PPIs for at least three months, in most cases after a year of therapy. Serious adverse events include tetany, arrhythmias, and seizures. In most patients, treatment of hypomagnesemia required magnesium replacement and discontinuation of the PPI.
For patients expected to be on prolonged treatment or who take PPIs with medications such as digoxin or drugs that may cause hypomagnesemia (e.g., diuretics), health care professionals may consider monitoring magnesium levels prior to initiation of PPI treatment and periodically [see Adverse Reactions (6.2)].

5.5   Concomitant Use of DEXILANT with Methotrexate
Literature suggests that concomitant use of PPIs with methotrexate (primarily at high dose; see methotrexate pre-

Table 2. Incidence of Adverse Reactions in Controlled Studies

Adverse Reaction	Placebo (N=896) %	DEXILANT 30 mg (N=455) %	DEXILANT 60 mg (N=2218) %	DEXILANT Total (N=2621) %	Lansoprazole 30 mg (N=1363) %
Diarrhea	2.9	5.1	4.7	4.8	3.2
Abdominal Pain	3.5	3.5	4.0	4.0	2.6
Nausea	2.6	3.3	2.8	2.9	1.8
Upper Respiratory Tract Infection	0.8	2.9	1.7	1.9	0.8
Vomiting	0.8	2.2	1.4	1.6	1.1
Flatulence	0.6	2.6	1.4	1.6	1.2

scribing information) may elevate and prolong serum levels of methotrexate and/or its metabolite, possibly leading to methotrexate toxicities. In high-dose methotrexate administration, a temporary withdrawal of the PPI may be considered in some patients [see Drug Interactions (7.5)].

6 ADVERSE REACTIONS

6.1 Clinical Trials Experience
Because clinical trials are conducted under widely varying conditions, adverse reaction rates observed in the clinical trials of a drug cannot be directly compared to rates in the clinical trials of another drug and may not reflect the rates observed in practice.

The safety of DEXILANT was evaluated in 4548 patients in controlled and uncontrolled clinical studies, including 863 patients treated for at least six months and 203 patients treated for one year. Patients ranged in age from 18 to 90 years (median age 48 years), with 54% female, 85% Caucasian, 8% Black, 4% Asian, and 3% other races. Six randomized controlled clinical trials were conducted for the treatment of EE, maintenance of healed EE, and symptomatic GERD, which included 896 patients on placebo, 455 patients on DEXILANT 30 mg, 2218 patients on DEXILANT 60 mg, and 1363 patients on lansoprazole 30 mg once daily.

Most Commonly Reported Adverse Reactions
The most common adverse reactions (≥2%) that occurred at a higher incidence for DEXILANT than placebo in the controlled studies are presented in Table 2.
[See table 2 above]

Adverse Reactions Resulting in Discontinuation
In controlled clinical studies, the most common adverse reaction leading to discontinuation from DEXILANT therapy was diarrhea (0.7%).

Other Adverse Reactions
Other adverse reactions that were reported in controlled studies at an incidence of less than 2% are listed below by body system:
Blood and Lymphatic System Disorders: anemia, lymphadenopathy
Cardiac Disorders: angina, arrhythmia, bradycardia, chest pain, edema, myocardial infarction, palpitation, tachycardia
Ear and Labyrinth Disorders: ear pain, tinnitus, vertigo
Endocrine Disorders: goiter
Eye Disorders: eye irritation, eye swelling
Gastrointestinal Disorders: abdominal discomfort, abdominal tenderness, abnormal feces, anal discomfort, Barrett's esophagus, bezoar, bowel sounds abnormal, breath odor, colitis microscopic, colonic polyp, constipation, dry mouth, duodenitis, dyspepsia, dysphagia, enteritis, eructation, esophagitis, gastric polyp, gastritis, gastroenteritis, gastrointestinal disorders, gastrointestinal hypermotility disorders, GERD, GI ulcers and perforation, hematemesis, hematochezia, hemorrhoids, impaired gastric emptying, irritable bowel syndrome, mucus stools, oral mucosal blistering, painful defecation, proctitis, paresthesia oral, rectal hemorrhage, retching
General Disorders and Administration Site Conditions: adverse drug reaction, asthenia, chest pain, chills, feeling abnormal, inflammation, mucosal inflammation, nodule, pain, pyrexia
Hepatobiliary Disorders: biliary colic, cholelithiasis, hepatomegaly
Immune System Disorders: hypersensitivity
Infections and Infestations: candida infections, influenza, nasopharyngitis, oral herpes, pharyngitis, sinusitis, viral infection, vulvo-vaginal infection
Injury, Poisoning and Procedural Complications: falls, fractures, joint sprains, overdose, procedural pain, sunburn
Laboratory Investigations: ALP increased, ALT increased, AST increased, bilirubin decreased/increased, blood creatinine increased, blood gastrin increased, blood glucose increased, blood potassium increased, liver function test abnormal, platelet count decreased, total protein increased, weight increase

Metabolism and Nutrition Disorders: appetite changes, hypercalcemia, hypokalemia
Musculoskeletal and Connective Tissue Disorders: arthralgia, arthritis, muscle cramps, musculoskeletal pain, myalgia
Nervous System Disorders: altered taste, convulsion, dizziness, headaches, migraine, memory impairment, paresthesia, psychomotor hyperactivity, tremor, trigeminal neuralgia
Psychiatric Disorders: abnormal dreams, anxiety, depression, insomnia, libido changes
Renal and Urinary Disorders: dysuria, micturition urgency
Reproductive System and Breast Disorders: dysmenorrhea, dyspareunia, menorrhagia, menstrual disorder
Respiratory, Thoracic and Mediastinal Disorders: aspiration, asthma, bronchitis, cough, dyspnoea, hiccups, hyperventilation, respiratory tract congestion, sore throat
Skin and Subcutaneous Tissue Disorders: acne, dermatitis, erythema, pruritis, rash, skin lesion, urticaria
Vascular Disorders: deep vein thrombosis, hot flush, hypertension

Additional adverse reactions that were reported in a long-term uncontrolled study and were considered related to DEXILANT by the treating physician included: anaphylaxis, auditory hallucination, B-cell lymphoma, bursitis, central obesity, cholecystitis acute, dehydration, diabetes mellitus, dysphonia, epistaxis, folliculitis, gout, herpes zoster, hyperlipidemia, hypothyroidism, increased neutrophils, MCHC decrease, neutropenia, rectal tenesmus, restless legs syndrome, somnolence, tonsillitis.

Other adverse reactions not observed with DEXILANT, but occurring with the racemate lansoprazole can be found in the lansoprazole prescribing information, ADVERSE REACTIONS section.

6.2 Postmarketing Experience
The following adverse reactions have been identified during post-approval of DEXILANT. As these reactions are reported voluntarily from a population of uncertain size, it is not always possible to reliably estimate their frequency or establish a causal relationship to drug exposure.
Blood and Lymphatic System Disorders: autoimmune hemolytic anemia, idiopathic thrombocytopenic purpura
Ear and Labyrinth Disorders: deafness
Eye Disorders: blurred vision
Gastrointestinal Disorders: oral edema, pancreatitis
General Disorders and Administration Site Conditions: facial edema
Hepatobiliary Disorders: drug-induced hepatitis
Immune System Disorders: anaphylactic shock (requiring emergency intervention), exfoliative dermatitis, Stevens-Johnson syndrome, toxic epidermal necrolysis (some fatal)
Infections and Infestations: Clostridium difficile associated diarrhea
Metabolism and Nutrition Disorders: hypomagnesemia, hyponatremia
Musculoskeletal System Disorders: bone fracture
Nervous System Disorders: cerebrovascular accident, transient ischemic attack
Renal and Urinary Disorders: acute renal failure
Respiratory, Thoracic and Mediastinal Disorders: pharyngeal edema, throat tightness
Skin and Subcutaneous Tissue Disorders: generalized rash, leukocytoclastic vasculitis

7 DRUG INTERACTIONS

7.1 Drugs with pH-Dependent Absorption Pharmacokinetics
DEXILANT causes inhibition of gastric acid secretion. DEXILANT is likely to substantially decrease the systemic concentrations of the HIV protease inhibitor atazanavir, which is dependent upon the presence of gastric acid for absorption, and may result in a loss of therapeutic effect of

atazanavir and the development of HIV resistance. Therefore, DEXILANT should not be co-administered with atazanavir.
DEXILANT may interfere with the absorption of other drugs where gastric pH is an important determinant of oral bioavailability (e.g., ampicillin esters, digoxin, iron salts, ketoconazole, erlotinib).

7.2 Warfarin
Co-administration of DEXILANT 90 mg and warfarin 25 mg did not affect the pharmacokinetics of warfarin or INR [see Clinical Pharmacology (12.3)]. However, there have been reports of increased INR and prothrombin time in patients receiving PPIs and warfarin concomitantly. Increases in INR and prothrombin time may lead to abnormal bleeding and even death. Patients treated with DEXILANT and warfarin concomitantly may need to be monitored for increases in INR and prothrombin time.

7.3 Tacrolimus
Concomitant administration of dexlansoprazole and tacrolimus may increase whole blood levels of tacrolimus, especially in transplant patients who are intermediate or poor metabolizers of CYP2C19.

7.4 Clopidogrel
Concomitant administration of dexlansoprazole and clopidogrel in healthy subjects had no clinically important effect on exposure to the active metabolite of clopidogrel or clopidogrel-induced platelet inhibition [see Clinical Pharmacology (12.3)]. No dose adjustment of clopidogrel is necessary when administered with an approved dose of DEXILANT.

7.5 Methotrexate
Case reports, published population pharmacokinetic studies, and retrospective analyses suggest that concomitant administration of PPIs and methotrexate (primarily at high dose; see methotrexate prescribing information) may elevate and prolong serum levels of methotrexate and/or its metabolite hydroxymethotrexate. However, no formal drug interaction studies of high-dose methotrexate with PPIs have been conducted [see Warnings and Precautions (5.5)].

8 USE IN SPECIFIC POPULATIONS

8.1 Pregnancy
Teratogenic Effects
Pregnancy Category B. There are no adequate and well-controlled studies with dexlansoprazole in pregnant women. There were no adverse fetal effects in animal reproduction studies of dexlansoprazole in rabbits. Because animal reproduction studies are not always predictive of human response, DEXILANT should be used during pregnancy only if clearly needed.

A reproduction study conducted in rabbits at oral dexlansoprazole doses up to approximately nine times the maximum recommended human dexlansoprazole dose (60 mg/day) revealed no evidence of impaired fertility or harm to the fetus due to dexlansoprazole. In addition, reproduction studies performed in pregnant rats with oral lansoprazole at doses up to 40 times the recommended human lansoprazole dose and in pregnant rabbits at oral lansoprazole doses up to 16 times the recommended human lansoprazole dose revealed no evidence of impaired fertility or harm to the fetus due to lansoprazole [see Nonclinical Toxicology (13.2)].

8.3 Nursing Mothers
It is not known whether dexlansoprazole is excreted in human milk. However, lansoprazole and its metabolites are present in rat milk following the administration of lansoprazole. As many drugs are excreted in human milk, and because of the potential for tumorigenicity shown for lansoprazole in rat carcinogenicity studies [see Nonclinical Toxicology (13.1)], a decision should be made whether to discontinue nursing or to discontinue the drug, taking into account the importance of the drug to the mother.

8.4 Pediatric Use
Safety and effectiveness of DEXILANT in pediatric patients (less than 18 years of age) have not been established.

8.5 Geriatric Use
In clinical studies of DEXILANT, 11% of patients were aged 65 years and over. No overall differences in safety or effectiveness were observed between these patients and younger patients, and other reported clinical experience has not identified significant differences in responses between geriatric and younger patients, but greater sensitivity of some older individuals cannot be ruled out [see Clinical Pharmacology (12.3)].

8.6 Renal Impairment
No dosage adjustment of DEXILANT is necessary in patients with renal impairment. The pharmacokinetics of dexlansoprazole in patients with renal impairment are not expected to be altered since dexlansoprazole is extensively metabolized in the liver to inactive metabolites, and no parent drug is recovered in the urine following an oral dose of dexlansoprazole [see Clinical Pharmacology (12.3)].

8.7 Hepatic Impairment
No dosage adjustment for DEXILANT is necessary for patients with mild hepatic impairment (Child-Pugh Class A).

DEXILANT 30 mg should be considered for patients with moderate hepatic impairment (Child-Pugh Class B). No studies have been conducted in patients with severe hepatic impairment (Child-Pugh Class C) *[see Clinical Pharmacology (12.3)]*.

10 OVERDOSAGE

There have been no reports of significant overdose of DEXILANT. Multiple doses of DEXILANT 120 mg and a single dose of DEXILANT 300 mg did not result in death or other severe adverse events. However, serious adverse events of hypertension have been reported in association with twice daily doses of DEXILANT 60 mg. Non-serious adverse reactions observed with twice daily doses of DEXILANT 60 mg include hot flashes, contusion, oropharyngeal pain, and weight loss. Dexlansoprazole is not expected to be removed from the circulation by hemodialysis. If an overdose occurs, treatment should be symptomatic and supportive.

11 DESCRIPTION

The active ingredient in DEXILANT (dexlansoprazole) delayed-release capsules, a proton pump inhibitor, is (+)-2-[(R)-{[3-methyl-4-(2,2,2-trifluoroethoxy)pyridin-2-yl] methyl} sulfinyl]-1H-benzimidazole, a compound that inhibits gastric acid secretion. Dexlansoprazole is the R-enantiomer of lansoprazole (a racemic mixture of the R- and S-enantiomers). Its empirical formula is: $C_{16}H_{14}F_3N_3O_2S$, with a molecular weight of 369.36. The structural formula is:

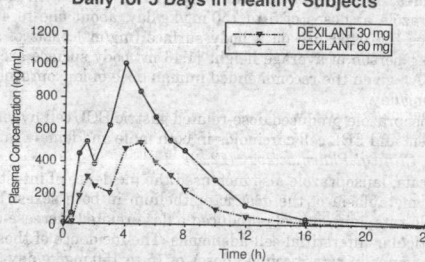

Dexlansoprazole is a white to nearly white crystalline powder which melts with decomposition at 140°C. Dexlansoprazole is freely soluble in dimethylformamide, methanol, dichloromethane, ethanol, and ethyl acetate; and soluble in acetonitrile; slightly soluble in ether; and very slightly soluble in water; and practically insoluble in hexane.

Dexlansoprazole is stable when exposed to light. Dexlansoprazole is more stable in neutral and alkaline conditions than acidic conditions.

DEXILANT is supplied as a dual delayed-release formulation in capsules for oral administration. The capsules contain dexlansoprazole in a mixture of two types of enteric-coated granules with different pH-dependent dissolution profiles *[see Clinical Pharmacology (12.3)]*.

DEXILANT is available in two dosage strengths: 30 mg and 60 mg, per capsule. Each capsule contains enteric-coated granules consisting of dexlansoprazole (active ingredient) and the following inactive ingredients: sugar spheres, magnesium carbonate, sucrose, low-substituted hydroxypropyl cellulose, titanium dioxide, hydroxypropyl cellulose, hypromellose 2910, talc, methacrylic acid copolymers, polyethylene glycol 8000, triethyl citrate, polysorbate 80, and colloidal silicon dioxide. The components of the capsule shell include the following inactive ingredients: hypromellose, carrageenan and potassium chloride. Based on the capsule shell color, blue contains FD&C Blue No. 2 aluminum lake; gray contains black ferric oxide; and both contain titanium dioxide.

12 CLINICAL PHARMACOLOGY

12.1 Mechanism of Action

Dexlansoprazole is a PPI that suppresses gastric acid secretion by specific inhibition of the (H⁺, K⁺)-ATPase in the gastric parietal cell. By acting specifically on the proton pump, dexlansoprazole blocks the final step of acid production.

12.2 Pharmacodynamics

Antisecretory Activity

The effects of DEXILANT 60 mg (n=20) or lansoprazole 30 mg (n=23) once daily for five days on 24 hour intragastric pH were assessed in healthy subjects in a multiple-dose crossover study. The results are summarized in Table 3.

Table 3. Effect on 24 Hour Intragastric pH on Day 5 After Administration of DEXILANT or Lansoprazole

DEXILANT 60 mg	Lansoprazole 30 mg
Mean Intragastric pH	
4.55	4.13
% Time Intragastric pH >4 (hours)	
71 (17 hours)	60 (14 hours)

Serum Gastrin Effects

The effect of DEXILANT on serum gastrin concentrations was evaluated in approximately 3460 patients in clinical trials up to eight weeks and in 1023 patients for up to six to 12 months. The mean fasting gastrin concentrations increased from baseline during treatment with DEXILANT 30 mg and 60 mg doses. In patients treated for more than six months, mean serum gastrin levels increased during approximately the first three months of treatment and were stable for the remainder of treatment. Mean serum gastrin levels returned to pre-treatment levels within one month of discontinuation of treatment.

Enterochromaffin-Like Cell (ECL) Effects

There were no reports of ECL cell hyperplasia in gastric biopsy specimens obtained from 653 patients treated with DEXILANT 30 mg, 60 mg or 90 mg for up to 12 months. During lifetime exposure of rats dosed daily with up to 150 mg/kg/day of lansoprazole, marked hypergastrinemia was observed followed by ECL cell proliferation and formation of carcinoid tumors, especially in female rats *[see Nonclinical Toxicology (13.1)]*.

Effect on Cardiac Repolarization

A study was conducted to assess the potential of DEXILANT to prolong the QT/QT_c interval in healthy adult subjects. DEXILANT doses of 90 mg or 300 mg did not delay cardiac repolarization compared to placebo. The positive control (moxifloxacin) produced statistically significantly greater mean maximum and time-averaged QT/QT_c intervals compared to placebo.

12.3 Pharmacokinetics

The dual delayed release formulation of DEXILANT results in a dexlansoprazole plasma concentration-time profile with two distinct peaks; the first peak occurs one to two hours after administration, followed by a second peak within four to five hours (see Figure 1). Dexlansoprazole is eliminated with a half-life of approximately one to two hours in healthy subjects and in patients with symptomatic GERD. No accumulation of dexlansoprazole occurs after multiple, once daily doses of DEXILANT 30 mg or 60 mg, although mean AUC_t and C_{max} values of dexlansoprazole were slightly higher (less than 10%) on Day 5 than on Day 1.

Figure 1: Mean Plasma Dexlansoprazole Concentration — Time Profile Following Oral Administration of 30 or 60 mg DEXILANT Once Daily for 5 Days in Healthy Subjects

The pharmacokinetics of dexlansoprazole are highly variable, with percent coefficient of variation (CV%) values for C_{max}, AUC, and CL/F of greater than 30% (see Table 4).

Table 4. Mean (CV%) Pharmacokinetic Parameters for Subjects on Day 5 After Administration of DEXILANT

Dose (mg)	C_{max} (ng/mL)	AUC_{24} (ng·h/mL)	CL/F (L/h)
30	658 (40%) (N=44)	3275 (47%) (N=43)	11.4 (48%) (N=43)
60	1397 (51%) (N=79)	6529 (60%) (N=73)	11.6 (46%) (N=41)

Absorption

After oral administration of DEXILANT 30 mg or 60 mg to healthy subjects and symptomatic GERD patients, mean C_{max} and AUC values of dexlansoprazole increased approximately dose proportionally (see Figure 1).

When granules of DEXILANT 60 mg are mixed with water and dosed via NG tube or orally via syringe, the bioavailability (C_{max} and AUC) of dexlansoprazole was similar to that when DEXILANT 60 mg was administered as an intact capsule.

Distribution

Plasma protein binding of dexlansoprazole ranged from 96.1% to 98.8% in healthy subjects and was independent of concentration from 0.01 to 20 mcg/mL. The apparent volume of distribution (V_z/F) after multiple doses in symptomatic GERD patients was 40.3 L.

Metabolism

Dexlansoprazole is extensively metabolized in the liver by oxidation, reduction, and subsequent formation of sulfate, glucuronide and glutathione conjugates to inactive metabolites. Oxidative metabolites are formed by the cytochrome P450 (CYP) enzyme system including hydroxylation mainly by CYP2C19, and oxidation to the sulfone by CYP3A4. CYP2C19 is a polymorphic liver enzyme which exhibits three phenotypes in the metabolism of CYP2C19 substrates; extensive metabolizers (*1/*1), intermediate metabolizers (*1/mutant) and poor metabolizers (mutant/mutant). Dexlansoprazole is the major circulating component in plasma regardless of CYP2C19 metabolizer status. In CYP2C19 intermediate and extensive metabolizers, the major plasma metabolites are 5-hydroxy dexlansoprazole and its glucuronide conjugate, while in CYP2C19 poor metabolizers dexlansoprazole sulfone is the major plasma metabolite.

Elimination

Following the administration of DEXILANT, no unchanged dexlansoprazole is excreted in urine. Following the administration of [14C] dexlansoprazole to six healthy male subjects, approximately 50.7% (standard deviation (SD): 9.0%) of the administered radioactivity was excreted in urine and 47.6% (SD: 7.3%) in the feces. Apparent clearance (CL/F) in healthy subjects was 11.4 to 11.6 L/h, respectively, after five days of 30 or 60 mg once daily administration.

Effect of Food on Pharmacokinetics and Pharmacodynamics

In food-effect studies in healthy subjects receiving DEXILANT under various fed conditions compared to fasting, increases in C_{max} ranged from 12% to 55%, increases in AUC ranged from 9% to 37%, and t_{max} varied (ranging from a decrease of 0.7 hours to an increase of three hours). No significant differences in mean intragastric pH were observed between fasted and various fed conditions. However, the percentage of time intragastric pH exceeded four over the 24 hour dosing interval decreased slightly when DEXILANT was administered after a meal (57%) relative to fasting (64%), primarily due to a decreased response in intragastric pH during the first four hours after dosing. Because of this, while DEXILANT can be taken without regard to food, some patients may benefit from administering the dose prior to a meal if post-meal symptoms do not resolve under post-fed conditions.

Special Populations

Pediatric Use

The pharmacokinetics of dexlansoprazole in patients under the age of 18 years have not been studied.

Geriatric Use

The terminal elimination half-life of dexlansoprazole is significantly increased in geriatric subjects compared to younger subjects (2.23 and 1.5 hours, respectively); this difference is not clinically relevant. Dexlansoprazole exhibited higher systemic exposure (AUC) in geriatric subjects (34.5% higher) than younger subjects. No dosage adjustment is needed in geriatric patients *[see Use in Specific Populations (8.5)]*.

Renal Impairment

Dexlansoprazole is extensively metabolized in the liver to inactive metabolites, and no parent drug is recovered in the urine following an oral dose of dexlansoprazole. Therefore, the pharmacokinetics of dexlansoprazole are not expected to be altered in patients with renal impairment, and no studies were conducted in subjects with renal impairment *[see Use in Specific Populations (8.6)]*. In addition, the pharmacokinetics of lansoprazole were studied in patients with mild, moderate or severe renal impairment; results demonstrated no need for a dose adjustment for this patient population.

Hepatic Impairment

In a study of 12 patients with moderately impaired hepatic function who received a single oral dose of DEXILANT 60 mg, plasma exposure (AUC) of bound and unbound dexlansoprazole in the hepatic impairment group was approximately two times greater compared to subjects with normal hepatic function. This difference in exposure was not due to a difference in protein binding between the two liver function groups. No adjustment for DEXILANT is necessary for patients with mild hepatic impairment (Child-Pugh Class A). DEXILANT 30 mg should be considered for patients with moderate hepatic impairment (Child-Pugh Class B). No studies have been conducted in patients with severe hepatic impairment (Child-Pugh Class C) *[see Use in Specific Populations (8.7)]*.

Gender

In a study of 12 male and 12 female healthy subjects who received a single oral dose of DEXILANT 60 mg, females had higher systemic exposure (AUC) (42.8% higher) than males. No dosage adjustment is necessary in patients based on gender.

Drug-Drug Interactions

Warfarin

In a study of 20 healthy subjects, co-administration of DEXILANT 90 mg once daily for 11 days with a single 25 mg oral dose of warfarin on Day 6 did not result in any

Table 5. EE Healing Rates*: All Grades

Study	Number of Patients (N)[†]	Treatment Group (daily)	Week 4 % Healed	Week 8[‡] % Healed	(95% CI) for the Treatment Difference (DEXILANT–Lansoprazole) by Week 8
1	657	DEXILANT 60 mg	70	87	(-1.5, 6.1)[§]
	648	Lansoprazole 30 mg	65	85	
2	639	DEXILANT 60 mg	66	85	(2.2, 10.5)[§]
	656	Lansoprazole 30 mg	65	79	

CI = Confidence interval
*Based on crude rate estimates, patients who did not have endoscopically documented healed EE and prematurely discontinued were considered not healed.
[†]Patients with at least one post baseline endoscopy
[‡]Primary efficacy endpoint
[§]Demonstrated non-inferiority to lansoprazole

Table 7. Median Percentage of 24 Hour Heartburn-Free Periods of the Maintenance of Healed EE Study

Treatment Group (daily)	Overall Treatment*		Month 1		Month 6	
	N	Heartburn-Free 24-hour Periods (%)	N	Heartburn-Free 24-hour Periods (%)	N	Heartburn-Free 24-hour Periods (%)
DEXILANT 30 mg	132	96.1[†]	126	96.7	80	98.3
Placebo	141	28.6	117	28.6	23	73.3

*Secondary efficacy endpoint
[†]Statistically significant vs placebo

significant differences in the pharmacokinetics of warfarin or INR compared to administration of warfarin with placebo. However, there have been reports of increased INR and prothrombin time in patients receiving PPIs and warfarin concomitantly [see Drug Interactions (7.2)].

Cytochrome P 450 Interactions
Dexlansoprazole is metabolized, in part, by CYP2C19 and CYP3A4 [see Clinical Pharmacology (12.3)].

In vitro studies have shown that dexlansoprazole is not likely to inhibit CYP isoforms 1A1, 1A2, 2A6, 2B6, 2C8, 2C9, 2D6, 2E1 or 3A4. As such, no clinically relevant interactions with drugs metabolized by these CYP enzymes would be expected. Furthermore, in vivo studies showed that DEXILANT did not have an impact on the pharmacokinetics of coadministered phenytoin (CYP2C9 substrate) or theophylline (CYP1A2 substrate). The subjects' CYP1A2 genotypes in the drug-drug interaction study with theophylline were not determined. Although in vitro studies indicated that DEXILANT has the potential to inhibit CYP2C19 in vivo, an in vivo drug-drug interaction study in mainly CYP2C19 extensive and intermediate metabolizers has shown that DEXILANT does not affect the pharmacokinetics of diazepam (CYP2C19 substrate).

Clopidogrel
Clopidogrel is metabolized to its active metabolite in part by CYP2C19. A study of healthy subjects who were CYP2C19 extensive metabolizers, receiving once daily administration of clopidogrel 75 mg alone or concomitantly with DEXILANT 60 mg (n=40), for nine days was conducted. The mean AUC of the active metabolite of clopidogrel was reduced by approximately 9% (mean AUC ratio was 91%, with 90% CI of 86-97%) when DEXILANT was coadministered compared to administration of clopidogrel alone. Pharmacodynamic parameters were also measured and demonstrated that the change in inhibition of platelet aggregation (induced by 5 mcM ADP) was related to the change in the exposure to clopidogrel active metabolite. The clinical significance of this finding is not clear.

12.5   Pharmacogenomics
Effect of CYP2C19 Polymorphism on Systemic Exposure of Dexlansoprazole
Systemic exposure of dexlansoprazole is generally higher in intermediate and poor metabolizers. In male Japanese subjects who received a single dose of DEXILANT 30 mg or 60 mg (N=2 to 6 subjects/group), mean dexlansoprazole C_{max} and AUC values were up to two times higher in intermediate compared to extensive metabolizers; in poor metabolizers, mean C_{max} was up to four times higher and mean AUC was up to 12 times higher compared to extensive metabolizers. Though such study was not conducted in Caucasians and African Americans, it is expected dexlansoprazole exposure in these races will be affected by CYP2C19 phenotypes as well.

13   NONCLINICAL TOXICOLOGY
13.1   Carcinogenesis, Mutagenesis, Impairment of Fertility
The carcinogenic potential of dexlansoprazole was assessed using lansoprazole studies. In two 24-month carcinogenicity studies, Sprague-Dawley rats were treated orally with lansoprazole at doses of 5 to 150 mg/kg/day, about one to 40 times the exposure on a body surface (mg/m²) basis of a 50 kg person of average height [1.46 m² body surface area (BSA)] given the recommended human dose of lansoprazole 30 mg/day.
Lansoprazole produced dose-related gastric ECL cell hyperplasia and ECL cell carcinoids in both male and female rats [see Clinical Pharmacology (12.2)].
In rats, lansoprazole also increased the incidence of intestinal metaplasia of the gastric epithelium in both sexes. In male rats, lansoprazole produced a dose-related increase of testicular interstitial cell adenomas. The incidence of these adenomas in rats receiving doses of 15 to 150 mg/kg/day (4 to 40 times the recommended human lansoprazole dose based on BSA) exceeded the low background incidence (range = 1.4 to 10%) for this strain of rat.
In a 24 month carcinogenicity study, CD-1 mice were treated orally with lansoprazole doses of 15 to 600 mg/kg/day, two to 80 times the recommended human lansoprazole dose based on BSA. Lansoprazole produced a dose-related increased incidence of gastric ECL cell hyperplasia. It also produced an increased incidence of liver tumors (hepatocellular adenoma plus carcinoma). The tumor incidences in male mice treated with 300 and 600 mg lansoprazole/kg/day (40 to 80 times the recommended human lansoprazole dose based on BSA) and female mice treated with 150 to 600 mg lansoprazole/kg/day (20 to 80 times the recommended human lansoprazole dose based on BSA) exceeded the ranges of background incidences in historical controls for this strain of mice. Lansoprazole treatment produced adenoma of rete testis in male mice receiving 75 to 600 mg/kg/day (10 to 80 times the recommended human lansoprazole dose based on BSA).
A 26 week p53 (+/-) transgenic mouse carcinogenicity study of lansoprazole was not positive.
Lansoprazole was positive in the Ames test and the in vitro human lymphocyte chromosomal aberration assay. Lansoprazole was not genotoxic in the ex vivo rat hepatocyte unscheduled DNA synthesis (UDS) test, the in vivo mouse micronucleus test or the rat bone marrow cell chromosomal aberration test.
Dexlansoprazole was positive in the Ames test and in the in vitro chromosome aberration test using Chinese hamster lung cells. Dexlansoprazole was negative in the in vivo mouse micronucleus test.
The potential effects of dexlansoprazole on fertility and reproductive performance were assessed using lansoprazole studies. Lansoprazole at oral doses up to 150 mg/kg/day (40 times the recommended human lansoprazole dose based on BSA) was found to have no effect on fertility and reproductive performance of male and female rats.

13.2   Animal Toxicology and/or Pharmacology
Reproductive Toxicology Studies
A reproduction study conducted in rabbits at oral dexlansoprazole doses up to 30 mg/kg/day (approximately nine times the maximum recommended human dexlansoprazole dose [60 mg/day] based on BSA) revealed no evidence of impaired fertility or harm to the fetus due to dexlansoprazole. In addition, reproduction studies performed in pregnant rats with oral lansoprazole at doses up to 150 mg/kg/day (40 times the recommended human lansoprazole dose based on BSA) and in pregnant rabbits at oral lansoprazole doses up to 30 mg/kg/day (16 times the recommended human lansoprazole dose based on BSA) revealed no evidence of impaired fertility or harm to the fetus due to lansoprazole.

14   CLINICAL STUDIES
14.1   Healing of Erosive Esophagitis
Two multi-center, double-blind, active-controlled, randomized, eight week studies were conducted in patients with endoscopically confirmed EE. Severity of the disease was classified based on the Los Angeles Classification Grading System (Grades A-D). Patients were randomized to one of the following three treatment groups: DEXILANT 60 mg daily, DEXILANT 90 mg daily or lansoprazole 30 mg daily. Patients who were H. pylori positive or who had Barrett's Esophagus and/or definite dysplastic changes at baseline were excluded from these studies. A total of 4092 patients were enrolled and ranged in age from 18 to 90 years (median age 48 years) with 54% male. Race was distributed as follows: 87% Caucasian, 5% Black and 8% other. Based on the Los Angeles Classification, 71% of patients had mild EE (Grades A and B) and 29% of patients had moderate to severe EE (Grades C and D) before treatment.
The studies were designed to test non-inferiority. If non-inferiority was demonstrated then superiority would be tested. Although non-inferiority was demonstrated in both studies, the finding of superiority in one study was not replicated in the other.
The proportion of patients with healed EE at Week 4 or 8 is presented below in Table 5.
[See table 5 above]
DEXILANT 90 mg was studied and did not provide additional clinical benefit over DEXILANT 60 mg.

14.2   Maintenance of Healed Erosive Esophagitis
A multi-center, double-blind, placebo-controlled, randomized study was conducted in patients who successfully completed an EE study and showed endoscopically confirmed healed EE. Maintenance of healing and symptom resolution over a six month period were evaluated with DEXILANT 30 mg or 60 mg once daily compared to placebo. A total of 445 patients were enrolled and ranged in age from 18 to 85 years (median age 49 years), with 52% female. Race was distributed as follows: 90% Caucasian, 5% Black and 5% other.
Sixty-six percent of patients treated with 30 mg of DEXILANT remained healed over the six-month time period as confirmed by endoscopy (see Table 6).

Table 6. Maintenance Rates* of Healed EE at Month 6

Number of Patients (N)[†]	Treatment Group (daily)	Maintenance Rate (%)
125	DEXILANT 30 mg	66.4[‡]
119	Placebo	14.3

*Based on crude rate estimates, patients who did not have endoscopically documented relapse and prematurely discontinued were considered to have relapsed.
[†]Patients with at least one post baseline endoscopy
[‡]Statistically significant vs placebo

DEXILANT 60 mg was studied and did not provide additional clinical benefit over DEXILANT 30 mg.
The effect of DEXILANT 30 mg on maintenance of relief of heartburn was also evaluated. Upon entry into the maintenance study, a majority of patients' baseline heartburn severity was rated as none. DEXILANT 30 mg demonstrated a statistically significantly higher percent of 24 hour heartburn-free periods compared to placebo over the six month treatment period (see Table 7). The majority of patients treated with placebo discontinued due to relapse of EE between month two and month six.
[See table 7 above]
14.3   Symptomatic Non-Erosive GERD
A multi-center, double-blind, placebo-controlled, randomized, four week study was conducted in patients with a di-

agnosis of symptomatic non-erosive GERD made primarily by presentation of symptoms. These patients who identified heartburn as their primary symptom, had a history of heartburn for 6 months or longer, had heartburn on at least four of seven days immediately prior to randomization and had no esophageal erosions as confirmed by endoscopy. However, patients with symptoms which were not acid-related may not have been excluded using these inclusion criteria. Patients were randomized to one of the following treatment groups: DEXILANT 30 mg daily, 60 mg daily, or placebo. A total of 947 patients were enrolled and ranged in age from 18 to 86 years (median age 48 years) with 71% female. Race was distributed as follows: 82% Caucasian, 14% Black and 4% other.

DEXILANT 30 mg provided statistically significantly greater percent of days with heartburn-free 24 hour periods over placebo as assessed by daily diary over four weeks (see Table 8). DEXILANT 60 mg was studied and provided no additional clinical benefit over DEXILANT 30 mg.

Table 8. Median Percentages of 24 Hour Heartburn-Free Periods During the 4 Week Treatment Period of the Symptomatic Non-Erosive GERD Study

N	Treatment Group (daily)	Heartburn-Free 24-hour Periods (%)
312	DEXILANT 30 mg	54.9*
310	Placebo	18.5

*Statistically significant vs placebo

A higher percentage of patients on DEXILANT 30 mg had heartburn-free 24 hour periods compared to placebo as early as the first three days of treatment and this was sustained throughout the treatment period (percentage of patients on Day 3: DEXILANT 38% versus placebo 15%; on Day 28: DEXILANT 63% versus placebo 40%).

16   HOW SUPPLIED/STORAGE AND HANDLING

DEXILANT delayed-release capsules, 30 mg, are opaque, blue and gray with TAP and "30" imprinted on the capsule and supplied as:

NDC Number	Size
64764-171-11	Unit dose package of 100
64764-171-30	Bottle of 30
64764-171-90	Bottle of 90
64764-171-19	Bottle of 1000

DEXILANT delayed-release capsules, 60 mg, are opaque, blue with TAP and "60" imprinted on the capsule and supplied as:

NDC Number	Size
64764-175-11	Unit dose package of 100
64764-175-30	Bottle of 30
64764-175-90	Bottle of 90
64764-175-19	Bottle of 1000

Store at 25°C (77°F); excursions permitted to 15 to 30°C (59 to 86°F) [see USP Controlled Room Temperature].

17   PATIENT COUNSELING INFORMATION

See FDA-approved patient labeling (Medication Guide and Instructions for Use)

To ensure the safe and effective use of DEXILANT, this information and instructions provided in the FDA-Approved Medication Guide should be discussed with the patient.

Inform the patient to watch for signs of an allergic reaction as these could be serious and may require that DEXILANT be discontinued.

Advise patients to immediately report and seek care for diarrhea that does not improve. This may be a sign of Clostridium difficile associated diarrhea [see Warnings and Precautions (5.2)].

Advise the patient to immediately report and seek care for any cardiovascular or neurological symptoms including palpitations, dizziness, seizures, and tetany as these may be signs of hypomagnesemia [see Warnings and Precautions (5.4)].

Advise the patient to tell their health care provider if they take atazanavir, tacrolimus, warfarin, methotrexate and drugs that are affected by gastric pH changes [see Drug Interactions (7)].

Advise the patient to follow the dosing instructions in the Medication Guide and inform the patient of the following administration options:
• DEXILANT is available as a delayed-release capsule.
• DEXILANT can be taken without regard to food.
• DEXILANT should be swallowed whole.
• DEXILANT should not be chewed.

Counsel patients who have difficulty swallowing capsules according to instructions provided in Dosage and Administration (2.3). Advise patients to follow the Instructions for Use that comes with the product.

MEDICATION GUIDE
DEXILANT (decks-i-launt)
(dexlansoprazole)
delayed-release capsules

Read this Medication Guide before you start taking DEXILANT and each time you get a refill. There may be new information. This information does not take the place of talking to your doctor about your medical condition or your treatment.

What is the most important information that I should know about DEXILANT?

DEXILANT may help your acid-related symptoms, but you could still have serious stomach problems. Talk with your doctor.

DEXILANT can cause serious side effects, including:
• **Diarrhea.** DEXILANT may increase your risk of getting severe diarrhea. This diarrhea may be caused by an infection (Clostridium difficile) in your intestines. Call your doctor right away if you have watery stool, stomach pain, and fever that does not go away.
• **Bone fractures.** People who take multiple daily doses of proton pump inhibitor medicines for a long period of time (a year or longer) may have an increased risk of fractures of the hip, wrist or spine. You should take DEXILANT exactly as prescribed, at the lowest dose possible for your treatment and for the shortest time needed. Talk to your doctor about your risk of bone fracture if you take DEXILANT.

DEXILANT can have other serious side effects. See "**What are the possible side effects of DEXILANT?**"

What is DEXILANT?

DEXILANT is a prescription medicine called a proton pump inhibitor (PPI). DEXILANT reduces the amount of acid in your stomach.

DEXILANT is used in adults:
• for up to 8 weeks to heal acid-related damage to the lining of the esophagus (called erosive esophagitis or EE).
• for up to 6 months to continue healing of erosive esophagitis and relief of heartburn.
• for 4 weeks to treat heartburn related to gastro-esophageal reflux disease (GERD).

GERD happens when acid from your stomach enters the tube (esophagus) that connects your mouth to your stomach. This may cause a burning feeling in your chest or throat, sour taste or burping.

It is not known if DEXILANT is safe and effective in children under 18 years of age.

Who should not take DEXILANT?

Do not take DEXILANT if you are allergic to dexlansoprazole or any of the other ingredients in DEXILANT. See the end of this Medication Guide for a complete list of ingredients in DEXILANT.

What should I tell my doctor before taking DEXILANT?

Before you take DEXILANT, tell your doctor if you:
• have been told that you have low magnesium levels in your blood
• have liver problems
• have any other medical conditions
• are pregnant or plan to become pregnant. It is not known if DEXILANT will harm your unborn baby.
• are breastfeeding or planning to breastfeed. It is not known if DEXILANT passes into your breast milk. You and your doctor should decide if you will take DEXILANT or breastfeed. You should not do both. Talk to your doctor about the best way to feed your baby if you take DEXILANT.

Tell your doctor about all the medicines you take, including prescription and non-prescription medicines, vitamins, and herbal supplements. DEXILANT may affect how other medicines work, and other medicines may affect how DEXILANT works.

Especially tell your doctor if you take:
• an antibiotic that contains ampicillin
• atazanavir (Reyataz)
• erlotinib (Tarceva)
• digoxin (Lanoxin)
• a product that contains iron
• ketoconazole (Nizoral)
• warfarin (Coumadin, Jantoven)
• tacrolimus (Prograf)
• methotrexate

Ask your doctor or pharmacist for a list of these medicines, if you are not sure.

Know the medicines that you take. Keep a list of them to show your doctor and pharmacist when you get a new medicine.

How should I take DEXILANT?
• Take DEXILANT exactly as prescribed by your doctor.
• Do not change your dose or stop taking DEXILANT without talking to your doctor first.
• You can take DEXILANT with or without food.
• Swallow DEXILANT capsules whole. Do not chew DEXILANT capsules or the granules that are in the capsules.

• If you have trouble swallowing DEXILANT capsules whole, you can open the capsules and sprinkle the contents on a tablespoon of applesauce.

See the "Instructions for Use" at the end of this Medication Guide for instructions about how to take DEXILANT capsules with applesauce, and how to give DEXILANT capsules using an oral syringe or through a nasogastric tube.
• If you forget to take a dose of DEXILANT, take it as soon as you remember. If it is almost time for your next dose, do not take the missed dose. Take the next dose on time. Do not take 2 doses at the same time to make up for the missed dose.
• If you take too much DEXILANT, call your doctor right away or go to the nearest hospital emergency room.

What are the possible side effects of DEXILANT?

DEXILANT may cause serious side effects, including:
• See "What is the most important information I should know about DEXILANT?"
• **Low magnesium levels in your body.** This problem can be serious. Low magnesium can happen in some people who take a proton pump inhibitor medicine for at least 3 months. If low magnesium levels happen, it is usually after a year of treatment. You may or may not have symptoms of low magnesium.

Tell your doctor right away if you develop any of these symptoms
  ○ seizures
  ○ dizziness
  ○ abnormal or fast heartbeat
  ○ jitteriness
  ○ jerking movements or shaking (tremors)
  ○ muscle weakness
  ○ spasms of the hands and feet
  ○ cramps or muscle aches
  ○ spasm of the voice box

Your doctor may check the level of magnesium in your body before you start taking DEXILANT, or during treatment, if you will be taking DEXILANT for a long period of time.

The most common side effects of DEXILANT include:
• diarrhea
• stomach pain
• nausea
• common cold
• vomiting
• gas

Other side effects:
• **Serious allergic reactions.** Tell your doctor if you get any of the following symptoms with DEXILANT:
  • rash
  • face swelling
  • throat tightness
  • difficulty breathing

Your doctor may stop DEXILANT if these symptoms happen.

Tell your doctor if you have any side effect that bothers you or that does not go away.

These are not all the possible side effects of DEXILANT. For more information, ask your doctor or pharmacist.

Call your doctor for medical advice about side effects. You may report side effects to FDA at 1-800-FDA-1088.

How should I store DEXILANT?
• Store DEXILANT at room temperature between 68°F to 77°F (20°C to 25°C).

Keep DEXILANT and all medicines out of the reach of children.

General information about DEXILANT

Medicines are sometimes prescribed for purposes other than those listed in a Medication Guide. Do not use DEXILANT for a condition for which it was not prescribed. Do not give DEXILANT to other people, even if they have the same symptoms you have. It may harm them.

This Medication Guide summarizes the most important information about DEXILANT. If you would like more information, talk with your doctor. You can ask your doctor or pharmacist for information about DEXILANT that is written for healthcare professionals.

For more information, go to www.DEXILANT.com or call 1-877-825-3327.

What are the ingredients in DEXILANT?

Active ingredient: dexlansoprazole.

Inactive ingredients: sugar spheres, magnesium carbonate, sucrose, low-substituted hydroxypropyl cellulose, titanium dioxide, hydroxypropyl cellulose, hypromellose 2910, talc, methacrylic acid copolymers, polyethylene glycol 8000, triethyl citrate, polysorbate 80, and colloidal silicon dioxide. The capsule shell is made of hypromellose, carrageenan and potassium chloride. Based on the capsule shell color, blue contains FD&C Blue No. 2 aluminum lake; gray contains black ferric oxide; and both contain titanium dioxide.

Instructions for Use
• DEXILANT may be taken with or without food.
• Swallow DEXILANT capsules whole.

- Do not chew DEXILANT capsules or the granules that are in the capsules.

If you have trouble swallowing DEXILANT capsules whole, you may take or give them as follows:

Taking DEXILANT with applesauce:
1. Place 1 tablespoon of applesauce into a clean container.
2. Carefully open the capsule and sprinkle the granules onto the applesauce.
3. Swallow the applesauce and granules right away. Do not chew the granules. Do not save the applesauce and granules for later use.

Giving DEXILANT with water using an oral syringe:
1. Place 20 mL of water into a clean container.
2. Carefully open the capsule and empty the granules into the container of water.
3. Use an oral syringe to draw up the water and granule mixture.
4. Gently swirl the syringe to keep the granules from settling.
5. Give the mixture into the mouth right away. Do not save the water and granule mixture for later use.
6. Refill the syringe with 10 mL of water and swirl gently. Give the water into the mouth.
7. Repeat step 6 above.

Giving DEXILANT with water through a nasogastric tube (NG tube):
For people who have a nasogastric (NG) tube that is **size 16 French or larger**, DEXILANT may be given as follows:
1. Place 20 mL of water into a clean container.
2. Carefully open the capsule and empty the granules into the container of water.
3. Use a 60 mL catheter-tip syringe to draw up the water and granule mixture.
4. Gently swirl the syringe to keep the granules from settling.
5. Connect the catheter-tip syringe to the nasogastric tube.
6. Give the mixture right away through the nasogastric tube into the stomach. Do not save the water and granule mixture for later use.
7. Refill the syringe with 10 mL of water and swirl gently. Flush the nasogastric tube with the water.
8. Repeat step 7 above.

This Medication Guide and Instructions for Use have been approved by the U.S. Food and Drug Administration.
Distributed by:
Takeda Pharmaceuticals America, Inc.
Deerfield, IL 60015
Revised: August 2013
DEXILANT is a trademark of Takeda Pharmaceuticals U.S.A., Inc. registered with the U. S. Patent and Trademark Office and used under license by Takeda Pharmaceuticals America, Inc.
All other trademark names are the property of their respective owners.
©2009-2013 Takeda Pharmaceuticals America, Inc.
DEX006 R20
Shown in Product Identification Guide, page 313

KAZANO   ℞
(alogliptin and metformin HCl)
tablets for oral administration

HIGHLIGHTS OF PRESCRIBING INFORMATION
These highlights do not include all the information needed to use KAZANO safely and effectively. See full prescribing information for KAZANO.
KAZANO (alogliptin and metformin HCl) tablets for oral administration
Initial U.S. Approval: 2013

> **WARNING: LACTIC ACIDOSIS**
> *See full prescribing information for complete boxed warning*
> - Lactic acidosis can occur due to metformin accumulation. The risk increases with conditions such as sepsis, dehydration, excess alcohol intake, hepatic impairment, renal impairment and acute congestive heart failure. (5.1)
> - Symptoms include malaise, myalgias, respiratory distress, increasing somnolence and nonspecific abdominal distress. Laboratory abnormalities include low pH, increased anion gap and elevated blood lactate. (5.1)
> - If acidosis is suspected, discontinue KAZANO and hospitalize the patient immediately. (5.1)

————INDICATIONS AND USAGE————
KAZANO is a dipeptidyl-peptidase-4 (DPP-4) inhibitor and a biguanide combination product indicated as an adjunct to diet and exercise to improve glycemic control in adults with type 2 diabetes mellitus. (1.1)

Important Limitation of Use: Not for treatment of type 1 diabetes or diabetic ketoacidosis. (1.2)

————DOSAGE AND ADMINISTRATION————
- Individualize the starting dose of KAZANO based on the patient's current regimen. (2.1)
- KAZANO should be taken twice daily with food. (2.1)
- May adjust the dosing based on effectiveness and tolerability while not exceeding the maximum recommended daily dose of 25 mg alogliptin and 2000 mg metformin HCl. (2.1)

————DOSAGE FORMS AND STRENGTHS————
Tablets: 12.5 mg alogliptin and 500 mg metformin HCl, 12.5 mg alogliptin and 1000 mg metformin HCl. (3)

————CONTRAINDICATIONS————
- Renal impairment. (4, 5.5)
- Metabolic acidosis, including diabetic ketoacidosis. (4, 5.1)
- History of a serious hypersensitivity reaction to alogliptin or metformin, components of KAZANO, such as anaphylaxis, angioedema or severe cutaneous adverse reactions. (4)

————WARNINGS AND PRECAUTIONS————
- Lactic acidosis: Warn against excessive alcohol intake. KAZANO is not recommended in hepatic impairment and is contraindicated in renal impairment. Ensure normal renal function before initiating and at least annually thereafter. (5.1)
- Acute pancreatitis: There have been postmarketing reports of acute pancreatitis. If pancreatitis is suspected, promptly discontinue KAZANO. (5.2)
- Hypersensitivity: There have been postmarketing reports of serious hypersensitivity reactions in patients treated with alogliptin such as anaphylaxis, angioedema and severe cutaneous adverse reactions. In such cases, promptly discontinue KAZANO, assess for other potential causes, institute appropriate monitoring and treatment and initiate alternative treatment for diabetes. (5.3)
- Hepatic effects: Postmarketing reports of hepatic failure, sometimes fatal. Causality cannot be excluded. If liver injury is detected, promptly interrupt KAZANO and assess patient for probable cause, then treat cause if possible, to resolution or stabilization. Do not restart KAZANO if liver injury is confirmed and no alternative etiology can be found. (5.4)
- Temporarily discontinue in patients undergoing radiologic studies with intravascular administration of iodinated contrast materials or any surgical procedures necessitating restricted intake of food and fluids. (5.5)
- Vitamin B_{12} deficiency: Metformin may lower vitamin B_{12} levels. Monitor hematologic parameters annually. (5.8)
- Hypoglycemia: When used with an insulin secretagogue (e.g., sulfonylurea) or with insulin, a lower dose of the insulin secretagogue or insulin may be required to reduce the risk of hypoglycemia. (5.9)
- Macrovascular outcomes: There have been no clinical studies establishing conclusive evidence of macrovascular risk reduction with KAZANO or any other antidiabetic drug. (5.10)

————ADVERSE REACTIONS————
Common adverse reactions reported in ≥4% of patients treated with coadministration of alogliptin with metformin were: upper respiratory tract infection, nasopharyngitis, diarrhea, hypertension, headache, back pain and urinary tract infection. (6.1)
To report SUSPECTED ADVERSE REACTIONS, contact Takeda Pharmaceuticals at 1-877-TAKEDA-7 or FDA at 1-800-FDA-1088 or www.fda.gov/medwatch.

————DRUG INTERACTIONS————
Cationic drugs eliminated by renal tubular secretion: Use with caution. (7.2)

————USE IN SPECIFIC POPULATIONS————
- Pregnancy Category B: There are no adequate and well-controlled studies in pregnant women. (8.1)
- Pediatrics: Safety and effectiveness of KAZANO in patients below the age of 18 have not been established. (8.4)
- Geriatric Use: Caution should be used when prescribing KAZANO to elderly patients because reduced renal functions are associated with increasing age. (8.5)

See 17 for PATIENT COUNSELING INFORMATION and FDA-approved patient labeling

Revised: 08/2013

FULL PRESCRIBING INFORMATION

> **WARNING: LACTIC ACIDOSIS**
> - Lactic acidosis is a rare but serious complication that can occur due to metformin accumulation. The risk increases with conditions such as sepsis, dehydration, excess alcohol intake, hepatic impairment, renal impairment and acute congestive heart failure *[see Warnings and Precautions (5.1)]*.
> - The onset is often subtle, accompanied only by nonspecific symptoms such as malaise, myalgias, respiratory distress, increasing somnolence and nonspecific abdominal distress. Laboratory abnormalities include low pH, increased anion gap and elevated blood lactate *[see Warnings and Precautions (5.1)]*.
> - If acidosis is suspected, KAZANO (alogliptin and metformin HCl) should be discontinued and the patient hospitalized immediately *[see Warnings and Precautions (5.1)]*.

1 INDICATIONS AND USAGE
1.1 Monotherapy and Combination Therapy
KAZANO is indicated as an adjunct to diet and exercise to improve glycemic control in adults with type 2 diabetes mellitus in multiple clinical settings when treatment with both alogliptin and metformin is appropriate *[see Clinical Studies (14)]*.

1.2 Limitation of Use
KAZANO should not be used in patients with type 1 diabetes mellitus or for the treatment of diabetic ketoacidosis, as it would not be effective in these settings.

2 DOSAGE AND ADMINISTRATION
2.1 Recommendations for All Patients
- Healthcare providers should individualize the starting dose of KAZANO based on the patient's current regimen.
- KAZANO should be taken twice daily with food with gradual dose escalation to reduce the gastrointestinal (GI) side effects due to metformin. KAZANO tablets must not be split before swallowing.
- Dosing may be adjusted based on effectiveness and tolerability while not exceeding the maximum recommended daily dose of 25 mg alogliptin and 2000 mg metformin HCl.
- The following doses are available:
  12.5 mg alogliptin and 500 mg metformin HCl
  12.5 mg alogliptin and 1000 mg metformin HCl

3 DOSAGE FORMS AND STRENGTHS
- 12.5 mg/500 mg tablets are pale yellow, oblong, film-coated tablets with "12.5/500" debossed on one side and "322M" debossed on the other side
- 12.5 mg/1000 mg tablets are pale yellow, oblong, film-coated tablets with "12.5/1000" debossed on one side and "322M" debossed on the other side

4 CONTRAINDICATIONS

KAZANO is contraindicated in patients with:

- Renal impairment (e.g., serum creatinine levels ≥1.5 mg/dL for men, ≥1.4 mg/dL for women or abnormal creatinine clearance), which may also result from conditions such as cardiovascular collapse (shock), acute myocardial infarction and septicemia [see Warnings and Precautions (5.5)].
- Acute or chronic metabolic acidosis, including diabetic ketoacidosis. Diabetic ketoacidosis should be treated with insulin.
- History of a serious hypersensitivity reaction to alogliptin or metformin, components of KAZANO, such as anaphylaxis, angioedema or severe cutaneous adverse reactions.

5 WARNINGS AND PRECAUTIONS

5.1 Lactic Acidosis

Lactic acidosis is a rare but serious metabolic complication that can occur due to metformin accumulation during treatment with KAZANO and is fatal in approximately 50% of cases. Lactic acidosis may also occur in association with a number of pathophysiologic conditions, including diabetes mellitus, and whenever there is significant tissue hypoperfusion and hypoxemia. Lactic acidosis is characterized by elevated blood lactate levels (more than 5 mmol/L), decreased blood pH, electrolyte disturbances with an increased anion gap, and an increased lactate/pyruvate ratio. When metformin is implicated as the cause of lactic acidosis, metformin plasma levels of more than 5 mcg/mL are generally found.

The reported incidence of lactic acidosis in patients receiving metformin HCl is very low (approximately 0.03 cases per 1000 patient-years, with approximately 0.015 fatal cases per 1000 patient-years). In more than 20,000 patient-years' exposure to metformin in clinical trials, there were no reports of lactic acidosis. Reported cases have occurred primarily in diabetic patients with significant renal impairment, including both intrinsic renal disease and renal hypoperfusion, often in the setting of multiple concomitant medical/surgical problems and multiple concomitant medications. Patients with congestive heart failure requiring pharmacologic management, particularly when accompanied by hypoperfusion and hypoxemia due to unstable or acute failure, are at increased risk of lactic acidosis. The risk of lactic acidosis increases with the degree of renal dysfunction and the patient's age. The risk of lactic acidosis may, therefore, be significantly decreased by regular monitoring of renal function in patients taking metformin. In particular, treatment of the elderly should be accompanied by careful monitoring of renal function. Metformin treatment should not be initiated in any patients unless measurement of creatinine clearance demonstrates that renal function is not reduced, as these patients are more susceptible to developing lactic acidosis. In addition, metformin should be promptly withheld in the presence of any condition associated with hypoxemia, dehydration or sepsis. Because impaired hepatic function may significantly limit the ability to clear lactate, metformin should generally be avoided in patients with clinical or laboratory evidence of hepatic impairment. Patients should be cautioned against excessive alcohol intake when taking metformin, because alcohol potentiates the effects of metformin on lactate metabolism. In addition, metformin should be temporarily discontinued prior to any intravascular radiocontrast study and for any surgical procedure necessitating restricted intake of food or fluids. Use of topiramate, a carbonic anhydrase inhibitor, in epilepsy and migraine prophylaxis may frequently cause dose-dependent metabolic acidosis (in controlled trials, 32% and 67% for adjunctive treatment in adult and pediatric patients, respectively, and 15% to 25% for monotherapy of epilepsy, with decrease in serum bicarbonate to less than 20 mEq/L; 3% and 11% for adjunctive treatment in adult and pediatric patients, respectively, and 1% to 7% for monotherapy of epilepsy, with decrease in serum bicarbonate to less than 17 mEq/L) and may exacerbate the risk of metformin-induced lactic acidosis [see Drug Interactions (7.1) and Clinical Pharmacology (12.3)].

The onset of lactic acidosis often is subtle and accompanied only by nonspecific symptoms such as malaise, myalgias, respiratory distress, increasing somnolence and nonspecific abdominal distress. There may be associated hypothermia, hypotension and resistant bradyarrhythmias with more marked acidosis.

Patients should be educated to promptly report these symptoms should they occur. If present, KAZANO should be withdrawn until lactic acidosis is ruled out. Serum electrolytes, ketones, blood glucose, blood pH, lactate levels and blood metformin levels may be useful. Once a patient is stabilized on any dose level of metformin, GI symptoms, which are common during initiation of therapy, are unlikely to recur. Later occurrence of GI symptoms could be due to lactic acidosis or other serious disease.

Levels of fasting venous plasma lactate above the upper limit of normal but less than 5 mmol/L in patients taking metformin do not necessarily indicate impending lactic acidosis and may be explainable by other mechanisms such as poorly controlled diabetes or obesity, vigorous physical activity or technical problems in sample handling.

Lactic acidosis should be suspected in any diabetic patient with metabolic acidosis lacking evidence of ketoacidosis (ketonuria and ketonemia).

Lactic acidosis is a medical emergency that must be treated in a hospital setting. In a patient with lactic acidosis who is taking metformin, the drug should be discontinued immediately and general supportive measures promptly instituted. Because metformin is dialyzable (with a clearance of up to 170 mL/min under good hemodynamic conditions), prompt hemodialysis is recommended to correct the acidosis and remove the accumulated metformin. Such management often results in prompt reversal of symptoms and recovery [see Contraindications (4)].

5.2 Pancreatitis

There have been postmarketing reports of acute pancreatitis in patients taking alogliptin. After initiation of KAZANO, patients should be observed carefully for signs and symptoms of pancreatitis. If pancreatitis is suspected, alogliptin should promptly be discontinued and appropriate management should be initiated. It is unknown whether patients with a history of pancreatitis are at increased risk for the development of pancreatitis while using KAZANO.

5.3 Hypersensitivity Reactions

There have been postmarketing reports of serious hypersensitivity reactions in patients treated with alogliptin. These reactions include anaphylaxis, angioedema and severe cutaneous adverse reactions, including Stevens-Johnson syndrome. If a serious hypersensitivity reaction is suspected, discontinue KAZANO, assess for other potential causes for the event and institute alternative treatment for diabetes [see Adverse Reactions (6.3)]. Use caution in patients with a history of angioedema to another DPP-4 inhibitor because it is unknown whether such patients will be predisposed to angioedema with KAZANO.

5.4 Hepatic Effects

There have been postmarketing reports of fatal and nonfatal hepatic failure in patients taking alogliptin, although the reports contain insufficient information necessary to establish the probable cause [see Adverse Reactions (6.3)]. In randomized controlled studies, serum alanine aminotransferase (ALT) elevations greater than three times the upper limit of normal (ULN) were observed: 1.3% in alogliptin-treated patients and 1.5% in all comparator-treated patients.

Patients with type 2 diabetes may have fatty liver disease, which may cause liver test abnormalities, and they may also have other forms of liver disease, many of which can be treated or managed. Therefore, obtaining a liver test panel and assessing the patient before initiating KAZANO therapy is recommended. Because impaired hepatic function has been associated with some cases of lactic acidosis with use of metformin, KAZANO should generally be avoided in patients with clinical or laboratory evidence of hepatic disease.

Measure liver tests promptly in patients who report symptoms that may indicate liver injury, including fatigue, anorexia, right upper abdominal discomfort, dark urine or jaundice. In this clinical context, if the patient is found to have clinically significant liver enzyme elevations and if abnormal liver tests persist or worsen, KAZANO should be interrupted and investigation done to establish the probable cause. KAZANO should not be restarted in these patients without another explanation for the liver test abnormalities.

5.5 Monitoring of Renal Function

Metformin is substantially excreted by the kidney, and the risk of metformin accumulation and lactic acidosis increases with the degree of impairment. Therefore, KAZANO is contraindicated in patients with renal impairment.

Before initiation of KAZANO therapy and at least annually thereafter, renal function should be assessed and verified as normal. In patients in whom development of renal dysfunction is anticipated, renal function should be assessed more frequently and KAZANO discontinued if evidence of renal impairment is present. Metformin treatment should not be initiated in patients ≥80 years of age unless measurement of creatinine clearance demonstrates that renal function is not reduced, as these patients are more susceptible to developing lactic acidosis.

Use of Concomitant Medications that May Affect Renal Function or Metformin Disposition

Concomitant medication(s) that may affect renal function or result in significant hemodynamic change or may interfere with the disposition of metformin, such as cationic drugs that are eliminated by renal tubular secretion [see Drug Interactions (7.2)], should be used with caution.

Radiological Studies and Surgical Procedures

Radiological studies involving the use of intravascular iodinated contrast materials (for example, intravenous urogram, intravenous cholangiography, angiography and computed tomography) can lead to acute alteration of renal function and have been associated with lactic acidosis in patients receiving metformin. Therefore, in patients in whom any such study is planned, KAZANO should be temporarily discontinued at the time of or prior to the procedure and withheld for 48 hours subsequent to the procedure and reinstituted only after renal function has been re-evaluated and found to be normal.

KAZANO therapy should be temporarily suspended for any surgical procedure (except minor procedures not associated with restricted intake of food and fluids) and should not be restarted until the patient's oral intake has resumed and renal function has been evaluated as normal.

5.6 Hypoxic States

Cardiovascular collapse (shock) from whatever cause, acute congestive heart failure, acute myocardial infarction and other conditions characterized by hypoxemia have been associated with lactic acidosis and may also cause prerenal azotemia. When such events occur in patients on KAZANO therapy, the drug should be promptly discontinued.

5.7 Alcohol Intake

Alcohol is known to potentiate the effect of metformin on lactate metabolism. Patients, therefore, should be warned against excessive alcohol intake while receiving KAZANO.

5.8 Vitamin B$_{12}$ Levels

In controlled, 29-week clinical trials of immediate-release metformin, a decrease to subnormal levels of previously normal serum vitamin B$_{12}$ levels, without clinical manifestations, was observed in approximately 7% of patients. Such decrease, possibly due to interference with B$_{12}$ absorption from the B$_{12}$-intrinsic factor complex is, however, very rarely associated with anemia and appears to be rapidly reversible with discontinuation of metformin or vitamin B$_{12}$ supplementation. Measurement of hematologic parameters on an annual basis is advised in patients on KAZANO, and any apparent abnormalities should be appropriately investigated and managed. Certain individuals (those with inadequate vitamin B$_{12}$ or calcium intake or absorption) appear to be predisposed to developing subnormal vitamin B$_{12}$ levels. In these patients, routine serum vitamin B$_{12}$ measurements at two- to three-year intervals may be useful.

5.9 Use with Medications Known to Cause Hypoglycemia

Alogliptin

Insulin and insulin secretagogues, such as sulfonylureas, are known to cause hypoglycemia. Therefore, a lower dose of insulin or insulin secretagogue may be required to reduce the risk of hypoglycemia when used in combination with KAZANO.

Metformin Hydrochloride

Hypoglycemia does not occur in patients receiving metformin alone under usual circumstances of use but could occur when caloric intake is deficient, when strenuous exercise is not compensated by caloric supplementation or during concomitant use with other glucose-lowering agents (such as sulfonylureas and insulin) or ethanol. Elderly, debilitated or malnourished patients and those with adrenal or pituitary insufficiency or alcohol intoxication are particularly susceptible to hypoglycemic effects. Hypoglycemia may be difficult to recognize in the elderly and in people who are taking β-adrenergic blocking drugs.

5.10 Macrovascular Outcomes

There have been no clinical studies establishing conclusive evidence of macrovascular risk reduction with KAZANO or any other antidiabetic drug.

6 ADVERSE REACTIONS

6.1 Clinical Studies Experience

Because clinical trials are conducted under widely varying conditions, adverse reaction rates observed in the clinical trials of a drug cannot be directly compared to rates in the clinical trials of another drug and may not reflect the rates observed in practice.

Alogliptin and Metformin Hydrochloride

Over 2700 patients with type 2 diabetes have received alogliptin coadministered with metformin in four large, randomized, double-blind controlled clinical trials. The mean exposure to KAZANO was 58 weeks, with more than 1400 subjects treated for more than one year. These included two 26-week placebo-controlled studies, one 52-week active control study and an interim analysis of a 104-week active-controlled study. In the KAZANO arm, the mean duration of diabetes was approximately six years, the mean body mass index (BMI) was 31 kg/m^2 (56% of patients had a BMI ≥30 kg/m^2) and the mean age was 55 years (18% of patients ≥65 years of age).

In a pooled analysis of these four controlled clinical studies, the overall incidence of adverse reactions was 74% in patients treated with KAZANO compared to 75% treated with placebo. Overall discontinuation of therapy due to adverse events was 6.2% with KAZANO compared to 1.9% in placebo, 6.4% in metformin and 5.0% in alogliptin.

Adverse reactions reported in ≥4% of patients treated with KAZANO and more frequently than in patients who received alogliptin, metformin or placebo are summarized in Table 1.

Table 1. Adverse Reactions Reported in ≥4% of Patients Treated with KAZANO and More Frequently than in Patients Receiving Either Alogliptin, Metformin or Placebo

	Number of Patients (%)			
	KAZANO*	Alogliptin†	Metformin‡	Placebo
	N=2794	N=222	N=1592	N=106
Upper respiratory tract infection	224 (8.0)	6 (2.7)	105 (6.6)	3 (2.8)
Nasopharyngitis	191 (6.8)	7 (3.2)	93 (5.8)	2 (1.9)
Diarrhea	155 (5.5)	4 (1.8)	105 (6.6)	3 (2.8)
Hypertension	154 (5.5)	5 (2.3)	96 (6.0)	6 (5.7)
Headache	149 (5.3)	11 (5.0)	74 (4.6)	3 (2.8)
Back pain	119 (4.3)	1 (0.5)	72 (4.5)	1 (0.9)
Urinary tract infection	116 (4.2)	4 (1.8)	59 (3.7)	2 (1.9)

* KAZANO – includes data pooled for patients receiving alogliptin 25 and 12.5 mg combined with various dose of metformin
† Alogliptin – includes data pooled for patients receiving alogliptin 25 and 12.5 mg
‡ Metformin – includes data pooled for patients receiving various doses of metformin

[See table 1 above]

Hypoglycemia
In a 26-week, double-blind, placebo-controlled study of alogliptin in combination with metformin, the number of patients reporting hypoglycemia was 1.9% in the alogliptin 12.5 mg with metformin HCl 500 mg, 5.3% in the alogliptin 12.5 mg with metformin HCl 1000 mg, 1.8% in the metformin HCl 500 mg and 6.3% in the metformin HCl 1000 mg treatment groups.
In a 26-week placebo-controlled study of alogliptin 25 mg administered once daily as add-on to metformin regimen, the number of patients reporting hypoglycemic events was 0% in the alogliptin with metformin and 2.9% in the placebo treatment groups.
In a 52-week, active-controlled, double-blind study of alogliptin once daily as add-on therapy to the combination of pioglitazone 30 mg and metformin compared to the titration of pioglitazone 30 mg to 45 mg and metformin, the number of patients reporting hypoglycemia was 4.5% in the alogliptin 25 mg with pioglitazone 30 mg and metformin group versus 1.5% in the pioglitazone 45 mg with metformin group.
In an interim analysis conducted in a 104-week, double-blind, active-controlled study of alogliptin 25 mg in combination with metformin, the number of patients reporting hypoglycemia was 1.4% in the alogliptin 25 mg with metformin group versus 23.8% in the glipizide with metformin group.

Alogliptin
Approximately 8500 patients with type 2 diabetes have been treated with alogliptin in 14 randomized, double-blind, controlled clinical trials with approximately 2900 subjects randomized to placebo and approximately 2200 to an active comparator. The mean exposure to alogliptin was 40 weeks, with more than 2400 subjects treated for more than one year. Among these patients, 63% had a history of hypertension, 51% had a history of dyslipidemia, 25% had a history of myocardial infarction, 8% had a history of unstable angina and 7% had a history of congestive heart failure. The mean duration of diabetes was seven years, the mean BMI was 31 kg/m² (51% of patients had a BMI ≥30 kg/m²) and the mean age was 57 years (24% of patients ≥65 years of age).
Two placebo-controlled monotherapy trials of 12 and 26 weeks of duration were conducted in patients treated with alogliptin 12.5 mg daily, alogliptin 25 mg daily and placebo. Four placebo-controlled add-on combination therapy trials of 26 weeks' duration were also conducted: with metformin, with a sulfonylurea, with a thiazolidinedione and with insulin.
Four placebo-controlled and one active-controlled trials of 16 weeks up through two years in duration were conducted in combination with metformin, in combination with pioglitazone and with pioglitazone added to a background of metformin therapy.
Three active-controlled trials of 52 weeks in duration were conducted in patients treated with pioglitazone and metformin, in combination with metformin and as monotherapy compared to glipizide.
In a pooled analysis of these 14 controlled clinical trials, the overall incidence of adverse events was 66% in patients treated with alogliptin 25 mg compared to 62% with placebo and 70% with active comparator. Overall discontinuation of therapy due to adverse events was 4.7% with alogliptin 25 mg compared to 4.5% with placebo or 6.2% with active comparator.

Adverse reactions reported in ≥4% of patients treated with alogliptin 25 mg and more frequently than in patients who received placebo are summarized in *Table 2*.

Table 2. Adverse Reactions Reported in ≥4% Patients Treated with Alogliptin 25 mg and More Frequently than in Patients Given Placebo in Pooled Studies

	Number of Patients (%)		
	Alogliptin 25 mg	Placebo	Active Comparator
	N=5902	N=2926	N=2257
Nasopharyngitis	257 (4.4)	89 (3.0)	113 (5.0)
Headache	247 (4.2)	72 (2.5)	121 (5.4)
Upper respiratory tract infection	247 (4.2)	61 (2.1)	113 (5.0)

Pancreatitis
In the clinical trial program, pancreatitis was reported in 11 of 5902 (0.2%) patients receiving alogliptin 25 mg daily compared to five of 5183 (<0.1%) patients receiving all comparators.

Hypersensitivity Reactions
In a pooled analysis, the overall incidence of hypersensitivity reactions was 0.6% with alogliptin 25 mg compared to 0.8% with all comparators. A single event of serum sickness was reported in a patient treated with alogliptin 25 mg.

Hypoglycemia
Hypoglycemic events were documented based upon a blood glucose value and/or clinical signs and symptoms of hypoglycemia.
In the monotherapy study, the incidence of hypoglycemia was 1.5% in patients treated with alogliptin compared to 1.6% with placebo. The use of alogliptin as add-on therapy to glyburide or insulin did not increase the incidence of hypoglycemia compared to placebo. In a monotherapy study comparing alogliptin to a sulfonylurea in elderly patients, the incidence of hypoglycemia was 5.4% with alogliptin compared to 26% with glipizide.

Metformin Hydrochloride

Table 3. Most Common Adverse Reactions (≥5%) in a Placebo-Controlled Clinical Study of Metformin Monotherapy*

	Metformin Monotherapy (n=141)	Placebo (n=145)
Adverse Reaction	% of Patients	
Diarrhea	53.2	11.7
Nausea/vomiting	25.5	8.3
Flatulence	12.1	5.5
Asthenia	9.2	5.5
Indigestion	7.1	4.1

Abdominal discomfort	6.4	4.8
Headache	5.7	4.8

* Reactions that were more common in metformin than placebo-treated patients

6.2 Laboratory Abnormalities
Alogliptin and Metformin Hydrochloride
No clinically meaningful differences were observed among treatment groups regarding hematology, serum chemistry or urinalysis results.
Alogliptin
No clinically meaningful changes in hematology, serum chemistry or urinalysis were observed in patients treated with alogliptin.
Metformin Hydrochloride
Metformin may lower serum vitamin B12 concentrations. Measurement of hematologic parameters on an annual basis is advised in patients on KAZANO, and any apparent abnormalities should be appropriately investigated and managed [see Warnings and Precautions (5.8)].

6.3 Postmarketing Experience
Alogliptin
The following adverse reactions have been identified during the postmarketing use of alogliptin outside the United States. Because these reactions are reported voluntarily from a population of uncertain size, it is not always possible to reliably estimate their frequency or establish a causal relationship to drug exposure.
Hypersensitivity reactions include anaphylaxis, angioedema, rash, urticaria, and severe cutaneous adverse reactions, including Stevens-Johnson syndrome, hepatic enzyme elevations, fulminant hepatic failure and acute pancreatitis.

7 DRUG INTERACTIONS
Alogliptin
Alogliptin is primarily renally excreted and CYP-related metabolism is negligible. No drug-drug interactions were observed with the CYP-substrates or inhibitors tested or with renally excreted drugs [see Clinical Pharmacology (12.3)].
Metformin Hydrochloride
7.1 Carbonic Anhydrase Inhibitors
Topiramate or other carbonic anhydrase inhibitors (e.g., zonisamide, acetazolamide or dichlorphenamide) frequently decrease serum bicarbonate and induce nonanion gap, hyperchloremic metabolic acidosis. Concomitant use of these drugs may induce metabolic acidosis. Use these drugs with caution in patients treated with metformin, as the risk of lactic acidosis may increase.
7.2 Cationic Drugs
Cationic drugs (e.g., amiloride, digoxin, morphine, procainamide, quinidine, quinine, ranitidine, triamterene, trimethoprim or vancomycin) that are eliminated by renal tubular secretion theoretically have the potential for interaction with metformin by competing for common renal tubular transport systems. Although such interactions remain theoretical (except for cimetidine), careful patient monitoring and dose adjustment of KAZANO and/or the interfering drug is recommended in patients who are taking cationic medications that are excreted via the proximal renal tubular secretory system.
7.3 The Use of Metformin with Other Drugs
Certain drugs tend to produce hyperglycemia and may lead to loss of glycemic control. These drugs include the thiazides and other diuretics, corticosteroids, phenothiazines, thyroid products, estrogens, oral contraceptives, phenytoin, nicotinic acid, sympathomimetics, calcium channel blocking drugs and isoniazid. When such drugs are administered to a patient receiving KAZANO, the patient should be closely observed for loss of blood glucose control. When such drugs are withdrawn from a patient receiving KAZANO, the patient should be observed closely for hypoglycemia.

8 USE IN SPECIFIC POPULATIONS
8.1 Pregnancy
Pregnancy Category B
Alogliptin and Metformin Hydrochloride
There are no adequate and well-controlled studies in pregnant women with KAZANO or its individual components. Based on animal data, KAZANO is not predicted to increase the risk of developmental abnormalities. Because animal reproduction studies are not always predictive of human risk and exposure, KAZANO, like other antidiabetic medications, should be used during pregnancy only if clearly needed.
No treatment-related fetal abnormalities occurred following concomitant administration of 100 mg/kg alogliptin with 150 mg/kg metformin to pregnant rats, or approximately 28 and two times the clinical dose of alogliptin (25 mg) and metformin (2000 mg), respectively (based on AUC).

Alogliptin
Alogliptin administered to pregnant rabbits and rats during the period of organogenesis was not teratogenic at doses of up to 200 and 500 mg/kg, or 149 times and 180 times, respectively, the clinical dose based on plasma drug exposure (AUC).

Doses of alogliptin up to 250 mg/kg (approximately 95 times clinical exposure based on AUC) given to pregnant rats from gestation Day 6 to lactation Day 20 did not harm the developing embryo or adversely affect growth and development of offspring.

Placental transfer of alogliptin into the fetus was observed following oral dosing to pregnant rats.

Metformin Hydrochloride
Metformin was not teratogenic in rats and rabbits at doses up to 600 mg/kg, which represents an exposure of about two and six times the MRHD dose of 2000 mg based on body surface area comparisons for rats and rabbits, respectively. Metformin HCl should not be used during pregnancy unless clearly needed.

8.3   Nursing Mothers
No studies have been conducted with the combined components of KAZANO. In studies performed with the individual components, both alogliptin and metformin are secreted in the milk of lactating rats. It is not known whether alogliptin and/or metformin are secreted in human milk. Because many drugs are excreted in human milk, caution should be exercised when KAZANO is administered to a nursing woman.

8.4   Pediatric Use
Safety and effectiveness of KAZANO in pediatric patients have not been established.

8.5   Geriatric Use
Alogliptin and Metformin Hydrochloride
Elderly patients are more likely to have decreased renal function. Because metformin is contraindicated in patients with renal impairment, carefully monitor renal function in the elderly and use KAZANO with caution as age increases [see Warnings and Precautions (5.5) and Clinical Pharmacology (12.3)].

Of the total number of patients (N = 2095) in clinical safety and efficacy studies, 343 (16.4%) patients were 65 years and older and 37 (1.8%) patients were 75 years and older. No overall differences in safety or effectiveness were observed between these patients and younger patients. While this and other reported clinical experiences have not identified differences in responses between the elderly and younger patients, greater sensitivity of some older individuals cannot be excluded.

Alogliptin
Of the total number of patients (N=8507) in clinical safety and efficacy studies treated with alogliptin, 2064 (24.3%) patients were 65 years and older and 341 (4%) patients were 75 years and older. No overall differences in safety or effectiveness were observed between patients 65 years and over and younger patients.

Metformin Hydrochloride
Controlled studies of metformin did not include sufficient numbers of subjects age 65 and over to determine whether they respond differently from younger patients. Other reported clinical experience has not identified differences in responses between the elderly and younger patients.
Metformin should only be used in patients with normal renal function. The initial and maintenance dosing of metformin should be conservative in patients with advanced age due to the potential for decreased renal function in this population [see Contraindications (4), Warnings and Precautions (5.5) and Clinical Pharmacology (12.3)].

10   OVERDOSAGE
Alogliptin
The highest doses of alogliptin administered in clinical trials were single doses of 800 mg to healthy subjects and doses of 400 mg once daily for 14 days to patients with type 2 diabetes (equivalent to 32 times and 16 times the recommended clinical dose, respectively). No dose-limiting adverse events were observed at these doses.

In the event of an overdose, it is reasonable to institute the necessary clinical monitoring and supportive therapy as dictated by the patient's clinical status. Per clinical judgment, it may be reasonable to initiate removal of unabsorbed material from the gastrointestinal tract.

Alogliptin is minimally dialyzable; over a three-hour hemodialysis session, approximately 7% of the drug was removed. Therefore, hemodialysis is unlikely to be beneficial in an overdose situation. It is not known if alogliptin is dialyzable by peritoneal dialysis.

Metformin Hydrochloride
Overdose of metformin has occurred, including ingestion of amounts greater than 50 grams. Hypoglycemia was reported in approximately 10% of cases, but no causal association with metformin has been established. Lactic acidosis has been reported in approximately 32% of metformin overdose cases [see Warnings and Precautions (5.1)]. Metformin

is dialyzable with a clearance of up to 170 mL/min under good hemodynamic conditions. Therefore, hemodialysis may be useful for removal of accumulated drug from patients in whom metformin overdosage is suspected.

11   DESCRIPTION
KAZANO tablets contain two oral antihyperglycemic drugs used in the management of type 2 diabetes: alogliptin and metformin hydrochloride.
Alogliptin
Alogliptin is a selective, orally bioavailable inhibitor of the enzymatic activity of dipeptidyl peptidase-4 (DPP-4). Chemically, alogliptin is prepared as a benzoate salt, which is identified as 2-({6-[(3R)-3-aminopiperidin-1-yl]-3-methyl-2,4-dioxo-3,4-dihydropyrimidin-1(2H)-yl]methyl}benzonitrile monobenzoate. It has a molecular formula of $C_{18}H_{21}N_5O_2 \cdot C_7H_6O_2$ and a molecular weight of 461.51 daltons; the structural formula is:

Alogliptin benzoate is a white to off-white crystalline powder, containing one asymmetric carbon in the aminopiperidine moiety. It is soluble in dimethylsulfoxide, sparingly soluble in water and methanol, slightly soluble in ethanol and very slightly soluble in octanol and isopropyl acetate.
Metformin Hydrochloride
Metformin hydrochloride (N,N-dimethylimidodicarbonimidic diamide hydrochloride) is not chemically or pharmacologically related to any other classes of oral antihyperglycemic agents. Metformin hydrochloride is a white to off-white crystalline compound with a molecular formula of $C_4H_{11}N_5 \cdot HCl$ and a molecular weight of 165.63. Metformin hydrochloride is freely soluble in water and is practically insoluble in acetone, ether and chloroform. The pKa of metformin is 12.4. The pH of a 1% aqueous solution of metformin hydrochloride is 6.68. The structural formula is as shown:

KAZANO is available as a tablet for oral administration containing 17 mg alogliptin benzoate equivalent to 12.5 mg alogliptin and:
• 500 mg metformin hydrochloride (12.5 mg/500 mg) or
• 1000 mg metformin hydrochloride (12.5 mg/1000 mg).
KAZANO tablets contain the following inactive ingredients: mannitol, microcrystalline cellulose, povidone, crospovidone, and magnesium stearate; the tablets are film-coated with hypromellose 2910, talc, titanium dioxide and ferric oxide yellow.

12   CLINICAL PHARMACOLOGY
12.1   Mechanism of Action
Alogliptin and Metformin Hydrochloride
KAZANO combines two antihyperglycemic agents with complementary and distinct mechanisms of action to improve glycemic control in patients with type 2 diabetes: alogliptin, a selective inhibitor of DPP-4, and metformin HCl, a member of the biguanide class.
Alogliptin
Increased concentrations of the incretin hormones such as glucagon-like peptide-1 (GLP-1) and glucose-dependent insulinotropic polypeptide (GIP) are released into the bloodstream from the small intestine in response to meals. These hormones cause insulin release from the pancreatic beta cells in a glucose-dependent manner but are inactivated by the DPP-4 enzyme within minutes. GLP-1 also lowers glucagon secretion from pancreatic alpha cells, reducing hepatic glucose production. In patients with type 2 diabetes, concentrations of GLP-1 are reduced but the insulin response to GLP-1 is preserved. Alogliptin is a DPP-4 inhibitor that slows the inactivation of the incretin hormones, thereby increasing their bloodstream concentrations and reducing fasting and postprandial glucose concentrations in a glucose-dependent manner in patients with type 2 diabetes mellitus. Alogliptin selectively binds to and inhibits DPP-4 but not DPP-8 or DPP-9 activity in vitro at concentrations approximating therapeutic exposures.
Metformin Hydrochloride
Metformin is a biguanide that improves glucose tolerance in patients with type 2 diabetes, lowering both basal and postprandial plasma glucose. Metformin decreases hepatic glucose production, decreases intestinal absorption of glucose

and improves insulin sensitivity by increasing peripheral glucose uptake and utilization. Metformin does not produce hypoglycemia in patients with type 2 diabetes or in healthy subjects except in special circumstances [see Warnings and Precautions (5.9)] and does not cause hyperinsulinemia. With metformin therapy, insulin secretion remains unchanged while fasting insulin levels and daylong plasma insulin response may actually decrease.

12.2   Pharmacodynamics
Alogliptin
Single-dose administration of alogliptin to healthy subjects resulted in a peak inhibition of DPP-4 within two to three hours after dosing. The peak inhibition of DPP-4 exceeded 93% across doses of 12.5 mg to 800 mg. Inhibition of DPP-4 remained above 80% at 24 hours for doses greater than or equal to 25 mg. Peak and total exposure over 24 hours to active GLP-1 were three- to four-fold greater with alogliptin (at doses of 25 to 200 mg) than placebo. In a 16-week, double-blind, placebo-controlled study, alogliptin 25 mg demonstrated decreases in postprandial glucagon while increasing postprandial active GLP-1 levels compared to placebo over an eight-hour period following a standardized meal. It is unclear how these findings relate to changes in overall glycemic control in patients with type 2 diabetes mellitus. In this study, alogliptin 25 mg demonstrated decreases in two-hour postprandial glucose compared to placebo (-30 mg/dL versus 17 mg/dL, respectively).
Multiple-dose administration of alogliptin to patients with type 2 diabetes also resulted in a peak inhibition of DPP-4 within one to two hours and exceeded 93% across all doses (25 mg, 100 mg and 400 mg) after a single dose and after 14 days of once-daily dosing. At these doses of alogliptin, inhibition of DPP-4 remained above 81% at 24 hours after 14 days of dosing.

12.3   Pharmacokinetics
Absorption and Bioavailability
Alogliptin and Metformin Hydrochloride
In bioequivalence studies of KAZANO, the area under the curve (AUC) and maximum concentration (C_{max}) of both the alogliptin and the metformin component following a single dose of the combination tablet were bioequivalent to the alogliptin 12.5 mg concomitantly administered with metformin HCl 500 or 1000 mg tablets under fasted conditions in healthy subjects. Administration of KAZANO with food resulted in no change in total exposure (AUC) of alogliptin and metformin. Mean peak plasma concentrations of alogliptin and metformin were decreased by 13% and 28%, respectively, when administered with food. There was no change in time to peak plasma concentrations (T_{max}) for alogliptin under fed conditions, however, there was a delayed T_{max} for metformin of 1.5 hours. These changes are not likely to be clinically significant.
Alogliptin
The absolute bioavailability of alogliptin is approximately 100%. Administration of alogliptin with a high-fat meal resulted in no change in total and peak exposure to alogliptin. Alogliptin may therefore be administered with or without food.
Metformin Hydrochloride
The absolute bioavailability of metformin following administration of a 500 mg metformin HCl tablet given under fasting conditions is approximately 50% to 60%. Studies using single oral doses of metformin HCl tablets 500 mg to 1500 mg and 850 mg to 2550 mg indicate that there is a lack of dose proportionality with increasing doses, which is due to decreased absorption rather than an alteration in elimination. Food decreases the extent of and slightly delays the absorption of metformin, as shown by approximately a 40% lower mean peak plasma concentration (C_{max}), a 25% lower area under the plasma concentration versus time curve (AUC), and a 35-minute prolongation of time to peak plasma concentration (T_{max}) following administration of a single 850 mg tablet of metformin HCl with food compared to the same tablet strength administered fasting. The clinical relevance of these decreases is unknown.
Distribution
Alogliptin
Following a single, 12.5 mg intravenous dose of alogliptin to healthy subjects, the volume of distribution during the terminal phase was 417 L, indicating that the drug is well distributed into tissues.
Alogliptin is 20% bound to plasma proteins.
Metformin Hydrochloride
The apparent volume of distribution (V/F) of metformin following single oral doses of immediate release metformin HCl tablets 850 mg averaged 654 ± 358 L. Metformin is negligibly bound to plasma proteins. Metformin partitions into erythrocytes, most likely as a function of time. At usual clinical doses and dosing schedules of metformin, steady-state plasma concentrations of metformin are reached within 24 to 48 hours and are generally less than 1 mcg/mL. During controlled clinical trials, which served as the basis for approval for metformin, maximum metformin plasma levels did not exceed 5 mcg/mL, even at maximum doses.

Figure 1. Effect of Alogliptin on the Pharmacokinetic Exposure to Other Drugs

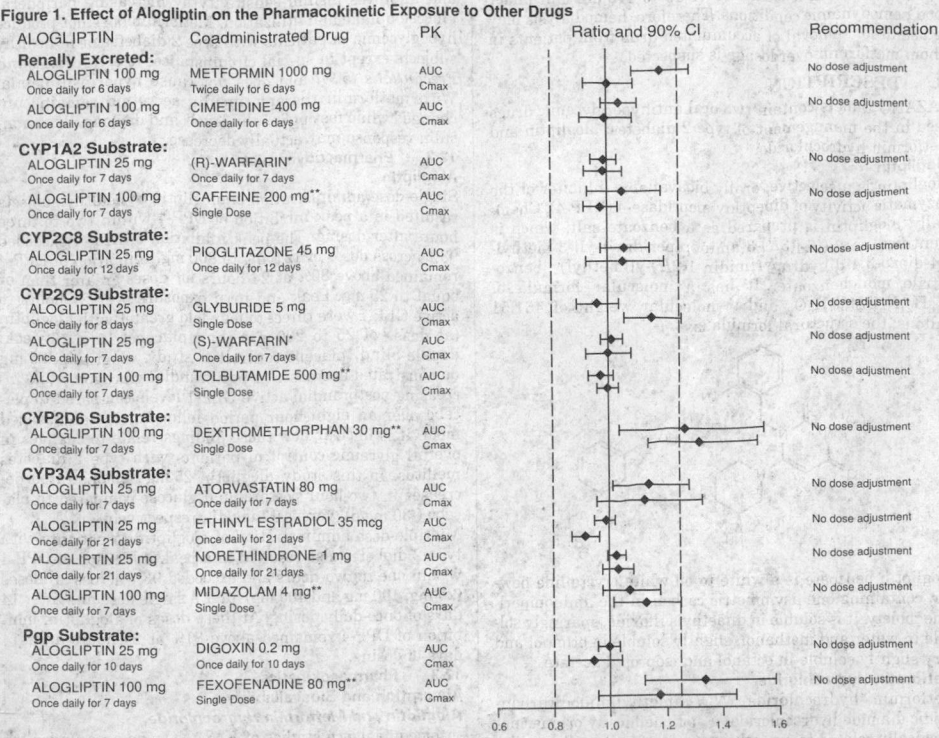

*Warfarin was given once daily at a stable dose in the range of 1 mg to 10 mg. Alogliptin had no significant effect on the prothrombin time (PT) or International Normalized Ratio (INR).

**Caffeine (1A2 substrate), tolbutamide (2C9 substrate), dextromethorphan (2D6 substrate), midazolam (3A4 substrate) and fexofenadine (P-gp substrate) were administered as a cocktail.

Figure 2. Effect of Other Drugs on the Pharmacokinetic Exposure of Alogliptin

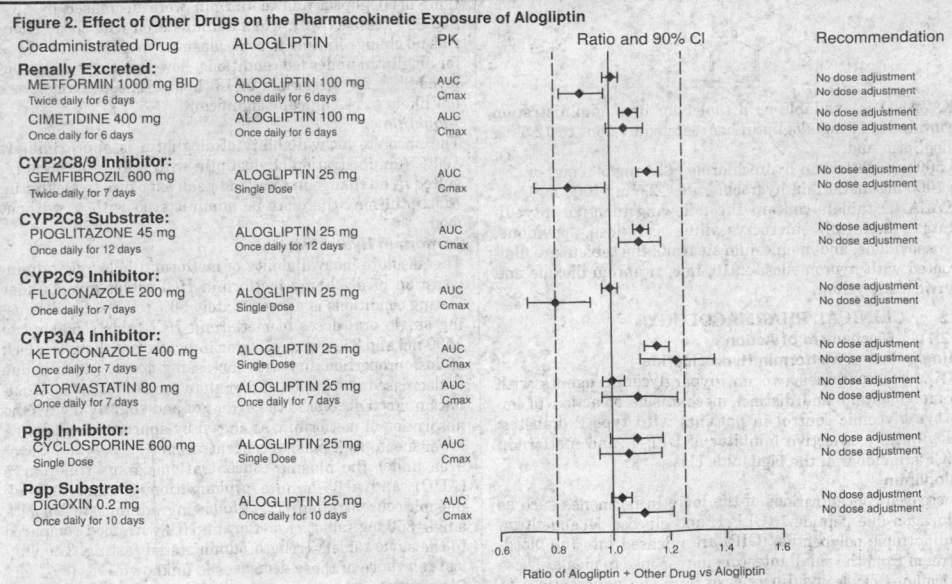

Metabolism

Alogliptin

Alogliptin does not undergo extensive metabolism and 60% to 71% of the dose is excreted as unchanged drug in the urine.

Two minor metabolites were detected following administration of an oral dose of [^{14}C] alogliptin, N-demethylated, M-I (less than 1% of the parent compound), and N-acetylated alogliptin, M-II (less than 6% of the parent compound). M-I is an active metabolite and is an inhibitor of DPP-4 similar to the parent molecule; M-II does not display any inhibitory activity toward DPP-4 or other DPP-related enzymes. In vitro data indicate that CYP2D6 and CYP3A4 contribute to the limited metabolism of alogliptin.

Alogliptin exists predominantly as the (R)-enantiomer (more than 99%) and undergoes little or no chiral conversion in vivo to the (S)-enantiomer. The (S)-enantiomer is not detectable at the 25 mg dose.

Metformin Hydrochloride

Intravenous single-dose studies in healthy subjects demonstrate that metformin is excreted unchanged in the urine and does not undergo hepatic metabolism (no metabolites have been identified in humans) or biliary excretion.

Excretion and Elimination

Alogliptin

The primary route of elimination of [^{14}C] alogliptin-derived radioactivity occurred via renal excretion (76%) with 13% recovered in the feces, achieving a total recovery of 89% of the administered radioactive dose. The renal clearance of alogliptin (9.6 L/hr) indicates some active renal tubular secretion and systemic clearance was 14.0 L/hr.

Metformin Hydrochloride

Renal clearance is approximately 3.5 times greater than creatinine clearance, which indicates that tubular secretion is the major route of metformin elimination. Following oral administration, approximately 90% of the absorbed drug is eliminated via the renal route within the first 24 hours, with a plasma elimination half-life of approximately 6.2 hours. In blood, the elimination half-life is approximately 17.6 hours, suggesting that the erythrocyte mass may be a compartment of distribution.

Special Populations

Renal Impairment

Alogliptin and Metformin Hydrochloride

Use of KAZANO in patients with renal impairment increases the risk for lactic acidosis. Because KAZANO contains metformin, KAZANO is contraindicated in patients with renal impairment [see Contraindications (4) and Warnings and Precautions (5.5)].

Hepatic Impairment

KAZANO is not recommended in patients with hepatic impairment. KAZANO contains metformin and use of metformin in patients with hepatic impairment has been associated with some cases of lactic acidosis [see Warnings and Precautions (5.4)].

Alogliptin

Total exposure to alogliptin was approximately 10% lower and peak exposure was approximately 8% lower in patients with moderate hepatic impairment (Child-Pugh Grade B) compared to healthy subjects. The magnitude of these reductions is not considered to be clinically meaningful. Patients with severe hepatic impairment (Child-Pugh Grade C) have not been studied.

Metformin Hydrochloride

No pharmacokinetic studies of metformin have been conducted in subjects with hepatic impairment.

Gender

Alogliptin

No dose adjustment is necessary based on gender. Gender did not have any clinically meaningful effect on the pharmacokinetics of alogliptin.

Metformin Hydrochloride

Metformin pharmacokinetic parameters did not differ significantly between normal subjects and patients with type 2 diabetes when analyzed according to gender. Similarly, in controlled clinical studies in patients with type 2 diabetes, the antihyperglycemic effect of metformin hydrochloride tablets was comparable in males and females.

Geriatric

KAZANO contains metformin, which is contraindicated in patients with renal impairment [see Warnings and Precautions (5.5)]. Due to declining renal function in the elderly, measurement of creatinine clearance should be obtained prior to initiation of therapy. Do not use KAZANO if renal function is not within normal range.

Alogliptin

No dose adjustment is necessary based on age. Age did not have any clinically meaningful effect on the pharmacokinetics of alogliptin.

Metformin Hydrochloride

Limited data from controlled pharmacokinetic studies of metformin in healthy elderly subjects suggest that total plasma clearance of metformin is decreased, the half-life is prolonged, and C_{max} is increased, compared to healthy young subjects. From these data it appears that the change in metformin pharmacokinetics with aging is primarily accounted for by a change in renal function.

Pediatrics

Studies characterizing the pharmacokinetics of alogliptin in pediatric patients have not been performed.

Race

Alogliptin

No dose adjustment of alogliptin is necessary based on race. Race (white, black and Asian) did not have any clinically meaningful effect on the pharmacokinetics of alogliptin.

Metformin Hydrochloride

No studies of metformin pharmacokinetic parameters according to race have been performed. In controlled clinical studies of metformin in patients with type 2 diabetes, the antihyperglycemic effect was comparable in whites (n=249), blacks (n=51) and Hispanics (n=24).

Drug Interactions

Alogliptin and Metformin Hydrochloride

Administration of alogliptin 100 mg once daily with metformin HCl 1000 mg twice daily for six days had no meaningful effect on the pharmacokinetics of alogliptin or metformin.

Specific pharmacokinetic drug interaction studies with KAZANO have not been performed, although such studies have been conducted with the individual components of KAZANO (alogliptin and metformin).

Alogliptin

In Vitro **Assessment of Drug Interactions**

In vitro studies indicate that alogliptin is neither an inducer of CYP1A2, CYP2B6, CYP2C9, CYP2C19 and CYP3A4, nor an inhibitor of CYP1A2, CYP2C8, CYP2C9, CYP2C19, CYP3A4 and CYP2D6 at clinically relevant concentrations.

In Vivo Assessment of Drug Interactions

Effects of Alogliptin on the Pharmacokinetics of Other Drugs

In clinical studies, alogliptin did not meaningfully increase the systemic exposure to the following drugs that are metabolized by CYP isozymes or excreted unchanged in urine (*Figure 1*). No dose adjustment of alogliptin is recommended based on results of the described pharmacokinetic studies.
[See figure 1 at top of previous page]

Effects of Other Drugs on the Pharmacokinetics of Alogliptin

There are no clinically meaningful changes in the pharmacokinetics of alogliptin when alogliptin is administered concomitantly with the drugs described below (*Figure 2*).
[See figure 2 at top of previous page]

Metformin Hydrochloride

Pharmacokinetic drug interaction studies have been performed on metformin (*Tables 4 and 5*).
[See table 4 above]
[See table 5 above]

13 NONCLINICAL TOXICOLOGY

13.1 Carcinogenesis, Mutagenesis, Impairment of Fertility

Alogliptin and Metformin Hydrochloride

No carcinogenicity, mutagenicity or impairment of fertility studies have been conducted with KAZANO. The following data are based on findings in studies performed with alogliptin or metformin individually.

Alogliptin

Rats were administered oral doses of 75, 400 and 800 mg/kg alogliptin for two years. No drug-related tumors were observed up to 75 mg/kg or approximately 32 times the maximum recommended clinical dose of 25 mg, based on AUC exposure. At higher doses (approximately 308 times the maximum recommended clinical dose of 25 mg), a combination of thyroid C-cell adenomas and carcinomas increased in male but not female rats. No drug-related tumors were observed in mice after administration of 50, 150 or 300 mg/kg alogliptin for two years, or up to approximately 51 times the maximum recommended clinical dose of 25 mg, based on AUC exposure.

Alogliptin was not mutagenic or clastogenic, with and without metabolic activation, in the Ames test with *S. typhimurium* and *E. coli* or the cytogenetic assay in mouse lymphoma cells. Alogliptin was negative in the *in vivo* mouse micronucleus study.

In a fertility study in rats, alogliptin had no adverse effects on early embryonic development, mating or fertility, at doses up to 500 mg/kg, or approximately 172 times the clinical dose based on plasma drug exposure (AUC).

Metformin Hydrochloride

Long-term carcinogenicity studies have been performed in rats (dosing duration of 104 weeks) and mice (dosing duration of 91 weeks) at doses up to and including 900 mg/kg and 1500 mg/kg, respectively. These doses are both approximately four times the maximum recommended human daily dose of 2000 mg based on body surface area comparisons. No evidence of carcinogenicity with metformin was found in either male or female mice. Similarly, there was no tumorigenic potential observed with metformin in male rats. There was an increased incidence of benign stromal uterine polyps in female rats treated with 900 mg/kg.

There was no evidence of a mutagenic potential of metformin in the following *in vitro* tests: Ames test (*S. typhimurium*), gene mutation test (mouse lymphoma cells) or chromosomal aberrations test (human lymphocytes). Results in the *in vivo* mouse micronucleus test were also negative.

Fertility of male or female rats was unaffected by metformin when administered at doses as high as 600 mg/kg, which is approximately three times the maximum recommended human daily dose based on body surface area comparisons.

14 CLINICAL STUDIES

The coadministration of alogliptin and metformin has been studied in patients with type 2 diabetes inadequately controlled on either diet and exercise alone, on metformin alone or metformin in combination with a thiazolidinedione.

There have been no clinical efficacy studies conducted with KAZANO; however, bioequivalence of KAZANO with coadministered alogliptin and metformin tablets was demonstrated, and efficacy of the combination of alogliptin and metformin has been demonstrated in three Phase 3 efficacy studies.

A total of 2095 patients with type 2 diabetes were randomized in three double-blind, placebo- or active-controlled clinical safety and efficacy studies conducted to evaluate the ef-

Table 4. Effect of Coadministered Drug on Plasma Metformin Systemic Exposure

Coadministered Drug	Dose of Coadministered Drug*	Dose of Metformin HCl*	Geometric Mean Ratio (ratio with/without coadministered drug) No effect = 1.00	
			AUC[†]	C_max
No dosing adjustments required for the following:				
Glyburide	5 mg	500 mg[‡]	0.98[§]	0.99[§]
Furosemide	40 mg	850 mg	1.09[§]	1.22[§]
Nifedipine	10 mg	850 mg	1.16	1.21
Propranolol	40 mg	850 mg	0.90	0.94
Ibuprofen	400 mg	850 mg	1.05[§]	1.07[§]
Cationic drugs eliminated by renal tubular secretion may reduce metformin elimination: use with caution [see *Warnings and Precautions (5)* and *Drug Interactions (7)*]				
Cimetidine	400 mg	850 mg	1.40	1.61
Carbonic anhydrase inhibitors may cause metabolic acidosis: use with caution [see *Warnings and Precautions (5)* and *Drug Interactions (7)*]				
Topiramate	100 mg[¶]	500 mg[¶]	1.25[¶]	1.17

* All metformin and coadministered drugs were given as single doses
† $AUC = AUC_{(0-\infty)}$
‡ Metformin hydrochloride extended-release tablets 500 mg
§ Ratio of arithmetic means
¶ At steady-state with topiramate 100 mg every 12 hours and metformin 500 mg every 12 hours; $AUC = AUC_{0-12h}$

Table 5. Effect of Metformin on Coadministered Drug Systemic Exposure

Coadministered Drug	Dose of Coadministered Drug*	Dose of Metformin HCl*	Geometric Mean Ratio (ratio with/without coadministered drug) No effect = 1.00	
			AUC[†]	C_max
No dosing adjustments required for the following:				
Glyburide	5 mg	500 mg[‡]	0.78[§]	0.63[§]
Furosemide	40 mg	850 mg	0.87[§]	0.69[§]
Nifedipine	10 mg	850 mg	1.10[‡]	1.08
Propranolol	40 mg	850 mg	1.01[‡]	0.94
Ibuprofen	400 mg	850 mg	0.97[‡]	1.01[¶]
Cimetidine	400 mg	850 mg	0.95[‡]	1.01

* All metformin and coadministered drugs were given as single doses
† $AUC = AUC_{(0-\infty)}$
‡ AUC_{0-24} hr reported
§ Ratio of arithmetic means, p-value of difference <0.05
¶ Ratio of arithmetic means

fects of KAZANO on glycemic control. The racial distribution of patients exposed to study medication was 69.2% white, 16.3% Asian, 6.5% black and 8.0% other racial groups. The ethnic distribution was 24.3% Hispanic. Patients had an overall mean age of approximately 54.4 years (range 22 to 80 years). In patients with type 2 diabetes, treatment with KAZANO produced clinically meaningful and statistically significant improvements in A1C versus comparator. As is typical for trials of agents to treat type 2 diabetes, the mean reduction in A1C with KAZANO appears to be related to the degree of A1C elevation at baseline.

Alogliptin and Metformin Coadministration in Patients with Type 2 Diabetes Inadequately Controlled on Diet and Exercise

In a 26-week, double-blind, placebo-controlled study, a total of 784 patients inadequately controlled on diet and exercise alone (mean baseline A1C = 8.4%) were randomized to one of seven treatment groups: placebo; metformin HCl 500 mg or metformin HCl 1000 mg twice daily, alogliptin 12.5 mg twice daily, or alogliptin 25 mg daily; alogliptin 12.5 mg in combination with metformin HCl 500 mg or metformin HCl 1000 mg twice daily. Both coadministration treatment arms (alogliptin 12.5 mg + metformin HCl 500 mg and alogliptin 12.5 mg + metformin HCl 1000 mg) resulted in significant improvements in A1C (*Figure 3*) and FPG when compared with their respective individual alogliptin and metformin component regimens (*Table 6*). Coadministration treatment arms demonstrated improvements in two-hour postprandial glucose (PPG) compared to alogliptin alone or metformin alone (*Table 6*). A total of 12% of patients receiving alogliptin 12.5 mg + metformin HCl 500 mg, 3% of patients receiving alogliptin 12.5 mg + metformin HCl 1000 mg, 17% of patients receiving alogliptin 12.5 mg, 23% of patients receiving metformin HCl 500 mg, 11% of patients receiving metformin HCl 1000 mg and 39% of patients receiving placebo required glycemic rescue.

Improvements in A1C were not affected by gender, age, race or baseline BMI. The mean decrease in body weight was similar between metformin alone and alogliptin when coadministered with metformin. Lipid effects were neutral.
[See table 6 on next page]
[See figure 3 at top of next column]

Alogliptin and Metformin Coadministration in Patients with Type 2 Diabetes Inadequately Controlled on Metformin Alone

In a 26-week, double-blind, placebo-controlled study, a total of 527 patients already on metformin (mean baseline A1C = 8%) were randomized to receive alogliptin 12.5 mg, alogliptin 25 mg, or placebo once daily. Patients were maintained on a stable dose of metformin HCl (median daily dose = 1700 mg) during the treatment period. Alogliptin 25 mg in combination with metformin resulted in statistically significant improvements from baseline in A1C and FPG at Week 26, when compared to placebo (*Table 7*). A total of 8% of patients receiving alogliptin 25 mg and 24% of patients receiving placebo required glycemic rescue. Improvements in A1C were not affected by gender, age, race, baseline BMI or baseline metformin dose.

Figure 3. Change from Baseline A1C at Week 26 with Alogliptin and Metformin Alone and Alogliptin in Combination with Metformin

Intent-to-treat population using last observation on study prior to discontinuation of double-blind study medication or sulfonylurea rescue therapy for patients needing rescue.
*P<0.001 when compared to metformin and alogliptin alone.

The mean decrease in body weight was similar between alogliptin 25 mg and placebo when given in combination with metformin. Lipid effects were also neutral.
[See table 7 at top of next page]

Alogliptin Add-On Therapy in Patients with Type 2 Diabetes Inadequately Controlled on the Combination of Metformin and Pioglitazone

In a 52-week, active-comparator study, a total of 803 patients inadequately controlled (mean baseline A1C = 8.2%) on a current regimen of pioglitazone 30 mg and metformin were randomized to either receive the addition of once-daily alogliptin 25 mg or the titration of pioglitazone 30 mg to 45 mg following a four-week single-blind, placebo run-in period. Patients were maintained on a stable dose of metformin HCl (median daily dose = 1700 mg). Patients who failed to meet prespecified hyperglycemic goals during the 52-week treatment period received glycemic rescue therapy.

In combination with pioglitazone and metformin, alogliptin 25 mg was shown to be statistically superior in lowering A1C and FPG compared with the titration of pioglitazone from 30 to 45 mg at Week 26 and at Week 52 (Table 8). A total of 11% of patients in the alogliptin 25 mg in combination with pioglitazone 30 mg and metformin treatment group and 22% of patients in the up titration of pioglitazone in combination with metformin treatment group required glycemic rescue. Improvements in A1C were not affected by gender, age, race or baseline BMI.

The mean increase in body weight was similar in both treatment arms. Lipid effects were neutral.
[See table 8 at top of next page]

16   HOW SUPPLIED/STORAGE AND HANDLING

KAZANO tablets are available in the following strengths and packages:

12.5 mg/500 mg tablet: pale yellow, oblong, film-coated tablets with "12.5/500" debossed on one side and "322M" debossed on the other side, available in:

NDC 64764-335-60	Bottles of 60 tablets
NDC 64764-335-80	Bottles of 180 tablets
NDC 64764-335-77	Bottles of 500 tablets

12.5 mg/1000 mg tablet: pale yellow, oblong, film-coated tablets with "12.5/1000" debossed on one side and "322M" debossed on the other side, available in:

NDC 64764-337-60	Bottles of 60 tablets
NDC 64764-337-80	Bottles of 180 tablets
NDC 64764-337-77	Bottles of 500 tablets

Storage

Store at 25°C (77°F); excursions permitted to 15° to 30°C (59° to 86°F) [see USP Controlled Room Temperature]. Keep container tightly closed.

17   PATIENT COUNSELING INFORMATION

See FDA-Approved Patient Labeling (Medication Guide).

17.1   Instructions

- Inform patients of the potential risks and benefits of KAZANO.
- The risks of lactic acidosis, its symptoms, and conditions that predispose to its development, as noted in *Warnings and Precautions (5.1)*, should be explained to patients. Patients should be advised to discontinue KAZANO immediately and to promptly notify their health practitioner if unexplained hyperventilation, myalgias, malaise, unusual somnolence or other non-specific symptoms occur. Once a patient is stabilized on any dose level of KAZANO, gastrointestinal symptoms, which are common during initiation of metformin ther-

Table 6. Glycemic Parameters at Week 26 for Alogliptin and Metformin Alone and in Combination in Patients with Type 2 Diabetes

	Placebo	Alogliptin 12.5 mg twice daily	Metformin HCl 500 mg twice daily	Metformin HCl 1000 mg twice daily	Alogliptin 12.5 mg + Metformin HCl 500 mg twice daily	Alogliptin 12.5 mg + Metformin HCl 1000 mg twice daily
A1C (%)*	N=102	N=104	N=103	N=108	N=102	N=111
Baseline (mean)	8.5	8.4	8.5	8.4	8.5	8.4
Change from baseline (adjusted mean[†])	0.1	-0.6	-0.7	-1.1	-1.2	-1.6
Difference from metformin (adjusted mean[†] with 95% confidence interval)	-	-	-	-	-0.6[‡] (-0.9, -0.3)	-0.4[‡] (-0.7, -0.2)
Difference from alogliptin (adjusted mean[†] with 95% confidence interval)	-	-	-	-	-0.7[‡] (-1.0, -0.4)	-1.0[‡] (-1.3, -0.7)
% of Patients (n/N) achieving A1C <7%[§]	4% (4/102)	20% (21/104)	27% (28/103)	34% (37/108)	47%[‡] (48/102)	59%[‡] (66/111)
FPG (mg/dL)*	N=105	N=106	N=106	N=110	N=106	N=112
Baseline (mean)	187	177	180	181	176	185
Change from baseline (adjusted mean[†])	12	-10	-12	-32	-32	-46
Difference from metformin (adjusted mean[†] with 95% confidence interval)	-	-	-	-	-20[‡] (-33, -8)	-14[‡] (-26, -2)
Difference from alogliptin (adjusted mean[†] with 95% confidence interval)	-	-	-	-	-22[‡] (-35, -10)	-36[‡] (-49, -24)
2-Hour PPG (mg/dL)[¶]	N=26	N=34	N=28	N=37	N=31	N=37
Baseline (mean)	263	272	247	266	261	268
Change from baseline (adjusted mean[†])	-21	-43	-49	-54	-68	-86[‡]
Difference from metformin (adjusted mean[†] with 95% confidence interval)	-	-	-	-	-19 (-49, 11)	-32[‡] (-58, -5)
Difference from alogliptin (adjusted mean[†] with 95% confidence interval)	-	-	-	-	-25 (-53, 3)	-43[‡] (-70, -16)

* Intent-to-treat population using last observation on study prior to discontinuation of double-blind study medication or sulfonylurea rescue therapy for patients needing rescue
† Least squares means adjusted for treatment, geographic region and baseline value
‡ p<0.05 when compared to metformin and alogliptin alone
§ Compared using logistic regression
¶ Intent-to-treat population using data available at Week 26

apy, are unlikely to recur. Later occurrence of gastrointestinal symptoms could be due to lactic acidosis or other serious disease.

- Patients should be informed that acute pancreatitis has been reported during use of alogliptin. Patients should be informed that persistent, severe abdominal pain, sometimes radiating to the back, which may or may not be accompanied by vomiting, is the hallmark symptom of acute pancreatitis. Patients should be instructed to promptly discontinue KAZANO and contact their physician if persistent severe abdominal pain occurs.
- Patients should be informed that allergic reactions have been reported during use of alogliptin and metformin. If symptoms of allergic reactions (including skin rash, hives and swelling of the face, lips, tongue and throat that may cause difficulty in breathing or swallowing) occur, patients should be instructed to discontinue KAZANO and seek medical advice promptly.
- Patients should be informed that postmarketing reports of liver injury, sometimes fatal, have been reported during use of alogliptin. If signs or symptoms of liver injury occur, patients should be instructed to discontinue KAZANO and seek medical advice promptly.
- Patients should be informed about the importance of regular testing of renal function and hematological parameters when receiving treatment with KAZANO.
- Patients should be counseled against excessive alcohol intake, either acute or chronic, while receiving KAZANO.
- Inform patients that hypoglycemia can occur, particularly when an insulin secretagogue or insulin is used in combination with KAZANO. Explain the risks, symptoms and appropriate management of hypoglycemia.
- Instruct patients to take KAZANO only as prescribed twice daily. KAZANO should be taken with food. If a dose is missed, advise patients not to double their next dose.
- Patients should be informed that the tablets must never be split.

Instruct patients to read the Medication Guide before starting KAZANO therapy and to reread each time the prescription is refilled. Instruct patients to inform their healthcare provider if an unusual symptom develops or if a symptom persists or worsens.

Revised: June 2013

ALM143P R3

MEDICATION GUIDE

KAZANO (Kah-ZAHN-oh)

(alogliptin and metformin HCl)

tablets

Read this Medication Guide carefully before you start taking KAZANO and each time you get a refill. There may be new information. This information does not take the place of talking with your doctor about your medical condition or treatment. If you have any questions about KAZANO, ask your doctor or pharmacist.

What is the most important information I should know about KAZANO?

KAZANO can cause serious side effects, including:

1. Lactic Acidosis. Metformin, one of the medicines in KAZANO, can cause a rare but serious condition called lactic acidosis (a buildup of an acid in the blood) that can cause death. Lactic acidosis is a medical emergency and must be treated in the hospital.

Stop taking KAZANO and call your doctor right away if you get any of the following symptoms of lactic acidosis:

- feel very weak or tired
- have unusual (not normal) muscle pain
- have trouble breathing
- have unusual sleepiness or sleep longer than usual
- have unexplained stomach or intestinal problems with nausea and vomiting, or diarrhea
- feel cold, especially in your arms and legs
- feel dizzy or lightheaded
- have a slow or irregular heartbeat

You have a higher chance for getting lactic acidosis with KAZANO if you:

- have kidney problems. People whose kidneys are not working properly should not take KAZANO
- have liver problems
- have congestive heart failure that requires treatment with medicines
- drink a lot of alcohol (very often or short-term "binge" drinking)
- get dehydrated (lose a large amount of body fluids). This can happen if you are sick with a fever, vomiting or diarrhea. Dehydration can also happen when you sweat a lot with activity or exercise and do not drink enough fluids
- have certain x-ray tests with injectable dyes or contrast agents
- have surgery
- have a heart attack, severe infection or stroke

Table 7. Glycemic Parameters at Week 26 in a Placebo-Controlled Study of Alogliptin as Add-on Therapy to Metformin*

	Alogliptin 25 mg + Metformin	Placebo + Metformin
A1C (%)	**N=203**	**N=103**
Baseline (mean)	7.9	8.0
Change from baseline (adjusted mean†)	-0.6	-0.1
Difference from placebo (adjusted mean† with 95% confidence interval)	-0.5‡ (-0.7, -0.3)	-
% of patients (n/N) achieving A1C ≤7%†	44% (92/207)‡	18% (19/104)
FPG (mg/dL)	**N=204**	**N=104**
Baseline (mean)	172	180
Change from baseline (adjusted mean†)	-17	0
Difference from placebo (adjusted mean† with 95% confidence interval)	-17‡ (-26, -9)	-

* Intent-to-treat population using last observation on study.
† Least squares means adjusted for treatment, baseline value, geographic region and baseline metformin dose.
‡ p<0.001 compared to placebo.

Table 8. Glycemic Parameters at Week 52 in an Active-Controlled Study of Alogliptin as Add-On Combination Therapy to Metformin and Pioglitazone*

	Alogliptin 25 mg + Pioglitazone 30 mg + Metformin	Pioglitazone 45 mg + Metformin
A1C (%)	**N=397**	**N=394**
Baseline (mean)	8.2	8.1
Change from baseline (adjusted mean†)	-0.7	-0.3
Difference from pioglitazone 45 mg + metformin* (adjusted mean† with 95% confidence interval)	-0.4‡ (-0.5, -0.3)	-
% of Patients (n/N) achieving A1C ≤7%	33% (134/404)§	21% (85/399)
FPG (mg/dL)‡	**N=399**	**N=396**
Baseline (mean)	162	162
Change from baseline (adjusted mean†)	-15	-4
Difference from pioglitazone 45 mg + metformin (adjusted mean† with 95% confidence interval)	-11§ (-16, -6)	-

* Intent-to-treat population using last observation on study
† Least squares means adjusted for treatment, baseline value, geographic region, and baseline metformin dose
‡ Non-inferior and statistically superior to metformin plus pioglitazone at the 0.025 one-sided significance level
§ p<0.001 compared to pioglitazone 45 mg + metformin

2. Inflammation of the pancreas (pancreatitis). Alogliptin, one of the medicines in KAZANO, may cause pancreatitis, which may be severe.

Certain medical conditions make you more likely to get pancreatitis.

Before you start taking KAZANO:

Tell your doctor if you have ever had:

- pancreatitis
- stones in your gallbladder (gallstones)
- a history of alcoholism
- kidney problems
- liver problems

Stop taking KAZANO and call your doctor right away if you have pain in your stomach area (abdomen) that is severe and will not go away. The pain may be felt going from your abdomen through to your back. The pain may happen with or without vomiting. These may be symptoms of pancreatitis.

What is KAZANO?

- KAZANO contains 2 prescription diabetes medicines, alogliptin (NESINA) and metformin hydrochloride.
- KAZANO is a prescription medicine used with diet and exercise to improve blood sugar (glucose) control in adults with type 2 diabetes.
- KAZANO is not for people with type 1 diabetes.
- KAZANO is not for people with diabetic ketoacidosis (increased ketones in blood or urine).

It is not known if KAZANO is safe and effective in children under the age of 18.

Who should not take KAZANO?

Do not take KAZANO if you:

- have kidney problems
- have a condition called metabolic acidosis or have had diabetic ketoacidosis (increased ketones in your blood or urine)

- are going to get an injection of dye or contrast agents for an x-ray procedure, KAZANO will need to be stopped for a short time. Talk to your doctor about when you should stop KAZANO and when you should start KAZANO again
- are allergic to alogliptin (NESINA) or metformin or any of the ingredients in KAZANO or have had a serious allergic (hypersensitivity) reaction to alogliptin or metformin. See the end of this Medication Guide for a complete list of the ingredients in KAZANO

Symptoms of a serious allergic reaction to KAZANO may include:

- ○ swelling of your face, lips, throat and other areas on your skin
- ○ difficulty with swallowing or breathing
- ○ raised, red areas on your skin (hives)
- ○ skin rash, itching, flaking or peeling

If you have any of these symptoms, stop taking KAZANO and contact your doctor right away or go to the nearest hospital emergency room.

What should I tell my doctor before and during treatment with KAZANO?

Before you take KAZANO, tell your doctor if you:

- have or have had inflammation of your pancreas (pancreatitis)
- have kidney or liver problems
- have heart problems, including congestive heart failure
- are older than 80 years, you should not take KAZANO unless your kidneys have been checked and they are normal
- drink alcohol very often or drink a lot of alcohol in short-term "binge" drinking
- have other medical conditions
- are pregnant or plan to become pregnant. It is not known if KAZANO will harm your unborn baby. Talk

with your doctor about the best way to control your blood sugar while you are pregnant or if you plan to become pregnant

- are breastfeeding or plan to breastfeed. It is not known whether KAZANO passes into your breast milk. Talk with your doctor about the best way to feed your baby if you are taking KAZANO

Tell your doctor about all the medicines you take, including prescription and nonprescription medicines, vitamins and herbal supplements. Know the medicines you take. Keep a list of them and show it to your doctor and pharmacist before you start any new medicine.

KAZANO may affect the way other medicines work, and other medicines may affect how KAZANO works. Contact your doctor before you start or stop other types of medicines.

How should I take KAZANO?

- Take KAZANO exactly as your doctor tells you to take it.
- Take KAZANO 2 times each day.
- Take KAZANO with food to lower your chances of having an upset stomach.
- Do not break or cut KAZANO tablets before swallowing.
- Your doctor may need to change your dose of KAZANO to control your blood glucose. Do not change your dose unless told to do so by your doctor.
- If you miss a dose, take it as soon as you remember. If you do not remember until it is time for your next dose, skip the missed dose, and take the next dose at your regular schedule. Do not take 2 doses of KAZANO at the same time.
- If you take too much KAZANO, call your doctor or go to the nearest hospital emergency room right away.
- If your body is under stress, such as from fever, infection, accident or surgery, the dose of your diabetes medicines may need to be changed. Call your doctor right away.
- Stay on your diet and exercise programs and check your blood sugar as your doctor tells you to.
- Your doctor may do certain blood tests before you start KAZANO and during treatment as needed. Your doctor may ask you to stop taking KAZANO based on the results of your blood tests due to how well your kidneys are working.
- Your doctor will check your diabetes with regular blood tests, including your blood sugar levels and your hemoglobin A1C.

What are the possible side effects of KAZANO?
KAZANO can cause serious side effects, including:

- See "What is the most important information I should know about KAZANO?"
- **Allergic (hypersensitivity) reactions,** such as:
  ○ swelling of your face, lips, throat and other areas on your skin
  ○ difficulty swallowing or breathing
  ○ raised, red areas on your skin (hives)
  ○ skin rash, itching, flaking or peeling
  If you have these symptoms, stop taking KAZANO and contact your doctor right away.
- **Liver problems.** Call your doctor right away if you have symptoms, such as:
  ○ nausea or vomiting
  ○ stomach pain
  ○ unusual or unexplained tiredness
  ○ loss of appetite
  ○ dark urine
  ○ yellowing of your skin or the whites of your eyes
- **Low blood sugar (hypoglycemia).** If you take KAZANO with another medicine that can cause low blood sugar, such as a sulfonylurea or insulin, your risk of getting low blood sugar is higher. The dose of your sulfonylurea medicine or insulin may need to be lowered while you take KAZANO. If you have symptoms of low blood sugar, you should check your blood sugar and treat if low, and then call your doctor. Signs and symptoms of low blood sugar may include:

- shaking or feeling jittery
- sweating
- fast heartbeat
- change in vision
- hunger
- headache
- change in mood
- confusion
- dizziness

The most common side effects of KAZANO include:
- cold-like symptoms (upper respiratory tract infection)
- stuffy or runny nose and sore throat
- diarrhea
- increase in blood pressure
- headache
- back pain
- urinary tract infection

Taking KAZANO with food can help lessen the common stomach side effects of metformin that usually happen at the beginning of treatment. If you have unexplained stomach problems, tell your doctor. Stomach problems that start later, during treatment, may be a sign of something more serious.

Tell your doctor if you have any side effect that bothers you or that does not go away.

These are not all the possible side effects of KAZANO. For more information, ask your doctor or pharmacist.

Call your doctor for medical advice about side effects. You may report side effects to FDA at 1-800-FDA-1088.

How should I store KAZANO?

- Store KAZANO at room temperature between 68°F to 77°F (20°C to 25°C).
- Keep the container of KAZANO tightly closed.

Keep KAZANO and all medicines out of the reach of children.

General information about the safe and effective use of KAZANO

Medicines are sometimes prescribed for purposes other than those listed in the Medication Guide. Do not take KAZANO for a condition for which it was not prescribed. Do not give KAZANO to other people, even if they have the same symptoms you have. It may harm them.

This Medication Guide summarizes the most important information about KAZANO. If you would like more information, talk with your doctor. You can ask your doctor or pharmacist for information about KAZANO that is written for health professionals.

For more information go to www.kazano.com or call 1-877-TAKEDA-7 (1-877-825-3327).

What are the ingredients in KAZANO?
Active ingredients: alogliptin and metformin hydrochloride

Inactive ingredients: mannitol, microcrystalline cellulose, povidone, crospovidone and magnesium stearate; the tablets are film-coated with hypromellose 2910, talc, titanium dioxide and ferric oxide yellow.

This Medication Guide has been approved by the U.S. Food and Drug Administration.

Distributed by:
Takeda Pharmaceuticals America, Inc.
Deerfield, IL 60015
Revised: June 2013
KAZANO and NESINA are trademarks of Takeda Pharmaceutical Company Limited registered with the U.S. Patent and Trademark Office and are used under license by Takeda Pharmaceuticals America, Inc.
©2013 Takeda Pharmaceuticals America, Inc.
ALM143P R3

Shown in Product Identification Guide, page 314

NESINA   ℞
(alogliptin)
tablets

HIGHLIGHTS OF PRESCRIBING INFORMATION
These highlights do not include all the information needed to use NESINA safely and effectively. See full prescribing information for NESINA.
NESINA (alogliptin) tablets
Initial U.S. Approval: 2013

————————**INDICATIONS AND USAGE**————————
NESINA is a dipeptidyl peptidase-4 (DPP-4) inhibitor indicated as an adjunct to diet and exercise to improve glycemic control in adults with type 2 diabetes mellitus. (1.1, 14)
Limitation of Use: Not for treatment of type 1 diabetes or diabetic ketoacidosis. (1.2)

————————**DOSAGE AND ADMINISTRATION**————————
- The recommended dose in patients with normal renal function or mild renal impairment is 25 mg once daily. (2.1)
- Can be taken with or without food. (2.1)
- Adjust dose if moderate or severe renal impairment or end-stage renal disease (ESRD). (2.2)

Degree of Renal Impairment	Creatinine Clearance (mL/min)	Recommended Dosing
Moderate	≥30 to <60	12.5 mg once daily
Severe/ESRD	<30	6.25 mg once daily

————**DOSAGE FORMS AND STRENGTHS**————
Tablets: 25 mg, 12.5 mg and 6.25 mg (3)

————————**CONTRAINDICATIONS**————————
History of a serious hypersensitivity reaction to alogliptin-containing products, such as anaphylaxis, angioedema or severe cutaneous adverse reactions. (4)

————————**WARNINGS AND PRECAUTIONS**————————
- Acute pancreatitis: There have been postmarketing reports of acute pancreatitis. If pancreatitis is suspected, promptly discontinue NESINA. (5.1)
- Hypersensitivity: There have been postmarketing reports of serious hypersensitivity reactions in patients treated with NESINA such as anaphylaxis, angioedema and severe cutaneous adverse reactions. In such cases, promptly discontinue NESINA, assess for other potential causes, institute appropriate monitoring and treatment and initiate alternative treatment for diabetes. (5.2)
- Hepatic effects: Postmarketing reports of hepatic failure, sometimes fatal. Causality cannot be excluded. If liver injury is detected, promptly interrupt NESINA and assess patient for probable cause, then treat cause if possible, to resolution or stabilization. Do not restart NESINA if liver injury is confirmed and no alternative etiology can be found. (5.3)
- Hypoglycemia: When an insulin secretagogue (e.g., sulfonylurea) or insulin is used in combination with NESINA, a lower dose of the insulin secretagogue or insulin may be required to minimize the risk of hypoglycemia. (5.4)
- Macrovascular outcomes: There have been no clinical studies establishing conclusive evidence of macrovascular risk reduction with NESINA or any other antidiabetic drug. (5.5)

————————**ADVERSE REACTIONS**————————
Common adverse reactions (reported in ≥4% of patients treated with NESINA 25 mg and more frequently than in patients who received placebo) are: nasopharyngitis, headache and upper respiratory tract infection. (6.1)

To report SUSPECTED ADVERSE REACTIONS, contact Takeda Pharmaceuticals at 1-877-TAKEDA-7 (1-877-825-3327) or FDA at 1-800-FDA-1088 or www.fda.gov/medwatch
See 17 for PATIENT COUNSELING INFORMATION and Medication Guide

Revised: 06/2013

FULL PRESCRIBING INFORMATION: CONTENTS*
1   INDICATIONS AND USAGE
  1.1   Monotherapy and Combination Therapy
  1.2   Limitation of Use
2   DOSAGE AND ADMINISTRATION
  2.1   Recommended Dosing
  2.2   Patients with Renal Impairment
3   DOSAGE FORMS AND STRENGTHS
4   CONTRAINDICATIONS
5   WARNINGS AND PRECAUTIONS
  5.1   Pancreatitis
  5.2   Hypersensitivity Reactions
  5.3   Hepatic Effects
  5.4   Use with Medications Known to Cause Hypoglycemia
  5.5   Macrovascular Outcomes

Table 1. Adverse Reactions Reported in ≥4% Patients Treated with NESINA 25 mg and More Frequently Than in Patients Given Placebo in Pooled Studies

	Number of Patients (%)		
	NESINA 25 mg	Placebo	Active Comparator
	N=5902	N=2926	N=2257
Nasopharyngitis	257 (4.4)	89 (3.0)	113 (5.0)
Headache	247 (4.2)	72 (2.5)	121 (5.4)
Upper Respiratory Tract Infection	247 (4.2)	61 (2.1)	113 (5.0)

FULL PRESCRIBING INFORMATION

1   INDICATIONS AND USAGE
1.1   Monotherapy and Combination Therapy
NESINA is indicated as an adjunct to diet and exercise to improve glycemic control in adults with type 2 diabetes mellitus in multiple clinical settings [see Clinical Studies (14)].
1.2   Limitation of Use
NESINA should not be used in patients with type 1 diabetes mellitus or for the treatment of diabetic ketoacidosis, as it would not be effective in these settings.

2   DOSAGE AND ADMINISTRATION
2.1   Recommended Dosing
The recommended dose of NESINA is 25 mg once daily. NESINA may be taken with or without food.
2.2   Patients with Renal Impairment
No dose adjustment of NESINA is necessary for patients with mild renal impairment (creatinine clearance [CrCl] ≥60 mL/min).
The dose of NESINA is 12.5 mg once daily for patients with moderate renal impairment (CrCl ≥30 to <60 mL/min).
The dose of NESINA is 6.25 mg once daily for patients with severe renal impairment (CrCl ≥15 to <30 mL/min) or with end-stage renal disease (ESRD) (CrCl <15 mL/min or requiring hemodialysis). NESINA may be administered without regard to the timing of dialysis. NESINA has not been studied in patients undergoing peritoneal dialysis [see Clinical Pharmacology (12.3)].
Because there is a need for dose adjustment based upon renal function, assessment of renal function is recommended prior to initiation of NESINA therapy and periodically thereafter.

3   DOSAGE FORMS AND STRENGTHS
• 25 mg tablets are light red, oval, biconvex, film-coated, with "TAK ALG-25" printed on one side.
• 12.5 mg tablets are yellow, oval, biconvex, film-coated, with "TAK ALG-12.5" printed on one side.
• 6.25 mg tablets are light pink, oval, biconvex, film-coated, with "TAK ALG-6.25" printed on one side.

4   CONTRAINDICATIONS
History of a serious hypersensitivity reaction to alogliptin-containing products, such as anaphylaxis, angioedema or severe cutaneous adverse reactions.

5   WARNINGS AND PRECAUTIONS
5.1   Pancreatitis
There have been postmarketing reports of acute pancreatitis in patients taking NESINA. After initiation of NESINA, patients should be observed carefully for signs and symptoms of pancreatitis. If pancreatitis is suspected, NESINA should promptly be discontinued and appropriate management should be initiated. It is unknown whether patients with a history of pancreatitis are at increased risk for the development of pancreatitis while using NESINA.
5.2   Hypersensitivity Reactions
There have been postmarketing reports of serious hypersensitivity reactions in patients treated with NESINA. These reactions include anaphylaxis, angioedema and severe cutaneous adverse reactions, including Stevens-Johnson syndrome. If a serious hypersensitivity reaction is suspected, discontinue NESINA, assess for other potential causes for the event and institute alternative treatment for diabetes [see Adverse Reactions (6.2)]. Use caution in a patient with a history of angioedema with another DPP-4 inhibitor because it is unknown whether such patients will be predisposed to angioedema with NESINA.

Table 2. Incidence and Rate of Hypoglycemia* in Placebo and Active-Controlled Studies when NESINA Was Used as Add-On Therapy to Glyburide, Insulin, Metformin, Pioglitazone or Compared to Glipizide

Add-On to Glyburide (26 Weeks)	NESINA 25 mg + Glyburide	Placebo + Glyburide
	N=198	N=99
Overall (%)	19 (9.6)	11 (11.1)
Severe (%)[†]	0	1 (1)
Add-On to Insulin (± Metformin) (26 Weeks)	**NESINA 25 mg + Insulin (± Metformin)**	**Placebo + Insulin (± Metformin)**
	N=129	N=129
Overall (%)	35 (27)	31 (24)
Severe (%)[†]	1 (0.8)	2 (1.6)
Add-On to Metformin (26 Weeks)	**NESINA 25 mg + Metformin**	**Placebo + Metformin**
	N=207	N=104
Overall (%)	0	3 (2.9)
Severe (%)[†]	0	0
Add-On to Pioglitazone (± Metformin or Sulfonylurea) (26 Weeks)	**NESINA 25 mg + Pioglitazone**	**Placebo + Pioglitazone**
	N=199	N=97
Overall (%)	14 (7.0)	5 (5.2)
Severe (%)[†]	0	1 (1)
Compared to Glipizide (52 Weeks)	**NESINA 25 mg**	**Glipizide**
	N=222	N=219
Overall (%)	12 (5.4)	57 (26)
Severe (%)[†]	0	3 (1.4)
Add-On to Metformin (26 Weeks)	**NESINA 25 mg**	**Metformin 500 mg twice daily**
	N=112	N=109
Overall (%)	2 (1.8)	2 (1.8)
Severe (%)[†]	0	0
Add-On to Metformin Compared to Glipizide (52 Weeks)	**NESINA 25 mg + Metformin**	**Glipizide + Metformin**
	N=877	N=869
Overall (%)	12 (1.4)	207 (23.8)
Severe (%)[†]	0	4 (0.5)

* Adverse reactions of hypoglycemia were based on all reports of symptomatic and asymptomatic hypoglycemia; a concurrent glucose measurement was not required; intent-to-treat population.
† Severe events of hypoglycemia were defined as those events requiring medical assistance or exhibiting depressed level or loss of consciousness or seizure.

5.3   Hepatic Effects
There have been postmarketing reports of fatal and nonfatal hepatic failure in patients taking NESINA, although some of the reports contain insufficient information necessary to establish the probable cause [see Adverse Reactions (6.2)]. In randomized controlled studies, serum alanine aminotransferase (ALT) elevations greater than three times the upper limit of normal (ULN) were observed: 1.3% in alogliptin-treated patients and 1.5% in all comparator-treated patients.
Patients with type 2 diabetes may have fatty liver disease, which may cause liver test abnormalities, and they may also have other forms of liver disease, many of which can be treated or managed. Therefore, obtaining a liver test panel and assessing the patient before initiating NESINA therapy is recommended. In patients with abnormal liver tests, NESINA should be initiated with caution.
Measure liver tests promptly in patients who report symptoms that may indicate liver injury, including fatigue, anorexia, right upper abdominal discomfort, dark urine or jaundice. In this clinical context, if the patient is found to have clinically significant liver enzyme elevations and if abnormal liver tests persist or worsen, NESINA should be interrupted and investigation done to establish the probable cause. NESINA should not be restarted in these patients without another explanation for the liver test abnormalities.
5.4   Use with Medications Known to Cause Hypoglycemia
Insulin and insulin secretagogues, such as sulfonylureas, are known to cause hypoglycemia. Therefore, a lower dose of insulin or insulin secretagogue may be required to minimize the risk of hypoglycemia when used in combination with NESINA.
5.5   Macrovascular Outcomes
There have been no clinical studies establishing conclusive evidence of macrovascular risk reduction with NESINA or any other antidiabetic drug.

Figure 1. Effect of Alogliptin on the Pharmacokinetic Exposure to Other Drugs

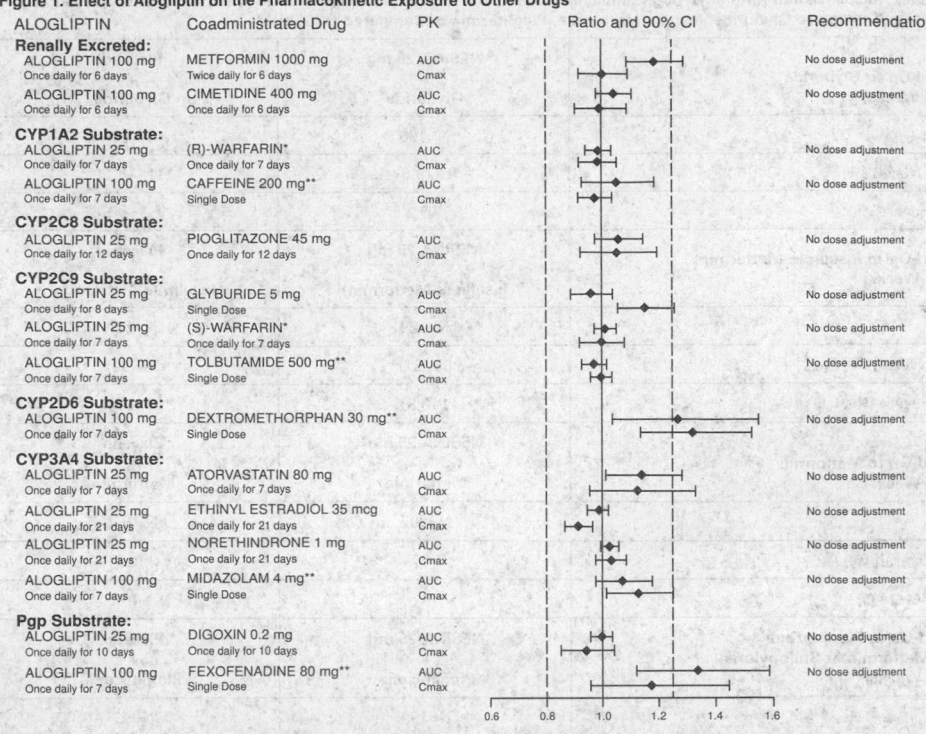

*Warfarin was given once daily at a stable dose in the range of 1 mg to 10 mg. Alogliptin had no significant effect on the prothrombin time (PT) or International Normalized Ratio (INR).

**Caffeine (1A2 substrate), tolbutamide (2C9 substrate), dextromethorphan (2D6 substrate), midazolam (3A4 substrate) and fexofenadine (P-gp substrate) were administered as a cocktail.

Figure 2. Effect of Other Drugs on the Pharmacokinetic Exposure of Alogliptin

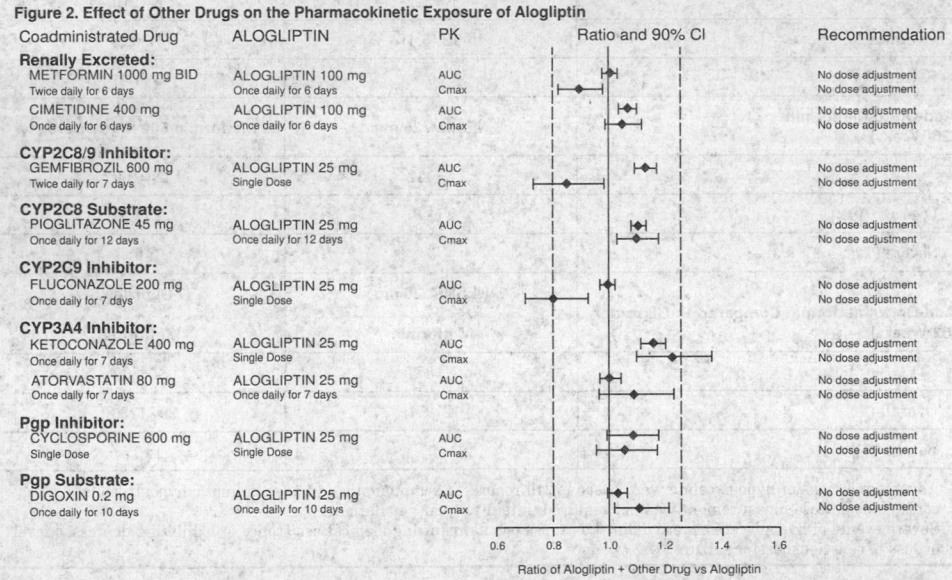

6 ADVERSE REACTIONS
6.1 Clinical Studies Experience
Because clinical trials are conducted under widely varying conditions, adverse reaction rates observed in the clinical trials of a drug cannot be directly compared to rates in the clinical trials of another drug and may not reflect the rates observed in clinical practice.

Approximately 8500 patients with type 2 diabetes have been treated with NESINA in 14 randomized, double-blind, controlled clinical trials with approximately 2900 subjects randomized to placebo and approximately 2200 to an active comparator. The mean exposure to NESINA was 40 weeks with more than 2400 subjects treated for more than one year. Among these patients, 63% had a history of hypertension, 51% had a history of dyslipidemia, 25% had a history of myocardial infarction, 8% had a history of unstable angina and 7% had a history of congestive heart failure. The mean duration of diabetes was seven years, the mean body mass index (BMI) was 31 kg/m^2 (51% of patients had a BMI ≥30 kg/m^2), and the mean age was 57 years (24% of patients ≥65 years of age).

Two placebo-controlled monotherapy trials of 12 and 26 weeks of duration were conducted in patients treated with NESINA 12.5 mg daily, NESINA 25 mg daily and placebo. Four placebo-controlled add-on combination therapy trials of 26 weeks duration were also conducted: with metformin, with a sulfonylurea, with a thiazolidinedione and with insulin.

Four placebo-controlled and one active-controlled trials of 16 weeks up through two years in duration were conducted in combination with metformin, in combination with pioglitazone and with pioglitazone added to a background of metformin therapy.

Three active-controlled trials of 52 weeks in duration were conducted in patients treated with pioglitazone and metformin, in combination with metformin and as monotherapy compared to glipizide.

In a pooled analysis of these 14 controlled clinical trials, the overall incidence of adverse events was 66% in patients treated with NESINA 25 mg compared to 62% with placebo and 70% with active comparator. Overall discontinuation of therapy due to adverse events was 4.7% with NESINA 25 mg compared to 4.5% with placebo or 6.2% with active comparator.

Adverse reactions reported in ≥4% of patients treated with NESINA 25 mg and more frequently than in patients who received placebo are summarized in *Table 1*.
[See table 1 at bottom of page 2284]

Pancreatitis
In the clinical trial program, pancreatitis was reported in 11 of 5902 (0.2%) patients receiving NESINA 25 mg daily compared to five of 5183 (<0.1%) patients receiving all comparators.

Hypersensitivity Reactions
In a pooled analysis, the overall incidence of hypersensitivity reactions was 0.6% with NESINA 25 mg compared to 0.8% with all comparators. A single event of serum sickness was reported in a patient treated with NESINA 25 mg.

Hypoglycemia
Hypoglycemic events were documented based upon a blood glucose value and/or clinical signs and symptoms of hypoglycemia.

In the monotherapy study, the incidence of hypoglycemia was 1.5% in patients treated with NESINA compared to 1.6% with placebo. The use of NESINA as add-on therapy to glyburide or insulin did not increase the incidence of hypoglycemia compared to placebo. In a monotherapy study comparing NESINA to a sulfonylurea in elderly patients, the incidence of hypoglycemia was 5.4% with NESINA compared to 26% with glipizide *(Table 2)*.
[See table 2 at top of previous page]

Vital Signs
No clinically meaningful changes in vital signs or in electrocardiograms were observed in patients treated with NESINA.

Laboratory Tests
No clinically meaningful changes in hematology, serum chemistry or urinalysis were observed in patients treated with NESINA.

6.2 Postmarketing Experience
The following adverse reactions have been identified during the postmarketing use of NESINA outside the United States. Because these reactions are reported voluntarily from a population of uncertain size, it is not always possible to reliably estimate their frequency or establish a causal relationship to drug exposure.

Hypersensitivity reactions including anaphylaxis, angioedema, rash, urticaria and severe cutaneous adverse reactions, including Stevens-Johnson syndrome, hepatic enzyme elevations, fulminant hepatic failure and acute pancreatitis.

7 DRUG INTERACTIONS
NESINA is primarily renally excreted. Cytochrome (CYP) P450-related metabolism is negligible. No significant drug-drug interactions were observed with the CYP-substrates or inhibitors tested or with renally excreted drugs *[see Clinical Pharmacology (12.3)]*.

8 USE IN SPECIFIC POPULATIONS
8.1 Pregnancy
Pregnancy Category B
No adequate or well-controlled studies in pregnant women have been conducted with NESINA. Based on animal data, NESINA is not predicted to increase the risk of developmental abnormalities. Because animal reproduction studies are not always predictive of human risk and exposure, NESINA, like other antidiabetic medications, should be used during pregnancy only if clearly needed.

Alogliptin administered to pregnant rabbits and rats during the period of organogenesis was not teratogenic at doses of up to 200 mg/kg and 500 mg/kg, or 149 times and 180 times, respectively, the clinical dose based on plasma drug exposure (AUC).

Doses of alogliptin up to 250 mg/kg (approximately 95 times clinical exposure based on AUC) given to pregnant rats from gestation Day 6 to lactation Day 20 did not harm the developing embryo or adversely affect growth and development of offspring.

Placental transfer of alogliptin into the fetus was observed following oral dosing to pregnant rats.

8.3 Nursing Mothers
Alogliptin is secreted in the milk of lactating rats in a 2:1 ratio to plasma. It is not known whether alogliptin is excreted in human milk. Because many drugs are excreted in human milk, caution should be exercised when NESINA is administered to a nursing woman.

8.4 Pediatric Use

Safety and effectiveness of NESINA in pediatric patients have not been established.

8.5 Geriatric Use

Of the total number of patients (N=8507) in clinical safety and efficacy studies treated with NESINA, 2064 (24.3%) patients were 65 years and older and 341 (4%) patients were 75 years and older. No overall differences in safety or effectiveness were observed between patients 65 years and over and younger patients. While this clinical experience has not identified differences in responses between the elderly and younger patients, greater sensitivity of some older individuals cannot be ruled out.

8.6 Hepatic Impairment

No dose adjustments are required in patients with mild to moderate hepatic impairment (Child-Pugh Grade A and B) based on insignificant change in systemic exposures (e.g., AUC) compared to subjects with normal hepatic function in a pharmacokinetic study. NESINA has not been studied in patients with severe hepatic impairment (Child-Pugh Grade C). Use caution when administering NESINA to patients with liver disease [see Warnings and Precautions (5.3)].

10 OVERDOSAGE

The highest doses of NESINA administered in clinical trials were single doses of 800 mg to healthy subjects and doses of 400 mg once daily for 14 days to patients with type 2 diabetes (equivalent to 32 times and 16 times the maximum recommended clinical dose of 25 mg, respectively). No serious adverse events were observed at these doses.

In the event of an overdose, it is reasonable to institute the necessary clinical monitoring and supportive therapy as dictated by the patient's clinical status. Per clinical judgment, it may be reasonable to initiate removal of unabsorbed material from the gastrointestinal tract.

Alogliptin is minimally dialyzable; over a three-hour hemodialysis session, approximately 7% of the drug was removed. Therefore, hemodialysis is unlikely to be beneficial in an overdose situation. It is not known if NESINA is dialyzable by peritoneal dialysis.

11 DESCRIPTION

NESINA tablets contain the active ingredient alogliptin, which is a selective, orally bioavailable inhibitor of the enzymatic activity of dipeptidyl peptidase-4 (DPP-4).

Chemically, alogliptin is prepared as a benzoate salt, which is identified as 2-({6-[(3R)-3-aminopiperidin-1-yl]-3-methyl-2,4-dioxo-3,4-dihydropyrimidin-1(2H)-yl}methyl)benzonitrile monobenzoate. It has a molecular formula of $C_{18}H_{21}N_5O_2 \cdot C_7H_6O_2$ and a molecular weight of 461.51 daltons. The structural formula is:

Alogliptin benzoate is a white to off-white crystalline powder containing one asymmetric carbon in the aminopiperidine moiety. It is soluble in dimethylsulfoxide, sparingly soluble in water and methanol, slightly soluble in ethanol and very slightly soluble in octanol and isopropyl acetate.

Each NESINA tablet contains 34 mg, 17 mg or 8.5 mg alogliptin benzoate, which is equivalent to 25 mg, 12.5 mg or 6.25 mg, respectively, of alogliptin and the following inactive ingredients: mannitol, microcrystalline cellulose, hydroxypropyl cellulose, croscarmellose sodium and magnesium stearate. In addition, the film coating contains the following inactive ingredients: hypromellose, titanium dioxide, ferric oxide (red or yellow) and polyethylene glycol, and is marked with printing ink (Gray F1).

12 CLINICAL PHARMACOLOGY

12.1 Mechanism of Action

Increased concentrations of the incretin hormones such as glucagon-like peptide-1 (GLP-1) and glucose-dependent insulinotropic polypeptide (GIP) are released into the bloodstream from the small intestine in response to meals. These hormones cause insulin release from the pancreatic beta cells in a glucose-dependent manner but are inactivated by the DPP-4 enzyme within minutes. GLP-1 also lowers glucagon secretion from pancreatic alpha cells, reducing hepatic glucose production. In patients with type 2 diabetes, concentrations of GLP-1 are reduced but the insulin response to GLP-1 is preserved. Alogliptin is a DPP-4 inhibitor that slows the inactivation of the incretin hormones, thereby increasing their bloodstream concentrations and reducing fasting and postprandial glucose concentrations in a glucose-dependent manner in patients with type 2 diabetes mellitus. Alogliptin selectively binds to and inhibits DPP-4 but not DPP-8 or DPP-9 activity in vitro at concentrations approximating therapeutic exposures.

12.2 Pharmacodynamics

Single-dose administration of NESINA to healthy subjects resulted in a peak inhibition of DPP-4 within two to three hours after dosing. The peak inhibition of DPP-4 exceeded 93% across doses of 12.5 mg to 800 mg. Inhibition of DPP-4 remained above 80% at 24 hours for doses greater than or equal to 25 mg. Peak and total exposure over 24 hours to active GLP-1 were three- to four-fold greater with NESINA (at doses of 25 to 200 mg) than placebo. In a 16-week, double-blind, placebo-controlled study, NESINA 25 mg demonstrated decreases in postprandial glucagon while increasing postprandial active GLP-1 levels compared to placebo over an eight-hour period following a standardized meal. It is unclear how these findings relate to changes in overall glycemic control in patients with type 2 diabetes mellitus. In this study, NESINA 25 mg demonstrated decreases in two-hour postprandial glucose compared to placebo (-30 mg/dL versus 17 mg/dL, respectively).

Multiple-dose administration of alogliptin to patients with type 2 diabetes also resulted in a peak inhibition of DPP-4 within one to two hours and exceeded 93% across all doses (25 mg, 100 mg and 400 mg) after a single dose and after 14 days of once-daily dosing. At these doses of NESINA, inhibition of DPP-4 remained above 81% at 24 hours after 14 days of dosing.

Cardiac Electrophysiology

In a randomized, placebo-controlled, four-arm, parallel-group study, 257 subjects were administered either alogliptin 50 mg, alogliptin 400 mg, moxifloxacin 400 mg or placebo once daily for a total of seven days. No increase in QTc was observed with either dose of alogliptin. At the 400 mg dose, peak alogliptin plasma concentrations were 19-fold higher than the peak concentrations following the maximum recommended clinical dose of 25 mg.

12.3 Pharmacokinetics

The pharmacokinetics of NESINA has been studied in healthy subjects and in patients with type 2 diabetes. After administration of single, oral doses up to 800 mg in healthy subjects, the peak plasma alogliptin concentration (median T_{max}) occurred one to two hours after dosing. At the maximum recommended clinical dose of 25 mg, NESINA was eliminated with a mean terminal half-life ($T_{1/2}$) of approximately 21 hours.

After multiple-dose administration up to 400 mg for 14 days in patients with type 2 diabetes, accumulation of alogliptin was minimal with an increase in total (i.e., AUC) and peak (i.e., C_{max}) alogliptin exposures of 34% and 9%, respectively. Total and peak exposure to alogliptin increased proportion-

Table 3. Glycemic Parameters at Week 26 in a Placebo-Controlled Monotherapy Study of NESINA*

	NESINA 25 mg	Placebo
A1C (%)	N=128	N=63
Baseline (mean)	7.9	8.0
Change from baseline (adjusted mean[†])	-0.6	0
Difference from placebo (adjusted mean[†] with 95% confidence interval)	-0.6[‡] (-0.8, -0.3)	-
% of patients (n/N) achieving A1C ≤7%	44% (58/131)[‡]	23% (15/64)
FPG (mg/dL)	N=129	N=64
Baseline (mean)	172	173
Change from baseline (adjusted mean[†])	-16	11
Difference from placebo (adjusted mean[†] with 95% confidence interval)	-28[‡] (-40, -15)	-

* Intent-to-treat population using last observation on study
† Least squares means adjusted for treatment, baseline value, geographic region and duration of diabetes
‡ p<0.01 compared to placebo

Table 4. Glycemic Parameters at Week 26 in an Active-Controlled Study of NESINA, Pioglitazone, and NESINA in Combination with Pioglitazone*

	NESINA 25 mg	Pioglitazone 30 mg	NESINA 25 mg + Pioglitazone 30 mg
A1C (%)	N=160	N=153	N=158
Baseline (mean)	8.8	8.8	8.8
Change from baseline (adjusted mean[†])	-1.0	-1.2	-1.7
Difference from NESINA 25 mg (adjusted mean[†] with 95% confidence interval)	-		-0.8[‡] (-1.0, -0.5)
Difference from pioglitazone 30 mg (adjusted mean[†] with 95% confidence interval)	-		-0.6[‡] (-0.8, -0.3)
% of patients (n/N) achieving A1C ≤7%	24% (40/164)	34% (55/163)	63% (103/164)[‡]
FPG (mg/dL)	N=162	N=157	N=162
Baseline (mean)	189	189	185
Change from baseline (adjusted mean[†])	-26	-37	-50
Difference from NESINA 25 mg (adjusted mean[†] with 95% confidence interval)	-		-24[‡] (-34, -15)
Difference from pioglitazone 30 mg (adjusted mean[†] with 95% confidence interval)	-		-13[‡] (-22, -4)

* Intent-to-treat population using last observation carried forward
† Least squares means adjusted for treatment, geographic region and baseline value
‡ p<0.01 compared to NESINA 25 mg or pioglitazone 30 mg

Table 5. Glycemic Parameters at Week 26 for NESINA and Metformin Alone and in Combination in Patients with Type 2 Diabetes

	Placebo	NESINA 12.5 mg Twice Daily	Metformin HCl 500 mg Twice Daily	Metformin HCl 1000 mg Twice Daily	NESINA 12.5 mg + Metformin HCl 500 mg Twice Daily	NESINA 12.5 mg + Metformin HCl 1000 mg Twice Daily
A1C (%)*	N=102	N=104	N=103	N=108	N=102	N=111
Baseline (mean)	8.5	8.4	8.5	8.4	8.5	8.4
Change from baseline (adjusted mean[†])	0.1	-0.6	-0.7	-1.1	-1.2	-1.6
Difference from metformin (adjusted mean[†] with 95% confidence interval)	-	-	-	-	-0.6[‡] (-0.9, -0.3)	-0.4[‡] (-0.7, -0.2)
Difference from NESINA (adjusted mean[†] with 95% confidence interval)	-	-	-	-	-0.7[‡] (-1.0, -0.4)	-1.0[‡] (-1.3, -0.7)
% of patients (n/N) achieving A1C <7%[§]	4% (4/102)	20% (21/104)	27% (28/103)	34% (37/108)	47%[‡] (48/102)	59%[‡] (66/111)
FPG (mg/dL)*	N=105	N=106	N=106	N=110	N=106	N=112
Baseline (mean)	187	177	180	181	176	185
Change from baseline (adjusted mean[†])	12	-10	-12	-32	-32	-46
Difference from metformin (adjusted mean[†] with 95% confidence interval)	-	-	-	-	-20[‡] (-33, -8)	-14[‡] (-26, -2)
Difference from NESINA (adjusted mean[†] with 95% confidence interval)	-	-	-	-	-22[‡] (-35, -10)	-36[‡] (-49, -24)
2-Hour PPG (mg/dL)[¶]	N=26	N=34	N=28	N=37	N=31	N=37
Baseline (mean)	263	272	247	266	261	268
Change from baseline (adjusted mean[†])	-21	-43	-49	-54	-68	-86[‡]
Difference from metformin (adjusted mean[†] with 95% confidence interval)					-19 (-49, 11)	-32[‡] (-58, -5)
Difference from NESINA (adjusted mean[†] with 95% confidence interval)					-25 (-53, -3)	-43[‡] (-70, -16)

* Intent-to-treat population using last observation on study prior to discontinuation of double-blind study medication or sulfonylurea rescue therapy for patients needing rescue
† Least squares means adjusted for treatment, geographic region and baseline value
‡ p<0.05 when compared to metformin and NESINA alone
§ Compared using logistic regression
¶ Intent-to-treat population using data available at Week 26

ally across single doses and multiple doses of alogliptin ranging from 25 mg to 400 mg. The intersubject coefficient of variation for alogliptin AUC was 17%. The pharmacokinetics of NESINA was also shown to be similar in healthy subjects and in patients with type 2 diabetes.

Absorption
The absolute bioavailability of NESINA is approximately 100%. Administration of NESINA with a high-fat meal results in no significant change in total and peak exposure to alogliptin. NESINA may therefore be administered with or without food.

Distribution
Following a single, 12.5 mg intravenous infusion of alogliptin to healthy subjects, the volume of distribution during the terminal phase was 417 L, indicating that the drug is well distributed into tissues.
Alogliptin is 20% bound to plasma proteins.

Metabolism
Alogliptin does not undergo extensive metabolism and 60% to 71% of the dose is excreted as unchanged drug in the urine.

Two minor metabolites were detected following administration of an oral dose of [^{14}C] alogliptin, N-demethylated, M-I (<1% of the parent compound), and N-acetylated alogliptin, M-II (<6% of the parent compound). M-I is an active metabolite and is an inhibitor of DPP-4 similar to the parent molecule; M-II does not display any inhibitory activity toward DPP-4 or other DPP-related enzymes. In vitro data indicate that CYP2D6 and CYP3A4 contribute to the limited metabolism of alogliptin.
Alogliptin exists predominantly as the (R)-enantiomer (>99%) and undergoes little or no chiral conversion in vivo to the (S)-enantiomer. The (S)-enantiomer is not detectable at the 25 mg dose.

Excretion
The primary route of elimination of [^{14}C] alogliptin-derived radioactivity occurs via renal excretion (76%) with 13% recovered in the feces, achieving a total recovery of 89% of the administered radioactive dose. The renal clearance of alogliptin (9.6 L/hr) indicates some active renal tubular secretion and systemic clearance was 14.0 L/hr.

Specific Populations
Renal Impairment
A single-dose, open-label study was conducted to evaluate the pharmacokinetics of alogliptin 50 mg in patients with chronic renal impairment compared with healthy subjects. In patients with mild renal impairment (creatinine clearance [CrCl] ≥60 to <90 mL/min), an approximate 1.2-fold increase in plasma AUC of alogliptin was observed. Because increases of this magnitude are not considered clinically relevant, dose adjustment for patients with mild renal impairment is not recommended.
In patients with moderate renal impairment (CrCl ≥30 to <60 mL/min), an approximate two-fold increase in plasma AUC of alogliptin was observed. To maintain similar systemic exposures of NESINA to those with normal renal function, the recommended dose is 12.5 mg once daily in patients with moderate renal impairment.
In patients with severe renal impairment (CrCl ≥15 to <30 mL/min) and ESRD (CrCl <15 mL/min or requiring dialysis), an approximate three- and four-fold increase in plasma AUC of alogliptin were observed, respectively. Dialysis removed approximately 7% of the drug during a three-hour dialysis session. NESINA may be administered without regard to the timing of the dialysis. To maintain similar systemic exposures of NESINA to those with normal renal function, the recommended dose is 6.25 mg once daily in patients with severe renal impairment, as well as in patients with ESRD requiring dialysis.

Hepatic Impairment
Total exposure to alogliptin was approximately 10% lower and peak exposure was approximately 8% lower in patients with moderate hepatic impairment (Child-Pugh Grade B) compared to healthy subjects. The magnitude of these reductions is not considered to be clinically meaningful. Patients with severe hepatic impairment (Child-Pugh Grade C) have not been studied. Use caution when administering NESINA to patients with liver disease [see Use in Specific Populations (8.6) and Warnings and Precautions (5.3)].

Gender
No dose adjustment of NESINA is necessary based on gender. Gender did not have any clinically meaningful effect on the pharmacokinetics of alogliptin.

Geriatric
No dose adjustment of NESINA is necessary based on age. Age did not have any clinically meaningful effect on the pharmacokinetics of alogliptin.

Pediatric
Studies characterizing the pharmacokinetics of alogliptin in pediatric patients have not been performed.

Race
No dose adjustment of NESINA is necessary based on race. Race (White, Black, and Asian) did not have any clinically meaningful effect on the pharmacokinetics of alogliptin.

Drug Interactions
In Vitro Assessment of Drug Interactions
In vitro studies indicate that alogliptin is neither an inducer of CYP1A2, CYP2B6, CYP2C9, CYP2C19 and CYP3A4, nor an inhibitor of CYP1A2, CYP2C8, CYP2C9, CYP2C19, CYP3A4 and CYP2D6 at clinically relevant concentrations.
In Vivo Assessment of Drug Interactions
Effects of Alogliptin on the Pharmacokinetics of Other Drugs
In clinical studies, alogliptin did not meaningfully increase the systemic exposure to the following drugs that are metabolized by CYP isozymes or excreted unchanged in urine (Figure 1). No dose adjustment of NESINA is recommended based on results of the described pharmacokinetic studies.
[See figure 1 at top of page 2286]
Effects of Other Drugs on the Pharmacokinetics of Alogliptin
There are no clinically meaningful changes in the pharmacokinetics of alogliptin when NESINA is administered concomitantly with the drugs described below (Figure 2).
[See figure 2 on page 2286]

13 NONCLINICAL TOXICOLOGY
13.1 Carcinogenesis, Mutagenesis, Impairment of Fertility
Rats were administered oral doses of 75, 400 and 800 mg/kg alogliptin for two years. No drug-related tumors were observed up to 75 mg/kg or approximately 32 times the maximum recommended clinical dose of 25 mg, based on AUC exposure. At higher doses (approximately 308 times the maximum recommended clinical dose of 25 mg), a combination of thyroid C-cell adenomas and carcinomas increased in male but not female rats. No drug-related tumors were observed in mice after administration of 50, 150 or 300 mg/kg alogliptin for two years, or up to approximately 51 times the maximum recommended clinical dose of 25 mg, based on AUC exposure.
Alogliptin was not mutagenic or clastogenic, with and without metabolic activation, in the Ames test with S. typhimurium and E. coli or the cytogenetic assay in mouse lymphoma cells. Alogliptin was negative in the in vivo mouse micronucleus study.

In a fertility study in rats, alogliptin had no adverse effects on early embryonic development, mating or fertility at doses up to 500 mg/kg, or approximately 172 times the clinical dose based on plasma drug exposure (AUC).

14 CLINICAL STUDIES

NESINA has been studied as monotherapy and in combination with metformin, a sulfonylurea, a thiazolidinedione (either alone or in combination with metformin or a sulfonylurea) and insulin (either alone or in combination with metformin).

A total of 8673 patients with type 2 diabetes were randomized in 10 double-blind, placebo- or active-controlled clinical safety and efficacy studies conducted to evaluate the effects of NESINA on glycemic control. The racial distribution of patients exposed to study medication was 68% Caucasian, 15% Asian, 7% Black and 9% other racial groups. The ethnic distribution was 30% Hispanic. Patients had an overall mean age of 55 years (range 21 to 80 years).

In patients with type 2 diabetes, treatment with NESINA produced clinically meaningful and statistically significant improvements in A1C compared to placebo. As is typical for trials of agents to treat type 2 diabetes, the mean reduction in A1C with NESINA appears to be related to the degree of A1C elevation at baseline.

NESINA had similar changes from baseline in serum lipids compared to placebo.

14.1 Patients with Inadequate Glycemic Control on Diet and Exercise

A total of 1768 patients with type 2 diabetes participated in three double-blind studies to evaluate the efficacy and safety of NESINA in patients with inadequate glycemic control on diet and exercise. All three studies had a four-week, single-blind, placebo run-in period followed by a 26-week randomized treatment period. Patients who failed to meet prespecified hyperglycemic goals during the 26-week treatment periods received glycemic rescue therapy.

In a 26-week, double-blind, placebo-controlled study, a total of 329 patients (mean baseline A1C = 8%) were randomized to receive NESINA 12.5 mg, NESINA 25 mg or placebo once daily. Treatment with NESINA 25 mg resulted in statistically significant improvements from baseline in A1C and fasting plasma glucose (FPG) compared to placebo at Week 26 *(Table 3)*. A total of 8% of patients receiving NESINA 25 mg and 30% of those receiving placebo required glycemic rescue therapy.

Improvements in A1C were not affected by gender, age or baseline BMI.

The mean change in body weight with NESINA was similar to placebo.

[See table 3 at top of page 2287]

In a 26-week, double-blind, active-controlled study, a total of 655 patients (mean baseline A1C = 8.8%) were randomized to receive NESINA 25 mg alone, pioglitazone 30 mg alone, NESINA 12.5 mg with pioglitazone 30 mg or NESINA 25 mg with pioglitazone 30 mg once daily. Coadministration of NESINA 25 mg with pioglitazone 30 mg resulted in statistically significant improvements from baseline in A1C and FPG compared to NESINA 25 mg alone and to pioglitazone 30 mg alone *(Table 4)*. A total of 3% of patients receiving NESINA 25 mg coadministered with pioglitazone 30 mg, 11% of those receiving NESINA 25 mg alone and 6% of those receiving pioglitazone 30 mg alone required glycemic rescue.

Improvements in A1C were not affected by gender, age or baseline BMI.

The mean increase in body weight was similar between pioglitazone alone and NESINA when coadministered with pioglitazone.

[See table 4 at top of page 2287]

In a 26-week, double-blind, placebo-controlled study, a total of 784 patients inadequately controlled on diet and exercise alone (mean baseline A1C = 8.4%) were randomized to one of seven treatment groups: placebo; metformin HCl 500 mg or metformin HCl 1000 mg twice daily; NESINA 12.5 mg twice daily; NESINA 25 mg daily; or NESINA 12.5 mg in combination with metformin HCl 500 mg or metformin HCl 1000 mg twice daily. Both coadministration treatment arms (NESINA 12.5 mg + metformin HCl 500 mg and NESINA 12.5 mg + metformin HCl 1000 mg) resulted in statistically significant improvements in A1C and FPG when compared with their respective individual alogliptin and metformin component regimens *(Table 5)*. Coadministration treatment arms demonstrated improvements in two-hour postprandial glucose (PPG) compared to NESINA alone or metformin alone *(Table 5)*. A total of 12.3% of patients receiving NESINA 12.5 mg + metformin HCl 500 mg, 2.6% of patients receiving NESINA 12.5 mg + metformin HCl 1000 mg, 17.3% of patients receiving NESINA 12.5 mg, 22.9% of patients receiving metformin HCl 500 mg, 10.8% of patients receiving metformin HCl 1000 mg and 38.7% of patients receiving placebo required glycemic rescue.

Improvements in A1C were not affected by gender, age, race or baseline BMI. The mean decrease in body weight was similar between metformin alone and NESINA when coadministered with metformin.

Table 6. Glycemic Parameters at Week 26 in a Placebo-Controlled Study of NESINA as Add-On Therapy to Metformin*

	NESINA 25 mg + Metformin	Placebo + Metformin
A1C (%)	N=203	N=103
Baseline (mean)	7.9	8.0
Change from baseline (adjusted mean†)	-0.6	-0.1
Difference from placebo (adjusted mean† with 95% confidence interval)	-0.5‡ (-0.7, -0.3)	-
% of patients (n/N) achieving A1C ≤7%	44% (92/207)‡	18% (19/104)
FPG (mg/dL)	N=204	N=104
Baseline (mean)	172	180
Change from baseline (adjusted mean†)	-17	0
Difference from placebo (adjusted mean† with 95% confidence interval)	-17‡ (-26, -9)	-

* Intent-to-treat population using last observation on study
† Least squares means adjusted for treatment, baseline value, geographic region and baseline metformin dose
‡ p<0.001 compared to placebo

[See table 5 at top of previous page]

14.2 Combination Therapy
Add-On Therapy to Metformin

A total of 2081 patients with type 2 diabetes participated in two 26-week, double-blind, placebo-controlled studies to evaluate the efficacy and safety of NESINA as add-on therapy to metformin. In both studies, patients were inadequately controlled on metformin at a dose of at least 1500 mg per day or at the maximum tolerated dose. All patients entered a four-week, single-blind placebo run-in period prior to randomization. Patients who failed to meet prespecified hyperglycemic goals during the 26-week treatment periods received glycemic rescue therapy.

In the first 26-week, placebo-controlled study, a total of 527 patients already on metformin (mean baseline A1C = 8%) were randomized to receive NESINA 12.5 mg, NESINA 25 mg or placebo. Patients were maintained on a stable dose of metformin (median dose = 1700 mg) during the treatment period. NESINA 25 mg in combination with metformin resulted in statistically significant improvements from baseline in A1C and FPG at Week 26, when compared to placebo *(Table 6)*. A total of 8% of patients receiving NESINA 25 mg and 24% of patients receiving placebo required glycemic rescue.

Improvements in A1C were not affected by gender, age, baseline BMI or baseline metformin dose.

The mean decrease in body weight was similar between NESINA and placebo when given in combination with metformin.

[See table 6 above]

In the second 26-week, double-blind, placebo-controlled study, a total of 1554 patients already on metformin (mean baseline A1C = 8.5%) were randomized to one of 12 double-blind treatment groups: placebo; 12.5 mg or 25 mg of NESINA alone; 15 mg, 30 mg or 45 mg of pioglitazone alone; or 12.5 mg or 25 mg of NESINA in combination with 15 mg, 30 mg or 45 mg of pioglitazone. Patients were maintained on a stable dose of metformin (median dose = 1700 mg) during the treatment period. Coadministration of NESINA and pioglitazone provided statistically significant improvements in A1C and FPG compared to placebo, to NESINA alone or to pioglitazone alone when added to background metformin therapy *(Table 7, Figure 3)*. In addition, improvements from baseline A1C were comparable between NESINA alone and pioglitazone alone (15 mg, 30 mg and 45 mg) at Week 26. A total of 4%, 5% or 2% of patients receiving NESINA 25 mg with 15 mg, 30 mg or 45 mg pioglitazone, 33% of patients receiving placebo, 13% of patients receiving NESINA 25 mg and 10%, 15% or 9% of patients receiving pioglitazone 15 mg, 30 mg or 45 mg alone required glycemic rescue.

Improvements in A1C were not affected by gender, age or baseline BMI.

The mean increase in body weight was similar between pioglitazone alone and NESINA when coadministered with pioglitazone.

[See table 7 at top of next page]
[See figure 3 at top of next column]

Add-On Therapy to a Thiazolidinedione

In a 26-week, placebo-controlled study, a total of 493 patients inadequately controlled on a thiazolidinedione alone or in combination with metformin or a sulfonylurea (10 mg) (mean baseline A1C = 8%) were randomized to receive NESINA 12.5 mg, NESINA 25 mg or placebo. Patients were maintained on a stable dose of pioglitazone (median dose =

Figure 3. Change from Baseline in A1C at Week 26 with NESINA and Pioglitazone Alone and NESINA in Combination with Pioglitazone When Added to Metformin

Intent-to-treat population using last observation on study.
*P≤0.001 compared to corresponding doses of NESINA alone or Pioglitazone alone.

30 mg) during the treatment period; those who were also previously treated on metformin (median dose = 2000 mg) or sulfonylurea (median dose = 10 mg) prior to randomization were maintained on the combination therapy during the treatment period. All patients entered into a four-week, single-blind placebo run-in period prior to randomization. Patients who failed to meet prespecified hyperglycemic goals during the 26-week treatment period received glycemic rescue therapy.

The addition of NESINA 25 mg once daily to pioglitazone therapy resulted in statistically significant improvements from baseline in A1C and FPG at Week 26, compared to placebo *(Table 8)*. A total of 9% of patients who were receiving NESINA 25 mg and 12% of patients receiving placebo required glycemic rescue.

Improvements in A1C were not affected by gender, age, baseline BMI or baseline metformin dose.

Clinically meaningful reductions in A1C were observed with NESINA compared to placebo regardless of whether subjects were receiving concomitant metformin or sulfonylurea (-0.2% placebo versus -0.9% NESINA) therapy or pioglitazone alone (0% placebo versus -0.52% NESINA).

The mean increase in body weight was similar between NESINA and placebo when given in combination with pioglitazone.

[See table 8 at top of page 2291]

Add-on Combination Therapy with Pioglitazone and Metformin

In a 52-week, active-comparator study, a total of 803 patients inadequately controlled (mean baseline A1C = 8.2%) on a current regimen of pioglitazone 30 mg and metformin at least 1500 mg per day or at the maximum tolerated dose were randomized to either receive the addition of NESINA 25 mg or the titration of pioglitazone 30 mg to 45 mg following a four-week, single-blind placebo run-in period. Patients were maintained on a stable dose of metformin (median dose = 1700 mg). Patients who failed to meet prespecified hyperglycemic goals during the 52-week treatment period received glycemic rescue therapy.

In combination with pioglitazone and metformin, NESINA 25 mg was shown to be statistically superior in lowering A1C and FPG compared with the titration of pioglitazone from 30 mg to 45 mg at Week 26 and at Week 52 *(Table 9; results shown only for Week 52)*. A total of 11% of patients in the NESINA 25 mg treatment group and 22% of patients in the pioglitazone up-titration group required glycemic rescue.

Table 7. Glycemic Parameters in a 26-Week Study of NESINA, Pioglitazone and NESINA in Combination with Pioglitazone when Added to Metformin*

	Placebo	NESINA 25 mg	Pioglitazone 15 mg	Pioglitazone 30 mg	Pioglitazone 45 mg	NESINA 25 mg + Pioglitazone 15 mg	NESINA 25 mg + Pioglitazone 30 mg	NESINA 25 mg + Pioglitazone 45 mg
A1C (%)	N=126	N=123	N=127	N=123	N=126	N=127	N=124	N=126
Baseline (mean)	8.5	8.6	8.5	8.5	8.5	8.5	8.5	8.6
Change from baseline (adjusted mean†)	-0.1	-0.9	-0.8	-0.9	-1.0	-1.3‡	-1.4‡	-1.6‡
Difference from pioglitazone (adjusted mean† with 95% confidence interval)	-	-	-	-	-	-0.5‡ (-0.7, -0.3)	-0.5‡ (-0.7, -0.3)	-0.6‡ (-0.8, -0.4)
Difference from NESINA (adjusted mean† with 95% confidence interval)	-	-	-	-	-	-0.4‡ (-0.6, -0.1)	-0.5‡ (-0.7, -0.3)	-0.7‡ (-0.9, -0.5)
Patients (%) achieving A1C ≤7%	6% (8/129)	27% (35/129)	26% (33/129)	30% (38/129)	36% (47/129)	55% (71/130)‡	53% (69/130)‡	60% (78/130)‡
FPG (mg/dL)	N=129	N=126	N=127	N=125	N=129	N=130	N=126	N=127
Baseline (mean)	177	184	177	175	181	179	179	178
Change from baseline (adjusted mean†)	7	-19	-24	-29	-32	-38‡	-42‡	-53‡
Difference from pioglitazone (adjusted mean† with 95% confidence interval)	-	-	-	-	-	-14‡ (-24, -5)	-13‡ (-23, -3)	-20‡ (-30, -11)
Difference from NESINA (adjusted mean† with 95% confidence interval)	-	-	-	-	-	-19‡ (-29, -10)	-23‡ (-33, -13)	-34‡ (-44, -24)

* Intent-to-treat population using last observation on study
† Least squares means adjusted for treatment, geographic region, metformin dose and baseline value
‡ p≤0.01 when compared to corresponding doses of pioglitazone and NESINA alone

Improvements in A1C were not affected by gender, age, race or baseline BMI.
The mean increase in body weight was similar in both treatment arms.
[See table 9 at top of next page]

Add-On Therapy to a Sulfonylurea
In a 26-week, placebo-controlled study, a total of 500 patients inadequately controlled on a sulfonylurea (mean baseline A1C = 8.1%) were randomized to receive NESINA 12.5 mg, NESINA 25 mg or placebo. Patients were maintained on a stable dose of glyburide (median dose = 10 mg) during the treatment period. All patients entered into a four-week, single-blind, placebo run-in period prior to randomization. Patients who failed to meet prespecified hyperglycemic goals during the 26-week treatment period received glycemic rescue therapy.
The addition of NESINA 25 mg to glyburide therapy resulted in statistically significant improvements from base-

line in A1C at Week 26 when compared to placebo (Table 10). Improvements in FPG observed with NESINA 25 mg were not statistically significant compared with placebo. A total of 16% of patients receiving NESINA 25 mg and 28% of those receiving placebo required glycemic rescue.
Improvements in A1C were not affected by gender, age, baseline BMI or baseline glyburide dose.
The mean change in body weight was similar between NESINA and placebo when given in combination with glyburide.
[See table 10 at top of page 2292]

Add-On Therapy to Insulin
In a 26-week, placebo-controlled study, a total of 390 patients inadequately controlled on insulin alone (42%) or in combination with metformin (58%) (mean baseline A1C = 9.3%) were randomized to receive NESINA 12.5 mg, NESINA 25 mg or placebo. Patients were maintained on their insulin regimen (median dose = 55 IU) upon random-

ization and those previously treated with insulin in combination with metformin (median dose = 1700 mg) prior to randomization continued on the combination regimen during the treatment period. Patients entered the trial on short-, intermediate- or long-acting (basal) insulin or premixed insulin. Patients who failed to meet prespecified hyperglycemic goals during the 26-week treatment period received glycemic rescue therapy.
The addition of NESINA 25 mg once daily to insulin therapy resulted in statistically significant improvements from baseline in A1C and FPG at Week 26, when compared to placebo (Table 11). A total of 20% of patients receiving NESINA 25 mg and 40% of those receiving placebo required glycemic rescue.
Improvements in A1C were not affected by gender, age, baseline BMI or baseline insulin dose. Clinically meaningful reductions in A1C were observed with NESINA compared to placebo regardless of whether subjects were receiving concomitant metformin and insulin (-0.2% placebo versus -0.8% NESINA) therapy or insulin alone (0.1% placebo versus -0.7% NESINA).
The mean increase in body weight was similar between NESINA and placebo when given in combination with insulin.
[See table 11 at top of page 2292]

16   HOW SUPPLIED/STORAGE AND HANDLING

NESINA tablets are available as film-coated tablets containing 25 mg, 12.5 mg or 6.25 mg of alogliptin as follows:
25 mg tablet: light red, oval, biconvex, film-coated, with "TAK ALG-25" printed on one side, available in:

NDC 64764-250-30	Bottles of 30 tablets
NDC 64764-250-90	Bottles of 90 tablets
NDC 64764-250-50	Bottles of 500 tablets

12.5 mg tablet: yellow, oval, biconvex, film-coated, with "TAK ALG-12.5" printed on one side, available in:

NDC 64764-125-30	Bottles of 30 tablets
NDC 64764-125-90	Bottles of 90 tablets
NDC 64764-125-50	Bottles of 500 tablets

6.25 mg tablet: light pink, oval, biconvex, film-coated, with "TAK ALG-6.25" printed on one side, available in:

NDC 64764-625-30	Bottles of 30 tablets
NDC 64764-625-90	Bottles of 90 tablets

Storage
Store at 25°C (77°F); excursions permitted to 15° to 30°C (59° to 86°F) [see USP Controlled Room Temperature].

17   PATIENT COUNSELING INFORMATION
See FDA-Approved Patient Labeling (Medication Guide)
17.1   Instructions
Inform patients of the potential risks and benefits of NESINA.
Patients should be informed that acute pancreatitis has been reported during use of NESINA. Patients should be informed that persistent, severe abdominal pain, sometimes radiating to the back, which may or may not be accompanied by vomiting, is the hallmark symptom of acute pancreatitis. Patients should be instructed to promptly discontinue NESINA and contact their physician if persistent severe abdominal pain occurs.
Patients should be informed that allergic reactions have been reported during use of NESINA. If symptoms of allergic reactions (including skin rash, hives and swelling of the face, lips, tongue and throat that may cause difficulty in breathing or swallowing) occur, patients should be instructed to discontinue NESINA and seek medical advice promptly.
Patients should be informed that postmarketing reports of liver injury, sometimes fatal, have been reported during use of NESINA. If signs or symptoms of liver injury occur, patients should be instructed to discontinue NESINA and seek medical advice promptly.
Inform patients that hypoglycemia can occur, particularly when an insulin secretagogue or insulin is used in combination with NESINA. Explain the risks, symptoms and appropriate management of hypoglycemia.
Instruct patients to take NESINA only as prescribed. If a dose is missed, advise patients not to double their next dose. Instruct patients to read the Medication Guide before starting NESINA therapy and to reread each time the prescription is refilled. Instruct patients to inform their healthcare provider if an unusual symptom develops or if a symptom persists or worsens.
Revised: June 2013
NES011 R3

MEDICATION GUIDE
NESINA (nes-see'-na)
(alogliptin)
tablets

Read this Medication Guide carefully before you start taking NESINA and each time you get a refill. There may be new information. This information does not take the place of talking with your doctor about your medical condition or treatment. If you have any questions about NESINA, ask your doctor or pharmacist.

What is the most important information I should know about NESINA?

Serious side effects can happen to people taking NESINA, including inflammation of the pancreas (pancreatitis), which may be severe.

Certain medical conditions make you more likely to get pancreatitis.

Before you start taking NESINA:

Tell your doctor if you have ever had:
- pancreatitis
- stones in your gallbladder (gallstones)
- a history of alcoholism
- kidney problems
- liver problems

Stop taking NESINA and call your doctor right away if you have pain in your stomach area (abdomen) that is severe and will not go away. The pain may be felt going from your abdomen through to your back. The pain may happen with or without vomiting. These may be symptoms of pancreatitis.

What is NESINA?
- NESINA is a prescription medicine used along with diet and exercise to improve blood sugar (glucose) control in adults with type 2 diabetes.
- NESINA is unlikely by itself to cause your blood sugar to be lowered to a dangerous level (hypoglycemia). However, hypoglycemia may still occur with NESINA.
- NESINA is not for people with type 1 diabetes.
- NESINA is not for people with diabetic ketoacidosis (increased ketones in blood or urine).

It is not known if NESINA is safe and effective in children under the age of 18.

Who should not take NESINA?

Do not take NESINA if you:
- Are allergic to any ingredients in NESINA or have had a serious allergic (hypersensitivity) reaction to NESINA. See the end of this Medication Guide for a complete list of the ingredients in NESINA.
- Symptoms of a serious allergic reaction to NESINA may include:
  ◦ swelling of your face, lips, throat and other areas on your skin
  ◦ difficulty with swallowing or breathing
  ◦ raised, red areas on your skin (hives)
  ◦ skin rash, itching, flaking or peeling

If you have any of these symptoms, stop taking NESINA and contact your doctor or go to the nearest hospital emergency room right away.

What should I tell my doctor before and during treatment with NESINA?

Before you take NESINA, tell your doctor if you:
- have or have had inflammation of your pancreas (pancreatitis)
- have kidney or liver problems
- have other medical conditions
- are pregnant or plan to become pregnant. It is not known if NESINA can harm your unborn baby. Talk with your doctor about the best way to control your blood sugar while you are pregnant or if you plan to become pregnant
- are breastfeeding or plan to breastfeed. It is not known whether NESINA passes into your breast milk. Talk with your doctor about the best way to feed your baby if you are taking NESINA

Tell your doctor about all the medicines you take, including prescription and nonprescription medicines, vitamins and herbal supplements.

Know the medicines you take. Keep a list of them and show it to your doctor and pharmacist before you start any new medicine.

NESINA may affect the way other medicines work, and other medicines may affect how NESINA works. Contact your doctor before you start or stop other types of medicines.

How should I take NESINA?
- Take NESINA exactly as your doctor tells you to take it.
- Take NESINA 1 time each day with or without food.
- If you miss a dose, take it as soon as you remember. If you do not remember until it is time for your next dose, skip the missed dose, and take the next dose at your regular time. **Do not** take 2 doses of NESINA at the same time
- If you take too much NESINA, call your doctor or go to the nearest hospital emergency room right away
- If your body is under stress, such as from fever, infection, accident or surgery, the dose of your diabetes medicines may need to be changed. Call your doctor right away

Table 8. Glycemic Parameters in a 26-Week, Placebo-Controlled Study of NESINA as Add-On Therapy to Pioglitazone*

	NESINA 25 mg + Pioglitazone ± Metformin ± Sulfonylurea	Placebo + Pioglitazone ± Metformin ± Sulfonylurea
A1C (%)	N=195	N=95
Baseline (mean)	8	8
Change from baseline (adjusted mean[†])	-0.8	-0.2
Difference from placebo (adjusted mean[†] with 95% confidence interval)	-0.6[‡] (-0.8, -0.4)	-
% of patients (n/N) achieving A1C ≤7%	49% (98/199)[‡]	34% (33/97)
FPG (mg/dL)	N=197	N=97
Baseline (mean)	170	172
Change from baseline (adjusted mean[†])	-20	-6
Difference from placebo (adjusted mean[†] with 95% confidence interval)	-14[‡] (-23, -5)	-

* Intent-to-treat population using last observation on study
† Least squares means adjusted for treatment, baseline value, geographic region, baseline treatment regimen (pioglitazone, pioglitazone + metformin or pioglitazone + sulfonylurea) and baseline pioglitazone dose
‡ p<0.01 compared to placebo

Table 9. Glycemic Parameters in a 52-Week, Controlled Study of NESINA as Add-On Combination Therapy with Pioglitazone and Metformin*

	NESINA 25 mg + Pioglitazone 30 mg + Metformin	Pioglitazone 45 mg + Metformin
A1C (%)	N=397	N=394
Baseline (mean)	8.2	8.1
Change from baseline (adjusted mean[†])	-0.7	-0.3
Difference from pioglitazone 45 mg + metformin (adjusted mean[†] with 95% confidence interval)	-0.4[‡] (-0.5, -0.3)	-
% of patients (n/N) achieving A1C≤7%	33% (134/404)[§]	21% (85/399)
Fasting Plasma Glucose (mg/dL)	N=399	N=396
Baseline (mean)	162	162
Change from baseline (adjusted mean[†])	-15	-4
Difference from pioglitazone 45 mg + metformin (adjusted mean[†] with 95% confidence interval)	-11[§] (-16, -6)	-

* Intent-to-treat population using last observation on study
† Least squares means adjusted for treatment, baseline value, geographic region and baseline metformin dose.
‡ Noninferior and statistically superior to metformin + pioglitazone at the 0.025 one-sided significance level
§ p<0.001 compared to pioglitazone 45 mg + metformin

- Stay on your diet and exercise programs and check your blood sugar as your doctor tells you to
- Your doctor may do certain blood tests before you start NESINA and during treatment as needed. Your doctor may change your dose of NESINA based on the results of your blood tests due to how well your kidneys are working
- Your doctor will check your diabetes with regular blood tests, including your blood sugar levels and your hemoglobin A1C

What are the possible side effects of NESINA?

NESINA can cause serious side effects, including:

See "What is the most important information I should know about NESINA?"
- **Allergic (hypersensitivity) reactions** such as:
  ◦ swelling of your face, lips, throat and other areas on your skin
  ◦ difficulty with swallowing or breathing
  ◦ raised, red areas on your skin (hives)
  ◦ skin rash, itching, flaking or peeling

If you have these symptoms, stop taking NESINA and contact your doctor right away.
- **Liver problems.** Call your doctor right away if you have unexplained symptoms, such as:
  ◦ nausea or vomiting
  ◦ stomach pain
  ◦ unusual or unexplained tiredness
  ◦ loss of appetite
  ◦ dark urine
  ◦ yellowing of your skin or the whites of your eyes
- **Low blood sugar (hypoglycemia).** If you take NESINA with another medicine that can cause low blood sugar, such as a sulfonylurea or insulin, your risk of getting low blood sugar is higher. The dose of your sulfonylurea medicine or insulin may need to be lowered while you take NESINA. If you have symptoms of low blood sugar, you should check your blood sugar and treat if low, then call your doctor. Signs and symptoms of low blood sugar include:

- shaking or feeling jittery
- sweating
- hunger
- headache
- change in mood
- fast heartbeat
- change in vision
- confusion
- dizziness

The most common side effects of NESINA include:
- stuffy or runny nose and sore throat
- headache
- cold-like symptoms (upper respiratory tract infection)

Tell your doctor if you have any side effect that bothers you or that does not go away.

Table 10. Glycemic Parameters in a 26-Week, Placebo-Controlled Study of NESINA as Add-On Therapy to Glyburide*

	NESINA 25 mg + Glyburide	Placebo + Glyburide
A1C (%)	N=197	N=97
Baseline (mean)	8.1	8.2
Change from baseline (adjusted mean[†])	-0.5	0
Difference from placebo (adjusted mean[†] with 95% confidence interval)	-0.5[‡] (-0.7, -0.3)	-
% of patients (n/N) achieving A1C ≤7%	35% (69/198)[‡]	18% (18/99)
FPG (mg/dL)	N=198	N=99
Baseline (mean)	174	177
Change from baseline (adjusted mean[†])	-8	2
Difference from placebo (adjusted mean[†] with 95% confidence interval)	-11 (-22, 1)	-

* Intent-to-treat population using last observation on study
† Least squares means adjusted for treatment, baseline value, geographic region and baseline glyburide dose
‡ p<0.01 compared to placebo

Table 11. Glycemic Parameters in a 26-Week, Placebo-Controlled Study of NESINA as Add-On Therapy to Insulin*

	NESINA 25 mg + Insulin ± Metformin	Placebo + Insulin ± Metformin
A1C (%)	N=126	N=126
Baseline (mean)	9.3	9.3
Change from baseline (adjusted mean[†])	-0.7	-0.1
Difference from placebo (adjusted mean[‡] with 95% confidence interval)	-0.6[‡] (-0.8, -0.4)	-
% of patients (n/N) achieving A1C ≤7%	8% (10/129)	1% (1/129)
FPG (mg/dL)	N=128	N=127
Baseline (mean)	186	196
Change from baseline (adjusted mean[†])	-12	6
Difference from placebo (adjusted mean[†] with 95% confidence interval)	-18[‡] (-33, -2)	-

* Intent-to-treat population using last observation on study
† Least squares means adjusted for treatment, baseline value, geographic region, baseline treatment regimen (insulin or insulin + metformin) and baseline daily insulin dose
‡ p<0.05 compared to placebo

These are not all the possible side effects of NESINA. For more information, ask your doctor or pharmacist.

Call your doctor for medical advice about side effects. You may report side effects to FDA at 1-800-FDA-1088.

How should I store NESINA?
Store NESINA at room temperature between 68°F to 77°F (20°C to 25°C).

Keep NESINA and all medicines out of the reach of children.

General information about the safe and effective use of NESINA
Medicines are sometimes prescribed for purposes other than those listed in the Medication Guide. Do not take NESINA for a condition for which it was not prescribed. Do not give NESINA to other people, even if they have the same symptoms you have. It may harm them.

This Medication Guide summarizes the most important information about NESINA. If you would like to know more information, talk with your doctor. You can ask your doctor or pharmacist for information about NESINA that is written for health professionals.

For more information go to www.NESINA.com or call 1-877-TAKEDA-7 (1-877-825-3327).

What are the ingredients in NESINA?
Active ingredient: alogliptin
Inactive ingredients: mannitol, microcrystalline cellulose, hydroxypropyl cellulose, croscarmellose sodium and magnesium stearate. In addition, the film-coating contains the following inactive ingredients: hypromellose, titanium dioxide, ferric oxide (red or yellow) and polyethylene glycol and is marked with gray F1 printing ink

This Medication Guide has been approved by the U.S. Food and Drug Administration.

Distributed by:
Takeda Pharmaceuticals America, Inc.
Deerfield, IL 60015
Revised: June 2013
NESINA is a trademark of Takeda Pharmaceutical Company Limited registered with the U.S. Patent and Trademark Office and is used under license by Takeda Pharmaceuticals America, Inc.
© 2013 Takeda Pharmaceuticals America, Inc.
NES011 R3
Shown in Product Identification Guide, page 314

OSENI
(alogliptin and pioglitazone)
tablets   ℞

HIGHLIGHTS OF PRESCRIBING INFORMATION
These highlights do not include all the information needed to use OSENI safely and effectively. See full prescribing information for OSENI.
OSENI (alogliptin and pioglitazone) tablets
Initial U.S. Approval: 2013

WARNING: CONGESTIVE HEART FAILURE
See full prescribing information for complete boxed warning
- **Thiazolidinediones, including pioglitazone, cause or exacerbate congestive heart failure in some patients. (5.1)**
- **After initiation of OSENI and after dose increases, monitor patients carefully for signs and symptoms of heart failure (e.g., excessive, rapid weight gain, dyspnea and/or edema). If heart failure develops, it**

---

should be managed according to current standards of care and discontinuation or dose reduction of pioglitazone in OSENI must be considered.
- **OSENI is not recommended in patients with symptomatic heart failure.**
- **Initiation of OSENI in patients with established New York Heart Association (NYHA) Class III or IV heart failure is contraindicated. (4, 5.1)**

——INDICATIONS AND USAGE——
OSENI is a dipeptidyl peptidase-4 inhibitor and thiazolidinedione combination product indicated as an adjunct to diet and exercise to improve glycemic control in adults with type 2 diabetes mellitus. (1.1)
Limitation of Use: Not for treatment of type 1 diabetes or diabetic ketoacidosis. (1.2)

——DOSAGE AND ADMINISTRATION——
- Individualize the starting dose of OSENI based on the patient's current regimen and concurrent medical condition but do not exceed a daily dose of alogliptin 25 mg and pioglitazone 45 mg.
- Can be taken with or without food. (2.1)
- Limit initial dose of pioglitazone to 15 mg once daily in patients with NYHA Class I or II heart failure. (2.1)
- Adjust dose if moderate renal impairment. (2.2)

Degree of Renal Impairment	Creatinine Clearance (mL/min)	Recommended Dosing
Moderate	≥30 to <60	12.5 mg/15 mg, 12.5 mg/30 mg or 12.5 mg/45 mg once daily

- OSENI is not recommended for patients with severe renal impairment or end-stage renal disease (ESRD) requiring dialysis. (2.2)
- The maximum recommended dose of pioglitazone is 15 mg once daily in patients taking strong CYP2C8 inhibitors (e.g., gemfibrozil). (2.3, 7.1)

——DOSAGE FORMS AND STRENGTHS——
Tablets:
25 mg alogliptin and 15 mg pioglitazone, 25 mg alogliptin and 30 mg pioglitazone, 25 mg alogliptin and 45 mg pioglitazone. (3)
12.5 mg alogliptin and 15 mg pioglitazone, 12.5 mg alogliptin and 30 mg pioglitazone, 12.5 mg alogliptin and 45 mg pioglitazone. (3)

——CONTRAINDICATIONS——
- History of a serious hypersensitivity reaction to alogliptin or pioglitazone, components of OSENI, such as anaphylaxis, angioedema or severe cutaneous adverse reactions. (4)
- Do not initiate OSENI in patients with established NYHA Class III or IV heart failure. (4)

——WARNINGS AND PRECAUTIONS——
- Congestive heart failure: Fluid retention may occur and can exacerbate or lead to congestive heart failure. Combination use with insulin and in congestive heart failure NYHA Class I and II may increase risk. Monitor patients for signs and symptoms. (5.1)
- Acute pancreatitis: There have been postmarketing reports of acute pancreatitis. If pancreatitis is suspected, promptly discontinue OSENI. (5.2)
- Hypersensitivity: There have been postmarketing reports of serious hypersensitivity reactions in patients treated with alogliptin such as anaphylaxis, angioedema and severe cutaneous adverse reactions. In such cases, promptly discontinue OSENI, assess for other potential causes, institute appropriate monitoring and treatment and initiate alternative treatment for diabetes. (5.3)
- Hepatic effects: Postmarketing reports of hepatic failure, sometimes fatal. Causality cannot be excluded. If liver injury is detected, promptly interrupt OSENI and assess patient for probable cause, then treat cause if possible, to resolution or stabilization. Do not restart OSENI if liver injury is confirmed and no alternative etiology can be found. Use with caution in patients with liver disease. (5.4)
- Edema: Dose-related edema may occur. (5.5)
- Fractures: Increased incidence in female patients. Apply current standards of care for assessing and maintaining bone health. (5.6)
- Bladder cancer: Preclinical and clinical trial data, and results from an observational study suggest an increased risk of bladder cancer in pioglitazone users. The observational data further suggest that the risk increases with duration of use. Do not use in patients with active bladder cancer. Use caution when using in patients with a prior history of bladder cancer. (5.7)

- Hypoglycemia: When an insulin secretagogue (e.g., sulfonylurea) or insulin is used in combination with OSENI, a lower dose of insulin secretagogue or insulin may be required to minimize the risk of hypoglycemia. (5.8)
- Macular edema: Postmarketing reports. Recommend regular eye exams in all patients with diabetes according to current standards of care with prompt evaluation for acute visual changes. (5.9)
- Macrovascular outcomes: There have been no clinical studies establishing conclusive evidence of macrovascular risk reduction with OSENI or any other antidiabetic drug. (5.11)

——————ADVERSE REACTIONS——————

Common adverse reactions reported in ≥4% of patients treated with coadministration of alogliptin 25 mg and pioglitazone 15 mg, 30 mg or 45 mg were nasopharyngitis, back pain and upper respiratory tract infection. (6.1)

To report SUSPECTED ADVERSE REACTIONS, contact Takeda Pharmaceuticals at 1-877-TAKEDA-7 (1-877-825-3327) or FDA at 1-800-FDA-1088 or www.fda.gov/medwatch.

——————DRUG INTERACTIONS——————

- Strong CYP2C8 inhibitors (e.g., gemfibrozil) increase pioglitazone concentrations. Limit the pioglitazone dose to 15 mg daily. (2.3, 7.1)
- CYP2C8 inducers (e.g., rifampin) may decrease pioglitazone concentrations. (7.2)

——————USE IN SPECIFIC POPULATIONS——————

- Nursing mothers: Discontinue drug or nursing, taking into consideration the importance of the drug to the mother. (8.3)

See 17 for PATIENT COUNSELING INFORMATION and Medication Guide

Revised: 07/2013

FULL PRESCRIBING INFORMATION

WARNING: CONGESTIVE HEART FAILURE

- **Thiazolidinediones, including pioglitazone, which is a component of OSENI, cause or exacerbate congestive heart failure in some patients** [see Warnings and Precautions (5.1)].
- **After initiation of OSENI and after dose increases, monitor patients carefully for signs and symptoms of heart failure (e.g., excessive, rapid weight gain, dyspnea and/or edema). If heart failure develops, it should be managed according to current standards of care and discontinuation or dose reduction of pioglitazone in OSENI must be considered.**
- **OSENI is not recommended in patients with symptomatic heart failure.**
- **Initiation of OSENI in patients with established New York Heart Association (NYHA) Class III or IV heart failure is contraindicated** [see Contraindications (4) and Warnings and Precautions (5.1)].

1 INDICATIONS AND USAGE

1.1 Monotherapy and Combination Therapy

OSENI is indicated as an adjunct to diet and exercise to improve glycemic control in adults with type 2 diabetes mellitus in multiple clinical settings when treatment with both alogliptin and pioglitazone is appropriate [see Clinical Studies (14)].

1.2 Limitation of Use

OSENI should not be used in patients with type 1 diabetes mellitus or for the treatment of diabetic ketoacidosis, as it would not be effective in these settings.

Use with caution in patients with liver disease [see Warnings and Precautions (5.4)].

2 DOSAGE AND ADMINISTRATION

2.1 Recommendations for All Patients

OSENI should be taken once daily and can be taken with or without food. The tablets must not be split before swallowing.

The recommended starting dose for OSENI (alogliptin and pioglitazone):

- for patients inadequately controlled on diet and exercise is 25 mg/15 mg or 25 mg/30 mg,
- for patients inadequately controlled on metformin monotherapy is 25 mg/15 mg or 25 mg/30 mg,
- for patients on alogliptin who require additional glycemic control is 25 mg/15 mg or 25 mg/30 mg,
- for patients on pioglitazone who require additional glycemic control is 25 mg/15 mg, 25 mg/30 mg or 25 mg/45 mg as appropriate based upon current therapy,
- for patients switching from alogliptin coadministered with pioglitazone, OSENI may be initiated at the dose of alogliptin and pioglitazone based upon current therapy,
- for patients with congestive heart failure (NYHA Class I or II) is 25 mg/15 mg.

The OSENI dose can be titrated up to a maximum of 25 mg/45 mg once daily based on glycemic response as determined by hemoglobin A1c (A1C).

After initiation of OSENI or with dose increase, monitor patients carefully for adverse reactions related to fluid retention as has been seen with pioglitazone (e.g., weight gain, edema and signs and symptoms of congestive heart failure) [see Boxed Warning and Warnings and Precautions (5.1)].

2.2 Patients with Renal Impairment

No dose adjustment of OSENI is necessary for patients with mild renal impairment (creatinine clearance [CrCl] ≥60 mL/min).

The dose of OSENI is 12.5 mg/15 mg, 12.5 mg/30 mg or 12.5 mg/45 mg once daily for patients with moderate renal impairment (CrCl ≥30 to <60 mL/min).

OSENI is not recommended for patients with severe renal impairment or ESRD [see Clinical Pharmacology (12.3)]. Coadministration of pioglitazone and alogliptin 6.25 mg once daily based on individual requirements may be considered in these patients.

Because there is a need for dose adjustment based upon renal function, assessment of renal function is recommended prior to initiation of OSENI therapy and periodically thereafter.

2.3 Coadministration with Strong CYP2C8 Inhibitors

Coadministration of pioglitazone and gemfibrozil, a strong CYP2C8 inhibitor, increases pioglitazone exposure approximately three-fold. Therefore, the maximum recommended dose of OSENI is 25 mg/15 mg daily when used in combination with gemfibrozil or other strong CYP2C8 inhibitors [see Drug Interactions (7.1) and Clinical Pharmacology (12.3)].

3 DOSAGE FORMS AND STRENGTHS

- 25 mg/15 mg tablets are yellow, round, biconvex, and film-coated, with both "A/P" and "25/15" printed on one side.
- 25 mg/30 mg tablets are peach, round, biconvex, and film-coated, with both "A/P" and "25/30" printed on one side.
- 25 mg/45 mg tablets are red, round, biconvex, and film-coated, with both "A/P" and "25/45" printed on one side.
- 12.5 mg/15 mg tablets are pale yellow, round, biconvex, and film-coated, with both "A/P" and "12.5/15" printed on one side.
- 12.5 mg/30 mg tablets are pale peach, round, biconvex, and film-coated, with both "A/P" and "12.5/30" printed on one side.
- 12.5 mg/45 mg tablets are pale red, round, biconvex, and film-coated, with both "A/P" and "12.5/45" printed on one side.

4 CONTRAINDICATIONS

History of a serious hypersensitivity reaction to alogliptin or pioglitazone, components of OSENI, such as anaphylaxis, angioedema or severe cutaneous adverse reactions.

Do not initiate in patients with NYHA Class III or IV heart failure [see Boxed Warning].

5 WARNINGS AND PRECAUTIONS

5.1 Congestive Heart Failure

Pioglitazone

Pioglitazone, like other thiazolidinediones, can cause dose-related fluid retention when used alone or in combination with other antidiabetic medications and is most common when pioglitazone is used in combination with insulin. Fluid retention may lead to or exacerbate congestive heart failure. Patients should be observed for signs and symptoms of congestive heart failure. If congestive heart failure develops, it should be managed according to current standards of care and discontinuation or dose reduction of pioglitazone must be considered [see Boxed Warning, Contraindications (4) and Adverse Reactions (6.1)].

5.2 Pancreatitis

There have been postmarketing reports of acute pancreatitis in patients taking alogliptin. After initiation of OSENI, patients should be observed carefully for signs and symptoms of pancreatitis. If pancreatitis is suspected, OSENI should promptly be discontinued and appropriate management should be initiated. It is unknown whether patients with a history of pancreatitis are at increased risk for the development of pancreatitis while using OSENI.

5.3 Hypersensitivity Reactions

There have been postmarketing reports of serious hypersensitivity reactions in patients treated with alogliptin. These reactions include anaphylaxis, angioedema and severe cutaneous adverse reactions, including Stevens-Johnson syndrome. If a serious hypersensitivity reaction is suspected, discontinue OSENI, assess for other potential causes for the event and institute alternative treatment for diabetes [see Adverse Reactions (6.3)]. Use caution in patients with a history of angioedema to another DPP-4 inhibitor because it is unknown whether such patients will be predisposed to angioedema with OSENI.

5.4 Hepatic Effects

There have been postmarketing reports of fatal and nonfatal hepatic events in patients taking pioglitazone or alogliptin, although the reports contain insufficient information necessary to establish the probable cause [see Adverse Reactions (6.3)]. There has been no evidence of drug-induced hepatotoxicity in the pioglitazone controlled clinical trial database to date [see Adverse Reactions (6.1)]. In randomized controlled studies of alogliptin, serum alanine aminotransferase (ALT) elevations greater than three times the upper limit of normal (ULN) were observed: 1.3% in alogliptin-treated patients and 1.5% in all comparator-treated patients.

Patients with type 2 diabetes may have fatty liver disease or cardiac disease with episodic congestive heart failure, both of which may cause liver test abnormalities, and they may also have other forms of liver disease, many of which can be treated or managed. Therefore, obtaining a liver test panel (ALT, aspartate aminotransferase [AST], alkaline phosphatase and total bilirubin) and assessing the patient is recommended before initiating OSENI therapy. In patients with abnormal liver tests, OSENI should be initiated with caution.

Measure liver tests promptly in patients who report symptoms that may indicate liver injury, including fatigue, anorexia, right upper abdominal discomfort, dark urine or jaundice. In this clinical context, if the patient is found to have abnormal liver tests (ALT greater than three times the upper limit of the reference range), OSENI treatment should be interrupted and an investigation done to establish the probable cause. OSENI should not be restarted in these patients without another explanation for the liver test abnormalities.

5.5 Edema

Pioglitazone

In controlled clinical trials, edema was reported more frequently in patients treated with pioglitazone than in placebo-treated patients and is dose-related [see Adverse Reactions (6.1)]. In postmarketing experience, reports of new onset or worsening of edema have been received.

Table 1. Adverse Reactions Reported in ≥4% of Patients Treated with OSENI and More Frequently than in Patients Receiving Either Alogliptin, Pioglitazone or Placebo

	Number of Patients (%)			
	OSENI*	Alogliptin[†]	Pioglitazone[‡]	Placebo
	N=1533	N=446	N=949	N=153
Nasopharyngitis	75 (4.9)	21 (4.7)	37 (3.9)	6 (3.9)
Back Pain	64 (4.2)	9 (2.0)	32 (3.4)	5 (3.3)
Upper Respiratory Tract Infection	63 (4.1)	19 (4.3)	26 (2.7)	5 (3.3)

* OSENI – includes data pooled for patients receiving alogliptin 25 mg and 12.5 mg combined with pioglitazone 15 mg, 30 mg and 45 mg
† Alogliptin – includes data pooled for patients receiving alogliptin 25 mg and 12.5 mg
‡ Pioglitazone – includes data pooled for patients receiving pioglitazone 15 mg, 30 mg and 45 mg

Table 2. Adverse Reactions Reported in ≥4% Patients Treated with Alogliptin 25 mg and More Frequently than in Patients Given Placebo in Pooled Studies

	Number of Patients (%)		
	Alogliptin 25 mg	Placebo	Active Comparator
	N=5902	N=2926	N=2257
Nasopharyngitis	257 (4.4)	89 (3.0)	113 (5.0)
Headache	247 (4.2)	72 (2.5)	121 (5.4)
Upper Respiratory Tract Infection	247 (4.2)	61 (2.1)	113 (5.0)

OSENI should be used with caution in patients with edema. Because thiazolidinediones, including pioglitazone, can cause fluid retention, which can exacerbate or lead to congestive heart failure, OSENI should be used with caution in patients at risk for congestive heart failure. Patients treated with OSENI should be monitored for signs and symptoms of congestive heart failure *[see Boxed Warning, Warnings and Precautions (5.1) and Patient Counseling Information (17.1)].*

5.6 Fractures
Pioglitazone
In PROactive (the Prospective Pioglitazone Clinical Trial in Macrovascular Events), 5238 patients with type 2 diabetes and a history of macrovascular disease were randomized to pioglitazone (N=2605), force-titrated up to 45 mg daily or placebo (N=2633) in addition to standard of care. During a mean follow-up of 34.5 months, the incidence of bone fracture in females was 5.1% (44/870) for pioglitazone versus 2.5% (23/905) for placebo. This difference was noted after the first year of treatment and persisted during the course of the study. The majority of fractures observed in female patients were nonvertebral fractures including lower limb and distal upper limb. No increase in the incidence of fracture was observed in men treated with pioglitazone (1.7%) versus placebo (2.1%). The risk of fracture should be considered in the care of patients, especially female patients, treated with pioglitazone and attention should be given to assessing and maintaining bone health according to current standards of care.

5.7 Urinary Bladder Tumors
Pioglitazone
Tumors were observed in the urinary bladder of male rats in the two-year carcinogenicity study *[see Nonclinical Toxicology (13.1)].* In two 3-year trials in which pioglitazone was compared to placebo or glyburide, there were 16/3656 (0.44%) reports of bladder cancer in patients taking pioglitazone compared to 5/3679 (0.14%) in patients not taking pioglitazone. After excluding patients in whom exposure to study drug was less than one year at the time of diagnosis of bladder cancer, there were six (0.16%) cases on pioglitazone and two (0.05%) cases on placebo.
A five-year interim report of an ongoing 10-year observational cohort study found a nonsignificant increase in the risk for bladder cancer in subjects ever exposed to pioglitazone, compared to subjects never exposed to pioglitazone (HR 1.2 [95% CI 0.9–1.5]). Compared to never exposure, a duration of pioglitazone therapy longer than 12 months was associated with an increase in risk (HR 1.4 [95% CI 0.9–2.1]), which reached statistical significance after more than 24 months of pioglitazone use (HR 1.4 [95% CI 1.03–2.0]). Interim results from this study suggested that taking pioglitazone longer than 12 months increased the relative risk of developing bladder cancer in any given year by 40%, which equates to an absolute increase of three cases in 10,000 (from approximately seven in 10,000 [without pioglitazone] to approximately 10 in 10,000 [with pioglitazone]).

There are insufficient data to determine whether pioglitazone is a tumor promoter for urinary bladder tumors. Consequently, pioglitazone should not be used in patients with active bladder cancer and the benefits of glycemic control versus unknown risks for cancer recurrence with pioglitazone should be considered in patients with a prior history of bladder cancer.

5.8 Use with Medications Known to Cause Hypoglycemia
Insulin and insulin secretagogues, such as sulfonylureas, are known to cause hypoglycemia. Therefore, a lower dose of insulin or insulin secretagogue may be required to minimize the risk of hypoglycemia when used in combination with OSENI.

5.9 Macular Edema
Pioglitazone
Macular edema has been reported in postmarketing experience in diabetic patients who were taking pioglitazone or another thiazolidinedione. Some patients presented with blurred vision or decreased visual acuity, but others were diagnosed on routine ophthalmologic examination.
Most patients had peripheral edema at the time macular edema was diagnosed. Some patients had improvement in their macular edema after discontinuation of their thiazolidinedione.
Patients with diabetes should have regular eye exams by an ophthalmologist according to current standards of care. Patients with diabetes who report any visual symptoms should be promptly referred to an ophthalmologist, regardless of the patient's underlying medications or other physical findings *[see Adverse Reactions (6.1)].*

5.10 Ovulation
Pioglitazone
Therapy with pioglitazone, like other thiazolidinediones, may result in ovulation in some premenopausal anovulatory women. As a result, these patients may be at an increased risk for pregnancy while taking OSENI *[see Use in Specific Populations (8.1)].* This effect has not been investigated in clinical trials, so the frequency of this occurrence is not known. Adequate contraception in all premenopausal women treated with OSENI is recommended.

5.11 Macrovascular Outcomes
There have been no clinical studies establishing conclusive evidence of macrovascular risk reduction with OSENI or any other antidiabetic drug.

6 ADVERSE REACTIONS
6.1 Clinical Studies Experience
Because clinical trials are conducted under widely varying conditions, adverse reaction rates observed in the clinical trials of a drug cannot be directly compared to rates in the clinical trials of another drug and may not reflect the rates observed in clinical practice.

Alogliptin and Pioglitazone
Over 1500 patients with type 2 diabetes have received alogliptin coadministered with pioglitazone in four large, randomized, double-blind, controlled clinical trials. The

mean exposure to OSENI was 29 weeks with more than 100 subjects treated for more than one year. The studies consisted of two placebo-controlled studies of 16 to 26 weeks in duration and two active-controlled studies of 26 weeks and 52 weeks in duration. In the OSENI arm, the mean duration of diabetes was approximately six years, the mean body mass index (BMI) was 31 kg/m^2 (54% of patients had a BMI ≥30 kg/m^2), and the mean age was 54 years (16% of patients ≥65 years of age).
In a pooled analysis of these four controlled clinical studies, the overall incidence of adverse events was 65% in patients treated with OSENI compared to 57% treated with placebo. Overall discontinuation of therapy due to adverse events was 2.5% with OSENI compared to 2.0% with placebo, 3.7% with pioglitazone or 1.3% with alogliptin.
Adverse reactions reported in ≥4% of patients treated with OSENI and more frequently than in patients who received alogliptin, pioglitazone or placebo are summarized in *Table 1.*
[See table 1 above]

Alogliptin Add-On Therapy to a Thiazolidinedione
In addition, in a 26-week, placebo-controlled, double-blind study, patients inadequately controlled on a thiazolidinedione alone or in combination with metformin or a sulfonylurea were treated with add-on alogliptin therapy or placebo; the adverse reactions reported in ≥5% of patients and more frequently than in patients who received placebo was influenza (alogliptin, 5.5%; placebo, 4.1%).

Hypoglycemia
In a 26-week, placebo-controlled factorial study with alogliptin in combination with pioglitazone on background therapy with metformin, the incidence of subjects reporting hypoglycemia was 0.8%, 0% and 3.8% for alogliptin 25 mg with pioglitazone 15 mg, 30 mg or 45 mg, respectively; 2.3% for alogliptin 25 mg; 4.7%, 0.8% and 0.8% for pioglitazone 15 mg, 30 mg or 45 mg, respectively; and 0.8% for placebo.
In a 26-week, active-controlled, double-blind study with alogliptin alone, pioglitazone alone or alogliptin coadministered with pioglitazone in patients inadequately controlled on diet and exercise, the incidence of hypoglycemia was 3% on alogliptin 25 mg with pioglitazone 30 mg, 0.6% on alogliptin 25 mg and 1.8% on pioglitazone 30 mg.
In a 52-week, active-controlled, double-blind study of alogliptin as add-on therapy to the combination of pioglitazone 30 mg and metformin compared to the titration of pioglitazone 30 mg to 45 mg and metformin, the incidence of subjects reporting hypoglycemia was 4.5% in the alogliptin 25 mg with pioglitazone 30 mg and metformin group versus 1.5% in the pioglitazone 45 mg and metformin group.

Alogliptin
Approximately 8500 patients with type 2 diabetes have been treated with alogliptin in 14 randomized, double-blind, controlled clinical trials with approximately 2900 subjects randomized to placebo and approximately 2200 to an active comparator. The mean exposure to alogliptin was 40 weeks with more than 2400 subjects treated for more than one year. Among these patients, 63% had a history of hypertension, 51% had a history of dyslipidemia, 25% had a history of myocardial infarction, 8% had a history of unstable angina and 7% had a history of congestive heart failure. The mean duration of diabetes was seven years, the mean BMI was 31 kg/m^2 (51% of patients had a BMI ≥30 kg/m^2) and the mean age was 57 years (24% of patients ≥65 years of age).
Two placebo-controlled monotherapy trials of 12 and 26 weeks in duration were conducted in patients treated with alogliptin 12.5 mg daily, alogliptin 25 mg daily and placebo. Four placebo-controlled add-on combination therapy trials of 26 weeks in duration were also conducted: with metformin, with a sulfonylurea, with a thiazolidinedione and with insulin.
Four placebo-controlled and one active-controlled trials of 16 weeks up through two years in duration were conducted in combination with metformin, in combination with pioglitazone and with pioglitazone added to a background of metformin therapy.
Three active-controlled trials of 52 weeks in duration were conducted in patients treated with pioglitazone and metformin, in combination with metformin and as monotherapy compared to glipizide.
In a pooled analysis of these 14 controlled clinical trials, the overall incidence of adverse events was 66% in patients treated with alogliptin 25 mg compared to 62% with placebo and 70% with active comparator. Overall discontinuation of therapy due to adverse events was 4.7% with alogliptin 25 mg compared to 4.5% with placebo or 6.2% with active comparator.
Adverse reactions reported in ≥4% of patients treated with alogliptin 25 mg and more frequently than in patients who received placebo are summarized in *Table 2.*
[See table 2 above]

Pancreatitis
In the clinical trial program, pancreatitis was reported in 11 of 5902 (0.2%) patients receiving alogliptin 25 mg daily compared to five of 5183 (<0.1%) patients receiving all comparators.

Hypersensitivity Reactions

In a pooled analysis, the overall incidence of hypersensitivity reactions was 0.6% with alogliptin 25 mg compared to 0.8% with all comparators. A single event of serum sickness was reported in a patient treated with alogliptin 25 mg.

Hypoglycemia

Hypoglycemic events were documented based upon a blood glucose value and/or clinical signs and symptoms of hypoglycemia.

In the monotherapy study, the incidence of hypoglycemia was 1.5% in patients treated with alogliptin compared to 1.6% with placebo. The use of alogliptin as add-on therapy to glyburide or insulin did not increase the incidence of hypoglycemia compared to placebo. In a monotherapy study comparing alogliptin to a sulfonylurea in elderly patients, the incidence of hypoglycemia was 5.4% with alogliptin compared to 26% with glipizide.

Pioglitazone

Over 8500 patients with type 2 diabetes have been treated with pioglitazone in randomized, double-blind, controlled clinical trials, including 2605 patients with type 2 diabetes and macrovascular disease treated with pioglitazone in the PROactive clinical trial. In these trials, over 6000 patients have been treated with pioglitazone for six months or longer, over 4500 patients have been treated with pioglitazone for one year or longer, and over 3000 patients have been treated with pioglitazone for at least two years.

Common Adverse Events: 16- to 26-Week Monotherapy Trials

A summary of the incidence and type of common adverse events reported in three pooled 16- to 26-week placebo-controlled monotherapy trials of pioglitazone is provided in *Table 3*. Terms that are reported represent those that occurred at an incidence of >5% and more commonly in patients treated with pioglitazone than in patients who received placebo. None of these adverse events were related to pioglitazone dose.

Table 3. Three Pooled 16- to 26-Week Placebo-Controlled Clinical Trials of Pioglitazone Monotherapy: Adverse Events Reported at an Incidence >5% and More Commonly in Patients Treated with Pioglitazone than in Patients Treated with Placebo

	% of Patients	
	Placebo N=259	Pioglitazone N=606
Upper Respiratory Tract Infection	8.5	13.2
Headache	6.9	9.1
Sinusitis	4.6	6.3
Myalgia	2.7	5.4
Pharyngitis	0.8	5.1

Congestive Heart Failure

A summary of the incidence of adverse events related to congestive heart failure for the 16- to 24-week add-on to sulfonylurea trials, for the 16- to 24-week add-on to insulin trials, and for the 16- to 24-week add-on to metformin trials were (at least one congestive heart failure, 0.2% to 1.7%; hospitalized due to congestive heart failure, 0.2% to 0.9%). None of the events were fatal.

Patients with type 2 diabetes and NYHA class II or early class III congestive heart failure were randomized to receive 24 weeks of double-blind treatment with either pioglitazone at daily doses of 30 mg to 45 mg (N=262) or glyburide at daily doses of 10 mg to 15 mg (N=256). A summary of the incidence of adverse events related to congestive heart failure reported in this study is provided in *Table 4*.

Table 4. Treatment-Emergent Adverse Events of Congestive Heart Failure (CHF) in Patients with NYHA Class II or III Congestive Heart Failure Treated with Pioglitazone or Glyburide

	Number (%) of Subjects	
	Pioglitazone N=262	Glyburide N=256
Death due to cardiovascular causes (adjudicated)	5 (1.9%)	6 (2.3%)
Overnight hospitalization for worsening CHF (adjudicated)	26 (9.9%)	12 (4.7%)
Emergency room visit for CHF (adjudicated)	4 (1.5%)	3 (1.2%)

Table 6. PROactive: Number of First and Total Events for Each Component Within the Cardiovascular Composite Endpoint

	Placebo N=2633		Pioglitazone N=2605	
Cardiovascular Events	First Events n (%)	Total Events n	First Events n (%)	Total Events n
Any Event	572 (21.7)	900	514 (19.7)	803
All-Cause Mortality	122 (4.6)	186	110 (4.2)	177
Nonfatal Myocardial Infarction (MI)	118 (4.5)	157	105 (4)	131
Stroke	96 (3.6)	119	76 (2.9)	92
Acute Coronary Syndrome	63 (2.4)	78	42 (1.6)	65
Cardiac Intervention (CABG/PCI)	101 (3.8)	240	101 (3.9)	195
Major Leg Amputation	15 (0.6)	28	9 (0.3)	28
Leg Revascularization	57 (2.2)	92	71 (2.7)	115

CABG=coronary artery bypass grafting; PCI=percutaneous intervention

Patients experiencing CHF progression during study	35 (13.4%)	21 (8.2%)

Congestive heart failure events leading to hospitalization that occurred during the PROactive trial are summarized in *Table 5*.

Table 5. Treatment-Emergent Adverse Events of Congestive Heart Failure (CHF) in PROactive Trial

	Number (%) of Patients	
	Placebo N=2633	Pioglitazone N=2605
At least one hospitalized congestive heart failure event	108 (4.1%)	149 (5.7%)
Fatal	22 (0.8%)	25 (1%)
Hospitalized, nonfatal	86 (3.3%)	124 (4.7%)

Cardiovascular Safety

In the PROactive trial, 5238 patients with type 2 diabetes and a history of macrovascular disease were randomized to pioglitazone (N=2605), force-titrated up to 45 mg daily or placebo (N=2633) in addition to standard of care. Almost all patients (95%) were receiving cardiovascular medications (beta blockers, ACE inhibitors, angiotensin II receptor blockers, calcium channel blockers, nitrates, diuretics, aspirin, statins and fibrates). At baseline, patients had a mean age of 62 years, mean duration of diabetes of 9.5 years and mean A1C of 8.1%. Mean duration of follow-up was 34.5 months.

The primary objective of this trial was to examine the effect of pioglitazone on mortality and macrovascular morbidity in patients with type 2 diabetes mellitus who were at high risk for macrovascular events. The primary efficacy variable was the time to the first occurrence of any event in a cardiovascular composite endpoint that included all-cause mortality, nonfatal myocardial infarction (MI) including silent MI, stroke, acute coronary syndrome, cardiac intervention including coronary artery bypass grafting or percutaneous intervention, major leg amputation above the ankle and bypass surgery or revascularization in the leg. A total of 514 (19.7%) patients treated with pioglitazone and 572 (21.7%) placebo-treated patients experienced at least one event from the primary composite endpoint (hazard ratio 0.90; 95% Confidence Interval: 0.80, 1.02; p=0.10).

Although there was no statistically significant difference between pioglitazone and placebo for the three-year incidence of a first event within this composite, there was no increase in mortality or in total macrovascular events with pioglitazone. The number of first occurrences and total individual events contributing to the primary composite endpoint is shown in *Table 6*.

[See table 6 above]

Weight Gain

Dose-related weight gain occurs when pioglitazone is used alone or in combination with other antidiabetic medications. The mechanism of weight gain is unclear but probably involves a combination of fluid retention and fat accumulation.

Edema

Edema induced from taking pioglitazone is reversible when pioglitazone is discontinued. The edema usually does not require hospitalization unless there is coexisting congestive heart failure.

Hepatic Effects

There has been no evidence of pioglitazone-induced hepatotoxicity in the pioglitazone controlled clinical trial database to date. One randomized, double-blind, three-year trial comparing pioglitazone to glyburide as add-on to metformin and insulin therapy was specifically designed to evaluate the incidence of serum ALT elevation to greater than three times the upper limit of the reference range, measured every eight weeks for the first 48 weeks of the trial then every 12 weeks thereafter. A total of 3/1051 (0.3%) patients treated with pioglitazone and 9/1046 (0.9%) patients treated with glyburide developed ALT values greater than three times the upper limit of the reference range. None of the patients treated with pioglitazone in the pioglitazone controlled clinical trial database to date have had a serum ALT greater than three times the upper limit of the reference range and a corresponding total bilirubin greater than two times the upper limit of the reference range, a combination predictive of the potential for severe drug-induced liver injury.

Hypoglycemia

In the pioglitazone clinical trials, adverse events of hypoglycemia were reported based on clinical judgment of the investigators and did not require confirmation with fingerstick glucose testing. In the 16-week add-on to sulfonylurea trial, the incidence of reported hypoglycemia was 3.7% with pioglitazone 30 mg and 0.5% with placebo. In the 16-week add-on to insulin trial, the incidence of reported hypoglycemia was 7.9% with pioglitazone 15 mg, 15.4% with pioglitazone 30 mg and 4.8% with placebo. The incidence of reported hypoglycemia was higher with pioglitazone 45 mg compared to pioglitazone 30 mg in both the 24-week add-on to sulfonylurea trial (15.7% versus 13.4%) and in the 24-week add-on to insulin trial (47.8% versus 43.5%). Three patients in these four trials were hospitalized due to hypoglycemia. All three patients were receiving pioglitazone 30 mg (0.9%) in the 24-week add-on to insulin trial. An additional 14 patients reported severe hypoglycemia (defined as causing considerable interference with patient's usual activities) that did not require hospitalization. These patients were receiving pioglitazone 45 mg in combination with sulfonylurea (N=2) or pioglitazone 30 mg or 45 mg in combination with insulin (N=12).

Urinary Bladder Tumors

Tumors were observed in the urinary bladder of male rats in the two-year carcinogenicity study *[see Nonclinical Toxicology (13.1)]*. In two 3-year trials in which pioglitazone was compared to placebo or glyburide, there were 16/3656 (0.44%) reports of bladder cancer in patients taking pioglitazone compared to 5/3679 (0.14%) in patients not taking pioglitazone. After excluding patients in whom exposure to study drug was less than one year at the time of diagnosis of bladder cancer, there were six (0.16%) cases on pioglitazone and two (0.05%) cases on placebo. There are too few events of bladder cancer to establish causality.

6.2 Laboratory Abnormalities

Alogliptin

No clinically meaningful changes in hematology, serum chemistry or urinalysis were observed in patients treated with alogliptin.

Pioglitazone

Hematologic Effects

Pioglitazone may cause decreases in hemoglobin and hematocrit. In placebo-controlled monotherapy trials, mean hemoglobin values declined by 2% to 4% in patients treated with pioglitazone compared with a mean change in hemoglobin of -1% to +1% in placebo-treated patients. These changes primarily occurred within the first four to 12 weeks of therapy and remained relatively constant thereafter. These changes may be related to increased plasma volume associated with pioglitazone therapy and are not likely to be associated with any clinically significant hematologic effects.

Creatine Phosphokinase

During protocol-specified measurement of serum creatine phosphokinase (CPK) in pioglitazone clinical trials, an isolated elevation in CPK to greater than 10 times the upper limit of the reference range was noted in nine (0.2%) patients treated with pioglitazone (values of 2150 to 11400 IU/L) and in no comparator-treated patients. Six of these nine patients continued to receive pioglitazone, two patients were noted to have the CPK elevation on the last day of dosing and one patient discontinued pioglitazone due to the elevation. These elevations resolved without any apparent clinical sequelae. The relationship of these events to pioglitazone therapy is unknown.

6.3 Postmarketing Experience

Alogliptin

The following adverse reactions have been identified during the postmarketing use of alogliptin outside the United States. Because these reactions are reported voluntarily from a population of uncertain size, it is not always possible to reliably estimate their frequency or establish a causal relationship to drug exposure.

Hypersensitivity reactions including anaphylaxis, angioedema, rash, urticaria and severe cutaneous adverse reactions, including Stevens-Johnson syndrome, hepatic enzyme elevations, fulminant hepatic failure and acute pancreatitis.

Pioglitazone

The following adverse reactions have been identified during the postmarketing use of pioglitazone. Because these reactions are reported voluntarily from a population of uncertain size, it is generally not possible to reliably estimate their frequency or establish a causal relationship to drug exposure.

New onset or worsening diabetic macular edema with decreased visual acuity *[see Warnings and Precautions (5.9)]*. Fatal and nonfatal hepatic failure *[see Warnings and Precautions (5.4)]*.

Postmarketing reports of congestive heart failure have been reported in patients treated with pioglitazone, both with and without previously known heart disease and both with and without concomitant insulin administration.

In postmarketing experience, there have been reports of unusually rapid increases in weight and increases in excess of that generally observed in clinical trials. Patients who experience such increases should be assessed for fluid accumulation and volume-related events such as excessive edema and congestive heart failure *[see Boxed Warning and Warnings and Precautions (5.1)]*.

7 DRUG INTERACTIONS

Alogliptin

Alogliptin is primarily renally excreted. Cytochrome (CYP) P450-related metabolism is negligible. No significant drug-drug interactions were observed with the CYP-substrates or inhibitors tested or with renally excreted drugs *[see Clinical Pharmacology (12.3)]*.

7.1 Strong CYP2C8 Inhibitors

Pioglitazone

An inhibitor of CYP2C8 (e.g., gemfibrozil) significantly increases the exposure (area under the concentration-time curve [AUC]) and half-life of pioglitazone. Therefore, the maximum recommended dose of pioglitazone is 15 mg daily if used in combination with gemfibrozil or other strong CYP2C8 inhibitors *[see Dosage and Administration (2.3) and Clinical Pharmacology (12.3)]*.

7.2 CYP2C8 Inducers

Pioglitazone

An inducer of CYP2C8 (e.g., rifampin) may significantly decrease the exposure (AUC) of pioglitazone. Therefore, if an inducer of CYP2C8 is started or stopped during treatment with OSENI, changes in diabetes treatment may be needed based on clinical response without exceeding the maximum recommended daily dose of 45 mg for pioglitazone *[see Clinical Pharmacology (12.3)]*.

8 USE IN SPECIFIC POPULATIONS

8.1 Pregnancy

Pregnancy Category C

Alogliptin and Pioglitazone

There are no adequate and well-controlled studies in pregnant women with OSENI or its individual components. Based on animal data, the likelihood that OSENI increases the risk of developmental abnormalities is predicted to be low. OSENI should be used during pregnancy only if the potential benefit justifies the potential risk to the fetus.

When administered to rats during organogenesis, the combination treatment with alogliptin and pioglitazone (100 mg/kg alogliptin plus 40 mg/kg pioglitazone) slightly augmented pioglitazone-related fetal effects of delayed development and reduced fetal weights but did not result in embryofetal mortality or teratogenicity.

Alogliptin

Alogliptin administered to pregnant rabbits and rats during the period of organogenesis was not teratogenic at doses of up to 200 and 500 mg/kg, or 149 times and 180 times, respectively, the clinical dose based on plasma drug exposure (AUC).

Doses of alogliptin up to 250 mg/kg (approximately 95 times clinical exposure based on AUC) given to pregnant rats from gestation Day 6 to lactation Day 20 did not harm the developing embryo or adversely affect growth and development of offspring.

Placental transfer of alogliptin into the fetus was observed following oral dosing to pregnant rats.

Pioglitazone

In animal reproductive studies, pregnant rats and rabbits received pioglitazone at doses up to approximately 17 (rat) and 40 (rabbit) times the MRHD based on body surface area (mg/m^2); no teratogenicity was observed. Increases in embryotoxicity (increased postimplantation losses, delayed development, reduced fetal weights and delayed parturition) occurred in rats that received oral doses approximately 10 or more times the MRHD (mg/m^2 basis). No functional or behavioral toxicity was observed in rat offspring. When pregnant rats received pioglitazone during late gestation and lactation, delayed postnatal development, attributed to decreased body weight, occurred in rat offspring at oral maternal doses approximately two or more times the MRHD (mg/m^2 basis). In rabbits, embryotoxicity occurred at oral doses approximately 40 times the MRHD (mg/m^2 basis).

8.3 Nursing Mothers

No studies have been conducted with the combined components of OSENI. In studies performed with the individual components, both alogliptin and pioglitazone are secreted in the milk of lactating rats. It is not known whether alogliptin and/or pioglitazone are secreted in human milk. Because many drugs are excreted in human milk, and because of the potential for OSENI to cause serious adverse reactions in nursing infants, a decision should be made to discontinue nursing or discontinue OSENI, taking into account the importance of OSENI to the mother.

8.4 Pediatric Use

Safety and effectiveness of OSENI in pediatric patients have not been established.

OSENI is not recommended for use in pediatric patients based on adverse effects observed in adults, including fluid retention and congestive heart failure, fractures and urinary bladder tumors *[see Warnings and Precautions (5.1, 5.5, 5.6, 5.7)]*.

8.5 Geriatric Use

Alogliptin and Pioglitazone

Of the total number of patients (N=1533) in clinical safety and efficacy studies treated with alogliptin and pioglitazone, 248 (16.2%) patients were 65 years and older and 15 (1%) patients were 75 years and older. No overall differences in safety or effectiveness were observed between these patients and younger patients. While this and other reported clinical experiences have not identified differences in responses between the elderly and younger patients, greater sensitivity of some older individuals cannot be excluded.

Alogliptin

Of the total number of patients (N=8507) in clinical safety and efficacy studies treated with alogliptin, 2064 (24.3%) patients were ≥65 years old and 341 (4%) patients were ≥75 years old. No overall differences in safety or effectiveness were observed between patients ≥65 years old and younger patients.

Pioglitazone

A total of 92 patients (15.2%) treated with pioglitazone in the three pooled, 16- to 26-week, double-blind, placebo-controlled, monotherapy trials were ≥65 years old and two patients (0.3%) were ≥75 years old. In the two pooled 16- to 24-week add-on to sulfonylurea trials, 201 patients (18.7%) treated with pioglitazone were ≥65 years old and 19 (1.8%) were ≥75 years old. In the two pooled 16- to 24-week add-on to metformin trials, 155 patients (15.5%) treated with pioglitazone were ≥65 years old and 19 (1.9%) were ≥75 years old. In the two pooled 16- to 24-week add-on to insulin trials, 272 patients (25.4%) treated with pioglitazone were ≥65 years old and 22 (2.1%) were ≥75 years old.

In PROactive, 1068 patients (41%) treated with pioglitazone were ≥65 years old and 42 (1.6%) were ≥75 years old.

In pharmacokinetic studies with pioglitazone, no significant differences were observed in pharmacokinetic parameters between elderly and younger patients. These clinical experiences have not identified differences in effectiveness and safety between the elderly (≥65 years) and younger patients although small sample sizes for patients ≥75 years old limit conclusions *[see Clinical Pharmacology (12.3)]*.

8.6 Hepatic Impairment

Alogliptin

No dose adjustments are required in patients with mild to moderate hepatic impairment (Child-Pugh Grade A and B) based on insignificant change in systemic exposures (e.g., AUC) compared to subjects with normal hepatic function in a pharmacokinetic study. Alogliptin has not been studied in patients with severe hepatic impairment (Child-Pugh Grade C). Use caution when administering alogliptin to patients with liver disease *[see Warnings and Precautions (5.4)]*.

Pioglitazone

No dose adjustments are required in patients with hepatic impairment (Child-Pugh Grade B and C) based on insignificant change in systemic exposures (e.g., AUC) compared to subjects with normal hepatic function in a pharmacokinetic study. However, use with caution in patients with liver disease *[see Warnings and Precautions (5.4)]*.

10 OVERDOSAGE

Alogliptin

The highest doses of alogliptin administered in clinical trials were single doses of 800 mg to healthy subjects and doses of 400 mg once daily for 14 days to patients with type 2 diabetes (equivalent to 32 times and 16 times the maximum recommended clinical dose of 25 mg, respectively). No serious adverse events were observed at these doses.

In the event of an overdose, it is reasonable to institute the necessary clinical monitoring and supportive therapy as dictated by the patient's clinical status. Per clinical judgment, it may be reasonable to initiate removal of unabsorbed material from the gastrointestinal tract.

Alogliptin is minimally dialyzable; over a three-hour hemodialysis session, approximately 7% of the drug was removed. Therefore, hemodialysis is unlikely to be beneficial in an overdose situation. It is not known if alogliptin is dialyzable by peritoneal dialysis.

Pioglitazone

During controlled clinical trials, one case of overdose with pioglitazone was reported. A male patient took 120 mg per day for four days, then 180 mg per day for seven days. The patient denied any clinical symptoms during this period.

In the event of overdosage, appropriate supportive treatment should be initiated according to patient's clinical signs and symptoms.

11 DESCRIPTION

OSENI tablets contain two oral antihyperglycemic drugs used in the management of type 2 diabetes: alogliptin and pioglitazone.

Alogliptin

Alogliptin is a selective, orally bioavailable inhibitor of the enzymatic activity of dipeptidyl peptidase-4 (DPP-4). Chemically, alogliptin is prepared as a benzoate salt, which is identified as 2-({6-[(3R)-3-aminopiperidin-1-yl]-3-methyl-2,4-dioxo-3,4-dihydropyrimidin-1(2H)-yl]methyl)-benzonitrile monobenzoate. It has a molecular formula of $C_{18}H_{21}N_5O_2 \bullet C_7H_6O_2$ and a molecular weight of 461.51 daltons. The structural formula is:

Alogliptin benzoate is a white to off-white crystalline powder that contains one asymmetric carbon in the aminopiperidine moiety. It is soluble in dimethylsulfoxide, sparingly soluble in water and methanol, slightly soluble in ethanol and very slightly soluble in octanol and isopropyl acetate.

Pioglitazone

Pioglitazone is an oral antihyperglycemic agent that acts primarily by decreasing insulin resistance. Chemically, pioglitazone is prepared as hydrochloride salt, which is identified as (±)-5-[[4-[2-(5-ethyl-2-pyridinyl)ethoxy]phenyl]methyl]-2,4-thiazolidinedione monohydrochloride. It has a molecular formula of $C_{19}H_{20}N_2O_3S \bullet HCl$ and a molecular weight of 392.90 daltons. The structural formula is:

Pioglitazone hydrochloride is an odorless white crystalline powder that contains one asymmetric carbon in the thiazolidinedione moiety. The synthetic compound is a racemate and the two enantiomers of pioglitazone interconvert *in vivo*. It is soluble in *N,N* dimethylformamide, slightly soluble in anhydrous ethanol, very slightly soluble in acetone and acetonitrile, practically insoluble in water and insoluble in ether.

OSENI is available as a fixed-dose combination tablet for oral administration containing 34 mg alogliptin benzoate equivalent to 25 mg alogliptin and any of the following strengths of pioglitazone hydrochloride:

- 16.53 mg pioglitazone hydrochloride equivalent to 15 mg pioglitazone (25 mg/15 mg)
- 33.06 mg pioglitazone hydrochloride equivalent to 30 mg pioglitazone (25 mg/30 mg)
- 49.59 mg pioglitazone hydrochloride equivalent to 45 mg pioglitazone (25 mg/45 mg)

OSENI is also available as a fixed-dose combination tablet for oral administration containing 17 mg alogliptin benzoate equivalent to 12.5 mg alogliptin and any of the following strengths of pioglitazone hydrochloride:

- 16.53 mg pioglitazone hydrochloride equivalent to 15 mg pioglitazone (12.5 mg/15 mg)
- 33.06 mg pioglitazone hydrochloride equivalent to 30 mg pioglitazone (12.5 mg/30 mg)
- 49.59 mg pioglitazone hydrochloride equivalent to 45 mg pioglitazone (12.5 mg/45 mg)

OSENI tablets contain the following inactive ingredients: mannitol, microcrystalline cellulose, hydroxypropyl cellulose, croscarmellose sodium, magnesium stearate and lactose monohydrate; the tablets are film-coated with hypromellose, polyethylene glycol, titanium dioxide, talc and ferric oxide (yellow and/or red) and are marked with printing ink (Red A1 or Gray F1).

12 CLINICAL PHARMACOLOGY

12.1 Mechanism of Action

OSENI combines two antihyperglycemic agents with complementary and distinct mechanisms of action to improve glycemic control in patients with type 2 diabetes: alogliptin, a selective inhibitor of DPP-4, and pioglitazone, a member of the TZD class.

Alogliptin

Increased concentrations of the incretin hormones such as glucagon-like peptide-1 (GLP-1) and glucose-dependent insulinotropic polypeptide (GIP) are released into the bloodstream from the small intestine in response to meals. These hormones cause insulin release from the pancreatic beta cells in a glucose-dependent manner but are inactivated by the DPP-4 enzyme within minutes. GLP-1 also lowers glucagon secretion from pancreatic alpha cells, reducing hepatic glucose production. In patients with type 2 diabetes, concentrations of GLP-1 are reduced but the insulin response to GLP-1 is preserved. Alogliptin is a DPP-4 inhibitor that slows the inactivation of the incretin hormones, thereby increasing their bloodstream concentrations and reducing fasting and postprandial glucose concentrations in a glucose-dependent manner in patients with type 2 diabetes mellitus. Alogliptin selectively binds to and inhibits DPP-4 but not DPP-8 or DPP-9 activity *in vitro* at concentrations approximating therapeutic exposures.

Pioglitazone

Pharmacologic studies indicate that pioglitazone improves insulin sensitivity in muscle and adipose tissue while inhibiting hepatic gluconeogenesis. Unlike sulfonylureas, pioglitazone is not an insulin secretagogue. Pioglitazone is an agonist for peroxisome proliferator-activated receptor-gamma (PPARγ). PPAR receptors are found in tissues important for insulin action such as adipose tissue, skeletal muscle and liver. Activation of PPARγ nuclear receptors modulates the transcription of a number of insulin-responsive genes involved in the control of glucose and lipid metabolism.

In animal models of diabetes, pioglitazone reduces the hyperglycemia, hyperinsulinemia and hypertriglyceridemia characteristic of insulin-resistant states such as type 2 diabetes. The metabolic changes produced by pioglitazone result in increased responsiveness of insulin-dependent tissues and are observed in numerous animal models of insulin resistance.

Because pioglitazone enhances the effects of circulating insulin (by decreasing insulin resistance), it does not lower blood glucose in animal models that lack endogenous insulin.

12.2 Pharmacodynamics

Alogliptin and Pioglitazone

In a 26-week, randomized, active-controlled study, patients with type 2 diabetes received alogliptin 25 mg coadministered with pioglitazone 30 mg, alogliptin 12.5 mg coadministered with pioglitazone 30 mg, alogliptin 25 mg alone or pioglitazone 30 mg alone. Patients who were randomized to alogliptin 25 mg with pioglitazone 30 mg achieved a 26.2% decrease in triglyceride levels from a mean baseline of 214.2 mg/dL compared to an 11.5% decrease for alogliptin alone and a 21.8% decrease for pioglitazone alone. In addition, a 14.4% increase in HDL cholesterol levels from a mean baseline of 43.2 mg/dL was also observed for alogliptin 25 mg with pioglitazone 30 mg compared to a

1.9% increase for alogliptin alone and a 13.2% increase for pioglitazone alone. The changes in measures of LDL cholesterol and total cholesterol were similar between alogliptin 25 mg with pioglitazone 30 mg versus alogliptin alone and pioglitazone alone. A similar pattern of lipid effects was observed in a 26-week, placebo-controlled factorial study.

Alogliptin

Single-dose administration of alogliptin to healthy subjects resulted in a peak inhibition of DPP-4 within two to three hours after dosing. The peak inhibition of DPP-4 exceeded 93% across doses of 12.5 mg to 800 mg. Inhibition of DPP-4 remained above 80% at 24 hours for doses greater than or equal to 25 mg. Peak and total exposure over 24 hours to active GLP-1 were three- to four-fold greater with alogliptin (at doses of 25 to 200 mg) than placebo. In a 16-week, double-blind, placebo-controlled study alogliptin 25 mg demonstrated decreases in postprandial glucagon while increasing postprandial active GLP-1 levels compared to placebo over an eight-hour period following a standardized meal. It is unclear how these findings relate to changes in overall glycemic control in patients with type 2 diabetes mellitus. In this study, alogliptin 25 mg alone demonstrated decreases in two-hour postprandial glucose compared to placebo (-30 mg/dL versus 17.3 mg/dL respectively).

Multiple-dose administration of alogliptin to patients with type 2 diabetes also resulted in a peak inhibition of DPP-4 within one to two hours and exceeded 93% across all doses (25 mg, 100 mg and 400 mg) after a single dose and after 14 days of once-daily dosing. At these doses of alogliptin, inhibition of DPP-4 remained above 81% at 24 hours after 14 days of dosing.

Pioglitazone

Clinical studies demonstrate that pioglitazone improves insulin sensitivity in insulin-resistant patients. Pioglitazone enhances cellular responsiveness to insulin, increases insulin-dependent glucose disposal, and improves hepatic sensitivity to insulin. In patients with type 2 diabetes, the decreased insulin resistance produced by pioglitazone results in lower plasma glucose concentrations, lower plasma insulin concentrations and lower A1C values. In controlled clinical trials, pioglitazone had an additive effect on glycemic control when used in combination with a sulfonylurea, metformin or insulin *[see Clinical Studies (14)]*. Patients with lipid abnormalities were included in clinical trials with pioglitazone. Overall, patients treated with pioglitazone had mean decreases in serum triglycerides, mean increases in HDL cholesterol and no consistent mean changes in LDL and total cholesterol. There is no conclusive evidence of macrovascular benefit with pioglitazone or any other antidiabetic medication *[see Warnings and Precautions (5,11) and Adverse Reactions (6.1)]*.

In a 26-week, placebo-controlled, dose-ranging monotherapy study, mean serum triglycerides decreased in the pioglitazone 15 mg, 30 mg and 45 mg dose groups compared to a mean increase in the placebo group. Mean HDL cholesterol increased to a greater extent in patients treated with pioglitazone than in the placebo-treated patients. There were no consistent differences for LDL and total cholesterol in patients treated with pioglitazone compared to placebo *(Table 7)*.

[See table 7 above]

In the two other monotherapy studies (16 weeks and 24 weeks) and in combination therapy studies with sulfonylurea (16 weeks and 24 weeks), metformin (16 weeks and 24 weeks) or insulin (16 weeks and 24 weeks), the lipid results were generally consistent with the data above.

12.3 Pharmacokinetics

Absorption and Bioavailability

Alogliptin and Pioglitazone

In bioequivalence studies of OSENI, the AUC and maximum concentration (C_{max}) of both the alogliptin and the pioglitazone component following a single dose of the combination tablet (12.5 mg/15 mg or 25 mg/45 mg) were bioequivalent to alogliptin (12.5 mg or 25 mg) concomitantly administered with pioglitazone (15 mg or 45 mg respectively) tablets under fasted conditions in healthy subjects. Administration of OSENI 25 mg/45 mg with food resulted in no significant change in overall exposure of alogliptin or pioglitazone. OSENI may therefore be administered with or without food.

Alogliptin

The absolute bioavailability of alogliptin is approximately 100%. Administration of alogliptin with a high-fat meal results in no significant change in total and peak exposure to alogliptin. Alogliptin may therefore be administered with or without food.

Pioglitazone

Following oral administration of pioglitazone hydrochloride, peak concentrations of pioglitazone were observed within two hours. Food slightly delays the time to peak serum concentration (T_{max}) to three to four hours but does not alter the extent of absorption (AUC).

Distribution

Alogliptin

Following a single, 12.5 mg intravenous infusion of alogliptin to healthy subjects, the volume of distribution during the terminal phase was 417 L, indicating that the drug is well distributed into tissues.

Alogliptin is 20% bound to plasma proteins.

Pioglitazone

The mean apparent V_d/F of pioglitazone following single-dose administration is 0.63 ± 0.41 (mean ± SD) L/kg of body weight. Pioglitazone is extensively protein bound (>99%) in human serum, principally to serum albumin. Pioglitazone also binds to other serum proteins, but with lower affinity. Metabolites M-III and M-IV also are extensively bound (>98%) to serum albumin.

Metabolism

Alogliptin

Alogliptin does not undergo extensive metabolism, and 60% to 71% of the dose is excreted as unchanged drug in the urine.

Two minor metabolites were detected following administration of an oral dose of [^{14}C] alogliptin, N-demethylated, M-I (<1% of the parent compound), and N-acetylated alogliptin, M-II (<6% of the parent compound). M-I is an active metabolite and is an inhibitor of DPP-4 similar to the parent molecule; M-II does not display any inhibitory activity toward DPP-4 or other DPP-related enzymes. *In vitro* data indicate that, CYP2D6 and CYP3A4 contribute to the limited metabolism of alogliptin.

Table 7. Lipids in a 26-Week, Placebo-Controlled, Monotherapy, Dose-Ranging Study

	Placebo	Pioglitazone 15 mg Once Daily	Pioglitazone 30 mg Once Daily	Pioglitazone 45 mg Once Daily
Triglycerides (mg/dL)	N=79	N=79	N=84	N=77
Baseline (mean)	263	284	261	260
Percent change from baseline (adjusted mean*)	4.8%	-9%†	-9.6%†	-9.3%†
HDL Cholesterol (mg/dL)	N=79	N=79	N=83	N=77
Baseline (mean)	42	40	41	41
Percent change from baseline (adjusted mean*)	8.1%	14.1%†	12.2%	19.1%†
LDL Cholesterol (mg/dL)	N=65	N=63	N=74	N=62
Baseline (mean)	139	132	136	127
Percent change from baseline (adjusted mean*)	4.8%	7.2%	5.2%	6%
Total Cholesterol (mg/dL)	N=79	N=79	N=84	N=77
Baseline (mean)	225	220	223	214
Percent change from baseline (adjusted mean*)	4.4%	4.6%	3.3%	6.4%

* Adjusted for baseline, pooled center and pooled center by treatment interaction
† p<0.05 versus placebo

Figure 1. Effect of Alogliptin on the Pharmacokinetic Exposure to Other Drugs

ALOGLIPTIN	Coadministered Drug	PK	Ratio and 90% CI	Recommendation
Renally Excreted:				
ALOGLIPTIN 100 mg Once daily for 6 days	METFORMIN 1000 mg Twice daily for 6 days	AUC Cmax		No dose adjustment
ALOGLIPTIN 100 mg Once daily for 6 days	CIMETIDINE 400 mg Once daily for 6 days	AUC Cmax		No dose adjustment
CYP1A2 Substrate:				
ALOGLIPTIN 25 mg Once daily for 7 days	(R)-WARFARIN* Once daily for 7 days	AUC Cmax		No dose adjustment
ALOGLIPTIN 100 mg Once daily for 7 days	CAFFEINE 200 mg** Single Dose	AUC Cmax		No dose adjustment
CYP2C8 Substrate:				
ALOGLIPTIN 25 mg Once daily for 12 days	PIOGLITAZONE 45 mg Once daily for 12 days	AUC Cmax		No dose adjustment
CYP2C9 Substrate:				
ALOGLIPTIN 25 mg Once daily for 8 days	GLYBURIDE 5 mg Single Dose	AUC Cmax		No dose adjustment
ALOGLIPTIN 25 mg Once daily for 7 days	(S)-WARFARIN* Once daily for 7 days	AUC Cmax		No dose adjustment
ALOGLIPTIN 100 mg Once daily for 7 days	TOLBUTAMIDE 500 mg** Single Dose	AUC Cmax		No dose adjustment
CYP2D6 Substrate:				
ALOGLIPTIN 100 mg Once daily for 7 days	DEXTROMETHORPHAN 30 mg** Single Dose	AUC Cmax		No dose adjustment
CYP3A4 Substrate:				
ALOGLIPTIN 25 mg Once daily for 7 days	ATORVASTATIN 80 mg Once daily for 7 days	AUC Cmax		No dose adjustment
ALOGLIPTIN 25 mg Once daily for 21 days	ETHINYL ESTRADIOL 35 mcg Once daily for 21 days	AUC Cmax		No dose adjustment
ALOGLIPTIN 25 mg Once daily for 21 days	NORETHINDRONE 1 mg Once daily for 21 days	AUC Cmax		No dose adjustment
ALOGLIPTIN 100 mg Once daily for 7 days	MIDAZOLAM 4 mg** Single Dose	AUC Cmax		No dose adjustment
Pgp Substrate:				
ALOGLIPTIN 25 mg Once daily for 10 days	DIGOXIN 0.2 mg Once daily for 10 days	AUC Cmax		No dose adjustment
ALOGLIPTIN 100 mg Once daily for 7 days	FEXOFENADINE 80 mg** Single Dose	AUC Cmax		No dose adjustment

0.6   0.8   1.0   1.2   1.4   1.6
Ratio of Alogliptin + Other Drug vs Other Drug

*Warfarin was given once daily at a stable dose in the range of 1 mg to 10 mg. Alogliptin had no significant effect on the prothrombin time (PT) or International Normalized Ratio (INR).

**Caffeine (1A2 substrate), tolbutamide (2C9 substrate), dextromethorphan (2D6 substrate), midazolam (3A4 substrate) and fexofenadine (P-gp substrate) were administered as a cocktail.

Alogliptin exists predominantly as the (R)-enantiomer (>99%) and undergoes little or no chiral conversion *in vivo* to the (S)-enantiomer. The (S)-enantiomer is not detectable at the 25 mg dose.

Pioglitazone

Pioglitazone is extensively metabolized by hydroxylation and oxidation; the metabolites also partly convert to glucuronide or sulfate conjugates. Metabolites M-III and M-IV are the major circulating active metabolites in humans. Following once-daily administration of pioglitazone, steady-state serum concentrations of both pioglitazone and its major active metabolites, M-III (keto derivative of pioglitazone) and M-IV (hydroxyl derivative of pioglitazone), are achieved within seven days. At steady-state, M-III and M-IV reach serum concentrations equal to or greater than that of pioglitazone. At steady-state, in both healthy volunteers and patients with type 2 diabetes, pioglitazone comprises approximately 30% to 50% of the peak total pioglitazone serum concentrations (pioglitazone plus active metabolites) and 20% to 25% of the total AUC.

Maximum serum concentration (C_{max}), AUC and trough serum concentrations (C_{min}) for pioglitazone and M-III and M-IV, increased proportionally with administered doses of 15 mg and 30 mg per day.

In vitro data demonstrate that multiple CYP isoforms are involved in the metabolism of pioglitazone. The cytochrome P450 isoforms involved are CYP2C8 and, to a lesser degree, CYP3A4 with additional contributions from a variety of other isoforms, including the mainly extrahepatic CYP1A1. *In vivo* studies of pioglitazone in combination with gemfibrozil, a strong CYP2C8 inhibitor, showed that pioglitazone is a CYP2C8 substrate *[see Dosage and Administration (2.3) and Drug Interactions (7)].* Urinary 6β-hydroxycortisol/cortisol ratios measured in patients treated with pioglitazone showed that pioglitazone is not a strong CYP3A4 enzyme inducer.

Excretion and Elimination

Alogliptin

The primary route of elimination of [^{14}C] alogliptin derived radioactivity occurred via renal excretion (76%), with 13% recovered in the feces, achieving a total recovery of 89% of the administered radioactive dose. The renal clearance of alogliptin (9.6 L/hr) indicates some active renal tubular secretion and systematic clearance was 14.0 L/hr.

Pioglitazone

Following oral administration, approximately 15% to 30% of the pioglitazone dose is recovered in the urine. Renal elimination of pioglitazone is negligible, and the drug is excreted primarily as metabolites and their conjugates. It is presumed that most of the oral dose is excreted into the bile either unchanged or as metabolites and eliminated in the feces.

The mean serum half-life of pioglitazone and its metabolites (M-III and M-IV) range from three to seven hours and 16 to 24 hours, respectively. Pioglitazone has an apparent clearance, CL/F, calculated to be 5 to 7 L/hr.

Special Populations

Renal Impairment

Alogliptin

A single-dose, open-label study was conducted to evaluate the pharmacokinetics of alogliptin 50 mg in patients with chronic renal impairment compared with healthy subjects. In patients with mild renal impairment (creatinine clearance [CrCl] ≥60 to <90 mL/min), an approximate 1.2-fold increase in plasma AUC of alogliptin was observed. Because increases of this magnitude are not considered clinically relevant, dose adjustment for patients with mild renal impairment is not recommended.

In patients with moderate renal impairment (CrCl ≥30 to <60 mL/min), an approximate two-fold increase in plasma AUC of alogliptin was observed. To maintain similar systemic exposures of OSENI to those with normal renal function, the recommended dose of OSENI is 12.5 mg/15 mg, 12.5 mg/30 mg or 12.5 mg/45 mg once daily in patients with moderate renal impairment.

In patients with severe renal impairment (CrCl ≥15 to <30 mL/min) and ESRD (CrCl <15 mL/min or requiring dialysis), approximate three- and four-fold increases in plasma AUC of alogliptin were observed. Dialysis removed approximately 7% of the drug during a three-hour dialysis session. OSENI is not recommended for patients with severe renal impairment or ESRD. Coadministration of pioglitazone and alogliptin 6.25 mg once daily based on individual requirements may be considered in these patients.

Pioglitazone

The serum elimination half-life of pioglitazone, M-III and M-IV remains unchanged in patients with moderate (creatinine clearance 30 to 50 mL/min) to severe (creatinine clearance <30 mL/min) renal impairment when compared to subjects with normal renal function. Therefore no dose adjustment in patients with renal impairment is required.

Hepatic Impairment

Alogliptin

Total exposure to alogliptin was approximately 10% lower and peak exposure was approximately 8% lower in patients with moderate hepatic impairment (Child-Pugh Grade B) compared to healthy subjects. The magnitude of these reductions is not considered to be clinically meaningful. Patients with severe hepatic impairment (Child-Pugh Grade C) have not been studied. Use caution when administering OSENI to patients with liver disease *[see Use in Specific Populations (8.6) and Warnings and Precautions (5.4)].*

Pioglitazone

Compared with healthy controls, subjects with impaired hepatic function (Child-Pugh Grade B and C) have an approximate 45% reduction in pioglitazone and total pioglitazone (pioglitazone, M-III and M-IV) mean peak concentrations but no change in the mean AUC values. Therefore, no dose adjustment in patients with hepatic impairment is required.

There are postmarketing reports of liver failure with pioglitazone and clinical trials have generally excluded patients with serum ALT >2.5 times the upper limit of the reference range. Use caution in patients with liver disease *[see Warnings and Precautions (5.4)].*

Gender

Alogliptin

No dose adjustment is necessary based on gender. Gender did not have any clinically meaningful effect on the pharmacokinetics of alogliptin.

Pioglitazone

The mean C_{max} and AUC values of pioglitazone were increased 20% to 60% in women compared to men. In controlled clinical trials, A1C decreases from baseline were generally greater for females than for males (average mean difference in A1C 0.5%). Because therapy should be individualized for each patient to achieve glycemic control, no dose adjustment is recommended based on gender alone.

Geriatric

Alogliptin

No dose adjustment is necessary based on age. Age did not have any clinically meaningful effect on the pharmacokinetics of alogliptin.

Pioglitazone

In healthy elderly subjects, peak serum concentrations of pioglitazone and total pioglitazone are not significantly different, but AUC values are approximately 21% higher than those achieved in younger subjects. The mean terminal half-life values of pioglitazone were also longer in elderly subjects (about 10 hours) as compared to younger subjects (about seven hours). These changes were not of a magnitude that would be considered clinically relevant.

Pediatrics

Alogliptin

Studies characterizing the pharmacokinetics of alogliptin in pediatric patients have not been performed.

Pioglitazone

Safety and efficacy of pioglitazone in pediatric patients have not been established. Pioglitazone is not recommended for use in pediatric patients *[see Use in Specific Populations (8.4)].*

Race and Ethnicity

Alogliptin

No dose adjustment is necessary based on race. Race (White, Black and Asian) did not have any clinically meaningful effect on the pharmacokinetics of alogliptin.

Pioglitazone

Pharmacokinetic data among various ethnic groups are not available.

Drug Interactions

Coadministration of alogliptin 25 mg once daily with a CYP2C8 substrate, pioglitazone 45 mg once daily for 12 days had no clinically meaningful effects on the pharmacokinetics of pioglitazone and its active metabolites.

Specific pharmacokinetic drug interaction studies with OSENI have not been performed, although such studies have been conducted with the individual components of OSENI (alogliptin and pioglitazone).

Alogliptin

In Vitro Assessment of Drug Interactions

In vitro studies indicate that alogliptin is neither an inducer of CYP1A2, CYP2B6, CYP2C9, CYP2C19 and CYP3A4, nor an inhibitor of CYP1A2, CYP2C8, CYP2C9, CYP2C19, CYP3A4 and CYP2D6 at clinically relevant concentrations.

In Vivo Assessment of Drug Interactions

Effects of Alogliptin on the Pharmacokinetics of Other Drugs

In clinical studies, alogliptin did not meaningfully increase the systemic exposure to the following drugs that are metabolized by CYP isozymes or excreted unchanged in urine (*Figure 1*). No dose adjustment of alogliptin is recommended based on results of the described pharmacokinetic studies. [See figure 1 above]

Effects of Other Drugs on the Pharmacokinetics of Alogliptin

There are no clinically meaningful changes in the pharmacokinetics of alogliptin when alogliptin is administered concomitantly with the drugs described below (*Figure 2*). [See figure 2 at top of next page]

Figure 2. Effect of Other Drugs on the Pharmacokinetic Exposure of Alogliptin

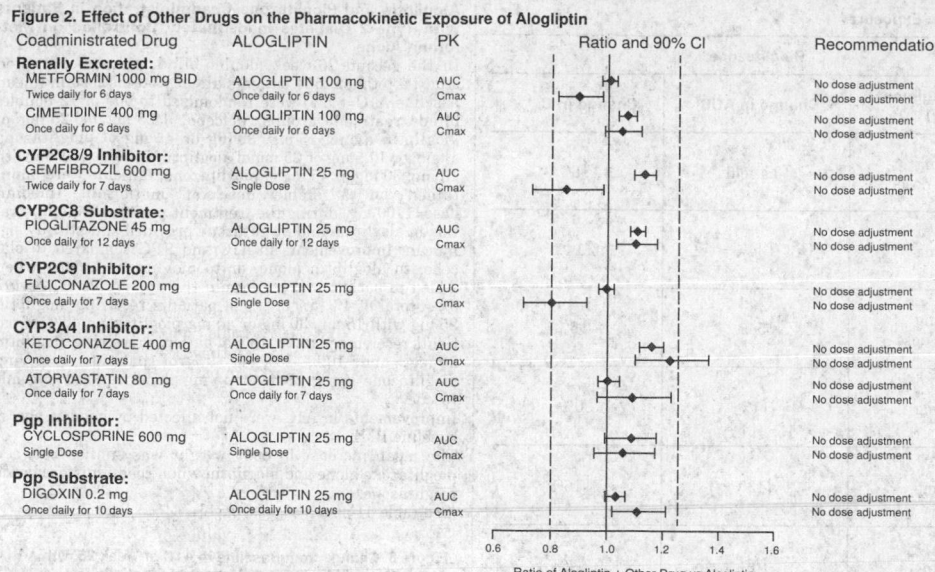

Coadministrated Drug	ALOGLIPTIN	PK	Ratio and 90% CI	Recommendation
Renally Excreted:				
METFORMIN 1000 mg BID Twice daily for 6 days	ALOGLIPTIN 100 mg Once daily for 6 days	AUC Cmax		No dose adjustment No dose adjustment
CIMETIDINE 400 mg Once daily for 6 days	ALOGLIPTIN 100 mg Once daily for 6 days	AUC Cmax		No dose adjustment No dose adjustment
CYP2C8/9 Inhibitor:				
GEMFIBROZIL 600 mg Twice daily for 7 days	ALOGLIPTIN 25 mg Single Dose	AUC Cmax		No dose adjustment No dose adjustment
CYP2C8 Substrate:				
PIOGLITAZONE 45 mg Once daily for 12 days	ALOGLIPTIN 25 mg Once daily for 12 days	AUC Cmax		No dose adjustment No dose adjustment
CYP2C9 Inhibitor:				
FLUCONAZOLE 200 mg Once daily for 7 days	ALOGLIPTIN 25 mg Single Dose	AUC Cmax		No dose adjustment No dose adjustment
CYP3A4 Inhibitor:				
KETOCONAZOLE 400 mg Once daily for 7 days	ALOGLIPTIN 25 mg Single Dose	AUC Cmax		No dose adjustment No dose adjustment
ATORVASTATIN 80 mg Once daily for 7 days	ALOGLIPTIN 25 mg Once daily for 7 days	AUC Cmax		No dose adjustment No dose adjustment
Pgp Inhibitor:				
CYCLOSPORINE 600 mg Single Dose	ALOGLIPTIN 25 mg Single Dose	AUC Cmax		No dose adjustment No dose adjustment
Pgp Substrate:				
DIGOXIN 0.2 mg Once daily for 10 days	ALOGLIPTIN 25 mg Once daily for 10 days	AUC Cmax		No dose adjustment No dose adjustment

0.6 0.8 1.0 1.2 1.4 1.6
Ratio of Alogliptin + Other Drug vs Alogliptin

Table 8. Effect of Pioglitazone Coadministration on Systemic Exposure of Other Drugs

Pioglitazone Dosage Regimen (mg)*	Coadministered Drug				
	Name and Dose Regimens	Change in AUC†		Change in C_{max}†	
45 mg (N=12)	**Warfarin‡** Daily loading then maintenance doses based PT and INR values Quick's Value=35 ± 5%	R-Warfarin	↓3%	R-Warfarin	↓2%
		S-Warfarin	↓1%	S-Warfarin	↑1%
45 mg (N=12)	**Digoxin** 0.200 mg twice daily (loading dose) then 0.250 mg daily (maintenance dose, 7 days)	↑15%		↑17%	
45 mg daily for 21 days (N=35)	**Oral Contraceptive** [Ethinyl Estradiol (EE) 0.035 mg plus Norethindrone (NE) 1 mg] for 21 days	EE	↓11%	EE	↓13%
		NE	↑3%	NE	↓7%
45 mg (N=23)	**Fexofenadine** 60 mg twice daily for 7 days	↑30%		↑37%	
45 mg (N=14)	**Glipizide** 5 mg daily for 7 days	↓3%		↓8%	
45 mg daily for 8 days (N=16)	**Metformin** 1000 mg single dose on 8 days	↓3%		↓5%	
45 mg (N=21)	**Midazolam** 7.5 mg single dose on day 15	↓26%		↓26%	
45 mg (N=24)	**Ranitidine** 150 mg twice daily for 7 days	↑1%		↓1%	
45 mg daily for 4 days (N=24)	**Nifedipine ER** 30 mg daily for 4 days	↓13%		↓17%	
45 mg (N=25)	**Atorvastatin Ca** 80 mg daily for 7 days	↓14%		↓23%	
45 mg (N=22)	**Theophylline** 400 mg twice daily for 7 days	↑2%		↑5%	

* Daily for seven days unless otherwise noted

† % change (with/without coadministered drug and no change=0%); symbols of ↑ and ↓ indicate the exposure increase and decrease, respectively

‡ Pioglitazone had no clinically significant effect on prothrombin time

Pioglitazone

[See table 8 below]
[See table 9 at top of next page]

13 NONCLINICAL TOXICOLOGY

13.1 Carcinogenesis, Mutagenesis, Impairment of Fertility

Alogliptin and Pioglitazone

No carcinogenicity, mutagenicity or impairment of fertility studies have been conducted with OSENI. The following data are based on findings in studies performed with alogliptin or pioglitazone individually.

Alogliptin

Rats were administered oral doses of 75, 400 and 800 mg/kg alogliptin for two years. No drug-related tumors were observed up to 75 mg/kg, or approximately 32 times the maximum recommended clinical dose of 25 mg, based on AUC exposure. At higher doses (approximately 308 times the maximum recommended clinical dose of 25 mg), a combination of thyroid C-cell adenomas and carcinomas increased in male but not female rats. No drug-related tumors were observed in mice after administration of 50, 150 or 300 mg/kg alogliptin for two years, or up to approximately 51 times the maximum recommended clinical dose of 25 mg, based on AUC exposure.

Alogliptin was not mutagenic or clastogenic, with and without metabolic activation, in the Ames test with *S. typhimurium* and *E. coli* or the cytogenetic assay in mouse lymphoma cells. Alogliptin was negative in the *in vivo* mouse micronucleus study.

In a fertility study in rats, alogliptin had no adverse effects on early embryonic development, mating or fertility at doses up to 500 mg/kg, or approximately 172 times the clinical dose based on plasma drug exposure (AUC).

Pioglitazone

A two-year carcinogenicity study was conducted in male and female rats at oral doses up to 63 mg/kg (approximately 14 times the MRHD of 45 mg based on mg/m²). Drug-induced tumors were not observed in any organ except for the urinary bladder. Benign and/or malignant transitional cell neoplasms were observed in male rats at 4 mg/kg and above (approximately equal to the MRHD based on mg/m²). A two-year carcinogenicity study was conducted in male and female mice at oral doses up to 100 mg/kg (approximately 11 times the MRHD based on mg/m²). No drug-induced tumors were observed in any organ.

Pioglitazone was not mutagenic in a battery of genetic toxicology studies, including the Ames bacterial assay, a mammalian cell forward gene mutation assay (CHO/HPRT and AS52/XPRT), an *in vitro* cytogenetics assay using CHL cells, an unscheduled DNA synthesis assay and an *in vivo* micronucleus assay.

No adverse effects upon fertility were observed in male and female rats at oral doses up to 40 mg/kg pioglitazone daily prior to and throughout mating and gestation (approximately nine times the MRHD based on mg/m²).

13.2 Animal Toxicology and/or Pharmacology

Pioglitazone

Heart enlargement has been observed in mice (100 mg/kg), rats (4 mg/kg and above) and dogs (3 mg/kg) treated orally with pioglitazone (approximately 11, one, and two times the MRHD for mice, rats and dogs, respectively, based on mg/m²). In a one-year rat study, drug-related early death due to apparent heart dysfunction occurred at an oral dose of 160 mg/kg (approximately 35 times the MRHD based on mg/m²). Heart enlargement was seen in a 13-week study in monkeys at oral doses of 8.9 mg/kg and above (approximately four times the MRHD based on mg/m²), but not in a 52-week study at oral doses up to 32 mg/kg (approximately 13 times the MRHD based on mg/m²).

14 CLINICAL STUDIES

The coadministration of alogliptin and pioglitazone has been studied in patients with type 2 diabetes inadequately controlled on either diet and exercise alone or on metformin alone.

There have been no clinical efficacy studies conducted with OSENI; however, bioequivalence of OSENI with coadministered alogliptin and pioglitazone tablets was demonstrated, and efficacy of the combination of alogliptin and pioglitazone has been demonstrated in four Phase 3 efficacy studies.

In patients with type 2 diabetes, treatment with OSENI produced clinically meaningful and statistically significant improvements in A1C compared to either alogliptin or pioglitazone alone. As is typical for trials of agents to treat type 2 diabetes, the mean reduction in A1C with OSENI appears to be related to the degree of A1C elevation at baseline.

Alogliptin and Pioglitazone Coadministration in Patients with Type 2 Diabetes Inadequately Controlled on Diet and Exercise

In a 26-week, double-blind, active-controlled study, a total of 655 patients inadequately controlled on diet and exercise alone (mean baseline A1C = 8.8%) were randomized to receive alogliptin 25 mg alone, pioglitazone 30 mg alone, alogliptin 12.5 mg with pioglitazone 30 mg or alogliptin 25 mg with pioglitazone 30 mg once daily. Coadministration

Table 9. Effect of Coadministered Drugs on Pioglitazone Systemic Exposure

Coadministered Drug and Dosage Regimen	Pioglitazone		
	Dose Regimen (mg)*	Change in AUC[†]	Change in C_{max}[†]
Gemfibrozil 600 mg twice daily for 2 days (N=12)	30 mg single dose	↑3.4-fold[‡]	↑6%
Ketoconazole 200 mg twice daily for 7 days (N=28)	45 mg	↑34%	↑14%
Rifampin 600 mg daily for 5 days (N=10)	30 mg single dose	↓54%	↓5%
Fexofenadine 60 mg twice daily for 7 days (N=23)	45 mg	↑1%	0%
Ranitidine 150 mg twice daily for 4 days (N=23)	45 mg	↓13%	↓16%
Nifedipine ER 30 mg daily for 7 days (N = 23)	45 mg	↑5%	↑4%
Atorvastatin Ca 80 mg daily for 7 days (N=24)	45 mg	↓24%	↓31%
Theophylline 400 mg twice daily for 7 days (N=22)	45 mg	↓4%	↓2%

* Daily for seven days unless otherwise noted
† Mean ratio (with/without coadministered drug and no change=one-fold) % change (with/without coadministered drug and no change=0%); symbols of ↑ and ↓ indicate the exposure increase and decrease, respectively
‡ The half-life of pioglitazone increased from 6.5 hours to 15.1 hours in the presence of gemfibrozil [see Dosage and Administration (2.3) and Drug Interactions (7)]

Table 10. Glycemic Parameters at Week 26 in a Coadministration Study of Alogliptin and Pioglitazone in Patients Inadequately Controlled on Diet and Exercise*

	Alogliptin 25 mg	Pioglitazone 30 mg	Alogliptin 25 mg + Pioglitazone 30 mg
A1C (%)	N=160	N=153	N=158
Baseline (mean)	8.8	8.8	8.8
Change from Baseline (adjusted mean[†])	-1	-1.2	-1.7
Difference from alogliptin 25 mg (adjusted mean[†] with 95% confidence interval)			-0.8[‡] (-1, -0.5)
Difference from pioglitazone 30 mg (adjusted mean[†] with 95% confidence interval)			-0.6[‡] (-0.8, -0.3)
% of Patients (n/N) achieving A1C ≤7%	24% (40/164)	34% (55/163)	63% (103/164)[‡]
FPG (mg/dL)	N=162	N=157	N=162
Baseline (mean)	189	189	185
Change from Baseline (adjusted mean[†])	-26	-37	-50
Difference from alogliptin 25 mg (adjusted mean[†] with 95% confidence interval)			-25[‡] (-34, -15)
Difference from pioglitazone 30 mg (adjusted mean[†] with 95% confidence interval)			-13[‡] (-22, -4)

* Intent-to-treat population using last observation carried forward
† Least squares means adjusted for treatment, geographic region and baseline value
‡ p<0.01 compared to alogliptin 25 mg or pioglitazone 30 mg

of alogliptin 25 mg with pioglitazone 30 mg resulted in statistically significant improvements from baseline in A1C and FPG compared to either alogliptin 25 mg alone or to pioglitazone 30 mg alone *(Table 10)*. Coadministration of alogliptin 25 mg with pioglitazone 30 mg once daily resulted in statistically significant reductions in fasting plasma glucose (FPG) starting from Week 2 through Week 26 compared to either alogliptin 25 mg or pioglitazone 30 mg alone. A total of 3% of patients receiving alogliptin 25 mg coadmin-

istered with pioglitazone 30 mg, 11% of those receiving alogliptin 25 mg alone, and 6% of those receiving pioglitazone 30 mg alone required glycemic rescue.
Improvements in A1C were not affected by gender, age or baseline BMI.
The mean increase in body weight was similar between pioglitazone alone and alogliptin when coadministered with pioglitazone.
[See table 10 above]

Alogliptin and Pioglitazone Coadministration in Patients with Type 2 Diabetes Inadequately Controlled on Metformin Alone

In the second 26-week, double-blind, placebo-controlled study, a total of 1554 patients already on metformin (mean baseline A1C=8.5%) were randomized to one of 12 double-blind treatment groups: placebo; 12.5 mg or 25 mg of alogliptin alone; 15 mg, 30 mg or 45 mg of pioglitazone alone; or 12.5 mg or 25 mg of alogliptin in combination with 15 mg, 30 mg or 45 mg of pioglitazone. Patients were maintained on a stable dose of metformin (median dose=1700 mg) during the treatment period. Coadministration of alogliptin and pioglitazone provided statistically significant improvements in A1C and FPG compared to placebo, to alogliptin alone, or to pioglitazone alone when added to background metformin therapy *(Table 11, Figure 3)*. A total of 4%, 5% or 2% of patients receiving alogliptin 25 mg with 15 mg, 30 mg or 45 mg pioglitazone, 33% of patients receiving placebo, 13% of patients receiving alogliptin 25 mg, and 10%, 15% or 9% of patients receiving pioglitazone 15 mg, 30 mg or 45 mg alone required glycemic rescue.
Improvements in A1C were not affected by gender, age or baseline BMI.
The mean increase in body weight was similar between pioglitazone alone and alogliptin when coadministered with pioglitazone.
[See table 11 at top of next page]

Figure 3. Change from Baseline in A1C at Week 26 with Alogliptin and Pioglitazone Alone and Alogliptin in Combination with Pioglitazone when Added to Metformin

Intent-to-treat population using last observation on study.
*P≤0.001 compared to corresponding doses of Alogliptin alone or Pioglitazone alone.

Alogliptin Add-On Therapy in Patients with Type 2 Diabetes Inadequately Controlled on Metformin in Combination with Pioglitazone

In a 52-week, active-comparator study, a total of 803 patients inadequately controlled (mean baseline A1C = 8.2%) on a current regimen of pioglitazone 30 mg and metformin at least 1500 mg per day or at the maximum tolerated dose were randomized to either receive the addition of alogliptin 25 mg or the titration of pioglitazone 30 mg to 45 mg following a four-week, single-blind, placebo run-in period. Patients were maintained on a stable dose of metformin (median dose = 1700 mg). Patients who failed to meet prespecified hyperglycemic goals during the 52-week treatment period received glycemic rescue therapy.
In combination with pioglitazone and metformin, alogliptin 25 mg was shown to be statistically superior in lowering A1C and FPG compared with the titration of pioglitazone from 30 mg to 45 mg at Week 26 and Week 52 *(Table 12, results shown only for Week 52)*. A total of 11% of patients who were receiving alogliptin 25 mg in combination with pioglitazone 30 mg and metformin and 22% of patients receiving a dose titration of pioglitazone from 30 mg to 45 mg in combination with metformin required glycemic rescue.
Improvements in A1C were not affected by gender, age, race or baseline BMI. The mean increase in body weight was similar in both treatment arms. Lipid effects were neutral.
[See table 12 at top of page 2302]

Alogliptin Add-On Therapy to a Thiazolidinedione

A 26-week, placebo-controlled study, was conducted to evaluate the efficacy and safety of alogliptin as add-on therapy to pioglitazone in patients with type 2 diabetes. A total of 493 patients inadequately controlled on a thiazolidinedione alone or in combination with metformin or a sulfonylurea (mean baseline A1C = 8%) were randomized to receive alogliptin 12.5 mg, alogliptin 25 mg or placebo. Patients were maintained on a stable dose of pioglitazone (median dose = 30 mg) during the treatment period and those who were also previously treated on metformin (median dose = 2000 mg) or sulfonylurea (median dose = 10 mg) prior to randomization were maintained on the combination therapy during the treatment period. All patients entered into a four-week, single-blind, placebo run-in period prior to randomization. Following randomization, all patients continued to receive instruction on diet and exercise. Patients who failed to meet prespecified hyperglycemic goals during the 26-week treatment period received glycemic rescue.
The addition of alogliptin 25 mg once daily to pioglitazone therapy resulted in significant improvements from baseline in A1C and FPG at Week 26 when compared to the addition of placebo *(Table 13)*. A total of 9% of patients who were receiving alogliptin 25 mg and 12% of patients receiving placebo required glycemic rescue.

Table 11. Glycemic Parameters at Week 26 for Alogliptin and Pioglitazone Alone and in Combination in Patients with Type 2 Diabetes*

	Placebo	Alogliptin 25 mg	Pioglitazone 15 mg	Pioglitazone 30 mg	Pioglitazone 45 mg	Alogliptin 25 mg + Pioglitazone 15 mg	Alogliptin 25 mg + Pioglitazone 30 mg	Alogliptin 25 mg + Pioglitazone 45 mg
A1C (%)	N=126	N=123	N=127	N=123	N=126	N=127	N=124	N=126
Baseline (mean)	8.5	8.6	8.5	8.5	8.5	8.5	8.5	8.6
Change from baseline (adjusted mean[†] with 95% confidence interval)	-0.1	-0.9	-0.8	-0.9	-1	-1.3[‡]	-1.4[‡]	-1.6[‡]
Difference from pioglitazone (adjusted mean[†] with 95% confidence interval)	-	-	-	-	-	-0.5[‡] (-0.7, -0.3)	-0.5[‡] (-0.7, -0.3)	-0.6[‡] (-0.8, -0.4)
Difference from alogliptin (adjusted mean[†] with 95% confidence interval)	-	-	-	-	-	-0.4[‡] (-0.6, -0.1)	-0.5[‡] (-0.7, -0.3)	-0.7[‡] (-0.9, -0.5)
Patients (%) achieving A1C ≤7%	6% (8/129)	27% (35/129)	26% (33/129)	30% (38/129)	36% (47/129)	55% (71/130)[‡]	53% (69/130)[‡]	60% (78/130)[‡]
FPG (mg/dL)	N=129	N=126	N=127	N=125	N=129	N=130	N=126	N=127
Baseline (mean)	177	184	177	175	181	179	179	178
Change from baseline (adjusted mean[†] with 95% confidence interval)	7	-19	-24	-29	-32	-38[‡]	-42[‡]	-53[‡]
Difference from pioglitazone (adjusted mean[†] with 95% confidence interval)	-	-	-	-	-	-14[‡] (-24, -5)	-13[‡] (-23, -3)	-20[‡] (-30, -11)
Difference from alogliptin (adjusted mean[†] with 95% confidence interval)	-	-	-	-	-	-19[‡] (-29, -10)	-23[‡] (-33, -13)	-34[‡] (-44, -24)

* Intent-to-treat population using last observation carried forward
† Least squares means adjusted for treatment, geographic region, metformin dose and baseline value
‡ p≤0.01 when compared to pioglitazone and alogliptin alone

The improvement in A1C was not affected by gender, age, baseline BMI or baseline pioglitazone dose. The mean increase in body weight was similar between alogliptin and placebo when given in combination with pioglitazone. Lipid effects were neutral.
[See table 13 at top of next page]

16 HOW SUPPLIED/STORAGE AND HANDLING

OSENI tablets are available in the following strengths and packages:
25 mg/15 mg tablet: yellow, round, biconvex and film-coated with both "A/P" and "25/15" printed on one side, available in:

NDC 64764-251-03	Bottles of 30 tablets
NDC 64764-251-04	Bottles of 90 tablets
NDC 64764-251-05	Bottles of 500 tablets

25 mg/30 mg tablet: peach, round, biconvex and film-coated with both "A/P" and "25/30" printed on one side, available in:

NDC 64764-253-03	Bottles of 30 tablets
NDC 64764-253-04	Bottles of 90 tablets
NDC 64764-253-05	Bottles of 500 tablets

25 mg/45 mg tablet: red, round, biconvex, film-coated and with both "A/P" and "25/45" printed on one side, available in:

NDC 64764-254-03	Bottles of 30 tablets
NDC 64764-254-04	Bottles of 90 tablets
NDC 64764-254-05	Bottles of 500 tablets

12.5 mg/15 mg tablet: pale yellow, round, biconvex and film-coated with both "A/P" and "12.5/15" printed on one side, available in:

NDC 64764-121-03	Bottles of 30 tablets
NDC 64764-121-04	Bottles of 90 tablets
NDC 64764-121-05	Bottles of 500 tablets

12.5 mg/30 mg tablet: pale peach, round, biconvex and film-coated with both "A/P" and "12.5/30" printed on one side, available in:

NDC 64764-123-03	Bottles of 30 tablets
NDC 64764-123-04	Bottles of 90 tablets
NDC 64764-123-05	Bottles of 500 tablets

12.5 mg/45 mg tablet: pale red, round, biconvex and film-coated with both "A/P" and "12.5/45" printed on one side, available in:

NDC 64764-124-03	Bottles of 30 tablets
NDC 64764-124-04	Bottles of 90 tablets
NDC 64764-124-05	Bottles of 500 tablets

Storage
Store at 25°C (77°F); excursions permitted to 15° to 30°C (59°to 86°F) [see USP Controlled Room Temperature]. Keep container tightly closed and protect from moisture and humidity.

17 PATIENT COUNSELING INFORMATION
See FDA-Approved Patient Labeling (Medication Guide).
17.1 Instructions
Inform patients of the potential risks and benefits of OSENI.
Patients who experience an unusually rapid increase in weight or edema or who develop shortness of breath or other symptoms of heart failure while on OSENI should immediately report these symptoms to their physician.
Patients should be informed that acute pancreatitis has been reported during use of alogliptin. Patients should be informed that persistent, severe abdominal pain, sometimes radiating to the back, which may or may not be accompanied by vomiting, is the hallmark symptom of acute pancreatitis. Patients should be instructed to promptly discontinue OSENI and contact their physician if persistent severe abdominal pain occurs.
Patients should be informed that allergic reactions have been reported during use of alogliptin and pioglitazone. If symptoms of allergic reactions (including skin rash, hives and swelling of the face, lips, tongue and throat that may cause difficulty in breathing or swallowing) occur, patients should be instructed to discontinue OSENI and seek medical advice promptly.
Patients should be informed that postmarketing reports of liver injury, sometimes fatal, have been reported during use of alogliptin and pioglitazone. If signs or symptoms of liver injury occur (e.g., unexplained nausea, vomiting, abdominal pain, fatigue, anorexia or dark urine), patients should be instructed to discontinue OSENI and seek medical advice promptly.
Tell patients to promptly report any sign of macroscopic hematuria or other symptoms such as dysuria or urinary urgency that develop or increase during treatment, as these may be due to bladder cancer.
Inform patients that hypoglycemia can occur, particularly when an insulin secretagogue or insulin is used in combination with OSENI. Explain the risks, symptoms and appropriate management of hypoglycemia.
Therapy with thiazolidinediones, including pioglitazone, which is one of the active components of OSENI, may result in ovulation in some premenopausal anovulatory women. As a result, these patients may be at an increased risk for pregnancy while taking OSENI. Therefore, adequate contraception should be recommended for all premenopausal women who are prescribed OSENI.

Table 12. Glycemic Parameters at Week 52 in an Active-Controlled Study of Alogliptin as Add-On Combination Therapy to Metformin and Pioglitazone*

	Alogliptin 25 mg + Pioglitazone 30 mg + Metformin	Pioglitazone 45 mg + Metformin
A1C (%)	N=397	N=394
Baseline (mean)	8.2	8.1
Change from Baseline (adjusted mean[†])	-0.7	-0.3
Difference from Pioglitazone 45 mg + Metformin (adjusted mean[†] with 95% confidence interval)	-0.4[‡] (-0.5, -0.3)	—
% of Patients (n/N) achieving A1C ≤7%	33% (134/404)[§]	21% (85/399)
FPG (mg/dL)	N=399	N=396
Baseline (mean)	162	162
Change from Baseline (adjusted mean[†])	-15	-4
Difference from Pioglitazone 45 mg + Metformin (adjusted mean[†] with 95% confidence interval)	-11[§] (-16, -6)	-

* Intent-to-treat population using last observation on study
† Least squares means adjusted for treatment, baseline value, geographic region and baseline metformin dose
‡ Noninferior and statistically superior to metformin plus pioglitazone at the 0.025 one-sided significance level
§ p<0.001 compared to pioglitazone 45 mg + metformin

Table 13. Glycemic Parameters at Week 26 in a Placebo-Controlled Study of Alogliptin as Add-On Therapy to Pioglitazone*

	Alogliptin 25 mg + Pioglitazone	Placebo + Pioglitazone
A1C (%)	N=195	N=95
Baseline (mean)	8	8
Change from baseline (adjusted mean[†])	-0.8	-0.2
Difference from placebo (adjusted mean[†] with 95% confidence interval)	-0.6[‡] (-0.8, -0.4)	-
% of patients (n/N) achieving A1C ≤7%	49% (98/199)[‡]	34% (33/97)
FPG (mg/dL)	N=197	N=97
Baseline (mean)	170	172
Change from baseline (adjusted mean[†])	-20	-6
Difference from placebo (adjusted mean[†] with 95% confidence interval)	-14[‡] (-23, -5)	-

* Intent-to-treat population using last observation on study
† Least squares means adjusted for treatment, baseline value, geographic region, baseline treatment regimen (pioglitazone, pioglitazone plus metformin or pioglitazone plus sulfonylurea) and baseline pioglitazone dose
‡ p<0.01 compared to placebo

Instruct patients to take OSENI only as prescribed daily. OSENI can be taken with or without meals. If a dose is missed, advise patients not to double their next dose.
Patients should be informed that the tablets must never be split.
Instruct patients to read the Medication Guide before starting OSENI therapy and to reread each time the prescription is refilled. Instruct patients to inform their healthcare provider if an unusual symptom develops or if a symptom persists or worsens.
Revised: June 2013
ALP008 R3
MEDICATION GUIDE
OSENI (OH-senn-ee)
(alogliptin and pioglitazone)
tablets
Read this Medication Guide carefully before you start taking OSENI and each time you get a refill. There may be new information. This information does not take the place of talking with your doctor about your medical condition or your treatment. If you have any questions about OSENI, ask your doctor or pharmacist.
What is the most important information I should know about OSENI?
OSENI can cause serious side effects, including:
1. New or worse heart failure: Pioglitazone, one of the medicines in OSENI, can cause your body to keep extra fluid (fluid retention), which leads to swelling (edema) and weight gain. Extra body fluid can make some heart problems worse or lead to heart failure. Heart failure means your heart does not pump blood well enough.
• Do not take OSENI if you have severe heart failure.

• If you have heart failure with symptoms (such as shortness of breath or swelling), even if these symptoms are not severe, OSENI may not be right for you.
Call your doctor right away if you have any of the following:
• swelling or fluid retention, especially in the ankles or legs
• shortness of breath or trouble breathing, especially when you lie down
• an unusually fast increase in weight
• unusual tiredness
2. Inflammation of the pancreas (pancreatitis): Alogliptin, one of the medicines in OSENI, may cause pancreatitis, which may be severe.
Certain medical conditions make you more likely to get pancreatitis.
Before you start taking OSENI:
Tell your doctor if you have ever had:
• pancreatitis
• stones in your gallbladder (gallstones)
• a history of alcoholism
• kidney problems
• liver problems
Stop taking OSENI and call your doctor right away if you have pain in your stomach area (abdomen) that is severe and will not go away. The pain may be felt going from your abdomen through to your back. The pain may happen with or without vomiting. These may be symptoms of pancreatitis.
What is OSENI?
• OSENI contains 2 prescription diabetes medicines, alogliptin (NESINA) and pioglitazone (ACTOS).

• OSENI is a prescription medicine used with diet and exercise to improve blood sugar (glucose) control in adults with type 2 diabetes.
• OSENI is not for people with type 1 diabetes.
• OSENI is not for people with diabetic ketoacidosis (increased ketones in blood or urine).
It is not known if OSENI is safe and effective in children under the age of 18. OSENI is not recommended for use in children.
Who should not take OSENI?
Do not take OSENI if you:
• have severe heart failure
• are allergic to alogliptin (NESINA), pioglitazone (ACTOS) or any ingredient in OSENI or have had a serious allergic (hypersensitivity) reaction to alogliptin or pioglitazone. See the end of this Medication Guide for a complete list of the ingredients in OSENI.
Symptoms of a serious allergic reaction to OSENI may include:
• swelling of your face, lips, throat and other areas on your skin
• difficulty with swallowing or breathing
• raised, red areas on your skin (hives)
• skin rash, itching, flaking or peeling
If you have these symptoms, stop taking OSENI and contact your doctor or go to the nearest hospital emergency room right away.
What should I tell my doctor before and during treatment with OSENI?
Before you start taking OSENI, tell your doctor if you:
• have heart failure
• have a type of diabetic eye disease that causes swelling of the back of the eye (macular edema)
• have kidney or liver problems
• have or have had inflammation of the pancreas (pancreatitis)
• have or have had cancer of the bladder
• have other medical conditions
• **are pregnant or plan to become pregnant.** It is not known if OSENI can harm your unborn baby. Talk to your doctor about the best way to control your blood sugar while you are pregnant or if you plan to become pregnant.
• **are a premenopausal woman who does not have periods regularly or at all.** OSENI may increase your chance of becoming pregnant. Talk to your doctor about birth control choices while taking OSENI. Tell your doctor right away if you become pregnant while taking OSENI.
• **are breastfeeding or plan to breastfeed.** It is not known whether OSENI passes into your breast milk and if it can harm your baby. You should not take OSENI if you breastfeed your baby. Talk with your doctor about the best way to feed your baby if you are taking OSENI.
Tell your doctor about all the medicines you take, including prescription and nonprescription medicines, vitamins and herbal supplements.
Know the medicines you take. Keep a list of them and show it to your doctor and pharmacist before you start a new medicine.
OSENI may affect the way other medicines work, and other medicines may affect how OSENI works. Contact your doctor before you start or stop other types of medicines.
How should I take OSENI?
• Take OSENI exactly as your doctor tells you to take it.
• Take OSENI 1 time each day with or without food.
• Do not break or cut OSENI tablets before swallowing.
• Your doctor may need to change your dose of OSENI to control your blood glucose. Do not change your dose unless told to do so by your doctor.
• If you miss a dose, take it as soon as you remember. If you do not remember until it is time for your next dose, skip the missed dose and take the next dose at your regular time. **Do not** take 2 doses of OSENI at the same time.
• If you take too much OSENI, call your doctor or go to the nearest hospital emergency room right away.
• If your body is under stress, such as from fever, infection, accident or surgery, the dose of your diabetes medicines may need to be changed. Call your doctor right away.
• Stay on your diet and exercise programs and check your blood sugar as your doctor tells you to.
• Your doctor may do certain blood tests before you start OSENI and during treatment as needed. Your doctor may change your dose of OSENI based on the results of your blood tests due to how well your kidneys are working.
• Your doctor will check your diabetes with regular blood tests, including your blood sugar levels and your hemoglobin A1C.
• Your doctor should check your eyes regularly while you take OSENI.
What are the possible side effects of OSENI?
OSENI can cause serious side effects, including:
• See "What is the most important information I should know about OSENI?"

- **Allergic (hypersensitivity) reactions,** such as:
  ○ swelling of your face, lips, throat and other areas on your skin
  ○ difficulty with swallowing or breathing
  ○ raised, red areas on your skin (hives)
  ○ skin rash, itching, flaking or peeling

If you have these symptoms, stop taking OSENI and contact your doctor right away.

- **Liver problems.** Call your doctor right away if you have unexplained symptoms such as:
  ○ nausea or vomiting
  ○ stomach pain
  ○ unusual or unexplained tiredness
  ○ loss of appetite
  ○ dark urine
  ○ yellowing of your skin or the whites of your eyes

- **Broken bones (fractures).** Usually in the hand, upper arm or foot in women. Talk to your doctor for advice on how to keep your bones healthy.

- **Bladder cancer.** There may be an increased chance of having bladder cancer when you take OSENI. You should not take OSENI if you are receiving treatment for bladder cancer. Tell your doctor right away if you have any of the following symptoms of bladder cancer:
  ○ blood or a red color in your urine
  ○ an increased need to urinate
  ○ pain while you urinate

- **Low blood sugar (hypoglycemia).** If you take OSENI with another medicine that can cause low blood sugar, such as a sulfonylurea or insulin, your risk of getting low blood sugar is higher. The dose of your sulfonylurea medicine or insulin may need to be lowered while you take OSENI. If you have symptoms of low blood sugar, you should check your blood sugar and treat if low, then call your doctor. Signs and symptoms of low blood sugar may include:

shaking or feeling jittery	headache
sweating	change in mood
fast heartbeat	confusion
change in vision	dizziness
hunger	

- **Diabetic eye disease with swelling in the back of the eye (macular edema).** Tell your doctor right away if you have any changes in your vision. Your doctor should check your eyes regularly.
- **Release of an egg from an ovary in a woman (ovulation) leading to pregnancy.** Ovulation may happen when premenopausal women who do not have regular monthly periods take OSENI. This can increase your chance of getting pregnant.

The most common side effects of OSENI include:
- stuffy or runny nose and sore throat
- back pain
- cold-like symptoms (upper respiratory tract infection)

Tell your doctor if you have any side effect that bothers you or that does not go away.

These are not all the possible side effects of OSENI. For more information, ask your doctor or pharmacist.

Call your doctor for medical advice about side effects. You may report side effects to FDA at 1-800-FDA-1088.

How should I store OSENI?
- Store OSENI at room temperature between 68°F to 77°F (20°C to 25°C).
- Keep container tightly closed and protect from moisture and humidity.

Keep OSENI and all medicines out of the reach of children.

General information about the safe and effective use of OSENI

Medicines are sometimes prescribed for purposes other than those listed in the Medication Guide. Do not take OSENI for a condition for which it was not prescribed. Do not give OSENI to other people, even if they have the same symptoms you have. It may harm them.

This Medication Guide summarizes the most important information about OSENI. If you would like more information, talk with your doctor. You can ask your doctor or pharmacist for information about OSENI that is written for health professionals.

For more information, go to www.oseni.com or call 1-877-TAKEDA-7 (1-877-825-3327).

What are the ingredients in OSENI?
Active ingredients: alogliptin and pioglitazone.
Inactive ingredients: mannitol, microcrystalline cellulose, hydroxypropyl cellulose, croscarmellose sodium, magnesium stearate, and lactose monohydrate; the tablets are film-coated with hypromellose, polyethylene glycol, titanium dioxide, talc and ferric oxide (yellow and/or red) and are marked with red A1 or gray F1 printing ink.

This Medication Guide has been approved by the U.S. Food and Drug Administration.

Distributed by:
Takeda Pharmaceuticals America, Inc.
Deerfield, IL 60015
Revised: June 2013
OSENI, NESINA and ACTOS are trademarks of Takeda Pharmaceutical Company Limited registered with the U.S. Patent and Trademark Office and are used under license by Takeda Pharmaceuticals America, Inc.
©2013 Takeda Pharmaceuticals America, Inc.
ALP008 R3

Shown in Product Identification Guide, page 314

ULORIC ℞
(febuxostat)
tablet for oral use

HIGHLIGHTS OF PRESCRIBING INFORMATION

These HIGHLIGHTS do not include all the information needed to use ULORIC safely and effectively. See full prescribing information for ULORIC.
ULORIC (febuxostat) tablet for oral use
Initial U.S. Approval: 2009

———RECENT MAJOR CHANGES———

Warnings and Precautions	
Hepatic Effects (5.3)	11/2012

———INDICATIONS AND USAGE———

ULORIC is a xanthine oxidase (XO) inhibitor indicated for the chronic management of hyperuricemia in patients with gout. (1)
ULORIC is not recommended for the treatment of asymptomatic hyperuricemia. (1)

———DOSAGE AND ADMINISTRATION———

- ULORIC is recommended at 40 mg or 80 mg once daily. The recommended starting dose of ULORIC is 40 mg once daily. For patients who do not achieve a serum uric acid (sUA) less than 6 mg/dL after 2 weeks with 40 mg, ULORIC 80 mg is recommended. (2.1)
- ULORIC can be administered without regard to food or antacid use. (2.1)
- No dose adjustment is necessary when administering ULORIC to patients with mild to moderate renal or hepatic impairment. (2.2)

———DOSAGE FORMS AND STRENGTHS———

Tablet: 40 mg, 80 mg. (3)

———CONTRAINDICATIONS———

ULORIC is contraindicated in patients being treated with azathioprine or mercaptopurine. (4)

———WARNINGS AND PRECAUTIONS———

- Gout Flare: An increase in gout flares is frequently observed during initiation of anti-hyperuricemic agents, including ULORIC. If a gout flare occurs during treatment, ULORIC need not be discontinued. Prophylactic therapy (i.e., non-steroidal anti-inflammatory drug [NSAID] or colchicine upon initiation of treatment) may be beneficial for up to six months. (2.4, 5.1)
- Cardiovascular Events: A higher rate of cardiovascular thromboembolic events was observed in patients treated with ULORIC than allopurinol in clinical trials. Monitor for signs and symptoms of MI and stroke. (5.2)
- Hepatic Effects: Postmarketing reports of hepatic failure, sometimes fatal. Causality cannot be excluded. If liver injury is detected, promptly interrupt ULORIC and assess patient for probable cause, then treat cause if possible, to resolution or stabilization. Do not restart ULORIC if liver injury is confirmed and no alternate etiology can be found. (5.3)

———ADVERSE REACTIONS———

Adverse reactions occurring in at least 1% of ULORIC-treated patients, and at least 0.5% greater than placebo, are liver function abnormalities, nausea, arthralgia, and rash. (6.1)

To report SUSPECTED ADVERSE REACTIONS, contact Takeda Pharmaceuticals at 1-877-TAKEDA-7 (1-877-825-3327) or FDA at 1-800-FDA-1088 or www.fda.gov/medwatch.

———DRUG INTERACTIONS———

Concomitant administration of ULORIC with XO substrate drugs, azathioprine or mercaptopurine could increase plasma concentrations of these drugs resulting in severe toxicity. (7)

———USE IN SPECIFIC POPULATIONS———

- There is insufficient data in patients with severe renal impairment. No studies have been conducted in patients with severe hepatic impairment. Caution should be exercised in these patients. (8.6, 8.7)

- No studies have been conducted in patients with secondary hyperuricemia (including patients being treated for Lesch-Nyhan syndrome or malignant disease, or in organ transplant recipients); therefore, ULORIC is not recommended for use in these patients. (8.8)

See 17 for PATIENT COUNSELING INFORMATION and FDA-approved patient labeling

Revised: 11/2013

———

FULL PRESCRIBING INFORMATION

1   INDICATIONS AND USAGE

ULORIC is a xanthine oxidase (XO) inhibitor indicated for the chronic management of hyperuricemia in patients with gout.
ULORIC is not recommended for the treatment of asymptomatic hyperuricemia.

2   DOSAGE AND ADMINISTRATION
2.1   Recommended Dose

For treatment of hyperuricemia in patients with gout, ULORIC is recommended at 40 mg or 80 mg once daily.
The recommended starting dose of ULORIC is 40 mg once daily. For patients who do not achieve a serum uric acid (sUA) less than 6 mg/dL after two weeks with 40 mg, ULORIC 80 mg is recommended.
ULORIC can be taken without regard to food or antacid use *[see Clinical Pharmacology (12.3)]*.

2.2   Special Populations

No dose adjustment is necessary when administering ULORIC in patients with mild to moderate renal impairment *[see Use in Specific Populations (8.6) and Clinical Pharmacology (12.3)]*. The recommended starting dose of ULORIC is 40 mg once daily. For patients who do not achieve a sUA less than 6 mg/dL after two weeks with 40 mg, ULORIC 80 mg is recommended.
No dose adjustment is necessary in patients with mild to moderate hepatic impairment *[see Use in Specific Populations (8.7) and Clinical Pharmacology (12.3)]*.

2.3   Uric Acid Level

Testing for the target serum uric acid level of less than 6 mg/dL may be performed as early as two weeks after initiating ULORIC therapy.

2.4   Gout Flares

Gout flares may occur after initiation of ULORIC due to changing serum uric acid levels resulting in mobilization of urate from tissue deposits. Flare prophylaxis with a non-steroidal anti-inflammatory drug (NSAID) or colchicine is

Table 1: Adverse Reactions Occurring in ≥1% of ULORIC-Treated Patients and at Least 0.5% Greater than Seen in Patients Receiving Placebo in Controlled Studies

Adverse Reactions	Placebo (N=134)	ULORIC 40 mg daily (N=757)	ULORIC 80 mg daily (N=1279)	allopurinol* (N=1277)
Liver Function Abnormalities	0.7%	6.6%	4.6%	4.2%
Nausea	0.7%	1.1%	1.3%	0.8%
Arthralgia	0%	1.1%	0.7%	0.7%
Rash	0.7%	0.5%	1.6%	1.6%

* Of the subjects who received allopurinol, 10 received 100 mg, 145 received 200 mg, and 1122 received 300 mg, based on level of renal impairment.

recommended upon initiation of ULORIC. Prophylactic therapy may be beneficial for up to six months [see Clinical Studies (14.1)].

If a gout flare occurs during ULORIC treatment, ULORIC need not be discontinued. The gout flare should be managed concurrently, as appropriate for the individual patient [see Warnings and Precautions (5.1)].

3 DOSAGE FORMS AND STRENGTHS

- 40 mg tablets, light green to green, round, debossed with "TAP" and "40"
- 80 mg tablets, light green to green, teardrop shaped, debossed with "TAP" and "80"

4 CONTRAINDICATIONS

ULORIC is contraindicated in patients being treated with azathioprine or mercaptopurine [see Drug Interactions (7)].

5 WARNINGS AND PRECAUTIONS

5.1 Gout Flare

After initiation of ULORIC, an increase in gout flares is frequently observed. This increase is due to reduction in serum uric acid levels, resulting in mobilization of urate from tissue deposits.

In order to prevent gout flares when ULORIC is initiated, concurrent prophylactic treatment with an NSAID or colchicine is recommended [see Dosage and Administration (2.4)].

5.2 Cardiovascular Events

In the randomized controlled studies, there was a higher rate of cardiovascular thromboembolic events (cardiovascular deaths, non-fatal myocardial infarctions, and non-fatal strokes) in patients treated with ULORIC (0.74 per 100 P-Y [95% Confidence Interval (CI) 0.36-1.37) than allopurinol (0.60 per 100 P-Y [95% CI 0.16-1.53) [see Adverse Reactions (6.1)]. A causal relationship with ULORIC has not been established. Monitor for signs and symptoms of myocardial infarction (MI) and stroke.

5.3 Hepatic Effects

There have been postmarketing reports of fatal and nonfatal hepatic failure in patients taking ULORIC, although the reports contain insufficient information necessary to establish the probable cause. During randomized controlled studies, transaminase elevations greater than three times the upper limit of normal (ULN) were observed (AST: 2%, 2%, and ALT: 3%, 2% in ULORIC and allopurinol-treated patients, respectively). No dose-effect relationship for these transaminase elevations was noted [see Clinical Pharmacology (12.3)].

Obtain a liver test panel (serum alanine aminotransferase [ALT], aspartate aminotransferase [AST], alkaline phosphatase, and total bilirubin) as a baseline before initiating ULORIC.

Measure liver tests promptly in patients who report symptoms that may indicate liver injury, including fatigue, anorexia, right upper abdominal discomfort, dark urine or jaundice. In this clinical context, if the patient is found to have abnormal liver tests (ALT greater than three times the upper limit of the reference range), ULORIC treatment should be interrupted and investigation done to establish the probable cause. ULORIC should not be restarted in these patients without another explanation for the liver test abnormalities.

Patients who have serum ALT greater than three times the reference range with serum total bilirubin greater than two times the reference range without alternative etiologies are at risk for severe drug-induced liver injury and should not be restarted on ULORIC. For patients with lesser elevations of serum ALT or bilirubin and with an alternate probable cause, treatment with ULORIC can be used with caution.

6 ADVERSE REACTIONS

6.1 Clinical Trials Experience

Because clinical trials are conducted under widely varying conditions, adverse reaction rates observed in the clinical trials of a drug cannot be directly compared to rates in the clinical trials of another drug and may not reflect the rates observed in practice.

A total of 2757 subjects with hyperuricemia and gout were treated with ULORIC 40 mg or 80 mg daily in clinical studies. For ULORIC 40 mg, 559 patients were treated for ≥6 months. For ULORIC 80 mg, 1377 subjects were treated for ≥6 months, 674 patients were treated for ≥1 year and 515 patients were treated for ≥2 years.

Most Common Adverse Reactions

In three randomized, controlled clinical studies (Studies 1, 2 and 3), which were six to 12 months in duration, the following adverse reactions were reported by the treating physician as related to study drug. Table 1 summarizes adverse reactions reported at a rate of at least 1% in ULORIC treatment groups and at least 0.5% greater than placebo.

[See table 1 above]

The most common adverse reaction leading to discontinuation from therapy was liver function abnormalities in 1.8% of ULORIC 40 mg, 1.2% of ULORIC 80 mg, and in 0.9% of allopurinol-treated subjects.

In addition to the adverse reactions presented in Table 1, dizziness was reported in more than 1% of ULORIC-treated subjects although not at a rate more than 0.5% greater than placebo.

Less Common Adverse Reactions

In Phase 2 and 3 clinical studies the following adverse reactions occurred in less than 1% of subjects and in more than one subject treated with doses ranging from 40 mg to 240 mg of ULORIC. This list also includes adverse reactions (less than 1% of subjects) associated with organ systems from Warnings and Precautions.

Blood and Lymphatic System Disorders: anemia, idiopathic thrombocytopenic purpura, leukocytosis/leukopenia, neutropenia, pancytopenia, splenomegaly, thrombocytopenia.

Cardiac Disorders: angina pectoris, atrial fibrillation/flutter, cardiac murmur, ECG abnormal, palpitations, sinus bradycardia, tachycardia.

Ear and Labyrinth Disorders: deafness, tinnitus, vertigo.

Eye Disorders: vision blurred.

Gastrointestinal Disorders: abdominal distention, abdominal pain, constipation, dry mouth, dyspepsia, flatulence, frequent stools, gastritis, gastroesophageal reflux disease, gastrointestinal discomfort, gingival pain, haematemesis, hyperchlorhydria, hematochezia, mouth ulceration, pancreatitis, peptic ulcer, vomiting.

General Disorders and Administration Site Conditions: asthenia, chest pain/discomfort, edema, fatigue, feeling abnormal, gait disturbance, influenza-like symptoms, mass, pain, thirst.

Hepatobiliary Disorders: cholelithiasis/cholecystitis, hepatic steatosis, hepatitis, hepatomegaly.

Immune System Disorder: hypersensitivity.

Infections and Infestations: herpes zoster.

Procedural Complications: contusion.

Metabolism and Nutrition Disorders: anorexia, appetite decreased/increased, dehydration, diabetes mellitus, hypercholesterolemia, hyperglycemia, hyperlipidemia, hypertriglyceridemia, hypokalemia, weight decreased/increased.

Musculoskeletal and Connective Tissue Disorders: arthritis, joint stiffness, joint swelling, muscle spasms/twitching/tightness/weakness, musculoskeletal pain/stiffness, myalgia.

Nervous System Disorders: altered taste, balance disorder, cerebrovascular accident, Guillain-Barré syndrome, headache, hemiparesis, hypoesthesia, hyposmia, lacunar infarction, lethargy, mental impairment, migraine, paresthesia, somnolence, transient ischemic attack, tremor.

Psychiatric Disorders: agitation, anxiety, depression, insomnia, irritability, libido decreased, nervousness, panic attack, personality change.

Renal and Urinary Disorders: hematuria, nephrolithiasis, pollakiuria, proteinuria, renal failure, renal insufficiency, urgency, incontinence.

Reproductive System and Breast Changes: breast pain, erectile dysfunction, gynecomastia.

Respiratory, Thoracic and Mediastinal Disorders: bronchitis, cough, dyspnea, epistaxis, nasal dryness, paranasal sinus hypersecretion, pharyngeal edema, respiratory tract congestion, sneezing, throat irritation, upper respiratory tract infection.

Skin and Subcutaneous Tissue Disorders: alopecia, angioedema, dermatitis, dermographism, ecchymosis, eczema, hair color changes, hair growth abnormal, hyperhidrosis, peeling skin, petechiae, photosensitivity, pruritus, purpura, skin discoloration/altered pigmentation, skin lesion, skin odor abnormal, urticaria.

Vascular Disorders: flushing, hot flush, hypertension, hypotension.

Laboratory Parameters: activated partial thromboplastin time prolonged, creatine increased, bicarbonate decreased, sodium increased, EEG abnormal, glucose increased, cholesterol increased, triglycerides increased, amylase increased, potassium increased, TSH increased, platelet count decreased, hematocrit decreased, hemoglobin decreased, MCV increased, RBC decreased, creatinine increased, blood urea increased, BUN/creatinine ratio increased, creatine phosphokinase (CPK) increased, alkaline phosphatase increased, LDH increased, PSA increased, urine output increased/decreased, lymphocyte count decreased, neutrophil count decreased, WBC increased/decreased, coagulation test abnormal, low density lipoprotein (LDL) increased, prothrombin time prolonged, urinary casts, urine positive for white blood cells and protein.

Cardiovascular Safety

Cardiovascular events and deaths were adjudicated to one of the pre-defined endpoints from the Anti-Platelet Trialists' Collaborations (APTC) (cardiovascular death, non-fatal myocardial infarction, and non-fatal stroke) in the randomized controlled and long-term extension studies. In the Phase 3 randomized controlled studies, the incidences of adjudicated APTC events per 100 patient-years of exposure were: Placebo 0 (95% CI 0.00-6.16), ULORIC 40 mg 0 (95% CI 0.00-1.08), ULORIC 80 mg 1.09 (95% CI 0.44-2.24), and allopurinol 0.60 (95% CI 0.16-1.53).

In the long-term extension studies, the incidences of adjudicated APTC events were: ULORIC 80 mg 0.97 (95% CI 0.57-1.56), and allopurinol 0.58 (95% CI 0.02-3.24).

Overall, a higher rate of APTC events was observed in ULORIC than in allopurinol-treated patients. A causal relationship with ULORIC has not been established. Monitor for signs and symptoms of MI and stroke.

6.2 Postmarketing Experience

Adverse reactions have been identified during postapproval use of ULORIC. Because these reactions are reported voluntarily from a population of uncertain size, it is not always possible to reliably estimate their frequency or establish a causal relationship.

Hepatobiliary Disorders: hepatic failure (some fatal), jaundice, serious cases of abnormal liver function test results, liver disorder.

Immune System Disorders: anaphylaxis, anaphylactic reaction.

Musculoskeletal and Connective Tissue Disorders: rhabdomyolysis.

Psychiatric Disorders: psychotic behavior including aggressive thoughts.

Renal and Urinary Disorders: tubulointerstitial nephritis.

Skin and Subcutaneous Tissue Disorders: generalized rash, Stevens Johnson Syndrome, hypersensitivity skin reactions.

7 DRUG INTERACTIONS

7.1 Xanthine Oxidase Substrate Drugs

ULORIC is an XO inhibitor. Based on a drug interaction study in healthy subjects, febuxostat altered the metabolism of theophylline (a substrate of XO) in humans [see Clinical Pharmacology (12.3)]. Therefore, use with caution when coadministering ULORIC with theophylline.

Drug interaction studies of ULORIC with other drugs that are metabolized by XO (e.g., mercaptopurine and azathioprine) have not been conducted. Inhibition of XO by ULORIC may cause increased plasma concentrations of these drugs leading to toxicity [see Clinical Pharmacology (12.3)]. ULORIC is contraindicated in patients being treated with azathioprine or mercaptopurine [see Contraindications (4)].

7.2 Cytotoxic Chemotherapy Drugs

Drug interaction studies of ULORIC with cytotoxic chemotherapy have not been conducted. No data are available regarding the safety of ULORIC during cytotoxic chemotherapy.

7.3 In Vivo Drug Interaction Studies

Based on drug interaction studies in healthy subjects, ULORIC does not have clinically significant interactions with colchicine, naproxen, indomethacin, hydrochlorothiazide, warfarin or desipramine *[see Clinical Pharmacology (12.3)]*. Therefore, ULORIC may be used concomitantly with these medications.

8 USE IN SPECIFIC POPULATIONS

8.1 Pregnancy
Pregnancy Category C: There are no adequate and well-controlled studies in pregnant women. ULORIC should be used during pregnancy only if the potential benefit justifies the potential risk to the fetus.

Febuxostat was not teratogenic in rats and rabbits at oral doses up to 48 mg/kg (40 and 51 times the human plasma exposure at 80 mg/day for equal body surface area, respectively) during organogenesis. However, increased neonatal mortality and a reduction in the neonatal body weight gain were observed when pregnant rats were treated with oral doses up to 48 mg/kg (40 times the human plasma exposure at 80 mg/day) during organogenesis and through lactation period.

8.3 Nursing Mothers
Febuxostat is excreted in the milk of rats. It is not known whether this drug is excreted in human milk. Because many drugs are excreted in human milk, caution should be exercised when ULORIC is administered to a nursing woman.

8.4 Pediatric Use
Safety and effectiveness in pediatric patients under 18 years of age have not been established.

8.5 Geriatric Use
No dose adjustment is necessary in elderly patients. Of the total number of subjects in clinical studies of ULORIC, 16% were 65 and over, while 4% were 75 and over. Comparing subjects in different age groups, no clinically significant differences in safety or effectiveness were observed but greater sensitivity of some older individuals cannot be ruled out. The C_{max} and AUC_{24} of febuxostat following multiple oral doses of ULORIC in geriatric subjects ($\geq$65 years) were similar to those in younger subjects (18 to 40 years) *[see Clinical Pharmacology (12.3)]*.

8.6 Renal Impairment
No dose adjustment is necessary in patients with mild or moderate renal impairment (Cl_{cr} 30 to 89 mL/min). The recommended starting dose of ULORIC is 40 mg once daily. For patients who do not achieve a sUA less than 6 mg/dL after two weeks with 40 mg, ULORIC 80 mg is recommended.

There are insufficient data in patients with severe renal impairment (Cl_{cr} less than 30 mL/min); therefore, caution should be exercised in these patients *[see Clinical Pharmacology (12.3)]*.

8.7 Hepatic Impairment
No dose adjustment is necessary in patients with mild or moderate hepatic impairment (Child-Pugh Class A or B). No studies have been conducted in patients with severe hepatic impairment (Child-Pugh Class C); therefore, caution should be exercised in these patients *[see Clinical Pharmacology (12.3)]*.

8.8 Secondary Hyperuricemia
No studies have been conducted in patients with secondary hyperuricemia (including organ transplant recipients); ULORIC is not recommended for use in patients whom the rate of urate formation is greatly increased (e.g., malignant disease and its treatment, Lesch-Nyhan syndrome). The concentration of xanthine in urine could, in rare cases, rise sufficiently to allow deposition in the urinary tract.

10 OVERDOSAGE
ULORIC was studied in healthy subjects in doses up to 300 mg daily for seven days without evidence of dose-limiting toxicities. No overdose of ULORIC was reported in clinical studies. Patients should be managed by symptomatic and supportive care should there be an overdose.

11 DESCRIPTION
ULORIC (febuxostat) is a xanthine oxidase inhibitor. The active ingredient in ULORIC is 2-[3-cyano-4-(2-methylpropoxy) phenyl]-4-methylthiazole-5-carboxylic acid, with a molecular weight of 316.38. The empirical formula is $C_{16}H_{16}N_2O_3S$. The chemical structure is:

Febuxostat is a non-hygroscopic, white crystalline powder that is freely soluble in dimethylformamide; soluble in dimethylsulfoxide; sparingly soluble in ethanol; slightly soluble in methanol and acetonitrile; and practically insoluble in water. The melting range is 205°C to 208°C.

ULORIC tablets for oral use contain the active ingredient, febuxostat, and are available in two dosage strengths, 40 mg and 80 mg. Inactive ingredients include lactose monohydrate, microcrystalline cellulose, hydroxypropyl cellulose, sodium croscarmellose, silicon dioxide and magnesium stearate. ULORIC tablets are coated with Opadry II, green.

12 CLINICAL PHARMACOLOGY

12.1 Mechanism of Action
ULORIC, a xanthine oxidase inhibitor, achieves its therapeutic effect by decreasing serum uric acid. ULORIC is not expected to inhibit other enzymes involved in purine and pyrimidine synthesis and metabolism at therapeutic concentrations.

12.2 Pharmacodynamics
Effect on Uric Acid and Xanthine Concentrations: In healthy subjects, ULORIC resulted in a dose dependent decrease in 24-hour mean serum uric acid concentrations and an increase in 24-hour mean serum xanthine concentrations. In addition, there was a decrease in the total daily urinary uric acid excretion. Also, there was an increase in total daily urinary xanthine excretion. Percent reduction in 24-hour mean serum uric acid concentrations was between 40% and 55% at the exposure levels of 40 mg and 80 mg daily doses.

Effect on Cardiac Repolarization: The effect of ULORIC on cardiac repolarization as assessed by the QTc interval was evaluated in normal healthy subjects and in patients with gout. ULORIC in doses up to 300 mg daily, at steady-state, did not demonstrate an effect on the QTc interval.

12.3 Pharmacokinetics
In healthy subjects, maximum plasma concentrations (C_{max}) and AUC of febuxostat increased in a dose proportional manner following single and multiple doses of 10 mg to 120 mg. There is no accumulation when therapeutic doses are administered every 24 hours. Febuxostat has an apparent mean terminal elimination half-life ($t_{1/2}$) of approximately 5 to 8 hours. Febuxostat pharmacokinetic parameters for patients with hyperuricemia and gout estimated by population pharmacokinetic analyses were similar to those estimated in healthy subjects.

Absorption: The absorption of radiolabeled febuxostat following oral dose administration was estimated to be at least 49% (based on total radioactivity recovered in urine). Maximum plasma concentrations of febuxostat occurred between 1 and 1.5 hours post-dose. After multiple oral 40 mg and 80 mg once daily doses, C_{max} is approximately 1.6 ± 0.6 mcg/mL (N=30), and 2.6 ± 1.7 mcg/mL (N=227), respectively. Absolute bioavailability of the febuxostat tablet has not been studied.

Following multiple 80 mg once daily doses with a high fat meal, there was a 49% decrease in C_{max} and an 18% decrease in AUC, respectively. However, no clinically significant change in the percent decrease in serum uric acid concentration was observed (58% fed vs. 51% fasting). Thus, ULORIC may be taken without regard to food.

Concomitant ingestion of an antacid containing magnesium hydroxide and aluminum hydroxide with an 80 mg single dose of ULORIC has been shown to delay absorption of febuxostat (approximately one hour) and to cause a 31% decrease in C_{max} and a 15% decrease in AUC_∞. As AUC rather than C_{max} was related to drug effect, change observed in AUC was not considered clinically significant. Therefore, ULORIC may be taken without regard to antacid use.

Distribution: The mean apparent steady state volume of distribution (V_{ss}/F) of febuxostat was approximately 50 L (CV ~40%). The plasma protein binding of febuxostat is approximately 99.2% (primarily to albumin), and is constant over the concentration range achieved with 40 mg and 80 mg doses.

Metabolism: Febuxostat is extensively metabolized by both conjugation via uridine diphosphate glucuronosyltransferase (UGT) enzymes including UGT1A1, UGT1A3, UGT1A9, and UGT2B7 and oxidation via cytochrome P450 (CYP) enzymes including CYP1A2, 2C8 and 2C9 and non-P450 enzymes. The relative contribution of each enzyme isoform in the metabolism of febuxostat is not clear. The oxidation of the isobutyl side chain leads to the formation of four pharmacologically active hydroxy metabolites, all of which occur in plasma of humans at a much lower extent than febuxostat.

In urine and feces, acyl glucuronide metabolites of febuxostat (~35% of the dose), and oxidative metabolites, 67M-1 (~10% of the dose), 67M-2 (~11% of the dose), and 67M-4, a secondary metabolite from 67M-1 (~14% of the dose), appeared to be the major metabolites of febuxostat *in vivo*.

Elimination: Febuxostat is eliminated by both hepatic and renal pathways. Following an 80 mg oral dose of ^{14}C-labeled febuxostat, approximately 49% of the dose was recovered in the urine as unchanged febuxostat (3%), the acyl glucuronide of the drug (30%), its known oxidative metabolites and their conjugates (13%), and other unknown metabolites

(3%). In addition to the urinary excretion, approximately 45% of the dose was recovered in the feces as the unchanged febuxostat (12%), the acyl glucuronide of the drug (1%), its known oxidative metabolites and their conjugates (25%), and other unknown metabolites (7%).

The apparent mean terminal elimination half-life ($t_{1/2}$) of febuxostat was approximately 5 to 8 hours.

Special Populations

Pediatric Use: The pharmacokinetics of ULORIC in patients under the age of 18 years have not been studied.

Geriatric Use: The C_{max} and AUC of febuxostat and its metabolites following multiple oral doses of ULORIC in geriatric subjects ($\geq$65 years) were similar to those in younger subjects (18 to 40 years). In addition, the percent decrease in serum uric acid concentration was similar between elderly and younger subjects. No dose adjustment is necessary in geriatric patients *[see Use in Specific Populations (8.5)]*.

Renal Impairment: Following multiple 80 mg doses of ULORIC in healthy subjects with mild (Cl_{cr} 50 to 80 mL/min), moderate (Cl_{cr} 30 to 49 mL/min) or severe renal impairment (Cl_{cr} 10 to 29 mL/min), the C_{max} of febuxostat did not change relative to subjects with normal renal function (Cl_{cr} greater than 80 mL/min). AUC and half-life of febuxostat increased in subjects with renal impairment in comparison to subjects with normal renal function, but values were similar among three renal impairment groups. Mean febuxostat AUC values were up to 1.8 times higher in subjects with renal impairment compared to those with normal renal function. Mean C_{max} and AUC values for three active metabolites increased up to 2- and 4-fold, respectively. However, the percent decrease in serum uric acid concentration for subjects with renal impairment was comparable to those with normal renal function (58% in normal renal function group and 55% in the severe renal function group).

No dose adjustment is necessary in patients with mild to moderate renal impairment *[see Dosage and Administration (2) and Use in Specific Populations (8.6)]*. The recommended starting dose of ULORIC is 40 mg once daily. For patients who do not achieve a sUA less than 6 mg/dL after two weeks with 40 mg, ULORIC 80 mg is recommended. There is insufficient data in patients with severe renal impairment; caution should be exercised in those patients *[see Use in Specific Populations (8.6)]*.

ULORIC has not been studied in end stage renal impairment patients who are on dialysis.

Hepatic Impairment: Following multiple 80 mg doses of ULORIC in patients with mild (Child-Pugh Class A) or moderate (Child-Pugh Class B) hepatic impairment, an average of 20% to 30% increase was observed for both C_{max} and AUC_{24} (total and unbound) in hepatic impairment groups compared to subjects with normal hepatic function. In addition, the percent decrease in serum uric acid concentration was comparable between different hepatic groups (62% in healthy group, 49% in mild hepatic impairment group, and 48% in moderate hepatic impairment group). No dose adjustment is necessary in patients with mild or moderate hepatic impairment. No studies have been conducted in subjects with severe hepatic impairment (Child-Pugh Class C); caution should be exercised in those patients *[see Use in Specific Populations (8.7)]*.

Gender: Following multiple oral doses of ULORIC, the C_{max} and AUC_{24} of febuxostat were 30% and 14% higher in females than in males, respectively. However, weight-corrected C_{max} and AUC were similar between the genders. In addition, the percent decrease in serum uric acid concentrations was similar between genders. No dose adjustment is necessary based on gender.

Race: No specific pharmacokinetic study was conducted to investigate the effects of race.

Drug-Drug Interactions

Effect of ULORIC on Other Drugs

Xanthine Oxidase Substrate Drugs-Azathioprine, Mercaptopurine, and Theophylline: Febuxostat is an XO inhibitor. A drug-drug interaction study evaluating the effect of ULORIC upon the pharmacokinetics of theophylline (an XO substrate) in healthy subjects showed that coadministration of febuxostat with theophylline resulted in an approximately 400-fold increase in the amount of 1-methylxanthine, one of the major metabolites of theophylline, excreted in the urine. Since the long-term safety of exposure to 1-methylxanthine in humans is unknown, use with caution when coadministering febuxostat with theophylline.

Drug interaction studies of ULORIC with other drugs that are metabolized by XO (e.g., mercaptopurine and azathioprine) have not been conducted. Inhibition of XO by ULORIC may cause increased plasma concentrations of these drugs leading to toxicity. ULORIC is contraindicated in patients being treated with azathioprine or mercaptopurine *[see Contraindications (4) and Drug Interactions (7)]*. Azathioprine and mercaptopurine undergo metabolism via three major metabolic pathways, one of which is mediated

Table 3: Proportion of Patients with Serum Uric Acid Levels less than 6 mg/dL at Final Visit

Study*	ULORIC 40 mg daily	ULORIC 80 mg daily	allopurinol	Placebo	Difference in Proportion (95% CI)	
					ULORIC 40 mg vs allopurinol	ULORIC 80 mg vs allopurinol
Study 1 (6 months) (N=2268)	45%	67%	42%		3% (-2%, 8%)	25% (20%, 30%)
Study 2 (6 months) (N=643)		72%	39%	1%		33% (26%, 42%)
Study 3 (12 months) (N=491)		74%	36%			38% (30%, 46%)

* Randomization was balanced between treatment groups, except in Study 2 in which twice as many patients were randomized to each of the active treatment groups compared to placebo.

by XO. Although ULORIC drug interaction studies with azathioprine and mercaptopurine have not been conducted, concomitant administration of allopurinol [a xanthine oxidase inhibitor] with azathioprine or mercaptopurine has been reported to substantially increase plasma concentrations of these drugs. Because ULORIC is a xanthine oxidase inhibitor, it could inhibit the XO-mediated metabolism of azathioprine and mercaptopurine leading to increased plasma concentrations of azathioprine or mercaptopurine that could result in severe toxicity.

P450 Substrate Drugs: In vitro studies have shown that febuxostat does not inhibit P450 enzymes CYP1A2, 2C9, 2C19, 2D6, or 3A4 and it also does not induce CYP1A2, 2B6, 2C9, 2C19, or 3A4 at clinically relevant concentrations. As such, pharmacokinetic interactions between ULORIC and drugs metabolized by these CYP enzymes are unlikely.

Effect of Other Drugs on ULORIC
Febuxostat is metabolized by conjugation and oxidation via multiple metabolizing enzymes. The relative contribution of each enzyme isoform is not clear. Drug interactions between ULORIC and a drug that inhibits or induces one particular enzyme isoform is in general not expected.

In Vivo Drug Interaction Studies
Theophylline: No dose adjustment is necessary for theophylline when coadministered with ULORIC. Administration of ULORIC (80 mg once daily) with theophylline resulted in an increase of 6% in C_{max} and 6.5% in AUC of theophylline. These changes were not considered statistically significant. However, the study also showed an approximately 400-fold increase in the amount of 1-methylxanthine (one of the major theophylline metabolites) excreted in urine as a result of XO inhibition by ULORIC. The safety of long-term exposure to 1-methylxanthine has not been evaluated. This should be taken into consideration when deciding to coadminister ULORIC and theophylline.

Colchicine: No dose adjustment is necessary for either ULORIC or colchicine when the two drugs are coadministered. Administration of ULORIC (40 mg once daily) with colchicine (0.6 mg twice daily) resulted in an increase of 12% in C_{max} and 7% in AUC_{24} of febuxostat. In addition, administration of colchicine (0.6 mg twice daily) with ULORIC (120 mg daily) resulted in a less than 11% change in C_{max} or AUC of colchicine for both AM and PM doses. These changes were not considered clinically significant.

Naproxen: No dose adjustment is necessary for ULORIC or naproxen when the two drugs are coadministered. Administration of ULORIC (80 mg once daily) with naproxen (500 mg twice daily) resulted in a 28% increase in C_{max} and a 40% increase in AUC of febuxostat. The increases were not considered clinically significant. In addition, there were no significant changes in the C_{max} or AUC of naproxen (less than 2%).

Indomethacin: No dose adjustment is necessary for either ULORIC or indomethacin when these two drugs are coadministered. Administration of ULORIC (80 mg once daily) with indomethacin (50 mg twice daily) did not result in any significant changes in C_{max} or AUC of febuxostat or indomethacin (less than 7%).

Hydrochlorothiazide: No dose adjustment is necessary for ULORIC when coadministered with hydrochlorothiazide. Administration of ULORIC (80 mg) with hydrochlorothiazide (50 mg) did not result in any clinically significant changes in C_{max} or AUC of febuxostat (less than 4%), and serum uric acid concentrations were not substantially affected.

Warfarin: No dose adjustment is necessary for warfarin when coadministered with ULORIC. Administration of ULORIC (80 mg once daily) with warfarin had no effect on the pharmacokinetics of warfarin in healthy subjects. INR and Factor VII activity were also not affected by the coadministration of ULORIC.

Desipramine: Coadministration of drugs that are CYP2D6 substrates (such as desipramine) with ULORIC are not ex-

pected to require dose adjustment. Febuxostat was shown to be a weak inhibitor of CYP2D6 in vitro and in vivo. Administration of ULORIC (120 mg once daily) with desipramine (25 mg) resulted in an increase in C_{max} (16%) and AUC (22%) of desipramine, which was associated with a 17% decrease in the 2-hydroxydesipramine to desipramine metabolic ratio (based on AUC).

13   NONCLINICAL TOXICOLOGY
13.1   Carcinogenesis, Mutagenesis, Impairment of Fertility
Carcinogenesis: Two-year carcinogenicity studies were conducted in F344 rats and B6C3F1 mice. Increased transitional cell papilloma and carcinoma of urinary bladder was observed at 24 mg/kg (25 times the human plasma exposure at maximum recommended human dose of 80 mg/day) and 18.75 mg/kg (12.5 times the human plasma exposure at 80 mg/day) in male rats and female mice, respectively. The urinary bladder neoplasms were secondary to calculus formation in the kidney and urinary bladder.
Mutagenesis: Febuxostat showed a positive mutagenic response in a chromosomal aberration assay in a Chinese hamster lung fibroblast cell line with and without metabolic activation in vitro. Febuxostat was negative in the in vitro Ames assay and chromosomal aberration test in human peripheral lymphocytes, and L5178Y mouse lymphoma cell line, and in vivo tests in mouse micronucleus, rat unscheduled DNA synthesis and rat bone marrow cells.
Impairment of Fertility: Febuxostat at oral doses up to 48 mg/kg/day (approximately 35 times the human plasma exposure at 80 mg/day) had no effect on fertility and reproductive performance of male and female rats.

13.2   Animal Toxicology
A 12-month toxicity study in beagle dogs showed deposition of xanthine crystals and calculi in kidneys at 15 mg/kg (approximately four times the human plasma exposure at 80 mg/day). A similar effect of calculus formation was noted in rats in a six-month study due to deposition of xanthine crystals at 48 mg/kg (approximately 35 times the human plasma exposure at 80 mg/day).

14   CLINICAL STUDIES
A serum uric acid level of less than 6 mg/dL is the goal of anti-hyperuricemic therapy and has been established as appropriate for the treatment of gout.

14.1   Management of Hyperuricemia in Gout
The efficacy of ULORIC was demonstrated in three randomized, double-blind, controlled trials in patients with hyperuricemia and gout. Hyperuricemia was defined as a baseline serum uric acid level ≥8 mg/dL.
Study 1 randomized patients to: ULORIC 40 mg daily, ULORIC 80 mg daily, or allopurinol (300 mg daily for patients with estimated creatinine clearance (Cl_{cr}) ≥60 mL/min or 200 mg daily for patients with estimated Cl_{cr} ≥30 mL/min and ≤59 mL/min). The duration of Study 1 was six months.
Study 2 randomized patients to: placebo, ULORIC 80 mg daily, ULORIC 120 mg daily, ULORIC 240 mg daily or allopurinol (300 mg daily for patients with a baseline serum creatinine ≤1.5 mg/dL or 100 mg daily for patients with a baseline serum creatinine greater than 1.5 mg/dL and ≤2 mg/dL). The duration of Study 2 was six months.
Study 3, a 1-year study, randomized patients to: ULORIC 80 mg daily, ULORIC 120 mg daily, or allopurinol 300 mg daily. Subjects who completed Study 2 and Study 3 were eligible to enroll in a phase 3 long-term extension study in which subjects received treatment with ULORIC for over three years.
In all three studies, subjects received naproxen 250 mg twice daily or colchicine 0.6 mg once or twice daily for gout flare prophylaxis. In Study 1 the duration of prophylaxis was six months; in Study 2 and Study 3 the duration of prophylaxis was eight weeks.

The efficacy of ULORIC was also evaluated in a four week dose ranging study which randomized patients to: placebo, ULORIC 40 mg daily, ULORIC 80 mg daily, or ULORIC 120 mg daily. Subjects who completed this study were eligible to enroll in a long-term extension study in which subjects received treatment with ULORIC for up to five years.
Patients in these studies were representative of the patient population for which ULORIC use is intended. Table 2 summarizes the demographics and baseline characteristics for the subjects enrolled in the studies.

Table 2: Patient Demographics and Baseline Characteristics in Study 1, Study 2 and Study 3

Male		95%
Race:	Caucasian	80%
	African American	10%
Ethnicity: Hispanic or Latino		7%
Alcohol User		67%
Mild to Moderate Renal Insufficiency (percent with estimated Cl_{cr} less than 90 mL/min)		59%
History of Hypertension		49%
History of Hyperlipidemia		38%
BMI ≥30 kg/m^2		63%
Mean BMI		33 kg/m^2
Baseline sUA ≥10 mg/dL		36%
Mean baseline sUA		9.7 mg/dL
Experienced a gout flare in previous year		85%

Serum Uric Acid Level less than 6 mg/dL at Final Visit: ULORIC 80 mg was superior to allopurinol in lowering serum uric acid to less than 6 mg/dL at the final visit. ULORIC 40 mg daily, although not superior to allopurinol, was effective in lowering serum uric acid to less than 6 mg/dL at the final visit (Table 3).
[See table 3 above]
In 76% of ULORIC 80 mg patients, reduction in serum uric acid levels to less than 6 mg/dL was noted by the Week 2 visit. Average serum uric acid levels were maintained at 6 mg/dL or below throughout treatment in 83% of these patients.
In all treatment groups, fewer subjects with higher baseline serum urate levels (≥10 mg/dL) and/or tophi achieved the goal of lowering serum uric acid to less than 6 mg/dL at the final visit; however, a higher proportion achieved a serum uric acid less than 6 mg/dL with ULORIC 80 mg than with ULORIC 40 mg or allopurinol.
Study 1 evaluated efficacy in patients with mild to moderate renal impairment (i.e., baseline estimated Cl_{cr} less than 90 mL/min). The results in this sub-group of patients are shown in Table 4.
[See table 4 at top of next page]

16   HOW SUPPLIED/STORAGE AND HANDLING
ULORIC 40 mg tablets are light green to green in color, round, debossed with "TAP" on one side and "40" on the other side and supplied as:

NDC Number	Size
64764-918-11	Hospital Unit Dose Pack of 100 Tablets
64764-918-30	Bottle of 30 Tablets
64764-918-90	Bottle of 90 Tablets
64764-918-18	Bottle of 500 Tablets

ULORIC 80 mg tablets are light green to green in color, teardrop shaped, debossed with "TAP" on one side and "80" on the other side and supplied as:

NDC Number	Size
64764-677-11	Hospital Unit Dose Pack of 100 Tablets
64764-677-30	Bottle of 30 Tablets
64764-677-13	Bottle of 100 Tablets
64764-677-19	Bottle of 1000 Tablets

Protect from light. Store at 25°C (77°F); excursions permitted to 15° to 30°C (59° to 86°F) [See USP Controlled Room Temperature].

Table 4: Proportion of Patients with Serum Uric Acid Levels less than 6 mg/dL in Patients with Mild or Moderate Renal Impairment at Final Visit

ULORIC 40 mg daily (N=479)	ULORIC 80 mg daily (N=503)	allopurinol* 300 mg daily (N=501)	Difference in Proportion (95% CI)	
			ULORIC 40 mg vs allopurinol	ULORIC 80 mg vs allopurinol
50%	72%	42%	7% (1%, 14%)	29% (23%, 35%)

* Allopurinol patients (n=145) with estimated Cl_{cr} ≥30 mL/min and Cl_{cr} ≤59 mL/min were dosed at 200 mg daily.

17 PATIENT COUNSELING INFORMATION

See FDA-Approved Patient Labeling (Patient Information)

17.1 General Information

Patients should be advised of the potential benefits and risks of ULORIC. Patients should be informed about the potential for gout flares, elevated liver enzymes and adverse cardiovascular events after initiation of ULORIC therapy. Concomitant prophylaxis with an NSAID or colchicine for gout flares should be considered.

Patients should be instructed to inform their healthcare professional if they develop a rash, chest pain, shortness of breath or neurologic symptoms suggesting a stroke. Patients should be instructed to inform their healthcare professional of any other medications they are currently taking with ULORIC, including over-the-counter medications.

Patient Information

ULORIC (U–'lor–ik)

(febuxostat) tablets

Read the Patient Information that comes with ULORIC before you start taking it and each time you get a refill. There may be new information. This information does not take the place of talking with your healthcare provider about your medical condition or your treatment.

What is ULORIC?

ULORIC is a prescription medicine called a xanthine oxidase (XO) inhibitor, used to lower blood uric acid levels in adults with gout.

It is not known if ULORIC is safe and effective in children under 18 years of age.

Who should not take ULORIC?

Do not take ULORIC if you:

• take azathioprine (Azasan, Imuran)

• take mercaptopurine (Purinethol)

It is not known if ULORIC is safe and effective in children under 18 years of age.

What should I tell my healthcare provider before taking ULORIC?

Before taking ULORIC tell your healthcare provider about all of your medical conditions, including if you:

• have liver or kidney problems

• have a history of heart disease or stroke

• are pregnant or plan to become pregnant. It is not known if ULORIC will harm your unborn baby. Talk with your healthcare provider if you are pregnant or plan to become pregnant.

• are breastfeeding or plan to breastfeed. It is not known if ULORIC passes into your breast milk. You and your healthcare provider should decide if you should take ULORIC while breastfeeding.

Tell your healthcare provider about all the medicines you take, including prescription and non-prescription medicines, vitamins, and herbal supplements. ULORIC may affect the way other medicines work, and other medicines may affect how ULORIC works.

Know the medicines you take. Keep a list of them and show it to your healthcare provider and pharmacist when you get a new medicine.

How should I take ULORIC?

• Take ULORIC exactly as your healthcare provider tells you to take it.

• ULORIC can be taken with or without food.

• ULORIC can be taken with antacids.

• Your gout may flare up when you start taking ULORIC, do not stop taking your ULORIC even if you have a flare. Your healthcare provider may give you other medicines to help prevent your gout flares.

• Your healthcare provider may do certain tests while you take ULORIC.

What are the possible side effects of ULORIC?

Heart problems. A small number of heart attacks, strokes and heart-related deaths were seen in clinical studies. It is not certain that ULORIC caused these events.

The most common side effects of ULORIC include:

• liver problems

• nausea

• gout flares

• joint pain

• rash

Tell your healthcare provider if you develop a rash, have any side effect that bothers you, or that does not go away. These are not all of the possible side effects of ULORIC. For more information, ask your healthcare provider or pharmacist.

Call your doctor for medical advice about side effects. You may report side effects to the FDA at 1-800-FDA-1088.

How should I store ULORIC?

Store ULORIC between 59°F and 86°F (15°C to 30°C).

Keep ULORIC out of the light.

Keep ULORIC and all medicines out of the reach of children.

General information about the safe and effective use of ULORIC.

Medicines are sometimes prescribed for purposes other than those listed in a patient information leaflet. Do not use ULORIC for a condition for which it was not prescribed. Do not give ULORIC to other people, even if they have the same symptoms that you have. It may harm them.

This patient information leaflet summarizes the most important information about ULORIC. If you would like more information about ULORIC talk with your healthcare provider. You can ask your healthcare provider or pharmacist for information about ULORIC that is written for health professionals. For more information go to www.uloric.com, or call 1-877-825-3327.

What are the ingredients in ULORIC?

Active Ingredient: febuxostat

Inactive ingredients include: lactose monohydrate, microcrystalline cellulose, hydroxypropyl cellulose, sodium croscarmellose, silicon dioxide, magnesium stearate, and Opadry II, green

Distributed by:

Takeda Pharmaceuticals America, Inc.

Deerfield, IL 60015

Revised: March 2013

ULORIC is a registered trademark of Teijin Limited registered in the U.S. Patent and Trademark Office and used under license by Takeda Pharmaceuticals America, Inc.

All other trademarks are the property of their respective owners.

©2009-2013 Takeda Pharmaceuticals America, Inc.

ULR015 R4

Shown in Product Identification Guide, page 314

Teva Respiratory, LLC.

425 PRIVET ROAD

HORSHAM, PA 19044

For All Inquiries Call:

1-888-482-9522

PROAIR HFA

(albuterol sulfate)

Inhalation Aerosol

℞

HIGHLIGHTS OF PRESCRIBING INFORMATION

These highlights do not include all the information needed to use PROAIR HFA safely and effectively. See full prescribing information for PROAIR HFA Inhalation Aerosol

PROAIR HFA (albuterol sulfate) INHALATION AEROSOL

Initial U.S. Approval: 1981

————RECENT MAJOR CHANGES————

Dosage and Administration (2.3)   03/12

————INDICATIONS AND USAGE————

PROAIR HFA Inhalation Aerosol is a beta₂-adrenergic agonist indicated for:

• Treatment or prevention of bronchospasm in patients 4 years of age and older with reversible obstructive airway disease. (1.1)

• Prevention of exercise-induced bronchospasm in patients 4 years of age and older. (1.2)

————DOSAGE AND ADMINISTRATION————

For oral inhalation only

• Treatment or prevention of bronchospasm in adults and children 4 years of age and older: 2 inhalations every 4 to 6 hours. In some patients, one inhalation every 4 hours may be sufficient. (2.1)

• Prevention of exercise-induced bronchospasm in adults and children 4 years of age and older: 2 inhalations 15 to 30 minutes before exercise. (2.2)

• Priming information: Prime PROAIR HFA before using for the first time, or when the inhaler has not been used for more than 2 weeks. To prime PROAIR HFA, release 3 sprays into the air away from the face. Shake well before each spray. (2.3)

• Cleaning information: At least once a week, wash the actuator with warm water, shake off excess, and air dry thoroughly. (2.3)

• PROAIR HFA inhaler should be discarded when the dose counter displays 0 or after the expiration date on the product, whichever comes first. (2.3)

————DOSAGE FORMS AND STRENGTHS————

Inhalation Aerosol: Each actuation delivers 108 mcg of albuterol sulfate from the actuator mouthpiece (equivalent to 90 mcg of albuterol base). Supplied in 8.5-g canister containing 200 actuations. (3)

————CONTRAINDICATIONS————

Hypersensitivity to albuterol and any other PROAIR HFA Inhalation Aerosol Components. (4)

————WARNINGS AND PRECAUTIONS————

• Life-threatening paradoxical bronchospasm may occur. Discontinue PROAIR HFA immediately and treat with alternative therapy. (5.1)

• Need for more doses of PROAIR HFA than usual may be a sign of deterioration of asthma and requires reevaluation of treatment. (5.2)

• PROAIR HFA is not a substitute for corticosteroids. (5.3)

• Cardiovascular effects may occur. Use with caution in patients sensitive to sympathomimetic drugs and patients with cardiovascular or convulsive disorders. (5.4, 5.7)

• Excessive use may be fatal. Do not exceed recommended dose. (5.5)

• Immediate hypersensitivity reactions may occur. Discontinue PROAIR HFA immediately. (5.6)

• Hypokalemia and changes in blood glucose may occur. (5.7, 5.8)

————ADVERSE REACTIONS————

Most common adverse reactions (≥3.0% and >placebo) are headache, tachycardia, pain, dizziness, pharyngitis, and rhinitis. (6.1)

To report SUSPECTED ADVERSE REACTIONS, contact Teva Respiratory, LLC at 1-888-482-9522 or FDA at 1-800-FDA-1088 or www.fda.gov/medwatch.

————DRUG INTERACTIONS————

• Other short-acting sympathomimetic aerosol bronchodilators and adrenergic drugs: May potentiate effect. (7)

• Beta-blockers: May decrease effectiveness of PROAIR HFA and produce severe bronchospasm. Patients with asthma should not normally be treated with beta-blockers. (7.1)

• Diuretics, or non-potassium sparing diuretics: May potentiate hypokalemia or ECG changes. Consider monitoring potassium levels. (7.2)

• Digoxin: May decrease serum digoxin levels. Consider monitoring digoxin levels. (7.3)

• Monoamine oxidase (MAO) inhibitors and tricyclic antidepressants: May potentiate effect of albuterol on the cardiovascular system. Consider alternative therapy in patients taking MAOs or tricyclic antidepressants. (7.4)

See 17 for PATIENT COUNSELING INFORMATION and FDA-approved patient labeling

Revised: 05/2012

FULL PRESCRIBING INFORMATION: CONTENTS*

FULL PRESCRIBING INFORMATION

1   INDICATIONS AND USAGE

1.1   Bronchospasm

PROAIR HFA Inhalation Aerosol is indicated for the treatment or prevention of bronchospasm in patients 4 years of age and older with reversible obstructive airway disease.

1.2   Exercise-Induced Bronchospasm

PROAIR HFA Inhalation Aerosol is indicated for the prevention of exercise-induced bronchospasm in patients 4 years of age and older.

2   DOSAGE AND ADMINISTRATION

2.1   Bronchospasm

For treatment of acute episodes of bronchospasm or prevention of symptoms associated with bronchospasm, the usual dosage for adults and children 4 years and older is two inhalations repeated every 4 to 6 hours. More frequent administration or a larger number of inhalations is not recommended. In some patients, one inhalation every 4 hours may be sufficient.

2.2   Exercise-Induced Bronchospasm

The usual dosage for adults and children 4 years of age or older is two inhalations 15 to 30 minutes before exercise.

2.3   Administration Information

Administer PROAIR HFA by oral inhalation only. Shake well before each spray. To maintain proper use of this product and to prevent medication build-up and blockage, it is important to follow the cleaning directions carefully.

Priming: Prime the inhaler before using for the first time and in cases where the inhaler has not been used for more than 2 weeks by releasing three sprays into the air, away from the face.

Cleaning: As with all HFA-containing albuterol inhalers, to maintain proper use of this product and to prevent medication build-up and blockage, it is important to clean the plastic mouthpiece regularly. The inhaler may cease to deliver medication if the plastic actuator mouthpiece is not properly cleaned and dried. To clean: Wash the plastic mouthpiece with warm running water for 30 seconds, shake off excess water, and air dry thoroughly at least once a week. If the patient has more than one PROAIR HFA inhaler, the patient should wash each one separately to prevent attaching the wrong canister to the wrong plastic actuator. In this way, the patient can be sure to always know the correct number of remaining doses. Never attach a canister of medication from any other inhaler to the PROAIR HFA actuator and never attach the PROAIR HFA canister to an actuator from any other inhaler. If the mouthpiece becomes blocked, washing the mouthpiece will remove the blockage. If it is necessary to use the inhaler before it is completely dry, shake off excess water, replace canister, spray twice into the air away from face, and take the prescribed dose. After such use, the mouthpiece should be re-washed and allowed to air dry thoroughly. *[see FDA-Approved Patient Labeling (17.9)]*.

Dose Counter: PROAIR HFA has a dose counter attached to the actuator. When the patient receives the inhaler, a black dot will appear in the viewing window until it has been primed 3 times, at which point the number 200 will be displayed. The dose counter will count down each time a spray is released. When the dose counter reaches 20, the color of the numbers will change to red to remind the patient to contact their pharmacist for a refill of medication or consult their physician for a prescription refill. When the dose counter reaches 0, the background will change to solid red. PROAIR HFA inhaler should be discarded when the dose counter displays 0 or after the expiration date on the product, whichever comes first.

3   DOSAGE FORMS AND STRENGTHS

PROAIR HFA is an inhalation aerosol. PROAIR HFA is supplied as an 8.5 g/200 actuations pressurized aluminum canister with a red plastic actuator with a dose counter and white dust cap each in boxes of one. Each actuation delivers 120 mcg of albuterol sulfate from the canister valve and 108 mcg of albuterol sulfate from the actuator mouthpiece (equivalent to 90 mcg of albuterol base).

4   CONTRAINDICATIONS

PROAIR HFA Inhalation Aerosol is contraindicated in patients with a history of hypersensitivity to albuterol and any other PROAIR HFA Inhalation Aerosol components. Rare cases of hypersensitivity reactions, including urticaria, angioedema, and rash have been reported after the use of albuterol sulfate *[see Warnings and Precautions (5.6)]*.

5   WARNINGS AND PRECAUTIONS

5.1   Paradoxical Bronchospasm

PROAIR HFA Inhalation Aerosol can produce paradoxical bronchospasm that may be life threatening. If paradoxical bronchospasm occurs, PROAIR HFA Inhalation Aerosol should be discontinued immediately and alternative therapy instituted. It should be recognized that paradoxical bronchospasm, when associated with inhaled formulations, frequently occurs with the first use of a new canister.

5.2   Deterioration of Asthma

Asthma may deteriorate acutely over a period of hours or chronically over several days or longer. If the patient needs more doses of PROAIR HFA Inhalation Aerosol than usual, this may be a marker of destabilization of asthma and requires re-evaluation of the patient and treatment regimen, giving special consideration to the possible need for anti-inflammatory treatment, e.g., corticosteroids.

5.3   Use of Anti-inflammatory Agents

The use of beta-adrenergic-agonist bronchodilators alone may not be adequate to control asthma in many patients. Early consideration should be given to adding anti-inflammatory agents, e.g., corticosteroids, to the therapeutic regimen.

5.4   Cardiovascular Effects

PROAIR HFA Inhalation Aerosol, like other beta-adrenergic agonists, can produce clinically significant cardiovascular effects in some patients as measured by pulse rate, blood pressure, and/or symptoms. Although such effects are uncommon after administration of PROAIR HFA Inhalation Aerosol at recommended doses, if they occur, the drug may need to be discontinued. In addition, beta-agonists have been reported to produce ECG changes, such as flattening of the T wave, prolongation of the QTc interval, and ST segment depression. The clinical significance of these findings is unknown. Therefore, PROAIR HFA Inhalation Aerosol, like all sympathomimetic amines, should be used with caution in patients with cardiovascular disorders, especially coronary insufficiency, cardiac arrhythmias, and hypertension.

5.5   Do Not Exceed Recommended Dose

Fatalities have been reported in association with excessive use of inhaled sympathomimetic drugs in patients with asthma. The exact cause of death is unknown, but cardiac arrest following an unexpected development of a severe acute asthmatic crisis and subsequent hypoxia is suspected.

5.6   Immediate Hypersensitivity Reactions

Immediate hypersensitivity reactions may occur after administration of albuterol sulfate, as demonstrated by rare cases of urticaria, angioedema, rash, bronchospasm, anaphylaxis, and oropharyngeal edema. The potential for hypersensitivity must be considered in the clinical evaluation of patients who experience immediate hypersensitivity reactions while receiving PROAIR HFA Inhalation Aerosol.

5.7   Coexisting Conditions

PROAIR HFA Inhalation Aerosol, like all sympathomimetic amines, should be used with caution in patients with cardiovascular disorders, especially coronary insufficiency, cardiac arrhythmias, and hypertension; in patients with convulsive disorders, hyperthyroidism, or diabetes mellitus; and in patients who are unusually responsive to sympathomimetic amines. Clinically significant changes in systolic and diastolic blood pressure have been seen in individual patients and could be expected to occur in some patients after use of any beta-adrenergic bronchodilator. Large doses of intravenous albuterol have been reported to aggravate preexisting diabetes mellitus and ketoacidosis.

5.8   Hypokalemia

As with other beta-agonists, PROAIR HFA Inhalation Aerosol may produce significant hypokalemia in some patients, possibly through intracellular shunting, which has the potential to produce adverse cardiovascular effects. The decrease is usually transient, not requiring supplementation.

6   ADVERSE REACTIONS

Use of PROAIR HFA may be associated with the following:
- Paradoxical bronchospasm *[see Warnings and Precautions (5.1)]*
- Cardiovascular Effects *[see Warnings and Precautions (5.4)]*
- Immediate hypersensitivity reactions *[see Warnings and Precautions (5.6)]*
- Hypokalemia *[see Warnings and Precautions (5.8)]*

6.1   Clinical Trials Experience

A total of 1090 subjects were treated with PROAIR HFA Inhalation Aerosol, or with the same formulation of albuterol as in PROAIR HFA Inhalation Aerosol, during the worldwide clinical development program.

Because clinical trials are conducted under widely varying conditions, adverse reaction rates observed in the clinical trials of a drug cannot be directly compared to rates in the clinical trials of another drug and may not reflect the rates observed in practice.

Adult and Adolescents 12 Years of Age and Older: The adverse reaction information presented in the table below concerning PROAIR HFA Inhalation Aerosol is derived from a 6-week, blinded study which compared PROAIR HFA Inhalation Aerosol (180 mcg four times daily) with a double-blinded matched placebo HFA-Inhalation Aerosol and an evaluator-blinded marketed active comparator HFA-134a albuterol inhaler in 172 asthmatic patients 12 to 76 years of age. The table lists the incidence of all adverse events (whether considered by the investigator drug related or unrelated to drug) from this study which occurred at a rate of 3% or greater in the PROAIR HFA Inhalation Aerosol treatment group and more frequently in the PROAIR HFA Inhalation Aerosol treatment group than in the matched placebo group. Overall, the incidence and nature of the adverse events reported for PROAIR HFA Inhalation Aerosol and the marketed active comparator HFA-134a albuterol inhaler were comparable.

[See table at top of next page]

Adverse events reported by less than 3% of the patients receiving PROAIR HFA Inhalation Aerosol but by a greater proportion of PROAIR HFA Inhalation Aerosol patients than the matched placebo patients, which have the potential to be related to PROAIR HFA Inhalation Aerosol, included chest pain, infection, diarrhea, glossitis, accidental injury (nervous system), anxiety, dyspnea, ear disorder, ear pain, and urinary tract infection.

In small cumulative dose studies, tremor, nervousness, and headache were the most frequently occurring adverse events.

Pediatric Patients 4 to 11 Years of Age: Adverse events reported in a 3-week pediatric clinical trial comparing the same formulation of albuterol as in PROAIR HFA Inhalation Aerosol (180 mcg albuterol four times daily) to a matching placebo HFA inhalation aerosol occurred at a low incidence rate (no greater than 2% in the active treatment group) and were similar to those seen in adult and adolescent trials.

6.2   Postmarketing Experience

The following adverse reactions have been identified during postapproval use of PROAIR HFA. Because these reactions are reported voluntarily from a population of uncertain size, it is not always possible to reliably estimate their frequency or establish a causal relationship to drug exposure. Reports have included rare cases of aggravated bronchospasm, lack of efficacy, asthma exacerbation (reported fatal in one case), muscle cramps, and various oropharyngeal side-effects such as throat irritation, altered taste, glossitis, tongue ulceration, and gagging.

The following adverse events have been observed in postapproval use of inhaled albuterol: urticaria, angioedema, rash, bronchospasm, hoarseness, oropharyngeal edema, and arrhythmias (including atrial fibrillation, supraventricular tachycardia, extrasystoles). In addition, albuterol, like other sympathomimetic agents, can cause adverse reactions such as: angina, hypertension or hypotension, palpitations, central nervous system stimulation, insomnia, headache, nervousness, tremor, muscle cramps, drying or irritation of the oropharynx, hypokalemia, hyperglycemia, and metabolic acidosis.

7 DRUG INTERACTIONS

Other short-acting sympathomimetic aerosol bronchodilators should not be used concomitantly with PROAIR HFA Inhalation Aerosol. If additional adrenergic drugs are to be administered by any route, they should be used with caution to avoid deleterious cardiovascular effects.

7.1 Beta-Blockers

Beta-adrenergic-receptor blocking agents not only block the pulmonary effect of beta-agonists, such as PROAIR HFA Inhalation Aerosol, but may produce severe bronchospasm in asthmatic patients. Therefore, patients with asthma should not normally be treated with beta-blockers. However, under certain circumstances, e.g., as prophylaxis after myocardial infarction, there may be no acceptable alternatives to the use of beta-adrenergic-blocking agents in patients with asthma. In this setting, consider cardioselective beta-blockers, although they should be administered with caution.

7.2 Diuretics

The ECG changes and/or hypokalemia which may result from the administration of non-potassium sparing diuretics (such as loop or thiazide diuretics) can be acutely worsened by beta-agonists, especially when the recommended dose of the beta-agonist is exceeded. Although the clinical significance of these effects is not known, caution is advised in the coadministration of beta-agonists with non-potassium sparing diuretics. Consider monitoring potassium levels.

7.3 Digoxin

Mean decreases of 16% and 22% in serum digoxin levels were demonstrated after single dose intravenous and oral administration of albuterol, respectively, to normal volunteers who had received digoxin for 10 days. The clinical significance of these findings for patients with obstructive airway disease who are receiving albuterol and digoxin on a chronic basis is unclear. Nevertheless, it would be prudent to carefully evaluate the serum digoxin levels in patients who are currently receiving digoxin and PROAIR HFA Inhalation Aerosol.

7.4 Monoamine Oxidase Inhibitors or Tricyclic Antidepressants

PROAIR HFA Inhalation Aerosol should be administered with extreme caution to patients being treated with monoamine oxidase inhibitors or tricyclic antidepressants, or within 2 weeks of discontinuation of such agents, because the action of albuterol on the cardiovascular system may be potentiated. Consider alternative therapy in patients taking MAO inhibitors or tricyclic antidepressants.

8 USE IN SPECIFIC POPULATIONS

8.1 Pregnancy

Teratogenic Effects: Pregnancy Category C:

There are no adequate and well-controlled studies of PROAIR HFA Inhalation Aerosol or albuterol sulfate in pregnant women. During worldwide marketing experience, various congenital anomalies, including cleft palate and limb defects, have been reported in the offspring of patients treated with albuterol. Some of the mothers were taking multiple medications during their pregnancies. No consistent pattern of defects can be discerned, and a relationship between albuterol use and congenital anomalies has not been established. Animal reproduction studies in mice and rabbits revealed evidence of teratogenicity. PROAIR HFA Inhalation Aerosol should be used during pregnancy only if the potential benefit justifies the potential risk to the fetus.

In a mouse reproduction study, subcutaneously administered albuterol sulfate produced cleft palate formation in 5 of 111 (4.5%) fetuses at an exposure approximately eight-tenths of the maximum recommended human dose (MRHD) for adults on a mg/m^2 basis and in 10 of 108 (9.3%) fetuses at approximately 8 times the MRHD. Similar effects were not observed at approximately one-thirteenth of the MRHD. Cleft palate also occurred in 22 of 72 (30.5%) fetuses from females treated subcutaneously with isoproterenol (positive control).

In a rabbit reproduction study, orally administered albuterol sulfate induced cranioschisis in 7 of 19 fetuses (37%) at approximately 630 times the MRHD.

In a rat reproduction study, an albuterol sulfate/HFA-134a formulation administered by inhalation did not produce any teratogenic effects at exposures approximately 65 times the MRHD *[see Nonclinical Toxicology (13.2)]*.

8.2 Labor and Delivery

Because of the potential for beta-agonist interference with uterine contractility, use of PROAIR HFA Inhalation Aerosol for relief of bronchospasm during labor should be restricted to those patients in whom the benefits clearly outweigh the risk. PROAIR HFA Inhalation Aerosol has not been approved for the management of pre-term labor. The benefit:risk ratio when albuterol is administered for tocolysis has not been established. Serious adverse reactions, including pulmonary edema, have been reported during or following treatment of premature labor with beta$_2$-agonists, including albuterol.

Adverse Experience Incidences (% of Patients) in a Six-Week Clinical Trial*

Body System/ Adverse Event (as Preferred Term)		PROAIR HFA Inhalation Aerosol (N = 58)	Marketed active comparator HFA-134a albuterol inhaler (N = 56)	Matched Placebo HFA-134a Inhalation Aerosol (N = 58)
Body as a Whole	Headache	7	5	2
Cardiovascular	Tachycardia	3	2	0
Musculoskeletal	Pain	3	0	0
Nervous System	Dizziness	3	0	0
Respiratory System	Pharyngitis	14	7	9
	Rhinitis	5	4	2

* This table includes all adverse events (whether considered by the investigator drug related or unrelated to drug) which occurred at an incidence rate of at least 3.0% in the PROAIR HFA Inhalation Aerosol group and more frequently in the PROAIR HFA Inhalation Aerosol group than in the placebo HFA Inhalation Aerosol group.

8.3 Nursing Mothers

Plasma levels of albuterol sulfate and HFA-134a after inhaled therapeutic doses are very low in humans, but it is not known whether the components of PROAIR HFA Inhalation Aerosol are excreted in human milk.

Caution should be exercised when PROAIR HFA Inhalation Aerosol is administered to a nursing woman. Because of the potential for tumorigenicity shown for albuterol in animal studies and lack of experience with the use of PROAIR HFA Inhalation Aerosol by nursing mothers, a decision should be made whether to discontinue nursing or to discontinue the drug, taking into account the importance of the drug to the mother.

8.4 Pediatric Use

The safety and effectiveness of PROAIR HFA Inhalation Aerosol for the treatment or prevention of bronchospasm in children 12 years of age and older with reversible obstructive airway disease is based on one 6-week clinical trial in 116 patients 12 years of age and older with asthma comparing doses of 180 mcg four times daily with placebo, and one single-dose crossover study comparing doses of 90, 180, and 270 mcg with placebo in 58 patients *[see Clinical Studies (14.1)]*. The safety and effectiveness of PROAIR HFA Inhalation Aerosol for treatment of exercise-induced bronchospasm in children 12 years of age and older is based on one single-dose crossover study in 24 adults and adolescents with exercise-induced bronchospasm comparing doses of 180 mcg with placebo *[see Clinical Studies (14.2)]*.

The safety of PROAIR HFA Inhalation Aerosol in children 4 to 11 years of age is based on one 3-week clinical trial in 50 patients 4 to 11 years of age with asthma using the same formulation of albuterol as in PROAIR HFA Inhalation Aerosol comparing doses of 180 mcg four times daily with placebo. The effectiveness of PROAIR HFA Inhalation Aerosol in children 4 to 11 years of age is extrapolated from clinical trials in patients 12 years of age and older with asthma and exercise-induced bronchospasm, based on data from a single-dose study comparing the bronchodilatory effect of PROAIR HFA 90 mcg and 180 mcg with placebo in 55 patients with asthma and a 3-week clinical trial using the same formulation of albuterol as in PROAIR HFA Inhalation Aerosol in 95 asthmatic children 4 to 11 years of age comparing a dose of 180 mcg albuterol four times daily with placebo *[see Clinical Studies (14.1)]*.

The safety and effectiveness of PROAIR HFA Inhalation Aerosol in pediatric patients below the age of 4 years have not been established.

8.5 Geriatric Use

Clinical studies of PROAIR HFA Inhalation Aerosol did not include sufficient numbers of patients aged 65 and over to determine whether they respond differently from younger patients. Other reported clinical experience has not identified differences in responses between elderly and younger patients. In general, dose selection for an elderly patient should be cautious, usually starting at the low end of the dosing range, reflecting the greater frequency of decreased hepatic, renal, or cardiac function, and of concomitant disease or other drug therapy *[see Warnings and Precautions (5.4, 5.7)]*.

All beta$_2$-adrenergic agonists, including albuterol, are known to be substantially excreted by the kidney, and the risk of toxic reactions may be greater in patients with impaired renal function. Because elderly patients are more likely to have decreased renal function, care should be taken in dose selection, and it may be useful to monitor renal function.

10 OVERDOSAGE

The expected symptoms with overdosage are those of excessive beta-adrenergic stimulation and/or occurrence or exaggeration of any of the symptoms listed under ADVERSE REACTIONS, e.g., seizures, angina, hypertension or hypotension, tachycardia with rates up to 200 beats per minute, arrhythmias, nervousness, headache, tremor, dry mouth, palpitation, nausea, dizziness, fatigue, malaise, and insomnia.

Hypokalemia may also occur. As with all sympathomimetic medications, cardiac arrest and even death may be associated with abuse of PROAIR HFA Inhalation Aerosol.

Treatment consists of discontinuation of PROAIR HFA Inhalation Aerosol together with appropriate symptomatic therapy. The judicious use of a cardioselective beta-receptor blocker may be considered, bearing in mind that such medication can produce bronchospasm. There is insufficient evidence to determine if dialysis is beneficial for overdosage of PROAIR HFA Inhalation Aerosol.

The oral median lethal dose of albuterol sulfate in mice is greater than 2,000 mg/kg (approximately 6,800 times the maximum recommended daily inhalation dose for adults on a mg/m^2 basis and approximately 3,200 times the maximum recommended daily inhalation dose for children on a mg/m^2 basis). In mature rats, the subcutaneous median lethal dose of albuterol sulfate is approximately 450 mg/kg (approximately 3,000 times the maximum recommended daily inhalation dose for adults on a mg/m^2 basis and approximately 1,400 times the maximum recommended daily inhalation dose for children on a mg/m^2 basis). In young rats, the subcutaneous median lethal dose is approximately 2,000 mg/kg (approximately 14,000 times the maximum recommended daily inhalation dose for adults on a mg/m^2 basis and approximately 6,400 times the maximum recommended daily inhalation dose for children on a mg/m^2 basis). The inhalation median lethal dose has not been determined in animals.

11 DESCRIPTION

The active ingredient of PROAIR HFA (albuterol sulfate) Inhalation Aerosol is albuterol sulfate, a racemic salt, of albuterol. Albuterol sulfate has the chemical name α^1-[(*tert*-butylamino) methyl]-4-hydroxy-*m*-xylene-α,α'-diol sulfate (2:1) (salt), and has the following chemical structure:

The molecular weight of albuterol sulfate is 576.7, and the empirical formula is $(C_{13}H_{21}NO_3)_2 \bullet H_2SO_4$. Albuterol sulfate is a white to off-white crystalline powder. It is soluble in water and slightly soluble in ethanol. Albuterol sulfate is the official generic name in the United States, and salbutamol sulfate is the World Health Organization recommended generic name. PROAIR HFA Inhalation Aerosol is a pressurized metered-dose aerosol unit with a dose counter. PROAIR HFA is for oral inhalation only. It contains a microcrystalline suspension of albuterol sulfate in propellant HFA-134a (1, 1, 1, 2-tetrafluoroethane) and ethanol.

Prime the inhaler before using for the first time and in cases where the inhaler has not been used for more than 2 weeks by releasing three sprays into the air, away from the face. After priming, each actuation delivers 108 mcg albuterol sulfate, from the actuator mouthpiece (equivalent to 90 mcg of albuterol base). Each canister provides 200 actuations (inhalations).

This product does not contain chlorofluorocarbons (CFCs) as the propellant.

12 CLINICAL PHARMACOLOGY

12.1 Mechanism of Action

Albuterol sulfate is a beta$_2$-adrenergic agonist. The pharmacologic effects of albuterol sulfate are attributable to activation of beta$_2$-adrenergic receptors on airway smooth muscle. Activation of beta$_2$-adrenergic receptors leads to the activation of adenylcyclase and to an increase in the intracellular concentration of cyclic-3', 5'-adenosine monophosphate (cyclic AMP). This increase of cyclic AMP is associated with the activation of protein kinase A, which in turn inhibits the phosphorylation of myosin and lowers intracellular ionic calcium concentrations, resulting in muscle relaxation. Albuterol relaxes the smooth muscle of all airways, from the trachea to the terminal bronchioles. Albuterol acts as a functional antagonist to relax the airway irrespective of the spasmogen involved, thus protecting against all bronchoconstrictor challenges. Increased cyclic AMP concentrations are also associated with the inhibition of release of mediators from mast cells in the airway. While it is recognized that $beta_2$-adrenergic receptors are the predominant receptors on bronchial smooth muscle, data indicate that there are beta-receptors in the human heart, 10% to 50% of which are cardiac $beta_2$-adrenergic receptors. The precise function of these receptors has not been established [see **Warnings and Precautions (5.4)**].

Albuterol has been shown in most controlled clinical trials to have more effect on the respiratory tract, in the form of bronchial smooth muscle relaxation, than isoproterenol at comparable doses while producing fewer cardiovascular effects. However, inhaled albuterol, like other beta-adrenergic agonist drugs, can produce a significant cardiovascular effect in some patients, as measured by pulse rate, blood pressure, symptoms, and/or electrocardiographic changes [see **Warnings and Precautions (5.4)**].

12.2 Pharmacokinetics

The systemic levels of albuterol are low after inhalation of recommended doses. In a crossover study conducted in healthy male and female volunteers, high cumulative doses of PROAIR HFA Inhalation Aerosol (1,080 mcg of albuterol base administered over one hour) yielded mean peak plasma concentrations (C_{max}) and systemic exposure (AUC_{inf}) of approximately 4,100 pg/mL and 28,426 pg/mL*hr, respectively compared to approximately 3,900 pg/mL and 28,395 pg/mL*hr, respectively following the same dose of an active HFA-134a albuterol inhaler comparator. The terminal plasma half-life of albuterol delivered by PROAIR HFA Inhalation Aerosol was approximately 6 hours. Comparison of the pharmacokinetic parameters demonstrated no differences between the products.

The pharmacokinetic profile of PROAIR HFA Inhalation Aerosol was evaluated in a two-way cross-over study in 11 healthy pediatric volunteers, 4 to 11 years of age. A single dose administration of PROAIR HFA Inhalation Aerosol (180 mcg albuterol base) yielded a least square mean (SE) C_{max} and $AUC_{0-\infty}$ of 1,100 (1.18) pg/mL and 5,120 (1.15) pg/mL*hr, respectively. The least square mean (SE) terminal plasma half-life of albuterol delivered by PROAIR HFA Inhalation Aerosol was 166 (7.8) minutes.

Metabolism and Elimination: Information available in the published literature suggests that the primary enzyme responsible for the metabolism of albuterol in humans is SULTIA3 (sulfotransferase). When racemic albuterol was administered either intravenously or via inhalation after oral charcoal administration, there was a 3- to 4-fold difference in the area under the concentration-time curves between the (R)- and (S)-albuterol enantiomers, with (S)-albuterol concentrations being consistently higher. However, without charcoal pretreatment, after either oral or inhalation administration the differences were 8- to 24-fold, suggesting that the (R)-albuterol is preferentially metabolized in the gastrointestinal tract, presumably by SULTIA3. The primary route of elimination of albuterol is through renal excretion (80% to 100%) of either the parent compound or the primary metabolite. Less than 20% of the drug is detected in the feces. Following intravenous administration of racemic albuterol, between 25% and 46% of the (R)-albuterol fraction of the dose was excreted as unchanged (R)-albuterol in the urine.

Geriatric, Pediatric, Hepatic/Renal Impairment: No pharmacokinetic studies for PROAIR HFA Inhalation Aerosol have been conducted in neonates or elderly subjects.

The effect of hepatic impairment on the pharmacokinetics of PROAIR HFA Inhalation Aerosol has not been evaluated.

The effect of renal impairment on the pharmacokinetics of albuterol was evaluated in 5 subjects with creatinine clearance of 7 to 53 mL/min, and the results were compared with those from healthy volunteers. Renal disease had no effect on the half-life, but there was a 67% decline in albuterol clearance. Caution should be used when administering high doses of PROAIR HFA Inhalation Aerosol to patients with renal impairment [see **Use in Specific Populations (8.5)**].

13 NONCLINICAL TOXICOLOGY

13.1 Carcinogenesis, Mutagenesis, Impairment of Fertility

In a 2-year study in Sprague-Dawley rats, albuterol sulfate caused a dose-related increase in the incidence of benign leiomyomas of the mesovarium at and above dietary doses of 2 mg/kg (approximately 15 times the maximum recommended daily inhalation dose for adults on a mg/m^2 basis

and approximately 6 times the maximum recommended daily inhalation dose for children on a mg/m^2 basis). In another study this effect was blocked by the coadministration of propranolol, a non-selective beta-adrenergic antagonist. In an 18-month study in CD-1 mice, albuterol sulfate showed no evidence of tumorigenicity at dietary doses of up to 500 mg/kg (approximately 1,600 times the maximum recommended daily inhalation dose for adults on a mg/m^2 basis and approximately 740 times the maximum recommended daily inhalation dose for children on a mg/m^2 basis). In a 22-month study in Golden Hamsters, albuterol sulfate showed no evidence of tumorigenicity at dietary doses of up to 50 mg/kg (approximately 210 times the maximum recommended daily inhalation dose for adults on a mg/m^2 basis and approximately 100 times the maximum recommended daily inhalation dose for children on a mg/m^2 basis).

Albuterol sulfate was not mutagenic in the Ames test or a mutation test in yeast. Albuterol sulfate was not clastogenic in a human peripheral lymphocyte assay or in an AH1 strain mouse micronucleus assay.

Reproduction studies in rats demonstrated no evidence of impaired fertility at oral doses up to 50 mg/kg (approximately 310 times the maximum recommended daily inhalation dose for adults on a mg/m^2 basis).

13.2 Animal Toxicology and/or Pharmacology

Preclinical: Intravenous studies in rats with albuterol sulfate have demonstrated that albuterol crosses the blood-brain barrier and reaches brain concentrations amounting to approximately 5% of the plasma concentrations. In structures outside the blood-brain barrier (pineal and pituitary glands), albuterol concentrations were found to be 100 times those in the whole brain.

Studies in laboratory animals (minipigs, rodents, and dogs) have demonstrated the occurrence of cardiac arrhythmias and sudden death (with histologic evidence of myocardial necrosis) when β-agonists and methylxanthines were administered concurrently. The clinical significance of these findings is unknown.

Propellant HFA-134a is devoid of pharmacological activity except at very high doses in animals (380 - 1300 times the maximum human exposure based on comparisons of AUC values), primarily producing ataxia, tremors, dyspnea, or salivation. These are similar to effects produced by the structurally related chlorofluorocarbons (CFCs), which have been used extensively in metered-dose inhalers.

In animals and humans, propellant HFA-134a was found to be rapidly absorbed and rapidly eliminated, with an elimination half-life of 3 - 27 minutes in animals and 5 - 7 minutes in humans. Time to maximum plasma concentration (T_{max}) and mean residence time are both extremely short leading to a transient appearance of HFA-134a in the blood with no evidence of accumulation.

Reproductive Toxicology Studies: A study in CD-1 mice given albuterol sulfate subcutaneously showed cleft palate formation in 5 of 111 (4.5%) fetuses at 0.25 mg/kg (less than the maximum recommended daily inhalation dose for adults on a mg/m^2 basis) and in 10 of 108 (9.3%) fetuses at 2.5 mg/kg (approximately 8 times the maximum recommended daily inhalation dose for adults on a mg/m^2 basis). The drug did not induce cleft palate formation at a dose of 0.025 mg/kg (less than the maximum recommended daily inhalation dose for adults on a mg/m^2 basis). Cleft palate also occurred in 22 of 72 (30.5%) fetuses from females treated subcutaneously with 2.5 mg/kg of isoproterenol (positive control).

A reproduction study in Stride Dutch rabbits revealed cranioschisis in 7 of 19 fetuses (37%) when albuterol sulfate was administered orally at 50 mg/kg (approximately 630 times the maximum recommended daily inhalation dose for adults on a mg/m^2 basis).

In an inhalation reproduction study in Sprague-Dawley rats, the albuterol sulfate/HFA-134a did not exhibit any teratogenic effects at 10.5 mg/kg (approximately 65 times the maximum recommended daily inhalation dose for adults on a mg/m^2 basis).

A study in which pregnant rats were dosed with radiolabeled albuterol sulfate demonstrated that drug-related material is transferred from the maternal circulation to the fetus.

14 CLINICAL STUDIES

14.1 Bronchospasm Associated with Asthma

Adult and Adolescent Patients 12 Years of Age and Older: In a 6-week, randomized, double-blind, placebo-controlled trial, PROAIR HFA Inhalation Aerosol (58 patients) was compared to a matched placebo HFA inhalation aerosol (58 patients) in asthmatic patients 12 to 76 years of age at a dose of 180 mcg albuterol four times daily. An evaluator-blind marketed active comparator HFA-134a albuterol inhaler arm (56 patients) was included.

Serial FEV$_1$ measurements, shown below as percent change from test-day baseline at Day 1 and at Day 43, demonstrated that two inhalations of PROAIR HFA Inhalation Aerosol produced significantly greater improvement in

FEV$_1$ over the pre-treatment value than the matched placebo, as well as a comparable bronchodilator effect to the marketed active comparator HFA-134a albuterol inhaler.

FEV$_1$ as Mean Percent Change from Test-Day Pre-Dose in a 6-Week Clinical Trial
Day 1

Day 43

In this study, 31 of 58 patients treated with PROAIR HFA Inhalation Aerosol achieved a 15% increase in FEV$_1$ within 30 minutes post-dose on Day 1. In these patients, the median time to onset, median time to peak effect, and median duration of effect were 8.2 minutes, 47 minutes, and approximately 3 hours, respectively. In some patients, the duration of effect was as long as 6 hours.

In a placebo-controlled, single-dose, crossover study, PROAIR HFA Inhalation Aerosol, administered at albuterol doses of 90, 180 and 270 mcg, produced bronchodilator responses significantly greater than those observed with a matched placebo HFA inhalation aerosol and comparable to a marketed active comparator HFA-134a albuterol inhaler.

Pediatric Patients 4 to 11 Years of Age: In a 3-week, randomized, double-blind, placebo-controlled trial, the same formulation of albuterol as in PROAIR HFA Inhalation Aerosol (50 patients) was compared to a matched placebo HFA inhalation aerosol (45 patients) in asthmatic children 4 to 11 years of age at a dose of 180 mcg albuterol four times daily. Serial FEV$_1$ measurements, expressed as the maximum percent change from test-day baseline in percent predicted FEV$_1$ at Day 1 and at Day 22 observed within two hours post-dose, demonstrated that two inhalations of HFA albuterol sulfate produced significantly greater improvement in FEV$_1$ over the pre-treatment value than the matched placebo.

In this study, 21 of 50 pediatric patients treated with the same formulation of albuterol as in PROAIR HFA Inhalation Aerosol achieved a 15% increase in FEV$_1$ within 30 minutes post-dose on Day 1. In these patients, the median time to onset, median time to peak effect and median duration of effect were 10 minutes, 31 minutes, and approximately 4 hours, respectively. In some pediatric patients, the duration of effect was as long as 6 hours.

In a placebo-controlled, single-dose, crossover study in 55 pediatric patients 4 to 11 years of age, PROAIR HFA Inhalation Aerosol, administered at albuterol doses of 90 and 180 mcg, was compared with a matched placebo HFA inhalation aerosol. Serial FEV$_1$ measurements, expressed as the baseline-adjusted percent predicted FEV$_1$ observed over 6 hours post-dose, demonstrated that one and two inhalations of PROAIR HFA Inhalation Aerosol produced significantly greater bronchodilator responses than the matched placebo.

14.2 Exercise-Induced Bronchospasm

In a randomized, single-dose, crossover study in 24 adults and adolescents with exercise-induced bronchospasm (EIB), two inhalations of PROAIR HFA taken 30 minutes before exercise prevented EIB for the hour following exercise (defined as maintenance of FEV_1 within 80% of post-dose, pre-exercise baseline values) in 83% (20 of 24) of patients as compared to 25% (6 of 24) of patients when they received placebo.

Some patients who participated in these clinical trials were using concomitant steroid therapy.

16 HOW SUPPLIED/STORAGE AND HANDLING

PROAIR HFA (albuterol sulfate) Inhalation Aerosol is supplied as a pressurized aluminum canister with a red plastic actuator with a dose counter and white dust cap each in boxes of one. Each canister contains 8.5 g of the formulation and provides 200 actuations (NDC 59310-579-22). Each actuation delivers 120 mcg of albuterol sulfate from the canister valve and 108 mcg of albuterol sulfate from the actuator mouthpiece (equivalent to 90 mcg of albuterol base).

SHAKE WELL BEFORE USE. Store between 15° and 25°C (59° and 77°F). Contents under pressure. Do not puncture or incinerate. Protect from freezing temperatures and prolonged exposure above direct sunlight. Exposure to temperatures above 120°F may cause bursting. For best results, canister should be at room temperature before use. Avoid spraying in eyes. Keep out of reach of children.

See **FDA-Approved Patient Labeling (17.9)** for priming and cleaning instructions.

The red actuator supplied with PROAIR HFA Inhalation Aerosol should not be used with the canister from any other inhalation aerosol products. The PROAIR HFA Inhalation Aerosol canister should not be used with the actuator from any other inhalation aerosol products.

PROAIR HFA inhaler has a dose counter attached to the actuator. Patients should never try to alter the numbers for the dose counter or tamper with the pin mechanism inside the actuator. Discard the PROAIR HFA inhaler when the counter displays 0 or after the expiration date on the product, whichever comes first. The labeled amount of medication in each actuation cannot be assured after the counter displays 0, even though the canister is not completely empty and will continue to operate. Never immerse the canister into water to determine how full the canister is ("float test"). PROAIR HFA Inhalation Aerosol does not contain chlorofluorocarbons (CFCs) as the propellant.

17 PATIENT COUNSELING INFORMATION

See **FDA-Approved Patient Labeling (17.9)**

Patients should be given the following information:

17.1 Frequency of Use

The action of PROAIR HFA Inhalation Aerosol should last for 4 to 6 hours. Do not use PROAIR HFA Inhalation Aerosol more frequently than recommended. Instruct patients to not increase the dose or frequency of doses of PROAIR HFA Inhalation Aerosol without consulting the physician. If patients find that treatment with PROAIR HFA Inhalation Aerosol becomes less effective for symptomatic relief, symptoms become worse, and/or they need to use the product more frequently than usual, they should seek medical attention immediately.

17.2 Priming and Cleaning

Priming: Priming is essential to ensure appropriate albuterol content in each actuation. Instruct patients to prime the inhaler before using for the first time and in cases where the inhaler has not been used for more than 2 weeks by releasing three sprays into the air, away from the face.

Cleaning: To ensure proper dosing and prevent actuator orifice blockage, instruct patients to wash the red plastic actuator mouthpiece and dry thoroughly at least once a week. Instruct patients that if they have more than one PROAIR HFA inhaler, they should wash each one at separate times to prevent attaching the wrong canister to the wrong plastic actuator. In this way, they can be sure they will always know the correct number of remaining doses. Patients should be instructed to never attach a canister of medicine from any other inhaler to the PROAIR HFA actuator and never attach the PROAIR HFA canister to an actuator from any other inhaler. Patients should not remove the canister from the actuator except during cleaning because reattachment may release a dose into the air and the dose counter will count down each time a spray is released. Detailed cleaning instructions are included in the illustrated Information for the Patient leaflet.

17.3 Dose Counter

Patients should be informed that PROAIR HFA has a dose counter attached to the actuator. When the patient receives the inhaler, a black dot will appear in the viewing window until it has been primed 3 times, at which point the number 200 will be displayed. The dose counter will count down each time a spray is released. The dose-counter window displays the number of sprays left in the inhaler in units of two (e.g., 200, 198, 196, etc). When the counter displays 20, the color of the numbers will change to red to remind the patient to contact their pharmacist for a refill of medication or consult their physician for a prescription refill. When the dose counter reaches 0, the background will change to solid red. Patients should be informed to discard PROAIR HFA inhaler when the dose counter displays 0 or after the expiration date on the product, whichever comes first.

17.4 Paradoxical Bronchospasm

Inform patients that PROAIR HFA Inhalation Aerosol can produce paradoxical bronchospasm. Instruct patients to discontinue PROAIR HFA Inhalation Aerosol if paradoxical bronchospasm occurs.

17.5 Concomitant Drug Use

While patients are taking PROAIR HFA Inhalation Aerosol, other inhaled drugs and asthma medications should be taken only as directed by a physician.

17.6 Common Adverse Events

Common adverse effects of treatment with inhaled albuterol include palpitations, chest pain, rapid heart rate, tremor, or nervousness.

17.7 Pregnancy

Patients who are pregnant or nursing should contact their physician about the use of PROAIR HFA Inhalation Aerosol.

17.8 General Information on Use

Effective and safe use of PROAIR HFA Inhalation Aerosol includes an understanding of the way that it should be administered.

Shake well before each spray.

Use PROAIR HFA Inhalation Aerosol only with the actuator supplied with the product. Discard the PROAIR HFA inhaler when the dose counter displays 0 or after the expiration date on the product, whichever comes first. Never immerse the canister in water to determine how full the canister is ("float test").

In general, the technique for administering PROAIR HFA Inhalation Aerosol to children is similar to that for adults. Children should use PROAIR HFA Inhalation Aerosol under adult supervision, as instructed by the patient's physician.

17.9 FDA-Approved Patient Labeling

See tear-off illustrated Information for the Patient leaflet.

Mktd by: Teva Respiratory, LLC
Horsham, PA 19044
Mfd by: IVAX Pharmaceuticals Ireland
Waterford, Ireland
Copyright ©2012, Teva Respiratory, LLC
All rights reserved.
PROAIR® is a registered trademark of Teva Respiratory, LLC
Manufactured In Ireland
PE 2557 05/12

Attention Pharmacist:
Detach Patient's Instructions for use from package insert and dispense with the product.

PATIENT INFORMATION

PROAIR® HFA (prō′ ār)
(albuterol sulfate)
Inhalation Aerosol

Read this Patient Information before you start using PROAIR HFA and each time you get a refill. There may be new information. This information does not take the place of talking to your doctor about your medical condition or your treatment.

What is PROAIR HFA?

PROAIR HFA is a prescription medicine used in people 4 years of age and older to:

• treat or prevent bronchospasm in people who have reversible obstructive airway disease
• prevent exercise induced bronchospasm

It is not known if PROAIR HFA is safe and effective in children under 4 years of age.

Who should not use PROAIR HFA?

Do not use PROAIR HFA if you are allergic to albuterol sulfate or any of the ingredients in PROAIR HFA. See the end of this leaflet for a complete list of ingredients in PROAIR HFA.

What should I tell my doctor before I use PROAIR HFA?
Before you use PROAIR HFA, tell your doctor if you:

• have heart problems
• have high blood pressure (hypertension)
• have convulsions (seizures)
• have thyroid problems
• have diabetes
• have low potassium levels in your blood
• are pregnant or plan to become pregnant. It is not known if PROAIR HFA will harm your unborn baby. Talk to your doctor if you are pregnant or plan to become pregnant.
• are breastfeeding or plan to breastfeed. It is not known if PROAIR HFA passes into your breast milk. Talk to your doctor about the best way to feed your baby if you are using PROAIR HFA.

Tell your doctor about all the medicines you take, including prescription and non-prescription medicines, vitamins, and herbal supplements.

PROAIR HFA and other medicines may affect each other and cause side effects. PROAIR HFA may affect the way other medicines work, and other medicines may affect the way PROAIR HFA works.

Especially tell your doctor if you take:

• other inhaled medicines or asthma medicines
• beta blocker medicines
• diuretics
• digoxin
• monoamine oxidase inhibitors
• tricyclic antidepressants

Ask your doctor or pharmacist for a list of these medicines if you are not sure.

Know the medicines you take. Keep a list of them to show your doctor and pharmacist when you get a new medicine.

How should I use PROAIR HFA?

• For detailed instructions, see **"Instructions for Use"** at the end of this Patient Information.
• Use PROAIR HFA exactly as your doctor tells you to use it.
• If your child needs to use PROAIR HFA, watch your child closely to make sure your child uses the inhaler correctly. Your doctor will show you how your child should use PROAIR HFA.
• Each dose of PROAIR HFA should last up to 4 hours to 6 hours.
• **Do not** increase your dose or take extra doses of PROAIR HFA without first talking to your doctor.
• Get medical help right away if PROAIR HFA no longer helps your symptoms.
• Get medical help right away if your symptoms get worse or if you need to use your inhaler more often.
• While you are using PROAIR HFA, **do not** use other inhaled rescue medicines and asthma medicines unless your doctor tells you to do so.
• Call your doctor if your asthma symptoms like wheezing and trouble breathing become worse over a few hours or days. Your doctor may need to give you another medicine (for example, corticosteroids) to treat your symptoms.

What are the possible side effects of PROAIR HFA?

PROAIR HFA may cause serious side effects, including:

• **worsening trouble breathing, coughing and wheezing (paradoxical bronchospasm).** If this happens stop using PROAIR HFA and call your doctor or get emergency help right away. Paradoxical bronchospasm is more likely to happen with your first use of a new canister of medicine.
• **heart problems including faster heart rate and higher blood pressure**
• **possible death in people with asthma who use too much PROAIR HFA**
• **allergic reactions.** Call your doctor right away if you have the following symptoms of an allergic reaction:
   ○ itchy skin
   ○ swelling beneath your skin or in your throat
   ○ rash
   ○ worsening trouble breathing
• **low potassium levels in your blood**
• **worsening of other medical problems in people who also use PROAIR HFA including increases in blood sugar**

The most common side effects of PROAIR HFA include:

• your heart feels like it is pounding or racing (palpitations)
• chest pain
• fast heart rate
• shakiness
• nervousness
• headache
• dizziness
• sore throat
• runny nose

Tell your doctor if you have any side effect that bothers you or that does not go away.

These are not all of the possible side effects of PROAIR HFA. For more information, ask your doctor or pharmacist. Call your doctor for medical advice about side effects. You may report side effects to FDA at 1-800-FDA-1088.

How should I store PROAIR HFA?

• Store PROAIR HFA at room temperature between 59° F and 77° F (15° C and 25° C).
• Avoid exposure to extreme heat and cold.
• Shake the PROAIR HFA canister well before use.
• **Do not** puncture the PROAIR HFA canister.
• **Do not** store the PROAIR HFA canister near heat or a flame. Temperatures above 120° F may cause the canister to burst.
• **Do not** throw the PROAIR HFA canister into a fire or an incinerator.
• Avoid spraying PROAIR HFA in your eyes.

Keep PROAIR HFA and all medicines out of the reach of children.

General Information about the safe and effective use of PROAIR HFA

Medicines are sometimes prescribed for purposes other than those listed in a Medication Guide. Do not use PROAIR HFA for a condition for which it was not prescribed. Do not give PROAIR HFA to other people, even if they have the same symptoms that you have. It may harm them.

This Patient Information summarizes the most important information about PROAIR HFA. If you would like more information, talk with your doctor. You can ask your pharmacist or doctor for information about PROAIR HFA that is written for health professionals.

For more information, go to www.ProAirHFA.com or call 1-888-482-9522.

What are the ingredients in PROAIR HFA?
Active ingredient: albuterol sulfate
Inactive ingredients: propellant HFA-134a and ethanol.

INSTRUCTIONS FOR USE
PROAIR® HFA *(prō' ār)*
(albuterol sulfate)
Inhalation Aerosol

Read this Instructions for Use before you start using PROAIR HFA and each time you get a refill. There may be new information. This information does not take the place of talking to your doctor about your medical condition or your treatment.

The Parts of Your PROAIR HFA Inhaler Device:
There are 2 main parts of your PROAIR HFA inhaler device including a:
• red plastic actuator that sprays the medicine from the canister. See Figure A.
• protective dust cap that covers the mouthpiece of the actuator. See Figure A.

There is also a metal canister that holds the medicine. See Figure A.

There is also a dose counter attached to the back of the actuator with a viewing window that shows you how many sprays of medicine you have left. See Figure B.

You will see a black dot in the viewing window on the actuator until the device has been primed 3 times. See Figure B and "**Priming Your PROAIR HFA Device**" below.

Figure A

Figure B

• **Do not** use the PROAIR HFA actuator with a canister of medicine from any other inhaler.
• **Do not** use a PROAIR HFA canister with an actuator from any other inhaler, including another PROAIR HFA inhaler.

Priming Your PROAIR HFA Device:
Your PROAIR device must be primed before you use it for the first time or if your device has not been used for more than 14 days in a row. **Do not** prime your PROAIR HFA device every day.
• Remove your PROAIR HFA device from its package.
• Remove the protective dust cap from the mouthpiece.
• Shake the inhaler well, and spray it into the air away from your face. See Figure C.

Figure C

• Shake and spray the inhaler like this 2 more times to finish priming it.
The dose counter on the actuator should display the number 200 after you prime the actuator for the first time. See Figure D.
[See figure D at top of next column.]

Each Time You Use Your PROAIR HFA Device:
• Make sure the canister fits firmly in the plastic actuator.
• Look into the mouthpiece to make sure there are no foreign objects there, especially if the cap has not been used to cover the mouthpiece.

Reading the Dose Counter on Your PROAIR HFA Actuator
• The dose counter will count down each time a spray is released. The dose counter window shows the number of sprays left in your inhaler in units of 2 sprays. For example, there are 190 sprays left if the arrow is exactly opposite the number 190, or 189 sprays left if the arrow points between 190 and 188. See Figure D.

Figure D

• When the dose counter reaches **0**, it will continue to show **0** and you should replace your PROAIR HFA device.
• The dose counter cannot be reset and is permanently attached to the actuator. **Never** change the numbers for the dose counter or touch the pin inside the actuator.
• **Do not** remove the canister from the plastic actuator except during cleaning. Reattaching the canister to the actuator may accidently release a dose of PROAIR HFA into the air. The dose counter will count down each time a spray is released.

Using Your PROAIR HFA Device:
Step 1. **Shake the inhaler well** before each spray. Take the cap off the mouthpiece of the actuator.
Step 2. Hold the inhaler with the mouthpiece down. See Figure E.

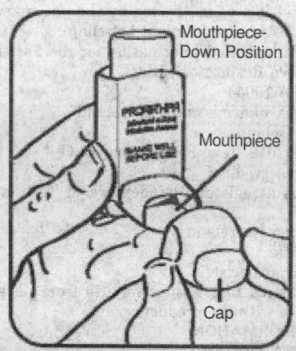

Mouthpiece-Down Position

Mouthpiece

Cap

Figure E

Step 3. **Breathe out through your mouth** and push as much air from your lungs as you can. Put the mouthpiece in your mouth and close your lips around it. See Figure F.
Step 4. **Push the top of the canister all the way down while you breathe in deeply and slowly through your mouth.** See Figure F.

Push down and breathe in.

Figure F

Step 5. Right after the spray comes out, take your finger off the canister. After you have breathed in all the way, take the inhaler out of your mouth and close your mouth.
Step 6. **Hold your breath as long as you can**, up to 10 seconds, then breathe normally.
If your doctor has told you to use more sprays, wait 1 minute and shake the inhaler again. Repeat Steps 2 through Step 6.
Step 7. Put the cap back on the mouthpiece after every time you use the inhaler. Make sure the cap snaps firmly into place.

Cleaning Your PROAIR HFA Device:
It is very important to keep the plastic actuator clean so the medicine will not build-up and block the spray. See Figure G and Figure H.

Figure G

Figure H

• **Do not try to clean the metal canister or let it get wet.** The inhaler may stop spraying if it is not cleaned correctly.
• If you have more than 1 PROAIR HFA inhaler, wash each device at separate times to prevent putting the wrong canister together with the wrong plastic actuator. This way you can be sure you will always know the correct number of remaining doses of PROAIR HFA.
• **Wash the actuator** at least 1 time each week as follows:
  ○ Take the canister out of the actuator, and take the cap off the mouthpiece.
  ○ Hold the actuator under the faucet and run warm water through it for about 30 seconds. See Figure I.

Wash mouthpiece under warm running water.

Figure I

○ Turn the actuator upside down and run warm water through the mouthpiece for about 30 seconds. See Figure J.

Figure J

○ Shake off as much water from the actuator as you can. Look into the mouthpiece to make sure any medicine build-up has been completely washed away. If there is any build-up, repeat the washing instructions.
○ Let the actuator air-dry completely, such as overnight. See Figure K.

Allow mouthpiece to dry, such as overnight.

Figure K

○ When the actuator is dry, put the canister in the actuator and make sure it fits firmly. Shake the inhaler well and spray it twice into the air away from your face. Put the cap back on the mouthpiece.
If you need to use your inhaler before the actuator is completely dry:
• Shake as much water off the actuator as you can.

- Put the canister in the actuator and make sure it fits firmly.
- Shake the inhaler well and spray it twice into the air away from your face.
- Take your PROAIR HFA dose as prescribed.
- Follow the Cleaning Instructions above.

Replacing Your PROAIR HFA Device

- **When the dose counter on the actuator says the number 20,** the color of the numbers will change to red. The red numbers are to remind you to refill your prescription or ask your doctor for another prescription for PROAIR HFA. When the dose counter reaches **0**, the background color will change to solid red.
- **Throw the PROAIR HFA inhaler away** as soon as the dose counter says **0** or after the expiration date on the PROAIR HFA packaging, whichever comes first. You should not keep using the inhaler after 200 sprays even though the canister may not be completely empty. You cannot be sure you will receive any medicine after using 200 sprays.
- **Do not use the inhaler** after the expiration date on the PROAIR HFA packaging.

This Patient Information and Instructions for Use has been approved by the U.S. Food and Drug Administration.

Marketed by Teva Respiratory, LLC
Horsham, PA 19044
Manufactured by IVAX Pharmaceuticals Ireland
Waterford, Ireland
Revised 05/12
PE2557

Shown in Product Identification Guide, page 314

Teva Select Brands

Division of Teva Pharmaceuticals USA
41 MOORES ROAD
FRAZER, PA 19355

Direct inquiries to:
800-292-4283

ADASUVE® ℞
[AD-uh-soov]
(loxapine)
inhalation powder, for oral inhalation use

HIGHLIGHTS OF PRESCRIBING INFORMATION
These highlights do not include all the information needed to use ADASUVE safely and effectively. See full prescribing information for ADASUVE.
ADASUVE® (loxapine) inhalation powder, for oral inhalation use
Initial U. S. Approval: 1975

WARNING: BRONCHOSPASM and
INCREASED MORTALITY IN ELDERLY PATIENTS WITH DEMENTIA-RELATED PSYCHOSIS
See full prescribing information for complete boxed warning.
Bronchospasm
- ADASUVE can cause bronchospasm that has the potential to lead to respiratory distress and respiratory arrest (4, 5.1)
- ADASUVE is available only through a restricted program under a Risk Evaluation and Mitigation Strategy (REMS) called the ADASUVE REMS (5.2)
- Administer ADASUVE only in an enrolled healthcare facility that has immediate access on-site to equipment and personnel trained to manage acute bronchospasm, including advanced airway management (intubation and mechanical ventilation) (5.1, 5.2)
Increased Mortality in Elderly Patients with Dementia-Related Psychosis
- Elderly patients with dementia-related psychosis treated with antipsychotic drugs are at an increased risk of death. ADASUVE is not approved for the treatment of patients with dementia-related psychosis (5.3)

INDICATIONS AND USAGE
ADASUVE is a typical antipsychotic indicated for the acute treatment of agitation associated with schizophrenia or bipolar I disorder in adults.
Efficacy was demonstrated in 2 trials in acute agitation: one in schizophrenia and one in bipolar I disorder (1, 14)
Limitations of Use:
ADASUVE must be administered only in an enrolled healthcare facility (1)

DOSAGE AND ADMINISTRATION
- Must be administered only by a healthcare professional (2.1)
- 10 mg by oral inhalation using an inhaler (2.1)
- Administer only a single dose within any 24-hour period (2.1)
- Prior to administering, screen all patients for a history of pulmonary disease, and examine patients (including chest auscultation) for respiratory abnormalities (e.g. wheezing) (2.2)
- Refer to Full Prescribing Information for important instructions on use of the ADASUVE inhaler (2.3)
- After administration, monitor patients for signs and symptoms of bronchospasm at least every 15 minutes for at least one hour (2.4)

DOSAGE FORMS AND STRENGTHS
- Inhalation powder: 10 mg unit in a single-use inhaler (3)

CONTRAINDICATIONS
- Current diagnosis or history of asthma, chronic obstructive pulmonary disease (COPD), or other lung disease associated with bronchospasm (4)
- Acute respiratory signs/symptoms (e.g., wheezing) (4)
- Current use of medications to treat airways disease, such as asthma or COPD (4)
- History of bronchospasm following ADASUVE treatment (4)
- Known hypersensitivity to loxapine or amoxapine (4)

WARNINGS AND PRECAUTIONS
- *Neuroleptic Malignant Syndrome:* May develop in patients treated with antipsychotic drugs. Discontinue treatment (5.4)
- *Hypotension and Syncope:* Use with caution in patients with known cardiovascular or cerebrovascular disease (5.5)
- *Seizure:* Use with caution in patients with a history of seizures or with conditions that lower the seizure threshold (5.6)
- *Potential for Cognitive and Motor Impairment:* Use caution when driving or operating machinery (5.7)
- *Cerebrovascular Adverse Reactions:* Increased incidence of stroke and transient ischemic attack in elderly patients with dementia-related psychosis treated with antipsychotic drugs (5.8)

ADVERSE REACTIONS
Most common adverse reactions (incidence ≥ 2% and greater than placebo) were dysgeusia, sedation, and throat irritation (6.1)

To report SUSPECTED ADVERSE REACTIONS contact Teva Pharmaceuticals at 1-888-483-8279- or FDA at 1-800-FDA-1088 or www.fda.gov/medwatch

---

USE IN SPECIFIC POPULATIONS
- Pregnancy: Based on animal data, may cause fetal harm (8.1)
- Nursing Mothers: Discontinue drug or nursing, taking into consideration importance of drug to mother (8.3)

See 17 for PATIENT COUNSELING INFORMATION and Medication Guide

Revised: 12/2013

FULL PRESCRIBING INFORMATION

WARNING: BRONCHOSPASM and INCREASED MORTALITY IN ELDERLY PATIENTS WITH DEMENTIA-RELATED PSYCHOSIS

Bronchospasm
ADASUVE can cause bronchospasm that has the potential to lead to respiratory distress and respiratory arrest. Administer ADASUVE only in an enrolled healthcare facility that has immediate access on-site to equipment and personnel trained to manage acute bronchospasm, including advanced airway management (intubation and mechanical ventilation) *[see Warnings and Precautions (5.1, 5.2)]*. Prior to administering ADASUVE, screen patients regarding a current diagnosis, history, or symptoms of asthma, COPD and other lung diseases, and examine (including chest auscultation) patients for respiratory signs. Monitor for signs and symptoms of bronchospasm following treatment with ADASUVE *[see Dosage and Administration (2.2, 2.4) and Contraindications (4)]*.

Because of the risk of bronchospasm, ADASUVE is available only through a restricted program under a Risk Evaluation and Mitigation Strategy (REMS) called the ADASUVE REMS *[see Warnings and Precautions (5.2)]*.

Increased Mortality in Elderly Patients with Dementia-Related Psychosis
Elderly patients with dementia-related psychosis treated with antipsychotic drugs are at an increased risk of death. ADASUVE is not approved for the treatment of patients with dementia-related psychosis *[see Warnings and Precautions (5.3)]*.

---

1   INDICATIONS AND USAGE
ADASUVE is a typical antipsychotic indicated for the acute treatment of agitation associated with schizophrenia or bipolar I disorder in adults.

"Psychomotor agitation" is defined in DSM-IV as "excessive motor activity associated with a feeling of inner tension." Patients experiencing agitation often manifest behaviors that interfere with their care (e.g., threatening behaviors, escalating or urgently distressing behavior, self-exhausting behavior), leading clinicians to the use of rapidly absorbed antipsychotic medications to achieve immediate control of the agitation *[see Clinical Studies (14)]*.

The efficacy of ADASUVE was established in one study of acute agitation in patients with schizophrenia and one study of acute agitation in patients with bipolar I disorder *[see Clinical Studies (14)]*.

Limitations of Use:
As part of the ADASUVE REMS Program to mitigate the risk of bronchospasm, ADASUVE must be administered only in an enrolled healthcare facility *[see Warnings and Precautions (5.2)]*.

2   DOSAGE AND ADMINISTRATION
2.1   Dosing Information
ADASUVE must be administered only by a healthcare professional. ADASUVE is administered by oral inhalation only. The recommended dose for acute agitation is 10 mg administered by oral inhalation, using a single-use inhaler. Administer only a single dose within a 24-hour period *[see Warnings and Precautions (5.1)]*.

2.2 Required Examination Prior to Dosing

Prior to administering ADASUVE, screen all patients for a history of asthma, COPD, or other pulmonary disease, and examine patients (including chest auscultation) for respiratory signs (e.g. wheezing) [see Warnings and Precautions (5.1)].

2.3 Important Administration Instructions

Read all of these instructions prior to administering ADASUVE.

Step 1. Open the Pouch

When ready to use, tear open the foil pouch and remove the inhaler from the package (see Figure 1).

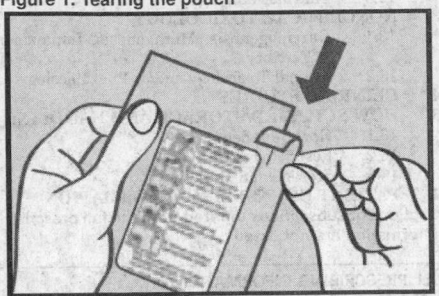

Figure 1. Tearing the pouch

When the ADASUVE inhaler is removed from the pouch, the indicator light is off (see Figure 2).

Figure 2. ADASUVE Inhaler with Indicator Light

Step 2. Pull Tab

Firmly pull the plastic tab from the rear of the inhaler (see Figure 3). Check that the green light turns on. This indicates that the inhaler is ready for use. Use the inhaler within 15 minutes after removing the tab to prevent automatic deactivation of the inhaler. The green light will turn off, indicating that the inhaler is not usable. Discard the inhaler after one use.

Figure 3.

Step 3. Explain Procedures to the Patient

- Explain the administration procedures to the patient prior to use, and advise the patient that it is important to follow the instructions. Inform the patient that the inhaler may produce a flash of light and a clicking sound, and it may become warm during use. These are normal.

Step 4. Instruct the Patient to Exhale

Instruct the patient to hold the inhaler away from the mouth and breathe out fully to empty the lungs (see Figure 4).

Figure 4. Exhale

Step 5. Instruct the Patient to Inhale

Instruct the patient to put the mouthpiece of the inhaler between the lips, close the lips, and inhale through the mouthpiece with a steady deep breath (see Figure 5). Check that the green light turns off indicating that the dose has been delivered.

Figure 5. Inhale

Step 6. Instruct the Patient to Hold Breath

Instruct the patient to remove the mouthpiece from the mouth and hold the breath for as long as possible, up to 10 seconds (see Figure 6).

Figure 6. Hold Breath

Important: If the green light remains on after the patient inhales, the dose of ADASUVE has NOT been delivered. Instruct the patient to repeat Step 4, Step 5, and Step 6 up to 2 additional times. If the green light still does not turn off, discard the inhaler and use a new one.

2.4 Monitoring to Assess Safety

Monitor the patient for signs and symptoms of bronchospasm after ADASUVE administration. Perform a physical examination, including chest auscultation, at least every 15 minutes for at least one hour after ADASUVE administration [see Warnings and Precautions (5.1)].

3 DOSAGE FORMS AND STRENGTHS

ADASUVE is an inhalation powder supplied in a single-use, disposable inhaler containing 10 mg of loxapine base.

4 CONTRAINDICATIONS

ADASUVE is contraindicated in patients with the following:

- Current diagnosis or history of asthma, COPD, or other lung disease associated with bronchospasm [see Warnings and Precautions (5.1)]
- Acute respiratory symptoms or signs (e.g., wheezing) [see Warnings and Precautions (5.1)]
- Current use of medications to treat airways disease, such as asthma or COPD [see Warnings and Precautions (5.1)]
- History of bronchospasm following ADASUVE treatment [see Warnings and Precautions (5.1)]

Known hypersensitivity to loxapine or amoxapine. Serious skin reactions have occurred with oral loxapine and amoxapine.

5 WARNINGS AND PRECAUTIONS

5.1 Bronchospasm

ADASUVE can cause bronchospasm that has the potential to lead to respiratory distress and respiratory arrest [see Adverse Reactions (6.1)]. Administer ADASUVE only in an enrolled healthcare facility that has immediate access onsite to equipment and personnel trained to manage acute bronchospasm, including advanced airway management (intubation and mechanical ventilation) [see Boxed Warning and Warnings and Precautions (5.2)].

Prior to administering ADASUVE, screen patients regarding a current diagnosis or history of asthma, COPD, and other lung disease associated with bronchospasm, acute respiratory symptoms or signs, current use of medications to treat airways disease, such as asthma or COPD; and examine patients (including chest auscultation) for respiratory abnormalities (e.g., wheezing) [See Dosage and Administration (2.2) and Contraindications (4)]. Monitor patients for symptoms and signs of bronchospasm (i.e., vital signs and chest auscultation) at least every 15 minutes for a minimum of one hour following treatment with ADASUVE [see Dosage and Administration (2.4)]. ADASUVE can cause sedation, which can mask the symptoms of bronchospasm.

Because clinical trials in patients with asthma or COPD demonstrated that the degree of bronchospasm, as indicated by changes in forced expiratory volume in 1 second (FEV1), was greater following a second dose of ADASUVE, limit ADASUVE use to a single dose within a 24 hour period.

Advise all patients of the risk of bronchospasm. Advise them to inform the healthcare professional if they develop any breathing problems such as wheezing, shortness of breath, chest tightness, or cough following treatment with ADASUVE.

5.2 ADASUVE REMS to Mitigate Bronchospasm

Because of the risk of bronchospasm, ADASUVE is available only through a restricted program under a REMS called the ADASUVE REMS. [see Boxed Warning and Warnings and Precautions (5.1)] Required components of the ADASUVE REMS are:

- Healthcare facilities that dispense and administer ADASUVE must be enrolled and comply with the REMS requirements. Certified healthcare facilities must have onsite access to equipment and personnel trained to provide advance airway management, including intubation and mechanical ventilation.
- Wholesalers and distributors that distribute ADASUVE must enroll in the program and distribute only to enrolled healthcare facilities.

Further information is available at www.adasuverems.com or 1-855-755-0492.

5.3 Increased Mortality in Elderly Patients with Dementia-Related Psychosis

Elderly patients with dementia-related psychosis treated with antipsychotic drugs are at increased risk of death. Analyses of 17 placebo-controlled trials (modal duration of 10 weeks), largely in patients taking atypical antipsychotic drugs, revealed a risk of death in drug-treated patients of 1.6 to 1.7 times the risk of death in placebo-treated patients. Over the course of a typical 10-week controlled trial, the rate of death in drug-treated patients was about 4.5%, compared to a rate of about 2.6% in the placebo group. Although the cases of death were varied, most of the deaths appeared to be either cardiovascular (e.g., heart failure, sudden death) or infectious (e.g., pneumonia) in nature. Observational studies suggest that, similar to atypical antipsychotic drugs, treatment with conventional antipsychotic drugs may increase mortality. The extent to which the findings of increased mortality in observational studies can be attributed to the antipsychotic drug as opposed to some characteristic(s) of the patients is not clear. ADASUVE is not approved for the treatment of elderly patients with dementia-related psychosis [see Boxed Warning].

5.4 Neuroleptic Malignant Syndrome

Antipsychotic drugs can cause a potentially fatal symptom complex termed Neuroleptic Malignant Syndrome (NMS). Clinical manifestations of NMS include hyperpyrexia, muscle rigidity, altered mental status, and autonomic instability (irregular pulse or blood pressure, tachycardia, diaphoresis, and cardiac dysrhythmia). Associated features can include elevated serum creatine phosphokinase (CPK) concentration, rhabdomyolysis, elevated serum and urine myoglobin concentration, and renal failure. NMS did not occur in the ADASUVE clinical program.

The diagnostic evaluation of patients with this syndrome is complicated. It is important to consider the presence of other serious medical conditions (e.g., pneumonia, systemic infection, heat stroke, primary CNS pathology, central anticholinergic toxicity, extrapyramidal symptoms, or drug fever).

The management of NMS should include: 1) immediate discontinuation of antipsychotic drugs and other drugs that may contribute to the underlying disorder, 2) intensive symptomatic treatment and medical monitoring, and 3) treatment of any concomitant serious medical problems. There is no general agreement about specific pharmacological treatment regimens for NMS.

If a patient requires antipsychotic drug treatment after recovery from NMS, the potential reintroduction of drug therapy should be carefully considered. The patient should be carefully monitored, since recurrences of NMS have been reported.

5.5 Hypotension and Syncope

ADASUVE can cause hypotension, orthostatic hypotension, and syncope. Use ADASUVE with caution in patients with known cardiovascular disease (history of myocardial infarction or ischemic heart disease, heart failure or conduction abnormalities), cerebrovascular disease, or conditions that would predispose patients to hypotension (dehydration, hypovolemia, or treatment with antihypertensive medications or other drugs that affect blood pressure or reduce heart rate).

In the presence of severe hypotension requiring vasopressor therapy, the preferred drugs may be norepinephrine or phenylephrine. Epinephrine should not be used, because beta stimulation may worsen hypotension in the setting of ADASUVE-induced partial alpha blockade.

In short-term (24-hour) placebo-controlled trials of patients with agitation associated with schizophrenia or bipolar I disorder, hypotension occurred in 0.4% and 0.8% in the ADASUVE 10 mg and placebo groups, respectively. There were no cases of orthostatic hypotension, postural symptoms, presyncope or syncope. A systolic blood pressure ≤ 90 mm Hg with a decrease of ≥ 20 mm Hg occurred in 1.5% and 0.8% of the ADASUVE 10 mg and placebo groups, respectively. A diastolic blood pressure ≤ 50 mm Hg with a decrease of ≥15 mmHg occurred in 0.8% and 0.4% of the ADASUVE 10 mg and placebo groups, respectively.

In 5 Phase 1 studies in normal volunteers, the incidence of hypotension was 3% and 0% in ADASUVE 10 mg and placebo groups, respectively. The incidence of syncope or presyncope in normal volunteers was 2.3% and 0% in the ADASUVE and placebo groups, respectively. In normal volunteers, a systolic blood pressure ≤ 90 mm Hg with a decrease of ≥ 20 mm Hg occurred in 5.3% and 1.1% in the ADASUVE and placebo groups, respectively. A diastolic blood pressure ≤ 50 mm Hg with a decrease of ≥ 15 mm Hg occurred in 7.5% and 3.3% in the ADASUVE and placebo groups, respectively.

5.6 Seizures

ADASUVE lowers the seizure threshold. Seizures have occurred in patients treated with oral loxapine. Seizures can occur in epileptic patients even during antiepileptic drug maintenance therapy. In short term (24 hour), placebo-controlled trials of ADASUVE, there were no reports of seizures.

5.7 Potential for Cognitive and Motor Impairment

ADASUVE can impair judgment, thinking, and motor skills. In short-term, placebo-controlled trials, sedation and/or somnolence were reported in 12% and 10% in the ADASUVE and placebo groups, respectively. No patients discontinued treatment because of sedation or somnolence. The potential for cognitive and motor impairment is increased when ADASUVE is administered concurrently with other CNS depressants [see Drug Interactions (7.1)]. Caution patients about operating hazardous machinery, including automobiles, until they are reasonably certain that therapy with ADASUVE does not affect them adversely.

5.8 Cerebrovascular Reactions, Including Stroke, in Elderly Patients with Dementia-Related Psychosis

In placebo-controlled trials with atypical antipsychotics in elderly patients with dementia-related psychosis, there was a higher incidence of cerebrovascular adverse reactions (stroke and transient ischemic attacks), including fatalities, compared to placebo-treated patients. ADASUVE is not approved for the treatment of patients with dementia-related psychosis [see Boxed Warning and Warnings and Precautions (5.3)].

5.9 Anticholinergic Reactions Including Exacerbation of Glaucoma and Urinary Retention

ADASUVE has anticholinergic activity, and it has the potential to cause anticholinergic adverse reactions including exacerbation of glaucoma or urinary retention. The concomitant use of other anticholinergic drugs (e.g., antiparkinson drugs) with ADASUVE could have additive effects.

6 ADVERSE REACTIONS

The following adverse reactions are discussed in more detail in other sections of the labeling:

- Hypersensitivity (serious skin reactions) [see Contraindications (4)]
- Bronchospasm [see Warnings and Precautions (5.1)]
- Increased Mortality in Elderly Patients with Dementia-Related Psychosis [see Warnings and Precautions (5.3)]
- Neuroleptic Malignant Syndrome [see Warnings and Precautions (5.4)]
- Hypotension and syncope [see Warnings and Precautions (5.5)]
- Seizure [see Warnings and Precautions (5.6)]
- Potential for Cognitive and Motor Impairment [see Warnings and Precautions (5.7)]
- Cerebrovascular Reactions, Including Stroke, in Elderly Patients with Dementia-Related Psychosis [see Warnings and Precautions (5.8)]
- Anticholinergic Reactions Including Exacerbation of Glaucoma and Urinary Retention [see Warnings and Precautions (5.9)]

6.1 Clinical Trials Experience

Because clinical trials are conducted under widely varying conditions, adverse reaction rates observed in the clinical trials of a drug cannot be directly compared to rates in the clinical trials of another drug and may not reflect the rates observed in clinical practice.

The following findings are based on pooled data from three short-term (24-hour), randomized, double-blind, placebo-controlled clinical trials (Studies 1, 2, and 3) of ADASUVE 10 mg in the treatment of patients with acute agitation associated with schizophrenia or bipolar I disorder. In the 3 trials, 259 patients received ADASUVE 10 mg, and 263 received placebo [see Clinical Studies (14)].

Commonly Observed Adverse Reactions: In the 3 trials in acute agitation, the most common adverse reactions were dysgeusia, sedation, and throat irritation. These reactions occurred at a rate of at least 2% of the ADASUVE group and at a rate greater than in the placebo group. (Refer to Table 1).

Table 1. Adverse Reactions in 3 Pooled Short-Term, Placebo-Controlled Trials (Studies 1, 2, and 3) in Patients with Schizophrenia or Bipolar Disorder

Adverse Reaction	Placebo (n = 263)	ADASUVE (n = 259)
Dysgeusia	5%	14%
Sedation	10%	12%
Throat Irritation	0%	3%

Airway Adverse Reactions in the 3 Trials in Acute Agitation Agitated patients with Schizophrenia or Bipolar Disorder: In the 3 short-term (24-hour), placebo-controlled trials in patients with agitation associated with schizophrenia or bipolar disorder (Studies 1, 2, and 3), bronchospasm (which includes reports of wheezing, shortness of breath and cough) occurred more frequently in the ADASUVE group, compared to the placebo group: 0% (0/263) in the placebo group and 0.8% (2/259) in the ADASUVE 10 mg group. One patient with schizophrenia, without a history of pulmonary disease, had significant bronchospasm requiring rescue treatment with a bronchodilator and oxygen.

Bronchospasm and Airway Adverse Reactions in Pulmonary Safety Trials

Clinical pulmonary safety trials demonstrated that ADASUVE can cause bronchospasm as measured by FEV1, and as indicated by respiratory signs and symptoms in the trials. In addition, the trials demonstrated that patients with asthma or other pulmonary diseases, such as COPD are at increased risk of bronchospasm. The effect of ADASUVE on pulmonary function was evaluated in 3 randomized, double-blind, placebo-controlled clinical pulmonary safety trials in healthy volunteers, patients with asthma, and patients with COPD. Pulmonary function was assessed by serial FEV1 tests, and respiratory signs and symptoms were assessed. In the asthma and COPD trials, patients with respiratory symptoms or FEV1 decrease of ≥ 20% were administered rescue treatment with albuterol (metered dose inhaler or nebulizer) as required. These patients were not eligible for a second dose; however, they had continued FEV1 monitoring in the trial.

Healthy Volunteers: In the healthy volunteer crossover trial, 30 subjects received 2 doses of either ADASUVE or placebo 8 hours apart, and 2 doses of the alternate treatment at least 4 days later. The results for maximum de-

Table 2: Maximum Decrease in FEV1 from Baseline in the Healthy Volunteer, Asthma, and COPD Trials

Maximum % FEV ↓	Healthy Volunteer Placebo n (%)	Healthy Volunteer ADASUVE 10 mg n (%)	Asthma Placebo n (%)	Asthma ADASUVE 10 mg n (%)	COPD Placebo n (%)	COPD ADASUVE 10 mg n (%)
After any Dose	N=26	N=26	N=26	N=26	N=27	N=25
≥10	7 (27)	7 (27)	3 (12)	22 (85)	18 (67)	20 (80)
≥15	1 (4)	5 (19)	1 (4)	16 (62)	9 (33)	14 (56)
≥20	0	1 (4)	1 (4)	11 (42)	3 (11)	10 (40)
After Dose 1	N=26	N=26	N=26	N=26	N=27	N=25
≥10	4 (15)	5 (19)	2 (8)	16 (62)	8 (30)	16 (64)
≥15	1 (4)	2 (8)	1 (4)	8 (31)	4 (15)	10 (40)
≥20	0	0	1 (4)	6 (23)	2 (7)	9 (36)
After Dose 2	N=26	N=25	N=25	N=17	N=26	N=19
≥10	5 (19)	6 (24)	3 (12)	12 (71)	15 (58)	12 (63)
≥15	0	5 (20)	1 (4)	9 (53)	6 (23)	10 (53)
≥20	0	1 (4)	1 (4)	5 (30)	1 (4)	5 (26)

crease in FEV1 are presented in Table 2. No subjects in this trial developed airway related adverse reactions (cough, wheezing, chest tightness, or dyspnea).

Asthma Patients: In the asthma trial, 52 patients with mild-moderate persistent asthma (with FEV1 ≥ 60% of predicted) were randomized to treatment with 2 doses of ADASUVE 10 mg or placebo. The second dose was to be administered 10 hours after the first dose. Approximately 67% of these patients had a baseline FEV1 ≥ 80% of predicted. The remaining patients had an FEV1 60-80% of predicted. Nine patients (17%) were former smokers. As shown in Table 2 and Figure 7, there was a marked decrease in FEV1 immediately following the first dose (maximum mean decreases in FEV1 and % predicted FEV1 were 303 mL and 9.1%, respectively). Furthermore, the effect on FEV1 was greater following the second dose (maximum mean decreases in FEV1 and % predicted FEV1 were 537 mL and 14.7 %, respectively). Respiratory-related adverse reactions (bronchospasm, chest discomfort, cough, dyspnea, throat tightness, and wheezing) occurred in 54% of ADASUVE-treated patients and 12% of placebo-treated patients. There were no serious adverse events. Nine of 26 (35%) patients in the ADASUVE group, compared to one of 26 (4%) in the placebo group, did not receive a second dose of study medication, because they had a ≥ 20% decrease in FEV1 or they developed respiratory symptoms after the first dose. Rescue medication (albuterol via metered dose inhaler or nebulizer) was administered to 54% of patients in the ADASUVE group [7 patients (27%) after the first dose and 7 of the remaining 17 patients (41%) after the second dose] and 12% in the placebo group (1 patient after the first dose and 2 patients after the second dose).

COPD Patients: In the COPD trial, 53 patients with mild to severe COPD (with FEV1 ≥ 40% of predicted) were randomized to treatment with 2 doses of ADASUVE 10 mg or placebo. The second dose was to be administered 10 hours after the first dose. Approximately 57% of these patients had moderate COPD [Global Initiative for Chronic Obstructive Lung Disease (GOLD) Stage II]; 32% had severe disease (GOLD Stage III); and 11% had mild disease (GOLD Stage I). As illustrated in Table 2 there was a decrease in FEV1 soon after the first dose (maximum mean decreases in FEV1 and % predicted FEV1 were 96 mL and 3.5%, respectively), and the effect on FEV1 was greater following the second dose (maximum mean decreases in FEV1 and % predicted FEV1 were 125 mL and 4.5%, respectively). Respiratory adverse reactions occurred more frequently in the ADASUVE group (19%) than in the placebo group (11%). There were no serious adverse events. Seven of 25 (28%) patients in the ADASUVE group and 1of 27 (4%) in the placebo group did not receive a second dose of study medication because of a ≥ 20% decrease in FEV1 or the development of respiratory symptoms after the first dose. Rescue medication (albuterol via MDI or nebulizer) was administered to 23% of patients in the ADASUVE group: 8% of patients after the first dose and 21% of patients after the second dose, and to 15% of patients in the placebo group.

[See table 2 above]

FEV1 categories are cumulative; i.e. a subject with a maximum decrease of 21% is included in all 3 categories. Patients with a ≥ 20% decrease in FEV1 did not receive a second dose of study drug.

[See figure 7 at top of next column]

Patients with a ≥ 20% decrease in FEV1 did not receive a second dose of study drug and are not included in the curves beyond hour 10.

Extrapyramidal Symptoms (EPS): Extrapyramidal reactions have occurred during the administration of oral loxapine. In most patients, these reactions involved parkinsonian symptoms such as tremor, rigidity, and masked facies. Akathisia (motor restlessness) has also occurred.

In the 3 short-term (24-hour), placebo-controlled trials of ADASUVE in 259 patients with agitation associated with

Figure 7: LS Mean Change from Baseline in FEV1 in Patients with Asthma

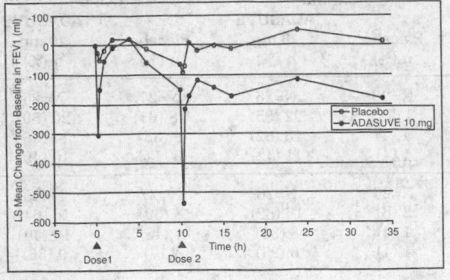

schizophrenia or bipolar disorder, extrapyramidal reactions occurred. One patient (0.4%) treated with ADASUVE developed neck dystonia and oculogyration. The incidence of akathisia was 0% and 0.4% in the placebo and ADASUVE groups, respectively.

Dystonia (Antipsychotic Class Effect): Symptoms of dystonia, prolonged abnormal contractions of muscle groups, may occur in susceptible individuals during treatment with ADASUVE. Dystonic symptoms include spasm of the neck muscles, sometimes progressing to tightness of the throat, difficulty swallowing or breathing, and/or protrusion of the tongue.

Acute dystonia tends to be dose-related, but can occur at low doses, and occurs more frequently with first generation antipsychotic drugs such as ADASUVE. The risk is greater in males and younger age groups.

Cardiovascular Reactions: Tachycardia, hypotension, hypertension, orthostatic hypotension, lightheadedness, and syncope have been reported with oral administration of loxapine.

7 DRUG INTERACTIONS
7.1 CNS Depressants
ADASUVE is a central nervous system (CNS) depressant. The concurrent use of ADASUVE with other CNS depressants (e.g., alcohol, opioid analgesics, benzodiazepines, tricyclic antidepressants, general anesthetics, phenothiazines, sedative/hypnotics, muscle relaxants, and/or illicit CNS depressants) can increase the risk of respiratory depression, hypotension, profound sedation, and syncope. Therefore, consider reducing the dose of CNS depressants if used concomitantly with ADASUVE.
7.2 Anticholinergic Drugs
ADASUVE has anticholinergic activity. The concomitant use of ADASUVE and other anticholinergic drugs can increase the risk of anticholinergic adverse reactions including exacerbation of glaucoma and urinary retention.

8 USE IN SPECIFIC POPULATIONS
In general, no dose adjustment for ADASUVE is required on the basis of a patient's age, gender, race, smoking status, hepatic function, or renal function.
8.1 Pregnancy
Pregnancy Category C
Risk Summary
There are no adequate and well-controlled studies of ADASUVE use in pregnant women. Neonates exposed to antipsychotic drugs during the third trimester of pregnancy are at risk for extrapyramidal and/or withdrawal symptoms following delivery. Loxapine, the active ingredient in ADASUVE, has demonstrated increased embryofetal toxicity and death in rat fetuses and offspring exposed to doses approximately 0.5-fold the maximum recommended human dose (MRHD) on a mg/m² basis. ADASUVE should be used during pregnancy only if the potential benefit justifies the potential risk to the fetus.
Human Data
Neonates exposed to antipsychotic drugs during the third trimester of pregnancy are at risk for extrapyramidal and/or withdrawal symptoms following delivery. There have been reports of agitation, hypertonia, hypotonia, tremor, somnolence, respiratory distress, and feeding disorders in these neonates. These complications have varied in severity; in some cases symptoms have been self-limited, but in other cases neonates have required intensive care unit support and prolonged hospitalization.
Animal Data
In rats, embryofetal toxicity (increased fetal resorptions, reduced weights, and hydronephrosis with hydroureter) was observed following oral administration of loxapine during the period of organogenesis at a dose of 1 mg/kg/day. This dose is equivalent to the MRHD of 10 mg/day on a mg/m² basis. In addition, fetal toxicity (increased prenatal death, decreased postnatal survival, reduced fetal weights, delayed ossification, and/or distended renal pelvis with reduced or absent papillae) was observed following oral administration

of loxapine from mid-pregnancy through weaning at doses of 0.6 mg/kg and higher. This dose is approximately half the MRHD of 10 mg/day on a mg/m² basis.

No teratogenicity was observed following oral administration of loxapine during the period of organogenesis in the rat, rabbit, or dog at doses up to 12, 60, and 10 mg/kg, respectively. These doses are approximately 12-, 120-, and 32-fold the MRHD of 10 mg/day on a mg/m² basis, respectively.

8.3 Nursing Mothers
It is not known whether ADASUVE is present in human milk. Loxapine and its metabolites are present in the milk of lactating dogs. Because many drugs are excreted in human milk and because of the potential for serious adverse reactions in nursing infants from ADASUVE, a decision should be made whether to discontinue nursing or discontinue ADASUVE, taking into account the importance of the drug to the mother.

8.4 Pediatric Use
The safety and effectiveness of ADASUVE in pediatric patients have not been established.

8.5 Geriatric Use
Elderly patients with dementia-related psychosis treated with antipsychotic drugs are at an increased risk of death *[see Boxed Warning and Warnings and Precautions (5.3)]*. ADASUVE is not approved for the treatment of dementia-related psychosis. Placebo-controlled studies of ADASUVE in patients with agitation associated with schizophrenia or bipolar disorder did not include patients over 65 years of age.

10 OVERDOSAGE
Signs and Symptoms of Overdosage
As would be expected from the pharmacologic actions of loxapine, the clinical findings may include CNS depression, unconsciousness, profound hypotension, respiratory depression, extrapyramidal symptoms, and seizure.
Management of Overdosage
For the most up to date information on the management of ADASUVE overdosage, contact a certified poison control center (1-800-222-1222 or www.poison.org). Provide supportive care including close medical supervision and monitoring. Treatment should consist of general measures employed in the management of overdosage with any drug. Consider the possibility of multiple drug overdosage. Ensure an adequate airway, oxygenation, and ventilation. Monitor cardiac rhythm and vital signs. Use supportive and symptomatic measures.

11 DESCRIPTION
ADASUVE, a typical antipsychotic, is an inhalation powder of loxapine supplied in a single-use, disposable inhaler containing 10 mg of loxapine base. ADASUVE is a drug-device combination product.
Active Ingredient: Loxapine (base). Loxapine, a dibenzoxazepine compound, represents a subclass of tricyclic antipsychotic agents, chemically distinct from the thioxanthenes, butyrophenones, and phenothiazines. Chemically, it is 2-Chloro-11-(4-methyl-1-piperazinyl) dibenz [b,f] [1,4] oxazepine.

$C_{18}H_{18}ClN_3O$

ADASUVE is a single-use, drug-device combination product that provides rapid systemic delivery by inhalation of a thermally-generated aerosol of loxapine. Oral inhalation through the product initiates the controlled rapid heating of a thin film of excipient-free loxapine to form a thermally-generated drug vapor. The vapor condenses into aerosol particles that are dispersed into the airstream created by the patient inhaling through the mouthpiece.

Each product is packaged inside a sealed foil pouch. The product is a white to off-white plastic unit, with a mouthpiece on one end and a pull-tab protruding from the other end.

Removal of a pull-tab from the product renders it ready for use, as indicated by illumination of a green light. After inhalation through the mouthpiece, successful dosing is signaled by the green light turning off.

Under standardized *in vitro* test conditions, ADASUVE, 10 mg delivers 9.1 mg loxapine out of the mouthpiece.

12 CLINICAL PHARMACOLOGY
12.1 Mechanism of Action
The mechanism of action of loxapine in the treatment of agitation associated with schizophrenia is unknown. However, its efficacy could be mediated through a combination of an-

tagonism of central dopamine D_2 and serotonin 5-HT$_{2A}$ receptors. The mechanism of action of loxapine in the treatment of agitation associated with bipolar I disorder is unknown.

12.2 Pharmacodynamics
Loxapine acts as an antagonist at central serotonin and dopamine receptors, with high affinity for serotonin 5-HT$_{2A}$ and dopamine D_1, D_2, D_3, and D_4 receptors (K_i values of 2 nM, 18 nM, 10 nM, 21 nM, 9 nM, respectively). Some of the adverse effects of loxapine may be related to the antagonism of histamine H_1 (somnolence), muscarinic M1 (anticholinergic), and adrenergic α_2 (orthostatic hypotension) receptors (K_i values of 15 nM, 117 nM and 250 nM, respectively).

Thorough QTc Study
ADASUVE did not prolong the QTc interval. The effect of ADASUVE on QTc prolongation was evaluated in a randomized, double-blinded, positive- (moxifloxacin 400 mg) and placebo-controlled parallel study in healthy subjects. A total of 48 healthy subjects were administered ADASUVE 10 mg. In this study with a demonstrated ability to detect small effects, the upper bound of the 90% confidence interval (CI) for the largest placebo-adjusted, baseline-corrected QTc based on individual correction method was below 10 milliseconds, the threshold for regulatory concern.

12.3 Pharmacokinetics
Absorption: The single-dose pharmacokinetic parameters of loxapine following administration of single doses of ADASUVE 10 mg in healthy adult subjects are presented in Table 3 and Figure 8.

Administration of ADASUVE resulted in rapid absorption of loxapine, with a median time of maximum plasma concentration (T_{max}) of 2 minutes. Loxapine exposure in the first 2 hours after administration (AUC_{0-2h}) was 66.7 ng•h/mL for the 10 mg dose. As a consequence of the very rapid absorption of loxapine after oral inhalation, there is substantial variability in the early plasma concentrations of loxapine. The mean plasma loxapine concentrations following administration of ADASUVE were linear over the clinical dose range. AUC_{0-2h}, AUC_{inf}, and C_{max} increased in a dose-dependent manner.

Table 3. Pharmacokinetics in Healthy Adult Subjects Administered a Single Dose of ADASUVE 10 mg

Parameter	Healthy Subjects ADASUVE 10 mg (N=114)
AUC_{0-2h} (ng•h/mL), mean ± SD	66.7 ± 18.2
AUC_{inf} (ng•h/mL), mean ± SD	188 ± 47
C_{max} (ng/mL), mean ± SD	257 ± 219
T_{max} (minutes), median (25%, 75%)	1.13 (1, 2)
Half-life(h), mean ± SD	7.61 ± 1.87

[See figure 8 at top of next page]

Distribution: Loxapine is removed rapidly from the plasma and distributed in tissues. Animal studies following oral administration suggest an initial preferential distribution in the lungs, brain, spleen, heart, and kidney. Loxapine is 96.6% bound to human plasma proteins.

Metabolism: Loxapine is metabolized extensively in the liver following oral administration, with multiple metabolites formed. The main metabolic pathways include: 1) hydroxylation to form 8-OH-loxapine by CYP1A2 and 7-OH-loxapine by CYP3A4 and CYP2D6, 2) N-oxidation to form loxapine N-oxide by flavanoid monoamine oxidases (FMOs), and 3) de-methylation to form amoxapine. Because there are multiple metabolic pathways, the risk of metabolic interactions caused by an effect on an individual isoform is minimal. For ADASUVE, the order of metabolites observed in humans (based on systemic exposure) was 8-OH-loxapine >> loxapine N-oxide, 7-OH-loxapine > amoxapine. Plasma levels of 8-OH-loxapine are similar to those of the parent compound.

Excretion: Excretion occurs mainly in the first 24 hours. Metabolites are excreted in the urine in the form of conjugates and in the feces unconjugated. The terminal elimination half-life ($T_{\frac{1}{2}}$) ranged from 6 to 8 hours.

Transporter Interaction: In vitro studies indicated that loxapine was not a substrate for p-glycoprotein (P-gp): however, loxapine inhibited P-gp.

Special Populations:
Pharmacokinetics in Smokers: Loxapine exposures in nonsmokers and smokers are similar, with geometric mean ratios of 92%, 85%, and 99% for AUC_{0-2h}, AUC_{inf}, and C_{max} respectively. No dosage adjustment is recommended based on smoking status.

Figure 8. Mean Plasma Concentrations of Loxapine following Single-Dose Administration ADASUVE 10 mg in Healthy Subjects

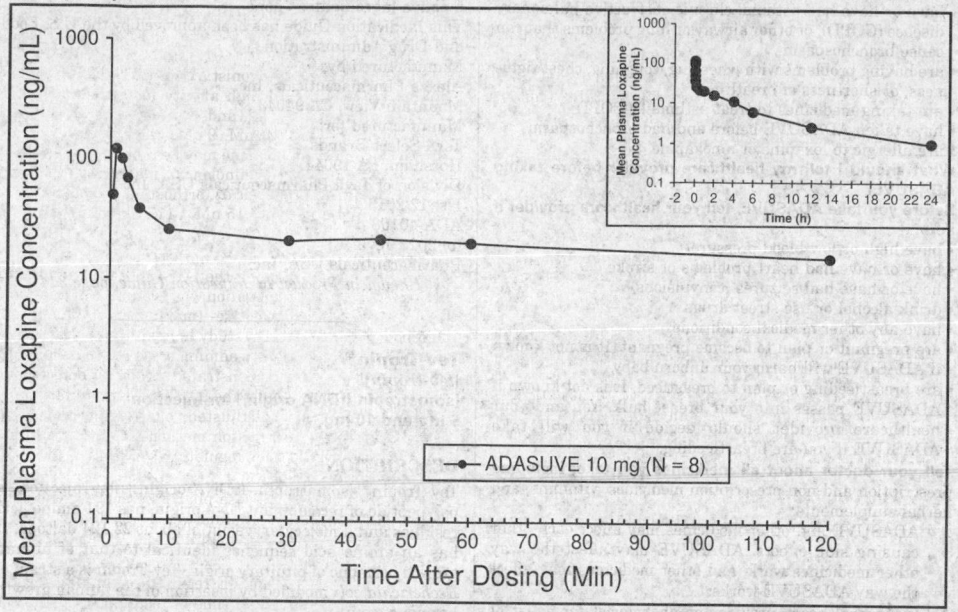

Examination of population subsets (age, race, and gender) on the primary endpoint did not reveal any differential responsiveness on the basis of these subgroupings.

Figures 9 and 10 show the decreases in PEC score at each time point assessed in the trials. In both trials, the decrease in agitation with ADASUVE was apparent at each time point tested (10, 20, 30, 45, 60, 90, and 120 minutes post-dose).

Figure 9. Mean Change from Baseline in PEC Score through 2 Hours after a Single Dose in Agitated Patients with Schizophrenia (Study 1)

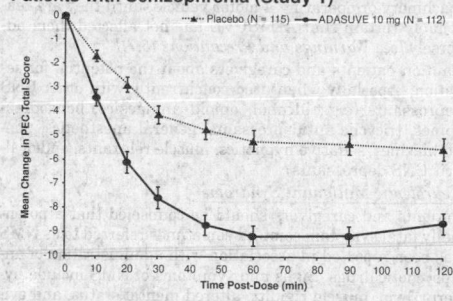

Figure 10. Mean Change from Baseline in PEC Score through 2 Hours after a Single Dose in Agitated Patients with Bipolar Disorder (Study 2)

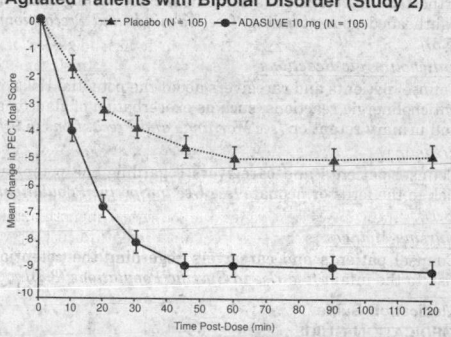

The results of the secondary endpoint, CGI-I scores, are shown in Table 5.

Table 5. CGI-I Score at 2 Hours Post-Dose in the Schizophrenia and Bipolar I Disorder Trials

	Placebo	ADASUVE
Study 1 (Schizophrenia)		
N	115	112
CGI-I score at 2 hours[a]	2.8	2.1
Difference from placebo (95% CI)	--	-0.8, (-1.1, -0.4)
p-value	--	< 0.0001
Study 2 (Bipolar Disorder)		
N	105	105
CGI-I score at 2 hours[a]	3.0	1.9
Difference from placebo (95% CI)[a]	--	-1.1 (-1.4, -0.8)
p-value	--	< 0.0001

[a] Least squares mean

Demographic Effects: There were no clinically significant differences in loxapine pharmacokinetics following administration of ADASUVE in subgroups based on age, weight, body mass index, gender, or race.

13 NONCLINICAL TOXICOLOGY

13.1 Carcinogenesis, Mutagenesis, Impairment of Fertility

Carcinogenesis: No adequate studies have been conducted.

Mutagenesis: Loxapine did not cause mutation or chromosomal aberration when tested *in vitro* and *in vivo*. Loxapine was negative in the Ames gene mutation assay, the human peripheral blood lymphocyte chromosomal aberration assay, and in the *in vivo* mouse bone marrow micronucleus assay up to 40 mg/kg (20-fold the MRHD on mg/m^2 basis). Loxapine metabolite 8-OH-loxapine was not mutagenic in the *in vitro* Ames reverse mutation assay and was not clastogenic in the *in vitro* human peripheral blood lymphocyte chromosomal aberration assay.

Impairment of Fertility: Loxapine had no effects on fertility or early embryonic development in male rats or in male and female rabbits following oral administration. Mating was decreased in female rats because these animals were in persistent diestrus, an expected pharmacologic effect for this class of compounds. This occurred at doses approximately 0.2- and 1-fold the MRHD of 10 mg/day on a mg/m^2 basis.

13.2 Animal Toxicology and/or Pharmacology

In the rat, minimal and reversible squamous metaplasia of the larynx was observed after daily inhalation exposure of loxapine for 14 days at 1.7 to 13 mg/kg/day (approximately 2- to 13-fold the MRHD of 10 mg/day on a mg/m^2 basis, respectively). This finding was considered a nonspecific particle impaction effect. Mammary hyperplasia in males and females and ovarian follicular cysts and mucification of vaginal epithelium in female rats were observed at all doses, with partial or complete recovery at the end of 14 days of treatment. In the dog, no effects on the respiratory tract or reproductive tissues were observed after inhalation exposure to loxapine for 28 days at doses up to 1.8 mg/kg/day (approximately 6-fold the MRHD of 10 mg/day on a mg/m^2 basis).

14 CLINICAL STUDIES

The efficacy of ADASUVE 10 mg in the acute treatment of agitation associated with schizophrenia or bipolar I disorder was established in two short-term (24-hour), randomized, double-blind, placebo-controlled, fixed-dose trials. Study 1 included 344 patients who met DSM-IV criteria for schizophrenia. Study 2 included 314 patients who met DSM-IV criteria for bipolar I disorder, manic or mixed episodes with or without psychotic features.

Patients were judged by the clinical investigators to be clinically agitated, with a level of agitation that met or exceeded a specific severity threshold as measured by the Positive and Negative Syndrome Scale-Excited Component (PEC). The PEC is an investigator-rated instrument consisting of 5 items: poor impulse control, tension, hostility, uncooperativeness, and excitement. Each item is scored on a scale

from 1 to 7 (1 = absent, 4 = moderate, 7 = extreme). Thus, the total PEC score can range from 5 to 35. For enrollment in the studies, patients had to have a PEC score of ≥ 14, with at least one individual item score ≥ 4.

Patients whose agitation was related to acute alcohol or drug intoxication were excluded. Patients with clinically significant acute or chronic pulmonary disease (e.g., asthma, COPD, chronic bronchitis, and emphysema) were excluded from the trials *[See Contraindications (4)]*.

The primary efficacy endpoint in both trials was the mean change from baseline in the PEC score, assessed 2 hours following dosing. The key secondary endpoint was the mean Clinical Global Impression Improvement (CGI-I) Scale score at two hours. The CGI-I is an investigator-rated global assessment of symptom improvement, scored on a scale of 1 to 7: 1 = very much improved; 4 = no change from baseline; 7 = very much worse.

In both studies, mean baseline PEC scores were similar in all treatment groups, averaging 17.3 to 17.7 (Table 4), with individual patient scores ranging from 14 to 31, indicating predominantly moderate levels of agitation. The mean baseline Clinical Global Impression Severity Scale (CGI-S) score in both studies was 4 (moderately ill). In Study 2, 69% of patients had a current manic episode, and 31% had a mixed/manic episode.

In Studies 1 and 2, treatment with ADASUVE was statistically significantly superior to placebo on the mean change in PEC score at 2 hours (Table 4). In both studies, the effect of ADASUVE was apparent at 10 minutes following dosing (Figures 9 and 10).

Table 4. Change from Baseline in the PEC Score at 2 Hours Post-Dose in the Schizophrenia (Study 1) and Bipolar I Disorder (Study 2) Trials

	Placebo	ADASUVE
Study 1 (Schizophrenia)		
N	115	112
PEC score		
Mean baseline	17.4	17.6
Change at 2 hours[a]	-5.8	-8.7
Difference from placebo (95% CI)[b]	--	-2.9 (-4.2, -1.6)
p-value	--	< 0.0001
Study 2 (Bipolar Disorder)		
N	105	105
PEC score		
Mean baseline	17.7	17.3
Change at 2 hours[a]	-4.7	-9.2
Difference from placebo (95% CI)[b]	--	-4.5 (-5.8, -3.1)
p-value	--	< 0.0001

[a] Least squares mean for the difference defined as the change from baseline

[b] Least squares mean for the difference defined as the change from baseline at hour 2 in the drug group minus that in the placebo group.

16 HOW SUPPLIED/STORAGE AND HANDLING

16.1 How Supplied

ADASUVE® (loxapine) inhalation powder is supplied as: ADASUVE 10 mg (NDC 57844-510-11) is a single-use, disposable inhaler containing 10 mg of loxapine, provided in a sealed foil pouch. ADASUVE, 10 mg is supplied in a carton of 5 units per carton (NDC 57844-510-55).

16.2 Restricted Access

ADASUVE is only available through a restricted program called the ADASUVE REMS Program *[see Warnings and Precautions (5.2)]*.

16.3 Storage and Handling

Store ADASUVE at room temperature, 15° to 30°C (59° to 86°F) [see USP Controlled Room Temperature].

Keep out of reach of children.

Keep ADASUVE in pouch until time of use.

ADASUVE contains a lithium battery. Dispose of ADASUVE in accordance with all federal, state and local laws.

17 PATIENT COUNSELING INFORMATION

See FDA-approved patient labeling (Medication Guide)

Bronchospasm

Advise patients and caregivers that there is a risk of bronchospasm. Advise patients to inform their healthcare professional if they develop any breathing problems such as wheezing, shortness of breath, chest tightness, or cough following treatment with ADASUVE *[see Boxed Warning and Warnings and Precautions (5.1)]*

Interference with Cognitive and Motor Performance

Caution patients and caregivers about performing activities requiring mental alertness, such as operating hazardous machinery or operating a motor vehicle, until they are reasonably certain that ADASUVE has not affected them adversely *[see Warnings and Precautions (5.7)]*.

Caution patients and caregivers about the potential for sedation, especially when used concurrently with other CNS depressants (e.g., alcohol, opioid analgesics, benzodiazepines, tricyclic antidepressants, general anesthetics, phenothiazines, sedative/hypnotics, muscle relaxants, and/or illicit CNS depressants).

Neuroleptic Malignant Syndrome

Patients and caregivers should be counseled that a potentially fatal symptom complex sometimes referred to as NMS has been reported in association with administration of antipsychotic drugs. Signs and symptoms of NMS include hyperpyrexia, muscle rigidity, altered mental status, and evidence of autonomic instability (irregular pulse or blood pressure, tachycardia, diaphoresis, and cardiac dysrhythmia) *[see Warnings and Precautions (5.4)]*.

Hypotension and Syncope

Advise patients and caregivers of the risk of hypotension or orthostatic hypotension (symptoms include feeling dizzy or lightheaded upon standing) *[see Warnings and Precautions (5.5)]*.

Anticholinergic Reactions

Counsel patients and caregivers about the potential risks of anticholinergic reactions, such as exacerbation of glaucoma and urinary retention *[see Warnings and Precautions (5.9)]*.

Pregnancy

Counsel patients and caregivers regarding the potential risk to the fetus or neonate *[see Use in Specific Populations (8.1)]*.

Nursing Mothers

Counsel patients and caregivers regarding the potential risk to the infant *[see Use in Specific Populations (8.3)]*.

Medication Guide

MEDICATION GUIDE

ADASUVE® (AD-uh-soov)

(loxapine)

Inhalation Powder

Read this Medication Guide before you start taking ADASUVE and each time it is given to you. There may be new information. This Medication Guide does not take the place of talking to your healthcare provider about your medical condition or your treatment. You should share this information with your family members and caregivers.

What is the most important information I should know about ADASUVE?

ADASUVE is available only through the ADASUVE Risk Evaluation and Mitigation Strategy (REMS) Program. The healthcare facility must be enrolled in the ADASUVE REMS Program before you can be given ADASUVE.

ADASUVE may cause serious side effects, including:

• **Narrowing of the airways (bronchospasm) that can cause you to have problems breathing or to stop breathing.** People who have asthma or other airway or lung problems, such as chronic obstructive pulmonary disease (COPD), have a higher risk of bronchospasm when taking ADASUVE. Symptoms of bronchospasm may include:
  ○ wheezing
  ○ coughing
  ○ chest tightness
  ○ shortness of breath

Tell your healthcare provider right away if you have any of these symptoms of bronchospasm after taking ADASUVE. Your healthcare provider should check you for breathing problems before and after you take ADASUVE.

• **Increased risk of death in elderly patients with dementia-related psychosis.** Medicines like ADASUVE can raise the risk of death in elderly people who have lost touch with reality (psychosis) due to confusion and memory loss (dementia). ADASUVE is not approved for the treatment of patients with dementia-related psychosis.

What is ADASUVE?

ADASUVE is a prescription medicine that is inhaled through your mouth and is used to treat acute agitation in adults with schizophrenia or bipolar I disorder.

It is not known if ADASUVE is safe and effective in children.

Who should not take ADASUVE?

Do not take ADASUVE if you:

• have or have had asthma, chronic obstructive pulmonary disease (COPD), or other airway or lung problems that can cause bronchospasm
• are having problems with wheezing, coughing, chest tightness, or shortness of breath
• are taking medicines to treat asthma or COPD
• have taken ADASUVE before and had bronchospasm
• are allergic to loxapine or amoxapine

What should I tell my healthcare provider before taking ADASUVE?

Before you take ADASUVE, tell your healthcare provider if you:

• have high or low blood pressure
• have or have had heart problems or stroke
• have or have had seizures (convulsions)
• drink alcohol or use street drugs
• have any other medical conditions
• are pregnant or plan to become pregnant. It is not known if ADASUVE will harm your unborn baby.
• are breastfeeding or plan to breastfeed. It is not known if ADASUVE passes into your breast milk. You and your healthcare provider should decide if you will take ADASUVE if you are breastfeeding.

Tell your doctor about all medicines you take, including prescription and non-prescription medicines, vitamins, and herbal supplements.
  ○ ADASUVE and other medicines may affect each other causing side effects. ADASUVE may affect the way other medicines work, and other medicines may affect the way ADASUVE works.

Ask your healthcare provider or pharmacist for a list of these medicines if you are not sure.

Know the medicines you take. Keep a list of them to show to your healthcare provider and pharmacist when you get a new medicine.

How should I take ADASUVE?

• Your healthcare provider will show you how to take ADASUVE right before you take it.
• Take ADASUVE exactly as your healthcare provider shows you to take it.
• ADASUVE is for oral inhalation only.

What should I avoid while taking ADASUVE?

• Do not drive, operate heavy machinery, or do other dangerous activities until you know how ADASUVE affects you.
• Do not drink alcohol while taking ADASUVE. It can increase your chances of getting serious side effects.

What are the possible side effects of ADASUVE?

ADASUVE can cause serious side effects, including:

• See "What is the most important information I should know about ADASUVE?"
• **neuroleptic malignant syndrome (NMS).** NMS is a rare but serious condition that may cause death. Symptoms of NMS may include:
  ○ high fever
  ○ stiff muscles
  ○ confusion
  ○ sweating
  ○ changes in pulse, heart rate, and blood pressure

Tell your healthcare provider right away if you have any of these symptoms of NMS after taking ADASUVE.

• **low blood pressure (hypotension), lightheadedness, or fainting**
• **seizures (convulsions)**
• **severe sleepiness and difficulty with potentially dangerous activities such as driving**
• **worsening of glaucoma**
• **difficulty urinating**

The most common side effects of ADASUVE include:
• bad, bitter, or metallic taste in your mouth (dysgeusia)
• sleepiness (especially when used with other drugs that cause sleepiness)
• sore throat

Tell your healthcare provider if you have any side effect that bothers you or that does not go away.

These are not all the possible side effects of ADASUVE. For more information ask your healthcare provider or pharmacist.

Call your doctor for medical advice about side effects. You may report side effects to FDA at 1-800-FDA-1088.

General information about the safe and effective use of ADASUVE.

Medicines are sometimes prescribed for purposes other than those listed in a Medication Guide.

This Medication Guide summarizes the most important information about ADASUVE. If you would like more information, talk to your healthcare provider. You can ask your pharmacist or healthcare provider for information about ADASUVE that is written for health professionals.

For more information, go to www.ADASUVE.com or call 1-888-483-8279.

What are the ingredients in ADASUVE?

Active Ingredient: loxapine

Inactive Ingredients: none

This Medication Guide has been approved by the U.S. Food and Drug Administration.

Manufactured by:
Alexza Pharmaceuticals, Inc.
Mountain View, CA 94043
Manufactured for:
Teva Select Brands
Horsham, PA 19044
Division of Teva Pharmaceuticals USA, Inc.
Iss. 12/2013
ADA-40198
(c) 2013 Teva
Pharmaceuticals USA, Inc.
Shown in Product Identification Guide, page 314

Tev-Tropin®   ℞

[tĕv-trō′pĭn]

[somatropin (rDNA origin)] for Injection

5 mg and 10 mg

DESCRIPTION

Tev-Tropin® [somatropin, (rDNA origin)] for Injection, a polypeptide of recombinant DNA origin, has 191 amino acid residues and a molecular weight of about 22,124 daltons. It has an amino acid sequence identical to that of human growth hormone of pituitary origin. Tev-Tropin is a strain of *Escherichia coli* modified by insertion of the human growth hormone gene.

Tev-Tropin is a sterile, white, lyophilized powder, intended for subcutaneous administration, after reconstitution with the accompanying diluent.

Tev-Tropin 5 mg vial contains recombinant somatropin 5 mg and mannitol 30 mg. The 5 mg vial is supplied in a combination package with an accompanying 5 mL vial of diluting solution. The diluent contains bacteriostatic 0.9% sodium chloride injection, USP, (normal saline), 0.9% benzyl alcohol as a preservative, and water for injection.

Tev-Tropin 10 mg vial contains recombinant somatropin 10 mg, mannitol 10 mg, disodium phosphate dodecahydrate 3.57 mg, and sodium dihydrogen phosphate dehydrate 0.79 mg. The 10 mg vial is supplied in a combination package with an accompanying 1 mL syringe of diluting solution. The diluent contains bacteriostatic water for injection with 0.33% metacresol as a preservative.

Tev-Tropin is a highly-purified preparation. Reconstituted solutions have a pH in the range of 7.0 to 9.0.

CLINICAL PHARMACOLOGY

Clinical trials have demonstrated that Tev-Tropin is equivalent in its therapeutic effectiveness and in its pharmacokinetic profile to those of human growth hormone of pituitary origin (somatropin). Tev-Tropin stimulates linear growth in children who lack adequate levels of endogenous growth hormone. Treatment of growth hormone-deficient children with Tev-Tropin produces increased growth rates and IGF-1 (Insulin-Like Growth Factor-1) concentrations that are similar to those seen after therapy with human growth hormone of pituitary origin.

Both Tev-Tropin and somatropin have also been shown to have other actions including:

A. *Tissue Growth*
  1. Skeletal Growth. Tev-Tropin stimulates skeletal growth in patients with growth hormone deficiency. The measurable increase in body length after administration of Tev-Tropin results from its effect on the epiphyseal growth plates of long bones. Concentration of IGF-1, which may play a role in skeletal growth, are low in the serum of growth hormone-deficient children but increase during treatment with Tev-Tropin. Mean serum alkaline phosphatase concentrations are increased.
  2. Cell Growth. It has been shown that there are fewer skeletal muscle cells in short statured children who lack endogenous growth hormone as compared with normal children. Treatment with somatropin results in an increase in both the number and size of muscle cells.
  3. Organ Growth. Somatropin influences the size of internal organs and it also increases red cell mass.

B. *Protein Metabolism*
  Linear growth is facilitated, in part, by increased cellular protein synthesis. Nitrogen retention, as demonstrated by decreased urinary nitrogen excretion and serum urea nitrogen, results from treatment with somatropin.

C. *Carbohydrate Metabolism*
  Children with hypopituitarism sometimes experience fasting hypoglycemia that is improved by treatment with somatropin. Large doses of somatropin may impair glucose tolerance.

D. *Lipid Metabolism*

Administration of somatropin to growth hormone-deficient patients mobilizes lipid, reduces body fat stores, and increases plasma fatty acids.

E. *Mineral Metabolism*

Sodium, potassium, and phosphorous are conserved by somatropin. Serum concentrations of inorganic phosphates increased in patients with growth hormone deficiency after therapy with Tev-Tropin or somatropin. Serum calcium concentrations are not significantly altered in patients treated with either somatropin or Tev-Tropin.

F. *Connective Tissue Metabolism*

Somatropin stimulates the synthesis of chondroitin sulfate and collagen as well as the urinary excretion of hydroxyproline.

PHARMACOKINETICS

Following intravenous administration of 0.1 mg/kg of Tev-Tropin, the elimination half-life was about 0.42 hours (approximately 25 minutes) and the mean plasma clearance ($\pm$SD) was 133 ($\pm$16) mL/min in healthy male volunteers. In the same volunteers, after a subcutaneous injection of 0.1 mg/kg Tev-Tropin to the forearm, the mean peak serum concentration ($\pm$SD) was 80 ($\pm$50) ng/mL which occurred approximately 7 hours post-injection and the apparent elimination half-life was approximately 2.7 hours. Compared to intravenous administration, the extent of systemic availability from subcutaneous administration was approximately 70%.

INDICATION AND USAGE

Tev-Tropin is indicated for the treatment of children who have growth failure due to an inadequate secretion of normal endogenous growth hormone.

CONTRAINDICATIONS

Tev-Tropin 5 mg reconstituted with bacteriostatic 0.9% sodium chloride injection, USP (normal saline) (benzyl alcohol preserved) should not be administered to patients with a known sensitivity to benzyl alcohol (see **WARNINGS**).

Tev-Tropin 10 mg reconstituted with bacteriostatic water for injection containing 0.33% metacresol should not be used if the patient is allergic to metacresol.

Somatropin should not be used for growth promotion in pediatric patients with closed epiphyses.

Somatropin is contraindicated in patients with active proliferative or severe non-proliferative diabetic retinopathy.

In general, somatropin is contraindicated in the presence of active malignancy. Any preexisting malignancy should be inactive and its treatment complete prior to instituting therapy with somatropin. Somatropin should be discontinued if there is evidence of recurrent activity. Since growth hormone deficiency may be an early sign of the presence of a pituitary tumor (or, rarely, other brain tumors), the presence of such tumors should be ruled out prior to initiation of treatment. Somatropin should not be used in patients with any evidence of progression or recurrence of an underlying intracranial tumor.

Treatment with pharmacologic amounts of somatropin is contraindicated in patients with acute critical illness due to complications following open heart surgery, abdominal surgery or multiple accidental trauma, or those with acute respiratory failure. Two placebo-controlled clinical trials in non-growth hormone deficient adult patients (n = 522) with these conditions in intensive care units revealed a significant increase in mortality (41.9% vs. 19.3%) among somatropin-treated patients (doses 5.3 to 8 mg/day) compared to those receiving placebo (see **WARNINGS**).

Somatropin is contraindicated in patients with Prader-Willi syndrome who are severely obese or have severe respiratory impairment (see **WARNINGS**). Tev-Tropin is not indicated for the treatment of pediatric patients who have growth failure due to genetically confirmed Prader-Willi syndrome.

WARNINGS

Increased mortality in patients with acute critical illness due to complications following open heart surgery, abdominal surgery or multiple accidental trauma, or those with acute respiratory failure has been reported after treatment with pharmacologic doses of somatropin (see **CONTRAINDICATIONS**). The safety of continuing somatropin treatment in patients receiving replacement doses for approved indications who concurrently develop these illnesses has not been established. Therefore, the potential benefit of treatment continuation with somatropin in patients experiencing acute critical illnesses should be weighed against the potential risk.

There have been reports of fatalities after initiating therapy with somatropin in pediatric patients with Prader-Willi syndrome who had one or more of the following risk factors: severe obesity, history of upper airway obstructions or sleep apnea, or unidentified respiratory infection. Male patients with one or more of these factors may be at greater risk than females. Patients with Prader-Willi syndrome should be evaluated for signs of upper airway obstruction and sleep

apnea before initiation of treatment with somatropin. If during treatment with somatropin, patients show signs of upper airway obstruction (including onset of or increased snoring) and/or new onset sleep apnea, treatment should be interrupted. All patients with Prader-Willi syndrome treated with somatropin should also have effective weight control and be monitored for signs of respiratory infection, which should be diagnosed as early as possible an treated aggressively (see **CONTRAINDICATIONS**). Tev-Tropin is not indicated for the treatment of pediatric patients who have growth failure due to genetically confirmed Prader-Willi syndrome.

Cases of pancreatitis have been reported rarely in children and adults receiving somatropin treatment, with some evidence supporting a greater risk in children compared with adults. Published literature indicates that girls who have Turner syndrome may be at greater risk than other somatropin-treated children. Pancreatitis should be considered in any somatropin-treated patient, especially a child, who develops persistent, severe abdominal pain.

Benzyl alcohol, a component used to reconstitute the Tev-Tropin 5 mg vial, has been associated with serious adverse events and death, particularly in pediatric patients. The "gasping syndrome," (characterized by central nervous system depression, metabolic acidosis, gasping respirations, and high levels of benzyl alcohol and its metabolites found in the blood and urine) has been associated with benzyl alcohol dosages >99 mg/kg/day in neonates and low-birth weight neonates. Additional symptoms may include gradual neurological deterioration, seizures, intracranial hemorrhage, hematologic abnormalities, skin breakdown, hepatic and renal failure, hypotension, bradycardia, and cardiovascular collapse. Practitioners administering this and other medications containing benzyl alcohol should consider the combined daily metabolic load of benzyl alcohol from all sources.

When administering Tev-Tropin 5 mg to newborns, reconstitute with sterile normal saline for injection, USP. WHEN RECONSTITUTING WITH STERILE NORMAL SALINE, USE ONLY ONE DOSE PER VIAL AND DISCARD THE UNUSED PORTION.

PRECAUTIONS

General

Tev-Tropin therapy should be carried out under the regular guidance of a physician who is experienced in the diagnosis and management of pediatric patients with growth hormone deficiency.

In childhood cancer survivors who were treated with radiation to the brain/head for their first neoplasm and who developed subsequent GHD and were treated with somatropin, an increased risk of a second neoplasm has been reported. Intracranial tumors, in particular meningiomas, were the most common of these second neoplasms. In adults, it is unknown whether there is any relationship between somatropin replacement therapy and CNS tumor recurrence [see **CONTRAINDICATIONS**]. Monitor all patients with a history of GHD secondary to an intracranial neoplasm routinely while on somatropin therapy for progression or recurrence of the tumor.

Because children with certain rare genetic causes of short stature have an increased risk of developing malignancies, practitioners should thoroughly consider the risks and benefits of starting somatropin in these patients. If treatment with somatropin is initiated, these patients should be carefully monitored for development of neoplasms.

Monitor patients on somatropin therapy carefully for increased growth, or potential malignant changes, or preexisting nevi.

Treatment with somatropin may decrease insulin sensitivity, particularly at higher doses in susceptible patients. As a result, previously undiagnosed impaired glucose tolerance and overt diabetes mellitus may be unmasked during somatropin treatment. New-onset type 2 diabetes mellitus has been reported in patients. Therefore, glucose levels should be monitored periodically in all patients treated with somatropin, especially in those with risk factors for diabetes mellitus, such as obesity, Turner syndrome, or a family history of diabetes mellitus. Patients with preexisting type 1 or type 2 diabetes mellitus or impaired glucose tolerance should be monitored closely during somatropin therapy. The doses of antihyperglycemic drugs (i.e., insulin or oral agents) may require adjustment when somatropin therapy is instituted in these patients.

In patients with hypopituitarism (multiple hormone deficiencies), standard hormonal replacement therapy should be monitored closely when somatropin therapy is administered. Undiagnosed/untreated hypothyroidism may prevent an optimal response to somatropin, in particular, the growth response in children. Patients with Turner syndrome have an inherently increased risk of developing autoimmune thyroid disease and primary hypothyroidism. In patients with growth hormone deficiency, central (secondary) hypothyroidism may first become evident or worsen

during somatropin treatment. Therefore, patients treated with somatropin should have periodic thyroid function tests and thyroid hormone replacement therapy should be initiated or appropriately adjusted when indicated.

Patients with endocrine disorders, including growth hormone deficiency, may have an increased incidence of slipped capital femoral epiphysis. Any child who develops a limp or complains of hip or knee pain during somatropin therapy should be evaluated.

Intracranial hypertension (IH) with papilledema, visual changes, headache, nausea and/or vomiting has been reported in a small number of patients treated with growth hormone products. IH has been reported more frequently after treatment with IGF-1. Symptoms usually occur within the first eight weeks after the initiation of growth hormone therapy. In all reported cases, IH-associated signs and symptoms resolved rapidly after temporary suspension or termination of therapy. Funduscopic examination should be performed routinely before initiating treatment with somatropin to exclude preexisting papilledema and periodically during the course of somatropin therapy. If papilledema is observed by funduscopy during somatropin treatment, treatment should be stopped. If somatropin induced idiopathic IH is diagnosed, treatment with somatropin can be restarted at a lower dose after IH-associated signs and symptoms have resolved.

Progression of scoliosis can occur in children who experience rapid growth. Because somatropin increases growth rate, patients with a history of scoliosis who are treated with somatropin should be monitored for progression of scoliosis. Bone age should be monitored periodically during somatropin administration, especially in patients who are pubertal and/or receiving concomitant thyroid hormone replacement therapy. Under these circumstances, epiphyseal maturation may progress rapidly.

When somatropin is administered subcutaneously at the same site over a long period of time, tissue atrophy may result. This can be avoided by rotating the injection site. As is the case with any protein, local or systemic allergic reactions may occur. Parents/Patient should be informed that such reactions are possible and that prompt medical attention should be sought if allergic reactions occur.

Information for Patients

Patients being treated with Tev-Tropin and/or their caregivers should be informed about the potential benefits and risks associated with treatment. See the patient information included with the product and/or injection device. This information is intended to aid in the safe and effective administration of the medication. It is not a disclosure of all possible adverse or intended effects.

Patients and caregivers who will administer Tev-Tropin should receive appropriate training and instruction on the proper use of Tev-Tropin from the physician or other suitable qualified health care professional. A puncture-resistant container for the disposal of used needles and syringes should be strongly recommended. Patients and/or caregivers should be thoroughly instructed in the importance of proper disposal, and cautioned against any reuse of needles and syringes.

Laboratory Tests

Serum levels of inorganic phosphorus, alkaline phosphatase, and IGF-1 may increase after somatropin therapy.

Drug Interactions

The microsomal enzyme 11β-hydroxysteroid dehydrogenase type 1 (11βHSD-1) is required for conversion of cortisone to its active metabolite, cortisol, in hepatic and adipose tissue. Growth hormone and somatropin inhibit 11βHSD-1. Consequently, individuals with untreated GH deficiency have relative increases in 11βHSD-1 and serum cortisol. Introduction of somatropin treatment may result in inhibition of 11βHSD-1 and reduced serum cortisol concentrations. As a consequence, previously undiagnosed central (secondary) hypoadrenalism may be unmasked and glucocorticoid replacement may be required in patients treated with somatropin. In addition, patients treated with glucocorticoid replacement for previously diagnosed hypoadrenalism may require an increase in their maintenance or stress doses following initiation of somatropin treatment; this may be especially true for patients treated with cortisone acetate and prednisone since conversion of these drugs to their biologically active metabolites is dependent on the activity of 11βHSD-1.

Pharmacologic glucocorticoid therapy and supraphysiologic glucocorticoid treatment may attenuate the growth promoting effects of somatropin in children. Therefore, glucocorticoid replacement dosing should be carefully adjusted in children receiving concomitant somatropin and glucocorticoid treatments to avoid both hypoadrenalism and an inhibitory effect on growth.

Limited published data indicate that somatropin treatment increases cytochrome P450 (CP450) mediated antipyrine clearance in man. These data suggest that somatropin administration may alter the clearance of compounds known to be metabolized by CP450 liver enzymes (e.g., corticosteroids, sex steroids, anticonvulsants, cyclosporine). Careful monitoring is advisable when somatropin is administered in combination with other drugs known to be metabolized by CP450 liver enzymes.

Carcinogenesis, Mutagenesis, Impairment of Fertility
Carcinogenesis, mutagenesis and reproduction studies have not been conducted with Tev-Tropin.

Pregnancy
Pregnancy Category C. Animal reproduction studies have not been conducted with Tev-Tropin. It is also not known whether Tev-Tropin can cause fetal harm when administered to a pregnant woman or can affect reproductive capacity. Tev-Tropin should be given to a pregnant woman only if clearly needed.

Nursing Mothers
It is not known whether this drug is excreted in human milk. Because many drugs are excreted in human milk, caution should be exercised when Tev-Tropin is administered to a nursing woman.

Geriatric Use
The safety and effectiveness of somatropin in patients aged 65 and over has not been evaluated in clinical studies. Elderly patients may be more sensitive to the action of somatropin, and may be more prone to develop adverse reactions.

ADVERSE REACTIONS
The following adverse reactions have been observed during appropriate use of somatropin: headaches (children and adults), gynecomastia (children) and pancreatitis (children and adults). See **WARNINGS** section.

As with all therapeutic proteins, there is potential for immunogenicity. The detection of antibody formation is highly dependent on the sensitivity and specificity of the assay. Additionally, the observed incidence of antibody (including neutralizing antibody) positivity in an assay may be influences by several factors including assay methodology, sample handling, timing of sample collection, concomitant medications, and underlying disease. For these reasons, comparison of the incidence of antibodies to Tev-Tropin with the incidence of antibodies to other products may be misleading. With respect to growth hormone, antibody binding capacities below 2 mg/L have not been associated with growth attenuation. In some cases, when binding capacity exceeds 2 mg/L, growth attenuation has been observed. None of the patients with anti-GH antibodies in the clinical studies experienced decreased linear growth response to Tev-Tropin or any other associated adverse event. Injection site reactions (e.g., pain, bruise) occurred in 8 of the 164 treated patients.

Leukemia has been reported in a small number of patients treated with other growth hormone products. It is uncertain whether this risk is related to the pathology of growth hormone deficiency itself, growth hormone therapy, or other associated treatments such as radiation therapy for intracranial tumors.

New-onset type 2 diabetes mellitus has been reported.

OVERDOSAGE
The recommended dosage of up to 0.1 mg/kg (0.3 IU/kg) of body weight 3 times per week should not be exceeded. Acute overdose could cause initial hypoglycemia and subsequent hyperglycemia. Repeated use of doses in excess of those recommended could result in signs and symptoms of gigantism and/or acromegaly consistent with the known effects of excess human growth hormone.

DOSAGE AND ADMINISTRATION
A dosage of up to 0.1 mg/kg (0.3 IU/kg) of body weight administered 3 times per week by subcutaneous injection is recommended.

Tev-Tropin 5 mg should be reconstituted with 1 to 5 mL of bacteriostatic 0.9% sodium chloride for injection, USP (benzyl alcohol preserved). Reconstituted Tev-Tropin 5 mg vials should not be used if the patient has a known sensitivity to benzyl alcohol. Benzyl alcohol as a preservative in bacteriostatic normal saline, USP, has been associated with toxicity in newborns. WHEN ADMINISTERING TEV-TROPIN TO NEWBORNS, RECONSTITUTE WITH STERILE NORMAL SALINE FOR INJECTION, USP.

Tev-Tropin 10 mg should be reconstituted with 1 mL syringe of bacteriostatic water for injection containing 0.33% metacresol as a preservative. Reconstituted Tev-Tropin 10 mg vials should not be used if the patient is allergic to metacresol.

The stream of normal saline should be aimed against the side of the vial to prevent foaming. Swirl the vial with a GENTLE rotary motion until the contents are completely dissolved and the solution is clear. DO NOT SHAKE. Since Tev-Tropin is a protein, shaking or vigorous mixing will cause the solution to be cloudy. If the resulting solution is cloudy or contains particulate matter, the contents MUST NOT be injected.

Occasionally, after refrigeration, some cloudiness may occur. This is not unusual for proteins like Tev-Tropin. Allow the product to warm to room temperature. If cloudiness persists or particulate matter is noted, the contents MUST NOT be used.

Before and after injection, the septum of the vial should be wiped with rubbing alcohol or an alcoholic antiseptic solution to prevent contamination of the contents by repeated needle insertions.

Tev-Tropin 5 mg can be administered using a standard sterile disposable syringe or a Tjet Needle-Free injection device. However, Tev-Tropin 10 mg can only be administered using a standard sterile disposable syringe. For proper use, please refer to the **User's Manual** provided with the administration device.

STABILITY AND STORAGE

Before Reconstitution
Vials of Tev-Tropin (5 and 10 mg) are stable when refrigerated at 36° to 46°F (2° to 8°C). Avoid freezing the accompanying diluent. Expiration dates are stated on the labels.

After Reconstitution
Tev-Tropin 5 mg is stable for up to 14 days when reconstituted with bacteriostatic 0.9% sodium chloride (normal saline), USP, and stored in a refrigerator at 36° to 46°F (2° to 8°C). Do not freeze the reconstituted solution.

Tev-Tropin 10 mg is stable for up to 28 days when reconstituted with 1 mL syringe of bacteriostatic water for injection containing 0.33% metacresol as a preservative, and stored in a refrigerator at 36° to 46°F (2° to 8°C). Do not freeze the reconstituted solution.

HOW SUPPLIED
Tev-Tropin [somatropin (rDNA origin)] for Injection is supplied as 5 mg and 10 mg of lyophilized, sterile somatropin per vial.

Tev-Tropin 5 mg carton contains one vial of Tev-Tropin (5 mg per vial) and one vial of diluent [5 mL of bacteriostatic 0.9% sodium chloride for injection, USP (benzyl alcohol preserved)], and is supplied in single cartons.

Tev-Tropin 10 mg carton contains one vial of Tev-Tropin (10 mg per vial), one syringe of diluent [1 mL of bacteriostatic water for injection with 0.33% metacresol as preservative] and a 25G reconstitution needle, and is supplied in single cartons.

Rx only.

Distributed by:

Teva Select Brands, Horsham, PA 19044

Division of Teva Pharmaceuticals USA, Inc.

Rev. 07/2014

6805-02

Tev-Tropin®

[somatropin (rDNA origin)] for Injection

5 mg & 10 mg

Information for the Patient or Parent

Read all instructions before proceeding.

Do not mix (reconstitute) the drug or inject it until you have been thoroughly trained in the proper techniques by your doctor. Use sterile techniques as instructed by your doctor. The first injection of Tev-Tropin should be given under the supervision of your doctor. Properly discard syringes and/or needles after each use.

PREPARATION
Your GROWTH HORMONE is supplied in a powder form that must be prepared for injection by mixing it with a *diluent* (a liquid, either Bacteriostatic 0.9% Sodium Chloride Injection, USP [5 mg vial] or Bacteriostatic Water for Injection with 0.33% Metacresol [10 mg vial]) prior to use. Only use the specific *diluent* that is supplied in the carton containing your growth hormone. Once you have reconstituted your growth hormone with the diluent, it is ready for injection. Your doctor will prescribe the exact amount of diluent and tell you the size of the syringe and needle to use. **Note:** The *diluents* are different for the 5 mg and 10 mg vials. Do not interchange the *diluents*.

Tev-Tropin should be kept refrigerated (36° to 46°F [2°to 8°C]) before and after reconstitution. Do not freeze.

Tev-Tropin 5 mg is supplied with a vial of liquid containing Bacteriostatic 0.9% Sodium Chloride Injection, USP (5 mL). After Tev-Tropin 5 mg vial is mixed with the *diluent*, the vial should be used within 14 days.

Tev-Tropin 10 mg is supplied with a syringe of liquid containing vial Bacteriostatic Water for Injection with 0.33% Metacresol as a preservative. After Tev-Tropin 10 mg vial is mixed with the *diluent*, the vial should be used within 28 days.

Before preparing your medication, be sure to wash your hands thoroughly with soap and water. This will help prevent infection.

Preparing Tev-Tropin 5 mg:
(1) Remove the hard plastic cap from the top of the *diluent* vial by gently pushing up on the edge of the cap. Do not remove the rubber stopper. Using an alcohol swab, wipe off the top of the *diluent* bottle. After cleansing, do not touch the rubber stopper.

(2) Carefully remove the needle cap from the syringe, taking care not to touch the needle. Do not discard the needle cap. Hold the barrel of the syringe with one hand and pull back on the plunger with the other, until you have drawn up the amount of air that is the same as the amount of diluent your doctor has ordered.

(3) Insert the needle into the *diluent* vial through the center of the cleansed rubber stopper. Push down on the plunger until all the air is released into the vial.

(4) Holding the vial with one hand, carefully turn it upside down making sure the syringe needle stays in the vial. The tip of the needle should be below the surface of the *diluent*. With your other hand, gently pull back the plunger until the amount of *diluent* your doctor has prescribed is in the syringe. Once the syringe is correctly filled with the *diluent*, remove the syringe and needle

Preparing Tev-Tropin 10 mg:
(1) Remove the syringe tip cap from the top of the pre-filled *diluent* syringe and attach the 25G mixing needle that is supplied in the carton.

DILUTING Tev-Tropin

Remove the hard plastic top of the growth hormone vial. Cleanse the top of the growth hormone vial with an alcohol swab. Remove the needle cap from the syringe filled with *diluent* and insert the needle into the center of the rubber stopper on the growth hormone vial from the vial and recap the needle.

(1) Point the needle toward the side of the vial and slowly push the plunger so that the *diluent* squirts onto the side of the vial, not directly onto the powder. When all the *diluent* is in the growth hormone vial, remove the needle from the vial, recap the needle and discard the syringe.

(2) To mix the growth hormone, hold the vial between your hands and gently roll it until the mixture is clear. NEVER SHAKE THE VIAL! Sometimes the vial may need to sit a few seconds before the mixture becomes clear. Do not use the mixture in the vial if it remains cloudy or you see particles floating in the mixture. If air bubbles appear, let the growth hormone sit for a while until they disappear.

Write the date you reconstitute the growth hormone on the vial label. The 5 mg vial must be used within 14 days whereas the 10 mg vial must be used within 28 days. Store reconstituted growth hormone along with all unopened vials of the growth hormone in a safe, clean place in the refrigerator. Do not freeze.

INJECTION

To prepare to give an injection of growth hormone, begin by thoroughly washing your hands with soap and water. Check that the vial of growth hormone you are using is clear and that the date of reconstitution is within 14 days (5 mg) or 28 days (10 mg).

(1) Cleanse the top of the growth hormone vial with an alcohol swab. After cleansing, do not touch the rubber stopper. Remove the needle cap from the syringe and insert the needle into the center of the rubber stopper on the growth hormone vial. Gently pull back the plunger until the amount of growth hormone solution your doctor has prescribed is in the syringe.

Once the needle is correctly filled with the solution, remove the needle from the vial. Recap the needle. If you are not experienced with filling a syringe, ask your doctor for a demonstration.

(2) Choose a site for your injection. Clean the injection site with an alcohol swab, using a circular pattern, and work from the injection site outward about 2 inches. Allow the alcohol to dry before giving the injection.

(3) Check that the correct dose is in the syringe and remove the needle cap. Hold the syringe the way you hold a pencil.

(4) With your free hand, pinch the cleansed skin between your fingers and quickly insert the needle into the skin at a 45° - 90° angle with a quick, firm wrist motion.

[See first figure at top of next column]

(5) Holding the syringe in place, pull back a little on the plunger and check to see if any blood flows into the syringe (vessel check). If you see blood in the syringe, remove the needle and syringe and discard. You will then need to prepare a new syringe for injection.

[See second figure at top of next column]

(6) If, during the vessel check, you see no blood, then slowly push down plunger until the syringe is completely empty.

(7) Quickly remove the needle from the skin and apply pressure to the injection site with a dry sterile gauze pad or cotton ball. A drop of blood may appear. Apply a small bandage if desired.

(8) Dispose of needle and syringe in a proper container identified by your physician or pharmacist. Never dispose of needles and syringes in your household trash.

INJECTION SITES

There are different sites you can use for your injections. These sites should be rotated.

If you notice any of the following signs, contact your physician:

- A lump, bruise or redness at the injection site that doesn't go away.
- Any sign of infection at the injection site (pus, redness, heat or persistent pain).
- Severe, sharp pain or persistent ache at injection site.
- Rash at injection site.

Distributed by:
Teva Select Brands, Horsham, PA 19044
Division of Teva Pharmaceuticals USA, Inc.
Rev. 07/2014
6805-02   TVT-40251
Shown in Product Identification Guide, page 314

The Medicines Company
8 Sylvan Way
Parsippany, NJ 07054
U.S.A.

Telephone:
973-290-6000
Medical Information: 1-888-977-6326

ORBACTIV™   Rx
(oritavancin)
for injection, for intravenous use

HIGHLIGHTS OF PRESCRIBING INFORMATION
These highlights do not include all the information needed to use ORBACTIV™ safely and effectively. See full prescribing information for ORBACTIV.
ORBACTIV (oritavancin) for injection, for intravenous use
Initial U.S. Approval: 2014

INDICATIONS AND USAGE

ORBACTIV is a lipoglycopeptide antibacterial drug indicated for the treatment of adult patients with acute bacterial skin and skin structure infections caused or suspected to be caused by susceptible isolates of designated Gram-positive microorganisms. (1.1)
To reduce the development of drug-resistant bacteria and maintain the effectiveness of ORBACTIV and other antibacterial drugs, ORBACTIV should be used only to treat infections that are proven or strongly suspected to be caused by susceptible bacteria. (1.2)

DOSAGE AND ADMINISTRATION

A 1200 mg single dose is administered by intravenous infusion over 3 hours. (2.1)

DOSAGE FORMS AND STRENGTHS

For injection: 400 mg of lyophilized powder in a single-use vial for reconstitution. (3)

CONTRAINDICATIONS

- Use of intravenous unfractionated heparin sodium is contraindicated for 48 hours after ORBACTIV administration. (4.1, 5.2)
- Known hypersensitivity to ORBACTIV (4.2, 5.3)

WARNINGS AND PRECAUTIONS

- Concomitant warfarin use: Co-administration of ORBACTIV and warfarin may result in higher exposure of warfarin, which may increase the risk of bleeding. Use ORBACTIV in patients on chronic warfarin therapy only when the benefits can be expected to outweigh the risk of bleeding. (5.1)
- Coagulation test interference: ORBACTIV has been shown to artificially prolong aPTT for up to 48 hours, and may prolong PT and INR for up to 24 hours. (5.2)
- Hypersensitivity reactions have been reported with the use of antibacterial agents including ORBACTIV. Discontinue infusion if signs of acute hypersensitivity occur. Monitor closely patients with known hypersensitivity to glycopeptides. (5.3)
- Infusion-related reactions have been reported. Slow the rate or interrupt infusion if infusion reaction develops. (5.4)
- *Clostridium difficile*-associated colitis: Evaluate patients if diarrhea occurs. (5.5)
- Osteomyelitis: Institute appropriate alternate antibacterial therapy in patients with confirmed or suspected osteomyelitis. (5.6)

ADVERSE REACTIONS

The most common adverse reactions (≥ 3%) in patients treated with ORBACTIV were headache, nausea, vomiting, limb and subcutaneous abscesses, and diarrhea. (6.1)

To report SUSPECTED ADVERSE REACTIONS, contact The Medicines Company at 1-888-977-6326 or FDA at 1-800-FDA-1088 or www.fda.gov/medwatch.

See 17 for PATIENT COUNSELING INFORMATION
Revised: 09/2014

FULL PRESCRIBING INFORMATION: CONTENTS*

* Sections or subsections omitted from the full prescribing information are not listed

FULL PRESCRIBING INFORMATION

1 INDICATIONS AND USAGE

1.1 Acute Bacterial Skin and Skin Structure Infections

ORBACTIV™ (Oritavancin) for injection is indicated for the treatment of adult patients with acute bacterial skin and skin structure infections (ABSSSI) caused by susceptible isolates of the following Gram-positive microorganisms: *Staphylococcus aureus* (including methicillin-susceptible and methicillin–resistant isolates), *Streptococcus pyogenes, Streptococcus agalactiae, Streptococcus dysgalactiae, Streptococcus anginosus* group (includes *S. anginosus, S. intermedius,* and *S. constellatus*), and *Enterococcus faecalis* (vancomycin-susceptible isolates only).

1.2 Usage

To reduce the development of drug-resistant bacteria and maintain the effectiveness of ORBACTIV and other antibacterial drugs, ORBACTIV should be used only to treat infections that are proven or strongly suspected to be caused by susceptible bacteria. When culture and susceptibility information are available, they should be considered in selecting or modifying antibacterial therapy. In the absence of such data, local epidemiology and susceptibility patterns may contribute to the empiric selection of therapy.

2 DOSAGE AND ADMINISTRATION

2.1 Recommended Dosage

The recommended dosing for ORBACTIV is a single 1200 mg dose administered by intravenous infusion over 3 hours in patients 18 years and older.

2.2 Preparation of ORBACTIV for Intravenous Infusion

ORBACTIV is intended for intravenous infusion, only after reconstitution and dilution.

Three ORBACTIV 400 mg vials need to be reconstituted and diluted to prepare a single 1200 mg intravenous dose.

Reconstitution: Aseptic technique should be used to reconstitute three ORBACTIV 400 mg vials.

• Add 40 mL of sterile water for injection (WFI) to reconstitute each vial to provide a 10 mg/mL solution per vial.

• For each vial, gently swirl to avoid foaming and ensure that all ORBACTIV powder is completely reconstituted in solution.

• Each vial should be inspected visually for particulate matter after reconstitution and should appear to be clear, colorless to pale yellow solution.

Dilution: Use ONLY 5% dextrose in sterile water (D5W) for dilution. Do NOT use Normal Saline for dilution as it is incompatible with ORBACTIV and may cause precipitation of the drug. Use aseptic technique to:

• Withdraw and discard 120 mL from a 1000 mL intravenous bag of D5W.

• Withdraw 40 mL from each of the three reconstituted vials and add to D5W intravenous bag to bring the bag volume to 1000 mL. This yields a concentration of 1.2 mg/mL.

Since no preservative or bacteriostatic agent is present in this product, aseptic technique must be used in preparing the final intravenous solution.

Diluted intravenous solution in an infusion bag should be used within 6 hours when stored at room temperature, or used within 12 hours when refrigerated at 2 to 8°C (36 to 46°F). The combined storage time (reconstituted solution in the vial and diluted solution in the bag) and 3 hour infusion time should not exceed 6 hours at room temperature or 12 hours if refrigerated.

2.3 Incompatibilities

ORBACTIV is administered intravenously. ORBACTIV should only be diluted in D5W. Do NOT use normal saline for dilution as it is incompatible with ORBACTIV and may cause precipitation of the drug. Therefore other intravenous substances, additives or other medications mixed in normal saline should not be added to ORBACTIV single-use vials or infused simultaneously through the same IV line or through a common intravenous port. In addition, drugs formulated at a basic or neutral pH may be incompatible with ORBACTIV. ORBACTIV should not be administered simultaneously with commonly used intravenous drugs through a common intravenous port. If the same intravenous line is used for sequential infusion of additional medications, the line should be flushed before and after infusion of ORBACTIV with D5W.

3 DOSAGE FORMS AND STRENGTHS

ORBACTIV is supplied as sterile, white to off-white lyophilized powder equivalent to 400 mg of oritavancin in a single use 50 mL clear glass vial.

4 CONTRAINDICATIONS

4.1 Intravenous Unfractionated Heparin Sodium

Use of intravenous unfractionated heparin sodium is contraindicated for 48 hours after ORBACTIV administration because the activated partial thromboplastin time (aPTT) test results are expected to remain falsely elevated for approximately 48 hours after ORBACTIV administration *[see Warnings and Precautions (5.2) and Drug Interactions (7.2)]*

4.2 Hypersensitivity

ORBACTIV is contraindicated in patients with known hypersensitivity to ORBACTIV.

5 WARNINGS AND PRECAUTIONS

5.1 Potential Risk of Bleeding with Concomitant Use of Warfarin

Co-administration of ORBACTIV and warfarin may result in higher exposure of warfarin, which may increase the risk of bleeding. Use ORBACTIV in patients on chronic warfarin therapy only when the benefits can be expected to outweigh the risk of bleeding. Frequently monitor for signs of bleeding. *[see Drug Interactions (7.1), Clinical Pharmacology (12.3)].*

ORBACTIV has been shown to artificially prolong PT and INR for up to 24 hours, making the monitoring of the anticoagulation effect of warfarin unreliable up to 24 hours after an ORBACTIV dose. *[see Warnings and Precautions (5.2)]*

5.2 Coagulation Test Interference

ORBACTIV has been shown to artificially prolong aPTT for 48 hours and the PT and INR for 24 hours by binding to and preventing action of the phospholipid reagents which activate coagulation in commonly used laboratory coagulation tests.

For patients who require aPTT monitoring within 48 hours of ORBACTIV dosing, a non-phospholipid dependent coagulation test such as a Factor Xa (chromogenic) assay or an alternative anticoagulant not requiring aPTT monitoring may be considered.

Effects by ORBACTIV on activated clotting time (ACT) are expected since the phospholipid reagents are also utilized in this coagulation test. ORBACTIV has no effect on the coagulation system. *[see Contraindications (4.1) and Drug Interactions (7.2)]*

5.3 Hypersensitivity

Serious hypersensitivity reactions have been reported with the use of ORBACTIV. If an acute hypersensitivity reaction occurs during ORBACTIV infusion, discontinue ORBACTIV immediately and institute appropriate supportive care. Before using ORBACTIV, inquire carefully about previous hypersensitivity reactions to glycopeptides. Due to the possibility of cross-sensitivity, carefully monitor for signs of hypersensitivity during ORBACTIV infusion in patients with a history of glycopeptide allergy. In the Phase 3 ABSSSI clinical trials, the median onset of hypersensitivity reactions in ORBACTIV-treated patients was 1.2 days and the median duration of these reactions was 2.4 days. *[see Adverse Reactions (6.1)]*

5.4 Infusion Related Reactions

Infusion related reactions have been reported with ORBACTIV including pruritus, urticaria or flushing. If reactions do occur, consider slowing or interrupting ORBACTIV infusion. *[see Adverse Reactions (6.1)]*

5.5 Clostridium difficile-associated Diarrhea

Clostridium difficile-associated diarrhea (CDAD) has been reported for nearly all systemic antibacterial drugs, including ORBACTIV, and may range in severity from mild diarrhea to fatal colitis. Treatment with antibacterial agents alters the normal flora of the colon and may permit overgrowth of *C. difficile.*

C. difficile produces toxins A and B which contribute to the development of CDAD. Hypertoxin-producing strains of *C. difficile* cause increased morbidity and mortality, as these infections can be refractory to antibacterial therapy and may require colectomy. CDAD must be considered in all patients who present with diarrhea following antibacterial use. Careful medical history is necessary because CDAD has been reported to occur more than 2 months after the administration of antibacterial agents.

If CDAD is suspected or confirmed, antibacterial use not directed against *C. difficile* may need to be discontinued. Appropriate fluid and electrolyte management, protein supplementation, antibacterial treatment of *C. difficile*, and surgical evaluation should be instituted as clinically indicated.

5.6 Osteomyelitis

In Phase 3 ABSSSI clinical trials, more cases of osteomyelitis were reported in the ORBACTIV treated arm than in the vancomycin-treated arm. Monitor patients for signs and symptoms of osteomyelitis. If osteomyelitis is suspected or diagnosed, institute appropriate alternate antibacterial therapy *[see Adverse Reactions (6.1)].*

5.7 Development of Drug Resistant Bacteria

Prescribing ORBACTIV in the absence of a proven or strongly suspected bacterial infection is unlikely to provide benefit to the patient and increases the risk of the development of drug-resistant bacteria *[see Patient Counseling Information (17)].*

6 ADVERSE REACTIONS

The following adverse reactions are also discussed in the Warnings and Precautions section of the label:

Hypersensitivity Reactions *[see Warnings and Precautions (5.3)]*

Infusion related reactions *[see Warnings and Precautions (5.4)]*

Clostridium difficile-associated diarrhea *[see Warnings and Precautions (5.5)]*

Osteomyelitis *[see Warnings and Precautions (5.6)]*

6.1 Clinical Trials Experience

Because clinical trials are conducted under widely varying conditions, adverse reaction rates observed in the clinical trials of ORBACTIV cannot be directly compared to rates in the clinical trials of another drug and may not reflect the rates observed in practice.

ORBACTIV has been evaluated in two, double-blind, controlled ABSSSI clinical trials, which included 976 adult patients treated with a single 1200 mg intravenous dose of ORBACTIV and 983 patients treated with intravenous vancomycin for 7 to 10 days. The median age of patients treated with ORBACTIV was 45.6 years, ranging between 18 and 89 years of age with 8.8% ≥65 years of age. Patients treated with ORBACTIV were predominantly male (65.4%), 64.4% were Caucasian, 5.8% were African American, and 28.1% were Asian. Safety was evaluated for up to 60 days after dosing.

In the pooled ABSSSI clinical trials, serious adverse reactions were reported in 57/976 (5.8%) patients treated with ORBACTIV and 58/983 (5.9%) treated with vancomycin. The most commonly reported serious adverse reaction was cellulitis in both treatment groups: 11/976 (1.1%) in ORBACTIV and 12/983 (1.2%) in the vancomycin arms, respectively.

The most commonly reported adverse reactions (≥3%) in patients receiving a single 1200 mg dose of ORBACTIV in the pooled ABSSSI clinical trials were: headache, nausea, vomiting, limb and subcutaneous abscesses, and diarrhea.

In the pooled ABSSSI clinical trials, ORBACTIV was discontinued due to adverse reactions in 36/976 (3.7%) of patients; the most common reported reactions leading to discontinuation were cellulitis (4/976, 0.4%) and osteomyelitis (3/976, 0.3%).

Table 1 provides selected adverse reactions occurring in ≥ 1.5% of patients receiving ORBACTIV in the pooled

ABSSSI clinical trials. There were 540 (55.3%) patients in the ORBACTIV arm and 559 (56.9%) patients in the vancomycin arm, who reported ≥1 adverse reaction.

Table 1: Incidence of Selected Adverse Reactions Occurring in ≥ 1.5% of Patients Receiving ORBACTIV in the Pooled ABSSSI Clinical Trials

Adverse Reactions	ORBACTIV N=976 (%)	Vancomycin N=983 (%)
Gastrointestinal disorders		
Diarrhea	36 (3.7)	32 (3.4)
Nausea	97 (9.9)	103 (10.5)
Vomiting	45 (4.6)	46 (4.7)
Nervous system disorders		
Dizziness	26 (2.7)	26 (2.6)
Headache	69 (7.1)	66 (6.7)
General disorders and administration		
Infusion site phlebitis	24 (2.5)	15 (1.5)
Infusion site reaction	19 (1.9)	34 (3.5)
Infections and infestations		
Abscess (limb and subcutaneous)	37 (3.8)	23 (2.3)
Investigations		
Alanine aminotransferase increased	27 (2.8)	15 (1.5)
Aspartate aminotransferase increased	18 (1.8)	15 (1.5)
Cardiac disorders		
Tachycardia	24 (2.5)	11 (1.1)

The following selected adverse reactions were reported in ORBACTIV-treated patients at a rate of less than 1.5%:
Blood and lymphatic system disorders: anemia, eosinophilia
General Disorders and administration site conditions: infusion site erythema, extravasation, induration, pruritus, rash, edema peripheral
Immune system disorders: hypersensitivity
Infections and infestations: osteomyelitis
Investigations: total bilirubin increased, hyperuricemia
Metabolism and nutrition disorders: hypoglycemia
Musculoskeletal and connective tissue disorders: tenosynovitis, myalgia
Respiratory, thoracic and mediastinal disorders: bronchospasm, wheezing
Skin and Subcutaneous Tissue Disorders: urticaria, angioedema, erythema multiforme, pruritus, leucocytoclastic vasculitis, rash.

7 DRUG INTERACTIONS
7.1 Effect of ORBACTIV on CYP Substrates
A cocktail drug-drug interaction study was conducted in healthy volunteers (n=16) evaluating the concomitant administration of a single 1200 mg dose of ORBACTIV with probe substrates for several CYP450 enzymes. ORBACTIV was found to be a nonspecific, weak inhibitor (CYP2C9 or CYP2C19) or inducer (CYP3A4 and CYP2D6) of several CYP isoforms [see Clinical Pharmacology (12.3)].
Caution should be used when administering ORBACTIV concomitantly with drugs with a narrow therapeutic window that are predominantly metabolized by one of the affected CYP450 enzymes (e.g., warfarin), as co-administration may increase (e.g. for CYP2C9 substrates) or decrease (e.g. for CYP2D6 substrates) concentrations of the narrow therapeutic range drug. Patients should be closely monitored for signs of toxicity or lack of efficacy if they have been given ORBACTIV while on a potentially affected compound (e.g. patients should be monitored for bleeding if concomitantly receiving ORBACTIV and warfarin) [see Warnings and Precautions (5.1)].
7.2 Drug-Laboratory Test Interactions
ORBACTIV has been shown to artificially prolong aPTT for 48 hours and PT and INR for up to 24 hours by binding to

and preventing action of the phospholipid reagents which activate coagulation in commonly used laboratory coagulation tests. Effects by ORBACTIV on ACT are expected since the phospholipid reagents are also utilized in this coagulation test. ORBACTIV has no effect on the coagulation system. [see Warnings and Precautions (5.2)].

8 USE IN SPECIFIC POPULATIONS
8.1 Pregnancy
Pregnancy Category C
Reproduction studies performed in rats and rabbits have revealed no evidence of harm to the fetus due to oritavancin at the highest concentrations administered, 30 mg/kg/day and 15 mg/kg/day, respectively. Those daily doses would be equivalent to a human dose of 300 mg, or 25% of the single clinical dose of 1200 mg. Higher doses were not evaluated in nonclinical developmental and reproductive toxicology studies.
There are no adequate and well-controlled trials in pregnant women. ORBACTIV should be used during pregnancy only if the potential benefit justifies the potential risk to the fetus.
8.3 Nursing Mothers
It is unknown whether oritavancin is excreted in human milk. Following a single intravenous infusion in lactating rats, radio-labeled [^{14}C]-oritavancin was excreted in milk and absorbed by nursing pups. Caution should be exercised when ORBACTIV is administered to a nursing woman.
8.4 Pediatric Use
Safety and effectiveness of ORBACTIV in pediatric patients (younger than 18 years of age) has not been studied.
8.5 Geriatric Use
The pooled Phase 3 ABSSSI clinical trials of ORBACTIV did not include sufficient numbers of subjects aged 65 and older to determine whether they respond differently from younger subjects. Other reported clinical experience has not identified differences in responses between the elderly and younger patients, but greater sensitivity of some older individuals cannot be ruled out.
8.6 Renal Impairment
No dosage adjustment of ORBACTIV is needed in patients with mild or moderate renal impairment [see Dosage and Administration (2.1), Clinical Pharmacology (12.3)]. The pharmacokinetics of ORBACTIV in severe renal impairment have not been evaluated. ORBACTIV is not removed from blood by hemodialysis.
8.7 Hepatic Impairment
No dosage adjustment of ORBACTIV is needed in patients with mild or moderate hepatic impairment. The pharmacokinetics of ORBACTIV in patients with severe hepatic insufficiency has not been studied [see Dosage and Administration (2.1), Clinical Pharmacology (12.3)].

•2H₃PO₄

10 OVERDOSAGE
In the ORBACTIV clinical program there was no incidence of accidental overdose of ORBACTIV.
Based on an in vitro hemodialysis study, ORBACTIV is unlikely to be removed from blood by hemodialysis. In the event of overdose, supportive measures should be taken.

11 DESCRIPTION
ORBACTIV (oritavancin) for injection contains oritavancin diphosphate, a semisynthetic lipoglycopeptide antibacterial drug.
The chemical name for oritavancin is [4";R]-22-O-(3-amino-2,3,6-trideoxy-3-C-methyl-α-L-arabino-hexopyranosyl)-N3"-[(4'-chloro[1,1'-biphenyl]-4-yl)methyl] vancomycin phosphate [1:2] (salt). The empirical formula of oritavancin diphosphate is $C_{86}H_{97}N_{10}O_{26}Cl_3 \bullet 2H_3PO_4$ and the molecular weight is 1989.09. The chemical structure is represented below:
[See figure above]
ORBACTIV is supplied as a sterile white to off-white lyophilized powder for intravenous infusion that contains oritavancin diphosphate, mannitol (an inactive ingredient) and phosphoric acid (to adjust pH 3.1 to 4.3). Each 50 ml capacity glass vial contains 449 mg oritavancin diphosphate (equivalent to 405 mg of oritavancin, 5 mg excess is to ensure withdrawal of 400 mg oritavancin), 400 mg oritavancin (free base equivalent).
Each vial is reconstituted with sterile water for injection and further diluted with 5% Dextrose in sterile Water for intravenous infusion. Both the reconstituted solution and the diluted solution for infusion should be clear, colorless to pale yellow solution [see Dosage and Administration (2.2)].

12 CLINICAL PHARMACOLOGY
12.1 Mechanism of Action
Oritavancin is an antibacterial drug [see Clinical Pharmacology (12.4)].
12.2 Pharmacodynamics
The antimicrobial activity of oritavancin appears to correlate with the ratio of area under the concentration-time curve to minimal inhibitory concentration (AUC/MIC) based on animal models of infection.
Exposure-response analyses from both preclinical and clinical studies support the treatment of clinically relevant Gram-positive microorganisms (e.g. S. aureus and S. pyogenes) causative of ABSSSI with a single 1200 mg dose of ORBACTIV.

Cardiac Electrophysiology
In a thorough QTc study of 135 healthy subjects at a dose 1.3 times the 1200 mg recommended dose, ORBACTIV did not prolong the QTc interval to any clinically relevant extent.

Figure 1: Population Mean Plasma Concentration-Time Profile after a Single 1200 mg dose of Oritavancin Administered Intravenously Over 3 Hours – Semi-Log Scale

Co-administration of ORBACTIV resulted in an increase of 18% in the ratio of 1-methylxanthine + 1 methylurate + 5-acetylamino-6-formylamino-3-methyluracil (1X + 1U + AFMU) to 1,7-dimethylurate (17U) concentrations in the urine after administration of caffeine (CYP1A2 probe substrate), and an increase of 16% in the ratio of AFMU to (1X +1U) concentrations in the urine after administration of caffeine (N-Acetyltransferase- 2 probe substrate). Co-administration of ORBACTIV did not change the mean systemic exposure of caffeine metabolite (Xanthine oxidase probe substrate).

12.4   Microbiology
ORBACTIV is a semi-synthetic, lipoglycopeptide antibacterial drug. ORBACTIV exerts a concentration-dependent bactericidal activity in vitro against *S. aureus, S. pyogenes,* and *E. faecalis.*

Mechanism of Action
Oritavancin has three mechanisms of action: (i) inhibition of the transglycosylation (polymerization) step of cell wall biosynthesis by binding to the stem peptide of peptidoglycan precursors; (ii) inhibition of the transpeptidation (crosslinking) step of cell wall biosynthesis by binding to the peptide bridging segments of the cell wall; and (iii) disruption of bacterial membrane integrity, leading to depolarization, permeabilization, and cell death. These multiple mechanisms contribute to the concentration-dependent bactericidal activity of oritavancin.

Mechanism of Resistance
In serial passage studies, resistance to oritavancin was observed in isolates of *S. aureus* and *E. faecalis.* Resistance to oritavancin was not observed in clinical studies.

Interaction with Other Antimicrobial Agents
In in vitro studies, oritavancin exhibits synergistic bactericidal activity in combination with gentamicin, moxifloxacin or rifampicin against isolates of methicillin-susceptible *S. aureus* (MSSA), with gentamicin or linezolid against isolates of heterogeneous vancomycin-intermediate *S. aureus* (hVISA), VISA, and vancomycin-resistant *S. aureus* (VRSA), and with rifampin against isolates of VRSA. In vitro studies demonstrated no antagonism between oritavancin and gentamicin, moxifloxacin, linezolid or rifampin.

Antibacterial Activity
Oritavancin has been shown to be active against most isolates of the following bacteria, both in vitro and in clinical infections as described in the Indications and Usage section *[see Indications and Usage (1.1)].*
Staphylococcus aureus (including methicillin-resistant isolates)
Streptococcus agalactiae
Streptococcus anginosus group (includes *S. anginosus, S. intermedius,* and *S. constellatus*)
Streptococcus dysgalactiae
Streptococcus pyogenes
Enterococcus faecalis (vancomycin-susceptible isolates only)
The following in vitro data are available but their clinical significance has not been established. At least 90% of isolates of the following microorganisms exhibit an in vitro minimum inhibitory concentration (MIC) less than or equal to 0.12 mcg/mL for oritavancin. However, the safety and effectiveness of oritavancin in treating clinical infections due to these bacteria have not been established in adequate and well-controlled clinical trials.
Enterococcus faecium (vancomycin-susceptible isolates only)

Susceptibility Testing Methods
When available, the clinical microbiology laboratory should provide cumulative results of in vitro susceptibility test results for antimicrobial drugs used in local hospitals and practice areas to the physician as periodic reports that describe the susceptibility profile of nosocomial and community-acquired pathogens. These reports should aid the physician in selecting the most effective antimicrobial drug for treatment.

Dilution technique
Quantitative methods are used to determine antimicrobial minimal inhibitory concentrations (MICs). These MICs provide estimates of the susceptibility of bacteria to antimicrobial compounds.[1] Oritavancin MICs should be determined using a standardized procedure which are based on a broth microdilution method or equivalent with standardized inoculum concentrations and standardized concentrations of oritavancin. Oritavancin powder is dissolved and diluted in the presence of 0.002% polysorbate 80 and broth test medium is supplemented with polysorbate 80 to a final concentration of 0.002%. The MIC values should be interpreted according to the criteria provided in the Table 3.

12.3   Pharmacokinetics
The population PK analysis was derived using data from the two Phase 3 ABSSSI clinical trials in 297 patients. The mean pharmacokinetic parameters of oritavancin in patients following a single 1200 mg dose are presented in Table 2.

Table 2: Mean PK parameters for patients receiving a single 1200 mg dose for ABSSSI (n=297)

Parameter	Mean (CV%)
C_{max} (μg/mL)	138 (23.0%)
AUC_{0-24} (μg•h/mL)	1110 (33.9%)
$AUC_{0-\infty}$ (μg•h/mL)	2800 (28.6%)
$T_{\frac{1}{2},\alpha}$ (h)	2.29 (49.8%)
$T_{\frac{1}{2},\beta}$ (h)	13.4 (10.5%)
$T_{\frac{1}{2},\gamma}$ (h)	245 (14.9%)

C_{max}, Maximum plasma concentration; AUC_{0-24}, Area under the plasma concentration-time curve from time zero to 24 hours, $AUC_{0-\infty}$ = Area under the plasma concentration time curve from time zero to infinity; $T_{\frac{1}{2},\alpha}$, Half-life for the alpha phase, $T_{\frac{1}{2},\beta}$, Half-life for the beta phase; $T_{\frac{1}{2},\gamma}$, Half-life for the gamma phase; CV% = Percent Coefficient of variation.

Oritavancin exhibits linear pharmacokinetics at a dose up to 1200 mg. The mean, population-predicted oritavancin concentration-time profile displays a multi-exponential decline with a long terminal plasma half-life as shown in Figure 1
[See figure 1 above]

Distribution
Oritavancin is approximately 85% bound to human plasma proteins.
Based on population PK analysis, the population mean total volume of distribution is estimated to be approximately 87.6 L, indicating oritavancin is extensively distributed into the tissues.
Exposures of oritavancin in skin blister fluid were approximately 20% of those in plasma (AUC_{0-24}) after single 800 mg dose in healthy subjects.

Metabolism/Excretion
Non-clinical studies including in vitro human liver microsome studies indicated that oritavancin is not metabolized. No mass balance study has been conducted in humans. In humans, oritavancin is slowly excreted unchanged in feces and urine with less than 1% and 5% of the dose recovered in feces and urine, respectively, after 2 weeks of collection.
Oritavancin has a terminal half-life of approximately 245 hours and a clearance of 0.445 L/h based on population pharmacokinetic analyses.

Specific Populations
No dosage adjustments of ORBACTIV are required for patients with mild to severe renal or mild to moderate hepatic impairment or other subpopulations including age, gender, race and weight.

Renal Impairment
The pharmacokinetics of oritavancin was examined in the Phase 3 ABSSSI trials in patients with normal renal function, CrCL ≥80 mL/min (n=238), mild renal impairment, CrCL 50-79 mL/min (n=48), and moderate renal impairment, CrCL 30-49 mL/min (n=11). Population pharmacokinetic analysis indicated that mild to moderate renal impairment had no clinically relevant effect on the exposure of oritavancin. No dedicated studies in dialysis patients have been conducted.
Dosage adjustment of ORBACTIV is not needed in patients with mild or moderate renal impairment. The pharmacokinetics of oritavancin in patients with severe renal impairment have not been evaluated.

Hepatic Impairment
The pharmacokinetics of oritavancin were evaluated in study of subjects with moderate hepatic impairment (Child-Pugh Class B) (n=20) and compared with healthy subjects (n=20) matched for gender, age and weight. There were no relevant changes in pharmacokinetics of oritavancin in subjects with moderate hepatic impairment.
Dosage adjustment of ORBACTIV is not needed in patients with mild or moderate hepatic impairment. The pharmacokinetics of oritavancin in patients with severe hepatic insufficiency has not been studied.

Pediatric
The pharmacokinetics of ORBACTIV in pediatric populations (<18 years of age) has not been studied *[see Use in Specific Populations (8.4)].*

Age, Gender, Weight and Race
Population pharmacokinetic analysis from the Phase 3 ABSSSI trials in patients indicated that gender, age, weight or race had no clinically relevant effect on the exposure of ORBACTIV. No dosage adjustment is warranted in these subpopulations.

Drug Interactions
In vitro studies with human liver microsomes showed that oritavancin inhibited the activities of cytochrome P450 (CYP) enzymes 1A2, 2B6, 2D6, 2C9, 2C19, and 3A4. The observed inhibition of multiple CYP isoforms by oritavancin in vitro is likely to be reversible and the mechanism of inhibition, noncompetitive. In vitro studies indicate that oritavancin is neither a substrate nor an inhibitor of the efflux transporter P-glycoprotein (P-gp).

Drugs that Inhibit or Induce CYP450 Enzymes
Results from a drug-drug interaction study in healthy volunteers (n=16) evaluating a single 1200 mg dose of ORBACTIV showed that ORBACTIV is a weak inducer of CYP3A4 (a decrease of 18% in the mean AUC of midazolam) and CYP2D6 (decrease of 31% in the ratio of dextromethorphan to dextrorphan concentrations in the urine after administration of dextromethorphan). ORBACTIV was also a weak inhibitor of CYP2C19 (increase of 15% in the ratio of omeprazole to 5-OH-omeprazole concentrations in the plasma after administration of omeprazole) and also showed to be a weak inhibitor of CYP2C9 (with an increase of 31% in the mean AUC of warfarin) *[see Warnings and Precautions (5.1), and Drug Interactions (7.1)].*

Table 3: Susceptibility Interpretive Criteria for ORBACTIV[a]

Microorganism	Minimum Inhibitory Concentration (MIC, mcg/mL)		
	S	I[b]	R[b]
Staphylococcus aureus (including methicillin-resistant isolates)	≤0.12	-	-

Streptococcus pyogenes, Streptococcus agalactiae, Streptococcus dysgalactiae, Streptococcus anginosus, Streptococcus constellatus, and Streptococcus intermedius.	≤0.25	-	-
Enterococcus faecalis (vancomycin-susceptible isolates only)	≤0.12	-	-

Abbreviations: MIC, minimum inhibitory concentration; S, Susceptible; I, intermediate; R, Resistant

[a] As determined by broth microdilution with 0.002% polysorbate-80 during oritavancin dissolution and dilution and in the final assay.

[b] The current absence of resistant isolates precludes defining any results other than "Susceptible". Isolates yielding test results other than "Susceptible" should be retested, and if the result is confirmed, the isolate should be submitted to a reference laboratory for further testing.

A report of "Susceptible" indicates that the antimicrobial drug is likely to inhibit growth of the microorganism if the antimicrobial drug reaches the concentration usually achievable at the site of infection.

Quality Control

Standardized susceptibility test procedures require the use of laboratory control microorganisms to monitor and ensure the accuracy and precision of supplies and reagents used in the assay and the techniques of the individuals performing the test. Acceptable oritavancin MIC ranges for the quality control strains are shown in Table 4.

Quality control microorganisms are specific strains of organisms with intrinsic biological properties, and are very stable strains that will give a standard and reproducible susceptibility pattern. The specific strains used for microbiological quality control are not clinically significant.

Table 4: Acceptable Quality Control Ranges for Oritavancin Susceptibility Testing[a]

Quality Control Organism	Minimum Inhibitory Concentration Range (MIC in mcg/mL)
Staphylococcus aureus ATCC 29213	0.015 – 0.12
Streptococcus pneumoniae ATCC 49619	0.001 – 0.004
Enterococcus faecalis ATCC 29212	0.008 – 0.03

ATCC = American Type Culture Collection.

[a] As determined by broth microdilution with 0.002% polysorbate-80 during oritavancin dissolution and dilution and in the final assay.[1,2]

Diffusion technique

The use of the disk diffusion method is not recommended since quality control ranges have not been defined for oritavancin.

13 NONCLINICAL TOXICOLOGY

13.1 Carcinogenesis, Mutagenesis, Impairment of Fertility

Long term studies in animals have not been conducted to determine the carcinogenic potential of oritavancin.

No mutagenic or clastogenic potential of oritavancin was found in a battery of tests, including an Ames assay, in vitro chromosome aberration assay in Chinese hamster ovary cells, in vitro forward mutation assay in mouse lymphoma cells and an in vivo mouse micronucleus assay.

Oritavancin did not affect the fertility or reproductive performance of male rats (exposed to daily doses up to 30 mg/kg for at least 4 weeks) and female rats (exposed to daily doses up to 30 mg/kg for at least 2 weeks prior to mating). Those daily doses would be equivalent to a human dose of 300 mg, or 25% of clinical dose. Higher doses were not evaluated in nonclinical fertility studies.

14 CLINICAL STUDIES

14.1 Acute Bacterial Skin and Skin Structure Infections (ABSSSI)

A total of 1987 adults with clinically documented ABSSSI suspected or proven to be due to Gram-positive pathogens were randomized into two identically designed, randomized, double-blind, multi-center, multinational, non-inferiority trials (Trial 1 and Trial 2) comparing a single 1200 mg intravenous dose of ORBACTIV to intravenous vancomycin (1 g or 15 mg/kg every 12 hours) for 7 to 10 days. The primary analysis population (modified intent to treat, mITT) included all randomized patients who received any study drug. Patients could receive concomitant aztreonam or metronidazole for suspected Gram-negative and anaerobic infection, respectively. Patient demographic and baseline characteristics were balanced between treatment groups. Approximately 64% of patients were Caucasian and 65% were males. The mean age was 45 years and the mean body mass index was 27 kg/m². Across both trials, approximately 60% of patients were enrolled from the United States and 27% of patients from Asia. A history of diabetes was present in 14% of patients. The types of ABSSSI across both trials included cellulitis/erysipelas (40%), wound infection (29%), and major cutaneous abscesses (31%). Median infection area at baseline across both trials was 266.6 cm².

The primary endpoint in both trials was early clinical response (responder), defined as cessation of spread or reduction in size of baseline lesion, absence of fever, and no rescue antibacterial drug at 48 to 72 hours after initiation of therapy. Table 5 provides the efficacy results for the primary endpoint in Trial 1 and Trial 2 in the primary analysis population.

Table 5: Clinical Response Rates in ABSSSI Trials using Responders[1,2] at 48-72 Hours after Initiation of Therapy

	ORBACTIV n/N (%)	Vancomycin n/N (%)	Difference (95% CI)[3]
Trial 1	391/475(82.3)	378/479(78.9)	3.4 (-1.6, 8.4)
Trial 2	403/503 (80.1)	416/502(82.9)	-2.7(-7.5, 2.0)

[1]Cessation of spread or reduction in size of baseline lesion, absence of fever (<37.7°C) and no rescue antibacterial drug at 48 to 72 hours.

[2]Patients who died at 48 to 72 hours, after initiation of therapy or who had increase in lesion size at 48 to 72 hours, after initiation of therapy or who used non-study antibacterial therapy during first 72 hours or who had an additional, unplanned, surgical procedure or who had missing measurements during the first 72 hours from initiation of study drug were classified as non-responders.

[3] 95% CI based on the Normal approximation to Binomial distribution.

Table 8: Outcomes by Baseline Pathogen (microITT)

	At 48-72 hours				Study day14 to 24	
	Early Clinical Responder[1]		≥ 20% reduction in lesion size[2]		Clinical Success[3]	
Pathogen[4]	ORBACTIV n/N (%)	Vancomycin n/N (%)	ORBACTIV n/N (%)	Vancomycin n/N (%)	ORBACTIV n/N (%)	Vancomycin n/N (%)
Staphylococcus aureus	388/472(82.2)	395/473(83.5)	421/472(89.2)	407/473(86.0)	390/472(82.6)	398/473 (84.1)
Methicillin-susceptible	222/268(82.8)	233/272(85.7)	231/268(86.2)	232/272(85.3)	220/268(82.1)	229/272(84.2)
Methicillin-resistant	166/204(81.4)	162/201(80.6)	190/204(93.1)	175/201(87.1)	170/204(83.3)	169/201(84.1)
Streptococcus pyogenes	21/31(67.7)	23/32(71.9)	24/31(77.4)	24/32(75.0)	25/31(80.6)	23/32(71.9)
Streptococcus agalactiae	7/8(87.5)	12/12(100.0)	8/8(100.0)	12/12(100.0)	7/8(87.5)	11/12(91.7)
Streptococcus dysgalactiae	7/9(77.8)	6/6(100.0)	6/9(66.7)	5/6(83.3)	7/9(77.8)	3/6(50.0)
Streptococcus anginosus group	28/33(84.8)	40/45(88.9)	29/33(87.9)	42/45(93.3)	25/33(75.8)	38/45(84.4)
Enterococcus faecalis	11/13(84.6)	10/12(83.3)	10/13(76.9)	8/12(66.7)	8/13(61.5)	9/12(75.0)

[1] Early clinical response defined as a composite of the cessation of spread or reduction in size of baseline lesion, absence of fever and no rescue antibacterial drug at 48-72 hours

[2] Patients achieving a 20% or greater reduction in lesion area from baseline at 48-72 hours after initiation of therapy

[3] Clinical success was defined if the patient experienced a complete or nearly complete resolution of baseline signs and symptoms as described above.

[4]Baseline bacteremia in the oritavancin arm with relevant microorganisms causing ABSSSI included four subjects with MSSA and seven subjects with MRSA. Eight of these eleven subjects were responders at 48 to 72 hours after initiation of therapy.

A key secondary endpoint in these two ABSSSI trials evaluated the percentage of patients achieving a 20% or greater reduction in lesion area from baseline at 48-72 hours after initiation of therapy. Table 6 summarizes the findings for this endpoint in the two ABSSSI trials.

Table 6: Clinical Response Rates[1] in ABSSSI Trials using Reduction in Lesion Area of 20% or Greater at 48-72 Hours after Initiation of Therapy

	ORBACTIV n /N(%)	Vancomycin n /N(%)	Difference (95% CI)[2]
Trial 1	413/ 475(86.9)	397/ 479(82.9)	4.1(-0.5, 8.6)
Trial 2	432/ 503(85.9)	428/ 502(85.3)	0.6(-3.7, 5.0)

[1]Patients who died at 48 to 72 hours, after initiation of therapy or who had increase in lesion size at 48 to 72 hours, after initiation of therapy or who used non-study antibacterial therapy during first 72 hours or who had an additional, unplanned, surgical procedure or who had missing measurements during the first 72 hours from initiation of study drug were classified as non-responders.

[2] 95% CI based on the Normal approximation to Binomial distribution.

Another secondary efficacy endpoint in the two trials was investigator-assessed clinical success at post therapy evaluation at day 14 to 24 (7 to 14 days from end of blinded therapy). A patient was categorized as a clinical success if the patient experienced a complete or nearly complete resolution of baseline signs and symptoms related to primary ABSSSI site (erythema, induration/edema, purulent drainage, fluctuance, pain, tenderness, local increase in heat/warmth) such that no further treatment with antibacterial drugs was needed.

Table 7 summarizes the findings for this endpoint in the mITT and clinically evaluable population in these two ABSSSI trials. Note that there are insufficient historical data to establish the magnitude of drug effect for antibacterial drugs compared with placebo at these therapy visits. Therefore, comparisons of ORBACTIV to vancomycin based on clinical success rates at these visits cannot be utilized to establish non-inferiority conclusions.

Table 7: Clinical Success Rates[1] in ABSSSI Trials at the Follow-Up Visit (7-14 days after end of therapy)

	ORBACTIV n /N(%)	Vancomycin n /N(%)	Difference (95% CI)[2]
Trial 1	378/475(79.6)	383/479(80.0)	-0.4 (-5.5, 4.7)
mITT	362/370(97.8)	370/397(93.2)	
CE	394(91.9)	397(93.2)	-1.3 (-5.0,2.3)
Trial 2	416/503(82.7)	404/502(80.5)	2.2 (-2.6, 7.0)
mITT	398/427(93.2)	387/408(94.9)	
CE	427(93.2)	408(94.9)	-1.6 (-4.9,1.6)

[1]Clinical success was defined if the patient experienced a complete or nearly complete resolution of baseline signs and symptoms as described above.
[2] 95% CI based on the Normal approximation to Binomial distribution
[3] mITT population consisted of all randomized patients who received study drug; CE population consisted of all mITT patients who did not have violations of inclusion and exclusion criteria, completed treatment and had investigator assessment at the Follow-Up Visit.

Outcomes by Baseline Pathogen: Table 8 shows outcomes in patients with an identified baseline pathogen in the microbiological Intent-to-Treat (microITT) population in a pooled analysis of Trial 1 and Trial 2. The outcomes shown in the table are clinical response rates at 48 to 72 hours and clinical success rates at follow-up study day14 to 24.
[See table 8 at top of previous page]

15   REFERENCES
1. Clinical and Laboratory Standards Institute (CLSI). *Methods for Dilution Antimicrobial Susceptibility Tests for Bacteria that Grow Aerobically; Approved Standard – Ninth Edition.* CLSI document M7-A09, Clinical and Laboratory Standards Institute, 950 West Valley Road, Suite 2500, Wayne, PA 19087, 2012.
2. Clinical and Laboratory Standards Institute (CLSI). *Performance Standards for Antimicrobial Susceptibility Testing; Twenty-fourth Informational Supplement,* CLSI document M100-S24, Clinical and Laboratory Standards Institute, 950 West Valley Road, Suite 2500, Wayne, Pennsylvania 19087, USA, 2014.

16   HOW SUPPLIED/STORAGE AND HANDLING
16.1   How Supplied/Storage
ORBACTIV is supplied as single use 50 mL capacity glass vials containing sterile lyophilized powder equivalent to 400 mg of oritavancin (NDC 65293-015-01). Three vials are packaged in a carton to supply for a single 1200 mg dose treatment (NDC 65293-015-03).
ORBACTIV vials should be stored at 20°C to 25°C (68°F to 77°F); excursions permitted to 15°C to 30°C (59°F to 86°F) [see USP, Controlled Room Temperature (CRT)].

17   PATIENT COUNSELING INFORMATION
Patients should be advised that allergic reactions, including serious allergic reactions, could occur and that serious reactions require immediate treatment. They should inform their healthcare provider about any previous hypersensitivity reactions to ORBACTIV, other glycopeptides (vancomycin, telavancin, or dalbavancin) or other allergens.
Patients should be advised that diarrhea is a common problem caused by antibacterial drugs including ORBACTIV, which usually resolves when the drug is discontinued. Sometimes, frequent watery or bloody diarrhea may occur and may be a sign of a more serious intestinal infection. If severe watery or bloody diarrhea develops, patients should contact their healthcare provider.
Marketed By:
The Medicines Company
Parsippany, NJ 07054 USA
Shown in Product Identification Guide, page 314

Look for PDR® services in your
EHR with PDR® BRIEF
and PDR®+ for Patients.

Vanda Pharmaceuticals, Inc.
2200 Pennsylvania Ave NW Suite 300E
Washington, DC 20037

Tel: 202-734-3400
Fax: 202-296-1450

HETLIOZ™   ℞
(tasimelteon)
capsules, for oral use

HIGHLIGHTS OF PRESCRIBING INFORMATION
These highlights do not include all the information needed to use HETLIOZ safely and effectively. See full prescribing information for HETLIOZ.
HETLIOZ™ (tasimelteon) capsules, for oral use
Initial U.S. Approval: 2014

——————INDICATIONS AND USAGE——————
HETLIOZ is a melatonin receptor agonist indicated for the treatment of Non-24-Hour Sleep-Wake Disorder (Non-24) (1)

——————DOSAGE AND ADMINISTRATION——————
• 20 mg prior to bedtime, at same time every night (2)
• Take without food (2)

——————DOSAGE FORMS AND STRENGTHS——————
Capsules: 20 mg (3)

——————CONTRAINDICATIONS——————
None (4)

——————WARNINGS AND PRECAUTIONS——————
May cause somnolence: After taking HETLIOZ, patients should limit their activity to preparing for going to bed, because HETLIOZ can impair the performance of activities requiring complete mental alertness (5.1)

——————ADVERSE REACTIONS——————
The most common adverse reactions (incidence >5% and at least twice as high on HETLIOZ than on placebo) were headache, increased alanine aminotransferase, nightmares or unusual dreams, and upper respiratory or urinary tract infection (6.1)
To report SUSPECTED ADVERSE REACTIONS, contact Vanda Pharmaceuticals Inc. at 1-844-438-5469 or www.hetlioz.com or FDA at 1-800-FDA-1088 or www.fda.gov/medwatch.

——————DRUG INTERACTIONS——————
• Strong CYP1A2 inhibitors (e.g., fluvoxamine): Avoid use of HETLIOZ in combination with strong CYP1A2 inhibitors because of increased exposure (7.1, 12.3)
• Strong CYP3A4 inducers (e.g., rifampin): Avoid use of HETLIOZ in combination with rifampin or other CYP3A4 inducers, because of decreased exposure (7.2, 12.3)

——————USE IN SPECIFIC POPULATIONS——————
• Pregnancy: Based on animal data, may cause fetal harm (8.1)
• Hepatic impairment: HETLIOZ has not been studied in patients with severe hepatic impairment and is not recommended in these patients (8.6)
See 17 for PATIENT COUNSELING INFORMATION
Revised: 01/2014

FULL PRESCRIBING INFORMATION: CONTENTS*

FULL PRESCRIBING INFORMATION

1.   INDICATIONS AND USAGE
HETLIOZ is indicated for the treatment of Non-24-Hour Sleep-Wake Disorder (Non-24).

2.   DOSAGE AND ADMINISTRATION
The recommended dosage of HETLIOZ is 20 mg per day taken before bedtime, at the same time every night.
Because of individual differences in circadian rhythms, drug effect may not occur for weeks or months.
HETLIOZ should be taken without food [see Clinical Pharmacology (12.3)].

3.   DOSAGE FORMS AND STRENGTHS
Capsules: 20 mg size 1 dark blue opaque, hard gelatin capsules printed with "VANDA 20 mg" in white.

4.   CONTRAINDICATIONS
None.

5.   WARNINGS AND PRECAUTIONS
5.1   Somnolence
After taking HETLIOZ, patients should limit their activity to preparing for going to bed. HETLIOZ can potentially impair the performance of activities requiring complete mental alertness.

6.   ADVERSE REACTIONS
6.1   Clinical Trial Experience
Because clinical trials are conducted under widely varying conditions, adverse reaction rates observed in the clinical trials of a drug cannot be directly compared to rates in the clinical trials of another drug and may not reflect the rates observed in clinical practice.
A total of 1346 subjects were treated with at least one dose of HETLIOZ, of which 139 were treated for > 26 weeks and 93 were treated for > 1 year.
A 26-week, parallel-arm placebo-controlled study (Study 1) evaluated HETLIOZ (n=42) compared to placebo (n=42) in patients with Non-24. A randomized-withdrawal, placebo-controlled study of 8 weeks duration (Study 2) also evaluated HETLIOZ (n=10), compared to placebo (n=10), in patients with Non-24.
In placebo-controlled studies, 6% of patients exposed to HETLIOZ discontinued treatment due to an adverse event, compared with 4% of patients who received placebo.
Table 1 shows the incidence of adverse reactions from Study 1.

Table 1: Adverse Reactions in Study 1

	HETLIOZ N=42	Placebo N=42
Headache	17 %	7 %
Alanine aminotransferase increased	10 %	5 %
Nightmare/abnormal dreams	10 %	0 %
Upper respiratory tract infection	7 %	0 %
Urinary tract infection	7 %	2 %

*Adverse reactions with an incidence > 5% and at least twice as high on HETLIOZ than on placebo are displayed.

7.   DRUG INTERACTIONS
7.1   Strong CYP1A2 Inhibitors (e.g., fluvoxamine)
Avoid use of HETLIOZ in combination with fluvoxamine or other strong CYP1A2 inhibitors because of a potentially large increase in tasimelteon exposure and greater risk of adverse reactions [see Clinical Pharmacology (12.3)].
7.2   Strong CYP3A4 Inducers (e.g., rifampin)
Avoid use of HETLIOZ in combination with rifampin or other CYP3A4 inducers because of a potentially large decrease in tasimelteon exposure with reduced efficacy [see Clinical Pharmacology (12.3)].

8.   USE IN SPECIFIC POPULATIONS
8.1   Pregnancy
Pregnancy Category C
There are no adequate and well-controlled studies of HETLIOZ in pregnant women. In animal studies, administration of tasimelteon during pregnancy resulted in devel-

opmental toxicity (embryofetal mortality, neurobehavioral impairment, and decreased growth and development in offspring) at doses greater than those used clinically. HETLIOZ should be used during pregnancy only if the potential benefit justifies the potential risks.

In pregnant rats administered tasimelteon at oral doses of 5, 50, or 500 mg/kg/day during the period of organogenesis, there were no effects on embryofetal development. The highest dose tested is approximately 240 times the recommended human dose (RHD) of 20 mg/day, on a mg/m² basis. In pregnant rabbits administered tasimelteon at oral doses of 5, 30, or 200 mg/kg/day during the period of organogenesis, embryolethality and embryofetal toxicity (reduced fetal body weight and delayed ossification) were observed at the highest dose tested. The highest dose not associated with adverse effects (30 mg/kg/day) is approximately 30 times the RHD on a mg/m² basis.

Oral administration of tasimelteon (50, 150, or 450 mg/kg/day) to rats throughout organogenesis and lactation resulted in persistent reductions in body weight, delayed sexual maturation and physical development, and neurobehavioral impairment in offspring at the highest dose tested. Reduced body weight in offspring was also observed at the mid-dose. The no effect dose (50 mg/kg/day) is approximately 25 times the RHD on a mg/m² basis.

8.3 Nursing Mothers
It is not known whether this drug is excreted in human milk. Because many drugs are excreted in human milk, caution should be exercised when HETLIOZ is administered to a nursing woman.

8.4 Pediatric Use
Safety and effectiveness in pediatric patients have not been established.

8.5 Geriatric Use
The risk of adverse reactions may be greater in elderly (>65 years) patients than younger patients because exposure to tasimelteon is increased by approximately 2-fold compared with younger patients.

8.6 Hepatic Impairment
Dose adjustment is not necessary in patients with mild or moderate hepatic impairment. HETLIOZ has not been studied in patients with severe hepatic impairment (Child-Pugh Class C). Therefore, HETLIOZ is not recommended for use in patients with severe hepatic impairment [see Clinical Pharmacology (12.3)].

8.7 Smokers
Smoking causes induction of CYP1A2 levels. The exposure of tasimelteon in smokers was lower than in non-smokers and therefore the efficacy of HETLIOZ may be reduced in smokers [see Clinical pharmacology (12.3)].

9. DRUG ABUSE AND DEPENDENCE
9.1 Controlled Substance
Tasimelteon is not a controlled substance under the Controlled Substances Act.

9.2 Abuse
Tasimelteon did not produce any abuse-related signals in animal behavioral studies. Rats did not self-administer tasimelteon, suggesting that the drug does not have rewarding properties. There were also no signs or symptoms indicative of abuse potential in clinical studies with HETLIOZ.

9.3 Dependence
Discontinuation of HETLIOZ in humans following chronic administration did not produce withdrawal signs. HETLIOZ does not appear to produce physical dependence.

10. OVERDOSAGE
There is limited premarketing clinical experience with the effects of an overdosage of HETLIOZ.

As with the management of any overdose, general symptomatic and supportive measures should be used, along with immediate gastric lavage where appropriate. Intravenous fluids should be administered as needed. Respiration, pulse, blood pressure, and other appropriate vital signs should be monitored, and general supportive measures employed.

While hemodialysis was effective at clearing HETLIOZ and the majority of its major metabolites in patients with renal impairment, it is not known if hemodialysis will effectively reduce exposure in the case of overdose.

As with the management of any overdose, the possibility of multiple drug ingestion should be considered. Contact a poison control center for current information on the management of overdose.

11. DESCRIPTION
HETLIOZ (tasimelteon) is a melatonin receptor agonist, chemically designated as (1R, 2R)-N-[2-(2,3-dihydrobenzofuran-4-yl)cyclopropylmethyl]propanamide, containing two chiral centers. The molecular formula is $C_{15}H_{19}NO_2$, and the molecular weight is 245.32. The structural formula is:

Tasimelteon is a white to off-white crystalline powder. It is very slightly soluble in cyclohexane, slightly soluble in water and 0.1 N hydrochloric acid, and freely soluble or very soluble in methanol, 95% ethanol, acetonitrile, isopropanol, polyethylene glycol 300, propylene glycol and ethyl acetate. HETLIOZ is available in 20 mg strength capsules for oral administration. Inactive ingredients are: lactose anhydrous, microcrystalline cellulose, croscarmellose sodium, colloidal silicon dioxide, and magnesium stearate. Each hard gelatin capsule consists of gelatin, titanium dioxide, FD&C Blue #1, FD&C Red #3, and FD&C Yellow #6.

12. CLINICAL PHARMACOLOGY
12.1 Mechanism of Action
The precise mechanism by which tasimelteon exerts its therapeutic effect in patients with Non-24 is not known. Tasimelteon is an agonist at melatonin MT_1 and MT_2 receptors. These receptors are thought to be involved in the control of circadian rhythms.

12.2 Pharmacodynamics
HETLIOZ is an agonist at MT_1 and MT_2 receptors. HETLIOZ exhibits a greater affinity for the MT_2 as compared to the MT_1 receptor. The most abundant metabolites of HETLIOZ have less than one-tenth of the binding affinity of the parent molecule for both the MT_1 and MT_2 receptors.

12.3 Pharmacokinetics
The pharmacokinetics of HETLIOZ is linear over doses ranging from 3 to 300 mg (0.15 to 15 times the recommended daily dosage). The pharmacokinetics of HETLIOZ and its metabolites did not change with repeated daily dosing.

Absorption

The peak concentration (T_{max}) of tasimelteon occurred approximately 0.5 to 3 hours after fasted oral administration. When administered with a high-fat meal, the C_{max} of tasimelteon was 44% lower than when given in a fasted state, and the median T_{max} was delayed by approximately 1.75 hours. Therefore, HETLIOZ should be taken without food.

Distribution

The apparent oral volume of distribution of tasimelteon at steady state in young healthy subjects is approximately 56 - 126 L. At therapeutic concentrations, tasimelteon is about 90% bound to proteins.

Metabolism

Tasimelteon is extensively metabolized. Metabolism of tasimelteon consists primarily of oxidation at multiple sites and oxidative dealkylation resulting in opening of the dihydrofuran ring followed by further oxidation to give a carboxylic acid. CYP1A2 and CYP3A4 are the major isozymes involved in the metabolism of tasimelteon.

Phenolic glucuronidation is the major phase II metabolic route.

Major metabolites had 13-fold or less activity at melatonin receptors compared to tasimelteon.

Elimination

Following oral administration of radiolabeled tasimelteon, 80% of total radioactivity was excreted in urine and approximately 4% in feces, resulting in a mean recovery of 84%. Less than 1% of the dose was excreted in urine as the parent compound.

The observed mean elimination half-life for tasimelteon is 1.3 ± 0.4 hours. The mean terminal elimination half-life ± standard deviation of the main metabolites ranges from 1.3 ± 0.5 to 3.7 ± 2.2.

Repeated once daily dosing with HETLIOZ does not result in changes in pharmacokinetic parameters or significant accumulation of tasimelteon.

Studies in Specific Populations

Elderly

In elderly subjects, tasimelteon exposure increased by approximately two-fold compared with non-elderly adults.

Gender

The mean overall exposure of tasimelteon was approximately 20-30% greater in female than in male subjects.

Race

The effect of race on exposure of HETLIOZ was not evaluated.

Hepatic Impairment

The pharmacokinetic profile of a 20 mg dose of HETLIOZ was compared among eight subjects with mild hepatic impairment (Child-Pugh Score ≥5 and ≤6 points), eight subjects with moderate hepatic impairment (Child-Pugh Score ≥7 and ≤9 points), and 13 healthy matched controls. Tasimelteon exposure was increased less than two-fold in subjects with moderate hepatic impairment. Therefore, no dose adjustment is needed in patients with mild or moder-

ate hepatic impairment. HETLIOZ has not been studied in patients with severe hepatic impairment (Child-Pugh Class C) and is not recommended in these patients.

Renal Impairment

The pharmacokinetic profile of a 20 mg dose of HETLIOZ was compared among eight subjects with severe renal impairment (estimated glomerular filtration rate [eGFR] ≤ 29 mL/min/1.73m²), eight subjects with end-stage renal disease (ESRD) (GFR < 15 mL/min/1.73m²) requiring hemodialysis, and sixteen healthy matched controls. There was no apparent relationship between tasimelteon CL/F and renal function, as measured by either estimated creatinine clearance or eGFR. Subjects with severe renal impairment had a 30% lower clearance, and clearance in subjects with ESRD was comparable to that of healthy subjects. No dose adjustment is necessary for patients with renal impairment.

Smokers (smoking is a moderate CYP1A2 inducer)

Tasimelteon exposure decreased by approximately 40% in smokers, compared to non- smokers [see Use in Specific Populations (8.7)].

Drug Interaction Studies

No potential drug interactions were identified in in vitro studies with CYP inducers or inhibitors of CYP1A1, CYP1A2, CYP2B6, CYP2C9/2C19, CYP2E1, CYP2D6 and transporters including P-glycoprotein, OATP1B1, OATP1B3, OCT2, OAT1 and OAT3.

Effect of Other Drugs on HETLIOZ

Drugs that inhibit CYP1A2 and CYP3A4 are expected to alter the metabolism of tasimelteon.

Fluvoxamine (strong CYP1A2 inhibitor): the AUC_{0-inf} and C_{max} of tasimelteon increased by 7-fold and 2-fold, respectively, when co-administered with fluvoxamine 50 mg (after 6 days of fluvoxamine 50 mg per day) [see Drug Interactions (7.1)].

Ketoconazole (strong CYP3A4 inhibitor): tasimelteon exposure increased by approximately 50% when co-administered with ketoconazole 400 mg (after 5 days of ketoconazole 400 mg per day) [see Drug Interactions (7.2)].

Rifampin (strong CYP3A4 and moderate CYP2C19 inducer): the exposure of tasimelteon decreased by approximately 90% when co-administered with rifampin 600 mg (after 11 days of rifampin 600 mg per day). Efficacy may be reduced when HETLIOZ is used in combination with strong CYP3A4 inducers, such as rifampin [see Drug Interactions (7.2)].

Effect of HETLIOZ on Other Drugs

Midazolam (CYP3A4 substrate): Administration of HETLIOZ 20 mg once a day for 14 days did not produce any significant changes in the T_{max}, C_{max}, or AUC of midazolam or 1-OH midazolam. This indicates there is no induction of CYP3A4 by tasimelteon at this dose.

Rosiglitazone (CYP2C8 substrate): Administration of HETLIOZ 20 mg once a day for 16 days did not produce any clinically significant changes in the T_{max}, C_{max}, or AUC of rosiglitazone after oral administration of 4 mg. This indicates that there is no induction of CYP2C8 by tasimelteon at this dose.

Effect of Alcohol on HETLIOZ

In a study of 28 healthy volunteers, a single dose of ethanol (0.6 g/kg for women and 0.7 g/kg for men) was co-administered with a 20 mg dose of HETLIOZ. There was a trend for an additive effect of HETLIOZ and ethanol on some psychomotor tests.

13. NONCLINICAL TOXICOLOGY
13.1 Carcinogenesis, Mutagenesis, Impairment of Fertility
Carcinogenesis

Tasimelteon was administered orally for up to two years to mice (30, 100, and 300 mg/kg/day) and rats (20, 100, and 250 mg/kg/day). No evidence of carcinogenic potential was observed in mice; the highest dose tested is approximately 75 times the recommended human dose (RHD) of 20 mg/day, on a mg/m² basis. In rats, the incidence of liver tumors was increased in males (adenoma and carcinoma) and females (adenoma) at 100 and 250 mg/kg/day; the incidence of tumors of the uterus (endometrial adenocarcinoma) and uterus and cervix (squamous cell carcinoma) were increased at 250 mg/kg/day. There was no increase in tumors at the lowest dose tested in rats, which is approximately 10 times the RHD on a mg/m² basis.

Mutagenesis

Tasimelteon was negative in an in vitro bacterial reverse mutation (Ames) assay, an in vitro cytogenetics assay in primary human lymphocytes, and an in vivo micronucleus assay in rats.

Impairment of Fertility

When male and female rats were given tasimelteon at oral doses of 5, 50, or 500 mg/kg/day prior to and throughout mating and continuing in females to gestation day 7, estrus cycle disruption and decreased fertility were observed at all but the lowest dose tested. The no-effect dose for effects on female reproduction (5 mg/kg/day) is approximately 2 times the RHD on a mg/m² basis.

Table 2: Effects of HETLIOZ 20 MG in Nightitme Sleep Time and Daytime Nap Time in Study 1 and Study 2

Change from Baseline	Study 1		Study 2	
	HETLIOZ 20 MG N=42	Placebo N=42	HETLIOZ 20 MG N=20	Placebo N=20
Nighttime sleep time on 25% most symptomatic nights (minutes)	50	22	-7	-74
Daytime nap time on 25% most symptomatic days (minutes)	-49	-22	-9	50

14. CLINICAL STUDIES

The effectiveness of HETLIOZ in the treatment of Non-24-Hour Sleep-Wake Disorder (Non-24) was established in two randomized double-masked, placebo-controlled, multi-center, parallel-group studies (Studies 1 and 2) in totally blind patients with Non-24.

In study 1, 84 patients with Non-24 (median age 54 years) were randomized to receive HETLIOZ 20 mg or placebo, one hour prior to bedtime, at the same time every night for up to 6 months.

Study 2 was a randomized withdrawal trial in 20 patients with Non-24 (median age 55 years) that was designed to evaluate the maintenance of efficacy of HETLIOZ after 12-weeks. Patients were treated for approximately 12 weeks with HETLIOZ 20 mg one hour prior to bedtime, at the same time every night. Patients in whom the calculated time of peak melatonin level (melatonin acrophase) occurred at approximately the same time of day (in contrast to the expected daily delay) during the run-in phase were randomized to receive placebo or continue treatment with HETLIOZ 20 mg for 8 weeks.

Study 1 and Study 2 evaluated the duration and timing of nighttime sleep and daytime naps via patient-recorded diaries. During Study 1, patient diaries were recorded for an average of 88 days during screening, and 133 days during randomization. During Study 2, patient diaries were recorded for an average of 57 days during the run-in phase, and 59 days during the randomized-withdrawal phase.

Because symptoms of nighttime sleep disruption and daytime sleepiness are cyclical in patients with Non-24, with severity varying according to the state of alignment of the individual patient's circadian rhythm with the 24-hour day (least severe when fully aligned, most severe when 12 hours out of alignment), efficacy endpoints for nighttime total sleep time and daytime nap duration were based on the 25% of nights with the least nighttime sleep, and the 25% of days with the most daytime nap time. In Study 1, patients in the HETLIOZ group had, at baseline, an average 195 minutes of nighttime sleep and 137 minutes of daytime nap time on the 25% of most symptomatic nights and days, respectively. Treatment with HETLIOZ resulted in a significant improvement, compared with placebo, for both of these endpoints in Study 1 and Study 2 (see Table 2).

[See table 2 above]

A responder analysis of patients with both ≥ 45 minutes increase in nighttime sleep and ≥ 45 minutes decrease in daytime nap time was conducted in Study 1: 29% (n=12) of patients treated with HETLIOZ, compared with 12% (n=5) of patients treated with placebo met the responder criteria. The efficacy of HETLIOZ in treating Non-24 may be reduced in subjects with concomitant administration of beta adrenergic receptor antagonists.

16. HOW SUPPLIED/STORAGE AND HANDLING

HETLIOZ 20 mg capsules are available as size 1, dark blue opaque, hard gelatin capsules printed with "VANDA 20 mg" in white, containing 20 mg of tasimelteon per capsule.
• NDC 43068-220-01   Bottles of 30

Storage

Store HETLIOZ 20 mg capsules at controlled room temperature, 25°C (77°F); excursions permitted to 15°C to 30°C (59°F to 86°F) [See USP Controlled Room Temperature]. Protect HETLIOZ 20 mg capsules from exposure to light and moisture.

17. PATIENT COUNSELING INFORMATION

Advise patients
• To take HETLIOZ before bedtime at the same time every night.
• To skip the dose that night if they cannot take HETLIOZ at approximately the same time on a given night.
• To limit their activities to preparing for going to bed after taking HETLIOZ because HETLIOZ can potentially impair the performance of activities requiring complete mental alertness.
• That because of individual differences in circadian rhythms, daily use for several weeks or months may be necessary before benefit from HETLIOZ is observed.
• To swallow the capsule whole.

Distributed by:
Vanda Pharmaceuticals Inc.
Washington, D.C. 20037 USA
www.hetlioz.com

Vanda and HETLIOZ are trademarks or registered trademarks of Vanda Pharmaceuticals Inc. in the United States and other countries.

Shown in Product Identification Guide, page 314

ViiV Healthcare Company
**FIVE MOORE DRIVE
RESEARCH TRIANGLE PARK, NC 27709**

For all inquiries, including adverse event and quality assurance reporting, contact the GSK Response Center at 1-888-825-5249.

For updates to the product information listed below, also consult www.gsk.com.

COMBIVIR   ℞
[kom' bə-vir]
(lamivudine and zidovudine)
Tablets 150 mg/300 mg

HIGHLIGHTS OF PRESCRIBING INFORMATION
These highlights do not include all the information needed to use COMBIVIR safely and effectively. See full prescribing information for COMBIVIR.
COMBIVIR (lamivudine and zidovudine) Tablets 150 mg/ 300 mg
Initial U.S. Approval: 1997

WARNING: RISK OF HEMATOLOGIC TOXICITY, MYOPATHY, LACTIC ACIDOSIS, EXACERBATIONS OF HEPATITIS B
See full prescribing information for complete boxed warning
• **Hematologic toxicity including neutropenia and anemia have been associated with the use of zidovudine, one of the components of COMBIVIR (5.1)**
• **Symptomatic myopathy associated with prolonged use of zidovudine. (5.2)**
• **Lactic acidosis and hepatomegaly with steatosis, including fatal cases, have been reported with the use of nucleoside analogues including zidovudine. Suspend treatment if clinical or laboratory findings suggestive of lactic acidosis or pronounced hepatotoxicity occur. (5.3)**
• **Severe, acute exacerbations of hepatitis B have been reported in patients who are co-infected with hepatitis B virus (HBV) and human immunodeficiency virus (HIV-1) and have discontinued lamivudine, a component of COMBIVIR. Monitor hepatic function closely in these patients and, if appropriate, initiate anti-hepatitis B treatment. (5.4)**

——INDICATIONS AND USAGE——
COMBIVIR, a combination of 2 nucleoside analogue reverse transcriptase inhibitors, is indicated in combination with other antiretroviral agents for the treatment of HIV-1 infection. (1)

——DOSAGE AND ADMINISTRATION——
• Adults and Adolescents weighing ≥30 kg: 1 tablet twice daily. (2.1)
• Pediatrics: Dosage should be based on body weight not to exceed adult doses. (2.2)
• COMBIVIR, a fixed-dose product, should not be prescribed for pediatric patients weighing less than 30 kg or patients requiring dosage adjustment, such as those with renal or hepatic impairment, or patients experiencing dose-limiting adverse reactions. (2.3)

——DOSAGE FORMS AND STRENGTHS——
Tablets: Scored 150 mg lamivudine and 300 mg zidovudine (3)

——CONTRAINDICATIONS——
COMBIVIR Tablets are contraindicated in patients with previously demonstrated clinically significant hypersensitivity (e.g., anaphylaxis, Stevens-Johnson syndrome). (4)

——WARNINGS AND PRECAUTIONS——
• See boxed warning for information about the following: hematologic toxicity, symptomatic myopathy, lactic acidosis and severe hepatotomegaly, and severe acute exacerbations of hepatitis B. (5.1, 5.2, 5.3, 5.4)
• COMBIVIR should not be administered with other lamivudine- or zidovudine-containing products or emtricitabine-containing products. (5.5)
• Hepatic decompensation, some fatal, has occurred in HIV-1/HCV co-infected patients receiving combination antiretroviral therapy and interferon alfa with/without ribavirin. Discontinue COMBIVIR as medically appropriate and consider dose reduction or discontinuation of interferon alfa, ribavirin, or both. (5.6)
• Exacerbation of anemia has been reported in HIV-1/HCV co-infected patients receiving ribavirin and zidovudine. Co-administration of ribavirin and zidovudine is not advised. (5.6)
• Pancreatitis: Use with caution in pediatric patients with a history of pancreatitis or other significant risk factors for pancreatitis. Discontinue treatment as clinically appropriate. (5.7)
• Immune reconstitution syndrome (5.8) and redistribution/ accumulation of body fat (5.9) have been reported in patients treated with combination antiretroviral therapy.

——ADVERSE REACTIONS——
• Most commonly reported adverse reactions (incidence greater than or equal to 15%) in adult and pediatric HIV-1 clinical trials of combination lamivudine and zidovudine were headache, nausea, malaise and fatigue, nasal signs and symptoms, diarrhea, and cough. (6.1)
To report SUSPECTED ADVERSE REACTIONS, contact ViiV Healthcare at 1-877-844-8872 or FDA at 1-800-FDA-1088 or www.fda.gov/medwatch.

——DRUG INTERACTIONS——
• Concomitant use with the following drugs should be avoided: stavudine (7.1), zalcitabine (7.1), doxorubicin (7.2).
• Bone marrow suppressive/cytotoxic agents: May increase the hematologic toxicity of zidovudine. (7.3)

——USE IN SPECIFIC POPULATIONS——
• Pregnancy: Physicians are encouraged to register patients in the Antiretroviral Pregnancy Registry by calling 1-800-258-4263. (8.1)
• Nursing Mothers: HIV-1 infected mothers in the United States should not breastfeed to avoid potential postnatal transmission of HIV-1. (8.3)

See 17 for PATIENT COUNSELING INFORMATION
Revised: 01/2013

FULL PRESCRIBING INFORMATION: CONTENTS*
WARNING: HEMATOLOGIC TOXICITY, MYOPATHY, LACTIC ACIDOSIS, EXACERBATIONS OF HEPATITIS B
1   INDICATIONS AND USAGE
2   DOSAGE AND ADMINISTRATION
    2.1   Adults and Adolescents Weighing ≥30 kg
    2.2   Pediatric Patients
    2.3   Patients Requiring Dosage Adjustment
3   DOSAGE FORMS AND STRENGTHS
4   CONTRAINDICATIONS
5   WARNINGS AND PRECAUTIONS
    5.1   Hemotologic Toxicity/Bone Marrow Suppression
    5.2   Myopathy
    5.3   Lactic Acidosis/Hepatomegaly With Steatosis
    5.4   Patients With HIV-1 and Hepatitis B Virus Co-infection
    5.5   Use With Other, Lamivudine-, Zidovudine-, and/or Emtricitabine-Containing Products
    5.6   Use With Interferon- and Ribavirin-Based Regimens
    5.7   Pancreatitis
    5.8   Immune Reconstitution Syndrome
    5.9   Fat Redistribution
6   ADVERSE REACTIONS
    6.1   Clinical Trials Experience
    6.2   Postmarketing Experience
7   DRUG INTERACTIONS
    7.1   Antiretroviral Agents
    7.2   Doxorubicin
    7.3   Hematologic/Bone Marrow Suppressive/Cytotoxic Agents
    7.4   Interferon- and Ribavirin-Based Regimens
    7.5   Trimethoprim/Sulfamethoxazole (TMP/SMX)
8   USE IN SPECIFIC POPULATIONS
    8.1   Pregnancy
    8.3   Nursing Mothers

FULL PRESCRIBING INFORMATION

WARNING: HEMATOLOGIC TOXICITY, MYOPATHY, LACTIC ACIDOSIS, EXACERBATIONS OF HEPATITIS B

Hematologic Toxicity: Zidovudine, one of the 2 active ingredients in COMBIVIR® (lamivudine and zidovudine) Tablets, has been associated with hematologic toxicity including neutropenia and anemia, particularly in patients with advanced HIV-1 disease *[see Warnings and Precautions (5.1)].*

Myopathy: Prolonged use of zidovudine has been associated with symptomatic myopathy *[see Warnings and Precautions (5.2)].*

Lactic Acidosis and Severe Hepatomegaly: Lactic acidosis and hepatomegaly with steatosis, including fatal cases, have been reported with the use of nucleoside analogues alone or in combination, including lamivudine, zidovudine, and other antiretrovirals. Suspend treatment if clinical or laboratory findings suggestive of lactic acidosis or pronounced hepatotoxicity occur *[see Warnings and Precautions (5.3)].*

Exacerbations of Hepatitis B: Severe, acute exacerbations of hepatitis B have been reported in patients who are co-infected with hepatitis B virus (HBV) and HIV-1 and have discontinued lamivudine, which is one component of COMBIVIR. Hepatic function should be monitored closely with both clinical and laboratory follow-up for at least several months in patients who discontinue COMBIVIR and are co-infected with HIV-1 and HBV. If appropriate, initiation of anti-hepatitis B therapy may be warranted *[see Warnings and Precautions (5.4)].*

1 INDICATIONS AND USAGE

COMBIVIR, a combination of 2 nucleoside analogues, is indicated in combination with other antiretrovirals for the treatment of HIV-1 infection.

2 DOSAGE AND ADMINISTRATION

2.1 Adults and Adolescents Weighing ≥30 kg

The recommended oral dose of COMBIVIR in HIV-1-infected adults and adolescents weighing greater than or equal to 30 kg is 1 tablet (containing 150 mg of lamivudine and 300 mg of zidovudine) twice daily.

2.2 Pediatric Patients

The recommended oral dosage of scored COMBIVIR Tablets for pediatric patients who weigh greater than or equal to 30 kg and for whom a solid oral dosage form is appropriate is 1 tablet administered twice daily.

Before prescribing COMBIVIR Tablets, children should be assessed for the ability to swallow tablets. If a child is unable to reliably swallow a COMBIVIR Tablet, the liquid oral formulations should be prescribed: EPIVIR® (lamivudine) Oral Solution and RETROVIR® (zidovudine) Syrup.

2.3 Patients Requiring Dosage Adjustment

Because COMBIVIR is a fixed-dose combination tablet, it should not be prescribed for pediatric patients weighing less than 30 kg or patients requiring dosage adjustment, such as those with reduced renal function (creatinine clearance less than 50 mL/min), patients with hepatic impairment, or patients experiencing dose-limiting adverse reactions. Liquid and solid oral formulations of the individual components of COMBIVIR are available for these populations.

3 DOSAGE FORMS AND STRENGTHS

COMBIVIR Tablets contain 150 mg of lamivudine and 300 mg of zidovudine. The tablets are white, scored, film-coated, modified capsule-shaped tablets, debossed on both tablet faces, such that when broken in half, the full "GX FC3" code is present on both halves of the tablet ("GX" on one face and "FC3" on the opposite face of the tablet).

4 CONTRAINDICATIONS

COMBIVIR Tablets are contraindicated in patients with previously demonstrated clinically significant hypersensitivity (e.g., anaphylaxis, Stevens-Johnson syndrome) to any of the components of the product.

5 WARNINGS AND PRECAUTIONS

5.1 Hematologic Toxicity/Bone Marrow Suppression

Zidovudine, a component of COMBIVIR, has been associated with hematologic toxicity including neutropenia and anemia, particularly in patients with advanced HIV-1 disease. COMBIVIR should be used with caution in patients who have bone marrow compromise evidenced by granulocyte count less than 1,000 cells/mm³ or hemoglobin less than 9.5 g/dL *[see Adverse Reactions (6.1)].*

Frequent blood counts are strongly recommended in patients with advanced HIV-1 disease who are treated with COMBIVIR. Periodic blood counts are recommended for other HIV-1-infected patients. If anemia or neutropenia develops, dosage interruption may be needed.

5.2 Myopathy

Myopathy and myositis, with pathological changes similar to that produced by HIV-1 disease, have been associated with prolonged use of zidovudine, and therefore may occur with therapy with COMBIVIR.

5.3 Lactic Acidosis/Hepatomegaly With Steatosis

Lactic acidosis and hepatomegaly with steatosis, including fatal cases, have been reported with the use of nucleoside analogues alone or in combination, including lamivudine, zidovudine, and other antiretrovirals. A majority of these cases have been in women. Obesity and prolonged nucleoside exposure may be risk factors. Particular caution should be exercised when administering COMBIVIR to any patient with known risk factors for liver disease; however, cases have also been reported in patients with no known risk factors. Treatment with COMBIVIR should be suspended in any patient who develops clinical or laboratory findings suggestive of lactic acidosis or pronounced hepatotoxicity (which may include hepatomegaly and steatosis even in the absence of marked transaminase elevations).

5.4 Patients With HIV-1 and Hepatitis B Virus Co-infection

Posttreatment Exacerbations of Hepatitis: In clinical trials in non-HIV-1-infected patients treated with lamivudine for chronic HBV, clinical and laboratory evidence of exacerbations of hepatitis have occurred after discontinuation of lamivudine. These exacerbations have been detected primarily by serum ALT elevations in addition to re-emergence of hepatitis B viral DNA (HBV DNA). Although most events appear to have been self-limited, fatalities have been reported in some cases. Similar events have been reported from post-marketing experience after changes from lamivudine-containing HIV-1 treatment regimens to non-lamivudine-containing regimens in patients infected with both HIV-1 and HBV. The causal relationship to discontinuation of lamivudine treatment is unknown. Patients should be closely monitored with both clinical and laboratory follow-up for at least several months after stopping treatment. There is insufficient evidence to determine whether re-initiation of lamivudine alters the course of posttreatment exacerbations of hepatitis.

Important Differences Among Lamivudine-Containing Products: COMBIVIR Tablets contain a higher dose of the same active ingredient (lamivudine) than EPIVIR-HBV® (lamivudine) Tablets and Oral Solution. EPIVIR-HBV was developed for treating chronic hepatitis B. Safety and efficacy of lamivudine have not been established for treatment of chronic hepatitis B in patients co-infected with HIV-1 and HBV.

Emergence of Lamivudine-Resistant HBV: In non-HIV-infected patients treated with lamivudine for chronic hepatitis B, emergence of lamivudine-resistant HBV has been detected and has been associated with diminished treatment response (see full prescribing information for EPIVIR-HBV for additional information). Emergence of hepatitis B virus variants associated with resistance to lamivudine has also been reported in HIV-1-infected patients who have received lamivudine-containing antiretroviral regimens in the presence of concurrent infection with hepatitis B virus.

5.5 Use With Other, Lamivudine-, Zidovudine-, and/or Emtricitabine-Containing Products

COMBIVIR is a fixed-dose combination of lamivudine and zidovudine. COMBIVIR should not be administered concomitantly with other lamivudine- or zidovudine-containing products including EPIVIR® (lamivudine) Tablets and Oral Solution; EPIVIR-HBV Tablets and Oral Solution; RETROVIR® (zidovudine) Tablets, Capsules, Syrup, and IV Infusion; EPZICOM® (abacavir sulfate and lamivudine) Tablets; or TRIZIVIR® (abacavir sulfate, lamivudine, and zidovudine) Tablets; or emtricitabine-containing products, including ATRIPLA® (efavirenz, emtricitabine, and tenofovir), EMTRIVA® (emtricitabine), TRUVADA® (emtricitabine and tenofovir), or COMPLERA® (rilpivirine/emtricitabine/tenofovir).

5.6 Use With Interferon- and Ribavirin-Based Regimens

In vitro studies have shown ribavirin can reduce the phosphorylation of pyrimidine nucleoside analogues such as lamivudine and zidovudine. Although no evidence of a pharmacokinetic or pharmacodynamic interaction (e.g., loss of HIV-1/HCV virologic suppression) was seen when ribavirin was coadministered with lamivudine or zidovudine in HIV-1/HCV co-infected patients *[see Clinical Pharmacology (12.3)],* hepatic decompensation (some fatal) has occurred in HIV-1/HCV co-infected patients receiving combination antiretroviral therapy for HIV-1 and interferon alfa with or without ribavirin. Patients receiving interferon alfa with or without ribavirin and COMBIVIR should be closely monitored for treatment-associated toxicities, especially hepatic decompensation, neutropenia, and anemia. Discontinuation of COMBIVIR should be considered as medically appropriate. Dose reduction or discontinuation of interferon alfa, ribavirin, or both should also be considered if worsening clinical toxicities are observed, including hepatic decompensation (e.g., Child-Pugh greater than 6) (see the complete prescribing information for interferon and ribavirin).

Exacerbation of anemia has been reported in HIV-1/HCV co-infected patients receiving ribavirin and zidovudine. Coadministration of ribavirin and zidovudine is not advised.

5.7 Pancreatitis

COMBIVIR should be used with caution in patients with a history of pancreatitis or other significant risk factors for the development of pancreatitis. Treatment with COMBIVIR should be stopped immediately if clinical signs, symptoms, or laboratory abnormalities suggestive of pancreatitis occur *[see Adverse Reactions (6.1)].*

5.8 Immune Reconstitution Syndrome

Immune reconstitution syndrome has been reported in patients treated with combination antiretroviral therapy, including COMBIVIR. During the initial phase of combination antiretroviral treatment, patients whose immune systems respond may develop an inflammatory response to indolent or residual opportunistic infections (such as *Mycobacterium avium* infection, cytomegalovirus, *Pneumocystis jirovecii* pneumonia [PCP], or tuberculosis), which may necessitate further evaluation and treatment.

Autoimmune disorders (such as Graves' disease, polymyositis, and Guillain-Barré syndrome) have also been reported to occur in the setting of immune reconstitution; however, the time to onset is more variable, and can occur many months after initiation of treatment.

5.9 Fat Redistribution

Redistribution/accumulation of body fat including central obesity, dorsocervical fat enlargement (buffalo hump), peripheral wasting, facial wasting, breast enlargement, and "cushingoid appearance" have been observed in patients receiving antiretroviral therapy. The mechanism and long-term consequences of these events are currently unknown. A causal relationship has not been established.

6 ADVERSE REACTIONS

The following adverse reactions are discussed in greater detail in other sections of the labeling:
- Hematologic toxicity, including neutropenia and anemia *[see Boxed Warning, Warnings and Precautions (5.1)].*
- Symptomatic myopathy *[see Boxed Warning, Warnings and Precautions (5.2)].*
- Lactic acidosis and hepatomegaly with steatosis *[see Boxed Warning, Warnings and Precautions (5.3)].*
- Acute exacerbations of hepatitis B *[see Boxed Warning, Warnings and Precautions (5.4)].*
- Hepatic decompensation in patients co-infected with HIV-1 and hepatitis C *[see Warnings and Precautions (5.6)].*
- Exacerbation of anemia in HIV-1/HCV co-infected patients receiving ribavirin and zidovudine *[see Warnings and Precautions (5.6)].*
- Pancreatitis *[see Warnings and Precautions (5.7)].*

6.1 Clinical Trials Experience

Because clinical trials are conducted under widely varying conditions, adverse reaction rates observed in the clinical trials of a drug cannot be directly compared with rates in the clinical trials of another drug and may not reflect the rates observed in practice.

Lamivudine Plus Zidovudine Administered As Separate Formulations: In 4 randomized, controlled trials of EPIVIR 300 mg per day plus RETROVIR 600 mg per day, the following selected adverse reactions and laboratory abnormalities were observed (see Tables 1 and 2).

Table 1. Selected Clinical Adverse Reactions (≥5% Frequency) in 4 Controlled Clinical Trials With EPIVIR 300 mg/day and RETROVIR 600 mg/day

Adverse Reaction	EPIVIR plus RETROVIR (n = 251)
Body as a whole	
Headache	35%
Malaise & fatigue	27%
Fever or chills	10%
Digestive	
Nausea	33%
Diarrhea	18%
Nausea & vomiting	13%
Anorexia and/or decreased appetite	10%
Abdominal pain	9%
Abdominal cramps	6%
Dyspepsia	5%
Nervous system	
Neuropathy	12%
Insomnia & other sleep disorders	11%
Dizziness	10%
Depressive disorders	9%
Respiratory	
Nasal signs & symptoms	20%
Cough	18%
Skin	
Skin rashes	9%
Musculoskeletal	
Musculoskeletal pain	12%
Myalgia	8%
Arthralgia	5%

Pancreatitis was observed in 9 of the 2,613 adult subjects (0.3%) who received EPIVIR in controlled clinical trials [see Warnings and Precautions (5.7)].
Selected laboratory abnormalities observed during therapy are listed in Table 2.

Table 2. Frequencies of Selected Laboratory Abnormalities Among Adults in 4 Controlled Clinical Trials of EPIVIR 300 mg/day plus RETROVIR 600 mg/day[a]

Test (Abnormal Level)	EPIVIR plus RETROVIR % (n)
Neutropenia (ANC<750/mm^3)	7.2% (237)
Anemia (Hgb<8.0 g/dL)	2.9% (241)
Thrombocytopenia (platelets<50,000/mm^3)	0.4% (240)
ALT (>5.0 × ULN)	3.7% (241)
AST (>5.0 × ULN)	1.7% (241)
Bilirubin (>2.5 × ULN)	0.8% (241)
Amylase (>2.0 × ULN)	4.2% (72)

ULN = Upper limit of normal.
ANC = Absolute neutrophil count.
n = Number of subjects assessed.
[a] Frequencies of these laboratory abnormalities were higher in subjects with mild laboratory abnormalities at baseline.

6.2   Postmarketing Experience
In addition to adverse reactions reported from clinical trials, the following reactions have been identified during postapproval use of EPIVIR, RETROVIR, and/or COMBIVIR. Because they are reported voluntarily from a population of unknown size, estimates of frequency cannot be made. These events have been chosen for inclusion due to a combination of their seriousness, frequency of reporting, or potential causal connection to EPIVIR, RETROVIR, and/or COMBIVIR.
Body as a Whole: Redistribution/accumulation of body fat [see Warnings and Precautions (5.9)].
Cardiovascular: Cardiomyopathy.
Endocrine and Metabolic: Gynecomastia, hyperglycemia.
Gastrointestinal: Oral mucosal pigmentation, stomatitis.
General: Vasculitis, weakness.
Hemic and Lymphatic: Anemia, (including pure red cell aplasia and anemias progressing on therapy), lymphadenopathy, splenomegaly.
Hepatic and Pancreatic: Lactic acidosis and hepatic steatosis, pancreatitis, posttreatment exacerbation of hepatitis B [see Boxed Warning, Warnings and Precautions (5.3), (5.4), (5.7)].
Hypersensitivity: Sensitization reactions (including anaphylaxis), urticaria.
Musculoskeletal: Muscle weakness, CPK elevation, rhabdomyolysis.

Nervous: Paresthesia, peripheral neuropathy, seizures.
Respiratory: Abnormal breath sounds/wheezing.
Skin: Alopecia, erythema multiforme, Stevens-Johnson syndrome.

7   DRUG INTERACTIONS
No drug interaction trials have been conducted using COMBIVIR Tablets [see Clinical Pharmacology (12.3)].
7.1   Antiretroviral Agents
Lamivudine: Zalcitabine: Lamivudine and zalcitabine may inhibit the intracellular phosphorylation of one another. Therefore, use of COMBIVIR in combination with zalcitabine is not recommended.
Zidovudine: Stavudine: Concomitant use of COMBIVIR with stavudine should be avoided since an antagonistic relationship with zidovudine has been demonstrated in vitro.
Nucleoside Analogues Affecting DNA Replication: Some nucleoside analogues affecting DNA replication, such as ribavirin, antagonize the in vitro antiviral activity of zidovudine against HIV-1; concomitant use of such drugs should be avoided.
7.2   Doxorubicin
Zidovudine: Concomitant use of COMBIVIR with doxorubicin should be avoided since an antagonistic relationship with zidovudine has been demonstrated in vitro.
7.3   Hematologic/Bone Marrow Suppressive/Cytotoxic Agents
Zidovudine: Coadministration of ganciclovir, interferon alfa, ribavirin, and other bone marrow suppressive or cytotoxic agents may increase the hematologic toxicity of zidovudine.
7.4   Interferon- and Ribavirin-Based Regimens
Lamivudine: Although no evidence of a pharmacokinetic or pharmacodynamic interaction (e.g., loss of HIV-1/HCV virologic suppression) was seen when ribavirin was coadministered with lamivudine in HIV-1/HCV co-infected patients, hepatic decompensation (some fatal) has occurred in HIV-1/HCV co-infected patients receiving combination antiretroviral therapy for HIV-1 and interferon alfa with or without ribavirin [see Warnings and Precautions (5.5), Clinical Pharmacology (12.3)].
7.5   Trimethoprim/Sulfamethoxazole (TMP/SMX)
Lamivudine: No change in dose of either drug is recommended. There is no information regarding the effect on lamivudine pharmacokinetics of higher doses of TMP/SMX such as those used to treat PCP.

8   USE IN SPECIFIC POPULATIONS
8.1   Pregnancy
Pregnancy Category C.
Fetal Risk Summary: There are no adequate and well-controlled trials of COMBIVIR (lamivudine and zidovudine) in pregnant women. Clinical trial data demonstrate that maternal zidovudine treatment during pregnancy reduces vertical transmission of HIV-1 infection to the fetus. Animal reproduction studies performed with lamivudine and zidovudine showed increased embryotoxicity and fetal malformations (zidovudine), and increased embryolethality (lamivudine). COMBIVIR should be used during pregnancy only if the potential benefit justifies the potential risk to the fetus.
Antiretroviral Pregnancy Registry: To monitor maternal-fetal outcomes of pregnant women exposed to COMBIVIR and other antiretroviral agents, an Antiretroviral Pregnancy Registry has been established. Physicians are encouraged to register patients by calling 1-800-258-4263.
Clinical Considerations: Treatment of HIV during pregnancy optimizes the health of both mother and fetus. Clinical trial data reviewed by FDA demonstrate that maternal zidovudine treatment significantly reduces vertical transmission of HIV-1 infection to the fetus [see Clinical Studies (14.2)]. Published data suggest that combination antiretroviral regimens may reduce the rate of vertical transmission even further.
Pharmacokinetics of lamivudine and zidovudine in pregnant women are similar to the pharmacokinetics in nonpregnant women. No dose adjustments are needed during pregnancy.
In a clinical trial, adverse events among HIV-1-infected women were not different among untreated women and women treated with zidovudine. It is not known whether risks of adverse events associated with lamivudine are altered in pregnant women compared with other HIV-1-infected patients (see Human data below).
Data: Human Data: Lamivudine: Lamivudine pharmacokinetics were studied in pregnant women during 2 clinical trials conducted in South Africa. The trial assessed pharmacokinetics in: 16 women at 36 weeks gestation using 150 mg lamivudine twice daily with zidovudine, 10 women at 38 weeks gestation using 150 mg lamivudine twice daily with zidovudine, and 10 women at 38 weeks gestation using lamivudine 300 mg twice daily without other antiretrovirals. Lamivudine pharmacokinetics in pregnant women were similar to those seen in nonpregnant adults

and in postpartum women. Lamivudine concentrations were generally similar in maternal, neonatal, and umbilical cord serum samples.
Zidovudine: A randomized, double-blind, placebo-controlled trial was conducted in HIV-1-infected pregnant women to determine the utility of zidovudine for the prevention of maternal-fetal HIV-1 transmission. Zidovudine treatment during pregnancy reduced the rate of maternal-fetal HIV-1 transmission from 24.9% for infants born to placebo-treated mothers to 7.8% for infants born to mothers treated with zidovudine. There were no differences in pregnancy-related adverse events between the treatment groups. Congenital abnormalities occurred with similar frequency between neonates born to mothers who received zidovudine and neonates born to mothers who received placebo. The observed abnormalities included problems in embryogenesis (prior to 14 weeks) or were recognized on ultrasound before or immediately after initiation of trial drug [see Clinical Studies (14.2)].
Zidovudine pharmacokinetics were studied in a Phase 1 trial of 8 women during the last trimester of pregnancy. As pregnancy progressed, there was no evidence of drug accumulation. The pharmacokinetics of zidovudine were similar to that of nonpregnant adults. Consistent with passive transmission of the drug across the placenta, zidovudine concentrations in neonatal plasma at birth were essentially equal to those in maternal plasma at delivery.
Animal Data: Lamivudine: Animal reproduction studies performed at oral doses up to 130 and 60 times the adult dose in rats and rabbits, respectively, revealed no evidence of teratogenicity due to lamivudine. Increased early embryolethality occurred in rabbits at exposure levels similar to those in humans. However, there was no indication of this effect in rats at exposure levels up to 35 times those in humans. Based on animal studies, lamivudine crosses the placenta and is transferred to the fetus [see Nonclinical Toxicology (13.2)].
Zidovudine: Increased fetal resorptions occurred in pregnant rats and rabbits treated with doses of zidovudine that produced drug plasma concentrations 66 to 226 times (rats) and 12 to 87 times (rabbits) the mean steady-state peak human plasma concentration following a single 100-mg dose of zidovudine. There were no other reported developmental anomalies. In another developmental toxicity study, pregnant rats received zidovudine up to near-lethal doses that produced peak plasma concentrations 350 times peak human plasma concentrations (300 times the daily exposure [AUC] in humans given 600 mg/day zidovudine). This dose was associated with marked maternal toxicity and an increased incidence of fetal malformations. However, there were no signs of teratogenicity at doses up to one-fifth the lethal dose [see Nonclinical Toxicology (13.2)].
8.3   Nursing Mothers
The Centers for Disease Control and Prevention recommend that HIV-1-infected mothers in the United States not breastfeed their infants to avoid risking postnatal transmission of HIV-1 infection. Because of both the potential for HIV-1 transmission and serious adverse reactions in nursing infants, mothers should be instructed not to breastfeed if they are receiving COMBIVIR.
Although no trials of COMBIVIR excretion in breast milk have been performed, lactation trials performed with lamivudine and zidovudine show that both drugs are excreted in human breast milk. Samples of breast milk obtained from 20 mothers receiving lamivudine monotherapy (300 mg twice daily) or combination therapy (150 mg lamivudine twice daily and 300 mg zidovudine twice daily) had measurable concentrations of lamivudine. In another trial, after administration of a single dose of 200 mg zidovudine to 13 HIV-1–infected women, the mean concentration of zidovudine was similar in human milk and serum.
8.4   Pediatric Use
COMBIVIR should not be administered to pediatric patients weighing less than 30 kg, because it is a fixed-dose combination that cannot be adjusted for this patient population.
8.5   Geriatric Use
Clinical trials of COMBIVIR did not include sufficient numbers of subjects aged 65 and over to determine whether they respond differently from younger subjects. In general, dose selection for an elderly patient should be cautious, reflecting the greater frequency of decreased hepatic, renal, or cardiac function, and of concomitant disease or other drug therapy. COMBIVIR is not recommended for patients with impaired renal function (i.e., creatinine clearance less than 50 mL/min) because it is a fixed-dose combination that cannot be adjusted.
8.6   Renal Impairment
Reduction of the dosages of lamivudine and zidovudine is recommended for patients with impaired renal function. Patients with creatinine clearance less than 50 mL/min should not receive COMBIVIR because it is a fixed-dose combination that cannot be adjusted.
8.7   Hepatic Impairment
A reduction in the daily dose of zidovudine may be necessary in patients with mild to moderate impaired hepatic function or liver cirrhosis. COMBIVIR is not recommended for patients with impaired hepatic function because it is a fixed-dose combination that cannot be adjusted.

10 OVERDOSAGE

COMBIVIR: There is no known antidote for COMBIVIR.
Lamivudine: One case of an adult ingesting 6 grams of lamivudine was reported; there were no clinical signs or symptoms noted and hematologic tests remained normal. Because a negligible amount of lamivudine was removed via (4-hour) hemodialysis, continuous ambulatory peritoneal dialysis, and automated peritoneal dialysis, it is not known if continuous hemodialysis would provide clinical benefit in a lamivudine overdose event.
Zidovudine: Acute overdoses of zidovudine have been reported in pediatric patients and adults. These involved exposures up to 50 grams. The only consistent findings were nausea and vomiting. Other reported occurrences included headache, dizziness, drowsiness, lethargy, confusion, and 1 report of a grand mal seizure. Hematologic changes were transient. All patients recovered. Hemodialysis and peritoneal dialysis appear to have a negligible effect on the removal of zidovudine, while elimination of its primary metabolite, 3'-azido-3'-deoxy-5'-O-β-D-glucopyranuronosylthymidine (GZDV), is enhanced.

11 DESCRIPTION

COMBIVIR: COMBIVIR Tablets are combination tablets containing lamivudine and zidovudine. Lamivudine (EPIVIR) and zidovudine (RETROVIR, azidothymidine, AZT, or ZDV) are synthetic nucleoside analogues with activity against HIV-1.
COMBIVIR Tablets are for oral administration. Each film-coated tablet contains 150 mg of lamivudine, 300 mg of zidovudine, and the inactive ingredients colloidal silicon dioxide, hypromellose, magnesium stearate, microcrystalline cellulose, polyethylene glycol, polysorbate 80, sodium starch glycolate, and titanium dioxide.
Lamivudine: The chemical name of lamivudine is (2R,cis)-4-amino-1-(2-hydroxymethyl-1,3-oxathiolan-5-yl)-(1H)-pyrimidin-2-one. Lamivudine is the (-)enantiomer of a dideoxy analogue of cytidine. Lamivudine has also been referred to as (-)2',3'-dideoxy, 3'-thiacytidine. It has a molecular formula of $C_8H_{11}N_3O_3S$ and a molecular weight of 229.3. It has the following structural formula:

Lamivudine is a white to off-white crystalline solid with a solubility of approximately 70 mg/mL in water at 20°C.
Zidovudine: The chemical name of zidovudine is 3'-azido-3'-deoxythymidine. It has a molecular formula of $C_{10}H_{13}N_5O_4$ and a molecular weight of 267.24. It has the following structural formula:

Zidovudine is a white to beige, odorless, crystalline solid with a solubility of 20.1 mg/mL in water at 25°C.

12 CLINICAL PHARMACOLOGY

12.1 Mechanism of Action

COMBIVIR is an antiviral agent [see Clinical Pharmacology (12.4)].

12.3 Pharmacokinetics

Pharmacokinetics in Adults: *COMBIVIR:* One COMBIVIR Tablet was bioequivalent to 1 EPIVIR Tablet (150 mg) plus 1 RETROVIR Tablet (300 mg) following single-dose administration to fasting healthy subjects (n = 24).
Lamivudine: The pharmacokinetic properties of lamivudine in fasting subjects are summarized in Table 3. Following oral administration, lamivudine is rapidly absorbed and extensively distributed. Binding to plasma protein is low. Approximately 70% of an intravenous dose of lamivudine is recovered as unchanged drug in the urine. Metabolism of lamivudine is a minor route of elimination. In humans, the only known metabolite is the trans-sulfoxide metabolite (approximately 5% of an oral dose after 12 hours).
Zidovudine: The pharmacokinetic properties of zidovudine in fasting subjects are summarized in Table 3. Following oral administration, zidovudine is rapidly absorbed and extensively distributed. Binding to plasma pro-

Table 3. Pharmacokinetic Parameters[a] for Lamivudine and Zidovudine in Adults

Parameter	Lamivudine		Zidovudine	
Oral bioavailability (%)	86 ± 16	N = 12	64 ± 10	n = 5
Apparent volume of distribution (L/kg)	1.3 ± 0.4	N = 20	1.6 ± 0.6	n = 8
Plasma protein binding (%)	<36		<38	
CSF:plasma ratio[b]	0.12 [0.04 to 0.47]	n = 38[c]	0.60 [0.04 to 2.62]	N = 39[d]
Systemic clearance (L/hr/kg)	0.33 ± 0.06	N = 20	1.6 ± 0.6	n = 6
Renal clearance (L/hr/kg)	0.22 ± 0.06	N = 20	0.34 ± 0.05	n = 9
Elimination half-life (hr)[e]	5 to 7		0.5 to 3	

[a] Data presented as mean ± standard deviation except where noted.
[b] Median [range].
[c] Children.
[d] Adults.
[e] Approximate range.

tein is low. Zidovudine is eliminated primarily by hepatic metabolism. The major metabolite of zidovudine is GZDV. GZDV area under the curve (AUC) is about 3-fold greater than the zidovudine AUC. Urinary recovery of zidovudine and GZDV accounts for 14% and 74% of the dose following oral administration, respectively. A second metabolite, 3'-amino-3'-deoxythymidine (AMT), has been identified in plasma. The AMT AUC was one fifth of the zidovudine AUC. [See table 3 above]
Effect of Food on Absorption of COMBIVIR: COMBIVIR may be administered with or without food. The lamivudine and zidovudine AUC following administration of COMBIVIR with food was similar when compared with fasting healthy subjects (n = 24).
Special Populations:
Pregnancy: See Use in Specific Populations (8.1).
COMBIVIR: No data are available.
Zidovudine: Zidovudine pharmacokinetics has been studied in a Phase 1 trial of 8 women during the last trimester of pregnancy. As pregnancy progressed, there was no evidence of drug accumulation. The pharmacokinetics of zidovudine was similar to that of nonpregnant adults. Consistent with passive transmission of the drug across the placenta, zidovudine concentrations in neonatal plasma at birth were essentially equal to those in maternal plasma at delivery. Although data are limited, methadone maintenance therapy in 5 pregnant women did not appear to alter zidovudine pharmacokinetics. In a nonpregnant adult population, a potential for interaction has been identified.
Nursing Mothers: See Use in Specific Populations (8.3).
Pediatric Patients: COMBIVIR should not be administered to pediatric patients weighing less than 30 kg.
Geriatric Patients: The pharmacokinetics of lamivudine and zidovudine have not been studied in patients over 65 years of age.
Gender: A pharmacokinetic trial in healthy male (n = 12) and female (n = 12) subjects showed no gender differences in zidovudine AUC_∞ or lamivudine AUC_∞ normalized for body weight.
Race: *Lamivudine:* There are no significant racial differences in lamivudine pharmacokinetics.
Zidovudine: The pharmacokinetics of zidovudine with respect to race have not been determined.
Drug Interactions: See Drug Interactions (7).
No drug interaction trials have been conducted using COMBIVIR Tablets. However, Table 4 presents drug interaction information for the individual components of COMBIVIR.
Lamivudine Plus Zidovudine: No clinically significant alterations in lamivudine or zidovudine pharmacokinetics were observed in 12 asymptomatic HIV-1-infected adult subjects given a single dose of zidovudine (200 mg) in combination with multiple doses of lamivudine (300 mg q 12 hr).
[See table 4 at top of next page]
Ribavirin: In vitro data indicate ribavirin reduces phosphorylation of lamivudine, stavudine, and zidovudine. However, no pharmacokinetic (e.g., plasma concentrations or intracellular triphosphorylated active metabolite concentrations) or pharmacodynamic (e.g., loss of HIV-1/HCV virologic suppression) interaction was observed when ribavirin and lamivudine (n = 18), stavudine (n = 10), or zidovudine (n = 6) were coadministered as part of a multidrug regimen to HIV-1/HCV co-infected subjects [see Warnings and Precautions (5.5)].

12.4 Microbiology

Mechanism of Action: *Lamivudine:* Intracellularly, lamivudine is phosphorylated to its active 5'-triphosphate metabolite, lamivudine triphosphate (3TC-TP). The principal mode of action of 3TC-TP is inhibition of reverse transcriptase (RT) via DNA chain termination after incorporation of the nucleotide analogue. 3TC-TP is a weak inhibitor of cellular DNA polymerases α, β, and γ.
Zidovudine: Intracellularly, zidovudine is phosphorylated to its active 5'-triphosphate metabolite, zidovudine triphos-

phate (ZDV-TP). The principal mode of action of ZDV-TP is inhibition of RT via DNA chain termination after incorporation of the nucleotide analogue. ZDV-TP is a weak inhibitor of the cellular DNA polymerases α and γ and has been reported to be incorporated into the DNA of cells in culture.
Antiviral Activity: *Lamivudine Plus Zidovudine:* In HIV-1-infected MT-4 cells, lamivudine in combination with zidovudine at various ratios exhibited synergistic antiretroviral activity.
Lamivudine: The antiviral activity of lamivudine against HIV-1 was assessed in a number of cell lines (including monocytes and fresh human peripheral blood lymphocytes) using standard susceptibility assays. EC_{50} values (50% effective concentrations) were in the range of 0.003 to 15 μM (1 μM = 0.23 mcg/mL). HIV-1 from therapy-naive subjects with no amino acid substitutions associated with resistance gave median EC_{50} values of 0.429 μM (range: 0.200 to 2.007 μM) from Virco (n = 92 baseline samples from COL40263) and 2.35 μM (1.37 to 3.68 μM) from Monogram Biosciences (n = 135 baseline samples from ESS30009). The EC_{50} values of lamivudine against different HIV-1 clades (A-G) ranged from 0.001 to 0.120 μM, and against HIV-2 isolates from 0.003 to 0.120 μM in peripheral blood mononuclear cells. Ribavirin (50 μM) decreased the anti-HIV-1 activity of lamivudine by 3.5 fold in MT-4 cells.
Zidovudine: The antiviral activity of zidovudine against HIV-1 was assessed in a number of cell lines (including monocytes and fresh human peripheral blood lymphocytes). The EC_{50} and EC_{90} values for zidovudine were 0.01 to 0.49 μM (1 μM = 0.27 mcg/mL) and 0.1 to 9 μM, respectively. HIV-1 from therapy-naive subjects with no amino acid substitutions associated with resistance gave median EC_{50} values of 0.011 μM (range: 0.005 to 0.110 μM) from Virco (n = 92 baseline samples from COL40263) and 0.0017 μM (0.006 to 0.0340 μM) from Monogram Biosciences (n = 135 baseline samples from ESS30009). The EC_{50} values of zidovudine against different HIV-1 clades (A-G) ranged from 0.00018 to 0.02 μM, and against HIV-2 isolates from 0.00049 to 0.004 μM. In cell culture drug combination studies, zidovudine demonstrates synergistic activity with the nucleoside reverse transcriptase inhibitors (NRTIs) abacavir, didanosine, lamivudine, and zalcitabine; the non-nucleoside reverse transcriptase inhibitors (NNRTIs) delavirdine and nevirapine; and the protease inhibitors (PIs) indinavir, nelfinavir, ritonavir, and saquinavir; and additive activity with interferon alfa. Ribavirin has been found to inhibit the phosphorylation of zidovudine in cell culture.
Resistance: *Lamivudine Plus Zidovudine Administered As Separate Formulations:* In subjects receiving lamivudine monotherapy or combination therapy with lamivudine plus zidovudine, HIV-1 isolates from most subjects became phenotypically and genotypically resistant to lamivudine within 12 weeks. In some subjects harboring zidovudine-resistant virus at baseline, phenotypic sensitivity to zidovudine was restored by 12 weeks of treatment with lamivudine and zidovudine. Combination therapy with lamivudine plus zidovudine delayed the emergence of amino acid substitutions conferring resistance to zidovudine.
HIV-1 strains resistant to both lamivudine and zidovudine have been isolated from subjects after prolonged lamivudine/zidovudine therapy. Dual resistance required the presence of multiple amino acid substitutions, the most essential of which may be G333E. The incidence of dual resistance and the duration of combination therapy required before dual resistance occurs are unknown.
Lamivudine: Lamivudine-resistant isolates of HIV-1 have been selected in cell culture and have also been recovered from subjects treated with lamivudine or lamivudine plus zidovudine. Genotypic analysis of isolates selected in cell culture and recovered from lamivudine-treated subjects showed that the resistance was due to a specific amino acid substitution in the HIV-1 reverse transcriptase at codon 184 changing the methionine to either isoleucine or valine (M184V/I).
Zidovudine: HIV-1 isolates with reduced susceptibility to zidovudine have been selected in cell culture and were also

recovered from subjects treated with zidovudine. Genotypic analyses of the isolates selected in cell culture and recovered from zidovudine–treated subjects showed substitutions in the HIV-1 RT gene resulting in 6 amino acid substitutions (M41L, D67N, K70R, L210W, T215Y or F, and K219Q) that confer zidovudine resistance. In general, higher levels of resistance were associated with greater number of amino acid substitutions.

Cross-Resistance: Cross-resistance has been observed among NRTIs.

Lamivudine Plus Zidovudine: Cross–resistance between lamivudine and zidovudine has not been reported. In some subjects treated with lamivudine alone or in combination with zidovudine, isolates have emerged with a substitution at codon 184, which confers resistance to lamivudine. Cross-resistance to abacavir, didanosine, tenofovir, and zalcitabine has been observed in some subjects harboring lamivudine–resistant HIV–1 isolates. In some subjects treated with zidovudine plus didanosine or zalcitabine, isolates resistant to multiple drugs, including lamivudine, have emerged (see under Zidovudine below).

Lamivudine: See Lamivudine Plus Zidovudine (above).

Zidovudine: In a trial of 167 HIV–1–infected subjects, isolates (n = 2) with multi–drug resistance to didanosine, lamivudine, stavudine, zalcitabine, and zidovudine were recovered from subjects treated for ≥1 year with zidovudine plus didanosine or zidovudine plus zalcitabine. The pattern of resistance–associated amino acid substitutions with such combination therapies was different (A62V, V75I, F77L, F116Y, Q151M) from the pattern with zidovudine mono–therapy, with the Q151M substitution being most commonly associated with multi–drug resistance. The substitution at codon 151 in combination with substitutions at 62, 75, 77, and 116 results in a virus with reduced susceptibility to didanosine, lamivudine, stavudine, zalcitabine, and zidovudine. Thymidine analogue mutations (TAMs) are selected by zidovudine and confer cross–resistance to abacavir, didanosine, stavudine, tenofovir, and zalcitabine.

13   NONCLINICAL TOXICOLOGY
13.1   Carcinogenesis, Mutagenesis, Impairment of Fertility
Carcinogenicity: *Lamivudine:* Long-term carcinogenicity studies with lamivudine in mice and rats showed no evidence of carcinogenic potential at exposures up to 10 times (mice) and 58 times (rats) those observed in humans at the recommended therapeutic dose for HIV-1 infection.

Zidovudine: Zidovudine was administered orally at 3 dosage levels to separate groups of mice and rats (60 females and 60 males in each group). Initial single daily doses were 30, 60, and 120 mg/kg/day in mice and 80, 220, and 600 mg/kg/day in rats. The doses in mice were reduced to 20, 30, and 40 mg/kg/day after day 90 because of treatment-related anemia, whereas in rats only the high dose was reduced to 450 mg/kg/day on day 91 and then to 300 mg/kg/day on day 279.

In mice, 7 late-appearing (after 19 months) vaginal neoplasms (5 nonmetastasizing squamous cell carcinomas, 1 squamous cell papilloma, and 1 squamous polyp) occurred in animals given the highest dose. One late-appearing squamous cell papilloma occurred in the vagina of a middle-dose animal. No vaginal tumors were found at the lowest dose.

In rats, 2 late-appearing (after 20 months), nonmetastasizing vaginal squamous cell carcinomas occurred in animals given the highest dose. No vaginal tumors occurred at the low or middle dose in rats. No other drug-related tumors were observed in either sex of either species.

At doses that produced tumors in mice and rats, the estimated drug exposure (as measured by AUC) was approximately 3 times (mouse) and 24 times (rat) the estimated human exposure at the recommended therapeutic dose of 100 mg every 4 hours.

It is not known how predictive the results of rodent carcinogenicity studies may be for humans.

Mutagenicity: *Lamivudine:* Lamivudine was mutagenic in an L5178Y/TK+/− mouse lymphoma assay and clastogenic in a cytogenetic assay using cultured human lymphocytes. Lamivudine was negative in a microbial mutagenicity assay, in an in vitro cell transformation assay, in a rat micronucleus test, in a rat bone marrow cytogenetic assay, and in an assay for unscheduled DNA synthesis in rat liver.

Zidovudine: Zidovudine was mutagenic in an L5178Y/TK+/− mouse lymphoma assay, positive in an in vitro cell transformation assay, clastogenic in a cytogenetic assay using cultured human lymphocytes, and positive in mouse and rat micronucleus tests after repeated doses. It was negative in a cytogenetic study in rats given a single dose.

Impairment of Fertility: *Lamivudine:* In a study of reproductive performance, lamivudine, administered to male and female rats at doses up to 130 times the usual adult dose based on body surface area considerations, revealed no evidence of impaired fertility (judged by conception rates) and no effect on the survival, growth, and development to weaning of the offspring.

Zidovudine: Zidovudine, administered to male and female rats at doses up to 7 times the usual adult dose based on body surface area considerations, had no effect on fertility judged by conception rates.

13.2   Reproductive and Developmental Toxicology Studies
Lamivudine: Reproduction studies have been performed in rats and rabbits at orally administered doses up to 4,000 mg/kg/day and 1,000 mg/kg/day, respectively, producing plasma levels up to approximately 35 times that for the adult HIV dose. No evidence of teratogenicity due to lamivudine was observed. Evidence of early embryolethality was seen in the rabbit at exposure levels similar to those observed in humans, but there was no indication of this effect in the rat at exposure levels up to 35 times those in humans. Studies in pregnant rats and rabbits showed that lamivudine is transferred to the fetus through the placenta.

Zidovudine: Oral teratology studies in the rat and in the rabbit at doses up to 500 mg/kg/day revealed no evidence of teratogenicity with zidovudine. Zidovudine treatment resulted in embryo/fetal toxicity as evidenced by an increase in the incidence of fetal resorptions in rats given 150 or 450 mg/kg/day and rabbits given 500 mg/kg/day. The doses used in the teratology studies resulted in peak zidovudine plasma concentrations (after one half of the daily dose) in rats 66 to 226 times, and in rabbits 12 to 87 times, mean steady-state peak human plasma concentrations (after one sixth of the daily dose) achieved with the recommended daily dose (100 mg every 4 hours). In an in vitro experiment with fertilized mouse oocytes, zidovudine exposure resulted in a dose-dependent reduction in blastocyst formation. In an additional teratology study in rats, a dose of 3,000 mg/kg/day (very near the oral median lethal dose in rats of 3,683 mg/kg) caused marked maternal toxicity and an increase in the incidence of fetal malformations. This dose resulted in peak zidovudine plasma concentrations 350 times peak human plasma concentrations. (Estimated AUC in rats at this dose level was 300 times the daily AUC in humans given 600 mg/day.) No evidence of teratogenicity was seen in this experiment at doses of 600 mg/kg/day or less.

14   CLINICAL STUDIES
There have been no clinical trials conducted with COMBIVIR. See *Clinical Pharmacology (12.3)* for information about bioequivalence. One COMBIVIR Tablet given twice daily is an alternative regimen to EPIVIR Tablets 150 mg twice daily plus RETROVIR 600 mg per day in divided doses.

14.1   Adults
Lamivudine Plus Zidovudine: The NUCB3007 (CAESAR) trial was conducted using EPIVIR 150–mg Tablets (150 mg twice daily) and RETROVIR 100–mg Capsules (2 × 100 mg 3 times daily). CAESAR was a multi-center, double-blind, placebo-controlled trial comparing continued current therapy (zidovudine alone [62% of subjects] or zidovudine with didanosine or zalcitabine [38% of subjects]) to the addition of EPIVIR or EPIVIR plus an investigational non-nucleoside reverse transcriptase inhibitor, randomized 1:2:1. A total of 1,816 HIV–1–infected adults with 25 to 250 (median 122) CD4 cells/mm³ at baseline were enrolled: median age was 36 years, 87% were male, 84% were nucleoside-experienced, and 16% were therapy–naive. The median duration on trial was 12 months. Results are summarized in Table 5.

[See table 5 at top of next page]

14.2   Prevention of Maternal-Fetal HIV-1 Transmission
The utility of zidovudine alone for the prevention of maternal-fetal HIV-1 transmission was demonstrated in a

Table 4. Effect of Coadministered Drugs on Lamivudine and Zidovudine AUC[a]

Note: ROUTINE DOSE MODIFICATION OF LAMIVUDINE AND ZIDOVUDINE IS NOT WARRANTED WITH COADMINISTRATION OF THE FOLLOWING DRUGS.

Drugs That May Alter Lamivudine Blood Concentrations

Coadministered Drug and Dose	Lamivudine Dose	n	Lamivudine Concentrations AUC	Variability	Concentration of Coadministered Drug
Nelfinavir 750 mg q 8 hr × 7 to 10 days	single 150 mg	11	↑AUC 10%	95% CI: 1% to 20%	↔
Trimethoprim 160 mg/Sulfamethoxazole 800 mg daily × 5 days	single 300 mg	14	↑AUC 43%	90% CI: 32% to 55%	↔

Drugs That May Alter Zidovudine Blood Concentrations

Coadministered Drug and Dose	Zidovudine Dose	n	Zidovudine Concentrations AUC	Variability	Concentration of Coadministered Drug
Atovaquone 750 mg q 12 hr with food	200 mg q 8 hr	14	↑AUC 31%	Range 23% to 78%[b]	↔
Clarithromycin 500 mg twice daily	100 mg q 4 hr × 7 days	4	↓AUC 12%	Range ↓34% to ↑14%	Not Reported
Fluconazole 400 mg daily	200 mg q 8 hr	12	↑AUC 74%	95% CI: 54% to 98%	Not Reported
Methadone 30 to 90 mg daily	200 mg q 4 hr	9	↑AUC 43%	Range 16% to 64%[b]	↔
Nelfinavir 750 mg q 8 hr × 7 to 10 days	single 200 mg	11	↓AUC 35%	Range 28% to 41%	↔
Probenecid 500 mg q 6 hr × 2 days	2 mg/kg q 8 hr × 3 days	3	↑AUC 106%	Range 100% to 170%[b]	Not Assessed
Rifampin 600 mg daily × 14 days	200 mg q 8 hr × 14 days	8	↓AUC 47%	90% CI: 41% to 53%	Not Assessed
Ritonavir 300 mg q 6 hr × 4 days	200 mg q 8 hr × 4 days	9	↓AUC 25%	95% CI: 15% to 34%	↔
Valproic acid 250 mg or 500 mg q 8 hr × 4 days	100 mg q 8 hr × 4 days	6	↑AUC 80%	Range 64% to 130%[b]	Not Assessed

↑ = Increase; ↓= Decrease; ↔ = no significant change; AUC = area under the concentration versus time curve; CI = confidence interval.
[a] This table is not all inclusive.
[b] Estimated range of percent difference.

Table 5. Number of Subjects (%) With At Least 1 HIV-1 Disease-Progression Event or Death

Endpoint	Current Therapy (n = 460)	EPIVIR plus Current Therapy (n = 896)	EPIVIR plus a NNRTI[a] plus Current Therapy (n = 460)
HIV-1 progression or death	90 (19.6%)	86 (9.6%)	41 (8.9%)
Death	27 (5.9%)	23 (2.6%)	14 (3.0%)

[a] An investigational non-nucleoside reverse transcriptase inhibitor not approved in the United States.

randomized, double-blind, placebo-controlled trial conducted in HIV-1-infected pregnant women with CD4+ cell counts of 200 to 1,818 cells/mm^3 (median in the treated group: 560 cells/mm^3) who had little or no previous exposure to zidovudine. Oral zidovudine was initiated between 14 and 34 weeks of gestation (median 11 weeks of therapy) followed by IV administration of zidovudine during labor and delivery. Following birth, neonates received oral zidovudine syrup for 6 weeks. The trial showed a statistically significant difference in the incidence of HIV-1 infection in the neonates (based on viral culture from peripheral blood) between the group receiving zidovudine and the group receiving placebo. Of 363 neonates evaluated in the trial, the estimated risk of HIV-1 infection was 7.8% in the group receiving zidovudine and 24.9% in the placebo group, a relative reduction in transmission risk of 68.7%. Zidovudine was well tolerated by mothers and infants. There was no difference in pregnancy-related adverse events between the treatment groups.

16 HOW SUPPLIED/STORAGE AND HANDLING

COMBIVIR Tablets, containing 150 mg lamivudine and 300 mg zidovudine, are white, scored, film-coated, modified-capsule-shaped tablets, debossed on both tablet faces, such that when broken in half, the full "GXFC3" code is present on both halves of the tablet ("GX" on one face and "FC3" on the opposite face of the tablet). They are available as follows:

60 Tablets/Bottle (NDC 49702-202-18).

Unit Dose Pack of 120 (NDC 49702-202-29).

Store between 2° and 30°C (36° and 86°F).

17 PATIENT COUNSELING INFORMATION

17.1 Advice for the Patient

Neutropenia and Anemia: Patients should be informed that the important toxicities associated with zidovudine are neutropenia and/or anemia. They should be told of the extreme importance of having their blood counts followed closely while on therapy, especially for patients with advanced HIV-1 disease [see Boxed Warning, Warnings and Precautions (5.1)].

Myopathy: Patients should be informed that myopathy and myositis with pathological changes, similar to that produced by HIV-1 disease, have been associated with prolonged use of zidovudine [see Warnings and Precautions (5.2)].

Lactic Acidosis/Hepatomegaly: Patients should be informed that some HIV medicines, including COMBIVIR, can cause a rare, but serious condition called lactic acidosis with liver enlargement (hepatomegaly) [see Warnings and Precautions (5.3)].

HIV-1/HBV Co-infection: Patients co-infected with HIV-1 and HBV should be informed that deterioration of liver disease has occurred in some cases when treatment with lamivudine was discontinued. Patients should be advised to discuss any changes in regimen with their physician [see Warnings and Precautions (5.4)].

Use With Other Lamivudine-, Zidovudine-, and/or Emtricitabine-Containing Products: COMBIVIR should not be coadministered with drugs containing lamivudine, zidovudine, or emtricitabine, including EPIVIR (lamivudine), EPIVIR-HBV (lamivudine), RETROVIR (zidovudine), EPZICOM (abacavir sulfate and lamivudine), TRIZIVIR (abacavir sulfate, lamivudine, and zidovudine), ATRIPLA (efavirenz, emtricitabine, and tenofovir), EMTRIVA (emtricitabine), TRUVADA (emtricitabine and tenofovir), or COMPLERA™ (rilpivirine/emtricitabine/tenofovir) [see Warnings and Precautions (5.5)].

HIV-1/HCV Co-Infection: Patients with HIV-1/HCV co-infection should be informed that hepatic decompensation (some fatal) has occurred in HIV-1/HCV co-infected patients receiving combination antiretroviral therapy for HIV-1 and interferon alfa with or without ribavirin [see Warnings and Precautions (5.6)].

Drug Interactions: Patients should be cautioned about the use of other medications, including ganciclovir, interferon alfa, and ribavirin, which may exacerbate the toxicity of zidovudine [see Drug Interactions (7.3)].

Redistribution/Accumulation of Body Fat: Patients should be informed that redistribution or accumulation of body fat may occur in patients receiving antiretroviral therapy and that the cause and long-term health effects of these conditions are not known at this time [see Warnings and Precautions (5.9)].

Information About HIV-1 Infection: COMBIVIR is not a cure for HIV-1 infection and patients may continue to experience illnesses associated with HIV-1 infection, including opportunistic infections. Patients should remain under the care of a physician when using COMBIVIR.

Patients should be advised to avoid doing things that can spread HIV-1 infection to others.

- **Do not share needles or other injection equipment.**
- **Do not share personal items that can have blood or body fluids on them, like toothbrushes and razor blades.**
- **Do not have any kind of sex without protection.** Always practice safe sex by using a latex or polyurethane condom or other barrier method to lower the chance of sexual contact with semen, vaginal secretions, or blood.
- **Do not breastfeed.** Lamivudine and zidovudine are excreted in human breast milk. Mothers with HIV-1 should not breastfeed because HIV-1 can be passed to the baby in the breast milk.

Patients should be informed to take all HIV medications exactly as prescribed.

EPIVIR, RETROVIR, EPZICOM, and TRIZIVIR are registered trademarks of ViiV Healthcare.

The other brands listed are trademarks of their respective owners and are not trademarks of ViiV Healthcare. The makers of these brands are not affiliated with and do not endorse ViiV Healthcare or its products.

Manufactured for:

ViiV Healthcare

Research Triangle Park, NC 27709

by GlaxoSmithKline

Research Triangle Park, NC 27709

Lamivudine is manufactured under agreement from

Shire Pharmaceuticals Group plc

Basingstoke, UK

©2013, ViiV Healthcare. All rights reserved.

CMB: 5PI

EPIVIR   ℞

[ĕp'ə-vir]

(lamivudine)

Tablets and Oral Solution

HIGHLIGHTS OF PRESCRIBING INFORMATION

These highlights do not include all the information needed to use EPIVIR safely and effectively. See full prescribing information for EPIVIR.

EPIVIR (lamivudine) Tablets and Oral Solution

Initial U.S. Approval: 1995

WARNING: LACTIC ACIDOSIS, POSTTREATMENT EXACERBATIONS OF HEPATITIS B IN CO-INFECTED PATIENTS, DIFFERENT FORMULATIONS OF EPIVIR

See full prescribing information for complete boxed warning

- Lactic acidosis and severe hepatomegaly with steatosis, including fatal cases, have been reported with the use of nucleoside analogues. Suspend treatment if clinical or laboratory findings suggestive of lactic acidosis or pronounced hepatotoxicity occur. (5.1)
- Severe acute exacerbations of hepatitis B have been reported in patients who are co-infected with hepatitis B virus (HBV) and human immunodeficiency virus (HIV-1) and have discontinued EPIVIR. Monitor hepatic function closely in these patients and, if appropriate, initiate anti-hepatitis B treatment. (5.2)
- Patients with HIV-1 infection should receive only dosage forms of EPIVIR appropriate for treatment of HIV-1. (5.2)

INDICATIONS AND USAGE

EPIVIR is a nucleoside analogue reverse transcriptase inhibitor indicated in combination with other antiretroviral agents for the treatment of HIV-1 infection. Limitation of Use: The dosage of this product is for HIV-1 and not for HBV. (1)

DOSAGE AND ADMINISTRATION

- Adults and adolescents aged >16 years: 300 mg daily, administered as either 150 mg twice daily or 300 mg once daily. (2.1)
- Pediatric patients aged 3 months 16 years: Dosage should be based on body weight. (2.2)
- Patients With Renal Impairment: Doses of EPIVIR must be adjusted in accordance with renal function. (2.3)

DOSAGE FORMS AND STRENGTHS

- Tablets: 300 mg (3)
- Tablets: Scored 150 mg (3)
- Oral Solution: 10 mg/mL (3)

CONTRAINDICATIONS

EPIVIR Tablets and Oral Solution are contraindicated in patients with previously demonstrated clinically significant hypersensitivity (e.g., anaphylaxis) to any of the components of the products. (4)

WARNINGS AND PRECAUTIONS

- Lactic acidosis and severe hepatomegaly with steatosis: Reported with the use of nucleoside analogues. Suspend treatment if clinical or laboratory findings suggestive of lactic acidosis or pronounced hepatoxicity occur. (5.1)
- Severe acute exacerbations of hepatitis: Reported in patients who are co-infected with hepatitis B virus and HIV-1 and discontinued EPIVIR. Monitor hepatic function closely in these patients and, if appropriate, initiate anti-hepatitis B treatment. (5.2)
- Patients with HIV-1 infection should receive only dosage forms of EPIVIR appropriate for treatment of HIV-1. (5.2)
- Co-infected HIV-1/HBV Patients: Emergence of lamivudine-resistant HBV variants associated with lamivudine-containing antiretroviral regimens has been reported. (5.2)
- Emtricitabine should not be administered concomitantly with lamivudine-containing products. (5.3)
- Hepatic decompensation (some fatal) has occurred in HIV-1/HCV co-infected patients receiving interferon and ribavirin-based regimens. Monitor for treatment-associated toxicities. Discontinue EPIVIR as medically appropriate and consider dose reduction or discontinuation of interferon alfa, ribavirin, or both. (5.4)
- Pancreatitis: Use with caution in pediatric patients with a history of pancreatitis or other significant risk factors for pancreatitis. Discontinue treatment as clinically appropriate. (5.5)
- Immune reconstitution syndrome (5.6) and redistribution/accumulation of body fat (5.7) have been reported in patients treated with combination antiretroviral therapy.

ADVERSE REACTIONS

- The most common reported adverse reactions (incidence ≥15%) in adults were headache, nausea, malaise and fatigue, nasal signs and symptoms, diarrhea, and cough. (6.1)
- The most common reported adverse reactions (incidence ≥15%) in pediatric subjects were fever and cough. (6.1)

To report SUSPECTED ADVERSE REACTIONS, contact ViiV Healthcare at 1-877-844-8872 or FDA at 1-800-FDA-1088 or www.fda.gov/medwatch.

DRUG INTERACTIONS

Zalcitabine is not recommended for use in combination with EPIVIR. (7.2)

USE IN SPECIFIC POPULATIONS

- Pregnancy: Physicians are encouraged to register patients in the Antiretroviral Pregnancy Registry by calling 1-800-258-4263. (8.1)

Revised: September 2010

See 17 for PATIENT COUNSELING INFORMATION

Revised: 01/2013

FULL PRESCRIBING INFORMATION: CONTENTS*

WARNING: RISK OF LACTIC ACIDOSIS, EXACERBATIONS OF HEPATITIS B IN CO-INFECTED PATIENTS UPON DISCONTINUATION OF EPIVIR®, DIFFERENT FORMULATIONS OF EPIVIR

1 INDICATIONS AND USAGE

2 DOSAGE AND ADMINISTRATION

    2.1 Adults and Adolescents >16 years of age

    2.2 Pediatric Patients

    2.3 Patients With Renal Impairment

3 DOSAGE FORMS AND STRENGTHS

4 CONTRAINDICATIONS

5 WARNINGS AND PRECAUTIONS

    5.1 Lactic Acidosis/Severe Hepatomegaly With Steatosis

    5.2 Patients With HIV-1 and Hepatitis B Virus Co-infection

    5.3 Use With Other Lamivudine- and Emtricitabine-Containing Products

    5.4 Use With Interferon- and Ribavirin-Based Regimens

    5.5 Pancreatitis

FULL PRESCRIBING INFORMATION

> **WARNING: RISK OF LACTIC ACIDOSIS, EXACERBATIONS OF HEPATITIS B IN CO-INFECTED PATIENTS UPON DISCONTINUATION OF EPIVIR®, DIFFERENT FORMULATIONS OF EPIVIR.**
>
> **Lactic Acidosis and Severe Hepatomegaly:** Lactic acidosis and severe hepatomegaly with steatosis, including fatal cases, have been reported with the use of nucleoside analogues alone or in combination, including lamivudine and other antiretrovirals. Suspend treatment if clinical or laboratory findings suggestive of lactic acidosis or pronounced hepatotoxicity occur *[see Warnings and Precautions (5.1)].*
>
> **Exacerbations of Hepatitis B:** Severe acute exacerbations of hepatitis B have been reported in patients who are co-infected with hepatitis B virus (HBV) and human immunodeficiency virus (HIV-1) and have discontinued EPIVIR. Hepatic function should be monitored closely with both clinical and laboratory follow-up for at least several months in patients who discontinue EPIVIR and are co-infected with HIV-1 and HBV. If appropriate, initiation of anti-hepatitis B therapy may be warranted *[see Warnings and Precautions (5.2)].*
>
> **Important Differences Among Lamivudine-Containing Products:** EPIVIR Tablets and Oral Solution (used to treat HIV-1 infection) contain a higher dose of the active ingredient (lamivudine) than EPIVIR-HBV® Tablets and Oral Solution (used to treat chronic HBV infection). Patients with HIV-1 infection should receive only dosage forms appropriate for treatment of HIV-1 *[see Warnings and Precautions (5.2)]*

1 INDICATIONS AND USAGE

EPIVIR is a nucleoside analogue indicated in combination with other antiretroviral agents for the treatment of human immunodeficiency virus (HIV-1) infection. Limitation of use: The dosage of this product is for HIV-1 and not for HBV.

2 DOSAGE AND ADMINISTRATION

2.1 Adults and Adolescents >16 years of age

The recommended oral dose of EPIVIR in HIV-1-infected adults and adolescents aged >16 years is 300 mg daily, administered as either 150 mg twice daily or 300 mg once daily, in combination with other antiretroviral agents. If lamivudine is administered to a patient infected with HIV-1 and HBV, the dosage indicated for HIV-1 therapy should be used as part of an appropriate combination regimen *[see Warnings and Precautions (5.2)].*

2.2 Pediatric Patients

The recommended oral dose of EPIVIR Oral Solution in HIV-1-infected pediatric patients aged 3 months to 16 years is 4 mg/kg twice daily (up to a maximum of 150 mg twice a day), administered in combination with other antiretroviral agents.

EPIVIR is also available as a scored tablet for HIV-1-infected pediatric patients who weigh ≥14 kg and for whom a solid dosage form is appropriate. Before prescribing EPIVIR Tablets, children should be assessed for the ability to swallow tablets. If a child is unable to reliably swallow EPIVIR Tablets, the oral solution formulation should be prescribed. The recommended oral dosage of EPIVIR Tablets for HIV-1-infected pediatric patients is presented in Table 1.

Table 1. Dosing Recommendations for EPIVIR Tablets in Pediatric Patients

Weight (kg)	Dosage Regimen Using Scored 150-mg Tablet		Total Daily Dose
	AM Dose	PM Dose	
14 to 21	½ tablet (75 mg)	½ tablet (75 mg)	150 mg
>21 to <30	½ tablet (75 mg)	1 tablet (150 mg)	225 mg
≥30	1 tablet (150 mg)	1 tablet (150 mg)	300 mg

2.3 Patients With Renal Impairment

Dosing of EPIVIR is adjusted in accordance with renal function. Dosage adjustments are listed in Table 2 *[see Clinical Pharmacology (12.3)].*

Table 2. Adjustment of Dosage of EPIVIR in Adults and Adolescents (≥30 kg) in Accordance With Creatinine Clearance

Creatinine Clearance (mL/min)	Recommended Dosage of EPIVIR
≥50	150 mg twice daily or 300 mg once daily
30-49	150 mg once daily
15-29	150 mg first dose, then 100 mg once daily
5-14	150 mg first dose, then 50 mg once daily
<5	50 mg first dose, then 25 mg once daily

No additional dosing of EPIVIR is required after routine (4-hour) hemodialysis or peritoneal dialysis.

Although there are insufficient data to recommend a specific dose adjustment of EPIVIR in pediatric patients with renal impairment, a reduction in the dose and/or an increase in the dosing interval should be considered.

3 DOSAGE FORMS AND STRENGTHS

• EPIVIR Scored Tablets

150 mg, are white, diamond-shaped, scored, film-coated tablets debossed with "GX CJ7" on both sides.

• EPIVIR Tablets

300 mg, are gray, modified diamond-shaped, film-coated tablets engraved with "GX EJ7" on one side and plain on the reverse side.

• EPIVIR Oral Solution

A clear, colorless to pale yellow, strawberry-banana flavored liquid, containing 10 mg of lamivudine per 1 mL.

4 CONTRAINDICATIONS

EPIVIR Tablets and Oral Solution are contraindicated in patients with previously demonstrated clinically significant hypersensitivity (e.g., anaphylaxis) to any of the components of the products.

5 WARNINGS AND PRECAUTIONS

5.1 Lactic Acidosis/Severe Hepatomegaly With Steatosis

Lactic acidosis and severe hepatomegaly with steatosis, including fatal cases, have been reported with the use of nucleoside analogues alone or in combination, including lamivudine and other antiretrovirals. A majority of these cases have been in women. Obesity and prolonged nucleoside exposure may be risk factors. Particular caution should be exercised when administering EPIVIR to any patient with known risk factors for liver disease; however, cases also have been reported in patients with no known risk factors. Treatment with EPIVIR should be suspended in any patient who develops clinical or laboratory findings suggestive of lactic acidosis or pronounced hepatotoxicity (which may include hepatomegaly and steatosis even in the absence of marked transaminase elevations).

5.2 Patients With HIV-1 and Hepatitis B Virus Co-infection

Posttreatment Exacerbations of Hepatitis: In clinical trials in non-HIV-1-infected patients treated with lamivudine for chronic hepatitis B, clinical and laboratory evidence of exacerbations of hepatitis have occurred after discontinuation of lamivudine. These exacerbations have been detected primarily by serum ALT elevations in addition to re-emergence of HBV DNA. Although most events appear to have been self-limited, fatalities have been reported in some cases. Similar events have been reported from postmarketing experience after changes from lamivudine-containing HIV-1 treatment regimens to non-lamivudine-containing regimens in patients infected with both HIV-1 and HBV. The causal relationship to discontinuation of lamivudine treatment is unknown. Patients should be closely monitored with both clinical and laboratory follow-up for at least several months after stopping treatment. There is insufficient evidence to determine whether re-initiation of lamivudine alters the course of posttreatment exacerbations of hepatitis.

Important Differences Among Lamivudine-Containing Products: EPIVIR Tablets and Oral Solution contain a higher dose of the same active ingredient (lamivudine) than EPIVIR-HBV Tablets and EPIVIR-HBV Oral Solution. EPIVIR-HBV was developed for patients with chronic hepatitis B. The formulation and dosage of lamivudine in EPIVIR-HBV are not appropriate for patients co-infected with HIV-1 and HBV. Safety and efficacy of lamivudine have not been established for treatment of chronic hepatitis B in patients co-infected with HIV-1 and HBV. If treatment with EPIVIR-HBV is prescribed for chronic hepatitis B for a patient with unrecognized or untreated HIV-1 infection, rapid emergence of HIV-1 resistance is likely to result because of the subtherapeutic dose and the inappropriateness of monotherapy HIV-1 treatment. If a decision is made to administer lamivudine to patients co-infected with HIV-1 and HBV, EPIVIR Tablets, EPIVIR Oral Solution, COMBIVIR® (lamivudine/zidovudine) Tablets, EPZICOM® (abacavir sulfate and lamivudine) Tablets, or TRIZIVIR® (abacavir sulfate, lamivudine, and zidovudine) Tablets should be used as part of an appropriate combination regimen.

Emergence of Lamivudine-Resistant HBV: In non–HIV-1-infected patients treated with lamivudine for chronic hepatitis B, emergence of lamivudine-resistant HBV has been detected and has been associated with diminished treatment response (see full prescribing information for EPIVIR-HBV for additional information). Emergence of hepatitis B virus variants associated with resistance to lamivudine has also been reported in HIV-1-infected patients who have received lamivudine-containing antiretroviral regimens in the presence of concurrent infection with hepatitis B virus.

5.3 Use With Other Lamivudine- and Emtricitabine-Containing Products

EPIVIR should not be administered concomitantly with other lamivudine-containing products including EPIVIR-HBV Tablets, EPIVIR Oral Solution, COMBIVIR (lamivudine/zidovudine) Tablets, EPZICOM (abacavir sulfate and lamivudine) Tablets, or TRIZIVIR (abacavir sulfate, lamivudine, and zidovudine) or emtricitabine-containing products, including ATRIPLA® (efavirenz, emtricitabine, and tenofovir), EMTRIVA® (emtricitabine), TRUVADA® (emtricitabine and tenofovir), or COMPLERA® (rilpivirine/emtricitabine/tenofovir).

5.4 Use With Interferon- and Ribavirin-Based Regimens

In vitro studies have shown ribavirin can reduce the phosphorylation of pyrimidine nucleoside analogues such as lamivudine. Although no evidence of a pharmacokinetic or pharmacodynamic interaction (e.g., loss of HIV-1/HCV virologic suppression) was seen when ribavirin was coadministered with lamivudine in HIV-1/HCV co-infected patients *[see Clinical Pharmacology (12.3)],* hepatic decompensation (some fatal) has occurred in HIV-1/HCV co-infected patients receiving combination antiretroviral therapy for HIV-1 and interferon alfa with or without ribavirin. Patients receiving interferon alfa with or without ribavirin and EPIVIR should be closely monitored for treatment-associated toxicities, especially hepatic decompensation. Discontinuation of EPIVIR should be considered as medically appropriate. Dose reduction or discontinuation of interferon alfa, ribavirin, or both should also be considered if worsening clinical toxicities are observed, including hepatic decompensation (e.g., Child-Pugh >6). See the complete prescribing information for interferon and ribavirin.

5.5 Pancreatitis

In pediatric patients with a history of prior antiretroviral nucleoside exposure, a history of pancreatitis, or other significant risk factors for the development of pancreatitis, EPIVIR should be used with caution. Treatment with EPIVIR should be stopped immediately if clinical signs, symptoms, or laboratory abnormalities suggestive of pancreatitis occur *[see Adverse Reactions (6.1)].*

5.6 Immune Reconstitution Syndrome

Immune reconstitution syndrome has been reported in patients treated with combination antiretroviral therapy, including EPIVIR. During the initial phase of combination antiretroviral treatment, patients whose immune system responds may develop an inflammatory response to indolent or residual opportunistic infections (such as *Mycobacterium avium* infection, cytomegalovirus, *Pneumocystis jirovecii* pneumonia [PCP], or tuberculosis), which may necessitate further evaluation and treatment.

Autoimmune disorders (such as Graves' disease, polymyositis, and Guillain-Barré syndrome) have also been reported to occur in the setting of immune reconstitution, however, the time to onset is more variable, and can occur many months after initiation of treatment.

5.7   Fat Redistribution
Redistribution/accumulation of body fat including central obesity, dorsocervical fat enlargement (buffalo hump), peripheral wasting, facial wasting, breast enlargement, and "cushingoid appearance" have been observed in patients receiving antiretroviral therapy. The mechanism and long-term consequences of these events are currently unknown. A causal relationship has not been established.

6   ADVERSE REACTIONS
The following adverse reactions are discussed in greater detail in other sections of the labeling:
- Lactic acidosis and severe hepatomegaly with steatosis [see Boxed Warning, Warnings and Precautions (5.1)].
- Severe acute exacerbations of hepatitis B [see Boxed Warning, Warnings and Precautions (5.2)].
- Hepatic decompensation in patients co-infected with HIV-1 and hepatitis C [see Warnings and Precautions (5.4)].
- Pancreatitis [see Warnings and Precautions (5.5)].

6.1   Clinical Trials Experience
Because clinical trials are conducted under widely varying conditions, adverse reaction rates observed in the clinical trials of a drug cannot be directly compared with rates in the clinical trials of another drug and may not reflect the rates observed in practice.
Adults - Clinical Trials in HIV-1:   The safety profile of EPIVIR in adults is primarily based on 3,568 HIV-1-infected subjects in 7 clinical trials.
The most common adverse reactions are headache, nausea, malaise, fatigue, nasal signs and symptoms, diarrhea and cough.
Selected clinical adverse reactions in ≥5% of subjects during therapy with EPIVIR 150 mg twice daily plus RETROVIR® 200 mg 3 times daily for up to 24 weeks are listed in Table 3.

Table 3. Selected Clinical Adverse Reactions (≥5% Frequency) in Four Controlled Clinical Trials (NUCA3001, NUCA3002, NUCB3001, NUCB3002)

Adverse Reaction	EPIVIR 150 mg Twice Daily plus RETROVIR (n = 251)	RETROVIR[a] (n = 230)
Body as a Whole		
Headache	35%	27%
Malaise & fatigue	27%	23%
Fever or chills	10%	12%
Digestive		
Nausea	33%	29%
Diarrhea	18%	22%
Nausea & vomiting	13%	12%
Anorexia and/or decreased appetite	10%	7%
Abdominal pain	9%	11%
Abdominal cramps	6%	3%
Dyspepsia	5%	5%
Nervous System		
Neuropathy	12%	10%
Insomnia & other sleep disorders	11%	7%
Dizziness	10%	4%
Depressive disorders	9%	4%
Respiratory		
Nasal signs & symptoms	20%	11%
Cough	18%	13%
Skin		
Skin rashes	9%	6%
Musculoskeletal		
Musculoskeletal pain	12%	10%
Myalgia	8%	6%
Arthralgia	5%	5%

[a] Either zidovudine monotherapy or zidovudine in combination with zalcitabine.

Pancreatitis: Pancreatitis was observed in 9 out of 2,613 adult subjects (0.3%) who received EPIVIR in controlled clinical trials EPV20001, NUCA3001, NUCB3001, NUCA3002, NUCB3002, and NUCB3007 [see Warnings and Precautions (5.5)].
EPIVIR 300 mg Once Daily: The types and frequencies of clinical adverse reactions reported in subjects receiving EPIVIR 300 mg once daily or EPIVIR 150 mg twice daily (in 3-drug combination regimens in EPV20001 and EPV40001) for 48 weeks were similar.
Selected laboratory abnormalities observed during therapy are summarized in Table 4.

Table 4. Frequencies of Selected Grade 3-4 Laboratory Abnormalities in Adults in Four 24-Week Surrogate Endpoint Trials(NUCA3001, NUCA3002, NUCB3001, NUCB3002) and a Clinical Endpoint Trial (NUCB3007)

Test (Threshold Level)	24-Week Surrogate Endpoint Trials[a]		Clinical Endpoint Trial[a]	
	EPIVIR plus RETROVIR	RETROVIR[b]	EPIVIR plus Current Therapy	Placebo plus Current Therapy[c]
Absolute neutrophil count (<750/mm³)	7.2%	5.4%	15%	13%
Hemoglobin (<8.0 g/dL)	2.9%	1.8%	2.2%	3.4%
Platelets (<50,000/mm³)	0.4%	1.3%	2.8%	3.8%
ALT (>5.0 × ULN)	3.7%	3.6%	3.8%	1.9%
AST (>5.0 × ULN)	1.7%	1.8%	4.0%	2.1%
Bilirubin (>2.5 × ULN)	0.8%	0.4%	ND	ND
Amylase (>2.0 × ULN)	4.2%	1.5%	2.2%	1.1%

[a] The median duration on study was 12 months.
[b] Either zidovudine monotherapy or zidovudine in combination with zalcitabine.
[c] Current therapy was either zidovudine, zidovudine plus didanosine, or zidovudine plus zalcitabine.
ULN = Upper limit of normal.
ND = Not done.

[See table 4 above]
The frequencies of selected laboratory abnormalities reported subjects receiving EPIVIR 300 mg once daily or EPIVIR 150 mg twice daily (in 3-drug combination regimens in EPV20001 and EPV40001) were similar.
Pediatric Subjects – Clinical Trials in HIV-1:   EPIVIR Oral Solution has been studied in 638 pediatric subjects aged 3 months to 18 years in 3 clinical trials.
Selected clinical adverse reactions and physical findings with a ≥5% frequency during therapy with EPIVIR 4 mg/kg twice daily plus RETROVIR 160 mg/m² 3 times daily in therapy-naive (≤56 days of antiretroviral therapy) pediatric subjects are listed in Table 5.

Table 5. Selected Clinical Adverse Reactions and Physical Findings (≥5% Frequency) in Pediatric Subjects in Trial ACTG300

Adverse Reaction	EPIVIR plus RETROVIR (n = 236)	Didanosine (n = 235)
Body as a Whole		
Fever	25%	32%
Digestive		
Hepatomegaly	11%	11%
Nausea & vomiting	8%	7%
Diarrhea	8%	6%
Stomatitis	6%	12%
Splenomegaly	5%	8%
Respiratory		
Cough	15%	18%
Abnormal breath sounds/wheezing	7%	9%
Ear, Nose, and Throat		
Signs or symptoms of ears[a]	7%	6%
Nasal discharge or congestion	8%	11%
Other		
Skin rashes	12%	14%
Lymphadenopathy	9%	11%

[a] Includes pain, discharge, erythema, or swelling of an ear.

Pancreatitis: Pancreatitis, which has been fatal in some cases, has been observed in antiretroviral nucleoside–experienced pediatric subjects receiving EPIVIR alone or in combination with other antiretroviral agents. In an open–label dose–escalation trial (NUCA2002), 14 subjects (14%) developed pancreatitis while receiving monotherapy with EPIVIR. Three of these subjects died of complications of pancreatitis. In a second open–label trial (NUCA2005), 12 subjects (18%) developed pancreatitis. In Trial ACTG300, pancreatitis was not observed in 236 subjects randomized to EPIVIR plus RETROVIR. Pancreatitis was observed in 1 subject in this trial who received open–label EPIVIR in combination with RETROVIR and ritonavir following discontinuation of didanosine monotherapy [see Warnings and Precautions (5.5)].
Paresthesias and Peripheral Neuropathies: Paresthesias and peripheral neuropathies were reported in 15 subjects (15%) in Trial NUCA2002, 6 subjects (9%) in Trial NUCA2005, and 2 subjects (<1%) in Trial ACTG300.
Selected laboratory abnormalities experienced by therapy–naive (56 days of antiretroviral therapy) pediatric subjects are listed in Table 6.

Table 6. Frequencies of Selected Grade 3-4 Laboratory Abnormalities in Pediatric Subjects in Trial ACTG300

Test (Threshold Level)	EPIVIR plus RETROVIR	Didanosine
Absolute neutrophil count (<400/mm³)	8%	3%
Hemoglobin (<7.0 g/dL)	4%	2%
Platelets (<50,000/mm³)	1%	3%
ALT (>10 × ULN)	1%	3%
AST (>10 × ULN)	2%	4%
Lipase (>2.5 × ULN)	3%	3%
Total Amylase (>2.5 × ULN)	3%	3%

ULN = Upper limit of normal.

Neonates - Clinical Trials in HIV-1:   Limited short-term safety information is available from 2 small, uncontrolled trials in South Africa in neonates receiving lamivudine with or without zidovudine for the first week of life following maternal treatment starting at Week 38 or 36 of gestation [see Clinical Pharmacology (12.3)]. Selected adverse reactions reported in these neonates included increased liver function tests, anemia, diarrhea, electrolyte disturbances, hypoglycemia, jaundice and hepatomegaly, rash, respiratory infections, and sepsis; 3 neonates died (1 from gastroenteritis with acidosis and convulsions, 1 from traumatic injury, and 1 from unknown causes). Two other nonfatal gastroenteritis or diarrhea cases were reported, including 1 with convulsions; 1 infant had transient renal insufficiency associated with dehydration. The absence of control groups limits assessments of causality, but it should be assumed that perinatally exposed infants may be at risk for adverse reactions comparable to those reported in pediatric and adult HIV-1-infected patients treated with lamivudine-containing combination regimens. Long-term effects of in utero and infant lamivudine exposure are not known.
6.2   Postmarketing Experience
In addition to adverse reactions reported from clinical trials, the following adverse reactions have been reported during postmarketing use of EPIVIR. Because these reactions are reported voluntarily from a population of unknown size, estimates of frequency cannot be made. These reactions have been chosen for inclusion due to a combination of their seriousness, frequency of reporting, or potential causal connection to lamivudine.
Body as a Whole: Redistribution/accumulation of body fat [see Warnings and Precautions (5.7)].
Endocrine and Metabolic: Hyperglycemia.
General: Weakness.
Hemic and Lymphatic: Anemia (including pure red cell aplasia and severe anemias progressing on therapy).
Hepatic and Pancreatic: Lactic acidosis and hepatic steatosis, posttreatment exacerbation of hepatitis B [see Boxed Warning, Warnings and Precautions (5.1, 5.2)].
Hypersensitivity: Anaphylaxis, urticaria.
Musculoskeletal: Muscle weakness, CPK elevation, rhabdomyolysis.
Skin: Alopecia, pruritus.

7   DRUG INTERACTIONS
Lamivudine is predominantly eliminated in the urine by active organic cationic secretion. The possibility of interactions with other drugs administered concurrently should be considered, particularly when their main route of elimination is active renal secretion via the organic cationic trans-

port system (e.g., trimethoprim). No data are available regarding interactions with other drugs that have renal clearance mechanisms similar to that of lamivudine.

7.1 Interferon- and Ribavirin-Based Regimens
Although no evidence of a pharmacokinetic or pharmacodynamic interaction (e.g., loss of HIV-1/HCV virologic suppression) was seen when ribavirin was coadministered with lamivudine in HIV-1/HCV co-infected patients, hepatic decompensation (some fatal) has occurred in HIV-1/HCV co-infected patients receiving combination antiretroviral therapy for HIV-1 and interferon alfa with or without ribavirin *[see Warnings and Precautions (5.4), Clinical Pharmacology (12.3)]*.

7.2 Zalcitabine
Lamivudine and zalcitabine may inhibit the intracellular phosphorylation of one another. Therefore, use of lamivudine in combination with zalcitabine is not recommended.

7.3 Trimethoprim/Sulfamethoxazole (TMP/SMX)
No change in dose of either drug is recommended. There is no information regarding the effect on lamivudine pharmacokinetics of higher doses of TMP/SMX such as those used to treat PCP.

7.4 Drugs with No Observed Interactions With EPIVIR
A drug interaction trial showed no clinically significant interaction between EPIVIR and zidovudine.

8 USE IN SPECIFIC POPULATIONS

8.1 Pregnancy
Pregnancy Category C. There are no adequate and well-controlled trials of EPIVIR in pregnant women. Animal reproduction studies in rats and rabbits revealed no evidence of teratogenicity. Increased early embryolethality occurred in rabbits at exposure levels similar to those in humans. EPIVIR should be used during pregnancy only if the potential benefit justifies the potential risk to the fetus.

Lamivudine pharmacokinetics were studied in pregnant women during 2 clinical trials conducted in South Africa. The trial assessed pharmacokinetics in: 16 women at 36 weeks gestation using 150 mg lamivudine twice daily with zidovudine, 10 women at 38 weeks gestation using 150 mg lamivudine twice daily with zidovudine, and 10 women at 38 weeks gestation using lamivudine 300 mg twice daily without other antiretrovirals. These trials were not designed or powered to provide efficacy information. Lamivudine pharmacokinetics in pregnant women were similar to those seen in non-pregnant adults and in postpartum women. Lamivudine concentrations were generally similar in maternal, neonatal, and umbilical cord serum samples. In a subset of subjects, lamivudine amniotic fluid specimens were collected following natural rupture of membranes. Amniotic fluid concentrations of lamivudine were typically 2 times greater than maternal serum levels and ranged from 1.2 to 2.5 mcg/mL (150 mg twice daily) and 2.1 to 5.2 mcg/mL (300 mg twice daily). It is not known whether risks of adverse events associated with lamivudine are altered in pregnant women compared with other HIV-1-infected patients.

Animal reproduction studies performed at oral doses up to 130 and 60 times the adult dose in rats and rabbits, respectively, revealed no evidence of teratogenicity due to lamivudine. Increased early embryolethality occurred in rabbits at exposure levels similar to those in humans. However, there was no indication of this effect in rats at exposure levels up to 35 times those in humans. Based on animal studies, lamivudine crosses the placenta and is transferred to the fetus *[see Nonclinical Toxicology (13.2)]*.

Antiretroviral Pregnancy Registry: To monitor maternal-fetal outcomes of pregnant women exposed to lamivudine, a Pregnancy Registry has been established. Physicians are encouraged to register patients by calling 1-800-258-4263.

8.3 Nursing Mothers
The Centers for Disease Control and Prevention recommend that HIV-1-infected mothers in the United States not breastfeed their infants to avoid risking postnatal transmission of HIV-1 infection. Because of the potential for serious adverse reactions in nursing infants and HIV-1 transmission, mothers should be instructed not to breastfeed if they are receiving lamivudine.

Lamivudine is excreted into human milk. Samples of breast milk obtained from 20 mothers receiving lamivudine monotherapy (300 mg twice daily) or combination therapy (150 mg lamivudine twice daily and 300 mg zidovudine twice daily) had measurable concentrations of lamivudine.

8.4 Pediatric Use
The safety and effectiveness of twice-daily EPIVIR in combination with other antiretroviral agents have been established in pediatric patients 3 months and older *[see Adverse Reactions (6.1), Clinical Pharmacology (12.3), Clinical Studies (14.2)]*.

8.5 Geriatric Use
Clinical trials of EPIVIR did not include sufficient numbers of subjects aged 65 and over to determine whether they respond differently from younger subjects. In general, dose se-

lection for an elderly patient should be cautious, reflecting the greater frequency of decreased hepatic, renal, or cardiac function, and of concomitant disease or other drug therapy. In particular, because lamivudine is substantially excreted by the kidney and elderly patients are more likely to have decreased renal function, renal function should be monitored and dosage adjustments should be made accordingly *[see Dosage and Administration (2.3), Clinical Pharmacology (12.3)]*.

8.6 Patients With Impaired Renal Function
Reduction of the dosage of EPIVIR is recommended for patients with impaired renal function *[see Dosage and Administration (2.3), Clinical Pharmacology (12.3)]*.

10 OVERDOSAGE
There is no known antidote for EPIVIR. One case of an adult ingesting 6 g of EPIVIR was reported; there were no clinical signs or symptoms noted and hematologic tests remained normal. Two cases of pediatric overdose were reported in Trial ACTG300. One case involved a single dose of 7 mg/kg of EPIVIR; the second case involved use of 5 mg/kg of EPIVIR twice daily for 30 days. There were no clinical signs or symptoms noted in either case. Because a negligible amount of lamivudine was removed via (4-hour) hemodialysis, continuous ambulatory peritoneal dialysis, and automated peritoneal dialysis, it is not known if continuous hemodialysis would provide clinical benefit in a lamivudine overdose event. If overdose occurs, the patient should be monitored, and standard supportive treatment applied as required.

11 DESCRIPTION
EPIVIR (also known as 3TC) is a brand name for lamivudine, a synthetic nucleoside analogue with activity against HIV-1 and HBV. The chemical name of lamivudine is (2R,cis)-4-amino-1-(2-hydroxymethyl-1,3-oxathiolan-5-yl)-(1H)-pyrimidin-2-one. Lamivudine is the (-)enantiomer of a dideoxy analogue of cytidine. Lamivudine has also been referred to as (-)2',3'-dideoxy, 3'-thiacytidine. It has a molecular formula of $C_8H_{11}N_3O_3S$ and a molecular weight of 229.3. It has the following structural formula:

Lamivudine is a white to off-white crystalline solid with a solubility of approximately 70 mg/mL in water at 20°C.

EPIVIR Tablets are for oral administration. Each scored 150-mg film-coated tablet contains 150 mg of lamivudine and the inactive ingredients hypromellose, magnesium stearate, microcrystalline cellulose, polyethylene glycol, polysorbate 80, sodium starch glycolate, and titanium dioxide.

Each 300-mg film-coated tablet contains 300 mg of lamivudine and the inactive ingredients black iron oxide, hypromellose, magnesium stearate, microcrystalline cellulose, polyethylene glycol, polysorbate 80, sodium starch glycolate, and titanium dioxide.

EPIVIR Oral Solution is for oral administration. One milliliter (1 mL) of EPIVIR Oral Solution contains 10 mg of lamivudine (10 mg/mL) in an aqueous solution and the inactive ingredients artificial strawberry and banana flavors, citric acid (anhydrous), methylparaben, propylene glycol, propylparaben, sodium citrate (dihydrate), and sucrose (200 mg).

12 CLINICAL PHARMACOLOGY

12.1 Mechanism of Action
Lamivudine is an antiviral agent *[see Clinical Pharmacology (12.4)]*.

12.3 Pharmacokinetics
Pharmacokinetics in Adults: The pharmacokinetic properties of lamivudine have been studied in asymptomatic, HIV-1-infected adult subjects after administration of single intravenous (IV) doses ranging from 0.25 to 8 mg/kg, as well as single and multiple (twice-daily regimen) oral doses ranging from 0.25 to 10 mg/kg.

The pharmacokinetic properties of lamivudine have also been studied as single and multiple oral doses ranging from 5 mg to 600 mg/day administered to HBV-infected subjects. The steady-state pharmacokinetic properties of the EPIVIR 300-mg tablet once daily for 7 days compared with the EPIVIR 150-mg tablet twice daily for 7 days were assessed in a crossover trial in 60 healthy subjects. EPIVIR 300 mg once daily resulted in lamivudine exposures that were similar to EPIVIR 150 mg twice daily with respect to plasma $AUC_{24,ss}$; however, $C_{max,ss}$ was 66% higher and the trough value was 53% lower compared with the 150-mg twice-daily regimen. Intracellular lamivudine triphosphate exposures in peripheral blood mononuclear cells were also similar with

respect to $AUC_{24,ss}$ and $C_{max24,ss}$; however, trough values were lower compared with the 150-mg twice-daily regimen. Inter-subject variability was greater for intracellular lamivudine triphosphate concentrations versus lamivudine plasma trough concentrations. The clinical significance of observed differences for both plasma lamivudine concentrations and intracellular lamivudine triphosphate concentrations is not known.

Absorption and Bioavailability: Lamivudine was rapidly absorbed after oral administration in HIV-1-infected subjects. Absolute bioavailability in 12 adult subjects was 86% ± 16% (mean ± SD) for the 150-mg tablet and 87% ± 13% for the oral solution. After oral administration of 2 mg/kg twice a day to 9 adults with HIV-1, the peak serum lamivudine concentration (C_{max}) was 1.5 ± 0.5 mcg/mL (mean ± SD). The area under the plasma concentration versus time curve (AUC) and C_{max} increased in proportion to oral dose over the range from 0.25 to 10 mg/kg.

The accumulation ratio of lamivudine in HIV-1-positive asymptomatic adults with normal renal function was 1.50 following 15 days of oral administration of 2 mg/kg twice daily.

Effects of Food on Oral Absorption: An investigational 25-mg dosage form of lamivudine was administered orally to 12 asymptomatic, HIV-1-infected subjects on 2 occasions, once in the fasted state and once with food (1,099 kcal; 75 grams fat, 34 grams protein, 72 grams carbohydrate). Absorption of lamivudine was slower in the fed state (T_{max}: 3.2 ± 1.3 hours) compared with the fasted state (T_{max}: 0.9 ± 0.3 hours); C_{max} in the fed state was 40% ± 23% (mean ± SD) lower than in the fasted state. There was no significant difference in systemic exposure (AUC_∞) in the fed and fasted states; therefore, EPIVIR Tablets and Oral Solution may be administered with or without food.

Distribution: The apparent volume of distribution after IV administration of lamivudine to 20 subjects was 1.3 ± 0.4 L/kg, suggesting that lamivudine distributes into extravascular spaces. Volume of distribution was independent of dose and did not correlate with body weight.

Binding of lamivudine to human plasma proteins is low (<36%). In vitro studies showed that over the concentration range of 0.1 to 100 mcg/mL, the amount of lamivudine associated with erythrocytes ranged from 53% to 57% and was independent of concentration.

Metabolism: Metabolism of lamivudine is a minor route of elimination. In man, the only known metabolite of lamivudine is the trans-sulfoxide metabolite. Within 12 hours after a single oral dose of lamivudine in 6 HIV-1-infected adults, 5.2% ± 1.4% (mean ± SD) of the dose was excreted as the trans-sulfoxide metabolite in the urine. Serum concentrations of this metabolite have not been determined.

Elimination: The majority of lamivudine is eliminated unchanged in urine by active organic cationic secretion. In 9 healthy subjects given a single 300-mg oral dose of lamivudine, renal clearance was 199.7 ± 56.9 mL/min (mean ± SD). In 20 HIV-1-infected subjects given a single IV dose, renal clearance was 280.4 ± 75.2 mL/min (mean ± SD), representing 71% ± 16% (mean ± SD) of total clearance of lamivudine.

In most single-dose trials in HIV-1-infected subjects, HBV-infected subjects, or healthy subjects with serum sampling for 24 hours after dosing, the observed mean elimination half-life (t½) ranged from 5 to 7 hours. In HIV-1-infected subjects, total clearance was 398.5 ± 69.1 mL/min (mean ± SD). Oral clearance and elimination half-life were independent of dose and body weight over an oral dosing range of 0.25 to 10 mg/kg.

Special Populations: Renal Impairment: The pharmacokinetic properties of lamivudine have been determined in a small group of HIV-1-infected adults with impaired renal function (Table 7).

[See table 7 at top of next page]

Exposure (AUC_∞), C_{max}, and half-life increased with diminishing renal function (as expressed by creatinine clearance). Apparent total oral clearance (Cl/F) of lamivudine decreased as creatinine clearance decreased. T_{max} was not significantly affected by renal function. Based on these observations, it is recommended that the dosage of lamivudine be modified in patients with renal impairment *[see Dosage and Administration (2.3)]*.

Based on a trial in otherwise healthy subjects with impaired renal function, hemodialysis increased lamivudine clearance from a mean of 64 to 88 mL/min; however, the length of time of hemodialysis (4 hours) was insufficient to significantly alter mean lamivudine exposure after a single-dose administration. Continuous ambulatory peritoneal dialysis and automated peritoneal dialysis have negligible effects on lamivudine clearance. Therefore, it is recommended, following correction of dose for creatinine clearance, that no additional dose modification be made after routine hemodialysis or peritoneal dialysis.

It is not known whether lamivudine can be removed by continuous (24-hour) hemodialysis.

The effects of renal impairment on lamivudine pharmacokinetics in pediatric patients are not known.

Hepatic Impairment: The pharmacokinetic properties of lamivudine have been determined in adults with impaired hepatic function. Pharmacokinetic parameters were not altered by diminishing hepatic function; therefore, no dose adjustment for lamivudine is required for patients with impaired hepatic function. Safety and efficacy of lamivudine have not been established in the presence of decompensated liver disease.

Pediatric Patients: In Trial NUCA2002, pharmacokinetic properties of lamivudine were assessed in a subset of 57 HIV-1-infected pediatric subjects (age range: 4.8 months to 16 years, weight range: 5 to 66 kg) after oral and IV administration of 1, 2, 4, 8, 12, and 20 mg/kg/day. In the 9 infants and children (age range: 5 months to 12 years) receiving oral solution 4 mg/kg twice daily (the usual recommended pediatric dose), absolute bioavailability was 66% ± 26% (mean ± SD), which was less than the 86% ± 16% (mean ± SD) observed in adults. The mechanism for the diminished absolute bioavailability of lamivudine in infants and children is unknown.

Systemic clearance decreased with increasing age in pediatric subjects, as shown in Figure 1.

Figure 1. Systemic Clearance (L/hr·kg) of Lamivudine in Relation to Age

After oral administration of lamivudine 4 mg/kg twice daily to 11 pediatric subjects ranging in age from 4 months to 14 years, C_{max} was 1.1 ± 0.6 mcg/mL and half-life was 2.0 ± 0.6 hours. (In adults with similar blood sampling, the half–life was 3.7 ± 1 hours.) Total exposure to lamivudine, as reflected by mean AUC values, was comparable between pediatric subjects receiving an 8-mg/kg/day dose and adults receiving a 4-mg/kg/day dose.

Distribution of lamivudine into cerebrospinal fluid (CSF) was assessed in 38 pediatric subjects after multiple oral dosing with lamivudine. CSF samples were collected between 2 and 4 hours postdose. At the dose of 8 mg/kg/day, CSF lamivudine concentrations in 8 subjects ranged from 5.6% to 30.9% (mean ± SD of 14.2% ± 7.9%) of the concentration in a simultaneous serum sample, with CSF lamivudine concentrations ranging from 0.04 to 0.3 mcg/mL.

Limited, uncontrolled pharmacokinetic and safety data are available from administration of lamivudine (and zidovudine) to 36 infants aged up to 1 week in 2 trials in South Africa. In these trials, lamivudine clearance was substantially reduced in 1-week-old neonates relative to pediatric subjects (aged >3 months) studied previously. There is insufficient information to establish the time course of changes in clearance between the immediate neonatal period and the age-ranges >3 months old *[see Adverse Reactions (6.1)]*.

Geriatric Patients: The pharmacokinetics of lamivudine after administration of EPIVIR to patients over 65 years have not been studied *[see Use in Specific Populations (8.5)]*.

Gender: There are no significant gender differences in lamivudine pharmacokinetics.

Race: There are no significant racial differences in lamivudine pharmacokinetics.

Drug Interactions: Interferon Alfa: There was no significant pharmacokinetic interaction between lamivudine and interferon alfa in a trial of 19 healthy male subjects *[see Warnings and Precautions (5.4)]*.

Ribavirin: In vitro data indicate ribavirin reduces phosphorylation of lamivudine, stavudine, and zidovudine. However, no pharmacokinetic (e.g., plasma concentrations or intracellular triphosphorylated active metabolite concentrations) or pharmacodynamic (e.g., loss of HIV-1/HCV virologic suppression) interaction was observed when ribavirin and lamivudine (n = 18), stavudine (n = 10), or zidovudine (n = 6) were coadministered as part of a multidrug regimen to HIV-1/HCV co-infected subjects *[see Warnings and Precautions (5.4)]*.

Trimethoprim/Sulfamethoxazole: Lamivudine and TMP/SMX were coadministered to 14 HIV-1-positive subjects in a single-center, open-label, randomized, crossover trial. Each subject received treatment with a single 300-mg dose of lamivudine and TMP 160 mg/SMX 800 mg once a day for 5 days with concomitant administration of lamivudine 300 mg with the fifth dose in a crossover design. Coadministration of TMP/SMX with lamivudine resulted in an increase of 43% ± 23% (mean ± SD) in lamivudine AUC∞, a decrease of 29% ± 13% in lamivudine oral clearance, and a decrease of 30% ± 36% in lamivudine renal clearance. The pharmacokinetic properties of TMP and SMX were not altered by coadministration with lamivudine *[see Drug Interactions (7.3)]*.

Zidovudine: No clinically significant alterations in lamivudine or zidovudine pharmacokinetics were observed in 12 asymptomatic HIV-1-infected adult subjects given a single dose of zidovudine (200 mg) in combination with multiple doses of lamivudine (300 mg q 12 hr) *[see Drug Interactions (7.4)]*.

12.4   Microbiology

Mechanism of Action: Intracellularly, lamivudine is phosphorylated to its active 5′-triphosphate metabolite, lamivudine triphosphate (3TC-TP). The principal mode of action of 3TC-TP is the inhibition of HIV-1 reverse transcriptase (RT) via DNA chain termination after incorporation of the nucleotide analogue into viral DNA. 3TC-TP is a weak inhibitor of mammalian DNA polymerases α, β, and γ.

Antiviral Activity: The antiviral activity of lamivudine against HIV-1 was assessed in a number of cell lines (including monocytes and fresh human peripheral blood lymphocytes) using standard susceptibility assays. EC_{50} values (50% effective concentrations) were in the range of 0.003 to 15 μM (1 μM = 0.23 mcg/mL). HIV-1 from therapy-naive subjects with no amino acid substitutions associated with resistance gave median EC_{50} values of 0.429 μM (range: 0.200 to 2.007 μM) from Virco (n = 92 baseline samples from COLA40263) and 2.35 μM (1.37 to 3.68 μM) from Monogram Biosciences (n = 135 baseline samples from ESS30009). The EC_{50} values of lamivudine against different HIV-1 clades (A-G) ranged from 0.001 to 0.120 μM, and against HIV-2 isolates from 0.003 to 0.120 μM in peripheral blood mononuclear cells. Ribavirin (50 μM) decreased the anti-HIV-1 activity of lamivudine by 3.5 fold in MT-4 cells. In HIV-1-infected MT-4 cells, lamivudine in combination with zidovudine at various ratios exhibited synergistic antiretroviral activity. Please see the full prescribing information for EPIVIR-HBV for information regarding the inhibitory activity of lamivudine against HBV.

Resistance: Lamivudine-resistant variants of HIV-1 have been selected in cell culture. Genotypic analysis showed that the resistance was due to a specific amino acid substitution in the HIV-1 reverse transcriptase at codon 184 changing the methionine to either isoleucine or valine (M184V/I).

HIV-1 strains resistant to both lamivudine and zidovudine have been isolated from subjects. Susceptibility of clinical isolates to lamivudine and zidovudine was monitored in controlled clinical trials. In subjects receiving lamivudine monotherapy or combination therapy with lamivudine plus zidovudine, HIV-1 isolates from most subjects became phenotypically and genotypically resistant to lamivudine within 12 weeks. In some subjects harboring zidovudine-resistant virus at baseline, phenotypic sensitivity to zidovudine was restored by 12 weeks of treatment with lamivudine and zidovudine. Combination therapy with lamivudine plus zidovudine delayed the emergence of mutations conferring resistance to zidovudine.

Lamivudine-resistant HBV isolates develop substitutions (rtM204V/I) in the YMDD motif of the catalytic domain of the viral reverse transcriptase. rtM204V/I substitutions are frequently accompanied by other substitutions (rtV173L, rtL180M) which enhance the level of lamivudine resistance or act as compensatory mutations improving replication efficiency. Other substitutions detected in lamivudine-resistant HBV isolates include: rtL80I and rtA181T. Similar HBV mutants have been reported in HIV-1-infected subjects who received lamivudine-containing antiretroviral regimens in the presence of concurrent infection with hepatitis B virus *[see Warnings and Precautions (5.2)]*.

Cross-Resistance: Lamivudine-resistant HIV-1 mutants were cross-resistant to didanosine (ddI) and zalcitabine (ddC). In some subjects treated with zidovudine plus didanosine or zalcitabine, isolates resistant to multiple reverse transcriptase inhibitors, including lamivudine, have emerged.

Genotypic and Phenotypic Analysis of On-Therapy HIV-1 Isolates From Subjects With Virologic Failure: Trial EPV20001: Fifty-three of 554 (10%) subjects enrolled in EPV20001 were identified as virologic failures (plasma HIV-1 RNA level 400 copies/mL) by Week 48. Twenty-eight subjects were randomized to the lamivudine once-daily treatment group and 25 to the lamivudine twice-daily treatment group. The median baseline plasma HIV-1 RNA levels of subjects in the lamivudine once-daily group and lamivudine twice-daily group were 4.9 $\log_{10}$ copies/mL and 4.6 $\log_{10}$ copies/mL, respectively.

Genotypic analysis of on-therapy isolates from 22 subjects identified as virologic failures in the lamivudine once-daily group showed that isolates from 0/22 subjects contained treatment-emergent amino acid substitutions associated with zidovudine resistance (M41L, D67N, K70R, L210W, T215Y/F, or K219Q/E), isolates from 10/22 subjects contained treatment-emergent amino acid substitutions associated with efavirenz resistance (L100I, K101E, K103N, V108I, or Y181C), and isolates from 8/22 subjects contained a treatment-emergent lamivudine resistance-associated substitution (M184I or M184V).

Genotypic analysis of on-therapy isolates from subjects (n = 22) in the lamivudine twice-daily treatment group showed that isolates from 1/22 subjects contained treatment-emergent zidovudine resistance substitutions, isolates from 7/22 contained treatment-emergent efavirenz resistance substitutions, and isolates from 5/22 contained treatment-emergent lamivudine resistance substitutions.

Phenotypic analysis of baseline-matched on-therapy HIV-1 isolates from subjects (n = 13) receiving lamivudine once daily showed that isolates from 12/13 subjects were susceptible to zidovudine; isolates from 8/13 subjects exhibited a 25- to 295-fold decrease in susceptibility to efavirenz, and isolates from 7/13 subjects showed an 85- to 299-fold decrease in susceptibility to lamivudine.

Phenotypic analysis of baseline-matched on-therapy HIV-1 isolates from subjects (n = 13) receiving lamivudine twice daily showed that isolates from all 13 subjects were susceptible to zidovudine; isolates from 3/13 subjects exhibited a 21- to 342-fold decrease in susceptibility to efavirenz, and isolates from 4/13 subjects exhibited a 29- to 159-fold decrease in susceptibility to lamivudine.

Trial EPV40001: Fifty subjects received zidovudine 300 mg twice daily plus abacavir 300 mg twice daily plus lamivudine 300 mg once daily and 50 subjects received zidovudine 300 mg plus abacavir 300 mg plus lamivudine 150 mg all twice-daily. The median baseline plasma HIV-1 RNA levels for subjects in the 2 groups were 4.79 $\log_{10}$ copies/mL and 4.83 $\log_{10}$ copies/mL, respectively. Fourteen of 50 subjects in the lamivudine once-daily treatment group and 9 of 50 subjects in the lamivudine twice-daily group were identified as virologic failures.

Genotypic analysis of on-therapy HIV-1 isolates from subjects (n = 9) in the lamivudine once-daily treatment group showed that isolates from 6 subjects had an abacavir and/or lamivudine resistance-associated substitution M184V alone. On-therapy isolates from subjects (n = 6) receiving lamivudine twice daily showed that isolates from 2 subjects had M184V alone, and isolates from 2 subjects harbored the M184V substitution in combination with zidovudine resistance-associated amino acid substitutions.

Phenotypic analysis of on-therapy isolates from subjects (n = 6) receiving lamivudine once daily showed that HIV-1 isolates from 4 subjects exhibited a 32- to 53-fold decrease in susceptibility to lamivudine. HIV-1 isolates from these 6 subjects were susceptible to zidovudine.

Phenotypic analysis of on-therapy isolates from subjects (n = 4) receiving lamivudine twice daily showed that HIV-1 isolates from 1 subject exhibited a 45-fold decrease in susceptibility to lamivudine and a 4.5-fold decrease in susceptibility to zidovudine.

Table 7. Pharmacokinetic Parameters (Mean ± SD) After a Single 300-mg Oral Dose of Lamivudine in 3 Groups of Adults With Varying Degrees of Renal Function

Parameter	Creatinine Clearance Criterion (Number of Subjects)		
	>60 mL/min (n = 6)	10-30 mL/min (n = 4)	<10 mL/min (n = 6)
Creatinine clearance (mL/min)	111 ± 14	28 ± 8	6 ± 2
C_{max} (mcg/mL)	2.6 ± 0.5	3.6 ± 0.8	5.8 ± 1.2
AUC∞ (mcg•hr/mL)	11.0 ± 1.7	48.0 ± 19	157 ± 74
Cl/F (mL/min)	464 ± 76	114 ± 34	36 ± 11

Table 8. Number of Subjects (%) With at Least One HIV-1 Disease Progression Event or Death

Endpoint	Current Therapy (n = 460)	EPIVIR plus Current Therapy (n = 896)	EPIVIR plus an NNRTI[a] plus Current Therapy (n = 460)
HIV-1 progression or death	90 (19.6%)	86 (9.6%)	41 (8.9%)
Death	27 (5.9%)	23 (2.6%)	14 (3.0%)

[a] An investigational non-nucleoside reverse transcriptase inhibitor not approved in the United States.

Table 9. Outcomes of Randomized Treatment Through 48 Weeks (Intent-to-Treat)

Outcome	EPIVIR 300 mg Once Daily plus RETROVIR plus Efavirenz (n = 278)	EPIVIR 150 mg Twice Daily plus RETROVIR plus Efavirenz (n = 276)
Responder[a]	67%	65%
Virologic failure[b]	8%	8%
Discontinued due to clinical progression	<1%	0%
Discontinued due to adverse events	6%	12%
Discontinued due to other reasons[c]	18%	14%

[a] Achieved confirmed plasma HIV-1 RNA <400 copies/mL and maintained through 48 weeks.
[b] Achieved suppression but rebounded by Week 48, discontinued due to virologic failure, insufficient viral response according to the investigator, or never suppressed through Week 48.
[c] Includes consent withdrawn, lost to followup, protocol violation, data outside the trial-defined schedule, and randomized but never initiated treatment.

13 NONCLINICAL TOXICOLOGY

13.1 Carcinogenesis, Mutagenesis, Impairment of Fertility

Long-term carcinogenicity studies with lamivudine in mice and rats showed no evidence of carcinogenic potential at exposures up to 10 times (mice) and 58 times (rats) those observed in humans at the recommended therapeutic dose for HIV-1 infection. Lamivudine was not active in a microbial mutagenicity screen or an in vitro cell transformation assay, but showed weak in vitro mutagenic activity in a cytogenetic assay using cultured human lymphocytes and in the mouse lymphoma assay. However, lamivudine showed no evidence of in vivo genotoxic activity in the rat at oral doses of up to 2,000 mg/kg, producing plasma levels of 35 to 45 times those in humans at the recommended dose for HIV-1 infection. In a study of reproductive performance, lamivudine administered to rats at doses up to 4,000 mg/kg/day, producing plasma levels 47 to 70 times those in humans, revealed no evidence of impaired fertility and no effect on the survival, growth, and development to weaning of the offspring.

13.2 Reproductive Toxicology Studies

Reproduction studies have been performed in rats and rabbits at orally administered doses up to 4,000 mg/kg/day and 1,000 mg/kg/day, respectively, producing plasma levels up to approximately 35 times that for the adult HIV dose. No evidence of teratogenicity due to lamivudine was observed. Evidence of early embryolethality was seen in the rabbit at exposure levels similar to those observed in humans, but there was no indication of this effect in the rat at exposure levels up to 35 times those in humans. Studies in pregnant rats and rabbits showed that lamivudine is transferred to the fetus through the placenta.

14 CLINICAL STUDIES

The use of EPIVIR is based on the results of clinical trials in HIV–1-infected subjects in combination regimens with other antiretroviral agents. Information from trials with clinical endpoints or a combination of CD4+ cell counts and HIV-1 RNA measurements is included below as documentation of the contribution of lamivudine to a combination regimen in controlled trials.

14.1 Adults

Clinical Endpoint Trial: NUCB3007 (CAESAR) was a multi-center, double-blind, placebo-controlled trial comparing continued current therapy (zidovudine alone [62% of subjects] or zidovudine with didanosine or zalcitabine [38% of subjects]) to the addition of EPIVIR or EPIVIR plus an investigational non-nucleoside reverse transcriptase inhibitor (NNRTI), randomized 1:2:1. A total of 1,816 HIV-1-infected adults with 25 to 250 CD4+ cells/mm[3] (median = 122 cells/mm[3]) at baseline were enrolled: median age was 36 years, 87% were male, 84% were nucleoside-experienced, and 16% were therapy-naive. The median duration on trial was 12 months. Results are summarized in Table 8.
[See table 8 above]
Surrogate Endpoint Trials: *Dual Nucleoside Analogue Trials:* Principal clinical trials in the initial development of lamivudine compared lamivudine/zidovudine combinations with zidovudine monotherapy or with zidovudine plus zalcitabine. These trials demonstrated the antiviral effect of lamivudine in a 2-drug combination. More recent uses of lamivudine in treatment of HIV-1 infection incorporate it into multiple-drug regimens containing at least 3 antiretroviral drugs for enhanced viral suppression.
Dose Regimen Comparison Surrogate Endpoint Trials in Therapy-Naive Adults: EPV20001 was a multi-center, double-blind, controlled trial in which subjects were randomized 1:1 to receive EPIVIR 300 mg once daily or EPIVIR 150 mg twice daily, in combination with zidovudine 300 mg twice daily and efavirenz 600 mg once daily. A total of 554 antiretroviral treatment-naive HIV-1-infected adults enrolled: male (79%), Caucasian (50%), median age of 35 years, baseline CD4+ cell counts of 69 to 1,089 cells/mm[3] (median = 362 cells/mm[3]), and median baseline plasma HIV-1 RNA of 4.66 log$_{10}$ copies/mL. Outcomes of treatment through 48 weeks are summarized in Figure 2 and Table 9.
[See table 9 above]

Figure 2. Virologic Response Through Week 48, EPV20001[ab](Intent-to-Treat)

[a] Roche AMPLICOR HIV-1 MONITOR.
[b] Responders at each visit are subjects who had achieved and maintained HIV-1 RNA <400 copies/mL without discontinuation by that visit.

The proportions of subjects with HIV-1 RNA <50 copies/mL (via Roche Ultrasensitive assay) through Week 48 were 61% for subjects receiving EPIVIR 300 mg once daily and 63% for subjects receiving EPIVIR 150 mg twice daily. Median increases in CD4+ cell counts were 144 cells/mm[3] at Week 48 in subjects receiving EPIVIR 300 mg once daily and 146 cells/mm[3] for subjects receiving EPIVIR 150 mg twice daily.
A small, randomized, open-label pilot trial, EPV40001, was conducted in Thailand. A total of 159 treatment-naive adult subjects (male 32%, Asian 100%, median age 30 years, baseline median CD4+ cell count 380 cells/mm[3], median plasma HIV-1 RNA 4.8 log$_{10}$ copies/mL) were enrolled. Two of the treatment arms in this trial provided a comparison between lamivudine 300 mg once daily (n = 54) and lamivudine 150 mg twice daily (n = 52), each in combination with zidovudine 300 mg twice daily and abacavir 300 mg twice daily.

In intent-to-treat analyses of 48-week data, the proportions of subjects with HIV-1 RNA below 400 copies/mL were 61% (33/54) in the group randomized to once-daily lamivudine and 75% (39/52) in the group randomized to receive all 3 drugs twice daily; the proportions with HIV-1 RNA below 50 copies/mL were 54% (29/54) in the once-daily lamivudine group and 67% (35/52) in the all-twice-daily group; and the median increases in CD4+ cell counts were 166 cells/mm[3] in the once-daily lamivudine group and 216 cells/mm[3] in the all-twice-daily group.

14.2 Pediatric Subjects

Clinical Endpoint Trial: ACTG300 was a multi-center, randomized, double-blind trial that provided for comparison of EPIVIR plus RETROVIR (zidovudine) with didanosine monotherapy. A total of 471 symptomatic, HIV-1-infected therapy-naive (56 days of antiretroviral therapy) pediatric subjects were enrolled in these 2 treatment arms. The median age was 2.7 years (range: 6 weeks to 14 years), 58% were female, and 86% were non-Caucasian. The mean baseline CD4+ cell count was 868 cells/mm[3] (mean: 1,060 cells/mm[3] and range:0 to 4,650 cells/mm[3] for subjects aged 5 years; mean: 419 cells/mm[3] and range: 0 to 1,555 cells/mm[3] for subjects aged >5 years) and the mean baseline plasma HIV-1 RNA was 5.0 log$_{10}$ copies/mL. The median duration on trial was 10.1 months for the subjects receiving EPIVIR plus RETROVIR and 9.2 months for subjects receiving didanosine monotherapy. Results are summarized in Table 10.

Table 10. Number of Subjects (%) Reaching a Primary Clinical Endpoint (Disease Progression or Death)

Endpoint	EPIVIR plus RETROVIR (n = 236)	Didanosine (n = 235)
HIV-1 disease progression or death (total)	15 (6.4%)	37 (15.7%)
Physical growth failure	7 (3.0%)	6 (2.6%)
Central nervous system deterioration	4 (1.7%)	12 (5.1%)
CDC Clinical Category C	2 (0.8%)	8 (3.4%)
Death	2 (0.8%)	11 (4.7%)

16 HOW SUPPLIED/STORAGE AND HANDLING

EPIVIR Scored Tablets, 150 mg
White, diamond-shaped, scored, film-coated tablets debossed with "GX CJ7" on both sides.
Bottle of 60 tablets (NDC 49702-203-18) with child-resistant closure.
EPIVIR Tablets, 300 mg
Gray, modified diamond-shaped, film-coated tablets engraved with "GX EJ7" on one side and plain on the reverse side.
Bottle of 30 tablets (NDC 49702-204-13) with child-resistant closure.
Recommended Storage:
Store EPIVIR Tablets at 25°C (77°F); excursions permitted to 15° to 30°C (59° to 86°F) [see USP Controlled Room Temperature].
EPIVIR Oral Solution, 10 mg/mL
A clear, colorless to pale yellow, strawberry-banana-flavored liquid, contains 10 mg of lamivudine in each 1 mL.
Plastic bottle of 240 mL (NDC 49702-205-48) with child-resistant closure. This product does not require reconstitution.
Recommended Storage:
Store in tightly closed bottles at 25°C (77°F) [see USP Controlled Room Temperature].

17 PATIENT COUNSELING INFORMATION

17.1 Advice for the Patient

Lactic Acidosis/Hepatomegaly: Patients should be informed that some HIV medicines, including EPIVIR, can cause a rare, but serious condition called lactic acidosis with liver enlargement (hepatomegaly) *[see Warnings and Precautions (5.1)].*
HIV/HBV Co-infection: Patients co-infected with HIV-1 and HBV should be informed that deterioration of liver disease has occurred in some cases when treatment with lamivudine was discontinued. Patients should be advised to discuss any changes in regimen with their physician *[see Warnings and Precautions (5.2)].*
Differences in Formulations of EPIVIR: Patients should be advised that EPIVIR Tablets and Oral Solution contain a higher dose of the same active ingredient (lamivudine) as EPIVIR-HBV Tablets and Oral Solution. If a decision is made to include lamivudine in the HIV-1 treatment regimen of a patient co-infected with HIV-1 and HBV, the formulation and dosage of lamivudine in EPIVIR (not EPIVIR-HBV) should be used *[see Warnings and Precautions (5.2)].*
Use With Other Lamivudine- and Emtricitabine-Containing Products: EPIVIR should not be coadministered with drugs containing lamivudine or emtricitabine, including

COMBIVIR (lamivudine/zidovudine) Tablets, EPZICOM (abacavir sulfate and lamivudine) Tablets, TRIZIVIR (abacavir sulfate, lamivudine, and zidovudine), ATRIPLA (efavirenz, emtricitabine, and tenofovir), EMTRIVA (emtricitabine), TRUVADA (emtricitabine and tenofovir), or COMPLERA (rilpivirine/emtricitabine/tenofovir) [see Warnings and Precautions (5.3)].

HIV-1/HCV Co-Infection: Patients with HIV-1/HCV co-infection should be informed that hepatic decompensation (some fatal) has occurred in HIV-1/HCV co-infected patients receiving combination antiretroviral therapy for HIV-1 and interferon alfa with or without ribavirin [see Warnings and Precautions (5.4)].

Risk of Pancreatitis: Parents or guardians should be advised to monitor pediatric patients for signs and symptoms of pancreatitis [see Warnings and Precautions (5.5)].

Redistribution/Accumulation of Body Fat: Patients should be informed that redistribution or accumulation of body fat may occur in patients receiving antiretroviral therapy, including EPIVIR, and that the cause and long-term health effects of these conditions are not known at this time [see Warnings and Precautions (5.7)].

Sucrose Content of EPIVIR Oral Solution: Diabetic patients should be advised that each 15-mL dose of EPIVIR Oral Solution contains 3 grams of sucrose [see Description (11)].

Information About HIV-1 Infection: EPIVIR is not a cure for HIV-1 infection and patients may continue to experience illnesses associated with HIV-1 infection, including opportunistic infections. Patients should remain under the care of a physician when using EPIVIR.

Patients should be advised to avoid doing things that can spread HIV-1 infection to others.

- **Do not share needles or other injection equipment.**
- **Do not share personal items that can have blood or body fluids on them, like toothbrushes and razor blades.**
- **Do not have any kind of sex without protection.** Always practice safe sex by using a latex or polyurethane condom or other barrier method to lower the chance of sexual contact with semen, vaginal secretions, or blood.
- **Do not breastfeed.** Lamivudine is excreted in human breast milk. Mothers with HIV-1 should not breastfeed because HIV-1 can be passed to the baby in the breast milk.

Patients should be informed to take all HIV medications exactly as prescribed.

COMBIVIR, EPIVIR, EPZICOM, RETROVIR, and TRIZIVIR are registered trademarks of ViiV Healthcare. The other brands listed are trademarks of their respective owners and are not trademarks of ViiV Healthcare. The makers of these brands are not affiliated with and do not endorse ViiV Healthcare or its products.

Manufactured for:
ViiV Healthcare
Research Triangle Park, NC 27709
by:
GlaxoSmithKline
Research Triangle Park, NC 27709
Manufactured under agreement from
Shire Pharmaceuticals Group plc
Basingstoke, UK
©2013, ViiV Healthcare. All rights reserved.
EPV:5PI

EPZICOM ℞

[ep' zih com]
(abacavir sulfate and lamivudine)
Tablets, for oral use

HIGHLIGHTS OF PRESCRIBING INFORMATION

These highlights do not include all the information needed to use EPZICOM safely and effectively. See full prescribing information for EPZICOM.

EPZICOM (abacavir sulfate and lamivudine) Tablets, for oral use

Initial U.S. Approval: 2004

WARNING: RISK OF HYPERSENSITIVITY REACTIONS, LACTIC ACIDOSIS AND SEVERE HEPATOMEGALY, AND EXACERBATIONS OF HEPATITIS B

See full prescribing information for complete boxed warning

- Serious and sometimes fatal hypersensitivity reactions have been associated with abacavir-containing products (5.1)
- Hypersensitivity to abacavir is a multi-organ clinical syndrome. (5.1)
- Patients who carry the HLA-B*5701 allele are at high risk for experiencing a hypersensitivity reaction to abacavir. (5.1)
- Discontinue EPZICOM as soon as a hypersensitivity reaction is suspected. Regardless of HLA-B*5701

---

status, permanently discontinue EPZICOM if hypersensitivity cannot be ruled out, even when other diagnoses are possible. (5.1)
- Following a hypersensitivity reaction to abacavir, NEVER restart EPZICOM or any other abacavir-containing product. (5.1)
- Lactic acidosis and severe hepatomegaly with steatosis, including fatal cases, have been reported with the use of nucleoside analogues. (5.2)
- Severe acute exacerbations of hepatitis B have been reported in patients who are co-infected with hepatitis B virus (HBV) and human immunodeficiency virus (HIV-1) and have discontinued lamivudine, a component of EPZICOM. Monitor hepatic function closely in these patients and, if appropriate, initiate anti-hepatitis B treatment. (5.3)

INDICATIONS AND USAGE

EPZICOM, a combination of abacavir and lamivudine, both nucleoside analogue HIV-1 reverse transcriptase inhibitors, is indicated in combination with other antiretroviral agents for the treatment of HIV-1 infection. (1)

DOSAGE AND ADMINISTRATION

- A medication guide and warning card should be dispensed with each new prescription and refill. (2)
- Adults: One tablet daily. (2.1)
- Do not prescribe for patients requiring a dosage adjustment or patients with hepatic impairment. (2.2)

DOSAGE FORMS AND STRENGTHS

Tablets contain 600 mg of abacavir and 300 mg of lamivudine. (3)

CONTRAINDICATIONS

- Previously demonstrated hypersensitivity to abacavir or any other component of the product. (4, 5.1)
- Hepatic impairment. (4)

WARNINGS AND PRECAUTIONS

- See boxed warning for information about the following: hypersensitivity reactions, lactic acidosis and severe hepatomegaly, and severe acute exacerbations of hepatitis B. (5.1, 5.2, 5.3)
- Hepatic decompensation, some fatal, has occurred in HIV-1/HCV co-infected patients receiving combination antiretroviral therapy and interferon alfa with or without ribavirin. Discontinue EPZICOM as medically appropriate and consider dose reduction or discontinuation of interferon alfa, ribavirin, or both. (5.4)
- Immune reconstitution syndrome (5.5) and redistribution/accumulation of body fat have been reported in patients treated with combination antiretroviral therapy. (5.6)
- EPZICOM should not be administered with other lamivudine- or zidovudine-containing products or emtricitabine-containing products. (5.8)

ADVERSE REACTIONS

The most commonly reported adverse reactions of at least moderate intensity (incidence >5%) in an adult HIV-1 clinical trial were drug hypersensitivity, insomnia, depression/depressed mood, headache/migraine, fatigue/malaise, dizziness/vertigo, nausea, and diarrhea. (6.1)

To report SUSPECTED ADVERSE REACTIONS, contact ViiV Healthcare at 1-877-844-8872 or FDA at 1-800-FDA-1088 or www.fda.gov/medwatch.

DRUG INTERACTIONS

- Ethanol: Decreases elimination of abacavir. (7.1)
- Methadone: An increased methadone dose may be required in a small number of patients. (7.3)

See 17 for PATIENT COUNSELING INFORMATION and Medication Guide

Revised: 09/2013

FULL PRESCRIBING INFORMATION: CONTENTS*

WARNING: RISK OF HYPERSENSITIVITY REACTIONS, LACTIC ACIDOSIS AND SEVERE HEPATOMEGALY, AND EXACERBATIONS OF HEPATITIS B

FULL PRESCRIBING INFORMATION

WARNING: RISK OF HYPERSENSITIVITY REACTIONS, LACTIC ACIDOSIS AND SEVERE HEPATOMEGALY, AND EXACERBATIONS OF HEPATITIS B

Hypersensitivity Reactions: Serious and sometimes fatal hypersensitivity reactions have been associated with abacavir sulfate, a component of EPZICOM® (abacavir sulfate and lamivudine) Tablets.

Hypersensitivity to abacavir is a multi-organ clinical syndrome usually characterized by a sign or symptom in 2 or more of the following groups: (1) fever, (2) rash, (3) gastrointestinal (including nausea, vomiting, diarrhea, or abdominal pain), (4) constitutional (including generalized malaise, fatigue, or achiness), and (5) respiratory (including dyspnea, cough, or pharyngitis). Discontinue EPZICOM as soon as a hypersensitivity reaction is suspected.

Patients who carry the HLA-B*5701 allele are at high risk for experiencing a hypersensitivity reaction to abacavir. Prior to initiating therapy with abacavir, screening for the HLA-B*5701 allele is recommended; this approach has been found to decrease the risk of hypersensitivity reaction. Screening is also recommended prior to reinitiation of abacavir in patients of unknown HLA-B*5701 status who have previously tolerated abacavir. HLA-B*5701-negative patients may develop a suspected hypersensitivity reaction to abacavir; however, this occurs significantly less frequently than in HLA-B*5701-positive patients.

Regardless of HLA-B*5701 status, permanently discontinue EPZICOM if hypersensitivity cannot be ruled out, even when other diagnoses are possible.

Following a hypersensitivity reaction to abacavir, NEVER restart EPZICOM or any other abacavir-containing product because more severe symptoms can occur within hours and may include life-threatening hypotension and death.

Reintroduction of EPZICOM or any other abacavir-containing product, even in patients who have no identified history or unrecognized symptoms of hypersensitivity to abacavir therapy, can result in serious or fatal hypersensitivity reactions. Such reactions can occur within hours [see Warnings and Precautions (5.1)].

Lactic Acidosis and Severe Hepatomegaly: Lactic acidosis and severe hepatomegaly with steatosis, including fatal cases, have been reported with the use of nucleoside analogues alone or in combination, including abacavir, lamivudine, and other antiretrovirals [see Warnings and Precautions (5.2)].

Exacerbations of Hepatitis B: Severe acute exacerbations of hepatitis B have been reported in patients who are co-infected with hepatitis B virus (HBV) and human immunodeficiency virus (HIV-1) and have discontinued lamivudine, which is one component of EPZICOM. Hepatic function should be monitored closely with both clinical and laboratory follow-up for at least several months in patients who discontinue EPZICOM and are co-infected with HIV-1 and HBV. If appropriate, initiation of anti-hepatitis B therapy may be warranted [see Warnings and Precautions (5.3)].

1 INDICATIONS AND USAGE

EPZICOM Tablets, in combination with other antiretroviral agents, are indicated for the treatment of HIV-1 infection. Additional important information on the use of EPZICOM for treatment of HIV-1 infection:

- EPZICOM is one of multiple products containing abacavir. Before starting EPZICOM, review medical history for prior exposure to any abacavir-containing product in order to avoid reintroduction in a patient with a history of hypersensitivity to abacavir [see Warnings and Precautions (5.1), Adverse Reactions (6)].
- As part of a triple-drug regimen, EPZICOM Tablets are recommended for use with antiretroviral agents from different pharmacological classes and not with other nucleoside/nucleotide reverse transcriptase inhibitors.

2 DOSAGE AND ADMINISTRATION

- A Medication Guide and Warning Card that provide information about recognition of hypersensitivity reactions should be dispensed with each new prescription and refill.
- EPZICOM can be taken with or without food.

2.1 Adult Patients

The recommended oral dose of EPZICOM for adults is one tablet daily, in combination with other antiretroviral agents.

2.2 Dosage Adjustment

Because it is a fixed-dose combination, EPZICOM should not be prescribed for:

- patients requiring dosage adjustment such as those with creatinine clearance <50 mL/min,
- patients with hepatic impairment.

Use of EPIVIR® (lamivudine) Oral Solution or Tablets and ZIAGEN® (abacavir sulfate) Oral Solution may be considered.

3 DOSAGE FORMS AND STRENGTHS

EPZICOM Tablets contain 600 mg of abacavir as abacavir sulfate and 300 mg of lamivudine. The tablets are modified capsule-shaped, orange, film-coated, and debossed with "GS FC2" on one side with no markings on the reverse side.

4 CONTRAINDICATIONS

EPZICOM Tablets are contraindicated in patients with:

- previously demonstrated hypersensitivity to abacavir or to any other component of the product. NEVER restart EPZICOM or any other abacavir-containing product following a hypersensitivity reaction to abacavir, regardless of HLA-B*5701 status [see Warnings and Precautions (5.1), Adverse Reactions (6)].
- hepatic impairment [see Use in Specific Populations (8.7)].

5 WARNINGS AND PRECAUTIONS

5.1 Hypersensitivity Reaction

Serious and sometimes fatal hypersensitivity reactions have been associated with EPZICOM and other abacavir-containing products. Patients who carry the HLA-B*5701 allele are at high risk for experiencing a hypersensitivity reaction to abacavir. Prior to initiating therapy with abacavir, screening for the HLA-B*5701 allele is recommended; this approach has been found to decrease the risk of a hypersensitivity reaction. Screening is also recommended prior to reinitiation of abacavir in patients of unknown HLA-B*5701 status who have previously tolerated abacavir. For HLA-B*5701-positive patients, treatment with an abacavir-containing regimen is not recommended and should be considered only with close medical supervision and under exceptional circumstances when the potential benefit outweighs the risk.

HLA-B*5701-negative patients may develop a hypersensitivity reaction to abacavir; however, this occurs significantly less frequently than in HLA-B*5701-positive patients. Regardless of HLA-B*5701 status, permanently discontinue EPZICOM if hypersensitivity cannot be ruled out, even when other diagnoses are possible.

Important information on signs and symptoms of hypersensitivity, as well as clinical management, is presented below.

Signs and Symptoms of Hypersensitivity: Hypersensitivity to abacavir is a multi-organ clinical syndrome usually characterized by a sign or symptom in 2 or more of the following groups.

Group 1: Fever

Group 2: Rash

Group 3: Gastrointestinal (including nausea, vomiting, diarrhea, or abdominal pain)

Group 4: Constitutional (including generalized malaise, fatigue, or achiness)

Group 5: Respiratory (including dyspnea, cough, or pharyngitis)

Hypersensitivity to abacavir following the presentation of a single sign or symptom has been reported infrequently.

Hypersensitivity to abacavir was reported in approximately 8% of 2,670 subjects (n = 206) in 9 clinical trials (range: 2% to 9%) with enrollment from November 1999 to February 2002. Data on time to onset and symptoms of suspected hypersensitivity were collected on a detailed data collection module. The frequencies of symptoms are shown in Figure 1. Symptoms usually appeared within the first 6 weeks of treatment with abacavir, although the reaction may occur at any time during therapy. Median time to onset was 9 days; 89% appeared within the first 6 weeks; 95% of subjects reported symptoms from 2 or more of the 5 groups listed above.

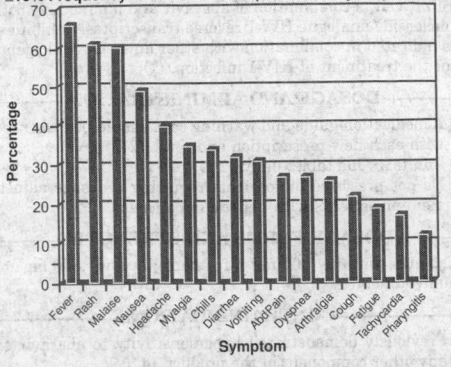

Figure 1: Hypersensitivity-Related Symptoms Reported With ≥10% Frequency in Clinical Trials (n = 206 Subjects)

Other less common signs and symptoms of hypersensitivity include lethargy, myolysis, edema, abnormal chest x-ray findings (predominantly infiltrates, which can be localized), and paresthesia. Anaphylaxis, liver failure, renal failure, hypotension, adult respiratory distress syndrome, respiratory failure, and death have occurred in association with hypersensitivity reactions. In one trial, 4 subjects (11%) receiving ZIAGEN 600 mg once daily experienced hypotension with a hypersensitivity reaction compared with 0 subjects receiving ZIAGEN 300 mg twice daily.

Physical findings associated with hypersensitivity to abacavir in some subjects include lymphadenopathy, mucous membrane lesions (conjunctivitis and mouth ulcerations), and rash. The rash usually appears maculopapular or urticarial, but may be variable in appearance. There have been reports of erythema multiforme. Hypersensitivity reactions have occurred without rash.

Laboratory abnormalities associated with hypersensitivity to abacavir in some subjects include elevated liver function tests, elevated creatine phosphokinase, elevated creatinine, and lymphopenia.

Clinical Management of Hypersensitivity: Discontinue EPZICOM as soon as a hypersensitivity reaction is suspected. To minimize the risk of a life-threatening hypersensitivity reaction, permanently discontinue EPZICOM if hypersensitivity cannot be ruled out, even when other diagnoses are possible (e.g., acute onset respiratory diseases such as pneumonia, bronchitis, pharyngitis, or influenza; gastroenteritis; or reactions to other medications).

Following a hypersensitivity reaction to abacavir, NEVER restart EPZICOM or any other abacavir-containing product because more severe symptoms can occur within hours and may include life-threatening hypotension and death.

When therapy with EPZICOM has been discontinued for reasons other than symptoms of a hypersensitivity reaction, and if reinitiation of EPZICOM or any other abacavir-containing product is under consideration, carefully evaluate the reason for discontinuation of EPZICOM to ensure that the patient did not have symptoms of a hypersensitivity reaction. If the patient is of unknown HLA-B*5701 status, screening for the allele is recommended prior to reinitiation of EPZICOM.

If hypersensitivity cannot be ruled out, DO NOT reintroduce EPZICOM or any other abacavir-containing product. Even in the absence of the HLA-B*5701 allele, it is important to permanently discontinue abacavir and not rechallenge with abacavir if a hypersensitivity reaction cannot be ruled out on clinical grounds, due to the potential for a severe or even fatal reaction.

If symptoms consistent with hypersensitivity are not identified, reintroduction can be undertaken with continued monitoring for symptoms of a hypersensitivity reaction. Make patients aware that a hypersensitivity reaction can occur with reintroduction of EPZICOM or any other abacavir-containing product and that reintroduction of

EPZICOM or introduction of any other abacavir-containing product needs to be undertaken only if medical care can be readily accessed by the patient or others.

Risk Factor: HLA-B*5701 Allele: Trials have shown that carriage of the HLA-B*5701 allele is associated with a significantly increased risk of a hypersensitivity reaction to abacavir.

CNA106030 (PREDICT-1), a randomized, double-blind trial, evaluated the clinical utility of prospective HLA-B*5701 screening on the incidence of abacavir hypersensitivity reaction in abacavir-naive HIV-1-infected adults (n = 1,650). In this trial, use of pre-therapy screening for the HLA-B*5701 allele and exclusion of subjects with this allele reduced the incidence of clinically suspected abacavir hypersensitivity reactions from 7.8% (66/847) to 3.4% (27/803). Based on this trial, it is estimated that 61% of patients with the HLA-B*5701 allele will develop a clinically suspected hypersensitivity reaction during the course of abacavir treatment compared with 4% of patients who do not have the HLA-B*5701 allele.

Screening for carriage of the HLA-B*5701 allele is recommended prior to initiating treatment with abacavir. Screening is also recommended prior to reinitiation of abacavir in patients of unknown HLA-B*5701 status who have previously tolerated abacavir. For HLA-B*5701-positive patients, initiating or reinitiating treatment with an abacavir-containing regimen is not recommended and should be considered only with close medical supervision and under exceptional circumstances where potential benefit outweighs the risk.

Skin patch testing is used as a research tool and should not be used to aid in the clinical diagnosis of abacavir hypersensitivity.

In any patient treated with abacavir, the clinical diagnosis of hypersensitivity reaction must remain the basis of clinical decision-making. Even in the absence of the HLA-B*5701 allele, it is important to permanently discontinue abacavir and not rechallenge with abacavir if a hypersensitivity reaction cannot be ruled out on clinical grounds, due to the potential for a severe or even fatal reaction.

5.2 Lactic Acidosis and Severe Hepatomegaly With Steatosis

Lactic acidosis and severe hepatomegaly with steatosis, including fatal cases, have been reported with the use of nucleoside analogues alone or in combination, including abacavir and lamivudine and other antiretrovirals. A majority of these cases have been in women. Obesity and prolonged nucleoside exposure may be risk factors. Particular caution should be exercised when administering EPZICOM to any patient with known risk factors for liver disease; however, cases have also been reported in patients with no known risk factors. Treatment with EPZICOM should be suspended in any patient who develops clinical or laboratory findings suggestive of lactic acidosis or pronounced hepatotoxicity (which may include hepatomegaly and steatosis even in the absence of marked transaminase elevations).

5.3 Patients With HIV-1 and Hepatitis B Virus Co-Infection

Posttreatment Exacerbations of Hepatitis: In clinical trials in non-HIV-1-infected subjects treated with lamivudine for chronic HBV, clinical and laboratory evidence of exacerbations of hepatitis have occurred after discontinuation of lamivudine. These exacerbations have been detected primarily by serum ALT elevations in addition to re-emergence of HBV DNA. Although most events appear to have been self-limited, fatalities have been reported in some cases. Similar events have been reported from post-marketing experience after changes from lamivudine-containing HIV-1 treatment regimens to non-lamivudine-containing regimens in patients infected with both HIV-1 and HBV. The causal relationship to discontinuation of lamivudine treatment is unknown. Patients should be closely monitored with both clinical and laboratory follow-up for at least several months after stopping treatment. There is insufficient evidence to determine whether re-initiation of lamivudine alters the course of posttreatment exacerbations of hepatitis.

Emergence of Lamivudine-Resistant HBV: Safety and efficacy of lamivudine have not been established for treatment of chronic hepatitis B in subjects dually infected with HIV-1 and HBV. In non–HIV-1-infected subjects treated with lamivudine for chronic hepatitis B, emergence of lamivudine-resistant HBV has been detected and has been associated with diminished treatment response (see full prescribing information for EPIVIR-HBV® [lamivudine] Tablets and Oral Solution for additional information). Emergence of hepatitis B virus variants associated with resistance to lamivudine has also been reported in HIV-1-infected subjects who have received lamivudine-containing antiretroviral regimens in the presence of concurrent infection with hepatitis B virus.

5.4 Use With Interferon- and Ribavirin-Based Regimens

In vitro studies have shown ribavirin can reduce the phosphorylation of pyrimidine nucleoside analogues such as lamivudine, a component of EPZICOM. Although no evidence of a pharmacokinetic or pharmacodynamic interaction (e.g., loss of HIV-1/HCV virologic suppression) was seen when ribavirin was coadministered with lamivudine in HIV-1/HCV co-infected subjects [see Clinical Pharmacology (12.3)], hepatic decompensation (some fatal) has occurred in HIV-1/HCV co-infected subjects receiving combination antiretroviral therapy for HIV-1 and interferon alfa with or without ribavirin. Patients receiving interferon alfa with or without ribavirin and EPZICOM should be closely monitored for treatment-associated toxicities, especially hepatic decompensation. Discontinuation of EPZICOM should be considered as medically appropriate. Dose reduction or discontinuation of interferon alfa, ribavirin, or both should also be considered if worsening clinical toxicities are observed, including hepatic decompensation (e.g., Child-Pugh >6) (see the complete prescribing information for interferon and ribavirin).

5.5 Immune Reconstitution Syndrome

Immune reconstitution syndrome has been reported in patients treated with combination antiretroviral therapy, including EPZICOM. During the initial phase of combination antiretroviral treatment, patients whose immune systems respond may develop an inflammatory response to indolent or residual opportunistic infections (such as *Mycobacterium avium* infection, cytomegalovirus, *Pneumocystis jirovecii* pneumonia [PCP], or tuberculosis), which may necessitate further evaluation and treatment.

Autoimmune disorders (such as Graves' disease, polymyositis, and Guillain-Barré syndrome) have also been reported to occur in the setting of immune reconstitution; however, the time to onset is more variable, and can occur many months after initiation of treatment.

5.6 Fat Redistribution

Redistribution/accumulation of body fat including central obesity, dorsocervical fat enlargement (buffalo hump), peripheral wasting, facial wasting, breast enlargement, and "cushingoid appearance" have been observed in patients receiving antiretroviral therapy. The mechanism and long-term consequences of these events are currently unknown. A causal relationship has not been established.

5.7 Myocardial Infarction

In a published prospective, observational, epidemiological trial designed to investigate the rate of myocardial infarction in patients on combination antiretroviral therapy, the use of abacavir within the previous 6 months was correlated with an increased risk of myocardial infarction (MI).[1] In a sponsor-conducted pooled analysis of clinical trials, no excess risk of MI was observed in abacavir-treated subjects as compared with control subjects. In totality, the available data from the observational cohort and from clinical trials are inconclusive.

As a precaution, the underlying risk of coronary heart disease should be considered when prescribing antiretroviral therapies, including abacavir, and action taken to minimize all modifiable risk factors (e.g., hypertension, hyperlipidemia, diabetes mellitus, smoking).

5.8 Use With Other Abacavir-, Lamivudine-, and/or Emtricitabine-Containing Products

EPZICOM contains fixed doses of 2 nucleoside analogues, abacavir and lamivudine, and should not be administered concomitantly with other abacavir-containing and/or lamivudine-containing products, including ZIAGEN (abacavir sulfate) Tablets and Oral Solution, EPIVIR (lamivudine) Tablets and Oral Solution, EPIVIR-HBV (lamivudine) Tablets and Oral Solution COMBIVIR® (lamivudine and zidovudine) Tablets, or TRIZIVIR® (abacavir sulfate, lamivudine, and zidovudine) Tablets; or emtricitabine-containing products, including ATRIPLA® (efavirenz/emtricitabine/tenofovir disoproxil fumarate) Tablets, EMTRIVA® (emtricitabine) Capsules and Oral Solution, TRUVADA® (emtricitabine/tenofovir disoproxil fumarate) Tablets, or COMPLERA® (emtricitabine/rilpivirine/tenofovir disoproxil fumarate) Tablets.

The complete prescribing information for all agents being considered for use with EPZICOM should be consulted before combination therapy with EPZICOM is initiated.

6 ADVERSE REACTIONS

The following adverse reactions are discussed in greater detail in other sections of the labeling:

- Serious and sometimes fatal hypersensitivity reaction. In one trial, once-daily dosing of abacavir was associated with more severe hypersensitivity reactions [see Boxed Warning, Warnings and Precautions (5.1)].
- Lactic acidosis and severe hepatomegaly [see Boxed Warning, Warnings and Precautions (5.2)].
- Acute exacerbations of hepatitis B [see Boxed Warning, Warnings and Precautions (5.3)].
- Hepatic decompensation in patients co-infected with HIV-1 and Hepatitis C [see Warnings and Precautions (5.4)].
- Immune reconstitution syndrome [see Warnings and Precautions (5.5)].

- Fat redistribution [see Warnings and Precautions (5.6)].
- Myocardial infarction [see Warnings and Precautions (5.7)].

6.1 Clinical Trials Experience

Because clinical trials are conducted under widely varying conditions, adverse reaction rates observed in the clinical trials of a drug cannot be directly compared to rates in the clinical trials of another drug and may not reflect the rates observed in clinical practice.

Therapy-Naive Adults: Treatment-emergent clinical adverse reactions (rated by the investigator as moderate or severe) with a ≥5% frequency during therapy with ZIAGEN 600 mg once daily or ZIAGEN 300 mg twice daily, both in combination with lamivudine 300 mg once daily and efavirenz 600 mg once daily, are listed in Table 1.

Table 1. Treatment-Emergent (All Causality) Adverse Reactions of at Least Moderate Intensity (Grades 2-4, ≥5% Frequency) in Therapy-Naive Adults (CNA30021) Through 48 Weeks of Treatment

Adverse Event	ZIAGEN 600 mg q.d. plus EPIVIR plus Efavirenz (n = 384)	ZIAGEN 300 mg b.i.d. plus EPIVIR plus Efavirenz (n = 386)
Drug hypersensitivity[a,b]	9%	7%
Insomnia	7%	9%
Depression/Depressed mood	7%	7%
Headache/Migraine	7%	6%
Fatigue/Malaise	6%	8%
Dizziness/Vertigo	6%	6%
Nausea	5%	6%
Diarrhea[a]	5%	6%
Rash	5%	5%
Pyrexia	5%	3%
Abdominal pain/gastritis	4%	5%
Abnormal dreams	4%	5%
Anxiety	3%	5%

[a]Subjects receiving ZIAGEN 600 mg once daily, experienced a significantly higher incidence of severe drug hypersensitivity reactions and severe diarrhea compared with subjects who received ZIAGEN 300 mg twice daily. Five percent (5%) of subjects receiving ZIAGEN 600 mg once daily had severe drug hypersensitivity reactions compared with 2% of subjects receiving ZIAGEN 300 mg twice daily. Two percent (2%) of subjects receiving ZIAGEN 600 mg once daily had severe diarrhea while none of the subjects receiving ZIAGEN 300 mg twice daily had this event.

[b]CNA30024 was a multi-center, double-blind, controlled trial in which 649 HIV-1-infected, therapy-naive adults were randomized and received either ZIAGEN (300 mg twice daily), EPIVIR (150 mg twice daily), and efavirenz (600 mg once daily); or zidovudine (300 mg twice daily), EPIVIR (150 mg twice daily), and efavirenz (600 mg once daily). CNA30024 used double-blind ascertainment of suspected hypersensitivity reactions. During the blinded portion of the trial, suspected hypersensitivity to abacavir was reported by investigators in 9% of 324 patients in the abacavir group and 3% of 325 patients in the zidovudine group.

Laboratory Abnormalities: Laboratory abnormalities observed in clinical trials of ZIAGEN were anemia, neutropenia, liver function test abnormalities, and elevations of CPK, blood glucose, and triglycerides. Additional laboratory abnormalities observed in clinical trials of EPIVIR were thrombocytopenia and elevated levels of bilirubin, amylase, and lipase.

The frequencies of treatment-emergent laboratory abnormalities were comparable between treatment groups in CNA30021.

Other Adverse Events: In addition to adverse reactions listed above, other adverse events observed in the expanded access program for abacavir were pancreatitis and increased GGT.

6.2 Postmarketing Experience

In addition to adverse reactions reported from clinical trials, the following reactions have been identified during postmarketing use of abacavir, lamivudine, and/or EPZICOM. Because they are reported voluntarily from a population of unknown size, estimates of frequency cannot be made. These reactions have been chosen for inclusion due to a combination of their seriousness, frequency of reporting, or potential causal connection to abacavir, lamivudine, and/or EPZICOM.

Abacavir: Cardiovascular: Myocardial infarction.

Skin: Suspected Stevens-Johnson syndrome (SJS) and toxic epidermal necrolysis (TEN) have been reported in pa-

tients receiving abacavir primarily in combination with medications known to be associated with SJS and TEN, respectively. Because of the overlap of clinical signs and symptoms between hypersensitivity to abacavir and SJS and TEN, and the possibility of multiple drug sensitivities in some patients, abacavir should be discontinued and not restarted in such cases.

There have also been reports of erythema multiforme with abacavir use.

Abacavir and Lamivudine: Body as a Whole: Redistribution/accumulation of body fat [see Warnings and Precautions (5.6)].

Digestive: Stomatitis.

Endocrine and Metabolic: Hyperglycemia.

General: Weakness.

Hemic and Lymphatic: Aplastic anemia, anemia (including pure red cell aplasia and severe anemias progressing on therapy), lymphadenopathy, splenomegaly.

Hepatic: Lactic acidosis and hepatic steatosis [see Warnings and Precautions (5.2)], posttreatment exacerbation of hepatitis B [see Warnings and Precautions (5.3)].

Hypersensitivity: Sensitization reactions (including anaphylaxis), urticaria.

Musculoskeletal: Muscle weakness, CPK elevation, rhabdomyolysis.

Nervous: Paresthesia, peripheral neuropathy, seizures.

Respiratory: Abnormal breath sounds/wheezing.

Skin: Alopecia, erythema multiforme, Stevens-Johnson syndrome.

7 DRUG INTERACTIONS

- No drug interaction trials have been conducted using EPZICOM Tablets [see Clinical Pharmacology (12.3)].

7.1 Ethanol

Abacavir: Abacavir has no effect on the pharmacokinetic properties of ethanol. Ethanol decreases the elimination of abacavir causing an increase in overall exposure [see Clinical Pharmacology (12.3)].

7.2 Interferon- and Ribavirin-Based Regimens

Lamivudine: Although no evidence of a pharmacokinetic or pharmacodynamic interaction (e.g., loss of HIV-1/HCV virologic suppression) was seen when ribavirin was coadministered with lamivudine in HIV-1/HCV co-infected subjects, hepatic decompensation (some fatal) has occurred in HIV-1/HCV co-infected subjects receiving combination antiretroviral therapy for HIV-1 and interferon alfa with or without ribavirin [see Warnings and Precautions (5.4), Clinical Pharmacology (12.3)].

7.3 Methadone

Abacavir: The addition of methadone has no clinically significant effect on the pharmacokinetic properties of abacavir. In a trial of 11 HIV-1-infected subjects receiving methadone-maintenance therapy with 600 mg of ZIAGEN twice daily (twice the currently recommended dose), oral methadone clearance increased [see Clinical Pharmacology (12.3)]. This alteration will not result in a methadone dose modification in the majority of patients; however, an increased methadone dose may be required in a small number of patients.

7.4 Trimethoprim/Sulfamethoxazole (TMP/SMX)

Lamivudine: No change in dose of either drug is recommended [see Clinical Pharmacology (12.3)]. There is no information regarding the effect on lamivudine pharmacokinetics of higher doses of TMP/SMX such as those used to treat PCP.

8 USE IN SPECIFIC POPULATIONS

8.1 Pregnancy

EPZICOM: Pregnancy Category C. There are no adequate and well-controlled studies of EPZICOM in pregnant women. Reproduction studies with abacavir and lamivudine have been performed in animals (see Abacavir and Lamivudine sections below). EPZICOM should be used during pregnancy only if the potential benefits outweigh the risks.

Abacavir: Studies in pregnant rats showed that abacavir is transferred to the fetus through the placenta. Fetal malformations (increased incidences of fetal anasarca and skeletal malformations) and developmental toxicity (depressed fetal body weight and reduced crown-rump length) were observed in rats at a dose which produced 35 times the human exposure, based on AUC. Embryonic and fetal toxicities (increased resorptions, decreased fetal body weights) and toxicities to the offspring (increased incidence of stillbirth and lower body weights) occurred at half of the above-mentioned dose in separate fertility studies conducted in rats. In the rabbit, no developmental toxicity and no increases in fetal malformations occurred at doses that produced 8.5 times the human exposure at the recommended dose based on AUC.

Lamivudine: Studies in pregnant rats showed that lamivudine is transferred to the fetus through the placenta. Reproduction studies with orally administered lamivudine have been performed in rats and rabbits at doses producing

Table 2. Pharmacokinetic Parameters[a] for Abacavir and Lamivudine in Adults

Parameter	Abacavir		Lamivudine	
Oral bioavailability (%)	86 ± 25	n = 6	86 ± 16	n = 12
Apparent volume of distribution (L/kg)	0.86 ± 0.15	n = 6	1.3 ± 0.4	n = 20
Systemic clearance (L/hr/kg)	0.80 ± 0.24	n = 6	0.33 ± 0.06	n = 20
Renal clearance (L/hr/kg)	.007 ± .008	n = 6	0.22 ± 0.06	n = 20
Elimination half-life (hr)	1.45 ± 0.32	n = 20	5 to 7[b]	

[a]Data presented as mean ± standard deviation except where noted.

[b]Approximate range.

plasma levels up to approximately 35 times that for the recommended adult HIV dose. No evidence of teratogenicity due to lamivudine was observed. Evidence of early embryolethality was seen in the rabbit at exposure levels similar to those observed in humans, but there was no indication of this effect in the rat at exposure levels up to 35 times those in humans.

Antiretroviral Pregnancy Registry: To monitor maternal-fetal outcomes of pregnant women exposed to EPZICOM or other antiretroviral agents, an Antiretroviral Pregnancy Registry has been established. Physicians are encouraged to register patients by calling 1-800-258-4263.

8.3   Nursing Mothers

The Centers for Disease Control and Prevention recommend that HIV-1-infected mothers not breastfeed their infants to avoid risking postnatal transmission of HIV-1 infection.

Abacavir: Abacavir is secreted into the milk of lactating rats.

Lamivudine: Lamivudine is excreted in human breast milk and into the milk of lactating rats.

Because of both the potential for HIV-1 transmission and the potential for serious adverse reactions in nursing infants, mothers should be instructed not to breastfeed if they are receiving EPZICOM.

8.4   Pediatric Use

Safety and effectiveness of EPZICOM in pediatric patients have not been established. EPZICOM is not recommended for use in patients younger than 18 years because it cannot be dose adjusted.

8.5   Geriatric Use

Clinical trials of abacavir and lamivudine did not include sufficient numbers of subjects aged 65 and over to determine whether they respond differently from younger subjects. In general, dose selection for an elderly patient should be cautious, reflecting the greater frequency of decreased hepatic, renal, or cardiac function, and of concomitant disease or other drug therapy [see Dosage and Administration (2.2), Use in Specific Populations (8.6, 8.7)].

8.6   Patients With Impaired Renal Function

EPZICOM is not recommended for patients with impaired renal function (creatinine clearance <50 mL/min) because EPZICOM is a fixed-dose combination and the dosage of the individual components cannot be adjusted.

8.7   Patients With Impaired Hepatic Function

EPZICOM is contraindicated for patients with hepatic impairment because EPZICOM is a fixed-dose combination and the dosage of the individual components cannot be adjusted.

10   OVERDOSAGE

Abacavir: There is no known antidote for abacavir. It is not known whether abacavir can be removed by peritoneal dialysis or hemodialysis.

Lamivudine: One case of an adult ingesting 6 grams of lamivudine was reported; there were no clinical signs or symptoms noted and hematologic tests remained normal. It is not known whether lamivudine can be removed by peritoneal dialysis or hemodialysis.

11   DESCRIPTION

EPZICOM: EPZICOM Tablets contain the following 2 synthetic nucleoside analogues: abacavir sulfate (ZIAGEN, also a component of TRIZIVIR) and lamivudine (also known as EPIVIR or 3TC) with inhibitory activity against HIV-1. EPZICOM Tablets are for oral administration. Each orange, film-coated tablet contains the active ingredients 600 mg of abacavir as abacavir sulfate and 300 mg of lamivudine, and the inactive ingredients magnesium stearate, microcrystalline cellulose, and sodium starch glycolate. The tablets are coated with a film (OPADRY® orange YS-1-13065-A) that is made of FD&C Yellow No. 6, hypromellose, polyethylene glycol 400, polysorbate 80, and titanium dioxide.

Abacavir Sulfate: The chemical name of abacavir sulfate is (1S,cis)-4-[2-amino-6-(cyclopropylamino)-9H-purin-9-yl]-2-cyclopentene-1-methanol sulfate (salt) (2:1). Abacavir sulfate is the enantiomer with 1S, 4R absolute configuration

on the cyclopentene ring. It has a molecular formula of $(C_{14}H_{18}N_6O)_2 \cdot H_2SO_4$ and a molecular weight of 670.76 daltons. It has the following structural formula:

Abacavir sulfate is a white to off-white solid with a solubility of approximately 77 mg/mL in distilled water at 25°C. In vivo, abacavir sulfate dissociates to its free base, abacavir. All dosages for abacavir sulfate are expressed in terms of abacavir.

Lamivudine: The chemical name of lamivudine is (2R,cis)-4-amino-1-(2-hydroxymethyl-1,3-oxathiolan-5-yl)-(1H)-pyrimidin-2-one. Lamivudine is the (-)enantiomer of a dideoxy analogue of cytidine. Lamivudine has also been referred to as (-)2′,3′-dideoxy, 3′-thiacytidine. It has a molecular formula of $C_8H_{11}N_3O_3S$ and a molecular weight of 229.3 daltons. It has the following structural formula:

Lamivudine is a white to off-white crystalline solid with a solubility of approximately 70 mg/mL in water at 20°C.

12   CLINICAL PHARMACOLOGY

12.1   Mechanism of Action

EPZICOM is an antiviral agent [see Clinical Pharmacology (12.4)].

12.3   Pharmacokinetics

Pharmacokinetics in Adults: EPZICOM: In a single-dose, 3-way crossover bioavailability trial of 1 EPZICOM Tablet versus 2 ZIAGEN Tablets (2 × 300 mg) and 2 EPIVIR Tablets (2 × 150 mg) administered simultaneously in healthy subjects (n = 25), there was no difference in the extent of absorption, as measured by the area under the plasma concentration-time curve (AUC) and maximal peak concentration (C_{max}), of each component.

Abacavir: Following oral administration, abacavir is rapidly absorbed and extensively distributed. After oral administration of a single dose of 600 mg of abacavir in 20 subjects, C_{max} was 4.26 ± 1.19 mcg/mL (mean ± SD) and AUC_∞ was 11.95 ± 2.51 mcg•h/mL. Binding of abacavir to human plasma proteins is approximately 50% and was independent of concentration. Total blood and plasma drug-related radioactivity concentrations are identical, demonstrating that abacavir readily distributes into erythrocytes. The primary routes of elimination of abacavir are metabolism by alcohol dehydrogenase to form the 5′-carboxylic acid and glucuronyl transferase to form the 5′-glucuronide.

Lamivudine: Following oral administration, lamivudine is rapidly absorbed and extensively distributed. After multiple-dose oral administration of lamivudine 300 mg once daily for 7 days to 60 healthy subjects, steady-state C_{max} ($C_{max,ss}$) was 2.04 ± 0.54 mcg/mL (mean ± SD) and the 24-hour steady-state AUC ($AUC_{24,ss}$) was 8.87 ± 1.83 mcg•h/mL. Binding to plasma protein is low. Approximately 70% of an intravenous dose of lamivudine is recovered as unchanged drug in the urine. Metabolism of

lamivudine is a minor route of elimination. In humans, the only known metabolite is the trans-sulfoxide metabolite (approximately 5% of an oral dose after 12 hours).

The steady-state pharmacokinetic properties of the EPIVIR 300-mg tablet once daily for 7 days compared with the EPIVIR 150-mg tablet twice daily for 7 days were assessed in a crossover trial in 60 healthy subjects. EPIVIR 300 mg once daily resulted in lamivudine exposures that were similar to EPIVIR 150 mg twice daily with respect to plasma $AUC_{24,ss}$; however, $C_{max,ss}$ was 66% higher and the trough value was 53% lower compared with the 150-mg twice-daily regimen. Intracellular lamivudine triphosphate exposures in peripheral blood mononuclear cells were also similar with respect to $AUC_{24,ss}$ and $C_{max24,ss}$; however, trough values were lower compared with the 150-mg twice-daily regimen. Inter-subject variability was greater for intracellular lamivudine triphosphate concentrations versus lamivudine plasma trough concentrations. The clinical significance of observed differences for both plasma lamivudine concentrations and intracellular lamivudine triphosphate concentrations is not known.

In humans, abacavir and lamivudine are not significantly metabolized by cytochrome P450 enzymes.

The pharmacokinetic properties of abacavir and lamivudine in fasting subjects are summarized in Table 2.
[See table 2 above]

Effect of Food on Absorption of EPZICOM: EPZICOM may be administered with or without food. Administration with a high-fat meal in a single-dose bioavailability trial resulted in no change in AUC_{last}, AUC_∞, and C_{max} for lamivudine. Food did not alter the extent of systemic exposure to abacavir (AUC_∞), but the rate of absorption (C_{max}) was decreased approximately 24% compared with fasted conditions (n = 25). These results are similar to those from previous trials of the effect of food on abacavir and lamivudine tablets administered separately.

Special Populations: Renal Impairment: EPZICOM: Because lamivudine requires dose adjustment in the presence of renal insufficiency, EPZICOM is not recommended for use in patients with creatinine clearance <50 mL/min [see Dosage and Administration (2.2)].

Hepatic Impairment: EPZICOM: EPZICOM is contraindicated for patients with hepatic impairment because EPZICOM is a fixed-dose combination and the dosage of the individual components cannot be adjusted. Abacavir is contraindicated in patients with moderate to severe hepatic impairment, and dose reduction is required in patients with mild hepatic impairment.

Pregnancy: See Use in Specific Populations (8.1).

Abacavir and Lamivudine: No data are available on the pharmacokinetics of abacavir or lamivudine during pregnancy.

Nursing Mothers: See Use in Specific Populations (8.3).

Abacavir: No data are available on the pharmacokinetics of abacavir in nursing mothers.

Lamivudine: Samples of breast milk obtained from 20 mothers receiving lamivudine monotherapy (300 mg twice daily) or combination therapy (150 mg lamivudine twice daily and 300 mg zidovudine twice daily) had measurable concentrations of lamivudine.

Pediatric Patients: EPZICOM: The pharmacokinetics of EPZICOM in pediatric subjects are under investigation. There are insufficient data at this time to recommend a dose.

Geriatric Patients: The pharmacokinetics of abacavir and lamivudine have not been studied in subjects over 65 years of age.

Gender: Abacavir: A population pharmacokinetic analysis in HIV-1-infected male (n = 304) and female (n = 67) subjects showed no gender differences in abacavir AUC normalized for lean body weight.

Lamivudine: A pharmacokinetic trial in healthy male (n = 12) and female (n = 12) subjects showed no gender differences in lamivudine AUC normalized for body weight.

Race: Abacavir: There are no significant differences between blacks and Caucasians in abacavir pharmacokinetics.

Lamivudine: There are no significant racial differences in lamivudine pharmacokinetics.

Drug Interactions: The drug interactions described are based on trials conducted with the individual nucleoside analogues. In humans, abacavir and lamivudine are not significantly metabolized by cytochrome P450 enzymes nor do they inhibit or induce this enzyme system; therefore, it is unlikely that clinically significant drug interactions will occur with drugs metabolized through these pathways.

Abacavir: Lamivudine and Zidovudine: Fifteen HIV-1-infected subjects were enrolled in a crossover-designed drug interaction trial evaluating single doses of abacavir (600 mg), lamivudine (150 mg), and zidovudine (300 mg) alone or in combination. Analysis showed no clinically relevant changes in the pharmacokinetics of abacavir with the addition of lamivudine or zidovudine or the combination of lamivudine and zidovudine. Lamivudine exposure (AUC decreased 15%) and zidovudine exposure (AUC increased 10%) did not show clinically relevant changes with concurrent abacavir.

Methadone: In a trial of 11 HIV-1-infected subjects receiving methadone-maintenance therapy (40 mg and 90 mg daily), with 600 mg of ZIAGEN twice daily (twice the currently recommended dose), oral methadone clearance increased 22% (90% CI: 6% to 42%) *[see Drug Interactions (7.3)].*

Lamivudine: Zidovudine: No clinically significant alterations in lamivudine or zidovudine pharmacokinetics were observed in 12 asymptomatic HIV-1-infected adult subjects given a single dose of zidovudine (200 mg) in combination with multiple doses of lamivudine (300 mg q 12 hr).

Ribavirin: In vitro data indicate ribavirin reduces phosphorylation of lamivudine, stavudine, and zidovudine. However, no pharmacokinetic (e.g., plasma concentrations or intracellular triphosphorylated active metabolite concentrations) or pharmacodynamic (e.g., loss of HIV-1/HCV virologic suppression) interaction was observed when ribavirin and lamivudine (n = 18), stavudine (n = 10), or zidovudine (n = 6) were coadministered as part of a multi-drug regimen to HIV-1/HCV co-infected subjects *[see Warnings and Precautions (5.4)].*

The effects of other coadministered drugs on abacavir or lamivudine are provided in Table 3.

[See table 3 above]

12.4 Microbiology

Mechanism of Action: *Abacavir:* Abacavir is a carbocyclic synthetic nucleoside analogue. Abacavir is converted by cellular enzymes to the active metabolite, carbovir triphosphate (CBV-TP), an analogue of deoxyguanosine-5'-triphosphate (dGTP). CBV-TP inhibits the activity of HIV-1 reverse transcriptase (RT) both by competing with the natural substrate dGTP and by its incorporation into viral DNA. The lack of a 3'-OH group in the incorporated nucleotide analogue prevents the formation of the 5' to 3' phosphodiester linkage essential for DNA chain elongation, and therefore, the viral DNA growth is terminated. CBV-TP is a weak inhibitor of cellular DNA polymerases α, β, and γ.

Lamivudine: Lamivudine is a synthetic nucleoside analogue. Intracellularly lamivudine is phosphorylated to its active 5'-triphosphate metabolite, lamivudine triphosphate (3TC-TP). The principal mode of action of 3TC-TP is inhibition of RT via DNA chain termination after incorporation of the nucleotide analogue. CBV-TP and 3TC-TP are weak inhibitors of cellular DNA polymerases α, β, and γ.

Antiviral Activity: *Abacavir:* The antiviral activity of abacavir against HIV-1 was evaluated against a T-cell tropic laboratory strain HIV-1$_{IIIB}$ in lymphoblastic cell lines, a monocyte/macrophage tropic laboratory strain HIV-1$_{BaL}$ in primary monocytes/macrophages, and clinical isolates in peripheral blood mononuclear cells. The concentration of drug necessary to effect viral replication by 50 percent (EC$_{50}$) ranged from 3.7 to 5.8 μM (1 μM = 0.28 mcg/mL) and 0.07 to 1.0 μM against HIV-1$_{IIIB}$ and HIV-1$_{BaL}$, respectively, and was 0.26 ± 0.18 μM against 8 clinical isolates. The EC$_{50}$ values of abacavir against different HIV-1 clades (A-G) ranged from 0.0015 to 1.05 μM, and against HIV-2 isolates, from 0.024 to 0.49 μM. Ribavirin (50 μM) had no effect on the anti–HIV-1 activity of abacavir in cell culture.

Lamivudine: The antiviral activity of lamivudine against HIV-1 was assessed in a number of cell lines (including monocytes and fresh human peripheral blood lymphocytes) using standard susceptibility assays. EC$_{50}$ values were in the range of 0.003 to 15 μM (1 μM = 0.23 mcg/mL). HIV-1 from therapy-naive subjects with no amino acid substitutions associated with resistance gave median EC$_{50}$ values of 0.429 μM (range: 0.200 to 2.007 μM) from Virco (n = 92 baseline samples from COLA40263) and 2.35 μM (1.37 to 3.68 μM) from Monogram Biosciences (n = 135 baseline samples from ESS30009). The EC$_{50}$ values of lamivudine against different HIV-1 clades (A-G) ranged from 0.001 to 0.120 μM, and against HIV-2 isolates from 0.003 to 0.120 μM in peripheral blood mononuclear cells. Ribavirin (50 μM) decreased the anti–HIV-1 activity of lamivudine by 3.5 fold in MT-4 cells.

The combination of abacavir and lamivudine has demonstrated antiviral activity in cell culture against non-subtype B isolates and HIV-2 isolates with equivalent antiviral activity as for subtype B isolates. Abacavir/lamivudine had additive to synergistic activity in cell culture in combination with the nucleoside reverse transcriptase inhibitors (NRTIs) emtricitabine, stavudine, tenofovir, zalcitabine, zidovudine; the non-nucleoside reverse transcriptase inhibitors (NNRTIs) delavirdine, efavirenz, nevirapine; the protease inhibitors (PIs) amprenavir, indinavir, lopinavir, nelfinavir, ritonavir, saquinavir; or the fusion inhibitor, enfuvirtide. Ribavirin, used in combination with interferon for the treatment of HCV infection, decreased the anti-HIV-1 potency of abacavir/lamivudine reproducibly by 2- to 6-fold in cell culture.

Resistance: HIV-1 isolates with reduced susceptibility to the combination of abacavir and lamivudine have been selected in cell culture and have also been obtained from subjects failing abacavir/lamivudine-containing regimens. Genotypic characterization of abacavir/lamivudine-resistant viruses selected in cell culture identified amino acid substitutions M184V/I, K65R, L74V, and Y115F in HIV-1 RT. Genotypic analysis of isolates selected in cell culture and recovered from abacavir-treated subjects demonstrated that amino acid substitutions K65R, L74V, Y115F, and M184V/I in HIV-1 RT contributed to abacavir resistance. Genotypic analysis of isolates selected in cell culture and recovered from lamivudine-treated subjects showed that the resistance was due to a specific amino acid substitution in HIV-1 RT at codon 184 changing the methionine to either isoleucine or valine (M184V/I). In a trial of therapy-naive adults receiving ZIAGEN 600 mg once daily (n = 384) or 300 mg twice daily (n = 386) in a background regimen of lamivudine 300 mg and efavirenz 600 mg once daily (CNA30021), the incidence of virologic failure at 48 weeks was similar between the 2 groups (11% in both arms). Genotypic (n = 38) and phenotypic analyses (n = 35) of virologic failure isolates from this trial showed that the RT substitutions that emerged during abacavir/lamivudine once-daily and twice-daily therapy were K65R, L74V, Y115F, and M184V/I. The abacavir- and lamivudine-associated resistance substitution M184V/I was the most commonly observed substitution in virologic failure isolates from subjects receiving abacavir/lamivudine once daily (56%, 10/18) and twice daily (40%, 8/20).

Thirty-nine percent (7/18) of the isolates from subjects who experienced virologic failure in the abacavir once-daily arm had a >2.5-fold decrease in abacavir susceptibility with a median-fold decrease of 1.3 (range: 0.5 to 11) compared with 29% (5/17) of the failure isolates in the twice-daily arm with a median-fold decrease of 0.92 (range: 0.7 to 13). Fifty-six percent (10/18) of the virologic failure isolates in the once-daily abacavir group compared with 41% (7/17) of the failure isolates in the twice-daily abacavir group had a >2.5-fold decrease in lamivudine susceptibility with median-fold changes of 81 (range 0.79 to >116) and 1.1 (range 0.68 to >116) in the once-daily and twice-daily abacavir arms, respectively.

Cross-Resistance: Cross-resistance has been observed among NRTIs. Viruses containing abacavir and lamivudine resistance-associated amino acid substitutions, namely, K65R, L74V, M184V, and Y115F, exhibit cross-resistance to didanosine, emtricitabine, lamivudine, tenofovir, and zalcitabine in cell culture and in subjects. The K65R substitution can confer resistance to abacavir, didanosine, emtricitabine, lamivudine, stavudine, tenofovir, and zalcitabine; the L74V substitution can confer resistance to abacavir, didanosine, and zalcitabine; and the M184V substitution can confer resistance to abacavir, didanosine, emtricitabine, lamivudine, and zalcitabine.

The combination of abacavir/lamivudine has demonstrated decreased susceptibility to viruses with the substitutions K65R with or without the M184V/I substitution, viruses with L74V plus the M184V/I substitution, and viruses with thymidine analog mutations (TAMs: M41L, D67N, K70R, L210W, T215Y/F, K219 E/R/H/Q/N) plus M184V. An increasing number of TAMs is associated with a progressive reduction in abacavir susceptibility.

13 NONCLINICAL TOXICOLOGY

13.1 Carcinogenesis, Mutagenesis, Impairment of Fertility

Carcinogenicity: *Abacavir:* Abacavir was administered orally at 3 dosage levels to separate groups of mice and rats in 2-year carcinogenicity studies. Results showed an increase in the incidence of malignant and non-malignant tumors. Malignant tumors occurred in the preputial gland of males and the clitoral gland of females of both species, and in the liver of female rats. In addition, non-malignant tumors also occurred in the liver and thyroid gland of female rats. These observations were made at systemic exposures in the range of 6 to 32 times the human exposure at the recommended dose.

Lamivudine: Long-term carcinogenicity studies with lamivudine in mice and rats showed no evidence of carcinogenic potential at exposures up to 10 times (mice) and 58 times (rats) those observed in humans at the recommended therapeutic dose for HIV-1 infection.

It is not known how predictive the results of rodent carcinogenicity studies may be for humans.

Mutagenicity: *Abacavir:* Abacavir induced chromosomal aberrations both in the presence and absence of metabolic activation in an in vitro cytogenetic study in human lymphocytes. Abacavir was mutagenic in the absence of metabolic activation, although it was not mutagenic in the presence of metabolic activation in an L5178Y mouse lymphoma assay. Abacavir was clastogenic in males and not clastogenic in females in an in vivo mouse bone marrow micronucleus assay. Abacavir was not mutagenic in bacterial mutagenicity assays in the presence and absence of metabolic activation.

Lamivudine: Lamivudine was mutagenic in an L5178Y mouse lymphoma assay and clastogenic in a cytogenetic assay using cultured human lymphocytes. Lamivudine was not mutagenic in a microbial mutagenicity assay, in an in vitro cell transformation assay, in a rat micronucleus test, in a rat bone marrow cytogenetic assay, and in an assay for unscheduled DNA synthesis in rat liver.

Impairment of Fertility: Abacavir or lamivudine induced no adverse effects on the mating performance or fertility of male and female rats at doses producing systemic exposure levels approximately 8 or 130 times, respectively, higher than those in humans at the recommended dose based on body surface area comparisons.

13.2 Animal Toxicology and/or Pharmacology

Myocardial degeneration was found in mice and rats following administration of abacavir for 2 years. The systemic exposures were equivalent to 7 to 24 times the expected systemic exposure in humans. The clinical relevance of this finding has not been determined.

14 CLINICAL STUDIES

EPZICOM: There have been no clinical trials conducted with EPZICOM. One EPZICOM Tablet given once daily is an alternative regimen to EPIVIR Tablets 300 mg once daily plus ZIAGEN Tablets 2 × 300 mg once daily as a component of antiretroviral therapy.

The following trial was conducted with the individual components of EPZICOM.

Therapy-Naive Adults: CNA30021 was an international, multi-center, double-blind, controlled trial in which 770 HIV-1-infected, therapy-naive adults were randomized and received either ZIAGEN 600 mg once daily or ZIAGEN 300 mg twice daily, both in combination with EPIVIR 300 mg once daily and efavirenz 600 mg once daily. The double-blind treatment duration was at least 48 weeks.

Table 3. Effect of Coadministered Drugs on Abacavir and Lamivudine AUC

Note: ROUTINE DOSE MODIFICATION OF ABACAVIR AND LAMIVUDINE IS NOT WARRANTED WITH COADMINISTRATION OF THE FOLLOWING DRUGS.

Drugs That May Alter Abacavir Blood Concentrations					
Coadministered Drug and Dose	Abacavir Dose	n	Abacavir Concentrations		Concentration of Coadministered Drug
			AUC	Variability	
Ethanol 0.7 g/kg	Single 600 mg	24	↑41%	90% CI: 35% to 48%	↔

Drugs That May Alter Lamivudine Blood Concentrations					
Coadministered Drug and Dose	Lamivudine Dose	n	Lamivudine Concentrations		Concentration of Coadministered Drug
			AUC	Variability	
Nelfinavir 750 mg q 8 hr × 7 to 10 days	Single 150 mg	11	↑10%	95% CI: 1% to 20%	↔
Trimethoprim 160 mg/ Sulfamethoxazole 800 mg daily × 5 days	Single 300 mg	14	↑43%	90% CI: 32% to 55%	↔

↑ = Increase; ↔ = no significant change; AUC = area under the concentration versus time curve; CI = confidence interval.

Trial participants had a mean age of 37 years; were male (81%), Caucasian (54%), black (27%), and American Hispanic (15%). The median baseline CD4+ cell count was 262 cells/mm^3 (range: 21 to 918 cells/mm^3) and the median baseline plasma HIV-1 RNA was 4.89 log$_{10}$ copies/mL (range: 2.60 to 6.99 log$_{10}$ copies/mL).

The outcomes of randomized treatment are provided in Table 4.

Table 4. Outcomes of Randomized Treatment Through Week 48 (CNA30021)

Outcome	ZIAGEN 600 mg q.d. plus EPIVIR plus Efavirenz (n = 384)	ZIAGEN 300 mg b.i.d. plus EPIVIR plus Efavirenz (n = 386)
Responder[a]	64% (71%)	65% (72%)
Virologic failure[b]	11% (5%)	11% (5%)
Discontinued due to adverse reactions	13%	11%
Discontinued due to other reasons[c]	11%	13%

[a]Subjects achieved and maintained confirmed HIV-1 RNA <50 copies/mL (<400 copies/mL) through Week 48 (Roche AMPLICOR Ultrasensitive HIV-1 MONITOR® standard test version 1.0).

[b]Includes viral rebound, failure to achieve confirmed <50 copies/mL (<400 copies/mL) by Week 48, and insufficient viral load response.

[c]Includes consent withdrawn, lost to follow-up, protocol violations, clinical progression, and other.

After 48 weeks of therapy, the median CD4+ cell count increases from baseline were 188 cells/mm^3 in the group receiving ZIAGEN once daily and 200 cells/mm^3 in the group receiving ZIAGEN 300 mg twice daily. Through Week 48, 6 subjects (2%) in the group receiving ZIAGEN 600 mg once daily (4 CDC classification C events and 2 deaths) and 10 subjects (3%) in the group receiving ZIAGEN 300 mg twice daily (7 CDC classification C events and 3 deaths) experienced clinical disease progression. None of the deaths were attributed to trial medications.

15　REFERENCES

1. Data Collection on Adverse Events of Anti-HIV Drugs (D:A:D) Study Group. *Lancet.* 2008;371 (9622):1417-1426.

16　HOW SUPPLIED/STORAGE AND HANDLING

EPZICOM is available as tablets. Each tablet contains 600 mg of abacavir as abacavir sulfate and 300 mg of lamivudine. The tablets are orange, film-coated, modified capsule-shaped, and debossed with GS FC2 on one side with no markings on the reverse side. They are packaged as follows:

Bottles of 30 Tablets (NDC 49702-206-13).

Store at 25°C (77°F); excursions permitted to 15° to 30°C (59° to 86°F) (see USP Controlled Room Temperature).

17　PATIENT COUNSELING INFORMATION

See FDA-approved patient labeling (Medication Guide)

Hypersensitivity Reaction:　Inform patients:

- that a Medication Guide and Warning Card summarizing the symptoms of the abacavir hypersensitivity reaction and other product information will be dispensed by the pharmacist with each new prescription and refill of EPZICOM, and encourage the patient to read the Medication Guide and Warning Card every time to obtain any new information that may be present about EPZICOM. (The complete text of the Medication Guide is reprinted at the end of this document.)
- to carry the Warning Card with them.
- how to identify a hypersensitivity reaction [see Warnings and Precautions (5.1), Medication Guide].
- that if they develop symptoms consistent with a hypersensitivity reaction they should call their doctor right away to determine if they should stop taking EPZICOM.
- that a hypersensitivity reaction can worsen and lead to hospitalization or death if EPZICOM is not immediately discontinued.
- that in one study, more severe hypersensitivity reactions were seen when ZIAGEN was dosed 600 mg once daily.
- to not restart EPZICOM or any other abacavir-containing product following a hypersensitivity reaction because more severe symptoms can occur within hours and may include life-threatening hypotension and death.
- that a hypersensitivity reaction is usually reversible if it is detected promptly and EPZICOM is stopped right away.
- that if they have interrupted EPZICOM for reasons other than symptoms of hypersensitivity (for example, those

who have an interruption in drug supply), a serious or fatal hypersensitivity reaction may occur with reintroduction of abacavir.

- to not restart EPZICOM or any other abacavir-containing product without medical consultation and that restarting abacavir needs to be undertaken only if medical care can be readily accessed by the patient or others.
- EPZICOM should not be administered concomitantly with ATRIPLA, COMBIVIR, COMPLERA, EMTRIVA, EPIVIR, EPIVIR-HBV, TRIZIVIR, TRUVADA, or ZIAGEN.

Lactic Acidosis/Hepatomegaly:　Inform patients that some HIV medicines, including EPZICOM, can cause a rare, but serious condition called lactic acidosis with liver enlargement (hepatomegaly) [see Warnings and Precautions (5.2)].

HIV-1/ HBV Co-infection:　Patients co-infected with HIV-1 and HBV should be informed that deterioration of liver disease has occurred in some cases when treatment with lamivudine was discontinued. Patients should be advised to discuss any changes in regimen with their physician [see Warnings and Precautions (5.3)].

HIV-1/HCV Co-Infection:　Patients with HIV-1/HCV co-infection should be informed that hepatic decompensation (some fatal) has occurred in HIV-1/HCV co-infected patients receiving combination antiretroviral therapy for HIV-1 and interferon alfa with or without ribavirin [see Warnings and Precautions (5.4)].

Redistribution/Accumulation of Body Fat:　Inform patients that redistribution or accumulation of body fat may occur in patients receiving antiretroviral therapy and that the cause and long-term health effects of these conditions are not known at this time [see Warnings and Precautions (5.6)].

Information About HIV-1 Infection:　EPZICOM is not a cure for HIV-1 infection and patients may continue to experience illnesses associated with HIV-1 infection, including opportunistic infections. Patients should remain under the care of a physician when using EPZICOM.

Patients should be advised to avoid doing things that can spread HIV-1 infection to others.

- Do not share needles or other injection equipment.
- Do not share personal items that can have blood or body fluids on them, like toothbrushes and razor blades.
- Do not have any kind of sex without protection. Always practice safe sex by using a latex or polyurethane condom to lower the chance of sexual contact with semen, vaginal secretions, or blood.
- Do not breastfeed. Lamivudine is excreted in human breast milk. It is not known if abacavir can be passed to your baby in your breast milk and whether it could harm your baby. Also, mothers with HIV-1 should not breastfeed because HIV-1 can be passed to the baby in the breast milk.

Patients should be informed to take all HIV medications exactly as prescribed.

COMBIVIR, EPIVIR, EPZICOM, TRIZIVIR, and ZIAGEN are registered trademarks of ViiV Healthcare.

The other brands listed are trademarks of their respective owners and are not trademarks of ViiV Healthcare. The makers of these brands are not affiliated with and do not endorse ViiV Healthcare or its products.

Manufactured for:

ViiV Healthcare
Research Triangle Park, NC 27709

by:

GlaxoSmithKline
Research Triangle Park, NC 27709

Lamivudine is manufactured under agreement from

Shire Pharmaceuticals Group plc
Basingstoke, UK

©2013, ViiV Healthcare. All rights reserved.

EPZ:9PI

MEDICATION GUIDE

EPZICOM® (ep' zih com)

(abacavir sulfate and lamivudine)

Tablets

Read this Medication Guide before you start taking EPZICOM and each time you get a refill. There may be new information. This information does not take the place of talking to your healthcare provider about your medical condition or your treatment. Be sure to carry your EPZICOM Warning Card with you at all times.

What is the most important information I should know about EPZICOM?

1. Serious allergic reaction (hypersensitivity reaction). EPZICOM contains abacavir (also contained in ZIAGEN® and TRIZIVIR®). Patients taking EPZICOM may have a serious allergic reaction (hypersensitivity reaction) that can cause death. Your risk of this allergic reaction is much higher if you have a gene variation called HLA-B*5701. Your healthcare provider can determine with a blood test if you have this gene variation.

If you get a symptom from 2 or more of the following groups while taking EPZICOM, call your healthcare provider right away to find out if you should stop taking EPZICOM.

	Symptom(s)
Group 1	Fever
Group 2	Rash
Group 3	Nausea, vomiting, diarrhea, abdominal (stomach area) pain
Group 4	Generally ill feeling, extreme tiredness, or achiness
Group 5	Shortness of breath, cough, sore throat

A list of these symptoms is on the Warning Card your pharmacist gives you. **Carry this Warning Card with you at all times.**

If you stop EPZICOM because of an allergic reaction, never take EPZICOM (abacavir sulfate and lamivudine) or any other abacavir-containing medicine (ZIAGEN and TRIZIVIR) again. If you take EPZICOM or any other abacavir-containing medicine again after you have had an allergic reaction, **within hours** you may get **life-threatening symptoms** that may include **very low blood pressure** or **death.** If you stop EPZICOM for any other reason, even for a few days, and you are not allergic to EPZICOM, talk with your healthcare provider before taking it again. Taking EPZICOM again can cause a serious allergic or life-threatening reaction, even if you never had an allergic reaction to it before.

If your healthcare provider tells you that you can take EPZICOM again, start taking it when you are around medical help or people who can call a healthcare provider if you need one.

2. Lactic Acidosis (buildup of acid in the blood). Some human immunodeficiency virus (HIV) medicines, including EPZICOM, can cause a rare but serious condition called lactic acidosis. Lactic acidosis is a serious medical emergency that can cause death and must be treated in the hospital. Call your healthcare provider right away if you get any of the following signs or symptoms of lactic acidosis:

- you feel very weak or tired
- you have unusual (not normal) muscle pain
- you have trouble breathing
- you have stomach pain with nausea and vomiting
- you feel cold, especially in your arms and legs
- you feel dizzy or light-headed
- you have a fast or irregular heartbeat

3. Serious liver problems. Some people who have taken medicines like EPZICOM have developed serious liver problems called hepatotoxicity, with liver enlargement (hepatomegaly) and fat in the liver (steatosis). Hepatomegaly with steatosis is a serious medical emergency that can cause death.

Call your healthcare provider right away if you get any of the following signs or symptoms of liver problems:

- your skin or the white part of your eyes turns yellow (jaundice)
- your urine turns dark
- your bowel movements (stools) turn light in color
- you don't feel like eating food for several days or longer
- you feel sick to your stomach (nausea)
- you have lower stomach area (abdominal) pain

You may be more likely to get lactic acidosis or serious liver problems if you are female, very overweight, or have been taking nucleoside analogue medicines for a long time.

4. Use with interferon and ribavirin-based regimens. Worsening of liver disease (sometimes resulting in death) has occurred in patients infected with both HIV and hepatitis C virus who are taking anti-HIV medicines and are also being treated for hepatitis C with interferon with or without ribavirin. If you are taking EPZICOM as well as interferon with or without ribavirin and you experience side effects, be sure to tell your healthcare provider.

5. If you have HIV and hepatitis B virus infection, your hepatitis B virus infection may get worse if you stop taking EPZICOM.

- Take EPZICOM exactly as prescribed.
- Do not run out of EPZICOM.
- Do not stop EPZICOM without talking to your healthcare provider.

Your healthcare provider should monitor your health and do regular blood tests to check your liver if you stop taking EPZICOM.

What is EPZICOM?

EPZICOM is a prescription medicine used to treat HIV infection. EPZICOM contains 2 medicines: abacavir (ZIAGEN) and lamivudine or 3TC (EPIVIR®). Both of these medicines are called nucleoside analogue reverse transcriptase inhibitors (NRTIs). When used together, they help lower the amount of HIV in your blood.

- **EPZICOM does not cure HIV infection or AIDS.**
- It is not known if EPZICOM will help you live longer or have fewer of the medical problems that people get with HIV or AIDS.
- It is very important that you see your healthcare provider regularly while you are taking EPZICOM.
- It is not known if EPZICOM is safe or effective in children under the age of 18.

Who should not take EPZICOM?

Do not take EPZICOM if you:

- are allergic to abacavir or any of the ingredients in EPZICOM. See the end of this Medication Guide for a complete list of ingredients in EPZICOM.
- have certain liver problems.

What should I tell my healthcare provider before taking EPZICOM?

Before you take EPZICOM tell your healthcare provider if you:

- **have been tested and know whether or not you have a particular gene variation called HLA-B*5701.**
- **have hepatitis B virus infection or have other liver problems.**
- **have kidney problems.**
- **have heart problems, smoke, or have diseases that increase your risk of heart disease such as high blood pressure, high cholesterol, or diabetes.**
- **are pregnant or plan to become pregnant.** It is not known if EPZICOM will harm your unborn baby. Talk to your healthcare provider if you are pregnant or plan to become pregnant.

Pregnancy Registry. If you take EPZICOM while you are pregnant, talk to your healthcare provider about how you can take part in the Pregnancy Registry for EPZICOM. The purpose of the pregnancy registry is to collect information about the health of you and your baby.

- **are breastfeeding or plan to breastfeed. Do not breastfeed.** Lamivudine is excreted in human breast milk. We do not know if abacavir can be passed to your baby in your breast milk and whether it could harm your baby. Also, mothers with HIV-1 should not breastfeed because HIV-1 can be passed to the baby in the breast milk.

Tell your healthcare provider about all the medicines you take, including prescription and nonprescription medicines, vitamins, and herbal supplements.

Especially tell your healthcare provider if you take:

- alcohol
- medicines used to treat hepatitis viruses such as interferon or ribavirin.
- methadone
- ATRIPLA® (efavirenz/emtricitabine/tenofovir disoproxil fumarate)
- COMBIVIR® (lamivudine and zidovudine)
- COMPLERA™ (emtricitabine/rilpivirine/tenofovir disoproxil fumarate)
- EMTRIVA® (emtricitabine)
- EPIVIR or EPIVIR-HBV® (lamivudine)
- TRIZIVIR (abacavir sulfate, lamivudine, and zidovudine)
- TRUVADA® (emtricitabine/tenofovir disoproxil fumarate)
- ZIAGEN (abacavir sulfate)

Ask your healthcare provider if you are not sure if you take one of the medicines listed above.

EPZICOM may affect the way other medicines work, and other medicines may affect how EPZICOM works.

Know the medicines you take. Keep a list of your medicines with you to show to your healthcare provider and pharmacist when you get a new medicine.

How should I take EPZICOM?

- **Take EPZICOM exactly as your healthcare provider tells you to take it.**
- EPZICOM may be taken with or without food.
- Do not skip doses.
- **Do not let your EPZICOM run out.**

If you stop your anti-HIV medicines, even for a short time, the amount of virus in your blood may increase and the virus may become harder to treat. If you take too much EPZICOM, call your healthcare provider or poison control center or go to the nearest hospital emergency room right away

What are the possible side effects of EPZICOM?

- **EPZICOM can cause serious side effects including allergic reactions, lactic acidosis, and liver problems. See "What is the most important information I should know about EPZICOM?"**
- **Changes in immune system (Immune Reconstitution Syndrome).** Your immune system may get stronger and begin to fight infections that have been hidden in your body for a long time. Tell your healthcare provider if you start having new or worse symptoms of infection after you start taking EPZICOM.
- **Changes in body fat (fat redistribution).** Changes in body fat (lipoatrophy or lipodystrophy) can happen in some people taking antiretroviral medicines including EPZICOM. These changes may include:

- more fat in or around your trunk, upper back and neck (buffalo hump), breast, or chest
- loss of fat in your legs, arms, or face
- **Heart attack (myocardial infarction).** Some HIV medicines including EPZICOM may increase your risk of heart attack.

The most common side effects of EPZICOM include:

- trouble sleeping
- depression
- headache
- tiredness
- dizziness
- nausea
- diarrhea
- rash
- fever

Tell your healthcare provider if you have any side effect that bothers you or that does not go away.

These are not all the possible side effects of EPZICOM. For more information, ask your healthcare provider or pharmacist.

Call your doctor for medical advice about side effects. You may report side effects to FDA at 1-800-FDA-1088.

How should I store EPZICOM?

Store EPZICOM at 59°F to 86°F (15°C to 30°C).

Keep EPZICOM and all medicines out of the reach of children.

General information for safe and effective use of EPZICOM.

Avoid doing things that can spread HIV infection to others.

- **Do not share needles or other injection equipment.**
- **Do not share personal items that can have blood or body fluids on them, like toothbrushes and razor blades.**
- **Do not have any kind of sex without protection.** Always practice safe sex by using a latex or polyurethane condom to lower the chance of sexual contact with semen, vaginal secretions, or blood.

Medicines are sometimes prescribed for purposes other than those listed in a Medication Guide. Do not use EPZICOM for a condition for which it was not prescribed. Do not give EPZICOM to other people, even if they have the same symptoms that you have. It may harm them.

This Medication Guide summarizes the most important information about EPZICOM. If you would like more information, talk with your healthcare provider. You can ask your healthcare provider or pharmacist for the information about EPZICOM that is written for health professionals.

For more information go to www.EPZICOM.com or call 1-877-844-8872.

What are the ingredients in EPZICOM?

Active ingredients: abacavir sulfate and lamivudine

Inactive ingredients: magnesium stearate, microcrystalline cellulose, sodium starch glycolate, and OPADRY® orange YS-1-13065-A, a film coating made of FD&C Yellow No. 6, hypromellose, polyethylene glycol 400, polysorbate 80, and titanium dioxide.

This Medication Guide has been approved by the US Food and Drug Administration.

COMBIVIR, EPIVIR, EPZICOM, TRIZIVIR, and ZIAGEN are registered trademarks of ViiV Healthcare.

The brands listed are trademarks of their respective owners and are not trademarks of ViiV Healthcare. The makers of these brands are not affiliated with and do not endorse ViiV Healthcare or its products.

Manufactured for:

ViiV Healthcare

Research Triangle Park, NC 27709

by:

GlaxoSmithKline

Research Triangle Park, NC 27709

Lamivudine is manufactured under agreement from

Shire Pharmaceuticals Group plc

Basingstoke, UK

©2012, ViiV Healthcare. All rights reserved.

May 2012

EPZ:8MG

LEXIVA   ℞

[lex-EE-vah]

(fosamprenavir calcium)

Tablets, for oral use

LEXIVA

(fosamprenavir calcium)

Oral Suspension

HIGHLIGHTS OF PRESCRIBING INFORMATION

These highlights do not include all the information needed to use LEXIVA safely and effectively. See full prescribing information for LEXIVA.

LEXIVA (fosamprenavir calcium) Tablets, for oral use
LEXIVA (fosamprenavir calcium) Oral Suspension
Initial U.S. Approval: 2003

---INDICATIONS AND USAGE---

LEXIVA is an HIV protease inhibitor indicated in combination with other antiretroviral agents for the treatment of HIV-1 infection. (1)

---DOSAGE AND ADMINISTRATION---

- Therapy-Naive Adults: LEXIVA 1,400 mg twice daily; LEXIVA 1,400 mg once daily plus ritonavir 200 mg once daily; LEXIVA 1,400 mg once daily plus ritonavir 100 mg once daily; LEXIVA 700 mg twice daily plus ritonavir 100 mg twice daily. (2.1)
- Protease Inhibitor-Experienced Adults: LEXIVA 700 mg twice daily plus ritonavir 100 mg twice daily. (2.1)
- Pediatric Patients (aged at least 4 weeks to 18 years): Dosage should be calculated based on body weight (kg) and should not exceed adult dose. (2.2)
- Hepatic Impairment: Recommended adjustments for patients with mild, moderate, or severe hepatic impairment. (2.3)

Dosing Considerations

- LEXIVA Tablets may be taken with or without food. (2)
- LEXIVA Suspension: Adults should take without food; pediatric patients should take with food. (2)

---DOSAGE FORMS AND STRENGTHS---

700 mg tablets and 50 mg per mL oral suspension (3)

---CONTRAINDICATIONS---

- Hypersensitivity to LEXIVA or amprenavir (e.g., Stevens-Johnson syndrome). (4)
- Drugs highly dependent on CYP3A4 for clearance and for which elevated plasma levels may result in serious and/or life-threatening events. (4)
- Review ritonavir contraindications when used in combination. (4)

---WARNINGS AND PRECAUTIONS---

- Certain drugs should not be coadministered with LEXIVA due to risk of serious or life-threatening adverse reactions. (5.1)
- LEXIVA should be discontinued for severe skin reactions including Stevens-Johnson syndrome. (5.2)
- LEXIVA should be used with caution in patients with a known sulfonamide allergy. (5.3)
- Use of higher than approved doses may lead to transaminase elevations. Patients with hepatitis B or C are at increased risk of transaminase elevations. (5.4)
- Patients receiving LEXIVA may develop new onset or exacerbations of diabetes mellitus, hyperglycemia (5.5), immune reconstitution syndrome (5.6), redistribution/accumulation of body fat (5.7), and elevated triglyceride and cholesterol concentrations (5.8). Monitor cholesterol and triglycerides prior to therapy and periodically thereafter.
- Acute hemolytic anemia has been reported with amprenavir. (5.9)
- Hemophilia: Spontaneous bleeding may occur, and additional factor VIII may be required. (5.10)
- Nephrolithiasis: Cases of nephrolithiasis have been reported with fosamprenavir. (5.11)

---ADVERSE REACTIONS---

- In adults the most common adverse reactions (incidence greater than or equal to 4%) are diarrhea, rash, nausea, vomiting, headache. (6.1)
- Vomiting and neutropenia were more frequent in pediatrics than in adults. (6.1)

To report SUSPECTED ADVERSE REACTIONS, contact ViiV Healthcare at 1-877-844-8872 or FDA at 1-800-FDA-1088 or www.fda.gov/medwatch.

---DRUG INTERACTIONS---

- Coadministration of LEXIVA with drugs that induce CYP3A4 may decrease amprenavir (active metabolite) concentrations leading to potential loss of virologic activity. (7, 12.3)
- Coadministration with drugs that inhibit CYP3A4 may increase amprenavir concentrations. (7, 12.3)
- Coadministration of LEXIVA and ritonavir may result in clinically significant interactions with drugs metabolized by CYP2D6. (7)

See 17 for PATIENT COUNSELING INFORMATION and FDA-approved patient labeling

Revised: 04/2013

FULL PRESCRIBING INFORMATION: CONTENTS*

Table 2. Drugs Contraindicated With LEXIVA. (Information in the table applies to LEXIVA with or without ritonavir, unless otherwise indicated.)

Drug Class/Drug Name	Clinical Comment
Alpha 1-adrenoreceptor antagonist: Alfuzosin	Potentially increased alfuzosin concentrations can result in hypotension.
Antiarrhythmics: Flecainide, propafenone	POTENTIAL for serious and/or life-threatening reactions such as cardiac arrhythmias secondary to increases in plasma concentrations of antiarrhythmics if LEXIVA is co-prescribed with **ritonavir**.
Antimycobacterials: Rifampin[a]	May lead to loss of virologic response and possible resistance to LEXIVA or to the class of protease inhibitors.
Ergot derivatives: Dihydroergotamine, ergonovine, ergotamine, methylergonovine	POTENTIAL for serious and/or life-threatening reactions such as acute ergot toxicity characterized by peripheral vasospasm and ischemia of the extremities and other tissues.
GI motility agents: Cisapride	POTENTIAL for serious and/or life-threatening reactions such as cardiac arrhythmias.
Herbal products: St. John's wort (*Hypericum perforatum*)	May lead to loss of virologic response and possible resistance to LEXIVA or to the class of protease inhibitors.
HMG co-reductase inhibitors: Lovastatin, simvastatin	POTENTIAL for serious reactions such as risk of myopathy including rhabdomyolysis.
Neuroleptic: Pimozide	POTENTIAL for serious and/or life-threatening reactions such as cardiac arrhythmias.
Non-nucleoside reverse transcriptase inhibitor: Delavirdine[a]	May lead to loss of virologic response and possible resistance to delavirdine.
PDE5 inhibitor: Sildenafil (REVATIO®) (for treatment of pulmonary arterial hypertension)	A safe and effective dose has not been established when used with LEXIVA. There is increased potential for sildenafil-associated adverse events (which include visual disturbances, hypotension, prolonged erection, and syncope).
Sedative/hypnotics: Midazolam, triazolam	POTENTIAL for serious and/or life-threatening reactions such as prolonged or increased sedation or respiratory depression.

[a] See Clinical Pharmacology (12.3) Tables 10, 11, 12, or 13 for magnitude of interaction.

Table 3. Selected Moderate/Severe Clinical Adverse Reactions Reported in Greater Than or Equal to 2% of Antiretroviral-Naive Adult Subjects

Adverse Reaction	APV30001[a]		APV30002[a]	
	LEXIVA 1,400 mg b.i.d. (n = 166)	Nelfinavir 1,250 mg b.i.d. (n = 83)	LEXIVA 1,400 mg q.d./ Ritonavir 200 mg q.d. (n = 322)	Nelfinavir 1,250 mg b.i.d. (n = 327)
Gastrointestinal				
Diarrhea	5%	18%	10%	18%
Nausea	7%	4%	7%	5%
Vomiting	2%	4%	6%	4%
Abdominal pain	1%	0%	2%	2%
Skin				
Rash	8%	2%	3%	2%
General disorders				
Fatigue	2%	1%	4%	2%
Nervous system				
Headache	2%	4%	3%	3%

[a]All subjects also received abacavir and lamivudine twice daily.

FULL PRESCRIBING INFORMATION

1 INDICATIONS AND USAGE

LEXIVA® is indicated in combination with other antiretroviral agents for the treatment of human immunodeficiency virus (HIV-1) infection.

The following points should be considered when initiating therapy with LEXIVA plus ritonavir in protease inhibitor-experienced patients:

- The protease inhibitor-experienced patient trial was not large enough to reach a definitive conclusion that LEXIVA plus ritonavir and lopinavir plus ritonavir are clinically equivalent [see Clinical Studies (14.2)].
- Once-daily administration of LEXIVA plus ritonavir is not recommended for adult protease inhibitor-experienced patients or any pediatric patients [see Dosage and Administration (2.1, 2.2), Clinical Studies (14.2, 14.3)].
- Dosing of LEXIVA plus ritonavir is not recommended for protease inhibitor-experienced pediatric patients younger than 6 months [see Clinical Pharmacology (12.3)].

2 DOSAGE AND ADMINISTRATION

LEXIVA Tablets may be taken with or without food. Adults should take LEXIVA Oral Suspension without food. Pediatric patients should take LEXIVA Oral Suspension with food [see Clinical Pharmacology (12.3)]. If emesis occurs within 30 minutes after dosing, re-dosing of LEXIVA Oral Suspension should occur.

Higher-than-approved dose combinations of LEXIVA plus ritonavir are not recommended due to an increased risk of transaminase elevations [see Overdosage (10)].

When LEXIVA is used in combination with ritonavir, prescribers should consult the full prescribing information for ritonavir.

2.1 Adults

Therapy-Naive Adults:

- LEXIVA 1,400 mg twice daily (without ritonavir).
- LEXIVA 1,400 mg once daily plus ritonavir 200 mg once daily.
- LEXIVA 1,400 mg once daily plus ritonavir 100 mg once daily.
  ◦ Dosing of LEXIVA 1,400 mg once daily plus ritonavir 100 mg once daily is supported by pharmacokinetic data [see Clinical Pharmacology (12.3)].
- LEXIVA 700 mg twice daily plus ritonavir 100 mg twice daily.
  ◦ Dosing of LEXIVA 700 mg twice daily plus 100 mg ritonavir twice daily is supported by pharmacokinetic and safety data [see Clinical Pharmacology (12.3)].

Protease Inhibitor-Experienced Adults:

- LEXIVA 700 mg twice daily plus ritonavir 100 mg twice daily.

2.2 Pediatric Patients (Aged at Least 4 Weeks to 18 Years)

The recommended dosage of LEXIVA in patients aged at least 4 weeks to 18 years should be calculated based on body weight (kg) and should not exceed the recommended adult dose (Table 1).

Table 1. Twice-Daily Dosage Regimens by Weight for Protease Inhibitor-Naive Pediatric Patients (Greater Than or Equal to 4 Weeks of Age) and for Protease Inhibitor-Experienced Pediatric Patients (Greater Than or Equal to 6 Months of Age) Using LEXIVA Oral Suspension With Concurrent Ritonavir

Weight	Twice-Daily Dosage Regimen
<11 kg	LEXIVA 45 mg/kg plus ritonavir 7 mg/kg[a]
11 kg - <15 kg	LEXIVA 30 mg/kg plus ritonavir 3 mg/kg[a]
15 kg - <20 kg	LEXIVA 23 mg/kg plus ritonavir 3 mg/kg[a]
≥20 kg	LEXIVA 18 mg/kg plus ritonavir 3 mg/kg[a]

[a]When dosing with ritonavir, do not exceed the adult dose of LEXIVA 700 mg/ritonavir 100 mg twice-daily dose.

Alternatively, protease inhibitor-naive children aged 2 years and older can be administered LEXIVA (without ritonavir) 30 mg per kg twice daily.

LEXIVA should only be administered to infants born at 38 weeks gestation or greater and who have attained a postnatal age of 28 days.

For pediatric patients, pharmacokinetic and clinical data:

- do not support once-daily dosing of LEXIVA alone or in combination with ritonavir [see Clinical Studies (14.3)].

- do not support administration of LEXIVA alone or in combination with ritonavir for protease inhibitor–experienced children younger than 6 months *[see Clinical Pharmacology (12.3)]*.
- do not support twice-daily dosing of LEXIVA without ritonavir in pediatric patients younger than 2 years *[see Clinical Pharmacology (12.3)]*.

Other Dosing Considerations:
- When administered without ritonavir, the adult regimen of LEXIVA Tablets 1,400 mg twice daily may be used for pediatric patients weighing at least 47 kg.
- When administered in combination with ritonavir, LEXIVA Tablets may be used for pediatric patients weighing at least 39 kg; ritonavir capsules may be used for pediatric patients weighing at least 33 kg.

2.3 Patients With Hepatic Impairment
See Clinical Pharmacology (12.3).
Mild Hepatic Impairment (Child-Pugh Score Ranging From 5 to 6): LEXIVA should be used with caution at a reduced dosage of 700 mg twice daily without ritonavir (therapy-naive) or 700 mg twice daily plus ritonavir 100 mg once daily (therapy-naive or protease inhibitor-experienced).
Moderate Hepatic Impairment (Child-Pugh Score Ranging From 7 to 9): LEXIVA should be used with caution at a reduced dosage of 700 mg twice daily without ritonavir (therapy-naive), or 450 mg twice daily plus ritonavir 100 mg once daily (therapy-naive or protease inhibitor-experienced).
Severe Hepatic Impairment (Child-Pugh Score Ranging From 10 to 15): LEXIVA should be used with caution at a reduced dosage of 350 mg twice daily without ritonavir (therapy-naive) or 300 mg twice daily plus ritonavir 100 mg once daily (therapy-naive or protease inhibitor-experienced).
There are no data to support dosing recommendations for pediatric patients with hepatic impairment.

3 DOSAGE FORMS AND STRENGTHS
LEXIVA Tablets, 700 mg, are pink, film-coated, capsule-shaped, biconvex tablets with "GX LL7" debossed on one face.
LEXIVA Oral Suspension, 50 mg per mL, is a white to off-white suspension that has a characteristic grape-bubblegum-peppermint flavor.

4 CONTRAINDICATIONS
LEXIVA is contraindicated:
- in patients with previously demonstrated clinically significant hypersensitivity (e.g., Stevens-Johnson syndrome) to any of the components of this product or to amprenavir.
- when coadministered with drugs that are highly dependent on cytochrome P450 3A4 (CYP3A4) for clearance and for which elevated plasma concentrations are associated with serious and/or life-threatening events (Table 2).
[See table 2 at top of previous page]
- when coadministered with ritonavir in patients receiving the antiarrhythmic agents, flecainide and propafenone. If LEXIVA is coadministered with ritonavir, reference should be made to the full prescribing information for ritonavir for additional contraindications.

5 WARNINGS AND PRECAUTIONS
5.1 Drug Interactions
See Table 2 for listings of drugs that are contraindicated due to potentially life-threatening adverse events, significant drug interactions, or loss of virologic activity *[see Contraindications (4), Drug Interactions (7.2)]*. See Table 7 for a listing of established and other potentially significant drug interactions *[see Drug Interactions (7.3)]*.
5.2 Skin Reactions
Severe and life-threatening skin reactions, including 1 case of Stevens-Johnson syndrome among 700 subjects treated with LEXIVA in clinical trials. Treatment with LEXIVA should be discontinued for severe or life-threatening rashes and for moderate rashes accompanied by systemic symptoms *[see Adverse Reactions (6)]*.
5.3 Sulfa Allergy
LEXIVA should be used with caution in patients with a known sulfonamide allergy. Fosamprenavir contains a sulfonamide moiety. The potential for cross-sensitivity between drugs in the sulfonamide class and fosamprenavir is unknown. In a clinical trial of LEXIVA used as the sole protease inhibitor, rash occurred in 2 of 10 subjects (20%) with a history of sulfonamide allergy compared with 42 of 126 subjects (33%) with no history of sulfonamide allergy. In 2 clinical trials of LEXIVA plus low-dose ritonavir, rash occurred in 8 of 50 subjects (16%) with a history of sulfonamide allergy compared with 50 of 412 subjects (12%) with no history of sulfonamide allergy.
5.4 Hepatic Toxicity
Use of LEXIVA with ritonavir at higher-than-recommended dosages may result in transaminase elevations and should not be used *[see Dosage and Administration (2), Overdosage (10)]*. Patients with underlying hepatitis B or C or marked elevations in transaminases prior to treatment may be at increased risk for developing or worsening of transaminase elevations. Appropriate laboratory testing should be conducted prior to initiating therapy with LEXIVA and patients should be monitored closely during treatment.
5.5 Diabetes/Hyperglycemia
New onset diabetes mellitus, exacerbation of pre-existing diabetes mellitus, and hyperglycemia have been reported during postmarketing surveillance in HIV-1-infected patients receiving protease inhibitor therapy. Some patients required either initiation or dose adjustments of insulin or oral hypoglycemic agents for treatment of these events. In some cases, diabetic ketoacidosis has occurred. In those patients who discontinued protease inhibitor therapy, hyperglycemia persisted in some cases. Because these events have been reported voluntarily during clinical practice, estimates of frequency cannot be made and causal relationships between protease inhibitor therapy and these events have not been established.
5.6 Immune Reconstitution Syndrome
Immune reconstitution syndrome has been reported in patients treated with combination antiretroviral therapy, including LEXIVA. During the initial phase of combination antiretroviral treatment, patients whose immune systems respond may develop an inflammatory response to indolent or residual opportunistic infections (such as *Mycobacterium avium* infection, cytomegalovirus, *Pneumocystis jirovecii* pneumonia [PCP], or tuberculosis), which may necessitate further evaluation and treatment.
Autoimmune disorders (such as Graves' disease, polymyositis, and Guillain-Barré syndrome) have also been reported to occur in the setting of immune reconstitution; however, the time to onset is more variable, and can occur many months after initiation of treatment.
5.7 Fat Redistribution
Redistribution/accumulation of body fat, including central obesity, dorsocervical fat enlargement (buffalo hump), peripheral wasting, facial wasting, breast enlargement, and "cushingoid appearance," have been observed in patients receiving antiretroviral therapy, including LEXIVA. The mechanism and long-term consequences of these events are currently unknown. A causal relationship has not been established.
5.8 Lipid Elevations
Treatment with LEXIVA plus ritonavir has resulted in increases in the concentration of triglycerides and cholesterol *[see Adverse Reactions (6)]*. Triglyceride and cholesterol testing should be performed prior to initiating therapy with LEXIVA and at periodic intervals during therapy. Lipid disorders should be managed as clinically appropriate *[see Drug Interactions (7)]*.
5.9 Hemolytic Anemia
Acute hemolytic anemia has been reported in a patient treated with amprenavir.
5.10 Patients With Hemophilia
There have been reports of spontaneous bleeding in patients with hemophilia A and B treated with protease inhibitors. In some patients, additional factor VIII was required. In many of the reported cases, treatment with protease inhibitors was continued or restarted. A causal relationship between protease inhibitor therapy and these episodes has not been established.
5.11 Nephrolithiasis
Cases of nephrolithiasis were reported during postmarketing surveillance in HIV-1-infected patients receiving LEXIVA. Because these events were reported voluntarily during clinical practice, estimates of frequency cannot be made. If signs or symptoms of nephrolithiasis occur, temporary interruption or discontinuation of therapy may be considered.
5.12 Resistance/Cross-Resistance
Because the potential for HIV cross-resistance among protease inhibitors has not been fully explored, it is unknown what effect therapy with LEXIVA will have on the activity of subsequently administered protease inhibitors. LEXIVA has been studied in patients who have experienced treatment failure with protease inhibitors *[see Clinical Studies (14.2)]*.

6 ADVERSE REACTIONS
- Severe or life-threatening skin reactions have been reported with the use of LEXIVA *[see Warnings and Precautions (5.2)]*.
- The most common moderate to severe adverse reactions in clinical trials of LEXIVA were diarrhea, rash, nausea, vomiting, and headache.
- Treatment discontinuation due to adverse events occurred in 6.4% of subjects receiving LEXIVA and in 5.9% of subjects receiving comparator treatments. The most common adverse reactions leading to discontinuation of LEXIVA (incidence less than or equal to 1% of subjects) included diarrhea, nausea, vomiting, AST increased, ALT increased, and rash.

6.1 Clinical Trials
Because clinical trials are conducted under widely varying conditions, adverse reaction rates observed in the clinical trials of a drug cannot be directly compared to rates in the clinical trials of another drug and may not reflect the rates observed in clinical practice.
Adult Trials: The data for the 3 active-controlled clinical trials described below reflect exposure of 700 HIV-1–infected subjects to LEXIVA Tablets, including 599 subjects exposed to LEXIVA for greater than 24 weeks, and 409 subjects exposed for greater than 48 weeks. The population age ranged from 17 to 72 years. Of these subjects, 26% were female, 51% Caucasian, 31% black, 16% American Hispanic, and 70% were antiretroviral-naive. Sixty-one percent received LEXIVA 1,400 mg once daily plus ritonavir 200 mg once daily; 24% received LEXIVA 1,400 mg twice daily; and 15% received LEXIVA 700 mg twice daily plus ritonavir 100 mg twice daily.
Selected adverse reactions reported during the clinical efficacy trials of LEXIVA are shown in Tables 3 and 4. Each table presents adverse reactions of moderate or severe intensity in subjects treated with combination therapy for up to 48 weeks.
[See table 3 at top of previous page]

Table 4. Selected Moderate/Severe Clinical Adverse Reactions Reported in Greater Than or Equal to 2% of Protease Inhibitor-Experienced Adult Subjects (Trial APV30003)

Adverse Reaction	LEXIVA 700 mg b.i.d./ Ritonavir 100 mg b.i.d.[a] (n = 106)	Lopinavir 400 mg b.i.d./ Ritonavir 100 mg b.i.d.[a] (n = 103)
Gastrointestinal		
Diarrhea	13%	11%
Nausea	3%	9%
Vomiting	3%	5%
Abdominal pain	<1%	2%
Skin		
Rash	3%	0%
Nervous system		
Headache	4%	2%

[a]All subjects also received 2 reverse transcriptase inhibitors.

Skin rash (without regard to causality) occurred in approximately 19% of subjects treated with LEXIVA in the pivotal

Table 5. Grade 3/4 Laboratory Abnormalities Reported in Greater Than or Equal to 2% of Antiretroviral-Naive Adult Subjects in Trials APV30001 and APV30002

Laboratory Abnormality	APV30001[a]		APV30002[a]	
	LEXIVA 1,400 mg b.i.d. (n = 166)	Nelfinavir 1,250 mg b.i.d. (n = 83)	LEXIVA 1,400 mg q.d./ Ritonavir 200 mg q.d. (n = 322)	Nelfinavir 1,250 mg b.i.d. (n = 327)
ALT (>5 × ULN)	6%	5%	8%	8%
AST (>5 × ULN)	6%	6%	6%	7%
Serum lipase (>2 × ULN)	8%	4%	6%	4%
Triglycerides[b] (>750 mg/dL)	0%	1%	6%	2%
Neutrophil count, absolute (<750 cells/mm^3)	3%	6%	3%	4%

[a]All subjects also received abacavir and lamivudine twice daily.
[b]Fasting specimens.
ULN = Upper limit of normal.

efficacy trials. Rashes were usually maculopapular and of mild or moderate intensity, some with pruritus. Rash had a median onset of 11 days after initiation of LEXIVA and had a median duration of 13 days. Skin rash led to discontinuation of LEXIVA in less than 1% of subjects. In some subjects with mild or moderate rash, dosing with LEXIVA was often continued without interruption; if interrupted, reintroduction of LEXIVA generally did not result in rash recurrence.

The percentages of subjects with Grade 3 or 4 laboratory abnormalities in the clinical efficacy trials of LEXIVA are presented in Tables 5 and 6.

[See table 5 at top of previous page]

The incidence of Grade 3 or 4 hyperglycemia in antiretroviral-naive subjects who received LEXIVA in the pivotal trials was less than 1%.

Table 6. Grade 3/4 Laboratory Abnormalities Reported in Greater Than or Equal to 2% of Protease Inhibitor-Experienced Adult Subjects in Trial APV30003

Laboratory Abnormality	LEXIVA 700 mg b.i.d./ Ritonavir 100 mg b.i.d.[a] (n = 104)	Lopinavir 400 mg b.i.d./ Ritonavir 100 mg b.i.d.[a] (n = 103)
Triglycerides[b] (>750 mg/dL)	11%[c]	6%[c]
Serum lipase (>2 × ULN)	5%	12%
ALT (>5 × ULN)	4%	4%
AST (>5 × ULN)	4%	2%
Glucose (>251 mg/dL)	2%[c]	2%[c]

[a]All subjects also received 2 reverse transcriptase inhibitors.
[b]Fasting specimens.
[c]n = 100 for LEXIVA plus ritonavir, n = 98 for lopinavir plus ritonavir.
ULN = Upper limit of normal.

Pediatric Trials: LEXIVA with and without ritonavir was studied in 237 HIV-1–infected pediatric subjects aged at least 4 weeks to 18 years in 3 open–label trials, APV20002, APV20003, and APV29005 [see Clinical Studies (14.3)]. Vomiting and neutropenia occurred more frequently in pediatric subjects compared to adults. Other adverse events occurred with similar frequency in pediatric subjects compared with adults.

The frequency of vomiting among pediatric subjects receiving LEXIVA twice daily with ritonavir was 20% in subjects aged at least 4 weeks to less than 2 years and 36% in subjects aged 2 to 18 years compared with 10% in adults. The frequency of vomiting among pediatric subjects receiving LEXIVA twice daily without ritonavir was 60% in subjects aged 2 to 5 years compared with 16% in adults.

The median duration of drug–related vomiting episodes in APV29005 was 1 day (range: 1 to 3 days), in APV20003 was 16 days (range: 1 to 38 days), and in APV20002 was 9 days (range: 4 to 13 days). Vomiting was treatment limiting in 4 pediatric subjects across all 3 trials.

The incidence of Grade 3 or 4 neutropenia (neutrophils less than 750 cells per mm³) seen in pediatric subjects treated with LEXIVA with and without ritonavir was higher (15%) than the incidence seen in adult subjects (3%). Grade 3/4 neutropenia occurred in 10% (5/51) of subjects aged at least 4 weeks to less than 2 years and 16% (28/170) of subjects aged 2 to 18 years.

6.2 Postmarketing Experience

In addition to adverse reactions reported from clinical trials, the following reactions have been identified during postapproval use of LEXIVA. Because they are reported voluntarily from a population of unknown size, estimates of frequency cannot be made. These reactions have been chosen for inclusion due to a combination of their seriousness, frequency of reporting, or potential causal connection to LEXIVA.

Cardiac Disorders: Myocardial infarction.
Metabolism and Nutrition Disorders: Hypercholesterolemia.
Nervous System Disorders: Oral paresthesia.
Skin and Subcutaneous Tissue Disorders: Angioedema.
Urogenital: Nephrolithiasis.

7 DRUG INTERACTIONS

See also Contraindications (4), Clinical Pharmacology (12.3).

If LEXIVA is used in combination with ritonavir, see full prescribing information for ritonavir for additional information on drug interactions.

7.1 Cytochrome P450 Inhibitors and Inducers

Amprenavir, the active metabolite of fosamprenavir, is an inhibitor of CYP3A4 metabolism and therefore should not

Table 7. Established and Other Potentially Significant Drug Interactions

Concomitant Drug Class: Drug Name	Effect on Concentration of Amprenavir or Concomitant Drug	Clinical Comment
HCV/HIV-Antiviral Agents		
HCV protease inhibitor: Telaprevir[a]	**LEXIVA/ritonavir:** ↓Amprenavir ↓Telaprevir	Coadministration of LEXIVA/ritonavir and telaprevir is not recommended.
HCV protease inhibitor: Boceprevir	**LEXIVA/ritonavir:** ↓Amprenavir (predicted) ↓Boceprevir (predicted)	Coadministration of LEXIVA/ritonavir and boceprevir is not recommended. A pharmacokinetic interaction has been reported between boceprevir and some HIV protease inhibitors in combination with ritonavir, leading to decreased HIV protease inhibitor concentrations and, in some cases, decreased boceprevir concentrations.
Non-nucleoside reverse transcriptase inhibitor: Efavirenz[a]	**LEXIVA:** ↓Amprenavir **LEXIVA/ritonavir:** ↓Amprenavir	Appropriate doses of the combinations with respect to safety and efficacy have not been established. An additional 100 mg/day (300 mg total) of ritonavir is recommended when efavirenz is administered with LEXIVA/ritonavir once daily. No change in the ritonavir dose is required when efavirenz is administered with LEXIVA plus ritonavir twice daily.
Non-nucleoside reverse transcriptase inhibitor: Nevirapine[a]	**LEXIVA:** ↓Amprenavir ↑Nevirapine **LEXIVA/ritonavir:** ↓Amprenavir ↑Nevirapine	Coadministration of nevirapine and LEXIVA without ritonavir is not recommended. No dosage adjustment required when nevirapine is administered with LEXIVA/ritonavir twice daily. The combination of nevirapine administered with LEXIVA/ritonavir once-daily regimen has not been studied.
HIV protease inhibitor: Atazanavir[a]	**LEXIVA:** Interaction has not been evaluated. **LEXIVA/ritonavir:** ↓Atazanavir ↔Amprenavir	Appropriate doses of the combinations with respect to safety and efficacy have not been established.
HIV protease inhibitors: Indinavir[a], nelfinavir[a]	**LEXIVA:** ↑Amprenavir Effect on indinavir and nelfinavir is not well established. **LEXIVA/ritonavir:** Interaction has not been evaluated.	Appropriate doses of the combinations with respect to safety and efficacy have not been established.
HIV protease inhibitors: Lopinavir/ritonavir[a]	↓Amprenavir ↓Lopinavir	An increased rate of adverse events has been observed. Appropriate doses of the combinations with respect to safety and efficacy have not been established.
HIV protease inhibitor: Saquinavir[a]	**LEXIVA:** ↓Amprenavir Effect on saquinavir is not well established. **LEXIVA/ritonavir:** Interaction has not been evaluated.	Appropriate doses of the combination with respect to safety and efficacy have not been established.
HIV integrase inhibitor: Raltegravir[a]	**LEXIVA:** ↓Amprenavir ↓Raltegravir **LEXIVA/ritonavir:** ↓Amprenavir ↓Raltegravir	Appropriate doses of the combination with respect to safety and efficacy have not been established.
HIV CCR5 co-receptor antagonist: Maraviroc[a]	**LEXIVA/ritonavir:** ↓Amprenavir ↑Maraviroc	No dosage adjustment required for LEXIVA/ritonavir. The recommended dose of maraviroc is 150 mg twice daily when coadministered with LEXIVA/ritonavir. LEXIVA should be given with ritonavir when coadministered with maraviroc.
Other Agents		
Antiarrhythmics: Amiodarone, bepridil, lidocaine (systemic), and quinidine	↑Antiarrhythmics	Use with caution. Increased exposure may be associated with life-threatening reactions such as cardiac arrhythmias. Therapeutic concentration monitoring, if available, is recommended for antiarrhythmics.
Anticoagulant: Warfarin		Concentrations of warfarin may be affected. It is recommended that INR (international normalized ratio) be monitored.
Anticonvulsants: Carbamazepine, phenobarbital, phenytoin Phenytoin[a]	**LEXIVA:** ↓Amprenavir **LEXIVA/ritonavir:** ↑Amprenavir ↓Phenytoin	Use with caution. LEXIVA may be less effective due to decreased amprenavir plasma concentrations in patients taking these agents concomitantly. Plasma phenytoin concentrations should be monitored and phenytoin dose should be increased as appropriate. No change in LEXIVA/ritonavir dose is recommended.

(Table continued on next page)

be administered concurrently with medications with narrow therapeutic windows that are substrates of CYP3A4. Data also suggest that amprenavir induces CYP3A4.

Amprenavir is metabolized by CYP3A4. Coadministration of LEXIVA and drugs that induce CYP3A4, such as rifampin, may decrease amprenavir concentrations and reduce its therapeutic effect. Coadministration of LEXIVA and drugs that inhibit CYP3A4 may increase amprenavir concentrations and increase the incidence of adverse effects.

The potential for drug interactions with LEXIVA changes when LEXIVA is coadministered with the potent CYP3A4 inhibitor ritonavir. The magnitude of CYP3A4-mediated drug interactions (effect on amprenavir or effect on coadministered drug) may change when LEXIVA is coadministered with ritonavir. Because ritonavir is a CYP2D6 inhibitor, clinically significant interactions with drugs metabolized by CYP2D6 are possible when coadministered with LEXIVA plus ritonavir.

There are other agents that may result in serious and/or life-threatening drug interactions [see Contraindications (4)].

7.2 Drugs That Should Not Be Coadministered With LEXIVA

See Contraindications (4).

7.3 Established and Other Potentially Significant Drug Interactions

Table 7 provides a listing of established or potentially clinically significant drug interactions. Information in the table applies to LEXIVA with or without ritonavir, unless otherwise indicated.

[See table 7 on pages 2348 through 2351]

8 USE IN SPECIFIC POPULATIONS

8.1 Pregnancy

Pregnancy Category C. Embryo/fetal development studies were conducted in rats (dosed from day 6 to day 17 of gestation) and rabbits (dosed from day 7 to day 20 of gestation). Administration of fosamprenavir to pregnant rats and rabbits produced no major effects on embryo-fetal development; however, the incidence of abortion was increased in rabbits that were administered fosamprenavir. Systemic exposures $(AUC_{0-24 \, hr})$ to amprenavir at these dosages were 0.8 (rabbits) to 2 (rats) times the exposures in humans following administration of the maximum recommended human dose (MRHD) of fosamprenavir alone or 0.3 (rabbits) to 0.7 (rats) times the exposures in humans following administration of the MRHD of fosamprenavir in combination with ritonavir. In contrast, administration of amprenavir was associated with abortions and an increased incidence of minor skeletal variations resulting from deficient ossification of the femur, humerus, and trochlea, in pregnant rabbits at the tested dose approximately one-twentieth the exposure seen at the recommended human dose.

The mating and fertility of the F_1 generation born to female rats given fosamprenavir was not different from control animals; however, fosamprenavir did cause a reduction in both pup survival and body weights. Surviving F_1 female rats showed an increased time to successful mating, an increased length of gestation, a reduced number of uterine implantation sites per litter, and reduced gestational body weights compared with control animals. Systemic exposure $(AUC_{0-24 \, hr})$ to amprenavir in the F_0 pregnant rats was approximately 2 times higher than exposures in humans following administration of the MRHD of fosamprenavir alone or approximately the same as those seen in humans following administration of the MRHD of fosamprenavir in combination with ritonavir.

There are no adequate and well-controlled studies in pregnant women. LEXIVA should be used during pregnancy only if the potential benefit justifies the potential risk to the fetus.

Antiretroviral Pregnancy Registry: To monitor maternal-fetal outcomes of pregnant women exposed to LEXIVA, an Antiretroviral Pregnancy Registry has been established. Physicians are encouraged to register patients by calling 1-800-258-4263.

8.3 Nursing Mothers

The Centers for Disease Control and Prevention recommend that HIV-infected mothers not breastfeed their infants to avoid risking postnatal transmission of HIV. Although it is not known if amprenavir is excreted in human milk, amprenavir is secreted into the milk of lactating rats. Because of both the potential for HIV transmission and the potential for serious adverse reactions in nursing infants, mothers should be instructed not to breastfeed if they are receiving LEXIVA.

8.4 Pediatric Use

The safety, pharmacokinetic profile, virologic, and immunologic responses of LEXIVA with and without ritonavir were evaluated in protease inhibitor-naive and –experienced HIV-1–infected pediatric subjects aged at least 4 weeks to less than 18 years and weighing at least 3 kg in 3 open-label trials [see Adverse Reactions (6.1), Clinical Pharmacology (12.3), Clinical Studies (14.3)]. Vomiting and neutropenia,

were more frequent in pediatrics than in adults [see Adverse Reactions (6.1)]. Other adverse events occurred with similar frequency in pediatric subjects compared with adults.

Treatment with LEXIVA is not recommended in protease inhibitor-experienced pediatric patients younger than 6 months. The pharmacokinetics, safety, tolerability, and effi-

cacy of LEXIVA in pediatric patients younger than 4 weeks have not been established [see Clinical Pharmacology (12.3)]. Available pharmacokinetic and clinical data do not support once-daily dosing of LEXIVA alone or in combination with ritonavir for any pediatrics or twice-daily dosing without ritonavir in pediatric patients younger than 2

Table 7 (cont.). Established and Other Potentially Significant Drug Interactions

Concomitant Drug Class: Drug Name	Effect on Concentration of Amprenavir or Concomitant Drug	Clinical Comment
Other Agents (cont.)		
Antidepressant: Paroxetine, trazodone	↓Paroxetine ↑Trazodone	Coadministration of paroxetine with LEXIVA/ritonavir significantly decreased plasma levels of paroxetine. Any paroxetine dose adjustment should be guided by clinical effect (tolerability and efficacy). Concomitant use of trazodone and LEXIVA with or without ritonavir may increase plasma concentrations of trazodone. Adverse events of nausea, dizziness, hypotension, and syncope have been observed following coadministration of trazodone and ritonavir. If trazodone is used with a CYP3A4 inhibitor such as LEXIVA, the combination should be used with caution and a lower dose of trazodone should be considered.
Antifungals: Ketoconazole[a], itraconazole	↑Ketoconazole ↑Itraconazole	Increase monitoring for adverse events. **LEXIVA:** Dose reduction of ketoconazole or itraconazole may be needed for patients receiving more than 400 mg ketoconazole or itraconazole per day. **LEXIVA/ritonavir:** High doses of ketoconazole or itraconazole (greater than 200 mg/day) are not recommended.
Anti-gout: Colchicine	↑Colchicine	Patients with renal or hepatic impairment should not be given colchicine with LEXIVA/ritonavir. **LEXIVA/ritonavir and coadministration of colchicine: Treatment of gout flares:** 0.6 mg (1 tablet) × 1 dose, followed by 0.3 mg (half tablet) 1 hour later. Dose to be repeated no earlier than 3 days. **Prophylaxis of gout flares:** If the original regimen was 0.6 mg twice a day, the regimen should be adjusted to 0.3 mg once a day. If the original regimen was 0.6 mg once a day, the regimen should be adjusted to 0.3 mg once every other day. **Treatment of familial Mediterranean fever (FMF):** Maximum daily dose of 0.6 mg (may be given as 0.3 mg twice a day). **LEXIVA and coadministration of colchicine: Treatment of gout flares:** 1.2 mg (2 tablets) × 1 dose. Dose to be repeated no earlier than 3 days. **Prophylaxis of gout flares:** If the original regimen was 0.6 mg twice a day, the regimen should be adjusted to 0.3 mg twice a day or 0.6 mg once a day. If the original regimen was 0.6 mg once a day, the regimen should be adjusted to 0.3 mg once a day. **Treatment of FMF:** Maximum daily dose of 1.2 mg (may be given as 0.6 mg twice a day).
Antimycobacterial: Rifabutin[a]	↑Rifabutin and rifabutin metabolite	A complete blood count should be performed weekly and as clinically indicated to monitor for neutropenia. **LEXIVA:** A dosage reduction of rifabutin by at least half the recommended dose is required. **LEXIVA/ritonavir:** Dosage reduction of rifabutin by at least 75% of the usual dose of 300 mg/day is recommended (a maximum dose of 150 mg every other day or 3 times per week).
Benzodiazepines: Alprazolam, clorazepate, diazepam, flurazepam	↑Benzodiazepines	Clinical significance is unknown. A decrease in benzodiazepine dose may be needed.
Calcium channel blockers: Diltiazem, felodipine, nifedipine, nicardipine, nimodipine, verapamil, amlodipine, nisoldipine, isradipine	↑Calcium channel blockers	Use with caution. Clinical monitoring of patients is recommended.
Corticosteroid: Dexamethasone	↓Amprenavir	Use with caution. LEXIVA may be less effective due to decreased amprenavir plasma concentrations.

(Table continued on next page)

Table 7 (cont.). Established and Other Potentially Significant Drug Interactions

Concomitant Drug Class: Drug Name	Effect on Concentration of Amprenavir or Concomitant Drug	Clinical Comment
Other Agents (cont.)		
Endothelin-receptor antagonists: Bosentan	↑Bosentan	Coadministration of bosentan in patients on LEXIVA: In patients who have been receiving LEXIVA for at least 10 days, start bosentan at 62.5 mg once daily or every other day based upon individual tolerability. Coadministration of LEXIVA in patients on bosentan: Discontinue use of bosentan at least 36 hours prior to initiation of LEXIVA. After at least 10 days following the initiation of LEXIVA, resume bosentan at 62.5 mg once daily or every other day based upon individual tolerability.
Histamine H_2-receptor antagonists: Cimetidine, famotidine, nizatidine, ranitidine[a]	**LEXIVA:** ↓Amprenavir **LEXIVA/ritonavir:** Interaction not evaluated	Use with caution. LEXIVA may be less effective due to decreased amprenavir plasma concentrations.
HMG-CoA reductase inhibitors: Atorvastatin[a]	↑Atorvastatin	Titrate atorvastatin dose carefully and use the lowest necessary dose; do not exceed atorvastatin 20 mg/day.
Immunosuppressants: Cyclosporine, tacrolimus, rapamycin	↑Immunosuppressants	Therapeutic concentration monitoring is recommended for immunosuppressant agents.
Inhaled beta-agonist: Salmeterol	↑Salmeterol	Concurrent administration of salmeterol with LEXIVA is not recommended. The combination may result in increased risk of cardiovascular adverse events associated with salmeterol, including QT prolongation, palpitations, and sinus tachycardia.
Inhaled/nasal steroid: Fluticasone	**LEXIVA:** ↑Fluticasone **LEXIVA/ritonavir:** ↑Fluticasone	Use with caution. Consider alternatives to fluticasone, particularly for long-term use. May result in significantly reduced serum cortisol concentrations. Systemic corticosteroid effects including Cushing's syndrome and adrenal suppression have been reported during postmarketing use in patients receiving ritonavir and inhaled or intranasally administered fluticasone. Coadministration of fluticasone and LEXIVA/ritonavir is not recommended unless the potential benefit to the patient outweighs the risk of systemic corticosteroid side effects.
Narcotic analgesic: Methadone	↓Methadone	Data suggest that the interaction is not clinically relevant; however, patients should be monitored for opiate withdrawal symptoms.
Oral contraceptives: Ethinyl estradiol/ norethindrone[a]	**LEXIVA:** ↓Amprenavir ↓Ethinyl estradiol **LEXIVA/ritonavir:** ↓Ethinyl estradiol	Alternative methods of non-hormonal contraception are recommended. May lead to loss of virologic response. [a] Increased risk of transaminase elevations. No data are available on the use of LEXIVA/ritonavir with other hormonal therapies, such as hormone replacement therapy (HRT) for postmenopausal women.

(Table continued on next page)

years[see Clinical Pharmacology (12.3), Clinical Studies (14.3)]. See Dosage and Administration (2.2) for dosing recommendations for pediatric patients.

8.5　Geriatric Use
Clinical studies of LEXIVA did not include sufficient numbers of patients aged 65 and over to determine whether they respond differently from younger adults. In general, dose selection for an elderly patient should be cautious, reflecting the greater frequency of decreased hepatic, renal, or cardiac function and of concomitant disease or other drug therapy.

8.6　Hepatic Impairment
Amprenavir is principally metabolized by the liver; therefore, caution should be exercised when administering LEXIVA to patients with hepatic impairment because amprenavir concentrations may be increased [see Clinical Pharmacology (12.3)]. Patients with impaired hepatic function receiving LEXIVA with or without concurrent ritonavir require dose reduction [see Dosage and Administration (2.3)].
There are no data to support dosing recommendations for pediatric subjects with hepatic impairment.

10　OVERDOSAGE
In a healthy volunteer repeat-dose pharmacokinetic trial evaluating high-dose combinations of LEXIVA plus ritonavir, an increased frequency of Grade 2/3 ALT elevations (greater than 2.5 × ULN) was observed with LEXIVA 1,400 mg twice daily plus ritonavir 200 mg twice daily (4 of 25 subjects). Concurrent Grade 1/2 elevations in AST

(greater than 1.25 × ULN) were noted in 3 of these 4 subjects. These transaminase elevations resolved following discontinuation of dosing.
There is no known antidote for LEXIVA. It is not known whether amprenavir can be removed by peritoneal dialysis or hemodialysis. If overdosage occurs, the patient should be monitored for evidence of toxicity and standard supportive treatment applied as necessary.

11　DESCRIPTION
LEXIVA (fosamprenavir calcium) is a prodrug of amprenavir, an inhibitor of HIV protease. The chemical name of fosamprenavir calcium is (3S)-tetrahydrofuran-3-yl (1S,2R)-3-[[(4-aminophenyl) sulfonyl](isobutyl)amino]-1-benzyl-2-(phosphonooxy) propylcarbamate monocalcium salt. Fosamprenavir calcium is a single stereoisomer with the (3S)(1S,2R) configuration. It has a molecular formula of $C_{25}H_{34}CaN_3O_9PS$ and a molecular weight of 623.7. It has the following structural formula:
[See chemical structure at top of next column]
Fosamprenavir calcium is a white to cream-colored solid with a solubility of approximately 0.31 mg per mL in water at 25°C.
LEXIVA Tablets are available for oral administration in a strength of 700 mg of fosamprenavir as fosamprenavir calcium (equivalent to approximately 600 mg of amprenavir). Each 700 mg tablet contains the inactive ingredients colloidal silicon dioxide, croscarmellose sodium, magnesium stearate, microcrystalline cellulose, and povidone K30. The

tablet film-coating contains the inactive ingredients hypromellose, iron oxide red, titanium dioxide, and triacetin. LEXIVA Oral Suspension is available in a strength of 50 mg per mL of fosamprenavir as fosamprenavir calcium equivalent to approximately 43 mg of amprenavir. LEXIVA Oral Suspension is a white to off-white suspension with a grape-bubblegum-peppermint flavor. Each one milliliter (1 mL) contains the inactive ingredients artificial grape-bubblegum flavor, calcium chloride dihydrate, hypromellose, methylparaben, natural peppermint flavor, polysorbate 80, propylene glycol, propylparaben, purified water, and sucralose.

12　CLINICAL PHARMACOLOGY
12.1　Mechanism of Action
Fosamprenavir is an antiviral agent [see Microbiology (12.4)].
12.3　Pharmacokinetics
The pharmacokinetic properties of amprenavir after administration of LEXIVA, with or without ritonavir, have been evaluated in both healthy adult volunteers and in HIV-1-infected subjects; no substantial differences in steady-state amprenavir concentrations were observed between the 2 populations.
The pharmacokinetic parameters of amprenavir after administration of LEXIVA (with and without concomitant ritonavir) are shown in Table 8.
[See table 8 at top of next page]
The mean plasma amprenavir concentrations of the dosing regimens over the dosing intervals are displayed in Figure 1.

Figure 1. Mean (SD) Steady-State Plasma Amprenavir Concentrations and Mean EC50 Values Against HIV from Protease Inhibitor-Naive Subjects (in the Absence of Human Serum)

Mean wild-type EC$_{50}$ = 0.0146 mcg/mL

- ▲- LEXIVA 1,400 mg once daily plus ritonavir 200 mg once daily (n = 22)
- ○- LEXIVA 700 mg twice daily plus ritonavir 100 mg twice daily (n = 24)
- ●- LEXIVA 1,400 mg twice daily (n = 22)
- △- LEXIVA 1,400 mg once daily plus ritonavir 100 mg once daily (n = 36)

Absorption and Bioavailability:　After administration of a single dose of LEXIVA to HIV-1–infected subjects, the time to peak amprenavir concentration (T_{max}) occurred between 1.5 and 4 hours (median 2.5 hours). The absolute oral bioavailability of amprenavir after administration of LEXIVA in humans has not been established.
After administration of a single 1,400-mg dose in the fasted state, LEXIVA Oral Suspension (50 mg per mL) and LEXIVA Tablets (700 mg) provided similar amprenavir exposures (AUC); however, the C_{max} of amprenavir after administration of the suspension formulation was 14.5% higher compared with the tablet.
Effects of Food on Oral Absorption:　Administration of a single 1,400-mg dose of LEXIVA Tablets in the fed state (standardized high-fat meal: 967 kcal, 67 grams fat, 33 grams protein, 58 grams carbohydrate) compared with the fasted state was associated with no significant changes in amprenavir C_{max}, T_{max}, or $AUC_{0-∞}$ [see Dosage and Administration (2)].
Administration of a single 1,400-mg dose of LEXIVA Oral Suspension in the fed state (standardized high-fat meal: 967 kcal, 67 grams fat, 33 grams protein, 58 grams carbohydrate) compared with the fasted state was associated with a

Table 7 (cont.). Established and Other Potentially Significant Drug Interactions

Concomitant Drug Class: Drug Name	Effect on Concentration of Amprenavir or Concomitant Drug	Clinical Comment
	Other Agents (cont.)	
PDE5 inhibitors: Sildenafil, tadalafil, vardenafil	↑Sildenafil ↑Tadalafil ↑Vardenafil	May result in an increase in PDE5 inhibitor-associated adverse events, including hypotension, syncope, visual disturbances, and priapism. Use of PDE5 inhibitors for pulmonary arterial hypertension (PAH): • Use of sildenafil (REVATIO) is contraindicated when used for the treatment of PAH [see Contraindications (4)]. • The following dose adjustments are recommended for use of tadalafil (ADCIRCA®) with LEXIVA: Coadministration of ADCIRCA in patients on LEXIVA: In patients receiving LEXIVA for at least one week, start ADCIRCA at 20 mg once daily. Increase to 40 mg once daily based upon individual tolerability. Coadministration of LEXIVA in patients on ADCIRCA: Avoid use of ADCIRCA during the initiation of LEXIVA. Stop ADCIRCA at least 24 hours prior to starting LEXIVA. After at least one week following the initiation of LEXIVA, resume ADCIRCA at 20 mg once daily. Increase to 40 mg once daily based upon individual tolerability. Use of PDE5 inhibitors for erectile dysfunction: **LEXIVA:** Sildenafil: 25 mg every 48 hours. Tadalafil: no more than 10 mg every 72 hours. Vardenafil: no more than 2.5 mg every 24 hours. **LEXIVA/ritonavir:** Sildenafil: 25 mg every 48 hours. Tadalafil: no more than 10 mg every 72 hours. Vardenafil: no more than 2.5 mg every 72 hours. Use with increased monitoring for adverse events.
Proton pump inhibitors: Esomeprazole[a], lansoprazole, omeprazole, pantoprazole, rabeprazole	**LEXIVA:** ↔Amprenavir ↑Esomeprazole **LEXIVA/ritonavir:** ↔Amprenavir ↔Esomeprazole	Proton pump inhibitors can be administered at the same time as a dose of LEXIVA with no change in plasma amprenavir concentrations.
Tricyclic antidepressants: Amitriptyline, imipramine	↑Tricyclics	Therapeutic concentration monitoring is recommended for tricyclic antidepressants.

[a] See Clinical Pharmacology (12.3) Tables 10, 11, 12, or 13 for magnitude of interaction.

Table 8. Geometric Mean (95% CI) Steady-State Plasma Amprenavir Pharmacokinetic Parameters in Adults

Regimen	C_{max} (mcg/mL)	T_{max} (hours)[a]	AUC_{24} (mcg•hr/mL)	C_{min} (mcg/mL)
LEXIVA 1,400 mg b.i.d.	4.82 (4.06-5.72)	1.3 (0.8-4.0)	33.0 (27.6-39.2)	0.35 (0.27-0.46)
LEXIVA 1,400 mg q.d. plus Ritonavir 200 mg q.d.	7.24 (6.32-8.28)	2.1 (0.8-5.0)	69.4 (59.7-80.8)	1.45 (1.16-1.81)
LEXIVA 1,400 mg q.d. plus Ritonavir 100 mg q.d.	7.93 (7.25-8.68)	1.5 (0.75-5.0)	66.4 (61.1-72.1)	0.86 (0.74-1.01)
LEXIVA 700 mg b.i.d. plus Ritonavir 100 mg b.i.d.	6.08 (5.38-6.86)	1.5 (0.75-5.0)	79.2 (69.0-90.6)	2.12 (1.77-2.54)

[a]Data shown are median (range).

Table 9. Geometric Mean (95% CI) Steady-State Plasma Amprenavir Pharmacokinetic Parameters by Weight in Pediatric and Adolescent Subjects Aged at Least 4 Weeks to 18 Years Receiving LEXIVA With Ritonavir

Weight	Recommended Dosage Regimen	C_{max}		AUC_{24}		C_{min}	
		n	(mcg/mL)	n	(mcg•hr/mL)	n	(mcg/mL)
<11 kg	LEXIVA 45 mg/kg plus Ritonavir 7 mg/kg b.i.d	12	6.00 (3.88, 9.29)	12	57.3 (34.1, 96.2)	27	1.65 (1.22, 2.24)
11 kg - <15 kg	LEXIVA 30 mg/kg plus Ritonavir 3 mg/kg b.i.d			Not studied[a]			
15 kg - <20 kg	LEXIVA 23 mg/kg plus Ritonavir 3 mg/kg b.i.d.	5	9.54 (4.63, 19.7)	5	121 (54.2, 269)	9	3.56 (2.33, 5.43)
>20 kg - <39 kg	LEXIVA 18 mg/kg plus Ritonavir 3 mg/kg b.i.d.	13	6.24 (5.01, 7.77)	12	97.9 (77.0, 124)	23	2.54 (2.11, 3.06)
≥39 kg	LEXIVA 700 mg plus Ritonavir 100 mg b.i.d.	15	5.03 (4.04, 6.26)	15	72.3 (59.6, 87.6)	42	1.98 (1.72, 2.29)

[a]Recommended dose for pediatric subjects weighing 11 kg to less than 15 kg is based on population pharmacokinetic analysis.

46% reduction in C_{max}, a 0.72-hour delay in T_{max}, and a 28% reduction in amprenavir $AUC_{0-\infty}$.

Distribution: In vitro, amprenavir is approximately 90% bound to plasma proteins, primarily to alpha₁-acid glycoprotein. In vitro, concentration-dependent binding was observed over the concentration range of 1 to 10 mcg per mL, with decreased binding at higher concentrations. The partitioning of amprenavir into erythrocytes is low, but increases as amprenavir concentrations increase, reflecting the higher amount of unbound drug at higher concentrations.

Metabolism: After oral administration, fosamprenavir is rapidly and almost completely hydrolyzed to amprenavir and inorganic phosphate prior to reaching the systemic circulation. This occurs in the gut epithelium during absorption. Amprenavir is metabolized in the liver by the CYP3A4 enzyme system. The 2 major metabolites result from oxidation of the tetrahydrofuran and aniline moieties. Glucuronide conjugates of oxidized metabolites have been identified as minor metabolites in urine and feces.

Amprenavir is both a substrate for and inducer of P-glycoprotein.

Elimination: Excretion of unchanged amprenavir in urine and feces is minimal. Unchanged amprenavir in urine accounts for approximately 1% of the dose; unchanged amprenavir was not detectable in feces. Approximately 14% and 75% of an administered single dose of ¹⁴C-amprenavir can be accounted for as metabolites in urine and feces, respectively. Two metabolites accounted for greater than 90% of the radiocarbon in fecal samples. The plasma elimination half-life of amprenavir is approximately 7.7 hours.

Special Populations: Hepatic Impairment: The pharmacokinetics of amprenavir have been studied after the administration of LEXIVA in combination with ritonavir to adult HIV-1–infected subjects with mild, moderate, and severe hepatic impairment. Following 2 weeks of dosing with LEXIVA plus ritonavir, the AUC of amprenavir was increased by approximately 22% in subjects with mild hepatic impairment, by approximately 70% in subjects with moderate hepatic impairment, and by approximately 80% in subjects with severe hepatic impairment compared with HIV-1–infected subjects with normal hepatic function. Protein binding of amprenavir was decreased in subjects with hepatic impairment. The unbound fraction at 2 hours (approximate C_{max}) ranged between a decrease of -7% to an increase of 57% while the unbound fraction at the end of the dosing interval (C_{min}) increased from 50% to 102% [see Dosage and Administration (2.3)].

The pharmacokinetics of amprenavir have been studied after administration of amprenavir given as AGENERASE® Capsules to adult subjects with hepatic impairment. Following administration of a single 600-mg oral dose, the AUC of amprenavir was increased by approximately 2.5-fold in subjects with moderate cirrhosis and by approximately 4.5-fold in subjects with severe cirrhosis compared with healthy volunteers [see Dosage and Administration (2.3)].

Renal Impairment: The impact of renal impairment on amprenavir elimination in adults has not been studied. The renal elimination of unchanged amprenavir represents approximately 1% of the administered dose; therefore, renal impairment is not expected to significantly impact the elimination of amprenavir.

Pediatric Patients: The pharmacokinetics of amprenavir following administration of LEXIVA Oral Suspension and LEXIVA Tablets, with or without ritonavir, have been studied in a total of 212 HIV-1–infected pediatric subjects enrolled in 3 trials. LEXIVA without ritonavir was administered as 30 or 40 mg per kg twice daily to children aged 2 to 5 years. LEXIVA with ritonavir was administered as LEXIVA 30 mg per kg plus ritonavir 6 mg per kg once daily to children aged 2 to 18 years and as LEXIVA 18 to 60 mg per kg plus ritonavir 3 to 10 mg per kg twice daily to children aged at least 4 weeks to 18 years; body weights ranged from 3 to 103 kg.

Amprenavir apparent clearance decreased with increasing weight. Weight-adjusted apparent clearance was higher in children younger than 4 years, suggesting that younger children require higher mg per kg dosing of LEXIVA.

The pharmacokinetics of LEXIVA Oral Suspension in protease inhibitor-naive infants younger than 6 months (n = 9) receiving LEXIVA 45 mg per kg plus ritonavir 10 mg per kg twice daily generally demonstrated lower AUC_{12} and C_{min} than adults receiving twice-daily LEXIVA 700 mg plus ritonavir 100 mg, the dose recommended for protease-experienced adults. The mean steady-state amprenavir AUC_{12}, C_{max}, and C_{min} were 26.6 mcg•hour per mL, 6.25 mcg per mL, and 0.86 mcg per mL, respectively. These data do not support twice-daily dosing of LEXIVA alone or in combination with ritonavir in protease inhibitor-experienced patients younger than 6 months. Because of ex-

Table 10. Drug Interactions: Pharmacokinetic Parameters for Amprenavir After Administration of LEXIVA in the Presence of the Coadministered Drug(s)

Coadministered Drug(s) and Dose(s)	Dose of LEXIVA[a]	n	% Change in Amprenavir Pharmacokinetic Parameters (90% CI)		
			C_{max}	AUC	C_{min}
Antacid (MAALOX TC®) 30 mL single dose	1,400 mg single dose	30	↓35 (↓24 to ↓42)	↓18 (↓9 to ↓26)	↑14 (↓7 to ↑39)
Atazanavir 300 mg q.d. for 10 days	700 mg b.i.d. plus ritonavir 100 mg b.i.d. for 10 days	22	↔	↔	↔
Atorvastatin 10 mg q.d. for 4 days	1,400 mg b.i.d. for 2 weeks	16	↓18 (↓34 to ↑1)	↓27 (↓41 to ↓12)	↓12 (↓27 to ↓6)
Atorvastatin 10 mg q.d. for 4 days	700 mg b.i.d. plus ritonavir 100 mg b.i.d. for 2 weeks	16	↔	↔	↔
Efavirenz 600 mg q.d. for 2 weeks	1,400 mg q.d. plus ritonavir 200 mg q.d. for 2 weeks	16	↔	↓13 (↓30 to 7)	↓36 (↓8 to ↓56)
Efavirenz 600 mg q.d. plus additional ritonavir 100 mg q.d. for 2 weeks	1,400 mg q.d. plus ritonavir 200 mg q.d. for 2 weeks	16	↑18 (↑1 to ↑38)	↑11 (0 to ↑24)	↔
Efavirenz 600 mg q.d. for 2 weeks	700 mg b.i.d. plus ritonavir 100 mg b.i.d. for 2 weeks	16	↔	↔	↓17 (↓4 to ↓29)
Esomeprazole 20 mg q.d. for 2 weeks	1,400 mg b.i.d. for 2 weeks	25	↔	↔	↔
Esomeprazole 20 mg q.d. for 2 weeks	700 mg b.i.d. plus ritonavir 100 mg b.i.d. for 2 weeks	23	↔	↔	↔
Ethinyl estradiol/ norethindrone 0.035 mg/0.5 mg q.d. for 21 days	700 mg b.i.d. plus ritonavir[b] 100 mg b.i.d. for 21 days	25	↔[c]	↔[c]	↔[c]
Ketoconazole[d] 200 mg q.d. for 4 days	700 mg b.i.d. plus ritonavir 100 mg b.i.d. for 4 days	15	↔	↔	↔
Lopinavir/ritonavir 533 mg/133 mg b.i.d.	1,400 mg b.i.d. for 2 weeks	18	↓13[e]	↓26[e]	↓42[e]
Lopinavir/ritonavir 400 mg/100 mg b.i.d. for 2 weeks	700 mg b.i.d. plus ritonavir 100 mg b.i.d. for 2 weeks	18	↓58 (↓42 to ↓70)	↓63 (↓51 to ↓72)	↓65 (↓54 to ↓73)
Maraviroc 300 mg b.i.d. for 10 days	700 mg b.i.d. plus ritonavir 100 mg b.i.d. for 20 days	14	↓34 (↓25 to ↓41)	↓35 (↓29 to ↓41)	↓36 (↓27 to ↓43)
Maraviroc 300 mg q.d. for 10 days	1,400 mg q.d. plus ritonavir 100 mg q.d. for 20 days	14	↓29 (↓20 to ↓38)	↓30 (↓23 to ↓36)	↓15 (↓3 to ↓25)
Methadone 70 to 120 mg q.d. for 2 weeks	700 mg b.i.d. plus ritonavir 100 mg b.i.d. for 2 weeks	19	↔[c]	↔[c]	↔[c]
Nevirapine 200 mg b.i.d. for 2 weeks[f]	1,400 mg b.i.d. for 2 weeks	17	↓25 (↓37 to ↓10)	↓33 (↓45 to ↓20)	↓35 (↓50 to ↓15)
Nevirapine 200 mg b.i.d. for 2 weeks[f]	700 mg b.i.d. plus ritonavir 100 mg b.i.d. for 2 weeks	17	↔	↓11 (↓23 to ↑3)	↓19 (↓32 to ↓4)

(Table continued on next page)

pected low amprenavir exposure and a requirement for large volume of drug, twice-daily dosing of LEXIVA alone (without ritonavir) in pediatric subjects younger than 2 years was not studied.

Pharmacokinetic parameters for LEXIVA administered with food and with ritonavir in this patient population at the recommended weight-band–based dosage regimens are provided in Table 9.

[See table 9 at bottom of previous page]

Subjects aged 2 to less than 6 years receiving LEXIVA 30 mg per kg twice daily without ritonavir achieved geometric mean (95% CI) amprenavir C_{max} (n = 9), AUC_{12} (n = 9), and C_{min} (n = 19) of 7.15 (5.05, 10.1), 22.3 (15.3, 32.6), and 0.513 (0.384, 0.686), respectively.

Geriatric Patients: The pharmacokinetics of amprenavir after administration of LEXIVA to patients older than 65 years have not been studied *[see Use in Specific Populations (8.5)].*

Gender: The pharmacokinetics of amprenavir after administration of LEXIVA do not differ between males and females.

Race: The pharmacokinetics of amprenavir after administration of LEXIVA do not differ between blacks and non-blacks.

Drug Interactions: *[See Contraindications (4), Warnings and Precautions (5.1), Drug Interactions (7).]*

Amprenavir, the active metabolite of fosamprenavir, is metabolized in the liver by the cytochrome P450 enzyme system. Amprenavir inhibits CYP3A4. Data also suggest that amprenavir induces CYP3A4. Caution should be used when coadministering medications that are substrates, inhibitors, or inducers of CYP3A4, or potentially toxic medications that are metabolized by CYP3A4. Amprenavir does not inhibit CYP2D6, CYP1A2, CYP2C9, CYP2C19, CYP2E1, or uridine glucuronosyltransferase (UDPGT).

Drug interaction trials were performed with LEXIVA and other drugs likely to be coadministered or drugs commonly used as probes for pharmacokinetic interactions. The effects of coadministration on AUC, C_{max}, and C_{min} values are summarized in Table 10 (effect of other drugs on amprenavir) and Table 12 (effect of LEXIVA on other drugs). In addition, since LEXIVA delivers comparable amprenavir plasma concentrations as AGENERASE, drug interaction data derived from trials with AGENERASE are provided in Tables 11 and 13. For information regarding clinical recommendations, *[see Drug Interactions (7)].*

[See table 10 above and on next page]
[See table 11 at top of page 2354]
[See table 12 on pages 2354 and 2355]
[See table 13 at top of page 2356]

12.4 Microbiology

Mechanism of Action: Fosamprenavir is a prodrug that is rapidly hydrolyzed to amprenavir by cellular phosphatases in the gut epithelium as it is absorbed. Amprenavir is an inhibitor of HIV-1 protease. Amprenavir binds to the active site of HIV-1 protease and thereby prevents the processing of viral Gag and Gag-Pol polyprotein precursors, resulting in the formation of immature non-infectious viral particles.

Antiviral Activity: Fosamprenavir has little or no antiviral activity in cell culture. The antiviral activity of amprenavir was evaluated against HIV-1 IIIB in both acutely and chronically infected lymphoblastic cell lines (MT-4, CEM-CCRF, H9) and in peripheral blood lymphocytes in cell culture. The 50% effective concentration (EC_{50}) of amprenavir ranged from 0.012 to 0.08 microM in acutely infected cells and was 0.41 microM in chronically infected cells (1 microM = 0.50 mcg per mL). The median EC_{50} value of amprenavir against HIV-1 isolates from clades A to G was 0.00095 microM in peripheral blood mononuclear cells (PBMCs). Similarly, the EC_{50} values for amprenavir against monocytes/macrophage tropic HIV-1 isolates (clade B) ranged from 0.003 to 0.075 microM in monocyte/macrophage cultures. The EC_{50} values of amprenavir against HIV-2 isolates grown in PBMCs were higher than those for HIV-1 isolates, and ranged from 0.003 to 0.11 microM. Amprenavir exhibited synergistic anti–HIV–1 activity in combination with the nucleoside reverse transcriptase inhibitors (NRTIs) abacavir, didanosine, lamivudine, stavudine, tenofovir, and zidovudine; the non-nucleoside reverse transcriptase inhibitors (NNRTIs) delavirdine and efavirenz; and the protease inhibitors atazanavir and saquinavir. Amprenavir exhibited additive anti–HIV–1 activity in combination with the NNRTI nevirapine, the protease inhibitors indinavir, lopinavir, nelfinavir, and ritonavir; and the fusion inhibitor enfuvirtide. These drug combinations have not been adequately studied in humans.

Resistance: HIV-1 isolates with decreased susceptibility to amprenavir have been selected in cell culture and obtained from subjects treated with fosamprenavir. Genotypic analysis of isolates from treatment-naive subjects failing amprenavir-containing regimens showed substitutions in the HIV-1 protease gene resulting in amino acid substitutions primarily at positions V32I, M46I/L, I47V, I50V, I54L/M, and I84V, as well as substitutions in the p7/p1 and p1/p6 Gag and Gag-Pol polyprotein precursor cleavage sites. Some of these amprenavir resistance-associated substitutions have also been detected in HIV-1 isolates from

antiretroviral-naive subjects treated with LEXIVA. Of the 488 antiretroviral-naive subjects treated with LEXIVA 1,400 mg twice daily or LEXIVA 1,400 mg plus ritonavir 200 mg once daily in Trials APV30001 and APV30002, respectively, 61 subjects (29 receiving LEXIVA and 32 receiving LEXIVA/ritonavir) with virologic failure (plasma HIV-1 RNA greater than 1,000 copies per mL on 2 occasions on or after Week 12) were genotyped. Five of the 29 antiretroviral-naive subjects (17%) receiving LEXIVA without ritonavir in Trial APV30001 had evidence of genotypic resistance to amprenavir: I54L/M (n = 2), I54L + L33F (n = 1), V32I + I47V (n = 1), and M46I + I47V (n = 1). No amprenavir resistance-associated substitutions were detected in antiretroviral-naive subjects treated with LEXIVA/ritonavir for 48 weeks in Trial APV30002. However, the M46I and I50V substitutions were detected in isolates from 1 virologic failure subject receiving LEXIVA/ritonavir once daily at Week 160 (HIV-1 RNA greater than 500 copies per mL). Upon retrospective analysis of stored samples using an ultrasensitive assay, these resistant substitutions were traced back to Week 84 (76 weeks prior to clinical virologic failure).
Cross-Resistance: Varying degrees of cross-resistance among HIV-1 protease inhibitors have been observed. An association between virologic response at 48 weeks (HIV-1 RNA level less than 400 copies per mL) and protease inhibitor-resistance substitutions detected in baseline HIV-1 isolates from protease inhibitor-experienced subjects receiving LEXIVA/ritonavir twice daily (n = 88), or lopinavir/ritonavir twice daily (n = 85) in Trial APV30003 is shown in Table 14. The majority of subjects had previously received either one (47%) or 2 protease inhibitors (36%), most commonly nelfinavir (57%) and indinavir (53%). Out of 102 subjects with baseline phenotypes receiving twice-daily LEXIVA/ritonavir, 54% (n = 55) had resistance to at least one protease inhibitor, with 98% (n = 54) of those having resistance to nelfinavir. Out of 97 subjects with baseline phenotypes in the lopinavir/ritonavir arm, 60% (n = 58) had resistance to at least one protease inhibitor, with 97% (n = 56) of those having resistance to nelfinavir.
[See table 14 on page 2356]
The virologic response based upon baseline phenotype was assessed. Baseline isolates from protease inhibitor-experienced subjects responding to LEXIVA/ritonavir twice daily had a median shift in susceptibility to amprenavir relative to a standard wild-type reference strain of 0.7 (range: 0.1 to 5.4, n = 62), and baseline isolates from individuals failing therapy had a median shift in susceptibility of 1.9 (range: 0.2 to 14, n = 29). Because this was a select patient population, these data do not constitute definitive clinical susceptibility break points. Additional data are needed to determine clinically relevant break points for LEXIVA.
Isolates from 15 of the 20 subjects receiving twice-daily LEXIVA/ritonavir up to Week 48 and experiencing virologic failure/ongoing replication were subjected to genotypic analysis. The following amprenavir resistance-associated substitutions were found either alone or in combination: V32I, M46I/L, I47V, I50V, I54L/M, and I84V. Isolates from 4 of the 16 subjects continuing to receive twice-daily LEXIVA/ritonavir up to Week 96 who experienced virologic failure underwent genotypic analysis. Isolates from 2 subjects contained amprenavir resistance-associated substitutions: V32I, M46I, and I47V in 1 isolate and I84V in the other.

13 NONCLINICAL TOXICOLOGY

13.1 Carcinogenesis, Mutagenesis, Impairment of Fertility

In long-term carcinogenicity studies, fosamprenavir was administered orally for up to 104 weeks at doses of 250, 400, or 600 mg per kg per day in mice and at doses of 300, 825, or 2,250 mg per kg per day in rats. Exposures at these doses were 0.3- to 0.7-fold (mice) and 0.7- to 1.4-fold (rats) those in humans given 1,400 mg twice daily of fosamprenavir alone, and 0.2- to 0.3-fold (mice) and 0.3- to 0.7-fold (rats) those in humans given 1,400 mg once daily of fosamprenavir plus 200 mg ritonavir once daily. Exposures in the carcinogenicity studies were 0.1- to 0.3-fold (mice) and 0.3- to 0.6-fold (rats) those in humans given 700 mg of fosamprenavir plus 100 mg ritonavir twice daily. There was an increase in hepatocellular adenomas and hepatocellular carcinomas at all doses in male mice and at 600 mg per kg per day in female mice, and in hepatocellular adenomas and thyroid follicular cell adenomas at all doses in male rats, and at 835 mg per kg per day and 2,250 mg per kg per day in female rats. The relevance of the hepatocellular findings in the rodents for humans is uncertain. Repeat dose studies with fosamprenavir in rats produced effects consistent with enzyme induction, which predisposes rats, but not humans, to thyroid neoplasms. In addition, in rats only there was an increase in interstitial cell hyperplasia at 825 mg per kg per day and 2,250 mg per kg per day, and an increase in uterine endometrial adenocarcinoma at 2,250 mg per kg per day. The incidence of endometrial findings was slightly increased over concurrent controls, but was within background range for female rats. The relevance of the uterine endometrial adenocarcinoma findings in rats for humans is uncertain.

Fosamprenavir was not mutagenic or genotoxic in a battery of in vitro and in vivo assays. These assays included bacterial reverse mutation (Ames), mouse lymphoma, rat micronucleus, and chromosome aberrations in human lymphocytes.

The effects of fosamprenavir on fertility and general reproductive performance were investigated in male (treated for 4 weeks before mating) and female rats (treated 2 weeks before mating through postpartum day 6). Systemic exposures ($AUC_{0-24\ hr}$) to amprenavir in these studies were 3 (males) to 4 (females) times higher than exposures in humans following administration of the MRHD of fosamprenavir alone or similar to those seen in humans fol-

Table 10 (cont.). Drug Interactions: Pharmacokinetic Parameters for Amprenavir After Administration of LEXIVA in the Presence of the Coadministered Drug(s)

Coadministered Drug(s) and Dose(s)	Dose of LEXIVA[a]	n	% Change in Amprenavir Pharmacokinetic Parameters (90% CI)		
			C_{max}	AUC	C_{min}
Phenytoin 300 mg q.d. for 10 days	700 mg b.i.d. plus ritonavir 100 mg b.i.d. for 10 days	13	↔	↑20 (↑8 to ↑34)	↑19 (↑6 to ↑33)
Raltegravir 400 mg b.i.d. for 14 days	1,400 mg b.i.d. for 14 days (fasted)	14	↓27 (↓46 to ↔)	↓36 (↓53 to ↓13)	↓43[g] (↓59 to ↓21)
	1,400 mg b.i.d. for 14 days[h]	14	↓15 (↓27 to ↓1)	↓17 (↓27 to ↓6)	↓32[g] (↓53 to ↓1)
	700 mg b.i.d. plus ritonavir 100 mg b.i.d. for 14 days (fasted)	14	↓14 (↓39 to ↑20)	↓17 (↓38 to ↑12)	↓20[g] (↓45 to ↑17)
	700 mg b.i.d. plus ritonavir 100 mg b.i.d. for 14 days[h]	12	↓25 (↓42 to ↓2)	↓25 (↓44 to ↔)	↓33[g] (↓52 to ↓7)
Raltegravir 400 mg b.i.d. for 14 days	1,400 mg q.d. plus ritonavir 100 mg q.d. for 14 days (fasted)	13	↓18 (↓34 to ↔)	↓24 (↓41 to ↔)	↓50[g] (↓64 to ↓31)
	1,400 mg q.d. plus ritonavir 100 mg q.d. for 14 days[h]	14	↑27 (↓1 to ↑62)	↑13 (↓7 to ↑38)	17[g] (↓45 to ↑26)
Ranitidine 300 mg single dose (administered 1 hour before fosamprenavir)	1,400 mg single dose	30	51 (↓43 to ↓58)	30 (↓22 to ↓37)	↔ (↓19 to ↑21)
Rifabutin 150 mg q.o.d. for 2 weeks	700 mg b.i.d. plus ritonavir 100 mg b.i.d. for 2 weeks	15	↑36[c] (↑18 to ↑55)	↑35[c] (↑17 to ↑56)	↑17[c] (↓1 to ↑39)
Telaprevir 750 mg q. 8 hr for 10 days	700 mg b.i.d. plus ritonavir 100 mg b.i.d. for 20 days	18	↓35 (↓30 to ↓41)	↓47 (↓42 to ↓51)	↓56 (↓50 to ↓60)
Telaprevir 1,125 mg q. 12 hr for 4 days	700 mg b.i.d. plus ritonavir 100 mg b.i.d. for 24 days	17	↓40[i] (↓33 to ↓45)	↓49[i] (↓45 to ↓53)	↓58[i] (↓53 to ↓63)
Tenofovir 300 mg q.d. for 4 to 48 weeks	700 mg b.i.d. plus ritonavir 100 mg b.i.d. for 4 to 48 weeks	45	NA	NA	↔[j]
Tenofovir 300 mg q.d. for 4 to 48 weeks	1,400 mg q.d. plus ritonavir 200 mg q.d. for 4 to 48 weeks	60	NA	NA	↔[j]

[a]Concomitant medication is also shown in this column where appropriate.
[b]Ritonavir C_{max}, AUC, and C_{min} increased by 63%, 45%, and 13%, respectively, compared with historical control.
[c]Compared with historical control.
[d]Subjects were receiving LEXIVA/ritonavir for 10 days prior to the 4-day treatment period with both ketoconazole and LEXIVA/ritonavir.
[e]Compared with LEXIVA 700 mg/ritonavir 100 mg b.i.d. for 2 weeks.
[f]Subjects were receiving nevirapine for at least 12 weeks prior to trial.
[g]C_{last} ($C_{12\ hr}$ or $C_{24\ hr}$).
[h]Doses of LEXIVA and raltegravir were given with food on pharmacokinetic sampling days and without regard to food all other days.
[i]N = 18 for C_{min}.
[j]Compared with parallel control group.
↑ = Increase; ↓ = Decrease; ↔ = No change (↑or ↓ less than or equal to 10%), NA = Not applicable.

Table 11. Drug Interactions: Pharmacokinetic Parameters for Amprenavir After Administration of AGENERASE in the Presence of the Coadministered Drug(s)

Coadministered Drug(s) and Dose(s)	Dose of AGENERASE[a]	n	% Change in Amprenavir Pharmacokinetic Parameters (90% CI)		
			C_{max}	AUC	C_{min}
Abacavir 300 mg b.i.d. for 2 to 3 weeks	900 mg b.i.d. for 2 to 3 weeks	4	↔[a]	↔[a]	↔[a]
Clarithromycin 500 mg b.i.d. for 4 days	1,200 mg b.i.d. for 4 days	12	↑15 (↑1 to ↑31)	↑18 (↑8 to ↑29)	↑39 (↑31 to ↑47)
Delavirdine 600 mg b.i.d. for 10 days	600 mg b.i.d. for 10 days	9	↑40[b]	↑130[b]	↑125[b]
Ethinyl estradiol/norethindrone 0.035 mg/1 mg for 1 cycle	1,200 mg b.i.d. for 28 days	10	↔	↓22 (↓35 to ↓8)	↓20 (↓41 to ↑8)
Indinavir 800 mg t.i.d. for 2 weeks (fasted)	750 or 800 mg t.i.d. for 2 weeks (fasted)	9	↑18 (↑13 to ↑58)	↑33 (↑2 to ↑73)	↑25 (↓27 to ↑116)
Ketoconazole 400 mg single dose	1,200 mg single dose	12	↓16 (↓25 to ↓6)	↑31 (↑20 to ↑42)	NA
Lamivudine 150 mg single dose	600 mg single dose	11	↔	↔	NA
Methadone 44 to 100 mg q.d. for >30 days	1,200 mg b.i.d. for 10 days	16	↓27[c]	↓30[c]	↓25[c]
Nelfinavir 750 mg t.i.d. for 2 weeks (fed)	750 or 800 mg t.i.d. for 2 weeks (fed)	6	↓14 (↓38 to ↑20)	↔	↑189 (↑52 to ↑448)
Rifabutin 300 mg q.d. for 10 days	1,200 mg b.i.d. for 10 days	5	↔	↓15 (↓28 to 0)	↓15 (↓38 to ↑17)
Rifampin 300 mg q.d. for 4 days	1,200 mg b.i.d. for 4 days	11	↓70 (↓76 to ↓62)	↓82 (↓84 to ↓78)	↓92 (↓95 to ↓89)
Saquinavir 800 mg t.i.d. for 2 weeks (fed)	750 or 800 mg t.i.d. for 2 weeks (fed)	7	↓37 (↓54 to ↓14)	↓32 (↓49 to ↓9)	↓14 (↓52 to ↑54)
Zidovudine 300 mg single dose	600 mg single dose	12	↔	↑13 (↓2 to ↑31)	NA

[a]Compared with parallel control group.
[b]Median percent change; confidence interval not reported.
[c]Compared with historical data.
↑ = Increase; ↓ = Decrease; ↔ = No change (↑or ↓ less than 10%); NA = C_{min} not calculated for single–dose trial.

Table 12. Drug Interactions: Pharmacokinetic Parameters for Coadministered Drug in the Presence of Amprenavir After Administration of LEXIVA

Coadministered Drug(s) and Dose(s)	Dose of LEXIVA[a]	n	% Change in Pharmacokinetic Parameters of Coadministered Drug (90% CI)		
			C_{max}	AUC	C_{min}
Atazanavir 300 mg q.d. for 10 days[b]	700 mg b.i.d. plus ritonavir 100 mg b.i.d. for 10 days	21	↓24 (↓39 to ↓6)	↓22 (↓34 to ↓9)	↔
Atorvastatin 10 mg q.d. for 4 days	1,400 mg b.i.d. for 2 weeks	16	↑304 (↑205 to ↑437)	↑130 (↑100 to ↑164)	↓10 (↓27 to ↑12)
Atorvastatin 10 mg q.d. for 4 days	700 mg b.i.d. plus ritonavir 100 mg b.i.d. for 2 weeks	16	↑184 (↑126 to ↑257)	↑153 (↑115 to ↑199)	↑73 (↑45 to ↑108)
Esomeprazole 20 mg q.d. for 2 weeks	1,400 mg b.i.d. for 2 weeks	25	↔	↑55 (↑39 to ↑73)	ND
Esomeprazole 20 mg q.d. for 2 weeks	700 mg b.i.d. plus ritonavir 100 mg b.i.d. for 2 weeks	23	↔	↔	ND
Ethinyl estradiol[c] 0.035 mg q.d. for 21 days	700 mg b.i.d. plus ritonavir 100 mg b.i.d. for 21 days	25	↓28 (↓21 to ↓35)	↓37 (↓30 to ↓42)	ND

(Table continued on next page)

lowing administration of fosamprenavir in combination with ritonavir. Fosamprenavir did not impair mating or fertility of male or female rats and did not affect the development and maturation of sperm from treated rats.

14   CLINICAL STUDIES

14.1   Therapy-Naive Adult Trials

APV30001: A randomized, open-label trial evaluated treatment with LEXIVA Tablets (1,400 mg twice daily) versus nelfinavir (1,250 mg twice daily) in 249 antiretroviral treatment-naive subjects. Both groups of subjects also received abacavir (300 mg twice daily) and lamivudine (150 mg twice daily).

The mean age of the subjects in this trial was 37 years (range: 17 to 70 years); 69% of the subjects were male, 20% were CDC Class C (AIDS), 24% were Caucasian, 32% were black, and 44% were Hispanic. At baseline, the median CD4+ cell count was 212 cells per mm[3] (range: 2 to 1,136 cells per mm[3]; 18% of subjects had a CD4+ cell count of less than 50 cells per mm[3] and 30% were in the range of 50 to less than 200 cells per mm[3]). Baseline median HIV-1 RNA was 4.83 $\log_{10}$ copies per mL (range: 1.69 to 7.41 $\log_{10}$ copies per mL; 45% of subjects had greater than 100,000 copies per mL).

The outcomes of randomized treatment are provided in Table 15.
[See table 15 at top of page 2357]
Treatment response by viral load strata is shown in Table 16.
[See table 16 at top of page 2357]
Through 48 weeks of therapy, the median increases from baseline in CD4+ cell counts were 201 cells per mm[3] in the group receiving LEXIVA and 216 cells per mm[3] in the nelfinavir group.

APV30002: A randomized, open-label trial evaluated treatment with LEXIVA Tablets (1,400 mg once daily) plus ritonavir (200 mg once daily) versus nelfinavir (1,250 mg twice daily) in 649 treatment-naive subjects. Both treatment groups also received abacavir (300 mg twice daily) and lamivudine (150 mg twice daily).

The mean age of the subjects in this trial was 37 years (range: 18 to 69 years); 73% of the subjects were male, 22% were CDC Class C, 53% were Caucasian, 36% were black, and 8% were Hispanic. At baseline, the median CD4+ cell count was 170 cells per mm[3] (range: 1 to 1,055 cells per mm[3]; 20% of subjects had a CD4+ cell count of less than 50 cells per mm[3] and 35% were in the range of 50 to less than 200 cells per mm[3]). Baseline median HIV-1 RNA was 4.81 $\log_{10}$ copies per mL (range: 2.65 to 7.29 $\log_{10}$ copies per mL; 43% of subjects had greater than 100,000 copies per mL).

The outcomes of randomized treatment are provided in Table 17.
[See table 17 on page 2357]
Treatment response by viral load strata is shown in Table 18.
[See table 18 on page 2357]
Through 48 weeks of therapy, the median increases from baseline in CD4+ cell counts were 203 cells per mm[3] in the group receiving LEXIVA and 207 cells per mm[3] in the nelfinavir group.

14.2   Protease Inhibitor-Experienced Adult Trials

APV30003: A randomized, open-label, multicenter trial evaluated 2 different regimens of LEXIVA plus ritonavir (LEXIVA Tablets 700 mg twice daily plus ritonavir 100 mg twice daily or LEXIVA Tablets 1,400 mg once daily plus ritonavir 200 mg once daily) versus lopinavir/ritonavir (400 mg/100 mg twice daily) in 315 subjects who had experienced virologic failure to 1 or 2 prior protease inhibitor-containing regimens.

The mean age of the subjects in this trial was 42 years (range: 24 to 72 years); 85% were male, 33% were CDC Class C, 67% were Caucasian, 24% were black, and 9% were Hispanic. The median CD4+ cell count at baseline was 263 cells per mm[3] (range: 2 to 1,171 cells per mm[3]). Baseline median plasma HIV-1 RNA level was 4.14 $\log_{10}$ copies per mL (range: 1.69 to 6.41 $\log_{10}$ copies per mL).

The median durations of prior exposure to NRTIs were 257 weeks for subjects receiving LEXIVA/ritonavir twice daily (79% had greater than or equal to 3 prior NRTIs) and 210 weeks for subjects receiving lopinavir/ritonavir (64% had greater than or equal to 3 prior NRTIs. The median durations of prior exposure to protease inhibitors were 149 weeks for subjects receiving LEXIVA/ritonavir twice daily (49% received greater than or equal to 2 prior protease inhibitors) and 130 weeks for subjects receiving lopinavir/ritonavir (40% received greater than or equal to 2 prior protease inhibitors).

The time-averaged changes in plasma HIV-1 RNA from baseline (AAUCMB) at 48 weeks (the endpoint on which the trial was powered) were -1.4 $\log_{10}$ copies per mL for twice-daily LEXIVA/ritonavir and -1.67 $\log_{10}$ copies per mL for the lopinavir/ritonavir group.

The proportions of subjects who achieved and maintained confirmed HIV-1 RNA less than 400 copies per mL (secondary efficacy endpoint) were 58% with twice-daily LEXIVA/ritonavir and 61% with lopinavir/ritonavir (95% CI for the difference: -16.6, 10.1). The proportions of subjects with HIV-1 RNA less than 50 copies per mL with twice-daily LEXIVA/ritonavir and with lopinavir/ritonavir were 46% and 50%, respectively (95% CI for the difference: -18.3, 8.9). The proportions of subjects who were virologic failures were 29% with twice-daily LEXIVA/ritonavir and 27% with lopinavir/ritonavir.

The frequency of discontinuations due to adverse events and other reasons, and deaths were similar between treatment arms.

Through 48 weeks of therapy, the median increases from baseline in CD4+ cell counts were 81 cells per mm^3 with twice-daily LEXIVA/ritonavir and 91 cells per mm^3 with lopinavir/ritonavir.

This trial was not large enough to reach a definitive conclusion that LEXIVA/ritonavir and lopinavir/ritonavir are clinically equivalent.

Once-daily administration of LEXIVA plus ritonavir is not recommended for protease inhibitor-experienced patients. Through Week 48, 50% and 37% of subjects receiving LEXIVA 1,400 mg plus ritonavir 200 mg once daily had plasma HIV-1 RNA less than 400 copies per mL and less than 50 copies per mL, respectively.

14.3 Pediatric Trials

Three open-label trials in pediatric subjects aged at least 4 weeks to 18 years were conducted. In one trial (APV29005), twice-daily dosing regimens (LEXIVA with or without ritonavir) were evaluated in combination with other antiretroviral agents in pediatric subjects aged 2 to 18 years. In a second trial (APV20002), twice-daily dosing regimens (LEXIVA with ritonavir) were evaluated in combination with other antiretroviral agents in pediatric subjects aged at least 4 weeks to less than 2 years. A third trial (APV20003) evaluated once-daily dosing of LEXIVA with ritonavir; the pharmacokinetic data from this trial did not support a once-daily dosing regimen in any pediatric patient population.

APV29005: LEXIVA: Twenty (18 therapy-naive and 2 therapy-experienced) pediatric subjects received LEXIVA Oral Suspension without ritonavir twice daily. At Week 24, 65% (13/20) achieved HIV-1 RNA less than 400 copies per mL, and the median increase from baseline in CD4+ cell count was 350 cells per mm^3.

LEXIVA plus Ritonavir: Forty-nine protease inhibitor-naive and 40 protease inhibitor-experienced pediatric subjects received LEXIVA Oral Suspension or Tablets with ritonavir twice daily. At Week 24, 71% of protease inhibitor-naive (35/49) and 55% of protease inhibitor-experienced (22/40) subjects achieved HIV-1 RNA less than 400 copies per mL; median increases from baseline in CD4+ cell counts were 184 cells per mm^3 and 150 cells per mm^3 in protease inhibitor-naive and experienced subjects, respectively.

APV20002: Fifty-four pediatric subjects (49 protease inhibitor-naive and 5 protease inhibitor-experienced) received LEXIVA Oral Suspension with ritonavir twice daily. At Week 24, 72% of subjects achieved HIV-1 RNA less than 400 copies per mL. The median increases from baseline in CD4+ cell counts were 400 cells per mm^3 in subjects aged at least 4 weeks to less than 6 months and 278 cells per mm^3 in subjects aged 6 months to 2 years.

16 HOW SUPPLIED/STORAGE AND HANDLING

LEXIVA Tablets, 700 mg, are pink, film-coated, capsule-shaped, biconvex tablets, with "GX LL7" debossed on one face.

Bottle of 60 with child-resistant closure (NDC 49702-207-18).

Store at controlled room temperature of 25°C (77°F); excursions permitted to 15° to 30°C (59° to 86°F) (see USP Controlled Room Temperature). Keep container tightly closed.

LEXIVA Oral Suspension, a white to off-white grape-bubble-gum-peppermint–flavored suspension, contains 50 mg of fosamprenavir as fosamprenavir calcium equivalent to approximately 43 mg of amprenavir in each 1 mL.

Bottle of 225 mL with child-resistant closure (NDC 49702-208-53).

This product does not require reconstitution.

Store in refrigerator or at room temperature (5° to 30°C; 41° to 86°F). Shake vigorously before using. Do not freeze.

17 PATIENT COUNSELING INFORMATION

See FDA-approved Patient Labeling (Patient Information)

17.1 Drug Interactions

A statement to patients and healthcare providers is included on the product's bottle label: ALERT: Find out about medicines that should NOT be taken with LEXIVA.

Table 12 (cont.). Drug Interactions: Pharmacokinetic Parameters for Coadministered Drug in the Presence of Amprenavir After Administration of LEXIVA

Coadministered Drug(s) and Dose(s)	Dose of LEXIVA[a]	n	% Change in Pharmacokinetic Parameters of Coadministered Drug (90% CI)		
			C_{max}	AUC	C_{min}
Ketoconazole[d] 200 mg q.d. for 4 days	700 mg b.i.d. plus ritonavir 100 mg b.i.d. for 4 days	15	↑25 (↑0 to ↑56)	↑169 (↑108 to ↑248)	ND
Lopinavir/ritonavir[e] 533 mg/133 mg b.i.d. for 2 weeks	1,400 mg b.i.d. for 2 weeks	18	↔[f]	↔[f]	↔[f]
Lopinavir/ritonavir[e] 400 mg/100 mg b.i.d. for 2 weeks	700 mg b.i.d. plus ritonavir 100 mg b.i.d. for 2 weeks	18	↑30 (↓15 to ↑47)	↑37 (↓20 to ↑55)	↑52 (↓28 to ↑82)
Maraviroc 300 mg b.i.d. for 10 days	700 mg b.i.d. plus ritonavir 100 mg b.i.d. for 20 days	14	↑52 (↑27 to ↑82)	↑149 (↑119 to ↑182)	↑374 (↑303 to ↑457)
Maraviroc 300 mg q.d. for 10 days	1,400 mg q.d. plus ritonavir 100 mg q.d. for 20 days	14	↑45 (↑20 to ↑74)	↑126 (↑99 to ↑158)	↑80 (↑53 to ↑113)
Methadone 70 to 120 mg q.d. for 2 weeks	700 mg b.i.d. plus ritonavir 100 mg b.i.d. for 2 weeks	19	R-Methadone (active)		
			↓21[g] (↓30 to ↓12)	↓18[g] (↓27 to ↓8)	↓11[g] (↓21 to ↑1)
			S-Methadone (inactive)		
			↓43[g] (↓49 to ↓37)	↓43[g] (↓50 to ↓36)	↓41[g] (↓49 to ↓31)
Nevirapine 200 mg b.i.d. for 2 weeks[h]	1,400 mg b.i.d. for 2 weeks	17	↑25 (↑14 to ↑37)	↑29 (↑19 to ↑40)	↑34 (↑20 to ↑49)
Nevirapine 200 mg b.i.d. for 2 weeks[h]	700 mg b.i.d. plus ritonavir 100 mg b.i.d. for 2 weeks	17	↑13 (↑3 to ↑24)	↑14 (↑5 to ↑24)	↑22 (↑9 to ↑35)
Norethindrone[c] 0.5 mg q.d. for 21 days	700 mg b.i.d. plus ritonavir 100 mg b.i.d. for 21 days	25	↓38 (↓32 to ↓44)	↓34 (↓30 to ↓37)	↓26 (↓20 to ↓32)
Phenytoin 300 mg q.d. for 10 days	700 mg b.i.d. plus ritonavir 100 mg b.i.d. for 10 days	14	↓20 (↓12 to ↓27)	↓22 (↓17 to ↓27)	↓29 (↓23 to ↓34)
Rifabutin 150 mg every other day for 2 weeks	700 mg b.i.d. plus ritonavir 100 mg b.i.d. for 2 weeks	15	↓14 (↓28 to ↑4)	↔	↑28 (↑12 to ↑46)
(25-O-desacetylrifabutin metabolite)			↑579 (↑479 to ↑698)	↑1,120 (↑965 to ↑1,300)	↑2,510 (↑1,910 to ↑3,300)
Rifabutin + 25-O-desacetylrifabutin metabolite			NA	↑64 (↑46 to ↑84)	NA
Rosuvastatin 10 mg single dose	700 mg b.i.d. plus ritonavir 100 mg b.i.d. for 7 days		↑45	↑8	NA
Telaprevir 750 mg q. 8 hr for 10 days	700 mg b.i.d. plus ritonavir 100 mg b.i.d. for 20 days	18	↓33 (↓29 to ↓37)	↓32 (↓28 to ↓37)	↓30 (↓23 to ↓36)

[a]Concomitant medication is also shown in this column where appropriate.
[b]Comparison arm of atazanavir 300 mg q.d. plus ritonavir 100 mg q.d. for 10 days.
[c]Administered as a combination oral contraceptive tablet: ethinyl estradiol 0.035 mg/norethindrone 0.5 mg.
[d]Subjects were receiving LEXIVA/ritonavir for 10 days prior to the 4-day treatment period with both ketoconazole and LEXIVA/ritonavir.
[e]Data represent lopinavir concentrations.
[f]Compared with lopinavir 400 mg/ritonavir 100 mg b.i.d. for 2 weeks.
[g]Dose normalized to methadone 100 mg. The unbound concentration of the active moiety, R–methadone, was unchanged.
[h]Subjects were receiving nevirapine for at least 12 weeks prior to trial.
[i]Comparison arm of rifabutin 300 mg q.d. for 2 weeks. AUC is $AUC_{(0\text{-}48\ hr)}$.
↑ = Increase; ↓= Decrease; ↔ = No change (↑or ↓less than 10%); ND = Interaction cannot be determined as C_{min} was below the lower limit of quantitation.

Table 13. Drug Interactions: Pharmacokinetic Parameters for Coadministered Drug in the Presence of Amprenavir After Administration of AGENERASE

Coadministered Drug(s) and Dose(s)	Dose of AGENERASE	n	C_{max}	AUC	C_{min}
Abacavir 300 mg b.i.d. for 2 to 3 weeks	900 mg b.i.d. for 2 to 3 weeks	4	↔[a]	↔[a]	↔[a]
Clarithromycin 500 mg b.i.d. for 4 days	1,200 mg b.i.d. for 4 days	12	↓10 (↓24 to ↑7)	↔	↔
Delavirdine 600 mg b.i.d. for 10 days	600 mg b.i.d. for 10 days	9	↓47[b]	↓61[b]	↓88[b]
Ethinyl estradiol 0.035 mg for 1 cycle	1,200 mg b.i.d. for 28 days	10	↔	↔	↑32 (↓3 to ↑79)
Indinavir 800 mg t.i.d. for 2 weeks (fasted)	750 mg or 800 mg t.i.d. for 2 weeks (fasted)	9	↓22[a]	↓38[a]	↓27[a]
Ketoconazole 400 mg single dose	1,200 mg single dose	12	↑19 (↑8 to ↑33)	↑44 (↑31 to ↑59)	NA
Lamivudine 150 mg single dose	600 mg single dose	11	↔	↔	NA
Methadone 44 to 100 mg q.d. for >30 days	1,200 mg b.i.d. for 10 days	16	R-Methadone (active)		
			↓25 (↓32 to ↓18)	↓13 (↓21 to ↓5)	↓21 (↓32 to ↓9)
			S-Methadone (inactive)		
			↓48 (↓55 to ↓40)	↓40 (↓46 to ↓32)	↓53 (↓60 to ↓43)
Nelfinavir 750 mg t.i.d. for 2 weeks (fed)	750 mg or 800 mg t.i.d. for 2 weeks (fed)	6	↑12[a]	↑15[a]	↑14[a]
Norethindrone 1 mg for 1 cycle	1,200 mg b.i.d. for 28 days	10	↔	↑18 (↑1 to ↑38)	↑45 (↑13 to ↑88)
Rifabutin 300 mg q.d. for 10 days	1,200 mg b.i.d. for 10 days	5	↑119 (↑82 to ↑164)	↑193 (↑156 to ↑235)	↑271 (↑171 to ↑409)
Rifampin 300 mg q.d. for 4 days	1,200 mg b.i.d. for 4 days	11	↔	↔	ND
Saquinavir 800 mg t.i.d. for 2 weeks (fed)	750 mg or 800 mg t.i.d. for 2 weeks (fed)	7	↑21[a]	↓19[a]	↓48[a]
Zidovudine 300 mg single dose	600 mg single dose	12	↑40 (↑14 to ↑71)	↑31 (↑19 to ↑45)	NA

[a]Compared with historical data.
[b]Median percent change; confidence interval not reported.
↑ = Increase; ↓ = Decrease; ↔ = No change (↑ or ↓ less than 10%); NA = C_{min} not calculated for single-dose trial; ND = Interaction cannot be determined as C_{min} was below the lower limit of quantitation.

Table 14. Responders at Trial Week 48 by Presence of Baseline Protease Inhibitor Resistance-Associated Substitutions[a]

Protease Inhibitor Resistance-Associated Substitutions[b]	LEXIVA/Ritonavir b.i.d. (n = 88)		Lopinavir/Ritonavir b.i.d. (n = 85)	
D30N	21/22	95%	17/19	89%
N88D/S	20/22	91%	12/12	100%
L90M	16/31	52%	17/29	59%
M46I/L	11/22	50%	12/24	50%
V82A/F/T/S	2/9	22%	6/17	35%
I54V	2/11	18%	6/11	55%
I84V	1/6	17%	2/5	40%

[a]Results should be interpreted with caution because the subgroups were small.
[b]Most subjects had greater than 1 protease inhibitor resistance-associated substitution at baseline.

LEXIVA may interact with many drugs; therefore, patients should be advised to report to their healthcare provider the use of any other prescription or nonprescription medication or herbal products, particularly St. John's wort.
Patients receiving PDE5 inhibitors should be advised that they may be at an increased risk of PDE5 inhibitor-associated adverse events, including hypotension, visual changes, and priapism, and should promptly report any symptoms to their healthcare provider.
Patients receiving hormonal contraceptives should be instructed to use alternate contraceptive measures during therapy with LEXIVA because hormonal levels may be al-tered, and if used in combination with LEXIVA and ritonavir, liver enzyme elevations may occur.

17.2   Sulfa Allergy
Patients should inform their healthcare provider if they have a sulfa allergy. The potential for cross-sensitivity between drugs in the sulfonamide class and fosamprenavir is unknown.

17.3   Redistribution/Accumulation of Body Fat
Patients should be informed that redistribution or accumulation of body fat may occur in patients receiving antiretroviral therapy, including LEXIVA, and that the cause and long-term health effects of these conditions are not known at this time.

17.4   Information About Therapy With LEXIVA
LEXIVA is not a cure for HIV-1 infection and patients may continue to experience illnesses associated with HIV-1 infection, including opportunistic infections. Patients should remain under the care of a physician when using LEXIVA. Patients should be advised to avoid doing things that can spread HIV-1 infection to others.
• **Do not share needles or other injection equipment.**
• **Do not share personal items** that can have blood or body fluids on them, like toothbrushes and razor blades.
• **Do not have any kind of sex without protection.** Always practice safe sex by using a latex or polyurethane condom to lower the chance of sexual contact with semen, vaginal secretions, or blood.
• **Do not breastfeed.** We do not know if LEXIVA can be passed to your baby in your breast milk and whether it could harm your baby. Also, mothers with HIV-1 should not breastfeed because HIV-1 can be passed to the baby in the breast milk.
Patients should be told that sustained decreases in plasma HIV-1 RNA have been associated with a reduced risk of progression to AIDS and death. Patients should be advised to take LEXIVA every day as prescribed. LEXIVA must always be used in combination with other antiretroviral drugs. Patients should not alter the dose or discontinue therapy without consulting their physician. If a dose is missed, patients should take the dose as soon as possible and then return to their normal schedule. However, if a dose is skipped, the patient should not double the next dose.

17.5   Oral Suspension
Patients should be instructed to shake the bottle vigorously before each use and that refrigeration of the oral suspension may improve the taste for some patients.
LEXIVA and AGENERASE are registered trademarks of ViiV Healthcare.
The brands listed are trademarks of their respective owners and are not trademarks of ViiV Healthcare. The makers of these brands are not affiliated with and do not endorse ViiV Healthcare or its products.
Manufactured for:

ViiV Healthcare   Vertex Pharmaceuticals
Research Triangle Park, NC   Incorporated
27709   Cambridge, MA 02139

by:
GlaxoSmithKline
Research Triangle Park, NC 27709
©2013, ViiV Healthcare. All rights reserved.
LXV:17PI
PHARMACIST-DETACH HERE AND GIVE INSTRUCTIONS TO PATIENT

PATIENT INFORMATION
LEXIVA® (lex-EE-vah)
(fosamprenavir calcium)
Tablets
and
Oral Suspension
Important: LEXIVA can interact with other medicines and cause serious side effects. It is important to know the medicines that should not be taken with LEXIVA. See the section "Who should not take LEXIVA?"
Read this Patient Information before you start taking LEXIVA and each time you get a refill. There may be new information. This information does not take the place of talking with your healthcare provider about your medical condition or treatment.

What is LEXIVA?
LEXIVA is a prescription anti-HIV medicine used with other anti-HIV medicines to treat human immunodeficiency

(HIV-1) infections in adults and children 4 weeks of age and older. LEXIVA is a type of anti-HIV medicine called a protease inhibitor. HIV-1 is the virus that causes AIDS (Acquired Immune Deficiency Syndrome).

When used with other anti-HIV medicines, LEXIVA may help:

1. Reduce the amount of HIV-1 in your blood. This is called "viral load".
2. Increase the number of white blood cells called CD4 (T) cells, which help fight off other infections. Reducing the amount of HIV-1 and increasing the CD4 (T) cell count may improve your immune system. This may reduce your risk of death or infections that can happen when your immune system is weak (opportunistic infections).

It is not known if LEXIVA is safe and effective in children less than 4 weeks of age.

LEXIVA does not cure HIV-1 infection or AIDS. People taking LEXIVA may develop infections or other conditions associated with HIV-1 infection, including opportunistic infections (for example, pneumonia and herpes virus infections). You should remain under the care of your healthcare provider when using LEXIVA.

Avoid doing things that can spread HIV-1 infection to others.

• **Do not share needles or other injection equipment.**
• **Do not share personal items that can have blood or body fluids on them, like toothbrushes and razor blades.**
• **Do not have any kind of sex without protection.** Always practice safe sex by using a latex or polyurethane condom to lower the chance of sexual contact with semen, vaginal secretions, or blood.

Ask your healthcare provider if you have any questions on how to prevent passing HIV to other people.

Who should not take LEXIVA?

Do not take LEXIVA if you take any of the following medicines:

• alfuzosin (UROXATRAL®)
• flecainide (TAMBOCOR™)
• propafenone (RYTHMOL SR®)
• rifampin (RIFADIN®, RIFAMATE®, RIFATER®, RIMACTANE®)
• ergot including:
   ○ dihydroergotamine mesylate (D.H.E. 45®, MIGRANAL®)
   ○ ergotamine tartrate (CAFERGOT®, MIGERGOT®, ERGOMAR®, MEDIHALER ERGOTAMINE®)
   ○ methylergonovine (METHERGINE®)
• St. John's wort (*Hypericum perforatum*)
• lovastatin (ADVICOR®, ALTOPREV®, MEVACOR®)
• simvastatin (ZOCOR®, VYTORIN®, SIMCOR®)
• pimozide (ORAP®)
• delavirdine mesylate (RESCRIPTOR®)
• sildenafil (REVATIO®), for treatment of pulmonary arterial hypertension
• triazolam (HALCION®)

Serious problems can happen if you or your child take any of the medicines listed above with LEXIVA.

Do not take LEXIVA if you are allergic to AGENERASE® (amprenavir), fosamprenavir calcium, or any of the ingredients in LEXIVA. See the end of this leaflet for a complete list of ingredients in LEXIVA.

What should I tell my healthcare provider before taking LEXIVA?

Before taking LEXIVA, tell your healthcare provider if you:

• are allergic to medicines that contain sulfa
• have liver problems, including hepatitis B or C
• have kidney problems
• have high blood sugar (diabetes)
• have hemophilia
• have any other medical condition
• are pregnant or plan to become pregnant. It is not known if LEXIVA will harm your unborn baby.

Pregnancy Registry. There is a pregnancy registry for women who take antiviral medicines during pregnancy. The purpose of the registry is to collect information about the health of you and your baby. Talk to your healthcare provider about how you can take part in this registry.

• **Do not breastfeed.** We do not know if LEXIVA can be passed to your baby in your breast milk and whether it could harm your baby. Also, mothers with HIV-1 should not breastfeed because HIV-1 can be passed to the baby in the breast milk.

Tell your healthcare provider about all prescription and non-prescription medicines you take. Also tell your healthcare provider about any vitamins , herbal supplements, and dietary supplements you are taking.

Taking LEXIVA with certain other medicines may cause serious side effects. LEXIVA may affect the way other medicines work, and other medicines may affect how LEXIVA works.

Especially tell your healthcare provider if you take estrogen-based contraceptives (birth control pills). LEXIVA may reduce effectiveness of estrogen-based contraceptives. During treatment with LEXIVA, you should use a different contraceptive method.

Know all the medicines that you take. Keep a list of them with you to show healthcare providers and pharmacists when you get a new medicine.

Table 15. Outcomes of Randomized Treatment Through Week 48 (APV30001)

Outcome (Rebound or discontinuation = failure)	LEXIVA 1,400 mg b.i.d. (n = 166)	Nelfinavir 1,250 mg b.i.d. (n = 83)
Responder[a]	66% (57%)	52% (42%)
Virologic failure	19%	32%
Rebound	16%	19%
Never suppressed through Week 48	3%	13%
Clinical progression	1%	1%
Death	0%	1%
Discontinued due to adverse reactions	4%	2%
Discontinued due to other reasons[b]	10%	10%

[a]Subjects achieved and maintained confirmed HIV-1 RNA less than 400 copies per mL (less than 50 copies per mL) through Week 48 (Roche AMPLICOR HIV-1 MONITOR Assay Version 1.5).
[b]Includes consent withdrawn, lost to follow up, protocol violations, those with missing data, and other reasons.

Table 16. Proportions of Responders Through Week 48 by Screening Viral Load (APV30001)

Screening Viral Load HIV-1 RNA (copies/mL)	LEXIVA 1,400 mg b.i.d.		Nelfinavir 1,250 mg b.i.d.	
	<400 copies/mL	n	<400 copies/mL	n
≤100,000	65%	93	65%	46
>100,000	67%	73	36%	37

Table 17. Outcomes of Randomized Treatment Through Week 48 (APV30002)

Outcome (Rebound or discontinuation = failure)	LEXIVA 1,400 mg q.d./ Ritonavir 200 mg q.d. (n = 322)	Nelfinavir 1,250 mg b.i.d. (n = 327)
Responder[a]	69% (58%)	68% (55%)
Virologic failure	6%	16%
Rebound	5%	8%
Never suppressed through Week 48	1%	8%
Death	1%	0%
Discontinued due to adverse reactions	9%	6%
Discontinued due to other reasons[b]	15%	10%

[a]Subjects achieved and maintained confirmed HIV-1 RNA less than 400 copies per mL (less than 50 copies per mL) through Week 48 (Roche AMPLICOR HIV-1 MONITOR Assay Version 1.5).
[b]Includes consent withdrawn, lost to follow up, protocol violations, those with missing data, and other reasons.

Table 18. Proportions of Responders Through Week 48 by Screening Viral Load (APV30002)

Screening Viral Load HIV-1 RNA (copies/mL)	LEXIVA 1,400 mg q.d./ Ritonavir 200 mg q.d.		Nelfinavir 1,250 mg b.i.d.	
	<400 copies/mL	n	<400 copies/mL	n
≤100,000	72%	197	73%	194
>100,000	66%	125	64%	133

How should I take LEXIVA?

• **Stay under the care of a healthcare provider while taking LEXIVA.**
• Take LEXIVA exactly as prescribed by your healthcare provider.
• Do not change your dose or stop taking LEXIVA without talking with your healthcare provider.
• If your child is taking LEXIVA, your child's healthcare provider will decide the right dose based on your child's weight.
• You can take LEXIVA Tablets with or without food.
• **Adults should take LEXIVA Oral Suspension without food.**
• **Children should take LEXIVA Oral Suspension with food.** If your child vomits within 30 minutes after taking a dose of LEXIVA, the dose should be repeated.
• Shake LEXIVA Oral Suspension well before each use.
• If you miss a dose of LEXIVA, take the next dose as soon as possible and then take your next dose at the regular time. Do not double the next dose. If you take too much LEXIVA, call your healthcare provider or go to the nearest hospital emergency room right away.

What are the possible side effects of LEXIVA?

LEXIVA may cause serious side effects including:

• **Severe skin rash.** LEXIVA may cause severe or life-threatening skin reactions or rash.

If you get a rash with any of the following symptoms, stop taking LEXIVA and call your healthcare provider or get medical help right away:

○ hives or sores in your mouth, or your skin blisters and peels
○ trouble swallowing or breathing
○ swelling of your face, eyes, lips, tongue, or throat

• **Liver problems.** Your healthcare provider should do blood tests before and during your treatment with LEXIVA to check your liver function. Some people with liver problems, including hepatitis B or C, may have an increased risk of developing worsening liver problem during treatment with LEXIVA.

• **Diabetes and high blood sugar (hyperglycemia).** Some people who take protease inhibitors, including LEXIVA, can get high blood sugar, develop diabetes, or your diabetes can get worse. Tell your healthcare provider if you notice an increase in thirst or urinate often while taking LEXIVA.

• **Changes in your immune system (Immune Reconstitution Syndrome)** can happen when you start taking HIV medicines. Your immune system may get stronger and begin to fight infections that have been hidden in your body for a long time. Call your healthcare provider right away if you start having new symptoms after starting your HIV medicine.

• **Changes in body fat.** These changes can happen in people who take antiretroviral therapy. The changes may include an increased amount of fat in the upper back and neck ("buffalo hump"), breast, and around the back, chest, and stomach area. Loss of fat from the legs, arms, and face may also happen. The exact cause and long-term health effects of these conditions are not known.

- **Changes in blood tests**. Some people have changes in blood tests while taking LEXIVA. These include increases seen in liver function tests, blood fat levels, and decreases in white blood cells. Your healthcare provider should do regular blood tests before and during your treatment with LEXIVA.
- **Increased bleeding problems in some people with hemophilia**. Some people with hemophilia have increased bleeding with protease inhibitors, including LEXIVA.
- **Kidney stones**. Some people have developed kidney stones while taking LEXIVA. Tell your healthcare provider right away if you develop signs or symptoms of kidney stones:
  - pain in your side
  - blood in your urine
  - pain when you urinate

The most common side effects of LEXIVA in adults include:
- nausea
- vomiting
- diarrhea
- headache

Vomiting is the most common side effect in children when taking LEXIVA.

Tell your healthcare provider about any side effect that bothers you or that does not go away.

These are not all the possible side effects of LEXIVA. For more information, ask your healthcare provider or pharmacist.

Call your doctor for medical advice about side effects. You may report side effects to FDA at 1-800-FDA-1088.

How should I store LEXIVA?
- Store LEXIVA Tablets at room temperature between 68°F to 77°F (20°C to 25°C).
- Keep the bottle of LEXIVA Tablets tightly closed.
- Store LEXIVA Oral Suspension between 41°F to 86°F (5°C to 30°C). Refrigeration of LEXIVA Oral Suspension may improve taste for some people.
- Do not freeze.
  Keep LEXIVA and all medicines out of the reach of children.

General information about LEXIVA
Medicines are sometimes prescribed for purposes other than those listed in a Patient Information leaflet. Do not use LEXIVA for a condition for which it was not prescribed. Do not give LEXIVA to other people, even if they have the same symptoms you have. It may harm them.

This leaflet summarizes the most important information about LEXIVA. If you would like more information, talk with your healthcare provider. You can ask your pharmacist or healthcare provider for information about LEXIVA that is written for health professionals.

For more information call 877-844-8872 or go to www.LEXIVA.com.

What are the ingredients in LEXIVA?
Tablets:
Active ingredient: fosamprenavir calcium
Inactive ingredients: colloidal silicon dioxide, croscarmellose sodium, magnesium stearate, microcrystalline cellulose, and povidone K30. The tablet film-coating contains the inactive ingredients hypromellose, iron oxide red, titanium dioxide, and triacetin.

Oral Suspension:
Active ingredient: fosamprenavir calcium
Inactive ingredients: artificial grape-bubblegum flavor, calcium chloride dihydrate, hypromellose, methylparaben, natural peppermint flavor, polysorbate 80, propylene glycol, propylparaben, purified water, and sucralose.

This Patient Information has been approved by the U.S. Food and Drug Administration.

LEXIVA and AGENERASE are registered trademarks of ViiV Healthcare.

The brands listed are trademarks of their respective owners and are not trademarks of ViiV Healthcare. The makers of these brands are not affiliated with and do not endorse ViiV Healthcare or its products.

Manufactured for:

ViiV Healthcare
Research Triangle Park, NC
27709

Vertex Pharmaceuticals
Incorporated
Cambridge, MA 02139

by:
GlaxoSmithKline
Research Triangle Park, NC 27709
©2013, ViiV Healthcare. All rights reserved.
February 2013
LXV:14PIL

RESCRIPTOR®
[ree-SKRIP-tor]
(delavirdine mesylate)
Tablets

Rx

DESCRIPTION
RESCRIPTOR Tablets contain delavirdine mesylate, a synthetic non-nucleoside reverse transcriptase inhibitor

Table 1. Pharmacokinetic Parameters for Coadministered Drugs in the Presence of Delavirdine

Coadministered Drug	Dose of Coadministered Drug	Dose of RESCRIPTOR	n	% Change in Pharmacokinetic Parameters of Coadministered Drug (90% CI)		
				C_{max}	AUC	C_{min}
HIV-Protease Inhibitors						
Indinavir	400 mg t.i.d. for 7 days	400 mg t.i.d. for 7 days	28	↓36[a] (↓52 to ↓14)	↔[a]	↑118[a] (↑16 to ↑312)
	600 mg t.i.d. for 7 days	400 mg t.i.d. for 7 days	28	↔	↑53[a] (↑7 to ↑120)	↑298[a] (↑104 to ↑678)
Nelfinavir[b]	750 mg t.i.d. for 14 days	400 mg t.i.d. for 7 days	12	↑88 (↑66 to ↑113)	↑107 (↑83 to ↑135)	↑136 (↑103 to ↑175)
Saquinavir	Soft gel capsule 1,000 mg t.i.d. for 28 days	400 mg t.i.d. for 28 days	20	↑98[c] (↑4 to ↑277)	↑121[c] (↑14 to ↑340)	↑199[c] (↑37 to ↑553)
Nucleoside Reverse Transcriptase Inhibitors						
Didanosine (buffered tablets)	125 or 250 mg b.i.d. for 28 days	400 mg t.i.d. for 28 days	9	↓20[d] (↓44 to ↑15)	↓21[d] (↓40 to ↑5)	-
Zidovudine	200 mg t.i.d. for >38 days	100 mg q.i.d. to 400 mg t.i.d. for 8 to 10 days	34	↔	↔	-
Anti-infective Agents						
Clarithromycin	500 mg b.i.d. for 15 days	300 mg t.i.d. for 30 days	6		↑100	
Rifabutin	300 mg q.d. for 15 to 99 days	400 to 1,000 mg t.i.d. for 45 to 129 days	5	↑128 (↑71 to ↑203)	↑230 (↑119 to ↑396)	↑452 (↑246 to ↑781)

↑ Indicates increase.
↓ Indicates decrease.
↔ Indicates no significant change.
- Indicates no data available.
[a] Relative to indinavir 800 mg t.i.d. without RESCRIPTOR.
[b] Plasma concentrations of the nelfinavir active metabolite (nelfinavir hydroxy-t-butylamide) were significantly reduced by delavirdine, which is more than compensated for by increased nelfinavir concentration.
[c] Saquinavir soft gel capsule 1,000 mg t.i.d. plus RESCRIPTOR 400 mg t.i.d. relative to saquinavir soft gel capsule 1,200 mg t.i.d. without RESCRIPTOR.
[d] RESCRIPTOR taken with didanosine (buffered tablets) relative to doses of RESCRIPTOR and didanosine (buffered tablets) separated by at least 1 hour.

(NNRTI) of the human immunodeficiency virus type 1 (HIV-1). The chemical name of delavirdine mesylate is piperazine, 1-[3-[(1-methyl-ethyl)amino]-2- pyridinyl]-4-[[5-[(methylsulfonyl)amino]-1H-indol-2-yl]carbonyl]-, mono-methanesulfonate. Its molecular formula is $C_{22}H_{28}N_6O_3S \cdot CH_4O_3S$, and its molecular weight is 552.68. The structural formula is:

• $CH_3 - SO_2 - OH$

Delavirdine mesylate is an odorless white-to-tan crystalline powder. The aqueous solubility of delavirdine free base at 23°C is 2,942 mcg/mL at pH 1.0, 295 mcg/mL at pH 2.0, and 0.81 mcg/mL at pH 7.4.

Each RESCRIPTOR Tablet, for oral administration, contains 100 or 200 mg of delavirdine mesylate (henceforth referred to as delavirdine). Inactive ingredients consist of carnauba wax, colloidal silicon dioxide, croscarmellose sodium, lactose, magnesium stearate, and microcrystalline cellulose. In addition, the 100-mg tablet contains Opadry White YS-1-7000-E and the 200-mg tablet contains hypromellose and Opadry White YS-1-18202-A.

MICROBIOLOGY
Mechanism of Action
Delavirdine is an NNRTI of HIV-1. Delavirdine binds directly to reverse transcriptase (RT) and blocks RNA-dependent and DNA-dependent DNA polymerase activities. Delavirdine does not compete with template:primer or deoxynucleoside triphosphates. HIV-2 RT and human cellular DNA polymerases α, γ, or δ are not inhibited by delavirdine. In addition, HIV-1 group O, a group of highly divergent strains that are uncommon in North America, may not be inhibited by delavirdine.

In Vitro HIV-1 Susceptibility: In vitro anti-HIV-1 activity of delavirdine was assessed by infecting cell lines of lympho-blastic and monocytic origin and peripheral blood lymphocytes with laboratory and clinical isolates of HIV-1. IC_{50} and IC_{90} values (50% and 90% inhibitory concentrations) for laboratory isolates (n = 5) ranged from 0.005 to 0.030 μM and 0.04 to 0.10 μM, respectively. Mean IC_{50} of clinical isolates (n = 74) was 0.038 μM (range: 0.001 to 0.69 μM); 73 of 74 clinical isolates had an IC_{50} ≤0.18 μM. The IC_{90} of 24 of these clinical isolates ranged from 0.05 to 0.10 μM. In drug combination studies of delavirdine with zidovudine, didanosine, zalcitabine, lamivudine, interferon-α, and protease inhibitors, additive to synergistic anti–HIV-1 activity was observed in cell culture. The relationship between the in vitro susceptibility of HIV-1 RT inhibitors and the inhibition of HIV replication in humans has not been established.

Drug Resistance: Phenotypic analyses of isolates from patients treated with RESCRIPTOR as monotherapy showed a 50- to 500-fold reduced susceptibility in 14 of 15 patients by Week 8 of therapy. Genotypic analysis of HIV-1 isolates from patients receiving RESCRIPTOR plus zidovudine combination therapy (n = 79) showed resistance-conferring mutations in all isolates by Week 24 of therapy. In patients treated with RESCRIPTOR, the mutations in RT occurred predominantly at amino acid positions 103 and less frequently at positions 181 and 236. In a separate study, an average of 86-fold increase in the zidovudine susceptibility of patient isolates (n = 24) was observed after 24 weeks of combination therapy with RESCRIPTOR and zidovudine. The clinical relevance of the phenotypic and the genotypic changes associated with therapy with RESCRIPTOR has not been established.

Cross-Resistance: RESCRIPTOR may confer cross-resistance to other NNRTIs when used alone or in combination. Mutations at positions 103 and/or 181 have been found in resistant virus during treatment with RESCRIPTOR and other NNRTIs. These mutations have been associated with cross-resistance among NNRTIs in vitro.

CLINICAL PHARMACOLOGY
Pharmacokinetics
Absorption and Bioavailability: Delavirdine is rapidly absorbed following oral administration, with peak plasma concentrations occurring at approximately 1 hour. Following administration of delavirdine 400 mg 3 times daily (n = 67,

HIV-1–infected patients), the mean ±SD steady-state peak plasma concentration (C_{max}) was 35 ± 20 μM (range: 2 to 100 μM), systemic exposure (AUC) was 180 ± 100 μM•hr (range: 5 to 515 μM•hr), and trough concentration (C_{min}) was 15 ± 10 μM (range: 0.1 to 45 μM). The single-dose bioavailability of delavirdine tablets relative to an oral solution was 85% ± 25% (n = 16, non-HIV–infected subjects). The single-dose bioavailability of delavirdine tablets (100-mg strength) was increased by approximately 20% when a slurry of drug was prepared by allowing delavirdine tablets to disintegrate in water before administration (n = 16, non-HIV–infected subjects). The bioavailability of the 200-mg strength delavirdine tablets has not been evaluated when administered as a slurry because they are not readily dispersed in water (see DOSAGE AND ADMINISTRATION). Delavirdine may be administered with or without food. In a multiple-dose, crossover study, delavirdine was administered every 8 hours with food or every 8 hours, 1 hour before or 2 hours after a meal (n = 13, HIV-1–infected patients). Patients remained on their typical diet throughout the study; meal content was not standardized. When multiple doses of delavirdine were administered with food, geometric mean C_{max} was reduced by approximately 25%, but AUC and C_{min} were not altered.

Distribution: Delavirdine is extensively bound (approximately 98%) to plasma proteins, primarily albumin. The percentage of delavirdine that is protein-bound is constant over a delavirdine concentration range of 0.5 to 196 μM. In 5 HIV-1–infected patients whose total daily dose of delavirdine ranged from 600 to 1,200 mg, cerebrospinal fluid concentrations of delavirdine averaged 0.4% ± 0.07% of the corresponding plasma delavirdine concentrations; this represents about 20% of the fraction not bound to plasma proteins. Steady-state delavirdine concentrations in saliva (n = 5, HIV-1–infected patients who received delavirdine 400 mg 3 times daily) and semen (n = 5 healthy volunteers who received delavirdine 300 mg 3 times daily) were about 6% and 2%, respectively, of the corresponding plasma delavirdine concentrations collected at the end of a dosing interval.

Metabolism and Elimination: Delavirdine is extensively converted to several inactive metabolites. Delavirdine is primarily metabolized by cytochrome P450 3A (CYP3A), but in vitro data suggest that delavirdine may also be metabolized by CYP2D6. The major metabolic pathways for delavirdine are N-desalkylation and pyridine hydroxylation. Delavirdine exhibits nonlinear steady-state elimination pharmacokinetics, with apparent oral clearance decreasing by about 22-fold as the total daily dose of delavirdine increases from 60 to 1,200 mg/day. In a study of ^{14}C-delavirdine in 6 healthy volunteers who received multiple doses of delavirdine tablets 300 mg 3 times daily, approximately 44% of the radiolabeled dose was recovered in feces, and approximately 51% of the dose was excreted in urine. Less than 5% of the dose was recovered unchanged in urine. The parent plasma half-life of delavirdine increases with dose; mean half-life following 400 mg 3 times daily is 5.8 hours, with a range of 2 to 11 hours.

In vitro and in vivo studies have shown that delavirdine reduces CYP3A activity and inhibits its own metabolism. In vitro studies have also shown that delavirdine reduces CYP2C9, CYP2D6, and CYP2C19 activity. Inhibition of hepatic CYP3A activity by delavirdine is reversible within 1 week after discontinuation of drug.

Special Populations

Hepatic or Renal Impairment: The pharmacokinetics of delavirdine in patients with hepatic or renal impairment have not been investigated (see PRECAUTIONS).

Age: The pharmacokinetics of delavirdine have not been adequately studied in patients aged <16 years or >65 years.

Gender: Data from population pharmacokinetics suggest that the plasma concentrations of delavirdine tend to be higher in females than in males. However, this difference is not considered to be clinically significant.

Race: No significant differences in the mean trough delavirdine concentrations were observed between different racial or ethnic groups.

Drug Interactions

(See also PRECAUTIONS: Drug Interactions.)

Specific drug interaction studies were performed with delavirdine and a number of drugs. Table 1 summarizes the effects of delavirdine on the geometric mean AUC, C_{max}, and C_{min} of coadministered drugs. Table 2 shows the effects of coadministered drugs on the geometric mean AUC, C_{max}, and C_{min} of delavirdine.

For information regarding clinical recommendations, see CONTRAINDICATIONS, WARNINGS, and PRECAUTIONS: Drug Interactions.

[See table 1 at top of previous page]
[See table 2 above]

INDICATIONS AND USAGE

RESCRIPTOR Tablets are indicated for the treatment of HIV-1 infection in combination with at least 2 other active antiretroviral agents when therapy is warranted.

Table 2. Pharmacokinetic Parameters for Delavirdine in the Presence of Coadministered Drugs

Coadministered Drug	Dose of Coadministered Drug	Dose of RESCRIPTOR	n	% Change in **Delavirdine** Pharmacokinetic Parameters (90% CI)		
				C_{max}	AUC	C_{min}
HIV-Protease Inhibitors						
Indinavir	400 or 600 mg t.i.d. for 7 days	400 mg t.i.d. for 7 days	81	No apparent changes based on a comparison to historical data		
Nelfinavir	750 mg t.i.d. for 7 days	400 mg t.i.d. for 14 days	7	↓27 (↓49 to ↑4)	↓31 (↓57 to ↑10)	↓33 (↓70 to ↑49)
Saquinavir	Soft gel capsule 1,000 mg t.i.d. for 28 days	400 mg t.i.d. for 7 to 28 days	23	No apparent changes based on a comparison to historical data		
Nucleoside Reverse Transcriptase Inhibitors						
Didanosine (buffered tablets)	125 or 200 mg b.i.d. for 28 days	400 mg t.i.d. for 28 days	9	↓32[a] (↓48 to ↓11)	↓19[a] (↓37 to ↑6)	↔[a]
Zidovudine	200 mg t.i.d. for ≥7 days	400 mg t.i.d. for 7 to 14 days	42	No apparent changes based on a comparison to historical data		
Anti-infective Agents						
Clarithromycin	500 mg b.i.d. for 15 days	300 mg t.i.d. for 30 days	6	↔	↔	↔
Fluconazole	400 mg q.d. for 15 days	300 mg t.i.d. for 30 days	8	↔	↔	↔
Ketoconazole	Various	200 to 400 mg t.i.d.	26	-	-	↑50[b]
Rifabutin	300 mg q.d. for 14 days	400 mg t.i.d. for 28 days	7	↓72 (↓61 to ↓80)	↓82 (↓74 to ↓88)	↓94 (↓90 to ↓96)
Rifampin	600 mg q.d. for 15 days	400 mg t.i.d. for 30 days	7	↓90 (↓94 to ↓83)	↓97 (↓98 to ↓95)	↓100
Sulfamethoxazole or Trimethoprim & Sulfamethoxazole	Various	200 to 400 mg t.i.d.	311	-	-	↔[b]
Other						
Antacid (Maalox® TC)	20 mL	300 mg single dose	12	↓52 (↓68 to ↓29)	↓44 (↓58 to ↓27)	-
Fluoxetine	Various	200 to 400 mg t.i.d.	36	-	-	↑50[b]
Phenytoin, Phenobarbital, Carbamazepine	Various	300 to 400 mg t.i.d.	8	-	-	↓90[b]

↑ Indicates increase.
↓ Indicates decrease.
↔ Indicates no significant change.
- Indicates no data available.
[a] RESCRIPTOR taken with didanosine (buffered tablets) relative to doses of RESCRIPTOR and didanosine (buffered tablets) separated by at least 1 hour.
[b] Population pharmacokinetic data from efficacy studies.

The following should be considered before initiating therapy with RESCRIPTOR in treatment-naive patients. There are insufficient data directly comparing antiretroviral regimens containing RESCRIPTOR with currently preferred 3-drug regimens for initial treatment of HIV. In studies comparing regimens consisting of 2 nucleoside reverse transcriptase inhibitors (NRTIs) (currently considered suboptimal) to RESCRIPTOR plus 2 NRTIs, the proportion of patients receiving the regimen containing RESCRIPTOR who achieved and sustained an HIV-1 RNA level <400 copies/mL over 1 year of therapy was relatively low (see DESCRIPTION OF CLINICAL STUDIES).

Resistant virus emerges rapidly when RESCRIPTOR is administered as monotherapy. Therefore, RESCRIPTOR should always be administered in combination with other antiretroviral agents.

DESCRIPTION OF CLINICAL STUDIES

For clinical Studies 21 Part II and 13C described below, efficacy was evaluated by the percentage of patients with a plasma HIV-1 RNA level <400 copies/mL through Week 52 as measured by the Roche Amplicor® HIV-1 Monitor (standard assay). An intent-to-treat analysis was performed where only subjects who achieved confirmed suppression and sustained it through Week 52 are regarded as responders. All other subjects (including never suppressed, discontinued, and those who rebounded after initial suppression of <400 copies/mL) are considered failures at Week 52. Results of an interim analysis of efficacy conducted for studies 21

Part II and 13C by independent Data and Safety Monitoring Boards (DSMBs) revealed that the triple-therapy arms in both studies produced significantly greater antiviral benefit than the dual-therapy arms, and early termination of the studies was recommended.

Study 21 Part II

Study 21 Part II was a double–blind, randomized, placebo–controlled trial comparing treatment with RESCRIPTOR (400 mg 3 times daily, zidovudine 200 mg 3 times daily, and lamivudine 150 mg twice daily versus RESCRIPTOR 400 mg 3 times daily and zidovudine 200 mg 3 times daily versus zidovudine 200 mg 3 times daily and lamivudine 150 mg twice daily in 373 HIV-1–infected patients (mean age 35 years [range: 17 to 67], 87% male, and 60% Caucasian) who were antiretroviral treatment naive (84%) or had limited nucleoside experience (16%). Mean baseline CD4+ cell count was 359 cells/mm[3] and mean baseline plasma HIV-1 RNA was 4.4 $\log_{10}$ copies/mL.

Results showed that the mean increases from baseline in CD4 cell counts at 52 weeks were 111 cells/mL for RESCRIPTOR + zidovudine + lamivudine, 27 cells/mL for RESCRIPTOR + zidovudine, and 74 cells/mL for zidovudine + lamivudine.

The results of the intent-to-treat analysis of the percentage of patients with a plasma HIV-1 RNA level <400 copies/mL are presented in Figure 1. HIV-1 RNA status and reasons for discontinuation of randomized treatment at 52 weeks are summarized in Table 3. Subjects who were never suppressed before discontinuation were placed in the discontinuation category.

Table 3. Outcomes of Randomized Treatment Through Week 52 for Protocol 21 Part II

Outcome	Zidovudine + Lamivudine (n = 124) %	RESCRIPTOR + Zidovudine (n = 125) %	RESCRIPTOR + Zidovudine + Lamivudine (n = 124) %
HIV-1 RNA <400 copies/mL[a]	14	2	45
HIV-1 RNA ≥400 copies/mL[b,c]	64	52	31
Discontinued due to adverse events[c]	8	13	10
Discontinued due to other reasons[c,d]	14	33	14

[a]Corresponds to rates at Week 52 in proportion curve.
[b]Virologic failures at or before Week 52.
[c]Considered to be treatment failure in the analysis.
[d] Includes discontinuations due to consent withdrawn, loss to follow-up, protocol violations, non-compliance, pregnancy, never treated, and other reasons.

Table 4. Outcomes of Randomized Treatment Through Week 54 for Protocol 13C

Outcome	Zidovudine + Didanosine or Zalcitabine or Lamivudine (n = 173) %	Zidovudine + Didanosine or Zalcitabine or Lamivudine + RESCRIPTOR (n = 172) %
HIV-1 RNA 400 copies/mL[a]	10	29
HIV-1 RNA 400 copies/mL[b,c]	69	42
Discontinued due to adverse events[c]	7	12
Discontinued due to other reasons[c,d]	14	17

[a]Corresponds to rates at Week 54 in proportion curve.
[b]Virologic failures at or before Week 54.
[c]Considered to be treatment failure in the analysis.
[d]Includes discontinuations due to consent withdrawn, loss to follow-up, protocol violations, non-compliance, pregnancy, never treated, and other reasons.

Figure 1. Percentage of Patients With HIV-1 RNA Below 400 copies/mL Standard PCR Assay Protocol 21 Part II: Intent-to-Treat Analysis

Figure 2. Percentage of Patients With HIV-1 RNA Below 400 copies/mL Standard PCR Assay Protocol 13C: Intent-to-Treat Analysis

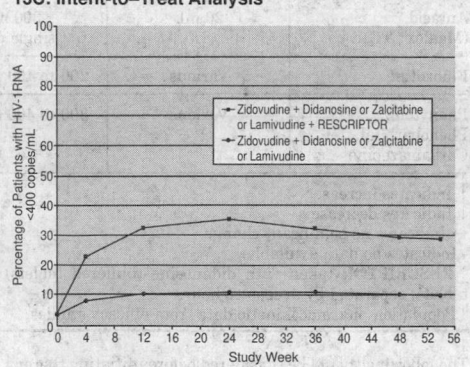

[See table 3 above]

Study 13C
Study 13C was a double–blind, randomized, placebo–controlled trial comparing treatment with RESCRIPTOR 400 mg 3 times daily, zidovudine 200 mg 3 times daily or 300 mg twice daily, and either didanosine 200 mg twice daily, zalcitabine 0.75 mg 3 times daily, or lamivudine 150 mg twice daily versus zidovudine 200 mg 3 times daily or 300 mg twice daily and either didanosine 200 mg twice daily, zalcitabine 0.75 mg 3 times daily, or lamivudine 150 mg twice daily in 345 HIV-1–infected patients (mean age 35.8 years [range: 18 to 72], 66% male, and 63% Caucasian) who were antiretroviral treatment naive (63%) or had limited antiretroviral experience (37%). Mean baseline CD4+ cell count was 210 cells/mm³ and mean baseline plasma HIV-1 RNA was 4.9 log₁₀ copies/mL.
Results showed that the mean increases from baseline in CD4+ cell counts at 54 weeks were 102 cells/mL for RESCRIPTOR + zidovudine + didanosine or zalcitabine or lamivudine, and 56 cells/mL for zidovudine + didanosine or zalcitabine or lamivudine.
The results of the intent–to–treat analysis of the percentage of patients with a plasma HIV–1 RNA level 400 copies/mL are presented in Figure 2. HIV–1 RNA status and reasons for discontinuation of randomized treatment at 54 weeks are summarized in Table 4. Subjects who were never suppressed before discontinuation were placed in the discontinuation category.

[See table 4 above]
Results from several smaller supportive studies evaluating the use of RESCRIPTOR in treatment-naive patients suggest that it may have activity when used in combination with protease inhibitors and NRTIs in 3- or 4-drug combinations.

CONTRAINDICATIONS
RESCRIPTOR Tablets are contraindicated in patients with known hypersensitivity to any of its ingredients. Coadministration of RESCRIPTOR is contraindicated with drugs that are highly dependent on CYP3A for clearance and for which elevated plasma concentrations are associated with serious and/or life-threatening events. These drugs are listed in Table 5. **Also, see PRECAUTIONS, Table 6, Drugs That Should Not Be Coadministered With RESCRIPTOR.**

Table 5. Drugs That Are Contraindicated With RESCRIPTOR

Drug Class	Drugs Within Class That Are Contraindicated With RESCRIPTOR
Antihistamines	Astemizole, terfenadine
Ergot derivatives	Dihydroergotamine, ergonovine, ergotamine, methylergonovine
GI motility agent	Cisapride
Neuroleptic	Pimozide
Sedative/hypnotics	Alprazolam, midazolam, triazolam

WARNINGS
ALERT: Find out about medicines that should NOT be taken with RESCRIPTOR. This statement is included on the product's bottle label.
Drug Interactions
Because delavirdine may inhibit the metabolism of many different drugs (e.g., antiarrhythmics, calcium channel blockers, sedative hypnotics, and others), **serious and/or life-threatening drug interactions could result from inappropriate coadministration of some drugs with delavirdine.** In addition, some drugs may markedly reduce delavirdine plasma concentrations, resulting in suboptimal antiviral activity and subsequent emergence of drug resistance. All prescribers should become familiar with the following tables in this package insert: **Table 5, Drugs That Are Contraindicated With RESCRIPTOR;Table 6, Drugs That Should Not Be Coadministered With RESCRIPTOR;and Table 7, Established and Other Potentially Significant Drug Interactions: Alteration in Dose or Regimen May Be Recommended Based on Drug Interaction Studies or Predicted Interaction.** Additional details on drug interactions can be found in Tables 1 and 2 under the CLINICAL PHARMACOLOGY section.
Concomitant use of lovastatin or simvastatin with RESCRIPTOR is not recommended. Caution should be exercised if RESCRIPTOR is used concurrently with other HMG-CoA reductase inhibitors that are also metabolized by the CYP3A4 pathway (e.g., atorvastatin or cerivastatin). The risk of myopathy including rhabdomyolysis may be increased when RESCRIPTOR is used in combination with these drugs.
Particular caution should be used when prescribing sildenafil in patients receiving RESCRIPTOR. Coadministration of sildenafil with RESCRIPTOR is expected to substantially increase sildenafil concentrations and may result in an increase in sildenafil-associated adverse events, including hypotension, visual changes, and priapism (see PRECAUTIONS: Drug Interactions and Information for Patients, and the complete prescribing information for sildenafil).
Concomitant use of St. John's wort (*Hypericum perforatum*) or St. John's wort-containing products and RESCRIPTOR is not recommended. Coadministration of St. John's wort with NNRTIs, including RESCRIPTOR, is expected to substantially decrease NNRTI concentrations and may result in suboptimal levels of RESCRIPTOR and lead to loss of virologic response and possible resistance to RESCRIPTOR or to the class of NNRTIs.

PRECAUTIONS
General
Delavirdine is metabolized primarily by the liver. Therefore, caution should be exercised when administering RESCRIPTOR Tablets to patients with impaired hepatic function.
Immune Reconstitution Syndrome
Immune reconstitution syndrome has been reported in patients treated with combination antiretroviral therapy, including RESCRIPTOR. During the initial phase of the combination antiretroviral treatment, patients whose immune systems respond may develop an inflammatory response to indolent or residual opportunistic infections (such as *Mycobacterium avium* infection, cytomegalovirus, *Pneumocystis jirovecii* pneumonia [PCP], or tuberculosis), which may necessitate further evaluation and treatment.
Autoimmune disorders (such as Graves' disease, polymyositis, and Guillain-Barré syndrome) have also been reported to occur in the setting of immune reconstitution; however, the time to onset is more variable, and can occur many months after initiation of treatment.
Resistance/Cross-Resistance
NNRTIs, when used alone or in combination, may confer cross-resistance to other NNRTIs.
Fat Redistribution
Redistribution/accumulation of body fat including central obesity, dorsocervical fat enlargement (buffalo hump), peripheral wasting, facial wasting, breast enlargement, and "cushingoid appearance" have been observed in patients receiving antiretroviral therapy. The mechanism and long-term consequences of these events are currently unknown. A causal relationship has not been established.
Skin Rash
Severe rash, including rare cases of erythema multiforme and Stevens-Johnson syndrome, has been reported in patients receiving RESCRIPTOR. Erythema multiforme and Stevens-Johnson syndrome were rarely seen in clinical trials and resolved after withdrawal of RESCRIPTOR. Any patient experiencing severe rash or rash accompanied by

symptoms such as fever, blistering, oral lesions, conjunctivitis, swelling, and muscle or joint aches should discontinue RESCRIPTOR and consult a physician. Two cases of Stevens-Johnson syndrome have been reported through postmarketing surveillance out of a total of 339 surveillance reports.

In Studies 21 Part II and 13C (see DESCRIPTION OF CLINICAL STUDIES), rash (including maculopapular rash) was reported in more patients who were treated with RESCRIPTOR 400 mg 3 times daily (35% and 32%, respectively) than in those who were not treated with RESCRIPTOR (21% and 16%, respectively). The highest intensity of rash reported in these studies was severe (Grade 3), which was observed in approximately 4% of patients treated with RESCRIPTOR in each study and in none of the patients who were not treated with RESCRIPTOR. Also in Studies 21 Part II and 13C, discontinuations due to rash were reported in more patients who received RESCRIPTOR 400 mg 3 times daily (3% and 4%, respectively) than in those who did not receive RESCRIPTOR (0% and 1%, respectively).

In most cases, the duration of the rash was less than 2 weeks and did not require dose reduction or discontinuation of RESCRIPTOR. Most patients were able to resume therapy after rechallenge with RESCRIPTOR following a treatment interruption due to rash. The distribution of the rash was mainly on the upper body and proximal arms, with decreasing intensity of the lesions on the neck and face, and progressively less on the rest of the trunk and limbs.

Occurrence of a delavirdine-associated rash after 1 month is uncommon. Symptomatic relief has been obtained using diphenhydramine hydrochloride, hydroxyzine hydrochloride, and/or topical corticosteroids.

Information for Patients

A statement to patients and healthcare providers is included on the product's bottle label: **ALERT: Find out about medicines that should NOT be taken with RESCRIPTOR.** A patient package insert (PPI) for RESCRIPTOR is available for patient information.

Patients should be informed that RESCRIPTOR is not a cure for HIV–1 infection and that patients may continue to experience illnesses associated with HIV–1 infection, including opportunistic infections. Patients should be advised to remain under the care of a physician while taking RESCRIPTOR.

Patients should be advised to avoid doing things that can spread HIV-1 infection to others.

• **Do not share needles or other injection equipment.**
• **Do not share personal items that can have blood or body fluids on them, like toothbrushes and razor blades.**
• **Do not have any kind of sex without protection.** Always practice safe sex by using a latex or polyurethane condom to lower the chance of sexual contact with semen, vaginal secretions, or blood.
• **Do not breastfeed.** We do not know if RESCRIPTOR can be passed to your baby in your breast milk and whether it could harm your baby. Also, mothers with HIV-1 should not breastfeed because HIV-1 can be passed to the baby in the breast milk.

Patients should be instructed that the major toxicity of RESCRIPTOR is rash and should be advised to promptly notify their physician should rash occur. The majority of rashes associated with RESCRIPTOR occur within 1 to 3 weeks after initiating treatment with RESCRIPTOR. The rash normally resolves in 3 to 14 days and may be treated symptomatically while therapy with RESCRIPTOR is continued. Any patient experiencing severe rash or rash accompanied by symptoms such as fever, blistering, oral lesions, conjunctivitis, swelling, and muscle or joint aches should discontinue medication and consult a physician.

Patients should be informed that redistribution or accumulation of body fat may occur in patients receiving antiretroviral therapy and that the cause and long-term health effects of these conditions are not known at this time.

Patients should be informed to take RESCRIPTOR every day as prescribed. Patients should not alter the dose of RESCRIPTOR without consulting their doctor. If a dose is missed, patients should take the next dose as soon as possible. However, if a dose is skipped, the patient should not double the next dose.

Patients with achlorhydria should take RESCRIPTOR with an acidic beverage (e.g., orange or cranberry juice). However, the effect of an acidic beverage on the absorption of delavirdine in patients with achlorhydria has not been investigated.

Patients taking both RESCRIPTOR and antacids should be advised to take them at least 1 hour apart.

Because RESCRIPTOR may interact with certain drugs, patients should be advised to report to their doctor the use of any prescription, nonprescription medication, or herbal products, particularly St. John's wort.

Patients receiving sildenafil and RESCRIPTOR should be advised that they may be at an increased risk of sildenafil–

Table 6. Drugs That Should Not Be Coadministered With RESCRIPTOR

Drug Class: Drug Name	Clinical Comment
Anticonvulsant agents: Phenytoin, phenobarbital, carbamazepine	May lead to loss of virologic response and possible resistance to RESCRIPTOR or to the class of NNRTIs.
Antihistamines: Astemizole, terfenadine	CONTRAINDICATED due to potential for serious and/or life-threatening reactions such as cardiac arrhythmias.
Antimycobacterials: Rifabutin,[a] rifampin [a]	May lead to loss of virologic response and possible resistance to RESCRIPTOR or to the class of NNRTIs or other coadministered antiviral agents.
Ergot Derivatives: Dihydroergotamine, ergonovine, ergotamine, methylergonovine	CONTRAINDICATED due to potential for serious and/or life-threatening reactions such as acute ergot toxicity characterized by peripheral vasospasm and ischemia of the extremities and other tissues.
GI motility agent: Cisapride	CONTRAINDICATED due to potential for serious and/or life-threatening reactions such as cardiac arrhythmias.
Herbal Products: St. John's wort (*Hypericum perforatum*)	May lead to loss of virologic response and possible resistance to RESCRIPTOR or to the class of NNRTIs.
HMG-CoA reductase inhibitors: Lovastatin, simvastatin	Potential for serious reactions such as risk of myopathy including rhabdomyolysis.
Neuroleptic: Pimozide	CONTRAINDICATED due to potential for serious and/or life-threatening reactions such as cardiac arrhythmias.
Sedative/hypnotics: Alprazolam, midazolam, triazolam	CONTRAINDICATED due to potential for serious and/or life-threatening reactions such as prolonged or increased sedation or respiratory depression.

[a]See CLINICAL PHARMACOLOGY for magnitude of interaction, Tables 1 and 2.

associated adverse events, including hypotension, visual changes, and prolonged penile erection, and should promptly report any symptoms to their doctor.

Drug Interactions

(See also CONTRAINDICATIONS, WARNINGS, and CLINICAL PHARMACOLOGY: Drug Interactions.)

Delavirdine is an inhibitor of CYP3A isoform and other CYP isoforms to a lesser extent including CYP2C9, CYP2D6, and CYP2C19. Coadministration of RESCRIPTOR and drugs primarily metabolized by CYP3A (e.g., HMG-CoA reductase inhibitors and sildenafil) may result in increased plasma concentrations of the coadministered drug that could increase or prolong both its therapeutic or adverse effects. Delavirdine is metabolized primarily by CYP3A, but in vitro data suggest that delavirdine may also be metabolized by CYP2D6. Coadministration of RESCRIPTOR and drugs that induce CYP3A, such as rifampin, may decrease delavirdine plasma concentrations and reduce its therapeutic effect. Coadministration of RESCRIPTOR and drugs that inhibit CYP3A may increase delavirdine plasma concentrations. **(See Table 6, Drugs That Should Not Be Coadministered With RESCRIPTOR, and Table 7, Established and Other Potentially Significant Drug Interactions: Alteration in Dose or Regimen May Be Recommended Based on Drug Interaction Studies or Predicted Interaction.)**

[See table 6 above]

[See table 7 on pages 2362 and 2363]

Carcinogenesis, Mutagenesis, Impairment of Fertility

Delavirdine was negative in a battery of genetic toxicology tests which included an Ames assay, an in vitro rat hepatocyte unscheduled DNA synthesis assay, an in vitro chromosome aberration assay in human peripheral lymphocytes, an in vitro mutation assay in Chinese hamster ovary cells, and an in vivo micronucleus test in mice.

Lifetime carcinogenicity studies were conducted in rats at doses of 10, 32, and 100 mg/kg/day and in mice at doses of 62.5, 250, and 500 mg/kg/day for males and 62.5, 125, and 250 mg/kg/day for females. In rats, delavirdine was noncarcinogenic at maximally tolerated doses that produced exposures (AUC) up to 12 (male rats) and 9 (female rats) times human exposure at the recommended clinical dose. In mice, delavirdine produced significant increases in the incidence of hepatocellular adenoma/adenocarcinoma in both males and females, hepatocellular adenoma in females, and mesenchymal urinary bladder tumors in males. The systemic drug exposures (AUC) in female mice were 0.5- to 3-fold and in male mice 0.2- to 4-fold of those in humans at the recommended clinical dose. Given the lack of genotoxic activity of delavirdine, the relevance of urinary bladder and hepatocellular neoplasm in delavirdine-treated mice to humans is not known.

Delavirdine at doses of 20, 100, and 200 mg/kg/day did not cause impairment of fertility in rats when males were treated for 70 days and females were treated for 14 days prior to mating.

Pregnancy

Pregnancy Category C. Delavirdine has been shown to be teratogenic in rats. Delavirdine caused ventricular septal defects in rats at doses of 50, 100, and 200 mg/kg/day when administered during the period of organogenesis. The lowest dose of delavirdine that caused malformations produced systemic exposures in pregnant rats equal to or lower than the expected human exposure to RESCRIPTOR (C_{min} 15 µM) at the recommended dose. Exposure in rats approximately 5-fold higher than the expected human exposure resulted in marked maternal toxicity, embryotoxicity, fetal developmental delay, and reduced pup survival. Additionally, reduced pup survival on postpartum day 0 occurred at an exposure (mean C_{min}) approximately equal to the expected human exposure. Delavirdine was excreted in the milk of lactating rats at a concentration 3 to 5 times that of rat plasma.

Delavirdine at doses of 200 and 400 mg/kg/day administered during the period of organogenesis caused maternal toxicity, embryotoxicity, and abortions in rabbits. The lowest dose of delavirdine that resulted in these toxic effects produced systemic exposures in pregnant rabbits approximately 6-fold higher than the expected human exposure to RESCRIPTOR (C_{min} 15 µM) at the recommended dose. The no-observed-adverse-effect dose in the pregnant rabbit was 100 mg/kg/day. Various malformations were observed at this dose, but the incidence of such malformations was not statistically significantly different from that observed in the control group. Systemic exposures in pregnant rabbits at a dose of 100 mg/kg/day were lower than those expected in humans at the recommended clinical dose. Malformations were not apparent at 200 and 400 mg/kg/day; however, only a limited number of fetuses were available for examination as a result of maternal and embryo death.

No adequate and well-controlled studies in pregnant women have been conducted. RESCRIPTOR should be used during pregnancy only if the potential benefit justifies the potential risk to the fetus. Of 9 pregnancies reported in premarketing clinical studies and postmarketing experience, a total of 10 infants were born (including 1 set of twins). Eight of the infants were born healthy. One infant was born HIV-positive but was otherwise healthy and with no congenital abnormalities detected, and 1 infant was born prematurely (34 to 35 weeks) with a small muscular ventricular septal defect that spontaneously resolved. The patient received approximately 6 weeks of treatment with delavirdine and zidovudine early in the course of the pregnancy.

Antiretroviral Pregnancy Registry: To monitor maternal-fetal outcomes of pregnant women exposed to RESCRIPTOR and other antiretroviral agents, an Antiretroviral Pregnancy Registry has been established. Physicians are encouraged to register patients by calling (800) 258-4263.

Nursing Mothers

The Centers for Disease Control and Prevention recommend that HIV-infected mothers not breastfeed their infants to avoid risking postnatal transmission of HIV. Because of both the potential for HIV transmission and any possible adverse reactions in nursing infants, **mothers should be instructed not to breastfeed if they are receiving RESCRIPTOR.**

Table 7. Established and Other Potentially Significant Drug Interactions: Alteration in Dose or Regimen May Be Recommended Based on Drug Interaction Studies or Predicted Interaction

Concomitant Drug Class: Drug Name	Effect on Concentration of Delavirdine or Concomitant Drug	Clinical Comment
HIV-Antiviral Agents: Nucleoside Reverse Transcriptase Inhibitor		
Didanosine[a]	↓Delavirdine ↓Didanosine	Administration of didanosine (buffered tablets) and RESCRIPTOR should be separated by at least 1 hour.
HIV-Antiviral Agents: Non-nucleoside Reverse Transcriptase Inhibitors		
NNRTI	↔Delavirdine ↑NNRTI	Combining NNRTIs has not been shown to be beneficial. RESCRIPTOR should not be coadministered with another NNRTI.
HIV-Antiviral Agents: Protease Inhibitors		
Indinavir[a]	↑Indinavir	A dose reduction of indinavir to 600 mg 3 times daily should be considered when RESCRIPTOR and indinavir are coadministered.
Lopinavir/Ritonavir	↑Lopinavir ↑Ritonavir	Appropriate doses of this combination with respect to safety, efficacy, and pharmacokinetics have not been established.
Nelfinavir[a]	↑Nelfinavir ↓Delavirdine	Appropriate doses of this combination with respect to safety, efficacy, and pharmacokinetics have not been established (see CLINICAL PHARMACOLOGY: Tables 1 and 2).
Ritonavir	↑Ritonavir	Appropriate doses of this combination with respect to safety, efficacy, and pharmacokinetics have not been established.
Saquinavir[a]	↑Saquinavir	A dose reduction of saquinavir (soft gelatin capsules) may be considered when RESCRIPTOR and saquinavir are coadministered (see CLINICAL PHARMACOLOGY: Table 1). Appropriate doses with respect to safety, efficacy, and pharmacokinetics have not been established.
HIV-Antiviral Agents: CCR5 Inhibitor		
Maraviroc	↑Maraviroc	Concomitant use of RESCRIPTOR and maraviroc has not been studied. However, RESCRIPTOR is a potent CYP3A4 inhibitor and the maraviroc dose should be reduced during coadministration. Refer to the full prescribing information for maraviroc (SELZENTRY) for dosing recommendations.
Other Agents		
Acid blockers: Antacids[a]	↓Delavirdine	Doses of an antacid and RESCRIPTOR should be separated by at least 1 hour, because the absorption of delavirdine is reduced when coadministered with antacids.
Histamine H₂-receptor antagonists: Cimetidine, famotidine, nizatidine, ranitidine	↓Delavirdine	These agents increase gastric pH and may reduce the absorption of delavirdine. Although the effect of these drugs on delavirdine absorption has not been evaluated, chronic use of these drugs with RESCRIPTOR is not recommended.
Proton pump inhibitors: Omeprazole, lansoprazole	↓Delavirdine	These agents increase gastric pH and may reduce the absorption of delavirdine. Although the effect of these drugs on delavirdine absorption has not been evaluated, chronic use of these drugs with RESCRIPTOR is not recommended.
Amphetamines	↑Amphetamines	Use with caution.
Antidepressant: Trazodone	↑Trazodone	Concomitant use of trazodone and RESCRIPTOR may increase plasma concentrations of trazodone. Adverse events of nausea, dizziness, hypotension, and syncope have been observed following coadministration of trazodone and ritonavir. If trazodone is used with a CYP3A4 inhibitor such as RESCRIPTOR, the combination should be used with caution and a lower dose of trazodone should be considered.

(Table continued on next page)

Pediatric Use
Safety and effectiveness of delavirdine in combination with other antiretroviral agents have not been established in HIV-1–infected individuals younger than 16 years of age.

Geriatric Use
Clinical studies of RESCRIPTOR did not include sufficient numbers of subjects aged 65 and over to determine whether they respond differently from younger subjects. In general, caution should be taken when dosing RESCRIPTOR in elderly patients due to the greater frequency of decreased hepatic, renal, or cardiac function and of concomitant disease or other drug therapy.

ADVERSE REACTIONS
The safety of RESCRIPTOR Tablets alone and in combination with other therapies has been studied in approximately 6,000 patients receiving RESCRIPTOR. The majority of adverse events were of mild or moderate (i.e., ACTG Grade 1 or 2) intensity. The most frequently reported drug-related adverse event (i.e., events considered by the investigator to be related to the blinded study medication or events with an unknown or missing causal relationship to the blinded medication) among patients receiving RESCRIPTOR was skin rash (see Table 8 and PRECAUTIONS: Skin Rash).
[See table 8 on next page]

Adverse events of moderate to severe intensity reported by at least 5% of evaluable patients in any treatment group in the pivotal trials, which includes patients receiving RESCRIPTOR in combination with zidovudine and/or lamivudine in Study 21 Part II for up to 98 weeks and in combination with zidovudine and either lamivudine, didanosine, or zalcitabine in Study 13C for up to 72 weeks are summarized in Table 9.
[See table 9 at top of page 2364]

Other Adverse Events in Phase II/III Studies
Other adverse events that occurred in patients receiving RESCRIPTOR (in combination treatment) in all Phase II and III studies, considered possibly related to treatment, and of at least ACTG Grade 2 in intensity are listed below by body system.

Body as a Whole: Abdominal cramps, abdominal distention, abdominal pain (localized), abscess, allergic reaction, chills, edema (generalized or localized), epidermal cyst, fever, infection, infection viral, lip edema, malaise, *Mycobacterium* tuberculosis infection, neck rigidity, sebaceous cyst, and redistribution/accumulation of body fat (see PRECAUTIONS: Fat Redistribution).

Cardiovascular System: Abnormal cardiac rate and rhythm, cardiac insufficiency, cardiomyopathy, hypertension, migraine, pallor, peripheral vascular disorder, and postural hypotension.

Digestive System: Anorexia, bloody stool, colitis, constipation, decreased appetite, diarrhea (*Clostridium difficile*), diverticulitis, dry mouth, dyspepsia, dysphagia, enteritis at all levels, eructation, fecal incontinence, flatulence, gagging, gastroenteritis, gastroesophageal reflux, gastrointestinal bleeding, gastrointestinal disorder, gingivitis, gum hemorrhage, hepatomegaly, increased appetite, increased saliva, increased thirst, jaundice, mouth or tongue inflammation or ulcers, nonspecific hepatitis, oral/enteric moniliasis, pancreatitis, rectal disorder, sialadenitis, tooth abscess, and toothache.

Hemic and Lymphatic System: Adenopathy, bruising, eosinophilia, granulocytosis, leukopenia, pancytopenia, purpura, spleen disorder, thrombocytopenia, and prolonged prothrombin time.

Metabolic and Nutritional Disorders: Alcohol intolerance, amylase increased, bilirubinemia, hyperglycemia, hyperkalemia, hypertriglyceridemia, hyperuricemia, hypocalcemia, hyponatremia, hypophosphatemia, increased AST (SGOT), increased gamma glutamyl transpeptidase, increased lipase, increased serum alkaline phosphatase, increased serum creatinine, and weight increase or decrease.

Musculoskeletal System: Arthralgia or arthritis of single and multiple joints, bone disorder, bone pain, myalgia, tendon disorder, tenosynovitis, tetany, and vertigo.

Nervous System: Abnormal coordination, agitation, amnesia, change in dreams, cognitive impairment, confusion, decreased libido, disorientation, dizziness, emotional lability, euphoria, hallucination, hyperesthesia, hyperreflexia, hypertonia, hypesthesia, impaired concentration, manic symptoms, muscle cramp, nervousness, neuropathy, nystagmus, paralysis, paranoid symptoms, restlessness, sleep cycle disorder, somnolence, tingling, tremor, vertigo, and weakness.

Respiratory System: Chest congestion, dyspnea, epistaxis, hiccups, laryngismus, pneumonia, and rhinitis.

Skin and Appendages: Angioedema, dermal leukocytoclastic vasculitis, dermatitis, desquamation, diaphoresis, discolored skin, dry skin, erythema, erythema multiforme, folliculitis, fungal dermatitis, hair loss, herpes zoster or simplex, nail disorder, petechiae, non-application site pruritus, seborrhea, skin hypertrophy, skin disorder, skin nodule, Stevens-Johnson syndrome, urticaria, vesiculobullous rash, and wart.

Special Senses: Blepharitis, blurred vision, conjunctivitis, diplopia, dry eyes, ear pain, parosmia, otitis media, photophobia, taste perversion, and tinnitus.

Urogenital System: Amenorrhea, breast enlargement, calculi of the kidney, chromaturia, epididymitis, hematuria, hemospermia, impaired urination, impotence, kidney pain, metrorrhagia, nocturia, polyuria, proteinuria, testicular pain, urinary tract infection, and vaginal moniliasis.

Postmarketing Experience
Adverse event terms reported from postmarketing surveillance that were not reported in the Phase II and III trials are presented below.

Digestive System: Hepatic failure.
Hemic and Lymphatic System: Hemolytic anemia.
Musculoskeletal System: Rhabdomyolysis.
Urogenital System: Acute kidney failure.

Laboratory Abnormalities
Marked laboratory abnormalities observed in at least 2% of patients during Studies 21 Part II and 13C are summarized in Table 10. Marked laboratory abnormalities are defined as any Grade 3 or 4 abnormality found in patients at any time during study.
[See table 10 at top of page 2365]

Table 7 (cont.). Established and Other Potentially Significant Drug Interactions: Alteration in Dose or Regimen May Be Recommended Based on Drug Interaction Studies or Predicted Interaction

Concomitant Drug Class: Drug Name	Effect on Concentration of Delavirdine or Concomitant Drug	Clinical Comment
Other Agents (cont.)		
Antiarrhythmics: Bepridil	↑Antiarrhythmics	Use with caution. Increased bepridil exposure may be associated with life–threatening reactions such as cardiac arrhythmias.
Amiodarone, lidocaine (systemic), quinidine, flecainide, propafenone		Caution is warranted and therapeutic concentration monitoring is recommended, if available, for antiarrhythmics when coadministered with RESCRIPTOR.
Anticoagulant: Warfarin	↑Warfarin	It is recommended that INR (international normalized ratio) be monitored.
Anti-infective: Clarithromycin[a]	↑Clarithromycin	When coadministered with RESCRIPTOR, clarithromycin should be adjusted in patients with impaired renal function: • For patients with CL_{CR} 30 to 60 mL/min the dose of clarithromycin should be reduced by 50%. • For patients with CL_{CR} <30 mL/min the dose of clarithromycin should be reduced by 75%.
Calcium channel blockers: Amlodipine, diltiazem, felodipine, isradipine, nifedipine, nicardipine, nimodipine, nisoldipine, verapamil	↑Calcium channel blockers	Caution is warranted and clinical monitoring of patients is recommended.
Corticosteroid: Dexamethasone	↓Delavirdine	Use with caution. RESCRIPTOR may be less effective due to decreased delavirdine plasma concentrations in patients taking these agents concomitantly.
Erectile dysfunction agents: Sildenafil	↑Sildenafil	Sildenafil should not exceed a maximum single dose of 25 mg in a 48–hour period.
HMG-CoA reductase inhibitors: Atorvastatin, cerivastatin, fluvastatin	↑Atorvastatin ↑Cerivastatin ↑Fluvastatin	Use lowest possible dose of atorvastatin or cerivastatin, or fluvastatin with careful monitoring, or consider other HMG-CoA reductase inhibitors such as pravastatin in combination with RESCRIPTOR.
Immunosuppressants: Cyclosporine, tacrolimus, rapamycin	↑Immunosuppressants	Therapeutic concentration monitoring is recommended for immunosuppressant agents when coadministered with RESCRIPTOR.
Inhaled/nasal steroid: Fluticasone	↑Fluticasone	Concomitant use of fluticasone and RESCRIPTOR may increase plasma concentrations of fluticasone. Use with caution. Consider alternatives to fluticasone, particularly for long-term use.
Narcotic analgesic: Methadone	↑Methadone	Dosage of methadone may need to be decreased when coadministered with RESCRIPTOR.
Oral contraceptives: Ethinyl estradiol	↑Ethinyl estradiol	Concentrations of ethinyl estradiol may increase. However, the clinical significance is unknown.

↑ Indicates increase.
↓ Indicates decrease.
[a]The interaction between RESCRIPTOR and the drug was evaluated in a clinical study. All other drug interactions shown are predicted.

Table 8. Percent of Patients With Treatment-Emergent Rash in Pivotal Trials (Studies 21 Part II and 13C)[a]

Percent of Patients With:	Description of Rash Grade[b]	RESCRIPTOR 400 mg t.i.d. (n = 412)	Control Group Patients (n = 295)
Grade 1 rash	Erythema, pruritus	69 (16.7%)	35 (11.9%)
Grade 2 rash	Diffuse maculopapular rash, dry desquamation	59 (14.3%)	17 (5.8%)
Grade 3 rash	Vesiculation, moist desquamation, ulceration	18 (4.4%)	0 (0.0%)
Grade 4 rash	Erythema multiforme, Stevens-Johnson syndrome, toxic epidermal necrolysis, necrosis requiring surgery, exfoliative dermatitis	0 (0.0%)	0 (0.0%)
Rash of any grade		146 (35.4%)	52 (17.6%)
Treatment discontinuation as a result of rash		13 (3.2%)	1 (0.3%)

[a]Includes events reported regardless of causality.
[b]ACTG Toxicity Grading System; includes events reported as "rash," "maculopapular rash," and "urticaria."

OVERDOSAGE

Human experience of acute overdose with RESCRIPTOR is limited.

Management of Overdosage

Treatment of overdosage with RESCRIPTOR should consist of general supportive measures, including monitoring of vital signs and observation of the patient's clinical status. There is no specific antidote for overdosage with RESCRIPTOR. If indicated, elimination of unabsorbed drug should be achieved by emesis or gastric lavage. Since delavirdine is extensively metabolized by the liver and is highly protein-bound, dialysis is unlikely to result in significant removal of the drug.

DOSAGE AND ADMINISTRATION

The recommended dosage for RESCRIPTOR Tablets is 400 mg (four 100-mg or two 200-mg tablets) 3 times daily. RESCRIPTOR should be used in combination with other antiretroviral therapy. The complete prescribing information for other antiretroviral agents should be consulted for information on dosage and administration.

The 100-mg RESCRIPTOR Tablets may be dispersed in water prior to consumption. To prepare a dispersion, add four 100-mg RESCRIPTOR Tablets to at least 3 ounces of water, allow to stand for a few minutes, and then stir until a uniform dispersion occurs (see CLINICAL PHARMACOLOGY: Pharmacokinetics: Absorption and Bioavailability). The dispersion should be consumed promptly. The glass should be rinsed with water and the rinse swallowed to insure the entire dose is consumed. **The 200-mg tablets should be taken as intact tablets, because they are not readily dispersed in water.** Note: The 200-mg tablets are approximately one-third smaller in size than the 100-mg tablets.

RESCRIPTOR Tablets may be administered with or without food (see CLINICAL PHARMACOLOGY: Pharmacokinetics: Absorption and Bioavailability). Patients with achlorhydria should take RESCRIPTOR with an acidic beverage (e.g., orange or cranberry juice). However, the effect of an acidic beverage on the absorption of delavirdine in patients with achlorhydria has not been investigated.

Patients taking both RESCRIPTOR and antacids should be advised to take them at least 1 hour apart.

HOW SUPPLIED

RESCRIPTOR Tablets are available as follows:
100-mg: white, capsule-shaped tablets marked with "U 3761"
Bottles of 360 tablets - NDC 49702-209-24.
200-mg: white, capsule-shaped tablets marked with "RES200"
Bottles of 180 tablets - NDC 49702-225-17.
Store at controlled room temperature 20° to 25°C (68° to 77°F) [see USP]. Keep container tightly closed. Protect from high humidity.

ANIMAL TOXICOLOGY

Toxicities among various organs and organ systems in rats, mice, rabbits, dogs, and monkeys were observed following the administration of delavirdine. Necrotizing vasculitis was the most significant toxicity that occurred in dogs when mean nadir serum concentrations of delavirdine were at least 7-fold higher than the expected human exposure to RESCRIPTOR (C_{min} 15 μM) at the recommended dose. Vasculitis in dogs was not reversible during a 2.5-month recovery period; however, partial resolution of the vascular lesion characterized by reduced inflammation, diminished necrosis, and intimal thickening occurred during this period. Other major target organs included the gastrointestinal tract, endocrine organs, liver, kidneys, bone marrow, lymphoid tissue, lung, and reproductive organs.

Manufactured for
ViiV Healthcare
Research Triangle Park, NC 27709
by
Pfizer Pharmaceuticals LLC
Vega Baja, Puerto Rico 00693
©2012, ViiV Healthcare. All rights reserved.
August 2012
RES: 3PI

Patient Information
RESCRIPTOR®
(ree-SKRIP-tor)
(delavirdine mesylate) Tablets
Generic name: delavirdine mesylate (de-LAH-vur-deen MESS-ihl-ate)
ALERT: Find out about medicines that should NOT be taken with RESCRIPTOR. Please also read the section "MEDICINES YOU SHOULD NOT TAKE WITH RESCRIPTOR."
Read this information carefully before taking RESCRIPTOR. Also, read this leaflet each time you renew the prescription, just in case anything has changed. This is a summary and not a replacement for a careful discussion with your healthcare provider (doctor, nurse, pharmacist). You and your healthcare provider should discuss RESCRIPTOR when you start taking this medication and at regular checkups. You should remain under a doctor's

Table 9. Treatment-Emergent Events Regardless of Causality, of Moderate-to-Severe or Life-Threatening Intensity Reported by at Least 5% of Evaluable[a] Patients in Any Treatment Group

	Study 21 Part II			Study 13C	
	Zidovudine + Lamivudine (n = 123)	400 mg t.i.d. RESCRIPTOR + Zidovudine (n = 123)	400 mg t.i.d. RESCRIPTOR + Zidovudine + Lamivudine (n = 119)	Zidovudine + Didanosine, Zalcitabine, or Lamivudine (n = 172)	400 mg t.i.d. RESCRIPTOR + Zidovudine + Didanosine, Zalcitabine, or Lamivudine (n = 170)
Adverse Events	% of pts. (n)	% of pts. (n)	% of pts. (n)	% of pts. (n)	% of pts. (n)
Body as a Whole					
Abdominal pain, generalized	2.4 (3)	3.3 (4)	5.0 (6)	1.7 (3)	2.4 (4)
Asthenia/fatigue	16.3 (20)	15.4 (19)	16.0 (19)	8.1 (14)	5.3 (9)
Fever	2.4 (3)	1.6 (2)	3.4 (4)	6.4 (11)	7.1 (12)
Flu syndrome	4.9 (6)	7.3 (9)	5.0 (6)	5.2 (9)	2.4 (4)
Headache	14.6 (18)	12.2 (15)	16.8 (20)	12.8 (22)	11.2 (19)
Localized pain	4.9 (6)	5.7 (7)	5.0 (6)	2.9 (5)	1.8 (3)
Digestive					
Diarrhea	8.1 (10)	2.4 (3)	4.2 (5)	8.1 (14)	5.9 (10)
Nausea	17.1 (21)	20.3 (25)	16.8 (20)	9.3 (16)	14.7 (25)
Vomiting	8.9 (11)	4.9 (6)	2.5 (3)	4.1 (7)	6.5 (11)
Nervous					
Anxiety	1.6 (2)	2.4 (3)	6.7 (8)	4.1 (7)	3.5 (6)
Depressive symptoms	6.5 (8)	4.9 (6)	12.6 (15)	3.5 (6)	5.9 (10)
Insomnia	4.9 (6)	4.9 (6)	5.0 (6)	2.9 (5)	1.2 (2)
Respiratory					
Bronchitis	4.1 (5)	6.5 (8)	6.7 (8)	3.5 (6)	3.5 (6)
Cough	9.8 (12)	4.1 (5)	5.0 (6)	5.2 (9)	3.5 (6)
Pharyngitis	6.5 (8)	1.6 (2)	5.0 (6)	4.1 (7)	3.5 (6)
Sinusitis	8.9 (11)	7.3 (9)	5.0 (6)	2.3 (4)	1.2 (2)
Upper respiratory infection	11.4 (14)	6.5 (8)	7.6 (9)	8.7 (15)	4.7 (8)
Skin					
Rashes	3.3 (4)	19.5 (24)	13.4 (16)	7.6 (13)	18.8 (32)

[a]Evaluable patients in Study 21 Part II were those who received at least 1 dose of study medication and returned for at least 1 clinic study visit. Evaluable patients in Study 13C were those who received at least 1 dose of study medication.

care when taking RESCRIPTOR and should not change or stop treatment without first talking with your healthcare provider.

What is RESCRIPTOR and how does it work?
RESCRIPTOR is a medicine used in combination with other anti-HIV medicines to treat people with HIV-1 infection. Infection with HIV-1 leads to the destruction of infection-fighting immune system cells (called CD4+ cells or T cells), which are important to the immune system. After a large number of CD4+ cells have been destroyed, the infected person develops acquired immune deficiency syndrome (AIDS). RESCRIPTOR helps to block HIV-1 reverse transcriptase, a chemical the virus uses to make more copies of itself. The main goals of anti-HIV medicines like RESCRIPTOR are to decrease the amount of virus in your blood (called viral load) and to increase the number of CD4+ cells as much as possible for as long as possible.
RESCRIPTOR, when taken with other anti-HIV medicines, lowers the HIV-1 viral load in patients. Patients who took RESCRIPTOR as part of combination therapy for HIV-1 also had increases in their CD4+ cell count.

General information about RESCRIPTOR
RESCRIPTOR does not cure HIV-1 or AIDS and you may continue to experience illnesses associated with HIV-1 infection, including opportunistic infections. You should remain under the care of a doctor when using RESCRIPTOR. Avoid doing things that can spread HIV-1 infection.

• Do not share needles or other injection equipment.
• Do not share personal items that can have blood or body fluids on them, like toothbrushes and razor blades.
• Do not have any kind of sex without protection. Always practice safe sex by using a latex or polyurethane condom to lower the chance of sexual contact with semen, vaginal secretions, or blood.

How should I take RESCRIPTOR?
• You should stay under a healthcare provider's care when taking RESCRIPTOR. Do not change your treatment or stop treatment without first talking with your healthcare provider.
• You must take RESCRIPTOR every day exactly as your healthcare provider prescribes it. Follow the directions from your healthcare provider, exactly as written on the label.
• **The usual dose of RESCRIPTOR is two 200–mg tablets 3 times a day or four 100–mg tablets 3 times a day, in combination with other anti-HIV-1 medicines. Either way, your total daily dose of RESCRIPTOR remains the same.**
• You can take RESCRIPTOR with or without food.
• If you have trouble swallowing tablets, the 100–mg RESCRIPTOR tablets may be dissolved in water. Place 4 tablets in at least 3 ounces of water and allow the tablets to sit in the water for a few minutes. Then, stir the water until the tablets have dissolved and drink the mixture right away. Add a little more water, swirl, and then drink

the rest of the mixture to be sure that you get all the medicine. **The 200–mg tablets must be swallowed whole. They cannot be dissolved in water.**
• Many people find it easier to take their RESCRIPTOR with breakfast, lunch, and dinner, since food does not interfere with RESCRIPTOR. It is a good idea to get into the habit of taking RESCRIPTOR on a regular schedule to make it easier to remember. Figure out things that happen every day at pill-taking time and take your tablets then. By taking your medicine along with activities you do every day, such as getting up in the morning, brushing your teeth, eating lunch, coming home from work in the evening, or watching a favorite TV show, you will find it easier to remember to take every dose.
• When your supply of RESCRIPTOR starts to run low, get more from your healthcare provider or pharmacy. This is very important because the amount of virus in your blood may increase if the medicine is stopped for even a short time. The virus may develop resistance to RESCRIPTOR and become harder to treat.
• Only take medicine that has been prescribed specifically for you. Do not give RESCRIPTOR to others or take medicine prescribed for someone else.

What should I do if I miss a dose of RESCRIPTOR?
If you forget to take a dose of RESCRIPTOR, take it as soon as possible. However, if you skip the dose entirely, do not double the next dose. If you forget a lot of doses, talk to your healthcare provider about how you should continue taking your medicine.

Who should not take RESCRIPTOR?
Together with your healthcare provider, you need to decide whether RESCRIPTOR is right for you.
• **Do not take RESCRIPTOR if you are taking certain medicines.** These could cause serious side effects that could cause death. Before you take RESCRIPTOR, you must tell your healthcare provider about all the medicines you are taking or are planning to take. These include other prescription and nonprescription medicines and herbal supplements.
For more information about medicines you should not take with RESCRIPTOR, please read the section titled "MEDICINES YOU SHOULD NOT TAKE WITH RESCRIPTOR."
• **Do not take RESCRIPTOR if you have an allergy to RESCRIPTOR.** Also tell your healthcare provider if you have any known allergies to other medicines, foods, preservatives, or dyes.
• **Tell your healthcare provider if you are pregnant or plan to become pregnant.** The effects of RESCRIPTOR on pregnant women or their unborn babies are not known.
• If you are breastfeeding, **do not breastfeed.** We do not know if RESCRIPTOR can be passed to your baby in your breast milk and whether it could harm your baby. Also, mothers with HIV-1 should not breastfeed because HIV-1 can be passed to the baby in the breast milk. Talk with your healthcare provider about the best way to feed your baby.
• **Talk with your healthcare provider if you have liver or kidney disease.** RESCRIPTOR has not been studied in people with liver or kidney disease.
• **Certain medical problems may affect the use of RESCRIPTOR.** Be sure to tell your healthcare provider of any other medical problems you may have.

Can I take RESCRIPTOR with other medicines?
RESCRIPTOR may interact with other medicines, including those you take without a prescription. You must tell your healthcare provider about all medicines you are taking or planning to take before you take RESCRIPTOR. It is a good idea to keep a complete list of all the medicines that you take, including nonprescription medicines, herbal remedies and supplements, and street drugs. Update this list when medicines are added or stopped. Give copies of this list to all of your healthcare providers **every** time you visit or fill a prescription.

MEDICINES YOU SHOULD NOT TAKE WITH RESCRIPTOR
Do not take the following medicines with RESCRIPTOR because they can cause serious problems or death if taken with RESCRIPTOR:
• VERSED® (midazolam) Injection and Syrup (for sedation)
• HALCION® (triazolam) Tablets (for sleep problems)
• XANAX® (alprazolam) Tablets (for anxiety)
• D.H.E. 45® Injection, ERGOMAR®, MIGRANAL®, WIGRAINE®, and CAFERGOT® (for migraine headaches)
• METHERGINE® (for bleeding after childbirth)
• ORAP® (pimozide) Tablets (for seizures)
• PROPULSID® (cisapride) Tablets and Suspension (for heartburn)
• HISMANAL® (astemizole) Tablets (for allergies)
• SELDANE® (terfenadine) Tablets (for allergies)
Do not take the following medicines when you take RESCRIPTOR. They may reduce the levels of RESCRIPTOR in the blood and make it less effective. Talk with your healthcare provider if you are currently taking these medicines because other medicines may have to be given to take their place:

Table 10. Marked Laboratory Abnormalities Reported by ≥2% of Patients

Adverse Events/Toxicity Limits	Study 21 Part II			Study 13C	
	Zidovudine + Lamivudine (n = 123)	400 mg t.i.d. RESCRIPTOR + Zidovudine (n = 123)	400 mg t.i.d. RESCRIPTOR + Zidovudine + Lamivudine (n = 119)	Zidovudine + Didanosine, Zalcitabine, or Lamivudine (n = 172)	400 mg t.i.d. RESCRIPTOR + Zidovudine + Didanosine, Zalcitabine, or Lamivudine (n = 170)
	% pts.	% pts.	% pts.	% pts.	% pts.
Hematology					
Hemoglobin <7 mg/dL	4.1	2.5	0.9	1.7	2.9
Neutrophils <750/mm³	5.7	4.9	3.4	10.4	7.6
Prothrombin time (PT) >1.5 × ULN	0	0	1.7	2.9	2.4
Activated partial thromboplastin (APTT) >2.33 × ULN	0	0.8	0	5.8	2.4
Chemistry					
Alananine aminotransferase (ALT/SGPT) >5 × ULN	2.5	4.1	5.1	3.5	4.1
Amylase >2 × ULN	0.8	2.5	2.6	3.5	2.9
Aspartate aminotransferase (AST/SGOT) >5 × ULN	1.6	2.5	3.4	3.5	2.3
Bilirubin >2.5 × ULN	0.8	2.5	1.7	1.2	0
Gamma glutamyl transferase (GGT) >5 × ULN	N/A	N/A	N/A	4.1	1.8
Glucose (hypo-/hyperglycemia) <40 mg/dL >250 mg/dL	4.1	0.8	1.7	1.2	0

N/A = not applicable because no predose values were obtained for patients.

- Rifampin (also known as RIMACTANE®, RIFADIN®, RIFATER®, RIFAMATE®) (to treat tuberculosis)
- Phenobarbital (for seizures)
- DILANTIN® (phenytoin) (for seizures)
- TEGRETOL® (carbamazepine) (for seizures)

Do not take RESCRIPTOR with St. John's wort (*Hypericum perforatum*), an herbal product sold as a dietary supplement, or products containing St. John's wort. Talk with your healthcare provider if you are taking or planning to take St. John's wort. Taking St. John's wort may decrease levels of RESCRIPTOR and lead to increased viral load and possible resistance to RESCRIPTOR or cross-resistance to other anti-HIV medicines.

Do not take RESCRIPTOR with cholesterol-lowering medicines MEVACOR® (lovastatin) or ZOCOR® (simvastatin) because of possible serious reactions. There is also an increased risk of drug interactions between RESCRIPTOR and LIPITOR® (atorvastatin), BAYCOL® (cerivastatin), and LESCOL® (fluvastatin); talk to your healthcare provider before you take any of these cholesterol-reducing medicines with RESCRIPTOR.

Medicines that require dosage adjustments:
It is possible that your healthcare provider may need to increase or decrease the dose of other medicines when you are taking RESCRIPTOR. Remember to tell your healthcare provider all the medicines you are taking or planning to take.

Before you take VIAGRA® (sildenafil) with RESCRIPTOR, talk to your healthcare provider about problems these 2 medicines can cause when taken together. You may get increased side effects of VIAGRA, such as low blood pressure, vision changes, and penis erection lasting more than 4 hours. If an erection lasts longer than 4 hours, get medical help right away to avoid permanent damage to your penis. Your healthcare provider can explain these symptoms to you.

- If you are taking both VIDEX® (didanosine, ddI) and RESCRIPTOR: Take VIDEX (buffered tablets) 1 hour before or 1 hour after you take RESCRIPTOR. Taking them together causes lower amounts of RESCRIPTOR in the blood, making both medicines less effective.
- **Protease inhibitors:** A number of healthy volunteers and HIV-1-infected patients were studied while taking RESCRIPTOR with one of these protease inhibitors: CRIXIVAN® (indinavir), INVIRASE® and FORTOVASE® (saquinavir), NORVIR® (ritonavir), or VIRACEPT® (nelfinavir). RESCRIPTOR was shown to increase the amount of these protease inhibitors in the blood. RESCRIPTOR is expected to increase the amount of AGENERASE® (amprenavir) and KALETRA® (lopinavir + ritonavir) in the blood. **As a result, your healthcare provider may choose to lower the dose of one of these medicines or monitor certain lab tests if these protease inhibitors are taken in combination with RESCRIPTOR.**
- **Antacids** should be taken at least 1 hour before or 1 hour after you take RESCRIPTOR because they can slow the absorption of RESCRIPTOR.

Based on your history of taking other anti-HIV medicine, your healthcare provider will direct you on how to take RESCRIPTOR and other anti-HIV medicines. These drugs should be taken in a certain order or at specific times. This will depend on how many times a day each medicine should be taken. It will also depend on whether the medicines should be taken with or without food.

What are the possible side effects of RESCRIPTOR?
- This list of side effects is not complete. If you have questions about side effects, ask your doctor, nurse, or pharmacist. You should report any new or continuing symptoms to your healthcare provider right away. Your healthcare provider may be able to help you manage these side effects.
- The most important common side effect seen in people taking RESCRIPTOR has been a skin rash. The rash occurs mainly on the upper body and upper arms, and sometimes on the neck and face. The rash appears as a red area on the skin with slight bumps, and it can be itchy. The rash tends to occur early, usually within 1 to 3 weeks after you

start taking RESCRIPTOR, and it usually lasts less than 2 weeks. Watch your rash carefully and talk to your healthcare provider about how to treat it. If the rash is going to be serious or severe (with fever, blistering, sores in the mouth, redness or swelling of the eyes, or muscle and joint aches), you and your healthcare provider will usually realize it during the first 3 days of the rash. If you have symptoms of a severe rash, you should stop taking RESCRIPTOR and speak with your healthcare provider as soon possible. Be prepared to explain where the rash is, your temperature, and whether or not you have other symptoms.
- Other side effects include headache, nausea, diarrhea, and tiredness. Of these, nausea was the most common.
- Changes in body fat have been seen in some patients taking antiretroviral therapy. These changes may include increased amount of fat in the upper back and neck ("buffalo hump"), breast, and around the trunk. Loss of fat from the legs, arms and face may also happen. The cause and long-term health effects of these conditions are not known at this time.
- Before you start using any medicine, talk with your healthcare provider about what to expect and discuss ways to reduce the side effects you may have.

How do I store RESCRIPTOR?
- Keep RESCRIPTOR and all other medicines out of the reach of children. Keep the bottle closed and store at room temperature (between 68°F and 77°F) away from sources of moisture such as a sink or other damp place. Heat and moisture may reduce the effectiveness of RESCRIPTOR.
- Do not keep medicine that is out of date or that you no longer need. Be sure that if you throw any medicine away, it is out of the reach of children.

General advice about prescription medicines:
Discuss all questions about your health with your healthcare provider. If you have questions about RESCRIPTOR or any other medicines you are taking, ask your healthcare provider. You can also call 1-877-844-8872 toll free.
AGENERASE and RESCRIPTOR are registered trademarks of ViiV Healthcare.
The brands listed are trademarks of their respective owners and are not trademarks of ViiV Healthcare. The makers of these brands are not affiliated with and do not endorse ViiV Healthcare or its products.
Manufactured for

ViiV Healthcare
Research Triangle Park, NC 27709
by
Pfizer Pharmaceuticals LLC
Vega Baja, Puerto Rico 00693
©2012, ViiV Healthcare. All rights reserved.
August 2012
RES: 3PIL

RETROVIR ℞

[*re′trō-vir*]
(zidovudine)
Tablets, Capsules, and Syrup

HIGHLIGHTS OF PRESCRIBING INFORMATION
These highlights do not include all the information needed to use RETROVIR safely and effectively. See full prescribing information for RETROVIR.
RETROVIR (zidovudine) Tablets, Capsules, and Syrup
Initial U.S. Approval: 1987

> **WARNING: RISK OF HEMATOLOGICAL TOXICITY, MYOPATHY, LACTIC ACIDOSIS**
> *See full prescribing information for complete boxed warning.*
> - **Hematologic toxicity including neutropenia and severe anemia have been associated with the use of zidovudine. (5.1)**
> - **Symptomatic myopathy associated with prolonged use of zidovudine. (5.2)**
> - **Lactic acidosis and severe hepatomegaly with steatosis, including fatal cases, have been reported with the use of nucleoside analogues including RETROVIR. Suspend treatment if clinical or laboratory findings suggestive of lactic acidosis or pronounced hepatotoxicity occur. (5.3)**

---INDICATIONS AND USAGE---

RETROVIR is a nucleoside analogue reverse transcriptase inhibitor indicated for:

- Treatment of Human Immunodeficiency Virus (HIV-1) infection in combination with other antiretroviral agents. (1.1)
- Prevention of maternal-fetal HIV-1 transmission. (1.2)

—————DOSAGE AND ADMINISTRATION—————

- Treatment of HIV-1 infection:
  Adults: 600 mg/day in divided doses with other antiretroviral agents.
  Pediatric patients (aged 4 weeks to <18 years): Dosage should be calculated based on body weight not to exceed adult dose. (2.1)
- Prevention of maternal-fetal HIV-1 transmission:
  Specific dosage instructions for mother and infant. (2.2)
- Patients with severe anemia and/or neutropenia:
  Dosage interruption may be necessary. (2.3)
- Renal impairment: Recommended dosage in hemodialysis or peritoneal dialysis patients is 100 mg every 6 to 8 hours. (2.4)

—————DOSAGE FORMS AND STRENGTHS—————

Tablets: 300 mg (3)
Capsules: 100 mg (3)
Syrup: 10 mg/mL (3)

—————————CONTRAINDICATIONS—————————

Hypersensitivity to zidovudine (e.g., anaphylaxis, Stevens-Johnson syndrome). (4)

—————WARNINGS AND PRECAUTIONS—————

- See boxed warning for information about the following: hematologic toxicity, myopathy, and lactic acidosis and severe hepatomegaly (5.1, 5.2, 5.3)
- Exacerbation of anemia has been reported in HIV-1/HCV co-infected patients receiving ribavirin and zidovudine. Coadministration of ribavirin and zidovudine is not advised. (5.4)
- Hepatic decompensation, (some fatal), has occurred in HIV-1/HCV co-infected patients receiving combination antiretroviral therapy and interferon alfa with/without ribavirin. Discontinue zidovudine as medically appropriate and consider dose reduction or discontinuation of interferon alfa, ribavirin, or both. (5.4)
- RETROVIR should not be administered with other zidovudine-containing combination products. (5.5)
- Immune reconstitution syndrome (5.6) and redistribution/accumulation of body fat (5.7) have been reported in patients treated with combination antiretroviral therapy.

—————————ADVERSE REACTIONS—————————

- Most commonly reported adverse reactions (incidence ≥15%) in adult HIV-1 clinical trials were headache, malaise, nausea, anorexia, and vomiting. (6.1)
- Most commonly reported adverse reactions (incidence ≥15%) in pediatric HIV-1 clinical trials were fever, cough, and digestive disorders. (6.1)
- Most commonly reported adverse reactions in neonates (incidence ≥15%) in the prevention of maternal-fetal transmission of HIV-1 clinical trial were anemia and neutropenia. (6.1)

To report SUSPECTED ADVERSE REACTIONS, contact ViiV Healthcare at 1-877-844-8872 or FDA at 1-800-FDA-1088 or www.fda.gov/medwatch.

—————————DRUG INTERACTIONS—————————

- Stavudine: Concomitant use with zidovudine should be avoided. (7.1)
- Doxorubicin: Use with zidovudine should be avoided. (7.2)
- Bone marrow suppressive/cytotoxic agents: May increase the hematologic toxicity of zidovudine. (7.3)

—————USE IN SPECIFIC POPULATIONS—————

Pregnancy: Physicians are encouraged to register patients in the Antiretroviral Pregnancy Registry by calling 1-800-258-4263. (8.1)
See 17 for PATIENT COUNSELING INFORMATION
Revised: 05/2013

FULL PRESCRIBING INFORMATION: CONTENTS*
WARNING: RISK OF HEMATOLOGICAL TOXICITY, MYOPATHY, LACTIC ACIDOSIS

FULL PRESCRIBING INFORMATION

> **WARNING: RISK OF HEMATOLOGICAL TOXICITY, MYOPATHY, LACTIC ACIDOSIS**
>
> **Hematologic Toxicity:** RETROVIR® (zidovudine) Tablets, Capsules, and Syrup have been associated with hematologic toxicity including neutropenia and severe anemia, particularly in patients with advanced HIV-1 disease *[see Warnings and Precautions (5.1)].*
>
> **Myopathy:** Prolonged use of RETROVIR has been associated with symptomatic myopathy *[see Warnings and Precautions (5.2)].*
>
> **Lactic Acidosis and Severe Hepatomegaly:** Lactic acidosis and severe hepatomegaly with steatosis, including fatal cases, have been reported with the use of nucleoside analogues alone or in combination, including RETROVIR and other antiretrovirals. Suspend treatment if clinical or laboratory findings suggestive of lactic acidosis or pronounced hepatotoxicity occur *[see Warnings and Precautions (5.3)].*

1   INDICATIONS AND USAGE
1.1   Treatment of HIV-1
RETROVIR, a nucleoside reverse transcriptase inhibitor, is indicated in combination with other antiretroviral agents for the treatment of HIV-1 infection.
1.2   Prevention of Maternal-Fetal HIV-1 Transmission
RETROVIR is indicated for the prevention of maternal-fetal HIV-1 transmission *[see Dosage and Administration (2.2)].* The indication is based on a dosing regimen that included 3 components:
1. antepartum therapy of HIV-1 infected mothers
2. intrapartum therapy of HIV-1 infected mothers
3. post-partum therapy of HIV-1 exposed neonate.
Points to consider prior to initiating RETROVIR in pregnant women for the prevention of maternal-fetal HIV-1 transmission include:
- In most cases, RETROVIR for prevention of maternal-fetal HIV-1 transmission should be given in combination with other antiretroviral drugs.

- Prevention of HIV-1 transmission in women who have received RETROVIR for a prolonged period before pregnancy has not been evaluated.
- Because the fetus is most susceptible to the potential teratogenic effects of drugs during the first 10 weeks of gestation and the risks of therapy with RETROVIR during that period are not fully known, women in the first trimester of pregnancy who do not require immediate initiation of antiretroviral therapy for their own health may consider delaying use; this indication is based on use after 14 weeks gestation.

2   DOSAGE AND ADMINISTRATION
2.1   Treatment of HIV-1 Infection
Adults: The recommended oral dose of RETROVIR is 600 mg/day in divided doses in combination with other antiretroviral agents.
Pediatric Patients (Aged 4 Weeks to <18 Years): Healthcare professionals should pay special attention to accurate calculation of the dose of RETROVIR, transcription of the medication order, dispensing information, and dosing instructions to minimize risk for medication dosing errors.
Prescribers should calculate the appropriate dose of RETROVIR for each child based on body weight (kg) and should not exceed the recommended adult dose.
Before prescribing RETROVIR Capsules or Tablets, children should be assessed for the ability to swallow capsules or tablets. If a child is unable to reliably swallow a RETROVIR Capsule or Tablet, the RETROVIR Syrup formulation should be prescribed.
The recommended dosage in pediatric patients aged 4 weeks to <18 years and weighing ≥4 kg is provided in Table 1. RETROVIR Syrup should be used to provide accurate dosage when whole tablets or capsules are not appropriate.

Table 1. Recommended Pediatric Dosage of RETROVIR

Body Weight (kg)	Total Daily Dose	Dosage Regimen and Dose	
		Twice Daily	Three Times Daily
4 to <9	24 mg/kg/day	12 mg/kg	8 mg/kg
≥9 to <30	18 mg/kg/day	9 mg/kg	6 mg/kg
≥30	600 mg/day	300 mg	200 mg

Alternatively, dosing for RETROVIR can be based on body surface area (BSA) for each child. The recommended oral dose of RETROVIR is 480 mg/m^2/day in divided doses (240 mg/m^2 twice daily or 160 mg/m^2 three times daily). In some cases the dose calculated by mg/kg will not be the same as that calculated by BSA.
2.2   Prevention of Maternal-Fetal HIV-1 Transmission
The recommended dosage regimen for administration to pregnant women (>14 weeks of pregnancy) and their neonates is:
Maternal Dosing: 100 mg orally 5 times per day until the start of labor *[see Clinical Studies(14.3)].* During labor and delivery, intravenous RETROVIR should be administered at 2 mg/kg (total body weight) over 1 hour followed by a continuous intravenous infusion of 1 mg/kg/hour (total body weight) until clamping of the umbilical cord.
Neonatal Dosing: Start neonatal dosing within 12 hours after birth and continue through 6 weeks of age. Neonates unable to receive oral dosing may be administered RETROVIR intravenously. See Table 2.

Table 2. Recommended Neonatal Dosages of RETROVIR

Route	Total Daily Dose	Dose and Dosage Regimen
Oral	8 mg/kg/day	2 mg/kg every 6 hours
IV	6 mg/kg/day	1.5 mg/kg infused over 30 minutes, every 6 hours

2.3   Patients With Severe Anemia and/or Neutropenia
Significant anemia (hemoglobin <7.5 g/dL or reduction >25% of baseline) and/or significant neutropenia (granulocyte count <750 cells/mm^3 or reduction >50% from baseline) may require a dose interruption until evidence of marrow recovery is observed *[see Warnings and Precautions (5.1)].* In patients who develop significant anemia, dose interruption does not necessarily eliminate the need for transfusion. If marrow recovery occurs following dose interruption, resumption in dose may be appropriate using adjunctive measures such as epoetin alfa at recommended doses, depending on hematologic indices such as serum erythropoietin level and patient tolerance.

2.4 Patients With Renal Impairment

End-Stage Renal Disease: In patients maintained on hemodialysis or peritoneal dialysis, the recommended dosage is 100 mg every 6 to 8 hours [see Clinical Pharmacology (12.3)].

2.5 Patients With Hepatic Impairment

There are insufficient data to recommend dose adjustment of RETROVIR in patients with mild to moderate impaired hepatic function or liver cirrhosis.

3 DOSAGE FORMS AND STRENGTHS

RETROVIR Tablets 300 mg (biconvex, white, round, film-coated) containing 300 mg zidovudine, one side engraved "GX CW3" and "300" on the other side.

RETROVIR Capsules 100 mg (white, opaque cap and body) containing 100 mg zidovudine and printed with "Wellcome" and unicorn logo on cap and "Y9C" and "100" on body.

RETROVIR Syrup (colorless to pale yellow, strawberry–flavored) containing 10 mg zidovudine in each mL.

4 CONTRAINDICATIONS

RETROVIR Tablets, Capsules, and Syrup are contraindicated in patients who have had potentially life-threatening allergic reactions (e.g., anaphylaxis, Stevens-Johnson syndrome) to any of the components of the formulations.

5 WARNINGS AND PRECAUTIONS

5.1 Hematologic Toxicity/Bone Marrow Suppression

RETROVIR should be used with caution in patients who have bone marrow compromise evidenced by granulocyte count <1,000 cells/mm[3] or hemoglobin <9.5 g/dL. Hematologic toxicities appear to be related to pretreatment bone marrow reserve and to dose and duration of therapy. In patients with advanced symptomatic HIV-1 disease, anemia and neutropenia were the most significant adverse events observed. In patients who experience hematologic toxicity, a reduction in hemoglobin may occur as early as 2 to 4 weeks, and neutropenia usually occurs after 6 to 8 weeks. There have been reports of pancytopenia associated with the use of RETROVIR, which was reversible in most instances after discontinuance of the drug. However, significant anemia, in many cases requiring dose adjustment, discontinuation of RETROVIR, and/or blood transfusions, has occurred during treatment with RETROVIR alone or in combination with other antiretrovirals.

Frequent blood counts are strongly recommended to detect severe anemia or neutropenia in patients with poor bone marrow reserve, particularly in patients with advanced HIV-1 disease who are treated with RETROVIR. For HIV-1-infected individuals and patients with asymptomatic or early HIV-1 disease, periodic blood counts are recommended. If anemia or neutropenia develops, dosage interruption may be needed [see Dosage and Administration (2.3)].

5.2 Myopathy

Myopathy and myositis with pathological changes, similar to that produced by HIV-1 disease, have been associated with prolonged use of RETROVIR.

5.3 Lactic Acidosis/Severe Hepatomegaly With Steatosis

Lactic acidosis and severe hepatomegaly with steatosis, including fatal cases, have been reported with the use of nucleoside analogues alone or in combination, including zidovudine and other antiretrovirals. A majority of these cases have been in women. Obesity and prolonged exposure to antiretroviral nucleoside analogues may be risk factors. Particular caution should be exercised when administering RETROVIR to any patient with known risk factors for liver disease; however, cases have also been reported in patients with no known risk factors. Treatment with RETROVIR should be suspended in any patient who develops clinical or laboratory findings suggestive of lactic acidosis or pronounced hepatotoxicity (which may include hepatomegaly and steatosis even in the absence of marked transaminase elevations).

5.4 Use With Interferon- and Ribavirin-Based Regimens in HIV-1/HCV Co-Infected Patients

In vitro studies have shown ribavirin can reduce the phosphorylation of pyrimidine nucleoside analogues such as zidovudine. Although no evidence of a pharmacokinetic or pharmacodynamic interaction (e.g., loss of HIV-1/HCV virologic suppression) was seen when ribavirin was coadministered with zidovudine in HIV-1/HCV co-infected subjects [see Clinical Pharmacology (12.3)], exacerbation of anemia due to ribavirin has been reported when zidovudine is part of the HIV regimen. Coadministration of ribavirin and zidovudine is not advised. Consideration should be given to replacing zidovudine in established combination HIV-1/HCV therapy, especially in patients with a known history of zidovudine-induced anemia.

Hepatic decompensation (some fatal) has occurred in HIV-1/HCV co-infected patients receiving combination antiretroviral therapy for HIV-1 and interferon alfa with or without ribavirin. Patients receiving interferon alfa with or without ribavirin and zidovudine should be closely monitored for treatment-associated toxicities, especially hepatic decompensation, neutropenia, and anemia.

Discontinuation of zidovudine should be considered as medically appropriate. Dose reduction or discontinuation of interferon alfa, ribavirin, or both should also be considered if worsening clinical toxicities are observed, including hepatic decompensation (e.g., Child-Pugh >6) (see the complete prescribing information for interferon and ribavirin).

5.5 Use With Other Zidovudine-Containing Products

RETROVIR should not be administered with combination products that contain zidovudine as one of their components (e.g., COMBIVIR® [lamivudine and zidovudine] Tablets or TRIZIVIR® [abacavir sulfate, lamivudine, and zidovudine] Tablets).

5.6 Immune Reconstitution Syndrome

Immune reconstitution syndrome has been reported in patients treated with combination antiretroviral therapy, including RETROVIR. During the initial phase of combination antiretroviral treatment, patients whose immune systems respond may develop an inflammatory response to indolent or residual opportunistic infections (such as Mycobacterium avium infection, cytomegalovirus, Pneumocystis jirovecii pneumonia [PCP], or tuberculosis), which may necessitate further evaluation and treatment.

Autoimmune disorders (such as Graves' disease, polymyositis, and Guillain-Barré syndrome) have also been reported to occur in the setting of immune reconstitution; however, the time to onset is more variable, and can occur many months after initiation of treatment.

5.7 Fat Redistribution

Redistribution/accumulation of body fat, including central obesity, dorsocervical fat enlargement (buffalo hump), peripheral wasting, facial wasting, breast enlargement, and "cushingoid appearance," have been observed in patients receiving antiretroviral therapy. The mechanism and long-term consequences of these events are currently unknown. A causal relationship has not been established.

6 ADVERSE REACTIONS

The following adverse reactions are discussed in greater detail in other sections of the labeling:

- Hematologic toxicity, including neutropenia and anemia [see Boxed Warning, Warnings and Precautions (5.1)].
- Symptomatic myopathy [see Boxed Warning, Warnings and Precautions (5.2)].
- Lactic acidosis and severe hepatomegaly with steatosis [see Boxed Warning, Warnings and Precautions (5.3)].
- Hepatic decompensation in patients co-infected with HIV-1 and hepatitis C [see Warnings and Precautions (5.4)].

6.1 Clinical Trials Experience

Because clinical trials are conducted under widely varying conditions, adverse reaction rates observed in the clinical trials of a drug cannot be directly compared with rates in the clinical trials of another drug and may not reflect the rates observed in practice.

Adults: The frequency and severity of adverse reactions associated with the use of RETROVIR are greater in patients with more advanced infection at the time of initiation of therapy.

Table 3 summarizes adverse reactions reported at a statistically significant greater incidence for subjects receiving RETROVIR in a monotherapy trial.

Table 3. Percentage (%) of Subjects With Adverse Reactions[a] in Asymptomatic HIV-1 Infection (ACTG 019)

Adverse Reaction	RETROVIR 500 mg/day (n = 453)	Placebo (n = 428)
Body as a whole		
Asthenia	9%[b]	6%
Headache	63%	53%
Malaise	53%	45%
Gastrointestinal		
Anorexia	20%	11%
Constipation	6%[b]	4%
Nausea	51%	30%
Vomiting	17%	10%

[a] Reported in ≥5% of trial population.
[b] Not statistically significant versus placebo.

In addition to the adverse reactions listed in Table 3, adverse reactions observed at an incidence of ≥5% in any treatment arm in clinical trials (NUCA3001, NUCA3002, NUCB3001, and NUCB3002) were abdominal cramps, abdominal pain, arthralgia, chills, dyspepsia, fatigue, insomnia, musculoskeletal pain, myalgia, and neuropathy. Additionally, in these trials hyperbilirubinemia was reported at an incidence of ≤0.8%.

Selected laboratory abnormalities observed during a clinical trial of monotherapy with RETROVIR are shown in Table 4.

Table 4. Frequencies of Selected (Grade 3/4) Laboratory Abnormalities in Subjects With Asymptomatic HIV-1 Infection (ACTG 019)

Test (Abnormal Level)	RETROVIR 500 mg/day (n = 453)	Placebo (n = 428)
Anemia (Hgb<8 g/dL)	1%	<1%
Granulocytopenia (<750 cells/mm[3])	2%	2%
Thrombocytopenia (platelets<50,000/mm[3])	0%	<1%
ALT (>5 × ULN)	3%	3%
AST (>5 × ULN)	1%	2%

ULN = Upper limit of normal.

Pediatrics: The clinical adverse reactions reported among adult recipients of RETROVIR may also occur in pediatric patients.

Trial ACTG 300: Selected clinical adverse reactions and physical findings with a ≥5% frequency during therapy with EPIVIR® (lamivudine) Oral Suspension 4 mg/kg twice daily plus RETROVIR 160 mg/m[2] 3 times daily compared with didanosine in therapy-naive (≤56 days of antiretroviral therapy) pediatric subjects are listed in Table 5.

Table 5. Selected Clinical Adverse Reactions and Physical Findings (≥5% Frequency) in Pediatric Subjects in Trial ACTG 300

Adverse Reaction	EPIVIR plus RETROVIR (n = 236)	Didanosine (n = 235)
Body as a whole		
Fever	25%	32%
Digestive		
Hepatomegaly	11%	11%
Nausea & vomiting	8%	7%
Diarrhea	8%	6%
Stomatitis	6%	12%
Splenomegaly	5%	8%
Respiratory		
Cough	15%	18%
Abnormal breath sounds/wheezing	7%	9%
Ear, Nose, and Throat		
Signs or symptoms of ears[a]	7%	6%
Nasal discharge or congestion	8%	11%
Other		
Skin rashes	12%	14%
Lymphadenopathy	9%	11%

[a] Includes pain, discharge, erythema, or swelling of an ear.

Selected laboratory abnormalities experienced by therapy-naive (≤56 days of antiretroviral therapy) pediatric subjects are listed in Table 6.

Table 6. Frequencies of Selected (Grade 3/4) Laboratory Abnormalities in Pediatric Subjects in Trial ACTG 300

Test (Abnormal Level)	EPIVIR plus RETROVIR	Didanosine
Neutropenia (ANC<400 cells/mm[3])	8%	3%
Anemia (Hgb<7.0 g/dL)	4%	2%
Thrombocytopenia (platelets<50,000/mm[3])	1%	3%
ALT (>10 × ULN)	1%	3%
AST (>10 × ULN)	2%	4%
Lipase (>2.5 × ULN)	3%	3%
Total amylase (>2.5 × ULN)	3%	3%

ULN = Upper limit of normal.
ANC = Absolute neutrophil count.

Macrocytosis was reported in the majority of pediatric subjects receiving RETROVIR 180 mg/m[2] every 6 hours in open-label trials. Additionally, adverse reactions reported at an incidence of <6% in these trials were congestive heart failure, decreased reflexes, ECG abnormality, edema, hematuria, left ventricular dilation, nervousness/irritability, and weight loss.

Use for the Prevention of Maternal-Fetal Transmission of HIV-1: In a randomized, double-blind, placebo-controlled trial in HIV-1-infected women and their neonates conducted to determine the utility of RETROVIR for the prevention of maternal-fetal HIV-1 transmission, RETROVIR Syrup at

2 mg/kg was administered every 6 hours for 6 weeks to neonates beginning within 12 hours following birth. The most commonly reported adverse reactions were anemia (hemoglobin <9.0 g/dL) and neutropenia (<1,000 cells/mm[3]). Anemia occurred in 22% of the neonates who received RETROVIR and in 12% of the neonates who received placebo. The mean difference in hemoglobin values was less than 1.0 g/dL for neonates receiving RETROVIR compared with neonates receiving placebo. No neonates with anemia required transfusion and all hemoglobin values spontaneously returned to normal within 6 weeks after completion of therapy with RETROVIR. Neutropenia in neonates was reported with similar frequency in the group that received RETROVIR (21%) and in the group that received placebo (27%). The long-term consequences of in utero and infant exposure to RETROVIR are unknown.

6.2   Postmarketing Experience
In addition to adverse reactions reported from clinical trials, the following reactions have been identified during postmarketing use of RETROVIR. Because they are reported voluntarily from a population of unknown size, estimates of frequency cannot be made. These reactions have been chosen for inclusion due to a combination of their seriousness, frequency of reporting, or potential causal connection to RETROVIR.

Body as a Whole: Back pain, chest pain, flu-like syndrome, generalized pain, redistribution/accumulation of body fat [see Warnings and Precautions (5.7)].
Cardiovascular: Cardiomyopathy, syncope.
Endocrine: Gynecomastia.
Eye: Macular edema.
Gastrointestinal: Dysphagia, flatulence, oral mucosa pigmentation, mouth ulcer.
General: Sensitization reactions including anaphylaxis and angioedema, vasculitis.
Hemic and Lymphatic: Aplastic anemia, hemolytic anemia, leukopenia, lymphadenopathy, pancytopenia with marrow hypoplasia, pure red cell aplasia.
Hepatobiliary Tract and Pancreas: Hepatitis, hepatomegaly with steatosis, jaundice, lactic acidosis, pancreatitis.
Musculoskeletal: Increased CPK, increased LDH, muscle spasm, myopathy and myositis with pathological changes (similar to that produced by HIV-1 disease), rhabdomyolysis, tremor.
Nervous: Anxiety, confusion, depression, dizziness, loss of mental acuity, mania, paresthesia, seizures, somnolence, vertigo.
Respiratory: Dyspnea, rhinitis, sinusitis.
Skin: Changes in skin and nail pigmentation, pruritus, Stevens-Johnson syndrome, toxic epidermal necrolysis, sweat, urticaria.
Special Senses: Amblyopia, hearing loss, photophobia, taste perversion.
Urogenital: Urinary frequency, urinary hesitancy.

7   DRUG INTERACTIONS
7.1   Antiretroviral Agents
Stavudine: Concomitant use of zidovudine with stavudine should be avoided since an antagonistic relationship has been demonstrated in vitro.
Nucleoside Analogues Affecting DNA Replication: Some nucleoside analogues affecting DNA replication, such as ribavirin, antagonize the in vitro antiviral activity of RETROVIR against HIV-1; concomitant use of such drugs should be avoided.
7.2   Doxorubicin
Concomitant use of zidovudine with doxorubicin should be avoided since an antagonistic relationship has been demonstrated in vitro.
7.3   Hematologic/Bone Marrow Suppressive/Cytotoxic Agents
Coadministration of ganciclovir, interferon alfa, ribavirin, and other bone marrow suppressive or cytotoxic agents may increase the hematologic toxicity of zidovudine.

8   USE IN SPECIFIC POPULATIONS
8.1   Pregnancy
Pregnancy Category C.
In humans, treatment with RETROVIR during pregnancy reduced the rate of maternal-fetal HIV-1 transmission from 24.9% for infants born to placebo-treated mothers to 7.8% for infants born to mothers treated with RETROVIR [see Clinical Studies (14.3)]. There were no differences in pregnancy-related adverse events between the treatment groups. Animal reproduction studies in rats and rabbits showed evidence of embryotoxicity and increased fetal malformations.
A randomized, double-blind, placebo-controlled trial was conducted in HIV-1-infected pregnant women to determine the utility of RETROVIR for the prevention of maternal-fetal HIV-1-transmission [see Clinical Studies (14.3)]. Congenital abnormalities occurred with similar frequency between neonates born to mothers who received RETROVIR and neonates born to mothers who received placebo. The observed abnormalities included problems in embryogenesis (prior to 14 weeks) or were recognized on ultrasound before or immediately after initiation of study drug.
Increased fetal resorptions occurred in pregnant rats and rabbits treated with doses of zidovudine that produced drug plasma concentrations 66 to 226 times (rats) and 12 to 87 times (rabbits) the mean steady-state peak human plasma concentration following a single 100-mg dose of zidovudine. There were no other reported developmental anomalies. In another developmental toxicity study, pregnant rats received zidovudine up to near-lethal doses that produced peak plasma concentrations 350 times peak human plasma concentrations (300 times the daily exposure [AUC] in humans given 600 mg/day zidovudine). This dose was associated with marked maternal toxicity and an increased incidence of fetal malformations. However, there were no signs of teratogenicity at doses up to one-fifth the lethal dose [see Nonclinical Toxicology (13.2)].
Antiretroviral Pregnancy Registry: To monitor maternal-fetal outcomes of pregnant women exposed to RETROVIR, an Antiretroviral Pregnancy Registry has been established. Physicians are encouraged to register patients by calling 1-800-258-4263.
8.3   Nursing Mothers
Zidovudine is excreted in human milk [see Clinical Pharmacology (12.3)].
The Centers for Disease Control and Prevention recommend that HIV-1-infected mothers in the United States not breastfeed their infants to avoid risking postnatal transmission of HIV-1 infection. Because of both the potential for HIV-1 transmission and the potential for serious adverse reactions in nursing infants, mothers should be instructed not to breastfeed if they are receiving RETROVIR.
8.4   Pediatric Use
RETROVIR has been studied in HIV-1-infected pediatric subjects aged ≥6 weeks who had HIV-1-related symptoms or who were asymptomatic with abnormal laboratory values indicating significant HIV-1-related immunosuppression. RETROVIR has also been studied in neonates perinatally exposed to HIV-1 [see Dosage and Administration (2.1), Adverse Reactions (6.1), Clinical Pharmacology (12.3), Clinical Studies (14.2), (14.3)].
8.5   Geriatric Use
Clinical studies of RETROVIR did not include sufficient numbers of subjects aged 65 and over to determine whether they respond differently from younger subjects. Other reported clinical experience has not identified differences in responses between the elderly and younger patients. In general, dose selection for an elderly patient should be cautious, reflecting the greater frequency of decreased hepatic, renal, or cardiac function, and of concomitant disease or other drug therapy.
8.6   Renal Impairment
In patients with severely impaired renal function (CrCl<15 mL/min), dosage reduction is recommended [see Dosage and Administration (2.4), Clinical Pharmacology (12.3)].
8.7   Hepatic Impairment
Zidovudine is eliminated from the body primarily by renal excretion following metabolism in the liver (glucuronidation). Although the data are limited, zidovudine concentrations appear to be increased in patients with severely impaired hepatic function, which may increase the risk of hematologic toxicity [see Dosage and Administration (2.5), Clinical Pharmacology (12.3)].

10   OVERDOSAGE
Acute overdoses of zidovudine have been reported in pediatric patients and adults. These involved exposures up to 50 grams. No specific symptoms or signs have been identified following acute overdosage with zidovudine apart from those listed as adverse events such as fatigue, headache, vomiting, and occasional reports of hematological disturbances. All patients recovered without permanent sequelae. Hemodialysis and peritoneal dialysis appear to have a negligible effect on the removal of zidovudine while elimination of its primary metabolite, 3'-azido-3'-deoxy-5'-O-β-D-glucopyranuronosylthymidine (GZDV), is enhanced.

11   DESCRIPTION
RETROVIR is the brand name for zidovudine (formerly called azidothymidine [AZT]), a pyrimidine nucleoside analogue active against HIV-1. The chemical name of zidovudine is 3'-azido-3'-deoxythymidine; it has the following structural formula:
[See chemical structure at top of next column]
Zidovudine is a white to beige, odorless, crystalline solid with a molecular weight of 267.24 and a solubility of 20.1 mg/mL in water at 25°C. The molecular formula is $C_{10}H_{13}N_5O_4$.
RETROVIR Tablets are for oral administration. Each film-coated tablet contains 300 mg of zidovudine and the inactive ingredients hypromellose, magnesium stearate, microcrystalline cellulose, polyethylene glycol, sodium starch glycolate, and titanium dioxide.

RETROVIR Capsules are for oral administration. Each capsule contains 100 mg of zidovudine and the inactive ingredients corn starch, magnesium stearate, microcrystalline cellulose, and sodium starch glycolate. The 100-mg empty hard gelatin capsule, printed with edible black ink, consists of black iron oxide, dimethylpolysiloxane, gelatin, pharmaceutical shellac, soya lecithin, and titanium dioxide.
RETROVIR Syrup is for oral administration. Each mL of RETROVIR Syrup contains 10 mg of zidovudine and the inactive ingredients sodium benzoate 0.2% (added as a preservative), citric acid, flavors, glycerin, and liquid sucrose. Sodium hydroxide may be added to adjust pH.

12   CLINICAL PHARMACOLOGY
12.1   Mechanism of Action
Zidovudine is an antiviral agent [see Clinical Pharmacology (12.4)].
12.3   Pharmacokinetics
Absorption and Bioavailability: In adults, following oral administration, zidovudine is rapidly absorbed and extensively distributed, with peak serum concentrations occurring within 0.5 to 1.5 hours. The AUC was equivalent when zidovudine was administered as RETROVIR Tablets or Syrup compared with RETROVIR Capsules. The pharmacokinetic properties of zidovudine in fasting adult subjects are summarized in Table 7.

Table 7. Zidovudine Pharmacokinetic Parameters in Fasting Adult Subjects

Parameter	Mean ± SD (except where noted)
Oral bioavailability (%)	64 ± 10 (n = 5)
Apparent volume of distribution (L/kg)	1.6 ± 0.6 (n = 8)
Plasma protein binding (%)	<38
CSF:plasma ratio[a]	0.6 [0.04 to 2.62] (n = 39)
Systemic clearance (L/h/kg)	1.6 ± 0.6 (n = 6)
Renal clearance (L/h/kg)	0.34 ± 0.05 (n = 9)
Elimination half-life (h)[b]	0.5 to 3 (n = 19)

[a] Median [range].
[b] Approximate range.

Distribution: The apparent volume of distribution of zidovudine, following oral administration, is 1.6 ± 0.6 L/kg; and binding to plasma protein is low, <38% (Table 7).
Metabolism and Elimination: Zidovudine is primarily eliminated by hepatic metabolism. The major metabolite of zidovudine is GZDV. GZDV AUC is about 3-fold greater than the zidovudine AUC. Urinary recovery of zidovudine and GZDV accounts for 14% and 74%, respectively, of the dose following oral administration. A second metabolite, 3'-amino-3'-deoxythymidine (AMT), has been identified in the plasma following single-dose intravenous (IV) administration of zidovudine. The AMT AUC was one-fifth of the zidovudine AUC. Pharmacokinetics of zidovudine were dose independent at oral dosing regimens ranging from 2 mg/kg every 8 hours to 10 mg/kg every 4 hours.
Effect of Food on Absorption: RETROVIR may be administered with or without food. The zidovudine AUC was similar when a single dose of zidovudine was administered with food.
Special Populations: Renal Impairment: Zidovudine clearance was decreased resulting in increased zidovudine and GZDV half-life and AUC in subjects with impaired renal function (n = 14) following a single 200-mg oral dose (Table 8). Plasma concentrations of AMT were not determined. A dose adjustment should not be necessary for patients with creatinine clearance (CrCl) ≥15 mL/min.

Table 8. Zidovudine Pharmacokinetic Parameters in Subjects With Severe Renal Impairment[a]

Parameter	Control Subjects (Normal Renal Function) (n = 6)	Subjects With Renal Impairment (n = 14)
CrCl (mL/min)	120 ± 8	18 ± 2
Zidovudine AUC (ng•h/mL)	1,400 ± 200	3,100 ± 300
Zidovudine half-life (h)	1.0 ± 0.2	1.4 ± 0.1

[a] Data are expressed as mean ± standard deviation.

Hemodialysis and Peritoneal Dialysis: The pharmacokinetics and tolerance of zidovudine were evaluated in a multiple-dose trial in subjects undergoing hemodialysis (n = 5) or peritoneal dialysis (n = 6) receiving escalating doses up to 200 mg 5 times daily for 8 weeks. Daily doses of 500 mg or less were well tolerated despite significantly elevated GZDV plasma concentrations. Apparent zidovudine oral clearance was approximately 50% of that reported in subjects with normal renal function. Hemodialysis and peritoneal dialysis appeared to have a negligible effect on the removal of zidovudine, whereas GZDV elimination was enhanced. A dosage adjustment is recommended for patients undergoing hemodialysis or peritoneal dialysis *[see Dosage and Administration (2.4)].*

Hepatic Impairment: Data describing the effect of hepatic impairment on the pharmacokinetics of zidovudine are limited. However, because zidovudine is eliminated primarily by hepatic metabolism, it is expected that zidovudine clearance would be decreased and plasma concentrations would be increased following administration of the recommended adult doses to patients with hepatic impairment *[see Dosage and Administration (2.5)].*

Pediatric Patients: Zidovudine pharmacokinetics have been evaluated in HIV-1-infected pediatric subjects (Table 9).

Patients Aged 3 Months to 12 Years: Overall, zidovudine pharmacokinetics in pediatric patients older than 3 months are similar to those in adult patients. Proportional increases in plasma zidovudine concentrations were observed following administration of oral solution from 90 to 240 mg/m² every 6 hours. Oral bioavailability, terminal half-life, and oral clearance were comparable to adult values. As in adult subjects, the major route of elimination was by metabolism to GZDV. After intravenous dosing, about 29% of the dose was excreted in the urine unchanged, and about 45% of the dose was excreted as GZDV *[see Dosage and Administration (2.1)].*

Patients Aged Less Than 3 Months: Zidovudine pharmacokinetics have been evaluated in pediatric subjects from birth to 3 months of life. Zidovudine elimination was determined immediately following birth in 8 neonates who were exposed to zidovudine in utero. The half-life was 13.0 ± 5.8 hours. In neonates ≤14 days old, bioavailability was greater, total body clearance was slower, and half-life was longer than in pediatric subjects older than 14 days. For dose recommendations for neonates *[see Dosage and Administration (2.2)].*

[See table 9 above]

Pregnancy: Zidovudine pharmacokinetics have been studied in a Phase I trial of 8 women during the last trimester of pregnancy. Zidovudine pharmacokinetics were similar to those of nonpregnant adults. Consistent with passive transmission of the drug across the placenta, zidovudine concentrations in neonatal plasma at birth were essentially equal to those in maternal plasma at delivery *[see Use in Specific Populations (8.1)].*

Although data are limited, methadone maintenance therapy in 5 pregnant women did not appear to alter zidovudine pharmacokinetics.

Nursing Mothers: The Centers for Disease Control and Prevention recommend that HIV-1-infected mothers not breastfeed their infants to avoid risking postnatal transmission of HIV-1. After administration of a single dose of 200 mg zidovudine to 13 HIV-1-infected women, the mean concentration of zidovudine was similar in human milk and serum *[see Use in Specific Populations (8.3)].*

Geriatric Patients: Zidovudine pharmacokinetics have not been studied in subjects over 65 years of age.

Gender: A pharmacokinetic trial in healthy male (n = 12) and female (n = 12) subjects showed no differences in zidovudine AUC when a single dose of zidovudine was administered as the 300-mg RETROVIR Tablet.

Table 9. Zidovudine Pharmacokinetic Parameters in Pediatric Subjects[a]

Parameter	Birth to 14 Days	Aged 14 Days to 3 Months	Aged 3 Months to 12 Years
Oral bioavailability (%)	89 ± 19 (n = 15)	61 ± 19 (n = 17)	65 ± 24 (n = 18)
CSF:plasma ratio	no data	no data	0.68 [0.03 to 3.25][b] (n = 38)
CL (L/h/kg)	0.65 ± 0.29 (n = 18)	1.14 ± 0.24 (n = 16)	1.85 ± 0.47 (n = 20)
Elimination half-life (h)	3.1 ± 1.2 (n = 21)	1.9 ± 0.7 (n = 18)	1.5 ± 0.7 (n = 21)

[a] Data presented as mean ± standard deviation except where noted.
[b] Median [range].

Table 10. Effect of Coadministered Drugs on Zidovudine AUC[a]

Note: ROUTINE DOSE MODIFICATION OF ZIDOVUDINE IS NOT WARRANTED WITH COADMINISTRATION OF THE FOLLOWING DRUGS.

Coadministered Drug and Dose	Zidovudine Dose	n	Zidovudine Concentrations AUC	Variability	Concentration of Coadministered Drug
Atovaquone 750 mg q 12 h with food	200 mg q 8 h	14	↑AUC 31%	Range 23% to 78%[b]	↔
Clarithromycin 500 mg twice daily	100 mg q 4 h × 7 days	4	↓AUC 12%	Range ↓34% to ↑14%	Not Reported
Fluconazole 400 mg daily	200 mg q 8 h	12	↑AUC 74%	95% CI: 54% to 98%	Not Reported
Lamivudine 300 mg q 12 h	single 200 mg	12	↑AUC 13%	90% CI: 2% to 27%	↔
Methadone 30 to 90 mg daily	200 mg q 4 h	9	↑AUC 43%	Range 16% to 64%[b]	↔
Nelfinavir 750 mg q 8 h × 7 to 10 days	single 200 mg	11	↓AUC 35%	Range 28% to 41%	
Probenecid 500 mg q 6 h × 2 days	2 mg/kg q 8 h × 3 days	3	↑AUC 106%	Range 100% to 170%[b]	Not Assessed
Rifampin 600 mg daily × 14 days	200 mg q 8 h × 14 days	8	↓AUC 47%	90% CI: 41% to 53%	Not Assessed
Ritonavir 300 mg q 6 h × 4 days	200 mg q 8 h × 4 days	9	↓AUC 25%	95% CI: 15% to 34%	↔
Valproic acid 250 mg or 500 mg q 8 h × 4 days	100 mg q 8 h × 4 days	6	↑AUC 80%	Range 64% to 130%[b]	Not Assessed

↑ = Increase; ↓ = Decrease; ↔ = no significant change; AUC = area under the concentration versus time curve; CI = confidence interval.
[a] This table is not all inclusive.
[b] Estimated range of percent difference.

Drug Interactions: *[See Drug Interactions (7)].*
[See table 10 above]

Phenytoin: Phenytoin plasma levels have been reported to be low in some patients receiving RETROVIR, while in one case a high level was documented. However, in a pharmacokinetic interaction trial in which 12 HIV-1-positive volunteers received a single 300-mg phenytoin dose alone and during steady-state zidovudine conditions (200 mg every 4 hours), no change in phenytoin kinetics was observed. Although not designed to optimally assess the effect of phenytoin on zidovudine kinetics, a 30% decrease in oral zidovudine clearance was observed with phenytoin.

Ribavirin: In vitro data indicate ribavirin reduces phosphorylation of lamivudine, stavudine, and zidovudine. However, no pharmacokinetic (e.g., plasma concentrations or intracellular triphosphorylated active metabolite concentrations) or pharmacodynamic (e.g., loss of HIV-1/HCV virologic suppression) interaction was observed when ribavirin and lamivudine (n = 18), stavudine (n = 10), or zidovudine (n = 6) were coadministered as part of a multidrug regimen to HIV-1/HCV co-infected subjects *[see Warnings and Precautions (5.4)].*

12.4 Microbiology

Mechanism of Action: Zidovudine is a synthetic nucleoside analogue. Intracellularly, zidovudine is phosphorylated to its active 5'-triphosphate metabolite, zidovudine triphosphate (ZDV-TP). The principal mode of action of ZDV-TP is inhibition of reverse transcriptase (RT) via DNA chain termination after incorporation of the nucleotide analogue.

ZDV-TP is a weak inhibitor of the cellular DNA polymerases α and γ and has been reported to be incorporated into the DNA of cells in culture.

Antiviral Activity: The antiviral activity of zidovudine against HIV-1 was assessed in a number of cell lines (including monocytes and fresh human peripheral blood lymphocytes). The EC_{50} and EC_{90} values for zidovudine were 0.01 to 0.49 μM (1 μM = 0.27 mcg/mL) and 0.1 to 9 μM, respectively. HIV-1 from therapy-naive subjects with no mutations associated with resistance gave median EC_{50} values of 0.011 μM (range: 0.005 to 0.110 μM) from Virco (n = 92 baseline samples from COL40263) and 0.0017 μM (0.006 to 0.0340 μM) from Monogram Biosciences (n = 135 baseline samples from ESS30009). The EC_{50} values of zidovudine against different HIV-1 clades (A-G) ranged from 0.00018 to 0.02 μM, and against HIV-2 isolates from 0.00049 to 0.004 μM. In cell culture drug combination studies, zidovudine demonstrates synergistic activity with the nucleoside reverse transcriptase inhibitors abacavir, didanosine, and lamivudine; the non-nucleoside reverse transcriptase inhibitors delavirdine and nevirapine; and the protease inhibitors indinavir, nelfinavir, ritonavir, and saquinavir; and additive activity with interferon alfa. Ribavirin has been found to inhibit the phosphorylation of zidovudine in cell culture.

Resistance: Genotypic analyses of the isolates selected in cell culture and recovered from zidovudine-treated subjects showed mutations in the HIV-1 RT gene resulting in 6 amino acid substitutions (M41L, D67N, K70R, L210W, T215Y or F, and K219Q) that confer zidovudine resistance. In general, higher levels of resistance were associated with greater number of amino acid substitutions. In some subjects harboring zidovudine-resistant virus at baseline, phenotypic sensitivity to zidovudine was restored by 12 weeks of treatment with lamivudine and zidovudine. Combination therapy with lamivudine plus zidovudine delayed the emergence of substitutions conferring resistance to zidovudine.

Cross-Resistance: In a study of 167 HIV-1-infected subjects, isolates (n = 2) with multi-drug resistance to didanosine, lamivudine, stavudine, zalcitabine, and zidovudine were recovered from subjects treated for ≥1 year with zidovudine plus didanosine or zidovudine plus zalcitabine. The pattern of resistance-associated amino acid substitutions with such combination therapies was different (A62V, V75I, F77L, F116Y, Q151M) from the pattern with zidovudine monotherapy, with the Q151M substitution being most commonly associated with multi-drug resistance. The substitution at codon 151 in combination with substitutions at 62, 75, 77, and 116 results in a virus with reduced susceptibility to didanosine, lamivudine, stavudine, zalcitabine, and zidovudine. Thymidine analogue mutations (TAMs) are selected by zidovudine and confer cross-resistance to abacavir, didanosine, stavudine, tenofovir, and zalcitabine.

13   NONCLINICAL TOXICOLOGY
13.1   Carcinogenesis, Mutagenesis, Impairment of Fertility
Zidovudine was administered orally at 3 dosage levels to separate groups of mice and rats (60 females and 60 males in each group). Initial single daily doses were 30, 60, and 120 mg/kg/day in mice and 80, 220, and 600 mg/kg/day in rats. The doses in mice were reduced to 20, 30, and 40 mg/kg/day after day 90 because of treatment-related anemia, whereas in rats only the high dose was reduced to 450 mg/kg/day on day 91 and then to 300 mg/kg/day on day 279.

In mice, 7 late-appearing (after 19 months) vaginal neoplasms (5 nonmetastasizing squamous cell carcinomas, 1 squamous cell papilloma, and 1 squamous polyp) occurred in animals given the highest dose. One late-appearing squamous cell papilloma occurred in the vagina of a middle-dose animal. No vaginal tumors were found at the lowest dose.

In rats, 2 late-appearing (after 20 months) nonmetastasizing vaginal squamous cell carcinomas occurred in animals given the highest dose. No vaginal tumors occurred at the low or middle dose in rats. No other drug-related tumors were observed in either sex of either species.

At doses that produced tumors in mice and rats, the estimated drug exposure (as measured by AUC) was approximately 3 times (mouse) and 24 times (rat) the estimated human exposure at the recommended therapeutic dose of 100 mg every 4 hours.

It is not known how predictive the results of rodent carcinogenicity studies may be for humans.

Zidovudine was mutagenic in a 5178Y/TK⁺/⁻ mouse lymphoma assay, positive in an in vitro cell transformation assay, clastogenic in a cytogenetic assay using cultured human lymphocytes, and positive in mouse and rat micronucleus tests after repeated doses. It was negative in a cytogenetic study in rats given a single dose.

Zidovudine, administered to male and female rats at doses up to 7 times the usual adult dose based on body surface area, had no effect on fertility judged by conception rates. Two transplacental carcinogenicity studies were conducted in mice. One study administered zidovudine at doses of 20 mg/kg/day or 40 mg/kg/day from gestation day 10 through parturition and lactation with dosing continuing in offspring for 24 months postnatally. The doses of zidovudine administered in this study produced zidovudine exposures approximately 3 times the estimated human exposure at recommended doses. After 24 months, an increase in incidence of vaginal tumors was noted with no increase in tumors in the liver or lung or any other organ in either gender. These findings are consistent with results of the standard oral carcinogenicity study in mice, as described earlier. A second study administered zidovudine at maximum tolerated doses of 12.5 mg/day or 25 mg/day (~1,000 mg/kg nonpregnant body weight or ~450 mg/kg of term body weight) to pregnant mice from days 12 through 18 of gestation. There was an increase in the number of tumors in the lung, liver, and female reproductive tracts in the offspring of mice receiving the higher dose level of zidovudine.

13.2   Reproductive and Developmental Toxicology Studies
Oral teratology studies in the rat and in the rabbit at doses up to 500 mg/kg/day revealed no evidence of teratogenicity with zidovudine. Zidovudine treatment resulted in embryo/fetal toxicity as evidenced by an increase in the incidence of fetal resorptions in rats given 150 or 450 mg/kg/day and rabbits given 500 mg/kg/day. The doses used in the teratol-

ogy studies resulted in peak zidovudine plasma concentrations (after one-half of the daily dose) in rats 66 to 226 times, and in rabbits 12 to 87 times, mean steady-state peak human plasma concentrations (after one-sixth of the daily dose) achieved with the recommended daily dose (100 mg every 4 hours). In an in vitro experiment with fertilized mouse oocytes, zidovudine exposure resulted in a dose-dependent reduction in blastocyst formation. In an additional teratology study in rats, a dose of 3,000 mg/kg/day (very near the oral median lethal dose of 3,683 mg/kg) caused marked maternal toxicity and an increase in the incidence of fetal malformations. This dose resulted in peak zidovudine plasma concentrations 350 times peak human plasma concentrations. (Estimated AUC in rats at this dose level was 300 times the daily AUC in humans given 600 mg/day.) No evidence of teratogenicity was seen in this experiment at doses of 600 mg/kg/day or less.

14   CLINICAL STUDIES
Therapy with RETROVIR has been shown to prolong survival and decrease the incidence of opportunistic infections in patients with advanced HIV-1 disease and to delay disease progression in asymptomatic HIV-1-infected patients.
14.1   Adults
Combination Therapy: RETROVIR in combination with other antiretroviral agents has been shown to be superior to monotherapy for one or more of the following endpoints: delaying death, delaying development of AIDS, increasing CD4+ cell counts, and decreasing plasma HIV-1 RNA.

The clinical efficacy of a combination regimen that includes RETROVIR was demonstrated in trial ACTG 320. This trial was a multi-center, randomized, double-blind, placebo-controlled trial that compared RETROVIR 600 mg/day plus EPIVIR 300 mg/day to RETROVIR plus EPIVIR plus indinavir 800 mg three times daily. The incidence of AIDS-defining events or death was lower in the triple-drug–containing arm compared with the 2-drug–containing arm (6.1% versus 10.9%, respectively).

Monotherapy: In controlled trials of treatment-naive subjects conducted between 1986 and 1989, monotherapy with RETROVIR, as compared with placebo, reduced the risk of HIV-1 disease progression, as assessed using endpoints that included the occurrence of HIV-1-related illnesses, AIDS-defining events, or death. These trials enrolled subjects with advanced disease (BW 002), and asymptomatic or mildly symptomatic disease in subjects with CD4+ cell counts between 200 and 500 cells/mm³ (ACTG 016 and ACTG 019). A survival benefit for monotherapy with RETROVIR was not demonstrated in the latter 2 trials. Subsequent trials showed that the clinical benefit of monotherapy with RETROVIR was time limited.

14.2   Pediatric Patients
ACTG 300 was a multi-center, randomized, double-blind trial that provided for comparison of EPIVIR plus RETROVIR to didanosine monotherapy. A total of 471 symptomatic, HIV-1-infected therapy-naive pediatric subjects were enrolled in these 2 treatment arms. The median age was 2.7 years (range: 6 weeks to 14 years), the mean baseline CD4+ cell count was 868 cells/mm³, and the mean baseline plasma HIV-1 RNA was 5.0 log₁₀ copies/mL. The median duration that subjects remained on trial was approximately 10 months. Results are summarized in Table 11.

Table 11. Number of Subjects (%) Reaching a Primary Clinical Endpoint (Disease Progression or Death)

Endpoint	EPIVIR plus RETROVIR (n = 236)	Didanosine (n = 235)
HIV disease progression or death (total)	15 (6.4%)	37 (15.7%)
Physical growth failure	7 (3.0%)	6 (2.6%)
Central nervous system deterioration	4 (1.7%)	12 (5.1%)
CDC Clinical Category C	2 (0.8%)	8 (3.4%)
Death	2 (0.8%)	11 (4.7%)

14.3   Prevention of Maternal-Fetal HIV-1 Transmission
The utility of RETROVIR for the prevention of maternal-fetal HIV-1 transmission was demonstrated in a randomized, double-blind, placebo-controlled trial (ACTG 076) conducted in HIV-1-infected pregnant women with CD4+ cell counts of 200 to 1,818 cells/mm³ (median in the treated group: 560 cells/mm³) who had little or no previous exposure to RETROVIR. Oral RETROVIR was initiated between 14 and 34 weeks of gestation (median 11 weeks of therapy) followed by IV administration of RETROVIR during labor and delivery. Following birth, neonates received oral

RETROVIR Syrup for 6 weeks. The trial showed a statistically significant difference in the incidence of HIV-1 infection in the neonates (based on viral culture from peripheral blood) between the group receiving RETROVIR and the group receiving placebo. Of 363 neonates evaluated in the trial, the estimated risk of HIV-1 infection was 7.8% in the group receiving RETROVIR and 24.9% in the placebo group, a relative reduction in transmission risk of 68.7%. RETROVIR was well tolerated by mothers and infants. There was no difference in pregnancy-related adverse events between the treatment groups.

16   HOW SUPPLIED/STORAGE AND HANDLING
RETROVIR Tablets 300 mg (biconvex, white, round, film-coated) containing 300 mg zidovudine, one side engraved "GX CW3" and "300" on the other side.
Bottle of 60 (NDC 49702-214-18).
Store at 15° to 25°C (59° to 77°F).
RETROVIR Capsules 100 mg (white, opaque cap and body) containing 100 mg zidovudine and printed with "Wellcome" and unicorn logo on cap and "Y9C" and "100" on body.
Bottles of 100 (NDC 49702-211-20).
Store at 15° to 25°C (59° to 77°F) and protect from moisture.
RETROVIR Syrup (colorless to pale yellow, strawberry-flavored) containing 10 mg zidovudine in each mL.
Bottle of 240 mL (NDC 49702-212-48) with child-resistant cap.
Store at 15° to 25°C (59° to 77°F).

17   PATIENT COUNSELING INFORMATION
17.1   Advice for the Patient
Neutropenia and Anemia: Patients should be informed that the major toxicities of RETROVIR are neutropenia and/or anemia. The frequency and severity of these toxicities are greater in patients with more advanced disease and in those who initiate therapy later in the course of their infection. Patients should be informed that if toxicity develops, they may require transfusions or drug discontinuation. Patients should be informed of the extreme importance of having their blood counts followed closely while on therapy, especially for patients with advanced symptomatic HIV-1 disease [see Boxed Warning, Warnings and Precautions (5.1)].

Myopathy: Patients should be informed that myopathy and myositis with pathological changes, similar to that produced by HIV-1 disease, have been associated with prolonged use of RETROVIR [see Boxed Warning, Warnings and Precautions (5.2)].

Lactic Acidosis/Hepatomegaly: Patients should be informed that some HIV medicines, including RETROVIR, can cause a rare, but serious condition called lactic acidosis with liver enlargement (hepatomegaly) [see Boxed Warning, Warnings and Precautions (5.3)].

HIV-1/HCV Co-Infection: Patients with HIV-1/HCV co-infection should be informed that hepatic decompensation (some fatal) has occurred in HIV-1/HCV co-infected patients receiving combination antiretroviral therapy for HIV-1 and interferon alfa with or without ribavirin [see Warnings and Precautions (5.4)].

Use With Other Zidovudine-Containing Products: RETROVIR should not be administered with combination products that contain zidovudine as one of their components (e.g., COMBIVIR [lamivudine and zidovudine] Tablets or TRIZIVIR [abacavir sulfate, lamivudine, and zidovudine] Tablets) [see Warnings and Precautions (5.5)].

Redistribution/Accumulation of Body Fat: Patients should be informed that redistribution or accumulation of body fat may occur in patients receiving antiretroviral therapy and that the cause and long-term health effects of these conditions are not known at this time [see Warnings and Precautions (5.7)].

Common Adverse Reactions: Patients should be informed that the most commonly reported adverse reactions in adult patients being treated with RETROVIR were headache, malaise, nausea, anorexia, and vomiting. The most commonly reported adverse reactions in pediatric patients receiving RETROVIR were fever, cough, and digestive disorders. Patients also should be encouraged to contact their physician if they experience muscle weakness, shortness of breath, symptoms of hepatitis or pancreatitis, or any other unexpected adverse events while being treated with RETROVIR [see Adverse Reactions (6)].

Drug Interactions: Patients should be cautioned about the use of other medications, including ganciclovir, interferon alfa, and ribavirin, which may exacerbate the toxicity of RETROVIR [see Drug Interactions (7)].

Pregnancy: Pregnant women considering the use of RETROVIR during pregnancy for prevention of HIV-1 transmission should be informed that transmission may still occur in some cases despite therapy. The long-term consequences of in utero and infant exposure to RETROVIR are unknown, including the possible risk of cancer [see Use in Specific Populations (8.1)].

HIV-1-infected pregnant women should be informed not to breastfeed to avoid postnatal transmission of HIV to a child who may not yet be infected [see Use in Specific Populations (8.3)].

Information About HIV-1 Infection: RETROVIR is not a cure for HIV-1 infection, and patients may continue to experience illnesses associated with HIV-1 infection, including opportunistic infections. Patients should remain under the care of a physician when using RETROVIR.

Patients should be advised to avoid doing things that can spread HIV-1 infection to others.

- **Do not share needles or other injection equipment.**
- **Do not share personal items that can have blood or body fluids on them, like toothbrushes and razor blades.**
- **Do not have any kind of sex without protection.** Always practice safe sex by using a latex or polyurethane condom or other barrier method to lower the chance of sexual contact with semen, vaginal secretions, or blood.
- **Do not breastfeed.** Zidovudine is excreted in human breast milk. Mothers with HIV-1 should not breastfeed because HIV-1 can be passed to the baby in the breast milk.

Patients should be informed to take all HIV medications exactly as prescribed.

RETROVIR, COMBIVIR, EPIVIR, and TRIZIVIR are registered trademarks of ViiV Healthcare.
Manufactured for:
ViiV Healthcare
Research Triangle Park, NC 27709
by:
GlaxoSmithKline
Research Triangle Park, NC 27709
©2013, ViiV Healthcare. All rights reserved.
RTT:8PI

RETROVIR®   ℞
[re'trō-vir]
(zidovudine)
IV Infusion
FOR INTRAVENOUS INFUSION ONLY

WARNING

RETROVIR (ZIDOVUDINE) HAS BEEN ASSOCIATED WITH HEMATOLOGIC TOXICITY, INCLUDING NEUTROPENIA AND SEVERE ANEMIA, PARTICULARLY IN PATIENTS WITH ADVANCED HUMAN IMMUNODEFICIENCY VIRUS (HIV) DISEASE (SEE WARNINGS). PROLONGED USE OF RETROVIR HAS BEEN ASSOCIATED WITH SYMPTOMATIC MYOPATHY.

LACTIC ACIDOSIS AND SEVERE HEPATOMEGALY WITH STEATOSIS, INCLUDING FATAL CASES, HAVE BEEN REPORTED WITH THE USE OF NUCLEOSIDE ANALOGUES ALONE OR IN COMBINATION, INCLUDING RETROVIR AND OTHER ANTIRETROVIRALS (SEE WARNINGS).

DESCRIPTION

RETROVIR is the brand name for zidovudine (formerly called azidothymidine [AZT]), a pyrimidine nucleoside analogue active against HIV. RETROVIR IV Infusion is a sterile solution for intravenous infusion only. Each mL contains 10 mg zidovudine in Water for Injection. Hydrochloric acid and/or sodium hydroxide may have been added to adjust the pH to approximately 5.5. RETROVIR IV Infusion contains no preservatives.

The chemical name of zidovudine is 3'-azido-3'-deoxythymidine; it has the following structural formula:

Zidovudine is a white to beige, odorless, crystalline solid with a molecular weight of 267.24 and a solubility of 20.1 mg/mL in water at 25°C. The molecular formula is $C_{10}H_{13}N_5O_4$.

MICROBIOLOGY
Mechanism of Action:
Zidovudine is a synthetic nucleoside analogue. Intracellularly, zidovudine is phosphorylated to its active 5'-triphosphate metabolite, zidovudine triphosphate (ZDV-TP). The principal mode of action of ZDV-TP is inhibition of reverse transcriptase (RT) via DNA chain termination after incorporation of the nucleotide analogue. ZDV-TP is a weak inhibitor of the cellular DNA polymerases α and γ and has been reported to be incorporated into the DNA of cells in culture.

Antiviral Activity:
Activity of zidovudine against HIV-1 was assessed in a number of cell lines (including monocytes and fresh human peripheral blood lymphocytes). The EC_{50} and EC_{90} values for zidovudine were 0.01 to 0.49 μM (1 μM = 0.27 mcg/mL) and 0.1 to 9 μM, respectively. HIV from therapy-naive subjects with no mutations associated with resistance gave median EC_{50} values of 0.011 μM (range: 0.005 to 0.110 μM) from Virco (n = 93 baseline samples from COLA40263) and 0.02 μM (0.01 to 0.03 μM) from Monogram Biosciences (n = 135 baseline samples from ESS30009). The EC_{50} values of zidovudine against different HIV-1 clades (A-G) ranged from 0.00018 to 0.02 μM, and against HIV-2 isolates from 0.00049 to 0.004 μM. In cell culture drug combination studies, zidovudine demonstrates synergistic activity with the nucleoside reverse transcriptase inhibitors (NRTIs) abacavir, didanosine, lamivudine, and zalcitabine; the nonnucleoside reverse transcriptase inhibitors (NNRTIs) delavirdine and nevirapine; and the protease inhibitors (PIs) indinavir, nelfinavir, ritonavir, and saquinavir; and additive activity with interferon alfa. Ribavirin has been found to inhibit the phosphorylation of zidovudine in cell culture.

Resistance:
Genotypic analyses of the isolates selected in cell culture and recovered from zidovudine-treated subjects showed mutations in the HIV-1 RT gene resulting in 6 amino acid substitutions (M41L, D67N, K70R, L210W, T215Y or F, and K219Q) that confer zidovudine resistance. In general, higher levels of resistance were associated with greater number of mutations. In some subjects harboring zidovudine-resistant virus at baseline, phenotypic sensitivity to zidovudine was restored by 12 weeks of treatment with lamivudine and zidovudine. Combination therapy with lamivudine plus zidovudine delayed the emergence of mutations conferring resistance to zidovudine.

Cross-Resistance:
In a trial of 167 HIV-infected subjects, isolates (n = 2) with multi-drug resistance to didanosine, lamivudine, stavudine, zalcitabine, and zidovudine were recovered from subjects treated for at least 1 year with zidovudine plus didanosine or zidovudine plus zalcitabine. The pattern of resistance-associated mutations with such combination therapies was different (A62V, V75I, F77L, F116Y, Q151M) from the pattern with zidovudine monotherapy, with the Q151M mutation being most commonly associated with multi-drug resistance. The mutation at codon 151 in combination with mutations at 62, 75, 77, and 116 results in a virus with reduced susceptibility to didanosine, lamivudine, stavudine, zalcitabine, and zidovudine. Thymidine analogue mutations (TAMs) are selected by zidovudine and confer cross-resistance to abacavir, didanosine, stavudine, tenofovir, and zalcitabine.

CLINICAL PHARMACOLOGY
Pharmacokinetics:
Adults: The pharmacokinetics of zidovudine have been evaluated in 22 adult HIV-infected subjects in a Phase 1 dose-escalation trial. Following intravenous (IV) dosing, dose-independent kinetics was observed over the range of 1 to 5 mg/kg. The major metabolite of zidovudine is 3'-azido-3'-deoxy-5'-*O*-β-*D*-glucopyranuronosylthymidine (GZDV). GZDV area under the curve (AUC) is about 3-fold greater than the zidovudine AUC. Urinary recovery of zidovudine and GZDV accounts for 18% and 60%, respectively, following IV dosing. A second metabolite, 3'-amino-3'-deoxythymidine (AMT), has been identified in the plasma following single-dose IV administration of zidovudine. The AMT AUC was one-fifth of the zidovudine AUC.

The mean steady-state peak and trough concentrations of zidovudine at 2.5 mg/kg every 4 hours were 1.06 and 0.12 mcg/mL, respectively.

The zidovudine cerebrospinal fluid (CSF)/plasma concentration ratio was determined in 39 subjects receiving chronic therapy with RETROVIR. The median ratio measured in 50 paired samples drawn 1 to 8 hours after the last dose of RETROVIR was 0.6.

Table 1. Zidovudine Pharmacokinetic Parameters Following Intravenous Administration in HIV-Infected Subjects

Parameter	Mean ± SD (except where noted)
Apparent volume of distribution (L/kg)	1.6 ± 0.6 (n = 11)
Plasma protein binding (%)	<38
CSF:plasma ratio[a]	0.6 [0.04 to 2.62] (n = 39)
Systemic clearance (L/hr/kg)	1.6 (0.8 to 2.7) (n =18)
Renal clearance (L/hr/kg)	0.34 ± 0.05 (n = 16)
Elimination half-life (hr)[b]	1.1 (0.5 to 2.9) (n = 19)

[a]Median [range].
[b]Approximate range.

Adults With Impaired Renal Function: Zidovudine clearance was decreased resulting in increased zidovudine and GZDV half-life and AUC in subjects with impaired renal function (n = 14) following a single 200-mg oral dose (Table 2). Plasma concentrations of AMT were not determined. A dose adjustment should not be necessary for patients with creatinine clearance (CrCl) ≥15 mL/min.

Table 2. Zidovudine Pharmacokinetic Parameters in Subjects With Severe Renal Impairment[a]

Parameter	Control Subjects (Normal Renal Function) (n = 6)	Subjects With Renal Impairment (n = 14)
CrCl (mL/min)	120 ± 8	18 ± 2
Zidovudine AUC (ng•hr/mL)	1,400 ± 200	3,100 ± 300
Zidovudine half-life (hr)	1.0 ± 0.2	1.4 ± 0.1

[a]Data are expressed as mean ± standard deviation.

The pharmacokinetics and tolerance of oral zidovudine were evaluated in a multiple-dose trial in subjects undergoing hemodialysis (n = 5) or peritoneal dialysis (n = 6) receiving escalating doses up to 200 mg 5 times daily for 8 weeks. Daily doses of 500 mg or less were well tolerated despite significantly elevated GZDV plasma concentrations. Apparent zidovudine oral clearance was approximately 50% of that reported in subjects with normal renal function. Hemodialysis and peritoneal dialysis appeared to have a negligible effect on the removal of zidovudine, whereas GZDV elimination was enhanced. A dosage adjustment is recommended for patients undergoing hemodialysis or peritoneal dialysis (see DOSAGE AND ADMINISTRATION: Dose Adjustment).

Adults With Impaired Hepatic Function: Data describing the effect of hepatic impairment on the pharmacokinetics of zidovudine are limited. However, because zidovudine is eliminated primarily by hepatic metabolism, it is expected that zidovudine clearance would be decreased and plasma concentrations would be increased following administration of the recommended adult doses to patients with hepatic impairment (see DOSAGE AND ADMINISTRATION: Dose Adjustment).

Pediatrics: Zidovudine pharmacokinetics have been evaluated in HIV-infected pediatric subjects (Table 3).

Patients Aged 3 Months to 12 Years: Overall, zidovudine pharmacokinetics in pediatric subjects older than 3 months are similar to those in adult subjects. Proportional increases in plasma zidovudine concentrations were observed following administration of oral solution from 90 to 240 mg/m² every 6 hours. Oral bioavailability, terminal half-life, and oral clearance were comparable to adult values. As in adult subjects, the major route of elimination was by metabolism to GZDV. After intravenous dosing, about 29% of the dose was excreted in the urine unchanged and about 45% of the dose was excreted as GZDV (see DOSAGE AND ADMINISTRATION: Pediatrics).

Patients Aged Less Than 3 Months: Zidovudine pharmacokinetics have been evaluated in pediatric subjects from birth to 3 months of life. Zidovudine elimination was determined immediately following birth in 8 neonates who were exposed to zidovudine in utero. The half-life was 13.0 ± 5.8 hours. In neonates from birth to 14 days old, bioavailability was greater, total body clearance was slower, and half-life was longer than in pediatric subjects older than 14 days. For dose recommendations for neonates, see DOSAGE AND ADMINISTRATION: Neonatal Dosing.
[See table 3 at top of next page]

Pregnancy: Zidovudine pharmacokinetics have been studied in a Phase 1 trial of 8 women during the last trimester of pregnancy. As pregnancy progressed, there was no evidence of drug accumulation. Zidovudine pharmacokinetics were similar to those of nonpregnant adults. Consistent with passive transmission of the drug across the placenta, zidovudine concentrations in neonatal plasma at birth were essentially equal to those in maternal plasma at delivery. Although data are limited, methadone maintenance ther-

Table 3. Zidovudine Pharmacokinetic Parameters in Pediatric Subjects[a]

Parameter	Birth to 14 Days	Aged 14 Days to 3 Months	Aged 3 Months to 12 Years
Oral bioavailability (%)	89 ± 19 (n = 15)	61 ± 19 (n = 17)	65 ± 24 (n = 18)
CSF:plasma ratio	no data	no data	0.26 ± 0.17[b] (n = 28)
CL (L/h/kg)	0.65 ± 0.29 (n = 18)	1.14 ± 0.24 (n = 16)	1.85 ± 0.47 (n = 20)
Elimination half-life (h)	3.1 ± 1.2 (n = 21)	1.9 ± 0.7 (n = 18)	1.5 ± 0.7 (n = 21)

[a]Data presented as mean ± standard deviation except where noted.
[b]CSF ratio determined at steady-state on constant intravenous infusion.

Table 4. Effect of Coadministered Drugs on Zidovudine AUC[a] Note: ROUTINE DOSE MODIFICATION OF ZIDOVUDINE IS NOT WARRANTED WITH COADMINISTRATION OF THE FOLLOWING DRUGS.

Coadministered Drug and Dose	Zidovudine Oral Dose	n	Zidovudine Concentrations		Concentration of Coadministered Drug
			AUC	Variability	
Atovaquone 750 mg q 12 h with food	200 mg q 8 h	14	↑AUC 31%	Range 23% to 78%[b]	↔
Fluconazole 400 mg daily	200 mg q 8 h	12	↑AUC 74%	95% CI: 54% to 98%	Not Reported
Methadone 30 to 90 mg daily	200 mg q 4 h	9	↑AUC 43%	Range 16% to 64%[b]	↔
Nelfinavir 750 mg q 8 h × 7 to 10 days	single 200 mg	11	↓AUC 35%	Range 28% to 41%	↔
Probenecid 500 mg q 6 h × 2 days	2 mg/kg q 8 h × 3 days	3	↑AUC 106%	Range 100% to 170%[b]	Not Assessed
Rifampin 600 mg daily × 14 days	200 mg q 8 h × 14 days	8	↓AUC 47%	90% CI: 41% to 53%	Not Assessed
Ritonavir 300 mg q 6 h × 4 days	200 mg q 8 h × 4 days	9	↓AUC 25%	95% CI: 15% to 34%	↔
Valproic acid 250 mg or 500 mg q 8 h × 4 days	100 mg q 8 h × 4 days	6	↑AUC 80%	Range 64% to 130%[b]	Not Assessed

↑ = Increase; ↓ = Decrease; ↔ = no significant change; AUC = area under the concentration versus time curve; CI = confidence interval.
[a]This table is not all inclusive.
[b]Estimated range of percent difference.

apy in 5 pregnant women did not appear to alter zidovudine pharmacokinetics. However, in another patient population, a potential for interaction has been identified (see PRECAUTIONS).

Nursing Mothers: The Centers for Disease Control and Prevention recommend that HIV-infected mothers not breastfeed their infants to avoid risking postnatal transmission of HIV. After administration of a single dose of 200 mg zidovudine to 13 HIV-infected women, the mean concentration of zidovudine was similar in human milk and serum (see PRECAUTIONS: Nursing Mothers).

Geriatric Patients: Zidovudine pharmacokinetics have not been studied in subjects over 65 years of age.

Gender: A pharmacokinetic trial in healthy male (n = 12) and female (n = 12) subjects showed no differences in zidovudine exposure (AUC) when a single dose of zidovudine was administered as the 300-mg RETROVIR Tablet.

Drug Interactions:
See Table 4 and PRECAUTIONS: Drug Interactions.

Zidovudine Plus Lamivudine: No clinically significant alterations in lamivudine or zidovudine pharmacokinetics were observed in 12 asymptomatic HIV-infected adult subjects given a single oral dose of zidovudine (200 mg) in combination with multiple oral doses of lamivudine (300 mg every 12 hours).
[See table 4 above]

Ribavirin: In vitro data indicate ribavirin reduces phosphorylation of lamivudine, stavudine, and zidovudine. However, no pharmacokinetic (e.g., plasma concentrations or intracellular triphosphorylated active metabolite concentrations) or pharmacodynamic (e.g., loss of HIV/HCV virologic suppression) interaction was observed when ribavirin and lamivudine (n = 18), stavudine (n = 10), or zidovudine (n = 6) were coadministered as part of a multi-drug regimen to HIV/HCV co-infected subjects (see WARNINGS).

INDICATIONS AND USAGE

RETROVIR IV Infusion in combination with other antiretroviral agents is indicated for the treatment of HIV infection.

Maternal-Fetal HIV Transmission:
RETROVIR is also indicated for the prevention of maternal-fetal HIV transmission as part of a regimen that includes oral RETROVIR beginning between 14 and 34 weeks of gestation, intravenous RETROVIR during labor, and administration of RETROVIR Syrup to the neonate after birth. The efficacy of this regimen for preventing HIV transmission in women who have received RETROVIR for a prolonged period before pregnancy has not been evaluated. The safety of RETROVIR for the mother or fetus during the first trimester of pregnancy has not been assessed (see Description of Clinical Studies).

Description of Clinical Studies:
Therapy with RETROVIR has been shown to prolong survival and decrease the incidence of opportunistic infections in subjects with advanced HIV disease at the initiation of therapy and to delay disease progression in asymptomatic HIV-infected subjects.

RETROVIR in combination with other antiretroviral agents has been shown to be superior to monotherapy in one or more of the following endpoints: delaying death, delaying development of AIDS, increasing CD4+ cell counts, and decreasing plasma HIV-1 RNA. The complete prescribing information for each drug should be consulted before combination therapy that includes RETROVIR is initiated.

Pregnant Women and Their Neonates: The utility of RETROVIR for the prevention of maternal-fetal HIV transmission was demonstrated in a randomized, double-blind, placebo-controlled trial (ACTG 076) conducted in HIV-infected pregnant women with CD4+ cell counts of 200 to 1,818 cells/mm[3] (median in the treated group: 560 cells/mm[3]) who had little or no previous exposure to

RETROVIR. Oral RETROVIR was initiated between 14 and 34 weeks of gestation (median 11 weeks of therapy) followed by intravenous administration of RETROVIR during labor and delivery. Following birth, neonates received oral RETROVIR Syrup for 6 weeks. The trial showed a statistically significant difference in the incidence of HIV infection in the neonates (based on viral culture from peripheral blood) between the group receiving RETROVIR and the group receiving placebo. Of 363 neonates evaluated in the trial, the estimated risk of HIV infection was 7.8% in the group receiving RETROVIR and 24.9% in the placebo group, a relative reduction in transmission risk of 68.7%. RETROVIR was well tolerated by mothers and infants. There was no difference in pregnancy-related adverse events between the treatment groups.

CONTRAINDICATIONS

RETROVIR IV Infusion is contraindicated for patients who have potentially life-threatening allergic reactions to any of the components of the formulation.

WARNINGS

COMBIVIR® (lamivudine and zidovudine) Tablets and TRIZIVIR® (abacavir sulfate, lamivudine, and zidovudine) Tablets are combination product tablets that contain zidovudine as one of their components. RETROVIR should not be administered concomitantly with COMBIVIR or TRIZIVIR.

The incidence of adverse reactions appears to increase with disease progression; patients should be monitored carefully, especially as disease progression occurs.

Bone Marrow Suppression:
RETROVIR should be used with caution in patients who have bone marrow compromise evidenced by granulocyte count <1,000 cells/mm[3] or hemoglobin <9.5 g/dL. In subjects with advanced symptomatic HIV disease, anemia and neutropenia were the most significant adverse events observed. There have been reports of pancytopenia associated with the use of RETROVIR, which was reversible in most instances, after discontinuance of the drug. However, significant anemia, in many cases requiring dose adjustment, discontinuation of RETROVIR, and/or blood transfusions, has occurred during treatment with RETROVIR alone or in combination with other antiretrovirals.

Frequent blood counts are strongly recommended in patients with advanced HIV disease who are treated with RETROVIR. For HIV-infected individuals and patients with asymptomatic or early HIV disease, periodic blood counts are recommended. If anemia or neutropenia develops, dosage adjustments may be necessary (see DOSAGE AND ADMINISTRATION).

Myopathy:
Myopathy and myositis with pathological changes, similar to that produced by HIV disease, have been associated with prolonged use of RETROVIR.

Lactic Acidosis/Severe Hepatomegaly with Steatosis:
Lactic acidosis and severe hepatomegaly with steatosis, including fatal cases, have been reported with the use of nucleoside analogues alone or in combination, including zidovudine and other antiretrovirals. A majority of these cases have been in women. Obesity and prolonged exposure to antiretroviral nucleoside analogues may be risk factors. Particular caution should be exercised when administering RETROVIR to any patient with known risk factors for liver disease; however, cases have also been reported in patients with no known risk factors. Treatment with RETROVIR should be suspended in any patient who develops clinical or laboratory findings suggestive of lactic acidosis or pronounced hepatotoxicity (which may include hepatomegaly and steatosis even in the absence of marked transaminase elevations).

Use With Interferon- and Ribavirin-Based Regimens:
In vitro studies have shown ribavirin can reduce the phosphorylation of pyrimidine nucleoside analogues such as zidovudine. Although no evidence of a pharmacokinetic or pharmacodynamic interaction (e.g., loss of HIV/HCV virologic suppression) was seen when ribavirin was coadministered with zidovudine in HIV/HCV co-infected subjects (see CLINICAL PHARMACOLOGY: Drug Interactions), **hepatic decompensation (some fatal) has occurred in HIV/HCV co-infected subjects receiving combination antiretroviral therapy for HIV and interferon alfa with or without ribavirin.** Patients receiving interferon alfa with or without ribavirin and RETROVIR should be closely monitored for treatment-associated toxicities, especially hepatic decompensation, neutropenia, and anemia. Discontinuation of RETROVIR should be considered as medically appropriate. Dose reduction or discontinuation of interferon alfa, ribavirin, or both should also be considered if worsening clinical toxicities are observed, including hepatic decompensation (e.g., Childs Pugh >6) (see the complete prescribing information for interferon and ribavirin).

PRECAUTIONS

General:
Zidovudine is eliminated from the body primarily by renal excretion following metabolism in the liver (glucuronida-

tion). In patients with severely impaired renal function (CrCl<15 mL/min), dosage reduction is recommended. Although the data are limited, zidovudine concentrations appear to be increased in subjects with severely impaired hepatic function, which may increase the risk of hematologic toxicity (see CLINICAL PHARMACOLOGY: Pharmacokinetics and DOSAGE AND ADMINISTRATION).

Immune Reconstitution Syndrome:

Immune reconstitution syndrome has been reported in patients treated with combination antiretroviral therapy, including RETROVIR. During the initial phase of combination antiretroviral treatment, patients whose immune system responds may develop an inflammatory response to indolent or residual opportunistic infections (such as *Mycobacterium avium* infection, cytomegalovirus, *Pneumocystis-jirovecii* pneumonia [PCP], or tuberculosis), which may necessitate further evaluation and treatment.

Autoimmune disorders (such as Graves' disease, polymyositis, and Guillain-Barré syndrome) have also been reported to occur in the setting of immune reconstitution, however, the time to onset is more variable, and can occur many months after initiation of treatment.

Information for Patients:

RETROVIR is not a cure for HIV-1 infection, and patients may continue to experience illnesses associated with HIV-1 infection, including opportunistic infections. Patients should remain under the care of a physician when using RETROVIR.

Patients should be advised to avoid doing things that can spread HIV-1 infection to others.

• **Do not share needles or other injection equipment.**

• **Do not share personal items that can have blood or body fluids on them, like toothbrushes and razor blades.**

• **Do not have any kind of sex without protection.** Always practice safe sex by using a latex or polyurethane condom or other barrier method to lower the chance of sexual contact with semen, vaginal secretions, or blood.

• **Do not breastfeed.** Zidovudine is excreted in human breast milk. Mothers with HIV-1 should not breastfeed because HIV-1 can be passed to the baby in the breast milk.

The safety and efficacy of RETROVIR in treating women, intravenous drug users, and racial minorities is not significantly different than that observed in white males.

Patients should be informed that the major toxicities of RETROVIR are neutropenia and/or anemia. The frequency and severity of these toxicities are greater in patients with more advanced disease and in those who initiate therapy later in the course of their infection. They should be told that if toxicity develops, they may require transfusions or drug discontinuation. They should be told of the extreme importance of having their blood counts followed closely while on therapy, especially for patients with advanced symptomatic HIV disease. They should be cautioned about the use of other medications, including ganciclovir and interferon alfa, which may exacerbate the toxicity of RETROVIR (see PRECAUTIONS: Drug Interactions). Patients should be informed that other adverse effects of RETROVIR include nausea and vomiting. Patients should also be encouraged to contact their physician if they experience muscle weakness, shortness of breath, symptoms of hepatitis or pancreatitis, or any other unexpected adverse events while being treated with RETROVIR.

Pregnant women considering the use of RETROVIR during pregnancy for prevention of HIV transmission to their infants should be advised that transmission may still occur in some cases despite therapy. The long-term consequences of in utero and neonatal exposure to RETROVIR are unknown, including the possible risk of cancer.

HIV-infected pregnant women should be advised not to breastfeed to avoid postnatal transmission of HIV to a child who may not yet be infected.

Drug Interactions:

See CLINICAL PHARMACOLOGY section (Table 4) for information on zidovudine concentrations when coadministered with other drugs. For patients experiencing pronounced anemia or other severe zidovudine-associated events while receiving chronic administration of zidovudine and some of the drugs (e.g., fluconazole, valproic acid) listed in Table 4, zidovudine dose reduction may be considered.

Antiretroviral Agents: Concomitant use of zidovudine with stavudine should be avoided since an antagonistic relationship has been demonstrated in vitro.

Some nucleoside analogues affecting DNA replication, such as ribavirin, antagonize the in vitro antiviral activity of RETROVIR against HIV; concomitant use of such drugs should be avoided.

Doxorubicin: Concomitant use of zidovudine with doxorubicin should be avoided since an antagonistic relationship has been demonstrated in vitro (see CLINICAL PHARMACOLOGY for additional drug interactions).

Phenytoin: Phenytoin plasma levels have been reported to be low in some patients receiving RETROVIR, while in 1 case a high level was documented. However, in a pharmacokinetic interaction trial in which 12 HIV-positive volunteers received a single 300-mg phenytoin dose alone and during steady-state zidovudine conditions (200 mg every 4 hours), no change in phenytoin kinetics was observed. Although not designed to optimally assess the effect of phenytoin on zidovudine kinetics, a 30% decrease in oral zidovudine clearance was observed with phenytoin.

Overlapping Toxicities: Coadministration of ganciclovir, interferon alfa, and other bone marrow suppressive or cytotoxic agents may increase the hematologic toxicity of zidovudine.

Carcinogenesis, Mutagenesis, Impairment of Fertility:

Zidovudine was administered orally at 3 dosage levels to separate groups of mice and rats (60 females and 60 males in each group). Initial single daily doses were 30, 60, and 120 mg/kg/day in mice and 80, 220, and 600 mg/kg/day in rats. The doses in mice were reduced to 20, 30, and 40 mg/kg/day after day 90 because of treatment-related anemia, whereas in rats only the high dose was reduced to 450 mg/kg/day on day 91, and then to 300 mg/kg/day on day 279.

In mice, 7 late-appearing (after 19 months) vaginal neoplasms (5 nonmetastasizing squamous cell carcinomas, 1 squamous cell papilloma, and 1 squamous polyp) occurred in animals given the highest dose. One late-appearing squamous cell papilloma occurred in the vagina of a middle-dose animal. No vaginal tumors were found at the lowest dose.

In rats, 2 late-appearing (after 20 months), nonmetastasizing vaginal squamous cell carcinomas occurred in animals given the highest dose. No vaginal tumors occurred at the low or middle dose in rats. No other drug-related tumors were observed in either sex of either species.

At doses that produced tumors in mice and rats, the estimated drug exposure (as measured by AUC) was approximately 3 times (mouse) and 24 times (rat) the estimated human exposure at the recommended therapeutic dose of 100 mg every 4 hours.

Two transplacental carcinogenicity studies were conducted in mice. One study administered zidovudine at doses of 20 mg/kg/day or 40 mg/kg/day from gestation day 10 through parturition and lactation with dosing continuing in offspring for 24 months postnatally. The doses of zidovudine employed in this study produced zidovudine exposures approximately 3 times the estimated human exposure at recommended doses. After 24 months, an increase in incidence of vaginal tumors was noted with no increase in tumors in the liver or lung or any other organ in either gender. These findings are consistent with results of the standard oral carcinogenicity study in mice, as described earlier. A second study administered zidovudine at maximum tolerated doses of 12.5 mg/day or 25 mg/day (~1,000 mg/kg nonpregnant body weight or ~450 mg/kg of term body weight) to pregnant mice from days 12 through 18 of gestation. There was an increase in the number of tumors in the lung, liver, and female reproductive tracts in the offspring of mice receiving the higher dose level of zidovudine. It is not known how predictive the results of rodent carcinogenicity studies may be for humans.

Zidovudine was mutagenic in a 5178Y/TK$^{+/-}$ mouse lymphoma assay, positive in an in vitro cell transformation assay, clastogenic in a cytogenetic assay using cultured human lymphocytes, and positive in mouse and rat micronucleus tests after repeated doses. It was negative in a cytogenetic study in rats given a single dose.

Zidovudine, administered to male and female rats at doses up to 7 times the usual adult dose based on body surface area considerations, had no effect on fertility judged by conception rates.

Pregnancy:

Pregnancy Category C. Oral teratology studies in the rat and in the rabbit at doses up to 500 mg/kg/day revealed no evidence of teratogenicity with zidovudine. Zidovudine treatment resulted in embryo/fetal toxicity as evidenced by an increase in the incidence of fetal resorptions in rats given 150 or 450 mg/kg/day and rabbits given 500 mg/kg/day. The doses used in the teratology studies resulted in peak zidovudine plasma concentrations (after one-half of the daily dose) in rats 66 to 226 times, and in rabbits 12 to 87 times, mean steady-state peak human plasma concentrations (after one-sixth of the daily dose) achieved with the recommended daily dose (100 mg every 4 hours). In an in vitro experiment with fertilized mouse oocytes, zidovudine exposure resulted in a dose-dependent reduction in blastocyst formation. In an additional teratology study in rats, a dose of 3,000 mg/kg/day (very near the oral median lethal dose in rats of 3,683 mg/kg) caused marked maternal toxicity and an increase in the incidence of fetal malformations. This dose resulted in peak zidovudine plasma concentrations 350 times peak human plasma concentrations. (Estimated area under the curve [AUC] in rats at this dose level

was 300 times the daily AUC in humans given 600 mg per day.) No evidence of teratogenicity was seen in this experiment at doses of 600 mg/kg/day or less.

Two rodent transplacental carcinogenicity studies were conducted (see Carcinogenesis, Mutagenesis, Impairment of Fertility).

A randomized, double-blind, placebo-controlled trial was conducted in HIV-infected pregnant women to determine the utility of RETROVIR for the prevention of maternal-fetal HIV transmission (see INDICATIONS AND USAGE: Description of Clinical Studies). Congenital abnormalities occurred with similar frequency between neonates born to mothers who received RETROVIR and neonates born to mothers who received placebo. Abnormalities were either problems in embryogenesis (prior to 14 weeks) or were recognized on ultrasound before or immediately after initiation of study drug.

Antiretroviral Pregnancy Registry: To monitor maternal-fetal outcomes of pregnant women exposed to RETROVIR, an Antiretroviral Pregnancy Registry has been established. Physicians are encouraged to register patients by calling 1-800-258-4263.

Nursing Mothers:

The Centers for Disease Control and Prevention recommend that HIV-infected mothers not breastfeed their infants to avoid risking postnatal transmission of HIV.

Zidovudine is excreted in human milk (see CLINICAL PHARMACOLOGY: Pharmacokinetics: Nursing Mothers). Because of both the potential for HIV transmission and the potential for serious adverse reactions in nursing infants, **mothers should be instructed not to breastfeed if they are receiving RETROVIR** (see Pediatric Use and INDICATIONS AND USAGE: Maternal-Fetal HIV Transmission).

Pediatric Use:

RETROVIR has been studied in HIV-infected pediatric subjects over 3 months of age who had HIV-related symptoms or who were asymptomatic with abnormal laboratory values indicating significant HIV-related immunosuppression. RETROVIR has also been studied in neonates perinatally exposed to HIV (see ADVERSE REACTIONS, DOSAGE AND ADMINISTRATION, INDICATIONS AND USAGE: Description of Clinical Studies, and CLINICAL PHARMACOLOGY: Pharmacokinetics).

Geriatric Use:

Clinical studies of RETROVIR did not include sufficient numbers of subjects aged 65 and over to determine whether they respond differently from younger subjects. Other reported clinical experience has not identified differences in responses between the elderly and younger patients. In general, dose selection for an elderly patient should be cautious, reflecting the greater frequency of decreased hepatic, renal, or cardiac function, and of concomitant disease or other drug therapy.

ADVERSE REACTIONS

The adverse events reported during intravenous administration of RETROVIR IV Infusion are similar to those reported with oral administration; neutropenia and anemia were reported most frequently. Long-term intravenous administration beyond 2 to 4 weeks has not been studied in adults and may enhance hematologic adverse events. Local reaction, pain, and slight irritation during intravenous administration occur infrequently.

Adults:

The frequency and severity of adverse events associated with the use of RETROVIR are greater in subjects with more advanced infection at the time of initiation of therapy.

Table 5 summarizes events reported at a statistically significantly greater incidence for subjects receiving RETROVIR orally in a monotherapy trial.

Table 5. Percentage (%) of Subjects with Adverse Events[a] in Asymptomatic HIV Infection (ACTG 019)

Adverse Event	RETROVIR 500 mg/day (n = 453)	Placebo (n = 428)
Body as a whole		
Asthenia	8.6%[b]	5.8%
Headache	62.5%	52.6%
Malaise	53.2%	44.9%
Gastrointestinal		
Anorexia	20.1%	10.5%
Constipation	6.4%[b]	3.5%
Nausea	51.4%	29.9%
Vomiting	17.2%	9.8%

[a] Reported in ≥5% of trial population.
[b] Not statistically significant versus placebo.

In addition to the adverse events listed in Table 5, other adverse events observed in clinical trials were abdominal cramps, abdominal pain, arthralgia, chills, dyspepsia, fatigue, hyperbilirubinemia, insomnia, musculoskeletal pain, myalgia, and neuropathy.

Selected laboratory abnormalities observed during a clinical trial of monotherapy with oral RETROVIR are shown in Table 6.

Table 6. Frequencies of Selected (Grade 3/4) Laboratory Abnormalities in Subjects with Asymptomatic HIV Infection (ACTG 019)

Adverse Event	RETROVIR 500 mg/day (n = 453)	Placebo (n = 428)
Anemia (Hgb<8 g/dL)	1.1%	0.2%
Granulocytopenia (<750 cells/mm³)	1.8%	1.6%
Thrombocytopenia (platelets <50,000/mm³)	0%	0.5%
ALT (>5 × ULN)	3.1%	2.6%
AST (>5 × ULN)	0.9%	1.6%
Alkaline phosphatase (>5 × ULN)	0%	0%

ULN = Upper limit of normal.

Pediatrics:

Trial ACTG300: Selected clinical adverse events and physical findings with a ≥5% frequency during therapy with EPIVIR® (lamivudine) 4 mg/kg twice daily plus RETROVIR 160 mg/m² orally 3 times daily compared with didanosine in therapy-naive (≤56 days of antiretroviral therapy) pediatric subjects are listed in Table 7.

Table 7. Selected Clinical Adverse Events and Physical Findings (≥5% Frequency) in Pediatric Subjects in Trial ACTG300

Adverse Event	EPIVIR plus RETROVIR (n = 236)	Didanosine (n = 235)
Body as a Whole		
Fever	25%	32%
Digestive		
Hepatomegaly	11%	11%
Nausea & vomiting	8%	7%
Diarrhea	8%	6%
Stomatitis	6%	12%
Splenomegaly	5%	8%
Respiratory		
Cough	15%	18%
Abnormal breath sounds/wheezing	7%	9%
Ear, Nose, and Throat		
Signs or symptoms of ears[a]	7%	6%
Nasal discharge or congestion	8%	11%
Other		
Skin rashes	12%	14%
Lymphadenopathy	9%	11%

[a]Includes pain, discharge, erythema, or swelling of an ear.

Selected laboratory abnormalities experienced by therapy-naive (≤56 days of antiretroviral therapy) pediatric subjects are listed in Table 8.

Table 8. Frequencies of Selected (Grade 3/4) Laboratory Abnormalities in Pediatric Subjects in Trial ACTG300

Test (Abnormal Level)	EPIVIR plus RETROVIR	Didanosine
Neutropenia (ANC<400 cells/mm³)	8%	3%
Anemia (Hgb<7.0 g/dL)	4%	2%
Thrombocytopenia (platelets<50,000/mm³)	1%	3%
ALT (>10 × ULN)	1%	3%
AST (>10 × ULN)	2%	4%
Lipase (>2.5 × ULN)	3%	3%
Total amylase (>2.5 × ULN)	3%	3%

ULN = Upper limit of normal.
ANC = Absolute neutrophil count.

Additional adverse events reported in open-label trials in pediatric subjects receiving RETROVIR 180 mg/m² every 6 hours were congestive heart failure, decreased reflexes, ECG abnormality, edema, hematuria, left ventricular dilation, macrocytosis, nervousness/irritability, and weight loss. The clinical adverse events reported among adult recipients of RETROVIR may also occur in pediatric patients.

Use for the Prevention of Maternal-Fetal Transmission of HIV:

In a randomized, double-blind, placebo-controlled trial in HIV-infected women and their neonates conducted to determine the utility of RETROVIR for the prevention of maternal-fetal HIV transmission, RETROVIR Syrup at 2 mg/kg was administered every 6 hours for 6 weeks to neonates beginning within 12 hours following birth. The most commonly reported adverse experiences were anemia (hemoglobin <9.0 g/dL) and neutropenia (<1,000 cells/mm³). Anemia occurred in 22% of the neonates who received RETROVIR and in 12% of the neonates who received placebo. The mean difference in hemoglobin values was less than 1.0 g/dL for neonates receiving RETROVIR compared to neonates receiving placebo. No neonates with anemia required transfusion and all hemoglobin values spontaneously returned to normal within 6 weeks after completion of therapy with RETROVIR. Neutropenia was reported with similar frequency in the group that received RETROVIR (21%) and in the group that received placebo (27%). The long-term consequences of in utero and infant exposure to RETROVIR are unknown.

Observed During Clinical Practice:

In addition to adverse events reported from clinical trials, the following events have been identified during use of RETROVIR in clinical practice. Because they are reported voluntarily from a population of unknown size, estimates of frequency cannot be made. These events have been chosen for inclusion due to either their seriousness, frequency of reporting, potential causal connection to RETROVIR, or a combination of these factors.

Body as a Whole: Back pain, chest pain, flu-like syndrome, generalized pain.

Cardiovascular: Cardiomyopathy, syncope.

Endocrine: Gynecomastia.

Eye: Macular edema.

Gastrointestinal: Constipation, dysphagia, flatulence, oral mucosal pigmentation, mouth ulcer.

General: Sensitization reactions including anaphylaxis and angioedema, vasculitis.

Hemic and Lymphatic: Aplastic anemia, hemolytic anemia, leukopenia, lymphadenopathy, pancytopenia with marrow hypoplasia, pure red cell aplasia.

Hepatobiliary Tract and Pancreas: Hepatitis, hepatomegaly with steatosis, jaundice, lactic acidosis, pancreatitis.

Musculoskeletal: Increased CPK, increased LDH, muscle spasm, myopathy and myositis with pathological changes (similar to that produced by HIV disease), rhabdomyolysis, tremor.

Nervous: Anxiety, confusion, depression, dizziness, loss of mental acuity, mania, paresthesia, seizures, somnolence, vertigo.

Respiratory: Cough, dyspnea, rhinitis, sinusitis.

Skin: Changes in skin and nail pigmentation, pruritus, rash, Stevens-Johnson syndrome, toxic epidermal necrolysis, sweat, urticaria.

Special Senses: Amblyopia, hearing loss, photophobia, taste perversion.

Urogenital: Urinary frequency, urinary hesitancy.

OVERDOSAGE

Acute overdoses of zidovudine have been reported in pediatric patients and adults. These involved exposures up to 50 grams. No specific symptoms or signs have been identified following acute overdosage with zidovudine apart from those listed as adverse events such as fatigue, headache, vomiting, and occasional reports of hematological disturbances. All patients recovered without permanent sequelae. Hemodialysis and peritoneal dialysis appear to have a negligible effect on the removal of zidovudine, while elimination of its primary metabolite, GZDV, is enhanced.

DOSAGE AND ADMINISTRATION

Adults:

The recommended intravenous dose is 1 mg/kg infused over 1 hour. This dose should be administered 5 to 6 times daily (5 to 6 mg/kg daily). The effectiveness of this dose compared with higher dosing regimens in improving the neurologic dysfunction associated with HIV disease is unknown. A small randomized trial found a greater effect of higher doses of RETROVIR on improvement of neurological symptoms in subjects with pre-existing neurological disease.

Patients should receive RETROVIR IV Infusion only until oral therapy can be administered. The intravenous dosing regimen equivalent to the oral administration of 100 mg every 4 hours is approximately 1 mg/kg intravenously every 4 hours.

Maternal-Fetal HIV Transmission:

The recommended dosing regimen for administration to pregnant women (>14 weeks of pregnancy) and their neonates is:

Maternal Dosing: 100 mg orally 5 times per day until the start of labor. During labor and delivery, intravenous RETROVIR should be administered at 2 mg/kg (total body weight) over 1 hour followed by a continuous intravenous infusion of 1 mg/kg/hour (total body weight) until clamping of the umbilical cord.

Neonatal Dosing: Start neonatal dosing within 12 hours after birth and continue through 6 weeks of age. Neonates unable to receive oral dosing may be administered RETROVIR intravenously. See Table 9. (See PRECAUTIONS if hepatic disease or renal insufficiency is present.)

Table 9. Recommended Neonatal Dosages of RETROVIR

Route	Total Daily Dose	Dose and Dosage Regimen
Oral	8 mg/kg/day	2 mg/kg every 6 hours
IV	6 mg/kg/day	1.5 mg/kg infused over 30 minutes, every 6 hours

Monitoring of Patients:

Hematologic toxicities appear to be related to pretreatment bone marrow reserve and to dose and duration of therapy. In patients with poor bone marrow reserve, particularly in patients with advanced symptomatic HIV disease, frequent monitoring of hematologic indices is recommended to detect serious anemia or neutropenia (see WARNINGS). In patients who experience hematologic toxicity, reduction in hemoglobin may occur as early as 2 to 4 weeks, and neutropenia usually occurs after 6 to 8 weeks.

Dose Adjustment:

Anemia: Significant anemia (hemoglobin of <7.5 g/dL or reduction of >25% of baseline) and/or significant neutropenia (granulocyte count of<750 cells/mm³ or reduction of >50% from baseline) may require a dose interruption until evidence of marrow recovery is observed (see WARNINGS). In patients who develop significant anemia, dose interruption does not necessarily eliminate the need for transfusion. If marrow recovery occurs following dose interruption, resumption in dose may be appropriate using adjunctive measures such as epoetin alfa at recommended doses, depending on hematologic indices such as serum erythropoietin level and patient tolerance.

For patients experiencing pronounced anemia while receiving chronic coadministration of zidovudine and some of the drugs (e.g., fluconazole, valproic acid) listed in Table 4, zidovudine dose reduction may be considered.

End-Stage Renal Disease: In patients maintained on hemodialysis or peritoneal dialysis (CrCl <15 mL/min), recommended dosing is 1 mg/kg every 6 to 8 hours (see CLINICAL PHARMACOLOGY: Pharmacokinetics).

Hepatic Impairment: There are insufficient data to recommend dose adjustment of RETROVIR in patients with mild to moderate impaired hepatic function or liver cirrhosis. Since RETROVIR is primarily eliminated by hepatic metabolism, a reduction in the daily dose may be necessary in these patients. Frequent monitoring of hematologic toxicities is advised (see CLINICAL PHARMACOLOGY: Pharmacokinetics and PRECAUTIONS: General).

Method of Preparation:

RETROVIR IV Infusion must be diluted prior to administration. The calculated dose should be removed from the 20-mL vial and added to 5% Dextrose Injection solution to achieve a concentration no greater than 4 mg/mL. Admixture in biologic or colloidal fluids (e.g., blood products, protein solutions, etc.) is not recommended.

After dilution, the solution is physically and chemically stable for 24 hours at room temperature and 48 hours if refrigerated at 2° to 8°C (36° to 46°F). Care should be taken during admixture to prevent inadvertent contamination. As an additional precaution, the diluted solution should be administered within 8 hours if stored at 25°C (77°F) or 24 hours if refrigerated at 2° to 8°C to minimize potential administration of a microbially contaminated solution.

Parenteral drug products should be inspected visually for particulate matter and discoloration prior to administration whenever solution and container permit. Should either be observed, the solution should be discarded and fresh solution prepared.

Administration:

RETROVIR IV Infusion is administered intravenously at a constant rate over 1 hour. Rapid infusion or bolus injection should be avoided. RETROVIR IV Infusion should not be given intramuscularly.

HOW SUPPLIED

RETROVIR IV Infusion, 10 mg zidovudine in each mL. 20-mL Single-Use Vial, Tray of 10 (NDC 49702-213-05). **Store vials at 15° to 25°C (59° to 77°F) and protect from light.**

RETROVIR, COMBIVIR, and TRIZIVIR are registered trademarks of the ViiV Healthcare group of companies.

Manufactured for:
ViiV Healthcare
Research Triangle Park, NC 27709
by:
GlaxoSmithKline
Research Triangle Park, NC 27709

©2013, ViiV Healthcare group of companies. All rights reserved.
October 2013
RTV: 4PI

SELZENTRY ℞
[sell-ZEN-tree]
(maraviroc)
Tablets, for oral use

HIGHLIGHTS OF PRESCRIBING INFORMATION
These highlights do not include all the information needed to use SELZENTRY safely and effectively. See full prescribing information for SELZENTRY.
SELZENTRY (maraviroc) tablets, for oral use
Initial U.S. Approval: 2007

> **WARNING: HEPATOTOXICITY**
> *See full prescribing information for complete boxed warning.*
> - Hepatotoxicity has been reported which may be preceded by severe rash or other features of a systemic allergic reaction (e.g., fever, eosinophilia, or elevated IgE).
> - Immediately evaluate patients with signs or symptoms of hepatitis or allergic reaction. (5.1)

——RECENT MAJOR CHANGES——

Dosage and Administration, Dose Recommendations for Patients With Normal Renal Function (2.1)	03/2014
Warnings and Precautions,Cardiovascular Events (5.3)	03/2014

——INDICATIONS AND USAGE——
SELZENTRY is a CCR5 co-receptor antagonist indicated for combination antiretroviral treatment of adults infected with only CCR5-tropic HIV-1.
- In treatment-naive subjects, more subjects treated with SELZENTRY experienced virologic failure and developed lamivudine resistance compared with efavirenz. (12.4,14.3)
- Tropism testing with a highly sensitive tropism assay is required for the appropriate use of SELZENTRY. (1)

——DOSAGE AND ADMINISTRATION——

When given with potent CYP3A inhibitors (with or without potent CYP3A inducers) including PIs (except tipranavir/ritonavir), delavirdine (2, 7.1)	150 mg twice daily
With NRTIs, tipranavir/ritonavir, nevirapine, raltegravir, and other drugs that are not potent CYP3A inhibitors or CYP3A inducers (2, 7.1)	300 mg twice daily
With potent CYP3A inducers including efavirenz (without a potent CYP3A inhibitor) (2, 7.1)	600 mg twice daily

A more complete list of coadministered drugs is listed in *Dosage and Administration (2)*.
Dose adjustment may be necessary in patients with renal impairment. (2.2)

——DOSAGE FORMS AND STRENGTHS——
Tablets: 150 mg and 300 mg (3)

——CONTRAINDICATIONS——
- SELZENTRY should not be used in patients with severe renal impairment or end-stage renal disease (ESRD) (CrCl <30 mL/min) who are taking potent CYP3A inhibitors or inducers. (4)

——WARNINGS AND PRECAUTIONS——
- Hepatotoxicity accompanied by severe rash or systemic allergic reaction, including potentially life-threatening events, has been reported. Hepatic laboratory parameters including ALT, AST, and bilirubin should be obtained prior to starting SELZENTRY and at other time points during treatment as clinically indicated. If rash or symptoms or signs of hepatitis or allergic reaction develop, hepatic laboratory parameters should be monitored and discontinuation of treatment should be considered. Use caution when administering SELZENTRY to patients with pre-existing liver dysfunction or who are co-infected with viral hepatitis B or C. (5.1)
- Severe and potentially life-threatening skin and hypersensitivity reactions have been reported in patients taking SELZENTRY. This includes cases of Stevens-Johnson syndrome, hypersensitivity reaction, and toxic epidermal necrolysis. Immediately discontinue SELZENTRY and other suspected agents if signs or symptoms of severe skin or hypersensitivity reactions develop and monitor clinical status, including liver aminotransferases, closely. (5.2)
- More cardiovascular events, including myocardial ischemia and/or infarction, were observed in treatment-experienced subjects who received SELZENTRY. Use with caution in patients at increased risk of cardiovascular events. (5.3)
- If patients with severe renal impairment or ESRD receiving SELZENTRY (without concomitant CYP3A inducers or inhibitors) experience postural hypotension, the dose of SELZENTRY should be reduced from 300 mg twice daily to 150 mg twice daily. (5.3)

——ADVERSE REACTIONS——
The most common adverse events in treatment-experienced subjects (>8% incidence) which occurred at a higher frequency compared with placebo are upper respiratory tract infections, cough, pyrexia, rash, and dizziness. (6)
To report SUSPECTED ADVERSE REACTIONS, contact ViiV Healthcare at 1-877-844-8872 or FDA at 1-800-FDA-1088 or www.fda.gov/medwatch

——DRUG INTERACTIONS——
- Coadministration with CYP3A inhibitors, including protease inhibitors (except tipranavir/ritonavir) and delavirdine, will increase the concentration of SELZENTRY. (7.1)
- Coadministration with CYP3A inducers, including efavirenz, may decrease the concentration of SELZENTRY. (7.1)

——USE IN SPECIFIC POPULATIONS——
- SELZENTRY should only be used in pregnant women if the potential benefit justifies the potential risk to the fetus. (8.1)
- There are no data available in pediatric patients; therefore, SELZENTRY should not be used in patients younger than 18 years. (8.4)
See 17 for PATIENT COUNSELING INFORMATION and Medication Guide

Revised: 03/2014

FULL PRESCRIBING INFORMATION

> **WARNING: HEPATOTOXICITY**
> Hepatotoxicity has been reported with use of SELZENTRY®. Severe rash or evidence of a systemic allergic reaction (e.g., fever, eosinophilia, or elevated IgE) prior to the development of hepatotoxicity may occur. Patients with signs or symptoms of hepatitis or allergic reaction following use of SELZENTRY should be evaluated immediately *[see Warnings and Precautions (5.1)]*.

1 INDICATIONS AND USAGE
SELZENTRY, in combination with other antiretroviral agents, is indicated for adult patients infected with only CCR5-tropic HIV-1.
This indication is based on analyses of plasma HIV-1 RNA levels in 2 controlled trials of SELZENTRY in treatment-experienced subjects and one trial in treatment-naive subjects. Both trials in treatment-experienced subjects were conducted in clinically advanced, 3-class antiretroviral-experienced (nucleoside reverse transcriptase inhibitor [NRTI], non-nucleoside reverse transcriptase inhibitor [NNRTI], protease inhibitor [PI], or enfuvirtide) adults with evidence of HIV-1 replication despite ongoing antiretroviral therapy.
The following points should be considered when initiating therapy with SELZENTRY:
- Adult patients infected with only CCR5-tropic HIV-1 should use SELZENTRY.
- Tropism testing must be conducted on a current sample with a highly sensitive tropism assay that has demonstrated the ability to identify patients appropriate for use of SELZENTRY. Outgrowth of pre-existing low-level CXCR4- or dual/mixed-tropic HIV-1 not detected by tropism testing at screening has been associated with virologic failure on SELZENTRY *[see Microbiology (12.4), Clinical Studies (14.3)]*.
- Use of SELZENTRY is not recommended in subjects with dual/mixed- or CXCR4-tropic HIV-1 as efficacy was not demonstrated in a Phase 2 trial of this patient group.
- The safety and efficacy of SELZENTRY have not been established in pediatric patients.
- In treatment-naive subjects, more subjects treated with SELZENTRY experienced virologic failure and developed lamivudine resistance compared with efavirenz *[see Microbiology (12.4), Clinical Studies (14.3)]*.

2 DOSAGE AND ADMINISTRATION
2.1 Dose Recommendations for Patients With Normal Renal Function
The recommended dose of SELZENTRY differs based on concomitant medications due to drug interactions (see Table 1). SELZENTRY can be taken with or without food. SELZENTRY must be given in combination with other antiretroviral medications.
Table 1 gives the recommended dose adjustments *[see Drug Interactions (7.1)]*.

Table 1. Recommended Dosing Regimen

Concomitant Medications	Dose of SELZENTRY
Potent CYP3A inhibitors (with or without a potent CYP3A inducer) including: • protease inhibitors (except tipranavir/ritonavir) • delavirdine • ketoconazole, itraconazole, clarithromycin • other potent CYP3A inhibitors (e.g., nefazodone, telithromycin) • boceprevir, telaprevir	150 mg twice daily
Other concomitant medications, including tipranavir/ritonavir, nevirapine, raltegravir, all NRTIs, and enfuvirtide	300 mg twice daily
Potent CYP3A inducers (without a potent CYP3A inhibitor) including: • efavirenz • rifampin • etravirine • carbamazepine, phenobarbital, and phenytoin	600 mg twice daily

Table 2. Recommended Dosing Regimens Based on Renal Function

Concomitant Medications[a]	Dose of SELZENTRY Based on Renal Function				
	Normal (CrCl >80 mL/min)	Mild (CrCl >50 and ≤80 mL/min)	Moderate (CrCl ≥30 and ≤50 mL/min)	Severe (CrCl <30 mL/min)	End-Stage Renal Disease On Regular Hemodialysis
Potent CYP3A inhibitors (with or without a CYP3A inducer)[a]	150 mg twice daily	150 mg twice daily	150 mg twice daily	NR	NR
Other concomitant medications[a]	300 mg twice daily	300 mg twice daily	300 mg twice daily	300 mg twice daily[b]	300 mg twice daily[b]
Potent CYP3A Inducers (without a potent CYP3A inhibitor)[a]	600 mg twice daily	600 mg twice daily	600 mg twice daily	NR	NR

NR = Not recommended.
[a]See Table 1 for the list of concomitant medications.
[b]The dose of SELZENTRY should be reduced to 150 mg twice daily if there are any symptoms of postural hypotension [see Warnings and Precautions (5.3)].

2.2 Dose Recommendations for Patients With Renal Impairment

Table 2 provides dosing recommendations for patients based on renal function and concomitant medications.
[See table 2 above]

3 DOSAGE FORMS AND STRENGTHS

- 150-mg blue, oval, film-coated tablets debossed with "MVC 150" on one side and plain on the other.
- 300-mg blue, oval, film-coated tablets debossed with "MVC 300" on one side and plain on the other.

4 CONTRAINDICATIONS

SELZENTRY should not be used in patients with severe renal impairment or end-stage renal disease (ESRD) (CrCl <30 mL/min) who are taking potent CYP3A inhibitors or inducers.

5 WARNINGS AND PRECAUTIONS

5.1 Hepatotoxicity

Hepatotoxicity with allergic features including life-threatening events has been reported in clinical trials and postmarketing. Severe rash or evidence of systemic allergic reaction including drug-related rash with fever, eosinophilia, elevated IgE, or other systemic symptoms have been reported in conjunction with hepatotoxicity [see Warnings and Precautions (5.2)]. These events occurred approximately 1 month after starting treatment. Among reported cases of hepatitis, some were observed in the absence of allergic features or with no pre-existing hepatic disease.

Appropriate laboratory testing including ALT, AST, and bilirubin should be conducted prior to initiating therapy with SELZENTRY and at other timepoints during treatment as clinically indicated. Hepatic laboratory parameters should be obtained in any patient who develops rash, or signs or symptoms of hepatitis, or allergic reaction. Discontinuation of SELZENTRY should be considered in any patient with signs or symptoms of hepatitis, or with increased liver transaminases combined with rash or other systemic symptoms.

Caution should be used when administering SELZENTRY to patients with pre-existing liver dysfunction or who are co-infected with viral hepatitis B or C. The safety and efficacy of SELZENTRY have not been specifically studied in patients with significant underlying liver disorders. In trials of treatment-experienced HIV-1-infected subjects, approximately 6% of subjects were co-infected with hepatitis B and approximately 6% were co-infected with hepatitis C. Due to the small number of co-infected subjects studied, no conclusions can be drawn regarding whether they are at an increased risk for hepatic adverse events with administration of SELZENTRY.

5.2 Severe Skin and Hypersensitivity Reactions

Severe, potentially life-threatening skin and hypersensitivity reactions have been reported in patients taking SELZENTRY, in most cases concomitantly with other drugs associated with these reactions. These include cases of Stevens-Johnson syndrome (SJS), toxic epidermal necrolysis (TEN), and drug rash with eosinophilia and systemic symptoms (DRESS) [see Adverse Reactions (6.2)]. The cases were characterized by features including rash, constitutional findings, and sometimes organ dysfunction, including hepatic failure. Discontinue SELZENTRY and other suspected agents immediately if signs or symptoms of severe skin or hypersensitivity reactions develop (including, but not limited to, severe rash or rash accompanied by fever, malaise, muscle or joint aches, blisters, oral lesions, conjunctivitis, facial edema, lip swelling, eosinophilia). Delay in stopping treatment with SELZENTRY or other suspect drugs after the onset of rash may result in a life-threatening reaction. Clinical status, including liver aminotransferases, should be monitored and appropriate therapy initiated.

5.3 Cardiovascular Events

Use with caution in patients at increased risk for cardiovascular events. Eleven subjects (1.3%) who received SELZENTRY had cardiovascular events, including myocardial ischemia and/or infarction, during the Phase 3 trials in treatment-experienced subjects (total exposure 609 patient-years [300 on SELZENTRY once daily + 309 on SELZENTRY twice daily]), while no subjects who received placebo had such events (total exposure 111 patient-years). These subjects generally had cardiac disease or cardiac risk factors prior to use of SELZENTRY, and the relative contribution of SELZENTRY to these events is not known.

In the Phase 2b/3 trial in treatment-naive subjects, 3 subjects (0.8%) who received SELZENTRY had events related to ischemic heart diseases and 5 subjects (1.4%) who received efavirenz had such events (total exposure 506 and 508 patient-years for SELZENTRY and efavirenz, respectively).

When SELZENTRY was administered to healthy volunteers at doses higher than the recommended dose, symptomatic postural hypotension was seen at a greater frequency than in placebo. However, when SELZENTRY was given at the recommended dose in HIV-1-infected subjects in Phase 3 trials, postural hypotension was seen at a rate similar to placebo (approximately 0.5%). Caution should be used when administering SELZENTRY in patients with a history of or risk factors for postural hypotension, cardiovascular comorbidities, or on concomitant medication known to lower blood pressure. Patients with cardiovascular comorbidities could be at increased risk of cardiovascular adverse events triggered by postural hypotension.

Postural Hypotension in Patients With Renal Impairment: An increased risk of postural hypotension may occur in patients with severe renal insufficiency or in those with ESRD due to increased maraviroc exposure in some patients. SELZENTRY should be used in patients with severe renal impairment or ESRD only if they are not receiving a concomitant potent CYP3A inhibitor or inducer. However, the use of SELZENTRY in these patients should only be considered when no alternative treatment options are available. If patients with severe renal impairment or ESRD experience any symptoms of postural hypotension while taking 300 mg twice daily, the dose should be reduced to 150 mg twice daily [see Dosage and Administration (2.2)].

5.4 Immune Reconstitution Syndrome

Immune reconstitution syndrome has been reported in patients treated with combination antiretroviral therapy, including SELZENTRY. During the initial phase of combination antiretroviral treatment, patients whose immune system responds may develop an inflammatory response to indolent or residual opportunistic infections (such as infection with Mycobacterium avium infection, cytomegalovirus, Pneumocystis jirovecii pneumonia [PCP], or tuberculosis, or reactivation of Herpes simplex and Herpes zoster), which may necessitate further evaluation and treatment.

Autoimmune disorders (such as Graves' disease, polymyositis, and Guillain-Barré syndrome) have also been reported to occur in the setting of immune reconstitution; however, the time to onset is more variable, and can occur many months after initiation of treatment.

5.5 Potential Risk of Infection

SELZENTRY antagonizes the CCR5 co-receptor located on some immune cells, and therefore could potentially increase the risk of developing infections. The overall incidence and severity of infection, as well as AIDS-defining category C infections, were comparable in the treatment groups during the Phase 3 treatment-experienced trials of SELZENTRY. While there was a higher rate of certain upper respiratory tract infections reported in the arm receiving SELZENTRY compared with placebo (23% versus 13%), there was a lower rate of pneumonia (2% versus 5%) reported in subjects receiving SELZENTRY. A higher incidence of Herpes virus infections (11 per 100 patient-years) was also reported in the arm receiving SELZENTRY when adjusted for exposure compared with placebo (8 per 100 patient-years).

In the Phase 2b/3 trial in treatment-naive subjects, the incidence of AIDS-defining Category C events when adjusted for exposure was 1.8 for SELZENTRY compared with 2.4 for efavirenz per 100 patient-years of exposure.

Patients should be monitored closely for evidence of infections while receiving SELZENTRY.

5.6 Potential Risk of Malignancy

While no increase in malignancy has been observed with SELZENTRY, due to this drug's mechanism of action it could affect immune surveillance and lead to an increased risk of malignancy.

The exposure-adjusted rate for malignancies per 100 patient-years of exposure in treatment-experienced trials was 4.6 for SELZENTRY compared with 9.3 on placebo. In treatment-naive subjects, the rates were 1.0 and 2.4 per 100 patient-years of exposure for SELZENTRY and efavirenz, respectively.

Long-term follow-up is needed to more fully assess this risk.

6 ADVERSE REACTIONS

The following adverse reactions are discussed in other sections of the labeling:
- Hepatotoxicity [see Boxed Warning, Warnings and Precautions (5.1)]
- Severe Skin and Hypersensitivity Reactions [see Warnings and Precautions (5.2)]
- Cardiovascular events [see Warnings and Precautions (5.3)]

6.1 Clinical Trials Experience

Because clinical trials are conducted under widely varying conditions, adverse reaction rates observed in the clinical trials of a drug cannot be directly compared with rates in the clinical trials of another drug and may not reflect the rates observed in practice.

Trials in Treatment-Experienced Subjects: The safety profile of SELZENTRY is primarily based on 840 HIV-1-infected subjects who received at least 1 dose of SELZENTRY during two Phase 3 trials. A total of 426 of these subjects received the indicated twice-daily dosing regimen.

Assessment of treatment-emergent adverse events is based on the pooled data from 2 trials in subjects with CCR5-tropic HIV-1 (A4001027 and A4001028). The median duration of therapy with SELZENTRY for subjects in these trials was 48 weeks, with the total exposure on SELZENTRY twice daily at 309 patient-years versus 111 patient-years on placebo + optimized background therapy (OBT). The population was 89% male and 84% white, with mean age of 46 years (range: 17 to 75 years). Subjects received dose equivalents of 300 mg maraviroc once or twice daily.

The most common adverse events reported with twice-daily therapy with SELZENTRY with frequency rates higher than placebo, regardless of causality, were upper respiratory tract infections, cough, pyrexia, rash, and dizziness. Additional adverse events that occurred with once-daily dosing at a higher rate than both placebo and twice-daily dosing were diarrhea, edema, influenza, esophageal candidiasis, sleep disorders, rhinitis, parasomnias, and urinary abnormalities. In these 2 trials, the rate of discontinuation due to adverse events was 5% for subjects who received SELZENTRY twice daily + OBT as well as those who received placebo + OBT. Most of the adverse events reported were judged to be mild to moderate in severity. The data described below occurred with twice-daily dosing of SELZENTRY.

The total number of subjects reporting infections were 233 (55%) and 84 (40%) in the group receiving SELZENTRY twice daily and the placebo group, respectively. Correcting for the longer duration of exposure on SELZENTRY compared with placebo, the exposure-adjusted frequency (rate per 100 subject-years) of these events was 133 for both SELZENTRY twice daily and placebo.

Dizziness or postural dizziness occurred in 8% of subjects on either SELZENTRY or placebo, with 2 subjects (0.5%) on SELZENTRY permanently discontinuing therapy (1 due to syncope, 1 due to orthostatic hypotension) versus 1 subject on placebo (0.5%) permanently discontinuing therapy due to dizziness.

Treatment-emergent adverse events, regardless of causality, from A4001027 and A4001028 are summarized in Table 3. Selected events occurring at ≥2% of subjects and at a numerically higher rate in subjects treated with SELZENTRY are included; events that occurred at the same or higher rate on placebo are not displayed.

[See table 3 above]
Laboratory Abnormalities: Table 4 shows the treatment-emergent Grade 3-4 laboratory abnormalities that occurred in >2% of subjects receiving SELZENTRY.
[See table 4 at top of next page]
Trial in Treatment-Naive Subjects: *Treatment-Emergent Adverse Events:* Treatment-emergent adverse events, regardless of causality, from Trial A4001026, a double-blind, comparative, controlled trial in which 721 treatment-naive subjects received SELZENTRY 300 mg twice daily (N = 360) or efavirenz (N = 361) in combination with zidovudine/lamivudine for 96 weeks, are summarized in Table 5. Selected events occurring in ≥2% of subjects and at a numerically higher rate in subjects treated with SELZENTRY are included; events that occurred at the same or higher rate on efavirenz are not displayed.
[See table 5 at top of next page]
Laboratory Abnormalities:
[See table 6 at top of page 2379]
Percentages based on total subjects evaluated for each laboratory parameter. If the same subject in a given treatment group had >1 occurrence of the same abnormality, only the most severe is counted.
Less Common Adverse Events in Clinical Trials: The following adverse events occurred in <2% of subjects treated with SELZENTRY. These events have been included because of their seriousness and either increased frequency on SELZENTRY or are potential risks due to the mechanism of action. Events attributed to the patient's underlying HIV infection are not listed.
Blood and Lymphatic System: Marrow depression and hypoplastic anemia.
Cardiac Disorders: Unstable angina, acute cardiac failure, coronary artery disease, coronary artery occlusion, myocardial infarction, myocardial ischemia.
Hepatobiliary Disorders: Hepatic cirrhosis, hepatic failure, cholestatic jaundice, portal vein thrombosis, hypertransaminasemia, jaundice.
Infections and Infestations: Endocarditis, infective myositis, viral meningitis, pneumonia, treponema infections, septic shock, *Clostridium* difficile colitis, meningitis.
Musculoskeletal and Connective Tissue Disorders: Myositis, osteonecrosis, rhabdomyolysis, blood CK increased.
Neoplasms Benign, Malignant, and Unspecified (Including Cysts and Polyps): Abdominal neoplasm, anal cancer, basal cell carcinoma, Bowen's disease, cholangiocarcinoma, diffuse large B-cell lymphoma, lymphoma, metastases to liver, esophageal carcinoma, nasopharyngeal carcinoma, squamous cell carcinoma, squamous cell carcinoma of skin, tongue neoplasm (malignant stage unspecified), anaplastic large cell lymphomas T- and null-cell types, bile duct neoplasms malignant, endocrine neoplasms malignant and unspecified.
Nervous System Disorders: Cerebrovascular accident, convulsions and epilepsy, tremor (excluding congenital), facial palsy, hemianopia, loss of consciousness, visual field defect.

6.2 Postmarketing Experience
The following events have been identified during postapproval use of SELZENTRY and are not listed above. Because these reactions are reported voluntarily from a population of unknown size, it is not possible to estimate their frequency or establish a causal relationship to exposure to SELZENTRY.
Skin and Subcutaneous Tissue Disorders: Stevens-Johnson syndrome (SJS), drug rash with eosinophilia and systemic symptoms (DRESS), toxic epidermal necrolysis (TEN).

7 DRUG INTERACTIONS
7.1 Effect of Concomitant Drugs on the Pharmacokinetics of Maraviroc
Maraviroc is a substrate of CYP3A and P-glycoprotein (P-gp) and hence its pharmacokinetics are likely to be modulated by inhibitors and inducers of these enzymes/transporters. Therefore, a dose adjustment may be required when maraviroc is coadministered with those drugs *[see Dosage and Administration (2)]*.
Concomitant use of maraviroc and St. John's wort (*Hypericum perforatum*) or products containing St. John's wort is not recommended. Coadministration of maraviroc with St. John's wort is expected to substantially decrease maraviroc concentrations and may result in suboptimal levels of maraviroc and lead to loss of virologic response and possible resistance to maraviroc.
For additional drug interaction information, see *Clinical Pharmacology (12.3)*.

8 USE IN SPECIFIC POPULATIONS
8.1 Pregnancy
Pregnancy Category B.
There are no adequate and well-controlled studies in pregnant women. Because animal reproduction studies are not always predictive of human response, SELZENTRY should be used during pregnancy only if the potential benefit justifies the potential risk to the fetus. To monitor maternal-fetal outcomes of pregnant women exposed to SELZENTRY and other antiretroviral agents, an Antiretroviral Pregnancy Registry has been established. Healthcare providers are encouraged to register patients by calling 1-800-258-4263.
Animal Data: The incidence of fetal variations and malformations was not increased in embryofetal toxicity studies performed with maraviroc in rats at exposures (AUC) approximately 20-fold higher and in rabbits at approximately 5-fold higher than human exposures at the recommended daily dose (up to 1,000 mg/kg/day in rats and 75 mg/kg/day in rabbits). During the pre- and postnatal development studies in the offspring, development of the offspring, including fertility and reproductive performance, was not affected by the maternal administration of maraviroc.

8.3 Nursing Mothers
The Centers for Disease Control and Prevention recommend that HIV-infected mothers not breastfeed their infants to avoid risking postnatal transmission of HIV infection. Studies in lactating rats indicate that maraviroc is extensively excreted in rat milk. It is not known whether maraviroc is excreted in human milk. Because of the potential for both HIV transmission and serious adverse reactions in nursing infants, mothers should be instructed not to breastfeed if they are receiving SELZENTRY.

8.4 Pediatric Use
The pharmacokinetics, safety and efficacy of maraviroc in patients younger than 18 years have not been established.

Table 3. Percentage of Subjects With Selected Treatment-Emergent Adverse Events (All Causality) ≥2% on SELZENTRY (and at a higher rate compared with placebo) Trials A4001027 and A4001028 (Pooled Analysis, 48 Weeks)

Body System/ Adverse Event	SELZENTRY Twice Daily[a]		Placebo	
	N = 426 (%)	Exposure-adjusted rate (per 100 pt-yrs) PYE = 309[b]	N = 209 (%)	Exposure-adjusted rate (per 100 pt-yrs) PYE = 111[b]
Eye Disorders				
Conjunctivitis	2	3	1	3
Ocular infections, inflammations, and associated manifestations	2	3	1	2
Gastrointestinal Disorders				
Constipation	6	9	3	6
General Disorders and Administration Site Conditions				
Pyrexia	13	20	9	17
Pain and discomfort	4	5	3	5
Infections and Infestations				
Upper respiratory tract infection	23	37	13	27
Herpes infection	8	11	4	8
Sinusitis	7	10	3	6
Bronchitis	7	9	5	9
Folliculitis	4	5	2	4
Pneumonia	2	3	5	10
Anogenital warts	2	3	1	3
Influenza	2	3	0.5	1
Otitis media	2	3	0.5	1
Metabolism and Nutrition Disorders				
Appetite disorders	8	11	7	13
Musculoskeletal and Connective Tissue Disorders				
Joint-related signs and symptoms	7	10	3	5
Muscle pains	3	4	0.5	1
Neoplasms Benign, Malignant, and Unspecified				
Skin neoplasms benign	3	4	1	3
Nervous System Disorders				
Dizziness/postural dizziness	9	13	8	17
Paresthesias and dysesthesias	5	7	3	6
Sensory abnormalities	4	6	1	3
Disturbances in consciousness	4	5	3	6
Peripheral neuropathies	4	5	3	6
Psychiatric Disorders				
Disturbances in initiating and maintaining sleep	8	11	5	10
Depressive disorders	4	6	3	5
Anxiety symptoms	4	5	3	7
Renal and Urinary Disorders				
Bladder and urethral symptoms	5	7	1	3
Urinary tract signs and symptoms	3	4	1	3
Respiratory, Thoracic, and Mediastinal Disorders				
Coughing and associated symptoms	14	21	5	10
Upper respiratory tract signs and symptoms	6	9	3	6
Nasal congestion and inflammations	4	6	3	5
Breathing abnormalities	4	5	2	5
Paranasal sinus disorders	3	4	0.5	1
Skin and Subcutaneous Tissue Disorders				
Rash	11	16	5	11
Apocrine and eccrine gland disorders	5	7	4	7.5
Pruritus	4	5	2	4
Lipodystrophies	3	5	0.5	1
Erythemas	2	3	1	2
Vascular Disorders				
Vascular hypertensive disorders	3	4	2	4

[a]300-mg dose equivalent.
[b]PYE = Patient-years of exposure.

Table 4. Maximum Shift in Laboratory Test Values (Without Regard to Baseline) Incidence ≥2% of Grade 3-4 Abnormalities (ACTG Criteria) Trials A4001027 and A4001028 (Pooled Analysis, 48 Weeks)

Laboratory Parameter Preferred Term	Limit	SELZENTRY Twice Daily + OBT (N = 421)[a] %	Placebo + OBT (N = 207)[a] %
Aspartate aminotransferase	>5.0 × ULN	4.8	2.9
Alanine aminotransferase	>5.0 × ULN	2.6	3.4
Total bilirubin	>2.5 × ULN	5.5	5.3
Amylase	>2.0 × ULN	5.7	5.8
Lipase	>2.0 × ULN	4.9	6.3
Absolute neutrophil count	<750/mm^3	4.3	2.4

[a]Percentages based on total subjects evaluated for each laboratory parameter.
ULN=upper limit of normal.

Table 5. Percentage of Subjects With Selected Treatment-Emergent Adverse Events (All Causality) (≥2% on SELZENTRY and at a higher rate compared with efavirenz) Trial A4001026 (96 Weeks)

Body System/ Adverse Event	SELZENTRY 300 mg Twice Daily + Zidovudine/Lamivudine (N = 360) %	Efavirenz 600 mg Once Daily + Zidovudine/Lamivudine (N = 361) %
Blood and Lymphatic System Disorders		
Anemias NEC	8	5
Neutropenias	4	3
Ear and Labyrinth Disorders		
Ear disorders NEC	3	2
Gastrointestinal Disorders		
Flatulence, bloating, and distention	10	7
Gastrointestinal atonic and hypomotility disorders NEC	9	5
Gastrointestinal signs and symptoms NEC	3	2
General Disorders and Administration Site Conditions		
Body temperature perception	3	1
Infections and Infestations		
Bronchitis	13	9
Herpes infection	7	6
Upper respiratory tract infection	32	30
Bacterial infections NEC	6	3
Herpes zoster/varicella	5	4
Lower respiratory tract and lung infections	3	2
Neisseria infections	3	0
Tinea infections	4	3
Viral infections NEC	3	2
Musculoskeletal and Connective Tissue Disorders		
Joint-related signs and symptoms	6	5
Nervous System Disorders		
Memory loss (excluding dementia)	3	1
Paresthesias and dysesthesias	4	3
Renal and Urinary Disorders		
Bladder and urethral symptoms	4	3
Reproductive System and Breast Disorders		
Erection and ejaculation conditions and disorders	3	2
Respiratory, Thoracic, and Mediastinal Disorders		
Upper respiratory tract signs and symptoms	9	5
Skin and Subcutaneous Disorders		
Acnes	3	2
Alopecias	2	1
Lipodystrophies	4	3
Nail and nail bed conditions (excluding infections and infestations)	6	2

Therefore, maraviroc should not be used in this patient population.

8.5   Geriatric Use
There were insufficient numbers of subjects aged 65 and over in the clinical trials to determine whether they respond differently from younger subjects. In general, caution should be exercised when administering SELZENTRY in elderly patients, also reflecting the greater frequency of decreased hepatic and renal function, of concomitant disease and other drug therapy.

8.6   Renal Impairment
Recommended doses of SELZENTRY for patients with impaired renal function (CrCl ≤80 mL/min) are based on the results of a pharmacokinetic trial conducted in healthy subjects with various degrees of renal impairment. The pharmacokinetics of maraviroc in subjects with mild and moderate renal impairment was similar to that in subjects with normal renal function [see Clinical Pharmacology (12.3)]. A limited number of subjects with mild and moderate renal impairment in the Phase 3 clinical trials (n = 131 and n = 12, respectively) received the same dose of SELZENTRY as that administered to subjects with normal renal function. In these subjects there was no apparent difference in the adverse event profile for maraviroc compared with subjects with normal renal function.

If patients with severe renal impairment or ESRD not receiving a concomitant potent CYP3A inhibitor or inducer experience any symptoms of postural hypotension while taking SELZENTRY 300 mg twice daily, the dose should be reduced to 150 mg twice daily. No trials have been performed in subjects with severe renal impairment or ESRD co-treated with potent CYP3A inhibitors or inducers. Hence, no dose of SELZENTRY can be recommended, and SELZENTRY is contraindicated for these patients [see Dosage and Administration (2.2), Contraindications (4), Warnings and Precautions (5.2), Clinical Pharmacology (12.3)].

8.7   Hepatic Impairment
Maraviroc is principally metabolized by the liver; therefore, caution should be exercised when administering this drug to patients with hepatic impairment, because maraviroc concentrations may be increased. Maraviroc concentrations are higher when SELZENTRY 150 mg is administered with a potent CYP3A inhibitor compared with following administration of 300 mg without a CYP3A inhibitor, so patients with moderate hepatic impairment who receive SELZENTRY 150 mg with a potent CYP3A inhibitor should be monitored closely for maraviroc-associated adverse events. Maraviroc has not been studied in subjects with severe hepatic impairment [see Warnings and Precautions (5.1), Clinical Pharmacology (12.3)].

8.8   Gender
Population pharmacokinetic analysis of pooled Phase 1/2a data indicated gender (female: n = 96, 23.2% of the total population) does not affect maraviroc concentrations. Dosage adjustment based on gender is not necessary.

8.9   Race
Population pharmacokinetic analysis of pooled Phase 1/2a data indicated exposure was 26.5% higher in Asians (n = 95) as compared with non-Asians (n = 318). However, a trial designed to evaluate pharmacokinetic differences between Caucasians (n = 12) and Singaporeans (n = 12) showed no difference between these 2 populations. No dose adjustment based on race is needed.

10   OVERDOSAGE
The highest single dose administered in clinical trials was 1,200 mg. The dose-limiting adverse event was postural hypotension, which was observed at 600 mg. While the recommended dose for SELZENTRY in patients receiving a CYP3A inducer without a CYP3A inhibitor is 600 mg twice daily, this dose is appropriate due to enhanced metabolism. Prolongation of the QT interval was seen in dogs and monkeys at plasma concentrations 6 and 12 times, respectively, those expected in humans at the intended exposure of 300 mg equivalents twice daily. However, no significant QT prolongation was seen in the trials in treatment-experienced subjects with HIV using the recommended doses of maraviroc or in a specific pharmacokinetic trial to evaluate the potential of maraviroc to prolong the QT interval [see Clinical Pharmacology (12.3)].

There is no specific antidote for overdose with maraviroc. Treatment of overdose should consist of general supportive measures including keeping the patient in a supine position, careful assessment of patient vital signs, blood pressure, and ECG.

If indicated, elimination of unabsorbed active maraviroc should be achieved by emesis. Administration of activated charcoal may also be used to aid in removal of unabsorbed drug. Hemodialysis had a minimal effect on maraviroc clearance and exposure in a trial in subjects with ESRD [see Clinical Pharmacology (12.3)].

11   DESCRIPTION
SELZENTRY (maraviroc) is a selective, slowly reversible, small molecule antagonist of the interaction between human CCR5 and HIV-1 gp120. Blocking this interaction prevents CCR5-tropic HIV-1 entry into cells.

SELZENTRY is available as film-coated tablets for oral administration containing either 150 or 300 mg of maraviroc and the following inactive ingredients: dibasic calcium phosphate (anhydrous), magnesium stearate, microcrystalline cellulose, and sodium starch glycolate. The film coat (Opadry® II Blue [85G20583]) contains FD&C blue #2 aluminum lake, soya lecithin, polyethylene glycol (macrogol 3350), polyvinyl alcohol, talc, and titanium dioxide.

Maraviroc is chemically described as 4,4-difluoro-N-[(1S)-3-[exo-3-(3-isopropyl-5-methyl-4H-1,2,4-triazol-4-yl)-8-azabicyclo[3.2.1]oct-8-yl]-1-phenylpropyl]cyclohexane-carboxamide.

The molecular formula is $C_{29}H_{41}F_2N_5O$ and the structural formula is:

Maraviroc is a white- to pale-colored powder with a molecular weight of 513.67. It is highly soluble across the physiological pH range (pH 1.0 to 7.5).

12 CLINICAL PHARMACOLOGY

12.1 Mechanism of Action
Maraviroc is an antiviral drug [see Microbiology (12.4)].

12.2 Pharmacodynamics
Exposure-Response Relationship in Treatment-Experienced Subjects: The relationship between maraviroc, modeled plasma trough concentration (C_{min}) (1 to 9 samples per subject taken on up to 7 visits), and virologic response was evaluated in 973 treatment-experienced HIV-1-infected subjects with varied optimized background antiretroviral regimens in Trials A4001027 and A4001028. The C_{min}, baseline viral load, baseline $CD4^+$ cell count, and overall sensitivity score (OSS) were found to be important predictors of virologic success (defined as viral load <400 copies/mL at 24 weeks). Table 7 illustrates the proportions of subjects with virologic success (%) within each C_{min} quartile for 150-mg twice-daily and 300-mg twice-daily groups.

[See table 7 above]

Exposure-Response Relationship in Treatment-Naive Subjects: The relationship between maraviroc, modeled plasma trough concentration (C_{min}) (1 to 12 samples per subject taken on up to 8 visits), and virologic response was evaluated in 294 treatment-naive HIV-1-infected subjects receiving maraviroc 300 mg twice daily in combination with zidovudine/lamivudine in Trial A4001026. Table 8 illustrates the proportion (%) of subjects with virologic success <50 copies/mL at 48 weeks within each C_{min} quartile for the 300-mg twice-daily dose.

Table 8. Treatment-Naive Subjects With Virologic Success by C_{min} Quartile (Q1-Q4)

	300 mg Twice Daily		
	N	Median C_{min}	% Subjects With Virologic Success
Q1	75	23	57.3
Q2	72	39	72.2
Q3	73	56	74.0
Q4	74	81	83.8

Eighteen of 75 (24%) subjects in Q1 had no measurable maraviroc concentration on at least one occasion versus 1 of 73 and 1 of 74 in Q3 and Q4, respectively.

Effects on Electrocardiogram: A placebo-controlled, randomized, crossover trial to evaluate the effect on the QT interval of healthy male and female volunteers was conducted with 3 single oral doses of maraviroc and moxifloxacin. The placebo-adjusted mean maximum (upper 1-sided 95% CI) increases in QTc from baseline after 100, 300, and 900 mg of maraviroc were −2 (0), -1 (1), and 1 (3) msec, respectively, and 13 (15) msec for moxifloxacin 400 mg. No subject in any group had an increase in QTc of ≥60 msec from baseline. No subject experienced an interval exceeding the potentially clinically relevant threshold of 500 msec.

12.3 Pharmacokinetics
[See table 9 above]

Absorption: Peak maraviroc plasma concentrations are attained 0.5 to 4 hours following single oral doses of 1 to 1,200 mg administered to uninfected volunteers. The pharmacokinetics of oral maraviroc are not dose proportional over the dose range.

The absolute bioavailability of a 100-mg dose is 23% and is predicted to be 33% at 300 mg. Maraviroc is a substrate for the efflux transporter P-gp.

Effect of Food on Oral Absorption: Coadministration of a 300-mg tablet with a high-fat breakfast reduced maraviroc C_{max} and AUC by 33% in healthy volunteers. There were no food restrictions in the trials that demonstrated the efficacy and safety of maraviroc [see Clinical Studies (14)]. Therefore, maraviroc can be taken with or without food at the recommended dose [see Dosage and Administration (2)].

Distribution: Maraviroc is bound (approximately 76%) to human plasma proteins, and shows moderate affinity for albumin and alpha-1 acid glycoprotein. The volume of distribution of maraviroc is approximately 194 L.

Metabolism: Trials in humans and in vitro studies using human liver microsomes and expressed enzymes have demonstrated that maraviroc is principally metabolized by the cytochrome P450 system to metabolites that are essentially inactive against HIV-1. In vitro studies indicate that CYP3A is the major enzyme responsible for maraviroc metabolism. In vitro studies also indicate that polymorphic enzymes CYP2C9, CYP2D6, and CYP2C19 do not contribute significantly to the metabolism of maraviroc.

Maraviroc is the major circulating component (~42% drug-related radioactivity) following a single oral dose of 300 mg [^{14}C]-maraviroc. The most significant circulating metabolite in humans is a secondary amine (~22% radioactivity) formed by N-dealkylation. This polar metabolite has no significant pharmacological activity. Other metabolites are products of mono-oxidation and are only minor components of plasma drug-related radioactivity.

Excretion: The terminal half-life of maraviroc following oral dosing to steady state in healthy subjects was 14 to 18 hours. A mass balance/excretion trial was conducted using a single 300-mg dose of ^{14}C-labeled maraviroc. Approximately 20% of the radiolabel was recovered in the urine and 76% was recovered in the feces over 168 hours. Maraviroc was the major component present in urine (mean of 8% dose) and feces (mean of 25% dose). The remainder was excreted as metabolites.

Hepatic Impairment: Maraviroc is primarily metabolized and eliminated by the liver. A trial compared the pharmacokinetics of a single 300-mg dose of SELZENTRY in subjects with mild (Child-Pugh Class A, n = 8), and moderate (Child-Pugh Class B, n = 8) hepatic impairment with pharmacokinetics in healthy subjects (n = 8). The mean C_{max} and AUC were 11% and 25% higher, respectively, for subjects with mild hepatic impairment, and 32% and 46% higher, respectively, for subjects with moderate hepatic impairment compared with subjects with normal hepatic function. These changes do not warrant a dose adjustment. Maraviroc concentrations are higher when SELZENTRY 150 mg is administered with a potent CYP3A inhibitor compared with following administration of 300 mg without a CYP3A inhibitor, so patients with moderate hepatic impairment who receive SELZENTRY 150 mg with a potent CYP3A inhibitor should be monitored closely for maraviroc-associated adverse events. The pharmacokinetics of maraviroc have not been studied in subjects with severe hepatic impairment [see Warnings and Precautions (5.1)].

Renal Impairment: A trial compared the pharmacokinetics of a single 300-mg dose of SELZENTRY in subjects with severe renal impairment (CLcr <30 mL/min, n = 6) and ESRD (n = 6) to healthy volunteers (n = 6). Geometric mean ratios for maraviroc C_{max} and AUC_{inf} were 2.4-fold and 3.2-fold higher, respectively, for subjects with severe renal impairment, and 1.7-fold and 2.0-fold higher, respectively, for subjects with ESRD as compared with subjects with normal renal function in this trial. Hemodialysis had a minimal effect on maraviroc clearance and exposure in subjects with ESRD. Exposures observed in subjects with severe renal impairment and ESRD were within the range observed in previous 300-mg single-dose trials of SELZENTRY in healthy volunteers with normal renal function. However, maraviroc

Table 6. Maximum Shift in Laboratory Test Values (Without Regard to Baseline) Incidence ≥2% of Grade 3-4 Abnormalities (ACTG Criteria) Trial A4001026 (96 Weeks)

Laboratory Parameter Preferred Term	Limit	SELZENTRY 300 mg Twice Daily + Zidovudine/Lamivudine (N = 353)[a] %	Efavirenz 600 mg Once Daily+ Zidovudine/Lamivudine (N = 350)[a] %
Aspartate aminotransferase	>5.0 × ULN	4.0	4.0
Alanine aminotransferase	>5.0 × ULN	3.9	4.0
Creatine kinase		3.9	4.8
Amylase	>2.0 × ULN	4.3	6.0
Absolute neutrophil count	<750/mm^3	5.7	4.9
Hemoglobin	<7.0 g/dL	2.9	2.3

[a]N = Total number of subjects evaluable for laboratory abnormalities.
ULN=upper limit of normal.

Table 7. Treatment-Experienced Subjects With Virologic Success by C_{min} Quartile (Q1-Q4)

	150 mg Twice Daily (With CYP3A Inhibitors)			300 mg Twice Daily (Without CYP3A Inhibitors)		
	N	Median C_{min}	% Subjects With Virologic Success	N	Median C_{min}	% Subjects With Virologic Success
Placebo	160	-	30.6	35	-	28.6
Q1	78	33	52.6	22	13	50.0
Q2	77	87	63.6	22	29	68.2
Q3	78	166	78.2	22	46	63.6
Q4	78	279	74.4	22	97	68.2

Table 9. Mean Maraviroc Pharmacokinetic Parameters

Patient Population	Maraviroc Dose	N	AUC_{12} (ng.h/mL)	C_{max} (ng/mL)	C_{min} (ng/mL)
Healthy volunteers (Phase 1)	300 mg twice daily	64	2,908	888	43.1
Asymptomatic HIV subjects (Phase 2a)	300 mg twice daily	8	2,550	618	33.6
Treatment-experienced HIV subjects (Phase 3)[a]	300 mg twice daily	94	1,513	266	37.2
	150 mg twice daily (+ CYP3A inhibitor)	375	2,463	332	101
Treatment-naive HIV subjects (Phase 2b/3)[a]	300 mg twice daily	344	1,865	287	60

[a]The estimated exposure is lower compared with other trials possibly due to sparse sampling, food effect, compliance, and concomitant medications.

Table 10. Effect of Coadministered Agents on the Pharmacokinetics of Maraviroc

Coadministered Drug and Dose	N	Dose of SELZENTRY	Ratio (90% CI) of Maraviroc Pharmacokinetic Parameters With/Without Coadministered Drug (No Effect = 1.00)		
			C_{min}	AUC_{tau}	C_{max}
CYP3A and/or P-gp Inhibitors					
Ketoconazole 400 mg q.d.	12	100 mg b.i.d.	3.75 (3.01, 4.69)	5.00 (3.98, 6.29)	3.38 (2.38, 4.78)
Ritonavir 100 mg b.i.d.	8	100 mg b.i.d.	4.55 (3.37, 6.13)	2.61 (1.92, 3.56)	1.28 (0.79, 2.09)
Saquinavir (soft gel capsules) /ritonavir 1,000 mg/100 mg b.i.d.	11	100 mg b.i.d.	11.3 (8.96, 14.1)	9.77 (7.87, 12.14)	4.78 (3.41, 6.71)
Lopinavir/ritonavir 400 mg/100 mg b.i.d.	11	300 mg b.i.d.	9.24 (7.98, 10.7)	3.95 (3.43, 4.56)	1.97 (1.66, 2.34)
Atazanavir 400 mg q.d.	12	300 mg b.i.d.	4.19 (3.65, 4.80)	3.57 (3.30, 3.87)	2.09 (1.72, 2.55)
Atazanavir/ritonavir 300 mg/100 mg q.d.	12	300 mg b.i.d.	6.67 (5.78, 7.70)	4.88 (4.40, 5.41)	2.67 (2.32, 3.08)
Darunavir/ritonavir 600 mg/100 mg b.i.d.	12	150 mg b.i.d.	8.00 (6.35, 10.1)	4.05 2.94, 5.59	2.29 (1.46, 3.59)
Boceprevir 800 mg t.i.d.	14	150 mg b.i.d.	2.78 (2.40, 3.23)	3.02 (2.53, 3.59)	3.33 (2.54, 4.36)
Telaprevir 750 mg t.i.d.[b]	13	150 mg b.i.d.	10.17 (8.73, 11.85)	9.49 (7.94, 11.34)	7.81 (5.92, 10.32)
CYP3A and/or P-gp Inducers					
Efavirenz 600 mg q.d.	12	100 mg b.i.d.	0.55 (0.43, 0.72)	0.55 (0.49, 0.62)	0.49 (0.38, 0.63)
Efavirenz 600 mg q.d.	12	200 mg b.i.d. (+ efavirenz): 100 mg b.i.d. (alone)	1.09 (0.89, 1.35)	1.15 (0.98, 1.35)	1.16 (0.87, 1.55)
Rifampicin 600 mg q.d.	12	100 mg b.i.d.	0.22 (0.17, 0.28)	0.37 (0.33, 0.41)	0.34 (0.26, 0.43)
Rifampicin 600 mg q.d.	12	200 mg b.i.d. (+ rifampicin): 100 mg b.i.d. (alone)	0.66 (0.54, 0.82)	1.04 (0.89, 1.22)	0.97 (0.72, 1.29)
Etravirine 200 mg b.i.d.	14	300 mg b.i.d.	0.61 (0.53, 0.71)	0.47 (0.38, 0.58)	0.40 (0.28, 0.57)
Nevirapine[a] 200 mg b.i.d. (+ lamivudine 150 mg b.i.d., tenofovir 300 mg q.d.)	8	300 mg single dose	-	1.01 (0.65, 1.55)	1.54 (0.94, 2.51)
CYP3A and/or P-gp Inhibitors and Inducers					
Lopinavir/ritonavir + efavirenz 400 mg/100 mg b.i.d. + 600 mg q.d.	11	300 mg b.i.d.	6.29 (4.72, 8.39)	2.53 (2.24, 2.87)	1.25 (1.01, 1.55)
Saquinavir (soft gel capsules) /ritonavir + efavirenz 1,000 mg/100 mg b.i.d. + 600 mg q.d.	11	100 mg b.i.d.	8.42 (6.46, 10.97)	5.00 (4.26, 5.87)	2.26 (1.64, 3.11)
Darunavir/ritonavir + etravirine 600 mg/100 mg b.i.d. + 200 mg b.i.d.	10	150 mg b.i.d.	5.27 (4.51, 6.15)	3.10 (2.57, 3.74)	1.77 (1.20, 2.60)
Fosamprenavir/ritonavir 700 mg/100 mg b.i.d.	14	300 mg b.i.d.	4.74 (4.03, 5.57)	2.49 (2.19, 2.82)	1.52 (1.27, 1.82)
Fosamprenavir/ritonavir 1,400 mg/100 mg q.d.	14	300 mg q.d.	1.80 (1.53, 2.13)	2.26 (1.99, 2.58)	1.45 (1.20, 1.74)
Tipranavir/ritonavir 500 mg/200 mg b.i.d.	12	150 mg b.i.d.	1.80 (1.55, 2.09)	1.02 (0.85, 1.23)	0.86 (0.61, 1.21)
Other					
Raltegravir 400 mg b.i.d.	17	300 mg b.i.d.	0.90 (0.85, 0.96)	0.86 (0.80, 0.92)	0.79 (0.67, 0.94)

[a]Compared with historical data.
[b]Conducted under fed conditions. The geometric mean C_{max} of maraviroc is 858 ng/mL when maraviroc is coadministered with telaprevir.

exposures in the subjects with normal renal function in this trial were 50% lower than that observed in previous trials.

Based on the results of this trial, no dose adjustment is recommended for patients with renal impairment receiving

SELZENTRY without a potent CYP3A inhibitor or inducer. However, if patients with severe renal impairment or ESRD experience any symptoms of postural hypotension while taking SELZENTRY 300 mg twice daily, their dose should be reduced to 150 mg twice daily [see Dosage and Administration (2.2), Warnings and Precautions (5.2)].

In addition, the trial compared the pharmacokinetics of multiple-dose SELZENTRY in combination with saquinavir/ritonavir 1,000/100 mg twice daily (a potent CYP3A inhibitor combination) for 7 days in subjects with mild renal impairment (CLcr >50 and ≤80 mL/min, n = 6) and moderate renal impairment (CLcr ≥30 and ≤50 mL/min, n = 6) with healthy volunteers with normal renal function (n = 6). Subjects received 150 mg of SELZENTRY at different dose frequencies (healthy volunteers – every 12 hours; mild renal impairment – every 24 hours; moderate renal impairment – every 48 hours). Compared with healthy volunteers (dosed every 12 hours), geometric mean ratios for maraviroc AUC_{tau}, C_{max}, and C_{min} were 50% higher, 20% higher, and 43% lower, respectively, for subjects with mild renal impairment (dosed every 24 hours). Geometric mean ratios for maraviroc AUC_{tau}, C_{max}, and C_{min} were 16% higher, 29% lower, and 85% lower, respectively, for subjects with moderate renal impairment (dosed every 48 hours) compared with healthy volunteers (dosed every 12 hours). Based on the data from this trial, no adjustment in dose is recommended for patients with mild or moderate renal impairment [see Dosage and Administration (2.2)].

Effect of Concomitant Drugs on the Pharmacokinetics of Maraviroc: Maraviroc is a substrate of CYP3A and P-gp and hence its pharmacokinetics are likely to be modulated by inhibitors and inducers of these enzymes/transporters. The CYP3A/P-gp inhibitors ketoconazole, telaprevir, boceprevir, lopinavir/ritonavir, ritonavir, darunavir/ritonavir, saquinavir/ritonavir, and atazanavir ± ritonavir all increased the C_{max} and AUC of maraviroc (see Table 10). The CYP3A inducers rifampin, etravirine, and efavirenz decreased the C_{max} and AUC of maraviroc (see Table 10). Tipranavir/ritonavir (net CYP3A inhibitor/P-gp inducer) did not affect the steady-state pharmacokinetics of maraviroc (see Table 10). Cotrimoxazole and tenofovir did not affect the pharmacokinetics of maraviroc.
[See table 10 above]

Effect of Maraviroc on the Pharmacokinetics of Concomitant Drugs: Maraviroc is unlikely to inhibit the metabolism of coadministered drugs metabolized by the following cytochrome P enzymes (CYP1A2, CYP2B6, CYP2C8, CYP2C9, CYP2C19, and CYP3A) because maraviroc did not inhibit activity of those enzymes at clinically relevant concentrations in vitro. Maraviroc does not induce CYP1A2 in vitro. In vitro results suggest that maraviroc could inhibit P-gp in the gut. However, maraviroc did not significantly affect the pharmacokinetics of digoxin in vivo, indicating maraviroc may not significantly inhibit or induce P-gp clinically.

Drug interaction trials were performed with maraviroc and other drugs likely to be coadministered or commonly used as probes for pharmacokinetic interactions (see Table 10). Coadministration of fosamprenavir 700 mg/ritonavir 100 mg twice daily and maraviroc 300 mg twice daily decreased the C_{min} and AUC of amprenavir by 36% and 35%, respectively. Coadministration of fosamprenavir 1,400 mg/ritonavir 100 mg once daily and maraviroc 300 mg once daily decreased the C_{min} and AUC by 15% and 30%, respectively. No dosage adjustment is necessary when SELZENTRY is dosed 150 mg twice daily in combination with fosamprenavir/ritonavir dosed once or twice daily. Fosamprenavir should be given with ritonavir when coadministered with SELZENTRY.

Maraviroc had no significant effect on the pharmacokinetics of boceprevir, telaprevir, zidovudine, or lamivudine. Maraviroc decreased the C_{min} and AUC of raltegravir by 27% and 37%, respectively, which is not clinically significant. Maraviroc had no clinically relevant effect on the pharmacokinetics of midazolam, the oral contraceptives ethinylestradiol and levonorgestrel, no effect on the urinary 6β-hydroxycortisol/cortisol ratio, suggesting no induction of CYP3A in vivo. Maraviroc had no effect on the debrisoquine metabolic ratio (MR) at 300 mg twice daily or less in vivo and did not cause inhibition of CYP2D6 in vitro until concentrations >100 μM. However, there was 234% increase in debrisoquine MR on treatment compared with baseline at 600 mg once daily, suggesting potential inhibition of CYP2D6 at higher dose.

12.4   Microbiology

Mechanism of Action: Maraviroc is a member of a therapeutic class called CCR5 co-receptor antagonists. Maraviroc selectively binds to the human chemokine receptor CCR5 present on the cell membrane, preventing the interaction of HIV-1 gp120 and CCR5 necessary for CCR5-tropic HIV-1 to enter cells. CXCR4-tropic and dual-tropic HIV-1 entry is not inhibited by maraviroc.

Antiviral Activity in Cell Culture: Maraviroc inhibits the replication of CCR5-tropic laboratory strains and primary isolates of HIV-1 in models of acute peripheral blood leukocyte infection. The mean EC$_{50}$ value (50% effective concentration) for maraviroc against HIV-1 group M isolates (subtypes A to J and circulating recombinant form AE) and group O isolates ranged from 0.1 to 4.5 nM (0.05 to 2.3 ng/mL) in cell culture.

When used with other antiretroviral agents in cell culture, the combination of maraviroc was not antagonistic with NNRTIs (delavirdine, efavirenz, and nevirapine), NRTIs (abacavir, didanosine, emtricitabine, lamivudine, stavudine, tenofovir, zalcitabine, and zidovudine), or protease inhibitors (amprenavir, atazanavir, darunavir, indinavir, lopinavir, nelfinavir, ritonavir, saquinavir, and tipranavir). Maraviroc was not antagonistic with the HIV fusion inhibitor enfuvirtide. Maraviroc was not active against CXCR4-tropic and dual-tropic viruses (EC$_{50}$ value >10 μM). The antiviral activity of maraviroc against HIV-2 has not been evaluated.

Resistance in Cell Culture: HIV-1 variants with reduced susceptibility to maraviroc have been selected in cell culture, following serial passage of 2 CCR5-tropic viruses (CC1/85 and RU570). The maraviroc-resistant viruses remained CCR5-tropic with no evidence of a change from a CCR5-tropic virus to a CXCR4-using virus. Two amino acid residue substitutions in the V3-loop region of the HIV-1 envelope glycoprotein (gp160), A316T, and I323V (HXB2 numbering), were shown to be necessary for the maraviroc-resistant phenotype in the HIV-1 isolate CC1/85. In the RU570 isolate a 3-amino acid residue deletion in the V3 loop, ΔQAI (HXB2 positions 315 to 317), was associated with maraviroc resistance. The relevance of the specific gp120 mutations observed in maraviroc-resistant isolates selected in cell culture to clinical maraviroc resistance is not known. Maraviroc-resistant viruses were characterized phenotypically by concentration-response curves that did not reach 100% inhibition in phenotypic drug assays, rather than increases in EC$_{50}$ values.

Cross-Resistance in Cell Culture: Maraviroc had antiviral activity against HIV-1 clinical isolates resistant to NNRTIs, NRTIs, PIs, and the fusion inhibitor enfuvirtide in cell culture (EC$_{50}$ values ranged from 0.7 to 8.9 nM (0.36 to 4.57 ng/mL). Maraviroc-resistant viruses that emerged in cell culture remained susceptible to the enfuvirtide and the protease inhibitor saquinavir.

Clinical Resistance: Virologic failure on maraviroc can result from genotypic and phenotypic resistance to maraviroc, through outgrowth of undetected CXCR4-using virus present before maraviroc treatment (see *Tropism* below), through resistance to background therapy drugs (Table 11), or due to low exposure to maraviroc *[see Clinical Pharmacology (12.2)].*

Antiretroviral Treatment-Experienced Subjects (Trials A4001027 and A4001028): Week 48 data from treatment-experienced subjects failing maraviroc-containing regimens with CCR5-tropic virus (n = 58) have identified 22 viruses that had decreased susceptibility to maraviroc characterized in phenotypic drug assays by concentration-response curves that did not reach 100% inhibition. Additionally, CCR5-tropic virus from 2 of these treatment-failure subjects had ≥3-fold shifts in EC$_{50}$ values for maraviroc at the time of failure.

Fifteen of these viruses were sequenced in the gp120 encoding region and multiple amino acid substitutions with unique patterns in the heterogeneous V3 loop region were detected. Changes at either amino acid position 308 or 323 (HXB2 numbering) were seen in the V3 loop in 7 of the subjects with decreased maraviroc susceptibility. Substitutions outside the V3 loop of gp120 may also contribute to reduced susceptibility to maraviroc.

Antiretroviral Treatment-Naive Subjects (Trial A4001026): Treatment-naive subjects receiving SELZENTRY had more virologic failures and more treatment-emergent resistance to the background regimen drugs compared with those receiving efavirenz (Table 11).

Table 11. Development of Resistance to Maraviroc or Efavirenz and Background Drugs in Antiretroviral Treatment-Naive Trial A4001026 for Patients with CCR5-Tropic Virus at Screening Using Enhanced Sensitivity TROFILE® Assay

	Maraviroc	Efavirenz
Total N in dataset (as-treated)	273	241
Total virologic failures (as-treated)	85 (31%)	56 (23%)
Evaluable virologic failures with post baseline genotypic and phenotypic data	73	43
• Lamivudine resistance	39 (53%)	13 (30%)
• Zidovudine resistance	2 (3%)	0
• Efavirenz resistance	--	23 (53%)
• Phenotypic resistance to maraviroc[a]	19 (26 %)	

[a]Includes subjects failing with CXCR4- or dual/mixed-tropism because these viruses are not intrinsically susceptible to maraviroc.

In an as-treated analysis of treatment-naive subjects at 96 weeks, 32 subjects failed a maraviroc-containing regimen with CCR5-tropic virus and had a tropism result at failure; 7 of these subjects had evidence of maraviroc phenotypic resistance defined as concentration-response curves that did not reach 95% inhibition. One additional subject had a ≥3-fold shift in the EC$_{50}$ value for maraviroc at the time of failure. A clonal analysis of the V3 loop amino acid envelope sequences was performed from 6 of the 7 subjects. Changes in V3 loop amino acid sequence differed between each of these different subjects, even for those infected with the same virus clade suggesting that that there are multiple diverse pathways to maraviroc resistance. The subjects who failed with CCR5-tropic virus and without a detectable maraviroc shift in susceptibility were not evaluated for genotypic resistance.

Of the 32 maraviroc virologic failures failing with CCR5-tropic virus, 20 (63%) also had genotypic and/or phenotypic resistance to background drugs in the regimen (lamivudine, zidovudine).

Tropism: In both treatment-experienced and treatment-naive subjects, detection of CXCR4-using virus prior to initiation of therapy has been associated with a reduced virologic response to maraviroc.

Antiretroviral Treatment-Experienced Subjects: In the majority of cases, treatment failure on maraviroc was associated with detection of CXCR4-using virus (i.e., CXCR4- or dual/mixed-tropic) which was not detected by the tropism assay prior to treatment. CXCR4-using virus was detected at failure in approximately 55% of subjects who failed treatment on maraviroc by Week 48, as compared with 9% of subjects who experienced treatment failure in the placebo arm. To investigate the likely origin of the on-treatment CXCR4-using virus, a detailed clonal analysis was conducted on virus from 20 representative subjects (16 subjects from the maraviroc arms and 4 subjects from the placebo arm) in whom CXCR4-using virus was detected at treatment failure. From analysis of amino acid sequence differences and phylogenetic data, it was determined that CXCR4-using virus in these subjects emerged from a low level of pre-existing CXCR4-using virus not detected by the tropism assay (which is population-based) prior to treatment rather than from a coreceptor switch from CCR5-tropic virus to CXCR4-using virus resulting from mutation in the virus.

Detection of CXCR4-using virus prior to initiation of therapy has been associated with a reduced virological response to maraviroc. Furthermore, subjects failing maraviroc twice daily at Week 48 with CXCR4-using virus had a lower median increase in CD4+ cell counts from baseline (+41 cells/mm^3) than those subjects failing with CCR5-tropic virus (+162 cells/mm^3). The median increase in CD4+ cell count in subjects failing in the placebo arm was +7 cells/mm^3.

Antiretroviral Treatment-Naive Subjects: In a 96-week trial of antiretroviral treatment-naive subjects, 14% (12/85) who had CCR5-tropic virus at screening with an enhanced sensitivity tropism assay (TROFILE) and failed therapy on maraviroc had CXCR4-using virus at the time of treatment failure. A detailed clonal analysis was conducted in 2 previously antiretroviral treatment-naive subjects enrolled in a Phase 2a monotherapy trial who had CXCR4-using virus detected after 10 days treatment with maraviroc. Consistent with the detailed clonal analysis conducted in treatment-experienced subjects, the CXCR4-using variants appear to emerge from outgrowth of a pre-existing undetected CXCR4-using virus. Screening with an enhanced sensitivity tropism assay reduced the number of maraviroc virologic failures with CXCR4- or dual/mixed-tropic virus at failure to 12 compared with 24 when screening with the original tropism assay. All but one (11/12; 92%) of the

Table 12. Demographic and Baseline Characteristics of Subjects in Trials A4001027 and A4001028

	SELZENTRY Twice Daily (N = 426)	Placebo (N = 209)
Age (years) Mean (range)	46.3 (21-73)	45.7 (29-72)
Sex		
Male	382 (89.7%)	185 (88.5%)
Female	44 (10.3%)	24 (11.5%)
Race		
White	363 (85.2%)	178 (85.2%)
Black	51 (12.0%)	26 (12.4%)
Other	12 (2.8%)	5 (2.4%)
Region		
U.S.	276 (64.8%)	135 (64.6%)
Non-U.S.	150 (35.2%)	74 (35.4%)
Subjects with previous enfuvirtide use	142 (33.3%)	62 (29.7%)
Subjects with enfuvirtide as part of OBT	182 (42.7%)	91 (43.5%)
Baseline plasma HIV-1 RNA (log$_{10}$ copies/mL) Mean (range)	4.85 (2.96-6.88)	4.86 (3.46-7.07)
Subjects with screening viral load ≥100,000 copies/mL	179 (42.0%)	84 (40.2%)
Baseline CD4+ cell count (cells/mm^3) Median (range)	167 (2-820)	171 (1-675)
Subjects with baseline CD4+ cell count ≤200 cells/mm^3)	250 (58.7%)	118 (56.5%)
Subjects with Overall Susceptibility Score (OSS):[a]		
0	57 (13.4%)	35 (16.7%)
1	136 (31.9%)	44 (21.1%)
2	104 (24.4%)	59 (28.2%)
≥3	125 (29.3%)	66 (31.6%)
Subjects with enfuvirtide resistance mutations	90 (21.2%)	45 (21.5%)
Median number of resistance-associated:[b]		
PI mutations	10	10
NNRTI mutations	1	1
NRTI mutations	6	6

[a]OSS - Sum of active drugs in OBT based on combined information from genotypic and phenotypic testing.
[b]Resistance mutations based on IAS guidelines.[1]

Table 13. Outcomes of Randomized Treatment at Week 48 Trials A4001027 and A4001028

Outcome	SELZENTRY Twice Daily (N = 426)	Placebo (N = 209)	Mean Difference
Mean change from Baseline to Week 48 in HIV-1 RNA ($\log_{10}$ copies/mL)	-1.84	-0.78	-1.05
<400 copies/mL at Week 48	239 (56%)	47 (22%)	34%
<50 copies/mL at Week 48	194 (46%)	35 (17%)	29%
Discontinuations			
Insufficient clinical response	97 (23%)	113 (54%)	
Adverse events	19 (4%)	11 (5%)	
Other	27 (6%)	18 (9%)	
Subjects with treatment-emergent CDC Category C events	22 (5%)	16 (8%)	
Deaths (during trial or within 28 days of last dose)	9 (2%)[a]	1 (0.5%)	

[a]One additional subject died while receiving open-label therapy with SELZENTRY subsequent to discontinuing double-blind placebo due to insufficient response.

Table 14. Demographic and Baseline Characteristics of Subjects in Trial A4001026

	SELZENTRY 300 mg Twice Daily + Zidovudine/Lamivudine (N = 360)	Efavirenz 600 mg Once Daily + Zidovudine/Lamivudine (N = 361)
Age (years)		
Mean	36.7	37.4
Range	20-69	18-77
Female, n%	104 (29)	102 (28)
Race, n%		
White	204 (57)	198 (55)
Black	123 (34)	133 (37)
Asian	6 (2)	5 (1)
Other	27 (8)	25 (7)
Median (range) CD4+ cell count (cells/µL)	241 (5-1,422)	254 (8-1,053)
Median (range) HIV-1 RNA ($\log_{10}$ copies/mL)	4.9 (3-7)	4.9 (3-7)

maraviroc failures failing with CXCR4 or dual/mixed-tropic virus also had genotypic and phenotypic resistance to the background drug lamivudine at failure and 33% (4 /12) developed zidovudine-associated resistance substitutions. Subjects who had CCR5-tropic virus at baseline and failed maraviroc therapy with CXCR4-using virus had a median increase in CD4+ cell counts from baseline of +113 cells/mm[3] while those subjects failing with CCR5-tropic virus had an increase of +135 cells/mm[3]. The median increase in CD4+ cell count in subjects failing in the efavirenz arm was + 95 cells/mm[3].

13 NONCLINICAL TOXICOLOGY

13.1 Carcinogenesis, Mutagenesis, Impairment of Fertility

Carcinogenesis: Long-term oral carcinogenicity studies of maraviroc were carried out in rasH2 transgenic mice (6 months) and in rats for up to 96 weeks (females) and 104 weeks (males). No drug-related increases in tumor incidence were found in mice at 1,500 mg/kg/day and in male and female rats at 900 mg/kg/day. The highest exposures in rats were approximately 11 times those observed in humans at the therapeutic dose of 300 mg twice daily for the treatment of HIV-1 infection.

Mutagenesis: Maraviroc was not genotoxic in the reverse mutation bacterial test (Ames test in Salmonella and E. coli), a chromosome aberration test in human lymphocytes and rat bone marrow micronucleus test.

Impairment of Fertility: Maraviroc did not impair mating or fertility of male or female rats and did not affect sperm of treated male rats at approximately 20-fold higher exposures (AUC) than in humans given the recommended 300-mg twice-daily dose.

14 CLINICAL STUDIES

The clinical efficacy and safety of SELZENTRY are derived from analyses of data from 3 trials in adult subjects infected with CCR5-tropic HIV-1: A4001027 and A4001028 in antiretroviral treatment-experienced adult subjects and A4001026 in treatment-naive subjects. These trials were supported by a 48-week trial in antiretroviral treatment-experienced adult subjects infected with dual/mixed-tropic HIV-1, A4001029.

14.1 Trials in CCR5-Tropic, Treatment-Experienced Subjects

Trials A4001027 and A4001028 were double-blind, randomized, placebo-controlled, multicenter trials in subjects in-

fected with CCR5-tropic HIV-1. Subjects were required to have an HIV-1 RNA greater than 5,000 copies/mL despite at least 6 months of prior therapy with at least 1 agent from 3 of the 4 antiretroviral drug classes (≥1 NRTI, ≥1 NNRTI, ≥2 PIs, and/or enfuvirtide) or documented resistance to at least 1 member of each class. All subjects received an optimized background regimen consisting of 3 to 6 antiretroviral agents (excluding low-dose ritonavir) selected on the basis of the subject's prior treatment history and baseline genotypic and phenotypic viral resistance measurements. In addition to the optimized background regimen, subjects were then randomized in a 2:2:1 ratio to SELZENTRY 300 mg once daily, SELZENTRY 300 mg twice daily, or placebo. Doses were adjusted based on background therapy as described in Dosing and Administration (2), Table 1.

In the pooled analysis for A4001027 and A4001028, the demographics and baseline characteristics of the treatment groups were comparable (Table 12). Of the 1,043 subjects with a CCR5 tropism result at screening, 7.6% had a dual/mixed-tropism result at the baseline visit 4 to 6 weeks later. This illustrates the background change from CCR5- to dual/mixed-tropism result over time in this treatment-experienced population, prior to a change in antiretroviral regimen or administration of a CCR5 co-receptor antagonist.

[See table 12 at top of previous page]

The Week 48 results for the pooled Trials A4001027 and A4001028 are shown in Table 13.

[See table 13 above]

After 48 weeks of therapy, the proportions of subjects with HIV-1 RNA <400 copies/mL receiving SELZENTRY compared with placebo were 56% and 22%, respectively. The mean changes in plasma HIV-1 RNA from baseline to Week 48 were −1.84 $\log_{10}$ copies/mL for subjects receiving SELZENTRY + OBT compared with −0.78 $\log_{10}$ copies/mL for subjects receiving OBT only. The mean increase in CD4+ cell count was higher on SELZENTRY twice daily + OBT (124 cells/mm[3]) than on placebo + OBT (60 cells/mm[3]).

14.2 Trial in Dual/Mixed-Tropic, Treatment-Experienced Subjects

Trial A4001029 was an exploratory, randomized, double-blind, multicenter trial to determine the safety and efficacy of SELZENTRY in subjects infected with dual/mixed coreceptor tropic HIV-1. The inclusion/exclusion criteria were similar to those for Trials A4001027 and A4001028 above

and the subjects were randomized in a 1:1:1 ratio to SELZENTRY once daily, SELZENTRY twice daily, or placebo. No increased risk of infection or HIV disease progression was observed in the subjects who received SELZENTRY. Use of SELZENTRY was not associated with a significant decrease in HIV-1 RNA compared with placebo in these subjects and no adverse effect on CD4+ cell count was noted.

14.3 Trial in Treatment-Naive Subjects

Trial A4001026 is an ongoing, randomized, double-blind, multicenter trial in subjects infected with CCR5-tropic HIV-1 classified by the original TROFILE tropism assay. Subjects were required to have plasma HIV-1 RNA ≥2,000 copies/mL and could not have: 1) previously received any antiretroviral therapy for >14 days, 2) an active or recent opportunistic infection or a suspected primary HIV-1 infection, or 3) phenotypic or genotypic resistance to zidovudine, lamivudine, or efavirenz. Subjects were randomized in a 1:1:1 ratio to SELZENTRY 300 mg once daily, SELZENTRY 300 mg twice daily, or efavirenz 600 mg once daily, each in combination with zidovudine/lamivudine. the efficacy and safety of SELZENTRY are based on the comparison of SELZENTRY twice daily versus efavirenz. In a pre-planned interim analysis at 16 weeks, SELZENTRY 300 mg once daily failed to meet the pre-specified criteria for demonstrating non-inferiority and was discontinued.

The demographic and baseline characteristics of the maraviroc and efavirenz treatment groups were comparable (Table 14). Subjects were stratified by screening HIV-1 RNA levels and by geographic region. The median CD4+ cell counts and mean HIV-1 RNA at baseline were similar for both treatment groups.

[See table 14 above]

The treatment outcomes at 96 weeks for Trial A4001026 are shown in Table 15. Treatment outcomes are based on reanalysis of the screening samples using a more sensitive tropism assay, enhanced sensitivity TROFILE HIV tropism assay, which became available after the Week 48 analysis, approximately 15% of the subjects identified as CCR5-tropic in the original analysis had dual/mixed- or CXCR4-tropic virus. Screening with enhanced sensitivity version of the TROFILE tropism assay reduced the number of maraviroc virologic failures with CXCR4- or dual/mixed-tropic virus at failure to 12 compared with 24 when screening with the original TROFILE HIV tropism assay.

[See table 15 at top of next page]

The median increase from baseline in CD4+ cell counts at Week 96 was 184 cells/mm[3] for the arm receiving SELZENTRY compared with 155 cells/mm[3] for the efavirenz arm.

15 REFERENCES

1. IAS-USA Drug Resistance Mutations Figures. http://www.iasusa.org/pub/topics/2006/issue3/125.pdf

16 HOW SUPPLIED/STORAGE AND HANDLING

SELZENTRY film-coated tablets are available as follows: 150- and 300-mg tablets are blue, biconvex, oval, film-coated tablets debossed with "MVC 150" or "MVC 300" on one side and plain on the other.

Bottle packs 150-mg tablets: 60 tablets (NDC 49702-223-18).

Bottle packs 300-mg tablets: 60 tablets (NDC 49702-224-18).

SELZENTRY film-coated tablets should be stored at 25°C (77°F); excursions permitted between 15°C and 30°C (59°F-86°F) [see USP Controlled Room Temperature].

17 PATIENT COUNSELING INFORMATION

Advise the patient to read the FDA-approved patient labeling (Medication Guide)

Patients should be informed that liver problems including life-threatening cases have been reported with SELZENTRY. Patients should be informed that if they develop signs or symptoms of hepatitis or allergic reaction following use of SELZENTRY (rash, skin or eyes look yellow, dark urine, vomiting, abdominal pain), they should stop SELZENTRY and seek medical evaluation immediately. Patients should understand that laboratory tests for liver enzymes and bilirubin will be ordered prior to starting SELZENTRY, at other times during treatment, and if they develop severe rash or signs and symptoms of hepatitis or an allergic reaction on treatment [see Warnings and Precautions (5.1), (5.2)].

Patients should be informed that SELZENTRY is not a cure for HIV-1 infection and patients may continue to experience illnesses associated with HIV-1 infection, including opportunistic infections.

Patients should remain under the care of a physician when using SELZENTRY.

Patients should be advised to avoid doing things that can spread HIV-1 infection to others.

• **Do not share needles or other injection equipment.**

• **Do not share personal items that can have blood or body fluids on them, like toothbrushes and razor blades.**

- **Do not have any kind of sex without protection.** Always practice safe sex by using a latex or polyurethane condom to lower the chance of sexual contact with semen, vaginal secretions, or blood.
- **Do not breastfeed.** We do not know if SELZENTRY can be passed to your baby in your breast milk and whether it could harm your baby. Also, mothers with HIV-1 should not breastfeed because HIV-1 can be passed to the baby in the breast milk.

Patients should be advised that it is important to take all their anti-HIV medicines as prescribed and at the same time(s) each day. SELZENTRY must always be used in combination with other antiretroviral drugs. Patients should not alter the dose or discontinue therapy without consulting their physician. If a dose is missed, patients should take the next dose of SELZENTRY as soon as possible and then take their next scheduled dose at its regular time. If it is less than 6 hours before their next scheduled dose, they should not take the missed dose and should instead wait and take the next dose at the regular time.

Patients should be advised that when their supply of SELZENTRY starts to run low, they should ask their doctor or pharmacist for a refill.

Caution should be used when administering SELZENTRY in patients with a history of postural hypotension or on concomitant medication known to lower blood pressure. Patients should be advised that if they experience dizziness while taking SELZENTRY, they should avoid driving or operating machinery.

SELZENTRY is a registered trademark of the ViiV Healthcare group of companies.

TROFILE is a registered trademark of Monogram Biosciences, Inc.

Manufactured for:
ViiV Healthcare
Research Triangle Park, NC 27709
by:
Pfizer Manufacturing Deutschland GmbH
Freiburg, Germany
©2014, the ViiV Healthcare group of companies. All rights reserved.
SEL:10PI
PHARMACIST-DETACH HERE AND GIVE MEDICATION GUIDE TO PATIENT

MEDICATION GUIDE
SELZENTRY® (sell-ZEN-tree) Tablets
(maraviroc)

Read the Medication Guide that comes with SELZENTRY before you start taking it and each time you get a refill. There may be new information. This information does not take the place of talking with your healthcare provider about your medical condition or treatment.

What is the most important information I should know about SELZENTRY?

Serious side effects have occurred with SELZENTRY, including liver problems (liver toxicity). An allergic reaction may happen before liver problems occur. Stop taking SELZENTRY and call your healthcare provider right away if you get any of the following symptoms:
- an itchy rash on your body (allergic reaction)
- yellowing of your skin or whites of your eyes (jaundice)
- dark (tea-colored) urine
- vomiting
- upper right stomach area (abdominal) pain

What is SELZENTRY?

SELZENTRY is an anti-HIV medicine called a CCR5 antagonist. HIV-1 (Human Immunodeficiency Virus) is the virus that causes AIDS (Acquired Immune Deficiency Syndrome). SELZENTRY is used with other anti-HIV medicines in adults with CCR5-tropic HIV-1 infection.

Use of SELZENTRY is not recommended in people with dual/mixed or CXCR4-tropic HIV-1.
- SELZENTRY will not cure HIV-1 infection.
- People taking SELZENTRY may still develop infections, including opportunistic infections or other conditions that happen with HIV-1 infection.
- It is very important that you stay under the care of your healthcare provider during treatment with SELZENTRY.
- The long-term effects of SELZENTRY are not known at this time.

SELZENTRY has not been studied in children less than 18 years of age.

General information about SELZENTRY

SELZENTRY does not cure HIV-1 infection and you may continue to experience illnesses associated with HIV-1 infection, including opportunistic infections. You should remain under the care of a doctor when using SELZENTRY.

Avoid doing things that can spread HIV-1 infection.
- **Do not share needles or other injection equipment.**
- **Do not share personal items that can have blood or body fluids on them, like toothbrushes and razor blades.**

Table 15: Trial Outcome (Snapshot) at Week 96 Using Enhanced Sensitivity Assay[a]

Outcome at Week 96[b]	SELZENTRY 300 mg Twice Daily + Zidovudine/Lamivudine N = 311 n (%)	Efavirenz 600 mg Once Daily + Zidovudine/Lamivudine N = 303 n (%)
Virologic Responders: (HIV-1 RNA <400 copies/mL)	199 (64)	195 (64)
Virologic Failure:		
• Non-sustained HIV-1 RNA suppression	39 (13)	22 (7)
• HIV-1 RNA never suppressed	9 (3)	1 (<1)
Virologic Responders: (HIV-1 RNA <50 copies/mL)	183 (59)	190 (63)
Virologic Failure:		
• Non-sustained HIV-1 RNA suppression	43 (14)	25 (8)
• HIV-1 RNA never suppressed	21 (7)	3 (1)
Discontinuations due to:		
• Adverse events	19 (6)	47 (16)
• Death	2 (1)	2 (1)
• Other[c]	43 (14)	36 (12)

[a]The total number of subjects (Ns) in Table 15 represents the subjects who had a CCR5-tropic virus in the reanalysis of screening samples using the more sensitive tropism assay. This reanalysis reclassified approximately 15% of subjects shown in Table 14 as having dual/mixed- or CXCR4-tropic virus. These numbers are different than those presented in Table 14 because the numbers in Table 14 reflect the subjects with CCR5-tropic virus according to the original tropism assay.
[b]Week 48 results: Virologic responders (<400): 228/311 (73%) in SELZENTRY, 219/303 (72%) in efavirenz; Virologic responders (<50): 213/311 (69 %) in SELZENTRY, 207/303 (68%) in efavirenz.
[c]Other reasons for discontinuation include lost to follow-up, withdrawn, protocol violation, and other.

- **Do not have any kind of sex without protection.** Always practice safe sex by using a latex or polyurethane condom to lower the chance of sexual contact with semen, vaginal secretions, or blood.

How does SELZENTRY work?

HIV-1 enters cells in your blood by attaching itself to structures on the surface of the cell called receptors. SELZENTRY blocks a specific receptor called CCR5 that CCR5-tropic HIV-1 uses to enter CD4 or T-cells in your blood. Your healthcare provider will do a blood test to see if you have been infected with CCR5-tropic HIV-1 before prescribing SELZENTRY for you.
- When used with other anti-HIV medicines, SELZENTRY may:
- reduce the amount of HIV-1 in your blood. This is called "viral load".
- increase the number of white blood cells called T (CD4) cells.

SELZENTRY does not work in all people with CCR5-tropic HIV-1 infection.

Who should not take SELZENTRY?

People with severe kidney problems or who are on hemodialysis and are taking certain other medications should not take SELZENTRY. Talk to your healthcare provider before taking this medicine if you have kidney problems.

What should I tell my healthcare provider before taking SELZENTRY?

Before you take SELZENTRY, tell your healthcare provider if you:
- have liver problems including a history of hepatitis B or C.
- have heart problems.
- have kidney problems.
- have low blood pressure or take medicines to lower blood pressure.
- have any other medical condition.
- are pregnant or plan to become pregnant. It is not known if SELZENTRY may harm your unborn baby.
  Antiretroviral Pregnancy Registry. There is a pregnancy registry for women who take antiviral medicines during pregnancy. The purpose of the registry is to collect information about the health of you and your baby. Talk to your healthcare provider about how you can take part in this registry.
- are breastfeeding or plan to breastfeed. **Do not breastfeed.** We do not know if SELZENTRY can be passed to your baby in your breast milk and whether it could harm your baby. Also, mothers with HIV-1 should not breastfeed because HIV-1 can be passed to the baby in the breast milk. Talk with your healthcare provider about the best way to feed your baby.

Tell your healthcare provider about all the medicines you take, including prescription and non-prescription medicines, vitamins, and herbal supplements. Certain other medicines may affect the levels of SELZENTRY in your blood. Your healthcare provider may need to change your dose of SELZENTRY when you take it with certain medicines.

The levels of SELZENTRY in your blood may change and your healthcare provider may need to adjust your dose of SELZENTRY when taking any of the following medications together with SELZENTRY:

- darunavir (PREZISTA®)	- delavirdine (RESCRIPTOR®)
- lopinavir/ritonavir (KALETRA®, NORVIR®)	- ketoconazole (NIZORAL®)
- atazanavir (REYATAZ®)	- itraconazole (SPORANOX®)
- saquinavir (INVIRASE®)	- clarithromycin (BIAXIN®)
- nelfinavir (VIRACEPT®)	- nefazodone
- indinavir (CRIXIVAN®)	- telithromycin (KETEK®)
- fosamprenavir (LEXIVA®)	- efavirenz (SUSTIVA®, ATRIPLA®)
- etravirine (INTELENCE®)	- rifampin (RIFADIN®, RIFATER®)
- carbamazepine (TEGRETOL®)	- phenobarbital
- phenytoin (DILANTIN®)	- boceprevir (VICTRELIS®)
- ritonavir (NORVIR®)	- telaprevir (INCIVEK™)

Do not take products that contain St. John's wort (*Hypericum perforatum*). St. John's wort may lower the levels of SELZENTRY in your blood so that it will not work to treat your CCR5-tropic HIV-1 infection.

Know the medicines you take. Keep a list of your medicines. Show the list to your healthcare provider and pharmacist when you get a new medicine.

How should I take SELZENTRY?

Take SELZENTRY exactly as prescribed by your healthcare provider. SELZENTRY comes in 150-mg and 300-mg tablets. Your healthcare provider will prescribe the dose that is right for you.
- Take SELZENTRY 2 times a day.
- Swallow SELZENTRY tablets whole. Do not chew the tablets.
- Take SELZENTRY tablets with or without food.
- Always take SELZENTRY with other anti-HIV drugs as prescribed by your healthcare provider.

Do not change your dose or stop taking SELZENTRY or your other anti-HIV medicines without first talking with your healthcare provider.
- If you take too much SELZENTRY, call your healthcare provider or the poison control center right away.
- If you forget to take SELZENTRY, take the next dose of SELZENTRY as soon as possible and then take your next scheduled dose at its regular time. If it is less than 6 hours before your next dose, do not take the missed dose. Wait and take the next dose at the regular time. Do not take a double dose to make up for a missed dose.

- It is very important to take all your anti-HIV medicines as prescribed. This can help your medicines work better. It also lowers the chance that your medicines will stop working to fight HIV-1 (drug resistance).
- When your SELZENTRY supply starts to run low, ask your healthcare provider or pharmacist for a refill. This is very important because the amount of virus in your blood may increase and SELZENTRY could stop working if it is stopped for even a short period of time.

What are the possible side effects of SELZENTRY?
There have been serious side effects when SELZENTRY has been given with other anti-HIV drugs including:
- **Liver problems.** See "What is the most important information I should know about SELZENTRY?"
- **Serious skin rash and allergic reactions.** Severe and potentially life-threatening skin reactions and allergic reactions have been reported in some patients taking SELZENTRY. If you develop a rash with any of the following symptoms, stop using SELZENTRY and contact your doctor right away:
  - fever
  - generally ill feeling
  - muscle aches
  - blisters or sores in your mouth
  - blisters or peeling of the skin
  - redness or swelling of the eyes
  - swelling of the mouth or face or lips
  - problems breathing
  - yellowing of the skin or whites of your eyes
  - dark or tea colored urine
  - pain, aching, or tenderness on the right side below the ribs
  - loss of appetite
  - nausea/vomiting
- **Heart problems** including heart attack.
- **Low blood pressure when standing up (postural hypotension).** Low blood pressure when standing up can cause dizziness or fainting. Do not drive a car or operate heavy machinery if you have dizziness while taking SELZENTRY.
- **Changes in your immune system.** A condition called Immune Reconstitution Syndrome can happen when you start taking HIV medicines. Your immune system may get stronger and could begin to fight infections that have been hidden in your body such as pneumonia, herpes virus, or tuberculosis. Tell your healthcare provider if you develop new symptoms after starting your HIV medicines.
- **Possible chance of infection or cancer.** SELZENTRY affects other immune system cells and therefore may possibly increase your chance for getting other infections or cancer.

The most common side effects of SELZENTRY include colds, cough, fever, rash, and dizziness.
Tell your healthcare provider about any side effect that bothers you or does not go away.
These are not all of the side effects with SELZENTRY. For more information, ask your healthcare provider or pharmacist.
Call your doctor for medical advice about side effects. You may report side effects to FDA at 1-800-FDA-1088.

How should I store SELZENTRY?
- Store SELZENTRY tablets at room temperature from 59°F to 86°F (15°C to 30°C).
- Safely throw away medicine that is out of date or that you no longer need.

Keep SELZENTRY and all medicines out of the reach of children.

General information about SELZENTRY
Medicines are sometimes prescribed for conditions that are not mentioned in Medication Guides. Do not use SELZENTRY for a condition for which it was not prescribed. Do not give SELZENTRY to other people, even if they have the same symptoms you have. It may harm them. This Medication Guide summarizes the most important information about SELZENTRY. If you would like more information, talk with your healthcare provider. You can ask your healthcare provider or pharmacist for more information about SELZENTRY that is written for health professionals.
For more information, go to www.selzentry.com.

What are the ingredients in SELZENTRY?
Active ingredient: maraviroc
Inactive ingredients: microcrystalline cellulose, dibasic calcium phosphate (anhydrous), sodium starch glycolate, magnesium stearate
Film-coat: FD&C blue #2 aluminum lake, soya lecithin, polyethylene glycol (macrogol 3350), polyvinyl alcohol, talc, and titanium dioxide
SELZENTRY is a registered trademark of the ViiV Healthcare group of companies.
The brands listed are the trademarks of their respective owners and are not trademarks of the ViiV Healthcare group of companies. The makers of these brands are not affiliated with and do not endorse the ViiV Healthcare group of companies or its products.

This Medication Guide has been approved by the US Food and Drug Administration.
Manufactured for:
ViiV Healthcare
Research Triangle Park, NC 27709
by:
Pfizer Manufacturing Deutschland GmbH
Freiburg, Germany
©2014, the ViiV Healthcare group of companies. All rights reserved.
March 2014
SEL:5MG

TIVICAY ℞
(dolutegravir)
Tablets for Oral Use

HIGHLIGHTS OF PRESCRIBING INFORMATION
These highlights do not include all the information needed to use TIVICAY safely and effectively. See full prescribing information for TIVICAY.
TIVICAY (dolutegravir) tablets for oral use
Initial U.S. Approval: 2013

———————INDICATIONS AND USAGE———————
TIVICAY is a human immunodeficiency virus type 1 (HIV-1) integrase strand transfer inhibitor (INSTI) indicated in combination with other antiretroviral agents for the treatment of HIV-1 infection in adults and children aged 12 years and older and weighing at least 40 kg. (1)
The following should be considered prior to initiating TIVICAY:
- Poor virologic response was observed in subjects treated with TIVICAY 50 mg twice daily with an INSTI-resistance Q148 substitution plus 2 or more additional INSTI-resistance substitutions including L74I/M, E138A/D/K/T, G140A/S, Y143H/R, E157Q, G163E/K/Q/R/S, or G193E/R. (12.4)

———————DOSAGE AND ADMINISTRATION———————
May be taken without regard to meals. (2)

Adult Population	Recommended Dose
Treatment-naïve or treatment-experienced INSTI-naïve	50 mg once daily
Treatment-naïve or treatment-experienced INSTI-naïve when coadministered with the following potent UGT1A/CYP3A inducers: efavirenz, fosamprenavir/ritonavir, tipranavir/ritonavir, or rifampin	50 mg twice daily
INSTI-experienced with certain INSTI-associated resistance substitutions or clinically suspected INSTI resistanceᵃ (12.4)	50 mg twice daily

ᵃ Alternative combinations that do not include metabolic inducers should be considered where possible.

Pediatric Patients: (Treatment-naïve or treatment-experienced, INSTI-naïve, aged 12 years and older, and weighing at least 40 kg). (2.2)
- The recommended dose is TIVICAY 50 mg once daily.
- If efavirenz, fosamprenavir/ritonavir, tipranavir/ritonavir, or rifampin are coadministered, then the dose is TIVICAY 50 mg twice daily.

———————DOSAGE FORMS AND STRENGTHS———————
Tablets: 50 mg (3)

———————CONTRAINDICATIONS———————
Coadministration with dofetilide is contraindicated. (4)

———————WARNINGS AND PRECAUTIONS———————
- Hypersensitivity reactions characterized by rash, constitutional findings, and sometimes organ dysfunction, including liver injury, have been reported. Discontinue TIVICAY and other suspect agents immediately if signs or symptoms of hypersensitivity reactions develop, as a delay in stopping treatment may result in a life-threatening reaction. TIVICAY should not be used in patients who have experienced a previous hypersensitivity reaction to TIVICAY. (5.1)
- Patients with underlying hepatitis B or C may be at increased risk for worsening or development of transaminase elevations with use of TIVICAY. Appropriate laboratory testing prior to initiating therapy and monitoring for

hepatotoxicity during therapy with TIVICAY is recommended in patients with underlying hepatic disease such as hepatitis B or C. (5.2)
- Redistribution/accumulation of body fat and immune reconstitution syndrome have been reported in patients treated with combination antiretroviral therapy. (5.3, 5.4)

———————ADVERSE REACTIONS———————
The most common adverse reactions of moderate to severe intensity and incidence ≥2% (in those receiving TIVICAY in any one adult trial) are insomnia and headache. (6.1)
To report SUSPECTED ADVERSE REACTIONS, contact ViiV Healthcare at 1-877-844-8872 or FDA at 1-800-FDA-1088 or www.fda.gov/medwatch

———————DRUG INTERACTIONS———————
- Drugs that are metabolic inducers may decrease the plasma concentrations of dolutegravir. (7.2, 7.3)
- TIVICAY should be taken 2 hours before or 6 hours after taking cation-containing antacids or laxatives, sucralfate, oral supplements containing iron or calcium, or buffered medications. Alternatively, TIVICAY and supplements containing calcium or iron can be taken together with food. (7.3)

———————USE IN SPECIFIC POPULATIONS———————
- Pregnancy: TIVICAY should be used during pregnancy only if the potential benefit justifies the potential risk. (8.1)
- Nursing mothers: Breastfeeding is not recommended due to the potential for HIV transmission. (8.3)
- Pediatric patients: Safety and efficacy of TIVICAY have not been established in pediatric patients younger than 12 years or weighing less than 40 kg, or in pediatric patients who are INSTI-experienced with documented or clinically suspected resistance to other INSTIs (raltegravir, elvitegravir). (8.4)
See 17 for PATIENT COUNSELING INFORMATION and FDA-approved patient labeling
Revised: 05/2014

FULL PRESCRIBING INFORMATION

1   INDICATIONS AND USAGE
TIVICAY® is indicated in combination with other antiretroviral agents for the treatment of human immunodeficiency virus type 1 (HIV-1) infection in adults and children aged 12 years and older and weighing at least 40 kg.

The following should be considered prior to initiating treatment with TIVICAY:

• Poor virologic response was observed in subjects treated with TIVICAY 50 mg twice daily with an integrase strand transfer inhibitor (INSTI)-resistance Q148 substitution plus 2 or more additional INSTI-resistance substitutions, including L74I/M, E138A/D/K/T, G140A/S, Y143H/R, E157Q, G163E/K/Q/R/S, or G193E/R [see Microbiology (12.4)].

2   DOSAGE AND ADMINISTRATION

TIVICAY tablets may be taken with or without food.

2.1   Adults

Table 1. Dosing Recommendations for TIVICAY in Adult Patients

Population	Recommended Dose
Treatment-naïve or treatment-experienced INSTI-naïve	50 mg once daily
Treatment-naïve or treatment-experienced INSTI-naïve when coadministered with the following potent UGT1A/CYP3A inducers: efavirenz, fosamprenavir/ritonavir, tipranavir/ritonavir, or rifampin	50 mg twice daily
INSTI-experienced with certain INSTI-associated resistance substitutions or clinically suspected INSTI resistanceᵃ [see Microbiology (12.4)]	50 mg twice daily

ᵃ Alternative combinations that do not include metabolic inducers should be considered where possible [see Drug Interactions (7)].

The safety and efficacy of doses above 50 mg twice daily have not been evaluated.

2.2   Pediatric Patients

Treatment-Naïve or Treatment-Experienced INSTI-Naïve: The recommended dose of TIVICAY in pediatric patients aged 12 years and older and weighing at least 40 kg is 50 mg administered orally once daily.

If efavirenz, fosamprenavir/ritonavir, tipranavir/ritonavir, or rifampin are coadministered, the recommended dose of TIVICAY is 50 mg twice daily.

Safety and efficacy of TIVICAY have not been established in pediatric patients younger than 12 years or weighing less than 40 kg, or in pediatric patients who are INSTI-experienced with documented or clinically suspected resistance to other INSTIs (raltegravir, elvitegravir).

3   DOSAGE FORMS AND STRENGTHS

TIVICAY 50-mg tablets are yellow, round, film-coated, biconvex tablets debossed with SV 572 on one side and 50 on the other side. Each tablet contains 50 mg of dolutegravir (as dolutegravir sodium) [see Description (11)].

4   CONTRAINDICATIONS

Coadministration of TIVICAY with dofetilide is contraindicated due to the potential for increased dofetilide plasma concentrations and the risk for serious and/or life-threatening events [see Drug Interactions (7)].

5   WARNINGS AND PRECAUTIONS

5.1   Hypersensitivity Reactions

Hypersensitivity reactions have been reported and were characterized by rash, constitutional findings, and sometimes organ dysfunction, including liver injury. The events were reported in <1% of subjects receiving TIVICAY in Phase 3 clinical trials. Discontinue TIVICAY and other suspect agents immediately if signs or symptoms of hypersensitivity reactions develop (including, but not limited to, severe rash or rash accompanied by fever, general malaise, fatigue, muscle or joint aches, blisters or peeling of the skin, oral blisters or lesions, conjunctivitis, facial edema, hepatitis, eosinophilia, angioedema, difficulty breathing). Clinical status, including liver aminotransferases, should be monitored and appropriate therapy initiated. Delay in stopping treatment with TIVICAY or other suspect agents after the onset of hypersensitivity may result in a life-threatening reaction. TIVICAY should not be used in patients who have experienced a previous hypersensitivity reaction to TIVICAY.

5.2   Effects on Serum Liver Biochemistries in Patients With Hepatitis B or C Co–infection

Patients with underlying hepatitis B or C may be at increased risk for worsening or development of transaminase elevations with use of TIVICAY [see Adverse Reactions (6.1)]. In some cases the elevations in transaminases were consistent with immune reconstitution syndrome or hepatitis B reactivation particularly in the setting where anti-hepatitis therapy was withdrawn. Appropriate laboratory testing prior to initiating therapy and monitoring for hepatotoxicity during therapy with TIVICAY are recommended in patients with underlying hepatic disease such as hepatitis B or C.

5.3   Fat Redistribution

Redistribution/accumulation of body fat, including central obesity, dorsocervical fat enlargement (buffalo hump), peripheral wasting, facial wasting, breast enlargement, and "cushingoid appearance" have been observed in patients receiving antiretroviral therapy. The mechanism and long-term consequences of these events are currently unknown. A causal relationship has not been established.

5.4   Immune Reconstitution Syndrome

Immune reconstitution syndrome has been reported in patients treated with combination antiretroviral therapy, including TIVICAY. During the initial phase of combination antiretroviral treatment, patients whose immune systems respond may develop an inflammatory response to indolent or residual opportunistic infections (such as Mycobacterium avium infection, cytomegalovirus, Pneumocystis jirovecii pneumonia [PCP], or tuberculosis), which may necessitate further evaluation and treatment.

Autoimmune disorders (such as Graves' disease, polymyositis, and Guillain-Barré syndrome) have also been reported to occur in the setting of immune reconstitution; however, the time to onset is more variable and can occur many months after initiation of treatment.

6   ADVERSE REACTIONS

The following adverse drug reactions (adverse events assessed as causally related by the investigator or ADRs) are discussed in other sections of the labeling:

• Hypersensitivity reactions [see Warnings and Precautions (5.1)].
• Effects on serum liver biochemistries in patients with hepatitis B or C co-infection [see Warnings and Precautions (5.2)].
• Fat Redistribution [see Warnings and Precautions (5.3)].
• Immune Reconstitution Syndrome [see Warnings and Precautions (5.4)].

Because clinical trials are conducted under widely varying conditions, adverse reaction rates observed in the clinical trials of a drug cannot be directly compared with rates in the clinical trials of another drug and may not reflect the rates observed in practice.

6.1   Clinical Trials Experience in Adult Subjects

Treatment–Emergent Adverse Drug Reactions (ADRs): Treatment-Naïve Subjects: The safety assessment of TIVICAY in HIV-1–infected treatment-naïve subjects is based on the analyses of 48-week data from 2 ongoing, international, multicenter, double-blind trials, SPRING-2 (ING113086) and SINGLE (ING114467).

In SPRING-2, 822 subjects were randomized and received at least 1 dose of either TIVICAY 50 mg once daily or raltegravir 400 mg twice daily, both in combination with fixed-dose dual nucleoside reverse transcriptase inhibitor (NRTI) treatment (either abacavir sulfate and lamivudine [EPZICOM®] or emtricitabine/tenofovir [TRUVADA®]). There were 808 subjects included in the efficacy and safety analyses. The rate of adverse events leading to discontinuation was 2% in both treatment arms.

Table 2. Treatment-Emergent Adverse Drug Reactions of at Least Moderate Intensity (Grades 2 to 4) and ≥2% Frequency in Treatment-Naïve Subjects in SPRING-2 and SINGLE Trials (Week 48 Analysis)

| System Organ Class/ Preferred Term | SPRING-2 | | SINGLE | |
	TIVICAY 50 mg Once Daily + 2 NRTIs (N = 403)	Raltegravir 400 mg Twice Daily + 2 NRTIs (N = 405)	TIVICAY 50 mg + EPZICOM Once Daily (N = 414)	ATRIPLA Once Daily (N = 419)
Psychiatric				
Insomnia	<1%	<1%	3%	2%
Abnormal dreams	<1%	<1%	<1%	2%
Nervous System				
Dizziness	<1%	<1%	<1%	5%
Headache	<1%	<1%	2%	2%
Gastrointestinal				
Nausea	1%	1%	<1%	3%
Diarrhea	<1%	<1%	<1%	2%
Skin and Subcutaneous Tissue				
Rashᵃ	0	<1%	<1%	6%
Ear and Labyrinth				
Vertigo	0	<1%		2%

ᵃIncludes pooled terms: rash, rash generalized, rash macular, rash maculo-papular, rash pruritic, and drug eruption.

In SINGLE, 833 subjects were randomized and received at least 1 dose of either TIVICAY 50 mg with fixed-dose abacavir sulfate and lamivudine (EPZICOM) once daily or fixed-dose efavirenz/emtricitabine/tenofovir (ATRIPLA®) once daily. The rates of adverse events leading to discontinuation were 2% in subjects receiving TIVICAY 50 mg once daily + EPZICOM and 10% in subjects receiving ATRIPLA once daily.

Treatment-emergent ADRs of moderate to severe intensity observed in ≥2% of subjects in either treatment arm are provided in Table 2. Side-by-side tabulation is to simplify presentation; direct comparisons across trials should not be made due to differing trial designs.

[See table 2 above]

In addition, Grade 1 insomnia was reported by 1% and <1% of subjects receiving TIVICAY and raltegravir, respectively, in SPRING-2; whereas in SINGLE the rates were 7% and 3% for TIVICAY and ATRIPLA, respectively. These events were not treatment limiting.

Treatment-Experienced, Integrase Strand Transfer Inhibitor-Naïve Subjects: In an international, multicenter, double-blind trial (ING111762, SAILING), 719 HIV-1–infected, antiretroviral treatment-experienced adults were randomized and received either TIVICAY 50 mg once daily or raltegravir 400 mg twice daily with investigator-selected background regimen consisting of up to 2 agents, including at least one fully active agent. At 24 weeks, the rates of adverse events leading to discontinuation were 2% in subjects receiving TIVICAY 50 mg once daily + background regimen and 4% in subjects receiving raltegravir 400 mg twice daily + background regimen.

The only treatment-emergent ADR of moderate to severe intensity with ≥2% frequency in either treatment group was diarrhea, 1% (5/354) in subjects receiving TIVICAY 50 mg once daily + background regimen and 2% (6/361) in subjects receiving raltegravir 400 mg twice daily + background regimen.

Treatment-Experienced, Integrase Strand Transfer Inhibitor-Experienced Subjects: In a multicenter, open-label, single-arm trial (ING112574, VIKING-3), 183 HIV-1–infected, antiretroviral treatment-experienced adults with virological failure and current or historical evidence of raltegravir and/or elvitegravir resistance received TIVICAY 50 mg twice daily with the current failing background regimen for 7 days and with optimized background therapy from Day 8. The rate of adverse events leading to discontinuation was 3% of subjects at Week 24.

Treatment-emergent ADRs in VIKING-3 were generally similar compared with observations with the 50-mg once-daily dose in adult Phase 3 trials.

Less Common Adverse Reactions Observed in Treatment-Naïve and Treatment-Experienced Trials: The following ADRs occurred in <2% of treatment-naïve or treatment-experienced subjects receiving TIVICAY in a combination regimen in any one trial. These events have been included because of their seriousness and assessment of potential causal relationship.

Gastrointestinal Disorders: Abdominal pain, abdominal discomfort, flatulence, upper abdominal pain, vomiting.

General Disorders: Fatigue.

Hepatobiliary Disorders: Hepatitis.

Musculoskeletal Disorders: Myositis.

Table 3. Selected Laboratory Abnormalities (Grades 2 to 4) in Treatment-Naïve Subjects in SPRING-2 and SINGLE Trials (Week 48 Analysis)

Laboratory Parameter Preferred Term	SPRING-2		SINGLE	
	TIVICAY 50 mg Once Daily + 2 NRTIs (N = 403)	Raltegravir 400 mg Twice Daily + 2 NRTIs (N = 405)	TIVICAY 50 mg + EPZICOM Once Daily (N = 414)	ATRIPLA Once Daily (N = 419)
ALT				
Grade 2 (>2.5-5.0 × ULN)	2%	3%	2%	5%
Grade 3 to 4 (>5.0 × ULN)	2%	1%	<1%	<1%
AST				
Grade 2 (>2.5-5.0 × ULN)	3%	3%	2%	3%
Grade 3 to 4 (>5.0 × ULN)	2%	2%	0	2%
Total Bilirubin				
Grade 2 (1.6-2.5 × ULN)	2%	2%	<1%	0
Grade 3 to 4 (>2.5 × ULN)	<1%	<1%	<1%	0
Creatine kinase				
Grade 2 (6.0-9.9 × ULN)	1%	3%	3%	1%
Grade 3 to 4 (≥10.0 × ULN)	4%	3%	3%	4%
Hyperglycemia				
Grade 2 (126-250 mg/dL)	5%	5%	7%	4%
Grade 3 (>251 mg/dL)	<1%	1%	1%	<1%
Lipase				
Grade 2 (>1.5-3.0 × ULN)	5%	6%	8%	7%
Grade 3 to 4 (>3.0 × ULN)	1%	3%	3%	2%
Total neutrophils				
Grade 2 (0.75-0.99 × 109)	3%	3%	2%	4%
Grade 3 to 4 (<0.75 × 109)	2%	1%	2%	3%

ULN = Upper limit of normal.

Table 4. Mean Change From Baseline in Fasted Lipid Values in Treatment-Naïve Subjects in SPRING-2 and SINGLE Trials (Week 48 Analysis)

Laboratory Parameter Preferred Term	SPRING-2		SINGLE	
	TIVICAY 50 mg Once Daily + 2 NRTIs (N = 403)	Raltegravir 400 mg Twice Daily + 2 NRTIs (N = 405)	TIVICAY 50 mg + EPZICOM Once Daily (N = 414)	ATRIPLA Once Daily (N = 419)
Cholesterol (mg/dL)	6.7	8.3	17.1	24.0
HDL cholesterol (mg/dL)	2.8	2.6	5.2	7.9
LDL cholesterol (mg/dL)	2.7	2.8	8.5	13.1
Triglycerides (mg/dL)	7.7	9.8	17.7	18.6

[a] Subjects on lipid-lowering agents at baseline were excluded from these analyses (19 subjects in each arm in SPRING-2, and in SINGLE: TIVICAY n = 27 and ATRIPLA n = 26). Forty-nine subjects initiated a lipid-lowering agent post-baseline; their last fasted on-treatment values (prior to starting the agent) were used regardless if they discontinued the agent (SPRING-2: TIVICAY n = 5, raltegravir n = 8; SINGLE: TIVICAY n = 19 and ATRIPLA: n = 17).

Renal and Urinary Disorders: Renal impairment.
Skin and Subcutaneous Tissue Disorders: Pruritus.
Laboratory Abnormalities: *Treatment-Naïve Subjects:* Selected laboratory abnormalities (Grades 2 to 4) with a worsening grade from baseline and representing the worst-grade toxicity in ≥2% of subjects are presented in Table 3. The mean change from baseline observed for selected lipid values is presented in Table 4. Side-by-side tabulation is to simplify presentation; direct comparisons across trials should not be made due to differing trial designs.
[See table 3 above]
[See table 4 above]
Treatment-Experienced, Integrase Strand Transfer Inhibitor-Naïve Subjects: Laboratory abnormalities observed in SAILING were generally similar compared with observations seen in the treatment-naïve (SPRING-2 and SINGLE) trials.
Treatment-Experienced, Integrase Strand Transfer Inhibitor-Experienced Subjects: The most common treatment-emergent laboratory abnormalities (>5% for Grades 2 to 4 combined) were elevated ALT (8%), AST (6%), cholesterol (8%), hyperglycemia (12%), and lipase (8%). Two percent (3/183) of subjects had a Grade 3 to 4, treatment-emergent hematology laboratory abnormality, with neutropenia (1% [2/183]) being the most frequently reported.
Hepatitis B and/or Hepatitis C Virus Co-infection: In Phase 3 trials, subjects with hepatitis B and/or C virus co-infection were permitted to enroll provided that baseline liver chemistry tests did not exceed 5 times the upper limit of normal. Overall, the safety profile in subjects with hepatitis B and/or C virus co-infection was similar to that ob-

served in subjects without hepatitis B or C co-infection, although the rates of AST and ALT abnormalities were higher in the subgroup with hepatitis B and/or C virus co-infection for all treatment groups. Grades 2 to 4 ALT abnormalities in hepatitis B and/or C co-infected compared with HIV mono-infected subjects receiving TIVICAY were observed in 16% vs. 2% with the 50-mg once-daily dose and 8% vs. 7% with the 50-mg twice-daily dose. Liver chemistry elevations consistent with immune reconstitution syndrome were observed in some subjects with hepatitis B and/or C at the start of therapy with TIVICAY, particularly in the setting where anti-hepatitis therapy was withdrawn *[see Warnings and Precautions (5.2)].*
Changes in Serum Creatinine: Dolutegravir has been shown to increase serum creatinine due to inhibition of tubular secretion of creatinine without affecting renal glomerular function *[see Clinical Pharmacology (12.2)].* Increases in serum creatinine occurred within the first 4 weeks of treatment and remained stable through 24 to 48 weeks. In treatment-naïve subjects, a mean change from baseline of 0.11 mg/dL (range: -0.60 mg/dL to 0.62 mg/dL) was observed after 48 weeks of treatment. Creatinine increases were comparable by background NRTIs and were similar in treatment-experienced subjects.
6.2   Clinical Trials Experience in Pediatric Subjects
IMPAACT P1093 is an ongoing multi-center, open-label, non-comparative trial of approximately 160 HIV–1–infected pediatric subjects aged 6 weeks to less than 18 years, of which 23 treatment-experienced, INSTI-naïve subjects aged 12 to less than 18 years were enrolled *[see Use in Specific Populations (8.4), Clinical Studies (14.2)].*

The adverse reaction profile was similar to that for adults. Grade 2 ADRs reported in at least 1 subject were rash (n = 1), abdominal pain (n = 1), and diarrhea (n = 1). No Grade 3 or 4 ADRs were reported. The Grade 3 laboratory abnormalities were elevated total bilirubin and lipase reported in 1 subject each. No Grade 4 laboratory abnormalities were reported. The changes in mean serum creatinine were similar to those observed in adults.

7   DRUG INTERACTIONS
Refer to Table 5 for established and other potentially significant drug-drug interactions.
7.1   Effect of Dolutegravir on the Pharmacokinetics of Other Agents
In vitro, dolutegravir inhibited the renal organic cation transporters, OCT2 (IC_{50} = 1.93 µM) and multidrug and toxin extrusion transporter (MATE) 1 (IC_{50} = 6.34 µM). In vivo, dolutegravir inhibits tubular secretion of creatinine by inhibiting OCT2 and potentially MATE1. Dolutegravir may increase plasma concentrations of drugs eliminated via OCT2 or MATE1 (dofetilide and metformin, Table 5) *[see Contraindications (4), Drug Interactions (7.3)].*
In vitro, dolutegravir inhibited the basolateral renal transporters, organic anion transporter (OAT) 1 (IC_{50} = 2.12 µM) and OAT3 (IC_{50} = 1.97 µM). However, in vivo, dolutegravir did not alter the plasma concentrations of tenofovir or para-amino hippurate, substrates of OAT1 and OAT3.
In vitro, dolutegravir did not inhibit (IC_{50} >50 µM) the following: cytochrome P450 (CYP)1A2, CYP2A6, CYP2B6, CYP2C8, CYP2C9, CYP2C19, CYP2D6, CYP3A, UGT1A1, UGT2B7, P-glycoprotein (P-gp), breast cancer resistance protein (BCRP), bile salt export pump (BSEP), organic anion transporter polypeptide (OATP)1B1, OATP1B3, OCT1, multidrug resistance protein (MRP)2 or MRP4. In vitro, dolutegravir did not induce CYP1A2, CYP2B6, or CYP3A4. Based on these data and the results of drug interaction trials, dolutegravir is not expected to affect the pharmacokinetics of drugs that are substrates of these enzymes or transporters.
In drug interaction trials, dolutegravir did not have a clinically relevant effect on the pharmacokinetics of the following drugs: tenofovir, methadone, midazolam, rilpivirine, and oral contraceptives containing norgestimate and ethinyl estradiol. Using cross-study comparisons to historical pharmacokinetic data for each interacting drug, dolutegravir did not appear to affect the pharmacokinetics of the following drugs: atazanavir, darunavir, efavirenz, etravirine, fosamprenavir, lopinavir, ritonavir, and telaprevir.
7.2   Effect of Other Agents on the Pharmacokinetics of Dolutegravir
Dolutegravir is metabolized by UGT1A1 with some contribution from CYP3A. Dolutegravir is also a substrate of UGT1A3, UGT1A9, BCRP, and P-gp in vitro. Drugs that induce those enzymes and transporters may decrease dolutegravir plasma concentration and reduce the therapeutic effect of dolutegravir.
Coadministration of dolutegravir and other drugs that inhibit these enzymes may increase dolutegravir plasma concentration.
Etravirine significantly reduced plasma concentrations of dolutegravir, but the effect of etravirine was mitigated by coadministration of lopinavir/ritonavir or darunavir/ritonavir, and is expected to be mitigated by atazanavir/ritonavir. (Table 5) *[see Drug Interactions (7.3), Clinical Pharmacology (12.3)].*
Darunavir/ritonavir, lopinavir/ritonavir, rilpivirine, tenofovir, boceprevir, telaprevir, prednisone, rifabutin, and omeprazole had no clinically significant effect on the pharmacokinetics of dolutegravir.
7.3   Established and Other Potentially Significant Drug Interactions
Table 5 provides clinical recommendations as a result of drug interactions with TIVICAY. These recommendations are based on either drug interaction trials or predicted interactions due to the expected magnitude of interaction and potential for serious adverse events or loss of efficacy. *[See Dosage and Administration (2), Clinical Pharmacology (12.3).]*
[See table 5 at top of next page]

8   USE IN SPECIFIC POPULATIONS
8.1   Pregnancy
Pregnancy Category B. There are no adequate and well-controlled studies in pregnant women. Because animal reproduction studies are not always predictive of human response, and dolutegravir was shown to cross the placenta in animal studies, this drug should be used during pregnancy only if clearly needed.
Antiretroviral Pregnancy Registry: To monitor maternal-fetal outcomes of pregnant women with HIV exposed to TIVICAY and other antiretroviral agents, an Antiretroviral Pregnancy Registry has been established. Physicians are encouraged to register patients by calling 1-800-258-4263.
Animal Data: Reproduction studies have been performed in rats and rabbits at doses up to 27 times the human dose of 50 mg twice daily and have revealed no evidence of impaired fertility or harm to the fetus due to TIVICAY.

Table 5. Established and Other Potentially Significant Drug Interactions: Alterations in Dose or Regimen May Be Recommended Based on Drug Interaction Trials or Predicted Interactions [see Dosage and Administration (2)]

Concomitant Drug Class: Drug Name	Effect on Concentration of Dolutegravir and/or Concomitant Drug	Clinical Comment
HIV-1 Antiviral Agents		
Non-nucleoside reverse transcriptase inhibitor: Etravirine[a]	↓Dolutegravir	TIVICAY should not be used with etravirine without coadministration of atazanavir/ritonavir, darunavir/ritonavir, or lopinavir/ritonavir.
Non-nucleoside reverse transcriptase inhibitor: Efavirenz[a]	↓Dolutegravir	A dose adjustment of TIVICAY to 50 mg twice daily is recommended in treatment-naïve or treatment-experienced, INSTI-naïve patients. Alternative combinations that do not include metabolic inducers should be considered where possible for INSTI-experienced patients with certain INSTI-associated resistance substitutions or clinically suspected INSTI resistance.[b]
Non-nucleoside reverse transcriptase inhibitor: Nevirapine	↓Dolutegravir	Coadministration with nevirapine should be avoided because there are insufficient data to make dosing recommendations.
Protease Inhibitor: Fosamprenavir/ritonavir[a] Tipranavir/ritonavir[a]	↓Dolutegravir	A dose adjustment of TIVICAY to 50 mg twice daily is recommended in treatment-naïve or treatment-experienced, INSTI-naïve patients. Alternative combinations that do not include metabolic inducers should be considered where possible for INSTI-experienced patients with certain INSTI-associated resistance substitutions or clinically suspected INSTI resistance.[b]
Other Agents		
Oxcarbazepine Phenytoin Phenobarbital Carbamazepine St. John's wort (*Hypericum perforatum*)	↓Dolutegravir	Coadministration with these metabolic inducers should be avoided because there are insufficient data to make dosing recommendations.
Medications containing polyvalent cations (e.g., Mg or Al) Cation-containing antacids[a] or laxatives Sucralfate Buffered medications	↓Dolutegravir	TIVICAY should be administered 2 hours before or 6 hours after taking medications containing polyvalent cations.
Oral calcium or iron supplements, including multivitamins containing calcium or iron[a]	↓Dolutegravir	TIVICAY should be administered 2 hours before or 6 hours after taking supplements containing calcium or iron. Alternatively, TIVICAY and supplements containing calcium or iron can be taken together with food.
Metformin	↑Metformin	Metformin dose reductions may be considered when coadministered with TIVICAY.
Rifampin[a]	↓Dolutegravir	A dose adjustment of TIVICAY to 50 mg twice daily is recommended in treatment-naïve or treatment-experienced, INSTI-naïve patients. Alternatives to rifampin should be used where possible for INSTI-experienced patients with certain INSTI-associated resistance substitutions or clinically suspected INSTI resistance.[b]

[a] *See Clinical Pharmacology (12.3) Table 9 for magnitude of interaction.*
[b] The lower dolutegravir exposures observed in INSTI-experienced patients (with certain INSTI-associated resistance substitutions or clinically suspected INSTI resistance [see Microbiology (12.4)]) upon coadministration with potent inducers may result in loss of therapeutic effect and development of resistance to TIVICAY or other coadministered antiretroviral agents.

Oral administration of dolutegravir to pregnant rats at doses up to 1,000 mg/kg daily, approximately 27 times the 50-mg twice-daily human clinical exposure based on AUC, from days 6 to 17 of gestation did not elicit maternal toxicity, developmental toxicity, or teratogenicity.

Oral administration of dolutegravir to pregnant rabbits at doses up to 1,000 mg/kg daily, approximately 0.4 times the 50-mg twice-daily human clinical exposure based on AUC, from days 6 to 18 of gestation did not elicit developmental toxicity or teratogenicity. In rabbits, maternal toxicity (decreased food consumption, scant/no feces/urine, suppressed body weight gain) was observed at 1,000 mg/kg.

8.3 Nursing Mothers
The Centers for Disease Control and Prevention recommend that HIV–1–infected mothers in the United States not breastfeed their infants to avoid risking postnatal transmission of HIV-1 infection. Studies in lactating rats and their offspring indicate that dolutegravir was present in rat milk. It is not known whether dolutegravir is excreted in human milk.

Because of both the potential for HIV transmission and the potential for adverse reactions in nursing infants, **mothers should be instructed not to breastfeed if they are receiving TIVICAY.**

8.4 Pediatric Use
TIVICAY is not recommended in pediatric patients younger than 12 years or weighing less than 40 kg. Safety and efficacy of TIVICAY have not been established in pediatric patients who are INSTI-experienced with documented or clinically suspected resistance to other INSTIs (raltegravir, elvitegravir).

The safety, virologic, and immunologic responses in subjects who received TIVICAY were evaluated in 23 treatment-experienced, INSTI-naïve, HIV–1–infected subjects aged 12 to less than 18 years in an open-label, multicenter, dose-finding clinical trial, IMPAACT P1093 [see Adverse Reactions (6.2), Clinical Pharmacology (12.3), Clinical Studies (14.2)]. Pharmacokinetic parameters, evaluated in 9 subjects weighing ≥40 kg receiving 50 mg daily and 1 subject (weighing 37 kg) receiving 35 mg once daily, were similar to adults receiving 50 mg once daily. See Dosage and Administration (2.2) for dosing recommendations for pediatric patients aged 12 years and older and weighing at least 40 kg. Frequency, type, and severity of adverse drug reactions in pediatric subjects were comparable to those observed in adults [see Adverse Reactions (6.2)].

8.5 Geriatric Use
Clinical trials of TIVICAY did not include sufficient numbers of subjects aged 65 and older to determine whether they respond differently from younger subjects. In general, caution should be exercised in the administration of TIVICAY in elderly patients reflecting the greater frequency of decreased hepatic, renal, or cardiac function, and of concomitant disease or other drug therapy [see Clinical Pharmacology (12.3)].

8.6 Hepatic Impairment
No clinically important pharmacokinetic differences between subjects with moderate hepatic impairment and matching healthy subjects were observed. No dosage adjustment is necessary for patients with mild to moderate hepatic impairment (Child-Pugh Score A or B). The effect of severe hepatic impairment (Child-Pugh Score C) on the pharmacokinetics of dolutegravir has not been studied. Therefore, TIVICAY is not recommended for use in patients with severe hepatic impairment [see Clinical Pharmacology (12.3)].

8.7 Renal Impairment
Dolutegravir plasma concentrations were decreased in subjects with severe renal impairment compared with those in matched healthy controls. However, no dosage adjustment is necessary for treatment-naïve or treatment-experienced and INSTI-naïve patients with mild, moderate, or severe renal impairment or for INSTI-experienced patients (with certain INSTI-associated resistance substitutions or clinically suspected INSTI resistance) with mild or moderate renal impairment. Caution is warranted for INSTI-experienced patients (with certain INSTI-associated resistance substitutions or clinically suspected INSTI resistance [see Microbiology (12.4)]) with severe renal impairment, as the decrease in dolutegravir concentrations may result in loss of therapeutic effect and development of resistance to TIVICAY or other coadministered antiretroviral agents [see Clinical Pharmacology (12.3)]. Dolutegravir has not been studied in patients on dialysis.

10 OVERDOSAGE
Limited experience with single higher doses (up to 250 mg in healthy subjects) revealed no specific symptoms or signs apart from those listed as adverse reactions. There is no known specific treatment for overdose with TIVICAY. If overdose occurs, the patient should be monitored and standard supportive treatment applied as required. As dolutegravir is highly bound to plasma proteins, it is unlikely that it will be significantly removed by dialysis.

11 DESCRIPTION
TIVICAY contains dolutegravir, as dolutegravir sodium, an HIV INSTI. The chemical name of dolutegravir sodium is sodium (4R,12aS)-9-{[(2,4-difluorophenyl)methyl]carbamoyl}-4-methyl-6,8-dioxo-3,4,6,8,12,12a-hexahydro-2H-pyrido[1',2':4,5]pyrazino[2,1-b][1,3]oxazin-7-olate. The empirical formula is $C_{20}H_{18}F_2N_3NaO_5$ and the molecular weight is 441.36 g/mol. It has the following structural formula:

Dolutegravir sodium is a white to light yellow powder and is slightly soluble in water.

Each film-coated tablet of TIVICAY for oral administration contains 52.6 mg of dolutegravir sodium, which is equivalent to 50 mg dolutegravir free acid, and the following inactive ingredients: D-mannitol, microcrystalline cellulose, povidone K29/32, sodium starch glycolate, and sodium stearyl fumarate. The tablet film-coating contains the inactive ingredients iron oxide yellow, macrogol/PEG, polyvinyl alcohol-part hydrolyzed, talc, and titanium dioxide.

12 CLINICAL PHARMACOLOGY
12.1 Mechanism of Action
Dolutegravir is an HIV-1 antiviral agent [see Microbiology (12.4)].

12.2 Pharmacodynamics
In a randomized, dose-ranging trial, HIV–1–infected subjects treated with dolutegravir monotherapy demonstrated rapid and dose-dependent antiviral activity with mean declines from baseline to Day 11 in HIV-1 RNA of 1.5, 2.0, and 2.5 $\log_{10}$ for dolutegravir 2 mg, 10 mg, and 50 mg once daily, respectively. This antiviral response was maintained for 3 to 4 days after the last dose in the 50-mg group.

Table 7. Dolutegravir Steady-State Pharmacokinetic Parameters in Pediatric Subjects

Age/Weight	Dose of TIVICAY[a]	Dolutegravir Pharmacokinetic Parameter Estimates Geometric Mean (%CV)		
		C_{max} (mcg/mL) (n = 10)	$AUC_{(0-24)}$ (mcg.h/mL) (n = 10)	C_{24} (mcg/mL) (n = 10)
12 to <18 years and ≥40 kg [a]	50 mg once daily	3.49 (38)	46 (43)	0.90 (59)

[a]One subject weighing 37 kg received TIVICAY 35 mg once daily.

Table 8. Summary of Effect of Dolutegravir on the Pharmacokinetics of Coadministered Drugs

Coadministered Drug(s) and Dose(s)	Dose of TIVICAY	n	Geometric Mean Ratio (90% CI) of Pharmacokinetic Parameters of Coadministered Drug With/Without Dolutegravir No Effect = 1.00		
			C_{max}	AUC	C_τ or C_{24}
Ethinyl estradiol 0.035 mg	50 mg twice daily	15	0.99 (0.91 to 1.08)	1.03 (0.96 to 1.11)	1.02 (0.93 to 1.11)
Methadone 16 to 150 mg	50 mg twice daily	11	1.00 (0.94 to 1.06)	0.98 (0.91 to 1.06)	0.99 (0.91 to 1.07)
Midazolam 3 mg	25 mg once daily	10	–	0.95 (0.79 to 1.15)	–
Norgestromin 0.25 mg	50 mg twice daily	15	0.89 (0.82 to 0.97)	0.98 (0.91 to 1.04)	0.93 (0.85 to 1.03)
Rilpivirine 25 mg once daily	50 mg once daily	16	1.10 (0.99 to 1.22)	1.06 (0.98 to 1.16)	1.21 (1.07 to 1.38)
Tenofovir disoproxil fumarate 300 mg once daily	50 mg once daily	15	1.09 (0.97 to 1.23)	1.12 (1.01 to 1.24)	1.19 (1.04 to 1.35)

Effects on Electrocardiogram: In a randomized, placebo-controlled, cross-over trial, 42 healthy subjects received single-dose oral administrations of placebo, dolutegravir 250-mg suspension (exposures approximately 3-fold of the 50-mg once-daily dose at steady state), and moxifloxacin 400 mg (active control) in random sequence. After baseline and placebo adjustment, the maximum mean QTc change based on Fridericia correction method (QTcF) for dolutegravir was 2.4 msec (1-sided 95% upper CI: 4.9 msec). TIVICAY did not prolong the QTc interval over 24 hours postdose.

Effects on Renal Function: The effect of dolutegravir on renal function was evaluated in an open-label, randomized, 3-arm, parallel, placebo-controlled trial in healthy subjects (n = 37) who received dolutegravir 50 mg once daily (n = 12), dolutegravir 50 mg twice daily (n = 13), or placebo once daily (n = 12) for 14 days. A decrease in creatinine clearance, as determined by 24-hour urine collection, was observed with both doses of dolutegravir after 14 days of treatment in subjects who received 50 mg once daily (9% decrease) and 50 mg twice daily (13% decrease). Neither dose of dolutegravir had a significant effect on the actual glomerular filtration rate (determined by the clearance of probe drug, iohexol) or effective renal plasma flow (determined by the clearance of probe drug, para-amino hippurate) compared with the placebo.

12.3 Pharmacokinetics

The pharmacokinetic properties of dolutegravir have been evaluated in healthy adult subjects and HIV–1–infected adult subjects. Exposure to dolutegravir was generally similar between healthy subjects and HIV–1–infected subjects. The non-linear exposure of dolutegravir following 50 mg twice daily compared with 50 mg once daily in HIV–1–infected subjects (Table 6) was attributed to the use of metabolic inducers in the background antiretroviral regimens of subjects receiving dolutegravir 50 mg twice daily in clinical trials. TIVICAY was administered without regard to food in these trials.

Table 6. Dolutegravir Steady-State Pharmacokinetic Parameter Estimates in HIV–1–Infected Adults

Parameter	50 mg Once Daily Geometric Mean[a] (%CV)	50 mg Twice Daily Geometric Mean[b] (%CV)
$AUC_{(0-24)}$ (mcg.h/mL)	53.6 (27)	75.1 (35)
C_{max} (mcg/mL)	3.67 (20)	4.15 (29)
C_{min} (mcg/mL)	1.11 (46)	2.12 (47)

[a]Based on population pharmacokinetic analyses using data from SPRING-1 and SPRING-2.
[b]Based on population pharmacokinetic analyses using data from VIKING (ING112961) and VIKING-3.

Absorption: Following oral administration of dolutegravir, peak plasma concentrations were observed 2 to 3 hours postdose. With once-daily dosing, pharmacokinetic steady state is achieved within approximately 5 days with average accumulation ratios for AUC, C_{max}, and $C_{24\ h}$ ranging from 1.2 to 1.5.

Dolutegravir plasma concentrations increased in a less than dose-proportional manner above 50 mg. Dolutegravir is a P-glycoprotein substrate in vitro. The absolute bioavailability of dolutegravir has not been established.

Effects of Food on Oral Absorption: TIVICAY may be taken with or without food. Food increased the extent of absorption and slowed the rate of absorption of dolutegravir. Low-, moderate-, and high-fat meals increased dolutegravir $AUC_{(0-\infty)}$ by 33%, 41%, and 66%; increased C_{max} by 46%, 52%, and 67%; and prolonged T_{max} to 3, 4, and 5 hours from 2 hours under fasted conditions, respectively.

Distribution: Dolutegravir is highly bound (≥98.9%) to human plasma proteins based on in vivo data and binding is independent of plasma concentration of dolutegravir. The apparent volume of distribution (Vd/F) following 50-mg once-daily administration is estimated at 17.4 L based on a population pharmacokinetic analysis.

Cerebrospinal Fluid (CSF): In 11 treatment-naïve subjects on dolutegravir 50 mg daily plus abacavir/lamivudine, the median dolutegravir concentration in CSF was 18 ng/mL (range: 4 ng/mL to 23.2 ng/mL) 2 to 6 hours postdose after 2 weeks of treatment. The clinical relevance of this finding has not been established.

Metabolism and Elimination: Dolutegravir is primarily metabolized via UGT1A1 with some contribution from CYP3A. After a single oral dose of [14C] dolutegravir, 53% of the total oral dose was excreted unchanged in feces. Thirty-one percent of the total oral dose was excreted in urine, represented by an ether glucuronide of dolutegravir (18.9% of total dose), a metabolite formed by oxidation at the benzylic carbon (3.0% of total dose), and its hydrolytic N-dealkylation product (3.6% of total dose). Renal elimination of unchanged drug was low (<1% of the dose). Dolutegravir has a terminal half-life of approximately 14 hours and an apparent clearance (CL/F) of 1.0 L/h based on population pharmacokinetic analyses.

Polymorphisms in Drug–Metabolizing Enzymes: In a meta-analysis of healthy subject trials, subjects with UGT1A1 (n = 7) genotypes conferring poor dolutegravir metabolism had a 32% lower clearance of dolutegravir and 46% higher AUC compared with subjects with genotypes associated with normal metabolism via UGT1A1 (n = 41).

Specific Populations: *Hepatic Impairment:* Dolutegravir is primarily metabolized and eliminated by the liver. In a trial comparing 8 subjects with moderate hepatic impairment (Child-Pugh Score B) with 8 matched healthy controls, exposure of dolutegravir from a single 50-mg dose was similar between the 2 groups. No dosage adjustment is necessary for patients with mild to moderate hepatic impairment (Child-Pugh Score A or B). The effect of severe hepatic impairment (Child-Pugh Score C) on the pharmacokinetics of dolutegravir has not been studied. Therefore, TIVICAY is not recommended for use in patients with severe hepatic impairment.

HBV/HCV Co-infection: Population analyses using pooled pharmacokinetic data from adult trials indicated no clinically relevant effect of HCV co-infection on the pharmacokinetics of dolutegravir. There were limited data on HBV co-infection.

Renal Impairment: Renal clearance of unchanged drug is a minor pathway of elimination for dolutegravir. In a trial comparing 8 subjects with severe renal impairment (CrCl <30 mL/min) with 8 matched healthy controls, AUC, C_{max}, and C_{24} of dolutegravir were decreased by 40%, 23%, and 43%, respectively, compared with those in matched healthy subjects. The cause of this decrease is unknown. Population pharmacokinetic analysis using data from SAILING and VIKING-3 trials indicated that mild and moderate renal impairment had no clinically relevant effect on the exposure of dolutegravir. No dosage adjustment is necessary for treatment-naïve or treatment-experienced and INSTI-naïve patients with mild, moderate, or severe renal impairment or for INSTI-experienced patients (with certain INSTI-associated resistance substitutions or clinically suspected INSTI resistance) with mild or moderate renal impairment. Caution is warranted for INSTI-experienced patients (with certain INSTI-associated resistance substitutions or clinically suspected INSTI resistance [see Microbiology (12.4)]) with severe renal impairment, as the decrease in dolutegravir concentrations may result in loss of therapeutic effect and development of resistance to TIVICAY or other coadministered antiretroviral agents. Dolutegravir has not been studied in patients requiring dialysis.

Gender: Population analyses using pooled pharmacokinetic data from adult trials indicated gender had no clinically relevant effect on the exposure of dolutegravir.

Race: Population analyses using pooled pharmacokinetic data from adult trials indicated race had no clinically relevant effect on the pharmacokinetics of dolutegravir.

Geriatric Patients: Population analyses using pooled pharmacokinetic data from adult trials indicated age had no clinically relevant effect on the pharmacokinetics of dolutegravir.

Pediatric Patients: The pharmacokinetics of dolutegravir in HIV–1–infected children (n = 10) aged 12 to less than 18 years were similar to those observed in HIV–1–infected adults who received dolutegravir 50 mg once daily (Table 7) [see Clinical Studies (14.2)].

[See table 7 above]

Drug Interactions: Drug interaction trials were performed with TIVICAY and other drugs likely to be coadministered or commonly used as probes for pharmacokinetic interactions. As dolutegravir is not expected to affect the pharmacokinetics of other drugs dependent on hepatic metabolism (Table 8) [see Drug Interactions (7.1)], the primary focus of these drug interaction trials was to evaluate the effect of coadministered drug on dolutegravir (Table 9).

Dosing or regimen recommendations as a result of established and other potentially significant drug-drug interactions with TIVICAY are provided in Table 5 [see Dosage and Administration (2.1), Drug Interactions (7.3)].

[See table 8 above]

[See table 9 on pages 2389 and 2390]

12.4 Microbiology

Mechanism of Action: Dolutegravir inhibits HIV integrase by binding to the integrase active site and blocking the strand transfer step of retroviral deoxyribonucleic acid (DNA) integration which is essential for the HIV replication cycle. Strand transfer biochemical assays using purified HIV-1 integrase and pre-processed substrate DNA resulted in IC_{50} values of 2.7 nM and 12.6 nM.

Antiviral Activity in Cell Culture: Dolutegravir exhibited antiviral activity against laboratory strains of wild-type HIV-1 with mean EC_{50} values of 0.5 nM (0.21 ng/mL) to 2.1 nM (0.85 ng/mL) in peripheral blood mononuclear cells (PBMCs) and MT-4 cells. Dolutegravir exhibited antiviral activity against 13 clinically diverse clade B isolates with a mean EC_{50} of 0.52 nM in a viral integrase susceptibility assay using the integrase coding region from clinical isolates. Dolutegravir demonstrated antiviral activity in cell culture against a panel of HIV-1 clinical isolates (3 in each group of M clades A, B, C, D, E, F, and G, and 3 in group O) with

Table 9. Summary of Effect of Coadministered Drugs on the Pharmacokinetics of Dolutegravir

Coadministered Drug(s) and Dose(s)	Dose of TIVICAY	n	Geometric Mean Ratio (90% CI) of Dolutegravir Pharmacokinetic Parameters With/Without Coadministered Drugs No Effect = 1.00		
			C_{max}	AUC	C_τ or C_{24}
Atazanavir 400 mg once daily	30 mg once daily	12	1.50 (1.40 to 1.59)	1.91 (1.80 to 2.03)	2.80 (2.52 to 3.11)
Atazanavir/ritonavir 300/100 mg once daily	30 mg once daily	12	1.34 (1.25 to 1.42)	1.62 (1.50 to 1.74)	2.21 (1.97 to 2.47)
Tenofovir 300 mg once daily	50 mg once daily	15	0.97 (0.87 to 1.08)	1.01 (0.91 to 1.11)	0.92 (0.82 to 1.04)
Darunavir/ritonavir 600/100 mg twice daily	30 mg once daily	15	0.89 (0.83 to 0.97)	0.78 (0.72 to 0.85)	0.62 (0.56 to 0.69)
Efavirenz 600 mg once daily	50 mg once daily	12	0.61 (0.51 to 0.73)	0.43 (0.35 to 0.54)	0.25 (0.18 to 0.34)
Etravirine 200 mg twice daily	50 mg once daily	16	0.48 (0.43 to 0.54)	0.29 (0.26 to 0.34)	0.12 (0.09 to 0.16)
Etravirine + darunavir/ ritonavir 200 mg + 600/100 mg twice daily	50 mg once daily	9	0.88 (0.78 to 1.00)	0.75 (0.69 to 0.81)	0.63 (0.52 to 0.76)
Etravirine + lopinavir/ ritonavir 200 mg + 400/100 mg twice daily	50 mg once daily	8	1.07 (1.02 to 1.13)	1.11 (1.02 to 1.20)	1.28 (1.13 to 1.45)
Fosamprenavir/ritonavir 700 mg/100 mg twice daily	50 mg once daily	12	0.76 (0.63 to 0.92)	0.65 (0.54 to 0.78)	0.51 (0.41 to 0.63)
Lopinavir/ritonavir 400/100 mg twice daily	30 mg once daily	15	1.00 (0.94 to 1.07)	0.97 (0.91 to 1.04)	0.94 (0.85 to 1.05)
Antacid (Maalox®) Simultaneous administration	50 mg single dose	16	0.28 (0.23 to 0.33)	0.26 (0.22 to 0.32)	0.26 (0.21 to 0.31)
Antacid (Maalox®) 2 hrs after dolutegravir	50 mg single dose	16	0.82 (0.69 to 0.98)	0.74 (0.62 to 0.90)	0.70 (0.58 to 0.85)
Calcium carbonate 1,200 mg simultaneous administration (fasted)	50 mg single dose	12	0.63 (0.50 to 0.81)	0.61 (0.47 to 0.80)	0.61 (0.47 to 0.80)
Calcium carbonate 1,200 mg simultaneous administration (fed)	50 mg single dose	11	1.07 (0.83 to 1.38)	1.09 (0.84 to 1.43)	1.08 (0.81 to 1.42)
Calcium carbonate 1,200 mg 2 h after dolutegravir	50 mg single dose	11	1.00 (0.78 to 1.29)	0.94 (0.72 to 1.23)	0.90 (0.68 to 1.19)
Ferrous fumarate 324 mg simultaneous administration (fasted)	50 mg single dose	11	0.43 (0.35 to 0.52)	0.46 (0.38 to 0.56)	0.44 (0.36 to 0.54)
Ferrous fumarate 324 mg simultaneous administration (fed)	50 mg single dose	11	1.03 (0.84 to 1.26)	0.98 (0/81 to 1.20)	1.00 (0.81 to 1.23)
Ferrous fumarate 324 mg 2 h after dolutegravir	50 mg single dose	10	0.99 (0.81 to 1.21)	0.95 (0.77 to 1.15)	0.92 (0.74 to 1.13)
Multivitamin (One-A-Day®) simultaneous administration	50 mg single dose	16	0.65 (0.54 to 0.77)	0.67 (0.55 to 0.81)	0.68 (0.56 to 0.82)
Omeprazole 40 mg once daily	50 mg single dose	12	0.92 (0.75 to 1.11)	0.97 (0.78 to 1.20)	0.95 (0.75 to 1.21)
Prednisone 60 mg once daily with taper	50 mg once daily	12	1.06 (0.99 to 1.14)	1.11 (1.03 to 1.20)	1.17 (1.06 to 1.28)

(Table continued on next page)

EC_{50} values ranging from 0.02 nM to 2.14 nM for HIV-1. Dolutegravir EC_{50} values against 3 HIV-2 clinical isolates in PBMC assays ranged from 0.09 nM to 0.61 nM.

Antiviral Activity in Combination With Other Antiviral Agents: The antiviral activity of dolutegravir was not antagonistic when combined with the INSTI, raltegravir; nonnucleoside reverse transcriptase inhibitors (NNRTIs), efavirenz or nevirapine; the nucleoside reverse transcriptase inhibitors (NRTIs), abacavir or stavudine; the protease inhibitors (PIs), amprenavir or lopinavir; the CCR5 coreceptor antagonist, maraviroc; or the fusion inhibitor, enfuvirtide. Dolutegravir antiviral activity was not antagonistic when combined with the HBV reverse transcriptase inhibitor, adefovir, or with the antiviral, ribavirin.

Resistance: *Cell Culture:* Dolutegravir-resistant viruses were selected in cell culture starting from different wildtype HIV-1 strains and clades. Amino acid substitutions E92Q, G118R, S153F or Y, G193E or R263K emerged in different passages and conferred decreased susceptibility to dolutegravir of up to 4-fold. Passage of mutant viruses containing the Q148R or Q148H substitutions selected for additional substitutions in integrase that conferred decreased susceptibility to dolutegravir (fold-change increase of 13 to 46). The additional integrase substitutions included T97A,

E138K, G140S, and M154I. Passage of mutant viruses containing both G140S and Q148H selected for L74M, E92Q, and N155H.

Treatment-Naïve Subjects: No subjects in the dolutegravir 50-mg once-daily treatment arms of treatment-naïve trials SPRING-2 and SINGLE had a detectable decrease in susceptibility to dolutegravir or background NRTIs in the resistance analysis subset (n = 6 with HIV-1 RNA >400 copies/mL at failure or last visit through Week 48 and having resistance data). One additional subject in SINGLE with 275 copies/mL HIV-1 RNA had a treatment-emergent INSTI-resistance substitution (E157Q/P) detected at Week 24, but no corresponding decrease in dolutegravir susceptibility. No treatment-emergent genotypic resistance to the background regimen was isolated in the dolutegravir arm in either the SPRING-2 or SINGLE trials.

Treatment-Experienced, Integrase Strand Transfer Inhibitor-Naïve Subjects: In SAILING, viruses from 5 of 15 subjects in the dolutegravir arm with post-baseline resistance data had evidence of treatment-emergent integrase substitutions (1 subject each with L74I/M, Q95Q/L, or V151V/I, and 2 subjects with R263K). However, none of these subjects' isolates had detectable phenotypic decreases in susceptibility to either dolutegravir or raltegravir. In the comparator raltegravir arm, 9 of 32 subjects with postbaseline resistance data had evidence of emergent INSTI-resistance substitutions (L74M, E92E/Q, Q95Q/R, T97A, G140A/S, Y143C/R, Q148H/R, V151I, N155H, E157E/Q, and G163G/R) and raltegravir phenotypic resistance.

Treatment-Experienced, Integrase Strand Transfer Inhibitor-Experienced Subjects: VIKING-3 examined the efficacy of dolutegravir 50 mg twice daily plus optimized background therapy in subjects with prior or current virologic failure on an INSTI- (elvitegravir or raltegravir) containing regimen.

Response by Baseline Genotype: Of the 183 subjects with baseline data, 30% harbored virus with a substitution at Q148, and 33% had no primary INSTI-resistance substitutions (T66A/I/K, E92Q/V, Y143C/H/R, Q148H/K/R, and N155H) at baseline, but had historical genotypic evidence of INSTI-resistance substitutions, phenotypic evidence of elvitegravir or raltegravir resistance, or genotypic evidence of INSTI-resistance substitutions at screening.

Response rates by baseline genotype were analyzed using a subset of subjects who had reached Week 24, as well as those who discontinued or rebounded before Week 24 (n = 124) (Table 10). The response rate at Week 24 for subjects with only historic evidence of INSTI-resistance at baseline was 75% (33/44). The response rate at Week 24 to dolutegravir-containing regimens was 36% (13/36) when Q148 substitutions were present at baseline; Q148 was always present with additional INSTI-resistance substitutions. Diminished virologic responses (25% [7/28]) were observed when ≥3 of the following INSTI-resistance substitutions were present at baseline: L74I/M, E138A/D/K/T, G140A/S, Y143H/R, Q148H/R, E157Q, G163E/K/Q/R/S, or G193E/R.

Table 10. Response by Baseline Integrase Genotype in Subjects with Prior Experience to an Integrase Strand Transfer Inhibitor in VIKING-3

Baseline Genotype	Response at Week 24 (<50 copies/mL) Subset N = 124
Overall Response	64% (79/124)
N155H without a Q148 substitution	80% (16/20)
Y143C/H/R without a Q148 substitution	56% (10/18)
Q148H/R + G140A/S without additional INSTI-resistance substitutions	56% (10/18)
Q148H/R + ≥2 INSTI-resistance substitutions[a,b]	18% (3/17)

[a]INSTI-resistance substitutions include L74I/M, E138A/D/K/T, G140A/S, Y143H/R, E157Q, G163E/K/Q/R/S, or G193E/R.

[b]The most common pathway with Q148H/R + ≥2 INSTI-resistance substitutions had Q148+G140+E138 substitutions (n = 12).

Response by Baseline Phenotype: Response rates by baseline phenotype were analyzed using a subset of subjects who had reached Week 24, as well as those who discontinued or rebounded before Week 24 (n = 120) (See Table 11). These baseline phenotypic groups are based on subjects enrolled in

VIKING-3 and are not meant to represent definitive clinical susceptibility cut points for dolutegravir. The data are provided to guide clinicians on the likelihood of virologic success based on pretreatment susceptibility to dolutegravir in INSTI-resistant patients.

Table 11. Response by Baseline Dolutegravir Phenotype (Fold-Change From Reference) in Subjects With Prior Experience to an Integrase Strand Transfer Inhibitor in VIKING-3

Baseline Dolutegravir Phenotype (Fold-Change From Reference)	Response at Week 24 (<50 copies/mL) Subset N = 120
Overall Response	63% (75/120)
<3-fold change	72% (63/87)
3- <10-fold change	42% (10/24)
≥10-fold change	22% (2/9)

Integrase Strand Transfer Inhibitor Treatment-Emergent Resistance: There were 40 subjects on the dolutegravir twice-daily regimen in VIKING-3 with HIV-1 RNA >400 copies/mL at Week 24, the failure timepoint, or the last timepoint on trial who were included in the Week 24 resistance analysis set. In the Week 24 resistance analysis set, 45% (18/40) of the subjects had treatment-emergent INSTI-resistance substitutions in their isolates. The most common treatment-emergent INSTI-resistance substitution was T97A. Other frequently emergent INSTI-resistance substitutions included E138K or A, G140S or A, or Q148H or R or K; substitutions at Q148 were detected in subjects with changes documented at or prior to enrollment in the trial. Substitutions L74M, E92Q, Y143H or C, S147G, V151A, M154I, and N155H each emerged in 1 or 2 subjects' isolates. At failure, the median dolutegravir fold-change from reference was 23-fold (range: 0.92 to 209) for isolates with emergent INSTI-resistance substitutions (n = 18).
Resistance to one or more background drugs in the dolutegravir twice-daily regimen also emerged in 30% (12/40) of the subjects in the Week 24 resistance analysis set.
Cross-Resistance: *Site-Directed Integrase Strand Transfer Inhibitor-Resistant Mutant HIV-1 and HIV-2 Strains*: The susceptibility of dolutegravir was tested against 60 INSTI-resistant site-directed mutant HIV-1 viruses (28 with single substitutions and 32 with 2 or more substitutions) and 6 INSTI-resistant site-directed mutant HIV-2 viruses. The single INSTI-resistance substitutions T66K, I151L, and S153Y conferred a >2-fold decrease in dolutegravir susceptibility (range: 2.3-fold to 3.6-fold from reference). Combinations of multiple substitutions T66K/L74M, E92Q/N155H, G140C/Q148R, G140S/Q148H, R or K, Q148R/N155H, T97A/G140S/Q148, and substitutions at E138/G140/Q148 showed a >2-fold decrease in dolutegravir susceptibility (range: 2.5-fold to 21-fold from reference). In HIV-2 mutants, combinations of substitutions A153G/N155H/S163G and E92Q/T97A/N155H/S163D conferred 4-fold decreases in dolutegravir susceptibility, and E92Q/N155H and G140S/Q148R showed 8.5-fold and 17-fold decreases in dolutegravir susceptibility, respectively.
Reverse Transcriptase Inhibitor- and Protease Inhibitor-Resistant Strains: Dolutegravir demonstrated equivalent antiviral activity against 2 NNRTI-resistant, 3 NRTI-resistant, and 2 PI-resistant HIV-1 mutant clones compared with the wild-type strain.

13 NONCLINICAL TOXICOLOGY
13.1 Carcinogenesis, Mutagenesis, Impairment of Fertility
Carcinogenesis: Two-year carcinogenicity studies in mice and rats were conducted with dolutegravir. Mice were administered doses of up to 500 mg/kg, and rats were administered doses of up to 50 mg/kg. In mice, no significant increases in the incidence of drug-related neoplasms were observed at the highest doses tested, resulting in dolutegravir AUC exposures approximately 14-fold higher than those in humans at the recommended dose of 50 mg twice daily. In rats, no increases in the incidence of drug-related neoplasms were observed at the highest dose tested, resulting in dolutegravir AUC exposures 10-fold and 15-fold higher in males and females, respectively, than those in humans at the recommended dose of 50 mg twice daily.
Mutagenesis: Dolutegravir was not genotoxic in the bacterial reverse mutation assay, mouse lymphoma assay, or in the in vivo rodent micronucleus assay.
Impairment of Fertility: In a study conducted in rats, there were no effects on mating or fertility with dolutegravir up to 1,000 mg/kg/day. This dose is associated with an exposure that is approximately 24 times higher than the exposure in humans at the recommended dose of 50 mg twice daily.

Table 9 (cont.). Summary of Effect of Coadministered Drugs on the Pharmacokinetics of Dolutegravir

Coadministered Drug(s) and Dose(s)	Dose of TIVICAY	n	Geometric Mean Ratio (90% CI) of Dolutegravir Pharmacokinetic Parameters With/Without Coadministered Drugs No Effect = 1.00		
			C_max	AUC	C_τ or C_24
Rifampin[a] 600 mg once daily	50 mg twice daily	11	0.57 (0.49 to 0.65)	0.46 (0.38 to 0.55)	0.28 (0.23 to 0.34)
Rifampin[b] 600 mg once daily	50 mg twice daily	11	1.18 (1.03 to 1.37)	1.33 (1.15 to 1.53)	1.22 (1.01 to 1.48)
Rifabutin 300 mg once daily	50 mg once daily	9	1.16 (0.98 to 1.37)	0.95 (0.82 to 1.10)	0.70 (0.57 to 0.87)
Rilpivirine 25 mg once daily	50 mg once daily	16	1.13 (1.06 to 1.21)	1.12 (1.05 to 1.19)	1.22 (1.15 to 1.30)
Tipranavir/ritonavir 500/200 mg twice daily	50 mg once daily	14	0.54 (0.50 to 0.57)	0.41 (0.38 to 0.44)	0.24 (0.21 to 0.27)
Telaprevir 750 mg every 8 hours	50 mg once daily	15	1.18 (1.11 to 1.26)	1.25 (1.19 to 1.31)	1.40 (1.29 to 1.51)
Boceprevir 800 mg every 8 hours	50 mg once daily	13	1.05 (0.96 to 1.15)	1.07 (0.95 to 1.20)	1.08 (0.91 to 1.28)

[a]Comparison is rifampin taken with dolutegravir 50 mg twice daily compared with dolutegravir 50 mg twice daily.
[b]Comparison is rifampin taken with dolutegravir 50 mg twice daily compared with dolutegravir 50 mg once daily.

Table 12. Virologic Outcomes of Randomized Treatment in SPRING-2 and SINGLE at Week 48 (Snapshot Algorithm)

	SPRING-2		SINGLE	
	TIVICAY 50 mg Once Daily + 2 NRTIs (N = 403)	Raltegravir 400 mg Twice Daily + 2 NRTIs (N = 405)	TIVICAY 50 mg + EPZICOM Once Daily (N = 414)	ATRIPLA Once Daily (N = 419)
HIV-1 RNA <50 copies/mL	88%	86%	88%	81%
Treatment difference[a]	2.6% (95% CI: -1.9%, 7.2%)		7.4% (95% CI: 2.5%, 12.3%)	
Virologic nonresponse[b]	5%	7%	5%	6%
No virologic data at Week 48 window	7%	7%	7%	13%
Reasons				
Discontinued study/study drug due to adverse event or death[c]	2%	1%	2%	10%
Discontinued study/study drug for other reasons[d]	5%	6%	5%	3%
Missing data during window but on study	0	0	0	<1%
Proportion (%) of Subjects With HIV-1 RNA <50 copies/mL at Week 48 by Baseline Category				
Plasma viral load (copies/mL)				
≤100,000	91%	90%	90%	83%
>100,000	82%	75%	83%	76%
Gender				
Male	89%	86%	88%	82%
Female	84%	82%	85%	75%
Race				
White	88%	86%	90%	84%
Non-white	85%	85%	84%	74%

[a]Adjusted for pre-specified stratification factors.
[b]Includes subjects who changed BR to new class or changed BR not permitted per protocol or due to lack of efficacy prior to Week 48 (for SPRING-2 only), subjects who discontinued prior to Week 48 for lack or loss of efficacy, and subjects who were HIV-1 RNA ≥50 copies/mL in the Week 48 window.
[c]Includes subjects who discontinued due to an adverse event or death at any time point from Day 1 through the Week 48 window if this resulted in no virologic data on treatment during the Week 48 window.
[d]Other includes reasons such as withdrew consent, loss to follow-up, moved, and protocol deviation.

SPRING-2: Virologic outcomes were also comparable across baseline characteristics including CD4+ cell count, age, and use of EPZICOM or TRUVADA as NRTI background regimen. The median change in CD4+ cell counts from baseline for both groups was +230 cells/mm³ at 48 weeks.
SINGLE: Treatment differences were maintained across baseline characteristics including HIV-1 RNA, CD4+ cell count, age, gender, and race.

14 CLINICAL STUDIES
The efficacy of TIVICAY is based on analyses of data from 2 trials, SPRING-2 (ING113086) and SINGLE (ING114467), in treatment-naïve, HIV-1–infected subjects (n = 1,641); one trial, SAILING (ING111762), in treatment-experienced, INSTI-naïve HIV-1–infected subjects (n = 715); and from VIKING-3 (ING112574) trial in INSTI-experienced HIV-1–infected subjects (n = 183). The use of TIVICAY in pediatric patients aged 12 years and older is based on evaluation of safety, pharmacokinetics, and efficacy through 24 weeks in a multi-center, open-label trial in subjects (n = 23) without INSTI resistance.

14.1 Adult Subjects

Treatment-Naïve Subjects: The efficacy of TIVICAY in HIV-1–infected treatment-naïve adults is based on the analyses of 48-week data from 2 randomized, international, multicenter, double-blind, active-controlled trials, SPRING-2 and SINGLE.

In SPRING-2, 822 subjects were randomized and received at least 1 dose of either TIVICAY 50 mg once daily or raltegravir 400 mg twice daily, both in combination with fixed-dose dual NRTI treatment (either abacavir sulfate and lamivudine [EPZICOM] or emtricitabine/tenofovir [TRUVADA]). There were 808 subjects included in the efficacy and safety analyses. At baseline, the median age of subjects was 36 years, 13% female, 15% non-white, 11% had hepatitis B and/or C virus co-infection, 2% were CDC Class C (AIDS), 28% had HIV-1 RNA >100,000 copies/mL, 48% had CD4+ cell count <350 cells/mm^3, and 39% received EPZICOM; these characteristics were similar between treatment groups.

In SINGLE, 833 subjects were randomized and received at least 1 dose of either TIVICAY 50 mg once daily with fixed-dose abacavir sulfate and lamivudine (EPZICOM) or fixed-dose efavirenz/emtricitabine/tenofovir (ATRIPLA). At baseline, the median age of subjects was 35 years, 16% female, 32% non-white, 7% had hepatitis C co-infection (hepatitis B virus co-infection was excluded), 4% were CDC Class C (AIDS), 32% had HIV-1 RNA >100,000 copies/mL, and 53% had CD4+ cell count <350 cells/mm^3; these characteristics were similar between treatment groups.

Week 48 outcomes for SPRING-2 and SINGLE are provided in Table 12. Side-by-side tabulation is to simplify presentation; direct comparisons across trials should not be made due to differing trial designs.

[See table 12 at top of previous page]

The adjusted mean changes in CD4+ cell counts from baseline were 267 cells/mm^3 in the group receiving TIVICAY + EPZICOM and 208 cells/mm^3 for the ATRIPLA group at 48 weeks. The adjusted difference between treatment arms and 95% CI was 58.9 cells/mm^3 (33.4 cells/mm^3, 84.4 cells/mm^3) (adjusted for pre-specified stratification factors: baseline HIV-1 RNA, baseline CD4+ cell count, and multiplicity).

Treatment-Experienced, Integrase Strand Transfer Inhibitor-Naïve Subjects: In the international, multicenter, double-blind trial (SAILING), 719 HIV-1– infected, antiretroviral treatment-experienced adults were randomized and received either TIVICAY 50 mg once daily or raltegravir 400 mg twice daily with investigator selected background regimen consisting of up to 2 agents, including at least 1 fully active agent. There were 715 subjects included in the efficacy and safety analyses. At baseline, the median age was 43 years, 32% were female, 50% non-white, 16% had hepatitis B and/or C virus co-infection, 46% were CDC Class C (AIDS), 20% had HIV-1 RNA >100,000 copies/mL, and 72% had CD4+ cell count <350 cells/mm^3; these characteristics were similar between treatment groups. All subjects had at least 2-class antiretroviral treatment resistance, and 49% of subjects had at least 3-class antiretroviral treatment resistance at baseline. Week 24 outcomes for SAILING are shown in Table 13.

Table 13. Virologic Outcomes of Randomized Treatment in SAILING at 24 Weeks (Snapshot Algorithm)

	TIVICAY 50 mg Once Daily + BR^a (N = 354)	Raltegravir 400 mg Twice Daily + BR^a (N = 361)
HIV-1 RNA <50 copies/mL	79%	70%
Adjusted^b treatment difference	9.7% (95% CI: 3.4%, 15.9%)	
Virologic nonresponse	15%	24%
No virologic data at Week 24 window Reasons	6%	6%
Discontinued study/study drug due to adverse event or death	2%	2%
Discontinued study/study drug for other reasons^c	3%	3%
Missing data during window but on study	<1%	<1%

Proportion (%) With HIV-1 RNA <50 copies/mL at Week 24 by Baseline Category

Plasma viral load (copies/mL)		
≤50,000 copies/mL	83%	77%
>50,000 copies/mL	70%	53%

Background regimen		
No darunavir use or use of darunavir with primary PI substitutions	79%	67%
Use of darunavir without primary PI substitutions	80%	81%
Gender		
Male	78%	70%
Female	83%	69%
Race		
White	79%	69%
Non-white	80%	71%

^{a}BR = Background regimen. Background regimen was restricted to ≤2 antiretroviral treatments with at least 1 fully active agent.
^{b}Adjusted for pre-specified stratification factors.
^{c}Other includes reasons such as withdrew consent, loss to follow-up, moved, and protocol deviation.

Treatment differences were maintained across the baseline characteristics including CD4+ cell count and age.

The mean changes in CD4+ cell counts from baseline were 114 cells/mm^3 in the group receiving TIVICAY and 106 cells/mm^3 in the raltegravir group.

Treatment-Experienced, Integrase Strand Transfer Inhibitor-Experienced Subjects: VIKING-3 examined the effect of TIVICAY 50 mg twice daily over 7 days of functional monotherapy, followed by optimized background therapy with continued treatment of TIVICAY 50 mg twice daily.

In the multicenter, open-label, single-arm VIKING-3 trial, 183 HIV-1–infected, antiretroviral treatment-experienced adults with virological failure and current or historical evidence of raltegravir and/or elvitegravir resistance received TIVICAY 50 mg twice daily with the current failing background regimen for 7 days, then received TIVICAY with optimized background therapy from Day 8. A total of 183 subjects enrolled: 133 subjects with INSTI resistance at screening and 50 subjects with only historical evidence of resistance (and not at screening). At baseline, median age of subjects was 48 years; 23% were female, 29% non-white, and 20% had hepatitis B and/or C virus co-infection. Median baseline CD4+ cell count was 140 cells/mm^3, median duration of prior antiretroviral treatment was 13 years, and 56% were CDC Class C. Subjects showed multiple-class antiretroviral treatment resistance at baseline: 79% had ≥2 NRTI, 75% ≥1 NNRTI, and 71% ≥2 PI major substitutions; 62% had non-R5 virus.

Mean reduction from baseline in HIV-1 RNA at Day 8 (primary endpoint) was 1.4 log$_{10}$ (95% CI: 1.3 log$_{10}$, 1.5 log$_{10}$). Response at Week 24 was affected by baseline INSTI substitutions [see Microbiology (12.4)].

After the functional monotherapy phase, subjects had the opportunity to re-optimize their background regimen when possible. Week 24 virologic outcomes for VIKING-3 are shown in Table 14.

Table 14. Virologic Outcomes of Treatment of VIKING-3 at 24 Weeks (Snapshot Algorithm)

	TIVICAY 50 mg Twice Daily + Optimized Background Therapy (N = 114)
HIV-1 RNA <50 copies/mL	63%
Virologic nonresponse No virologic data at Week 24 Reasons	32%
Discontinued study/study drug due to adverse event or death	4%

Proportion (%) With HIV-1 RNA <50 copies/mL at Week 24 by Baseline Category

Gender	
Male	64%
Female	60%
Race	
White	67%
Non-white	52%

Subjects harboring virus with Q148 and with additional Q148-associated secondary substitutions also had a reduced response at Week 24 in a stepwise fashion [see Microbiology (12.4)].

The median change in CD4+ cell count from baseline was 65 cells/mm^3 at Week 24.

14.2 Pediatric Subjects

IMPAACT P1093 is a Phase 1/2, 48-week, multicenter, open-label trial to evaluate the pharmacokinetic parameters, safety, tolerability, and efficacy of TIVICAY in combination treatment regimens in HIV-1–infected infants, children, and adolescents.

The initial dose-finding stage included intensive pharmacokinetic evaluation in 10 INSTI-naïve subjects (aged 12 to 18 years). Dose selection was based upon achieving similar dolutegravir plasma exposure and trough concentration as seen in adults. After dose selection, an additional 13 subjects were enrolled for evaluation of long-term safety, tolerability, and efficacy.

These 23 subjects had a mean age of 14 years (range: 12 to 17), were 78% female and 52% black. At baseline, mean plasma HIV-1 RNA was 4.3 log$_{10}$ copies/mL, median CD4+ cell count was 466 cells/mm3 (range: 11 to 1,025), and median CD4+% was 22% (range: 1% to 39%). Overall, 17% had baseline plasma HIV-1 RNA >50,000 copies/mL and 39% had a CDC HIV clinical classification of category C. Most subjects had previously used at least 1 NNRTI (52%) or 1 PI (78%).

At 24 weeks, 70% of subjects treated with TIVICAY once daily (35 mg: n = 4, 50 mg: n = 19) plus optimized background therapy achieved a viral load <50 copies/mL. The median CD4+ cell count (percent) increase from baseline to Week 24 was 63 cells/mm3 (5%).

16 HOW SUPPLIED/STORAGE AND HANDLING

TIVICAY Tablets, 50 mg, are yellow, round, film-coated, biconvex tablets debossed with SV 572 on one side and 50 on the other side.

Bottle of 30 tablets with child-resistant closure NDC 49702-228-13.

Store at 25°C (77°F); excursions permitted 157° to 30°C (59° to 86°F) [See USP Controlled Room Temperature].

17 PATIENT COUNSELING INFORMATION

Advise the patient to read the FDA-approved patient labeling (Patient Information).

Drug Interactions: TIVICAY should not be coadministered with dofetilide because interactions between these drugs can result in potentially life-threatening adverse events [see Contraindications (4)].

Hypersensitivity Reactions: Patients should be advised to immediately contact their healthcare provider if they develop rash. Instruct patients to immediately stop taking TIVICAY and other suspect agents, and seek medical attention if they develop a rash associated with any of the following symptoms, as it may be a sign of a more serious reaction such as severe hypersensitivity: fever; generally ill feeling; extreme tiredness; muscle or joint aches; blisters or peeling of the skin; oral blisters or lesions; eye inflammation; facial swelling; swelling of the eyes, lips, tongue, or mouth; breathing difficulty; and/or signs and symptoms of liver problems (e.g., yellowing of the skin or whites of the eyes, dark or tea-colored urine, pale-colored stools or bowel movements, nausea, vomiting, loss of appetite, or pain, aching, or sensitivity on the right side below the ribs). Patients should understand that if hypersensitivity occurs, they will be closely monitored, laboratory tests will be ordered, and appropriate therapy will be initiated. Patients should also be told that it is very important that they remain under a physician's care during treatment with TIVICAY [see Warnings and Precautions (5.1)].

Effects on Serum Liver Biochemistries in Patients With Hepatitis B or C Co-infection: Patients with underlying hepatitis B or C may be at increased risk for worsening or development of transaminase elevations with use of TIVICAY and should be advised that they are recommended to have laboratory testing before and during therapy [see Warnings and Precautions (5.2)].

Fat Redistribution: Patients should be informed that redistribution or accumulation of body fat may occur in patients receiving antiretroviral therapy and that the cause and long–term health effects of these conditions are not known at this time [see Warnings and Precautions (5.3)].

Immune Reconstitution Syndrome: In some patients with advanced HIV infection, signs and symptoms of inflammation from previous infections may occur soon after anti-HIV treatment is started. It is believed that these symptoms are due to an improvement in the body's immune response, enabling the body to fight infections that may have been present with no obvious symptoms. Patients should be advised to inform their healthcare provider immediately of any symptoms of infection [see Warnings and Precautions (5.4)].

Information About HIV–1 Infection: TIVICAY is not a cure for HIV–1 infection and patients may continue to experience illnesses associated with HIV–1 infection, including opportunistic infections. Patients must remain on continuous HIV therapy to control HIV infection and decrease HIV-related illness. Patients should be told that sustained decreases in plasma HIV RNA have been associated with a reduced risk of progression to AIDS and death. Patients should remain under the care of a physician when using TIVICAY.

Patients should be informed to take all HIV medications exactly as prescribed.

Patients should be advised to avoid doing things that can spread HIV-1 infection to others.

- **Do not re-use or share needles or other injection equipment.**
- **Do not share personal items that can have blood or body fluids on them, like toothbrushes and razor blades.**
- Continue to practice safe sex by using a latex or polyurethane condom to lower the chance of sexual contact with semen, vaginal secretions, or blood.
- Female patients should be advised not to breastfeed because it is not known if TIVICAY can be passed to the baby in your breast milk and whether it could harm the baby. Mothers with HIV-1 should not breastfeed because HIV-1 can be passed to the baby in the breast milk.

Physicians should instruct their patients to read the Patient Information before starting TIVICAY and to reread it each time the prescription is renewed. Patients should be instructed to inform their physician or pharmacist if they develop any unusual symptom, or if any known symptom persists or worsens.

Physicians should instruct their patients that if they miss a dose, they should take it as soon as they remember. If they do not remember until it is within 4 hours of the time for the next dose, they should be instructed to skip the missed dose and go back to the regular schedule. Patients should not double their next dose or take more than the prescribed dose.

TIVICAY and EPZICOM are registered trademarks of the ViiV Healthcare group of companies.

The other brands listed are trademarks of their respective owners and are not trademarks of the ViiV Healthcare group of companies. The makers of these brands are not affiliated with and do not endorse the ViiV Healthcare group of companies or its products.

Manufactured for:

ViiV Healthcare

Research Triangle Park, NC 27709

by:

GlaxoSmithKline

Research Triangle Park, NC 27709

©2014, the ViiV Healthcare group of companies. All rights reserved.

TVC:2PI

Patient Information

TIVICAY® (TIV-eh-kay)

(dolutegravir)

Tablets

Read this Patient Information before you start taking TIVICAY and each time you get a refill. There may be new information. This information does not take the place of talking with your healthcare provider about your medical condition or treatment.

What is TIVICAY?

TIVICAY is a prescription HIV medicine that is used with other antiretroviral medicines to treat Human Immunodeficiency Virus-1 (HIV-1) infections in adults and children 12 years of age and older and weighing at least 88 pounds.

HIV-1 is the virus that causes Acquired Immune Deficiency Syndrome (AIDS).

It is not known if TIVICAY is safe and effective in children under 12 years of age or who weigh less than 88 pounds.

When used with other HIV-1 medicines to treat HIV-1 infection, TIVICAY may help:

- Reduce the amount of HIV-1 in your blood. This is called "viral load".
- Increase the number of white blood cells called CD4+ (T) cells in your blood, which help fight off other infections.
- Reduce the amount of HIV-1 and increase the CD4+ (T) cells in your blood which may help improve your immune system. This may reduce your risk of death or getting infections that can happen when your immune system is weak (opportunistic infections).

TIVICAY does not cure HIV-1 infection or AIDS. You must stay on continuous HIV-1 therapy to control HIV-1 infection and decrease HIV-related illnesses.

Avoid doing things that can spread HIV-1 infection to others.

- Do not share or re-use needles or other injection equipment.
- Do not share personal items that can have blood or body fluids on them, like toothbrushes and razor blades.
- Do not have any kind of sex without protection. Always practice safe sex by using a latex or polyurethane condom

to lower the chance of sexual contact with any body fluids such as semen, vaginal secretions, or blood.

Ask your healthcare provider if you have any questions about how to prevent passing HIV to other people.

Who should not take TIVICAY?

Do not take TIVICAY if you take dofetilide. Taking TIVICAY and dofetilide can cause side effects that may be life-threatening.

What should I tell my healthcare provider before taking TIVICAY?

Before you take TIVICAY, tell your healthcare provider if you:

- have ever had an allergic reaction to TIVICAY
- have or had liver problems, including hepatitis B or C infection
- have any other medical condition
- are pregnant or plan to become pregnant. It is not known if TIVICAY will harm your unborn baby. Tell your healthcare provider if you become pregnant while taking TIVICAY.

Pregnancy Registry. There is a pregnancy registry for women who take antiviral medicines during pregnancy. The purpose of the registry is to collect information about the health of you and your baby. Talk to your healthcare provider about how you can take part in this registry.

- are breastfeeding or plan to breastfeed. **Do not breastfeed if you take TIVICAY.**
  - You should not breastfeed if you have HIV-1 because of the risk of passing HIV-1 to your baby.
  - It is not known if TIVICAY passes into your breast milk.
  - Talk to your healthcare provider about the best way to feed your baby.

Tell your healthcare provider about the medicines you take, including prescription and over-the-counter medicines, vitamins, or herbal supplements.

TIVICAY and other medicines may affect each other causing side effects. TIVICAY may affect the way other medicines work, and other medicines may affect how TIVICAY works. Especially tell your healthcare provider if you take:

- other HIV-1 medicines including: efavirenz (SUSTIVA®), etravirine (INTELENCE®), fosamprenavir (LEXIVA®)/ritonavir (NORVIR®), nevirapine (VIRAMUNE®), or tipranavir (APTIVUS®)/ritonavir (NORVIR).
- antacids or laxatives that contain aluminum, magnesium, sucralfate (CARAFATE®), or buffered medicines. TIVICAY should be taken at least 2 hours before or 6 hours after you take these medicines.
- iron or calcium supplements. Supplements including multivitamins containing calcium or iron may be taken at the same time with TIVICAY if taken with food. Otherwise, TIVICAY should be taken at least 2 hours before or 6 hours after you take these medicines.
- anti-seizure medicines:
  - oxcarbazepine (TRILEPTAL®)
  - phenytoin (DILANTIN®, DILANTIN®-125, PHENYTEK®)
  - phenobarbital (LUMINAL®)
  - carbamazepine (CARBATROL®, EQUETRO®, TEGRETOL®, TEGRETOL®-XR, TERIL®, EPITOL®)
- St. John's wort (*Hypericum perforatum*)
- a medicine that contains metformin
- rifampin (RIFATER®, RIFAMATE®, RIMACTANE®, RIFADIN®)

Ask your healthcare provider or pharmacist if you are not sure if your medicine is one that is listed above.

Know the medicines you take. Keep a list of them to show your healthcare provider and pharmacist when you get a new medicine.

How should I take TIVICAY?

- Take TIVICAY exactly as your healthcare provider tells you.
- Do not change your dose or stop taking TIVICAY without talking with your healthcare provider.
- Stay under the care of a healthcare provider while taking TIVICAY.
- You can take TIVICAY with or without food.
- If you miss a dose of TIVICAY, take it as soon as you remember. If it is within 4 hours of your next dose, skip the missed dose and take the next dose at your regular time. Do not take 2 doses at the same time. If you are not sure about your dosing, call your healthcare provider.
- If you take too much TIVICAY, call your healthcare provider or go to the nearest hospital emergency room right away.
- Do not run out of TIVICAY. The virus in your blood may become resistant to other HIV-1 medicines if TIVICAY is stopped for even a short time. When your supply starts to run low, get more from your healthcare provider or pharmacy.

What are the possible side effects of TIVICAY?

TIVICAY may cause serious side effects, including:

- **Allergic reactions.** Call your healthcare provider right away if you develop a rash with TIVICAY. **Stop taking TIVICAY and get medical help right away if you:**

- develop a rash with any of the following signs or symptoms:
  - fever
  - generally ill feeling
  - extreme tiredness
  - muscle or joint aches
  - blisters or sores in mouth
  - blisters or peeling of the skin
  - redness or swelling of the eyes
  - swelling of the mouth, face, lips, or tongue
  - problems breathing
- develop any of the following signs or symptoms of liver problems:
  - yellowing of the skin or whites of the eyes
  - dark or tea-colored urine
  - pale-colored stools or bowel movements
  - nausea or vomiting
  - loss of appetite
  - pain, aching, or tenderness on the right side below the ribs
- **Changes in liver tests.** People with a history of hepatitis B or C virus may have an increased risk of developing new or worsening changes in certain liver tests during treatment with TIVICAY. Your healthcare provider may do tests to check your liver function before and during treatment with TIVICAY.
- **Changes in body fat** can happen in people who take HIV-1 medicines. These changes may include increased amount of fat in the upper back and neck ("buffalo hump"), breast, and around the middle of your body (trunk). Loss of fat from the legs, arms, and face may also happen. The exact cause and long-term health effects of these problems are not known.
- **Changes in your immune system (Immune Reconstitution Syndrome)** can happen when you start taking HIV-1 medicines. Your immune system may get stronger and begin to fight infections that have been hidden in your body for a long time. Tell your healthcare provider right away if you start having new symptoms after starting your HIV-1 medicine.

The most common side effects of TIVICAY include:

- trouble sleeping
- headache

Tell your healthcare provider about any side effect that bothers you or that does not go away.

These are not all the possible side effects of TIVICAY. For more information, ask your healthcare provider or pharmacist.

Call your doctor for medical advice about side effects. You may report side effects to FDA at 1–800–FDA–1088.

How should I store TIVICAY?

- Store TIVICAY at room temperature between 68°F to 77°F (20°C to 25°C).

Keep TIVICAY and all medicines out of the reach of children.

General information about TIVICAY

Medicines are sometimes prescribed for purposes other than those listed in a Patient Information leaflet. Do not use TIVICAY for a condition for which it was not prescribed. Do not give TIVICAY to other people, even if they have the same symptoms you have. It may harm them.

You can ask your pharmacist or healthcare provider for information about TIVICAY that is written for health professionals.

For more information call 1-877-844-8872 or go to www.TIVICAY.com.

What are the ingredients in TIVICAY?

Active ingredient: dolutegravir sodium

Inactive ingredients: d-mannitol, microcrystalline cellulose, povidone K29/32, sodium starch glycolate, and sodium stearyl fumarate. The tablet film-coating contains the inactive ingredients iron oxide yellow, macrogol/PEG, polyvinyl alcohol-part hydrolyzed, talc, and titanium dioxide.

This Patient Information has been approved by the U.S. Food and Drug Administration.

Manufactured for:

ViiV Healthcare

Research Triangle Park, NC 27709

by:

GlaxoSmithKline

Research Triangle Park, NC 27709

May 2014

TVC:2PIL

©2014, the ViiV Healthcare group of companies. All rights reserved.

TIVICAY and LEXIVA are registered trademarks of the ViiV Healthcare group of companies.

The brands listed are trademarks of their respective owners and are not trademarks of the ViiV Healthcare group of companies. The makers of these brands are not affiliated with and do not endorse the ViiV Healthcare group of companies or its products.

TRIUMEQ
(abacavir, dolutegravir, and lamivudine)
tablets for oral use

℞

HIGHLIGHTS OF PRESCRIBING INFORMATION
These highlights do not include all the information needed to use TRIUMEQ safely and effectively. See full prescribing information for TRIUMEQ.
TRIUMEQ (abacavir, dolutegravir, and lamivudine) tablets for oral use
Initial U.S. Approval: 2014

WARNING: HYPERSENSITIVITY REACTIONS, LACTIC ACIDOSIS AND SEVERE HEPATOMEGALY, AND EXACERBATIONS OF HEPATITIS B
See full prescribing information for complete boxed warning.
- Serious and sometimes fatal hypersensitivity reactions have been associated with abacavir-containing products. (5.1)
- Hypersensitivity to abacavir is a multi-organ clinical syndrome. (5.1)
- Patients who carry the HLA–B*5701 allele are at high risk for experiencing a hypersensitivity reaction to abacavir. (5.1)
- Discontinue TRIUMEQ as soon as a hypersensitivity reaction is suspected. Regardless of HLA-B*5701 status, permanently discontinue TRIUMEQ if hypersensitivity cannot be ruled out, even when other diagnoses are possible. (5.1)
- Following a hypersensitivity reaction to abacavir, NEVER restart TRIUMEQ or any other abacavir–containing product. (5.1)
- Lactic acidosis and severe hepatomegaly with steatosis, including fatal cases, have been reported with the use of nucleoside analogues. (5.2)
- Severe acute exacerbations of hepatitis B have been reported in patients who are co–infected with hepatitis B virus (HBV) and human immunodeficiency virus (HIV–1) and have discontinued lamivudine, a component of TRIUMEQ. Monitor hepatic function closely in these patients and, if appropriate, initiate anti-hepatitis B treatment. (5.3)

——INDICATIONS AND USAGE——
TRIUMEQ, a combination of dolutegravir (integrase strand transfer inhibitor [INSTI]), abacavir, and lamivudine (both nucleoside analogue reverse transcriptase inhibitors) is indicated for the treatment of HIV-1 infection. (1)
Limitations of Use:
- TRIUMEQ alone is not recommended for use in patients with current or past history of resistance to any components of TRIUMEQ. (12.4)
- TRIUMEQ alone is not recommended in patients with resistance-associated integrase substitutions or clinically suspected integrase strand transfer inhibitor resistance because the dose of dolutegravir in TRIUMEQ is insufficient in these subpopulations. See the dolutegravir prescribing information. (1)

——DOSAGE AND ADMINISTRATION——
- Before initiating TRIUMEQ, screen for the HLA-B*5701 allele because TRIUMEQ contains abacavir. (2.1)
- Adults: One tablet daily. May be taken with or without food. (2.2)
- Dosing with certain concomitant medications: If efavirenz, fosamprenavir/ritonavir, tipranavir/ritonavir, or rifampin are coadministered, then the recommended dolutegravir dosage regimen is 50 mg twice daily. An additional 50-mg dose of dolutegravir, separated by 12 hours from TRIUMEQ, should be taken. (2.3)

——DOSAGE FORMS AND STRENGTHS——
Tablets: 600 mg of abacavir, 50 mg of dolutegravir, and 300 mg of lamivudine. (3)

——CONTRAINDICATIONS——
- Presence of HLA-B*5701 allele. (4)
- Previous hypersensitivity reaction to abacavir, dolutegravir, or lamivudine. (4)
- Coadministration with dofetilide. (4)
- Moderate or severe hepatic impairment. (4, 8.7)

——WARNINGS AND PRECAUTIONS——
- Patients with underlying hepatitis B or C may be at increased risk for worsening or development of transaminase elevations with use of TRIUMEQ. Appropriate laboratory testing prior to initiating therapy and monitoring for hepatotoxicity during therapy with TRIUMEQ is recommended in patients with underlying hepatic disease such as hepatitis B or C. (5.3)
- Hepatic decompensation, some fatal, has occurred in HIV-1/HCV co–infected patients receiving combination antiretroviral therapy and interferon alfa with or without ribavirin. Discontinue TRIUMEQ as medically appropriate and consider dose reduction or discontinuation of interferon alfa, ribavirin, or both. (5.4)
- Immune reconstitution syndrome and redistribution/accumulation of body fat have been reported in patients treated with combination antiretroviral therapy. (5.5, 5.6)
- Administration of TRIUMEQ is not recommended in patients receiving other products containing abacavir, or lamivudine. (5.8)

——ADVERSE REACTIONS——
The most commonly reported adverse reactions of at least moderate intensity and incidence at least 2% (in those receiving TRIUMEQ) were insomnia, headache and fatigue. (6.1)
To report SUSPECTED ADVERSE REACTIONS, contact ViiV Healthcare at 1-877-844-8872 or FDA at 1-800-FDA-1088 or www.fda.gov/medwatch

——DRUG INTERACTIONS——
Coadministration of TRIUMEQ with other drugs can alter the concentration of other drugs and other drugs may alter the concentrations of TRIUMEQ. The potential drug-drug interactions must be considered prior to and during therapy. (4, 7, 12.3)

——USE IN SPECIFIC POPULATIONS——
- Pregnancy: TRIUMEQ should be used during pregnancy only if the potential benefit justifies the potential risk. (8.1)
- Nursing mothers: Breastfeeding is not recommended due to the potential for HIV transmission. (8.3)
- TRIUMEQ is not recommended in patients with creatinine clearance less than 50 mL per min. (8.6)
- If a dose reduction of abacavir, a component of TRIUMEQ, is required for patients with mild hepatic impairment, then the individual components should be used. (8.7)

See 17 for PATIENT COUNSELING INFORMATION and Medication Guide

Revised: 08/2014

FULL PRESCRIBING INFORMATION: CONTENTS*

FULL PRESCRIBING INFORMATION

WARNING: HYPERSENSITIVITY REACTIONS, LACTIC ACIDOSIS AND SEVERE HEPATOMEGALY, AND EXACERBATIONS OF HEPATITIS B

Hypersensitivity Reactions
Serious and sometimes fatal hypersensitivity reactions, with multiple organ involvement, have been associated with abacavir, a component of TRIUMEQ®. Patients who carry the HLA–B*5701 allele are at a higher risk of a hypersensitivity reaction to abacavir; although, hypersensitivity reactions have occurred in patients who do not carry the HLA–B*5701 allele. *[see Warnings and Precautions (5.1)]*.
All patients should be screened for the HLA-B*5701 allele prior to initiating therapy with TRIUMEQ or re-initiation of therapy with TRIUMEQ unless patients have had an HLA-B*5701 allele assessment. Discontinue TRIUMEQ if a hypersensitivity reaction is suspected. TRIUMEQ is contraindicated in patients who have the HLA-B*5701 allele or in patients with a prior hypersensitivity reaction to abacavir *[see Contraindications (4), Warnings and Precautions (5.1)]*. Reintroduction of TRIUMEQ or any other abacavir-containing product can result in life-threatening or fatal hypersensitivity reactions, even in patients who have no history of hypersensitivity to abacavir therapy. Such reactions can occur within hours *[see Warnings and Precautions (5.1)]*.

Lactic Acidosis and Severe Hepatomegaly
Lactic acidosis and severe hepatomegaly with steatosis, including fatal cases, have been reported with the use of nucleoside analogues alone or in combination, including abacavir, lamivudine, and other antiretrovirals. Discontinue TRIUMEQ if clinical or laboratory findings suggestive of lactic acidosis or pronounced hepatotoxicity occur *[see Warnings and Precautions (5.2)]*.

Exacerbations of Hepatitis B
Severe acute exacerbations of hepatitis B have been reported in patients who are co–infected with hepatitis B virus (HBV) and human immunodeficiency virus (HIV-1) and have discontinued lamivudine, one component of TRIUMEQ. Hepatic function should be monitored closely with both clinical and laboratory follow-up for at least several months in patients who discontinue TRIUMEQ and are co-infected with HIV-1 and HBV. If appropriate, initiation of anti–hepatitis B therapy may be warranted *[see Warnings and Precautions (5.3)]*.

---

1   INDICATIONS AND USAGE
TRIUMEQ is indicated for the treatment of human immunodeficiency virus type 1 (HIV-1) infection.
Limitations of Use:
- TRIUMEQ alone is not recommended for use in patients with current or past history of resistance to any components of TRIUMEQ *[see Microbiology (12.4)]*.
- TRIUMEQ alone is not recommended in patients with resistance-associated integrase substitutions or clinically suspected integrase strand transfer inhibitor resistance because the dose of dolutegravir in TRIUMEQ is insufficient in these subpopulations. See full prescribing information for dolutegravir.

2   DOSAGE AND ADMINISTRATION
2.1   Screening for HLA–B*5701 Allele Prior to Starting TRIUMEQ
Screen for the HLA–B*5701 allele prior to initiating therapy with TRIUMEQ *[see Boxed Warning, Warnings and Precautions (5.1)]*.
2.2   Recommended Dosage
TRIUMEQ is a fixed-dose combination product containing 600 mg of abacavir, 50 mg of dolutegravir, and 300 mg of lamivudine. The recommended dosage regimen of TRIUMEQ in adults is one tablet once daily orally with or without food.
2.3   Dosage Recommendation with Certain Concomitant Medications
The dolutegravir dose (50 mg) in TRIUMEQ is insufficient when coadministered with medications listed in Table 1 that may decrease dolutegravir concentrations; the following dolutegravir dosage regimen is recommended.

Table 1. Dosing Recommendations for TRIUMEQ with Coadministered Medications

Coadministered Drug	Dosing Recommendation
Efavirenz, fosamprenavir/ ritonavir, tipranavir/ ritonavir, or rifampin	The recommended dolutegravir dosage regimen is 50 mg twice daily. An additional dolutegravir 50-mg tablet, separated by 12 hours from TRIUMEQ, should be taken.

3 DOSAGE FORMS AND STRENGTHS

TRIUMEQ tablets are purple, biconvex, oval, and debossed with "572 Tri" on one side. Each film-coated tablet contains abacavir sulfate equivalent to 600 mg of abacavir, dolutegravir sodium equivalent to 50 mg of dolutegravir, and 300 mg of lamivudine [see Description (11)].

4 CONTRAINDICATION

TRIUMEQ is contraindicated in patients:
- who have the HLA-B*5701 allele [see Warnings and Precautions (5.1)].
- with previous hypersensitivity reaction to abacavir. Before starting TRIUMEQ, review medical history for prior exposure to any abacavir-containing product. NEVER restart TRIUMEQ or any other abacavir-containing product following a hypersensitivity reaction to abacavir, regardless of HLA-B*5701 status [see Warnings and Precautions (5.1)].
- with previous hypersensitivity reaction to dolutegravir [see Warnings and Precautions (5.1)] or lamivudine.
- receiving dofetilide, due to the potential for increased dofetilide plasma concentrations and the risk for serious and/or life-threatening events with concomitant use of dolutegravir [see Drug Interactions (7)].
- with moderate or severe hepatic impairment [see Use in Specific Populations (8.7)].

5 WARNINGS AND PRECAUTIONS

5.1 Hypersensitivity Reaction

Hypersensitivity reactions have been reported with the use of abacavir or dolutegravir, components of TRIUMEQ.

Abacavir: Serious and sometimes fatal hypersensitivity reactions have been associated with abacavir-containing regimens. See full prescribing information for ZIAGEN® (abacavir). Patients who carry the HLA-B*5701 allele are at high risk for experiencing a hypersensitivity reaction to abacavir. All patients should be screened for the HLA-B*5701 allele prior to initiating therapy with abacavir or reinitiation of abacavir therapy unless HLA-B*5701 information is available. Do not treat HLA-B*5701-positive patients with an abacavir-containing regimen [see Contraindications (4)].

HLA-B*5701-negative patients may develop a hypersensitivity reaction to abacavir; however, this occurs significantly less frequently than in HLA-B*5701-positive patients. Regardless of HLA-B*5701 status, permanently discontinue TRIUMEQ if hypersensitivity cannot be ruled out, even when other diagnoses are possible.

Symptoms indicating a multi-organ clinical syndrome usually appear within the first 6 weeks of treatment with abacavir (median time to onset was 9 days), although the reaction may occur at any time during therapy. The reaction is typically characterized by the presentation of key signs or symptoms in 2 or more of the following groups: (1) fever; (2) rash; (3) gastrointestinal (including nausea, vomiting, diarrhea, or abdominal pain); (4) constitutional (including generalized malaise, fatigue, or achiness); (5) respiratory (including dyspnea, cough, or pharyngitis).

Other signs and symptoms of hypersensitivity include lethargy, headache, myolysis, edema, abnormal chest x-ray findings (predominantly infiltrates, which can be localized), arthralgia, and paresthesia. Anaphylaxis, liver failure, renal failure, hypotension, adult respiratory distress syndrome, respiratory failure, and death have occurred in association with hypersensitivity reactions. Physical findings associated with hypersensitivity to abacavir in some subjects include lymphadenopathy, mucous membrane lesions (conjunctivitis and mouth ulcerations), and rash. The rash usually appears maculopapular or urticarial, but may be variable in appearance. There have been reports of erythema multiforme. Hypersensitivity reactions have occurred without rash.

Laboratory abnormalities associated with hypersensitivity to abacavir in some subjects include elevated liver function tests, elevated creatine phosphokinase, elevated creatinine, and lymphopenia.

Clinical Management of Abacavir Hypersensitivity: Discontinue TRIUMEQ as soon as a hypersensitivity reaction is suspected. To minimize the risk of a life-threatening hypersensitivity reaction, permanently discontinue TRIUMEQ if hypersensitivity cannot be ruled out, even when other diagnoses are possible (e.g., acute onset respiratory diseases such as pneumonia, bronchitis, pharyngitis, or influenza; gastroenteritis; or reactions to other medications).

Following a hypersensitivity reaction to abacavir, NEVER restart TRIUMEQ or any other abacavir-containing product because more severe symptoms can occur within hours and may include life-threatening hypotension and death.

When therapy with TRIUMEQ has been discontinued for reasons other than symptoms of a hypersensitivity reaction, and if reinitiation of TRIUMEQ or any other abacavir-containing product is under consideration, carefully evaluate the reason for discontinuation of TRIUMEQ to ensure that the patient did not have symptoms of a hypersensitivity reaction.

If hypersensitivity cannot be ruled out, DO NOT reintroduce TRIUMEQ or any other abacavir-containing product.

If symptoms consistent with abacavir hypersensitivity are not identified, reintroduction can be undertaken with continued monitoring for symptoms of a hypersensitivity reaction. Make patients aware that a hypersensitivity reaction can occur with reintroduction of TRIUMEQ or any other abacavir-containing product and that reintroduction of TRIUMEQ or introduction of any other abacavir-containing product needs to be undertaken only if medical care can be readily accessed by the patient or others.

In any patient treated with abacavir, the clinical diagnosis of hypersensitivity reaction must remain the basis of clinical decision-making. Even in the absence of the HLA-B*5701 allele, it is important to permanently discontinue abacavir and not rechallenge with abacavir if a hypersensitivity reaction cannot be ruled out on clinical grounds, due to the potential for a severe or even fatal reaction.

Dolutegravir: Hypersensitivity reactions have been reported and were characterized by rash, constitutional findings, and sometimes organ dysfunction, including liver injury. The events were reported in less than 1% of subjects receiving TIVICAY® in Phase 3 clinical trials. Discontinue TRIUMEQ and other suspect agents immediately if signs or symptoms of hypersensitivity reactions develop (including, but not limited to, severe rash or rash accompanied by fever, general malaise, fatigue, muscle or joint aches, blisters or peeling of the skin, oral blisters or lesions, conjunctivitis, facial edema, hepatitis, eosinophilia, angioedema, difficulty breathing). Clinical status, including liver aminotransferases, should be monitored and appropriate therapy initiated. Delay in stopping treatment with TRIUMEQ or other suspect agents after the onset of hypersensitivity may result in a life-threatening reaction.

Clinically, it is not possible to determine whether a hypersensitivity reaction with TRIUMEQ would be caused by abacavir or dolutegravir. Therefore, never restart TRIUMEQ or any other abacavir- or dolutegravir-containing product in patients who have stopped therapy with TRIUMEQ due to a hypersensitivity reaction.

5.2 Lactic Acidosis and Severe Hepatomegaly with Steatosis

Lactic acidosis and severe hepatomegaly with steatosis, including fatal cases, have been reported with the use of nucleoside analogues and other antiretrovirals. See full prescribing information for ZIAGEN (abacavir) and EPIVIR® (lamivudine). Treatment with TRIUMEQ should be suspended in any patient who develops clinical or laboratory findings suggestive of lactic acidosis or pronounced hepatotoxicity (which may include hepatomegaly and steatosis even in the absence of marked transaminase elevations).

5.3 Patients with Hepatitis B or C Virus Co-infection

Effects on Serum Liver Biochemistries: Patients with underlying hepatitis B or C may be at increased risk for worsening or development of transaminase elevations with use of TRIUMEQ [see Adverse Reactions (6.1)]. See full prescribing information for TIVICAY (dolutegravir). In some cases the elevations in transaminases were consistent with immune reconstitution syndrome or hepatitis B reactivation particularly in the setting where anti-hepatitis therapy was withdrawn. Appropriate laboratory testing prior to initiating therapy and monitoring for hepatotoxicity during therapy with TRIUMEQ are recommended in patients with underlying hepatic disease such as hepatitis B or C.

Posttreatment-exacerbations of Hepatitis: Clinical and laboratory evidence of exacerbations of hepatitis have occurred after discontinuation of lamivudine. See full prescribing information for EPIVIR (lamivudine). Patients should be closely monitored with both clinical and laboratory follow-up for at least several months after stopping treatment.

Emergence of Lamivudine-resistant HBV: Safety and efficacy of lamivudine have not been established for treatment of chronic hepatitis B in subjects dually infected with HIV-1 and HBV. Emergence of hepatitis B virus variants associated with resistance to lamivudine has also been reported in HIV-1-infected subjects who have received lamivudine-containing antiretroviral regimens in the presence of concurrent infection with hepatitis B virus. See full prescribing information for EPIVIR (lamivudine).

5.4 Use with Interferon- and Ribavirin-based Regimens

Patients receiving interferon alfa with or without ribavirin and TRIUMEQ should be closely monitored for treatment-associated toxicities, especially hepatic decompensation. See full prescribing information for EPIVIR (lamivudine). Discontinuation of TRIUMEQ should be considered as medically appropriate. Dose reduction or discontinuation of interferon alfa, ribavirin, or both should also be considered if worsening clinical toxicities are observed, including hepatic decompensation (e.g., Child-Pugh greater than 6) (see full prescribing information for interferon and ribavirin).

5.5 Immune Reconstitution Syndrome

Immune reconstitution syndrome has been reported in patients treated with combination antiretroviral therapy, including TRIUMEQ. During the initial phase of combination antiretroviral treatment, patients whose immune systems respond may develop an inflammatory response to indolent or residual opportunistic infections (such as Mycobacterium avium infection, cytomegalovirus, Pneumocystis jirovecii pneumonia [PCP], or tuberculosis), which may necessitate further evaluation and treatment.

Autoimmune disorders (such as Graves' disease, polymyositis, and Guillain-Barré syndrome) have also been reported to occur in the setting of immune reconstitution; however, the time to onset is more variable, and can occur many months after initiation of treatment.

5.6 Fat Redistribution

Redistribution/accumulation of body fat including central obesity, dorsocervical fat enlargement (buffalo hump), peripheral wasting, facial wasting, breast enlargement, and "cushingoid appearance" have been observed in patients receiving antiretroviral therapy. The mechanism and long-term consequences of these events are currently unknown. A causal relationship has not been established.

5.7 Myocardial Infarction

In a published prospective, observational, epidemiological trial designed to investigate the rate of myocardial infarction (MI) in patients on combination antiretroviral therapy, the use of abacavir within the previous 6 months was correlated with an increased risk of MI. In a sponsor-conducted pooled analysis of clinical trials, no excess risk of MI was observed in abacavir-treated subjects as compared with control subjects. In totality, the available data from the observational cohort and from clinical trials are inconclusive.

As a precaution, the underlying risk of coronary heart disease should be considered when prescribing antiretroviral therapies, including abacavir, and action taken to minimize all modifiable risk factors (e.g., hypertension, hyperlipidemia, diabetes mellitus, smoking).

5.8 Related Products that are Not Recommended

TRIUMEQ contains fixed doses of an INSTI (dolutegravir) and 2 nucleoside analogue reverse transcriptase inhibitors (abacavir and lamivudine); concomitant administration of TRIUMEQ with other products containing abacavir or lamivudine is not recommended.

6 ADVERSE REACTIONS

The following adverse reactions are discussed in other sections of the labeling:
- Serious and sometimes fatal hypersensitivity reaction [see Boxed Warning, Warnings and Precautions (5.1)].
- Lactic acidosis and severe hepatomegaly [see Boxed Warning, Warnings and Precautions (5.2)].
- Effects on serum liver biochemistries in patients with hepatitis B or C co-infection [see Warnings and Precautions (5.3)].
- Exacerbations of hepatitis B [see Boxed Warning, Warnings and Precautions (5.3)].
- Hepatic decompensation in patients co-infected with HIV-1 and Hepatitis C [see Warnings and Precautions (5.4)].
- Immune reconstitution syndrome [see Warnings and Precautions (5.5)].
- Fat redistribution [see Warnings and Precautions (5.6)].
- Myocardial infarction [see Warnings and Precautions (5.7)].

6.1 Clinical Trials Experience

Because clinical trials are conducted under widely varying conditions, adverse reaction rates observed in the clinical trials of a drug cannot be directly compared with rates in the clinical trials of another drug and may not reflect the rates observed in clinical practice.

Treatment-emergent Adverse Drug Reactions (ADRs): The safety assessment of TRIUMEQ is primarily based on the analyses of data from a randomized, international, multicenter, double-blind, active-controlled trial, SINGLE (ING114467) and supported by data in treatment-experienced, INSTI-naïve subjects from SAILING (ING111762) and by data from other treatment-naïve trials. See full prescribing information for TIVICAY.

Treatment-naïve Subjects: In SINGLE, 833 adult subjects were randomized and received at least one dose of either dolutegravir (TIVICAY) 50 mg with fixed-dose abacavir sulfate and lamivudine (EPZICOM®) once daily (n = 414) or fixed-dose efavirenz/emtricitabine/tenofovir (ATRIPLA®) once daily (n = 419). Through 96 weeks, the rate of adverse events leading to discontinuation was 3% in subjects receiving TIVICAY + EPZICOM and 12% in subjects receiving ATRIPLA once daily.

Treatment-emergent ADRs of moderate to severe intensity observed in at least 2% of subjects in either treatment arm of SINGLE are provided in Table 2.

Table 2. Treatment-emergent Adverse Drug Reactions of at Least Moderate Intensity (Grades 2 to 4) and at Least 2% Frequency in Treatment-naïve Subjects in SINGLE (Week 96 Analysis)

Adverse Reaction	TIVICAY + EPZICOM Once Daily (N = 414)	ATRIPLA Once Daily (N = 419)
Psychiatric		
Insomnia	3%	2%
Depression	1%	2%
Abnormal dreams	<1%	2%
Nervous System		
Dizziness	<1%	5%
Headache	2%	2%
Gastrointestinal		
Nausea	<1%	3%
Diarrhea	<1%	2%
General Disorders		
Fatigue	2%	2%
Skin and Subcutaneous Tissue		
Rash[a]	<1%	6%
Ear and Labyrinth		
Vertigo	0	2%

[a] Includes pooled terms: rash, rash generalized, rash macular, rash maculo-papular, rash pruritic, and drug eruption.

Treatment-experienced Subjects: SAILING is an international, double-blind trial in INSTI-naive, antiretroviral treatment-experienced adult subjects. Subjects were randomized and received either TIVICAY 50 mg once daily or raltegravir 400 mg twice daily with investigator-selected background regimen consisting of up to 2 agents, including at least one fully active agent. At 48 weeks, the rate of adverse events leading to discontinuation was consistent with that seen in the overall treatment-naïve patient population. See full prescribing information for TIVICAY.

The ADRs observed in the subset of subjects who received TIVICAY + EPZICOM were generally consistent with those seen in the overall treatment-naïve patient population.

Less Common Adverse Reactions Observed in Clinical Trials: The following adverse reactions occurred in less than 2% of treatment-naïve or treatment-experienced subjects in any one trial. These events have been included because of their seriousness and/or assessment of potential causal relationship.

Gastrointestinal Disorders: Abdominal pain, abdominal distention, abdominal discomfort, dyspepsia, flatulence, gastroesophageal reflux disease, upper abdominal pain, vomiting.

General Disorders: Fever, lethargy.

Hepatobiliary Disorders: Hepatitis.

Metabolism and Nutrition Disorders: Anorexia, hypertriglyceridemia.

Musculoskeletal Disorders: Arthralgia, myositis.

Nervous: Somnolence.

Psychiatric: Nightmare and sleep disorder.

Renal and Urinary Disorders: Renal impairment.

Skin and Subcutaneous Tissue Disorders: Pruritus.

Laboratory Abnormalities: Treatment-naïve Subjects: Selected laboratory abnormalities (Grades 2 to 4) with a worsening grade from baseline and representing the worst-grade toxicity in at least 2% of subjects in SINGLE are presented in Table 3. The mean change from baseline observed for selected lipid values is presented in Table 4.

Table 3. Selected Laboratory Abnormalities (Grades 2 to 4) in Treatment-naïve Subjects in SINGLE (Week 96 Analysis)

Laboratory Abnormality	TIVICAY + EPZICOM Once Daily (N = 414)	ATRIPLA Once Daily (N = 419)
ALT		
Grade 2 (>2.5-5.0 × ULN)	2%	5%
Grade 3 to 4 (>5.0 × ULN)	<1%	<1%
AST		
Grade 2 (>2.5-5.0 × ULN)	3%	3%
Grade 3 to 4 (>5.0 × ULN)	<1%	3%
Creatine kinase		
Grade 2 (6.0-9.9 × ULN)	4%	1%
Grade 3 to 4 (≥10.0 × ULN)	5%	7%
Hyperglycemia		
Grade 2 (126-250 mg/dL)	7%	5%
Grade 3 (>250 mg/dL)	2%	<1%
Lipase		
Grade 2 (>1.5-3.0 × ULN)	9%	9%
Grade 3 to 4 (>3.0 ULN)	4%	3%
Total neutrophils		
Grade 2 (0.75-0.99 × 10⁹)	3%	5%
Grade 3 to 4 (<0.75 × 10⁹)	2%	3%

ULN = Upper limit of normal.

Table 4. Mean Change from Baseline in Fasted Lipid Values in Treatment-naïve Subjects in SINGLE (Week 96 Analysis[a])

Lipid	TIVICAY + EPZICOM Once Daily (N = 414)	ATRIPLA Once Daily (N = 419)
Cholesterol (mg/dL)	23.2	28.0
HDL cholesterol (mg/dL)	5.2	7.4
LDL cholesterol (mg/dL)	14.5	18.0
Triglycerides (mg/dL)	17.2	17.4

[a] Subjects on lipid-lowering agents at baseline were excluded from these analyses (TIVICAY n = 30 and ATRIPLA n = 27). Fifty-five subjects initiated a lipid-lowering agent post-baseline; their last fasted on-treatment values (prior to starting the agent) were used regardless if they discontinued the agent (SINGLE: TIVICAY n = 25 and ATRIPLA: n = 30).

Treatment-experienced Subjects: Laboratory abnormalities observed in SAILING were generally similar compared with observations seen in the treatment-naïve trials.

Hepatitis C Virus Co-infection: In SINGLE, the pivotal Phase 3 trial, subjects with hepatitis C virus co-infection were permitted to enroll provided that baseline liver chemistry tests did not exceed 5 times the upper limit of normal; subjects with hepatitis B co-infection were excluded. Overall, the safety profile in subjects with hepatitis C virus co-infection was similar to that observed in subjects without hepatitis C co-infection, although the rates of AST and ALT abnormalities were higher in the subgroup with hepatitis C virus co-infection for both treatment groups. Grades 2 to 4 ALT abnormalities in hepatitis C co-infected compared with HIV mono-infected subjects receiving TRIUMEQ were observed in 15% and 2% (vs. 24% and 4% of subjects treated with ATRIPLA), respectively [see Warnings and Precautions (5.3)]. See also full prescribing information for TIVICAY.

Changes in Serum Creatinine: Dolutegravir has been shown to increase serum creatinine due to inhibition of tubular secretion of creatinine without affecting renal glomerular function [see Clinical Pharmacology (12.2)]. Increases in serum creatinine occurred within the first 4 weeks of treatment and remained stable through 24 to 96 weeks. In SINGLE, a mean change from baseline of 0.14 mg per dL (range: -0.32 mg per dL to 0.59 mg per dL) was observed after 96 weeks of treatment. Creatinine increases were similar in treatment-experienced subjects.

Abacavir Sulfate and Lamivudine: Laboratory abnormalities observed in clinical trials of ZIAGEN (in combination with other antiretroviral treatment) were anemia, neutropenia, liver function test abnormalities, and elevations of CPK, blood glucose, and triglycerides. Additional laboratory abnormalities observed in clinical trials of EPIVIR (in combination with other antiretroviral treatment) were thrombocytopenia and elevated levels of bilirubin, amylase, and lipase.

6.2 Postmarketing Experience

In addition to adverse reactions reported from clinical trials, the following adverse reactions have been identified during postmarketing use. Because these reactions are reported voluntarily from a population of uncertain size, it is not always possible to reliably estimate their frequency or establish a causal relationship to drug exposure.

Abacavir and/or Lamivudine:

Digestive: Stomatitis.

Gastrointestinal: Pancreatitis.

General: Weakness.

Blood and Lymphatic Systems: Aplastic anemia, anemia (including pure red cell aplasia and severe anemias progressing on therapy), lymphadenopathy, splenomegaly.

Hypersensitivity: Sensitization reactions (including anaphylaxis), urticaria.

Metabolism and Nutrition Disorders: Hyperlactemia.

Musculoskeletal: Muscle weakness, CPK elevation, rhabdomyolysis.

Nervous: Paresthesia, peripheral neuropathy, seizures.

Respiratory: Abnormal breath sounds/wheezing.

Skin: Alopecia, erythema multiforme. Suspected Stevens-Johnson syndrome (SJS) and toxic epidermal necrolysis (TEN) have been reported in patients receiving abacavir primarily in combination with medications known to be associated with SJS and TEN, respectively. Because of the overlap of clinical signs and symptoms between hypersensitivity to abacavir and SJS and TEN, and the possibility of multiple drug sensitivities in some patients, abacavir should be discontinued and not restarted in such cases.

7 DRUG INTERACTIONS

7.1 Effect of Dolutegravir on the Pharmacokinetics of Other Agents

In vitro, dolutegravir inhibited the renal organic cation transporters, OCT2 (IC_{50} = 1.93 µM) and multidrug and toxin extrusion transporter (MATE) 1 (IC_{50} = 6.34 µM). In vivo, dolutegravir inhibits tubular secretion of creatinine by inhibiting OCT2 and potentially MATE1. Dolutegravir may increase plasma concentrations of drugs eliminated via OCT2 or MATE1 (dofetilide and metformin) [see Contraindications (4), Drug Interactions (7.3)].

In vitro, dolutegravir inhibited the basolateral renal transporters, organic anion transporter (OAT) 1 (IC_{50} = 2.12 µM) and OAT3 (IC_{50} = 1.97 µM). However, in vivo, dolutegravir did not alter the plasma concentrations of tenofovir or para-amino hippurate, substrates of OAT1 and OAT3.

In vitro, dolutegravir did not inhibit (IC_{50} greater than 50 µM) the following: cytochrome P450 (CYP)1A2, CYP2A6, CYP2B6, CYP2C8, CYP2C9, CYP2C19, CYP2D6, CYP3A, UGT1A1, UGT2B7, P-glycoprotein (P-gp), breast cancer resistance protein (BCRP), bile salt export pump (BSEP), organic anion transporter polypeptide (OATP)1B1, OATP1B3, OCT1, or multidrug resistance protein (MRP)2, or MRP4. In vitro, dolutegravir did not induce CYP1A2, CYP2B6, CYP3A4. Based on these data and the results of drug interaction trials, dolutegravir is not expected to affect the pharmacokinetics of drugs that are substrates of these enzymes or transporters.

In drug interaction trials, dolutegravir did not have a clinically relevant effect on the pharmacokinetics of the following drugs: tenofovir, methadone, midazolam, rilpivirine, and oral contraceptives containing norgestimate and ethinyl estradiol. Using cross-study comparisons to historical pharmacokinetic data for each interacting drug, dolutegravir did not appear to affect the pharmacokinetics of the following drugs: atazanavir, darunavir, efavirenz, etravirine, fosamprenavir, lopinavir, ritonavir, and telaprevir.

7.2 Effect of Other Agents on the Pharmacokinetics of Dolutegravir

Dolutegravir is metabolized by UGT1A1 with some contribution from CYP3A. Dolutegravir is also a substrate of UGT1A3, UGT1A9, BCRP, and P-gp in vitro. Drugs that induce those enzymes and transporters may decrease dolutegravir plasma concentrations and reduce the therapeutic effect of dolutegravir.

Coadministration of dolutegravir and other drugs that inhibit these enzymes may increase dolutegravir plasma concentrations.

Etravirine significantly reduced plasma concentrations of dolutegravir, but the effect of etravirine was mitigated by coadministration of lopinavir/ritonavir or darunavir/ritonavir, and is expected to be mitigated by atazanavir/ritonavir (Table 5) [see Drug Interactions (7.3), Clinical Pharmacology (12.3)].

Darunavir/ritonavir, lopinavir/ritonavir, rilpivirine, tenofovir, boceprevir, telaprevir, prednisone, rifabutin, and omeprazole had no clinically significant effect on the pharmacokinetics of dolutegravir.

Table 5. Established and Other Potentially Significant Drug Interactions for Dolutegravir: Alterations in Dose May Be Recommended Based on Drug Interaction Trials or Predicted Interactions

Concomitant Drug Class: Drug Name	Effect on Concentration	Clinical Comment
HIV-1 Antiviral Agents		
Non-nucleoside reverse transcriptase inhibitor: Etravirine[a]	↓Dolutegravir	Use of TRIUMEQ with etravirine without coadministration of atazanavir/ritonavir, darunavir/ritonavir, or lopinavir/ritonavir is not recommended.
Non-nucleoside reverse transcriptase inhibitor: Efavirenz[a]	↓Dolutegravir	Adjust dolutegravir dose to 50 mg twice daily. An additional 50-mg dose of dolutegravir should be taken, separated by 12 hours from TRIUMEQ.
Non-nucleoside reverse transcriptase inhibitor: Nevirapine	↓Dolutegravir	Avoid coadministration with TRIUMEQ because there are insufficient data to make dosing recommendations.
Protease inhibitor: Fosamprenavir/ritonavir[a] Tipranavir/ritonavir[a]	↓Dolutegravir	Adjust dolutegravir dose to 50 mg twice daily. An additional dolutegravir 50-mg dose should be taken, separated by 12 hours from TRIUMEQ.
Other Agents		
Oxcarbazepine Phenytoin Phenobarbital Carbamazepine St. John's wort (*Hypericum perforatum*)	↓Dolutegravir	Avoid coadministration with TRIUMEQ because there are insufficient data to make dosing recommendations.
Medications containing polyvalent cations (e.g., Mg or Al): Cation-containing antacids[a] or laxatives Sucralfate Buffered medications	↓Dolutegravir	Administer TRIUMEQ 2 hours before or 6 hours after taking medications containing polyvalent cations.
Oral calcium and iron supplements, including multivitamins containing calcium or iron[a]	↓Dolutegravir	Administer TRIUMEQ 2 hours before or 6 hours after taking supplements containing calcium or iron. Alternatively, TRIUMEQ and supplements containing calcium or iron can be taken together with food.
Metformin	↑Metformin	Consider metformin dose reductions when coadministered with TRIUMEQ.
Rifampin[a]	↓Dolutegravir	Adjust dolutegravir dose to 50 mg twice daily. An additional 50-mg dose of dolutegravir should be taken, separated by 12 hours from TRIUMEQ.

[a]*See Clinical Pharmacology (12.3) Table 9 for magnitude of interaction.*

7.3 Established and Other Potentially Significant Drug Interactions

There were no drug-drug interaction trials conducted with the abacavir, dolutegravir, and lamivudine fixed-dose combination tablets.

Information regarding potential drug interactions with dolutegravir (Table 5) and abacavir are provided below. These recommendations are based on either drug interaction trials or predicted interactions due to the expected magnitude of interaction and potential for serious adverse events or loss of efficacy. [*See Clinical Pharmacology (12.3).*] [See table 5 above]

Ethanol: *Abacavir:* Abacavir has no effect on the pharmacokinetic properties of ethanol. Ethanol decreases the elimination of abacavir causing an increase in overall exposure [*see Clinical Pharmacology (12.3)*].

Methadone: *Abacavir:* The addition of methadone has no clinically significant effect on the pharmacokinetic properties of abacavir. In a trial of 11 HIV-1-infected subjects receiving methadone-maintenance therapy with 600 mg of abacavir twice daily (twice the currently recommended dose), oral methadone clearance increased [*see Clinical Pharmacology (12.3)*]. This alteration will not result in a methadone dose modification in the majority of patients; however, an increased methadone dose may be required in a small number of patients. The addition of methadone had no clinically significant effect on the pharmacokinetic properties of abacavir.

8 USE IN SPECIFIC POPULATIONS
8.1 Pregnancy
Pregnancy Category C. There are no adequate and well-controlled trials in pregnant women. Reproduction studies with the components of TRIUMEQ have been performed in animals (see Dolutegravir, Abacavir, and Lamivudine sections below). Animal reproduction studies are not always predictive of human response. TRIUMEQ should be used during pregnancy only if the potential benefit outweigh the risks.

Antiretroviral Pregnancy Registry: To monitor maternal–fetal outcomes of pregnant women exposed to TRIUMEQ or other antiretroviral agents, an Antiretroviral Pregnancy Registry has been established. Physicians are encouraged to register patients by calling 1–800–258–4263.

Animal Data: *Dolutegravir:* Reproduction studies performed in rats and rabbits at doses up to 50 times the human dose of 50 mg once daily have revealed no evidence of impaired fertility or harm to the fetus due to dolutegravir. Oral administration of dolutegravir to pregnant rats at doses up to 1,000 mg per kg daily, approximately 50 times the 50-mg once-daily human clinical exposure based on AUC, from days 6 to 17 of gestation did not elicit maternal toxicity, developmental toxicity, or teratogenicity. Oral administration of dolutegravir to pregnant rabbits at doses up to 1,000 mg per kg daily, approximately 0.74 times the 50-mg once-daily human clinical exposure based on AUC, from days 6 to 18 of gestation did not elicit developmental toxicity or teratogenicity. In rabbits, maternal toxicity (decreased food consumption, scant/no feces/urine, suppressed body weight gain) was observed at 1,000 mg per kg. *Abacavir:* Studies in pregnant rats showed that abacavir is transferred to the fetus through the placenta. Fetal malformations (increased incidences of fetal anasarca and skeletal malformations) and developmental toxicity (depressed fetal body weight and reduced crown–rump length) were observed in rats at a dose which produced 28 times the human exposure for a dose of 600 mg based on AUC. Embryonic and fetal toxicities (increased resorptions, decreased fetal body weights) and toxicities to the offspring (increased incidence of stillbirth and lower body weights) occurred at half of the above-mentioned dose in separate fertility studies conducted in rats. In the rabbit, no developmental toxicity and no increases in fetal malformations occurred at doses that produced 7 times the human exposure at the recommended dose based on AUC.

Lamivudine: Studies in pregnant rats showed that lamivudine is transferred to the fetus through the placenta. Reproduction studies with orally administered lamivudine have been performed in rats and rabbits at doses producing plasma levels up to approximately 32 times the human exposure for a dose of 300 mg. No evidence of teratogenicity due to lamivudine was observed. Evidence of early embryo-lethality was seen in the rabbit at exposure levels similar to those observed in humans, but there was no indication of this effect in the rat at plasma levels up to 32 times those in humans.

8.3 Nursing Mothers
The Centers for Disease Control and Prevention recommend that HIV-1-infected mothers in the United States not breastfeed their infants to avoid risking postnatal transmission of HIV-1 infection.

Because of both the potential for HIV-1 transmission and the potential for serious adverse reactions in nursing infants, instruct **mothers not to breastfeed**.

Dolutegravir: Studies in lactating rats and their offspring indicate that dolutegravir was present in rat milk. It is not known whether dolutegravir is excreted in human breast milk.

Abacavir: Abacavir is excreted in the milk of lactating rats.

Lamivudine: Lamivudine is excreted in human breast milk.

8.4 Pediatric Use
Safety and effectiveness of TRIUMEQ in pediatric patients have not been established [*see Clinical Pharmacology (12.3)*].

8.5 Geriatric Use
Clinical trials of abacavir, dolutegravir, or lamivudine did not include sufficient numbers of subjects aged 65 and over to determine whether they respond differently from younger subjects. In general, caution should be exercised in the administration of TRIUMEQ in elderly patients reflecting the greater frequency of decreased hepatic, renal, or cardiac function, and of concomitant disease or other drug therapy [*see Clinical Pharmacology (12.3)*].

8.6 Patients with Impaired Renal Function
TRIUMEQ is not recommended for patients with impaired renal function (creatinine clearance less than 50 mL per min) because TRIUMEQ is a fixed-dose combination and the dosage of the individual components cannot be adjusted. If a dose reduction of lamivudine, a component of TRIUMEQ, is required for patients with creatinine clearance less than 50 mL per min, then the individual components should be used [*see Clinical Pharmacology (12.3)*].

8.7 Patients with Impaired Hepatic Function
TRIUMEQ is a fixed-dose combination and the dosage of the individual components cannot be adjusted. If a dose reduction of abacavir, a component of TRIUMEQ, is required for patients with mild hepatic impairment (Child-Pugh Score A), then the individual components should be used [*see Clinical Pharmacology (12.3)*].

The safety, efficacy, and pharmacokinetic properties of abacavir have not been established in patients with moderate (Child-Pugh Score B) or severe (Child-Pugh Score C) hepatic impairment; therefore, TRIUMEQ is contraindicated in these patients.

10 OVERDOSAGE
There is no known specific treatment for overdose with TRIUMEQ. If overdose occurs, the patient should be monitored and standard supportive treatment applied as required.

Dolutegravir: As dolutegravir is highly bound to plasma proteins, it is unlikely that it will be significantly removed by dialysis.

Abacavir: It is not known whether abacavir can be removed by peritoneal dialysis or hemodialysis.

Lamivudine: Because a negligible amount of lamivudine was removed via (4-hour) hemodialysis, continuous ambulatory peritoneal dialysis, and automated peritoneal dialysis, it is not known if continuous hemodialysis would provide clinical benefit in a lamivudine overdose event. If overdose occurs, the patient should be monitored, and standard supportive treatment applied as required.

11 DESCRIPTION
TRIUMEQ: TRIUMEQ contains an INSTI (dolutegravir) and 2 nucleoside analogues (abacavir and lamivudine) with inhibitory activity against HIV.

Each film-coated tablet contains abacavir sulfate equivalent to 600 mg of abacavir, dolutegravir sodium equivalent to 50 mg of dolutegravir, and 300 mg of lamivudine. TRIUMEQ tablets are purple, biconvex, oval, debossed with "572 Tri" on one side and contain the inactive ingredients D-mannitol, magnesium stearate, microcrystalline cellulose, povidone, and sodium starch glycolate. The tablet film-coating (OPADRY® II Purple 85F90057) contains the inactive ingredients iron oxide black, iron oxide red, macrogol/PEG, polyvinyl alcohol-part hydrolyzed, talc, and titanium oxide.

Abacavir: The chemical name of abacavir sulfate is (1S,cis)-4-[2-amino-6-(cyclopropylamino)-9H-purin-9-yl]-2-cyclopentene-1-methanol sulfate (salt) (2:1). It has a molecular formula of $(C_{14}H_{18}N_6O)_2 \cdot H_2SO_4$ and a molecular weight of 670.76 g per mol. It has the following structural formula:

Abacavir sulfate is a white to off-white solid and is soluble in water.

Dolutegravir: The chemical name of dolutegravir sodium is sodium (4R,12aS)-9-[[(2,4-difluorophenyl)methyl]carbamoyl]-4-methyl-6,8-dioxo-3,4,6,8,12,12a-hexahydro-2H-pyrido[1',2':4,5]pyrazino[2,1-b][1,3]oxazin-7-olate. The empirical formula is $C_{20}H_{18}F_2N_3NaO_5$ and the molecular weight is 441.36 g per mol. It has the following structural formula:

Dolutegravir sodium is a white to light yellow powder and is slightly soluble in water.

Lamivudine: The chemical name of lamivudine is (2R,cis)-4-amino-1-(2-hydroxymethyl-1,3-oxathiolan-5-yl)-(1H)-pyrimidin-2-one. Lamivudine is the (-)enantiomer of a dideoxy analogue of cytidine. Lamivudine has also been referred to as (-)2',3'-dideoxy, 3'-thiacytidine. It has a molecular formula of $C_8H_{11}N_3O_3S$ and a molecular weight of 229.3 g per mol. It has the following structural formula:

Lamivudine is a white to off-white crystalline solid and is soluble in water.

12   CLINICAL PHARMACOLOGY

12.1   Mechanism of Action

TRIUMEQ is an HIV-1 antiviral agent [see Microbiology (12.4)].

12.2   Pharmacodynamics

Effects on Electrocardiogram: A thorough QT trial has been conducted for dolutegravir. Neither the effects of abacavir nor lamivudine as single entities or the combination of abacavir, dolutegravir, and lamivudine on the QT interval have been evaluated.

In a randomized, placebo-controlled, cross-over trial, 42 healthy subjects received single-dose oral administrations of placebo, dolutegravir 250-mg suspension (exposures approximately 3-fold of the 50-mg once-daily dose at steady state), and moxifloxacin 400 mg (active control) in random sequence. After baseline and placebo adjustment, the maximum mean QTc change based on Fridericia correction method (QTcF) for dolutegravir was 2.4 msec (1-sided 95% upper CI: 4.9 msec). Dolutegravir did not prolong the QTc interval over 24 hours postdose.

Effects on Renal Function: The effect of dolutegravir on renal function was evaluated in an open-label, randomized, 3-arm, parallel, placebo-controlled trial in healthy subjects (n = 37) who received dolutegravir 50 mg once daily (n = 12), dolutegravir 50 mg twice daily (n = 13), or placebo once daily (n = 12) for 14 days. A decrease in creatinine clearance, as determined by 24-hour urine collection, was observed with both doses of dolutegravir after 14 days of treatment in subjects who received 50 mg once daily (9% decrease) and 50 mg twice daily (13% decrease). Neither dose of dolutegravir had a significant effect on the actual glomerular filtration rate (determined by the clearance of probe

drug, iohexol) or effective renal plasma flow (determined by the clearance of probe drug, para-amino hippurate) compared with the placebo.

12.3   Pharmacokinetics

Pharmacokinetics in Adults: One TRIUMEQ tablet was bioequivalent to one dolutegravir (TIVICAY) tablet (50 mg) plus one abacavir and lamivudine fixed-dose combination tablet (EPZICOM) under fasted conditions in healthy subjects (n = 62).

Abacavir: Following oral administration, abacavir is rapidly absorbed and extensively distributed. After oral administration of a single dose of 600 mg of abacavir in 20 subjects, C_{max} was 4.26 ± 1.19 mcg per mL (mean ± SD) and AUC_∞ was 11.95 ± 2.51 mcg•hour per mL. Binding of abacavir to human plasma proteins is approximately 50% and was independent of concentration. Total blood and plasma drug-related radioactivity concentrations are identical, demonstrating that abacavir readily distributes into erythrocytes. The primary routes of elimination of abacavir are metabolism by alcohol dehydrogenase to form the 5'-carboxylic acid and glucuronyl transferase to form the 5'-glucuronide. In single-dose trials, the observed elimination half-life ($t_{1/2}$) was 1.54 ± 0.63 hours. After intravenous administration, total clearance was 0.80 ± 0.24 L per hour per kg (mean ± SD).

Dolutegravir: Following oral administration of dolutegravir, peak plasma concentrations were observed 2 to 3 hours postdose. With once-daily dosing, pharmacokinetic steady state is achieved within approximately 5 days with average accumulation ratios for AUC, C_{max}, and $C_{24\,h}$ ranging from 1.2 to 1.5. Dolutegravir is a P-glycoprotein substrate in vitro. The absolute bioavailability of dolutegravir has not been established. Dolutegravir is highly bound (greater than or equal to 98.9%) to human plasma proteins based on in vivo data and binding is independent of plasma concentration of dolutegravir. The apparent volume of distribution (Vd/F) following 50-mg once-daily administration is estimated at 17.4 L based on a population pharmacokinetic analysis.

Dolutegravir is primarily metabolized via UGT1A1 with some contribution from CYP3A. After a single oral dose of [^{14}C] dolutegravir, 53% of the total oral dose is excreted unchanged in the feces. Thirty-one percent of the total oral dose is excreted in the urine, represented by an ether glucuronide of dolutegravir (18.9% of total dose), a metabolite formed by oxidation at the benzylic carbon (3.0% of total dose), and its hydrolytic N-dealkylation product (3.6% of total dose). Renal elimination of unchanged drug was less than 1% of the dose. Dolutegravir has a terminal half-life of approximately 14 hours and an apparent clearance (CL/F) of 1.0 L per hour based on population pharmacokinetic analyses.

The pharmacokinetic properties of dolutegravir have been evaluated in healthy adult subjects and HIV–1–infected adult subjects. Exposure to dolutegravir was generally similar between healthy subjects and HIV–1–infected subjects.

Cerebrospinal Fluid (CSF): In 11 treatment-naïve subjects on dolutegravir 50 mg daily plus abacavir/lamivudine, the median dolutegravir concentration in CSF was 18 ng per mL (range: 4 ng per mL to 23.2 ng per mL) 2 to 6 hours postdose after 2 weeks of treatment. The clinical relevance of this finding has not been established.

Lamivudine: Following oral administration, lamivudine is rapidly absorbed and extensively distributed. After multiple-dose oral administration of lamivudine 300 mg once daily for 7 days to 60 healthy subjects, steady-state C_{max} ($C_{max,ss}$) was 2.04 ± 0.54 mcg per mL (mean ± SD) and the 24-hour steady-state AUC ($AUC_{24,ss}$) was 8.87 ± 1.83 mcg•hour per mL. Binding to plasma protein is low. Approximately 70% of an intravenous dose of lamivudine is recovered as unchanged drug in the urine. Metabolism of lamivudine is a minor route of elimination. In humans, the only known metabolite is the trans-sulfoxide metabolite (approximately 5% of an oral dose after 12 hours). In most single-dose trials in HIV–1-infected subjects, HBV-infected subjects, or healthy subjects with serum sampling for 24 hours after dosing, the observed mean elimination half-life ($t_{1/2}$) ranged from 5 to 7 hours. In HIV-1-infected subjects, total clearance was 398.5 ± 69.1 mL per min (mean ± SD).

Effect of Food on Oral Absorption: TRIUMEQ may be taken with or without food. Overall, when compared with fasted conditions, administration of TRIUMEQ to healthy adult subjects with a high-fat meal (53% fat, 869 calories) resulted in decreased C_{max} for abacavir and increased C_{max} and AUC for dolutegravir. Lamivudine exposures were not affected by food. With a high-fat meal, the C_{max} of abacavir decreased 23% and the C_{max} and AUC of dolutegravir increased 37% and 48%, respectively.

Special Populations: Renal Impairment: The effect of renal impairment on the combination of abacavir, dolutegravir, and lamivudine has not been evaluated.

Abacavir: The pharmacokinetic properties of abacavir have not been determined in patients with impaired renal function.

Dolutegravir: In a trial comparing 8 subjects with severe renal impairment (CrCl less than 30 mL per min) with 8 matched healthy controls, AUC, C_{max}, and C_{24} of dolutegravir were decreased by 40%, 23%, and 43%, respectively, compared with those in matched healthy subjects. The cause of this decrease is unknown. Population pharmacokinetic analysis indicated that mild and moderate renal impairment had no clinically relevant effect on the exposure of dolutegravir.

Lamivudine: The pharmacokinetic properties of lamivudine have been determined in a small group of HIV-1-infected adults with impaired renal function (Table 7).

Table 8. Summary of Effect of Dolutegravir on the Pharmacokinetics of Coadministered Drugs

Coadministered Drug(s) and Dose(s)	Dose of Dolutegravir	n	Geometric Mean Ratio (90% CI) of Pharmacokinetic Parameters of Coadministered Drug with/without Dolutegravir No Effect = 1.00		
			C_{max}	AUC	C_τ or C_{24}
Ethinyl estradiol 0.035 mg	50 mg twice daily	15	0.99 (0.91 to 1.08)	1.03 (0.96 to 1.11)	1.02 (0.93 to 1.11)
Methadone 16 to 150 mg	50 mg twice daily	11	1.00 (0.94 to 1.06)	0.98 (0.91 to 1.06)	0.99 (0.91 to 1.07)
Midazolam 3 mg	25 mg once daily	10	—	0.95 (0.79 to 1.15)	—
Norelgestromin 0.25 mg	50 mg twice daily	15	0.89 (0.82 to 0.97)	0.98 (0.91 to 1.04)	0.93 (0.85 to 1.03)
Rilpivirine 25 mg once daily	50 mg once daily	16	1.10 (0.99 to 1.22)	1.06 (0.98 to 1.16)	1.21 (1.07 to 1.38)
Tenofovir disoproxil fumarate 300 mg once daily	50 mg once daily	15	1.09 (0.97 to 1.23)	1.12 (1.01 to 1.24)	1.19 (1.04 to 1.35)

Table 6. Dolutegravir Steady-state Pharmacokinetic Parameter Estimates in HIV-1– Infected Adults

Parameter	50 mg Once Daily Geometric Mean (%CV)
$AUC_{(0-24)}$ (mcg•h/mL)	53.6 (27)
C_{max} (mcg/mL)	3.67 (20)
C_{min} (mcg/mL)	1.11 (46)

Table 7. Pharmacokinetic Parameters (Mean ± SD) After a Single 300-mg Oral Dose of Lamivudine in 3 Groups of Adults with Varying Degrees of Renal Function

Parameter	Creatinine Clearance Criterion (Number of Subjects)		
	>60 mL/min (n = 6)	10-30 mL/min (n = 4)	<10 mL/min (n = 6)
Creatinine clearance (mL/min)	111 ± 14	28 ± 8	6 ± 2

Table 9. Summary of Effect of Coadministered Drugs on the Pharmacokinetics of Dolutegravir

Coadministered Drug(s) and Dose(s)	Dose of Dolutegravir	n	Geometric Mean Ratio (90% CI) of Dolutegravir Pharmacokinetic Parameters with/without Coadministered Drugs No Effect = 1.00		
			C_{max}	AUC	C_τ or C_{24}
Atazanavir 400 mg once daily	30 mg once daily	12	1.50 (1.40 to 1.59)	1.91 (1.80 to 2.03)	2.80 (2.52 to 3.11)
Atazanavir/ritonavir 300/100 mg once daily	30 mg once daily	12	1.34 (1.25 to 1.42)	1.62 (1.50 to 1.74)	2.21 (1.97 to 2.47)
Tenofovir 300 mg once daily	50 mg once daily	15	0.97 (0.87 to 1.08)	1.01 (0.91 to 1.11)	0.92 (0.82 to 1.04)
Darunavir/ritonavir 600/100 mg twice daily	30 mg once daily	15	0.89 (0.83 to 0.97)	0.78 (0.72 to 0.85)	0.62 (0.56 to 0.69)
Efavirenz 600 mg once daily	50 mg once daily	12	0.61 (0.51 to 0.73)	0.43 (0.35 to 0.54)	0.25 (0.18 to 0.34)
Etravirine 200 mg twice daily	50 mg once daily	16	0.48 (0.43 to 0.54)	0.29 (0.26 to 0.34)	0.12 (0.09 to 0.16)
Etravirine + darunavir/ritonavir 200 mg + 600/100 mg twice daily	50 mg once daily	9	0.88 (0.78 to 1.00)	0.75 (0.69 to 0.81)	0.63 (0.52 to 0.76)
Etravirine + lopinavir/ritonavir 200 mg + 400/100 mg twice daily	50 mg once daily	8	1.07 (1.02 to 1.13)	1.11 (1.02 to 1.20)	1.28 (1.13 to 1.45)
Fosamprenavir/ ritonavir 700 mg/100 mg twice daily	50 mg once daily	12	0.76 (0.63 to 0.92)	0.65 (0.54 to 0.78)	0.51 (0.41 to 0.63)
Lopinavir/ritonavir 400/100 mg twice daily	30 mg once daily	15	1.00 (0.94 to 1.07)	0.97 (0.91 to 1.04)	0.94 (0.85 to 1.05)
Antacid (Maalox®) simultaneous administration	50 mg single dose	16	0.28 (0.23 to 0.33)	0.26 (0.22 to 0.32)	0.26 (0.21 to 0.31)
Antacid (Maalox®) 2 h after dolutegravir	50 mg single dose	16	0.82 (0.69 to 0.98)	0.74 (0.62 to 0.90)	0.70 (0.58 to 0.85)
Calcium carbonate 1,200 mg simultaneous administration (fasted)	50 mg single dose	12	0.63 (0.50 to 0.81)	0.61 (0.47 to 0.80)	0.61 (0.47 to 0.80)
Calcium carbonate 1,200 mg simultaneous administration (fed)	50 mg single dose	11	1.07 (0.83 to 1.38)	1.09 (0.84 to 1.43)	1.08 (0.81 to 1.42)
Calcium carbonate 1,200 mg 2 h after dolutegravir	50 mg single dose	11	1.00 (0.78 to 1.29)	0.94 (0.72 to 1.23)	0.90 (0.68 to 1.19)

(Table continued on next page)

C_{max} (mcg/mL)	2.6 ± 0.5	3.6 ± 0.8	5.8 ± 1.2
AUC∞ (mcg•h/mL)	11.0 ± 1.7	48.0 ± 19	157 ± 74
Cl/F (mL/min)	464 ± 76	114 ± 34	36 ± 11

Hepatic Impairment: The effect of hepatic impairment on the combination of abacavir, dolutegravir, and lamivudine has not been evaluated.

Abacavir: The pharmacokinetics of abacavir have been studied in subjects with mild hepatic impairment (Child-Pugh score 5 to 6). Results showed that there was a mean increase of 89% in the abacavir AUC and an increase of 58% in the half-life of abacavir after a single dose of 600 mg of abacavir. The AUCs of the metabolites were not modified by mild liver disease; however, the rates of formation and elimination of the metabolites were decreased. The safety, efficacy, and pharmacokinetics of abacavir have not been studied in patients with moderate or severe hepatic impairment.

Dolutegravir: In a trial comparing 8 subjects with moderate hepatic impairment (Child-Pugh Score B) with 8 matched healthy controls, exposure of dolutegravir from a single 50-mg dose was similar between the 2 groups. The effect of severe hepatic impairment (Child-Pugh Score C) on the pharmacokinetics of dolutegravir has not been studied.

Lamivudine: The pharmacokinetic properties of lamivudine have been determined in adults with impaired hepatic function. Pharmacokinetic parameters were not altered by diminishing hepatic function. Safety and efficacy of lamivudine have not been established in the presence of decompensated liver disease.

Pediatric Patients: The pharmacokinetics of the combination of abacavir, dolutegravir, and lamivudine in pediatric subjects have not been established.

Geriatric Patients: Population analyses using pooled pharmacokinetic data from adult trials indicated age had no clinically relevant effect on the pharmacokinetics of dolutegravir. The pharmacokinetics of abacavir or lamivudine have not been studied in subjects older than 65 years.

Gender: There are no significant or clinically relevant gender differences in the pharmacokinetics of the individual components (dolutegravir, abacavir, or lamivudine) based on the available information that was analyzed for each of the individual components.

Race: There are no significant or clinically relevant racial differences in pharmacokinetics of the individual compo-

nents (dolutegravir, abacavir, or lamivudine) based on the available information that was analyzed for each of the individual components.

Drug Interactions: The drug interaction trials described were conducted with dolutegravir, abacavir, and/or lamivudine as single entities; no drug interaction trials have been conducted using the combination of abacavir, dolutegravir, and lamivudine. No clinically significant drug interactions are expected between dolutegravir, abacavir, and lamivudine.

Dosing recommendations as a result of established and other potentially significant drug-drug interactions with dolutegravir or abacavir are provided in Section 7.3 *[see Drug Interactions (7)].*

[See table 8 at top of previous page]

[See table 9 above and on next page]

Abacavir or Lamivudine: The drug interactions described are based on trials conducted with abacavir or lamivudine as single entities.

Interferon Alfa: There was no significant pharmacokinetic interaction between lamivudine and interferon alfa in a trial of 19 healthy male subjects.

Methadone: In a trial of 11 HIV–1–infected subjects receiving methadone-maintenance therapy (40 mg and 90 mg daily), with 600 mg of abacavir twice daily (twice the currently recommended dose), oral methadone clearance increased 22% (90% CI: 6% to 42%) *[see Drug Interactions (7.3)].*

Ribavirin: In vitro data indicate ribavirin reduces phosphorylation of lamivudine, stavudine, and zidovudine. However, no pharmacokinetic (e.g., plasma concentrations or intracellular triphosphorylated active metabolite concentrations) or pharmacodynamic (e.g., loss of HIV-1/HCV virologic suppression) interaction was observed when ribavirin and lamivudine (n = 18), stavudine (n = 10), or zidovudine (n = 6) were coadministered as part of a multidrug regimen to HIV-1/HCV co-infected subjects *[see Warnings and Precautions (5.4)].*

Abacavir, Lamivudine, Zidovudine: Fifteen HIV–1–infected subjects were enrolled in a crossover-designed drug interaction trial evaluating single doses of abacavir (600 mg), lamivudine (150 mg), and zidovudine (300 mg) alone or in combination. Analysis showed no clinically relevant changes in the pharmacokinetics of abacavir with the addition of lamivudine or zidovudine or the combination of lamivudine and zidovudine. Lamivudine exposure (AUC decreased 15%) and zidovudine exposure (AUC increased 10%) did not show clinically relevant changes with concurrent abacavir.

Lamivudine and Zidovudine: No clinically significant alterations in lamivudine or zidovudine pharmacokinetics were observed in 12 asymptomatic HIV–1–infected adult patients given a single dose of zidovudine (200 mg) in combination with multiple doses of lamivudine (300 mg every 12 h).

The effects of other coadministered drugs on abacavir or lamivudine are provided in Table 10.

[See table 10 on next page]

12.4   Microbiology

Mechanism of Action: *Dolutegravir:* Dolutegravir inhibits HIV integrase by binding to the integrase active site and blocking the strand transfer step of retroviral DNA integration which is essential for the HIV replication cycle. Strand transfer biochemical assays using purified recombinant HIV-1 integrase and pre-processed substrate DNA resulted in IC_{50} values of 2.7 nM and 12.6 nM.

Abacavir: Abacavir is a carbocyclic synthetic nucleoside analogue. Abacavir is converted by cellular enzymes to the active metabolite, carbovir triphosphate (CBV-TP), an analogue of deoxyguanosine-5'-triphosphate (dGTP). CBV-TP inhibits the activity of HIV-1 reverse transcriptase (RT) both by competing with the natural substrate dGTP and by its incorporation into viral DNA.

Lamivudine: Lamivudine is a synthetic nucleoside analogue. Intracellularly lamivudine is phosphorylated to its active 5'-triphosphate metabolite, lamivudine triphosphate (3TC-TP). The principal mode of action of 3TC-TP is inhibition of RT via DNA chain termination after incorporation of the nucleotide analogue.

Antiviral Activity in Cell Culture: *Dolutegravir:* Dolutegravir exhibited antiviral activity against laboratory strains of wild-type HIV-1 with mean concentration of drug necessary to effect viral replication by 50 percent (EC_{50}) values of 0.5 nM (0.21 ng per mL) to 2.1 nM (0.85 ng per mL) in peripheral blood mononuclear cells (PBMCs) and MT-4 cells. Dolutegravir exhibited antiviral activity against 13 clinically diverse clade B isolates with a median EC_{50} value of 0.54 nM (range: 0.41 to 0.60 nM) in a viral susceptibility assay using the integrase coding region from clinical isolates. Dolutegravir demonstrated antiviral activity in cell culture against a panel of HIV–1 clinical isolates with median EC_{50} values of 0.18 nM (n = 3, range: 0.09 to 0.5 nM), 0.08 nM (n = 5, range: 0.05 to 2.14 nM) 0.12 nM (n = 4, range: 0.05 to 0.51 nM), 0.17 nM (n = 3, range: 0.16 to

0.35 nM), 0.24 nM (n = 3, range: 0.09 to 0.32 nM), 0.17 nM (range: 0.07 to 0.44 nM), 0.2 nM (n = 3, range: 0.02 to 0.87 nM), and 0.42 nM (n = 3, range: 0.41 to 1.79 nM) for clades A, B, C, D, E, F, and G, and group O viruses, respectively. Dolutegravir EC_{50} values against three HIV-2 clinical isolates in PBMC assays ranged from 0.09 nM to 0.61 nM.

Abacavir: The antiviral activity of abacavir against HIV-1 was assessed in a number of cell lines including in primary monocytes/macrophages and PBMCs. EC_{50} values ranged from 3.7 to 5.8 µM (1 µM = 0.28 mcg per mL) and 0.07 to 1.0 µM against HIV-1$_{IIIB}$ and HIV-1$_{BaL}$, respectively, and was 0.26 ± 0.18 µM against 8 clinical isolates. The median EC_{50} values of abacavir were 344 nM (range: 14.8 to 676 nM), 16.9 nM (range: 5.9 to 27.9 nM), 8.1 nM (range: 1.5 to 16.7 nM), 356 nM (range: 35.7 to 396 nM), 105 nM (range: 28.1 to 168 nM), 47.6 nM (range: 5.2 to 200 nM), 51.4 nM (range: 7.1 to 177 nM), and 282 nM (range: 22.4 to 598 nM) against HIV-1 clades A-G and group O viruses (n = 3 except n = 2 for clade B), respectively. The EC_{50} values against HIV-2 isolates (n = 4), ranged from 0.024 to 0.49 µM.

Lamivudine: The antiviral activity of lamivudine against HIV-1 was assessed in a number of cell lines including monocytes and PBMCs using standard susceptibility assays. EC_{50} values were in the range of 0.003 to 15 µM (1 µM = 0.23 mcg per mL). The median EC_{50} values of lamivudine were 60 nM (range: 20 to 70 nM), 35 nM (range: 30 to 40 nM), 30 nM (range: 20 to 90 nM), 20 nM (range: 3 to 40 nM), 30 nM (range: 1 to 60 nM), 30 nM (range: 20 to 70 nM), 30 nM (range: 3 to 70 nM), and 30 nM (range: 20 to 90 nM) against HIV-1 clades A-G and group O viruses (n = 3 except n = 2 for clade B) respectively. The EC_{50} values against HIV-2 isolates (n = 4) from 0.003 to 0.120 µM in PBMCs.

Antiviral Activity in Combination with Other Antiviral Agents: Neither dolutegravir, abacavir, nor lamivudine were antagonistic to all tested anti-HIV agents. See full prescribing information for ZIAGEN (abacavir), TIVICAY (dolutegravir), and EPIVIR (lamivudine).

Resistance in Cell Culture: *Dolutegravir:* Dolutegravir-resistant viruses were selected in cell culture starting from different wild-type HIV-1 strains and clades. Amino acid substitutions E92Q, G118R, S153F or Y, G193E or R263K emerged in different passages and conferred decreased susceptibility to dolutegravir of up to 4-fold.

Abacavir and Lamivudine: HIV-1 isolates with reduced susceptibility to the combination of abacavir and lamivudine have been selected in cell culture with amino acid substitutions M184V/I, K65R, L74V, and Y115F in HIV-1 RT. Substitution at M184I or V causes high-level resistance to lamivudine and approximately 2-fold decreased susceptibility to abacavir. Substitutions K65R, L74M, or Y115F with M184I or V conferred a 7-fold to 8-fold reduction in abacavir susceptibility, and combinations of three substitutions were required to confer more than an 8-fold reduction in susceptibility.

Resistance in Clinical Subjects: *Dolutegravir:* No subjects in the treatment arm receiving dolutegravir + EPZICOM of SINGLE (treatment-naïve trial) had a detectable decrease in susceptibility to dolutegravir or background NRTIs in the resistance analysis subset (n = 9 with HIV-1 RNA greater than 400 copies per mL at failure or last visit through Week 96 and having resistance data). One subject in SINGLE with 275 copies per mL HIV-1 RNA had a treatment-emergent integrase substitution (E157Q/P) detected at Week 24, but no corresponding decrease in dolutegravir susceptibility. No treatment-emergent genotypic resistance to abacavir and lamivudine, components of TRIUMEQ, was observed in the arm receiving dolutegravir + EPZICOM in the SINGLE trial.

Cross Resistance: *Dolutegravir:* The single INSTI-resistance substitutions T66K, I151L, and S153Y conferred a greater than 2-fold decrease in dolutegravir susceptibility (range: 2.3-fold to 3.6-fold from reference). Combinations of multiple substitutions T66K/L74M, E92Q/N155H, G140C/ Q148R, G140S/Q148H, R or K, Q148R/N155H, T97A/ G140S/Q148, and substitutions at E138/G140/Q148 showed a greater than 2-fold decrease in dolutegravir susceptibility (range: 2.5-fold to 21-fold from reference). In HIV-2 mutants, combinations of substitutions A153G/N155H/S163G and E92Q/T97A/N155H/S163D conferred 4-fold decreases in dolutegravir susceptibility, and E92Q/N155H and G140S/ Q148R showed 8.5-fold and 17-fold decreases in dolutegravir susceptibility, respectively.

Abacavir and Lamivudine: Cross-resistance has been observed among NRTIs. The combination of abacavir/lamivudine has demonstrated decreased susceptibility to viruses with the substitutions K65R with or without the M184V/I substitution, viruses with L74V plus the M184V/I substitution, and viruses with thymidine analog mutations (TAMs: M41L, D67N, K70R, L210W, T215Y/F, K219 E/R/H/Q/N) plus M184V. An increasing number of TAMs is associated with a progressive reduction in abacavir susceptibility.

Table 9 (cont.). Summary of Effect of Coadministered Drugs on the Pharmacokinetics of Dolutegravir

Coadministered Drug(s) and Dose(s)	Dose of Dolutegravir	n	Geometric Mean Ratio (90% CI) of Dolutegravir Pharmacokinetic Parameters with/without Coadministered Drugs No Effect = 1.00		
			C_{max}	AUC	C_τ or C_{24}
Ferrous fuarate 324 mg simultaneous administration (fasted)	50 mg single dose	11	0.43 (0.35 to 0.52)	0.46 (0.38 to 0.56)	0.44 (0.36 to 0.54)
Ferrous fuarate 324 mg simultaneous administration (fed)	50 mg single dose	11	1.03 (0.84 to 1.26)	0.98 (0.81 to 1.20)	1.00 (0.81 to 1.23)
Ferrous fuarate 324 mg 2 h after dolutegravir	50 mg single dose	10	0.99 (0.81 to 1.21)	0.95 (0.77 to 1.15)	0.92 (0.74 to 1.13)
Multivitamin (One-A-Day®) simultaneous administration	50 mg single dose	16	0.65 (0.54 to 0.77)	0.67 (0.55 to 0.81)	0.68 (0.56 to 0.82)
Omeprazole 40 mg once daily	50 mg single dose	12	0.92 (0.75 to 1.11)	0.97 (0.78 to 1.20)	0.95 (0.75 to 1.21)
Prednisone 60 mg once daily with taper	50 mg once daily	12	1.06 (0.99 to 1.14)	1.11 (1.03 to 1.20)	1.17 (1.06 to 1.28)
Rifampin[a] 600 mg once daily	50 mg twice daily	11	0.57 (0.49 to 0.65)	0.46 (0.38 to 0.55)	0.28 (0.23 to 0.34)
Rifampin[b] 600 mg once daily	50 mg twice daily	11	1.18 (1.03 to 1.37)	1.33 (1.15 to 1.53)	1.22 (1.01 to 1.48)
Rifabutin 300 mg once daily	50 mg once daily	9	1.16 (0.98 to 1.37)	0.95 (0.82 to 1.10)	0.70 (0.57 to 0.87)
Rilpivirine 25 mg once daily	50 mg once daily	16	1.13 (1.06 to 1.21)	1.12 (1.05 to 1.19)	1.22 (1.15 to 1.30)
Tipranavir/ritonavir 500/200 mg twice daily	50 mg once daily	14	0.54 (0.50 to 0.57)	0.41 (0.38 to 0.44)	0.24 (0.21 to 0.27)
Telaprevir 750 mg every 8 hours	50 mg once daily	15	1.18 (1.11 to 1.26)	1.25 (1.19 to 1.31)	1.40 (1.29 to 1.51)
Boceprevir 800 mg every 8 hours	50 mg once daily	13	1.05 (0.96 to 1.15)	1.07 (0.95 to 1.20)	1.08 (0.91 to 1.28)

[a] Comparison is rifampin taken with dolutegravir 50 mg twice daily compared with dolutegravir 50 mg twice daily.
[b] Comparison is rifampin taken with dolutegravir 50 mg twice daily compared with dolutegravir 50 mg once daily.

Table 10. Effect of Coadministered Drugs on Abacavir or Lamivudine

Coadministered Drug and Dose	Drug and Dose	n	Concentrations of Abacavir or Lamivudine		Concentration of Coadministered Drug
			AUC	Variability	
Ethanol 0.7 g/kg	Abacavir Single 600 mg	24	↑41%	90% CI: 35% to 48%	↔[a]
Nelfinavir 750 mg every 8 h × 7 to 10 days	Lamivudine Single 150 mg	11	↑10%	95% CI: 1% to 20%	↔
Trimethoprim 160 mg/ Sulfamethoxazole 800 mg daily × 5 days	Lamivudine Single 300 mg	14	↑43%	90% CI: 32% to 55%	↔

↑ = Increase; ↔ = no significant change; AUC = area under the concentration versus time curve; CI = confidence interval.
[a] The drug-drug interaction was only evaluated in males.

13 NONCLINICAL TOXICOLOGY

13.1 Carcinogenesis, Mutagenesis, Impairment of Fertility

Carcinogenicity: *Dolutegravir:* Two-year carcinogenicity studies in mice and rats were conducted with dolutegravir. Mice were administered doses of up to 500 mg per kg, and rats were administered doses of up to 50 mg per kg. In mice, no significant increases in the incidence of drug-related neoplasms were observed at the highest doses tested, resulting in dolutegravir AUC exposures approximately 26-fold higher than those in humans at the recommended dose of 50 mg once daily. In rats, no increases in the incidence of drug-related neoplasms were observed at the highest dose tested, resulting in dolutegravir AUC exposures 17-fold and 30-fold higher in males and females, respectively, than those in humans at the recommended dose of 50 mg once daily.

Abacavir: Abacavir was administered orally at 3 dosage levels to separate groups of mice and rats in 2-year carcinogenicity studies. Results showed an increase in the incidence of malignant and non-malignant tumors. Malignant tumors occurred in the preputial gland of males and the clitoral gland of females of both species, and in the liver of female rats. In addition, non-malignant tumors also occurred in the liver and thyroid gland of female rats. These observations were made at systemic exposures in the range of 7 to 28 times the human exposure at the recommended dose of 600 mg.

Lamivudine: Long–term carcinogenicity studies with lamivudine in mice and rats showed no evidence of carcinogenic potential at exposures up to 12 times (mice) and 57 times (rats) the human exposures at the recommended dose of 300 mg.

Mutagenicity: *Dolutegravir:* Dolutegravir was not genotoxic in the bacterial reverse mutation assay, mouse lymphoma assay, or in the in vivo rodent micronucleus assay.

Abacavir: Abacavir induced chromosomal aberrations both in the presence and absence of metabolic activation in an in vitro cytogenetic study in human lymphocytes. Abacavir was mutagenic in the absence of metabolic activation, although it was not mutagenic in the presence of metabolic activation in an L5178Y mouse lymphoma assay. Abacavir was clastogenic in males and not clastogenic in females in an in vivo mouse bone marrow micronucleus assay. Abacavir was not mutagenic in bacterial mutagenicity assays in the presence and absence of metabolic activation.

Lamivudine: Lamivudine was mutagenic in an L5178Y mouse lymphoma assay and clastogenic in a cytogenetic assay using cultured human lymphocytes. Lamivudine was not mutagenic in a microbial mutagenicity assay, in an in vitro cell transformation assay, in a rat micronucleus test, in a rat bone marrow cytogenetic assay, and in an assay for unscheduled DNA synthesis in rat liver.

Impairment of Fertility: Dolutegravir, abacavir, or lamivudine did not affect male or female fertility in rats at doses associated with exposures approximately 44, 9, or 112 times (respectively) higher than the exposures in humans at the doses of 50 mg, 600 mg, and 300 mg (respectively).

13.2 Animal Toxicology and/or Pharmacology

Myocardial degeneration was found in mice and rats following administration of abacavir for 2 years. The systemic exposures were equivalent to 7 to 21 times the expected systemic exposure in humans at a dose of 600 mg. The clinical relevance of this finding has not been determined.

14 CLINICAL STUDIES
14.1 Adult Subjects

The efficacy of TRIUMEQ is supported by data from a randomized, controlled trial in antiretroviral treatment-naïve subjects, SINGLE (ING114467) and other trials in treatment-naïve subjects. See full prescribing information for TIVICAY. The efficacy of dolutegravir, in combination with at least two active background regimens in treatment-experienced, INSTI-naïve subjects is supported by data from SAILING (ING111762) (refer to the prescribing information for TIVICAY).

Treatment-naïve Subjects: In SINGLE, 833 subjects were randomized and received at least 1 dose of either TIVICAY 50 mg once daily with fixed-dose abacavir and lamivudine (EPZICOM) or fixed-dose efavirenz/emtricitabine/tenofovir disoproxil fumarate (ATRIPLA). At baseline, the median age of subjects was 35 years, 16% female, 32% non-white, 7% had hepatitis C co-infection (hepatitis B virus co-infection was excluded), 4% were CDC Class C (AIDS), 32% had HIV–1 RNA greater than 100,000 copies per mL, and 53% had CD4+ cell count less than 350 cells per mm³; these characteristics were similar between treatment groups. Week 96 outcomes for SINGLE are provided in Table 11.

Table 11. Virologic Outcomes of Randomized Treatment in SINGLE at 96 Weeks (Snapshot Algorithm)

	TIVICAY + EPZICOM Once Daily (N = 414)	ATRIPLA Once Daily (N = 419)
HIV–1 RNA <50 copies/mL	80%	72%
Treatment difference[a]	8.0% (95% CI: 2.3%, 13.8%)	
Virologic nonresponse[b]	7%	8%
No virologic data	12%	20%
Reasons		
Discontinued study/study drug due to adverse event or death[c]	3%	11%
Discontinued study/study drug for other reasons[d]	9%	8%
Missing data during window but on study	<1%	0

Proportion (%) of Subjects with HIV–1 RNA <50 copies/mL by Baseline Category

Plasma viral load (copies/mL)[e]		
≤100,000	85%	73%
>100,000	71%	72%
Gender		
Male	81%	75%
Female	76%	56%
Race		
White	79%	77%
African-American/African Heritage/Other	83%	62%

[a] Adjusted for pre-specified stratification factors.
[b] Includes subjects who discontinued prior to Week 96 for lack or loss of efficacy, and subjects who were HIV-1 RNA greater than or equal to 50 copies per mL in the Week 96 window.
[c] Includes subjects who discontinued due to an adverse event or death at any time point from Day 1 through the Week 96 window if this resulted in no virologic data on treatment during the Week 96 window.
[d] Other includes reasons such as withdrew consent, loss to follow-up, moved, and protocol deviation.
[e] The proportion of subjects who had no virologic data due to reasons such as withdrew consent, lost to follow-up, moved, and protocol deviation was 10% (TIVICAY + EPZICOM) and 6% (ATRIPLA) in the greater than 100,000–copies-per-mL group and 8% and 9% (respectively) in the less than or equal to 100,000–copies-per-mL group.

Treatment differences were maintained across baseline characteristics including CD4+ cell count, age, gender, and race. The adjusted mean changes in CD4+ cell counts from baseline were 325 cells per mm³ in the group receiving TIVICAY + EPZICOM and 281 cells per mm³ for the ATRIPLA group at 96 weeks. The adjusted difference between treatment arms and 95% CI was 44.0 cells per mm³ (14.3 cells per mm³, 73.6 cells per mm³) (adjusted for pre-specified stratification factors: baseline HIV–1 RNA, baseline CD4+ cell count, and multiplicity).

Treatment-experienced: In SAILING, there were 715 subjects included in the efficacy and safety analyses (see full prescribing information for TIVICAY). At Week 48, 71% of subjects randomized to TIVICAY plus background regimen versus 64% of subjects randomized to raltegravir plus background regimen had HIV–1 RNA less than 50 copies per mL [treatment difference and 95% CI: 7.4% (0.7%, 14.2%)].

16 HOW SUPPLIED/STORAGE AND HANDLING

TRIUMEQ tablets, 600 mg of abacavir as abacavir sulfate, 50 mg of dolutegravir as dolutegravir sodium, and 300 mg lamivudine, are purple, oval, film-coated, biconvex tablets debossed with "572 Tri" on one side.

Bottle of 30 with child-resistant closure NDC 49702-231-13. Store and dispense in the original package, protect from moisture, and keep the bottle tightly closed. Do not remove desiccant.

Store at 25°C (77°F); excursions permitted 15° to 30°C (59° to 86°F). [See USP Controlled Room Temperature].

17 PATIENT COUNSELING INFORMATION

Advise the patient to read the FDA-approved patient labeling (Medication Guide).

Drug Interactions: Do not coadminister TRIUMEQ with dofetilide (TIKOSYN®) because the interaction between dofetilide and dolutegravir can result in potentially life-threatening adverse events [see Contraindications (4)]. Patients should be advised to report to their healthcare provider the use of any other prescription or nonprescription medication or herbal products.

Hypersensitivity Reaction: Inform patients:

- that a Medication Guide and Warning Card summarizing the symptoms of the abacavir hypersensitivity reaction and other product information will be dispensed by the pharmacist with each new prescription and refill of TRIUMEQ, and instruct the patient to read the Medication Guide and Warning Card every time to obtain any new information that may be present about TRIUMEQ. (The complete text of the Medication Guide is reprinted at the end of this document.)
- to carry the Warning Card with them.
- how to identify a hypersensitivity reaction [see Warnings and Precautions (5.1), Medication Guide].
- that if they develop symptoms consistent with a hypersensitivity reaction they should call their doctor right away to determine if they should stop taking TRIUMEQ.
- that a hypersensitivity reaction can worsen and lead to hospitalization or death if TRIUMEQ is not immediately discontinued.

- to not restart TRIUMEQ or any other abacavir-containing product following a hypersensitivity reaction because more severe symptoms can occur within hours and may include life–threatening hypotension and death.
- that a hypersensitivity reaction is usually reversible if it is detected promptly and TRIUMEQ is stopped right away.
- that if they have interrupted TRIUMEQ for reasons other than symptoms of hypersensitivity (for example, those who have an interruption in drug supply), a serious or fatal hypersensitivity reaction may occur with reintroduction of abacavir.
- to not restart TRIUMEQ or any other abacavir–containing product without medical consultation and only if medical care can be readily accessed by the patient or others.
- to not restart TRIUMEQ or any other dolutegravir-containing product following a hypersensitivity reaction to TRIUMEQ.

Inform patients that they should not take TRIUMEQ with ATRIPLA, COMBIVIR®, COMPLERA®, EMTRIVA®, EPIVIR, EPIVIR–HBV®, EPZICOM®, STRIBILD®, TRIZIVIR, TRUVADA®, or ZIAGEN.

Lactic Acidosis/Hepatomegaly: Inform patients that some HIV medicines, including TRIUMEQ, can cause a rare, but serious condition called lactic acidosis with liver enlargement (hepatomegaly) [see Warnings and Precautions (5.2)].

Patients with Hepatitis B or C Co-infection: Patients with underlying hepatitis B or C may be at increased risk for worsening or development of transaminase elevations with use of TRIUMEQ and advise patients to have laboratory testing before and during therapy [see Warnings and Precautions (5.3)].

Advise patients co-infected with HIV–1 and HBV that worsening of liver disease has occurred in some cases when treatment with lamivudine was discontinued. Advise patients to discuss any changes in regimen with their physician [see Warnings and Precautions (5.3)].

Inform patients with HIV– 1/HCV co-infection that hepatic decompensation (some fatal) has occurred in HIV– 1/HCV co-infected patients receiving combination antiretroviral therapy for HIV– 1 and interferon alfa with or without ribavirin [see Warnings and Precautions (5.4)].

Immune Reconstitution Syndrome: In some patients with advanced HIV infection, signs and symptoms of inflammation from previous infections may occur soon after anti-HIV treatment is started. It is believed that these symptoms are due to an improvement in the body's immune response, enabling the body to fight infections that may have been present with no obvious symptoms. Advise patients to inform their healthcare provider immediately of any symptoms of infection [see Warnings and Precautions (5.5)].

Redistribution/Accumulation of Body Fat: Inform patients that redistribution or accumulation of body fat may occur in patients receiving antiretroviral therapy and that the cause and long-term health effects of these conditions are not known at this time [see Warnings and Precautions (5.6)].

Information About HIV–1 Infection: TRIUMEQ is not a cure for HIV–1 infection and patients may continue to experience illnesses associated with HIV–1 infection, including opportunistic infections. Patients must remain on continuous HIV therapy to control HIV–1infection and decrease HIV-related illness. Inform patients that sustained decreases in plasma HIV RNA have been associated with a reduced risk of progression to AIDS and death.

Advise patients to remain under the care of a physician when using TRIUMEQ.

Advise patients to take all HIV medications exactly as prescribed.

Advise patients to avoid doing things that can spread HIV–1 infection to others.

Advise patients not to re-use or share needles or other injection equipment.

Advise patients not to share personal items that can have blood or body fluids on them, like toothbrushes and razor blades.

Always practice safer sex by using a latex or polyurethane condom to lower the chance of sexual contact with semen, vaginal secretions, or blood.

Female patients should be advised not to breastfeed because it is not known if TRIUMEQ can be passed to your baby in your breast milk and whether it could harm your baby. Mothers with HIV–1 should not breastfeed because HIV-1 can be passed to the baby in the breast milk.

Instruct patients to read the Medication Guide before starting TRIUMEQ and to reread it each time the prescription is renewed. Instruct patients to inform their physician or pharmacist if they develop any unusual symptom, or if any known symptom persists or worsens.

Instruct patients that if they miss a dose, they should take it as soon as they remember. If they do not remember until it is within 4 hours of the time for the next dose, they should be instructed to skip the missed dose and go back to the regular schedule. Patients should not double their next dose or take more than the prescribed dose.

Instruct patients to store TRIUMEQ in the original package, protect from moisture, and keep the bottle tightly closed. Do not remove desiccant.

COMBIVIR, EPIVIR, EPZICOM, TIVICAY, TRIUMEQ, TRIZIVIR, and ZIAGEN are registered trademarks of the ViiV Healthcare group of companies.

EPIVIR-HBV is a registered trademark of the GSK group of companies.

The other brands listed are trademarks of their respective owners and are not trademarks of the ViiV Healthcare group of companies. The makers of these brands are not affiliated with and do not endorse the ViiV Healthcare group of companies or its products.

Manufactured for:
ViiV Healthcare
Research Triangle Park, NC 27709
by:
GlaxoSmithKline
Research Triangle Park, NC 27709
Lamivudine is manufactured under agreement from
Shire Pharmaceuticals Group plc
Basingstoke, UK
©2014, the ViiV Healthcare group of companies. All rights reserved.
TRM:1PI

MEDICATION GUIDE
TRIUMEQ® (TRI-u-meck)
(abacavir, dolutegravir, and lamivudine)
Tablets

Read this Medication Guide before you start taking TRIUMEQ and each time you get a refill. There may be new information. This information does not take the place of talking to your healthcare provider about your medical condition or your treatment. Be sure to carry your TRIUMEQ Warning Card with you at all times.

What is the most important information I should know about TRIUMEQ?

• **Serious allergic reaction (hypersensitivity reaction).** TRIUMEQ contains abacavir (also contained in EPZICOM®, TRIZIVIR®, and ZIAGEN®). Patients taking TRIUMEQ may have a serious allergic reaction (hypersensitivity reaction) that can cause death. Your risk of this allergic reaction to abacavir is much higher if you have a gene variation called HLA-B*5701. Your healthcare provider can determine with a blood test if you have this gene variation.

If you get a symptom from 2 or more of the following groups while taking TRIUMEQ, call your healthcare provider right away to find out if you should stop taking TRIUMEQ.

	Symptom(s)
Group 1	Fever
Group 2	Rash
Group 3	Nausea, vomiting, diarrhea, abdominal (stomach area) pain
Group 4	Generally ill feeling, extreme tiredness, or achiness
Group 5	Shortness of breath, cough, sore throat

A list of these symptoms is on the Warning Card your pharmacist gives you. **Carry this Warning Card with you at all times.**

If you stop TRIUMEQ because of an allergic reaction, never take TRIUMEQ or any other medicines that contain abacavir or dolutegravir (EPZICOM, ZIAGEN, TRIZIVIR, or TIVICAY®) again. If you take TRIUMEQ or any other abacavir–containing medicine again after you have had an allergic reaction, **within hours** you may get **life–threatening symptoms** that may include **very low blood pressure** or **death**. If you stop TRIUMEQ for any other reason, even for a few days, and you are not allergic to TRIUMEQ, talk with your healthcare provider before taking it again. Taking TRIUMEQ again can cause a serious allergic or life–threatening reaction, even if you never had an allergic reaction to it before.

If your healthcare provider tells you that you can take TRIUMEQ again, start taking it when you are around medical help or people who can call a healthcare provider if you need one.

• **Build-up of acid in your blood (lactic acidosis).** Lactic acidosis can happen in some people who take TRIUMEQ. Lactic acidosis is a serious medical emergency that can lead to death.

Lactic acidosis can be hard to identify early, because the symptoms could seem like symptoms of other health problems.

Call your healthcare provider right away if you get the following symptoms that could be signs of lactic acidosis:

• feel very weak or tired
• have unusual (not normal) muscle pain
• have trouble breathing
• have stomach pain with nausea and vomiting
• feel cold, especially in your arms and legs
• feel dizzy or lightheaded
• have a fast or irregular heartbeat
• **Severe liver problems.** Severe liver problems can happen in people who take TRIUMEQ. In some cases these severe liver problems can lead to death. Your liver may become large (hepatomegaly) and you may develop fat in your liver (steatosis).

Call your healthcare provider right away if you get any of the following signs or symptoms of liver problems:

• your skin or the white part of your eyes turns yellow
• dark "tea-colored" urine
• light colored stools (bowel movements)
• nausea
• itching
• stomach-area pain

You may be more likely to get lactic acidosis or serious liver problems if you are female, very overweight, or have been taking nucleoside analogue medicines for a long time.

• **Worsening of hepatitis B virus in people who have HIV-1 infection.** If you have HIV-1 and hepatitis B virus infections, your hepatitis virus infection may get worse if you stop taking TRIUMEQ. To help avoid this: Take TRIUMEQ exactly as prescribed.

• Do not run out of TRIUMEQ.
• Do not stop taking TRIUMEQ without talking to your healthcare provider.
• Your healthcare provider should monitor your health and do regular blood tests to check your liver for at least several months if you stop taking TRIUMEQ.

• **Resistant Hepatitis B Virus (HBV).** If you have HIV-1 and hepatitis B, the hepatitis B virus can change (mutate) during your treatment with TRIUMEQ and become harder to treat (resistant).

• **Use with interferon and ribavirin–based regimens.** Worsening of liver disease has happened in people infected with HIV-1 and hepatitis C virus who are taking anti–HIV medicines and are also being treated for hepatitis C with interferon with or without ribavirin. If you are taking TRIUMEQ and interferon with or without ribavirin, tell your healthcare provider if you have any new symptoms.

What is TRIUMEQ?

TRIUMEQ is a prescription medicine used to treat HIV–1 (Human Immunodeficiency Virus-type 1) infection. TRIUMEQ contains 3 prescription medicines: abacavir (ZIAGEN), dolutegravir (TIVICAY), and lamivudine (EPIVIR®).

• TRIUMEQ is not for use by itself in people who have or have had resistance to abacavir, dolutegravir, or lamivudine.

It is not known if TRIUMEQ is safe and effective in children.

TRIUMEQ may help:

• reduce the amount of HIV–1 in your blood. This is called "viral load".

• increase the number of white blood cells called CD4+ (T) cells in your blood, which help fight off other infections.

Reducing the amount of HIV-1 and increasing the CD4+ (T) cells in your blood may help improve your immune system. This may reduce your risk of death or getting infections that can happen when your immune system is weak (opportunistic infections).

TRIUMEQ does not cure HIV-1 infection or AIDS. You must stay on continuous HIV–1 therapy to control HIV–1 infection and decrease HIV-related illnesses.

Avoid doing things that can spread HIV–1 infection to others.

• Do not share or re-use needles or other injection equipment.
• Do not share personal items that can have blood or body fluids on them, like toothbrushes and razor blades.
• Do not have any kind of sex without protection. Always practice safer sex by using a latex or polyurethane condom to lower the chance of sexual contact with semen, vaginal secretions, or blood.

Ask your healthcare provider if you have any questions about how to prevent passing HIV to other people.

Who should not take TRIUMEQ?

Do not take TRIUMEQ if you:

• have a certain type of gene variation called the HLA-B*5701 allele. Your healthcare provider will test you for this before prescribing treatment with TRIUMEQ.
• have ever had an allergic reaction to abacavir, dolutegravir, or lamivudine
• take dofetilide (TIKOSYN®). Taking TRIUMEQ and dofetilide (TIKOSYN) can cause side effects that may be life-threatening.
• have certain liver problems

What should I tell my healthcare provider before taking TRIUMEQ?

Before you take TRIUMEQ, tell your healthcare provider if you:

• have been tested and know whether or not you have a particular gene variation called HLA-B*5701
• have or had liver problems, including hepatitis B or C virus infection
• have kidney problems
• have heart problems, smoke, or have diseases that increase your risk of heart disease such as high blood pressure, high cholesterol, or diabetes
• drink alcoholic beverages
• have any other medical condition
• are pregnant or plan to become pregnant. It is not known if TRIUMEQ will harm your unborn baby. Tell your healthcare provider if you become pregnant while taking TRIUMEQ.

Pregnancy Registry. There is a pregnancy registry for women who take antiviral medicines during pregnancy. The purpose of the registry is to collect information about the health of you and your baby. Talk to your healthcare provider about how you can take part in this registry.

• **are breastfeeding or plan to breastfeed. Do not breastfeed** if you take TRIUMEQ. You should not breastfeed because of the risk of passing HIV–1 to your baby. It is not known if abacavir or dolutegravir passes into your breast milk. Lamivudine can pass into your breast milk and may harm your baby. Talk to your healthcare provider about the best way to feed your baby.

Tell your healthcare provider about all the medicines you take, including prescription and over-the-counter medicines, vitamins, and herbal supplements. TRIUMEQ may affect the way other medicines work, and other medicines may affect how TRIUMEQ works.

You should not take TRIUMEQ if you also take:

• abacavir (EPZICOM, TRIZIVIR, or ZIAGEN)
• lamivudine (COMBIVIR®, EPIVIR, EPIVIR-HBV®, EPZICOM, or TRIZIVIR)
• emtricitabine (EMTRIVA®, ATRIPLA®, COMPLERA®, STRIBILD®, TRUVADA®)

Tell your healthcare provider if you take:

• antacids, laxatives or other medicines that contain aluminum, magnesium, sucralfate (CARAFATE®), or buffered medicines. TRIUMEQ should be taken at least 2 hours before or 6 hours after you take these medicines.
• anti-seizure medicines:
  • oxcarbazepine (TRILEPTAL®)
  • phenytoin (DILANTIN®, DILANTIN®-125, PHENYTEK®)
  • phenobarbital
  • carbamazepine (CARBATROL®, EQUETRO®, TEGRETOL®, TEGRETOL®-XR, TERIL®, EPITOL®)
• any other medicine to treat HIV-1
• iron or calcium supplements taken by mouth. Supplements containing calcium or iron may be taken at the same time with TRIUMEQ if taken with food. Otherwise, TRIUMEQ should be taken at least 2 hours before or 6 hours after you take these medicines.
• medicines used to treat hepatitis virus infections, such as interferon or ribavirin
• a medicine that contains metformin
• methadone
• rifampin (RIFATER®, RIFAMATE®, RIMACTANE®, RIFADIN®)
• St. John's wort (Hypericum perforatum)

Know the medicines you take. Keep a list of your medicines with you to show to your healthcare provider and pharmacist when you get a new medicine.

Ask your healthcare provider or pharmacist if you are not sure if you take one of the medicines listed above.

How should I take TRIUMEQ?

• **Take TRIUMEQ exactly as your healthcare provider tells you.**
• Do not change your dose or stop taking TRIUMEQ without talking with your healthcare provider.
• Stay under the care of a healthcare provider while taking TRIUMEQ.
• You can take TRIUMEQ with or without food.
• If you miss a dose of TRIUMEQ, take it as soon as you remember. If it is within 4 hours of your next dose, skip the missed dose and take the next dose at your regular time. Do not take 2 doses at the same time. If you are not sure about your dosing, call your healthcare provider.
• Do not run out of TRIUMEQ. The virus in your blood may become resistant to other HIV-1 medicines if TRIUMEQ is stopped for even a short time. When your supply starts to run low, get more from your healthcare provider or pharmacy.
• If you take too much TRIUMEQ, call your healthcare provider or go to the nearest hospital emergency room right away.

What are the possible side effects of TRIUMEQ?
TRIUMEQ can cause serious side effects including:
- See "What is the most important information I should know about TRIUMEQ?"
- **Changes in liver tests.** People with a history of hepatitis B or C virus may have an increased risk of developing new or worsening changes in certain liver tests during treatment with TRIUMEQ. Your healthcare provider may do tests to check your liver function before and during treatment with TRIUMEQ.
- **Changes in your immune system (Immune Reconstitution Syndrome)** can happen when you start taking HIV-1 medicines. Your immune system may get stronger and begin to fight infections that have been hidden in your body for a long time. Tell your healthcare provider right away if you start having new symptoms after starting your HIV-1 medicine.
- **Changes in body fat (fat redistribution)** can happen in people who take HIV-1 medicines. These changes may include increased amount of fat in the upper back and neck ("buffalo hump"), breast, and around the middle of your body (trunk). Loss of fat from the legs, arms, and face may also happen. The exact cause and long-term health effects of these problems are not known.
- **Heart attack (myocardial infarction).** Some HIV medicines including TRIUMEQ may increase your risk of heart attack.

The most common side effects of TRIUMEQ include:
- trouble sleeping
- headache
- tiredness

Tell your healthcare provider if you have any side effect that bothers you or that does not go away.
These are not all the possible side effects of TRIUMEQ. For more information, ask your healthcare provider or pharmacist.
Call your doctor for medical advice about side effects. You may report side effects to FDA at 1–800–FDA–1088.

How should I store TRIUMEQ?
- Store TRIUMEQ at room temperature between 68°F to 77°F (20°C to 25°C).
- Store TRIUMEQ in the original bottle.
- Keep the bottle of TRIUMEQ tightly closed and protect from moisture.
- The bottle of TRIUMEQ contains a desiccant packet to help keep your medicine dry (protect it from moisture). Keep the desiccant packet in the bottle. Do not remove the desiccant packet.

Keep TRIUMEQ and all medicines out of the reach of children.

General information about the safe and effective use of TRIUMEQ
Medicines are sometimes prescribed for purposes other than those listed in a Medication Guide. Do not use TRIUMEQ for a condition for which it was not prescribed. Do not give TRIUMEQ to other people, even if they have the same symptoms that you have. It may harm them.
This Medication Guide summarizes the most important information about TRIUMEQ. If you would like more information, talk with your healthcare provider. You can ask your healthcare provider or pharmacist for information about TRIUMEQ that is written for health professionals.
For more information go to www.TRIUMEQ.com or call 1-877-844-8872.

What are the ingredients in TRIUMEQ?
Active ingredients: abacavir, dolutegravir, and lamivudine.
Inactive ingredients: D-mannitol, magnesium stearate, microcrystalline cellulose, povidone, and sodium starch glycolate. The tablet film–coating contains iron oxide black, iron oxide red, macrogol/PEG, polyvinyl alcohol–part hydrolyzed, talc, and titanium oxide.
This Medication Guide has been approved by the U.S. Food and Drug Administration.
Manufactured for:
ViiV Healthcare
Research Triangle Park, NC 27709
by:
GlaxoSmithKline
Research Triangle Park, NC 27709
Lamivudine is manufactured under agreement from
Shire Pharmaceuticals Group plc
Basingstoke, UK
COMBIVIR, EPIVIR, EPZICOM, TIVICAY, TRIUMEQ, TRIZIVIR, and ZIAGEN are registered trademarks of the ViiV Healthcare group of companies.
EPIVIR-HBV is a registered trademark of the GSK group of companies.
The other brands listed are trademarks of their respective owners and are not trademarks of the ViiV Healthcare group of companies. The makers of these brands are not affiliated with and do not endorse the ViiV Healthcare group of companies or its products.

©2014, the ViiV Healthcare group of companies. All rights reserved.
Issued: August 2014
TRM:1MG

TRIZIVIR   ℞
[trī' zə-vir]
(abacavir sulfate, lamivudine, and zidovudine)
Tablets, for oral use

HIGHLIGHTS OF PRESCRIBING INFORMATION
These highlights do not include all the information needed to use TRIZIVIR safely and effectively. See full prescribing information for TRIZIVIR.
TRIZIVIR (abacavir sulfate, lamivudine, and zidovudine)
Tablets, for oral use
Initial U.S. Approval: 2000

> **WARNING: RISK OF HYPERSENSITIVITY REACTIONS, HEMATOLOGIC TOXICITY, MYOPATHY, LACTIC ACIDOSIS AND SEVERE HEPATOMEGALY, EXACERBATIONS OF HEPATITIS B**
> *See full prescribing information for complete boxed warning.*
> - Serious and sometimes fatal hypersensitivity reactions have been associated with abacavir-containing products. (5.1)
> - Hypersensitivity to abacavir is a multi-organ clinical syndrome. (5.1)
> - Patients who carry the HLA-B*5701 allele are at high risk for experiencing a hypersensitivity reaction to abacavir. (5.1)
> - Discontinue TRIZIVIR as soon as a hypersensitivity reaction is suspected. Regardless of HLA-B*5701 status, permanently discontinue TRIZIVIR if hypersensitivity cannot be ruled out. (5.1)
> - Following a hypersensitivity reaction to abacavir, NEVER restart TRIZIVIR or any other abacavir-containing product. (5.1)
> - Hematologic toxicity, including neutropenia and anemia, has been associated with the use of zidovudine, a component of TRIZIVIR. (5.2)
> - Symptomatic myopathy associated with prolonged use of zidovudine. (5.3)
> - Lactic acidosis and severe hepatomegaly with steatosis, including fatal cases, have been reported with the use of nucleoside analogues. (5.4)
> - Severe acute exacerbations of hepatitis B have been reported in patients who are co-infected with hepatitis B virus (HBV) and human immunodeficiency virus (HIV-1) and have discontinued lamivudine, a component of TRIZIVIR. Monitor hepatic function closely in these patients and, if appropriate, initiate anti-hepatitis B treatment. (5.5)

INDICATIONS AND USAGE
TRIZIVIR, a combination of abacavir, lamivudine, and zidovudine, each nucleoside analogue HIV-1 reverse transcriptase inhibitors, is indicated in combination with other antiretroviral agents for the treatment of HIV-1 infection. (1)

DOSAGE AND ADMINISTRATION
- A medication guide and warning card should be dispensed with each new prescription and refill. (2)
- Adults and Adolescents: 1 tablet twice daily. (2.1)
- Not recommended in adolescents who weigh less than 40 kg. (2.1)
- Do not prescribe for patients requiring dosage adjustment or patients with hepatic impairment. (2.2)

DOSAGE FORMS AND STRENGTHS
Tablets contain 300 mg abacavir, 150 mg of lamivudine, and 300 mg of zidovudine. (3)

CONTRAINDICATIONS
- Previously demonstrated hypersensitivity to abacavir or any other component of the product. (4, 5.1, 6)
- Hepatic impairment. (4)

WARNINGS AND PRECAUTIONS
- See boxed warning for information about the following: hypersensitivity reactions, hematologic toxicity, myopathy, lactic acidosis and severe hepatomegaly, and severe acute exacerbations of hepatitis B. (5.1, 5.2, 5.3, 5.4, 5.5)
- Hepatic decompensation, some fatal, has occurred in HIV-1/HCV co-infected patients receiving combination antiretroviral therapy and interferon alfa with or without ribavirin. Discontinue TRIZIVIR as medically appropriate and consider dose reduction or discontinuation of interferon alfa, ribavirin, or both. (5.6)

- Exacerbation of anemia has been reported in HIV-1/HCV co-infected patients receiving ribavirin and zidovudine. Coadministration of ribavirin and zidovudine is not advised. (5.6)
- Immune reconstitution syndrome (5.7) and redistribution/accumulation of body fat (5.8) have been reported in patients treated with combination antiretroviral therapy.
- TRIZIVIR should not be administered with other products containing abacavir, lamivudine, or zidovudine; or with emtricitabine. (5.11)

ADVERSE REACTIONS
The most commonly reported adverse reactions (incidence ≥10%) in clinical trials were nausea, headache, malaise and fatigue, and nausea and vomiting. (6.1)
To report SUSPECTED ADVERSE REACTIONS, contact ViiV Healthcare at 1-877-844-8872 or FDA at 1-800-FDA-1088 or www.fda.gov/medwatch.

DRUG INTERACTIONS
- Concomitant use with the following drugs should be avoided: stavudine (7.1), doxorubicin (7.2).
- Ethanol: Decreases the elimination of abacavir. (7.3)
- Bone marrow suppressive/cytotoxic agents: May increase the hematologic toxicity of zidovudine. (7.4)
- Methadone: An increased methadone dose may be required in a small number of patients. (7.6)

See 17 for PATIENT COUNSELING INFORMATION and Medication Guide

Revised: 05/2013

FULL PRESCRIBING INFORMATION

> **WARNING: RISK OF HYPERSENSITIVITY RE-ACTIONS, HEMATOLOGIC TOXICITY, MYOPATHY, LACTIC ACIDOSIS AND SEVERE HEPATOMEGALY, EXACERBATIONS OF HEPATITIS B**
>
> **Hypersensitivity Reactions:** Serious and sometimes fatal hypersensitivity reactions have been associated with abacavir sulfate, a component of TRIZIVIR. Hypersensitivity to abacavir is a multi-organ clinical syndrome usually characterized by a sign or symptom in 2 or more of the following groups: (1) fever, (2) rash, (3) gastrointestinal (including nausea, vomiting, diarrhea, or abdominal pain), (4) constitutional (including generalized malaise, fatigue, or achiness), and (5) respiratory (including dyspnea, cough, or pharyngitis). Discontinue TRIZIVIR as soon as a hypersensitivity reaction is suspected.
>
> Patients who carry the HLA-B*5701 allele are at high risk for experiencing a hypersensitivity reaction to abacavir. Prior to initiating therapy with abacavir, screening for the HLA-B*5701 allele is recommended; this approach has been found to decrease the risk of hypersensitivity reaction. Screening is also recommended prior to reinitiation of abacavir in patients of unknown HLA-B*5701 status who have previously tolerated abacavir. HLA-B*5701-negative patients may develop a suspected hypersensitivity reaction to abacavir; however, this occurs significantly less frequently than in HLA-B*5701-positive patients. Regardless of HLA-B*5701 status, permanently discontinue TRIZIVIR if hypersensitivity cannot be ruled out, even when other diagnoses are possible.
>
> Following a hypersensitivity reaction to abacavir, NEVER restart TRIZIVIR or any other abacavir-containing product because more severe symptoms can occur within hours and may include life-threatening hypotension and death.
>
> Reintroduction of TRIZIVIR or any other abacavir-containing product, even in patients who have no identified history or unrecognized symptoms of hypersensitivity to abacavir therapy, can result in serious or fatal hypersensitivity reactions. Such reactions can occur within hours *[see Warnings and Precautions (5.1)]*.
>
> **Hematologic Toxicity:** Zidovudine, a component of TRIZIVIR, has been associated with hematologic toxicity, including neutropenia and severe anemia, particularly in patients with advanced Human Immunodeficiency Virus (HIV-1) disease *[see Warnings and Precautions (5.2)]*.
>
> **Myopathy:** Prolonged use of zidovudine has been associated with symptomatic myopathy *[see Warnings and Precautions (5.3)]*.
>
> **Lactic Acidosis and Severe Hepatomegaly:** Lactic acidosis and severe hepatomegaly with steatosis, including fatal cases, have been reported with the use of nucleoside analogues alone or in combination, including abacavir, lamivudine, zidovudine, and other antiretrovirals *[see Warnings and Precautions (5.4)]*.
>
> **Exacerbations of Hepatitis B:** Severe acute exacerbations of hepatitis B have been reported in patients who are co-infected with hepatitis B virus (HBV) and HIV-1 and have discontinued lamivudine, which is one component of TRIZIVIR. Hepatic function should be monitored closely with both clinical and laboratory follow-up for at least several months in patients who discontinue TRIZIVIR and are co-infected with HIV-1 and HBV. If appropriate, initiation of anti-hepatitis B therapy may be warranted *[see Warnings and Precautions (5.5)]*.

1 INDICATIONS AND USAGE

TRIZIVIR is indicated in combination with other antiretrovirals or alone for the treatment of HIV-1 infection.

Additional important information on the use of TRIZIVIR for treatment of HIV-1 infection:

• TRIZIVIR is one of multiple products containing abacavir. Before starting TRIZIVIR, review medical history for prior exposure to any abacavir-containing product in order to avoid reintroduction in a patient with a history of hypersensitivity to abacavir *[see Warnings and Precautions (5.1), Adverse Reactions (6)]*.

• TRIZIVIR is a fixed-dose combination of 3 nucleoside analogues: abacavir, lamivudine, and zidovudine and is intended only for patients whose regimen would otherwise include these 3 components.

• Limited data exist on the use of TRIZIVIR alone in patients with higher baseline viral load levels (>100,000 copies/mL) *[see Clinical Studies (14)]*.

2 DOSAGE AND ADMINISTRATION

• A Medication Guide and Warning Card that provide information about recognition of hypersensitivity reactions should be dispensed with each new prescription and refill.

• TRIZIVIR can be taken with or without food.

2.1 Adults and Adolescent Patients

The recommended oral dose of TRIZIVIR is one tablet twice daily.

TRIZIVIR is not recommended in adolescents who weigh less than 40 kg because it is a fixed-dose tablet and cannot be dose adjusted.

2.2 Dosage Adjustment

Because it is a fixed-dose combination, TRIZIVIR should not be prescribed for:

• patients requiring dosage adjustment such as those with creatinine clearance <50 mL/min.

• patients with hepatic impairment.

3 DOSAGE FORMS AND STRENGTHS

TRIZIVIR Tablets contain 300 mg of abacavir as abacavir sulfate, 150 mg of lamivudine, and 300 mg of zidovudine. The tablets are blue-green, capsule-shaped, film-coated, and imprinted with "GX LL1" on one side with no markings on the reverse side.

4 CONTRAINDICATIONS

TRIZIVIR Tablets are contraindicated in patients with:

• previously demonstrated hypersensitivity to abacavir or any other component of the product. NEVER restart TRIZIVIR or any other abacavir-containing product following a hypersensitivity reaction to abacavir, regardless of HLA-B*5701 status *[see Warnings and Precautions (5.1), Adverse Reactions (6)]*.

• hepatic impairment *[see Use in Specific Populations (8.7)]*.

5 WARNINGS AND PRECAUTIONS

5.1 Hypersensitivity Reaction

Serious and sometimes fatal hypersensitivity reactions have been associated with TRIZIVIR and other abacavir-containing products. Patients who carry the HLA-B*5701 allele are at high risk for experiencing a hypersensitivity reaction to abacavir. Prior to initiating therapy with abacavir, screening for the HLA-B*5701 allele is recommended; this approach has been found to decrease the risk of a hypersensitivity reaction. Screening is also recommended prior to reinitiation of abacavir in patients of unknown HLA-B*5701 status who have previously tolerated abacavir. For HLA-B*5701-positive patients, treatment with an abacavir-containing regimen is not recommended and should be considered only with close medical supervision and under exceptional circumstances when the potential benefit outweighs the risk.

HLA-B*5701-negative patients may develop a hypersensitivity reaction to abacavir; however, this occurs significantly less frequently than in HLA-B*5701-positive patients. Regardless of HLA-B*5701 status, permanently discontinue TRIZIVIR if hypersensitivity cannot be ruled out, even when other diagnoses are possible.

Important information on signs and symptoms of hypersensitivity, as well as clinical management, is presented below.

Signs and Symptoms of Hypersensitivity: Hypersensitivity to abacavir is a multi-organ clinical syndrome usually characterized by a sign or symptom in 2 or more of the following groups:

Group 1: Fever

Group 2: Rash

Group 3: Gastrointestinal (including nausea, vomiting, diarrhea, or abdominal pain)

Group 4: Constitutional (including generalized malaise, fatigue, or achiness)

Group 5: Respiratory (including dyspnea, cough, or pharyngitis)

Hypersensitivity to abacavir following the presentation of a single sign or symptom has been reported infrequently.

Hypersensitivity to abacavir was reported in approximately 8% of 2,670 subjects (n = 206) in 9 clinical trials (range: 2% to 9%) with enrollment from November 1999 to February 2002. Data on time to onset and symptoms of suspected hypersensitivity were collected on a detailed data collection module. The frequencies of symptoms are shown in Figure 1. Symptoms usually appeared within the first 6 weeks of treatment with abacavir, although the reaction may occur at any time during therapy. Median time to onset was 9 days; 89% appeared within the first 6 weeks; 95% of subjects reported symptoms from 2 or more of the 5 groups listed above.

A trial with ZIAGEN® (abacavir sulfate) used double-blind ascertainment of suspected hypersensitivity reactions. During the blinded portion of the trial, suspected hypersensitivity to abacavir was reported by investigators in 9% of 324 subjects in the abacavir group and 3% of 325 subjects in the zidovudine group.

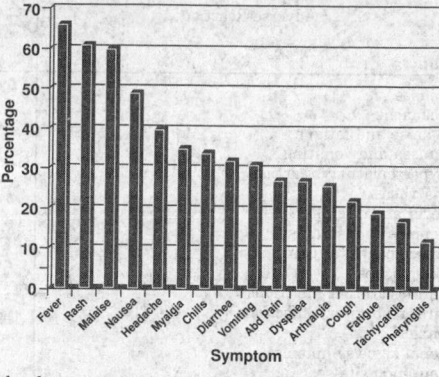

Figure 1. Hypersensitivity-Related Symptoms Reported With ≥10% Frequency in Clinical Trials (n = 206 Subjects)

Other less common signs and symptoms of hypersensitivity include lethargy, myolysis, edema, abnormal chest x-ray findings (predominantly infiltrates, which can be localized), and paresthesia. Anaphylaxis, liver failure, renal failure, hypotension, adult respiratory distress syndrome, respiratory failure, and death have occurred in association with hypersensitivity reactions.

Physical findings associated with hypersensitivity to abacavir in some subjects include lymphadenopathy, mucous membrane lesions (conjunctivitis and mouth ulcerations), and rash. The rash usually appears maculopapular or urticarial, but may be variable in appearance. There have been reports of erythema multiforme. Hypersensitivity reactions have occurred without rash.

Laboratory abnormalities associated with hypersensitivity to abacavir in some subjects include elevated liver function tests, elevated creatinine phosphokinase, elevated creatinine, and lymphopenia.

Clinical Management of Hypersensitivity: Discontinue TRIZIVIR as soon as a hypersensitivity reaction is suspected. To minimize the risk of a life-threatening hypersensitivity reaction, permanently discontinue TRIZIVIR if hypersensitivity cannot be ruled out, even when other diagnoses are possible (e.g., acute onset respiratory diseases such as pneumonia, bronchitis, pharyngitis, or influenza; gastroenteritis; or reactions to other medications).

Following a hypersensitivity reaction to abacavir, NEVER restart TRIZIVIR or any other abacavir-containing product because more severe symptoms can occur within hours and may include life-threatening hypotension and death.

When therapy with TRIZIVIR has been discontinued for reasons other than symptoms of a hypersensitivity reaction, and if reinitiation of abacavir is under consideration, carefully evaluate the reason for discontinuation to ensure that the patient did not have symptoms of a hypersensitivity reaction. If the patient is of unknown HLA-B*5701 status, screening for the allele is recommended prior to reinitiation of TRIZIVIR.

If hypersensitivity cannot be ruled out, DO NOT reintroduce TRIZIVIR or any other abacavir-containing product. Even in the absence of the HLA-B*5701 allele, it is important to permanently discontinue abacavir and not rechallenge with abacavir if a hypersensitivity reaction cannot be ruled out on clinical grounds, due to the potential for a severe or even fatal reaction.

If symptoms consistent with hypersensitivity are not identified, reintroduction can be undertaken with continued monitoring for symptoms of a hypersensitivity reaction. Make patients aware that a hypersensitivity reaction can occur with reintroduction of abacavir and that abacavir reintroduction needs to be undertaken only if medical care can be readily accessed by the patient or others.

Risk Factor: HLA-B*5701 Allele: Trials have shown that carriage of the HLA-B*5701 allele is associated with a significantly increased risk of a hypersensitivity reaction to abacavir.

CNA106030 (PREDICT-1), a randomized, double-blind trial, evaluated the clinical utility of prospective HLA-B*5701 screening on the incidence of abacavir hypersensitivity reaction in abacavir-naive HIV-1-infected adults (n = 1,650). In this trial, use of pre-therapy screening for the HLA-B*5701 allele and exclusion of subjects with this allele reduced the incidence of clinically suspected abacavir hypersensitivity reactions from 7.8% (66/847) to 3.4% (27/803). Based on this trial, it is estimated that 61% of patients with the HLA-B*5701 allele will develop a clinically suspected hypersensitivity reaction during the course of abacavir treatment compared with 4% of patients who do not have the HLA-B*5701 allele.

Screening for carriage of the HLA-B*5701 allele is recommended prior to initiating treatment with abacavir. Screening is also recommended prior to reinitiation of abacavir in

Table 1. Treatment-Emergent (All Causality) Adverse Reactions of at Least Moderate Intensity (Grades 2-4, ≥5% Frequency) in Therapy-Naive Adults (CNA3005) Through 48 Weeks of Treatment

Adverse Reaction	ZIAGEN plus Lamivudine/Zidovudine (n = 262)	Indinavir plus Lamivudine/Zidovudine (n = 264)
Nausea	19%	17%
Headache	13%	9%
Malaise and fatigue	12%	12%
Nausea and vomiting	10%	10%
Hypersensitivity reaction	8%	2%
Diarrhea	7%	5%
Fever and/or chills	6%	3%
Depressive disorders	6%	4%
Musculoskeletal pain	5%	7%
Skin rashes	5%	4%
Ear/nose/throat infections	5%	4%
Viral respiratory infections	5%	5%
Anxiety	5%	3%
Renal signs/symptoms	<1%	5%
Pain (non-site-specific)	<1%	5%

patients of unknown HLA-B*5701 status who have previously tolerated abacavir. For HLA-B*5701-positive patients, initiating or reinitiating treatment with an abacavir-containing regimen is not recommended and should be considered only with close medical supervision and under exceptional circumstances where potential benefit outweighs the risk.

Skin patch testing is used as a research tool and should not be used to aid in the clinical diagnosis of abacavir hypersensitivity.

In any patient treated with abacavir, the clinical diagnosis of hypersensitivity reaction must remain the basis of clinical decision-making. Even in the absence of the HLA-B*5701 allele, it is important to permanently discontinue abacavir and not rechallenge with abacavir if a hypersensitivity reaction cannot be ruled out on clinical grounds, due to the potential for a severe or even fatal reaction.

5.2 Hematologic Toxicity/Bone Marrow Suppression

Zidovudine, a component of TRIZIVIR, has been associated with hematologic toxicity including neutropenia and anemia, particularly in patients with advanced HIV-1 disease. TRIZIVIR should be used with caution in patients who have bone marrow compromise evidenced by granulocyte count less than 1,000 cells/mm^3 or hemoglobin less than 9.5 g/dL. Frequent blood counts are strongly recommended in patients with advanced HIV-1 disease who are treated with TRIZIVIR. Periodic blood counts are recommended for other HIV-1-infected patients. If anemia or neutropenia develops, dosage interruption may be needed.

5.3 Myopathy

Myopathy and myositis, with pathological changes similar to that produced by HIV-1 disease, have been associated with prolonged use of zidovudine, and therefore may occur with therapy with TRIZIVIR.

5.4 Lactic Acidosis/Hepatomegaly With Steatosis

Lactic acidosis and severe hepatomegaly with steatosis, including fatal cases, have been reported with the use of nucleoside analogues alone or in combination, including abacavir, lamivudine, zidovudine, and other antiretrovirals. A majority of these cases have been in women. Obesity and prolonged nucleoside exposure may be risk factors. Particular caution should be exercised when administering TRIZIVIR to any patient with known risk factors for liver disease; however, cases have also been reported in patients with no known risk factors. Treatment with TRIZIVIR should be suspended in any patient who develops clinical or laboratory findings suggestive of lactic acidosis or pronounced hepatotoxicity (which may include hepatomegaly and steatosis even in the absence of marked transaminase elevations).

5.5 Patients With HIV-1 and Hepatitis B Virus Co-infection

Posttreatment Exacerbations of Hepatitis: In clinical trials in non-HIV-1-infected subjects treated with lamivudine for chronic HBV, clinical and laboratory evidence of exacerbations of hepatitis have occurred after discontinuation of lamivudine. These exacerbations have been detected primarily by serum ALT elevations in addition to re-emergence of hepatitis B viral DNA (HBV DNA). Although most events appear to have been self-limited, fatalities have been reported in some cases. Similar events have been reported from post-marketing experience after changes from lamivudine-containing HIV-1 treatment regimens to non-lamivudine-containing regimens in patients infected with both HIV-1 and HBV. The causal relationship to discontinuation of lamivudine treatment is unknown. Patients should be closely monitored with both clinical and laboratory follow-up for at least several months after stopping treat-

ment. There is insufficient evidence to determine whether reinitiation of lamivudine alters the course of posttreatment exacerbations of hepatitis.

Emergence of Lamivudine-Resistant HBV: Safety and efficacy of lamivudine have not been established for treatment of chronic hepatitis B in subjects dually infected with HIV-1 and HBV. In non-HIV-infected subjects treated with lamivudine for chronic hepatitis B, emergence of lamivudine-resistant HBV has been detected and has been associated with diminished treatment response (see full prescribing information for EPIVIR-HBV® [lamivudine] for additional information). Emergence of hepatitis B virus variants associated with resistance to lamivudine has also been reported in HIV-1-infected subjects who have received lamivudine-containing antiretroviral regimens in the presence of concurrent infection with hepatitis B virus.

5.6 Use With Interferon- and Ribavirin-Based Regimens

In vitro studies have shown ribavirin can reduce the phosphorylation of pyrimidine nucleoside analogues such as lamivudine and zidovudine. Although no evidence of a pharmacokinetic or pharmacodynamic interaction (e.g., loss of HIV-1/HCV virologic suppression) was seen when ribavirin was coadministered with lamivudine or zidovudine in HIV-1/HCV co-infected subjects [see Clinical Pharmacology (12.3)], hepatic decompensation (some fatal) has occurred in HIV-1/HCV co-infected subjects receiving combination antiretroviral therapy for HIV-1 and interferon alfa with or without ribavirin. Patients receiving interferon alfa with or without ribavirin and TRIZIVIR should be closely monitored for treatment-associated toxicities, especially hepatic decompensation, neutropenia, and anemia. Discontinuation of TRIZIVIR should be considered as medically appropriate. Dose reduction or discontinuation of interferon alfa, ribavirin, or both should also be considered if worsening clinical toxicities are observed, including hepatic decompensation (e.g., Child-Pugh greater than 6) (see the complete prescribing information for interferon and ribavirin).

Exacerbation of anemia has been reported in HIV-1/HCV co-infected patients receiving ribavirin and zidovudine. Coadministration of ribavirin and TRIZIVIR is not advised.

5.7 Immune Reconstitution Syndrome

Immune reconstitution syndrome has been reported in patients treated with combination antiretroviral therapy, including TRIZIVIR. During the initial phase of combination antiretroviral treatment, patients whose immune systems respond may develop an inflammatory response to indolent or residual opportunistic infections (such as Mycobacterium avium infection, cytomegalovirus, Pneumocystis jirovecii pneumonia [PCP], or tuberculosis), which may necessitate further evaluation and treatment.

Autoimmune disorders (such as Graves' disease, polymyositis, and Guillain-Barré syndrome) have also been reported to occur in the setting of immune reconstitution; however, the time to onset is more variable, and can occur many months after initiation of treatment.

5.8 Fat Redistribution

Redistribution/accumulation of body fat including central obesity, dorsocervical fat enlargement (buffalo hump), peripheral wasting, facial wasting, breast enlargement, and "cushingoid appearance" have been observed in patients receiving antiretroviral therapy. The mechanism and long-term consequences of these events are currently unknown. A causal relationship has not been established.

5.9 Myocardial Infarction

In a published prospective, observational, epidemiological trial designed to investigate the rate of myocardial infarction in patients on combination antiretroviral therapy, the use of abacavir within the previous 6 months was correlated

with an increased risk of myocardial infarction (MI).[1] In a sponsor-conducted pooled analysis of clinical trials, no excess risk of myocardial infarction was observed in abacavir-treated subjects as compared with control subjects. In totality, the available data from the observational cohort and from clinical trials are inconclusive.

As a precaution, the underlying risk of coronary heart disease should be considered when prescribing antiretroviral therapies, including abacavir, and action taken to minimize all modifiable risk factors (e.g., hypertension, hyperlipidemia, diabetes mellitus, smoking).

5.10 Therapy Experienced Patients

In clinical trials, subjects with prolonged prior nucleoside reverse transcriptase inhibitor (NRTI) exposure or who had HIV-1 isolates that contained multiple mutations conferring resistance to NRTIs had limited response to abacavir. The potential for cross-resistance between abacavir and other NRTIs should be considered when choosing new therapeutic regimens in therapy-experienced patients [see Clinical Pharmacology (12.4)].

5.11 Use With Other Abacavir-, Lamivudine-, Zidovudine-, and/or Emtricitabine Containing Products

TRIZIVIR is a fixed-dose combination of abacavir, lamivudine, and zidovudine and is intended only for patients whose regimen would otherwise include these 3 components. TRIZIVIR should not be administered concomitantly with other abacavir-, lamivudine-, or zidovudine-containing products including ZIAGEN (abacavir sulfate) Tablets and Oral Solution, EPIVIR® (lamivudine) Tablets and Oral Solution, EPIVIR-HBV (lamivudine) Tablets and Oral Solution, RETROVIR® (zidovudine) Tablets, Capsules, Syrup, and IV Infusion, COMBIVIR® (lamivudine and zidovudine) Tablets, EPZICOM® (abacavir sulfate and lamivudine) Tablets; or emtricitabine-containing products, including ATRIPLA® (efavirenz/emtricitabine/tenofovir disoproxil fumarate) Tablets, EMTRIVA® (emtricitabine) Capsules and Oral Solution, TRUVADA® (emtricitabine/tenofovir disoproxil fumarate) Tablets, or COMPLERA® (emtricitabine/rilpivirine/tenofovir disoproxil fumarate) Tablets.

The complete prescribing information for all agents being considered for use with TRIZIVIR should be consulted before combination therapy with TRIZIVIR is initiated.

6 ADVERSE REACTIONS

The following adverse reactions are discussed in greater detail in other sections of the labeling:

- Serious and sometimes fatal hypersensitivity reactions [see Boxed Warning, Warnings and Precautions (5.1)].
- Hematologic toxicity, including neutropenia and anemia [see Boxed Warning, Warnings and Precautions (5.2)].
- Symptomatic myopathy [see Boxed Warning, Warnings and Precautions (5.3)].
- Lactic acidosis and severe hepatomegaly with steatosis [see Boxed Warning, Warnings and Precautions (5.4)].
- Acute exacerbations of hepatitis B [see Boxed Warning, Warnings and Precautions (5.5)].
- Hepatic decompensation in patients co-infected with HIV-1 and hepatitis C [see Warnings and Precautions (5.6)].
- Exacerbation of anemia in HIV-1/HCV co-infected patients receiving ribavirin and zidovudine [see Warnings and Precautions (5.6)].
- Immune reconstitution syndrome [see Warnings and Precautions (5.7)].
- Fat redistribution [see Warnings and Precautions (5.8)].
- Myocardial infarction [see Warnings and Precautions (5.9)].

6.1 Clinical Trials Experience

Because clinical trials are conducted under widely varying conditions, adverse reaction rates observed in the clinical trials of a drug cannot be directly compared with rates in the clinical trials of another drug and may not reflect the rates observed in clinical practice.

Treatment-emergent clinical adverse reactions (rated by the investigator as moderate or severe) with a frequency greater than or equal to 5% during therapy with abacavir 300 mg twice daily, lamivudine 150 mg twice daily, and zidovudine 300 mg twice daily compared with indinavir 800 mg 3 times daily, lamivudine 150 mg twice daily, and zidovudine 300 mg twice daily from CNA3005 are listed in Table 1.

[See table 1 above]

Five subjects receiving abacavir in CNA3005 experienced worsening of pre-existing depression compared to none in the indinavir arm. The background rates of pre-existing depression were similar in the 2 treatment arms.

Laboratory Abnormalities: Laboratory abnormalities in CNA3005 are listed in Table 2.

[See table 2 at top of next page]

Other Adverse Events: In addition to adverse reactions in Tables 1 and 2, other adverse events observed in the expanded access program for abacavir were pancreatitis and increased GGT.

6.2 Postmarketing Experience

In addition to adverse reactions reported from clinical trials, the following reactions have been identified during postmarketing use of abacavir, lamivudine, and/or zidovudine. Because they are reported voluntarily from a population of unknown size, estimates of frequency cannot be made. These reactions have been chosen for inclusion due to a combination of their seriousness, frequency of reporting, or potential causal connection to abacavir, lamivudine and/or zidovudine.

Abacavir:

Cardiovascular: Myocardial infarction.

Skin: Suspected Stevens-Johnson syndrome (SJS) and toxic epidermal necrolysis (TEN) have been reported in patients receiving abacavir primarily in combination with medications known to be associated with SJS and TEN, respectively. Because of the overlap of clinical signs and symptoms between hypersensitivity to abacavir and SJS and TEN, and the possibility of multiple drug sensitivities in some patients, abacavir should be discontinued and not restarted in such cases.

There have also been reports of erythema multiforme with abacavir use.

Abacavir, Lamivudine, and/or Zidovudine:

Body as a Whole: Redistribution/accumulation of body fat [see Warnings and Precautions (5.8)].

Cardiovascular: Cardiomyopathy.

Digestive: Stomatitis.

Endocrine and Metabolic: Gynecomastia, hyperglycemia.

Gastrointestinal: Anorexia and/or decreased appetite, abdominal pain, dyspepsia, oral mucosal pigmentation.

General: Vasculitis, weakness.

Hemic and Lymphatic: Aplastic anemia, anemia (including pure red cell aplasia and severe anemias progressing on therapy), lymphadenopathy, splenomegaly, thrombocytopenia.

Hepatic: Lactic acidosis and hepatic steatosis [see Warnings and Precautions (5.4)], elevated bilirubin, elevated transaminases, posttreatment exacerbation of hepatitis B [see Warnings and Precautions (5.5)].

Hypersensitivity: Sensitization reactions (including anaphylaxis), urticaria.

Musculoskeletal: Arthralgia, myalgia, muscle weakness, CPK elevation, rhabdomyolysis.

Nervous: Dizziness, paresthesia, peripheral neuropathy, seizures.

Psychiatric: Insomnia and other sleep disorders.

Respiratory: Abnormal breath sounds/wheezing.

Skin: Alopecia, erythema multiforme, Stevens-Johnson syndrome.

7 DRUG INTERACTIONS

• No drug interaction trials have been conducted using TRIZIVIR Tablets [see Clinical Pharmacology (12.3)].

7.1 Antiretroviral Agents

Zidovudine: Stavudine: Concomitant use of zidovudine with stavudine should be avoided since an antagonistic relationship has been demonstrated in vitro.

Nucleoside Analogues Affecting DNA Replication: Some nucleoside analogues affecting DNA replication, such as ribavirin, antagonize the in vitro antiviral activity of zidovudine against HIV-1; concomitant use of such drugs should be avoided.

7.2 Doxorubicin

Zidovudine: Concomitant use of zidovudine with doxorubicin should be avoided since an antagonistic relationship has been demonstrated in vitro.

7.3 Ethanol

Abacavir: Abacavir has no effect on the pharmacokinetic properties of ethanol. Ethanol decreases the elimination of abacavir causing an increase in overall exposure [see Clinical Pharmacology (12.3)].

7.4 Hematologic/Bone Marrow Suppressive/Cytotoxic Agents

Zidovudine: Coadministration of ganciclovir, interferon alfa, ribavirin, and other bone marrow suppressive or cytotoxic agents may increase the hematologic toxicity of zidovudine.

7.5 Interferon- and Ribavirin-Based Regimens

Lamivudine: Although no evidence of a pharmacokinetic or pharmacodynamic interaction (e.g., loss of HIV-1/HCV virologic suppression) was seen when ribavirin was coadministered with lamivudine in HIV-1/HCV co-infected subjects, hepatic decompensation (some fatal) has occurred in HIV-1/HCV co-infected subjects receiving combination antiretroviral therapy for HIV-1 and interferon alfa with or without ribavirin [see Warnings and Precautions (5.6), Clinical Pharmacology (12.3)].

7.6 Methadone

Abacavir: The addition of methadone has no clinically significant effect on the pharmacokinetic properties of abacavir. In a trial of 11 HIV-1-infected subjects receiving methadone-maintenance therapy with 600 mg of ZIAGEN twice daily (twice the currently recommended dose), oral

methadone clearance increased [see Clinical Pharmacology (12.3)]. This alteration will not result in a methadone dose modification in the majority of patients; however, an increased methadone dose may be required in a small number of patients.

7.7 Trimethoprim/Sulfamethoxazole (TMP/SMX)

Lamivudine: No change in dose of either drug is recommended [see Clinical Pharmacology (12.3)]. There is no information regarding the effect on lamivudine pharmacokinetics of higher doses of TMP/SMX such as those used to treat PCP.

8 USE IN SPECIFIC POPULATIONS

8.1 Pregnancy

TRIZIVIR: Pregnancy Category C. There are no adequate and well-controlled studies of TRIZIVIR in pregnant women. Reproduction studies with abacavir, lamivudine, and zidovudine have been performed in animals (see Abacavir, Lamivudine, and Zidovudine sections below). TRIZIVIR should be used during pregnancy only if the potential benefits outweigh the risks.

Abacavir: Studies in pregnant rats showed that abacavir is transferred to the fetus through the placenta. Fetal malformations (increased incidences of fetal anasarca and skeletal malformations) and developmental toxicity (depressed fetal body weight and reduced crown-rump length) were observed in rats at a dose which produced 35 times the human exposure, based on AUC. Embryonic and fetal toxicities (increased resorptions, decreased fetal body weights) and toxicities to the offspring (increased incidence of stillbirth and lower body weights) occurred at half of the above-mentioned dose in separate fertility studies conducted in rats. In the rabbit, no developmental toxicity and no increases in fetal malformations occurred at doses that produced 8.5 times the human exposure at the recommended dose based on AUC.

Lamivudine: Studies in pregnant rats showed that lamivudine is transferred to the fetus through the placenta. Reproduction studies with orally administered lamivudine have been performed in rats and rabbits at doses producing plasma levels up to approximately 35 times that for the recommended adult HIV dose. No evidence of teratogenicity due to lamivudine was observed. Evidence of early embryolethality was seen in the rabbit at exposure levels similar to those observed in humans, but there was no indication of this effect in the rat at exposure levels up to 35 times those in humans.

Zidovudine: Reproduction studies with orally administered zidovudine in the rat and in the rabbit at doses up to 500 mg/kg/day revealed no evidence of teratogenicity with zidovudine. Zidovudine treatment resulted in embryo/fetal toxicity as evidenced by an increase in the incidence of fetal resorptions in rats given 150 or 450 mg/kg/day and rabbits given 500 mg/kg/day. The doses used in the teratology studies resulted in peak zidovudine plasma concentrations (after one half of the daily dose) in rats 66 to 226 times, and in rabbits 12 to 87 times, mean steady-state peak human plasma concentrations (after one sixth of the daily dose) achieved with the recommended daily dose (100 mg every 4 hours). In an additional teratology study in rats, a dose of 3,000 mg/kg/day (very near the oral median lethal dose in rats of approximately 3,700 mg/kg) caused marked maternal toxicity and an increase in the incidence of fetal malformations. This dose resulted in peak zidovudine plasma concentrations 350 times peak human plasma concentrations. No evidence of teratogenicity was seen in this experiment at doses of 600 mg/kg/day or less. Two rodent carcinogenicity studies were conducted [see Nonclinical Toxicology (13.1)].

Antiretroviral Pregnancy Registry: To monitor maternal-fetal outcomes of pregnant women exposed to TRIZIVIR or other antiretroviral agents, an Antiretroviral Pregnancy Registry has been established. Physicians are encouraged to register patients by calling 1-800-258-4263.

8.3 Nursing Mothers

The Centers for Disease Control and Prevention recommend that HIV-1-infected mothers not breastfeed their infants to avoid risking postnatal transmission of HIV infection. Abacavir, Lamivudine, and Zidovudine: Lamivudine and zidovudine are excreted in human breast milk; abacavir and lamivudine are secreted into the milk of lactating rats. Because of both the potential for HIV-1 transmission and the potential for serious adverse reactions in nursing infants, mothers should be instructed not to breastfeed if they are receiving TRIZIVIR.

8.4 Pediatric Use

TRIZIVIR is not intended for use in pediatric patients and is not recommended in adolescents who weigh less than 40 kg because it is a fixed-dose tablet that cannot be adjusted for these patient populations.

Therapy-Experienced Pediatric Trial: A randomized, double-blind trial, CNA3006, compared ZIAGEN plus lamivudine and zidovudine versus lamivudine and zidovudine in pediatric subjects, most of whom were extensively pretreated with nucleoside analogue antiretroviral agents. Subjects in this trial had a limited response to abacavir.

8.5 Geriatric Use

Clinical studies of abacavir, lamivudine, and zidovudine did not include sufficient numbers of subjects aged 65 and over to determine whether they respond differently from younger subjects. In general, dose selection for an elderly patient should be cautious, reflecting the greater frequency of decreased hepatic, renal, or cardiac function, and of concomitant disease or other drug therapy [see Dosage and Administration (2.3), Use in Specific Populations (8.6)].

8.6 Patients With Impaired Renal Function

TRIZIVIR is not recommended for patients with impaired renal function (i.e., creatinine clearance <50 mL/min) because TRIZIVIR is a fixed-dose combination and the dosage of the individual components cannot be adjusted.

8.7 Patients With Impaired Hepatic Function

TRIZIVIR is contraindicated for patients with hepatic impairment because TRIZIVIR is a fixed-dose combination and the dosage of the individual components cannot be adjusted.

10 OVERDOSAGE

Abacavir: There is no known antidote for abacavir. It is not known whether abacavir can be removed by peritoneal dialysis or hemodialysis.

Lamivudine: One case of an adult ingesting 6 grams of lamivudine was reported; there were no clinical signs or symptoms noted and hematologic tests remained normal. It is not known whether lamivudine can be removed by peritoneal dialysis or hemodialysis.

Zidovudine: Acute overdoses of zidovudine have been reported in pediatric patients and adults. These involved exposures up to 50 grams. The only consistent findings were nausea and vomiting. Other reported occurrences included headache, dizziness, drowsiness, lethargy, and confusion. Hematologic changes were transient. All patients recovered. Hemodialysis and peritoneal dialysis appear to have a negligible effect on the removal of zidovudine, while elimination of its primary metabolite, 3'-azido-3'-deoxy-5'-O-β-D-glucopyranuronosylthymidine (GZDV), is enhanced.

11 DESCRIPTION

TRIZIVIR: TRIZIVIR Tablets contain the following 3 synthetic nucleoside analogues: abacavir sulfate (ZIAGEN), lamivudine (also known as EPIVIR or 3TC), and zidovudine (also known as RETROVIR, azidothymidine, or ZDV) with inhibitory activity against HIV-1.

TRIZIVIR Tablets are for oral administration. Each film-coated tablet contains the active ingredients 300 mg of abacavir as abacavir sulfate, 150 mg of lamivudine, and 300 mg of zidovudine, and the inactive ingredients magne-

Table 2. Treatment-Emergent Laboratory Abnormalities (Grades 3/4) in CNA3005

Grade 3/4 Laboratory Abnormalities	Number of Subjects by Treatment Group	
	ZIAGEN plus Lamivudine/Zidovudine (n = 262)	Indinavir plus Lamivudine/Zidovudine (n = 264)
Elevated CPK (>4 × ULN)	18 (7%)	18 (7%)
ALT (>5.0 × ULN)	16 (6%)	16 (6%)
Neutropenia (<750/mm³)	13 (5%)	13 (5%)
Hypertriglyceridemia (>750 mg/dL)	5 (2%)	3 (1%)
Hyperamylasemia (>2.0 × ULN)	5 (2%)	1 (<1%)
Hyperglycemia (>13.9 mmol/L)	2 (<1%)	2 (<1%)
Anemia (Hgb ≤6.9 g/dL)	0 (0%)	3 (1%)

ULN = Upper limit of normal.
n = Number of patients assessed.

Table 3. Pharmacokinetic Parameters[a] for Abacavir, Lamivudine, and Zidovudine in Adults

Parameter	Abacavir		Lamivudine		Zidovudine	
Oral bioavailability (%)	86 ± 25	n = 6	86 ± 16	n = 12	64 ± 10	n = 5
Apparent volume of distribution (L/kg)	0.86 ± 0.15	n = 6	1.3 ± 0.4	n = 20	1.6 ± 0.6	n = 8
Systemic clearance (L/h/kg)	0.80 ± 0.24	n = 6	0.33 ± 0.06	n = 20	1.6 ± 0.6	n = 6
Renal clearance (L/h/kg)	.007 ± .008	n = 6	0.22 ± 0.06	n = 20	0.34 ± 0.05	n = 9
Elimination half-life (h)	1.45 ± 0.32	n = 20	5 to 7[b]		0.5 to 3[b]	

[a] Data presented as mean ± standard deviation except where noted.
[b] Approximate range.

sium stearate, microcrystalline cellulose, and sodium starch glycolate. The tablets are coated with a film (OPADRY® green 03B11434) that is made of FD&C Blue No. 2, hypromellose, polyethylene glycol, titanium dioxide, and yellow iron oxide.

Abacavir Sulfate: The chemical name of abacavir sulfate is (1S,cis)-4-[2-amino-6-(cyclopropylamino)-9H-purin-9-yl]-2-cyclopentene-1-methanol sulfate (salt) (2:1). Abacavir sulfate is the enantiomer with 1S, 4R absolute configuration on the cyclopentene ring. It has a molecular formula of $(C_{14}H_{18}N_6O_2)_2 \cdot H_2SO_4$ and a molecular weight of 670.76 daltons. It has the following structural formula:

Abacavir sulfate is a white to off-white solid with a solubility of approximately 77 mg/mL in distilled water at 25°C. In vivo, abacavir sulfate dissociates to its free base, abacavir. In this insert, all dosages for ZIAGEN (abacavir sulfate) are expressed in terms of abacavir.

Lamivudine: The chemical name of lamivudine is (2R,cis)-4-amino-1-(2-hydroxymethyl-1,3-oxathiolan-5-yl)-(1H)-pyrimidin-2-one. Lamivudine is the (-)enantiomer of a dideoxy analogue of cytidine. Lamivudine has also been referred to as (-)2',3'-dideoxy, 3'-thiacytidine. It has a molecular formula of $C_8H_{11}N_3O_3S$ and a molecular weight of 229.3 daltons. It has the following structural formula:

Lamivudine is a white to off-white crystalline solid with a solubility of approximately 70 mg/mL in water at 20°C.

Zidovudine: The chemical name of zidovudine is 3'-azido-3'-deoxythymidine. It has a molecular formula of $C_{10}H_{13}N_5O_4$ and a molecular weight of 267.24 daltons. It has the following structural formula:

Zidovudine is a white to beige, crystalline solid with a solubility of 20.1 mg/mL in water at 25°C.

12 CLINICAL PHARMACOLOGY

12.1 Mechanism of Action
TRIZIVIR is an antiviral agent [see Clinical Pharmacology (12.4)].

12.3 Pharmacokinetics
Pharmacokinetics in Adults: TRIZIVIR: In a single-dose, 3-way crossover bioavailability trial of 1 TRIZIVIR Tablet versus 1 ZIAGEN Tablet (300 mg), 1 EPIVIR Tablet (150 mg), plus 1 RETROVIR Tablet (300 mg) administered simultaneously in healthy subjects (n = 24), there was no difference in the extent of absorption, as measured by the area under the plasma concentration-time curve (AUC) and maximal peak concentration (C_{max}), of all 3 components. One TRIZIVIR Tablet was bioequivalent to 1 ZIAGEN Tablet (300 mg), 1 EPIVIR Tablet (150 mg), plus 1 RETROVIR Tablet (300 mg) following single-dose administration to fasting healthy subjects (n = 24).

Abacavir: Following oral administration, abacavir is rapidly absorbed and extensively distributed. Binding of abacavir to human plasma proteins is approximately 50%. Binding of abacavir to plasma proteins was independent of concentration. Total blood and plasma drug-related radioactivity concentrations are identical, demonstrating that abacavir readily distributes into erythrocytes. The primary routes of elimination of abacavir are metabolism by alcohol dehydrogenase to form the 5'-carboxylic acid and glucuronyl transferase to form the 5'-glucuronide.

Lamivudine: Following oral administration, lamivudine is rapidly absorbed and extensively distributed. Binding to plasma protein is low. Approximately 70% of an intravenous dose of lamivudine is recovered as unchanged drug in the urine. Metabolism of lamivudine is a minor route of elimination. In humans, the only known metabolite is the transsulfoxide metabolite (approximately 5% of an oral dose after 12 hours).

Zidovudine: Following oral administration, zidovudine is rapidly absorbed and extensively distributed. Binding to plasma protein is low. Zidovudine is eliminated primarily by hepatic metabolism. The major metabolite of zidovudine is GZDV. GZDV AUC is about 3-fold greater than the zidovudine AUC. Urinary recovery of zidovudine and GZDV accounts for 14% and 74% of the dose following oral administration, respectively. A second metabolite, 3'-amino-3'-deoxythymidine (AMT), has been identified in plasma. The AMT AUC was one-fifth of the zidovudine AUC.

In humans, abacavir, lamivudine, and zidovudine are not significantly metabolized by cytochrome P450 enzymes.

The pharmacokinetic properties of abacavir, lamivudine, and zidovudine in fasting subjects are summarized in Table 3.

[See table 3 above]

Effect of Food on Absorption of TRIZIVIR: Administration with food in a single-dose bioavailability trial resulted in lower C_{max}, similar to results observed previously for the reference formulations. The average [90% CI] decrease in abacavir, lamivudine, and zidovudine C_{max} was 32% [24% to 38%], 18% [10% to 25%], and 28% [13% to 40%], respectively, when administered with a high-fat meal, compared with administration under fasted conditions. Administration of TRIZIVIR with food did not alter the extent of abacavir, lamivudine, and zidovudine absorption (AUC), as compared with administration under fasted conditions (n = 24) [see Dosage and Administration (2.1)].

Special Populations: Renal Impairment: TRIZIVIR: Because lamivudine and zidovudine require dose adjustment in the presence of renal insufficiency, TRIZIVIR is not recommended for use in patients with creatinine clearance <50 mL/min [see Use in Specific Populations (8.6)].

Hepatic Impairment: TRIZIVIR: TRIZIVIR is contraindicated for patients with impaired hepatic function because TRIZIVIR is a fixed-dose combination and the dosage of the individual components cannot be adjusted. Abacavir is contraindicated in patients with moderate to severe hepatic impairment and dose reduction is required in patients with mild hepatic impairment.

Pregnancy: See Use in Specific Populations (8.1).
Abacavir and Lamivudine: No data are available on the pharmacokinetics of abacavir or lamivudine during pregnancy.
Zidovudine: Zidovudine pharmacokinetics have been studied in a Phase 1 trial of 8 women during the last trimester of pregnancy. As pregnancy progressed, there was no evidence of drug accumulation. The pharmacokinetics of zidovudine were similar to that of nonpregnant adults. Consistent with passive transmission of the drug across the placenta, zidovudine concentrations in neonatal plasma at birth were essentially equal to those in maternal plasma at delivery. Although data are limited, methadone maintenance therapy in 5 pregnant women did not appear to alter zidovudine pharmacokinetics. In a nonpregnant adult population, a potential for interaction has been identified [see Use in Specific Populations (8.1)].

Nursing Mothers: See Use in Specific Populations (8.3).
Abacavir: No data are available on the pharmacokinetics of abacavir in nursing mothers.
Lamivudine: Samples of breast milk obtained from 20 mothers receiving lamivudine monotherapy (300 mg twice daily) or combination therapy (150 mg lamivudine twice daily and 300 mg zidovudine twice daily) had measurable concentrations of lamivudine.
Zidovudine: After administration of a single dose of 200 mg zidovudine to 13 HIV-1-infected women, the mean concentration of zidovudine was similar in human milk and serum [see Use in Specific Populations (8.3)].

Pediatric Patients: TRIZIVIR is not intended for use in pediatric patients. TRIZIVIR is not recommended in adolescents who weigh less than 40 kg because it is a fixed-dose tablet that cannot be dose adjusted for this patient population.

Geriatric Patients: The pharmacokinetics of abacavir, lamivudine, and zidovudine have not been studied in subjects over 65 years of age.

Gender:
Abacavir: A population pharmacokinetic analysis in HIV-1-infected male (n = 304) and female (n = 67) subjects showed no gender differences in abacavir AUC normalized for lean body weight.
Lamivudine and Zidovudine: A pharmacokinetic trial in healthy male (n = 12) and female (n = 12) subjects showed no gender differences in zidovudine exposure (AUC_∞) or lamivudine (AUC_∞) normalized for body weight.

Race:
Abacavir: There are no significant differences between blacks and Caucasians in abacavir pharmacokinetics.
Lamivudine: There are no significant racial differences in lamivudine pharmacokinetics.
Zidovudine: The pharmacokinetics of zidovudine with respect to race have not been determined.

Drug Interactions: The drug interactions described below are based on trials conducted with the individual nucleoside analogues.
Cytochrome P450: In humans, abacavir, lamivudine, and zidovudine are not significantly metabolized by cytochrome P450 enzymes; therefore, it is unlikely that clinically significant drug interactions will occur with drugs metabolized through these pathways.
Glucuronyl Transferase: Due to the common metabolic pathways of abacavir and zidovudine via glucuronyl transferase, 15 HIV-1-infected subjects were enrolled in a crossover trial evaluating single doses of abacavir (600 mg), lamivudine (150 mg), and zidovudine (300 mg) alone or in combination. Analysis showed no clinically relevant changes in the pharmacokinetics of abacavir with the addition of lamivudine or zidovudine or the combination of lamivudine and zidovudine. Lamivudine exposure (AUC decreased 15%) and zidovudine exposure (AUC increased 10%) did not show clinically relevant changes with concurrent abacavir.
Lamivudine and Zidovudine: No clinically significant alterations in lamivudine or zidovudine pharmacokinetics were observed in 12 asymptomatic HIV-1-infected adult subjects given a single dose of zidovudine (200 mg) in combination with multiple doses of lamivudine (300 mg q 12 h).
Methadone: In a trial of 11 HIV-1-infected subjects receiving methadone-maintenance therapy (40 mg and 90 mg daily), with 600 mg of ZIAGEN twice daily (twice the currently recommended dose), oral methadone clearance increased 22% (90% CI: 6% to 42%) [see Drug Interactions (7.6)].
Ribavirin: In vitro data indicate ribavirin reduces phosphorylation of lamivudine, stavudine, and zidovudine. However, no pharmacokinetic (e.g., plasma concentrations or intracellular triphosphorylated active metabolite concentrations) or pharmacodynamic (e.g., loss of HIV-1/HCV virologic suppression) interaction was observed when ribavirin and lamivudine (n = 18), stavudine (n = 10), or zidovudine (n = 6) were coadministered as part of a multi-drug regimen to HIV-1/HCV co-infected subjects [see Warnings and Precautions (5.6)].

The effects of other coadministered drugs on abacavir, lamivudine, or zidovudine are provided in Table 4.
[See table 4 at top of next page]

12.4 Microbiology
Mechanism of Action: Abacavir: Abacavir is a carbocyclic synthetic nucleoside analogue. Abacavir is converted by cellular enzymes to the active metabolite, carbovir triphosphate (CBV-TP), an analogue of deoxyguanosine-5'-triphosphate (dGTP). CBV-TP inhibits the activity of HIV-1 reverse transcriptase (RT) both by competing with the natural substrate dGTP and by its incorporation into viral DNA. The lack of a 3'-OH group in the incorporated nucleotide analogue prevents the formation of the 5' to 3' phos-

phodiester linkage essential for DNA chain elongation, and therefore, the viral DNA growth is terminated. CBV-TP is a weak inhibitor of cellular DNA polymerases α, β, and γ.

Lamivudine: Lamivudine is a synthetic nucleoside analogue. Intracellularly, lamivudine is phosphorylated to its active 5'-triphosphate metabolite, lamivudine triphosphate (3TC-TP). The principal mode of action of 3TC-TP is inhibition of RT via DNA chain termination after incorporation of the nucleotide analogue. 3TC-TP is a weak inhibitor of cellular DNA polymerases α, β, and γ.

Zidovudine: Zidovudine is a synthetic nucleoside analogue. Intracellularly, zidovudine is phosphorylated to its active 5'-triphosphate metabolite, zidovudine triphosphate (ZDV-TP). The principal mode of action of ZDV-TP is inhibition of RT via DNA chain termination after incorporation of the nucleotide analogue. ZDV-TP is a weak inhibitor of the cellular DNA polymerases α and γ and has been reported to be incorporated into the DNA of cells in culture.

Antiviral Activity: Abacavir: The antiviral activity of abacavir against HIV-1 was evaluated against a T-cell tropic laboratory strain HIV-1$_{IIIB}$ in lymphoblastic cell lines, a monocyte/macrophage tropic laboratory strain HIV-1$_{BaL}$ in primary monocytes/macrophages, and clinical isolates in peripheral blood mononuclear cells. The concentration of drug necessary to effect viral replication by 50 percent (EC$_{50}$) ranged from 3.7 to 5.8 μM (1 μM = 0.28 mcg/mL) and 0.07 to 1.0 μM against HIV-1$_{IIIB}$ and HIV-1$_{BaL}$, respectively, and was 0.26 ± 0.18 μM against 8 clinical isolates. The EC$_{50}$ values of abacavir against different HIV-1 clades (A-G) ranged from 0.0015 to 1.05 μM, and against HIV-2 isolates, from 0.024 to 0.49 μM. Abacavir had synergistic activity in cell culture in combination with the NRTI zidovudine, the non-nucleoside reverse transcriptase inhibitor (NNRTI) nevirapine, and the protease inhibitor (PI) amprenavir; and additive activity in combination with the NRTIs didanosine, emtricitabine, lamivudine, stavudine, tenofovir, and zalcitabine. Ribavirin (50 μM) had no effect on the anti–HIV-1 activity of abacavir in cell culture.

Lamivudine: The antiviral activity of lamivudine against HIV-1 was assessed in a number of cell lines (including monocytes and fresh human peripheral blood lymphocytes) using standard susceptibility assays. EC$_{50}$ values (50% effective concentrations) were in the range of 0.003 to 15 μM (1 μM = 0.23 mcg/mL). HIV-1 from therapy-naive subjects with no amino acid substitutions associated with resistance gave median EC$_{50}$ values of 0.429 μM (range: 0.200 to 2.007 μM) from Virco (n = 92 baseline samples from COLA40263) and 2.35 μM (1.37 to 3.68 μM) from Monogram Biosciences (n = 135 baseline samples from ESS30009). The EC$_{50}$ values of lamivudine against different HIV-1 clades (A-G) ranged from 0.001 to 0.120 μM, and against HIV-2 isolates from 0.003 to 0.120 μM in peripheral blood mononuclear cells. Ribavirin (50 μM) decreased the anti-HIV-1 activity of lamivudine by 3.5-fold in MT-4 cells.

Zidovudine: The antiviral activity of zidovudine against HIV-1 was assessed in a number of cell lines (including monocytes and fresh human peripheral blood lymphocytes). The EC$_{50}$ and EC$_{90}$ values for zidovudine were 0.01 to 0.49 μM (1 μM = 0.27 mcg/mL) and 0.1 to 9 μM, respectively. HIV-1 from therapy-naive subjects with no amino acid substitutions associated with resistance gave median EC$_{50}$ values of 0.011 μM (range: 0.005 to 0.110 μM) from Virco (n = 92 baseline samples from COLA40263) and 0.0017 μM (0.006 to 0.0340 μM) from Monogram Biosciences (n = 135 baseline samples from ESS30009). The EC$_{50}$ values of zidovudine against different HIV-1 clades (A-G) ranged from 0.00018 to 0.02 μM, and against HIV-2 isolates from 0.00049 to 0.004 μM. In cell culture drug combination studies, zidovudine demonstrates synergistic activity with the NRTIs abacavir, didanosine, lamivudine, and zalcitabine; the NNRTIs delavirdine and nevirapine; and the PIs indinavir, nelfinavir, ritonavir, and saquinavir; and additive activity with interferon alfa. Ribavirin has been found to inhibit the phosphorylation of zidovudine in cell culture.

Resistance: HIV-1 isolates with reduced sensitivity to abacavir, lamivudine, or zidovudine have been selected in cell culture and were also obtained from subjects treated with abacavir, lamivudine, and zidovudine, or the combination of lamivudine and zidovudine.

Abacavir: Genotypic analysis of isolates selected in cell culture and recovered from abacavir-treated subjects demonstrated that amino acid substitutions K65R, L74V, Y115F, and M184V/I in HIV-1 RT contributed to abacavir resistance. In a trial of subjects receiving abacavir once or twice daily in combination with lamivudine and efavirenz once daily, 39% (7/18) of the isolates from subjects who experienced virologic failure in the abacavir once-daily arm had a >2.5-fold decrease in abacavir susceptibility with a median-fold decrease of 1.3 (range: 0.5 to 11) compared with 29% (5/17) of the failure isolates in the twice-daily arm with a median-fold decrease of 0.92 (range: 0.7 to 13).

Lamivudine: Genotypic analysis of isolates selected in cell culture and recovered from lamivudine-treated subjects showed that the resistance was due to a specific amino acid substitution in the HIV-1 RT at codon 184 changing the methionine to either valine or isoleucine (M184V/I).

Table 4. Effect of Coadministered Drugs on Abacavir, Lamivudine, and Zidovudine AUC[a] Note: ROUTINE DOSE MODIFICATION OF ABACAVIR, LAMIVUDINE, AND ZIDOVUDINE IS NOT WARRANTED WITH COADMINISTRATION OF THE FOLLOWING DRUGS.

Drugs That May Alter Lamivudine Blood Concentrations

Coadministered Drug and Dose	Lamivudine Dose	n	Lamivudine Concentrations		Concentration of Coadministered Drug
			AUC	Variability	
Nelfinavir 750 mg q 8 h × 7 to 10 days	single 150 mg	11	↑10%	95% CI: 1% to 20%	↔
Trimethoprim 160 mg/ Sulfamethoxazole 800 mg daily × 5 days	single 300 mg	14	↑43%	90% CI: 32% to 55%	↔

Drugs That May Alter Zidovudine Blood Concentrations

Coadministered Drug and Dose	Zidovudine Dose	n	Zidovudine Concentrations		Concentration of Coadministered Drug
			AUC	Variability	
Atovaquone 750 mg q 12 h with food	200 mg q 8 h	14	↑31%	Range 23% to 78%[b]	↔
Clarithromycin 500 mg twice daily	100 mg q 4 h × 7 days	4	↓12%	Range ↓34% to ↑14%	Not Reported
Fluconazole 400 mg daily	200 mg q 8 h	12	↑74%	95% CI: 54% to 98%	Not Reported
Methadone 30 to 90 mg daily	200 mg q 4 h	9	↑43%	Range 16% to 64%[b]	↔
Nelfinavir 750 mg q 8 h × 7 to 10 days	single 200 mg	11	↓35%	Range 28% to 41%	↔
Probenecid 500 mg q 6 h × 2 days	2 mg/kg q 8 h × 3 days	3	↑106%	Range 100% to 170%[b]	Not Assessed
Rifampin 600 mg daily × 14 days	200 mg q 8 h × 14 days	8	↓47%	90% CI: 41% to 53%	Not Assessed
Ritonavir 300 mg q 6 h × 4 days	200 mg q 8 h × 4 days	9	↓25%	95% CI: 15% to 34%	↔
Valproic acid 250 mg or 500 mg q 8 h × 4 days	100 mg q 8 h × 4 days	6	↑80%	Range 64% to 130%[b]	Not Assessed

Drugs That May Alter Abacavir Blood Concentrations

Coadministered Drug and Dose	Abacavir Dose	n	Abacavir Concentrations		Concentration of Coadministered Drug
			AUC	Variability	
Ethanol 0.7 g/kg	single 600 mg	24	↑41%	90% CI: 35% to 48%	↔

↑ = Increase; ↓ = Decrease; ↔ = no significant change; AUC = area under the concentration versus time curve; CI = confidence interval.
[a] See *Drug Interactions (7)* for additional information on drug interactions.
[b] Estimated range of percent difference.

Zidovudine: Genotypic analyses of the isolates selected in cell culture and recovered from zidovudine-treated subjects showed mutations in the HIV-1 RT gene resulting in 6 amino acid substitutions (M41L, D67N, K70R, L210W, T215Y or F, and K219Q) that confer zidovudine resistance. In general, higher levels of resistance were associated with greater number of mutations. In some subjects harboring zidovudine-resistant virus at baseline, phenotypic sensitivity to zidovudine was restored by 12 weeks of treatment with lamivudine and zidovudine. Combination therapy with lamivudine plus zidovudine delayed the emergence of substitutions conferring resistance to zidovudine.

Cross-Resistance: Cross-resistance has been observed among NRTIs.

Abacavir: Isolates containing abacavir resistance-associated amino acid substitutions, namely, K65R, L74V, Y115F, and M184V, exhibited cross-resistance to didanosine, emtricitabine, lamivudine, tenofovir, and zalcitabine in cell culture and in subjects. The K65R substitution can confer resistance to abacavir, didanosine, emtricitabine, lamivudine, stavudine, tenofovir, and zalcitabine; the L74V substitution can confer resistance to abacavir, didanosine, and zalcitabine; and the M184V substitution can confer resistance to abacavir, didanosine, emtricitabine, lamivudine, and zalcitabine. An increasing number of thymidine analogue mutations (TAMs: M41L, D67N, K70R, L210W, T215Y/F, K219E/R/H/Q/N) is associated with a progressive reduction in abacavir susceptibility.

Lamivudine: Cross-resistance to abacavir, didanosine, tenofovir, and zalcitabine has been observed in some sub-jects harboring lamivudine-resistant HIV-1 isolates. In some subjects treated with zidovudine plus didanosine or zalcitabine, isolates resistant to multiple drugs, including lamivudine, have emerged (see under Zidovudine below). Cross-resistance between lamivudine and zidovudine has not been reported.

Zidovudine: In a trial of 167 HIV-infected subjects, isolates (n = 2) with multi-drug resistance to didanosine, lamivudine, stavudine, zalcitabine, and zidovudine were recovered from subjects treated for ≥1 year with zidovudine plus didanosine or zidovudine plus zalcitabine. The pattern of resistance-associated amino acid substitutions with such combination therapies was different (A62V, V75I, F77L, F116Y, Q151M) from the pattern with zidovudine monotherapy, with the Q151M substitution being most commonly associated with multi-drug resistance. The substitution at codon 151 in combination with substitutions at 62, 75, 77, and 116 results in a virus with reduced susceptibility to didanosine, lamivudine, stavudine, zalcitabine, and zidovudine. TAMs are selected by zidovudine and confer cross-resistance to abacavir, didanosine, stavudine, tenofovir, and zalcitabine.

13 NONCLINICAL TOXICOLOGY

13.1 Carcinogenesis, Mutagenesis, Impairment of Fertility

Carcinogenicity:

Abacavir: Abacavir was administered orally at 3 dosage levels to separate groups of mice and rats in 2-year carcino-

Table 5. Outcomes of Randomized Treatment Through Week 48 (CNA3005)

Outcome	ZIAGEN plus Lamivudine/Zidovudine (n = 262)	Indinavir plus Lamivudine/Zidovudine (n = 265)
Responder[a]	49%	50%
Virologic failure[b]	31%	28%
Discontinued due to adverse reactions	10%	12%
Discontinued due to other reasons[c]	11%	10%

[a] Patients achieved and maintained confirmed HIV-1 RNA <400 copies/mL.
[b] Includes viral rebound and failure to achieve confirmed <400 copies/mL by Week 48.
[c] Includes consent withdrawn, lost to follow-up, protocol violations, those with missing data, clinical progression, and other.

Table 6. Proportions of Responders Through Week 48 By Screening Plasma HIV-1 RNA Levels (CNA3005)

Screening HIV-1 RNA (copies/mL)	ZIAGEN plus Lamivudine/Zidovudine (n = 262)		Indinavir plus Lamivudine/Zidovudine (n = 265)	
	<400 copies/mL	n	<400 copies/mL	N
≥10,000 - ≤100,000	50%	166	48%	165
>100,000	48%	96	52%	100

genicity studies. Results showed an increase in the incidence of malignant and non-malignant tumors. Malignant tumors occurred in the preputial gland of males and the clitoral gland of females of both species, and in the liver of female rats. In addition, non-malignant tumors also occurred in the liver and thyroid gland of female rats. These observations were made at systemic exposures in the range of 6 to 32 times the human exposure at the recommended dose. It is not known how predictive the results of rodent carcinogenicity studies may be for humans.

Lamivudine: Long-term carcinogenicity studies with lamivudine in mice and rats showed no evidence of carcinogenic potential at exposures up to 10 times (mice) and 58 times (rats) those observed in humans at the recommended therapeutic dose for HIV-1 infection.

Zidovudine: Zidovudine was administered orally at 3 dosage levels to separate groups of mice and rats (60 females and 60 males in each group). Initial single dose doses were 30, 60, and 120 mg/kg/day in mice and 80, 220, and 600 mg/kg/day in rats. The doses in mice were reduced to 20, 30, and 40 mg/kg/day after day 90 because of treatment-related anemia, whereas in rats only the high dose was reduced to 450 mg/kg per day on day 91 and then to 300 mg/kg/day on day 279.

In mice, 7 late-appearing (after 19 months) vaginal neoplasms (5 nonmetastasizing squamous cell carcinomas, 1 squamous cell papilloma, and 1 squamous polyp) occurred in animals given the highest dose. One late-appearing squamous cell papilloma occurred in the vagina of a middle-dose animal. No vaginal tumors were found at the lowest dose.

In rats, 2 late-appearing (after 20 months), nonmetastasizing vaginal squamous cell carcinomas occurred in animals given the highest dose. No vaginal tumors occurred at the low or middle dose in rats. No other drug-related tumors were observed in either sex of either species.

At doses that produced tumors in mice and rats, the estimated drug exposure (as measured by AUC) was approximately 3 times (mouse) and 24 times (rat) the estimated human exposure at the recommended therapeutic dose of 100 mg every 4 hours.

Two transplacental carcinogenicity studies were conducted in mice. One study administered zidovudine at doses of 20 mg/kg/day or 40 mg/kg/day from gestation day 10 through parturition and lactation with dosing continuing in offspring for 24 months postnatally. At these doses, exposures were approximately 3 times the estimated human exposure at the recommended doses. After 24 months at the 40-mg/kg/day dose, an increase in incidence of vaginal tumors was noted with no increase in tumors in the liver or lung or any other organ in either gender. These findings are consistent with results of the standard oral carcinogenicity study in mice, as described earlier. A second study administered zidovudine at maximum tolerated doses of 12.5 mg/day or 25 mg/day (~1,000 mg/kg nonpregnant body weight or ~450 mg/kg of term body weight) to pregnant mice from days 12 through 18 of gestation. There was an increase in the number of tumors in the lung, liver, and female reproductive tracts in the offspring of mice receiving the higher dose level of zidovudine.

It is not known how predictive the results of rodent carcinogenicity studies may be for humans.

Mutagenicity:

Abacavir: Abacavir induced chromosomal aberrations both in the presence and absence of metabolic activation in an in vitro cytogenetic study in human lymphocytes.

Abacavir was mutagenic in the absence of metabolic activation, although it was not mutagenic in the presence of metabolic activation in an L5178Y/TK+/- mouse lymphoma assay. Abacavir was clastogenic in males and not clastogenic in females in an in vivo mouse bone marrow micronucleus assay. Abacavir was not mutagenic in bacterial mutagenicity assays in the presence and absence of metabolic activation.

Lamivudine: Lamivudine was mutagenic in an L5178Y/TK+/- mouse lymphoma assay and clastogenic in a cytogenetic assay using cultured human lymphocytes. Lamivudine was negative in a microbial mutagenicity assay, in an in vitro cell transformation assay, in a rat micronucleus test, in a rat bone marrow cytogenetic assay, and in an assay for unscheduled DNA synthesis in rat liver.

Zidovudine: Zidovudine was mutagenic in an L5178Y/TK+/- mouse lymphoma assay, positive in an in vitro cell transformation assay, clastogenic in a cytogenetic assay using cultured human lymphocytes, and positive in mouse and rat micronucleus tests after repeated doses. It was negative in a cytogenetic study in rats given a single dose.

Impairment of Fertility:

Abacavir: Abacavir had no adverse effects on the mating performance or fertility of male and female rats at a dose approximately 8 times the human exposure at the recommended dose based on body surface area comparisons.

Lamivudine: In a study of reproductive performance, lamivudine, administered to male and female rats at doses up to 130 times the usual adult dose based on body surface area considerations, revealed no evidence of impaired fertility judged by conception rates and no effect on the survival, growth, and development to weaning of the offspring.

Zidovudine: Zidovudine, administered to male and female rats at doses up to 7 times the usual adult dose based on body surface area considerations, had no effect on fertility judged by conception rates.

13.2 Animal Toxicology and/or Pharmacology

Myocardial degeneration was found in mice and rats following administration of abacavir for 2 years. The systemic exposures were equivalent to 7 to 24 times the expected systemic exposure in humans. The clinical relevance of this finding has not been determined.

14 CLINICAL STUDIES

The following trial was conducted with the individual components of TRIZIVIR [see Clinical Pharmacology (12.3)].

CNA3005 was a multicenter, double-blind, controlled trial in which 562 HIV-1-infected, therapy-naive adults were randomized to receive either ZIAGEN (300 mg twice daily) plus COMBIVIR (lamivudine 150 mg/zidovudine 300 mg twice daily), or indinavir (800 mg 3 times a day) plus COMBIVIR twice daily. The trial was stratified at randomization by pre-entry plasma HIV-1 RNA 10,000 to 100,000 copies/mL and plasma HIV-1 RNA >100,000 copies/mL. Trial participants were male (87%), Caucasian (73%), black (15%), and Hispanic (9%). At baseline the median age was 36 years, the median pretreatment CD4+ cell count was 360 cells/mm³, and median plasma HIV-1 RNA was 4.8 $\log_{10}$ copies/mL. Proportions of subjects with plasma HIV-1 RNA <400 copies/mL (using Roche AMPLICOR HIV-1 MONITOR® Test) through 48 weeks of treatment are summarized in Table 5.
[See table 5 above]
Treatment response by plasma HIV-1 RNA strata is shown in Table 6.
[See table 6 above]

In subjects with baseline viral load >100,000 copies/mL, percentages of subjects with HIV-1 RNA levels <50 copies/mL were 31% in the group receiving abacavir vs. 45% in the group receiving indinavir.

Through Week 48, an overall mean increase in CD4+ cell count of about 150 cells/mm³ was observed in both treatment arms. Through Week 48, 9 subjects (3.4%) in the group receiving abacavir sulfate (6 CDC classification C events and 3 deaths) and 3 subjects (1.5%) in the group receiving indinavir (2 CDC classification C events and 1 death) experienced clinical disease progression.

15 REFERENCES

• Data Collection on Adverse Events of Anti-HIV Drugs (D:A:D) Study Group. *Lancet.* 2008;371 (9622):1417-1426.

16 HOW SUPPLIED/STORAGE AND HANDLING

TRIZIVIR is available as tablets. Each tablet contains 300 mg of abacavir as abacavir sulfate, 150 mg of lamivudine, and 300 mg of zidovudine. The tablets are blue-green capsule-shaped, film-coated, and imprinted with GX LL1 on one side with no markings on the reverse side. They are packaged as follows:
Bottles of 60 Tablets (NDC 49702-217-18).
Store at 25°C (77°F); excursions permitted to 15° to 30°C (59° to 86°F) (see USP Controlled Room Temperature).

17 PATIENT COUNSELING INFORMATION

See FDA-approved patient labeling (Medication Guide)
Hypersensitivity Reaction: Inform patients:
• that a Medication Guide and Warning Card summarizing the symptoms of the abacavir hypersensitivity reaction and other product information will be dispensed by the pharmacist with each new prescription and refill of TRIZIVIR, and encourage the patient to read the Medication Guide and Warning Card every time to obtain any new information that may be present about TRIZIVIR. (The complete text of the Medication Guide is reprinted at the end of this document).
• to carry the Warning Card with them.
• how to identify a hypersensitivity reaction [see Warnings and Precautions (5.1), Medication Guide].
• that if they develop symptoms consistent with a hypersensitivity reaction they should call their doctor right away to determine if they should stop taking TRIZIVIR.
• that a hypersensitivity reaction can worsen and lead to hospitalization or death if TRIZIVIR is not immediately discontinued.
• to not restart TRIZIVIR or any other abacavir-containing product following a hypersensitivity reaction because more severe symptoms can occur within hours and may include life-threatening hypotension and death.
• that a hypersensitivity reaction is usually reversible if it is detected promptly and TRIZIVIR is stopped right away.
• that if they have interrupted TRIZIVIR for reasons other than symptoms of hypersensitivity (for example, those who have an interruption in drug supply), a serious or fatal hypersensitivity reaction may occur with reintroduction of abacavir.
• to not restart TRIZIVIR or any other abacavir-containing product without medical consultation and that restarting abacavir needs to be undertaken only if medical care can be readily accessed by the patient or others.
• TRIZIVIR should not be coadministered with ATRIPLA, COMBIVIR, COMPLERA, EMTRIVA, EPIVIR, EPIVIR-HBV, EPZICOM, RETROVIR (zidovudine), TRUVADA, or ZIAGEN.

Neutropenia and Anemia: Patients should be informed that the important toxicities associated with zidovudine are neutropenia and/or anemia. They should be told of the extreme importance of having their blood counts followed closely while on therapy, especially for patients with advanced HIV-1 disease [see Warnings and Precautions (5.2)].
Myopathy: Patients should be informed that myopathy and myositis with pathological changes, similar to that produced by HIV-1 disease, have been associated with prolonged use of zidovudine [see Warnings and Precautions (5.3)].
Lactic Acidosis/Hepatomegaly: Inform patients that some HIV medicines, including TRIZIVIR, can cause a rare, but serious condition called lactic acidosis with liver enlargement (hepatomegaly) [see Warnings and Precautions (5.4)].
HIV-1/ HBV Co-Infection: Patients co-infected with HIV-1 and HBV should be informed that deterioration of liver disease has occurred in some cases when treatment with lamivudine was discontinued. Patients should be advised to discuss any changes in regimen with their physician [see Warnings and Precautions (5.5)].
HIV-1/HCV Co-Infection: Patients with HIV-1/HCV co-infection should be informed that hepatic decompensation (some fatal) has occurred in HIV-1/HCV co-infected patients receiving combination antiretroviral therapy for HIV-1 and interferon alfa with or without ribavirin [see Warnings and Precautions (5.6)].

Redistribution/Accumulation of Body Fat: Inform patients that redistribution or accumulation of body fat may occur in patients receiving antiretroviral therapy and that the cause and long-term health effects of these conditions are not known at this time [see Warnings and Precautions (5.8)].

Information About HIV-1 Infection: TRIZIVIR is not a cure for HIV-1 infection and patients may continue to experience illnesses associated with HIV-1 infection, including opportunistic infections. Patients should remain under the care of a physician when using TRIZIVIR.

Patients should be advised to avoid doing things that can spread HIV-1 infection to others.

- Do not share needles or other injection equipment.
- Do not share personal items that can have blood or body fluids on them, like toothbrushes and razor blades.
- Do not have any kind of sex without protection. Always practice safe sex by using a latex or polyurethane condom to lower the chance of sexual contact with semen, vaginal secretions, or blood.
- Do not breastfeed. Lamivudine and zidovudine are excreted in human breast milk. It is not known if abacavir can be passed to your baby in your breast milk and whether it could harm your baby. Also, mothers with HIV-1 should not breastfeed because HIV-1 can be passed to the baby in the breast milk.

Patients should be informed to take all HIV medications exactly as prescribed.

COMBIVIR, EPIVIR, EPZICOM, RETROVIR, TRIZIVIR, and ZIAGEN are registered trademarks of ViiV Healthcare. Other brands are trademarks of their respective owners and are not trademarks of ViiV Healthcare. The makers of these brands are not affiliated with and do not endorse ViiV Healthcare or its products.

Manufactured for:
ViiV Healthcare
Research Triangle Park, NC 27709
by:
GlaxoSmithKline
Research Triangle Park, NC 27709
Lamivudine is manufactured under agreement from
Shire Pharmaceuticals Group plc
Basingstoke, UK
©2013, ViiV Healthcare. All rights reserved.
TRZ: 7PI

MEDICATION GUIDE
TRIZIVIR® (TRY-zih-veer)
(abacavir sulfate, lamivudine, and zidovudine
Tablets

Read this Medication Guide before you start taking TRIZIVIR and each time you get a refill. There may be new information. This information does not take the place of talking to your healthcare provider about your medical condition or your treatment. Be sure to carry your TRIZIVIR Warning Card with you at all times.

What is the most important information I should know about TRIZIVIR?

1. Serious allergic reaction (hypersensitivity reaction). TRIZIVIR contains abacavir (also contained in ZIAGEN® and EPZICOM®). Patients taking TRIZIVIR may have a serious allergic reaction (hypersensitivity reaction) that can cause death. Your risk of this allergic reaction is much higher if you have a gene variation called HLA-B*5701. Your healthcare provider can determine with a blood test if you have this gene variation.

If you get a symptom from 2 or more of the following groups while taking TRIZIVIR, call your healthcare provider right away to find out if you should stop taking TRIZIVIR.

	Symptom(s)
Group 1	Fever
Group 2	Rash
Group 3	Nausea, vomiting, diarrhea, abdominal (stomach area) pain
Group 4	Generally ill feeling, extreme tiredness, or achiness
Group 5	Shortness of breath, cough, sore throat

A list of these symptoms is on the Warning Card your pharmacist gives you. **Carry this Warning Card with you at all times.**

If you stop TRIZIVIR because of an allergic reaction, never take TRIZIVIR(abacavir sulfate, lamivudine, and zidovudine)or any other abacavir-containing medicine (ZIAGEN and EPZICOM) again. If you take TRIZIVIR or any other abacavir-containing medicine again after you have had an allergic reaction, **within hours** you may get **life-threatening symptoms** that may include **very low blood pressure** or **death.** If you stop TRIZIVIR, for any other reason, even for a few days, and you are not allergic to TRIZIVIR, talk with your healthcare provider before taking it again. Taking TRIZIVIR again can cause a serious allergic or life-threatening reaction, even if you never had an allergic reaction to it before.

If your healthcare provider tells you that you can take TRIZIVIR again, start taking it when you are around medical help or people who can call a healthcare provider if you need one.

2. Blood problems. RETROVIR®, one of the medicines in TRIZIVIR, can cause serious blood cell problems. These include reduced numbers of white blood cells (neutropenia) and extremely reduced numbers of red blood cells (anemia). These blood cell problems are especially likely to happen in patients with advanced human immunodeficiency virus (HIV) disease or AIDS. Your doctor should be checking your blood cell counts regularly while you are taking TRIZIVIR. This is especially important if you have advanced HIV or AIDS. This is to make sure that any blood cell problems are found quickly.

3. Lactic Acidosis (buildup of acid in the blood). Some human immunodeficiency virus (HIV) medicines, including TRIZIVIR, can cause a rare but serious condition called lactic acidosis. Lactic acidosis is a serious medical emergency that can cause death and must be treated in the hospital. **Call your healthcare provider right away if you get any of the following signs or symptoms of lactic acidosis:**

- you feel very weak or tired
- you have unusual (not normal) muscle pain
- you have trouble breathing
- you have stomach pain with nausea and vomiting
- you feel cold, especially in your arms and legs
- you feel dizzy or light-headed
- you have a fast or irregular heartbeat

4. Serious liver problems. Some people who have taken medicines like TRIZIVIR have developed serious liver problems called hepatotoxicity, with liver enlargement (hepatomegaly) and fat in the liver (steatosis). Hepatomegaly with steatosis is a serious medical emergency that can cause death.

Call your healthcare provider right away if you get any of the following signs or symptoms of liver problems:

- your skin or the white part of your eyes turns yellow (jaundice)
- your urine turns dark
- your bowel movements (stools) turn light in color
- you don't feel like eating food for several days or longer
- you feel sick to your stomach (nausea)
- you have lower stomach area (abdominal) pain

You may be more likely to get lactic acidosis or serious liver problems if you are female, very overweight, or have been taking nucleoside analogue medicines for a long time.

5. Use with interferon and ribavirin-based regimens. Worsening of liver disease (sometimes resulting in death) has occurred in patients infected with both HIV and hepatitis C virus who are taking anti-HIV medicines and are also being treated for hepatitis C with interferon with or without ribavirin. If you are taking TRIZIVIR as well as interferon with or without ribavirin and you experience side effects, be sure to tell your healthcare provider.

6. If you have HIV and hepatitis B virus infection, your hepatitis B virus infection may get worse if you stop taking TRIZIVIR.

- Take TRIZIVIR exactly as prescribed.
- Do not run out of TRIZIVIR.
- Do not stop TRIZIVIR without talking to your healthcare provider.

Your healthcare provider should monitor your health and do regular blood tests to check your liver if you stop taking TRIZIVIR.

7. Muscle weakness (myopathy). RETROVIR, one of the medicines in TRIZIVIR, can cause muscle weakness. This can be a serious problem.

What is TRIZIVIR?

TRIZIVIR is a prescription medicine used to treat HIV infection. TRIZIVIR contains 3 medicines: abacavir (ZIAGEN), lamivudine or 3TC (EPIVIR®), and zidovudine, AZT, or ZDV (RETROVIR). All 3 of these medicines are called nucleoside analogue reverse transcriptase inhibitors (NRTIs). When used together, they help lower the amount of HIV in your blood.

- TRIZIVIR does not cure HIV infection or AIDS.
- It is not known if TRIZIVIR will help you live longer or have fewer of the medical problems that people get with HIV or AIDS.
- It is very important that you see your healthcare provider regularly while you are taking TRIZIVIR.

Who should not take TRIZIVIR?

Do not take TRIZIVIR if you:

- are allergic to abacavir or any of the ingredients in TRIZIVIR. See the end of this Medication Guide for a complete list of ingredients in TRIZIVIR.
- have certain liver problems.
- are an adolescent who weighs less than 90 pounds.

What should I tell my healthcare provider before taking TRIZIVIR?

Before you take TRIZIVIR, tell your healthcare provider if you:

- have been tested and know whether or not you have a particular gene variation called HLA-B*5701.
- have hepatitis B virus infection or have other liver problems.
- have kidney problems.
- have low blood cell counts (bone marrow problem). Ask your doctor if you are not sure.
- have heart problems, smoke, or have diseases that increase your risk of heart disease such as high blood pressure, high cholesterol, or diabetes.
- are pregnant or plan to become pregnant. It is not known if TRIZIVIR will harm your unborn baby. Talk to your healthcare provider if you are pregnant or plan to become pregnant.

Pregnancy Registry. If you take TRIZIVIR while you are pregnant, talk to your healthcare provider about how you can take part in the Pregnancy Registry for TRIZIVIR. The purpose of the pregnancy registry is to collect information about the health of you and your baby.

- are breastfeeding or plan to breastfeed. Do not breastfeed. Lamivudine and zidovudine are excreted in human breast milk. We do not know if abacavir can be passed to your baby in your breast milk and whether it could harm your baby. Also, mothers with HIV-1 should not breastfeed because HIV-1 can be passed to the baby in the breast milk.

Tell your healthcare provider about all the medicines you take, including prescription and nonprescription medicines, vitamins, and herbal supplements.

Especially tell your healthcare provider if you take:

- alcohol
- medicines used to treat hepatitis viruses such as interferon or ribavirin
- methadone
- BACTRIM®, SEPTRA® (trimethoprim [TMP/sulfamethoxazole SMX])
- CYTOVENE®, DHPG (ganciclovir)
- interferon-alfa
- ADRIAMYCIN® (doxorubicin)
- COPEGUS®, REBETOL®, VIRAZOLE® (ribavirin)
- any bone marrow suppressive medicines or cytotoxic medicines. Ask your doctor if you are not sure.
- ATRIPLA® (efavirenz/emtricitabine/tenofovir disoproxil fumarate)
- COMBIVIR® (lamivudine and zidovudine)
- COMPLERA® (emtricitabine/rilpivirine/tenofovir disoproxil fumarate)
- EMTRIVA® (emtricitabine)
- EPIVIR or EPIVIR-HBV® (lamivudine)
- EPZICOM (abacavir sulfate and lamivudine)
- RETROVIR (zidovudine)
- TRUVADA® (emtricitabine/tenofovir disoproxil fumarate)
- ZERIT® (stavudine)
- ZIAGEN (abacavir sulfate)

Ask your healthcare provider if you are not sure if you take one of the medicines listed above.

TRIZIVIR may affect the way other medicines work, and other medicines may affect how TRIZIVIR works.

Know the medicines you take. Keep a list of your medicines with you to show to your healthcare provider and pharmacist when you get a new medicine.

How should I take TRIZIVIR?

- Take TRIZIVIR exactly as your healthcare provider tells you to take it.
- TRIZIVIR may be taken with or without food.
- Do not skip doses.
- Do not let your TRIZIVIR run out.

If you stop your anti-HIV medicines, even for a short time, the amount of virus in your blood may increase and the virus may become harder to treat. If you take too much TRIZIVIR, call your healthcare provider or poison control center or go to the nearest hospital emergency room right away.

What are the possible side effects of TRIZIVIR?

TRIZIVIR can cause serious side effects including allergic reactions, lactic acidosis, and liver problems. See "What is the most important information I should know about TRIZIVIR?"

- Blood problems.
- Muscle weakness.
- Changes in immune system (Immune Reconstitution Syndrome). Your immune system may get stronger and begin to fight infections that have been hidden in your body for a long time. Tell your healthcare provider if you start having new or worse symptoms of infection after you start taking TRIZIVIR.
- Changes in body fat (fat redistribution). Changes in body fat (lipoatrophy or lipodystrophy) can happen in some people taking antiretroviral medicines including TRIZIVIR.

These changes may include:
- more fat in or around your trunk, upper back and neck (buffalo hump), breast or chest
- more fat in or around your trunk, upper back and neck (buffalo hump), breast or chest
- loss of fat in your legs, arms, or face
- **Heart attack (myocardial infarction).** Some HIV medicines including TRIZIVIR may increase your risk of heart attack.

The most common side effects of TRIZIVIR include:
- nausea
- headache
- weakness or tiredness
- vomiting
- diarrhea
- fever and/or chills
- depression
- muscle and joint pain
- skin rashes
- ear, nose, throat infections
- cold symptoms
- nervousness

Tell your healthcare provider if you have any side effect that bothers you or that does not go away.

These are not all the possible side effects of TRIZIVIR. For more information, ask your healthcare provider or pharmacist.

Call your doctor for medical advice about side effects. You may report side effects to FDA at 1-800-FDA-1088.

How should I store TRIZIVIR?
- Store TRIZIVIR at 59°F to 86°F (15°C to 30°C).
- **Keep TRIZIVIR and all medicines out of the reach of children.**

General information for safe and effective use of TRIZIVIR.
Avoid doing things that can spread HIV-1 infection to others.
- **Do not share needles or other injection equipment.**
- **Do not share personal items that can have blood or body fluids on them, like toothbrushes and razor blades.**
- **Do not have any kind of sex without protection.** Always practice safe sex by using a latex or polyurethane condom to lower the chance of sexual contact with semen, vaginal secretions, or blood.

Medicines are sometimes prescribed for purposes other than those listed in a Medication Guide. Do not use TRIZIVIR for a condition for which it was not prescribed. Do not give TRIZIVIR to other people, even if they have the same symptoms that you have. It may harm them.

This Medication Guide summarizes the most important information about TRIZIVIR. If you would like more information, talk with your healthcare provider. You can ask your healthcare provider or pharmacist for the information about TRIZIVIR that is written for healthcare professionals.

For more information go to www.TRIZIVIR.com or call 1-877-844-8872.

What are the ingredients in TRIZIVIR?
Active ingredients: abacavir sulfate, lamivudine, and zidovudine
Inactive ingredients: magnesium stearate, microcrystalline cellulose, sodium starch glycolate, and OPADRY® green 03B11434, a film coating made of FD&C Blue No. 2, hypromellose, polyethylene glycol, titanium dioxide, and yellow iron oxide.

This Medication Guide has been approved by the US Food and Drug Administration.

COMBIVIR, EPIVIR, EPZICOM, RETROVIR, TRIZIVIR, and ZIAGEN are registered trademarks of ViiV Healthcare. The brands listed are trademarks of their respective owners and are not trademarks of ViiV Healthcare. The makers of these brands are not affiliated with and do not endorse ViiV Healthcare or its products.
Manufactured for:
ViiV Healthcare
Research Triangle Park, NC 27709
by:
GlaxoSmithKline
Research Triangle Park, NC 27709
Lamivudine is manufactured under agreement from
Shire Pharmaceuticals Group plc
Basingstoke, UK
©2013, ViiV Healthcare. All rights reserved.
May 2013
TRZ:7MG

ZIAGEN
[zī'ə-jin]
(abacavir sulfate)
Tablets, for oral use
ZIAGEN
(abacavir sulfate)
Oral Solution

HIGHLIGHTS OF PRESCRIBING INFORMATION
These highlights do not include all the information needed to use ZIAGEN safely and effectively. See full prescribing information for ZIAGEN.

ZIAGEN (abacavir sulfate) Tablets, for oral use
ZIAGEN (abacavir sulfate) Oral Solution
Initial U.S. Approval: 1998

WARNING: HYPERSENSITIVITY REACTIONS, LACTIC ACIDOSIS, AND SEVERE HEPATOMEGALY
See full prescribing information for complete boxed warning.
- **Serious and sometimes fatal hypersensitivity reactions have been associated with ZIAGEN (abacavir sulfate). (5.1)**
- **Hypersensitivity to abacavir is a multi-organ clinical syndrome. (5.1)**
- **Patients who carry the HLA-B*5701 allele are at high risk for experiencing a hypersensitivity reaction to abacavir. (5.1)**
- **Discontinue ZIAGEN as soon as a hypersensitivity reaction is suspected. Regardless of HLA-B*5701 status, permanently discontinue ZIAGEN if hypersensitivity cannot be ruled out, even when other diagnoses are possible. (5.1)**
- **Following a hypersensitivity reaction to abacavir, NEVER restart ZIAGEN or any other abacavir-containing product. (5.1)**
- **Lactic acidosis and severe hepatomegaly with steatosis, including fatal cases, have been reported with the use of nucleoside analogues. (5.2)**

INDICATIONS AND USAGE
ZIAGEN, a nucleoside analogue, is indicated in combination with other antiretroviral agents for the treatment of HIV-1 infection. (1)

DOSAGE AND ADMINISTRATION
- A medication guide and warning card should be dispensed with each new prescription and refill. (2)
- Adults: 600 mg daily, administered as either 300 mg twice daily or 600 mg once daily. (2.1)
- Pediatric Patients Aged 3 Months and Older: Dose should be calculated on body weight (kg) and should not exceed 300 mg twice daily. (2.2)
- Patients With Hepatic Impairment: Mild hepatic impairment – 200 mg twice daily; moderate/severe hepatic impairment – contraindicated. (2.3)

DOSAGE FORMS AND STRENGTHS
Tablets: 300 mg, scored; Oral Solution: 20 mg/mL (3)

CONTRAINDICATIONS
- Previously demonstrated hypersensitivity to abacavir. (4, 5.1)
- Moderate or severe hepatic impairment. (4)

WARNINGS AND PRECAUTIONS
- Hypersensitivity: Serious and sometimes fatal hypersensitivity reactions have been associated with ZIAGEN and other abacavir-containing products. Read full prescribing information section 5.1 before prescribing ZIAGEN. (5.1)
- Lactic acidosis and severe hepatomegaly with steatosis have been reported with the use of nucleoside analogues. (5.2)
- Immune reconstitution syndrome (5.3) and redistribution/accumulation of body fat have been reported in patients treated with combination antiretroviral therapy. (5.4)

ADVERSE REACTIONS
- The most commonly reported adverse reactions of at least moderate intensity (incidence ≥10%) in adult HIV-1 clinical trials were nausea, headache, malaise and fatigue, nausea and vomiting, and dreams/sleep disorders. (6.1)
- The most commonly reported adverse reactions of at least moderate intensity (incidence ≥5%) in pediatric HIV-1 clinical trials were fever and/or chills, nausea and vomiting, skin rashes, and ear/nose/throat infections. (6.1)
To report SUSPECTED ADVERSE REACTIONS, contact ViiV Healthcare at 1-877-844-8872 or FDA at 1-800-FDA-1088 or .

DRUG INTERACTIONS
- Ethanol: Decreases elimination of abacavir. (7.1)
- Methadone: An increased methadone dose may be required in a small number of patients. (7.2)
See 17 for PATIENT COUNSELING INFORMATION and Medication Guide

Revised: 09/2013

FULL PRESCRIBING INFORMATION: CONTENTS*
WARNING: RISK OF HYPERSENSITIVITY REACTIONS, LACTIC ACIDOSIS, AND SEVERE HEPATOMEGALY
1   INDICATIONS AND USAGE

FULL PRESCRIBING INFORMATION

WARNING: RISK OF HYPERSENSITIVITY REACTIONS, LACTIC ACIDOSIS, AND SEVERE HEPATOMEGALY

Hypersensitivity Reactions: Serious and sometimes fatal hypersensitivity reactions have been associated with ZIAGEN® (abacavir sulfate).
Hypersensitivity to abacavir is a multi-organ clinical syndrome usually characterized by a sign or symptom in 2 or more of the following groups: (1) fever, (2) rash, (3) gastrointestinal (including nausea, vomiting, diarrhea, or abdominal pain), (4) constitutional (including generalized malaise, fatigue, or achiness), and (5) respiratory (including dyspnea, cough, or pharyngitis). Discontinue ZIAGEN as soon as a hypersensitivity reaction is suspected.
Patients who carry the HLA-B*5701 allele are at high risk for experiencing a hypersensitivity reaction to abacavir. Prior to initiating therapy with abacavir, screening for the HLA-B*5701 allele is recommended; this approach has been found to decrease the risk of hypersensitivity reaction. Screening is also recommended prior to reinitiation of abacavir in patients of unknown HLA-B*5701 status who have previously tolerated abacavir. HLA-B*5701-negative patients may develop a suspected hypersensitivity reaction to abacavir; however, this occurs significantly less frequently than in HLA-B*5701-positive patients.
Regardless of HLA-B*5701 status, permanently discontinue ZIAGEN if hypersensitivity cannot be ruled out, even when other diagnoses are possible.
Following a hypersensitivity reaction to abacavir, NEVER restart ZIAGEN or any other abacavir-containing product because more severe symptoms can occur within hours and may include life-threatening hypotension and death.
Reintroduction of ZIAGEN or any other abacavir-containing product, even in patients who have no identified history or unrecognized symptoms of hypersensitivity to abacavir therapy, can result in serious or fatal hypersensitivity reactions. Such reactions can occur within hours *[see Warnings and Precautions (5.1)]*.
Lactic Acidosis and Severe Hepatomegaly: Lactic acidosis and severe hepatomegaly with steatosis, including fatal cases, have been reported with the use of nucleoside analogues alone or in combination, including ZIAGEN and other antiretrovirals *[see Warnings and Precautions (5.2)]*.

1 INDICATIONS AND USAGE

ZIAGEN Tablets and Oral Solution, in combination with other antiretroviral agents, are indicated for the treatment of human immunodeficiency virus (HIV-1) infection.

Additional important information on the use of ZIAGEN for treatment of HIV-1 infection:

ZIAGEN is one of multiple products containing abacavir. Before starting ZIAGEN, review medical history for prior exposure to any abacavir-containing product in order to avoid reintroduction in a patient with a history of hypersensitivity to abacavir *[see Warnings and Precautions (5.1), Adverse Reactions (6)]*.

2 DOSAGE AND ADMINISTRATION

• A Medication Guide and Warning Card that provide information about recognition of hypersensitivity reactions should be dispensed with each new prescription and refill.
• ZIAGEN may be taken with or without food.

2.1 Adult Patients

The recommended oral dose of ZIAGEN for adults is 600 mg daily, administered as either 300 mg twice daily or 600 mg once daily, in combination with other antiretroviral agents.

2.2 Pediatric Patients

The recommended oral dose of ZIAGEN Oral Solution in HIV-1-infected pediatric patients aged 3 months and older is 8 mg/kg twice daily (up to a maximum of 300 mg twice daily) in combination with other antiretroviral agents.

ZIAGEN is also available as a scored tablet for HIV-1-infected pediatric patients weighing greater than or equal to 14 kg for whom a solid dosage form is appropriate. Before prescribing ZIAGEN Tablets, children should be assessed for the ability to swallow tablets. If a child is unable to reliably swallow ZIAGEN Tablets, the oral solution formulation should be prescribed. The recommended oral dosage of ZIAGEN Tablets for HIV-1-infected pediatric patients is presented in Table 1.

Table 1. Dosing Recommendations for ZIAGEN Tablets in Pediatric Patients

Weight (kg)	Dosage Regimen Using Scored Tablet		Total Daily Dose
	AM Dose	PM Dose	
14 to 21	½ tablet (150 mg)	½ tablet (150 mg)	300 mg
>21 to <30	½ tablet (150 mg)	1 tablet (300 mg)	450 mg
≥30	1 tablet (300 mg)	1 tablet (300 mg)	600 mg

2.3 Patients With Hepatic Impairment

The recommended dose of ZIAGEN in patients with mild hepatic impairment (Child-Pugh score 5 to 6) is 200 mg twice daily. To enable dose reduction, ZIAGEN Oral Solution (10 mL twice daily) should be used for the treatment of these patients. The safety, efficacy, and pharmacokinetic properties of abacavir have not been established in patients with moderate to severe hepatic impairment; therefore, ZIAGEN is contraindicated in these patients.

3 DOSAGE FORMS AND STRENGTHS

ZIAGEN Tablets contain 300 mg of abacavir as abacavir sulfate. The tablets are yellow, biconvex, scored, capsule-shaped, film-coated, and imprinted with "GX 623" on both sides.

ZIAGEN Oral Solution contains 20 mg/mL of abacavir as abacavir sulfate. The solution is a clear to opalescent, yellowish, strawberry-banana-flavored liquid.

4 CONTRAINDICATIONS

ZIAGEN is contraindicated in patients with:

• previously demonstrated hypersensitivity to abacavir or any other component of the products. NEVER restart ZIAGEN or any other abacavir-containing product following a hypersensitivity reaction to abacavir, regardless of HLA-B*5701 status *[see Warnings and Precautions (5.1), Adverse Reactions (6)]*.
• moderate or severe hepatic impairment *[see Dosage and Administration (2.3)]*.

5 WARNINGS AND PRECAUTIONS

5.1 Hypersensitivity Reaction

Serious and sometimes fatal hypersensitivity reactions have been associated with ZIAGEN and other abacavir-containing products. Patients who carry the HLA-B*5701 allele are at high risk for experiencing a hypersensitivity reaction to abacavir. Prior to initiating therapy with abacavir, screening for the HLA-B*5701 allele is recommended; this approach has been found to decrease the risk of a hypersensitivity reaction. Screening is also recommended prior to reinitiation of abacavir in patients of unknown HLA-B*5701 status who have previously tolerated abacavir. For HLA-B*5701-positive patients, treatment with an abacavir-containing regimen is not recommended and should be considered only with close medical supervision and under exceptional circumstances when the potential benefit outweighs the risk.

HLA-B*5701-negative patients may develop a hypersensitivity reaction to abacavir; however, this occurs significantly less frequently than in HLA-B*5701-positive patients. Regardless of HLA-B*5701 status, permanently discontinue ZIAGEN if hypersensitivity cannot be ruled out, even when other diagnoses are possible.

Important information on signs and symptoms of hypersensitivity, as well as clinical management, is presented below.

Signs and Symptoms of Hypersensitivity: Hypersensitivity to abacavir is a multi-organ clinical syndrome usually characterized by a sign or symptom in 2 or more of the following groups:

Group 1: Fever
Group 2: Rash
Group 3: Gastrointestinal (including nausea, vomiting, diarrhea, or abdominal pain)
Group 4: Constitutional (including generalized malaise, fatigue, or achiness)
Group 5: Respiratory (including dyspnea, cough, or pharyngitis).

Hypersensitivity to abacavir following the presentation of a single sign or symptom has been reported infrequently.

Hypersensitivity to abacavir was reported in approximately 8% of 2,670 subjects (n = 206) in 9 clinical trials (range: 2% to 9%) with enrollment from November 1999 to February 2002. Data on time to onset and symptoms of suspected hypersensitivity were collected on a detailed data collection module. The frequencies of symptoms are shown in Figure 1. Symptoms usually appeared within the first 6 weeks of treatment with abacavir, although the reaction may occur at any time during therapy. Median time to onset was 9 days; 89% appeared within the first 6 weeks; 95% of subjects reported symptoms from 2 or more of the 5 groups listed above.

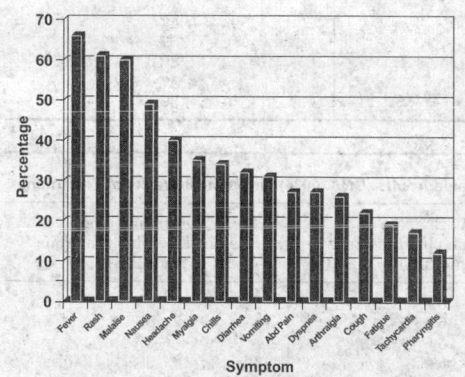

Figure 1. Hypersensitivity-Related Symptoms Reported With ≥10% Frequency in Clinical Trials (n = 206 Subjects)

Other less common signs and symptoms of hypersensitivity include lethargy, myolysis, edema, abnormal chest x-ray findings (predominantly infiltrates, which can be localized), and paresthesia. Anaphylaxis, liver failure, renal failure, hypotension, adult respiratory distress syndrome, respiratory failure, and death have occurred in association with hypersensitivity reactions. In one trial, 4 subjects (11%) receiving ZIAGEN 600 mg once daily experienced hypotension with a hypersensitivity reaction compared with 0 subjects receiving ZIAGEN 300 mg twice daily.

Physical findings associated with hypersensitivity to abacavir in some patients include lymphadenopathy, mucous membrane lesions (conjunctivitis and mouth ulcerations), and rash. The rash usually appears maculopapular or urticarial, but may be variable in appearance. There have been reports of erythema multiforme. Hypersensitivity reactions have occurred without rash.

Laboratory abnormalities associated with hypersensitivity to abacavir in some patients include elevated liver function tests, elevated creatine phosphokinase, elevated creatinine, and lymphopenia.

Clinical Management of Hypersensitivity: Discontinue ZIAGEN as soon as a hypersensitivity reaction is suspected. To minimize the risk of a life-threatening hypersensitivity reaction, permanently discontinue ZIAGEN if hypersensitivity cannot be ruled out, even when other diagnoses are possible (e.g., acute onset respiratory diseases such as pneumonia, bronchitis, pharyngitis, or influenza; gastroenteritis; or reactions to other medications).

Following a hypersensitivity reaction to abacavir, NEVER restart ZIAGEN or any other abacavir-containing product because more severe symptoms can occur within hours and may include life-threatening hypotension and death.

When therapy with ZIAGEN has been discontinued for reasons other than symptoms of a hypersensitivity reaction, and if reinitiation of ZIAGEN or any other abacavir-containing product is under consideration, carefully evaluate the reason for discontinuation of ZIAGEN to ensure that the patient did not have symptoms of a hypersensitivity reaction. If the patient is of unknown HLA-B*5701 status, screening for the allele is recommended prior to reinitiation of ZIAGEN.

If hypersensitivity cannot be ruled out, DO NOT reintroduce ZIAGEN or any other abacavir-containing product. Even in the absence of the HLA-B*5701 allele, it is important to permanently discontinue abacavir and not rechallenge with abacavir if a hypersensitivity reaction cannot be ruled out on clinical grounds, due to the potential for a severe or even fatal reaction.

If symptoms consistent with hypersensitivity are not identified, reintroduction can be undertaken with continued monitoring for symptoms of a hypersensitivity reaction. Make patients aware that a hypersensitivity reaction can occur with reintroduction of ZIAGEN or any other abacavir-containing product and that reintroduction of ZIAGEN or any other abacavir-containing product needs to be undertaken only if medical care can be readily accessed by the patient or others.

Risk Factor: *HLA-B*5701 Allele:* Trials have shown that carriage of the HLA-B*5701 allele is associated with a significantly increased risk of a hypersensitivity reaction to abacavir.

CNA106030 (PREDICT-1), a randomized, double-blind trial, evaluated the clinical utility of prospective HLA-B*5701 screening on the incidence of abacavir hypersensitivity reaction in abacavir-naive HIV-1-infected adults (n = 1,650). In this trial, use of pre-therapy screening for the HLA-B*5701 allele and exclusion of subjects with this allele reduced the incidence of clinically suspected abacavir hypersensitivity reactions from 7.8% (66/847) to 3.4% (27/803). Based on this trial, it is estimated that 61% of patients with the HLA-B*5701 allele will develop a clinically suspected hypersensitivity reaction during the course of abacavir treatment compared with 4% of patients who do not have the HLA-B*5701 allele.

Screening for carriage of the HLA-B*5701 allele is recommended prior to initiating treatment with abacavir. Screening is also recommended prior to reinitiation of abacavir in patients of unknown HLA-B*5701 status who have previously tolerated abacavir. For HLA-B*5701-positive patients, initiating or reinitiating treatment with an abacavir-containing regimen is not recommended and should be considered only with close medical supervision and under exceptional circumstances where potential benefit outweighs the risk.

Skin patch testing is used as a research tool and should not be used to aid in the clinical diagnosis of abacavir hypersensitivity.

In any patient treated with abacavir, the clinical diagnosis of hypersensitivity reaction must remain the basis of clinical decision-making. Even in the absence of the HLA-B*5701 allele, it is important to permanently discontinue abacavir and not rechallenge with abacavir if a hypersensitivity reaction cannot be ruled out on clinical grounds, due to the potential for a severe or even fatal reaction.

5.2 Lactic Acidosis/Severe Hepatomegaly With Steatosis

Lactic acidosis and severe hepatomegaly with steatosis, including fatal cases, have been reported with the use of nucleoside analogues alone or in combination, including abacavir and other antiretrovirals. A majority of these cases have been in women. Obesity and prolonged nucleoside exposure may be risk factors. Particular caution should be exercised when administering ZIAGEN to any patient with known risk factors for liver disease; however, cases have also been reported in patients with no known risk factors. Treatment with ZIAGEN should be suspended in any patient who develops clinical or laboratory findings suggestive of lactic acidosis or pronounced hepatotoxicity (which may include hepatomegaly and steatosis even in the absence of marked transaminase elevations).

5.3 Immune Reconstitution Syndrome

Immune reconstitution syndrome has been reported in patients treated with combination antiretroviral therapy, including ZIAGEN. During the initial phase of combination

Table 2. Treatment-Emergent (All Causality) Adverse Reactions of at Least Moderate Intensity (Grades 2-4, ≥5% Frequency) in Therapy-Naive Adults (CNA30024[a]) Through 48 Weeks of Treatment

Adverse Reaction	ZIAGEN plus Lamivudine plus Efavirenz (n = 324)	Zidovudine plus Lamivudine plus Efavirenz (n = 325)
Dreams/sleep disorders	10%	10%
Drug hypersensitivity	9%	<1%[b]
Headaches/migraine	7%	11%
Nausea	7%	11%
Fatigue/malaise	7%	10%
Diarrhea	7%	6%
Rashes	6%	12%
Abdominal pain/gastritis/gastrointestinal signs and symptoms	6%	8%
Depressive disorders	6%	6%
Dizziness	6%	6%
Musculoskeletal pain	6%	5%
Bronchitis	4%	5%
Vomiting	2%	9%

[a] This trial used double-blind ascertainment of suspected hypersensitivity reactions. During the blinded portion of the trial, suspected hypersensitivity to abacavir was reported by investigators in 9% of 324 subjects in the abacavir group and 3% of 325 subjects in the zidovudine group.

[b] Ten (3%) cases of suspected drug hypersensitivity were reclassified as not being due to abacavir following unblinding.

Table 3. Treatment-Emergent (All Causality) Adverse Reactions of at Least Moderate Intensity (Grades 2-4, ≥5% Frequency) in Therapy-Naive Adults (CNA3005) Through 48 Weeks of Treatment

Adverse Reaction	ZIAGEN plus Lamivudine/Zidovudine (n = 262)	Indinavir plus Lamivudine/Zidovudine (n = 264)
Nausea	19%	17%
Headache	13%	9%
Malaise and fatigue	12%	12%
Nausea and vomiting	10%	10%
Hypersensitivity reaction	8%	2%
Diarrhea	7%	5%
Fever and/or chills	6%	3%
Depressive disorders	6%	4%
Musculoskeletal pain	5%	7%
Skin rashes	5%	4%
Ear/nose/throat infections	5%	4%
Viral respiratory infections	5%	5%
Anxiety	5%	3%
Renal signs/symptoms	<1%	5%
Pain (non-site-specific)	<1%	5%

Table 4. Laboratory Abnormalities (Grades 3-4) in Therapy-Naive Adults (CNA30024) Through 48 Weeks of Treatment

Grade 3/4 Laboratory Abnormalities	ZIAGEN plus Lamivudine plus Efavirenz (n = 324)	Zidovudine plus Lamivudine plus Efavirenz (n = 325)
Elevated CPK (>4 × ULN)	8%	8%
Elevated ALT (>5 × ULN)	6%	6%
Elevated AST (>5 × ULN)	6%	5%
Hypertriglyceridemia (>750 mg/dL)	6%	5%
Hyperamylasemia (>2 × ULN)	4%	5%
Neutropenia (ANC <750/mm^3)	2%	4%
Anemia (Hgb ≤6.9 gm/dL)	<1%	2%
Thrombocytopenia (Platelets <50,000/mm^3)	1%	<1%
Leukopenia (WBC ≤1,500/mm^3)	<1%	2%

ULN = Upper limit of normal.
n = Number of subjects assessed.

antiretroviral treatment, patients whose immune systems respond may develop an inflammatory response to indolent or residual opportunistic infections (such as *Mycobacterium avium* infection, cytomegalovirus, *Pneumocystis jirovecii* pneumonia [PCP], or tuberculosis), which may necessitate further evaluation and treatment.

Autoimmune disorders (such as Graves' disease, polymyositis, and Guillain-Barré syndrome) have also been reported to occur in the setting of immune reconstitution; however, the time to onset is more variable and can occur many months after initiation of treatment.

5.4   Fat Redistribution
Redistribution/accumulation of body fat including central obesity, dorsocervical fat enlargement (buffalo hump), peripheral wasting, facial wasting, breast enlargement, and "cushingoid appearance" have been observed in patients receiving antiretroviral therapy. The mechanism and long-term consequences of these events are currently unknown. A causal relationship has not been established.

5.5   Myocardial Infarction
In a published prospective, observational, epidemiological trial designed to investigate the rate of myocardial infarction in patients on combination antiretroviral therapy, the use of abacavir within the previous 6 months was correlated with an increased risk of myocardial infarction (MI).[1] In a sponsor-conducted pooled analysis of clinical trials, no excess risk of myocardial infarction was observed in abacavir-treated subjects as compared with control subjects. In totality, the available data from the observational cohort and from clinical trials are inconclusive.

As a precaution, the underlying risk of coronary heart disease should be considered when prescribing antiretroviral therapies, including abacavir, and action taken to minimize all modifiable risk factors (e.g., hypertension, hyperlipidemia, diabetes mellitus, smoking).

6   ADVERSE REACTIONS
The following adverse reactions are discussed in greater detail in other sections of the labeling:

- Serious and sometimes fatal hypersensitivity reaction. In one trial, once-daily dosing of abacavir was associated with more severe hypersensitivity reactions [see Boxed Warning, Warnings and Precautions (5.1)].
- Lactic acidosis and severe hepatomegaly [see Boxed Warning, Warnings and Precautions (5.2)].
- Immune reconstitution syndrome [see Warnings and Precautions (5.3)].
- Fat redistribution [see Warnings and Precautions (5.4)].
- Myocardial infarction [see Warnings and Precautions (5.5)].

6.1   Clinical Trials Experience
Because clinical trials are conducted under widely varying conditions, adverse reaction rates observed in the clinical trials of a drug cannot be directly compared with rates in the clinical trials of another drug and may not reflect the rates observed in practice.

Adults: *Therapy-Naive Adults:* Treatment-emergent clinical adverse reactions (rated by the investigator as moderate or severe) with a greater than or equal to 5% frequency during therapy with ZIAGEN 300 mg twice daily, lamivudine 150 mg twice daily, and efavirenz 600 mg daily compared with zidovudine 300 mg twice daily, lamivudine 150 mg twice daily, and efavirenz 600 mg daily from CNA30024 are listed in Table 2.
[See table 2 above]

Treatment-emergent clinical adverse reactions (rated by the investigator as moderate or severe) with a greater than or equal to 5% frequency during therapy with ZIAGEN 300 mg twice daily, lamivudine 150 mg twice daily, and zidovudine 300 mg twice daily compared with indinavir 800 mg 3 times daily, lamivudine 150 mg twice daily, and zidovudine 300 mg twice daily from CNA3005 are listed in Table 3.
[See table 3 above]

Five subjects receiving ZIAGEN in CNA3005 experienced worsening of pre-existing depression compared with none in the indinavir arm. The background rates of pre-existing depression were similar in the 2 treatment arms.

ZIAGEN Once Daily Versus ZIAGEN Twice Daily (CNA30021): Treatment-emergent clinical adverse reactions (rated by the investigator as at least moderate) with a greater than or equal to 5% frequency during therapy with ZIAGEN 600 mg once daily or ZIAGEN 300 mg twice daily, both in combination with lamivudine 300 mg once daily and efavirenz 600 mg once daily from CNA30021, were similar. For hypersensitivity reactions, subjects receiving ZIAGEN once daily showed a rate of 9% in comparison with a rate of 7% for subjects receiving ZIAGEN twice daily. However, subjects receiving ZIAGEN 600 mg once daily, experienced a significantly higher incidence of severe drug hypersensitivity reactions and severe diarrhea compared with subjects who received ZIAGEN 300 mg twice daily. Five percent (5%) of subjects receiving ZIAGEN 600 mg once daily had severe drug hypersensitivity reactions compared with 2% of subjects receiving ZIAGEN 300 mg twice daily. Two percent (2%) of subjects receiving ZIAGEN 600 mg once daily had severe diarrhea while none of the subjects receiving ZIAGEN 300 mg twice daily had this event.

Laboratory Abnormalities: Laboratory abnormalities (Grades 3-4) in therapy-naive adults during therapy with ZIAGEN 300 mg twice daily, lamivudine 150 mg twice daily, and efavirenz 600 mg daily compared with zidovudine 300 mg twice daily, lamivudine 150 mg twice daily, and efavirenz 600 mg daily from CNA30024 are listed in Table 4.
[See table 4 above]

Laboratory abnormalities in CNA3005 are listed in Table 5.
[See table 5 at top of next page]

The frequencies of treatment-emergent laboratory abnormalities were comparable between treatment groups in CNA30021.

Pediatric Trials: *Therapy-Experienced Pediatric Subjects:* Treatment-emergent clinical adverse reactions (rated by the investigator as moderate or severe) with a greater than or equal to 5% frequency during therapy with ZIAGEN 8 mg/kg twice daily, lamivudine 4 mg/kg twice daily, and zidovudine 180 mg/m^2 twice daily compared with lamivudine 4 mg/kg twice daily and zidovudine 180 mg/m^2 twice daily from CNA3006 are listed in Table 6.
[See table 6 at top of next page]

Laboratory Abnormalities: In CNA3006, laboratory abnormalities (anemia, neutropenia, liver function test abnormalities, and CPK elevations) were observed with similar frequencies as in a trial of therapy-naive adults (CNA30024). Mild elevations of blood glucose were more frequent in pediatric subjects receiving ZIAGEN (CNA3006) as compared with adult subjects (CNA30024).

Other Adverse Events: In addition to adverse reactions and laboratory abnormalities reported in Tables 2, 3, 4, 5, and 6, other adverse reactions observed in the expanded access program were pancreatitis and increased GGT.

6.2 Postmarketing Experience

In addition to adverse reactions reported from clinical trials, the following reactions have been identified during postmarketing use of ZIAGEN. Because they are reported voluntarily from a population of unknown size, estimates of frequency cannot be made. These reactions have been chosen for inclusion due to a combination of their seriousness, frequency of reporting, or potential causal connection to ZIAGEN.

Body as a Whole: Redistribution/accumulation of body fat.

Cardiovascular: Myocardial infarction.

Hepatic: Lactic acidosis and hepatic steatosis.

Skin: Suspected Stevens-Johnson syndrome (SJS) and toxic epidermal necrolysis (TEN) have been reported in patients receiving abacavir primarily in combination with medications known to be associated with SJS and TEN, respectively. Because of the overlap of clinical signs and symptoms between hypersensitivity to abacavir and SJS and TEN, and the possibility of multiple drug sensitivities in some patients, abacavir should be discontinued and not restarted in such cases.

There have also been reports of erythema multiforme with abacavir use.

7 DRUG INTERACTIONS

7.1 Ethanol

Abacavir has no effect on the pharmacokinetic properties of ethanol. Ethanol decreases the elimination of abacavir causing an increase in overall exposure *[see Clinical Pharmacology (12.3)]*.

7.2 Methadone

The addition of methadone has no clinically significant effect on the pharmacokinetic properties of abacavir. In a trial of 11 HIV-1-infected subjects receiving methadone-maintenance therapy with 600 mg of ZIAGEN twice daily (twice the currently recommended dose), oral methadone clearance increased *[see Clinical Pharmacology (12.3)]*. This alteration will not result in a methadone dose modification in the majority of patients; however, an increased methadone dose may be required in a small number of patients.

8 USE IN SPECIFIC POPULATIONS

8.1 Pregnancy

Pregnancy Category C. Studies in pregnant rats showed that abacavir is transferred to the fetus through the placenta. Fetal malformations (increased incidences of fetal anasarca and skeletal malformations) and developmental toxicity (depressed fetal body weight and reduced crown-rump length) were observed in rats at a dose which produced 35 times the human exposure based on AUC. Embryonic and fetal toxicities (increased resorptions, decreased fetal body weights) and toxicities to the offspring (increased incidence of stillbirth and lower body weights) occurred at half of the above-mentioned dose in separate fertility studies conducted in rats. In the rabbit, no developmental toxicity and no increases in fetal malformations occurred at doses that produced 8.5 times the human exposure at the recommended dose based on AUC.

There are no adequate and well-controlled studies in pregnant women. ZIAGEN should be used during pregnancy only if the potential benefits outweigh the risk.

Antiretroviral Pregnancy Registry: To monitor maternal-fetal outcomes of pregnant women exposed to ZIAGEN, an Antiretroviral Pregnancy Registry has been established. Physicians are encouraged to register patients by calling 1-800-258-4263.

8.3 Nursing Mothers

The Centers for Disease Control and Prevention recommend that HIV-1-infected mothers not breastfeed their infants to avoid risking postnatal transmission of HIV-1 infection.

Although it is not known if abacavir is excreted in human milk, abacavir is secreted into the milk of lactating rats. Because of both the potential for HIV-1 transmission and the potential for serious adverse reactions in nursing infants, mothers should be instructed not to breastfeed if they are receiving ZIAGEN.

8.4 Pediatric Use

The safety and effectiveness of ZIAGEN have been established in pediatric patients 3 months to 13 years of age. Use of ZIAGEN in these age-groups is supported by pharmacokinetic trials and evidence from adequate and well-controlled trials of ZIAGEN in adults and pediatric patients *[see Dosage and Administration (2.2), Clinical Pharmacology (12.3), Clinical Studies (14.2)]*.

8.5 Geriatric Use

Clinical studies of ZIAGEN did not include sufficient numbers of patients aged 65 and over to determine whether they respond differently from younger patients. In general, dose selection for an elderly patient should be cautious, reflecting the greater frequency of decreased hepatic, renal, or cardiac function, and of concomitant disease or other drug therapy.

10 OVERDOSAGE

There is no known antidote for ZIAGEN. It is not known whether abacavir can be removed by peritoneal dialysis or hemodialysis.

11 DESCRIPTION

ZIAGEN is the brand name for abacavir sulfate, a synthetic carbocyclic nucleoside analogue with inhibitory activity against HIV-1. The chemical name of abacavir sulfate is (1S,cis)-4-[2-amino-6-(cyclopropylamino)-9H-purin-9-yl]-2-cyclopentene-1-methanol sulfate (salt) (2:1). Abacavir sulfate is the enantiomer with 1S, 4R absolute configuration on the cyclopentene ring. It has a molecular formula of $(C_{14}H_{18}N_6O)_2 \cdot H_2SO_4$ and a molecular weight of 670.76 daltons. It has the following structural formula:

Abacavir sulfate is a white to off-white solid with a solubility of approximately 77 mg/mL in distilled water at 25°C. It has an octanol/water (pH 7.1 to 7.3) partition coefficient (log P) of approximately 1.20 at 25°C.

ZIAGEN Tablets are for oral administration. Each tablet contains abacavir sulfate equivalent to 300 mg of abacavir as active ingredient and the following inactive ingredients: colloidal silicon dioxide, magnesium stearate, microcrystalline cellulose, and sodium starch glycolate. The tablets are coated with a film that is made of hypromellose, polysorbate 80, synthetic yellow iron oxide, titanium dioxide, and triacetin.

ZIAGEN Oral Solution is for oral administration. Each milliliter (1 mL) of ZIAGEN Oral Solution contains abacavir sulfate equivalent to 20 mg of abacavir (i.e., 20 mg/mL) as active ingredient and the following inactive ingredients: artificial strawberry and banana flavors, citric acid (anhydrous), methylparaben and propylparaben (added as preservatives), propylene glycol, saccharin sodium, sodium citrate (dihydrate), sorbitol solution, and water.

In vivo, abacavir sulfate dissociates to its free base, abacavir. All dosages for ZIAGEN are expressed in terms of abacavir.

12 CLINICAL PHARMACOLOGY

12.1 Mechanism of Action

Abacavir is an antiviral agent *[See Clinical Pharmacology (12.4)]*.

12.3 Pharmacokinetics

Pharmacokinetics in Adults: The pharmacokinetic properties of abacavir have been studied in asymptomatic, HIV-1-infected adult subjects after administration of a single intravenous (IV) dose of 150 mg and after single and multiple oral doses. The pharmacokinetic properties of abacavir were independent of dose over the range of 300 to 1,200 mg/day.

Absorption and Bioavailability: Abacavir was rapidly and extensively absorbed after oral administration. The geometric mean absolute bioavailability of the tablet was 83%. After oral administration of 300 mg twice daily in 20 subjects, the steady-state peak serum abacavir concentration (C_{max}) was 3.0 ± 0.89 mcg/mL (mean $\pm$ SD) and $AUC_{(0-12\ hr)}$ was 6.02 ± 1.73 mcg•hr/mL. After oral administration of a single dose of 600 mg of abacavir in 20 subjects, C_{max} was 4.26 ± 1.19 mcg/mL (mean $\pm$ SD) and AUC_∞ was 11.95 ± 2.51 mcg•hr/mL.

Distribution: The apparent volume of distribution after IV administration of abacavir was 0.86 ± 0.15 L/kg, suggesting that abacavir distributes into extravascular space. In 3 subjects, the $CSF\ AUC_{(0-6\ hr)}$ to plasma abacavir $AUC_{(0-6\ hr)}$ ratio ranged from 27% to 33%.

Binding of abacavir to human plasma proteins is approximately 50%. Binding of abacavir to plasma proteins was independent of concentration. Total blood and plasma drug-related radioactivity concentrations are identical, demonstrating that abacavir readily distributes into erythrocytes.

Metabolism: In humans, abacavir is not significantly metabolized by cytochrome P450 enzymes. The primary routes of elimination of abacavir are metabolism by alcohol dehydrogenase (to form the 5'-carboxylic acid) and glucuronyl transferase (to form the 5'-glucuronide). The metabolites do not have antiviral activity. In vitro experiments reveal that abacavir does not inhibit human CYP3A4, CYP2D6, or CYP2C9 activity at clinically relevant concentrations.

Elimination: Elimination of abacavir was quantified in a mass balance trial following administration of a 600-mg dose of ^{14}C-abacavir: 99% of the radioactivity was recovered, 1.2% was excreted in the urine as abacavir, 30% as the 5'-carboxylic acid metabolite, 36% as the 5'-glucuronide metabolite, and 15% as unidentified minor metabolites in the urine. Fecal elimination accounted for 16% of the dose.

In single-dose trials, the observed elimination half-life ($t_{1/2}$) was 1.54 ± 0.63 hours. After intravenous administration, total clearance was 0.80 ± 0.24 L/hr/kg (mean $\pm$ SD).

Effects of Food on Oral Absorption: Bioavailability of abacavir tablets was assessed in the fasting and fed states. There was no significant difference in systemic exposure (AUC_∞) in the fed and fasting states; therefore, ZIAGEN Tablets may be administered with or without food. Systemic exposure to abacavir was comparable after administration of ZIAGEN Oral Solution and ZIAGEN Tablets. Therefore, these products may be used interchangeably.

Special Populations: *Renal Impairment:* The pharmacokinetic properties of ZIAGEN have not been determined in

Table 5. Treatment-Emergent Laboratory Abnormalities (Grades 3-4) in CNA3005

Grade 3/4 Laboratory Abnormalities	Number of Subjects by Treatment Group	
	ZIAGEN plus Lamivudine/Zidovudine (n = 262)	Indinavir plus Lamivudine/Zidovudine (n = 264)
Elevated CPK (>4 × ULN)	18 (7%)	18 (7%)
ALT (>5.0 × ULN)	16 (6%)	16 (6%)
Neutropenia (<750/mm³)	13 (5%)	13 (5%)
Hypertriglyceridemia (>750 mg/dL)	5 (2%)	3 (1%)
Hyperamylasemia (>2.0 × ULN)	5 (2%)	1 (<1%)
Hyperglycemia (>13.9 mmol/L)	2 (<1%)	2 (<1%)
Anemia (Hgb ≤6.9 g/dL)	0 (0%)	3 (1%)

ULN = Upper limit of normal.
n = Number of subjects assessed.

Table 6. Treatment-Emergent (All Causality) Adverse Reactions of at Least Moderate Intensity (Grades 2-4, ≥5% Frequency) in Therapy-Experienced Pediatric Subjects (CNA3006) Through 16 Weeks of Treatment

Adverse Reaction	ZIAGEN plus Lamivudine plus Zidovudine (n = 102)	Lamivudine plus Zidovudine (n = 103)
Fever and/or chills	9%	7%
Nausea and vomiting	9%	2%
Skin rashes	7%	1%
Ear/nose/throat infections	5%	1%
Pneumonia	4%	5%
Headache	1%	5%

Table 7. Outcomes of Randomized Treatment Through Week 48 (CNA30024)

Outcome	ZIAGEN plus Lamivudine plus Efavirenz (n = 324)	Zidovudine plus Lamivudine plus Efavirenz (n = 325)
Responder[a]	69% (73%)	69% (71%)
Virologic failures[b]	6%	4%
Discontinued due to adverse reactions	14%	16%
Discontinued due to other reasons[c]	10%	11%

[a] Subjects achieved and maintained confirmed HIV-1 RNA ≤50 copies/mL (<400 copies/mL) through Week 48 (Roche AMPLICOR Ultrasensitive HIV-1 MONITOR® standard test 1.0 PCR).
[b] Includes viral rebound, insufficient viral response according to the investigator, and failure to achieve confirmed ≤50 copies/mL by Week 48.
[c] Includes consent withdrawn, lost to follow up, protocol violations, those with missing data, clinical progression, and other.

Table 8. Outcomes of Randomized Treatment Through Week 48 (CNA3005)

Outcome	ZIAGEN plus Lamivudine/Zidovudine (n = 262)	Indinavir plus Lamivudine/Zidovudine (n = 265)
Responder[a]	49%	50%
Virologic failure[b]	31%	28%
Discontinued due to adverse reactions	10%	12%
Discontinued due to other reasons[c]	11%	10%

[a] Subjects achieved and maintained confirmed HIV-1 RNA <400 copies/mL.
[b] Includes viral rebound and failure to achieve confirmed <400 copies/mL by Week 48.
[c] Includes consent withdrawn, lost to follow up, protocol violations, those with missing data, clinical progression, and other.

patients with impaired renal function. Renal excretion of unchanged abacavir is a minor route of elimination in humans.

Hepatic Impairment: The pharmacokinetics of abacavir have been studied in subjects with mild hepatic impairment (Child-Pugh score 5 to 6). Results showed that there was a mean increase of 89% in the abacavir AUC and an increase of 58% in the half-life of abacavir after a single dose of 600 mg of abacavir. The AUCs of the metabolites were not modified by mild liver disease; however, the rates of formation and elimination of the metabolites were decreased. A dose of 200 mg (provided by 10 mL of ZIAGEN Oral Solution) administered twice daily is recommended for patients with mild liver disease. The safety, efficacy, and pharmacokinetics of abacavir have not been studied in patients with moderate or severe hepatic impairment; therefore, ZIAGEN is contraindicated in these patients.

Pediatric Patients: The pharmacokinetics of abacavir have been studied after either single or repeat doses of ZIAGEN in 68 pediatric subjects. Following multiple-dose administration of ZIAGEN 8 mg/kg twice daily, steady-state $AUC_{(0-12\ hr)}$ and C_{max} were 9.8 ± 4.56 mcg•hr/mL and 3.71 ± 1.36 mcg/mL (mean ± SD), respectively *[see Use in Specific Populations (8.4)]*. In addition, to support dosing of ZIAGEN scored tablet (300 mg) for pediatric patients 14 kg to greater than 30 kg, analysis of actual and simulated pharmacokinetic data indicated comparable exposures are expected following administration of 300 mg scored tablet and the 8 mg/kg dosing regimen using oral solution.

Geriatric Patients: The pharmacokinetics of ZIAGEN have not been studied in patients over 65 years of age.

Gender: A population pharmacokinetic analysis in HIV-1-infected male (n = 304) and female (n = 67) subjects showed no gender differences in abacavir AUC normalized for lean body weight.

Race: There are no significant differences between blacks and Caucasians in abacavir pharmacokinetics.

Drug Interactions: In human liver microsomes, abacavir did not inhibit cytochrome P450 isoforms (2C9, 2D6, 3A4). Based on these data, it is unlikely that clinically significant drug interactions will occur between abacavir and drugs metabolized through these pathways.

Lamivudine and/or Zidovudine: Due to the common metabolic pathways of abacavir and zidovudine via glucuronyl transferase, 15 HIV-1-infected subjects were enrolled in a crossover trial evaluating single doses of abacavir (600 mg), lamivudine (150 mg), and zidovudine (300 mg) alone or in combination. Analysis showed no clinically relevant changes in the pharmacokinetics of abacavir with the addition of lamivudine or zidovudine or the combination of lamivudine and zidovudine. Lamivudine exposure (AUC decreased 15%) and zidovudine exposure (AUC increased 10%) did not show clinically relevant changes with concurrent abacavir.

Ethanol: Due to the common metabolic pathways of abacavir and ethanol via alcohol dehydrogenase, the pharmacokinetic interaction between abacavir and ethanol was studied in 24 HIV-1-infected male subjects. Each subject received the following treatments on separate occasions: a single 600-mg dose of abacavir, 0.7 g/kg ethanol (equivalent to 5 alcoholic drinks), and abacavir 600 mg plus 0.7 g/kg ethanol. Coadministration of ethanol and abacavir resulted in a 41% increase in abacavir AUC_∞ and a 26% increase in abacavir $t_{1/2}$. In males, abacavir had no effect on the pharmacokinetic properties of ethanol, so no clinically significant interaction is expected in men. This interaction has not been studied in females.

Methadone: In a trial of 11 HIV-1-infected subjects receiving methadone-maintenance therapy (40 mg and 90 mg daily), with 600 mg of ZIAGEN twice daily (twice the currently recommended dose), oral methadone clearance increased 22% (90% CI: 6% to 42%). This alteration will not result in a methadone dose modification in the majority of patients; however, an increased methadone dose may be required in a small number of patients. The addition of methadone had no clinically significant effect on the pharmacokinetic properties of abacavir.

12.4   Microbiology

Abacavir is a carbocyclic synthetic nucleoside analogue. Abacavir is converted by cellular enzymes to the active metabolite, carbovir triphosphate (CBV-TP), an analogue of deoxyguanosine-5′-triphosphate (dGTP). CBV-TP inhibits the activity of HIV-1 reverse transcriptase (RT) both by competing with the natural substrate dGTP and by its incorporation into viral DNA. The lack of a 3′-OH group in the incorporated nucleotide analogue prevents the formation of the 5′ to 3′ phosphodiester linkage essential for DNA chain elongation, and therefore, the viral DNA growth is terminated. CBV-TP is a weak inhibitor of cellular DNA polymerases α, β, and γ.

Antiviral Activity: The antiviral activity of abacavir against HIV-1 was evaluated against a T-cell tropic laboratory strain HIV-1$_{IIIB}$ in lymphoblastic cell lines, a monocyte/macrophage tropic laboratory strain HIV-1$_{BaL}$ in primary monocytes/macrophages, and clinical isolates in peripheral blood mononuclear cells. The concentration of drug necessary to effect viral replication by 50 percent (EC_{50}) ranged from 3.7 to 5.8 µM (1 µM = 0.28 mcg/mL) and 0.07 to 1.0 µM against HIV-1$_{IIIB}$ and HIV-1$_{BaL}$, respectively, and was 0.26 ± 0.18 µM against 8 clinical isolates. The EC_{50} values of abacavir against different HIV-1 clades (A-G) ranged from 0.0015 to 1.05 µM, and against HIV-2 isolates, from 0.024 to 0.49 µM. The antiviral activity of abacavir in cell culture was not antagonized when combined with the nucleoside reverse transcriptase inhibitors (NRTIs) didanosine, emtricitabine, lamivudine, stavudine, zalcitabine or zidovudine, the non-nucleoside reverse transcriptase inhibitor

(NNRTI) nevirapine, or the protease inhibitor (PI) amprenavir. Ribavirin (50 µM) had no effect on the anti–HIV-1 activity of abacavir in cell culture.

Resistance: HIV-1 isolates with reduced susceptibility to abacavir have been selected in cell culture and were also obtained from subjects treated with abacavir. Genotypic analysis of isolates selected in cell culture and recovered from abacavir-treated subjects demonstrated that amino acid substitutions K65R, L74V, Y115F, and M184V/I in RT contributed to abacavir resistance. In a trial of therapy-naive adults receiving ZIAGEN 600 mg once daily (n = 384) or 300 mg twice daily (n = 386), in a background regimen of lamivudine 300 mg once daily and efavirenz 600 mg once daily (CNA30021), the incidence of virologic failure at 48 weeks was similar between the 2 groups (11% in both arms). Genotypic (n = 38) and phenotypic analyses (n = 35) of virologic failure isolates from this trial showed that the RT substitutions that emerged during abacavir once-daily and twice-daily therapy were K65R, L74V, Y115F, and M184V/I. The substitution M184V/I was the most commonly observed substitution in virologic failure isolates from subjects receiving abacavir once daily (56%, 10/18) and twice daily (40%, 8/20).

Thirty-nine percent (7/18) of the isolates from subjects who experienced virologic failure in the abacavir once-daily arm had a greater than 2.5-fold decrease in abacavir susceptibility with a median-fold decrease of 1.3 (range: 0.5 to 11) compared with 29% (5/17) of the failure isolates in the twice-daily arm with a median-fold decrease of 0.92 (range: 0.7 to 13).

Cross-Resistance: Cross-resistance has been observed among NRTIs. Isolates containing abacavir resistance-associated substitutions, namely, K65R, L74V, Y115F, and M184V, exhibited cross-resistance to didanosine, emtricitabine, lamivudine, tenofovir, and zalcitabine in cell culture and in subjects. The K65R substitution can confer resistance to abacavir, didanosine, emtricitabine, lamivudine, stavudine, tenofovir, and zalcitabine; the L74V substitution can confer resistance to abacavir, didanosine, and zalcitabine; and the M184V substitution can confer resistance to abacavir, didanosine, emtricitabine, lamivudine, and zalcitabine. An increasing number of thymidine analogue mutations (TAMs: M41L, D67N, K70R, L210W, T215Y/F, K219E/R/H/Q/N) is associated with a progressive reduction in abacavir susceptibility.

13   NONCLINICAL TOXICOLOGY

13.1   Carcinogenesis, Mutagenesis, Impairment of Fertility

Carcinogenicity: Abacavir was administered orally at 3 dosage levels to separate groups of mice and rats in 2-year carcinogenicity studies. Results showed an increase in the incidence of malignant and non-malignant tumors. Malignant tumors occurred in the preputial gland of males and the clitoral gland of females of both species, and in the liver of female rats. In addition, non-malignant tumors also occurred in the liver and thyroid gland of female rats. These observations were made at systemic exposures in the range of 6 to 32 times the human exposure at the recommended dose. It is not known how predictive the results of rodent carcinogenicity studies may be for humans.

Mutagenicity: Abacavir induced chromosomal aberrations both in the presence and absence of metabolic activation in an in vitro cytogenetic study in human lymphocytes. Abacavir was mutagenic in the absence of metabolic activation, although it was not mutagenic in the presence of metabolic activation in an L5178Y mouse lymphoma assay. Abacavir was clastogenic in males and not clastogenic in females in an in vivo mouse bone marrow micronucleus assay. Abacavir was not mutagenic in bacterial mutagenicity assays in the presence and absence of metabolic activation.

Impairment of Fertility: Abacavir had no adverse effects on the mating performance or fertility of male and female rats at a dose approximately 8 times the human exposure at the recommended dose based on body surface area comparisons.

13.2   Animal Toxicology and/or Pharmacology

Myocardial degeneration was found in mice and rats following administration of abacavir for 2 years. The systemic exposures were equivalent to 7 to 24 times the expected systemic exposure in humans. The clinical relevance of this finding has not been determined.

14   CLINICAL STUDIES

14.1   Adults

Therapy-Naive Adults: CNA30024 was a multicenter, double-blind, controlled trial in which 649 HIV-1-infected, therapy-naive adults were randomized and received either ZIAGEN (300 mg twice daily), lamivudine (150 mg twice daily), and efavirenz (600 mg once daily); or zidovudine

(300 mg twice daily), lamivudine (150 mg twice daily), and efavirenz (600 mg once daily). The duration of double-blind treatment was at least 48 weeks. Trial participants were male (81%), Caucasian (51%), black (21%), and Hispanic (26%). The median age was 35 years; the median pretreatment CD4+ cell count was 264 cells/mm³, and median plasma HIV-1 RNA was 4.79 log₁₀ copies/mL. The outcomes of randomized treatment are provided in Table 7.

[See table 7 at top of previous page]

After 48 weeks of therapy, the median CD4+ cell count increases from baseline were 209 cells/mm³ in the group receiving ZIAGEN and 155 cells/mm³ in the zidovudine group. Through Week 48, 8 subjects (2%) in the group receiving ZIAGEN (5 CDC classification C events and 3 deaths) and 5 subjects (2%) on the zidovudine arm (3 CDC classification C events and 2 deaths) experienced clinical disease progression.

CNA3005 was a multicenter, double-blind, controlled trial in which 562 HIV-1-infected, therapy-naive adults were randomized to receive either ZIAGEN (300 mg twice daily) plus COMBIVIR® (lamivudine 150 mg/zidovudine 300 mg twice daily), or indinavir (800 mg 3 times a day) plus COMBIVIR twice daily. The trial was stratified at randomization by pre-entry plasma HIV-1 RNA 10,000 to 100,000 copies/mL and plasma HIV-1 RNA greater than 100,000 copies/mL. Trial participants were male (87%), Caucasian (73%), black (15%), and Hispanic (9%). At baseline the median age was 36 years; the median baseline CD4+ cell count was 360 cells/mm³, and median baseline plasma HIV-1 RNA was 4.8 log₁₀ copies/mL. Proportions of subjects with plasma HIV-1 RNA less than 400 copies/mL (using Roche AMPLICOR HIV-1 MONITOR Test) through 48 weeks of treatment are summarized in Table 8.

[See table 8 at top of previous page]

Treatment response by plasma HIV-1 RNA strata is shown in Table 9.

[See table 9 above]

In subjects with baseline viral load greater than 100,000 copies/mL, percentages of subjects with HIV-1 RNA levels less than 50 copies/mL were 31% in the group receiving abacavir versus 45% in the group receiving indinavir.

Through Week 48, an overall mean increase in CD4+ cell count of about 150 cells/mm³ was observed in both treatment arms. Through Week 48, 9 subjects (3.4%) in the group receiving abacavir sulfate (6 CDC classification C events and 3 deaths) and 3 subjects (1.5%) in the group receiving indinavir (2 CDC classification C events and 1 death) experienced clinical disease progression.

CNA30021 was an international, multicenter, double-blind, controlled trial in which 770 HIV-1-infected, therapy-naive adults were randomized and received either abacavir 600 mg once daily or abacavir 300 mg twice daily, both in combination with lamivudine 300 mg once daily and efavirenz 600 mg once daily. The double-blind treatment duration was at least 48 weeks. Trial participants had a mean age of 37 years; were male (81%), Caucasian (54%), black (27%), and American Hispanic (15%). The median baseline CD4+ cell count was 262 cells/mm³ (range 21 to 918 cells/mm³) and the median baseline plasma HIV-1 RNA was 4.89 log₁₀ copies/mL (range: 2.60 to 6.99 log₁₀ copies/mL).

The outcomes of randomized treatment are provided in Table 10.

[See table 10 above]

After 48 weeks of therapy, the median CD4+ cell count increases from baseline were 188 cells/mm³ in the group receiving abacavir 600 mg once daily and 200 cells/mm³ in the group receiving abacavir 300 mg twice daily. Through Week 48, 6 subjects (2%) in the group receiving ZIAGEN 600 mg once daily (4 CDC classification C events and 2 deaths) and 10 subjects (3%) in the group receiving ZIAGEN 300 mg twice daily (7 CDC classification C events and 3 deaths) experienced clinical disease progression. None of the deaths were attributed to trial medications.

14.2   Pediatric Trials

Therapy-Experienced Pediatric Subjects: CNA3006 was a randomized, double-blind trial comparing ZIAGEN 8 mg/kg twice daily plus lamivudine 4 mg/kg twice daily plus zidovudine 180 mg/m² twice daily versus lamivudine 4 mg/kg twice daily plus zidovudine 180 mg/m² twice daily. Two hundred and five therapy-experienced pediatric subjects were enrolled: female (56%), Caucasian (17%), black (50%), Hispanic (30%), median age of 5.4 years, baseline CD4+ cell percent greater than 15% (median = 27%), and median baseline plasma HIV-1 RNA of 4.6 log₁₀ copies/mL. Eighty percent and 55% of subjects had prior therapy with zidovudine and lamivudine, respectively, most often in combination. The median duration of prior nucleoside analogue therapy was 2 years. At 16 weeks the proportion of subjects responding based on plasma HIV-1 RNA less than or equal

Table 9. Proportions of Responders Through Week 48 By Screening Plasma HIV-1 RNA Levels (CNA3005)

Screening HIV-1 RNA (copies/mL)	ZIAGEN plus Lamivudine/Zidovudine (n = 262)		Indinavir plus Lamivudine/Zidovudine (n = 265)	
	<400 copies/mL	n	<400 copies/mL	n
≥10,000 - ≤100,000	50%	166	48%	165
>100,000	48%	96	52%	100

Table 10. Outcomes of Randomized Treatment Through Week 48 (CNA30021)

Outcome	ZIAGEN 600 mg q.d. plus EPIVIR plus Efavirenz (n = 384)	ZIAGEN 300 mg b.i.d. plus EPIVIR plus Efavirenz (n = 386)
Responder[a]	64% (71%)	65% (72%)
Virologic failure[b]	11% (5%)	11% (5%)
Discontinued due to adverse reactions	13%	11%
Discontinued due to other reasons[c]	11%	13%

[a] Subjects achieved and maintained confirmed HIV-1 RNA <50 copies/mL (<400 copies/mL) through Week 48 (Roche AMPLICOR Ultrasensitive HIV-1 MONITOR standard test version 1.0).
[b] Includes viral rebound, failure to achieve confirmed <50 copies/mL (<400 copies/mL) by Week 48, and insufficient viral load response.
[c] Includes consent withdrawn, lost to follow up, protocol violations, clinical progression, and other.

to 400 copies/mL was significantly higher in subjects receiving ZIAGEN plus lamivudine plus zidovudine compared with subjects receiving lamivudine plus zidovudine, 13% versus 2%, respectively. Median plasma HIV-1 RNA changes from baseline were -0.53 log₁₀ copies/mL in the group receiving ZIAGEN plus lamivudine plus zidovudine compared with -0.21 log₁₀ copies/mL in the group receiving lamivudine plus zidovudine. Median CD4+ cell count increases from baseline were 69 cells/mm³ in the group receiving ZIAGEN plus lamivudine plus zidovudine and 9 cells/mm³ in the group receiving lamivudine plus zidovudine.

15   REFERENCES

1. Data Collection on Adverse Events of Anti-HIV Drugs (D:A:D) Study Group. *Lancet.* 2008;371 (9622):1417-1426.

16   HOW SUPPLIED/STORAGE AND HANDLING

ZIAGEN Tablets, containing abacavir sulfate equivalent to 300 mg abacavir are yellow, biconvex, scored, capsule-shaped, film-coated, and imprinted with "GX 623" on both sides. They are packaged as follows:

Bottles of 60 tablets (NDC 49702-221-18).

Unit dose blister packs of 60 tablets (NDC 49702-221-44). Each pack contains 6 blister cards of 10 tablets each.

Store at controlled room temperature of 20° to 25°C (68° to 77°F) (see USP).

ZIAGEN Oral Solution is a clear to opalescent, yellowish, strawberry-banana-flavored liquid. Each mL of the solution contains abacavir sulfate equivalent to 20 mg of abacavir. It is packaged in plastic bottles as follows:

Bottles of 240 mL (NDC 49702-222-48) with child-resistant closure. This product does not require reconstitution.

Store at controlled room temperature of 20° to 25°C (68° to 77°F) (see USP). DO NOT FREEZE. May be refrigerated.

17   PATIENT COUNSELING INFORMATION

See FDA-approved patient labeling (Medication Guide)

17.1   Information About Therapy With ZIAGEN

Hypersensitivity Reaction: Inform patients:

• that a Medication Guide and Warning Card summarizing the symptoms of the abacavir hypersensitivity reaction and other product information will be dispensed by the pharmacist with each new prescription and refill of ZIAGEN, and encourage the patient to read the Medication Guide and Warning Card every time to obtain any new information that may be present about ZIAGEN. (The complete text of the Medication Guide is reprinted at the end of this document.)
• to carry the Warning Card with them.
• how to identify a hypersensitivity reaction *[see Medication Guide].*
• that if they develop symptoms consistent with a hypersensitivity reaction they should call their doctor right away to determine if they should stop taking ZIAGEN.
• that a hypersensitivity reaction can worsen and lead to hospitalization or death if ZIAGEN is not immediately discontinued.
• that in one trial, more severe hypersensitivity reactions were seen when ZIAGEN was dosed 600 mg once daily.

• to not restart ZIAGEN or any other abacavir-containing product following a hypersensitivity reaction because more severe symptoms can occur within hours and may include life-threatening hypotension and death.
• that a hypersensitivity reaction is usually reversible if it is detected promptly and ZIAGEN is stopped right away.
• that if they have interrupted ZIAGEN for reasons other than symptoms of hypersensitivity (for example, those who have an interruption in drug supply), a serious or fatal hypersensitivity reaction may occur with reintroduction of abacavir.
• to not restart ZIAGEN or any other abacavir-containing product without medical consultation and that restarting abacavir needs to be undertaken only if medical care can be readily accessed by the patient or others.
• ZIAGEN should not be coadministered with EPZICOM® (abacavir sulfate and lamivudine) Tablets or TRIZIVIR® (abacavir sulfate, lamivudine, and zidovudine) Tablets.

Lactic Acidosis/Hepatomegaly: Inform patients that some HIV medicines, including ZIAGEN, can cause a rare, but serious condition called lactic acidosis with liver enlargement (hepatomegaly) *[see Boxed Warning, Warnings and Precautions (5.2)].*

Redistribution/Accumulation of Body Fat: Inform patients that redistribution or accumulation of body fat may occur in patients receiving antiretroviral therapy and that the cause and long-term health effects of these conditions are not known at this time *[see Warnings and Precautions (5.4)].*

Information About HIV-1 Infection: ZIAGEN is not a cure for HIV-1 infection and patients may continue to experience illnesses associated with HIV-1 infection, including opportunistic infections. Patients should remain under the care of a physician when using ZIAGEN.

Patients should be advised to avoid doing things that can spread HIV-1 infection to others.

• Do not share needles or other injection equipment.
• Do not share personal items that can have blood or body fluids on them, like toothbrushes and razor blades.
• Do not have any kind of sex without protection. Always practice safe sex by using a latex or polyurethane condom to lower the chance of sexual contact with semen, vaginal secretions, or blood.
• Do not breastfeed. We do not know if ZIAGEN can be passed to your baby in your breast milk and whether it could harm your baby. Also, mothers with HIV-1 should not breastfeed because HIV-1 can be passed to the baby in the breast milk.

Patients should be informed to take all HIV medications exactly as prescribed.

COMBIVIR, EPIVIR, EPZICOM, TRIZIVIR, and ZIAGEN are registered trademarks of ViiV Healthcare.

Manufactured for:
ViiV Healthcare
Research Triangle Park, NC 27709
by:
GlaxoSmithKline
Research Triangle Park, NC 27709
©2013, ViiV Healthcare. All rights reserved.
ZGN:7PI

MEDICATION GUIDE
ZIAGEN® (ZY-uh-jen)
(abacavir sulfate)
Tablets and Oral Solution

Read this Medication Guide before you start taking ZIAGEN and each time you get a refill. There may be new information. This information does not take the place of talking to your healthcare provider about your medical condition or your treatment. Be sure to carry your ZIAGEN Warning Card with you at all times.

What is the most important information I should know about ZIAGEN?

1. **Serious allergic reaction (hypersensitivity reaction).** ZIAGEN contains abacavir (also contained in EPZICOM® and TRIZIVIR®). Patients taking ZIAGEN may have a serious allergic reaction (hypersensitivity reaction) that can cause death. Your risk of this allergic reaction is much higher if you have a gene variation called HLA-B*5701. Your healthcare provider can determine with a blood test if you have this gene variation.

If you get a symptom from 2 or more of the following groups while taking ZIAGEN, call your healthcare provider right away to find out if you should stop taking ZIAGEN.

	Symptom(s)
Group 1	Fever
Group 2	Rash
Group 3	Nausea, vomiting, diarrhea, abdominal (stomach area) pain
Group 4	Generally ill feeling, extreme tiredness, or achiness
Group 5	Shortness of breath, cough, sore throat

A list of these symptoms is on the Warning Card your pharmacist gives you. **Carry this Warning Card with you at all times.**

If you stop ZIAGEN because of an allergic reaction, never take ZIAGEN (abacavir sulfate) or any other abacavir-containing medicine (EPZICOM and TRIZIVIR) again. If you take ZIAGEN or any other abacavir-containing medicine again after you have had an allergic reaction, **within hours** you may get **life-threatening symptoms** that may include **very low blood pressure** or **death.** If you stop ZIAGEN, for any other reason, even for a few days, and you are not allergic to ZIAGEN, talk with your healthcare provider before taking it again. Taking ZIAGEN again can cause a serious allergic or life-threatening reaction, even if you never had an allergic reaction to it before.

If your healthcare provider tells you that you can take ZIAGEN again, start taking it when you are around medical help or people who can call a healthcare provider if you need one.

2. **Lactic Acidosis (buildup of acid in the blood).** Some human immunodeficiency virus (HIV) medicines, including ZIAGEN, can cause a rare but serious condition called lactic acidosis. Lactic acidosis is a serious medical emergency that can cause death and must be treated in the hospital.

Call your healthcare provider right away if you get any of the following signs or symptoms of lactic acidosis:
• you feel very weak or tired
• you have unusual (not normal) muscle pain
• you have trouble breathing
• you have stomach pain with nausea and vomiting
• you feel cold, especially in your arms and legs
• you feel dizzy or light-headed
• you have a fast or irregular heartbeat

3. **Serious liver problems.** Some people who have taken medicines like ZIAGEN have developed serious liver problems called hepatotoxicity, with liver enlargement (hepatomegaly) and fat in the liver (steatosis). Hepatomegaly with steatosis is a serious medical emergency that can cause death. Call your healthcare provider right away if you get any of the following signs or symptoms of liver problems:
• your skin or the white part of your eyes turns yellow (jaundice)
• your urine turns dark
• your bowel movements (stools) turn light in color
• you don't feel like eating food for several days or longer
• you feel sick to your stomach (nausea)
• you have lower stomach area (abdominal) pain

You may be more likely to get lactic acidosis or serious liver problems if you are female, very overweight, or have been taking nucleoside analogue medicines for a long time.

What is ZIAGEN?

ZIAGEN is a prescription medicine used to treat HIV infection. ZIAGEN is a medicine called a nucleoside analogue reverse transcriptase inhibitor (NRTI). ZIAGEN is always used with other anti-HIV medicines. When used in combination with these other medicines, ZIAGEN helps lower the amount of HIV in your blood.

• **ZIAGEN does not cure HIV infection or AIDS.**
• It is not known if ZIAGEN will help you live longer or have fewer of the medical problems that people get with HIV or AIDS.
• It is very important that you see your doctor regularly while you are taking ZIAGEN.

Who should not take ZIAGEN?

Do not take ZIAGEN if you:
• are allergic to abacavir or any of the ingredients in ZIAGEN. See the end of this Medication Guide for a complete list of ingredients in ZIAGEN.
• have certain liver problems.

What should I tell my healthcare provider before taking ZIAGEN?

Before you take ZIAGEN, tell your healthcare provider if you:
• have been tested and know whether or not you have a particular gene variation called HLA-B*5701.
• have hepatitis B virus infection or have other liver problems.
• have heart problems, smoke, or have diseases that increase your risk of heart disease such as high blood pressure, high cholesterol, or diabetes.
• are pregnant or plan to become pregnant. It is not known if ZIAGEN will harm your unborn baby. Talk to your healthcare provider if you are pregnant or plan to become pregnant.
Pregnancy Registry. If you take ZIAGEN while you are pregnant, talk to your healthcare provider about how you can take part in the Pregnancy Registry for ZIAGEN. The purpose of the pregnancy registry is to collect information about the health of you and your baby.
• are breastfeeding or plan to breastfeed. Do not breastfeed. We do not know if ZIAGEN can be passed to your baby in your breast milk and whether it could harm your baby. Also, mothers with HIV-1 should not breastfeed because HIV-1 can be passed to the baby in the breast milk.

Tell your healthcare provider about all the medicines you take, including prescription and nonprescription medicines, vitamins, and herbal supplements.

Especially tell your healthcare provider if you take:
• alcohol
• methadone
• TRIZIVIR (abacavir sulfate, lamivudine, and zidovudine)
• EPZICOM (abacavir sulfate and lamivudine)

Ask your healthcare provider if you are not sure if you take one of the medicines listed above.

ZIAGEN may affect the way other medicines work, and other medicines may affect how ZIAGEN works.

Know the medicines you take. Keep a list of your medicines with you to show to your healthcare provider and pharmacist when you get a new medicine.

How should I take ZIAGEN?

• **Take ZIAGEN exactly as your healthcare provider tells you to take it.**
• **ZIAGEN is taken by mouth as a tablet or a strawberry- and banana-flavored liquid.**
• ZIAGEN may be taken with or without food.
• Do not skip doses.
• Children aged 3 months and older can also take ZIAGEN. The child's healthcare provider will decide the right dose and whether the child should take the tablet or liquid, based on the child's weight. The dose should not be more than the recommended adult dose.
• **Do not let your ZIAGEN run out.**
If you stop your anti-HIV medicines, even for a short time, the amount of virus in your blood may increase and the virus may become harder to treat. If you take too much ZIAGEN, call your healthcare provider or poison control center or go to the nearest hospital emergency room right away.

What are the possible side effects of ZIAGEN?

• ZIAGEN can cause serious side effects including allergic reactions, lactic acidosis, and liver problems. See "What is the most important information I should know about ZIAGEN?"
• **Changes in immune system (Immune Reconstitution Syndrome).** Your immune system may get stronger and begin to fight infections that have been hidden in your body for a long time. Tell your healthcare provider if you start having new or worse symptoms of infection after you start taking ZIAGEN.
• **Changes in body fat (fat redistribution).** Changes in body fat (lipoatrophy or lipodystrophy) can happen in some people taking antiretroviral medicines including ZIAGEN. These changes may include:
• more fat in or around your trunk, upper back and neck (buffalo hump), breast, or chest
• loss of fat in your legs, arms, or face

• **Heart attack (myocardial infarction).** Some HIV medicines including ZIAGEN may increase your risk of heart attack.

The most common side effects of ZIAGEN in adults include:
• bad dreams or sleep problems
• nausea
• headache
• tiredness
• vomiting

The most common side effects of ZIAGEN in children include:
• fever and chills
• nausea
• vomiting
• rash
• ear, nose, or throat infections

Tell your healthcare provider if you have any side effect that bothers you or that does not go away.

These are not all the possible side effects of ZIAGEN. For more information, ask your healthcare provider or pharmacist.

Call your doctor for medical advice about side effects. You may report side effects to FDA at 1-800-FDA-1088.

How should I store ZIAGEN?

• Store ZIAGEN at room temperature, between 68°F to 77°F (20°C to 25°C).
• Do not freeze ZIAGEN.
• **Keep ZIAGEN and all medicines out of the reach of children.**

General information for safe and effective use of ZIAGEN

Avoid doing things that can spread HIV infection to others.
• **Do not share needles or other injection equipment.**
• **Do not share personal items that can have blood or body fluids on them, like toothbrushes and razor blades.**
• **Do not have any kind of sex without protection.** Always practice safe sex by using a latex or polyurethane condom to lower the chance of sexual contact with semen, vaginal secretions, or blood.

Medicines are sometimes prescribed for purposes other than those listed in a Medication Guide. Do not use ZIAGEN for a condition for which it was not prescribed. Do not give ZIAGEN to other people, even if they have the same symptoms that you have. It may harm them.

This Medication Guide summarizes the most important information about ZIAGEN. If you would like more information, talk with your healthcare provider. You can ask your healthcare provider or pharmacist for the information that is written for healthcare professionals.

For more information go to www.ZIAGEN.com or call 1-877-844-8872.

What are the ingredients in ZIAGEN?

Tablets
Active ingredient: abacavir sulfate
Inactive ingredients: colloidal silicon dioxide, magnesium stearate, microcrystalline cellulose, and sodium starch glycolate, and a film-coating made of hypromellose, polysorbate 80, synthetic yellow iron oxide, titanium dioxide, and triacetin.

Oral Solution
Active ingredient: abacavir sulfate
Inactive ingredients: artificial strawberry and banana flavors, citric acid (anhydrous), methylparaben and propylparaben (added as preservatives), propylene glycol, saccharin sodium, sodium citrate (dihydrate), sorbitol solution, and water.

This Medication Guide has been approved by the US Food and Drug Administration.

EPZICOM and TRIZIVIR are registered trademarks of ViiV Healthcare.

Manufactured for:
ViiV Healthcare
Research Triangle Park, NC 27709
by:

GlaxoSmithKline
Research Triangle Park, NC 27709
©2012, ViiV Healthcare. All rights reserved.
May 2012
ZGN:5MG

The PDR® is always within reach with PDR.net online, PDR® BRIEF in your EHR, *mobile*PDR® on your wireless device, and now as a convenient eBook.

AHC Ventures Inc. (Corp)

5415 NW 24th St, Suite 103
Margate, FL 33063

Direct Inquiries to:
Phone - 954-978-9290
Fax - 954-978-9130

Bioease®   **OTC**
Pain Relieving Gel

Active Ingredients: Menthol 3.5% and Camphor 0.2%
Inactive Ingredients: Water, Isopropyl Alcohol, Herbal Extract (ILEX Paraguariensis), Carbomer, Triethanolamine, Silicon Dioxide, Methylparaben, FD&C Yellow #4, FD&C Blue #1
Indications: Temporary relief from minor aches and pains of muscles and joints due to arthritis, backache, strains and sprains.
Warnings: For external use only. Ask a doctor before use if you have sensitive skin. Keep away from excessive heat or open flame. Avoid contact with the eyes or mucous membranes. Do not apply to wounds or damaged skins. Do not use with other ointments, creams, sprays or liniments. Do not apply to irritated skin or if excessive irritation develops. Do not bandage. Wash hands after use. If pregnant or breast-feeding, ask a health professional before use. Keep out of reach of children. If accidentally ingested, get medical help or contact a Poison Control Center.
Directions: Adults and children 2.5 years of age and older: Apply to the affected areas not more than 3 to 4 times daily. Children under 2.5 years of age: Consult physician.
How Supplied: 4 oz, tube, 3 oz, roll-on, 5 gram packet, 16 oz, 32 oz, and 1 gallon.

Concordia Pharmaceuticals, Inc.

5 Canewood Industrial Park
St. Michael, Barbados
BB11128

Phone:
(246)-621-1861
Fax: (246)-621-1860
Email: info@concordiarx.com

DONNATAL® TABLETS   ℞

Rx Only
REV 0213

DESCRIPTION: DONNATAL® TABLETS:
Each Donnatal® Tablet contains:

Phenobarbital, USP	16.2 mg
Hyoscyamine Sulfate, USP	0.1037 mg
Atropine Sulfate, USP	0.0194 mg
Scopolamine Hydrobromide, USP	0.0065 mg

INACTIVE INGREDIENTS: Anhydrous Lactose, Calcium Stearate, Colloidal Silicon Dioxide, Corn Starch, and Microcrystalline Cellulose.

INDICATIONS AND USAGE: Based on a review of this drug by the National Academy of Sciences-National Research Council and/or other information, FDA has classified the following indications as "possibly" effective: For use as adjunctive therapy in the treatment of irritable bowel syndrome (irritable colon, spastic colon, mucous colitis) and acute enterocolitis. May also be useful as adjunctive therapy in the treatment of duodenal ulcer. IT HAS NOT BEEN SHOWN CONCLUSIVELY WHETHER ANTICHOLINERGIC/ANTISPASMODIC DRUGS AID IN THE HEALING OF A DUODENAL ULCER, DECREASE THE RATE OF RECURRENCES OR PREVENT COMPLICATIONS.

CLINICAL PHARMACOLOGY: This drug combination provides natural belladonna alkaloids in a specific, fixed ratio combined with phenobarbital to provide peripheral anticholinergic/antispasmodic action and mild sedation.
CONTRAINDICATIONS: Glaucoma, obstructive uropathy (for example, bladder neck obstruction due to prostatic hypertrophy); obstructive disease of the gastrointestinal tract (as in achalasia, pyloroduodenal stenosis, etc.); paralytic ileus, intestinal atony of the elderly or debilitated patient; unstable cardiovascular status in acute hemorrhage; severe ulcerative colitis especially if complicated by toxic megacolon; myasthenia gravis; hiatal hernia associated with reflux esophagitis.
Donnatal® is contraindicated in patients with known hypersensitivity to any of the ingredients. Phenobarbital is contraindicated in acute intermittent porphyria and in those patients in whom phenobarbital produces restlessness and/or excitement.
WARNINGS: In the presence of a high environmental temperature, heat prostration can occur with belladonna alkaloids (fever and heatstroke due to decreased sweating). Diarrhea may be an early symptom of incomplete intestinal obstruction, especially in patients with ileostomy or colostomy. In this instance, treatment with this drug would be inappropriate and possibly harmful. Donnatal® may produce drowsiness or blurred vision. The patient should be warned, should these occur, not to engage in activities requiring mental alertness, such as operating a motor vehicle or other machinery, and not to perform hazardous work. Phenobarbital may decrease the effect of anticoagulants, and necessitate larger doses of the anticoagulant for optimal effect. When the phenobarbital is discontinued, the dose of the anticoagulant may have to be decreased. Phenobarbital may be habit forming and should not be administered to individuals known to be addiction prone or to those with a history of physical and/or psychological dependence upon drugs. Since barbiturates are metabolized in the liver, they should be used with caution and initial doses should be small in patients with hepatic dysfunction.
PRECAUTIONS: GENERAL: Use with caution in patients with: autonomic neuropathy, hepatic or renal disease, hyperthyroidism, coronary heart disease, congestive heart failure, cardiac arrhythmias, tachycardia, and hypertension. Belladonna alkaloids may produce a delay in gastric emptying (antral stasis) which would complicate the management of gastric ulcer. Do not rely on the use of the drug in the presence of complication of biliary tract disease. Theoretically, with overdosage, a curare-like action may occur.
CARCINOGENESIS, MUTAGENESIS, IMPAIRMENT OF FERTILITY: Long-term studies in animals have not been performed to evaluate carcinogenic potential.
PREGNANCY: PREGNANCY CATEGORY C: Animal reproduction studies have not been conducted with Donnatal®. It is not known whether Donnatal® can cause fetal harm when administered to a pregnant woman or can affect reproduction capacity. Donnatal® should be given to a pregnant woman only if clearly needed.
NURSING MOTHERS It is not known whether this drug is excreted in human milk. Because many drugs are excreted in human milk, caution should be exercised when Donnatal® is administered to a nursing woman.
ADVERSE REACTIONS: Adverse reactions may include xerostomia; urinary hesitancy and retention; blurred vision; tachycardia; palpitation; mydriasis; cycloplegia; increased ocular tension; loss of taste sense; headache; nervousness; drowsiness; weakness; dizziness; insomnia; nausea; vomiting; impotence; suppression of lactation; constipation; bloated feeling; musculoskeletal pain; severe allergic reaction or drug idiosyncrasies, including anaphylaxis, urticaria and other dermal manifestations; and decreased sweating. Acquired hypersensitivity to barbiturates consists chiefly in allergic reactions that occur especially in persons who tend to have asthma, urticaria, angioedema and similar conditions. Hypersensitivity reactions in this category include localized swelling, particularly of the eyelids, cheeks, or lips, and erythematous dermatitis. Rarely, exfoliative dermatitis (e.g. Stevens-Johnson syndrome and toxic epidermal necrolysis) may be caused by phenobarbital and can prove fatal. The skin eruption may be associated with fever, delirium, and marked degenerative changes in the liver and other parenchymatous organs. In a few cases, megaloblastic anemia has been associated with the chronic use of phenobarbital. Elderly patients may react with symptoms of excitement, agitation, drowsiness, and other untoward manifestations to even small doses of the drug. Phenobarbital may produce excitement in some patients, rather than a sedative effect. In patients habituated to barbiturates, abrupt withdrawal may produce delirium or convulsions.
To report SUSPECTED ADVERSE REACTIONS, contact the IriSys Inc at 1-858-623-1520 or the FDA at 1-800-FDA-1088 or www.fda.gov/medwatch.
OVERDOSAGE: The signs and symptoms of overdose are headache, nausea, vomiting, blurred vision, dilated pupils, hot and dry skin, dizziness, dryness of the mouth, difficulty in swallowing, and CNS stimulation. Treatment should consist of gastric lavage, emetics, and activated charcoal. If indicated, parenteral cholinergic agents such as physostigmine or bethanechol chloride should be used.
DOSAGE AND ADMINISTRATION: The dosage of Donnatal® should be adjusted to the needs of the individual patient to assure symptomatic control with a minimum of adverse effects.

Donnatal® Tablets - Adults: One or two Donnatal® tablets three or four times a day according to condition and severity of symptoms.
HOW SUPPLIED: Donnatal® Tablets are supplied as: White, D-shaped tablets debossed "D" on one side and "Donnatal" on the other side.
• Bottles of 100 tablets- NDC 59212-425-10.
• Bottles of 1000 tablets- NDC 59212-425-11.
AVOID FREEZING
Store at 20-25°C (68-77°F) [See USP Controlled Room Temperature]. Protect from light and moisture. Dispense in a tight, light-resistant container as defined in the USP using a child-resistant closure. Use safety closures when dispensing this product unless otherwise directed by a physician or requested by purchaser.
Also available: Donnatal® Elixir, grape and/or mint flavored liquid, in 4 fl oz (118mL) and 1 pint (473mL) bottles
Manufactured For:
Concordia Pharmaceutical, Inc.
St. Michael, Barbados, BB11128
www.concordiarx.com
Manufactured By:
IriSys Inc.
San Diego, CA 92121
8181603
Rev 02/13
R0
Shown in Product Identification Guide, page 306

Edgemont Pharmaceuticals

1250 CAPITAL OF TEXAS HIGHWAY, SOUTH
BUILDING 3, SUITE 400
AUSTIN, TX 78746

Toll Free: (888) 594-4332
Fax: (512) 329-2094

FLUOXETINE   ℞
tablets for oral use

HIGHLIGHTS OF PRESCRIBING INFORMATION
These highlights do not include all the information needed to use FLUOXETINE safely and effectively. See full prescribing information for FLUOXETINE.
FLUOXETINE tablets for oral use
Initial U.S. Approval: 1987

> **WARNING: SUICIDALITY AND ANTIDEPRESSANT DRUGS**
> *See full prescribing information for complete boxed warning.*
> **Increased risk of suicidal thinking and behavior in children, adolescents,**
> **and young adults taking antidepressants for Major Depressive Disorder (MDD) and other psychiatric disorders (5.1).**

——————RECENT MAJOR CHANGES——————

Warnings and Precautions (5.8)	06/2014

——————INDICATIONS AND USAGE——————

Fluoxetine is a selective serotonin reuptake inhibitor indicated for the treatment of:
• Major Depressive Disorder (MDD) (1.1)
  Adults: Efficacy was established in one 5 week trial, three 6 week trials, and one maintenance study (14.1)
  Pediatrics: Efficacy was established in two 8 to 9 week trials of patients aged 8 to 18 years (14.1)
• Obsessive Compulsive Disorder (OCD) (1.2)
  Adults: Efficacy was established in two 13 week trials (14.2)
  Pediatrics: Efficacy was established in one 13 week trial in patients aged 7 to 17 years (14.2)
• Bulimia Nervosa (1.3)
  Adults: Efficacy was established in two 8 week trials and one 16 week trial (14.3)
• Panic Disorder, with or without agoraphobia (1.4)
  Adults: Efficacy was established in two 12 week trials (14.4)

——————DOSAGE AND ADMINISTRATION——————

• Use another fluoxetine product for initial doses of 10 to 20 mg/day or for doses other than 30 mg or 60 mg:

Indication	Adult	Pediatric
MDD (2.1)	20 mg/day in morning (initial dose) 20 mg/day (target dose) 80 mg/day (maximum dose studied)	10 to 20 mg/day (initial dose)* *This product has not been studied in doses greater than 20 mg/day in pediatric MDD.
OCD (2.2)	20 mg/day in morning (initial dose) 20 to 60 mg/day (target dose)	10 mg/day (initial dose) 10 to 60 mg/day (target dose)
Bulimia Nervosa (2.3)	60 mg/day in morning	-
Panic Disorder (2.4)	10 mg/day (initial dose) 20 mg/day (target dose) 60 mg/day (maximum dose studied)	-

- No additional benefits seen at higher doses above 20 mg/day in MDD (2.1, 14.1)
- Consider tapering the dose of fluoxetine for pregnant women during the third trimester (2.5, 8.1)
- Use a lower or less frequent dosage in patients with hepatic impairment, the elderly, and for patients with concurrent disease or on multiple concomitant medications (2.5, 8.6)

─────DOSAGE FORMS AND STRENGTHS─────

- Tablets: 60 mg, functionally scored (3)

─────────CONTRAINDICATIONS─────────

- Monoamine Oxidase Inhibitors (MAOI): Do not use with an MAOI or within 14 days of discontinuing an MAOI. Do not start an MAOI until at least 5 weeks after stopping fluoxetine (4, 7.1)
- Pimozide (4, 7.8)
- Thioridazine: Do not use concomitantly with or within 5 weeks of discontinuing fluoxetine (4, 7.8)
- Known hypersensitivity to fluoxetine products (4, 5.3)

──────WARNINGS AND PRECAUTIONS──────

- *Clinical Worsening and Suicide Risk:* Monitor for clinical worsening and suicidal thinking and behavior (5.1)
- *Serotonin Syndrome or Neuroleptic Malignant Syndrome (NMS)-Like Reactions:* Have been reported with fluoxetine. Discontinue fluoxetine and initiate supportive treatment (5.2)
- *Activation of Mania/Hypomania:* Screen for Bipolar Disorder and monitor for mania/hypomania (5.4)
- *Abnormal Bleeding:* May increase the risk of bleeding. Use with NSAIDs, aspirin, warfarin, or drugs that affect coagulation may potentiate the risk of gastrointestinal or other bleeding (5.7, 7.6)
- *Angle Closure Glaucoma:* Angle closure glaucoma has occurred in patients with untreated anatomically narrow angles treated with antidepressants (5.9)
- *Hyponatremia:* Has been reported with fluoxetine in association with syndrome of inappropriate antidiuretic hormone (SIADH) (5.9)
- *Long Half-Life:* Changes in dose will not be fully reflected in plasma for several weeks (5.13)

────────────ADVERSE REACTIONS────────────

Most common adverse reactions (≥5% and at least twice that for placebo):
abnormal dreams, abnormal ejaculation, anorexia, anxiety, asthenia, diarrhea, dry mouth, dyspepsia, flu syndrome, impotence, insomnia, libido decreased, nausea, nervousness, pharyngitis, rash, sinusitis, somnolence, sweating, tremor, vasodilatation, and yawn (6.1)

To report SUSPECTED ADVERSE REACTIONS, contact Edgemont Pharmaceuticals, LLC, at 1-888-594-4332 or FDA at 1-800-FDA-1088 or www.fda.gov/medwatch.

─────────DRUG INTERACTIONS─────────

- *Serotonergic Drugs:* Potential for Serotonin Syndrome (5.2, 7.3)
- *Triptans:* There have been rare postmarketing reports of Serotonin Syndrome with use of an SSRI and a triptan (5.2, 7.4)
- *Tryptophan:* Concomitant use with tryptophan is not recommended (5.2, 7.5)

- *Drugs Metabolized by CYP2D6:* Fluoxetine is a potent inhibitor of CYP2D6 enzyme pathway (7.8)
- *Tricyclic Antidepressants (TCAs):* Monitor TCA levels during coadministration with fluoxetine or when fluoxetine has been recently discontinued (7.8)
- *Benzodiazepines:* Diazepam – increased t½, alprazolam – further psychomotor performance decrement due to increased levels (7.8)
- *Antipsychotics:* Potential for elevation of haloperidol and clozapine levels (7.8)
- *Anticonvulsants:* Potential for elevated phenytoin and carbamazepine levels and clinical anticonvulsant toxicity (7.8)

────────USE IN SPECIFIC POPULATIONS────────

- *Pregnancy:* Fluoxetine should be used during pregnancy only if the potential benefit justifies the potential risks to the fetus (8.1)
- *Nursing Mothers:* Breast feeding is not recommended (8.3)

See 17 for PATIENT COUNSELING INFORMATION and Medication Guide

Revised: 06/2014

FULL PRESCRIBING INFORMATION: CONTENTS*
WARNING: SUICIDALITY AND ANTIDEPRESSANT DRUGS

FULL PRESCRIBING INFORMATION

> **WARNING: SUICIDALITY AND ANTIDEPRESSANT DRUGS**
>
> Antidepressants increased the risk compared to placebo of suicidal thinking and behavior (suicidality) in children, adolescents, and young adults in short-term studies of Major Depressive Disorder (MDD) and other psychiatric disorders. Anyone considering the use of fluoxetine tablets or any other antidepressant in a child, adolescent, or young adult must balance this risk with the clinical need. Short-term studies did not show an increase in the risk of suicidality with antidepressants compared to placebo in adults beyond age 24; there was a reduction in risk with antidepressants compared to placebo in adults aged 65 and older. Depression and certain other psychiatric disorders are themselves associated with increases in the risk of suicide. Patients of all ages who are started on antidepressant therapy should be monitored appropriately and observed closely for clinical worsening, suicidality, or unusual changes in behavior. Families and caregivers should be advised of the need for close observation and communication with the prescriber. Fluoxetine is approved for use in pediatric patients with MDD and Obsessive Compulsive Disorder (OCD) [*see Warnings and Precautions (5.1) and Use in Specific Populations (8.4)*].

1   INDICATIONS AND USAGE
1.1   Major Depressive Disorder
Fluoxetine is indicated for the treatment of Major Depressive Disorder (MDD) [*see Clinical Studies (14.1)*]. The efficacy of fluoxetine in MDD was established in one 5 week trial, three 6 week trials, and one maintenance study in adults. The efficacy of fluoxetine was also established in two 8 to 9 week trials in pediatric patients aged 8 to 18 years; doses greater than 20 mg/day have not been studied in pediatric patients with MDD.
The usefulness of the drug in adult and pediatric patients receiving fluoxetine for extended periods should periodically be re-evaluated [*see Dosage and Administration (2.1)*].
1.2   Obsessive Compulsive Disorder
Fluoxetine is indicated for the treatment of Obsessive Compulsive Disorder (OCD) [*see Clinical Studies (14.2)*]. The efficacy of fluoxetine in OCD was demonstrated in two 13 week trials in adults and one 13 week trial in pediatric patients aged 7 to 17 years.
The effectiveness of fluoxetine in long-term use, i.e., for more than 13 weeks, has not been systematically evaluated in placebo-controlled trials. Therefore, the physician who elects to use fluoxetine for extended periods should periodically re-evaluate the long-term usefulness of the drug for the individual patient [*see Dosage and Administration (2.2)*].
1.3   Bulimia Nervosa
Fluoxetine is indicated for the treatment of moderate to severe Bulimia Nervosa [*see Clinical Studies (14.3)*]. The efficacy of fluoxetine in Bulimia was demonstrated in two 8 week trials and one 16 week trial in adults.
The physician who elects to use fluoxetine for extended periods should periodically re-evaluate the long-term usefulness of the drug for the individual patient [*see Dosage and Administration (2.3)*].
1.4   Panic Disorder
Fluoxetine is indicated for the treatment of Panic Disorder, with or without agoraphobia [*see Clinical Studies (14.4)*]. The efficacy of fluoxetine in Panic Disorder was demonstrated in two 12 week trials in adults.

The effectiveness of fluoxetine in long-term use, i.e., for more than 12 weeks, has not been established in placebo-controlled trials. Therefore, the physician who elects to use fluoxetine for extended periods should periodically re-evaluate the long-term usefulness of the drug for the individual patient [see Dosage and Administration (2.4)].

2 DOSAGE AND ADMINISTRATION

This product is only available in a 60 mg dosage form. A 30 mg dose may be achieved with one-half of the scored tablet. Use of this product requires initial titration with another fluoxetine product according to the dosing guidelines indicated below.

2.1 Major Depressive Disorder

Initial Treatment

Adult — In controlled trials used to support the efficacy of fluoxetine, patients were administered morning doses ranging from 20 to 80 mg/day. Studies comparing fluoxetine 20, 40, and 60 mg/day to placebo indicate that 20 mg/day is sufficient to obtain a satisfactory response in MDD in most cases. Consequently, a dose of 20 mg/day, administered in the morning, is recommended as the initial dose. A dose increase may be considered after several weeks if insufficient clinical improvement is observed. Doses above 20 mg/day may be administered on a once daily (morning) or twice daily schedule (i.e., morning and noon) and should not exceed a maximum dose of 80 mg/day.

Pediatric (children and adolescents) — In the short-term (8 to 9 week) controlled clinical trials of fluoxetine supporting its effectiveness in the treatment of MDD, patients were administered fluoxetine doses of 10 to 20 mg/day [see Clinical Studies (14.1)]. Treatment should be initiated with a dose of 10 or 20 mg/day. After 1 week at 10 mg/day, the dose should be increased to 20 mg/day. However, due to higher plasma levels in lower weight children, the starting and target dose in this group may be 10 mg/day. A dose increase to 20 mg/day may be considered after several weeks if insufficient clinical improvement is observed. This product is only available in a 60 mg dosage form. Administration of doses with demonstrated efficacy of fluoxetine 10 to 20 mg/day in pediatric MDD requires the use of another formulation.

All patients — As with other drugs effective in the treatment of MDD, the full effect may be delayed until 4 weeks of treatment or longer.

Maintenance/Continuation/Extended Treatment — It is generally agreed that acute episodes of MDD require several months or longer of sustained pharmacologic therapy. Whether the dose needed to induce remission is identical to the dose needed to maintain and/or sustain euthymia is unknown.

Daily Dosing — Systematic evaluation of fluoxetine in adult patients has shown that its efficacy in MDD is maintained for periods of up to 38 weeks following 12 weeks of open-label acute treatment (50 weeks total) at a dose of 20 mg/day [see Clinical Studies (14.1)].

Switching Patients to a Tricyclic Antidepressant (TCA) — Dosage of a TCA may need to be reduced, and plasma TCA concentrations may need to be monitored temporarily when fluoxetine is coadministered or has been recently discontinued [see Drug Interactions (7.8)].

Switching Patients to or From a Monoamine Oxidase Inhibitor (MAOI) — At least 14 days should elapse between discontinuation of an MAOI and initiation of therapy with fluoxetine. In addition, at least 5 weeks, perhaps longer, should be allowed after stopping fluoxetine before starting an MAOI [see Contraindications (4) and Drug Interactions (7.1)].

2.2 Obsessive Compulsive Disorder

Initial Treatment

Adults — In the controlled clinical trials of fluoxetine supporting its effectiveness in the treatment of OCD, patients were administered fixed daily doses of 20, 40, or 60 mg of fluoxetine or placebo [see Clinical Studies (14.2)]. In one of these studies, no dose-response relationship for effectiveness was demonstrated. Consequently, a dose of 20 mg/day, administered in the morning, is recommended as the initial dose. Since there was a suggestion of a possible dose-response relationship for effectiveness in the second study, a dose increase may be considered after several weeks if insufficient clinical improvement is observed. The full therapeutic effect may be delayed until 5 weeks of treatment or longer.

Doses above 20 mg/day may be administered on a once daily (i.e., morning) or twice daily schedule (i.e., morning and noon). A dose range of 20 to 60 mg/day is recommended; however, doses of up to 80 mg/day have been well tolerated in open studies of OCD. The maximum fluoxetine dose should not exceed 80 mg/day.

Pediatric (children and adolescents) — In the controlled clinical trial of fluoxetine supporting its effectiveness in the treatment of OCD, patients were administered fluoxetine doses in the range of 10 to 60 mg/day [see Clinical Studies (14.2)].

In adolescents and higher weight children, treatment should be initiated with a dose of 10 mg/day. After 2 weeks, the dose should be increased to 20 mg/day. Additional dose increases may be considered after several more weeks if insufficient clinical improvement is observed. A dose range of 20 to 60 mg/day is recommended.

In lower weight children, treatment should be initiated with a dose of 10 mg/day. Additional dose increases may be considered after several more weeks if insufficient clinical improvement is observed. A dose range of 20 to 30 mg/day is recommended. Experience with daily doses greater than 20 mg is very minimal, and there is no experience with doses greater than 60 mg.

Maintenance/Continuation Treatment — While there are no systematic studies that answer the question of how long to continue fluoxetine, OCD is a chronic condition and it is reasonable to consider continuation for a responding patient. Although the efficacy of fluoxetine after 13 weeks has not been documented in controlled trials, adult patients have been continued in therapy under double-blind conditions for up to an additional 6 months without loss of benefit. However, dosage adjustments should be made to maintain the patient on the lowest effective dosage, and patients should be periodically reassessed to determine the need for treatment.

2.3 Bulimia Nervosa

Initial Treatment — In the controlled clinical trials of fluoxetine supporting its effectiveness in the treatment of Bulimia Nervosa, patients were administered fixed daily fluoxetine doses of 20 or 60 mg, or placebo [see Clinical Studies (14.3)]. Only the 60 mg dose was statistically significantly superior to placebo in reducing the frequency of binge-eating and vomiting. Consequently, the recommended dose is 60 mg/day, administered in the morning. For some patients it may be advisable to titrate up to this target dose over several days. Fluoxetine doses above 60 mg/day have not been systematically studied in patients with bulimia.

Maintenance/Continuation Treatment — Systematic evaluation of continuing fluoxetine 60 mg/day for periods of up to 52 weeks in patients with bulimia who have responded while taking fluoxetine 60 mg/day during an 8 week acute treatment phase has demonstrated a benefit of such maintenance treatment [see Clinical Studies (14.3)]. Nevertheless, patients should be periodically reassessed to determine the need for maintenance treatment.

2.4 Panic Disorder

Initial Treatment — In the controlled clinical trials of fluoxetine supporting its effectiveness in the treatment of Panic Disorder, patients were administered fluoxetine doses in the range of 10 to 60 mg/day [see Clinical Studies (14.4)]. Treatment should be initiated with a dose of 10 mg/day. After one week, the dose should be increased to 20 mg/day. The most frequently administered dose in the 2 flexible-dose clinical trials was 20 mg/day. A dose increase may be considered after several weeks if no clinical improvement is observed. Fluoxetine doses above 60 mg/day have not been systematically evaluated in patients with Panic Disorder.

Maintenance/Continuation Treatment — While there are no systematic studies that answer the question of how long to continue fluoxetine, panic disorder is a chronic condition and it is reasonable to consider continuation for a responding patient. Nevertheless, patients should be periodically reassessed to determine the need for continued treatment.

2.5 Dosing in Specific Populations

Treatment of Pregnant Women During the Third Trimester — When treating pregnant women with fluoxetine during the third trimester, the physician should carefully consider the potential risks and potential benefits of treatment. Neonates exposed to SNRIs or SSRIs late in the third trimester have developed complications requiring prolonged hospitalization, respiratory support, and tube feeding. The physician may consider tapering fluoxetine in the third trimester [see Use in Specific Populations (8.1)].

Geriatrics — A lower or less frequent dosage should be considered for the elderly [see Use in Specific Populations (8.5)].

Hepatic Impairment — As with many other medications, a lower or less frequent dosage should be used in patients with hepatic impairment [see Clinical Pharmacology (12.3) and Use in Specific Populations (8.6)].

3 DOSAGE FORMS AND STRENGTHS

Fluoxetine tablets, USP 60 mg, are available as 60 mg (fluoxetine base equivalent), film coated, functionally scored, capsule-shaped, white tablets debossed with "FL 60" on one side ("FL" above the score and "60" below the score).

4 CONTRAINDICATIONS

The use of fluoxetine is contraindicated with the following:
• Monoamine Oxidase Inhibitors: Do not use with an MAOI or within 14 days of discontinuing an MAOI due to risk of drug interaction. At least 5 weeks should be allowed after stopping fluoxetine before treatment with a MAOI [see Drug Interactions (7.1)]
• Pimozide: Do not use with pimozide due to risk of QTc prolongation [see Drug Interactions (7.8)].

• Thioridazine: Do not use with thioridazine due to QTc interval prolongation. Do not use thioridazine within 5 weeks of discontinuing fluoxetine [see Drug Interactions (7.8)].
• Known hypersensitivity to fluoxetine: Do not use this product in patients with known hypersensitivity to fluoxetine due to risk of anaphylactoid reactions, including bronchospasm, angioedema, laryngospasm, and urticaria [see Warnings and Precautions (5.3)].

5 WARNINGS AND PRECAUTIONS

5.1 Clinical Worsening and Suicide Risk

Patients with MDD, both adult and pediatric, may experience worsening of their depression and/or the emergence of suicidal ideation and behavior (suicidality) or unusual changes in behavior, whether or not they are taking antidepressant medications, and this risk may persist until significant remission occurs. Suicide is a known risk of depression and certain other psychiatric disorders, and these disorders themselves are the strongest predictors of suicide. There has been a long-standing concern, however, that antidepressants may have a role in inducing worsening of depression and the emergence of suicidality in certain patients during the early phases of treatment. Pooled analyses of short-term placebo-controlled trials of antidepressant drugs (SSRIs and others) showed that these drugs increase the risk of suicidal thinking and behavior (suicidality) in children, adolescents, and young adults (ages 18 to 24) with MDD and other psychiatric disorders. Short-term studies did not show an increase in the risk of suicidality with antidepressants compared to placebo in adults beyond age 24; there was a reduction with antidepressants compared to placebo in adults aged 65 and older.

The pooled analyses of placebo-controlled trials in children and adolescents with MDD, OCD, or other psychiatric disorders included a total of 24 short-term trials of 9 antidepressant drugs in over 4400 patients. The pooled analyses of placebo-controlled trials in adults with MDD or other psychiatric disorders included a total of 295 short-term trials (median duration of 2 months) of 11 antidepressant drugs in over 77,000 patients. There was considerable variation in risk of suicidality among drugs, but a tendency toward an increase in the younger patients for almost all drugs studied. There were differences in absolute risk of suicidality across the different indications, with the highest incidence in MDD. The risk differences (drug versus placebo), however, were relatively stable within age strata and across indications. These risk differences (drug-placebo difference in the number of cases of suicidality per 1000 patients treated) are provided in *Table 1*.

Table 1. Suicidality per 1000 Patients Treated

Age Range	Drug-Placebo Difference in Number of Cases of Suicidality per 1000 Patients Treated
	Increases Compared to Placebo
<18	14 additional cases
18–24	5 additional cases
	Decreases Compared to Placebo
25–64	1 fewer case
≥65	6 fewer cases

No suicides occurred in any of the pediatric trials. There were suicides in the adult trials, but the number was not sufficient to reach any conclusion about drug effect on suicide.

It is unknown whether the suicidality risk extends to longer-term use, i.e., beyond several months. However, there is substantial evidence from placebo-controlled maintenance trials in adults with depression that the use of antidepressants can delay the recurrence of depression.

All patients being treated with antidepressants for any indication should be monitored appropriately and observed closely for clinical worsening, suicidality, and unusual changes in behavior, especially during the initial few months of a course of drug therapy, or at times of dose changes, either increases or decreases.

The following symptoms, anxiety, agitation, panic attacks, insomnia, irritability, hostility, aggressiveness, impulsivity, akathisia (psychomotor restlessness), hypomania, and mania, have been reported in adult and pediatric patients being treated with antidepressants for MDD as well as for other indications, both psychiatric and nonpsychiatric. Although a causal link between the emergence of such symptoms and either the worsening of depression and/or the emergence of suicidal impulses has not been established, there is concern that such symptoms may represent precursors to emerging suicidality.

Consideration should be given to changing the therapeutic regimen, including possibly discontinuing the medication,

Table 2. Most Common Adverse Reactions: Incidence in Major Depressive Disorder, Obsessive-Compulsive Disorder, Bulimia, and Panic Disorder Placebo-Controlled Clinical Trials

Body System/ Adverse Reaction	MDD Fluoxetine (N = 1728)	MDD Placebo (N = 975)	OCD Fluoxetine (N = 266)	OCD Placebo (N = 89)	Bulimia Fluoxetine (N = 450)	Bulimia Placebo (N = 267)	Panic Disorder Fluoxetine (N = 425)	Panic Disorder Placebo (N = 342)
Body as a Whole								
Asthenia	9	5	15	11	21	9	7	7
Flu Syndrome	3	4	10	7	8	3	5	5
Cardiovascular System								
Vasodilatation	3	2	5	--	2	1	1	--
Digestive System								
Nausea	21	9	26	13	29	11	12	7
Diarrhea	12	8	18	13	8	6	9	4
Anorexia	11	2	17	10	8	4	4	1
Dry Mouth	10	7	12	3	9	6	4	4
Dyspepsia	7	5	10	4	10	6	6	2
Nervous System								
Insomnia	16	9	28	22	33	13	10	7
Anxiety	12	7	14	7	15	9	6	2
Nervousness	14	9	14	15	11	5	8	6
Somnolence	13	6	17	7	13	5	5	2
Tremor	10	3	9	1	13	1	3	1
Libido Decreased	3	--	11	2	5	1	1	2
Abnormal Dreams	1	1	5	2	5	3	1	1
Respiratory System								
Pharyngitis	3	3	11	9	10	5	3	3
Sinusitis	1	4	5	2	6	4	2	3
Yawn	--	--	7	--	11	--	1	--
Skin and Appendages								
Sweating	8	3	7	--	8	3	2	2
Rash	4	3	6	3	4	4	2	2
Urogenital System								
Impotence[a]	2	--	--	--	7	--	1	--
Abnormal Ejaculation[a]	--	--	7	--	7	--	2	1

Note: Includes U.S. data for MDD, OCD, bulimia, and Panic Disorder clinical trials, plus non-U.S. data for Panic Disorder clinical trials.

[a] = Denominator used was for males only (N= 690 fluoxetine MDD; N= 410 placebo MDD; N= 116 fluoxetine OCD; N= 43 placebo OCD; N= 14 fluoxetine Bulimia; N= 1 placebo Bulimia; N= 162 fluoxetine Panic Disorder; N= 121 placebo Panic Disorder).

-- = Incidence less than 1%.

in patients whose depression is persistently worse, or who are experiencing emergent suicidality or symptoms that might be precursors to worsening depression or suicidality, especially if these symptoms are severe, abrupt in onset, or were not part of the patient's presenting symptoms.

If the decision has been made to discontinue treatment, medication should be tapered, as rapidly as is feasible, but with recognition that abrupt discontinuation can be associated with certain symptoms [see Warnings and Precautions (5.14)].

Families and caregivers of patients being treated with antidepressants for MDD or other indications, both psychiatric and nonpsychiatric, should be alerted about the need to monitor patients for the emergence of agitation, irritability, unusual changes in behavior, and the other symptoms described above, as well as the emergence of suicidality, and to report such symptoms immediately to health care providers. Such monitoring should include daily observation by fami-lies and caregivers. Prescriptions for fluoxetine should be written for the smallest quantity of tablets consistent with good patient management, in order to reduce the risk of overdose.

It should be noted that fluoxetine is approved in the pediatric population only for MDD and OCD.

5.2   Serotonin Syndrome or Neuroleptic Malignant Syndrome (NMS)-Like Reactions

The development of a potentially life-threatening serotonin syndrome or neuroleptic malignant syndrome (NMS)-like reactions have been reported with SNRIs and SSRIs alone, including fluoxetine treatment, but particularly with con-comitant use of serotonergic drugs (including triptans) with drugs which impair metabolism of serotonin (including MAOIs), or with antipsychotics or other dopamine antagonists. Serotonin syndrome symptoms may include mental status changes (e.g., agitation, hallucinations, coma), autonomic instability (e.g., tachycardia, labile blood pressure, hyperthermia), neuromuscular aberrations (e.g., hyperreflexia, incoordination) and/or gastrointestinal symptoms (e.g., nausea, vomiting, diarrhea). Serotonin syndrome, in its most severe form can resemble neuroleptic malignant syndrome, which includes hyperthermia, muscle rigidity, autonomic instability with possible rapid fluctuation of vital signs, and mental status changes. Patients should be monitored for the emergence of serotonin syndrome or NMS-like signs and symptoms.

The concomitant use of fluoxetine with MAOIs intended to treat depression is contraindicated [see Contraindications (4) and Drug Interactions (7.1)].

If concomitant treatment of fluoxetine with a 5-hydroxytryptamine receptor agonist (triptan) is clinically warranted, careful observation of the patient is advised, particularly during treatment initiation and dose increases [see Drug Interactions (7.4)].

The concomitant use of fluoxetine with serotonin precursors (such as tryptophan) is not recommended [see Drug Interactions (7.3)].

Treatment with fluoxetine and any concomitant serotonergic or antidopaminergic agents, including antipsychotics, should be discontinued immediately if the above reactions occur, and supportive symptomatic treatment should be initiated.

5.3   Allergic Reactions and Rash

In U.S. fluoxetine clinical trials, 7% of 10,782 patients developed various types of rashes and/or urticaria. Among the cases of rash and/or urticaria reported in premarketing clinical trials, almost a third were withdrawn from treatment because of the rash and/or systemic signs or symptoms associated with the rash. Clinical findings reported in association with rash include fever, leukocytosis, arthralgias, edema, carpal tunnel syndrome, respiratory distress, lymphadenopathy, proteinuria, and mild transaminase elevation. Most patients improved promptly with discontinuation of fluoxetine and/or adjunctive treatment with antihistamines or steroids, and all patients experiencing these reactions were reported to recover completely.

In premarketing clinical trials, 2 patients are known to have developed a serious cutaneous systemic illness. In neither patient was there an unequivocal diagnosis, but one was considered to have a leukocytoclastic vasculitis, and the other, a severe desquamating syndrome that was considered variously to be a vasculitis or erythema multiforme. Other patients have had systemic syndromes suggestive of serum sickness.

Since the introduction of fluoxetine, systemic reactions, possibly related to vasculitis and including lupus-like syndrome, have developed in patients with rash. Although these reactions are rare, they may be serious, involving the lung, kidney, or liver. Death has been reported to occur in association with these systemic reactions.

Anaphylactoid reactions, including bronchospasm, angioedema, laryngospasm, and urticaria alone and in combination, have been reported.

Pulmonary reactions, including inflammatory processes of varying histopathology and/or fibrosis, have been reported rarely. These reactions have occurred with dyspnea as the only preceding symptom.

Whether these systemic reactions and rash have a common underlying cause or are due to different etiologies or pathogenic processes is not known. Furthermore, a specific underlying immunologic basis for these reactions has not been identified. Upon the appearance of rash or of other possibly allergic phenomena for which an alternative etiology cannot be identified, fluoxetine should be discontinued.

5.4   Screening Patients for Bipolar Disorder and Monitoring for Mania/Hypomania

A major depressive episode may be the initial presentation of Bipolar Disorder. It is generally believed (though not established in controlled trials) that treating such an episode with an antidepressant alone may increase the likelihood of precipitation of a mixed/ manic episode in patients at risk for Bipolar Disorder. Whether any of the symptoms described for clinical worsening and suicide risk represent such a conversion is unknown. However, prior to initiating treatment with an antidepressant, patients with depressive symptoms should be adequately screened to determine if they are at risk for Bipolar Disorder; such screening should include a detailed psychiatric history, including a family history of suicide, Bipolar Disorder, and depression. It should be noted that fluoxetine monotherapy is not approved for use in treating Bipolar I Disorder.

In U.S. placebo-controlled clinical trials for MDD, mania/hypomania was reported in 0.1% of patients treated with fluoxetine and 0.1% of patients treated with placebo. Activation of mania/hypomania has also been reported in a small proportion of patients with Major Affective Disorder treated with other marketed drugs effective in the treatment of MDD [see Use in Specific Populations (8.4)].

In U.S. placebo-controlled clinical trials for OCD, mania/hypomania was reported in 0.8% of patients treated with fluoxetine and no patients treated with placebo. No patients reported mania/hypomania in U.S. placebo-controlled clinical trials for bulimia. In all U.S. fluoxetine clinical trials, 0.7% of 10,782 patients reported mania/hypomania [see Use in Specific Populations (8.4)].

5.5 Seizures

In U.S. placebo-controlled clinical trials for MDD, convulsions (or reactions described as possibly having been seizures) were reported in 0.1% of patients treated with fluoxetine and 0.2% of patients treated with placebo. No patients reported convulsions in U.S. placebo-controlled clinical trials for either OCD or bulimia. In all U.S. fluoxetine clinical trials, 0.2% of 10,782 patients reported convulsions. The percentage appears to be similar to that associated with other marketed drugs effective in the treatment of MDD. Fluoxetine should be introduced with care in patients with a history of seizures. There have been rare reports of prolonged seizures in patients on fluoxetine receiving ECT treatment.

5.6 Altered Appetite and Weight

Significant weight loss, especially in underweight depressed or bulimic patients, may be an undesirable result of treatment with fluoxetine.

In U.S. placebo-controlled clinical trials for MDD, 11% of patients treated with fluoxetine and 2% of patients treated with placebo reported anorexia (decreased appetite). Weight loss was reported in 1.4% of patients treated with fluoxetine and in 0.5% of patients treated with placebo. However, only rarely have patients discontinued treatment with fluoxetine because of anorexia or weight loss [see Use in Specific Populations (8.4)].

In U.S. placebo-controlled clinical trials for OCD, 17% of patients treated with fluoxetine and 10% of patients treated with placebo reported anorexia (decreased appetite). One patient discontinued treatment with fluoxetine because of anorexia [see Use in Specific Populations (8.4)].

In U.S. placebo-controlled clinical trials for Bulimia Nervosa, 8% of patients treated with fluoxetine 60 mg and 4% of patients treated with placebo reported anorexia (decreased appetite). Patients treated with fluoxetine 60 mg on average lost 0.45 kg compared with a gain of 0.16 kg by patients treated with placebo in the 16 week double-blind trial. Weight change should be monitored during therapy.

5.7 Abnormal Bleeding

SNRIs and SSRIs, including fluoxetine, may increase the risk of bleeding reactions. Concomitant use of aspirin, nonsteroidal anti-inflammatory drugs, warfarin, and other anticoagulants may add to this risk. Case reports and epidemiological studies (case-control and cohort design) have demonstrated an association between use of drugs that interfere with serotonin reuptake and the occurrence of gastrointestinal bleeding. Bleeding reactions related to SNRIs and SSRIs use have ranged from ecchymoses, hematomas, epistaxis, and petechiae to life-threatening hemorrhages. Patients should be cautioned about the risk of bleeding associated with the concomitant use of fluoxetine and NSAIDs, aspirin, warfarin, or other drugs that affect coagulation [see Drug Interactions (7.6)].

5.8 Angle Closure Glaucoma

The pupillary dilation that occurs following use of many antidepressant drugs including fluoxetine may trigger an angle closure attack in a patient with anatomically narrow angles who does not have a patent iridectomy.

5.9 Hyponatremia

Hyponatremia has been reported during treatment with SNRIs and SSRIs, including fluoxetine. In many cases, this hyponatremia appears to be the result of the syndrome of inappropriate antidiuretic hormone secretion (SIADH). Cases with serum sodium lower than 110 mmol/L have been reported and appeared to be reversible when fluoxetine was discontinued. Elderly patients may be at greater risk of developing hyponatremia with SNRIs and SSRIs. Also, patients taking diuretics or who are otherwise volume-depleted may be at greater risk [see Use in Specific Populations (8.5)]. Discontinuation of fluoxetine should be considered in patients with symptomatic hyponatremia and appropriate medical intervention should be instituted.

Signs and symptoms of hyponatremia include headache, difficulty concentrating, memory impairment, confusion, weakness, and unsteadiness, which may lead to falls. More severe and/or acute cases have been associated with hallucination, syncope, seizure, coma, respiratory arrest, and death.

5.10 Anxiety and Insomnia

In U.S. placebo-controlled clinical trials for MDD, 12% to 16% of patients treated with fluoxetine and 7% to 9% of patients treated with placebo reported anxiety, nervousness, or insomnia.

In U.S. placebo-controlled clinical trials for OCD, insomnia was reported in 28% of patients treated with fluoxetine and in 22% of patients treated with placebo. Anxiety was reported in 14% of patients treated with fluoxetine and in 7% of patients treated with placebo.

In U.S. placebo-controlled clinical trials for Bulimia Nervosa, insomnia was reported in 33% of patients treated with fluoxetine 60 mg, and 13% of patients treated with placebo. Anxiety and nervousness were reported, respectively, in 15% and 11% of patients treated with fluoxetine 60 mg and in 9% and 5% of patients treated with placebo.

Among the most common adverse reactions associated with discontinuation (incidence at least twice that for placebo and at least 1% for fluoxetine in clinical trials collecting only a primary reaction associated with discontinuation) in U.S. placebo-controlled fluoxetine clinical trials were anxiety (2% in OCD), insomnia (1% in combined indications and 2% in bulimia), and nervousness (1% in MDD) [see Adverse Reactions (6.1)].

5.11 Use in Patients with Concomitant Illness

Clinical experience with fluoxetine in patients with concomitant systemic illness is limited. Caution is advisable in using fluoxetine in patients with diseases or conditions that could affect metabolism or hemodynamic responses.

Cardiovascular — Fluoxetine has not been evaluated or used to any appreciable extent in patients with a recent history of myocardial infarction or unstable heart disease. Patients with these diagnoses were systematically excluded from clinical studies during the product's premarket testing. However, the electrocardiograms of 312 patients who received fluoxetine in double-blind trials were retrospec-

Table 3. Adverse Reactions: Incidence in Major Depressive Disorder, Obsessive-Compulsive Disorder, Bulimia, and Panic Disorder Placebo-Controlled Clinical Trials

Body System/Adverse Reaction	Percentage of Patients Reporting Event	
	MDD, OCD, Bulimia, and Panic Disorder Combined	
	Fluoxetine (N = 2869)	Placebo (N = 1673)
Body as a Whole		
Headache	21	19
Asthenia	11	6
Flu Syndrome	5	4
Fever	2	1
Cardiovascular System		
Vasodilatation	2	1
Digestive System		
Nausea	22	9
Diarrhea	11	7
Anorexia	10	3
Dry Mouth	9	6
Dyspepsia	8	4
Constipation	5	4
Flatulence	3	2
Vomiting	3	2
Metabolic and Nutritional Disorders		
Weight Loss	2	1
Nervous System		
Insomnia	19	10
Nervousness	13	8
Anxiety	12	6
Somnolence	12	5
Dizziness	9	6
Tremor	9	2
Libido Decreased	4	1
Thinking Abnormal	2	1
Respiratory System		
Yawn	3	--
Skin and Appendages		
Sweating	7	3
Rash	4	3
Pruritus	3	2
Special Senses		
Abnormal Vision	2	1

Note: Includes U.S. data for MDD, OCD, bulimia, and Panic Disorder clinical trials, plus non-U.S. data for Panic Disorder clinical trials.
-- = Incidence less than 1%.

Table 4. Most Common Adverse Reactions Associated with Discontinuation in Major Depressive Disorder, Obsessive-Compulsive Disorder, Bulimia, and Panic Disorder Placebo-Controlled Clinical Trials

MDD, OCD, Bulimia, and Panic Disorder Combined (N = 1533)	MDD (N = 392)	OCD (N = 266)	Bulimia (N = 450)	Panic Disorder (N = 425)
Anxiety (1%)	--	Anxiety (2%)	--	Anxiety (2%)
--	--	--	Insomnia (2%)	--
--	Nervousness (1%)	--	--	Nervousness (1%)
--	--	Rash (1%)	--	--

Note: Includes U.S. data for MDD, OCD, Bulimia, and Panic Disorder clinical trials, plus non-U.S. data for Panic Disorder clinical trials.

tively evaluated; no conduction abnormalities that resulted in heart block were observed. The mean heart rate was reduced by approximately 3 beats/min.

Glycemic Control — In patients with diabetes, fluoxetine may alter glycemic control. Hypoglycemia has occurred during therapy with fluoxetine, and hyperglycemia has developed following discontinuation of the drug. As is true with many other types of medication when taken concurrently by patients with diabetes, insulin and/or oral hypoglycemic, dosage may need to be adjusted when therapy with fluoxetine is instituted or discontinued.

5.12   Potential for Cognitive and Motor Impairment
As with any CNS-active drug, fluoxetine has the potential to impair judgment, thinking, or motor skills. Patients should be cautioned about operating hazardous machinery, including automobiles, until they are reasonably certain that the drug treatment does not affect them adversely.

5.13   Long Elimination Half-Life
Because of the long elimination half-lives of the parent drug and its major active metabolite, changes in dose will not be fully reflected in plasma for several weeks, affecting both strategies for titration to final dose and withdrawal from treatment. This is of potential consequence when drug discontinuation is required or when drugs are prescribed that might interact with fluoxetine and norfluoxetine following the discontinuation of fluoxetine [see *Clinical Pharmacology* (12.3)].

5.14   Discontinuation of Treatment
During marketing of fluoxetine, SNRIs, and SSRIs, there have been spontaneous reports of adverse reactions occurring upon discontinuation of these drugs, particularly when abrupt, including the following: dysphoric mood, irritability, agitation, dizziness, sensory disturbances (e.g., paresthesias such as electric shock sensations), anxiety, confusion, headache, lethargy, emotional lability, insomnia, and hypomania. While these reactions are generally self-limiting, there have been reports of serious discontinuation symptoms. Patients should be monitored for these symptoms when discontinuing treatment with fluoxetine. A gradual reduction in the dose rather than abrupt cessation is recommended whenever possible. If intolerable symptoms occur following a decrease in the dose or upon discontinuation of treatment, then resuming the previously prescribed dose may be considered. Subsequently, the physician may continue decreasing the dose but at a more gradual rate. Plasma fluoxetine and norfluoxetine concentration decrease gradually at the conclusion of therapy which may minimize the risk of discontinuation symptoms with this drug.

6   ADVERSE REACTIONS
6.1   Clinical Trials Experience
Because clinical trials are conducted under widely varying conditions, adverse reaction rates observed in the clinical trials of a drug cannot be directly compared to rates in the clinical trials of another drug and may not reflect or predict the rates observed in practice.
Multiple doses of fluoxetine had been administered to 10,782 patients with various diagnoses in U.S. clinical trials. In addition, there have been 425 patients administered fluoxetine in panic clinical trials. Adverse reactions were recorded by clinical investigators using descriptive terminology of their own choosing. Consequently, it is not possible to provide a meaningful estimate of the proportion of individuals experiencing adverse reactions without first grouping similar types of reactions into a limited (i.e., reduced) number of standardized reaction categories.
In the tables and tabulations that follow, COSTART Dictionary terminology has been used to classify reported adverse reactions. The stated frequencies represent the proportion of individuals who experienced, at least once, an adverse reaction of the type listed. An adverse reaction was included if it occurred for the first time or worsened while receiving therapy following baseline evaluation. It is important to emphasize that adverse reactions reported during therapy were not necessarily caused by it.

The prescriber should be aware that the figures in the tables and tabulations cannot be used to predict the incidence of adverse reactions in the course of usual medical practice where patient characteristics and other factors differ from those that prevailed in the clinical trials. Similarly, the cited frequencies cannot be compared with figures obtained from other clinical investigations involving different treatments, uses, and investigators. The cited figures, however, do provide the prescribing physician with some basis for estimating the relative contribution of drug and nondrug factors to the side effect incidence rate in the population studied.

Incidence in MDD, OCD, bulimia, and Panic Disorder placebo-controlled clinical trials (excluding data from extensions of trials) — Table 2 enumerates the most common adverse reactions associated with the use of fluoxetine (incidence of at least 5% for fluoxetine and at least twice that for placebo within at least 1 of the indications) for the treatment of MDD, OCD, and bulimia in U.S. controlled clinical trials and Panic Disorder in U.S. plus non-U.S. controlled trials. *Table 3* provides combined data for the pool of studies that are provided separately by indication in *Table 2*.
[See table 2 at top of page 2420]
[See table 3 at top of previous page]

Associated with discontinuation in MDD, OCD, bulimia, and Panic Disorder placebo-controlled clinical trials (excluding data from extensions of trials) — Table 4 lists the adverse reactions associated with discontinuation of fluoxetine treatment (incidence at least twice that for placebo and at least 1% for fluoxetine in clinical trials collecting only a primary reaction associated with discontinuation) in MDD, OCD, bulimia, and Panic Disorder clinical trials, plus non-U.S. Panic Disorder clinical trials.
[See table 4 above]

Other adverse reactions in pediatric patients (children and adolescents) — Adverse reactions were collected in 322 pediatric patients (180 fluoxetine-treated, 142 placebo-treated). The overall profile of adverse reactions was generally similar to that seen in adult studies, as shown in Table 2 and Table 3. However, the following adverse reactions (excluding those which appear in the body or footnotes of Table 2 and Table 3 and those for which the COSTART terms were uninformative or misleading) were reported at an incidence of at least 2% for fluoxetine and greater than placebo: thirst, hyperkinesia, agitation, personality disorder, epistaxis, urinary frequency, and menorrhagia.
The most common adverse reaction (incidence at least 1% for fluoxetine and greater than placebo) associated with discontinuation in 3 pediatric placebo-controlled trials (N = 418 randomized; 228 fluoxetine-treated; 190 placebo-treated) was mania/hypomania (1.8% for fluoxetine-treated, 0% for placebo-treated). In these clinical trials, only a primary reaction associated with discontinuation was collected.

Male and female sexual dysfunction with SSRIs — Although changes in sexual desire, sexual performance, and sexual satisfaction often occur as manifestations of a psychiatric disorder, they may also be a consequence of pharmacologic treatment. In particular, some evidence suggests that SSRIs can cause such untoward sexual experiences. Reliable estimates of the incidence and severity of untoward experiences involving sexual desire, performance, and satisfaction are difficult to obtain, however, in part because patients and physicians may be reluctant to discuss them. Accordingly, estimates of the incidence of untoward sexual experience and performance, cited in product labeling, are likely to underestimate their actual incidence. In patients enrolled in U.S. MDD, OCD, and bulimia placebo-controlled clinical trials, decreased libido was the only sexual side effect reported by at least 2% of patients taking fluoxetine (4% fluoxetine, <1% placebo). There have been spontaneous reports in women taking fluoxetine of orgasmic dysfunction, including anorgasmia.
There are no adequate and well-controlled studies examining sexual dysfunction with fluoxetine treatment.

Symptoms of sexual dysfunction occasionally persist after discontinuation of fluoxetine treatment.
Priapism has been reported with all SSRIs.
While it is difficult to know the precise risk of sexual dysfunction associated with the use of SSRIs, physicians should routinely inquire about such possible side effects.

Other Adverse Reactions Observed During the Premarketing Evaluation of Fluoxetine—Following is a list of adverse reactions reported by patients treated with fluoxetine in clinical trials. This listing is not intended to include reactions (1) already listed in previous tables or elsewhere in labeling, (2) for which a drug cause was remote, (3) which were so general as to be uninformative, (4) which were not considered to have significant clinical implications, or (5) which occurred at a rate equal to or less than placebo.
Reactions are classified by body system using the following definitions: frequent adverse reactions are those occurring in at least 1/100 patients; infrequent adverse reactions are those occurring in 1/100 to 1/1000 patients; rare reactions are those occurring in fewer than 1/1000 patients.

Body as a Whole — *Frequent:* chills; *Infrequent:* suicide attempt; *Rare:* acute abdominal syndrome, photosensitivity reaction.
Cardiovascular System — *Frequent:* palpitation; *Infrequent:* arrhythmia, hypotension[1].
Digestive System — *Infrequent:* dysphagia, gastritis, gastroenteritis, melena, stomach ulcer; *Rare:* bloody diarrhea, duodenal ulcer, esophageal ulcer, gastrointestinal hemorrhage, hematemesis, hepatitis, peptic ulcer, stomach ulcer hemorrhage.
Hemic and Lymphatic System — *Infrequent:* ecchymosis; *Rare:* petechia, purpura.
Nervous System — *Frequent:* emotional lability; *Infrequent:* akathisia, ataxia, balance disorder[1], bruxism[1], buccoglossal syndrome, depersonalization, euphoria, hypertonia, libido increased, myoclonus, paranoid reaction; *Rare:* delusions.
Respiratory System — *Rare:* larynx edema.
Skin and Appendages — *Infrequent:* alopecia; *Rare:* purpuric rash.
Special Senses — *Frequent:* taste perversion; *Infrequent:* mydriasis.
Urogenital System — *Frequent:* micturition disorder; *Infrequent:* dysuria, gynecological bleeding[2].
[1]MedDRA dictionary term from integrated database of placebo-controlled trials of 15,870 patients, of which 9,673 received fluoxetine.
[2]Group term that includes individual MedDRA terms: cervix hemorrhage uterine, dysfunctional uterine bleeding, genital hemorrhage, menometrorrhagia, menorrhagia, metrorrhagia, polymenorrhea, postmenopausal hemorrhage, uterine hemorrhage, vaginal hemorrhage. Adjusted for gender.

6.2   Postmarketing Experience
The following adverse reactions have been identified during post approval use of fluoxetine. Because these reactions are reported voluntarily from a population of uncertain size, it is difficult to reliably estimate their frequency or evaluate a causal relationship to drug exposure.
Voluntary reports of adverse reactions temporally associated with fluoxetine that have been received since market introduction and that may have no causal relationship with the drug include the following: aplastic anemia, atrial fibrillation[1], cataract, cerebrovascular accident[1], cholestatic jaundice, dyskinesia (including, for example, a case of buccal-lingual-masticatory syndrome with involuntary tongue protrusion reported to develop in a 77-year-old female after 5 weeks of fluoxetine therapy and which completely resolved over the next few months following drug discontinuation), eosinophilic pneumonia[1], epidermal necrolysis, erythema multiforme, erythema nodosum, exfoliative dermatitis, gynecomastia, heart arrest[1], hepatic failure/necrosis, hyperprolactinemia, hypoglycemia, immune-related hemolytic anemia, kidney failure, memory impairment, movement disorders developing in patients with risk factors including drugs associated with such reactions and worsening of preexisting movement disorders, optic neuritis, pancreatitis[1], pancytopenia, pulmonary embolism, pulmonary hypertension, QT prolongation, Stevens-Johnson syndrome, thrombocytopenia[1], thrombocytopenic purpura, ventricular tachycardia (including torsade de pointes-type arrhythmias), vaginal bleeding, and violent behaviors[1].
[1]These terms represent serious adverse events, but do not meet the definition for adverse drug reactions. They are included here because of their seriousness.

7   DRUG INTERACTIONS
As with all drugs, the potential for interaction by a variety of mechanisms (e.g., pharmacodynamic, pharmacokinetic drug inhibition or enhancement, etc.) is a possibility.
7.1   Monoamine Oxidase Inhibitors (MAOI)
There have been reports of serious, sometimes fatal, reactions (including hyperthermia, rigidity, myoclonus, autonomic instability with possible rapid fluctuations of vital

signs, and mental status changes that include extreme agitation progressing to delirium and coma) in patients receiving fluoxetine in combination with a monoamine oxidase inhibitor (MAOI), and in patients who have recently discontinued fluoxetine and are then started on an MAOI. Some cases presented with features resembling neuroleptic malignant syndrome. Therefore, fluoxetine should not be used in combination with an MAOI, or within a minimum of 14 days of discontinuing therapy with an MAOI [see Contraindications (4)]. Since fluoxetine and its major metabolite have very long elimination half-lives, at least 5 weeks perhaps longer, especially if fluoxetine has been prescribed chronically and/or at higher doses should be allowed after stopping fluoxetine before starting an MAOI [see Clinical Pharmacology (12.3)].

7.2 CNS Acting Drugs

Caution is advised if the concomitant administration of fluoxetine and such drugs is required. In evaluating individual cases, consideration should be given to using lower initial doses of the concomitantly administered drugs, using conservative titration schedules, and monitoring of clinical status [see Clinical Pharmacology (12.3)].

7.3 Serotonergic Drugs

Based on the mechanism of action of SNRIs and SSRIs, including fluoxetine, and the potential for serotonin syndrome, caution is advised when fluoxetine is coadministered with other drugs that may affect the serotonergic neurotransmitter systems, such as triptans, linezolid (an antibiotic which is a reversible non-selective MAOI), lithium, tramadol, or St. John's Wort [see Warnings and Precautions (5.2)]. The concomitant use of fluoxetine with SNRIs, SSRIs, or tryptophan is not recommended [see Drug Interactions (7.4), (7.5)].

7.4 Triptans

There have been rare postmarketing reports of serotonin syndrome with use of an SSRI and a triptan. If concomitant treatment of fluoxetine with a triptan is clinically warranted, careful observation of the patient is advised, particularly during treatment initiation and dose increases [see Warnings and Precautions (5.2) and Drug Interactions (7.3)].

7.5 Tryptophan

Five patients receiving fluoxetine in combination with tryptophan experienced adverse reactions, including agitation, restlessness, and gastrointestinal distress. The concomitant use with tryptophan is not recommended [see Warnings and Precautions (5.2) and Drug Interactions (7.3)].

7.6 Drugs That Interfere With Hemostasis (e.g., NSAIDS, Aspirin, Warfarin)

Serotonin release by platelets plays an important role in hemostasis. Epidemiological studies of the case-control and cohort design that have demonstrated an association between use of psychotropic drugs that interfere with serotonin reuptake and the occurrence of upper gastrointestinal bleeding have also shown that concurrent use of an NSAID or aspirin may potentiate this risk of bleeding.

Altered anticoagulant effects, including increased bleeding, have been reported when SNRIs or SSRIs are coadministered with warfarin. Patients receiving warfarin therapy should be carefully monitored when fluoxetine is initiated or discontinued [see Warnings and Precautions (5.7)].

7.7 Potential for Other Drugs to Affect Fluoxetine

Drugs Tightly Bound to Plasma Proteins – Because fluoxetine is tightly bound to plasma protein, adverse effects may result from displacement of protein-bound fluoxetine by other tightly-bound drugs [see Clinical Pharmacology (12.3)].

7.8 Potential for Fluoxetine to Affect Other Drugs

Pimozide – Concomitant use in patients taking pimozide is contraindicated. Clinical studies of pimozide with other antidepressants demonstrate an increase in drug interaction or QTc prolongation. While a specific study with pimozide and fluoxetine has not been conducted, the potential for drug interactions or QTc prolongation warrants restricting the concurrent use of pimozide and fluoxetine [see Contraindications (4)].

Thioridazine – Thioridazine should not be administered with fluoxetine or within a minimum of 5 weeks after fluoxetine has been discontinued [see Contraindications (4)]. In a study of 19 healthy male subjects, which included 6 slow and 13 rapid hydroxylators of debrisoquin, a single 25 mg oral dose of thioridazine produced a 2.4 fold higher C_{max} and a 4.5-fold higher AUC for thioridazine in the slow hydroxylators compared with the rapid hydroxylators. The rate of debrisoquin hydroxylation is felt to depend on the level of CYP2D6 isozyme activity. Thus, this study suggests that drugs which inhibit CYP2D6, such as certain SSRIs, including fluoxetine, will produce elevated plasma levels of thioridazine.

Thioridazine administration produces a dose-related prolongation of the QTc interval, which is associated with serious ventricular arrhythmias, such as torsade de pointes-type arrhythmias, and sudden death. This risk is expected to increase with fluoxetine-induced inhibition of thioridazine metabolism.

Drugs Metabolized by CYP2D6 – Fluoxetine inhibits the activity of CYP2D6, and may make individuals with normal CYP2D6 metabolic activity resemble a poor metabolizer. Coadministration of fluoxetine with other drugs that are metabolized by CYP2D6, including certain antidepressants (e.g., TCAs), antipsychotics (e.g., phenothiazines and most atypicals), and antiarrhythmics (e.g., propafenone, flecainide, and others) should be approached with caution. Therapy with medications that are predominantly metabolized by the CYP2D6 system and that have a relatively narrow therapeutic index (see list below) should be initiated at the low end of the dose range if a patient is receiving fluoxetine concurrently or has taken it in the previous 5 weeks. Thus, his/her dosing requirements resemble those of poor metabolizers. If fluoxetine is added to the treatment regimen of a patient already receiving a drug metabolized by CYP2D6, the need for decreased dose of the original medication should be considered. Drugs with a narrow therapeutic index represent the greatest concern (e.g., flecainide, propafenone, vinblastine, and TCAs). Due to the risk of serious ventricular arrhythmias and sudden death potentially associated with elevated plasma levels of thioridazine, thioridazine should not be administered with fluoxetine or within a minimum of 5 weeks after fluoxetine has been discontinued [see Contraindications (4)].

Tricyclic Antidepressants (TCAs) — In 2 studies, previously stable plasma levels of imipramine and desipramine have increased greater than 2 to 10 fold when fluoxetine has been administered in combination. This influence may persist for 3 weeks or longer after fluoxetine is discontinued. Thus, the dose of TCAs may need to be reduced and plasma TCA concentrations may need to be monitored temporarily when fluoxetine is coadministered or has been recently discontinued [see Clinical Pharmacology (12.3)].

Benzodiazepines — The half-life of concurrently administered diazepam may be prolonged in some patients [see Clinical Pharmacology (12.3)]. Coadministration of alprazolam and fluoxetine has resulted in increased alprazolam plasma concentrations and in further psychomotor performance decrement due to increased alprazolam levels.

Antipsychotics — Some clinical data suggests a possible pharmacodynamic and/or pharmacokinetic interaction between SSRIs and antipsychotics. Elevation of blood levels of haloperidol and clozapine has been observed in patients receiving concomitant fluoxetine [see Contraindications (4)].

Anticonvulsants — Patients on stable doses of phenytoin and carbamazepine have developed elevated plasma anticonvulsant concentrations and clinical anticonvulsant toxicity following initiation of concomitant fluoxetine treatment.

Lithium — There have been reports of both increased and decreased lithium levels when lithium was used concomitantly with fluoxetine. Cases of lithium toxicity and increased serotonergic effects have been reported. Lithium levels should be monitored when these drugs are administered concomitantly.

Drugs Tightly Bound to Plasma Proteins — Because fluoxetine is tightly bound to plasma protein, the administration of fluoxetine to a patient taking another drug that is tightly bound to protein (e.g., Coumadin, digitoxin) may cause a shift in plasma concentrations potentially resulting in an adverse effect [see Clinical Pharmacology (12.3)].

Drugs Metabolized by CYP3A4 — In an in vivo interaction study involving coadministration of fluoxetine with single doses of terfenadine (a CYP3A4 substrate), no increase in plasma terfenadine concentrations occurred with concomitant fluoxetine. Additionally, in vitro studies have shown ketoconazole, a potent inhibitor of CYP3A4 activity, to be at least 100 times more potent than fluoxetine or norfluoxetine as an inhibitor of the metabolism of several substrates for this enzyme, including astemizole, cisapride, and midazolam. These data indicate that fluoxetine's extent of inhibition of CYP3A4 activity is not likely to be of clinical significance.

Olanzapine — Fluoxetine (60 mg single dose or 60 mg daily dose for 8 days) causes a small (mean 16%) increase in the maximum concentration of olanzapine and a small (mean 16%) decrease in olanzapine clearance. The magnitude of the impact of this factor is small in comparison to the overall variability between individuals, and therefore dose modification is not routinely recommended.

8 USE IN SPECIFIC POPULATIONS

8.1 Pregnancy

Pregnancy Category C — Fluoxetine should be used during pregnancy only if the potential benefit justifies the potential risk to the fetus. All pregnancies have a background risk of birth defects, loss, or other adverse outcome regardless of drug exposure.

Treatment of Pregnant Women During the First Trimester— There are no adequate and well-controlled clinical studies on the use of fluoxetine in pregnant women. Results of a number of published epidemiological studies assessing the risk of fluoxetine exposure during the first trimester of pregnancy have demonstrated inconsistent results. More than

10 cohort studies and case-control studies failed to demonstrate an increased risk for congenital malformations overall. However, one prospective cohort study conducted by the European Network of Teratology Information Services reported an increased risk of cardiovascular malformations in infants born to women (N = 253) exposed to fluoxetine during the first trimester of pregnancy compared to infants of women (N = 1,359) who were not exposed to fluoxetine. There was no specific pattern of cardiovascular malformations. Overall, however, a causal relationship has not been established.

Treatment of Pregnant Women During the Third Trimester — Neonates exposed to fluoxetine, SNRIs, or SSRIs, late in the third trimester have developed complications requiring prolonged hospitalization, respiratory support, and tube feeding. Such complications can arise immediately upon delivery. Reported clinical findings have included respiratory distress, cyanosis, apnea, seizures, temperature instability, feeding difficulty, vomiting, hypoglycemia, hypotonia, hypertonia, hyperreflexia, tremor, jitteriness, irritability, and constant crying. These features are consistent with either a direct toxic effect of SNRIs and SSRIs or, possibly, a drug discontinuation syndrome. It should be noted that, in some cases, the clinical picture is consistent with serotonin syndrome.

Infants exposed to SSRIs in late pregnancy may have an increased risk for persistent pulmonary hypertension of the newborn (PPHN). PPHN occurs in 1 to 2 per 1000 live births in the general population and is associated with substantial neonatal morbidity and mortality. In a retrospective case-control study of 377 women whose infants were born with PPHN and 836 women whose infants were born healthy, the risk for developing PPHN was approximately 6-fold higher for infants exposed to SSRIs after the 20th week of gestation compared to infants who had not been exposed to antidepressants during pregnancy. There is currently no corroborative evidence regarding the risk for PPHN following exposure to SSRIs in pregnancy; this is the first study that has investigated the potential risk. The study did not include enough cases with exposure to individual SSRIs to determine if all SSRIs posed similar levels of PPHN risk.

Clinical Considerations — When treating pregnant women with fluoxetine during the third trimester, the physician should carefully consider both the potential risks and potential benefits of treatment, taking into account the risk of untreated depression during pregnancy. Physicians should note that in a prospective longitudinal study of 201 women with a history of major depression who were euthymic at the beginning of pregnancy, women who discontinued antidepressant medication during pregnancy were more likely to experience a relapse of major depression than women who continued antidepressant medication.

The physician may consider tapering fluoxetine in the third trimester [see Dosage and Administration (2.5)].

Animal Data—In embryo-fetal development studies in rats and rabbits, there was no evidence of teratogenicity following administration of up to 12.5 and 15 mg/kg/day, respectively (1.5 and 3.6 times, respectively, the maximum recommended human dose (MRHD) of 80 mg on a mg/m² basis) throughout organogenesis. However, in rat reproduction studies, an increase in stillborn pups, a decrease in pup weight, and an increase in pup deaths during the first 7 days postpartum occurred following maternal exposure to 12 mg/kg/day (1.5 times the MRHD on a mg/m² basis) during gestation or 7.5 mg/kg/day (0.9 times the MRHD on a mg/m² basis) during gestation and lactation. There was no evidence of developmental neurotoxicity in the surviving offspring of rats treated with 12 mg/kg/day during gestation. The no-effect dose for rat pup mortality was 5 mg/kg/day (0.6 times the MRHD on a mg/m² basis).

8.2 Labor and Delivery

The effect of fluoxetine on labor and delivery in humans is unknown. However, because fluoxetine crosses the placenta and because of the possibility that fluoxetine may have adverse effects on the newborn, fluoxetine should be used during labor and delivery only if the potential benefit justifies the potential risk to the fetus.

8.3 Nursing Mothers

Because fluoxetine is excreted in human milk, nursing while on fluoxetine is not recommended. In one breast-milk sample, the concentration of fluoxetine plus norfluoxetine was 70.4 ng/mL. The concentration in the mother's plasma was 295.0 ng/mL. No adverse effects on the infant were reported. In another case, an infant nursed by a mother on fluoxetine developed crying, sleep disturbance, vomiting, and watery stools. The infant's plasma drug levels were 340 ng/mL of fluoxetine and 208 ng/mL of norfluoxetine on the second day of feeding.

8.4 Pediatric Use

The efficacy of fluoxetine for the treatment of MDD was demonstrated in two 8 to 9 week placebo-controlled clinical trials with 315 pediatric outpatients ages 8 to ≤18 [see Clinical Studies (14.1)]. Doses greater than 20 mg/day have not been studied in pediatric patients with MDD.

The efficacy of fluoxetine for the treatment of OCD was demonstrated in one 13 week placebo-controlled clinical trial with 103 pediatric outpatients ages 7 to <18 [see *Clinical Studies (14.2)*].

The safety and effectiveness in pediatric patients <8 years of age in MDD and <7 years of age in OCD have not been established.

Fluoxetine pharmacokinetics were evaluated in 21 pediatric patients (ages 6 to ≤18) with MDD or OCD [see *Clinical Pharmacology (12.3)*].

The acute adverse reaction profiles observed in the 3 studies (N = 418 randomized; 228 fluoxetine-treated, 190 placebo-treated) were generally similar to that observed in adult studies with fluoxetine. The longer-term adverse reaction profile observed in the 19 week MDD study (N = 219 randomized; 109 fluoxetine-treated, 110 placebo-treated) was also similar to that observed in adult trials with fluoxetine [see *Adverse Reactions (6.1)*].

Manic reaction, including mania and hypomania, was reported in 6 (1 mania, 5 hypomania) out of 228 (2.6%) fluoxetine-treated patients and in 0 out of 190 (0%) placebo-treated patients. Mania/hypomania led to the discontinuation of 4 (1.8%) fluoxetine-treated patients from the acute phases of the 3 studies combined. Consequently, regular monitoring for the occurrence of mania/hypomania is recommended.

As with other SSRIs, decreased weight gain has been observed in association with the use of fluoxetine in children and adolescent patients. After 19 weeks of treatment in a clinical trial, pediatric subjects treated with fluoxetine gained an average of 1.1 cm less in height and 1.1 kg less in weight than subjects treated with placebo. In addition, fluoxetine treatment was associated with a decrease in alkaline phosphatase levels. The safety of fluoxetine treatment for pediatric patients has not been systematically assessed for chronic treatment longer than several months in duration. In particular, there are no studies that directly evaluate the longer-term effects of fluoxetine on the growth, development and maturation of children and adolescent patients. Therefore, height and weight should be monitored periodically in pediatric patients receiving fluoxetine [see *Warnings and Precautions (5.6)*].

Fluoxetine is approved for use in pediatric patients with MDD and OCD [see *Boxed Warning and Warnings and Precautions (5.1)*].

Anyone considering the use of fluoxetine in a child or adolescent must balance the potential risks with the clinical need.

Significant toxicity, including myotoxicity, long-term neurobehavioral and reproductive toxicity, and impaired bone development, has been observed following exposure of juvenile animals to fluoxetine. Some of these effects occurred at clinically relevant exposures. In a study in which fluoxetine (3, 10, or 30 mg/kg) was orally administered to young rats from weaning (Postnatal Day 21) through adulthood (Day 90), male and female sexual development was delayed at all doses, and growth (body weight gain, femur length) was decreased during the dosing period in animals receiving the highest dose. At the end of the treatment period, serum levels of creatine kinase (marker of muscle damage) were increased at the intermediate and high doses, and abnormal muscle and reproductive organ histopathology (skeletal muscle degeneration and necrosis, testicular degeneration and necrosis, epididymal vacuolation and hypospermia) was observed at the high dose. When animals were evaluated after a recovery period (up to 11 weeks after cessation of dosing), neurobehavioral abnormalities (decreased reactivity at all doses and learning deficit at the high dose) and reproductive functional impairment (decreased mating at all doses and impaired fertility at the high dose) were seen; in addition, testicular and epididymal microscopic lesions and decreased sperm concentrations were found in the high dose group, indicating that the reproductive organ effects seen at the end of treatment were irreversible. The reversibility of fluoxetine-induced muscle damage was not assessed. Adverse effects similar to those observed in rats treated with fluoxetine during the juvenile period have not been reported after administration of fluoxetine to adult animals. Plasma exposures (AUC) to fluoxetine in juvenile rats receiving the low, intermediate, and high dose in this study were approximately 0.1 to 0.2, 1 to 2, and 5 to 10 times, respectively, the average exposure in pediatric patients receiving the maximum recommended dose (MRD) of 20 mg/day. Rat exposures to the major metabolite, norfluoxetine, were approximately 0.3 to 0.8, 1 to 8, and 3 to 20 times, respectively, pediatric exposure at the MRD.

A specific effect of fluoxetine on bone development has been reported in mice treated with fluoxetine during the juvenile period. When mice were treated with fluoxetine (5 or 20 mg/kg, intraperitoneal) for 4 weeks starting at 4 weeks of age, bone formation was reduced resulting in decreased bone mineral content and density. These doses did not affect overall growth (body weight gain or femoral

length). The doses administered to juvenile mice in this study are approximately 0.5 and 2 times the MRD for pediatric patients on a body surface area (mg/m^2) basis.

In another mouse study, administration of fluoxetine (10 mg/kg intraperitoneal) during early postnatal development (Postnatal Days 4 to 21) produced abnormal emotional behaviors (decreased exploratory behavior in elevated plus-maze, increased shock avoidance latency) in adulthood (12 weeks of age). The dose used in this study is approximately equal to the pediatric MRD on a mg/m^2 basis. Because of the early dosing period in this study, the significance of these findings to the approved pediatric use in humans is uncertain.

8.5 Geriatric Use

U.S. fluoxetine clinical trials included 687 patients ≥65 years of age and 93 patients ≥75 years of age. The efficacy in geriatric patients has been established [see *Clinical Studies (14.1)*]. For pharmacokinetic information in geriatric patients, [see *Clinical Pharmacology (12.3)*]. No overall differences in safety or effectiveness were observed between these subjects and younger subjects, and other reported clinical experience has not identified differences in responses between the elderly and younger patients, but greater sensitivity of some older individuals cannot be ruled out. SNRIs and SSRIs, including fluoxetine, have been associated with cases of clinically significant hyponatremia in elderly patients, who may be at greater risk for this adverse reaction [see *Warnings and Precautions (5.9)*].

8.6 Hepatic Impairment

In subjects with cirrhosis of the liver, the clearances of fluoxetine and its active metabolite, norfluoxetine, were decreased, thus increasing the elimination half-lives of these substances. A lower or less frequent dose of fluoxetine should be used in patients with cirrhosis. Caution is advised when using fluoxetine in patients with diseases or conditions that could affect its metabolism [see *Dosage and Administration (2.5) and Clinical Pharmacology (12.3)*].

9 DRUG ABUSE AND DEPENDENCE

9.3 Dependence

Fluoxetine has not been systematically studied, in animals or humans, for its potential for abuse, tolerance, or physical dependence. While the premarketing clinical experience with fluoxetine did not reveal any tendency for a withdrawal syndrome or any drug seeking behavior, these observations were not systematic and it is not possible to predict on the basis of this limited experience the extent to which a CNS active drug will be misused, diverted, and/or abused once marketed. Consequently, physicians should carefully evaluate patients for history of drug abuse and follow such patients closely, observing them for signs of misuse or abuse of fluoxetine (e.g., development of tolerance, incrementation of dose, drug-seeking behavior).

10 OVERDOSAGE

10.1 Human Experience

Worldwide exposure to fluoxetine hydrochloride is estimated to be over 38 million patients (circa 1999). Of the 1578 cases of overdose involving fluoxetine hydrochloride, alone or with other drugs, reported from this population, there were 195 deaths.

Among 633 adult patients who overdosed on fluoxetine hydrochloride alone, 34 resulted in a fatal outcome, 378 completely recovered, and 15 patients experienced sequelae after overdose, including abnormal accommodation, abnormal gait, confusion, unresponsiveness, nervousness, pulmonary dysfunction, vertigo, tremor, elevated blood pressure, impotence, movement disorder, and hypomania. The remaining 206 patients had an unknown outcome. The most common signs and symptoms associated with nonfatal overdosage were seizures, somnolence, nausea, tachycardia, and vomiting. The largest known ingestion of fluoxetine hydrochloride in adult patients was 8 grams in a patient who took fluoxetine alone and who subsequently recovered. However, in an adult patient who took fluoxetine alone, an ingestion as low as 520 mg has been associated with lethal outcome, but causality has not been established.

Among pediatric patients (ages 3 months to 17 years), there were 156 cases of overdose involving fluoxetine alone or in combination with other drugs. Six patients died, 127 patients completely recovered, 1 patient experienced renal failure, and 22 patients had an unknown outcome. One of the six fatalities was a 9-year-old boy who had a history of OCD, Tourette's syndrome with tics, attention deficit disorder, and fetal alcohol syndrome. He had been receiving 100 mg of fluoxetine daily for 6 months in addition to clonidine, methylphenidate, and promethazine. Mixed-drug ingestion or other methods of suicide complicated all 6 overdoses in children that resulted in fatalities. The largest ingestion in pediatric patients was 3 grams which was nonlethal.

Other important adverse reactions reported with fluoxetine overdose (single or multiple drugs) include coma, delirium, ECG abnormalities (such as QT interval prolongation and

ventricular tachycardia, including torsade de pointes-type arrhythmias), hypotension, mania, neuroleptic malignant syndrome-like reactions, pyrexia, stupor, and syncope.

10.2 Animal Experience

Studies in animals do not provide precise or necessarily valid information about the treatment of human overdose. However, animal experiments can provide useful insights into possible treatment strategies.

The oral median lethal dose in rats and mice was found to be 452 and 248 mg/kg, respectively. Acute high oral doses produced hyperirritability and convulsions in several animal species.

Among 6 dogs purposely overdosed with oral fluoxetine, 5 experienced grand mal seizures. Seizures stopped immediately upon the bolus intravenous administration of a standard veterinary dose of diazepam. In this short-term study, the lowest plasma concentration at which a seizure occurred was only twice the maximum plasma concentration seen in humans taking 80 mg/day, chronically.

In a separate single-dose study, the ECG of dogs given high doses did not reveal prolongation of the PR, QRS, or QT intervals. Tachycardia and an increase in blood pressure were observed. Consequently, the value of the ECG in predicting cardiac toxicity is unknown. Nonetheless, the ECG should ordinarily be monitored in cases of human overdose [see *Overdosage (10.3)*].

10.3 Management of Overdose

Treatment should consist of those general measures employed in the management of overdosage with any drug effective in the treatment of MDD.

Ensure an adequate airway, oxygenation, and ventilation. Monitor cardiac rhythm and vital signs. General supportive and symptomatic measures are also recommended. Induction of emesis is not recommended. Gastric lavage with a large-bore orogastric tube with appropriate airway protection, if needed, may be indicated if performed soon after ingestion, or in symptomatic patients.

Activated charcoal should be administered. Due to the large volume of distribution of this drug, forced diuresis, dialysis, hemoperfusion, and exchange transfusion are unlikely to be of benefit. No specific antidotes for fluoxetine are known.

A specific caution involves patients who are taking or have recently taken fluoxetine and might ingest excessive quantities of a TCA. In such a case, accumulation of the parent tricyclic and/or an active metabolite may increase the possibility of clinically significant sequelae and extend the time needed for close medical observation [see *Drug Interactions (7.8)*].

Based on experience in animals, which may not be relevant to humans, fluoxetine-induced seizures that fail to remit spontaneously may respond to diazepam.

In managing overdosage, consider the possibility of multiple drug involvement. The physician should consider contacting a poison control center for additional information on the treatment of any overdose.

11 DESCRIPTION

Fluoxetine hydrochloride is a selective serotonin reuptake inhibitor for oral administration. It is designated (±)-*N*-methyl-3-phenyl-3-[(α,α,α-trifluoro-*p*-tolyl)oxy]propylamine hydrochloride and has the molecular formula of $C_{17}H_{18}F_3NO \cdot HCl$. Its molecular weight is 345.79. The structural formula is:

Fluoxetine hydrochloride is a white to off-white crystalline solid with a solubility of 14 mg/mL in water.

Each scored tablet contains fluoxetine hydrochloride equivalent to 60 mg (194 µmol) of fluoxetine. In addition, each scored tablet also contains the following inactive ingredients: mannitol, microcrystalline cellulose, maize starch, povidone, hypromellose, magnesium stearate, titanium dioxide, sucrose, glycerol, and polysorbate.

12 CLINICAL PHARMACOLOGY

12.1 Mechanism of Action

Although the exact mechanism of fluoxetine is unknown, it is presumed to be linked to its inhibition of CNS neuronal uptake of serotonin.

12.2 Pharmacodynamics

Studies at clinically relevant doses in man have demonstrated that fluoxetine blocks the uptake of serotonin into human platelets. Studies in animals also suggest that fluoxetine is a much more potent uptake inhibitor of serotonin than of norepinephrine. Antagonism of muscarinic, histaminergic, and α1-adrenergic receptors has been hypothesized to be associated with various anticholinergic, sedative, and cardiovascular effects of classical tricyclic antidepressant (TCA) drugs. Fluoxetine binds to these and other membrane receptors from brain tissue much less potently *in vitro* than do the tricyclic drugs.

12.3 Pharmacokinetics

Systemic Bioavailability — In man, following a single, oral dose of fluoxetine 60 mg tablet, USP, the peak plasma concentration of fluoxetine and time to achieve peak plasma concentration were 49.6 ± 10.0 ng/mL, and 7.20 ± 1.41 hours, respectively (both values are mean ± SD).

The capsule, tablet, and oral solution dosage forms of fluoxetine are bioequivalent. The exposure (C_{max}, AUC) to fluoxetine was similar after administration of either 1 × 60 mg fluoxetine tablet USP or 3 × 20 mg fluoxetine tablets. Food does not appear to affect the systemic bioavailability of fluoxetine, although it may delay its absorption by 1 to 2 hours, which is probably not clinically significant. Thus, fluoxetine may be administered with or without food.

Protein Binding — Over the concentration range from 200 to 1000 ng/mL, approximately 94.5% of fluoxetine is bound *in vitro* to human serum proteins, including albumin and α1-glycoprotein. The interaction between fluoxetine and other highly protein-bound drugs has not been fully evaluated, but may be important.

Enantiomers — Fluoxetine is a racemic mixture (50/50) of R-fluoxetine and S-fluoxetine enantiomers. In animal models, both enantiomers are specific and potent serotonin uptake inhibitors with essentially equivalent pharmacologic activity. The S-fluoxetine enantiomer is eliminated more slowly and is the predominant enantiomer present in plasma at steady state.

Metabolism — Fluoxetine is extensively metabolized in the liver to norfluoxetine and a number of other unidentified metabolites. The only identified active metabolite, norfluoxetine, is formed by demethylation of fluoxetine. In animal models, S-norfluoxetine is a potent and selective inhibitor of serotonin uptake and has activity essentially equivalent to R- or S-fluoxetine. R-norfluoxetine is significantly less potent than the parent drug in the inhibition of serotonin uptake. The primary route of elimination appears to be hepatic metabolism to inactive metabolites excreted by the kidney.

Variability in Metabolism — A subset (about 7%) of the population has reduced activity of the drug metabolizing enzyme cytochrome P450 2D6 (CYP2D6). Such individuals are referred to as "poor metabolizers" of drugs such as debrisoquin, dextromethorphan, and the TCAs. In a study involving labeled and unlabeled enantiomers administered as a racemate, these individuals metabolized S-fluoxetine at a slower rate and thus achieved higher concentrations of S-fluoxetine. Consequently, concentrations of S-norfluoxetine at steady state were lower. The metabolism of R-fluoxetine in these poor metabolizers appears normal. When compared with normal metabolizers, the total sum at steady state of the plasma concentrations of the 4 active enantiomers was not significantly greater among poor metabolizers. Thus, the net pharmacodynamic activities were essentially the same. Alternative, nonsaturable pathways (non 2D6) also contribute to the metabolism of fluoxetine. This explains how fluoxetine achieves a steady-state concentration rather than increasing without limit.

Because fluoxetine's metabolism, like that of a number of other compounds including TCAs and other selective serotonin reuptake inhibitors (SSRIs), involves the CYP2D6 system, concomitant therapy with drugs also metabolized by this enzyme system (such as the TCAs) may lead to drug interactions [*see Drug Interactions (7.8)*].

Accumulation and Slow Elimination — The relatively slow elimination of fluoxetine (elimination half-life of 1 to 3 days after acute administration and 4 to 6 days after chronic administration) and its active metabolite, norfluoxetine (elimination half-life of 4 to 16 days after acute and chronic administration), leads to significant accumulation of these active species in chronic use and delayed attainment of steady state, even when a fixed dose is used [*see Warnings and Precautions (5.13)*]. After 30 days of dosing at 40 mg/day, plasma concentrations of fluoxetine in the range of 91 to 302 ng/mL and norfluoxetine in the range of 72 to 258 ng/mL have been observed. Plasma concentrations of fluoxetine were higher than those predicted by single-dose studies, because fluoxetine's metabolism is not proportional to dose. Norfluoxetine, however, appears to have linear pharmacokinetics. Its mean terminal half-life after a single dose was 8.6 days and after multiple dosing was 9.3 days. Steady-state levels after prolonged dosing are similar to levels seen at 4 to 5 weeks.

The long elimination half-lives of fluoxetine and norfluoxetine assure that, even when dosing is stopped, active drug substance will persist in the body for weeks (primarily depending on individual patient characteristics, previous dosing regimen, and length of previous therapy at discontinuation). This is of potential consequence when drug discontinuation is required or when drugs are prescribed that might interact with fluoxetine and norfluoxetine following the discontinuation of fluoxetine.

Liver Disease—As might be predicted from its primary site of metabolism, liver impairment can affect the elimination of fluoxetine. The elimination half-life of fluoxetine was prolonged in a study of cirrhotic patients, with a mean of 7.6 days compared with the range of 2 to 3 days seen in subjects without liver disease; norfluoxetine elimination was also delayed, with a mean duration of 12 days for cirrhotic patients compared with the range of 7 to 9 days in normal subjects. This suggests that the use of fluoxetine in patients with liver disease must be approached with caution. If fluoxetine is administered to patients with liver disease, a lower or less frequent dose should be used [*see Dosage and Administration (2.5) and Use in Specific Populations (8.6)*].

Renal Disease—In depressed patients on dialysis (N = 12), fluoxetine administered as 20 mg once daily for 2 months produced steady-state fluoxetine and norfluoxetine plasma concentrations comparable with those seen in patients with normal renal function. While the possibility exists that renally excreted metabolites of fluoxetine may accumulate to higher levels in patients with severe renal dysfunction, use of a lower or less frequent dose is not routinely necessary in renally impaired patients.

Geriatric Pharmacokinetics—The disposition of single doses of fluoxetine in healthy elderly subjects (>65 years of age) did not differ significantly from that in younger normal subjects. However, given the long half-life and nonlinear disposition of the drug, a single-dose study is not adequate to rule out the possibility of altered pharmacokinetics in the elderly, particularly if they have systemic illness or are receiving multiple drugs for concomitant diseases. The effects of age upon the metabolism of fluoxetine have been investigated in 260 elderly but otherwise healthy depressed patients (≥60 years of age) who received 20 mg fluoxetine for 6 weeks. Combined fluoxetine plus norfluoxetine plasma concentrations were 209.3 ± 85.7 ng/mL at the end of 6 weeks. No unusual age-associated pattern of adverse reactions was observed in those elderly patients.

Pediatric Pharmacokinetics (children and adolescents)—Fluoxetine pharmacokinetics were evaluated in 21 pediatric patients (10 children ages 6 to <13, 11 adolescents ages 13 to <18) diagnosed with MDD or OCD. Fluoxetine 20 mg/day was administered for up to 62 days. The average steady-state concentrations of fluoxetine in these children were 2 fold higher than in adolescents (171 and 86 ng/mL, respectively). The average norfluoxetine steady-state concentrations in these children were 1.5 fold higher than in adolescents (195 and 113 ng/mL, respectively). These differences can be almost entirely explained by differences in weight. No gender-associated differences in fluoxetine pharmacokinetics was observed. Similar ranges of fluoxetine and norfluoxetine plasma concentrations were observed in another study in 94 pediatric patients (ages 8 to <18) diagnosed with MDD.

Higher average steady-state fluoxetine and norfluoxetine concentrations were observed in children relative to adults; however, these concentrations were within the range of concentrations observed in the adult population. As in adults, fluoxetine and norfluoxetine accumulated extensively following multiple oral dosing; steady-state concentrations were achieved within 3 to 4 weeks of daily dosing.

13 NONCLINICAL TOXICOLOGY

13.1 Carcinogenesis, Mutagenesis, Impairment of Fertility

Carcinogenicity — The dietary administration of fluoxetine to rats and mice for 2 years at doses of up to 10 and 12 mg/kg/day, respectively [approximately 1.2 and 0.7 times, respectively, the maximum recommended human dose (MRHD) of 80 mg on a mg/m^2 basis], produced no evidence of carcinogenicity.

Mutagenicity — Fluoxetine and norfluoxetine have been shown to have no genotoxic effects based on the following assays: bacterial mutation assay, DNA repair assay in cultured rat hepatocytes, mouse lymphoma assay, and *in vivo* sister chromatid exchange assay in Chinese hamster bone marrow cells.

Impairment of Fertility — Two fertility studies conducted in adult rats at doses of up to 7.5 and 12.5 mg/kg/day (approximately 0.9 and 1.5 times the MRHD on a mg/m^2 basis) indicated that fluoxetine had no adverse effects on fertility. However, adverse effects on fertility were seen when juvenile rats were treated with fluoxetine [*see Use in Specific Populations (8.4)*].

13.2 Animal Toxicology and/or Pharmacology

Phospholipids are increased in some tissues of mice, rats, and dogs given fluoxetine chronically. This effect is reversible after cessation of fluoxetine treatment. Phospholipid accumulation in animals has been observed with many cationic amphiphilic drugs, including fenfluramine, imipramine, and ranitidine. The significance of this effect in humans is unknown.

14 CLINICAL STUDIES

14.1 Major Depressive Disorder

Daily Dosing

Adult—The efficacy of fluoxetine was studied in 5 and 6 week placebo-controlled trials with depressed adult and geriatric outpatients (≥18 years of age) whose diagnoses corresponded most closely to the DSM-III (currently DSM-IV) category of MDD. Fluoxetine was shown to be significantly more effective than placebo as measured by the Hamilton Depression Rating Scale (HAM-D). Fluoxetine was also significantly more effective than placebo on the HAM-D subscores for depressed mood, sleep disturbance, and the anxiety subfactor.

Two 6 week controlled studies (N = 671, randomized) comparing fluoxetine 20 mg and placebo have shown fluoxetine 20 mg daily to be effective in the treatment of elderly patients (≥60 years of age) with MDD. In these studies, fluoxetine produced a significantly higher rate of response and remission as defined, respectively, by a 50% decrease in the HAM-D score and a total endpoint HAM-D score of ≤8. Fluoxetine was well tolerated and the rate of treatment discontinuations due to adverse reactions did not differ between fluoxetine (12%) and placebo (9%).

A study was conducted involving depressed outpatients who had responded (modified HAMD-17 score of ≤7 during each of the last 3 weeks of open-label treatment and absence of MDD by DSM-III-R criteria) by the end of an initial 12 week open-treatment phase on fluoxetine 20 mg/day. These patients (N = 298) were randomized to continuation on double-blind fluoxetine 20 mg/day or placebo. At 38 weeks (50 weeks total), a statistically significantly lower relapse rate (defined as symptoms sufficient to meet a diagnosis of MDD for 2 weeks or a modified HAMD-17 score of ≥14 for 3 weeks) was observed for patients taking fluoxetine compared with those on placebo.

Pediatric (children and adolescents)—The efficacy of fluoxetine 20 mg/day in children and adolescents (N = 315 randomized; 170 children ages 8 to <13, 145 adolescents ages 13 to ≤18) was studied in two 8 to 9 week placebo-controlled clinical trials in depressed outpatients whose diagnoses corresponded most closely to the DSM-III-R or DSM-IV category of MDD. In both studies independently, fluoxetine produced a statistically significantly greater mean change on the Childhood Depression Rating Scale-Revised (CDRS-R) total score from baseline to endpoint than did placebo.

Subgroup analyses on the CDRS-R total score did not suggest any differential responsiveness on the basis of age or gender.

14.2 Obsessive Compulsive Disorder

Adult — The effectiveness of fluoxetine for the treatment of OCD was demonstrated in two 13 week, multicenter, parallel group studies (Studies 1 and 2) of adult outpatients who received fixed fluoxetine doses of 20, 40, or 60 mg/day (on a once-a-day schedule, in the morning) or placebo. Patients in both studies had moderate to severe OCD (DSM-III-R), with mean baseline ratings on the Yale-Brown Obsessive Compulsive Scale (YBOCS, total score) ranging from 22 to 26. In Study 1, patients receiving fluoxetine experienced mean reductions of approximately 4 to 6 units on the YBOCS total score, compared with a 1 unit reduction for placebo patients. In Study 2, patients receiving fluoxetine experienced mean reductions of approximately 4 to 9 units on the YBOCS total score, compared with a 1 unit reduction for placebo patients. While there was no indication of a dose-response relationship for effectiveness in Study 1, a dose-response relationship was observed in Study 2, with numerically better responses in the 2 higher dose groups. *Table 5* provides the outcome classification by treatment group on the Clinical Global Impression (CGI) improvement scale for Studies 1 and 2 combined:

[See table 5 at top of next page]

Exploratory analyses for age and gender effects on outcome did not suggest any differential responsiveness on the basis of age or sex.

Pediatric (children and adolescents) — In one 13 week clinical trial in pediatric patients (N = 103 randomized; 75 children ages 7 to <13, 28 adolescents ages 13 to <18) with OCD (DSM-IV), patients received fluoxetine 10 mg/day for 2 weeks, followed by 20 mg/day for 2 weeks. The dose was then adjusted in the range of 20 to 60 mg/day on the basis of clinical response and tolerability. Fluoxetine produced a statistically significantly greater mean change from baseline to endpoint than did placebo as measured by the Children's Yale-Brown Obsessive Compulsive Scale (CY-BOCS).

Subgroup analyses on outcome did not suggest any differential responsiveness on the basis of age or gender.

14.3 Bulimia Nervosa

The effectiveness of fluoxetine for the treatment of bulimia was demonstrated in two 8 week and one 16 week, multicenter, parallel group studies of adult outpatients meeting DSM-III-R criteria for bulimia. Patients in the 8 week studies received either 20 or 60 mg/day of fluoxetine or placebo in the morning. Patients in the 16 week study received a

Table 5. Outcome Classification (%) on CGI Improvement Scale for Completers in Pool of Two OCD Studies

Outcome Classification	Placebo	Fluoxetine		
		20 mg	40 mg	60 mg
Worse	8%	0%	0%	0%
No change	64%	41%	33%	29%
Minimally improved	17%	23%	28%	24%
Much improved	8%	28%	27%	28%
Very much improved	3%	8%	12%	19%

fixed fluoxetine dose of 60 mg/day (once a day) or placebo. Patients in these 3 studies had moderate to severe bulimia with median binge-eating and vomiting frequencies ranging from 7 to 10 per week and 5 to 9 per week, respectively. In these 3 studies, fluoxetine 60 mg, but not 20 mg, was statistically significantly superior to placebo in reducing the number of binge-eating and vomiting episodes per week. The statistically significantly superior effect of 60 mg versus placebo was present as early as Week 1 and persisted throughout each study.

The fluoxetine-related reduction in bulimic episodes appeared to be independent of baseline depression as assessed by the Hamilton Depression Rating Scale. In each of these 3 studies, the treatment effect, as measured by differences between fluoxetine 60 mg and placebo on median reduction from baseline in frequency of bulimic behaviors at endpoint, ranged from 1 to 2 episodes per week for binge-eating and 2 to 4 episodes per week for vomiting. The size of the effect was related to baseline frequency, with greater reductions seen in patients with higher baseline frequencies. Although some patients achieved freedom from binge-eating and purging as a result of treatment, for the majority, the benefit was a partial reduction in the frequency of binge-eating and purging.

In a longer-term trial, 150 patients meeting DSM-IV criteria for Bulimia Nervosa, purging subtype, who had responded during a single-blind, 8 week acute treatment phase with fluoxetine 60 mg/day, were randomized to continuation of fluoxetine 60 mg/day or placebo, for up to 52 weeks of observation for relapse. Response during the single-blind phase was defined by having achieved at least a 50% decrease in vomiting frequency compared with baseline. Relapse during the double-blind phase was defined as a persistent return to baseline vomiting frequency or physician judgment that the patient had relapsed. Patients receiving continued fluoxetine 60 mg/day experienced a significantly longer time to relapse over the subsequent 52 weeks compared with those receiving placebo.

14.4 Panic Disorder

The effectiveness of fluoxetine in the treatment of Panic Disorder was demonstrated in 2 double-blind, randomized, placebo-controlled, multicenter studies of adult outpatients who had a primary diagnosis of Panic Disorder (DSM-IV), with or without agoraphobia.

Study 1 ($N = 180$ randomized) was a 12 week flexible-dose study. Fluoxetine was initiated at 10 mg/day for the first week, after which patients were dosed in the range of 20 to 60 mg/day on the basis of clinical response and tolerability. A statistically significantly greater percentage of fluoxetine-treated patients were free from panic attacks at endpoint than placebo-treated patients, 42% versus 28%, respectively.

Study 2 ($N = 214$ randomized) was a 12 week flexible-dose study. Fluoxetine was initiated at 10 mg/day for the first week, after which patients were dosed in a range of 20 to 60 mg/day on the basis of clinical response and tolerability. A statistically significantly greater percentage of fluoxetine-treated patients were free from panic attacks at endpoint than placebo-treated patients, 62% versus 44%, respectively.

16 HOW SUPPLIED/STORAGE AND HANDLING

16.1 How Supplied

Fluoxetine tablets, USP 60 mg, are available as 60 mg (fluoxetine base equivalent), film coated, functional scored, capsule-shaped, white tablets debossed with "FL 60" on one side ("FL" above the score and "60" below the score) in bottles of 30 tablets (NDC 49909-005-30).

16.2 Storage and Handling

Store at 20 °C to 25 °C (68 °F to 77 °F) [See USP Controlled Room Temperature]. Protect from light.

17 PATIENT COUNSELING INFORMATION

See FDA-approved patient labeling (Medication Guide).
Patients should be advised of the following issues and asked to alert their prescriber if these occur while taking fluoxetine.

17.1 Information on Medication Guide and Benefits/Risks of Fluoxetine

Healthcare providers should instruct their patients to read the Medication Guide before starting therapy with fluoxetine tablets and to reread it each time the prescription is renewed.

Healthcare providers should inform patients, their families, and their caregivers about the benefits and risks associated with treatment with fluoxetine tablets and should counsel them in its appropriate use. Healthcare providers should instruct patients, their families, and their caregivers to read the Medication Guide and should assist them in understanding its contents. Patients should be given the opportunity to discuss the contents of the Medication Guide and to obtain answers to any questions they may have.

Patients should be advised of the following issues and asked to alert their healthcare provider if these occur while taking fluoxetine tablets.

17.2 Clinical Worsening and Suicide Risk

Patients, their families, and their caregivers should be encouraged to be alert to the emergence of anxiety, agitation, panic attacks, insomnia, irritability, hostility, aggressiveness, impulsivity, akathisia (psychomotor restlessness), hypomania, mania, other unusual changes in behavior, worsening of depression, and suicidal ideation, especially early during antidepressant treatment and when the dose is adjusted up or down. Families and caregivers of patients should be advised to look for the emergence of such symptoms on a day-to-day basis, since changes may be abrupt. Such symptoms should be reported to the patient's prescriber or health professional, especially if they are severe, abrupt in onset, or were not part of the patient's presenting symptoms. Symptoms such as these may be associated with an increased risk for suicidal thinking and behavior and indicate a need for very close monitoring and possibly changes in the medication [see Boxed Warning and Warnings and Precautions (5.1)].

17.3 Serotonin Syndrome or Neuroleptic Malignant Syndrome (NMS)-Like Reactions

Patients should be cautioned about the risk of serotonin syndrome or NMS-like reactions with the concomitant use of fluoxetine and triptans, tramadol, or other serotonergic agents [see Warnings and Precautions (5.2) and Drug Interactions (7.3)].

Patients should be advised of the signs and symptoms associated with serotonin syndrome or NMS-like reactions that may include mental status changes (e.g., agitation, hallucinations, coma), autonomic instability (e.g., tachycardia, labile blood pressure, hyperthermia), neuromuscular aberrations (e.g., hyperreflexia, incoordination) and/or gastrointestinal symptoms (e.g., nausea, vomiting, diarrhea). Serotonin syndrome, in its most severe form can resemble neuroleptic malignant syndrome, in which the symptoms may include hyperthermia, muscle rigidity, autonomic instability with possible rapid fluctuation of vital signs, and mental status changes. Patients should be cautioned to seek medical care immediately if they experience these symptoms.

17.4 Allergic Reactions and Rash

Patients should be advised to notify their physician if they develop a rash or hives [see Warnings and Precautions (5.3)]. Patients should also be advised of the signs and symptoms associated with a severe allergic reaction, including swelling of the face, eyes, or mouth, or have trouble breathing. Patients should be cautioned to seek medical care immediately if they experience these symptoms.

17.5 Abnormal Bleeding

Patients should be cautioned about the concomitant use of fluoxetine and NSAIDs, aspirin, warfarin, or other drugs that affect coagulation since combined use of psychotropic drugs that interfere with serotonin reuptake and these agents have been associated with an increased risk of bleeding [see Warnings and Precautions (5.7) and Drug Interactions (7.6)]. Patients should be advised to call their doctor if they experience any increased or unusual bruising or bleeding while taking fluoxetine.

17.6 Angle Closure Glaucoma

Patients should be advised that taking fluoxetine can cause mild pupillary dilation, which in susceptible individuals, can lead to an episode of angle closure glaucoma. Pre-existing glaucoma is almost always open-angle glaucoma because angle closure glaucoma, when diagnosed, can be treated definitively with iridectomy. Open-angle glaucoma is not a risk factor for angle closure glaucoma. Patients may wish to be examined to determine whether they are susceptible to angle closure, and have a prophylactic procedure (e.g., iridectomy), if they are susceptible. [see Warning and Precautions (5.8)]

17.7 Hyponatremia

Patients should be advised that hyponatremia has been reported as a result of treatment with SNRIs and SSRIs, including fluoxetine. Signs and symptoms of hyponatremia include headache, difficulty concentrating, memory impairment, confusion, weakness, and unsteadiness, which may lead to falls. More severe and/or acute cases have been associated with hallucination, syncope, seizure, coma, respiratory arrest, and death [see Warnings and Precautions (5.9)].

17.8 Potential for Cognitive and Motor Impairment

Fluoxetine may impair judgment, thinking, or motor skills. Patients should be advised to avoid driving a car or operating hazardous machinery until they are reasonably certain that their performance is not affected [see Warnings and Precautions (5.12)].

17.9 Use of Concomitant Medications

Patients should be advised to inform their physician if they are taking, or plan to take, any prescription medication, including Prozac® (fluoxetine hydrochloride), Symbyax® (olanzapine and fluoxetine hydrochloride capsules), Sarafem® (fluoxetine tablets), or over-the-counter drugs, including herbal supplements or alcohol. Patients should also be advised to inform their physicians if they plan to discontinue any medications while they are taking while on fluoxetine.

17.10 Discontinuation of Treatment

Patients should be advised to take fluoxetine exactly as prescribed, and to continue taking fluoxetine as prescribed even after their symptoms improve. Patients should be advised that they should not alter their dosing regimen, or stop taking fluoxetine without consulting their physician [see Warnings and Precautions (5.14)]. Patients should be advised to consult with their healthcare provider if their symptoms do not improve with fluoxetine.

17.11 Use in Specific Populations

Pregnancy — Patients should be advised to notify their physician if they become pregnant or intend to become pregnant during therapy. Fluoxetine should be used during pregnancy only if the potential benefit justifies the potential risk to the fetus [see Use in Specific Populations (8.1)].

Nursing Mothers — Patients should be advised to notify their physician if they intend to breast-feed an infant during therapy. Because fluoxetine is excreted in human milk, nursing while taking fluoxetine is not recommended [see Use in Specific Populations (8.3)].

Pediatric Use — Fluoxetine is approved for use in pediatric patients with MDD and OCD [see Boxed Warning and Warnings and Precautions (5.1)]. Limited evidence is available concerning the longer-term effects of fluoxetine on the development and maturation of children and adolescent patients. Height and weight should be monitored periodically in pediatric patients receiving fluoxetine. Doses greater than 20 mg/day have not been studied in pediatric patients with MDD.

Symbyax and Prozac are registered trademarks of Eli Lilly and Company.

Sarafem is a registered trademark of Warner Chilcott.

Manufactured and packaged for:
Edgemont Pharmaceuticals, LLC
Austin, TX 78746
Manufactured by:
Orion Pharmaceuticals
FIN-02200
Espoo, Finland
Packaged by:
Patheon Puerto Rico, Inc.
Manati, Puerto Rico 00674
Revised June 2014
FXT_V3

MEDICATION GUIDE
FLUOXETINE TABLETS

Read the Medication Guide that comes with fluoxetine before you start taking it and each time you get a refill. There may be new information. This Medication Guide does not take the place of talking to your healthcare provider about your medical condition or treatment. Talk with your healthcare provider if there is something you do not understand or want to learn more about.

What is the most important information I should know about fluoxetine?

Fluoxetine and other antidepressant medicines may cause serious side effects, including:

1. Suicidal thoughts or actions:

- **Fluoxetine and other antidepressant medicines may increase suicidal thoughts or actions** in some children, teenagers, or young adults within the **first few months of treatment or when the dose is changed.**
- Depression or other serious mental illnesses are the most important causes of suicidal thoughts or actions.
- Watch for these changes and call your healthcare provider right away if you notice:
  - New or sudden changes in mood, behavior, actions, thoughts, or feelings, especially if severe.
  - Pay particular attention to such changes when fluoxetine is started or when the dose is changed.

Keep all follow-up visits with your healthcare provider and call between visits if you are worried about symptoms.

Call your healthcare provider right away if you have any of the following symptoms, or call 911 if an emergency, especially if they are new, worse, or worry you:

- attempts to commit suicide
- acting on dangerous impulses
- acting aggressive or violent
- thoughts about suicide or dying
- new or worse depression
- new or worse anxiety or panic attacks
- feeling agitated, restless, angry or irritable
- trouble sleeping
- an increase in activity or talking more than what is normal for you
- other unusual changes in behavior or mood

Call your healthcare provider right away if you have any of the following symptoms, or call 911 if an emergency. Fluoxetine may be associated with these serious side effects:

2. Serotonin Syndrome or Neuroleptic Malignant Syndrome-like reactions. This condition can be life-threatening and may include:

- agitation, hallucinations, coma or other changes in mental status
- coordination problems or muscle twitching (overactive reflexes)
- racing heartbeat, high or low blood pressure
- sweating or fever
- nausea, vomiting, or diarrhea
- muscle rigidity

3. Severe allergic reactions:

- trouble breathing
- swelling of the face, tongue, eyes or mouth
- rash, itchy welts (hives) or blisters, alone or with fever or joint pain

4. Abnormal bleeding: Fluoxetine and other antidepressant medicines may increase your risk of bleeding or bruising, especially if you take the blood thinner warfarin (Coumadin®, Jantoven®), a non-steroidal anti-inflammatory drug (NSAIDs, like ibuprofen or naproxen), or aspirin.

5. Visual problems

- eye pain
- changes in vision
- swelling or redness in or around the eye

Only some people are at risk for these problems. You may want to undergo an eye examination to see if you are at risk and receive preventative treatment if you are.

6. Seizures or convulsions

7. Manic episodes:

- greatly increased energy
- severe trouble sleeping
- racing thoughts
- reckless behavior
- unusually grand ideas
- excessive happiness or irritability
- talking more or faster than usual

8. Changes in appetite or weight. Children and adolescents should have height and weight monitored during treatment.

9. Low salt (sodium) levels in the blood. Elderly people may be at greater risk for this. Symptoms may include:

- headache
- weakness or feeling unsteady
- confusion, problems concentrating or thinking or memory problems

Do not stop fluoxetine without first talking to your healthcare provider. Stopping fluoxetine too quickly may cause serious symptoms including:

- anxiety, irritability, high or low mood, feeling restless or changes in sleep habits
- headache, nausea, dizziness
- electric shock-like sensations, shaking, confusion

What is fluoxetine?

Fluoxetine is a prescription medicine used to treat depression. It is important to talk with your healthcare provider about the risks of treating depression and also the risks of not treating it. You should discuss all treatment choices with your healthcare provider.

Fluoxetine is used to treat:

- Major Depressive Disorder (MDD)
- Obsessive Compulsive Disorder (OCD)
- Bulimia Nervosa*
- Panic Disorder*
- Depressive episodes associated with Bipolar I Disorder, taken with olanzapine (Zyprexa)*
- Treatment Resistant Depression (depression that has not gotten better with at least 2 other treatments), taken with olanzapine (Zyprexa)*

*Not approved for use in children.

Talk to your healthcare provider if you do not think that your condition is getting better with fluoxetine treatment.

Who should not take fluoxetine?

Do not take fluoxetine if you:

- are allergic to fluoxetine hydrochloride or any of the ingredients in fluoxetine. See the end of this Medication Guide for a complete list of ingredients in fluoxetine.
- take a Monoamine Oxidase Inhibitor (MAOI). Ask your healthcare provider or pharmacist if you are not sure if you take an MAOI.
  - Do not take an MAOI within 5 weeks of stopping fluoxetine.
  - Do not start fluoxetine if you stopped taking an MAOI in the last 2 weeks.

People who take fluoxetine close in time to an MAOI may have serious or even life-threatening side effects. Get medical help right away if you have any of these symptoms:

  - high fever
  - uncontrolled muscle spasms
  - stiff muscles
  - rapid changes in heart rate or blood pressure
  - confusion
  - loss of consciousness (pass out)

- take Mellaril® (thioridazine). **Do not take Mellaril with in 5 weeks of stopping fluoxetine because** this can cause **serious heart rhythm problems or sudden** death.
- take the antipsychotic medicine pimozide (Orap®) be cause this can cause serious heart problems.

What should I tell my healthcare provider before taking fluoxetine? Ask if you are not sure.

Before starting fluoxetine, tell your healthcare provider if you:

- are taking certain drugs or treatments such as:
  - Triptans used to treat migraine headache
  - Medicines used to treat mood, anxiety, psychotic or thought disorders, including tricyclics, lithium, SSRIs, SNRIs, MAOIs (including linezolid, an antibiotic), or antipsychotics
  - Tramadol
  - Over-the-counter supplements such as tryptophan or St. John's Wort
  - Electroconvulsive therapy (ECT)
- have liver problems
- have kidney problems
- have heart problems
- have or had seizures or convulsions
- have bipolar disorder or mania
- have low sodium levels in your blood
- have a history of a stroke
- have high blood pressure
- have or had bleeding problems
- are pregnant or plan to become pregnant. It is not known if fluoxetine will harm your unborn baby. Talk to your healthcare provider about the benefits and risks of treating depression during pregnancy.
- are breast-feeding or plan to breast-feed. Some fluoxetine may pass into your breast milk. Talk to your healthcare provider about the best way to feed your baby while taking fluoxetine.

Tell your healthcare provider about all the medicines that you take, including prescription and non-prescription medicines, vitamins, and herbal supplements. Fluoxetine and some medicines may interact with each other, may not work as well, or may cause serious side effects.

Your healthcare provider or pharmacist can tell you if it is safe to take fluoxetine with your other medicines. Do not start or stop any medicine while taking fluoxetine without talking to your healthcare provider first.

> If you take fluoxetine, you should not take any other medicines that contain fluoxetine hydrochloride including:
> - Symbax® (olanzapine and fluoxetine hydrochloride)
> - Sarafem® (fluoxetine)
> - Prozac®
> - Prozac® Weekly™

How should I take fluoxetine?

- Take fluoxetine exactly as prescribed. Your healthcare provider may need to change the dose of fluoxetine until it is the right dose for you. Each tablet can be broken in half (along the functional score).
- Fluoxetine may be taken with or without food.
- If you miss a dose of fluoxetine, take the missed dose as soon as you remember. If it is almost time for the next dose, skip the missed dose and take your next dose at the regular time. Do not take two doses of fluoxetine at the same time.
- If you take too much fluoxetine, call your healthcare provider or poison control center right away, or get emergency treatment.

What should I avoid while taking fluoxetine?

Fluoxetine can cause sleepiness or may affect your ability to make decisions, think clearly, or react quickly. You should not drive, operate heavy machinery, or do other dangerous activities until you know how fluoxetine affects you. Do not drink alcohol while using fluoxetine.

What are the possible side effects of fluoxetine?

Fluoxetine may cause serious side effects, including:

- See "What is the most important information I should know about fluoxetine?"
- **Problems with blood sugar control.** People who have diabetes and take fluoxetine may have problems with low blood sugar while taking fluoxetine. High blood sugar can happen when fluoxetine is stopped. Your healthcare provider may need to change the dose of your diabetes medicines when you start or stop taking fluoxetine.
- **Feeling anxious or trouble sleeping**

Common possible side effects in people who take fluoxetine include:

- unusual dreams
- sexual problems
- loss of appetite, diarrhea, indigestion, nausea or vomiting, weakness, or dry mouth
- flu symptoms
- feeling tired or fatigued
- change in sleep habits
- yawning
- sinus infection or sore throat
- tremor or shaking
- sweating
- feeling anxious or nervous
- hot flashes
- rash

Other side effects in children and adolescents include:

- increased thirst
- abnormal increase in muscle movement or agitation
- nose bleed
- urinating more often
- heavy menstrual periods
- possible slowed growth rate and weight change. Your child's height and weight should be monitored during treatment with fluoxetine.

Tell your healthcare provider if you have any side effect that bothers you or that does not go away. These are not all the possible side effects of fluoxetine. For more information, ask your healthcare provider or pharmacist.

Call your doctor for medical advice about side effects. You may report side effects to the FDA at 1-800-FDA-1088.

How should I store fluoxetine?

- Store fluoxetine at room temperature between 68 °F and 77 °F (20 °C to 25 °C).
- Keep fluoxetine away from light.
- Keep fluoxetine bottle closed tightly.

Keep fluoxetine and all medicines out of the reach of children.

General information about fluoxetine

Medicines are sometimes prescribed for purposes other than those listed in a Medication Guide. Do not use fluoxetine for a condition for which it was not prescribed. Do not give fluoxetine to other people, even if they have the same condition. It may harm them.

This Medication Guide summarizes the most important information about fluoxetine. If you would like more information, talk with your healthcare provider. You may ask your healthcare provider or pharmacist for information about fluoxetine that is written for healthcare professionals.

For more information about fluoxetine call 1-888-594-4332.

What are the ingredients in fluoxetine tablets, 60 mg?

Active ingredient: fluoxetine hydrochloride

Inactive ingredients: mannitol, microcrystalline cellulose, maize starch, povidone, hypromellose, magnesium stearate, titanium dioxide, sucrose, glycerol, and polysorbate.

This Medication Guide has been approved by the U.S. Food and Drug Administration.

Symbyax and Prozac are registered trademarks of Eli Lilly and Company.

Prozac Weekly is a registered trademark of Eli Lilly and Company.

Sarafem is a registered trademark of Warner Chilcott.

Mellaril is a registered trademark of Novartis AG Corporation.

Orap is a registered trademark of Teva Pharmaceuticals USA.

Coumadin is a registered trademark of Bristol Myers Squibb.

Jantoven is a registered trademark of Upsher-Smith Laboratories Inc.

Manufactured and packaged for:
Edgemont Pharmaceuticals, LLC
Austin, TX 78746
Manufactured by:
Orion Pharmaceuticals
FIN-02200
Espoo, Finland
Packaged by:
Patheon Puerto Rico, Inc.
Manati, Puerto Rico 00674
Revised June 2014
FXT_V3
Shown in Product Identification Guide, page 306

FORFIVO XL   ℞
(bupropion hydrochloride extended-release tablets) for oral use

HIGHLIGHTS OF PRESCRIBING INFORMATION
These highlights do not include all the information needed to use FORFIVO XL safely and effectively. See full prescribing information for FORFIVO XL.
FORFIVO XL (bupropion hydrochloride extended-release tablets), for oral use
Initial U.S. Approval: 1985

RECENT MAJOR CHANGES

Warnings and Precautions (5.6)   06/2014

WARNING: SUICIDALITY and ANTIDEPRESSANT DRUGS; PSYCHIATRIC EVENTS and SMOKING CESSATION
See full prescribing information for complete boxed warning
- **Increased risk of suicidal thinking and behavior in children, adolescents, and young adults taking antidepressants for Major Depressive Disorder (MDD) and other psychiatric disorders. Closely monitor for clinical worsening and suicidal thinking and behavior (5.1).**
- **Serious neuropsychiatric events, including depression, suicidal ideation, suicide attempt, and completed suicide have been reported in patients taking bupropion for smoking cessation. Stop bupropion and contact a healthcare provider immediately if agitation, hostility, depressed mood, or changes in thinking or behavior that are not typical for the patient are observed, or if the patient develops suicidal ideation or suicidal behavior (5.2).**

INDICATIONS AND USAGE

FORFIVO XL is an aminoketone indicated for the treatment of major depressive disorder (1). The efficacy was established in two 4 week trials, one 6 week trial with bupropion immediate release formulation and one maintenance trial with bupropion sustained-release formulation, all in adults (14).

DOSAGE AND ADMINISTRATION

- Use one tablet (450 mg) once daily without regard to food (2.1).
- Swallow the tablet whole. Do not chew, divide, or crush (2.1).
- Do not initiate treatment with FORFIVO XL. Use another bupropion formulation for initial dose titration (2.2).
- Can be used in patients who are receiving 300 mg/day of another bupropion formulation for at least 2 weeks, and require a dosage of 450 mg/day (2.2).
- Patients who are currently being treated with other bupropion products at 450 mg/day can be switched to equivalent dose of FORFIVO XL once daily (2.2).

DOSAGE FORMS AND STRENGTHS

- Extended-release tablets: 450 mg (3)

CONTRAINDICATIONS

- Seizure disorder (4)
- Current use of other bupropion products (4)
- Current or prior diagnosis of bulimia or anorexia nervosa (4)
- Abrupt discontinuation of alcohol or sedatives (4)
- Use with monoamine oxidase (MAO) inhibitor: stop at least 2 weeks prior to bupropion use (4)
- Known hypersensitivity to bupropion or other ingredients of FORFIVO XL. (4, 5.10)

WARNINGS AND PRECAUTIONS

- Activation of mania/ hypomania: Screen patients for bipolar disorder and monitor for manic symptoms. (5.3)
- Seizure risk: The risk is dose-dependent. Discontinue if seizure occurs (4, 5.4, 7.6)
- Psychosis and other neuropsychiatric events: Discontinue if these events occur. (5.5)
- Angle Closure Glaucoma: Angle closure glaucoma has occurred in patients with untreated anatomically narrow angles treated with antidepressants (5.6)
- Severe hypertension: Monitor blood pressure periodically. (5.7)

ADVERSE REACTIONS

Most common adverse reactions are (incidence ≥ 5%; ≥ 2 times placebo rate): Dry mouth, nausea, insomnia, dizziness, pharyngitis, abdominal pain, agitation, anxiety, tremor, palpitation, sweating, tinnitus, myalgia, anorexia, urinary frequency, rash (6.1)
To report SUSPECTED ADVERSE REACTIONS, contact Edgemont Pharmaceuticals, LLC at 1-888- 594-4332 or FDA at 1-800-FDA-1088 or www.fda.gov/medwatch.

DRUG INTERACTIONS

- Ticlopidine or clopidogrel: May increase bupropion exposure. Coadministration of FORFIVO XL with ticlopidine or clopidogrel is not recommended (7.1)
- Drugs metabolized by CYP2D6 (e.g., desipramine, paroxetine, fluoxetine, sertraline, venlafaxine): Consider dose reduction when using with bupropion. Bupropion & hydroxybupropion inhibit CYP2D6 (7.2)
- Nicotine transdermal system: Monitor for severe hypertension (5.7, 7.3)
- Drug laboratory test interactions: May cause false-positive urine immunoassay screening test results for amphetamines (7.4).

USE IN SPECIFIC POPULATIONS

- Pregnancy: Use only if the potential benefit justifies the potential risk to the fetus (8.1)
- Nursing: Can be secreted in human milk. A decision whether to discontinue nursing or to discontinue the drug, should be made taking into account the importance of the drug to the mother. (8.3).
- Renal Impairment: Since there is no lower dose strength for FORFIVO XL, FORFIVO XL is not recommended in patients with renal impairment (8.6)
- Hepatic Impairment: Since there is no lower dose strength for FORFIVO XL, FORFIVO XL is not recommended in patients with hepatic impairment (8.7)

See 17 for PATIENT COUNSELING INFORMATION and Medication Guide

Revised: 09/2014

FULL PRESCRIBING INFORMATION: CONTENTS*

FULL PRESCRIBING INFORMATION

WARNING: SUICIDALITY and ANTIDEPRESSANT DRUGS; PSYCHIATRIC EVENTS and SMOKING CESSATION

SUICIDALITY and ANTIDEPRESSANT DRUGS:
Antidepressants increased the risk compared to placebo of suicidal thinking and behavior (suicidality) in children, adolescents, and young adults in short-term studies of major depressive disorder (MDD) and other psychiatric disorders. Anyone considering the use of FORFIVO XL or any other antidepressant in a child, adolescent, or young adult must balance this risk with the clinical need. Short-term studies did not show an increase in the risk of suicidality with antidepressants compared to placebo in adults beyond age 24; there was a reduction in risk with antidepressants compared to placebo in adults aged 65 and older. Depression and certain other psychiatric disorders are themselves associated with increases in the risk of suicide. Patients of all ages who are started on antidepressant therapy should be monitored appropriately and observed closely for clinical worsening, suicidality, or unusual changes in behavior. Families and caregivers should be advised of the need for close observation and communication with the prescriber. FORFIVO XL is not approved for use in pediatric patients [*see Warnings and Precautions (5.1)*].

PSYCHIATRIC EVENTS and SMOKING CESSATION:
FORVIVO XL is not approved for smoking cessation treatment, but bupropion under the name ZYBAN® is approved for this use. Serious neuropsychiatric events, including but not limited to depression, suicidal ideation, suicide attempt, and completed suicide have been reported in patients taking bupropion for smoking cessation. Some cases may have been complicated by the symptoms of nicotine withdrawal in patients who stopped smoking. Depressed mood may be a symptom of nicotine withdrawal. Depression, rarely including suicidal ideation, has been reported in smokers undergoing a smoking cessation attempt without medication. However, some of these symptoms have occurred in patients taking bupropion who continued to smoke.
All patients being treated with bupropion for smoking cessation treatment should be observed for neuropsychiatric symptoms including changes in behavior, hostility, agitation, depressed mood, and suicide-related events, including ideation, behavior, and attempted suicide. These symptoms, as well as worsening of pre-existing psychiatric illness and completed suicide have been reported in some patients attempting to quit smoking while taking ZYBAN in the postmarketing experience. When symptoms were reported, most were during treatment with ZYBAN, but some were following discontinuation of treatment with ZYBAN. These events have occurred in patients with and without pre-existing psychiatric disease; some have experienced worsening of their psychiatric illnesses. Patients with serious psychiatric illness such as schizophrenia, bipolar disorder, and major depressive disorder did not participate in the premarketing studies of ZYBAN.

Advise patients and caregivers that the patient using bupropion for smoking cessation should stop taking bupropion and contact a healthcare provider immediately if agitation, hostility, depressed mood, or changes in thinking or behavior that are not typical for the patient are observed, or if the patient develops suicidal ideation or suicidal behavior. In many post-marketing cases, resolution of symptoms after discontinuation of ZYBAN was reported, although in some cases the symptoms persisted; therefore, ongoing monitoring and supportive care should be provided until symptoms resolve.

The risks of using bupropion for smoking cessation should be weighed against the benefits of its use. ZYBAN has been demonstrated to increase the likelihood of abstinence from smoking for as long as 6 months compared to treatment with placebo. The health benefits of quitting smoking are immediate and substantial [see *Warnings and Precautions (5.2)* and *Patient Counseling Information (17)*].

1 INDICATIONS AND USAGE

FORFIVO XL (bupropion hydrochloride extended-release tablets) is indicated for the treatment of major depressive disorder (MDD).

The efficacy in the treatment of MDD was established in two 4-week and one 6-week and one maintenance trial in adult patients whose diagnoses corresponded most closely to the Major Depression category of the APA Diagnostic and Statistical Manual (DSM) [see *Clinical Studies (14)*].

A major depressive episode (DSM-IV) implies the presence of 1) depressed mood or 2) loss of interest or pleasure; in addition, at least 5 of the following symptoms have been present during the same 2-week period and represent a change from previous functioning: depressed mood, markedly diminished interest or pleasure in usual activities, significant change in weight and/or appetite, insomnia or hypersomnia, psychomotor agitation or retardation, increased fatigue, feelings of guilt or worthlessness, slowed thinking or impaired concentration, a suicide attempt, or suicidal ideation.

The efficacy of bupropion in pediatric population has not been established.

The physician who elects to use FORFIVO XL for extended periods should periodically reevaluate the long-term usefulness of the drug for the individual patient.

2 DOSAGE AND ADMINISTRATION

2.1 Instructions for Use

One tablet (450 mg) of FORFIVO XL should be taken once daily without regard to meals. FORFIVO XL tablet should be swallowed whole and not crushed, divided, or chewed.

2.2 Initial Treatment with FORFIVO XL

Do not initiate treatment with FORFIVO XL because 450 mg tablet is the only available dose formulation. Use another bupropion formulation for initial dose titration (referring to prescribing information of other bupropion products).

FORFIVO XL can be used in patients who are receiving 300 mg/day of another bupropion formulation for at least 2 weeks, and require a dosage of 450 mg/day.

Patients who are currently being treated with other bupropion products at 450 mg/day can be switched to equivalent dose of FORFIVO XL once daily.

2.3 Maintenance Treatment with FORFIVO XL

It is generally agreed that acute episodes of depression require several months or longer of sustained pharmacological therapy beyond response to the acute episode. It is unknown whether or not the 450 mg dose needed to achieve an initial response is identical to the dose needed for maintenance treatment. Patients should be periodically reassessed to determine the need for maintenance treatment and the appropriate dose for such treatment.

2.4 Patients with Impaired Hepatic Function

Since there is no lower dose strength for FORFIVO XL, FORFIVO XL is not recommended in patients with hepatic impairment [see *Use in Specific Population (8.7) and Clinical Pharmacology (12.3)*].

2.5 Patients with Impaired Renal Function

Since there is no lower dose strength for FORFIVO XL, FORFIVO XL is not recommended in patients with renal impairment [see *Use in Specific Populations (8.6) and Clinical Pharmacology (12.3)*].

3 DOSAGE FORMS AND STRENGTHS

FORFIVO XL Extended-Release Tablets, 450 mg of bupropion hydrochloride, are white to off white, oval tablets with the logo "Forfivo" printed on one side.

4 CONTRAINDICATIONS

FORFIVO XL is contraindicated in patients with the following:

• Seizure disorder because these patients may have a lower seizure threshold.
• Treated currently with other bupropion products because the incidence of seizure is dose dependent.
• Current or prior diagnosis of bulimia or anorexia nervosa because of a higher incidence of seizures noted in patients treated for bulimia with the immediate-release formulation of bupropion in a pre-marketing clinical trial.
• Undergoing abrupt discontinuation of alcohol or sedatives because of a lower seizure threshold in these conditions.
• Concurrent administration of monoamine oxidase (MAO) inhibitors because MAOIs potentially can enhance the CNS toxicity. At least 14 days should elapse between discontinuation of an MAO inhibitor and initiation of treatment with FORFIVO XL.
• Known hypersensitivity to bupropion or the other ingredients of FORFIVO XL tablets Anaphylactoid/anaphylactic reactions and Stevens-Johnson syndrome have been reported [see *Warnings and Precautions (5.10)*].

5 WARNINGS AND PRECAUTIONS

5.1 Clinical Worsening and Suicide Risk in Treating Psychiatric Disorder

Patients with major depressive disorder (MDD), both adult and pediatric, may experience worsening of their depression and/or the emergence of suicidal ideation and behavior (suicidality) or unusual changes in behavior, whether or not they are taking antidepressant medications, and this risk may persist until significant remission occurs. Suicide is a known risk of depression and certain other psychiatric disorders, and these disorders themselves are the strongest predictors of suicide. There has been a long-standing concern that antidepressants may have a role in inducing worsening of depression and the emergence of suicidality in certain patients during the early phases of treatment. Pooled analyses of short-term placebo-controlled trials of antidepressant drugs (SSRIs and others) show that these drugs increase the risk of suicidal thinking and behavior (suicidality) in children, adolescents, and young adults (ages 18-24) with major depressive disorder (MDD) and other psychiatric disorders. Short-term studies did not show an increase in the risk of suicidality with antidepressants compared to placebo in adults beyond age 24; there was a reduction with antidepressants compared to placebo in adults aged 65 and older.

The pooled analyses of placebo-controlled trials in children and adolescents with MDD, obsessive compulsive disorder (OCD), or other psychiatric disorders included a total of 24 short-term trials of 9 antidepressant drugs in over 4,400 patients. The pooled analyses of placebo-controlled trials in adults with MDD or other psychiatric disorders included a total of 295 short-term trials (median duration of 2 months) of 11 antidepressant drugs in over 77,000 patients. There was considerable variation in risk of suicidality among drugs, but a tendency toward an increase in the younger patients for almost all drugs studied. There were differences in absolute risk of suicidality across the different indications, with the highest incidence in MDD. The risk differences (drug vs. placebo), however, were relatively stable within age strata and across indications. These risk differences (drug-placebo difference in the number of cases of suicidality per 1,000 patients treated) are provided in **Table 1**.

Table 1. Drug-Placebo Difference in Number of Cases of Suicidality per 1,000 Patients Treated

Age Range	
	Increases Compared to Placebo
<18	14 additional cases
18-24	5 additional cases
	Decreases Compared to Placebo
25-64	1 fewer case
≥65	6 fewer cases

No suicides occurred in any of the pediatric trials. There were suicides in the adult trials, but the number was not sufficient to reach any conclusion about drug effect on suicide.

It is unknown whether the suicidality risk extends to longer-term use, i.e., beyond several months. However, there is substantial evidence from placebo-controlled maintenance trials in adults with depression that the use of antidepressants can delay the recurrence of depression.

All patients being treated with antidepressants for any indication should be monitored appropriately and observed closely for clinical worsening, suicidality, and unusual changes in behavior, especially during the initial few months of a course of drug therapy, or at times of dose changes, either increases or decreases [see *Boxed Warning and Use in Specific Populations (8.4)*].

The following symptoms, anxiety, agitation, panic attacks, insomnia, irritability, hostility, aggressiveness, impulsivity, akathisia (psychomotor restlessness), hypomania, and mania, have been reported in adult and pediatric patients being treated with antidepressants for major depressive disorder as well as for other indications, both psychiatric and nonpsychiatric. Although a causal link between the emergence of such symptoms and either the worsening of depression and/or the emergence of suicidal impulses has not been established, there is concern that such symptoms may represent precursors to emerging suicidality.

Consideration should be given to changing the therapeutic regimen, including possibly discontinuing the medication, in patients whose depression is persistently worse, or who are experiencing emergent suicidality or symptoms that might be precursors to worsening depression or suicidality, especially if these symptoms are severe, abrupt in onset, or were not part of the patient's presenting symptoms.

Families and caregivers of patients being treated with antidepressants for major depressive disorder or other indications, both psychiatric and nonpsychiatric, should be alerted about the need to monitor patients for the emergence of agitation, irritability, unusual changes in behavior, and the other symptoms described above, as well as the emergence of suicidality, and to report such symptoms immediately to health care providers. Such monitoring should include daily observation by families and caregivers [see *Patient Counseling Information (17)*]. Prescription for FORFIVO XL should be written for the smallest quantity of tablets consistent with good patient management, in order to reduce the risk of overdose.

5.2 Neuropsychiatric Symptoms and Suicide Risk in Smoking Cessation Treatment

FORFIVO XL is not approved forsmoking cessation treatment, but bupropion under the name ZYBAN is approved for this use. Serious neuropsychiatric symptoms have been reported in patients taking bupropion for smoking cessation [see *Boxed Warning and Adverse Reactions (6)*]. These have included changes in mood (including depression and mania), psychosis, hallucinations, paranoia, delusions, homicidal ideation, hostility, agitation, aggression, anxiety, and panic, as well as suicidal ideation, suicide attempt, and completed suicide [see *Patient Counseling Information (17)*].

5.3 Activation of Mania/Hypomania

A major depressive episode may be the initial presentation of bipolar disorder. It is generally believed (though not established in controlled trials) that treating such an episode with an antidepressant alone may increase the likelihood of precipitation of a mixed/manic episode in patients at risk for bipolar disorder. Prior to initiating treatment with an antidepressant, patients with depressive symptoms should be adequately screened to determine if they are at risk for bipolar disorder; such screening should include a detailed psychiatric history, including a family history of suicide, bipolar disorder, and depression. It should be noted that FORFIVO XL is not approved for use in treating bipolar depression.

5.4 Seizures

Bupropion is associated with a dose-related risk of seizures. The risk of seizures is also related to patient factors, clinical situations, and concomitant medications, which must be considered in selection of patients for therapy with FORFIVO XL. FORFIVO XL should be discontinued and not restarted in patients who experience a seizure while on treatment.

Dose

At doses up to 300 mg/day of the sustained-release formulation of bupropion hydrochloride (WELLBUTRIN SR®), the incidence of seizure is approximately 0.1% (1/1,000).

Data for the immediate-release formulation of bupropion hydrochloride revealed a seizure incidence of approximately 0.4% (i.e., 13 of 3,200 patients followed prospectively) in patients treated at doses in a range of 300 to 450 mg/day. This seizure incidence (0.4%) may exceed that of some other marketed antidepressants.

Additional data accumulated for the immediate-release formulation of bupropion hydrochloride suggested that the estimated seizure incidence increases almost tenfold between 450 and 600 mg/day. The 600 mg dose is twice the usual adult dose and one and one-third the maximum recommended daily dose (450 mg) of FORFIVO XL. This disproportionate increase in seizure incidence with dose incrementation calls for caution in dosing.

Patient Factors

Predisposing factors that may increase the risk of seizure with bupropion use include history of head trauma or prior seizure, central nervous system (CNS) tumor, the presence of severe hepatic cirrhosis, and concomitant medications that lower seizure threshold.

Clinical Situations

Circumstances associated with an increased seizure risk include, among others, excessive use of alcohol or sedatives;

addiction to opiates, cocaine, or stimulants; use of over-the-counter stimulants and anorectics; and diabetes treated with oral hypoglycemics or insulin.

Concomitant Medications

Many medications (e.g., antipsychotics, antidepressants, theophylline, and systemic steroids) are known to lower seizure threshold.

Recommendations for Reducing the Risk of Seizure:

Retrospective analysis of clinical experience gained during the development of bupropion suggests that the risk of seizure may be minimized if

- the total daily dose of bupropion does *not* exceed 450 mg;
- the rate of incrementation of the bupropion dose is gradual.

5.5 Psychosis and Other Neuropsychiatric Events

Depressed patients treated with bupropion have been reported to show a variety of neuropsychiatric signs and symptoms, including delusions, hallucinations, psychosis, concentration disturbance, paranoia, and confusion. In some cases, these symptoms abated upon dose reduction and/or withdrawal of treatment. It is recommended stopping bupropion when the symptoms occurred.

5.6 Angle Closure Glaucoma

Angle Closure Glaucoma: The pupillary dilation that occurs following use of many antidepressant drugs including FORFIVO XL may trigger an angle closure attack in a patient with anatomically narrow angles who does not have a patent iridectomy.

5.7 Severe Hypertension

In clinical practice, hypertension, in some cases severe, requiring acute treatment, has been reported in patients receiving bupropion alone and in combination with nicotine replacement therapy. These reactions have been observed in both patients with and without evidence of preexisting hypertension.

Data from a comparative study of the sustained-release formulation of bupropion hydrochloride (ZYBAN® Sustained-Release Tablets), nicotine transdermal system (NTS), the combination of sustained-release bupropion hydrochloride plus NTS, and placebo as an aid to smoking cessation suggest a higher incidence of treatment-emergent hypertension in patients treated with the combination of sustained-release bupropion hydrochloride and NTS. Monitoring of blood pressure is recommended in patients who receive the combination of bupropion and nicotine replacement.

There is no clinical experience establishing the safety of FORFIVO XL tablets in patients with a recent history of myocardial infarction or unstable heart disease. Therefore, care should be exercised if it is used in these groups.

Bupropion was well tolerated in depressed patients who had previously developed orthostatic hypotension while receiving tricyclic antidepressants, and was also generally well tolerated in a group of 36 depressed inpatients with stable congestive heart failure (CHF). However, bupropion was associated with a rise in supine blood pressure in the study of patients with CHF, resulting in discontinuation of treatment in 2 patients for exacerbation of baseline hypertension.

5.8 Agitation and Insomnia

Increased restlessness, agitation, anxiety, and insomnia, especially shortly after initiation of treatment, have been associated with treatment with bupropion.

Patients in placebo-controlled trials of major depressive disorder with sustained-release formulation of bupropion hydrochloride, experienced agitation, anxiety, and insomnia as shown in **Table 2**.

Table 2. Incidence of Agitation, Anxiety, and Insomnia in Placebo-Controlled Trials of Bupropion HCl Sustained-release Tablets for Major Depressive Disorder

Adverse Reactions Term	Bupropion HCl 300 mg/day (n = 376)	Bupropion HCl 400 mg/day (n = 114)	Placebo (n = 385)
Agitation	3%	9%	2%
Anxiety	5%	6%	3%
Insomnia	11%	16%	6%

In clinical studies of major depressive disorder, these symptoms were sometimes of sufficient magnitude to require treatment with sedative/hypnotic drugs.

Symptoms in these studies were sufficiently severe to require discontinuation of treatment in 1% and 2.6% of patients treated with 300 and 400 mg/day, respectively, of bupropion hydrochloride sustained-release tablets and 0.8% of patients treated with placebo.

5.9 Altered Appetite and Weight

In placebo-controlled short-term studies of major depressive disorder using the sustained-release formulation of bupropion hydrochloride, patients experienced weight gain or weight loss as shown in **Table 3**.

Table 3. Incidence of Weight Gain and Weight Loss in Placebo-Controlled Trials of Bupropion Hydrochloride Sustained-release tablets for Major Depressive Disorder

Weight Change	Bupropion HCl 300 mg/day (n = 339)	Bupropion HCl 400 mg/day (n = 112)	Placebo (n = 347)
Gained >5 lbs	3%	2%	4%
Lost >5 lbs	14%	19%	6%

In studies conducted with the immediate-release formulation of bupropion hydrochloride, 35% of patients receiving tricyclic antidepressants gained weight, compared to 9% of patients treated with the immediate-release formulation of bupropion hydrochloride. If weight loss is a major presenting sign of a patient's depressive illness, the anorectic and/or weight-reducing potential of FORFIVO XL tablets should be considered.

5.10 Hypersensitivity Reactions

Anaphylactoid/anaphylactic reactions characterized by symptoms such as pruritus, urticaria, angioedema, and dyspnea requiring medical treatment have been reported in clinical trials with bupropion. In addition, there have been rare spontaneous postmarketing reports of erythema multiforme, Stevens-Johnson syndrome, and anaphylactic shock associated with bupropion. A patient should stop taking FORFIVO XL and consult a doctor if experiencing allergic or anaphylactoid/anaphylactic reactions (e.g., skin rash, pruritus, hives, chest pain, edema, and shortness of breath) during treatment.

Arthralgia, myalgia, and fever with rash and other symptoms suggestive of delayed hypersensitivity have been reported in association with bupropion. These symptoms may resemble serum sickness [see **Contraindications (4)**].

6 ADVERSE REACTIONS

The following risks are discussed in greater detail in other sections of the labeling:

- Clinical worsening and suicide risk [see **Warnings and Precautions (5.1)**]
- Neuropsychiatric symptoms and suicide risk in smoking cessation treatment [see **Warnings and Precautions (5.2)**]
- Activation of mania or hypomania [see **Warnings and Precautions (5.3)**]
- Seizures [see **Warnings and Precautions (5.4)**]
- Psychosis, and other neuropsychiatric events [see **Warnings and Precautions (5.5)**]
- Angle Closure Glaucoma [see **Warnings and precautions (5.6)**]
- Severe hypertension [see **Warnings and Precautions (5.7)**]
- Agitation and insomnia [see **Warnings and Precautions (5.8)**]
- Altered appetite and weight [see **Warnings and Precautions (5.9)**]
- Hypersensitivity reactions [see **Warnings and Precautions (5.10)**]

6.1 Clinical Trials Experience

Commonly Observed Adverse Reactions in Controlled Clinical Trials

Because clinical trials are conducted under widely varying conditions, adverse reaction rates observed in the clinical trials of a drug cannot be directly compared to rates in the clinical trials of another drug and may not reflect the rates observed in clinical practice.

Adverse reactions from **Table 5** occurring in at least 5% of patients treated with the sustained-release formulation of bupropion hydrochloride and at a rate at least twice the placebo rate are listed below for the 300- and 400-mg/day dose groups.

300 mg/day of bupropion sustained release: Anorexia, dry mouth, rash, sweating, tinnitus, and tremor.

400 mg/day of bupropion sustained release: Abdominal pain, agitation, anxiety, dizziness, dry mouth, insomnia, myalgia, nausea, palpitation, pharyngitis, sweating, tinnitus, and urinary frequency.

FORFIVO XL is bioequivalent to three 150 mg tablets of WELLBUTRIN XL®, which has been demonstrated to have similar bioavailability both to the immediate-release formulation of bupropion and to the sustained-release formulation of bupropion. The information included under this subsection and under subsections **6.2** and **6.3** is based primarily on data from controlled clinical trials with the sustained-release formulation of bupropion hydrochloride.

Adverse Reactions Leading to Discontinuation of Treatment with Bupropion Immediate Release or Bupropion Sustained Release

In placebo-controlled clinical trials, 9% and 11% of patients treated with 300 and 400 mg/day, respectively, of the sustained-release formulation of bupropion hydrochloride

and 4% of patients treated with placebo discontinued treatment due to adverse reactions. The specific adverse reactions in these trials that led to discontinuation in at least 1% of patients treated with either 300 mg/day or 400 mg/day of the sustained-release formulation of bupropion hydrochloride, and at a rate at least twice the placebo rate are listed in **Table 4**.

Table 4. Treatment Discontinuations Due to Adverse Reactions in Placebo-Controlled Trials for Major Depressive Disorder using Bupropion Hydrochloride Sustained Release Formulation

Adverse Reaction	Bupropion HCl 300 mg/day (n = 376)	Bupropion HCl 400 mg/day (n = 114)	Placebo (n = 385)
Rash	2.4%	0.9%	0.0%
Nausea	0.8%	1.8%	0.3%
Agitation	0.3%	1.8%	0.3%
Migraine	0.0%	1.8%	0.3%

In clinical trials with the immediate-release formulation of bupropion, 10% of patients and volunteers discontinued due to an adverse reaction. Reactions resulting in discontinuation, in addition to those listed above for the sustained-release formulation of bupropion hydrochloride, include vomiting, seizures, and sleep disturbances.

Adverse Reactions Occurring at an Incidence of 1% or More Among Patients Treated With Bupropion Immediate Release or Bupropion Sustained Release

Table 5 enumerates adverse reactions that occurred among patients treated with 300 and 400 mg/day of the sustained-release formulation of bupropion hydrochloride and with placebo in controlled trials. Reactions that occurred in either the 300- or 400-mg/day group at an incidence of 1% or more and were more frequent than in the placebo group are included. Reported adverse reactions were classified using a COSTART-based Dictionary.

Accurate estimates of the incidence of adverse reactions associated with the use of any drug are difficult to obtain. Estimates are influenced by drug dose, detection technique, setting, physician judgments, etc. The figures cited cannot be used to predict precisely the incidence of untoward reactions in the course of usual medical practice where patient characteristics and other factors differ from those that prevailed in the clinical trials. These incidence figures also cannot be compared with those obtained from other clinical studies involving related drug products as each group of drug trials is conducted under a different set of conditions. Finally, it is important to emphasize that the tabulation does not reflect the relative severity and/or clinical importance of the reactions. A better perspective on the serious adverse reactions associated with the use of bupropion is provided in the **Warnings and Precautions (5)**.

Table 5. Adverse Reactions in Placebo-Controlled Trials* for Major Depressive Disorder

Body System/ Adverse Reaction	Bupropion HCl 300 mg/ day (n = 376)	Bupropion HCl 400 mg/ day (n = 114)	Placebo (n = 385)
Body (General)			
Headache	26%	25%	23%
Infection	8%	9%	6%
Abdominal pain	3%	9%	2%
Asthenia	2%	4%	2%
Chest pain	3%	4%	1%
Pain	2%	3%	2%
Fever	1%	2%	—
Cardiovascular			
Palpitation	2%	6%	2%
Flushing	1%	4%	—
Migraine	1%	4%	1%
Hot flashes	1%	3%	1%
Digestive			
Dry mouth	17%	24%	7%
Nausea	13%	18%	8%
Constipation	10%	5%	7%
Diarrhea	5%	7%	6%
Anorexia	5%	3%	2%
Vomiting	4%	2%	2%
Dysphagia	0%	2%	0%
Musculoskeletal			
Myalgia	2%	6%	3%
Arthralgia	1%	4%	1%
Arthritis	0%	2%	0%
Twitch	1%	2%	—
Nervous system			
Insomnia	11%	16%	6%
Dizziness	7%	11%	5%
Agitation	3%	9%	2%

Anxiety	5%	6%	3%
Tremor	6%	3%	1%
Nervousness	5%	3%	3%
Somnolence	2%	3%	2%
Irritability	3%	2%	2%
Memory decreased	—	3%	1%
Paresthesia	1%	2%	1%
Central nervous system stimulation	2%	1%	1%
Respiratory			
Pharyngitis	3%	11%	2%
Sinusitis	3%	1%	2%
Increased cough	1%	2%	1%
Skin			
Sweating	6%	5%	2%
Rash	5%	4%	1%
Pruritus	2%	4%	2%
Urticaria	2%	1%	0%
Special senses			
Tinnitus	6%	6%	2%
Taste perversion	2%	4%	—
Blurred vision or diplopia	3%	2%	2%
Urogenital			
Urinary frequency	2%	5%	2%
Urinary urgency	—	2%	0%
Vaginal hemorrhage†	0%	2%	—
Urinary tract infection	1%	0%	—

— Hyphen denotes adverse reactions occurring in greater than 0 but less than 0.5% of patients.

*Adverse reactions that occurred in at least 1% of patients treated with either 300 or 400 mg/day of the sustained-release formulation of bupropion hydrochloride, but equally or more frequently in the placebo group, were: abnormal dreams, accidental injury, acne, appetite increased, back pain, bronchitis, dysmenorrhea, dyspepsia, flatulence, flu syndrome, hypertension, neck pain, respiratory disorder, rhinitis, and tooth disorder.
†Incidence based on the number of female patients.

Additional reactions to those listed in **Table 5** that occurred at an incidence of at least 1% in controlled clinical trials of the immediate-release formulation of bupropion hydrochloride (300 to 600 mg/day) and that were numerically more frequent than placebo were: cardiac arrhythmias (5% vs. 4%), hypertension (4% vs. 2%), hypotension (3% vs. 2%), tachycardia (11% vs. 9%), appetite increase (4% vs. 2%), dyspepsia (3% vs. 2%), menstrual complaints (5% vs. 1%), akathisia (2% vs. 1%), impaired sleep quality (4% vs. 2%), sensory disturbance (4% vs. 3%), confusion (8% vs. 5%), decreased libido (3% vs. 2%), hostility (6% vs. 4%), auditory disturbance (5% vs. 3%), and gustatory disturbance (3% vs. 1%).

Other adverse reactions occurring < 1% in clinical trials: Chills, facial edema, postural hypotension, stroke, syncope, bruxism, gastric reflux, gingivitis, glossitis, increased salivation, mouth ulcers, stomatitis, edema of tongue, ecchymosis, edema, abnormal coordination, decreased libido, depersonalization, emotional lability, hyperkinesia, hypertonia, hypesthesia, ataxia, and derealization, bronchospasm, accommodation abnormality, dry eye, impotence, and prostate disorder.

6.2 Postmarketing Experience
The following adverse reactions have been identified during post-approval use of Bupropion hydrochloride. Because these reactions are reported voluntarily from a population of uncertain size, it is not always possible to reliably estimate their frequency or establish a causal relationship to drug exposure.

Only those adverse reactions not previously listed for bupropion are included. The extent to which these reactions may be associated with FORFIVO XL is unknown.
Cardiovascular—complete atrioventricular block, extrasystoles, myocardial infarction, phlebitis, and pulmonary embolism.
Gastrointestinal—colitis, esophagitis, gastrointestinal hemorrhage, gum hemorrhage, intestinal perforation, pancreatitis, and stomach ulcer.
Endocrine—hyperglycemia, hypoglycemia, and syndrome of inappropriate antidiuretic hormone.
Hemic and Lymphatic—anemia, leukocytosis, leukopenia, lymphadenopathy, pancytopenia, and thrombocytopenia.
Metabolic and Nutritional—glycosuria.
Musculoskeletal—muscle rigidity/fever/rhabdomyolysis and muscle weakness.
Nervous System—abnormal electroencephalogram (EEG), aggression, akinesia, aphasia, coma, delirium, dysarthria, dyskinesia, dystonia, extrapyramidal syndrome, hypokinesia, increased libido, neuralgia, neuropathy, and unmasking tardive dyskinesia.

Skin—alopecia, exfoliative dermatitis, and hirsutism.
Eye—mydriasis.
Urogenital—abnormal ejaculation, cystitis, dyspareunia, dysuria, gynecomastia, painful erection, salpingitis, urinary incontinence, and urinary retention.

7 DRUG INTERACTIONS
Few systemic data have been collected on the metabolism of bupropion following concomitant administration with other drugs or, alternatively, the effect of concomitant administration of bupropion on the metabolism of other drugs.

7.1 Potential for Other Drugs to Affect FORFIVO XL
Because bupropion is extensively metabolized, the coadministration of other drugs may affect its clinical activity.
Substrates or Inhibitors/Inducers of Cytochrome P450IIB6 (CYP2B6): In vitro studies indicate that bupropion is primarily metabolized to hydroxybupropion by the CYP2B6 isoenzyme. Therefore, the potential exists for a drug interaction between FORFIVO XL and drugs that are substrates or inhibitors/inducers of the CYP2B6 isoenzyme (e.g., orphenadrine, thiotepa, cyclophosphamide, ticlopidine and clopidogrel). In addition, in vitro studies suggest that paroxetine, sertraline, norfluoxetine, and fluvoxamine as well as nelfinavir, inhibit the hydroxylation of bupropion.

Ticlopidine, Clopidogrel: In a study in healthy male volunteers, 75 mg clopidogrel once daily or 250 mg ticlopidine twice daily increased exposures (Cmax and AUC) of bupropion by 40% and 60% for clopidogrel, by 38% and 85% for ticlopidine, respectively. The exposures of hydroxybupropion were decreased. This effect is thought to be due to the inhibition of the CYP2B6-catalyzed bupropion hydroxylation. Coadministration of FORFIVO XL with ticlopidine or clopidogrel is not recommended.
Prasugrel: Prasugrel is a weak inhibitor of CYP2B6. In healthy subjects, prasugrel increased C_{max} and AUC values of bupropion by 14% and 18%, respectively, and decreased C_{max} and AUC values of hydroxybupropion, an active metabolite of bupropion, by 32% and 24%, respectively. The inhibition of prasugrel on bupropion metabolism is not considered clinically significant.
Ritonavir, Lopinavir, Efavirenz: In a series of studies in healthy volunteers, ritonavir (100 mg twice daily or 600 mg twice daily) or ritonavir 100 mg plus lopinavir (KALETRA) 400 mg twice daily reduced the exposure of bupropion and its major metabolites in a dose dependent manner by approximately 20% to 80%. Similarly, efavirenz 600 mg once daily for 2 weeks reduced the exposure of bupropion by approximately 55%. This effect is thought to be due to the induction of bupropion metabolism. Patients receiving any of these drugs with bupropion may need increased doses of bupropion, but the maximum recommended dose of bupropion should not be exceeded [see **Clinical Pharmacology (12.3)**].
Cimetidine: The threohydrobupropion metabolite of bupropion does not appear to be produced by the cytochrome P450 isoenzymes. The effects of concomitant administration of cimetidine on the pharmacokinetics of bupropion and its active metabolites were studied in 24 healthy young male volunteers. Following oral administration of two 150-mg tablets of the sustained-release formulation of bupropion hydrochloride with and without 800 mg of cimetidine, the pharmacokinetics of bupropion and hydroxybupropion were unaffected. However, there were 16% and 32% increases in the AUC and C_{max}, respectively, of the combined moieties of threohydrobupropion and erythrohydrobupropion.
Carbamazepine, Phenobarbital, Phenytoin: While not systematically studied, these drugs may induce the metabolism of bupropion.

7.2 Potential for FORFIVO XL to Affect Other Drugs
Animal data indicated that bupropion may be an inducer of drug-metabolizing enzymes in humans. In one study, following chronic administration of bupropion hydrochloride, 100 mg 3 times daily to 8 healthy male volunteers for 14 days, there was no evidence of induction of its own metabolism. Nevertheless, there may be the potential for clinically important alterations of blood levels of coadministered drugs.
Lamotrigine: Multiple oral doses of bupropion had no statistically significant effects on the single dose pharmacokinetics of lamotrigine in 12 healthy volunteers.
Drugs Metabolized by Cytochrome P450IID6 (CYP2D6)
Many drugs, including most antidepressants (SSRIs, many tricyclics), beta-blockers, antiarrhythmics, and antipsychotics are metabolized by the CYP2D6 isoenzyme. Although bupropion is not metabolized by this isoenzyme, bupropion and hydroxybupropion are inhibitors of the CYP2D6 isoenzyme in vitro. In a study of 15 male subjects (ages 19 to 35 years) who were extensive metabolizers of the CYP2D6 isoenzyme, daily doses of bupropion hydrochloride given as 150 mg twice daily followed by a single dose of 50 mg desipramine increased the C_{max}, AUC, and t1/2 of desipramine by an average of approximately 2-, 5-, and 2-fold, respectively. The effect was present for at least 7 days after the

last dose of bupropion. Concomitant use of bupropion with other drugs metabolized by CYP2D6 has not been formally studied.
Therefore, coadministration of bupropion with drugs that are metabolized by the CYP2D6 isoenzyme including certain antidepressants (e.g., venlafaxine, nortriptyline, imipramine, desipramine, paroxetine, fluoxetine, and sertraline), antipsychotics (e.g., haloperidol, risperidone, and thioridazine), beta-blockers (e.g., metoprolol), and Type 1C antiarrhythmics (e.g., propafenone, and flecainide), should be approached with caution and should be initiated at the lower end of the dose range of the concomitant medication. If bupropion is added to the treatment regimen of a patient already receiving a drug metabolized by CYP2D6, the need to decrease the dose of the original medication should be considered, particularly for those concomitant medications with a narrow therapeutic index.
CYP2D6 in order to be effective (e.g., tamoxifen) theoretically could have reduced efficacy when administered concomitantly with inhibitors of CYP2D6 such as bupropion. Although citalopram is not primarily metabolized by CYP2D6, in one study bupropion increased the C_{max} and AUC of citalopram by 30% and 40%, respectively. Citalopram did not affect the pharmacokinetics of bupropion and its three metabolites.

7.3 Nicotine Transdermal System
Data from a smoking cessation study suggest that a higher incidence of hypertension in patients who received the combination of sustained-release bupropion hydrochloride and nicotine transdermal system (NTS). Monitoring of blood pressure is recommended in patients who receive the combination of bupropion and nicotine replacement [see **Warnings and Precautions (5.7)**].

7.4 Drug Laboratory Test Interactions
False-positive urine immunoassay screening tests for amphetamines have been reported in patients taking bupropion. This is due to lack of specificity of some screening tests. False-positive test results may result even following discontinuation of bupropion therapy. Confirmatory test such as gas chromatography/mass spectrometry, will distinguish bupropion from amphetamines.

7.5 MAO Inhibitors
Studies in animals demonstrate that the acute toxicity of bupropion is enhanced by the MAO inhibitor phenelzine [see **Contraindications (4)**].

7.6 Drugs that Lower Seizure Threshold
Since there is no lower strength for FORFIVO XL, concurrent administration of FORFIVO XL tablets and agents (e.g., antipsychotics, other antidepressants, theophylline, systemic steroids, etc.) that lower seizure threshold should be undertaken only with caution [see **Warnings and Precautions (5.4)**].

7.7 Alcohol
In postmarketing experience, there have been rare reports of adverse neuropsychiatric events or reduced alcohol tolerance in patients who were drinking alcohol during treatment with bupropion. Alcohol increased the release rate of FORFIVO XL in vitro. The consumption of alcohol during treatment with FORFIVO XL should be avoided.

7.8 Levodopa and Amantadine
Limited clinical data suggest a higher incidence of adverse experiences in patients receiving bupropion concurrently with either levodopa or amantadine. Since there is no lower strength for FORFIVO XL, administration of FORFIVO XL tablets to patients receiving either levodopa or amantadine concurrently should be undertaken with caution.

8 USE IN SPECIFIC POPULATIONS
8.1 Pregnancy
Teratogenic Effects
Pregnancy Category C. In studies conducted in rats and rabbits, bupropion hydrochloride was administered orally at doses up to 450 and 150 mg/kg/day, respectively (approximately 11 and 7 times the maximum recommended human dose [MRHD], respectively, on a mg/m^2 basis), during the period of organogenesis. No clear evidence of teratogenic activity was found in either species; however, in rabbits, slightly increased incidences of fetal malformations and skeletal variations were observed at the lowest dose tested (25 mg/kg/day, approximately equal to the MRHD on a mg/m^2 basis) and greater. Decreased fetal weights were seen at 50 mg/kg and greater.
When rats were administered bupropion hydrochloride at oral doses of up to 300 mg/kg/day (approximately 7 times the MRHD on a mg/m^2 basis) prior to mating and throughout pregnancy and lactation, there were no apparent adverse effects on offspring development.
One study has been conducted in pregnant women. This retrospective, managed-care database study assessed the risk of congenital malformations overall, and cardiovascular malformations specifically, following exposure to bupropion in the first trimester compared to the risk of these malformations following exposure to other antidepressants in the first trimester and bupropion outside of the first trimester.

This study included 7,005 infants with antidepressant exposure during pregnancy, 1,213 of whom were exposed to bupropion in the first trimester. The study showed no greater risk for congenital malformations overall, or cardiovascular malformations specifically, following first trimester bupropion exposure compared to exposure to all other antidepressants in the first trimester, or bupropion outside of the first trimester. The results of this study have not been corroborated. FORFIVO XL should be used during pregnancy only if the potential benefit justifies the potential risk to the fetus.

8.3 Nursing Mothers

Like many other drugs, bupropion and its metabolites are secreted in human milk. Because of the potential for serious adverse reactions in nursing infants from FORFIVO XL tablets, a decision should be made whether to discontinue nursing or to discontinue the drug, taking into account the importance of the drug to the mother.

8.4 Pediatric Use

Safety and effectiveness in pediatric patients have not been established. Anyone considering the use of FORFIVO XL in a child or adolescent must balance the potential risks with the clinical need.

8.5 Geriatric Use

Of the approximately 6,000 patients who participated in clinical trials with bupropion hydrochloride sustained-release tablets (depression and smoking cessation studies), 275 were 65 years old and over and 47 were 75 years old and over. In addition, several hundred patients 65 and over participated in clinical trials using the immediate-release formulation of bupropion hydrochloride (depression studies). No overall differences in safety or effectiveness were observed between these subjects and younger subjects. Reported clinical experience has not identified differences in responses between the elderly and younger patients, but greater sensitivity of some older individuals cannot be ruled out.

A single-dose pharmacokinetic study demonstrated that the disposition of bupropion and its metabolites in elderly subjects was similar to that of younger subjects; however, another pharmacokinetic study, single and multiple dose, has suggested that the elderly are at increased risk for accumulation of bupropion and its metabolites [see *Clinical Pharmacology (12.3)*].

Bupropion is extensively metabolized in the liver to active metabolites, which are further metabolized and excreted by the kidneys. The risk of toxic reaction to this drug may be greater in patients with impaired renal function. Because elderly patients are more likely to have decreased renal function, care should be taken in dose selection, and it may be useful to monitor renal function [see *Dosage and Administration (2.5) and Use in Specific Populations (8.6)*].

8.6 Renal Impairment

Since there is no lower dose strength for FORFIVO XL, FORFIVO XL is not recommended in patients with renal impairment [see *Clinical Pharmacology (12.3)*].

8.7 Hepatic Impairment

Since there is no lower dose strength for FORFIVO XL, FORFIVO XL is not recommended in patients with hepatic impairment [see *Clinical Pharmacology (12.3)*].

9 DRUG ABUSE AND DEPENDENCE

9.1 Controlled Substance

Bupropion is not a controlled substance.

9.2 Abuse

Humans

Controlled clinical studies of bupropion hydrochloride (immediate-release formulation) conducted in normal volunteers, in subjects with a history of multiple drug abuse, and in depressed patients showed some increase in motor activity and agitation/excitement.

In a population of individuals experienced with drugs of abuse, a single dose of 400 mg of bupropion hydrochloride produced mild amphetamine-like activity as compared to placebo on the Morphine-Benzedrine Subscale of the Addiction Research Center Inventories (ARCI), and a score intermediate between placebo and amphetamine on the Liking Scale of the ARCI. These scales measure general feelings of euphoria and drug desirability.

Findings in clinical trials, however, are not known to reliably predict the abuse potential of drugs. Nonetheless, evidence from single-dose studies does suggest that the recommended daily dosage of bupropion when administered in divided doses is not likely to be especially reinforcing to amphetamine or stimulant abusers. However, higher doses that could not be tested because of the risk of seizure might be modestly attractive to those who abuse stimulant drugs.

Animals

Studies in rodents and primates have shown that bupropion exhibits some pharmacologic actions common to psychostimulants. In rodents, it has been shown to increase locomotor activity, elicit a mild stereotyped behavioral response, and increase rates of responding in several schedule-controlled behavior paradigms. In primate models to assess the positive reinforcing effects of psychoactive drugs, bupropion was self-administered intravenously. In rats, bupropion produced amphetamine-like and cocaine-like discriminative stimulus effects in drug discrimination paradigms used to characterize the subjective effects of psychoactive drugs.

10 OVERDOSAGE

10.1 Human Overdose Experience

Overdoses of up to 30 g or more of bupropion have been reported. Seizure was reported in approximately one third of all cases. Other serious reactions reported with overdoses of bupropion alone included hallucinations, loss of consciousness, sinus tachycardia, and ECG changes such as conduction disturbances or arrhythmias. Fever, muscle rigidity, rhabdomyolysis, hypotension, stupor, coma, and respiratory failure have been reported mainly when bupropion was part of multiple drug overdoses.

Although most patients recovered without sequelae, deaths associated with overdoses of bupropion alone have been reported in patients ingesting large doses of the drug. Multiple uncontrolled seizures, bradycardia, cardiac failure, and cardiac arrest prior to death were reported in these patients.

10.2 Overdosage Management

Ensure an adequate airway, oxygenation, and ventilation. Monitor cardiac rhythm and vital signs. EEG monitoring is also recommended for the first 48 hours post-ingestion. General supportive and symptomatic measures are also recommended. Induction of emesis is not recommended. Gastric lavage with a large-bore orogastric tube with appropriate airway protection, if needed, may be indicated if performed soon after ingestion or in symptomatic patients. Activated charcoal should be administered. There is no experience with the use of forced diuresis, dialysis, hemoperfusion, or exchange transfusion in the management of bupropion overdoses. No specific antidotes for bupropion are known.

Due to the dose-related risk of seizures with FORFIVO XL, hospitalization following suspected overdose should be considered. Based on studies in animals, it is recommended that seizures be treated with intravenous benzodiazepine administration and other supportive measures, as appropriate.

In managing overdosage, consider the possibility of multiple drug involvement. The physician should consider contacting a poison control center for additional information on the treatment of any overdose. Telephone numbers for certified poison control centers are listed in the *Physicians' Desk Reference* (PDR).

11 DESCRIPTION

FORFIVO XL (bupropion hydrochloride), an antidepressant of the aminoketone class, is chemically unrelated to tricyclic, tetracyclic, selective serotonin re-uptake inhibitor, or other known antidepressant agents. Its structure closely resembles that of diethylpropion; it is related to phenylethylamines. It is designated as (±)-2-(tert-Butylamino)-3'-chloropropiophenone hydrochloride. The molecular weight is 276.2. The empirical formula is $C_{13}H_{18}ClNO \cdot HCl$. Bupropion hydrochloride powder is white or almost white, crystalline, and soluble in water. It has a bitter taste and produces the sensation of local anesthesia on the oral mucosa. The structural formula is:

FORFIVO XL tablets are supplied for oral administration of 450 mg of bupropion hydrochloride as white to off white extended-release tablets. Each film coated tablet contains the labeled amount of bupropion hydrochloride and the inactive ingredients: hydroxypropyl cellulose, hydrochloric acid, polyvinyl pyrrolidone and polyvinyl acetate blend, polyethylene oxide, stearic acid, colloidal silicon dioxide, magnesium stearate, hydroxypropylmethyl cellulose, triacetin, talc, methacrylic acid copolymer, polyethylene glycol 8000, titanium dioxide and carboxymethyl cellulose sodium. The logo "Forfivo" is printed on one side of the tablet with edible black ink.

12 CLINICAL PHARMACOLOGY

12.1 Mechanism of Action

The mechanism of action of bupropion is unknown, as is the case with other antidepressants. However, it is presumed that this action is mediated by noradrenergic and/or dopaminergic mechanisms.

12.2 Pharmacodynamics

Bupropion is a relatively weak inhibitor of the neuronal uptake of norepinephrine and dopamine, and does not inhibit monoamine oxidase or the re-uptake of serotonin.

12.3 Pharmacokinetics

Bupropion is a racemic mixture. The pharmacologic activity and pharmacokinetics of the individual enantiomers have not been studied.

Following single dosing under fasted conditions of FORFIVO XL tablets, the maximum peak plasma concentration (C_{max}), and the area under the plasma concentration vs. time curve of bupropion from zero to infinity (AUC_{inf}), were 207.46 (±59.40) ng/mL, and 2147.53 (±664.12) ng•hr/mL, respectively. The elimination half-life (±SD) of bupropion after a single dose was 14.44 (±5.00) hours.

In a single dose study under fasting conditions, one FORFIVO XL tablet given once daily and three Wellbutrin XL® 150 mg tablets once daily were evaluated. Equivalence was demonstrated for peak concentration and area under the curve for bupropion and the 3 metabolites (hydroxybupropion, erythrhydrobupropion, and threohydrobupropion).

Absorption

Following single oral administration of FORFIVO XL tablets to healthy volunteers, the median time to peak plasma concentrations for bupropion was approximately 5 hours under fasted conditions, and 12 hours under fed conditions. The presence of food did not affect the maximum peak plasma concentration for bupropion, however, mean systemic exposure to bupropion was increased by 25% when FORFIVO XL tablet was taken with food. The food effect is not considered clinically significant and FORFIVO XL can be taken with or without food.

Distribution

In vitro tests show that bupropion is 84% bound to human plasma proteins at concentrations up to 200 mcg/mL. The extent of protein binding of the hydroxybupropion metabolite is similar to that for bupropion, whereas the extent of protein binding of the threohydrobupropion metabolite is about half that seen with bupropion.

Metabolism

Bupropion is extensively metabolized in humans. Three metabolites have been shown to be active: hydroxybupropion, which is formed via hydroxylation of the *tert*-butyl group of bupropion, and the amino-alcohol isomers threohydrobupropion and erythrohydrobupropion, which are formed via reduction of the carbonyl group. In vitro findings suggest that cytochrome P450IIB6 (CYP2B6) is the principal isoenzyme involved in the formation of hydroxybupropion, while cytochrome P450 isoenzymes are not involved in the formation of threohydrobupropion. Oxidation of the bupropion side chain results in the formation of a glycine conjugate of metachlorobenzoic acid, which is then excreted as the major urinary metabolite. The potency and toxicity of the metabolites relative to bupropion have not been fully characterized. However, it has been demonstrated in an antidepressant screening test in mice that hydroxybupropion is one half as potent as bupropion, while threohydrobupropion and erythrohydrobupropion are 5-fold less potent than bupropion. This may be of clinical importance because the plasma concentrations of the metabolites are as high or higher than those of bupropion.

Because bupropion is extensively metabolized, there is the potential for drug-drug interactions, particularly with those agents that are metabolized by the cytochrome P450IIB6 (CYP2B6) isoenzyme, such as ritonavir or efavirenz. In a healthy volunteer study, ritonavir at a dose of 100 mg twice daily reduced the AUC and C_{max} of bupropion by 22% and 21%, respectively. The exposure of the hydroxybupropion metabolite was decreased by 23%, the threohydrobupropion metabolite decreased by 38% and the erythrohydrobupropion metabolite decreased by 48%.

In a second healthy volunteer study, ritonavir at a dose of 600 mg twice daily decreased the AUC and the C_{max} of bupropion by 66% and 62%, respectively. The exposure of the hydroxybupropion metabolite was decreased by 78%, the threohydrobupropion decreased by 50% and the erythrohydrobupropion decreased by 68%.

In another healthy volunteer study, KALETRA® (lopinavir 400 mg/ritonavir 100 mg twice daily) decreased bupropion AUC and C_{max} by 57%. The AUC and C_{max} of hydroxybupropion were decreased by 50% and 31%, respectively [see *Drug Interactions (7)*].

In a study in healthy volunteers, efavirenz 600 mg once daily for 2 weeks reduces the AUC and C_{max} of bupropion by approximately 55% and 34%, respectively. The AUC of hydroxybupropion was unchanged, whereas C_{max} of hydroxybupropion was increased by 50%.

Although bupropion is not metabolized by cytochrome P450IID6 (CYP2D6), there is the potential for drug-drug interactions when bupropion is coadministered with drugs metabolized by this isoenzyme [see *Drug Interactions (7.2)*].

In humans, peak plasma concentrations of hydroxybupropion occur approximately 10 hours after administration of single dose of FORFIVO XL under fasted conditions and 16 hours under fed conditions. Following administration of WELLBUTRIN XL, peak plasma concentrations of hydroxybupropion are approximately 7 times the peak level of the parent drug at steady state. The elimination half-life of hydroxybupropion is approximately 20 (±5) hours, and its AUC at steady state is about 13 times that of bupropion. The times to peak concentrations for the erythrohydrobupropion and threohydrobupropion metabolites are similar to that of the hydroxybupropion metabolite. However, their elimination half-lives are longer, approximately 33 (±10) and 37 (±13) hours, respectively, and steady-state AUCs are 1.4 and 7 times that of bupropion, respectively.

Bupropion and its metabolites exhibit linear kinetics following chronic administration of 300 to 450 mg/day of bupropion hydrochloride.

Elimination

Following oral administration of 200 mg of ^{14}C-bupropion in humans, 87% and 10% of the radioactive dose were recovered in the urine and feces, respectively. However, the fraction of the oral dose of bupropion excreted unchanged was only 0.5%, a finding consistent with the extensive metabolism of bupropion.

Population Subgroups

Factors or conditions altering metabolic capacity (e.g., liver disease, congestive heart failure [CHF], age, concomitant medications, etc.) or elimination may be expected to influence the degree and extent of accumulation of the active metabolites of bupropion. The elimination of the major metabolites of bupropion may be affected by reduced renal or hepatic function because they are moderately polar compounds and are likely to undergo further metabolism or conjugation in the liver prior to urinary excretion.

Hepatic

The effect of hepatic impairment on the pharmacokinetics of bupropion was characterized in 2 single-dose studies, one in patients with alcoholic liver disease and one in patients with mild to severe cirrhosis. The first study showed that the half-life of hydroxybupropion was significantly longer in 8 patients with alcoholic liver disease than in 8 healthy volunteers (32±14 hours versus 21±5 hours, respectively). Although not statistically significant, the AUCs for bupropion and hydroxybupropion were more variable and tended to be greater (by 53% to 57%) in patients with alcoholic liver disease. The differences in half-life for bupropion and the other metabolites in the 2 patient groups were minimal.

The second study showed no statistically significant differences in the pharmacokinetics of bupropion and its active metabolites in 9 patients with mild to moderate hepatic cirrhosis compared to 8 healthy volunteers. However, more variability was observed in some of the pharmacokinetic parameters for bupropion (AUC, C_{max}, and T_{max}) and its active metabolites (t½) in patients with mild to moderate hepatic cirrhosis. In addition, in patients with severe hepatic cirrhosis, the bupropion C_{max} and AUC were substantially increased (mean difference: by approximately 70% and 3-fold, respectively) and more variable when compared to values in healthy volunteers; the mean bupropion half-life was also longer (29 hours in patients with severe hepatic cirrhosis vs. 19 hours in healthy subjects). For the metabolite hydroxybupropion, the mean C_{max} was approximately 69% lower. For the combined amino-alcohol isomers threohydrobupropion and erythrohydrobupropion, the mean Cmax was approximately 31% lower. The mean AUC increased by about 1½-fold for hydroxybupropion and about 2½-fold for threo/erythrohydrobupropion. The median T_{max} was observed 19 hours later for hydroxybupropion and 31 hours later for threo/erythrohydrobupropion. The mean half-lives for hydroxybupropion and threo/erythrohydrobupropion were increased 5- and 2-fold, respectively, in patients with severe hepatic cirrhosis compared to healthy volunteers [see *Dosage and Administration (2.4) and Use in Specific Populations (8.7)*].

Renal

There is limited information on the pharmacokinetics of bupropion in patients with renal impairment. An inter-study comparison between normal subjects and patients with end-stage renal failure demonstrated that the parent drug C_{max} and AUC values were comparable in the 2 groups, whereas the hydroxybupropion and threohydrobupropion metabolites had a 2.3- and 2.8-fold increase, respectively, in AUC for patients with end-stage renal failure. The elimination of the major metabolites of bupropion may be reduced by impaired renal function. A second study, comparing normal subjects and patients with moderate-to-severe renal impairment (GFR 30.9 ± 10.8 mL/min) showed that exposure to a single 150 mg dose sustained-release bupropion was approximately 2-fold higher in patients with impaired renal function while levels of the hydroxybupropion and threo/erythrohydrobupropion (combined) metabolites were similar in the 2 groups. The elimination of bupropion and/or the major metabolites of bupropion may be reduced by impaired renal function [see *Dosage and Administration (2.5) and Use in Specific Populations (8.6)*].

Left Ventricular Dysfunction

During a chronic dosing study with bupropion in 14 depressed patients with left ventricular dysfunction (history of CHF or an enlarged heart on x-ray), no apparent effect on the pharmacokinetics of bupropion or its metabolites was revealed, compared to healthy volunteers.

Age

The effects of age on the pharmacokinetics of bupropion and its metabolites have not been fully characterized, but an exploration of steady-state bupropion concentrations from several depression efficacy studies involving patients dosed in a range of 300 to 750 mg/day, on a 3 times daily schedule, revealed no relationship between age (18 to 83 years) and plasma concentration of bupropion. A single-dose pharmacokinetic study demonstrated that the disposition of bupropion and its metabolites in elderly subjects was similar to that of younger subjects. These data suggest there is no prominent effect of age on bupropion concentration; however, another pharmacokinetic study, single and multiple dose, has suggested that the elderly are at increased risk for accumulation of bupropion and its metabolites [see *Use in Specific Populations (8.5)*].

Gender

A single-dose study involving 12 healthy male and 12 healthy female volunteers revealed no sex-related differences in the pharmacokinetic parameters of bupropion.

Smokers

The effects of cigarette smoking on the pharmacokinetics of bupropion hydrochloride were studied in 34 healthy male and female volunteers; 17 were chronic cigarette smokers and 17 were nonsmokers. Following oral administration of a single 150-mg dose of bupropion, there was no statistically significant difference in C_{max}, half-life, T_{max}, AUC, or clearance of bupropion or its active metabolites between smokers and nonsmokers.

13 NONCLINICAL TOXICOLOGY

13.1 Carcinogenesis, Mutagenesis, Impairment of Fertility

Lifetime carcinogenicity studies were performed in rats and mice at doses up to 300 and 150 mg/kg/day bupropion hydrochloride, respectively. These doses are approximately 7 and 2 times the maximum recommended human dose (MRHD), respectively, on a mg/m^2 basis. In the rat study there was an increase in nodular proliferative lesions of the liver at doses of 100 to 300 mg/kg/day of bupropion hydrochloride (approximately 2 to 7 times the MRHD on a mg/m^2 basis); lower doses were not tested. The question of whether or not such lesions may be precursors of neoplasms of the liver is currently unresolved. Similar liver lesions were not seen in the mouse study, and no increase in malignant tumors of the liver and other organs was seen in either study.

Bupropion produced a positive response (2 to 3 times control mutation rate) in 2 of 5 strains in one Ames bacterial mutagenicity assay, but was negative in another. Bupropion produced an increase in chromosomal aberrations in 1 of 3 in vivo rat bone marrow cytogenetic studies.

A fertility study in rats at doses up to 300 mg/kg/day revealed no evidence of impaired fertility.

14 CLINICAL STUDIES

The efficacy of bupropion as a treatment for major depressive disorder was established with the immediate-release formulation of bupropion hydrochloride in two 4-week, placebo-controlled trials in adult inpatients and in one 6-week, placebo-controlled trial in adult outpatients. In the first study, patients were titrated in a bupropion hydrochloride dose range of 300 to 600 mg/day of the immediate-release formulation on a 3 times daily schedule; 78% of patients received maximum doses of 450 mg/day or less. This trial demonstrated the effectiveness of bupropion on the Hamilton Depression Rating Scale (HDRS) total score, the depressed mood item (item 1) from that scale, and the Clinical Global Impressions (CGI) severity score. A second study included 2 fixed doses of the immediate-release formulation of bupropion hydrochloride (300 and 450 mg/day) and placebo. This trial demonstrated the effectiveness of bupropion, but only at the 450 mg/day dose of the immediate-release formulation; the results were positive for the HDRS total score and the CGI severity score, but not for HDRS item 1. In the third study, outpatients received 300 mg/day of the immediate-release formulation of bupropion hydrochloride. This study demonstrated the effectiveness of bupropion on the HDRS total score, HDRS item 1, the Montgomery-Asberg Depression Rating Scale, the CGI severity score, and the CGI improvement score.

In a longer-term study, outpatients meeting DSM-IV criteria for major depressive disorder, recurrent type, who had responded during an 8-week open trial on bupropion hydrochloride (150 mg twice daily of the sustained-release formulation) were randomized to continuation of their same dose of bupropion or placebo, for up to 44 weeks of observation for relapse. Response during the open phase was defined as CGI Improvement score of 1 (very much improved) or 2 (much improved) for each of the final 3 weeks. Relapse during the double-blind phase was defined as the investigator's judgment that drug treatment was needed for worsening depressive symptoms. Patients receiving continued bupropion treatment experienced significantly lower relapse rates over the subsequent 44 weeks compared to those receiving placebo.

Although there are no independent trials demonstrating the antidepressant effectiveness of bupropion extended release studies have demonstrated similar bioavailability of bupropion extended-release to both the immediate-release formulation and to the sustained-release formulation of bupropion under steady-state conditions, i.e., WELLBUTRIN XL® 300 mg once daily was shown to have bioavailability that was similar to that of 100 mg 3 times daily of the immediate-release formulation of bupropion and to that of 150 mg 2 times daily of the sustained-release formulation of bupropion, with regard to both peak plasma concentration and extent of absorption, for parent drug and metabolites. Further, it has been demonstrated that FORFIVO XL is bioequivalent to WELLBUTRIN XL®.

16 HOW SUPPLIED/STORAGE AND HANDLING

FORFIVO XL Extended-Release Tablets, 450 mg of bupropion hydrochloride, are white to off white, oblong shaped tablets printed with the "Forfivo" logo on one side supplied in bottles of 30 tablets
(NDC 49909-010-30).

Store at 20 °C to 25 °C (68 °F to 77 °F) [See USP Controlled Room Temperature].

17 PATIENT COUNSELING INFORMATION

See FDA-approved patient labeling (Medication Guide).

17.1 Information for Patients

Prescribers or other health professionals should inform patients, their families, and their caregivers about the benefits and risks associated with treatment with FORFIVO XL and should counsel them in its appropriate use. A patient Medication Guide about "Antidepressant Medicines, Depression and Other Serious Mental Illnesses, and Suicidal Thoughts or Actions", "Quitting Smoking, Quit-Smoking Medication, Changes in Thinking and Behavior, Depression, and Suicidal Thoughts or Actions" and "What Other Important Information Should I Know about FORFIVO XL" is available for FORFIVO XL. The prescriber or health professional should instruct patients, their families, and their caregivers to read the Medication Guide and should assist them in understanding its contents. Patients should be given the opportunity to discuss the contents of the Medication Guide and to obtain answers to any questions they may have. The complete text of the Medication Guide is reprinted at the end of this document. Patients should be advised of the following issues and asked to alert their prescriber if these occur while taking FORFIVO XL.

Clinical Worsening and Suicide Risk in Treating Psychiatric Disorders: Patients, their families, and their caregivers should be encouraged to be alert to the emergence of anxiety, agitation, panic attacks, insomnia, irritability, hostility, aggressiveness, impulsivity, akathisia (psychomotor restlessness), hypomania, mania, other unusual changes in behavior, worsening of depression, and suicidal ideation, especially early during antidepressant treatment and when the dose is adjusted up or down. Families and caregivers of patients should be advised to observe for the emergence of such symptoms on a day-to-day basis, since changes may be abrupt. Such symptoms should be reported to the patient's prescriber or health professional, especially if they are severe, abrupt in onset, or were not part of the patient's presenting symptoms. Symptoms such as these may be associated with an increased risk for suicidal thinking and behavior and indicate a need for very close monitoring and possibly changes in the medication.

Neuropsychiatric Symptoms and Suicide Risk in Smoking Cessation Treatment: Although FORFIVO XL is not indicated for smoking cessation treatment, it contains the same active ingredient as ZYBAN which is approved for this use. Patients should be informed that quitting smoking, with or without ZYBAN, may be associated with nicotine withdrawal symptoms (including depression or agitation), or exacerbation of pre-existing psychiatric illness. Furthermore, some patients have experienced changes in mood (including depression and mania), psychosis, hallucinations, paranoia, delusions, homicidal ideation, aggression, anxiety, and panic, as well as suicidal ideation and completed suicide when attempting to quit smoking while taking ZYBAN.

Bupropion-Containing Products: Patients should be made aware that FORFIVO XL contains the same active ingredient (bupropion) found in ZYBAN, which is used as an aid to smoking cessation treatment, and that FORFIVO XL should not be used in combination with ZYBAN or any other medications that contain bupropion hydrochloride (such as WELLBUTRIN XL®, the extended-release formulation, WELLBUTRIN SR, the sustained-release formulation, WELLBUTRIN, the immediate-release formulation) or APLENZIN, Extended Release tablet.

Patients should be told that FORFIVO XL should be discontinued and not restarted if they experience a seizure while on treatment.

Patients should be told that any CNS-active drug like FORFIVO XL tablets may impair their ability to perform tasks requiring judgment or motor and cognitive skills. Consequently, until they are reasonably certain that FORFIVO XL tablets do not adversely affect their performance, they should refrain from driving an automobile or operating complex, hazardous machinery.

Patients should be told that the excessive use or abrupt discontinuation of alcohol or sedatives (including benzodiazepines) may alter the seizure threshold. Some patients have reported lower alcohol tolerance during treatment with bupropion. Patients should be advised that the consumption of alcohol should be minimized or avoided.

Patients should be advised that taking FORFIVO XL can cause mild pupillary dilation, which in susceptible individuals, can lead to an episode of angle closure glaucoma. Pre-existing glaucoma is almost always open-angle glaucoma because angle closure glaucoma, when diagnosed, can be treated definitively with iridectomy. Open-angle glaucoma is not a risk factor for angle closure glaucoma. Patients may wish to be examined to determine whether they are susceptible to angle closure, and have a prophylactic procedure (e.g., iridectomy), if they are susceptible [see *Warnings and Precautions (5.6)*].

Patients should be advised to notify their physicians if they are taking or plan to take any prescription or over-the-counter drugs. Concern is warranted because FORFIVO XL tablets and other drugs may affect each other's metabolism. Patients should be advised to notify their physicians if they become pregnant or intend to become pregnant during therapy.

Patients should be advised to swallow FORFIVO XL tablets whole so that the release rate is not altered. Do not chew, divide, or crush tablets, as this may lead to an increased risk of adverse effects, including seizures.

The following are registered trademarks of their respective manufacturers: WELLBUTRIN® and WELLBUTRIN XL®/GlaxoSmithKline; ZYBAN® /GlaxoSmithKline; KALETRA®/Abbott Laboratories.

Manufactured by:
Pillar5 Pharma Inc.
Arnprior, Ontario, K7S 0C9
Canada
For:
Edgemont Pharmaceuticals, LLC
Austin, TX 78746
Revised June 2014
FFO_V3

MEDICATION GUIDE

FORFIVO XL
Fore fye' voe Eks el
(bupropion hydrochloride extended-release tablets)

Read this Medication Guide carefully before you start using FORFIVO XL and each time you get a refill. There may be new information. This information does not take the place of talking with your healthcare provider about your medical condition or your treatment. If you have any questions about FORFIVO XL, ask your healthcare provider or pharmacist.

IMPORTANT: Be sure to read the three sections of this Medication Guide. The first section is about the risk of suicidal thoughts and actions with antidepressant medicines; the second section is about the risk of changes in thinking and behavior, depression and suicidal thoughts or actions with medicines used to quit smoking; and the third section is entitled "What other important information should I know about FORFIVO XL?"

Antidepressant Medicines, Depression and Other Serious Mental Illnesses, and Suicidal Thoughts or Actions

This section of the Medication Guide is only about the risk of suicidal thoughts and actions with antidepressant medicines. **Talk to your, healthcare provider or your family member's healthcare provider about:**

- all risks and benefits of treatment with antidepressant medicines
- all treatment choices for depression or other serious mental illness

What is the most important information I should know about antidepressant medicines, depression and other serious mental illnesses, and suicidal thoughts or actions?

1. **Antidepressant medicines may increase suicidal thoughts or actions in some children, teenagers, and young adults within the first few months of treatment.**
2. **Depression and other serious mental illnesses are the most important causes of suicidal thoughts and actions. Some people may have a particularly high risk of having suicidal thoughts or actions. These include people who have (or have a family history of) bipolar illness (also called manic-depressive illness) or suicidal thoughts or actions.**

3. **How can I watch for and try to prevent suicidal thoughts and actions in myself or a family member?**
   - Pay close attention to any changes, especially sudden changes in mood, behaviors, thoughts, or feelings. This is very important when an antidepressant medicine is started or when the dose is changed.
   - Call the healthcare provider right away to report new or sudden changes in mood, behavior, thoughts, or feelings.
   - Keep all follow-up visits with the healthcare provider as scheduled. Call the healthcare provider between visits as needed, especially if you have concerns about symptoms.

Call a healthcare provider right away if you or your family member has any of the following symptoms, especially if they are new, worse, or worry you:

- thoughts about suicide or dying
- attempts to commit suicide
- new or worse depression
- new or worse anxiety
- feeling very agitated or restless
- panic attacks
- trouble sleeping (insomnia)
- new or worse irritability
- acting aggressive, being angry, or violent
- acting on dangerous impulses
- an extreme increase in activity and talking (mania)
- other unusual changes in behavior or mood

What else do I need to know about antidepressant medicines?

- **Never stop an antidepressant medicine without first talking to a healthcare provider.** Stopping an antidepressant medicine suddenly can cause other symptoms.
- **Antidepressants are medicines used to treat depression and other illnesses.** It is important to discuss all the risks of treating depression and also the risks of not treating it. Patients and their families or other caregivers should discuss all treatment choices with the healthcare provider, not just the use of antidepressants.
- **Antidepressant medicines have other side effects.** Talk to the healthcare provider about the side effects of the medicine prescribed for you or your family member.
- **Antidepressant medicines can interact with other medicines.** Know all of the medicines that you or your family member takes. Keep a list of all medicines to show the healthcare provider. Do not start new medicines without first checking with your healthcare provider.
- **Not all antidepressant medicines prescribed for children are FDA approved for use in children.** Talk to your child's healthcare provider for more information.

It is not known if FORFIVO XL is safe and effective in children.

Quitting Smoking, Quit-Smoking Medications, Changes in Thinking and Behavior, Depression, and Suicidal Thoughts or Actions

This section of the Medication Guide is only about the risk of changes in thinking and behavior, depression and suicidal thoughts or actions with drugs used to quit smoking.

Although FORFIVO XL is not a treatment for quitting smoking, it contains the same active ingredient (bupropion hydrochloride) as ZYBAN® which is used to help patients quit smoking.

Some people have had changes in behavior, hostility, agitation, depression, suicidal thoughts or actions while taking bupropion to help them quit smoking. These symptoms can develop during treatment with bupropion or after stopping treatment with bupropion.

If you, your family member, or your caregiver notice agitation, hostility, depression or changes in thinking or behavior that are not typical for you, or you have any of the following symptoms, stop taking bupropion and call your healthcare provider right away:

- thoughts about suicide or dying
- attempts to commit suicide
- new or worse depression
- new or worse anxiety
- panic attacks
- feeling very agitated or restless
- acting aggressive, being angry, or violent
- acting on dangerous impulses
- an extreme increase in activity and talking (mania)
- abnormal thoughts or sensations
- seeing or hearing things that are not there (hallucinations)
- feeling people are against you (paranoia)
- feeling confused
- other unusual changes in behavior or mood

When you try to quit smoking, with or without bupropion, you may have symptoms that may be due to nicotine withdrawal, including urge to smoke, depressed mood, trouble sleeping, irritability, frustration, anger, feeling anxious, difficulty concentrating, restlessness, decreased heart rate, and increased appetite or weight gain.

Some people have even experienced suicidal thoughts when trying to quit smoking without medication. Sometimes quitting smoking can lead to worsening of mental health problems that you already have, such as depression.

Before taking bupropion, tell your healthcare provider if you have ever had depression or other mental illnesses. You should also tell your healthcare provider about any symptoms you had during other times you tried to quit smoking, with or without bupropion.

WHAT OTHER IMPORTANT INFORMATION SHOULD I KNOW ABOUT FORFIVO XL?

- **Activation of mania/hypomania:** Depression may be the early symptom of bipolar disorder. Using FORFIVO XL can trigger mania/hypomania if you have bipolar disorder. Tell your healthcare provider all of your symptoms, and if you or a family member has ever had depression, suicidal thoughts or actions, bipolar disorder or other mental health problems. Your healthcare provider may check you for bipolar disorder.
- **Seizures: There is a chance of having a seizure (convulsion, fit) with FORFIVO XL, especially in people:**
  - with certain medical problems.
  - who take certain medicines.

For more information, see the sections "Who should not take FORFIVO XL?" and "What should I tell my healthcare provider before using FORFIVO XL?" Tell your healthcare provider about all of your medical conditions and all the medicines you take. **Do not take any other medicines while you are using FORFIVO XL unless your healthcare provider has said it is okay to take them.**

If you have a seizure while taking FORFIVO XL, stop taking the tablets and call your healthcare provider right away. Do not take FORFIVO XL again if you have a seizure.

- **High blood pressure (hypertension):** Some people get high blood pressure that can be severe, while taking FORFIVO XL. The chance of high blood pressure may be higher if you also use nicotine replacement therapy (such as a nicotine patch) to help you stop smoking.
- **Severe allergic reactions:** Some people have severe allergic reactions to FORFIVO XL. Stop taking FORFIVO XL and call your healthcare provider right away if you get a rash, itching, hives, fever, swollen lymph glands, painful sores in the mouth or around the eyes, swelling of the lips or tongue, chest pain, or have trouble breathing. These could be signs of a serious allergic reaction.
- **Unusual thoughts or behaviors:** Some patients have unusual thoughts or behaviors while taking FORFIVO XL, including delusions (believe you are someone else), hallucinations (seeing or hearing things that are not there), paranoia (feeling that people are against you), or feeling confused. If this happens to you, call your healthcare provider.
- **Visual problems:**
  - eye pain
  - changes in vision
  - swelling or redness in or around the eye

    Only some people are at risk for these problems. You may want to undergo an eye examination to see if you are at risk and receive preventative treatment if you are.

What is FORFIVO XL?

FORFIVO XL is a prescription medicine used to treat adults with a certain type of depression called major depressive disorder.

Who should not take FORFIVO XL?

Do not take FORFIVO XL if you:

- have or had a seizure disorder or epilepsy.
- **are taking ZYBAN® (used to help people stop smoking) or any other medicines that contain bupropion, such as WELLBUTRIN® Tablets, or WELLBUTRIN SR® Sustained-Release Tablets, or WELLBUTRIN XL® Extended-Release Tablets or APLENZIN EXTENDED-RELEASE TABLETS.** Bupropion is the same active ingredient that is in FORFIVO XL.
- abruptly stop drinking, or use medicines called sedatives (these make you sleepy) or benzodiazepines and you stop using them all of a sudden.
- have taken within the last 14 days medicine for depression called a monoamine oxidase inhibitor (MAOI), such as NARDIL® (phenelzine sulfate), PARNATE® (tranylcypromine sulfate), or MARPLAN® (isocarboxazid).
- have or had an eating disorder such as anorexia nervosa or bulimia.
- are allergic to the active ingredient in FORFIVO XL, bupropion, or to any of the inactive ingredients. See the end of this leaflet for a complete list of ingredients in FORFIVO XL.

What should I tell my healthcare provider before using FORFIVO XL?

- Tell your healthcare provider if you have ever had depression, suicidal thoughts or actions, or other mental health problems. See "Antidepressant Medicines, Depression and Other Serious Mental Illnesses, and Suicidal Thoughts or Actions."

- Tell your healthcare provider about your other medical conditions. Tell your healthcare provider if you:
  ◦ are pregnant or plan to become pregnant. It is not known if FORFIVO XL can harm your unborn baby.
  ◦ are breastfeeding. FORFIVO XL passes through your milk. It is not known if FORFIVO XL can harm your baby.
  ◦ have liver problems, especially cirrhosis of the liver.
  ◦ have kidney problems.
  ◦ have an eating disorder such as anorexia nervosa or bulimia.
  ◦ have had a head injury.
  ◦ have had a seizure (convulsion, fit).
  ◦ have a tumor in your nervous system (brain or spine).
  ◦ have had a heart attack, heart problems, or high blood pressure.
  ◦ are a diabetic taking insulin or other medicines to control your blood sugar.
  ◦ drink alcohol.
  ◦ abuse prescription medicines or street drugs.
- Tell your healthcare provider about all the medicines you take, including prescription and non-prescription medicines, vitamins and herbal supplements. Many medicines increase your chances of having seizures or other serious side effects if you take them while you are using FORFIVO XL.

How should I take FORFIVO XL?
- Take FORFIVO XL exactly as prescribed by your doctor.
- Do not chew, cut, or crush FORFIVO XL tablets. If you do, the medicine will be released into your body too quickly. If this happens, you may be more likely to get side effects including seizures. You must swallow the tablets whole. Tell your healthcare provider if you cannot swallow medicine tablets.
- You may take FORFIVO XL with or without food.
- If you take too much FORFIVO XL, or overdose, call your healthcare provider or go to the nearest hospital emergency room right away.
- Do not take any other medicines while using FORFIVO XL unless your healthcare provider has told you it is okay.
- If you are taking FORFIVO XL for the treatment of major depressive disorder, it may take several weeks for you to feel that FORFIVO XL is working. Once you feel better, it is important to keep taking FORFIVO XL exactly as directed by your doctor. Call your healthcare provider if you do not feel FORFIVO XL is working for you.
- Do not change your dose or stop taking FORFIVO XL without talking with your healthcare provider first.

What should I avoid while taking FORFIVO XL?
- Do not drink alcohol while taking FORFIVO XL.
- Do not drive a car or use heavy machinery until you know how FORFIVO XL affects you. FORFIVO XL can impair your ability to perform these tasks.

What are possible side effects of FORFIVO XL?
FORFIVO XL can cause serious side effects, including:
- See "What is the most important information I should know about FORFIVO XL?"

The most common side effects of FORFIVO XL include:

- dry mouth
- nausea
- trouble sleeping
- dizziness
- sore throat
- stomach pain
- agitation
- anxiety
- shakiness
- fast heart beat
- sweating
- ringing in the ears
- muscle pain
- anorexia
- urinating more often than normal for you
- rash

If you have nausea, take your medicine with food. If you have trouble sleeping, do not take your medicine too close to bedtime.
Tell your healthcare provider right away about any side effects that bother you.
These are not all the side effects of FORFIVO XL. For a complete list, ask your healthcare provider or pharmacist. Call your healthcare provider for medical advice about side effects. You may report side effects to FDA at 1-800-FDA-1088.

How should I store FORFIVO XL?
- Store FORFIVO XL between 68 °F to 77 °F (20 °C to 25 °C).

Keep FORFIVO XL and all medicines out of the reach of children.

General Information about FORFIVO XL.
Medicines are sometimes prescribed for purposes other than those listed in a Medication Guide. Do not use FORFIVO XL for a condition for which it was not prescribed. Do not give FORFIVO XL to other people, even if they have the same symptoms you have. It may harm them.
If you take a urine drug screening test, FORFIVO XL may make the test result positive for amphetamines. If you tell

the person giving you the drug screening test that you are taking FORFIVO XL, they can do a more specific drug screening test that should not have this problem.
This Medication Guide summarizes important information about FORFIVO XL. For more information, talk with your healthcare provider. You can ask your healthcare provider or pharmacist for information about FORFIVO XL that is written for health professionals.
For more information, call 1-888-594-4332.
What are the ingredients in FORFIVO XL?
Active ingredient: bupropion hydrochloride.
Inactive ingredients: hydroxypropyl cellulose, hydrochloric acid, polyvinyl pyrrolidone and polyvinyl acetate blend, polyethylene oxide, stearic acid, colloidal silicon dioxide, magnesium stearate, hydroxypropylmethyl cellulose, triacetin, talc, methacrylic acid copolymer, polyethylene glycol 8000, titanium dioxide and carboxymethyl cellulose sodium. The tablets are printed with edible black ink.
The following are registered trademarks of their respective manufacturers: WELLBUTRIN® and WELLBUTRIN XL®/GlaxoSmithKline; ZYBAN® /GlaxoSmithKline; PARNATE® / GlaxoSmithKline; NARDIL®/Warner Lambert Company; MARPLAN®/ Validus Pharmaceuticals LLC; KALETRA®/Abbott Laboratories.
Rx only
This Medication Guide has been approved by the U.S. Food and Drug Administration.
Manufactured by:
Pillar5 Pharma Inc.
Arnprior, Ontario, K7S 0C9
Canada
For:
Edgemont Pharmaceuticals, LLC
Austin, TX 78746
Revised June 2014
FFO_V3

Shown in Product Identification Guide, page 306

Novartis Pharmaceuticals Corporation
ONE HEALTH PLAZA
EAST HANOVER, NJ 07936
(for branded products)

For Information Contact (branded products):
Customer Interaction Center
(888) NOW-NOVA [888-669-6682]
www.pharma.us.novartis.com

XOLAIR®
[zō-lər]
(omalizumab)
For injection, for subcutaneous use

℞

The following prescribing information is based on official labeling in effect July 2014.
HIGHLIGHTS OF PRESCRIBING INFORMATION
These highlights do not include all the information needed to use XOLAIR safely and effectively. See full prescribing information for XOLAIR.
XOLAIR® (omalizumab) for injection, for subcutaneous use
Initial U.S. Approval: 2003

WARNING: ANAPHYLAXIS
See full prescribing information for complete boxed warning.
Anaphylaxis, presenting as bronchospasm, hypotension, syncope, urticaria, and/or angioedema of the throat or tongue, has been reported to occur after administration of Xolair. Anaphylaxis has occurred after the first dose of Xolair but also has occurred beyond 1 year after beginning treatment. Closely observe patients for an appropriate period of time after Xolair administration and be prepared to manage anaphylaxis that can be life-threatening. Inform patients of the signs and symptoms of anaphylaxis and have them seek immediate medical care should symptoms occur. (5.1)

——RECENT MAJOR CHANGES——
Indications and Usage (1.2) 3/2014
Dosage and Administration (2.2) 3/2014
Warnings and Precautions (5.2) 9/2014
——INDICATIONS AND USAGE——
Xolair is an anti-IgE antibody indicated for:
- Moderate to severe persistent asthma in patients (12 years of age and above) with a positive skin test or in

vitro reactivity to a perennial aeroallergen and symptoms that are inadequately controlled with inhaled corticosteroids (1.1)
- Chronic idiopathic urticaria in adults and adolescents (12 years of age and above) who remain symptomatic despite H1 antihistamine treatment (1.2)
Limitations of use:
- Not indicated for other allergic conditions or other forms of urticaria. (1.1, 1.2,)
- Not indicated for acute bronchospasm or status asthmaticus. (1.1, 5.3)
——DOSAGE AND ADMINISTRATION——
For subcutaneous (SC) administration only. (2.1, 2.2)
Divide doses of more than 150 mg among more than one injection site to limit injections to not more than 150 mg per site. (2.4)
- Asthma: Xolair 150 to 375 mg SC every 2 or 4 weeks. Determine dose (mg) and dosing frequency by serum total IgE level (IU/mL), measured before the start of treatment, and body weight (kg). See the dose determination charts. (2.1)
- Chronic Idiopathic Urticaria: Xolair 150 or 300 mg SC every 4 weeks. Dosing in CIU is not dependent on serum IgE level or body weight. (2.2)
——DOSAGE FORMS AND STRENGTHS——
- For injection: Lyophilized, sterile powder in a single-use 5mL vial, 150 mg. (3)
——CONTRAINDICATIONS——
- Severe hypersensitivity reaction to Xolair or any ingredient of Xolair. (4, 5.1)
——WARNINGS AND PRECAUTIONS——
- Anaphylaxis: Administer only in a healthcare setting prepared to manage anaphylaxis that can be life-threatening and observe patients for an appropriate period of time after administration. (5.1)
- Malignancy: Malignancies have been observed in clinical studies. (5.2)
- Acute Asthma Symptoms: Do not use for the treatment of acute bronchospasm or status asthmaticus. (5.3)
- Corticosteroid Reduction: Do not abruptly discontinue corticosteroids upon initiation of Xolair therapy. (5.4)
- Fever, Arthralgia, and Rash: Stop Xolair if patients develop signs and symptoms similar to serum sickness. (5.6)
- Eosinophilic Conditions: Be alert to eosinophilia, vasculitic rash, worsening pulmonary symptoms, cardiac complications, and/or neuropathy, especially upon reduction of oral corticosteroids. (5.5)
——ADVERSE REACTIONS——
- Asthma: The most common adverse reactions (≥1% more frequent in Xolair-treated patients) in clinical studies were arthralgia, pain (general), leg pain, fatigue, dizziness, fracture, arm pain, pruritus, dermatitis, and earache. (6.1)
- Chronic Idiopathic Urticaria: The most common adverse reactions (≥2% Xolair-treated patients and more frequent than in placebo) included the following: nausea, nasopharyngitis, sinusitis, upper respiratory tract infection, viral upper respiratory tract infection, arthralgia, headache, and cough. (6.1)
To report SUSPECTED ADVERSE REACTIONS, contact Genentech at 1-888-835-2555 or FDA at 1-800-FDA-1088 or www.fda.gov/medwatch.
——DRUG INTERACTIONS——
- No formal drug interaction studies have been performed. (7)
See 17 for PATIENT COUNSELING INFORMATION and Medication Guide.

Revised: 9/2014

FULL PRESCRIBING INFORMATION: CONTENTS*
WARNING: ANAPHYLAXIS
1 INDICATIONS AND USAGE
  1.1 Asthma
  1.2 Chronic Idiopathic Urticaria (CIU)
2 DOSAGE AND ADMINISTRATION
  2.1 Dosage for Asthma
  2.2 Dosage for Chronic Idiopathic Urticaria
  2.3 Reconstitution
  2.4 Administration
3 DOSAGE FORMS AND STRENGTHS
4 CONTRAINDICATIONS
5 WARNINGS AND PRECAUTIONS
  5.1 Anaphylaxis
  5.2 Malignancy
  5.3 Acute Asthma Symptoms
  5.4 Corticosteroid Reduction
  5.5 Eosinophilic Conditions
  5.6 Fever, Arthralgia, and Rash
  5.7 Parasitic (Helminth) Infection
  5.8 Laboratory Tests
6 ADVERSE REACTIONS
  6.1 Clinical Trials Experience
  6.2 Immunogenicity
  6.3 Postmarketing Experience

Table 1. Subcutaneous Xolair Doses Every 4 Weeks for Patients 12 Years of Age and Older with Asthma

Pre-treatment Serum IgE	Body Weight			
	30–60 kg	> 60–70 kg	> 70–90 kg	> 90–150 kg
≥ 30–100 IU/mL	150 mg	150 mg	150 mg	300 mg
> 100–200 IU/mL	300 mg	300 mg	300 mg	
> 200–300 IU/mL	300 mg			
> 300–400 IU/mL		SEE TABLE 2		
> 400–500 IU/mL				
> 500–600 IU/mL				

Table 2. Subcutaneous Xolair Doses Every 2 Weeks for Patients 12 Years of Age and Older with Asthma

Pre-treatment Serum IgE	Body Weight			
	30–60 kg	> 60–70 kg	> 70–90 kg	> 90–150 kg
≥ 30-100 IU/mL	SEE TABLE 1			
> 100-200 IU/mL				225 mg
> 200-300 IU/mL		225 mg	225 mg	300 mg
> 300-400 IU/mL	225 mg	225 mg	300 mg	
> 400-500 IU/mL	300 mg	300 mg	375 mg	
> 500-600 IU/mL	300 mg	375 mg	DO NOT DOSE	
> 600-700 IU/mL	375 mg			

7 **DRUG INTERACTIONS**
8 **USE IN SPECIFIC POPULATIONS**
    8.1 Pregnancy
    8.3 Nursing Mothers
    8.4 Pediatric Use
    8.5 Geriatric Use
10 **OVERDOSAGE**
11 **DESCRIPTION**
12 **CLINICAL PHARMACOLOGY**
    12.1 Mechanism of Action
    12.2 Pharmacodynamics
    12.3 Pharmacokinetics
13 **NONCLINICAL TOXICOLOGY**
    13.1 Carcinogenesis, Mutagenesis, Impairment of Fertility
14 **CLINICAL STUDIES**
    14.1 Asthma
    14.2 Chronic Idiopathic Urticaria
16 **HOW SUPPLIED/STORAGE AND HANDLING**
17 **PATIENT COUNSELING INFORMATION**
* Sections or subsections omitted from the full prescribing information are not listed.

FULL PRESCRIBING INFORMATION

WARNING: ANAPHYLAXIS

Anaphylaxis presenting as bronchospasm, hypotension, syncope, urticaria, and/or angioedema of the throat or tongue, has been reported to occur after administration of Xolair. Anaphylaxis has occurred as early as after the first dose of Xolair, but also has occurred beyond 1 year after beginning regularly administered treatment. Because of the risk of anaphylaxis, observe patients closely for an appropriate period of time after Xolair administration. Health care providers administering Xolair should be prepared to manage anaphylaxis that can be life-threatening. Inform patients of the signs and symptoms of anaphylaxis and instruct them to seek immediate medical care should symptoms occur [see Warnings and Precautions (5.1) and Adverse Reactions (6.3)].

---

1 **INDICATIONS AND USAGE**
1.1 **Asthma**
Xolair is indicated for adults and adolescents (12 years of age and above) with moderate to severe persistent asthma who have a positive skin test or in vitro reactivity to a perennial aeroallergen and whose symptoms are inadequately controlled with inhaled corticosteroids.
Xolair has been shown to decrease the incidence of asthma exacerbations in these patients.

Limitations of Use:
• Xolair is not indicated for the relief of acute bronchospasm or status asthmaticus.
• Xolair is not indicated for treatment of other allergic conditions.

1.2 **Chronic Idiopathic Urticaria (CIU)**
Xolair is indicated for the treatment of adults and adolescents (12 years of age and above) with chronic idiopathic urticaria who remain symptomatic despite H1 antihistamine treatment.
Limitation of Use:
• Xolair is not indicated for treatment of other forms of urticaria.

2 **DOSAGE AND ADMINISTRATION**
2.1 **Dosage for Asthma**
Administer Xolair 150 to 375 mg by subcutaneous injection every 2 or 4 weeks. Determine doses (mg) and dosing frequency by serum total IgE level (IU/mL), measured before the start of treatment, and body weight (kg) (see Table 1 and 2).
Adjust doses for significant changes in body weight (see Table 1 and 2).
Total IgE levels are elevated during treatment and remain elevated for up to one year after the discontinuation of treatment. Therefore, re-testing of IgE levels during Xolair treatment cannot be used as a guide for dose determination.
• Interruptions lasting less than one year: Dose based on serum IgE levels obtained at the initial dose determination.
• Interruptions lasting one year or more: Re-test total serum IgE levels for dose determination.
Periodically reassess the need for continued therapy based upon the patient's disease severity and level of asthma control.
[See table 1 above]
[See table 2 above]
2.2 **Dosage for Chronic Idiopathic Urticaria**
Administer Xolair 150 or 300 mg by subcutaneous injection every 4 weeks.
Dosing of Xolair in CIU patients is not dependent on serum IgE (free or total) level or body weight.
The appropriate duration of therapy for CIU has not been evaluated. Periodically reassess the need for continued therapy.
2.3 **Reconstitution**
The supplied Xolair lyophilized powder must be reconstituted with Sterile Water for Injection (SWFI) USP, using the following instructions:
1. Before reconstitution, determine the number of vials that will need to be reconstituted (each vial delivers 150 mg of Xolair) [see Dosage and Administration (2.1, 2.2)].

2. Draw 1.4 mL of SWFI, USP, into a 3 mL syringe equipped with a 1 inch, 18-gauge needle.
3. Place the vial upright on a flat surface and using standard aseptic technique, insert the needle and inject the SWFI, USP, directly onto the product.
4. Keeping the vial upright, gently swirl the upright vial for approximately 1 minute to evenly wet the powder. Do not shake.
5. Gently swirl the vial for 5 to 10 seconds approximately every 5 minutes in order to dissolve any remaining solids. **The lyophilized product takes 15 to 20 minutes to dissolve.** If it takes longer than 20 minutes to dissolve completely, gently swirl the vial for 5 to 10 seconds approximately every 5 minutes until there are no visible gel-like particles in the solution. Do not use if the contents of the vial do not dissolve completely by 40 minutes.
6. After reconstitution, Xolair solution is somewhat viscous and will appear clear or slightly opalescent. It is acceptable if there are a few small bubbles or foam around the edge of the vial; there should be no visible gel-like particles in the reconstituted solution. Do not use if foreign particles are present.
7. Invert the vial for 15 seconds in order to allow the solution to drain toward the stopper.
8. **Use the Xolair solution within 8 hours following reconstitution when stored in the vial at 2 to 8°C (36 to 46°F), or within 4 hours of reconstitution when stored at room temperature.** Reconstituted Xolair vials should be protected from sunlight.
9. Using a new 3 mL syringe equipped with a 1-inch, 18-gauge needle, insert the needle into the inverted vial. Position the needle tip at the very bottom of the solution in the vial stopper when drawing the solution into the syringe. The reconstituted product is somewhat viscous; in order to obtain the full 1.2 mL dose, **all of the product must be withdrawn** from the vial before expelling any air or excess solution from the syringe. Before removing the needle from the vial, pull the plunger all the way back to the end of the syringe barrel in order to remove all of the solution from the inverted vial.
10. Replace the 18-gauge needle with a 25-gauge needle for subcutaneous injection.
11. Expel air, large bubbles, and any excess solution in order to obtain the required 1.2 mL dose. A thin layer of small bubbles may remain at the top of the solution in the syringe.

2.4 **Administration**
Administer Xolair by subcutaneous injection. The injection may take 5-10 seconds to administer because the solution is slightly viscous. Do not administer more than 150 mg (contents of one vial) per injection site. Divide doses of more than 150 mg among two or more injection sites (Table 3).

Table 3. Number of Injections and Total Injection Volumes

Xolair Dose*	Number of Injections	Total Volume Injected
150 mg	1	1.2 mL
225 mg	2	1.8 mL
300 mg	2	2.4 mL
375 mg	3	3.0 mL

* All doses in the table are approved for use in asthma patients. The 150 mg and 300 mg Xolair doses are intended for use in CIU patients.

3 **DOSAGE FORMS AND STRENGTHS**
For injection: 150 mg of omalizumab as lyophilized, sterile powder in a single-dose 5 mL vial.

4 **CONTRAINDICATIONS**
The use of Xolair is contraindicated in the following:
Severe hypersensitivity reaction to Xolair or any ingredient of Xolair [see Warnings and Precautions (5.1)].

5 **WARNINGS AND PRECAUTIONS**
5.1 **Anaphylaxis**
Anaphylaxis has been reported to occur after administration of Xolair in premarketing clinical trials and in postmarketing spontaneous reports [see Boxed Warning and Adverse Reactions (6.3)]. Signs and symptoms in these reported cases have included bronchospasm, hypotension, syncope, urticaria, and/or angioedema of the throat or tongue. Some of these events have been life-threatening. In premarketing clinical trials in patients with asthma, anaphylaxis was reported in 3 of 3507 (0.1%) patients. Anaphylaxis occurred with the first dose of Xolair in two patients and with the fourth dose in one patient. The time to onset of anaphylaxis was 90 minutes after administration in two patients and 2 hours after administration in one patient. In postmarketing spontaneous reports, the frequency of anaphylaxis attributed to Xolair use was estimated to be at

least 0.2% of patients based on an estimated exposure of about 57,300 patients from June 2003 through December 2006. Anaphylaxis has occurred as early as after the first dose of Xolair, but also has occurred beyond one year after beginning regularly scheduled treatment.

Administer Xolair only in a healthcare setting by healthcare providers prepared to manage anaphylaxis that can be life-threatening. Observe patients closely for an appropriate period of time after administration of Xolair, taking into account the time to onset of anaphylaxis seen in premarketing clinical trials and postmarketing spontaneous reports [see Adverse Reactions (6)]. Inform patients of the signs and symptoms of anaphylaxis, and instruct them to seek immediate medical care should signs or symptoms occur. Discontinue Xolair in patients who experience a severe hypersensitivity reaction [see Contraindications (4)].

5.2 Malignancy

Malignant neoplasms were observed in 20 of 4127 (0.5%) Xolair-treated patients compared with 5 of 2236 (0.2%) control patients in clinical studies of adults and adolescents (≥ 12 years of age) with asthma and other allergic disorders. The observed malignancies in Xolair-treated patients were a variety of types, with breast, non-melanoma skin, prostate, melanoma, and parotid occurring more than once, and five other types occurring once each. The majority of patients were observed for less than 1 year. The impact of longer exposure to Xolair or use in patients at higher risk for malignancy (e.g., elderly, current smokers) is not known. In a subsequent observational study of 5007 Xolair-treated and 2829 non-Xolair-treated patients with moderate to severe persistent asthma and a positive skin test reaction or in vitro reactivity to a perennial aeroallergen, patients were followed for up to 5 years. In this study, the incidence rates of primary malignancies (per 1000 patient years) were similar among Xolair-treated (12.3) and non-Xolair-treated patients (13.0) [see Adverse Reactions (6)]. However, study limitations preclude definitively ruling out a malignancy risk with Xolair. Study limitations include: the observational study design, the bias introduced by allowing enrollment of patients previously exposed to Xolair (88%), enrollment of patients (56%) while a history of cancer or a premalignant condition were study exclusion criteria, and the high study discontinuation rate (44%).

5.3 Acute Asthma Symptoms

Xolair has not been shown to alleviate asthma exacerbations acutely. Do not use Xolair to treat acute bronchospasm or status asthmaticus.

5.4 Corticosteroid Reduction

Do not discontinue systemic or inhaled corticosteroids abruptly upon initiation of Xolair therapy for asthma. Decrease corticosteroids gradually under the direct supervision of a physician. In CIU patients, the use of Xolair in combination with corticosteroids has not been evaluated.

5.5 Eosinophilic Conditions

In rare cases, patients with asthma on therapy with Xolair may present with serious systemic eosinophilia sometimes presenting with clinical features of vasculitis consistent with Churg-Strauss syndrome, a condition which is often treated with systemic corticosteroid therapy. These events usually, but not always, have been associated with the reduction of oral corticosteroid therapy. Physicians should be alert to eosinophilia, vasculitic rash, worsening pulmonary symptoms, cardiac complications, and/or neuropathy presenting in their patients. A causal association between Xolair and these underlying conditions has not been established.

5.6 Fever, Arthralgia, and Rash

In post-approval use, some patients have experienced a constellation of signs and symptoms including arthritis/arthralgia, rash, fever and lymphadenopathy with an onset 1 to 5 days after the first or subsequent injections of Xolair. These signs and symptoms have recurred after additional doses in some patients. Although circulating immune complexes or a skin biopsy consistent with a Type III reaction were not seen with these cases, these signs and symptoms are similar to those seen in patients with serum sickness. Physicians should stop Xolair if a patient develops this constellation of signs and symptoms [see Adverse Reactions (6.3)].

5.7 Parasitic (Helminth) Infection

Monitor patients at high risk of geohelminth infection while on Xolair therapy. Insufficient data are available to determine the length of monitoring required for geohelminth infections after stopping Xolair treatment.

In a one-year clinical trial conducted in Brazil in patients at high risk for geohelminthic infections (roundworm, hookworm, whipworm, threadworm), 53% (36/68) of Xolair-treated patients experienced an infection, as diagnosed by standard stool examination, compared to 42% (29/69) of placebo controls. The point estimate of the odds ratio for infection was 1.96, with a 95% confidence interval (0.88, 4.36) indicating that in this study a patient who had an infection was anywhere from 0.88 to 4.36 times as likely to have received Xolair than a patient who did not have an infection.

Response to appropriate anti-geohelminth treatment of infection as measured by stool egg counts was not different between treatment groups.

5.8 Laboratory Tests

Serum total IgE levels increase following administration of Xolair due to formation of Xolair:IgE complexes [see Clinical Pharmacology (12.2)]. Elevated serum total IgE levels may persist for up to 1 year following discontinuation of Xolair. Do not use serum total IgE levels obtained less than 1 year following discontinuation to reassess the dosing regimen for asthma patients, because these levels may not reflect steady state free IgE levels.

6 ADVERSE REACTIONS

Use of Xolair has been associated with:
- Anaphylaxis [see Boxed Warning and Warnings and Precautions (5.1)]
- Malignancies [see Warnings and Precautions (5.2)]

6.1 Clinical Trials Experience

Because clinical trials are conducted under widely varying conditions, adverse reaction rates observed in the clinical trials of a drug cannot be directly compared to rates in the clinical trials of another drug and may not reflect the rates observed in clinical practice.

Adverse Reactions from Clinical Studies in Patients with Asthma

The data described below reflect Xolair exposure for 2076 adult and adolescent patients ages 12 and older, including 1687 patients exposed for six months and 555 exposed for one year or more, in either placebo-controlled or other controlled asthma studies. The mean age of patients receiving Xolair was 42 years, with 134 patients 65 years of age or older; 60% were women, and 85% Caucasian. Patients received Xolair 150 to 375 mg every 2 or 4 weeks or, for patients assigned to control groups, standard therapy with or without a placebo.

The adverse events most frequently resulting in clinical intervention (e.g., discontinuation of Xolair, or the need for concomitant medication to treat an adverse event) were injection site reaction (45%), viral infections (23%), upper respiratory tract infection (20%), sinusitis (16%), headache (15%), and pharyngitis (11%). These events were observed at similar rates in Xolair-treated patients and control patients.

Table 4 shows adverse reactions from four placebo-controlled asthma trials that occurred ≥ 1% and more frequently in patients receiving Xolair than in those receiving placebo. Adverse events were classified using preferred terms from the International Medical Nomenclature (IMN) dictionary. Injection site reactions were recorded separately from the reporting of other adverse events.

Table 4. Adverse Reactions ≥ 1% More Frequent in Xolair-Treated Adult or Adolescent Patients 12 years of Age and Older in Four Placebo-controlled Asthma Trials

Adverse reaction	Xolair n = 738	Placebo n = 717
Body as a whole		
Pain	7%	5%
Fatigue	3%	2%
Musculoskeletal system		
Arthralgia	8%	6%
Fracture	2%	1%
Leg pain	4%	2%
Arm pain	2%	1%
Nervous system		
Dizziness	3%	2%
Skin and appendages		
Pruritus	2%	1%
Dermatitis	2%	1%
Special senses		
Earache	2%	1%

There were no differences in the incidence of adverse reactions based on age (among patients under 65), gender or race.

Injection Site Reactions

Injection site reactions of any severity occurred at a rate of 45% in Xolair-treated patients compared with 43% in placebo-treated patients. The types of injection site reactions included: bruising, redness, warmth, burning, stinging, itching, hive formation, pain, indurations, mass, and inflammation.

Severe injection site reactions occurred more frequently in Xolair-treated patients compared with patients in the placebo group (12% versus 9%).

The majority of injection site reactions occurred within 1 hour-post injection, lasted less than 8 days, and generally decreased in frequency at subsequent dosing visits.

Adverse Reactions from Clinical Studies in Patients with Chronic Idiopathic Urticaria (CIU)

The safety of Xolair for the treatment of CIU was assessed in three placebo-controlled, multiple-dose clinical trials of 12 weeks' (CIU Trial 2) and 24 weeks' duration (CIU Trials 1 and 3). In CIU Trials 1 and 2, patients received Xolair 75, 150, or 300 mg or placebo every 4 weeks in addition to their baseline level of H1 antihistamine therapy throughout the treatment period. In CIU Trial 3 patients were randomized to Xolair 300 mg or placebo every 4 weeks in addition to their baseline level of H1 antihistamine therapy. The data described below reflect Xolair exposure for 733 patients enrolled and receiving at least one dose of Xolair in the three clinical trials, including 684 patients exposed for 12 weeks and 427 exposed for 24 weeks. The mean age of patients receiving Xolair 300 mg was 43 years, 75% were women, and 89% were white. The demographic profiles for patients receiving Xolair 150 mg and 75 mg were similar.

Table 5 shows adverse reactions that occurred in ≥ 2% of patients receiving Xolair (150 or 300 mg) and more frequently than those receiving placebo. Adverse reactions are pooled from Trial 2 and the first 12 weeks of Trials 1 and 3. [See table 5 above]

Additional reactions reported during the 24 week treatment period in Trials 1 and 3 [≥2% of patients receiving Xolair (150 or 300 mg) and more frequently than those receiving placebo] included: toothache, fungal infection, urinary tract infection, myalgia, pain in extremity, musculoskeletal pain, peripheral edema, pyrexia, migraine, sinus headache, anxiety, oropharyngeal pain, asthma, urticaria, and alopecia.

Injection Site Reactions

Injection site reactions of any severity occurred during the studies in more Xolair-treated patients [11 patients (2.7%) at 300 mg, 1 patient (0.6%) at 150 mg] compared with 2 placebo-treated patients (0.8%). The types of injection site reactions included: swelling, erythema, pain, bruising, itching, bleeding and urticaria. None of the events resulted in study discontinuation or treatment interruption.

Cardiovascular and Cerebrovascular Events from Clinical Studies in Patients with Asthma

A 5-year observational cohort study was conducted in patients ≥ 12 years old with moderate to severe persistent asthma and a positive skin test reaction to a perennial aeroallergen to evaluate the long term safety of Xolair, including the risk of malignancy [see Warnings and Precau-

Table 5. Adverse Reactions Occurring in ≥2 % in Xolair-Treated Patients and More Frequently than in Patients Treated with Placebo (Day 1 to Week 12) in CIU Trials

Adverse Reactions*	CIU Trials 1, 2 and 3 Pooled		
	150mg (n=175)	300mg (n=412)	Placebo (n=242)
Gastrointestinal disorders			
Nausea	2 (1.1%)	11 (2.7%)	6 (2.5%)
Infections and infestations			
Nasopharyngitis	16 (9.1%)	27 (6.6%)	17 (7.0%)
Sinusitis	2 (1.1%)	20 (4.9%)	5 (2.1%)
Upper respiratory tract infection	2 (1.1%)	14 (3.4%)	5 (2.1%)
Viral upper respiratory tract infection	4 (2.3%)	2 (0.5%)	(0.0%)
Musculoskeletal and connective tissue disorders			
Arthralgia	5 (2.9%)	12 (2.9%)	1 (0.4%)
Nervous system disorders			
Headache	21 (12.0%)	25 (6.1%)	7 (2.9%)
Respiratory, thoracic, and mediastinal disorders			
Cough	2 (1.1%)	9 (2.2%)	3 (1.2%)

* by MedDRA (15.1) System Organ Class and Preferred Term

tions (5.2)]. A total of 5007 Xolair-treated and 2829 non-Xolair-treated patients enrolled in the study. Similar percentages of patients in both cohorts were current (5%) or former smokers (29%). Patients had a mean age of 45 years and were followed for a mean of 3.7 years. More Xolair-treated patients were diagnosed with severe asthma (50%) compared to the non-Xolair-treated patients (23%) and 44% of patients prematurely discontinued the study. Additionally, 88% of patients in the Xolair-treated cohort had been previously exposed to Xolair for a mean of 8 months.

A higher incidence rate (per 1000 patient-years) of overall cardiovascular and cerebrovascular serious adverse events (SAEs) was observed in Xolair-treated patients (13.4) compared to non-Xolair-treated patients (8.1). Increases in rates were observed for transient ischemic attack (0.7 versus 0.1), myocardial infarction (2.1 versus 0.8), pulmonary hypertension (0.5 versus 0), pulmonary embolism/venous thrombosis (3.2 versus 1.5), and unstable angina (2.2 versus 1.4), while the rates observed for ischemic stroke and cardiovascular death were similar among both study cohorts. The results suggest a potential increased risk of serious cardiovascular and cerebrovascular events in patients treated with Xolair. However, the observational study design, the inclusion of patients previously exposed to Xolair (88%), baseline imbalances in cardiovascular risk factors between the treatment groups, an inability to adjust for unmeasured risk factors, and the high study discontinuation rate limit the ability to quantify the magnitude of the risk.

A pooled analysis of 25 randomized double-blind, placebo-controlled clinical trials of 8 to 52 weeks in duration was conducted to further evaluate the imbalance in cardiovascular and cerebrovascular SAEs noted in the above observational cohort study. A total of 3342 Xolair-treated patients and 2895 placebo-treated patients were included in the pooled analysis. The patients had a mean age of 38 years, and were followed for a mean duration of 6.8 months. No notable imbalances were observed in the rates of cardiovascular and cerebrovascular SAEs listed above. However, the results of the pooled analysis were based on a low number of events, slightly younger patients, and shorter duration of follow-up than the observational cohort study; therefore, the results are insufficient to confirm or reject the findings noted in the observational cohort study.

6.2 Immunogenicity

Antibodies to Xolair were detected in approximately 1/1723 (< 0.1%) of patients treated with Xolair in the clinical studies for approval of asthma. There were no detectable antibodies in the patients treated in the phase 3 CIU clinical trials, but due to levels of Xolair at the time of anti-therapeutic antibody sampling and missing samples for some patients, antibodies to Xolair could only have been determined in 88% of the 733 patients treated in these clinical studies. The data reflect the percentage of patients whose test results were considered positive for antibodies to Xolair in ELISA assays and are highly dependent on the sensitivity and specificity of the assays. Additionally, the observed incidence of antibody positivity in the assay may be influenced by several factors including sample handling, timing of sample collection, concomitant medications, and underlying disease. Therefore, comparison of the incidence of antibodies to Xolair with the incidence of antibodies to other products may be misleading.

6.3 Postmarketing Experience

The following adverse reactions have been identified during post-approval use of Xolair in adult and adolescent patients 12 years of age and older. Because these reactions are reported voluntarily from a population of uncertain size, it is not always possible to reliably estimate their frequency or establish a causal relationship to drug exposure.

Anaphylaxis: Based on spontaneous reports and an estimated exposure of about 57,300 patients from June 2003 through December 2006, the frequency of anaphylaxis attributed to Xolair use was estimated to be at least 0.2% of patients. Diagnostic criteria of anaphylaxis were skin or mucosal tissue involvement, and, either airway compromise, and/or reduced blood pressure with or without associated symptoms, and a temporal relationship to Xolair administration with no other identifiable cause. Signs and symptoms in these reported cases included bronchospasm, hypotension, syncope, urticaria, angioedema of the throat or tongue, dyspnea, cough, chest tightness, and/or cutaneous angioedema. Pulmonary involvement was reported in 89% of the cases. Hypotension or syncope was reported in 14% of cases. Fifteen percent of the reported cases resulted in hospitalization. A previous history of anaphylaxis unrelated to Xolair was reported in 24% of the cases.

Of the reported cases of anaphylaxis attributed to Xolair, 39% occurred with the first dose, 19% occurred with the second dose, 10% occurred with the third dose, and the rest after subsequent doses. One case occurred after 39 doses (after 19 months of continuous therapy, anaphylaxis occurred when treatment was restarted following a 3 month gap). The time to onset of anaphylaxis in these cases was up to 30 minutes in 35%, greater than 30 and up to 60 minutes in 16%, greater than 60 and up to 90 minutes in 2%, greater than 90 and up to 120 minutes in 6%, greater than 2 hours and up to 6 hours in 5%, greater than 6 hours and up to 12 hours in 14%, greater than 12 hours and up to 24 hours in 8%, and greater than 24 hours and up to 4 days in 5%. In 9% of cases the times to onset were unknown.

Twenty-three patients who experienced anaphylaxis were rechallenged with Xolair and 18 patients had a recurrence of similar symptoms of anaphylaxis. In addition, anaphylaxis occurred upon rechallenge with Xolair in 4 patients who previously experienced urticaria only.

Eosinophilic Conditions: Eosinophilic conditions have been reported [see Warnings and Precautions (5.5)].

Fever, Arthralgia, and Rash: A constellation of signs and symptoms including arthritis/arthralgia, rash (urticaria or other forms), fever and lymphadenopathy similar to serum sickness have been reported in post-approval use of Xolair [see Warnings and Precautions (5.6)].

Hematologic: Severe thrombocytopenia has been reported.

Skin: Hair loss has been reported.

7 DRUG INTERACTIONS

No formal drug interaction studies have been performed with Xolair.

In patients with asthma the concomitant use of Xolair and allergen immunotherapy has not been evaluated.

In patients with CIU the use of Xolair in combination with immunosuppressive therapies has not been studied.

8 USE IN SPECIFIC POPULATIONS

8.1 Pregnancy

Pregnancy Category B

Pregnancy Exposure Registry

There is a pregnancy exposure registry that monitors pregnancy outcomes in women exposed to Xolair during pregnancy. Encourage patients to call 1-866-4XOLAIR (1-866-496-5247) or visit www.xolairpregnancyregistry.com for information about the pregnancy exposure registry and the enrollment procedure.

Risk Summary

Adequate and well-controlled studies with Xolair have not been conducted in pregnant women. All pregnancies, regardless of drug exposure, have a background rate of 2 to 4% for major malformations, and 15 to 20% for pregnancy loss. In animal reproduction studies, no evidence of fetal harm was observed in Cynomolgus monkeys with subcutaneous doses of omalizumab up to 10 times the maximum recommended human dose (MRHD). Because animal reproduction studies are not always predictive of human response, Xolair should be used during pregnancy only if clearly needed.

Clinical Considerations

In general, monoclonal antibodies are transported across the placenta in a linear fashion as pregnancy progresses, with the largest amount transferred during the third trimester.

Data

Animal Data

Reproductive studies have been performed in Cynomolgus monkeys at subcutaneous doses of omalizumab up to 75 mg/kg (approximately 10 times the MRHD on a mg/kg basis). No evidence of maternal toxicity, embryotoxicity, or teratogenicity was observed when omalizumab was administered throughout organogenesis. Omalizumab did not elicit adverse effects on fetal or neonatal growth when administered throughout late gestation, delivery and nursing. Neonatal serum levels of omalizumab after in utero exposure and 28 days of nursing were between 11% and 94% of the maternal serum level. Levels of omalizumab in milk were 0.15% of maternal serum concentration.

8.3 Nursing Mothers

It is not known whether Xolair is present in human breast milk; however, IgG is present in human milk in small amounts. In Cynomolgus monkeys, milk levels of omalizumab were measured at 0.15% of the maternal serum concentration [see Use in Specific Populations (8.1)]. The developmental and health benefits of breastfeeding should be considered along with the mother's clinical need for Xolair and any potential adverse effects on the breastfed child from Xolair or from the underlying maternal condition. Exercise caution when administering Xolair to a nursing woman.

8.4 Pediatric Use

Asthma

Safety and effectiveness of Xolair for asthma were evaluated in 2 trials in 926 (Xolair 624; placebo 302) pediatric patients 6 to <12 years of age moderate to severe persistent asthma who had a positive skin test or in vitro reactivity to a perennial aeroallergen. One trial was a pivotal trial of similar design and conduct to that of adult and adolescent Asthma Trials 1 and 2 [see Clinical Studies (14.1)]. The other trial was primarily a safety study and included evaluation of efficacy as a secondary outcome. In the pivotal trial, Xolair-treated patients had a statistically significant reduction in the rate of exacerbations (exacerbation was defined as worsening of asthma that required treatment with systemic corticosteroids or a doubling of the baseline ICS dose), but other efficacy variables such as nocturnal symptom scores, beta-agonist use, and measures of airflow (FEV$_1$) were not significantly different in Xolair-treated patients compared to placebo. Considering the risk of anaphylaxis and malignancy seen in Xolair-treated patients ≥ 12 years old and the modest efficacy of Xolair in the pivotal pediatric trial, the risk-benefit assessment does not support the use of Xolair in patients 6 to <12 years of age. Although patients treated with Xolair in these two trials did not develop anaphylaxis or malignancy, the trials are not adequate to address these concerns because patients with a history of anaphylaxis or malignancy were excluded, and the duration of exposure and sample size were not large enough to exclude these risks in patients 6 to <12 years of age. Furthermore, there is no reason to expect that younger pediatric patients would not be at risk of anaphylaxis and malignancy seen in adult and adolescent patients with Xolair [see Warnings and Precautions (5.1) (5.2) and Adverse Reactions (6)].

Trials in patients 0-5 years of age were not performed because of the safety concerns of anaphylaxis and malignancy associated with the use of Xolair in adults and adolescents.

Chronic Idiopathic Urticaria

The safety and effectiveness of Xolair for adolescent patients with CIU were evaluated in 39 patients 12 to 17 years of age (Xolair 29, placebo 10) included in three randomized, placebo-controlled CIU trials. A numerical decrease in weekly itch score was observed, and adverse reactions were similar to those reported in patients 18 years and older. Clinical trials with Xolair have not been conducted in CIU patients below the age of 12 years. Considering the risk of anaphylaxis and malignancy seen in Xolair-treated patients ≥ 12 years old, the risk-benefit assessment does not support the use of Xolair in patients <12 years of age. Therefore, the use of Xolair in this patient population is not recommended.

8.5 Geriatric Use

In clinical studies 134 asthma patients and 37 CIU phase 3 study patients 65 years of age or older were treated with Xolair. Although there were no apparent age-related differences observed in these studies, the number of patients aged 65 and over is not sufficient to determine whether they respond differently from younger patients.

10 OVERDOSAGE

The maximum tolerated dose of Xolair has not been determined. Single intravenous doses of up to 4,000 mg have been administered to patients without evidence of dose limiting toxicities. The highest cumulative dose administered to patients was 44,000 mg over a 20 week period, which was not associated with toxicities.

11 DESCRIPTION

Xolair is a recombinant DNA-derived humanized IgG1κ monoclonal antibody that selectively binds to human immunoglobulin E (IgE). The antibody has a molecular weight of approximately 149 kiloDaltons. Xolair is produced by a Chinese hamster ovary cell suspension culture in a nutrient medium containing the antibiotic gentamicin. Gentamicin is not detectable in the final product.

Xolair is a sterile, white, preservative free, lyophilized powder contained in a single use vial that is reconstituted with Sterile Water for Injection (SWFI), USP, and administered as a subcutaneous (SC) injection. Each 202.5 mg vial of omalizumab also contains L-histidine (1.8 mg), L-histidine hydrochloride monohydrate (2.8 mg), polysorbate 20 (0.5 mg) and sucrose (145.5 mg) and is designed to deliver 150 mg of omalizumab in 1.2 mL after reconstitution with 1.4 mL SWFI, USP.

12 CLINICAL PHARMACOLOGY

12.1 Mechanism of Action

Asthma

Omalizumab inhibits the binding of IgE to the high-affinity IgE receptor (FcεRI) on the surface of mast cells and basophils. Reduction in surface-bound IgE on FcεRI-bearing cells limits the degree of release of mediators of the allergic response. Treatment with Xolair also reduces the number of FcεRI receptors on basophils in atopic patients.

Chronic Idiopathic Urticaria

Omalizumab binds to IgE and lowers free IgE levels. Subsequently, IgE receptors (FcεRI) on cells down-regulate. The mechanism by which these effects of omalizumab result in an improvement of CIU symptoms is unknown.

12.2 Pharmacodynamics

Asthma

In clinical studies, serum free IgE levels were reduced in a dose dependent manner within 1 hour following the first dose and maintained between doses. Mean serum free IgE decrease was greater than 96% using recommended doses. Serum total IgE levels (i.e., bound and unbound) increased after the first dose due to the formation of omalizumab:IgE complexes, which have a slower elimination rate compared with free IgE. At 16 weeks after the first dose, average serum total IgE levels were five-fold higher compared with pre-treatment when using standard assays. After discontinuation of Xolair dosing, the Xolair-induced increase in total IgE and decrease in free IgE were reversible, with no observed rebound in IgE levels after drug washout. Total IgE levels did not return to pre-treatment levels for up to one year after discontinuation of Xolair.

Chronic Idiopathic Urticaria

In clinical studies in CIU patients, Xolair treatment led to a dose-dependent reduction of serum free IgE and an increase of serum total IgE levels, similar to the observations in asthma patients. Maximum suppression of free IgE was observed 3 days following the first subcutaneous dose. After repeat dosing once every 4 weeks, predose serum free IgE levels remained stable between 12 and 24 weeks of treatment. Total IgE levels in serum increased after the first dose due to the formation of omalizumab-IgE complexes which have a slower elimination rate compared with free IgE. After repeat dosing once every 4 weeks at 75 mg up to 300 mg, average predose serum total IgE levels at Week 12 were two-to three-fold higher compared with pre-treatment levels, and remained stable between 12 and 24 weeks of treatment. After discontinuation of Xolair dosing, free IgE levels increased and total IgE levels decreased towards pre-treatment levels over a 16-week follow-up period.

12.3 Pharmacokinetics

After SC administration, omalizumab was absorbed with an average absolute bioavailability of 62%. Following a single SC dose in adult and adolescent patients with asthma, omalizumab was absorbed slowly, reaching peak serum concentrations after an average of 7-8 days. In patients with CIU, the peak serum concentration was reached at a similar time after a single SC dose. The pharmacokinetics of omalizumab was linear at doses greater than 0.5 mg/kg. In patients with asthma, following multiple doses of Xolair, areas under the serum concentration-time curve from Day 0 to Day 14 at steady state were up to 6-fold of those after the first dose. In patients with CIU, omalizumab exhibited linear pharmacokinetics across the dose range of 75 mg to 600 mg given as single SC dose. Following repeat dosing from 75 to 300 mg every 4 weeks, trough serum concentrations of omalizumab increased proportionally with the dose levels.

In vitro, omalizumab formed complexes of limited size with IgE. Precipitating complexes and complexes larger than 1 million daltons in molecular weight were not observed in vitro or in vivo. Tissue distribution studies in Cynomolgus monkeys showed no specific uptake of ^{125}I-omalizumab by any organ or tissue. The apparent volume of distribution of omalizumab in patients with asthma following SC administration was 78 ± 32 mL/kg. In patients with CIU, based on population pharmacokinetics, distribution of omalizumab was similar to that in patients with asthma.

Clearance of omalizumab involved IgG clearance processes as well as clearance via specific binding and complex formation with its target ligand, IgE. Liver elimination of IgG included degradation in the liver reticuloendothelial system (RES) and endothelial cells. Intact IgG was also excreted in bile. In studies with mice and monkeys, omalizumab:IgE complexes were eliminated by interactions with Fcγ receptors within the RES at rates that were generally faster than IgG clearance. In asthma patients omalizumab serum elimination half-life averaged 26 days, with apparent clearance averaging 2.4 ± 1.1 mL/kg/day. Doubling body weight approximately doubled apparent clearance. In CIU patients, at steady state, based on population pharmacokinetics, omalizumab serum elimination half-life averaged 24 days and apparent clearance averaged 240 mL/day (corresponding to 3.0 mL/kg/day for an 80 kg patient).

Special Populations

Asthma

The population pharmacokinetics of omalizumab was analyzed to evaluate the effects of demographic characteristics in patients with asthma. Analyses of these data suggested that no dose adjustments are necessary for age (12-76 years), race, ethnicity, or gender.

Chronic Idiopathic Urticaria

The population pharmacokinetics of omalizumab was analyzed to evaluate the effects of demographic characteristics and other factors on omalizumab exposure in patients with CIU. Covariate effects were evaluated by analyzing the relationship between omalizumab concentrations and clinical responses. These analyses demonstrate that no dose adjustments are necessary for age (12 to 75 years), race/ethnicity, gender, body weight, body mass index or baseline IgE level.

13 NONCLINICAL TOXICOLOGY

13.1 Carcinogenesis, Mutagenesis, Impairment of Fertility

No long-term studies have been performed in animals to evaluate the carcinogenic potential of Xolair.

There were no effects on fertility and reproductive performance in male and female Cynomolgus monkeys that re-

Table 6. Frequency of Asthma Exacerbations per Patient by Phase in Trials 1 and 2

| | Stable Steroid Phase (16 wks) | | | |
| | Asthma Trial 1 | | Asthma Trial 2 | |
Exacerbations per patient	Xolair N = 268	Placebo N = 257	Xolair N = 274	Placebo N = 272
0	85.8%	76.7%	87.6%	69.9%
1	11.9%	16.7%	11.3%	25.0%
≥ 2	2.2%	6.6%	1.1%	5.1%
p-Value	0.005		< 0.001	
Mean number exacerbations/patient	0.2	0.3	0.1	0.4

| | Steroid Reduction Phase (12 wks) | | | |
	Xolair N = 268	Placebo N = 257	Xolair N = 274	Placebo N = 272
Exacerbations per patient				
0	78.7%	67.7%	83.9%	70.2%
1	19.0%	28.4%	14.2%	26.1%
≥ 2	2.2%	3.9%	1.8%	3.7%
p-Value	0.004		< 0.001	
Mean number exacerbations/patient	0.2	0.4	0.2	0.3

Table 7. Asthma Symptoms and Pulmonary Function During Stable Steroid Phase of Trial 1

	Xolair N = 268*		Placebo N = 257*	
Endpoint	Mean Baseline	Median Change (Baseline to Wk 16)	Mean Baseline	Median Change (Baseline to Wk 16)
Total asthma symptom score	4.3	−1.5[†]	4.2	−1.1[†]
Nocturnal asthma score	1.2	−0.4[†]	1.1	−0.2[†]
Daytime asthma score	2.3	−0.9[†]	2.3	−0.6[†]
FEV_1 % predicted	68	3[†]	68	0[†]

Asthma symptom scale: total score from 0 (least) to 9 (most); nocturnal and daytime scores from 0 (least) to 4 (most symptoms).

* Number of patients available for analysis ranges 255-258 in the Xolair group and 238-239 in the placebo group.

† Comparison of Xolair versus placebo (p < 0.05).

ceived Xolair at subcutaneous doses up to 75 mg/kg/week (approximately 10 times the maximum recommended human dose on a mg/kg basis).

14 CLINICAL STUDIES

14.1 Asthma

Adult and Adolescent Patients 12 Years of Age and Older

The safety and efficacy of Xolair were evaluated in three randomized, double-blind, placebo-controlled, multicenter trials.

The trials enrolled patients 12 to 76 years old, with moderate to severe persistent (NHLBI criteria) asthma for at least one year, and a positive skin test reaction to a perennial aeroallergen. In all trials, Xolair dosing was based on body weight and baseline serum total IgE concentration. All patients were required to have a baseline IgE between 30 and 700 IU/mL and body weight not more than 150 kg. Patients were treated according to a dosing table to administer at least 0.016 mg/kg/IU (IgE/mL) of Xolair or a matching volume of placebo over each 4-week period. The maximum Xolair dose per 4 weeks was 750 mg.

In all three trials an exacerbation was defined as a worsening of asthma that required treatment with systemic corticosteroids or a doubling of the baseline ICS dose. Most exacerbations were managed in the out-patient setting and the majority were treated with systemic steroids. Hospitalization rates were not significantly different between Xolair and placebo-treated patients; however, the overall hospitalization rate was small. Among those patients who experienced an exacerbation, the distribution of exacerbation severity was similar between treatment groups.

Asthma Trials 1 and 2

At screening, patients in Asthma Trials 1 and 2 had a forced expiratory volume in one second (FEV_1) between 40% and 80% predicted. All patients had a FEV_1 improvement of at least 12% following beta$_2$-agonist administration. All patients were symptomatic and were being treated with inhaled corticosteroids (ICS) and short acting beta$_2$-agonists. Patients receiving other concomitant controller medications were excluded, and initiation of additional controller medications while on study was prohibited. Patients currently smoking were excluded.

Each trial was comprised of a run-in period to achieve a stable conversion to a common ICS (beclomethasone dipropionate), followed by randomization to Xolair or placebo. Patients received Xolair for 16 weeks with an unchanged corticosteroid dose unless an acute exacerbation

necessitated an increase. Patients then entered an ICS reduction phase of 12 weeks during which ICS dose reduction was attempted in a step-wise manner.

The distribution of the number of asthma exacerbations per patient in each group during a study was analyzed separately for the stable steroid and steroid-reduction periods. In both Asthma Trials 1 and 2 the number of exacerbations per patient was reduced in patients treated with Xolair compared with placebo (Table 6).

Measures of airflow (FEV_1) and asthma symptoms were also evaluated in these trials. The clinical relevance of the treatment-associated differences is unknown. Results from the stable steroid phase Asthma Trial 1 are shown in Table 7. Results from the stable steroid phase of Asthma Trial 2 and the steroid reduction phases of both Asthma Trials 1 and 2 were similar to those presented in Table 7.

[See table 6 above]

[See table 7 above]

Asthma Trial 3

In Asthma Trial 3, there was no restriction on screening FEV_1, and unlike Asthma Trials 1 and 2, long-acting beta$_2$-agonists were allowed. Patients were receiving at least 1000 µg/day fluticasone propionate and a subset was also receiving oral corticosteroids. Patients receiving other concomitant controller medications were excluded, and initiation of additional controller medications while on study was prohibited. Patients currently smoking were excluded.

The trial was comprised of a run-in period to achieve a stable conversion to a common ICS (fluticasone propionate), followed by randomization to Xolair or placebo. Patients were stratified by use of ICS-only or ICS with concomitant use of oral steroids. Patients received Xolair for 16 weeks with an unchanged corticosteroid dose unless an acute exacerbation necessitated an increase. Patients then entered an ICS reduction phase of 16 weeks during which ICS or oral steroid dose reduction was attempted in a step-wise manner.

The number of exacerbations in patients treated with Xolair was similar to that in placebo-treated patients (Table 8). The absence of an observed treatment effect may be related to differences in the patient population compared with Asthma Trials 1 and 2, study sample size, or other factors.

[See table 8 at top of next page]

In all three of the trials, a reduction of asthma exacerbations was not observed in the Xolair-treated patients who had $FEV_1 > 80\%$ at the time of randomization. Reductions in exacerbations were not seen in patients who required oral steroids as maintenance therapy.

Table 8. Percentage of Patients with Asthma Exacerbations by Subgroup and Phase in Trial 3

| | Stable Steroid Phase (16 wks) | | | |
| | Inhaled Only | | Oral + Inhaled | |
	Xolair N = 126	Placebo N = 120	Xolair N = 50	Placebo N = 45
% Patients with ≥ 1 exacerbations	15.9%	15.0%	32.0%	22.2%
Difference (95% CI)	0.9 (−9.7, 13.7)		9.8 (−10.5, 31.4)	

| | Steroid Reduction Phase (16 wks) | | | |
	Xolair N = 126	Placebo N = 120	Xolair N = 50	Placebo N = 45
% Patients with ≥ 1 exacerbations	22.2%	26.7%	42.0%	42.2%
Difference (95% CI)	−4.4 (−17.6, 7.4)		−0.2 (−22.4, 20.1)	

Table 9. Change from Baseline to Week 12 in Weekly Itch Severity Score and Weekly Hive Count Score in CIU Trial 1*

	Xolair 75mg	Xolair 150mg	Xolair 300mg	Placebo
n	77	80	81	80
Weekly Itch Severity Score				
Mean Baseline Score (SD)	14.5 (3.6)	14.1 (3.8)	14.2 (3.3)	14.4 (3.5)
Mean Change Week 12(SD)	−6.46 (6.14)	−6.66 (6.28)	−9.40 (5.73)	−3.63 (5.22)
Difference in LS means vs. placebo	−2.96	−2.95	−5.80	
95% CI for difference	−4.71, −1.21	−4.72, −1.18	−7.49, −4.10	-
Weekly Hive Count Score †				
Mean Baseline Score (SD)	17.2 (4.2)	16.2 (4.6)	17.1 (3.8)	16.7 (4.4)
Mean Change Week 12(SD)	−7.36 (7.52)	−7.78 (7.08)	−11.35 (7.25)	−4.37 (6.60)
Difference in LS means vs. placebo	−2.75	−3.44	−6.93	
95% CI for difference	−4.95, −0.54	−5.57, −1.32	−9.10, −4.76	-

* Modified intent-to-treat (mITT) population: all patients who were randomized and received at least one dose of study medication.
† Score measured on a range of 0–21

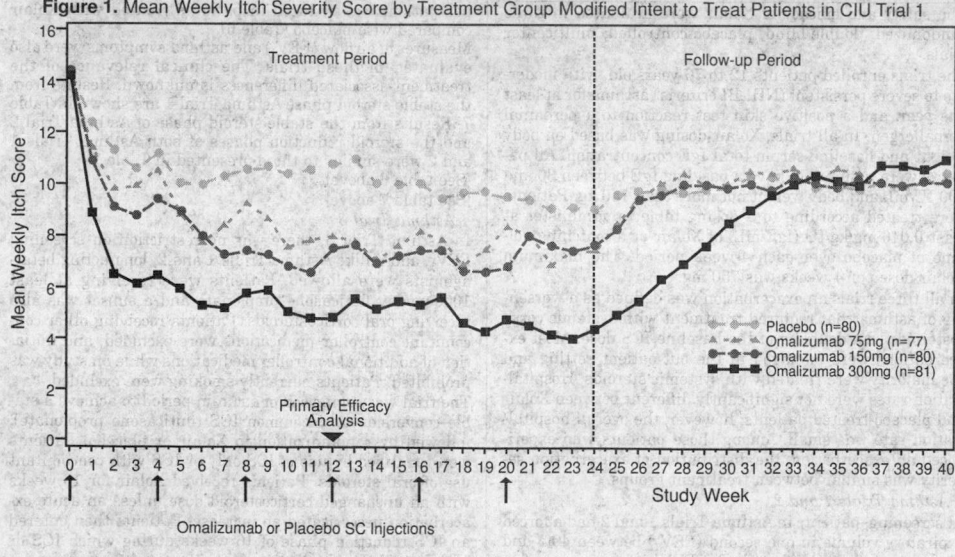

Figure 1. Mean Weekly Itch Severity Score by Treatment Group Modified Intent to Treat Patients in CIU Trial 1

Treatment Period   Follow-up Period

Primary Efficacy Analysis

Placebo (n=80)
Omalizumab 75mg (n=77)
Omalizumab 150mg (n=80)
Omalizumab 300mg (n=81)

Study Week

Omalizumab or Placebo SC Injections

Pediatric Patients 6 to < 12 Years of Age
Clinical trials with Xolair in pediatric patients 6 to 11 years of age have been conducted [see Use in Specific Populations (8.4)]

Pediatric Patients <6 Years of Age
Clinical trials with Xolair in pediatric patients less than 6 years of age have not been conducted [see Use in Specific Populations (8.4)]

14.2   Chronic Idiopathic Urticaria
Adult and Adolescent Patients 12 Years of Age and Older
The safety and efficacy of Xolair for the treatment of CIU was assessed in two placebo-controlled, multiple-dose clinical trials of 24 weeks' duration (CIU Trial 1; n= 319) and 12 weeks' duration (CIU Trial 2; n=322). Patients received Xolair 75, 150, or 300 mg or placebo by SC injection every 4 weeks in addition to their baseline level of H1 antihistamine therapy for 24 or 12 weeks, followed by a 16-week

---

washout observation period. A total of 640 patients (165 males, 475 females) were included for the efficacy analyses. Most patients were white (84%) and the median age was 42 years (range 12–72).

Disease severity was measured by a weekly urticaria activity score (UAS7, range 0–42), which is a composite of the weekly itch severity score (range 0–21) and the weekly hive count score (range 0–21). All patients were required to have a UAS7 of ≥ 16, and a weekly itch severity score of ≥ 8 for the 7 days prior to randomization, despite having used an H1 antihistamine for at least 2 weeks.

The mean weekly itch severity scores at baseline were fairly balanced across treatment groups and ranged between 13.7 and 14.5 despite use of an H1 antihistamine at an approved dose. The reported median durations of CIU at enrollment across treatment groups were between 2.5 and 3.9 years (with an overall subject-level range of 0.5 to 66.4 years).

In both CIU Trials 1 and 2, patients who received Xolair 150 mg or 300 mg had greater decreases from baseline in weekly itch severity scores and weekly hive count scores than placebo at Week 12. Representative results from CIU Trial 1 are shown (Table 9); similar results were observed in CIU Trial 2. The 75-mg dose did not demonstrate consistent evidence of efficacy and is not approved for use.
[See table 9 above]

The mean weekly itch severity score at each study week by treatment groups is shown in Figure 1. Representative results from CIU Trial 1 are shown; similar results were observed in CIU Trial 2. The appropriate duration of therapy for CIU with Xolair has not been determined.
[See figure 1 above]

In CIU Trial 1, a larger proportion of patients treated with Xolair 300 mg (36%) reported no itch and no hives (UAS7=0) at Week 12 compared to patients treated with Xolair 150 mg (15%), Xolair 75 mg (12%), and placebo group (9%). Similar results were observed in CIU Trial 2.

16   HOW SUPPLIED/STORAGE AND HANDLING

Xolair is supplied as a lyophilized, sterile powder in a single-use, 5 mL vial without preservatives. Each vial delivers 150 mg of Xolair upon reconstitution with 1.4 mL SWFI, USP. Each carton contains one single-use vial of Xolair® (omalizumab) NDC 50242-040-62.

Xolair should be shipped at controlled ambient temperature (≤ 30°C [≤ 86°F]). Store Xolair under refrigerated conditions 2 to 8°C (36 to 46°F). Do not use beyond the expiration date stamped on carton.

Use the solution for subcutaneous administration within 8 hours following reconstitution when stored in the vial at 2 to 8°C (36 to 46°F), or within 4 hours of reconstitution when stored at room temperature.

Reconstituted Xolair vials should be protected from direct sunlight.

17   PATIENT COUNSELING INFORMATION

See FDA-approved patient labeling (Medication Guide)
Information for Patients
Provide and instruct patients to read the accompanying Medication Guide before starting treatment and before each subsequent treatment. The complete text of the Medication Guide is reprinted at the end of this document.

Inform patients of the risk of life-threatening anaphylaxis with Xolair including the following points [see Boxed Warning and Warnings and Precautions (5.1)]:
• There have been reports of anaphylaxis occurring up to 4 days after administration of Xolair
• Xolair should only be administered in a healthcare setting by healthcare providers
• Patients should be closely observed following administration
• Patients should be informed of the signs and symptoms of anaphylaxis
• Patients should be instructed to seek immediate medical care should such signs or symptoms occur

Instruct patients receiving Xolair not to decrease the dose of, or stop taking any other asthma or CIU medications unless otherwise instructed by their physician. Inform patients that they may not see immediate improvement in their asthma or CIU symptoms after beginning Xolair therapy.

Pregnancy Exposure Registry
Encourage pregnant women exposed to Xolair to enroll in the Xolair Pregnancy Exposure Registry [1-866-4XOLAIR (1-866-496-5247)] or visit www.xolairpregnancyregistry.com [see Use in Specific Populations (8.1)].

MEDICATION GUIDE
XOLAIR® (ZOHL-air)
(omalizumab)
Injection
Read this Medication Guide before you start receiving and before each dose of Xolair. This Medication Guide does not take the place of talking with your healthcare provider about your medical condition or your treatment.

What is the most important information I should know about Xolair?
A severe allergic reaction called anaphylaxis can happen when you receive Xolair. The reaction can occur after the first dose, or after many doses. It may also occur right after a Xolair injection or days later. Anaphylaxis is a life-

threatening condition and can lead to death. Go to the nearest emergency room right away if you have any of these symptoms of an allergic reaction:
• wheezing, shortness of breath, cough, chest tightness, or trouble breathing
• low blood pressure, dizziness, fainting, rapid or weak heartbeat, anxiety, or feeling of "impending doom"
• flushing, itching, hives, or feeling warm
• swelling of the throat or tongue, throat tightness, hoarse voice, or trouble swallowing

Your healthcare provider will monitor you closely for symptoms of an allergic reaction while you are receiving Xolair and for a period of time after your injection. Your healthcare provider should talk to you about getting medical treatment if you have symptoms of an allergic reaction after leaving the healthcare provider's office or treatment center.

What is Xolair?
Xolair is an injectable prescription medicine used to treat adults and children 12 years of age and older with:
• moderate to severe persistent asthma whose asthma symptoms are not controlled by asthma medicines called inhaled corticosteroids. A skin or blood test is performed to see if you have allergies to year-round allergens.
• chronic idiopathic urticaria (CIU; chronic hives without a known cause) who continue to have hives that are not controlled by H1 antihistamine treatment.
Xolair is not used to treat other allergic conditions, other forms of urticaria, acute bronchospasm or status asthmaticus.

Do not receive Xolair if you:
• are allergic to omalizumab or any of the ingredients in Xolair. See the end of this Medication Guide for a complete list of ingredients in Xolair.

Before receiving Xolair, tell your healthcare provider about all of your medical conditions, including if you:
• have any other allergies (such as food allergy or seasonal allergies)
• have sudden breathing problems (bronchospasm)
• have ever had a severe allergic reaction called anaphylaxis
• have or have had a parasitic infection
• have or have had cancer
• are pregnant or plan to become pregnant. It is not known if Xolair may harm your unborn baby.
• if you become pregnant while taking Xolair, talk to your healthcare provider about registering with the Xolair Pregnancy Registry. You can get more information and register by calling 1-866-4XOLAIR (1-866-496-5247) or visit www.xolairpregnancyregistry.com. The purpose of this registry is to monitor pregnancy outcomes in women receiving Xolair during pregnancy.
• are breastfeeding or plan to breastfeed. It is not known if Xolair passes into your breast milk. Talk with your healthcare provider about the best way to feed your baby while you receive Xolair.

Tell your healthcare provider about all the medicines you take, including prescription and over-the-counter medicines, vitamins, or herbal supplements.

How should I receive Xolair?
• Xolair should be given by your healthcare provider, in a healthcare setting.
• Xolair is given in 1 or more injections under the skin (subcutaneous), 1 time every 2 or 4 weeks.
• In asthma patients, a blood test for a substance called IgE must be performed prior to starting Xolair to determine the appropriate dose and dosing frequency.
• In patients with chronic hives, a blood test is not necessary to determine the dose or dosing frequency.
• Do not decrease or stop taking any of your other asthma or hive medicine unless your healthcare providers tell you to.
• You may not see improvement in your symptoms right away after Xolair treatment.

What are the possible side effects of Xolair?
Xolair may cause serious side effects, including:
• See, "What is the most important information I should know about Xolair?"
• **Cancer.** People who receive treatment with Xolair may have a higher chance for getting certain types of cancer.
• **Fever, muscle aches, and rash.** Some people who take Xolair get these symptoms 1 to 5 days after receiving a Xolair injection. If you have any of these symptoms, tell your healthcare provider.
• **Parasitic infection.** Some people who are at a high risk for parasite (worm) infections, get a parasite infection after receiving Xolair. Your healthcare provider can test your stool to check if you have a parasite infection.
• Some people who receive Xolair have had chest pain, heart attack, blood clots in the lungs or legs, or temporary symptoms of weakness on one side of the body, slurred speech, or altered vision. It is not known whether this is caused by Xolair.

The most common side effects of Xolair:
• In people with asthma: pain especially in your arms and legs, dizziness, feeling tired, skin rash, bone fractures, and pain or discomfort of your ears.

• In people with chronic idiopathic urticaria: nausea, headaches, swelling of the inside of your nose, throat or sinuses, cough, joint pain, and upper respiratory tract infection.
These are not all the possible side effects of Xolair. Call your doctor for medical advice about side effects. You may report side effects to FDA at 1-800-FDA-1088.

General information about the safe and effective use of Xolair.
Medicines are sometimes prescribed for purposes other than those listed in a Medication Guide. You can ask your pharmacist or healthcare provider for information about Xolair that is written for health professionals. Do not use Xolair for a condition for which it was not prescribed.
For more information, go to www.xolair.com or call 1-866-4XOLAIR (1-866-496-5247).
What are the ingredients in Xolair?
Active ingredient: omalizumab
Inactive ingredients: L-histidine, L-histidine hydrochloride monohydrate, polysorbate 20 and sucrose

Manufactured by: **Genentech, Inc.**
A Member of the Roche Group
1 DNA Way
South San Francisco, CA 94080-4990

Jointly marketed by:
Genentech USA, Inc.
A Member of the Roche Group,
1 DNA Way
South San Francisco, CA 94080-4990
Novartis Pharmaceuticals Corporation
One Health Plaza
East Hanover, NJ 07936-1080

Initial US Approval: June 2003
Revision Date: September 2014
Xolair® is a registered trademark of Novartis AG.
©2014 Genentech USA, Inc

This Medication Guide has been approved by the U.S. Food and Drug Administration.
Shown in Product Identification Guide, page 311

Otsuka America Pharmaceutical, Inc.
2440 RESEARCH BOULEVARD
ROCKVILLE, MD 20850

Direct Inquiries to:
Medical Affairs
Otsuka America Pharmaceutical, Inc.
(800) 441-6763
FAX: 301-212-8634
To Request Routine or Emergency Medical Information, or to Report an Adverse Experience:
(800) 438-9927

SAMSCA® ℞
(tolvaptan)
tablets for oral use

HIGHLIGHTS OF PRESCRIBING INFORMATION
These highlights do not include all the information needed to use SAMSCA safely and effectively. See full prescribing information for SAMSCA.
SAMSCA® (tolvaptan) tablets for oral use
Initial U.S. Approval: 05/2009

WARNING: INITIATE AND RE-INITIATE IN A HOSPITAL AND MONITOR SERUM SODIUM
See full prescribing information for complete boxed warning.
• SAMSCA should be initiated and re-initiated in patients only in a hospital where serum sodium can be monitored closely.
• Too rapid correction of hyponatremia (e.g., >12 mEq/L/24 hours) can cause osmotic demyelination resulting in dysarthria, mutism, dysphagia, lethargy, affective changes, spastic quadriparesis, seizures, coma and death. In susceptible patients, including those with severe malnutrition, alcoholism or advanced liver disease, slower rates of correction may be advisable.

RECENT MAJOR CHANGES
Contraindications
  Hypersensitivity (4.6)   02/2014
Warnings and Precautions
  Liver Injury (5.2)   04/2013

INDICATIONS AND USAGE
SAMSCA is a selective vasopressin V_2-receptor antagonist indicated for the treatment of clinically significant hypervolemic and euvolemic hyponatremia [serum sodium <125 mEq/L or less marked hyponatremia that is symptomatic and has resisted correction with fluid restriction], including patients with heart failure and Syndrome of Inappropriate Antidiuretic Hormone (SIADH) (1)
Important Limitations:
• Patients requiring intervention to raise serum sodium urgently to prevent or to treat serious neurological symptoms should not be treated with SAMSCA (1)
• It has not been established that SAMSCA provides a symptomatic benefit to patients (1)

DOSAGE AND ADMINISTRATION
• SAMSCA should be initiated and re-initiated in a hospital (2.1)
• The recommended starting dose is 15 mg once daily. Dosage may be increased at intervals ≥24 hr to 30 mg once daily, and to a maximum of 60 mg once daily as needed to raise serum sodium. (2.1)

DOSAGE FORMS AND STRENGTHS
• Tablets: 15 mg and 30 mg (3)

CONTRAINDICATIONS
• Need to raise serum sodium acutely (4.1)
• Patients who are unable to respond appropriately to thirst (4.2)
• Hypovolemic hyponatremia (4.3)
• Concomitant use of strong CYP 3A inhibitors (4.4)
• Anuria (4.5)
• Hypersensitivity (4.6)

WARNINGS AND PRECAUTIONS
• Liver injury: Limit treatment duration to 30 days. If hepatic injury is suspected, discontinue SAMSCA. Avoid use in patients with underlying liver disease. (5.2)
• Dehydration and hypovolemia may require intervention (5.3)
• Avoid use with hypertonic saline (5.4)
• Avoid use with CYP 3A inducers and moderate CYP 3A inhibitors (5.5)
• Consider dose reduction if co-administered with P-gp inhibitors (5.5)
• Monitor serum potassium in patients with potassium >5 mEq/L or on drugs known to increase potassium (5.6)

ADVERSE REACTIONS
Most common adverse reactions (≥5% placebo) are thirst, dry mouth, asthenia, constipation, pollakiuria or polyuria, and hyperglycemia (6.1)
To report SUSPECTED ADVERSE REACTIONS, contact Otsuka at 1-877-726-7220 or FDA at 1-800-FDA-1088 (*www.fda.gov/medwatch*).

USE IN SPECIFIC POPULATIONS
• Pregnancy: Based on animal data, may cause fetal harm (8.1)
• Nursing mothers: Discontinue drug or nursing taking into consideration importance of drug to mother (8.3)
• Pediatric Use: There are no studies (8.4)
See 17 for PATIENT COUNSELING INFORMATION and Medication Guide

Revised: 02/2014

FULL PRESCRIBING INFORMATION: CONTENTS*
WARNING: INITIATE AND RE-INITIATE IN A HOSPITAL AND MONITOR SERUM SODIUM

FULL PRESCRIBING INFORMATION

WARNING: INITIATE AND RE-INITIATE IN A HOSPITAL AND MONITOR SERUM SODIUM

SAMSCA should be initiated and re-initiated in patients only in a hospital where serum sodium can be monitored closely.

Too rapid correction of hyponatremia (e.g., >12 mEq/L/24 hours) can cause osmotic demyelination resulting in dysarthria, mutism, dysphagia, lethargy, affective changes, spastic quadriparesis, seizures, coma and death. In susceptible patients, including those with severe malnutrition, alcoholism or advanced liver disease, slower rates of correction may be advisable.

1   INDICATIONS AND USAGE

SAMSCA® is indicated for the treatment of clinically significant hypervolemic and euvolemic hyponatremia (serum sodium <125 mEq/L or less marked hyponatremia that is symptomatic and has resisted correction with fluid restriction), including patients with heart failure and Syndrome of Inappropriate Antidiuretic Hormone (SIADH).

Important Limitations

Patients requiring intervention to raise serum sodium urgently to prevent or to treat serious neurological symptoms should not be treated with SAMSCA.

It has not been established that raising serum sodium with SAMSCA provides a symptomatic benefit to patients.

2   DOSAGE AND ADMINISTRATION

2.1   Usual Dosage in Adults

Patients should be in a hospital for initiation and re-initiation of therapy to evaluate the therapeutic response and because too rapid correction of hyponatremia can cause osmotic demyelination resulting in dysarthria, mutism, dysphagia, lethargy, affective changes, spastic quadriparesis, seizures, coma and death.

The usual starting dose for SAMSCA is 15 mg administered once daily without regard to meals. Increase the dose to 30 mg once daily, after at least 24 hours, to a maximum of 60 mg once daily, as needed to achieve the desired level of serum sodium. Do not administer SAMSCA for more than 30 days to minimize the risk of liver injury [see Warnings and Precautions (5.2)].

During initiation and titration, frequently monitor for changes in serum electrolytes and volume. Avoid fluid restriction during the first 24 hours of therapy. Patients receiving SAMSCA should be advised that they can continue ingestion of fluid in response to thirst [see Warnings and Precautions (5.1)].

2.2   Drug Withdrawal

Following discontinuation from SAMSCA, patients should be advised to resume fluid restriction and should be monitored for changes in serum sodium and volume status.

2.3   Co-Administration with CYP 3A Inhibitors, CYP 3A Inducers and P-gp Inhibitors

CYP 3A Inhibitors

Tolvaptan is metabolized by CYP 3A, and use with strong CYP 3A inhibitors causes a marked (5–fold) increase in exposure [see Contraindications (4.4)]. The effect of moderate CYP 3A inhibitors on tolvaptan exposure has not been assessed. Avoid co-administration of SAMSCA and moderate CYP 3A inhibitors [see Warnings and Precautions (5.5), Drug Interactions (7.1)].

CYP 3A Inducers

Co-administration of SAMSCA with potent CYP 3A inducers (e.g., rifampin) reduces tolvaptan plasma concentrations by 85%. Therefore, the expected clinical effects of SAMSCA may not be observed at the recommended dose. Patient response should be monitored and the dose adjusted accordingly [see Warnings and Precautions (5.5), Drug Interactions (7.1)].

P-gp Inhibitors

Tolvaptan is a substrate of P-gp. Co-administration of SAMSCA with inhibitors of P-gp (e.g., cyclosporine) may necessitate a decrease in SAMSCA dose [see Warnings and Precautions (5.5), Drug Interactions (7.1)].

3   DOSAGE FORMS AND STRENGTHS

SAMSCA (tolvaptan) is available in 15 mg and 30 mg tablets [see How Supplied/Storage and Handling (16)].

4   CONTRAINDICATIONS

SAMSCA is contraindicated in the following conditions:

4.1   Urgent need to raise serum sodium acutely

SAMSCA has not been studied in a setting of urgent need to raise serum sodium acutely.

4.2   Inability of the patient to sense or appropriately respond to thirst

Patients who are unable to auto-regulate fluid balance are at substantially increased risk of incurring an overly rapid correction of serum sodium, hypernatremia and hypovolemia.

4.3   Hypovolemic hyponatremia

Risks associated with worsening hypovolemia, including complications such as hypotension and renal failure, outweigh possible benefits.

4.4   Concomitant use of strong CYP 3A inhibitors

Ketoconazole 200 mg administered with tolvaptan increased tolvaptan exposure by 5–fold. Larger doses would be expected to produce larger increases in tolvaptan exposure. There is not adequate experience to define the dose adjustment that would be needed to allow safe use of tolvaptan with strong CYP 3A inhibitors such as clarithromycin, ketoconazole, itraconazole, ritonavir, indinavir, nelfinavir, saquinavir, nefazodone, and telithromycin.

4.5   Anuric patients

In patients unable to make urine, no clinical benefit can be expected.

4.6   Hypersensitivity

SAMSCA is contraindicated in patients with hypersensitivity (e.g. anaphylactic shock, rash generalized) to tolvaptan or any component of the product [see Adverse Reactions (6.2)].

5   WARNINGS AND PRECAUTIONS

5.1   Too Rapid Correction of Serum Sodium Can Cause Serious Neurologic Sequelae (see BOXED WARNING)

Osmotic demyelination syndrome is a risk associated with too rapid correction of hyponatremia (e.g., >12 mEq/L/24 hours). Osmotic demyelination results in dysarthria, mutism, dysphagia, lethargy, affective changes, spastic quadriparesis, seizures, coma or death. In susceptible patients, including those with severe malnutrition, alcoholism or advanced liver disease, slower rates of correction may be advisable. In controlled clinical trials in which tolvaptan was administered in titrated doses starting at 15 mg once daily, 7% of tolvaptan-treated subjects with a serum sodium <130 mEq/L had an increase in serum sodium greater than 8 mEq/L at approximately 8 hours and 2% had an increase greater than 12 mEq/L at 24 hours. Approximately 1% of placebo-treated subjects with a serum sodium <130 mEq/L had a rise greater than 8 mEq/L at 8 hours and no patient had a rise greater than 12 mEq/L/24 hours. Osmotic demyelination syndrome has been reported in association with SAMSCA therapy [see Adverse Reactions (6.2)]. Patients treated with SAMSCA should be monitored to assess serum sodium concentrations and neurologic status, especially during initiation and after titration. Subjects with SIADH or very low baseline serum sodium concentrations may be at greater risk for too-rapid correction of serum sodium. In patients receiving SAMSCA who develop too rapid a rise in serum sodium, discontinue or interrupt treatment with SAMSCA and consider administration of hypotonic fluid.

Fluid restriction during the first 24 hours of therapy with SAMSCA may increase the likelihood of overly-rapid correction of serum sodium, and should generally be avoided.

5.2   Liver Injury

SAMSCA can cause serious and potentially fatal liver injury. In a placebo-controlled and open label extension study of chronically administered tolvaptan in patients with autosomal dominant polycystic kidney disease, cases of serious liver injury attributed to tolvaptan were observed. An increased incidence of ALT greater than three times the upper limit of normal was associated with tolvaptan (42/958 or 4.4%) compared to placebo (5/484 or 1.0%). Cases of serious liver injury were generally observed starting 3 months after initiation of tolvaptan although elevations of ALT occurred prior to 3 months.

Patients with symptoms that may indicate liver injury, including fatigue, anorexia, right upper abdominal discomfort, dark urine or jaundice should discontinue treatment with SAMSCA.

Limit duration of therapy with SAMSCA to 30 days. Avoid use in patients with underlying liver disease, including cirrhosis, because the ability to recover from liver injury may be impaired [see Adverse Reactions (6.1)].

5.3   Dehydration and Hypovolemia

SAMSCA therapy induces copious aquaresis, which is normally partially offset by fluid intake. Dehydration and hypovolemia can occur, especially in potentially volume-depleted patients receiving diuretics or those who are fluid restricted. In multiple-dose, placebo-controlled trials in which 607 hyponatremic patients were treated with tolvaptan, the incidence of dehydration was 3.3% for tolvaptan and 1.5% for placebo-treated patients. In patients receiving SAMSCA who develop medically significant signs or symptoms of hypovolemia, interrupt or discontinue SAMSCA therapy and provide supportive care with careful management of vital signs, fluid balance and electrolytes. Fluid restriction during therapy with SAMSCA may increase the risk of dehydration and hypovolemia. Patients receiving SAMSCA should continue ingestion of fluid in response to thirst.

5.4   Co-administration with Hypertonic Saline

Concomitant use with hypertonic saline is not recommended.

5.5   Drug Interactions

Other Drugs Affecting Exposure to Tolvaptan

CYP 3A Inhibitors

Tolvaptan is a substrate of CYP 3A. CYP 3A inhibitors can lead to a marked increase in tolvaptan concentrations [see Dosage and Administration (2.3), Drug Interactions (7.1)]. Do not use SAMSCA with strong inhibitors of CYP 3A [see Contraindications (4.4)] and avoid concomitant use with moderate CYP 3A inhibitors.

CYP 3A Inducers

Avoid co-administration of CYP 3A inducers (e.g., rifampin, rifabutin, rifapentin, barbiturates, phenytoin, carbamazepine, St. John's Wort) with SAMSCA, as this can lead to a reduction in the plasma concentration of tolvaptan and decreased effectiveness of SAMSCA treatment. If co-administered with CYP 3A inducers, the dose of SAMSCA may need to be increased [see Dosage and Administration (2.3), Drug Interactions (7.1)].

P-gp Inhibitors

The dose of SAMSCA may have to be reduced when SAMSCA is co-administered with P-gp inhibitors, e.g., cyclosporine [see Dosage and Administration (2.3), Drug Interactions (7.1)].

5.6   Hyperkalemia or Drugs that Increase Serum Potassium

Treatment with tolvaptan is associated with an acute reduction of the extracellular fluid volume which could result in increased serum potassium. Serum potassium levels should be monitored after initiation of tolvaptan treatment in patients with a serum potassium >5 mEq/L as well as those who are receiving drugs known to increase serum potassium levels.

6   ADVERSE REACTIONS

6.1   Clinical Trials Experience

Because clinical trials are conducted under widely varying conditions, adverse reactions rates observed in the clinical trials of a drug cannot be directly compared to rates in the clinical trials of another drug and may not reflect the rates observed in practice. The adverse event information from clinical trials does, however, provide a basis for identifying the adverse events that appear to be related to drug use and for approximating rates.

In multiple-dose, placebo-controlled trials, 607 hyponatremic patients (serum sodium <135 mEq/L) were treated with SAMSCA. The mean age of these patients was 62 years; 70% of patients were male and 82% were Caucasian. One hundred eighty nine (189) tolvaptan-treated patients had a serum sodium <130 mEq/L, and 52 patients had a serum sodium <125 mEq/L. Hyponatremia was attributed to cirrhosis in 17% of patients, heart failure in 68% and

SIADH/other in 16%. Of these patients, 223 were treated with the recommended dose titration (15 mg titrated to 60 mg as needed to raise serum sodium).

Overall, over 4,000 patients have been treated with oral doses of tolvaptan in open-label or placebo-controlled clinical trials. Approximately 650 of these patients had hyponatremia; approximately 219 of these hyponatremic patients were treated with tolvaptan for 6 months or more.

The most common adverse reactions (incidence ≥5% more than placebo) seen in two 30–day, double-blind, placebo-controlled hyponatremia trials in which tolvaptan was administered in titrated doses (15 mg to 60 mg once daily) were thirst, dry mouth, asthenia, constipation, pollakiuria or polyuria and hyperglycemia. In these trials, 10% (23/223) of tolvaptan-treated patients discontinued treatment because of an adverse event, compared to 12% (26/220) of placebo-treated patients; no adverse reaction resulting in discontinuation of trial medication occurred at an incidence of >1% in tolvaptan-treated patients.

Table 1 lists the adverse reactions reported in tolvaptan-treated patients with hyponatremia (serum sodium <135 mEq/L) and at a rate at least 2% greater than placebo-treated patients in two 30–day, double-blind, placebo-controlled trials. In these studies, 223 patients were exposed to tolvaptan (starting dose 15 mg, titrated to 30 and 60 mg as needed to raise serum sodium). Adverse events resulting in death in these trials were 6% in tolvaptan-treated-patients and 6% in placebo-treated patients.

Table 1. Adverse Reactions (>2% more than placebo) in Tolvaptan-Treated Patients in Double-Blind, Placebo-Controlled Hyponatremia Trials

System Organ Class MedDRA Preferred Term	Tolvaptan 15 mg/day-60 mg/day (N = 223) n (%)	Placebo (N = 220) n (%)
Gastrointestinal Disorders		
Dry mouth	28 (13)	9 (4)
Constipation	16 (7)	4 (2)
General Disorders and Administration Site Conditions		
Thirst*	35 (16)	11 (5)
Asthenia	19 (9)	9 (4)
Pyrexia	9 (4)	2 (1)
Metabolism and Nutrition Disorders		
Hyperglycemia†	14 (6)	2 (1)
Anorexia‡	8 (4)	2 (1)
Renal and Urinary Disorders		
Pollakiuria or polyuria§	25 (11)	7 (3)

The following terms are subsumed under the referenced ADR in Table 1:
* polydipsia;
† diabetes mellitus;
‡ decreased appetite;
§ urine output increased, micturition urgency, nocturia

In a subgroup of patients with hyponatremia (N = 475, serum sodium <135 mEq/L) enrolled in a double-blind, placebo-controlled trial (mean duration of treatment was 9 months) of patients with worsening heart failure, the following adverse reactions occurred in tolvaptan-treated patients at a rate at least 2% greater than placebo: mortality (42% tolvaptan, 38% placebo), nausea (21% tolvaptan, 16% placebo), thirst (12% tolvaptan, 2% placebo), dry mouth (7% tolvaptan, 2% placebo) and polyuria or pollakiuria (4% tolvaptan, 1% placebo).

Gastrointestinal bleeding in patients with cirrhosis
In patients with cirrhosis treated with tolvaptan in the hyponatremia trials, gastrointestinal bleeding was reported in 6 out of 63 (10%) tolvaptan-treated patients and 1 out of 57 (2%) placebo treated patients.

The following adverse reactions occurred in <2% of hyponatremic patients treated with SAMSCA and at a rate greater than placebo in double-blind placebo-controlled trials (N = 607 tolvaptan; N = 518 placebo) or in <2% of patients in an uncontrolled trial of patients with hyponatremia (N = 111) and are not mentioned elsewhere in the label.

Blood and Lymphatic System Disorders: Disseminated intravascular coagulation

Cardiac Disorders: Intracardiac thrombus, ventricular fibrillation

Investigations: Prothrombin time prolonged
Gastrointestinal Disorders: Ischemic colitis
Metabolism and Nutrition Disorders: Diabetic ketoacidosis
Musculoskeletal and Connective Tissue Disorders: Rhabdomyolysis
Nervous System: Cerebrovascular accident
Renal and Urinary Disorders: Urethral hemorrhage
Reproductive System and Breast Disorders (female): Vaginal hemorrhage
Respiratory, Thoracic, and Mediastinal Disorders: Pulmonary embolism, respiratory failure
Vascular disorder: Deep vein thrombosis

6.2 Postmarketing Experience
The following adverse reactions have been identified during post-approval use of SAMSCA. Because these reactions are reported voluntarily from a population of an unknown size, it is not always possible to reliably estimate their frequency or establish a causal relationship to drug exposure.

Neurologic: Osmotic demyelination syndrome
Investigations: Hypernatremia

Removal of excess free body water increases serum osmolality and serum sodium concentrations. All patients treated with tolvaptan, especially those whose serum sodium levels become normal, should continue to be monitored to ensure serum sodium remains within normal limits. If hypernatremia is observed, management may include dose decreases or interruption of tolvaptan treatment, combined with modification of free-water intake or infusion. During clinical trials of hyponatremic patients, hypernatremia was reported as an adverse event in 0.7% of patients receiving tolvaptan vs. 0.6% of patients receiving placebo; analysis of laboratory values demonstrated an incidence of hypernatremia of 1.7% in patients receiving tolvaptan vs. 0.8% in patients receiving placebo.

Immune System Disorders: Hypersensitivity reactions including anaphylactic shock and rash generalized *[see Contraindications (4.6)].*

7 DRUG INTERACTIONS
7.1 Effects of Drugs on Tolvaptan
Ketoconazole and Other Strong CYP 3A Inhibitors
SAMSCA is metabolized primarily by CYP 3A. Ketoconazole is a strong inhibitor of CYP 3A and also an inhibitor of P-gp. Co-administration of SAMSCA and ketoconazole 200 mg daily results in a 5–fold increase in exposure to tolvaptan. Co-administration of SAMSCA with 400 mg ketoconazole daily or with other strong CYP 3A inhibitors (e.g., clarithromycin, itraconazole, telithromycin, saquinavir, nelfinavir, ritonavir and nefazodone) at the highest labeled dose would be expected to cause an even greater increase in tolvaptan exposure. Thus, SAMSCA and strong CYP 3A inhibitors should not be co-administered *[see Dosage and Administration (2.3) and Contraindications (4.4)].*

Moderate CYP 3A Inhibitors
The impact of moderate CYP 3A inhibitors (e.g., erythromycin, fluconazole, aprepitant, diltiazem and verapamil) on the exposure to co-administered tolvaptan has not been assessed. A substantial increase in the exposure to tolvaptan would be expected when SAMSCA is co-administered with moderate CYP 3A inhibitors. Co-administration of SAMSCA with moderate CYP3A inhibitors should therefore generally be avoided *[see Dosage and Administration (2.3) and Warnings and Precautions (5.5)].*

Grapefruit Juice
Co-administration of grapefruit juice and SAMSCA results in a 1.8–fold increase in exposure to tolvaptan *[see Dose and Administration (2.3) and Warnings and Precautions (5.5)].*

P-gp Inhibitors
Reduction in the dose of SAMSCA may be required in patients concomitantly treated with P-gp inhibitors, such as e.g., cyclosporine, based on clinical response *[see Dose and Administration (2.3) and Warnings and Precautions (5.5)].*

Rifampin and Other CYP 3A Inducers
Rifampin is an inducer of CYP 3A and P-gp. Co-administration of rifampin and SAMSCA reduces exposure to tolvaptan by 85%. Therefore, the expected clinical effects of SAMSCA in the presence of rifampin and other inducers (e.g., rifabutin, rifapentin, barbiturates, phenytoin, carbamazepine and St. John's Wort) may not be observed at the usual dose levels of SAMSCA. The dose of SAMSCA may have to be increased *[Dosage and Administration (2.3) and Warnings and Precautions (5.5)].*

Lovastatin, Digoxin, Furosemide, and Hydrochlorothiazide
Co-administration of lovastatin, digoxin, furosemide, and hydrochlorothiazide with SAMSCA has no clinically relevant impact on the exposure to tolvaptan.

7.2 Effects of Tolvaptan on Other Drugs
Digoxin
Digoxin is a P-gp substrate. Co-administration of SAMSCA with digoxin increased digoxin AUC by 20% and Cmax by 30%.

Warfarin, Amiodarone, Furosemide, and Hydrochlorothiazide
Co-administration of tolvaptan does not appear to alter the pharmacokinetics of warfarin, furosemide, hydrochlorothiazide, or amiodarone (or its active metabolite, desethylamiodarone) to a clinically significant degree.

Lovastatin
SAMSCA is a weak inhibitor of CYP 3A. Co-administration of lovastatin and SAMSCA increases the exposure to lovastatin and its active metabolite lovastatin-β hydroxyacid by factors of 1.4 and 1.3, respectively. This is not a clinically relevant change.

Pharmacodynamic Interactions
Tolvaptan produces a greater 24 hour urine volume/excretion rate than does furosemide or hydrochlorothiazide. Concomitant administration of tolvaptan with furosemide or hydrochlorothiazide results in a 24 hour urine volume/excretion rate that is similar to the rate after tolvaptan administration alone.

Although specific interaction studies were not performed, in clinical studies tolvaptan was used concomitantly with beta-blockers, angiotensin receptor blockers, angiotensin converting enzyme inhibitors and potassium sparing diuretics. Adverse reactions of hyperkalemia were approximately 1-2% higher when tolvaptan was administered with angiotensin receptor blockers, angiotensin converting enzyme inhibitors and potassium sparing diuretics compared to administration of these medications with placebo. Serum potassium levels should be monitored during concomitant drug therapy.

As a V_2-receptor antagonist, tolvaptan may interfere with the V_2-agonist activity of desmopressin (dDAVP). In a male subject with mild Von Willebrand (vW) disease, intravenous infusion of dDAVP 2 hours after administration of oral tolvaptan did not produce the expected increases in vW Factor Antigen or Factor VIII activity. It is not recommended to administer SAMSCA with a V_2-agonist.

8 USE IN SPECIFIC POPULATIONS
There is no need to adjust dose based on age, gender, race, or cardiac function *[see Clinical Pharmacology (12.3)].*

8.1 Pregnancy
Pregnancy Category C.
There are no adequate and well controlled studies of SAMSCA use in pregnant women. In animal studies, cleft palate, brachymelia, microphthalmia, skeletal malformations, decreased fetal weight, delayed fetal ossification, and embryo-fetal death occurred. SAMSCA should be used during pregnancy only if the potential benefit justifies the potential risk to the fetus.

In embryo-fetal development studies, pregnant rats and rabbits received oral tolvaptan during organogenesis. Rats received 2 to 162 times the maximum recommended human dose (MRHD) of tolvaptan (on a body surface area basis). Reduced fetal weights and delayed fetal ossification occurred at 162 times the MRHD. Signs of maternal toxicity (reduction in body weight gain and food consumption) occurred at 16 and 162 times the MRHD. When pregnant rabbits received oral tolvaptan at 32 to 324 times the MRHD (on a body surface area basis), there were reductions in maternal body weight gain and food consumption at all doses, and increased abortions at the mid and high doses (about 97 and 324 times the MRHD). At 324 times the MRHD, there were increased rates of embryo-fetal death, fetal microphthalmia, open eyelids, cleft palate, brachymelia and skeletal malformations *[see Nonclinical Toxicology (13.3)].*

8.2 Labor and Delivery
The effect of SAMSCA on labor and delivery in humans is unknown.

8.3 Nursing Mothers
It is not known whether SAMSCA is excreted into human milk. Tolvaptan is excreted into the milk of lactating rats. Because many drugs are excreted into human milk and because of the potential for serious adverse reactions in nursing infants from SAMSCA, a decision should be made to discontinue nursing or SAMSCA, taking into consideration the importance of SAMSCA to the mother.

8.4 Pediatric Use
Safety and effectiveness of SAMSCA in pediatric patients have not been established.

8.5 Geriatric Use
Of the total number of hyponatremic subjects treated with SAMSCA in clinical studies, 42% were 65 and over, while 19% were 75 and over. No overall differences in safety or effectiveness were observed between these subjects and younger subjects, and other reported clinical experience has not identified differences in responses between the elderly and younger patients, but greater sensitivity of some older individuals cannot be ruled out. Increasing age has no effect on tolvaptan plasma concentrations.

8.6 Use in Patients with Hepatic Impairment
Moderate and severe hepatic impairment do not affect exposure to tolvaptan to a clinically relevant extent. Avoid use of tolvaptan in patients with underlying liver disease.

8.7 Use in Patients with Renal Impairment

No dose adjustment is necessary based on renal function. There are no clinical trial data in patients with CrCl <10 mL/min, and, because drug effects on serum sodium levels are likely lost at very low levels of renal function, use in patients with a CrCl <10 mL/min is not recommended. No benefit can be expected in patients who are anuric [see Contraindications (4.5) and Clinical Pharmacology (12.3)].

8.8 Use in Patients with Congestive Heart Failure

The exposure to tolvaptan in patients with congestive heart failure is not clinically relevantly increased. No dose adjustment is necessary.

10 OVERDOSAGE

Single oral doses up to 480 mg and multiple doses up to 300 mg once daily for 5 days have been well tolerated in studies in healthy subjects. There is no specific antidote for tolvaptan intoxication. The signs and symptoms of an acute overdose can be anticipated to be those of excessive pharmacologic effect: a rise in serum sodium concentration, polyuria, thirst, and dehydration/hypovolemia.

The oral LD_{50} of tolvaptan in rats and dogs is >2000 mg/kg. No mortality was observed in rats or dogs following single oral doses of 2000 mg/kg (maximum feasible dose). A single oral dose of 2000 mg/kg was lethal in mice, and symptoms of toxicity in affected mice included decreased locomotor activity, staggering gait, tremor and hypothermia.

If overdose occurs, estimation of the severity of poisoning is an important first step. A thorough history and details of overdose should be obtained, and a physical examination should be performed. The possibility of multiple drug involvement should be considered.

Treatment should involve symptomatic and supportive care, with respiratory, ECG and blood pressure monitoring and water/electrolyte supplements as needed. A profuse and prolonged aquaresis should be anticipated, which, if not matched by oral fluid ingestion, should be replaced with intravenous hypotonic fluids, while closely monitoring electrolytes and fluid balance.

ECG monitoring should begin immediately and continue until ECG parameters are within normal ranges. Dialysis may not be effective in removing tolvaptan because of its high binding affinity for human plasma protein (>99%). Close medical supervision and monitoring should continue until the patient recovers.

11 DESCRIPTION

Tolvaptan is (±)-4'-[(7-chloro-2,3,4,5-tetrahydro-5-hydroxy-1H-1-benzazepin-1-yl) carbonyl]-o-tolu-m-toluidide. The empirical formula is $C_{26}H_{25}ClN_2O_3$. Molecular weight is 448.94. The chemical structure is:

SAMSCA tablets for oral use contain 15 mg or 30 mg of tolvaptan. Inactive ingredients include corn starch, hydroxypropyl cellulose, lactose monohydrate, low-substituted hydroxypropyl cellulose, magnesium stearate and microcrystalline cellulose and FD&C Blue No. 2 Aluminum Lake as colorant.

12 CLINICAL PHARMACOLOGY

12.1 Mechanism of Action

Tolvaptan is a selective vasopressin V_2-receptor antagonist with an affinity for the V_2-receptor that is 1.8 times that of native arginine vasopressin (AVP). Tolvaptan affinity for the V_2-receptor is 29 times greater than for the V_{1a}-receptor. When taken orally, 15 to 60 mg doses of tolvaptan antagonize the effect of vasopressin and cause an increase in urine water excretion that results in an increase in free water clearance (aquaresis), a decrease in urine osmolality, and a resulting increase in serum sodium concentrations. Urinary excretion of sodium and potassium and plasma potassium concentrations are not significantly changed. Tolvaptan metabolites have no or weak antagonist activity for human V_2-receptors compared with tolvaptan.

Plasma concentrations of native AVP may increase (avg. 2-9 pg/mL) with tolvaptan administration.

12.2 Pharmacodynamics

In healthy subjects receiving a single dose of SAMSCA 60 mg, the onset of the aquaretic and sodium increasing effects occurs within 2 to 4 hours post-dose. A peak effect of about a 6 mEq increase in serum sodium and about 9 mL/min increase in urine excretion rate is observed between 4 and 8 hours post-dose; thus, the pharmacological activity lags behind the plasma concentrations of tolvaptan. About 60% of the peak effect on serum sodium is sustained at 24 hours post-dose, but the urinary excretion rate is no longer elevated by this time. Doses above 60 mg tolvaptan do not increase aquaresis or serum sodium further. The effects of tolvaptan in the recommended dose range of 15 to 60 mg once daily appear to be limited to aquaresis and the resulting increase in sodium concentration.

In a parallel-arm, double-blind (for tolvaptan and placebo), placebo- and positive-controlled, multiple dose study of the effect of tolvaptan on the QTc interval, 172 healthy subjects were randomized to tolvaptan 30 mg, tolvaptan 300 mg, placebo, or moxifloxacin 400 mg once daily. At both the 30 mg and 300 mg doses, no significant effect of administering tolvaptan on the QTc interval was detected on Day 1 and Day 5. At the 300 mg dose, peak tolvaptan plasma concentrations were approximately 4–fold higher than the peak concentrations following a 30 mg dose. Moxifloxacin increased the QT interval by 12 ms at 2 hours after dosing on Day 1 and 17 ms at 1 hour after dosing on Day 5, indicating that the study was adequately designed and conducted to detect tolvaptan's effect on the QT interval, had an effect been present.

12.3 Pharmacokinetics

In healthy subjects the pharmacokinetics of tolvaptan after single doses of up to 480 mg and multiple doses up to 300 mg once daily have been examined. Area under the curve (AUC) increases proportionally with dose. After administration of doses ≥60 mg, however, Cmax increases less than proportionally with dose. The pharmacokinetic properties of tolvaptan are stereospecific, with a steady-state ratio of the S-(-) to the R-(+) enantiomer of about 3. The absolute bioavailability of tolvaptan is unknown. At least 40% of the dose is absorbed as tolvaptan or metabolites. Peak concentrations of tolvaptan are observed between 2 and 4 hours post-dose. Food does not impact the bioavailability of tolvaptan. In vitro data indicate that tolvaptan is a substrate and inhibitor of P-gp. Tolvaptan is highly plasma protein bound (99%) and distributed into an apparent volume of distribution of about 3 L/kg. Tolvaptan is eliminated entirely by non-renal routes and mainly, if not exclusively, metabolized by CYP 3A. After oral dosing, clearance is about 4 mL/min/kg and the terminal phase half-life is about 12 hours. The accumulation factor of tolvaptan with the once-daily regimen is 1.3 and the trough concentrations amount to ≤16% of the peak concentrations, suggesting a dominant half-life somewhat shorter than 12 hours. There is marked inter-subject variation in peak and average exposure to tolvaptan with a percent coefficient of variation ranging between 30 and 60%.

In patients with hyponatremia of any origin the clearance of tolvaptan is reduced to about 2 mL/min/kg. Moderate or severe hepatic impairment or congestive heart failure decrease the clearance and increase the volume of distribution of tolvaptan, but the respective changes are not clinically relevant. Exposure and response to tolvaptan in subjects with creatinine clearance ranging between 79 and 10 mL/min and patients with normal renal function are not different.

In a study in patients with creatinine clearances ranging from 10-124 mL/min administered a single dose of 60 mg tolvaptan, AUC and Cmax of plasma tolvaptan were less than doubled in patients with severe renal impairment relative to the controls. The peak increase in serum sodium was 5-6 mEq/L, regardless of renal function, but the onset and offset of tolvaptan's effect on serum sodium were slower in patients with severe renal impairment [see Use in Special Populations (8.7)].

13 NONCLINICAL TOXICOLOGY

13.1 Carcinogenesis, Mutagenesis, Impairment of Fertility

Up to two years of oral administration of tolvaptan to male and female rats at doses up to 1000 mg/kg/day (162 times the maximum recommended human dose [MRHD] on a body surface area basis), to male mice at doses up to 60 mg/kg/day (5 times the MRHD) and to female mice at doses up to 100 mg/kg/day (8 times the MRHD) did not increase the incidence of tumors.

Tolvaptan tested negative for genotoxicity in in vitro (bacterial reverse mutation assay and chromosomal aberration test in Chinese hamster lung fibroblast cells) and in vivo (rat micronucleus assay) test systems.

In a fertility study in which male and female rats were orally administered tolvaptan at 100, 300 or 1000 mg/kg/day, the highest dose level was associated with significantly fewer corpora lutea and implants than control.

13.3 Reproductive and Developmental Toxicology

In pregnant rats, oral administration of tolvaptan at 10, 100 and 1000 mg/kg/day during organogenesis was associated

Table 2. Effects of Treatment with Tolvaptan 15 mg/day to 60 mg/day

	Tolvaptan 15 mg/day-60 mg/day	Placebo	Estimated Effect (95% CI)
Subjects with Serum Sodium <135 mEq/L (ITT population)			
Change in average daily serum [Na+] AUC baseline to Day 4 (mEq/L) Mean (SD) N	4.0 (2.8) 213	0.4 (2.4) 203	3.7 (3.3-4.2) p <0.0001
Change in average daily serum [Na+] AUC baseline to Day 30 (mEq/L) Mean (SD) N	6.2 (4.0) 213	1.8 (3.7) 203	4.6 (3.9-5.2) p <0.0001
Percent of Patients Needing Fluid Restriction*	14% 30/215	25% 51/206	p =0.0017
Subgroup with Serum Sodium <130 mEq/L			
Change in average daily serum [Na+] AUC baseline to Day 4 (mEq/L) Mean (SD) N	4.8 (3.0) 110	0.7 (2.5) 105	4.2 (3.5-5.0) p <0.0001
Change in average daily serum [Na+] AUC baseline to Day 30 (mEq/L) Mean (SD) N	7.9 (4.1) 110	2.6 (4.2) 105	5.5 (4.4-6.5) p <0.0001
Percent of Patients Needing Fluid Restriction*	19% 21/110	36% 38/106	p <0.01
Subgroup with Serum Sodium <125 mEq/L			
Change in average daily serum [Na+] AUC baseline to Day 4 (mEq/L) Mean (SD) N	5.7 (3.8) 26	1.0 (1.8) 30	5.3 (3.8-6.9) p <0.0001
Change in average daily serum [Na+] AUC baseline to Day 30 (mEq/L) Mean (SD) N	10.0 (4.8) 26	4.1 (4.5) 30	5.7 (3.1-8.3) p <0.0001
Percent of Patients Needing Fluid Restriction*	35% 9/26	50% 15/30	p = 0.14

*Fluid Restriction defined as <1L/day at any time during treatment period.

with a reduction in maternal body weight gain and food consumption at 100 and 1000 mg/kg/day, and reduced fetal weight and delayed ossification of fetuses at 1000 mg/kg/day (162 times the MRHD on a body surface area basis). Oral administration of tolvaptan at 100, 300 and 1000 mg/kg/day to pregnant rabbits during organogenesis was associated with reductions in maternal body weight gain and food consumption at all doses, and abortions at mid- and high-doses. At 1000 mg/kg/day (324 times the MRHD), increased incidences of embryo-fetal death, fetal microphthalmia, open eyelids, cleft palate, brachymelia and skeletal malformations were observed. There are no adequate and well-controlled studies of SAMSCA in pregnant women. SAMSCA should be used in pregnancy only if the potential benefit justifies the risk to the fetus.

14   CLINICAL STUDIES

14.1   Hyponatremia

In two double-blind, placebo-controlled, multi-center studies (SALT-1 and SALT-2), a total of 424 patients with euvolemic or hypervolemic hyponatremia (serum sodium <135 mEq/L) resulting from a variety of underlying causes (heart failure, liver cirrhosis, syndrome of inappropriate antidiuretic hormone [SIADH] and others) were treated for 30 days with tolvaptan or placebo, then followed for an additional 7 days after withdrawal. Symptomatic patients, patients likely to require saline therapy during the course of therapy, patients with acute and transient hyponatremia associated with head trauma or postoperative state and patients with hyponatremia due to primary polydipsia, uncontrolled adrenal insufficiency or uncontrolled hypothyroidism were excluded. Patients were randomized to receive either placebo (N = 220) or tolvaptan (N = 223) at an initial oral dose of 15 mg once daily. The mean serum sodium concentration at study entry was 129 mEq/L. Fluid restriction was to be avoided if possible during the first 24 hours of therapy to avoid overly rapid correction of serum sodium, and during the first 24 hours of therapy 87% of patients had no fluid restriction. Thereafter, patients could resume or initiate fluid restriction (defined as daily fluid intake of ≤1.0 liter/day) as clinically indicated.

The dose of tolvaptan could be increased at 24 hour intervals to 30 mg once daily, then to 60 mg once daily, until either the maximum dose of 60 mg or normonatremia (serum sodium >135 mEq/L) was reached. Serum sodium concentrations were determined at 8 hours after study drug initiation and daily up to 72 hours, within which time titration was typically completed. Treatment was maintained for 30 days with additional serum sodium assessments on Days 11, 18, 25 and 30. On the day of study discontinuation, all patients resumed previous therapies for hyponatremia and were reevaluated 7 days later. The primary endpoint for these studies was the average daily AUC for change in serum sodium from baseline to Day 4 and baseline to Day 30 in patients with a serum sodium less than 135 mEq/L. Compared to placebo, tolvaptan caused a statistically greater increase in serum sodium ($p < 0.0001$) during both periods in both studies (see Table 2). For patients with a serum sodium of <130 mEq/L or <125 mEq/L, the effects at Day 4 and Day 30 remained significant (see Table 2). This effect was also seen across all disease etiology subsets (e.g., CHF, cirrhosis, SIADH/other).

[See table 2 at top of previous page]

In patients with hyponatremia (defined as <135 mEq/L), serum sodium concentration increased to a significantly greater degree in tolvaptan-treated patients compared to placebo-treated patients as early as 8 hours after the first dose, and the change was maintained for 30 days. The percentage of patients requiring fluid restriction (defined as ≤1 L/day at any time during the treatment period) was also significantly less (p =0.0017) in the tolvaptan-treated group (30/215, 14%) as compared with the placebo-treated group (51/206, 25%).

Figure 1 shows the change from baseline in serum sodium by visit in patients with serum sodium <135 mEq/L. Within 7 days of tolvaptan discontinuation, serum sodium concentrations in tolvaptan-treated patients declined to levels similar to those of placebo-treated patients.

[See figure 1 at top of next column]
[See figure 2 at top of next column]

In the open-label study SALTWATER, 111 patients, 94 of them hyponatremic (serum sodium <135 mEq/L), previously on tolvaptan or placebo therapy were given tolvaptan as a titrated regimen (15 to 60 mg once daily) after having returned to standard care for at least 7 days. By this time, their baseline mean serum sodium concentration had fallen to between their original baseline and post-placebo therapy level. Upon initiation of therapy, average serum sodium concentrations increased to approximately the same levels as observed for those previously treated with tolvaptan, and

Figure 1: Pooled SALT Studies: Analysis of Mean Serum Sodium (± SD, mEq/L) by Visit - Patients with Baseline Serum Sodium <135 mEq/L

*p-value <0.0001 for all visits during tolvaptan treatment compared to placebo

Figure 2: Pooled SALT Studies: Analysis of Mean Serum Sodium (± SD, mEq/L) by Visit - Patients with Baseline Serum Sodium <130 mEq/L

*p-value <0.0001 for all visits during tolvaptan treatment compared to placebo

were sustained for at least a year. Figure 3 shows results from 111 patients enrolled in the SALTWATER Study.

Figure 3: SALTWATER: Analysis of Mean Serum Sodium (± SD, mEq/L) by Visit

*p-value <0.0001 for all visits during tolvaptan treatment compared to baseline

14.2   Heart Failure

In a phase 3 double-blind, placebo-controlled study (EVEREST), 4133 patients with worsening heart failure were randomized to tolvaptan or placebo as an adjunct to standard of care. Long-term tolvaptan treatment (mean duration of treatment of 0.75 years) had no demonstrated effect, either favorable or unfavorable, on all-cause mortality [HR (95% CI): 0.98 (0.9, 1.1)] or the combined endpoint of CV mortality or subsequent hospitalization for worsening HF [HR (95% CI): 1.0 (0.9, 1.1)].

16   HOW SUPPLIED/STORAGE AND HANDLING

How Supplied

SAMSCA® (tolvaptan) tablets are available in the following strengths and packages.

SAMSCA 15 mg tablets are non-scored, blue, triangular, shallow-convex, debossed with "OTSUKA" and "15" on one side.

Blister of 10   NDC 59148-020-50

SAMSCA 30 mg tablets are non-scored, blue, round, shallow-convex, debossed with "OTSUKA" and "30" on one side.

Blister of 10   NDC 59148-021-50

Storage and Handling

Store at 25 °C (77 °F), excursions permitted between 15 °C and 30 °C (59 °F to 86 °F) [see USP controlled Room Temperature].

Keep out of reach of children.

17   PATIENT COUNSELING INFORMATION

As a part of patient counseling, healthcare providers must review the SAMSCA Medication Guide with every patient [see FDA-Approved Medication Guide (17.3)].

17.1   Concomitant Medication

Advise patients to inform their physician if they are taking or plan to take any prescription or over-the-counter drugs since there is a potential for interactions.

Strong and Moderate CYP 3A inhibitors and P-gp inhibitors

Advise patients to inform their physician if they use strong (e.g., ketoconazole, itraconazole, clarithromycin, telithromycin, nelfinavir, saquinavir, indinavir, ritonavir) or moderate CYP 3A inhibitors (e.g., aprepitant, erythromycin, diltiazem, verapamil, fluconazole) or P-gp inhibitors (e.g., cyclosporine) [see Dosage and Administration (2.3), Contraindications (4.4), Warnings and Precautions (5.5) and Drug Interactions (7.1)].

17.2   Nursing

Advise patients not to breastfeed an infant if they are taking SAMSCA [see Use In Specific Populations (8.3)].

Manufactured by Otsuka Pharmaceutical Co., Ltd., Tokyo, 101-8535 Japan

Distributed and marketed by Otsuka America Pharmaceutical, Inc., Rockville, MD 20850

SAMSCA is a registered trademark of Otsuka Pharmaceutical Co., Ltd., Tokyo, 101-8535 Japan

© 2014 Otsuka Pharmaceutical Co., Ltd.

17.3   FDA-Approved Medication Guide

MEDICATION GUIDE

SAMSCA® (sam-sca)

tolvaptan

Tablets

Read the Medication Guide that comes with SAMSCA before you take it and each time you get a new prescription. There may be new information. This Medication Guide does not take the place of talking to your healthcare provider about your medical condition or your treatment. Share this important information with members of your household.

What is the most important information I should know about SAMSCA?

1) **SAMSCA may make the salt (sodium) level in your blood rise too fast.** This can increase your risk of a serious condition called osmotic demyelination syndrome (ODS). ODS can lead to coma or death. ODS can also cause new symptoms such as:
• trouble speaking
• swallowing trouble or feeling like food or liquid gets stuck while swallowing
• drowsiness
• confusion
• mood changes
• trouble controlling body movement (involuntary movement) and weakness in muscles of the arms and legs
• seizures

You or a family member should tell your healthcare provider right away if you have any of these symptoms even if they begin later in treatment. Also tell you healthcare provider about any other new symptoms while taking SAMSCA.

You may be more at risk for ODS if you have:
• liver disease
• not eaten enough for a long period of time (malnourished)
• very low sodium level in your blood
• been drinking large amounts of alcohol for a long period of time (chronic alcoholism)

To lessen your risk of ODS while taking SAMSCA:
• **Treatment with SAMSCA should be started and restarted only in a hospital, where the sodium levels in your blood can be checked closely.**
• Do not take SAMSCA if you can not tell if you are thirsty.
• To prevent losing too much body water (dehydration), have water available to drink at all times while taking SAMSCA. Unless your healthcare provider tells you otherwise, drink when you are thirsty.
• If your healthcare provider tells you to keep taking SAMSCA after you leave a hospital, it is important that you do not stop and re-start SAMSCA on your own. You may need to go back to a hospital to re-start SAMSCA. Talk to your healthcare provider right away if you stop taking SAMSCA for any reason.
• It is important to stay under the care of your healthcare provider while taking SAMSCA and follow their instructions.

2) **SAMSCA may cause liver problems, including life-threatening liver failure.** SAMSCA should not be taken

for more than 30 days. Tell your doctor right away if you develop or have worsening of any of these signs and symptoms of liver problems:
• Loss of appetite, nausea, vomiting
• Fever, feeling unwell, unusual tiredness
• Itching
• Yellowing of the skin or the whites of the eyes (jaundice)
• Unusual darkening of the urine
• Right upper stomach area pain or discomfort

What is SAMSCA?

SAMSCA is a prescription medicine used to help increase low sodium levels in the blood, in adults with conditions such as heart failure and certain hormone imbalances. SAMSCA helps raise salt levels in your blood by removing extra body water as urine.

It is not known if SAMSCA is safe or works in children.

Who should not take SAMSCA?

Do not take SAMSCA if:
• you are allergic to tolvaptan or any of the ingredients in SAMSCA. See the end of this Medication Guide for a complete list of ingredients in SAMSCA.
• the sodium level in your blood must be increased right away.
• you cannot replace fluids by drinking or you can not feel if you are thirsty.
• you are dizzy, faint, or your kidneys are not working normally because you have lost too much body fluid.
• you take certain medicines. These medicines could cause you to have too much SAMSCA in your blood:
  ■ the antibiotic medicines, clarithromycin (Biaxin, Biaxin XL) or telithromycin (Ketek)
  ■ the antifungal medicines, ketoconazole (Nizoral) or itraconazole (Sporonox)
  ■ the anti-HIV medicines, ritonavir (Kaletra, Norvir), indinavir (Crixivan), nelfinavir (Viracept), and saquinavir (Invirase)
  ■ the antidepressant medicine, nefazodone hydrochloride
• your body is not able to make urine. SAMSCA will not help your condition.

What should I tell my healthcare provider before taking SAMSCA?

Tell your healthcare provider about all your medical conditions, including if you:
• have kidney problems and your body can not make urine.
• have liver problems
• can not feel if you are thirsty. See "What is the most important information I should know about SAMSCA?"
• have any allergies. See the end of this Medication Guide for a list of the ingredients in SAMSCA.

• are pregnant or plan to become pregnant. It is not known if SAMSCA will harm your unborn baby.
• are breast-feeding. It is not known if SAMSCA passes into your breast milk. You and your healthcare provider should decide if you will take SAMSCA or breast-feed. You should not do both.
• are taking desmopressin (dDAVP).

Tell your healthcare provider about all the medicines you take, including prescription and non-prescription medicines, vitamins, and herbal supplements.

Using SAMSCA with certain medicines could cause you to have too much SAMSCA in your blood. See "Who should not take SAMSCA?"

SAMSCA may affect the way other medicines work, and other medicines may affect how SAMSCA works.

Know the medicines you take. Keep a list of them and show it to your healthcare provider and pharmacist when you get a new medicine.

How should I take SAMSCA?

• See "What is the most important information I should know about SAMSCA?"
• Take SAMSCA exactly as prescribed by your healthcare provider.
• Take SAMSCA one time each day.
• You can take SAMSCA with or without food.
• Do not drink grapefruit juice during treatment with SAMSCA. This could cause you to have too much SAMSCA in your blood.
• Certain medicines or illnesses may keep you from drinking fluids or may cause you to lose too much body fluid, such as vomiting or diarrhea. If you have these problems, call your healthcare provider right away.
• Do not miss or skip doses of SAMSCA. If you miss a dose, take it as soon as you remember. If it is near the time of the next dose, skip the missed dose. Just take the next dose at your regular time. Do not take 2 doses at the same time.
• **If you take too much SAMSCA, call your healthcare provider right away.** If you take an overdose of SAMSCA, you may need to go to a hospital.
• If your healthcare provider tells you to stop taking SAMSCA, follow their instructions about limiting the amount of fluid you should drink.

What are the possible side effects of SAMSCA?

SAMSCA can cause serious side effects including:
• **See "What is the most important information I should know about SAMSCA?"**
• **Loss of too much body fluid (dehydration).** Tell your healthcare provider if you:

  ■ have vomiting or diarrhea, and cannot drink normally.
  ■ feel dizzy or faint. These may be symptoms that you have lost too much body fluid.

Call your healthcare provider right away, if you have any of these symptoms.

The most common side effects of SAMSCA are:
■ thirst
■ dry mouth
■ weakness
■ constipation
■ making large amounts of urine and urinating often
■ increased blood sugar levels

These are not all the possible side effects of SAMSCA. Talk to your healthcare provider about any side effect that bothers you or that does not go away while taking SAMSCA.

Call your doctor for medical advice about side effects. You may report side effects to FDA at 1-800-FDA-1088.

How should I store SAMSCA?

Store SAMSCA between 59 °F to 86 °F (15 °C to 30 °C).

Keep SAMSCA and all medicines out of the reach of children.

General Information about SAMSCA

Medicines are sometimes prescribed for purposes other than those listed in a Medication Guide. Do not use SAMSCA for a condition for which it was not prescribed. Do not give SAMSCA to other people, even if they have the same symptoms you have. It may harm them.

This Medication Guide summarizes the most important information about SAMSCA. If you would like more information, talk with your healthcare provider. You can ask your healthcare provider or pharmacist for information about SAMSCA that is written for healthcare professionals. For more information about SAMSCA, call 1-877-726-7220 or go to www.samsca.com.

What are the ingredients in SAMSCA?

Active ingredient: tolvaptan.

Inactive ingredients: corn starch, hydroxypropyl cellulose, lactose monohydrate, low-substituted hydroxypropyl cellulose, magnesium stearate and microcrystalline cellulose, and FD&C Blue No. 2 Aluminum Lake as colorant.

SAMSCA is a registered trademark of Otsuka Pharmaceutical Co., Ltd., Tokyo, 101-8535 Japan

07US14L-0919

Rev. 02, 2014

This Medication Guide has been approved by the U.S. Food and Drug Administration.

© 2014 Otsuka Pharmaceutical Co., Ltd.

Shown in Product Identification Guide, page 311

DIETARY SUPPLEMENTS

This section presents information on natural remedies and nutritional supplements marketed under the Dietary Supplement Health and Education Act (DSHEA) of 1994. The information on each product described has been provided by the manufacturer and contains the latest information available when the *PDR®* went to press. Listings are arranged alphabetically by manufacturer.

The function of PDR Network® is solely the compilation, organization, and distribution of this information on natural remedies and nutritional supplements. PDR Network does not assume, and expressly disclaims, any obligation to obtain and include any information on natural remedies and nutritional supplements other than that provided to it by the manufacturers. It should be understood that by making this material available, PDR Network is not advocating the use of any product described herein, nor is PDR Network responsible for misuse of a product due to typographical error. Additional information on any natural remedy and/or nutritional supplement product may be obtained from the manufacturer.

Products found in this section include herbal preparations, vitamins, minerals, and other substances intended to supplement the diet. The descriptions of these products are designed to provide the information necessary for informed use. Dietary supplements marketed under the DSHEA do not receive formal evaluation or approval from the FDA. The following disclaimer applies to all product information listed in this section, as mandated by the federal government: *These statements have not been evaluated by the Food and Drug Administration. This product is not intended to diagnose, treat, cure, or prevent any disease.*

4Life Research USA, LLC

9850 SOUTH 300 WEST
SANDY, UT 84070

Direct Inquiries to:
(801) 562-3600
productsupport@4life.com
www.4life.com

4LIFE TRANSFER FACTOR® **DS**
TRI-FACTOR® FORMULA

PRODUCT DESCRIPTION

4Life Transfer Factor Tri-Factor Formula combines proprietary transfer factors and NanoFactor® molecules extracted from bovine colostrum and chicken egg yolk sources. These molecules contain antigen information which educates, enhances, and helps maintain immune system balance.

TECHNICAL DESCRIPTION

Transfer factors are molecules that communicate antigenic immunological information intercellularly and from a donor to a recipient. They support immune function through cell mediated immunity. Transfer factors, which carry antigen specific information to which all tested immune cells respond, are produced by mononuclear cells and serve to support and improve immune mediated pathways. Mammalian transfer factors, including those of humans are small molecules between 3,500 and 10,000 daltons. (1; 2) Transfer factors are polypeptides that consist of 40 to 44 amino acids (3) and have a conserved region and a variable region. From a molecular biological standpoint, these two properties are analogous to antibodies; however transfer factor's functions of cell mediated immunity (CMI) and non-specific immunological activity differ almost completely from the functions of antibodies. The molecules that have a molecular weight of less than 3,500 daltons modulate immune response but they do not transfer delayed-type hypersensitivity (DTH). (1)

4Life's transfer factors are sourced from the ultra-filtration of colostrum and from egg yolks. (4; 5) The molecules obtained from the spray dried ultra-filtrate of bovine colostrum are of two classes; the transfer factors present in the ultra-filtrate of ≤10,000 daltons and the nanofraction molecules that are present in the nano-filtrate of ≤3,500 daltons.

Transfer factors were first discovered in 1949 by H. Sherwood Lawrence when he demonstrated that CMI could be transferred from one individual to another by way of low molecular weight extracts of white blood cells. Transfer factors could transfer DTH of a specific form from a skin test positive individual to a skin test negative individual who subsequent to the transfer would skin test positive for that antigen. (6) In a subsequent study in 1955 he demonstrated that DTH could be passed serially, first from a skin test positive individual to a test negative individual, who became test positive, then 6 months later from the second individual to another test negative individual who became test positive. (7) At the time antibodies were the focus of immune research and little was known of the importance of DTH and of the involvement of T-cells in immune response. Transfer factors promote wellness via cell mediated immunity. These compounds are components of colostrum, an infant's first meal. They bridge the generational gap by passing cell mediated immunity from mother to infant.

BIOLOGICAL AND PHYSIOLOGICAL ACTION

Transfer factors' preparations contain more than 200 different moieties of polypeptide molecules with a molecular weight of <10,000 daltons; each moiety potentially having a great number of epitotic variations. These antigen specific factors are synthesized in monocytes and stored in the cytoplasm or on the cell membrane. A significant body of evidence indicates that the primary biological function of transfer factors is to recruit and specifically sensitize previously uncommitted lymphocytes. These sensitized T-lymphocytes initiate the events of cell-mediated immunity, thereby, promoting immunity not only at the site of antigen challenge but also throughout the body. (8) The effect of transfer factors on antigen mediated immunity, via B-cells, is not completely understood; however, a clinical test has reported an increase in particular antibodies, such as IgA and IgG, during transfer factor administration. Clinical studies have demonstrated that transfer factors' unique ability to express DTH and promote cell-mediated immunity can be transferred from a sensitized donor to a non-immune recipient. (1; 9) This antigen specific effect is well documented and is likely produced through activation of the CD3-antigen site of T-cells, increased macrophage activation, and interleukin production—which can also enhance natural killer cell function. (1; 10)

Although the exact mechanism of action is unknown, research has shown that transfer factors will bind to antigens. However, the antigen specificity that is "transferred" to recipients is mediated by T-lymphocytes. (3) Current structure function models propose that transfer factors have a variable region and a conserved amino acid region, which determines the antigenic specificity for an estimated 8^{18} epitopes (1) and serves as a binding target for immune cell receptors respectively. (2; 11) These highly conserved regions presumably allow transfer factors to be administered across a species barrier without any loss of potency. In fact, research has demonstrated that bovine transfer factors are structurally analogous to human-derived transfer factors with equivalent physiological activity. This is further supported by several studies, which used transfer factors extracted from bovine lymph nodes and colostrum to confer cell-mediated immunity to specific antigens in animals and human recipients. (12; 13)

Although most clinical trials with transfer factors have used parental administration; oral administration has also demonstrated successful transfer of DTH and cell mediated immunity I recipients. (14) Dose response studies, which compare in various routes of administration, have been performed in both human and animals. Results of these experiments refute any arguments that the acidic or enzymatic environment of gastrointestinal tract effects oral administration of transfer factors. (14)

CLINICAL AND EXPERIMENTAL STUDIES

Natural Killer Cell Activity

Peripheral blood mononuclear cells were isolated and pooled from several healthy donors. Sixty thousand cells were added to each well of 96-well microtiter plate. Various immune modulating ingredients, including 4Life Transfer Factor Tri-Factor Formula, were added to select wells on the plate and 48 hour incubation started. At the end of the incubation period 30 thousand K562 cells were added to each well. MTT assay techniques were used to determine the cytotoxic index. The various 4Life Transfer Factor products resulted in cytotoxic indices of 80-98%. By comparison, mononuclear cells incubated with IL-2 for the same 48 hour period produced a cytotoxic index of 88%.

CD4 T Helper Cell Research

Multiple studies were performed using the FDA-approved diagnostic CD4 T Helper cell assay kit and/or a T Cell Memory (CD8) assay kit under development by the same company. Similar to the NK cell research described above these in vitro studies were preformed on 96-well microtiter plates measuring ATP production via a luciferase-based luminescence reaction.

The CD4 assay utilizes PHA-stimulated cells isolated from whole blood via the use of Dynabeads™. An 18 hour incubation of these isolated, stimulated CD4 cells with the 4Life Transfer Factor products has resulted in a modulation of immune cell activity as exhibited by a decrease in ATP production without a negative impact on cell viability. It is hypothesized that this reduction on ATP production is a result of a redirection in immune cell focus, essentially diminishing the distraction induced by the addition of PHA to the microtiter wells.

Salivary Secretory IgA-Preliminary Investigation

Twenty-four subjects naïve to transfer factor supplementation were enrolled in a small-scale, preliminary test. Twenty-one were included in the final analysis. Salivary samples were collected from each subject weekly at roughly the same time of day and day of the week. Saliva was collected over a 5 minute period via passive drool while subjects chewed on a piece of Parafilm™. The samples were put on ice and then frozen at -70°C until assay. The commercial Salimetrics™ salivary IgA assay kit was used for analysis. Subjects were given 4Life Transfer Factor Tri-Factor Formula at 2 capsules per day for two weeks and then transitioned to 4Life Transfer Factor RioVida Tri-Factor Formula at 60ml per day for an additional 2 weeks. At the end of the 4 week supplementation period the group showed an average 73% increase in salivary secretory IgA (SIgA) production over their baseline value. Furthermore, none of the 21 subjects showed SIgA production rate less than their baseline value at the end of the test.

Wellness Research

A study conducted with 30 college students found that either 15 or 30 days of transfer factor administered according to label dose helped them maintain their health. Those that took the product for 30 days showed prolonged health maintenance than those who took it for only 15 days. (15)

Longevity Studies

Two studies on the effects of 4Life Transfer Factor products on longevity were conducted. An initial, preliminary study was done on mice. This was followed up with a more intricate study on a small group of older men.

Groups of 20 mice each were compared in terms of organ weights, serum immune parameters, strength (dynamometer and hanging time), and isoproterenol-induced salivary hyperplasia. One group was injected with 4mg/kg of a product containing transfer factors. The treatment group showed improvements in all the aforementioned parameters. Isoproterenol-induced salivary gland hyperplasia declines with age. This diminished response is thought to be a consequence of decreased lymphoid cellular regulation of somatic tissue growth. The increased hyperplasia seen in the treatment animals approximated that seen in the treatment animals approximated that seen in younger, untreated mice. There were no significant changes noted in height, weight, or rectal temperature between the two groups. (16) Based on the results of this study an additional study was undertaken in 11 older men aged 55-73. Subjects were given 3 capsules per day of a product containing transfer factors 5 days a week for 6 weeks. At the end of the six week study period a determination of biological age using the Kiev method (17; 18) showed a reduction of approximately four years. There were significant improvements in several parameters of cardiovascular function, hearing, balance, vital lung capacity, ability to hold their breath, and some subjective measures. (16)

Safety

In a study of acute toxicity rats were assessed for fourteen days following a single gavage of 4Life Transfer Factor. Five female SD rats were each gavaged with a dose of 2,000mg/kg. No treatment-related mortalities occurred and there were no clinical signs of toxicity. No significant difference in body weight occurred. No gross lesions were found at necropsy in any of the animals. Thus, acute toxicity is considered to be greater than 2,000mg/kg.

Since the discovery of transfer factors in 1949 there have been no reports of allergic reactions (1) or of any side effects resulting from long-term use of 10 years or more. The use of transfer factors is contraindicated in person receiving immunosuppressive therapy, though actual interactions have not been documented.

How Supplied

4Life Transfer Factor® can be found in the following products:

4Life Transfer Factor® Tri-Factor® Formula
4Life® Transfer Factor Plus® Tri-Factor® Formula
4Life Transfer Factor® RioVida Tri-Factor® Formula
4Life Transfer Factor Renuvo®
4Life Transfer Factor® Chewable Tri-Factor® Formula
4Life Transfer Factor® Classic
4Life Transfer Factor® Immune Spray
4Life Transfer Factor® KBU®
4Life Transfer Factor® Kids
4Life Transfer Factor® Belle Vie®
4Life Transfer Factor® Cardio
4Life Transfer Factor® GluCoach®
4Life Transfer Factor® MalePro®
4Life Transfer Factor® ReCall®
4Life Transfer Factor Vista®
4Life RiteStart® Men
4Life RiteStart® Women

REFERENCES

1. *Progress in Drug Research.* Fundenberg, H. and G. Pizza. 1994, Vol. 42. 309-400.
2. **Lawrence, H.S. and W. Borkowsjy.** (1-3), 1996, Biotherapy, Vol. 9, pp. 1-5.
3. **Kirkpatrick, C.H.** 4, 2000, Mol Med, Vol. 6, pp. 332-41.
4. **Hennen, W. and D. Lisonbee.** s.l. : U.P. Office, Editor., 2002, 4Life Research, LC:USA.
5. **Wilson, G. and G. Paddock.** s.l. : U.P. Office, Editor., 1989, Amtron, Inc: USA.
6. **Lawrence, H.S.** 4, 1949, Proc Soc Exp Biol Med, Vol. 71, pp. 516-22.
7. **Lawrence, H.S.** 2, 1955, J Clin Invest, Vol. 34, pp. 219-30.
8. **Levin, A.S., L.E. Spitler, and H.H. Fundenberg.** 1973, Annu Rev Med, Vol. 24, pp. 175-208.
9. **Fudenberg, H. and H. Fudenberg.** 1989, Ann Rev Pharmacol Toxicol, Vol. 29, pp. 475-516.
10. **See, D., S. Mason, and R. Roshan.** 2, 2002, Immunol Invest, Vol. 31, pp. 137-53.
11. *Transfer factor in the age of molecular biology: A review.* Dwyer, John M. 1-3, 1996, Biotherapy, Vol. 9, pp. 7-11.
12. **Wilson, G.B., R.T. Newell, and N.M. Burdash.** 1, 1979, Cell Immunol, Vol. 47, pp. 1-18.
13. **Radosevich, J.K., G.H. Scott, and G.B. Olson.** 4, 1985, Am J Vet Res, Vol. 46, pp. 875-8.
14. *Activities and characteristics of transfer factors.* **Kirkpatrick, C.H.** 1-3, 1996, Biotherapy, Vol. 9, pp. 13-6.
15. *in Euromedica Hanover.* **Chizhov, A. et al.** Hanover, Germany : s.n., 2007.
16. *in Euromedica Hannover 2004.* **Klimov, V. and E. Oganova.** Hannover, Germany : s.n., 2004. pp. 15-16.
17. **Agadzhanian, N., et al.** 1996, ATMA.
18. **Chebotarev, D.** 1984, Annals of Gerontology and Geriatrics.

These statements have not been evaluated by the Food and Drug Administration. This product is not intended to diagnose, treat, cure of prevent any disease.

Shown in Product Identification Guide, page 303

A&Z Pharmaceutical Inc.
180 OSER AVENUE, SUITE 300
HAUPPAUGE, NY 11788

Direct Inquiries to:
Telephone: (631) 952-3800
Fax: (631) 952-3900
E-Mail: info@azpharmaceutical.com
Website: www.azpharmaceutical.com

D-CAL   OTC
Calcium Supplement / Antacid
Calcium 300 mg
Vitamin D₃ 100IU

Supplement Facts

	Adults	Children
▪ Serving size	2	1
▪ Servings per Container	30	60
▪ Amount per Serving		
Calories:	4	2
Calcium (as calcium carbonate)	600 mg (60%DV)	300 mg (37.5%DV)
Vitamin D₃	200 IU (50%DV)	100 IU (25%DV)

Drug Facts

Active ingredient (in each tablet)	Purpose
Calcium Carbonate 750 mg	Antacid

Uses

relieves ▪ heartburn ▪ acid indigestion ▪ sour stomach ▪ upset stomach due to these symptoms

Warnings

Ask a doctor or pharmacist before use if you are taking a prescription drug. Antacids may interact with certain prescription drugs.

When using this product ▪ do not take more than 10 tablets for adults and 5 tablets for chidren in a 24 hour period.
Keep out of reach of children.

Directions

▪ **Adults:** chew 2 tablets daily. ▪ **Children:** chew 1 tablet daily.
If symptoms persist, ask a doctor.

Other Information

▪ store in a dry place
▪ do not use if imprinted seal under cap is torn or open
Inactive ingredients cholecalciferol, D&C red #27, flavors, magnesium stearate, maltodextrin, mineral oil, sorbitol
How supplied: bottles of 60 tablets
A&Z Pharmaceutical, Inc
Hauppauge, NY 11788

Shown in Product Identification Guide, page 303

D-CAL® KIDS   OTC
Calcium Supplement / Antacid
Granules
Calcium 300mg
Vitamin D₃ 100 IU

Supplement Facts

▪ Serving size	1g
▪ Servings per Container	10
▪ Amount per Serving	
Calories: 1	
Calcium (as calcium carbonate)	300 mg (37.5%DV)

Drug Facts

Active Ingredient (in each pouch)	Purpose
Calcium Carbonate 750 mg	Antacid

Uses relieves ▪ heartburn ▪ acid indigestion ▪ sour stomach ▪ upset stomach due to these symptoms

Warnings

Ask a doctor or pharmacist before use if you are taking a prescription drug. Antacids may interact with certain prescription drugs.

When using this product ▪ do not take more than 1 pouch in a 24 hour period
Keep out of reach of children.

Directions

▪ find the right dose on chart below based on weight, otherwise use age.
▪ pour powder into cup and add 15ml (0.51 oz.) of water, stir and drink.

Dosing Chart

Weight (lbs)	Age	Dose
Under 24	Under 2 yrs	Ask a doctor
24-47	2-5 yrs	1/2 pouch
48-95	6-11 yrs	1 pouch

Other Information

▪ store in a dry place ▪ do not use if pouch is open or torn
Inactive Ingredients cholecalciferol, dextrose, maltodextrin, sodium citrate
How supplied: 10 1g pouches per carton
A&Z Pharmaceutical, Inc
Hauppauge, NY 11788

Shown in Product Identification Guide, page 303

Alto Pharmaceuticals, Inc.
P.O. BOX 271150
TAMPA, FL 33688-1150
3172 LAKE ELLEN DRIVE
TAMPA, FL 33618
www.altopharm.com

Direct Inquiries to:
John J. Cullaro
Customer Service
JOHNC@ALTOPHARM.COM
(813) 968-0522
Fax (813) 968-0527

ZINC-220®   DS
DIETARY SUPPLEMENT
(Zinc Sulfate 220 mg. USP)

UNIT DOSE
100 CAPSULES

Supplement Facts
Serving Size 1 Capsule

Amount Per Serving	% Daily Value*
Zinc	50mg 333%

(From Zinc Sulfate Heptahydrate 220mg)

INGREDIENTS: Each blue and pink capsule contains 50 mg. of elemental zinc. Zinc-220 capsules are gluten free and do not contain dextrose or glucose. Inactive ingredients: rice flour, magnesium stearate, D&C red #22, D&C red #28, FD&C blue #1, titanium dioxide and gelatin (capsule shell).
ACTION AND USES: Zinc-220® Capsules are indicated as a dietary supplement. Normal growth and tissue repair are directly dependent upon an adequate supply of zinc in the diet. Zinc functions as an integral part of a number of enzymes important to protein and carbohydrate metabolism. Zinc-220® Capsules are recommended for deficiencies or the prevention of deficiencies of zinc.
WARNINGS: Zinc-220® if administered in stat dosages of 2 grams (9 capsules) will cause an emetic effect. As with any supplement, if you are pregnant, nursing or taking medication, consult your physician before use.
PRECAUTION: It is recommended that Zinc-220® Capsules be taken with meals to avoid gastric distress.
ADULTS: Take one capsule daily with meals or as directed by a physician.
ALTO®
Pharmaceuticals, Inc.
Tampa, Florida 33688
For Customer Service: 1-813-968-0522
Dist. U.S.A   REV 3/11

Shown in Product Identification Guide, page 305

Andorra Life Corporation
555 QUINCE ORCHARD ROAD, SUITE 500C
GAITHERSBURG, MD 20878

Direct Inquiries to:
(Tel): 1-855-558-8088
(Email): info@andorralife.com

ADVANCED BLOOD SUGAR CONTROL   DS

Benefits:
• Helps Maintain Healthy Blood Sugar Levels
• Supports Healthy Blood Vessels
• Supports Sensory/Nerve Function
Why high blood sugar level is bad for you?
Balanced blood sugar is critical for our bodies to function; it is important for healthy blood vessels, optimal circulation and nerve functions. Persistently elevated blood sugar level leads to Diabetes. Diabetes damages the body and can lead to the multiple health problems.
A normal sugar level is currently considered to be less than 100 mg/dL when fasting and less than 140 mg/dL two hours after eating. But in most healthy people, sugar levels are even lower. During the day, our blood glucose levels tend to be at their lowest just before meals. For most people without diabetes, blood sugar levels before meals hover around 70 to 80 mg/dL. In some, 60 is normal; in others, 90. Again, anything less than 100 mg/dL while fasting is considered normal by today's standards.
High blood sugar (Hyperglycemia) is caused by many factors:
• Type I Diabetes: The body does not produce insulin.
• Type II Diabetes: The body does not produce enough insulin for proper function. (most common)
• Gestational Diabetes: This type affects about 9.2% of females during pregnancy.
People with Diabetes are in special need to lower their blood sugar levels. People who have irregular life styles are also in need to regulate their blood sugar levels. Stress, lack of exercise and eating more than planned, all trigger high blood glucose.
Why choose Andorra Life?
Andorra's Advanced Blood Sugar Control uses the finest ingredients which are specially formulated to keep your blood sugar level in line.
Premium Pine Bark:
Advanced scientific research has revealed that pine bark has potent blood sugar benefits, including lowering fasting and post-meal glucose levels as well as promoting insulin sensitivity. Pine bark can significantly lowered fasting and post meal blood glucose levels compared to baseline. Furthermore, insulin levels remained unchanged at all doses, indicating Pine bark facilitated blood sugar uptake by previously insulin resistant cells. In another study Pine bark was shown to significantly lower fasting blood glucose.
Alpha Lipoic Acid (ALA):
Studies have shown that ALA significantly improves insulin stimulated glucose uptake in patients with type II diabetes. Not only does it help lower blood sugar levels by reducing the secretion of insulin, it also increases insulin sensitivity at the cell level and thus, even LESS insulin is required.
Cinnamon Powder:
Cinnamon powders may help improve glucose and lipids levels in patients with type 2 diabetes, according to a study published in Diabetics Care.
The study authors concluded that consuming up to 6 grams of cinnamon per day "reduces serum glucose, triglyceride, LDL cholesterol, and total cholesterol in people with type 2 diabetes." and that "the inclusion of cinnamon in the diet of people with type 2 diabetes will reduce risk factors associated with diabetes and cardiovascular diseases."
In addition, cinnamon extract can reduce fasting blood sugar levels in patients, researchers reported in the European Journal of Clinical Investigation.
Berberine:
A plant alkaloid and naturally occurring compound found in the roots, rhizomes, and stem bark of various plants, berberine works by targeting a key regulator of metabolism, the AMP-activated protein kinase (AMPK) enzyme. AMPK regulates glucose uptake and the synthesis of glucose transporters— which move glucose out of your blood and into your cells, where it is converted to energy. Berberine may also increase the number and activity of the insulin receptors, promoting insulin sensitivity. On top of that, AMPK facilitates the burning of fatty acids in your cells, which is why it is a powerful tool for helping keep blood lipid levels in check.
Chromium:
This essential trace element is required for normal fat and carbohydrate metabolism and healthy glucose tolerance.

Help Patients Save on Rx Drugs: PDR.net/PharmacyDiscountCard

Chromium may help promote insulin sensitivity by increasing the number of insulin binding sites on cells, which allow for better transport of glucose into cells for energy.

Vitamin B6:
Pyridoxamine is a specialized form of vitamin B6 easily converted in the body to pyridoxal 5-phosphate (PLP), the active form of the vitamin. Pyridoxamine may help prevent diabetic complications by blocking formation of advanced glycation end products (AGEs) and advanced lipoxidation end products (ALEs) underlying loss of structure and function accompanying aging. AGEs are implicated in diabetes-related conditions including kidney disease (nephropathy), visual loss (retinopathy), and neuropathy. It has been described as "the most potent natural substance for inhibiting AGE formation."

Vitamin B12:
Vitamin B12 supports the digestive system in keeping glucose levels stable. Vitamin B12 is bound to protein in food. The activity of hydrochloric acid and gastric protease in the stomach releases vitamin B12 from its protein. Once it is released, vitamin B12 begins to work quickly. B12 deficiency can cause permanent nerve damage. Neuropathy is a common problem for people with diabetes, who experience pain, tingling, and numbness in their arms, hands, legs, and feet, resulting in sores.

Supplement Facts Serving Size: 1 capsule	Per Serving
Servings Per Container: 30	
Vitamin B6	10 mg
Vitamin B12	100 mcg
Chromium	200 mcg
Cinnamon Bark	200 mg
Alpha Lipoic Acid	50 mg
Pine Bark Extract	50 mg
Berberine	200 mg

Free of: milk or milk by-products, egg or egg by-products, fish or fish by-products, shellfish and by-products, tree nuts, peanut or peanut by-products, wheat or wheat by-products, soybeans and soy byproducts.

Suggested Use: take one (1) capsule daily as a dietary supplement or as recommended by your healthcare professional.

• **KEEP OUT OF REACH OF CHILDREN.**
• Consult your doctor before use if you are pregnant, nursing or taking medication.
• Keep tightly closed at a cool dry place.
• Store at Room temperature.
• For your protection, do not use if imprinted safety seal under cap is broken or missing.

Manufactured in a FDA Licensed cGMP facility.

REFERENCES
1. Alam Khan, MS, PHD, Mahpara Safdar, MS, Mohammad Muzaffar Ali Khan, MS, PHD, Khan Nawaz Khattak, MS and Richard A. Anderson, PHD. *"Cinnamon Improves Glucose and Lipids of People With Type 2 Diabetes"*. *Diabetes Care*. December 2003 vol. 26 no. 12 3215-3218. Accessed October 14th 2013.
2. Cameron NE, Gibson TM, Nangle MR, Cotter MA. Inhibitors of advanced glycation end product formation and neurovascular dysfunction in experimental diabetes. Ann NY Acad Sci. 2005 Jun;1043:784-92.
3. Giusti C, Gargiulo P. Advances in biochemical mechanisms of diabetic retinopathy. Eur Rev Med Pharmacol Sci. 2007 May;11(3):155-63.
4. Head KA. Peripheral neuropathy: pathogenic mechanisms and alternative therapies. Altern Med Rev. 2006 Dec;11(4):294-329.
5. Karachalias N, Babaei-Jadidi R, Ahmed N, Thornalley PJ. Accumulation of fructosyl-lysine and advanced glycation end products in the kidney, retina and peripheral nerve of streptozotocin-induced diabetic rats. Biochem Soc Trans. 2003 Dec;31(Pt 6):1423-5.
6. Ahmed N, Thornalley PJ. Advanced glycation endproducts: what is their relevance to diabetic complications? Diabetes Obes Metab. 2007 May;9(3):233-45.
7. Vasdev S, Gill V, Singal P. Role of advanced glycation end products in hypertension and atherosclerosis: therapeutic implications. Cell Biochem Biophys. 2007;49(1):48-63.
8. Theodoratou E, Farrington SM, Tenesa A, et al. Dietary vitamin B6 intake and the risk of colorectal cancer. Cancer Epidemiol Biomarkers Prev. 2008 Jan;17(1):171-82.
9. Nawale RB, Mourya VK, Bhise SB. Non-enzymatic glycation of proteins: a cause for complications in diabetes. Indian J Biochem Biophys. 2006 Dec;43(6):337-44.
10. Perricone N. Ageless Face, Ageless Mind. New York, New York: Ballantine Books; 2007.
11. Chetyrkin SV, Mathis ME, Ham AJ, et al. Propagation of protein glycation damage involves modification of tryptophan residues via reactive oxygen species: inhibition by pyridoxamine. Free Radic Biol Med. 2008 Apr 1;44(7):1276-85.
12. Ahmed N, Thornalley PJ. Advanced glycation endproducts: what is their relevance to diabetic complications? Diabetes Obes Metab. 2007 May;9(3):233-45.
13. Voziyan PA, Metz TO, Baynes JW, Hudson BG. A post-Amadori inhibitor pyridoxamine also inhibits chemical modification of proteins by scavenging carbonyl intermediates of carbohydrate and lipid degradation. J Biol Chem. 2002 Feb 1;277(5):3397-403.
14. Chetyrkin SV, Zhang W, Hudson BG, Serianni AS, Voziyan PA. Pyridoxamine protects proteins from functional damage by 3-deoxyglucosone: mechanism of action of pyridoxamine. Biochemistry. 2008 Jan 22;47(3):997-1006.
15. Jain SK, Lim G. Pyridoxine and pyridoxamine inhibits superoxide radicals and prevents lipid peroxidation, protein glycosylation, and (Na+ + K+)-ATPase activity reduction in high glucose-treated human erythrocytes. Free Radic Biol Med. 2001 Feb 1;30(3):232-7.
16. Metz TO, Alderson NL, Thorpe SR, Baynes JW. Pyridoxamine, an inhibitor of advanced glycation and lipoxidation reactions: a novel therapy for treatment of diabetic complications. Arch Biochem Biophys. 2003 Nov 1;419(1):41-9.
17. Onorato JM, Jenkins AJ, Thorpe SR, Baynes JW. Pyridoxamine, an inhibitor of advanced glycation reactions, also inhibits advanced lipoxidation reactions. Mechanism of action of pyridoxamine. J Biol Chem. 2000 Jul 14;275(28):21177-84.
18. Higuchi O, Nakagawa K, Tsuzuki T, et al. Aminophospholipid glycation and its inhibitor screening system: a new role of pyridoxal 5'-phosphate as the inhibitor. J Lipid Res. 2006 May;47(5):964-74.
19. Takatori A, Ishii Y, Itagaki S, Kyuwa S, Yoshikawa Y. Amelioration of the beta-cell dysfunction in diabetic APA hamsters by antioxidants and AGE inhibitor treatments. Diabetes Metab Res Rev. 2004 May;20(3):211-8.
20. Alderson NL, Chachich ME, Youssef NN, et al. The AGE inhibitor pyridoxamine inhibits lipemia and development of renal and vascular disease in Zucker obese rats. Kidney Int. 2003 Jun;63(6):2123- 33.
21. Araghi-Niknam M, Hosseini S, Larson D, Rohdewald P, Watson RR. Pine bark extract reduces platelet aggregation. *Integr Med*. 2000;2:73-77.
22. Summary of data for chemical selection: oligomeric proanthocyanidins from grape seeds and pine bark. National Toxicology Program Web site. Accessed at http://ntp.niehs.nih.gov/ntp/htdocs/Chem_Background/ExSumPdf/GrapeSeeds_PineBark.pdf on June 6, 2008.
23. Devaraj S, Vega-López S, Kaul N, et al. Supplementation with a pine bark extract rich in polyphenols increase plasma antioxidant capacity and alters the plasma lipoprotein profile. Lipids. 2002;37:931-934.

Shown in Product Identification Guide, page 305

ADVANCED LUNG CLEANSE   DS

Benefits:
• Supports Healthy Respiration
• Supports Healthy Bronchial Sinus Function
• Maintain Healthy Lung Function

Why our lungs need protection?
The lungs are different from most of the other organs in our bodies because their delicate tissues are directly connected to the outside environment. Anything we breathe in can affect the lungs. Germs, tobacco smoke and other harmful substances can cause damage to the airways and threaten the lungs ability to work properly.

Our bodies have the natural defense systems designed to protect the lungs. This works very well most of the time to keep out dirt and fight off germs. But there are some important things we have to do to reduce the risk of lung disease. Cigarette smoking, Secondhand smoke, outdoor air pollution, chemicals in the home and workplace, and radon can all cause or worsen lung disease. Regular check-ups are an important part of disease prevention, even when you are feeling well. This is especially true for lung disease, which sometimes goes undetected until it is serious.

Without any extra effort, our lungs are in a near-constant state of inhaling and exhaling. Like all active areas of our bodies, the lungs require a fair share of vitamins to help them create new cells, repair DNA and fight damage from oxidation. In addition to a healthy diet, consuming the best vitamins for lungs can help promote lung health.

Why choose Andorra Life?
Andorra's Lung Cleanse is scientifically formulated and tested to shield your lung from air pollutants, smoking damages, detoxifies, and promotes the healthy lung blood circulation.

N-Acetyl Cysteine (NAC):
NAC is a compound that is converted by the body into the naturally occurring amino acid cysteine. NAC has been shown to lower blood levels of homocysteine, an effect that is potentially beneficial for heart disease prevention.
NAC also can break up trapped mucus and enhance its clearance from the bronchial passages, thereby improving the flow of air in and out of the lungs in people with COPD. In addition, NAC is the precursor of glutathione, one of the major antioxidants in lung tissue. Although the mucus-clearing effect of NAC occurs mainly when the compound is administered by inhalation, oral NAC has repeatedly been shown to prevent flare-ups in people with chronic bronchitis.
Supplementing with N-Acetylcysteine (NAC) can reduce the need for hospitalization among people suffering from chronic obstructive pulmonary disease (COPD), according to a study in the *European Respiratory Journal* (2003;21:795-8).
In the study, 1,219 people who had been hospitalized for COPD were observed for an average of nine months after they were discharged from the hospital. Those who were prescribed NAC were approximately one-third less likely to be readmitted to the hospital, compared with those who were not given NAC. The risk of hospitalization decreased with increasing doses of NAC. Excluding those who were prescribed less than 400 mg per day, treatment with NAC was associated with an 85% reduction in the rate of readmission.
A large number of studies have used 600 mg per day of NAC for prevention of chronic bronchitis. Although a few of participants in some studies experienced side effects, including nausea, vomiting, abdominal pain, indigestion, dyspepsia, dry mouth, headache, dizziness, or abnormal taste, most people tolerated the treatment well. Long-term use of NAC has the potential to increase the requirement for zinc and copper. Some doctors, therefore, advise people who are taking NAC also to take a multivitaminmineral preparation that provides approximately 15 mg of zinc and 2 mg of copper per day.

Vitamin A:
Vitamin A is the name of a group of fat-soluble retinoids, including retinol, retinal, retinoic acid, and retinyl esters. Vitamin A is involved in immune function, vision, reproduction, and cellular communication . Vitamin A is critical for vision as an essential component of rhodopsin, a protein that absorbs light in the retinal receptors, and because it supports the normal differentiation and functioning of the conjunctival membranes and cornea. Vitamin A also supports cell growth and differentiation, playing a critical role in the normal formation and maintenance of the heart, lungs, kidneys, and other organs.
One of the most important functions of vitamin A is to repair and re-build all the internal mucosal membranes, from the top orifice to the bottom one. Thus Vitamin A is recommended for sinus problems, leaky gut syndrome and even interstitial cystitis. Vitamin A is helpful for anything that has to do with internal mucous membranes.
In these days of constantly increasing air pollution, and the spread of airborne bacteria and viruses, it is important to realize that the lining of the sinuses and lungs are the first line of defense. Thus vitamin A is essential for protection against colds, influenza and infections of the kidneys, bladder, lungs and mucous membranes.

Vitamin B-6 and Vitamin B-12:
Vitamin B6 is also called pyridoxine. Vitamin B6 has been studied for the treatment of many conditions, including anemia (low amounts of healthy red blood cells). A new study has shown that to have higher blood levels of vitamin B6 and the amino acid methionine both appear to reduce lung cancer risk in smokers and nonsmokers alike.
Vitamin B12 is a B vitamin. It can be found in foods such as meat, fish, and dairy products. Vitamin B12 is used for treating and preventing vitamin B12 deficiency that could cause pernicious anemia. Vitamin B12 is also used for asthma, allergies and skin infections.

Vitamin C:
Vitamin C was identified in the early 1900s in the search for a deficient substance responsible for scurvy, which was a serious disease of sailors in the Age of Sail. Starting in the 1930s, some German and US physicians proposed that vitamin C would be beneficial in the treatment of pneumonia. Although the burden of pneumonia has decreased dramatically in developed countries during the past century, lung infections are still a leading cause of mortality and morbidity globally. Many infections, including pneumonia, lead to reduced vitamin C levels in plasma, leukocytes and urine. Because of these changes in metabolism, vitamin C might

have a therapeutic effect on pneumonia patients. Thus there is a biological rationale to examine the effect of vitamin C on infections in humans.

The researchers agreed that a diet rich in the foods that provide vitamin C is likely to be beneficial for lung health. By reducing the amount of decline in lung function over time, consuming ample amounts of these foods could lower the risk of COPD - a COPD can be due to chronic bronchitis, emphysema, or both. Risk factors for COPD include history of smoking or passive smoke exposure, allergy and asthma, exposure to environmental pollution, recurrent respiratory illness, or a family history of chronic bronchitis or emphysema.

Vitamin D:

Many people associate vitamin D strictly with the health of their bones. However, vitamin D is also important for immune health, hormone production and lung function. According to research published in the May 2011 "American Journal of Respiratory and Critical Care Medicine," vitamin D deficiency can lead to poor lung function.

Coenzyme Q10, Ginger Extract and Tumeric Extract:

Coenzyme Q10 (CoQ10) is a substance similar to a vitamin. It is found in every cell of the body. The body makes CoQ10, and the cells use it to produce energy that the body needs for cell growth and maintenance. It also functions as an antioxidant, which protects the body from damage caused by harmful molecules known as free radicals.

Ginger is an herb. The rhizome (underground stem) is used as a spice and also as a medicine to improve conditions on many diseases. Ginger is used here for its anti inflammation effect on upper respiratory tract infections, cough, and bronchitis.

Turmeric is a plant. It has a warm, bitter taste and is frequently used to flavor or color curry powders, mustards, butters, and cheeses. But the root of turmeric is also used widely to make medicine. Turmeric is used for arthritis, heartburn (dyspepsia), stomach pain, bronchitis, colds, lung infections, fibromyalgia, leprosy, and fever. Turmeric has also been recognized for its anti inflammatory effect.

Hawthorn Berry Extract and Elecampane Root:

Hawthorn is used for Cadiovascular health and a powerfully antioxidant. Hawthorn can help improve the amount of blood pumped out of the heart during contractions, widen the blood vessels, and increase the transmission of nerve signals. It can relax the tiniest lung blood vessels hence increased blood flow farther from the heart, due to a component in hawthorn called proanthocyanidin.

Elecampane, also known as horse heal and marchalan, is a plant common in Great Britain, central and southern Europe, and Asia. Elecampane, has been long valued as an effective respiratory support herb, even being listed in the U.S. Pharmacopeia. Traditional Chinese and Indian Ayurvedic medicine use elecampane for bronchitis and asthma, as did ancient Greeks and Romans. In the 1800's, lozenges, candy, and cough drops were all produced from elecampane root.

Elecampane has actions, which are expectorant, antitussive, sedative, anti-fungal, relaxing, warming, and antimicrobial. Elecampane can soothe bronchial tube linings and act as an expectorant for lung cleansing. For this reason, elecampane is beneficial in supporting any respiratory condition which produces copious mucus discharge.

Supplement Facts Serving Size: 2 Capsules Servings Per Container: 30	Per Serving
Vitamin A	5000 IU
Vitamin C	250 mg
Vitamin D	400 IU
Vitamin B-6 (Pyridoxine)	10 mg
Vitamin B-12	100 mcg
Calcium	94 mg
Coenzyme Q10	10 mg
Ginger Extract	50 mg
Hawthorn Berry Extract	25 mg
N-Acetyl Cysteine	200 mg
Tumeric Extract (Curcumin)	10 mg
Elecampane Root Extract	100 mg

Free of: milk or milk by-products, egg or egg by-products, fish or fish by-products, shellfish and by-products, tree nuts, peanut or peanut by-products, wheat or wheat by-products, soybeans and soy by-products.

Suggested Use: take two (2) capsules daily as a dietary supplement or as recommended by your healthcare professional.

• **KEEP OUT OF REACH OF CHILDREN.**
• Consult your doctor before use if you are pregnant, nursing or taking medication.
• Keep tightly closed at a cool dry place.
• Store at Room temperature.
• For your protection, do not use if imprinted safety seal under cap is broken or missing.

Manufactured in a FDA Licensed cGMP facility.

REFERENCES

1. Tokarski S, Rutkowski M, Godala M, Mejer A, Kowalski J. [The impact of ascorbic acid on the concentrations of antioxidative vitamins in the plasma of patients with non-small cell lung cancer undergoing first-line chemotherapy]. Pol Merkur Lekarski. 2013 Sep;35(207):136-40. Polish.

2. Cheng TY, Lacroix AZ, Beresford SA, Goodman GE, Thornquist MD, Zheng Y, Chlebowski RT, Ho GY, Neuhouser ML. Vitamin D intake and lung cancer risk in the Women's Health Initiative. Am J Clin Nutr. 2013 Oct;98(4):1002-11. doi: 10.3945/ajcn.112.055905. Epub 2013 Aug 21.

3. Arrieta Ó, Hernández-Pedro N, Fernández-González-Aragón MC, Saavedra-Pérez D, Campos- Parra AD, Ríos-Trejo MÁ, Cerón-Lizárraga T, Martínez-Barrera L, Pineda B, Ordóñez G, Ortiz-Plata A, Granados-Soto V, Sotelo J. Retinoic acid reduces chemotherapy-induced neuropathy in an animal model and patients with lung cancer. Neurology. 2011 Sep 6;77(10):987-95. doi: 10.1212/WNL.0b013e31822e045c. Epub 2011 Aug 24.

4. Neuhouser ML, Barnett MJ, Kristal AR, Ambrosone CB, King IB, Thornquist M, Goodman GG. Dietary supplement use and prostate cancer risk in the Carotene and Retinol Efficacy Trial. Cancer Epidemiol Biomarkers Prev. 2009 Aug;18(8):2202-6. doi: 10.1158/1055-9965.EPI-09-0013.

5. Ito Y, Wakai K, Suzuki K, Ozasa K, Watanabe Y, Seki N, Ando M, Nishino Y, Kondo T, Ohno Y, Tamakoshi A; JACC Study Group. Lung cancer mortality and serum levels of carotenoids, retinol, tocopherols, and folic acid in men and women: a case-control study nested in the JACC Study. J Epidemiol. 2005 Jun;15 Suppl 2:S140-9.

6. Galluzzi L, Vitale I, Senovilla L, Olaussen KA, Pinna G, Eisenberg T, Goubar A, Martins I, Michels J, Kratassiouk G, Carmona-Gutierrez D, Scoazec M, Vacchelli E, Schlemmer F, Kepp O, Shen S, Tailler M, Niso-Santano M, Morselli E, Criollo A, Adjemian S, Jemaà M, Chaba K, Pailleret C, Michaud M, Pietrocola F, Tajeddine N, de La Motte Rouge T, Araujo N, Morozova N, Robert T, Ripoche H, Commo F, Besse B, Validire P, Fouret P, Robin A, Dorvault N, Girard P, Gouy S, Pautier P, Jägemann N, Nickel AC, Marsili S, Paccard C, Servant N, Hupé P, Behrens C, Behnam-Motlagh P, Kohno K, Cremer I, Damotte D, Alifano M, Midttun O, Ueland PM, Lazar V, Dessen P, Zischka H, Chatelut E, Castedo M, Madeo F, Barillot E, Thomale J, Wistuba II, Sautès-Fridman C, Zitvogel L, Soria JC, Harel-Bellan A, Kroemer G. Prognostic impact of vitamin B6 metabolism in lung cancer. Cell Rep. 2012 Aug 30;2(2):257-69. doi: 10.1016/j.celrep.2012.06.017. Epub 2012 Jul 26.

7. Mooney LA, Madsen AM, Tang D, Orjuela MA, Tsai WY, Garduno ER, Perera FP. Antioxidant vitamin supplementation reduces benzo(a)pyrene-DNA adducts and potentialcancer risk in female smokers. Cancer Epidemiol Biomarkers Prev. 2005 Jan;14(1):237-42.

8. Yang TY, Chang GC, Hsu SL, Huang YR, Chiu LY, Sheu GT. Effect of folic acid and vitamin B12 on pemetrexed antifolate chemotherapy in nutrientlung cancer cells. Biomed Res Int. 2013;2013:389046. doi: 10.1155/2013/389046. Epub 2013 Jul 31.

9. Takata Y, Cai Q, Beeghly-Fadiel A, Li H, Shrubsole MJ, Ji BT, Yang G, Chow WH, Gao YT, Zheng W, Shu XO. Dietary B vitamin and methionine intakes and lung cancer risk among female never smokers in China. Cancer Causes Control. 2012 Dec;23(12):1965-75. doi: 10.1007/s10552-012-0074-z. Epub 2012 Oct 12.

10. Cobanoglu U, Demir H, Cebi A, Sayir F, Alp HH, Akan Z, Gur T, Bakan E. Lipid peroxidation, DNA damage and coenzyme Q10 in lung cancer patients--markers for risk assessment? Asian Pac J Cancer Prev. 2011;12(6):1399-403.

11. Miyamae T, Seki M, Naga T, Uchino S, Asazuma H, Yoshida T, Iizuka Y, Kikuchi M, Imagawa T, Natsumeda Y, Yokota S, Yamamoto Y. Increased oxidative stress and coenzyme Q10 deficiency in juvenile fibromyalgia: amelioration of hypercholesterolemia and fatigue by ubiquinol-10 supplementation. Redox Rep. 2013;18(1):12-9. doi: 10.1179/1351000212Y.0000000036.

12. Cooney RV, Dai Q, Gao YT, Chow WH, Franke AA, Shu XO, Li H, Ji B, Cai Q, Chai W, Zheng W. Low plasma coenzyme Q(10) levels and breast cancer risk in Chinese women. Cancer Epidemiol Biomarkers Prev. 2011 Jun;20(6):1124-30. doi: 10.1158/1055-9965.EPI-10-1261. Epub 2011 Apr 5.

13. Ryan JL, Heckler CE, Roscoe JA, Dakhil SR, Kirshner J, Flynn PJ, Hickok JT, Morrow GR. Ginger (Zingiber officinale) reduces acute chemotherapy-induced nausea: a URCC CCOP study of 576 patients. Support Care Cancer. 2012 Jul;20(7):1479-89. doi: 10.1007/s00520-011-1236-3. Epub 2011 Aug 5.

14. Walker AF, Marakis G, Morris AP, Robinson PA. Promising hypotensive effect of hawthorn extract: a randomized double-blind pilot study of mild, essential hypertension. Phytother Res. 2002 Feb;16(1):48-54.

15. De Backer J, Vos W, Van Holsbeke C, Vinchurkar S, Claes R, Parizel PM, De Backer W. Effect of high-dose N-acetylcysteine on airway geometry, inflammation, and oxidative stress in COPD patients. Int J Chron Obstruct Pulmon Dis. 2013;8:569-79. doi: 10.2147/COPD.S49307. Epub 2013 Nov 22.

16. Tse HN, Raiteri L, Wong KY, Yee KS, Ng LY, Wai KY, Loo CK, Chan MH. High-dose N-acetylcysteine in stable COPD: the 1-year, double-blind, randomized, placebo-controlled HIACE study. Chest. 2013 Jul;144(1):106-18. doi: 10.1378/chest.12-2357.

17. Stav D, Raz M. Effect of N-acetylcysteine on air trapping in COPD: a randomized placebocontrolled study. Chest. 2009 Aug;136(2):381-6. doi: 10.1378/chest.09-0421. Epub 2009 May 15.

18. Moradi M, Mojtahedzadeh M, Mandegari A, Soltan-Sharifi MS, Najafi A, Khajavi MR, Hajibabayee M, Ghahremani MH. The role of glutathione-S-transferase polymorphisms on clinical outcome of ALI/ARDS patient treated with N-acetylcysteine. Respir Med. 2009 Mar;103(3):434-41. doi: 10.1016/j.rmed.2008.09.013. Epub 2008 Nov 7.

19. Panahi Y, Sahebkar A, Parvin S, Saadat A. A randomized controlled trial on the anti-inflammatory effects of curcumin in patients with chronic sulphur mustard-induced cutaneous complications. Ann Clin Biochem. 2012 Nov;49(Pt 6):580-8. doi: 10.1258/acb.2012.012040. Epub 2012 Oct 4.

20. Pinsornsak P, Niempoog S. The efficacy of Curcuma Longa L. extract as an adjuvant therapy in primary knee osteoarthritis: a randomized control trial. J Med Assoc Thai. 2012 Jan;95 Suppl 1:S51-8.

21. Satoskar RR, Shah SJ, Shenoy SG. Evaluation of anti-inflammatory property of curcumin (diferuloyl methane) in patients with postoperative inflammation. Int J Clin Pharmacol Ther Toxicol. 1986 Dec;24(12):651-4.

22. Lim SS, Kim JR, Lim HA, Jang CH, Kim YK, Konishi T, Kim EJ, Park JH, Kim JS. Induction of detoxifying enzyme by sesquiterpenes present in Inula helenium. J Med Food. 2007 Sep;10(3):503-10. Erratum in: J Med Food. 2007 Dec;10(4):739. Lim, Soon Sung.

23. Supplementing with N-Acetylcysteine (NAC) can reduce the need for hospitalization among people suffering from chronic obstructive pulmonary disease (COPD), *European Respiratory Journal* (2003;21:795-8).

Shown in Product Identification Guide, page 305

CHOLESTERIGHT   DS

Benefits:
• Reduces the Risk of Coronary Heart Disease
• Supports Healthy Cholesterol, LDL & Triglyceride Levels
• Natural Formula

What is Cholesterol?

Cholesterol is an important substance made by the liver. It is necessary for the production of hormones, bile that is necessary for digestion, and maintains cell membranes within the body.

Cholesterol moves around in the body is special molecules called lipoproteins. The low density lipoproteins (LDL) bring cholesterol from the liver to the rest of the body. The high density lipoproteins (HDL) carry excess cholesterol back to the liver. Both are critical for a normal functioning body.

However, it is important to regulate lipoprotein levels and rations to maintain a healthy cardiovascular system. Ideally you should maintain LDL cholesterol under 130 and HDL cholesterol at 60 or above. While your genetics plays a big role in determining your cholesterol levels, a diet high in certain fats (mainly saturated and trans fats) is a significant factor as well.

Changing your diet and getting enough exercise is the first step toward maintaining healthy cholesterol levels, but for those who need extra support, nature has several solutions with scientific research showing their benefits.

Why choose Andorra Life?

Andorra Life's Cholesteright fights cholesterol powerfully. The ingredients in Cholesteright are tested to be effective in helping you reach and maintain healthy cholesterol levels - without medication.

A daily serving of Two Cholesteright includes:

800mg of Phytosterols Concentrate:

Phytosterols Concentrate is a source of plant sterols including beta sitosterol, campesterol and stigmasterol, it helps absorb excess cholesterol from the diet so it can be excreted.

800mg is the effective dosage that can help our bodies to fight off the bad Cholesterol and to reduce risk of coronary heart disease.

Policosanol:
Helps to lower LDL cholesterol ("bad" cholesterol) and increase HDL cholesterol ("good" or "healthy" cholesterol) and to help prevent atherosclerosis (thickening of the arteries).

Vitamin C
Is superb at fighting free radicals—one of the main contributors to LDL cholesterol oxidation. It also helps to reduce lipid peroxidation, including that of cholesterol and unsaturated fatty acids, such as EPA and DHA, which make up cell membranes. Vitamin C helps maintain healthy blood vessels, another important factor for total cholesterol health.

Tocotrienols Complex:
In nature, there are eight types of Vitamin E, 4 types of tocopherols and 4 types of tocotrienols. They differ in cellular uptake and bioavailability. Tocotrienols are mainly transported in triglyceride-rich particles such as very low density lipoproteins (VLDLs) and chylomicrons. Tocopherols are mainly transported in low-density lipoproteins (LDLs). Most importantly, tocotrienols have unique and additional health properties with a much more potent antioxidant effect than the more "common" forms of tocopherols. It is also believed that tocotrienols may help reduce serum cholesterol and reverse arterial blockage in Carotid Stenosis patients. These unique additional health benefits are not associated with the use of alpha-tocopherol by itself.

Supplement Facts Serving Size: 2 capsules Servings Per Container: 30	Per Serving
Vitamin C	50 mg
Vitamin E (Tocotrienols Complex)	10 mg
Phytosterols	800 mg
Policosanol	10 mg

Free of: milk or milk by-products, egg or egg by-products, fish or fish by-products, shellfish and by-products, tree nuts, peanut or peanut by-products, wheat or wheat by-products, soybeans and soy by-products.

Suggested Use: take two (2) capsules daily as a dietary supplement or as recommended by your healthcare professional.
• **KEEP OUT OF REACH OF CHILDREN.**
• Consult your doctor before use if you are pregnant, nursing or taking medication.
• Keep tightly closed at a cool dry place.
• Store at Room temperature.
• For your protection, do not use if imprinted safety seal under cap is broken or missing.
Manufactured in a FDA Licensed cGMP facility.

REFERENCES

1. Desvarieux M, Demmer RT, Jacobs DR, Papapanou PN, Sacco RL, Rundek T. Changes in clinical and microbiological periodontal profiles relate to progression of carotid intima-media thickness: the oral infections and vascular disease epidemiology study. J Am Heart Assoc. 2013 Oct 28
2. Mathunjwa M, Semple S, Preez Cd. The effect of 10-week tae-bo intervention programme on physical fitness and health related risk factors in overweight/obese females. Br J Sports Med. 2013 Nov
3. Burg VK, Grimm HS, Rothhaar TL, Grösgen S, Hundsdörfer B, Haupenthal VJ, Zimmer VC, Mett J, Weingärtner O, Laufs U, Broersen LM, Tanila H, Vanmierlo T, Lütjohann D, Hartmann T, Grimm MO. Plant sterols the better cholesterol in Alzheimer's disease? A mechanistical study. J Neurosci. 2013 Oct 9
4. Nunes D, Eskinazi B, Camboim Rockett F, Delgado VB, Schweigert Perry ID. Nutritional status, food intake and cardiovascular disease risk in individuals with schizophrenia in southern Brazil: A case-control study. Rev Psiquiatr Salud Ment. 2013 Sep 17.
5. Barbosa SP, Lins LC, Fonseca FA, Matos LN, Aguirre AC, Bianco HT, Amaral JB, França CN, Santana JM, Izar MC. Effects of ezetimibe on markers of synthesis and absorption of cholesterol in high-risk patients with elevated C-reactive protein. Life Sci. 2013 May 2
6. Grattan BJ Jr. Plant sterols as anticancer nutrients: evidence for their role in breast cancer. Nutrients. 2013 Jan 31;5(2):359-87.
7. Tang M, Wu SZ, Gong X. Effects of policosanol combined with simvastatin on serum lipids and sex hormones in male patients with hyperlipidemia. Zhonghua Xin Xue Guan Bing Za Zhi. 2013 Jun;41(6):488-92.
8. Zanardi M, Quirico E, Benvenuti C, Pezzana A. Use of a lipid-lowering food supplement in patients on hormone therapy following breast cancer. Minerva Ginecol. 2012 Oct;64(5):431-5.

9. Becker DJ, Gordon RY, Morris PB, et al. Simvastatin vs therapeutic lifestyle changes and supplements: randomized primary prevention trial. Mayo Clin Proc. 2008 Jul;83(7):758-64.
10. Li JJ, Lu ZL, Kou WR, et al. Beneficial Impact of Xuezhikang on Cardiovascular Events and Mortality in Elderly Hypertensive Patients With Previous Myocardial Infarction From the China Coronary Secondary Prevention Study (CCSPS). J Clin Pharmacol. 2009;49:947-56.
11. Lu Z, Kou W, Du B, et al. Effect of Xuezhikang, an extract from red yeast Chinese rice, on coronary events in a Chinese population with previous myocardial infarction. Am J Cardiol. 2008;101:1689-93.
12. Keithley JK, Swanson B, Sha BE, Zeller JM, Kessler HA, Smith KY. A pilot study of the safety and efficacy of cholestin in treating HIV-related dyslipidemia. Nutrition. 2002;18:201-4.
13. Liu J, Zhang J, Shi Y, et al. Chinese red yeast rice (Monascus purpureus) for primary hyperlipidemia: a meta-analysis of randomized controlled trials. Chin Med. 2006;1:4.
14. Becker DJ, Gordon RY, et al. Red yeast rice for dyslipidemia in statin-intolerant patients. Annals Int Med. 2009 Jun;150(16):830-9.
15. Zhao SP, Liu L, Cheng YC, Li YL. Effect of xuezhikang, a cholestin extract, on reflecting postprandial triglyceridemia after a high-fat meal in patients with coronary heart disease. Atherosclerosis. 2003;168:375-80.
16. Binaghi P, Cellina G, Lo Cicero G, Bruschi F, Porcaro E, Penotti M. Evaluation of the cholesterol-lowering effectiveness of pantethine in women in perimenopausal age. Minerva Med. 1990;81:475-9.
17. Bertolini S, Donati C, Elicio N, et al. Lipoprotein changes induced by pantethine in hyperlipoproteinemic patients: adults and children. Int J Clin Pharmacol Ther Toxicol. 1986;24:630-7.
18. Gensini GF, Prisco D, Rogasi PG, Matucci M, Neri Serneri GG. Changes in fatty acid composition of the single platelet phospholipids induced by pantethine treatment. Int J Clin Pharmacol Res. 1985;5:309-18.
19. Lau VW, Journoud M, Jones PJ. Plant sterols are efficacious in lowering plasma LDL and non-HDL cholesterol in hypercholesterolemic type 2 diabetic and nondiabetic persons. Am J Clin Nutr. 2005 Jun;81(6):1351-8.
20. Law MR. Plant sterol and stanol margarines and health. West J Med. 2000 Jul;173(1):43-7.
21. Bouic PJ. The role of phytosterols and phytosterolins in immune modulation: a review of the past 10 years. Curr Opin Clin Nutr Metab Care. 2001 Nov;4(6):471-5.
22. Bouic PJ, Clark A, Lamprecht J, et al. The effects of β-itosterol (BSS) and—sitosterol glucoside (BSSG) mixture on selected immune parameters of marathon runners: inhibition of post marathon immune suppression and inflammation. Int J Sports Med. 1999;20:258-62.
23. Castaño G, Fernández L, Mas R, et al. Effects of addition of policosanol and omega-3 fatty acid therapy on the lipid profile of patients with type II hypercholesterolaemia. Drugs R D. 2005;6(4):207-19.
24. Kassis AN, Marinangeli CP, Jain D, Ebine N, Jones PJ. Lack of effect of sugar cane policosanol on plasma cholesterol in Golden Syrian hamsters. Atherosclerosis. 2007;194:153-8.
25. Gamez R, Maz, R, Arruzazabala ML, Mendoza S, Castano G. Effects of concurrent therapy with policosanol and omega-3 fatty acids on lipid profile and platelet aggregation in rabbits. Drugs R D. 2005;6(1):11-9.
26. Hanai J, Cao P, Tanksale P, et al. The muscle-specific ubiquitin ligase atrogin-1/MAFbx mediates statin-induced muscle toxicity. J Clin Invest. 2007 Dec;117(12):3940-51.
27. King DS, Wilburn AJ, Wofford MR, Harrell TK, Lindley BJ, Jones DW. Cognitive impairment associated with atorvastatin and simvastatin. Pharmacotherapy. 2003;23:1663-7.
28. Fraunfelder FW, Richards AB. Diplopia, blepharoptosis, and ophthalmoplegia and 3-hydroxy-3-methyl-glutaryl-CoA reductase inhibitor use. Ophthalmology. 2008;115:2282-5.
29. Gaist D, García Rodríguez LA, Huerta C, Hallas J, Sindrup SH. Are users of lipid-lowering drugs at increased risk of peripheral neuropathy? Eur J Clin Pharmacol. 2001;56:931-3.
30. de Langen JJ, van Puijenbroek EP. HMG-CoA-reductase inhibitors and neuropathy: reports to the Netherlands Pharmacovigilance Centre. Neth J Med. 2006;64:334-8.
31. Chong PH, Boskovich A, Stevkovic N, Bartt RE. Statin-associated peripheral neuropathy: review of the literature. Pharmacotherapy. 2004;24:1194-203.
32. Yang HT, Lin SH, Huang SY, Chou HJ. Acute administration of red yeast rice (Monascus purpureus) depletes tissue coenzyme Q(10) levels in ICR mice. Br J Nutr. 2005;93:131-5.
33. Prasad GV, Wong T, Meliton G, et al. Rhabdomyolysis due to red yeast rice (Monascus purpureus) in a renal transplant recipient. Transplantation. 2002;74:1200-1.

34. Yang HT, Lin SH, Huang SY, et al. Acute administration of red yeast rice (Monascus purpureus) depletes tissue coenzyme Q(10) levels in ICR mice. Br J Nutr. 2005;93:131-5.
Shown in Product Identification Guide, page 305

OPC SUPREME   DS

Benefits:
• Mega Antioxidant Blends of Supreme Ingredients
• Supports Energy and Overall Health
• Anti-stress, Anti-aging

Why we need antioxidants?
Antioxidants are natural compounds found in some foods that help neutralize free radicals in our bodies.
Free radicals are substances that occur naturally in our bodies that attack the fats, protein and the DNA in our cells, ultimately causing different types of diseases by accelerating the aging process. Therefore, antioxidants play an important role in our overall health.

Why choose Andorra Life?
Andorra's OPC Supreme contains 4 types natural's most powerful antioxidants extract.

Grapeseed extract:
Grapeseed extract is an excellent source of specific polyphenol antioxidants called OPCs, which have been clinically proven to fight free radicals and provide many healthy-aging benefits. Grapeseed extract supports production and stability of collagen and elastin, the two proteins which are very important to connective tissue health. Grapeseed extract also supports cardiovascular health and a healthy immune system.
All parts of red grapes contain some proanthocyanidins, including the juice, skins and seeds, and the highest source of small molecule and highly bioactive oligomeric proanthocyanidins (OPCs) are found in red grape seeds. Misleading marketers market their white grape products and lower quality red grape products as red grape seed extracts. For the purpose of dietary supplements, only red grape seed extracts have the overwhelming science behind them.

Vitamin C:
Vitamin C is an essential nutrient for humans and certain other animal species. Vitamin C is a cofactor in at least eight enzymatic reactions, including several collagen synthesis reactions. Ascorbate (a form of Vitamin C) may also act as an antioxidant against oxidative stress, it is required for a range of essential metabolic reactions in all animals and plants. It is made internally by almost all organisms but not humans. Humans absorb Vitamin C from the diet. A major deficiency of vitamin c can cause the most severe symptoms of scurvy.
Andorra Life's Nature C is the new form of Vitamin C, clinically proven superior to standard vitamin c supplements. It contains vitamin C-lipid metabolites for enhanced delivery, absorption and utilization throughout your body. Nature C also improves blood plasma and tissue retention of vitamin C.

Green Tea Extract:
A green tea extract is an herbal derivative from green tea leaves. Containing antioxidant ingredients - mainly green tea catechins (GTC) - green tea and its derivatives are sought-after amongst people who pursue good health. The Indian and Chinese have used the green tea for hundreds of years for a wide variety of health related functions. These cultures have used green tea to treat headaches, aching body parts to improve life expectancy and more.

Pine Bark Extract:
Pine bark extract is made from the bark of the maritime pine tree, which contains naturally occurring OPCs. Pine bark extract is used for its antioxidant properties and multiple anti-aging benefits, such as improving the hearts condition, providing joint support, skin care, eye and vision support, and to ameliorate the condition of chronic venous insufficiency (blood circulation).

Andorra's OPC Supreme brings you:
• Highest quality ingredients: All Natural, Non GMO
• Maximum Strength and science based grapeseed extract formulation for optimal health
• Made in the USA in an FDA inspected and registered facility to meet the stringent standards of US Pharmacopeia (USP) for quality, purity and potency.

Supplement Facts Serving Size: 2 capsules Servings Per Container: 60	Per Serving
Vitamin C	500 mg
Grape Seed Extract	250 mg
Green Tea Extract	50 mg
Pine Bark Extract	20 mg

Free of: milk or milk by-products, egg or egg by-products, fish or fish by-products, shellfish and by-products, tree nuts, peanut or peanut by-products, wheat or wheat by-products, soybeans and soy by-products.

Suggested Use: take two (2) capsules daily as a dietary supplement or as recommended by your healthcare professional.

- **KEEP OUT OF REACH OF CHILDREN.**
- Consult your doctor before use if you are pregnant, nursing or taking medication.
- Keep tightly closed at a cool dry place.
- Store at Room temperature.
- For your protection, do not use if imprinted safety seal under cap is broken or missing.

Manufactured in a FDA Licensed cGMP facility.

REFERENCES

1. Araghi-Niknam M, Hosseini S, Larson D, Rohdewald P, Watson RR. Pine bark extract reduces platelet aggregation. *Integr Med.* 2000;2:73-77.
2. Summary of data for chemical selection: oligomeric proanthocyanidins from grape seeds and pine bark. National Toxicology Program Web site. Accessed at http://ntp.niehs.nih.gov/ntp/htdocs/Chem_Background/ExSumPdf/GrapeSeeds_PineBark.pdf on June 6, 2008.
3. Devaraj S, Vega-López S, Kaul N, et al. Supplementation with a pine bark extract rich in polyphenols increase plasma antioxidant capacity and alters the plasma lipoprotein profile. Lipids. 2002;37:931-934.
4. Downs AM, Sansom JE. Colophony allergy: a review. *Contact Dermatitis.*1999;41:305-310.
5. Fetrow CW, Avila JR. *Professional's Handbook of Complementary & Alternative Medicines.* Springhouse, PA: Springhouse Corp; 1999.
6. Pine Bark. PDRhealth Web site. Accessed at www.pdrhealth.com/drugs/altmed/altmedmono.aspx?contentFileName=ame0425.xml&contentName=Pine+Bark+ on June 6, 2008.
7. Kushi LH, Doyle C, McCullough M, et al; American Cancer Society 2010 Nutrition and Physical Activity Guidelines Advisory Committee. American Cancer Society guidelines on Nutrition and Physical Activity for cancer prevention: reducing the risk of cancer with healthy food choices and physical activity. *CA Cancer J Clin.* 2012;62:30-67.
8. McEvoy CT, Schilling D, Clay N, Jackson K, Go MD, Spitale P, Bunten C, Leiva M, Gonzales D, Hollister-Smith J, Durand M, Frei B, Buist AS, Peters D, Morris CD, Spindel ER. Vitamin C supplementation for pregnant smoking women and pulmonary function in their newborn infants: a randomized clinical trial. JAMA. 2014 May;311(20):2074-82. doi: 10.1001/jama.2014.5217.
9. Jubiz W, Ramirez M. Effect of vitamin C on the absorption of levothyroxine in patients with hypothyroidism and gastritis. J Clin Endocrinol Metab. 2014 Jun;99(6):E1031-4. doi: 10.1210/jc.2013-4360. Epub 2014 Mar 6.
10. Mazloom Z, Ekramzadeh M, Hejazi N. Pak. Efficacy of supplementary vitamins C and E on anxiety, depression and stress in type 2 diabetic patients: a randomized, single-blind, placebo-controlled trial. J Biol Sci. 2013 Nov 15;16(22):1597-600.
11. Hong YH, Jung EY, Shin KS, Yu KW, Chang UJ, Suh HJ. Tannase-converted green tea catechins and their anti-wrinkle activity in humans. J Cosmet Dermatol. 2013 Jun;12(2):137-43. doi: 10.1111/jocd.12038.
12. Basu A, Betts NM, Mulugeta A, Tong C, Newman E, Lyons TJ. Green tea supplementation increases glutathione and plasma antioxidant capacity in adults with the metabolic syndrome. Nutr Res. 2013 Mar;33(3):180-7. doi: 10.1016/j.nutres.2012.12.010. Epub 2013 Jan 30.
13. Bogdanski P, Suliburska J, Szulinska M, Stepien M, Pupek-Musialik D, Jablecka A. Green tea extract reduces blood pressure, inflammatory biomarkers, and oxidative stress and improves parameters associated with insulin resistance in obese, hypertensive patients. Nutr Res. 2012 Jun;32(6):421-7. doi: 10.1016/j.nutres.2012.05.007. Epub 2012 Jun 20.
14. Razavi SM, Gholamin S, Eskandari A, Mohsenian N, Ghorbanihaghjo A, Delazar A, Rashtchizadeh N, Keshtkar-Jahromi M, Argani H. Red grape seed extract improves lipid profiles and decreases oxidized low-density lipoprotein in patients with mild hyperlipidemia. J Med Food. 2013 Mar;16(3):255-8. doi: 10.1089/jmf.2012.2408. Epub 2013 Feb 25.
15. De Groote D, Van Belleghem K, Devière J, Van Brussel W, Mukaneza A, Amininejad L. Effect of the intake of resveratrol, resveratrol phosphate, and catechin-rich grape seed extract on markers of oxidative stress and gene expression in adult obese subjects. Ann Nutr Metab. 2012;61(1):15-24. doi: 10.1159/000338634. Epub 2012 Jul 5.
16. Sano A, Tokutake S, Seo A. Proanthocyanidin-rich grape seed extract reduces leg swelling in healthy women during prolonged sitting. J Sci Food Agric. 2013 Feb;93(3):457-62. doi: 10.1002/jsfa.5773. Epub 2012 Jul 2.
17. Kar P, Laight D, Rooprai HK, Shaw KM, Cummings M. Effects of grape seed extract in Type 2 diabetic subjects at high cardiovascular risk: a double blind randomized placebo controlled trial examining metabolic markers, vascular tone, inflammation, oxidative stress and insulin sensitivity. Diabet Med. 2009 May;26(5):526-31. doi: 10.1111/j.1464-5491.2009.02727.x.
18. Yubero N, Sanz-Buenhombre M, Guadarrama A, Villanueva S, Carrión JM, Larrarte E, Moro C. LDL cholesterol-lowering effects of grape extract used as a dietary supplement on healthy volunteers. Int J Food Sci Nutr. 2013 Jun;64(4):400-6. doi: 10.3109/09637486.2012.753040. Epub 2012 Dec 19.

Shown in Product Identification Guide, page 305

Ariix
563 West 500 South, Suite 300
Bountiful, UT 84010

Direct Inquiries to:
Telephone: 1-801-813-3000 Toll Free: 855-GO-ARIIX (855-462-7449)
Fax: 801.813.3001

OPTIMALS   DS
OPTIMAL-V™
OPTIMAL-M™

Overall Support For Your Body And Life

Nutrifii Optimals contain a comprehensive array of vitamins, minerals and antioxidants, including nutrients and other beneficial ingredients which university studies have shown to be critical in maintaining healthy cellular function, support heart, eye, skin and lung function, as well as promoting improved bone, muscle and nerve health.[1]

[1]These statements have not been evaluated by the Food and Drug Administration. These products are not intended to diagnose, treat, cure, or prevent any disease.

FOR YOUR VISION

Studies have shown the effectiveness of vitamins and minerals such as beta carotene, vitamin C, E, zinc and lutein in supporting the maintenance of healthy vision.[1]

FOR YOUR HEART AND LUNGS

Both B and E vitamins, plus an arsenal of antioxidants in our special blends, work together to complement your diet in supporting a healthy cardiovascular system. Also antioxidants vitamin C and E, combined with carotenoids, have been shown to help support healthy pulmonary and respiratory function.[1]

FOR YOUR BONES AND JOINTS

Getting enough calcium in your diet is crucial for bone health. While bones increase in size and mass during your childhood and adolescence, as you age, your bones naturally become more fragile. Nutrifii Optimals support bone and joint health with a signature blend of calcium, vitamin C, manganese, magnesium, vitamin D, vitamin K, and silicon.[1]

FOR YOUR LIFE

The benefits of ensuring that essential vitamins are in your diet can make a very long list. As a few examples, vitamin C plays a vital role in protecting cells and tissues from damaging oxidation. Studies have also shown that it plays an important role in retaining sound cardiovascular function. Vitamin E is a family of essential nutrients that act as powerful antioxidants. Vitamin B is also known for improving mental function, especially in the elderly.[1]

Optimal-V

Supplement Facts
Serving Size: 3 Capsules Twice Daily
Servings Per Container: 56

	Amount Per Serving	%DV
Vitamin A (as beta-carotene)	7500 IU	150%
Vitamin C (as calcium ascorbate, magnesium ascorbate, zinc ascorbate, potassium ascorbate, acerola cherry)	650 mg	1083%
Vitamin D3 (as cholecalciferol)	1000 IU	250%
Vitamin E (as D alpha tocopheryl succinate, mixed tocopherols 50 mg)	150 IU	500%
Vitamin K (as phylloquinone)	45 mcg	57%
Thiamin (as thiamin HCl)	14 mg	900%
Riboflavin	14 mg	794%
Niacin (50% as niacinamide)	20 mg	100%
Vitamin B6 (as pyridoxine HCl)	16 mg	750%
Folate (folic acid)	500 mcg	125%
Vitamin B12 (as methylcobalamin)	200 mcg	3333%
Biotin	150 mcg	50%
Pantothenic Acid (as D calcium pantothenate)	45 mg	450%
Calcium (as calcium ascorbate)	75 mg	8%
Molybdenum (as molybdenum citrate complex)	25 mcg	33%
Inositol	75 mg	*
Grape Seed Extract (95% anthocyanins)	50 mg	*
Bromelain	25 mg	*
Vegetable Blend	10 mg	*

(broccoli leaf and flower, carrot, tomato, beet root, spinach leaf, cucumber, brussels sprout, cabbage leaf, celery leaf, kale leaf, asparagus shoot, green bell pepper, cauliflower, parsley, wheat grass)

*Daily Value (DV) Not Established.

Other Ingredients: Gelatin, rice bran, mica, sodium copper chlorophyllin.

Optimal-M

Supplement Facts
Serving Size: 2 Capsules Twice Daily
Servings Per Container: 56

	Amount Per Serving	%DV
Calcium (as calcium citrate)	75 mg	8%
Iodine (as potassium iodide)	150 mcg	100%
Magnesium (as magnesium amino acid chelate)	100 mg	25%
Zinc (as zinc citrate)	10 mg	67%
Selenium (as selenomethionine, selenium methionate)	100 mcg	142%
Copper (as copper gluconate)	1 mg	50%
Manganese (as manganese gluconate)	2.5 mg	125%
Chromium (as chromium niacinate)	200 mcg	167%
Citrus bioflavonoids	100 mg	*
N-Acetyl Cysteine	50 mg	*
Rutin	30 mg	*
Resveratrol	15 mg	*
Green Tea Leaf Extract (90% polyphenols / 50% EGCG)	20 mg	*
Quercetin	6 mg	*
Hesperidin	6 mg	*
Pomegranate Fruit Extract (40% ellagic acid)	5 mg	*

Choline (as choline bitartrate)	50 mg	*
Alpha Lipoic Acid	50 mg	*
Inland Sea Trace Minerals*	1500 mcg	*
Boron (as boron citrate)	1.5 mg	*
Superplant Blend	98 mg	*

(broccoli leaf and flower, carrot, tomato, beet root, spinach leaf, cucumber, brussels sprout, cabbage leaf, celery leaf, kale leaf, asparagus shoot, green bell pepper, cauliflower, parsley, wheat grass, rosemary leaf extract, olive leaf extract, cinnamon bark extract, lutein, lycopene)

*Daily Value (DV) Not Established.

Other Ingredients: Gelatin, rice bran, mica.
Shown in Product Identification Guide, page 305

AwarenessLife/PureTrim
**25 SOUTH ARIZONA PLACE, SUITE 320
CHANDLER, AZ 85225**

Direct Inquiries to:
800-69AWARE
http://www.puretrim.net

EXPERIENCE DS

Description:
Promotes Regularity and Cleanses the Colon.*
Ingredients:
A Mediterranean Proprietary Blend of Senna (leaf), Psyllium (Blonde) Seed Husk, Fennel (Seed), Kelp (entire plant), Cornsilk (stigmas), Polygonatum (many flower Solomon's seal) (rhizome), Black Seed (Nigella sativa), Rhubarb (root).
Directions:
Take 1 capsule with a full glass of water before bedtime. Increase your serving size by one capsule every other day until you achieve your desired results.
Warnings:
Do not use if pregnant or nursing. Keep out of reach of children.
If you are under 18, consult your physician before use.
How Supplied:
90 Capsules per bottle.
Shown in Product Identification Guide, page 305

LIQUID DAILY COMPLETE DS

Description
Mediterranean Liquid Supplement. 243 Vitamins, Minerals & Special Nutrients which Provide Energy, Reduce Stress & Support Healthy Joints*. Contains 100% RDA of key Vitamins and Minerals, and other Nutrients.

Ingredients
A Food-based Blend of Organic Mediterranean Super Seed Blend, Organic Fruit & Vegetable Whole Juice Complex, 100% RDA Of Essential Vitamins & Minerals, With Vitamins D3 & K1, Antioxidants With Resveratrol & Acai Berry, Whole Superfood Green Complex, Proprietary Ocean Blend With Pure Phytoplankton, Ionic Plant Minerals, 34 Mediterranean Herbal Ingredients, Essential Fatty Acid Complex, Vegetarian Wellness Formula

Directions
Take 1 ounce (2 tbsp) only once per day, during or immediately after a meal. Less than 4 calories per ounce, less than 1 gram of sugar.

Warnings
Do not use if Pregnant. Keep out of reach of children.

How Supplied
30 ounces per bottle.
Shown in Product Identification Guide, page 305

LIVERMASTER DS

Cleanses and supports a healthy liver, thyroid, and pancreas.

Mediterranean Ingredients
Proprietary Mediterranean
Liver/Thyroid/Pancreas Blend

Milk thistle seed extract, Blessed thistle, Milk thistle seed, Chlorophyll, Eucommia leaf extract, Cordyceps extract, N-acetyl-L-tyrosine, Red beet root extract, Artichoke leaf extract, Enzyme concentrate (a proprietary blend of cellulases, hemicellulase, invertase, alpha-galactosidase, amylase, protease and lipase), Bacillus coagulans (Lactospore® probiotic, 100 million CFU), Black pepper extract, Organic blend [Organic Acai fruit (Euterpe oleracea), Organic Alfalfa grass (leaf), Organic Amla fruit, Organic Burdock root, Organic Carrot root, Organic Chlorella (cracked cell wall), Organic Ginger root extract, Organic Lycium (goji) fruit, Organic Kale (aerial parts), Organic Kelp (Ascophylium nodosum), Organic Moringa leaf, Organic Nopal (cladode), Organic Oat grass, Organic Pomegranate fruit, Organic Purple corn, Organic Spirulina (whole algae)], Organic Rosemary leaf extract, Pycnogenol® French Maritime pine tree bark extract.

Directions
1 capsule with water right after your morning meal then take 1 capsule with water right after your evening meal. Take Liver Master for 90 days. You can do up to two 90 day cleanses a year.

Warnings
Do not use if Pregnant. Keep out of reach of children.

How Supplied
60 capsules per box
Shown in Product Identification Guide, page 305

PURETRIM MEDITERRANEAN WELLNESS SHAKES DS

Description
Natural, Vegetarian Weight Loss Shake, High Protein, Low Carbs, Less than 1 gram of Sugar. No Soy, No Whey, No Dairy, and No Aspartame. Less than 200 calories per shake.

Ingredients
21 Gram Protein Blend: NON-GMO Vegetable Pea, Organic Brown Rice, Organic Lentil, and Organic Flaxseed. Blend of Antioxidants, Prebiotics, 500mg of Plant Calcium, 8000mg of Essential Fatty Acids & 1100mg of Super Raw Greens Blend.

Directions
Mix contents of shake in 10-12 oz. of chilled water.
Have 2 shakes a day (one for breakfast & one for your evening meal.) Drink 2 glasses of water after you drink your shake for best results. Once weight loss is achieved, reduce to 1 shake a day for maintenance.

Warnings
Do not use if you are pregnant or nursing. Must be 18 years or older to use. Do not use as a replacement for more than two meals per day.

How Supplied
10 Packets (Net Weight 500g)
Shown in Product Identification Guide, page 305

PURETRIM MEDITERRANEAN TRUFFLES DS

Description
Helps lipid fat binding in the body to promote weight loss. Comes in Sea Salt Caramel or Milk Chocolate flavors. Only 25 calories per Truffle, less than 1 gram of sugar. Helps to control cravings, naturally.

Ingredients
Organic Prickly-pear (Opuntia ficus-indica) [Fruit], Organic Pomegranate (Punica granatum) [Fruit], Organic Thyme (Thymus vulgaris) [Leaf], Organic Cinnamon (Cinnamomum aromaticum) [Bark], Organic Black Seed (Nigella sativa), Organic Milk Thistle (Silybum marianum) [Seed], Organic Olive (Olea europaea) [Leaf], Organic Artichoke (Cynara cardunculus), Organic Lemon Balm (Melissa officinalis) [Herb Top], Organic Sage (Salvia sclarea) [Leaves], Organic Fennel (Foeniculum vulgare) [Leaf], Organic Fenugreek (Trigonella foenum-graecum) [Seed]

Directions
As a dietary supplement, eat 1 Truffle with a FULL glass of water twice daily, any time you feel hungry or start to feel a craving coming on. Do not exceed 4 truffles a day.

Warnings
Do not use if under the age of 18. Do not use if you are pregnant or breastfeeding.

How Supplied
30 Truffles, individually wrapped.
Shown in Product Identification Guide, page 305

Essentia Water, LLC
**22833 Bothell Everett Hwy., Ste 220
Bothell, WA 98021**

For general inquiries
425.402.9555 or toll free 877.293.2239

Essentia® Water OTC
Reduced Alkalinized Water

PRODUCT CLASS
Water (Reduced Alkalinized Water)

INGREDIENTS
Purified water, sodium bicarbonate, dipotassium phosphate, magnesium sulfate and calcium chloride (electrolyte sources added for taste)

DEA CLASS
N/A

INDICATIONS
For hydration of healthy adults

PEDIATRIC DOSAGE
Pediatrics: ≥1 yr.: Consume 32-64 fl. oz./day for rehydration. Take as frequently as desired.

HOW SUPPLIED
20 ounce with Sports cap, 1.0 liter (33.8 oz.) and 1.5 liter (50.7oz) PET bottles

WARNINGS/PRECAUTIONS
Notify and use only under medical supervision if experiencing vomiting, fever, and/or diarrhea.

PREGNANCY
Safe for pregnancy/nursing. Category A

MECHANISM OF ACTION
Hydration. In randomized, double-blind, parallel arm study of the effect of Essentia Water, an electrolyzed high-pH bottled water, on serial blood viscosity (SBV) and other hydration biomarkers in healthy subjects, Essentia® demonstrated 87.5% greater rehydration overall when compared with the leading brand of bottled water.

ASSESSMENT
Assess hydration status.

MONITORING
Monitor for dehydration, vomiting, fever, and persistence of diarrhea.

PATIENT COUNSELING
Advise to notify physician if diarrhea continues beyond 24 hrs or if vomiting or fever occurs.

ADMINISTRATION/STORAGE
Administration: Oral route. See label for directions for use.
Storage: Store unopened product in a cool place. Do not reuse plastic bottle. Avoid excessive heat. After opening, replace cap, and refrigerate to chill if desired.
Shown in Product Identification Guide, page 306

Immunotec Inc.
**300 JOSEPH CARRIER
VAUDREUIL-DORION, QC
CANADA J7V 5V5**

For Direct Inquiries Contact:
450-424-9992 Ext 4453

IMMUNOCAL® DS
**Nutraceutical
Glutathione precursor (Bonded cysteine™ supplement)
Powder Sachets**

DESCRIPTION and CLINICAL PHARMACOLOGY
IMMUNOCAL® is a U.S. patented natural food protein isolate in the FDA category of GRAS (generally recognized as safe) which assists the body in maintaining optimal concentrations of glutathione (GSH) by supplying the precursors required for intracellular glutathione synthesis. It is clinically proven to raise glutathione values.
Glutathione is a tripeptide made intracellularly from its constituent amino acids L-glutamate, L-cysteine and glycine. The sulfhydryl (thiol) group (SH) of cysteine is respon-

sible for the biological activity of glutathione. Provision of this amino acid is the rate-limiting factor in glutathione synthesis since bioavailable cysteine is relatively rare in foodstuffs.

Immunocal® is a bovine whey protein isolate specially prepared so as to provide a rich source of bioavailable cysteine. Immunocal® can thus be viewed as a cysteine delivery system.

The disulphide bond in cystine is pepsin and trypsin resistant but may be split by heat, low pH or mechanical stress releasing free cysteine. When subject to heat or shearing forces (inherent in most extraction processes), the fragile disulfide bonds within the peptides are broken and the bioavailablility of cysteine is greatly diminished.

Glutathione is a tightly regulated intracellular constituent and is limited in its production by negative feedback inhibition of its own synthesis through the enzyme gamma-glutamylcysteine synthetase, thus greatly minimizing any possibility of overdosage.

Glutathione has multiple functions:

1. It is the major endogenous antioxidant produced by the cells, participating directly in the neutralization of free radicals and reactive oxygen compounds, as well as maintaining exogenous antioxidants such as vitamins C and E in their reduced (active) forms.
2. Through direct conjugation, it detoxifies many xenobiotics (foreign compounds) and carcinogens, both organic and inorganic.
3. It is essential for the immune system to exert its full potential, e.g. (1) modulating antigen presentation to lymphocytes, thereby influencing cytokine production and type of response (cellular or humoral) that develops, (2) enhancing proliferation of lymphocytes thereby increasing magnitude of response, (3) enhancing killing activity of cytotoxic T cells and NK cells, and (4) regulating apoptosis, thereby maintaining control of the immune response.
4. It plays a fundamental role in numerous metabolic and biochemical reactions such as DNA synthesis and repair, protein synthesis, prostaglandin synthesis, amino acid transport and enzyme activation. Thus, most systems in the body can be affected by the state of the glutathione system, especially the immune system, the nervous system, the gastrointestinal system and the lungs.

INDICATIONS AND USAGE

IMMUNOCAL® is a natural food supplement and as such is limited from stating medical claims per se. Statements have not been evaluated by the FDA. As such, this product is thus not intended to diagnose, cure, prevent or treat any disease. Glutathione augmentation is a strategy developed to address states of glutathione deficiency, high oxidative stress, immune deficiency, and xenobiotic overload in which glutathione plays a part in the detoxification of the xenobiotic in question. Glutathione deficiency states include, but are not limited to: HIV/AIDS, infectious hepatitis, certain types of cancers, cataracts, Alzheimer's Disease, Parkinsons, chronic obstructive pulmonary disease, asthma, radiation, poisoning by acetominophen and related agents, malnutritive states, arduous physical stress, aging, and has been associated with sub-optimal immune response. Many clinical pathologies are associated with oxidative stress and are elaborated upon in numerous medical references.

Low glutathione is also strongly implicated in wasting and negative nitrogen balance, notably as seen in cancer, AIDS, sepsis, trauma, burns and even athletic overtraining. Cysteine supplementation can oppose this process and in AIDS, for example, result in improved survival rates.

CONTRAINDICATIONS

IMMUNOCAL® is contraindicated in individuals who develop or have known hypersensitivity to specific milk proteins.

PRECAUTIONS

Each sachet of IMMUNOCAL® contains nine grams of protein. Patients on a protein-restricted diet need to take this into account when calculating their daily protein load. Although a bovine milk derivative, IMMUNOCAL® contains less than 1% lactose and therefore is generally well tolerated by lactose-intolerant individuals.

WARNINGS

Patients undergoing immunosuppressive therapy should discuss the use of this product with their health professional. Individuals with the autosomal-recessive metabolic disorder cystinuria, are at higher risk of developing cysteine nephrolithiasis (1–2% of renal calculi).

ADVERSE REACTIONS

Gastrointestinal bloating and cramps if not sufficiently rehydrated. Transient urticarial-like rash in rare individuals undergoing severe detoxification reaction. Rash abates when product intake stopped or reduced.

OVERDOSAGE

Overdosing on IMMUNOCAL® has not been reported.

DOSAGE AND ADMINISTRATION

For mild to moderate health challenges, 20 grams per day is recommended. Clinical trials in patients with AIDS, COPD, cancer and chronic fatigue syndrome have used 30–40 grams per day without ill effect. IMMUNOCAL® is best administered on an empty stomach or with a light meal. Concomitant intake of another high protein load may adversely affect absorption.

RECONSTITUTION

IMMUNOCAL® is a dehydrated powdered protein isolate. It must be appropriately rehydrated before use. Ideally consumed after mixing. If it is premixed for later consumption, it should be refrigerated and consumed shortly after mixing. DO NOT heat or use a hot liquid to rehydrate the product. DO NOT use a high-speed blender for reconstitution. These methods will decrease the activity of the product.

Proper mixing is imperative. Consult instructions included in packaging.

HOW SUPPLIED

10 grams of bovine milk protein isolate powder per sachet. 30 sachets per box.

STORAGE

Store in a cool dry environment. Refrigeration is not necessary.

REFERENCES

1. Baruchel S, Viau G, Olivier R. et al. Nutraceutical modulation of glutathione with a humanized native milk serum protein isolate, Immunocal®: application in AIDS and cancer. In: Oxidative Stress in Cancer, AIDS and Neurodegenerative Diseases. Ed.; Montagnier L, Olivier R, Pasquier C. Marcel Dekker Inc. New York, 447–461, 1998
2. Bounous G, Kongshavn P. Influence of protein type in nutritionally adequate diets on the development of immunity. In Absorption and Utilization of Amino Acids Vol.II. Ed. M. Friedman. CRC Press, Inc., Fla. 2:219–32, 1989
3. Bounous G, Gold P. The biological activity of undenatured whey proteins: role of glutathione. Clin Invest Med 14:296–309, 1991
4. Bounous G, Baruchel S, Falutz J. Gold P. Whey proteins as a food supplement in HIV-seropositive individuals. Clin Invest Med. 16:3; 204–209, 1992
5. Bounous G. Whey protein concentrate (WPC) and glutathione modulation in cancer treatment. Anticancer Res. 20:4785–4792, 2000
6. Bounous G. Immunoenhancing properties of undenatured milk serum protein isolate in HIV patients. Int. Dairy Fed: Whey: 293–305, 1998
7. Bray T, Taylor C. Enhancement of tissue glutathione for antioxidant and immune functions in malnutrition. Biochem. Pharmacol. 47:2113–2123, 1994.
8. Dröge W, Holm E. Role of cysteine and glutathione in HIV infection and other diseases associated with muscle wasting and immunological dysfunction. FASEB J: 11(13):1077–1089, 1997
9. Herzenberg LA, De Rosa SC, Dubs JG et al. Glutathione deficiency is associated with impaired survival in HIV disease. Proc Natl Acad Sci 94:1967–72, 1997
10. Kennedy R, Konok G, Bounous G et al.. The use of a whey protein concentrate in the treatment of patients with metastatic carcinoma: A phase 1-II clinical study. Anticancer Res. 15:2643–50, 1995
11. Lands LC, Grey VL, Smountas AA. Effect of supplementation with a cysteine donor on muscular performance. J. Appl. Physiol. 87:1381–1385, 1999
12. Locigno R, Castronovo V. Reduced glutathione System: Role in cancer development, prevention and treatment. International Journal of Oncology 19:221–236, 2001
13. Lomaestro B, Malone M. Glutathione in health and disease: pharmacotherapeutic issues. Ann Pharmacother 29: 1263–73, 1995
14. Lothian B, Grey V, Kimoff RJ, Lands. Treatment of obstructive airway disease with a cysteine donor protein supplement: a case report. Chest 117:914–916, 2000
15. Meister A. Glutathione. Ann Rev Biochem 52:711–60, 1983
16. Peterson JD, Herzenberg LA, Vasquez KK, Waltenbaugh C. Glutathione levels in antigen-presenting cells modulate Th1 versus Th2 response patterns. Proc. Natl. Acad. Sci. 95:3071–3076, 1998
17. Tozer RG, Tai P, Falconer W, Ducruet T, Karabadjian A, Bounous G, Molson J, Dröge W. Cysteine-rich protein reverses weight loss in lung cancer patients receiving chemotherapy or radiotherapy. Antioxidants & redox signalling. 10: 395–402, 2008.
18. Watanabe A, Higachi K, Yasumura S. et al. Nutritional modulation of glutathione level and cellular immunity in chronic hepatitis B and C. Hepatology. 24:597A, 1996
19. Witschi A, Reddy S, Stofer B, Lauterberg B. The systemic availability of oral glutathione. Eur. J. Clin. Pharmacol. 43:667–669, 1992.

Manufactured by Immunotec Inc.
Tel: 450-424-9992 Ext. 4453
www.immunocal.com

LifePharm Global Network

32 Rancho Circle
Lake Forest, CA 92630
United States of America

Phone:
949.216.9600 • 800.400.1287
Fax: 949.216.9601
Email: CustomerService@LifePharmGlobal.com

Laminine® DS

LifePharm Global Network

RECOMMENDED USE

Laminine® is a dietary supplement intended for anti-aging. Laminine® capsules are to be administered orally. Recommended usage for adults is 1 to 4 capsules daily.

Do not take if you have a known allergy to eggs or fish.

If you are pregnant or nursing do NOT consume this product.

PRODUCT DESCRIPTION

Ingredients & Supplement Facts

Serving size: 1 capsule
Serving per container: 30

	Amount Per Serving	% Daily Value
OPT9 Proprietary Blend	620 mg	*

(Fertilized Avian Egg Extract, Marine Protein, Phyto Protein)

*Daily Value (%DV) Not Established

The proprietary formula in Laminine® is called OPT9™. This formula is composed of three (3) ingredients: Fertilized Avian Egg Extract (FAEE), Phyto Proteins, and Marine Proteins.

Other Ingredients

Laminine® contains the following inactive carriers: Vegetable Capsule, Silicon Dioxide, and Magnesium Stearate.

PRODUCT DESCRIPTION

Laminine® contains the proprietary process of fertilized avian egg extract, along with a blend of marine and phyto proteins added to make it unique with all essential amino acids.

TECHNICAL DESCRIPTION

The health benefits of the hen egg have been known for centuries. Investigation of the mechanism of the development of an egg after fertilization revealed certain health benefits. In earlier studies, whilst monitoring weight gain of the egg during their development, scientists (1) found very little gain in the first 9-10 days (7.5%), and then a sharp increase (1190% by day 23), suggesting rapid development of a body. The potency of the nutrients available to the fertilized avian egg at this stage has always been assumed to be high, but it was only recently that the chemical structure of the original egg solids for these critical stages, termed blastodermal to protoembryoinic stages was obtained. During the blastodermal to protoembryonic stages of embryogenesis, oligopeptides with molecular weights from 0.5 to 1.0 kD were identified. Oligopeptides are compounds, which have 2 to 20 amino acids joined by a peptide bond. These short chains of amino acids are able to cross the digestive barrier without breaking down or changing the ratios and proportions (2). Peptides are far more potent than other neurotransmitters, requiring only small amounts to produce a profound effect. Additionally, the uptake of the Fibroblast Growth Factor (FGF) (present in the protoembryonic fluid) and other bioactive peptides by the developing avian egg sharply increases between days 11 & 12. These peptides and the FGF have been isolated through a proprietary process precisely at the right stage of development, using a proprietary drying technique to bring the health benefits to humans. The extract is termed Fertilized Avian Egg Extract (FAEE).

In 1929, John R. Davidson, a Canadian Doctor, discovered an extract derived from fertilized avian eggs when they were at a critical stage of development. He used this extract to restore health in his patients. Dr. Davidson spent well

Help Patients Save on Rx Drugs: PDR.net/PharmacyDiscountCard

over a decade developing and researching his theory. However, when Dr. Davidson passed away in 1943, his research on fertilized avian eggs was not passed on and was soon forgotten. Nearly 50 years later, the pursuit of fertilized avian egg extract was revived by Norway's foremost expert on egg research: Dr. Bjoedne Eskeland. He took Dr. Davidson's original research a step further and hypothesized that fertilized avian eggs contained a special combination of amino acids, peptides and protein fractions that could help provide an incredible array of health benefits when consumed by humans. This included vitamins, minerals and proteins, as well as important defense elements, growth factors, hormones and other biologically active components.

MECHANISM OF ACTION

The bioactive peptides in Laminine stimulate the dormant stem cells to utilize the phyto amino acids and marine protein to repair damaged aged cells.

Drying the protoembryonic fluid before the peptides are "used up" to build organs and bones, allows us to provide this building, repairing, maintenance mechanism of perfectly balanced amino acids, peptides and growth factors to humans.

Nature has devised an extremely versatile mechanism to provide nutrition with miraculous precision to the embryo of living creatures. The precise blend of oligopeptides may be seen as building blocks, without a bridge, or a director. The role of such a director is fulfilled by a growth factor known as the Fibroblast Growth Factor, or FGF, also a bioactive peptide. FGF is prolific in protoembryonic liquid as well as the human placenta. On the 11th day of the incubation cycle of a chicken egg, the chicken tissue shows a steep increase in these bioactive peptides, with the appropriate peptides to form the solid organs and bones (3). A detailed day-by-day study was performed in 1988 (5; 7). Discovered only in the seventies, FGF and bioactive peptides are critical in the development of embryos, including humans.

Bioactive peptides are responsible for building the linings in the blood vessels, creating the infrastructure for the nutrients to flow to critical areas of the brain and organs. Research credits bioactive peptides with the potential to directly affect many neuro disorders because of clear results of the ability of bioactive peptides to affect the growth of neurites (4). Neurites are signal senders (Axons) and signal receivers (dendrites) attached to the brain neurons.

Research (6) has also shown clearly that new cell cultures show a dramatic increase in peptide and amino acid uptake in the presence of FGF. This result gives credence to the hypothesis that embryonic growth is influenced by a very precise mechanism, which combines unique combinations of amino acids, peptides and FGF.

BENEFITS

The beneficial impacts of Laminine® are: positive effects on memory, skin, libido, energy, joints, muscles, stress, sleep and emotional stability.

CLINICAL AND EXPERIMENTAL STUDIES
Wound Healing Activity

In a 1997 study, immediately following surgery, (animal) subjects were randomized to receive either an amino acid diet or a peptide diet for 10 days and the strength of the wound was measured. Wound bursting pressure was found to be significantly higher in subjects receiving the peptide diets than in those just receiving amino acid diets. The authors suggest that dietary peptides may stimulate the production of growth factors such as growth hormone, insulin, or insulin growth factor (IGF-1). They also postulate that it is possible that the amino acid entry into the cell via peptide transporters is more efficient for stimulation of protein synthesis than entry in the form of just amino acids. Other possible mechanisms suggested by the authors for the increased wound healing with peptide versus non peptide diets include stimulation of collagen synthesis, increased blood flow to the wound, free radical scavenging, and generation of cytokine profiles which better support wound healing.

Cortisol Study

This study was designed to ascertain the effect of the nutritional supplement, Laminine on cortisol levels in the body. During the experiment, 28 subjects, 16 women and 12 men, between the ages of 36 and 83 took part in the study. Salivary cortisol level content of each participant was measured prior to him/her taking part in the study. This figure is known as "pre-Laminine usage level." The salivary cortisol level was also measured every fifth day three times throughout the study when each participant's intake amount was changed. Overall, study participants' cortisol levels were reduced by an average of 23.7 percent, where 16 started on a higher intake of Laminine—four capsules, twice a day—and 12 started on one capsule twice per day. Participants that initially started on a higher intake of Laminine saw their cortisol level reduced significantly over the first four days as compared to subjects that began the study with a lower usage amount. However, at the end of

the study, there was a small, although insignificant, difference in favor of the high initial intake. The total cortisol reduction by the end of the study was 27.3 percent in women and 19.2 percent in men.

CLINICAL EXPERIENCE
Cholesterol and Blood Pressure Studies

The study was designed to test the effects of the nutritional supplement, Laminine, independently and in combination with Laminine OMEGA+++, on cholesterol, low density lipoproteins (LDL), high density lipoproteins (HDL), triglycerides and blood pressure. There were 15 individuals in the study, broken into three groups of five. This was a double-blind placebo-controlled study that took place over a total period of 12 weeks.

The study took place during two phases. The first lasted eight weeks and included Groups A, B, and C. Cholesterol serum profiles and blood pressure were taken from participants in each group at the start of week one and at the conclusion of week eight. During this phase of the study, participants took a total of four supplements a day—two in the morning and two in the evening. The second phase of the study only included participants from Group A and lasted an additional four weeks, after which time cholesterol serum profiles were measured again. During phase II, participants in Group A consumed eight supplements a day—four in the morning and four in the evening.

During the first phase of the study, results showed that the average cholesterol drop in Group B was about 9.8 percent, compared to 11.5 percent in Group C. Meanwhile, cholesterol levels in Group A actually increased by 1.0 percent over the first eight weeks but dropped by 12 percent between weeks eight and 12. Results for LDL and triglycerides generally followed a similar pattern.

Phase I	CHOLESTEROL*	LDL*	TRIGLYCERIDES*
GROUP A (Placebo/Placebo)	↑ 1.04%	↓ 9.7%	↑ 140.3%
GROUP B (Laminine OMEGA+++/Placebo)	↓ 9.8%	↓ 19.6%	↓ 32.2%
GROUP C (Laminine/Laminine OMEGA+++)	↓ 11.5%	↓ 20.9%	↓ 16.7%

* Measured in mg/dl
Percentages reflect average change after eight weeks

Phase II	CHOLESTEROL*	LDL*	TRIGLYCERIDES*
GROUP A (Laminine/Laminine OMEGA+++)	↓ 11%	↓ 2.6%	↓ 58.2%

* Measured in mg/dl
Percentages reflect average change after eight weeks

Subjects in Group A were also given a subjective survey at the conclusion of Phase II, when they were asked to rate improvement in their joints, memory, skin, sexual drive, muscle tone and strength, stress levels, sleep and emotional wellbeing. Of the five subjects in Group A, only four chose to be a part of the survey. After Phase II, the average improvement in all categories was about 5.75 on a scale of 0-10, with zero representing no change and 10 representing a significant improvement. These are subjective results but nonetheless notable.

	AVERAGE IMPROVEMENT AT WEEK 12
JOINTS	5.8
MEMORY	6
SKIN	5.8
SEXUAL DRIVE	5.8
MUSCLE TONE AND STRENGTH	5.5
STRESS	5
SLEEP	6.2
EMOTIONAL WELL-BEING	6.2

Cholesterol and Blood Pressure Studies Discussion

Triglyceride levels in Group A dropped by 267 mg/dl or 58.2 percent during Phase II, the most substantial change throughout the duration of the study. However, participants in Group C experienced the best and most consistent overall results. HDL levels were within normal limits both at the beginning and end of the study for all participants.

Although participants in Group A took double the Laminine and Laminine OMEGA+++ during Phase II, results were not drastic enough to recommend doubling the suggested usage for Laminine OMEGA+++ for all individuals. The decrease in LDL was not significant in Group A during Phase II as compared to Group C during Phase I. Nevertheless, for individuals that do have high triglycerides, doubling the intake of Laminine and Laminine OMEGA+++ can yield a drastic improvement in a short period of time.

From these data, we can conclude that Laminine OMEGA+++ helps to lower cholesterol, LDL and triglyceride and blood pressure levels (Group B), but when taken with Laminine, the decreases are more significant as a whole (Group C after Phase I and Group A after Phase II).

Safety

People with egg allergies should consult a physician before taking Laminine®. Pregnant women should consult with a physician before taking Laminine®.

How Supplied

The Fertilized Avian Egg Extract in Laminine® is also contained in:
Laminine® OMEGA+++

PRODUCT PHOTO

NOTE: These photos can be used only for identification by shape, color, and imprint. They do not depict actual or relative size.

REFERENCES
1. **Roberts, Pamela R,** et al. Nutrition Vol. 14, No. 3, 1998.
2. **Arvanitakis, Constantine.** Am. Jour. of Physiology, Vol. 231, No. 1, July 1976.
3. **Joseph-Silverstein, Jacquelyn,** et al (June 1989) Basic Fibroblast Growth Factor in the Chick Embryo: Immunolocalization to Striated Muscle Cells and Their Precursors. The Journal of Cell Biology, 108: 2459-2466.
4. **Hatten, M. E.,** et al (1988) In Vitro Neurite Extension by Granule Neurons is Dependent upon Astroglial-Derived Fibroblast Growth Factor. Developmental Biology, 125:280-289.
5. **Seed, Jennifer,** et al (1988) Fibroblast Growth Factor Levels in the Whole Embryo and Limb Bud during Chick Development. Developmental Biology, 128:50-57.
6. **Gospodarowicz, D,** et al (1986) Molecular and Biological Characterization of Fibroblast Growth Factor, an Angiogenic Factor Which Also Controls the Proliferation and Differentiation of Mesoderm and Neuroectoderm Derived Cells. Cell Differentiation, 19: 1-17.
7. **Seed, Jennifer,** et al (1988) Fibroblast Growth Factor Levels in the Whole Embryo and Limb Bud during Chick Development. Developmental Biology, 128:50-57.

SUMMARY

Laminine®
OPT9™ Proprietary Blend – LifePharm Global Network (LPGN)
THERAPEUTIC CLASS
Dietary supplement
INDICATIONS
Dietary management of aging
ADULT USAGE
1 to 4 capsules daily
HOW SUPPLIED
One 620 mg capsule in 15-count blister cards, 30-count bottles, and 120-count bottles
WARNINGS AND PRECAUTIONS
Do not take if you have a known allergy to eggs or fish.
If you are pregnant or nursing, do NOT consume this product.
ADVERSE REACTIONS
None known
DRUG INTERACTIONS
None known
MECHANISM OF ACTION
This FGF and bioactive peptides in the FAEE stimulates stem cells to repair aged damaged cells. This anti-aging effect is accomplished by the stem cells utilizing the phyto amino acids and marine proteins.
STORAGE
Store in a dry, cool place and avoid excessive heat. Keep out of reach of children. Do not use if seal is broken.
Shown in Product Identification Guide, page 307

Help your patients save on prescription drugs with the PDR® Pharmacy Discount Card.
For more, visit PDR.net/PharmacyDiscountCard.

NSE Products, Inc. (Pharmanex)
75 WEST CENTER STREET
PROVO, UT 84601

For Information and Product Support:
Phone: 1-800-487-1000
Website: www.nuskin.com

ageLOC R²   DS

Description

ageLOC® R² is delivered as alternating Day and Night formulas to help balance two interconnected aspects of youthfulness. ageLOC R² Day resets youthful gene expression related to cellular energy production while ageLOC R² Night resets youthful gene expression related to cellular purification. Together, ageLOC R² targets aging at its source to promote physical vigor, mental acuity, and sexual health, as well as to support the body's ability to neutralize and remove cellular waste and metabolic byproducts.*

Benefits

ageLOC R² Day and Night were developed to address cellular energy production (primarily mitochondrial functions) and cellular purification mechanisms. The cellular mechanisms of energy production and cellular purification are mutually supporting. ageLOC R² Day and Night work synergistically by targeting both mechanisms of cellular energy production and mechanisms of cellular purification.*

Ingredients

Each ageLOC R² Day capsule provides 378 mg of a proprietary blend of Cordyceps Cs-4 Mushroom Mycelia (*Cordyceps sinensis* [Berk.] Sacc.), Pomegranate (*Punica granatum*) Fruit Extract, and Pharmanex Asian Ginseng Rb1 (*Panax ginseng*) Root Extract. Each ageLOC R² Night capsule provides 225 mg of a proprietary blend of Grape (*Vitis vinifera L.*) Seed Extract, Red Orange (*Citrus sinensis*) Fruit Extract, and Broccoli (*Brassica oleracea italica*) Seed Extract.

Recommended Use

Take six (6) ageLOC R² Day capsules in the morning, and take two (2) ageLOC R² Night capsules in the evening. May be taken with or without meals.

Warnings

Keep this product out of reach of children. Consult a physician prior to use if pregnant or lactating, or taking a prescription medication. Discontinue use of this product 2 weeks prior to and after surgery. Discontinue use and consult a physician if any adverse reactions occur. May contain soy and/or peanuts.

How Supplied

One box of ageLOC R² delivers 180 capsules of ageLOC R² Day, and 60 capsules of ageLOC R² Night, providing a 30 day supply of each.

*These statements have not been evaluated by the Food and Drug Administration. This product is not intended to diagnose, treat, cure or prevent any disease.

ageLOC® TR90™   DS

Description

The ageLOC TR90 program is a weight management system which consists of three dietary supplements, protein shake formulations, a simple eating plan, and physical activity recommendations. The ageLOC TR90 product regimen includes a powder mix-in beverage supplement known as ageLOC TR90 JumpStart, two encapsulated dietary supplements known as ageLOC TR90 Fit and ageLOC TR90 Control, and ageLOC TR90 TrimShakes formulated to meet specific protein requirements. ageLOC TR90 JumpStart is used during the first 15 days of the program. The eating plan provides optimal portions of protein, fruits, vegetables, and complex carbohydrates based on hand sizes so intake is proportional to an individual's body size. The central design of the eating plan is to create a caloric deficit without creating a protein deficit, with the intent to minimize diet-induced lean muscle loss, and increase healthy metabolism. Emerging weight management research indicates that most westernized diets consume adequate daily protein but only with the largest meal of the day (typically dinner). Key points of the TR90 eating plan include: 1) equal distribution of protein intake among each of three daily meals (approximately 30 grams of protein per meal), 2) limiting intake of excess carbohydrate including grains, pastas, and breads, 3) consuming small healthy snacks two to three times each day, 4) consuming large portion sizes of fruits and vegetables to remain in line with recommended intakes of 5-9 servings of fruits and vegetables per day. Exercise recommendations strive for regular physical activity from aerobic and resistance training.

Benefits

ageLOC TR90 is a program designed to create a healthy body transformation. The ageLOC TR90 program helps support the maintenance of lean muscle, increase healthy metabolism, and improve mood and mindset while reducing cravings. The TR90 dietary supplements were formulated using typical dietary supplement methodologies as well as gene expression research. ageLOC TR90 supplements, including ageLOC TR90 JumpStart, Control and Fit, provide ingredients designed to support appetite control, healthy metabolism, and lean muscle to optimize weight management.* The ageLOC TR90 TrimShakes provide high-quality protein and help reduce calories and control appetite.* The ageLOC TR90 eating plan and exercise programs are complementary to the benefits of the supplements and are essential to the program.

Ingredients

Each ageLOC TR90 JumpStart packet provides 2000 mg of Prickly Pear (Opuntia ficus-indica) fruit powder, 177 mg of Satiereal® Saffron (Crocus sativus L.) stigma extract, 150 mg of Pomegranate (Punica granatum) fruit extract, and 125 mg of Red Orange (Citrus sinensis) fruit extract. Each ageLOC TR90 Fit capsule provides 83.3 mg of Red Orange (Citrus sinensis) fruit extract, 83.3 mg of Brown Seaweed (Undaria pinnatifida) Extract, 50 mg of Green Tea (Camellia sinensis) leaf extract, 33.3 mg of Citrus Bioflavonoids (from citrus fruits), 25 mg of Quercetin (from Onion (Allium cepa alliaceae) bulb extract), and 16.7 mg of Cayenne (Capsicum annum L.) fruit powder. Each ageLOC TR90 Control capsule provides 187.5 mg of Cocoa (Theobroma Cacao) bean powder, 75 mg of Tart Cherry (Prunus cerasus) fruit powder, 62.5 mg of Pomegranate (Punica granatum) fruit extract, and 107.5 mg of Green Tea (Camellia sinensis) leaf extract with added L-Theanine. Each TR90 TrimShake serving provides 15 grams of Protein, 0 grams of Total fat, and 10-11 grams of Total Carbohydrate including 3 grams of dietary fiber and 6 grams of sugar.

Recommended Use

Exact dosage varies from market to market. Please consult local labels for instructions.

ageLOC TR90 Fit and TR90 Control usage instructions:

ageLOC TR90 Fit and ageLOC TR90 Control should be taken 15 to 20 minutes prior to meals, per label instructions. 90 count bottles recommend taking one (1) capsule 15 to 20 minutes before meals three times per day, while 120 count bottles recommend taking two (2) capsules 15 to 20 minutes before meals twice per day.

ageLOC TR90 JumpStart usage instructions:

Mix packet with 2-8 ounces (60-240 mL) of water or other beverage. Drink each morning for the first 15 days of the ageLOC TR90 program.

ageLOC TR90 TrimShakes:

ageLOC TR90 TrimShakes can be taken one or two times per day. Each serving provides one portion of six daily portions of protein.

Warnings

Keep out of reach of children. Pregnant or lactating women and people with known medical conditions should consult a physician prior to use. Discontinue use and consult a physician if any adverse reactions occur. If you have any questions or concerns or any medical conditions you should consult your physician prior to starting any diet or change in exercise program.

*These statements have not been evaluated by the Food and Drug Administration. This product is not intended to diagnose, treat, cure or prevent any disease.

CORDYMAX® CS-4®   DS

Description

CordyMax® Cs-4® is a dietary supplement used to reduce symptoms of fatigue and to promote vitality and overall well-being.* It is an exclusive fermentation product derived from the renowned *Cordyceps sinensis* mushroom.

Benefits

Numerous scientific studies suggest that CordyMax Cs-4 may promote natural vitality and reduce fatigue.* Cordyceps has been shown in third party research to reduce oxidative stress by scavenging oxygen free radicals in mitochondria, promote efficient utilization of oxygen, elevate energy states (ATP) in organs, redistribute blood flow to essential organs, improve liver and kidney functions through metabolizing and excreting toxic substances, and provide a positive benefit for sexual health.*

CordyMax Cs-4, also known as Jin Shui Bao in Chinese, is a cultivated strain of the principle Cordyceps fungal mycelia developed to provide similar benefits delivered by the wild mushroom. It has been profiled extensively by chemical and pharmacological methods. Cs-4 closely mimics the wild mushroom in the temperatures used during fermentation, the similarity of its outward appearance when allowed to grow to maturity, the similarity of its chemical components, and in its beneficial actions as an herbal supplement. Studies have shown that Cs-4® has, in some instances, proven more effective than the wild form.

Ingredients

Each capsule contains 525 mg *Cordyceps sinensis* (Berk.) Sacc. Mycelia (*Paecilomyces hepialid* Chen, Cs-4), standardized 0.14% adenosine and 6% mannitol.

Recommended Use

Take 2 capsules bid or tid with water and food.

Warnings

Keep out of reach of children. Consult a physician prior to use if pregnant or lactating, or using prescription medication. Discontinue use of this product 2 weeks prior to and after surgery. Discontinue use and consult a physician if any adverse reactions occur. May contain soy and/or peanuts.

How Supplied

20-30 day supply, 120 count bottle.

Research using Pharmanex CordyMax Cs-4

CordyMax Cs-4 has been used as the source of Cordyceps in over 11 published studies. Contact Nu Skin for a list of references of studies which have used Pharmanex CordyMax Cs-4.

*These statements have not been evaluated by the Food and Drug Administration. This product is not intended to diagnose, treat, cure or prevent any disease.

LIFEPAK® ANTI-AGING FORMULA   DS

Description

LifePak® is a comprehensive nutritional wellness program, delivering the optimum types and amounts of vitamins, minerals, trace elements, antioxidants, and phytonutrients for general health and well-being. LifePak addresses all common nutrient deficiencies, and provides key anti-aging nutrients that promote cellular protection. Additionally, it supports cardiovascular health, bone nutrition, nutrient metabolism, and normal immune function.*

Benefits

Addresses common nutrient deficiencies: LifePak was formulated in consideration of typical dietary intakes, and when consumed with a typical diet ensures meeting the RDAs for all vitamins and minerals.
Provides ingredients that promote cellular protection: LifePak, with its broad spectrum of vitamins and phytonutrients, is optimally formulated to provide comprehensive protection of cellular and mitochondrial DNA as well as the body's lipids and proteins.
Supports cardiovascular health: LifePak addresses many aspects of cardiovascular health by offering the recommended amounts of key cardiovascular nutrients, including vitamin E, vitamin C, carotenoids, flavonoids, B vitamins, magnesium, and calcium.
Supports bone nutrition: LifePak addresses bone health with a comprehensive array of bone nutrients, including nutritionally significant amounts of calcium, magnesium, and vitamin D.
Supports nutrient metabolism: LifePak provides nutritionally meaningful amounts of vitamins and minerals that promote normal glucose metabolism and insulin function, including chromium, zinc, and antioxidants.
Supports normal immune function: LifePak provides nutritionally significant amounts of vitamins A, C, E, and B₆, zinc and selenium. Since the immune system depends on adequate nutritional status of these nutrients, it is expected that LifePak effectively promotes healthy immune function in multiple ways. Deficiency of single nutrients results in altered immune responses, which can be observed even when the deficiency state is relatively mild.
Protects cells with a powerful antioxidant network: LifePak contains more than 40 antioxidants for cell health, including both water- and fat-soluble antioxidants. As part of this antioxidant support, LifePak provides a balanced carotenoid combination in amounts similar to those provided by diets high in fruits and vegetables.
Pharmanex BioPhotonic Scanner:
The BioPhotonic Scanner program may be used in conjunction with LifePak usage. Nu Skin has licensed a scientifi-

cally validated method to non-invasively measure the levels of carotenoids present in the skin. These fat-soluble carotenoids have been shown in third party literature to be a reliable indicator of overall antioxidant status. The BioPhotonic Scanner can be used to track overall antioxidant status over time as well as track the effect of LifePak on an individual's skin carotenoid status.

Ingredients

LifePak provides an optimal blend of vitamins, minerals, trace elements, antioxidants, and phytonutrients.
Each LifePak packet contains 1 vitamin capsule, two mineral capsules, and 1 phytonutrient capsule, together providing 1250 IU Vitamin A, 6250 IU Beta Carotene, 200 mg Vitamin C, 200 IU Vitamin D, 75 IU Vitamin E, 20 mcg Vitamin K, 3.75 mg Thiamin, 4.25 mg Riboflavin, 17.5 mg Niacin, 5 mg Vitamin B6, 300 mcg Folate, 15 mcg Vitamin B12, 75 mcg Biotin, 15 mg Pantothenic acid, 250 mg Calcium, 50 mcg Iodine, 125 mg Magnesium, 7.5 mg Zinc, 70 mcg Selenium, 0.5 mg Copper, 1 mg Manganese, 100 mcg Chromium, 37.5 mcg Molybdenum, 45 mg Catechins (from green tea), 25 mg Quercetin, 12.5 mg Grape Seed Extract, 12.5 mg Citrus Bioflavonoids, 2.5 mg Resveratrol, 37.5 mg Gamma Tocopherol, 16 mg Beta- and Delta-Tocopherols, 15 mg Alpha-Lipoic Acid, 5 mg Inositol, 2.5 mg Lycopene, 1 mg Alpha Carotene, 1 mg Lutein, 1.5 mg Boron, and 10 mcg Vanadium.

Recommended Use

Take 1 packet bid with water and food.

Warnings

Keep this product out of reach of children. Consult a physician prior to use if pregnant or lactating, or taking a prescription medication. Discontinue use of this product 2 weeks prior to and after surgery. Discontinue use and consult a physician if any adverse reactions occur.

How Supplied

60 individual packets, 30 day supply. Additional LifePak® products include: LifePak® Nano, LifePak Prime, LifePak Women, LifePak Prenatal, LifePak Teen, and Jungamals.

Research using Pharmanex LifePak

LifePak has been used in over 13 published studies. Contact Nu Skin for a list of references of studies which have used Pharmanex LifePak.

*These statements have not been evaluated by the Food and Drug Administration. This product is not intended to diagnose, treat, cure or prevent any disease.

MARINEOMEGA   DS

Description

MarineOmega is a blend of ultra-pure oils from anchovies and krill; both a source of EPA, DHA and other omega-3 fatty acids. Vitamin E is included to protect important fatty acids against oxidation. Oil derived from wild-caught anchovies delivers omega-3 fatty acids in triglyceride form, and both oils are tested free of harmful levels of toxins PCB's and heavy metals.
Euphasia superba, commonly known as krill, are small shrimp-like crustaceans. Krill oil is rich in EPA and DHA in a unique phospholipid form targeted for use in the brain and in cell membranes throughout the body. Krill oil also contains a unique flavonoid (yet unnamed) and the carotenoid antioxidant astaxanthin.
MarineOmega is delivered in vanilla-infused softgels.

Benefits

Balanced essential fatty acid nutrition is important for normal immune function, cardiovascular health, joint mobility, brain function, and skin health.*
Krill oil provides phospholipids high in EPA and DHA and offers a high ratio of omega-3 to omega-6 fatty acids (15:1) to help compensate for modern diets which significantly favor the omega-6 type.*
Phospholipids are an essential component of cell membranes in every cell of the body. They are essential for all vital cell processes and are indispensable nutrients for proper brain function. Krill oil naturally contains 40% phospholipids, while most fish oil sources do not provide any phospholipids.*

Ingredients

Each softgel capsule contains 1,100 mg of Marine Lipid Concentrate (150 mg of EPA, 100 mg DHA, and 50 mg of other Omega-3 Fatty Acids), 50 mg of krill oil, and 5 IU of Vitamin E (as Natural Mixed Tocopherols).

Recommended Use

Take 2 softgel capsules bid with water and food.

Warnings

Keep this product out of reach of children. Consult a physician if pregnant or lactating, taking anticoagulants, or taking any other prescription medication. Discontinue use of this product 2 weeks prior to and after surgery. Discontinue use and consult a physician if any adverse reactions occur. Contains shellfish.

How Supplied

30 day supply, 120 count bottle.
*These statements have not been evaluated by the Food and Drug Administration. This product is not intended to diagnose, treat, cure or prevent any disease.

REISHIMAX GLp®   DS

Description

ReishiMax GLp® is a proprietary, standardized extract of reishi (*Ganoderma lucidum*) mushroom. This standardized product also incorporates cracked spores, a novel technology that releases reishi's active ingredient, providing unique immune activity.*
ReishiMax is produced through solid wood log cultivation. This method is preferred to sawdust and liquid cultivation because it yields both polysaccharides and triterpenes from the fruiting body and is less prone to contamination and quality control issues than other methods.
Reishi spores are minute reproductive cells that are released by the mushroom at maturity. The spores are protected by an extremely hard shell, which prevents the polysaccharides and triterpenes contained in the spore from being absorbed. Pharmanex uses technology which mechanically 'cracks' the spores, making the active ingredients bioavailable.

Benefits

ReishiMax has been demonstrated to support healthy immune system function by stimulating cell-mediated immunity. According to the results of animal and *in vitro* studies, ReishiMax has been demonstrated to stimulate the formation of antibodies, stimulate the proliferation of immune cells, and modulate the functions of T cells. ReishiMax is intended for adults who wish to maintain a healthy immune system.*
In addition to animal and *in vitro* studies conducted with ReishiMax, third party clinical studies have established the ability of reishi mushroom to support immune function in humans.*

Ingredients

Each capsule contains 495 mg of standardized reishi mushroom extract and 5 mg of reishi cracked spores and is standardized to 6% triterpenes and 13.5% polysaccharides.

Warnings

Keep out of reach of children. If you are pregnant or nursing, or taking a prescription medication, including immunosuppressive therapies, consult a physician before using this product. Discontinue use of this product 2 weeks prior to and after surgery. Discontinue use and consult a physician if any adverse reactions occur.

Recommended Use

Take 1-2 capsules bid with water and food.

How Supplied

15-30 day supply, 60 count bottle.

Research using Pharmanex ReishiMax Glp

ReishiMax has been used as the source of reishi mushroom in over 29 published studies. Contact Nu Skin for a list of references of studies which have used Pharmanex ReishiMax Glp.

*These statements have not been evaluated by the Food and Drug Administration. This product is not intended to diagnose, treat, cure or prevent any disease.

TEGREEN 97   DS

Description

Tegreen® is a standardized, decaffeinated polyphenol extract of fresh green tea leaves, with proven free radical scavenging and antioxidant properties.*

Benefits

Studies have demonstrated that the polyphenols in green tea, particularly the catechin component, offer potent antioxidant activity through the scavenging of free radicals. More specifically, numerous experiments and studies indicate that green tea polyphenols, especially EGCg, may help block the formation of some potentially toxic compounds such as nitrosamines, suppress the activation of free radicals, detoxify or trap free radicals, inhibit spontaneous and photo-enhanced lipid peroxidation, and increase the activity of natural antioxidants and detoxifying enzymes (e.g., glutathione peroxidase and catalase).*
Antioxidant supplementation may also offer some protective benefits to the skin from free radical damage and the effects of ultraviolet rays. Among the polyphenols that are antioxidants in green tea, EGCg and ECG show the strongest effect in reducing collagenase activity—an enzyme that breaks down collagen.*
Additional third party research shows that green tea supplementation may help improve lipid and glucose metabolism, maintain normal insulin sensitivity, and support a healthy metabolic rate.*

Ingredients

Each capsule contains 250 mg of extract of green tea leaves (*Camellia sinensis*) standardized to a minimum 97% pure polyphenols including 162 mg catechins, of which 95 mg is EGCg.

Recommended Use

Take 1-2 capsules bid with water and food. Maximum recommended dose of 4 capsules daily (1,000 mg). Do not exceed 1,200 mg green tea extract in combination with other green tea-containing supplements.

Warnings

Keep out of reach of children. Consult a physician prior to use if pregnant or lactating, taking anticoagulants, or taking any other prescription medications. Discontinue use of this product 2 weeks prior to and after surgery. Discontinue use and consult a physician if any adverse reactions occur.

How Supplied

30-day supply, 30 and 120 count bottles.

Research using Pharmanex Tegreen 97

Tegreen 97 has been used as the source of green tea in over 13 published studies. Contact Nu Skin for a list of references of studies which have used Pharmanex Tegreen 97.
* These statements have not been evaluated by the Food and Drug Administration. This product is not intended to diagnose, treat, cure or prevent any disease.

Perque Integrative Health
44621 GUILFORD DRIVE, SUITE 150
ASHBURN, VA 20147

Telephone:
1-(800)-525-7372

PERQUE LIFE GUARD™   DS
Tabsules

40 Essential Nutrients Protects Heart, Body, and Brain
Full Disclosure Label
(no hidden or inactive ingredients)
Directions: As a dietary supplement, take two (2) tabsules with meals or as directed by your health professional. *Best if taken with meals.* Alternative daily doses as follows:

Low stress, healthy   1-2 tabsules/day
Moderate stress, unwell   3-4 tabsules/day
High stress, training   5-6 tabsules/day

SUPPLEMENT FACTS
Serving size: 2 Tabsules
Servings per container: 90

Energized Nutrients	Amount per serving	% Daily Value
Vitamins:		
Vitamin A (beta-carotene)	5,000 IU	100
Vitamin B-1 (thiamine HCl)	100 mg.	6,666
Vitamin B-2 (riboflavin 40 mg: riboflavin 5'-phosphate, 10 mg)	50 mg.	2,941
Vitamin B-3 (niacin)	25 mg.	125
Vitamin B-3 (niacinamide)	75 mg.	375
Vitamin B-5 (calcium d-pantothenate)	100 mg.	1,000
Vitamin B-6 (pyridoxine HCl, 160 mg. pyridoxol 5'-phosphate, 40 mg	200 mg.	10,000
Vitamin B-12 (hydroxocobalamin)	200 mcg	3,333
Folinate (as calcium folinate)	200 mcg	100
(6S)-5-Methyltetrahydrofolate (as Quatrefolic™)	200 mcg	
PABA (para-aminobenzoic acid)	30 mg.	*

	Amount per serving	% Daily Value
Biotin (pure crystalline)	500 mcg	166
Vitamin C (100% l-ascorbate, fully reduced, corn free)	150 mg.	250
Vitamin D-3 (cholecalciferol)	400 IU	100
Vitamins E (from mixed natural tocopherols)	200 IU	667
Vitamin K-1 (phylloquinone)	500 mcg	625
Elemental Minerals:		
Potassium (as citrate)	99 mg.	3
Calcium (as ascorbate, pantothenate, citrate, fumarate, malate and succinate)	50 mg.	5
Magnesium (as C16 and C18 alkyls†)	100 mg.	25
Zinc (as picolinate)	25 mg.	167
Boron (as ascorbate)	2 mg	*
Chromium (as picolinate 50%, ascorbate 50%)	200 mcg	167
Manganese (as ascorbate)	15 mg.	750
Molybdenum (as ascorbate)	100 mcg	133
Selenium (as l-selenomethionine)	50 mcg	71
Vanadium (as ascorbate)	100 mcg	*
Active Cofactors:		
Quercetin dihydrate (water-soluble bioflavonoid)	100 mg.	*
L-aspartic acid (magnesium aspartate)	50 mg.	*
Trimethylglycine (betaine HCl)	50 mg.	*
Tocotrienols:		
Triacontanol (polycosonol)	774 mcg	*
Hexacosanol (polycosonol)	33 mcg	*
Tetracosanol (polycosonol)	193 mcg	*
Octacosanol (polycosonol)	500 mcg	*
Citrate	59 mg.	*
Fumarate	59 mg.	*
Malate	59 mg.	*
Succinate	59 mg.	*
Vegetable fiber (organic croscarmellose)	170 mg.	*
Natural Vanilla	120 mg.	*

†from whole, untreated palm fruit and leaf

*Daily value not established by FDA

OTHER INGREDIENTS: None

KEEP OUT OF REACH OF CHILDREN. Must be stored with cap on tightly in a cool, dry place . Do not use product if the tamper-resist shrink band around the cap or the inner seal beneath the cap appears to have been tampered with or is missing.

WARNING: Pregnant and nursing mothers need to check with their health professional before taking supplements.

How Supplied: 180 Count
Patents Pending
Researched, uniquely formulated,
& exclusively distributed by:
PERQUE Integrative Health, USA
These statements have not been evaluated by the Food and Drug Administration. This product is not intended to diagnose, treat, cure, or prevent any disease.

PERQUE POTENT C GUARD™   DS
Buffered Ascorbate Powder

Enhances Cell Energy and Helps Reduce Oxidative Stress
Full Disclosure Label
(no hidden or inactive ingredients)
Directions: Take one (1) rounded half-teaspoon mixed with two (2) to four (4) ounces of liquid or as directed by your health professional. Use only **dry** transfer spoons to remove powder from bottle. Keep tightly capped and moisture free. Please take a few deep, relaxing breaths while the natural effervescence subsides (~1 min.). May be kept on the counter, in refrigerator or freezer to maintain dryness.

SUPPLEMENT FACTS
Serving Size: 1 Rounded Half-Teaspoon
Servings per container: 287

Energized Nutrients	Amount per serving	% Daily Value
Vitamin C (as 100% l-ascorbates, fully reduced and buffered)	1,584 mg.	2,640
Potassium (as ascorbate)	99 mg.	3
Calcium (as ascorbate)	40 mg.	5
Magnesium (as ascorbate)	16 mg.	4
Zinc (as ascorbate)	600 mcg	4

Other Ingredients: None
3/13
KEEP OUT OF REACH OF CHILDREN. Must be stored with cap on tightly in a cool, dry place. Do not use product if the

---

tamper-resist shrink band around the cap or the inner seal beneath the cap appears to have been tampered with or is missing.

WARNING: Pregnant and nursing mothers need to check with their health professional before taking supplements.
How Supplied: 16 oz./454 grams net weight
Patents Pending
Researched, uniquely formulated,
& exclusively distributed by:
PERQUE Integrative Health, USA
These statements have not been evaluated by the Food and Drug Administration. This product is not intended to diagnose, treat, cure, or prevent any disease.

PERQUE REPAIR GUARD™   DS
Tabsules

Eases Oxidative Stress, Pain, and Inflammation
Full Disclosure Label
(no hidden or inactive ingredients)
Directions:
Mild condition: 1 tabsule daily
Moderate condition: 2-4 tabsules daily
Severe condition: 4-12 tabsules daily

SUPPLEMENT FACTS
Serving size:1 Tabsule
Servings per container: 180

Energized Nutrients	Amount per serving	% Daily Value
Quercetin dihydrate (water-soluble bioflavonoid)	1,000 mg.	*
Pomegranate juice powder (high ORAC)	60 mg.	*
OPC (soluble LMW ActiVin®1294™)	10 mg.	*
Magnesium (as c16 and C18 alkyls from whole, untreated palm fruit and leaf)	35 mg.	*
Vegetable fiber (organic croscarmellose)	10 mg.	*
Chlorophyll	100 mcg	*
Turmeric	4 mcg	*

* Daily value not established by FDA

Other Ingredients: None
3/13
KEEP OUT OF REACH OF CHILDREN. Must be stored with cap on tightly in a cool, dry place. Do not use product if the tamper-resist shrink band around the cap or the inner seal beneath the cap appears to have been tampered with or is missing.

WARNING: Pregnant and nursing mothers need to check with their health professional before taking supplements.
How Supplied: 180 Count
U.S Pat. No. 6,620,798
Researched, uniquely formulated,
& exclusively distributed by:
PERQUE Integrative Health, USA
These statements have not been evaluated by the Food and Drug Administration. This product is not intended to diagnose, treat, cure, or prevent any disease.

PERQUE VESSEL HEALTH GUARD™   DS

90 LOZENGES
Promotes Healthy
Homocysteine Levels
Full disclosure label (no hidden or inactive ingredients)
Directions: As a dietary supplement, take one (1) to six (6) lozenges daily or as directed by your health professional.

SUPPLEMENT FACTS
Serving size:1 Lozenge
Servings per container: 90

Energized Nutrients	Amount per serving	% Daily Value
B-12 (hydroxocobalamin)	2 mg.	33,330
Folinate (as calcium folinate)	2.5 mg.	625
Magnesium ascorbate	50 mg.	13
B-6 (pyridoxine)	10 mg.	500
Mannitol	198 mg.	*
Magnesium (as C16 and C18 alkyls†)	3 mg.	1
100% Whole cherry fruit extract	10 mg.	*

	Amount	% Daily Value
Sucanat® (organic, whole cane juice)	5 mg	*
Xylitol	20 mg.	*

† from whole, untreated palm fruit and leaf
* Daily value not established by FDA

KEEP OUT OF REACH OF CHILDREN. Must be stored with cap on tightly in a cool, dry place. Do not use product if the tamper-resist shrink band around the cap or the inner seal beneath the cap appears to have been tampered with or is missing. **WARNING:** Pregnant and nursing mothers need to check with their health professional before taking supplements.

Unique PERQUE Features
Pure, hypoallergenic components • Organic base •Biochemically formulated • Includes cofactors that are usable in generating high-energy compounds •Vitamins, minerals, synergistic cofactors • **DOES NOT CONTAIN:** citrus, MSG, wheat, gluten, corn, starch, sugar, soy, yeast, zein, sulfate, phosphates (other than coenzymes), preservatives, casein or other milk derivatives • No GMOs
Dietary Supplement
90 Lozenges
Patents Pending
Researched, uniquely formulated, & exclusively distributed by:
PERQUE LLC
Ashburn, VA 20147
These statements have not been evaluated by the Food and Drug Administration. This product is not intended to diagnose, treat, cure, or prevent any disease.

PERQUE WHEY GUARD REPAIR

100 Percent Native Whey Protein
Contains Quercetin Dihydrate and OPC
Directions for Use:
Replace 1 meal per day (or as directed by your healthcare practitioner) with 1 serving of PERQUE Whey Guard REPAIR. Add 2 scoops (40g) of powder to 6-8 oz. of cold water and shake or blend. May also be mixed with milk, juice or fruit smoothie of your choice.

Nutrition Facts
Serving Size: 2 scoops (40g)
Servings Per Container: 14

Amount Per Serving

Calories 150		Calories from Fat 13
	Amt	% Daily Value*
Total Fat	14 g	2%
Saturated Fat	0.5 g	3%
Trans Fats	0 g	0%
Cholesterol	42.5 mg	14%
Sodium	85.8 mg	4%
Potassium	179.4 mg	5%
Total Carbohydrates	18.7 g	6%
Dietary Fiber	10.3 g	41%
Sugars	8 g	
Protein	15.4 g	
Quercetin dihydrate (water soluble bioflavonoid)	500 mg	
OPC (ActiVin®)	500 mg	

* Percent Daily Values are based on a 2,000 calorie diet. Calories per gram: Fat – 9 Carbohydrate – 4 Protein – 4

Native Whey Protein Concentrate by Cross Flow, fibers (dahlian, guar gum, xanthan gum), sugars (organic evaporated cane juice, maple flakes), natural vanilla extract, quercetin dihydrate, OPC (ActiVin®), milk buds, potassium chloride, natural cream extract (butyrate rich butter fat), cinnamon, nutmeg, monk fruit concentrate, Equisetum arvense (natural silica), MCT (from raw coconut and palm)

Actual Amino Acid Profile*

in mg per serving (40g)

Branch chain amino acid; BCAA

Isoleucine (enhanced alertness; BCAA)	2567
Leucine (enhanced alertness; BCAA)	4278
Valine (enhanced alertness; BCAA)	3935

Communication, detox, energy and neurochemicals

Alanine (energy source)	1344
Aspartate (nerve energy source)	2394
Arginine (nitric oxide [NO] source)	295
Cysteine/Cystine (detox sulfur source)	1170
Glutamine/Glutamate (energy source)	9036
Glycine (detox & soothing neurotransmitter)	539
Methionine (detox sulfur source)	1240
Phenylalanine (noradrenaline source)	1113
Serine (phosphoserine source)	1317
Threonine (phosphothreonine source)	1912
Tyrosine (adrenaline source)	1234

Specialized functions

Histidine (stomach digestive source)	518
Lysine (collagen cross link source)	1938
Proline (structure source)	4223

Analysis by H. Stone (BUMC) April 2010. Data on file.

PERQUE Whey Guard REPAIR contains NO:

Corn	Phthalates	Melamine
Soy	GMOs	Toxic Metals
Eggs	BSE	Pesticide Residues
Gluten	BPA	Solvent Residues

KEEP OUT OF REACH OF CHILDREN.
Must be stored with cap on tightly in a cool, dry place Do not use product if the tamper-resistant shrink band around the cap or the inner seal beneath the cap appears to have been tampered with or is missing.
14 servings
NET WT.
20 oz. 573g
Vanilla flavored
These statements have not been evaluated by the Food and Drug Administration. This product is not intended to diagnose, treat, cure or prevent any disease.

Synergy WorldWide
1955 West Grove Parkway, Suite 100
Pleasant Grove, Utah 84062

(801) 769-7800

PROARGI-9+   DS
L-arginine Complexer
Dietary Supplement

ProArgi-9+ is the highest quality l-arginine supplement in the world. This proprietary formulation combines the powerful cardiovascular benefits of l-arginine with a variety of superior heart health ingredients to give your cardiovascular system optimum support.
ProArgi-9+ was formulated in collaboration with leading scientists and cardiovascular specialists who have conducted extensive research on the proper application of l-arginine in promoting heart health. With ProArgi-9+, you're giving your heart the supplementation it needs for a long, healthy life.*
These statements have not been evaluated by the Food and Drug Administration. This product is not intended to diagnose, treat, cure or prevent any disease.

Supplement Facts
Serving Size: 10.5 g (approx. 1 level scoop)
Servings per container: 30

Amount Per Serving		% Daily Value
Calories 15		
Total Carbohydrate	5 g	2%*
Vitamin C (Ascorbic Acid)	60 mg	100%
Vitamin D3 (Cholecalciferol)	2,500 IU	625%
Vitamin K (Menaquinone)	20 mcg	25%
Vitamin B6 (Pyridoxine HCl)	2 mg	100%
Folate (Folic Acid)	200 mcg	50%
Vitamin B12 (Cyanocobalamin)	6 mcg	100%
Proprietary Blend	6.5 g	**

L-arginine, xylitol, pomegranate fruit concentrate (*Punica granatum*), L-citrulline, d-ribose, grape skin extract (*Vitis vinifera*), red wine extract

*Percent daily values are based on a 2,000 calorie diet.
**Daily value not established.

Other Ingredients: Citric Acid, Malic Acid, Natural Citrus Sweetener, Silicon Dioxide, Natural Citrus and Huckleberry Flavors, Stevia leaf extract (*Stevia rebaudiana*).
DIRECTIONS: Mix 1 serving (1 scoop providing 5 g pure, free form L-arginine) with 4-8 oz. water (depending on individual taste). Stir to dissolve. If water is very cold, mixture will take about one minute to dissolve. One serving (1 scoop) may be taken twice per day.
Store in a cool, dry place. Slight color changes may occur over time due to the natural fruit flavor. There is no change in the efficacy or potency of the product.
Shake Well Before Dispensing
Consult your physician prior to use if you have a preexisting medical condition including: myocardial infarction (heart attack), cardiovascular disease or diabetes, or take medications for any reasons including erectile dysfunction. Not recommended for use in children or pregnant or lactating women.
Manufactured Exclusively for Synergy Worldwide®
Pleasant Grove, UT 84062 • (801) 769-7700
www.synergyworldwide.com
Item Code: Isu74154 ©2012 Made in U.S.A. REV1112
Shown in Product Identification Guide, page 313

TriVita, Inc.
16100 N GREENWAY HAYDEN LP.
SUITE #950
SCOTTSDALE, AZ 85260

PH: 1.800.991.7116
Fax: 1.480.778.2992

NOPALEA™ SUPERFRUIT FOR WELLNESS   DS
Daily Dietary Supplement

SUPPLEMENT FACTS
Serving Size 2 tbsp (1 fl oz)(30 mL)
Servings per Container 32

	Amount per Serving	% Daily Value*
Calories	13	
Calories from Fat	0	
Total Fat	0 g	0%
Saturated Fat	0 g	0%
Cholesterol	0 g	0%
Sodium	2 mg	0%
Total Carbohydrate	3.1 g	1%
Dietary Fiber	0 g	0%
Sugars	2.27 g	
Protein	41 mg	0%
Vitamin A	6.8 IU	0%
Vitamin C	1.4 mg	0%
Calcium	3.4 mg	0%
Iron	.04 mg	0%

Proprietary Blend (Nopalea Sonoran Bloom™) Total 907.15 g   †
Water (filtered), Nopal fruit puree (Opuntia ficus indica), Clarified Agave syrup, Beet juice (Beta vulgaris), Cranberry powder (Vaccinium macrocarpon), Papaya powder (Carica papaya fruit with papain), Orange juice crystals (Citrus sinensis), Tomato concentrate (Solanum lycopersicon), Strawberry powder concentrate (Fragaria sp.), Apple powder (Malus domestica), Guava powder (Psidium guajava), Peach fruit powder (Prunus persica), Mango fruit powder (Mangifera indca), Apricot extract (Prunus armeniaca), Acerola powdered extract (Malpighia emarginata), Raspberry powder (Rubus ideaus), Kiwi fruit powder (Actinidia deliciosa), Lemon juice crystals (Citrus limon), Papain from papaya (Carica papaya), Green Tea extract (Camellia sinensis), Grape Seed extract (Vitis vinifera), Pomegranate extract (Punica granatum with ellagic acid and punicaligans), Bromelain from pineapple (Ananas comosus), Cellulase, Amylase, Protease, Lipase, Maltodextrin, Stevia powder (Stevia rebaudiana), Natural flavors, Guar gum, Silicon dioxide, Cherry Powder, Citric acid, Xanthan gum

* Percent Daily Values are based on a 2,000 calorie diet.
† Daily Value not established.

SUGGESTED USE
When taking Nopalea for the first time, drink 3 to 6 ounces each day, for 30 days. For maintenance, drink 1 to 3 ounces daily depending on your body's inflammation-fighting needs. May be mixed with water or your favorite beverage.
KEEP REFRIGERATED – SHAKE WELL BEFORE USING – PRESERVATIVE FREE
To maintain freshness: Don't drink directly from the container and consume within 30 days of opening. Do not use if safety seal under cap is broken or missing.
To report a serious adverse event or obtain product information, contact: 800.991.7116
Children, women who are pregnant or nursing and all individuals allergic to any food/ingredients should consult their healthcare provider before use.
You should not stop taking any medication without first consulting with a healthcare provider.
What's in Nopalea (Nō-pah lay' uh)
Nopalea is a delicious, nutrient-rich drink liquid that features the Superfruit of the Nopal cactus. Nopalea supports the normal and essential anti-inflammatory function performed by the immune system using a powerful class of nutrients called Bioflavonoids, which have been proven to help the body detoxify, and promote optimal cellular health.

These statements have not been evaluated by the Food and Drug Administration.
This product is not intended to diagnose, treat, cure or prevent any disease.

TRIVITA®
Experience wellness
Manufactured for and distributed by TriVita, Inc.
16100 N Greenway Hayden Loop, Suite 950 Scottsdale, AZ 85260 USA
© 2012 TriVita, Inc.
www.trivita.com
Item 30710 L1204-01
Shown in Product Identification Guide, page 314

For the first time, the trusted *Physicians' Desk Reference®* is now available as a convenient eBook. Visit PDR.net to download your free copy today.

Unicity International, Inc.
THE MAKE LIFE BETTER COMPANY
1201 NORTH 800 EAST
OREM, UT 84097

Direct Inquiries to:
(801) 226-2600
www.unicity.com
science.unicity@unicity.com
Products of Unicity International, Inc. are distributed through independent distributors.

BIO-C™   DS
[bī̄o sē]

DESCRIPTION
Bio-C™ is a vitamin C nutritional supplement.
Bio-C™ is a yellow, water-soluble, crystalline powder pressed into a tablet. Each Bio-C™ tablet consists of a proprietary blend of ascorbyl palmitate, calcium ascorbate, ascorbic acid, magnesium ascorbate, and 37.5 mg of citrus bioflavonoids. In addition to the active ingredients, each tablet contains cellulose, stearic acid, silicon dioxide, croscarmellose sodium, and magnesium stearate.

BENEFITS AND RESEARCH
Vitamin C (ascorbic acid) is a water-soluble vitamin that is used in the body to form cartilage, collagen, muscles, and blood vessels. Vitamin C is a potent antioxidant that can protect small molecules such as proteins, carbohydrates, nucleic acids, and lipids from damage caused by free radicals that are generated through the course of normal metabolism or through exposure to external toxins and pollutants (e.g. ultraviolet radiation from the sun or smoking). Vitamin C can also regenerate other antioxidants like vitamin E. Additionally, vitamin C is required for the synthesis of carnitine, a molecule involved in the transport of fats across the mitochondrial membrane, as well as the synthesis of norepinephrine, a neurotransmitter.[1]

USAGE
Take one tablet morning and night with a meal.

SAFETY AND WARNINGS
Bio-C™ is well tolerated. Some gastrointestinal discomfort may be experienced as with any dietary supplement.

HOW SUPPLIED
Available in tablets.

REFERENCES
Carr, AC and Frei B. (1999), American Journal of Clinical Nutrition 96: 1086-1107.
Jacob, RA and Sotoudeh G. (2002), Nutrition in Clinical Care 5: 66-74.
Deruelle F, Baron B. (2008), Journal of Alternative and Complementary Medicine 14:1291-1298.
Levine M, Rumsey SC, Daruwala R, Park JB, Wang Y. (1999), The Journal of the American Medical Association 281: 1415-1423.

[1] THESE STATEMENTS HAVE NOT BEEN EVALUATED BY THE FOOD AND DRUG ADMINISTRATION. THIS PRODUCT IS NOT INTENDED TO DIAGNOSE, TREAT, CURE, OR PREVENT ANY DISEASE.

BIOS LIFE® CARDIO   DS
[bī-ōs līf kärd-ē-ō]
Advanced Fiber and Nutrient Drink

DESCRIPTION
Bios Life® Cardio is a fiber-based, vitamin rich dietary supplement. Bios Life® Cardio contains a blend of soluble and insoluble fibers, phytosterols, policosanol, an extract of *Chrysanthemum morifolium*, vitamins, and minerals that when combined with a healthy diet and exercise may lower total serum cholesterol and triglyceride levels.
Bios Life® Cardio is light orange in color. It is a hygroscopic crystalline powder that is generally soluble in water. Each serving of Bios Life® Cardio contains 3 g of fiber, 1 g of phytosterols, 6 mg of policosanol, and 12.5 mg of an extract of *Chrysamthemum morifolium*. In addition to these active ingredients, each serving of Bios Life® Cardio contains maltodextrin, citric acid, orange juice powder, sucralose, and orange flavor.

BENEFITS AND RESEARCH
It's estimated that Americans consume 10-12 g of total fiber per day, less than half the amount of the recommended daily intake. Epidemiological and clinical studies have correlated high daily fiber intake with an improvement in overall health.

Bios Life® Cardio is a dietary supplement designed to increased daily fiber intake. Each serving of Bios Life® Cardio contains three grams of dietary fiber. When taken three times daily, Bios Life® Cardio contributes nearly half of the recommended daily value of fiber. Fiber supplementation has been shown to decrease preprandial and postprandial glucose levels and lower LDL cholesterol and apolipoprotein B levels.
In addition to fiber supplementation, Bios Life® Cardio contains a patented blend of phytosterols, policosanol, *Chrysanthemum morifolium*, vitamins, and minerals. This blend of ingredients optimizes cholesterol levels through a combination of four mechanisms. First, the soluble fiber matrix prevents cholesterol reabsorption in the gastrointestinal tract through bile-acid sequestration. Second, the phytosterols reduce dietary absorption of cholesterol. Third, policosanol inhibits hepatic synthesis of cholesterol mediated through HMG-CoA reductase. Fourth, *Chrysanthemum morifolium* provides phytonutrients that enhance conversion of cholesterol to 7-α-hydryoxycholesterol. The four mechanisms provide a synergistic approach to optimizing cholesterol levels.

SUGGESTED USAGE
Dissolve the contents of one packet or one scoop into 8 to 10 fl. oz. of liquid (water or juice) and stir vigorously. Drink immediately. Use 15-20 minutes prior to meals up to three times daily.

SAFETY AND WARNINGS
Bios Life® Cardio is well tolerated. There may be mild gastrointestinal discomfort, such as increased flatulence or loose stools, during the first month of initial use due to the increased uptake of dietary fiber. This GI disturbance usually disappears within the first thirty days. If the GI discomfort persists, reduce the number of servings of Bios Life® Cardio. If the GI discomfort further persists, stop taking the product and consult your physician. Taking this product without adequate liquid can result in complications.

HOW SUPPLIED
Bios Life® Cardio is packaged in single-serving foil packets or in bulk canisters.

REFERENCES
Sprecher, DL and Pearce GL (2002), Metabolism 51: 1166–70.
Verdegem, PJE; Freed, S and Joffe D (2005), American Diabetes Assocation 65th Scientific Sessions, San Diego, CA.
Duenas, V; Duenas, J; Burke, E and Verdegem, PJE (2006), 7th International Conference on Arteriosclerosis, Thrombosis, and Vascular Biology, American Heart Association, Denver, CO.
Verdegem, PJE (2007), Current Topics in Nutraceutical Research 5: 1-6
US Patent 6,933,291.
* THESE STATEMENTS HAVE NOT BEEN EVALUATED BY THE FOOD AND DRUG ADMINISTRATION. THIS PRODUCT IS NOT INTENDED TO DIAGNOSE, TREAT, CURE, OR PREVENT ANY DISEASE.
Shown in Product Identification Guide, page 314

BIOS LIFE PROBIONIC®   OTC

Description
ProBionic® contains four strands of live, healthy bacteria that enter the digestive system and help balance bacterial populations in the intestinal tract. This supplement is for individuals with symptoms of poor digestive health such as constipation, diarrhea, bloating, and inflammation.
ProBionic® is a water-soluble, light-pink crystalline powder. The proprietary encapsulation used for ProBionic® allows the healthy bacteria to be delivered to the small intestines alive, ensuring the bacteria can confer health benefits for the user. Each packet of ProBionic® contains a 100 mg Probiotic Blend of *Lactobacillus acidophilus LA 02*, *Lactobacillus rhamnosus LR 04*, *Bifidobacterium breve BR 03*, and *Bifidobacterium lactis BS 01*, with a total of 5 billion cells. In addition to these live bacteria, each 2 g packet also contains xylitol, natural berry flavor, citric acid, and silica.

Benefits and Research
Your body needs good bacteria to help with detoxification, food digestion, waste removal, production of vitamins, and protection from harmful organisms. When the intestinal bacteria is imbalanced and unhealthy bacteria dominate, the body is less able to fight off infection resulting in inflammation. The individual strains used in ProBionic® are helpful for maintaining overall gut health.
The proprietary encapsulation used in ProBionic® allows healthy strains of bacteria to be delivered to the digestive system alive and undisturbed. This also ensures the bacteria will remain alive throughout their shelf life.

Suggested Use
The contents of the packet can be taken dry, or they can be mixed with 8-10 fl. oz. of liquid (water or juice) and consumed. Use one packet daily

Safety and Warnings
ProBionic® is generally well tolerated. As with any dietary supplement, some gastrointestinal discomfort may be experienced.

How Supplied
ProBionic® is packaged in single-serve foil packets.

References
Saggioro A. Probiotics in the treatment of Irritable Bowel Syndrome. Journal of Clinical Gastroenterology, 2004; 38(8): S104-106.
Del Piano M, Carmagnola S, Andorno S, Pagliarulo M, Tari R, Mogna L, Strozzi GP, Sforza F, Capurso L. Evaluation of the intestinal colonization by microencapsulated probiotic bacteria in comparison to the same uncoated strains. Under pubblication in supplement of the Journal of Clinical Gastroenterology.
Del Piano M, Carmagnola S, Anderloni A, Andorno S, Ballare M, Balzarini M, Montino F, Orsello M, Pagliarulo M, Stratori M, Tari R, Sforza F, Capurso L. The use of probiotics in healthy volunteers with evacuation disorders and hard stools. A double blind, randomized, placebo-controlled study. Under pubblication in a supplement of the Journal of Clinical Gastroenterology.
Pregliasco F., Anselmi G., Fonte L., Giussani F., Schieppati S., Soletti L. A New Chance of Preventing Winter Diseases by the Administration of Symbiotic Formulations. Journal of Clinical Gastroenterology, 2008; 42(2): 224-233.
* THESE STATEMENTS HAVE NOT BEEN EVALUATED BY THE FOOD AND DRUG ADMINISTRATION. THIS PRODUCT IS NOT INTENDED TO DIAGNOSE, TREAT, CURE, OR PREVENT ANY DISEASE.

BIOS LIFE® VISION ESSENTIALS™   DS
[bī-ōs līf vizh-uhn ē-sen-shuhls]

Clinically proven to support healthy eyes and vision.*

DESCRIPTION
Bios Life® Vision Essentials™ is a nutritional supplement for maintaining healthy eyes. Bios Life® Vision Essentials™ contains the following active ingredients: vitamin C, vitamin E, zinc, natural beta carotene, lutein, zeaxanthin, and anthocyanidins from wild bilberry, wild blueberry, strawberry, cranberry, grape seed extract, elderberry, and raspberries.
Bios Life® Vision Essentials™ is a purple crystalline powder that is water-soluble. In addition to the active ingredients, each capsule contains silicon dioxide, microcrystalline cellulose, and is packaged in vegetarian capsules.

BENEFITS AND RESEARCH
Antioxidants from the carotenoid chemical family, such as beta carotene, lutein, and zeaxanthin, play an important role in eye health. Clinical studies have demonstrated that lutein and zeaxanthin are concentrated to the retina and lens of the eye. Supplementation with high levels of lutein can restore the lutein concentration in the retina. Further supplementation of vitamins C, E, and A (in the form of beta-carotene) along with zinc and copper aid with the healthy function of the eyes. Additional support for the eyes comes from a proprietary berry blend included in Bios Life® Vision Essentials™. This proprietary berry blend contains anthocyanidins, antioxidant compounds that support the vasculature within the eye.

USAGE
Take two capsules per day with a meal.

SAFETY AND WARNINGS
Bios Life® Vision Essentials™ is well tolerated. As with any dietary supplement, some gastrointestinal discomfort may be experienced.

HOW SUPPLIED
Available in vegetarian capsules.

REFERENCES
Krishnadev N, Meleth AD, Chew EY (2010) "Nutritional supplements for age-related macular degeneration." Current Opinion in Opthamology 21:184-189.
Ma L, Lin XM, Zou ZY, Xu XR, Li Y, Xu R. (2009) "A 12-week lutein supplementation improves visual function in Chinese people with long-term computer display light exposure." British Journal of Nutrition 102: 186-190.
Yagi, A, Fujimoto, K, Michihiro, K, Goh, B, Tsi, D, Nagai, H, (2009) "The effect of lutein supplementation on visual fatigue: A psychophysiological analysis". Applied Ergonomics 40:1047-1054.
Age Related Eye Disease Study Group, (2001) "A randomized, placebo-controlled, clinical trial of high-dose supple-

mentation with vitamins C and E, beta carotene, and zinc for age-related macular degeneration and vision loss: AREDS report no. 8". Archives of Ophthalmology. 10: 1417-36.

* THESE STATEMENTS HAVE NOT BEEN EVALUATED BY THE FOOD AND DRUG ADMINISTRATION. THIS PRODUCT IS NOT INTENDED TO DIAGNOSE, TREAT CURE, OR PREVENT ANY DISEASE.

BONEMATE® PLUS   DS
[bŏn-māt plŭs]
For Strong Bones and Healthy Teeth[1]

DESCRIPTION
BoneMate® Plus is specially formulated to help maintain optimal bone health.[1] It contains three forms of calcium and vitamin D to maximize absorption and aid in the support of healthy bones, teeth, nerves, heart, and muscle tissue. BoneMate® Plus is a light gray in color and is soluble in water. Each serving of BoneMate® Plus contains the following active ingredients: 600 mg of calcium, 300 mg of magnesium, 30 mg of vitamin C, 2000 IU of vitamin D, 0.5 mg of boron, 5 mg of zinc, 1 mg of manganese, 1 mg of copper, and 20 mcg of vitamin K. In addition, it also contains the inactive ingredients microcrystalline cellulose, croscarmellose sodium, magnesium stearate, hypromellose, hydroxypropylcellulose, and stearic acid.

BENEFITS AND RESEARCH
Calcium is the most common mineral in the body. Almost 99% of the calcium in our body is found in the bones and teeth. Bone is a dynamic tissue that is constantly being remodeled throughout our lives. A chronically low calcium intake in growing individuals may prevent the attainment of optimal peak bone mass. Once peak bone mass has been achieved, inadequate calcium intake may contribute to accelerated bone loss.
Vitamin D, a secosteroid that is produced by the body upon exposure to the sun, is required for optimal calcium absorption. To ensure that calcium absorption is not limited by inadequate vitamin D levels, BoneMate® Plus contains 2000 IU of vitamin D per serving. In addition to facilitating calcium absorption, vitamin D has been shown to target over 2,000 different genes in the body. Vitamin D is needed to maintain overall bone and heart health.

USAGE
Take two tablets twice daily with a meal.

SAFETY AND WARNINGS
BoneMate® Plus is well tolerated. As with any dietary supplement, some gastrointestinal discomfort may be experienced. The Food and Nutrition Board of the Institute of Medicine has set the tolerable upper level (UL) of intake for calcium in adults at 2,500 milligrams (mg) of calcium/day.

HOW SUPPLIED
Available as tablets.

REFERENCES
Weaver CM, Heaney RP. Calcium. In: Shils M, Olson JA, Shike M, Ross AC, eds. Modern Nutrition in Health and Disease. 9th ed. Baltimore: Williams & Wilkins; 1999:141-155.
Heaney RP. Calcium, dairy products and osteoporosis. J Am Coll Nutr. 2000;19(2 Suppl):83S-99S.
Food and Nutrition Board, Institute of Medicine. Calcium. Dietary Reference Intakes: Calcium, Phosphorus, Magnesium, Vitamin D, and Fluoride. Washington, D.C.: National Academy Press; 1997:71-145.
Reid IR. Therapy of osteoporosis: calcium, vitamin D, and exercise. Am J Med Sci 1996;312:278-86. Food and Nutrition Board, Institute of Medicine. Calcium. Dietary Reference Intakes: Calcium, Phosphorus, Magnesium, Vitamin D, and Fluoride. Washington, D.C.: National Academy Press; 1997:71-145.

[1] THESE STATEMENTS HAVE NOT BEEN EVALUATED BY THE FOOD AND DRUG ADMINISTRATION. THIS PRODUCT IS NOT INTENDED TO DIAGNOSE, TREAT, CURE, OR PREVENT ANY DISEASE.

CARDIO-BASICS™   DS
Essential Cardiovascular Nutrients*

DESCRIPTION
Cardio-Basics™ is a nutritional supplement that combines multivitamins, minerals, and antioxidants to support the cardiovascular system.
Cardio-Basics™ is a light orange, water-soluble powder pressed into tablets. Each tablet of Cardio-Basics™ contains the following vitamins, minerals, amino acids, and antioxidants: beta-carotene (vitamin A), thiamine (vitamin B1), riboflavin (vitamin B2), niacin (vitamin B3), calcium d-pantothenate (vitamin B5), pyridoxine hydrochloride (vitamin B6), folate (vitamin B9), cyanocobalamin (vitamin B12), ascorbic acid and ascorbyl palmitate (vitamin C), cholecalciferol (vitamin D), d-alpha-tocopherol (vitamin E), biotin, calcium, chromium, copper, magnesium, manganese, molybdenum, phosphorus, potassium, selenium, sodium, zinc, L-arginine, L-carnitine, L-cysteine, L-lysine, L-proline, inositol, coenzyme Q10, and maritime pine extract. In addition to those active ingredients, each tablet also contains cellulose, croscarmellose sodium, stearic acid, silicon dioxide, and magnesium stearate.

BENEFITS AND RESEARCH
Cardio-Basics™ provides the vitamins, minerals, and antioxidants needed for a healthy heart. In clinical studies, participants using Cardio-Basics™ and Bio-C™ saw a significant reduction in arterial wall thickness and removal of calcification deposits when compared to the placebo group. Cardio-Basics™ provides the body with the necessary vitamins and minerals needed to support a healthy vascular system.*

SUGGESTED USE
Take two tablets daily with food.

SAFETY AND WARNINGS
Cardio-Basics™ is well tolerated. Contains chromium and niacin. Do not use if pregnant, nursing, diabetic, or when taking other niacin-containing supplements.

HOW SUPPLIED
Available in tablets

REFERENCES
Niedzwieckci A, Rath, M. (1996) Journal of Applied Nutrition, 48: 67-78.
Jeejeebhoy F, Keith M, Freeman M, Barr A, McCall M, Kurian R, Mazer D, Errett L, (2002), American Heart Journal 143: 1092-1100.
Verdgem PJE, Lonky S, Curley S. (2005) 7th Conference on Arteriosclerosis, Thrombosis and Vascular Biology.
Lloyd-Jones D, Adams R, Carnethon M, DeSimone G, Ferguson TB, Flegal K, Ford E, Furie K, Go A, Greenlund K, Haase N, Hailpern S, Ho M, Howard V, Kissela B, Kittner S, Lackland D, Lisabeth L, Marelli A, McDermott M, Meigs J, Mozaffarian D, Nichol G, O'Donnell C, Roger V, Rosamond W, Sacco R, Sorlie P, Stafford R, Steinberger J, Hong Y; (2009) Circulation, 119: 480-486.

* THESE STATEMENTS HAVE NOT BEEN EVALUATED BY THE FOOD AND DRUG ADMINISTRATION. THIS PRODUCT IS NOT INTENDED TO DIAGNOSE, TREAT, CURE, OR PREVENT ANY DISEASE.

CARDIO-ESSENTIALS™   DS
Caring for your heart*

DESCRIPTION
Cardio-Essentials™ is a dietary supplement for the heart. Cardio-Essentials™ contains Coenzyme Q-10, L-carnitine, L-taurine, and Hawthorn berry.
Cardio-Essentials™ is a light tan, water-soluble powder. Each serving of Cardio-Essentials™ contains 100 mg of Coenzyme Q-10 and 3.5 g of a blend of L-carnitine, L-taurine, and Hawthorn berry. In addition to these active ingredients, each capsule also contains silicon dioxide, stearic acid, and calcium silicate.

BENEFITS AND RESEARCH
The ventricles of the heart requires specific nutrients to maintain overall health. These important nutrients are included in Cardio-Essentials™: Coenzyme Q10, L-carnitine, and L-taurine. In a clinical study, the combination of L-carnitine, L-taurine, and Coenzyme Q10 was shown to reduce the size of the left ventricle, which is important to maintain heart health. These ingredients are known to be important in providing adequate energy for heart muscle. Cardio-Essentials™ provides adequate amounts of these ingredients, i.e. 100 mg of CoQ10. Hawthorn extract is traditionally used in supporting the heart function.

SUGGESTED USE
Take three capsules twice daily with food.

SAFETY AND WARNINGS
Cardio-Essentials™ is well tolerated. As with any dietary supplement, some gastrointestinal discomfort may be experienced.

HOW SUPPLIED
Available in capsules.

REFERENCES
Lee, JH. et al. (2011) Congestive Heart Failure 4 199-203.
* THESE STATEMENTS HAVE NOT BEEN EVALUATED BY THE FOOD AND DRUG ADMINISTRATION. THIS PRODUCT IS NOT INTENDED TO DIAGNOSE, TREAT, CURE, OR PREVENT ANY DISEASE.

CM PLEX® AND CM PLEX® CREAM   DS
[CM plĕks]
Supports Joint Health and Mobility*

DESCRIPTION
CM Plex® and CM Plex® Cream are a softgel and topical cream, respectively, that contain a proprietary blend of cetylated fatty acids, soy, and fish oil.
CM Plex® is an opaque oil that is insoluble in water. One softgel capsule of CM Plex® contains 350 mg of cetylated fatty acids, 160 mg of soy oil, and 25 mg of salmon oil. In addition to these active ingredients, each softgel capsule contains glycerin and St. John's Bread.
CM Plex® Cream is an off-white cream that is insoluble in water. One gram of CM Plex® Cream contains 7.7 mg of cetylated fatty acids and olive oil. In addition to these active ingredients, CM Plex® Cream also contains glyceryl stearate, glycerin, lecithin, tocopheryl acetate, benzyl alcohol, phenoxyethanol, carbomer, PEG-100 stearate, sodium hydroxide, methylparaben, propylparaben, butylparaben, ethylparaben, isobutylparaben,and citrus aurantium bergamia (Bergamot) fruit oil.

BENEFITS AND RESEARCH
Cetyl myristoleate and related fatty acids have been proven to improve joint health through their anti-inflammatory effects. A clinical study indicated that subjects exhibited improvements in knee flexion compared to placebo. A second study indicated the cream is effective for improving knee range of motion, ability to climb stairs, rise from a chair and walk, balance, strength, and endurance.*

SUGGESTED USE
Softgels: Take one to two softgels three times daily with meals.
Cream: Apply generously onto clean skin and gently massage until the cream disappears. Repeat 3 to 4 times daily as necessary. For maximum results, use both products concurrently.

SAFETY AND WARNINGS
CM Plex® Softgels and Cream are well tolerated. As with any dietary supplement, some gastrointestinal discomfort may be experienced with CM Plex® Softgels.

HOW SUPPLIED
CM Plex® is available in softgels and as a topical cream.

REFERENCES
Hesslink, R et al (2002), Journal of Rheumatology 29, 1708–1712.
Kraemer, WJ et al (2004), Journal of Rheumatology 31, 767–774.
* THESE STATEMENTS HAVE NOT BEEN EVALUATED BY THE FOOD AND DRUG ADMINISTRATION. THIS PRODUCT IS NOT INTENDED TO DIAGNOSE, TREAT, CURE, OR PREVENT ANY DISEASE.
Shown in Product Identification Guide, page 314

IMMUNIZEN®   DS
[ĭm mōō nĭ zĕn]

DESCRIPTION
Immunizen® is a dietary supplement for strengthening and fortifying the immune system.
Immunizen® is a modestly water-soluble, white crystalline powder. Immunizen® consists of a proprietary ingredient blend of colostrum, arabinogalactan, 1,3, 1,6 yeast betaglucans, and lactoferrin. In addition to the active ingredients, each 835 mg capsule of Immunizen® contains natural gelatin, stearic acid, and silicon dioxide.

BENEFITS AND RESEARCH
Immunizen® combines the positive immune modulating effects of colostrum, arabinogalactans, yeast beta-glucans, and lactoferrin to boost your body's natural defenses to foreign antigens. Colostrum is composed of immunoglobulins that bolster the body's immune system by providing immunity against various pathogens.
Beta-glucans are generally derived from the cell walls of the yeast species *Saccharomyces cerevisiae*. Beta-glucans are potent immuno-modulating agents that prime both the innate and adaptive immune systems.

USAGE
As a dietary supplement, take two capsules daily with water one to two hours before a meal.

SAFETY AND WARNINGS
Immunizen® is well tolerated. As with any dietary supplement, some gastrointestinal discomfort may be experienced.

HOW SUPPLIED

Available in capsules.

REFERENCES

Lilius EM, Marnila P. (2001), Current Opinion in Infectious Diseases 14:295-300.

Hammarström L, Weiner CK. (2008), Advances in Experimental Medicine and Biology 606: 321-343.

Chan GC, Chan WK, Sze DM. (2009), The Journal of Hematology and Oncology, 2: 25-

* THESE STATEMENTS HAVE NOT BEEN EVALUATED BY THE FOOD AND DRUG ADMINISTRATION. THIS PRODUCT IS NOT INTENDED TO DIAGNOSE, TREAT, CURE, OR PREVENT ANY DISEASE.

JOINT MOBILITY™　　　　　　　　　　DS
capsule

Description

Joint Mobility is a nutritional supplement for overall joint health.

Joint Mobility contains Undenatured Type II Collagen, Turmeric Extract (95% Curcumin), Boswellia Extract and Vitamin D3 as active ingredients, and also includes microcrystalline cellulose and silicon dioxide. This supplement is for individuals with joint pain and discomfort caused from normal wear and tear.

Joint Mobility is a powder filled capsule that takes on the yellow color of Turmeric. Compared to more traditional joint supplements, Joint Mobility is a small dose at just 881 mg per day. These smaller capsules are ideal for individuals who have trouble taking large capsules or pills.

Benefits and Research

Many people suffer daily from joint pain and discomfort caused from years of overuse or from being overweight or obese. Joint pain and a loss of mobility can dramatically affect quality of life, making simple everyday activity difficult and painful. The ingredients contained in Joint Mobility work in several different ways to help maintain overall joint health. Curcumin and Boswellia extract have been shown to downregulate the genes involved in chronic inflammation. Vitamin D3 has been shown to help increase collagen production which is needed to maintain overall joint health. Joint Mobility works in several different ways for a multifaceted approach to joint health. The ingredients contained have been shown to inhibit proinflammatory pathways, and also help to prevent the breakdown of joint collagen allowing the body to repair and heal itself.[1]

Usage

Take two capsules daily.

Safety and Warnings

Joint Mobility is generally well tolerated. As with any dietary supplement, some gastrointestinal discomfort may be experienced.

How Supplied

Available in capsules.

References

Crowley DC, Lau FC, Sharma P, *et al.*: Safety and efficacy of undenatured type II collagen in the treatment of osteoarthritis of the knee: a clinical trial. Int J Med Sci 2009, 6:312-321.

Chandran B, Goel A.: A randomized, pilot study to assess the efficacy and safety of curcumin in patients with active rheumatoid arthritis. Phytother Res. 2012 Nov; 26(11): 1719-25. Doi: 10.1002/ptr.4639.Epub 2012 Mar 9.

Dobak J1, Grzybowski J, et al.: 1,25-Dihydroxyvitamin D3 increases collagen production in dermal fibroblasts. J Dermatol Sci. 1994 Aug;8(1):18-24.

Kimmatkar N, Thawani V, et al.: Efficacy and tolerability of Boswellia serrate extract in treatment of osteoarthritis of knee—a randomized double bling placebo controlled trial. Phytomedicine 2003 Jan; 10(1):3-7.

Reuter S, Gupta S, et al.: Epigenetic changes induced by curcumin and other natural compounds. Genes Nutr (2011) 6:93–108.

Takada Y, Ichikawa H, et al.: Acetyl-11-Keto-β-Boswellic Acid Potentiates Apoptosis, Inhibits Invasion, and Abolishes Osteoclastogenesis by Suppressing NF-κB and NF-κB-Regulated Gene Expression. J Immunol 2006; 176:3127-3140.

[1]THESE STATEMENTS HAVE NOT BEEN EVALUATED BY THE FOOD AND DRUG ADMINISTRATION. THIS PRODUCT IS NOT INTENDED TO DIAGNOSE, TREAT, CURE OR PREVENT ANY DISEASE.

Shown in Product Identification Guide, page 314

OMEGALIFE-3™　　　　　　　　　　　DS
[ōmĕgā-līf 3]
Omega-3 Fatty Acid Supplementation

DESCRIPTION

OmegaLife-3™ is a blend of omega-3 fatty acids designed to help maintain healthy cardiovascular and cerebral function. OmegaLife-3™ is an amber-colored, semi-viscous, fat-soluble liquid. Each serving of OmegaLife-3™ contains the following active ingredients: 800 mg eicosapentaenoic acid (EPA), 400 mg docosahexaenoic acid (DHA), and vitamin E. In addition, it also contains the inactive ingredients gelatin, glycerin, purified water, and orange oil. OmegaLife-3™ has been molecularly distilled to ensure exceptionally pure oil and includes orange oil to prevent a fishy aftertaste.

BENEFITS AND RESEARCH

Clinical research suggests fish oil can help support proper brain and visual function. In 2002 the FDA approved supplementation of DHA in infant formula. DHA is potentially important in fetal and infant neural development, in that DHA and arachidonic acid have been shown to be incorporated into brain and retinal cell membranes—particularly during the third trimester of pregnancy and early infant life.

DHA is the predominant structural fatty acid in the central nervous system and in the retina of the eyes.

EPA supports the synthesis of important compounds in the body. EPA is the precursor of thromboxane and leukotriene, compounds involved in supporting healthy circulation. They also promote healthy blood vessels.

Evidence is accumulating that increasing intakes of EPA and DHA can decrease the risk thrombosis, decrease triglyceride levels, and decrease inflammation.[1]

The U.S. Food and Drug Administration (FDA) has stated, "Supportive but not conclusive research shows that consumption of EPA and DHA omega-3 fatty acids may reduce the risk of coronary heart disease."

USAGE

Take two softgels twice daily with a meal.

SAFETY AND WARNINGS

OmegaLife-3™ is well tolerated. As with any dietary supplement, some gastrointestinal discomfort may be experienced. Common side effects include a "fishy" taste upon eructation.

HOW SUPPLIED

Available in softgels.

REFERENCES

Barter P, Ginsberg HN. Effectiveness of combined statin plus omega-3 fatty acid therapy for mixed dyslipidemia. Am J Cardiol. 2008 Oct 15:102(8):1040-5

Lee JH, Harris WS, et al. Omega-3 fatty acids for cardioprotection. Mayo Clin Proc. 2008 Mar;83(3):324-32.

SanGiovanni JP, Chew EY, Sperduto RD, et al. The relationship of dietary omega-3 long-chain polyunsaturated fatty acid intake with incident age-related macular degeneration: AREDS report no. 23. Arch Ophthalmol. 2008 Sep;126(9):1274-9.

SanGiovanni JP, Parra-Cabrera S, Colditz GA, Berkey CS, Dwyer JT. Meta-analysis of dietary essential fatty acids and long-chain polyunsaturated fatty acids as they relate to visual resolution acuity in healthy preterm infants. Pediatrics 2000;105:1292-8.

Kris-Etherton PM, Harris WS, Appel LJ. Omega-3 fatty acids and cardiovascular disease: new recommendations from the American Heart Association. Arterioscler Thromb Vasc Biol. 2003;23(2):151-152.

[1] THESE STATEMENTS HAVE NOT BEEN EVALUATED BY THE FOOD AND DRUG ADMINISTRATION. THIS PRODUCT IS NOT INTENDED TO DIAGNOSE, TREAT, CURE, OR PREVENT ANY DISEASE.

UNICITY BALANCE™　　　　　　　　　DS
(Also known as Bios Life® Slim or Bios Life® S)
Formula for Healthy Cholesterol Support

DESCRIPTION

Unicity Balance™ (also known as Bios Life® Slim or Bios Life® S) is a fiber-based, vitamin-rich nutritional supplement. Unicity Balance™ contains a blend of soluble and insoluble fibers, Unicity® 7× technology, phytosterols, policosanol, an extract of *Chrysanthemum morifolium*, vitamins, and minerals that when combined with a healthy diet and exercise may lower total serum cholesterol, and help achieve and maintain a healthy body weight.

Unicity Balance™ is light orange in color. It is a hygroscopic crystalline powder that is generally soluble in water. Each serving of Unicity Balance™ contains 4 g of fiber, 1 g of phytosterols, 750 mg of Unicity 7×, 6 mg of policosanol, and 12.5 mg of an extract of *Chrysanthemum morifolium*. In ad-

dition to these active ingredients, each serving of Balance™ contains maltodextrin, citric acid, orange powder, sweeteners, and orange flavor.

BENEFITS AND RESEARCH

It's estimated that Americans consume 10-12 g of total fiber per day, less than half the amount of the recommended daily intake. Epidemiological and clinical studies have correlated high daily fiber intake with an improvement in overall health.

Unicity Balance™ is a nutritional supplement designed to increase fiber intake. Each serving of Unicity Balance™ contains four grams of fiber. When taken three times daily, Unicity Balance™ contributes half of the recommended daily value of fiber. Fiber supplementation has been shown to decrease preprandial and postprandial glucose levels, lower LDL cholesterol and apolipoprotein B levels, increase satiety, and facilitate weight loss.

In addition to fiber supplementation, Unicity Balance™ contains a patented blend of phytosterols, policosanol, *Chrysanthemum morifolium*, vitamins, and minerals. Unicity Balance™ facilitates weight loss through five distinct mechanisms. First, the soluble fiber matrix promotes an increase in satiety. Second, Unicity Balance™ improves cholesterol levels. Reduction in LDL content removes a potent inhibitor of lipolysis. Third, Unicity Balance™ improves blood glucose levels. Appropriate serum glucose levels help maintain many metabolic processes in the body. Reducing insulin levels permits fatty acid oxidation to occur. Fourth, Unicity Balance™ restores appropriate leptin signaling. Lastly, Unicity Balance™ reduces triglyceride levels allowing for leptin to cross the blood-brain barrier and affect its mechanism of action.

SUGGESTED USAGE

Dissolve the contents of one packet or one scoop into 8 to 10 fl. oz. of liquid (water or juice) and stir vigorously. Drink immediately. Use 15-20 minutes before meals up to three times daily.

SAFETY AND WARNINGS

Unicity Balance™ is well tolerated. There may be mild gastrointestinal discomfort, such as increased flatulence or loose stools, during the first month of initial use due to the increased uptake of dietary fiber. This GI disturbance usually disappears within the first thirty days. If the GI discomfort persists, reduce the number of servings of Unicity Balance™. If the GI discomfort further persists, stop taking the product and consult your physician. Taking this product without adequate liquid can result in complications.

HOW SUPPLIED

Unicity Balance™ is packaged in single-serving foil packets or in bulk canisters.

REFERENCES

Sprecher, DL and Pearce GL (2002), Metabolism 51: 1166-70.

Verdegem, PJE; Freed, S and Joffe D (2005), American Diabetes Assocation 65th Scientific Sessions, San Diego, CA.

Slavin, JL, (2005) Nutrition 21: 411-418.

Delzenne NM, Cani PD, (2005) Current Opinion Clincal Nutrition & Metabolic Care 8: 636-640

Duenas, V; Duenas, J; Burke, E and Verdegem, PJE (2006), 7th International Conference on Arteriosclerosis, Thrombosis, and Vascular Biology, American Heart Association, Denver, CO.

Verdegem, PJE (2007), Current Topics in Nutraceutical Research 5: 1-6

US Patent 6,933,291.

* THESE STATEMENTS HAVE NOT BEEN EVALUATED BY THE FOOD AND DRUG ADMINISTRATION. THIS PRODUCT IS NOT INTENDED TO DIAGNOSE, TREAT, CURE, OR PREVENT ANY DISEASE.

Shown in Product Identification Guide, page 314

Register at PDR.net to receive free PDR® Drug Alerts, monthly Drug Updates, and FDA-required Drug Safety Alerts via email from PDR Network.

USANA Health Sciences, Inc.
3838 WEST PARKWAY BOULEVARD
SALT LAKE CITY, UT 84120-6336

Direct Inquiries to:
Ph: (801) 954 7860
Fax: (801) 954 7658

ACTIVE CALCIUM™ DS

COMPOSITION

Each Active Calcium contains the following minerals:

Vitamin D3 (as Cholecalciferol)	100 IU
Vitamin K (as Phylloquinone)	15 mcg
Calcium (as Calcium Citrate and Carbonate)	200 mg
Magnesium (as Magnesium Citrate, Amino Acid Chelate and Oxide)	100 mg
Boron (as Boron Citrate)	0.33 mg
Silicon (as Silicon Amino Acid Complex)	2.25 mg

ADVANTAGES

Each tablet contains a balanced blend of calcium, magnesium, vitamin D, vitamin K, boron and silicon; six nutrients required for bone development, bone remodeling and skeletal health. This non-prescription product meets USP guidelines for potency (as applicable), uniformity and disintegration, and is manufactured according to pharmaceutical cGMP standards.

RECOMMENDED USE

Take 4 tablets by mouth daily, preferably with meals.

SUPPLIED

Capsule-shaped tablet, mottled greenish-white color, with clear film coating, and with USANA imprint. In bottle of 112 tablets.

CHELATED MINERAL DS
[key'-lā-tĕd]
mineral

COMPOSITION

Each Chelated Mineral contains the following minerals:

Calcium (As Calcium Citrate and Carbonate)	67.5 mg
Iodine (As Potassium Iodide)	75 mcg
Magnesium (As Magnesium Citrate and Amino Acid Chelate)	75 mg
Zinc (As Zinc Citrate)	5 mg
Selenium (As L-selenomethionine and Amino Acid Complex)	50 mcg
Copper (As Copper Gluconate)	0.5 mg
Manganese (As Manganese Gluconate)	1.25 mg
Chromium (As Chromium Polynicotinate and Picolinate**)	75 mcg
Molybdenum (As Molybdenum Citrate)	12.5 mcg
Boron (As Boron Citrate)	0.75 mg
Silicon (As Silicon Amino Acid Complex)	1 mg
Vanadium (As Vanadium Citrate)	10 mcg
Ultra trace Minerals	0.75 mg

**Licensed under U.S. Patent 4,315,927.

ADVANTAGES

Each tablet contains a complete and balanced blend of essential minerals in bioavailable forms. The Chelated Mineral is designed to be taken with USANA's Mega Antioxidant to provide a full complement of essential nutrients required for health. This non-prescription product meets USP guidelines for potency (as applicable), uniformity and disintegration, and is manufactured according to pharmaceutical cGMP standards.

RECOMMENDED USE

Take two (2) tablets twice daily, preferably with food.

SUPPLIED

Oblong shaped tablets, off-white color, with clear film coating with USANA imprint. In bottle of 112 tablets

COQUINONE® 30 DS
[cō'-kwi-nōn]

COMPOSITION

Each CoQuinone 30 capsule contains the following:

Coenzyme Q10	30 mg
Alpha Lipoic Acid	12.5 mg

ADVANTAGES

CoQuinone 30 contains a hydrosoluble form of Coenzyme Q10 (CoQ10) that is 2.5 times more bioavailable than material supplied in dry tablet/capsule formulas. The higher blood levels of CoQ10 supplied enhance mitochondrial production of ATP. CoQ10 is a rate-limiting factor in the electron transport chain involved in mitochondrial production of ATP. It is also involved in neutralizing free radicals generated during ATP production. As such, CoQ10 helps the body maintain healthy skeletal and cardiac muscle. Alpha lipoic acid is included in the formula as a lipid-soluble antioxidant to recycle CoQ10 from the prooxidant form to the antioxidant form. This non-prescription product meets USP guidelines for potency (where applicable), uniformity and disintegration, and is manufactured according to cGMP standards.

RECOMMENDED USE

Take 1 or 2 capsules by mouth daily.

SUPPLIED

Oval shaped, soft gelatin capsule, annatto-colored, opaque. Capsules contain an orange colored liquid. In bottle of 56 soft-gel capsules.

MEGA ANTIOXIDANT DS
[mĕ-gă aenti-ŏx'-si-dĕnt]

COMPOSITION

Each Mega Antioxidant contains the following vitamins and Minerals:

Vitamin A (as Beta Carotene)	3,750 IU
Vitamin C (as Calcium, Potassium, Magnesium, & Zinc Ascorbates)	325 mg
Vitamin D3 (as Cholecalciferol)	450 IU
Vitamin E (as D-alpha Tocopheryl Succinate)	100 IU
Vitamin K (as Phylloquinone)	15 mcg
Thiamin (as Thiamine HCL)	6.75 mg
Riboflavin	6.75 mg
Niacin and Niacinamide	10 mg
Vitamin B6 (as Pyridoxine HCL)	8 mg
Folate (as Folic Acid)	250 mcg
Vitamin B12 (as Cyanocobalamin)	50 mcg
Biotin	75 mcg
Pantothenic Acid (as D-Calcium Pantothenate)	22.5 mg
Olivol ® (Olive Extract)	7.5 mg
Mixed Natural Tocopherols (D-gamma, D-delta, D-beta Tocopherol)	8.5 mg
Bioflavonoid complex (Rutin, Quercetin, Hesperidin, Green Tea Extract-Decaffeinated, Pomegranate Extract, Cinnamon Extract, Bilberry Extract)	49.5 mg
Inositol	37.5 mg
Choline Bitartrate	25 mg
N-Acetyl L-Cysteine	25 mg
Alpha-Lipoic Acid	5 mg
Coenzyme Q10	3 mg
Turmeric Extract	3.75 mg
Lutein	150 mcg
Lycopene	250 mcg

ADVANTAGES

A comprehensive and balanced formula containing the essential vitamins and antioxidants at levels substantially higher than RDA amounts. In addition to the traditionally recognized essential nutrients, the formula contains a unique blend of dietary antioxidants including carotenoids, a bioflavonoid complex, a glutathione complex, and USANA's patented Olivol™ to provide full-spectrum antioxidant protection. This formula is designed to be taken with USANA's Chelated Mineral to provide a full compliment of essential nutrients required for health. This non-prescription product meets USP guidelines for potency (as applicable), uniformity and disintegration, and is manufactured according to pharmaceutical cGMP standards.

RECOMMENDED USE

Take two (2) tablets twice daily, preferably with food.

SUPPLIED

Oblong shaped tablets, mottled orange-brown color, with clear film coating with USANA imprint. In bottle of 112 tablets.

PROCOSA DS

COMPOSITION

Each Procosa tablet contains the following:

Vitamin C (As Calcium Ascorbate)	75 mg
Manganese (As Manganese Gluconate)	1.67 mg
Glucosamine HCL (Vegetarian)	500 mg
Potassium (As Potassium Sulphate)	31.4 mg
Magnesium (As Magnesium Sulphate)	14.5 mg
Meriva Bioavailable Curcumin Complex	82.5 mg

ADVANTAGES

USANA's Procosa is comprehensive joint health formula with a blend of glucosamine, manganese, vitamin C, and silicon — building blocks for healthy cartilage. The combination of glucosamine with Meriva® bioavailable curcumin complex, manganese, vitamin C, and silicon represents a more comprehensive approach to joint health. Over the long term, these ingredients help retain healthy cartilage. Meriva, the new curcumin phytosome used in Procosa, dramatically increases human absorption of curcumin, delivering the same effectiveness at a much lower dose.

RECOMMENDED USE

Take three (3) tablets daily, preferably with meals

SUPPLIED

Modified rectangle, orange-colored tablet, scored on one side. In bottle of 84 tablets.

PROFLAVANOL® C 100 DS
[prō-flă' vi-nol]

COMPOSITION

Each Proflavanol C 100 tablet contains the following:

Vitamin C (As Calcium, Potassium, Magnesium, Zinc Ascorbates)	300 mg
Grape Seed Extract (*Vitis Vinifera L.*, Seeds)	100 mg

ADVANTAGES

A potent antioxidant formula combining the proanthocyanidins (bioflavonoids) from standardized grape seed extract with vitamin C in the form of ascorbate salts and ascorbyl palmitate. Proflavanol C 100 is designed to be taken as a stand-alone antioxidant, or preferably in combination with USANA's Mega Antioxidant and Chelated Mineral to provide additional antioxidant protection. This non-prescription product meets USP guidelines for potency (where applicable), uniformity and disintegration, and is manufactured according to pharmaceutical cGMP standards.

RECOMMENDED USE

Adults, take two (2) to four (4) tablets daily, preferably with meals.

SUPPLIED

Oblong, bilayer tablet, with clear film coating, with USANA imprint, with bisect. In bottles of 56 tablets.

USANA BabyCare Prenatal Essentials DS

USANA BabyCare Prenatal Essentials are multivitamin and mineral supplements for women who are pregnant, want to become pregnant, or who have recently given birth. BabyCare Prenatal Essentials are comprised of two products:

- **BabyCare Prenatal Chelated Mineral** is a speckled off-white, water-soluble tablet that contains calcium, iodine, magnesium, zinc, copper, iron. In addition to these active ingredients, each tablet also contains manganese, selenium, molybdenum, and vanadium.
- **BabyCare Prenatal Mega Antioxidant** is an amber color, water-soluble tablet that contains a balanced blend of vitamins A (as beta carotene), C, D, E, B6, B12, folate, thiamin, riboflavin, niacin, biotin, and pantothenic acid. In addition to these active ingredients, each tablet also contains additional natural antioxidant extracts, inositol, choline, and vitamin K.

BabyCare Prenatal Chelated Mineral Tablets OTC

SUPPLEMENT FACTS

SERVING SIZE: 2 TABLETS

AMOUNT PER SERVING		%DV*
CALCIUM (AS CALCIUM CITRATE AND CALCIUM CARBONATE)	135 mg	10%
IODINE (AS POTASSIUM IODIDE)	150 μg	100%
MAGNESIUM (AS MAGNESIUM CITRATE AND MAGNESIUM AMINO ACID CHELATE)	150 mg	35%

ZINC (AS ZINC CITRATE)	10 mg	70%
COPPER (AS COPPER GLUCONATE)	1 mg	50%
IRON (AS FERROUS FUMERATE USP)	14 mg	80%

*%DV FOR PREGNANT WOMEN

OTHER INGREDIENTS

MICROCRYSTALLINE CELLULOSE, HYDROXYPROPYL CELLULOSE, CROSCARMALLOSE SODIUM, ASCORBYL PALMITATE, MANGANESE GLUCONATE, SELENIUM AMINO ACID COMPLEX, PREGELATINIZED STARCH, SILICON DIOXIDE, DEXTRIN, L-SELENOMETHIONINE, CALCIUM SILICATE, HYDROLIZED RICE PROTEIN, VANADIUM CITRATE, MOLYBDENUM CITRATE, DEXTROSE, SOY LECITHIN, CHROMIUM POLYNICOTINATE, ULTRA TRACE MINERALS, VANILLA EXTRACT, SODIUM CARBOXYMETHYL CELLULOSE, SODIUM CITRATE.

INDICATIONS

USANA PRENATAL CHELATED MINERAL IS A MULTI-MINERAL SUPPLEMENT INDICATED TO IMPROVE THE NUTRITIONAL NEEDS OF WOMEN DURING PREGNANCY. IT ALSO IMPROVES THE NUTRITIONAL BALANCE DURING A MOTHER'S POST NATAL PERIOD FOR LACTATING AND NON-LACTATING WOMEN.

DIRECTIONS

TAKE TWO (2) TABLETS TWICE DAILY WITH FOOD.

WARNINGS

WARNING: ACCIDENTAL OVERDOSE OF IRON CONTAINING PRODUCTS IS A LEADING CAUSE OF FATAL POISONING IN CHILDREN UNDER 6. KEEP THIS PRODUCT OUT OF REACH OF CHILDREN. IN CASE OF ACCIDENTAL OVERDOSE, CALL A DOCTOR OR POISON CONTROL CENTER IMMEDIATELY.
CONSULT YOUR PHYSICIAN IF YOU ARE PREGNANT, NURSING, TAKING A PRESCRIPTION DRUG , OR HAVE A MEDICAL CONDITION.
DO NOT USE IF SAFETY SEAL UNDER CAP IS BROKEN OR MISSING.

STORAGE

STORE BELOW 25° C.

QUESTIONS OR COMMENTS?
FOR INFORMATION, CONTACT 1-800-950-9595

BabyCare Prenatal Mega Antioxidant TABLETS   DS

SUPPLEMENT FACTS
SERVING SIZE: 2 TABLETS

AMOUNT PER SERVING		%DV*
VITAMIN A (AS BETA CAROTENE)	7,500 IU	90%
VITAMIN C (AS CALCIUM, POTASSIUM, MAGNESIUM, & ZINC ASCORBATES)	650 mg	1080%
VITAMIN D3 (AS CHOLECALCIFEROL)	900 IU	225%
VITAMIN E (AS D-ALPHA TOCOPHERYL SUCCINATE)	200 IU	670%
THIAMIN (AS THIAMIN HCL)	13.5 mg	790%
RIBOFLAVIN	13.5 mg	675%
NIACIN (AS NIACIN AND NIACINAMIDE)	20 mg	100%
VITAMIN B6 (AS PYRIDOXINE HCL)	16 mg	640%
FOLATE (AS FOLIC ACID)	500 µg	60%
VITAMIN B12 (AS CYANOCOBALAMIN)	100 µg	1250%
BIOTIN	150 µg	50%
PANTOTHENIC ACID (AS D-CALCIUM PANTOTHENATE)	45 mg	450%

*%DV For Pregnant Women.

OTHER INGREDIENTS

MICROCRYSTALLINE CELLULOSE, INOSITOL, PREGELATINIZED STARCH, RUTIN, MIXED TOCOPHEROLS, CROSCARMALLOSE SODIUM, CHOLINE BITARTRATE, N-ACETYL L-CYSTEINE, HESPERIDIN, OLIVOL®OLEA EUROPAEA (OLIVE FRUIT) EXTRACT[1], ASCORBYL PALMITATE, DEXTRIN, QUERCETIN, ALPHA LIPOIC ACID, SILICON DIOXIDE, CAMELIA SINENSIS (GREEN TEA) EXTRACT, CURCUMA LONGA (TURMERIC) EXTRACT, LUTEIN, COENZYME Q-10, PUNICA GRANATUM (POMEGRANATE) EXTRACT, LYCOPENE, VITAMIN K, DEXTROSE, SOY LECITHIN, CINNAMOMUM CASSIA (CINNAMON) EXTRACT, SODIUM CARBOXYMETHYLCELLULOSE, VACCINIUM MYRTILLUS L. (BILBERRY) EXTRACT, SODIUM CITRATE.

[1]PROTECTED UNDER US PATENTS 6,358,542 OR 6,361,803.

INDICATIONS

USANA PRENATAL MEGA ANTIOXIDANT IS A MULTI-VITAMIN SUPPLEMENT INDICATED TO IMPROVE THE NUTRITIONAL NEEDS OF WOMEN DURING PREGNANCY. IT ALSO IMPROVES THE NUTRITIONAL BALANCE DURING A MOTHER'S POST NATAL PERIOD FOR LACTATING AND NON-LACTATING WOMEN.

DIRECTIONS

TAKE TWO (2) TABLETS TWICE DAILY WITH FOOD.

PRECAUTIONS/WARNINGS

FOLIC ACID IS IMPROPER THERAPY IN THE TREATMENT OF PERNICIOUS ANEMIA AND OTHER MEGALOBLASTIC ANEMIAS WHERE VITAMIN B12 IS DEFICIENT. FOLIC ACID ABOVE 1MG DAILY MAY OBSCURE PERNICIOUS ANEMIA IN THAT HEMATOLOGIC REMISSION CAN OCCUR WHILE NEUROLOGICAL MANIFISTATIONS PROGRESS.
KEEP OUT OF REACH OF CHILDREN. CONSULT YOUR PHYSICIAN IF YOU ARE PREGNANT, NURSING, TAKING A PRESCRIPTION DRUG, OR HAVE A MEDICAL CONDITION.
DO NOT USE IF SAFETY SEAL UNDER CAP IS BROKEN OR MISSING.

STORAGE

STORE BELOW 25°C

QUESTIONS OR COMMENTS?

FOR INFORMATION, CONTACT 1-800-950-9595

DRUGS THAT SHOULD NOT BE USED IN PREGNANCY

The following list is not comprehensive; generic forms and alternate brands of some products may be available. When recommending drugs to pregnant or nursing patients, always check labeling for specific precautions.

Abiraterone acetate
Acetohydroxamic acid
Acitretin
Ambrisentan
Amlodipine besylate/ Atorvastatin calcium
Anastrozole
Aspirin
Atorvastatin calcium
Atorvastatin/Ezetimibe
Benzphetamine hydrochloride
Bexarotene
Bicalutamide
Boceprevir
Bosentan
Caffeine
Cetrorelix acetate
Chenodiol
Cholecalciferol
Choriogonadotropin alfa
Chorionic gonadotropin
Clomiphene citrate
Danazol
Degarelix
Denosumab
Desogestrel/Ethinyl estradiol
Diclofenac sodium/Misoprostol
Dihydroergotamine mesylate
Dronedarone
Drospirenone/Ethinyl estradiol
Dutasteride
Dutasteride/Tamsulosin hydrochloride
Enzalutamide
Ergotamine tartrate
Estazolam
Estradiol
Estradiol valerate
Estradiol/Norethindrone acetate
Estrogens, Conjugated, Synthetic B
Estropipate
Ethinyl estradiol
Ethinyl estradiol/Ethynodiol diacetate

Ethinyl estradiol/Etonogestrel
Ethinyl estradiol/Ferrous fumarate/ Norethindrone acetate
Ethinyl estradiol/Levonorgestrel
Ethinyl estradiol/Norelgestromin
Ethinyl estradiol/Norethindrone
Ethinyl estradiol/Norgestimate
Ethinyl estradiol/Norgestrel
Exemestane
Ezetimibe/Simvastatin
Finasteride
Fluorouracil
Fluoxymesterone
Fluvastatin sodium
Follitropin alfa
Follitropin beta
Ganirelix acetate
Genistein aglycone
Goserelin acetate
Histrelin acetate
Iodine I 131 tositumomab
Isotretinoin
Leflunomide
Lenalidomide
Letrozole
Leuprolide acetate
Leuprolide acetate/ Norethindrone acetate
Levonorgestrel
Lomitapide
Lorcaserin hydrochloride
Lovastatin
Lovastatin/Niacin
Lutropin alfa
Macitentan
Medroxyprogesterone acetate
Megestrol acetate
Menotropins
Mequinol/Tretinoin
Mestranol/Norethindrone
Methotrexate
Methyltestosterone

Mifepristone
Miglustat
Misoprostol
Mitomycin
Nafarelin acetate
Niacin/Simvastatin
Norethindrone
Orlistat
Ospemifene
Oxandrolone
Phendimetrazine tartrate
Phentermine hydrochloride
Phentermine/Topiramate
Pitavastatin
Pomalidomide
Pravastatin sodium
Radium Ra 223 dichloride
Raloxifene hydrochloride
Ribavirin
Riociguat
Rosuvastatin calcium
Simeprevir
Simvastatin
Simvastatin/Sitagliptin
Sofosbuvir
Tazarotene
Telaprevir
Temazepam
Teriflunomide
Tesamorelin
Testosterone
Testosterone cypionate
Testosterone enanthate
Thalidomide
Triazolam
Triptorelin pamoate
Ulipristal acetate
Urofollitropin
Vitamin A palmitate
Warfarin sodium
Zinc bisglycinate

PREGNANCY CATEGORY X

Studies in animals or humans, or investigational or postmarketing reports, have demonstrated fetal risk, which clearly outweighs any possible benefit to the patient.

DRUGS THAT SHOULD NOT BE CRUSHED

Listed below are various slow-release as well as enteric-coated products that should not be crushed or chewed. Slow-release (sr) represents products that are controlled-release, extended-release, long-acting, or timed-release. Enteric-coated (ec) represents products that are delayed release.

In general, capsules containing slow-release or enteric-coated particles may be opened and their contents administered on a spoonful of soft food. Instruct patients not to chew particles, though. (Patients should, in fact, be discouraged from chewing any medication unless it is specifically formulated for that purpose.)

This list should not be considered all-inclusive. Generic and alternate brands of some products may exist. Tablets intended for sublingual or buccal administration (not included in this list) should be administered only as intended, in an intact form.

DRUG	MANUFACTURER	FORM	DRUG	MANUFACTURER	FORM
Aciphex	Eisai	ec	Cardizem CD	Biovail	sr
Actoplus Met XR	Takeda	sr	Cardizem LA	Abbott	sr
Adalat CC	Bayer Healthcare	sr	Cardura XL	Pfizer	sr
Adderall XR	Shire U.S.	sr	Cartia XT	Actavis	sr
Adenovirus Type 4 and Type 7 Vaccine	Teva Women's Health, Inc.	ec	Chlor-Trimeton Allergy	Schering Plough	sr
			Cipro XR	Schering Plough	sr
Advicor	Abbott	sr	Clarinex-D 12 Hour	Schering Plough	sr
Afeditab CR	Watson	sr	Clarinex-D 24 Hour	Schering Plough	sr
Aggrenox	Boehringer Ingelheim	sr	Claritin-D 12 Hour	Schering	sr
Aleve-D Cold & Sinus	Bayer Healthcare	sr	Claritin-D 24 Hour	Schering	sr
Aleve-D Sinus & Headache	Bayer Healthcare	sr	Cometriq	Exelixis, Inc	sr
Allegra-D 12 Hour	sanofi-aventis	sr	Concerta	Ortho-McNeil-Janssen	sr
Allegra-D 24 Hour	sanofi-aventis	sr	Coreg CR	GlaxoSmithKline	sr
Alophen	Numark	ec	Covera-HS	Pfizer	sr
Altoprev	Watson	sr	Creon	Abbott	ec
Ambien CR	sanofi-aventis	sr	Cymbalta	Eli Lilly	ec
Ampyra ER	Acorda Therapeutics	sr	Dairycare	Plainview	ec
Amrix	Cephalon	sr	Deconex DM	Poly	sr
Aplenzin	sanofi-aventis	sr	Delzicol	Warner Chilcott	ec
Apriso	Salix	sr	Depakote	Abbott	ec
Arthrotec	Pfizer	ec	Depakote ER	Abbott	sr
Asacol	Procter & Gamble	ec	Depakote Sprinkles	Abbott	ec
Asacol HD	Procter & Gamble	ec	Detrol LA	Pfizer	sr
Astagraf XL	Astellas	sr	Dexedrine Spansules	GlaxoSmithKline	sr
Augmentin XR	GlaxoSmithKline	sr	Dexilant	Takeda	sr
Avinza	King	sr	Diamox Sequels	Duramed	sr
Azulfidine EN-tabs	Pfizer	ec	Diclegis	Duchesnay USA	sr
Bayer Aspirin Regimen	Bayer Healthcare	ec	Dilacor XR	Watson	sr
Biaxin XL	Abbott	sr	Dilantin	Pfizer	sr
Bontril Slow-Release	Valeant	sr	Dilantin Kapseals	Pfizer	sr
Budeprion SR	Teva	sr	Dilatrate-SR	UCB	sr
Calan SR	Pfizer	sr	Diltia XT	Watson	sr
Campral	Forest	ec	Dilt-CD	Apotex	sr
Carbatrol	Shire U.S.	sr	Ditropan XL	Ortho-McNeil Janssen	sr
Cardene SR	EKR Therapeutics	sr	Donnatal Extentabs	PBM	sr
			Doryx	Mayne	ec

(Continued)

DRUG	MANUFACTURER	FORM	DRUG	MANUFACTURER	FORM
Duavee	Wyeth	ec	K-Tab	Abbott	sr
Dulcolax	Boehringer Ingelheim	ec	Lamictal XR	GlaxoSmithKline	sr
EC Naprosyn	Genentech	ec	Lescol XL	Novartis	sr
Ecotrin 81 mg	GlaxoSmithKline	ec	Levbid	Meda	sr
Ecotrin 325 mg	GlaxoSmithKline	ec	Lialda	Shire	ec
Effexor-XR	Wyeth	sr	Liptruzet	Merck	ec
Embeda	King	sr	Lithobid	Noven Therapeutics	sr
Enablex	Novartis Consumer	sr	Luvox CR	Jazz Pharmaceuticals	sr
Entocort EC	Prometheus	ec	Mag64	Rising	ec
Equetro	Validus	sr	MagDelay	Major	ec
ERYC	Mayne	sr	Mag-Tab SR	Niche	sr
Ery-Tab	Abbott	ec	Maxifed	MCR American	sr
Exalgo	Mallinckrodt	sr	Maxifed DM	MCR American	sr
Ferro-Sequels	Inverness Medical	sr	Maxifed DMX	MCR American	sr
Fetzima	Forest	sr	Maxifed-G	MCR American	sr
Flagyl ER	Pfizer	sr	Menopause Relief Trio	Mason Vitamins	sr
Fleet Bisacodyl	Fleet, C.B.	ec	Mestinon Timespan	Valeant	sr
Focalin XR	Novartis	sr	Metadate CD	UCB	sr
Folitab 500	Rising	sr	Metadate ER	UCB	sr
Forfivo XL	IntelGenx	sr	Methylin ER	Mallinckrodt	sr
Fortamet	Shionogi Pharma	sr	Micro-K	Ther-Rx	sr
Fulyzaq	Salix	ec	Micro-K 10	Ther-Rx	sr
Fumatinic	Laser	sr	Mild-C	Carlson, J.R.	sr
Galzin	Gate	ec	Mirapex ER	Boehringer Ingelheim	sr
Gilphex TR	Gil	sr	Moxatag	Victory	sr
Glucophage XR	Bristol-Myers-Squibb	sr	MS Contin	Purdue	sr
Glucotrol XL	Pfizer	sr	Mucinex	Reckitt Benckiser	sr
Glumetza	Depomed	sr	Mucinex D	Reckitt Benckiser	sr
Hemax	Pronova	sr	Mucinex DM	Reckitt Benckiser	sr
Horizant	GlaxoSmithKline	sr	Myfortic	Novartis	ec
Imbruvica	Pharmacyclics	ec	Myrbetriq	Astellas	sr
Inderal LA	Akrimax	sr	Namenda XR	Forest	sr
Innopran XL	GlaxoSmithKline	sr	Naprelan	Victory	sr
Intuniv	Shire	sr	Nexium	AstraZeneca	ec
Invega	Ortho-McNeil-Janssen	sr	Niaspan	Abbott	sr
Janumet XR	Merck Sharp & Dohme Corp.	sr	Nifediac CC	Teva	sr
			Nifedical XL	Teva	sr
Kadian	Actavis	sr	Nitro-Time	Time-Cap	sr
Kapvay ER	Shionogi	sr	Norel SR	U.S. Pharmaceutical	sr
Keppra XR	UCB	sr	Norpace CR	Pfizer	sr
Khedezla ER	Par	sr	Nucynta ER	Janssen	sr
Klor-Con 8	Upsher-Smith	sr	Oleptro	LaboPharm	sr
Klor-Con 10	Upsher-Smith	sr	Olysio	Janssen	ec
Klor-Con M10*	Upsher-Smith	sr	Opana ER	Endo	sr
Klor-Con M15*	Upsher-Smith	sr	Opsumit	Actelion	ec
Klor-Con M20*	Upsher-Smith	sr	Oracea	Galderma	ec
Kombiglyze XR	BMS/AstraZeneca	sr			

DRUG	MANUFACTURER	FORM
Orenitram	United Therapeutics Corp.	sr
Oxtellar XR	Supernus	sr
Oxycontin	Purdue	sr
Pancreaze	Ortho-McNeil-Janssen	ec
Paser	Jacobus	ec
Paxil CR	GlaxoSmithKline	sr
PCE Dispertab	Arbor	sr
Pentasa	Shire U.S.	sr
Pentoxil	Upsher-Smith	sr
Phenytek	Mylan	sr
Poly Hist Forte	Poly	sr
Poly-Vent	Poly	sr
Prevacid	Takeda	ec
Prilosec	AstraZeneca	ec
Prilosec OTC	Procter & Gamble	sr
Pristiq	Wyeth	sr
Procardia XL	Pfizer	sr
Protonix	Wyeth	ec
Prozac Weekly	Eli Lilly	ec
Qsymia	Vivus	sr
Ranexa	Gilead	sr
Rayos	Horizon	ec
Razadyne ER	Ortho-McNeil-Janssen	sr
Requip XL	GlaxoSmithKline	sr
Rescon-Jr	Capellon	sr
Ritalin LA	Novartis	sr
Ritalin-SR	Novartis	sr
Rodex Forte	Legere	sr
Rythmol SR	GlaxoSmithKline	sr
SAM-e	Pharmavite	ec
Sanctura XR	Allergan	sr
Seroquel XR	AstraZeneca	sr
Simcor	Abbott	sr
Sinemet CR	Bristol-Myers Squibb	sr
Sitavig	Farmea	ec
Slo-Niacin	Upsher-Smith	sr
Slow Fe	Novartis Consumer	sr
Slow-Mag	Purdue	ec
Solodyn	Medicis	sr
St. Joseph Pain Reliever	McNeil Consumer	ec
Stavzor	Noven	ec
Sudafed 12 hour	McNeil Consumer	sr
Sudafed 24 hour	McNeil Consumer	sr
Sular	Shionogi Pharma	sr
Sulfazine EC	Qualitest	ec

DRUG	MANUFACTURER	FORM
Synax Duotab	Caellon	
Symax-SR	Capllon	
Tafinlar	GlaxoSmith	
Tarka	Abbott	
Taztia XT	Watson	
Tecfidera	biogen	
Tegretol-XR	Novartis	
Theo-24	UCB	
Tiazac	Forest	sr
Toprol XL†	AstraZeneca	sr
Totalday	National Vitamin	
Toviaz	Pfizer	sr
Trental	sanofi-aventis	sr
Treximet	GlaxoSmithKline	ec
Trilipix	Abbott	ec
Trokendi XR	Supernus	sr
Tussicaps	Mallinckrodt	sr
Tylenol Arthritis	McNeil Consumer	sr
Uceris	Santarus, Inc.	sr
Ultram ER	Valeant	sr
Urocit-K	Mission	sr
Uroxatral	sanofi-aventis	sr
Verelan	UCB	sr
Verelan PM	UCB	sr
Videx EC	Bristol-Myers-Squibb	ec
Vimovo	AstraZeneca	ec
Voltaren-XR	Novartis	sr
Vospire ER	Dava	sr
Votrient	GlaxoSmithKline	ec
Wellbutrin SR	GlaxoSmithKline	sr
Wellbutrin XL	GlaxoSmithKline	sr
Wobenzym N	Marlyn	ec
Xanax XR	Pfizer	sr
Zenpep	Eurand	ec
Zohydro ER	Zogenix	sr
Zyban	GlaxoSmithKline	sr
Zyflo CR	Cornerstone	sr
Zyrtec-D	McNeil Consumer	sr

*May split in half or dissolve in water.
† May divide tablet.

PDR.net®: Your Online Home of the PDR®

Trusted Drug Information Online

A web portal designed specifically for prescribers, providing trusted, professional drug information, including full FDA-approved labeling as well as concise point-of-care prescribing information. PDR.net offers online access to authoritative drug information to support treatment decisions.

©2014 PDR Network, LLC. All Rights Reserved. *PDR, PDR.net,* and *PDR Network* are registered trademarks of PDR Network, LLC.

Coming Soon: Updated & Expanded
*mobile*PDR®

*mobile*PDR has always been the source for FDA-approved full product labeling and concise point-of-care drug information from PDR for your mobile device. This spring, PDR Network will release a new version of *mobile*PDR. Developed with the prescriber in mind, this new platform will deliver more robust drug information to your mobile device than ever before.

Coming this Spring!

Reserve Now
Visit PDR.net/GetMobile for more information and to pre-register

***mobile*PDR** is free for U.S.-based MDs, DOs, NPs, and PAs in full-time patient practice and can be downloaded for all major mobile platforms.

©2014 PDR Network, LLC. All Rights Reserved. *PDR*, *PDR.net*, and *PDR Network* are registered trademarks of PDR Network, LLC.